NATURAL MEDICINES
COMPREHENSIVE DATABASE

Seventh Edition

Published by Therapeutic Research Faculty

3120 W. March Lane • PO Box 8190 • Stockton CA 95208
phone (209) 472-2244 • fax (209) 472-2249
mail@naturaldatabase.com • www.naturaldatabase.com

Compiled by the Editors of:

PHARMACIST'S LETTER®

PRESCRIBER'S LETTER®

When referencing this *Database*, use the following format for the citation:

Jellin JM, Gregory PJ, Batz F, Hitchens, K, et al. *Pharmacist's Letter/ Prescriber's Letter Natural Medicines Comprehensive Database*.7th ed. Stockton, CA: Therapeutic Research Faculty; 2005:pg xx-xx.

For information on obtaining additional copies of this edition, or access to the Web version or the PDA Handheld version of *Natural Medicines Comprehensive Database,* or for a subscription to *Prescriber's Letter* or *Pharmacist's Letter*, see the last pages of this book, or contact:
Therapeutic Research Faculty, 3120 W. March Lane,
PO Box 8190, Stockton, CA 95208
TEL: 209-472-2244 • FAX: 209-472-2249
E-MAIL: mail@NaturalDatabase.com • WEBSITE: www.NaturalDatabase.com

---

Printed in the United States of America
ISBN #0-9747062-2-1

NATURAL MEDICINES
COMPREHENSIVE DATABASE

Table of Contents

Letter from Editor-In-Chief i

Research and Writing Team iii

How to get data from this *Database* v

Data on Natural Medicines 1

References 1376

Brand Names Index 1615

Chart: Herbs and Supplements with Therapeutic Efficacy 2089

Chart: Drug/Natural Medicines Interactions 2105

Chart: Natural Medicines/Drug Interactions 2121

Chart: Drug Influences on Nutrient Levels and Depletion 2137

General Index 2153

NATURAL MEDICINES
COMPREHENSIVE DATABASE

Dear User:

What makes this 7th edition different from previous editions, and different from other books on this subject?

Natural Medicines Comprehensive Database provides users with scientifically reliable evidence-based data presented in an easy-to-use manner. This *Database* neither advocates for or against the use of natural medicines. This *Database* is intended to provide objective, scientific data in a format that facilitates access and use of the data. No other resource makes such a comprehensive collection of data as scientifically reliable and as easy to use.

This *Database* was created by the editors of *Pharmacist's Letter* and *Prescriber's Letter*. These seasoned drug information professionals have been analyzing drug information and publishing drug advisory *Letters* for 20 years. Hundreds of thousands of pharmacists, physicians, and others subscribe to these *Letters* for trustworthy advice about drug therapy.

The first edition of this *Database* was released in September 1999. Seven new editions have been released in the span of six years. *Natural Medicines Comprehensive Database* has grown not only in volume, but also in recognition. It is now recognized as the scientific gold standard for evidence-based information on this topic. Leaders in conventional medicine as well as complementary, alternative, and integrative medicine recognize the *Database* as the go-to resource. This *Database* is in wide use throughout the English speaking world, by a variety of medical professionals.

In recent years the effectiveness section of this *Database* has been completely reformatted to allow easier use. Additionally, the entire *Database* has been re-edited to make it more current and consistent. Many new monographs have been added…many new references are cited…new drug interactions have been added…and the safety and effectiveness ratings have been altered for several products based on important new findings. We also continue to add many new brand name products in the brand name listings. In some sections readers are referred to use the website. This is due to the simple fact that we can not fit any more pages into this volume.

As good as this book is, it can not compare to the website version of *Natural Medicines Comprehensive Database* (www.naturaldatabase.com). Thousands of users are transitioning to the web or PDA versions. By using the *Database* on the web, users are able to do fast, easy, and highly sophisticated searches, and get information that is updated daily by our researchers. Users of the web-based *Database* also get the complete patient education series providing a patient education monograph for each product in the *Database*. There is far more data on the website than can be fit into this volume.

The website now also has a *"Natural Product Effectiveness Checker"* to see the effectiveness of each product... *"Natural Product / Drug Interaction Checker"* that checks each ingredient of each natural product... *"Disease / Medical Condition Checker"* to find products that might be effective for a condition. The entire website has recently been named one of the 12 most trusted medical websites.

Subscribers to the website also get emailed updates and continuing education that is fully accredited for physicians, pharmacists, nurse practitioners, physician assistants, and dietitians.

There is now a new consumer website, *Natural Medicines Comprehensive Database - CONSUMER VERSION* that is licensed by health care organizations who wish to provide their members with trustworthy information on natural medicines.

We hope you enjoy this new edition. If you have suggestions, comments, or inquiries, please don't hesitate to contact us: e-mail: mail@NaturalDatabase.com; phone: (209) 472-2244.

Sincerely,

Jeff M. Jellin, Pharm.D.
Editor-in-Chief

Natural Medicines Comprehensive Database Team

Natural Medicines Comprehensive Database Team

How to Get Data From *Natural Medicines Comprehensive Database*

Monograph Name

Every one of the 1000 plus monographs in the *Natural Medicines Comprehensive Database* is given a name based on the most widely used or most recognized name. These appear in ALL CAPS at the top of every monograph.

Also Known As

Many natural medicines go by a variety of names. The most common name is chosen as the name of the monograph. Other colloquial, non-scientific names are included in this section. These names are all indexed at the end of the book for easy reference. This makes finding a natural medicine by any of its names quick and easy.

In many cases, different natural medicines may have similar sounding names. For example, there are numerous varieties of ginseng: Siberian ginseng, American ginseng, Panax ginseng, and others. The *Database* has a separate monograph for each of these. This section will alert you when there are other monographs that have similar names.

Scientific Names

This section contains all botanical, chemical, or other scientific names. Often there is not just one botanical or scientific name for a natural medicine. In these cases, we have provided as many scientific names as are known. We have also included any synonyms. For plants, a family name is also listed.

People Use This For

There are a wide variety of uses for most natural medicines. Not all uses have been validated through scientific study. In this field, ALL known uses are listed without regard for scientific evidence of effectiveness. A use listed in this section does NOT mean the product is effective for that use. Efficacy is discussed in the Effectiveness section (see below).

Safety

For each natural medicine in the *Database* you get an evidence-based safety rating.

These are PRACTICAL ratings that are STANDARDIZED throughout the *Natural Medicines Comprehensive Database*.

You will see that different routes of administration of a product often get different safety ratings. For example, camphor is rated "LIKELY SAFE" when used topically, but it is rated "UNSAFE" when used orally.

Questions often come up about using products during pregnancy or lactation, or in children. If there are safety considerations that apply specifically to children, a special mention in the safety field will address the concern. Every listing includes a rating for safety in PREGNANCY and LACTATION.

Our team has been very meticulous in analyzing the medical literature and applying principles of evidence-based medicine to assign the safety ratings. Each rating is assigned according to specific criteria:

LIKELY SAFE = The product has undergone a rigorous scientific evaluation equivalent to a review by the FDA, Health Canada, or other governmental authority and has been found to be safe when used appropriately. Or reputable references generally agree that the product is safe when used appropriately based on two or more randomized, controlled, clinical trials involving several hundred to several thousand patients and published in refereed journals; or based on large-scale post-marketing surveillance showing a low incidence of significant adverse effects.

POSSIBLY SAFE = Reputable references agree that the product might be safe when used appropriately, and there are sufficiently rigorous human studies reporting no serious adverse effects.

POSSIBLY UNSAFE = There is some evidence suggesting that use of the product might be unsafe.

LIKELY UNSAFE = Reputable references or reliable literature report that the product can be harmful, based on human studies or reliable case reports of significant adverse effects.

UNSAFE = The product has undergone a rigorous scientific evaluation or a review by a reliable regulatory agency and found to often cause clinically significant harm to humans. Or large-scale post-marketing surveillance shows a high incidence of significant adverse effects.

Effectiveness

For each natural medicine in the *Database* you get an evidence-based effectiveness rating.

These are PRACTICAL ratings that are STANDARDIZED throughout the *Natural Medicines Comprehensive Database*.

The "effectiveness" rating differs depending on the use, so you will often see more than one rating for a product.

Our team has been very meticulous in analyzing the medical literature, and applying principles of evidence-based medicine to assign the efficacy ratings. Each product is rated by the following scale:

EFFECTIVE = The product has passed a rigorous scientific review equivalent to a review by the FDA, Health Canada, or other governmental authority and has been found to be effective for a specific indication as an OTC drug, orphan drug, or prescription drug product.

LIKELY EFFECTIVE = Reputable references generally agree that the product is effective for the given indication, based on two or more randomized, controlled, clinical trials involving several hundred to several thousand patients, giving positive results for clinically relevant end-points and published in established, refereed journals.

POSSIBLY EFFECTIVE = Reputable references suggest that the product might work for the given indication based on one or more clinical trials giving positive results for clinically relevant end-points.

POSSIBLY INEFFECTIVE = Reputable references suggest that the product might not work for the given indication based on one human study giving negative results for clinically relevant end-points.

LIKELY INEFFECTIVE = Reputable references generally agree that the product is not effective for the given indication, based on two or more randomized, controlled, clinical trials giving negative results for clinically relevant end-points and published in established, refereed journals.

INEFFECTIVE = Most reputable references agree that the product is not effective for the given indication, or multiple high-quality studies resulted in negative results; there are no equally reliable human studies offering convincing contradictory data.

When possible, we have included one very useful bit of information in the Effectiveness section. This section includes the SPECIFIC FORMULA OR EXTRACT that was used in studies that found the product to be effective or ineffective. This information is not easily found elsewhere, but it is very important. For example, a significant study was published in the *Journal of the American Medical Association* providing evidence that ginkgo has a positive role in delaying the progression of Alzheimer's disease. Its effects have been likened to *Aricept*. Many published works, and many ginkgo manufacturers have since stated ginkgo's effectiveness in this area. But this information is not useful without knowing what formulation of ginkgo was shown to have a positive effect. The *Natural Medicines Comprehensive Database* states that the formulations of ginkgo that contain Egb 761 (Tanakan) or LI 1370 (Lichtwer Pharma), consisting of 24-25% flavone glycosides and 6% terpene lactones, are the formulations in the prominent studies that were shown to have beneficial effect. It cannot be inferred from this that other formulations of ginkgo will also have the same effect.

Mechanism of Action and Active Ingredients

In this field you will find a description of the known constituents and pharmacological actions that might be attributable to these constituents. Keep in mind that most natural medicines are used because people have observed, or think they observed, some benefit to using the product. In many cases there has been relatively little scientific inquiry into the active ingredients and the exact mechanism of action. Also recognize that most herbal medicines are combinations of many constituents. It is quite possible that herbal medicines work by the combined effects of multiple constituents, and the concept of identifying a single specific active ingredient is flawed. Even when a single, specific active ingredient is identified, it is possible that other active ingredients may be discovered later. For example, authorities used to think that St. John's wort exerted its effect due to hypericin content. More recent findings suggest that hyperforin exerts significant activity.

Adverse Reactions

In this field you get information about all the known adverse reactions and side effects associated with the product. These are typically derived from the side effects reported in clinical trials and from reliable case reports regarding adverse effects. In some cases, certain adverse reactions are suspected based on pharmacological properties of the product. Information about suspected adverse reactions and documented adverse reactions is clearly distinguished.

Known allergies are also listed. This can help you anticipate potential problems. For example, people who are allergic to one herb coming from the asteraceae family might also be allergic to other herbs in the same family.

Interactions

There are five separate fields listing different categories of possible interactions. For each product, this *Database* lists Possible Interactions with...

Herbs and Other Dietary Supplements
Drugs
Foods
Lab Tests
Diseases and Conditions

This is a very important part of the *Database*. There are hundreds of potential interactions...and many practitioners are not on the look-out for them. The usual computerized checking systems do not have all this info...and patients do not recognize the potential problems like they do with regular drugs. To use the information in these interaction fields, it is important to understand the origin of the data. In some cases, it comes from documented reports. In other cases, the data are theoretical, based on the pharmacological profile of the natural medicine. For example, horse chestnut seed contains coumarin derivatives and theoretically increases bleeding time. At this point in time, there are very few well-documented interactions. Much of the information regarding potential interactions is theoretical. A synopsis of documented reports and theoretical predictions appears in this field. We have also prepared a separate pair of charts in the back of the book to give you a listing of the potential interactions between drugs and natural medicines.

Drug Influences on Nutrient Levels and Depletion

Some nutrients are thought to be depleted from the body by certain drugs. Data about nutrient depletion appear in this field. This is the only field in the *Database* that appears ONLY for those natural medicines that are involved in nutrient depletion interactions. Most of these include vitamins and minerals. The natural medicines listed in this *Database* are typically the substances that are being depleted, and are not the entities causing the depletion. For this reason, the editors have chosen to only list this field when there are important data to present.

Dosage and Administration

The dosages in this field are not necessarily recommended doses, safe doses, or efficacious doses. If clinical trials have been conducted, then the doses used in the studies are listed. Other doses listed are the common or traditional doses or those typically used in supplements. Many products included in this *Database* may not be safe or effective. This needs to be considered even when a typical dose is listed.

Comments

This field presents a potpourri of info. For example, the comments on Siberian ginseng point out that it is a completely different herb than American or Panax ginseng. American or Panax ginseng is considerably more expensive. It is said that the Soviet Union wanted to provide its athletes with any advantage offered by ginseng but wanted a less expensive version. Therefore, Siberian ginseng became popular, and this is why most studies on Siberian ginseng are written in Russian.

Scattered throughout the *Database* you will see statements like, "None known." This means that data do not exist, or the literature is too contradictory, or the studies are not of high enough quality. This information is valuable because it is important for practitioners to know what is NOT known. Many references state that certain products are effective, or safe, etc. when data do not exist to support this conclusion. This *Database* states when there is insufficient information to meet the reliability standards of this *Database*.

References

This *Database* is thoroughly referenced with thousands of reference citations. In each monograph you will see numbers in parentheses appearing at the end of statements. These refer to reference citations that are listed in the back of the book in numerical order. The fact that so many references were used to create this *Database* allows this *Database* to be both a scientific consensus of clinical information and a comprehensive collection of data on natural medicines.

Brand Names Listing

There are really two separate databases of natural products within the *Natural Medicines Comprehensive Database*. There is a compilation of over 1000 monographs on natural medicines or ingredients. There is another database consisting of several thousand brand name products and their ingredients. Each brand name listing provides the name of the manufacturer and all of the ingredients. This information is towards the back of the book following the reference citations.

Within the Brand Name listing, you will sometimes find the term "**Editor's Comment.**" In these instances there will be some important commentary from the editors related to the particular brand name product. For example, the listing of all the ingredients in a brand name product may serve to answer some questions about the product, but the use of all these ingredients in COMBINATION form may require additional commentary. Or, there may be some data related to this particular brand that the editors wish for you to know about. For example, some brand name products contain substances derived from animal organs. Since there is some theoretical risk of contamination with diseased animal tissue (e.g., mad cow disease), our editors have included an "Editor's Comment" about this risk.

Keep in mind that manufacturers can change the ingredients of their brand name products at any time. This has been creating problems for years. Remember when *Ex-Lax* contained phenolphthalein? Some people did not realize that it was changed to contain sennosides and docusate sodium. The same thing happens frequently with natural medicines.

"Tell The Editors" Form

It is unrealistic to believe that all clinicians, researchers, and other experts will always agree with every statement in this *Database*. The Editors recognize that new information is surfacing all the time and new interpretations develop all the time. A team of researchers and editors work full-time to constantly update this *Database*. These editors respect intelligent differences of opinion, and in fact, invite and encourage any professional user of this *Database* to share new knowledge or new interpretations with us. If you recommend a change to any statement in this *Database*, please use the form at the back of the book and send it to us. Please include the reference citation. The Editors review all suggestions. We thank you for helping to make this the best resource possible.

General Index

There are a couple of different ways you can find data on a particular product in this *Database*. One way is to just flip to the listing…it's all in alphabetical order based on the most common name. If you don't see a listing for the product you want, you can use the index in the back of the book. The index is very complete. It allows you to search by scientific name, common names, and botanical name of every product in the *Database*. Keep in mind that the index does NOT include brand names. These are listed in the brand name section in alphabetical order.

Differences between the Book and Web versions of *Natural Medicines Comprehensive Database*:

Everything in this Book version of the *Database* is also contained in the Web site (www.NaturalDatabase.com). In addition, the Web version has many added features and information.

Updated Daily

The Web version of the *Database* is updated daily. Our team of editors and researchers work full-time to continuously add the latest data.

Searchability

Web version features easy, fast, sophisticated searching. You can find any data very quickly and easily. For example you can use:

Natural Product Effectiveness Checker to find the effectiveness rating of any product for any condition.
Diseases/Medical Condition Search to find which products are effective for any given condition.
Natural Product/Drug Interaction Checker to find any potential interactions between any natural products, (including all ingredients of the natural brand name products), and any conventional drug.

Patient Education

The Web version provides a full set of patient education handouts covering all of the monographs in the book. This allows you to provide patient-friendly information to all of your patients interested in these products. The patient information is updated right along with the professional monographs, so your patients get the most up-to-date information. And the Web version can pull in the health organization's name and logo to add to the patient handouts.

Research Abstracts

The *Natural Medicines Comprehensive Database* is a great clinical tool. It's also an efficient research tool. The *Database* is completely referenced with several thousand reference citations from the primary peer-reviewed literature. New citations are added all the time. Citations are typically linked directly to the original abstract so you can see the original research publication.

Colleagues Interact

Connect with your colleagues. *Colleagues Interact* is an online discussion group that allows users to post questions and discuss interesting cases.

Emailed Updates

Web users can also elect to receive emailed updates about the latest additions to the *Database*.

Continuing Education

The Web version provides complete continuing education courses that compare conventional and natural treatments for various conditions. This is fully accredited for physicians, pharmacists, nurse practitioners, nurses, physician assistants, and dietitians.

Whether you get the Book version, the Web version, or both depends on your specific needs. The Book version allows you to quickly flip through a few pages to find the answers you need. Some practitioners like to keep a copy handy so they can go over the info face-to-face with their patients.

The Web version offers the same great content with some additional capabilities that can only be made available in the dynamic online format.

Many practitioners choose to get BOTH the Book and Web versions...the best of both worlds.

Tell the Editors

Users of the *Natural Medicines Comprehensive Database* website can instantly click and send comments to the Editors. This is useful to suggest changes to the *Database* or to point out interesting findings to the Editors.

PDA Version

In addition to the Book and Web versions of *Natural Medicines Comprehensive Database*, you can obtain this *Database* on a PDA version for your handheld Palm or Pocket PC computer.

5-HTP

Also Known As
L-5 HTP, Oxitriptan.
CAUTION: See separate listing for L-tryptophan.

Scientific Names
5-hydroxytryptophan; L-5 hydroxytryptophan.

People Use This For
Orally, 5-HTP is used for sleep disorders, depression, anxiety, migraine and tension-type headaches, fibromyalgia, binge eating associated with obesity, attention deficit disorder (ADD), cerebellar ataxia, Ramsey-Hunt syndrome, Down syndrome, and as adjunctive therapy in seizure disorder and Parkinson's disease.
In combination with carbidopa, 5-HTP is used for treating intention myoclonus and as an orphan drug for treating post-anoxia myoclonus.

Safety
POSSIBLY UNSAFE ...when used orally. There is a lot of controversy about the safety of 5-HTP. There is some concern that 5-HTP might cause eosinophilia myalgia syndrome (EMS) (902,919,7067,10084). However, there is speculation that only certain contaminated 5-HTP products may cause this serious adverse effect. So far, there is not enough evidence to know if EMS is caused by 5-HTP, contaminants, or other unknown factors (919,7067,10084). Until more is known, advise patients against using 5-HTP.
PREGNANCY AND LACTATION: POSSIBLY UNSAFE ...when used orally (919); avoid using.

Effectiveness
POSSIBLY EFFECTIVE

Cerebellar ataxia. Taking 5-HTP orally seems to help decrease cerebellar ataxia (916).

Depression. Taking 5-HTP orally seems to significantly improve symptoms of depression (903,10853), including in patients with treatment-resistant depression (904). There is evidence that 5-HTP might be comparable to the conventional antidepressants fluvoxamine (Luvox) and imipramine (Tofranil) (904,2203).

Fibromyalgia. Taking 5-HTP orally appears to improve symptoms of primary fibromyalgia syndrome (PFS), including pain severity, morning stiffness, and sleeplessness (913,10285,10286).

Obesity. Taking 5-HTP orally seems to help reduce appetite, caloric intake, and weight in obese patients (914).

Palatal myoclonus. Taking 5-HTP orally seems to help reduce contractions in patients with palatal myoclonus (917).

POSSIBLY INEFFECTIVE

Alzheimer's disease. Taking 5-HTP orally doesn't seem to improve symptoms of Alzheimer's disease (918).

Tension headache. Taking 5-HTP orally doesn't seem to reduce pain intensity or the number of days with headache in patients with chronic tension-type headaches (2204).

INSUFFICIENT RELIABLE EVIDENCE to RATE

Anxiety. There's preliminary evidence that taking 5-HTP orally might help reduce symptoms of anxiety disorders (915). More evidence is needed to rate 5-HTP for this use.

Mechanism of Action
5-HTP (5-hydroxytryptophan) is related to both L-tryptophan and serotonin. In the body, L-tryptophan is converted to 5-HTP, which can then be converted to serotonin. 5-HTP readily crosses the blood-brain barrier and increases central nervous system (CNS) synthesis of serotonin (10853). Serotonin can affect sleep, appetite, temperature, sexual behavior, and pain sensation. Serotonin also has a significant role in depression, anxiety, and aggression (901). Since 5-HTP can increase synthesis of serotonin, 5-HTP is used for several disease states where serotonin is believed to play a significant role including depression, insomnia, obesity, and numerous other conditions.

Adverse Reactions
Orally, 5-HTP can cause gastrointestinal (GI) side effects such as heartburn, stomach pain, belching and flatulence, nausea, vomiting, diarrhea, and anorexia (2203,10858). There is also concern that 5-HTP, like L-tryptophan, can cause asymptomatic eosinophilia and eosinophilia myalgia syndrome (EMS) (902,919,7067). There is speculation that many commercial 5-HTP products may contain contaminants from the peak X family, a group of impurities that might cause EMS (919,10084). However, the presence of the peak X family or other contaminants has not been verified in all cases of EMS. So far, there is not enough evidence to determine if 5-HTP, a contaminant, or some other factor is responsible for EMS (902,919,7067,10084). Until more is known, tell patients to avoid taking 5-HTP supplements.

Interactions with Herbs & Other Dietary Supplements

HERBS AND SUPPLEMENTS WITH SEROTONERGIC PROPERTIES: Theoretically, 5-HTP might increase the therapeutic and adverse effects of products that increase serotonin levels, including Hawaiian baby woodrose, L-tryptophan, S-adenosylmethionine (SAMe), and St. John's wort (901).

Interactions with Drugs

ANTIDEPRESSANT DRUGS: Combining serotonergic antidepressants with 5-HTP might increase the risk of serotonergic side effects including serotonin syndrome and cerebral vasoconstrictive disorders such as Call-Fleming syndrome (8056). These drugs include the selective serotonin reuptake inhibitors (SSRIs) such as fluoxetine (Prozac), paroxetine (Paxil), sertraline (Zoloft), and others; and tricyclic and atypical antidepressants such as amitriptyline (Elavil), clomipramine (Anafranil), imipramine (Tofranil), and others.
CARBIDOPA (Lodosyn): Combining 5-HTP and carbidopa can increase the risk of serotonergic side effects. Carbidopa is sometimes used with 5-HTP to minimize peripheral 5-HTP metabolism and boost the amount that reaches the brain. But this combination might also increase the risk of some side effects including hypomania, restlessness, rapid speech, anxiety, insomnia, and aggressiveness. Combining carbidopa and 5-HTP might also cause an eosinophilia myalgia syndrome (EMS)-like reaction including scleroderma-like skin changes. It is suspected that a decrease in 5-HTP metabolism and an increase in either serotonin or a metabolite, kynurenine, are responsible for this adverse effect (1403,1404).
DEXTROMETHORPHAN (Robitussin DM, and others): Combining serotonergic drugs such as dextromethorphan with 5-HTP might increase the risk of serotonergic side effects including serotonin syndrome and cerebral vasoconstrictive disorders such as Call-Fleming syndrome (8056).
MEPERIDINE (Demerol): Combining serotonergic drugs such as meperidine with 5-HTP might increase the risk of serotonergic side effects including serotonin syndrome and cerebral vasoconstrictive disorders such as Call-Fleming syndrome (8056).
MONOAMINE OXIDASE INHIBITORS (MAOIs): Combining serotonergic drugs such as one of the MAOIs with 5-HTP might increase the risk of serotonergic side effects including serotonin syndrome and cerebral vasoconstrictive disorders such as Call-Fleming syndrome (8056).
PENTAZOCINE (Talwin): Combining serotonergic drugs such as pentazocine with 5-HTP might increase the risk of serotonergic side effects including serotonin syndrome and cerebral vasoconstrictive disorders such as Call-Fleming syndrome (8056).
TRAMADOL (Ultram): Combining serotonergic drugs such as tramadol with 5-HTP might increase the risk of serotonergic side effects including serotonin syndrome and cerebral vasoconstrictive disorders such as Call-Fleming syndrome (8056).

Interactions with Foods

None known.

Interactions with Lab Tests

None known.

Interactions with Diseases or Conditions

DOWN SYNDROME: 5-HTP is reported to cause seizures in some patients with Down syndrome. In one case series, 15% of patients receiving long-term 5-HTP treatment experienced seizures (5050).

Dosage and Administration

ORAL: For depression, the typical dose of 5-HTP is 150-300 mg daily (903,2203). For the treatment of primary fibromyalgia syndrome (PFS), 5-HTP 100 mg 3 times daily has been used for up to 1 month (10286). For post-anoxic myoclonus, 5-HTP has an orphan drug status. The sponsor of the orphan drug is Circa Pharmaceuticals (phone: 516-842-8383).

Comments

5-HTP is often produced commercially from the seeds of the African plant Griffonia simplicifolia.

7-KETO-DHEA

Also Known As

5-androsten-3-beta-17-one-DHEA, 7-ODA, 7-oxo-dehydroepiandrosterone-3-acetate, 7-oxo-DHEA, 7-oxo-DHEA-acetate.
CAUTION: See separate listing for DHEA.

Scientific Names

3-acetyl-7-oxo-dehydroepiandrosterone; 3beta-acetoxy-androst-5-ene-7,17-dione.

People Use This For
Orally, 7-keto-DHEA is used to increase metabolism and thermogenesis and promote weight loss, to improve lean body mass and build muscle, to increase activity of the thyroid gland and immune system, to boost memory, and to reduce aging.

Safety
There is insufficient reliable information available about the safety of 7-keto-DHEA.
Pregnancy and Lactation: Insufficient reliable information available; avoid using.

Effectiveness
INSUFFICIENT RELIABLE EVIDENCE to RATE

Obesity. There is preliminary evidence that 7-keto-DHEA might significantly decrease body weight and fat composition in obese females (5842). More evidence is needed to rate 7-keto-DHEA for this use.

Mechanism of Action
7-keto-DHEA is a metabolite of dehydroepiandrosterone (DHEA), which is formed in the body (5837). Unlike DHEA, 7-keto-DHEA is not converted to androgens and estrogens (5837,5840,5842). Oral or topical administration of 7-keto-DHEA does not affect plasma levels of steroid hormones (10404,10405). Similarly to DHEA, 7-keto-DHEA is rapidly converted to the sulfated form, known as 7-keto-DHEAS (10404).
7-keto-DHEA is thought to be beneficial in weight loss by increasing metabolism and thermogenesis. Early evidence in animals suggests 7-keto-DHEA can increase thermogenesis, possibly by stimulation of thermogenic enzymes in the liver (5837); however this effect has not yet been reported in humans. Clinical evidence suggests 7-keto-DHEA might increase basal metabolism.
In obese patients, 7-keto-DHEA can significantly increase the thyroid hormone triiodothyronine (T3) when used over 4 weeks (5842). Other preliminary evidence suggests that 7-keto-DHEA improves chemically-induced and age-related memory impairment (5839). 7-keto-DHEA may have immunomodulatory effects by stimulating interleukin-2 production by human lymphocytes in vitro (5841).
After oral administration, 7-keto-DHEA is not found in blood. It is rapidly converted to 7-keto-DHEAS, the primary form in which it is found. The half-life of 7-keto-DHEAS is about 2.17 hours, the time to peak plasma levels is about 2.2 hours, and the apparent volume of distribution is about 540 L (10404).

Adverse Reactions
None reported.

Interactions with Herbs & Other Dietary Supplements
None known.

Interactions with Drugs
None known.

Interactions with Foods
None known.

Interactions with Lab Tests
TRIIODOTHYROXINE (T3): In obese patients, 7-keto-DHEA may increase T3 levels (5842).

Interactions with Diseases or Conditions
None known.

Dosage and Administration
ORAL: For weight loss, 100 mg twice daily has been used (5842).

ABSCESS ROOT

Also Known As
American Greek Valerian, Blue Bells, False Jacob's Ladder, Sweatroot.
CAUTION: See separate listing for Jacob's Ladder.

Scientific Names
Polemonium reptans.
Family: Polemoniaceae.

People Use This For
Orally, abscess root is used to reduce fever, reduce inflammation, stimulate sweating, as an astringent, and an expectorant.

Safety
There is insufficient reliable information available about the safety of abscess root.
Pregnancy and Lactation: Insufficient reliable information available; avoid using.

Effectiveness
There is insufficient reliable information available about the effectiveness of abscess root.

Mechanism of Action
Abscess root contains triterpene saponins. These substances are from colloidal solutions in water that foam when they are shaken. They are often irritating to mucous membranes and could cause symptoms such as sneezing and GI irritation (18,4077).

Adverse Reactions
Orally, abscess root can irritate the GI tract. It might cause sneezing and GI upset (18,4077).

Interactions with Herbs & Other Dietary Supplements
None known.

Interactions with Drugs
None known.

Interactions with Foods
None known.

Interactions with Lab Tests
None known.

Interactions with Diseases or Conditions
None known.

Dosage and Administration
ORAL: A tea is made from the ground root (18).

Comments
Abscess root is also called false Jacob's ladder because it has astringent activity similar to Jacob's ladder (see separate listing). These two plants are used in similar ways, but differ chemically. Be cautious with use, because one can be confused with the other (18).

ABUTA

Also Known As
Bejunco de Cerca, Butua, False Pareira, Pareira, Patacon, Velvetleaf.
CAUTION: See separate listing for Pareira.

Scientific Names
Cissampelos pareira.
Family: Menispermaceae.

Comments
At the date of publication, there was very little scientific information available about this product. Our staff is continually analyzing the available information on natural medicines and will add data to the online version of *Natural Medicines Comprehensive Database* as it becomes available. See www.naturaldatabase.com.

ACACIA

Also Known As

Arabic Gum, Gomme Arabique, Gomme de Senegal, Gum Acacia, Gum Arabic, Gum Senegal, Gummae Mimosae, Kher.
CAUTION: See separate listing for Cassie Absolute.

Scientific Names

Acacia senegal, synonyms Acacia verek, Mimosa senegal, Senegalia senegal.
Family: Fabaceae/Leguminosae.

People Use This For

Orally, acacia is used to reduce cholesterol levels.
In manufacturing, acacia is used as a pharmaceutical ingredient in making emulsions and troches, a demulcent for throat or stomach inflammation, a masking agent for acrid substances (e.g., capsicum), and as a film-forming agent in peel-off skin masks.

Safety

LIKELY SAFE ...when used orally and appropriately in amounts commonly found in foods. Acacia has Generally Recognized As Safe (GRAS) status in the US (4912).
POSSIBLY SAFE ...when used orally and appropriately in medicinal amounts (11).
PREGNANCY AND LACTATION: Insufficient reliable information available; avoid using.

Effectiveness

POSSIBLY INEFFECTIVE

Hypercholesterolemia. Taking acacia orally doesn't seem to reduce cholesterol levels. Five grams twice daily for 4 weeks doesn't seem to affect any plasma lipid levels (8072).

There is insufficient reliable information available about the effectiveness of acacia for its other uses.

Mechanism of Action

Acacia is the gum that is exuded from the acacia tree. Acacia gum is a water-soluble dietary fiber. It consists mostly of arabic acid which becomes arabinose, galactose, and arabinosic acid when hydrolyzed. It is almost completely soluble in twice its weight of water (16,8072).

Adverse Reactions

Orally, acacia can cause minor gastrointestinal disturbances such as gas, bloating, and loose stools. These effects may subside with continued use (8072).
Allergy to acacia dust manifests as skin lesions and severe asthmatic attacks (11).

Interactions with Herbs & Other Dietary Supplements

None known.

Interactions with Drugs

ALCOHOL (Ethanol): Mixing acacia with a substance containing greater than 50% concentration of ethyl alcohol can cause acacia to become insoluble (19).
ORAL DRUGS: The fiber in acacia can impair absorption of oral drugs (19).

Interactions with Foods

None known.

Interactions with Lab Tests

None known.

Interactions with Diseases or Conditions

None known.

Dosage and Administration

ORAL: Acacia is usually dissolved in water to make a mucilage. The usual dose is 1 to 4 teaspoons (5263).

Comments

Avoid confusion with sweet acacia (Acacia farnesiana).

ACEROLA

Also Known As

Barbados Cherry, Puerto Rican Cherry, West Indian Cherry.
CAUTION: See separate listings for Cherokee Rosehip, Rose Hip, and Vitamin C.

Scientific Names

Malpighia glabra; Malpighia punicifolia.
Family: Malpighiaceae.

People Use This For

Orally, acerola is used to treat or prevent scurvy, colds, heart disease, cancer, pressure sores, retinal hemorrhages, tooth decay, gum infections, atherosclerosis, depression, hay fever, for preventing blood clots, collagen disorders, and to enhance physical endurance.

Safety

POSSIBLY SAFE ...when used orally (6,15).
PREGNANCY AND LACTATION: Insufficient reliable information available; avoid using.

Effectiveness

POSSIBLY EFFECTIVE

Scurvy. Taking acerola orally might prevent scurvy due to its vitamin C content (6,15).

There is insufficient reliable information available about the effectiveness of acerola for its other uses.

Mechanism of Action

The applicable part of acerola is the fruit. Acerola contains 1000-2330 mg of vitamin C per 100 grams (6). Vitamin C is an essential coenzyme required for normal metabolic function. It is important for collagen formation and tissue repair. Vitamin C is involved in tyrosine metabolism, folic acid conversion, carbohydrate metabolism, synthesis of lipids and proteins, iron metabolism, resistance to infections, and cellular respiration. Vitamin C also acts as an antioxidant (6,15). It regenerates and restores oxidized vitamin E (127,128). Acerola fruit also contains vitamin A, thiamine, riboflavin, and niacin (6).

Adverse Reactions

Orally, the vitamin C in acerola can cause nausea, abdominal cramps, fatigue, insomnia, and sleepiness. Doses greater than 1 gram might cause diarrhea (15).

Interactions with Herbs & Other Dietary Supplements

VITAMIN C SUPPLEMENTS: Due to vitamin C content in acerola, concomitant use of acerola with vitamin C supplements might increase the risk of adverse effects associated with vitamin C.

Interactions with Drugs

ESTROGENS: Concomitant use of estrogens with acerola might increase absorption and therapeutic effects due to vitamin C content (129,130).
FLUPHENAZINE (Prolixin): Concomitant use with acerola decreases blood levels due to vitamin C content (15).
WARFARIN (Coumadin): Concomitant use with acerola can reduce anticoagulant activity of warfarin due to its vitamin C content (506).

Interactions with Foods

IRON: Concomitant use of iron with acerola increases GI absorption of iron from foods (ferric) but not from supplements (ferrous) due to vitamin C content (15).

Interactions with Lab Tests

STOOL OCCULT BLOOD TESTS: The vitamin C in acerola can cause false-negative results if it is ingested 48-72 hours before amine-dependent tests (506).
URINE GLUCOSE TESTS: Doses of vitamin C greater than 500 mg can cause false-decreases with glucose oxidase tests (e.g., Clinistix). The vitamin C in acerola might also cause false increases with cupric sulfate tests (e.g., Clinitest) (15).

Interactions with Diseases or Conditions

GOUT: The vitamin C in acerola might increase uric acid levels (15).
KIDNEY STONES: The vitamin C in acerola in large doses might cause precipitation of urate, cystine, or oxalate stones (15).

Dosage and Administration

No typical dosage.

ACETYL-L-CARNITINE

Also Known As

Acetyl-Levocarnitine, Acetyl Carnitine, ALC, ALCAR, Carnitine Acetyl Ester, Gamma-Trimethyl-Beta-Acetylbutyrobetaine, L-Acetylcarnitine, Levacecarnine, N-Acetyl-Carnitine, N-Acetyl-L-Carnitine, ST-200, Vitamin B(t) Acetate.
CAUTION: See separate listings for L-Carnitine and Propionyl-L-Carnitine.

Scientific Names

2-(acetyloxy)-3-carboxy-N,N,N-trimethyl-1-propanaminium inner salt; (3-carboxy-2-hydroxy-propyl)trimethylammonium hydroxide inner salt acetate.

People Use This For

Orally, acetyl-L-carnitine is used for Alzheimer's disease, age-related memory deficits, senile depression, Down syndrome, alcoholism-related cognitive deficits, and cerebrovascular insufficiency after stroke. It is also used for peripheral neuropathies, diabetic neuropathy, neuropathy due to anti-viral drugs used in the treatment of AIDS, facial paralysis, male infertility, symptoms of male aging, and Peyronie's disease.
Intravenously, acetyl-L-carnitine is used for dementia and cerebral ischemia.
Intramuscularly, acetyl-L-carnitine is used for peripheral neuropathy with pain.

Safety

POSSIBLY SAFE ...when used orally and appropriately. Periodic monitoring of blood cell counts and liver and renal function has been recommended during acetyl-L-carnitine therapy (42,1589,1594,1595,1596,1597,1598,1599,3600,3601,9105,9791,10076,10391). ...when used parenterally and appropriately under medical supervision (1591,1592).
PREGNANCY AND LACTATION: Insufficient reliable information available; avoid using.

Effectiveness

POSSIBLY EFFECTIVE

Age-related cognitive impairment. Taking acetyl-L-carnitine orally seems to improve some measures of cognitive function and memory in elderly people with age-related mental impairment (42,3600,3601).
Alzheimer's disease. Acetyl-L-carnitine might slow the rate of disease progression, improve memory, and improve some measures of cognitive function and behavioral performance in some patients with Alzheimer's disease. It is more likely to show some effect in those with early onset Alzheimer's disease who are less than 66 years of age and have a faster rate of disease progression and mental decline (1594,1595,1596,1597,1598,1599,9105,10391). Acetyl-L-carnitine has not been compared with cholinesterase inhibitors such as donepezil (Aricept).
Chronic cerebral ischemia. Administering a single does of acetyl-L-carnitine intravenously seems to produce short-term improvements in cerebral blood flow in people with chronic cerebral ischemia after single doses (1591,1592).
Cognitive impairment. Taking acetyl-L-carnitine orally seems to improve memory and visuospatial capacity in 30 to 60 year-old chronic alcoholics with cognitive impairment (1589).
Infertility. Taking acetyl-L-carnitine orally, in combination with L-carnitine for 6 months seems to increase sperm motility in men with infertility (12352). Taking acetyl-L-carnitine orally in combination with L-carnitine and nonsteroidal anti-inflammatory drugs (NSAIDs) seems to improve male infertility caused by abacterial prostatovesiculoepididymitis, an inflammation of the prostate gland, seminal vesicles, and epididymis. The carnitines increase sperm count and motility. The carnitines are used following 2 months of treatment with NSAIDs (9791).
Male aging. Taking acetyl-L-carnitine orally in combination with propionyl-L-carnitine seems to help symptoms of androgen decline in older men. The combination taken for 6 months seems to be similar to testosterone for improving sexual dysfunction, depression and fatigue (12353).
Peyronie's disease. Taking acetyl-L-carnitine orally seems to help treat acute and early chronic Peyronie's disease (10076). Acetyl-L-carnitine appears to be more effective than tamoxifen for reducing pain and inhibiting disease progression.

INSUFFICIENT RELIABLE EVIDENCE to RATE

Depression. Some clinical research suggests acetyl-L-carnitine might decrease symptoms of dysthymia and depression in elderly people (3602,3603,3604). More evidence is needed to rate acetyl-L-carnitine for this use.

Mechanism of Action

Acetyl-L-carnitine occurs naturally in the body. It is an ester of L-carnitine, and is converted to L-carnitine in the body by carnitine acetyltransferase.

Acetyl-L-carnitine is structurally related to acetylcholine. It also serves as a precursor to acetyl coenzyme A, and contributes acetyl groups to acetylcholine (10395). It also seems to promote acetylcholine release and increases choline acetyltransferase activity (44). These effects have lead to the study of acetyl-L-carnitine in Alzheimer's disease, in which there is substantial cholinergic neuronal loss and acetylcholine depletion (1594).

Acetyl-L-carnitine also participates in cellular energy production by acting as a shuttle between the cytoplasm and mitochondria for long-chain fatty acids (1594).

In HIV patients, acetyl-L-carnitine might slow the loss of CD4 lymphocytes by reducing apoptosis and increasing the serum level of insulin-like growth factor 1 which protects against apoptosis (3605). Lower plasma levels of acetyl-L-carnitine are also associated with neuropathy in people who take HIV drugs (3606).

Acetyl-L-carnitine and L-carnitine are present in human sperm and seminal fluid (3607). Their levels increase in sperm during the maturation process in the epididymis and coincide with the acquisition of progressive motility (3608,3609). Levels of acetyl-L-carnitine, and the ratio of acetyl-L-carnitine to L-carnitine, have been reported to be lower in infertile semen and sperm samples with low motility (3610,3611), and an increase in sperm motility is seen in vitro when acetyl-L-carnitine or L-carnitine is added to the sample (3612).

Adverse Reactions

Orally, acetyl-L-carnitine is generally well tolerated (10391). It may cause nausea, vomiting, and agitation (restlessness and motor overactivity) (1596,1599). Side effects reported in people with Alzheimer's disease include psychiatric disturbances, such as depression, mania, confusion and aggression, but it is not clear whether these are due to acetyl-L-carnitine or the disease itself (1594,1595,1596,1597,1598,1599,9105,10391).

Acetyl-L-carnitine is used for male aging. Unlike testosterone, it doesn't cause prostate enlargement or increase prostate-specific antigen when taken orally for 6 months (12353).

Interactions with Herbs & Other Dietary Supplements

None known.

Interactions with Drugs

None known.

Interactions with Foods

None known.

Interactions with Lab Tests

None known.

Interactions with Diseases or Conditions

None known.

Dosage and Administration

ORAL: In Alzheimer's disease, 1500-4000 mg daily has been used, usually divided into two or three doses during the day (1594,1595,1599). In age-related memory impairment, 1500-2000 mg daily has been used (3601). For depression in the elderly, 1500-3000 mg daily in divided doses has been used (3602,3603). In some infertile men, 4000 mg daily has been used to improve sperm function (3607). For Peyronie's disease, 1 gram twice daily for 3 months has been used (10076). For male infertility, 1 gram of acetyl-L-carnitine plus 2 grams of L-carnitine daily has been used (12352). For male infertility secondary to abacterial prostatovesiculoepididymitis, acetyl-L-carnitine 500 mg plus carnitine 1 gram every 12 hours has been used following 2 months of treatment with nonsteroidal anti-inflammatory drugs (9791). For symptoms of male aging, 2 grams of acetyl-L-carnitine plus 2 grams of propionyl-L-carnitine daily has been used (12353).

INTRAVENOUS: Single doses of 1500 mg have been used in people with chronic cerebral ischemia (1591,1592).

INTRAMUSCULAR: In people with peripheral neuropathy, 500-1000 mg daily has been used (1593).

ACKEE

Also Known As
Akee, Aki, Arbre Fricasse, Seso Vegetal.

Scientific Names
Blighia sapida, synonym Cupania sapida.
Family: Sapindaceae.

People Use This For
Orally, ackee is used as a treatment for colds, fever, edema, and epilepsy.
For food uses, the ripe fruit is eaten.

Safety
LIKELY SAFE ...when the ripe fruit is used in traditional Jamaican cooking (6).
UNSAFE ...when the unripe fruit and seeds are ingested. It can cause severe hypoglycemia, convulsions, and death (6).
CHILDREN: UNSAFE ...when the unripe fruit and seeds are ingested. Children are more sensitive to the toxic effects of ackee than adults (6). There is insufficient reliable information available about the safety of the ripe fruit for children.
PREGNANCY AND LACTATION: UNSAFE ...when the unripe fruit and seeds are ingested (6). There is insufficient reliable information available about the safety of the ripe fruit during pregnancy and breast-feeding.

Effectiveness
There is insufficient reliable information available about the effectiveness of ackee.

Mechanism of Action
The applicable parts of ackee are the seed and fruit. Unripe fruit and seeds contain liver toxins (hypoglycin A, hypoglycin B). By inactivating flavoprotein acyl-CoA dehydrogenases and inhibiting the oxidation of long-chain fatty acids, the toxins inhibit gluconeogenesis and induce hypoglycemia (5609,5610).

Adverse Reactions
Orally, there are two forms of toxicity that can occur from ingestion of the unripe fruit and seeds of ackee. One form is referred to as "vomiting sickness". The symptoms include vomiting, remission for 8-10 hours, renewed vomiting, convulsions, and eventually coma. The second type of toxicity includes convulsions and coma at the onset. Both forms lead to severe hypoglycemia (6) known as toxic hypoglycemic syndrome (THS) (5602). Electrolyte and fluid disturbances may occur due to vomiting (6). Urticaria and anaphylaxis has been reported after ingestion of ackee (5610).

Interactions with Herbs & Other Dietary Supplements
None known.

Interactions with Drugs
ANTIDIABETES DRUGS: Monitor blood glucose levels closely due to claims that ackee has hypoglycemic effects (19).

Interactions with Foods
None known.

Interactions with Lab Tests
None known.

Interactions with Diseases or Conditions
DIABETES: Monitor blood glucose levels closely due to claims that ackee has hypoglycemic effects (19).

Dosage and Administration
No typical dosage.

Comments

Ackee was brought to Jamaica from West Africa during the end of the 18th century, and the ripe fruit has since become a common ingredient in traditional Jamaican cooking (6). Avoid use of unripe fruit and seeds or water in which unripe ackee has been cooked due to toxicity (5602). Ackee is also found in southern Florida, Central America, and Africa (5602,5609).

ACONITE

Also Known As

Aconiti Tuber, Autumn Monkshood, Blue Monkshood Root, Chuan-wu, Monkshood, Monkshood Tuber, Wolfsbane.

Scientific Names

Aconitum napellus; Aconitum species.
Family: Ranunculaceae.

People Use This For

Orally, aconite is used for pain, facial paralysis, joint pain, arthritis, gout, rheumatic complaints, inflammation, pleurisy, pericarditis sicca, fever, skin and mucosal diseases, disinfection, and wound treatment. Aconite is also used orally as a cardiac depressant and an agent to induce mild sweating.
Topically, aconite is used as a counterirritant in liniment. Aconite is also used topically for facial neuralgia, rheumatism, and sciatica.

Safety

UNSAFE ...when used orally. Aconite root is a strong, fast-acting poison that affects the heart and CNS (11). All species of this herb are dangerous. Severe poisoning has been reported after ingestion of 0.2 mg of aconitine or 6 grams of processed and cured aconite (3490). Even when used in the therapeutic dose range, aconite can cause toxicity including nausea, vomiting, dizziness, muscle spasms, hypothermia, paralysis of respiratory system, and heart rhythm disorders (2,11). ...when used topically. Aconite can be absorbed through the skin and cause significant toxicity (12).
PREGNANCY AND LACTATION: UNSAFE ...when used orally or topically (11,12); avoid using.

Effectiveness

There is insufficient reliable information available about the effectiveness of aconite.

Mechanism of Action

The applicable part of aconite is the root. Aconite contains alkaloids including aconitine, mesoconitine, and hypaconitine, which have widespread effects on cardiac, neural, and muscle tissue by activating sodium channels (559,3490). In the heart muscle, this activation enhances inward currents during the plateau phase of the cardiac action potential, prolonging repolarization, and inducing afterdepolarization, leading to tachyarrhythmias (2634).

Adverse Reactions

Orally, aconite causes symptoms of intoxication including nausea, vomiting, weakness, sweating, restlessness, dizziness, numbness, paresthesias (beginning in the mouth and then spreading to the limbs), hypotension, palpitations, hypokalemia, metabolic and/or respiratory acidosis, cardiac toxicity (sustained ventricular tachycardia, ventricular fibrillation), reduced consciousness, and death (558,559,561,562,563,3490). Symptoms of intoxication usually begin 30 minutes after ingestion of aconite (559). Life-threatening symptoms and fatalities have been reported after aconite ingestion (3490,3491). No specific antidote is available. Cardioversion has been reported to be ineffective, but the use of antiarrhythmic agents such as amiodarone has been successful in some cases (2634,3490). Some Chinese medicine practitioners still commonly use aconite rootstocks in their preparations. They cure the rootstocks of aconite by soaking in water (with frequent changes to fresh water) and then boiling or steaming for prolonged periods of time. The process hydrolyzes the aconite alkaloids into less toxic derivatives, but toxicities and fatalities can also occur after ingestion of these cured and processed aconite roots (2634,3490). Aconite is also a common ingredient in numerous homeopathic products. Since most homeopathic products are so diluted that they contain virtually no active molecules, these products are not likely to have any pharmacological or toxic effects.

Interactions with Herbs & Other Dietary Supplements

None known.

Interactions with Drugs

None known.

Interactions with Foods
None known.

Interactions with Lab Tests
None known.

Interactions with Diseases or Conditions
None known.

Dosage and Administration
ORAL: No typical dosage. But people have used homeopathic preparations of aconite of 6c to 30c potency strength. A 6c potency is made by diluting one part of aconite tincture to 99 parts of water or alcohol. One part of the resulting solution is taken and diluted again with 99 parts of water or alcohol. The process done six times resulting in a 6c potency (5011).
TOPICAL: No typical dosage.

ACTIVATED CHARCOAL

Also Known As
Animal Charcoal, Charcoal, Gas Black, Lamp Black, Medicinal Charcoal.
CAUTION: See separate listing for Coffee Charcoal.

Scientific Names
Carbon.

People Use This For
Orally, activated charcoal is used as an antiflatulent, for reducing blood lipid levels, acute management of poisonings, and cholestasis of pregnancy.

Safety
LIKELY SAFE ...when used orally short-term (6).
PREGNANCY AND LACTATION: POSSIBLY SAFE ...when used orally short-term (126).

Effectiveness
LIKELY EFFECTIVE

Poisoning. Taking activated charcoal orally is effective when used as part of a standard treatment for some acute poisonings (15).

POSSIBLY EFFECTIVE

Cholestasis. Taking activated charcoal orally seems to help treat cholestasis of pregnancy (126).
Flatulence. Taking activated charcoal orally seems to act as an antiflatulent and reduce gas (15).
Hypercholesterolemia. Taking activated charcoal orally seems to reduce serum cholesterol levels (6).

Mechanism of Action
Activated charcoal has a very large surface area which adsorbs chemicals and therefore prevents their systemic absorption. Activated charcoal may interrupt enterohepatic recirculation of drugs and other compounds that are excreted into the bile (6).

Adverse Reactions
Orally, activated charcoal can cause GI obstruction, pulmonary aspiration, hypernatremic dehydration, and prolonged GI transit time (6). Be cautious when using activated charcoal along with an emetic. There is a risk of pulmonary aspiration (6).

Interactions with Herbs & Other Dietary Supplements
MICRONUTRIENTS: Activated charcoal may cause reduced absorption of micronutrients (15).

Interactions with Drugs
ORAL DRUGS: Activated charcoal may reduce or prevent absorption of drugs including acetaminophen, barbiturates, carbamazepine, digoxin, furosemide, glutethimide, hydantoins, methotrexate, nizatidine, phenothiazines, phenylbutazones, propoxyphene, salicylates, sulfones, sulfonylureas, tetracyclines, theophyllines, tricyclic antidepressants, and valproic acid (506); avoid co-administration.
SYRUP OF IPECAC: Activated charcoal adsorbs and inactivates syrup of ipecac; avoid co-administration (506).

Interactions with Foods
MICRONUTRIENTS: Activated charcoal can reduce absorption of micronutrients (15).
MILK, ICE CREAM OR SHERBET AND OTHER DAIRY PRODUCTS: Co-administration of these foods along with activated charcoal may decrease the adsorptive capacity of activated charcoal (506).

Interactions with Lab Tests
SERUM CHOLESTEROL: Activated charcoal can reduce serum total cholesterol and LDL cholesterol concentrations and test results (6).

Interactions with Diseases or Conditions
GI OBSTRUCTION: Avoid using activated charcoal in conditions of GI obstruction.

Dosage and Administration
ORAL: The usual antiflatulent dose is 520-975 mg after meals or at first sign of discomfort. Separate activated charcoal doses from other drugs by at least two hours to avoid interaction.

Comments
In case of POISONING, use caution if an emetic is given, due to the risk of pulmonary aspiration. Laxatives are often co-administered to reduce GI transit time and speed removal of poison from the body (6).

ADENOSINE

Also Known As
A5MP, Adenine Nucleoside, Adenine Riboside, Adenosine Phosphate, ADP, AMP, ATP.

Scientific Names
Adenosine; Adenosine Monophosphate (AMP); Adenosine-5-monophosphate (A5MP); Adenosine Diphosphate (ADP); Adenosine Triphosphate (ATP).

People Use This For
Orally, adenosine monophosphate (AMP) is used for treating herpes zoster and porphyria cutanea tarda.
Sublingually, adenosine triphosphate (ATP) is used to increase physical energy.
Intravenously, adenosine is used for treating surgical and neuropathic pain, pulmonary hypertension, supraventricular tachycardia, and controlling blood pressure during anesthesia and surgery. It is also used for pharmacological cardiac stress tests.
Intrathecally, adenosine is used to treat neuropathic pain.
Intramuscularly, adenosine phosphate is used for treating varicose veins, bursitis, tendonitis, tenosynovitis, pruritus, multiple sclerosis, neuropathy, herpes zoster and herpes simplex infections, and improving coronary and peripheral blood flow.
Intravenously, adenosine triphosphate is used for treating acute renal failure, multiple organ failure, pulmonary hypertension, cystic fibrosis, lung cancer, cachexia associated with cancer, and controlling blood pressure during anesthesia and surgery. It is also used for pharmacological cardiac stress tests.

Safety
LIKELY SAFE ...when adenosine is used intravenously and appropriately. Adenosine (Adenocard, Adenoscan) is an FDA-approved prescription drug (15). ...when adenosine monophosphate (adenosine phosphate, AMP) is used intramuscularly and appropriately. Adenosine monophosphate is an FDA-approved prescription drug (15).
POSSIBLY SAFE ...when adenosine triphosphate (ATP) is used intravenously and appropriately. ATP appears to be safe when up to 75 mcg/kg per minute is given intravenously for 30 hours every 2 weeks for 28 weeks, although doses higher than 50 mcg/kg per minute cause a higher incidence of adverse effects (9149,9154).
PREGNANCY AND LACTATION: Insufficient reliable information available; avoid using.

Effectiveness
EFFECTIVE

Paroxysmal supraventricular tachycardia. Administering adenosine intravenously improves paroxysmal supraventricular tachycardia (15).

POSSIBLY EFFECTIVE

Cachexia. Administering adenosine triphosphate (ATP) given intravenously every 2 to 4 weeks at a dose of up to 75 mcg/kg per minute over 30 hours seems to stabilize body composition, appetite, and dietary intake, and to improve quality of life in people with advanced non-small-cell lung cancer and other tumors (9149,9151,9152).
Venous stasis ulcers. Administering adenosine monophosphate intramuscularly might relieve edema, pruritus,

dermatitis, and erythema of varicose ulcers (15).

INSUFFICIENT RELIABLE EVIDENCE to RATE

Herpes zoster (shingles). There is preliminary clinical research that suggests adenosine monophosphate given intramuscularly might be useful for herpes zoster (shingles) infection and to treat and prevent post-herpetic neuralgia (9155,10067). Intramuscular adenosine monophosphate might also be useful for treating other kinds of herpes infections, according to limited clinical research (9590).

Lung cancer. Preliminary clinical studies suggest that adenosine triphosphate (ATP) is not effective for treating non-small-cell lung cancer (9151,9154).

Neuropathic pain. Some clinical research suggests that adenosine given intrathecally might relieve neuropathic pain (9157).

More evidence is needed to rate adenosine for these uses.

Mechanism of Action

Adenosine is a purine nucleotide that is present in all human cells. It contains a purine base, adenine; plus a ribose sugar; and can have one to three phosphate groups (9148). Adenosine is used pharmacologically as an adenosine base, and as the mono- and triphosphate salts. Adenosine is involved in many physiological processes including cellular metabolism, nucleic acid synthesis, neurotransmission, muscle contraction, cardiac function, platelet function, vasodilation, and liver glycogen metabolism (9148,9150). Adenosine triphosphate (ATP) is broken down to adenosine diphosphate (ADP), then to adenosine monophosphate (AMP), and then to adenosine. The ultimate metabolite of adenosine is uric acid. This conversion occurs rapidly. The half-life of adenosine and ATP given by rapid intravenous injection is 0.6 to 1.5 seconds (9148).

Adenosine and ATP both have negative inotropic, dromotropic, and chronotropic effects on the heart. Adenosine and ATP, after degradation to adenosine, stimulate the release of potassium in the sinoatrial (SA) and atrioventricular (AV) nodal cells, which depresses cardiac conduction (9148). Adenosine and ATP given intravenously works for paroxysmal supraventricular tachycardia by causing a transient AV block, and therefore preventing re-entrant atrial tachyarrhythmias (15).

ATP and its degradation products, ADP and adenosine, may help attenuate ischemic tissue trauma. These compounds seem to slow the progression of ischemia involved in alterations of cellular energy and depletion of ATP stores (10066). ATP might also prevent cachexia in people with cancer by crossing the cell membrane and changing metabolic activity. Weight loss seems to occur due to conversion of glucose to lactate in peripheral tissues followed by gluconeogenesis from lactate in the liver. ATP seems to inhibit gluconeogenesis, which might contribute to maintenance of body fat and cell mass in people with cancer (9149,9151,9153,9159).

During intravenous infusion of 25 to 75 mcg/kg per minute, ATP is taken up by the erythrocytes and reaches dose-dependent plateau levels that are 1.5 to 1.7 times higher than baseline within 24 hours. After the infusion is stopped, the half-life of ATP in erythrocytes is 6 hours (9158). Preclinical research suggests that ATP might be active orally (9160).

Adverse Reactions

Intravenously, adenosine can cause general discomfort, breathing more deeply or frequently, headache, flushing, chest pressure or pain, and nausea. Sinus bradycardia and atrial fibrillation can also occur. Adenosine given by rapid intravenous injection can cause small but significant decreases in blood pressure and mean arterial pressure (9148). Intravenously, adenosine triphosphate (ATP) commonly causes dyspnea (sometimes severe) and chest pain, particularly at doses greater than 50 mcg/kg per minute (9154). Headache, palpitations, hypotension, nausea, sweating, flushing, lightheadedness, insomnia, coughing, and anxiety can also occur (9148,9151,9152,9154,9158). When given by rapid intravenous injection, adenosine and ATP adverse effects are likely to be mild and transient because of their extremely short half-lives (9148). Following intramuscular injection, adenosine monophosphate (AMP) can cause local erythema, rash, slight flushing, dizziness, diuresis, and palpitations. Hypotension, dyspnea, epigastric discomfort, and nausea may also occur. Anaphylactic reactions have also been reported (15).

Interactions with Herbs & Other Dietary Supplements

CAFFEINE-CONTAINING HERBS/SUPPLEMENTS: Concomitant use can decrease therapeutic effects of adenosine. Methylxanthines, such as caffeine, are competitive antagonists of adenosine on cell surface receptors (9157). It is recommended that caffeine-containing herbs be stopped 24 hours prior to pharmacological stress tests (11770). However, caffeine appears more likely to interfere with dipyridamole (Persantine) than adenosine-induced stress testing (11771). Herbs that contain caffeine include coffee, black tea, green tea, guarana, mate, and cola.

Interactions with Drugs

ANTIGOUT DRUGS: Adenosine triphosphate (ATP) can cause hyperuricemia and uricosuria, and might reduce the effectiveness of drugs used to prevent and treat gout (9152,9158). Some of these drugs are allopurinol (Zyloprim), colchicine, and probenecid (Benemid).

CARBAMAZEPINE (Tegretol): Carbamazepine given concurrently with adenosine might have an additive effect on heart block (15).

DIPYRIDAMOLE (Persantine): Dipyridamole decreases the metabolism of adenosine and might increase its pharmacologic and toxic effects (15).

METHYLXANTHINES: Aminophylline, caffeine, and theophylline might block the effects of adenosine since methylxanthines are competitive antagonists of adenosine on cell surface receptors (9157). It is recommended that methylxanthines and methylxanthine-containing products be stopped 24 hours prior to pharmacological stress tests (11770). However, methylxanthines appear more likely to interfere with dipyridamole (Persantine) than adenosine-induced stress testing (11771).

Interactions with Foods

CAFFEINE: Caffeine might decrease the effectiveness of adenosine since caffeine and other methylxanthines are competitive antagonists for adenosine receptors (9157). It is recommended that caffeine-containing foods and beverages be stopped 24 hours prior to pharmacological stress tests (11770). However, caffeine appears more likely to interfere with dipyridamole (Persantine) than adenosine-induced stress testing (11771).

Interactions with Lab Tests

ELECTROCARDIOGRAM (ECG,EKG): Adenosine triphosphate (ATP) can cause EKG changes such as ST and T wave changes, which can indicate cardiac ischemia (9152).
URIC ACID: Adenosine triphosphate (ATP) can cause hyperuricemia and uricosuria (9152,9158).

Interactions with Diseases or Conditions

GOUT: Adenosine triphosphate (ATP) can cause hyperuricemia and uricosuria, and might precipitate gout (9152,9158).
HEART DISEASE: Adenosine triphosphate (ATP) can cause cardiac ischemia and chest pain. It might worsen symptoms in patients with heart diseases such as angina and myocardial infarction (9152).

Dosage and Administration

INTRAMUSCULAR: For symptomatic relief of varicose vein complications, adenosine monophosphate 25 mg once or twice weekly followed by 25 mg two to three times weekly has been used (15). For bursitis and tendonitis, adenosine monophosphate 20 mg one to three times daily or every hour for five doses on each of the first three days, followed by 20 mg daily as needed thereafter has been used. Alternatively, 100 mg daily for the first three days, followed by alternate day injections has been used (15).
INTRAVENOUS: For paroxysmal supraventricular tachycardia, adenosine 6 mg given rapidly over 1 to 2 minutes is used. If not effective within 1 to 2 minutes, 12 mg can be given and repeated if necessary. For use with thallium in pharmacologic cardiac stress testing, adenosine is given at a dose of 140 mcg/kg per minute over 6 minutes (total dose of 0.84 mg/kg) (15). For preventing cachexia in patients with advanced cancer, adenosine triphosphate (ATP) has been given every 2 to 4 weeks at a dose of up to 75mcg/kg per minute over 30 hours (9149,9151,9152).

Comments

Adenosine is used pharmacologically as adenosine base, and as the mono- and triphosphate salts. Do not confuse adenosine (Adenocard) with adenosine phosphate. They cannot be used interchangeably (15).

ADRENAL EXTRACT

Also Known As

ACE, Adrenal Complex, Adrenal Cortex Extract, Adrenal Factors, Adrenal Substance, Glandular, Whole Adrenal Extract.

Scientific Names

None.

People Use This For

Orally, adrenal extract is used for low adrenal function; fatigue; stress; impaired resistance to illness; and for treating severe allergies, asthma, eczema, psoriasis, rheumatoid arthritis, and other inflammatory conditions.
Sublingually, adrenal extract is used for stress induced fatigue or exhaustion, poor stress tolerance, general fatigue, allergies, auto-immune disorders, depression, physical or emotional stress, inflammation, low blood pressure, hypoglycemia, drug and alcohol withdrawal, and discontinuing cortisone drugs.
Intravenously, adrenal extract has been used for treating adrenal cortical insufficiency, hyperkalemia, ulcerative colitis, status thymicolymphaticus, and preventing spontaneous abortion.

Safety

LIKELY UNSAFE ...when used parenterally. Use of injectable adrenal extract has been associated with at least 50 cases of serious bacterial infections at injection sites (6620). Adrenal extracts are derived from animals so there is concern about contamination with diseased animal parts. So far, there are no reports of disease transmission to humans due to use of contaminated adrenal extracts.

There is insufficient reliable information available about the safety of adrenal extract for its other uses.
PREGNANCY AND LACTATION: Insufficient reliable information available; avoid using.

Effectiveness
There is insufficient reliable information available about the effectiveness of adrenal extract.

Mechanism of Action
Adrenal extracts are derived from raw cow, pig, or sheep adrenal glands gathered from slaughterhouses (6620). No human studies are reported regarding the absorption or efficacy of adrenal extracts.

Adverse Reactions
Orally, no adverse reactions have been reported; however, adrenal extracts are derived from raw cow, pig, or sheep adrenal glands gathered from slaughterhouses and possibly from sick or diseased animals (6620). Products made from contaminated or diseased organs might present a human health hazard. There is also some concern that adrenal extracts produced from cows in countries where bovine spongiform encephalitis (BSE) has been reported might be contaminated with diseased tissue. Countries where BSE has been reported include Great Britain, France, The Netherlands, Portugal, Luxembourg, Ireland, Switzerland, Oman, and Belgium (1825); however, there have been no reports of BSE transfer to humans from contaminated adrenal extract products. Until more is known, tell patients to avoid these products unless country of origin can be determined. Patients should avoid products that are produced in countries where BSE has been found.
Intravenously, adrenal extract can cause infection and abscess at the site of injection (6620). In 1996, the FDA issued a nationwide alert regarding an injectable adrenal cortex extract after more than 50 cases of serious bacterial infections at injection sites were reported (6620).

Interactions with Herbs & Other Dietary Supplements
None known.

Interactions with Drugs
None known.

Interactions with Foods
None known.

Interactions with Lab Tests
None known.

Interactions with Diseases or Conditions
IMMUNODEFICIENCY: Theoretically, adrenal extracts might increase the risk of infection. Adrenal extracts might harbor pathogens. Injectable adrenal extract reportedly caused more than 50 serious infections at injection sites (6620); avoid using.

Dosage and Administration
No typical dosage.

ADRUE

Also Known As
Chintul, Guinea Rush, Jointed Flat Sedge, Piripiri.

Scientific Names
Cyperus articulatus, synonym Cyperus corymbosus.
Family: Cyperaceae.

Comments
At the date of publication, this product was not a common ingredient used in brand name supplements marketed to consumers. Details about this product are available at the online version of *Natural Medicines Comprehensive Database*. See www.naturaldatabase.com.

AFRICAN WILD POTATO

Also Known As

Bantu Tulip, Hypoxis Plant, South African Star Grass, Sterretjie.
CAUTION: See separate listing for Potato.

Scientific Names

Hypoxis hemerocallidea, synonym Hypoxis rooperi.
Family: Hypoxidaceae or Liliaceae

People Use This For

Orally, the African wild potato is used for bladder and urinary disorders including cystitis, prostate problems including prostatic hyperplasia and prostate cancer, lung disease, and cancer. It is also used in maintaining health in individuals who are HIV positive, for TB, "yuppie flu," arthritis, and psoriasis.
Topically, the African wild potato is used for wound healing.

Safety

POSSIBLY SAFE ...when used orally and appropriately. African wild potato has been taken with apparent safety for up to 18 months (5327,5328,7198).
PREGNANCY AND LACTATION: Insufficient reliable information available; avoid using.

Effectiveness

POSSIBLY EFFECTIVE

Benign prostatic hyperplasia (BPH). African wild potato taken orally, alone or in combination with other beta-sitosterol sources, seems to reduce urinary symptoms and improve quality of life (5327,5328,7198).

There is insufficient reliable information available about the effectiveness of African wild potato for its other uses.

Mechanism of Action

The African wild potato tuber contains 3.5%-4.5% lignans, particularly norlignan glucoside (5944). Preliminary human trials indicate the African wild potato glucoside constituent is non-toxic (4284). It also contains beta-sitosterol and beta-sitosterolin, and is sometimes used as a source of beta-sitosterol (5327,5328,7198). The activity of the African wild potato is attributed to the phytosterols that inhibit the production of prostaglandin synthase (5944). Animal research suggests that African wild potato might lower blood glucose levels, but this hasn't been seen in humans (11236).

Adverse Reactions

Orally, the African wild potato is usually well tolerated. In some patients it can cause nausea, indigestion, gas, diarrhea, or constipation (5327,5328). The beta-sitosterol constituent has been associated with erectile dysfunction and loss of libido (5942).

Interactions with Herbs & Other Dietary Supplements

CAROTENE, VITAMIN E: The beta-sitosterol may reduce absorption and blood levels of alpha- and beta-carotene and vitamin E (5814).
CHOLESTEROL LOWERING HERBS/SUPPLEMENTS: The beta-sitosterol constituent of African wild potato might have additive effects with herbs and supplements that also lower cholesterol levels (5331,5336). Some of these herbs and supplements include chromium, flaxseed, garlic, guar gum, niacin, oat bran, psyllium, red yeast, and others.

Interactions with Drugs

None known.

Interactions with Foods

CAROTENE, VITAMIN E: The beta-sitosterol constituent of African wild potato may reduce absorption and blood levels of alpha- and beta-carotene and vitamin E (5814).

Interactions with Lab Tests

CHOLESTEROL: The beta-sitosterol constituent of African wild potato may decrease total serum cholesterol and low-density lipoprotein (LDL) levels (5331,5336).

Interactions with Diseases or Conditions

SITOSTEROLEMIA (Phytosterolemia): The beta-sitosterol constituent of African wild potato can exacerbate sitosterolemia, a rare inherited lipid storage disease (5326,10305). People with this disorder have increased absorption of cholesterol and beta-sitosterol from the diet, and decreased clearance of beta-sitosterol. Total body stores of beta-sitosterol are increased up to 17-fold. Elevated hepatic beta-sitosterol levels competitively inhibit cholesterol catabolism, contributing to hypercholesterolemia (3663). Patients with sitosterolemia are prone to premature coronary artery disease and xanthomas (3661,3662). Beta-sitosterol and its glycoside sitosterolin are contraindicated in patients with sitosterolemia. However, beta-sitosterol appears to be safe for heterozygous carriers of sitosterolemia (10457).

Dosage and Administration

ORAL: For benign prostatic hyperplasia (BPH), African wild potato containing 60 to 130 mg of beta-sitosterol divided into 2-3 doses daily has been used (5327,5328).

Comments

The African wild potato is native to South Africa (5944).

AGA

Also Known As

Fly Agaric, Soma.

Scientific Names

Amanita muscaria.
Family: Amanitaceae.

People Use This For

Orally, aga is used as a hallucinogen. It is also used orally in homeopathic dilutions for nerve pain, fever, anxiety, alcohol poisoning, and joint pains.

Safety

UNSAFE ...when used orally (18).
PREGNANCY AND LACTATION: UNSAFE ...when used orally due to its toxicity (18); avoid using.

Effectiveness

There is insufficient reliable information available about the effectiveness of aga.

Mechanism of Action

The applicable part of aga is the fruiting body. Aga is not a true hallucinogen. The illusions that occur with aga ingestion are a misinterpretation of sensory stimuli. These mind altering effects are due to the isoxazoles ibotenic acid, muscimol, muscazone, and traces of muscarine (18).

Adverse Reactions

Orally, people develop symptoms within 30-90 minutes of using aga. The effects peak at 2-3 hours. Toxicity can occur after ingesting a single aga mushroom. Mind-altering effects have occurred with ingestion of 2-4 mushrooms, and 20 large mushrooms have been ingested with survival. Death due to aga ingestion is rare, less than 1%. The mushrooms can cause drowsiness, confusion, illusions, and mania (18).

Interactions with Herbs & Other Dietary Supplements

None known.

Interactions with Drugs

None known.

Interactions with Foods

None known.

Interactions with Lab Tests

None known.

Interactions with Diseases or Conditions

None known.

Dosage and Administration

No typical dosage.

Comments
Aga is a mushroom with a red cap that is spotted with white. It grows in sandy, acidic soils in the US. It is known as "fly agaric" because ibotenic acid and muscimol are toxic to the common housefly.

AGAR

Also Known As
Agar-Agar, Agarweed, Chinese Gelatin, Colle du Japon, Gelosa, Japanese Isinglas, Layor Carang, Vegetable Gelatin.

Scientific Names
Gelidiella acerosa; Gelidium amanasii; Gelidium cartilagineum; Gelidium crinale; Gelidium divaricatum; Gelidium pacificum; Gelidium vagum; Garacilaria confervoides.
Family: Sphaerococcaceae. Species of the genera Pterocladia; Ahnfeltia; Acanthopeltis; Suhria.

People Use This For
Orally, agar is used as a bulk laxative for chronic constipation.
In dentistry, agar is used to make dental impressions.
In manufacturing processes, agar is used as an ingredient in emulsions, suspensions, gels, and hydrophilic suppositories.

Safety
LIKELY SAFE ...when used orally with at least 250 mL of water (12).
PREGNANCY AND LACTATION: Insufficient reliable information available.

Effectiveness
EFFECTIVE
Constipation. Taking agar orally seems to help decrease constipation by producing a bulk laxative effect (11).

Mechanism of Action
Agar consists of two major polysaccharides, neutral agarose and charged agaropectin. Agarose is the gelling fraction (11).

Adverse Reactions
Potential to cause esophageal or bowel obstruction if taken with insufficient volume of water (12). Possibly can increase cholesterol levels (11).

Interactions with Herbs & Other Dietary Supplements
None known.

Interactions with Drugs
ORAL DRUGS: The fiber in agar can impair absorption of oral drugs (19).

Interactions with Foods
None known.

Interactions with Lab Tests
None known.

Interactions with Diseases or Conditions
BOWEL OBSTRUCTION OR DIFFICULTY SWALLOWING: Contraindicated (12).

Dosage and Administration
ORAL: A typical dose is 4-16 grams, one to two times daily (12). Take each dose with at least 250 mL of water (11).

Comments
OTC products must be labeled: "Warning, taking this product without adequate fluid may cause it to swell and block your throat or esophagus and may cause choking. Do not take this product if you have difficulty swallowing. If you experience chest pain, vomiting, or difficulty swallowing or breathing after using this product, seek immediate medical attention" (12).

AGRIMONY

Also Known As

Ackerkraut, Agrimoniae herba, Agromonia, Cocklebur, Fragrant Agrimony, Funffing, Funffingerkraut, Herba eupatoriae, Herbe d'Aigremoine, Herbe de Saint-Guillaume, Liverwort, Stickwort.
CAUTION: See separate listings for Liverwort and Potentilla.

Scientific Names

Agrimonia eupatoria; Agrimonia procera, synonym Agrimonia odorata.
Family: Rosaceae.

People Use This For

Orally, agrimony is used for sore throat, upset stomach, mild diarrhea, gallbladder disorders, tuberculosis, bleeding, corns, warts, as a gargle, antitumor agent, cardiotonic, diuretic, sedative, and antihistamine.
Topically, agrimony is used as a mild astringent and for mild skin inflammation. The ethanolic extracts of agrimony are used for their antiviral properties.

Safety

LIKELY SAFE ...when the dried above ground parts are used orally and appropriately short-term (2,12). ...when used topically (2).
POSSIBLY UNSAFE ...when used orally or topically in excessive doses due to its high tannin content (12).
PREGNANCY AND LACTATION: POSSIBLY UNSAFE ...when used orally because of the possible effects on the menstrual cycle (4,12).

Effectiveness

There is insufficient reliable information available about the effectiveness of agrimony.

Mechanism of Action

The applicable parts of agrimony are the dried, above ground parts. The aerial plant parts contain 4-10% condensed tannins which can account for its astringent properties (6). Because of the tannin content and astringent properties of agrimony, it is thought to be helpful for gastrointestinal conditions such as diarrhea.

Adverse Reactions

The use of agrimony can cause photodermatitis and can affect blood pressure (6).

Interactions with Herbs & Other Dietary Supplements

None known.

Interactions with Drugs

ANTIDIABETES DRUGS: Monitor blood glucose levels closely due to claims that agrimony has hypoglycemic effects (19).

Interactions with Foods

None known.

Interactions with Lab Tests

None known.

Interactions with Diseases or Conditions

None known.

Dosage and Administration

ORAL: The typical dose of agrimony is 3 grams per day (2).
TOPICAL: A poultice is commonly applied several times daily using approximately 10% water extract, which is prepared by boiling the herb at low heat for 10-20 minutes (8).

ALCHEMILLA

Also Known As

Feuilles d'Alchemille, Frauenmantelkraut, Lady's Mantle, Leontopodium, Lion's Foot, Marienmantel, Nine Hooks, Silerkraut, Stellaria.
CAUTION: See separate listing for Alpine Lady's Mantle.

Scientific Names

Alchemilla xanthochlora; Alchemilla vulgaris.
Family: Rosaceae.

People Use This For

Orally, alchemilla is used for mild diarrhea, heavy menstrual flow, diabetes, menopausal complaints, painful menses, gastrointestinal disorders, as a relaxant for muscle spasms, an anti-inflammatory, a diuretic, and as a gargle for mouth and throat inflammation.
Topically, alchemilla is used as an astringent for bleeding, to improve wound healing, for ulcers, eczema, skin rashes, and as a bath additive for treating lower-abdominal ailments.

Safety

POSSIBLY SAFE ...when used orally and appropriately. Alchemilla has been used for many years without reports of significant toxicity (6,8,12).
There is insufficient reliable information available about the safety of the topical use of alchemilla.
PREGNANCY AND LACTATION: Insufficient reliable information available; avoid using.

Effectiveness

There is insufficient reliable information available about the effectiveness of alchemilla.

Mechanism of Action

The applicable parts of alchemilla are the above ground parts. Alchemilla contains 6-8% tannins (8), which might account for its perceived astringent activity (6). An aqueous extract of Alchemilla xanthochlora demonstrates lipid peroxidation and superoxide anion scavenging activity (6). Flavonoid extracts inhibit proteolytic enzymes, including elastase, trypsin, and alpha-chymotrypsin. This property suggests alchemilla might have a role in protecting conjunctive and elastic tissues (6).

Adverse Reactions

Rarely, alchemilla can cause liver damage (8).

Interactions with Herbs & Other Dietary Supplements

None known.

Interactions with Drugs

None known.

Interactions with Foods

None known.

Interactions with Lab Tests

None known.

Interactions with Diseases or Conditions

None known.

Dosage and Administration

ORAL: For diarrhea, a typical dose is one cup tea, prepared by steeping 1-4 grams above ground parts in boiling water for 10 minutes and then straining (8), used up to three times per day between meals. The average amount used per day is 5-10 grams. Equivalent preparations can also be used (2). Diarrhea persisting for more than 3-4 days should be medically evaluated (8).
TOPICAL: No typical dosage.

Comments

Although the German Standard License warns about possible liver damage, some experts consider the concern to be exaggerated (8).

ALDER BUCKTHORN

Also Known As

Alder Dogwood, Arrow Wood, Black Dogwood, Buckthorn, Dog Wood, Frangula, Frangulae Cortex, Glossy Buckthorn.
CAUTION: See separate listings for European Buckthorn, Sea Buckthorn, and Cascara.

Scientific Names

Frangula alnus, synonym Rhamnus frangula.
Family: Rhamnaceae.

People Use This For

Orally, alder buckthorn is used as a laxative, as a tonic, and as a component in the Hoxsey cancer formula.

Safety

LIKELY SAFE ...when used orally and appropriately for no more than 8 to 10 days (12). Only properly aged bark should be used, and the recommended dose should not be exceeded (12).
POSSIBLY UNSAFE ...when used orally for more than 8 to 10 days (12).
CHILDREN: LIKELY UNSAFE ...when used orally in children younger than 12 years of age (12); avoid using.
PREGNANCY AND LACTATION: LIKELY UNSAFE ...when used orally (12); avoid using.

Effectiveness

LIKELY EFFECTIVE

Constipation. Taking alder buckthorn orally seems to relieve constipation (3,4,7,12). Alder buckthorn has laxative effects comparable to cascara (3).

There is insufficient reliable information available about the effectiveness of alder buckthorn for its other uses.

Mechanism of Action

The applicable part of alder buckthorn is the bark. The anthraglycosides and particularly the diglycosides are cathartic in the large intestine (1,8,11). They can increase intestinal motility by inhibiting stationary contractions, stimulating propulsive contractions, stimulating active chloride secretion, and increasing water and electrolytes in the intestinal contents (2). The fresh bark contains free anthrone, which can cause severe vomiting and is destroyed by aging the bark naturally for one year or artificially with heat and aeration (2). Anthroid laxative use is not associated with an increased risk of developing colorectal adenoma or carcinoma (6138).

Adverse Reactions

Orally, alder buckthorn can cause cramp-like discomfort (2). Chronic use can cause pseudomelanosis coli (pigment spots in intestinal mucosa) which is harmless, usually reverses with discontinuation (2), and is not associated with an increased risk of developing colorectal adenoma or carcinoma (6138). Chronic use or abuse of the bark can lead to potassium depletion, albuminuria, and hematuria. Potassium depletion can lead to disturbed heart function and muscle weakness (2). The fresh or improperly aged bark can cause severe vomiting due to the presence of the free anthrone, an emetic constituent.

Interactions with Herbs & Other Dietary Supplements

LICORICE: Concomitant use of alder buckthorn with licorice can increase the risk of potassium depletion (2).
POTASSIUM DEPLETING HERBS: Theoretically, concomitant use of alder buckthorn with horsetail plant or licorice rhizome increases the risk of potassium depletion.
STIMULANT LAXATIVE HERBS: Theoretically, concomitant use of alder buckthorn with other stimulant laxative herbs can increase the risk of potassium depletion. Stimulant laxative herbs include aloe dried leaf sap, wild cucumber fruit (Ecballium elaterium), blue flag rhizome, butternut bark, cascara bark, castor oil, colocynth fruit pulp, gamboge bark exudate, jalap root, black root, manna bark exudate, podophyllum root, rhubarb root, senna leaves and pods, and yellow dock root (19).

Interactions with Drugs

CORTICOSTEROIDS: Concomitant use of corticosteroids with alder buckthorn can increase the risk of potassium depletion (2).
DIGOXIN (Lanoxin): Theoretically, overuse or abuse of alder buckthorn can increase the risk of adverse effects from cardiac glycoside drugs (19).
DIURETIC DRUGS: Overuse of alder buckthorn might compound diuretic-induced potassium loss (19).
There is some concern that people taking alder buckthorn along with potassium depleting diuretics might have an increased risk for hypokalemia. Initiation of potassium supplementation or an increase in potassium supplement dose may be necessary for some patients. Some diuretics that can deplete potassium include chlorothiazide (Diuril), chlorthalidone (Thalitone), furosemide (Lasix), and hydrochlorothiazide (HCTZ,

HydroDIURIL, Microzide), and others.
ORAL DRUGS: Theoretically, alder buckthorn can reduce absorption of some drugs due to reduced gastrointestinal transit time (19).
STIMULANT LAXATIVES: Concomitant use might compound fluid and electrolyte loss (19).

Interactions with Foods

None known.

Interactions with Lab Tests

COLORIMETRIC TESTS: Alder buckthorn can discolor urine (pink, red, purple, orange, rust), interfering with diagnostic tests that depend on a color change, due to its anthraquinone content (1,12,275).
POTASSIUM: Excessive use of alder buckthorn can cause potassium depletion, reducing serum potassium concentrations and test results (1,2,4,12,19).

Interactions with Diseases or Conditions

GI CONDITIONS: Alder buckthorn is contraindicated in individuals with intestinal obstruction; abdominal pain of unknown origin; and intestinal inflammation, including appendicitis, Crohn's disease, irritable bowel syndrome (IBS), and ulcerative colitis (12).

Dosage and Administration

ORAL: The typical dose of alder buckthorn is 0.5-2.5 grams of the dried bark (4) or as a tea, which is prepared by steeping 2 grams of the herb in 150 mL boiling water for 5-10 minutes and then straining (12). The average dose per day of the bark is 1 gram (3) or 20-30 mg of the hydoxyanthracene derivatives calculated as glycofrangulin A (2). The common dose of the liquid extract: (1:1 in 25% alcohol) is 2-5 mL three times daily (2). The individual dose of the bark is the minimum amount required to produce a soft stool (2). Limit its use to a maximum of seven to ten days. This preparation should be used only if no effect can be obtained through change of diet or the use of bulk-forming laxative products (2).

Comments

Avoid confusion with European buckthorn. The American Herbal Products Association (AHPA) recommends the following label statement: "Do not use this product if you have abdominal pain or diarrhea. Consult a healthcare provider prior to use if you are pregnant or nursing. Discontinue use in the event of diarrhea or watery stools. Do not exceed dose. Not for long-term use." (12). Today, alder buckthorn is primarily used as a dye.

ALETRIS

Also Known As

Ague, Aloerot, Blazing Star, Colic Root, Crow Corn, Devil's-bit, Stargrass, Starwort, True Unicorn Root, Whitetube Stargrass.

Scientific Names

Aletris farinosa.
Family: Liliaceae or Nartheciaceae.

People Use This For

Orally, aletris is used for rheumatism, as a general tonic, a sedative, to relieve menstrual disorders, as a laxative, an antiflatulent, an antispasmodic, for colic, as an antidiarrheal, and a diuretic. It is also used orally for infertility, dyspepsia, and to prevent miscarriage.

Safety

POSSIBLY SAFE ...when used orally and appropriately (6,12).
PREGNANCY AND LACTATION: POSSIBLY UNSAFE ...when used orally due to the possibility that aletris contains components that cause estrogenic activity (11) and oxytocin (Pitocin) antagonism (12); avoid using.

Effectiveness

There is insufficient reliable information available about the effectiveness of aletris.

Mechanism of Action

Some aletris constituents may have estrogenic activity (6).

Adverse Reactions

Orally, small doses of aletris may induce colic, stupefaction, and vertigo (6).

Interactions with Herbs & Other Dietary Supplements

None known.

Interactions with Drugs

ANTACIDS: Theoretically, due to reports that aletris increases stomach acid, aletris might decrease the effectiveness of antacids (19).
H2-BLOCKERS: Theoretically, due to reports that aletris increases stomach acid, aletris might decrease the effectiveness of H2-blockers (19). The H2 blockers include cimetidine (Tagamet), ranitidine (Zantac), nizatidine (Axid), and famotidine (Pepcid).
PROTON PUMP INHIBITORS (PPIs): Theoretically, due to reports that aletris increases stomach acid, aletris might decrease the effectiveness of PPIs (19). PPIs include omeprazole (Prilosec), lansoprazole (Prevacid), rabeprazole (Aciphex), pantoprazole (Protonix), and esomeprazole (Nexium).

Interactions with Foods

None known.

Interactions with Lab Tests

None known.

Interactions with Diseases or Conditions

GASTROINTESTINAL (GI) DISEASES: Aletris can irritate the GI tract. It is contraindicated in individuals with infectious or inflammatory GI conditions (19).
HORMONE SENSITIVE CANCERS/CONDITIONS: Aletris might have estrogenic effects (6). Women with hormone sensitive conditions should avoid aletris. Some of these conditions include breast cancer, uterine cancer, ovarian cancer, endometriosis, and uterine fibroids.

Dosage and Administration

ORAL: Aletris is typically used as the powdered root, a liquid extract, and an infusion (18). One common dosage recommendation is 0.3 to 0.6 grams three times daily (18). The infusion is prepared by adding 1.5 grams of aletris to 100 mL of water, and the fluid extract (1:1) is commonly produced with 45% ethanol water (18).

ALFALFA

Also Known As

Feuille De Luzerne, Lucerne, Medicago, Phytoestrogen, Purple Medick.

Scientific Names

Medicago sativa.
Family: Fabaceae/Leguminosae.

People Use This For

Orally, alfalfa is used as a diuretic, for kidney conditions, bladder and prostate conditions, asthma, arthritis, rheumatoid arthritis, diabetes, indigestion, and thrombocytopenic purpura. It is also used orally as a source of vitamins A, C, E, and K4; and minerals calcium, potassium, phosphorous, and iron.

Safety

LIKELY SAFE ...when the above ground parts are used orally and appropriately (4,6,12).
LIKELY UNSAFE ...when excessive amounts of seeds are used. The seed have been associated with pancytopenia (5,6).
PREGNANCY AND LACTATION: POSSIBLY UNSAFE ...when used orally in medicinal amounts. Alfalfa contains constituents with possible estrogenic activity (4,11).

Effectiveness

POSSIBLY EFFECTIVE

Hypercholesterolemia. Taking alfalfa seeds orally seems to lower total cholesterol and low-density lipoprotein (LDL) cholesterol in patients with high cholesterol levels (5816).

There is insufficient reliable information available about the effectiveness of alfalfa for its other uses.

Mechanism of Action

The applicable parts of alfalfa are the above ground parts. The alfalfa leaf contains saponins which appear to decrease plasma cholesterol without creating a change in HDL levels (4). Constituents of alfalfa seem to decrease cholesterol absorption, and increase excretion of neutral steroids and bile acids (4,6). Alfalfa contains manganese which might be responsible for hypoglycemic effects (4). Alfalfa contains medicagol which appears to have antifungal properties. Alfalfa also contains isoflavonoids including coumetrol, genistein, biochanin A, and daidzein which all seem to have estrogenic properties (11).

Adverse Reactions

Alfalfa might cause photosensitivity (605). Ingestion of ground alfalfa seeds is associated with a case of pancytopenia (381). Stems and leaves are reportedly free of systemic lupus erythematosus (SLE) triggering substance(s) found in seeds (4). There is one case report of listeriosis traced to the consumption of contaminated alfalfa tablets from which Listeria monocytogenes was isolated (5600).

Interactions with Herbs & Other Dietary Supplements

HERBS WITH CLOTTING POTENTIAL: Excessive use of herbs that contain vitamin K, an essential coagulation factor, can increase the risk of clotting in people using anticoagulants. These herbs include alfalfa, parsley, nettle, plantain, and others.
VITAMIN E: Alfalfa contains saponins which interfere with the absorption or activity of vitamin E (11).

Interactions with Drugs

CONTRACEPTIVE DRUGS: Excessive doses of alfalfa may interfere with contraceptive drugs. Alfalfa contains isoflavonoids with estrogenic effects (4).
ESTROGENS: Excessive doses of alfalfa may interfere with hormone therapy due to estrogenic effects of isoflavonoids alfalfa (4).
PHOTOSENSITIZING DRUGS: Excessive doses of alfalfa may potentiate drug-induced photosensitivity (605).
WARFARIN (Coumadin): Alfalfa contains large amount of vitamin K (4,6). Concomitant use can reduce the anticoagulant activity of warfarin.

Interactions with Foods

None known.

Interactions with Lab Tests

CHOLESTEROL: Alfalfa seed might lower serum cholesterol concentrations and test results in individuals with type II hyperlipoproteinemia (4).

Interactions with Diseases or Conditions

DIABETES: Alfalfa might reduce blood sugar levels; monitor closely (4).
HORMONE SENSITIVE CANCERS/CONDITIONS: Because alfalfa seems to have estrogenic effects (11), women with hormone sensitive conditions should avoid alfalfa. Some of these conditions include breast, uterine, and ovarian cancer, and endometriosis and uterine fibroids.
KIDNEY TRANSPLANT: There is one report of acute kidney transplant rejection in a patient who took black cohosh and an alfalfa supplement together. The mechanism for this disease interaction is not known, but it is more likely due to alfalfa than black cohosh. Alfalfa is thought to have immune-stimulating effects that might counteract the immunosuppressant effects of cyclosporine (12174).
SYSTEMIC LUPUS ERYTHEMATOSUS (SLE): Consumption of seeds (not stems/leaves) might reactivate latent disease (6,605).

Dosage and Administration

ORAL: A typical dosage is 5-10 grams, or as steeped strained tea, three times a day (4). Liquid extract (1:1 in 25% alcohol) 5-10 mL three times a day has also been used (4).

ALGIN

Also Known As

Alginates, Sodium Alginate.
CAUTION: See separate listings for Laminaria and Bladderwrack.

Scientific Names

Ascophyllum nodosum; Laminaria digitata; Macrocystis pyrifera.
Family: Lessoniaceae.

People Use This For

Orally, algin is used to lower serum cholesterol levels and to reduce absorption of strontium, barium, tin, cadmium, manganese, zinc, and mercury. Algin is also orally for the prevention and treatment of hypertension.

In foods, algin is used in candy, gelatins, puddings, condiments, relishes, processed vegetables, fish products, and imitation dairy products.
In manufacturing, algin is used as a binding and disintegrating agent in tablets, as binding and demulcent in lozenges, and as film in peel-off facial masks.

Safety
LIKELY SAFE ...when used orally in amounts typically found in foods.
PREGNANCY AND LACTATION: Insufficient reliable information available.

Effectiveness
There is insufficient reliable information available about the effectiveness of algin.

Mechanism of Action
Algin is the purified carbohydrate product extracted from brown seaweed by use of dilute alkali. Algin is comprised of the sodium salt of alginic acid, a linear polymer of L-guluronic and D-mannuronic acid. Although mannuronic acid is the major component, there is variation depending on the algal source (13). Cholesterol lowering effects may be related to viscosity of gel and inhibiting cholesterol absorption (11). Hypotensive effects may be due to laminine dioxalate (11). Algin is believed, but not confirmed, to be indigestible (11).

Adverse Reactions
None reported.

Interactions with Herbs & Other Dietary Supplements
None known.

Interactions with Drugs
ORAL DRUGS: The fiber in algin can impair absorption of oral drugs (19).

Interactions with Foods
None known.

Interactions with Lab Tests
BLOOD PRESSURE: Theoretically, algin might lower blood pressure and blood pressure readings (11).
CHOLESTEROL: Theoretically, algin might reduce serum cholesterol concentrations and test results (11).

Interactions with Diseases or Conditions
None known.

Dosage and Administration
No typical dosage.

Comments
Algin is isolated from a variety of brown algae (seaweeds, Class: Phaeophyceae), particularly from the genera Ascophyllum, Macrocystis, and Laminaria (11).

ALKANNA

Also Known As
Alkanet, Alkanna Radix, Anchusa, Dyer's Bugloss, Henna, Orchanet, Radix Anchusae.
CAUTION: See separate listing for Henna.

Scientific Names
Alkanna tinctoria, synonyms Alkanna lehmanii, Alkanna tuberculata, Anchusa bracteolata, Anchusa tuberculata, Lithospermum lehmanii.
Family: Boraginaceae.

People Use This For
Orally, alkanna is used for diarrhea.
Topically, alkanna is used to heal skin wounds, as an astringent, and for skin diseases.

Safety

POSSIBLY UNSAFE ...when the root preparations are used topically on broken or abraded skin (12) because they contain toxic unsaturated pyrrolizidine alkaloids (UPAs) that might be absorbed systemically.
LIKELY UNSAFE ...when used orally. Repeated exposure to low concentrations of UPAs is linked to serious liver toxicity (4,12). UPAs are also thought to be carcinogenic and mutagenic (12).
There is insufficient reliable information available about the safety of alkanna used topically on unbroken skin.
PREGNANCY: POSSIBLY UNSAFE ...when used topically (12). LIKELY UNSAFE ...when used orally because it contains UPAs (4,12).
LACTATION: POSSIBLY UNSAFE ...when used topically (12). LIKELY UNSAFE ...when used orally. There is concern that UPAs could be excreted in breast milk (4,12,18).

Effectiveness

There is insufficient reliable information available about the effectiveness of alkanna.

Mechanism of Action

The applicable part of alkanna is the root. Alkanna contains napthazarine esters, pyrrolizidine alkaloids, and tannins (18). Some pyrrolizidine alkaloids have shown carcinogenic and mutagenic properties, and there are reports of renal toxicity. However, the primary concern is veno-occlusive disease (12). Unsaturated pyrrolizidine alkaloids (UPAs) are known to be hepatotoxic (4). The color of alkanna comes from a mixture of 5-6% red pigments which consist mainly of fat-soluble naphthazarin (6).

Adverse Reactions

Chronic exposure to plants containing unsaturated pyrrolizidine alkaloids (UPAs) have been associated with veno-occlusive disease (4021). Symptoms of acute veno-occlusive disease are characterized by a dull, dragging ache in the right upper abdomen and marked distention of the abdomen. These symptoms are sometimes accompanied by reduced urine output. Subacute veno-occlusive disease is associated with vague symptoms and persistent liver enlargement (4021).

Interactions with Herbs & Other Dietary Supplements

EUCALYPTUS: Theoretically, concomitant use might increase the risk of unsaturated pyrrolizidine alkaloid toxicity due to enzyme induction by eucalyptus (19).
UNSATURATED PYRROLIZIDINE ALKALOID (UPA)-CONTAINING HERBS: Concomitant use of these plants is contraindicated due to the risk of additive toxicity. Herbs that contain UPAs include alkanna, borage, gravel root, hemp agrimony, hound's tongue, petasites, comfrey, coltsfoot; and the Senecio species including dusty miller, alpine ragwort, groundsel, golden ragwort, and tansy ragwort (12,19,271).

Interactions with Drugs

None known.

Interactions with Foods

None known.

Interactions with Lab Tests

None known.

Interactions with Diseases or Conditions

LIVER DISEASE: Alkanna is contraindicated due to hepatotoxic potential (19).

Dosage and Administration

No typical dosage.

Comments

Although alkanna is used as a reddish pigment in foods and cosmetics, many countries have banned its use in food (8).

ALLSPICE

Also Known As
Aqua Pimentae, Clove Pepper, Jamaica Pepper, Kiln-Dried Allspice, Pimenta, Pimento, Pimento Oil, Pimento Water, Spanish Pimienta, Water of Pimento.

Scientific Names
Pimenta dioica, synonyms Pimenta officinalis, Eugenia pimenta.
Family: Myrtaceae.

People Use This For
Orally, allspice is used for indigestion, flatulence, menorrhagia, vomiting, diarrhea, fever, colds, and as a purgative.
Topically, allspice is used for muscle pain, toothache, and as an antiseptic.
In dentistry, some dentists use eugenol, a constituent of allspice, as a local antiseptic for teeth and gums.
For food uses, allspice is used as an aromatic spice.
In manufacturing, it is used in toothpaste as a flavoring.

Safety
LIKELY SAFE ...when used orally in amounts commonly found in foods. Allspice has Generally Recognized As Safe status (GRAS) for use in foods in the US (4912).
PREGNANCY AND LACTATION: There is insufficient reliable information available about the safety of allspice when used in medicinal amounts during pregnancy and breast-feeding.

Effectiveness
There is insufficient reliable information available about the effectiveness of allspice.

Mechanism of Action
The applicable parts of allspice are the unripe fruit and leaf. The eugenol constituent in allspice may explain this product's effects on the digestive system and its pain relief properties. Eugenol seems to decrease intestinal pain by depressing the CNS and inhibiting prostaglandin activity in the human colon mucosa (11). It also increases the activity of some digestive enzymes, including trypsin (6002). Eugenol may be responsible for allspice's anesthetic effects when the crushed berries are applied topically.

Adverse Reactions
Orally, excessive doses of allspice may cause nausea, vomiting, CNS depression, and convulsions due to eugenol content (6).
Topically, allspice may irritate mucous membranes (6).

Interactions with Herbs & Other Dietary Supplements
None known.

Interactions with Drugs
ANTICOAGULANT/ANTIPLATELET DRUGS: Eugenol, a constituent of allspice, inhibits platelet activity. Individuals on anticoagulant or antiplatelet therapy who choose to use this product should use caution (4).

Interactions with Foods
None known.

Interactions with Lab Tests
None known.

Interactions with Diseases or Conditions
None known.

Dosage and Administration
ORAL: A typical dose for flatulence is 0.05-0.2 mL allspice oil (11).
TOPICAL: No typical dosage.

Comments
The commercially available allspice powder consists of whole ground dried fruit (6).

ALOE gel

Also Known As

Aloe Africana, Aloe Arborescens Natalenis, Aloe Barbadensis, Aloe Capensis, Aloe Ferox, Aloe Perfoliata, Aloe Perryi, Aloe Spicata, Ghrita-Kumari, Kanya, Kumari.
CAUTION: See separate listing for Aloe latex.

Scientific Names

Aloe vera, synonyms Aloe barbadensis, Aloe indica; Aloe africana; Aloe arborescens, synonyms Aloe natalenis, Aloe frutescens, Aloe ucriae; Aloe ferox, synonym Aloe supralaevis; Aloe perryi; Aloe spicata.
Family: Aloaceae or Asphodelaceae.

People Use This For

Orally, aloe gel is used for inflammation, osteoarthritis, inflammatory bowel diseases including ulcerative colitis, fever, itching, as a general tonic, antiseptic, and moisturizer. Aloe gel is also used orally for gastroduodenal ulcers, diabetes, asthma, and radiation-related mucositis.
Topically, aloe gel is used for burns and wound healing, psoriasis, sunburn, frostbite, inflammation, osteoarthritis, and cold sores.

Safety

POSSIBLY SAFE ...when used orally and topically (11982,11984).
PREGNANCY AND LACTATION: Insufficient reliable information available; avoid using.

Effectiveness

POSSIBLY EFFECTIVE

Psoriasis. Applying aloe extract 0.5% cream topically three times daily for four weeks significantly improves and increases the resolution of psoriatic plaques compared to placebo (101,12096). Aloe extract cream seems to reduce desquamation, erythema, and infiltration (12096).

INSUFFICIENT RELIABLE EVIDENCE to RATE

Burns. Applying aloe gel topically seems to enhance healing of partial thickness burns (101).
Diabetes. Preliminary evidence suggests that taking one tablespoon (15 mL) of aloe gel daily for 42 days can significantly decrease blood glucose levels in women with type 2 diabetes (12164).
Frostbite. Applying aloe gel topically seems to enhance tissue survival following frostbite injury (101).
Genital herpes. There is some evidence that applying aloe vera extract 0.5% cream three times daily increases healing rates compared to aloe gel or placebo. Some patients heal within five days of use compared to 12 days with placebo (12164).
Hyperlipidemia. Preliminary evidence suggests that taking 10 mL or 20 mL of aloe vera orally daily for 12 weeks can reduce total cholesterol by about 15%, low-density lipoprotein (LDL) cholesterol by about 18%, and triglycerides by about 25% to 30% in patients with hyperlipidemia (12164).
Pressure ulcers. Preliminary evidence suggests that applying aloe gel does not improve the healing rate of pressure ulcers compared to management with moist saline gauze (12160).
Radiation-induced skin toxicity. Radiation therapy for cancer often causes erythema, skin desquamation, and itching. Applying topically a 98% aloe gel three times daily throughout radiation treatment and after treatment does not seem to reduce these radiation-related side effects in patients being treated for breast cancer (12098,12163). Applying a 100% aloe gel 6-8 times per day also does not seem to reduce these radiation related side effects in people treated for other cancers. But there is some evidence that aloe gel might prolong the time before radiation-related side effects occur (12159).
Ulcerative colitis. Preliminary evidence suggests that some patients with mild to moderate ulcerative colitis who take aloe gel 25-50 mL twice daily have significantly reduced symptoms (11984).
Wound healing. Applying aloe gel extract (Carrington Dermal Wound Gel) to surgical wounds seems to delay wound healing (11982).
More evidence is needed to rate aloe gel for these uses.

Mechanism of Action

Aloe gel is the clear, jelly-like substance found in the thin-walled, sticky cells of the inner portion of the aloe leaf. The active constituents include aloe emodin anthrone, dithranol, chrysarobin, and allantoin (10377,11982).
The carboxypeptidase and salicylate components of aloe gel can inhibit bradykinin, a pain-producing agent. The magnesium lactate component can inhibit histamine, which may reduce itching (101). The component C-glucosyl chromone appears to reduce topical inflammation (8223).
Aloe gel might inhibit the synthesis of thromboxane A2, which is a potent vasoconstrictor. By inhibiting thromboxane A2, aloe gel is thought to increase microcirculation and prevent ischemia in the wound area, which may speed the healing of burns and frostbite (101,8224,12161,12162).
Aloe gel also seems to have antibacterial and antifungal properties (101).

In vitro, aloe gel seems to have an antioxidant effect and decrease levels of colorectal prostaglandin E2 and interleukin-8. These effects may explain why aloe gel seems to help some patients with inflammatory bowel disease (12158).

Preliminary research suggests that aloe gel might have hypoglycemic effects (11983).

In animal models, aloe seems to prevent the inhibition of wound contraction caused by silver sulfadiazine (SSD). SSD is often applied to wounds, especially burn wounds, to prevent infection. But SSD seems to slow wound healing by inhibiting contraction and epithelialization. Applying aloe in conjunction with SSD seems to improve the speed of wound healing compared to SSD alone (12097). However, there is also evidence SSD improves the rate of wound healing better than aloe when each product is used alone (12161). This suggests that there might be a synergistic effect when SSD and aloe are used together.

In animal models of frostbite, aloe gel seems to be more effective for improving tissue survival than pentoxifylline. The combination of pentoxifylline plus aloe gel seems to be better than either agent alone (12162).

When applied to psoriatic plaques, aloe extract cream seems to reduce cellular desquamation, erythema, and infiltration. This results in reduction or resolution of the plaques (12096).

Adverse Reactions

Orally and topically, aloe gel is well tolerated (11982,11984).

Interactions with Herbs & Other Dietary Supplements

HERBS & SUPPLEMENTS WITH HYPOGLYCEMIC POTENTIAL: Preliminary research suggests aloe gel can lower blood glucose levels (11983) and might have additive effects when used with other herbs and supplements that also lower glucose levels. This might increase the risk of hypoglycemia in some patients. Some herbs and supplements with hypoglycemic effects include alpha-lipoic acid, bitter melon, chromium, devil's claw, fenugreek, garlic, guar gum, horse chestnut, Panax ginseng, psyllium, Siberian ginseng, and others.

Interactions with Drugs

ANTIDIABETES DRUGS: Preliminary research suggests aloe gel can lower blood glucose levels (11983) and might have additive effects when used with antidiabetes drugs. This might increase the risk of hypoglycemia in some patients. Monitor blood glucose levels closely. Some antidiabetes drugs include glimepiride (Amaryl), glyburide (DiaBeta, Glynase PresTab, Micronase), insulin, metformin (Glucophage), pioglitazone (Actos), rosiglitazone (Avandia), and others.

Interactions with Foods

None known.

Interactions with Lab Tests

BLOOD GLUCOSE: Preliminary research suggests aloe gel can lower blood glucose levels (11983).

Interactions with Diseases or Conditions

DIABETES: Preliminary research suggests aloe gel can lower blood glucose levels (11983). Monitor blood glucose levels closely.

Dosage and Administration

ORAL: For ulcerative colitis, 100 mL of a 50% solution has been used twice daily (11984).

TOPICAL: For psoriasis, aloe extract 0.5% cream applied 3 times daily has been used (12096).

Comments

Avoid confusion with aloe juice or latex, which is obtained from the cells beneath the plant's skin and contains cathartic laxative anthraquinones (101).

The FDA required manufacturers to remove or reformulate all over-the-counter (OTC) laxative products containing aloe from the US market by November 5th, 2002. The FDA previously requested safety data, but the manufacturers decided it was not worth the expense of conducting studies (8229,8443).

ALOE latex

Also Known As

Aloe Capensis, Aloe Dried Juice from Leaf, Aloe Juice, Burn Plant, Cape Aloe, Elephant's Gall, Ghrita-Kumari, Hsiang-Dan, Kanya, Kumari, Lily of the Desert, Lu-Hui, Miracle Plant, Plant of Immortality.
CAUTION: See separate listing for Aloe gel.

Scientific Names

Aloe vera, synonyms Aloe barbadensis, Aloe indica; Aloe africana; Aloe arborescens, synonyms Aloe natalenis, Aloe frutescens, Aloe ucriae; Aloe ferox, synonym Aloe supralaevis; Aloe perryi; Aloe spicata.
Family: Aloaceae or Asphodelaceae.

People Use This For

Orally, aloe latex is used as a laxative or cathartic. It is also used orally for seizures, asthma, colds, ulcers, bleeding, amenorrhea, colitis, depression, diabetes, glaucoma, multiple sclerosis, hemorrhoids, peptic ulcers, varicose veins, bursitis, arthritis, and vision problems.

Safety

POSSIBLY SAFE ...when used orally and appropriately, short-term (12).
LIKELY UNSAFE ...when used orally, in high doses (8,8961). Doses of 1 gram per day for several days can cause nephritis, acute renal failure, and death.
CHILDREN: LIKELY UNSAFE ...when used orally in children (4). Children younger than 12 years may experience abdominal pain, cramps, and diarrhea.
PREGNANCY: LIKELY UNSAFE ...when used orally (19). Aloe latex can induce abortions and stimulate menstruation.
LACTATION: LIKELY UNSAFE ...when used orally (4,19). Genotoxic aloe-emodin might pass into milk; avoid using.

Effectiveness

LIKELY EFFECTIVE

Constipation. Taking aloe latex orally as a stimulant laxative seems to be effective for relieving constipation due to the cathartic effects of the anthraquinones in the aloe (4,5,8).

There is insufficient reliable information available about the effectiveness of aloe latex for its other uses.

Mechanism of Action

Aloe latex is the dried juice that is obtained from the cells beneath the epidermis of the aloe leaf (101). Aloe latex belongs to the anthraquinone family of laxatives and contains a tricyclic anthracene nucleus (16). It is likely that the anthracene derivatives are cleaved into aloe-emodin anthrone in the colon. Anthrones irritate mucous membranes, causing increased mucous secretion and peristalsis. Aloe latex increases motility of the colon and therefore, increases propulsion and reduces transit time. It also causes fluids and electrolytes to be secreted in the lumen. The effects of aloe cause a feeling of distention. These cathartic effects happen within about ten hours of taking the dose. Water and electrolyte reabsorption are inhibited (8). Aloe latex causes loss of potassium, which paralyzes the intestinal muscles. With continued use, the dose must be increased to maintain a laxative effect (8). Anthroid laxative use is not associated with an increased risk of developing colorectal adenoma or carcinoma (6138).

Adverse Reactions

Orally, aloe latex occasionally leads to abdominal pain and cramps (4). Aloe latex might increase blood to the uterus if used orally during menstruation (8), or if used by women who have bleeding between periods (19). Long-term use or abuse of aloe can cause diarrhea, sometimes with blood and sometimes without blood; potassium depletion; albuminuria; hematuria; muscle weakness; weight loss; heart disturbance; and pseudomelanosis coli (4).
Aloe latex can cause pseudomelanosis coli (pigment spots in intestinal mucosa). This condition is believed to be harmless, and it usually reverses with discontinuation of aloe. It is not directly associated with an increased risk of developing colorectal adenoma or carcinoma (6138). The loss of potassium through increased excretion can paralyze the intestinal muscle. With continued use, the dose of aloe latex must be increased to maintain the laxative effect (8). There is also concern that aloe latex might adversely affect the kidneys. Nephritis and acute renal failure are primarily associated with prolonged use of very high doses (8961).

Interactions with Herbs & Other Dietary Supplements

CARDIAC GLYCOSIDE-CONTAINING HERBS: Theoretically, overuse of aloe can increase the risk of cardiac glycoside toxicity. Watch for possible interactions with herbs that contain cardiac glycosides such as black hellebore, Canadian hemp roots, digitalis leaf, hedge mustard, figwort, lily of the valley roots, motherwort, oleander leaf, pheasant's eye plant, pleurisy root, squill bulb leaf scales, and strophanthus seeds (19).
LICORICE/HORSETAIL: Theoretically, concomitant use of aloe with horsetail plant or licorice rhizome increases

the risk of potassium depletion (19).
STIMULANT LAXATIVE HERBS: Theoretically, concomitant use of aloe with other stimulant laxative herbs may increase the risk of potassium depletion. Stimulant laxative herbs include wild cucumber fruit (Ecballium elaterium), blue flag rhizome, alder buckthorn, European buckthorn, butternut bark, cascara bark, castor oil, colocynth fruit pulp, gamboge bark exudate, jalap root, black root, manna bark exudate, podophyllum root, rhubarb root, senna leaves and pods, and yellow dock root (19).

Interactions with Drugs
CORTICOSTEROIDS: Overuse of aloe can compound potassium loss (2).
DIGOXIN (Lanoxin): Theoretically, overuse of aloe increases the risk of adverse effects from the cardiac glycoside drugs. Overuse of aloe, along with drugs that contain cardiac glycosides (19), can increase the risk of toxicity from increased cardiac glycoside effects.
DIURETIC DRUGS: Overuse of aloe might compound diuretic-induced potassium loss (19). There is some concern that people taking aloe along with potassium depleting diuretics might have an increased risk for hypokalemia. Initiation of potassium supplementation or an increase in potassium supplement dose may be necessary for some patients. Some diuretics that can deplete potassium include chlorothiazide (Diuril), chlorthalidone (Thalitone), furosemide (Lasix), hydrochlorothiazide (HCTZ, HydroDIURIL, Microzide), and others.
STIMULANT LAXATIVES: Concomitant use might compound fluid and electrolyte loss (19).
ORAL DRUGS: Aloe can reduce drug absorption of some other drugs because aloe causes shorter GI transit time (19).

Interactions with Foods
None known.

Interactions with Lab Tests
BLOOD GLUCOSE: Small amounts of aloe latex might reduce blood glucose concentrations and test results (4).
COLORIMETRIC DIAGNOSTIC TESTS: Aloe latex discolors alkaline urine (red) and can interfere with diagnostic tests that depend on a color change (4).
SERUM POTASSIUM: Excessive use of aloe latex can cause potassium depletion, reducing serum potassium concentrations and test results (19).

Interactions with Diseases or Conditions
GI CONDITIONS: Contraindicated in individuals with intestinal obstruction, acute intestinal inflammation (Crohn's disease, ulcerative colitis, appendicitis), ulcers, abdominal pain of unknown origin, nausea, or vomiting (4) due to the irritating effect of anthranoid aloins (19).
HEART CONDITIONS: Theoretically, overuse of aloe latex might lead to potassium depletion (8).
HEMORRHOIDS: Contraindicated due to the possibility of causing stenosis, thrombosis or prolapse (19).
KIDNEY DISORDERS: Contraindicated; theoretically, excessive doses can cause nephritis (19).

Dosage and Administration
ORAL: The common laxative dose is 100-200 mg aloe or 50 mg aloe extract taken in the evening (8).

Comments
Aloe latex is obtained from the cells beneath the plant's skin and contains cathartic laxative anthraquinones (101). Avoid confusion with aloe gel, which is obtained from the thin-walled mucilaginous cells of the inner central zone of the leaf. Aloe gel products sold for internal consumption might be contaminated with aloe latex, which can cause cathartic laxative effects (5). Aloe of the Bible is an unrelated fragrant wood used as incense (5).
The FDA required manufacturers to remove or reformulate all over-the-counter (OTC) laxative products containing aloe from the US market by November 5th, 2002. The FDA previously requested safety data, but the manufacturers decided it was not worth the expense of conducting studies (8229,8443).

ALPHA-GPC

Also Known As
Alpha-glycerylphosphorylcholine, Choline Alphoscerate, Glycerophosphorylcholine, GPC, GroPCho.
CAUTION: See separate listings for Choline, Lecithin, Phosphatidylcholine, and Soy.

Scientific Names
L-alpha-glycerylphosphorylcholine.

People Use This For
Orally and intramuscularly, alpha-GPC is used for Alzheimer's disease, vascular dementia, ischemic dementia, multi-infarct dementia, stroke, transient ischemic attack (TIA), improving memory and cognitive function, and learning.

Safety
POSSIBLY SAFE ...when used orally and appropriately. There is some evidence that taking alpha-GPC 400 mg three times daily (1200 mg/day) seems to be safe when used for up to 6 months (12102,12176). ...when used intramuscularly and appropriately. There is some evidence that administering alpha-GPC from 1000-1200 mg/day intramuscularly seems to be safe when used for 28 to 90 days (12100,12102).
PREGNANCY AND LACTATION: Insufficient reliable information available; avoid using.

Effectiveness
INSUFFICIENT RELIABLE EVIDENCE to RATE

Alzheimer's disease. Preliminary evidence suggests that taking alpha-GPC 1200 mg/day significantly improves cognitive function in Alzheimer's patients after 3 and 6 months of treatment (12176).
Dementia. Giving alpha-GPC intramuscularly might improve symptoms of vascular (multi-infarct) dementia. These patients who get a prescription only formulation of alpha-GPC (Delecit; not available in the US) 1000 mg/day intramuscularly seem to have improved cognitive function, behavior, mood, and functionality (12101).
Stroke. Stroke and transient ischemic attack (TIA) patients who receive alpha-GPC within 10 days post-stroke might have improved outcomes. Preliminary evidence suggests that these patients who get alpha-GPC 1200 mg/day intramuscularly for 28 days, followed by 400 mg three times daily (1200 mg/day) orally for 6 months, have improved recovery including improved cognitive and behavioral function (12102).
More evidence is needed to rate alpha-GPC for these uses.

Mechanism of Action
Alpha-GPC is a breakdown product of phosphatidylcholine derived from plant sources such as soy.
Following administration, alpha-GPC is rapidly metabolized by glycerylphosphorylcholine diesterase to form glycerophosphate and choline (12100).
Alpha-GPC is thought to work for dementia and improving memory and learning because it increases plasma levels of choline and therefore also increase production of acetylcholine and phosphatidylcholine (12100). Alpha-GPC is also a precursor to membrane phospholipids. Therefore, alpha-GPC might improve neuronal functioning by improving neuronal membrane fluidity (12101).
After intramuscular injection of alpha-GPC 1000 mg (405 mg of choline), plasma choline levels significantly increase by about 27% within 30 minutes. Choline levels quickly fall after this peak, following a first order pharmacokinetic process. After 6 hours, choline plasma levels return to normal endogenous amounts, which is about 9.7 micromoles/L (12100).
Levels of alpha-GPC-derived choline in the brain are thought to increase much more slowly, but also remain elevate for longer period of time (12100).
The cholinergic effects of alpha-GPC seem to counteract the attention and memory impairment effects of cause by the anticholinergic drug scopolamine (12103).

Adverse Reactions
Orally, alpha-GPC seems to be well tolerated. Some patients can experience heartburn or upset stomach, nausea, diarrhea, dizziness, skin rash, and headache (12102).
Intramuscularly, alpha-GPC can cause headache, heartburn, diarrhea, insomnia or excitation, flushing, confusion, and erythema at the injection site (12101).

Interactions with Herbs & Other Dietary Supplements
None known.

Interactions with Drugs
SCOPOLAMINE: Alpha-GPC seems to partially counteract the attention and memory impairment effects caused by scopolamine given intramuscularly (12103). It is not known if alpha-GPC is capable of decreasing the beneficial anti-motion sickness effects of the scopolamine patch (Transderm Scop).

Interactions with Foods
None known.

Interactions with Lab Tests
None known.

Interactions with Diseases or Conditions
None known.

Dosage and Administration

ORAL: For Alzheimer's disease, a prescription only formulation of alpha-GPC (Gliatilin; not available in the US) 1200 mg/day has been used (12176).
For stroke and transient ischemic attacks (TIA), alpha-GPC 1200 mg/day intramuscularly starting within 10 days post-stroke, followed by 400 mg three times daily orally has been used (12103).
INTRAMUSCULAR: For vascular dementia, a prescription only formulation of alpha-GPC (Delecit; not available in the US) 1000 mg/day given intramuscularly has been used (12101).
For stroke and transient ischemic attacks (TIA), alpha-GPC 1200 mg/day intramuscularly starting within 10 days post-stroke, followed by 400 mg three times daily orally has been used (12103).

Comments

Alpha-GPC is regulated as a prescription drug used for Alzheimer's disease in European countries. It is known as brand names Gliatilin and Delecit and generic name choline alphoscerate. In the United States alpha-GPC is only available as a dietary supplement, mostly in products promoted to improve memory.

ALPHA HYDROXY ACIDS

Also Known As

AHA, Alpha-hydroxyethanoic Acid, Apple Acid, Citric Acid, Dihydroxysuccinic Acid, Gluconolactone, Glycolic Acid, Hydroxyacetic Acid, Hydroxycaprylic Acid, Hydroxypropionic Acid, Hydroxysuccinic Acid, Lactic Acid, Malic Acid, Mixed Fruit Acid, Monohydroxysuccinic Acid, Tartaric Acid.

Scientific Names

Hydroxysuccinic acid; Monohydroxysuccinic acid (Malic acid); 2-hydroxypropionic acid (Lactic acid); Hydroxyacetic acid (Glycolic acid); Dihydroxysuccinic acid (Tartaric acid); Gluconolactone.

People Use This For

Orally, malic acid (an alpha hydroxy acid) is used with magnesium for treating pain and tenderness associated with fibromyalgia.
Topically, alpha hydroxy acids are used for moisturizing and removing dead skin cells, for treating acne and improving the appearance of atrophic acne scars, improving the appearance of photo-aged skin, and firming and smoothing skin. Alpha hydroxy acids are also used to treat xerosis (pathologic dry skin), ichthyosis (disorder with hyperkeratinization and scaling of skin), and decreasing hyperpigmentation associated with melasma.

Safety

LIKELY SAFE ...when used topically and appropriately (947,949,952,10101). Preparations containing concentrations of 10% or less can be safely used for self-treatment if used appropriately (6079,10102). However, higher concentrations should only be used under the supervision of a dermatologist (6079,10101,10103).
POSSIBLY SAFE ...when malic acid (an alpha hydroxy acid) is used orally and appropriately. Malic acid has been safely used for up to 6 months (3262).
POSSIBLY UNSAFE ...when used topically and inappropriately. Inappropriate use of high concentrations of alpha hydroxy acids can cause skin burns (10103).
PREGNANCY AND LACTATION: LIKELY SAFE ...when used topically and appropriately (947,949,952). There is insufficient reliable information available about the safety of the oral use of malic acid during pregnancy and lactation; avoid using.

Effectiveness

LIKELY EFFECTIVE

Dry skin. Applying alpha hydroxy acids in a lotion or cream daily can improve dry skin (949,955).
Wrinkled skin. Applying alpha hydroxy acids in a lotion, cream, or solution daily can decrease wrinkles and other signs of photo-damaged skin (952,953,954,8011). However, applying alpha hydroxy acids in short-contact skin peels is not effective (953).

POSSIBLY EFFECTIVE

Acne. Applying alpha hydroxy acids seems to help reduce acne (947).
Atrophic acne scars. Applying glycolic acid, an alpha hydroxy acid, as a facial peel or lotion seems to improve the appearance of atrophic acne scars. Serial applications of 70% glycolic acid can significantly improve the appearance of atrophic acne scars when compared to daily usage of 15% glycolic acid lotion. However, 15% glycolic acid lotion seems to be moderately effective in persons who can not tolerate facial peeling (10101).
Fibromyalgia. Malic acid, an alpha hydroxy acid, used orally with magnesium hydroxide (Super Malic tablets) seems to help reduce pain and tenderness associated with fibromyalgia (3262).
Melasma. Applying 10% glycolic acid, an alpha hydroxy acid, as a lotion for 2 weeks followed by a facial peeling program using 50% glycolic acid every month for 3 consecutive months seems to reduce pigmentation in

patients with epidermal-type and mixed-type melasma. However, dermal-type melasma does not appear to respond to glycolic acid facial peels (10102).

INSUFFICIENT RELIABLE EVIDENCE to RATE

Ichthyosis. There is some preliminary evidence that alpha hydroxy acid preparations, such as lactic acid at 8-12% concentration or glycolic acid, mandelic acid and others at 5-10% concentration, might be useful for treating ichthyosis. These alpha hydroxy acids used daily for 1 to 3 weeks might improve the appearance of skin (10104).
More evidence is needed to rate alpha hydroxy acids for this use.

Mechanism of Action

Alpha hydroxy acids are a group of natural acids found in foods including citric acid (citrus fruits), glycolic acid (sugarcane), lactic acid (sour milk), malic acid (apples), tartaric acid (grapes), gluconolactone, and others (6064,10104). Hyperkeratinization is thought to contribute to acne, dry skin, and photo-aging. Alpha hydroxy acids work by exfoliating the top layers of dead skin cells (948,950,6064,6079). Alpha hydroxy acids seem to improve the appearance of aging skin by increasing smoothness and reducing dark spots (6064). The degree of exfoliation is determined by the type, concentration, and pH of the alpha hydroxy acid; and other ingredients in the product. The lower the pH of the alpha hydroxy acid, the more rapidly it is absorbed into the skin (6079). Alpha hydroxy acids that are small in molecular size per volume are more active and penetrate the skin more deeply than larger-size alpha hydroxy acids. Glycolic acid is smallest in molecular size followed by lactic, pyruvic, malic, tartaric, and citric acid (10102). Glycolic acid reverses photodamage to the skin by increasing glycosaminoglycans, including hyaluronic acid, collagen and its precursors, and factor 13A. This contributes to epidermal and dermal growth factors and mast cell degranulation, resulting in the production of thicker and less fragmented elastic fibers and an increase in epidermal volume and tightening of superficial skin layers. There is also preliminary evidence that glycolic acid stimulates fibroblasts and increases cell proliferation in a dose-dependent manner to produce a new zone of collagen (10101). Lactic acid solutions increase skin firmness by increasing the thickness of the epidermal and dermal layers. This effect is concentration dependent; a 5% solution acts at the epidermal layer, while a 12% solution increases the thickness of both layers (8011).

The exfoliating action of alpha hydroxy acids reduces the thickness of the stratum corneum by diminishing corneocyte cohesion at the lower, newly forming levels, but not the mature upper levels, of the stratum corneum. This improves the flexibility of the stratum corneum and the skin surface. The exact mechanism of this effect is unknown. However, some researchers think alpha hydroxy acids interfere with the function of the enzymes involved in the formation of ionic sulfate and phosphate bonds in the stratum corneum (10104). There is concern, however, that the barrier function of the stratum corneum may be reduced, but current evidence suggests alpha hydroxy acids either have no effect or slightly increase the barrier function of the stratum corneum (951,7842).

A combination of the alpha hydroxy acid, malic acid, plus magnesium hydroxide seem to decrease pain and tenderness in patients with fibromyalgia, but the mechanism is not known (3262).

Adverse Reactions

Orally, the alpha hydroxy acid, malic acid, seems to be well tolerated. Some patients can experience gastrointestinal upset including diarrhea and nausea (3262).

Topically, alpha hydroxy acids are generally well tolerated when used in concentrations at or below 10% (947,949,952,10101,10102). However, these products can increase sensitivity to the sun and ultraviolet (UV) light. This can increase damage to the skin, and after long-term use might increase the risk of skin cancer. Advise patients to protect themselves from the sun by using sunscreen and/or protective clothing.

Also, tell patients to test the product on a small area of skin before applying it to a larger area. Adverse reactions can range from mild irritation, a tingling sensation, and stinging to severe redness, swelling, itching, blistering, bleeding, rash, burns, and skin discoloration (6079,6080,10101). Higher concentrations can cause severe skin irritation, burning, sloughing, and limited frosting and whitening to scar areas which sometimes results in transient hyperpigmentation (10101,10102).

There is a report of first and second degree burns with airway compromise resulting after an application of a 10% citric acid facial peel that was left on the face for four hours. After treatment, the patient had permanent facial and neck scars (10103).

Interactions with Herbs & Other Dietary Supplements

MAGNESIUM: Malic acid (an alpha hydroxy acid) is used with magnesium hydroxide for reducing pain and tenderness associated with fibromyalgia (3262).

Interactions with Drugs

None known.

Interactions with Foods

None known.

Interactions with Lab Tests
None known.

Interactions with Diseases or Conditions
INDIVIDUALS WITH SENSITIVE SKIN: Alpha hydroxy acids can worsen skin conditions by causing skin irritation and sloughing (6079,6080,10101).

Dosage and Administration
ORAL: For reducing pain and tenderness associated with fibromyalgia, malic acid (an alpha hydroxy acid) 800-1200 mg per day orally with magnesium hydroxide 200-300 mg twice daily, equivalent to 4-6 Super Malic tablets twice daily, has been used (3262).
TOPICAL: For treating photo-aged skin, alpha hydroxy acid products are typically used in a concentration of 8% as lactic acid, tartaric acid, gluconolactone, or glycolic acid. They are usually applied to facial or other photo-aged skin twice daily (950,952). The alpha hydroxy acid glucolactone has also been used in a 14% solution. For increasing skin firmness and smoothness, solutions and lotions containing 5 to 12% lactic acid have been used on the face two times daily for up to 16 weeks (955,8011). For improving the appearance of atrophic acne scars, serial glycolic acid (GA) facial peels of 20%, 35%, 50%, and 70% are applied biweekly. Peels are applied first for 2 minutes and then the exposure time is gradually increased up to 4-5 minutes as tolerated with each application before applying the next stronger solution. Repetitive use of 70% GA at least 6 times is usually needed before improvement is seen. For patients unable to tolerate facial peels, long-term daily use of 15% GA lotion has been used (10101).
For decreasing pigmentation associated with melasma, a 10% lotion of the glycolic acid (GA) is applied with a sunscreen to facial skin nightly for 2 weeks followed by a facial peeling program. A 50% GA peel is applied three times to the face and left on for a period of 2-5 minutes each time (first peel 2 minutes, second peel 4 minutes, and third peel 5 minutes). The peeling program is done monthly for 3 consecutive months (10102).

Comments
Alpha hydroxy acid-containing cosmetic products may lack concentration information on labeling. Try to use products that identify the concentration of active ingredients.

ALPHA-KETOGLUTARATE

Also Known As
A-Ketoglutaric Acid, AKG, Alpha Ketoglutaric Acid, Alpha-Ketoglutarates, Alpha-Ketoglutaric Acid, Alpha KG.

Scientific Names
2-Oxopentanedoicic acid, 2-Oxoglutaric acid.

People Use This For
Orally, alpha-ketoglutarate is used for treating chronic kidney and gastrointestinal dysfunction, bacterial overgrowth, intestinal toxemia, liver dysfunction, and chronic candidiasis. It is also used as an adjunct to diet and training for improving peak athletic performance, and improving amino acid metabolism in hemodialysis patients.
Intravenously, alpha-ketoglutarate is used for preventing ischemic injury during heart surgery, improving renal blood flow after heart surgery, and preventing muscle protein depletion after surgery or trauma.

Safety
POSSIBLY SAFE ...when used orally and appropriately (5311). ...when used intravenously and appropriately (5308,5309,5310,5311,5312,5313).
PREGNANCY AND LACTATION: Insufficient reliable information available; avoid using.

Effectiveness
POSSIBLY EFFECTIVE

Ischemic reperfusion injury. Intravenous use of alpha-ketoglutarate seems to help decrease ischemic injury during heart surgery (5312,5313).

Muscle catabolism. Alpha-ketoglutarate seems to help reduce muscle protein depletion after surgery or trauma (5309,5310).

There is insufficient reliable information available about the effectiveness of alpha-ketoglutarate for its other uses.

Mechanism of Action
Alpha-ketoglutarate, the carbon skeleton of glutamate and glutamine, is an intermediate compound in the Krebs cycle (5308). As a precursor of glutamate, alpha-ketoglutarate is taken up by fibroblasts involved in wound healing (5314). The availability of alpha-ketoglutarate determines the recovery of muscle protein synthesis after surgical

trauma (5309). Some evidence suggests that rapidly growing cells use alpha-ketoglutarate when cellular glutamine uptake is limited (5314). Hemodialysis patients who take alpha-ketoglutarate with calcium carbonate have improved amino acid metabolism and reduced hyperphosphatemia (5311).

Adverse Reactions
None reported.

Interactions with Herbs & Other Dietary Supplements
None known.

Interactions with Drugs
None known.

Interactions with Foods
None known.

Interactions with Lab Tests
None known.

Interactions with Diseases or Conditions
None known.

Dosage and Administration
ORAL: To improve amino acid metabolism in hemodialysis patients, 1.187 grams are typically used three times daily (5311).
INTRAVENOUS: For cardiac surgery, a dose of 28 grams of alpha-ketoglutarate has been added to blood cardioplegia (5312,5313). For preventing muscle protein depletion after surgery or trauma, 280 mg/kg of body weight is added to parenteral nutrition (5310).

Comments
Suppliers of athletic nutritional supplements claim alpha-ketoglutaric acid may be an important adjunct to proper diet and training for the athlete desiring peak performance. They base this claim on studies that show excessive ammonia in the body can combine with alpha-ketoglutarate to reduce ammonia toxicity. So far, the only studies that show alpha-ketoglutarate can reduce ammonia toxicity have been performed in hemodialysis patients (5311).

ALPHA-LINOLENIC ACID

Also Known As
ALA, Alpha Linolenic Acid, Essential Fatty Acid, LNA, n-3 Fatty Acid, n-3 Polyunsaturated Fatty Acid, Omega-3 Fatty Acids, Omega-3 Polyunsaturated Fatty Acid.
CAUTION: See separate listings for Blue-Green Algae, Chasteberry, DHA, Emu Oil, English Walnut, EPA, Fish Oils, Flaxseed Oil, Gamma-Linolenic Acid, Lecithin, Safflower, Sea Buckthorn, and Sour Cherry.

Scientific Names
Alpha-Linolenic Acid.

People Use This For
Orally, alpha-linolenic acid is used to treat hypertension, rheumatoid arthritis (RA), multiple sclerosis (MS), lupus, diabetes, hypercholesterolemia, renal disease, ulcerative colitis, and Crohn's disease. It is also used to treat chronic obstructive pulmonary disease (COPD), migraine headache, skin cancer, depression, and allergic and inflammatory conditions such as psoriasis and eczema. Alpha-linolenic acid is also used to prevent cardiovascular disease, cancer, the common cold, and upper respiratory tract infections.

Safety
LIKELY SAFE ...when used orally in amounts typically found in foods (7141,7142,7144). There is insufficient reliable information available about the safety of alpha-linolenic acid when used in amounts exceeding those typically found in foods.
PREGNANCY AND LACTATION: LIKELY SAFE ...when used orally in amounts typically found in foods (7141,7142,7145). There is insufficient reliable information available about the safety of alpha-linolenic acid during pregnancy and lactation when used in amounts exceeding those typically found in foods; avoid using.

Effectiveness

POSSIBLY EFFECTIVE

Cardiovascular disease. High dietary intake of alpha-linolenic acid over a period of 6 years seems to reduce the risk of a first myocardial infarction (MI) by as much as 59% in both men and women (7152). In women, a high dietary intake of alpha-linolenic acid over 10 years seems to reduce the risk of fatal ischemic heart disease by 65% (7153). For prevention of secondary MI, starting a Mediterranean diet rich in alpha-linolenic acid and low in saturated fat and cholesterol after an initial MI can significantly reduce the rate of occurrence of a second MI and death rate. Over a 27 month period, patients using this diet seem to be 73% less likely to have a second MI and 70% less likely to die from any cause, compared to the standard postinfarction diet (7150).

It is not known if alpha-linolenic acid supplements have these same benefits.

INSUFFICIENT RELIABLE EVIDENCE to RATE

Respiratory infections. Preliminary clinical research suggests alpha-linolenic in combination with linoleic acid might reduce the number of recurrent respiratory infections in children (10785). More evidence is needed to rate alpha-linolenic acid for this use.

Mechanism of Action

Alpha-linolenic acid is an essential omega-3 fatty acid. Dietary alpha-linolenic acid is found primarily in vegetable oils such as flaxseed (linseed) oil, canola (rapeseed) oil, and soybean oil; and also in red meat and dairy products (1337). It is also found in margarines and salad dressings that contain vegetable oils (7141,7142). Walnuts and other edible nuts also contain significant amounts of alpha-linolenic acid. Alpha-linolenic acid is found in smaller amounts in green leafy vegetables, and chocolate (7141). Alpha-linolenic acid is also a component of human breast milk, infant formulas, and intravenous fat emulsions (7143). The body converts some alpha-linolenic acid into longer and more unsaturated omega-3 fatty acids, such as eicosapentaenoic (EPA) and docosahexaenoic acids (DHA); however, the effects of EPA and DHA are not duplicated by alpha-linolenic acid, even at high doses (7141,7165). In some disease states, such as type 1 diabetes, chronic alcoholism, and schizophrenia, the amount of alpha-linolenic acid converted to longer chain fatty acids is reduced (7165); however, the reason for this is not known.

Omega-6 fatty acids, such as linoleic acid, that are found in corn, safflower, sunflower, and peanut oils compete for enzyme systems that elongate alpha-linolenic acid into EPA and DHA (7142). The Western diet, including vegetarian diets, usually provides a disproportionate amount of omega-6 fatty acids. For example, the typical Western diet often includes an omega-6 to omega-3 fatty acid ratio of 20-30:1 (7148,7149). There is some concern that a diet high in omega-6 fatty acids can lead to long-chain omega-3 fatty acid deficiency and produce a physiologic state that is favorable for platelet aggregation and clot formation and an increased risk of heart disease (7141,7142). The ideal omega-6 to omega-3 fatty acid ratio in the diet should probably be no more than 4:1 (7141,7148). Some researchers theorize that adding omega-3 fatty acids, such as alpha-linolenic acid, can normalize this ratio and therefore decrease the risk of heart disease. Dietary alpha-linolenic acid significantly increases the concentrations of omega-3 fatty acids such as EPA and DHA in platelet phospholipids and plasma lipids (7149,7166).

Although alpha-linolenic acid seems to have beneficial effects on the cardiovascular system and might reduce risk of heart disease, it does not appear to have a significant effect on cholesterol or triglyceride levels (7146,7165). Alpha-linolenic acid does seem to increase arterial compliance and decrease cardiac workload (7165). There is also some evidence that alpha-linolenic acid has antiarrhythmic effects, but researchers are not sure if this is due to alpha-linolenic acid itself, or due to the longer-chain fatty acids EPA and DHA, to which alpha-linolenic acid is converted (7153,7156). Alpha-linolenic acid does not affect measures of coagulation or serum activity of factors associated with coagulation (10323).

Some researchers are interested in alpha-linolenic acid for prevention of breast cancer. There is some evidence that women with higher levels of alpha-linolenic acid in breast adipose tissue have a lower risk of breast cancer. Fatty acid composition of adipose tissue is thought to reflect past dietary intake, so researchers think high intake of alpha-linolenic acid might have a cancer protective effect (7168). However, there is some concern that high dietary intake of alpha-linolenic acid might actually increase risk for prostate cancer (1334,1336,2558,2559,7147,7823,7824). Typical figures reported are that men with the highest intakes of alpha-linolenic acid have 2 to 4 times the risk of prostate cancer than men with the lowest intake (1336,2558,7147,7824). It's been suggested that alpha-linolenic acid could increase sex hormone levels or formation of free radicals in prostate cell membranes (2558,7823), but these mechanisms haven't been confirmed. Also, it's been found that alpha-linolenic acid levels in biopsy samples are actually lower in more aggressive tumors (7167). Of the food sources of alpha-linolenic acid, prostate cancer risk is most strongly associated with red meat intake (1336,1337,2558,7823). Therefore, alpha-linolenic acid may be only a marker for other carcinogenic substances present in red meat, or formed during cooking (1337,7823). There aren't any studies which have investigated whether alpha-linolenic acid supplements affect prostate cancer risk.

There is some evidence that alpha-linolenic acid might have a beneficial effect on immune function (10785). However, in adults, dietary fatty acids don't seem to affect immune response (10786).

Adverse Reactions

Orally, alpha-linolenic acid from dietary sources is very well tolerated; however, alpha-linolenic acid is high in calories and may result in weight gain if consumed in excess. Patients should be advised that it's best to substitute alpha-linolenic acid in the diet for other sources of fat, such as saturated fats. Very high intake of alpha-linolenic acid from some dietary sources, such as margarine, which also contain high concentrations of linoleic and trans-fatty acids, can increase the risk of heart disease and myocardial infarction. This effect is probably attributable to trans-fatty acid content, and not alpha-linolenic acid (7155).

There is also some concern that high dietary intake of alpha-linolenic acid might increase risk for prostate cancer, but this is probably attributable to high intake of red meat (see Mechanism of Action) (1337,2558). Tell men not to be concerned about moderate dietary intake of alpha-linolenic acid from other sources (e.g., canola, soybean, and flaxseed oils), especially if this replaces intake of oils rich in omega-6 fatty acids.

Interactions with Herbs & Other Dietary Supplements

None known.

Interactions with Drugs

None known.

Interactions with Foods

None known.

Interactions with Lab Tests

BLOOD PRESSURE: Alpha-linolenic acid might decrease diastolic blood pressure in patients with hypertension when consumed in place of dietary linoleic acid (7151).

Interactions with Diseases or Conditions

ALCOHOLISM: The synthesis of long-chain omega-3 fatty acids from alpha-linolenic acid may be reduced in chronic alcohol abuse (7165).

DIABETES: Diabetes may reduce the synthesis of long-chain omega-3 fatty acids from alpha-linolenic acid (7141,7165).

SCHIZOPHRENIA: The synthesis of long-chain omega-3 fatty acids from alpha-linolenic acid may be reduced in people with schizophrenia (7165).

Dosage and Administration

ORAL: For primary prevention of coronary heart disease, approximately 1.2-2 grams per day from dietary sources seems to be associated with the greatest benefit (7152,7153,7156). For secondary prevention of coronary heart disease, approximately 1.6 grams per day as part of a Mediterranean diet appears to be beneficial (7150). Fatty acid dosing is often done based on percentage of daily calories it provides. Some researchers suggest that alpha-linolenic acid should make up roughly 1% of daily calories. This comes to approximately 2 grams based on a 2000 kilocalorie diet (149,7165).

Comments

Use caution in extrapolating information about other omega-3 fatty acids, including EPA and DHA, to alpha-linolenic acid. Although some alpha-linolenic acid is converted to long-chain fatty acids, clinical effects may be different.

ALPHA-LIPOIC ACID

Also Known As

a-Lipoic Acid, Acetate Replacing Factor, ALA, Alpha-Lipoic Acid Extract, Biletan, Lipoic Acid, Lipoicin, Thioctacid, Thioctan, Thioctic Acid.

Scientific Names

Alpha Lipoic Acid; 1,2-dithiolane-3-pentanoic acid; 1,2-dithiolane-3-valeric acid; 6,8-thioctic acid; 5-(1,2-dithiolan-3-yl) valeric acid; 6,8-dithiooctanoic acid.

People Use This For

Orally, alpha-lipoic acid is for diabetes, peripheral neuropathy, cardiac autonomic neuropathy, retinopathy, cataracts, and glaucoma. Alpha-lipoic acid is also used orally for dementia, HIV/AIDS, cancer, liver disease, Wilson's disease, cardiovascular disease, and lactic acidosis caused by inborn errors of metabolism. Intravenously, alpha-lipoic acid is used for improving insulin-resistance and glucose disposal in type 2 diabetes, diabetic neuropathy, and Amanita mushroom poisoning.

Safety

POSSIBLY SAFE ...when used orally and appropriately. Oral alpha-lipoic acid has been used safely in clinical trials lasting from 4 months to 2 years (3540,3541,3542,10148). ...when used intravenously and appropriately. Intravenous alpha-lipoic acid has been used safely in clinical trials lasting up to

3 weeks (3540,3557,10148,12106).
PREGNANCY AND LACTATION: Insufficient reliable information available; avoid using.

Effectiveness

POSSIBLY EFFECTIVE

Diabetes. Alpha-lipoic acid used orally or intravenously seems to improve insulin sensitivity and glucose disposal in patients with type 2 diabetes (3545,3874,3875,3876). Patients who took alpha-lipoic acid 600 to 1800 mg orally or 500 to 1000 mg intravenously daily had significant improvement in insulin resistance and glucose effectiveness after four weeks of oral treatment or after 1 to 10 days of intravenous administration (3545,3874,3875,3876). However, alpha-lipoic acid doesn't seem to lower glycosylated hemoglobin (HgbA1c) levels in patients with type 2 diabetes.

Peripheral neuropathy. Giving alpha-lipoic acid orally or intravenously 600 mg to 1200 mg/day seems to reduce symptoms of peripheral neuropathy in diabetes patients. Alpha-lipoic acid seems to improve neuropathic sensory symptoms such as burning, pain, numbness, and prickling of the feet and legs. It also seems to improve objective measures such as ratings of neurological deficit and disability. Onset of symptom improvement occurs within 3 to 5 weeks with oral and intravenous dosing (3540,3541,3557,3868,10148,12106). However, lower doses have not been shown to be effective (3869).

POSSIBLY INEFFECTIVE

Alcohol-related liver disease. People with alcohol-related liver disease taking alpha-lipoic acid orally 300 mg per day for six months did not demonstrate significant improvement compared to placebo (3880).

Cardiac autonomic neuropathy. Taking alpha-lipoic acid orally appears to improve autonomic nerve function indices, measured by ECG, in patients with cardiac autonomic neuropathy, but symptoms don't seem to significantly improve (3542).

HIV-related dementia. Taking alpha-lipoic acid orally had no effect on HIV-associated cognitive impairment in a small trial comparing alpha-lipoic acid alone or in combination with selegiline (Deprenyl) and placebo (1556).

INSUFFICIENT RELIABLE EVIDENCE to RATE

Amanita mushroom poisoning. Alpha-lipoic acid has been used orally in combination with other treatments for Amanita mushroom poisoning. Its use is controversial. Reports are anecdotal, and experimental evidence does not support its effectiveness. Some researchers recommend against its use (105,1548,1549,3871,3879).

Dementia. Preliminary evidence suggests that taking alpha-lipoic acid might decrease the decline in cognitive function in patients with various subtypes of dementia when used over a period of about 337 days (12152).

More evidence is needed to rate alpha-lipoic acid for these uses.

Mechanism of Action

Alpha-lipoic acid was identified as a vitamin when it was isolated 50 years ago, but was reclassified upon the finding that it is synthesized in humans and animals (3871). Endogenous alpha-lipoic acid is a coenzyme that, together with pyrophosphatase, is involved in carbohydrate metabolism and production of adenosine triphosphate (ATP). Exogenous alpha-lipoic acid and the metabolite, dihydrolipoic acid (DHLA), have antioxidant activity and can scavenge free radicals both intra- and extra-cellularly (3871). Alpha-lipoic acid is both water and fat soluble and can regenerate endogenous antioxidants, such as vitamin E, vitamin C, and glutathione, and prevent oxidative damage (1547,1550,3546,3871). Alpha-lipoic acid is about 30% absorbed from dietary or supplemental sources, and is reduced to DHLA in many tissues (1561,3871,3872). Preliminary data suggests that these antioxidant effects might provide protection in cerebral ischemia, excitotoxic amino acid brain injury, mitochondrial dysfunction, diabetes, diabetic neuropathy, and other causes of damage to brain or neural tissue (1561,3546,3871,10148). In experimental diabetic models, alpha-lipoic acid increases neuronal blood flow, improves neuronal glucose uptake, increases amounts of reduced glutathione in neurons, and improves neuronal conduction velocity (3873,3878). Preliminary evidence suggests that DHLA in combination with vitamin E might prevent oxidative stress in cardiac ischemia-reperfusion injury (3871,3877). The antioxidant effects of alpha-lipoic acid might be beneficial in liver diseases in which oxidative stress is a factor (3879). Alpha-lipoic acid has shown promise in experimental models to prevent aminoglycoside-induced cochlear damage, and metal (lead, arsenic, cadmium, mercury) and chemical (hexachlorobenzene, n-hexane) poisoning (3871,3879,3881,3882,3883,3884). Children treated with alpha-lipoic acid, alone or in combination with vitamin E, showed normalized organ function and lessened indices of oxidative damage following radiation exposure in the Chernobyl accident (3871). Case reports indicate that it may be helpful in various inborn errors of metabolism which result in lactic acidosis (1554,1555,1557). Preliminary data suggests that alpha-lipoic acid can inhibit replication of the human immunodeficiency virus (HIV) by inhibiting reverse transcriptase (1280,3871). Reactive oxygen species may act as intracellular messengers for HIV gene expression and transcription, and the antioxidant effects of alpha-lipoic acid could inhibit this process (1562,1563). Alpha-lipoic acid supplementation might improve blood antioxidant status and blood peroxidation products, and increase T-helper lymphocytes and T-helper to T-helper suppressor cell ratio, based on a small open trial in HIV positive patients (3885).

Adverse Reactions

Orally, skin rash has been reported after use of alpha-lipoic acid.

Intravenously, local allergic reactions have occurred at the injection site (1547). Paresthesias have been reported to worsen temporarily at the beginning of therapy. Alpha-lipoic acid can cause gastrointestinal upset, including nausea and vomiting, and headache. Adverse effects are more common in patients receiving higher intravenous doses (3557).

Laboratory studies suggest that very large doses of alpha-lipoic acid can cause fatal toxicity in thiamine deficient animals. For people who are taking high doses of alpha-lipoic acid and are at risk for thiamine deficiency (e.g. alcoholics), thiamine supplementation may be warranted (3871).

Interactions with Herbs & Other Dietary Supplements

HERBS WITH HYPERGLYCEMIC POTENTIAL: Theoretically, herbs that increase blood glucose levels might antagonize the antidiabetic effects of alpha-lipoic acid (3545). Herbs with hyperglycemic potential include ephedra, ginger, gotu kola, and the above ground parts of the stinging nettle.
HERBS WITH HYPOGLYCEMIC POTENTIAL: Theoretically, alpha-lipoic acid might have additive effects with herbs that decrease blood glucose levels (3545). Herbs with hypoglycemic potential include devil's claw, fenugreek, garlic, guar gum, horse chestnut, Panax ginseng, psyllium, and Siberian ginseng.

Interactions with Drugs

ANTIDIABETES DRUGS: Theoretically, concomitant use might cause additive hypoglycemic effects (3545). Dosing adjustments for insulin or oral hypoglycemic agents may be necessary; however, in one study, co-administration of single doses of alpha-lipoic acid and glyburide or acarbose (Precose, Prandase) did not cause detectable drug interactions in healthy volunteers (3870).
CHEMOTHERAPY: Theoretically, concomitant use might decrease the effectiveness of chemotherapy. Preliminary evidence from an unpublished study suggests antioxidants may decrease the effectiveness of chemotherapy (391).

Interactions with Foods

None known.

Interactions with Lab Tests

BLOOD GLUCOSE: Alpha-lipoic acid might decrease blood glucose levels and test results in patients with type 2 diabetes. Alpha-lipoic acid reduces insulin resistance and improves blood glucose disposal in patients with type 2 diabetes (3545); however, alpha-lipoic acid has no effect on glycosylated hemoglobin (HgbA1c) levels (3540,3557).
T HELPER/SUPPRESSOR LYMPHOCYTE RATIO: Alpha-lipoic acid might increase the T helper/suppressor ratio in patients infected with the human immunodeficiency virus (HIV) (3885).
TRIIODOTHYROXINE (T3): Preliminary evidence suggests alpha-lipoic acid might lower T3 levels (8946), but effects on thyroid function have not been reported in clinical trials (3540,3541,3542).

Interactions with Diseases or Conditions

DIABETES: Alpha-lipoic acid can decrease blood glucose levels (3545). Dosing adjustments for insulin or oral hypoglycemic agents may be necessary.
THIAMINE DEFICIENCY: Laboratory studies suggest that very large doses of alpha-lipoic acid can cause fatal toxicity in thiamine deficient animals. Supplementation might be needed for people taking high-dose alpha-lipoic acid who have thiamine-depleting conditions such as alcoholism (3871).
THYROID DISORDERS: Theoretically, concomitant use might interfere with therapy for hyperthyroid or hypothyroid conditions; monitor use (8946).

Dosage and Administration

ORAL: For treatment of diabetes and peripheral neuropathy, doses of 600 and 1200 mg daily has been used (3540,3541,3868). For cardiac autonomic neuropathy in patients with type 2 diabetes, 800 mg daily has been used (3542).
INTRAVENOUS: For peripheral neuropathy in patients with type 2 diabetes, doses 600 mg and 1200 mg daily has been used (3540,3541,3557,10148).

Comments

High doses of alpha-lipoic acid are approved in Germany for the treatment of diabetic neuropathy (3871).

ALPINE CRANBERRY

Also Known As

Cowberry, Dry Ground Cranberry, Foxberry, Lingen, Lingenberry, Lingon, Lingonberry, Lowbush Cranberry, Moss Cranberry, Partridgeberry, Red Bilberry, Redberries, Red Whortleberry, Rock Cranberry, Shore Cranberry, Vine of Mount Ida.
CAUTION: See separate listings for Cranberry, Cramp Bark, and Uva Ursi.

Scientific Names

Vaccinium vitis-idaea.
Family: Ericaceae.

People Use This For
Orally, alpine cranberry is used for urinary tract irritation, gout, arthritis and kidney stones. It is also used orally as a urinary tract disinfectant, diuretic, and antiviral.

Safety
LIKELY UNSAFE ...when the preparations of the leaves are used orally long-term because the arbutin constituent could be toxic (18).
There is insufficient reliable information available about the safety of the short-term oral use of alpine cranberry leaf.
CHILDREN: LIKELY UNSAFE ...when used orally in children under 12 years of age because alpine cranberry might be hepatotoxic (18).
PREGNANCY AND LACTATION: LIKELY UNSAFE ...when used orally because constituents have mutagenic effects (18); avoid using.

Effectiveness
There is insufficient reliable information available about the effectiveness of alpine cranberry.

Mechanism of Action
The applicable part of alpine cranberry is the leaf or berry. When ingested, alpine cranberry releases hydroquinones. In alkaline urine, the hydroquinones act as a disinfectant. Because hydroquinones can cause liver damage, long-term use is not recommended. There is also concern about long-term use because the constituents, arbutin and hydrochinon, are mutagenic and carcinogenic (18).

Adverse Reactions
Orally, alpine cranberry may cause nausea and vomiting due to its high tannin content (18).

Interactions with Herbs & Other Dietary Supplements
None known.

Interactions with Drugs
None known.

Interactions with Foods
None known.

Interactions with Lab Tests
None known.

Interactions with Diseases or Conditions
LIVER DISEASE: Theoretically, the hydroquinones in alpine cranberry may worsen liver disease (18).

Dosage and Administration
ORAL: The typical daily dose is 2 grams of dried leaf or one cup of tea taken orally. The tea is prepared by steeping 2 grams dried leaf in 150 mL of boiling water for 10-15 minutes and straining (18).

Comments
Alpine cranberry leaves are sometimes used as a substitute for bearberry (uva ursi) leaves (18).

ALPINE LADY'S MANTLE

Also Known As
Alchemillae alpinae herba, Alpine Ladys Mantle.
CAUTION: See separate listing for Alchemilla (Lady's Mantle).

Scientific Names
Alchemilla alpina.
Family: Rosaceae.

People Use This For
Orally, alpine lady's mantle is used as a diuretic, antispasmodic, and cardioactive agent. It is also used orally for unspecific female complaints.

Safety
There is insufficient reliable information available about the safety of alpine lady's mantle.
Pregnancy and Lactation: Insufficient reliable information available; avoid using.

Effectiveness
There is insufficient reliable information available about the effectiveness of alpine lady's mantle.

Mechanism of Action
There is insufficient reliable information available about the possible mechanism of action and active ingredients.

Adverse Reactions
None reported.

Interactions with Herbs & Other Dietary Supplements
None known.

Interactions with Drugs
None known.

Interactions with Foods
None known.

Interactions with Lab Tests
None known.

Interactions with Diseases or Conditions
None known.

Dosage and Administration
No typical dosage.

Comments
Avoid confusion with alchemilla (lady's mantle).

ALPINE RAGWORT

Also Known As
Life Root, Liferoot, Senecio Herb, Squawweed, Squaw Weed.
CAUTION: See separate listing for Golden Ragwort (Senecio aureus).

Scientific Names
Senecio nemorensis.
Family: Asteraceae/Compositae.

People Use This For
Orally, alpine ragwort is used for diabetes mellitus, hemorrhage, high blood pressure, spasms, and as a uterine stimulant.
Alpine ragwort is also used orally to control bleeding after tooth extraction.

Safety
LIKELY UNSAFE ...when used orally, due to the potential for liver toxicity and possible carcinogenicity and mutagenicity (12,18).
PREGNANCY AND LACTATION: LIKELY UNSAFE ...when used orally due to hepatotoxic pyrrolizidine alkaloids constituents (2). Pyrrolizidine alkaloids might also be excreted in breast milk (19).

Effectiveness
There is insufficient reliable information available about the effectiveness of alpine ragwort.

Mechanism of Action
The applicable parts of alpine ragwort are the above ground parts. Alpine ragwort contains the pyrrolizidine alkaloids senecionine, fuschsisencionine, 7-angeloylretronecin, bulgarsenine, nemorensin, platyphyllin, and sarracin (18).

Hepatotoxicity and carcinogenicity may be attributed to the unsaturated pyrrolizidine alkaloids (UPAs) and associated unsaturated parent compounds (18). Some UPAs have shown carcinogenic and mutagenic properties; there are also reports of associated renal toxicity. However, the primary concern with UPAs is veno-occlusive liver disease (12). UPAs are known to be hepatotoxic in animals and humans (4).

Adverse Reactions

Chronic exposure to plants containing UPA constituents has been associated with veno-occlusive disease (4021). Symptoms of acute veno-occlusive disease are characterized by a dull, dragging ache in the right upper abdomen and marked distention of the abdomen. These symptoms are sometimes accompanied by reduced urine output. Subacute veno-occlusive disease is associated with vague symptoms and persistent liver enlargement (4021). Alpine ragwort can cause an allergic reaction in individuals sensitive to the Asteraceae/Compositae family. Members of this family include ragweed, chrysanthemums, marigolds, daisies, and many other herbs.

Interactions with Herbs & Other Dietary Supplements

EUCALYPTUS: Theoretically, concomitant use may increase the risk of UPA toxicity due to enzyme induction by eucalyptus (19).
UNSATURATED PYRROLIZIDINE ALKALOID-CONTAINING HERBS (UPAs): Concomitant use is contraindicated due to the risk of additive toxicity (12,19,271). Herbs containing UPAs include alkanna, borage, gravel root, hemp agrimony, hound's tongue, petasites, comfrey, coltsfoot; and the Senecio species plants dusty miller, alpine ragwort, groundsel, golden ragwort, and tansy ragwort.

Interactions with Drugs

None known.

Interactions with Foods

None known.

Interactions with Lab Tests

None known.

Interactions with Diseases or Conditions

CROSS-ALLERGENICITY: Alpine ragwort may cause an allergic reaction in individuals sensitive to the Asteraceae/Compositae family. Members of this family include ragweed, chrysanthemums, marigolds, daisies, and many other herbs.
LIVER DISEASE: Contraindicated due to hepatotoxic potential (19).

Dosage and Administration

No typical dosage.

Comments

Avoid confusion with golden ragwort (Senecio aureus) also referred to as squaw weed.

ALPINIA

Also Known As

Catarrh Root, China Root, Chinese Ginger, Colic Root, East India Catarrh Root, East India Root, Galanga, Galangal, Galangal Officinal, Galangal Root, Galgant, Gargaut, Gao Liang, India Root, Lesser Galangal, Rasna, Rhizome Galangae.

Scientific Names

Alpinia officinarum, synonym Languas officinarum.
Family: Zingiberaceae.

People Use This For

Orally, alpinia is used as a stimulant, antiflatulent, antibacterial, antispasmodic, anti-inflammatory agent, and for fever.

Safety

LIKELY SAFE ...when used orally in amounts found in foods. Alpinia has Generally Recognized As Safe (GRAS) status in the US (4912).
POSSIBLY SAFE ...when used orally and appropriately in medicinal amounts (12).

PREGNANCY AND LACTATION: There is insufficient reliable information available about the safety of alpinia when used in medicinal amounts during pregnancy and lactation; avoid using.

Effectiveness

There is insufficient reliable information available about the effectiveness of alpinia.

Mechanism of Action

The applicable part of alpinia is the rhizome. Alpinia is related to ginger in its botanical and pharmacological properties. The gingerols and diaryheptanoids constituents are potent inhibitors of PG synthetase (prostaglandin biosynthesizing enzyme). Their structures indicate they can also be active against 5-lipoxygenase, an enzyme involved in leukotriene biosynthesis (6). Some constituents possess antifungal activity while others inhibit prostaglandin biosynthesis and can inhibit leukotriene biosynthesis. The other Alpinia genus plants are also pharmacologically active (6).

Adverse Reactions

None reported.

Interactions with Herbs & Other Dietary Supplements

None known.

Interactions with Drugs

ANTACIDS: Theoretically, due to reports that alpinia increases stomach acid, alpinia might decrease the effectiveness of antacids (19).
H2-BLOCKERS: Theoretically, due to reports that alpinia increases stomach acid, alpinia might decrease the effectiveness of H2-blockers (19). The H2 blockers include cimetidine (Tagamet), ranitidine (Zantac), nizatidine (Axid), and famotidine (Pepcid).
PROTON PUMP INHIBITORS (PPIs): Theoretically, due to reports that alpinia increases stomach acid, alpinia might decrease the effectiveness of PPIs (19). PPIs include omeprazole (Prilosec), lansoprazole (Prevacid), rabeprazole (Aciphex), pantoprazole (Protonix), and esomeprazole (Nexium).

Interactions with Foods

None known.

Interactions with Lab Tests

None known.

Interactions with Diseases or Conditions

None known.

Dosage and Administration

ORAL: The typical dose of alpinia is 2-4 grams of the herb per day or one cup of the tea 30 minutes before meals (18). The tea is prepared by steeping 0.5-1 grams in 150 mL hot water for 10 minutes and then straining.

AMARANTH

Also Known As

Chua, Huantli, Lady Bleeding, Love-Lies-Bleeding, Lovely Bleeding, Ramdana, Pilewort, Prince's Feather, Red Cockscomb, Ramdana, Velvet Flower.
CAUTION: See separate listings for Bulbous Buttercup, Lesser Celandine, and Potentilla.

Scientific Names

Amaranthus hypochondriacus, synonyms Amaranthus frumentaceus, Amaranthus leucocarpus.
Family: Amaranthaceae or Chenopodiaceae.

People Use This For

Orally, amaranth is used for ulcers, diarrhea, and inflammation of the mouth and throat.
In foods, amaranth is used similarly to wheat as a cereal grain.

Safety

There is insufficient reliable information available about the safety of amaranth.
Pregnancy and Lactation: Insufficient reliable information available; avoid using.

Effectiveness

POSSIBLY INEFFECTIVE

Hypercholesterolemia. Amaranth muffins added to a National Cholesterol Education Program (NCEP) step-one low-fat diet failed to reduce cholesterol levels in a group of hypercholesterolemic adults beyond the reduction achieved by a group who ate only the low-fat diet (6188).

There is insufficient reliable information available about the effectiveness of amaranth for its other uses.

Mechanism of Action

The applicable part of amaranth is the whole plant. Amaranth is considered an astringent (18). The leaf contains a small amount of vitamin C (3833). There is preliminary evidence that suggests that amaranth seed can reduce serum cholesterol. It seems to reduce total cholesterol and low density lipoprotein (LDL) cholesterol, while increasing high density lipoprotein (HDL) cholesterol. Additionally, it seems to have a minimal effect on very low density lipoprotein (VLDL) cholesterol (5063).

Adverse Reactions

None reported.

Interactions with Herbs & Other Dietary Supplements

None known.

Interactions with Drugs

None known.

Interactions with Foods

None known.

Interactions with Lab Tests

None known.

Interactions with Diseases or Conditions

None known.

Dosage and Administration

ORAL: People typically prepare amaranth as a tea, adding 1 teaspoon of leaves to 1 cup of cold water. The tea is taken cold, 1 to 2 cups a day. As a tincture amaranth is dosed up to 1 teaspoon (5263).

Comments

Avoid confusion with bulbous buttercup (Ranunculus bulbosus) or lesser celandine (Ranunculus ficaria), also known as pilewort.

AMBRETTE

Also Known As

Abelmosk, Ambretta, Egyptian Alcee, Gandapura, Kasturidana, Kasturilatika, Latakasthuri, Latakasturi, Lathakasthuri, Muskadana, Muskmallow, Musk Seed, Okra, Target-Leaved Hibiscus.

Scientific Names

Abelmoschus moschatus, synonym Hibiscus abelmoschus.
Family: Malvaceae.

Comments

At the date of publication, there was very little scientific information about this product. Our staff is continually analyzing the available information on natural medicines and will add data to the online version of *Natural Medicines Comprehensive Database* as it becomes available. See www.naturaldatabase.com.

AMERICAN ADDER'S TONGUE

Also Known As
American Adders Tongue, Dog's Tooth Violet, Dogs Tooth Voilet, Erythronium, Lamb's Tongue, Lambs Tongue, Rattlesnake Violet, Serpent's Tongue, Serpents Tongue, Snake Leaf, Yellow Snakeleaf, Yellow Snowdrop.
CAUTION: See separate listing for English Adder's Tongue.

Scientific Names
Erythronium americanum.
Family: Liliaceae.

People Use This For
Topically, American adder's tongue is used for ulcers.

Safety
There is insufficient reliable information available about the safety of American adder's tongue.
Pregnancy and Lactation: Insufficient reliable information available; avoid using.

Effectiveness
There is insufficient reliable information available about the effectiveness of American adder's tongue.

Mechanism of Action
The applicable parts of American adder's tongue are the leaves and tubers. The leaves can have emollient effects and treat skin ulcers when applied as a poultice. Used internally, they act as an emetic (18).

Adverse Reactions
Cross-sensitivity can occur with the use of American adder's tongue in individuals allergic to tulip, fritallaria, lily, alstroemeria, or Bomarea (18).

Interactions with Herbs & Other Dietary Supplements
None known.

Interactions with Drugs
None known.

Interactions with Foods
None known.

Interactions with Lab Tests
None known.

Interactions with Diseases or Conditions
PLANT ALLERGIES: Cross-sensitivity can occur in individuals allergic to tulip, fritallaria, lily, alstroemeria, or Bomarea (18).

Dosage and Administration
TOPICAL: The fresh leaves of American adder's tongue are commonly applied as a poultice (18).

Comments
Avoid confusion with English adder's tongue.

AMERICAN BITTERSWEET

Also Known As
False Bittersweet, Waxwork.

Scientific Names
Celastrus scandens.
Family: Celastraceae.

Comments

At the date of publication, this product was not a common ingredient used in brand name supplements marketed to consumers. Details about this product are available at the online version of *Natural Medicines Comprehensive Database*. See www.naturaldatabase.com.

AMERICAN CHESTNUT

Also Known As

None.
CAUTION: See separate listing for European Chestnut.

Scientific Names

Castanea dentata, synonym Castanea americana.
Family: Fagaceae.

People Use This For

Orally, American chestnut is used for cough, pertussis, respiratory ailments, as an antirheumatic, sedative, tonic, and astringent agent.
Topically, American chestnut is used for pharyngitis.
In foods, an extract of American chestnut is used in beverages.

Safety

LIKELY SAFE ...when used orally in amounts commonly found in foods. American chestnut has Generally Recognized As Safe (GRAS) status in the US (4912).
There is insufficient reliable information available about the safety of the oral or topical use of American chestnut for medicinal purposes.
PREGNANCY AND LACTATION: Insufficient reliable information available; avoid using.

Effectiveness

There is insufficient reliable information available about the effectiveness of American chestnut.

Mechanism of Action

American chestnut contains 8-9% tannins (11), which exerts an astringent effect on the mucosal tissue. This effect dehydrates the tissue, reducing internal secretions and forming external cells into a protective layer (12).

Adverse Reactions

Orally, though no cases have been reported, adverse effects from the use of American chestnut are theoretically possible. Plants with at least 10% tannins may cause gastrointestinal disturbances, kidney damage, and necrotic conditions of the liver (12). Some animal experiments show that tannins may cause cancer; others show they may prevent it (12). Regular consumption of herbs with high tannin concentrations correlates with increased incidence of esophageal or nasal cancer (12).

Interactions with Herbs & Other Dietary Supplements

TANNIN-CONTAINING HERBS: Herbs that contain high percentages of tannins (such as American chestnut) may cause precipitation alkaloid constituents of other herbs (19).

Interactions with Drugs

ORAL DRUGS: Theoretically, concomitant oral administration may cause precipitation of some drugs due to the high tannin content of American chestnut. Separate administration of oral drugs and tannin-containing herbs by the longest period of time practical (19).

Interactions with Foods

None known.

Interactions with Lab Tests

None known.

Interactions with Diseases or Conditions

None known.

Dosage and Administration
ORAL: People typically prepare American chestnut as a tea with 1 teaspoon of leaves and bark boiled in a covered container with 2 cups of water for 30 minutes. The liquid is cooled slowly in the closed container and taken cold, 1 to 2 cups per day (5254).

Comments
American chestnut (Castanea dentata) has been devastated by fungal disease. Chestnut leaves used in commerce usually come from European chestnut (Castanea sativa) or other Castanea species (11).

AMERICAN DOGWOOD

Also Known As
Bitter Redberry, Box Tree, Boxwood, Budwood, Cornel, Cornelian Tree, Dog-Tree, Dogwood, False Box, Green Ozier, Osier, Rose Willow, Silky Cornel, Swamp Dogwood.
CAUTION: See separate listing for Jamaican Dogwood.

Scientific Names
Cornus florida.
Family: Cornaceae.

People Use This For
Orally, American dogwood is used for headaches and fatigue. It is also used orally to increase strength, for fever, chronic diarrhea and to stimulate appetite. It is also used orally as a tonic.
Topically, American dogwood is used as an astringent for boils and wounds.
Historically, American dogwood was used orally as a substitute for quinine.

Safety
There is insufficient reliable information available about the safety of American dogwood.
Pregnancy and Lactation: Insufficient reliable information available; avoid using.

Effectiveness
There is insufficient reliable information available about the effectiveness of American dogwood.

Mechanism of Action
The applicable part of American dogwood is the bark. American dogwood destroys the snails that carry the tropical human parasite species Schistosoma. A methanol extract has a dose-dependent inhibiting effect on heart activity, and stops the heartbeat at high doses. Animal data suggests the water-insoluble fraction of American dogwood has antimalarial effects comparable to quinine and sulfadiazine (18).

Adverse Reactions
None reported.

Interactions with Herbs & Other Dietary Supplements
None known.

Interactions with Drugs
None known.

Interactions with Foods
None known.

Interactions with Lab Tests
None known.

Interactions with Diseases or Conditions
None known.

Dosage and Administration
No typical dosage.

Comments
American dogwood is rarely used. Be careful not to confuse it with Jamaican dogwood (18).

AMERICAN ELDER

Also Known As
American Elderberry, Common Elderberry, Elder Flower, Elderberry, Sambucus, Sweet Elder.
CAUTION: See separate listings for Dwarf Elder, Elderberry, and Elderflower.

Scientific Names
Sambucus canadensis.
Family: Adoxaceae/Sambucaceae or Caprifoliaceae.

People Use This For
Orally, American elder is used for asthma, bronchitis, bruises, cancer, flatulence, colds, edema associated with weak heart function, epilepsy, fever, gout, headache, neuralgia, psoriasis, rheumatism, to stimulate healing, for sore throat, sores, swelling, syphilis, toothache, as a cathartic laxative, as a diaphoretic, as a diuretic, emetic, eye wash, mouthwash, poultice, "purifier", and stimulant.
In foods, American elder is cooked and eaten and used to make elderberry wine. American elder is also used as a flavor component in foods and beverages.
In manufacturing, extracts of American elder are used in perfumes.

Safety
LIKELY SAFE ...when the flower is used in amounts found in foods. The flowers have Generally Recognized As Safe (GRAS) status in the US (4912). Cooked, ripe fruit has few if any adverse effects (6).
POSSIBLY SAFE ...when flowers are used orally for medicinal purposes (12).
POSSIBLY UNSAFE ...when leaves, stems, or unripe fruit are used. All these parts contain cyanogenic glycosides (12). Limit juice consumption to avoid toxicity (6).
PREGNANCY AND LACTATION: LIKELY UNSAFE ...when the leaves, stems, or unripe fruit are used (6). There is insufficient reliable information available about the safety of the flower or cooked fruit; avoid using.

Effectiveness
There is insufficient reliable information available about the effectiveness of American elder.

Mechanism of Action
The applicable parts of American elder are the flower and ripe fruit. Elder flowers are believed to have diuretic and laxative effects (6). They are a rich source of vitamin C (19). Elder leaves (6) and unripe berries (12) contain cyanogenic glycosides. If ingested, the leaves or unripe berries can cause cyanide poisoning (6). Sambucus species contain plant lectins with hemagglutinin characteristics that might be useful in blood typing and other blood testing (11).

Adverse Reactions
Orally, ingesting several glasses of American elderberry juice can cause nausea, vomiting, weakness, dizziness, numbness and stupor (6).

Interactions with Herbs & Other Dietary Supplements
None known.

Interactions with Drugs
CYTOCHROME P450 3A4 (CYP3A4) SUBSTRATES: There is preliminary evidence that American elder can inhibit the cytochrome P450 3A4 (CYP3A4) enzymes (6450). Theoretically, American elder might increase levels of drugs metabolized by CYP3A4; however, this interaction has not been reported in humans. Some drugs metabolized by CYP3A4 include lovastatin (Mevacor), ketoconazole (Nizoral), itraconazole (Sporanox), fexofenadine (Allegra), triazolam (Halcion), and numerous others. Use American elder cautiously or avoid in patients taking these drugs.

Interactions with Foods
None known.

Interactions with Lab Tests
None known.

Interactions with Diseases or Conditions
None known.

Dosage and Administration
No typical dosage.

Comments
Though making a pea shooter from an American elder stem seems innocuous, it is not a good idea. The stem contains cyanogenic glycosides and has been reported to cause toxicity in children (6).

AMERICAN HELLEBORE

Also Known As
American Veratrum, American White Hellebore, Bugbane, Devil's Bite, Earth Gall, False Hellebore, Green Hellebore, Green Veratrum, Indian Poke, Itchweed, Tickleweed, Veratro Verde.
CAUTION: See separate listings for Black Hellebore, Pheasant's Eye, and White Hellebore.

Scientific Names
Veratrum viride, synonym Veratrum eschscholtzii.
Family: Liliaceae or Melanthiaceae.

People Use This For
Orally, American hellebore has been used as an antispasmodic, diuretic, sedative, antipyretic, and for hypertension. In manufacturing, American hellebore has been used as an insecticide.

Safety
LIKELY UNSAFE ...when used orally (18,1502) or topically. The alkaloids can be absorbed through unbroken skin and should be avoided (18).
UNSAFE ...when used orally in large amounts. American hellebore can cause death (18).
PREGNANCY AND LACTATION: LIKELY UNSAFE ...when used orally or topically; avoid using.

Effectiveness
There is insufficient reliable information available about the effectiveness of American hellebore.

Mechanism of Action
The applicable part of American hellebore is the rhizome and root. The principal active constituents are steroid ester alkaloids (13,18), which reduce blood pressure even in small doses (13,18,1502). At therapeutic dosages, they have cardiac depressant, bradycardic, and sedative effects (13,18). The alkaloids inhibit inactivation of sodium-ion channels in excitable cells, especially those regulating cardiac activity (18).

Adverse Reactions
Orally, American hellebore in therapeutic amounts can cause numerous adverse effects, including irritation of mucous membranes and cardiac depression (18). Large doses can cause sneezing, lacrimation, salivation, vomiting, diarrhea, burning sensations in the mouth and pharynx, dysphagia, paresthesias, vertigo, possible blindness, paralysis, mild convulsions, bradycardia, arrhythmias, hypotension, and death due to cardiac arrest or asphyxiation (17,18).

Interactions with Herbs & Other Dietary Supplements
None known.

Interactions with Drugs
None known.

Interactions with Foods
None known.

Interactions with Lab Tests
None known.

Interactions with Diseases or Conditions
CARDIAC DISEASE: Theoretically, American hellebore can worsen cardiac disease by depressing cardiac activity or causing bradycardia (13,18).

GI IRRITATION: American hellebore can irritate the gastrointestinal tract and is contraindicated in individuals with infectious or inflammatory gastrointestinal conditions (19).

Dosage and Administration
No typical dosage.

Comments
Avoid confusion with European hellebore and pheasant's eye.

AMERICAN IVY

Also Known As
American Woodbine, Creeper, False Grapes, Five Leaves, Ivy, Virginia Creeper, Wild Woodbine, Wild Woodvine, Woody Climber.
CAUTION: See separate listings for Gelsemium, Honeysuckle, and Woodbine.

Scientific Names
Parthenocissus quinquefolia.
Family: Vitaceae.

People Use This For
Orally, American ivy is used for digestive disorders. It is also used orally to stimulate sweating, as an astringent, and a tonic.

Safety
There is insufficient reliable information available about the safety of American ivy.
Pregnancy and Lactation: Insufficient reliable information available; avoid using.

Effectiveness
There is insufficient reliable information available about the effectiveness of American ivy.

Mechanism of Action
The applicable part of American ivy is the bark. There is insufficient reliable information available about the possible mechanism of action and active ingredients.

Adverse Reactions
Orally, ingestion of the berries, containing 2% oxalic acid, is considered poisonous. There is one case of a child's death following ingestion of the berries (18).

Interactions with Herbs & Other Dietary Supplements
None known.

Interactions with Drugs
None known.

Interactions with Foods
None known.

Interactions with Lab Tests
None known.

Interactions with Diseases or Conditions
None known.

Dosage and Administration
ORAL: People typically drink a tea made from the ground bark (18).

Comments
Avoid confusion with woodbine (Clematis virginiana). Also, avoid confusing American ivy with gelsemium or honeysuckle, which are also known as woodbine.

AMERICAN MISTLETOE

Also Known As
Eastern Mistletoe, Mistletoe.
CAUTION: See separate listing for European Mistletoe.

Scientific Names
Phoradendron leucarpum, synonyms Phoradendron flavescens, Phoradendron serontium, and Viscum leucarpum; Phoradendron macrophyllum; Phoradendron tomentosum.
Family: Viscaceae.

People Use This For
Orally, American mistletoe is used as a smooth muscle stimulant to increase blood pressure, and to increase uterine and intestinal contractions. It is also used as an abortifacient.

Safety
LIKELY UNSAFE ...when the flower, fruit, leaf, or stem are used orally (6,515). All American mistletoe plant parts are considered toxic (6).
PREGNANCY: LIKELY UNSAFE ...when used orally. American mistletoe is considered an abortifacient (19).
LACTATION: LIKELY UNSAFE ...when used orally (6,515); avoid using.

Effectiveness
There is insufficient reliable information available about the effectiveness of American mistletoe.

Mechanism of Action
The applicable parts of American mistletoe are the flower, fruit, leaf, and stem. The constituent phoratoxins produce dose-dependent hypertension or hypotension, bradycardia, and increased uterine and intestinal motility. Phoratoxins can cause contraction of smooth muscle, vasoconstriction, and cardiac arrest, similar to the cardiotoxins from cobra venom (6).

Adverse Reactions
Some people who have ingested American mistletoe have reported nausea, bradycardia, hypertension, delirium, hallucinations, vasoconstriction, and cardiac arrest. Diarrhea and vomiting from ingestion of this product can lead to dehydration, hypovolemic shock, and cardiovascular collapse. Acute gastroenteritis has occurred following ingestion of a few berries. Deaths have been reported after ingestion of teas used as an abortifacient (mistletoe species not identified) (6). However, no fatalities were reported in a review of 1754 accidental American mistletoe exposures extracted from the American Association of Poison Control Centers national data collection system from 1985-1992. Ingestion of one to three berries or one or two leaves of American mistletoe is unlikely to result in any significant toxicity (3706).

Interactions with Herbs & Other Dietary Supplements
None known.

Interactions with Drugs
None known.

Interactions with Foods
None known.

Interactions with Lab Tests
None known.

Interactions with Diseases or Conditions
HEART DISEASE: Avoid in individuals with heart disease; theoretically, may exacerbate.

Dosage and Administration
No typical dosage.

Comments
American mistletoe is considered likely unsafe; avoid using. Avoid confusion with European mistletoe, as well as mistletoe from Australia, Korea, New Zealand, and other areas. Mistletoe is a parasite. Some Australian mistletoe species are reported to extract toxic constituents from the host plant on

which they grow (515), suggesting the importance of identifying the host plant before use of mistletoe is considered.

AMERICAN PAWPAW

Also Known As
Custard Apple, Dog-Banana, Pawpaw.
CAUTION: See separate listings for Papaya and Papain.

Scientific Names
Asimina triloba, synonym Annona triloba.
Family: Annonaceae.

People Use This For
Orally, in homeopathy, American pawpaw is used for treating fever, vomiting, and inflammation of the mouth and throat.

Safety
There is insufficient reliable information available about the safety of American pawpaw.
Pregnancy and Lactation: Insufficient reliable information available; avoid using.

Effectiveness
There is insufficient reliable information available about the effectiveness of American pawpaw.

Mechanism of Action
The applicable parts of American pawpaw are the bark, leaf, and seed. American pawpaw contains multiple acetogenin constituents; of these asimin, asiminacin and asininecin are reported to be highly cytotoxic (258). Based on preliminary animal studies and in vitro studies of human cancer lines, scientists report some acetogenins show activity against certain lung and breast cancers (256). An acetogenin mixture also demonstrates pesticide activity (257).

Adverse Reactions
Topically, American pawpaw extract can cause contact dermatitis (1525).

Interactions with Herbs & Other Dietary Supplements
None known.

Interactions with Drugs
None known.

Interactions with Foods
None known.

Interactions with Lab Tests
None known.

Interactions with Diseases or Conditions
None known.

Dosage and Administration
No typical dosage.

AMERICAN SPIKENARD

Also Known As
Indian Root, Life of Man, Life-of-Man, Old Man's Root, Pettymorell, Small Spikenard, Spignet, Spikenard.

Scientific Names
Aralia racemosa.
Family: Araliaceae.

Comments
At the date of publication, there was very little scientific information available about this product. Our staff is continually analyzing the available information on natural medicines and will add data to the online version of *Natural Medicines Comprehensive Database* as it becomes available. See www.naturaldatabase.com.

AMERICAN WHITE POND LILY

Also Known As
Cow Cabbage, Pond Lily, Water Cabbage, Water Lily, Water Nymph.

Scientific Names
Nymphaea odorata, synonyms Nymphaea maximilianii, Nymphaea rosea.
Family: Nymphaeaceae.

Comments
At the date of publication, this product was not a common ingredient used in brand name supplements marketed to consumers. Details about this product are available at the online version of *Natural Medicines Comprehensive Database*. See www.naturaldatabase.com.

ANDIROBA

Also Known As
Andiroba-Saruba, Bastard Mahogany, Brazilian Mahogany, Carapa, Cedro, Crabwood, Iandirova, Mahogany, Requia.

Scientific Names
Carapa guianensis.
Family: Meliaceae.

Comments
At the date of publication, there was very little scientific information about this product. Our staff is continually analyzing the available information on natural medicines and will add data to the online version of *Natural Medicines Comprehensive Database* as it becomes available. See www.naturaldatabase.com.

ANDRACHNE

Also Known As
None.

Scientific Names
Andrachne aspera; Andrachne cordifolia; Andrachne phyllanthoides
Family: Euphorbiaceae.

Comments
At the date of publication, this product was not a common ingredient used in brand name supplements marketed to consumers. There was also very little scientific information available about this product. Our staff is continually analyzing the available information on natural medicines and will add data to the online version of *Natural Medicines Comprehensive Database* as it becomes available. See www.naturaldatabase.com.

ANDROGRAPHIS

Also Known As
Andrographolide, Bhunimba, Bidara, Carmantina, Chiretta, Chuan Xin Lian, Chuan Xin Lin, Creat, Fa-Tha-Lai-Jone, Gubak, Indian Echinacea, Kalamegha, Kariyat, King of Bitters, Kirta, Nabin Chanvandi, Poogiphalam, Sadilata, Sambilata, Shivaphala, Supari, Takila, Vizra Ufar, Yavatikta.

Scientific Names
Andrographis paniculata, synonym Justicia paniculata.
Family: Acanthaceae.

People Use This For
Orally, andrographis is used for preventing and treating the common cold, influenza, pharyngotonsillitis, allergies, sinusitis, and to treat HIV/AIDS. Andrographis is also used orally for anorexia, atherosclerosis, snake and insect bites, bronchitis, cachexia, prevention of cardiovascular disease, cholera, colic, diabetes, diarrhea, flatulence, gastritis, gonorrhea, hemorrhoids, hepatomegaly, drug-induced hepatotoxicity, and other hepatic disorders. Other uses include myocardial ischemia, jaundice, leprosy, leptospirosis, malaria, familial Mediterranean fever, pharyngitis, pneumonia, pruritus, pyelonephritis, rabies, skin wounds, skin diseases, syphilis, tuberculosis, tonsillitis, and ulcers. Andrographis is also used as an astringent, antiseptic, antidote, analgesic, antipyretic, anti-inflammatory, antithrombotic, expectorant, anthelmintic, laxative, and tonic.

Safety
POSSIBLY SAFE ...when used orally and appropriately, short-term. Andrographis extracts have been shown to be safe in one clinical trial using low doses lasting 3 months and in others using higher doses lasting 4-7 days (2744,2748,2772,2773,2774).
There is insufficient reliable information available about the safety of augmented andrographis preparations which contain elevated concentrations of the constituent andrographolide.
CHILDREN: POSSIBLY SAFE ...when used orally and appropriately, short-term. Andrographis, in combination with Siberian ginseng and other herbs, has been given to children with apparent safety for up to one month (12381,12382).
PREGNANCY: LIKELY UNSAFE ...when used orally due to abortifacient effects; avoid using (12).
LACTATION: Insufficient reliable information available; avoid using.

Effectiveness
POSSIBLY EFFECTIVE

Common cold. Taking andrographis orally seems to significantly improve symptoms of the common cold when started within 72 hours of symptom onset. Some symptoms can improve after 2 days of treatment (2744,2773), but it typically takes 4-5 days of treatment before there is maximal symptom relief (2744,2773,2774,5784,10795,12380). Andrographis is often given in combination with Siberian ginseng for treating colds (12380). Some research suggests this combination relieves cold symptoms better than echinacea or placebo in children (12381). There is some preliminary evidence that taking andrographis prophylactically might decrease the risk of developing a cold by about 50% after 2 months of continuous treatment (2772), but more evidence is needed.

Pharyngotonsillitis. There is some evidence that high doses of andrographis are comparable to acetaminophen after 3 and 7 days of treatment for fever and sore throat associated with pharyngotonsillitis (2748).

Most clinical trials used Andrographis paniculata dried extract (Kan Jang, Swedish Herbal Institute), standardized to contain 4-5.6 mg of the constituent andrographolide per tablet (2744,2772,2773,2774,5784).

INSUFFICIENT RELIABLE EVIDENCE to RATE

Familial Mediterranean fever. Preliminary clinical research suggests a combination of andrographis, Siberian ginseng, schisandra, and licorice reduces the duration, frequency, and severity of attacks of familial Mediterranean fever in children (12382). More evidence is needed to rate andrographis for this use.

Mechanism of Action
The applicable parts of andrographis are the leaf and rhizome (12,2758,2767). Several active constituents have been identified, including andrographolide, deoxyandrographolide, and other diterpenes (2750,2760,2768,2771). Although andrographis is used for a wide variety of indications in Ayurvedic and herbal medicine, clinical evidence of effectiveness in humans is limited to the common cold. People use andrographis for the common cold because it is thought to have immunostimulant properties. There is some preliminary evidence that it might increase antibody activity and phagocytosis by macrophages (2766). Preliminary evidence also suggests that andrographis might have mast cell-stabilizing and antiallergy activity (2750,2751). People use andrographis for HIV/AIDS because some of its constituents have been found to have anti-HIV in vitro (2765). High doses of the purified andrographolide constituent can also increase CD4+ cell counts in HIV patients. Andrographolide is thought to work through correction of T-lymphocyte function rather than by direct inhibition of viral replication (6767). Andrographis might also have leukemia cell differentiation-inducing activity (2766,2768). Possible analgesic, antipyretic, and anti-ulcerogenic effects

of andrographis have been described (2753,2754). Andrographis has traditionally been used for infectious diseases. Antibacterial activity was not detected by one group of investigators, but preliminary evidence suggests potential use against bacteria in raw water, human roundworm (Ascaris lumbricoides), Toxoplasma gondii, malaria, and E. coli enterotoxin secretion (2752,2753,2764,2767,2777,2779,2780,2781). Andrographis might protect the liver against hepatotoxic drugs (e.g., acetaminophen) and chemicals possibly by increasing bile flow, bile salt, and bile acids (2761,2762,2763,2778). The andrographis constituent, andrographolide, is a more potent hepatoprotectant than silymarin, an active constituent of milk thistle (Silybum marianum) (2762,2778). Andrographis may be beneficial in cardiovascular disease. Early evidence suggests that andrographis might lower blood pressure, prevent arteriosclerosis, inhibit platelet aggregation, and reduce myocardial ischemia and reperfusion injury (2755,2756,2757,2758,2759,2760,2782,2783). Andrographis is reported to have abortifacient activity (12). The mechanism of abortifacient action is unknown (2771). Preliminary evidence suggests that andrographis might also have detrimental effects on male and female fertility. In animals, andrographis decreased fertility of both males and females (2769,2770,2776); however, this has not been demonstrated in humans.

Adverse Reactions

Orally, andrographis is generally well tolerated (12380,12381,12382). Large doses of andrographis are reported to cause gastrointestinal (GI) distress, anorexia, and emesis (2743). Urticaria has also been reported (2743,2773). Preliminary evidence suggests that andrographis might inhibit male and female fertility (2769,2770,2776), but this has not been demonstrated in humans. High doses of the purified andrographolide constituent, 5 mg/kg three times daily, have caused headache, fatigue, rash, abnormal taste, diarrhea, itching, lymphadenopathy, and anaphylactic reactions. The andrographolide constituent may also cause dose-related increases in liver enzymes such as ALT, which return to normal when andrographolide is discontinued (6767); however, these effects have not yet been reported.

Interactions with Herbs & Other Dietary Supplements

HERBS & SUPPLEMENTS WITH HYPOTENSIVE ACTIVITY: Theoretically, concomitant use with andrographis might enhance therapeutic effects and increase the risk of hypotension (2755,2760).
HERBS WITH ANTICOAGULANT/ANTIPLATELET POTENTIAL: Theoretically, concomitant use of andrographis with herbs that have anticoagulant or antiplatelet activity might enhance therapeutic effects and increase the risk of bleeding (2758,2759). These include angelica, clove, danshen, garlic, ginger, ginkgo, Panax ginseng, horse chestnut, red clover, turmeric, and others.

Interactions with Drugs

ANTICOAGULANT/ANTIPLATELET DRUGS: Theoretically, concomitant use with andrographis might enhance therapeutic effects and increase the risk of bleeding (2758,2759).
ANTIHYPERTENSIVE DRUGS: Theoretically, concomitant use with andrographis might enhance therapeutic effects and increase the risk of hypotension (2755,2760).
IMMUNOSUPPRESSANTS: Theoretically, andrographis might interfere with immunosuppressive drugs because of its immunostimulant activity (2766). Immunosuppressant drugs include azathioprine (Imuran), basiliximab (Simulect), cyclosporine (Neoral, Sandimmune), daclizumab (Zenapax), muromonab-CD3 (OKT3, Orthoclone OKT3), mycophenolate (CellCept), tacrolimus (FK506, Prograf), sirolimus (Rapamune), prednisone (Deltasone, Orasone), and other corticosteroids (glucocorticoids).

Interactions with Foods

None known.

Interactions with Lab Tests

None known.

Interactions with Diseases or Conditions

BLEEDING DISORDERS: Theoretically, andrographis might have antiplatelet activity and increase the risk of bleeding in patients with bleeding disorders (2758,2759).
HYPOTENSION: Theoretically, andrographis might lower blood pressure and exacerbate hypotension (2755,2760).
INFERTILITY: Theoretically, andrographis might have detrimental effects on male and female fertility (2769,2770,2776). Avoid in couples with infertility.

Dosage and Administration

ORAL: Most of the clinical trials have used andrographis dried extract (Kan Jang, Swedish Herbal Institute), standardized to contain 4-5.6 mg andrographolide. For decreasing symptoms of the common cold, 400 mg three times daily has been used (2744,2773,2774,5784). For preventing the common cold, a dose of 200 mg daily for 5 days each week has been used (2772). For relieving fever and sore throat in pharyngotonsillitis, doses of 3 grams and 6 grams daily has been used (2748).

Comments
Andrographis is native to Asian countries such as India and Sri Lanka, and is cultivated and naturalized in other areas of the world. Andrographis products have reportedly been used in Scandinavia for more than a decade (2772). One writer credits Andrographis with arresting the 1919 flu epidemic in India, although this has not been verified (2774).
Some Internet vendors offer andrographis augmented to contain up to 30% andrographolide (2746). The safety and effectiveness of andrographis preparations with augmented andrographolide content is unknown.

ANDROSTENEDIOL

Also Known As
4-AD, 4-Androstenediol, 5-AD, 5-Androstenediol, Androdiol.
CAUTION: See separate listing for Androstenedione.

Scientific Names
4-androstene-3beta,17beta-diol; 5-androstene-3beta,17beta-diol.

People Use This For
Orally, androstenediol is used to increase endogenous testosterone production to increase energy, enhance recovery and growth from exercise, heighten sexual arousal and function, and to promote a greater sense of well being.

Safety
POSSIBLY UNSAFE ...when used orally; the potency and purity of androstenediol products can differ significantly from the product label (10641).
PREGNANCY AND LACTATION: Insufficient reliable information available; avoid using.

Effectiveness
POSSIBLY INEFFECTIVE

Athletic conditioning. Androstenediol taken orally, 100 mg twice per day, does not seem to add any significant increase in muscle strength or size when used for 12 weeks in conjunction with high-intensity resistance training (1905).

There is insufficient reliable information available about the effectiveness of androstenediol for its other uses.

Mechanism of Action
Androstenediol, a prohormone, is a weak steroid hormone and is a direct precursor of testosterone (1905).
Androstenediol can be converted to estradiol, estrone, dehydroepiandrosterone (DHEA), and testosterone; and may increase levels of these hormones (1905,10162).
Androstenediol also decreases high-density lipoprotein cholesterol (HDL-C) levels. It also increases low-density lipoprotein cholesterol LDL-C/HDL-C and apolipoprotein A/apolipoprotein B lipid ratio, which are considered to be indicators of coronary heart disease risk (1905).

Adverse Reactions
Orally, androstenediol can increase endogenous testosterone production and increase levels of estrone and estradiol (1905,10162). Theoretically, androstenediol may cause masculinization and increased growth of facial hair in women.

Interactions with Herbs & Other Dietary Supplements
None known.

Interactions with Drugs
ESTROGENS: Intake of androstenediol can increase levels of the estrogens, estradiol, and estrone (1905). Theoretically, concomitant use with androstenediol might increase therapeutic and adverse effects of estrogens. Some of these drugs include CombiPatch, Estraderm Transdermal, Kestrone, Vivelle Transdermal, and others.
TESTOSTERONE: Androstenediol is a precursor to testosterone and can increase levels of testosterone (1905). Theoretically, concomitant use with androstenediol might increase therapeutic and adverse effects of testosterone. Some of these drugs include Androderm Transdermal, AndroGel, Depo-Testosterone, Testex, Testoderm, and others.

Interactions with Foods
None known.

Interactions with Lab Tests
ESTRADIOL AND ESTRONE ASSAYS: Androstenediol can increase levels of estrone and estradiol (1905).

HIGH DENSITY LIPOPROTEIN (HDL) CHOLESTEROL: Androstenediol can lower HDL levels (1905).
TESTOSTERONE: Androstenediol is a precursor to testosterone and can increase levels of testosterone (1905).

Interactions with Diseases or Conditions

BREAST CANCER: Androstenediol can increase levels of estrone and estradiol (1905). Theoretically, use of androstenediol might increase the risk of hormone-sensitive cancers such as breast cancer.
HEART DISEASE: There is some concern that androstenediol might increase the risk of coronary heart disease (1905).
HORMONE SENSITIVE CANCERS/CONDITIONS: Androstenediol can increase levels of estrone, estradiol, and testosterone (1905). Theoretically, androstenediol might increase the risk of or aggravate hormone sensitive conditions. Some of these conditions include endometriosis, uterine fibroids, uterine cancer, and ovarian cancer.
PROSTATE CANCER/CONDITIONS: Androstenediol can increase levels of testosterone (1905). There is also preliminary evidence that androstenediol might stimulate prostate cancer cell growth (10161). There is concern androstenediol might aggravate prostate conditions such as benign prostate hypertrophy (BPH) or prostate cancer (10161,10162).

Dosage and Administration

For improving muscle strength and size of weight trainers, 100 mg twice daily has been used (1905).

ANDROSTENEDIONE

Also Known As

Andro, Androstene.
CAUTION: See separate listings for Androstenediol and Androstenetrione.

Scientific Names

4-androstene-3,17-dione; Androst-4-ene-3,17-dione.

People Use This For

Orally, androstenedione is used to increase endogenous testosterone production to enhance athletic performance, increase energy, keep red blood cells healthy, enhance recovery and growth from exercise, and to heighten sexual arousal and function.

Safety

POSSIBLY UNSAFE ...when used orally. Androstenedione has been associated with significant side effects, including increased risk of breast, pancreatic, and prostate cancer (672,3861,6000). In addition, there are safety concerns that the potency and purity of androstenedione products can differ significantly from the product labeling (10641).
CHILDREN: LIKELY UNSAFE ...when used orally. Androstenedione could potentially cause premature closure of the bone growth plates (674).
PREGNANCY: LIKELY UNSAFE ...when used orally. Androstenedione might induce labor (673).
LACTATION: Insufficient reliable information available; avoid using.

Effectiveness

LIKELY INEFFECTIVE

Athletic conditioning. Taking androstenedione orally in doses of 100-300 mg per day does not significantly increase muscle strength, muscle size, or lean body mass when used for 2-3 months in conjunction with weight training (1365,1905,6000,7514).

There is insufficient reliable information available about the effectiveness of androstenedione for its other uses.

Mechanism of Action

Androstenedione is a steroid hormone produced by the adrenal glands, testes, and ovaries (3861). It is a direct precursor of testosterone and estrone in both men and women (674). Androstenedione production peaks in the mid-twenties and declines steadily after age 30 (1365). A lot of people use it as an alternative to anabolic steroids to increase testosterone levels, improve athletic performance, and build muscle. Short-term use (less than one month) can sometimes increase testosterone levels (1905,3861,10696); however, with continued use, testosterone levels return to normal (1365,1905,6000,7236,7514,10696). The acute pharmacokinetic response seems to diminish after 28 days of supplementation (10696). When used for longer than one month, luteinizing hormone secretion seems to decline by about a third, and dehydroepiandrosterone (DHEA) concentrations rise (1905,8138,10696). This suggests androstenedione might actually down-regulate testosterone synthesis (1905,10696). Androstenedione also does not seem to have anabolic effects and does not significantly affect markers of muscle anabolism or growth; increase lean body mass or physical strength; or produce any perceived changes in mood, health, or libido (1365,1905,3862,7236).

Furthermore, androstenedione consistently increases estrogen levels (1905,3861,3862,6000,7236,8138). This might increase the risk of estrogenic side effects in both men and women using androstenedione (674,6000). Androstenedione also lowers high-density lipoprotein (HDL) cholesterol (1905,8138). Some androstenedione products are combined with herbal aromatase and 5-alpha-reductase inhibitors to prevent these adverse effects on hormones and lipids. However, these combinations don't seem to help (8138).

Adverse Reactions

Orally, side effects can be different for men and women. In men, androstenedione might decrease endogenous testosterone production and increase estrogen. Theoretically, androstenedione might cause decreased spermatogenesis, acne, testicular atrophy, gynecomastia, behavioral changes, and potentially increase the risk of pancreatic and prostate cancer (672,674,6000). There is preliminary evidence that androstenedione might stimulate prostate cancer cell growth (672). There is also some concern that androstenedione might increase risk of heart disease in men. Androstenedione decreases high-density lipoprotein (HDL) cholesterol (1905,6000). Some androstenedione products are combined with other supplements such as dehydroepiandrosterone, puncture vine, saw palmetto, indole-3-carbinol, and chrysin (DION) to lessen the adverse effects of androstenedione, lipids, and on hormones such as increased estradiol and dihydrotestosterone (DHT), which is associated with increased prostate cancer risk. However, this combination does not seem to help (8138). Some male patients might also be at risk for developing priapism. There is one case report of two episodes of priapism associated with androstenedione use in a 30-year-old man (5089). In women, androstenedione theoretically might cause masculinization with the deepening of voice, hirsutism, acne, clitoral hypertrophy, menorrhea, male-pattern baldness, and coarsening of the skin (674). There is also some concern that androstenedione might cause or worsen depression in women. Some women with severe major depression seem to have increased endogenous androstenedione concentrations; however, it is not known if supplements can actually cause this adverse effect (6796).

In children, androstenedione might cause premature bone growth plate closure and decrease adult height (674). Androstenedione might cause early development of secondary sex characteristics in boys; and acne, oligomenorrhea or amenorrhea, hirsutism, and virilization in girls. Testosterone derivatives similar to androstenedione have also been associated with hepatic toxicity (3861). Consider monitoring liver function tests (LFTs) in patients using androstenedione.

Interactions with Herbs & Other Dietary Supplements

None known.

Interactions with Drugs

ESTROGENS: There is some concern that taking androstenedione with estrogens might increase estrogenic effects and potential side effects. Androstenedione is a precursor to estrogen and seems to increase estrogen levels (674).

Interactions with Foods

None known.

Interactions with Lab Tests

ESTRONE ASSAYS: Androstenedione is a precursor to estrone and might increase results of estrone assays (674,1905).

HIGH DENSITY LIPOPROTEIN (HDL) CHOLESTEROL: Androstenedione can lower HDL levels (7236).

NANDROLONE: Trace contamination of androstenedione with 19-norandrostenedione can result in positive urine test results for nandrolone use (1906).

TESTOSTERONE: Androstenedione is a precursor to testosterone and can increase results of total and free testosterone assays during the first month of androstenedione use. However, testosterone levels tend to normalize when androstenedione is used for longer than 1 month (674,1905).

Interactions with Diseases or Conditions

DEPRESSION: Theoretically, androstenedione supplementation might cause or worsen depression in women. There is evidence that some women with severe major depression have elevated endogenous androstenedione levels (6796). However, it is not known if taking androstenedione supplements causes this adverse effect.

HORMONE SENSITIVE CANCERS/CONDITIONS: Androstenedione is a precursor to testosterone and estrogen and seems to increase estrogen levels (674). Men and women with hormone sensitive conditions should avoid androstenedione. Some of these conditions include breast, uterine, ovarian and prostate cancer; endometriosis; and uterine fibroids.

LIVER DISEASE: There is some concern that androstenedione might adversely affect the liver. So far there are no cases of this adverse effect, but steroids similar to androstenedione have been associated with liver abnormalities. Androstenedione should be avoided by people with hepatic disease (3861). Consider checking liver function tests (LFTs) in patients taking androstenedione.

PROSTATE CANCER: There is some concern that androstenedione might increase the risk of developing prostate cancer. There is preliminary evidence that androstenedione can stimulate human prostate tumor cell growth (672). Avoid using in patients with prostate cancer.

Dosage and Administration

ORAL: For improving muscle strength and size in weight trainers, 50-150 mg twice daily has been used in studies. However, androstenedione does not seem to be effective for this use (1365,1905,3861,6000,7514).

Comments

Androstenedione gained popularity as the supplement used by home run hitter Mark McGwire. Androstenedione is not prohibited by Major League Baseball, but is banned by the International Olympics Committee (IOC), the National Collegiate Athletic Association (NCAA), the National Basketball Association (NBA), the National Football League (NFL), and the World Natural Body Building Federation.

California is considering legislation that would ban the sale of androstenedione and other supplements frequently used in sports performance-enhancing products to anyone under the age of 18. The bill, which received California Senate approval and is now in the Assembly, would also require warning labels about the adverse effects of androstenedione (8639).

ANDROSTENETRIONE

Also Known As

6-Oxo, ADT.

CAUTION: See separate listing for Androstenedione.

Scientific Names

4-androstene-3,6,17-trione, synonym androst-4- ene-3,6,17-trione.

People Use This For

Orally, androstenetrione is used to increase testosterone levels and improve athletic performance.

Safety

POSSIBLY UNSAFE ...when used orally. There is no scientifically reliable information about androstenetrione. However, promoters indicate that it can increase testosterone levels. If this is true, this product may not be safe due to the adverse effects associated with elevated testosterone levels.

PREGNANCY AND LACTATION: POSSIBLY UNSAFE ...when used orally. There is no scientifically reliable information about using androstenetrione during pregnancy or lactation. Promoters indicate that it can increase testosterone levels. If this is true, this product may not be safe due to the adverse effects associated with elevated testosterone levels; avoid using.

Effectiveness

There is insufficient reliable information available about the effectiveness of androstenetrione.

Mechanism of Action

Androstenetrione is an aromatase inhibitor. It blocks conversion of testosterone to estrogen (12167,12168). Theoretically, as a result of falling estrogen levels, the body is thought to compensate by further increasing testosterone levels.

Promoters of androstenetrione say that it increases total testosterone by 188% and free testosterone by 226% over 3 weeks of use. Despite this claim by marketers of androstenetrione, there is no scientifically reliable research in humans that validates this information.

Adverse Reactions

There is no data regarding oral use of androstenetrione in humans. However, androstenetrione might increase testosterone levels. Theoretically, androstenetrione might cause testosterone-like side effects including spermatogenesis and infertility, acne, testicular atrophy, gynecomastia, behavioral changes, cardiovascular disease, and potentially increase the risk of pancreatic and prostate cancer.

Interactions with Herbs & Other Dietary Supplements

None known.

Interactions with Drugs

None known.

Interactions with Foods

None known.

Interactions with Lab Tests

ESTRONE ASSAYS: Androstenetrione is thought to have aromatase inhibitor activity. Theoretically, this could cause decreased estrogen levels.
TESTOSTERONE: Androstenetrione is thought to have aromatase inhibitor activity. Theoretically, this could cause increased testosterone levels.

Interactions with Diseases or Conditions

HORMONE SENSITIVE CANCERS/CONDITIONS: Androstenetrione is thought to have aromatase inhibitor activity. This might decrease estrogen levels and increase testosterone levels. Men with hormone sensitive conditions such as prostate cancer should avoid androstenetrione.
LIVER DISEASE: Androstenetrione is thought to have aromatase inhibitor activity. This might decrease estrogen levels and increase testosterone levels. Increased testosterone is associated with liver abnormalities. Androstenetrione should be avoided by people with hepatic disease. Consider checking liver function tests (LFTs) in patients who take androstenetrione.
PROSTATE CANCER: Androstenetrione is thought to have aromatase inhibitor activity. This might decrease estrogen levels and increase testosterone levels. Men with hormone sensitive conditions such as prostate cancer should avoid androstenetrione.

Dosage and Administration

No typical dosage.

Comments

Androstenetrione is promoted as an alternative to "prohormones" such as androstenedione. Marketers claim that androstenetrione increases the body's natural testosterone levels and therefore is free from the negative side effects of prohormones. There is no reliable evidence to substantiate these claims.

ANGEL'S TRUMPET

Also Known As

Devil's Trumpet.
CAUTION: See separate listing for Jimson Weed (Datura stramonium).

Scientific Names

Brugmansia suaveolens, synonym Datura suaveolens.
Family: Solanaceae.

People Use This For

Orally, Angel's trumpet is used to induce hallucinations and euphoria; and to treat asthma.

Safety

UNSAFE ...when used orally (5624,5625,5626,5627). All parts of the plant contain tropane alkaloids and are considered poisonous (5624,5625,5627); the foliage and seeds contain the highest concentration of toxic alkaloids (5627).
CHILDREN: UNSAFE ...when used orally (5624,5625,5626,5627). Severe toxicity has occurred in cases of accidental ingestion and in teenagers experimenting with Angel's trumpet for recreational use (5626).
PREGNANCY AND LACTATION: UNSAFE ...when used orally. The entire plant is considered poisonous (5624,5627); avoid using.

Effectiveness

There is insufficient reliable information available about the effectiveness of Angel's trumpet.

Mechanism of Action

The applicable parts of Angel's trumpet are the leaf and flower. Angel's trumpet contains tropane alkaloids, particularly atropine, hyoscyamine, and hyoscine (scopolamine), which are responsible for the anticholinergic effects and toxicity (5625,5627).

Adverse Reactions

Orally, Angel's trumpet can cause severe toxicity. Ingestion of Angel's trumpet can cause acute anticholinergic poisoning, which often requires medical attention (5624,5625,5626,5627). Oral use has been associated with delirium, dilated pupils, hyperactivity, disorientation, intense thirst, dry skin and mucous membranes, flushing, fever, widened pulse pressure, systolic hypertension, tachycardia (5624,5625), audio-visual disassociation (5627), hyperexcitability, visual hallucinations, anxiety, amnesia, combativeness, ataxia, clonus, muscular weakness, expressive aphasia, muscular paralysis, seizure, urinary retention (5624,5625), decreased GI motility (5627), alternating levels of consciousness, convulsions, and coma (5624,5625). Death may result from respiratory arrest (5624). Each flower contains approximately 0.20 mg of atropine and 0.65 mg of scopolamine. Reports suggest ingestion of tea made from 3-6 flowers can produce hallucinations, and 9 flowers can produce total paralysis (5624).

Interactions with Herbs & Other Dietary Supplements

None known.

Interactions with Drugs

ANTICHOLINERGIC DRUGS: Concomitant use may increase anticholinergic effects and adverse effects. Drugs include amantadine, atropine, belladonna alkaloids, phenothiazines, scopolamine, and tricyclic antidepressants (506).

Interactions with Foods

None known.

Interactions with Lab Tests

None known.

Interactions with Diseases or Conditions

CONGESTIVE HEART FAILURE (CHF): Angel's trumpet might cause tachycardia and exacerbate CHF due to its hyoscyamine (atropine) and scopolamine content (5625).
CONSTIPATION: Angel's trumpet might cause constipation due to its hyoscyamine (atropine) and scopolamine content (5625,5627).
DOWN SYNDROME: Caution, patients with Down syndrome might be hypersensitive to the antimuscarinic effects (mydriasis, positive chronotropic heart effects, etc.) of hyoscyamine (atropine) and scopolamine contained in Angel's trumpet (15).
ESOPHAGEAL REFLUX: Angel's trumpet might delay gastric emptying due to anticholinergic effects, exacerbating reflux (5626).
FEVER: Angel's trumpet might increase the risk of hyperthermia in patients with fever due to its hyoscyamine (atropine) and scopolamine content (5624).
GASTRIC ULCER: Angel's trumpet might delay gastric emptying and exacerbate gastric ulcers due to anticholinergic effects of hyoscyamine (atropine) and scopolamine content (5626,5627).
NARROW-ANGLE GLAUCOMA: Angel's trumpet might increase ocular tension in patients with narrow-angle (angle-closure) glaucoma due to anticholinergic effects of hyoscyamine (atropine) and scopolamine (5627).
OBSTRUCTIVE GI TRACT DISEASE: Angel's trumpet might exacerbate obstructive GI tract diseases (including atony, paralytic ileus, and stenosis) due to its hyoscyamine (atropine) and scopolamine content (15).
TACHYARRHYTHMIAS: Angel's trumpet might cause tachycardia due to its hyoscyamine (atropine) and scopolamine content (5625).
ULCERATIVE COLITIS: Angel's trumpet might suppress intestinal motility, which might produce paralytic ileus and precipitate toxic megacolon, due to its hyoscyamine (atropine) and scopolamine content (5626).
URINARY RETENTION: Angel's trumpet might increase urinary retention due to its hyoscyamine (atropine) and scopolamine content (5625,5627).

Dosage and Administration

No typical dosage.

Comments

Angel's trumpet is usually cultivated as an ornamental plant in the southeastern United States (5625,5626) and may be confused with jimson weed which grows wild throughout the United States (5621,5622).

ANGELICA herb, seed

Also Known As

Angelicae, Angelicae Fructus, Angelicae Herba.
CAUTION: See separate listings for Angelica root and Dong Quai.

Scientific Names

Angelica archangelica, synonyms Angelica officinalis, Archangelica officinalis.
Family: Apiaceae/Umbelliferae.

People Use This For

Orally, angelica herb and seed are used as a diuretic and as a diaphoretic.
In food, angelica herb and seed are used in candied products to decorate cakes and pastries.

Safety

LIKELY UNSAFE ...when used orally due to the furocoumarins contained in the stem and other plant parts (2,12). Angelica contains a volatile oil. The furocoumarins are angelicin, bergapten, imperatorin, and xanthotoxin. These are photosensitizers and photocarcinogenic (5,8).
PREGNANCY AND LACTATION: UNSAFE ...when used orally because it seems to be a menstrual and uterine stimulant (12); avoid using.

Effectiveness

There is insufficient reliable information available about the effectiveness of angelica herb and seed.

Mechanism of Action

Angelica herb and seed contain a volatile oil. It contains furocoumarin which consists of angelicin, bergapten, imperatorin, and xanthotoxin which can make the skin more photosensitive (2).

Adverse Reactions

Orally, angelica herb and seed may cause photosensitivity (2,6,12).
Topically, photodermatitis is possible following contact with plant juice (18).

Interactions with Herbs & Other Dietary Supplements

HERBS WITH ANTICOAGULANT/ANTIPLATELET POTENTIAL: Theoretically, concomitant use with herbs that have antiplatelet/anticoagulant activity might increase the risk of bleeding in some people.

Interactions with Drugs

ANTACIDS: Theoretically, due to reports that angelica increases stomach acid, angelica might decrease the effectiveness of antacids (19).
ANTICOAGULANT/ANTIPLATELET DRUGS: Excessive doses of angelica herb and seed can potentiate therapeutic effects and adverse effects of anticoagulants (4).
H2-BLOCKERS: Theoretically, due to reports that angelica increases stomach acid, angelica might decrease the effectiveness of H2-blockers (19). The H2 blockers include cimetidine (Tagamet), ranitidine (Zantac), nizatidine (Axid), and famotidine (Pepcid).
PROTON PUMP INHIBITORS (PPIs): Theoretically, due to reports that angelica increases stomach acid, angelica might decrease the effectiveness of PPIs (19). PPIs include omeprazole (Prilosec), lansoprazole (Prevacid), rabeprazole (Aciphex), pantoprazole (Protonix), and esomeprazole (Nexium).

Interactions with Foods

None known.

Interactions with Lab Tests

None known.

Interactions with Diseases or Conditions

None known.

Dosage and Administration

ORAL: People typically use 1 teaspoon of the powdered seeds or leaves in 1 cup boiling water and drink as a tea twice daily. As a tincture, angelica is dosed up to 1 teaspoon up to twice a day (5250).

Comments

There has been confusion in the past between angelica and water hemlock. Water hemlock is highly toxic (6).

ANGELICA root

Also Known As

Dang Gui, European Angelica, Garden Angelica, Root of the Holy Ghost, Wild Angelica.
CAUTION: See separate listings for Angelica seed, herb, and Dong Quai.

Scientific Names

Angelica archangelica, synonyms Angelica officinalis, Archangelica officinalis; Angelica atropurpurea; Angelica sylvestris; Angelica curtisi; Angelica rosaefolia; Angelica pubescens.
Family: Apiaceae/Umbelliferae.

People Use This For

Orally, angelica root is used for loss of appetite, gastrointestinal spasms, the feeling of fullness, and flatulence. It is also used to promote menstrual flow; and as an abortifacient, antiseptic, expectorant, diuretic, and cure for the plague.
Topically, angelica root is used to create warmth in neuralgia and rheumatism, and for skin disorders. It is also used as part of a multi-ingredient preparation for treating premature ejaculation.

Safety

POSSIBLY SAFE ...when the root is used as a medicinal tea or a steam-distilled oil. Although the root contains furanocoumarin constituents that can be phototoxic, photomutagenic, and carcinogenic when exposed to UV light; these compounds are only slightly soluble in water (8), and absent in the steam-distilled oil (11). ...when used orally in amounts commonly found in foods. Angelica has Generally Recognized As Safe (GRAS) status in the US, but Canada does not allow Archangelica as a food ingredient (12,4912). ...when used topically, short-term as part of a multi-ingredient preparation (SS Cream). This preparation was used safely for premature ejaculation in a clinical trial where the cream was applied and left on the glans penis for 1 hour (2537). Further evaluation is needed to determine its safety after prolonged, repetitive use.
POSSIBLY UNSAFE ...when the root or root extracts are used orally in medicinal amounts (2). Angelica root contains photosensitizing furanocoumarin constituents. ...when applied topically in medicinal amounts. The International Fragrance Association recommends limiting angelica root to a maximum of 0.78% in products to be applied to the skin and exposed to the sun (4,8).
LIKELY UNSAFE ...when used orally in large amounts angelica root preparations can cause poisoning (5). ...when used topically in high concentrations.
PREGNANCY: LIKELY UNSAFE ...when used orally angelica can have an abortifacient effect (4,12); avoid using. POSSIBLY UNSAFE ...when used topically; avoid using.
LACTATION: POSSIBLY UNSAFE ...when used topically; avoid using. There is insufficient reliable information available about the safety of oral use during lactation; avoid using.

Effectiveness

POSSIBLY EFFECTIVE

Premature ejaculation. In one controlled clinical trial, a multi-ingredient cream preparation containing Panax ginseng root, Angelica root, Cistanches deserticola, Zanthoxyl species, Torlidis seed, clove flower, Asiasari root, cinnamon bark, and toad venom (SS Cream) was applied to the glans penis one-hour prior to intercourse and washed off immediately before intercourse. Men suffering from premature ejaculation who were treated with the cream had significantly improved ejaculatory latency compared to placebo (2537).

There is insufficient reliable information available about the effectiveness of angelica root for its other uses.

Mechanism of Action

The constituent alpha-angelica lactone may have calcium antagonist effects (11). The furanocoumarins in angelica are responsible for its phototoxicity (12). Volatile emissions from the angelica root can have fungistatic activity (6). The coumarin constituents of related Angelica species can inhibit human platelet aggregation in vitro (736). The related species, Angelica sinensis, can lower prothrombin time in rabbits when coadministered with warfarin (737). The multi-ingredient preparation containing Angelica root is thought to work in premature ejaculation by increasing the penile vibratory threshold and reducing the amplitude of penile somatosensory evoked potentials (2537).

Adverse Reactions

Angelica is a photosensitizer; prolonged exposure to sunlight should be avoided (2,12). Severe poisoning can occur from large doses (5). When the multi-ingredient cream preparation (SS Cream) is applied topically to the glans penis, sporadic erectile dysfunction, excessively delayed ejaculation, mild pain, local irritation, and burning has occurred (2537).

Interactions with Herbs & Other Dietary Supplements

HERBS WITH ANTICOAGULANT/ANTIPLATELET POTENTIAL: Concomitant use of herbs that have constituents that might affect platelet aggregation could theoretically increase the risk of bleeding in some people. These herbs include clove, danshen, garlic, ginger, ginkgo, Panax ginseng, red clover, turmeric, and others.

Interactions with Drugs

ANTACIDS: Theoretically, due to reports that angelica increases stomach acid, angelica might decrease the effectiveness of antacids (19).
ANTICOAGULANT/ANTIPLATELET DRUGS: Concomitant use of the angelica root can potentiate anticoagulant and antiplatelet effects (736,737).
H2-BLOCKERS: Theoretically, due to reports that angelica increases stomach acid, angelica might decrease the effectiveness of H2-blockers (19). The H2 blockers include cimetidine (Tagamet), ranitidine (Zantac), nizatidine (Axid), and famotidine (Pepcid).
PHOTOSENSITIZING DRUGS: Theoretically, angelica can increase photosensitization and side effects; concomitant use with these drugs should be avoided.
PROTON PUMP INHIBITORS (PPIs): Theoretically, due to reports that angelica increases stomach acid, angelica might decrease the effectiveness of PPIs (19). PPIs include omeprazole (Prilosec), lansoprazole (Prevacid), rabeprazole (Aciphex), pantoprazole (Protonix), and esomeprazole (Nexium).

Interactions with Foods

None known.

Interactions with Lab Tests

None known.

Interactions with Diseases or Conditions

None known.

Dosage and Administration

ORAL: The typical dose of angelica is 4.5 grams per day of the crude root or equivalent preparations for appetite loss, digestive problems, mild GI tract spasms, and flatulence (2). The dose of the 1:1 fluid extract is commonly 1.5-3 grams per day (2). The 1:5 tincture is usually dosed at 1.5 grams per day (2). Do not store angelica root preparations in plastic, because plastic can react with the essential oil (8).

Comments

According to legend, humans began to use the angelica root after an angel explained to them that the plant was a cure for the plague (6). Angelica is often planted in herb gardens as a decorative border and to protect other herbs from the wind (6).

ANGOSTURA

Also Known As

Angustura, Carony Bark, Cusparia, Cusparia Bark, True Angostura.

Scientific Names

Angostura trifoliata, synonyms Galipea officinalis, Bonplandia trifoliata, Cusparia febrifuga, Cusparia trifoliata. Family: Rutaceae.

Comments

At the date of publication, this product was not a common ingredient used in brand name supplements marketed to consumers. Details about this product are available at the online version of *Natural Medicines Comprehensive Database*. See www.naturaldatabase.com.

ANISE

Also Known As
Aniseed, Anisi Fructus, Phytoestrogen, Semen Anisi, Sweet Cumin.

Scientific Names
Pimpinella anisum.
Family: Apiaceae/Umbelliferae.

People Use This For
Orally, anise is used for dyspepsia and as a pediatric antiflatulent and expectorant. Anise is also used orally to increase lactation, induce menstruation, facilitate birth, increase libido; and to alleviate the symptoms of male climacteric, which is the period of life after reproduction functions stop.
Topically, anise is used for lice, scabies, and psoriasis treatment.
In foods, anise is used as a flavoring agent, and has a sweet, aromatic taste characteristic of black licorice. It is commonly used in alcohols and liqueurs, such as Ouzo, Benedictine, Boonekamp, and Danziger Goldwasser. It is also used in dairy products, gelatins, meats, candies, breath fresheners.
In manufacturing, anise is often used as a fragrance in soap, creams, perfumes, and sachets.

Safety
LIKELY SAFE ...when used orally in amounts commonly found in food. Anise and anise oil have Generally Recognized As Safe (GRAS) status in the US (4912).
POSSIBLY UNSAFE ...when used topically. Anise contains furanocoumarin constituents that may cause photosensitivity reactions when skin is exposed to UV light. The constituent bergapten is also believed to be carcinogenic (4).
LIKELY UNSAFE ...when the undiluted oil is used orally. Ingestion of 1-5 mL can cause nausea, vomiting, seizures, and pulmonary edema (4).
PREGNANCY: POSSIBLY UNSAFE ...when used orally in medicinal amounts due to possible abortifacient activity (4,12).
LACTATION: POSSIBLY UNSAFE ...when used orally in medicinal amounts (4). Anise has traditionally been used to promote lactation; however the safety has not been established.

Effectiveness
There is insufficient reliable information available about the effectiveness of anise.

Mechanism of Action
The applicable parts of anise are the dried fruit, seed, and oil. Anise seed is rich in calcium and iron (19). Trans-anethole is a major component of the anise oil, and is responsible for its characteristic taste, smell, and medicinal properties. Anethole has a structure that is similar to catecholamines including adrenaline, noradrenaline, and dopamine; and to the hallucinogenic compound myristicin as well (4). Anethole and the anethole polymers, dianethole and photoanethole might be responsible for the estrogenic activity (4,11). The constituent bergapten can cause photosensitivity and may be carcinogenic (6). Anise also includes the furanocoumarins umbelliferone, umbelliprenine, bergapten, and scopoletin (6).

Adverse Reactions
Allergic reactions to anise may include reactions of the skin, respiratory, and GI tract, and photosensitivity. Anise is not considered a primary irritant, but its use has been associated with skin and mouth irritation and sensitization. Excessive doses of anise can cause adverse neurological effects. The ingestion of 1-5 mL of the oil can cause nausea, vomiting, seizures, and pulmonary edema (4).

Interactions with Herbs & Other Dietary Supplements
None known.

Interactions with Drugs
CONTRACEPTIVE DRUGS: Theoretically, concomitant use of large amounts of anise might interfere with contraceptive drugs through competition for estrogen receptors (4).
ESTROGENS: Theoretically, concomitant use of large amounts of anise might interfere with hormone replacement therapy through competition for estrogen receptors (4).
MONOAMINE OXIDASE INHIBITORS (MAOIs): Theoretically, large doses of anise might interfere with MAOI therapy (4).
TAMOXIFEN (Nolvadex): Theoretically, large doses of anise might interfere with tamoxifen because of its potential estrogenic effects (4).

Interactions with Foods
None known.

Interactions with Lab Tests
BLOOD PRESSURE: Theoretically, anise might increase blood pressure and blood pressure readings, due to the catecholamine activity of the constituent anethole (4,11).
HEART RATE: Theoretically, anise might increase heart rate and pulse rate due to the catecholamine activity of the constituent anethole (4,11).

Interactions with Diseases or Conditions
HORMONE SENSITIVE CANCERS/CONDITIONS: Because anise might have estrogenic effects (4,11), women with hormone sensitive conditions should avoid using it. Some of these conditions include breast cancer, uterine cancer, ovarian cancer, endometriosis, and uterine fibroids.
SKIN CONDITIONS: Anise oil can be potentially irritating and photosensitizing. Avoid anise in cases of dermatitis and inflammatory or allergic skin reactions (4).

Dosage and Administration
ORAL: The typical dose of anise is 0.5-1 grams of the dried fruit or .05-.2 mL of the essential oil, three times per day (4). The tea is prepared by steeping 1-2 teaspoons of the crushed seed for 10-15 minutes and then straining (4). As an expectorant, one cup of tea is commonly taken in the morning and/or at night. As an antiflatulent, 1 tablespoon of the tea is usually taken several times a day. For nursing babies and infants, the typical dose is one teaspoon of the tea (8).

ANNATTO

Also Known As
Achiote, Achiotillo, Annato, Annotta, Arnotta, Bija, Lipstick Tree, Roucou.

Scientific Names
Bixa orellana.
Family: Bixaceae.

People Use This For
Orally, annatto is used to treat diabetes, diarrhea, fevers, heartburn, malaria, hepatitis; and as an antioxidant, diuretic, and purgative.
Topically, annatto is used for burns, vaginitis, and as an insect repellent.
In foods, annatto is used as a coloring agent.

Safety
LIKELY SAFE ...when used orally in amounts commonly found in foods. Annatto has Generally Recognized As Safe (GRAS) status in the US (4912).
PREGNANCY AND LACTATION: There is insufficient reliable information available about the safety of annatto during pregnancy and breast-feeding.

Effectiveness
There is insufficient reliable information available about the effectiveness of annatto.

Mechanism of Action
The applicable part of annatto is the seed. Researchers think the coloring principles are carotenoids, mostly bixin and norbixin (11), which do not have vitamin A activity (11).

Adverse Reactions
None reported.

Interactions with Herbs & Other Dietary Supplements
None known.

Interactions with Drugs
ANTIDIABETES DRUGS: Monitor blood glucose levels closely due to claims that annatto has hyperglycemic effects (19).

Interactions with Foods
None known.

Interactions with Lab Tests
None known.

Interactions with Diseases or Conditions
None known.

Dosage and Administration
ORAL: People typically use 1 to 2 grams of powdered leaf in tablets or capsules twice daily. Annatto is also used as a 4:1 tincture in a dose of 2 to 4 mL twice daily (5255).

Comments
This product is used commercially as a food coloring agent (11).

APPLE

Also Known As
Apples.

Scientific Names
Malus sylvestris
Family: Rosaceae.

People Use This For
Orally, apples are used to control diarrhea or constipation; and for the softening, passage, and collection of gallstones. Apples are also used for treating cancer, diabetes, dysentery, fever, heart ailments, scurvy, warts, and cleaning teeth.

Safety
LIKELY SAFE ...when used orally in food amounts. Tell patients to avoid eating apple seeds, which can be toxic (6).
PREGNANCY AND LACTATION: There is insufficient reliable information about the safety of apple in medicinal amounts during pregnancy and lactation; avoid using.

Effectiveness
INSUFFICIENT RELIABLE EVIDENCE to RATE

Gallbladder disease. There is some preliminary evidence apple juice used orally for seven days, with olive oil used on the seventh day before going to bed, might be effective for the softening, passage, and collection of gallstones in the stool (3472).

Lung cancer. There is some preliminary evidence that increasing apple consumption might decrease the risk of developing lung cancer (3470).

More evidence is needed to rate apple for these uses.

Mechanism of Action
The applicable part of apple is the fruit. The pectin in apples probably accounts for their effect on diarrhea and constipation. Pectin absorbs water in the gastrointestinal (GI) tract and swells to a gummy mass. The mass provides bulk which tends to normalize bowel function (6). Apples also contain phloretin, which has antibacterial activity (6). There is some interest in using apples for improving lung function. There is some evidence that consuming 5 or more apples per week can improve lung function as measured by maximum forced expiration in one second (FEV1) (3469). The constituent quercetin is an antioxidant flavonoid found in high concentrations in apples. Quercetin is thought to be responsible for apples potential benefit in preventing lung cancer (3469,3470).

Adverse Reactions
No adverse reactions are generally known or predicted to occur with apple fruit. However, one death is attributed to ingestion of a large amount (a cupful) of apple seeds, which contain hydrogen cyanide (HCN) (6). Ingestion of large amounts of seeds may cause cyanide poisoning, leading to death. To release cyanide, seeds must be hydrolyzed in the stomach, and several hours may elapse before poisoning symptoms occur (6). Patients allergic to other fruits in the Rosaceae family can also be allergic to apples. Cross-reactivity among the apple fruit and other members of the Rosaceae family, including apricot, almond, plum, peach, pear, and strawberry, has been demonstrated (7129).

Interactions with Herbs & Other Dietary Supplements
None known.

Interactions with Drugs
FEXOFENADINE (Allegra): Apple juice can significantly decrease oral absorption and blood levels of fexofenadine when used together. Apple juice decreases bioavailability of fexofenadine by about 78%. Apple juice seems to inhibit organic anion transporting polypeptide (OATP), which is involved in drug uptake in the gut, liver, and kidney (7046). It's not yet known how long apple juice inhibits OATP. Separating administration times might not prevent this interaction. Tell patients it's best to take their medications with a plain glass of water.

Interactions with Foods
CROSS-ALLERGENICITY: Patients allergic to other fruits in the Rosaceae family can also be allergic to apples. Cross-reactivity among the apple fruit and other members of the Rosaceae family, including apricot, almond, plum, peach, pear, and strawberry, has been demonstrated (7129).

Interactions with Lab Tests
None known.

Interactions with Diseases or Conditions
CROSS-ALLERGENICITY: Patients allergic to other fruits in the Rosaceae family can also be allergic to apples. Cross-reactivity among the apple fruit and other members of the Rosaceae family, including apricot, almond, plum, peach, pear, and strawberry, has been demonstrated (7129).

Dosage and Administration
ORAL: People typically use 500 mg apple pectin capsules daily as a supplement. Dried apple peels are used to make a tea: 1 to 2 teaspoons with 1 cup simmering water. The usual dose is from 1 to 3 cups per day (5250,5263,6006). For the softening of gallstones, one liter of apple juice used daily for seven days with 1 cup of olive oil used on the seventh day before going to bed has been used (3472).

APPLE CIDER VINEGAR

Also Known As
Applecider Vinegar, Cider Vinegar.
CAUTION: See separate listing for Apple.

Scientific Names
Malus sylvestris.
Family: Rosaceae.

People Use This For
Orally, apple cider vinegar is used alone or with honey for weight loss, leg cramps and pain, upset stomach, sore throats, sinus problems, high blood pressure, arthritis, to help rid the body of toxins, stimulate thinking, slow the aging process, regulate blood pressure, reduce cholesterol, fight infection, and osteoporosis.
Topically, apple cider vinegar is used for acne, as a skin toner, as an ingredient in hair rinse, to soothe sunburn, for shingles, insect bites, and to prevent dandruff. It is also used in the bath for vaginitis.
In foods, apple cider vinegar is used as a flavoring agent.

Safety
LIKELY SAFE ...when used orally as a food flavoring. ...when used topically, diluted.
POSSIBLY UNSAFE ...when used orally in amounts of 250 mL per day long-term. There is one report of an individual who developed hypokalemia, elevated renin levels, and osteoporosis after 6 years of ingesting 250 mL apple cider vinegar per day (5911).
There is insufficient reliable information available about the safety of apple cider vinegar for its other uses.
PREGNANCY AND LACTATION: There is insufficient reliable information available about the safety of apple cider vinegar in medicinal amounts during pregnancy and lactation.

Effectiveness
There is insufficient reliable information available about the effectiveness of apple cider vinegar.

Mechanism of Action
Cider vinegar is fermented juice from crushed apples. Like apple juice, it probably contains some pectin; vitamins B1, B2, and B6; biotin; folic acid; niacin; pantothenic acid; and vitamin C. It also contains small amounts of the minerals sodium, phosphorous, potassium, calcium, iron, and magnesium (5912).

Adverse Reactions
Orally, there has been one published report of an individual who developed hypokalemia, high renin levels, and osteoporosis after ingesting 250 mL apple cider vinegar daily for 6 years.

Interactions with Herbs & Other Dietary Supplements
HERBS WITH CARDIAC ACTIVITY: Theoretically, the overuse of apple cider vinegar can increase the risk of cardiotoxicity due to potassium depletion. Cardioactive herbs include digitalis, lily-of-the-valley, pheasant's eye, and squill.
HORSETAIL, LICORICE: Theoretically, overuse of apple cider vinegar can increase the risk of potassium depletion from overuse of horsetail or licorice.
STIMULANT LAXATIVE HERBS: Theoretically, overuse of apple cider vinegar and stimulant laxative herbs can increase the risk of potassium depletion. Stimulant laxative herbs include aloe vera, alder buckthorn, European buckthorn, cascara sagrada, castor oil, rhubarb, and senna.

Interactions with Drugs
DIGOXIN (Lanoxin): Theoretically, overuse of apple cider vinegar could decrease potassium levels, increasing the risk of toxicity for cardiovascular drugs such as digoxin (Lanoxin) (5911).
DIURETIC DRUGS: Overuse of apple cider vinegar might compound diuretic-induced potassium loss (5911). There is some concern that people taking apple cider vinegar along with potassium depleting diuretics might have an increased risk for hypokalemia. Initiation of potassium supplementation or an increase in potassium supplement dose may be necessary for some patients. Some diuretics that can deplete potassium include chlorothiazide (Diuril), chlorthalidone (Thalitone), furosemide (Lasix), hydrochlorothiazide (HCTZ, HydroDIURIL, Microzide), and others.
INSULIN: Theoretically, overuse of apple cider vinegar concomitantly with insulin might cause hypokalemia (5911).

Interactions with Foods
None known.

Interactions with Lab Tests
POTASSIUM LEVEL: Theoretically, long-term use or high doses can reduce serum potassium level and increase urine potassium level (5911).
URINARY ANION GAP: In one case report, long-term use of 250 mL apple cider vinegar per day was associated with high positive urinary anion gap (5911).

Interactions with Diseases or Conditions
DIABETES: Theoretically, long-term use or high doses of apple cider vinegar might increase potassium loss of individuals using insulin.
OSTEOPOROSIS: Theoretically, long-term use or high doses might cause osteoporosis (5911).

Dosage and Administration
TOPICAL: For vaginitis add 3 cups of apple cider vinegar to hot bath and soak, spreading legs to allow water into vagina (5910).

APRICOT

Also Known As
Amygdaloside, Apricots, Armeniaca, Chinese Almond, Laetrile, Madelonitrile, Vitamin B17.

Scientific Names
Prunus armeniaca, synonyms Amygdalus armeniaca, Armeniaca vulgaris.
Family: Rosaceae.

People Use This For
Orally, apricot is used for asthma, cough, constipation, hemorrhage, infertility, eye inflammation, spasm, and vaginal infections. Laetrile, the semi-synthetic derivative of amygdalin constituent, has been fraudulently acclaimed as a cancer treatment.
In manufacturing, apricot oil is used in cosmetics or as a vehicle for pharmaceutical preparations.

Safety

POSSIBLY SAFE ...when apricot oil is used topically (6).
LIKELY UNSAFE ...when apricot kernels are taken orally because they are a source of cyanide. Acute poisonings may progress to respiratory failure, coma and death within 15 minutes (4). The lethal dose is 50-60 kernels (12) but amount may vary (4). Chronic poisoning can also occur (4).
CHILDREN: POSSIBLY SAFE ...when apricot oil is used topically (6). LIKELY UNSAFE ...when apricot kernels are ingested. The lethal dose is 7-10 kernels (12) but amount may vary (4).
PREGNANCY AND LACTATION: POSSIBLY SAFE ...when apricot oil is used topically (6). LIKELY UNSAFE ...when apricot kernels are ingested (4,12).

Effectiveness

INEFFECTIVE

Cancer. Taking apricot orally is not effective for treating cancer (4,5).

There is insufficient reliable information available about the effectiveness of apricot for its other uses.

Mechanism of Action

The applicable parts of apricot are the kernel and oil. Apricot contains fruit acids, a variety of sugars, vitamins C and K, beta-carotene, thiamine, niacin, and iron. The seed contains the glycoside amygdalin which yields laetrile and hydrocyanic acid (6). Related glucosides include prunasin, sambunigrin and prulaurasin (6673). Several popular theories that have now been disproved claimed preferential uptake and conversion of amygdalin to hydrogen cyanide in tumor cells. Actually, research shows that amygdalin is slowly hydrolyzed to HCN in the stomach, rapidly absorbed via the GI tract, and then diffused through the body (4).

Adverse Reactions

Apricot may cause acute poisoning, with symptoms including dizziness, headache, nausea, vomiting, drowsiness, dyspnea, palpitations, marked hypotension, convulsions, paralysis, coma, and death (4). Apricot may also cause chronic poisoning, with symptoms of increased blood thiocyanate, goiter, thyroid cancer, optic nerve lesions, blindness, ataxia, hypertonia, cretinism and mental retardation. Demyelinating lesions and neuromyopathies reportedly occur secondary to chronic exposure, including long-term therapy (4).

Interactions with Herbs & Other Dietary Supplements

None known.

Interactions with Drugs

None known.

Interactions with Foods

None known.

Interactions with Lab Tests

None known.

Interactions with Diseases or Conditions

None known.

Dosage and Administration

No typical dosage.

Comments

The apricot seed constituent, amygdalin, is the generic name for laetrile, which is also referred to as amygdaloside, madelonitrile, or vitamin B17 (6673). In 1984, amygdalin, was classified prescription-only to protect the general public (4). In 1987, laetrile was ruled to be an unapproved drug and its importation into the USA under an affidavit system created in 1977 ended (6672).
The FDA is seeking a permanent injunction against three corporations for unlawfully promoting and marketing laetrile (injectable and oral) and apricot seeds for treating cancer on their Internet websites (6669). The companies named in the action are Without Cancer, Inc. and The Health World International, Inc. both located in Florida, and Health Genesis Corporation located in Arizona.

ARECA

Also Known As
Areca Nut, Betel Nut, Betel Quid, Gubak, Pinag, Pinlag, Poogiphalam, Puga, Supari, Tantusara.

Scientific Names
Areca catechu.
Family: Arecaceae/Palmae.

People Use This For
Orally, areca is used as a recreational drug because of its central nervous system (CNS) stimulating properties. It is also used orally for treatment of schizophrenia, glaucoma, as a mild stimulant, and digestive aid.

In veterinary medicine, an extract of areca is used for expelling tapeworms in cattle, dogs, and horses; as a cathartic; and for treating intestinal colic in horses.

Safety
LIKELY UNSAFE ...when used orally, long-term or in high doses. Constituents of areca have documented carcinogenic potential and have been commonly associated with precancerous lesions and squamous cell carcinoma in long-term users (6,17). Other constituents are poisonous. Ingesting 8-30 grams of areca nut can cause death (6). There is insufficient reliable information available about the safety of short-term use of areca.

PREGNANCY AND LACTATION: LIKELY UNSAFE ...when used orally. Areca has carcinogenic potential as well as central nervous system (CNS) stimulant and cholinergic properties and might adversely affect pregnancy and nursing infants (6,17); avoid using.

Effectiveness
INSUFFICIENT RELIABLE EVIDENCE to RATE

Schizophrenia. There is preliminary evidence that areca might be helpful for schizophrenia. Some patients with schizophrenia who chew areca nut seem to have less severe symptoms (6081). More evidence is needed to rate areca for this use.

Mechanism of Action
The applicable part of areca is the nut. Researchers think alkaloid components have cholinergic action similar to pilocarpine, but with greater central nervous system (CNS) action (6). The most abundant alkaloid is arecoline (6081). Arecoline's cholinergic effects are thought to be the reason for improvement in psychotic symptoms in patients with schizophrenia who chew areca nut (6081). Arecoline also has anthelmintic activity (6). The constituents arecaidine, and arecoline have carcinogenic potential (6); and chewing areca nut has been associated with oral cancer (329). Areca was also historically tried for glaucoma due to its cholinergic effects.

Adverse Reactions
Orally, areca may cause pupil dilation, increased salivation, vomiting, diarrhea, gingivitis, and periodontitis (6). High doses can cause convulsions and death (6). Chewing areca nut results in red-stained mouth, lips, and feces (18). Chewing areca quids is likely to produce central nervous system (CNS) stimulation similar to caffeine and tobacco (6). Areca quid chewing can cause oral submucous fibrosis in susceptible individuals (327,328,329). Chronic use of areca has also been associated with cardiovascular disease, diabetes, asthma (326), and oral cancer (329).

Interactions with Herbs & Other Dietary Supplements
None known.

Interactions with Drugs
ANTICHOLINERGIC DRUGS: Theoretically, due to cholinergic effects areca nut can interfere with anti-cholinergic drug therapy (6). Avoid concomitant use.

CHOLINERGIC DRUGS: Theoretically, due to cholinergic effects areca nut can increase the effects and risk of side effects of cholinergic drugs (6). Avoid concomitant use.

PROCYCLIDINE: Concomitant use can reduce anticholinergic effects of procyclidine (Kemadrin) given to treat the extrapyramidal effects of fluphenazine (19).

Interactions with Foods
None known.

Interactions with Lab Tests
FECAL LAB TESTS: Chewing areca nuts stains feces red (18). This coloration may interfere with fecal lab tests.

Interactions with Diseases or Conditions
ASTHMA: Areca may aggravate asthma (6).

Dosage and Administration
ORAL: An average of approximately 11 whole nuts per day is commonly used (6081).

Comments
Areca nut is chewed alone or in the form of quids, a mixture of tobacco, powdered or sliced areca nut, and slaked lime wrapped in the leaf of "betel" vine (Piper betel) (6).

ARENARIA RUBRA

Also Known As
Common Sandspurry, Sabline Rouge, Sandwort.

Scientific Names
Spergularia rubra.
Family: Caryophyllaceae.

Comments
At the date of publication, this product was not a common ingredient used in brand name supplements marketed to consumers. Details about this product are available at the online version of *Natural Medicines Comprehensive Database*. See www.naturaldatabase.com.

ARISTOLOCHIA

Also Known As
Birthwort, Long Birthwort, Pelican Flower, Red River Snakeroot, Sangree Root, Sangrel, Serpentaria, Snakeroot, Snakeweed, Texas Snakeroot, Virginia Serpentary, Virginia Snakeroot.

Scientific Names
Aristolochia auricularia; Aristolochia clematitis; Aristolochia fangchi; Aristolochia heterophylla; Aristolochia kwangsiensis; Aristolochia moupinensis; Aristolochia reticulata; Aristolochia serpentaria; other Aristolochia species.
Family: Aristolochiaceae.

People Use This For
Orally, aristolochia is used as an aphrodisiac, anticonvulsant, immune stimulant, and to promote menstruation. It is also used orally to treat allergic gastrointestinal colic and gallbladder colic.

Safety
UNSAFE ...when used orally. Aristolochia contains aristolochic acid, which is nephrotoxic and carcinogenic (18,6073,6118). The FDA considers all products containing aristolochic acid to be unsafe and adulterated (6118).
PREGNANCY AND LACTATION: UNSAFE ...when used orally; avoid using (6118).

Effectiveness
There is insufficient reliable information available about the effectiveness of aristolochia.

Mechanism of Action
The applicable parts of aristolochia are the above ground parts and root. Aristolochia contains aristolochic acid which is nephrotoxic and carcinogenic. Aristolochic acid has been associated with cancers of the kidney, bladder, stomach, lung, and lymphoma in rodents and cancers of the bladder, ureter, and/or renal pelvis in people with aristolochic acid-associated nephropathy (6118).

Adverse Reactions
Orally, use of aristolochia can cause vomiting, gastroenteritis, spasms, severe kidney damage, and death (18). There have been more than 100 cases of nephropathy, referred to as "Chinese herb nephropathy," characterized by interstitial fibrosis and associated with tea believed adulterated with aristolochia. Of these cases, 43 progressed to end stage renal failure requiring dialysis or transplantation (564,6073) and 18 developed urothelial carcinomas of the bladder, ureter, and/or renal pelvis (6073). The risk of developing urothelial carcinoma seems to be related to cumulative intake of the herb (6073).

Interactions with Herbs & Other Dietary Supplements
None known.

Interactions with Drugs
ANTACIDS: Theoretically, due to reports that aristolochia increases stomach acid, aristolochia might decrease the effectiveness of antacids (19).
H2-BLOCKERS: Theoretically, due to reports that aristolochia increases stomach acid, aristolochia might decrease the effectiveness of H2-blockers (19). The H2 blockers include cimetidine (Tagamet), ranitidine (Zantac), nizatidine (Axid), and famotidine (Pepcid).
PROTON PUMP INHIBITORS (PPIs): Theoretically, due to reports that aristolochia increases stomach acid, aristolochia might decrease the effectiveness of PPIs (19). PPIs include omeprazole (Prilosec), lansoprazole (Prevacid), rabeprazole (Aciphex), pantoprazole (Protonix), and esomeprazole (Nexium).

Interactions with Foods
None known.

Interactions with Lab Tests
KIDNEY FUNCTION TESTS: Aristolochia can cause nephropathy and abnormal kidney function results (564).

Interactions with Diseases or Conditions
GASTROINTESTINAL (GI) IRRITATION: Aristolochia can irritate the GI tract. It is contraindicated in individuals with infectious or inflammatory GI conditions (19).

Dosage and Administration
ORAL: When the plant is in flower, the entire plant is used. The root alone is also used. A liquid preparation of aristolochia is prepared by adding 2 teaspoons of the fresh plant or root to 1 cup of water and boiling for 10 minutes. A cold extract is prepared by adding 2 teaspoons of the plant or root to 1 cup cold water, which is allowed to stand for 6 to 8 hours. Sources warn against the toxicity of aristolochia and suggest that a dosage should be obtained from a health care professional (5263).

Comments
The FDA considers all products containing aristolochic acid to be unsafe and adulterated (6118). The FDA intends to automatically detain, without physical examination, any product which contains plants known or suspected to contain aristolochic acid, or which might be adulterated with plants known to contain aristolochic acid. Each detained product will be released only after the responsible party provides direct analytical evidence that it is free of aristolochic acid (6118). Aristolochia is also banned in Germany, Austria, France, Great Britain, Belgium, and Japan (367).
Health Canada, the Canadian health authority, removed five aristolochia-containing Chinese herbal medicine products from sale. The products include, Touku Natural Herbal Rheumatic Pills, two brands of Tri-Snakegall & Fritillary Powder, Tracheitis Pills, and Gastropathy Capsules (367).

ARNICA

Also Known As
Arnica Flos, Arnica Flower, Arnikablüten, Bergwohlverleih, Fleurs d'Arnica, Kraftwurz, Leopard's Bane, Mountain Tobacco, Wolf's Bane, Wundkraut.

Scientific Names
Arnica montana; Arnica fulgens; Arnica sororia; Arnica latifolia; Arnica cordifolia.
Family: Asteraceae/Compositae.

People Use This For
Topically, arnica is used for the inflammation and immune system stimulation associated with bruises, aches, and sprains. It is also used orally for mouth and throat inflammation, insect bites, superficial phlebitis, and as an abortifacient.
In foods, arnica is a flavor ingredient in alcoholic beverages, nonalcoholic beverages, frozen dairy desserts, candy, baked goods, gelatins, and puddings.
In manufacturing, arnica is used in hair tonics and anti-dandruff preparations. The oil is used in perfumes and other cosmetic preparations.

Safety

POSSIBLY SAFE ...when used in amounts commonly found in foods. Arnica has Generally Recognized As Safe (GRAS) status in the US (4912), although Canadian regulations do not allow its use as a food ingredient (12). ...when used topically for short-term use on unbroken skin (12).

LIKELY UNSAFE ...when taken orally. Arnica is considered poisonous and has caused severe or fatal poisonings (5). It can be cardiotoxic and cause large increases in blood pressure (5,17). Arnica is irritating to mucous membranes and can cause gastroenteritis, muscle paralysis (voluntary and cardiac), an increase or decrease in pulse rate, heart palpitations, shortness of breath, and death (4,17).

PREGNANCY AND LACTATION: LIKELY UNSAFE ...when used orally or topically; avoid using (12).

Effectiveness

POSSIBLY INEFFECTIVE

Wisdom tooth extraction. Taking arnica orally doesn't seem to reduce the postsurgical complications of third molar extraction. Arnica does not appear to improve pain, swelling, or wound infection associated with wisdom tooth removal (10630).

There is insufficient reliable information available about the effectiveness of arnica for its other uses.

Mechanism of Action

The applicable part of arnica is the flowerhead. The sesquiterpene lactones of arnica are the active constituents and produce anti-inflammatory and analgesic effects (102). They also can have some antibiotic activity (5). Two constituents of arnica, helenalin and 11 alpha,13-dihyrohelenalin, have been shown to inhibit human platelet function (104).

Adverse Reactions

Arnica taken orally can cause irritation of mucous membranes, drowsiness, stomach pain, vomiting, diarrhea, tachycardia, shortness of breath, coma, and death (4,6,11). Arnica can cause an allergic reaction in individuals sensitive to the Asteraceae/Compositae family. Members of this family include ragweed, chrysanthemums, marigolds, daisies, and many other herbs. Topically, arnica can cause contact dermatitis and mucous membrane irritation (6,11).

Interactions with Herbs & Other Dietary Supplements

None known.

Interactions with Drugs

ANTICOAGULANT/ANTIPLATELET DRUGS: There is some concern that arnica might potentiate the effects of anticoagulant and antiplatelet drugs and possibly increase the risk of bleeding. Constituents of arnica can decrease platelet aggregation in vitro (104). However, this effect has not yet been demonstrated in humans. Until more is known, use cautiously in patients taking anticoagulant or antiplatelet drugs. Some of these drugs include aspirin, clopidogrel (Plavix), dalteparin (Fragmin), enoxaparin (Lovenox), heparin, ticlopidine (Ticlid), warfarin (Coumadin), and others.

Interactions with Foods

None known.

Interactions with Lab Tests

PLATELET FUNCTION: Theoretically, arnica might inhibit platelet function and test results (104).

Interactions with Diseases or Conditions

BROKEN SKIN: Avoid the use of arnica on broken or damaged skin (2,4).

CROSS-ALLERGENICITY: Arnica can cause reactions in individuals allergic to plants in the Asteraceae/Compositae family. Members of this family include ragweed, chrysanthemums, marigolds, daisies, and many other herbs (12,17).

GASTROINTESTINAL (GI) IRRITATION: Arnica can irritate the gastrointestinal (GI) tract. Arnica is contraindicated in individuals with infectious or inflammatory GI conditions (19).

Dosage and Administration

TOPICAL: The typical dose of arnica is 2 grams of the flowerheads in 100 mL of water (8). As a poultice, the tincture of arnica is diluted three to ten times with water (8). As a mouthwash, the tincture is diluted ten times (8); the mouthwash should not be swallowed. Ointments commonly contain a maximum of 20-25% of the tincture or 15% of the oil (8). The tincture is usually 1:10 (2), and the oil is usually 1:5 in vegetable fixed oil (2,8).

ARRACH

Also Known As
Dog's Arrach, Goat's Arrach, Goosefoot, Netchweed, Oraches, Stinking Arrach, Stinking Goosefoot, Stinking Motherwort.

Scientific Names
Chenopodium vulvaria.
Family: Chenopodiaceae or Amaranthaceae.

Comments
At the date of publication, this product was not a common ingredient used in brand name supplements marketed to consumers. Details about this product are available at the online version of *Natural Medicines Comprehensive Database*. See www.naturaldatabase.com.

ARROWROOT

Also Known As
Maranta.

Scientific Names
Maranta arundinacea.
Family: Marantaceae.

People Use This For
Orally, arrowroot is used as a nutritional food for infants and convalescents. Babies cut teeth on arrowroot cookies. It is also used as a dietary aid in gastrointestinal disorders and acute diarrhea.
Topically, arrowroot is used as a soothing agent for painful, irritated or inflamed mucous membranes.
In foods, arrowroot is used as an ingredient in cooking.

Safety
LIKELY SAFE ...when the starch from the root or rhizome are used orally in amounts found in foods (12).
POSSIBLY SAFE ...when used orally or topically in medicinal amounts (12).
PREGNANCY AND LACTATION: POSSIBLY SAFE ...when used in amounts found in foods. There is insufficient reliable information available about the safety of larger amounts used during pregnancy and lactation; avoid using.

Effectiveness
There is insufficient reliable information available about the effectiveness of arrowroot.

Mechanism of Action
The applicable part of arrowroot is the starch from the root and rhizome. Animal data suggests that arrowroot may reduce deposited cholesterol in the aorta and heart muscle. This may be due to an increase in the elimination of cholesterol in the form of bile acids (18).

Adverse Reactions
None reported.

Interactions with Herbs & Other Dietary Supplements
None known.

Interactions with Drugs
None known.

Interactions with Foods
None known.

Interactions with Lab Tests
None known.

Interactions with Diseases or Conditions
None known.

Dosage and Administration
ORAL: Arrowroot starch is extracted from the chopped root and rhizome by a specific process using water. The powdered starch is usually boiled with water and used orally (18).

Comments
Arrowroot is often replaced with cheaper starches, including potato, corn, wheat, or rice starch (18).

ARTICHOKE

Also Known As
Alcachofa, Alcaucil, Artichaut Commun, Artichoke Extract, Artichoke Leaf, Artichoke Leaf Extract, Artischocke, Cardo, Cardo de Comer, Cardon d'Espagne, Cardoon, Garden Artichoke, Gemuseartischocke, Globe Artichoke, Kardone, Tyosen-Azami.

Scientific Names
Cynara cardunculus, synonym Cynara scolymus.
Family: Asteraceae/Compositae.

People Use This For
Orally, artichoke is used for dyspepsia, hyperlipidemia, nausea, alcohol-induced hangover, and irritable bowel syndrome (IBS). It is also used orally as a diuretic and choleretic. Artichoke is also used orally for treating snakebites, renal insufficiency, anemia, edema, arthritis, cystitis, liver dysfunction, preventing gallstones, lowering blood pressure, as a hypoglycemic, stimulant, and a tonic.
In foods, artichoke leaves and extracts are used as flavoring agents in beverages. The constituents, cynarin and chlorogenic acid, are sometimes used as sweeteners.

Safety
LIKELY SAFE ...when used orally in amounts commonly found in foods. Artichoke is has Generally Recognized As Safe (GRAS) status in the US (4912).
POSSIBLY SAFE ...when used orally and appropriately in therapeutic amounts (2056,11773). Artichoke extract appears to be safe for up to 23 months (11773).
PREGNANCY AND LACTATION: There is insufficient reliable information about the safety of therapeutic amounts of artichoke used during pregnancy or lactation; avoid using.

Effectiveness
POSSIBLY EFFECTIVE

Dyspepsia. Artichoke leaf extract seems to significantly reduce symptoms such as nausea, vomiting, flatulence, and abdominal pain in idiopathic dyspepsia and dyspepsia associated with biliary disease. Improvement can take up to 2 to 8 weeks of treatment (2056,11429).

Hyperlipidemia. Artichoke extract seems to modestly reduce total and low-density lipoprotein (LDL) cholesterol, and the LDL/high density lipoprotein (HDL) ratio over 6 to 12 weeks of treatment. Artichoke extract may work better in people with higher cholesterol levels (6282,11773).

Irritable bowel syndrome (IBS). There is some evidence that artichoke extract might significantly reduce abdominal pain and cramping, bloating, flatulence, and constipation associated with IBS after 6 weeks of treatment (2562).

POSSIBLY INEFFECTIVE

Hangover. Artichoke extract doesn't seem to prevent alcohol-induced hangover (11774).

There is insufficient reliable information available about the effectiveness of artichoke for its other uses.

Mechanism of Action
The applicable parts of artichoke are the leaf, stem, and root. The primary constituents include up to 2% phenolic acids, primarily chlorogenic acid, cynarin, and caffeic acid. Artichoke also contains up to 4% sesquiterpene lactones, and 1% flavonoids including scolymoside, cynaroside, and luteolin (2056). Artichoke's therapeutic benefit in dyspepsia has centered around its choleretic effects, or ability to stimulate bile flow, which has been demonstrated in several studies (2056). This might explain its use as a hangover remedy (11774). Constituents responsible for this effect are thought to be cynarin, chlorogenic acid, and scolymoside (2056).
Antiemetic, spasmolytic, and carminative effects of artichoke have also been described. These effects may be responsible for the potential beneficial effects in patients with irritable bowel syndrome (IBS) (2562). Cynarin and chlorogenic acid may also have cholesterol-lowering effects, although studies with cynarin for hyperlipidemia have

produced mixed results (1423,1424).
Artichoke might reduce cholesterol synthesis (11773). Cynaroside and its derivative, luteolin, might also indirectly inhibit HMG-CoA reductase (1425,1426,2056). Several constituents are reported to have antioxidant activity (1422). Preliminary research suggests that artichoke leaf extract might also protect liver cells from damage (1421,1422,2056,3269). A mixture of polyphenols and flavonoids including caffeic acid, chlorogenic acid, cynarin, luteolin-7-O-glycoside (cynaroside), and luteolin might contribute to hepatoprotective activity (3269,2056).

Adverse Reactions
Orally, artichoke extract might increase flatulence in some patients (2562). Artichoke can also cause an allergic reaction in some patients. Patients sensitive to the Asteraceae/Compositae family may be at the greatest risk. Members of this family include ragweed, chrysanthemums, marigolds, daisies, and many other herbs.
Topically, allergic contact dermatitis can occur with the use of artichoke. This has been attributed to the constituent cynaropicrin (11).

Interactions with Herbs & Other Dietary Supplements
None known.

Interactions with Drugs
None known.

Interactions with Foods
None known.

Interactions with Lab Tests
None known.

Interactions with Diseases or Conditions
BILE DUCT OBSTRUCTION: Theoretically, artichoke might worsen bile duct obstruction by increasing bile flow (2056); avoid using.
CROSS-ALLERGENICITY: Artichoke might cause an allergic reaction in individuals sensitive to Asteraceae/Compositae family plants. Members of this family include ragweed, chrysanthemums, marigolds, daisies, and many other herbs (2056).
GALLSTONES: Theoretically, artichoke might worsen gallstones by increasing bile flow (2056); use with caution.

Dosage and Administration
ORAL: For irritable bowel syndrome (IBS), 640 mg leaf extract three times daily has been used (2562). For dyspepsia, 320 mg to 640 mg artichoke leaf extract daily has been used (11429). For lowering serum cholesterol, an artichoke extract 1800 to 1920 mg per day in 2 to 3 divided doses has been used. The isolated constituent cynarin 60-1500 mg per day has also been used to lower cholesterol (1423,1424,2056,11773). For extract preparations, appropriate dosing will vary depending on the specific extract being used.

Comments
Avoid confusion with Jerusalem artichoke (Helianthus tuberosus).

ARUM

Also Known As
Adder's Root, Bobbins, Cocky Baby, Cuckoo Pint, Cypress Powder, Dragon Root, Friar's Cowl, Gaglee, Kings and Queens, Ladysmock, Lords and Ladies, Parson and Clerk, Portland Arrowroot, Quaker, Ramp, Starchwort, Wake Robin.
CAUTION: See separate listing for Beth Root.

Scientific Names
Arum maculatum.
Family: Araceae.

People Use This For
Orally, arum is used for colds and inflammation of the throat. It is also used orally to stimulate sweating and as an expectorant.

Safety
UNSAFE ...when used orally (18).
PREGNANCY AND LACTATION: UNSAFE ...when used orally because of its toxicity (18); avoid using.

Effectiveness
There is insufficient reliable information available about the effectiveness of arum.

Mechanism of Action
The applicable part of arum is the root. Arum can cause severe mucous membrane irritation and bleeding. This is probably due to sharp oxalate crystals present in the root. These injure the mucous membranes, and may also introduce impurities into the wounds. Arum also contains cyanogenic glycosides, but the levels are probably too low to cause poisoning (18).

Adverse Reactions
Orally, arum can cause swelling of the tongue, bloody vomiting, and bloody diarrhea (18).

Interactions with Herbs & Other Dietary Supplements
CALCIUM, IRON, ZINC: Concurrent use might decrease mineral absorption. Arum contains oxalate (18), which can bind multivalent metal ions in the gastrointestinal tract and decrease mineral absorption.

Interactions with Drugs
None known.

Interactions with Foods
CALCIUM, IRON, ZINC: Concurrent use might decrease mineral absorption from foods. Arum contains oxalate (18), which can bind multivalent metal ions in the gastrointestinal tract and decrease mineral absorption.

Interactions with Lab Tests
None known.

Interactions with Diseases or Conditions
None known.

Dosage and Administration
No typical dosage.

ASAFOETIDA

Also Known As
Asa Foetida, Asafetida, Assant, Devil's Dung, Food of the Gods, Fum, Giant Fennel, Heeng.

Scientific Names
Ferula assa-foetida; Ferula foetida; Ferula pseudalliacea, synonym Ferula rubricaulis.
Family: Apiaceae/Umbelliferae.

People Use This For
Orally, asafoetida is used for chronic bronchitis, asthma, pertussis, hoarseness, hysteria, flatulent colic, chronic gastritis, dyspepsia, irritable colon, convulsions, as a nerve stimulant in treating neurasthenia. It is also used orally for amenorrhea, croup, insanity, and sarcomas.
Topically, asafoetida is used for corns and calluses.
In manufacturing, asafoetida is used as a fragrance or fixative in cosmetics, and it is used as a flavoring ingredient in foods and beverages.
Other uses for asafoetida include its use as a cat, dog, and wildlife repellent.

Safety
LIKELY SAFE ...when used orally in amounts commonly found in foods. Asafoetida has Generally Recognized As Safe (GRAS) status in the US (4912).
POSSIBLY SAFE ...when used orally and appropriately (12).
CHILDREN: UNSAFE ...when used orally in infants due to the possible risk of methemoglobinemia (4).
PREGNANCY: UNSAFE ...when used orally in medicinal amounts; asafoetida might cause abortion (4).
LACTATION: UNSAFE ...when used orally due to possible risk of methemoglobinemia in infants (4).

Effectiveness
There is insufficient reliable information available about the effectiveness of asafoetida.

Mechanism of Action
The applicable part of asafoetida is the root resin. Asafoetida may contain sulfur compounds in its volatile oil which may protect against fat-induced hyperlipidemia. Asafoetida may contain coumarin constituents with anticoagulant activity (4). There is some evidence to suggest that its constituents treat irritable bowel syndrome (IBS) (4).

Adverse Reactions
Orally, 50-100 mg of asafoetida may cause convulsions in people with nervousness (12). There is one report of methemoglobinemia in an infant (4). Large amounts are reported to cause swelling of the lips, belching, flatulence, diarrhea, headache, or convulsions (18).
Topically, genital organ swelling was reported after external use of asafoetida on the abdomen (18).

Interactions with Herbs & Other Dietary Supplements
None known.

Interactions with Drugs
ANTICOAGULANT/ANTIPLATELET DRUGS: Theoretically, asafoetida might increase the risk of bleeding (4).
ANTIHYPERTENSIVE DRUGS: Theoretically, concomitant use may increase therapeutic effects of antihypertensive therapy due to hypotensive activity of asafoetida (4).

Interactions with Foods
None known.

Interactions with Lab Tests
None known.

Interactions with Diseases or Conditions
BLEEDING DISORDERS: Theoretically, asafoetida might increase the risk of bleeding (4).
CENTRAL NERVOUS SYSTEM (CNS) CONDITIONS: Asafoetida is contraindicated in people with CNS conditions that could result in convulsions (12).
GASTROINTESTINAL (GI) IRRITATION: Asafoetida can irritate GI tract. It is contraindicated in individuals with infectious or inflammatory gastrointestinal conditions (19).
HYPERTENSION: Theoretically, asafoetida might interfere with blood pressure control (4).
HYPOTENSION: Theoretically, asafoetida might interfere with blood pressure control (4).

Dosage and Administration
ORAL: A typical dose is 300-1000 mg powdered resin three times daily (4). Tincture of asafoetida (concentration unspecified), 2-4 mL (4), or 20 drops as a single dose (18) have also been used.
TOPICAL: No typical dosage.

Comments
Asafoetida resin is produced by solidifying juice exuded from incisions in living roots of Ferula foetida and other Ferula species. Asafoetida is known to have putrid odor and tastes bitter. The acrid taste is the basis for its name, devil's dung (6). Various species of this plant have somewhat different constituents. The related species Ferula communis, contains toxic coumarin constituents. Other related species are Ferula galbaniflua and Ferula rubricaulis. These seem to cause contact dermatitis (4).

ASARABACCA

Also Known As
Asaroun, Asarum, Azarum, False Coltsfoot, Hazelwort, Public House Plant, Snakeroot, Wild Ginger, Wild Nard.
CAUTION: See separate listings for Bitter Milkwort , Coltsfoot, and Senega.

Scientific Names
Asarum europaeum.
Family: Aristolochiaceae.

People Use This For

Orally, asarabacca is used for acute and chronic bronchitis, bronchial spasms, and bronchial asthma. It is also used orally as an emetic; antitussive; menstrual stimulant; abortifacient; and to treat pneumonia, angina pectoris, migraines, liver disease, jaundice, and dehydration.

Safety

POSSIBLY SAFE ...when used orally and appropriately short-term (12).
POSSIBLY UNSAFE ...when used orally in large amounts or long-term (12). Large doses have been associated with significant side effects, including burning tongue, gastroenteritis, diarrhea, skin rashes, and partial paralysis (18). ...when the essential oil is taken orally. The essential oil contains a potential hepatocarcinogenic constituent, beta-asarone (12).
UNSAFE ...when aristolochic acid-contaminated asarabacca is used orally. Asarabacca is commonly contaminated with aristolochic acid, which is nephrotoxic and carcinogenic. The FDA considers all products containing aristolochic acid to be unsafe and adulterated. Only products analytically verified to be aristolochic acid-free should be used (6118).
PREGNANCY: LIKELY UNSAFE ...when used orally. Asarabacca might act as a menstrual or uterine stimulant (12); contraindicated.
LACTATION: Insufficient reliable information available; avoid using.

Effectiveness

There is insufficient reliable information available about the effectiveness of asarabacca.

Mechanism of Action

The applicable part of asarabacca is the rhizome. The constituent phenylpropanol may be responsible for the effects of asarabacca on bronchitis/bronchial asthma. Some products are standardized for content of this constituent (18). The emetic and spasmolytic effects may be due to the constituent trans-isoasarone (18). Local anesthetic effect demonstrated in humans may be due to constituents, trans-isoasarone and trans-isomethyleugenol (18).

Adverse Reactions

Orally, asarabacca may cause nausea and vomiting (12). Severe poisoning has also been reported (553). Symptoms of poisoning include burning of tongue, gastroenteritis, diarrhea, skin rashes, and partial paralysis (18). Asarabacca is commonly contaminated with aristolochic acid, which is nephrotoxic and carcinogenic (6118).

Interactions with Herbs & Other Dietary Supplements

None known.

Interactions with Drugs

None known.

Interactions with Foods

None known.

Interactions with Lab Tests

None known.

Interactions with Diseases or Conditions

GASTROINTESTINAL (GI) IRRITATION: Asarabacca can irritate the GI tract; contraindicated in individuals with infectious or inflammatory GI conditions (19).

Dosage and Administration

ORAL: Typically, 30 mg of the extract made from dried asarabacca is used in adults and children over 13 years old (18).

Comments

Asarabacca has been reported as obsolete for medicinal use (18); safer alternatives are available. Avoid confusion with bitter milkwort (Polygala amara), or senega (Polygala senega) also known as snakeroot.
Asarabacca is frequently contaminated with aristolochic acid, which is nephrotoxic and carcinogenic. The FDA considers all products containing aristolochic acid to be unsafe and adulterated (6118). The FDA intends to automatically detain, without physical examination, any product which contains plants known or suspected to contain aristolochic acid, or which might be adulterated with plants known to contain aristolochic acid. Each detained product will be released only after the responsible party provides direct analytical evidence that it is free of aristolochic acid (6118).

ASH

Also Known As

Bird's Tongue, Common Ash, European Ash, Weeping Ash, White Ash.
CAUTION: See separate listings for Northern Prickly Ash and Southern Prickly Ash.

Scientific Names

Fraxinus americana; Fraxinus excelsior.
Family: Oleaceae.

Comments

At the date of publication, there was very little scientific information about this product. Our staff is continually analyzing the available information on natural medicines and will add data to the online version of *Natural Medicines Comprehensive Database* as it becomes available. See www.naturaldatabase.com.

ASHWAGANDHA

Also Known As

Ajagandha, Amangura, Amukkirag, Asan, Asgand, Asgandh, Asgandha, Ashagandha, Ashvagandha, Ashwaganda, Asoda, Asundha, Asvagandha, Aswagandha, Avarada, Ayurvedic Ginseng, Clustered Wintercherry, Ghoda Asoda, Indian Ginseng, Kanaje Hindi, Kuthmithi, Samm Al Ferakh, Turangi-Ghanda, Winter Cherry, Withania.
CAUTION: See separate listings for Blue Cohosh, Canaigre, Codonopsis, Ginseng American, Ginseng Panax, Ginseng Siberian, and Winter Cherry.

Scientific Names

Withania somnifera, synonym Physalis somnifera.
Family: Solanaceae.

People Use This For

Orally, ashwagandha is used for arthritis, anxiety, insomnia, tumors, tuberculosis, and chronic liver disease. Ashwagandha is also used as an "adaptogen" to increase resistance to environmental stress, and as a general tonic. It is also used orally for immunomodulatory effects, improving cognitive function, decreasing inflammation, preventing the effects of aging, for emaciation, infertility in men and women, menstrual disorders, and hiccups. It is also used orally as an aphrodisiac, and emmenagogue; and for treating asthma, leukoderma, bronchitis, backache, and arthritis.
Topically, ashwagandha is used for treating ulcerations, backache, and hemiplegia.

Safety

POSSIBLY SAFE ...when used orally and appropriately, short-term (3710,11301).
There is insufficient reliable information available about the safety of ashwagandha when used long-term or topically.
PREGNANCY: LIKELY UNSAFE ...when used orally. Ashwagandha has abortifacient effects (12).
LACTATION: Insufficient reliable information available; avoid using.

Effectiveness

There is insufficient reliable information available about the effectiveness of ashwagandha.

Mechanism of Action

The applicable parts of ashwagandha are the root and berry. Ashwagandha contains several active constituents including alkaloids (isopelletierine, anaferine), steroidal lactones (withanolides, withaferins), and saponins (4116,11301). Ashwagandha does not contain nicotine as some researchers have reported (3710). Preliminary animal evidence suggests ashwagandha may have a variety of pharmacological effects including analgesic, antipyretic, anxiolytic, immunomodulatory, sedative, hypotensive, anti-inflammatory, and antioxidant effects (3710,3711,4113,4116,11301). It might also stimulate respiratory function, cause smooth muscle relaxation, and stimulate thyroid synthesis and/or secretion (3710).
Some researchers think ashwagandha has a so-called "anti-stressor" effect. Preliminary evidence suggests ashwagandha might suppress stress-induced increases of dopamine receptors in the corpus striatum of the brain (3710). It also appears to reduce stress-induced increases of plasma corticosterone, blood urea nitrogen, and blood lactic acid (11301). Ashwagandha might also have anxiolytic effects, possibly by acting as a gamma-aminobutyric acid (GABA) mimetic agent. It might also have anticonvulsant activity, by binding to the GABA receptor (3710). Ashwagandha and its constituents also seem to have immunomodulatory effects. The withanolides and sitoindosides

seem to cause a mobilization of macrophages, phagocytosis, and lysosomal enzymes (11301). Preliminary evidence suggests ashwagandha might reduce cyclophosphamide-induced immunosuppression and leukopenia (3711,4114). Ashwagandha also seems to increase bone marrow cell and white blood cell count in radiation-treated animals (3711). It remains unclear, however, what net effect whole ashwagandha preparations have on the immune system (3710,3711).

Adverse Reactions

Orally, ashwagandha seems to be well tolerated at typical doses. Large doses may cause gastrointestinal (GI) upset, diarrhea, and vomiting secondary to irritation of the mucous and serous membranes (3710).

Interactions with Herbs & Other Dietary Supplements

HERBS/SUPPLEMENTS WITH SEDATIVE PROPERTIES: Theoretically, concomitant use with herbs that have sedative properties might enhance therapeutic and adverse effects (11301). Some of these include 5-HTP, calamus, California poppy, catnip, hops, Jamaican dogwood, kava, St. John's wort, scullcap, valerian, yerba mansa, and others.

Interactions with Drugs

BENZODIAZEPINES: Theoretically, ashwagandha might increase the effects of benzodiazepines (3710). There is preliminary evidence that ashwagandha might have an additive effect with diazepam (Valium) and clonazepam (Klonopin) (3710). This may also occur with other benzodiazepines such as alprazolam (Xanax), flurazepam (Dalmane), lorazepam (Ativan), and midazolam (Versed).
CNS DEPRESSANTS: Theoretically, ashwagandha's sedative effect may potentiate the effects of barbiturates, other sedatives, and anxiolytics (3710).
IMMUNOSUPPRESSANTS: Theoretically, ashwagandha might decrease the effectiveness of immunosuppressant therapy because of its potential immunostimulating effects. There is preliminary evidence that ashwagandha might decrease immunosuppression caused by cyclophosphamide (3711,4114). It might also decrease the effectiveness of other immunosuppressant drugs such as azathioprine (Imuran), basiliximab (Simulect), cyclosporine (Neoral, Sandimmune), daclizumab (Zenapax), muromonab-CD3 (OKT3, Orthoclone OKT3), mycophenolate (CellCept), tacrolimus (FK506, Prograf), sirolimus (Rapamune), prednisone (Deltasone, Orasone), and other corticosteroids (glucocorticoids).
THYROID HORMONE: Theoretically, ashwagandha might have additive effects when used with thyroid supplements. There is preliminary evidence that ashwagandha might boost thyroid hormone synthesis and/or secretion (3710).

Interactions with Foods

None known.

Interactions with Lab Tests

THYROID FUNCTION TESTS: Theoretically, ashwagandha might suppress thyroid stimulating hormone (TSH) or increase triiodothyronine (T3) or thyroxine (T4) values. There is some evidence that ashwagandha might stimulate thyroid hormone synthesis or secretion (3710).

Interactions with Diseases or Conditions

PEPTIC ULCER DISEASE: Theoretically, ashwagandha should be avoided by people with peptic ulcer disease because of its irritant effect on the gastrointestinal (GI) tract (3710).

Dosage and Administration

ORAL: People typically use 1 to 6 grams daily of the whole herb in capsule or tea form (3710). The tea is prepared by boiling ashwagandha roots in water for 15 minutes and cooled. The usual dose is 3 cups daily. Tincture or fluid extracts are dosed 2 to 4 mL 3 times per day.
TOPICAL: No typical dosage.

Comments

The name Ashwagandha is from the Sanskrit language and is a combination of the word ashva, meaning horse, and gandha, meaning smell. The root has a strong aroma that is described as "horse-like" (3710). In Ayurvedic, Indian, and Unani medicine, ashwagandha is described as "Indian ginseng". Ashwagandha is sometimes substituted or adulterated with a similar plant, Withania coagulans (3710). Avoid confusing ashwagandha with Physalis alkekengi, also known as winter cherry.

ASPARAGUS

Also Known As
Asparagi Rhizoma Root, Asperge, Garden Asparagus, Sativari, Shatavari, Spargelkraut, Spargelwurzelstock, Sparrow Grass.

Scientific Names
Asparagus officinalis, synonym Asparagus longifolius.
Family: Asparagaceae or Liliaceae.

People Use This For
Orally, asparagus is used along with copious fluid consumption as "irrigation therapy" to increase urine output. It is also used orally for treating urinary tract infections and other inflammatory conditions of the urinary tract, preventing kidney and bladder stones, rheumatic joint pain and swelling, female hormone imbalances, dryness in the lungs and throat, AIDS, to prevent anemia due to folic acid deficiency, as a laxative, for neuritis, and for treating parasitic diseases and cancer.
Topically, asparagus is used for cleaning the face, drying sores, and acne.
In foods, the newly-formed shoots, or spears, are eaten as a vegetable. The seed and root extracts of asparagus are used in alcoholic beverages.

Safety
LIKELY SAFE ...when used in amounts commonly found in foods. Asparagus seed and root extract have Generally Recognized As Safe (GRAS) status in the US (4912).
POSSIBLY SAFE ...when used orally and appropriately for medicinal purposes (2,12).
There is insufficient reliable information available about the safety of the topical uses of asparagus.
PREGNANCY: POSSIBLY UNSAFE ...when used for medicinal purposes; asparagus extracts have been used as a contraceptive (6); avoid using.
LACTATION: There is insufficient reliable information available about the safety of asparagus in medicinal amounts during breast-feeding.

Effectiveness
There is insufficient reliable information available about the effectiveness of asparagus.

Mechanism of Action
The applicable parts of asparagus are the rhizome and root. Asparagus is a vitamin E rich plant source (19). The asparagus root has diuretic effects in animal experiments (2). Asparagus also has hypotensive, antibacterial, and antiviral effects in vitro (11). Fibers from the plant can have mutagen-adsorbing (cancer-preventing) activity (11). The saponin constituents can irritate mucous membranes and can be cytotoxic (6,3901). Asparagus can also cause urinary tract irritation (19).

Adverse Reactions
Orally, asparagus can cause mucous membrane irritation (3901).
Topically, asparagus can cause allergic skin reactions (2).

Interactions with Herbs & Other Dietary Supplements
None known.

Interactions with Drugs
None known.

Interactions with Foods
None known.

Interactions with Lab Tests
None known.

Interactions with Diseases or Conditions
EDEMA: Irrigation therapy with asparagus is contraindicated in individuals with edema caused by heart or kidney disorders (2).
KIDNEY DISEASE: Asparagus is contraindicated in individuals with inflammatory kidney disease because the mucosal irritant effect of asparagus can exacerbate this condition (2,6,12).

Dosage and Administration

ORAL: Typically, asparagus is used daily as a tea prepared by steeping 40-60 grams of the cut rhizome or root in 150 mL of boiling water for 5-10 minutes and then straining (2). Ensure ample fluid intake when used as "irrigation therapy" (2,18).
TOPICAL: No typical dosage.

Comments

Asparagus seeds are used medicinally in a few cultures. The consumption of asparagus spears produces a pungent odor in the urine of some people.

ASPARTATES

Also Known As

Aspartate Chelated Minerals, Aspartate Mineral Chelates, Aspartic Acid, Mineral Aspartates.
CAUTION: See separate listing for Chelated Minerals.

Scientific Names

None.

People Use This For

Orally, aspartates are used to increase absorption of mineral supplements and enhance athletic performance.

Safety

There is insufficient reliable information available about the safety of aspartates.
Pregnancy and Lactation: Insufficient reliable information available; avoid using.

Effectiveness

INSUFFICIENT RELIABLE EVIDENCE to RATE

Hepatic encephalopathy. Preliminary clinical research suggests an L-ornithine-L-aspartate infusion might reduce hepatic encephalopathy in some patients with hepatic cirrhosis (10655). More evidence is needed to rate aspartates for this use.

Mechanism of Action

Aspartate is an amino acid that is metabolized in resting muscles (5141). People theorize that aspartate mineral salts of copper, iron, magnesium, manganese, potassium, or zinc have better absorption or improve athletic ability. There is no evidence to suggest that this is true (5133). Except in cases of mineral deficiency, such as iron-deficiency anemia, a well-balanced diet typically provides the RDA of minerals (5133).

Adverse Reactions

None reported.

Interactions with Herbs & Other Dietary Supplements

None known.

Interactions with Drugs

None known.

Interactions with Foods

None known.

Interactions with Lab Tests

None known.

Interactions with Diseases or Conditions

None known.

Dosage and Administration

No typical dosage.

ASPEN

Also Known As
American Aspen, European Aspen, Populi Cortex, Populi Folium, Trembling Aspen, Quaking Aspen, Zitter-Pappel.

Scientific Names
Populus tremuloides; Populus tremula.
Family: Salicaceae.

People Use This For
Orally, aspen is used as a component in various medicinal herbal combinations for treating rheumatic disorders, prostate discomforts, sciatica, neuralgia, and bladder problems.

Safety
There is insufficient reliable information available about the safety of aspen.
Pregnancy and Lactation: Insufficient reliable information available; avoid using.

Effectiveness
There is insufficient reliable information available about the effectiveness of aspen.

Mechanism of Action
The applicable parts of aspen are the bark and leaf. Aspen contains salicin, a precursor to salicylate (3700), and therefore aspen may have anti-inflammatory activity (2,7).

Adverse Reactions
Topically, salicin is associated with skin rashes (4). Pollen sensitization and allergic contact dermatitis may occur following contact with the bud resin (2).

Interactions with Herbs & Other Dietary Supplements
SALICYLATE-CONTAINING HERBS: Theoretically, concomitant use with aspen may potentiate effects of other herbs that contain salicylates (19).

Interactions with Drugs
None known.

Interactions with Foods
ALCOHOL: Theoretically, concomitant use with aspen increases the incidence, severity, and risk of salicylate-induced gastrointestinal bleeding (15).

Interactions with Lab Tests
Theoretically, salicylate-containing herbs may interfere with lab tests affected by salicylates, such as serum uric acid, urine glucose, vanillylmandelic acid (VMA), and 5-HIAA tests.

Interactions with Diseases or Conditions
SALICYLATE HYPERSENSITIVITY: Theoretically contraindicated, due to salicylate (salicin) content. Avoid or use aspen with caution in people with active peptic ulcer disease, diabetes, gout, hemophilia, hypoprothrombinemia, kidney, or liver disease (15).

Dosage and Administration
ORAL: People typically use 1 to 5 grams of powdered aspen bark. A liquid is prepared using 1 to 2 teaspoons of the bark simmered in a cup of water for 10 to 15 minutes. This is taken three times daily. The liquid extract is commonly dosed 1 to 5 mL (223,5253).

ASTAXANTHIN

Also Known As

Microalgae, Ovoester.
CAUTION: See separate listing for Beta-Carotene.

Scientific Names

3,3'-dihydroxy-4,4'-diketo-beta-carotene; 3S,3'S-astaxanthin; 3R,3'R-astaxanthin; 3R,3'S-astaxanthin.

People Use This For

Orally, astaxanthin is used for macular degeneration, Alzheimer's and Parkinson's disease, stroke, cancer, and hypercholesterolemia.
Topically, astaxanthin is used for sunburn.

Safety

LIKELY SAFE ...when used in amounts found in foods. Astaxanthin has Generally Recognized As Safe (GRAS) status in the US (4912). There is insufficient reliable information available about the safety of oral use of astaxanthin supplements or the topical use of astaxanthin.
PREGNANCY AND LACTATION: Insufficient reliable information available; avoid using.

Effectiveness

There is insufficient reliable information available about the effectiveness of astaxanthin.

Mechanism of Action

Astaxanthin is a reddish carotenoid pigment found in the microalgae Haematococcus pluvialis. Salmon, trout, red sea bream, shrimp, lobster, fish eggs, and many bird species also contain substantial amounts of astaxanthin (4326,4332). It is a powerful antioxidant that is structurally similar to beta-carotene (8467). Astaxanthin contains the highest relative antioxidant activity when compared with alpha-tocopherol, alpha-carotene, beta-carotene, lutein, and lycopene (10634). The concentration of astaxanthin is 1% to 3% in microalgae. A 4-ounce portion of farmed Atlantic salmon contains about 0.5 to 1.1 mg of astaxanthin; 4 ounces of sockeye salmon contains about 4.5 mg (8467).
Preliminary data suggests astaxanthin may decrease the oxidative liver damage caused by carbon tetrachloride. It seems to decrease oxidative consumption of glutathione (GSH) and increase hepatoprotective antioxidant activity (8454). There is also preliminary data that suggests that astaxanthin might have gastroprotective effects against Helicobacter pylori, possibly by inhibiting inflammation and acting as an antioxidant (4341).
Evidence also suggests that astaxanthin might stimulate immunity (4335,4336). Additional animal research suggests astaxanthin might protect against mammary cancer, liver cancer, bladder cancer, and oral cancer (4337,4338,4339,4340). It seems to suppress the growth of tumor cells by increasing concentrations of gamma-interferon and increasing the activity of cytotoxic T lymphocytes. It appears that astaxanthin needs to be part of the diet prior to tumor development to inhibit tumor growth (8453).
Preliminary research also suggests that astaxanthin may be able to prevent the oxidative damage caused by ultraviolet (UVA) light (8490).

Adverse Reactions

None reported. However, another carotenoid substance that is chemically related to astaxanthin, canthaxanthin, caused crystals in the retina and loss of visual acuity in one patient (8455). This effect has not been observed with astaxanthin, but patients who have visual changes while taking astaxanthin should stop taking it immediately.

Interactions with Herbs & Other Dietary Supplements

CAROTENOIDS: Other carotenoids may decrease the absorption of astaxanthin, by competing for absorption in the gastrointestinal tract. Carotenoids include beta-carotene, lutein, canthaxanthin, and lycopene (8456).

Interactions with Drugs

None known.

Interactions with Foods

CAROTENOID-CONTAINING FOODS: Carotenoids present in food may decrease the absorption of astaxanthin (8456). Carotenoids are found in a wide variety of vegetables and have high concentrations in carrots and tomatoes.

Interactions with Lab Tests

None known.

Interactions with Diseases or Conditions
None known.

Dosage and Administration
No typical dosage.

ASTRAGALUS

Also Known As
Astragali, Beg Kei, Bei Qi, Buck Qi, Huang Qi, Hwanggi, Membranous Milk Vetch, Milk Vetch, Mongolian Milk, Ogi.
CAUTION: See separate listing for Tragacanth.

Scientific Names
Astragalus membranaceus, synonym Phaca membranacea; Astragalus mongholicus.
Family: Fabaceae/Leguminosae or Papilionaceae.

People Use This For
Orally, astragalus is used for treating the common cold and upper respiratory infections; to strengthen and regulate the immune system; and to increase the production of blood cells particularly in individuals with chronic degenerative disease or in individuals with cancer undergoing chemotherapy or radiation therapy. It is also used orally for chronic nephritis, diabetes, as an antibacterial, antiviral, tonic, liver protectant, anti-inflammatory, antioxidant, as a diuretic, vasodilator, and as a hypotensive agent.
Topically, astragalus is used as a vasodilator and to speed healing.
In combination with Ligustrum lucidum (glossy privet), astragalus is used orally for treating breast cancer, cervical cancer, and lung cancer.

Safety
POSSIBLY SAFE ...when used orally and appropriately (12). Significant toxic reactions have not been reported (11,303); however, specific safety evaluations have not been performed. ...when used topically (12).
PREGNANCY AND LACTATION: Insufficient reliable information available.

Effectiveness
INSUFFICIENT RELIABLE EVIDENCE to RATE

Breast cancer and lung cancer. There is preliminary evidence that adjunctive use of astragalus in combination with glossy privet (Ligustrum lucidum) might increase survival rates in patients being treated conventionally for breast or lung cancer (303).
Common cold. There is preliminary evidence that long-term ingestion of astragalus might reduce the risk of catching the common cold (303).
Hepatitis. There is preliminary evidence that intravenous use of astragalus might be beneficial for patients with chronic hepatitis (303).
More evidence is needed to rate astragalus for these uses.

Mechanism of Action
The applicable part of astragalus is the root. Astragalus contains a variety of active constituents including more than 40 saponins such as astragaloside, several flavonoids, polysaccharides, multiple trace minerals, amino acids, and coumarins (11,303). Astragalus is an antioxidant. It inhibits free radical production, increases superoxide dismutase, and decreases lipid peroxidation (303). Astragalus is often promoted for its effects on the immune system, liver, and cardiovascular system. Astragalus seems to improve the immune response by potentiating the effects of interferon, and increasing antibody levels of IgA and IgG in nasal secretions (303). It also seems to improve the response of mononuclear cells and stimulate lymphocyte production (10777). Additionally, there is preliminary evidence that astragalus extracts can restore or improve immune function in cases of immune deficiency (423,3713). For example, astragalus seems to restore suppressed T-cell function in cancer patients (423). In animal models, an astragalus extract can reverse cyclophosphamide-induced immune deficiency (3713). Lower doses of astragalus appear to stimulate the immune system, but doses in excess of 28 grams might suppress immunity (303). When administered intravenously, some evidence suggests astragalus extract might increase proliferation and differentiation of bone marrow stem cells and progenitor cells (303). Astragalus also shows evidence of broad-spectrum antibiotic activity (303). In individuals with chronic hepatitis, astragalus seems to improve liver function as demonstrated by improvement in serum glutamate pyruvate transaminase (SGPT) levels (303). Astragalus is also thought to cause vasodilation and increase cardiac output which might be beneficial in angina, congestive heart failure, and post-myocardial infarction (303).

Adverse Reactions
The toxicity of astragalus root is reportedly "very low" (11). Although side effects have not been reported, doses greater than 28 grams might cause immunosuppression (303).

Interactions with Herbs & Other Dietary Supplements
None known.

Interactions with Drugs
CYCLOPHOSPHAMIDE: Some evidence suggests astragalus might reduce immunosuppression caused by cyclophosphamide (Cytoxan, Neosar) (303,3713).
IMMUNOSUPPRESSANTS: Theoretically, concurrent use might interfere with immunosuppressive therapy (303); avoid concurrent use. Immunosuppressant drugs include azathioprine (Imuran), basiliximab (Simulect), cyclosporine (Neoral, Sandimmune), daclizumab (Zenapax), muromonab-CD3 (OKT3, Orthoclone OKT3), mycophenolate (CellCept), tacrolimus (FK506, Prograf), sirolimus (Rapamune), prednisone (Deltasone, Orasone), and other corticosteroids (glucocorticoids).

Interactions with Foods
None known.

Interactions with Lab Tests
None known.

Interactions with Diseases or Conditions
AUTO-IMMUNE DISORDERS: Astragalus might increase immune system activity and may not be appropriate for individuals with auto-immune disorders (303).
ORGAN TRANSPLANT RECIPIENTS: Astragalus might interfere with immunosuppressive therapy; avoid concurrent use (303).

Dosage and Administration
ORAL: Astragalus powder 1-30 grams per day is typically used (11,303). For enhancing immune function for prevention of the common cold, 4-7 grams per day is commonly used (303). In some cases, people have used astragalus powder 30-60 grams per day (303). However, this should be avoided because some research suggests that doses greater than 28 grams per day offers no additional benefit and might even cause immune suppression (303). Astragalus decoction 0.5-1 L per day (maximum of 120 grams of whole root per liter of water) has been used (303). As a soup, mix 30 grams in 3.5 L of soup and simmer with other food ingredients (303).
TOPICAL: No typical dosage.

Comments
Astragalus is most commonly used in combination with other herbs (303).

AUTUMN CROCUS

Also Known As
Colchicum, Crocus, Fall Crocus, Meadow Saffran, Meadow Saffron, Mysteria, Naked Ladies, Upstart, Vellorita, Wonder Bulb.
CAUTION: See separate listing for Saffron.

Scientific Names
Colchicum autumnale; Colchicum speciosum; Colchicum vernum.
Family: Colchicaceae or Liliaceae.

People Use This For
Orally, autumn crocus is used for arthritis, gout, and familial Mediterranean fever.

Safety
UNSAFE ...when used orally for self-medication because it is a potential poison (6,500). Human intoxication can occur when corms, which are the underground bulb-like stems, are mistaken for onions and ingested (6).
PREGNANCY AND LACTATION: UNSAFE ...when used orally because autumn crocus is a potential mutagen and toxin (500); avoid using.

Effectiveness
There is insufficient reliable information available about the effectiveness of autumn crocus.

Mechanism of Action
The applicable parts of autumn crocus are the seed, tuber, and flower. The seeds of this plant contain at least 0.4% colchicine, which is the constituent responsible for its therapeutic benefit (2).

Adverse Reactions
Orally, autumn crocus can cause burning of the mouth and throat, thirst, nausea, vomiting, diarrhea, liver necrosis, hypovolemic shock, kidney impairment, multiorgan failure, and death (6,553). Long-term use of colchicine is associated with agranulocytosis, aplastic anemia, and peripheral neuritis (6). Human intoxication can occur when corms, which are the underground bulb-like stems, are mistaken for onions or when contaminated milk is ingested (6).
Topically, handling fresh corm slices can cause finger numbness (6).

Interactions with Herbs & Other Dietary Supplements
None known.

Interactions with Drugs
COLCHICINE: Avoid concomitant use of autumn crocus with colchicine because it can increase therapeutic and adverse effects (2).

Interactions with Foods
None known.

Interactions with Lab Tests
URIC ACID: Autumn crocus can lower serum uric acid concentrations and test results due to its colchicine content (8).

Interactions with Diseases or Conditions
None known.

Dosage and Administration
ORAL: Dosing is related to the colchicine content (2). Due to its toxic potential, use the standardized, FDA-approved colchicine. Gout and familial Mediterranean fever require diagnosis, treatment, and monitoring by a medical professional.

Comments
Colchicine is available by prescription and used to treat acute gout attacks and familial Mediterranean fever (506).

AVENS

Also Known As
Benedict's Herb, Bennet's Root, Colewort, Geum, Herb Bennet.

Scientific Names
Geum urbanum.
Family: Rosaceae.

People Use This For
Orally, avens is used to treat diarrhea, catarrhal colitis, uterine bleeding, intermittent fevers, and ulcerative colitis.
In foods, avens is used as a source of food flavoring.

Safety
LIKELY SAFE ...when used in amounts typically found in foods. The Council of Europe allows avens as a natural source of food flavoring (4).
There is insufficient reliable information available about the safety of avens for its other uses.
PREGNANCY AND LACTATION: POSSIBLY UNSAFE ...when used orally because avens seems to have an affect on the menstrual cycle (4); avoid using.

Effectiveness
There is insufficient reliable information available about the effectiveness of avens.

Mechanism of Action
The applicable parts of avens are the above ground parts. The tannin-type constituents of avens have an astringent action; this supports the traditional use of avens for treating diarrhea (4).

Adverse Reactions
None reported.

Interactions with Herbs & Other Dietary Supplements
None known.

Interactions with Drugs
None known.

Interactions with Foods
None known.

Interactions with Lab Tests
None known.

Interactions with Diseases or Conditions
None known.

Dosage and Administration
ORAL: People typically use 1-4 grams steeped in boiling water, strained, three times a day (4). Liquid extract (1:1 in 25% alcohol) 1-4 mL three times a day has also been used (4).

Comments
Avens is very rarely used medicinally today (18).

AVOCADO

Also Known As
Abokado, Ahuacate, Alligator Pear, Avocato.

Scientific Names
Persea americana; Persea americana var. americana, synonyms Laurus persea, Persea gratissima, Persea leiogyna, Persea persea.
Family: Lauraceae.

People Use This For
Orally, avocado fruit is used to reduce serum cholesterol levels, as an aphrodisiac and to stimulate menstrual flow. Unsaponifiable fractions of the oil are used to treat osteoarthritis. The seeds, leaves, and bark are used for dysentery and diarrhea.
Topically, avocado oil is applied to soothe and heal skin, treat sclerosis of the skin, pyorrhea, and arthritis. The fruit pulp is used topically to promote hair growth and hasten wound healing. The seeds, leaves, and bark are used to relieve toothache.
In foods, avocado fruit is edible.

Safety
LIKELY SAFE ...when the fruit is consumed in amounts commonly found in foods (668,669,670,671).
POSSIBLY SAFE ...when unsaponifiable fractions of avocado oil are used orally and appropriately in medicinal amounts. Unsaponifiable fractions of avocado oil appear to be safe for up to 6 months (10693).
There is insufficient reliable information available about the safety of avocado for its other uses.
PREGNANCY AND LACTATION: There is insufficient reliable information available about the safety of avocado used in medicinal amounts during pregnancy and lactation.

Effectiveness

POSSIBLY EFFECTIVE

Hypercholesterolemia. An avocado-enriched diet high in monounsaturated fatty acids seems to lower total serum cholesterol, low-density lipoprotein (LDL) cholesterol, and apolipoprotein B. It may also increase high-density lipoprotein (HDL) serum cholesterol levels (668,669,670,671).

Osteoarthritis. Taking unsaponifiable fractions of avocado and soybean oils orally appears to significantly improve pain and overall disability. It seems to be more effective for hip than knee osteoarthritis (10693).

There is insufficient reliable information available about the effectiveness of avocado for its other uses.

Mechanism of Action

The applicable parts of avocado are the fruit, leaves, and seed. Among fruits, avocado contains more protein and fiber than most. It also contains manganese, phosphorous, iron, potassium, vitamin E, vitamin C, Beta-carotene, thiamin, riboflavin, nicotinic acid, and folate. It is relatively low in sodium and simple sugars. Avocado is rich in oil (15-30 g/100 g fresh fruit) that is mainly monounsaturated. It is a good source of linoleic acid. Its high fiber content might be responsible for its cholesterol-lowering effects (11010).

Unsaponifiable fractions of avocado and soybean oils may reduce the progression of joint space loss in patients with osteoarthritis who have advanced joint space narrowing of the hip (10694). Preliminary evidence suggests this combination can inhibit cartilage degradation and promote cartilage repair in osteoarthritic chondrocytes (10695).

Adverse Reactions

Allergic cross-sensitivity may be seen in latex-sensitive individuals (6197,7853).

Interactions with Herbs & Other Dietary Supplements

None known.

Interactions with Drugs

WARFARIN (Coumadin): Avocado may antagonize the anticoagulant effects of warfarin, but there has been only one case report of this interaction (667).

Interactions with Foods

None known.

Interactions with Lab Tests

CHOLESTEROL: Avocado can lower serum total cholesterol, LDL cholesterol, and apolipoprotein B concentrations and test results. Avocado can increase serum HDL cholesterol concentrations and test results (668,669,670,671).

Interactions with Diseases or Conditions

LATEX ALLERGY: People who are allergic to latex should avoid eating avocado because of the possibility of cross hypersensitivity between latex and avocado (6197,7853).

Dosage and Administration

ORAL: For lowering cholesterol, avocado is dosed in relation to dietary calorie content or fat intake (668,669,670,671,675). For osteoarthritis, 300 mg daily (a combination of one-third avocado and two-thirds soybean unsaponifiables) has been used (10693).

BA JI TIAN

Also Known As

Bi Ji, Indian Mulberry, Morinda, Morinda Root, Morindae officinalis, Morindae radix, Noni.
CAUTION: See separate listing for Morinda.

Scientific Names

Morinda officinalis.
Family: Rubiaceae.

People Use This For

Orally, ba ji tian is used for cancer, cholecystitis, debility, enuresis, polyuria, hernia, impotence, premature ejaculation, back pain, depression, increasing white blood cell count, stimulating the endocrine system, improving kidney function, strengthening the skeletal and nervous systems, and as a kidney tonic to strengthen the yang.

Safety

LIKELY SAFE ...when used orally and appropriately (12).
PREGNANCY AND LACTATION: Insufficient reliable information available; avoid using.

Effectiveness

There is insufficient reliable information available about the effectiveness of ba ji tian.

Mechanism of Action

The applicable part of ba ji tian is the root. The root contains several active constituents, including an iridoid lactone called morindolide, iridoid glucosides including morofficinaloside, anthraquinones, a monoterpene glycoside, sterols including beta-sitosterol, an ursane-type triterpene, a lactone compound, and 24-ethylcholesterol (448,451,452). However, the roles of specific constituents have not been described. Constituents reported to have antidepressant activity have been isolated (succinic acid, nystose, 1F-fructofuranosylnystose, inulin-type hexasaccharide, and heptasaccharide) (449). Ba ji tian is thought to work in depression by increasing serotonergic effects (3558). A study in mice reported that ba ji tian had anti-fatigue properties, reversed radiation-induced leukopenia, and reduced excitability of the parasympathetic nervous system associated with hypothyroidism (453).

Adverse Reactions

None reported.

Interactions with Herbs & Other Dietary Supplements

None known.

Interactions with Drugs

None known.

Interactions with Foods

None known.

Interactions with Lab Tests

None known.

Interactions with Diseases or Conditions

DYSURIA: Theoretically, ba ji tian may exacerbate urinary difficulties. Ba ji tian is reported to stimulate the kidneys. Use with caution (12).

Dosage and Administration

No typical dosage.

Comments

In some commercial preparations, Morinda officinalis is combined with Morinda citrifolia.

BAEL

Also Known As

Bel, Bengal Quince, Bilva, Bilwa, Indian Bael, Shivaphala.

Scientific Names

Aegle marmelos.
Family: Rutaceae.

Comments

At the date of publication, there was very little scientific information about this product. Our staff is continually analyzing the available information on natural medicines and will add data to the online version of *Natural Medicines Comprehensive Database* as it becomes available. See www.naturaldatabase.com.

BAIKAL SKULLCAP

Also Known As

Baikal Scullcap, Baikal Skullcap Root, Chinese Scullcap, Chinese Skullcap, Huang Qin, Huangquin, Hwanggum, Ogon, Ou-gon, Scullcap, Scute, Skullcap, Wogon.
CAUTION: See separate listing for Skullcap.

Scientific Names

Scutellaria baicalensis, synonym Scutellaria macrantha.
Family: Lamiaceae/Labiatae.

People Use This For

Orally, Baikal skullcap is used to treat respiratory and gastrointestinal infections, allergic rhinitis, jaundice, viral hepatitis, nephritis, pelvic inflammation, sores or swelling, and fever. It is also used orally for scarlet fever, headache, irritability, red eyes, flushed face, seizures, epilepsy, hysteria, nervous tension, and a bitter taste in the mouth.
In combination with shung hua, the Baikal skullcap constituent baicalin is used to treat upper respiratory tract infections. In combination with other herbs, Baikal skullcap is used to treat minimal brain dysfunction, prostate cancer, and hemorrhoids.

Safety

POSSIBLY SAFE ...when used orally and appropriately (5549,5550,5551).
PREGNANCY AND LACTATION: Insufficient reliable information available; avoid using.

Effectiveness

There is insufficient reliable information available about the effectiveness of Baikal skullcap.

Mechanism of Action

The applicable parts of Baikal skullcap are the root and to a lesser extent the above ground parts. Most pharmacological activity has been attributed to flavonoid constituents, including baicalin, baicalein, wogonin, and scutellarein. These flavonoids all appear to bind to GABA receptors with possibly benzodiazepine-like effects (6290,6291). The constituent baicalein has weak antipyretic properties and might also have antimutagenic (6294) alpha-glucosidase (6292) activity, according to preliminary evidence.
Baicalin, a glycoside constituent, has potent anti-inflammatory and antitumor properties (5541). Some evidence suggests it can inhibit tumor growth and suppress carcinoma cell proliferation (5541). Baicalin also shows evidence that it might inhibit HIV-1 infection and replication by inhibiting HIV reverse transcriptase (5541). Baicalein and baicalin are reported to be more active free-radical scavengers than alpha-tocopherol (vitamin E) (5541,6293) Baikal skullcap also appears to have antibacterial and antiviral properties, as well as antifungal activity, particularly against Candida albicans (5541,6295). It also might have diuretic and antihypertensive properties (5541).

Adverse Reactions

Orally, Baikal skullcap is generally well tolerated. However, several case reports implicate Baikal skullcap in hepatotoxicity (4284). Baikal skullcap can cause pneumonitis (9185). Use of Baikal skullcap as an intramuscular injection can cause fever and a sudden drop in the leukocyte count (5541). Theoretically, Baikal skullcap could cause sedation (6290,6291).

Interactions with Herbs & Other Dietary Supplements

HERBS WITH SEDATIVE PROPERTIES: Theoretically, concomitant use with herbs that have sedative properties might enhance therapeutic and adverse effects (6290,6291). Some of these include 5-HTP, calamus, California poppy, catnip, hops, Jamaican dogwood, kava, St. John's wort, scullcap, valerian, yerba mansa, and others.

Interactions with Drugs

ALCOHOL (Ethanol): Theoretically, Baikal skullcap can potentiate the sedative effects of alcohol (6290,6291); use with caution.
ANTIDIABETES DRUGS: Theoretically, concomitant use might enhance blood glucose lowering effects due to alpha-glucosidase inhibitor activity of the constituent baicalein (6292). Monitor blood glucose levels closely.
BENZODIAZEPINES: Theoretically, concomitant use with benzodiazepines can cause additive therapeutic and adverse effects (6290,6291); use with caution.
CNS DEPRESSANTS: Theoretically, concomitant use of Baikal skullcap and drugs with sedative properties can cause additive therapeutic and adverse effects (6290,6291); use with caution.

Interactions with Foods

None known.

Interactions with Lab Tests

BLOOD GLUCOSE: Theoretically, Baikal skullcap might reduce postprandial blood glucose concentrations and test results due to alpha-glucosidase activity (6292).

Interactions with Diseases or Conditions

DIABETES: Theoretically, Baikal skullcap could have hypoglycemic activity (6292). Use in diabetics might increase the risk of hypoglycemic episodes; use with caution.
STOMACH DYSFUNCTION: Baikal skullcap should not be used by individuals with stomach or spleen dysfunction (5544).

Dosage and Administration

ORAL: A typical dose is 6-15 grams of Baikal skullcap, toasted to moderate the effect (5544). A typical dose of the Baikal skullcap constituent baicalin to treat viral hepatitis is 500 mg three times daily (5541). A typical dose to treat an upper respiratory tract infection is a tablet containing 50 mg of the Baikal skullcap constituent baicalin in combination with 100 mg of shung hua. Two to three tablets are taken four to six times per day (5541).

Comments

Common substitutions for Scutellaria baicalensis (Baikal scullcap) in Chinese medicine include Scutellaria viscidula, Scutellaria amonea, and Scutellaria ikoninikovii (5541).

BAMBOO

Also Known As

Arrow Bamboo, Yadake.

Scientific Names

Pseudosasa japonica, synonyms Arundinaria japonica, Sasa japonica.
Family: Poaceae/Gramineae.

Comments

At the date of publication, there was very little scientific information about this product. Our staff is continually analyzing the available information on natural medicines and will add data to the online version of *Natural Medicines Comprehensive Database* as it becomes available. See www.naturaldatabase.com.

BANABA

Also Known As

Corosolic Acid, Crape Myrtle, Crepe Myrtle, Pride-of-India, Pyinma, Queen's Crape Myrtle.

Scientific Names

Lagerstroemia speciosa; synonyms Lagerstroemia flos-reginae, Munchausia speciosa.
Family: Lythraceae.

People Use This For

Orally, banaba is used for diabetes and weight loss.

Safety

POSSIBLY SAFE ...when banaba extract is used orally for 15 days (11954). The safety of long-term use is unknown.
PREGNANCY AND LACTATION: Insufficient reliable information available; avoid using.

Effectiveness

INSUFFICIENT RELIABLE EVIDENCE to RATE

Diabetes. Preliminary clinical research suggests that orally administered banaba extract, standarized to 1% corosolic acid, might lower blood sugar in people with type 2 diabetes (11954). More evidence is needed to rate banaba for this use.

Mechanism of Action

The applicable part of the banaba tree is the leaf. Active constituents include corosolic acid and the ellagitannins lagerstroemin, flosin B, and reginin A (11954,11955,11956). In diabetic animals and in humans with type 2 diabetes, banaba extract lowers blood glucose (11954,11955). In vitro research suggests that the ellagitannins have an insulin-like

effect (11956). Research on lagerstroemin suggests that it might activate insulin receptors (11957).
The banaba constituent valoneic acid seems to have xanthine oxidase activity similar to or better than allopurinol, according to in vitro research (11958).
In genetically diabetic obese mice, banaba seems to suppress weight gain (11959). However, this antiobesity effect has not been tested in nondiabetic animals or humans.

Adverse Reactions
None reported.

Interactions with Herbs & Other Dietary Supplements
HERBS WITH HYPOGLYCEMIC POTENTIAL: Theoretically, banaba might have additive effects with herbs that decrease blood glucose levels (11954). Herbs with hypoglycemic potential include alpha-lipoic acid, devil's claw, fenugreek, garlic, guar gum, horse chestnut, Panax ginseng, psyllium, and Siberian ginseng.

Interactions with Drugs
ANTIDIABETES DRUGS: Theoretically, banaba might enhance the blood glucose-lowering effects of hypoglycemic drugs (11954). Monitor blood glucose levels closely. Some antidiabetes drugs include glimepiride (Amaryl), glyburide (Diabeta, Glynase PresTabs, Micronase), insulin, metformin (Glucophage), pioglitazone (Actos), rosiglitazone (Avandia), and others.

Interactions with Foods
None known.

Interactions with Lab Tests
BLOOD GLUCOSE: Banaba can lower blood sugar resulting in lower blood glucose test results (11954).

Interactions with Diseases or Conditions
DIABETES: Banaba can affect blood sugar control, and blood glucose levels should be monitored closely (11954).

Dosage and Administration
ORAL: For lowering blood sugar in people with type 2 diabetes, 16 to 48 mg per day has been used (11954).

Comments
Banaba is the Tagalog name for a species of crepe myrtle that is native to the Philippines and Southeast Asia (11954).

BARLEY

Also Known As
Cereal Fiber, Dietary Fiber, Hordeum, Mai Ya, Pearl Barley, Pot Barley, Scotch Barley.

Scientific Names
Hordeum vulgare; Hordeum distychum.
Family: Poaceae/Gramineae.

People Use This For
Orally, barley is used for bronchitis, diarrhea, gastritis, inflammatory bowel conditions, and cancer prevention. It is also used for lowering blood sugar, blood pressure, and cholesterol, and for promoting weight loss. It is also used for increasing strength and stamina.
Topically, barley is used for treating boils.
In foods, barley is utilized as a source of vitamins, carbohydrates, proteins, and fatty oils.
In manufacturing, barley is used as a food grain, natural sweetener, and as an ingredient for brewing beer and making alcoholic beverages.

Safety
POSSIBLY SAFE ...when used orally in medicinal amounts (11463).
PREGNANCY: LIKELY SAFE ...when used in moderate amounts as a food (19). POSSIBLY UNSAFE ...when barley sprouts are consumed in relatively high doses. Excessive amounts of barley sprouts should not be consumed during pregnancy (19).
LACTATION: Insufficient reliable information available; avoid using.

Effectiveness

POSSIBLY EFFECTIVE

Gastric cancer. Epidemiologic evidence suggests that dietary fiber consumed in the diet might reduce the incidence of stomach cancer (10435).

Hypercholesterolemia. Taking barley orally seems to reduce total cholesterol and low-density lipoprotein (LDL) cholesterol when added to the National Cholesterol Education Program's Step I diet (11134,11986). The effect of barley on cholesterol appears to be dose dependent. Taking 0.4, 3, or 6 grams of soluble fiber from barley daily reduces total cholesterol by 14%, 17%, and 20% respectively. LDL is lowered by 17% to 24%. Barley also seems to lower triglycerides by 6% to 16% and increase high density lipoprotein (HDL) cholesterol by 9% to 18% (11986). However, barley that is highly enriched with beta-glucan doesn't seem to affect cholesterol. This lack of effect seems to be the result of processing the barley into a highly enriched beta-glucan product (10166). Taking barley orally also seems to produce modest, but significant reductions in systolic, diastolic, and mean arterial blood pressures in non-hypertensive patients with moderate hypercholesterolemia (11463).

POSSIBLY INEFFECTIVE

Colorectal cancer. Dietary cereal fiber, including barley fiber, doesn't seem to the reduce the risk of colorectal cancer (160,4819,4820,4821,5104).

There is insufficient reliable information available about the effectiveness of barley for its other uses.

Mechanism of Action

The applicable part of barley is the grain. Barley contains 5% to 10% beta-glucan, a soluble fiber (10166). The fiber content of barley is likely responsible for the observed reduction of cholesterol levels in healthy and hypercholesterolemic people (11134). Researchers think soluble fiber such as barley might increase the excretion of bile acids or neutral sterols (cholesterol precursors), increase catabolism of low-density lipoprotein (LDL) cholesterol, and reduce fat absorption (11986).

Researchers also think that the beta-glucan contained in barley helps control appetite by slowing stomach emptying, prolonging the feeling of fullness, and stabilizing blood sugar (11135). Several mechanisms have been proposed for reducing blood pressure, including an increase in electrolyte and water excretion, alteration of gastric emptying time, and an increase in fecal mineral loss (11463).

Barley contains hordenine, a sympathomimetic. There have been no reports of stimulant effects in humans (11136). The enzyme, diastase, is responsible for barley's ability to ferment (216).

Adverse Reactions

Orally, beer made with barley can cause anaphylaxis in sensitive individuals (317). Occupational exposure to barley flour can cause asthma (1300).

Interactions with Herbs & Other Dietary Supplements

HERBS AND SUPPLEMENTS WITH HYPOGLYCEMIC EFFECTS: There is some evidence that barley might lower blood glucose (11135). Theoretically, concomitant use with other herbs and supplements that decrease blood glucose levels might increase the risk of hypoglycemia. Some of these products include bitter melon, ginger, goat's rue, fenugreek, kudzu, willow bark, and others.

Interactions with Drugs

ANTIDIABETES DRUGS: Theoretically, concomitant use might enhance blood glucose lowering effects (11135). Monitor blood glucose levels closely. Some antidiabetes drugs include glimepiride (Amaryl), glyburide (DiaBeta, Glynase PresTab, Micronase), insulin, pioglitazone (Actos), rosiglitazone (Avandia), and others.

ORAL DRUGS: Theoretically, fiber can reduce the absorption of some drugs by reducing the gastrointestinal transit time (11135).

Interactions with Foods

None known.

Interactions with Lab Tests

CHOLESTEROL: Barley might reduce serum total cholesterol and LDL cholesterol concentrations and test results (11134).

GLUCOSE: Barley might reduce blood glucose concentrations and test results (11135).

URINE DRUG SCREENS: The barley constituent, hordenine, can yield false-positive test results with ELISA, RIA and TLC urine assays for a number of opiate drugs. Positive urine test results should be confirmed with the more sensitive GC/MS or HPLC assay (1302).

Interactions with Diseases or Conditions

CELIAC DISEASE: The gluten content in barley can exacerbate celiac disease (11137); avoid using.

Dosage and Administration

ORAL: For lowering cholesterol, 3 grams of barley oil extract or 30 grams of barley bran flour or 0.4 to 6 grams of soluble fiber from barley added to a National Cholesterol Education Program (NCEP) Step I diet has been used (11134,11986). For reducing blood pressure, 3-6 grams barley flakes, barley flour, or pearled barley daily, combined with a National Cholesterol Education Program (NCEP) Step I diet has been used in non-hypertensive patients with moderate hypercholesterolemia (11463).

Comments

Barley is a common grain that is used world-wide as a food and in the brewing processes of alcoholic beverages. Avoid confusion with malt extract products that do not contain the enzyme diastase and are intended for use as bulk laxatives (13).

BASIL

Also Known As

Basilici Herba, Common Basil, Garden Basil, Munjariki, St. Josephwort, Surasa, Sweet Basil, Vanatulasi, Varvara.

Scientific Names

Ocimum basilicum.
Family: Lamiaceae/Labiatae.

People Use This For

Orally, basil is used for stomach spasms, kidney conditions, before and after childbirth to promote blood circulation, and to treat snakebites and insect bites. It is also used orally as an appetite stimulant, antiflatulent, diuretic, lactation stimulant, gargle and mouth astringent, and in maggot-infested nasal disease. Basil is also used to treat head colds, worms and warts.
In foods, basil is used as an oil or oleoresin at levels usually below 0.005%.

Safety

LIKELY SAFE ...when used orally in amounts commonly found in foods. Basil has Generally Recognized As Safe (GRAS) status in the US (4912).
POSSIBLY SAFE ...when the above ground parts are used orally and appropriately short-term (2,8,12).
POSSIBLY UNSAFE ...when the above ground parts of basil are used orally long-term. ...when the oil of basil is used orally (12). Both the above ground parts and the oil contain estragole which shows evidence that it might be hepatocarcinogenic (8) and mutagenic (2).
CHILDREN: LIKELY SAFE ...when the above ground parts are used as a spice. POSSIBLY UNSAFE ...when used orally in larger amounts due to the estragole constituents (2,8).
PREGNANCY AND LACTATION: LIKELY SAFE ...when the above ground parts are used as a spice. POSSIBLY UNSAFE ...when used in larger amounts due to the estragole constituent of the essential oil. Estragole might have mutagenic effects (2,12).

Effectiveness

There is insufficient reliable information available about the effectiveness of basil.

Mechanism of Action

The applicable parts of basil are the above ground plant parts. The basil plant is a rich source of vitamin C, calcium, magnesium, potassium, and iron (19). The basil constituents methyl cinnamate, methyl chavicol, ocimene, cineole, and linalool have insecticidal activities (11). The volatile oil of basil can have antagonistic activity on worms (11). The essential oil contains up to 85% estragole (2) (methyl chavicol), which can produce liver tumors in mice (11). The constituent, xanthomicrol, can have cytotoxic and antineoplastic activities (11).

Adverse Reactions

Orally, basil is known to cause hypoglycemia (6002). Due to the adverse effects of the constituents of basil, CAUTION should be used in long-term treatment, which may be unsafe (12).

Interactions with Herbs & Other Dietary Supplements

None known.

Interactions with Drugs

None known.

Interactions with Foods
None known.

Interactions with Lab Tests
None known.

Interactions with Diseases or Conditions
None known.

Dosage and Administration
ORAL: The typical dose of basil leaf for distention or flatulence is 1 cup of the fresh brewed tea 2-3 times a day between meals. The tea is prepared by steeping 2-4 grams in 150 mL boiling water for 10-15 minutes and straining (8). For chronic flatulence the usual oral dose is 1 cup 2-3 times daily between meals for 8 days, then stopped for 14 days, and resumed for another 8 days (8).

Comments
Due to the carcinogenic potential of basil oil; avoid using (18).

BAYBERRY

Also Known As
Candleberry, Myrica, Southern Bayberry, Southern Wax Myrtle, Tallow Shrub, Vegetable Tallow, Wax Myrtle, Waxberry.
CAUTION: See separate listings for Sweet Gale and Tung Seed.

Scientific Names
Morella cerifera, synonyms Myrica cerifera, Myrica pumila; Morella caroliniensis, synonyms Myrica pensylvanica, Morella pensylvanica, Myrica caroliniensis, Myrica heterophylla.
Family: Myricaceae.

People Use This For
Orally, bayberry is used for head colds, mucous colitis, diarrhea, as an antipyretic, a circulatory stimulant, and an emetic in large doses.
Topically, bayberry is used as a gargle for sore throat, as a douche for leukorrhea (vaginal discharge), for indolent ulcers, and wound healing.

Safety
POSSIBLY UNSAFE ...when used orally. The root bark and berries contain high amounts of tannins (6). Large doses may have mineralocorticoid activity (4). Root bark can also contain a carcinogen (5).
There is insufficient reliable information available about the safety of bayberry for its other uses.
PREGNANCY AND LACTATION: POSSIBLY UNSAFE ...when used orally or topically because of possible carcinogenic, or mineralocorticoid activities; avoid using (4,5).

Effectiveness
There is insufficient reliable information available about the effectiveness of bayberry.

Mechanism of Action
The applicable parts of bayberry are the root bark and berry. The tannin constituents of bayberry are responsible for its astringent action (4).

Adverse Reactions
Orally, bayberry can cause gastrointestinal irritation, vomiting, liver damage (possibly due to tannin content), and can act as an irritant and sensitizer (6).

Interactions with Herbs & Other Dietary Supplements
None known.

Interactions with Drugs
None known.

Interactions with Foods
None known.

Interactions with Lab Tests
None known.

Interactions with Diseases or Conditions
HYPERTENSION: Consuming large amounts of tannin-containing herbs such as bayberry can cause sodium and water retention and possibly increase blood pressure (4).

Dosage and Administration
ORAL: The typical dose of bayberry is 0.6-2 grams powdered bark, steeped in boiling water and strained, used three times a day (4). The liquid extract of bayberry (1:1 in 45% alcohol) is typically used 0.6-2 mL three times a day (4).
TOPICAL: No typical dosage.

Comments
Bayberry is a shrub that is commonly found in Texas and the eastern US. The wax extract taken from the berries is used in fragrances and candles.

BEAN POD

Also Known As
Cannelli Beans, Common Bean, Green Bean, Legume, Navy Bean, Phaseoli fructus, Pinto Bean, Seed-Free Bean Pods, Sine Semine, Snap Bean, Starch Blocker, String Bean, Wax Bean, White Kidney Bean.

Scientific Names
Phaseolus vulgaris; Phaseolus vulgaris varieties.
Family: Fabaceae/Leguminosae.

People Use This For
Orally, bean pod is used for urinary tract infections, kidney or bladder stones, and for the promotion of urine flow. It is also as a diuretic and for diabetes.

Safety
POSSIBLY SAFE ...when the ripe, dried pods are used orally and appropriately in medicinal amounts (18).
POSSIBLY UNSAFE ...when large amounts of fresh bean husks are ingested. Raw bean husks contain lectins that can cause gastrointestinal upset. Cooking destroys lectins (18).
PREGNANCY AND LACTATION: Insufficient reliable information available; avoid using.

Effectiveness
INSUFFICIENT RELIABLE EVIDENCE to RATE

Hypercholesterolemia. There is preliminary clinical evidence that a bean pod and carob extract might modestly decrease cholesterol levels and excretion of fat in feces of overweight and obese patients (10633). More evidence is needed to rate bean pod for this use.

Mechanism of Action
The applicable part of bean pod is the pod without the seeds. Bean pod is a source of dietary fiber, which suggests it might modestly reduce lipids. It might also bind cholic acids and fat, thereby reducing fat absorption (10633).

Adverse Reactions
Orally, large amounts of green bean husks, or raw green beans, can cause vomiting, diarrhea, and gastroenteritis due to the content of the plant protein lectin. Cooking usually destroys lectins (18).

Interactions with Herbs & Other Dietary Supplements
None known.

Interactions with Drugs
ANTIDIABETES DRUGS: Monitor blood glucose levels closely due to claims that bean pod has hypoglycemic effects (19).

Interactions with Foods
None known.

Interactions with Lab Tests
None known.

Interactions with Diseases or Conditions
DIABETES: Monitor blood glucose level closely due to claims that bean pod has hypoglycemic effects (19).

Dosage and Administration
ORAL: For improvement of lipid profiles and excretion of fat in feces, bean pod (Phaseolus vulgaris, kidney bean) 300-600 mg three times daily, combined with carob gum 50-100 mg three times daily, has been used (10633).

BEAR'S GARLIC

Also Known As
Bears Garlic, Broad-leaved Garlic, Ramsons, Wild Garlic.

Scientific Names
Allium ursinum.
Family: Liliaceae or Alliaceae.

Comments
At the date of publication, this product was not a common ingredient used in brand name supplements marketed to consumers. Details about this product are available at the online version of *Natural Medicines Comprehensive Database*. See www.naturaldatabase.com.

BEE POLLEN

Also Known As
Bee Pollen Extract, Buckwheat Pollen, Honeybee Pollen, Honey Bee Pollen, Maize Pollen, Pine Pollen, Pollen, Pollen D'Abeille.
CAUTION: See separate listings for Bee Venom, Honey, and Royal Jelly.

Scientific Names
None.

People Use This For
Orally, bee pollen is used for nutrition, as an appetite stimulant, to improve stamina and athletic performance, for premature aging, premenstrual syndrome (PMS), hay fever or allergic rhinitis, mouth sores, rheumatism, painful urination, prostate conditions, and radiation sickness. It is also used orally for bleeding problems including coughing or vomiting blood, bloody diarrhea, nosebleed, cerebral hemorrhage, and menstrual problems. Bee pollen is also used for gastrointestinal (GI) problems including constipation, diarrhea, enteritis, colitis, as a general tonic, diuretic, and for alcohol intoxication.
Topically, bee pollen is used for skin care in skin softening products, and for treating eczema, pustular eruptions, and diaper rash.

Safety
POSSIBLY SAFE ...when used orally and appropriately, short-term (7062,7063,12008). There is some evidence that taking bee pollen extracts for up to approximately 30 days is safe (7063). There is also preliminary evidence that taking 2 tablets twice daily of a specific combination product containing royal jelly 6 mg, bee pollen extract 36 mg, and bee pollen plus pistil extract 120 mg (Femal, Natumin Pharma) per tablet for up to 2 months seems to be safe (12008).
PREGNANCY: POSSIBLY UNSAFE ...when used orally. There is some concern that bee pollen might have uterine stimulant effects (5,6,11); avoid using.
LACTATION: Insufficient reliable information available; avoid using.

Effectiveness

POSSIBLY INEFFECTIVE

Athletic performance. Taking bee pollen orally doesn't seem to increase athletic performance or stamina (7062,7063).

INSUFFICIENT RELIABLE EVIDENCE to RATE

Premenstrual syndrome (PMS). Preliminary evidence suggests that a specific combination product (Femal, Natumin Pharma) seems to decrease some symptoms of PMS including irritability, weight increases, and edema when given over a period of 2 menstrual cycles. This product contains royal jelly 6 mg, bee pollen extract 36 mg, and bee pollen plus pistil extract 120 mg per tablet. It is given as 2 tablets twice daily (12008). More evidence is needed to rate bee pollen for this use.

Mechanism of Action

Bee pollen refers to the pollen from flowers that collects on the legs and bodies of worker bees. It can also include amounts of nectar and bee saliva. Bee pollen composition varies depending on plant source and geographic region. Up to 50% of bee pollen may be polysaccharides. The other constituents include lipids, protein, simple sugars, vitamin C, and carotenoids (5). Proponents often claim that enzymes in bee pollen provide a variety of therapeutic benefits. However, any enzymes in bee pollen are likely to be digested in the gastrointestinal (GI) tract. There is no reliable evidence indicating that bee pollen enzymes or other constituents in bee pollen offer any therapeutic benefit.

Adverse Reactions

Orally, bee pollen seems to be well tolerated in most patients. There is one report of dizziness in a patient who took a combination product containing royal jelly, bee pollen extract, and a bee pollen plus pistil extract (12008).
Patients with pollen allergies are at risk for serious allergic reactions. Allergic reactions can include itching, swelling, shortness of breath, light headedness, and anaphylaxis. Chronic allergy symptoms due to bee pollen include gastrointestinal (GI) and neurologic symptoms and eosinophilia (5,6,11). There have also been two cases of acute hepatitis associated with bee pollen use. One case involved ingestion of two tablespoons of pure bee pollen daily for several months. Another case involved ingestion of 14 tablets per day of a combination herbal product containing bee pollen, chaparral, and 19 other herbs for 6 weeks (1351). In this case it is not known if bee pollen or another herb might have caused the adverse event.

Interactions with Herbs & Other Dietary Supplements

None known.

Interactions with Drugs

None known.

Interactions with Foods

None known.

Interactions with Lab Tests

LIVER FUNCTION TESTS: Bee pollen might increase alkaline phosphatase (Alk Phos), alanine aminotransferase (ALT), aspartate aminotransferase (AST), lactate dehydrogenase (LDH), total bilirubin, prothrombin time (PT), and test results. Bee pollen has been associated with two cases of acute hepatitis and abnormally high results for these tests (1351).

Interactions with Diseases or Conditions

LIVER DISEASE: Use of bee pollen has been associated with two cases of acute hepatitis (1351). Avoid using in patients with existing liver disease.
POLLEN ALLERGY: Patients with pollen allergies are at risk for serious allergic reactions. Allergic reactions can include itching, swelling, shortness of breath, light headedness, and anaphylaxis (5,6).

Dosage and Administration

ORAL: For premenstrual syndrome (PMS), two tablets twice daily of a specific combination containing royal jelly 6 mg, bee pollen extract 36 mg, and bee pollen plus pistil extract 120 mg (Femal, Natumin Pharma) per tablet for 2 menstrual cycles has been used (12008).

Comments

Pollens come from various plants, including buckwheat, maize, pine (songhuafen), rape, and typha (puhuang) (11). Avoid confusion with bee venom, honey, and royal jelly.

BEE VENOM

Also Known As

Apis Venenum Purum, Apitoxin, Bald-Faced Hornet, Bee Sting Venom, Bumblebee Venom, Honeybee Venom, Mixed Vespids, Pure Bee Venom, Wasp Venom, White-Faced Hornet, Yellow Hornet, Yellow-Jacket Venom. CAUTION: See separate listings for Bee Pollen, Honey, and Royal Jelly.

Scientific Names

Apis mellifera (Honeybee); Bombus terrestis (Bumblebee); Vespula maculata (Hornet, Wasp). Family: Apidae; Vespidae.

People Use This For

Parenterally, bee venom is used for rheumatoid arthritis, neuralgias, multiple sclerosis, desensitization to bee stings (venom immunotherapy), tendonitis and tendosynovitis, and muscle conditions such as fibromyositis and enthesitis.

Safety

LIKELY SAFE ...when used by subcutaneous injection by a trained medical professional (2619,6070). Purified bee venom for subcutaneous injection is an FDA approved product (2619).
PREGNANCY AND LACTATION: POSSIBLY SAFE ...when used by subcutaneous injection by a trained medical professional. Significant adverse effects to fetus or mother have not been reported. However, some clinicians decrease maintenance dose by half during pregnancy (2619). POSSIBLY UNSAFE ...when used by subcutaneous injection in high doses. High doses of bee venom can increase release of histamine, which can cause uterine contraction (2619); avoid using in high doses.

Effectiveness

LIKELY EFFECTIVE

Bee sting allergy. Subcutaneous use of bee venom seems to be effective for bee sting desensitization in patients with severe allergy to bee stings. Bee venom immunotherapy provides 98-99% protection from systemic reactions to bee stings. Once immunotherapy is stopped, the risk of a systemic reaction over the next 5 to 10 years is about 5-15% (6043,6075,6076). Bee venom is an FDA-approved subcutaneous injectable product for the treatment of severe allergies to bee stings (2619).

POSSIBLY INEFFECTIVE

Osteoarthritis. Some early reports seemed to indicate a possible benefit of injected bee venom in the treatment of arthritis; however, results are conflicting and most clinical studies do not show a benefit (6045).

There is insufficient reliable information available about the effectiveness of bee venom for its other uses.

Mechanism of Action

Bee venom contains several physiologically active components. Two of the most toxic compounds are melittin and phospholipase A2 (PLA2). Melittin constitutes 30-50% of dry bee venom (6041,6045,6046), and PLA2 makes up about 10-12% of bee venom (6041). Mellitin is a potent hemolytic (6042,6045) that causes mast cell degranulation and activates PLA2 (6045). Other constituents in bee venom include hyaluronidase, apamin, mast cell degranulating peptide (MCD peptide), procamine, secapin, tertiapin, and other small peptides including adolapin (6). Some other components are histamine, dopamine, and noradrenaline (6041). In desensitization to bee stings, hymenoptera venom stimulates an allergenic response, decreases leukocyte sensitivity to the allergen, and increases the number of T-suppressor cells (2619). There were early suggestions that bee venom could be a useful treatment in patients with arthritis. This theory was largely due to purported anti-inflammatory effects of bee venom, and the observation that many beekeepers don't develop arthritis (6). While some components in bee venom have been shown to have anti-inflammatory effects, studies have also shown that some components of bee venom are pro-inflammatory. For example, activators of PLA2 such as melittin, are thought to cause an increase in the synthesis of cytokines (tumor necrosis factor and interleukin 1) and stimulate arachidonic acid release resulting in an immune or inflammatory response (6044,6071).
PLA2 is an enzyme which catalyzes the hydrolysis of phospholipid bonds, destroying the major component of cell membranes and leading to cell death (6041,6046). PLA2 causes smooth muscle contraction, blood pressure reduction, increased capillary permeability, and mast cell destruction. PLA2 also reduces blood coagulation, possibly by reducing the activity of coagulation factors II, V, and VIII (6046). Melittin might also be partially responsible for bee venom's anticoagulant effects (6046). Some components in bee venom seem to cause neutrophil degranulation and superoxide production (6,6044), but other actions of bee venom components seem to decrease superoxide production (6,6041,6045,6072). The formation of superoxide anions can be destructive to tissues. The melittin component of bee venom possesses antimicrobial activity, but due to its hemolytic effects, melittin is unsuitable as a treatment for infections (6042). Hyaluronidase is an enzyme which hydrolyzes hyaluronic acid. The adhesive properties of hyaluronic acid hold cells together, so once hydrolyzed, other venom components can penetrate into the cell. For this reason, hyaluronidase is termed a spreading factor (6041). Apamin is a neurotoxin (6045). It blocks many inhibitory effects, including alpha-adrenergic, cholinergic, and neurotensin-induced relaxation, by blocking calcium-dependent potassium channels (6041). MCD peptide is chemically similar to apamin. It causes mast cell degranulation and

release of histamine at extremely low concentrations. Histamine causes dilation and increased permeability of capillaries (6041). The constituent adolapin inhibits inflammation and the prostaglandin-synthase system (6). In animals, whole bee venom, melittin, and apamin have also been shown to cause increases in cortisol levels (6039,6040). The mechanism of other peptides is not yet understood (6041).

Adverse Reactions

Parenterally, local erythema and swelling at the injection site are the most common reactions to bee venom treatment (1343). Less common adverse effects ranging from itching, urticaria, edema, malaise, and anxiety to anaphylaxis occur in about 20% of patients (1343). Adverse reactions most often occur during the dose increase phase of immunotherapy, particularly with rapid dose increases (1343,6077). Risk of adverse effects seems to be increased in people treated with honeybee venom (1343,6077). Women seem to have more severe and more frequent adverse effects (1343). Anaphylaxis is most likely to occur in extremely sensitive individuals or in the case of an overdose (2169,6074,6077). Other adverse reactions include chest tightness, palpitations, dizziness, nausea, vomiting, diarrhea, somnolence, respiratory distress, hypotension, confusion, fainting, and laryngeal edema or asthma (1343,2619,6070,6078). Uncommon reactions are abdominal pain, incontinence, chest pain, or visual disturbances (6078). Rarely, coagulation abnormalities can occur, and are usually associated with severe reactions to bee stings (6046).

Interactions with Herbs & Other Dietary Supplements

None known.

Interactions with Drugs

None known.

Interactions with Foods

None known.

Interactions with Lab Tests

PROTHROMBIN TIME (PT): Bee venom might increase the prothrombin time (PT) and partial thromboplastin time (PTT) (6046). The PLA2 component of bee venom seems to reduce the activity of clotting factors II, V, and VIII (6046).

Interactions with Diseases or Conditions

None known.

Dosage and Administration

PARENTERAL: Bee venom is used subcutaneously, intradermally, and intra-arterially for these uses. For arthritis, purified, sterile bee toxin (apitoxin 2 mg/mL) has been used starting with 0.05-0.1 mL. The dose is gradually increased to 0.25 mL, 0.5 mL, and 1 mL, with dose intervals usually from 5 to 7 days. For bee venom immunotherapy in people hypersensitive to bee stings, increased doses of venom are given at selected intervals, usually weekly (6078). There are many possible protocols for immunotherapy. Some start with 0.0001 or 0.001 mcg of venom extract (6077). This is continued until a maintenance dose is achieved, usually 100 micrograms per venom. Once the maintenance dose is achieved, therapy can continue for years. Patients have varying sensitivities to venom and tolerability to immunotherapy, so it is not possible to provide a general dosing schedule for all patients. Venom immunotherapy should only be done by physicians thoroughly familiar with the use of these products, including the treatment of anaphylactic and other adverse reactions. It is also advised to have injectable epinephrine and emergency facilities nearby in case an anaphylactic reaction occurs (2619,6074,6078). Alcohol and tincture of iodine rapidly destroy the activity of bee venom and should not be applied at the site of injection. In China, bee venom is also commonly administered by electrophoresis, ultrasonophoresis, and acupuncture.

Comments

Avoid confusion with bee pollen, honey, and royal jelly. Other venoms are derived from related members of the insect order, Hymenoptera (6).

BEER

Also Known As

Alcohol, Ethanol.
CAUTION: See separate listings for Barley, Hops, Wine, and Yeast.

Scientific Names

None.

People Use This For

Orally, beer is used for reducing the risk of cardiovascular disease, including coronary heart disease, atherosclerosis, heart failure, and myocardial infarction (MI), and for reducing the risk of ischemic stroke and type 2 diabetes. It is also used to reduce the risk of mortality after an acute MI and in people with ischemic left ventricular (LV) dysfunction. Additionally, beer is used orally for preventing cognitive decline in later life, Alzheimer's disease, loss of bone mineral density, cancer, gallstones, kidney stones, and Helicobacter pylori (H. pylori) infection. Beer is also used orally as an appetite and digestive stimulant, and to promote lactation.

Safety

LIKELY SAFE ...when used orally in moderation. Beer seems to be safe when 24 oz or less is consumed daily (2060).
POSSIBLY UNSAFE ...when consumed in large amounts. More than 24 oz per day can cause significant adverse effects (2060,6840).
PREGNANCY: LIKELY UNSAFE ...when used orally. Alcohol is a teratogen. Use during pregnancy, especially during the first two months after conception, is associated with significant risk of spontaneous abortion, fetal alcohol syndrome, and developmental and behavioral dysfunction in infants and children exposed to alcohol in utero (8100); avoid using.
LACTATION: LIKELY UNSAFE ...when used orally. Alcohol is secreted in breast milk. Chronic use can cause abnormal psychomotor development, and disrupt the infant's sleep wake pattern. Alcohol also seems to reduce milk production (11878); avoid using.

Effectiveness

LIKELY EFFECTIVE

Cardiovascular disease. Consumption of alcoholic drinks, including beer, by otherwise healthy people seems to reduce the risk of developing cardiovascular disease. Moderate alcohol use (one to two drinks per day) reduces the risk of coronary heart disease, atherosclerosis, and myocardial infarction (MI), by approximately 30-50% when compared with nondrinkers (2267,2268,2271,6888,6892,8648,8649,10128,11879). Alcohol reduces the risk of ischemic stroke, but increase the risk of hemorrhagic stroke. Light to moderate alcohol consumption reduces ischemic stroke risk (2271,2279,6834,6842,6893). However, there is evidence that consuming any amount of alcohol can increase the risk of hemorrhagic stroke (841,2271,6842). There is some evidence that light to moderate consumption of alcoholic drinks can reduce the risk of all-cause mortality in people who are middle-aged or older (2058,6823,6837,6843). Light to moderate consumption of alcohol might also reduce the risk of cardiovascular mortality in otherwise healthy people (2058,2270,6835,6837). Light to moderate alcohol consumption in the year prior to first acute MI is associated with a reduced cardiovascular and all-cause mortality risk compared with non-drinkers (8650). Consumption of one alcoholic beverage per day or consuming alcohol on at least 3 to 4 days per week is a good rule of thumb for people who drink alcohol. Tell patients not to exceed two drinks per day. More than two drinks daily can increase the risk of cardiovascular and overall mortality (841,2060,2261,6173,6890,8648,11879). In men with established coronary heart disease (CHD), consumption of 1-14 alcoholic drinks per week, including beer, doesn't seem to have any effect on cardiovascular disease or all-cause mortality compared with men who drink less than one drink per week. Consuming three or more drinks per day is associated with increased mortality in men with a history of heart attacks (6173).

POSSIBLY EFFECTIVE

Cognitive function. Elderly men who have a history of consuming one alcoholic drink per day seem to maintain better general cognitive function during their late 70s and 80s compared to non-drinkers (6824,6829). However, consumption of more than four drinks per day during middle age seems to be associated with significantly poorer cognitive function later in life (6824).

Diabetes. People who consume alcohol in moderate amounts seem to have a lower risk of developing type 2 diabetes (6172,6891). Diabetes patients who consume alcohol in moderate amounts seem to have a reduced risk of coronary heart disease compared with non-drinkers with type 2 diabetes. The risk reduction is similar to that found in healthy people who consume light to moderate amounts of alcohol (8653,8654).

Heart failure. There is some evidence that consuming one to four alcoholic drinks per day reduces the risk of heart failure in persons aged 65 years or older (8104).

Helicobacter pylori (H pylori). There is evidence that suggests that moderate to high consumption of alcohol, more than 75 grams, per week from beverages such as beer and wine can reduce the risk of H. pylori infection (8034).

POSSIBLY INEFFECTIVE

Cancer. Although wine consumption has been associated with some reductions in cancer mortality, beer consumption does not seem to have this effect (2058). In fact, there is some evidence that beer consumption might slightly increase cancer-related mortality (6823,6843). There is some evidence that consumption of one or more alcoholic drinks might increase mortality from breast cancer (6843).

INSUFFICIENT RELIABLE EVIDENCE to RATE

Alzheimer's disease. There is preliminary evidence that suggests one to two alcoholic drinks per day can reduce the risk of Alzheimer's disease in both men and women compared to non-drinkers (6603).

Anxiety. The effect of alcohol on anxiety is complex and may be affected by the psychological state of the user. It

sometimes reduces anxiety, sometimes increases it, and sometimes has no effect (2266).
Bone mineral density. There is also preliminary evidence that suggests moderate alcohol consumption in postmenopausal women is associated with increased bone mineral density in the trochanter, femoral neck, midradius, and lumbar spine (6825,6836,8655). Alcohol intake of one-half to one drink per day seems to have the greatest effect on bone mineral density compared with non-drinkers and heavy drinkers of alcohol (8655).
More evidence is needed to rate beer for these uses.

Mechanism of Action

Beers vary in ethanol content between 2-6%, with typical American beers averaging 4-5% ethanol by volume (17). Ethanol is a central nervous system (CNS) depressant (2263).
Several mechanisms have been proposed for the protective effects of alcohol against coronary heart disease. One to two alcoholic drinks per day increases HDL cholesterol by about 12% (6892) and apolipoprotein A-I by about 2.2% (8649). The increase in HDL cholesterol levels might account for approximately 50% of the cardioprotective effect of moderate alcohol consumption (2261,6838,6841). Moderate alcohol consumption also decreases LDL cholesterol by 5-17%, triglycerides by 5-10%, and apolipoprotein B levels by 3.7% (6841,8649). There is concern that moderate alcohol consumption can increase systolic blood pressure (6841). However, there is evidence light to moderate alcohol consumption does not increase the risk of hypertension and may actually decrease the risk (8102).
Effects of alcohol on blood clotting include a reduction in clotting potential and enhancement of clot breakdown (2261). Alcohol consumption decreases platelet aggregation, possibly via inhibition of prostaglandin synthesis (6892). Moderate alcohol consumption is also associated with an increase in plasma levels of tissue-type plasminogen activator, an indicator of fibrinolytic capacity (6894). Light to moderate alcohol consumption produces a reduction in coronary narrowing due to atherosclerosis (2261,6840,8652).
High levels of homocysteine are a risk factor for cardiovascular disease. Homocysteine breakdown and removal requires folate and vitamin B6, and alcohol is an antagonist of folate metabolism (8101). However, there is evidence that an increased intake of dietary folate or the use if supplemental folate, 400 mcg/day, in moderate alcohol users can lower homocysteine levels compared to nonusers of alcohol (8101). However, beer contains folate and vitamin B6 (pyridoxine), and its presence may explain why the increase in plasma homocysteine levels seen with other alcoholic beverages is not seen with beer (6832).
Dark beers contain flavonoids (6892). These polyphenolic compounds, which are found in higher concentrations in red wine, have antioxidant properties and may contribute to protection against CHD by reducing oxidation of LDL cholesterol (2268).
Possible mechanisms by which alcohol could have a protective effect against ischemic stroke include increasing HDL and prostacyclin, decreasing fibrinogen, and inhibiting platelet aggregation (6842). There is evidence that suggests that moderate intake of alcohol increases cerebral blood flow (8651). Moderate alcohol consumption is associated with a lower prevalence of white matter changes and brain infarcts on magnetic resonance imaging in adults 65 years of age or older compared to non-drinkers and heavy drinkers (8651).
The protective effect of alcohol against cardiovascular disease is lost at higher intakes of alcohol (greater than 1-2 drinks per day). High alcohol consumption can cause increased homocysteine levels, hypertension, hemorrhagic stroke, fatal arrhythmias, and direct damage to heart muscle (alcoholic cardiomyopathy) (2060,2261,2267,2270,8101,8102,8103). Certain alcoholic beverages, in particular red wine, may be more protective than other alcoholic beverages such as beer. However, a difference in lifestyle among wine, beer, and other alcohol beverage drinkers, including diet and social class, might also explain why some alcoholic beverages appear to offer more protection than others against coronary heart disease (10129).
Moderate alcohol intake may be protective against the development of type 2 diabetes due to an increase in insulin sensitivity (6891).
Moderate alcohol consumption may be protective against postmenopausal bone loss due to an increase in estrogen levels, increased calcitonin secretion, and reduced parathyroid hormone secretion (6825,6836,8655). However, heavy and chronic alcohol consumption reduces bone mineral density, possibly due to increased calcium and magnesium excretion, increased cortisol secretion, and reduced osteoblast activity (6836,8656). Chronic alcoholics also often have other risk factors for osteoporosis, including poor nutrition, smoking, sedentary lifestyle, and lower body weight (6825,6836).
Preliminary studies suggest that substances in beer may have inhibitory effects on heterocyclic amines, which are carcinogenic substances formed during cooking of some foods (6833).
Beer stimulates gastric acid secretions and gastrin release. This may explain why moderate to high alcohol consumption from beverages such as beer seems to prevent Helicobacter pylori infection (8034).

Adverse Reactions

Orally, beer can cause a variety of side effects due to the alcohol content. The side effects depend on the amount ingested and can vary among individuals. Some common side effects include flushing, confusion, emotional lability, perceptual and sensational disturbances, blackouts, lack of coordination and trouble walking, central nervous system (CNS) depression, drowsiness, respiratory depression, hypothermia, hypoglycemia, nausea, vomiting, diarrhea, abdominal pain, and others. Chronic heavy ethanol ingestion (three or more alcoholic drinks per day) can lead to physical dependence, malnutrition, amnesia, dementia, somnolence, cardiac myopathy, hepatotoxicity, and cirrhosis. Other effects of chronic abuse are pancreatitis, hypomagnesemia, skeletal myopathies, Wernicke's encephalopathy,

Korsakoff's psychosis, chronic cerebellar syndrome, mouth cancer, esophageal cancer, pharyngeal cancer, laryngeal cancer, and liver cancer (6843,9004). There is evidence heavy alcohol consumption is associated with the mutation of the p53 gene in individuals with esophageal carcinoma (9005). There is also some evidence that heavy consumption of wine is associated with the highest risk of esophageal cancer compared with heavy consumption of beer and spirits (9004). Chronic intake of three or more drinks per day is associated with an increased risk of all-cause mortality, ischemic stroke, and hypertension (2261,6892,8102). Heavy alcohol consumption (fifteen or more drinks per week) is also associated with a higher percentage of white matter changes and larger ventricular and sulcal size on magnetic resonance imaging of the brain, suggesting heavy alcohol consumption decreases cerebral blood flow and may contribute to brain atrophy (8651).

Consumption of any amount of alcohol can increase the risk of hemorrhagic stroke (841,2271). Daily consumption of one or more alcoholic drinks in women might increase the risk of breast cancer by 2-15% and increase mortality from breast cancer by as much as 30% (6843,8100,9006). There is also evidence suggesting that women who consume alcohol daily have an increased risk of developing breast cancer increases when the daily intake of folate is 300 mcg or less (9006).

Beer made with barley can cause anaphylaxis in sensitive individuals (317). There have been occasional reports of asthma triggered by beer consumption (6174).

Some research suggests an association between alcohol consumption and an increased risk for pancreatic cancer, but other studies do not support this association (8038).

Study results of a possible association between beer consumption and increased waist-to-hip ratio are inconsistent. There is evidence that suggests that consumption of more than six beers per week is associated with a larger waist-to-hip ratio than those consuming an equivalent amount of hard liquor or wine. However, an association between moderate alcohol intake equivalent to approximately 3 beers per week or less and waist-to-hip ratio does not seem to exist (10164,10165). It also is unclear whether waist-to-hip ratios associated with the intake of wine, beer, or other alcoholic beverages have any clinical significance (9007).

Interactions with Herbs & Other Dietary Supplements

HERBS/SUPPLEMENTS WITH SEDATIVE PROPERTIES: Theoretically, concomitant use of beer with herbs that have sedative properties might enhance adverse effects (2262). Some of these include 5-HTP, calamus, California poppy, catnip, hops, Jamaican dogwood, kava, St. John's wort, scullcap, valerian, yerba mansa, and others.

Interactions with Drugs

ASPIRIN: Concomitant use of aspirin with alcohol can increase the risk of gastrointestinal (GI) bleeding (2262).

BARBITURATES: Concomitant consumption of large amounts of alcohol may decrease metabolism of barbiturates (2262). Some of these sedative medications include pentobarbital (Nembutal), phenobarbital (Luminal), secobarbital (Seconal), and others.

BENZODIAZEPINES: Concomitant consumption of large amounts of alcohol may decrease metabolism of benzodiazepines (2262).

CEFAMANDOLE (Mandol): Cefamandole antibiotics can cause a disulfiram-like reaction when taken with alcohol (2262).

CEFOPERAZONE (Cefobid): Cefoperazone can cause a disulfiram-like reaction when taken with alcohol (2262).

CHLORPROPAMIDE (Diabinese): Chlorpropamide can cause a disulfiram-like reaction when taken with alcohol (506).

CISAPRIDE (Propulsid): Concomitant use of beer with cisapride (Propulsid) might increase blood alcohol levels and effects (2262).

CNS DEPRESSANTS: Concomitant use of beer with antihistamines, barbiturates, benzodiazepines, and tricyclic antidepressants may increase sedative and other adverse effects (2262).

DISULFIRAM (Antabuse): The alcohol content of beer can cause a disulfiram reaction when taken within 12 hours of disulfiram (2262). Patients taking disulfiram should not drink any alcoholic beverages including beer.

ERYTHROMYCIN: Concomitant use of erythromycin with alcohol can increase blood alcohol levels and effects (2262).

GRISEOFULVIN (Fulvicin): Griseofulvin can cause a disulfiram-like reaction when taken with alcohol (2262).

H2-BLOCKERS: Concomitant use of cimetidine (Tagamet) and ranitidine (Zantac) with alcohol may increase blood alcohol levels and adverse effects (2262).

HEPATOTOXIC DRUGS: Concomitant use of beer with acetaminophen, isoniazid, or phenylbutazone can increase the risk of hepatotoxicity (2262).

METFORMIN (Glucophage): Concomitant consumption of large amounts of alcohol may increase the risk of lactic acidosis with metformin (Glucophage) (2262).

METRONIDAZOLE (Flagyl): Metronidazole can cause a disulfiram-like reaction when taken with alcohol (2262).

NARCOTIC DRUGS: Concomitant consumption of large amounts of alcohol may decrease metabolism of narcotics (2262).

NONSTEROIDAL ANTI-INFLAMMATORY DRUGS (NSAIDs): Concomitant use of nonsteroidal anti-inflammatory drugs with alcohol can increase the risk of gastrointestinal (GI) bleeding (2262).

PHENYTOIN (Dilantin): Concomitant consumption of large amounts of alcohol may induce metabolism, reducing therapeutic effectiveness of phenytoin (Dilantin) (2262).

SULFONAMIDE ANTIBIOTICS: Sulfonamide antibiotics can cause a disulfiram-like reaction when taken with alcohol (2262).
TOLBUTAMIDE (Orinase): Tolbutamide can cause a disulfiram-like reaction when taken with alcohol (2262).
WARFARIN (Coumadin): Acute alcohol intoxication can decrease metabolism and increase effects of warfarin (Coumadin) (2262). In contrast, chronic intoxication can induce metabolism of warfarin, reducing therapeutic effectiveness (2262).

Interactions with Foods

FOOD: Chronic use of alcohol might interfere with absorption of B vitamins and other nutrients (2263).

Interactions with Lab Tests

FOLATE: Chronic alcohol ingestion may decrease folate levels and test results (2263).
LIVER FUNCTION TESTS: Chronic alcohol ingestion can increase alkaline phosphatase (Alk phos), alanine aminotransferase (ALT), aspartate aminotransferase (AST), gamma-glutamyltransferase (GGT), and bilirubin test results (2263).
MEAN CORPUSCULAR VOLUME (MCV): Chronic alcohol ingestion can increase MCV (2263).
TRIGLYCERIDES: Chronic alcohol ingestion can increase triglycerides (2263).

Interactions with Diseases or Conditions

ASTHMA: There have been occasional reports of asthma triggered by beer consumption (6174).
GOUT: Alcohol use can exacerbate gout (2263).
HEART CONDITIONS: Alcohol use can exacerbate variant angina, congestive heart failure (2261,2263,6889), and idiopathic cardiomyopathy (6889).
HIGH BLOOD PRESSURE: Consuming three or more alcoholic drinks a day can increase blood pressure and exacerbate hypertension (2261).
HYPERTRIGLYCERIDEMIA: Alcohol ingestion can exacerbate hypertriglyceridemia (2261,2263,6892).
INSOMNIA: Alcohol use may exacerbate insomnia (2263).
LIVER DISEASE: Alcohol use can exacerbate liver disease (2261).
NEUROLOGICAL CONDITIONS: Alcohol use can exacerbate degenerative neurological conditions (6889).
PANCREATITIS: Alcohol use can exacerbate pancreatitis (2261).
PEPTIC ULCER DISEASE (PUD)/GASTROESOPHAGEAL REFLUX DISEASE (GERD): Alcohol use can exacerbate PUD and GERD (2261,2263).
PORPHYRIA: Alcohol use can exacerbate porphyria (2261).
PSYCHIATRIC DISORDERS: Consuming three or more drinks of alcohol a day can also exacerbate psychiatric disorders and increase cognitive impairment (2261).

Dosage and Administration

ORAL: For reducing the risk of cardiovascular disease, and ischemic stroke one or two drinks, 12 oz, per day has been used (2261,2271,6835,6837,6840,6841,6842,6888,6892,6893,8648,8649,8650,10128). Up to four glasses per day has been associated with reducing the risk for heart failure (8104). Up to one drink per day has been associated with less cognitive decline in older men (6824,6829). Three drinks per day to two drinks per week and have been associated with reduced risk of type 2 diabetes in healthy men (6172,6891). Up to seven drinks per week has been associated with reducing the risk of coronary heart disease in people with type 2 diabetes (8653,8654). Consumption of more than 75 grams of alcohol from beverages such as beer has been associated with reducing the risk of Helicobacter pylori infection (8034). Alcohol intake is often measured in number of "drinks." One drink is equivalent to a 4 oz or a 120 mL glass of wine, 12 oz of beer, or 1 oz of spirits.

BEESWAX

Also Known As

Bees Wax, Bleached Beeswax, White Beeswax, White Wax, Yellow Beeswax, Yellow Wax.

Scientific Names

Apis cerana; Apis mellifera.
Family: Apidae.

People Use This For

Orally, beeswax is used for lowering lipids, as an anti-inflammatory, anti-ulcer, for diarrhea, hiccups, and pain relief.
In foods and beverages, white beeswax and beeswax absolute are utilized as stiffening agents.
In manufacturing, yellow and white beeswax are used as thickeners, emulsifiers, and as stiffening agents in cosmetics. Beeswax absolute is used as a fragrance ingredient in soaps and perfumes. White beeswax and beeswax absolute are also used as tablet polishing components in pharmaceutical products.

Safety

LIKELY SAFE ...when used orally in amounts commonly found in foods. Beeswax has Generally Recognized As Safe (GRAS) status in the US (4912). ...when used orally as a medicinal agent (11). ...when used topically (11).
PREGNANCY AND LACTATION: There is insufficient reliable information available about the safety of medicinal amounts of beeswax during pregnancy and lactation.

Effectiveness

There is insufficient reliable information available about the effectiveness of beeswax.

Mechanism of Action

A natural mixture of high molecular weight alcohols isolated and purified from beeswax, termed D-002, had mild anti-inflammatory effects in experimental animals (4052). In rats, injected D-002 partially inhibited experimentally-induced gastric damage (4053,4054). Concomitant use of beeswax and nonsteroidal anti-inflammatory drugs (NSAIDs) may protect against NSAID-induced ulcers (4053,4054).

Adverse Reactions

Orally, beeswax may cause allergic reactions (11).

Interactions with Herbs & Other Dietary Supplements

None known.

Interactions with Drugs

None known.

Interactions with Foods

None known.

Interactions with Lab Tests

None known.

Interactions with Diseases or Conditions

None known.

Dosage and Administration

No typical dosage.

Comments

The three major beeswax products are yellow beeswax, white beeswax, and beeswax absolute. Yellow beeswax is the crude product obtained from the honeycomb. White beeswax is derived from yellow beeswax by bleaching, and beeswax absolute is derived from yellow beeswax by extraction with alcohol. Beeswax is obtained from the honeycomb of the honeybee (Apis mellifera) and other Apis species.

BEET

Also Known As

Beets, Fodder Beet, Garden Beet, Mangel, Mangold, Red Beet, Sugarbeet, Yellow Beet.

Scientific Names

Beta vulgaris.
Family: Chenopodiaceae.

People Use This For

Orally, beets are used as a supportive therapy in the treatment of liver diseases and fatty liver.

Safety

LIKELY SAFE ...when used in amounts commonly found in foods.
There is insufficient reliable information available about the safety of medicinal use of beets.
PREGNANCY AND LACTATION: There is insufficient reliable information available about the safety of medicinal amounts of beets during pregnancy and breast-feeding.

Effectiveness
There is insufficient reliable information available about the effectiveness of beets.

Mechanism of Action
The applicable part of beet is the root. Animal data suggests that beets may be effective against fat deposition in the liver. A component called betaine may play a role (18).

Adverse Reactions
Orally, ingestion of large quantities of beets could lead to hypocalcemia and kidney damage because of the oxaluric acid content (18).

Interactions with Herbs & Other Dietary Supplements
None known.

Interactions with Drugs
None known.

Interactions with Foods
None known.

Interactions with Lab Tests
None known.

Interactions with Diseases or Conditions
KIDNEY DISEASE: Ingestion of large quantities of beets could worsen kidney disease (18).

Dosage and Administration
ORAL: Beet is used as a standardized granular powder (18).

BELLADONNA

Also Known As
Belladone, Deadly Nightshade, Devil's Cherries, Devil's Herb, Divale, Dwale, Dwayberry, Great Morel, Indian Belladonna, Naughty Man's Cherries, Poison Black Cherries.
CAUTION: See separate listings for Bittersweet Nightshade, Henbane, and Scopolia.

Scientific Names
Atropa belladonna; Atropa acuminata.
Family: Solanaceae.

People Use This For
Orally, belladonna is used as a sedative, as an antispasmodic in bronchial asthma and whooping cough, and as a cold and hay fever remedy, for Parkinson's disease, intestinal and biliary colic, motion sickness, and as anesthetic.
Topically, belladonna is used in liniments for rheumatism, sciatica, and neuralgia; and in medicinal plasters for treating psychiatric disorders, hyperkinesis, hyperhidrosis, and bronchial asthma.
Rectally, belladonna is used in hemorrhoid suppositories.

Safety
POSSIBLY SAFE ...when the standardized extract is used orally and appropriately under the supervision of a medical professional trained in the use of belladonna (2). Belladonna is available as a prescription drug in the US and has a narrow therapeutic index.
LIKELY UNSAFE ...when the standardized extract is used orally without professional medical supervision (12). ...when the unstandardized leaf, root, or other preparation is used orally (12).
There is insufficient reliable information available about the safety of belladonna for its other uses.
CHILDREN: POSSIBLY SAFE ...when used orally in children older than 6 years old only under professional medical supervision. LIKELY UNSAFE ...when the leaf, root, or extract is used orally in children under 6 years old (12). There is insufficient reliable information available about the safety of the topical or rectal use of belladonna in children.
PREGNANCY: LIKELY UNSAFE ...when the leaf or root are used orally without medical supervision. There is insufficient reliable information about the safety of belladonna for its other uses during pregnancy.
LACTATION: LIKELY UNSAFE ...when the leaf, root, standardized extract, or other preparation are used orally.

Use should be avoided because it can reduce milk production and is secreted into breast milk (15). There is insufficient reliable information available about the safety of belladonna for its other uses during lactation.

Effectiveness

There is insufficient reliable information available about the effectiveness of belladonna.

Mechanism of Action

The applicable parts of belladonna are the leaf and root. Its anticholinergic activity is due to the 0.3%-0.5% tropane alkaloid constituents; mainly l-hyoscyamine, but it also contains traces of l-scopolamine and atropine (dl-hyoscyamine) (11). On extraction, most of the l-hyoscyamine is racemized to atropine (11).

Adverse Reactions

Orally, belladonna can cause dry mouth, decreased perspiration, dilation of pupils, blurred vision, red dry skin, hyperthermia, tachycardia, difficulty urinating, hallucinations, spasms, acute psychosis, convulsions, and coma (2,11,553).

Interactions with Herbs & Other Dietary Supplements

None known.

Interactions with Drugs

ANTICHOLINERGIC DRUGS: Belladonna can increase the anticholinergic effects and adverse effects of amantadine, antihistamines, phenothiazines, procainamide, quinidine, tricyclic antidepressants, and others (2).

Interactions with Foods

None known.

Interactions with Lab Tests

None known.

Interactions with Diseases or Conditions

CONGESTIVE HEART FAILURE (CHF): Belladonna might cause tachycardia and exacerbate CHF due to its hyoscyamine (atropine) and scopolamine content (15).
CONSTIPATION: Belladonna might cause constipation due to its hyoscyamine (atropine) and scopolamine content (15).
DOWN SYNDROME: Caution, patients with Down syndrome might be hypersensitive to the antimuscarinic effects (mydriasis, positive chronotropic heart effects, etc.) of hyoscyamine (atropine) and scopolamine contained in belladonna (15).
ESOPHAGEAL REFLUX: Belladonna might delay gastric emptying and decrease lower esophageal pressure, promoting gastric retention and exacerbating reflux due to its hyoscyamine (atropine) and scopolamine content (15).
FEVER: Belladonna might increase the risk of hyperthermia in patients with fever due to its hyoscyamine (atropine) and scopolamine content (15).
GASTRIC ULCER: Belladonna might delay gastric emptying and exacerbate gastric ulcers due to its hyoscyamine (atropine) and scopolamine content (15).
GASTROINTESTINAL (GI) INFECTIONS: Belladonna might suppress GI motility causing retention of infecting organisms or toxins due to its hyoscyamine (atropine) and scopolamine content (15).
HIATAL HERNIA: Belladonna might delay gastric emptying and decrease lower esophageal pressure, promoting gastric retention and exacerbating reflux due to its hyoscyamine (atropine) and scopolamine content (15).
NARROW-ANGLE GLAUCOMA: Belladonna might increase ocular tension in patients with narrow-angle (angle-closure) glaucoma due to its hyoscyamine (atropine) and scopolamine content (2,15).
OBSTRUCTIVE GASTROINTESTINAL (GI) TRACT DISEASE: Belladonna might exacerbate obstructive GI tract diseases (including atony, paralytic ileus, and stenosis) due to its hyoscyamine (atropine) and scopolamine content (15).
TACHYARRHYTHMIAS: Belladonna might cause tachycardia due to its hyoscyamine (atropine) and scopolamine content (2,15).
TOXIC MEGACOLON: Belladonna might suppress intestinal motility, which might produce paralytic ileus and exacerbate toxic megacolon, due to its hyoscyamine (atropine) and scopolamine content (2,15).
ULCERATIVE COLITIS: Belladonna might suppress intestinal motility, which might produce paralytic ileus and precipitate toxic megacolon, due to its hyoscyamine (atropine) and scopolamine content (15).
URINARY RETENTION: Belladonna might increase urinary retention due to its hyoscyamine (atropine) and scopolamine content (2,15).

Dosage and Administration

ORAL: The belladonna leaf powder is typically an average single dose of 50-100 mg. The maximum single dose is 200 mg, which is equivalent to 0.6 mg total alkaloids, calculated as hyoscyamine. The maximum daily dose is

600 mg, which is equivalent to 1.8 mg total alkaloids, calculated as hyoscyamine. The root powder is commonly used in an average single dose of 50 mg. The maximum single dose is 100 mg, which is equivalent to 0.5 mg total alkaloids, calculated as hyoscyamine. The maximum daily dose of the root powder is 300 mg, equivalent to 1.5 mg total alkaloids calculated as hyoscyamine. The belladonna extract has an average single dose of 10 mg. The maximum single dose is 50 mg, equivalent to 0.73 mg total alkaloids calculated as hyoscyamine, and the maximum daily dosage is 150 mg, equivalent to 2.2 mg total alkaloids calculated as hyoscyamine (2).
TOPICAL: No typical dosage.
RECTAL: No typical dosage.

Comments
The name, belladonna, means beautiful lady. The belladonna berry juice has been used historically in Italy to dilate the pupils of women giving them a striking appearance (11). Avoid confusion with bittersweet nightshade (Solanum dulcamara) and henbane (nightshade).

BENZOIN

Also Known As
Benzoe, Gum Benjamin, Gum Benzoin, Sumatra Benzoin.

Scientific Names
Styrax benzoin; Styrax paralleloneurum.
Family: Styracaceae.

People Use This For
Orally, benzoin is used for throat and bronchial inflammation.
Topically, benzoin is used as an antiseptic, astringent, skin protectant, and styptic on small cuts. Benzoin is also used topically for skin ulcers, bedsores, cracked nipples, and fissures of the lips and anus.
By inhalation, benzoin is used to treat laryngitis, croup, and other respiratory conditions.
In combination with other herbs, benzoin tincture (benzoin, aloe, storax, and tolu balsam) is used as a skin protectant.
In dentistry, benzoin is used for gum inflammation and oral herpes lesions.
In manufacturing, benzoin is used in making pharmaceutical preparations.

Safety
POSSIBLY SAFE ...when preparations of the gum resin are used orally for medicinal purposes (12). ...when used topically (11). Tincture of benzoin can cause contact dermatitis.
There is insufficient reliable information available about the safety of benzoin for its other uses.
PREGNANCY AND LACTATION: Insufficient reliable information available; avoid using.

Effectiveness
There is insufficient reliable information available about the effectiveness of benzoin.

Mechanism of Action
The applicable part of benzoin is the gum resin. Benzoin has antiseptic, stimulant, expectorant, astringent, diuretic, and skin protectant effects (11,13).

Adverse Reactions
Topically, the compound benzoin tincture (benzoin, aloe, storax, and tolu balsam) can cause contact dermatitis (11) and should be avoided in sensitive individuals.

Interactions with Herbs & Other Dietary Supplements
None known.

Interactions with Drugs
None known.

Interactions with Foods
None known.

Interactions with Lab Tests
None known.

Interactions with Diseases or Conditions

SENSITIVE INDIVIDUALS: Avoid contact with benzoin and the compound benzoin tincture due to contact dermatitis (11).

Dosage and Administration

ORAL: No typical dosage.
TOPICAL: A typical dosage is a few drops of compound benzoin tincture (USP) every two hours (6002). Compound benzoin tincture contains 100 grams of benzoin powder, 20 grams of aloe powder, 80 grams of storax, and 40 grams of tolu balsam per 1000 mL of tincture (16).
INHALATION: People typically add 5 mL of a compound benzoin tincture (USP) to 473 mL of hot water or place the tincture directly on a handkerchief (6002).

Comments

Benzoin is the gum resin of Styrax species trees. Avoid confusion with Siam benzoin (Styrax tonikensis), which is used only in manufacturing and has no medicinal uses (11,13).

BERGAMOT OIL

Also Known As

Bergamot, Bergamot Orange, Bergamota, Bergamotier, Bergamoto, Bergamotte, Bergamotto Bigarade Orange, Oleum Bergamotte.
CAUTION: See separate listings for Bitter Orange and Sweet Orange.

Scientific Names

Citrus bergamia, synonym Citrus aurantium var. bergamia.
Family: Rutaceae.

People Use This For

Topically, bergamot oil is used to treat psoriasis in conjunction with long-wave ultraviolet light. Bergamot oil is also used topically for vitiligo, mycosis fungoides, and as an insecticide to protect the body against lice and other vermin.
By inhalation, bergamot oil is used as aromatherapy for anxiety.
In foods, bergamot oil is widely used as a citrus flavoring agent, up to 0.02% in gelatins and puddings.
In manufacturing of cosmetics, bergamot oil is used (up to 3% in perfumes and 0.25% in creams and lotions), in soaps, and suntan oils.

Safety

LIKELY SAFE ...when bergamot oil is used orally in amounts commonly found in foods (4912).
POSSIBLY UNSAFE ...when used topically. Bergamot oil can act as a photosensitizer and can induce malignant changes (6).
CHILDREN: POSSIBLY UNSAFE ...when large amounts are ingested. Bergamot oil can cause intestinal colic, convulsions, and death (12).
PREGNANCY AND LACTATION: POSSIBLY UNSAFE ...when used topically (6).

Effectiveness

INSUFFICIENT RELIABLE EVIDENCE to RATE

Anxiety. There's preliminary evidence that suggests using bergamot oil as aromatherapy does not help reduce anxiety in patients receiving concurrent radiotherapy (11452). More evidence is needed to rate bergamot oil for this use.

Mechanism of Action

Bergamot oil is obtained from the peel of Citrus bergamia. The photosensitivity of bergamot oil is linked to the furocoumarin constituents, bergapten (5-methoxypsoralen) (11019), and xanthotoxin (8-methoxypsoralen) (6).

Adverse Reactions

Frequent contact with the peel or oil of bergamot can cause erythema, blisters, pustules, dermatoses leading to scab formation, and pigment spots (18).
Topically, photosensitivity can also occur, especially in fair-skinned people (11909).

Interactions with Herbs & Other Dietary Supplements

None known.

Interactions with Drugs

PHOTOSENSITIZING DRUGS: Topically due to bergapten content use of bergamot oil can compound photosensitizing effects and increase the risk of side effects (11909). Concomitant use should be avoided.

Interactions with Foods

None known.

Interactions with Lab Tests

None known.

Interactions with Diseases or Conditions

None known.

Dosage and Administration

No typical dosage.

BETA-CAROTENE

Also Known As

A-Beta-Carotene, Carotenes, Carotenoids, Provitamin A.
CAUTION: See separate listings for Astaxanthin and Vitamin A.

Scientific Names

Beta-carotene.

People Use This For

Orally, beta-carotene is taken as a dietary source of vitamin A; and to reduce photosensitivities, including erythropoietic protoporphyria (EPP) and polymorphous light eruption. Beta-carotene is also used orally for decreasing exercise-induced asthma; and to reduce the risk of some cancers, cardiovascular disease, cataracts, and age related macular degeneration. Additionally, beta-carotene is used to treat AIDS, alcoholism, Alzheimer's disease, depression, epilepsy, headache, heartburn, hypertension, infertility, Parkinson's disease, psoriasis, rheumatoid arthritis, schizophrenia, and vitiligo.

Safety

LIKELY SAFE ...when used orally and appropriately in amounts commonly found in foods (139,4844,6393).
POSSIBLY SAFE ...when used orally as a dietary supplement. Doses up to 300 mg per day have been used with apparent safety for conditions such as erythropoietic protoporphyria (11793). However, doses as low as 20 mg per day have been associated with increased risk of lung and prostate cancer in people who smoke. Although there is no evidence of significant adverse effects of beta-carotene in nonsmokers, the mechanism for cancer promotion is unknown. If beta-carotene supplements are used, it may be prudent to limit daily consumption to 7 mg per day until more is known about its long-term toxicity (11786).
POSSIBLY UNSAFE ...when used orally in people who smoke or have a history of asbestos exposure. Supplemental beta-carotene 20 mg daily for 5-8 years seems to increase the risk of lung cancer, prostate cancer, intracerebral hemorrhage, and cardiovascular and total mortality in people who smoke cigarettes or have a history of high-level exposure to asbestos (1371,3359,3937,3959,6393,11786). Beta-carotene from foods does not seem to have this effect.
CHILDREN: LIKELY SAFE ...when used orally in amounts commonly found in foods (4844). POSSIBLY SAFE ...when used orally as a dietary supplement. High doses (greater than 60 mg per day) have been used with apparent safety for conditions such as erythropoietic protoporphyria (11793). However, doses as low as 20 mg per day have been associated with increased risk of lung and prostate cancer in adults who smoke. Although there is no evidence of significant adverse effects of beta-carotene in nonsmokers, the mechanism for cancer promotion is unknown. Supplemental beta-carotene in children should be limited to specific medical indications.
PREGNANCY AND LACTATION: LIKELY SAFE ...when used orally and appropriately in amounts commonly found in foods (139,6393,4844). POSSIBLY SAFE ...when used orally as a dietary supplement. Although there is no evidence of significant adverse effects of beta-carotene in nonsmokers, the mechanism for promotion of some cancers is unknown. If used, it may be prudent to limit daily consumption of supplemental beta-carotene to 7 mg per day until more is known about its long-term toxicity (11786). There is insufficient reliable information available about the safety of large doses of beta-carotene in pregnancy and lactation.

Effectiveness

EFFECTIVE

Erythropoietic protoporphyria (EPP). Taking beta-carotene orally can reduce photosensitivity in patients with EPP, a genetic disorder resulting in defective porphyrin metabolism (11793).

POSSIBLY EFFECTIVE

Age-related macular degeneration (AMD). Taking beta-carotene orally 15 mg, combined with vitamin C 500 mg, vitamin E 400 IU, and elemental zinc 80 mg daily seems to provide a risk reduction of 27% for visual acuity loss and a risk reduction of 25% for progression of AMD in patients with advanced AMD (7303,11326). Patients with monocular or binocular intermediate AMD or monocular advanced AMD are at high risk for advanced AMD. Theoretically, these patients may also benefit from beta-carotene and antioxidant-zinc supplementation (11326). There isn't enough evidence to know if this combination is beneficial for people with less advanced macular disease. Supplemental beta-carotene with antioxidants, but without zinc, doesn't seem to have any significant effect on AMD (7303,7304). Additionally, there is preliminary evidence that a high dietary intake of beta-carotene might decrease the risk of AMD (5922). Other dietary carotenoids such as lycopene, lutein, and zeaxanthin may provide greater protection from radiation and oxidative damage in the retina than beta-carotene (6110,8446).

Breast cancer. There is some evidence that a diet rich in beta-carotene may reduce the risk of breast cancer in premenopausal women, especially those at high risk due to family history or high alcohol intake (1444,10132).

Chronic obstructive pulmonary disease (COPD). The prevalence of bronchitis and dyspnea in male smokers with chronic obstructive pulmonary disorder (COPD) seems to be lower in those patients who consume a diet containing high amounts of beta-carotene (2580). But taking beta-carotene supplements doesn't seem to help (2580).

Colorectal cancer. There is epidemiologic evidence that higher dietary content of beta-carotene can decrease the incidence of colorectal cancer (10244).

Exercise-induced asthma. Taking a mixture of beta-carotene isomers orally seems to prevent exercise-induced asthma (1474).

Gastric cancer. Taking beta-carotene orally, 30 mg daily, seems to increase the rate of regression of premalignant gastric lesions in patients at risk for gastric cancer (2579). Taking beta-carotene orally with other antioxidants seems to prevent gastric cancer in malnourished, high risk patients. There is some evidence that beta-carotene 15 mg daily plus vitamin E and selenium can decrease gastric cancer incidence by 21% in the high-risk, malnourished Chinese population (2658).

Oral leukoplakia. Taking beta-carotene orally seems to induce remission in patients with oral leukoplakia. There's an increased risk of disease progression over 12 months if beta-carotene is stopped (1472).

Osteoarthritis. Taking beta-carotene orally doesn't seem to prevent osteoarthritis, but it might slow progression of the disease (5881).

Ovarian cancer. There is some evidence a diet rich in carotenoids, including beta-carotene and especially alpha-carotene, can decrease the risk of ovarian cancer in postmenopausal women (10133).

Post-partum complications. Taking beta carotene orally seems to reduce the occurrence of post-partum diarrhea and fever in malnourished women. All-trans beta-carotene (synthetic beta-carotene) taken weekly before, during, and after pregnancy reduces, but does not eliminate, the occurrence of post partum diarrhea and fever (2581).

Pregnancy-related complications. Taking beta-carotene orally seems to reduce pregnancy-related maternal mortality and night blindness in malnourished women. All-trans beta-carotene (synthetic beta-carotene) taken weekly before, during, and after pregnancy seems to reduce pregnancy-related mortality and night blindness (6153,6154). But synthetic beta-carotene does not reduce fetal and early infant mortality (6152).

Prostate cancer. Taking beta-carotene orally seems to reduce the risk of prostate cancer in men who have plasma beta-carotene concentrations less than 153.25 ng/mL (1473). However, dietary or supplemental beta-carotene doesn't seem to help prevent prostate cancer in men with plasma beta-carotene concentrations greater than 153.25 ng/mL (148,1473,2406,7895).

Sunburn. Taking beta-carotene orally seems to modestly reduce the risk of sunburn in individuals who are sensitive to sun exposure. There is some evidence that 25 mg of mixed beta-carotene daily for 12 weeks reduces skin redness after exposure to UV light in sun-sensitive individuals (6134). However, beta-carotene is unlikely to have much effect on sunburn risk in most people (11792). Also, it doesn't seem to reduce the incidence of solar keratoses or skin cancers associated with sun exposure (1297,2599,11302).

POSSIBLY INEFFECTIVE

Alzheimer's disease. Intake of dietary or supplemental beta-carotene doesn't seem to have any effect on Alzheimer's disease risk (10131).

Cataracts. Taking elemental beta-carotene orally 15 mg, in combination with vitamin C 500 mg, vitamin E 400 IU, and zinc 80 mg daily for 6.3 years does not seem to have any effect on the development or progression of age-related lens opacities (cataracts) or the need for cataract surgery in well-nourished people 55-80 years of age. However, it is unknown whether earlier intervention and/or a longer period of treatment with supplements would have any effect on cataracts (7304).

Stroke. Taking all-trans beta-carotene (synthetic beta-carotene) orally, 20 mg/day for a median of six years may have no effect on the overall incidence of stroke in male smokers (1371). Additionally, there is some evidence that beta-carotene actually increases the risk of intracerebral hemorrhage by 62% in patients who also drink alcohol (1371,3359).

LIKELY INEFFECTIVE

Cancer. Beta-carotene 20-50 mg daily, or 50 mg on alternate days, does not affect the incidence of a variety of cancers in adults, including uterine cancer, cervical cancer, thyroid cancer, bladder cancer, skin cancers (melanoma, basal cell carcinoma, squamous cell carcinoma) brain cancer, pancreatic cancer, and blood cancer (140,1297,1448,2599,2642,2646,2657,3949). Dietary beta-carotene intake also doesn't seem to affect colon cancer risk (3962).

Cardiovascular disease. Taking beta-carotene orally doesn't reduce the risk of heart disease and cardiovascular mortality. Large population studies of dietary or supplemental beta-carotene show mixed results (3933,7386,7387), but large-scale controlled clinical trials are more definitive. In male and female patients with no history of cardiovascular disease, dietary beta-carotene and beta-carotene 20-50 mg daily or every other day has no effect on death rates from cardiovascular causes (1448,2646,2657,3935,10130). In people with coronary heart disease, beta-carotene 25 mg daily in combination with selenium and vitamin C and vitamin E doesn't seem to protect from cardiovascular disease progression and related events such as myocardial infarction (MI) (7388). In people who smoke, beta-carotene 20-30 mg daily actually increases cardiovascular mortality by 12% to 26% (2642,3949). In men who smoke and have had a prior MI, the risk of fatal coronary heart disease increases by as much as 43% with beta-carotene 20 mg daily (3937). These adverse effects do not seem to occur in people who eat foods high in beta-carotene content (1440,2657,7714,7715,7716). A Science Advisory from the American Heart Association states that the evidence does not justify use of antioxidants such as beta-carotene for reducing the risk of cardiovascular disease (12142).

Lung cancer. Taking beta-carotene 20 to 30 mg daily actually seems to increase the risk of lung cancer by 18-28%, in people who smoke (especially those smoking more than 20 cigarettes per day), former smokers, people exposed to asbestos, and those who ingest significant amounts of alcohol (one or more drinks per day) in addition to smoking (139,1471,2582,2642,3949,11303,11786). However, beta-carotene from food does not seem to have this adverse effect.

INSUFFICIENT RELIABLE EVIDENCE to RATE

Chemotherapy toxicity. Observational research suggests that greater dietary intake of beta-carotene appears to lower the incidence of adverse effects in children undergoing chemotherapy for lymphoblastic leukemia (11997). More evidence is needed to rate beta-carotene for this use.

Mechanism of Action

Beta-carotene belongs to a class of red, orange, and yellow pigments called carotenoids. There are hundreds of varieties of provitamin A carotenoids, which are present in many fruits, grains, oils, and vegetables (2628,8044). Commercially available beta-carotene is produced synthetically or from palm oil, algae, or fungi (11786).

Beta carotene is converted to retinal, which is essential for vision and is subsequently converted to retinoic acid, which is used for processes involving growth and cell differentiation (7135,8044). The typical dietary intake of beta-carotene in American adults varies from 0.5 to 6.5 mg per day (2628). Beta-carotene is closely related to alpha-carotene; both are precursors for vitamin A (2628). Beta-carotene and other carotenoids provide approximately 50% of the vitamin A needed in the American diet (8044).

Absorption of beta-carotene is variable. The intestine has a limited capacity to absorb intact beta-carotene (8044). The amount of beta-carotene absorbed from food is only about 5% to 30% of that from synthetic supplements due to complexes it forms with proteins and fiber. Heating food may break down these complexes (2628). Carotenoid absorption is improved by dietary fat. Carotenoids are mainly carried in the blood on low-density lipoproteins (LDLs) (2628). The amount of beta-carotene absorbed and converted to vitamin A also depends upon the individual's vitamin A status, beta-carotene body stores, and the amount of beta-carotene ingested (2628,8044). Some of the ingested beta-carotene is converted to vitamin A in the intestinal mucosa (2628). Although beta-carotene is partly metabolized to vitamin A, high intake of beta-carotene does not result in vitamin A toxicity because the proportion converted to vitamin A decreases as beta-carotene intake increases (8044). Beta-carotene also has activity independent of its conversion to vitamin A (139,1470).

Beta-carotene consists of a number of isomers. Synthetic beta-carotene, the form used in most of the clinical studies, is composed of the all-trans form. Natural beta-carotene sources contain 9-cis-, 13-cis-, and 15-cis-beta-carotene (1474). The 9-cis-beta-carotene isomer is poorly absorbed, and most of it is converted to all-trans-beta-carotene in the intestine (2628). The cis isomers account for less than 5% of carotenoids in plasma, but 10-25% of carotenoids in the tissues are beta-carotene cis isomers (2628). Little is known about the pharmacology of beta-carotene and the differences that may exist between the various isomers and the natural and synthetic forms (2628).

Beta-carotene seems to have antioxidant activities and prevent lipid peroxidation (139). Serum beta-carotene levels seem to be inversely related to C-reactive protein levels and the white blood count. These markers are markers of inflammation and are associated with tumor recurrence and arteriosclerotic cardiovascular disease events (10135). It has been proposed that the antioxidant effects may help prevent cancer by reducing free radical-induced DNA damage (2592,2599). There seems to be an inverse relationship between dietary carotenoid intake, or serum beta-carotene levels, and the incidence of various cancers. In-vitro studies show that beta-carotene inhibits tumor cell growth (2592,2628). There is preliminary evidence that carotenoids, including beta-carotene, can inhibit breast cancer cell growth regardless of estrogen receptor status (8045). However, dietary beta-carotene is not substantially concentrated in breast adipose tissue. Breast adipose tissue concentrations are only slightly higher than serum concentrations (10243). There is also evidence that the inhibitory effect on cancer cell growth by certain statin drugs with a closed ring structure, such as mevastatin and lovastatin (Mevacor), may be enhanced when used with carotenoids (8046). However, anticancer effects of beta-carotene supplementation have not been effectively demonstrated in humans.

There is some concern that beta-carotene metabolites with pharmacological activity can accumulate and have carcinogenic effects (6377,6393). Components of cigarette smoke can degrade beta-carotene, and lower concentrations of beta-carotene have been reported in both active and passive smokers (2592,2593). Smoking might enhance production of carcinogenic beta-carotene oxidation metabolites which, if not neutralized by other antioxidants (such as tocopherol and ascorbate, which are also often depleted in smokers), could lead to increased risk of lung cancer (2628,6377). In addition, beta-carotene metabolites might increase the binding of carcinogenic metabolites to DNA and inhibit gap-junction communication between normal cells and tumor cells. Beta-carotene itself might also increase the levels of certain cytochrome P450 (CYP450) dependent enzymes that can hydroxylate and activate certain compounds into their highly carcinogenic forms (6393), as well as increase catabolism of retinoic acid, which controls lung epithelial cell proliferation and differentiation (2592).

Adverse Reactions

Orally, beta-carotene is typically well tolerated and safe when used in appropriate amounts. High doses can cause yellow or orange skin pigmentation called carotenoderma (11786). Although beta-carotene is partly metabolized to vitamin A, high intake of beta-carotene does not result in vitamin A toxicity because the proportion converted to vitamin A decreases as beta-carotene intake increases (8044).

Advise smokers and people with a history of asbestos exposure not to use beta-carotene supplements. Beta-carotene in doses of 20 mg per day for 5-8 years has been associated with an increased risk of lung and prostate cancer and increased total mortality in people who smoke cigarettes, and in people with a history of high-level asbestos exposure (3959,6393,11303,11786). In people who smoke, beta-carotene 20 to 30 mg daily also seems to increase cardiovascular mortality by 12% to 26% (2642,3949). In men who smoke and have had a prior myocardial infarction (MI), the risk of fatal coronary heart disease increases by as much as 43% with beta-carotene 20 mg daily (3937). These adverse effects do not seem to occur in people who eat foods high in beta-carotene content (1440,2657).

There is some evidence that beta-carotene in combination with selenium and vitamin C and vitamin E might lower high-density lipoprotein 2 (HDL2) by 15%, which is considered to be the most cardioprotective component of HDL (7388). Beta-carotene 20 mg daily increases serum concentrations of beta-carotene and alpha-carotene, beta-cryptoxanthin, and retinal. Additionally, beta-carotene supplementation lowers serum lutein concentrations. Increased or decreased levels of carotenoids may be responsible for the untoward effects of beta-carotene supplementation (10134). More research is needed to determine the mechanism of the adverse effects of beta-carotene supplements.

Interactions with Herbs & Other Dietary Supplements

None known.

Interactions with Drugs

HMG-CoA REDUCTASE INHIBITORS ("Statins"): Concomitant use of beta-carotene in combination with selenium, vitamin C, and vitamin E appears to decrease the effectiveness of the combination of simvastatin (Zocor) and niacin (7388). This combination of antioxidants can lower high-density lipoprotein 2 (HDL-2) levels by 15% and reduce the HDL-2-raising effects of HMG-CoA reductase inhibitors and niacin by more than 50% in people with heart disease (7388). Theoretically, beta-carotene could reduce the effectiveness of other HMG-CoA reductase inhibitors such as atorvastatin (Lipitor), fluvastatin (Lescol), lovastatin (Mevacor), and pravastatin (Pravachol).

NIACIN: Concomitant use of beta-carotene in combination with selenium, vitamin C, and vitamin E appears to decrease the effectiveness of the combination of niacin and simvastatin (Zocor) (7388). This combination of antioxidants can lower high-density lipoprotein 2 (HDL-2) levels by 15% and reduce the HDL-2-raising effects of HMG-CoA reductase inhibitors and niacin by more than 50% in people with heart disease (7388).

Drug Influences on Nutrient Levels and Depletion

SOME DRUGS CAN AFFECT BETA-CAROTENE LEVELS:

BILE ACID SEQUESTRANTS: Cholestyramine (Questran) and colestipol (Colestid) can reduce absorption of fat-soluble vitamins, including beta-carotene (4457,4461,4454,4458,5919). Serum levels of beta-carotene can be reduced (4457,4461), but this is probably only in proportion to the lowering of cholesterol (on which beta-carotene is transported). Supplements aren't usually needed (4461).

COLCHICINE: Colchicine can cause disruption of intestinal mucosal function, resulting in malabsorption (4543). Limited evidence suggests that short-term treatment with colchicine 1.9 to 3.9 mg/day can reduce absorption and serum levels of beta-carotene (4543). Long-term use of 1 to 2 mg/day does not affect beta-carotene levels (5921). Advise patients that this is unlikely to be clinically significant.

MINERAL OIL: Mineral oil reduces absorption of fat-soluble vitamins, including beta-carotene (4454,4495,4496). This isn't likely to be clinically significant when mineral oil is used for four months or less (4496).

NEOMYCIN: Oral neomycin sulfate in doses of 4 to 12 grams per day can reduce beta-carotene absorption, but this isn't likely to be clinically significant with short-term use (5916).

ORLISTAT (Xenical): Orlistat can decrease absorption of beta-carotene and other fat soluble vitamins (6001). Recommend that patients take a multivitamin supplement, and separate the dosing time by at least two hours from orlistat (6001).

PROTON PUMP INHIBITORS: Loss of stomach acid can reduce absorption of a single dose of beta-carotene (31), but it isn't known if this is clinically significant, or if it occurs with dietary beta-carotene. Some of these drugs include Lansoprazole (Prevacid), Omeprazole (Prilosec, Losec), Rabeprazole (Aciphex), and Pantoprazole (Protonix, Pantoloc).

Interactions with Foods

ALCOHOL (Ethanol): High consumption of alcohol can decrease serum concentrations of beta-carotene and other carotenoids such as alpha-carotene and beta-cryptoxanthin, and increase serum concentrations of retinol. Researchers are concerned increased retinol concentrations might promote carcinogenesis (10134). Further study is needed to determine whether this effect actually occurs.

OLESTRA (fat substitute): Olestra may interfere with supplemental beta-carotene activity. Olestra lowers serum beta-carotene concentrations in healthy people by 27% (2392).

Interactions with Lab Tests

HIGH-DENSITY LIPOPROTEIN 2 (HDL-2): Beta-carotene in combination with selenium, vitamins C, and vitamin E seems to lower HDL-2 levels (7388). This combination can lower HDL-2 levels by 15% in people with heart disease (7388).

Interactions with Diseases or Conditions

ANGIOPLASTY: There is some concern that when antioxidant vitamins, including beta-carotene, are used together they might have harmful effects in patients after angioplasty. A combination of beta-carotene 30,000 IU, vitamin C 500 mg, and vitamin E 700 IU daily started 30 days before angioplasty, and continued for 6 months thereafter, seems to prevent beneficial vascular remodeling in patients after angioplasty by promoting fibrosis at the site of angioplastic intervention (11000). Tell patients to avoid taking supplements of these vitamins immediately before and following angioplasty without the supervision of a healthcare professional.

SMOKERS: Cigarette smoking decreases serum concentrations of beta-carotene and other carotenoids, and depletes body stores of beta-carotene (7722,10134). However, beta-carotene supplementation should not be recommended because supplemental beta-carotene in doses greater than 20 mg per day is associated with a significantly higher risk of lung and prostate cancer in smokers (139,3949,3959,6382,6393). Tell smokers to avoid taking beta-carotene supplements.

Dosage and Administration

ORAL: For erythropoietic protoporphyria (EPP), dosage is based on age. For age 1 to 4, the daily dose is 60-90 mg; age 5 to 8 years, 90-120 mg; age 9 to 12 years, 120-150 mg; age 13 to 16 years, 150-180 mg; and age 16 and older, 180 mg. If adequate photoprotection is not provided by theses doses, beta-carotene can be increased by 30-60 mg per day for children under 16 years old, and up to a total of 300 mg per day for people older than age 16 (11793). For decreasing the risk of prostate cancer in men with plasma beta-carotene concentrations less than 153.25 ng/mL, 50 mg every other day has been used (1473). For oral leukoplakia, 30 mg orally twice daily for a total of 6 months has been used (1472). For preventing sunburn in sun-sensitive people, beta-carotene 25 mg orally daily has been used (6134). For preventing gastric cancer in people at high risk, 15-30 mg daily has been used (2579,2658). For treating age-related macular degeneration (AMD), beta-carotene 15 mg plus vitamin C 500 mg, zinc oxide 80 mg, and vitamin E 400 IU has been given daily (7303).

The Institute of Medicine has reviewed beta-carotene, but did not make recommendations for daily intake, citing lack of sufficient evidence. Consuming 5 servings of fruit and vegetables daily provides 6-8 mg of beta-carotene. Routine use of beta-carotene supplements is not necessary in the general population (4844). Beta-carotene requires some dietary fat for absorption, but supplemental beta-carotene is similarly absorbed when taken with high-fat (36 grams fat) or low-fat (3 grams fat) meals (2628,6133).

Beta-carotene supplements are available in both oil matrix gelatin capsules and water-miscible forms. Some clinical trials have used water-miscible beta-carotene (10%) beadlets. The water miscible form seems to produce a significantly higher response in plasma beta-carotene (approximately 47% to 50%) than oil matrix gelatin capsules (10136).

Comments

The American Heart Association recommends obtaining antioxidants, including beta-carotene, from a diet high in fruits, vegetables and whole grains rather than through supplements until more information is known from randomized clinical trials (1440). Similar statements have been released by the American Cancer Society, the World Cancer Research Institute in association with the American Institute for Cancer Research, and the World Health Organization's International Agency for Research on Cancer (1470).

BETA GLUCANS

Also Known As

Beta Glucan, Beta 1,3 Glucans, Beta-Glucan, Beta-Glucans, Beta Glycans, Beta-Glycans, Grifolan (GRN), Lentinan, PGG Glucan, PGG-Glucan, Poly-[1-6]-Beta-D-Glucopyranosyl-[1-3]-Beta-D-Glucopyranose, Schizophyllan (SPG), SSG, Yeast-Derived Beta Glucan.

CAUTION: See separate listings for Barley, Brewer's Yeast, Maitake Mushroom, Oat above ground parts, Oat Bran, Oats, Saccharomyces Boulardii, Salep, and Shiitake Mushroom.

Scientific Names

1-3,1-6-beta-glucan; beta-1,3-D-glucan; beta-1-6,1,3-beta-glucan.

People Use This For

Orally, beta glucans are used for hypercholesterolemia, diabetes, cancer, and HIV/AIDS. Beta glucans are also used orally as an immunostimulant in people with conditions that may compromise their immune system such as chronic fatigue syndrome, physical and emotional stress, and patients receiving chemotherapy or radiation treatment. It is also used orally for colds (common cold), flu (influenza), allergies, hepatitis, Lyme disease, asthma, ear infections, aging, ulcerative colitis and Crohn's disease, fibromyalgia, rheumatoid arthritis, and multiple sclerosis.

Topically, beta glucans are used for dermatitis, eczema, wrinkles, bedsores, wounds, burns, diabetic ulcers, and radiation burns.

Intravenously and intramuscularly, beta glucans are used for treating cancer and as an immunostimulant in patients with HIV/AIDS and AIDS-related disorders. It is also used intravenously for preventing sepsis in trauma patients after undergoing exploratory laparotomy or thoracotomy and for preventing infection in surgical patients.

Subcutaneously, beta glucans are used for treating and reducing the size of subcutaneous tumors resulting from malignant metastatic disease.

In manufacturing, beta glucans are used as a food additive in products such as salad dressings, frozen desserts, sour cream, and cheese spreads.

Safety

LIKELY SAFE ...when used orally in amounts commonly found in foods. Beta glucans derived from baker's yeast or brewer's yeast (Saccharomyces cerevisiae) have Generally Recognized As Safe (GRAS) status in the US (4912).

POSSIBLY SAFE ...when used orally and appropriately, short-term in medicinal amounts. There is some evidence that yeast-derived beta-glucans 15 grams per day can be used safely for up to 8 weeks (7272). ...when used intravenously or intramuscularly and appropriately. Both yeast and fungal beta-glucans seem to be safe when soluble forms are used (7261,7263,7264,7266,7267,7269,7270,7271). Particulate beta glucans may not be safe. There is preliminary evidence that intravenous beta glucans in the microparticulate form might cause serious side effects such as hepatosplenomegaly, granuloma formation, and microembolization (7241). Most studies evaluating parenteral use of beta glucans have used specific forms including PGG-glucan (Betafectin) from a proprietary strain of Saccharomyces cerevisiae (7269,7270,7271) and specific fungal-derived beta glucans lentinan and schizophyllan (SPG) (7261,7263,7264,7266,7267). Lentinan and SPG have been safely used in studies lasting for up to 12 months (7263,7264,7267). PGG-glucan has been safely used in studies when given 24 hours prior to surgery and lasting up to 96 hours after surgery (7269,7270,7271).

There is insufficient reliable information available about the safety of beta glucans when used subcutaneously or topically.

PREGNANCY AND LACTATION: Insufficient reliable information available; avoid using.

Effectiveness

POSSIBLY EFFECTIVE

Cancer. Giving the specific fungal beta glucans lentinan and schizophyllan intravenously or intramuscularly seems to prolong survival time of cancer patients when used in addition to conventional cancer treatment regimens. Lentinan 1-2 mg once or twice weekly for at least 1 year increases survival time by 6-9 months in people with advanced (stage III or IV) unresectable cancers (7266). Schizophyllan 20-40 mg once or twice weekly for at least 1 year significantly improves 4-5 year survival rates in people with cervical cancer and head and neck cancer (7261,7263,7264).

HIV/AIDS. There is preliminary evidence that giving the specific fungal beta glucans lentinan 2-10 mg once or twice weekly intravenously can increase levels of CD4 cells by 5.5-18% and decrease p24 antigen levels (a marker of viral replication) by 11.5% after 12-20 weeks of treatment in asymptomatic patients with HIV (7267).

Hypercholesterolemia. Taking yeast-derived beta glucans 7.5 grams twice daily appears to reduce serum total cholesterol concentrations by 6-8% in patients with hypercholesterolemia after 7-8 weeks of treatment (7272). However, barley that is highly enriched (75% by weight) with beta glucan doesn't seem to affect cholesterol. This lack of effect seems to be the result of processing the barley into a highly enriched beta glucan product (10166). More research is needed to determine if improved processing methods can produce beta-glucan enriched products that can lower cholesterol.

Postoperative infection. A proprietary beta glucans preparation from Saccharomyces cerevisiae called PGG-glucan given intravenously 12-24 hours before and 4-96 hours after surgery at 0.5-1 mg/kg per dose reduces the occurrence of postoperative infection by 10-16%, decreases the number of days of intravenous antibiotic use by 10 days, and shortens the length of stay in the intensive care unit (ICU) by 3 days in surgical patients at high risk for infection (7269,7271). Administering beta glucans intravenously also seems to help prevent sepsis in trauma patients following exploratory laparotomy or thoracotomy. There is some evidence that intravenous soluble yeast-derived beta glucans 50 mg/M2 daily for 7 days decreases the rate of septic morbidity by 39.5% in trauma patients following exploratory surgical procedures (7268).

There is insufficient reliable information available about the effectiveness of beta glucans for their other uses.

Mechanism of Action

Beta glucans are polysaccharides that consist of (1-3)-beta-D-linked polymers of glucose that are either non-branched or with 1-6-beta-branches (3394,7242). Beta glucans are primary components in cell walls of bacteria, fungi, yeasts, algae, lichens, plants such as oats and barley, and are excreted extracellularly by various fungi (3394,7242,7250). The beta glucans most extensively studied to date are yeast-derived beta glucans from Saccharomyces cerevisiae; the fungal-derived beta glucans such as lentinan from Lentinus edodes, gifolan (GRN) from Grifola frondosa, schizophyllan (SPG) from Schizophyllum commune, SSG from Sclerotinia sclerotiorum; and beta glucans from oats (7241,7248,7273). Mammals cannot digest and absorb beta glucans because they lack the enzyme beta-1-3-glucanase needed to break down large beta glucan molecules. Since beta glucans cannot be absorbed orally, clinical studies have usually administered beta glucans by the parenteral route (3393). Beta glucans seem to have antibacterial, antiviral, antifungal, antiparasitic, and antitumor activity; and might promote recovery from sepsis and immunosuppression associated with various disease states or conditions such as HIV infection or whole body radiation (7238,7243,7250). Laboratory findings suggest beta glucans specifically bind to monocyte and macrophage cell lines, increase the proliferation and activation of macrophages, and increase the production of cytokine interleukin-1 (IL-1) by macrophages which in turn promotes the release of IL-2 by T-cells (7243,7248,7249,7250,7252,7268). Beta glucans also seem to have anticancer effects. Beta glucans don't seem to have direct antitumor or antibacterial activity, but are thought to act as biological response modifiers (BRMs) that restore or enhance humoral and cell-mediated immune responses (3394,7237,7251). Beta glucans increase macrophage phagocytosis of tumor cells, increase the cytotoxicity of natural killer cells (NK), and stimulate the release of interleukin-1 (IL-1) and tumor necrosis factor (TNF) (7237,7238,7240,7265). Beta glucans bind to a beta glucan receptor on macrophages, neutrophils, and NK cells and seem to activate a complement receptor on the cells which bind to tumor or bacterial cells that are opsonized with complement and antibodies (7237,7239,7248,7269,7270,7271). Many cells, including cancer cells and bacteria, can acquire mechanisms to resist the action of complement, but there is some evidence that beta glucans can override this mechanism and allow the phagocytosis to occur (7237).

For wound healing after surgery, there is some evidence beta glucans can decrease inflammation, and accelerate the repair of surgical wounds by stimulating macrophages and increasing macrophage infiltration, causing increased tissue granulation and enhanced re-epithelization of tissue (7246).

For hypercholesterolemia, beta glucans are thought to lower cholesterol by forming a layer adjacent to the intestinal mucosa that delays or prevents cholesterol absorption (7273,10166). Beta glucans might also bind bile acids in the intestinal lumen (7272,10166).

Adverse Reactions

Orally, yeast-derived beta glucans seem to be well-tolerated. No adverse effects have been reported (7272). Intravenously, beta glucans can cause chills and fever (7267,7271), redness, pain and swelling at the injection site, lymph node swelling (7261,7263), joint pain, lower back pain, headache, diarrhea, dizziness, flushing (7267), hypotension, hypertension, vasodilation, nausea, vomiting, leukocytosis (7270,7271), hives (7267), maculopapular rash (7270,7271), and excessive urination (7267).

Interactions with Herbs & Other Dietary Supplements

None known.

Interactions with Drugs

IMMUNOSUPPRESSANTS: Theoretically, beta glucans might decrease the effects of immunosuppressants because of its immunostimulant effects (7243,7248,7249,7250,7252,7268). Immunosuppressant drugs include azathioprine (Imuran), basiliximab (Simulect), cyclosporine (Neoral, Sandimmune), daclizumab (Zenapax), muromonab-CD3 (OKT3, Orthoclone OKT3), mycophenolate (CellCept), tacrolimus (FK506, Prograf), sirolimus (Rapamune), prednisone (Deltasone, Orasone), and other corticosteroids (glucocorticoids).

Interactions with Foods

None known.

Interactions with Lab Tests

WHITE BLOOD CELL COUNT: Beta glucans can cause a transient increase in the number of white cells (leukocytosis) (7270).

Interactions with Diseases or Conditions

ACQUIRED IMMUNODEFICIENCY SYNDROME (AIDS) or AIDS-RELATED COMPLEX (ARC): Keratoderma of the palms and soles can develop in patients with AIDS/HIV or ARC who are receiving yeast beta glucans. The condition can begin during the first two weeks of therapy and resolves two to four weeks after discontinuation of beta glucans (7252).

Dosage and Administration

ORAL: For hypercholesterolemia, 7.5 grams twice daily of yeast-derived beta glucans fiber added to juice has been used (7272).

INTRAVENOUS: For HIV infection, 1-10 mg of the fungal beta glucan lentinan, administered over 10-30 minutes and given once to twice weekly has been used (7267). To prolong survival time in patients with cancer, 1-2 mg of the fungal beta glucan lentinan or 20-40 mg of the fungal beta glucan schizophyllan (SPG) administered once or twice weekly for at least one year has been used (3393,7261,7263,7264,7266). To prevent infection in trauma patients undergoing exploratory surgical procedures, 50 mg/M2 of soluble yeast-derived beta-glucan per day for 7 days has been used (7268). In surgical patients at high-risk for infection, 0.5-2 mg/kg of PGG-glucan given 1-6 hours before surgery and then repeated 4 hours, 48 hours, and 96 hours after surgery has been used (7270,7271).

Comments

There are several beta glucan supplement products that claim beta glucan taken orally can only be absorbed if the product is prepared by a special patented process that micronizes beta glucan particles to a size of 1 micron or less. However, there is no reliable evidence to support such a claim.

BETA-SITOSTEROL

Also Known As

24-ethyl-cholesterol, Angelicin, B-sitosterol 3-B-D-glucoside, B-sitosterolin, Beta sitosterin, Beta Sitosterol, Beta-sitosterol glucoside, Beta-sitosterol glycoside, Betasitosterol, Cinchol, Cupreol, Phytosterols, Plant Sterols, Quebrachol, Rhamnol, Sitosterin, Sitosterol, Sitosterolins, Sitosterols, Sterinol, Sterolins.
CAUTION: See separate listing for Sitostanol.

Scientific Names

22,23-dihydrostigmasterol; 24-beta-ethyl-delta-5-cholesten-3beta-ol; 24-ethyl-cholesterol; 3-beta-stigmast-5-en-3-ol.

People Use This For

Orally, beta-sitosterol is used for coronary heart disease and hypercholesterolemia, benign prostatic hyperplasia (BPH) and prostatitis, and gallstones. It is also used orally for enhancing sexual activity and for preventing colon cancer. Beta-sitosterol is also used orally for boosting the immune system, preventing immune suppression and inflammation following participation in a marathon, common cold and flu (influenza), HIV/AIDS, rheumatoid arthritis, tuberculosis, psoriasis, allergies, cervical cancer, fibromyalgia, systemic lupus erythematosus, asthma, alopecia, bronchitis, idiopathic thrombocytopenia purpura (ITP), migraine headache, chronic fatigue syndrome, and symptoms of menopause.
In foods, beta-sitosterol is added to some margarines designed for use as part of a cholesterol-lowering diet and for preventing heart disease.

Safety

LIKELY SAFE ...when used orally and appropriately. Beta-sitosterol has been safely used in studies lasting up to 18 months (5327,5328,5329,5330,5331,5332,5333,5334,5336,5337,5338,5339,7198,10638).

PREGNANCY AND LACTATION: Insufficient reliable information available; avoid using.

Effectiveness

LIKELY EFFECTIVE

Benign prostatic hyperplasia (BPH). Taking beta-sitosterol orally significantly improves urinary symptoms, increases maximum urinary flow, and decreases postvoid residual urine volume; however, it does not affect prostate size (5327,5328,5329,7195,7198).

Hypercholesterolemia. Taking beta-sitosterol orally significantly reduces total and low-density lipoprotein (LDL) cholesterol levels, but has little or no effect on high-density lipoprotein (HDL) cholesterol levels (5330,5331,5332,5333,5334,5336,6668,7195,8528,10638).

POSSIBLY INEFFECTIVE

Tuberculosis. There is some evidence that taking beta-sitosterol orally as an adjunct to conventional treatment for tuberculosis can increase lymphocyte counts; however, beta-sitosterol does not seem to decrease the time to cure based on negative sputum culture (5337).

LIKELY INEFFECTIVE

Gallbladder disease. Taking beta-sitosterol orally isn't effective for treating gallstones (5338,5339).

There is insufficient reliable information available about the effectiveness of beta-sitosterol for its other uses.

Mechanism of Action

Beta-sitosterol is a plant sterol. It has a chemical structure similar to cholesterol with an ethyl group added at position 24. The average diet provides about 175-200 mg of beta-sitosterol, but less than 5% is actually absorbed when consumed orally. Therefore these plant sterols do not cause some of the atherogenic adverse effects associated with cholesterol from animal products. Beta-sitosterol is commonly added to margarines as a cholesterol reducing aid. Fats are needed to solubilize plant sterols so margarines are an ideal vehicle. Soybean phytosterols containing 48% beta-sitosterol, 26% campesterol, and 21% stigmasterol have been added to ground beef (8528). Capsules containing beta-sitosterol may not disperse properly in the gut, limiting their ability to reduce cholesterol absorption (5814). Beta-sitosterol actually inhibits intestinal absorption of cholesterol by competing for the limited space in mixed micelles, which decreases cholesterol absorption by about 50% (5814). Because there is less cholesterol available in the body, compensatory mechanisms kick in and increase cholesterol synthesis in the liver (5814).

For prostatic hyperplasia, animal research suggests that beta-sitosterol might inhibit 5-alpha-reductase activity, although finasteride (Proscar) appears to be more potent (11739). Laboratory research suggests beta-sitosterol might have antiproliferative effects on the prostate, possibly by inhibiting growth factors (11234). In animals, beta-sitosterol shrinks the prostate, but this has not been shown in humans (11759).

There is some preliminary evidence that beta-sitosterol might also have anticancer and immunostimulant effects. Beta-sitosterol can inhibit the growth of human colon cancer cells in vitro (3667,3668). Mixtures of beta-sitosterol and its glycoside sitosterolin seem to also enhance proliferative responses of T-cells in vitro (3669,5342). Beta-sitosterol might also reduce the mild immune suppression and inflammation seen in marathon runners after a race (5335).

Adverse Reactions

Orally, beta-sitosterol is usually well tolerated. In some patients it can cause nausea, indigestion, gas, diarrhea, or constipation (5327,5328).

Interactions with Herbs & Other Dietary Supplements

CAROTENE, VITAMIN E: Beta-sitosterol may reduce absorption and blood levels of alpha- and beta-carotene and vitamin E (5814).

CHOLESTEROL LOWERING HERBS/SUPPLEMENTS: Beta-sitosterol might have additive effects with herbs and supplements that also lower cholesterol levels. Some of these herbs and supplements include chromium, flaxseed, garlic, guar gum, niacin, oat bran, psyllium, red yeast, and others.

Interactions with Drugs

EZETIMIBE (Zetia): Ezetimibe inhibits intestinal absorption of beta-sitosterol and reduces plasma concentrations in people with and without sitosterolemia. In people with mild to moderate hypercholesterolemia, ezetimibe reduces beta-sitosterol levels by 41% (11985,11989).

PRAVASTATIN (Pravachol): There is some evidence that pravastatin can lower blood levels of beta-sitosterol (3672). Theoretically, this might occur with other HMG-CoA reductase inhibitors ("statins"); however, simvastatin (Zocor) does not seem to affect beta-sitosterol levels (3673). Other statin drugs include atorvastatin (Lipitor), cerivastatin (Baycol), fluvastatin (Lescol), and lovastatin (Mevacor).

Interactions with Foods

CAROTENE, VITAMIN E: Beta-sitosterol may reduce absorption and blood levels of alpha- and beta-carotene and vitamin E (5814).

Interactions with Lab Tests

CHOLESTEROL: Beta-sitosterol decreases total serum cholesterol and low-density lipoprotein (LDL) levels (5331,5336).

Interactions with Diseases or Conditions

SITOSTEROLEMIA (Phytosterolemia): Taking beta-sitosterol can exacerbate sitosterolemia, a rare inherited lipid storage disease (5326,10305). People with this disorder have increased absorption of cholesterol and beta-sitosterol from the diet, and decreased clearance of beta-sitosterol. Total body stores of beta-sitosterol are increased up to 17-fold. Elevated hepatic beta-sitosterol levels competitively inhibit cholesterol catabolism, contributing to hypercholesterolemia (3663). Patients with sitosterolemia are prone to premature coronary artery disease and xanthomas (3661,3662). Beta-sitosterol and its glycoside sitosterolin are contraindicated in patients with sitosterolemia. However, beta-sitosterol appears to be safe for heterozygous carriers of sitosterolemia (10457).

Dosage and Administration

ORAL: For benign prostatic hyperplasia (BPH) and prostatitis, a typical dose is 60 to 130 mg of beta-sitosterol divided into 2-3 doses daily (5327,5328,5329). For hypercholesterolemia, the usual dose is 800 mg to 6 grams per day divided and given before meals. Beta-sitosterol is typically given in conjunction with a low-fat diet (5327,5328,5329,5330,5331,5332,5333,5334,5336,5337,5338,5339,10638). One supplier suggests that doses should be taken at least 30 minutes, but not more than 90 minutes, before meals for maximum effect on cholesterol absorption (3658).

Comments

Beta-sitosterol is a supplement that is also found in the functional food product Take Control. The FDA authorized the use of labeling health claims for foods containing plant sterol esters, including beta-sitosterol, for reducing the risk of coronary heart disease (CHD) (6668). This rule is based on the FDA's conclusion that plant sterol esters may reduce the risk of CHD by lowering blood cholesterol levels. Although there is plenty of evidence that beta-sitosterol does lower cholesterol levels, there is no proof that long-term use actually lowers the risk of developing CHD. Avoid confusing beta-sitosterol with sitostanol, the saturated beta-sitosterol derivative contained in Benecol (5340). Both sitostanol and beta-sitosterol are used for lowering cholesterol levels in people with hypercholesterolemia and appear to be equally effective (7196).

BETAINE ANHYDROUS

Also Known As

Betaine, Cystadane, Trimethyl Glycine, Trimethylglycine, TMG.
CAUTION: See separate listing for Betaine Hydrochloride.

Scientific Names

Trimethylglycine anhydrous.

People Use This For

Orally, betaine anhydrous is used for homocystinuria caused by cystathionine beta-synthase deficiency, 5,10-methylenetetrahydrofolate reductase deficiency, or cobalamin cofactor metabolism defect. It is also used orally for hyperhomocysteinemia, homocystinuria not responsive to pyridoxine, and nonalcoholic steatohepatitis.
Topically, betaine anhydrous is used as an ingredient in toothpastes to reduce the subjective symptoms of dry mouth.

Safety

LIKELY SAFE ...when used orally and appropriately (698,10631). Betaine anhydrous is an FDA-approved prescription product.
PREGNANCY AND LACTATION: Insufficient reliable information available; avoid using.

Effectiveness

EFFECTIVE

Homocystinuria. Betaine anhydrous reduces plasma homocysteine levels by 20-30% (15). Betaine anhydrous is FDA-approved for this indication.

POSSIBLY EFFECTIVE

Dry mouth. Applying betaine anhydrous topically as an ingredient of toothpastes seems to reduce the subjective symptoms of dry mouth (6812).

INSUFFICIENT RELIABLE EVIDENCE to RATE

Cardiovascular disease. There is some evidence that betaine supplementation for 3 weeks can produce a small, 5.5% to 8%, decrease in plasma homocysteine levels in people with normal homocysteine levels, <15 micromol/L. It is not clear whether this reduction results in a decreased risk for cardiovascular disease (6810).

Steatohepatitis. Preliminary evidence suggests that betaine supplementation might be useful for nonalcoholic steatohepatitis. Use for 12 months seems to normalize liver enzymes and improve the degree of steatosis, necroinflammatory grade, and stage of fibrosis (10631).

More evidence is needed to rate betaine anhydrous for these uses.

Mechanism of Action

Betaine anhydrous occurs naturally in the body. It is the major metabolite of choline. It is present in small amounts in foods such as beets, spinach, cereals, seafood, and wine. Betaine is a methyl group donor. It reduces homocysteine levels by remethylating homocysteine to methionine (15). Elevated homocysteine levels can be reduced by two mechanisms: trans-sulfuration to cysteine using pyridoxine as a cofactor, or remethylation to methionine. This latter reaction uses either 5-methyltetrahydrofolate derived from folic acid as a methyl donor, and either vitamin B12 or betaine anhydrous as a cofactor (6810). In patients with homocystinuria, total plasma homocysteine concentrations are very high, >50 micromol/L, compared to normal levels in the population of 5 to 15 micromol/L (3047,6810). Levels greater than 15 micromol/L are referred to as hyperhomocysteinemia and have been identified as a risk factor for cardiovascular disease (3047). The potential role of betaine anhydrous in lowering normal or slightly elevated homocysteine levels in order to reduce the risk of cardiovascular disease is not known. It has been suggested that the betaine content of wine may contribute to the lower incidence of cardiovascular disease in countries with a high wine consumption such as France, but it is not known whether the levels present, approximately 3 mg per glass, have any significant effect (6811). Preliminary studies suggest that betaine supplementation may increase methionine and S-adenosyl-L-methionine (SAMe) synthesis from homocysteine in the liver when these compunds have been inhibited by ethanol; betaine may also reduce ethanol-induced liver damage (6813). Topically, betaine anhydrous has been reported to reduce the irritant effects of sodium lauryl sulfate on the skin and oral mucosa, and may reduce subjective symptoms of dry mouth (6812).

Adverse Reactions
Orally, betaine anhydrous can cause nausea, GI distress, diarrhea, and body odor (698,10631).

Interactions with Herbs & Other Dietary Supplements
None known.

Interactions with Drugs
None known.

Interactions with Foods
None known.

Interactions with Lab Tests
None known.

Interactions with Diseases or Conditions
None known.

Dosage and Administration
ORAL: For homocystinuria, a maintenance dose of 3 grams is typically taken twice daily in both adults and children. Dose titration is preferable in children. For children under three years old, the starting dose is 100 mg/kg per day, increased in weekly intervals in increments of 100 mg/kg daily. All patients can receive dose increases until plasma homocysteine concentrations are undetectable or very low, which can require doses up to 20 grams per day. Dissolve the powder in water immediately before administration (15). For reducing plasma homocysteine levels, 3 grams betaine anhydrous twice daily orally has been used (6810). For nonalcoholic steatohepatitis, 20 grams daily, in two divided doses has been used (10631).
TOPICAL: Betaine anhydrous has been added to toothpastes in a concentration of 4% for treatment of symptoms of dry mouth (6812).

Comments
Betaine anhydrous has Orphan Drug status in the US. Avoid confusion with betaine hydrochloride, a dietary supplement with variable purity and potency that has not been demonstrated safe or effective for treating homocystinuria.

BETAINE HYDROCHLORIDE

Also Known As
Betaine, Betaine HCl, Trimethyl Glycine, Trimethylglycine, TMG.
CAUTION: See separate listing for Betaine Anhydrous.

Scientific Names
Trimethylglycine hydrochloride.

People Use This For
Orally, betaine hydrochloride is used as a supplemental source of hydrochloric acid, to treat hypokalemia, and as a liver protectant. It is also used for allergic rhinitis, anemia, asthma, atherosclerosis, candidiasis, diarrhea, food allergies, gallstones, inner ear infection, rheumatoid arthritis, and thyroid disorders.

Safety
There is insufficient reliable information available about the safety of betaine hydrochloride.
Pregnancy and Lactation: Insufficient reliable information available; avoid using.

Effectiveness
There is insufficient reliable information available about the effectiveness of betaine hydrochloride.

Mechanism of Action
Betaine hydrochloride is a source of hydrochloric acid (9). Some people use it due to inaccurate claims that many conditions are due to inadequate gastric acid.

Adverse Reactions
Orally, betaine hydrochloride can theoretically irritate gastric or duodenal ulcers or impede ulcer healing by increasing gastric acid. Theoretically, it might also cause heartburn (9).

Interactions with Herbs & Other Dietary Supplements
None known.

Interactions with Drugs
None known.

Interactions with Foods
None known.

Interactions with Lab Tests
None known.

Interactions with Diseases or Conditions
GASTRIC AND DUODENAL ULCERS: Theoretically, betaine hydrochloride can irritate ulcers or impede healing by increasing gastric acid; avoid using in patients with gastric or duodenal ulcers (9).

Dosage and Administration
No typical dosage.

Comments
Avoid confusion with betaine anhydrous. Betaine is manufactured in various salt forms around the world, including betaine hydrochloride. The purity and potency of these dietary supplement products can vary. There are no data to support the effectiveness of betaine hydrochloride in any condition, including homocystinuria. Use only the FDA-approved betaine anhydrous for the treatment of homocystinuria (see separate listing for betaine anhydrous).

BETH ROOT

Also Known As
Birthroot, Coughroot, Ground Lily, Jew's Harp Plant, Indian Balm, Indian Shamrock, Lamb's Quarters, Milk Ipecac, Pariswort, Rattlesnake Root, Snakebite, Stinking Benjamin, Three-Leafed Nightshade, Wake Robin.
CAUTION: See separate listing for Arum.

Scientific Names
Trillium erectum.
Family: Liliaceae or Trilliaceae.

People Use This For
Orally, beth root is used for long, heavy menstruation and pain relief. It is also used orally as an astringent and expectorant.
Topically, beth root is used for varicose veins and ulcers, hematomas, and hemorrhoid bleeding.

Safety
POSSIBLY UNSAFE ...when used orally. Beth root is a gastrointestinal irritant (12).
There is insufficient reliable information available about the safety of beth root for its other uses.
PREGNANCY AND LACTATION: LIKELY UNSAFE ...when used orally; avoid using. Beth root might have menstrual or uterine stimulant activity (12,18).

Effectiveness
There is insufficient reliable information available about the effectiveness of beth root.

Mechanism of Action
The applicable parts of beth root are the rhizome, and dried root and leaf. There is insufficient reliable information about the possible mechanism of action or active ingredients.

Adverse Reactions
Orally, ingestion of large amounts of the plant or volatile oil might produce GI irritation severe enough to cause vomiting (12,18). In pregnant women, the drastic purgative effects can cause reflex uterine contractions.
Topically, beth root causes extreme irritation (18).

Interactions with Herbs & Other Dietary Supplements
None known.

Interactions with Drugs
None known.

Interactions with Foods
None known.

Interactions with Lab Tests
None known.

Interactions with Diseases or Conditions
CARDIAC CONDITIONS: Due to potential cardiotoxicity from the convallamarin-like glycoside, patients with a cardiac condition should be cautioned against the use of this herb (6002).

Dosage and Administration
ORAL: No typical dosage.
TOPICAL: The ground plant parts are used as a poultice (18).

BETONY

Also Known As
Bishopswort, Bishop Wort, Hedge Nettles, Wood Betony.

Scientific Names
Stachys officinalis, synonyms Betonica officinalis, Stachys betonica.
Family: Lamiaceae/Labiatae.

People Use This For
Orally, betony is used to treat diarrhea, irritation of mucous membranes, stress and tension, headache, facial pain, coughs as an expectorant, bronchitis, asthma, as an antiflatulent, and as a sedative. It is also used orally to treat heartburn, gout, nervousness, bladder and kidney stones, and for bladder inflammation.
In combination with other herbs, betony is used to treat neuralgia and anxiety.

Safety
POSSIBLY SAFE ...when the dried above ground parts are used orally in medicinal amounts (5,6,12).
POSSIBLY UNSAFE ...when used in large amounts because it contains 15% tannins and these can cause gastrointestinal irritation (5,12).
PREGNANCY: POSSIBLY UNSAFE ...when used orally; avoid using (6).
LACTATION: Insufficient reliable information available; avoid using.

Effectiveness
There is insufficient reliable information available about the effectiveness of betony.

Mechanism of Action
The applicable parts of betony are the dried above ground parts. The high tannin content (15%) is responsible for its astringent properties (5). The glycoside mixture can have a hypotensive effect, possibly explaining its effectiveness in mild anxiety states and headache (5,6). One constituent, stachydrine, is a systolic depressant that is also active against rheumatism (6).

Adverse Reactions
Large doses can cause significant GI irritation due to the tannin component (5,6).

Interactions with Herbs & Other Dietary Supplements
None known.

Interactions with Drugs

ANTIHYPERTENSIVE DRUGS: Theoretically, betony might have additive effects with blood pressure lowering drugs due to hypotensive activity of the glycosides found in betony. It might also interfere with the activity of pressor drugs (5,6).

Interactions with Foods

None known.

Interactions with Lab Tests

None known.

Interactions with Diseases or Conditions

None known.

Dosage and Administration

ORAL: Betony is typically taken as a tea or an infusion (6002). Use small doses to avoid gastrointestinal (GI) irritation.

BHT (BUTYLATED HYDROXYTOLUENE)

Also Known As

Butylated Hydroxytoluene, Butylhydroxytoluene, Dibutylated Hydroxytoluene.

Scientific Names

2,6-di-tert-butyl-p-creosol.

People Use This For

Orally, BHT is used for genital herpes and acquired immunodeficiency syndrome (AIDS).
Topically, BHT is used for herpes simplex labialis.
In foods, BHT is used as an antioxidant.

Safety

LIKELY SAFE ...when used orally as a food additive (10292,10293). BHT has Generally Recognized As Safe (GRAS) status for food use in the US (4912).
There is insufficient reliable information available about the safety of BHT for its other uses.
CHILDREN: LIKELY SAFE ...when used orally as a food additive (10292).
PREGNANCY AND LACTATION: LIKELY SAFE ...when used orally as a food additive (10292).

Effectiveness

INSUFFICIENT RELIABLE EVIDENCE to RATE

Herpes labialis (cold sores). There is preliminary evidence that suggests that topical application of BHT might be helpful for herpes simplex labialis. Topical application of BHT may decrease the time from lesion formation to dry crust formation by about 0.4 days; and it may decrease the duration of the vesicle-ulcer stage by about 0.8 days (10294). More evidence is needed to rate BHT for this use.

Mechanism of Action

BHT is a synthetic phenolic, hydrophobic chemical that is used extensively as an antioxidant in foods, pharmaceutical preparations, and other manufacturing processes (10293,10697). BHT may exert antiviral effects by interfering with membrane function in viruses that have a lipid envelope. BHT is lipid soluble and remains in highly lipid soluble regions, such as membranes (10295,10697). However, BHT does not appear to affect plaque diameter in cells infected with herpes simplex virus (HSV) (10295).

Adverse Reactions

Orally, BHT can cause severe gastritis characterized by severe epigastric pain, nausea, and vomiting. Symptoms may progress to weakness, dizziness, confusion, slurred speech, unsteady gait, and loss of consciousness (10303,10698,10699). BHT is highly lipid soluble. It may cross the blood brain barrier, causing psychotropic symptoms (10303). BHT has been associated with development of cancer; however, BHT does not appear to increase the incidence of cancer in the amounts consumed in the diet. Some evidence suggests that BHT may actually decrease the formation of cancer (10292,10293).

Interactions with Herbs & Other Dietary Supplements
None known.

Interactions with Drugs
None known.

Interactions with Foods
None known.

Interactions with Lab Tests
None known.

Interactions with Diseases or Conditions
None known.

Dosage and Administration
ORAL: No typical dosage. However, the typical dietary consumption of BHT is less than 0.1 mg/kg/day (10292).
TOPICAL: For treating herpes simplex labialis, BHT 15% in mineral oil applied 4 times daily for 5 days has been used (10294).

BIFIDOBACTERIA

Also Known As
B. bifidum, Bifido, Bifidobacteria bifidus, Bifidobacterium, Bifidum, Probiotics.
CAUTION: See separate listings for Lactobacillus, Saccharomyces Boulardii, and Yogurt.

Scientific Names
Bifidobacterium adolescentis; Bifidobacterium bifidum; Bifidobacterium breve; Bifidobacterium infantis; Bifidobacterium lactis; Bifidobacterium longum.
Family: Actinomycetaceae.

People Use This For
Orally, bifidobacteria are used for preventing acute diarrhea in infants and children; preventing necrotizing enterocolitis in neonates; treating atopic eczema in infants; preventing traveler's diarrhea; improving immune function; and replenishing intestinal normal flora depleted by diarrhea, radiation, chemotherapy, antibiotics, or other causes. Bifidobacteria are also used orally for candidiasis, the common cold and flu (influenza), hepatitis, hypercholesterolemia, lactose intolerance, mastitis, mumps, and cancer. They are also used orally to treat ulcerative colitis and pouchitis following surgery for ulcerative colitis.

Safety
POSSIBLY SAFE ...when used orally and appropriately. Bifidobacteria seem to be safe when used for up to 9 months (162,6087).
CHILDREN: POSSIBLY SAFE ...when used orally and appropriately. Bifidobacteria seem to be safe in children including those under two years of age and critically ill neonates when used for up to 8 months (161,3162,3169,3458).
PREGNANCY AND LACTATION: Insufficient reliable information available; avoid using.

Effectiveness
POSSIBLY EFFECTIVE

Antibiotic-induced gastrointestinal adverse effects. Ingestion of Bifidobacterium longum can reduce stool frequency, abdominal discomfort, and stool clostridial spore count when used in patients concurrently taking erythromycin (1233).

Atopic dermatitis (eczema). Giving infants Bifidobacterium lactis orally seems to help reduce the severity of atopic eczema and the markers for allergic responses including soluble CD4 in serum and eosinophilic protein X in urine (3458).

Chronic pouchitis. Taking bifidobacteria orally seems to help treat chronic pouchitis, a complication of surgery for ulcerative colitis. A combination of Bifidobacterium longum, Bifidobacterium breve, Lactobacillus species, and Streptococcus thermophilus seems to prevent chronic pouchitis flare-ups (6087). Daily consumption of bifidobacteria is usually required to maintain effectiveness, although effects may persist a week after discontinuation (1731).

Necrotizing enterocolitis (NEC). Bifidobacterium infantis in combination with Lactobacillus acidophilus seems to reduce the incidence of NEC and NEC-associated mortality in critically ill neonates (3162).

Rotaviral diarrhea. Bifidobacterium bifidum combined with Streptococcus thermophilus or the Bifidobacterium Bb12 strain appears to reduce the incidence of diarrhea and rotavirus shedding in infants (153,161,3169).
Traveler's diarrhea. Bifidobacterium in combination with Lactobacillus acidophilus, Lactobacillus bulgaricus, or Streptococcus thermophilus seems to decrease the chance of developing traveler's diarrhea (155).
Ulcerative colitis. In patients intolerant to 5-aminosalicylic acid, bifidobacteria plus lactobacilli and Streptococcus thermophilus seems to prevent increases in pathogenic bacteria and relapse in some patients with ulcerative colitis (3261).

INSUFFICIENT RELIABLE EVIDENCE to RATE

Radiation sickness. There is preliminary evidence that antibiotic-resistant Bifidobacterium longum can help improve short-term survival in the treatment of radiation sickness. In combination with prophylactic antibiotics, bifidobacteria appear to inhibit colonization and overgrowth of intestinal opportunistic pathogens, preventing post-irradiation sepsis (3457). More evidence is needed to rate bifidobacteria for this use.

Mechanism of Action

Bifidobacteria are anaerobic, rod-shaped, Gram-positive bacteria that normally colonize in the human colon (1060,1137). Bifidobacteria belong to a group of bacteria called lactic acid bacteria. Lactic acid bacteria, which also include the lactobacilli species, are found in fermented foods like yogurt and cheese (1055,3589). Bifidobacteria are used therapeutically as so-called probiotics, the opposite of antibiotics. They are considered "friendly" bacteria and are used with the purpose of re-colonizing areas of the body where they normally would occur. The human body relies on the normal flora for several functions, including metabolizing foods, absorbing nutrients, and preventing colonization by pathogenic bacteria. Probiotics such as bifidobacteria are typically used in cases when a disease occurs or might occur due to depleted normal flora. For example, treatment with antibiotics can kill off pathogenic bacteria and also the normal flora of the gastrointestinal and genitourinary tracts. The theory is that taking Bifidobacterium probiotics during antibiotic treatment can prevent or minimize normal flora depletion and pathogenic bacteria colonization. Bifidobacteria given in combination with lactobacillus concurrently with clindamycin seem to prevent increases in the number of Bacteroides fragilis bacteria (1055,3589,11382).
Bifidobacteria, especially Bifidobacterium bifidum, are the predominant intestinal flora of breast-fed infants (161). Bifidobacteria might contribute to the protection that breast-feeding provides against gastrointestinal infections in infants (1060). Bifidobacteria appear to produce antimicrobial substances that protect the intestine (1060). Bifidobacteria are also in the adult colon, but are less predominant (1060). When used orally, some species of bifidobacteria, such as Bifidobacterium infantis, and some strains of Bifidobacterium breve and Bifidobacterium longum, pass through the gut and bind to the intestinal mucosa, preventing attachment of pathogenic coliform bacteria (1137,1731). Bifidobacteria disappear from the feces within 2 weeks of discontinuation of bifidobacteria, suggesting that there is no long-term colonization (1117,4363). For continued effect, bifidobacteria must be used regularly.
In addition to acting as a barrier to pathogenic bacterial adhesion, some researchers think bifidobacteria and other probiotics might have immunomodulating effects (1137). Quantitative differences in the composition of intestinal microflora appear to affect immunological homeostasis (3458). Bifidobacteria seem to modulate non-specific cellular and humoral immunity possibly by stimulating lymphocyte and macrophage activity and cytokine production by mononuclear cells (6099). Due to these immunomodulating effects, some researchers think bifidobacteria and other probiotics might not only fight intestinal pathogens, but might also be helpful for conditions such as inflammatory bowel disease and pouchitis (6087). The addition of Bifidobacterium lactis to milk enhances cellular immunity in healthy middle-aged and elderly people, improving phagocyte function and natural killer cell activity, and increasing production of interferon-alpha (1055,1117). In infants, bacterial colonization appears to be essential in the development of oral tolerance instead of sensitization to dietary antigens (3458).
There is also some preliminary evidence that bifidobacteria and other probiotics might help protect against cancer. Bifidobacteria decrease fecal enzymes such as beta-glucuronidase, beta-glucosidase, nitroreductase, and urease, which are involved in the metabolic activation of some mutagens and carcinogens (6099). Bifidobacteria might also fight cancer by alteration of colonic physiochemical conditions and production of antitumorigenic or antimutagenic compounds in the colon (1154). Most researchers agree that the effectiveness of bifidobacteria and other probiotics for all indications depends on their ability to colonize an area of tissue. To do this, bifidobacteria preparations must contain live and viable organisms. Products stored for long periods of time or stored improperly may contain few live and active organisms to start with. For oral preparations, bacteria must also remain viable after passing through the gut (3589). Bifidobacterium longum is particularly resistant to gastric acid (3589). They must also be able to latch on to the intestinal epithelium. Bifidobacteria strains might vary in their effectiveness due to differences in their ability to adhere to epithelial cells (1137). Complex sugars, such as fructo-oligosaccharides, inulin, and oligofructose, are selectively fermented by bifidobacteria in the colon, and increase indigenous bifidobacteria quantities (4363). The addition of oligosaccharides to bifidobacteria also seems to enhance the activity of bifidobacteria (1117). However, there are no trials confirming the clinical benefit of combining bifidobacteria with complex sugars.

Adverse Reactions

Orally, bifidobacteria seem to be well tolerated by most people. In children, bifidobacteria can cause diarrhea (3169). Adverse effects from ingestion of bifidobacteria have not been reported; however, with other probiotics, patients can sometimes experience gastrointestinal upset including bloating and flatulence. This effect is usually mild and typically subsides with continued use. Most bifidobacteria species are considered nonpathogenic and nontoxigenic; however, the Bifidobacterium dentium species, has been associated with dental caries (1137,1236). Sepsis with the Bifidobacterium longum species has occurred in one patient following acupuncture. This was likely due to needle contamination. This effect would not be expected to occur from taking oral bifidobacteria supplements in most healthy patients (1236).

Interactions with Herbs & Other Dietary Supplements

None known.

Interactions with Drugs

ANTIBIOTIC DRUGS: There is some concern that concomitant administration of antibiotics might decrease the effectiveness of bifidobacteria. Since bifidobacteria preparations usually contain live and active organisms, simultaneously taking antibiotics might kill a significant number of the organisms (1740). Tell patients to separate administration of antibiotics and bifidobacteria preparations by at least 2 hours.

Interactions with Foods

None known.

Interactions with Lab Tests

None known.

Interactions with Diseases or Conditions

IMMUNODEFICIENCY: There is some concern that bifidobacteria preparations might cause pathogenic colonization in patients who are immunocompromised. Although this has not occurred specifically with bifidobacteria, there have been rare cases involving other probiotic species such as lactobacillus. Pathogenic colonization seems to be more likely to occur in severely immunocompromised patients (4380,4391,4393,4398). Use with caution in these patients.

Dosage and Administration

ORAL: The strength of bifidobacteria preparations is usually quantified by the number of living organisms per capsule. People typically take 1 to 10 billion viable cells daily in 3 to 4 divided doses (5009).

BILBERRY

Also Known As

Airelle, Bilberry Fruit, Bilberry Leaf, Black Whortles, Bleaberry, Blueberry, Burren Myrtle, Dwarf Bilberry, Dyeberry, Huckleberry, Hurtleberry, Myrtilli Fructus, Trackleberry, Whortleberry, Wineberry.
CAUTION: See separate listings for Blueberry and Bog Bilberry.

Scientific Names

Vaccinium myrtillus.
Family: Ericaceae.

People Use This For

Orally, bilberry is used to improve visual acuity including night vision, and to treat degenerative retinal conditions, varicose veins, atherosclerosis, venous insufficiency, and hemorrhoids. It is also used orally for angina; diabetes; arthritis; gout; dermatitis; and prevention and treatment of gastrointestinal (GI), kidney, and urinary tract symptoms and diseases.
Topically, it is used for mild inflammation of the mouth and throat mucous membranes.

Safety

LIKELY SAFE ...when the fruit is used in amounts commonly found in foods. Bilberry has Generally Recognized As Safe (GRAS) status in the US (4912).
POSSIBLY UNSAFE ...when the leaves are used orally in high doses or for prolonged use. Death can occur with chronic use of 1.5 g/kg/day (2).
PREGNANCY AND LACTATION: There is insufficient reliable information available about the safety of bilberry fruit used in medicinal amounts during pregnancy and lactation.

Effectiveness

POSSIBLY EFFECTIVE

Retinopathy. Taking bilberry fruit orally seems to improve retinal lesions from diabetic or hypertensive retinopathy (39,40). Clinical studies of bilberry's effectiveness have used formulations containing 25% of the bioflavonoid complex anthocyanoside.

POSSIBLY INEFFECTIVE

Night vision. Bilberry fruit extract 160 mg taken three times daily for 21 days does not seem to improve night visual acuity and contrast sensitivity in men with good vision and normal night vision (8139). A single dose of anthocyanosides, the active constituents of bilberry, does not significantly improve night vision (9738,9739).

There is insufficient reliable information available about the effectiveness of bilberry for its other uses.

Mechanism of Action

The applicable parts of bilberry are the fruit and leaf. Astringent tannin components of bilberry dried, ripe fruit are responsible for the potential benefits in diarrhea and irritation of the mouth and throat mucosa. Anthocyanadin (anthocyanoside) constituents increase the synthesis of glycosaminoglycans, decrease vascular permeability, reduce basement membrane thickness, and aid in the redistribution of microvascular blood flow and the formation of interstitial fluid. An anthocyanadin pigment found in bilberry fruit might have anti-ulcer and gastroprotective effects (6). Preliminary evidence indicates these constituents are widely distributed in the body after oral administration and are eliminated by the kidneys (8140). Laboratory research also suggests that anthocyanadins have anti-inflammatory and anti-edema effects (8141). Bilberry leaves contain polyphenols, tannins, flavonoids (1265) and a relatively high concentration of chromium (9.0 ppm) (8). Preliminary evidence suggests that a bilberry leaf extract might have blood glucose, triglyceride, and cholesterol lowering effects (1264). The chromium in bilberry leaf is theorized to play a role in potential blood glucose lowering activity (8). Bilberry leaf also contains a glucokinin, neomirtilline, that seems to lower blood glucose (1264). Some researchers think that flavonoids in bilberry leaf might also be useful for diabetic circulatory disorders (8).

Adverse Reactions

None reported.

Interactions with Herbs & Other Dietary Supplements

HERBS WITH HYPOGLYCEMIC POTENTIAL: Theoretically, bilberry leaf might have additive effects with herbs that decrease blood glucose levels (1264). Herbs with hypoglycemic potential include devil's claw, fenugreek, garlic, guar gum, horse chestnut, Panax ginseng, psyllium, Siberian ginseng, and others.

Interactions with Drugs

ANTIDIABETES DRUGS: Theoretically, concomitant use of bilberry leaf might require dosing adjustment of antidiabetes drugs. Preliminary evidence suggests that bilberry leaf extract might have blood glucose lowering activity (1264); monitor closely.

Interactions with Foods

None known.

Interactions with Lab Tests

BLOOD GLUCOSE: Theoretically, bilberry leaf might lower blood glucose and test results. Preliminary evidence suggests that a bilberry leaf extract might have blood glucose lowering activity (1264).

TRIGLYCERIDES: Theoretically, bilberry leaf might lower serum triglycerides and test results. Preliminary evidence suggests that a bilberry leaf extract might have triglyceride lowering activity (1264).

Interactions with Diseases or Conditions

DIABETES: Theoretically, bilberry leaf might lower blood glucose. Preliminary evidence suggests that a bilberry leaf extract might have blood glucose lowering activity (1264); monitor closely.

Dosage and Administration

ORAL: The typical dose of the dried, ripe berries is 20-60 grams daily. People also drink a decoction of the berries, which is prepared by adding 5-10 grams, 1-2 teaspoons, of mashed berries in cold water, bringing the water to a simmer for 10 minutes, and then straining. A dose of 160 mg of bilberry extract taken twice daily has been used in patients with retinopathy (39). Clinical studies of bilberry's effectiveness have used formulations containing 25% of the bioflavonoid complex anthocyanoside. Bilberry leaf is commonly used as a tea. The tea is prepared by steeping 1 gram, 1-2 teaspoons, finely chopped dried leaf in 150 mL boiling water for 5-10 minutes, then straining; avoid prolonged use (8). For improving night vision, anthocyanosides have been used as a single dose of 12, 24, or 36 mg or as 12 or 24 mg 2 times daily for 4 days (9738,9739).

TOPICAL: The berries are usually applied as a 10% decoction, made by boiling the dried berries in water for 10 minutes and straining (2).

Comments

During World War II, British pilots in the Royal Air Force ate bilberry jam to improve their night vision; however, subsequent clinical studies indicate that bilberry probably doesn't help night vision (8139).

BIOTIN

Also Known As
Coenzyme R, D-Biotin, Vitamin H, W Factor.

Scientific Names
Cis-hexahydro-2-oxo-1H-thieno[3,4-d]-imidazole-4-valeric acid.

People Use This For
Orally, biotin is used for preventing and treating biotin deficiency associated with pregnancy, long-term parenteral nutrition, malnutrition, rapid weight loss, and multiple carboxylase deficiency. It is also used orally for hair loss, brittle nails, seborrheic dermatitis of infancy, diabetes, and mild depression.

Safety
LIKELY SAFE ...when used orally and appropriately (1900,8468).
CHILDREN: POSSIBLY SAFE ...when used orally and appropriately (173).
PREGNANCY AND LACTATION: POSSIBLY SAFE ...when used orally and appropriately (1901).

Effectiveness
LIKELY EFFECTIVE

Biotin deficiency. Taking biotin orally is effective for preventing or treating biotin deficiency (1901).

POSSIBLY EFFECTIVE

Brittle nails. Taking biotin orally seems to increase the thickness of fingernails and toenails in people with brittle nails (171).

POSSIBLY INEFFECTIVE

Seborrheic dermatitis. Taking biotin orally doesn't seem to improve seborrheic dermatitis of infancy (8469).

INSUFFICIENT RELIABLE EVIDENCE to RATE

Alopecia areata. There is some preliminary evidence that biotin given orally in combination with zinc and topical clobetasol propionate (Olux, Temovate) might be helpful for alopecia areata (6932).

Peripheral neuropathy. There is preliminary evidence that intramuscular or oral biotin might help decrease symptoms of peripheral neuropathy in diabetic patients (8468).

More evidence is needed to rate biotin for these uses.

Mechanism of Action
Biotin is a vitamin that is found in small amounts in numerous foods. In food, biotin is protein bound and is cleaved by the enzyme biotinidase. Biotin is also synthesized in animals by intestinal microflora. Researchers think biotin is stored in the mitochondria, and that it acts as a coenzyme in bicarbonate-dependent carboxylation reactions (6243). Biotin-containing enzymes are involved in gluconeogenesis, fatty acid synthesis, propionate metabolism, and the catabolism of leucine in mammals (173). Pyruvate decarboxylase is a biotin-dependent enzyme. Decreased activity of this enzyme during biotin deficiency may result in accumulation of pyruvate or decreased aspartate concentration (8468).

Biotin deficiency is difficult to detect because of the lack of assay techniques to determine biotin concentrations in blood (8501). Symptoms of deficiency include thinning of the hair, frequently with loss of hair color, and red scaly rash around the eyes, nose, and mouth. Neurological symptoms, including depression, lethargy, hallucinations, and paresthesias of the extremities, are also common in biotin deficiency (6243). Biotin deficiency is most likely to occur in people with congenital biotinidase deficiency, malabsorption syndromes, such as short-gut syndrome, during pregnancy, and in people receiving long-term parenteral nutrition (6243,7878,8501). There is some evidence that diabetes may produce a biotin-deficient state (8468).

Biotin supplementation can reduce the activity of interleukins and interferons and reduce the number of lymphocytes (7879). Blood glucose concentrations decrease as plasma and tissue concentrations of biotin increase in people with and without diabetes, but this effect is far more dramatic in people with diabetes (7880).

After oral administration, biotin is completely absorbed. About half of the dose of biotin is excreted within 24 hours (8758). Biotin is recycled endogenously. This may be the reason why deficiency symptoms take a long time to develop and are rarely seen in humans (173).

Adverse Reactions
Orally, there is one case of eosinophilic pleuropericardial effusion with high-dose biotin 10 mg per day in combination with pantothenic acid 300 mg for 2 months (3914). Whether eosinophilia in this case is related to high-dose biotin use is unknown. However, biotin is well tolerated when used at recommended dosages (6243). Biotin in doses of 10 mg per day have been taken without adverse effects (6243).

Interactions with Herbs & Other Dietary Supplements
None known.

Interactions with Drugs
None known.

Drug Influences on Nutrient Levels and Depletion
SOME DRUGS CAN AFFECT BIOTIN LEVELS:
CARBAMAZEPINE: Taking carbamazepine can reduce biotin absorption (172,176).
PHENOBARBITAL: Taking phenobarbital can reduce biotin levels (175,176).
PHENYTOIN: Taking phenytoin can reduce biotin levels (175,176).
PRIMIDONE: Taking primidone can reduce biotin absorption (172,176).

Interactions with Foods
EGG WHITES: Consumption of large amounts of egg whites can cause biotin deficiency (173,6243).

Interactions with Lab Tests
FREE THYROXINE (FT4): There is one report of a false-high FT4 on the assay by the Boehringer Mannheim ES 700 analyzer due to high serum biotin levels in a neonate (170).
THYROID STIMULATING HORMONE (TSH): There is one report of a false-low TSH on the assay by the Boehringer Mannheim ES 700 analyzer due to high serum biotin levels in a neonate (170).

Interactions with Diseases or Conditions
BIOTINIDASE DEFICIENCY: Biotin requirements may be higher in people with genetic biotinidase deficiency (6243).
RENAL DIALYSIS: Biotin requirements may be higher in people receiving hemodialysis or peritoneal dialysis (6243).

Dosage and Administration
ORAL: There is no recommended dietary allowance (RDA) established for biotin. The adequate intakes (AI) for biotin are 7 mcg for infants 0-12 months, 8 mcg for children 1-3 years, 12 mcg for children 4-8 years, 20 mcg for children 9-13 years, 25 mcg for adolescents 14-18 years, 30 mcg for adults over 18 years and pregnant women, and 35 mcg for lactating women (6243). In the treatment of diabetic peripheral neuropathy, oral biotin 5 mg daily has been used for up to 130 weeks. This was preceded by 12 weeks of intramuscular treatment (8468).
INTRAMUSCULAR: In the treatment of diabetic peripheral neuropathy, intramuscular biotin 10 mg daily for six weeks, then three times weekly for six weeks, followed by an oral dose has been used (8468).

BIRCH

Also Known As
Betula, Betulae folium, Downy Birch, Silver Birch, White Birch.

Scientific Names
Betula pendula, synonym Betula verrucosa; Betula pubescens, synonym Betula alba.
Family: Betulaceae.

People Use This For
Orally, birch is used as a diuretic, for rheumatic ailments, "irrigation therapy" (use of a mild diuretic along with copious fluid intake to increase urine flow), to treat pyelonephritis, ureteritis, cystitis, urethritis, for arthritis, rheumatism, loss of hair, skin rashes, and in "spring cures" for "purifying the blood."

Safety
LIKELY SAFE ...when used orally and appropriately as irrigation therapy (2,12).
PREGNANCY AND LACTATION: Insufficient reliable information available; avoid using.

Effectiveness
There is insufficient reliable information available about the effectiveness of birch.

Mechanism of Action
The applicable part of birch is the leaf. The aquaretic and possibly saluretic effects are due to the flavonoid constituents of the birch leaf. Aquaretics increase urine volume (water loss) but not electrolyte excretion (512). The high vitamin C content of the leaf can enhance the effect (8).

Adverse Reactions
None reported.

Interactions with Herbs & Other Dietary Supplements
None known.

Interactions with Drugs
DIURETIC DRUGS: Theoretically, birch might interfere with diuretic therapy (512).

Interactions with Foods
None known.

Interactions with Lab Tests
None known.

Interactions with Diseases or Conditions
EDEMA DUE TO HEART OR KIDNEY CONDITIONS: Irrigation therapy is contraindicated (2).
HYPERTENSION: Theoretically, birch leaf might increase sodium retention and worsen hypertension (512).
URINARY TRACT INFECTIONS (UTIs): Herbal "irrigation therapy" can be insufficient and requires the addition of an antibacterial agent and close monitoring (8).

Dosage and Administration
ORAL: The typical dose of birch leaf is several times daily as a tea, which is prepared by steeping 2-3 grams of finely cut dried leaf in 150 mL boiling water for 10-15 minutes and straining (2,8). The tea should be taken with plenty of water (8).

BISHOP'S WEED

Also Known As
Ajava Seeds, Ajowan, Ajowan Caraway, Ajowan Seed, Ajowanj, Bishop's Flower, Bishops Weed, Bullwort, Carum, Flowering Ammi, Omum, Yavani.
CAUTION: See separate listings for Goutweed and Khella.

Scientific Names
Ammi majus, synonym Ammi glaucifolium.
Family: Apiaceae/Umbelliferae.

People Use This For
Orally, bishop's weed is used for digestive disorders, asthma, angina, kidney stones, and as a diuretic.
Topically, bishop's weed is used for psoriasis and vitiligo.

Safety
There is insufficient reliable information available about the safety of bishop's weed.
PREGNANCY: LIKELY UNSAFE ...when used orally. The active constituent, khellin, has uterine stimulant activity (19); avoid using.
LACTATION: Insufficient reliable information available; avoid using.

Effectiveness
There is insufficient reliable information available about the effectiveness of bishop's weed.

Mechanism of Action
The applicable parts of bishop's weed are the seeds (7161). Bishop's weed contains several active ingredients including khellin, 8-methoxsalen, xanthotoxin, bergapten, and umbelliferone (1332,7162). The constituent, khellin, seems to have calcium channel blocking effects. There is some evidence it might also increase high-density lipoprotein (HDL) levels without affecting total cholesterol or triglyceride concentrations (2522,7162). The 8-methoxsalen (8-MOP, methoxypsoralen) constituent is one of the first agents used along with ultraviolet-A (UVA) radiation to treat psoriasis. It binds pyrimidine bases in DNA and suppresses cell division. This constituent also seems to contribute to the phototoxicity caused by bishop's weed (15,2528). Another constituent, xanthotoxin, also seems to have antipsoriatic activity (7162). The bergapten (5-methoxypsoralen) has antipsoriatic activity and antiplatelet activity (7162). Bergapten also appears to inhibit the cytochrome P450 3A4 (CYP3A4) system, which might lead to numerous interactions with drugs metabolized by this system (7029). The umbelliferone constituent is a hydroxycoumarin. Some researchers are

interested in coumarins such as umbelliferone from bishop's weed because of in vitro evidence that they can inhibit reverse transcriptase in human immunodeficiency virus (HIV) replication (1332,1333). Further research is being done to see if these constituents have this effect in humans. Although people use bishop's weed for kidney stones, animal models show that it does not seem to decrease calcium oxalate deposition in the kidneys (2526).

Adverse Reactions

Orally, bishop's weed can cause nausea, vomiting, and headache (7161). Bishop's weed can also cause allergic reactions including rhinitis and urticaria in sensitive patients (2520). There is some concern that bishop's weed might increase liver enzymes. The isolated constituent khellin can increase transaminase levels (2522); however, so far this effect has not been reported for bishop's weed. Bishop's weed might also cause photosensitivity due to the 8-MOP constituent. In some patients bishop's weed can also cause contact dermatitis (2520,2521). There is also concern based on preliminary evidence that bishop's weed might cause ophthalmic changes, such as pigmentary retinopathy (2527). Topically, bishop's weed might cause skin malignancies in patients predisposed to cancer (6002).

Interactions with Herbs & Other Dietary Supplements

HEPATOTOXIC HERBS: Theoretically, bishop's weed might have additive effects with herbs that cause hepatotoxicity. The khellin constituent can cause elevated transaminase levels in some patients (2522). Other products that might affect the liver include borage, chaparral, uva ursi, and others (2,2522).
HERBS WITH ANTICOAGULANT/ANTIPLATELET POTENTIAL: Concomitant use of herbs that affect platelet aggregation might increase the risk of bleeding. These herbs include angelica, anise, arnica, asafoetida, bogbean, boldo, capsicum, celery, chamomile, clove, fenugreek, feverfew, garlic, ginger, ginkgo, Panax ginseng, horse chestnut, horseradish, licorice, meadowsweet, onion, prickly ash, papain, passionflower, poplar, quassia, red clover, turmeric, wild carrot, wild lettuce, willow, and others (7162).
PHOTOSENSITIZING HERBS: Theoretically, bishop's weed might have an additive effect with products that increase sun sensitivity, such as St. John's wort (2521,7162).

Interactions with Drugs

ANTICOAGULANT/ANTIPLATELET DRUGS: There is some concern that bishop's weed might have additive effects with anticoagulant or antiplatelet drugs and possibly increase the risk of bleeding. The bergapten constituent of bishop's weed has antiplatelet effects. Some anticoagulant or antiplatelet drugs include aspirin, clopidogrel (Plavix), dalteparin (Fragmin), enoxaparin (Lovenox), heparin, ticlopidine (Ticlid), warfarin (Coumadin), and others (7162).
CYTOCHROME P450 3A4 (CYP3A4) SUBSTRATES: Theoretically, bishop's weed might inhibit elimination and increase blood levels of drugs metabolized by cytochrome P450 3A4 (CYP3A4) isoenzymes (7029). The bergapten constituent of bishop's weed is the same constituent as in bitter orange, which inhibits CYP3A4. Some drugs metabolized by CYP3A4 include alprazolam (Xanax), amitriptyline (Elavil), amiodarone (Cordarone), buspirone (Buspar), cerivastatin (Baycol), citalopram (Celexa), felodipine (Plendil), fexofenadine (Allegra), itraconazole (Sporanox), ketoconazole (Nizoral), lansoprazole (Prevacid), losartan (Cozaar), lovastatin (Mevacor), ondansetron (Zofran), prednisone (Deltasone, Orasone), sertraline (Zoloft), sibutramine (Meridia), sildenafil (Viagra), simvastatin (Zocor), verapamil (Calan, Covera-HS, Isoptin), and many others.
HEPATOTOXIC DRUGS: Theoretically, bishop's weed might have additive adverse effects on the liver when used with hepatotoxic drugs. The khellin constituent of bishop's weed can increase liver transaminases (2,2522). Some drugs that can adversely affect the liver include acetaminophen (Tylenol), amiodarone (Cordarone), carbamazepine (Tegretol), isoniazid (INH), methotrexate (Rheumatrex), methyldopa (Aldomet), and many others.
PHOTOSENSITIZING DRUGS: Theoretically, concomitant use might result in increased photosensitivity. Bishop's weed constituents seem to cause photosensitivity (2521,7162). Some drugs that cause photosensitivity include amitriptyline (Elavil), quinolones (Ciprofloxacin, others), sulfa drugs (Septra, Bactrim, others), and tetracycline.

Interactions with Foods

None known.

Interactions with Lab Tests

HIGH-DENSITY LIPOPROTEIN (HDL): Theoretically, bishop's weed might increase HDL levels. The isolated bishop's weed constituent, khellin, seems to increase in HDL levels without affecting total cholesterol or triglycerides (2522).
LIVER FUNCTION TESTS: There is some concern that bishop's weed might increase liver function tests in some patients. It is known that the isolated constituent khellin can increase aspartic acid transaminase (AST) and alanine aminotransferase (ALT, SGPT) (2522). However, this effect has not yet been reported specifically for bishop's weed.

Interactions with Diseases or Conditions

LIVER DISEASE: Theoretically, bishop's weed might exacerbate liver dysfunction in patients with liver disease. The isolated khellin constituent of bishop's weed is known to increase liver enzymes in some patients (2522).

Dosage and Administration
No typical dosage.

Comments
The prescription drug methoxsalen (Oxasoralen, Methoxypsoralen) was originally prepared from bishop's weed, but is now made synthetically (9,15). Bishop's weed is sometimes confused with its more used relative, khella (Ammi visnaga). The two species do have some common chemical constituents and pharmacological effects. Bishop's weed is more commonly used for dermatological conditions, and khella is usually used for cardiac and pulmonary conditions (7161). The isolated active constituent, khellin, is also used medicinally for angina pectoris, asthma, in conjunction with phototherapy for vitiligo, psoriasis, and alopecia areata (9,560,849,868).

BISTORT

Also Known As
Adderwort, Dragonwort, Easter Giant, Easter Mangiant, Oderwort, Osterick, Patience Dock, Red Legs, Snakeweed, Sweet Dock.

Scientific Names
Polygonum bistorta.
Family: Polygonaceae.

People Use This For
Orally, bistort is used for digestive disorders, particularly diarrhea.
Topically, bistort is used for mouth and throat infections, and for wounds.

Safety
There is insufficient reliable information available about the safety of bistort.
Pregnancy and Lactation: Insufficient reliable information available; avoid using.

Effectiveness
There is insufficient reliable information available about the effectiveness of bistort.

Mechanism of Action
The applicable parts of bistort are the rhizome and root. Bistort contains 15-21% tannins, which have astringent effects. Tannins work internally by dehydrating mucosal tissue, which reduces secretions. Externally, tannin astringent effects result in a protective layer of constricted, harder cells. Plants with at least 10% tannins can cause gastrointestinal upset, kidney damage, and liver damage. Animal data conflicts with respect to the carcinogenicity of tannins. They may be carcinogenic or may have anti-carcinogenic effects. An increased risk of esophageal or nasal cancer may be linked to people who regularly ingest herbs with high tannin concentrations (12).

Adverse Reactions
None reported.

Interactions with Herbs & Other Dietary Supplements
TANNIN-CONTAINING HERBS: Theoretically, herbs that contain high percentages of tannins, such as bistort, may cause precipitation of constituents of other herbs (19).

Interactions with Drugs
ORAL DRUGS: Theoretically, concomitant use may cause precipitation of some drugs due to the high tannin content of bistort (19). Separate administration of oral drugs and tannin-containing herbs by the longest period of time practical (19).

Interactions with Foods
None known.

Interactions with Lab Tests
None known.

Interactions with Diseases or Conditions
None known.

Dosage and Administration
ORAL: The rhizome and root are powdered and used to make an infusion (18).
TOPICAL: The powdered root is used as an extract or ointment (18).

BITTER ALMOND

Also Known As
Amygdala Amara, Badama, Bitter Almond Oil, Vatadha, Vathada, Volatile Almond Oil.
CAUTION: See separate listing for Sweet Almond Oil.

Scientific Names
Prunus dulcis, synonyms Prunus amygdalus, Amygdalus communis, Amygdalus dulcis, Prunus communis, Prunus dulcis var. amara.
Family: Rosaceae.

People Use This For
Orally, bitter almond is used as an antispasmodic, local anesthetic, for its narcotic properties, as a cough suppressant, and as an antipruritic.

Safety
POSSIBLY SAFE ...when the HCN (hydrocyanic acid)-free oil is used orally in amounts commonly found in foods. HCN free oil is also known as FFPA (free form prussic acid). FFPA bitter almond oil has Generally Recognized As Safe (GRAS) status in the US (4912).
LIKELY UNSAFE ...when the volatile oil containing HCN is used orally (11,12). ...when large amounts of HCN-free volatile oil are used orally. Ingesting 50-60 mL benzaldehyde can cause fatal CNS depression and respiratory failure (11).
PREGNANCY AND LACTATION: LIKELY UNSAFE ...when the volatile oil containing HCN is used orally (11). There is insufficient reliable information available about the safety of the oral of the HCN-free oil during pregnancy and breast-feeding; avoid using.

Effectiveness
There is insufficient reliable information available about the effectiveness of bitter almond.

Mechanism of Action
The applicable part of bitter almond is the volatile oil. The bitter almond kernel contains 3-4% amygdalin, which is hydrolyzed to poisonous hydrocyanic acid (HCN, prussic acid). The volatile oil contains 95% benzaldehyde and 2-4% HCN. For food and flavor use, HCN is removed. High doses of benzaldehyde can have narcotic properties and the potential for adverse reactions (11).

Adverse Reactions
Orally, 50-60 mL of benzaldehyde (sole constituent of HCN-free oil) can have high toxicity and be fatal due to CNS depression with respiratory failure (11). There is a report of one death of an adult after ingestion of 7.5 mL of the volatile oil (11).

Interactions with Herbs & Other Dietary Supplements
None known.

Interactions with Drugs
CNS DEPRESSANTS: Theoretically, bitter almond oil use with CNS depressants increases the risk of severe or fatal CNS and respiratory depression.

Interactions with Foods
None known.

Interactions with Lab Tests
None known.

Interactions with Diseases or Conditions
None known.

Dosage and Administration
No typical dosage.

Comments
The volatile oil of bitter almond contains 95% benzaldehyde and 2-4% poisonous HCN. It is made by water maceration and steam distillation of partially defatted bitter almond (Prunus amygdalus amara), apricot (Prunus armeniaca), peach (Prunus persica), and plum (Prunus domestica) kernels. The fixed almond oil (sweet almond oil) is prepared by pressing the kernels of both sweet almond and bitter almond and contains no benzaldehyde or hydrocyanic acid (HCN). Sweet almond does not yield a volatile oil (11). Bitter almond volatile oil consists of distilled, partially defatted oil of the kernels of bitter almond (Prunus amygdalus amara) and kernels of other Prunus species.

BITTER MELON

Also Known As
African Cucumber, Balsam Pear, Balsam-Apple, Balsambirne, Balsamo, Bitter Apple, Bitter Cucumber, Bitter Gourd, Bittergurke, Carilla Gourd, Cerasee, Chinli-Chih, Cundeamor, Karavella, Kathilla, Karela, Kerala, Kuguazi, K'u-Kua, Lai Margose, Momordique, Pepino Montero, P'u-T'ao, Sorosi, Sushavi, Wild Cucumber.

Scientific Names
Momordica charantia, synonym Momordica murcata.
Family: Cucurbitaceae.

People Use This For
Orally, bitter melon is used to treat diabetes, psoriasis, gastrointestinal upset, ulcers, colitis, constipation, intestinal worms, urinary tract stones (kidney stones), fever, and hepatic disease. It is also used orally to induce menstruation and as supportive therapy for patients with AIDS/HIV.
Topically, bitter melon is used for skin abscesses and wounds, and anorectal herpes lesions.

Safety
POSSIBLY SAFE ...when used orally and appropriately, short-term. Extract of bitter melon fruit appears to be safe for up to 7 weeks (36).
There is insufficient reliable information available about the safety of bitter melon when used topically.
PREGNANCY: LIKELY UNSAFE ...when used orally. Bitter melon juice can stimulate menstruation and cause abortion (19).
LACTATION: Insufficient reliable information available; avoid using.

Effectiveness
INSUFFICIENT RELIABLE EVIDENCE to RATE

Diabetes. Bitter melon fruit, fruit juice, and extract seems to improve glucose tolerance, reduce blood glucose levels, and lower glycosylated hemoglobin (HbA1c) in patients with type 2 diabetes (34,35,36). More evidence is needed to rate bitter melon for this use.

Mechanism of Action
The applicable parts of bitter melon are the fruit and seeds, and less commonly the leaves and roots. The bitter melon fruit and fruit extracts seem to have hypoglycemic activity in humans and animal models of diabetes (34,35,36,3762,3763,3764,3765,7700,8179). Bitter melon fruit extract might also protect against hyperinsulinemia (7700). Bitter melon contains an insulin-like polypeptide called polypeptide P, plant insulin, or p-insulin. P-insulin has pharmacologic effects similar to bovine insulin with an onset of action between 30 and 60 minutes, and a peak effect at about four hours (37,38). Preliminary evidence suggests that an aqueous extract of bitter melon fruit can slow the progression of microalbuminuria and diabetic nephropathy (8179).
Bitter melon contains several other constituents with a variety of pharmacological effects. Flavonoids in bitter melon seem to have a cholesterol lowering effect. There's also some preliminary evidence that they might raise hemoglobin, and increase white and red blood cell counts (8180). Constituents called alpha- and beta-momorcharin seem to have immunosuppressive activity in vitro and in animal models (3724). However, other constituents have antitumor, antileukemia, and antiviral activity (3722,3723). A bitter melon protein from the seed and fruit called momordica anti-human immunodeficiency virus (HIV) protein (MAP30) has antiviral and antitumor activity in vitro (3720,3721,7540). It inhibits HIV and herpes simplex viruses, including acyclovir-resistant strains (7539,7540). It appears to inhibit HIV by inhibiting reverse transcriptase. MAP30 is also a N-glucosidase, which inhibits HIV ribosomal protein synthesis and might make viral and plasmid DNA inactive (7542,7543). MAP30 also seems to inhibit HIV integrase, which prevents integration of viral DNA into the genetic material of healthy cells (7542).
Another protein, MRK29, found in the seed and fruit of a smaller variety of bitter melon found in Thailand, appears

to inhibit HIV reverse transcriptase and to increase tumor necrosis factor (TNF) activity (7541). There's some preliminary evidence that an ethanolic extract of bitter melon seed might also have antispermatogenic and androgenic properties, suggesting potential use as a male contraceptive (7538).

Adverse Reactions
None reported.

Interactions with Herbs & Other Dietary Supplements
HERBS & SUPPLEMENTS WITH HYPOGLYCEMIC POTENTIAL: Bitter melon can lower blood glucose levels (34,35,36) and might have additive effects when used with other herbs and supplements that also lower glucose levels. This might increase the risk of hypoglycemia in some patients. Some herbs and supplements with hypoglycemic effects include alpha-lipoic acid, chromium, devil's claw, fenugreek, garlic, guar gum, horse chestnut seed, Panax ginseng, psyllium, Siberian ginseng, and others.

Interactions with Drugs
ANTIDIABETES DRUGS: Bitter melon can lower blood glucose levels (34,35,36) and might have additive effects when used with antidiabetes drugs. This might increase the risk of hypoglycemia in some patients. Monitor blood glucose levels closely. An additive effect of chlorpropamide (Diabinese) and bitter melon has been reported (8181). Some antidiabetes drugs include glimepiride (Amaryl), glyburide (Diabeta, Glynase PresTabs, Micronase), insulin, metformin (Glucophage), pioglitazone (Actos), rosiglitazone (Avandia), and others.

Interactions with Foods
None known.

Interactions with Lab Tests
BLOOD GLUCOSE: Bitter melon extracts, fruits, and fruit juice can lower blood glucose and test results in patients with type 2 diabetes (34,35,36).
GLYCOSYLATED HEMOGLOBIN (HbA1c): Bitter melon extract can lower HbA1c in type 2 diabetes patients after 7 weeks of treatment (36).

Interactions with Diseases or Conditions
DIABETES: Bitter melon can lower blood glucose levels (34,35,36) and might have additive effects when used with antidiabetes drugs. This might increase the risk of hypoglycemia in some patients. Monitor blood glucose levels closely.

Dosage and Administration
No typical dosage.

Comments
Bitter melon is used as a vegetable in India and other Asian countries (7538,7541). Bitter melon is used as an ingredient in some kinds of curries. A reduction in blood sugar after eating foods spiced with curry has been described in a patient taking chlorpropamide (Diabenese) (8181).

BITTER MILKWORT

Also Known As
European Bitter Polygala, European Senega, Evergreen Snakeroot, Flowering Wintergreen, Little Pollom, Snakeroot.
CAUTION: See separate listings for Asarabacca and Senega.

Scientific Names
Polygala amara.
Family: Polygalaceae.

Comments
At the date of publication, this product was not a common ingredient used in brand name supplements marketed to consumers. Details about this product are available at the online version of *Natural Medicines Comprehensive Database*. See www.naturaldatabase.com.

BITTER ORANGE

Also Known As

Aurantii Pericarpium, Green Orange, Kijitsu, Neroli Oil, Seville Orange, Shangzhou Zhiqiao, Sour Orange, Synephrine, Zhi Qiao, Zhi Shi.
CAUTION: See separate listings for Bergamot Oil, Oswego Tea, and Sweet Orange.

Scientific Names

Citrus aurantium, synonyms Citrus amara, Citrus bigarradia, Citrus vulgaris.
Family: Rutaceae.

People Use This For

Orally, bitter orange peel is used as an appetite stimulant and for dyspepsia. Bitter orange fruit and peel are also used orally for weight loss and nasal congestion. The bitter orange flower and its oil are used orally for gastrointestinal (GI) disturbances, duodenal ulcers, constipation, regulating blood lipid levels, lowering blood sugar in diabetes, blood purification, functional disorders of liver and gallbladder, stimulation of the heart and circulation, frostbite, as a sedative for sleep disorders, for kidney and bladder diseases, general feebleness, anemia, imbalances of mineral metabolism, impurities of the skin, hair loss, as a tonic, antiflatulent, and for cancer. Other uses include prolapsed uterus, prolapsed anus or rectum, diarrhea, and blood in the stools.
Topically, bitter orange peel is used for inflammation of the eyelid, conjunctiva, and retina. It is also used for retinal hemorrhage, exhaustion accompanying colds, headaches, neuralgia, muscular pain, rheumatic discomfort, bruises, phlebitis, and bed sores.
In aromatherapy, the essential oil of bitter orange is used topically and by inhalation as an analgesic.
In foods, bitter orange oil is used as a flavoring agent.
In manufacturing, bitter orange oil is used in pharmaceuticals, cosmetics, and soaps.

Safety

LIKELY SAFE ...when used orally in the amounts found in foods. Bitter orange has Generally Recognized As Safe (GRAS) status in the US (4912).
POSSIBLY SAFE ...when used orally and appropriately for medicinal purposes (2040,11269). ...when the essential oil is used topically or by inhalation as aromatherapy (6972,7107).
POSSIBLY UNSAFE ...when used orally in high doses. Bitter orange fruit, peel, and juice contain the stimulant synephrine. In high doses or when used in combination with other stimulants such as ephedra, it might cause cardiotoxicity (2040,6979). There is insufficient reliable information available about the safety of other forms of bitter orange when used orally for medicinal purposes.
CHILDREN: POSSIBLY UNSAFE ...when used orally in high doses. High doses of bitter orange peel have been linked to intestinal colic, convulsions, and death in some children (11). There is insufficient reliable information available about the safety of moderate doses of bitter orange peel or the safety of other forms of bitter orange in children.
PREGNANCY AND LACTATION: Insufficient reliable information available; avoid using.

Effectiveness

POSSIBLY EFFECTIVE

Tinea corporis, tinea cruris, and tinea pedis. Applying bitter orange oil seems to help treat tinea corporis, cruris, or pedis (6972).

INSUFFICIENT RELIABLE EVIDENCE to RATE

Obesity. Preliminary clinical research suggests that a combination of bitter orange, caffeine, and St. John's wort may be helpful for weight reduction when used with caloric restriction and exercise (11268). More evidence is needed to rate bitter orange for this use.

Mechanism of Action

The applicable parts of bitter orange are the peel, flower, leaf, and fruit. Bitter orange has numerous active constituents and pharmacological effects; however, the amount of each constituent can vary depending on the part of the plant used. For example, the flavonoid content is higher in the flowers than the leaves (6971). The fruit and peel of bitter orange contain the sympathetic alpha-adrenergic agonists phenylephrine and synephrine (2080,4800,11267). It also contains octopamine, which is similar to norepinephrine, and the amino acid tyramine. Like tyramine, octopamine and synephrine are substrates of monoamine oxidase. Laboratory research suggests that octopamine might stimulate fat cell lipolysis and stimulate glucose update by fat cells (11995,12378). Trace amounts of synephrine and octopamine are part of the pool of circulating amines in humans (12379). Their physiological function is unclear. Preliminary research suggests that migraine and cluster headaches might be related to excess levels of synephrine and octopamine (11996).
Commercially available bitter orange extracts usually contain from 1% to 6% synephrine. But some manufacturers boost synephrine content to as much as 30%. Bitter orange preparations are often promoted for weight loss due to

purported thermogenic effects (4800). In animal models, synephrine causes weight loss, but also increases cardiovascular toxicity (6969). There is some evidence that bitter orange can cause vasoconstriction and increase mean arterial pressure (MAP), but reduce portal pressure (6975). Bitter orange plus a synthetic preparation of the active components synephrine and N-methyltyramine have been used successfully to treat infectious shock in preliminary research. N-methyltyramine seems to increase blood pressure by increasing norepinephrine release (6978). Bitter orange peel is also commonly used for dyspepsia due to spasmolytic effects. Bitter orange peel might also have anti-inflammatory activity, which might be due to the flavonoids naringin and nobiletin (1281). Limonene is the most abundant monoterpene in bitter orange juice (4946).

Bitter orange preparations have a variety of antimicrobial properties. The oil of the bitter orange peel seems to have insecticidal activity (6973). Two flavonoids of the bitter orange fruit, neohesperidin and hesperidin, also seem to have antiviral activity against rotavirus infection (6976). Early research indicates that compounds found in bitter orange, auraptene, marmin, tangeretin, nobiletin, and a psoralen compound, might have antitumor effects (6974).

Preliminary research suggests that synephrine, a constituent of bitter orange, might have antidepressant effects, possibly by promoting norepinephrine release (12376,12377).

The furocoumarins bergapten and oxypeucedanin in bitter orange oil are photosensitizing (11019). The furocoumarins bergamottin, dihydroxybergamottin, and bergapten in the fruit and juice can inhibit the cytochrome P450 3A4 (CYP3A4) isoenzyme (7029). Bitter orange appears to selectively inhibit intestinal CYP3A4, but not hepatic CYP3A4 (7029,11269). These are the same constituents found in grapefruit that are responsible for numerous drug interactions. However, grapefruit juice contains a significantly higher concentration of these constituents than bitter orange juice (7029). Research on the effects of bitter orange on P-glycoprotein is conflicting (7029,11269,11270,11362). Dihydroxybergamottin appears to inhibit CYP3A4, but not P-glycoprotein (11270).

Adverse Reactions

Orally, bitter orange, which contains the adrenergic agent synephrine and N-methyltyramine, might cause hypertension and cardiovascular toxicity (2040,6969,6979). Synephrine is similar to phenylephrine and the ephedrine contained in the herb ephedra. Theoretically, synephrine might cause similar side effects as ephedra such as myocardial infarction, stroke, seizure, and other serious side effects.

There is a one documented case of myocardial infarction in a patient without a history of cardiovascular disease who took a supplement containing 300 mg of bitter orange for a year. The supplement also contained guarana and green tea, both of which are sources of caffeine (12030). Photosensitivity can also occur, especially in fair-skinned people (11909).

The ingestion of large amounts of bitter orange peel in children can cause intestinal colic, convulsions, and death (11).

Interactions with Herbs & Other Dietary Supplements

STIMULANTS: Theoretically, herbs and supplements with stimulant properties, such as caffeine, coffee, cola nut, ephedra, guarana, and mate, might increase the risk of hypertension and adverse cardiovascular effects with bitter orange fruit or peel due to synephrine content (6979).

Interactions with Drugs

CYTOCHROME P450 3A4 (CYP3A4) SUBSTRATES: Bitter orange juice can inhibit cytochrome P450 3A4 (CYP3A4) metabolism of drugs (7029), causing increased drug levels and potentially increasing the risk of adverse effects. But the extent of the effect of bitter orange on drug interactions is unknown. Bitter orange selectively inhibits intestinal CYP3A4, but not hepatic CYP3A4. Its effect on P-glycoprotein, which strongly overlaps with CYP3A4 interactions, is unclear (7029,11269,11270,11362). It has no effect on cyclosporin which seems to be more dependent on hepatic CYP3A4 and P-glycoprotein than intestinal CYP3A4 (11270). Some possible drug interactions with bitter orange include calcium channel blockers (diltiazem, nicardipine, verapamil), chemotherapeutic agents (etoposide, paclitaxel, vinblastine, vincristine, vindesine), antifungals (ketoconazole, itraconazole), glucocorticoids, cisapride (Propulsid), losartan (Cozaar), fexofenadine (Allegra), and numerous others.

DEXTROMETHORPHAN (Robitussin DM, and others): Bitter orange juice can inhibit cytochrome P450 3A4 (CYP3A4) metabolism (11362), causing increased dextromethorphan levels and potentially increasing the risk of adverse effects.

FELODIPINE (Plendil): Consumption of bitter orange juice 240 mL can significantly increase felodipine levels. Bitter orange juice inhibits cytochrome P450 3A4 (CYP3A4) metabolism of felodipine (7029).

INDINAVIR (Crixivan): Bitter orange juice slightly increases indinavir levels, but this effect is likely to be clinically insignificant. Bitter orange selectively inhibits intestinal cytochrome P450 3A4 (CYP3A4). The metabolism of indinavir seems to be more dependent on hepatic CYP3A4 (11269). The effect of bitter orange on other protease inhibitors has not been studied.

MIDAZOLAM (Versed): Bitter orange juice can significantly inhibit cytochrome P450 3A4 (CYP3A4) metabolism of the midazolam, and potentially increase drug levels and adverse effects (7029).

MONOAMINE OXIDASE INHIBITORS (MAOIs): Theoretically, concurrent use of MAOIs with synephrine-containing bitter orange preparations might increase the blood pressure raising effects of synephrine and potentially cause hypertensive crisis. Bitter orange contains tyramine, octopamine, and synephrine, which are MAO substrates (11267,11995,12378). Tell patients taking MAOIs to avoid using bitter orange. Some MAOIs include phenelzine (Nardil), tranylcypromine (Parnate), and others (2040).

STIMULANT DRUGS: Theoretically, drugs with CNS stimulant properties, such as phenylpropanolamine, pseudoephedrine, and caffeine, might increase the risk of hypertension and adverse cardiovascular effects of bitter orange fruit, peel, or juice due to synephrine content (2040,6979).

Interactions with Foods

CAFFEINE: Theoretically, large amounts of caffeine-containing beverages might increase the risk of hypertension and adverse cardiovascular effects with bitter orange fruit or peel due to synephrine content (6979).

Interactions with Lab Tests

None known.

Interactions with Diseases or Conditions

HEADACHE: Theoretically, bitter orange might trigger migraine or cluster headache due to its synephrine and octopamine content (11996).
HYPERTENSION: Theoretically, bitter orange fruit, peel, or juice might worsen hypertension due to synephrine content (2040,6979).
NARROW-ANGLE GLAUCOMA: Theoretically, bitter orange fruit, peel, or juice might worsen narrow-angle glaucoma due to synephrine content (2040,6979).
TACHYARRHYTHMIAS: Theoretically, bitter orange fruit, peel, or juice might worsen tachyarrhythmias due to synephrine content (2040,6979).

Dosage and Administration

ORAL: For weight loss, bitter orange extract 975 mg in combination with St. John's wort 900 mg and caffeine 528 mg per day has been used (11268). Bitter orange extracts commonly contain from 1.5% to 6% synephrine (6969).
TOPICAL: For treatment of fungal skin infections, pure oil of bitter orange has been applied once daily for 1-3 weeks (6972).

BITTERSWEET NIGHTSHADE

Also Known As

Bitter Nightshade, Bittersweet, Blue Nightshade, Common Nightshade, Deadly Nightshade, Dulcarara, Fellen, Fellonwood, Felonwort, Fever Twig, Mortal, Scarlet Berry, Snake Berry, Staff Vine, Violet Bloom, Woody, Woody Nightshade.
CAUTION: See separate listings for Belladonna and Henbane.

Scientific Names

Solanum dulcamara.
Family: Solanaceae.

People Use This For

Orally, bittersweet nightshade is used for chronic eczema, itchy skin conditions, acne, furuncles, skin abrasions, warts, as an antirheumatic, diuretic, narcotic, sedative, and for inflammation.
Topically, bittersweet nightshade is used for chronic eczema.

Safety

POSSIBLY SAFE ...when used orally or topically and appropriately (2,18).
LIKELY UNSAFE ...when the leaves or berries are used orally. The plant contains the toxic compounds solanine, solanidine, and dulcamarin (6).
CHILDREN: LIKELY UNSAFE ...when used orally; unripe berries have caused poisonings. A lethal dose is estimated to be 200 berries (18). There is insufficient reliable information available about the safety of bittersweet nightshade when used topically in children; avoid using.
PREGNANCY: LIKELY UNSAFE ...when used orally. The alkaloids of the plant, solasodine, soladulcine, and related compounds have been linked to malformations in animals (6); avoid using. There is insufficient reliable information available about the safety of bittersweet nightshade when used topically during pregnancy; avoid using.
LACTATION: LIKELY UNSAFE ...when orally; avoid using. There is insufficient reliable information available about the safety of bittersweet nightshade when used topically; avoid using.

Effectiveness

There is insufficient reliable information available about the effectiveness of bittersweet nightshade.

Mechanism of Action

The applicable part of bittersweet nightshade is the stem. It has astringent, antimicrobial, and mucous membrane-irritating actions (2). The steroidal alkaloid constituents of the stem can have anticholinergic effects (2). The component, solasodin, can prevent inflammation (2).

Adverse Reactions

Orally, the bittersweet nightshade plant can cause the symptoms of solanine poisoning, commonly associated with old potatoes. Symptoms include scratchy throat, headache, vertigo, dilated pupils, speech difficulties, subnormal temperature, vomiting, diarrhea, GI bleeding, cyanosis, convulsions, circulatory and respiratory depression, and even death (6). The ingestion of unripe berries can cause poisoning in children (18).

Interactions with Herbs & Other Dietary Supplements

None known.

Interactions with Drugs

None known.

Interactions with Foods

None known.

Interactions with Lab Tests

None known.

Interactions with Diseases or Conditions

GI IRRITATION: Bittersweet nightshade can irritate the gastrointestinal tract. It is contraindicated in individuals with infectious or inflammatory gastrointestinal conditions (19).

Dosage and Administration

ORAL: The typical dose of the bittersweet nightshade stem is 1-3 grams of the dried herb per day, and can be taken as a tea, which is prepared by steeping the herb in 150 mL boiling water for 5-10 minutes and straining (2).
TOPICAL: The stem is used as a compress prepared by steeping 1-2 grams of the dried herb in 250 mL boiling water for 5-10 minutes and straining (2).

Comments

Bittersweet nightshade is a perennial vine-like plant that is found throughout the United States, Canada, and Eurasia and is a member of the same family that includes tomatoes and potatoes.

BLACK ALDER

Also Known As

Betula Alnus, Common Alder, English Alder, European Alder, European Black Alder, Owler.

Scientific Names

Alnus glutinosa, synonyms Betula glutinosa, Alnus barbata.
Family: Betulaceae.

Comments

At the date of publication, this product was not a common ingredient used in brand name supplements marketed to consumers. Details about this product are available at the online version of *Natural Medicines Comprehensive Database*. See www.naturaldatabase.com.

BLACK BRYONY

Also Known As

Black Bindweed, Blackeye Root, Lady's-Seal.

Scientific Names

Dioscorea communis, synonyms Tamus communis, Tamus edulis.
Family: Dioscoreaceae.

People Use This For

Orally, black bryony is used as an emetic.
Topically, black bryony is used as a counterirritant, to treat bruises, strains, torn muscles, gout, rheumatic disorders, hair loss, and for improving blood circulation to the scalp.

Safety

POSSIBLY UNSAFE ...when the fresh root is used topically. Skin contact can cause severe skin irritation (3829).
UNSAFE ...when used orally. Black bryony can cause seizures, respiratory and kidney failure (18).
PREGNANCY AND LACTATION: Insufficient reliable information; avoid using.

Effectiveness

There is insufficient reliable information available about the effectiveness of black bryony.

Mechanism of Action

The applicable part of black bryony is the root. It can stimulate external nerve endings. Applied topically, it acts as a mechanical irritant, penetrating the skin with tiny, needle-like crystals of calcium oxalate (3829). The rhizome contains histamine (3829), which can have a role in producing skin irritation (3829). In rats, an ethanolic extract of the root exhibited local anti-inflammatory activity (3828).

Adverse Reactions

Orally, black bryony can cause severe mouth, pharyngeal and GI irritation, as well as vomiting, diarrhea, spasms, colic, decreased kidney function, and respiratory depression (18).
Topically, the fresh root can cause reddening of skin (18). The fresh plant used topically can cause skin irritation, rash, swelling, pustules, wheals, and mucous membrane irritation (18).

Interactions with Herbs & Other Dietary Supplements

None known.

Interactions with Drugs

None known.

Interactions with Foods

None known.

Interactions with Lab Tests

None known.

Interactions with Diseases or Conditions

None known.

Dosage and Administration

ORAL: No typical dosage.
TOPICAL: The fresh root is scraped and the pulp rubbed into affected areas (223).

BLACK COHOSH

Also Known As

Baneberry, Black Snakeroot, Bugbane, Bugwort, Cimicifuga, Macrotys, Phytoestrogen, Rattle Root, Rattle Top, Rattlesnake Root, Rattleweed, Snakeroot, Squaw Root.
CAUTION: See separate listings for Blue Cohosh and White Cohosh.

Scientific Names

Actaea racemosa, synonym Cimicifuga racemosa; Actaea macrotys.
Family: Ranunculaceae.

People Use This For

Orally, black cohosh is used for symptoms of menopause, inducing labor in pregnant women, premenstrual syndrome (PMS), dysmenorrhea, nervous tension, dyspepsia, rheumatism, fever, sore throat, cough, as an insect repellent, and as a mild sedative.
Topically, black cohosh is used for rattlesnake bites.

Safety

POSSIBLY SAFE ...when used orally and appropriately. Black cohosh has been safely used in studies lasting up to 6 months (141,4614,4620,7054,9437,9494). But there is concern that black cohosh might cause liver damage in some patients. There are a few case reports that link black cohosh to liver failure and autoimmune hepatitis (4383,10692,12006,11906). There is no conclusive evidence that black cohosh is the cause of liver damage in these patients. Until more is known, monitor liver function in patients who take black cohosh.
PREGNANCY: LIKELY UNSAFE ...when used orally in pregnant women who are not at term. Black cohosh has menstrual and uterine stimulant effects, which can increase the risk of miscarriage (3382); contraindicated. There is insufficient reliable information about the safety of black cohosh for labor induction. Some midwives use black cohosh to induce labor in pregnant women at term. Observational reports suggest that this practice does not appear to adversely affect the mother or fetus, but there are no clinical trials to support the safety of this practice (1122).
LACTATION: POSSIBLY UNSAFE ...when used orally. There is some concern that black cohosh, particularly in large doses, may adversely affect a nursing child (3382). Until more is known, tell nursing mothers to avoid taking black cohosh.

Effectiveness

POSSIBLY EFFECTIVE

Menopausal symptoms. Taking black cohosh orally seems to significantly reduce symptoms of menopause, such as hot flashes, in perimenopausal women. Some research suggests it can be as effective as estrogen replacement for some patients. Treatment for 4 weeks is usually required before there is significant improvement in symptoms (4620,9437,10987,11913). Black cohosh does not seem to reduce hot flashes in breast cancer survivors (7054).

Most clinical studies on the effectiveness of black cohosh have used a specific black cohosh formulation standardized to contain 1 mg triterpene glycosides, calculated as 27-deoxyacetin (Remifemin, GlaxoSmithKline).

There is insufficient reliable information available about the effectiveness of black cohosh for its other uses.

Mechanism of Action

The applicable parts of black cohosh are the rhizome and root. The active constituents of black cohosh include phytosterin; isoferulic acid; fukinolic acid; caffeic acid, salicylic acid; sugars; tannins; long-chain fatty acids; and triterpene glycosides, including acetin, cimicifugoside, and 27-deoxyacetin (4618,9432).
Fukinolic acid is a potent inhibitor of neutrophil elastase, which is important in inflammatory responses. Inhibition of neutrophil elastase is a possible mechanism by which black cohosh exerts anti-inflammatory action (9432).
The presence of an isoflavone, formononetin, is doubtful (1122,4616,9431). Earlier reports of isoflavone content may have been a result of contamination with other similar plant species (4615).
Black cohosh has estrogen-like effects that are exerted by an unknown mechanism (4618,4619). Clinically, it doesn't appear to affect endometrial tissue or hormone levels such as estradiol, luteinizing hormone (LH), follicle-stimulating hormone (FSH), and prolactin (9437,10987). Laboratory research suggests that extracts of black cohosh don't bind to estrogen receptors, up-regulate estrogen-dependent genes, or stimulate the growth of estrogen-dependent tumors in experimental animals (4619,7860,9996,9998). But there is some evidence from animal studies that black cohosh can suppress pituitary secretion of luteinizing hormone (LH) (12064). Preliminary clinical evidence also suggests that black cohosh might increase osteoblast activity (10987).
Its thought that black cohosh might have selective estrogen receptor modulating (SERM) effects and therefore have estrogenic effects in some tissues and antiestrogenic effects in other tissues. For example, in animal models, there is preliminary evidence that black cohosh might have a modest estrogenic effect on bone and suppress LH, but it doesn't seem to stimulate an increase in uterine weight (12064).
Research on breast cancer cells suggests that black cohosh doesn't promote tumor growth (9435,9436,11911). Some constituents of black cohosh seem to inhibit breast cancer cell growth (11912). Animal research suggests that black cohosh doesn't increase or decrease risk of breast cancer (9999). But black cohosh does seem to increase metastatic cancer in animals with existing cancer (9999). Therefore, black cohosh shouldn't be used by women with existing breast cancer or women with a high risk of developing breast cancer.
In vitro research suggests black cohosh might increase the toxicity of the chemotherapy drugs doxorubicin (Adriamycin) and docetaxel (Taxotere). Theoretically, it could also make these agents more effective in eliminating cancerous cells (10000).

Adverse Reactions

Orally, black cohosh can commonly cause gastrointestinal upset (3382,4383,4615,4616). Other potential adverse effects include rash, headache, dizziness, weight gain, feeling of heaviness in the legs, and cramping (3382,7054,10987).
There is concern that black cohosh might cause liver disease. Less than a dozen cases of liver toxicity have been described in women taking black cohosh products alone or in combination with other herbs. In some cases, women developed liver failure and required immediate liver transplantation. In one case, a women developed autoimmune hepatitis after 3 weeks of taking black cohosh. Symptoms resolved 2 weeks after discontinuing black cohosh (4383,10692,12006,11906,11909). Hepatitis can occur with no identifiable cause, raising the possibility that black cohosh and hepatitis might have been coincidental. Also, plant misidentification can occur, resulting in accidental substitution of a hepatotoxic plant (11910,11911). These cases do not provide conclusive evidence that black cohosh is responsible for liver disease. Until more is known, monitor liver function in patients who take black cohosh.

Some patients taking tamoxifen plus black cohosh have experienced endometrial hyperplasia and vaginal bleeding. However, these effects are more likely due to tamoxifen than black cohosh (7054).
There is one case report of seizures in a woman who used black cohosh, evening primrose oil, and chasteberry (10988).
There has been a case report of severe complications, including seizures, renal failure, and respiratory distress, in an infant whose mother was given an unknown dose of black and blue cohosh at 42 weeks gestation to induce labor (1122,9492,9493). However, this adverse effect may have been attributable to blue cohosh.
Studies on black cohosh mutagenicity, teratogenicity, and carcinogenicity have been negative (4615).

Interactions with Herbs & Other Dietary Supplements

HEPATOTOXIC HERBS AND SUPPLEMENTS: There is some concern that black cohosh can adversely affect the liver (4383,10692,12006,11906,11909). Theoretically, concomitant use with other potentially hepatotoxic products might increase the risk of developing liver damage. Some of these products include androstenedione, chaparral, comfrey, DHEA, germander, kava, niacin, pennyroyal oil, red yeast, and others.

Interactions with Drugs

HEPATOTOXIC DRUGS: There is concern that black cohosh might be linked to cases of liver failure and autoimmune hepatitis (4383,10692,12006,11906,11909). Theoretically, taking black cohosh with hepatotoxic drugs might increase the risk of liver damage. Advise patients against combining black cohosh with potentially hepatotoxic drugs. Some drugs that can adversely affect the liver include acetaminophen (Tylenol), amiodarone (Cordarone), càrbamazepine (Tegretol), isoniazid (INH), methotrexate (Rheumatrex), methyldopa (Aldomet), and many others.

Interactions with Foods

None known.

Interactions with Lab Tests

None known.

Interactions with Diseases or Conditions

BREAST CANCER: Preliminary evidence suggests that black cohosh might increase the risk of metastasis in existing breast cancer. Women with a history of breast cancer or women at risk for breast cancer should avoid black cohosh (9999).
HORMONE-SENSITIVE CANCERS/CONDITIONS: Black cohosh doesn't seem to affect estrogen receptors, but it hasn't been studied for longer than 2 months in women with hormone-sensitive conditions (7054). Until more is known, women with hormone-sensitive conditions should avoid black cohosh. Some of these conditions include uterine cancer, ovarian cancer, endometriosis, and uterine fibroids.
KIDNEY TRANSPLANT: There is one report of acute kidney transplant rejection in a patient who took black cohosh and an alfalfa supplement together. The mechanism for this disease interaction is not known, but it is more likely due to alfalfa than black cohosh. Alfalfa is thought to have immune-stimulating effects that might counteract the immunosuppressant effects of cyclosporine (12174).
LIVER DISEASE: There is concern that black cohosh might be linked to cases of liver failure and autoimmune hepatitis (4383,10692,12006,11906,11909). Theoretically, black cohosh might exacerbate liver problems in patients with existing liver disease such as hepatitis. Advise these patients to avoid taking black cohosh.

Dosage and Administration

ORAL: For menopause and premenstrual syndrome (PMS), most clinical studies have used a specific black cohosh extract (Remifemin, Enzymatic Therapy, and Phytopharmica) standardized to contain 1 mg triterpene glycosides, calculated as 27-deoxyacetin, per 20 mg tablet. Most studies used doses of 40-80 mg twice daily, providing 4-8 mg triterpene glycosides for up to 6 months (141,4614,4620,7054,9437,9494). The manufacturer now claims that improvement in the extraction process permits using their currently recommended lower dose of 20 mg twice daily, providing 2 mg triterpene glycosides (4615). An isopropanolic aqueous extract of black cohosh 39 to 127.3 mg daily has also been used to treat postmenopausal symptoms (9437).

Comments

Black cohosh was first used medicinally by Native Americans who introduced it to European colonists (9997). It was introduced into Germany in the late 19th century. Remifemin, a branded black cohosh product, has been used in Germany since the mid-1950s to manage menopause (141). Black cohosh was also used as the main ingredient in Lydia Pinkham's Vegetable Compound (3382).
One clinical study used the product Menofem (Pharmaton) which contains 20 mg black cohosh extract per dose (10987). This product is not available in the US or Canada. Another product called Menofem (Vitamin Plus Company) contains unspecified quantities of black cohosh and a variety of other ingredients. These products are not interchangeable.
The genus name of black cohosh, cimicifuga, comes from the Latin words for "bedbug" and "repel." Although less fragrant than other species of the genus, black cohosh was used as an insect repellent,

hence the common name "bugbane." Do not confuse black cohosh with two unrelated plants, blue cohosh and white cohosh.

BLACK CURRANT

Also Known As

Cassis, European Black Currant, Ribes Nigri Folium (black currant leaf), Ribes Nero.
CAUTION: See separate listings for Borage Seed Oil, Evening Primrose Oil, Gamma Linolenic Acid (GLA), and Omega-6 Fatty Acids.

Scientific Names

Ribes nigrum.
Family: Grossulariaceae.

People Use This For

Orally, black currant seed oil is used for menopausal symptoms, premenstrual syndrome, dysmenorrhea, mastodynia, and for boosting immunity. Black currant berry is used orally for coughs. Black currant dried leaf is used orally for arthritis, gout, rheumatism, diarrhea, colic, hepatitis, liver ailments, convulsions, and inflammatory disorders of the mouth and throat. Black currant dried leaf is also used for coughs and colds, whooping cough, disinfecting the urine, promoting diuresis, treating bladder stones, and as a cleansing tea.
Topically, black currant leaf is used for the treatment of wounds and insect bites.
In foods, black currant berry is utilized as a flavor component in liqueurs, for flavorings, and as a food.

Safety

LIKELY SAFE ...when used in amounts commonly found in foods. Black currant juice, leaves, and flower have Generally Recognized As Safe (GRAS) status in the US (4912).
POSSIBLY SAFE ...when black currant berry or seed oil is used orally and appropriately in medicinal amounts (12,4016).
There is insufficient reliable information available about the safety of black currant dried leaf.
PREGNANCY AND LACTATION: Insufficient reliable information available; avoid using.

Effectiveness

There is insufficient reliable information available about the effectiveness of black currant.

Mechanism of Action

The applicable parts of black currant are the seed oil, berry, flower, and leaf.
Black currant seed oil is obtained by pressing the seeds found in the fruit of black currant. Black currant seed oil contains 6-19% gamma-linolenic acid (GLA), an omega-6 fatty acid, and approximately 13% alpha-linolenic acid (ALA), an omega-3 fatty acid (512,515,4016). GLA may be beneficial for people who are unable to metabolize cis-linolenic acid to GLA, and produce adequate prostaglandin E1 (PGE-1). People with this condition have an imbalance in the ratio of inflammatory to non-inflammatory prostaglandins. GLA is thought to improve this ratio (512,4016). The volatile oil contains trace amounts of ascorbic acid (18).
Black currant seed oil may increase immune response in healthy elderly people by reducing prostaglandin E2 (PGE-2) production, which contributes to the decline in T cell-mediated function associated with aging. Black currant seed oil supplementation improves delayed-type hypersensitivity skin testing response and improves immune response in peripheral blood mononuclear cells (4016). However, whether black currant seed oil supplementation results in better health in elderly people is unknown.
There is also evidence that GLA may be a good source of nutrition in critical care patients and neonates who might have low stores of essential fatty acids (9238).
Preliminary evidence suggests GLA might have an antiestrogenic effect and might hasten the response to tamoxifen (Nolvadex) in women with estrogen-sensitive breast cancer (5902). GLA also seems to modulate the sensitivity of breast cancer cells to paclitaxel (Taxol) and fulvestrant (Faslodex), enhancing malignant cell killing without adverse effects on normal cells (8133,11791). However, other research suggests that taking GLA alone might stimulate the growth of breast cancer cells at low concentrations and inhibit growth at higher concentrations (11339).
Black currant leaves can have diuretic, hypotensive, and cooling effects (18). The leaves of black currant contain flavonoids, including astragalin, isoquercitrin, and rutin.
Preliminary research suggests that a hydroalcoholic extract of black currant leaves has anti-inflammatory action. The active component that causes this action has not been identified (9239).

Adverse Reactions

None reported.

Interactions with Herbs & Other Dietary Supplements
None known.

Interactions with Drugs
None known.

Interactions with Foods
None known.

Interactions with Lab Tests
None known.

Interactions with Diseases or Conditions
None known.

Dosage and Administration
ORAL: Three to four cups of black currant dried leaf tea has traditionally been used. The tea is prepared by adding 2-4 grams of the black currant leaves to 150 mL of boiling water (18).
TOPICAL: No typical dosage.

BLACK HAW

Also Known As
Blackhaw, Nanny Bush, Southern Black Haw, Stag Bush, Viburnum.

Scientific Names
Viburnum prunifolium; Viburnum lentago; Viburnum rufidulum.
Family: Adoxaceae/Viburnaceae or Caprifoliaceae.

People Use This For
Orally, black haw is used as a tonic, uterine sedative, antidiarrheal, diuretic, antispasmodic, to treat painful menses, preventing miscarriage, asthma, and as a postpartum antispasmodic.

Safety
LIKELY SAFE ...when the stem bark is used orally in amounts commonly found in foods. Black haw has Generally Recognized As Safe (GRAS) status in the US (4912).
POSSIBLY SAFE ...when the root bark is used orally and appropriately in medicinal amounts (12).
PREGNANCY: POSSIBLY UNSAFE ...when used orally. Some evidence suggests black haw has uterine relaxant effects (11); avoid using.
LACTATION: Insufficient reliable information available.

Effectiveness
There is insufficient reliable information available about the effectiveness of black haw.

Mechanism of Action
The applicable parts of black haw are the root bark and stem bark. The root bark has several active constituents, including scopoletin, tannins, oxalic acid, salicin, salicylic acid biflavone, iridoid glycosiders, coumarins, urolic acid, and oleanolic acid (11,296,9241). Scopoletin is thought to be a uterine relaxant (11).
Black haw has spasmolytic activity in the uterus and other smooth muscle. It has been reported to cause vasoconstriction (9241).

Adverse Reactions
None reported.

Interactions with Herbs & Other Dietary Supplements
CALCIUM, IRON, ZINC: Concurrent use might decrease mineral absorption. Black haw contains oxalic acid (oxalate) (11,296), which can bind multivalent metal ions in the gastrointestinal (GI) tract and decrease mineral absorption.

Interactions with Drugs
None known.

Interactions with Foods
CALCIUM, IRON, ZINC: Concurrent use might decrease mineral absorption from foods. Black haw contains oxalic acid (oxalate) (11,296), which can bind multivalent metal ions in the gastrointestinal (GI) tract and decrease mineral absorption.

Interactions with Lab Tests
None known.

Interactions with Diseases or Conditions
ASPIRIN ALLERGY: Theoretically, the salicylate constituents in black haw could trigger allergic reaction in individuals with aspirin allergy or asthma.
HISTORY OF KIDNEY STONES: Avoid the use of black haw because it contains oxalic acid and might increase stone formation in individuals with a history of kidney stones (11,12).

Dosage and Administration
ORAL: People typically use 2 teaspoons of the dried bark in 1 cup of water, boiled and simmered for 10 minutes. This is taken three times daily. In tincture form, black haw is taken 5 to 10 mL three times daily (5253).

Comments
Black haw is a shrub that has serrated oval leaves, clusters of white flowers, and blue-black berries. It is native to the woodlands of central and southern North America (4201).

BLACK HELLEBORE

Also Known As
Christe Herbe, Christmas Rose, Christmas Rose Plant, Melampode.
CAUTION: See separate listings for American Hellebore, Pheasant's Eye, and White Hellebore.

Scientific Names
Helleborus niger.
Family: Ranunculaceae.

People Use This For
Orally, black hellebore is used for nausea, worm infestations, regulating menstruation, acute nephritis, head colds, as a laxative, and as an abortifacient.

Safety
LIKELY UNSAFE ...when used orally. Black hellebore contains cardiac glycosides with structure, activity, and adverse effects similar to digitalis (3).
PREGNANCY: LIKELY UNSAFE ...when used orally because it can have menstrual stimulant (19) or abortifacient effects (18); avoid using.
LACTATION: LIKELY UNSAFE ...when used orally (3); avoid using.

Effectiveness
There is insufficient reliable information available about the effectiveness of black hellebore.

Mechanism of Action
Black hellebore root contains cardioactive glycosides with digitalis-like effects (18). It also contains saponins that irritate mucous membranes and can cause toxicity (18). Black hellebore is a GI irritant (19), and the fresh plant has local irritant properties (19).

Adverse Reactions
Orally, black hellebore can cause GI irritation (19). The symptoms of poisoning from black hellebore include scratchy throat or mouth, salivation, nausea, vomiting, diarrhea, dizziness, shortness of breath, spasm, and asphyxiation (18). Topically, the fresh plant may cause irritation or inflammation when handled (19).

Interactions with Herbs & Other Dietary Supplements
CARDIAC GLYCOSIDE-CONTAINING HERBS: Contraindicated; concomitant use can increase the risk of cardiac glycoside toxicity. Cardiac glycoside-containing herbs, including black hellebore, Canadian hemp roots, digitalis leaf, hedge mustard, figwort, lily of the valley roots, motherwort, oleander leaf, pheasant's eye plant, pleurisy root, squill bulb leaf scales, and strophanthus seeds (19).

LICORICE/HORSETAIL: Theoretically, overuse/misuse of licorice rhizome or horsetail plant with cardiac glycoside-containing herbs increases the risk of toxicity due to potassium depletion (19).
OTHER CARDIOACTIVE HERBS: Avoid concomitant use with other cardioactive herbs due to unpredictability of effects and adverse effects. Other cardioactive herbs include calamus, cereus, cola, coltsfoot, devil's claw, European mistletoe, fenugreek, fumitory, ginger, Panax ginseng, hawthorn, white horehound, mate, parsley, quassia, scotch broom flower, shepherd's purse, and wild carrot (4).
STIMULANT LAXATIVE HERBS: Theoretically, overuse or misuse of stimulant laxatives with cardiac glycoside-containing herbs increases the risk of cardiac toxicity due to potassium depletion. Stimulant laxative herbs include aloe dried leaf sap, blue flag rhizome, alder buckthorn, European buckthorn, butternut bark, cascara bark, castor oil, colocynth fruit pulp, gamboge bark exudate, jalap root, black root, manna bark exudate, podophyllum root, rhubarb root, senna leaves and pods, wild cucumber fruit (Ecballium elaterium), and yellow dock root (19).

Interactions with Drugs

DIGOXIN (Lanoxin): Black hellebore contains cardiac glycosides. Using black hellebore in combination with digoxin might have additive effects and increase the risk of toxicity (18,19).
DIURETIC DRUGS: Theoretically, concomitant use of potassium depleting diuretics and black hellebore can increase the risk of cardiac glycoside toxicity due to potassium depletion (506). Some diuretics that can deplete potassium include chlorothiazide (Diuril), chlorthalidone (Thalitone), furosemide (Lasix), hydrochlorothiazide (HCTZ, HydroDIURIL, Microzide), and others.
MACROLIDE ANTIBIOTICS: Theoretically, concomitant use might increase risk of cardiac glycoside toxicity (17). Some of these drugs include erythromycin, azithromycin, and clarithromycin.
QUININE: Theoretically, concomitant use of quinine and black hellebore can increase the risk of cardiac glycoside toxicity (506).
STIMULANT LAXATIVES: Theoretically, overuse or misuse of stimulant laxatives can increase the risk of cardiac glycoside toxicity due to potassium depletion (19,506).
TETRACYCLINE ANTIBIOTICS: Theoretically, concomitant use might increase risk of cardiac glycoside toxicity (17).

Interactions with Foods

None known.

Interactions with Lab Tests

None known.

Interactions with Diseases or Conditions

GASTROINTESTINAL (GI) INFLAMMATION: Black hellebore can aggravate gastrointestinal inflammation, contraindicated (19).
HEART DISEASE: Self-medication is contraindicated; requires diagnosis, treatment, and monitoring (515).

Dosage and Administration

No typical dosage.

Comments

Avoid confusion with white hellebore (Veratrum album). Black hellebore is an obsolete and dangerous natural product (18).

BLACK HOREHOUND

Also Known As

Ballota, Black Stinking Horehound.
CAUTION: See separate listing for White Horehound.

Scientific Names

Ballota nigra.
Family: Lamiaceae/Labiatae.

People Use This For

Orally, black horehound is used for nausea, vomiting, sedation in hysteria and hypochondria, nervous dyspepsia increasing bile flow, whooping cough, and as an antispasmodic. It is also used orally for symptomatic relief of nervous disorders in adults and children, especially mild sleep disorders, and for cough.
Topically, black horehound is used as a mild astringent and for gout.
Rectally, black horehound is used as an enema against ascaridae, or intestinal worms.

Safety

POSSIBLY SAFE ...when the above ground parts are used orally and appropriately in medicinal amounts (12). There is insufficient reliable information available about the safety of topical or rectal use of black horehound.
PREGNANCY: LIKELY UNSAFE ...when used orally; black horehound may affect the menstrual cycle (4). There is insufficient reliable information available about the safety of black horehound used topically or rectally during pregnancy.
LACTATION: Insufficient reliable information available; avoid using.

Effectiveness

There is insufficient reliable information available about the effectiveness of black horehound.

Mechanism of Action

The applicable parts of black horehound are the above ground parts. Chemicals isolated from black horehound include flavonoids (apigenin-7-glucoside, vicenin-2, tangeretin), diterpenoids (ballotinone, ballonigrine, 7-alpha-acetoxymarrubiin, ballotenol, preleosibirin, 13-hydroxyballonigrinolide), and phenylpropanoids (caffeoyl-L-malic acid, verbascoside, forsythoside B, arenarioside, ballotetroside, alyssonoside, lavandulifolioside, angoroside A). In vitro studies indicate that caffeoyl-L-malic acid, verbascoside, forsythoside B, and arenarioside are able to bind to dopaminergic D2, benzodiazepine and morphine (mu) receptors. Verbascoside, forsythoside B, caffeoyl-L-malic acid, arenarioside, and ballotetroside (in order of decreasing potency) also have antioxidant properties, as demonstrated by scavenging of reactive oxygen species and reducing their release from polymorphonuclear neutrophils in vitro (5880). Black horehound also has antiemetic (4,18), sedative, mild astringent (4), antispasmodic, and stimulant effects (18). Preliminary evidence suggests that the aqueous extracts of black horehound may reduce arterial blood pressure and heart rate and increase gallbladder secretions (18).

Adverse Reactions

None reported.

Interactions with Herbs & Other Dietary Supplements

None known.

Interactions with Drugs

DOPAMINE AGONISTS: Theoretically, black horehound might have additive effects when used with dopamine agonists. Some constituents of black horehound bind to dopamine D2 receptors in vitro (5880); however, this has not yet been reported in humans. Some dopamine agonists include bromocriptine (Parlodel), levodopa (Dopar, component of Sinemet), pramipexole (Mirapex), ropinirole (Requip), and others.

Interactions with Foods

None known.

Interactions with Lab Tests

None known.

Interactions with Diseases or Conditions

PARKINSON'S DISEASE: Theoretically, black horehound might affect therapy for Parkinson's disease. Some constituents of black horehound bind to dopamine D2 receptors in vitro (5880); however, this has not yet been reported in humans.
SCHIZOPHRENIA, PSYCHOTIC DISORDERS: Theoretically, black horehound might adversely affect people with schizophrenia and psychotic disorders. Some constituents of black horehound bind to dopamine D2 receptors in vitro (5880); however, this has not yet been reported in humans.

Dosage and Administration

ORAL: The typical dose of black horehound is 2-4 grams of the above ground parts or one cup of tea three times daily (4). The tea is prepared by steeping 2-4 grams of the above ground parts in 150 mL boiling water for 10-15 minutes and then straining. The usual dose of the liquid extract, 1:1 in 25% alcohol, is 1-3 mL three times daily (4). The common dose of the tincture,1:10 in 45% alcohol, is 1-2 mL three times daily (4).
TOPICAL: No typical dosage.

Comments

Avoid confusion with white horehound.

BLACK MULBERRY

Also Known As
Mulberry, Purple Mulberry.

Scientific Names
Morus nigra.
Family: Moraceae.

People Use This For
Orally, black mulberry is used as a laxative and for chronic rhinitis.

Safety
There is insufficient reliable information available about the safety of black mulberry.
Pregnancy and Lactation: Insufficient reliable information available; avoid using.

Effectiveness
There is insufficient reliable information available about the effectiveness of black mulberry.

Mechanism of Action
The applicable parts of black mulberry are the ripe berry and root bark. The fruit contains small amounts of vitamin C (0.17%), rutin, and pectin (18). The pectin may have laxative activity (7).

Adverse Reactions
None reported.

Interactions with Herbs & Other Dietary Supplements
None known.

Interactions with Drugs
ANTIDIABETES DRUGS: Monitor blood glucose levels closely due to claims that some species of mulberry leaves have hypoglycemic effects (19).

Interactions with Foods
None known.

Interactions with Lab Tests
None known.

Interactions with Diseases or Conditions
None known.

Dosage and Administration
ORAL: The average amount used daily is 2-4 mL of syrup (18).

BLACK MUSTARD OIL

Also Known As
Mustard Oil.
CAUTION: See separate listings for Black Mustard seed, Hedge Mustard, and White Mustard.

Scientific Names
Brassica nigra, synonym Sinapis nigra.
Family: Brassicaceae/Cruciferae.

People Use This For
Topically, black mustard oil is used for symptoms of the common cold including pulmonary congestion, rheumatism and arthritis, as a counterirritant, and in footbaths for aching feet. In foods and beverages, black mustard oil is used as a flavoring agent. In manufacturing, black mustard oil is used as a lubricant and illuminant in soap and an ingredient in cat and dog repellents.

Safety

LIKELY SAFE ...when used orally in the amounts commonly found in foods. Mustard oil has Generally Recognized As Safe (GRAS) status in the US (4912).
POSSIBLY SAFE ...when used topically in concentrations of 0.5-5% applied 3-4 times daily (3,272).
LIKELY UNSAFE ...when used orally, undiluted. Black mustard oil is an extremely powerful topical irritant and ingesting large amounts can cause irritant poisoning (12). ...when inhaled (11).
CHILDREN: LIKELY UNSAFE ...when used orally in children under 6 years of age (12,19); avoid using. There is insufficient reliable information available about the safety of the topical use of black mustard oil in children.
PREGNANCY: LIKELY UNSAFE ...when used orally because it might have abortifacient and menstrual stimulant effects (19); avoid using. There is insufficient reliable information available about the safety of the topical use of black mustard oil during pregnancy; avoid using.
LACTATION: Insufficient reliable information available; avoid using.

Effectiveness

There is insufficient reliable information available about the effectiveness of black mustard oil.

Mechanism of Action

Black mustard oil consists mainly of allyl isothiocyanate, which is produced after the glucosinolate sinigrin is hydrolyzed and distilled (3,6,11). The allyl isothiocyanate of black mustard oil has strong antimicrobial (bacterial and fungi) properties (11), lacrimatory effects, and can act as a counterirritant when diluted (1:50) (6,11). Black mustard oil has powerful irritant properties that can cause pain and increased inflammation of the skin (6,11).

Adverse Reactions

Orally, large amounts of black mustard oil can lead to vomiting, stomach pain, diarrhea, somnolence, cardiac failure, breathing difficulties, coma, and possibly death (18). Rarely, black mustard oil exacerbates stomach and intestinal ulcers (18,19) and causes kidney irritation (19). The isothiocyanate constituents can cause endemic goiters (6,11). Topically, the oil can cause skin blistering and necroses (6,11), and can rarely cause contact allergies (18).

Interactions with Herbs & Other Dietary Supplements

None known.

Interactions with Drugs

ANTACIDS: Theoretically, due to reports that black mustard oil increases stomach acid, black mustard oil might decrease the effectiveness of antacids (19).
H2-BLOCKERS: Theoretically, due to reports that black mustard oil increases stomach acid, black mustard oil might decrease the effectiveness of H2-blockers (19). The H2 blockers include cimetidine (Tagamet), ranitidine (Zantac), nizatidine (Axid), and famotidine (Pepcid).
PROTON PUMP INHIBITORS (PPIs): Theoretically, due to reports that black mustard oil increases stomach acid, black mustard oil might decrease the effectiveness of PPIs (19). PPIs include omeprazole (Prilosec), lansoprazole (Prevacid), rabeprazole (Aciphex), pantoprazole (Protonix), and esomeprazole (Nexium).

Interactions with Foods

None known.

Interactions with Lab Tests

None known.

Interactions with Diseases or Conditions

GASTROINTESTINAL ULCERS: Black mustard oil can exacerbate stomach and intestinal ulcers by irritating the mucus membranes (19).

Dosage and Administration

TOPICAL: As a counterirritant, black mustard oil is typically used in concentrations from 0.5-5% and as frequently as 3-4 times daily (3,272).

Comments

Avoid confusion with black mustard seed, hedge mustard (Sisymbrium officinale), and white mustard (Sinapis alba). Derivatives of mustard oil (allyl isothiocyanate) have formed the basis for toxic agents such as the "mustard gases" and antineoplastic agents (11). The volatile oil of mustard is prepared by steam distillation from brown or black mustard after expressing the fixed oil and macerating in water to allow hydrolysis of sinigrin by enzyme myrosin. The volatile oil mainly consists of allyl isothiocyanate.

BLACK MUSTARD seed

Also Known As
Mustard.
CAUTION: See separate listings for Black Mustard oil, Hedge Mustard, and White Mustard.

Scientific Names
Brassica nigra, synonym Sinapis nigra.
Family: Brassicaceae/Cruciferae.

People Use This For
Orally, black mustard seed is used as an emetic, diuretic, and appetite stimulant.
Topically, black mustard seed is used as a poultice for bronchial pneumonia, pleurisy, arthritis, lumbago, aching feet, for rheumatism, and as a counterirritant.
In foods, black mustard seed is a flavoring agent in condiments, foods, and beverages; and is a culinary spice.

Safety
LIKELY SAFE ...when used orally in the amounts commonly found in foods. Black mustard seed has Generally Recognized As Safe (GRAS) status in the US (4912).
POSSIBLY SAFE ...when used topically and appropriately for less than 2 weeks (18).
LIKELY UNSAFE ...when used orally as an emetic. Black mustard seed is an irritant and when used as an emetic, it re-exposes the esophageal tissue to its corrosive effects (19). Ingesting a large amount can cause irritant poisoning (12). ...when pure mustard powder is applied topically for more than 15-30 minutes, it can cause severe burns (12). ...when it is used topically for more than 2 weeks (18).
CHILDREN: LIKELY UNSAFE ...when used orally; contraindicated for use in children under 6 years of age (12,19). There is insufficient reliable information available about the safety of the topical use of black mustard seed in children.
PREGNANCY: LIKELY UNSAFE ...when used orally because it might have abortifacient and menstrual stimulant effects (19). There is insufficient reliable information available about the safety of the topical use of black mustard seed during pregnancy; avoid using.
LACTATION: Insufficient reliable information available; avoid using.

Effectiveness
There is insufficient reliable information available about the effectiveness of black mustard seed.

Mechanism of Action
Black mustard powder contains the glucosinolate sinigrin, which produces allyl isothiocyanate when mixed with warm water (3,6,11,18). Allyl isothiocyanate has strong antimicrobial (bacterial and fungi) properties (11), lacrimatory effects, and can act as a counterirritant when diluted (1:50) (6,11). Mustard oil (produced from powder by hydrolysis) is absorbed through the skin and eliminated through the lungs. This could explain its inclusion in liniment preparations to treat lung congestion (11). Black mustard has powerful irritant properties that can cause pain and increased inflammation of the skin (6,11,18). Sinigrin can be toxic to certain insect larvae (11). The glucosinolate products can have protective effects against carcinogens (11).

Adverse Reactions
Orally, large amounts of black mustard seed can lead to vomiting, stomach pain, diarrhea, somnolence, cardiac failure, breathing difficulties, coma, and possibly death (18). The isothiocyanate constituents can cause endemic goiters (6,11).
Topically, the allyl isothiocyanate found in black mustard seed can cause skin blistering and necroses (6,11,18) but rarely cause contact allergies (18).

Interactions with Herbs & Other Dietary Supplements
None known.

Interactions with Drugs
ANTACIDS: Theoretically, due to reports that black mustard seed increases stomach acid, black mustard oil might decrease the effectiveness of antacids (19).
H2-BLOCKERS: Theoretically, due to reports that black mustard oil increases stomach acid, black mustard seed might decrease the effectiveness of H2-blockers (19). The H2 blockers include cimetidine (Tagamet), ranitidine (Zantac), nizatidine (Axid), and famotidine (Pepcid).
PROTON PUMP INHIBITORS (PPIs): Theoretically, due to reports that black mustard oil increases stomach acid, black mustard seed might decrease the effectiveness of PPIs (19). PPIs include omeprazole (Prilosec), lansoprazole (Prevacid), rabeprazole (Aciphex), pantoprazole (Protonix), and esomeprazole (Nexium).

Interactions with Foods
None known.

Interactions with Lab Tests
None known.

Interactions with Diseases or Conditions
ASTHMA: Coughing, sneezing, and possible asthma attacks can result from handling mustard flour (18).
GI IRRITATION: Can irritate gastrointestinal tract. Contraindicated in individuals with infectious or inflammatory gastrointestinal conditions (19).

Dosage and Administration
TOPICAL: To prepare a mustard plaster, typically 100 grams of mustard flour (ground mustard) is mixed with warm water to make a paste. The paste is packed in linen and applied to the affected area for 10 minutes (3-5 minutes for children over 6 years old) (18). Mustard plaster applied for longer than 15-30 minutes is associated with severe burns and skin necroses (12). Treatment should not exceed two weeks (19).

Comments
Avoid confusion with black mustard oil, hedge mustard (Sisymbrium officinale), and white mustard (Sinapis alba).

BLACK NIGHTSHADE

Also Known As
Garden Nightshade, Houndsberry, Kakamachi, Petty Morel, Poisonberry.

Scientific Names
Solanum nigrum.
Family: Solanaceae.

People Use This For
Orally, black nightshade is used for gastric irritation, cramps, as an antispasmodic, pain reliever, sedative, and narcotic.
Topically, black nightshade is used for psoriasis, hemorrhoids, and abscesses. The bruised, fresh leaves are used topically to treat inflammation, burns, and ulcers.

Safety
LIKELY UNSAFE ...when used orally (4009).
There is insufficient reliable information available about the safety of black nightshade for its other uses.
PREGNANCY AND LACTATION: LIKELY UNSAFE ...when used orally because of concerns it could be teratogenic (4009); avoid using.

Effectiveness
There is insufficient reliable information available about the effectiveness of black nightshade.

Mechanism of Action
Most of the toxic effects of black nightshade can be attributed to the solanine constituent. The green fruits have higher solanine concentrations and are therefore more toxic than the other plant parts. However, among plant strains, toxicity varies widely (4009).

Adverse Reactions
Orally, ingestion of large quantities of the green berries or fresh foliage with high alkaloid content can result in overdose. Symptoms include nausea, vomiting, headache, and in rare cases, dilation of the pupils (18). At doses of 200-400 mg, solanine can cause gastroenteritis, tachycardia, dyspnea, vertigo, drowsiness, lethargy, twitches of the arms and legs, and cramping. Other symptoms of poisoning include diarrhea, panic, excitation, coma, hyperthermia. This is followed later by a dazed state, paralysis, and rarely, death due to respiratory arrest and hypothermia (4009).

Interactions with Herbs & Other Dietary Supplements
None known.

Interactions with Drugs
None known.

Interactions with Foods
None known.

Interactions with Lab Tests
None known.

Interactions with Diseases or Conditions
None known.

Dosage and Administration
ORAL: No typical dosage.
TOPICAL: A handful of herb is placed in boiling water for 10 minutes, and used as a compress or a rinse (18).

Comments
Black nightshade is sometimes referred to as petty morel. This name is a corruption of the original, petit morel. Originally, black nightshade was called petit morel to differentiate it from the more poisonous species, deadly nightshade that is known as great morel. Black nightshade has a musk-like fragrance when wilting (18).

BLACK PEPPER AND WHITE PEPPER

Also Known As
Black Pepper, Blanc Poivre, Kosho, Krishna, Maricha, Pepe, Pepper, Pepper Extract, Pepper Plant, Peppercorn, Pfeffer, Pimenta, Pimienta, Piper, Piperine, Poivre, Poivre Noir, Vellaja, White Pepper.

Scientific Names
Piper nigrum.
Family: Piperaceae.

People Use This For
Orally, black pepper is used for stomach upset, bronchitis, and cancer. White pepper is used orally for stomach upset, malaria, cholera, and cancer.
Topically, black pepper is used for treating neuralgia and scabies. Black and white pepper are also used topically as a counterirritant for pain.
In foods and beverages, black pepper, white pepper, and pepper oil are used as flavoring agents.

Safety
LIKELY SAFE ...when used orally in amounts commonly found in foods. Black and white pepper have Generally Recognized As Safe (GRAS) status in the US (4912).
POSSIBLY SAFE ...when used orally and appropriately in medicinal amounts (12). ...when black pepper oil is used topically. Black pepper oil is nonirritating and is typically well tolerated (11).
CHILDREN: LIKELY SAFE ...when used orally in amounts commonly found in foods (11). POSSIBLY UNSAFE ...when used orally in large amounts. Fatal cases of pepper aspiration have been reported in some patients (5619,5620). There is insufficient reliable information available about the safety of topical pepper oil when used in children.
PREGNANCY: LIKELY SAFE ...when used orally in amounts commonly found in foods (11). LIKELY UNSAFE ...when used orally in large amounts. Black pepper might have abortifacient effects (11,19); contraindicated. There is insufficient reliable information available about the safety of topical pepper when used during pregnancy.
LACTATION: LIKELY SAFE ...when used orally in amounts commonly found in foods (11). There is insufficient reliable information available about the safety of black and white pepper when used in medicinal amounts during breast-feeding.

Effectiveness
There is insufficient reliable information available about the effectiveness of black pepper and white pepper.

Mechanism of Action
The applicable part of black pepper and white pepper is the fruit. Piper nigrum is said to have antiflatulent and diuretic properties (11), antimicrobial and insecticidal effects (18). It is thought to influence liver and metabolic functions (11), stimulate thermal receptors, induce sweating, and stimulate taste buds causing a reflex increase in gastric secretions (18). It might also have lipolytic activity related to the outer layer of the fruit (11). Piper nigrum contains piperine which increases oral absorption of drugs and other substances, possibly by modulating intestinal membrane dynamics (3757). Some evidence suggests piper nigrum might protect against colon cancer (3761); however, other evidence suggests black pepper might induce hepatic enzymes (3760) or cause liver tumors (3759).

Adverse Reactions
Orally, pepper can cause a burning aftertaste.
Topically, eye contact with ground pepper can cause redness of eyes and swelling of eyelids (5619). Deaths due to aspiration of large amounts of pepper have been reported (5619,5620).

Interactions with Herbs & Other Dietary Supplements
SPARTEINE: Piperine increases the bioavailability of sparteine, a constituent of scotch broom (19).

Interactions with Drugs
PHENYTOIN (Dilantin): Concomitant administration speeds absorption and slows elimination of phenytoin (Dilantin) (537).
PROPRANOLOL (Inderal): Concomitant administration speeds and increases absorption, and increases serum concentrations of propranolol (Inderal) (538).
THEOPHYLLINE: Concomitant administration increases absorption and serum concentrations of theophylline (Theo-Dur) (538).

Interactions with Foods
None known.

Interactions with Lab Tests
SERUM DRUG ASSAYS: Black pepper and white pepper can increase phenytoin, propranolol, and theophylline serum concentrations and test results (537,538).

Interactions with Diseases or Conditions
None known.

Dosage and Administration
ORAL: A typical dose of black pepper and white pepper ranges from 300-600 mg (18); up to 1.5 grams per day have been used (18).
TOPICAL: No typical dosage.

Comments
Black pepper is the dried, full grown but unripe fruit of Piper nigrum (11). White pepper is the dried ripe fruit of Piper nigrum with the outer covering that is known as a pericarp removed (11). Pepper oil is distilled from black pepper (11). Indian long pepper contains higher concentrations of piperine. Red pepper and cayenne contain no piperine.

BLACK PSYLLIUM

Also Known As
Brown Psyllium, Dietary Fiber, Fleaseed, Fleawort, French Psyllium, Plantain, Psyllion, Psyllios, Psyllium Seed, Spanish Psyllium.
CAUTION: See separate listings for Blond Psyllium, Buckhorn Plantain, Great Plantain, and Water Plantain.

Scientific Names
Plantago psyllium, synonym Psyllium afra; Psyllium indica, synonym Psyllium arenaria.
Family: Plantaginaceae.

People Use This For
Orally, black psyllium is used for chronic constipation and for softening stools in conditions such as hemorrhoids, anal fissures, anorectal surgery, and pregnancy. It is also used for diarrhea, irritable bowel syndrome (IBS), reducing elevated cholesterol, dysentery, and treating cancer.

Safety
LIKELY SAFE ...when used orally with appropriate fluid intake (4,12,272).
LIKELY UNSAFE ...when used orally without adequate fluid intake because it can cause esophageal obstruction (2,4,18). ...when the seeds of non-commercial preparations of black psyllium are chewed, crushed, or ground because they release a pigment that deposits in renal tubules (11) and can be nephrotoxic (6). This pigment has been removed from most commercial products (6).
PREGNANCY AND LACTATION: LIKELY SAFE ...when used orally with appropriate fluid intake (272).

Effectiveness

EFFECTIVE

Constipation. Taking black psyllium orally works as a bulk laxative and reduces constipation (272).

POSSIBLY EFFECTIVE

Hypercholesterolemia. Taking black psyllium orally seems to reduce total and LDL cholesterol, and the LDL:HDL ratio (6,11).

There is insufficient reliable information available about the effectiveness of black psyllium for its other uses.

Mechanism of Action

The applicable part of black psyllium is the seed. Its constituents are not absorbed and have no systemic effects (1). Black psyllium seed forms a mucilaginous mass when mixed with water and has a bulk laxative effect (1,4,6). In people with diarrhea, the mucilage absorbs water, provides mass, and prolongs gastrointestinal transit (1,6). In individuals with constipation, the mucilage absorbs water, swells, and stimulates peristalsis, reducing gastrointestinal transit time (1,4,6). Black psyllium can decrease abdominal pain in people with irritable bowel syndrome (IBS) by reducing rectosigmoidal pressure (405). Psyllium reduces peak blood glucose levels by slowing carbohydrate absorption (1,6) and can decrease cholesterol by absorbing dietary fats in the gastrointestinal tract, thereby preventing systemic absorption. It can also increase cholesterol elimination in the fecal bile acids (1,6,11,12). Chewing or crushing the seeds can release a pigment that deposits in renal tubules (11) and can be nephrotoxic (6). This pigment is removed from most commercial products (6).

Adverse Reactions

Orally, black psyllium can cause transient flatulence and abdominal distention (4). When consumed without water, it can cause esophageal (4) and bowel obstruction (4,604). Chewing or crushing the seeds can release a pigment that deposits in the renal tubules (11) and can be nephrotoxic (6). This pigment is removed from most commercial products (6). Allergic reactions to black psyllium include allergic rhinitis, conjunctivitis, urticaria, and asthma (18). Occupational exposure to black psyllium can cause sensitization, of which symptoms include sneezing, watery eyes, chest congestion, and anaphylactoid reaction (6).

Interactions with Herbs & Other Dietary Supplements

VITAMIN/MINERAL SUPPLEMENTS: The long-term use of black psyllium with vitamin or mineral supplements can reduce the absorption of calcium, iron, zinc, and vitamin B12 (1,12). Supplements should be taken one hour before or four hours after black psyllium to avoid this interaction (4,12).

Interactions with Drugs

ANTIDIABETES DRUGS: Black psyllium can reduce blood glucose levels in patients with type 2 diabetes (10091) and might have additive effects on glucose levels when used with antidiabetes drugs. Monitor blood glucose levels closely. Medication dose adjustments may be necessary. Some antidiabetes drugs include glimepiride (Amaryl), glyburide (Diabeta, Glynase PresTab, Micronase), insulin, pioglitazone (Actos), rosiglitazone (Avandia), and others.

CARBAMAZEPINE (Tegretol): Black psyllium can reduce carbamazepine absorption (539).

DIGOXIN (Lanoxin): Concomitant use might reduce digoxin absorption (1), requiring dose adjustment (12).

LITHIUM: Black psyllium use can reduce serum lithium levels (540). The fiber in lithium might decrease the absorption of lithium.

ORAL DRUGS: Oral drugs should be administered one hour before or four hours after black psyllium to avoid decreased or delayed absorption (4,12).

WARFARIN (Coumadin): Concomitant use might reduce warfarin absorption (1), requiring dose adjustment (12).

Interactions with Foods

NUTRIENT ABSORPTION: The long-term use of black psyllium with meals can reduce nutrient absorption requiring vitamin or mineral supplementation (12).

Interactions with Lab Tests

BLOOD GLUCOSE: Theoretically, black psyllium might lower postprandial blood glucose levels and test results (1,6,1405).

SERUM CHOLESTEROL: Black psyllium can lower total cholesterol and LDL cholesterol levels, LDL:HDL ratio, and test results (1,6,1405).

Interactions with Diseases or Conditions

DIABETES: Black psyllium can lower blood glucose levels in people with type 2 diabetes by retarding carbohydrate absorption (1405,8064). Monitor blood glucose levels closely. Doses of conventional antidiabetes medications may require adjustment. Also, warn patients with diabetes that some commercial blond psyllium products can contain added sugars and other absorbable carbohydrates which might increase blood glucose levels.

GI CONDITIONS: Black psyllium is contraindicated in people with fecal impaction, GI atony (1), GI tract narrowing, and obstruction or conditions that can lead to obstruction, such as spastic bowel (1,2,4,12,18).

HYPERSENSITIVITY: Some patients can have severe hypersensitivity reactions to black psyllium. This is more likely to occur in patients with previous occupation exposure to black psyllium (2328,2329,2330,8079,9246). Blond psyllium is contraindicated in these patients.
PHENYLKETONURIA: Avoid products containing aspartame (Nutrasweet) (272).
SWALLOWING DISORDERS: Patients with swallowing disorders might be at greater risk for esophageal obstruction when using blond psyllium. Blond psyllium is contraindicated in these patients (8080,8081).

Dosage and Administration

The amount of black psyllium seed required for an individual can vary. For best results, start with small amounts and increase to the desired response. Follow the package labeling when available.
ORAL: As a laxative, the typical dose of black psyllium seed is 10-30 grams per day (2,18), in divided amounts. Mix 10 grams seed in 100 mL water, to be followed by at least 200 mL water (18). Avoid chewing or crushing the seeds which can release a pigment that deposits in renal tubules (11). Adequate fluid intake is necessary and should be at least 150 mL water for each 5 grams of drug. The FDA labeling recommends at least 8 ounces (a full glass) of water or other fluid with each dose. Taking this product without enough liquid can cause choking (12). Black psyllium should be taken 30-60 minutes after a meal or the administration of other drugs (272).

Comments

Black psyllium is an aggressive-growing, perennial weed found throughout the world. The plant was spread with the colonization of the New World and was nicknamed "Englishman's foot" by the North American Indians.
The FDA requires that psyllium be labeled: "WARNING: Taking this product without adequate fluid may cause it to swell and block your throat or esophagus and may cause choking. Do not take this product if you have difficulty in swallowing. If you experience chest pain, vomiting, or difficulty in swallowing or breathing after taking this product, seek immediate medical attention" (12).

BLACK ROOT

Also Known As

Beaumont Root, Bowman's Root, Culvers, Culveris Root, Culver's Physic, Culver's Root, Hini, Oxadoddy, Physic Root, Purple Leptandra, Tall Speedwell, Tall Veronica, Veronica Virginica Root, Veronicastrum Virginicum, Whorlywort.
CAUTION: See separate listings for Brooklime (Veronica beccabungo), Veronica (Veronica officinalis), Indian Physic, and Comfrey.

Scientific Names

Veronicastrum virginicum, synonyms Leptandra virginica, Veronica virginica.
Family: Scrophulariaceae.

People Use This For

Orally, black root is used for chronic constipation and disorders of the liver and gallbladder. It has also been used as an emetic and to treat bilious fever.

Safety

POSSIBLY SAFE ...when the dried root is used orally (12). The dried root has a milder action than the fresh root (18).
POSSIBLY UNSAFE ...when the fresh root is used orally (12).
PREGNANCY: LIKELY UNSAFE ...when the fresh root is used orally because it has abortifacient and teratogenic effects (19). There is insufficient reliable information available about the safety of the dried root, avoid using.
LACTATION: Insufficient reliable information available; avoid using.

Effectiveness

There is insufficient reliable information available about the effectiveness of black root.

Mechanism of Action

The applicable parts of black root are the rhizome and root. Black root is stated to have antiflatulent, laxative, and bowel evacuant properties (18). It can stimulate bile flow into the duodenum and induce sweating. It contains tannic acid, which has astringent properties that act on the GI mucosa. Tannic acid can also form insoluble complexes with alkaloids, glycosides, and certain heavy metals (6002).

Adverse Reactions

Orally, black root can cause abdominal pain or cramps, changes in stool color or odor, drowsiness, headache, nausea, and vomiting. Hepatotoxicity has been reported after ingestion of large amounts (6002).

Interactions with Herbs & Other Dietary Supplements

POTASSIUM DEPLETING HERBS: Theoretically, concomitant use with horsetail plant or the licorice rhizome can increase the risk of potassium depletion (19).
STIMULANT LAXATIVE HERBS: Theoretically, concomitant use with other stimulant laxative herbs can increase the risk of potassium depletion. Stimulant laxative herbs include aloe dried leaf sap, wild cucumber fruit (Ecballium elaterium), blue flag rhizome, alder buckthorn, European buckthorn, butternut bark, cascara bark, castor oil, colocynth fruit pulp, gamboge bark exudate, jalap root, manna bark exudate, podophyllum root, rhubarb root, senna leaves and pods, and yellow dock root (19).

Interactions with Drugs

DIGOXIN (Lanoxin): Theoretically, the overuse or abuse of black root can increase the risk of adverse effects of cardiac glycoside drugs. Black root chemically binds with the glycosides while in the gastrointestinal (GI) tract, which may reduce their effectiveness if used concomitantly (6002).
DIURETIC DRUGS: Overuse of black root might compound diuretic-induced potassium loss (19).There is some concern that people taking black root along with potassium depleting diuretics might have an increased risk for hypokalemia. Initiation of potassium supplementation or an increase in potassium supplement dose may be necessary for some patients. Some diuretics that can deplete potassium include chlorothiazide (Diuril), chlorthalidone (Thalitone), furosemide (Lasix), hydrochlorothiazide (HCTZ, HydroDIURIL, Microzide), and others.

Interactions with Foods

None known.

Interactions with Lab Tests

None known.

Interactions with Diseases or Conditions

GALLSTONES/BILE DUCT OBSTRUCTION: Black root is contraindicated, because it theoretically has bile stimulatory effects and could aggravate these conditions (19).
GASTROINTESTINAL (GI) INFLAMMATION: Black root is contraindicated in individuals with inflammation of the GI tract due to the irritant, emetic, and stimulant laxative effects (19).
HEMORRHOIDS/ MENSTRUATION: Theoretically, black root is contraindicated due to its cathartic properties (19).

Dosage and Administration

ORAL: People typically use 1 teaspoon of dried black root in 1 cup boiling water, which is allowed to steep for 30 minutes, to make a tea. The suggested dose is 1/3 cup before each meal. A black root tincture is taken as 2 to 4 drops in water. The powdered root bark is taken in a dose of 1 to 4 grams (223,5263).

Comments

Black root grows in the United States and Canada and has a bitter and nauseous taste.

BLACK SEED

Also Known As

Ajenuz, Arañuel, Baraka, Black Cumin, Black Caraway, Charnuska, Cominho Negro, Cominho-Negro, Fennel Flower, Fennel-Flower, Fitch, Kalajaji, Kalajira, Kalonji, Love in a Mist, Mugrela, Nigelle de Crète, Nutmeg Flower, Nutmeg-Flower, Roman-Coriander, Schwarzkümmel, Toute Épice.
CAUTION: See separate listings for Caraway, Coriander, Cumin, Fennel, and Nutmeg.

Scientific Names

Nigella sativa.
Family: Ranunculaceae.

People Use This For

Orally, black seed is used for treating gastrointestinal conditions including gas, colic, diarrhea, dysentery, constipation and hemorrhoids. It is also used orally for respiratory conditions, including asthma, allergies, cough, bronchitis, emphysema, flu and congestion. Additionally, it is used orally as an antihypertensive, immunoprotectant, anticancer agent, and vermifuge. It is used orally for women's health: including as a contraceptive, for stimulation of menstruation, and increasing milk flow.
Topically, black seed is used for inflammatory conditions including rheumatism, headache and skin conditions.
Traditionally, black seed has been used for headache, toothache, nasal congestion, and intestinal worms. It has also

been used for conjunctivitis, abscesses, and parasites.
In combination with cysteine, vitamin E, and saffron, black seed is used to decrease cisplatin-induced side effects.
In foods, black seed is used as a flavoring or spice.

Safety

LIKELY SAFE ...when used orally in amounts found in foods (6).
There is insufficient reliable information available about the safety of black seed for its other uses.
PREGNANCY: LIKELY UNSAFE ...when used orally in amounts exceeding those found in food. Black seed may decrease or inhibit uterine contractions (241) and may have contraceptive activity (242).
LACTATION: Insufficient reliable information available; avoid using.

Effectiveness

There is insufficient reliable information available about the effectiveness of black seed.

Mechanism of Action

In allergic conditions, black seed might have antihistamine effects. Although not yet demonstrated in humans, low concentration of the constituent nigellone has been shown to inhibit the release of histamine from mast cells in animals (233). Black seed is thought to have immunoprotectant effects. Preliminary evidence suggests it may help minimize chemotherapy-induced decreases in hemoglobin and leukocyte counts. It may also enhance the production of certain human interleukins and alter macrophages (234). Black seed is also used as an anticancer agent. According to preliminary studies, black seed may inhibit stomach tumors, carcinoma, and Ehrlich ascites carcinoma (236,239). The black seed constituents thymoquinone and dithymoquinone are actually cytotoxic toward human cells (238). Although some evidence suggests thymoquinone may offer protection against chemically induced hepatotoxicity (237,240), a study in rats indicates that black seed may actually be hepatotoxic. A fixed oil from black seed is reported to have anti-eicosanoid and antioxidant effects, which may support anti-inflammatory activity (235), but this effect has not been studied in humans. The essential oil may have antimicrobial and anthelmintic activity, particularly against staphylococcus as well as other gram-positive and gram-negative bacteria (243,1516). Black seed may have anti-oxytocic potential, and may inhibit spontaneous contractions (241). It may also have contraceptive activity (242).

Adverse Reactions

Topically, black seed oil can cause allergic contact dermatitis (6). Black seed may be associated with hepatotoxicity based on preliminary animal research (245).

Interactions with Herbs & Other Dietary Supplements

None known.

Interactions with Drugs

None known.

Interactions with Foods

None known.

Interactions with Lab Tests

None known.

Interactions with Diseases or Conditions

None known.

Dosage and Administration

No typical dosage.

Comments

Black seed is reported to have been used for over 2000 years. Recordings mention it as far back as 1400 years. Black seed was found in the tomb of King Tutankhamen (6).
An issued patent covers the use of black seed to stimulate immune-competent cells in humans; however, this should not be taken as evidence for the safety and efficacy of black seed as an immunostimulant (246).

BLACK TEA

Also Known As

Black Leaf Tea, English Tea, Tea.
CAUTION: See separate listings for Caffeine and Green Tea.

Scientific Names

Camellia sinensis, synonyms Camellia thea, Camellia theifera, Thea bohea, Thea sinensis, Thea viridis.
Family: Theaceae.

People Use This For

Orally, black tea is used for improving mental alertness, and cognitive performance. It is also used for headache, hypotension, atherosclerosis, and myocardial infarction; preventing Parkinson's disease; and reducing the risk of gastrointestinal cancer, ovarian cancer, and breast cancer. It is also used for stomach disorders, vomiting, diarrhea, preventing dental caries and kidney stones, and as a diuretic. In combination with various other products, black tea is used orally for weight loss.
In foods, black tea is consumed as a hot or cold beverage.

Safety

LIKELY SAFE ...when used orally in moderate amounts (9222,9223,9224,9228,9233,9234,9235,9236).
POSSIBLY UNSAFE ...when used orally long term or in high doses. Black tea contains a significant amount of caffeine. Chronic use, especially in large amounts, can produce tolerance, habituation, psychological dependence, and other significant adverse effects. Doses greater than 250-300 mg per day have been associated with significant adverse effects such as tachyarrhythmias and sleep disturbances (11832).
These effects would not be expected to occur with the consumption of decaffeinated black tea.
LIKELY UNSAFE ...when used orally in very high doses. The fatal acute oral dose of caffeine is estimated to be 10-14 grams (150-200 mg per kilogram). Serious toxicity can occur at lower doses depending on variables in caffeine sensitivity such as smoking, age, prior caffeine use, etc (11832).
CHILDREN: POSSIBLY SAFE ...when used in food and beverage amounts (4912,11833).
PREGNANCY: POSSIBLY SAFE ...when used orally in moderate amounts. Due to the caffeine content of black tea, mothers should closely monitor their intake to ensure moderate consumption. Fetal blood concentrations of caffeine approximate maternal concentrations (4260). Use of caffeine in pregnancy is controversial; however, moderate consumption has not been associated with clinically important adverse fetal effects (2708,2709,2710,2711,9606). Caffeine crosses the human placenta, but is not considered a teratogen. Mothers should keep caffeine consumption below 200 mg per day. This is similar to the amount of caffeine found in 1-2 cups of coffee or tea (2708).
POSSIBLY UNSAFE ...when used orally in large amounts. Caffeine crosses the placenta, producing fetal blood concentrations similar to maternal levels (4260). Mothers should avoid consuming more than 200 mg of caffeine daily or more than 1-2 cups of tea or black tea per day (2708). Maternal doses of greater than 200 mg per day throughout pregnancy have resulted in symptoms of caffeine withdrawal in newborn infants (9891). High doses of caffeine have been associated with spontaneous abortion, premature delivery, and low birth weight (2709,2711). Fetal birth weight is reduced by 28 grams for every 100 mg-per-day of caffeine consumed during pregnancy. But this is unlikely to be clinically important except for women consuming more than 600 mg of caffeine daily (9606).
LACTATION: POSSIBLY SAFE ...when used orally in moderate amounts. Due to the caffeine content of black tea, nursing mothers should closely monitor caffeine intake. Breast milk concentrations of caffeine are thought to be approximately 50% of maternal serum concentrations. Minimal consumption would likely result in limited exposure to a nursing infant (9892). POSSIBLY UNSAFE ...when used orally in large amounts. Consumption of black tea might cause irritability and increased bowel activity in nursing infants (6026). Large doses or excessive intake of black tea should be avoided during lactation.

Effectiveness

LIKELY EFFECTIVE

Mental alertness. Consumption of black tea and other caffeinated beverages seems to prevent a decline in alertness and cognitive capacity when consumed throughout the day (4221,4224).Caffeine can improve mental performance and alertness following prolonged sleep deprivation (10205). Combining caffeine with taurine seems to provide a small improvement in mental performance (9899).

POSSIBLY EFFECTIVE

Atherosclerosis. Epidemiological evidence shows that black tea consumption seems to reduce the risk of severe aortic atherosclerosis, especially in women (3450).

Hypotension. Consuming caffeinated beverages seems to increase blood pressure in elderly people with postprandial hypotension (11834,11835).

Kidney stones (nephrolithiasis). Women consuming black tea seem to have an 8% decreased risk of developing kidney stones (4216).

Myocardial infarction (MI). There is some evidence that people who consume black tea have a lower risk of MI (4222,8119,8121). Consuming black tea for at least one year before a heart attack also seems to reduce the risk of subsequent death (8120).

Parkinson's disease. There is some evidence from large-scale epidemiological studies that people who consume caffeinated beverages such as coffee, tea, and cola have a decreased risk of Parkinson's disease. For men, the effects seem to be dose related. For example, men consuming a total of 421-2716 mg of caffeine from any source daily seem to have the greatest reduction in risk. However, there seems to be a significant reduction in risk even with consumption of as little as 124-208 mg caffeine per day (6022). In women, the effects do not seem to be dose related. Moderate consumption of caffeine (equivalent to one to four cups black tea daily) seems to provide the most reduction in risk (1238). Drinking black tea appears to reduce the incidence of Parkinson's disease among people who smoke (9236).

POSSIBLY INEFFECTIVE

Breast cancer. People who drink black tea do not seem to have a lower risk of breast cancer (9235).

Gastrointestinal cancer. People who drink black tea do not seem to have a lower risk of colon cancer, stomach cancer, or rectal cancer (9222,9223,9224,9233,9234).

Ovarian cancer. People who drink black tea do not seem to have a lower risk of ovarian cancer (9228).

INSUFFICIENT RELIABLE EVIDENCE to RATE

Osteoporosis. There is some preliminary evidence that black tea might be beneficial for preventing osteoporosis by improving bone mineral density (6404). More evidence is needed to rate black tea for this use.

Mechanism of Action

The applicable parts of black tea are the leaf and stem. Black tea is different than green and oolong teas. Black tea is fully fermented tea. Oolong tea is partially fermented. Green tea is not fermented.

Polyphenols such as flavonoids including catechins, thearubigins, and theaflavins are abundant in black tea, and are thought to be responsible for many of its proposed benefits as an antioxidant (6032,6033,9232). Black tea contains 2% to 4% caffeine (519). Black tea also contains significant amounts of gallic acid, an antioxidant with antimutagenic and anticarcinogenic activities (8123).

It's often thought that green tea has more polyphenols, and therefore greater potential health benefits, than black tea. But there is some evidence that suggests there is no difference in quantity and quality of polyphenols between green and black teas (12087).

Theaflavins are effective antioxidants, which may be beneficial for preventing atherosclerosis and cardiovascular disease (9232). Consumption of a theaflavin-enriched green tea extract has been shown to produce mild reductions in low-density lipoprotein (LDL) levels (11308). In addition, a single dose of black tea can increase the concentration of antioxidants in serum (6032,6033). However, drinking black tea on a regular basis does not appear to significantly reduce lipoprotein oxidation (9230,9231). Preliminary evidence suggests that consumption of four cups of black tea might restore blood vessel dilation to near-normal in people with heart disease. Constituents other than caffeine are thought to be responsible for this effect. Acute or chronic consumption of black tea does not seem to inhibit platelet aggregation in people with coronary heart disease and is unlikely to be responsible for the reported beneficial effect of black tea on heart disease (8905). Earlier conflicting evidence had suggested that an inhibitory effect on platelets resulted from a higher concentration of flavonoids than is attainable with oral intake (8028,8029).

Black tea might also have a negative effect on a cardiac risk factor. There is evidence suggesting that black tea increases homocysteine levels, possibly due to the high concentration of polyphenols in tea (8035). It is unknown whether this effect decreases any of the benefits black tea may have in reducing cardiovascular disease.

Caffeine, a constituent of black tea, has been reported to cause increases and decreases in blood glucose. In people with type 2 diabetes, acute administration of caffeine impairs postprandial glucose metabolism, while acute abstention from caffeine reduces postprandial glucose levels by 21%. Whether these effects also occur with caffeinated beverages and herbs is unknown (12374). Other research in obese people suggests that caffeine ingestion may contribute to insulin resistance (12375). However, one study found that type 1 diabetics taking 200 mg of caffeine twice daily had increased frequency and intensity of warning signs of hypoglycemia. This may be due to a reduction in blood flow to the brain and an increase in glucose utilization by the brain (6024).

For osteoporosis, the mechanism is not known, but it is thought that isoflavonoids in black tea have weak estrogenic effects that might be beneficial for postmenopausal women with low endogenous estrogen levels (6404). Tea consumption seems to raise prolactin levels in women (an indicator of estrogen activity) in a dose-dependent manner (8122).

The caffeine in black tea stimulates the central nervous system (CNS), heart, muscles, and possibly the pressor centers that control blood pressure (2722). Possible mechanisms include adenosine receptor blockade and phosphodiesterase inhibition (2722). By blocking adenosine receptors, caffeine is thought to increase the release of neurotransmitters such as dopamine (6370). Caffeine also decreases airway resistance and stimulates respiration, via adenosine receptor blockade and phosphodiesterase inhibition (11836). It has also been proposed that caffeine may decrease GABA and serotonin signaling (6370). Caffeine stimulates gastric acid secretion, and increases plasma catecholamine levels (11837). Caffeine can have positive inotropic and chronotropic effects on the heart (11836). Caffeine can also acutely elevate both diastolic and systolic blood pressure, but might not have this effect in habitual users (2722).

Caffeine exerts a diuretic effect, with water losses estimated at 1.17 mL per milligram of caffeine (2712). Tachyphylaxis to the diuretic effect develops rapidly, diminishing fluid losses associated with caffeine intake (10206).

Caffeine-containing beverages consumed during moderate endurance exercise do not appear to compromise bodily hydration status (2713). Caffeine does not substantially affect the fluid status of people who drink caffeinated beverages on a regular basis (10206). The caffeine content is also thought to be responsible for black tea's effects on cognitive performance (4221,4224).

For prevention of Parkinson's disease, caffeine in black tea may prevent adenosine's inhibition of dopaminergic transmission. This may result in a reduction in the clinical expression of Parkinsonism (6022).

Adverse Reactions

Orally, black tea, due to its caffeine content, can cause insomnia, nervousness, restlessness, gastric irritation, nausea, vomiting, tachycardia, quickened respiration, tremors, delirium, convulsions, and diuresis. Large doses can produce headache, anxiety, agitation, ringing in the ears, premature heartbeat, and arrhythmia (11832,11838).

In fatal overdose, the cause of death is usually ventricular fibrillation (11838). In infants, black tea can cause microcytic anemia (631). The caffeine in black tea may exacerbate sleep disturbances in patients with acquired immunodeficiency syndrome (AIDS) (10204).

Although acute administration of black tea can cause increased blood pressure, regular consumption does not seem to increase either blood pressure or pulse, even in mildly hypertensive patients (1451,1452,2722).

Tolerance to caffeine is a widely held belief, but there is little supportive clinical evidence. If it exists, it appears to be of little clinical significance (11839). Withdrawal symptoms such as irritability, sleepiness, delirium, nausea, vomiting, rhinorrhea, nervousness, restlessness, anxiety, muscle tension, muscle pains, and flushed face have been described. However, these symptoms may be from nonpharmacological factors related to knowledge and expectation of effects. Clinically significant symptoms caused by caffeine withdrawal may be uncommon (2723,11839).

Some evidence shows caffeine is associated with fibrocystic breast disease, breast cancer, and endometriosis in women; however, this is controversial since findings are conflicting (8043). Restricting caffeine in women with fibrocystic breast conditions doesn't seem to affect breast nodularity, swelling, or pain (8996).

There is evidence that daily consumption of strong black tea (2 liters) or black tea solids (4 grams) can raise plasma homocysteine levels; however it is unclear if lower doses have this effect (8035). There is also some evidence consumption of black tea (greater than 1 cup per day) may increase the risk of colon cancer (8041).

Epidemiological evidence regarding the relationship between use of caffeine, a constituent of black tea, and the risk for osteoporosis is contradictory. Caffeine can increase urinary excretion of calcium (2669,10202,11317). Women identified with a genetic variant of the vitamin D receptor appear to be at an increased risk for the detrimental effect of caffeine on bone mass (2669). However, moderate caffeine intake, less than 300 mg per day, does not seem to significantly increase osteoporosis risk in most postmenopausal women with normal calcium intake (2669,6025,10202,11317).

Combining ephedra with caffeine or caffeinated beverages can increase the risk of adverse effects. Jitteriness, hypertension, seizures, temporary loss of consciousness, and hospitalization requiring life support have been associated with the combined use of ephedra and caffeine (2729). There is also a report of ischemic stroke in an athlete who consumed ephedra 40-60 mg, creatine monohydrate 6 grams, caffeine 400-600 mg, and a variety of other supplements daily for six weeks (1275).

The caffeine in black tea can cause anaphylaxis in sensitive individuals, although true IgE-mediated caffeine allergy seems to be relatively rare (11315).

Interactions with Herbs & Other Dietary Supplements

CAFFEINE-CONTAINING HERBS/SUPPLEMENTS: Concomitant use can increase caffeine therapeutic and adverse effects. Natural products that contain caffeine include coffee, tea (black or green), guarana, mate, and cola.

CALCIUM: High caffeine intake from foods and beverages including black tea increases urinary calcium excretion (2570).

CREATINE: There is some concern that combining caffeine, a constituent of black tea, with ephedra, and creatine might increase the risk of serious adverse effects. There is a report of ischemic stroke in an athlete who consumed creatine monohydrate 6 grams, caffeine 400-600 mg, ephedra 40-60 mg, and a variety of other supplements daily for 6 weeks (1275). Caffeine might also decrease creatine's possible beneficial effects on athletic performance. Some researchers think caffeine can inhibit phosphocreatine resynthesis (2117,4575).

EPHEDRA (ma huang): Use of ephedra with black tea can increase the risk of stimulatory adverse effects due to its caffeine content. There is evidence that using ephedra with caffeine might increase the risk of serious life-threatening or debilitating adverse effects such as hypertension, myocardial infarction, stroke, seizures, and death (6486,10307). Tell patients to avoid taking black tea with ephedra and other stimulants.

IRON: Black tea appears to reduce absorption of non-heme iron from foods (8904). Infants given tea to drink have an increased risk of microcytic anemia (631). Theoretically, black tea might reduce the absorption of iron supplements. For most patients, this effect will not be clinically significant. Advise patients with iron deficiency to consume tea between meals rather than with meals to lessen this interaction (8904).

MAGNESIUM: Consuming large amounts of black tea can increase excretion of magnesium (11939).

Interactions with Drugs

ADENOSINE (Adenocard): The caffeine in black tea is a competitive inhibitor of adenosine at the cellular level. However, caffeine doesn't seem to affect supplemental adenosine because high interstitial levels of adenosine overcome the antagonistic effects of caffeine (11771). It is recommended that methylxanthines and methylxanthine-containing products be stopped 24 hours prior to pharmacological stress tests (11770). However, methylxanthines appear more likely to interfere with dipyridamole (Persantine) than adenosine-induced stress testing (11771).

ALCOHOL (Ethanol): Concomitant use of alcohol can increase caffeine serum concentrations and the risk of caffeine adverse effects. Alcohol reduces caffeine metabolism (6370).

ANTICOAGULANT/ANTIPLATELET DRUGS: Theoretically, the caffeine in black tea might increase the risk of bleeding when used concomitantly with these agents. Caffeine is reported to have antiplatelet activity (8028,8029); however, this interaction has not been reported in humans. Antiplatelet agents include aspirin, clopidogrel (Plavix), dipyridamole (Persantine), ticlopidine (Ticlid), and others. Anticoagulant agents include heparin and warfarin (Coumadin).

ANTIDIABETES DRUGS: Theoretically, concomitant use of caffeine, because of its caffeine content, and diabetes drugs might interfere with blood glucose control. Data are conflicting. Reports claim that caffeine might increase or decrease blood sugar (6024,8646).

CIMETIDINE (Tagamet): Cimetidine interacts with the caffeine in black tea and decreases caffeine clearance by 31-42% (11736).

CLOZAPINE (Clozaril): The caffeine in black tea might interact with clozapine and cause acute exacerbation of psychotic symptoms. Caffeine can increase effects and toxicity of clozapine. Caffeine doses of 400-1000 mg per day inhibit clozapine metabolism (5051).

CONTRACEPTIVE DRUGS: Theoretically, concomitant use might increase caffeine concentrations and the risk adverse effects, due to the caffeine contained in black tea. Contraceptive drugs decrease the rate of caffeine clearance by 40-65% (2714,11737).

DIPYRIDAMOLE (Persantine): The caffeine in black tea might inhibit dipyridamole-induced vasodilation (11770,11772). It is recommended that methylxanthines and methylxanthine-containing products be stopped 24 hours prior to pharmacological stress tests (11770). Methylxanthines appear more likely to interfere with dipyridamole (Persantine) than adenosine-induced stress testing (11771).

DISULFIRAM (Antabuse): Concomitant use can decrease clearance and increase the half-life of caffeine, increasing effects and risk of adverse effects (11840).

EPHEDRINE: Use of ephedrine with caffeine-containing products can increase the risk of stimulatory adverse effects. There is evidence that using ephedrine with caffeine might increase the risk of serious life-threatening or debilitating adverse effects such as hypertension, myocardial infarction, stroke, seizures, and death (6486,10307). Tell patients to avoid taking caffeine with ephedrine and other stimulants.

ESTROGENS: Concomitant use can increase serum concentrations of caffeine, a constituent of black tea, and the risk of caffeine adverse effects. Estrogen inhibits caffeine metabolism (2714).

FLUCONAZOLE (Diflucan): Concomitant use might increase the effects of caffeine in black tea. Fluconazole decreases caffeine clearance by approximately 25% (11022).

FLUVOXAMINE (Luvox): Concomitant use can increase serum concentrations of caffeine, a constituent of black tea, and the risk of caffeine adverse effects. Fluvoxamine reduces caffeine metabolism (6370).

LITHIUM: Abrupt withdrawal of the caffeine in black tea can increase serum lithium levels (609), worsening lithium tremor (610).

MEXILETINE (Mexitil): Concomitant use might increase the effects and adverse effects of caffeine in black tea. Mexiletine can decrease caffeine elimination by 50% (1260,11741).

MONOAMINE OXIDASE INHIBITORS (MAOIs): Theoretically, concomitant intake of large amounts of black tea with MAOIs might precipitate a hypertensive crisis, due to the caffeine contained in black tea. This is based on the claim that intake of large amounts of caffeine with MAOIs might precipitate a hypertensive crisis (15).

PHENOTHIAZINES: The tannins in black tea might cause precipitation of solutions of fluphenazine (Permitil, Prolixin), chlorpromazine (Thorazine), haloperidol (Haldol), prochlorperazine (Compazine), thioridazine (Mellaril), and trifluoperazine (Stelazine) (626,627).

PHENYLPROPANOLAMINE: Concomitant use of phenylpropanolamine and black tea might cause an additive increase in blood pressure due to the caffeine in black tea (11738).

QUINOLONE ANTIBIOTICS: Concomitant use can decrease caffeine clearance and increase effects and risk of adverse effects (606,607,608). Quinolones include ciprofloxacin (Cipro), enoxacin (Penetrex), norfloxacin (Chibroxin, Noroxin), sparfloxacin (Zagam), trovafloxacin (Trovan), and grepafloxacin (Raxar).

RILUZOLE (Rilutek): Theoretically, concomitant use of riluzole and caffeinated beverages such as black tea might increase serum caffeine and riluzole concentrations and the risk of adverse effects of both caffeine and riluzole. Caffeine and riluzole are both metabolized by cytochrome P450 1A2, and concomitant use might reduce metabolism of one or both agents (11739).

STIMULANT DRUGS: Due to the CNS stimulant effects of the caffeine constituent of black tea, concomitant use can increase the risk of adverse effects (11832). Some stimulant drugs include diethylpropion (Tenuate), epinephrine, phentermine (Ionamin), pseudoephedrine (Sudafed), and many others.

TERBINAFINE (Lamisil): Theoretically, concomitant use of terbinafine and caffeinated beverages such as black tea might increase serum caffeine concentrations and the risk of adverse effects. Terbinafine decreases the rate of caffeine clearance (11740).

THEOPHYLLINE: The caffeine in black tea can increase theophylline levels (11862).

TRICYCLIC ANTIDEPRESSANTS (TCAs): The tannins in black tea might cause precipitation of solutions of

amitriptyline (Elavil) or imipramine (Tofranil, Janimine) (626,627).
VERAPAMIL (Calan, Covera, Isoptin, Verelan): Theoretically, concomitant use of verapamil and caffeinated beverages such as black tea might increase plasma caffeine concentrations and the risk of adverse effects. Verapamil increases plasma caffeine concentrations by 25% (11741).

Interactions with Foods

IRON: Black tea may interfere with the absorption of iron in the diet. People who are iron-deficient should not drink black tea. Black tea doesn't seem to affect iron status in people with normal iron stores (631,9237).
MILK: When taken together, milk might bind the antioxidants in black tea and reduce their beneficial effects (220); however, in one study this interaction did not occur (6032).

Interactions with Lab Tests

5-HYDROXYINDOLEACETIC ACID: Black tea might increase urine 5-hydroxyindoleacetic acid concentrations and test results, due to its caffeine content. Caffeine can increase urine catecholamine concentrations (15).
BLEEDING TIME: Theoretically, black tea might increase bleeding time. Caffeine is reported to have antiplatelet activity (8028,8029). However, the significance of these effects in humans is not known.
CATECHOLAMINE: Caffeine can increase plasma catecholamine levels (8646).
CREATINE: The caffeine in black tea can increase urine creatine levels (1701).
DIPYRIDAMOLE THALLIUM IMAGING: Black tea might interfere with dipyridamole thallium imaging studies, due to its caffeine content. Caffeine attenuates the characteristic cardiovascular responses to dipyridamole and has altered test results (11742).
FERRITIN: Drinking black tea may cause a reduction in serum ferritin in iron-deficient people (631,9237).
GLUCOSE: Caffeine, a constituent of black tea, has been reported to cause increases and decreases in blood glucose (8646).
HEMOGLOBIN: Drinking black tea may cause a reduction in hemoglobin in iron-deficient people (631,9237).
IRON: In people with iron deficiency, black tea may further reduce the concentration of serum iron (631,9237).
LACTATE: The combination of ephedrine, a constituent of ephedra, and caffeine, a constituent of black tea, can increase blood lactate levels (8646).
NEUROBLASTOMA TESTS: Black tea (due to its caffeine content) might cause false-positive diagnosis of neuroblastoma, when diagnosis is based on tests of urine vanillylmandelic acid (VMA) or catecholamine concentrations. Caffeine can increase urine catecholamine and VMA concentrations (15).
PHARMACOLOGICAL STRESS TESTS: The caffeine in black tea is a competitive antagonist for adenosine receptors (11771). It is recommended that caffeine and caffeine-containing products be stopped 24 hours prior to pharmacological stress tests (11770). However, caffeine appears more likely to interfere with dipyridamole (Persantine) than adenosine (Adenocard) stress testing (11771). The interaction between caffeine and dipyridamole is unlikely to be significant in stress testing if the heart rate increase is greater than 5% after dipyridamole infusion (11772).
PHEOCHROMOCYTOMA TESTS: Black tea (due to its caffeine content) might cause false-positive diagnosis of pheochromocytoma, when diagnosis is based on tests of urine vanillylmandelic acid (VMA) or catecholamine concentrations. Caffeine can increase urine catecholamine and VMA concentrations (15).
PULMONARY FUNCTION TESTS: People may need to avoid caffeine and caffeinated beverages such as black tea for at least four hours prior to lung function testing. Forced expiratory volume in one minute (FEV1) seems to show a small improvement up to two hours after caffeine use. Mid-expiratory flow rates may also improve with caffeine for up to four hours (9607).
URATE: Black tea might falsely increase serum urate test results determined by the Bittner method, due to its caffeine content. Caffeine causes false elevations in serum urate test results determined by the Bittner method (11844).
URINARY CALCIUM: Caffeine, a constituent of black tea, can increase urinary calcium levels (11317).
VANILLYLMANDELIC ACID (VMA): Black tea might increase urine VMA concentrations and test results, due to its caffeine content. Caffeine can increase urine VMA concentrations (15).

Interactions with Diseases or Conditions

ANEMIA: Drinking black tea may worsen anemia in people with iron deficiency (631,9237).
ANXIETY DISORDERS: The caffeine in black tea might aggravate anxiety disorders (11743).
BLEEDING DISORDERS: Theoretically, caffeine in black tea might aggravate these conditions. Caffeine is reported to have antiplatelet activity (8028,8029); however, this interaction has not been reported in humans. Caffeine can prolong bleeding time and increase the results of a bleeding time test (1701).
CARDIAC CONDITIONS: Caffeine in black tea can induce cardiac arrhythmias in sensitive individuals (11845); use with caution.
DIABETES: Some research suggests that caffeine (a constituent of black tea) may impair postprandial glucose metabolism in people with diabetes and contribute to insulin resistance. The effect of caffeinated beverages such as black tea and herbs has not been studied (12374,12375). Caffeine in black tea may enhance the frequency and intensity of hypoglycemic warning symptoms in type 1 diabetics. This may increase the ability of diabetics to detect and treat hypoglycemia early. However, it might also increase the frequency of hypoglycemic events (6024); use with caution. Caffeine has been reported to cause increases and decreases in blood glucose (8646); use with caution.

GLAUCOMA: Drinking caffeinated black tea increases intraocular pressure. The increase occurs within 30 minutes and persists for at least 90 minutes (8540).
HORMONE-SENSITIVE CANCERS/CONDITIONS: Because black tea might have weak estrogenic effects (6404), women with hormone-sensitive conditions should avoid high doses of black tea. Some of these conditions include breast, uterine, and ovarian cancer, and endometriosis and uterine fibroids.
HYPERTENSION: The caffeine in black tea might increase blood pressure in people with high blood pressure. However, this doesn't seem to occur in people who consume black tea or other caffeinated products regularly (1451,1452,2722).
OSTEOPOROSIS: Consuming caffeinated black tea can increase urinary excretion of calcium. Caffeine consumption should be limited to less than 300 mg per day (approximately 2-3 cups of black tea). Adequate calcium supplementation may partially compensate for calcium losses (2669,10202,11317). Postmenopausal women identified with a genetic variant of the vitamin D receptor should use caffeine with caution (2669).

Dosage and Administration

ORAL: A typical dose as a stimulant is several cups per day. The typical dose of caffeine for headache or restoring mental alertness is up to 250 mg per day (2718,11743). For reducing the risk of heart attack and kidney stones, a dose of at least one cup per day has been used (4216,4222,4224). For preventing atherosclerosis, consumption of 125-500 mL (1-4 cups) of brewed black tea daily has been used (3450). For preventing Parkinson's disease, men consuming 421-2716 mg total caffeine (approximately 5-33 cups of black tea) daily have the lowest risk of developing Parkinson's disease. However, a significantly lower risk is also associated with consumption of as little as 124-208 mg of caffeine (approximately 1-3 cups of black tea) daily (6022). In women, more moderate caffeine consumption seems to be best; equivalent to approximately 1-4 cups of black tea per day (1238).

Comments

Camellia sinensis leaves and stems are used to manufacture green tea (non-fermented), oolong tea (partially fermented), and black tea (fermented) (4218). Black tea is the more frequently ingested variety. Leaves used for green tea are prepared immediately after harvest, which limits enzymatic changes. Leaves used for black tea are fermented before preparation, promoting enzymatic changes. Consequently, black tea and green tea have different chemical constituents (8115).

BLACK WALNUT

Also Known As

Nogal Americano, Nogueira-preta, Noyer Noir, Schwarze Walnuss.
CAUTION: See separate listing for English Walnut hull and English Walnut leaf.

Scientific Names

Juglans nigra.
Family: Juglandaceae.

People Use This For

Orally, black walnut is used for diphtheria, leukemia, syphilis, and as an anthelmintic.
Topically, black walnut is used as a gargle, hair dye, insecticide, and for wounds.

Safety

POSSIBLY SAFE ...when used orally and appropriately, short-term (12).
POSSIBLY UNSAFE ...when used topically because it contains the constituent juglone (2). Daily use of the juglone-containing bark of a related species (English walnut) is associated with increased risk of tongue cancer and lip leukoplakia (2,12).
PREGNANCY AND LACTATION: POSSIBLY UNSAFE ...when used topically (12); avoid using. There is insufficient reliable information about the safety of the oral use of black walnut during pregnancy or lactation; avoid using.

Effectiveness

There is insufficient reliable information available about the effectiveness of black walnut.

Mechanism of Action

The applicable part of black walnut is the hull. Black walnut hulls contain approximately 45% tannins (19) which exert an astringent effect on the mucosal tissue. Tannins work internally by dehydrating mucosal tissue, which reduces secretions.
Externally, tannin astringent effects result in a protective layer of constricted, harder cells. Plants with at least 10% tannins can cause gastrointestinal upset, kidney damage, and liver damage. Animal data conflicts

with respect to the carcinogenicity of tannins. They may be carcinogenic or may even have anti-carcinogenic effects. An increased risk of esophageal or nasal cancer may be linked with people who regularly ingest herbs with high tannin concentrations (12).

Adverse Reactions
None reported.

Interactions with Herbs & Other Dietary Supplements
TANNIN-CONTAINING HERBS: Theoretically, herbs such as black walnut contain high percentages of tannins, which might cause precipitation of constituents of other herbs (19).

Interactions with Drugs
ORAL DRUGS: Theoretically, concomitant oral administration might cause precipitation of some drugs due to the high tannin content of black walnut hulls (19). Separate administration of oral drugs and tannin-containing herbs by the longest period of time practical (19).

Interactions with Foods
None known.

Interactions with Lab Tests
None known.

Interactions with Diseases or Conditions
None known.

Dosage and Administration
No typical dosage.

BLACKBERRY

Also Known As
Black Berry, Bramble, Dewberry, Goutberry, Rubi Fruticosi Folium, Rubi Fruticosi Radix, Thimbleberry.
CAUTION: See separate listing for Raspberry.

Scientific Names
Rubus plicatus, synonyms Rubus fruticosus, Rubus affinis.
Family: Rosaceae.

People Use This For
Orally, blackberry is used diarrhea and edema.
Topically, blackberry is used as a mouth rinse for mild inflammation of the mucosa of the oral cavity and throat.

Safety
POSSIBLY SAFE ...when used orally, short-term (12).
There is insufficient reliable information available about the safety blackberry for its other uses.
PREGNANCY AND LACTATION: Insufficient reliable information available; avoid using.

Effectiveness
There is insufficient reliable information available about the effectiveness of blackberry.

Mechanism of Action
The applicable part s of blackberry are the leaf and root. Tannin constituents in the leaf have an astringent effect and are thought to help relieve mucosal inflammation and diarrhea (12).

Adverse Reactions
None reported.

Interactions with Herbs & Other Dietary Supplements
None known.

Interactions with Drugs
None known.

Interactions with Foods
None known.

Interactions with Lab Tests
None known

Interactions with Diseases or Conditions
None known.

Dosage and Administration
No typical dosage.

BLACKTHORN berry

Also Known As
Blackthorn Fruit, Pruni Spinosae Fructus, Sloe, Sloe Berry.
CAUTION: See separate listing for Blackthorn flower.

Scientific Names
Prunus spinosa.
Family: Rosaceae.

People Use This For
Orally, the syrup and wine of the blackthorn berry are used for purging the bowels and as a diuretic. The berry marmalade is used for dyspepsia.
Topically, blackthorn berry is used as a mouth rinse (gargle) for mild inflammation of the oral and pharyngeal mucosa.

Safety
LIKELY SAFE ...when used topically and appropriately as a mouth rinse, short-term (2,12).
POSSIBLY UNSAFE ...when used orally; not recommended for long-term use (12).
PREGNANCY AND LACTATION: Insufficient reliable information available; avoid using.

Effectiveness
There is insufficient reliable information available about the effectiveness of blackthorn berry.

Mechanism of Action
The astringent properties of the tannin constituents can contribute to the reduction of mucous membrane inflammation (2,7).

Adverse Reactions
None reported.

Interactions with Herbs & Other Dietary Supplements
None known.

Interactions with Drugs
None known.

Interactions with Foods
None known.

Interactions with Lab Tests
None known.

Interactions with Diseases or Conditions
None known.

Dosage and Administration
ORAL: The blackthorn berry is typically used as a mouth rinse up to two times per day. The rinse is obtained from the tea, which is prepared by steeping 1-2 grams in 150 mL boiling water for 10-15 minutes and then straining (2,12).

BLACKTHORN flower

Also Known As
Pruni Spinosae Llos, Sloe Flower, Wild Plum Flower.
CAUTION: See separate listing for Blackthorn berry.

Scientific Names
Prunus spinosa.
Family: Rosaceae.

People Use This For
Orally, blackthorn flower is used for common colds, ailments of the respiratory tract, bloating, general exhaustion, dyspepsia, kidney and bladder ailments, and to treat and prevent gastric spasms. The blackthorn flower is also used orally as a laxative, diuretic, diaphoretic, expectorant, and as a component in "blood cleansing" teas.
Topically, blackthorn flower is used for rashes, skin impurities, and "blood purification."
In foods, blackthorn flower is utilized in herbal teas as a coloring agent.

Safety
POSSIBLY UNSAFE ...when used orally. Contains cyanogenic glycosides that could be toxic (12).
LIKELY UNSAFE ...when used orally long-term or in excessive amounts (12).
There is insufficient reliable information available about the safety of blackthorn flower for its other uses.
PREGNANCY AND LACTATION: LIKELY UNSAFE ...when used orally; avoid using. Blackthorn flower contains cyanogenic glycosides that can be teratogenic (12).

Effectiveness
There is insufficient reliable information available about the effectiveness of blackthorn flower.

Mechanism of Action
There is insufficient reliable information available about the possible mechanism of action and active ingredients.

Adverse Reactions
None reported.

Interactions with Herbs & Other Dietary Supplements
None known.

Interactions with Drugs
None known.

Interactions with Foods
None known.

Interactions with Lab Tests
None known.

Interactions with Diseases or Conditions
None known.

Dosage and Administration
ORAL: Blackthorn flower is usually taken as a tea, 1-2 cups during the day or 2 cups in the evening. The tea is prepared by steeping 1-2 heaping teaspoons (1-2 grams) in 150 mL boiling water for 5-10 minutes and then straining (18). Blackthorn is for short-term use only (12).

Comments
Blackthorn can be stored for up to one year away from light and moisture (18).

BLADDERWORT

Also Known As
None.
CAUTION: See separate listing for Bladderwrack.

Scientific Names
Utricularia vulgaris.
Family: Lentibulariaceae.

People Use This For
Orally, bladderwort is used for urinary tract disorders including kidney stones and urinary tract infections (UTIs). It is also used orally for weight loss, as a diuretic, antispasmodic, anti-inflammatory, and to stimulate gall bladder secretions.
Topically, bladderwort is used for burns and skin and mucous membrane inflammation.

Safety
There is insufficient reliable information available about the safety of bladderwort.
Pregnancy and Lactation: Insufficient reliable information available; avoid using.

Effectiveness
There is insufficient reliable information available about the effectiveness of bladderwort.

Mechanism of Action
There is insufficient reliable information available about the possible mechanism of action and active ingredients.

Adverse Reactions
None reported.

Interactions with Herbs & Other Dietary Supplements
None known.

Interactions with Drugs
None known.

Interactions with Foods
None known.

Interactions with Lab Tests
None known.

Interactions with Diseases or Conditions
None known.

Dosage and Administration
ORAL: As a diuretic, two cups are taken daily. The tea is prepared by steeping 2 grams dried leaf in 100 mL of boiling water for 10-15 minutes and then straining.
TOPICAL: As an anti-inflammatory, a tea is used in mouthwashes, cleansers, cosmetic, and medical packs. The tea is prepared by steeping 6 grams dried leaf in 100 mL of boiling water for 10-15 minutes and then straining (18).

Comments
Bladderwort use is nearly obsolete in Germany. It continues to be used in other countries (18).

BLADDERWRACK

Also Known As

Black Tang, Bladder Fucus, Bladder Wrack, Blasentang, Cutweed, Fucus, Kelp, Kelp-Ware, Kelpware, Knotted Wrack, Meereiche, Quercus Marina, Rockweed, Rockwrack, Schweintang, Seawrack, Tang, Varech.
CAUTION: See separate listings for Algin, Bladderwort, and Laminaria.

Scientific Names

Fucus vesiculosus; Ascophyllum nodosum; other Fucus species.
Family: Fucaceae.

People Use This For

Orally, bladderwrack is used for thyroid disorders, iodine deficiency, lymphadenoid goiter, myxedema, obesity, arthritis, and rheumatism. Bladderwrack is also used orally for arteriosclerosis, digestive disorders, "blood cleansing," constipation, bronchitis, emphysema, genitourinary disorders, decreased resistance to disease, and anxiety.
Topically, bladderwrack is used for skin diseases, burns, and insect bites.

Safety

POSSIBLY UNSAFE ...when used orally; one gram of bladderwrack might contain as much as 600 mcg iodine (12). Ingesting more than 150 mcg iodine per day can cause hyperthyroidism or exacerbate existing hyperthyroidism (2). Heavy metal poisoning has also been reported (645).
PREGNANCY AND LACTATION: LIKELY UNSAFE ...when used orally (4,12); avoid using.

Effectiveness

There is insufficient reliable information available about the effectiveness of bladderwrack.

Mechanism of Action

Iodine is an essential substrate for thyroid hormone, in bladderwrack concentrations vary from 0.03-1.0% (18). The constituent algin (sodium alginate) has bulk laxative and demulcent (soothing) effects (4,5). The isolated fraction, fucoidin, has 40-50% of the blood anticoagulant activity of heparin (4). Bladderwrack can concentrate heavy metals (4).

Adverse Reactions

Orally, bladderwrack can induce or exacerbate hyperthyroidism (2,12) and acne (4). Prolonged ingestion can reduce iron absorption (4). High sodium content can adversely affect individuals with restricted sodium intake (5). Iodine can cause idiosyncratic or allergic reactions (2,18). There is one case report of heavy metal poisoning where arsenic poisoning occurred with ingestions of a contaminated kelp product (645).

Interactions with Herbs & Other Dietary Supplements

IRON: Prolonged ingestion of bladderwrack can reduce iron absorption (4).

Interactions with Drugs

ANTICOAGULANT/ANTIPLATELET DRUGS: Theoretically, concomitant use might increase bleeding risk (4).
DIURETIC DRUGS: Bladderwrack can decrease the effectiveness of diuretics due to high sodium content (5).
LITHIUM: Theoretically, concomitant use might enhance hypothyroid activity due to high iodine content in bladderwrack (19).
THYROID HORMONE: The high iodine content of bladderwrack might interfere with thyroid hormone replacement therapy (4).

Interactions with Foods

IRON: Prolonged ingestion of bladderwrack can reduce iron absorption (4).

Interactions with Lab Tests

ACTIVATED PARTIAL THROMBOPLASTIN TIME (aPTT): Theoretically, bladderwrack might increase aPTT test results due to the heparin-like activity of one of its constituents (4).
RADIOACTIVE IODINE UPTAKE: Theoretically, bladderwrack might interfere with the results of thyroid function tests using radioactive iodine uptake (15).
THYROID STIMULATING HORMONE (TSH): Theoretically, bladderwrack might increase serum TSH levels and test results (1701).
THYROXINE (T4): Theoretically, bladderwrack might increase serum T4 levels and test results (1701).

Interactions with Diseases or Conditions
ACNE: Bladderwrack can exacerbate acne (4).
CONDITIONS REQUIRING SODIUM RESTRICTION: The high sodium content can exacerbate these conditions (5).
HYPERTHYROIDISM: Bladderwrack can exacerbate hyperthyroidism (2,12).
IODINE ALLERGY: Avoid bladderwrack use in people sensitive to iodine (2,18).
IRON DEFICIENCY: Bladderwrack can exacerbate iron deficiency by reducing absorption (4).

Dosage and Administration
ORAL: The usual dose is 5-10 grams of the plant or as a tea three times a day. The tea is prepared by steeping the herb in 150 mL boiling water for 5-10 minutes and then straining (4). The typical dose of the liquid extract (1:1) is 4-8 mL three times a day. Bladderwrack can contain over 600 mcg iodine per gram seaweed (12).

Comments
Avoid confusion with bladderwort.

BLESSED THISTLE

Also Known As
Carbenia Benedicta, Cardo Santo, Carduus, Carduus Benedictus, Cnici Benedicti Herba, Cnicus, Holy Thistle, St. Benedict Thistle, Spotted Thistle.
CAUTION: See separate listing for Milk Thistle.

Scientific Names
Cnicus benedictus.
Family: Asteraceae/Compositae.

People Use This For
Orally, blessed thistle is used for loss of appetite and indigestion; and as an antidiarrheal, expectorant, antibiotic, and diruetic. It is also used orally for promoting lactation, and for treating colds and fever.
Topically, blessed thistle is used as a poultice for boils, wounds, and ulcers.
In manufacturing, blessed thistle is used as a flavoring in alcoholic beverages.

Safety
LIKELY SAFE ...when used orally in amounts commonly found in foods. Blessed thistle has Generally Recognized As Safe (GRAS) status in the US (4912).
POSSIBLY SAFE ...when used orally and appropriately (12).
PREGNANCY: LIKELY UNSAFE ...when used orally (4,12); avoid using.
LACTATION: Insufficient reliable information available; avoid using.

Effectiveness
There is insufficient reliable information available about the effectiveness of blessed thistle.

Mechanism of Action
The applicable parts of blessed thistle are the flowering tops, leaves, and upper stems. Blessed thistle may have bacteriostatic properties due to the volatile oil content. The sesquiterpene lactone constituent, cnicin, may have antibacterial and antitumor activity (11). Metabolism of the constituents, arctiin and tracheoloside, following oral ingestion results in compounds that inhibit cyclic-AMP phosphodiesterase and histamine release from mast cells (11). Blessed thistle contains 8% tannins (4).

Adverse Reactions
Orally, when blessed thistle is used in high doses (greater than five grams per cup of tea), it can cause stomach irritation and vomiting (12). Blessed thistle may cause an allergic reaction in individuals sensitive to the Asteraceae/Compositae family. Members of this family include ragweed, chrysanthemums, marigolds, daisies, and many other herbs.

Interactions with Herbs & Other Dietary Supplements
None known.

Interactions with Drugs

ANTACIDS: Theoretically, due to reports that blessed thistle increases stomach acid, blessed thistle might decrease the effectiveness of antacids (19).
H2-BLOCKERS: Theoretically, due to reports that blessed thistle increases stomach acid, blessed thistle might decrease the effectiveness of H2-blockers (19). The H2 blockers include cimetidine (Tagamet), ranitidine (Zantac), nizatidine (Axid), and famotidine (Pepcid).
PROTON PUMP INHIBITORS (PPIs): Theoretically, due to reports that blessed thistle increases stomach acid, blessed thistle might decrease the effectiveness of PPIs (19). PPIs include omeprazole (Prilosec), lansoprazole (Prevacid), rabeprazole (Aciphex), pantoprazole (Protonix), and esomeprazole (Nexium).

Interactions with Foods

None known.

Interactions with Lab Tests

None known.

Interactions with Diseases or Conditions

CROSS-ALLERGENICITY: Blessed thistle may cause an allergic reaction in individuals sensitive to the Asteraceae/Compositae family. Members of this family include ragweed, chrysanthemums, marigolds, daisies, and many other herbs.
GASTROINTESTINAL (GI) IRRITATION: Blessed thistle may irritate the GI tract. It is contraindicated in individuals with infectious or inflammatory GI conditions (19).

Dosage and Administration

ORAL: The typical dose of the dried, flowering tops is 1.5-3 grams as a tea three times daily. The tea is prepared by steeping the dried, flowering tops in boiling water and then straining. 1.5-3 mL of the liquid extract, 1:1 in 25% alcohol, is commonly taken three times daily (4).
TOPICAL: No typical dosage.

Comments

Blessed thistle was commonly used during the Middle Ages to treat the bubonic plague and as a tonic for monks. Avoid confusion with milk thistle (Silybum marianum).

BLOND PSYLLIUM

Also Known As

Blond Plantago, Blonde Psyllium, Dietary Fiber, Englishman's Foot, Indian Plantago, Ispaghula, Ispagol, Pale Psyllium, Plantaginis ovatae semen, Plantaginis ovatae testa, Psyllium, Sand Plantain, Spogel.
CAUTION: See separate listings for Black Psyllium, Buckhorn Plantain, Great Plantain, and Water Plantain.

Scientific Names

Plantago ovata, synonyms Plantago fastigiata, Plantago insularis, Plantago ispaghula, Plantago decumbens.
Family: Plantaginaceae.

People Use This For

Orally, blond psyllium is used for constipation, softening stools in patients with hemorrhoids, anal fissures, post-anorectal surgery, and during pregnancy. It is also used for diarrhea, irritable bowel syndrome (IBS), hypercholesterolemia, hypertension, diabetes, dysentery, cancer, ulcerative colitis, weight control, and end-stage renal disease.
Topically, blond psyllium is used as a poultice for furunculosis (boils).
In food manufacturing, blond psyllium is used as a thickener or stabilizer in some frozen dairy desserts.

Safety

LIKELY SAFE ...when used orally and appropriately. Commercial blond psyllium preparations have been safely used in doses up to 20 grams per day for up to 6 months (1376,8423,9422).
PREGNANCY AND LACTATION: LIKELY SAFE ...when used orally and appropriately (272).

Effectiveness

EFFECTIVE

Constipation. Taking blond psyllium orally is effective as a bulk laxative for reducing constipation or softening stools (8424,9423,10092). Some evidence suggests that blond psyllium alone can relieve constipation and improve stool consistency as effectively as preparations containing blond psyllium plus senna (8424) or docusate sodium (10088).

LIKELY EFFECTIVE

Hypercholesterolemia. Taking blond psyllium orally reduces cholesterol levels in patients with mild to moderate hypercholesterolemia. Blond psyllium seed husk or seed added to food or as a separate supplement in a dose of approximately 10-12 grams daily, in combination with a low-fat or a high-fat diet, can reduce levels of total cholesterol by 3-14%, low density lipoprotein (LDL) cholesterol by 5-10%, and apolipoprotein B by 8.8% after seven weeks or greater of treatment. It also significantly reduces the LDL to high-density lipoprotein (HDL) ratio after six months of treatment (1376,2324,2327,6261,6262,8060,8061,8066,10095). There is evidence the LDL:HDL ratio can be reduced further when psyllium is consumed with a diet containing approximately 12% of energy as monounsaturated fatty acids, 29% of total fat (8067). There is evidence psyllium seed might be more effective than the seed husk in lowering serum cholesterol (8069). Psyllium seems to lower LDL cholesterol levels to a lesser degree in patients aged 60 years or older than in patients less than 60 years of age (2326). Blond psyllium does not significantly increase HDL levels and may actually lower HDL cholesterol levels. However, the magnitude of change in the HDL level is much less than changes in total and LDL cholesterol levels (1376,8433,10095). Blond psyllium seems to be most effective when consumed with foods at mealtime (8062). Breakfast cereal containing blond psyllium can modestly decrease total cholesterol and LDL cholesterol, by 5% and 9% respectively (1584,6263,8060,8061). Blond psyllium in combination with pectin, guar gum, and locust bean gum in a dose of 15 grams daily with a low-fat diet, reduces total cholesterol by 6.4% and LDL cholesterol by 10.5% after six months of treatment (8431). A combination of blond psyllium with colestipol, at half their usual doses seems to be as effective as colestipol alone (8432). Blond psyllium also seems to reduce colestipol and cholestyramine side effects such as constipation and abdominal pain (8432,9424). In children with hypercholesterolemia, psyllium supplementation can further decrease LDL cholesterol levels by 7-15% when added to a low fat, low cholesterol diet, National Cholesterol Education Program (NCEP) Step 1 diet. However, psyllium supplementation added to a more stringent low fat, low cholesterol diet, NCEP Step 2 diet, may have less of an additional effect in lowering LDL cholesterol (8073,8074,8075,8076).

POSSIBLY EFFECTIVE

Diabetes. There is some evidence that blond psyllium seed husk taken orally can significantly reduce postprandial serum glucose, insulin levels, serum total cholesterol, and low-density lipoprotein (LDL) cholesterol levels in patients with type 2 diabetes and hypercholesterolemia (1405,8058,8064,10091,10099). Blond psyllium's maximum effect on the glycemic index occurs when psyllium is mixed and consumed with carbohydrate foods (8064,10091). However, blond psyllium does not lower postprandial glucose in people without diabetes (9249).

Diarrhea. Taking blond psyllium orally seems to delay gastric emptying, slow colonic transit, increase fecal viscosity, and improve fecal consistency in patients with diarrhea (5246,8419,8420,8421). Psyllium is also used in combination with calcium carbonate and calcium phosphate, weight ratio 4:1:1, and seems to be as effective as loperamide in reducing the frequency and urgency associated with diarrhea (8422). In patients receiving enteral tube feedings, psyllium does not decrease the frequency of stools, but it may decrease the number of liquid stools (8423,9422). Preliminary clinical evidence suggests blond psyllium might also be useful in treating postcholecystectomy diarrhea (10097). Taking blond psyllium orally seems to reduce diarrhea associated with the use of misoprostol (Cytotec). There is preliminary evidence that blond psyllium relieves diarrhea associated with misoprostol use and prevents its reoccurrence when used throughout misoprostol therapy (8429).

Hemorrhoids. Taking blond psyllium orally, with micronized purified flavonidic fraction (MPFF, Daflon), seems to help to relieve bleeding from nonprolapsed hemorrhoids. Psyllium husk used with micronized purified flavonidic fraction relieves bleeding more rapidly than psyllium husk used alone or psyllium husk used with rubber band ligation (8077).

Hypertension. Taking psyllium fiber (husks) orally, with soy protein, seems to help reduce systolic blood pressure by about 8 mmHg and diastolic blood pressure by about 2 mmHg in adult men and women (10458).

Irritable bowel syndrome (IBS). Taking blond psyllium orally seems to improve some symptoms of IBS. There is some controversy about the clinical benefits of blond psyllium seed husk for IBS. There is evidence that shows no benefit (8425), but the majority of evidence shows that blond psyllium seed husk can relieve constipation and improve abdominal pain, diarrhea, and overall well-being (2316,8426,8427,8428). There is also some evidence that a combination of blond psyllium and propantheline (Pro-Banthine) relieves constipation, incomplete bowel evacuation, abdominal pain, constipation, and straining associated with IBS. Patients typically experience relief after four weeks of treatment (8428).

Orlistat (Xenical) side effects. Taking blond psyllium orally with each dose of orlistat seems to relieve orlistat side effects such as flatulence, borborygmi, abdominal cramps, oily spotting, and fecal incontinence without decreasing the weight-reducing effect of orlistat (5245).

Ulcerative colitis. There is some evidence 10 grams of blond psyllium seeds taken orally twice daily might be as effective as 500 mg of mesalamine (Asacol) taken three times daily in preventing the relapse of ulcerative colitis (2385). Blond psyllium also appears to relieve gastrointestinal symptoms in adult patients with ulcerative colitis in remission, including abdominal pain, diarrhea, loose stools, urgency, bloating, incomplete evacuation, mucus discharge, and constipation (10086). However, in patients with juvenile ulcerative colitis in remission, blond psyllium does not appear to have an effect on fecal bile acid excretion, an indicator of disease progression (10090).

POSSIBLY INEFFECTIVE

Colorectal adenoma. Taking blond psyllium orally 3.5 grams per day does not seem to reduce the risk of colorectal adenoma recurrence. There is some evidence that it might actually increase the risk of adenoma recurrence, particularly in people with high dietary calcium intake. However, more evidence is needed to determine the relationship of psyllium and calcium to colorectal adenoma (7585).

End-stage renal disease (ESRD). Taking blond psyllium orally does not seem to reduce potassium, phosphate, or ammonia concentrations in patients with ESRD (9248).

There is insufficient reliable information available about the effectiveness of blond psyllium for its other uses.

Mechanism of Action

The applicable parts of blond psyllium are the seed and seed husk. The blond psyllium husk and intact seed contain water-soluble fibers that form a viscous gel in the intestine (2387). Most commercial preparations contain purified seed husk. The inner seed components, the endosperm and the plant embryo, are responsible for the majority of the allergic reactions to blond psyllium. The inner seed parts, which sometimes contaminate commercially produced psyllium seed husks, seem to be responsible for allergenicity, rather than the husk itself (9245). There is some evidence that the soluble fibers undergo partial fermentation by bacteria in the colon (2393,5246,8071), but the bulking effect of psyllium is primarily a result of intact material (10096). When psyllium seed husk is mixed with water, the mucilage has a bulk laxative effect and stimulates peristalsis, which decreases gastrointestinal transit time (8421). In patients with diarrhea, the mucilage increases the water-holding capacity and viscosity of stools, which delays gastric emptying and improves stool consistency (5246,8420,8421). It also prolongs gastrointestinal transit time, possibly by delaying the production of gaseous fermentation products (5246). The polysaccharides in psyllium that form into a gel in the intestine also lubricate stool contents and provide greater ease during defecation (8421). In patients with irritable bowel syndrome (IBS), blond psyllium is thought to normalize bowel function and relieve symptoms of abdominal pain by reducing rectosigmoidal pressure (405). Blond psyllium is also thought to maintain remission in adult patients with ulcerative colitis since fermentation of blond psyllium in the colon yields butyrate, a short-chain fatty acid known to inhibit cytokine production and have an anti-inflammatory effect (2385).

Blond psyllium seems to decrease serum cholesterol levels by adsorbing dietary fats in the gastrointestinal tract and decreasing systemic absorption of the fat. Cholesterol elimination in fecal bile acids also seems to be increased by blond psyllium (1376,8065,8070,8072). Increasing elimination of bile acids increases their production and turnover in the liver, which lowers serum cholesterol. Blond psyllium does not bind to cholesterol or bile acids, but they probably become trapped in the mucilloid matrix and are then expelled. This mechanism also seems to inhibit cholesterol stone formation. Because bile acid sequestrants work by different mechanisms than blond psyllium, together their effects on cholesterol is additive (2387,9425,9426).

There seems to be an inverse relationship between cholesterol and blood urea nitrogen (BUN) levels (8068). This may explain why psyllium is not useful for lowering BUN in end-stage renal disease (ESRD).

Psyllium, by itself, does not affect the absorption of carcinogens in the gastrointestinal tract. The soluble fiber formed by psyllium does not bind to carcinogens. However, wheat bran, which provides insoluble fiber does bind carcinogens. Some evidence suggests that psyllium might improve the chemoprotective effect of wheat bran (9250). A diet that includes an equal combination of psyllium and wheat bran might decrease the risk of breast and colon cancer. In addition, psyllium might help maintain normal cell proliferation in the colon (8082,8083).

In patients with diabetes, blond psyllium reduces postprandial blood glucose levels, probably by delaying the rate of digestion and absorption of carbohydrates (1405,8064). However, psyllium does not seem to reduce postprandial blood glucose when it is given to people without diabetes (9249).

Adverse Reactions

Orally, blond psyllium can cause transient flatulence, abdominal pain, diarrhea, constipation, dyspepsia, and nausea (1376). Starting with a low dose and slowly titrating to the desired dose can often minimize gastrointestinal side effects. There is some concern that blond psyllium can cause esophageal or bowel obstruction when consumed without water or in patients with swallowing disorders (604,8080,8081). Tell patients to consume plenty of water when taking blond psyllium. Suggest at least 240 mL of fluid for every 3.5-5 grams of seed husk or 7 grams of seed (1376,8080,8081). Occasionally, headache, backache, rhinitis, increased cough, and sinusitis have also been reported in patients taking psyllium (1376). Some patients can have an allergic response to blond psyllium. Allergy symptoms include allergic rhinitis, sneezing, conjunctivitis, urticarial rash, itching, flushing, and dyspnea. More serious symptoms include wheezing, facial and body swelling, chest congestion, chest and throat tightness, cough, diarrhea, hypotension, loss of consciousness, and anaphylactic shock. Occupational exposure or repeated ingestion of psyllium can cause sensitization, which can lead to serious allergic reactions (2328,2329,2330,8079,9246). Severe allergic reactions may occur after eating a small quantity of cereal that contains blond psyllium. At least one cereal (Heartwise, Kellogg Co.) has increased the purity of the psyllium it contains, which has decreased the incidence of allergic reactions (9244). A warning of the potential for allergic reactions is on the label of all cereals that contain psyllium (9247). Patients hypersensitive to psyllium usually have marked eosinophilia and an elevated psyllium-specific IgE antibody serum level (2328,2329). There is concern that individuals allergic to English plantain weed, Plantain lanceolata, pollen might also react to psyllium husk dust; however, it appears that there is little cross-allergenicity between these plants and is probably of no clinical significance (8057,9244).

Blond psyllium has a tendency to plug feeding tubes. This can be avoided if blond psyllium is mixed with water and pushed through the feeding tube in less than 5 minutes (8423).

Interactions with Herbs & Other Dietary Supplements

IRON SUPPLEMENTS: Use of blond psyllium with iron supplements can reduce iron absorption (2340,2367,10089). There is some evidence that blond psyllium decreases the absorption of iron by forming a highly stable complex in the intestine (2340,2367). Take supplements one hour before or four hours after psyllium to avoid this interaction.
RIBOFLAVIN SUPPLEMENTS: Psyllium seems to slightly reduce the absorption of riboflavin by about 5%, but this is unlikely to be clinically significant (10094).

Interactions with Drugs

ANTIDIABETES DRUGS: Blond psyllium can reduce blood glucose levels in patients with type 2 diabetes (1405) and might have additive effects on glucose levels when used with antidiabetes drugs. Monitor blood glucose levels closely. Medication dose adjustments may be necessary. Some antidiabetes drugs include glimepiride (Amaryl), glyburide (Diabeta, Glynase PresTab, Micronase), insulin, pioglitazone (Actos), rosiglitazone (Avandia), and others.
CARBAMAZEPINE (Tegretol): Blond psyllium can reduce carbamazepine absorption and serum levels (539).
DIGOXIN (Lanoxin): Theoretically, psyllium might reduce digoxin absorption. However, some evidence suggests that the effect of psyllium on digoxin absorption is not clinically significant (10098).
LITHIUM: There is one case report of reduced serum lithium levels associated with psyllium use. This was reversed when psyllium was stopped (540). The fiber in lithium might decrease the absorption of lithium.
ORAL DRUGS: Due to fiber content blond psyllium may decrease absorption of drugs taken orally. As a general rule take oral drugs one hour before or four hours after blond psyllium to avoid decreased or delayed absorption.
WARFARIN (Coumadin): Blond psyllium may reduce warfarin absorption (12).

Interactions with Foods

NUTRIENT ABSORPTION: Despite concern that long-term use of psyllium with meals can reduce nutrient absorption, possibly requiring vitamin or mineral supplementation, use of blond psyllium husk for up to six months did not clinically alter vitamin or mineral status in a review of eight human trials (1376). Blond psyllium does not reduce the absorption of calcium (9243).

Interactions with Lab Tests

CHOLESTEROL: Blond psyllium reduces serum total cholesterol and LDL cholesterol levels, LDL:HDL ratio, and test results (1405,1376).
GLUCOSE: Blond psyllium can reduce postprandial blood glucose levels and test results (1405).

Interactions with Diseases or Conditions

DIABETES: Blond psyllium can lower blood glucose levels in people with type 2 diabetes by retarding carbohydrate absorption (1405,8064). Monitor blood glucose levels closely. Doses of conventional antidiabetes medications may require adjustment. Also, warn patients with diabetes that some commercial blond psyllium products can contain added sugars and other absorbable carbohydrates which might increase blood glucose levels.
GASTROINTESTINAL CONDITIONS: Blond psyllium is contraindicated in people with fecal impaction, GI tract narrowing, obstruction, or conditions that can lead to obstruction, such as spastic bowel (12).
HYPERSENSITIVITY: Some patients can have severe hypersensitivity reactions to blond psyllium. This is more likely to occur in patients with previous occupation exposure to blond psyllium (2328,2329,2330,8079,9246). Blond psyllium is contraindicated in these patients.
PHENYLKETONURIA: Some blond psyllium preparations are sweetened with aspartame (Nutrasweet) and should be avoided in patients with phenylketonuria (272).
SWALLOWING DISORDERS: Patients with swallowing disorders might be at greater risk for esophageal obstruction when using blond psyllium. Blond psyllium is contraindicated in these patients (8080,8081).

Dosage and Administration

ORAL: As a bulk laxative for constipation, blond psyllium seed 7-40 grams per day, in 2-4 divided doses is commonly used (6248,9423,10088). For diarrhea, 7-18 grams of blond psyllium, in 2-3 divided doses, has been used (8419,8420) or 5 grams of a combination of blond psyllium, calcium carbonate, and calcium phosphate, weight ratio 4:1:1, has been used twice daily (8422). For decreasing diarrhea in patients receiving tube feedings, up to 30 grams of blond psyllium has been used daily in divided doses of 2.5-7.5 grams per dose. It may be given through the feeding tube, mixed with the enteral feeding, or by bolus followed by a flush with water. However, psyllium may cause clogging of the feeding tube when either of these techniques is used (8423,9422). For chronic diarrhea associated with postcholecystectomy diarrhea, blond psyllium 6.5 grams three times daily has been used (10097). For irritable bowel syndrome (IBS), blond psyllium seed husk, 10-30 grams in two to three divided doses, has been used daily (2316,8426,8427,8428). Blond psyllium seed husk 10 grams twice daily with propantheline 15 mg three times daily has also been used (8428). For diarrhea associated with the use of misoprostol, blond psyllium 3.4 grams twice daily has been used (8429). For reducing the gastrointestinal (GI) side effects of orlistat, 6 grams three times daily with each orlistat dose has been used (5245). For maintaining remission in patients with ulcerative colitis, 10 grams of blond psyllium seeds, taken twice daily, has been used (2385). For relieving bleeding from nonprolapsed hemorrhoids, 3.5 grams of psyllium seed husk, twice daily for three months, has been used in addition to treatment with micronized purified flavonidic fraction (MPFF, Daflon) 1500 mg twice daily for five days, followed by 1000 mg twice daily for three weeks (8077). For lowering serum cholesterol, blond psyllium seed husk 3.4 grams three times daily or 5.1 grams twice daily has been used (2324,8433,6261,6262,6264,8066,10095). However, doses up to 20.4 grams per day have been tried (1376). Psyllium-enriched cereal containing 12 grams of soluble fiber per day has been also used (1584,6263,8060,8061). A mixture of 2.1 grams of psyllium, 1.3 grams of pectin, 1.1 grams of guar gum and 0.5 grams of locust bean gum has been used three times daily (8431). A combination of 2.5 grams of blond psyllium powder (Metamucil) with 2.5 grams of colestipol, taken three times daily, has also been used (8432). In children with hypercholesterolemia, psyllium-enriched cereal containing 5-10 grams of psyllium has been used daily (8073,8075,8076). For type 2 diabetes and hypercholesterolemia, blond psyllium 15 grams in three divided doses has been used (10099). For reducing the glycemic index of food in patients with type 2 diabetes, blond psyllium 15 grams in three divided doses with a carbohydrate meal has been used (10091). For treating end-stage renal disease (ESRD), 8.7 grams daily of blond psyllium has been used (9248). For hypertension, blond psyllium husks 15 grams daily has been used for 8 weeks (10458). Tell patients to ensure adequate fluid intake. Inadequate fluid intake can lead to choking and esophageal or bowel obstruction. Suggest a minimum of 240 mL per 5 grams or less of blond psyllium husk or 7 grams of blond psyllium seed (1376,8080,8081). To minimize some of the common gastrointestinal side effects, suggest that patients start with a low dose and titrate slowly to the desired dose.

Comments

There are some blond psyllium-containing foods with labeling that claim these foods, when consumed as part of a low-fat diet, may reduce the risk of coronary heart disease (CHD) (6264). It is true that blond psyllium can help lower cholesterol levels; however, there is not yet proof that taking blond psyllium reduces the risk of developing heart disease. Despite its effectiveness in lowering cholesterol levels, blond psyllium has not yet been included in the stepwise approaches to dietary therapy such as the American Heart Association Step I or Step II diets for hypercholesterolemia (2321,8430). Most clinical studies have used a specific blond psyllium powder preparation (Metamucil) (1376,6261) or psyllium seed husk-containing foods such as cereals, breads, or snack bars (8433,6262). The FDA allows foods containing at least 1.7 grams of psyllium per serving to be labeled with the claim that it may reduce the risk of heart disease when it is consumed as part of a diet low in fat and cholesterol (11018).

BLOODROOT

Also Known As

Bloodwort, Blood Root, Coon Root, Indian Plant, Indian Red Paint, Pauson, Red Indian Paint, Red Puccoon, Red Root, Sanguinaria, Snakebite, Sweet Slumber, Tetterwort.
CAUTION: See Separate listing for Yarrow.

Scientific Names

Sanguinaria canadensis.
Family: Papaveraceae.

People Use This For

Orally, bloodroot is used as an emetic, cathartic, antispasmodic, and expectorant. Bloodroot is also used orally for bronchitis, asthma, croup, laryngitis, pharyngitis, deficient capillary circulation, nasal polyps, rheumatism, warts, cancer (Fell technique), dental analgesic, fever, and as a general tonic.
Topically, bloodroot is used as an irritant and debriding agent.
In dentistry, bloodroot is used topically to reduce plaque.

Safety

POSSIBLY SAFE ...when used orally and appropriately short-term (4).
POSSIBLY UNSAFE ...when excessive doses are used orally; sanguinarine, although thought to be poorly absorbed, is a toxic alkaloid (6,12).
There is insufficient reliable information available about the safety of bloodroot for its other uses.
PREGNANCY: LIKELY UNSAFE ...when used orally (12); avoid using.
LACTATION: POSSIBLY UNSAFE ...when used orally (4); avoid using.

Effectiveness

There is insufficient reliable information available about the effectiveness of bloodroot.

Mechanism of Action

The applicable part of bloodroot is the rhizome. The isoquinolone alkaloid constituents, primarily sanguinarine, appear to have antimicrobial, antifungal, anti-inflammatory, and antihistamine activity (11446,11448). The negative ion of sanguinarine can bind to dental plaque and exert antiplaque activity (11446). Bloodroot also seems to exhibit cardiotonic (exerts a favorable effect on the heart) actions, possibly by inhibiting Na/K-ATPase activity and producing a positive inotropic effect (11447).

Adverse Reactions

Orally, bloodroot may cause nausea, vomiting (12), slight central nervous system (CNS) depression, and narcosis (6). High doses may cause hypotension, shock, coma, and glaucoma (6).
Topically, skin contact with fresh bloodroot can cause irritation or contact dermatitis (19). Avoid contact with the eyes and mucous membranes because of its irritant properties.

Interactions with Herbs & Other Dietary Supplements

None known.

Interactions with Drugs

None known.

Interactions with Foods

None known.

Interactions with Lab Tests

None known.

Interactions with Diseases or Conditions

GASTROINTESTINAL (GI) IRRITATION: Bloodroot can irritate the GI tract and is contraindicated in individuals with infectious or inflammatory gastrointestinal conditions (19).
GLAUCOMA: Bloodroot might affect glaucoma treatment. Do not exceed the recommended dose (12).

Dosage and Administration

ORAL: The typical dose of the bloodroot rhizome is 60-500 mg three times a day (4). The usual dose of the liquid extract, 1:1 in 60% alcohol, is 0.06-0.3 mL three times a day (4). The tincture, 1:5 in 60% alcohol, is dosed at 0.3-2 mL three times a day (4).
TOPICAL: No typical dosage.
EMETIC DOSE: As an emetic, 1-2 g of the rhizome; 1-2 mL of the liquid extract, 1:1 in 60% alcohol; or 2-8 mL of the tincture, 1:5 in 60% alcohol have been used (4).

Comments

During the mid-1800s, topical preparations of the bloodroot extracts were used in the Fell Technique for treatment of breast tumors (6).

BLUE COHOSH

Also Known As

Blue Ginseng, Caulophyllum, Papoose Root, Squaw Root, Yellow Ginseng.
CAUTION: See separate listings for Black Cohosh, White Cohosh, Ginseng American, Canaigre, Codonopsis, Ginseng Siberian, Ginseng Panax, and Ashwaganda.

Scientific Names

Caulophyllum thalictroides.
Family: Berberidaceae or Leonticaceae.

People Use This For

Orally, blue cohosh is used for stimulating the uterus and inducing labor, inducing menstruation, as an antispasmodic, as a laxative, and for colic, sore throat, cramps, hiccups, epilepsy, hysterics, inflammation of the uterus, and rheumatic conditions.
In foods, the roasted seeds of blue cohosh are used as a coffee substitute.

Safety

LIKELY UNSAFE ...when used orally (4,12). Poisonings have occurred after ingestion of blue cohosh leaf or seeds (4).
PREGNANCY AND LACTATION: LIKELY UNSAFE ...when used orally. Blue cohosh is a uterine stimulant and can induce labor (12047). Several blue cohosh constituents are potentially teratogenic and might cause congenital malformations in newborns (1122,7110). Use of blue cohosh near term can cause life-threatening toxicity

in the infant (1207,9492,9493,12047). Many midwives still use blue cohosh to facilitate delivery. This dangerous practice should be avoided (1122,1207).

Effectiveness

There is insufficient reliable information available about the effectiveness of blue cohosh.

Mechanism of Action

The applicable parts of blue cohosh are the rhizome and root. Blue cohosh has several pharmacological effects. However, most of these effects are undesirable. Blue cohosh constricts coronary arteries and seems to decrease the flow of oxygen to the heart (3383). Blue cohosh also contains several alkaloid constituents that are suspected teratogens. There is some evidence that the constituent anagyrine might cause birth defects in humans (7110). Another constituent, N-methylcytosine also seems to be teratogenic (7110). N-methylcytosine seems to act similarly to nicotine, which can increase blood pressure, stimulate the small intestine, and produce hyperglycemia the developing fetus (7110). Blue cohosh also contains taspine, which is chemically related to morphine and its congeners (7110). Taspine seems to be cytotoxic and lethal to embryos even at very low concentrations (7110). There is preliminary evidence that blue cohosh might have estrogenic effects. A blue cohosh extract seems to enhance estradiol binding to estrogen receptors and increase estradiol-induced transcription activity in estrogen-responsive cells (6180). In animal models, it also decreases luteinizing hormone (LH) levels and increases serum ceruloplasmin oxidase activity, which is a measure of estrogenic activity in the liver (6180).

Adverse Reactions

Orally, blue cohosh can cause significant adverse effects including mucous membrane irritation, stomach upset including diarrhea and cramping, chest pain (angina), hypertension, and hyperglycemia (6002).
Neonatal acute myocardial infarction (MI), congestive heart failure (CHF), and shock has occurred following maternal use of a blue cohosh combination product one month before delivery (566,3383). There is also a case report of severe complications, including seizures, renal failure, and respiratory distress, in an infant whose mother was given an unknown dose of black and blue cohosh at 42-weeks gestation to induce labor (1122,9492,9493). In another case, a mother was advised to drink a blue cohosh tea to induce labor. The infant experienced a seizure during delivery and 2 days later it was discovered that the infant was experiencing an evolving ischemic stroke (12047).
Due to these life-threatening side effects pregnant women should be advised not to ingest any blue cohosh product during pregnancy.

Interactions with Herbs & Other Dietary Supplements

None known.

Interactions with Drugs

ANTIDIABETES DRUGS: There is some concern that blue cohosh might increase blood glucose levels (6002). Theoretically, it might decrease the effectiveness of medicines used for diabetes.
ANTIHYPERTENSIVE DRUGS: Constituents in blue cohosh might increase blood pressure by causing coronary vasoconstriction (6002). Theoretically, this might decrease the effectiveness of drugs used for angina and high blood pressure.
NICOTINE: Blue cohosh can increase the effects of nicotine (6002).

Interactions with Foods

None known.

Interactions with Lab Tests

None known.

Interactions with Diseases or Conditions

CARDIOVASCULAR CONDITIONS: There is some concern that blue cohosh might worsen cardiovascular conditions such as angina and hypertension. There is evidence that blue cohosh can cause coronary vasoconstriction and decrease oxygen flow to the heart. It might also increase blood pressure (6002). Avoid using in these patients.
DIABETES: There is some concern that blue cohosh might worsen diabetes. It can increase blood glucose levels in some patients (6002).
DIARRHEA: Blue cohosh might worsen symptoms in patients with diarrhea (4). Blue cohosh seems to increase gastrointestinal motility (5).
HORMONE SENSITIVE CANCERS/CONDITIONS: Because blue cohosh might have estrogenic effects (6180), women with hormone sensitive conditions should avoid blue cohosh. Some of these conditions include breast cancer, uterine cancer, ovarian cancer, endometriosis, and uterine fibroids.

Dosage and Administration

ORAL: The typical dose of the dried rhizome or root is 0.3-1 grams or as a tea three times daily. The tea is prepared by steeping the herb in 150 mL boiling water and then straining. The usual dose of the liquid extract (1:1 in 70% alcohol) is 0.5-1.0 mL three times daily (4).

Comments

Cohosh is from the Algonquin word "rough," referring to the appearance of the roots (7110). Blue cohosh was listed in the US Pharmacopoeia from 1882 to 1905 for inducing labor (7110).

BLUE FLAG

Also Known As

Iris, Sweet Flag, Water Flag.
CAUTION: See separate listing for Orris.

Scientific Names

Iris versicolor; Iris caroliniana; Iris virginica.
Family: Iridaceae.

People Use This For

Orally, blue flag is used as a laxative and diuretic and for dermatological, anti-inflammatory, and antiemetic uses. It is also used as a bile stimulant, for liver dysfunction, and specifically for skin eruptions.

Safety

LIKELY UNSAFE ...when used orally; contraindicated in all but small doses (4). The fresh root can cause nausea, vomiting, and mucosal irritation (4,12). The blue flag oil is a mucous membrane irritant (4).
PREGNANCY AND LACTATION: LIKELY UNSAFE ...when used orally (4,12); avoid using.

Effectiveness

There is insufficient reliable information available about the effectiveness of blue flag.

Mechanism of Action

The applicable part of blue flag is the rhizome. There is insufficient reliable information available about the possible mechanism of action and active ingredients. Some related species can be toxic (4).

Adverse Reactions

Orally, blue flag can cause nausea and vomiting, and the fresh root can irritate mucosa or skin (4,19). The volatile oil constituent irritates mucous membranes and can cause lacrimation, eye inflammation, irritation of the throat, and headache (4).

Interactions with Herbs & Other Dietary Supplements

POTASSIUM DEPLETING HERBS: Theoretically, concomitant use with horsetail plant or the licorice rhizome increases the risk of potassium depletion.
STIMULANT LAXATIVE HERBS: Theoretically, concomitant use of blue flag with other stimulant laxative herbs can increase the risk of potassium depletion. Stimulant laxative herbs include aloe dried leaf sap, wild cucumber fruit (Ecballium elaterium), alder buckthorn, European buckthorn, butternut bark, cascara bark, castor oil, colocynth fruit pulp, gamboge bark exudate, jalap root, black root, manna bark exudate, podophyllum root, rhubarb root, senna leaves and pods, and yellow dock root (19).

Interactions with Drugs

DIGOXIN (Lanoxin): Theoretically, overuse or abuse of this product increases the risk of adverse effects from cardiac glycoside drugs.
DIURETIC DRUGS: Overuse of blue flag might compound diuretic-induced potassium loss (19). There is some concern that people taking blue flag along with potassium depleting diuretics might have an increased risk for hypokalemia. Initiation of potassium supplementation or an increase in potassium supplement dose may be necessary for some patients. Some diuretics that can deplete potassium include chlorothiazide (Diuril), chlorthalidone (Thalitone), furosemide (Lasix), hydrochlorothiazide (HCTZ, HydroDIURIL, Microzide), and others.

Interactions with Foods

None known.

Interactions with Lab Tests
None known.

Interactions with Diseases or Conditions
GASTROINTESTINAL IRRITATION: Blue flag can irritate the GI tract and is contraindicated in individuals with infectious or inflammatory gastrointestinal conditions (19).

Dosage and Administration
No typical dosage.

Comments
Little is known about blue flag's phytochemical, pharmacological, or toxicological properties, or those of its constituents. Some related species can be toxic (4). Though orris root is sometimes used as a common name for blue flag, it is also used to describe the Iris species.

BLUE-GREEN ALGAE

Also Known As
AFA, BGA, Cyanobacteria, Dihe, Klamath Blue/Green Algae, Blue-Green Micro-Algae, Spirulina, Tecuitlatl.

Scientific Names
Microcystis aeruginosa; Microcystis wesenbergii; other Microcystis species; Spirulina maxima; Spirulina platensis;, Spirulina pacifica; other Spirulina species; Anabaena species; Lyngbya wollei; Aphanizomenon flos-aquae.

People Use This For
Orally, blue-green algae is used as a source of dietary protein, B-vitamins, and iron. It is also used orally for weight loss, oral leukoplakia, and obstetric and gynecological disorders. Blue-green algae is also used orally for attention deficit-hyperactivity disorder (ADHD), premenstrual syndrome, allergic rhinitis, diabetes, stimulating the immune system, stress, fatigue, anxiety, depression, improving memory, increasing energy and metabolism, lowering cholesterol, decreasing cardiovascular disease, wound healing, and for promoting digestion and bowel health.

Safety
POSSIBLY SAFE ...when non-contaminated, non-microcystin containing species of blue-green algae are used orally (9171).
POSSIBLY UNSAFE ...when contaminated blue-green algae are used orally. Blue-green algae can be contaminated with microbes, heavy metals (including mercury, cadmium, lead, or arsenic), and radioactive divalent and trivalent metal ions (6).
LIKELY UNSAFE ...when any microcystin-containing blue-green algae products are used orally (3535,3536,9171); avoid using all untested blue-green algae products.
CHILDREN: LIKELY UNSAFE ...when any microcystin-containing blue-green algae products are used orally. Children are more sensitive to poisoning by microcystins produced by blue-green algae (3536).
PREGNANCY AND LACTATION: Insufficient reliable information available; avoid using.

Effectiveness
POSSIBLY EFFECTIVE
Oral leukoplakia. Taking spirulina blue-green algae orally seems to reduce oral leukoplakia in people who chew tobacco (6).
POSSIBLY INEFFECTIVE
Weight loss. Taking spirulina blue-green algae doesn't seem to help reduce weight (6).
There is insufficient reliable information available about the effectiveness of blue-green algae for its other uses.

Mechanism of Action
Blue-green algae are a mixture of single celled organisms that have biochemical and cellular similarities to both plant and animal species. While these organisms have the ability to perform photosynthesis like plants, they lack a cell wall. Like animal species, they form many complex glycoproteins. Spirulina and aphanizomenon are the species that have been studied most intensively. Spirulina blue-green algae consists of approximately 65% crude protein, high concentrations of B vitamins, phenylalanine, and iron and other minerals (6). The B vitamins are thought to be analogs of vitamin B12 and nutritionally insignificant (6). The phenylalanine content is promoted as being responsible for reducing appetite and causing weight loss (6). The FDA reviewed this claim and found no evidence to support using blue-green algae for weight loss (6). The iron in spirulina blue-green algae has been found to be highly

bioavailable in humans (6). As much as 1.5-2 mg of iron can be absorbed from a dose of 10 grams of blue-green algae (6).

Spirulina blue-green algae has a high concentration of vitamin B12. However, consumption of spirulina does not appear to decrease mean corpuscular volume (MCV) when added to a vegetarian diet (9467). For reasons that are not clear, the vitamin B12 in spirulina is not bioactive (9477).

A constituent called C- phycocyanin that is found in some species of blue-green algae may have anti-inflammatory actions. In addition, it may bind to reactive oxygen species (ROS), such as hydroxyl free radicals, resulting in antioxidant effects (9468,9469). Preliminary evidence suggests that the antioxidant effect may decrease the toxicity of lead (9470). Evidence suggests that spirulina blue-green algae might reduce serum lipids, liver triglycerides, and gastric secretions (6). It might also protect against the effects of gamma radiation, enhance the regression of oral carcinoma, and have antiviral effects (6).

Blue-green algae seems to have immunomodulatory effects. The blue-green algae species Spirulina platensis may increase the concentration of immune globulin A (IgA) in the gastrointestinal tract, without increasing concentrations of IgG or IgE. This effect may decrease the risk of food allergies (9434,10267). Preliminary research suggests that Spirulina species can inhibit mast cell-mediated allergic reactions (9173). Spirulina platensis also appears to increase immune function by increasing the activity of macrophages, increase phagocytosis, and increase the concentration of interleukin-1 (IL1) (10267). The species of blue-green algae Aphanizomenon flos-aquae (AFA) may stimulate the immune system by stimulating the activity and motility of T lymphocytes, B lymphocytes and natural killer cells. AFA slightly increases the phagocytic activity of polymorphonuclear (PMN) leucocytes (2534).

AFA contains 1.9-2.9 times less of the polyunsaturated fatty acids (PUFA), alpha-linolenic acid, and 32-44 times less linoleic acid than soybean oil. Preliminary evidence suggests that an AFA-supplemented diet may be more effective than the soybean oil-supplemented diet at lowering triglycerides and total cholesterol (2535). Preliminary research suggests that AFA might improve utilization of proteins and increase synthesis of enzymes involved with digestion and nutrient utilization (9242).

Researchers at the National Cancer Institute have isolated an antiviral protein, cyanovirin-N (CV-N), which might prove useful in treating human immunodeficiency virus (HIV) infection. Isolated from the blue-green algae Nostoc ellipsosporum, CV-N binds irreversibly to sites on the viral envelope, inactivating HIV and inhibiting its entry into cells. CV-N has unique temperature (heat and cold) stability which might allow for its use in applications not typical for proteins. The researchers hypothesize that, attached to a solid matrix, CV-N might be used to adsorb and remove HIV from infected blood products. This unpublished research was presented at the Microbicides 2000 International Conference (1375).

Adverse Reactions

Orally, blue-green algae appear to cause few adverse effects when non-contaminated products are used. Blue-green algae can be contaminated with the toxic blue-green algae species Microcystis aeruginosa, which produces potent hepatotoxins called microcystins (9171). Microcystin-containing blue-green algae products can cause hepatotoxicity, jaundice, abdominal pain and distention, nausea, vomiting, weakness, excessive thirst, rapid and weak pulse, shock, and death (3535,9172). Symptoms of poisoning usually occur 30 minutes to 24 hours after ingestion (3535). Children are more sensitive to microcystin poisoning than adults (3536).

There is concern that blue-green algae might cause or worsen autoimmune disorders due to its immune-stimulating effects. In one case a patient with pemphigus vulgaris had a disease flare after taking a supplement containing spirulina blue-green algae. In another case, a woman developed dermatomyositis within 1-2 days after taking a supplement containing blue-green algae (12171). More evidence is needed to determine if blue-green algae is responsible for these effects.

Interactions with Herbs & Other Dietary Supplements

None known.

Interactions with Drugs

None known.

Interactions with Foods

None known.

Interactions with Lab Tests

LIVER FUNCTION TESTS: Increases in liver function tests, ALT (alanine aminotransferase, formerly SGPT), and AST (aspartate aminotransferase, formerly SGOT), suggest possible consumption of microcystin-contaminated blue-green algae (9172).

Interactions with Diseases or Conditions

PEMPHIGUS VULGARIS: In one case, a patient with well-controlled pemphigus vulgaris took a supplement containing spirulina blue-green algae and within 7-10 days developed a disease flare. The immunostimulatory effects of spirulina blue-green algae are thought to exacerbate this and other autoimmune disorders (12171).

PHENYLKETONURIA: Theoretically, the phenylalanine content of Spirulina species blue-green algae products might exacerbate phenylketonuria (6); avoid Spirulina species blue-green algae products (6).

Dosage and Administration

ORAL: The typical dose of spirulina blue-green algae is 3-5 grams daily before meals (6002).

Comments

Blue-green algae are commonly found in tropical or subtropical alkaline waters that have a high-salt content, but some species such as Aphanizomenon grow in large fresh water lakes (6002,9171). The natural color of these algae can give bodies of water a dark-green appearance (6). Blue-green algae (cyanophyta) comprises thousands of species, including Spirulina species of blue-green algae and non-Spirulina species of blue-green algae (3536). Most commercial products contain Aphanizomenon flos-aquae, Spirulina maxima, or Spirulina platensis. The altitude, temperature, and sun exposure where the blue-green algae are grown dramatically influence the constituents and the species mixture (9242). Commercial Spirulina species of blue-green algae are usually grown under controlled conditions while some non-spirulina blue-green algae (Klamath blue-green algae and others) are grown in natural setting (lakes, etc.) where contamination and microcystin production may be more likely (3536). Hepatotoxic microcystins have been found in both Spirulina and non-Spirulina products (3536,9171). Select blue-green algae products that have been tested for contamination with heavy metals, microbes, or microcystins (3536). While blue-green algae products are promoted as an excellent source of dietary protein, they are no better than meat or milk and are estimated to cost more than 30 times as much as beef on a per gram basis (6).

BLUEBERRY

Also Known As

Blueberries, Highbush Blueberry, Hillside Blueberry, Lowbush Blueberry, Rabbiteye Blueberry.
Caution: See separate listing for Bilberry (Vaccinium myrtillus).

Scientific Names

Vaccinium angustifolium, synonyms Vaccinium brittonii, Vaccinium lamarckii, Vaccinium pensylvanicum; Vaccinium virgatum, synonyms Vaccinium ashei, Vaccinium amoenum; Vaccinium corymbosum, synonym Vaccinium constablaei; Vaccinium pallidum, synonyms Vaccinium altomontanum, Vaccinium vacillans.
Family: Ericaceae.

People Use This For

Orally, blueberry is used for preventing cataracts and glaucoma, ulcers, urinary tract infections (UTIs), multiple sclerosis, fever, varicose veins, hemorrhoids, improving circulation, and as a laxative. It is also used for colic, labor pain, and as a tonic after miscarriage. The dried fruit and leaves are used for diarrhea. Tea made from the dried leaves is used for sore throat and other inflammations of the mouth or mucous membranes of the throat. Blueberry juice is used as a contrast agent in magnetic resonance imaging (MRI).
By inhalation, fumes of burning dried blueberry flowers are inhaled for treatment of insanity.

Safety

LIKELY SAFE ...when used orally and appropriately (12).
PREGNANCY AND LACTATION: Insufficient reliable information available; avoid using.

Effectiveness

There is insufficient reliable information available about the effectiveness of blueberry.

Mechanism of Action

The applicable parts of the blueberry are the fruit and leaves. Blueberry fruit is high in fiber and vitamin C. Blueberries also contain anthocyanins and proanthocyanidins, which appear to have antioxidant activity (900,907,908). Ethyl acetate extracts of blueberry fruit inhibit ornithine decarboxylase, which is a key enzyme in tumor progression (888). Preliminary research from animal models suggests that the antioxidant effects of blueberry extracts might have anticancer activity and potentially reduce normal oxidative cellular damage that occurs with aging (888,908,1419,9429). Blueberry, like its relative, the cranberry, also appears to prevent bacterial adhesion to the bladder and bacterial colonization (2813,6757); however, clinical studies have not yet been performed.

Adverse Reactions

None reported.

Interactions with Herbs & Other Dietary Supplements

None known.

Interactions with Drugs
ANTIDIABETES DRUGS: Theoretically, blueberry leaf might lower blood glucose (909); however, this effect has not yet been reported in humans. Until more is known, monitor blood glucose levels more closely in patients with diabetes who are taking blueberry. Dose adjustments may be necessary in patients taking diabetes medications.

Interactions with Foods
None known.

Interactions with Lab Tests
BLOOD GLUCOSE: Theoretically, blueberry leaf might lower blood glucose and test results (909); however, this effect has not yet been reported in humans.
MAGNETIC RESONANCE IMAGING (MRI): Because of the high concentration of manganese in blueberry juice, it may act as a negative contrast agent in MRI of the gastrointestinal tract (9427).
TRIGLYCERIDES: Theoretically, blueberry leaf, which is related to the bilberry, might lower serum triglycerides and test results (909); however, this effect has not yet been reported in humans.

Interactions with Diseases or Conditions
DIABETES: Theoretically, blueberry leaf might lower blood glucose (909); however, this effect has not yet been reported in humans. Until more is known, monitor blood glucose levels more closely in patients with diabetes who are taking blueberry. Dose adjustments may be necessary in patients taking diabetes medications.

Dosage and Administration
No typical dosage.

Comments
Don't confuse blueberry with bilberry. Blueberry in the US refers to the species of Vaccinium listed in this monograph. However, elsewhere in the world, blueberry may refer to the European plant, Vaccinium myrtillus, which is called bilberry in the US.

BOG BILBERRY

Also Known As
Moosbeere, Western-Huckleberry.
CAUTION: See separate listing for Bilberry.

Scientific Names
Vaccinium uliginosum, synonyms Vaccinium gaultherioides, Vaccinium occidentale.
Family: Ericaceae.

People Use This For
Orally, bog bilberry is used for mucous membrane inflammation of the gastric and intestinal tract, diarrhea, and bladder complaints.

Safety
POSSIBLY UNSAFE ...when used orally in large amounts. Poisoning has been reported when individuals ingest fruit from fungus-infested plants (18).
There is insufficient reliable information available about the safety of dried bog bilberry fruit used in medicinal amounts.
PREGNANCY AND LACTATION: POSSIBLY UNSAFE ...when used orally in large amounts; avoid using (18).

Effectiveness
There is insufficient reliable information available about the effectiveness of bog bilberry.

Mechanism of Action
The applicable part of bog bilberry is the dried, ripe fruit. The active constituents of bog bilberry are tannins, anthocyanoside, and flavonoids (18).

Adverse Reactions
Orally, poisonings from the ingestion of large quantities of the bog bilberry fruit are rare and could have been due to contamination with a fungus, Sclerroyina megalospora (18). The symptoms of poisoning include queasiness, vomiting, states of intoxication, feelings of weakness, and visual disorders (18).

Interactions with Herbs & Other Dietary Supplements
None known.

Interactions with Drugs
None known.

Interactions with Foods
None known.

Interactions with Lab Tests
None known.

Interactions with Diseases or Conditions
None known.

Dosage and Administration
ORAL: The usual dose of bog bilberry is one cup of the unsweetened tea once or twice daily (18). The tea is prepared by steeping 2 heaping teaspoons of the dried, ripe fruit in 250 mL cold water for 10-12 hours and then straining.

Comments
Avoid confusion with bilberry fruit or bilberry leaf.

BOGBEAN

Also Known As
Buckbean, Marsh Trefoil, Menyanthes, Water Shamrock.

Scientific Names
Menyanthes trifoliata.
Family: Menyanthaceae.

People Use This For
Orally, bogbean is used for rheumatism, rheumatoid arthritis, loss of appetite, and dyspepsia.
In food manufacturing, bogbean is used as a flavoring agent.

Safety
LIKELY SAFE ...when used orally in amounts commonly found in foods. The Council of Europe lists bogbean as a natural food flavoring (4).
POSSIBLY SAFE ...when used orally in medicinal amounts (12).
POSSIBLY UNSAFE ...when used orally in excessive amounts. Bogbean leaf preparations can irritate the GI tract (4).
PREGNANCY AND LACTATION: POSSIBLY UNSAFE ...when used orally due to the lack of toxicity information and its possible purgative action (4); avoid using.

Effectiveness
There is insufficient reliable information available about the effectiveness of bogbean.

Mechanism of Action
The applicable part of bogbean is the leaf. The bitter principles, or iridoids, can stimulate saliva and gastric juices (2,4). Bogbean can have purgative actions (4). An unidentified constituent has hemolytic activity (4).

Adverse Reactions
Orally, excessive doses of bogbean can irritate the GI tract, and cause diarrhea, pain, nausea, and vomiting. Theoretically, it can cause bleeding (4).

Interactions with Herbs & Other Dietary Supplements
None known.

Interactions with Drugs
ANTICOAGULANT/ANTIPLATELET DRUGS: Theoretically, bogbean can increase the risk of bleeding.

Interactions with Foods
None known.

Interactions with Lab Tests
None known.

Interactions with Diseases or Conditions
DIARRHEA, DYSENTERY, COLITIS: Contraindicated (12).
PEOPLE AT RISK FOR BLEEDING: Theoretically, bogbean can increase bleeding risk.

Dosage and Administration
ORAL: The typical dose of bogbean is 1-3 grams of the dried leaf three times daily or as a tea three times daily. The tea is prepared by steeping 1-3 grams of the dried leaf in 150 mL boiling water for 5-10 minutes and then straining (2,4). The common dose of the liquid extract (1:1 in 25% alcohol) is 1-2 mL three times daily (4). The tincture (1:5 in 45% alcohol) is usually given as 1-3 mL three times daily (4).

Comments
The bogbean fruit resembles a small bean and is commonly found in swamps or bogs, which is the reason for its name (6002).

BOIS DE ROSE OIL

Also Known As
Cayenne Rosewood Oil, Distilled Oil from Aniba Rosaeodora Wood, Rosewood Oil.

Scientific Names
Aniba rosaeodora, synonym Aniba duckei.
Family: Lauraceae.

Comments
At the date of publication, there was very little scientific information about this product. Our staff is continually analyzing the available information on natural medicines and will add data to the online version of *Natural Medicines Comprehensive Database* as it becomes available. See www.naturaldatabase.com.

BOLDO

Also Known As
Boldine, Boldo Folium, Boldoak Boldea, Boldus, Boldus Boldus.

Scientific Names
Peumus boldus, synonyms Boldea fragrans, Peumus fragrans.
Family: Monimiaceae.

People Use This For
Orally, boldo is used for mild gastrointestinal (GI) spasms, gallstones, rheumatism, cystitis, hepatic disease, and gonorrhea. It is also used as a diuretic, sedative, bile stimulant, and antiseptic.

Safety
LIKELY SAFE ...when used in amounts commonly found in foods. Boldo has Generally Recognized As Safe (GRAS) status in the US (4912).
LIKELY UNSAFE ...when used excessively for oral medicinal purposes; the volatile oil (2.5% in leaf) contains ascaridole (4). If taken by mouth, ascaridole-free preparations should be used (2).
PREGNANCY AND LACTATION: UNSAFE ...when the volatile oil is used orally, due to ascaridole (4).

Effectiveness
There is insufficient reliable information available about the effectiveness of boldo.

Mechanism of Action

The applicable part of boldo is the leaf. The alkaloidal constituents are responsible for actions that include stimulating bile and bile flow, stimulating stomach function, and diuresis (4). The diuretic and mild urinary antiseptic properties probably result from the irritant volatile oil (4). There's some evidence that the boldine constituent may inhibit thromboxane A2 production, resulting in antiplatelet activity (5191).

Adverse Reactions

Orally, boldo can cause convulsions.
Topically, boldo can irritate the skin (4).

Interactions with Herbs & Other Dietary Supplements

None known.

Interactions with Drugs

ANTICOAGULANT/ANTIPLATELET DRUGS: There is some concern that boldo might have additive effects when used with anticoagulant or antiplatelet drugs and increase the risk of bruising and bleeding. Boldo constituents may have antiplatelet effects (5191). Some of these drugs include aspirin, clopidogrel (Plavix), nonsteroidal anti-inflammatory drugs (NSAIDs) such as diclofenac (Voltaren, Cataflam, others), ibuprofen (Advil, Motrin, others), naproxen (Anaprox, Naprosyn, others), dalteparin (Fragmin), enoxaparin (Lovenox), heparin, and others.
WARFARIN (Coumadin): Boldo may have additive effects with warfarin and increase the international normalized ratio (INR). Boldo constituents may have antiplatelet activity (5191).

Interactions with Foods

None known.

Interactions with Lab Tests

None known.

Interactions with Diseases or Conditions

BILE DUCT OBSTRUCTION: Contraindicated (12).
GALLSTONES: Boldo should not be used for self-medication of gallstones, which requires monitoring (12).
KIDNEY DISORDERS: Avoid boldo products which are not certified as ascaridole-free (4).
LIVER DISEASE: Contraindicated (8,12).

Dosage and Administration

ORAL: The typical dose of boldo is 60-200 mg of the dried leaf three times daily or as a tea three times a day. The tea is prepared by steeping 1 gram of the dried leaf in 150 mL boiling water for 5-10 minutes and then straining (2,4). The common dose of the liquid extract, 1:1 in 45% alcohol, is 0.1-0.3 mL three times daily (4). The tincture, 1:10 in 60% alcohol, is usually given as 0.5-2 mL three times daily (4). The average daily dose of the boldo leaf by infusion is 3 grams (2).

Comments

Fossilized boldo leaves that are over thirteen thousand years old have been found in Chile with the imprints of human teeth on them (6002).

BONESET

Also Known As

Agueweed, Crosswort, Feverwort, Indian Sage, Sweating Plant, Teasel, Thoroughwort, Vegetable Antimony.
CAUTION: See separate listings for Gravel Root and Sage.

Scientific Names

Eupatorium perfoliatum.
Family: Asteraceae/Compositae.

People Use This For

Orally, boneset is used as an antipyretic, diuretic, laxative, emesis, and cathartic.
Boneset is also used to treat influenza (especially with aching muscles), acute bronchitis, nasal inflammation, rheumatism, edema, dengue fever, and pneumonia; and as a stimulant and a diaphoretic.

Safety

POSSIBLY UNSAFE ...when used orally in excessive amounts. Large doses are both cathartic and emetic. Though the alkaloids have not been characterized, hepatotoxic unsaturated pyrrolizidine alkaloids (UPAs) are common in this genus (12).

PREGNANCY AND LACTATION: POSSIBLY UNSAFE ...when used orally (12); avoid using.

Effectiveness

There is insufficient reliable information available about the effectiveness of boneset.

Mechanism of Action

The applicable parts of boneset are the dried leaf and flowering parts. Researchers think the sesquiterpene lactones may have immunostimulant activity (4).

Adverse Reactions

Orally, boneset can cause an allergic reaction in individuals sensitive to the Asteraceae/Compositae family. Members of this family include ragweed, chrysanthemums, marigolds, daisies, and many other herbs.

Interactions with Herbs & Other Dietary Supplements

None known.

Interactions with Drugs

None known.

Interactions with Foods

None known.

Interactions with Lab Tests

None known.

Interactions with Diseases or Conditions

CROSS-ALLERGENICITY: Boneset can cause an allergic reaction in individuals sensitive to the Asteraceae/Compositae family. Members of this family include ragweed, chrysanthemums, marigolds, daisies, and many other herbs.

Dosage and Administration

ORAL: One cup of tea, prepared by steeping 1-2 grams herb in 150 mL boiling water 5-10 minutes, has been used three times daily (4). The typical dosage for the liquid extract, 1:1 in 25% alcohol, is 1-2 mL three times daily (4). 1-4 mL of the tincture, 1:5 in 45% alcohol, has also been used three times daily (4).

Comments

Avoid confusion with gravel root (Eupatorium purpureum) also known as boneset. Snakeroot is a common name used for poisonous Eupatorium species (4).

BORAGE flower, dried above ground parts

Also Known As

Bee Plant, Beebread, Borago, Burrage, Common Borage, Common Bugloss, Cool Tankard, Ox's Tongue, Talewort.
CAUTION: See separate listing for Borage Seed Oil.

Scientific Names

Borago officinalis.
Family: Boraginaceae.

People Use This For

Orally, borage is used for fever, cough, depression, arthritis, pain relief, phlebitis, inflammation, and menopausal disorders. Borage is also used to restore the adrenal cortex, for "blood purification", as a diuretic, as a preventative for inflammation of lungs and peritoneum, as a cardiac tonic, as a sedative, to induce sweating, and to increase circulatory capacity. Borage is also used orally to promote "happiness and courage"; increase breast milk production; and to treat rheumatism, bronchitis, colds, breast cancer, and facial cancer.
Topically, borage is used as a poultice and as an emollient.

In foods, borage is in various products including preserved leaves, salads, and soups.
In manufacturing, borage is used in skin care products.

Safety

POSSIBLY SAFE ...when used orally in amounts commonly found in foods (6).
LIKELY UNSAFE ...when used orally for medicinal uses. Borage flower and dried above ground parts contain hepatotoxic unsaturated pyrrolizidine alkaloids (UPAs) (4,12). Excessive doses or long-term use increases risk of adverse effects (2,4,12).
PREGNANCY AND LACTATION: LIKELY UNSAFE ...when used orally (4,12); avoid using.

Effectiveness

There is insufficient reliable information available about the effectiveness of borage flower and dried above ground parts.

Mechanism of Action

Borage flower and dried above ground parts contain tannins which are thought to give it astringent properties. The mucilage content may contribute to reported expectorant effects. Malic acid and potassium nitrate constituents may have a diuretic effects (6). Borage contains variable amounts of toxic unsaturated pyrrolizidine alkaloids (UPAs) which are organotoxic, hepatotoxic, and carcinogenic in animal models (2). Unlike borage seed, the above ground parts of the plant do not contain gamma-linolenic acid (GLA) (7162).

Adverse Reactions

Orally, use of borage can cause constipation (5,6). The potential for hepatotoxicity, due to unsaturated pyrrolizidine alkaloid (UPA) content, increases with larger doses and longer periods of use (4,12).

Interactions with Herbs & Other Dietary Supplements

EUCALYPTUS: Theoretically, concomitant use might increase the risk of unsaturated pyrrolizidine alkaloid (UPA) toxicity due to enzyme induction by eucalyptus (19).
UNSATURATED PYRROLIZIDINE ALKALOID (UPA)-CONTAINING HERBS: Concomitant use is contraindicated due to the risk of additive toxicity. Herbs containing UPAs include alkanna, gravel root, hemp agrimony, hound's tongue, petasites, comfrey, coltsfoot; and Senecio species, dusty miller, alpine ragwort, groundsel, golden ragwort, and tansy ragwort (4,12,19,271).

Interactions with Drugs

HEPATOTOXIC DRUGS: Theoretically, borage flower and dried above ground parts could have additive toxicity with drugs with hepatotoxic potential (2). Some of these drugs are amidarone (Codarone), fluconazole (Diflucan), itraconazole (Sporanox), carbamazepine (Tegretol), erythromycin (Erythrocin, Illosone, others), estrogens, isoniazid (INH), phenytoin (Dilantin), lovastatin (Mevacor), pravastatin (Pravachol), simvastatin (Zocor), and others.

Interactions with Foods

None known.

Interactions with Lab Tests

None known.

Interactions with Diseases or Conditions

HEPATIC DISEASE: Theoretically, borage flower and dried above ground parts could worsen hepatic disease. Borage flower and dried above ground parts contain hepatotoxic unsaturated pyrrolizidine alkaloids (UPAs) (2).

Dosage and Administration

No typical dosage.

Comments

Avoid confusion with borage seed oil.

BORAGE SEED OIL

Also Known As

Borage Oil, Bugloss, Burage, Burrage, Huile De Bourrache, Starflower.
CAUTION: See separate listings for Borage flower, Black Currant, Evening Primrose Oil, Gamma Linolenic Acid, and Omega-6 Fatty Acids.

Scientific Names

Borago officinalis.
Family: Boraginaceae.

People Use This For

Orally, borage seed oil is used for rheumatoid arthritis, neurodermatitis, stress, atopic eczema, and infantile seborrheic dermatitis. It is also used for premenstrual syndrome (PMS), diabetes, attention deficit-hyperactivity disorder (ADHD), acute respiratory distress syndrome (ARDS), alcoholism, inflammation, and for preventing heart disease and stroke.

Safety

POSSIBLY SAFE ...when used orally and appropriately. Only products that are certified and labeled as unsaturated pyrrolizidine alkaloids (UPA)-free should be used (8458).
LIKELY UNSAFE ...when products containing UPAs are used orally. UPAs are hepatotoxic (7631,11882,11883). Although borage seed oil is reported to contain only small amounts of UPAs (502), therapeutic doses of borage seed oil can provide UPA amounts that can reach toxic levels (6002).
PREGNANCY AND LACTATION: Insufficient reliable information available; avoid using.

Effectiveness

POSSIBLY EFFECTIVE

Acute respiratory distress syndrome (ARDS). There is some evidence that borage seed oil might reduce the days in the intensive care unit (ICU) and the duration of ventilator requirement in patients with ARDS when used orally in combination with eicosapentaenoic acid (EPA) (7629).
Rheumatoid arthritis (RA). There is some evidence that taking borage seed oil in combination with conventional analgesics or anti-inflammatory agents might help decrease symptoms of RA after six weeks of treatment. The improvement appears to be sustained for up to 24 weeks. Borage seed oil can decrease the number of tender joints by 36%, the tender joint score by 45%, the number of swollen joints by 28%, and the swollen joint score by 41% (1985,8458).

POSSIBLY INEFFECTIVE

Atopic dermatitis (eczema). Taking borage seed oil orally 500-2000 mg daily for up to 24 weeks does not seem to improve symptoms of atopic dermatitis in adults or children (7632,7633,11341).

INSUFFICIENT RELIABLE EVIDENCE to RATE

Dermatitis. There is some preliminary evidence that topical application of borage seed oil might be helpful for infantile seborrheic dermatitis (7630). More evidence is needed to rate borage seed oil for this use.

Mechanism of Action

Borage seed oil is the fatty oil of the seeds of Borago officinalis. Borage oil contains 18% to 26% of the essential fatty acid gamma-linolenic acid (GLA) (8013). GLA is rapidly metabolized to dihomogammalinolenic acid (DGLA). DGLA is a precursor to prostaglandin E1 (PGE1), which has potent anti-inflammatory properties (6002,8013,12088,12089).
Borage seed oil, in combination with fish oil, modulates the immune system by decreasing the serum activity of interleukin 10 (IL-10) and interleukin 4 (IL-4) and changing the activity of other cytokines (7635). Borage seed oil can decrease the activity of tumor necrosis factor (8459).
The GLA constituent of borage seed oil also seems to lower plasma triglycerides, increase high-density lipoprotein (HDL) levels, decrease blood pressure, and prolong bleeding time (1979,7634,8470). GLA in borage seed oil may reduce the growth of tumors. In addition, metastatic extension of tumors may be reduced by increasing tumor cell adhesion locally and reducing endothelium adhesion at distant metastatic sites (8013).
GLA might have an antiestrogenic effect. It seems to modulate the sensitivity of breast cancer cells to paclitaxel (Taxol) and fulvestrant (Faslodex), enhancing malignant cell-killing without adverse effects on normal cells (8133,11791). However, other research suggests that GLA alone can stimulate the growth of breast cancer cells at low concentrations and inhibit growth at higher concentrations (11339).
It has been theorized that low arachidonic acid levels in breast milk of atopic mothers might increase the risk for development of atopy in infants; however, maternal oral supplementation with borage seed oil does not increase the concentration of arachidonic acid in breast milk (6106).
Some borage seed oil preparations contain toxic constituents known as unsaturated pyrrolizidine alkaloids (UPAs). The main liver injury induced by UPAs is veno-occlusive disease. Hepatotoxicity may result form biotransformation

by cytochrome P450 (CYP450) enzymes of UPAs into unstable toxic metabolites, which may then serve as alkylating agents (11882).

Adverse Reactions

Orally, borage seed oil may cause soft stools, diarrhea, belching, and bloating (8013,11341). Gamma linolenic acid (GLA), a component of borage seed oil, can prolong bleeding time (1979).
Hepatotoxicity, renal toxicity, and carcinogenicity may be caused by unsaturated pyrrolizidine alkaloids (UPAs) in some preparations of borage seed oil (7631). Tell patients to use only borage seed oil preparations that are certified and labeled as UPA-free.

Interactions with Herbs & Other Dietary Supplements

HERBS WITH ANTICOAGULANT/ANTIPLATELET POTENTIAL: Theoretically, concomitant use of herbs that have constituents that might affect platelet aggregation could increase the risk of bleeding in some people (1979). These herbs include angelica, clove, danshen, garlic, ginger, ginkgo, ginseng Panax, red clover, turmeric, and others.
UNSATURATED PYRROLIZIDINE ALKALOID-CONTAINING HERBS: Concomitant use is contraindicated due to the risk of additive toxicity (11882). Herbs containing unsaturated pyrrolizidine alkaloids (UPAs) include alkanna, gravel root, hemp agrimony, hound's tongue, petasites, comfrey, coltsfoot, and the Senecio species plants; dusty miller, alpine ragwort, groundsel, golden ragwort, and tansy ragwort.

Interactions with Drugs

ANESTHESIA: Theoretically, concomitant use can increase the risk of seizures based on one case report of evening primrose oil (another source of gamma linolenic acid) and possibly other drugs (613).
ANTICOAGULANT/ANTIPLATELET DRUGS: Borage seed oil, which contains gamma linolenic acid (GLA), could have anticoagulant effects (1979). Theoretically, taking borage seed oil with other anticoagulant or antiplatelet drugs might increase the risk of bruising and bleeding. Some of these drugs include aspirin; clopidogrel (Plavix); nonsteroidal anti-inflammatory drugs (NSAIDs) such as diclofenac (Voltaren, Cataflam, others), ibuprofen (Advil, Motrin, others), and naproxen (Anaprox, Naprosyn, others); dalteparin (Fragmin); enoxaparin (Lovenox); heparin, warfarin (Coumadin); and others.
NONSTEROIDAL ANTI-INFLAMMATORY DRUGS (NSAIDs): Theoretically, concomitant use of nonsteroidal anti-inflammatory drugs (NSAIDs) with borage seed oil might decrease the anti-inflammatory effect of borage seed oil (8459). However, borage seed oil is used commonly with NSAIDs in rheumatoid arthritis, so the clinical significance of this potential interaction is uncertain (1985,8458).

Interactions with Foods

None known.

Interactions with Lab Tests

BLEEDING TIME: Borage seed oil might prolong bleeding time. Borage seed oil contains gamma linolenic acid (GLA), which can inhibit platelet aggregation (1979).
LIPID PROFILE: Borage seed oil might affect lipid levels. Borage seed oil contains gamma linolenic acid (GLA), which can lower plasma triglycerides and increase high-density lipoprotein (HDL) cholesterol (1979).

Interactions with Diseases or Conditions

BLEEDING DISORDERS: There is some concern that borage seed oil might prolong bleeding time and increase the risk of bruising and bleeding. Borage seed oil contains gamma linolenic acid (GLA), which can inhibit platelet aggregation (1979).
LIVER DISEASE: Borage seed oil might exacerbate liver disease. Borage seed oil can contain hepatotoxic unsaturated pyrrolizidine alkaloids (UPAs) (7631). Tell patients with liver disease to only use products certified and labeled as unsaturated pyrrolizidine alkaloid (UPA)-free.

Dosage and Administration

ORAL: For rheumatoid arthritis, studies have used either 1.1 or 1.4 grams borage seed oil daily for up to 24 weeks (8458). For atopic dermatitis, 500-2000 mg borage seed oil daily has been used for up to 24 weeks (7632,11341).
TOPICAL: For infantile seborrheic dermatitis, 0.5 mL of borage seed oil applied two times daily for 10 to 12 days, has been used. After the lesions resolve, borage seed oil has been applied two to three times each week until the infants reach six to seven months of age (7630).

Comments

Some sources have suggested that borage seed oil could be used as an alternative to evening primrose oil because both are good sources of gamma-linolenic acid (GLA) (6002).

BORON

Also Known As
Borate, Borates, Boric Acid, Boric Anhydride, Boric Tartrate, Sodium Borate.

Scientific Names
Boron; B; atomic number 5.

People Use This For
Orally, boron is used for promoting bone health, treating osteoarthritis, as an aid for building muscles and increasing testosterone levels, and for enhancing cognitive function and fine motor skills.
Topically, boric acid, the most common form of boron, is used as an astringent, to prevent skin infection, and as an ophthalmological irrigant.

Safety
LIKELY SAFE ...when used orally and appropriately. Boron is safe in amounts that do not exceed 20 mg per day, the Tolerable Upper Intake Level (UL) (7135). ...when used topically and appropriately. Boric acid, the most common form of boron, can be safely applied to non-broken skin (6).
POSSIBLY UNSAFE ...when used orally in high doses. Tell patients to avoid exceeding the UL of 20 mg per day. Higher doses might theoretically cause adverse effects on the testes and male fertility (7135). Poisoning has occurred after ingestion of equivalent of 2.12 grams boron per day for 3-4 weeks (17).
CHILDREN: LIKELY SAFE ...when used orally and appropriately. Boron is safe in children in amounts that do not exceed the UL of 3 mg per day in children 1 to 3 years; 6 mg per day in children 4 to 8 years; 11 mg per day in children 9 to 13 years; 17 mg per day in adolescents 14 years or older (7135). The UL for infants has not been determined (7135). POSSIBLY UNSAFE ...when used orally in high doses. Tell patients to avoid exceeding the UL of 3 mg per day in children 1 to 3 years; 6 mg per day in children 4 to 8 years; 11 mg per day in children 9 to 13 years; and 17 mg per day in adolescents 14 years or older (7135). Higher doses might theoretically cause adverse effects on the testes and male fertility (7135).
PREGNANCY AND LACTATION: LIKELY SAFE ...when used orally and appropriately. Boron is safe in amounts that do not exceed the UL of 20 mg per day for pregnant or lactating women 19-50 years, or 17 mg per day for pregnant or lactating women ages 14 to 18 (7135). POSSIBLY UNSAFE ...when used orally in high doses. Tell patients to avoid exceeding the UL of 20 mg per day for pregnant or lactating women 19-50 years, or 17 mg per day for pregnant or lactating women ages 14 to 18 (7135). Higher doses might theoretically cause adverse effects in the developing fetus (7135).

Effectiveness
POSSIBLY INEFFECTIVE

Athletic conditioning. Taking boron orally doesn't seem to help increase lean body mass, muscle mass, or testosterone levels (944).

INSUFFICIENT RELIABLE EVIDENCE to RATE

Cognitive function. There is preliminary evidence that taking boron orally might improve cognitive function and fine motor skills in older people (943).

Osteoarthritis. Preliminary evidence suggests that boron might be useful for decreasing symptoms of osteoarthritis (941).

More evidence is needed to rate boron for these uses.

Mechanism of Action
Boron is a trace mineral for which a clear biological function in humans has not been established. There is some evidence, though, that boron might have a role in reproduction and development (945,7135). Boron is well absorbed from dietary beverages including prune and grape juice; wine; coffee; milk; and in some geographical locations, water (7135). Avocados, peanuts, pecans, apples, dried beans, and potatoes also contain boron (7135). Boron is excreted unchanged in the urine, with a half-life of 21 hours (7135).
Boron seems to be important in mineral metabolism and membrane function (943). Diets higher in boron seem to increase serum 17-beta-estradiol levels in postmenopausal women using estrogen replacement therapy (945). Supplemental boron may increase serum estradiol levels in postmenopausal women (945) and healthy men (937). Boron together with exercise seems to result in lower serum magnesium levels and modestly lower serum phosphorus concentrations (942). The lower serum phosphorus concentrations are diminished by exercise (940). Preliminary evidence suggests that boron may have a role in hand-eye coordination, attention span, and short-term memory (7135).

Adverse Reactions
Orally, boron appears to have a low toxicity (7135). Adverse reactions in doses below 10 mg per day (937) are unlikely. Chronic use of 1 gram daily of boric acid or 25 grams daily of boric tartrate can cause dermatitis, alopecia, anorexia,

and indigestion (7135). Boric acid/borate can be fatal when taken orally in doses of 300 mg/kg (6).
Large doses can result in acute poisoning. Children who have ingested 5 grams or more of borates can have persistent nausea, vomiting, and diarrhea leading to acute dehydration, shock, and coma. Adults who have ingested 15-20 grams of borate can exhibit nausea, vomiting, diarrhea, epigastric pain, hematemesis, and a blue-green discoloration of feces and vomit (17). Poisoning symptoms in adults and children may also include skin erythema, desquamation, exfoliation, hyperexcitability, irritability, tremors, convulsions, weakness, lethargy, headaches, and depression (17).

Interactions with Herbs & Other Dietary Supplements

MAGNESIUM: Boron supplements can reduce urinary excretion of magnesium and increase serum levels in women (940,9529,9623). In young women, age 18 to 25 years, the effect appears to be greater in sedentary than athletic women (940). In postmenopausal women, the effect is more marked in women with low dietary magnesium intake (9623). The clinical significance of these effects, and whether they occur in men, isn't known.
PHOSPHORUS: Supplemental boron might reduce serum phosphorus concentrations in some individuals (942).

Interactions with Drugs

ESTROGENS: Concomitant administration may increase serum estrogen levels (945).

Interactions with Foods

None known.

Interactions with Lab Tests

BONE MINERAL DENSITY (BMD): Supplemental boron may increase BMD and BMD measurements in young athletic females (942).
MAGNESIUM: Supplemental boron may reduce magnesium excretion and increase magnesium levels in women (940,9529,9623). Whether this occurs in men is unknown.
PHOSPHORUS: Supplemental boron might reduce serum phosphorus concentrations and test results in some individuals (942).

Interactions with Diseases or Conditions

HORMONE SENSITIVE CANCERS/CONDITIONS: Because boron might have estrogenic effects (945), women with hormone sensitive conditions should avoid supplemental boron or high amounts of boron from foods. Some of these conditions include breast cancer, uterine cancer, ovarian cancer, endometriosis, and uterine fibroids.
KIDNEY DISEASE/IMPAIRED KIDNEY FUNCTION: Theoretically, avoid supplements; boron appears to be largely excreted by kidneys (939).

Dosage and Administration

ORAL: There is no RDA for boron since an essential biological role for it has not been identified (7135). Dietary intake of boron varies. Diets considered to be high in boron provide approximately 3.25 mg boron per 2000 kcal/day. Diets considered to be low in boron provide 0.25 mg boron per 2000 kcal/day (943).
The Tolerable Upper Intake Level (UL), the maximum dose at which no adverse effects would be expected, is 20 mg per day for adults and pregnant or lactating women over 19 years (7135). For adolescents 14 to 18 years and pregnant or lactating women 14 to 18 years, the UL is 17 mg per day (7135). For children 9 to 13 years, the UL is 11 mg per day; children 4 to 8 years, 6 mg per day; and children 1 to 3 years, 3 mg per day. A UL has not been established for infants (7135).

Comments

Boron was used as a food preservative between 1870 and 1920, and during World Wars I and II (945).

BOVINE CARTILAGE

Also Known As

Antitumor Angiogenesis Factor (anti-TAF), Bovine Tracheal Cartilage (BTC), Catrix, Catrix-S, Glycosaminoglycan Polysulphuric Acid Complex, Processed Bovine Cartilage, Psoriacin, Psoriacin-T, Rumalon.
CAUTION: See separate listings for Shark Cartilage and Chondroitin Sulfate.

Scientific Names

None.

People Use This For

Orally, bovine cartilage is used for rheumatoid arthritis, osteoarthritis, ulcerative colitis, scleroderma, psoriasis, allergic reactions caused by chemical toxins, herpes infection, glioblastoma multiforme, and cancer.

Topically, bovine cartilage is used for non-healing ulcerated wounds, moist lesions including pruritus ani, external hemorrhoids, acne, poison oak or poison ivy dermatitis, mandibular alveolitis (dry socket), and psoriasis.
Rectally, bovine cartilage is used for internal hemorrhoids and anal fissures.
Subcutaneously, bovine cartilage is used for osteoarthritis; rheumatoid arthritis; psoriasis; ulcerative colitis; regional enteritis; progressive systemic sclerosis; glioblastoma multiforme; inoperable squamous cancer of the nose; and cancers of the pancreas, lung, ovary, rectum, prostate, cervix, and thyroid.
Intramuscularly, bovine cartilage is used for osteoarthritis.

Safety

POSSIBLY SAFE ...when used orally, topically, subcutaneously, or intramuscularly and appropriately. Bovine cartilage has been used orally, topically, subcutaneously, and intramuscularly for up to five years without significant adverse effects (2009,2010,8242). Orally, up to 20 kg total have been used without evidence of toxicity. Subcutaneously, up to 40 grams per week and 300 grams total have been injected without evidence of toxicity. Intramuscularly, a complex including bovine cartilage and bone marrow (Rumalon) has been used safely when given in a total of ten treatment courses over five years. However, since these preparations are derived from animals, there is concern about contamination with diseased animal parts (1825). So far, there are no reports of disease transmission to humans due to use of contaminated bovine cartilage.
PREGNANCY AND LACTATION: Insufficient reliable information available; avoid using.

Effectiveness

POSSIBLY EFFECTIVE

Acne. Applying bovine cartilage topically seems to help reduce acne (2009).
Anal fissures. Rectal use of bovine cartilage seems to help treat anal fissures (2009).
Anal pruritus. Applying a 5% bovine cartilage cream topically at least twice daily seems to help relieve itching within three days (2009).
Hemorrhoids. Rectal use of bovine cartilage seems to be help reduce hemorrhoids (2009).
Mandibular alveolitis. Applying bovine cartilage topically seems to be help treat mandibular alveolitis (2009).
Osteoarthritis. Administering bovine cartilage subcutaneously seems to help reduce symptoms of osteoarthritis (2009). However, intramuscular administration does not seem to be beneficial (8242).
Poison oak and poison ivy dermatitis. Applying a 5% bovine cartilage cream topically seems to help resolve dermatitis within one to two weeks (2009).
Psoriasis. There is some evidence that bovine cartilage can help patients with psoriasis when used topically or subcutaneously. However, churning symptoms, the appearance of new papules as the original lesions fade, may occur for three to six weeks during treatment. These are thought to result from release of psoriagens from present lesions. Eventually, these psoriagens seem to be excreted or metabolized, and then symptoms improve (2009).
Rheumatoid arthritis (RA). Administering bovine cartilage subcutaneously seems to help reduce symptoms of RA (2009).

There is insufficient reliable information available about the effectiveness of bovine cartilage for its other uses.

Mechanism of Action

Bovine cartilage is typically derived from bovine trachea rings. Some researchers think that bovine cartilage provides the needed biochemical components to support resynthesis of cartilage in individuals with osteoarthritis. It might also have anti-inflammatory effects (2009). Bovine cartilage is also thought to have immunoregulatory, hygroscopic-drying, and wound-healing activity (2009).

Adverse Reactions

Orally, bovine cartilage can cause osmotic diarrhea, nausea, and scrotal edema (2009). Subcutaneously, bovine cartilage might initially cause local redness, swelling, and itching (2010). To minimize initial local allergic reaction after subcutaneous administration, the first treatment dose should be limited to 2.5 grams, and administered in combination with oral diphenhydramine 25 mg for the first four treatments (2010). The appearance of new psoriatic papules (2009) and nephrotic syndrome (2011) has also occurred with use of bovine cartilage. Intramuscularly, bovine cartilage might initially cause local redness, rash, swelling, and itching (8242). Bovine cartilage can also cause local allergic reaction (2010). Since these products are derived from bovine tissues, there is some concern about the transmission of bovine spongiform encephalopathy to humans (1825). However, transmission of bovine disease to humans has not been reported with these products.

Interactions with Herbs & Other Dietary Supplements

None known.

Interactions with Drugs

None known.

Interactions with Foods

None known.

Interactions with Lab Tests
None known.

Interactions with Diseases or Conditions
None known.

Dosage and Administration
ORAL: For ulcerative colitis, a dose of 3 grams four times daily has been used (2009).
TOPICAL: For anal pruritus, a 5% cream applied two or more times daily has been used (2009). For poison ivy/oak dermatitis, a 5% cream has been applied every two hours initially and less frequently as itching is controlled (2009). For acne, a 5% cream has been applied at least twice daily after washing (2009). For mandibular alveolitis, powdered bovine cartilage mixed with saline to form a paste, packed into the dry socket following tooth extraction has been used (2009). For psoriasis, parenteral therapy followed by 5% ointment applied two to three times daily after bathing has been used (2009).
RECTAL: As a stool softener for hemorrhoids and anal fissures, bovine cartilage 2.2 grams in the form of a 2% suppository administered at least three times daily with oral dioctyl sodium sulfosuccinate (DSS) 100 mg twice daily has been used (2009).
SUBCUTANEOUS (SC): In general, 5-25 grams is usually given weekly or biweekly for most indications. An exception is osteoarthritis, where doses up to 40 grams have been used. For psoriasis, doses of up to 75 grams have been used. For cancer, doses of 100-300 grams have been used, followed by an oral maintenance dose of 3 grams every eight hours for a maximum dose for the course of treatment of 20 kilograms. Bovine cartilage solutions for subcutaneous injection are usually prepared in a concentration of 50 mg/mL (diluted 1:10 with 1% lidocaine to alleviate discomfort). Doses of 25-50 mL (1.25-2.5 grams) are slowly injected in different sites with an 18-gauge needle until the total dose (e.g., 5-300 grams) is reached. Common sites of administration include the flanks, anterior thorax, abdomen, or anterior thighs, where subcutaneous space is readily distensible (2009,2010). To minimize initial local allergic reaction, the first treatment dose should be limited to 2.5 grams, and administered with oral diphenhydramine 25 mg for the first four treatments (2010).
INTRAMUSCULAR (IM): For osteoarthritis, a complex including bovine cartilage and bone marrow (Rumalon) has been used. It has been given in a total of ten treatment courses over five years. Each course consists of 15 total injections of 2 mL of the complex, administered twice weekly. Two courses are given each year (8242).

Comments
Catrix is a name which refers to activated acid-pepsin-digested bovine tracheal cartilage of calf origin (2009).

BOXWOOD

Also Known As
Boxwood Extract, Bush Tree, Buxaceae, Buxus, Dudgeon, SPV 30, SPV-30, SPV30.

Scientific Names
Buxus sempervirens, synonyms Buxus colchica, Buxus hyrcana.
Family: Buxaceae.

People Use This For
Orally, boxwood is used to treat HIV/AIDS and to boost immunity. Boxwood is also used for arthritis and as a "blood detoxifying agent."

Safety
POSSIBLY SAFE ...when the leaf extract is used orally and appropriately. There is some evidence that the boxwood leaf extract can be used safely for up to 16 months (5643).
LIKELY UNSAFE ...when the whole leaf is used orally (12,18). The whole boxwood leaf can cause life threatening side effects including seizures, paralysis, and death by asphyxiation (18).
PREGNANCY AND LACTATION: LIKELY UNSAFE ...when the whole leaf is used orally (12,18); avoid using. There is insufficient reliable information available about the safety of the boxwood leaf extract when used during pregnancy and lactation; avoid using.

Effectiveness
INSUFFICIENT RELIABLE EVIDENCE to RATE

HIV/AIDS. There is preliminary evidence that a specific boxwood leaf extract (SPV30) 990 mg per day might delay disease progression in HIV-infected patients. It seems to delay decreases in CD4 cell counts, increases in viral load, and/or progression to AIDS in asymptomatic patients with CD4 counts greater than 350 cells per microliter and a relatively low viral load. A higher dose of 1980 mg per day does not seem to be effective possibly due to oxidative stress induced by flavonoids in the extract (5643). More evidence is needed to rate boxwood for this use.

Mechanism of Action
The applicable part of boxwood is the leaf. More than 20 steroidal alkaloids and four steroidal alkamines have been isolated from the boxwood extract. The extract containing cyclobuxine D and buxamine appears to be active against HIV; however, the mechanism is not known (4447). There is some speculation that flavonoids in the boxwood extract inhibit viral replication; however, there is not yet scientific evidence to support this.

Adverse Reactions
Orally, boxwood leaf extract can cause diarrhea and abdominal cramps. Ingestion of whole-leaf boxwood can cause serious side effects including vomiting, diarrhea, severe clonic spasms, paralysis and death secondary to asphyxiation (18). The extract, however, does not seem to have these effects (5643).
Topically, the fresh plant can also cause contact dermatitis (18).

Interactions with Herbs & Other Dietary Supplements
None known.

Interactions with Drugs
None known.

Interactions with Foods
None known.

Interactions with Lab Tests
None known.

Interactions with Diseases or Conditions
None known.

Dosage and Administration
ORAL: For HIV, a specific boxwood leaf extract (SPV30) 330 mg every 8 hours has been used (5643). Higher doses do not appear to be effective (5643).

Comments
Boxwood extract (SPV 30) is not usually found on store shelves. Most users get it through Internet sources or AIDS buyers' clubs.

BRAHMI

Also Known As
Bacopa, Jalanimba, Jalnaveri, Nira-Brahmi, Sambrani Chettu, Thyme-Leave Gratiola.
CAUTION: See separate listing for Gotu Kola.

Scientific Names
Bacopa monnieri, synonym Bacopa monniera; Herpestis monniera; Moniera cuneifolia.
Family: Scrophulariaceae.

People Use This For
Orally, brahmi is used to aid learning, and for anxiety, memory problems, attention deficit-hyperactivity disorder (ADHD), allergic conditions, and irritable bowel syndrome. Brahmi has also been used orally for treating backache, hoarseness, mental illness, epilepsy, rheumatism, sexual dysfunction in both men and women, as a nerve tonic, cardiotonic, and as a diuretic.

Safety
POSSIBLY SAFE ...when used orally and appropriately for up to 12 weeks (10058).
PREGNANCY AND LACTATION: Insufficient reliable information available; avoid using.

Effectiveness
POSSIBLY EFFECTIVE

Cognitive function. Taking 300 mg brahmi extract per day for 12 weeks seems to improve verbal learning, memory, and information processing in healthy men and women (10058).

POSSIBLY INEFFECTIVE

Irritable bowel syndrome (IBS). Brahmi appears to be no more effective than placebo in preventing relapse of IBS (10059).

There is insufficient reliable information available about the effectiveness of brahmi for its other uses.

Mechanism of Action

The applicable part of brahmi is the leaf. Pharmacological activity of brahmi is attributed to the saponin bacoside and bacopasaponin constituents (10060,10061). Some evidence suggests purified bacosides A and B may facilitate learning ability and cognitive performance. Possible mechanisms for cognitive improvement include modulation of acetylcholine release, choline acetylase activity, and muscarinic cholinergic receptor binding (10058). Brahmi may also act as a mast cell stabilizer for allergic conditions (10060).

Adverse Reactions

Orally, brahmi can cause nausea, dry mouth, and fatigue (10058).

Interactions with Herbs & Other Dietary Supplements

None known.

Interactions with Drugs

None known.

Interactions with Foods

None known.

Interactions with Lab Tests

None known.

Interactions with Diseases or Conditions

None known.

Dosage and Administration

ORAL: For cognitive function improvement, a dosage of 300 mg brahmi extract per day has been used (10058).

Comments

Brahmi is a well-known herb in India and is frequently used in Ayurvedic herbal preparations. The name "brahmi" is derived from Brahma, a mystical creator of the Hindu pantheon. Centella asiatica (gotu kola) and Merremia gangetica have also been referred to by the name "brahmi," but most authorities associate brahmi with Bacopa monnieri (10061).

BRANCHED-CHAIN AMINO ACIDS

Also Known As

BCAA, Isoleucine, Leucine, L-Isoleucine, L-Leucine, L-Valine, Valine.
CAUTION: See separate listing for Whey Protein.

Scientific Names

2-amino-3-methylvaleric acid; 2-amino-4-methylvaleric acid; 2-amino-3-methylbutanoic acid.

People Use This For

Orally, branched-chain amino acids are used to enhance exercise performance, prevent fatigue, improve concentration, and reduce protein and muscle breakdown during intense exercise. They are also used for amyotrophic lateral sclerosis (ALS, Lou Gehrig's disease), latent portosystemic encephalopathy, and chronic hepatic encephalopathy. Branched-chain amino acids have also been used orally to treat anorexia in cancer patients, tardive dyskinesia, McArdle's disease (a genetic glycogen metabolic disorder), spinocerebellar degeneration, and to attenuate muscle-wasting during bed rest.

Intravenously, branched-chain amino acids are used for acute hepatic encephalopathy and in conditions of high metabolic stress due to severe trauma or sepsis.

Safety

LIKELY SAFE ...when used intravenously and appropriately. Branched-chain amino acids are an FDA-approved injectable product (15).

POSSIBLY SAFE ...when used orally and appropriately, short-term. Branched-chain amino acids have not been associated with significant adverse effects in studies lasting from 1-2 weeks up to 6 months (68,72,73,74,10117,10146,10147).

PREGNANCY AND LACTATION: Insufficient reliable information available; avoid using.

Effectiveness

POSSIBLY EFFECTIVE

Anorexia. Taking branched-chain amino acids orally seems to reduce anorexia and improve the overall nutritional status in elderly malnourished hemodialysis patients. A combination of branched-chain amino acids consisting of valine, leucine, and isoleucine may rapidly improve appetite and caloric intake, increasing plasma albumin levels and anthropometric measurements (10147). There is also some preliminary evidence that oral branched-chain amino acids might be helpful for anorexia in cancer patients (71).

Hepatic encephalopathy. Taking branched-chain amino acids orally can improve liver function tests and nitrogen balance in patients with chronic hepatic encephalopathy (68,69,82,690). Oral branched-chain amino acids are recommended for malnourished chronic hepatic encephalopathy patients who cannot tolerate protein supplementation (69,4274). When the enteral route is unavailable and in patients who cannot tolerate general purpose amino acid solutions, intravenous solutions with branched-chain amino acids can be used for nutritional support; however, most patients can tolerate standard amino acid mixtures (4274). In patients with latent hepatic encephalopathy taking branched-chain amino acids orally long-term seems to help improve psychomotor function and driving ability (684,685). There is also some preliminary evidence that intravenous branched-chain amino acids might be helpful for reversing coma in acute hepatic encephalopathy. So far, findings are conflicting (66,81,686,687,688,689,4274).

Mania. A tyrosine-free amino acid drink containing leucine, isoleucine, and valine, seems to diminish acute manic symptoms within 6 hours. When taken daily for 7 days, it seems to continue to improve symptoms over a 2-week period (10117).

Muscle breakdown. Taking branched-chain amino acids orally seems to reduce muscle breakdown during exercise (694).

Tardive dyskinesia. Taking branched-chain amino acids orally seems to reduce symptoms of tardive dyskinesia (72,10146). A branched-chain amino acid drink containing valine, isoleucine, and leucine seems to reduce tardive dyskinesia movements by 30-60% in patients receiving antipsychotic treatment (10146).

POSSIBLY INEFFECTIVE

Athletic performance. Taking branched-chain amino acids orally doesn't seem to enhance exercise or athletic performance (692).

LIKELY INEFFECTIVE

Amyotrophic lateral sclerosis (ALS, Lou Gehrig's disease). Early studies indicated that taking branched-chain amino acids orally are effective for ALS; however, more recent studies show no benefit and possibly excess loss of pulmonary function and mortality among patients using branched-chain amino acids (678,679,680,681).

INSUFFICIENT RELIABLE EVIDENCE to RATE

Diabetes. There is some preliminary evidence that ingestion of carbohydrates with an amino acid/protein mixture consisting of leucine 25%, phenylalanine 25%, and a wheat protein hydrolysate 50%, may increase the insulin response in patients with type 2 diabetes. Whether dietary supplementation of such a mixture can increase the efficacy of glucose-lowering medications or reduce dependency on insulin is unknown (10118).

Spinocerebellar degeneration (SCD). There is some preliminary clinical evidence that oral branched-chain amino acids might have a beneficial effect on symptoms of SCD (73).

More evidence is needed to rate branched-chain amino acids for these uses.

Mechanism of Action

Branched-chain amino acids are essential amino acids, including leucine, isoleucine, and valine (15,66,10116).

Branched-chain amino acids are found in dietary protein, such as meat, dairy products, and legumes, and account for 15-25% of the total daily intake of protein (10116). Branched-chain amino acids act in numerous metabolic processes as modulators of protein synthesis, as substrates for protein synthesis, and as precursors in the synthesis of alanine and glutamine (10110,10116).

Branched-chain amino acids, in particular leucine, act as signaling molecules to stimulate protein synthesis (10110).

Branched-chain amino acids seem to simulate pancreatic islet cells to release insulin, which is required for maximal stimulation of protein synthesis (10105,10108,10109,10110,10112,10113,10114). Skeletal muscle is the major site where branched-chain amino acids stimulate protein synthesis and are metabolized (78,10110). Branched-chain amino acids also stimulate protein synthesis in the adipose tissue and liver but not in the heart or kidney (10111). Evidence indicates most, if not all, of the effects of protein synthesis in skeletal muscle is attributable to leucine alone (10108). The brain and kidney are involved in branched-chain amino acid metabolism but to a lesser degree than skeletal muscle (78). The sensitivity of branched-chain amino acids to stimulate protein synthesis appears to decline with age (10110).

The metabolism and degradation of branched-chain amino acids is linked to the production of alanine and glutamine and the maintenance of glucose homeostasis. The relationship between branched-chain amino acids and glucose metabolism is that they are associated with the glucose-alanine cycle. Branched-chain amino acids are continuously released from the liver and transported to skeletal muscle. Uptake of branched-chain amino acids by the muscle stimulates the transamination of branched-chain amino acids, which results in the production of glutamine and also the transfer of nitrogen from BCAA to pyruvate to produce alanine. Alanine circulates to the liver to support hepatic gluconeogenesis. The glucose-alanine cycle might account for greater than 40% of the glucose produced during prolonged exercise (10116).

The oral administration of branched-chain amino acids before exercise increases serum ammonia levels during exercise (693,694); and appears to decrease muscle breakdown (694) and inhibit muscle glycogen degradation during exercise (77).

Branched-chain amino acids also cross the blood brain barrier rapidly. Branched-chain amino acids play a role in the oxidation and synthesis of the excitatory neurotransmitter glutamate. Researchers think that dietary intake of branched-chain amino acids may be necessary to maintain pools of glutamate in the central nervous system (10107). Increased intake of branched-chain amino acids seems to decrease the synthesis of amine neurotransmitters such as dopamine, noradrenaline, and serotonin. Branched-chain amino acids decrease peripheral levels of aromatic amino acids, which are precursors of amine neurotransmitters, and reduce the amount of aromatic amino acids that is available for transport to the brain. An excess of neurotransmitters is associated with disorders such as tardive dyskinesia (10146). Branched-chain amino acids also compete with aromatic amino acids such as tryptophan, tyrosine, phenylalanine, and methionine for access to the neural amino acid transport system that allows amino acid entry into the brain (66,79,80,2719,10146). This competitive inhibition is used therapeutically for amino acid imbalances that produce false neurotransmitters in pathologic conditions such as hepatic encephalopathy (66,2719). Branched-chain amino acids are also used in hepatic encephalopathy as an energy source to prevent endogenous catabolism of proteins and reduce ammonia detoxification in the brain by increasing ammonia metabolism in skeletal muscle (69).

There is preliminary evidence diets deficient in branched-chain amino acids, including leucine, might be associated with decreased appetite and the development of anorexia. Continued consumption of such a diet is thought to cause a conditioned taste aversion and involve several neurotransmitters in the brain, including norepinephrine, GABA, serotonin, dopamine, and nitric oxide. However, the exact mechanism for this is unknown (10115). Supplementation of malnourished elderly patients with branched-chain amino acids seems to reduce anorexia and improve nutritional indices. Branched-chain amino acids might compete with tryptophan, a precursor for serotonin, for uptake across the blood brain barrier. By decreasing the synthesis of serotonin, branched-chain amino acids might increase appetite (10147).

There is some evidence daily administration of branched-chain amino acids containing leucine, isoleucine, and valine can decrease acute symptoms of mania, possibly by attenuating central dopaminergic overactivity and neurotransmission (10117).

There is evidence that ingestion of carbohydrates with an amino acid/protein mixture consisting of leucine, phenylalanine, and a wheat protein hydrolysate can increase the insulin response in type 2 diabetic patients. This suggests that amino acids might stimulate pancreatic beta cells to secrete insulin, independent of glucose stimulation (10118).

Adverse Reactions

Orally and intravenously, branched-chain amino acids can increase plasma ammonia levels (693,694), which can lead to fatigue and loss of motor coordination. Branched-chain amino acids can also cause nausea (10117). Short term use of 60 grams of branched-chain amino acids containing leucine, isoleucine, and valine for 7 days in patients with normal metabolic function seems to increase levels of ammonia, but not to toxic plasma levels (10117). Liver function should be monitored if high doses or long-term use of branched-chain amino acids is used (10117). Branched-chain amino acids should be used cautiously before or during activities where performance depends on motor coordination (75).

Orally, there has been one case report of hepatic encephalopathy in a chronic alcoholic. This resolved when dietary branched-chain amino acids were discontinued and recurred with rechallenge (691).

Increased mortality was reported in one study using branched-chain amino acids in the treatment of amyotrophic lateral sclerosis (ALS) (679).

Interactions with Herbs & Other Dietary Supplements

None known.

Interactions with Drugs

ANTIDIABETES DRUGS: Some evidence suggests that branched-chain amino acids might stimulate insulin release (10105,10110,10113,10114,10118). Theoretically, branched-chain amino acids might have an additive hypoglycemic effect with antidiabetic medications such as chlorpropamide (Diabinese), glipizide (Glucotrol), glyburide (DiaBeta), insulin, tolbutamide (Orinase), and others.

LEVODOPA: Theoretically, branched-chain amino acids may compete with levodopa for transport systems in the intestine and brain and decrease the effectiveness of levodopa (66,2719).

Drug Influences on Nutrient Levels and Depletion

SOME DRUGS CAN AFFECT BRANCHED-CHAIN AMINO ACID LEVELS:

DIAZOXIDE (Hyperstat, Proglycem): Theoretically, the use of diazoxide might decrease the stimulation of protein synthesis by branched-chain amino acids (10110,10114). The significance of this and how muscle mass might be

affected requires further study.
GLUCOCORTICOIDS (Decadron, Solu-Medrol, Deltasone): Theoretically, the use of glucocorticoids, such as dexamethasone, methylprednisolone, and prednisone, might decrease the stimulation of protein synthesis by branched-chain amino acids and increase the metabolism of branched-chain amino acids (10106). The significance of this and how muscle mass might be affected requires further study.
THYROID HORMONE (Cytomel, Triostat): There is evidence the use of some thyroid hormones (T3, L-triiodothyronine, liothyronine) can decrease metabolism of branched-chain amino acids. The significance of this and how muscle mass might be affected requires further study (10106).

Interactions with Foods

None known.

Interactions with Lab Tests

None known.

Interactions with Diseases or Conditions

AMYOTROPHIC LATERAL SCLEROSIS (ALS, Lou Gehrig's disease): The use of branched-chain amino acids has been associated with accelerated pulmonary failure and increased mortality when used in patients with ALS (679,681).
BRANCHED-CHAIN KETO ACIDURIA: Patients with branched-chain keto-aciduria are unable to effectively oxidize branched-chain amino acids, resulting in increased blood concentrations of branched-chain amino acids and branched-chain alpha-keto acids. Seizures and severe mental and physical retardation can result without proper dietary modification or if intake of branched-chain amino acids is increased (10107).
CHRONIC ALCOHOLISM: Dietary use of branched-chain amino acids in alcoholics has been associated with hepatic encephalopathy (691).
IDIOPATHIC HYPOGLYCEMIA: Intake of leucine has been reported to precipitate hypoglycemia in infants with idiopathic hypoglycemia. Some research suggests leucine stimulates the release of insulin (10105).

Dosage and Administration

ORAL: For latent or chronic hepatic encephalopathy, 240 mg/kg/day up to 25 grams of branched-chain amino acids have been used (68,685,690). For decreasing acute symptoms of mania, a 60 gram branched-chain amino acid drink containing valine, isoleucine, and leucine in a ratio of 3:3:4 has been used every morning for 7 days (10117). For reducing tardive dyskinesia movements, a branched-chain amino acid drink containing valine, isoleucine, and leucine at a dose of 222 mg/kg taken three times daily for 3 weeks has been used (10146). For reducing anorexia and improving the overall nutritional status in elderly malnourished hemodialysis patients, granules of branched-chain amino acids consisting of valine, leucine, and isoleucine at a dose of 4 grams taken three times daily has been used (10147).
INTRAVENOUS (IV): For all types of hepatic encephalopathy in patients who are intolerant to standard amino acid solutions and cannot take oral therapy, a typical dose of commercially available branched-chain amino acid solution (e.g., Hepatamine) is 80-120 grams per day, which provides 28-43 grams of branched-chain amino acids per day (68,266,687,689).

BREWER'S YEAST

Also Known As

Baker's Yeast, Brewers Yeast, Faex Medicinalis, Levure De Biere, Medicinal Yeast.
CAUTION: See separate listing for Saccharomyces boulardii.

Scientific Names

Saccharomyces cerevisiae.
Family: Saccharomycetaceae.
Candida utilis.
Family: Candidaceae.

People Use This For

Orally, brewer's yeast is used for diarrhea, loss of appetite, chronic acne, premenstrual syndrome, furunculosis, and high chromium type diabetes. It has also been used as a source of B vitamins and protein.

Safety

POSSIBLY SAFE ...when used orally and appropriately, short-term.
There is insufficient reliable information available about the safety of the long-term use of brewer's yeast.
CHILDREN: POSSIBLY SAFE ...when used orally and appropriately; however, diarrhea should be evaluated by a

medical professional before using brewer's yeast (2).
PREGNANCY AND LACTATION: Insufficient reliable information available; avoid using.

Effectiveness

POSSIBLY EFFECTIVE

Premenstrual syndrome (PMS). There is some evidence that taking a specific brewer's yeast preparation orally in combination with vitamins and minerals (Sillix Donna, Giuliani) might help reduce symptoms of PMS (7845).

INSUFFICIENT RELIABLE EVIDENCE to RATE

Clostridium difficile colitis. There is a case report of resolution of recurrent Clostridium difficile colitis after use of brewer's yeast for four months in combination with a 30-day course of vancomycin. Before this treatment, the patient experienced four relapses; after this treatment, there were no further relapses (6432). It is not clear what benefit, if any, the yeast product provided in the treatment. More evidence is needed to rate brewer's yeast for this use.

Mechanism of Action

Brewer's yeast can have some action against C. difficile and enterotoxic E. coli. It reduces water and electrolyte influx into the intestines stimulated by the C. vibrio toxin. Brewer's yeast can increase the activity of intestinal disaccharidases, saccharidases, maltase, and lactase to alleviate diarrhea symptoms (2). Preliminary evidence suggests that brewer's yeast can reduce infection caused by Brucella species, by increasing activity of phagocytic cells (7846). It can also increase insulin release (6004).

Adverse Reactions

Orally, brewer's yeast can cause migraine-like headaches in sensitive individuals, intestinal discomfort, and flatulence (2). Allergic reactions to brewer's yeast can occur in hypersensitive individuals. Symptoms include itching, urticaria, local or general exanthemas, and Quincke's edema (2). Crohn's disease can be exacerbated by brewer's yeast with dietary or occupational exposure (7645).

Interactions with Herbs & Other Dietary Supplements

None known.

Interactions with Drugs

ANTIFUNGALS: These drugs can reduce yeast activity (2).
MONOAMINE OXIDASE INHIBITORS (MAOIs): Brewer's yeast is contraindicated, because concomitant use can increase blood pressure (2).

Interactions with Foods

None known.

Interactions with Lab Tests

ANTIMICROBIAL TESTS: Brewer's yeast can confound results. Report the use of brewer's yeast to the lab (2).

Interactions with Diseases or Conditions

CROHN'S DISEASE: Dietary intake of Brewer's yeast can increase the severity of Crohn's disease (7645).

Dosage and Administration

ORAL: The typical dose is 6 grams of brewer's yeast per day (2).

Comments

Brewer's yeast is obtained as a by-product from the brewing of beer made from an extract of grains and hops.

BROMELAIN

Also Known As

Bromelains, Bromelainum, Bromelin, Pineapple Enzyme, Plant Protease Concentrate.
CAUTION: See separate listing for Papain.

Scientific Names

Ananas comosus (Pineapple), synonyms Ananas ananas, Ananas duckei, Ananas sativus, Bromelia ananas, Bromelia comosa.
Family: Bromeliaceae.

People Use This For

Orally, bromelain is used for acute postoperative and post-traumatic conditions of swelling, especially of the nasal and paranasal sinuses. It is also used orally for burn debridement, anti-inflammatory action, allergic rhinitis, prevention of epinephrine-induced pulmonary edema, smooth muscle relaxation, stimulation of muscle contractions, inhibition of blood platelet aggregation, enhanced antibiotic absorption, cancer prevention, shortening of labor, and enhanced excretion of fat. Bromelain is also used orally for mild ulcerative colitis.

In combination with trypsin and rutin, bromelain is used orally for osteoarthritis.

Safety

POSSIBLY SAFE ...when used orally and appropriately (960,6252).

PREGNANCY AND LACTATION: Insufficient reliable information available; avoid using.

Effectiveness

POSSIBLY EFFECTIVE

Osteoarthritis. Taking bromelain orally as a specific combination with trypsin and rutin (Phlogenzym) seems to reduce pain and improve knee function in patients with osteoarthritis. This bromelain combination product seems to be comparable to diclofenac (Voltaren) 50 mg three times daily for one week, then twice daily for 2 weeks (6252).

POSSIBLY INEFFECTIVE

Myalgia. Bromelain 300 mg three times daily, immediately following an intense exercise regimen, does not seem to delay onset of muscle soreness and has no effect on pain, flexibility, or skeletal weakness (10622).

INSUFFICIENT RELIABLE EVIDENCE to RATE

Knee pain. There's some evidence that taking bromelain orally can reduce mild acute (duration of less than 3 months) knee pain in otherwise healthy patients. Doses of 400 mg bromelain daily seem to be more effective than 200 mg daily in relieving pain, stiffness, and physical function of the knee (11457).

Trauma. Preliminary clinical research suggests bromelain might reduce swelling and pain after surgery or trauma (960); but it doesn't seem to reduce swelling after oral surgery (957).

Ulcerative colitis. Anecdotal evidence suggests that bromelain might improve some symptoms of ulcerative colitis in people with persistent disease despite standard therapy (6253).

More evidence is needed to rate bromelain for these uses.

Mechanism of Action

Bromelain is a general name for proteolytic enzymes obtained from the stem and fruit of the pineapple (9183). Bromelain contains constituents that interfere with the growth of malignant cells and inhibit platelet aggregation. It also possesses fibrinolytic activity and skin debridement properties (10639). The platelet aggregation inhibition action may be related to proteolytic activity. Fibrinolytic activity and an increase in adenosine monophosphate (AMP) may be key in the anti-cancer properties (10639). Bromelain might also exert an anti-inflammatory effect by altering leukocyte migration and activation. However, there is some question whether bromelain reaches concentrations required for anti-inflammatory activity outside of the gastrointestinal tract. Plasma contains proteinase inhibitors that may inactivate bromelain (9183). A polyenzyme preparation containing bromelain can increase the release of reactive oxygen species by polymorphonuclear neutrophils in healthy people (962).

Adverse Reactions

Orally, bromelain may cause gastrointestinal (GI) disturbances or diarrhea. Immunoglobulin E (IgE)-mediated allergic reactions to bromelain may occur and include a cross-allergenicity between bromelain and wheat flour, celery, papain, carrot, fennel, cypress pollen, and grass pollen. Cross-allergenicity may also occur with members of the Asteraceae/Compositae plant family. Some of these herbs include ragweed, chrysanthemums, marigolds, daisies, echinacea, and many other herbs (959,9184).

Interactions with Herbs & Other Dietary Supplements

HERBS WITH ANTICOAGULANT/ANTIPLATELET POTENTIAL: Theoretically, bromelain can increase the risk of bleeding when used concomitantly with herbs that have anticoagulant or antiplatelet potential (10639). Some of these herbs include alfalfa, angelica, aniseed, arnica, asafoetida, celery, chamomile, clove, fenugreek, feverfew, fucus, garlic, ginger, horse chestnut, licorice, meadowsweet, poplar, northern and southern prickly ash, quassia, red clover, and willow.

MAGNESIUM: Acts as a reducing agent and activates bromelain (11).

ZINC (an oxidizing agent): Concomitant use inhibits bromelain activity (11).

Interactions with Drugs

ANTICOAGULANT/ANTIPLATELET DRUGS: Theoretically, concomitant use might cause additive anticoagulant/antiplatelet effects and increase the risk of bleeding (10639).

TETRACYCLINE ANTIBIOTICS: Concomitant therapy increases plasma and urine tetracycline levels (2).

Interactions with Foods

POTATO PROTEIN and SOYBEAN: These foods can inhibit bromelain activity (958,961).

Interactions with Lab Tests

None known.

Interactions with Diseases or Conditions

PINEAPPLE ALLERGY: People allergic to pineapple might also have allergic reactions to bromelain (959).

Dosage and Administration

ORAL: For osteoarthritis, a combination enzyme product (Phlogenzym), which contains rutin 100 mg, trypsin 48 mg, and bromelain 90 mg, given 2 tablets 3 times daily has been used (6252). For delayed onset muscle soreness, bromelain 300 mg three times daily immediately following an intense exercise regimen has been used (10622). For acute knee pain, bromelain 200 mg to 400 mg daily for 30 days has been used (11457).

BROOKLIME

Also Known As

Beccabunga, Mouth-Smart, Neckweed, Speedwell, Water Pimpernel, Water Purslane.
CAUTION: See separate listings for Black Root and Veronica.

Scientific Names

Veronica beccabunga.

Comments

At the date of publication, there was very little scientific information about this product. Our staff is continually analyzing the available information on natural medicines and will add data to the online version of *Natural Medicines Comprehensive Database* as it becomes available. See www.naturaldatabase.com.

BROOM CORN

Also Known As

Darri, Durri, Guinea Corn, Sorghum.

Scientific Names

Sorghum bicolor, synonyms Sorghum vulgare, Andropogon sorghum, Holcus bicolor, Milium nigricans, Panicum caffrorum.
Family: Poaceae/Gramineae.

People Use This For

Orally, broom corn is used for digestive disorders.
In foods, broom corn is used as a cereal grain.

Safety

LIKELY SAFE ...when consumed in food amounts (18). Although the fruit contains cyanogenic glycosides, the concentrations are very low (18).
There is insufficient reliable information available about the safety of broom corn used in amounts larger than those found in foods.
PREGNANCY AND LACTATION: Insufficient reliable information available.

Effectiveness

There is insufficient reliable information available about the effectiveness of broom corn.

Mechanism of Action

The applicable part of broom corn is the seed. Broom corn contains a high percentage of starch and a small amount of protein and fatty oil. It also contains thiamine and riboflavin. Dhurrin, a cyanogenic glycoside, is present in a very low amount in the fruit, 0.005-5 mg per 100 grams. In contrast, the foliage contains a much higher level, 250-700 mg per 100 grams. Broom corn is thought to have a soothing effect on the alimentary tract (18).

Adverse Reactions
None reported.

Interactions with Herbs & Other Dietary Supplements
None known.

Interactions with Drugs
None known.

Interactions with Foods
None known.

Interactions with Lab Tests
None known.

Interactions with Diseases or Conditions
None known.

Dosage and Administration
No typical dosage.

BRYONIA

Also Known As
Bryoniae Radix, Devil's Turnip, English Mandrake, Ladies' Seal, Tamus, Tetterberry, White Bryony, Wild Hops, Wild Nep, Wild Vine, Wood Vine.
CAUTION: See separate listings for European Mandrake and Podophyllum (American mandrake).

Scientific Names
Bryonia cretica; Bryonia alba.
Family: Cucurbitaceae.

People Use This For
Orally, bryonia is used as a laxative, emetic, diuretic, for gastrointestinal diseases, respiratory tract diseases, arthritis, liver disease, metabolic disorders, and for prophylaxis against infections.

Safety
LIKELY UNSAFE ...when the root is used orally (2). ...when the berries are ingested; 40 berries might be fatal (18).
CHILDREN: LIKELY UNSAFE ...when the berries are ingested; 15 berries can be fatal (18). ...when the root is used orally (2).
PREGNANCY: UNSAFE ...when the root is used orally because it can cause abortion (2). ...when the berries are ingested (2).
LACTATION: LIKELY UNSAFE ...when the root is used orally (2). ...when the berries are ingested (2).

Effectiveness
There is insufficient reliable information available about the effectiveness of bryonia.

Mechanism of Action
The applicable part of bryonia is the root. The resin from bryonia has strong purgative effects (18). Some evidence suggests the aqueous extract might be effective against tumors (18). Other evidence suggests the methanol extract could have hypoglycemic effects (18).

Adverse Reactions
Orally, bryonia can cause dizziness, vomiting, convulsions, colic, bloody diarrhea, abortion, nervous excitement, and kidney damage (2). Large doses can cause anuria, collapse, spasms, paralysis, and death (2).
Topically, skin contact with fresh bryonia may cause irritation (19). Ingestion of 15 berries is likely to be fatal to a child. Ingestion of 40 berries is likely to be fatal for adults (18).

Interactions with Herbs & Other Dietary Supplements
None known.

Interactions with Drugs
None known.

Interactions with Foods
None known.

Interactions with Lab Tests
None known.

Interactions with Diseases or Conditions
GASTROINTESTINAL (GI) IRRITATION: Bryonia may irritate the GI tract. It is contraindicated in individuals with infectious or inflammatory GI conditions (19).

Dosage and Administration
No typical dosage.

Comments
Bryonia is no longer used as an emetic or laxative due to safety concerns (2).

BUCHU

Also Known As
Barosmae Folium, Bookoo, Bucco, Bucku, Diosma, Round Buchu, Short Buchu.

Scientific Names
Agathosma betulina, synonyms Barosma betulina, Hartogia betulin, Parapetalifera betulina; Agathosma crenulata, synonyms Barosma crenulata, Diosma crenulata, Parapetalifera crenulata, Parapetalifera odorata; Agathosma serratifolia, synonyms Barosma serratifolia, Diosma serratifolia, Parapetalifera serrata, Parapetalifera serratifolia.
Family: Rutaceae.

People Use This For
Orally, buchu is used as a urinary tract disinfectant in cystitis, urethritis, prostatitis, acute cystitis, kidney infections, and venereal disease.
In manufacturing, the oil from buchu is used to give a fruit flavor (often black currant) to foods.

Safety
LIKELY SAFE ...when the leaf is used in amounts commonly found in foods. Buchu has Generally Recognized As Safe (GRAS) status in the US (4912).
POSSIBLY SAFE ...when the leaf is used orally and appropriately in medicinal amounts (2,12).
POSSIBLY UNSAFE ...when excessive amounts of buchu leaf are taken orally or when the oil is ingested. Buchu contains pulegone, a known hepatotoxin (4). Pulegone is a major component of the oil.
PREGNANCY: LIKELY UNSAFE ...when used in medicinal amounts; buchu is reported to be an abortifacient (4).
LACTATION: POSSIBLY SAFE ...when used in food amounts. There is insufficient reliable information available about the safety of using larger amounts; avoid using.

Effectiveness
There is insufficient reliable information available about the effectiveness of buchu.

Mechanism of Action
The applicable part of buchu is the leaf. Buchu camphor (also known as diosphenol) is the principal constituent of the oil. Researchers believe this constituent may be responsible for buchu's reported diuretic and antiseptic effects (5).

Adverse Reactions
Orally, buchu leaf can cause GI and kidney irritation (4,6) and increase menstrual flow (6). Buchu is also a reported abortifacient (4).

Interactions with Herbs & Other Dietary Supplements
None known.

Interactions with Drugs
ANTICOAGULANT/ANTIPLATELET DRUGS: May possibly enhance the effects of anticoagulants (6002).

Interactions with Foods
None known.

Interactions with Lab Tests
None known.

Interactions with Diseases or Conditions
KIDNEY INFECTION: Contraindicated (4,12).
URINARY TRACT INFLAMMATION: Contraindicated (4,12).

Dosage and Administration
ORAL: The typical dose is 1 cup of tea (steep 1 gram dry leaf in 150 mL boiling water 5-10 minutes, strain) several times per day (8).

Comments
Liver function should be monitored in people who use buchu because of its potential hepatotoxicity.

BUCKHORN PLANTAIN

Also Known As
Buckhorn, Chimney-Sweeps, English Plantain, Headsman, Hoary Plantain, Plantaginis lanceolatae herba, Plantain, Ribgrass, Ribwort, Ribwort Plantain, Ripplegrass, Soldier's Herb, Spitzwegerichkraut.
CAUTION: See separate listings for Great Plantain, Blond Psyllium, Black Psyllium, and Water Plantain.

Scientific Names
Plantago lanceolata.
Family: Plantaginaceae.

People Use This For
Orally, buckhorn plantain is used to treat inflammation of mucous membranes in the respiratory tract, for the common cold, cough, bronchitis, and fevers.
Topically, buckhorn plantain is used for pharyngeal mucous membrane inflammation, inflammation of the skin, wound healing, and to arrest hemorrhages.

Safety
POSSIBLY SAFE ...when used orally and appropriately (2). ...when used topically (2).
PREGNANCY AND LACTATION: LIKELY UNSAFE ...when used orally or topically. Some evidence suggests buckhorn plantain affects muscle tone of the uterus (4275).

Effectiveness
There is insufficient reliable information available about the effectiveness of buckhorn plantain.

Mechanism of Action
The applicable parts of buckhorn plantain are the above ground parts. The tannin constituents have an astringent and antibacterial effect (18). Mucilage constituents are believed to be responsible for reducing local irritation and protecting mucous membranes from irritants (7).

Adverse Reactions
Buckhorn plantain is an allergen and a common problem in the early spring (3901).

Interactions with Herbs & Other Dietary Supplements
None known.

Interactions with Drugs
None known.

Interactions with Foods
None known.

Interactions with Lab Tests
None known.

Interactions with Diseases or Conditions
None known.

Dosage and Administration
ORAL: People typically use one cup tea (steep 2-3 grams chopped plant parts in 150 mL boiling water for 10 minutes, strain) several times daily (8,18); average amount is 3-6 grams per day (2).
TOPICAL: No typical dosage.

Comments
Avoid confusion with common plantain (Plantago major). CAUTION: Digitalis leaves resemble plantain leaves; adulteration of plantain with digitalis has been reported (3905). Be careful not to confuse buckhorn plantain with digitalis which is an unsafe product (2,12).

BUCKWHEAT

Also Known As
Buchweizen, Grano Turco, Sarrasin, Silverhull Buckwheat.

Scientific Names
Fagopyrum esculentum, synonyms Fagopyrum sagittatum, Fagopyrum vulgare; Fagopyrum tataricum, synonym Polygonum tataricum.
Family: Polygonaceae.

People Use This For
Orally, buckwheat is used to improve venous and capillary tone, to prevent hardening of the arteries, and for diabetes. It is also used orally to alleviate venous stasis and varicose veins.

Safety
POSSIBLY SAFE ...when used orally and appropriately (11438,11442).
PREGNANCY AND LACTATION: Insufficient reliable information available; avoid using.

Effectiveness
INSUFFICIENT RELIABLE EVIDENCE to RATE

Diabetes. Preliminary evidence suggests that consuming dietary buckwheat may improve long-term glucose tolerance in patients with diabetes (11438,11442). More evidence is needed to rate buckwheat for this use.

Mechanism of Action
The applicable parts of buckwheat are the leaves and flowers (18). The active constituents of buckwheat include the tocopherols, phenolic acids, and flavonoids. Many flavonoids including rutin, orientin, quercetin, quercitrin, isoorientin, isovitexin, and vitexin have been isolated in buckwheat grain (11431,11439). Buckwheat contains naphthadianthrones, which have photosensitizing effects. Phototoxicity has occurred in animals that ingest large quantities of buckwheat (18).
Dietary buckwheat is largely consumed as flour, used as an ingredient in foods such as bread, pancakes, and noodles. Buckwheat flour contains up to 12% protein, 69% carbohydrates, 3% lipids, and 14% water; as well as a well-balanced composition of amino acids. A buckwheat protein product, extracted from buckwheat flour, contains up to 66% protein, 6% carbohydrates, 22% lipids, and 3% water; as well as an unchanged well-balanced composition of amino acids (11434).
Buckwheat may improve overall glucose tolerance in diabetes by increasing the sensitivity of beta cells to glucose (11438,11442). Buckwheat is reported to have antioxidant activity, possibly through free radical scavenger and anti-lipid peroxidation activities (11432,11444). Preliminary animal research suggests this antioxidant activity might reduce the progression of renal failure (11433). Animal evidence also suggests buckwheat may possess anti-allergenic properties. Although the mechanism is not completely understood, the anti-allergenic action may be associated with histamine release inhibition and cytokine expression in mast cells (11441).

Adverse Reactions
Orally, allergic reactions to buckwheat in adults and children can include skin sensitization, allergic rhinitis, asthma, and anaphylaxis (11435,11436,11437). Occupational exposure to buckwheat, or household exposure through sleeping on a buckwheat husk stuffed-pillow can cause sensitization, of which symptoms include allergic rhinitis and asthma (11437,11443).

Interactions with Herbs & Other Dietary Supplements
None known.

Interactions with Drugs
None known.

Interactions with Foods
None known.

Interactions with Lab Tests
None known.

Interactions with Diseases or Conditions
BUCKWHEAT ALLERGY: Patients with buckwheat allergies are at risk for serious allergic reactions. Allergic reactions can include skin sensitization, allergic rhinitis, asthma, and anaphylaxis (11435,11437).
CELIAC DISEASE: Although some debate exists over the safety of buckwheat in a gluten-free diet, both the Celiac Disease Foundation and the Gluten Intolerance Group consider buckwheat an acceptable food item (11440,11445).

Dosage and Administration
ORAL: For diabetes, 70-100 g buckwheat flour or grain daily has been used (11438,11442).

BUGLE

Also Known As
Ajuga, Bugula, Carpenter's Herb, Middle Comfrey, Middle Confound, Sicklewort.

Scientific Names
Ajuga reptans.
Family: Lamiaceae/Labiatae.

Comments
At the date of publication, this product was not a common ingredient used in brand name supplements marketed to consumers. Details about this product are available at the online version of *Natural Medicines Comprehensive Database*. See www.naturaldatabase.com.

BUGLEWEED

Also Known As
Archangle, Ashangee, Bugle Weed, Green Wolf's Foot, Gypsy Weed, Gypsywort, Hoarhound, Lycopi Herba, Paul's Betony, Sweet Bugle, Virginia Water Horehound, Water Bugle, Water Hoarhound, Water Horehound, Wolfstrapp.
CAUTION: See separate listings for Horehound, Black Horehound, and Veronica.

Scientific Names
Lycopus americanus; Lycopus europaeus; Lycopus virginicus.
Family: Lamiaceae/Labiatae.

People Use This For
Orally, bugleweed is used for mild hyperthyroidism; premenstrual syndrome; breast pain; nervousness; insomnia; and bleeding, especially nosebleeds and heavy bleeding during menses.

Safety
POSSIBLY SAFE ...when used orally and appropriately (12).
PREGNANCY: LIKELY UNSAFE ...when used orally (12,19). It has anti-gonadotropic and anti-thyrotropic activity (7,19); avoid using.
LACTATION: LIKELY UNSAFE ...when used orally (12,19). It might have anti-prolactin activity (7,19); avoid using.

Effectiveness
There is insufficient reliable information available about the effectiveness of bugleweed.

Mechanism of Action

The applicable parts of bugleweed are the above ground parts. Bugleweed demonstrates anti-gonadotropic and anti-thyrotropic activity. It also seems to lower serum prolactin levels (7) and inhibit peripheral deiodination of T4 (2). Bugleweed can also have hypoglycemic activity (19).

Adverse Reactions

Orally, bugleweed rarely can cause thyroid enlargement during extended therapy or with large amounts (7). The sudden discontinuation of bugleweed can result in a sudden increase in thyroid function (2) and prolactin secretion (7).

Interactions with Herbs & Other Dietary Supplements

THYROID-SUPPRESSING HERBS: Theoretically, concomitant use of bugleweed with other thyroid suppressing herbs can have additive therapeutic and adverse effects (19). Herbs with thyroid-suppressing effects include balm leaf and the wild thyme plant (19).

Interactions with Drugs

ANTIDIABETES DRUGS: Theoretically, concomitant use of bugleweed can increase the risk of hypoglycemia (19). Blood glucose levels should be monitored closely.
THYROID HORMONE: Concomitant use of bugleweed is contraindicated because bugleweed may reduce the effects of thyroid hormones by blocking peripheral conversion of thyroxin to T3 (19).

Interactions with Foods

None known.

Interactions with Lab Tests

RADIOACTIVE ISOTOPES: Bugleweed can interfere with diagnostic procedures using radioactive isotopes (2).
THYROID FUNCTION TESTS: Bugleweed might improve thyroid function and test results in mildly hyperthyroid patients (2).

Interactions with Diseases or Conditions

DIABETES: Theoretically, bugleweed can interfere with blood glucose control and increase the risk of hypoglycemia (19). Blood glucose levels should be monitored closely while using bugleweed in diabetic patients.
THYROID DISEASE: Bugleweed is contraindicated in thyroid enlargement, thyroid hypofunction (2,12,19), and during administration of other thyroid treatments (12).

Dosage and Administration

ORAL: The typical dose of bugleweed is 0.2-2 grams per day of the above ground parts or equivalent preparations (7). The dose must be carefully individualized, taking age and weight into consideration (2).

BULBOUS BUTTERCUP

Also Known As

Crowfoot, Cuckoo Buds, Frogsfoot, Frogwort, Goldcup, King's Cup, Meadowbloom, Pilewort, St. Anthony's Turnip.
CAUTION: See separate listings for Buttercup and Poisonous Buttercup.

Scientific Names

Ranunculus bulbosus.
Family: Ranunculaceae.

People Use This For

Orally, bulbous buttercup is used for skin diseases, arthritis, gout, neuralgia, influenza, and meningitis.

Safety

LIKELY UNSAFE ...when used orally or topically because it can cause severe local irritation (18).
PREGNANCY AND LACTATION: LIKELY UNSAFE ...when used orally or topically (18); avoid using.

Effectiveness

There is insufficient reliable information available about the effectiveness of bulbous buttercup.

Mechanism of Action

The applicable parts of bulbous buttercup are the latex and the whole fresh flowering plant. When the fresh plant is crushed or cut into small pieces, the glycoside ranunculin is enzymatically changed into a severely irritating protoanemonin, which, in turn, rapidly degrades into the less toxic anemonin (18). Both protoanemonin and ranunculin are destroyed to an unknown extent during the drying process (2). The constituents ranunculin, protoanemonin, anemonin, and labenzym can cause drowsiness, fatigue and depressive moods. Protoanemonin present in the freshly harvested, bruised plant is severely irritating to skin and mucous membranes (18).

Adverse Reactions

Orally, ingestion of bulbous buttercup can cause severe irritation of the gastrointestinal tract, with colic and diarrhea (18).
Topically, irritation of the urinary tract can also occur. Skin contact can cause blisters and burns which are difficult to heal (18).

Interactions with Herbs & Other Dietary Supplements

None known.

Interactions with Drugs

None known.

Interactions with Foods

None known.

Interactions with Lab Tests

None known.

Interactions with Diseases or Conditions

None known.

Dosage and Administration

No typical dosage.

Comments

This product is rarely used. Avoid confusing bulbous buttercup with lesser celandine and amaranth; these plants are also referred to as pilewort (18).

BUPLEURUM

Also Known As

Bei Chai Hu, Chi Hu, Chinese Thoroughwax, Hare's Ear Root, Sho-saiko-to, Shrubby Hare's-ear, Sickle-leaf Hare's-ear, Thoroughwax.

Scientific Names

Bupleurum chinense; Bupleurum exaltatum; Bupleurum falcatum; Bupleurum fruticosum; Bupleurum longifolium; Bupleurum multinerve; Bupleurum octoradiatum; Bupleurum rotundifolium; Bupleurum scorzonerifolium.
Family: Apiaceae/Umbelliferae.

People Use This For

Orally, bupleurum is used for fevers, flu, the common cold, cough, fatigue, headache, tinnitus, liver disorders, premenstrual syndrome (PMS), dysmenorrhea, depression, anorexia, cancer, inflammation, lung congestion, malaria, angina, epilepsy, pain, muscle cramps, rheumatism, asthma, bronchitis, indigestion, ulcers, hemorrhoids, diarrhea, constipation, as a sedative, antioxidant, antiseptic, antifungal, antiviral, as an immune stimulant, and for reducing cholesterol and triglyceride levels. It is also used orally for increasing sweating, as a protectant against kidney problems, a liver tonic, and a spleen and stomach toner.
In combination, bupleurum is used in many herbal formulas. It is included in a Chinese herbal formula used for treating thrombocytopenic purpura and in a Japanese herbal formula (Sho-saiko-to, TJ-9, Xiao-chai-hu-tang) used for various chronic liver diseases. Bupleurum is used orally in combination with Panax ginseng and licorice to help stimulate adrenal gland function, particularly in patients with a history of long-term corticosteroid use.

Safety

There is insufficient reliable information available about the safety of bupleurum.
Pregnancy and Lactation: Insufficient reliable information available; avoid using.

Effectiveness

There is insufficient reliable information available about the effectiveness of bupleurum.

Mechanism of Action

The applicable part of bupleurum is the root (12). Compounds isolated from Bupleurum species used in traditional Chinese medicine include saikosaponins, polysaccharides, and polyacetylenes. Saikosaponins are triterpenoid saponins, known as saikosides (6). While the saikosaponin content of some species is very similar (3151), that of other species varies considerably, as well as pharmacologic activity (3152). The saikosaponin content is highest in Bupleurum falcatum (2-8%) and Bupleurum chinense (1.7%). For infections, including the flu and the common cold, bupleurum is theorized to work by improving immune function. Bupleurum falcatum is reported to cause proliferation of B-lymphocytes and stimulate them to produce immunoglobulins in vitro. It is also reported to stimulate in vitro macrophage activity, possibly by increasing the number of antibody-binding sites on the cell surface (2598). The constituent saikosaponin-d has immunoregulatory actions on T-lymphocytes, including promotion of interleukin-2 (IL-2) production and IL-2 receptor expression (3160). It also increases macrophage activity, IL-1 production and antibody response (3161). Bupleurum also is reported to have antitussive properties (6). For peptic ulcers, bupleurum is thought to decrease gastric acid and pepsin secretion and have mucosal protecting effects (3154,3155). Bupleurum is also reported to have antitumor (3157), antibacterial (3170), anti-inflammatory (2597,3166,3167,3168), antispasmodic (3167), antioxidant (3154,3155,3156), antiplatelet (3159), and hepatoprotectant effects (3163,3164,3165); however these effects have not been demonstrated in humans.

Adverse Reactions

Orally, bupleurum can cause increased bowel movements, flatulence, and sedation (3148). The Japanese herbal formula, Sho-saiko-to, which contains bupleurum, has been associated with eosinophilic pneumonia (354), pulmonary edema (361), and multiple cases of pneumonitis (355,356,357). Sho-saiko-to, used in combination with interferon-alpha in people with chronic active hepatitis, has been associated with multiple cases of pneumonitis (358,359,360).

Interactions with Herbs & Other Dietary Supplements

None known.

Interactions with Drugs

None known.

Interactions with Foods

None known.

Interactions with Lab Tests

None known.

Interactions with Diseases or Conditions

None known.

Dosage and Administration

ORAL: A dose of 1.5 to 6 grams per day of bupleurum root has been used (3148). As a fluid extract (1:2), 1.5-3 mL daily, up to 25-60 mL per week has been used (3148).

Comments

The Japanese herbal formula, Sho-saiko-to, which contains bupleurum, enhances the anti-HIV-1 activity of lamivudine (Epivir, 3TC) in vitro (362).

BURDOCK

Also Known As

Arctium, Bardana, Bardanae Radix, Bardane, Beggar's Buttons, Burr Seed, Clotbur, Cocklebur, Cockle Buttons, Edible Burdock, Fox's Clote, Gobo, Great Bur, Great Burdocks, Happy Major, Hardock, Harebur, Lappa, Love Leaves, Personata, Philanthropium, Thorny Burr.

Scientific Names

Arctium lappa; Arctium minus; Arctium tomentosum.
Family: Asteraceae/Compositae.

People Use This For

Orally, burdock is used as a diuretic, "blood purifier", antimicrobial, antipyretic. It is also used to treat anorexia nervosa, gastrointestinal (GI) complaints, rheumatism, gout, cystitis, syphilitic disorders, and chronic skin conditions including acne and psoriasis.

Burdock is also used for treating colds, catarrh, cancers, and as an aphrodisiac.
Topically, burdock is used for dry skin (ichthyosis) and eczema.
The root of burdock is consumed as a food.

Safety

LIKELY SAFE ...when used in amounts commonly found in foods. Burdock is listed as a food flavoring by the Council of Europe (4).
POSSIBLY SAFE ...when used orally and appropriately in medicinal amounts (12).
PREGNANCY: LIKELY UNSAFE ...when used orally. Burdock may cause uterine stimulation (4,19); avoid using.
LACTATION: Insufficient reliable information available; avoid using.

Effectiveness

There is insufficient reliable information available about the effectiveness of burdock.

Mechanism of Action

The applicable part of burdock is the root, leaf, and flower. The leaf and flower have Gram-positive and Gram-negative antibacterial activity; the root is active against Gram-negative bacteria. The constituent arctiopiricin is active against Gram-positive bacteria. In vivo, burdock has uterine stimulant activity in animals. It may also have some antimutagenic and antitumor activity (4).

Adverse Reactions

Orally, burdock can cause an allergic reaction in individuals sensitive to the Asteraceae/Compositae family. Members of this family include ragweed, chrysanthemums, marigolds, daisies, and many other herbs.
Topically, sensitization may occur via skin contact (18).

Interactions with Herbs & Other Dietary Supplements

None known.

Interactions with Drugs

ANTIDIABETES DRUGS: Theoretically, large amounts of burdock might cause hypoglycemia (4).
INSULIN: Concomitant use might require insulin dosage adjustment due to hypoglycemic effect (19).

Interactions with Foods

None known.

Interactions with Lab Tests

None known.

Interactions with Diseases or Conditions

CROSS-ALLERGENICITY: Burdock may cause an allergic reaction in individuals sensitive to the Asteraceae/Compositae family. Members of this family include ragweed, chrysanthemums, marigolds, daisies, and many other herbs.
DIABETES: Theoretically, large amounts of burdock may affect blood sugar control (4).

Dosage and Administration

ORAL: A typical dosage is 2-6 grams of the dried root used three times daily, or 1 cup of the tea (steep 1-2 grams dried root in 150 mL boiling water for 5-10 minutes) three times daily (4). For the liquid extract 2-8 mL (1:1 in 25% alcohol), and for the tincture (1:10 in 45% alcohol) 8-12 mL are typically used three times daily (4).

Comments

Burdock has been associated with atropine poisoning as a result of being adulterated with root of belladonna or deadly nightshade (4,5).

BURNING BUSH leaf

Also Known As

Adiptam, Burnet Saxifrage, Dictamo Blanco, Dittany, Fraxinella, Gas Plant, Herba dictamni herba.
CAUTION: See separate listing for Burning Bush root.

Scientific Names

Dictamnus albus, synonyms Dictamnus caucasicus, Dictamnus fraxinellus.
Family: Rutaceae.

People Use This For
Orally, burning bush leaf is used for cramps, stomach disorders, worm infestations, epilepsy, as a stimulant, tonic, diuretic, to promote menstruation and aid in the expulsion of the afterbirth.
Topically, burning bush leaf is used for treating wounds and rheumatism.

Safety
POSSIBLY UNSAFE ...when used topically because it can cause photosensitivity (18).
There is insufficient reliable information available about the safety of burning bush leaf for its other uses.
PREGNANCY AND LACTATION: POSSIBLY UNSAFE ...when used topically (18). There is insufficient reliable information available about the safety of burning bush leaf used orally during pregnancy or lactation; avoid using.

Effectiveness
There is insufficient reliable information available about the effectiveness of burning bush leaf.

Mechanism of Action
There is evidence to support the use of burning bush leaf in treating worm infestations. It decreases the ability of a tropical liver fluke called Clonorchis sinensis to lay eggs. This same liver fluke can occur in sushi if the fish has been imported from Asia. Burning bush leaf contains psoralen, xanthotoxin, auraptene, and bergapten. These furocoumarins can cause phototoxic reactions when they are applied topically (18).

Adverse Reactions
Topically, skin contact can cause phototoxicity (18).

Interactions with Herbs & Other Dietary Supplements
None known.

Interactions with Drugs
None known.

Interactions with Foods
None known.

Interactions with Lab Tests
None known.

Interactions with Diseases or Conditions
None known.

Dosage and Administration
ORAL: The typical dose is 1 cup of tea taken orally 3 times daily. One cup of tea is also taken after main meals twice daily. The tea is prepared by steeping 20 grams of dried leaf in 1 L of boiling water for 10-15 minutes and straining. Alternately, 1 gram of fresh or 2 grams of dried herb is added to 1 cup of water (18).
TOPICAL: No typical dosage.

Comments
Avoid confusion with Euonymus, which has also been referred to as burning bush. Euonymus is the dried bark of the root of Euonymus atropurpureus (Fam. Celastracaea). Burning bush has a distinctive lemon or cinnamon scent. Its oil is easily flammable (18).

BURNING BUSH root

Also Known As
Adiptam, Burnet Saxifrage, Dittany, Fraxinella, Gas Plant, Herba Dictamni Herba.
CAUTION: See separate listing for Burning Bush leaf.

Scientific Names
Dictamnus albus, synonyms Dictamnus caucasicus, Dictamnus fraxinellus.
Family: Rutaceae.

People Use This For
Orally, burning bush root is used for digestive and urogenital disorders, to promote hair growth, as diuretic and spasmolytic, for desiccation, epilepsy, hysteria, worm infestations, to promote menstruation, and as birth control. Topically, burning bush root is used for eczema, impetigo, scabies, for arthritis, fever, hepatitis, skin inflammation, thread fungus, uterine hemorrhages, to calm children crying as a result of a nervous state, and as a sedative and tonic.

Safety
POSSIBLY UNSAFE ...when used topically (18).
There is insufficient reliable information available about the safety of burning bush root for its other uses.
PREGNANCY AND LACTATION: POSSIBLY UNSAFE ...when used topically. There is insufficient reliable information available about the safety of burning bush root used orally during pregnancy or lactation; avoid using.

Effectiveness
There is insufficient reliable information available about the effectiveness of burning bush root.

Mechanism of Action
There is insufficient reliable information available about the possible mechanism of action and active ingredients.

Adverse Reactions
Topically, skin contact can cause phototoxicity (18).

Interactions with Herbs & Other Dietary Supplements
None known.

Interactions with Drugs
None known.

Interactions with Foods
None known.

Interactions with Lab Tests
None known.

Interactions with Diseases or Conditions
None known.

Dosage and Administration
ORAL: Tea is commonly used over the course of one day. The tea is prepared by steeping 1 teaspoon dried root in 2 glasses of hot water for 10-15 minutes and straining . It is also occasionally used in tea mixtures and in Swedish herb mixtures (18).
TOPICAL: No typical dosage.

Comments
Sources report confusion with Carophyllaceen roots. Avoid confusion with Euonymus, which has also been referred to as burning bush. Euonymus is the dried bark of the root of Euonymus atropurpureus (Fam. Celastracaea). Burning bush has a distinctive lemon or cinnamon scent. Its oil is easily flammable. Its use is mostly obsolete (18).

BURR MARIGOLD

Also Known As
Water Agrimony.

Scientific Names
Bidens tripartita.
Family: Asteraceae/Compositae.

Comments
At the date of publication, this product was not a common ingredient used in brand name supplements marketed to consumers. Details about this product are available at the online version of *Natural Medicines Comprehensive Database*. See www.naturaldatabase.com.

BUTANEDIOL (BD)

Also Known As
1,4-BD, 1,4-butylene glycol, 1,4-dihydroxybutane, 1,4-tetramethylene glycol, 2(3H)-Furanone di-dihydro, BD, BDO, Butane-1,4-diol, Butylene glycol, Tetramethylene glycol, Tetramethylene-1,4-diol.
CAUTION: See separate listings for Gamma Hydroxybutyrate (GHB) and Gamma Butyrolactone (GBL).

Scientific Names
1,4-butanediol.

People Use This For
Orally, butanediol has been used to stimulate growth hormone production and muscle growth, for bodybuilding, weight loss, and insomnia.

Safety
UNSAFE ...when used orally. Butanediol, and the closely related products gamma hydroxybutyrate (GHB) and gamma butyrolactone (GBL) have been linked to at least 131 serious illnesses, including 5 deaths (1318,3678,10640).
PREGNANCY AND LACTATION: UNSAFE ...when used orally (1318,3678).

Effectiveness
There is insufficient reliable information available about the effectiveness of butanediol.

Mechanism of Action
Butanediol is converted to gamma hydroxybutyrate (GHB, see separate listing) in the body (3678,5813). It is a powerful hypnotic, producing potentially dangerous sedative effects (3679). GHB can be converted in the brain to the neurotransmitter gamma aminobutyric acid (GABA) (3699), and specific GHB uptake systems, transport systems, and receptors have also been identified (713,3699,5800,5801). Stimulation of GHB receptors reduces dopamine release in the brain (713,3699,5801), and GHB has also been reported to affect the endogenous opioid system, raising dynorphin levels (3682,5803). GHB induces REM and non-REM sleep, hypothermia, abnormalities on the EEG similar to those seen in petit mal epilepsy (5800,5803); and it stimulates growth hormone secretion (5804).

Adverse Reactions
Orally, butanediol, like gamma butyrolactone (GBL), is metabolized to gamma hydroxybutyrate (GHB), and therefore causes similar toxic effects, including breathing problems, respiratory depression requiring intubation, coma, amnesia, combativeness, confusion, agitation, vomiting, urinary and fecal incontinence, seizures, bradycardia, and death (1318,3678,3679,10640). Butanediol, GHB, and GBL have been linked to at least 131 serious illnesses, including 5 deaths (1318,3678,10640). Non-fatal toxicity has been reported with doses of 1 to 14 grams. Death has occurred with doses of 5 to 20 grams (1318). Withdrawal symptoms, including insomnia, tremor, anxiety, hallucinations, and delirium can occur in chronic users of butanediol and GBL, as well as GHB (1430,10375). GHB-like withdrawal has also occurred in a patient who presented with butanediol toxicity (1318).

Interactions with Herbs & Other Dietary Supplements
None known.

Interactions with Drugs
ALCOHOL (Ethanol): Concomitant use with butanediol and its metabolite GHB may increase the risk of serious CNS and respiratory depression (1430,3678).
AMPHETAMINES: Concomitant use with GHB (a metabolite of butanediol) has been associated with severe side effects. Theoretically, concomitant use may also antagonize the effects of GHB (3682).
ANTICONVULSANTS: Theoretically, GHB (a metabolite of butanediol) may antagonize the effects of GHB (3682).
ANTIPSYCHOTIC DRUGS: Concomitant use with GHB (a metabolite of butanediol) has been associated with severe side effects. Antipsychotics can potentiate the effects of GHB (3682).
BENZODIAZEPINES: Concomitant use with GHB (a metabolite of butanediol) has been associated with severe side effects Benzodiazepines can potentiate the effects of GHB (3682).
CNS DEPRESSANTS: Concomitant use with GHB (a metabolite of butanediol) has been associated with severe side effects. Additive sedative effects with butanediol may occur (3682,3679).
HALOPERIDOL (Haldol): Theoretically, Haloperidol may antagonize the effects of GHB (a metabolite of butanediol) (3682).
NALOXONE (Narcan): Theoretically, concomitant use with GHB (a metabolite of butanediol) may antagonize the effects of GHB (3682).
NARCOTIC DRUGS: Concomitant use with GHB (a metabolite of butanediol) has been associated with severe side effects. Concomitant use of GHB with narcotic drugs can potentiate the therapeutic and adverse effects of narcotic analgesics (3682,3679).

RITONAVIR (Norvir): Concomitant use of the protease inhibitor-type antiretroviral drugs ritonavir and saquinavir with GHB (a metabolite of butanediol) reportedly caused a near-fatal reaction, probably due to inhibition of GHB metabolism (1431).
SAQUINAVIR (Fortovase, Invirase): Concomitant use of the protease inhibitor-type antiretroviral drugs ritonavir and saquinavir with GHB (a metabolite of butanediol) reportedly caused a near-fatal reaction, probably due to inhibition of GHB metabolism (1431).
SKELETAL MUSCLE RELAXANTS: Concomitant use with GHB (a metabolite of butanediol) has been associated with severe side effects. Concomitant use with GHB can potentiate the therapeutic and adverse effects of skeletal muscle relaxants (3682).

Interactions with Foods
ALCOHOL: Concomitant use with butanediol and its metabolite GHB may increase the risk of serious CNS and respiratory depression (1430,3678).

Interactions with Lab Tests
None known.

Interactions with Diseases or Conditions
BRADYCARDIA: GHB (a metabolite of butanediol) should be avoided since it can cause bradycardia conditions (4259).
EPILEPSY: GHB (a metabolite of butanediol) should be avoided due to its possible capacity to induce seizures (10658).
HYPERTENSION: GHB (a metabolite of butanediol) should be avoided since it may increase blood pressure (10658).

Dosage and Administration
ORAL: Doses of 0.25 to 1 gram butanediol have been used for stimulating growth hormone release and muscle growth and treating insomnia, but are considered unsafe (3678).

Comments
Butanediol is used industrially to make floor stripper, paint thinner, and other solvent products (3678). It is illegal to sell any product for human consumption containing butanediol (3678). Some manufacturers have substituted butanediol in products previously containing GHB or GBL, but the effects of butanediol are just as dangerous (3679). GBL, GHB, and BD are associated with at least 122 reports of serious adverse effects including dangerously low respiratory rates (intubation might be required), unconsciousness, coma, vomiting, seizures, slowed heart rate, and death (4259).

BUTCHER'S BROOM

Also Known As
Box Holly, Butchers Broom, Butchers' Broom, Butcherbroom, Jew's Myrtle, Kneeholm, Knee Holly, Pettigree, Sweet Broom, Rusci Aculeati, Rusci Aculeati Rhizoma.
CAUTION: See separate listings for Scotch Broom flower, Scotch Broom herb, and Spanish Broom.

Scientific Names
Ruscus aculeatus.
Family: Ruscaceae.

People Use This For
Orally, butcher's broom is used for hemorrhoids, gallstones, atherosclerosis, and for symptoms of chronic venous insufficiency such as pain, heaviness, leg cramps, leg edema, varicose veins, peripheral vascular disease, itching, and swelling. Butcher's broom is also used as a laxative, diuretic, an anti-inflammatory, and to facilitate the healing of fractures.
As food, the rhizome shoots are eaten in some cultures in a manner similar to asparagus.

Safety
POSSIBLY SAFE ...when used orally and appropriately short-term (9932,10068,10069,10070). The use of butcher's broom is not associated with any significant toxicity for up to 3 months of use.
PREGNANCY AND LACTATION: Insufficient reliable information available; avoid using.

Effectiveness

POSSIBLY EFFECTIVE

Chronic venous insufficiency. Taking butcher's broom orally alone, or in combination with vitamin C and hesperidin, seems to relieve chronic venous insufficiency symptoms including pain, heaviness, leg cramps, itching, and swelling (9932,10068,10070).

INSUFFICIENT RELIABLE EVIDENCE to RATE

Orthostatic hypotension. Some clinical research suggests that butcher's broom taken orally might relieve orthostatic hypotension (10069). More evidence is needed to rate butcher's broom for this use.

Mechanism of Action

The applicable parts of butcher's broom are the rhizomes and roots. The steroidal saponin constituents, ruscogenin and neoruscogenin, produce vasoconstrictive effects by direct activation of alpha-adrenergic receptors. This activation, in turn, stimulates the release of noradrenaline at the vascular wall (10069). Butcher's broom appears to have venotonic properties that reduce venous capacity and pooling of blood in the legs. It also seems to have a protective effect on capillaries, vascular endothelium, and smooth muscle (10068,10070). The flavonoid content might help strengthen blood vessels, lessen capillary fragility, and sustain healthy circulation (10069).

Adverse Reactions

Orally, butcher's broom can cause nausea, gastritis, and diarrhea (10068).

Interactions with Herbs & Other Dietary Supplements

HERBS WITH ALPHA-ADRENERGIC AGONIST ACTIVITY: Theoretically, butcher's broom might have an additive effect on herbs and supplements with alpha-agonist properties (10069). Some of these include bitter orange and ephedra.

HERBS WITH ALPHA-ADRENERGIC ANTAGONIST ACTIVITY: Theoretically, butcher's broom might reduce the effects of herbs and supplements with alpha-antagonist properties (10069). Some of these include yohimbe and saw palmetto.

Interactions with Drugs

ALPHA-ADRENERGIC AGONISTS: Theoretically, butcher's broom might have an additive effect on drugs with alpha-agonist properties (10069). Some of these include pseudoephedrine (Sudafed), phenylpropanolamine (Afrin, Drixoral Non-Drowsy), and others.

ALPHA-ADRENERGIC ANTAGONISTS: Theoretically, butcher's broom might reduce the effects of drugs with alpha-antagonist properties (10069). Some of these include doxazosin (Cardura), terazosin (Hytrin), yohimbine (Aphrodyne), and others.

Interactions with Foods

None known.

Interactions with Lab Tests

None known.

Interactions with Diseases or Conditions

None known.

Dosage and Administration

ORAL: For relieving symptoms of chronic venous insufficiency, butcher's broom 150 mg root extract, combined with 150 mg hesperidin and 100 mg ascorbic acid, has been used twice daily (10068).

BUTTERBUR

Also Known As

Blatterdock, Bog Rhubarb, Bogshorns, Butter Bur, Butterburr, Butter-Dock, Butterfly Dock, Capdockin, Exwort, Flapperdock, Langwort, Petasites, Petasites flower, Petasites leaf, Petasites rhizome, Petasites root, Petasitidis folium, Petasitidis rhizoma, Petasitidis hybridus, Umbrella Leaves.

Scientific Names

Petasites hybridus, synonyms Petasites officinalis, Tussilago hybrida.
Family: Asteraceae/Compositae.

People Use This For

Orally, butterbur is used for pain, stomach upset, gastric ulcers, headaches including migraine headaches, chronic cough, chills, anxiety, plague, fever, insomnia whooping cough, asthma, allergic rhinitis (hay fever), and for irritable bladder and urinary tract spasms. It is also used orally as an antispasmodic and appetite stimulant.
Topically, butterbur is used to improve wound healing.

Safety

POSSIBLY SAFE ...when used orally and appropriately. Rhizome extracts that are free of unsaturated pyrrolizidine alkaloid (UPA) constituents seem to be safe when used for up to 12 weeks (7230). Tell patients not to use butterbur products that are not certified and labeled as UPA free. Preparations containing UPAs are likely unsafe.
LIKELY UNSAFE ...when products containing UPAs are used orally (19). Repeated exposure to low concentrations of UPAs can cause severe veno-occlusive disease (12). UPAs might also be carcinogenic and mutagenic (12). Tell patients not to use butterbur preparations that are not certified and labeled as UPA free. ...when products containing UPAs are used topically on abraded or broken skin. Absorption of UPAs through broken skin can lead to systemic toxicities (12). Tell patients not to use topical butterbur preparations that are not certified and labeled as UPA free. There is insufficient reliable information available about the safety of topical UPA free butterbur on unbroken skin.
PREGNANCY: LIKELY UNSAFE ...when used orally. Butterbur preparations containing UPAs might be teratogenic and hepatotoxic (19). There is insufficient reliable information available about the safety of UPA free butterbur preparations during pregnancy.
LACTATION: POSSIBLY UNSAFE ...when used orally. UPA constituents in butterbur might be excreted in milk (19). There is insufficient reliable information available about the safety of UPA free butterbur preparations during lactation.

Effectiveness

POSSIBLY EFFECTIVE

Allergic rhinitis (hayfever). Taking petasins, isolated from butterbur, may decrease symptoms of allergic rhinitis. In addition, petasins can decrease concentrations of inflammatory mediators (7595,10336,10337).
Some research suggests that butterbur petasins may be as effective as cetirizine (Zyrtec) (7595). Whole butterbur root extract that is not standardized for petasin content (Petaforce) seems to reduce response to adenosine monophosphate challenge in patients with allergic rhinitis (11941). But this extract doesn't seem to improve peak nasal inspiratory flow, nasal and eye symptoms, or quality of life any better than placebo when taken for 2 weeks (11942).

Migraine headache. Taking butterbur orally seems to prevent migraine headache. There's some evidence that a specific butterbur rhizome extract standardized to 7.5 mg of the constituents petasin and isopetasin (Petadolex), and unsaturated pyrrolizidine alkaloids (UPAs) free, can reduce the frequency, intensity, and duration of migraine headache (7230).

INSUFFICIENT RELIABLE EVIDENCE to RATE

Respiratory conditions. There is some preliminary evidence that butterbur might be helpful for treating asthma and chronic bronchitis (7596). More evidence is needed to rate butterbur for this use.

Mechanism of Action

The applicable parts of butterbur are the leaf, rhizome, and root. The active constituents of butterbur are the sesquiterpene compounds, petasin, and isopetasin. Butterbur extracts also contain volatile oils, flavonoids, tannins, and pyrrolizidine alkaloids. Some butterbur extracts are standardized to contain a minimum of 7.5 mg petasin and isopetasin (7229).
Butterbur is thought to have antispasmodic effects on smooth muscle and vascular walls. It might also exert anti-inflammatory effects by inhibiting leukotriene synthesis (7229,7597).
In allergic rhinitis (hayfever), butterbur and purified petasin decrease blood concentrations of histamine and leukotrienes (10336). They also appear to decrease priming of mast cells in response to contact with allergens (10337).
Pyrrolizidine alkaloids that are unsaturated (UPAs) can cause serious toxicity. They are considered hepatotoxic, carcinogenic, mutagenic, and renal toxic (12). They can also cause veno-occlusive disease (12). Methods to remove UPAs from butterbur extracts are available (7231). However, it is not known if commercial products containing butterbur commonly remove UPAs.

Adverse Reactions

Orally, butterbur can cause headache, itchy eyes, diarrhea, asthma, pruritus, stomach upset, fatigue, and drowsiness. However, it seems to cause less drowsiness and fatigue than cetirizine (Zyrtec) (7595).The major concern about butterbur preparations is the unsaturated pyrrolizidine alkaloid (UPA) content. These constituents are considered hepatotoxic, carcinogenic, mutagenic, and renal toxic (12). Chronic exposure to other plants containing UPA constituents is associated with veno-occlusive disease (4021). Subacute veno-occlusive disease causes vague symptoms with persistent liver enlargement (4021). Symptoms of acute veno-occlusive disease include a dull, dragging ache in the right upper abdomen and distention of the abdomen. These symptoms are sometimes accompanied by reduced urine output. Butterbur can cause an allergic reaction in individuals sensitive to the Asteraceae/Compositae family.

Interactions with Herbs & Other Dietary Supplements
UNSATURATED PYRROLIZIDINE ALKALOID (UPA)-CONTAINING HERBS: Concomitant use is contraindicated due to the risk of additive toxicity. Herbs containing UPAs include alkanna, borage, gravel root, hemp agrimony, hound's tongue, comfrey, coltsfoot; and the Senecio species plants dusty miller, alpine ragwort, groundsel, golden ragwort, and tansy ragwort (4,12,19,271).

Interactions with Drugs
None known.

Interactions with Foods
None known.

Interactions with Lab Tests
LIVER FUNCTION TESTS (LFTs): Butterbur can cause increases in liver enzyme activity (7595).

Interactions with Diseases or Conditions
CROSS-ALLERGENICITY: Butterbur may cause an allergic reaction in individuals sensitive to the Asteraceae/Compositae family. Members of this family include ragweed, chrysanthemums, marigolds, daisies, and many other herbs.
LIVER DISEASE: Contraindicated due to hepatotoxic potential (19).

Dosage and Administration
ORAL: For migraine headache prophylaxis, a pyrrolizidine alkaloid free butterbur rhizome extract standardized to 7.5 mg petasin and isopetasin has been used in doses of 50 to 100 mg twice daily with meals (7230). Some researchers suggest taking the extract for 4 to 6 months, then tapering the dose until migraine incidence begins to increase (7229). For seasonal allergic rhinitis, an extract of butterbur (ZE 339, Zeller AG) standardized to 8 to16 mg of petasin has been used 3 to 4 times daily (7595,10336). Whole butterbur root extract (Petaforce) 50 mg twice daily has also been used for allergic rhinitis (11941).

BUTTERCUP

Also Known As
Acrid Crowfoot, Batchelor's Buttons, Blisterweed, Burrwort, Globe Amaranth, Gold Cup, Meadowbloom, Meadow Buttercup, Tall Buttercup, Yellows, Yellowweed.
CAUTION: See separate listings for Poisonous Buttercup, Bulbous Buttercup, Cornflower, and Feverfew.

Scientific Names
Ranunculus acris; Ranunculus acris subsp. friesianus, synonym Ranunculus friesianus.
Family: Ranunculaceae.

People Use This For
Orally, buttercup is used for arthritis, blisters, bronchitis, chronic skin complaints, and nerve pain.

Safety
LIKELY UNSAFE ...when the fresh plant is used orally or topically because it can cause severe local irritation (18). There is insufficient reliable information about the safety of the medicinal use of the dried, cut above ground parts of buttercup.
PREGNANCY AND LACTATION: LIKELY UNSAFE ...when the fresh plant is used orally or topically (18). Buttercup might also stimulate uterine contractions (19). There is insufficient reliable information about the safety of buttercup used during pregnancy and lactation.

Effectiveness
There is insufficient reliable information available about the effectiveness of buttercup.

Mechanism of Action
The applicable parts of buttercup are the fresh above ground parts. When the fresh plant is crushed or cut into small pieces, the glycoside ranunculin is enzymatically changed into a severely irritating protoanemonin, which, in turn, rapidly degrades into the less toxic anemonin (18). Both protoanemonin and ranunculin are destroyed to an unknown extent during the drying process (2).

Adverse Reactions
Orally, ingestion of buttercup may cause severe irritation of the gastrointestinal tract, with colic and diarrhea. Irritation of the urinary tract can also occur.
Topically, skin contact may cause blisters and burns which are difficult to heal (18). Buttercup can also cause phototoxic skin reactions (19).

Interactions with Herbs & Other Dietary Supplements
None known.

Interactions with Drugs
None known.

Interactions with Foods
None known.

Interactions with Lab Tests
None known.

Interactions with Diseases or Conditions
None known.

Dosage and Administration
No typical dosage.

BUTTERNUT

Also Known As
Butternussbaum, Lemon Walnut, Nogal Ceniciento, Noyer Cerdré, Oil Nut, White Walnut.

Scientific Names
Juglans cinerea.
Family: Juglandaceae.

People Use This For
Orally, butternut is used for gallbladder disorders, hemorrhoids, and skin diseases. It is also used orally as a stimulant laxative, antimicrobial, antineoplastic, antiparasitic, and tonic.

Safety
POSSIBLY SAFE ...when used orally and appropriately (12).
PREGNANCY AND LACTATION: LIKELY UNSAFE ...when used orally in large amounts, it can be cathartic (12); avoid using.

Effectiveness
There is insufficient reliable information available about the effectiveness of butternut.

Mechanism of Action
The applicable part of butternut is the bark. It is reported to have cathartic properties (12,19).

Adverse Reactions
Orally, butternut can cause diarrhea and gastrointestinal irritation (19).

Interactions with Herbs & Other Dietary Supplements
CARDIAC GLYCOSIDE-CONTAINING HERBS: Stimulant laxative herbs such as butternut can cause potassium depletion increasing the risk of cardiac toxicity. Cardiac glycoside-containing herbs include black hellebore, Canadian hemp roots, digitalis leaf, hedge mustard, figwort, lily of the valley roots, motherwort, oleander leaf, pheasant's eye plant, pleurisy root, squill bulb leaf scales, and strophanthus seeds (18,19).
LICORICE/HORSETAIL: Theoretically, concomitant use with horsetail plant or licorice rhizome increases the risk of potassium depletion (19).
STIMULANT LAXATIVE HERBS: Theoretically, concomitant use with other stimulant laxative herbs may increase the risk of potassium depletion. Stimulant laxative herbs include aloe dried leaf sap, blue flag rhizome, alder buckthorn, European buckthorn, cascara bark, castor oil, colocynth fruit pulp, gamboge bark exudate, jalap root,

black root, manna bark exudate, podophyllum root, rhubarb root, senna leaves and pods, wild cucumber fruit (Ecballium elaterium), and yellow dock root (19).

Interactions with Drugs

CORTICOSTEROIDS: Overuse of butternut might compound corticosteroid-induced potassium loss (2).
DIGOXIN (Lanoxin): Theoretically, overuse of butternut bark increases the risk of adverse effects of cardiac glycoside drugs, including digoxin (Lanoxin).
DIURETIC DRUGS: Overuse of butternut might compound diuretic-induced potassium loss (19). There is some concern that people receiving butternut along with potassium-depleting diuretics might be at an increased risk for hypokalemia. Initiation of potassium supplementation or an increase in potassium supplement dose may be necessary for some patients. Some diuretics that can deplete potassium include chlorothiazide (Diuril), chlorthalidone (Thalitone), furosemide (Lasix), hydrochlorothiazide (HCTZ, HydroDIURIL, Microzide), and others.
ORAL DRUGS: Concomitant use with butternut bark might reduce absorption of drugs due to reduced gastrointestinal transit time (19).
STIMULANT LAXATIVES: Concomitant use might compound fluid and electrolyte loss (19).

Interactions with Foods

None known.

Interactions with Lab Tests

None known.

Interactions with Diseases or Conditions

None known.

Dosage and Administration

No typical dosage.

CABBAGE

Also Known As

Colewort, Kale, Red Cabbage, White Cabbage.

Scientific Names

Brassica oleracea; Brassica oleracea var. capitata.
Family: Brassicaceae/Cruciferae.

People Use This For

Orally, cabbage is used for gastritis, gastric and duodenal ulcers, gastric pain, gastric hyperacidity, and Roemheld syndrome. Cabbage is also used orally to treat asthma, morning sickness, and prevent osteoporosis. It is also used orally to prevent lung cancer, stomach cancer, colorectal cancer, breast cancer, and other cancers.
Topically, cabbage leaves and cabbage leaf extracts are used to relieve swelling and to reduce breast engorgement.

Safety

LIKELY SAFE ...when used orally in amounts commonly found in foods. ...when used topically and appropriately, short-term. Significant side effects have not been reported in short-term studies (6781,6782,6783,6784).
POSSIBLY SAFE ...when used orally and appropriately in medicinal amounts (18).
PREGNANCY: There is insufficient reliable information available about using cabbage in medicinal amounts during pregnancy; avoid using.
LACTATION: LIKELY SAFE ...when used topically and appropriately, short-term. Significant adverse effects have not been reported in short-term studies (6781,6782,6783,6784). POSSIBLY UNSAFE ...when used orally in amounts commonly found in foods. There is some evidence that exclusively breast-fed infants develop colic if mothers consume cabbage as little as once per week (6789).

Effectiveness

POSSIBLY EFFECTIVE

Breast engorgement. Whole cabbage leaves seem to produce subjective relief similar to the standard practice of applying chilled gel-packs to the engorged breast of lactating women (6781,6784). Both chilled and room temperature cabbage leaves seem to provide the same relief (6782). A cabbage leaf extract applied as a cream has also been tried. The cabbage leaf extract cream seems to provide subjective relief, but not significantly better than a placebo cream (6783).

INSUFFICIENT RELIABLE EVIDENCE to RATE
Cancer. There is some evidence that people who consume large amounts of cabbage and other Brassica vegetables such as kale, broccoli, and cauliflower have a lower risk of developing some cancers, such as lung cancer, stomach cancer, and rectal cancer (6790,6792,6793). More evidence is needed to rate cabbage for this use.

Mechanism of Action

The applicable part of cabbage is the leaf. Cabbage, like other dark leafy vegetables, contains high amounts of vitamin K1 (11285). Cabbage contains modest amounts of calcium, vitamin C, vitamin A, vitamin E, and several B vitamins. Cabbage also contains other active constituents including chlorogenic acid, caffeic acid, and goitrin. These constituents seem to have antithyroid effects, possibly by inhibiting iodine uptake (7162). There is some interest in cabbage for breast cancer prevention because it contains constituents called glucosinolates such as indole-3-carbinol. Indole-3-carbinol is released from cabbage when it is chewed and is thought to change how estrogen is metabolized. Estrogen can be converted to either 16-alpha-hydroxyestrone or 2-alpha-hydroxyestrone. The 16-alpha-hydroxyestrone metabolite is thought to have a role in developing cancer. The 2-alpha-hydroxyestrone seems to protect against breast cancer. Indole-3-carbinol induces cytochrome P450 1A1 (CYP1A1) and 1A2 (CYP1A2), which shifts metabolism away from 16-alpha-hydroxyestrone in favor of 2-alpha-hydroxyestrone (7175,7176,7177,7179,7180,7181,7182,7187). This means that indole-3-carbinol might boost levels of a protective estrogen metabolites and decrease levels of a harmful ones. Indole-3-carbinol and other glucosinolates, including S-methyl cysteine sulfoxide, might also have anticarcinogenic properties. These constituents seem to inhibit the enzymatic transformation of pro-mutagens (6790). Cabbage also has antioxidant effects (5234,6791).

Adverse Reactions

None reported.

Interactions with Herbs & Other Dietary Supplements

None known.

Interactions with Drugs

ACETAMINOPHEN (Tylenol, Others): Cabbage can increase metabolism and decrease levels of acetaminophen. A diet that includes daily consumption of cabbage and Brussels sprouts decreases acetaminophen levels by as much as 16%. Cabbage seems to boost elimination through glucuronide conjugation (3952).
CYTOCHROME P450 1A2 (CYP1A2) SUBSTRATES: There is some concern that cabbage might decrease the effectiveness of numerous drugs. Cabbage might increase drug metabolism and elimination by stimulating cytochrome P450 1A2 (CYP1A2) activity (7176,7187). Some drugs metabolized by CYP1A2 include clozapine (Clozaril), cyclobenzaprine (Flexeril), fluvoxamine (Luvox), haloperidol (Haldol), imipramine (Tofranil), mexiletine (Mexitil), olanzapine (Zyprexa), pentazocine (Talwin), propranolol (Inderal), tacrine (Cognex), theophylline, zileuton (Zyflo), zolmitriptan (Zomig), and others.
GLUCURONIDATED DRUGS: Cabbage seems to boost elimination through glucuronide conjugation (3952). Theoretically, cabbage might also lower levels of other drugs that are metabolized through glucuronide conjugation including acetaminophen (Tylenol, others) and oxazepam (Serax), haloperidol (Haldol), lamotrigine (Lamictal), morphine (MS Contin, Roxanol), zidovudine (AZT, Retrovir), and others.
OXAZEPAM (Serax): Cabbage can increase metabolism and decrease levels of oxazepam. A diet that includes daily consumption of cabbage and Brussels sprouts decreases oxazepam levels by as much as 17%. Cabbage seems to boost elimination through glucuronide conjugation (3952). Theoretically, cabbage might also lower levels of other drugs that are metabolized through glucuronide conjugation including acetaminophen (Tylenol, others) and oxazepam (Serax), haloperidol (Haldol), lamotrigine (Lamictal), morphine (MS Contin, Roxanol), zidovudine (AZT, Retrovir), and others.
WARFARIN (Coumadin): Cabbage might decrease the anticoagulant effects of warfarin due to its high vitamin K content (19).

Interactions with Foods

None known.

Interactions with Lab Tests

INTERNATIONAL NORMALIZED RATIO (INR)/PROTHROMBIN TIME (PT): Theoretically, cabbage might decrease coagulation test results due to high vitamin K content (11285).
THYROID STIMULATING HORMONE (TSH): Ingesting large quantities of cabbage juice might elevate TSH test results (7162).

Interactions with Diseases or Conditions

HYPOTHYROIDISM: There is some concern that cabbage might worsen hypothyroidism. Cabbage constituents have antithyroid properties and there is some evidence that cabbage can boost TSH levels (7162); avoid using.

Dosage and Administration

ORAL: Cabbage is typically chopped and pressed for its juice. For augmenting the diet, 1 liter of juice has been consumed daily. For gastric pain and hyperacidity, people typically use 1 teaspoon of the juice 3 times daily before meals (18).

TOPICAL: For breast engorgement, cabbage leaves were prepared in clinical studies by stripping out the large vein of the cabbage leaf, cutting a hole for the nipple, and then rinsing and chilling the leaf. The chilled cabbage leaf is worn inside the bra or as a compress under a cool towel until the cabbage leaf reaches body temperature (approximately 20 minutes). This procedure is repeated 1-4 times daily for 1-2 days (6781,6784).

CADE OIL

Also Known As

Alquitran de Enebro, Goudron de Cade, Juniper Tar, Juniper Tar Oil, Kadeol, Oil of Cade, Oil of Juniper Tar, Oleum Cadinum, Oleum Juniperi Empyreumaticum, Pix Cadi, Pix Juniper, Pix Oxycedri, Pyroleum Juniperi, Pyroleum Oxycedri, Wacholderteer.

CAUTION: See separate listing for Juniper.

Scientific Names

Juniperus oxycedrus.

Family: Cupressaceae or Pinaceae.

People Use This For

Topically, cade oil is used for itching, psoriasis, eczema and seborrhea, parasitic skin conditions, hair loss, scalp conditions, cancers, as an antiseptic in wound dressings, and in analgesic and antipruritic preparations.

In manufacturing, cade oil is an ingredient in dermatologic creams and ointments, and in anti-dandruff shampoos.

Safety

There is insufficient reliable information available about the safety of cade oil.

Pregnancy and Lactation: Insufficient reliable information available; avoid using.

Effectiveness

There is insufficient reliable information available about the effectiveness of cade oil.

Mechanism of Action

Cade oil contains volatile oils with several constituents. Cade oil is thought to have antipruritic and keratolytic activity, and antimicrobial activity in vitro (11).

Adverse Reactions

None known.

Interactions with Herbs & Other Dietary Supplements

None known.

Interactions with Drugs

None known.

Interactions with Foods

None known.

Interactions with Lab Tests

None known.

Interactions with Diseases or Conditions

None known.

Dosage and Administration

No typical dosage.

Comments

Avoid confusion with juniper berry (Juniperus communis). Cade oil is obtained by distilling the wood of the juniper tree (Juniperus oxycedrus).

CAFFEINE

Also Known As

Anhydrous Caffeine, Caffeine and Sodium Benzoate, Caffeine Anhydrous, Caffeine Citrate, Citrated Caffeine, Methylxanthine, Methylxanthines.
CAUTION: See separate listings for Black Tea, Green Tea, Coffee, Cola Nut, Guarana, and Mate.

Scientific Names

1,3,7-trimethylxanthine.

People Use This For

Orally, caffeine is used in combination with analgesics and ergotamine for treating migraine headaches. It is used orally with analgesics for simple headaches and preventing and treating postoperative and postdural puncture headaches. It is also used orally for asthma, gallbladder disease, attention-deficit hyperactivity disorder (ADHD), neonatal apnea, increasing blood pressure in hypotension, increasing mental alertness, and enhancing athletic performance. In combination, caffeine is used with ephedrine or other stimulants and diuretics for weight loss. Very high doses are used as euphoriants, often in combination with ephedrine as an alternative to illicit stimulants.
Topically, caffeine cream preparations have been used for reducing erythema and itching in dermatitis.
Rectally, caffeine is used in combination with ergotamine for migraine headaches.
Parenterally, caffeine is used for postoperative and postdural puncture headache, neonatal apnea, acute respiratory depression, and as a diuretic. It is also used for extending the length of seizure with electroconvulsive therapy.
In foods, caffeine is used as an ingredient in soft drinks, energy drinks, and other beverages.

Safety

LIKELY SAFE ...when used orally, parenterally, or rectally and appropriately. Caffeine has Generally Recognized As Safe (GRAS) status in the US (4912). Caffeine is an FDA-approved product and a component of several over-the-counter and prescription products (4912,11832).
POSSIBLY UNSAFE ...when used orally, long term or in high doses. Chronic use, especially in large amounts, can produce tolerance, habituation, psychological dependence, and other significant adverse effects. Doses greater than 250-300 mg per day have been associated with significant adverse effects such as tachyarrhythmias and sleep disturbances (11832).
LIKELY UNSAFE ...when used orally in very high doses. The fatal acute oral dose of caffeine is estimated to be 10-14 grams (150-200 mg per kilogram). Serious toxicity can occur at lower doses depending on variables in caffeine sensitivity such as smoking, age, prior caffeine use, etc (11832).
CHILDREN: POSSIBLY SAFE ...when used orally or intravenously and appropriately in neonates (6371). ...when used in amounts commonly found in foods and beverages (4912,11833).
PREGNANCY: POSSIBLY SAFE ...when used orally amounts commonly found in foods. Mothers should closely monitor their intake of caffeine. Use of caffeine in pregnancy is controversial; however, moderate consumption has not been associated with clinically important adverse fetal effects (2708,2709,2710,2711,9606). Caffeine crosses the human placenta, but is not considered a teratogen. Fetal blood and tissue levels are similar to maternal concentrations (4260). Mothers should keep caffeine consumption below 200 mg per day. This is similar to the amount of caffeine found in 1-2 cups of coffee or tea (2708). POSSIBLY UNSAFE ...when used orally in large amounts. Caffeine crosses the placenta, producing fetal blood concentrations similar to maternal levels (4260). Mothers should avoid consuming more than 200 mg of caffeine daily or more than 1-2 cups of tea or coffee per day (2708). Maternal doses of greater than 200 mg per day throughout pregnancy have resulted in symptoms of caffeine withdrawal in newborn infants (9891). High doses of caffeine have been associated with spontaneous abortion, premature delivery, and low birth weight (2709,2711). Fetal birth weight is reduced by 28 grams for every 100 mg per day of caffeine consumed during pregnancy. But this is unlikely to be clinically significant except for women consuming more than 600 mg of caffeine daily (9606).
LACTATION: POSSIBLY SAFE ...when used orally in amounts commonly found in foods. Nursing mothers should closely monitor caffeine intake. Breast milk concentrations of caffeine are thought to be approximately 50% of maternal serum concentrations. Minimal consumption would likely result in limited exposure to a nursing infant (9892). POSSIBLY UNSAFE ...when used orally in large amounts. Caffeine is excreted slowly in infants and may accumulate. Caffeine can cause sleep disturbances, irritability, and increased bowel activity in breast-fed infants exposed to caffeine (2708,6026).

Effectiveness

EFFECTIVE

Headache. Taking caffeine orally in combination with analgesics is effective for treating simple headache. Caffeine is an FDA-approved product for use with analgesics for improving pain relief (2718,11832).

Migraine headache. Taking caffeine orally in combination with acetaminophen and aspirin is effective for treating migraine headache. Caffeine is an FDA-approved product for use with analgesics for the treatment of migraine (2715,2716,2717).

Postoperative headache. Using caffeine orally or intravenously is effective for preventing postoperative headache (2725,2726). Caffeine is an FDA-approved product for preventing headache in postoperative patients who regularly consume caffeinated products.

LIKELY EFFECTIVE

Mental alertness. Consumption of caffeinated beverages seems to prevent a decline in alertness and cognitive capacity when consumed throughout the day (4221,4224). Caffeine can improve mental performance and alertness following prolonged sleep deprivation (10205). Combining caffeine with taurine seems to provide a small improvement in mental performance (9899).

POSSIBLY EFFECTIVE

Asthma. Taking caffeine orally appears to improve airway function modestly in people with asthma for up to four hours (9607).

Athletic performance. Caffeine seems to increase physical endurance (11832) and may increase the time to exhaustion during physical exertion (10203). Caffeine doesn't seem to affect activity requiring high exertion over a short period of time such as sprinting and lifting (11832).

Gallbladder disease. Consumption of caffeinated beverages that provide 400 mg or greater of caffeine per day, is associated with significantly reducing the risk of developing symptomatic gallstone disease (3345,8032). The effect seems to be dose-dependent. Consumption of 800 mg caffeine per day has the greatest reduction in risk (3345).

Hypotension. Consuming caffeinated beverages seems to increase blood pressure in elderly people with postprandial hypotension (11834,11835).

Neonatal apnea. Using caffeine orally or intravenously seems to improve neonatal apnea of prematurity in infants 28-32 weeks postconception (6023,6371). Caffeine citrate seems to reduce the number of apnea episodes by at least 50% over 7-10 days of treatment (6371).

Parkinson's disease. There is some evidence from large-scale epidemiological studies that suggests people who consume caffeinated beverages such as coffee, tea, and cola have a decreased risk of Parkinson's disease. Men consuming 3-4 cups (28 oz) of caffeinated coffee per day, or 421-2716 mg total caffeine, had the lowest risk of developing Parkinson's disease. However, a significantly lower risk was also associated with consumption of as little as 124-208 mg of caffeine (6022). In women, more moderate caffeinated coffee consumption seems to be best; 1-3 cups per day (1238). Caffeine does not appear to provide additional protection from Parkinson's disease in cigarette smokers (9236).

Postdural puncture headache. Using caffeine orally or intravenously seems to help prevent postdural puncture headache (2727,2728).

Weight loss. Taking caffeine orally in combination with ephedrine seems to help reduce weight, short-term (695,696,1704,8647). Caffeine 192 mg in combination with ephedra 90 mg per day for 6 months, seems to cause a modest weight reduction (5.3 kg) in people with a body mass index (BMI) between 25-40 kg per meter squared. This combination, along with limiting fat intake to 30 percent of calories and moderate exercise, also seems to reduce body fat, decrease low-density lipoprotein (LDL) cholesterol, and increase high-density lipoprotein (HDL) cholesterol. Even in carefully screened and monitored otherwise healthy adults, caffeine/ephedra combinations can cause small changes in blood pressure and heart rate (8647).

POSSIBLY INEFFECTIVE

Attention deficit-hyperactivity disorder (ADHD). Most research suggests caffeine doesn't significantly reduce ADHD symptoms in children when used at tolerable doses (10755,10756,10757,10758,10759,10760). The use of caffeine in adolescents and adults with ADHD hasn't been studied.

Mechanism of Action

Caffeine is a methylxanthine compound and is structurally related to theophylline, theobromine, and uric acid (6372). It is 100% bioavailable after oral administration and is metabolized principally in the liver to paraxanthine, theophylline, and theobromine (6370). The half-life of caffeine is about six hours (8644).

Caffeine stimulates the central nervous system (CNS), heart, muscles, and possibly the pressor centers that control blood pressure (2722). Possible mechanisms include adenosine receptor blockade and phosphodiesterase inhibition (2722). By blocking adenosine receptors, caffeine is thought to increase the release of neurotransmitters such as dopamine (6370). Caffeine also decreases airway resistance and stimulates respiration, via adenosine receptor blockade and phosphodiesterase inhibition (11836). It has also been proposed that caffeine may decrease GABA and serotonin signaling (6370). Caffeine stimulates gastric acid secretion, and increases plasma catecholamine levels (11837). Caffeine can have positive inotropic and chronotropic effects on the heart (11836). Caffeine can also acutely elevate both diastolic and systolic blood pressure, but might not have this effect in habitual users (2722).

Caffeine exerts a diuretic effect, with water losses estimated at 1.17 mL per milligram of caffeine (2712). Tachyphylaxis to the diuretic effect develops rapidly, diminishing fluid losses associated with caffeine intake (10206). Caffeine-containing beverages consumed during moderate endurance exercise do not appear to compromise bodily hydration status (2713). Caffeine does not substantially affect the fluid status of people who drink caffeinated beverages on a regular basis (10206). Caffeine's CNS stimulant effects are thought to improve vigilance and psychomotor performance (2720,10205). For improving athletic performance, caffeine has been shown to decrease perceived levels of exertion, which enables the athlete to feel less tired and increase their performance (6370). Caffeine alone or in combination with ephedrine can improve anaerobic exercise performance. Caffeine seems to enhance muscle metabolism and increases time to exhaustion and oxygen deficit, which may lead to better performance (8646). Studies have also suggested caffeine possibly influences cardiovascular stress reactivity, either by potentiating the stress response itself or adding to the level reached during stress (6372). Caffeine may cause a slight decrease in heart rate after consumption and appears to raise blood pressure during psychological stress (6372). Large amounts of caffeine, >10 mg/kg/day, can also produce tachycardia and premature ventricular contractions (6372). Caffeine has been reported to cause increases and decreases in blood glucose. In people with type 2 diabetes, acute administration of caffeine impairs postprandial glucose metabolism, while acute abstention from caffeine reduces postprandial glucose levels by 21%. Whether these effects also occur with caffeinated beverages and herbs is unknown (12374). Other research in obese people suggests that caffeine ingestion may contribute to insulin resistance (12375). However, one study found that type 1 diabetics taking 200 mg of caffeine twice daily had increased frequency and intensity of warning signs of hypoglycemia. This may be due to a reduction in blood flow to the brain and an increase in glucose utilization by the brain (6024). For preventing Parkinson's disease, caffeine may protect dopaminergic neurons in the brain. This effect appears to be related to modulation of adenosine receptors (10201). This may result in a reduction in the clinical expression of Parkinsonism (6022). Evidence suggests that tolerance to caffeine's neuroendocrine and cardiovascular effects may develop during consumption throughout the day, but tolerance appears to be lost during overnight abstinence of caffeine (6372). Preliminary evidence also suggests caffeine may increase plasma levels of cortisol and adrenocorticotrophic hormone (ACTH), decrease levels of extracellular potassium, and increase levels of intracellular calcium in skeletal muscle; but the mechanisms are poorly understood (6370). Caffeine may be beneficial in the prevention of cardiovascular disease. There is evidence caffeine inhibits platelet aggregation and suppresses thromboxane formation during blood clotting (8028,8029). There is also evidence caffeine might be associated with decreased levels of testosterone and increased levels of estrone and sex-hormone binding globulin. These findings might explain why some studies have reported associations between caffeine and hormone-dependent conditions such as fibrocystic disease, osteoporosis, breast cancer, and endometriosis (8043).

Caffeine in green tea seems to work synergistically with other constituents such as catechins and theanine to produce weight loss in animals (11960). Caffeine is often used in combination with ephedra for weight loss and seems to have additive pharmacodynamic effects. A single dose of ephedra in combination with caffeine can increase heart rate from 67 beats per minute to 82 beats per minute in young, healthy people. The combination also increases systolic blood pressure and to a lesser extent, diastolic pressure (8644). Caffeine in combination with ephedra also increases oxygen consumption. Whether the increased oxygen consumption is an indication of a significant increase in metabolism and contributes to weight loss is unknown (8645).

Adverse Reactions

Orally, caffeine can cause insomnia, nervousness, restlessness, gastric irritation, nausea, vomiting, tachycardia, quickened respiration, tremors, delirium, convulsions, and diuresis. Large doses can produce headache, anxiety, agitation, ringing in the ears, premature heartbeat, and arrhythmia (11832,11838). In fatal caffeine overdose, the cause of death is usually ventricular fibrillation (11838). Insomnia is a frequent adverse effect in children (10755). Caffeine may cause feeding intolerance and gastrointestinal irritation in infants (6023). Caffeine may exacerbate sleep disturbances in patients with acquired immunodeficiency syndrome (AIDS) (10204).

Some evidence shows caffeine is associated with fibrocystic breast disease, breast cancer, and endometriosis in women; however, this is controversial since findings are conflicting (8043). Restricting caffeine in women with fibrocystic breast conditions doesn't seem to affect breast nodularity, swelling, or pain (8996).

Although acute administration of caffeine can cause increased blood pressure, regular consumption does not seem to increase either blood pressure or pulse, even in mildly hypertensive patients (1451,1452,2722).

Tolerance to caffeine is a widely held belief, but there is little supportive clinical evidence. If it exists, it appears to be of little clinical significance (11839). Withdrawal symptoms such as irritability, sleepiness, delirium, nausea, vomiting, rhinorrhea, nervousness, restlessness, anxiety, muscle tension, muscle pains, and flushed face have been described. However, these symptoms may be from nonpharmacological factors related to knowledge and expectation of effects. Clinically significant symptoms caused by caffeine withdrawal may be uncommon (2723,11839).

Epidemiological evidence regarding the relationship between caffeine use and the risk for osteoporosis is contradictory. Caffeine can increase urinary excretion of calcium (2669,10202,11317). Women identified with a genetic variant of the vitamin D receptor appear to be at an increased risk for the detrimental effect of caffeine on bone mass (2669). However, moderate caffeine intake, less than 300 mg per day, does not seem to significantly increase osteoporosis risk in most postmenopausal women with normal calcium intake (2669,6025,10202,11317).

Combining ephedra with caffeine can increase the risk of adverse effects. Jitteriness, hypertension, seizures, temporary loss of consciousness, and hospitalization requiring life support has been associated with the combined use of ephedra and caffeine (2729). There is also a report of ischemic stroke in an athlete who consumed ephedra 40-60 mg, creatine monohydrate 6 grams, caffeine 400-600 mg, and a variety of other supplements daily for six weeks (1275).

Caffeine can cause anaphylaxis in sensitive individuals, although true IgE-mediated caffeine allergy seems to be relatively rare (11315).

Interactions with Herbs & Other Dietary Supplements

CAFFEINE-CONTAINING HERBS/SUPPLEMENTS: Concomitant use can increase the therapeutic and adverse effects. Natural products that contain caffeine include coffee, black or green tea, guarana, mate, and cola nut.

CALCIUM: High caffeine intake from foods and beverages increases urinary calcium excretion (2570).
CREATINE: There is some concern that combining caffeine, ephedra, and creatine might increase the risk of serious adverse effects. There is a report of ischemic stroke in an athlete who consumed creatine monohydrate 6 grams, caffeine 400-600 mg, ephedra 40-60 mg, and a variety of other supplements daily for 6 weeks (1275). Caffeine might also decrease creatine's possible beneficial effects on athletic performance. Some researchers think caffeine can inhibit phosphocreatine resynthesis (2117,4575).
EPHEDRA (Ma Huang): Use of ephedra with caffeine can increase the risk of stimulatory adverse effects. There is evidence that using ephedra with caffeine might increase the risk of serious life-threatening or debilitating adverse effects such as hypertension, myocardial infarction, stroke, seizures, and death (1275,6486,10307). Tell patients to avoid taking caffeine with ephedra and other stimulants.

Interactions with Drugs

ADENOSINE (Adenocard): Caffeine is a competitive inhibitor of adenosine at the cellular level. However, caffeine doesn't seem to affect supplemental adenosine because high interstitial levels of adenosine overcome the antagonistic effects of caffeine (11771). It is recommended that methylxanthines and methylxanthine-containing products be stopped 24 hours prior to pharmacological stress tests (11770). However, methylxanthines appear more likely to interfere with dipyridamole (Persantine) than adenosine-induced stress testing (11771).
ALCOHOL (Ethanol): Concomitant use of alcohol can increase caffeine serum concentrations and the risk of caffeine adverse effects. Alcohol reduces caffeine metabolism (6370).
ANTICOAGULANT/ANTIPLATELET DRUGS: Theoretically, caffeine might increase the risk of bleeding when used concomitantly with these agents. Caffeine is reported to have antiplatelet activity (8028,8029); however, this interaction has not been reported in humans. Antiplatelet agents include aspirin, clopidogrel (Plavix), dipyridamole (Persantine), ticlopidine (Ticlid), and others. Anticoagulant agents include heparin and warfarin (Coumadin).
ANTIDIABETES DRUGS: Theoretically, concomitant use of caffeine and diabetes drugs might interfere with blood glucose control. Data are conflicting. Reports claim that caffeine might increase or decrease blood sugar (6024,8646).CIMETIDINE (Tagamet): Concomitant use can increase serum caffeine concentrations, and the risk of caffeine adverse effects. Cimetidine decreases the rate of caffeine clearance by 31% to 42% (11736).
CLOZAPINE (Clozaril): Co-administration can acutely exacerbate psychotic symptoms. Caffeine can also increase the effects and toxicity of clozapine. Caffeine doses of 400-1000 mg per day inhibit clozapine metabolism (5051).
CONTRACEPTIVE DRUGS: Theoretically, concomitant use might increase caffeine concentrations and the risk adverse effects. Oral contraceptives decrease the rate of caffeine clearance by 40-65% (2714,11737).
DIPYRIDAMOLE (Persantine): Caffeine inhibits dipyridamole-induced vasodilation (11770,11772). It is recommended that methylxanthines and methylxanthine-containing products be stopped 24 hours prior to pharmacological stress tests (11770). Methylxanthines appear more likely to interfere with dipyridamole (Persantine) than adenosine-induced stress testing (11771).
DISULFIRAM (Antabuse): Concomitant use can increase caffeine serum concentrations, and the risk of adverse effects. Disulfiram decreases the rate of caffeine clearance (11840).
EPHEDRINE: Use of ephedrine with caffeine can increase the risk of stimulatory adverse effects. There is evidence that using ephedrine with caffeine might increase the risk of serious life-threatening or debilitating adverse effects such as hypertension, myocardial infarction, stroke, seizures, and death (1275,6486,10307). Tell patients to avoid taking caffeine with ephedrine and other stimulants.
ESTROGENS: Concomitant use can increase serum caffeine concentrations and the risk of caffeine adverse effects. Estrogen inhibits caffeine metabolism (2714).
FLUCONAZOLE (Diflucan): Concomitant use might increase the effects of caffeine. Fluconazole decreases caffeine clearance by approximately 25% (11022).
FLUVOXAMINE (Luvox): Concomitant use can increase caffeine serum concentrations, and the risk of caffeine adverse effects. Fluvoxamine reduces caffeine metabolism (6370).
LITHIUM: Abrupt caffeine withdrawal might increase serum lithium levels (609). There are two case reports of lithium tremor that worsened upon abrupt coffee withdrawal (610).
MEXILETINE (Mexitil): Concomitant use can increase serum caffeine concentrations and the risk of caffeine adverse effects. Mexiletine reduces caffeine metabolism (1260,11741).
MONOAMINE OXIDASE INHIBITORS (MAOIs): Theoretically, concomitant intake of large amounts of caffeine with MAOIs might precipitate a hypertensive crisis (15).
PHENYLPROPANOLAMINE: Concomitant use of phenylpropanolamine and caffeine might cause an additive increase in blood pressure (11738).
QUINOLONE ANTIBIOTICS: Concomitant use can increase serum caffeine concentrations and the risk of caffeine adverse effects. Quinolones decrease caffeine clearance (606,607,608). Quinolones (fluoroquinolones) include ciprofloxacin (Cipro), enoxacin (Penetrex), gatifloxacin (Tequin), levofloxacin (Levaquin), lomefloxacin (Maxaquin), moxifloxacin (Avelox), norfloxacin (Noroxin), ofloxacin (Floxin), sparfloxacin (Zagam), and trovafloxacin (Trovan).
RILUZOLE (Rilutek): Theoretically, concomitant use might increase serum caffeine and riluzole concentrations and the risk of adverse effects of both caffeine and riluzole. Caffeine and riluzole are both metabolized by cytochrome P450 1A2, and concomitant use might reduce metabolism of one or both agents (11739).
STIMULANT DRUGS: Due to the CNS stimulant effects of caffeine concomitant use can increase the risk of

adverse effects (11832). Some stimulant drugs include diethylpropion (Tenuate), epinephrine, phentermine (Ionamin), pseudoephedrine (Sudafed), and many others.
TERBINAFINE (Lamisil): Concomitant use can increase serum caffeine concentrations and the risk of caffeine adverse effects. Terbinafine decreases the clearance of intravenous caffeine by 19% (11740).
THEOPHYLLINE: Theoretically, concomitant use might increase serum theophylline concentrations and the risk of adverse effects. Large amounts of caffeine might inhibit theophylline metabolism (11741).
VERAPAMIL (Calan, Covera, Isoptin, Verelan): Theoretically, concomitant use might increase plasma caffeine concentrations and the risk of adverse effects. Verapamil increases plasma caffeine concentrations by 25% (11741).

Interactions with Foods

None known.

Interactions with Lab Tests

5-HYDROXYINDOLEACETIC ACID: Caffeine might increase urine 5-hydroxyindoleacetic acid concentrations and test results. Caffeine can increase urine catecholamine concentrations (15).
BLEEDING TIME: Caffeine is reported to have antiplatelet activity and theoretically affect bleeding time (8028,8029). However, the significance of these effects in humans is not known.
CATECHOLAMINE: Caffeine can increase plasma catecholamine levels (8646).
CREATINE: Caffeine can increase urine creatine levels (1701).
DIPYRIDAMOLE THALLIUM IMAGING: Caffeine might interfere with dipyridamole thallium imaging studies. Caffeine attenuates the characteristic cardiovascular responses to dipyridamole and has altered test results (11742).
GLUCOSE: Caffeine has been reported to cause increases and decreases in blood glucose (8646).
LACTATE: The combination of ephedrine, a constituent of ephedra, and caffeine can increase blood lactate levels (8646).
NEUROBLASTOMA TESTS: Caffeine might cause false-positive diagnosis of neuroblastoma, when diagnosis is based on tests of urine vanillylmandelic acid (VMA) or catecholamine concentrations. Caffeine can increase urine catecholamine and VMA concentrations (15).
PHARMACOLOGICAL STRESS TESTS: Caffeine is a competitive antagonist for adenosine receptors (11771). It is recommended that caffeine and caffeine-containing products be stopped 24 hours prior to pharmacological stress tests (11770). However, caffeine appears more likely to interfere with dipyridamole (Persantine) than adenosine (Adenocard) stress testing (11771). The interaction between caffeine and dipyridamole is unlikely to be significant in stress testing if the heart rate increase is greater than 5% after dipyridamole infusion (11772).
PHEOCHROMOCYTOMA TESTS: Caffeine might cause false-positive diagnosis of pheochromocytoma, when diagnosis is based on tests of urine vanillylmandelic acid (VMA) or catecholamine concentrations. Caffeine can increase urine catecholamine and VMA concentrations (15).
PULMONARY FUNCTION TESTS: People may need to avoid caffeine for at least four hours prior to lung function testing. Forced expiratory volume in one minute (FEV1) seems to show a small improvement up to two hours after caffeine use. Mid-expiratory flow rates may also improve with caffeine for up to four hours (9607).
URATE: Caffeine might falsely increase serum urate test results determined by the Bittner method. Caffeine causes false elevations in serum urate test results determined by the Bittner method (11844).
URINARY CALCIUM: Caffeine can increase urinary calcium levels (11317).
VANILLYLMANDELIC ACID (VMA): Caffeine might increase urine VMA concentrations and test results. Caffeine can increase urine VMA concentrations (15).

Interactions with Diseases or Conditions

ANXIETY DISORDERS: Caffeine might aggravate anxiety disorders (11743).
BLEEDING DISORDERS: Theoretically, caffeine might aggravate bleeding disorders. Caffeine is reported to have antiplatelet activity (8028,8029); however, this interaction has not been reported in humans. Caffeine can prolong bleeding time and increase the results of a bleeding time test (1701).
CARDIAC CONDITIONS: Caffeine can induce cardiac arrhythmias in sensitive individuals (11845); use with caution.
DIABETES: Some research suggests that caffeine may impair postprandial glucose metabolism in people with diabetes and contribute to insulin resistance. The effect of caffeinated beverages and herbs has not been studied (12374,12375). Caffeine may enhance the frequency and intensity of hypoglycemic warning symptoms in type 1 diabetics. This may increase the ability of diabetics to detect and treat hypoglycemia early. However, it might also increase the frequency of hypoglycemic events (6024); use with caution. Caffeine has been reported to cause increases and decreases in blood glucose (8646); use with caution.
GLAUCOMA: Caffeine increases intraocular pressure. The increase occurs within 30 minutes and persists for at least 90 minutes after drinking caffeinated beverages (8540).
HYPERTENSION: Consuming caffeine might increase blood pressure in people with high blood pressure. However, this effect might be less in habitual caffeine users (2722).
OSTEOPOROSIS: Caffeine can increase urinary excretion of calcium. Caffeine consumption should be limited to less than 300 mg per day (approximately 2-3 cups of coffee). Adequate calcium supplementation may partially

compensate for calcium losses (2669,10202,11317). Postmenopausal women identified with a genetic variant of the vitamin D receptor should use caffeine with caution (2669).

Dosage and Administration

ORAL: The typical dose of caffeine for headache or restoring mental alertness is up to 250 mg per day (2718,11743). For fatigue, the common dose is 150-600 mg (11832). For increasing exercise performance, 2-10 mg/kg or more has been used. However, doses in excess of 10 mg/kg can result in urine levels greater than the 12 mcg/mL allowed by the International Olympic Committee and the National Collegiate Athletic Association (6370). For weight loss, the ephedrine and caffeine combination products are commonly dosed 20 mg/200 mg three times per day (695,696,1704). For postdural puncture headache, 300 mg orally has been used (2727,2728). For preventing symptomatic gallstone disease, consumption of 400 mg or greater of caffeine per day has been used for risk reduction (3345,8032). For preventing Parkinson's disease, men consuming 3-4 cups (28 oz) of caffeinated coffee per day or 421-2716 mg total caffeine had the lowest risk of developing Parkinson's disease. However, a significantly lower risk was also associated with consumption of as little as 124-208 mg of caffeine (6022). In women, more moderate caffeinated coffee consumption seems to be best; 1-3 cups per day (1238).
INTRAVENOUS: For apnea in infants, one study used an initial intravenous dose of caffeine benzoate of 10 mg/kg. Some infants required a second dose of 5 mg/kg 18-24 hours later (6023). Another study used a 20 mg/kg loading dose of caffeine citrate intravenously followed by a daily dose of 2.5 mg/kg intravenously or orally for 10 days for maintenance (6371). For postdural puncture headache, 500 mg caffeine sodium benzoate in 1000 mL normal saline infused over 90 minutes following anesthesia has been used (2727,2728).

Comments

People with voice disorders, singers, and other voice professionals are often advised against the use of caffeine; however, this recommendation has been based on anecdotal evidence. Now preliminary research seems to indicate that caffeine ingestion may actually adversely affect subjective voice quality. Further study is necessary to confirm these preliminary findings (2724). The use of caffeine in combination with ephedra for weight loss is controversial. Some authorities think the combination of caffeine and ephedra should only be used with physician supervision (8640). Others call for FDA licensing as a prescription drug (8641). One cup of coffee, tea, and cocoa contain approximately 75-200 mg, 50 mg, and 5 mg of caffeine respectively (6372). A 12 oz bottle of cola drink contains approximately 30-50 mg caffeine (6372).

CAJEPUT OIL

Also Known As

Cajuput, Cajeputi Aetheroleum, Paperbark Tree Oil, Punk Tree.
CAUTION: See separate listings for Niauli Oil and Tea Tree Oil.

Scientific Names

Melaleuca leucadendra, synonym Kajuputi leucadendra, Myrtus leucadendra; Melaleuca quinquenervia.
Family: Myrtaceae.

People Use This For

Orally, cajeput oil is used as an expectorant, tonic, to treat colds, headaches, toothache, and indolent tumors.
Topically, cajeput is used for its anti-parasitic effect in scabies and tinea versicolor. Cajeput oil is also used either alone or in combination with other ingredients in commercially available antiseptic liniments to treat rheumatic and neuralgic discomforts.
As an inhalant, it is used as an expectorant and tonic.
In dentistry, cajeput oil is used to relieve dry socket discomfort.
In food and beverages, it is used as a flavoring in very small amounts.

Safety

LIKELY SAFE ...when cajeput oil is used orally in amounts commonly found in foods. Cajeput oil has Generally Recognized As Safe (GRAS) status in the US (4912).
POSSIBLY SAFE ...when used topically on unbroken skin (2,7).
POSSIBLY UNSAFE ...when inhaled. Inhalation can cause bronchospasm (7).
There is insufficient reliable information available about the safety of cajeput oil for its other uses or in amounts exceeding those found in food.
CHILDREN: LIKELY UNSAFE ...when used topically on facial areas, especially the nose (2,7) because it might cause bronchospasm.
PREGNANCY AND LACTATION: Insufficient reliable information available; avoid using.

Effectiveness
There is insufficient reliable information available about the effectiveness of cajeput oil.

Mechanism of Action
Cajeput oil contains 14-65% cineole (7,11), which is reported to have antispasmodic, antimicrobial and fungicidal properties (7). Cineole may act as a counterirritant (7). Cineole is identical to eucalyptol (215).

Adverse Reactions
Orally, use of cajeput oil can lead to dyspepsia (7).
Topically, use can produce hypersensitivity, allergic reactions and irritation of mucous membranes (7).
Inhalation can cause bronchospasm (7).

Interactions with Herbs & Other Dietary Supplements
None known.

Interactions with Drugs
None known.

Interactions with Foods
None known.

Interactions with Lab Tests
None known.

Interactions with Diseases or Conditions
ASTHMA: Inhalation of cajeput oil may provoke bronchospasm (7).

Dosage and Administration
No typical dosage.

Comments
Avoid confusion with tea tree oil (Maleleuca alternifolia) and niauli oil (Malaleuca viridiflora). Cajeput oil is produced by steam distillation of fresh leaves and twigs of Melaleuca leucadendra and Melaleuca quinquenervia.

CALABAR BEAN

Also Known As
Chop Nut, Esere Nut, Faba Calabarica, Legume, Ordeal Bean, Physotigma.

Scientific Names
Physostigma venenosum.
Family: Fabaceae/Leguminosae.

People Use This For
Orally, calabar bean is used for visual disorders, constipation, epilepsy, cholera, and tetanus. Calabar bean is a source of the prescription drug physostigmine (Isopto Eserine, Antilirium).

Safety
UNSAFE ...when used orally. The calabar bean is extremely toxic. Its active constituent, physostigmine, can cause death by impairing heart contractility and causing respiratory paralysis (6).
PREGNANCY AND LACTATION: UNSAFE ...when used orally (6); avoid using.

Effectiveness
There is insufficient reliable information available about the effectiveness of calabar bean.

Mechanism of Action
The applicable part of calabar bean is the dried, ripe seed. The major constituent, physostigmine, prolongs activity of neurotransmitter acetylcholine (6). It increases parasympathetic nervous system and striated muscle tone, stimulates glandular secretions, increases GI peristalsis, reduces heart rate, and causes pupil contraction leading to a reduction in intraocular pressure (18).

Adverse Reactions
Orally, overdose of physostigmine, the constituent of calabar bean, causes cholinergic crisis characterized by excessive salivation and sweating, constricted pupils of eye, nausea, vomiting, diarrhea, bradycardia or tachycardia, hypotension or hypertension, confusion, seizures, coma, severe muscle weakness, paralysis, and death (15).

Interactions with Herbs & Other Dietary Supplements
None known.

Interactions with Drugs
ANTICHOLINERGIC DRUGS: Physostigmine, a constituent of calabar bean, reverses the effect of belladonna and other drugs with anticholinergic action. These drugs include antihistamines, some emetics, some anti-Parkinson agents, and phenothiazines (15).

Interactions with Foods
None known.

Interactions with Lab Tests
None known.

Interactions with Diseases or Conditions
Avoid in patients with Parkinson's disease, bradycardia, asthma, gangrene, diabetes, cardiovascular disease, and mechanical obstruction of intestinal or urogenital tract.

Dosage and Administration
No typical dosage.

Comments
Historically, African tribes used calabar bean, the "ordeal bean," to identify witches and people possessed by evil spirits. They believed that people who regurgitated the bean and lived were innocent. Ritual uses continue in Africa despite being outlawed (6). Subjects of the "ordeal" can increase their chance of survival by not chewing the bean and swallowing it whole. Chewing releases the toxic constituents.

CALAMINT

Also Known As
Basil Thyme, Lesser Calamint, Mill Mint, Mountain Balm, Mountain Mint.

Scientific Names
Calamintha nepeta, synonyms Clinopodium nepeta, Melissa nepeta, Satureja calamintha, Satureja nepeta.
Family: Lamiaceae/Labiatae.

Comments
At the date of publication, this product was not a common ingredient used in brand name supplements marketed to consumers. Details about this product are available at the online version of *Natural Medicines Comprehensive Database*. See www.naturaldatabase.com.

CALAMUS

Also Known As
Bach, Cinnamon Sedge, Flagroot, Gladdon, Grass Myrtle, Kalmus, Myrtle Flag, Myrtle Sedge, Sadgrantha, Sweet Cane, Sweet Cinnamon, Sweet Calamus, Sweet Flag, Sweet Grass, Sweet Myrtle, Sweet Root, Sweet Rush, Sweet Sedge, Ugragandha, Vacha, Vayambur.

Scientific Names
Acorus calamus; Acorus americanus; Acorus gramineus; Acorus sp.
Family: Acoraceae.

People Use This For

Orally, calamus is used for digestive disorders including ulcers, gastritis, and flatulence, acute and chronic dyspepsia, anorexia; and to stimulate appetite and digestion. Calamus is also used orally as a sedative, to induce sweating, and for rheumatoid arthritis, and stroke.
Calamus is also chewed to remove the smell of tobacco, as a stimulant, as a euphoric, and as a hallucinogen.
Topically calamus is used for skin disease.
In foods, calamus is utilized in cooking as a spice.

Safety

LIKELY UNSAFE ...when used orally. The FDA prohibits calamus use in food products (4912) due to the presence of the carcinogenic constituent, beta-isoasarone in three of the four distinct species. However, the beta-isoasarone content can vary widely among species, from 0% to 96%, (6); some products may be safer than others.
PREGNANCY AND LACTATION: LIKELY UNSAFE ...when used orally; avoid using (4,500).

Effectiveness

There is insufficient reliable information available about the effectiveness of calamus.

Mechanism of Action

The applicable part of calamus is the rhizome. The constituent asarone, which is chemically related to reserpine, may explain calamus' sedative effects (6). It is not known exactly which constituent is responsible for calamus' ability to relieve smooth muscle spasms, though it is probably not isoasarone, because preparations without isoasarone have a measurable spasmolytic effect (6).

Adverse Reactions

Calamus oil may contain beta-isoasarone, a known carcinogen associated with kidney damage, tremors, and convulsions.

Interactions with Herbs & Other Dietary Supplements

HERBS WITH SEDATIVE PROPERTIES: Theoretically, concomitant use with supplements that have sedative properties might enhance therapeutic and adverse effects or calamus. Some of these include 5-HTP, calamus, California poppy, catnip, hops, Jamaican dogwood, kava, St. John's wort, scullcap, valerian, yerba mansa, and others.

Interactions with Drugs

ANTACIDS: Theoretically, due to reports that calamus increases stomach acid, calamus might decrease the effectiveness of antacids (19).
CNS DEPRESSANTS: Theoretically, concomitant use with drugs with sedative properties can cause additive effects and side effects (4).
H2-BLOCKERS: Theoretically, due to reports that calamus increases stomach acid, calamus might decrease the effectiveness of H2-blockers (19). The H2 blockers include cimetidine (Tagamet), ranitidine (Zantac), nizatidine (Axid), and famotidine (Pepcid).
MONOAMINE OXIDASE INHIBITORS (MAOIs): Theoretically, calamus might potentiate the effects and adverse effects of monoamine oxidase inhibitor drugs (4).
PROTON PUMP INHIBITORS (PPIs): Theoretically, due to reports that calamus increases stomach acid, calamus might decrease the effectiveness of PPIs (19). PPIs include omeprazole (Prilosec), lansoprazole (Prevacid), rabeprazole (Aciphex), pantoprazole (Protonix), and esomeprazole (Nexium).

Interactions with Foods

None known.

Interactions with Lab Tests

None known.

Interactions with Diseases or Conditions

None known.

Dosage and Administration

ORAL: 1-3 grams of the rhizome has been used three times daily (4). As a tea one cup tea, prepared by steeping 1-3 grams of the rhizome in 150 mL of boiling water for 5-10 minutes, has been used three times daily (4). 1-3 mL of the liquid extract, 1:1 in 60% alcohol, has been used three times daily (4). 2-4 mL of the tincture, 1:5 in 60% alcohol, has been used three times daily (4).

Comments
Four different species of Calamus exist, each in a different geographic region of the world. The North American variety is isoasarone free and the European form contains less than 10% isoasarone in the volatile oil. Others contain up to 96% carcinogenic beta-isoasarone in the volatile oil (5).

CALCIUM

Also Known As
Bone Meal, Calcium Acetate, Calcium Aspartate, Calcium Carbonate, Calcium Chelate, Calcium Chloride, Calcium Citrate, Calcium Gluconate, Calcium Lactate, Calcium Lactogluconate, Calcium Orotate, Calcium Phosphate, Di-calcium Phosphate, Heated Oyster Shell-Seaweed Calcium, Hydroxyapatite, Oyster Shell Calcium, Tricalcium Phosphate.
CAUTION: See separate listing for Dolomite.

Scientific Names
Calcium; Ca; atomic number 20.

People Use This For
Orally, calcium is used for treatment and prevention of hypocalcemia, osteoporosis, rickets, and latent tetany. It is also used orally for hypoparathyroidism, osteomalacia, premenstrual syndrome (PMS), leg cramps associated with pregnancy, and reducing the risk of colorectal cancer. Calcium is also used orally for diarrhea and rectal epithelial hyperproliferation following intestinal bypass, hypertension, elevated levels of low-density lipoprotein (LDL), elevated fluoride levels in children, and elevated lead levels. Calcium carbonate is used orally as an antacid. Calcium carbonate and calcium acetate are also used orally as phosphate binders in renal failure.
Intravenously, calcium gluconate, acetate, gluceptate and chloride are used for severe hypocalcemia and hypocalcemic tetany, and during cardiopulmonary resuscitation. Calcium gluconate and gluceptate are also given intramuscularly when intravenous administration is not possible.

Safety
LIKELY SAFE ...when used orally and appropriately. Calcium is safe when used in doses that do not exceed the tolerable upper intake level (UL) of 2.5 grams (7555). Although higher doses have been used safely, taking doses that exceed the UL are more likely to cause side effects. ...when used intravenously and appropriately (15).
POSSIBLY UNSAFE ...when used orally in high doses. Doses that exceed 2.5 grams of elemental calcium are more likely to cause side effects (7555). ...when calcium chloride is used orally. Ingestion of calcium chloride has been reported to cause gastrointestinal hemorrhage (15).
PREGNANCY AND LACTATION: LIKELY SAFE ...when used orally and appropriately (945,1586,3263,3264). There is insufficient reliable information available about the safety of the intravenous use of calcium during pregnancy and lactation.

Effectiveness
EFFECTIVE

Dyspepsia. Taking calcium carbonate orally as an antacid is effective for treating dyspepsia (9,15).

Hypocalcemia. Taking calcium orally is effective for treating and preventing hypocalcemia (15). Intravenous calcium gluconate, acetate, gluceptate, or chloride is effective for severe hypocalcemia or hypocalcemic tetany (15).

Renal failure. Taking calcium carbonate or calcium acetate orally is effective as a phosphate binder in renal failure (9). Calcium citrate is not recommended for this purpose because it increases aluminum absorption.

LIKELY EFFECTIVE

Corticosteroid-induced osteoporosis. Taking calcium in combination with vitamin D as adjunctive therapy seems to be effective for reducing bone mineral density loss in people using corticosteroids long-term (982,1046,1830,1831,1832,4462,4463,4464,4465,4466,4467).

Fetal bone mineralization. Calcium supplementation in pregnant women who have low dietary calcium intake (less than 562 mg elemental calcium per day), increases fetal bone mineralization and density. However, in women with adequate dietary intake, calcium supplementation doesn't offer any additional benefit (3263,3264).

Hyperparathyroidism. Taking calcium orally reduces parathyroid hormone levels in patients with chronic renal failure and secondary hyperparathyroidism (1827,1828,1829). In elderly women, the combination of calcium and vitamin D reverses secondary hyperparathyroidism and reduces hip fracture risk (8818).

Osteoporosis. Taking calcium orally is effective for preventing and treating bone loss and osteoporosis. Maximal bone growth occurs in the teenage years, then bone density in women remains relatively constant until age 30 to 40. After age 40, bone loss typically occurs at rates of 0.5% to 1% per year. In men, this occurs several decades later. Bone loss is more pronounced if dietary calcium intake is below the RDA, which is the case for many Americans (2571,2578). This bone loss in premenopausal women over 40 can be reduced significantly by supplementing with 1000 mg calcium per day (2578). In the 5 years immediately after menopause, calcium supplementation has very little effect on bone loss (2569,2570,2575,2576). The rapid loss of estrogen causes a very high bone resorption rate, which increases serum calcium levels and inhibits intestinal absorption of calcium (2570). After this period, calcium supplementation has a significant benefit on bone loss. The typical rate of bone loss in postmenopausal women who are not taking calcium supplements is 2% per year (2572,2576). Calcium 1000 to 1600 mg per day (as carbonate, citrate, lactate gluconate, or citrate malate) decreases this rate by 0.25% to 1% annually (977,979,981,2569,2571,2572,2575,2576,2578,6850). The greatest reductions (1% or more) are seen in the first one to two years of supplementation when bone remodeling foci can be filled in (2569,2576). After this period, the differences in rate of loss between supplemented and unsupplemented women are closer to 0.25% per year (2569,2577). Despite the "first year effect" it is estimated that 30 years of continuous calcium supplementation after menopause might result in a 10% improvement in bone mineral density, and a 50% overall reduction in fracture rates, compared with women who do not take calcium supplements (2570). Most studies show that long-term calcium supplementation decreases fracture rates for specific bones by 30% to 35% for vertebral bone and 25% for hip bone (2576). Supplements must be continued indefinitely since the effects of two years of calcium supplements on bone mineral density are largely lost within two years after discontinuing the supplements (981,2576,6853). Calcium supplementation also seems to reduce bone turnover during weight reduction in postmenopausal women (987). The usefulness of calcium in preventing osteoporosis in men is not as well-studied as in women. Some evidence suggests calcium 1 gram per day taken for 2 years might improve trabecular or cortical bone mass by 2% to 4% (980,8827,8873). Dietary supplementation with calcium and vitamin D seems to moderately reduce bone loss measured in the femoral neck, spine, and total body, and seems to reduce the incidence of nonvertebral fractures (980). Calcium has additive effects on bone density with other agents such as vitamin D, estrogens, or calcitonin. Whereas calcium alone generally reduces or prevents loss of bone density, combination with other agents can produce small increases in bone density ranging from 0.3% to 3.3% depending on the combination and doses used (978,980,1836,2570,2571,2572,2576). The full potential of osteoporosis treatments cannot be realized without adequate calcium intake (2569,2570,2571,2572). Advise patients taking agents such as estrogens, calcitonin, bisphosphonates, or raloxifene (Evista) to ensure that their daily calcium intake meets the RDA. Use supplements if necessary. Higher calcium intake is associated with higher radial bone mineral content, but is not associated with higher tibial bone mineral content. The non-weight bearing radial bone of the arm seems to benefit more from high calcium intake than physical activity. The weight-bearing tibial bone of the leg seems to benefit more from physical activity than calcium intake (8819). However, calcium supplements don't seem to be effective for preventing bone mineral density loss in lactating women (988), after bone marrow transplantation (1817), or for preventing bone loss associated with renal transplantation (4823).

Premenstrual syndrome (PMS). There seems to be a link between low dietary calcium intake and symptoms of PMS (6847). Taking calcium 1-1.2 grams daily seems to significantly reduce depressed mood, water retention, and pain associated with PMS (1822,1823,1824). Calcium seems to decrease symptom scores by about 18% compared to placebo (1822).

POSSIBLY EFFECTIVE

Colorectal cancer. High intake of dietary or supplemental calcium seems to reduce the risk of adenoma recurrence and colorectal cancer (970,994,1047,8820,12118,12120). Vitamin D might be an important factor. People with lower than average vitamin D levels don't seem to get any benefit from calcium supplements (12118).

Fluorosis. Taking calcium orally in combination with ascorbic acid (vitamin C) and vitamin D supplements seems to be effective for reducing excessive fluoride levels in children and improving symptoms of fluorosis (990).

Hypercholesterolemia. Taking calcium orally in conjunction with a low-fat diet seems to be effective for treating mild to moderate hypercholesterolemia. Calcium carbonate 400 mg three times daily produced a 4.4% reduction in low-density lipoprotein (LDL) cholesterol and a 4.1% increase in high-density lipoprotein (HDL) after six weeks of treatment when used in combination with a low-fat diet (American Heart Association step 1) starting eight weeks prior to calcium carbonate (2557).

Hypertension. Calcium supplementation produces a very modest reduction in blood pressure, usually around 2 mmHg. However, it may be more effective for certain subpopulations of patients, such as salt-sensitive people and African-American patients with low dietary calcium intake (945,972,974,976,984,1818,1819,1820,1821,6852). Taking calcium orally also seems to be effective for reducing blood pressure in individuals with end-stage renal disease (975).

Ischemic stroke. There is some evidence that increasing dietary calcium intake might decrease the relative risk of ischemic stroke in women (4822).

Pregnancy-related complications. Taking calcium orally seems to be effective for reducing pregnancy-related hypertension and pre-eclampsia in women with insufficient dietary calcium intake (971,973,1833,1834,8828). Calcium 2 grams daily appears to reduce pre-eclampsia occurrences up to sevenfold among women at high risk. Supplementation in women with adequate dietary intake does not seem to affect pre-eclampsia. There is also some evidence that calcium 1 gram twice daily (as a mixture of salts) can reduce pregnancy-related leg cramps during the second half of pregnancy (2567).

Tooth retention. Taking calcium and vitamin D orally appear to beneficially affect tooth retention in the elderly population (8816).

Weight loss. Adults and children with low calcium intake are more likely to gain weight, have a higher body mass index (BMI), and be overweight or obese compared to people with high calcium intake (8824,12124,12125,12126,12127). Increasing calcium consumption from dairy products seems to increase weight reduction in people on a calorie restricted diet (8824,8830,12128). Increasing calcium from dairy products such as yogurt to a total calcium intake from 800-1100 mg seems to result in more weight and body fat loss than consuming less calcium. An increase in calcium consumption of 900 mg to 1000 mg/day seems to be associated with an 8-9 kilogram reduction in body weight (8824,12050,12051,12127). But increasing calcium from supplements might not be as beneficial (12051,12052).

POSSIBLY INEFFECTIVE

Elevated lead concentrations. Taking calcium orally doesn't seem to reduce lead concentrations in lactating women. Lead is mobilized along with calcium from bone during pregnancy and lactation, resulting in increased serum concentrations of lead. Calcium supplementation does not significantly decrease these elevated lead concentrations (1586).

INSUFFICIENT RELIABLE EVIDENCE to RATE

Seizures. Preliminary clinical evidence suggests calcium might help control seizures resulting from sudden declines in serum ionized calcium (8835). More evidence is needed to rate calcium for this use.

Mechanism of Action

The bones and teeth contain greater than 99% of the calcium in the human body. Calcium in bone is present mainly as hydroxyapatite (1834).

Calcium is also present in blood, extracellular fluid, muscle, and other tissues. It is essential for nerve transmission, muscle contraction, vascular contraction, vasodilation, glandular secretion, cell membrane and capillary permeability, enzyme reactions, respiration, renal function, and blood coagulation. It also plays a role in neurotransmitter and hormone release and storage, uptake and binding of amino acids, cyanocobalamin (vitamin B12) absorption, and gastrin secretion (15).

Calcium in bone is a reserve source of calcium that can be mobilized to maintain extracellular calcium concentrations. About half of serum calcium is bound to plasma proteins. The free or ionized calcium is tightly regulated and is a useful clinical indicator of calcium status (1834).

Calcium balance is generally positive during growth, neutral in the mature adult, and negative in older adults. Calcium is lost in varying amounts through the feces, urine, sweat, and sloughed skin cells. Reduced estrogen levels in women result in reduced calcium absorption and retention, increased bone turnover, and lower bone mass (1834,8833,8838,8839).

Calcium absorption varies with age, environmental and dietary conditions, and race (1837,8870). People of Asian and African descent absorb calcium more efficiently than Caucasians (1837). Elderly women, in general, have an impaired intestinal response to vitamin D. This impairment can further contribute to negative calcium balance and bone loss (8833,8838). In healthy premenopausal women, the proportion of dietary calcium absorbed varies from 10-60%, and is positively correlated with body mass index, dietary fat, and serum vitamin D level (6851). It is inversely correlated with total dietary calcium, dietary fiber, alcohol intake, and physical activity (6851). There is a link between a low fat, high fiber diet and poor calcium absorption, possibly due to a faster rate of intestinal transit (6851).

There is also a link between weight loss and calcium absorption. Weight loss of 5% or greater is associated with decreased bone mass and increased risk of fracture. Weigh loss seems to decrease calcium absorption and increase parathyroid hormone. Taking calcium supplements during weight loss seems to suppress the increased bone resorption (12117).

Calcium exhibits threshold absorption. Below the threshold, an increase in calcium intake results in improved response; above the threshold, increased calcium intake has no effect. The many variables of calcium absorption complicate interpretation of calcium absorption studies (1834,8823). Some evidence suggests that calcium citrate and heated oyster shell-seaweed calcium are absorbed better than calcium carbonate, while other research indicates similar bioavailability (1838,1839,1840,1841,1842,1847,8832).

Calcium carbonate absorption is decreased by estrogen or vitamin D deficiency (8823).

Preliminary evidence suggests that calcium-rich mineral waters appear to have similar bioavailability when compared to oral calcium supplements (8836).

Calcium absorption is not impaired due to lactose intolerance. However, lactose intolerance could limit dairy calcium intake (8837).

Contrary to laboratory evidence, lactose does not enhance calcium bioavailability in lactose tolerant people (4824).

Calcium is sometimes used for renal patients because it can bind with phosphate in the gut, preventing its absorption and reducing the hyperphosphatemia associated with renal failure. Calcium carbonate and calcium acetate are used for this purpose. Calcium citrate is not recommended because it increases aluminum absorption. Conversely, hypophosphatemia causes an increase in intestinal calcium absorption and increased calcium in the blood, which can inhibit formation of new bone (3372,8821), and potentially lead to a greater risk of renal calcium stone formation (3372).

Calcium may help to lower serum cholesterol levels by forming insoluble complexes with saturated fatty acids in the gut, causing them to be excreted in the feces without being absorbed (2557).

For weight loss, calcium seems to modulate diet-related adiposity by inhibiting lipogenesis, increasing lipolysis, and promoting fat loss. Increasing dietary calcium intake may result in reduced body weight, primarily by reducing fat mass (8824,8825,8870). Calcium seems to repartition dietary energy from adipose tissue to lean body mass (12119).

Dairy products containing calcium seem to be more effective at regulating adiposity than elemental calcium supplements (12121).

Evidence also suggests that inadequate dietary intake of calcium can play a role in the development of hypertension, stroke, and cardiovascular disease (8817). Calcium might lower blood pressure by increasing renal sodium excretion (12122).

In women, calcium levels may be lower in the premenstrual period (due to effects of variations in estrogen levels on calcium absorption and metabolism), which may contribute to the mood changes and other symptoms associated with premenstrual syndrome (PMS) (2639,6847).

There is also interest in using calcium for cancer prevention. Preliminary evidence suggests calcium may have an antiproliferative effect on colorectal cancer cells (8820,8870,10019). Calcium taken orally also seems to reverse rectal epithelial hyperproliferation caused by excessive output of fecal bile acids and lipids after intestinal bypass (1826).

Adverse Reactions

Orally, calcium can cause gastrointestinal irritation, belching, and flatulence (1843). Although constipation is frequently cited as an adverse effect of calcium, there is no scientific substantiation of this side effect (1843,1844,1845). Calcium chloride can cause gastrointestinal hemorrhage when taken orally (15). Extended use of calcium carbonate for gastric hyperacidity can cause acid rebound (9). Prolonged ingestion of large amounts of calcium carbonate (usually greater than 20 grams per day) can cause hypercalcemia, milk-alkali syndrome (1843,6123), nephrocalcinosis, and renal insufficiency (6122). In patients with impaired renal function, doses as low as 4 grams per day might cause hypercalcemia and milk-alkali syndrome (1843,6849). There is concern that calcium supplements, both oyster shell and refined calcium products, can be contaminated with lead (997,6459,6460). In one report, 8 of 23 nationally available calcium carbonate products contained small amounts of lead (6459). However, these findings are likely clinically insignificant. The amount of lead in these calcium supplements is substantially less than that found in common foods, such as green salads, grapes, and wine. Also, calcium significantly decreases lead absorption. Small amounts of lead in a calcium supplement would not likely be significantly absorbed or achieve clinically relevant levels in the body (6460). So far, there have not been reports of significant lead toxicity from appropriate use of calcium supplements (996). Epidemiological evidence suggests that a high intake of dietary calcium might increase the risk for prostate cancer (4825).

Interactions with Herbs & Other Dietary Supplements

VITAMIN D: Concomitant administration with vitamin D increases active absorption of calcium in the small intestine (945).

Interactions with Drugs

BISPHOSPHONATES: Calcium supplements decrease absorption of bisphosphonates. Advise patients to take bisphosphonates at least 30 minutes before calcium, but preferably at a different time of day (15,506). The bisphosphonates include alendronate (Fosamax), etidronate (Didronel), risedronate (Actonel), and tiludronate (Skelid).

CALCIUM CHANNEL BLOCKERS: Calcium, particularly when given intravenously, may decrease the effects of calcium channel blockers. It is used in the management of calcium channel blocker overdose (15,506). The calcium channel blockers include nifedipine (Adalat, Procardia), verapamil (Calan, Isoptin, Verelan), diltiazem (Cardizem), isradipine (DynaCirc), felodipine (Plendil), amlodipine (Norvasc), and others. Intravenous calcium gluconate has been used before intravenous verapamil (Isoptin) to prevent or reduce the hypotensive effects without affecting the antiarrhythmic effects (6124).

ESTROGENS: Estrogen increases supplemental calcium absorption in postmenopausal women (995).

LEVOTHYROXINE (Synthroid, Levothroid, Levoxyl, and others): Calcium reduces levothyroxine absorption, probably by forming insoluble complexes (5082). Calcium carbonate supplements reduce effectiveness of levothyroxine in patients with hypothyroid (5081,5082,6137). Advise patients to take levothyroxine and calcium supplements at least four hours apart.

QUINOLONE ANTIBIOTICS: Taking calcium at the same time as quinolones reduces quinolone absorption. Calcium forms insoluble complexes with quinolones (4412,10339). Advise patients to take these drugs at least 2 hours before, or four to six hours after calcium supplements (10339). Quinolones include ciprofloxacin (Cipro), levofloxacin (Levaquin), ofloxacin (Floxin), moxifloxacin (Avelox), gatifloxacin (Tequin), gemifloxacin (Factive), and others.

SOTALOL (Betapace): Calcium appears to reduce the absorption of sotalol, probably by forming insoluble complexes (10018). Advise patients to separate doses by at least two hours before or four to six hours after dolomite.

TETRACYCLINE ANTIBIOTICS: Calcium decreases the absorption of tetracyclines by forming insoluble complexes (9). Advise patients to take these drugs at least two hours before, or four to six hours after calcium supplements. Tetracyclines include demeclocycline (Declomycin), doxycycline (Vibramycin), and minocycline (Minocin).

THIAZIDE DIURETICS: Thiazides reduce calcium excretion by the kidneys (1902). Using thiazides along with moderately large amounts of calcium carbonate increases the risk of milk-alkali syndrome (hypercalcemia, metabolic alkalosis, renal failure). Advise patients to consult their physician about appropriate calcium doses, and to have their serum calcium levels and/or parathyroid function monitored regularly. These diuretics include chlorothiazide (Diuril), hydrochlorothiazide (HydroDIURIL, Esidrix), indapamide (Lozol), metolazone (Zaroxolyn), chlorthalidone (Hygroton), etc.

Drug Influences on Nutrient Levels and Depletion

SOME DRUGS CAN AFFECT CALCIUM LEVELS:

ALUMINUM SALTS: Large doses of aluminum salts (aluminum hydroxide 1 to 3 grams four times daily, e.g., 90 to 260 mL Maalox daily) bind dietary phosphate, causing hypophosphatemia. This induces movement of calcium from bone into the blood, increasing urinary calcium excretion (4400). There are reports of negative calcium balance after short-term use of large doses of aluminum-containing antacids, and of osteomalacia after prolonged use of large doses, especially in people with a low dietary phosphate intake, or a low dietary calcium intake (less than 250 mg per day) (4400,5979). Advise patients to avoid taking large doses of aluminum-containing antacids for prolonged periods, unless they are taking them for hyperphosphatemia associated with chronic renal failure.

ANTICONVULSANTS: Phenytoin (Dilantin), fosphenytoin (Cerebyx), phenobarbital, and carbamazepine (Tegretol) decrease calcium absorption by increasing metabolism of vitamin D, which is needed for calcium absorption (2675). Hypocalcemia and osteomalacia have occurred, especially with prolonged therapy and use of more than one of these drugs concurrently (2675). Advise patients taking these medications for six months or more that they may also need vitamin D and calcium supplements. Other anticonvulsants such as gabapentin (Neurontin), felbamate (Felbatol), lamotrigine (Lamictal), levetiracetam (Keppra), tiagabine (Gabitril), and topiramate (Topamax) do not have these effects.

CHOLESTYRAMINE (Questran): Cholestyramine can reduce absorption of vitamin D, which in turn reduces absorption of calcium. Occasionally this can lead to osteomalacia, usually in patients receiving large doses of cholestyramine (more than 32 grams per day), or prolonged therapy (more than two years). It can also occur in the presence of additional risk factors such as ileal resection or primary biliary cirrhosis (which deplete the bile acids needed for vitamin D absorption) (4458,5655,5809,5838). Supplements of vitamin D, and sometimes calcium, are necessary in these patients. Use of cholestyramine (24 grams/day) for treatment of hyperlipidemia in otherwise healthy men doesn't seem to affect vitamin D and calcium levels, and supplements aren't necessary (2672).

CORTICOSTEROIDS: Corticosteroids, in daily doses equivalent to 7.5 mg prednisone or more, cause significant bone loss, osteoporosis, and increased risk of fractures. The severity increases with duration of therapy. Mechanisms include decreased absorption and increased excretion of calcium, reduction in sex hormones, and inhibition of bone formation. Advise adults taking prednisone 7.5 mg/day (or equivalent doses of other corticosteroids) for six months or longer to maintain a daily calcium intake of 1500 mg/day. They may also need a vitamin D supplement (e.g., 800 IU/day). Monitor serum calcium (1832,4462,4463,4464,4465,4466,4467).

DIURETICS: Loop diuretics increase urinary calcium excretion and may reduce serum calcium levels, especially at higher doses (1902,4412). Loop diuretics include furosemide (Lasix), bumetanide (Bumex), ethacrynic acid (Edecrin), and torsemide (Demadex).

FLUOROQUINOLONES: Fluoroquinolones form complexes with calcium in the gastrointestinal tract, which could reduce absorption of both the fluoroquinolone and calcium if taken at the same time (4412). Significant effects on calcium levels are unlikely when fluoroquinolones are taken at least two hours before, or four to six hours after calcium supplements or calcium-containing foods. Fluoroquinolones include ciprofloxacin (Cipro), levofloxacin (Levaquin), ofloxacin (Floxin), moxifloxacin (Avelox), gatifloxacin (Tequin), and others.

H2 BLOCKERS and PROTON PUMP INHIBITORS (PPIs): Absorption of some calcium supplements, especially calcium carbonate, is reduced when gastric acid is reduced (15,506). However, there isn't any evidence that acid suppressive drugs reduce serum calcium levels. There also isn't any evidence that cimetidine affects parathyroid hormone (PTH) or calcium levels in healthy people, but there are conflicting reports about cimetidine's effect on PTH and calcium levels in people with primary hyperparathyroidism (2738,4330,4331,5060). H2 blockers include cimetidine (Tagamet), ranitidine (Zantac), nizatidine (Axid), and famotidine (Pepcid). PPIs include omeprazole (Prilosec), lansoprazole (Prevacid), rabeprazole (Aciphex), pantoprazole (Protonix), and esomeprazole (Nexium).

LEVOTHYROXINE: Levothyroxine (Synthroid, Levothroid, Levoxyl) may accelerate bone remodeling and turnover, increase the rate of bone loss at several sites including the spine and hips, and cause a negative calcium balance (27,2685,2695,2697,2721). This is most likely when high doses are used for suppressive therapy in thyroid cancer, nodules, or goiter, rather than replacement doses for hypothyroidism. Clinically significant bone loss is most likely in postmenopausal women, but negative effects have also been reported in premenopausal women and men (28,29,2685,2695). Advise patients to have regular thyroid function tests to monitor for appropriate levothyroxine dose (2684,2695,2698,2721). Also check to see patients daily intakes of calcium and vitamin D meet the recommendations for their age and gender (2684).

MAGNESIUM SALTS: Large doses of magnesium salts may cause hypocalcemia. This is most likely with intravenous doses sufficient to produce hypermagnesemia, such as in the treatment of acute myocardial infarction or premature labor (2730,2731). High magnesium levels increase urinary calcium excretion, possibly due to changes in the renal threshold for calcium absorption, or reduced parathyroid hormone secretion (2730,2731). Calcium supplementation is unlikely to be needed with short-term, intravenous magnesium therapy. Oral magnesium supplements (e.g., magnesium oxide 576 mg/day) do not affect calcium absorption (4623).

MINERAL OIL: Mineral oil can interfere with calcium utilization and retention by reducing absorption of both calcium and vitamin D (4495). Advise patients against regular or long-term use of mineral oil.

STIMULANT LAXATIVES: Prolonged use of high doses of stimulant laxatives can reduce dietary calcium and vitamin D absorption, and possibly lead to osteomalacia (15,506). Advise patients to limit stimulant laxatives to

short-term use of recommended doses. Some stimulant laxatives include cascara (CitraMax Plus), senna (Senokot), bisacodyl (Dulcolax), and others.
TETRACYCLINES: Tetracyclines form complexes with calcium in the gastrointestinal tract, which could reduce absorption of both the tetracycline and calcium if taken at the same time (4412). Significant effects on calcium levels are unlikely when tetracyclines are taken at least two hours before, or four to six hours after calcium supplements or calcium-containing foods. Tetracyclines include demeclocycline (Declomycin), doxycycline (Vibramycin), and minocycline (Minocin).

Interactions with Foods

CAFFEINE: High caffeine intake from foods and beverages increases urinary calcium excretion (2570). Intake of more than 300 mg/day (three to four cups of coffee, or six 12 oz cola drinks) is linked to increased bone loss and increased fracture rates in elderly women, especially when calcium intake is low (2669,2670). Advise patients to ensure that their calcium intake from food and supplements is at the recommended level for their age and sex.
FIBER: Certain constituents of dietary fiber inhibit calcium absorption. These include phytic acid (found in wheat bran), oxalic acid (found in spinach and rhubarb), and uronic acid (a common plant fiber constituent) (945). Separate administration of calcium supplements from these foods by two hours.
IRON, ZINC, MAGNESIUM: Calcium supplements may decrease the absorption of dietary iron, zinc, and magnesium. However, in people with adequate stores of these minerals, this doesn't have any clinically significant effect on the long-term status of iron, zinc, or magnesium in the body (1848,1849,1850,7135,7308,8822,8831). Advise people at high risk for deficiency of these minerals to take calcium supplements at bedtime, instead of with meals, to avoid inhibiting dietary mineral absorption (7308).
SODIUM: High sodium intake from foods increases urinary calcium excretion (1834,2570). A calcium intake of 1000 mg/day is needed to prevent bone loss in postmenopausal women ingesting 2000 mg sodium chloride daily. About 1500 mg/day calcium is needed if sodium chloride intake is 3000 mg/day (2570).

Interactions with Lab Tests

11-HYDROXYCORTICOSTEROIDS: Calcium gluconate given intravenously may increase plasma 11-hydroxycorticosteroid concentrations and test results (275).
17-HYDROXYCORTICOSTEROIDS: Calcium gluconate may reduce urinary 17-hydroxycorticosteroid concentrations and test results. One case of this interaction is reported (275).
BONE MINERAL DENSITY (BMD): Supplemental calcium taken orally may prevent or reduce the rate of bone mineral loss as reflected in BMD measures (977,978,981).
GASTRIN: Calcium carbonate may increase serum gastrin concentrations and test results within 30-75 minutes after calcium carbonate ingestion (275).
GLUCOSE: Calcium gluconate may decrease serum glucose concentrations and test results. This interaction was reported in newborns (275).
I-131 UPTAKE: Calcium gluconate may decrease serum uptake of I-131 (275).
INSULIN: Calcium gluconate may increase plasma insulin concentrations and test results. This interaction was reported in newborns (275).
LIPASE: Calcium ions may falsely decrease test results when measuring serum lipase concentrations greater than 5 mmol/L using the method of Teitz (275). Calcium ions do not affect test results when measuring serum lipase concentrations up to 5 mmol/L using the method of Teitz (275).
MAGNESIUM: Calcium gluconate can falsely decrease test results for serum magnesium measured by titan-yellow, but will not affect test results measured by the dihydroxyazobenzene method (275). Calcium gluconate can falsely decrease test results for urine magnesium measured by titan-yellow (275).

Interactions with Diseases or Conditions

HYPERCALCIURIA (CALCIUM OXALATE STONES): Restricting intake of animal protein and salt, combined with a normal dietary calcium intake, appears to provide greater protection from recurrent kidney stones than a low-calcium diet (8826).
HYPERPARATHYROIDISM: Hyperparathyroid activity predisposes individuals to increased calcium absorption (945).
HYPERPHOSPHATEMIA: Use cautiously in patients with high serum phosphate levels. The product of serum phosphate and calcium levels should not exceed 60 to prevent precipitation of calcium phosphate and soft tissue calcification (6479).
HYPOPHOSPHATEMIA: Use cautiously in patients with low serum phosphate levels. If calcium intake increases without a concurrent increase in phosphorus intake, phosphorus absorption can decrease, worsening phosphorus deficiency (8821).
HYPOTHYROIDISM: Patients taking levothyroxine (L-thyroxine, Levothroid, Synthroid) replacement therapy should separate administration of levothyroxine and calcium carbonate by four hours. Calcium carbonate reduces levothyroxine absorption and effectiveness in hypothyroid patients on levothyroxine replacement therapy (5081,5082,6137).
RENAL INSUFFICIENCY: Calcium carbonate supplementation increases the risk of hypercalcemia and alkalosis (9). Renal insufficiency predisposes individuals to reduced calcium absorption (945).

SARCOIDOSIS: This condition results in increased risk of excessive calcium absorption and hypercalcemia (945).
SMOKING: Cigarette smoking decreases intestinal calcium absorption (1846).

Dosage and Administration

ORAL: For preventing hypocalcemia 1 gram elemental calcium daily is typically used (15). Calcium replacement requirements in people with hypocalcemia can be estimated by clinical condition or serum calcium determinations, but a typical starting dose is 1 to 2 grams daily (15).
For heartburn, calcium carbonate as an antacid is usually 0.5 to 1.5 grams as needed (15).
For hyperphosphatemia in adults with chronic renal failure, the initial dose of calcium acetate is 1.334 grams (338 mg elemental calcium) with each meal, increasing to 2 to 2.67 grams (500-680 mg elemental calcium) with each meal if necessary (15).
For prevention of osteoporosis in postmenopausal women, doses of 1 to 1.6 grams elemental calcium daily in divided doses (as carbonate, citrate, lactate gluconate, or citrate malate) have been used (977,979,981,2569,2571,2575,2576,2578,8838,8871), and should be chosen to bring the total daily calcium intake from diet and supplements up to the relevant dietary reference intake (see below) (981,2569,2571,2575,2578,8838,8870).
For prevention of bone loss in premenopausal women over 40, a dose of 1 gram daily has been used (2578).
For pregnant women with low dietary calcium intake, the dose for increasing fetal bone density ranges from 300-1300 mg/day beginning at gestation week 20-22 (3263,3264). A dose of 1 to 1.2 grams calcium per day as calcium carbonate has reduced symptoms of premenstrual syndrome (PMS) (1822,1824).
For treatment of secondary hyperparathyroidism in people with chronic renal failure, doses of 2 to 21 grams calcium carbonate daily have been used (1827,1828,1829).
For treatment of secondary hyperparathyroidism in elderly women, elemental calcium 1200 mg daily, combined with 800 IU vitamin D daily, has been used (8818).
To prevent bone loss associated with chronic corticosteroid therapy, a dose of 1.5 grams elemental calcium daily has been recommended (15).
For reducing the risk of recurrence of colorectal adenomas, calcium carbonate 3 to 4 grams (1.2 to 1.6 grams calcium) daily has been used (970,994,1047,8820,12118).
As an adjunct to other treatments for hypertension, 1 to 1.5 grams calcium daily has been used (945,972,974,976,984,1818,1819,1820,1821,6852). Typical doses used to reduce the risk of preeclampsia are 1 to 2 grams elemental calcium daily as calcium carbonate (971,973,1833,1834,8828).
For treating diarrhea and rectal epithelial hyperproliferation due to intestinal bypass, a dose of 2.4 to 3.6 grams daily calcium as calcium carbonate has been used (1826).
For hypercholesterolemia, 400 mg calcium (as calcium carbonate) three times daily has been used in conjunction with a low-fat diet (2557).
High serum fluoride levels and symptoms of fluorosis in children have been reduced with calcium 125 mg twice daily, in combination with ascorbic acid and vitamin D (990).
For weight loss, increasing calcium consumption from dairy products to a total consumption of 800 mg to 1000 mg/day in combination a calorie-restricted diet seems to increase weight loss (12050,12051,12052).
Calcium carbonate and calcium citrate are the two most commonly used forms of calcium (945,8832). Calcium carbonate contains 400 mg calcium/gram and calcium citrate contains 211 mg calcium/gram (15) (1000 mg elemental calcium = 2500 mg calcium carbonate = 4700 mg calcium citrate). Absorption of calcium from supplements is greatest when taken with food in doses of 500 mg or less since the active transport system for calcium in the small bowel is easily saturated (6122,8832). Calcium supplements are usually divided into two doses daily (8871). Calcium citrate may be preferable in people with achlorhydria or taking drugs that reduce gastric acidity (e.g., H2 antagonists, proton pump inhibitors) (1816,8832).
The daily Dietary Reference Intakes (DRI) for elemental calcium are: Age 1-3 years, 500 mg; 4-8 years, 800 mg; 9-18 years, 1300 mg; 19-50 years, 1000 mg; 51+ years, 1200 mg; Pregnant or Lactating (under 19 years), 1300 mg; Pregnant or Lactating (19-50 years), 1000 mg (7555,8839). The daily upper intake level (UL) for calcium is 2.5 grams for everyone over one year of age (3094).
INTRAVENOUS: Calcium injections are prescription products which must be administered slowly (maximum rate of 1.8 mEq/minute) (15) and under medical supervision. The usual initial dose for severe hypocalcemia is 7 to 14 mEq elemental calcium (1 mEq = 20 mg elemental calcium) (15). Subsequent doses are given according to the patient's response and serum calcium levels. For hypocalcemic tetany, 4.5 to 16 mEq doses are given until a response occurs (15). Doses of calcium used in cardiopulmonary resuscitation are 0.027 to 0.054 mEq/kg calcium chloride, 4.5 to 6.3 mEq calcium gluceptate, or 2.3 to 3.7 mEq calcium gluconate (15).

Comments

Calcium-rich foods include milk and dairy products, kale and broccoli, as well as the calcium-enriched citrus juices, mineral water (6356), canned fish with bones, and soy products processed with calcium.
In the US and Canada, foods containing at least 200 mg calcium with less phosphorus content than calcium are allowed to be labeled with a health claim for osteoporosis. In the US, the health claim may read "Regular exercise and a healthy diet with enough calcium helps teen and young adult white and Asian women maintain good bone health and may reduce their high risk of osteoporosis later in life." Canada recently updated its health claim wording to emphasize the importance of vitamin D and to broaden the claim to beyond women: "A healthy diet with adequate

calcium and vitamin D, and regular physical activity, help to achieve strong bones and may reduce the risk of osteoporosis" (11940).

CALCIUM D-GLUCARATE

Also Known As
Calcium Glucarate, Calcium-D Glucarate, Calcium-D-Glucarate, D-Glucarate (GA).
CAUTION: See separate listing for Calcium.

Scientific Names
D-glucaro-1,4-lactone (1,4 GL).

People Use This For
Orally, calcium D-glucarate is used for preventing breast, prostate, and colon cancer; and for removing carcinogens, toxins, and steroid hormones from the body.

Safety
There is insufficient reliable information available about the safety of calcium D-glucarate.
Pregnancy and Lactation: Insufficient reliable information available; avoid using.

Effectiveness
There is insufficient reliable information available about the effectiveness of calcium D-glucarate.

Mechanism of Action
Glucaric acid is combined with calcium to form calcium D-glucarate. Glucaric acid is found in tissues and body fluids. Glucaric acid is also found in foods such as fruits and vegetables including oranges, apples, Brussels sprouts, broccoli, and cabbage (772,3952). Dietary sources provide from 1.12-1.73 mg/100 grams (broccoli and potatoes) to a high of 4.53 mg/100 grams (oranges) (772).
There is a lot of interest in using calcium D-glucarate for preventing estrogen-related cancer such as breast cancer and other hormone-related cancers. Calcium D-glucarate is thought to decrease estrogen levels by affecting estrogen's elimination. Estrogen is normally metabolized hepatically in phase II metabolism by combining with glucuronic acid. It's then excreted in the bile, but a bacterial enzyme in the intestine called beta-glucuronidase normally breaks the estrogen-glucuronide bond, allowing estrogen to be reabsorbed. Calcium D-glucarate works at this step by inhibiting beta-glucuronidase. Blocking this enzyme is thought to decrease the amount of estrogen that is reabsorbed and lower circulating estrogen levels. There is some evidence that beta-glucuronidase activity might be increased in patients with hormone-dependent cancers like breast and prostate cancer (773,774). Dietary glucarate can inhibit beta-glucuronidase activity and inhibits animal models of mammary tumor development (775). In vitro, D-glucarate decreases tumor cell proliferation (776). Urinary excretion of D-glucaric acid may be an indicator of drug metabolizing enzyme activity in people with impaired renal function (778).

Adverse Reactions
None reported.

Interactions with Herbs & Other Dietary Supplements
None known.

Interactions with Drugs
ALCOHOL (Ethanol): Theoretically, concomitant use with alcohol might decrease calcium D-glucarate activity. There is some evidence that urinary excretion of D-glucarate is increased in people consuming alcohol (779).
GLUCURONIDATED DRUGS: Theoretically, calcium D-glucarate might increase the clearance of drugs that undergo glucuronidation. Some of these drugs include acetaminophen, atorvastatin (Lipitor), diazepam (Valium), digoxin, entacapone (Comtan), estrogen, irinotecan (Camptosar), lamotrigine (Lamictal), lorazepam (Ativan), lovastatin (Mevacor), meprobamate, morphine, oxazepam (Serax), and others (772,3952).
KANAMYCIN: Theoretically, D-glucarate may increase the rate of kanamycin elimination and possibly reduce the risk of drug-induced renal impairment (777).

Interactions with Foods
ALCOHOL (Ethanol): Theoretically, concomitant use with alcohol might decrease calcium D-glucarate activity. There is some evidence that urinary excretion of D-glucarate is increased in people consuming alcohol (779).

Interactions with Lab Tests
None known.

Interactions with Diseases or Conditions
None known.

Dosage and Administration
No typical dosage.

CALENDULA

Also Known As
Garden Marigold, Gold-Bloom, Holligold, Marigold, Marybud, Pot Marigold, Zergul.
CAUTION: See separate listing for Tagetes.

Scientific Names
Calendula officinalis.
Family: Asteraceae/Compositae.

People Use This For
Orally, calendula flower is used as an antispasmodic, to initiate menstrual periods, to reduce fever, for treating cancer, and for inflammation of oral and pharyngeal mucosa. Calendula has also been used orally for gastric and duodenal ulcers and dysmenorrhea.
Topically, calendula is used as an anti-inflammatory and for poorly healing wounds and leg ulcers. It is also used topically for nosebleeds, varicose veins, hemorrhoids, proctitis, and conjunctivitis.

Safety
LIKELY SAFE ...when the flower preparations are used orally or topically and appropriately (4).
PREGNANCY: LIKELY UNSAFE ...when used orally; contraindicated due to spermatocide, antiblastocyst, and abortifacient effects. There is insufficient reliable information available about the safety of the topical use of calendula during pregnancy (4).
LACTATION: Insufficient reliable information available; avoid using.

Effectiveness
There is insufficient reliable information available about the effectiveness of calendula.

Mechanism of Action
The applicable part of calendula is the flower. Calendula is used for wound healing due to potential anti-inflammatory effects. The faradiol monoester is believed to play an important role in the anti-inflammatory activity. Some evidence suggests the water-soluble flavonoids might be responsible for the wound-healing effects (515). Preliminary data suggests that calendula may inhibit human immunodeficiency virus (HIV) replication (11455). Calendula also shows some evidence of antibacterial and antitumor activity (4).

Adverse Reactions
Orally, calendula can cause allergic reactions.
Topically, calendula can cause eczematous allergic reactions. Calendula-specific patch testing is recommended prior to usage to determine allergenic potential. Testing is particularly necessary in individuals sensitive to the Asteraceae/Compositae family (10691,11458). Members of this family include ragweed, chrysanthemums, marigolds, daisies, and many other herbs. Despite the widespread use of calendula and the occurrence of allergies to other family members, there has been only one report of anaphylaxis (11152).

Interactions with Herbs & Other Dietary Supplements
None known.

Interactions with Drugs
CNS DEPRESSANTS: Theoretically, concomitant use of calendula with drugs having sedative properties might cause additive therapeutic and adverse effects. A saponoside constituent in Calendula has been reported to increase hexobarbital sleep time in animals (19).

Interactions with Foods
None known.

Interactions with Lab Tests
None known.

Interactions with Diseases or Conditions
CROSS-ALLERGENICITY: Calendula may cause an eczematous allergic reaction in individuals sensitive to the Asteraceae/Compositae family (10691,11458). Members of this family include ragweed, chrysanthemums, marigolds, daisies, and many other herbs.

Dosage and Administration
ORAL: One cup of the tea is commonly taken three times daily; the tea is prepared by steeping 1-2 grams of the dried flowers in 150 mL boiling water for 5-10 minutes and then straining (2,4). The typical dose of the liquid extract, 1:1 in 40% alcohol, is 0.5-1 mL three times daily (4). The tincture, 1:5 in 90% alcohol, is usually given as 0.3-1.2 mL three times daily (4).
TOPICAL: The tea is commonly used as a gargle, mouthwash, or poured over an absorbent cloth and applied as a poultice to skin ailments (3). For topical use, 2-4 mL of the tincture is usually diluted into 0.25-0.5 L water. Ointments typically contain 2-5 grams of the herb in 100 grams ointment (2).

Comments
Avoid confusion with ornamental marigolds of the Tagets genus, which are commonly grown in vegetable gardens (11).

CALIFORNIA POPPY

Also Known As
California Poppies, Poppy California.
CAUTION: See separate listing for Corn Poppy.

Scientific Names
Eschscholzia californica.
Family: Papaveraceae.

People Use This For
Orally, California poppy is used for insomnia, sedation, aches, nervous agitation, enuresis in children, and diseases of the bladder and liver.
In combination with other herbs, California poppy is used orally for depression, neurasthenia, neuropathy, various psychiatric conditions, foehn illness (sleep and mood disturbance associated with strong, warm wind in the Alps), vasomotor dysfunction, sensitivity to weather changes, and sedation.

Safety
POSSIBLY UNSAFE ...when used orally. Although only the dried aerial parts are used medicinally, the freshly harvested plant contains cyanogenic glycosides that could potentially cause cyanide poisoning (18).
PREGNANCY AND LACTATION: POSSIBLY UNSAFE ...when used orally; avoid using (18).

Effectiveness
There is insufficient reliable information available about the effectiveness of California poppy.

Mechanism of Action
The applicable parts of California poppy are the dried, above ground parts. The active constituents are thought to be isoquinoline alkaloids (2,18). One alkaloid, cryptonine, may have uterine stimulating activity in guinea pigs (2). The tincture is reported to prolong pentobarbital-induced sleep in mice and to prevent chemically-induced spasms in rat jejunum (2).

Adverse Reactions
None reported.

Interactions with Herbs & Other Dietary Supplements
HERBS WITH SEDATIVE PROPERTIES: Theoretically, concomitant use with supplements that have sedative properties might enhance therapeutic and adverse effects of California poppy. Some of these supplements include 5-HTP, calamus, California poppy, catnip, hops, Jamaican dogwood, kava, St. John's wort, scullcap, valerian, yerba mansa, and others.

Interactions with Drugs
CNS DEPRESSANTS: Theoretically, concomitant use of California poppy with drugs with sedative properties may cause additive effects and side effects (19).

Interactions with Foods
ALCOHOL: Theoretically, California poppy may increase the risk of drowsiness and impair motor skills; avoid concomitant use.

Interactions with Lab Tests
None known.

Interactions with Diseases or Conditions
None known.

Dosage and Administration
ORAL: People typically drink 1 cup tea (made by steeping 2 grams herb in 150 mL boiling water 10-15 minutes, strain) up to four times daily (12). Liquid extract, 1-2 mL per day (18).

Comments
Avoid use of the freshly harvested plant due to presence of cyanogenic glycosides. Avoid confusion with corn poppy (Papaver rhoeas). The California poppy (Eschscholzia californica) is sometimes confused with the opium poppy (Papaver somniferum). Both are members of the Papaveraceae family, but they are members of a different genera. They are distant relatives and the California poppy does not provide opium like the opium poppy.

CALOTROPIS

Also Known As
Ak, Akada, Alarka, Arka, Mudar Bark, Muder Yercum, Sodom-Apple.

Scientific Names
Calotropis procera, synonym Asclepias procera.
Family: Apocynaceae or Asclepiadaceae.

People Use This For
Orally, calotropis is used for toothache, syphilis, digestive disorders, diarrhea, boils, ulcers, swellings, rheumatism, epilepsy, hysteria, cramps, fever, joint pain, muscular spasm, and constipation, cancer, warts, leprosy, elephantiasis, worms, fever, gout, and snake bites.
In inhalation therapy, smoke from the bark is inhaled for coughs, asthma, and to induce sweating.

Safety
LIKELY UNSAFE ...when used orally, especially in high doses. Calotropis contains cardiac glycosides. High doses can cause vomiting, diarrhea, bradycardia, convulsions, and death (18).
There is insufficient reliable information available about the safety of calotropis for its other uses.
PREGNANCY AND LACTATION: LIKELY UNSAFE ...when used orally (18); avoid using.

Effectiveness
There is insufficient reliable information available about the effectiveness of calotropis.

Mechanism of Action
Calotropis contains cardioactive glycosides (cardenolides) (13,18) that show some antitumor effects on human cells in vitro (18). Calotropis also has expectorant and diuretic properties (18). Animal studies of calotropis extract have shown anti-inflammatory (3823), antibacterial (3824), antipyretic, analgesic, and neuromuscular blocking activity (3822). In one animal study, the extract produced contractions that were blocked by atropine; this supports a use in constipation (3822). In another animal study, an extract of the root showed significant anti-ulcer activity against aspirin, indomethacin, ethanol, indomethacin + ethanol, or stress-induced ulcerations. This anti-ulcer activity may be attributable to the inhibition of 5-lipoxygenase (3825).

Adverse Reactions
Orally, high doses can cause vomiting, diarrhea, bradycardia, convulsions, and death (18).

Interactions with Herbs & Other Dietary Supplements

CARDIAC GLYCOSIDE-CONTAINING HERBS: Concomitant use can increase the risk of cardiac glycoside toxicity. Cardiac glycoside-containing herbs include black hellebore, Canadian hemp roots, digitalis leaf, hedge mustard, figwort, lily of the valley roots, motherwort, oleander leaf, pleurisy root, squill bulb leaf scales, strophanthus seeds, and uzara (19).
CARDIOACTIVE HERBS: Avoid concomitant use with cardioactive herbs due to unpredictability of effects and adverse effects. These include calamus, cereus, cola, coltsfoot, devil's claw, European mistletoe, fenugreek, fumitory, ginger, Panax ginseng, hawthorn, white horehound, maté, parsley, quassia, scotch broom flower, shepherd's purse, and wild carrot (4).
LICORICE/HORSETAIL: Theoretically, the overuse or misuse of licorice rhizome or horsetail plant increases the risk of toxicity due to potassium depletion (19).
STIMULANT LAXATIVE HERBS: Theoretically, the overuse or misuse of stimulant laxatives increases the risk of cardiac toxicity due to potassium depletion. Stimulant laxative herbs include aloe dried leaf sap, blue flag rhizome, alder buckthorn, European buckthorn, butternut bark, cascara bark, castor oil, colocynth fruit pulp, gamboge bark exudate, jalap root, black root, manna bark exudate, podophyllum root, rhubarb root, senna leaves and pods, wild cucumber fruit (Ecballium elaterium), and yellow dock root (19).

Interactions with Drugs

DIGOXIN (Lanoxin): Theoretically, concomitant use with calotropis increases the risk of cardiac glycoside toxicity.
DIURETIC DRUGS: Theoretically, concomitant use of calotropis and potassium-depleting diuretics can increase the risk of cardiac glycoside toxicity due to potassium depletion (13,18). Some diuretics that can deplete potassium include chlorothiazide (Diuril), chlorthalidone (Thalitone), furosemide (Lasix), hydrochlorothiazide (HCTZ, HydroDIURIL, Microzide), and others.
STIMULANT LAXATIVES: Theoretically, concomitant use with calotropis may increase risk of cardiac glycoside toxicity due to potassium loss.

Interactions with Foods

None known.

Interactions with Lab Tests

None known.

Interactions with Diseases or Conditions

None known.

Dosage and Administration

ORAL: As an expectorant or diuretic, 200 to 600 mg daily; as an emetic, 2-4 grams daily has been used (18).
TOPICAL: Calotropis is applied as a powder (18).

Comments

In India, calotropis has been used as a suicidal and infanticidal poison (215).

CAMPHOR

Also Known As

Camphora, Camphor Tree, Cemphire, Gum Camphor, Karpoora, Laurel Camphor.

Scientific Names

Cinnamomum camphora, synonym Laurus camphora.
Family: Lauraceae.

People Use This For

Topically, camphor is used to relieve pain. It has been used to treat warts, cold sores, hemorrhoids, and osteoarthritis. It has also been applied topically as an analgesic and an antipruritic. It has been used as a counterirritant, and to increase local blood flow. Camphor has frequently been used topically to treat respiratory tract diseases involving mucous membrane inflammation. It is sometimes used topically to treat cardiac symptoms. Camphor is also used topically as an eardrop, and for treating minor burns.
In inhalation therapy, camphor is used as an antitussive.
Orally, camphor is used as an expectorant, antiflatulent, and for treating respiratory tract diseases.

Safety

LIKELY SAFE ...when used topically in low concentrations, short-term. Concentrations ranging from 0.1%-11% seem to be safe for short-term topical use on intact skin (272,10327). ...when used by inhalation, appropriately (272).
POSSIBLY SAFE ...when used topically and appropriately short term. Camphor in combination with glucosamine, shark cartilage, and chondroitin appears to be safe when applied topically on an as-needed basis for up to eight weeks (10327).
LIKELY UNSAFE ...when used topically on broken or injured skin. Application of camphor to broken skin can result in systemic absorption and toxicity (272).
UNSAFE ...when used orally. Ingestion of camphor can cause significant toxicity including death (12). Oral preparations of camphor are no longer available in the US (159).
CHILDREN: POSSIBLY UNSAFE ...when used topically (4814). Young children might be more susceptible to the adverse effects associated with even minor systemic absorption of camphor. UNSAFE ...when used orally. Ingestion of camphor can cause significant toxicity including death (4814).
PREGNANCY AND LACTATION: UNSAFE ...when used orally. Ingestion of camphor can cause serious toxicity including death (17). There is insufficient reliable information available about the safety of camphor when used topically during pregnancy and lactation.

Effectiveness

EFFECTIVE

Cough. Camphor is FDA-approved as a topical antitussive (chest rub) in concentrations less than 11% (4814).
Pain. Camphor is FDA-approved for topical use as an analgesic and anesthetic in concentrations of 3% to 11% (272,4814). It is in many topical products for cold sores, insect stings and bites, minor burns, and hemorrhoids (272).
Pruritus (itching). Camphor is FDA-approved for topical use as an antipruritic agent in concentrations of 3% to 11% (272,4814).

POSSIBLY EFFECTIVE

Osteoarthritis. A topical cream containing camphor, glucosamine sulfate, and chondroitin sulfate seems to reduce the severity of symptoms of osteoarthritis by about half. Symptom relief is most likely due to the counterirritant effect of camphor and not the other ingredients (10327).

There is insufficient reliable information available about the effectiveness of camphor for its other uses.

Mechanism of Action

The applicable part of camphor is the wood distillate. Camphor seems to exert its effect as a nasal decongestant by inducing local vasoconstriction (16). Camphor's counterirritant action is also due to vasoconstriction, which often improves local circulation, and therefore provides analgesic and antipruritic effects (16). Camphor also has weak expectorant effects.

Adverse Reactions

Orally, camphor can cause significant toxicity. Symptoms of camphor toxicity occur rapidly and start with nausea and vomiting, oral and intestinal burning, feeling of warmth, and headache. This can progress to confusion, vertigo, excitement, restlessness, delirium, hallucinations, muscular excitability, tremors, jerky movements, epileptiform convulsions, and depression. This is sometimes followed by central nervous system depression and coma. Death can occur from respiratory failure or status epilepticus (17). Other adverse effects that can occur after oral ingestion include tachycardia, mydriasis, visual disturbances, urinary retention, albuminuria, mild transient elevations of aspartate dehydrogenase and lactic dehydrogenase (LDH), and rarely, hepatic failure (17). While adults have recovered after ingesting as much as 42 grams of camphor, as little as 2 grams is usually enough to produce significant toxic effects. Much less is required to cause toxicity in children. In children, ingestion of as little as 700-1000 mg of camphor has been fatal. For example, 20 mL of a 5% camphor product can be lethal in a child (4814). In patients who survive camphor ingestion, recovery from toxicity is usually slow.
Although topical application of camphor is not as likely to cause adverse effects, some camphor can be absorbed through intact skin. A considerable amount of camphor can also be absorbed when used by inhalation. Excessive use of camphor either topically or by inhalation can result in the development of symptoms of toxicity (17). Topical use of camphor has also been associated with contact eczema (12). There is also a report of increased liver enzymes in an infant who received a camphor-containing topical cold remedy. The liver enzymes normalized after stopping treatment (4608). Camphor products can contain safrole, which has been found to be a mild carcinogen in vitro (12); however, carcinogenic effects due to use of safrole-containing camphor preparations have not yet been reported in humans (12).
Due to the potential risk, camphor products should only be used short-term.

Interactions with Herbs & Other Dietary Supplements

None known.

Interactions with Drugs

None known.

Interactions with Foods
None known.

Interactions with Lab Tests
LIVER FUNCTION TESTS: Oral use of camphor can cause transient elevations of liver enzymes in both adults and children. There is also a report of increased liver enzymes in an infant who received a camphor-containing topical cold remedy. The enzymes affected included aspartate aminotransferase (AST), alanine aminotransferase (ALT), alkaline phosphatase, and lactate dehydrogenase (LDH). The liver enzymes normalized after stopping the topical cold formula (4608).

Interactions with Diseases or Conditions
GASTROINTESTINAL (GI) IRRITATION: Camphor might irritate the GI tract, and is contraindicated in individuals with infectious or inflammatory GI conditions (19).

Dosage and Administration
TOPICAL: For itching, cold sores, and hemorrhoids, a 0.1%-3% ointment is typically used three to four times daily (272). As an counterirritant, a 3%-11% ointment is typically used three to four times daily (272). As an antitussive, a thick layer of 4.7%-5.3% camphor ointment is applied to the throat and chest as a thick layer. The area may be covered with a warm, dry cloth or left uncovered (272). For osteoarthritis, a topical cream containing camphor (32 mg/g), glucosamine sulfate (30 mg/g), and chondroitin sulfate (50 mg/g), has been used as needed on sore joints for up to 8 weeks (10327).
INHALATION: 1 tablespoon of solution per quart of water is placed directly into a hot steam vaporizer, bowl, or washbasin. Sometimes 1.5 teaspoons of solution are added to a pint of water and boiled. The medicated vapors are breathed. This inhalation may be repeated up to three times a day (272).
ORAL: Camphor is unsafe for oral use (12).

Comments
Camphor is a well-established folk remedy and is commonly used. The American Academy of Pediatrics recommends non-prescription camphor products should not exceed 11% strength. They also recommend that camphor not be used in treating children (4814). Camphorated oil (20% camphor in cottonseed oil) was removed from the US market due to toxicity in the 1980s.

CANADA BALSAM

Also Known As
Balm of Gilead, Balsam, Balsam Canada, Balsam Fir, Balsam Fir Canada, Balsam of Fir, Canada Turpentine, Canadian Balsam, Eastern Fir.
CAUTION: See separate listing for Oregon Fir Balsam.

Scientific Names
Abies balsamea, synonym Pinus balsamea.
Family: Pinaceae.

People Use This For
Topically, Canada balsam is used for hemorrhoids and as an antiseptic.
In dentistry, Canada balsam is used in root canal sealers and dentifrices.
Historically, Canada balsam has been used for burns, sores, cuts, tumors, heart and chest pains, cancer, mucous membrane inflammation, colds, coughs, warts, wounds, urogenital complaints, and as a pain-reliever.
In foods, Canada balsam is an ingredient in foods and beverages.
In manufacturing, Canada balsam is used in cosmetics as a fixative and fragrance and in ointments and creams. It is also used as a cement for lenses and prepared microscope slides.

Safety
LIKELY SAFE ...when used orally in amounts commonly found in foods. Canada balsam has Generally Recognized As Safe (GRAS) status in the US (4912).
POSSIBLY SAFE ...when used topically (11).
There is insufficient reliable information available about the safety of Canada balsam used orally in medicinal amounts.
PREGNANCY AND LACTATION: Insufficient reliable information available; avoid using.

Effectiveness
There is insufficient reliable information available about the effectiveness of Canada balsam.

Mechanism of Action
There is insufficient reliable information available about the possible mechanism of action and active ingredients.

Adverse Reactions
None reported.

Interactions with Herbs & Other Dietary Supplements
None known.

Interactions with Drugs
None known.

Interactions with Foods
None known.

Interactions with Lab Tests
None known.

Interactions with Diseases or Conditions
None known.

Dosage and Administration
ORAL: People typically take 2 to 6 tablespoons of weak tea of Canada balsam. As a tincture (1:5 with 50% ethanol), Canada balsam is usually dosed 5 to 20 drops.
TOPICAL: A weak liquid is usually applied to affected areas (5276).

Comments
Avoid confusion with poplar (Populus tacamahacca, P. balsamifera, P. candicans) or spruce (Picea excelsa) also known as balm of Gilead. Oregon fir balsam (Pseudotsuga menziesii) has been detected as an adulterant in Canada balsam (Abies balsamea) (11). Canada balsam is an oleoresin (rather than a true balsam) collected from punctures in the bark of the Canadian balsam tree (Abies balsamea).

CANADIAN FLEABANE

Also Known As
Butterweed, Canadian Horseweed, Canadian-Fleabane, Canadian Trailing Arbutus, Coltstail, Flea Wort, Hogweed, Horsewood, Prideweed.

Scientific Names
Conyza canadensis, synonym Erigeron canadensis.
Family: Asteraceae/Compositae.

Comments
At the date of publication, there was very little scientific information about this product. Our staff is continually analyzing the available information on natural medicines and will add data to the online version of *Natural Medicines Comprehensive Database* as it becomes available. See www.naturaldatabase.com.

CANADIAN HEMP

Also Known As
Bitter Root, Catchfly, Dogbane, Fly-Trap, Honeybloom, Indian Physic, Indian-Hemp, Milk Ipecac, Milkweed, Wallflower, Wild Cotton.
CAUTION: See separate listings for Gentian and Indian Physic.

Scientific Names
Apocynum cannabinum. Family: Apocynaceae.

People Use This For
Orally, Canadian hemp is used for arthritis, asthma, coughs, edema, and syphilis. It is also used orally for valvular insufficiency, senile heart, and to strengthen weak heart muscles following pneumonia. Canadian hemp is also used orally as a diuretic.
Topically, the fresh juice of Canadian hemp is used for warts.

Safety
LIKELY UNSAFE ...when used orally. Contains digitalis-like cardiac glycosides that can cause toxicity (18).
There is insufficient reliable information available about the safety of Canadian hemp for its other uses.
PREGNANCY AND LACTATION: LIKELY UNSAFE ...when used orally due to toxic potential of digitalis-like cardiac glycosides (18); avoid using.

Effectiveness
There is insufficient reliable information available about the effectiveness of Canadian hemp.

Mechanism of Action
The applicable part of Canadian hemp is the root. Canadian hemp contains cardenolide or digitalis-type glycosides, including cymine. These may cause bradycardia with low blood pressure, increased heart contractions, and reflex hypertension. It also may increase diuresis. It is more irritating to the intestinal mucosa than digitalis and strophanthus preparations. It has a lower therapeutic effect on atrial fibrillation than digitalis (18).

Adverse Reactions
Canadian hemp causes topical irritation of the gastrointestinal mucous membranes. This can cause nausea and vomiting more commonly than in other cardenolide glycoside containing plants (such as digitalis). It can also cause bradycardia with low blood pressure, increased heart contractions, and reflex hypertension (18).

Interactions with Herbs & Other Dietary Supplements
CARDIAC GLYCOSIDE-CONTAINING HERBS: Canadian hemp is contraindicated with these herbs, and concomitant use can increase the risk of cardiac glycoside toxicity. Cardiac glycoside containing herbs include black hellebore, digitalis leaf, hedge mustard, figwort, lily of the valley roots, motherwort, oleander leaf, pheasant's eye plant, pleurisy root, squill bulb leaf scales, strophanthus seeds, and uzara (19).

Interactions with Drugs
DIGOXIN (Lanoxin): Theoretically, concomitant use of Canadian hemp with digoxin (Lanoxin) might increase therapeutic effects and adverse effects (19).
DIURETIC DRUGS: Theoretically, concomitant use of potassium depleting diuretics and Canadian hemp can increase the risk of cardiac glycoside toxicity due to potassium depletion (19). Some diuretics that can deplete potassium include chlorothiazide (Diuril), chlorthalidone (Thalitone), furosemide (Lasix), hydrochlorothiazide (HCTZ, HydroDIURIL, Microzide), and others.

Interactions with Foods
None known.

Interactions with Lab Tests
None known.

Interactions with Diseases or Conditions
None known.

Dosage and Administration
ORAL: Some people take 10 to 30 drops of the liquid extract three times daily or 0.3 to 0.6 mL of the tincture (1:10) (18).
TOPICAL: No typical dosage.

Comments
The tough, fibrous barks of both Canadian hemp and Indian hemp have been used as a substitute for hemp; hence, both are known as hemp (18).

CANAIGRE

Also Known As

Red American Ginseng, Wild Red American Ginseng, Wild Red Desert Ginseng.
CAUTION: See separate listings for Ashwaganda, Blue Cohosh, Codonopsis, Ginseng American, Ginseng Panax, and Ginseng Siberian.

Scientific Names

Rumex hymenosepalus.
Family: Polygonaceae.

People Use This For

Orally, canaigre is used for improving physical and athletic stamina, cognitive function and concentration, and work efficiency or athletic stamina; and as a general tonic to improve well-being. It is also used orally for soothing irritated or inflamed tissues, as a diuretic, as an antidepressant, as an astringent, and to treat leprosy.
In manufacturing, it is used for tanning leather and dying wool.

Safety

LIKELY SAFE ...when used orally (12). The petioles, or stems, are edible like rhubarb (6). There is some speculation that the high tannin content may be carcinogenic (5,6); avoid excessive amounts.
PREGNANCY AND LACTATION: Insufficient reliable information available; avoid using.

Effectiveness

There is insufficient reliable information available about the effectiveness of canaigre.

Mechanism of Action

The applicable part of canaigre is the root. The high tannin content, 25%, has astringent effects when applied topically. The leucoanthocyanin fraction may have antitumor activity (6).

Adverse Reactions

None reported.

Interactions with Herbs & Other Dietary Supplements

None known.

Interactions with Drugs

None known.

Interactions with Foods

None known.

Interactions with Lab Tests

None known.

Interactions with Diseases or Conditions

None known.

Dosage and Administration

No typical dosage.

Comments

Avoid confusion with Panax ginseng, Siberian ginseng, and American ginseng. Canaigre root is botanically unrelated to the ginsengs. A 1976 Herb Trade Association policy states that "any herb products consisting of whole or part of Rumex hymenosepalus should not be labeled as containing 'ginseng' " (5).

CANANGA OIL

Also Known As
None.
CAUTION: See separate listing for Ylang Ylang Oil.

Scientific Names
Cananga odorata forma. macrophylla, synonym Canangium odoratum forma. macrophylla.
Family: Annonaceae.

People Use This For
In foods, cananga oil is used as a flavoring agent in gelatins, puddings, and beverages.
In manufacturing, cananga oil is used to make fragrances in cosmetics and soaps.

Safety
LIKELY SAFE ...when used orally in amounts commonly found in foods. Cananga oil has Generally Recognized As Safe (GRAS) status in the US (4912).
POSSIBLY SAFE ...when used topically (11).
PREGNANCY AND LACTATION: Insufficient reliable information available; avoid using.

Effectiveness
There is insufficient reliable information available about the effectiveness of cananga oil.

Mechanism of Action
There insufficient reliable information available about the possible mechanism of action and active ingredients.

Adverse Reactions
Cananga oil can cause allergic skin reactions in sensitive people (5244).

Interactions with Herbs & Other Dietary Supplements
None known.

Interactions with Drugs
None known.

Interactions with Foods
None known.

Interactions with Lab Tests
None known.

Interactions with Diseases or Conditions
None known.

Dosage and Administration
No typical dosage.

Comments
Cananga oil is used predominately as a food and cosmetic ingredient. Avoid confusion with ylang ylang oil (oil from Canangium odorata genuina).

CANELLA

Also Known As
Barbasco, Curbana, Macambo, White Cinnamon, White Wood, Wild Cinnamon.

Scientific Names
Canella winteriana, synonyms Canella alba, Laurus winteriana, Winterana canella.
Family: Canellaceae.

Comments
At the date of publication, there was very little scientific information about this product. Our staff is continually analyzing the available information on natural medicines and will add data to the online version of *Natural Medicines Comprehensive Database* as it becomes available. See www.naturaldatabase.com.

CANTHAXANTHIN

Also Known As
Canthaxanthine, Carophyll Red, CI Food Orange 8, Colour Index No. 40850, E161, Roxanthin Red 10.
CAUTION: See separate listing for Beta-carotene.

Scientific Names
4,4-diketo-beta-carotene; Beta,beta-carotene-4,4-dione;Canthaxanthin.

People Use This For
Orally, canthaxanthin is used to reduce photosensitivity associated with erythropoietic protoporphyria (EPP); and light-sensitive skin diseases including polymorphous light eruptions, drug-induced photosensitivity and solar urticaria. It is also used orally to color the skin and produce an artificial suntan.
In foods, canthaxanthin is used as a food coloring additive and added to animal feed to enhance the color of chicken skins, egg yolks, salmon, and trout.
In manufacturing, canthaxanthin has been used in cosmetics and as a tablet excipient.

Safety
LIKELY SAFE ...when used orally in amounts commonly found in foods. Canthaxanthin has Generally Recognized As Safe (GRAS) status in the US (4912), but is not to exceed 30 mg per pint of liquid food or per pound of solid or semisolid food (5630).
POSSIBLY UNSAFE ...when used orally in doses to treat and reduce photosensitivities. Development of retinal changes has been reported in patients with erythropoietic protoporphyria (EPP) being treated with canthaxanthin to prevent photosensitization, including deposition of crystals around the macula of the retina (5644), slowing of dark-adaptation curves, and decreased amplitudes in electroretinograms (1326,5632,5638). Deposition of retinal crystals appears dose related (5638). Evidence suggests individuals taking a cumulative dose of 37 grams will have retinal changes 50% of the time, while those taking a total cumulative dose of 60 grams of canthaxanthin will demonstrate definite retinal changes upon examination (5636,5641).
LIKELY UNSAFE ...when used orally in large amounts to color and produce an artificial tan (5628,5629). Retinal changes have been reported in individuals ingesting large amounts of canthaxanthin chronically for tanning purposes (5636,5639,5641). Altered eye function, decreased visual acuity (5639), and aplastic anemia (5635) have also been reported.
PREGNANCY AND LACTATION: POSSIBLY UNSAFE ...when consumed in doses to treat and reduce photosensitivities due to reported retinal changes with use (5632); avoid using. LIKELY UNSAFE ...when used orally in large amounts for artificial tanning purposes due to reported retinal changes with use (5639); avoid using.

Effectiveness
POSSIBLY EFFECTIVE

Erythropoietic protoporphyria (EPP). Taking canthaxanthin orally seems to reduce photosensitivity reactions in EPP (rash, itching, or eczema) due to sunlight exposure (1326,5644).

There is insufficient reliable information available about the effectiveness of canthaxanthin for its other uses.

Mechanism of Action
Canthaxanthin is a carotenoid that is found naturally and produced synthetically (5637). It is not a precursor of vitamin A, has no vitamin A activity, is highly lipid soluble (5635), and accumulates in fatty tissue (5632). Oral canthaxanthin is thought to color the skin by accumulating in the epidermis and subcutaneous fat tissue (5635). Evidence suggests canthaxanthin and other carotenoids protect against photosensitization due to their antioxidant activity against reactive oxygen species by deactivating electronically excited molecules or acting as chain-breaking agents (1326,5649). In vitro and in vivo animal studies suggest canthaxanthin may inhibit the growth and transformation of tumor cells (5642,5647,5648) by inducing the gap junctional communication between cells (5649).

Adverse Reactions
Orally, large amounts of canthaxanthin can cause orange-brown coloration of the skin (5632), brick-red coloration of stools (5631), orange discoloration of plasma (5632), discolored body secretions (5634), diarrhea, nausea, stomach cramps, dry and itchy skin (5634), urticaria (5637), welts, gold and yellow crystalline deposits around the macula of the retina (5632,5635,5636,5638,5639,5640,5641), and hepatitis (5635). Decreased visual acuity (5639), diminished retinal sensitivity (5641), and aplastic anemia (5635) have been associated with large doses of canthaxanthin ingestion. A fatal case of aplastic anemia (5635) associated with the ingestion of

canthaxanthin for tanning purposes has been reported. The patient refused treatment with human blood products due to religious beliefs and died (5635).

Interactions with Herbs & Other Dietary Supplements
None known.

Interactions with Drugs
None known.

Interactions with Foods
None known.

Interactions with Lab Tests
VITAMIN A ASSAYS: Canthaxanthin can interfere with carotene and vitamin A laboratory assays (5634).

Interactions with Diseases or Conditions
VITAMIN A HYPERSENSITIVITY: Individuals with known hypersensitivities to vitamin A and carotenoids might also be hypersensitive to canthaxanthin.

Dosage and Administration
ORAL: The typical dose for reducing and treating photosensitivities associated with erythropoietic protoporphyria (EPP) is 60 to 90 mg daily on average for three to five months per year (5640). The typical dose for artificial tanning is 120 mg per day for several days (5633).

Comments
Orobronze (canthaxanthin) is sold in Canada as a nonprescription drug for artificial tanning purposes as 30 mg oral capsules (5631,5633). Oral tanning preparations containing canthaxanthin have been found to be readily available to consumers in the United States through mail order and tanning salons despite the FDA warning (5635,5638). A combination product containing beta-carotene and canthaxanthin (Phenoro: 10 mg beta-carotene and 15 mg canthaxanthin) is used in Europe for treatment of photosensitivities associated with EPP (5637). Other combination products containing beta-carotene and canthaxanthin are manufactured (Carotinoid-N, Apotrin), but are not available in the US (1326,5628).

CAPERS

Also Known As
Cabra, Cappero, Himsra.

Scientific Names
Capparis spinosa, synonym Capparis rupestris.
Family: Brassicaceae/Cruciferae.

People Use This For
Topically, capers are used for skin disorders, improving the function of enlarged capillaries, and dry skin.
Capers are consumed as food, and used as a flavoring.

Safety
LIKELY SAFE ...when used orally in amounts commonly found in foods. The pickled flower buds are commonly used without reports of adverse effects.
There is insufficient reliable information available about the safety of the topical use of capers. Compresses soaked in fluid containing capers can cause contact dermatitis (6).
PREGNANCY AND LACTATION: LIKELY SAFE ...when used orally in amounts typically found in foods; avoid large amounts. There is insufficient reliable information available about the safety of the topical use of capers during pregnancy and lactation.

Effectiveness
There is insufficient reliable information available about the effectiveness of capers.

Mechanism of Action
The applicable part of capers is the unopened flower bud. Some evidence suggests that unknown constituents of caper extract may improve dry skin and functioning of enlarged capillaries (6).

Adverse Reactions
Topically, capers can cause contact dermatitis (6).

Interactions with Herbs & Other Dietary Supplements
None known.

Interactions with Drugs
None known.

Interactions with Foods
None known.

Interactions with Lab Tests
None known.

Interactions with Diseases or Conditions
PEOPLE WITH SENSITIVE SKIN: Capers may cause skin irritation (6); avoid topical use.

Dosage and Administration
No typical dosage.

Comments
CAUTION: Leaves of related species (Capparis fasicularis, Capparis tumentosa) are reported to be poisonous (6).

CAPSICUM

Also Known As
African Chillies, African Pepper, Bird Pepper, Capsaicin, Capsicum Fruit, Cayenne, Chili Pepper, Garden Pepper, Goat's Pod, Grains Of Paradise, Green Bell Pepper, Green Chili Pepper, Hot Pepper, Hungarian Pepper, Ici Fructus, Katuvira, Louisiana Long Pepper, Louisiana Sport Pepper, Mexican Chilies, Mirchi, Paprika, Pimento, Red Pepper, Sweet Pepper, Tabasco Pepper, Zanzibar Pepper.
CAUTION: See separate listing for Grains of Paradise.

Scientific Names
Capsicum frutescens; Capsicum annuum; Capsicum chinense; Capsicum baccatum; Capsicum pubscens; and other Capsicum species.
Family: Solanaceae.

People Use This For
Orally, capsicum is used to stimulate digestion, as an antiflatulent, for colic, diarrhea, cramps, toothache, to improve peripheral circulation, for reducing blood clotting tendencies, seasickness, alcoholism, malarial fever, yellow and other fevers, for reducing cholesterol, and preventing arteriosclerosis and heart disease.
Topically, capsicum is used for the pain of shingles; and for post-herpetic, trigeminal, diabetic, post-mastectomy, and post-surgical neuralgias; prurigo nodularis; HIV-associated peripheral neuropathy; and fibromyalgia. It is also used as a counterirritant to desensitize nerves and to create a feeling of warmth. Capsicum is also used to relieve muscle spasms, as a gargle for laryngitis, and as a deterrent to thumb-sucking or nail biting.
As an inhalational provocation test, capsicum is used to distinguish sensory hyperreactivity of the airways from asthma.
In foods, capsicum is used as a condiment.
In manufacturing, capsicum is the main ingredient used in many self-defense sprays, also referred to as pepper spray.

Safety
LIKELY SAFE ...when used orally in amounts typically found in food. Capsicum has Generally Recognized As Safe (GRAS) status in the US (4912). ...when used topically and appropriately. The active capsicum constituent capsaicin used in topical preparations is an FDA-approved over-the-counter product (272).
POSSIBLY SAFE ...when used orally and appropriately, short-term in medicinal amounts (4,12). ...when used topically and appropriately (7038,10650).
POSSIBLY UNSAFE ...when used orally, long-term or in high doses. Long-term use or use of excessive doses can sometimes cause hepatic or renal damage (4,12).
CHILDREN: POSSIBLY UNSAFE ...when used topically in children under 2 years old (272,506). There is insufficient reliable information available about the safety of oral use in children.

PREGNANCY: LIKELY SAFE ...when used topically and appropriately (272). There is insufficient reliable information available about the safety of capsicum during pregnancy when used orally in medicinal amounts.
LACTATION: LIKELY SAFE ...when used topically and appropriately (272). POSSIBLY UNSAFE ...when used orally. Dermatitis can sometimes occur in breast-fed infants when mothers ingest foods heavily spiced with capsicum peppers (739).

Effectiveness

LIKELY EFFECTIVE

Pain. Applying capsicum topically temporarily relieves pain from rheumatoid arthritis (RA), osteoarthritis, and neuralgias including shingles and diabetic neuropathy. The active capsicum constituent capsaicin used in topical preparations is FDA-approved for these uses (272,506).

POSSIBLY EFFECTIVE

Fibromyalgia. Applying cream containing 0.025% of the active capsicum constituent capsaicin 4 times daily to tender points for 4 weeks seems to reduce tenderness in patients with fibromyalgia (7038).

Prurigo nodularis. Applying a cream containing 0.025%-0.3% of the active capsicum constituent capsaicin 4-6 times daily seems to relieve burning sensations, erythema, pruritus, and healing of skin lesions over a period of 2 weeks to 33 months. Symptoms, however, may return after discontinuation of therapy (10650).

POSSIBLY INEFFECTIVE

HIV-associated peripheral neuropathy. Applying capsaicin topically does not seem to relieve symptoms of HIV-associated peripheral neuropathy (3891).

INSUFFICIENT RELIABLE EVIDENCE to RATE

Peptic ulcers. There is preliminary evidence that suggests people who eat capsicum fruit (chili) an average of 24 times per month appear to be less likely to have an ulcer than people who eat chili an average of 8 times per month. This applies to chili in the form of chili powder, chili sauce, curry powder, and other chili-containing foods (12053). More evidence is needed to rate capsicum for this use.

Mechanism of Action

The applicable part of capsicum is the fruit. Capsicum contains capsaicinoid constituents which stimulate digestion and therefore are said to aid in digestion (4).
When used topically, the capsaicin constituent causes the release of substance P in the nerves. This initially causes pain, but after repeated applications, substance P is depleted. This reduces the ability of the nerves to transmit sensations and reduces pain (506).
Capsaicin also stimulates the unmyelinated slow C-fibers of the sensory nervous system, which can induce cough, dyspnea, nasal congestion, and eye irritation after inhalation (5885). Some evidence shows the crude juice of fresh capsicum has antibacterial properties (11). Capsicum might also increase glucose-6-phosphate dehydrogenase and adipose lipase activity (4).
Some researchers theorize that the capsaicin constituent might also have gastroprotective effects. Preliminary evidence suggests that capsicum protects against alcohol and non-steroidal anti-inflammatory drug (NSAID) damage to the GI mucosa. This has also led to the hypothesis that capsaicin might decrease the risk of peptic ulcer disease (12053).

Adverse Reactions

Orally, capsicum can cause gastrointestinal (GI) irritation (4). Sweating and flushing of the head and neck, lacrimation, and rhinorrhea have also been reported (7005). Excessive amounts of capsicum can lead to gastroenteritis and hepatic or renal damage (4). There are also reports of dermatitis in breast-fed infants whose mothers' food is heavily spiced with capsicum (739). Capsicum can also decrease blood coagulation (7006).
Topically, capsicum can cause burning and urticaria. Skin contact with fresh capsicum fruit can cause irritation or contact dermatitis (19). Inhalation of capsicum can cause cough, dyspnea, nasal congestion, eye irritation, and allergic alveolitis (5885). Capsicum can be extremely irritating to the eyes and mucous membranes.

Interactions with Herbs & Other Dietary Supplements

COCA: Theoretically, concomitant use of capsicum (including exposure to the capsicum in pepper spray) and coca might increase the effects and risk of adverse effects of the cocaine in coca (1394).

Interactions with Drugs

ACE INHIBITORS (ACEIs): There is one case report of a topically applied cream containing capsaicin contributing to the cough reflex in a patient using an ACE inhibitor (7002). But it is unclear if this interaction is clinically significant.
ANTACIDS: Theoretically, due to reports that capsicum increases stomach acid, capsicum might decrease the effectiveness of antacids (19).
ANTICOAGULANT/ANTIPLATELET DRUGS: Theoretically, capsicum might increase the effects and adverse effects of antiplatelet drugs (19).
CNS DEPRESSANTS: Theoretically, concomitant use of capsicum and drugs with sedative activity might enhance sedative effects and the risk of adverse effects (19).

COCAINE: Theoretically, concomitant use of capsicum (including exposure to the capsicum in pepper spray) and cocaine might increase cocaine effects and the risk of adverse effects, including death (1394).
H2-BLOCKERS: Theoretically, due to reports that capsicum increases stomach acid, capsicum might decrease the effectiveness of H2-blockers (19). The H2 blockers include cimetidine (Tagamet), ranitidine (Zantac), nizatidine (Axid), and famotidine (Pepcid).
PROTON PUMP INHIBITORS (PPIs): Theoretically, due to reports that capsicum increases stomach acid, capsicum might decrease the effectiveness of PPIs (19). PPIs include omeprazole (Prilosec), lansoprazole (Prevacid), rabeprazole (Aciphex), pantoprazole (Protonix), and esomeprazole (Nexium).
THEOPHYLLINE: Theoretically, oral administration of capsicum before or at the same time as theophylline might enhance theophylline absorption (19).

Interactions with Foods
None known.

Interactions with Lab Tests
None known.

Interactions with Diseases or Conditions
DAMAGED SKIN: Capsicum is contraindicated in situations involving injured skin. Do not apply capsicum if the skin is open.
GI IRRITATION: Contraindicated in individuals with infectious or inflammatory gastrointestinal conditions (19).

Dosage and Administration
ORAL: The capsicum fruit is usually used in doses of 30-120 mg three times daily (4). The tincture is usually given in doses of 0.0.6-2 mL (4). Capsicum is also sometimes administered as an oleoresin in doses of 0.6-2 mg (4).
TOPICAL: For pain syndromes, including rheumatoid and osteo-arthritis, neuropathy, and fibromyalgia, creams contain the active capsicum constituent capsaicin and are typically applied 3-4 times daily. It can take up to 14 days for the full analgesic effect. Most creams contain 0.025% to 0.075% capsaicin concentrations. Higher potency preparations may be used for diabetic neuropathy (272,506). For prurigo nodularis, 0.025%-0.3% of the active capsicum constituent capsaicin 4-6 times daily has been used (10650). Tell patients to make sure they wash their hands after applying capsaicin cream (506). Tell patients they can use a diluted vinegar solution to remove capsicum cream. The active constituent, capsaicin is not water washable (5). Warn against using capsicum preparations near the eyes or on sensitive skin (5).

Comments
In nature, capsaicin occurs only as a trans stereoisomer. However, civamide, the cis isomer also has activity. Products labeled capsaicin sometimes include nonivamide which is an adulterant or pelargonic acid vanillylamide, referred to as "synthetic capsaicin" (7007). Capsaicin is being studied for use in treating urinary urgency as an intravesical injection (6002). Capsicum powder has been reported to prevent radiation-induced damage to bacterial DNA and thereby protect certain bacteria (Escherichia coli, Bacillus megaterium, and Bacillus pumilus spores) from gamma irradiation used to preserve some foods (5886).

CARAWAY dried fruit, seed

Also Known As
Anis des Vosges, Apium carvi, Carvi Fructus, Cumin des Pres, Haravi, Krishan Jeeraka, Krishnajiraka, Kummel, Kummich, Semen Cumini Pratensis, Semences de Carvi, Wiesen-Feldkummel.
CAUTION: See separate listing for Caraway Oil.

Scientific Names
Carum carvi, synonym Carum velenovskyi.
Family: Apiaceae/Umbelliferae.

People Use This For
Orally, the dried fruit and seed of caraway is used for dyspepsia, distention, flatulence, mild spastic conditions of the gastrointestinal tract, as an expectorant, to promote lactation, to relieve menstrual discomforts, for incontinence, and as a mouthwash. It is also used orally as an antibacterial, laxative, and digestive aid.
In foods, caraway is used as a cooking spice.

Safety

LIKELY SAFE ...when consumed in amounts commonly found in foods. Caraway has Generally Recognized As Safe (GRAS) status in the US (4912). ...when used orally for medicinal purposes in appropriate amounts (12).
There is insufficient reliable information available about the safety of caraway in large amounts.
PREGNANCY AND LACTATION: LIKELY SAFE ...when used orally in the amounts commonly found in food.

Effectiveness

There is insufficient reliable information available about the effectiveness of caraway dried fruit and seed.

Mechanism of Action

Caraway produces a warm sensation and promotes postprandial gas elimination (7). The caraway fruits contain 2-7% volatile oil, consisting mainly of carvone and limonene (7). Carvone induces glutathione S-transferase (GST) in mouse tissues, which can inhibit carcinogenesis (11). There is some evidence that caraway oil has antispasmodic effects, but they are probably weak. There may also be some antihistaminic activity. It is possible that the antispasmodic effects are slightly more pronounced with the alcoholic extract, and less pronounced with the essential oil (7,11).

Adverse Reactions

Topically, caraway can cause contact dermatitis (19).

Interactions with Herbs & Other Dietary Supplements

None known.

Interactions with Drugs

None known.

Interactions with Foods

None known.

Interactions with Lab Tests

None known.

Interactions with Diseases or Conditions

None known.

Dosage and Administration

ORAL: The typical dose of caraway is 1.5-6 grams of the dried fruit per day or one cup of the freshly prepared tea two to four times daily between meals (8). The tea is prepared by steeping 1-2 teaspoons of the freshly crushed fruit in 150 mL boiling water for 5-10 minutes and then straining. The dose for infants and small children is usually one teaspoonful of the tea, and if necessary, given in a bottle (8).

Comments

Superstitions held that caraway had the power to prevent the theft of any object that contained the seed and to keep lovers from losing interest with one another (6002). Avoid confusion with caraway oil (distilled oil of caraway fruit/seed).

CARAWAY OIL

Also Known As

Roman Cumin, Wild Cumin.
CAUTION: See separate listing for Caraway dried fruit, seed.

Scientific Names

Carum carvi, synonym Apium carvi.
Family: Apiaceae/Umbelliferae.

People Use This For

Orally, caraway oil is used for digestive problems including mild gastrointestinal (GI) spasms, flatulence, fullness, and dyspepsia. Caraway oil is also used to stimulate menstruation, relieve menstrual cramps, and to increase milk flow in nursing mothers.
Topically, it has been used as a component of mouthwashes and in skin rubs to improve local blood flow.

In manufacturing, caraway oil is used as a flavoring agent in pharmaceutical compounding. It is a fragrance commonly utilized in the manufacturing of toothpaste, soap, and cosmetics.

Safety

LIKELY SAFE ...when used orally in amounts commonly found in foods. Caraway oil has Generally Recognized As Safe (GRAS) status in the US (4912).
POSSIBLY SAFE ...when used orally in medicinal amounts (6740,6741,6742,10075).
PREGNANCY: POSSIBLY UNSAFE ...when used in medicinal amounts (4912,6746). Caraway has been used to stimulate menstruation (6746); avoid using.
LACTATION: There is insufficient reliable information available about the safety of caraway oil in medicinal amounts during breast-feeding.

Effectiveness

POSSIBLY EFFECTIVE

Dyspepsia. Taking caraway oil orally as a specific combination with peppermint oil (Enteroplant) seems to relieve non-ulcerative dyspepsia, including symptoms of fullness and mild gastrointestinal (GI) spasms (6740,6741,10075). This combination of enteric-coated peppermint oil 90 mg and caraway oil 50 mg twice daily seems to be comparable to cisapride 10 mg three times daily for relieving dyspepsia.

There is insufficient reliable information available about the effectiveness of caraway oil for its other uses.

Mechanism of Action

Caraway oil is obtained from the distilled oil of caraway fruit and seed. Caraway oil has antibacterial, antifungal, and larvicidal activity in vitro (11). Some experts believe that caraway oil has antispasmodic effects; however this is controversial (11,512). There's preliminary evidence that peppermint oil in combination with caraway oil can reduce gastroduodenal motility when administered orally in enteric-coated capsules (6742). Preliminary evidence also indicates that the constituent carvone induces glutathione S-transferase (GST), which might inhibit carcinogenesis (11,911). Topically applied caraway oil has shown activity against skin tumors in early laboratory research (6745).

Adverse Reactions

Orally, caraway oil when used in combination with peppermint oil may cause a substernal burning sensation, belching, nausea, and vomiting (6741,6742,10075).
Topically, caraway oil can also cause contact dermatitis when used topically (19).

Interactions with Herbs & Other Dietary Supplements

None known.

Interactions with Drugs

None known.

Interactions with Foods

None known.

Interactions with Lab Tests

None known.

Interactions with Diseases or Conditions

None known.

Dosage and Administration

ORAL: For non-ulcerative dyspepsia, caraway oil 50-100 mg per day has been used in combination with peppermint oil (6740,6741,10075).

Comments

Caraway has been used as a love potion, because people superstitiously believed that it had a power of retention and could prevent lovers from losing interest in one another (6002).

CARDAMOM

Also Known As

Bai Dou Kou, Cardamon, Cardomomi Fructus, Ela.

Scientific Names
Elettaria cardamomum, synonym Amomum cardamomum.
Family: Zingiberaceae.

People Use This For
Orally, cardamom is used for dyspepsia, intestinal spasm, irritable bowel syndrome (IBS), common cold, cough, bronchitis, inflammation of the mouth and pharynx, liver and gallbladder complaints, loss of appetite, and tendency toward infection. It is also used as an antiflatulent, laxative, and as a stimulant and for urinary problems.
In foods, cardamom is consumed as a spice in many parts of the world.

Safety
LIKELY SAFE ...when used orally and appropriately (2).
PREGNANCY AND LACTATION: Insufficient reliable information available; avoid using amounts greater than those used in food.

Effectiveness
There is insufficient reliable information available about the effectiveness of cardamom.

Mechanism of Action
The applicable part of cardamom is the seed. The active principals of cardamom are thought to be volatile oils, including cineole (2,11). Volatile oils are believed to have antispasmodic (11), antiflatulent, virustatic (2,18), and motility-enhancing effects (18).

Adverse Reactions
None reported.

Interactions with Herbs & Other Dietary Supplements
None known.

Interactions with Drugs
None known.

Interactions with Foods
None known.

Interactions with Lab Tests
None known.

Interactions with Diseases or Conditions
GALLSTONES: The cardamom seed can trigger gallstone colic (spasmodic pain) (18) and is not recommended for self-medication in patients with gallstones (2).

Dosage and Administration
ORAL: The typical dose of cardamom is 1.5 grams of the ground seeds per day. The usual dose of the tincture is 1-2 grams per day (2).

CARLINA

Also Known As
Carlinae Radix, Dwarf Carline, Eberwurz, Ground Thistle, Racine de Carline Acaule, Radix Cardopatiae, Radix Chamaeleontis Albae, Silberdistelwurz, Stemless Carlina Root, Southernwood Root.

Scientific Names
Carlina acaulis.
Family: Asteraceae/Compositae.

People Use This For
Orally, carlina is used for gallbladder disease, poor digestion, alimentary tract spasms, and catarrh. It has also been used as a diuretic, tonic, gargle, and to induce sweating. Topically, carlina is used for dermatosis, rinsing wounds and ulcers, and to alleviate cancer of the tongue. Acetic extracts are used for herpes eruptions, skin pustules, and toothaches. In combination herbal products, carlina is used for gallbladder disorders and gastrointestinal spasms.

Safety
There is insufficient reliable information available about the safety of carlina.
Pregnancy and Lactation: Insufficient reliable information available; avoid using.

Effectiveness
There is insufficient reliable information available about the effectiveness of carlina.

Mechanism of Action
The applicable part of carlina is the root. Acetone extracts and the essential oil have shown antibacterial activity; however the aqueous extract has not (8).

Adverse Reactions
Orally, carlina may cause an allergic reaction in individuals sensitive to the Asteraceae/Compositae family. Members of this family include ragweed, chrysanthemums, marigolds, daisies, and many other herbs.

Interactions with Herbs & Other Dietary Supplements
None known.

Interactions with Drugs
None known.

Interactions with Foods
None known.

Interactions with Lab Tests
None known.

Interactions with Diseases or Conditions
CROSS-ALLERGENICITY: Carlina may cause an allergic reaction in individuals sensitive to the Asteraceae/Compositae family. Members of this family include ragweed, chrysanthemums, marigolds, daisies, and many other herbs.

Dosage and Administration
ORAL: One cup tea, prepared by steeping 1.5-3 grams of finely cut dried root in 150 mL of boiling water for 5-10 minutes, has been used three times daily between meals (8,18). 40-50 drops of the tincture, 1:4 in 60% alcohol, has been used four to five times daily (18). Carlina has also been used as a wine, prepared by combining 50 grams of root in 1 L of white wine for a minimum of 12 days, one small glass has been taken before mealtime (18).
TOPICAL: The tea, prepared by simmering 30 grams of root in 1 L of boiling water for 5-10 minutes, has been used externally (18).

Comments
Carlina is rarely used today (8).

CARNOSINE

Also Known As
B-alanyl-L-histidine, B-alanyl histidine, L-carnosine.
CAUTION: See separate listing for L-Carnitine.

Scientific Names
Beta-alanyl-L-histidine.

People Use This For
Orally, carnosine is used to prevent aging and for preventing or treating complications of diabetes such as neuropathy, cataracts, and renal dysfunction.

Safety
There is insufficient reliable information available about the safety of carnosine.
Pregnancy and Lactation: Insufficient reliable information available; avoid using.

Effectiveness
There is insufficient reliable information available about the effectiveness of carnosine.

Mechanism of Action
Carnosine is a naturally occurring di-peptide found in skeletal muscle, heart, brain and other innervated tissues. Carnosine is formed by a process involving the enzyme carnosine synthetase, which bonds the amino acids beta-alanine and L-histidine. The enzyme carnosinase maintains the carnosine equilibrium by inactivating carnosine located in tissues or blood (3381,3391). Carnosine seems to be concentrated in actively contracting muscles. In patients with muscular dystrophies carnosine levels may be lower. The concentration of carnosine in muscles also appears to correlate with age. Older patients have lower muscle carnosine levels (3391). Preliminary information also suggests that carnosine may play a role in the regulation of intracellular calcium and contractility in cardiac tissue (3390).
Carnosine is of interest as an anti-aging product because of its effects on advance glycosylation end-products (AGEs). AGEs are abnormal, cross-linked, and oxidized proteins that might play a role in the aging process. Animal studies show carnosine may diminish the glycosylation of these proteins, preventing them from inducing cellular damage (3364,10210,10645). Because carnosine appears to diminish the effects of protein glycosylation, there is some interest in using carnosine for complications of diabetes such as cataracts, neuropathy, and kidney failure, which arise from glycosylation (3364).
There is some animal evidence that carnosine can help prevent lipid peroxidation within the cell membranes. Carnosine may block malondialdehyde (MDA) production, which is a toxic lipid peroxidation end-product. Animal studies show carnosine can inhibit MDA-induced protein changes and MDA-induced toxicity (3364,3381,10644). Blocking MDA might decrease oxidative damage to lipids, as well as to enzymes and DNA. This raises the question of whether carnosine might play a role in preventing atherosclerosis, joint inflammation, and cataract formation (3364,3381).
Carnosine may also play a role in the prevention of Alzheimer's disease. The anti-glycating and antioxidant activities of carnosine are both implicated in the neuronal and endothelial cell damage of Alzheimer's disease (10645). Carnosine binds heavy metals and may provide some protection from zinc and copper mediated neurotoxicity (7219). The ability of carnosine to bind heavy metals may also be important in its ability to act as an antioxidant (10211).

Adverse Reactions
None reported.

Interactions with Herbs & Other Dietary Supplements
None known.

Interactions with Drugs
None known.

Interactions with Foods
None known.

Interactions with Lab Tests
None known.

Interactions with Diseases or Conditions
None known.

Dosage and Administration
No typical dosage.

Comments
There is very little scientific information about this product. Our staff is continually analyzing the available information on natural medicines and will add data here as it becomes available.

CAROB

Also Known As
Locust Bean, Locust Pods, St. John's Bread, Sugar Pods.

Scientific Names
Ceratonia siliqua.
Family: Fabaceae/Leguminosae.

People Use This For

Orally, carob is used for acute nutritional disorders, celiac disease, obesity, diarrhea, dyspepsia, enterocolitis, vomiting during pregnancy, and sprue. It is also used for improvement of lipid profiles and excretion of fat in feces. In infants, it is used for vomiting, retching cough, and diarrhea.
In foods and beverages, carob is used as a flavoring agent and as a chocolate substitute. Carob flour and extracts are also used as ingredients in food products.

Safety

LIKELY SAFE ...when used orally in amounts commonly found in foods. Carob has Generally Recognized As Safe (GRAS) status (4912). ...when used orally in medicinal amounts (12).
PREGNANCY AND LACTATION: Insufficient reliable information available; avoid using.

Effectiveness

INSUFFICIENT RELIABLE EVIDENCE to RATE

Obesity. There is preliminary clinical evidence that a carob and bean pod extract might modestly improve lipid profiles and excretion of fat in feces of overweight and obese patients (10633). More evidence is needed to rate carob for this use.

Mechanism of Action

The applicable part of carob is the fruit. Tannins contained in carob strongly inhibit digestive enzymes. Animal data suggest that a 15% carob gum diet fed for 2-6 weeks may result in weight loss. Decreases in blood glucose levels, decreases in cholesterol plasma levels, decreases in insulin levels, and an increases in glucose tolerance are also suggested (11).

Adverse Reactions

None reported.

Interactions with Herbs & Other Dietary Supplements

None known.

Interactions with Drugs

None known.

Interactions with Foods

None known.

Interactions with Lab Tests

None known.

Interactions with Diseases or Conditions

None known.

Dosage and Administration

ORAL: For improvement of lipid profiles and excretion of fat in feces, carob gum 50-100 mg three times daily, combined with bean pod (Phaseolus vulgaris, kidney bean) 300-600 mg three times daily, has been used (10633).

Comments

Avoid confusing carob with carob tree, Jacaranda procera and Jacaranda caroba. The term "carat" evolved from the use of carob seeds as weight units for measuring gold (6).

CARRAGEENAN

Also Known As

Carrageenin, Carragheenan, Chondrus Extract, Irish Moss, Irish Moss Extract, Mousse D'Irlande.

Scientific Names

Chondrus crispus; Euchema species; Gigartina mamillosa and other Gigartina species; related red algae.
Family: Gigartinaceae.

People Use This For

Orally, carrageenan is used to soothe mucous membranes irritated by coughs, bronchitis, tuberculosis, and intestinal problems. The French use a form that has been degraded by low pH and high temperatures to treat peptic ulcers, and as a bulk laxative; this degraded form has lost the gelling properties of the original product.
Topically, carrageenan is used for anorectal symptoms.
In manufacturing, carrageenan is used as a binder, emulsifier, thickening agent, and as a stabilizer in pharmaceuticals, foods, and toothpaste. Carrageenan is also an ingredient in weight loss products.

Safety

LIKELY SAFE ...when used orally in food amounts (11).
POSSIBLY UNSAFE ...when the degraded form is used orally. The degraded form is broken down into a lower molecular weight product that is partially absorbed. There is concern about the safety of this form because it has been linked to lesions in the colons of animals (11).
PREGNANCY AND LACTATION: LIKELY SAFE ...when used in food amounts (11). There is insufficient reliable information available about the safety of using larger amounts; avoid using.

Effectiveness

There is insufficient reliable information available about the effectiveness of carrageenan.

Mechanism of Action

Carrageenan has been reported to lower blood cholesterol, reduce gastrointestinal (GI) secretions and food absorption, and increase water content of the gut when large amounts are given. Parenterally it has shown anticoagulant, hypotensive, and immunosuppressive activities; it may also have anti-inflammatory properties (11).

Adverse Reactions

None known.

Interactions with Herbs & Other Dietary Supplements

None known.

Interactions with Drugs

ANTICOAGULANT/ANTIPLATELET DRUGS: Carrageenan may increase the risk of bleeding in patients taking anticoagulants (6002).
ANTIHYPERTENSIVE DRUGS: Carrageenan may enhance hypotensive effects of antihypertensive agents (6002).
ORAL DRUGS: Carrageenan can impair gastrointestinal (GI) absorption of oral drugs (6002).

Interactions with Foods

None known.

Interactions with Lab Tests

None known.

Interactions with Diseases or Conditions

None known.

Dosage and Administration

ORAL: One cup of the decoction of Irish moss is sometimes used two to three times daily. The decoction is prepared by adding 1 ounce of the dried plant in 1-1.5 pints boiling water, simmer and strain. The decoction can be sweetened with lemon, honey, or cinnamon (6002).

Comments

Carrageenan consists of hydrocolloids from various red algae or seaweeds.

CASCARA

Also Known As

Bitter Bark, Buckthorn, California Buckthorn, Cascara Sagrada, Chittem Bark, Dogwood Bark, Purshiana Bark, Rhamni Purshianae Cortex, Sacred Bark, Sagrada Bark, Yellow Bark.

Scientific Names

Frangula purshiana, synonym Rhamnus purshiana. Family: Rhamnaceae.

People Use This For

Orally, cascara is used for constipation, as a laxative, for gallstones, liver ailments, cancer, as a bitter tonic.
In foods and beverages, a bitterless extract of cascara is sometimes used as a flavoring agent.
In manufacturing, cascara is used in the processing of some sunscreens.

Safety

POSSIBLY SAFE ...when used orally and appropriately, short term. Cascara seems to be safe when used for less than one week (272). Cascara was formerly FDA-approved as safe and effective, but this designation was removed in 2002 because of lack of supporting evidence (8229).
POSSIBLY UNSAFE ...when used orally, long term. Using cascara for more than one to two weeks can lead to dependence and electrolyte loss, specifically low levels of potassium (272).
CHILDREN: POSSIBLY UNSAFE ...when used orally in children. Cascara should be used cautiously in children due to the risk of electrolyte loss, specifically low levels of potassium (272).
PREGNANCY: Insufficient reliable information available (4258); avoid using.
LACTATION: POSSIBLY UNSAFE ...when used orally. Cascara is excreted into breast milk and might cause diarrhea (272).

Effectiveness

LIKELY EFFECTIVE

Constipation. Taking cascara orally has laxative effects and helps for treating constipation (272). Cascara was formerly FDA-approved as safe and effective, but this designation was removed in 2002 because of lack of supporting evidence (8229).

There is insufficient reliable information available about the effectiveness of cascara for its other uses.

Mechanism of Action

The applicable part of cascara is the dried bark. The anthraglycoside constituents in cascara are cascarosides A and B. These stimulate peristalsis and evacuation leading to its stimulant laxative effect (6). Cascara exerts its effect on the large intestine and does not have much effect on the small intestine. Bacteria in the intestine are required to transform the anthraglycosides into stimulant laxatives. The fresh bark contains free anthrone which is an emetic compound that can cause severe vomiting. But the free anthrone is destroyed by aging the bark for at least one year, or by artificial aging with heat and aeration (2). Anthroid laxative use is not associated with an increased risk of developing colorectal adenoma or carcinoma (6138).

Adverse Reactions

Orally, cascara can commonly cause mild abdominal discomfort, colic, and cramps. Long-term use can lead to potassium depletion, albuminuria, hematuria, disturbed heart function, muscle weakness, finger clubbing, and cachexia (4). In some cases, chronic use can also cause pseudomelanosis coli. Pseudomelanosis coli (pigment spots in intestinal mucosa) is believed to be harmless, usually reverses with discontinuation, and is not directly associated with an increased risk of developing colorectal adenoma or carcinoma (6138). Fresh or improperly aged cascara bark can cause severe vomiting due to the presence of free anthrone constituents. There is also some concern about potential liver problems. In one case, cascara aged bark 425 mg (containing approximately 21 mg cascaroside) three times daily for three days resulted in cholestatic hepatitis, ascites, and portal hypertension. Symptoms resolved over about three months following discontinuation of cascara (6895). This adverse effect is suspected to be the result of a hypersensitivity reaction.

Interactions with Herbs & Other Dietary Supplements

DIGITALIS, LILY OF THE VALLEY, SQUILL: Overuse of cascara can increase the risk of cardiac toxicity; these herbs are also cardiac glycoside-containing herbs (19), and because of potassium loss (4).
LICORICE: Using cascara concomitantly with licorice can increase the risk of potassium depletion (2).
POTASSIUM DEPLETING HERBS: Theoretically, concomitant use of cascara along with horsetail plant or licorice rhizome can increase the risk of potassium depletion.
STIMULANT LAXATIVE HERBS: Theoretically, cascara used concomitantly with other herbs that are stimulant laxatives can increase the risk of potassium depletion. Stimulant laxative herbs include aloe, wild cucumber fruit (Ecballium elaterium), blue flag rhizome, alder buckthorn, European buckthorn, butternut bark, castor oil, colocynth fruit pulp, gamboge bark exudate, jalap root, black root, manna bark exudate, podophyllum root, rhubarb root, senna leaves and pods, and yellow dock root (19).

Interactions with Drugs

CORTICOSTEROIDS: Concomitant use of corticosteroids along with cascara can increase the risk of potassium depletion (2).
DIGOXIN (Lanoxin): Theoretically, overuse of cascara increases the risk of adverse effects of cardiac glycoside drugs.
DIURETIC DRUGS: Overuse of cascara might compound diuretic-induced potassium loss (19). There is some

concern that people taking cascara along with potassium depleting diuretics might have an increased risk for hypokalemia. Initiation of potassium supplementation or an increase in potassium supplement dose may be necessary for some patients. Some diuretics that can deplete potassium include chlorothiazide (Diuril), chlorthalidone (Thalitone), furosemide (Lasix), hydrochlorothiazide (HCTZ, HydroDIURIL, Microzide), and others.
ORAL DRUGS: Theoretically, cascara can reduce the absorption of some drugs due to the reduced transit time through the GI tract (19).
STIMULANT LAXATIVES: Concomitant use of cascara along with other laxatives can cause electrolyte and fluid depletion.

Interactions with Foods
None known.

Interactions with Lab Tests
COLORIMETRIC TESTS: Cascara can discolor urine (pink, red, purple, orange, rust), interfering with diagnostic tests that depend on a color change, due to its anthraquinone content (275).
POTASSIUM: Excessive use of cascara can cause potassium depletion, reducing serum potassium concentrations and test results (19).

Interactions with Diseases or Conditions
GASTROINTESTINAL (GI) CONDITIONS: Cascara is contraindicated in people with intestinal obstruction, or acute intestinal inflammation. This includes people with Crohn's disease, ulcerative colitis, and appendicitis. It is also contraindicated for people who have ulcers, and abdominal pain of unknown origin (2,4,8).

Dosage and Administration
ORAL: 20-30 mg per day of the active ingredient, hyroxyanthracene derivatives, has been used. This is calculated as cascaroside A, from the cut bark, powder, or extracts (2). A typical dose includes 1 cup of tea which is made by steeping 2 grams of finely chopped bark in 150 mL of boiling water for 5-10 minutes, and then straining (18). The cascara liquid extract is given in a dose of 2-5 mL three times daily (4). The appropriate amount of cascara is the smallest dose that is necessary to maintain soft stools (2).

Comments
Cascara is no longer an FDA-approved drug. It may be sold as a dietary supplement, but not as a drug. The FDA notified manufacturers to remove or reformulate all over-the-counter (OTC) laxative products containing cascara from the US market by November 5, 2002, citing lack of safety and efficacy studies. The FDA gave manufacturers the chance to submit safety and efficacy data; however, the companies decided the expense of conducting safety and efficacy studies exceeded potential profits (8229,8442,8443).

CASCARILLA

Also Known As
Bahama Cascarilla, Sweet Bark, Sweet Wood Bark.

Scientific Names
Croton eluteria, synonym Clutia eluteria.
Family: Euphorbiaceae.

People Use This For
Orally, cascarilla is used for digestive disorders, diarrhea, and vomiting.

Safety
There is insufficient reliable information available about the safety of cascarilla.
Pregnancy and Lactation: Insufficient reliable information available; avoid using.

Effectiveness
There is insufficient reliable information available about the effectiveness of cascarilla.

Mechanism of Action
The applicable part of cascarilla is the bark. The constituents are reported to have stimulant and tonic properties (18).

Adverse Reactions
None reported.

Interactions with Herbs & Other Dietary Supplements
None known.

Interactions with Drugs
None known.

Interactions with Foods
None known.

Interactions with Lab Tests
None known.

Interactions with Diseases or Conditions
None known.

Dosage and Administration
No typical dosage.

Comments
In the past, cascarilla was added to tobacco before smoking, due to its pleasant odor when burned. It also produced vertigo and intoxication during this process (215).

CASHEW

Also Known As
East Indian Almond.

Scientific Names
Anacardium occidentale.
Family: Anarcardiaceae.

People Use This For
Orally, cashew is used for gastrointestinal ailments.
Topically, cashew is used as a skin stimulant and cauterizing agent for ulcers, warts and corns.
Cashew is also consumed as a food.

Safety
LIKELY SAFE ...when used in amounts commonly found in foods. Cashew has Generally Recognized As Safe (GRAS) status in the US (4912).
There is insufficient reliable information available about the safety of cashew when used in medicinal amounts.
PREGNANCY AND LACTATION: There is insufficient reliable information available about the safety of medicinal amounts of cashew during pregnancy and lacation.

Effectiveness
There is insufficient reliable information available about the effectiveness of cashew.

Mechanism of Action
The applicable part of cashew is the nut. A dried ethanolic extract is effective in vitro against gram-positive bacteria Bacillus subtilis and Staphylococcus aureus. Alkyl phenols contained in the cashew nut shell are strong skin irritants. Cashew contains alkyl phenols that are chemically related to constituents in poison ivy, poison oak, mango, and ginkgo. The adverse reactions resulting from cashew are related to the adverse reactions that sometimes occur with these other irritants. Roasted cashew nuts are free of the alkyl phenols (18).

Adverse Reactions
Topically, contact can lead to redness and nodule and blister formation.

Interactions with Herbs & Other Dietary Supplements
None known.

Interactions with Drugs
None known.

Interactions with Foods
None known.

Interactions with Lab Tests
None known.

Interactions with Diseases or Conditions
None known.

Dosage and Administration
No typical dosage.

Comments
Acajou oil, oleum anacardiae, and fatty oil are extracted from cashew nuts (18).

CASSIA AURICULATA

Also Known As
Avaram, Avari Panchaga Choornam, Kalpa Herbal Tea, Ranawara, Tanner's Cassia.

Scientific Names
Cassia auriculata, synonym Senna auriculata.
Family: Cesalpiniaceae.

People Use This For
Orally, cassia auriculata is used for diabetes, conjunctivitis, rheumatism, constipation, jaundice, liver disease, and urinary tract disorders.

Safety
There is insufficient reliable information available about the safety of cassia auriculata.
Pregnancy and Lactation: Insufficient reliable information available; avoid using.

Effectiveness
There is insufficient reliable information available about the effectiveness of cassia auriculata.

Mechanism of Action
The applicable parts of cassia auriculata are the flower, seed, leaves, root, bark, and unripe fruit. The flower is most commonly used. Animal research suggests that cassia auriculata flower alone or in combination with other herbs has antihyperglycemic activity, reducing blood glucose and glycosylated hemoglobin, and increasing insulin levels. It may act by stimulating beta-cells to release more insulin (12366,12370). It seems to be similar to acarbose (Precose) in alpha-glucosidase inhibitory activity (12369). Cassia auriculata flower also seems to have antihyperlipidemic and antioxidant effects in diabetic animals (12367,12371). Cassia auriculata leaf extract also reduces blood sugar in normal and diabetic animals (12368).

Cassia auriculata leaf extract shows potential use for liver disease. In animal models of alcoholism, it protects against free radical damage. It restores hepatic levels of glutathione, which is involved in protective antioxidant activity, and serum vitamin E and C levels. It also lowers hepatic enzymes, suggesting that it prevents damage to hepatic parenchymal cells (12372).

There is no reliable published research in humans.

Adverse Reactions
None reported.

Interactions with Herbs & Other Dietary Supplements
HERBS WITH HYPOGLYCEMIC POTENTIAL: Theoretically, cassia auriculata might have additive effects with herbs that decrease blood glucose levels (12366,12370). Herbs with hypoglycemic potential include devil's claw, fenugreek, guar gum, Panax ginseng, and Siberian ginseng.

Interactions with Drugs
ANTIDIABETES DRUGS: Theoretically, cassia auriculata may reduce blood glucose levels (12366,12370) and might have additive effects on glucose levels when used with antidiabetes drugs. Monitor blood glucose levels closely. Medication dose adjustments may be necessary. Some antidiabetes drugs include glimepiride (Amaryl), glyburide

(DiaBeta, Glynase PresTab, Micronase), insulin, pioglitazone (Actos), rosiglitazone (Avandia), and others.
CARBAMAZEPINE (Tegretol): Theoretically, cassia auriculata flower may increase carbamazepine levels. Research in animals suggests that concurrent administration may cause a significant rise in carbamazepine blood levels. The mechanism of this interaction is unknown (12373).

Interactions with Foods
None known.

Interactions with Lab Tests
None known.

Interactions with Diseases or Conditions
None known.

Dosage and Administration
No typical dosage.

Comments
Cassia auriculata is an evergreen shrub that grows widely in India and other parts of Asia. It is used in Ayurvedic medicine (12366).

CASSIA CINNAMON

Also Known As
Bastard Cinnamon, Canton Cassia, Cassia, Cassia Aromaticum, Cassia Bark, Cassia Lignea, Chinese Cinnamon, Cinnamomum, Cinnamon, Cinnamon Flos, Cinnamomi Cassiae Cortex, Cortex Cinnamomi, False Cinnamon, Nees, Rou Gui, Sthula Tvak, Taja, Zimbluten.
CAUTION: See separate listing for Cinnamon bark.

Scientific Names
Cinnamomum aromaticum, synonym Cinnamomum cassia.
Family: Lauraceae.

People Use This For
Orally, cassia cinnamon is used for type 2 diabetes, gas (flatulence), muscle and gastrointestinal spasms, preventing nausea and vomiting, diarrhea, infections, the common cold, and loss of appetite. It is also used for impotence, enuresis, rheumatic conditions, testicle hernia, menopausal symptoms, amenorrhea, and as an abortifacient. Cassia cinnamon is also used orally for angina, kidney disorders, hypertension, cramps, cancer, and as a blood purifier.
Topically, cassia cinnamon is used in suntan lotions, nasal sprays, mouthwashes, gargles, toothpaste, and as a counterirritant in liniments.
In food and beverages, cassia cinnamon is used as a flavoring agent.

Safety
LIKELY SAFE ...when used orally in amounts commonly found in foods. Cassia cinnamon has Generally Recognized As Safe (GRAS) status in the US (4912).
POSSIBLY SAFE ...when used orally and appropriately in medicinal doses (11347).
PREGNANCY AND LACTATION: There is insufficient reliable information available about the safety of cassia cinnamon when used in medicinal amounts during pregnancy and breast-feeding; avoid using.

Effectiveness
POSSIBLY EFFECTIVE

Diabetes. Taking cassia cinnamon orally seems to improve type 2 diabetes. Some research suggests that taking cassia cinnamon 1 to 6 grams for 40 days can lower fasting serum glucose by 18-29%, triglycerides by 23-30%, low-density lipoprotein (LDL) cholesterol by 7-27%, and total cholesterol by 12-26% (11347).

There is insufficient reliable information available about the effectiveness of cassia cinnamon for its other uses.

Mechanism of Action
The applicable parts of cassia cinnamon are the bark and flower. Cinnamaldehyde is found in the volatile oil fraction of cassia cinnamon. The cassia cinnamon bark contains about 1400 to 1900 ppm cinnamaldehyde (3919).
Cinnamaldehyde seems to have antibacterial activity (11244). It may also have immunomodulating, anti-tumor, and antioxidant activity (11245,11246,11247).
Polyphenolic polymers such as hydroxychalcone found in cassia cinnamon seem to potentiate insulin action. These

compounds seem to increase phosphorylation of the insulin receptor, which increases insulin sensitivity. Increased insulin sensitivity may improve blood glucose control and lipid levels. Cinnamon extracts also seem to activate glycogen synthetase and increase glucose uptake (11247,11248,11249,11973).

Adverse Reactions

Topically, allergic skin reactions and stomatitis from toothpaste flavored with cassia cinnamon have been reported (11915,11920).

Interactions with Herbs & Other Dietary Supplements

HERBS & SUPPLEMENTS WITH HYPOGLYCEMIC POTENTIAL: Cassia cinnamon can lower blood glucose levels (11347) and might have additive effects when used with other herbs and supplements that also lower glucose levels. This might increase the risk of hypoglycemia in some patients. Some herbs and supplements with hypoglycemic effects include alpha-lipoic acid, bitter melon, chromium, devil's claw, fenugreek, garlic, guar gum, horse chestnut, Panax ginseng, psyllium, Siberian ginseng, and others.

Interactions with Drugs

ANTIDIABETES DRUGS: Cassia cinnamon may lower blood glucose levels, and have additive effects in patients treated with antidiabetic agents; use with caution (11347). Dose adjustments to diabetes medications might be necessary. Some antidiabetes drugs include glimepiride (Amaryl), glyburide (DiaBeta, Glynase PresTab, Micronase), insulin, metformin (Glucophage), pioglitazone (Actos), rosiglitazone (Avandia), and others.

Interactions with Foods

None known.

Interactions with Lab Tests

BLOOD GLUCOSE: Cassia cinnamon might lower blood glucose levels in some patients (11347).

Interactions with Diseases or Conditions

DIABETES: Cassia cinnamon might lower blood glucose in patients with type 2 diabetes (11347). Tell patients with diabetes to use cassia cinnamon products cautiously and monitor blood glucose levels very closely. Dose adjustments to diabetes medications might be necessary.

Dosage and Administration

ORAL: For type 2 diabetes, 1 to 6 grams (about 1/2 teaspoon) of cassia cinnamon daily for 40 days has been used (11347).

Comments

There are a lot of different types of cinnamon. Cinnamon verum (Ceylon cinnamon) is the type used most commonly in the Western world. Cinnamomum aromaticum (Cassia cinnamon or Chinese cinnamon) is also commonly used. In many cases, the cinnamon spice purchased in food stores contains a combination of these different types of cinnamon. So far, only cassia cinnamon has been shown to have any effect on blood glucose in humans. However, cinnamon verum also contains the hydroxychalcone polymer thought to be responsible for lower blood sugar (11247).

CASSIE ABSOLUTE

Also Known As

Huisache, Popinac Absolute, Sweet Acacia.

Scientific Names

Acacia farnesiana, synonyms Acacia smallii, Mimosa farnesiana.
Family: Fabaceae/Leguminosae.

People Use This For

Orally, cassie absolute is used as an antispasmodic, antidiarrheal, stimulant, aphrodisiac, to treat fever, rheumatoid arthritis (RA), pulmonary tuberculosis, and stomach cancer.
Topically, cassie absolute is used for dry skin and as an insecticide.
In India, tea made from cassie absolute leaves is used for gonorrhea, and the root is chewed for sore throat.
In foods, cassie absolute is a flavor ingredient in foods and beverages.
In manufacturing, cassie absolute is used as a fragrance in perfumes.

Safety

LIKELY SAFE ...when used orally in amounts commonly found in foods. Cassie absolute has Generally Recognized As Safe (GRAS) status in the US (4912).

There is insufficient reliable information available about the safety of cassie absolute used in medicinal amounts.

PREGNANCY AND LACTATION: Insufficient reliable information available; avoid using.

Effectiveness

There is insufficient reliable information available about the effectiveness of cassie absolute.

Mechanism of Action

Cassie absolute is reported to have antispasmodic, aphrodisiac, astringent, demulcent, antidiarrheal, antipyretic, antirheumatic and stimulant properties (11). It contains glycosides which reportedly have anti-inflammatory and bronchodilator effects (1505).

Adverse Reactions

None reported.

Interactions with Herbs & Other Dietary Supplements

None known.

Interactions with Drugs

None known.

Interactions with Foods

None known.

Interactions with Lab Tests

None known.

Interactions with Diseases or Conditions

None known.

Dosage and Administration

No typical dosage.

Comments

Cassie absolute is an extract of Acacia farnesiana flowers. Limited pharmacologic and toxicologic information is available (11).

CASTOR OIL

Also Known As

African Coffee Tree, Bofareira, Castor, Castor Oil Plant, Eranda, Gandharva Hasta, Mexico Weed, Palma Christi, Tangantangan Oil Plant, Wonder Tree.

CAUTION: See separate listing for Castor seed.

Scientific Names

Ricinus communis; Ricinus sanguines.

Family: Euphorbiaceae.

People Use This For

Orally, castor oil is used as a stimulant laxative, to stimulate labor, and to promote the flow of breast milk.

In combination, castor oil is used with quinine sulfate or alone to induce labor at term.

Topically, castor oil is used as an emollient and to dissolve cysts, growths, or warts, and to soften bunions and corns. It is also applied topically as a cervical abortifacient and vaginal contraceptive. Castor oil is used in the eyes to soothe the irritated conjunctiva after the presence of foreign bodies.

Safety

LIKELY SAFE ...when used orally and appropriately, short-term (16).

POSSIBLY UNSAFE ...when used orally in high doses or for extended periods. Taking castor oil for greater than one week or exceeding the recommended dose of 15 to 60 mL per day can increase the risk of fluid and electrolyte

disturbances (272).
CHILDREN: LIKELY SAFE ...when used orally and appropriately, short-term (16). POSSIBLY UNSAFE ...when used orally in high doses or for extended periods. Taking castor oil for greater than one week or exceeding the recommended dose of 1-15 mL, depending on age, can increase the risk of fluid and electrolyte disturbances (272).
PREGNANCY: POSSIBLY SAFE ...when used orally for inducing labor in pregnant women at term. Midwives routinely use castor oil for labor induction in pregnant women at term. This practice does not appear to adversely affect the mother or fetus (1122,7191). However, castor oil should not be used without the supervision of a clinician. LIKELY UNSAFE ...when used orally in pregnant women who are not at term. Castor oil might induce premature labor and induce miscarriage (12,18); avoid using.
LACTATION: Insufficient reliable information available; avoid using.

Effectiveness

LIKELY EFFECTIVE

Constipation. Taking castor oil orally is effective as a stimulant laxative for reducing constipation (272).

POSSIBLY EFFECTIVE

Parturition. A single 60 mL dose of castor oil appears to stimulate labor within 24 hours in at least 50% of women at term pregnancy with no prior signs of labor (7191). There is also some evidence that women at term pregnancy with premature membrane rupture who take castor oil have a higher incidence of labor onset and a lower incidence of cesarean section than women who take no medication (1122).

There is insufficient reliable information available about the effectiveness of castor oil for its other uses.

Mechanism of Action

Castor oil is produced by cold pressing ripe seeds of Ricinus communis. Unlike the seeds from this plant, castor oil does not contain the deadly poison ricin (16,17). Castor oil is a glyceride that can be absorbed from the intestine and metabolized as a fatty acid (272). Castor oil is hydrolyzed in the duodenum by pancreatic lipase to release ricinoleic acid, which might have stimulant laxative effects (6,272). Although the exact mechanism of ricinoleic acid is unknown, the laxative effect appears to result from fluid secretion induced by cyclic adenosine monophosphate, rather than the increased peristalsis due to an irritant effect (272). Onset of bowel evacuant action is usually within 2 hours, but sometimes can take up to 6 hours (16). In pregnancy, castor oil is thought to induce labor by producing hyperemia in the intestinal tract, which causes reflex stimulation of the uterus (16). Castor oil might also increase prostaglandin production, which stimulates uterine activity (7191).

Adverse Reactions

Orally, castor oil, like all stimulant laxatives, can cause abdominal discomfort, cramping, nausea, and faintness (15,272). Nausea can also occur because of the unpleasant taste of castor oil (7191). Using flavored products might reduce this effect. Castor oil can also cause fluid and electrolyte loss, particularly potassium, which can result in hypokalemia. It can also cause malabsorption from intestinal hypermotility (15,272). Chronic ingestion over long periods of time can lead to cathartic colon (15). There is some concern that castor oil might cause amniotic fluid embolism. There is one case of amniotic fluid embolism and cardiopulmonary arrest within one hour of ingestion of 30 mL of castor oil at full-term pregnancy (1219).

Interactions with Herbs & Other Dietary Supplements

CARDIAC GLYCOSIDE-CONTAINING HERBS: Theoretically, castor oil can increase the risk of cardiac glycoside toxicity (19).
LICORICE/HORSETAIL: Theoretically, concomitant use with horsetail plant or licorice rhizome increases the risk of potassium depletion (18).
MALE FERN: Concomitant use with oil-soluble anthelmintic herbs, such as the male fern, should be avoided due to enhanced absorption of castor oil (19).
STIMULANT LAXATIVE HERBS: Theoretically, concomitant use with other stimulant laxative herbs might increase the risk of potassium depletion (19).
WORMSEED: Concomitant use with wormseed oil might reduce both toxicity and efficacy of wormseed oil (19).

Interactions with Drugs

CORTICOSTEROIDS: Concomitant use of corticosteroids and castor oil may increase the risk of potassium depletion (18).
DIGOXIN (Lanoxin): Theoretically, concomitant use can increase the risk of adverse effects of cardiac glycoside drugs due to fluid and electrolyte loss.
DIURETIC DRUGS: Overuse of castor oil might compound diuretic-induced potassium loss (19). There is some concern that people taking castor oil along with potassium depleting diuretics might have an increased risk for hypokalemia. Initiation of potassium supplementation or an increase in potassium supplement dose may be necessary for some patients. Some diuretics that can deplete potassium include chlorothiazide (Diuril), chlorthalidone (Thalitone), furosemide (Lasix), hydrochlorothiazide (HCTZ, HydroDIURIL, Microzide), and others.
ORAL DRUGS: Theoretically, castor oil may reduce absorption of drugs due to reduced transit time (19).

STIMULANT LAXATIVES: Concomitant use of castor oil and laxatives may lead to electrolyte and fluid depletion (19).

Interactions with Foods

None known.

Interactions with Lab Tests

None known.

Interactions with Diseases or Conditions

INTESTINAL DISORDERS: Contraindicated in intestinal obstruction (appendicitis, Crohn's disease, irritable bowel syndrome (IBS), ulcerative colitis), abdominal pain of unknown origin (18), abdominal pain of unknown origin (18), biliary tract obstruction and other biliary disorders (7).

Dosage and Administration

ORAL: For constipation, 15 mL is commonly used (15). For total colonic evacuation, such as before surgery, or radiologic or colonoscopic procedures, the dose for adults and children over 12 is 15-60 mL given 16 hours prior to surgery or colonic examination (15). For children age 2 to 11 years, 5-15 mL is typically used. In children younger than 2 years, 1-5 mL is commonly used. For induction of labor, a variety of dosage regimens have been used (1122). Single doses vary from 5-120 mL (1122). A one-time dose of 60 mL in fruit juice is a commonly used regimen (7191). Other regimens that have been used include 5 mL in peppermint tea every 2 hours, 15 mL three times daily, 30 mL every 2 hours, 30 mL every 6 hours, 30 mL every 3 hours for 3 doses, 60 ml daily, and 60 ml daily for 2 days (1122). Castor oil is most effective when taken on an empty stomach (7).

Comments

Castor oil has been used medicinally for centuries and was mentioned in the Ebers Papyrus (16). The taste of castor oil is bland, followed by a slightly bitter and usually nauseating taste (16). Castor oil is sometimes flavored with cinnamon, peppermint, or other flavorings to mask the unpleasant taste (16).

CASTOR seed

Also Known As

African Coffee Tree, Bofareira, Castor Bean, Eranda, Gandharva Hasta, Mexico Weed, Palma Christi, Ricin, Tangantangan Oil Plant, Wonder Tree.
CAUTION: See separate listing for Castor Oil.

Scientific Names

Ricinus communis; Ricinus sanguines.
Family: Euphorbiaceae.

People Use This For

Orally, castor seeds are used as a birth control, a laxative, for leprosy, and syphilis.
Topically, castor seed paste is used as a poultice for inflammatory skin disorders, boils, carbuncles, abscesses, inflammation of the middle ear, and migraines.

Safety

POSSIBLY SAFE ...when the hulled seed is used orally and appropriately, short-term. There is some evidence that a single dose of castor seed with the outer coat removed (hulled) can be used safely (7127,7128).
UNSAFE ...when the whole seed is used orally. Safety depends on whether or not the seed is chewed or if the outer coat is ruptured. Chewing as few as 1-6 whole seeds can be lethal in an adult. If the seed is swallowed intact, poisoning is less likely (6,5611); however, prompt medical attention should be sought after ingestion of any whole castor seed (5611).
There is insufficient reliable information available about the safety of castor seed when applied topically.
CHILDREN: UNSAFE ...when the whole seed is used orally. The chewed or uncoated seeds can cause severe toxic effects (5611,5612) and death (5611). There is insufficient reliable information available about the safety of the hulled seed or topical use in children.
PREGNANCY AND LACTATION: UNSAFE ...when the whole seed is used orally. The chewed or uncoated seeds can cause severe toxic effects, including death (6,5611); avoid using. There is insufficient reliable information available about the safety of the hulled seed or topical use during pregnancy and lactation.

Effectiveness

POSSIBLY EFFECTIVE

Contraception. Taking the hulled castor seed orally seems to be effective as a contraceptive. There is some evidence that a single dose of seeds with the outer coat removed (hulled) can work as a contraceptive for up to 8-12 months (7127,7128).

There is insufficient reliable information available about the effectiveness of castor seed for its other uses.

Mechanism of Action

Castor seeds are the seeds of the evergreen castor shrub (7122). The seeds are used to produce castor oil. Castor seeds are best known for their toxic effects. They contain the toxic glycoprotein ricin. Ricin can be fatal when ingested, inhaled, or given intravenously. Ricin is an N-glycosidase that affects an RNA subunit and interferes with protein synthesis, causing cell death (6,5611). Toxic effects typically occur 2-5 days after ingestion (5611). There is some preliminary evidence that ricin might also have analgesic effects and activity against leukemia (6). It is unclear how castor seeds work as a contraceptive; however, its effects do not seem to be hormonally mediated (7127,7128).

Adverse Reactions

Orally, castor seed can cause severe toxicity. Chewing whole seeds can cause nausea, vomiting, diarrhea, abdominal pain, dehydration, shock, hemolysis, severe fluid and electrolyte disturbances, peripheral vascular collapse, renal failure secondary to hypovolemia, and death. Cellular damage to liver, kidneys, and pancreas typically occurs 2-5 days after ingestion (5611,5612). As few as 1-6 seeds can be lethal in humans (6,5611). Rupture of the seed hull seems to be necessary to cause toxicity. Swallowing seeds whole, without chewing, is less likely to cause toxic effects; however, prompt medical attention should be received after ingestion of any whole seed. Serum chemistries should be monitored for at least 5 days after ingestion in symptomatic patients (5611). Hulled castor seeds, with the outer coat carefully removed, seem to be well-tolerated, and without toxic side effects (7127,7128); however, some patients taking hulled seeds can have transient anorexia and weight loss (1727).

Topically, the castor plant, crushed seeds, or seed dust can cause dermatitis in some patients (5611).

Castor seed is also an inhalant allergen in workers in the coffee industry (6). Anaphylaxis can occur in these patients after exposure to castor beans, plants, or dust (5611).

Interactions with Herbs & Other Dietary Supplements

None known.

Interactions with Drugs

None known.

Interactions with Foods

None known.

Interactions with Lab Tests

None known.

Interactions with Diseases or Conditions

None known.

Dosage and Administration

ORAL: No typical dosage.

TOPICAL: Paste made with ground seeds applied to affected skin twice daily has been used; treatment takes up to 15 days (18). For use on intact skin; avoid use on broken or damaged skin.

Comments

The plant is used mainly for ornamental purposes. Because of its toxic effects, the castor seed constituent, ricin, is used as a chemical warfare agent.

CASTOREUM

Also Known As

Canadian Beaver, European Beaver, Siberian Beaver.

Scientific Names

Castor canadensis; Castor fiber.

Family: Castoridae.

People Use This For

Orally, castoreum is used for absence of menstrual periods, painful menses, hysteria, restless sleep, and as a calming and restorative agent.
In foods and beverages, castoreum extract is used as a flavoring agent.
In manufacturing, castoreum tincture is used as a fragrance or fixative in cosmetics and soaps.

Safety

LIKELY SAFE ...when used in amounts commonly found in foods. Castoreum has Generally Recognized As Safe (GRAS) status in the US (4912). ...when used topically. Castoreum tincture is reported to be nontoxic in dermatological tests (11).
There is insufficient reliable information available about the safety of castoreum for its other uses.
PREGNANCY AND LACTATION: Insufficient reliable information available; avoid using.

Effectiveness

There is insufficient reliable information available about the effectiveness of castoreum.

Mechanism of Action

Castoreum is reported to have calming and sedating effects (11).

Adverse Reactions

None reported.

Interactions with Herbs & Other Dietary Supplements

None known.

Interactions with Drugs

None known.

Interactions with Foods

None known.

Interactions with Lab Tests

None known.

Interactions with Diseases or Conditions

None known.

Dosage and Administration

No typical dosage.

Comments

Castoreum is a secretion collected from scent glands of Canadian, European, and Siberian beavers. Castoreum from the Canadian beaver is considered superior in quality to that of the Siberian beaver (11).

CAT'S CLAW

Also Known As

Cats Claw, Griffe Du Chat, Life-Giving Vine of Peru, Samento, Uña De Gato, Una De Gato.
CAUTION: See separate listing for Cat's Foot.

Scientific Names

Uncaria guianensis; Uncaria tomentosa.
Family: Rubiaceae.

People Use This For

Orally, cat's claw is used for diverticulitis, peptic ulcers, colitis, gastritis, hemorrhoids, parasites, Alzheimer's disease, and leaky bowel syndrome. Cat's claw is also used orally viral infections including herpes zoster, herpes simplex, and human immunodeficiency virus (HIV). It is also used orally for wound healing, arthritis, asthma, allergic rhinitis, cancer (especially urinary tract cancer), gonorrhea, dysentery, birth control, bone pains, and "cleansing" the kidneys.

Safety

POSSIBLY SAFE ...when used orally, short-term. A specific freeze-dried aqueous extract seems to be safe when used for up to four weeks (7317). Another extract of cat's claw, free of tetracyclic oxindole alkaloids, seems to be safe when used for up to 24 weeks (8661).
PREGNANCY: POSSIBLY UNSAFE ...when used orally. There is concern that cat's claw might be unsafe based on its use as a contraceptive (12); avoid using.
LACTATION: Insufficient reliable information available; avoid using.

Effectiveness

POSSIBLY EFFECTIVE

Osteoarthritis. Taking a specific freeze-dried cat's claw extract (Uncaria guianensis) orally appears to relieve knee pain related to physical activity within one week of treatment, but it does not decrease pain at rest or decrease knee swelling (7317).

Rheumatoid arthritis (RA). Taking a specific cat's claw extract (Uncaria tomentosa) orally, containing pentacyclic oxindole alkaloids but free of tetracyclic oxindole alkaloids, appears to modestly improve symptoms of RA. Taken orally in combination with sulfasalazine or hydroxychloroquine for 24 weeks, cat's claw seems to reduce the number of painful and swollen joints (8661).

There is insufficient reliable information available about the effectiveness of cat's claw for its other uses.

Mechanism of Action

The applicable part of cat's claw is the root and bark. The major alkaloid of cat's claw is rhynchophylline. There is some evidence that it might have cardiovascular effects including dilating peripheral blood vessels, lowering heart rate, and possibly lowering blood cholesterol. Rhynchophylline might also inhibit sympathetic nervous system activity (6).
Cat's claw is thought to work for osteoarthritis due to anti-inflammatory effects. It seems to inhibit the production of prostaglandin E2 and tumor necrosis factor-alpha (TNF-alpha) (7317). There is interest in using cat's claw for rheumatoid arthritis. The pentacyclic oxindole alkaloids found in cat's claw seem to exhibit immunomodulatory effects, enhancing phagocytosis and altering lymphocyte activity. However, these effects appear to be antagonized by the tetracyclic oxindole alkaloids also found in cat's claw, suggesting greater effectiveness of extracts without this alkaloid (8661).
There is also interest in cat's claw for cancer and viral infections because some of its constituents seem to have antioxidant, immunostimulant, and antiviral effects (7225,7317). These constituents include quinovic acid alkaloids and the alkaloids pteropodine and isopteropodine (7225). Extracts of cat's claw also might have antimutagenic activity. There is preliminary evidence that cat's claw extracts can induce tumor cell death (apoptosis) (7224,8969), and inhibit proliferation of leukemia and lymphoma cells (7225). However, cat's claw does not appear to be cytotoxic to normal cells (7227,8969). Cat's claw may also exert antiestrogenic effects, although the mechanism is not yet completely understood (8660).
Some cat's claw alkaloids may have a beneficial effect on memory loss caused by cholinergic dysfunction. These alkaloids seem to enhance central cholinergic transmission by increasing acetylcholine levels or by affecting dopaminergic systems that can enhance cholinergic function (7226). Another constituent, uncarine E, might also affect the glutamateric system, which might also play a critical role in memory and cognition (7226).

Adverse Reactions

Orally, cat's claw can cause headache, dizziness, and vomiting (7317).

Interactions with Herbs & Other Dietary Supplements

None known.

Interactions with Drugs

ANTIHYPERTENSIVE DRUGS: Since cat's claw may lower blood pressure, exercise caution when using cat's claw with antihypertensive drugs.
CYTOCHROME P450 3A4 (CYP3A4) SUBSTRATES: There's preliminary evidence that cat's claw can inhibit cytochrome P450 3A4 (CYP3A4) enzymes (6450). Theoretically, cat's claw might increase levels of drugs metabolized by CYP3A4; however, so far, this interaction has not been reported in humans. Some drugs metabolized by CYP3A4 include lovastatin (Mevacor), ketoconazole (Nizoral), itraconazole (Sporanox), fexofenadine (Allegra), triazolam (Halcion), and numerous others. Use cat's claw cautiously or avoid in patients taking these drugs.
IMMUNOSUPPRESSANTS: Theoretically, cat's claw may interfere with immunosuppressant therapy (7225) due to immunostimulating activity. It stimulates phagocytosis and increases respiratory cellular activity and the mobility of leukocytes. Immunosuppressant drugs include azathioprine (Imuran), basiliximab (Simulect), cyclosporine (Neoral, Sandimmune), daclizumab (Zenapax), muromonab-CD3 (OKT3, Orthoclone OKT3), mycophenolate (CellCept), tacrolimus (FK506, Prograf), sirolimus (Rapamune), prednisone (Deltasone, Orasone), and other corticosteroids (glucocorticoids).

Interactions with Foods
None known.

Interactions with Lab Tests
None known.

Interactions with Diseases or Conditions
AUTOIMMUNE DISEASES: There is some concern that cat's claw might adversely affect patients with autoimmune disorders because of its immune stimulating effects (7225). Avoid using in patients with multiple sclerosis, systemic lupus erythematosus (SLE), or other autoimmune disorders without the advice of a healthcare professional.
HYPOTENSION: Cat's claw might reduce blood pressure and exacerbate hypotension (6).

Dosage and Administration
ORAL: For osteoarthritis of the knee, 100 mg daily of a specific freeze-dried aqueous cat's claw extract has been used (7317). For rheumatoid arthritis, 60 mg daily in three divided doses of a specific cat's claw extract (free of tetracyclic oxindole alkaloids) has been used (8661).

Comments
Cat's claw was ranked as the seventh most popular herb in US sales in 1997 (2). Two species of cat's claw are of primary interest for medicinal use: Uncaria tomentosa and Uncaria guianensis. Uncaria tomentosa is most commonly used in the US, and Uncaria guianensis is typically used in Europe (6).

CAT'S FOOT

Also Known As
Antennariase Dioicae Flos, Cats Ear Flower, Cat's Ear Flower, Cats Foot, Cudweed, Katsenpfotchenbluten, Life Everlasting, Mountain Everlasting.
CAUTION: See separate listings for Cudweed, Cat's Claw, and Ground Ivy.

Scientific Names
Antennaria dioica, synonym Gnaphalium dioicum.
Family: Asteraceae/Compositae.

People Use This For
Orally, cat's foot is used to treat intestinal disease; and as a diuretic.

Safety
There is insufficient reliable information available about the safety of cat's foot.
Pregnancy and Lactation: Insufficient reliable information available; avoid using.

Effectiveness
There is insufficient reliable information available about the effectiveness of cat's foot.

Mechanism of Action
The applicable part of cat's foot is the fresh or dried flowers. Mild spasmolytic and choleric effects have been reported in animals (18).

Adverse Reactions
Orally, cat's foot can cause an allergic reaction in individuals sensitive to the Asteraceae/Compositae family. Members of this family include ragweed, chrysanthemums, marigolds, daisies, and many other herbs.

Interactions with Herbs & Other Dietary Supplements
None known.

Interactions with Drugs
None known.

Interactions with Foods
None known.

Interactions with Lab Tests
None known.

Interactions with Diseases or Conditions
CROSS-ALLERGENICITY: Cat's foot may cause an allergic reaction in individuals sensitive to the Asteraceae/Compositae family. Members of this family include ragweed, chrysanthemums, marigolds, daisies, and many other herbs.

Dosage and Administration
ORAL: The fluid extract of cat's foot is sometimes taken as 14-28 grains three times daily (6002).

Comments
Avoid confusion with ground ivy, which is also sometimes referred to as cat's foot (6002).

CATECHU

Also Known As
Black Catechu: Acacia Catechu Heartwood Extract, Black Cutch, Cachou, Cashou, Catechu nigrum, Cutch, Dark Catechu, Khair, Khadira, Pegu Catechu.
Pale Catechu: Cube Gambir, Gambier, Gambir, Gambir Catechu, Terra Japonica, Uncaria Gambier Leaf/Twig Extract.

Scientific Names
Black catechu: Acacia catechu, synonym Mimosa catechu.
Family: Fabaceae/Leguminosae.
Pale catechu: Uncaria gambir, synonyms Nauclea gambir, Ourouparia gambir.
Family: Rubiaceae.

People Use This For
Orally, catechu is used for diarrhea, chronic mucous membrane inflammation, dysentery, colitis, bleeding, indigestion, and cancer. Catechu is used orally in some parts of the world as an anti-fertility drug.
Topically, catechu is used for skin diseases, hemorrhoids, traumatic injuries, to stop bleeding, and for dressing wounds. Catechu is included in mouthwashes and gargles for gingivitis, stomatitis, pharyngitis, and oral ulcers.
In foods and beverages, catechu is used as a flavoring agent.

Safety
LIKELY SAFE ...when used orally in amounts commonly found in foods. Catechu has Generally Recognized As Safe (GRAS) status in the US (4912).
POSSIBLY UNSAFE ...when used in medicinal amounts. Catechu contains tannins with possible carcinogenic and hepatotoxic properties (11). Another constituent, (+)-catechin (cianidanol), is associated with fatal hemolytic anemia (9).
There is insufficient reliable information available about the safety of the topical use of catechu.
PREGNANCY AND LACTATION: POSSIBLY UNSAFE ...when used orally (9); avoid using.

Effectiveness
There is insufficient reliable information available about the effectiveness of catechu.

Mechanism of Action
Both black and pale catechu are applicable. Researchers think the astringent and antibacterial properties of catechu result from its high tannin content (11). Gambrine (in pale catechu) has hypotensive effects (11). D-catechin (in black and pale catechu) causes blood vessel constriction (11). Fisetin (in black catechu) and (+)-catechin (in black and pale catechu) and may protect against liver damage; (+)-catechin (cianidanol) is also thought to protect against experimentally-induced ulcers in animals (11); (+)-catechin (cianidanol) is associated with fatal hemolytic anemia (9). Methylcatechin, which is one of the major metabolites of (+)-catechin, inhibits the binding of monocytes to vascular endothelial cells. This suggests that the catechins found in catechu may reduce atherosclerosis (9444).

Adverse Reactions
None reported.

Interactions with Herbs & Other Dietary Supplements
None known.

Interactions with Drugs
None known.

Interactions with Foods
None known.

Interactions with Lab Tests
None known.

Interactions with Diseases or Conditions
None known.

Dosage and Administration
ORAL: Typical dose ranges 0.3-2 grams three times daily, or a single 500 mg dose (18).
TOPICAL: Catechu tincture, 20 drops in a glass of lukewarm water (mouth rinse) or applied undiluted with a toothbrush has been used (18).

Comments
Though black catechu and pale catechu differ somewhat chemically, they are used for the same purposes at the same dose (11). Unstandardized products may contain high amounts of aflatoxin, a metabolite of Aspergillus, which is toxic and may lead to certain cancers.

CATNIP

Also Known As
Catmint, Catnep, Catswort, Field Balm, Menta De Gato.

Scientific Names
Nepeta cataria.
Family: Lamiaceae/Labiatae.

People Use This For
Orally, catnip is used for insomnia; migraine headaches; cold; flu; fever; hives; and gastrointestinal (GI) upset, including indigestion, colic, cramping, and flatulence. It is also used orally for conditions associated with anxiety, diuresis, as a tonic, for upper respiratory tract infections, and headaches. Additionally, catnip is also used orally for lung and uterine congestion, eradicating worms, and for initiating menses in girls with delayed onset of menstruation.
Topically, catnip has been used for arthritis, hemorrhoids, and as a poultice to relieve swelling.
As an inhalant, catnip is smoked for respiratory conditions and recreationally for inducing a euphoric high.
In manufacturing, catnip is used as a pesticide and insecticide.

Safety
POSSIBLY SAFE ...when used orally and appropriately (6,12). Significant adverse effects have not been reported when catnip tea is used in cupful amounts (6).
POSSIBLY UNSAFE ...when used orally in excessive doses. Higher doses may be associated with significant adverse effects (6). ...when inhaled by smoking dried leaves. Smoking the dried leaves of catnip has been associated with a euphoric high (6), which might impair judgment; however, whether catnip can truly produce this effect in humans remains controversial (6).
There is insufficient reliable information available about the safety of topically applied catnip.
CHILDREN: POSSIBLY UNSAFE ...when used orally. One child developed stomach pain and irritability followed by lethargy and hypnotic state after ingesting catnip leaves and tea (5,2596).
PREGNANCY: LIKELY UNSAFE ...when used orally. Catnip tea has been reported to have uterine stimulant properties (12); avoid using.
LACTATION: Insufficient reliable information available; avoid using.

Effectiveness
There is insufficient reliable information available about the effectiveness of catnip.

Mechanism of Action
The applicable part of catnip is the flowering tops. The pharmacological effect that catnip is famous for is the euphoric state it induces in cats. It is thought that the constituent cis-trans-nepetalcatone produces the characteristic stimulation in cats only when they smell it (5). Although humans have used catnip to induce a euphoric high, whether

or not this effect actually occurs in humans is controversial. In humans, the constituent nepetalactone is thought to be responsible for catnip's calming effects in insomnia, anxiety, gastrointestinal (GI) conditions, and migraine headache. Nepetalactone is the major component (80-95%) of the volatile oil of catnip and is structurally related to the valepotriates found in valerian. Catnip provides approximately 0.2-1% volatile oil. Catnip reportedly also has antipyretic and diaphoretic effects, which have been attributed to its use for colds, flu, and fever. Other reported pharmacological effects, include diuretic and stimulation of gallbladder activity (6).

Adverse Reactions

Catnip abuse may result in headache and malaise. Large amounts of tea may cause vomiting (6). One case report exists of a nineteen-month-old child who developed a stomachache and irritability, followed by lethargy and a hypnotic state after ingesting raisins soaked in catnip tea and chewing on the tea bag (5,2596).

Interactions with Herbs & Other Dietary Supplements

HERBS WITH SEDATIVE PROPERTIES: Theoretically, concomitant use of catnip with herbs that have sedative properties might enhance therapeutic and adverse effects. Some of these supplements include 5-HTP, calamus, California poppy, catnip, hops, Jamaican dogwood, kava, St. John's wort, sculleap, valerian, yerba mansa, and others.

Interactions with Drugs

CNS DEPRESSANTS: Theoretically, concomitant use with drugs with sedative properties may cause additive effects and side effects (19).

Interactions with Foods

None known.

Interactions with Lab Tests

None known.

Interactions with Diseases or Conditions

PELVIC INFLAMMATORY DISEASE (PID) and MENORRHAGIA: Because catnip is also used to stimulate menstruation, theoretically it is contraindicated in pelvic inflammatory disease (PID) and excessive menstrual bleeding (12).

Dosage and Administration

ORAL: People typically use two 380 mg capsules three times daily at meals or prepared as a tea using 1 to 2 teaspoons in 6 ounces of boiling water (6006).

CATUABA

Also Known As

Caramuru, Catuaba Casca, Chuchuhuasha, Golden Trumpet, Pau De Reposta, Piratancara, Tatuaba.

Scientific Names

Erythroxylum catuaba.
Family: Erythroxylaceae.

Comments

At the date of publication, there was very little scientific information about this product. Our staff is continually analyzing the available information on natural medicines and will add data to the online version of *Natural Medicines Comprehensive Database* as it becomes available. See www.naturaldatabase.com.

CEDAR leaf

Also Known As

American Arborvitae, Arborvitae, Eastern Arborvitae, Eastern White Cedar, Hackmatack, Northern White Cedar, Swamp Cedar, Thuga, Thuja, Tree of Life, White Cedar.
CAUTION: See separate listings for Cedar Leaf Oil, Cedarwood Oil, and Cedarwood.

Scientific Names

Thuja occidentalis.
Family: Cupressaceae.

People Use This For

Orally, cedar leaf is used to treat respiratory tract infections, in conjunction with antibiotics for bacterial skin infections and herpes simplex, for bronchitis, rheumatism, trigeminal neuralgia, and strep throat. It is also used as an abortifacient.

Topically, cedar leaf is used to manage joint pain, arthritis, and muscle rheumatism.

Safety

LIKELY SAFE ...when used orally in amounts commonly found in foods if thujone-free (12).

POSSIBLY SAFE ...when used orally as a medicinal for occasional use in recommended amounts (12); not for long-term use.

There is insufficient reliable information available about the safety of cedar leaf for its other uses.

PREGNANCY: UNSAFE ...when used orally due to abortifacient activity (12); avoid using.

LACTATION: Insufficient reliable information available; avoid using.

Effectiveness

There is insufficient reliable information available about the effectiveness of cedar leaf.

Mechanism of Action

Cedar leaf is reported to be a urinary irritant (19), a uterine stimulant, and affect menstrual cycle (12). Thujone, a constituent, is a neurotoxin that can cause convulsions (1304). The glycoprotein and polysaccharide fractions have been used therapeutically (18). Some evidence suggests the polysaccharides might have antiviral and immunostimulating (1305) properties, and might inhibit HIV-1-specific antigens and reverse transcriptase activity (1306).

Adverse Reactions

Orally, symptoms of overdose include queasiness, vomiting, painful diarrhea, and mucous membrane hemorrhage. Deaths have been reported (18). Other side effects include asthma, CNS stimulation, and seizures (6002).

Interactions with Herbs & Other Dietary Supplements

THUJONE CONTAINING HERBS: Avoid; concomitant use may increase the risk of thujone toxicity. Thujone-containing herbs include oak moss, oriental arborvitae, sage, tansy, tree moss, and wormwood (2,4,12).

Interactions with Drugs

ANTICONVULSANTS: Cedar leaf may lower the seizure threshold in those individuals taking anti-convulsants (6002).

Interactions with Foods

None known.

Interactions with Lab Tests

None known.

Interactions with Diseases or Conditions

GI CONDITIONS: Cedar leaf can irritate gastrointestinal tract. Contraindicated in individuals with infectious or inflammatory gastrointestinal conditions (19).

Dosage and Administration

ORAL: The typical dose of liquid extract (unspecified concentration) is 2-4 mL only for occasional use (12).

TOPICAL: No typical dosage.

Comments

Avoid confusion with other Thuja species.

CEDAR LEAF OIL

Also Known As

American Arborvitae, Arborvitae, Eastern Arborvitae, Eastern White Cedar, Hackmatack, Northern White Cedar, Swamp Cedar, Thuja, Thuja Oil, Tree of Life, White Cedar.
CAUTION: See separate listings for Cedar leaf, Cedarwood Oil, and Cedarwood.

Scientific Names

Thuja occidentalis.
Family: Cupressaceae.

People Use This For

Orally, cedar leaf oil is used as an immune stimulant, expectorant, and diuretic.
Topically, cedar leaf oil is used to treat skin diseases, condyloma, cancers, as an insect repellent, and as a counterirritant to treat warts.
In foods and beverages, cedar leaf oil is used as a flavoring.
In manufacturing, cedar leaf oil is used as a fragrance in cosmetics and soaps.

Safety

LIKELY SAFE ...when used orally in amounts commonly found in foods. Cedar leaf oil that is thujone-free has Generally Recognized As Safe (GRAS) status in the US (4912).
POSSIBLY SAFE ...when used topically (11).
UNSAFE ...when used orally for medicinal use (11). A constituent, thujone, is a neurotoxin (1304).
PREGNANCY: UNSAFE ...when used orally or topically due to toxicity and uterine stimulant activity (11); avoid using.
LACTATION: UNSAFE ...when used orally or topically due to toxicity (11); avoid using.

Effectiveness

There is insufficient reliable information available about the effectiveness of cedar leaf oil.

Mechanism of Action

Thujone, a constituent of cedar leaf oil, is a neurotoxin that can cause convulsions (1304). Polysaccharides have demonstrated in vitro antiviral, immunostimulating (1305), inhibition of HIV-1-specific antigens and reverse transcriptase activity (1306).

Adverse Reactions

Orally, use of cedar leaf oil can result in poisoning. Symptoms of thujone poisoning include hypotension, convulsion, and death (11). Other side effects include asthma, CNS stimulation, and seizures (6002).

Interactions with Herbs & Other Dietary Supplements

THUJONE CONTAINING HERBS: Avoid; concomitant use may increase the risk of thujone toxicity. Thujone-containing herbs include oak moss, oriental arborvitae, sage, tansy, tree moss, and wormwood (2,4,12).

Interactions with Drugs

ANTICONVULSANTS: Cedar leaf oil may lower the threshold in those individuals taking anti-convulsants (6002).

Interactions with Foods

None known.

Interactions with Lab Tests

None known.

Interactions with Diseases or Conditions

None known.

Dosage and Administration

ORAL: People typically use 2 to 4 mL of the liquid extract (5263).
TOPICAL: No typical dosage.

Comments

Cedar leaf oil is produced by steam distillation of Thuja occidentalis leaves and twigs (11).

CEDARWOOD

Also Known As
Ashe Juniper, Cedar, Eastern Red Cedar, Red Cedarwood, Red Juniper, Texas Cedarwood, Virginia Cedarwood.
CAUTION: See separate listings for Cedar Leaf Oil, Cedar leaf, and Cedarwood Oil.

Scientific Names
Juniperus virginiana.
Family: Cupressaceae.

People Use This For
Orally, cedarwood is used for cough, bronchitis, rheumatism, venereal warts, and skin rash.

Safety
POSSIBLY SAFE ...when the berry or leaf is used orally (12).
There is insufficient reliable information available about the safety of the oral or topical use of the bark, seed or twig.
PREGNANCY AND LACTATION: LIKELY UNSAFE ...when the berry or leaf are used orally. Virginia cedarwood berry or leaf is contraindicated in pregnancy (12). There is insufficient reliable information available about the safety of the oral or topical use of cedarwood bark, seed, or twig; avoid using.

Effectiveness
There is insufficient reliable information available about the effectiveness of cedarwood.

Mechanism of Action
Steam distillation of Virginia cedarwood produces an oil that contains alpha- and beta-cedrene, cedrol, and cedreol. It also contains the toxic constituent thujone (11).

Adverse Reactions
None reported.

Interactions with Herbs & Other Dietary Supplements
THUJONE CONTAINING HERBS: Avoid; concomitant use may increase the risk of thujone toxicity. Thujone-containing herbs include oak moss (12), oriental arborvitae (12), sage (2,4,12), tansy (2,4,12), tree moss (12), and wormwood (2,12).

Interactions with Drugs
BARBITURATES: Theoretically, inhaling red cedar chip fragrance might reduce efficacy of hexobarbital or pentobarbital (19). Some of these sedative medications include pentobarbital (Nembutal), phenobarbital (Luminal), secobarbital (Seconal), and others.

Interactions with Foods
None known.

Interactions with Lab Tests
None known.

Interactions with Diseases or Conditions
None known.

Dosage and Administration
No typical dosage.

Comments
Avoid confusion with cedarwood oil.

CEDARWOOD OIL

Also Known As

None.
CAUTION: See separate listings for Cedar leaf, Cedar Leaf Oil, and Cedarwood.

Scientific Names

Juniperus ashei, synonym Juniperus mexicana (Cedarwood Oil Texas); Juniperus virginiana (Cedarwood Oil Virginia).
Family: Cupressaceae.
Cedrus atlantica (Cedarwood Oil Atlas).
Family: Pinaceae.

People Use This For

Topically, cedarwood oil is used for alopecia areata. It is also used topically as an insect repellent.
In manufacturing, cedarwood oils are used as fragrance or fixatives in cosmetics, soaps, and perfumes.

Safety

POSSIBLY SAFE ...when used topically and appropriately. Cedarwood oil (Cedrus atlantica) has been used safely for up to 7 months (5177). The maximum use level in perfumes is 0.8%.
PREGNANCY AND LACTATION: Insufficient reliable information available; avoid using.

Effectiveness

POSSIBLY EFFECTIVE

Alopecia areata. Applying cedarwood oil topically in combination with other essential oils seems to be effective for treating alopecia areata. Cedarwood oil (Cedrus atlantica) in combination with the essential oils from thyme, lavender, and rosemary seem to improve hair growth by 44% after 7 months of treatment (5177).

There is insufficient reliable information available about the effectiveness of cedarwood oil for its other uses.

Mechanism of Action

Steam distillation of Virginia cedarwood produces an oil that contains alpha- and beta-cedrene, cedrol, and cedreol. It also contains the constituent thujone (11). It's not clear how cedarwood oil (Cedrus atlantica) works in alopecia areata, but it may have a stimulatory effect on hair growth (5177). Dermatological studies have shown that all three cedarwood oils (Virginia, Texas, Atlas) are generally non-toxic (11); however, there is other evidence that cedarwood oil (probably Virginia) can produce tumors on mouse skin (11).

Adverse Reactions

There is some evidence that cedarwood oil (Virginia and/or Texas) is an allergenic and is a local irritant (11).

Interactions with Herbs & Other Dietary Supplements

THUJONE CONTAINING HERBS: Avoid; concomitant use may increase the risk of thujone toxicity. Thujone-containing herbs include oak moss (12), oriental arborvitae (12), sage (2,4,12), tansy (2,4,12), tree moss (12), and wormwood (2,12).

Interactions with Drugs

None known.

Interactions with Foods

None known.

Interactions with Lab Tests

None known.

Interactions with Diseases or Conditions

None known.

Dosage and Administration

TOPICAL: For the treatment of alopecia areata, a combination of the essential oils including cedarwood (Cedrus atlantica) 2 drops or 94 mg, rosemary 3 drops or 114 mg, thyme 2 drops or 88 mg, and lavender 3 drops or 108 mg, all mixed with 3 mL jojoba oil and 20 mL grapeseed oil has been used. Each night, the mixture is massaged into the scalp for 2 minutes with a warm towel placed around the head to increase absorption (5177).

Comments

There are several cedarwood oils with different physical and chemical properties, each produced by steam distillation of wood from various trees. The most common are: cedarwood oil Virginia (synonym cedar oil, red cedarwood oil), cedarwood oil Atlas (synonym cedarwood oil Moroccan), and cedarwood oil Texas (cedarwood oil mountain, Mexican). Avoid confusion with cedar leaf, cedar leaf oil, or cedarwood.

CELERY

Also Known As

Ache des Marais, Ajamoda, Apii Fructus, Celery Fruit, Celery Seed, Fruit de Celeri, Smallage, Selleriefruchte, Selleriesamen.

Scientific Names

Apium graveolens.
Family: Apiaceae/Umbelliferae.

People Use This For

Orally, celery is used to treat rheumatism, gout, hysteria, nervousness, headache, weight loss due to malnutrition, loss of appetite, and exhaustion. Celery is also used as a sedative, mild diuretic, urinary antiseptic, digestive aid, menstrual stimulant, antiflatulent, aphrodisiac, to reduce lactation, for regulating bowel movements, stimulating glands, and for blood purification.

Safety

LIKELY SAFE ...when the oil or seeds are consumed in amounts commonly found in foods. Celery seed has Generally Recognized As Safe (GRAS) status in the US (4912).
POSSIBLY SAFE ...when used orally and appropriately in medicinal amounts (12).
PREGNANCY: LIKELY UNSAFE ...when the oil or seeds are used orally in larger amounts; celery might have uterine stimulant or abortifacient effects (4,19).
LACTATION: There is insufficient reliable information available about the safety of medicinal amounts of celery during lactation; avoid using.

Effectiveness

There is insufficient reliable information available about the effectiveness of celery.

Mechanism of Action

The applicable parts of celery are the fruit and seed. Sedative, diuretic, and antispasmodic effects of celery seed may be due to phthalide constituents (d-limonene, selinene, and related phthalides) (4,6). Celery plant extracts have hypotensive and hypoglycemic effects (4). In preliminary research, 5 of 23 celery-based preparations displayed antiarthritis effects; none of the extracts displayed anti-inflammatory or antipyretic effects. The activity of celery seed is thought to be dependent on processing at low temperatures (6131). Another constituent, apiogenin, has shown evidence of antiplatelet activity. The essential oil can increase kidney inflammation by irritating epithelial tissue (8). Celery juice has been reported to have bile stimulating activity (4). Celery seed oil has shown bacteriostatic effects (4). Celery also contains the furocoumarins bergapten and celereodise, a dihydrofurocoumarin glycoside (isoquercitrin), and the coumarin glycoside apiumoside (6). Celery is a rich plant source of calcium, magnesium, and iron (19).

Adverse Reactions

Topically, celery can cause contact dermatitis (19). Allergic and anaphylactic reactions have also been documented (4,6). Cross-allergenicity is possible between celery and carrots, dandelion, or wild carrot (4,6). Consuming large amounts of celery seed oil can induce CNS depression (6). Contact with celery stems could lead to photosensitivity (4).

Interactions with Herbs & Other Dietary Supplements

None known.

Interactions with Drugs

CNS DEPRESSANTS: Theoretically, concomitant use with these drugs may cause additive effects (4).
PHOTOSENSITIZING DRUGS: Theoretically, concomitant use might result in increased photosensitivity (6178). Some drugs that cause photosensitivity include amitriptyline (Elavil), quinolones (Ciprofloxacin, others), sulfa drugs (Septra, Bactrim, others), and tetracycline.
LEVOTHYROXINE (Synthroid, Levothroid, Levoxyl, and others): Celery seed might decrease the effects of levothyroxine replacement therapy (10646). The mechanism for this interaction is unknown.

Interactions with Foods
None known.

Interactions with Lab Tests
THYROXINE (T-4): Celery seed might decrease thyroxine (T-4) serum levels and test results (10646). The mechanism for this interaction is unknown.

Interactions with Diseases or Conditions
KIDNEY CONDITIONS: Contraindicated in kidney disorders; celery might increase inflammation (8).

Dosage and Administration
ORAL: 0.5-2 grams of dried fruit three times daily has been used. One cup of tea, prepared by simmering 1 gram of fresh crushed dried fruit in 150 mL boiling water 5-10 minutes, has been used three times daily (4,8). 0.3-1.2 mL of the liquid extract, 1:1 in 60% alcohol, has been used three times daily (4).

Comments
Furocoumarin (a potential carcinogen) content increases 100-fold in injured or diseased celery (6). Celery is available in capsule form, containing 450 or 505 mg of the oil. The ancient Greeks used celery to make wine, which was served as an award at athletic games (6002).

CENTAURY

Also Known As
Bitter Herb, Common Centaury, Drug Centaurium, Lesser Centauru, Minor Centaury.

Scientific Names
Centaurium erythraea, synonyms Erythraea centaurium, Centaurium minus, Centaurium umbellatum.
Family: Gentianaceae.

People Use This For
Orally, centaury is used orally for anorexia and dyspepsia.
In beverages, it is used as a flavoring.

Safety
LIKELY SAFE ...when used orally in amounts commonly found in foods. Centaury has Generally Recognized As Safe (GRAS) status in the US (4912).
POSSIBLY SAFE ...when used orally in medicinal amounts (12). There is no documented toxicity (4).
PREGNANCY AND LACTATION: Insufficient reliable information available; avoid the use of centaury in amounts greater than those commonly found in foods.

Effectiveness
There is insufficient reliable information available about the effectiveness of centaury.

Mechanism of Action
The applicable parts of centaury are the dried, above ground parts. The bitter constituents amarogentin, gentiopicroside, swertiamarin, and the related bitters (3,7) can act as an appetite stimulant, although with less activity than comparable bitter herbs (4). Its antipyretic activity can result from the phenolic acid constituents. The constituent, gentiopicrin, can have antimalarial properties. Animal evidence suggests that centaury has anti-inflammatory activity (4).

Adverse Reactions
None reported.

Interactions with Herbs & Other Dietary Supplements
None known.

Interactions with Drugs
None known.

Interactions with Foods
None known.

Interactions with Lab Tests
None known.

Interactions with Diseases or Conditions
None known.

Dosage and Administration
ORAL: The typical dose of centaury is 2-4 grams or as a tea three times daily. The tea is prepared by steeping 2-4 grams in 150 mL boiling water (4). The average daily dose of centaury is 6 grams (2). The usual dose of the liquid extract (1:1 in 25% alcohol) is 2-4 mL three times daily (4).

CEREUS

Also Known As
Night Blooming Cereus, Sweet Scented Cactus.

Scientific Names
Selenicereus grandiflorus, synonyms Cereus grandiflorus, Cactus grandiflorus.
Family: Cactaceae.

People Use This For
Orally, cereus is used for angina pectoris, edema associated with weak heart function, and as a cardiac stimulant (sometimes instead of digitalis). Cereus is also used orally for urinary ailments, hemoptysis, menorrhagia, dysmenorrhea, hemorrhage, cystitis, and shortness of breath.
Topically, cereus is used as a skin stimulant for rheumatism.

Safety
POSSIBLY SAFE ...when the flower or stem is used orally for non-cardiac conditions (12). Although it contains cactine, which may have a digitalis-like effect, there are no reports of human toxicity (12).
POSSIBLY UNSAFE ...when used orally to self-medicate for cardiac conditions.
There is insufficient reliable information available about the safety of cereus for its other uses.
PREGNANCY AND LACTATION: Insufficient reliable information available; avoid using.

Effectiveness
There is insufficient reliable information available about the effectiveness of cereus.

Mechanism of Action
The applicable parts of cereus are the flower, stem, and young shoots. There is some evidence that cereus can stimulate the heart and dilate peripheral vessels (18), as well as stimulate spinal cord motor neurons (18). Researchers think tyramine, a cardiotonic amine, can strengthen heart muscle action (4). The reputed digitalis effect of cereus is claimed to be non-cumulative (12).

Adverse Reactions
Orally, fresh cereus juice may cause burning of the mouth, queasiness, nausea, vomiting, and diarrhea (4,18).
Topically, it may cause itching and skin pustules (18).

Interactions with Herbs & Other Dietary Supplements
None known.

Interactions with Drugs
DIGOXIN (Lanoxin): Cereus may potentiate the actions of cardiac glycosides and may enhance the effect of other cardiac drugs (6002).
MONOAMINE OXIDASE INHIBITORS (MAOIs): Theoretically, excessive doses of cereus may interact with MAOIs, because of the tyramine content (4).

Interactions with Foods
None known.

Interactions with Lab Tests
None known.

Interactions with Diseases or Conditions

HEART CONDITIONS: Theoretically, cereus may affect individuals with existing heart conditions or interfere with therapy (4).

Dosage and Administration

ORAL: Typical doses are fluid extract (1:1) 0.6 mL one to ten times daily (4,18), tincture of cereus (1:10) 0.12-2 mL two to three times daily (4,18), or tincture in sweetened water (1:10) 10 drops three to five times daily (18). Should not be used as self-medication for cardiac conditions.

CESIUM

Also Known As

Caesium, Cesium-137, Cesium Chloride, CsCl, High pH Therapy.

Scientific Names

Cesium; Cs; atomic number 55.

People Use This For

Orally, cesium is used for treating cancer and depression.
Radioactive cesium (cesium-137) is used as radiation therapy in cancer patients.
In industry, radioactive cesium is also used in instruments that measure thickness, moisture, and liquid flow.

Safety

POSSIBLY UNSAFE ...when used orally in large doses. There is no reliable evidence about the safety of cesium from clinical trials. There is a case report of life-threatening hypokalemia, hypotensive syncope, and prolonged QT interval on electrocardiogram (ECG) in a patient who took cesium 3 grams/day for several weeks (12178). The safety of lower doses is not known.
PREGNANCY AND LACTATION: Insufficient reliable information available; avoid using.

Effectiveness

INSUFFICIENT RELIABLE EVIDENCE to RATE

Cancer. Preliminary evidence suggests that cesium in combination with other vitamins and minerals might reduce mortality rate in some patients with various types of cancer (7613). More evidence is needed to rate cesium for this use.

Mechanism of Action

Cesium is an alkali metal element, structurally similar to lithium, sodium, and potassium (Group 1A on the periodic table). It is stable in its naturally occurring state. Unstable or radioactive cesium is formed by nuclear fission of uranium and plutonium (3894).
Preliminary research on breast and skin cancer cells suggests that cesium might have an anti-tumor effect. It might also stimulate the release of catecholamines (7612).

Adverse Reactions

Orally, cesium can cause nausea, diarrhea, and anorexia. Tingling of the lips, hands, and feet may also occur (7671). In one case, a female patient who took cesium 3 grams/day for several weeks experienced repeated episodes of diarrhea and then numbness or tingling of the lips. The patient was later admitted to the emergency room after having an episode of hypotensive syncope. She was found to be hypokalemic, disoriented, and had a prolonged cardiac QT interval on electrocardiogram ECG). Symptoms reemerged on rechallenge and resolved gradually over several days when cesium was discontinued (12178). It is not known if these symptoms developed due to potassium loss related to diarrhea or due to a direct effect of cesium on potassium channels.
Cesium-137 in high exposures can cause serious burns and death (3894).

Interactions with Herbs & Other Dietary Supplements

None known.

Interactions with Drugs

CORTICOSTEROIDS: Theoretically, drugs that deplete potassium, such as corticosteroids, in combination with cesium might lower serum potassium levels and test results (7670,7671).
DIURETIC DRUGS: Theoretically, people taking cesium along with potassium depleting diuretics might have lower serum potassium levels and test results (7670,7671). Initiation of potassium supplementation or an increase in potassium supplement dose may be necessary for some patients. Some diuretics that can deplete potassium include

chlorothiazide (Diuril), chlorthalidone (Thalitone), furosemide (Lasix), hydrochlorothiazide (HCTZ, HydroDIURIL, Microzide), and others.

Interactions with Foods
None known.

Interactions with Lab Tests
POTASSIUM: Theoretically, cesium might lower potassium levels (7670,7671).

Interactions with Diseases or Conditions
None known.

Dosage and Administration
ORAL: A typical dosage is 6 to 9 grams in 3 divided doses (7613).

Comments
Cesium therapy is sometimes called "high pH therapy." According to proponents, oral administration of cesium chloride increases the pH of tumor cells, which are described as very acidic. There is no scientific research that indicates tumor cells differ in pH from normal cells or that cesium affects the pH of tumor or normal cells. Tell patients these are claims without supporting research.

CETYLATED FATTY ACIDS

Also Known As
Cerasomal-cis-9-cetylmyristoleate, Cetyl Laureate, Cetyl Myristate, Cetyl Myristoleate, Cetyl Oleate, Cetyl Palmitate, Cetyl Palmitoleate, Cetylated Fatty Acids, Cetylated Monounsaturated Fatty Acids, Cetylmyristoleate, CM, CMO.

Scientific Names
Cis-9-cetylmyristoleate.

People Use This For
Orally, cetylated fatty acids are used for rheumatoid arthritis (RA), osteoarthritis, systemic lupus erythematosus (SLE), multiple sclerosis (MS), ankylosing spondylitis, Reiter's syndrome, Behcet's syndrome, Sjogren's syndrome, psoriasis, fibromyalgia, emphysema, benign prostate hyperplasia (BPH), silicone breast disease, leukemia and other cancers, and relief of various types of back pain.
Topically, cetylated fatty acids are used for osteoarthritis.

Safety
POSSIBLY SAFE ...when used orally or topically and appropriately. A blend of cetylated fatty acids (Celadrin, Imagenetix, Inc.) has been used safely when taken orally for 68 days (8924). A topical cream containing a cetylated fatty acid blend (Celadrin, Imagenetix, Inc.) has been safely used when applied twice daily for up to 30 days (12076).
PREGNANCY AND LACTATION: Insufficient reliable information available; avoid using.

Effectiveness
INSUFFICIENT RELIABLE EVIDENCE to RATE

Osteoarthritis. Some preliminary clinical research suggests that taking a blend of cetylated fatty acids (Celadrin, Imagenetix, Inc.) orally or applying the same blend topically might improve knee range of motion and function in patients with knee osteoarthritis (8924,12076). More evidence is needed to rate cetylated fatty acids for this use.

Mechanism of Action
Cetylated fatty acids include cetyl myristoleate, cetyl myristate, cetyl palmitoleate, cetyl laureate, cetyl palmitate, and cetyl oleate. Many products that contain cetyl myristoleate also contain a mixture of these other cetylated fatty acids.
There is interest in cetyl myristoleate for osteoarthritis because it is a substance isolated from mice that are immune to chemically-induced arthritis (677). Researchers also hypothesize that cetyl myristoleate and other cetylated fatty acids might have surfactant effects. These fatty acids might cause lubrication of joints and muscles, softening of tissues, and increased pliability. It is thought that they might also be a modulator of the immune system and a mediator of inflammatory process. Another proposed mechanism of action is possible inhibition of 5-lipoxygenase, a mediator of inflammation (8924,12076). But the evidence to back these theories is very preliminary.

Adverse Reactions
None reported.

Interactions with Herbs & Other Dietary Supplements
None known.

Interactions with Drugs
None known.

Interactions with Foods
None known.

Interactions with Lab Tests
None known.

Interactions with Diseases or Conditions
None known.

Dosage and Administration
No typical dosage.

Comments
There is very little scientific information about this product. Our staff is continually analyzing the available information on natural medicines and will add data here as it becomes available.

CHANCA PIEDRA

Also Known As
Chanca-Piedra Blanca, Chancapiedra, Child Pick-a-Back, Derriere Dos, Derrière-Dos, Des Dos, Dukong Anak, Feuilles la Fievre, Memeniran, Meniran, Niruri, Pitirishi, Quebra Pedra, Quebrapedra, Quinina Criolla, Quinine Créole, Rami Buah, Sacha Foster, Sasha Foster, Seed on the Leaf, Shatter Stone, Stone Breaker, Stonebreaker, Tamalaka, Turi Hutan.

Scientific Names
Phyllanthus niruri.
Family: Euphorbiaceae.

People Use This For
Orally, chanca piedra is used for urinary tract infections and inflammation, kidney stones, urethral or vaginal mucous discharge, as a diuretic, an antiflatulent, aperitif, appetite stimulant, liver tonic, and blood purifier. It is also used orally for diabetes, gallstones, colic, stomachache, dyspepsia, intestinal infections, constipation, dysentery, flu, tenesmus, jaundice, hepatitis B, abdominal tumors, fever, pain, venereal problems, syphilis, gonorrhea, malaria, tumors, caterpillar stings, cough, edema, itching, miscarriage, rectitis, tremors, typhoid, vaginitis, anemia, asthma, bronchitis, thirst, tuberculosis, and vertigo.

Safety
There is insufficient reliable information available about the safety of chanca piedra.
Pregnancy and Lactation: Insufficient reliable information available; avoid using.

Effectiveness
POSSIBLY INEFFECTIVE

Hepatitis B. Taking chanca piedra orally doesn't seem to be effective for treating hepatitis B (3924,3925).

There is insufficient reliable information available about the effectiveness of chanca piedra for its other uses.

Mechanism of Action
Chanca piedra is thought to have multiple properties; antispasmodic, antiviral, bactericidal, antipyretic, and diuretic. It is also thought that chanca piedra reduces blood sugar and protects the liver (517); however, not all of these properties are supported by scientific evidence. In vitro, the constituent niuriside, inhibits specific HIV-protein binding activity, but does not protect cells from acute HIV infection (3927). In isolated animal tissue, an extract from the related plant, Phyllanthus sellowianus, has antispasmodic activity (3921). Preliminary studies in humans show the related species, Phyllanthus amarus, has diuretic, hypotensive and hypoglycemic effects (3928).

Adverse Reactions
None reported.

Interactions with Herbs & Other Dietary Supplements
None known.

Interactions with Drugs
ANTIDIABETES DRUGS: Monitor blood glucose levels closely due to claims that chanca piedra has hypoglycemic effects (19).

Interactions with Foods
None known.

Interactions with Lab Tests
None known.

Interactions with Diseases or Conditions
None known.

Dosage and Administration
ORAL: People typically use 1 to 2 grams of powdered herb in tablets or capsules twice daily. Chanca piedra is also taken as a 4:1 tincture in a dose of 1 to 3 mL twice daily (5255).

Comments
Older studies published in India were reportedly conducted with Phyllanthus niruri, which is thought to be indigenous to the West Indies (271). A report from India mentions Phyllanthus niruri is a synonym for Phyllanthus amarus (3928); however, these appear to be different species (513,816).

CHAPARRAL

Also Known As
Creosote Bush, Greasewood, Hediondilla, Jarilla, Larreastat.

Scientific Names
Larrea divaricata; Larrea tridentata, synonyms Larrea mexicana, Zygophyllum tridentatum.
Family: Zygophyllaceae.

People Use This For
Orally, chaparral is used for cancer, arthritis, venereal disease, tuberculosis, bowel cramps, colds, and chronic cutaneous disorders. It is also used orally for weight loss, as a tonic, antiparasitic, antiflatulent, "blood purifier" for genitourinary and respiratory tract infections, and a treatment for musculoskeletal inflammation, skin diseases, GI conditions, CNS conditions, chickenpox and snakebite pain.

Safety
LIKELY UNSAFE ...when used orally; avoid using. There are reports of serious poisoning, acute hepatitis, kidney and liver damage, and irreversible renohepatic failure (568,569,570,571,3497,11121,11122,11129).
PREGNANCY AND LACTATION: LIKELY UNSAFE ...when used orally; avoid using. There are reports of serious poisoning, acute hepatitis, kidney and liver damage, and irreversible renohepatic failure (568,569,570,571,3497,11121,11122,11129).

Effectiveness
There is insufficient reliable information available about the effectiveness of chaparral.

Mechanism of Action
The applicable part of chaparral is the leaf. Nordihydroguaiaretic acid (NDGA), a constituent of chaparral, may have antioxidant properties and also selectively inhibits lipoxygenases. It is also involved with platelet -derived growth factor receptors and the protein kinase C intracellular signally family, which suggests it might have anticancer activity. It may also induce apoptosis (cellular death) in tumor cells (11123,11124). NGDA might also be responsible for the nephropathy and hepatotoxicity associated with chaparral. The exact mechanism of toxicity is unknown (11125). NDGA might also have antifungal and antiviral activity (11126,11127).
Preliminary research suggests NGDA undergoes glucuronidation in the liver (11125).

Adverse Reactions

Orally, chaparral can cause symptoms of hepatoxicity including jaundice, fatigue, abdominal pain (right upper quadrant), dark urine, light stools, nausea, diarrhea, weight loss, fever, and anorexia. It can cause cirrhosis, cholestasis, cholangitis, acute hepatitis, kidney and liver failure (3497) There are multiple reports of hepatotoxicity, including at least two requiring liver transplant (568,569,570,571,3497,11121,11122). Consumption of chaparral tea has been associated with cystic renal disease and cystic adenocarcinoma of the kidney (11129). Preliminary information suggests low doses of chaparral can be used safely (10417). Tell patients until further information is available, chaparral should be considered unsafe.

Topically, chaparral can cause contact dermatitis (11128).

Interactions with Herbs & Other Dietary Supplements

HEPATOTOXIC HERBS: Theoretically, chaparral might have additive effects with herbs that cause hepatotoxicity (568,569,570,571,3497,11121,11122). Other products that might affect the liver include bishop's weed, borage, uva ursi, and others.

Interactions with Drugs

HEPATOTOXIC DRUGS: Theoretically, chaparral might have additive adverse effects on the liver when used with hepatotoxic drugs (568,569,570,571,3497,11121,11122). Some drugs that can adversely affect the liver include acetaminophen (Tylenol), amiodarone (Cordarone), carbamazepine (Tegretol), isoniazid (INH), methotrexate (Rheumatrex), methyldopa (Aldomet), and many others.

Interactions with Foods

None known.

Interactions with Lab Tests

LIVER FUNCTION TESTS: As a hepatotoxin, chaparral might increase liver function tests including alkaline phosphatase, aspartic acid transaminase (AST,SGOT) alanine aminotransferase (ALT, SGPT), total bilirubin, gamma-glutamyltransferase, and lactate dehydrogenase, (568,569,570,571,3497,11121,11122).

Interactions with Diseases or Conditions

LIVER DISEASE: Theoretically, chaparral might exacerbate liver dysfunction in patients with liver disease (568,569,570,571,3497,11121,11122).

Dosage and Administration

No typical dosage.

Comments

Herp-Eeze is a dietary supplement promoted for preventing and treating herpes infections. The manufacturer states that a patented manufacturing process renders the product nontoxic. However, toxicity information about this product is limited to the manufacturer's claims (267).

CHASTEBERRY

Also Known As

Agnolyt, Agnus Castus, Agnus-Castus, Chaste Berry, Chaste Tree, Chaste Tree Berry, Chastetree, Gattilier, Hemp Tree, Monk's Pepper, Vitex, Vitex Agnus Castus.

Scientific Names

Vitex agnus-castus.
Family: Verbenaceae.

People Use This For

Orally, chasteberry is used for menstrual irregularities including dysmenorrhea, secondary amenorrhea, metrorrhagia, oligomenorrhea, and polymenorrhea. Chasteberry is also used for symptoms of menopause, for symptoms of premenstrual syndrome (PMS) including cyclical mastalgia, luteal-phase dysfunction (corpus luteum insufficiency), and other symptoms. It is also used orally for treating female infertility, preventing miscarriage in patients with progesterone insufficiency, controlling postpartum bleeding, aiding expulsion of the placenta, increasing lactation, and treating fibrocystic breasts. It is used for promoting urination, treating benign prostatic hyperplasia (BPH), and reducing sexual desire. Chasteberry is also used for acne, nervousness, dementia, rheumatic conditions, colds, dyspepsia, spleen disorders, headaches, body inflammation and swelling, and insect bites and stings.

Safety

LIKELY SAFE ...when used orally and appropriately. Chasteberry has been used safely in studies, lasting from 3 months up to 1.5 years (6500,6557,7055,7076,7077,7078,7079).
PREGNANCY: LIKELY UNSAFE ...when used orally. Chasteberry can have uterine-stimulant properties and should be avoided during all stages of pregnancy (6557). Some clinicians use chasteberry during the first trimester of pregnancy to prevent miscarriage in patients with progesterone insufficiency (6500). However, because it is not known if chasteberry is helpful or safe in these patients, avoid using.
LACTATION: POSSIBLY UNSAFE ...when used orally. Chasteberry is thought to be a dopamine agonist and inhibit prolactin secretion. This might result in decreased breast milk production (6500). However, this is controversial. Some clinicians actually use low doses of chasteberry to increase milk production with some reports of benefit (6500,6557). Until more is known, avoid using chasteberry in breast-feeding mothers.

Effectiveness

POSSIBLY EFFECTIVE

Acne. There is some evidence that chasteberry can significantly improve acne in up to 70% of patients treated. Treatment for at least 6 months is usually required before there is significant improvement (6500).
Infertility. There is some preliminary clinical evidence that taking chasteberry orally can increase the chance of getting pregnant in women who are infertile due to relative progesterone deficiency. However, chasteberry does not seem to work quickly. It can take from 3-7 months of treatment to achieve pregnancy (6500,7012,7077).
Menstrual disorders (amenorrhea, polymenorrhea, oligomenorrhea, menorrhagia). There is some evidence that taking chasteberry orally might normalize menstruation in patients with secondary amenorrhea, polymenorrhea (short cycle), oligomenorrhea (infrequent menstruation), and menorrhagia (prolonged menstruation). Chasteberry might be most effective in patients with low levels of progesterone (6500). Use for at least 8 weeks or more is often required before there is significant improvement (6557).
Premenstrual syndrome (PMS). Taking chasteberry orally seems to decrease some symptoms of PMS, especially breast pain or tenderness (mastalgia), edema, constipation, irritability, depressed mood or mood alterations, anger, and headache (6500,6557,7055,7076,7078,7079). In some patients these symptoms can be decreased by as much as 50% (7055). Chasteberry may not be as effective for symptoms of bloating (7055) or in patients with a specific type of PMS with symptoms consisting mostly of craving sweets, sweating, palpitations, and dizziness (6500). Some evidence suggests that women who have PMS primarily due to low progesterone levels and higher estrogen levels are most likely to respond to treatment with chasteberry (6500,6557). Patients may not respond to therapy immediately. Treatment for 4-12 weeks can be required before there is significant improvement in symptoms (6557).
Some clinical studies have used a specific extract of chasteberry (Agnolyt) standardized to contain 6% of the constituent agnoside. In the US, this formulation is found in the brand product Femaprin (Nature's Way).

INSUFFICIENT RELIABLE EVIDENCE to RATE

Lactation. There is some preliminary evidence that chasteberry might increase breast milk production in lactating women when used in low doses (6500,7012,7013). More evidence is needed to rate chasteberry for this use.

Mechanism of Action

The applicable part of the chasteberry tree is the fruit. The active constituents of chasteberries are the essential oils, iridoid glycosides, flavonoids, and diterpenes (7012,7013,10121). The primary essential oils consist of limonene, cineol, pinene, and sabinene (7013). The primary flavonoids include casticin, kaempferol, quercetagetin, orientin, and isovitexin (6500,7013). The primary diterpenes include vitexilactone, rotundifuran, and 6-beta,7 beta-diacetoxy-13-hydroxy-labda-8,14-dien (10121,10122). The relevant iridoid glycosides are aucubin and agnoside (6500,10121). Many chasteberry extracts are standardized to contain 6% agnoside (7012). However, there is increasing evidence that part of the activity of chasteberry fruit is associated with the diterpenes and the flavonoid casticin, which are thought to be a more appropriate marker for the effectiveness of chasteberry preparations (10121). Although not generally considered key constituents, chasteberries also contain several essential fatty acids, including oleic acid, linolenic acid, palmitic acid, and stearic acid (7012).
The therapeutic effects of chasteberry have primarily been attributed to its indirect effects on various neurotransmitters and hormones. Chasteberry seems to affect dopamine, and possibly acetylcholine and opioid receptors (7014,7015,10122). Chasteberry extracts contain multiple active constituents that seem to have agonistic effects at pituitary dopamine (D2) receptors when used in higher doses. This dopaminergic activity inhibits basal and thyrotropin-releasing hormone (TRH)-stimulated prolactin release (7014,7015,11456). In women with hyperprolactinemia, chasteberry seems to suppress prolactin release. This may normalize luteal phase defects in the menstrual cycle (9988). In healthy men, chasteberry's hormonal effects seem to be dose dependent. Lower doses of chasteberry extract of approximately 120 mg per day seem to increase prolactin release. Higher doses seem to suppress prolactin release (7016). Chasteberry doesn't appear to affect testosterone (7016).
Preliminary research suggests chasteberry also might have estrogen and progestin activity (10979,11456). Chasteberry appears to be selective for beta estrogen receptors. The beta estrogen receptor predominates in the heart, vasculature, bone, and bladder (11456). Other preliminary research suggests that chasteberry might inhibit the growth of breast cancer cells and other cancer cells such as ovarian, cervical, gastric, colon, and lung (9990,9991). However, due to the possible estrogenic effect of chasteberry, the safety chasteberry in estrogen-sensitive conditions is unknown.

In addition to hormonal effects, essential oils of chasteberry also seem to have antibacterial and antifungal effects. Extracts of chasteberry have in vitro activity against Staphylococcus aureus, Streptococcus faecalis, Escherichia coli, Bacillus anthracoides, Candida species, Trichophyton mentagrophytes, Epidermophyton floccosum, Microsporum species, and Penicillium virdicatum (6500).

Adverse Reactions

Orally, chasteberry is usually well tolerated. However, some patients can experience gastrointestinal upset, headache, nausea, itching and urticaria, rash, acne, and intramenstrual bleeding (6500,7055,7076,10121). Some patients have also had alopecia, headaches, fatigue, agitation, tachycardia, and dry mouth while taking chasteberry (6500). Side effects are relatively rare, occurring in approximately 2-5% of patients (6557). Changes in menstrual flow can also occur when chasteberry is first started (6557). Allergic reactions can occur in some patients, but typically resolve spontaneously when chasteberry is stopped.

Interactions with Herbs & Other Dietary Supplements

None known.

Interactions with Drugs

ANTIPSYCHOTIC DRUGS: Theoretically, chasteberry might interfere with the action of dopamine antagonists such as antipsychotic drugs due to dopaminergic effects of chasteberry (7014,7015).
CONTRACEPTIVE DRUGS: Theoretically, chasteberry can interfere with the efficacy of oral contraceptives because chasteberry seems to have hormone modulating activity (19).
DOPAMINE AGONISTS: Theoretically, chasteberry might potentiate the actions of dopaminergic agonists due to dopaminergic effects of chasteberry (10122). Some of these drugs include bromocriptine (Parlodel), levodopa (Dopar, component of Sinemet), pramipexole (Mirapex) ropinirole (Requip), and others.
ESTROGENS: Theoretically, chasteberry can interfere with the efficacy of hormone replacement therapy because chasteberry seems to have hormone modulating activity (19).
METOCLOPRAMIDE (Reglan): Theoretically, chasteberry might interfere with the action of dopamine antagonists such as metoclopramide due to dopaminergic effects of chasteberry (7014,7015).

Interactions with Foods

None known.

Interactions with Lab Tests

None known.

Interactions with Diseases or Conditions

HORMONE SENSITIVE CANCERS/CONDITIONS: Because chasteberry seems to have hormonal effects and might affect estrogen levels (6180), women with hormone sensitive conditions should avoid chasteberry. Some of these conditions include breast, uterine, and ovarian cancer, and endometriosis and uterine fibroids.
IN VITRO FERTILIZATION: There is some evidence that using chasteberry during in vitro fertilization procedures might prevent an ensuing pregnancy despite having a viable embryo. In one case, a woman undergoing in vitro fertilization began taking chasteberry. During her fourth in vitro fertilization treatment cycle she was found to have signs of ovarian hyperstimulation syndrome and a viable embryo did not result in pregnancy (6556).

Dosage and Administration

ORAL: For premenstrual syndrome (PMS) and other conditions doses vary considerably. The dosing regimen used depends on the formulation of chasteberry. In one study a specific chasteberry extract (Ze440) 20 mg per day has been used (7055). In a study using a different specific chasteberry extract (Agnolyt), 4 mg daily has been used (7076). One capsule (Femicur) containing 1.6-3.0 mg of dried fruit extract (6.7-12.5:1) has been used twice daily (7079). Crude herb extracts are typically used in doses of 20-240 mg per day up to 1800 mg per day in 2-3 divided doses (6500,7055). Chasteberry fluid extract 40 drops daily has also been used (6500). A dose of 35-45 drops (approximately 1 mL) of chasteberry tincture (1:5-1:2) three times daily has been used (10121).
Some experts suggest that chasteberry should be taken on an empty stomach and in the morning for the most benefit (6500); however, potential benefits of this administration schedule have not been verified.

Comments

Historians say that monks chewed chaste tree parts to make it easier to maintain their celibacy.

CHAULMOOGRA

Also Known As
Gynocardia Oil, Hydnocarp, Hydnocarpus, Oleum Chaulmoograe.

Scientific Names
Hydnocarpus kurzii, synonym Taraktogenos kurzii; Hydnocarpus anthelminthicus; Hydnocarpus species.
Family: Flacourtiaceae.

People Use This For
Topically, chaulmoogra is used for skin disorders, psoriasis, and eczema.
Parenterally, chaulmoogra is used for leprosy.

Safety
LIKELY UNSAFE ...when used orally. The seeds are considered very toxic due to their cyanogenic glycoside content (18).
There is insufficient reliable information available about the safety of chaulmoogra for its other uses.
PREGNANCY AND LACTATION: Insufficient reliable information available; avoid using.

Effectiveness
There is insufficient reliable information available to rate the effectiveness of chaulmoogra.

Mechanism of Action
The applicable part of chaulmoogra is the seed. Chaulmoogra is thought to have sedative, antipyretic, and skin effects (18). In mice, intraperitoneal and subcutaneous administration of chaulmoogra fatty acids demonstrated antimicrobial activity against Mycobacterium leprae (3826). The cyanogenic glycoside content of the seeds renders them extremely poisonous (18).

Adverse Reactions
Orally, ingestion of the seed can cause cough, dyspnea, laryngospasms, nephrotoxicity, visual disorders, head and muscle pain, and central paralysis (18).
Topically, use can cause skin irritation (18).

Interactions with Herbs & Other Dietary Supplements
None known.

Interactions with Drugs
None known.

Interactions with Foods
None known.

Interactions with Lab Tests
None known.

Interactions with Diseases or Conditions
None known.

Dosage and Administration
ORAL: No typical dosage.
TOPICAL: People typically use chaulmoogra as a powder, oil, emulsion, or in ointments (18).
PARENTERAL: No typical dosage.

Comments
Chaulmoogra seeds provided the elemental materials for synthesizing the first antileprostatic agents (6002).

CHEKEN

Also Known As
Arryan, Chekan, Myrtus.

Scientific Names
Luma chequen, synonyms Eugenia chequen, Myrtus chequen.
Family: Myrtaceae.

Comments
At the date of publication, this product was not a common ingredient used in brand name supplements marketed to consumers. Details about this product are available at the online version of *Natural Medicines Comprehensive Database*. See www.naturaldatabase.com.

CHELATED MINERALS

Also Known As
Chelated Boron, Chelated Calcium, Chelated Chromium, Chelated Cobalt, Chelated Copper, Chelated Iron, Chelated Magnesium, Chelated Manganese, Chelated Molybdenum, Chelated Potassium, Chelated Selenium, Chelated Trace Minerals, Chelated Vanadium, Chelated Zinc.
CAUTION: See separate listings for Aspartates and individual minerals.

Scientific Names
Mineral-amino acid complex.

People Use This For
Orally, chelated minerals are used as dietary mineral supplements (marketed to be more bioavailable than non-chelated minerals), for supporting normal growth, stabilizing bipolar disorder, building strong muscles and bones, and improving immune function and overall health.

Safety
There is insufficient reliable information available about the safety of chelated minerals.
Pregnancy and Lactation: Insufficient reliable information available; avoid using.

Effectiveness
INSUFFICIENT RELIABLE EVIDENCE to RATE

Bipolar disorder. There is preliminary evidence that suggests that some cases of bipolar disorder may be stabilized with a chelated mineral supplement. A randomized, placebo-controlled trial in adults with bipolar disorder is presently underway (10651,10660). More evidence is needed to rate chelated minerals for this use.

Mechanism of Action
The term, chelated mineral, refers to the formation of a complex between a mineral and an amino acid. Evidence supports the importance of chelated minerals in the central nervous system (CNS), citing a beneficial psychotropic effect, although the exact mechanism is not fully understood (10651,10660).

Adverse Reactions
Orally, chelated minerals can cause nausea (10660). Fatty liver-hemorrhagic syndrome is reported in commercial chickens that are fed diets containing chelated minerals (1162).

Interactions with Herbs & Other Dietary Supplements
None known.

Interactions with Drugs
None known.

Interactions with Foods
None known.

Interactions with Lab Tests
None known.

Interactions with Diseases or Conditions
None known.

Dosage and Administration
See separate listings for specific minerals.

Comments
There is very little scientific information about this product. Our staff is continually analyzing the available information on natural medicines and will add data here as it becomes available.

CHENOPODIUM OIL

Also Known As
Epazote, Jesuit Tea, Mexican Tea.
CAUTION: See separate listings for Wormseed, Wormwood Oil, and Wormwood.

Scientific Names
Chenopodium ambrosioides; Chenopodium anthelminticum.
Family: Chenopodiaceae.

People Use This For
Orally, chenopodium oil has been used as an oral antiparasitic against roundworms and hookworms.

Safety
UNSAFE ...when used orally due to toxicity (11).
PREGNANCY AND LACTATION: UNSAFE ...when used orally due to toxicity (11).

Effectiveness
There is insufficient reliable information available about the effectiveness of chenopodium oil.

Mechanism of Action
The constituent ascaridole is thought to paralyze roundworms, hookworms, and dwarf tapeworms but not large tapeworms within the intestines (11). However, toxicity precludes its clinical use for these helminth infections. Chenopodium oil may explode when heated or treated with acids due to high ascaridole content (11). Handle with caution.

Adverse Reactions
Orally, chenopodium oil can cause skin and mucous membrane irritation, vomiting, headache, vertigo/dizziness, kidney and liver damage, temporary deafness, convulsions, circulatory collapse, paralysis, and death (11).

Interactions with Herbs & Other Dietary Supplements
None known.

Interactions with Drugs
PHOTOSENSITIZING DRUGS: Theoretically, concomitant use of chenopodium oil can increase risk of adverse effects. Chenopodium species are associated with photosensitivity (19).

Interactions with Foods
None known.

Interactions with Lab Tests
None known.

Interactions with Diseases or Conditions
None known.

Dosage and Administration
No typical dosage.

Comments
Authorities disagree on whether chenopodium oil is the distilled oil of fresh above ground flowering and fruiting parts (11) or seed oil (18) of Chenopodium ambrosioides.

CHEROKEE ROSEHIP

Also Known As
Chinese Rosehip, Fructus Rosae Laevigatae, Jinyingzi.
CAUTION: See separate listings for Acerola, Vitamin C, and Rose Hip.

Scientific Names
Rosa laevigata, synonym Rosa cherokeensi; Rosa chinensis, synonyms Rosa sinica, Rosa indica, Rosa roulettii; Rosa ternata; Rosa nivea; Rosa camellia.
Family: Rosaceae.

People Use This For
Orally, Cherokee rosehip is used for male sexual dysfunction (nocturnal emission, spermatorrhea, neurasthenia), gynecologic problems (leukorrhea, uterine bleeding), night sweats, polyuria, enuresis, chronic diarrhea, chronic cough, hypertension, and enteritis.

Safety
POSSIBLY SAFE ...when used orally and appropriately. It contains vitamin C as a major constituent (11).
POSSIBLY UNSAFE ...when used orally in large amounts. Hyperoxaluria, hyperuricosuria, hematuria, and crystalluria can occur in some people taking 1 gram of vitamin C (67 grams of Cherokee rosehip) or more per day (3042). Prolonged use of large amounts of vitamin C can increase its metabolism, and scurvy might occur when intake is reduced (15).
PREGNANCY: POSSIBLY UNSAFE ...when used orally in large doses because it is associated with newborn scurvy (15). There is insufficient reliable information available about the safety of smaller amounts.
LACTATION: Insufficient reliable information available.

Effectiveness
There is insufficient reliable information available about the effectiveness of Cherokee rosehip.

Mechanism of Action
Cherokee rosehip contains vitamin C (approximately 1.5%) (11). An antidiarrheal effect occurs in humans (11).

Adverse Reactions
Orally, the vitamin C in Cherokee rosehip may cause nausea, abdominal cramps, fatigue, insomnia, and sleepiness. Doses greater than 1 gram may cause diarrhea (15).

Interactions with Herbs & Other Dietary Supplements
VITAMIN CONTAINING HERBS: Due to the vitamin C content, concomitant use of Cherokee rosehip with other products containing vitamin C increases total dose of vitamin C and may increase risk of adverse effects.

Interactions with Drugs
ALUMINUM: Concomitant use interacts with the vitamin C in Cherokee rose hip and can increase aluminum absorption, but the clinical significance of this is unknown (3046). Administer Cherokee rose hip with vitamin C two hours before or four hours after antacids (3046).
ASPIRIN: Theoretically, the vitamin C in large amounts of Cherokee rosehip might decrease excretion of aspirin (15).
CHOLINE MAGNESIUM TRISALICYLATE (Trilisate): The vitamin C in Cherokee rose hip can increase urinary excretion of ascorbic acid and decrease excretion of salicylates such as choline magnesium trisalicylate. But this may not have a clinically significant effect on salicylate plasma levels (3046).
ESTROGENS: Theoretically, the vitamin C in large amounts of Cherokee rosehip might increase absorption and effects of estrogen (129,130).
FLUPHENAZINE (Prolixin): Concomitant use with Cherokee rosehip decreases blood levels due to vitamin C content (15).
WARFARIN (Coumadin): Theoretically, the vitamin C in large amounts of Cherokee rosehip might reduce anticoagulant activity (506).

Interactions with Foods
IRON: Theoretically, the vitamin C in Cherokee rosehip might increase GI absorption of food iron (ferric) but not supplement iron (ferrous) (15).

Interactions with Lab Tests
STOOL OCCULT BLOOD TESTS: Theoretically, large amounts of Cherokee rosehip may cause a false-negative result if ingested 48-72 hours before amine-dependent tests due to vitamin C content (506).
URINE GLUCOSE TESTS: Theoretically, large amounts of Cherokee rosehip (containing greater than 500 mg vitamin C) may cause false decreases with glucose oxidase tests (e.g., Clinistix) and may cause false increases with cupric sulfate tests (e.g., Clinitest) (15).

Interactions with Diseases or Conditions
DIABETES: Large amounts may affect blood sugar control because of the vitamin C content (15).
GOUT: Theoretically, the vitamin C in large amounts of Cherokee rosehip might increase uric acid levels (15).
KIDNEY STONE FORMING TENDENCY: Theoretically, the vitamin C in large amounts of Cherokee rosehip might cause precipitation of urate, cystine, or oxalate stones (15).

Dosage and Administration
No typical dosage.

Comments
Cherokee rosehip contains vitamin C (approximately 1.5%) (11).

CHERRY LAUREL WATER

Also Known As
Common Cherry Laurel, Laurocerasus Leaves.
CAUTION: See separate listing for Wild Cherry.

Scientific Names
Prunus laurocerasus, synonyms Laurocerasus officinalis, Cerasus laurocerasus, Laurocerasus ottinii, Laurocerasus vulgaris, Prunus grandifolia.
Family: Rosaceae.

People Use This For
Orally, cherry laurel water is used as a sedative, pain reliever, antispasmodic, for treating cough, colds, insomnia, stomach and intestinal spasms, vomiting, and cancer.
Topically, cherry laurel water is used in eye lotions.
As an inhalant, cherry laurel water is used as an aromatic, and breathing stimulant.

Safety
POSSIBLY SAFE ...when used orally and appropriately (18).
LIKELY UNSAFE ...when use orally in high doses. Cherry laurel water contains 0.1% hydrocyanic acid (11). Overdose can be fatal (18).
PREGNANCY AND LACTATION: Insufficient reliable information available; avoid using.

Effectiveness
There is insufficient reliable information available about the effectiveness of cherry laurel water.

Mechanism of Action
Contains prunasin, a cyanogenic glycoside (11,18).

Adverse Reactions
Orally, adverse effects have not been reported with typical doses. However, cherry laurel water contains 0.1% hydrocyanic acid (11), and overdoses can cause significant toxicity and death (18).

Interactions with Herbs & Other Dietary Supplements
None known.

Interactions with Drugs
None known.

Interactions with Foods
None known.

Interactions with Lab Tests
None known.

Interactions with Diseases or Conditions
None known.

Dosage and Administration
ORAL: People typically use a dose of 2 to 8 mL cherry laurel water (223,5267).

Comments
Cherry laurel water is produced by water distillation of cherry laurel (Prunus laurocerasus) leaves. Avoid confusion with wild cherry bark, sweet bay leaf (laurel).

CHERVIL

Also Known As
Garden Chervil, Salad Chervil.

Scientific Names
Anthriscus cerefolium, synonyms Anthriscus longirostris, Scandix cerefolium.
Family: Apiaceae/Umbelliferae.

People Use This For
Orally, chervil is used as a diuretic, expectorant, digestive aid, and an antihypertensive. Juice from fresh chervil is used for eczema, gout, and abscesses.
In foods and beverages, chervil is used as a flavoring agent.

Safety
LIKELY SAFE ...when used orally in amounts commonly found in foods. Chervil and chervil extract have Generally Recognized As Safe (GRAS) status in the US (4912).
There is insufficient reliable information available about the safety of the oral use of chervil in medicinal amounts.
PREGNANCY AND LACTATION: LIKELY UNSAFE ...when used orally in medicinal amounts. Chervil contains estragole which might be mutagenic (12).

Effectiveness
There is insufficient reliable information available about the effectiveness of chervil.

Mechanism of Action
The applicable parts of chervil are the dried flowering parts and leaf. Chervil is a plant source rich in calcium and potassium (19). Estragole, the major constituent of the volatile oil, is reported to produce tumors in mice (11).

Adverse Reactions
None reported.

Interactions with Herbs & Other Dietary Supplements
None known.

Interactions with Drugs
None known.

Interactions with Foods
None known.

Interactions with Lab Tests
None known.

Interactions with Diseases or Conditions
None known.

Dosage and Administration

ORAL: Chervil is typically prepared by adding 1 teaspoon of fresh or dried herb to water. The dose is up to 1 cup a day, unsweetened, consumed a mouthful at a time (5263).

CHICKEN COLLAGEN

Also Known As

Chicken Type II Collagen, Type II Collagen.

Scientific Names

Chicken collagen type II.

People Use This For

Orally, chicken collagen is used to treat pain syndromes associated with rheumatoid arthritis, osteoarthritis, gouty arthritis, juvenile rheumatoid arthritis, post-surgical joint pain, post-traumatic pain, fibrositis, back pain, and neck pain.

Safety

There is insufficient reliable information available about the safety of chicken collagen.
Pregnancy and Lactation: Insufficient reliable information available; avoid using.

Effectiveness

There is insufficient reliable information available about the effectiveness of chicken collagen.

Mechanism of Action

The rationale of using chicken collagen for pain syndromes is based on the theory of oral tolerance. This theory hypothesizes that oral administration of small quantities of antigens causes biological processes that suppress inflammation at the cellular level, suppress response to delayed-hypersensitivity antigens, and eliminate the cells that respond to antigens. Although evidence suggests this theory might be true in animals, it is unproven in humans (3126). Based on the theory of oral tolerance, when individuals with rheumatoid arthritis take oral collagen, the collagen should cause certain areas of the gut to generate T-cells that are absorbed by the body. Then, in the body, these T-cells are activated by joint collagen and they secrete cytokines that suppress inflammation. Cytokines thought to be involved include interleukin 4, 10, and transforming growth factor beta (3111,3112,3125). Oral administration of collagen is also believed to decrease the expression of pro-inflammatory cytokines including interleukins 1, 2, 6, and 8; tumor necrosis factor alpha; and interferon gamma (3111). So far, the studies determining the efficacy of chicken collagen demonstrate conflicting results (3125,3112), but these studies have used microgram doses.

Adverse Reactions

Although no significant adverse effects have been reported in the small trials of chicken collagen (3111,3112), allergic reactions to other collagen products have occurred, e.g., bovine collagen used in corneal shields, catgut suture for eye surgery, and dietary collagen in the form of gelatin (3127). If large doses are used, side effects associated with glucosamine sulfate or chondroitin might occur. These include nausea, heartburn, diarrhea and constipation, drowsiness, skin reactions, and headache (2608).

Interactions with Herbs & Other Dietary Supplements

None known.

Interactions with Drugs

None known.

Interactions with Foods

None known.

Interactions with Lab Tests

None known.

Interactions with Diseases or Conditions

ALLERGIES: Theoretically, individuals who are allergic to chicken or eggs should not use chicken collagen. Collagen products have been associated with allergic reactions (e.g., bovine collagen used in corneal shields, catgut suture for eye surgery, and dietary collagen in the form of gelatin) (3127).

Dosage and Administration

ORAL: For rheumatoid arthritis, doses of 20 to 2500 mcg per day of chicken collagen have been used. For juvenile arthritis, doses of 100 mcg per day for the first month then 500 mcg per day thereafter have been used (3111,3112).

Comments

The manufacturer of Colloral, an oral chicken collagen product, stopped product development because it failed to demonstrate efficacy in humans (3128). Bovine collagen products have also been used in the treatment of rheumatoid arthritis.

CHICKWEED

Also Known As

Star Chickweed, Starweed.

Scientific Names

Stellaria media, synonym Alsine media.
Family: Caryophyllaceae.

People Use This For

Orally, chickweed is used for constipation, bronchial asthma, stomach and bowel problems, blood disorders, lung disease, obesity, scurvy, psoriasis, rabies, itching, and muscle and joint pain.
Topically, chickweed is used for skin problems including boils, abscesses, and ulcers.
In foods, chickweed is eaten in salads or served as cooked greens.

Safety

LIKELY SAFE ...when used orally (12).
There is insufficient reliable information available about the safety of the topical use of chickweed.
PREGNANCY AND LACTATION: Insufficient reliable information available; avoid using in amounts greater than those found in food.

Effectiveness

There is insufficient reliable information available about the effectiveness of chickweed.

Mechanism of Action

The applicable part of chickweed is the leaf. There is no indication that any of the constituents have therapeutic value (5,6). While chickweed does contain some vitamin C, the concentrations are too small to be effective (6).

Adverse Reactions

Orally, chickweed is generally well-tolerated (6). There are, however, some poorly documented human cases of paralysis from consumptions of large amounts of chickweed tea (6). There is one case of alleged nitrate toxicity leading to paralysis, but the chickweed implicated in this case may have been contaminated (12).

Interactions with Herbs & Other Dietary Supplements

None known.

Interactions with Drugs

None known.

Interactions with Foods

None known.

Interactions with Lab Tests

None known.

Interactions with Diseases or Conditions

None known.

Dosage and Administration

ORAL: People typically use 1155 to 3450 mg per day in 2 to 3 divided doses. One chickweed supplier suggests three daily doses based on body weight: under 100 pounds, 385 mg per dose; 100 to 175 pounds, 770 mg; and over 175 pounds, 1155 mg. Chickweed is also prepared as a tea with 1 to 2 teaspoons in 6 ounces of boiling water.

Chickweed is available as a tincture of unspecified concentration with a typical dose of 1 to 5 mL per day (6006).
TOPICAL: No typical dosage.

CHICORY

Also Known As
Blue Sailors, Cichorii Herba, Cichorii Radix, Common Chicory Root, Hendibeh, Kasani, Succory, Wild Chicory.
CAUTION: See separate listing for Inulin.

Scientific Names
Cichorium intybus.
Family: Asteraceae/Compositae.

People Use This For
Orally, chicory is used as a tonic, diuretic, laxative, liver protectant, to balance the stimulant effect of coffee, for loss of appetite, dyspepsia, liver and gallbladder disorders, cancer, and tachycardia.
Topically, chicory leaves are used as a poultice for swelling and inflammation.
In foods, chicory leaves are often eaten like celery, and the roots are boiled and eaten. Chicory is used as a culinary spice, and the leaf buds and roots are eaten as vegetables.
In food manufacturing, chicory is used as a flavoring component in foods and beverages. The roasted root is also ground and used in coffee mixes to enhance richness and as a coffee substitute.

Safety
LIKELY SAFE ...when consumed in amounts commonly found in food. Chicory and chicory extract have Generally Recognized As Safe (GRAS) status in the US (4912).
POSSIBLY SAFE ...when used orally in medicinal amounts (2,12).
There is insufficient reliable information available about the safety of chicory for its other uses.
PREGNANCY: LIKELY UNSAFE ...when used orally due to concerns that chicory can induce menstruation or miscarriage (19).
LACTATION: Insufficient reliable information available; avoid using.

Effectiveness
There is insufficient reliable information available about the effectiveness of chicory.

Mechanism of Action
The applicable parts of chicory are the root and dried above ground parts. Chicory root has a mild laxative effect and stimulates bile production. It is also believed to slow the heart rate (2,11), perhaps due to the presence of a digitalis-like compound (5). Chicory has a sedative effect that has been attributed to the constituent lactucopicrin (5) and other water-soluble components (6). The sedative effect antagonizes the stimulant effects of coffee and tea (6). The sesquiterpene alkaloid constituents show evidence of bacteriostatic properties (11). The extracts seem to have anti-inflammatory activity (11). Chicory is a rich source of beta-carotene (19).

Adverse Reactions
Topically, chicory can cause contact dermatitis (6,11). It can cause an allergic reaction in individuals sensitive to the Asteraceae/Compositae family. Members of this family include ragweed, chrysanthemums, marigolds, daisies, and many other herbs.

Interactions with Herbs & Other Dietary Supplements
None known.

Interactions with Drugs
None known.

Interactions with Foods
None known.

Interactions with Lab Tests
None known.

Interactions with Diseases or Conditions
CHICORY ALLERGY: Contraindicated (11).
CROSS-ALLERGENICITY: Chicory may cause an allergic reaction in individuals sensitive to the

Asteraceae/Compositae family. Members of this family include ragweed, chrysanthemums, marigolds, daisies, and many other herbs.
GALLSTONES: Chicory should be used with medical supervison due to chicory's bile stimulating effects (2,6,11).

Dosage and Administration

ORAL: The typical dose of chicory is one cup of the tea, which is prepared by steeping 2-4 grams of the root in 150 mL boiling water for 10 minutes and then straining (18). The average dose of chicory is 3-5 grams of the root per day (18).
TOPICAL: No typical dosage.

Comments

Chicory can be contaminated with bacteria (6,3807) or foreign substances, including fungicides (6).

CHINESE CLUB MOSS

Also Known As

Huperazon, Qian Ceng Ta.
CAUTION: See separate listing for Huperzine A.

Scientific Names

Huperzia serrata.
Family: Lycopodiaceae.

People Use This For

Orally, Chinese club moss is used for Alzheimer's disease, general memory disorders, fever, inflammation, blood loss, irregular menstruation, and as a diuretic.

Safety

There is insufficient reliable information available about the safety of Chinese club moss.
Pregnancy and Lactation: Insufficient reliable information available; avoid using.

Effectiveness

There is insufficient reliable information available about the effectiveness of Chinese club moss.

Mechanism of Action

Chinese club moss contains the alkaloid huperzine A, a reversible acetylcholinesterase (AChE) inhibitor which crosses the blood-brain barrier (3082).

Adverse Reactions

None reported with Chinese club moss.
Orally, huperzine A which is found in Chinese club moss can cause dizziness, nausea and sweating (3140).

Interactions with Herbs & Other Dietary Supplements

None known.

Interactions with Drugs

ACETYLCHOLINESTERASE (AChE) INHIBITORS: Theoretically, concurrent use with Chinese club moss might have additive effects with drugs that promote acetylcholine activity because huperzine A has AChE inhibitor properties (3082). AChE inhibitors and cholinergic drugs include bethanechol (Urecholine), donepezil (Aricept), echothiophate (Phospholine Iodide), edrophonium (Enlon, Reversol, Tensilon), neostigmine (Prostigmin), physostigmine (Antilirium), pyridostigmine (Mestinon, Regonol), succinylcholine (Anectine, Quelicin), and tacrine (Cognex).
ANTICHOLINERGIC DRUGS: Theoretically, concurrent use of anticholinergic drugs and Chinese club moss might decrease the effectiveness of Chinese club moss or the anticholinergic drug. In an animal model, huperzine A, an active constituent of Chinese club moss, reversed cognitive deficits induced by scopolamine (3135). Anticholinergic drugs include atropine, benztropine (Cogentin), biperiden (Akineton), procyclidine (Kemadrin), and trihexyphenidyl (Artane).
CHOLINERGIC DRUGS: Theoretically, concurrent use with Chinese club moss might have additive effects with drugs that promote acetylcholine activity because huperzine A has AChE inhibitor properties (3082). AChE inhibitors and cholinergic drugs include bethanechol (Urecholine), donepezil (Aricept), echothiophate (Phospholine Iodide), edrophonium (Enlon, Reversol, Tensilon), neostigmine (Prostigmin), physostigmine (Antilirium), pyridostigmine (Mestinon, Regonol), succinylcholine (Anectine, Quelicin), and tacrine (Cognex).

Interactions with Foods
None known.

Interactions with Lab Tests
None known.

Interactions with Diseases or Conditions
VARIOUS DISEASES: Acetylcholinesterase (AChE) inhibitors are used with caution or are contraindicated in people with asthma, chronic obstructive pulmonary disease, cardiovascular disease, obstruction of the intestinal or urogenital tracts, gastrointestinal ulcer disease, or seizures (15). Avoid using Chinese club moss in people with these conditions until more is known about its effects in humans.

Dosage and Administration
ORAL: Currently available products contain isolated huperzine A extracted from Chinese club moss (see separate listing for Huperzine A).

Comments
Be careful not to confuse club moss and Chinese club moss. Only Chinese club moss contains huperzine A.

CHINESE CUCUMBER fruit

Also Known As
Chinese Snake Gourd, Compound Q, Gua Lou, Gua-Lou, Trichosanthes, Trichosanthes Fruit Peel.
CAUTION: See separate listings for Chinese Cucumber root and Chinese Cucumber seed.

Scientific Names
Trichosanthes kirilowii, synonym Trichosanthes japonica.
Family: Curcurbitaceae.

People Use This For
Orally, Chinese cucumber fruit is used for coughing, reducing fever, swelling, tumors, and diabetes.
Intravaginally, Chinese cucumber fruit is used as an abortifacient.

Safety
POSSIBLY SAFE ...when used orally and appropriately (12).
There is insufficient reliable information available about the safety of the intravaginal use of Chinese cucumber fruit.
PREGNANCY: LIKELY UNSAFE ...when used orally because it might induce abortion (6).
LACTATION: Insufficient reliable information available; avoid using.

Effectiveness
There is insufficient reliable information available about the effectiveness of Chinese cucumber fruit.

Mechanism of Action
Some evidence suggests a 50% ethanolic extract might have protective effects against ulcers (4044). A sponge containing Chinese cucumber juice might induce abortions when inserted intravaginally (6).

Adverse Reactions
Orally, Chinese cucumber fruit may cause mild diarrhea and gastric discomfort (12).

Interactions with Herbs & Other Dietary Supplements
None known.

Interactions with Drugs
None known.

Interactions with Foods
None known.

Interactions with Lab Tests
None known.

Interactions with Diseases or Conditions
None known.

Dosage and Administration
No typical dosage.

CHINESE CUCUMBER root

Also Known As
Chinese Snake Gourd, Compound Q, Tian Hua Fen, Tian-Hua-Fen, Trichosanthes.
CAUTION: See separate listings for Chinese Cucumber fruit and Chinese Cucumber seed.

Scientific Names
Trichosanthes kirilowii, synonym Trichosanthes japonica.
Family: Curcurbitaceae.

People Use This For
Orally, Chinese cucumber root is used to treat HIV infection, coughs, fever, swelling, tumors and diabetes. A starch extract is used for treating abscesses, amenorrhea, jaundice, frequent urination, and tumors. Intramuscularly, Chinese cucumber root is used to induce abortions (by intramuscular injection).

Safety
LIKELY UNSAFE ...when used orally or by injection for self-medication; requires monitoring (6). Extracts of Chinese cucumber can be very toxic (6).
PREGNANCY: LIKELY UNSAFE ...when used orally or by injection due to abortifacient effects and possible teratogenicity (6,12).
LACTATION: LIKELY UNSAFE ...when used orally or by injection (6); avoid using.

Effectiveness
POSSIBLY EFFECTIVE
Abortion. Administering Chinese cucumber root parenterally seems to be effective as an abortifacient (6).
There is insufficient reliable information available about the effectiveness of Chinese cucumber root for its other uses.

Mechanism of Action
Chinese cucumber root contains several constituents that demonstrate anti-HIV activity. Trichosanthin and protein "TAP 29" can block HIV replication and some evidence suggests they might selectively kill HIV infected cells in the immune system. Other constituents of the root, trichosanthin and momorcharin, can have abortifacient effects. Trichosanthin injected intramuscularly or extra-amniotically can induce first-trimester abortions. It has also been used to terminate ectopic pregnancies (6). Some evidence suggests trichosanthin and momorcharin might cause birth defects (12). Trichosanthin also shows antitumor activity. It has been used to treat invasive moles and certain types of liver tumors. Some evidence suggests that a water extract of the root might have hypoglycemic activity in individuals with normal blood glucose. Subsequent fractionation of the extract yielded five compounds. The activity of one of these suggests it might be useful in reducing blood sugars in individuals with diabetes (4045).

Adverse Reactions
Chinese cucumber root extracts are extremely toxic, particularly when they are injected. Trichosanthin injections can be fatal. They can also cause severe reactions including seizures, fever, lung and cerebral edema, cerebral hemorrhage, and heart damage. People receiving trichosanthin injections to cause abortion can develop a severe allergy. After a single exposure, the risk of anaphylaxis from a second exposure can persist for more than a decade (6).

Interactions with Herbs & Other Dietary Supplements
ANTIDIABETES HERBS: Theoretically, concomitant use may potentiate effects of other herbs with hypoglycemic effects (6,4045).

Interactions with Drugs
ANTIDIABETES DRUGS: Theoretically, concomitant use with Chinese cucumber root may have additive effects and adverse effects (6,4045). Monitor blood glucose levels closely, dose adjustment may be needed.

Interactions with Foods
None known.

Interactions with Lab Tests
BLOOD GLUCOSE: Theoretically, may decrease blood glucose levels and test results (6,4045).

Interactions with Diseases or Conditions
DIABETES: Theoretically, use of Chinese cucumber root may alter blood glucose control (6,4045).

Dosage and Administration
ORAL: People typically use 9 to 15 grams of the root (5268).

Comments
Avoid confusion with Chinese cucumber fruit and Chinese cucumber seed.

CHINESE CUCUMBER seed

Also Known As
Chinese Snake Gourd, Compound Q, Gua Luo Ren, Gua-Luo-Ren, Trichosanthes.
CAUTION: See separate listings for Chinese Cucumber root and Chinese Cucumber fruit.

Scientific Names
Trichosanthes kirilowii, synonym Trichosanthes japonica.
Family: Curcurbitaceae.

People Use This For
Orally, Chinese cucumber seed is used for coughs, reducing fever, swelling, tumors, and diabetes.

Safety
POSSIBLY SAFE ...when used orally (12).
PREGNANCY AND LACTATION: Insufficient reliable information available; avoid using.

Effectiveness
There is insufficient reliable information available about the effectiveness of Chinese cucumber seed.

Mechanism of Action
Some evidence suggests three triterpene compounds isolated from the seed might have anti-inflammatory effects (4042). Other information suggests that a 50% ethanolic seed extract might have anti-inflammatory and analgesic effects (4043).

Adverse Reactions
None reported.

Interactions with Herbs & Other Dietary Supplements
None known.

Interactions with Drugs
None known.

Interactions with Foods
None known.

Interactions with Lab Tests
None known.

Interactions with Diseases or Conditions
None known.

Dosage and Administration
No typical dosage.

CHIRATA

Also Known As
Bitter Stick, Bitterstick, Chirayta, Chiretta, East Indian Balmony, Indian Bolonong, Indian Gentian, Kairata, Kirata, Yin Du Zhang Ya Cai.

Scientific Names
Swertia chirayita, Swertia chirata, Gentiana chirata, Gentiana chirayita.
Family: Gentianaceae.

People Use This For
Orally, chirata is used as a bitter tonic, antipyretic, laxative, anthelmintic, for dyspepsia, loss of appetite, skin diseases, and cancer.
In India, it has been used as an anti-malarial, combined with the seeds of Guilandina Bonducella.
In manufacturing, chirata is used for alcoholic and non-alcoholic beverages.

Safety
LIKELY SAFE ...when used orally in amounts commonly found in foods. Chirata has Generally Recognized As Safe (GRAS) status in the US (4912).
There is insufficient reliable information available about the safety of chirata in medicinal amounts.
PREGNANCY AND LACTATION: Insufficient reliable information available; avoid using.

Effectiveness
There is insufficient reliable information available about the effectiveness of chirata.

Mechanism of Action
The applicable parts of chirata are the above ground parts. The extract is reported to have anti-inflammatory activity in animals (11). Constituents and their reported activity include chirata stimulates gastric juice secretion (18); swerchirin has antimalarial activity (in vivo) (11); amarogentin has hepatoprotective activity (in vitro) (11); xanthones claimed to have antituberculous activity (11).

Adverse Reactions
None reported.

Interactions with Herbs & Other Dietary Supplements
None known.

Interactions with Drugs
None known.

Interactions with Foods
None known.

Interactions with Lab Tests
None known.

Interactions with Diseases or Conditions
DUODENAL ULCERS: May exacerbate (18); avoid using.

Dosage and Administration
ORAL: People typically use 0.5 to 2 grams of the powdered herb or 2 to 4 mL of the liquid extract (223).

Comments
Adulteration reported with Andrographis paniculata, roots of Rubia cordifolia, and Swertia species, including Swertia angustifolia (11).

CHITOSAN

Also Known As

Chitosan Ascorbate, Mono-carboxymethylated chitosan, N-Carboxybutyl Chitosan, N,O-Sulfated Chitosan, O-Sulfated N-Acetylchitosan, Sulfated N-Carboxymethylchitosan, Sulfated O-Carboxymethylchitosan, Trimethyl chitosan chloride.

Scientific Names

Chitosan.

People Use This For

Orally, chitosan is used for weight loss. It is also used orally by some people with renal failure on chronic hemodialysis for reducing high cholesterol, improving anemia, enhancing physical strength, appetite, and sleep. Chitosan is also used for Crohn's disease.
Topically, chitosan is used for treating periodontitis and promoting donor site tissue regeneration in plastic surgery.
In pharmaceutical manufacturing, chitosan is used as an excipient in tablets, as a disintegrant to improve drug dissolution, as a vehicle for parenteral drug delivery devices, and as a carrier in controlled release drug systems.

Safety

POSSIBLY SAFE ...when used orally for up to 4 weeks (1942,9609,9610,10022,10023,10024,10025,11307). ...when used topically (1944,1945,4269,4270).
PREGNANCY AND LACTATION: Insufficient reliable information available; avoid using.

Effectiveness

POSSIBLY EFFECTIVE

Periodontitis. Applying chitosan ascorbate topically seems to help in the treatment of periodontitis (1945).
Plastic surgery. Applying N-carboxybutyl chitosan topically seems to help promote donor site tissue regeneration in plastic surgery (1944).
Renal failure. Taking chitosan orally, by patients with renal failure on chronic hemodialysis, seems to be effective for reducing high cholesterol; improving anemia; and enhancing physical strength, appetite, and sleep (1942).

POSSIBLY INEFFECTIVE

Weight loss. Taking chitosan orally, without a reduction in food intake, doesn't seem to cause weight loss in healthy people (3243,3244,9986). It doesn't seem to have any effect on fecal fat excretion (9987,10020). Some studies suggest that chitosan can help reduce weight when used in combination with a 1000 to 1200 calorie per day diet; but these studies have methodological flaws and are unreliable (9610,10022,10023,10024,10025).

INSUFFICIENT RELIABLE EVIDENCE to RATE

Crohn's disease. Preliminary clinical research suggests a combination of chitosan and ascorbic acid taken orally might help Crohn's disease. This combination seems to increase fecal excretion of fat, which might decrease intestinal inflammation (9609).
Hypercholesterolemia. The effect of chitosan on cholesterol is controversial. Some studies show a modest decrease in cholesterol, while others show no effect (1942,3243,3244,9986,11307).
More evidence is needed to rate chitosan for these uses.

Mechanism of Action

Chitosan is the N-deacetylated form of chitin that is extracted from the shells of crustaceans (9987). It is a polysaccharide containing copolymers of glucosamine and N-acetylglucosamine (10021). Reported hemostatic and wound-healing activity is believed to be due to an enhancement of macrophages, fibroblasts, and polymorphonuclear leukocytes; this appears to be independent of the classical coagulation cascade (1943,9608). Chitosan ascorbate acts as a surgical cement in treatment of periodontitis, protecting periodontal pockets from oxygen and allowing for proliferation of periodontal tissues (1945).
For weight loss chitosan is promoted as a fat blocker, similar to orlistat (Xenical). When taken orally, chitosan is positively charged. In theory, it binds to negatively charged dietary fat in the intestine, decreasing absorption. However, studies in healthy humans suggest chitosan doesn't affect fat excretion (9987,10020). In patients with Crohn's disease, chitosan seems to increase fat excretion when combined with ascorbic acid (9609). For reduction of cholesterol, some evidence suggests that positively charged chitosan might bind to negatively charged bile acids, thus lowering cholesterol levels (10743). However, the effect of chitosan on cholesterol in humans is variable (1942,3243,3244,9986).
Scientists are interested in the potential for chitosan to enhance absorption of drugs, such as peptides, that normally can't cross the intestinal mucosa. In laboratory research, chitosan appears to increase permeation and intestinal absorption of hydrophilic macromolecules, such as low molecular weight heparin (10021).

Adverse Reactions
People with shellfish allergies should use chitosan with caution (9987).

Interactions with Herbs & Other Dietary Supplements
None known.

Interactions with Drugs
None known.

Interactions with Foods
None known.

Interactions with Lab Tests
CHOLESTEROL: Chitosan may reduce serum cholesterol levels, and test results in patients with renal failure on chronic hemodialysis (1942).
HEMOGLOBIN: Chitosan may increase serum hemoglobin levels, and test results in patients with renal failure on chronic hemodialysis (1942).
UREA/CREATININE: Chitosan may reduce blood urea and creatinine levels, and test results in patients with renal failure on chronic hemodialysis (1942).

Interactions with Diseases or Conditions
RENAL FAILURE: Chitosan may reduce serum cholesterol, urea, and creatinine levels; and increase hemoglobin levels in patients on chronic hemodialysis (1942).

Dosage and Administration
ORAL: For treating renal failure with chronic hemodialysis, 1.35 grams has been used three times daily (1942).
TOPICAL: No typical dosage.

Comments
Chitosan is a mucopolysaccharide component of crab, lobster, shrimp, and other marine organism exoskeletons.

CHIVE

Also Known As
Chives, Cives.

Scientific Names
Allium schoenoprasum, synonym Allium sibiricum.
Family: Liliaceae or Alliaceae.

People Use This For
Orally, chive is used to expel parasitic worms.
In foods, chives are used commonly as a food flavoring agent.

Safety
LIKELY SAFE ...when used orally in amounts commonly found in food amounts. Chives have Generally Recognized As Safe (GRAS) status in the US (4912).
POSSIBLY SAFE ...when used orally in medicinal amounts (12).
PREGNANCY AND LACTATION: There is insufficient reliable information about the safety of medicinal amounts of chive during pregnancy and breast-feeding; avoid using.

Effectiveness
There is insufficient reliable information available about the effectiveness of chive.

Mechanism of Action
The applicable parts of chive are the above ground parts. There is insufficient reliable information available about the possible mechanism of action and active ingredients.

Adverse Reactions
Orally, intake of large quantities of chives can lead to dyspepsia (18).

Interactions with Herbs & Other Dietary Supplements
None known.

Interactions with Drugs
None known.

Interactions with Foods
None known.

Interactions with Lab Tests
None known.

Interactions with Diseases or Conditions
None known.

Dosage and Administration
No typical dosage.

CHLORELLA

Also Known As
Bulgarian Chlorella, Bulgarian Green Algae, Freshwater Green Algae, Freshwater Seaweed, Green Alga, Green Algae, Seaweed.

Scientific Names
Chlorella pyrenoidosa; Chlorella vulgaris; other Chlorella species.

People Use This For
Orally, chlorella is used as a food supplement and source of nutrients, including protein, nucleic acids, fiber, vitamins, and minerals. Chlorella is also used orally for cancer prevention, stimulating the immune system, improving response to flu vaccine, increasing white blood cell counts (e.g., in people with HIV infection or cancer), preventing colds, to protect the body from the effects of radiation (e.g., during cancer therapy), to protect the body from toxic metals such as lead and mercury, and to slow aging. It is also used orally to increase beneficial flora in the gastrointestinal tract in order to improve digestion, and to help treat ulcers, colitis, Crohn's disease, and diverticulosis. Chlorella is also promoted for the prevention of stress-induced ulcers; treatment of constipation, bad breath, and hypertension; as an antioxidant; to reduce serum cholesterol; to increase energy; to detoxify the body; and as a source of magnesium to promote mental health, relieve premenstrual syndrome (PMS), and reduce asthma attacks. It is also used orally for fibromyalgia.
Topically, chlorella is used for treating ulcers, postirradiation dermatitis, vulval leukoplakias, and trichomoniasis.

Safety
POSSIBLY SAFE ...when used orally and appropriately short-term. Chlorella appears to be safe for up to 2 months (5890,10388).
There is insufficient reliable information about the safety of chlorella for its other uses.
PREGNANCY AND LACTATION: Insufficient reliable information available; avoid using.

Effectiveness
INSUFFICIENT RELIABLE EVIDENCE to RATE

Fibromyalgia. Preliminary clinical research shows subjective improvements in general symptom and pain scores in people with fibromyalgia taking chlorella tablets plus a liquid extract containing malic acid daily for two months (5890).

Glioma. Early research suggests chlorella tablets plus chlorella liquid extract might help people with glioma better tolerate chemotherapy and radiotherapy, possibly by improving immune system function; however, there appears to be no effect on tumor progression or survival (6804).

More evidence is needed to rate chlorella for these uses.

Mechanism of Action
Chlorella is a single-celled, freshwater green alga, also referred to as seaweed (5850). The whole plant is processed for medicinal use and is a rich source of chlorophyll. The cell wall must be broken down before it can be digested by humans (5890). Chlorella contains significant amounts of protein, lipid, carbohydrates, fiber, nucleic acids, vitamins, and minerals (5890). There is some evidence that consuming chlorella can increase serum vitamin B12 levels (5848).

However, it has been suggested that the vitamin B12 found in chlorella might be in an inactive form which can raise serum levels without contributing biological activity (5849).
In vitro and animal research indicates that substances in chlorella might have antitumor, antibacterial, antifungal, and antiviral activities (5850,5891,5892,10388).
Chlorella might stimulate the immune system by increasing the number and activity of macrophages and polymorphonuclear leukocytes. It might also stimulate interleukin production (10388). A polysaccharide from the cell wall of chlorella might also induce production of interferon (6804). However, chlorella doesn't seem to affect antibody response to influenza vaccine in humans (10388). The photosensitizing components in chlorella have been identified as pheophorbides (5847).

Adverse Reactions

Orally, chlorella can cause diarrhea, abdominal cramping, flatus, and nausea, especially during the first week of treatment (5890,6804). It can also cause fatigue (10388). Green discoloration of the feces has also been reported, presumably due to the chlorophyll content of chlorella (6804). Allergic reactions, including asthma and anaphylaxis, have been reported in people taking chlorella, and in those preparing chlorella tablets (3900,5847). Photosensitivity reactions have also occurred following ingestion of chlorella (3900,5852). Rarely, chlorella and other algae causes infections in humans (11011).

Interactions with Herbs & Other Dietary Supplements

None known.

Interactions with Drugs

WARFARIN (Coumadin): Chlorella contains significant amounts of vitamin K, which may inhibit the anticoagulant activity of warfarin (Coumadin) and related drugs (3900).

Interactions with Foods

None known.

Interactions with Lab Tests

None known.

Interactions with Diseases or Conditions

ALLERGIES, INCLUDING IODINE SENSITIVITY: Chlorella has been associated with significant allergic reactions (5847), and is also reported to contain iodine (10275).
IMMUNODEFICIENCY: Chlorella preparations might cause pathogenic colonization, particularly in patients who are immunocompromised (11011). Use with caution in these patients.

Dosage and Administration

ORAL: For fibromyalgia, doses of 10 gram tablets plus 100 mL liquid extract (Wakasa Gold) daily have been used (5890). For improving tolerability of chemotherapy and radiotherapy in people with brain tumors, chlorella tablets, up to 20 grams daily, plus 150 mL liquid extract daily have been used (6804).
TOPICAL: No typical dosage.

Comments

Since chlorella is a naturally occurring organism, its content can vary with growing, harvesting, and processing conditions. By varying the cultivation conditions, it has been reported that a dried preparation of chlorella can contain from 7-88% protein, 6-38% carbohydrate, and 7-75% fat (5851). Most chlorella sold in the United States is cultivated in Japan or Taiwan (3900). Processing of the chlorella cultures includes destroying the cell walls, dehydration and sterilization (5851). Commercially available products include tablets and liquid extracts. The latter contain "chlorella growth factor", described as a water soluble extract of chlorella, containing amino acids, peptides, proteins, vitamins, sugars, and nucleic acids (5890).

CHLOROPHYLL

Also Known As

None.
CAUTION: See separate listing for Chlorophyllin.

Scientific Names

Chlorophyll a; Chlorophyll b; Chlorophyll c; Chlorophyll d.

People Use This For
Orally, chlorophyll is used for reducing colostomy odor, bad breath, constipation, detoxification, and wound healing. Intravenously, chlorophyll is used for treating chronic relapsing pancreatitis.

Safety
LIKELY SAFE ...when used orally (1324).
POSSIBLY SAFE ...when used intravenously (1324).
PREGNANCY AND LACTATION: POSSIBLY SAFE ...when used orally. There is insufficient reliable information available about the safety of the intravenous use of chlorophyll during pregnancy and lactation.

Effectiveness
POSSIBLY EFFECTIVE

Pancreatitis. Administering chlorophyll intravenously seems to help reduce pain and other symptoms in patients with chronic relapsing pancreatitis (1324).

POSSIBLY INEFFECTIVE

Colostomy odor. Taking chlorophyll orally doesn't seem to reduce colostomy odor (1322).

There is insufficient reliable information available about the effectiveness of chlorophyll for its other uses.

Mechanism of Action
Chlorophyll contains components that are activated by light. It appears that chlorophyll can cause a photosensitization when it is taken internally (1326). Derivatives of chlorophyll which have been extracted from silkworm droppings seem to have a cytotoxic effect on certain cancer cells (1314,1315). Certain carotenoids such as beta-carotene and canthaxanthin seem to prevent or lessen the photosensitivity that results from taking chlorophyll (1326).

Adverse Reactions
None reported.

Interactions with Herbs & Other Dietary Supplements
CAROTENOIDS (Beta-carotene, Canthaxanthin): Theoretically, carotenoids may prevent or lessen chlorophyll-induced photosensitivity (1326).

Interactions with Drugs
PHOTOSENSITIZING DRUGS: Theoretically, concomitant use may exacerbate effects (1326).

Interactions with Foods
None known.

Interactions with Lab Tests
None known.

Interactions with Diseases or Conditions
None known.

Dosage and Administration
ORAL: No typical dosage.
INTRAVENOUS: For pancreatitis; infusion of 5-20 mg water soluble chlorophyll-a per day for 1-2 weeks, followed by intermittent administration has been used (1324).

Comments
Avoid confusion with chlorophyllin, a semisynthetic derivative of chlorophyll. Commercial sources of chlorophyll include alfalfa (Medicago sativa) and silk worm droppings (11). Chlorophyll is a group of related green pigments found in photosynthetic organisms including Chlorophyll a (found in higher plants, red and green algae), Chlorophyll b (found in higher plants), Chlorophyll c (found in brown algae, diatoms, flagellates), and Chlorophyll d (found in red algae).

CHLOROPHYLLIN

Also Known As
None.
CAUTION: See separate listing for Chlorophyll.

Scientific Names
Chlorophyllin.

People Use This For
Orally, chlorophyllin is used for controlling body, fecal, and urine odors, and for treating constipation and flatulence.

Safety
POSSIBLY SAFE ...when used orally (1321,1323).
PREGNANCY AND LACTATION: Insufficient reliable information available; avoid using.

Effectiveness
POSSIBLY INEFFECTIVE

Urinary odor. Taking chlorophyllin orally doesn't seem to be effective for controlling urinary odor in incontinent geriatric patients with indwelling catheters (1323).

INSUFFICIENT RELIABLE EVIDENCE to RATE

Body and fecal odor. Preliminary evidence suggests that taking chlorophyllin orally might help reduce body and fecal odors in geriatric patients (1321).

Constipation. Preliminary evidence suggests that taking chlorophyllin orally might reduce constipation in geriatric patients (1321).

Flatulence. Preliminary evidence suggests that taking chlorophyllin orally might reduce flatulence in geriatric patients (1321).

More evidence is needed to rate chlorophyllin for these uses.

Mechanism of Action
Chlorophyllin has antimutagenic activity in human lymphocytes (in vitro) (1312). Mechanisms may include reduced carcinogen DNA-binding (in fish) (1309), reduced chromosome damage (in vitro) (1311), and reduced carcinogen-induced cell transformation (in vitro) (1307). Bacteriologic studies failed to confirm reports of antibacterial properties for chlorophyllin (1321).

Adverse Reactions
None reported.

Interactions with Herbs & Other Dietary Supplements
None known.

Interactions with Drugs
None known.

Interactions with Foods
None known.

Interactions with Lab Tests
None known.

Interactions with Diseases or Conditions
None known.

Dosage and Administration
ORAL: Typically, 100 mg per day is used for controlling urinary odor in incontinent geriatric patients with indwelling catheters (1323).

Comments
Avoid confusion with Chlorophyll.

CHOLINE

Also Known As

Choline Bitartrate, Choline Chloride, Intrachol, Lipotropic Factor, Methylated Phosphatidylethanolamine.
CAUTION: See separate listings for Alpha-GPC, Lecithin, and Phosphatidylcholine.

Scientific Names

Trimethylethanolamine; (beta-hydroxyethyl) trimethylammonium hydroxide.

People Use This For

Orally, choline is used for liver disease including chronic hepatitis and cirrhosis, hypercholesterolemia, depression, memory loss, Alzheimer's disease and dementia, and schizophrenia. It is also used orally for body building, delaying fatigue in endurance sports, Huntington's chorea, Tourette's disease, cerebellar ataxia, complex partial seizures, asthma, and as a supplement in infant formulas.
Intravenously, choline has orphan drug status for TPN-associated hepatic steatosis.

Safety

LIKELY SAFE ...when used orally and appropriately (3094). ...when used intravenously and appropriately (5173,5174).
POSSIBLY UNSAFE ...when used orally in excessive doses. High doses can increase the risk of adverse effects. Tell patients not to exceed 3.5 grams per day for adults over age 18 (3094).
CHILDREN: LIKELY SAFE ...when used orally and appropriately (3094). POSSIBLY UNSAFE ...when used orally in excessive doses. High doses can increase the risk of adverse effects. Tell patients not to exceed 1 gram daily for children 1-8 years of age, 2 grams daily for children 9-13 years of age, and 3 grams daily for children 14-18 years of age (3094).
PREGNANCY AND LACTATION: LIKELY SAFE ...when used orally and appropriately. Doses up to 3 grams daily for pregnant and lactating women up to 18 years of age, and 3.5 grams daily for women 19 years and older are not likely to cause adverse effects (3094). There is insufficient reliable information about the safety of choline used in pregnant or lactating women.

Effectiveness

LIKELY EFFECTIVE

Hepatic steatosis. Administering choline intravenously is effective for treating total parenteral nutrition-associated hepatic steatosis in patients with choline deficiency (5163,5174).

POSSIBLY EFFECTIVE

Asthma. Taking choline orally seems to decrease the severity of symptoms, number of symptomatic days (5165), and the need to use bronchodilators (5166) in patients with asthma. There is some evidence that higher doses of 3 grams daily might be more effective than lower doses of 1.5 grams daily (5165).

POSSIBLY INEFFECTIVE

Alzheimer's disease. Taking choline orally does not reduce symptoms of Alzheimer's disease (5170).

Athletic performance. Taking choline orally doesn't seem to be effective for delaying fatigue in endurance sports (5164).

Cerebellar ataxia. Taking choline orally doesn't seem to reduce cerebellar ataxia (5161,5173).

LIKELY INEFFECTIVE

Age-related memory impairment. Taking choline orally does not improve memory in elderly people with memory loss (5170).

Schizophrenia. Taking choline orally does not reduce symptoms of schizophrenia (5171,5172).

INSUFFICIENT RELIABLE EVIDENCE to RATE

Complex partial seizures. There is anecdotal evidence that high doses of choline, 12-16 grams daily, might be helpful for some patients with complex partial seizures (5162). More evidence is needed to rate choline for this use.

Mechanism of Action

Choline has traditionally been considered a B vitamin. However, this is controversial because choline can be synthesized by the human body (5139). Choline is produced in the liver via the methylation of phosphatidylethanolamine. S-adenosylmethionine is the methyl donor for this reaction (1949). Choline is also readily available in the typical diet (5139). Foods that supply large amounts of choline are liver, muscle meats, fish, nuts, beans, peas, eggs, and others. A typical diet provides 200-600 mg daily. Deficiency of choline is uncommon except in people receiving long-term total parenteral nutrition (TPN) (5139,5174). Choline deficiency related to long-term TPN use can result in fatty liver and liver damage. Adding choline to the TPN solution usually resolves liver abnormalities (1949). This indicates that dietary choline is required in addition to the choline normally synthesized by the body (5139,5174). Human breast milk contains choline. Choline is added to infant formulas from cow milk and soy (3094). Choline, or its metabolites, are needed for the synthesis of cell membrane phospholipids and as methyl donors for the synthesis of other compounds (1949). For example, the choline metabolite betaine is a methyl donor during the methylation of homocysteine to form methionine (1949). Choline concentrates in nervous tissue (272). There is preliminary evidence that supplemental choline during pregnancy and lactation probably affects the birth, death, and migration of cells in the hippocampus during fetal brain development and possibly changes the distribution and morphology of neurons responsible for memory function in the brain (1949).

Some researchers are interested in choline for Alzheimer's disease because it is a precursor to acetylcholine. However, there is evidence that oral choline does not affect concentrations of choline metabolites such as acetylcholine in the brain. This might be the reason oral choline does not seem to be effective for neurodegenerative disorders of cholinergic transmission (5175). In asthma, choline is thought to have anti-inflammatory effects by lowering lipophosphatidylcholine levels (5165). Some researchers speculate that choline might also have a role in cancer prevention (5178,5179,5180). In animal models, long-term withdrawal of choline from the diet can cause hepatocarcinoma (5178,5180).

Adverse Reactions

Orally, adverse reactions can include sweating, a fishy body odor, gastrointestinal distress, and vomiting (5160,5163). Large doses can cause diarrhea (272).

Interactions with Herbs & Other Dietary Supplements

None known.

Interactions with Drugs

None known.

Interactions with Foods

None known.

Interactions with Lab Tests

None known.

Interactions with Diseases or Conditions

None known.

Dosage and Administration

ORAL: For asthma, 500-1000 mg three times daily has been used (5165,5166). An average diet supplies 200-600 mg of choline daily (272). Adequate Intake (AI), as established by the Food and Nutrition Board of the National Institute of Medicine, for adults is 550 mg per day for males and lactating women; females, 425 mg per day; pregnant females, 450 mg per day (3094). For children 1-3 years the AI is 200 mg per day; 4-8 years, 250 mg per day; 9-13 years, 375 mg per day (3094); for infants less than 6 months, 125 mg per day; infants 7-12 months, 150 mg per day (3094). Daily Upper Intake Levels (UL, the highest level of intake that is likely to pose no risk of adverse effects) for choline are 1 gram daily for children 1-8 years, 2 grams for children 9-13 years, 3 grams for children 14-18 years, and 3.5 grams for adults over 18 years of age (3094).

Comments

Many people think choline, phosphatidylcholine, and lecithin are synonymous. Choline is a component of phosphatidylcholine, which is a component of lecithin. Although closely related, these terms are not synonymous. See separate listings for Phosphatidylcholine and Lecithin.

CHONDROITIN SULFATE

Also Known As

CDS, Chondroitin, Chondroitin Polysulfate, Chondroitin Sulfates, Chondroitin Sulfate B, Chondroitin Sulfate C, Chondroitin Sulphate A Sodium, CS, CPS, CSA, CSC, GAG, Galactosaminoglucuronoglycan Sulfate.

Scientific Names

Chondroitin 4-sulfate; chondroitin 4- and 6-sulfate.

People Use This For

Orally, chondroitin sulfate is used for osteoarthritis. Chondroitin sulfate is frequently used in combination with other products, including manganese ascorbate, glucosamine sulfate, glucosamine hydrochloride, or N-acetyl glucosamine for osteoarthritis. Chondroitin sulfate is also used orally for ischemic heart disease, osteoporosis, and hyperlipidemia. Chondroitin is also used in a complex with iron for treating iron-deficiency anemia.

Intramuscularly, chondroitin sulfate is used for osteoarthritis.

Topically, chondroitin sulfate is used for keratoconjunctivitis sicca (dry eyes), as a viscoelastic agent in cataract surgery, and as a medium for preservation of corneas used for transplantation. Chondroitin sulfate is also used topically in combination with other products for osteoarthritis.

Safety

LIKELY SAFE ...when used orally and appropriately. Chondroitin sulfate has been used safely in studies lasting from 2 months to 6 years (1342,1955,1970,1971,1972,2533). However, since chondroitin is often derived from bovine cartilage there is some concern about contamination with diseased animal parts (1825). So far, there are no reports of disease transmission to humans due to use of contaminated chondroitin preparations. ...when used topically and appropriately as an ophthalmic product, which is an FDA-approved prescription-only product that also contains sodium hyaluronate (Viscoat).

POSSIBLY SAFE ...when used intramuscularly (10149). ...when used topically and appropriately short term. Chondroitin in combination with glucosamine, shark cartilage, and camphor appears to be safe when applied topically on an as-needed basis for up to eight weeks (10327).

PREGNANCY AND LACTATION: Insufficient reliable information available; avoid using.

Effectiveness

LIKELY EFFECTIVE

Eye surgery. Applying chondroitin sulfate topically, in combination with sodium hyaluronate, to the eye is effective as a surgical aid in cataract extraction or lens implantation. A combination product containing chondroitin sulfate and sodium hyaluronate (Viscoat) is an FDA-approved, prescription ophthalmic product (266).

Osteoarthritis. Taking chondroitin sulfate orally seems to relieve symptoms of osteoarthritis. Treatment with chondroitin sulfate for 2-4 months is usually required before significant improvement is experienced (1342). Chondroitin doesn't seem to prevent osteoarthritis, but might help slow progression of established disease. Adding chondroitin sulfate to conventional analgesics or nonsteroidal anti-inflammatory drugs (NSAIDs) is significantly more effective than analgesics or NSAIDs alone for reducing pain and improving functionality indices in patients with osteoarthritis of the hip and knee. Some evidence suggests that chondroitin may allow dosage lowering or discontinuation of NSAIDs after 6 to 8 weeks (322,323,324,1342,1970,1971,1972,2533,4237,7256,10149,10150,10310).

Intermittent treatment with chondroitin might also be effective. Patients who take chondroitin sulfate 800 mg/day for 3 months followed by 3 months of no treatment and then again for 3 months seem to have significantly reduced symptoms. Chondroitin dosed intermittently also seems to prevent joint space narrowing compared to placebo. This suggests that intermittent dosing can also slow disease progression (12148).

Chondroitin sulfate combined with glucosamine HCl and manganese ascorbate (Cosamin-DS) is also effective, but it is not known if this combination is more effective than the individual components alone (4237). A topical preparation of chondroitin sulfate in combination with glucosamine sulfate, shark cartilage, and camphor also seems to reduce arthritis symptoms. But any symptom relief is most likely due to the counterirritant effect of camphor and not the other ingredients (10327). There's no research showing that chondroitin is absorbed topically. Don't recommend topical chondroitin products.

POSSIBLY EFFECTIVE

Dry eyes. Administering chondroitin sulfate as an ophthalmic preparation seems to lessen dry eyes (1974).

INSUFFICIENT RELIABLE EVIDENCE to RATE

Myocardial infarction (MI). There is some preliminary evidence that oral chondroitin sulfate might lower the risk of MI; or reduce the recurrence of MI in people who have previously had a MI or who have unstable angina (1955,8126). More evidence is needed to rate chondroitin sulfate for this use.

Mechanism of Action

Chondroitin sulfate belongs to a class of very large molecules called glucosaminoglycans (GAGs), which are made up of glucuronic acid and galactosamine. Chondroitin is manufactured from natural sources, such as shark and bovine cartilage. Pure chondroitin is a relatively large molecule, weighing about 16,900 daltons. The species or tissue of origin, and the extraction method used, can affect the size of the molecule (8128). People use chondroitin for osteoarthritis because it is endogenously found in cartilaginous tissues of most mammals and serves as a substrate for the formation of the joint matrix structure (1972,1973,6738). There is some evidence that chondroitin sulfate protects cartilage against degradation by inhibiting the action of the enzyme leukocyte elastase, by decreasing the migration of polymorphonuclear leukocytes, and by increasing the synthesis of proteoglycans and hyaluronic acid (6738,7256). Some researchers think chondroitin might have cardiovascular applications due to potential antiatherogenic properties; laboratory studies suggest that chondroitin might protect against atherosclerosis (1955,8125).

Chondroitin might be useful in cancer monitoring. There is evidence that measurements of endogenous chondroitin sulfate in the peritumoral stromal tissue of the prostate can be a useful biomarker in the disease progression of prostate cancer. The concentration of chondroitin sulfate is increased in the prostate tissue of men with prostate cancer when compared to tissue samples of cancer-free men. When used with the Gleason score and the prostate-specific antigen (PSA) level, the peritumoral chondroitin sulfate measurement can allow practitioners to more accurately assess the progression of prostate cancer (8962).

Preliminary evidence suggests that chondroitin or other GAGs might prevent calcium oxalate crystallization in the urinary tract (8127). Since chondroitin is a minor component, approximately 4%, of the low molecular weight heparinoid mixture, danaparoid (Orgaran), some concern has been expressed about possible anticoagulant activity of

chondroitin sulfate. However, significant hematological changes have not been found in studies (760).
Early evidence suggesting that chondroitin is not absorbed orally (4202,10315) has been refuted by more recent studies. Studies show that people absorb 8-18% of orally administered chondroitin (3242,4203,4205,4237). Lower molecular weight derivatives of chondroitin formed in the gastrointestinal tract are more readily absorbed and might also contribute to the pharmacological activity of orally administered chondroitin (3242).
Early evidence suggesting chondroitin might show promise as an HIV therapy adjunct has been refuted. More recent laboratory information suggests that chondroitin does not have anti-HIV activity (1263,1335,8662). However, preliminary research suggests that the chemically oversulfated form of chondroitin has activity against HIV, herpes simplex virus, and human cytomegalovirus (10616).

Adverse Reactions

Orally, chondroitin sulfate is usually well-tolerated. Some patients can have epigastric pain and nausea. Diarrhea, constipation, eyelid edema, lower limb edema, alopecia, and extrasystoles have also been reported in clinical trials (322,323,324,1342,1970,1971,1972,2533,4237,7256,10149,10150,10310), but it's not known if chondroitin sulfate is the cause of these adverse events.
Concern has been expressed about possible anticoagulant activity of chondroitin sulfate. However, hematological changes have not occurred in patients taking chondroitin sulfate in clinical trials (760).
Since chondroitin is usually produced from bovine cartilage, typically the trachea, there is some concern about the potential risk of contamination with diseased animals and transmission of bovine spongiform encephalopathy (BSE, mad cow disease) and other diseases. Although bovine trachea tissue does not seem to carry a high risk of BSE disease infectivity, in some cases manufacturing methods might lead to contamination with other diseased animal tissues. So far there are no reports of BSE or other disease transmission to humans from dietary supplements containing animal materials and the risk of potential disease transmission is thought to be low.

Interactions with Herbs & Other Dietary Supplements

None known.

Interactions with Drugs

WARFARIN (Coumadin): There is concern that high-dose chondroitin sulfate (2400 mg per day) combined with high-dose glucosamine (3000 mg per day) may enhance the effects of warfarin (Coumadin) as measured by the INR (11389). Chondroitin is a small component of a heparinoid and might have weak anticoagulant activity. Glucosamine is also a small component of heparin, but it does not seem to have anticoagulant activity. Interactions with warfarin have not been reported at recommended dosages of chondroitin or glucosamine.

Interactions with Foods

None known.

Interactions with Lab Tests

ANTI-FACTOR Xa: Theoretically, because chondroitin is a component of danaparoid, chondroitin sulfate administered by injection might increase the anti-factor Xa level and test results. No significant hematological changes were noted in a group of patients during six months of oral chondroitin therapy (760).
INTERNATIONAL NORMALIZED RATIO (INR), PROTHROMBIN TIME (PT): High dose chondroitin sulfate (2400 mg per day), combined with high dose glucosamine (3000 mg per day), may increase the INR in patients anticoagulated with warfarin (Coumadin). There is one case report of an increased INR associated with concomitant use of warfarin a glucosamine-chondroitin supplement that was taken above recommended dosages (11389).

Interactions with Diseases or Conditions

ASTHMA: Chondroitin might exacerbate asthma possibly by an unidentified allergic mechanism. Use chondroitin cautiously in patients with asthma (10002).
COAGULATION DISORDERS: Theoretically, parenterally administered chondroitin sulfate might affect coagulation and increase the risk of bleeding when used in patients with clotting disorders; avoid use.
PROSTATE CANCER: Preliminary clinical research suggests that chondroitin may cause the spread or recurrence of prostate cancer (8962). The chondroitin sulfate proteoglycan, versican, seems to facilitate invasion of cancer cells into the prostate stroma (11761). This effect has not been shown with supplemental chondroitin sulfate. But until more is known, advise men with prostate cancer or those at increased risk for prostate cancer to avoid chondroitin.

Dosage and Administration

ORAL: For osteoarthritis, the typical dose of chondroitin sulfate is 200-400 mg two to three times daily (1970,1971,1972,4237,10149) or 1000-1200 mg as a single daily dose (1971,7256). Intermittent dosing also seems to be effective. One study has used 800 mg/day for 3 months followed by 3 months of no treatment, and then 3 months of treatment again (12148).
For prevention of recurrent myocardial infarction (MI), 10 grams daily in 3 divided doses for 3 months, followed by 1.5 grams in 3 divided doses as maintenance therapy has been used (1955).

TOPICAL: For osteoarthritis, topical administration of a cream containing 50 mg/g of chondroitin sulfate, 30 mg/g of glucosamine sulfate, 140 mg/g of shark cartilage, and 32 mg/g of camphor has been used as needed for sore joints for up to 8 weeks (10327).
INTRAMUSCULAR: For osteoarthritis, chondroitin polysulfate 50 mg twice weekly for 8 weeks every 4 months has been used (10149). Parenteral chondroitin sulfate products are not available in the US.

Comments

Although chondroitin sulfate and glucosamine sulfate are frequently marketed together in combination products (760), there is no evidence that the combination has greater benefit than either product alone. There is great variability among chondroitin and chondroitin plus glucosamine products. Actual content versus label claim varies from 0 to 115%. Low-cost chondroitin products (less than $1 per 1200 mg chondroitin) seem to contain little chondroitin, but some higher-priced products may also contain less chondroitin than claimed (8128).
The National Institutes of Health (NIH) is sponsoring a clinical trial of chondroitin sulfate and glucosamine sulfate. The 24-week, parallel group, double-blind RCT includes five separate treatment arms, in which patients will ingest: placebo, glucosamine sulfate 500 mg three times per day, chondroitin 400 mg three times per day, a combination of glucosamine sulfate and chondroitin, or celecoxib (Celebrex) (11012).
Tell patients to look out for chondroitin plus glucosamine combination products that also contain manganese (e.g., CosaminDS). Remind patients to adhere to product directions. When taken at doses slightly higher than the recommended dose, these products can sometimes supply greater than the tolerable upper limit (UL) for manganese of 11 mg per day. Ingestion of more than 11 mg per day of manganese might cause significant central nervous system toxicity (7135).

CHROMIUM

Also Known As

Chromic Chloride, Chromium Acetate, Chromium Chloride, Chromium Nicotinate, Chromium Picolinate, Chromium Polynicotinate, Chromium Trichloride, Chromium Tripicolinate, Chromium III, Chromium III Picolinate, Chromium 3+, Cr III, Cr3+, Glucose Tolerance Factor, Glucose Tolerance Factor-Cr, GTF, GTF-Cr, GTF Cr, Trivalent Chromium.

Scientific Names

Chromium; Cr; atomic number 24.

People Use This For

Orally, chromium is used for improving glycemic control in type 1 and 2 diabetes, corticosteroid-induced hyperglycemia and reactive hypoglycemia, for hypercholesterolemia, and for increasing high-density lipoprotein (HDL) cholesterol levels in patients taking beta-blockers. It is also used orally for weight loss, to increase muscle mass and fat-free mass, and decrease body fat. Chromium is also used orally to enhance athletic performance, to increase energy and vigor, and to treat dysthymic disorder (a mild form of depression) and atypical depression.
Intravenously, chromium is used as a supplement in total parenteral nutrition (TPN).

Safety

LIKELY SAFE ...when used orally and appropriately. Chromium is safe in amounts found in foods or supplemental amounts not exceeding adequate intake (AI) levels. The AI for chromium is different based on gender and age. For men aged 14 to 50, the AI is 35 mcg per day. For men aged 51 and older, the AI is 30 mcg. For women aged 19 to 50 years, the AI is 25 mcg per day. For women aged 51 and older, the AI is 20 mcg (7135).
POSSIBLY SAFE ...when used orally and appropriately, short-term in amounts greater than adequate intake (AI) levels. Short-term, chromium picolinate has been safely used in doses up to 1000 mcg per day (1934,6867,7135,7137); however, there is insufficient information to establish safe and tolerable upper intake levels (7135). There is also some concern that long-term supplemental use may not be safe due to potential mutagenic effects (6863,6869). Until more is known, tell patients not to take chromium supplements long-term.
CHILDREN: LIKELY SAFE ...when used orally and appropriately. Chromium is safe in amounts not exceeding the adequate intake (AI) levels (7135). For infants 0 to 6 months, the AI is 0.2 mcg per day; 7 to 12 months, 5.5 mcg. For children 1 to 3 years, the AI is 11 mcg; 4 to 8 years, 15 mcg. For boys 9 to 13 years, the AI is 25 mcg. For girls 9 to 13 years, the AI is 21 mcg; 14 to 18 years, 24 mcg. There is insufficient reliable information available about the safety of chromium in higher amounts when used in children.
PREGNANCY: LIKELY SAFE ...when used orally and appropriately. Chromium is safe in amounts not exceeding adequate intake (AI) levels. The AI for pregnant women aged 14 to 18 years is 29 mcg per day. For pregnant women aged 19 to 50 years, it is 30 mcg per day (7135). POSSIBLY SAFE ...when used orally in amounts exceeding the adequate intake (AI) levels. There is some evidence that pregnant patients with gestational diabetes can safely use chromium in doses of 4-8 mcg per kilogram (1953); however, patients should not take chromium supplements during pregnancy without medical supervision.

LACTATION: LIKELY SAFE ...when used orally and appropriately. Chromium is safe in amounts not exceeding adequate intake (AI) levels. The AI for lactating women aged 14 to 18 years is 44 mcg per day. For lactating women aged 19 to 50 years it is 45 mcg per day (7135). Chromium supplements do not seem to increase normal chromium concentration in human breast milk (1937). There is insufficient reliable information available about the safety of chromium in higher amounts when used in breast-feeding women.

Effectiveness

POSSIBLY EFFECTIVE

Beta blocker-induced dyslipidemia. Taking chromium 600 mcg daily for 2 months seems to increase high-density lipoprotein (HDL) levels by 16% in men who take beta-blockers (5040).

Diabetes. There is some evidence that taking chromium picolinate orally can decrease fasting blood glucose and insulin levels, and decrease glycosylated hemoglobin (HbA1c) in people with type 2 diabetes (6862,6867,7137). Higher doses might be more effective and work more quickly. Taking 500 mcg twice daily significantly decreases HbA1c after 2 months of treatment. Taking 100 mcg twice daily can take up to 4 months to decrease HbA1c levels. Higher doses of 200 mcg three times daily or 500 mcg twice daily also seem to reduce triglyceride and total serum cholesterol levels after 2 to 4 months of treatment. This suggests that chromium might also be beneficial for patients with metabolic syndrome (syndrome X) (1934,6867). But there is speculation that chromium supplements might only help patients with low chromium levels. It doesn't seem to help all patients with type 2 diabetes (8927). It only seems to have a blood glucose-lowering effect in 40% to 80% of people with elevated blood glucose (6858). Chromium levels are sometimes below normal in patients with diabetes (7058). There is preliminary evidence that chromium picolinate might also have the same benefits in patients with type 1 diabetes (1935) and in patients who have diabetes secondary to corticosteroid use (5039).

There isn't enough evidence to recommend chromium for all diabetes patients. Consider trial use in interested patients to see if it helps. Use chromium picolinate preparations; chromium chloride may not be as effective (7060). Remind patients that chromium is not an alternative to conventional medicines and should not be used in place of conventional treatments.

Hypoglycemia. Taking chromium orally seems to help prevent reactive hypoglycemia. Treatment for 3 months with chromium chloride 200 mg daily seems to improve symptoms and increase blood glucose levels in patients with reactive hypoglycemia following an oral glucose load (6859).

Obesity. Taking chromium picolinate orally might help with weight loss in obese people (body mass index 30 to 32). Studies have not consistently found benefit, but overall, research suggests chromium picolinate might produce modest weight loss, about a 1.1 kg greater weight loss than placebo over 72 to 90 days (6860,11962).

POSSIBLY INEFFECTIVE

Athletic conditioning. Taking chromium orally doesn't seem to enhance body building, strength or lean body mass. There is some evidence that suggests taking chromium can increase weight loss, body fat loss, and lean body mass in people taking chromium picolinate 200-400 mcg per day in conjunction with resistance training (6860,6861,6868). But the results of these studies are unreliable due to questionable methods (6861). More reliable studies show that adding chromium picolinate or chloride 177-200 mcg daily to a weight-training program has no additional beneficial effect on body composition (6861,6862).

INSUFFICIENT RELIABLE EVIDENCE to RATE

Atypical depression. Preliminary clinical research suggests chromium picolinate might help atypical depression (10309).

Dysthymia. There is some preliminary evidence that chromium might improve the response to antidepressants in people with dysthymic disorder (a mild form of depression). Chromium picolinate or chromium polynicotinate 200 mcg once or twice daily appears to improve mood in patients who have only a partial response to antidepressants such as sertraline or nortriptyline (2659).

More evidence is needed to rate chromium for these uses.

Mechanism of Action

Chromium is an essential trace element. The activity of chromium depends on its valance state. Metallic chromium, or chromium 0, has no activity. The other two common forms, chromium III (Cr III) and chromium VI (Cr VI), have different activities. Cr VI is typically used in chemical and welding industries and is carcinogenic to humans. Cr III is the form found in foods and supplements. Chromium is sometimes referred to as glucose tolerance factor (GTF), but GTF is actually a complex of molecules found in the body that includes chromium bound to single molecules of glycine, cysteine, glutamic acid, and two molecules of nicotinic acid. Chromium is thought to be the active component of the complex. Some dietary sources of chromium include canned foods (due to chromium leaching from the can), meats and animal fats, fish, brown sugar, coffee, tea, some spices, calf liver, whole wheat bread, rye bread, and brewer's yeast (7061).

Symptomatic chromium deficiency is rare. When it does occur, it is most often due to malnutrition, pregnancy, stress, or long-term use of chromium deficient total parenteral nutrition (TPN) (6863). Other people might also be at risk for low chromium levels. Although not yet confirmed, some researchers suspect that tissue levels of chromium might decline with age (6863). Some athletes might also be at risk for low chromium levels since strenuous aerobic exercise seems to increase urinary excretion of chromium (6860,6861). However, exercise-induced losses seem to be less in those who regularly exercise (6862). People doing strength training seem to have increased absorption of chromium (7136). It is difficult to measure chromium status to determine who might require supplementation. Blood chromium levels are not in equilibrium with chromium stores and, therefore, do not provide a good indicator of chromium status (6859). However, elevated blood chromium levels may indicate excessive chromium exposure (11786). Levels in the urine and hair do not reflect overall chromium status (6867). There is no reliable method available to diagnose chromium deficiency, other than observing outcome following supplementation in patients suspected of being deficient (3859,6869). Symptoms of chromium deficiency can include impaired insulin function and glucose tolerance, increased serum cholesterol and triglycerides, neuropathy, weight loss, decreased respiratory function, and nitrogen metabolism abnormalities (6863,6869,11786).

Discovery of the role of chromium in insulin function occurred when patients on long-term TPN, developed symptoms of diabetes that did not respond to insulin, but were reversed by chromium (6869). Because of the symptoms associated with chromium deficiency, researchers have speculated that chromium supplementation might be an effective treatment for diabetes and hypercholesterolemia. Chromium has a normal role in insulin function, so it might help patients with diabetes who are chromium deficient. There is some evidence that patients with diabetes might have lower than normal levels of chromium due to increased chromium excretion (6858). However, patients with diabetes also seem to have increased gastrointestinal absorption of chromium. It's also theorized that patients with diabetes may not be able to adequately convert chromium from the diet to a usable form in the body (6867). Chromium seems to be transported to insulin-sensitive cells by transferrin, in response to increases in plasma insulin levels (6869). It is suspected to potentiate insulin by increasing receptor numbers and affinity, and increasing insulin binding to cells (6859,6867). In animal models, a chromium-containing peptide called chromodulin has been identified, which potentiates the actions of insulin at its receptors, including activation of receptor tyrosine kinase activity (6869). In patients with diabetes, these actions seem to translate into decreased insulin resistance, improved glucose tolerance, and lower blood glucose levels (6862). Researchers are interested in chromium for treatment of obesity and metabolic syndrome (syndrome X) due to its potential effects on lipids and body composition.

Some research suggests that chromium might also sensitize insulin-sensitive glucoreceptors in the brain, resulting in appetite suppression, activation of the sympathetic nervous system and stimulation of thermogenesis, and down-regulation of insulin secretion (6170,6860). It is also theorized that chromium might enhance glucose utilization in the brain and stimulate norepinephrine release (2659). Preliminary clinical research suggests that chromium decreases endocrine responses to serotonin receptor stimulation, which could produce antidepressant activity (8929). Chromium is also hypothesized to increase muscle mass by increasing amino acid uptake into muscle cells via potentiation of insulin activity (6862).

Chromium supplements come in several salt forms. The most common are chromium picolinate, chromium nicotinate, and chromium chloride. Chromium picolinate is a complex of chromium and picolinic acid, which is a naturally occurring metabolic derivative of tryptophan. Adding the picolinate or nicotinate salt increases absorption, retention and accumulation of chromium compared to inorganic salts such as chromium chloride (6861,6864,9141). When ingested, most chromium is excreted unabsorbed in the feces. The small percentage that is absorbed, typically 0.4% to 2.5%, is rapidly excreted in the urine (7135). Once absorbed, chromium concentrates in the kidney, heart, liver, brain, muscle, spleen, testes, epididymis, and lungs (6863). Chromium picolinate seems to be handled differently in the body than dietary chromium (6869). There is some evidence that chromium picolinate can enter cells unchanged and then produce hydroxyl radicals when the chromium is released, which might cause DNA damage (1299,6869). This may be due to its higher solubility and lipophilicity compared with other chromium compounds (11786). The clinical significance of this potential harmful effect is not known.

Adverse Reactions

Orally, chromium in the trivalent form (Cr III) is generally well tolerated. However, some patients can experience cognitive, perceptual, and motor dysfunction at doses as low as 200-400 mcg per day of chromium picolinate (1935). Chromium picolinate has also been associated with weight gain in young women who do not exercise and in those on a weight-lifting program (1938). Some patients can also experience headaches, insomnia, sleep disturbances, irritability, and mood changes (6860). Acute chromium toxicity can cause vomiting, diarrhea, hemorrhage and blood loss into the gastrointestinal tract resulting in cardiogenic shock (11786).

Chronic use of chromium picolinate in higher doses might cause significant adverse effects. In some cases, doses of 600-2400 mcg per day can cause anemia, thrombocytopenia, hemolysis, hepatic dysfunction, and renal failure in some patients (554); however, it is not clear if chromium is responsible for these effects. For example, chromium picolinate has been associated with chronic interstitial nephritis in two case reports, but contradictory laboratory evidence shows that chromium does not seem to cause kidney tissue damage even after long-term, high dose exposure (7135). Toxic hepatitis has been reported in a patient taking 200 mcg chromium polynicotinate daily for 5 months (9141). Although there are reports of severe adverse events in people taking chromium supplements, in most instances it is unclear if chromium was actually responsible for the adverse event. Furthermore, there does not appear to be any dose-effect relationship for severe adverse effects. A sports supplement containing caffeine, ephedrine, and chromium picolinate (Hydroxycut) has been associated with seizures (10307). The role of chromium in this adverse effect is unclear.

Hexavalent chromium (CR VI) is 100 times more toxic than trivalent chromium. It can cause hepatic, renal, and cardiac failure (9141). Occupational inhalation of hexavalent chromium can cause ulceration of the nasal mucosa and perforation of the nasal septum, and has been associated with pneumoconiosis, allergic asthma, and increased susceptibility to respiratory tract carcinomas. Industrial hexavalent chromium is considered

cytotoxic and genotoxic (6863). It penetrates the cells easily (unlike trivalent chromium) and appears to induce oxidative damage to DNA (7326).
Intravenously, chromium is associated with decreased glomerular filtration rate (GFR) in children who receive long-term chromium-containing total parenteral nutrition (TPN) (11787).

Interactions with Herbs & Other Dietary Supplements

CHROMIUM-CONTAINING HERBS: Herbs that contain chromium, such as horsetail (Equisetum arvense) and cascara (Rhamus purshiana), can increase the risk of chromium toxicity when taken chronically, or when taken with chromium supplements (9141).
IRON: Chromium competes with iron for binding to the transport protein, transferrin, and could predispose people to iron deficiency. This effect is unlikely to be clinically significant at usual supplemental doses of chromium (6861,6865,6866).
VITAMIN C: Concomitant vitamin C use might increase chromium absorption (7135).
ZINC: Theoretically, co-administration might decrease absorption of both chromium and zinc (1950).

Interactions with Drugs

INSULIN: Theoretically, concomitant use might increase the risk of hypoglycemia (1952).
NONSTEROIDAL ANTI-INFLAMMATORY DRUGS (NSAIDs): There is some evidence that NSAIDs might increase chromium levels by increasing chromium absorption and retention. Drugs that are prostaglandin inhibitors seem to increase chromium absorption and retention (7135). Some of these drugs include ibuprofen (Advil, Motrin, Nuprin, others), indomethacin (Indocin), naproxen (Aleve, Anaprox, Naprelan, Naprosyn), piroxicam (Feldene), aspirin, and others.

Drug Influences on Nutrient Levels and Depletion

SOME DRUGS CAN AFFECT CHROMIUM LEVELS:
ANTACIDS: There is some evidence that antacids might decrease chromium levels by inhibiting absorption of chromium, but the clinical significance of this isn't clear. Increasing gastric pH seems to decrease chromium absorption due to formation of less soluble chromium salts (7135).
CORTICOSTEROIDS: Use of corticosteroids can increase urinary chromium excretion, which might lead to chromium deficiency and/or corticosteroid-induced hyperglycemia (5039).
H2-BLOCKERS: There is some evidence that H2-blockers might decrease chromium levels by inhibiting absorption of chromium, but the clinical significance of this isn't clear. Increasing gastric pH seems to decrease chromium absorption due to formation of less soluble chromium salts (7135). The H2 blockers include cimetidine (Tagamet), ranitidine (Zantac), nizatidine (Axid), and famotidine (Pepcid).
PROTON PUMP INHIBITORS (PPIs): There is some evidence that PPIs might decrease chromium levels by inhibiting chromium absorption, but the clinical significance of this isn't clear. Increasing gastric pH might decrease chromium absorption due to formation of less soluble chromium salts (7135). PPIs include omeprazole (Prilosec), lansoprazole (Prevacid), rabeprazole (Aciphex), pantoprazole (Protonix, Pantoloc), and esomeprazole (Nexium).

Interactions with Foods

None known.

Interactions with Lab Tests

None known.

Interactions with Diseases or Conditions

BEHAVIORAL AND PSYCHIATRIC DISORDERS: Theoretically, chromium picolinate preparations might affect behavioral and psychiatric conditions. Picolinic acid in chromium picolinate preparations can alter serotonin, dopamine, and norepinephrine metabolism in the central nervous system (1935).
CHROMATE/LEATHER CONTACT ALLERGY: Oral chromium supplements can cause allergic reactions in people with chromate or leather contact allergy, including dermatitis, erythema, and scaling on the extremities (6624).
DIABETES: Chromium might lower blood glucose levels (1939); monitor closely.
RENAL INSUFFICIENCY: Chromium supplements might exacerbate renal insufficiency (1951). Tell patients with renal dysfunction to avoid chromium supplements.

Dosage and Administration

ORAL: For lowering blood glucose and lipid levels in patients with type 2 diabetes, 200 to 1000 mcg daily in divided dose has been used (1934,6867). For increasing serum HDL cholesterol in men taking beta-blockers, 200 mcg three times daily has been used (5040). For corticosteroid-induced hyperglycemia or exacerbation of pre-existing diabetes, 400 mcg per day or 200 mcg three times daily has been used (5039). Chromium picolinate has been used in most studies. For preventing reactive hypoglycemia, 200 mcg daily of chromium chloride has been used (6859). For treating dysthymic disorder (mild depression), 200 mcg once or twice daily of chromium picolinate or polynicotinate has been used (2659). Daily adequate intake (AI) levels for chromium have been established: Infants 0 to 6 months, 0.2 mcg; 7 to 12 months, 5.5 mcg; children 1 to 3 years, 11 mcg; 4 to 8 years, 15 mcg; boys 9 to 13 years, 25 mcg;

men 14 to 50 years, 35 mcg; men 51 and older, 30 mcg; girls 9 to 13 years, 21 mcg; 14 to 18 years, 24 mcg; women 19 to 50 years, 25 mcg; women 51 and older, 20 mcg; pregnant women 14 to 18 years, 29 mcg; 19 to 50 years, 30 mcg; lactating women 14 to 18 years, 44 mcg; 19 to 50 years, 45 mcg. Sometimes chromium amounts are listed in micromols. The conversion factor to micrograms is: 1.92 micromol Cr = 100 mcg (6867).
INTRAVENOUS: No typical dosage.

Comments
Chromium was discovered in France in the late 1790s, but it took until the 1960s before it was recognized as being an important trace element and important for insulin function (7058).

CHRYSANTHEMUM

Also Known As
Florist's Chrysanthemum, Ju Hua, Mum.

Scientific Names
Chrysanthemum morifolium, synonyms Anthemis grandiflorum, Anthemis stipulacea, Chrysanthemum sinense, Chrysanthemum stipulaceum, Dendranthema grandiflorum, Dendranthema morifolium, Matricaria morifolia.
Family: Asteraceae/Compositae.

People Use This For
Orally, chrysanthemum is used to treat angina, hypertension, type 2 diabetes, fever, cold, headache, dizziness, and swelling.
In combination with other herbs, chrysanthemum is used orally to treat prostate cancer. In combination with licorice (Glycyrrhiza uralensis) and Panax notoginseng, it is used to treat precancerous lesions.
As a beverage, chrysanthemum is very popular as a summertime tea in southern China.

Safety
There is insufficient reliable information available about the safety of chrysanthemum.
Pregnancy and Lactation: Insufficient reliable information available; avoid using.

Effectiveness
There is insufficient reliable information available about the effectiveness of chrysanthemum.

Mechanism of Action
The dried chrysanthemum flower contains the essential oil bornol, chrysantheonon, camphor, the alkaloid stachydrine, and several glycosides. It also contains adenine, choline, B vitamins, and substances similar to vitamin A. Some evidence suggests that chrysanthemum might increase coronary vasodilatation and blood flow without increasing coronary contractility or oxygen consumption. Chrysanthemum may also have antibacterial and antipyretic effects. It may also reduce the capillary permeability induced by histamine (5545). Preliminary information suggests the chrysanthemum product Jiangtangkang used by individuals with non-insulin dependent diabetes might improve insulin sensitivity and decrease blood viscosity (5546). A preliminary trial suggests Hua-sheng-ping, a combination of chrysanthemum, licorice (Glycyrrhiza uralensis), and Panax notoginseng can reverse precancerous gastrointestinal lesions (5555). The chrysanthemum constituents chrysin and acetin-7-O-beta-D-galactopyranoside inhibit HIV replication in vitro (5545,5547).

Adverse Reactions
Chrysanthemum flowers may cause photosensitivity and contact dermatitis (5552,5553,5554,5556,5557). Chrysanthemum flowers may cause an allergic reaction in individuals sensitive to the Asteraceae/Compositae family. Members of this family include ragweed, chrysanthemums, marigolds, daisies and many other herbs.

Interactions with Herbs & Other Dietary Supplements
None known.

Interactions with Drugs
None known.

Interactions with Foods
None known.

Interactions with Lab Tests
None known.

Interactions with Diseases or Conditions
None known.

Dosage and Administration
ORAL: To make the concentrated water extract, 300 mg of the dried chrysanthemum flower are condensed into 500 mL water. A typical dose is 25 mL three times daily or as a tea (5545).

Comments
The name chrysanthemum is from the Greek words for "gold" and "flower."

CHRYSIN

Also Known As
5,7-Chrysin, 5,7-Dihydroxyflavone, Flavone X, Flavonoid, Galangin Flavanone.
CAUTION: See separate listings for Diosmin, Hesperidin, Methoxylated Flavones, Passionflower, Quercetin, and Rutin.

Scientific Names
Chrysin.

People Use This For
Orally, chrysin is used for bodybuilding, anxiety, inflammation, gout, HIV/AIDS, impotence, baldness, and preventing cancer.

Safety
POSSIBLY SAFE ...when used orally and appropriately, short term. Chrysin 300 mg daily seems to be safe when taken for up to 8 weeks (7514).
PREGNANCY AND LACTATION: Insufficient reliable information available; avoid using.

Effectiveness
POSSIBLY INEFFECTIVE

Athletic conditioning. Taking chrysin orally, in combination with androgen precursors, doesn't seem to be effective for enhancing resistance training in athletes. The combination of chrysin 300 mg with androstenedione, dehydroepiandrosterone (DHEA), puncture vine, indole-3-carbinole, and saw palmetto taken daily for eight weeks does not appear to increase testosterone concentrations, reduce the estrogenic effects of androstenedione, change body composition, or increase strength in response to resistance training (7514).

There is insufficient reliable information available about the effectiveness of chrysin for its other uses.

Mechanism of Action
Chrysin is a flavonoid that occurs naturally in plants such as the passionflower, silver linden, some geranium species, and in honey and bee propolis (4001,7501,7502). Athletes are interested in chrysin for bodybuilding due to its potential effect on testosterone levels. In vitro research shows that chrysin might inhibit aromatase and decrease aromatization of androstenedione and testosterone to estrogen and dihydrotestosterone (7506), but research in humans shows that chrysin does not increase testosterone levels when used in combination with androgen precursors such as androstenedione and dehydroepiandrosterone (DHEA) (7514).

Researchers are also interested in chrysin due to several potential anticancer properties. Chrysin seems to increase glucuronidation by inducing UDP-glucuronosyltransferase 1A1 (UGT1A1), which might reduce the bioavailability of dietary carcinogens (7504,8170). Chrysin might also might inhibit cytochrome P450 1A1 (CYP1A1) and 1A2 (CYP1A2), which could prevent activation of potentially carcinogenic food-derived heterocyclic aromatic amines (7503,8172). There is also preliminary evidence that chrysin might decrease estrogen synthesis by acting as an aromatase (estrogen synthetase) inhibitor, similar to the breast cancer drugs anastrozole (Arimidex) and letrozole (Femara) (7507,7508).

Chrysin might also have antioxidant properties (7509). Chrysin appears to inhibit xanthine oxidase, suggesting potential use for preventing oxidative injury in ischemia-reperfusion and treating gout (7510).

Chrysin might have activity against the human immunodeficiency virus (HIV). It appears to block HIV transcriptional activation, possibly by blocking casein kinase II (CKII), an enzyme that seems to regulate HIV transcription (7512,8171).

There's also some evidence that chrysin might act as a sunscreen. Chrysin-fed experimental animals are protected from contact hypersensitivity induced by ultraviolet (UV) radiation (7511).

There is some preliminary evidence that chrysin can bind benzodiazepine receptors and might have some anxiolytic effects. Some researchers call it a partial benzodiazepine agonist because it does not seem to affect memory and does not have anticonvulsant, muscle relaxant, or sedative activity (4001,8165,8166,8167).

Some chrysin derivatives appear to have hypoglycemic activity, unlike chrysin, which seems to inhibit insulin release (8169).
The oral bioavailability of chrysin is low. Since it induces the enzyme UGT, specifically UGT1A1, chrysin appears to induce its own elimination (7513). Most chrysin is deactivated by presystemic intestinal as well as hepatic glucuronidation and sulfonation (8168). There is some speculation that the therapeutic usefulness of chrysin might be negligible due to limited systemic bioavailability (7502,7504,7505).

Adverse Reactions

None reported.

Interactions with Herbs & Other Dietary Supplements

ANDROSTENEDIONE: Preliminary research showed that chrysin might increase androstenedione levels and its conversion to testosterone by inhibiting aromatization of androstenedione to estrogen and dihydrotestosterone (7506). However, research in humans shows that chrysin has no effect on androstenedione metabolism and does not increase testosterone levels (7514).

Interactions with Drugs

AROMATASE INHIBITORS: Theoretically, chrysin may have an additive effect on other aromatase inhibitors such as aminoglutethimide (Cytadren), anastrozole (Arimidex), exemestane (Aromasin), and letrozole (Femara) (7507,7508).
CYTOCHROME P450 1A2 (CYP1A2) SUBSTRATES: There is some preliminary evidence that chrysin inhibits CYP1A2 isozymes (7503,8172). Theoretically, chrysin might decrease the metabolism of CYP1A2 substrates and increase serum concentrations. Some substrates of CYP1A2 include clozapine (Clozaril), cyclobenzaprine (Flexeril), fluvoxamine (Luvox), haloperidol (Haldol), imipramine (Tofranil), mexiletine (Mexitil), olanzapine (Zyprexa), pentazocine (Talwin), propranolol (Inderal), tacrine (Cognex), theophylline, zileuton (Zyflo), zolmitriptan (Zomig), and others.
GLUCURONIDATED DRUGS: There is some preliminary evidence that chrysin might induce UDP-glucuronosyltransferase 1A1 (UGT1A1) (7504,7513,8170). Theoretically, chrysin might increase the clearance of drugs that are UGT1A1 substrates, such as acetaminophen (Tylenol), estrogens (Estrace, Premarin, others) and oral contraceptives, entacapone (Comtan), irinotecan (Camptosar), and others.

Interactions with Foods

None known.

Interactions with Lab Tests

None known.

Interactions with Diseases or Conditions

None known.

Dosage and Administration

ORAL: For bodybuilding, chrysin 300 mg daily has been taken as a component of a combination product (Andro-6) that also includes androstenedione, DHEA, puncture vine (Tribulus terrestris), indole-3-carbinole, and saw palmetto (7514).

CHYMOTRYPSIN

Also Known As

A-Chymotrypsin, Alpha-Chymotrypsin, Chymotrypsin A, Chymotrypsin B, Chymotrypsinum, Quimotripsina.

Scientific Names

Alpha-chymotrypsin; chymotrypsinum.

People Use This For

Orally, chymotrypsin is used for reducing inflammation and edema associated with abscesses, ulcers, surgery or traumatic injuries; as an expectorant in asthma, bronchitis, pulmonary diseases, and sinusitis. It is used in minimizing initial rise in serum liver enzymes in burn patients, reducing liver stress, and associated degradative changes during wound repair.
Topically, chymotrypsin is used for inflammatory and infectious disorders.
As an inhalant, chymotrypsin is used for inflammatory and infectious disorders.
Intramuscularly, chymotrypsin is used to reduce inflammation and edema associated with abscesses, ulcers, surgery or traumatic injuries, and as an expectorant in asthma, bronchitis, pulmonary diseases, and sinusitis, and for

inflammatory and infectious disorders.
Ophthalmalgically, chymotrypsin is used as an adjunct in cataract surgery to reduce trauma to the eye.

Safety
LIKELY SAFE ...when used ophthalmically, as approved by the FDA.
POSSIBLY SAFE ...when used orally for inflammation due to surgery or trauma injuries (717,718). ...when used topically for treating burns (716).
There is insufficient reliable information available about the safety of chymotrypsin for its other uses.
PREGNANCY AND LACTATION: Insufficient reliable information available; avoid using.

Effectiveness
EFFECTIVE

Cataracts. Chymotrypsin is effective when used as an adjunct in cataract surgery according to FDA-approved prescription product labeling (9,509).

POSSIBLY EFFECTIVE

Burns. There is some evidence that chymotrypsin might decrease tissue destruction in burn patients (716).
Fractures. Taking chymotrypsin orally seems to be effective for reducing inflammation and edema associated with hand fractures (717,718).

There is insufficient reliable information available about the effectiveness of chymotrypsin for its other uses.

Mechanism of Action
Chymotrypsin has ingredients that have proteolytic, anti-inflammatory, and antioxidant activities that reduce tissue destruction (715).

Adverse Reactions
Orally, anaphylactic reaction (rare) is characterized by dyspnea, urticaria, edema of the glottis or lip, shock and vascular collapse, loss of consciousness, and death (9,509). If hypersensitivity is suspected, a sensitivity test should be performed before administration (9).
Opthamalmically, chymotrypsin leads to increased intraocular pressure (9,509), corneal edema, striation, moderate uveitis (9), iridoplegia, and filamentary keratitis (509).

Interactions with Herbs & Other Dietary Supplements
None known.

Interactions with Drugs
None known.

Interactions with Foods
None known.

Interactions with Lab Tests
None known.

Interactions with Diseases or Conditions
Contraindicated in ocular surgery cases involving congenital cataracts, high vitreous pressure and a gaping incisional wound, or if individual is 20 years of age or younger (9).

Dosage and Administration
ORAL: For inflammation, edema and respiratory secretions, 6:1 ratio (trypsin: chymotrypsin) in a combined amount of 100,000 units USP four times daily has been used (717,718). For burns, as 6:1 ratio (trypsin:chymotrypsin) in a combined amount of 200,000 units USP four times daily for 10 days has been used (716).
INTRAMUSCULAR: For inflammation, edema and respiratory secretions: 5000 USP units one to three times daily has been used (9).
OPHTHALMIC: As an adjunct in cataract surgery, 1:5000 or 1:10,000 solution of chymotrypsin in sterile sodium chloride injection (0.9%) injected to irrigate the posterior chamber has been used (9).
TOPICAL: No typical dosage.

CIGUATERA

Also Known As
Ciguatera, Ciguatera Poisoning.

Scientific Names
Gambierdiscus toxicus (dinoflagellate).

People Use This For
There are no medicinal uses for this product, but it may be encountered inadvertently by eating tainted fish.

Safety
UNSAFE ...when ingested. Up to 20% mortality has been reported (6). A single bite of fish contaminated with this toxin will produce symptoms (6).
PREGNANCY: UNSAFE ...when ingested. There has been one report of a fetus being aborted during acute phase of maternal poisoning. However, no lasting adverse effects have been reported in liveborn infants (6).
LACTATION: UNSAFE ...when ingested. Ciguatera is excreted in breast milk; GI symptoms and itching reported in infants breast-fed by symptomatic mothers; infant symptoms resolved with discontinuation of breast-feeding (6).

Effectiveness
There is insufficient reliable information available about the effectiveness of ciguatera.

Mechanism of Action
The applicable part of ciguatera is the toxin. Ciguatoxin increases cell permeability to sodium, causing sustained depolarization (6). Action in humans is dependent on anti-cholinesterase activity and also to a transmitter-like cholinomimetic activity (6).

Adverse Reactions
Poisoning has many different manifestations. But in general, poisoning is characterized by abdominal cramps, nausea, vomiting, diarrhea within 1-6 hours of ingestion; itching, numbness of lips, tongue, throat, paresthesias, blurred vision, hypotension, bradycardia; reversal of hot and cold sensations, and coma (rarely). In severe cases, shock, muscular paralysis, and death are possible (6). GI symptoms usually resolve within 24 hours. Muscle weakness/numbness may last weeks to months (6). Tumultuous fetal movements and intermittent fetal shivering have been reported with maternal poisoning. There has been one case of a fetus aborted during the acute phase of maternal poisoning (6).

Interactions with Herbs & Other Dietary Supplements
None known.

Interactions with Drugs
None known.

Interactions with Foods
None known.

Interactions with Lab Tests
None known.

Interactions with Diseases or Conditions
None known.

Dosage and Administration
No typical dosage.

Comments
Ciguatera poisoning is caused by eating normally safe, bottom-feeding, coral-reef fish that have accumulated ciguatoxin via the marine food chain (6). The red snapper, barracuda, and grouper are most often involved. Florida and Hawaii have the greatest incidence of ciguatera poisoning. Avoid consumption of fish in areas of recently disturbed coral reefs (includes waterfront construction). Ciguatoxic fish appear normal, including smell and taste. Local "rules of thumb" for detection are unsubstantiated. Testing for ciguatoxin is available in some areas (6).
Over 400 (normally safe) fish species may contain toxin, including red snapper, barracuda, parrotfish, jacks and grouper (6).

CINCHONA

Also Known As

Chinarinde, Ecorce de Quina, Fieberrinde, Jesuit's Bark, Peruvian Bark, Quinine, Red Cinchona Bark.

Scientific Names

Cinchona calisaya, synonyms Cinchona ledgeriana, Cinchona carabayensis, Cinchona officinalis;
Cinchona pubescens, synonym Cinchona succirubra.
Family: Rubiaceae.

People Use This For

Orally, cinchona is used for stimulating appetite, promoting GI secretions, bloating and fullness, hemorrhoids, varicose veins, colds, and leg cramps. It is also used orally for mild attacks of influenza, malaria, fever, cancer, mouth and throat diseases, enlarged spleen, muscle cramps, and gastric disorders.
Topically, cinchona is used in eye lotions for astringent, bactericidal, and anesthetic effects. Cinchona extract is also used topically for hemorrhoids, stimulating hair growth, and managing varicose veins.

Safety

POSSIBLY SAFE ...when used orally and appropriately (12).
LIKELY UNSAFE ...when excessive amounts are used orally. 2 to 8 grams of the quinine constituent (505) or 2.5-8 grams quinidine constituent (17) can cause serious toxicity including death (505); however, the amount of these constituents varies according to the cinchona species (13).
PREGNANCY: LIKELY UNSAFE ...when used orally; avoid using (12).
LACTATION: Insufficient reliable information available; avoid using.

Effectiveness

There is insufficient reliable information available about the effectiveness of cinchona.

Mechanism of Action

The applicable part of cinchona is the bark. The cinchona bark can stimulate saliva and gastric juice secretion (2). The antimalarial effects can be attributed to quinine, an alkaloid constituent. The constituents, quinidine and quinine, have cardiac depressant properties (11).

Adverse Reactions

Orally, cinchona can cause thrombocytopenia, bleeding, and hypersensitivity reactions, including hives and fever (2). Overdose or hypersensitivity to cinchona can cause cinchonism; symptoms include headache (505), nausea, diarrhea, vomiting, ringing in the ears (6), and vision disturbance (8,505).
Topically, the cinchona bark can cause contact dermatitis (11).

Interactions with Herbs & Other Dietary Supplements

HERBS WITH ANTICOAGULANT/ANTIPLATELET POTENTIAL: Theoretically, concomitant use of cinchona bark with herbs that might have anticoagulant or antiplatelet properties might increase the risk of bleeding in some people. These herbs include alfalfa, angelica, clove, garlic, ginger, Panax ginseng, horse chestnut, red clover, and others.

Interactions with Drugs

ANTACIDS: Theoretically, due to reports that cinchona increases stomach acid, cinchona might decrease the effectiveness of antacids (19).
ANTICOAGULANT/ANTIPLATELET DRUGS: Cinchona can increase the drug effects and risk of bleeding due to its quinine content (2).
CARBAMAZEPINE (Tegretol): Cinchona can increase serum drug levels of carbamazepine due to its quinine content (11016).
H2-BLOCKERS: Theoretically, due to reports that cinchona increases stomach acid, cinchona might decrease the effectiveness of H2-blockers (19). The H2 blockers include cimetidine (Tagamet), ranitidine (Zantac), nizatidine (Axid), and famotidine (Pepcid).
PHENOBARBITAL (Luminal): Cinchona can increase serum drug levels of phenobarbital due to its quinine content (504).
PROTON PUMP INHIBITORS (PPIs): Theoretically, due to reports that cinchona increases stomach acid, cinchona might decrease the effectiveness of PPIs (19). PPIs include omeprazole (Prilosec), lansoprazole (Prevacid), rabeprazole (Aciphex), pantoprazole (Protonix), and esomeprazole (Nexium).
QUINIDINE: Cinchona contains quinidine; concomitant use with cinchona can increase the therapeutic and adverse effects of quinidine (505).

QUININE: Cinchona contains quinine; concomitant use with cinchona can increase the therapeutic and adverse effects of quinine (505).

Interactions with Foods
None known.

Interactions with Lab Tests
None known.

Interactions with Diseases or Conditions
GASTRIC OR INTESTINAL ULCERS: Cinchona is contraindicated (8,12) in conditions with an increased risk of bleeding.

Dosage and Administration
ORAL: The typical dose of cinchona is one cup of the tea up to three times daily (18). The tea is prepared by steeping 500 mg of the dried bark in 150 mL boiling water for 5-10 minutes and then straining. The maximum amount of cinchona is 1-3 grams of the bark per day (18) or 0.05-0.2 grams of the essential oil per day (12). The usual dose of the cinchona liquid extract (4-5% total alkaloids) is 0.6-3 grams per day (18). The cinchona extract (15-20% total alkaloids) is commonly given as 0.15-0.6 grams per day (18).

Comments
Cinchona bark contains quinine and related alkaloids, including quinidine (a cardiac depressant) and cinchotannic acid (can cause constipation). While quinine is effective for preventing or suppressing malaria caused by susceptible organisms (15), people treated with cinchona bark are exposed to the risks of quinidine, cinchotannic acid, and other alkaloid constituents. It is recommended that only purified quinine, or other appropriate antimalarial agents, be used to prevent or suppress malaria (15). US drug regulations require products containing cinchona derivatives to contain the labeling, "Discontinue use if ringing in the ears, deafness, skin rash or visual disturbances occur" (12).

CINNAMON bark

Also Known As
Batavia Cassia, Batavia Cinnamon, Cannelier de Ceylan, Ceylon Cinnamon, Ceylonzimt, Ceylonzimtbaum, Cinnamomum, Madagascar Cinnamon, Padang-Cassia, Panang Cinnamon, Sri Lanka Cinnamon, Thwak, Tvak.
CAUTION: See separate listings for Cassia Cinnamon.

Scientific Names
Cinnamomum verum, synonyms Cinnamomum zeylanicum, Laurus cinnamomum.
Family: Lauraceae.

People Use This For
Orally, cinnamon bark is used as an antispasmodic, antiflatulent, appetite stimulant, antidiarrheal, antimicrobial, anthelmintic; and for treating the common cold and influenza, gastrointestinal (GI) upset, diabetes, and dysmenorrhea.
Topically, cinnamon bark is used as part of a multi-ingredient preparation for treating premature ejaculation.
In foods, cinnamon is commonly consumed as a spice and as a flavoring agent in beverages.
In manufacturing, the volatile oil is commonly used in small amounts in toothpaste, mouthwashes, gargles, lotions, liniments, soaps, detergents, and other pharmaceutical products and cosmetics.

Safety
LIKELY SAFE ...when consumed in amounts commonly found in foods. Cinnamon bark has Generally Recognized As Safe (GRAS) status in the US (4912).
POSSIBLY SAFE ...when used orally and appropriately in medicinal amounts (4,12). ...when used topically, short-term as part of a multi-ingredient preparation (SS Cream). This preparation was used safely in a clinical trial where the cream was applied and left on the glans penis for 1-hour (2537). Further evaluation is needed to determine its safety after prolonged, repetitive use.
POSSIBLY UNSAFE ...when used orally in excessive amounts or long-term (4,12). Consumption of up to 700 mcg per kilogram of the constituent, cinnamaldehyde, is considered the highest acceptable level (4).
PREGNANCY: LIKELY SAFE ...when consumed in amounts commonly found in foods (4912). LIKELY UNSAFE ...when used orally in amounts greater than those found in foods (4,12).
LACTATION: LIKELY SAFE ...when consumed in amounts commonly found in foods (4912). There is insufficient reliable information available about using cinnamon bark in amounts greater than those found in foods; avoid using amounts greater than those found in foods.

Effectiveness

POSSIBLY EFFECTIVE

Premature ejaculation. Applying cinnamon bark topically, as part of a multi-ingredient preparation, seems to be helpful for treating premature ejaculation. In one controlled clinical trial, a multi-ingredient cream preparation (SS Cream) containing Panax ginseng root, Angelica root, Cistanches deserticola, Zanthoxyl species, Torlidis seed, clove flower, Asiasari root, cinnamon bark, and toad venom was applied to the glans penis one hour prior to intercourse and washed off immediately before intercourse. Men suffering from premature ejaculation who were treated with the cream had significantly improved ejaculatory latency compared to placebo (2537).

There is insufficient reliable information available about the effectiveness of cinnamon bark for its other uses.

Mechanism of Action

The volatile oils of cinnamon bark are thought to be the active constituents of cinnamon. They seem to be responsible for the proposed antispasmodic, antiflatulent, and appetite stimulating effects (4).

There are approximately 6000 to 30,000 ppm of cinnamaldehyde in cinnamon bark (3919). Cinnamaldehyde makes up 60% to 80% of the volatile oil from the bark (4800). Cinnamaldehyde is thought to have central nervous system (CNS) stimulant effects at low doses and sedative effects at high doses. It is also thought to have hypothermic, antipyretic, antibacterial, and antifungal activity. Cinnamaldehyde might also increase peripheral blood flow, slow heart rate, reduce blood pressure, and possibly affect blood sugar levels (4). However, these pharmacological effects are thought to be fairly weak. Furthermore, much of the active volatile oil in cinnamon is thought to evaporate away when the cinnamon is prepared as a tea (4).

The tannin constituents in cinnamon bark have astringent properties and are thought to be responsible for an antidiarrheal effect (4). A multi-ingredient topical preparation containing cinnamon bark and several other herbs (SS Cream) is thought to work in premature ejaculation by increasing the penile vibratory threshold and reducing the amplitude of penile somatosensory-evoked potentials (2537). There is some preliminary research that suggests the cinnamon bark constituent, methylhydroxychalcone polymer (MHCP), might improve insulin sensitivity. It seems to mimic the activity of insulin, stimulating glucose metabolism. It also appears to work synergistically with insulin, possibly by improving insulin signaling pathways and alternative pathways that cause increased cellular glucose uptake. It may also have antioxidant effects (11247,11248,11973). An extract from Cinnamon cassia, a cinnamon species that also contains MHCP, lowers blood glucose, triglycerides, and total and low-density lipoprotein (LDL) cholesterol in people with type II diabetes (11347).

Adverse Reactions

Orally, no adverse reactions tend to occur with the use of the cinnamon bark; however, the oil can irritate mucous membranes and is a skin irritant and sensitizer.

Topically, preparations in concentrations greater than 0.01% may cause allergic dermatitis in sensitive individuals (4). When the multi-ingredient cream preparation (SS Cream) has been applied topically to the glans penis, sporadic erectile dysfunction, excessively delayed ejaculation, mild pain, and local irritation and burning has occurred (2537).

Interactions with Herbs & Other Dietary Supplements

HERBS & SUPPLEMENTS WITH HYPOGLYCEMIC POTENTIAL: Cinnamon bark can lower blood glucose levels (11247,11248,11973) and might have additive effects when used with other herbs and supplements that also lower glucose levels. This might increase the risk of hypoglycemia in some patients. Some herbs and supplements with hypoglycemic effects include alpha-lipoic acid, bitter melon, chromium, devil's claw, fenugreek, garlic, guar gum, horse chestnut, Panax ginseng, psyllium, Siberian ginseng, and others.

Interactions with Drugs

ANTIDIABETES DRUGS: Theoretically, cinnamon bark may lower blood glucose levels, and have additive effects in patients treated with antidiabetic agents; use with caution (11247,11248,11973). Dose adjustments to diabetes medications might be necessary. Some antidiabetes drugs include glimepiride (Amaryl), glyburide (DiaBeta, Glynase PresTab, Micronase), insulin, metformin (Glucophage), pioglitazone (Actos), rosiglitazone (Avandia), and others.

Interactions with Foods

None known.

Interactions with Lab Tests

BLOOD GLUCOSE: Theoretically, cinnamon bark may lower blood glucose levels in some patients (11247,11248,11973).

Interactions with Diseases or Conditions

CARDIOVASCULAR CONDITIONS: There is concern that cinnamon bark might adversely affect patients with cardiovascular conditions such as high or low blood pressure or congestive heart failure. Some constituents in cinnamon bark seem to slow heart rate and might lower blood pressure (4). However, the clinical significance of these effects in patients is not known. Until more is known, advise patients with cardiovascular conditions to avoid

or use cinnamon bark preparations cautiously.
DIABETES: Theoretically, cinnamon bark might lower blood glucose in patients with type 2 diabetes (11247,11248,11973). Tell patients with diabetes to use cinnamon bark products cautiously and monitor blood glucose levels very closely. Dose adjustments to diabetes medications might be necessary.

Dosage and Administration

No typical dosage.

Comments

Cinnamon is getting a lot of attention as a treatment for diabetes. There is preliminary evidence that it can lower blood glucose and cholesterol levels in people with type 2 diabetes. So far this benefit has only been found with Cassia Cinnamon (Chinese Cinnamon) in humans (11347). See separate listing for Cassia Cinnamon. There are lots of different types of cinnamon. Cinnamon verum (Ceylon cinnamon) is the type used most commonly in the Western world. Cinnamomum aromaticum (Cassia cinnamon or Chinese cinnamon) is also commonly used. In many cases, the cinnamon spice purchased in food stores contains a combination of these different types of cinnamon.

CITICOLINE

Also Known As

CDP-Choline, Cytidine 5-diphosphocholine, Cytidine diphosphate choline.
CAUTION: See separate listings for Choline and Phosphatidylcholine.

Scientific Names

Cytidine 5'-diphosphocholine, synonyms 5'-Cytidine diphosphate choline, Cytidine (5') diphosphocholine.

People Use This For

Orally or parenterally, citicoline is used for Alzheimer's disease and other types of dementia, head trauma, cerebrovascular disease such as stroke, age-related memory loss, Parkinson's disease, and glaucoma.

Safety

POSSIBLY SAFE ...when used orally and appropriately, short-term. Taking citicoline in doses of 1000-2000 mg/day seems to be safe when used for 60 to 90 days (12130).
PREGNANCY AND LACTATION: Insufficient reliable information available; avoid using.

Effectiveness

POSSIBLY EFFECTIVE

Age-related cognitive impairment. People aged 50 to 85 years with poor memory, taking citicoline 1000-2000 mg daily, seem to have improved verbal memory (12130).

Cerebrovascular disease. There is some evidence that citicoline taken orally or given intramuscularly or by intravenous infusion might improve memory and behavior in patients with chronic cerebrovascular diseases, such as stroke (12131).

Ischemic stroke. Stroke patients who receive citicoline 500-2000 mg/day orally within 24 hours of acute ischemic stroke are more likely to have a complete recovery within 3 months compared to placebo (12139).

INSUFFICIENT RELIABLE EVIDENCE to RATE

Alzheimer's disease. Preliminary evidence suggests that taking citicoline 1000 mg/day orally might improve cognitive function in patients with mild to moderate Alzheimer's disease (12131).

Glaucoma. Preliminary evidence suggests that citicoline 1000 mg/day intramuscularly might improve vision in patients with open-angle glaucoma (12132). Taking 1000 mg/day orally also seems to improve visual evoked potentials in patients with glaucoma (12173).

Parkinson's disease. Preliminary evidence suggests that patients who receive citicoline 500 mg/day intramuscularly in conjunction with conventional treatment might have improved rigidity and bradykinesia. But citicoline does not seem to improve tremor (12132).

Vascular dementia. Preliminary evidence indicates that citicoline 500 mg twice daily (1000 mg/day) does not seem to improve symptoms in patients with vascular dementia (12135).

More evidence is needed to rate citicoline for these uses.

Mechanism of Action

Citicoline is an intermediate compound that is formed endogenously in the process of synthesizing phosphatidylcholine from choline (12129,12140).
When taken orally, citicoline is metabolized in the gut to cytidine and choline. Both compounds are absorbed independently and taken up by brain cells. Within the brain cell cytidine is converted to cytidine monophosphate, cytidine diphosphate, and cytidine triphosphate. Choline is phosphorylated to form phosphocholine. Phosphocholine

combines with cytidine triphosphate to reform citicoline. Citicoline then rapidly combines with diacylglycerol to from phosphatidylcholine (12129,12140).

In animal models, orally administered citicoline increases brain phosphatidylcholine levels by 23% after 42 days and 30% after 90 days. In humans, a single dose of citicoline increases brain choline levels by about 18% in younger adults. But in older adults, brain choline levels don't seem to increase significantly. It's thought that choline uptake in the brain decreases with age, but cytidine uptake does not decrease (12129).

Age-related cognitive dysfunction, dementia, and other brain disorders have been linked to decreases in cholinergic neurons, decreases in acetylcholine, and alterations in cell membrane composition, including decreases in choline-containing phospholipids (12129). During episodes of cerebral ischemia and brain trauma, phosphatidylcholine is degraded to free radicals and free fatty acids (12131).

Citicoline also seems to decrease generation of reactive oxygen species (12134).

It's thought that citicoline's potential benefits for central nervous system disorders such as dementia, brain trauma, and other conditions is related to citicoline's effects on brain acetylcholine and phosphatidylcholine levels (12129,12130).

Citicoline might also affect dopamine levels. In animal models, citicoline increases retinal dopamine levels. Therefore, there is interest in using citicoline for glaucoma and Parkinson's disease (12132).

Citicoline might also help for Parkinson's disease by improving dopaminergic cell survival. Patients with Parkinson's disease tend to have a degeneration of dopaminergic cells over time. Citicoline also seems to increase levels of reduced glutathione, a potent antioxidant. Glutathione levels are found to be decreased in the substantia nigra of Parkinson's patients (12133,12140).

In animal models of brain trauma, citicoline reduces neuronal death, cortical contusion volume, and improves neurological recovery (12137).

In animal models of ischemic stroke, citicoline seems to help reduce neuronal damage, possibly by decreasing neuronal apoptosis (12138).

Citicoline seems to have a pressor effect. In animal models of hemorrhagic shock, intravenous administration of citicoline reverses hypotension. In normotensive rats, intravenous administration of citicoline increases blood pressure (12136). It's not known if therapeutic doses of citicoline affect blood pressure in humans.

Citicoline is readily absorbed when taken orally. Less than 1% is excreted unchanged in the feces. Citicoline has a biphasic peak. The first peak occurs at 1 hour after administration, followed by a higher peak 24-hours post-dose. Citicoline is primarily eliminated through the kidneys. It's half-life is 71 hours (12132).

Adverse Reactions

Orally, citicoline seems to be well-tolerated (12131). The most common side effects appear to be nausea and diarrhea. Some people who take citicoline also experience insomnia, constipation, headache, blurred vision, chest pain, palpitations, hypotension, bradycardia, tachycardia, and skin rash (12130,12132). But these adverse reactions do not appear to occur more often than in people taking placebo (12131).

Interactions with Herbs & Other Dietary Supplements

None known.

Interactions with Drugs

None known.

Interactions with Foods

None known.

Interactions with Lab Tests

None known.

Interactions with Diseases or Conditions

None known.

Dosage and Administration

ORAL: For age-related cognitive impairment, citicoline 1000-2000 mg/day has been used (12130).

For Alzheimer's disease, citicoline 1000 mg/day has been used (12131).

For chronic cerebrovascular diseases, 600 mg/day has been used (12131).

For acute ischemic stroke, citicoline 500-2000 mg/day starting within 24 hours of stroke has been used (12139).

For glaucoma, 1000 mg/day has been used (12173).

PARENTERAL: For age-related cognitive impairment, citicoline 1000 mg/day intravenous infusion has been used (12131).

For Alzheimer's disease, citicoline 200-1000 mg/day intramuscularly has been used (12131).

For chronic cerebrovascular diseases, 200-1000 mg/day intramuscularly or by intravenous infusion has been used (12131).

For glaucoma, 1000 mg/day intramuscularly has been used (12132).

Comments

Citicoline was originally developed in Japan for acute cerebrovascular events. Citicoline was eventually introduced as a prescription drug in many European countries. In these countries it is now frequently prescribed for cognitive impairment related to chronic cerebrovascular disease (12131). In the US citicoline is marketed as a dietary supplement and is often promoted for age-related cognitive impairment.

CITRONELLA OIL

Also Known As

Ceylon Citronella, Java Citronella.
CAUTION: See separate listings for Lemongrass and Stone Root.

Scientific Names

Cymbopogon nardus, synonyms Andropogon nardus, Cymbopogon afronardus, Cymbopogon validus; Cymbopogon winterianus.
Family: Poaceae/Graminaea.

People Use This For

Orally, citronella oil is used as a vermifuge, diuretic, antispasmodic, and digestive stimulant.
Topically, citronella oil is used as an insect repellent for people and pets.
In foods and beverages, citronella oil is used as a flavoring agent.
In manufacturing, citronella oil is used as a fragrance in cosmetics and soaps.

Safety

LIKELY SAFE ...when used orally in amounts commonly found in foods. Citronella oil has Generally Recognized As Safe (GRAS) status in the US (4912).
LIKELY UNSAFE ...when used orally in large amounts (6,11). ...when inhaled. There have been reports of toxic alveolitis (2).
CHILDREN: LIKELY UNSAFE ...when used orally. There are reports of poisoning in children and one toddler died after ingesting insect repellent that contained citronella oil (2,6,17).
PREGNANCY AND LACTATION: Insufficient reliable information available; avoid using.

Effectiveness

There is insufficient reliable information available about the effectiveness of citronella oil.

Mechanism of Action

There is insufficient reliable information available about the possible mechanism of action or active ingredients.

Adverse Reactions

Orally, there has been at least one report of death following ingestion of insect repellent containing citronella oil (2).
Topically, citronella oil has caused contact dermatitis (6,11).
By inhalation, citronella oil has caused toxic alveolitis (2).

Interactions with Herbs & Other Dietary Supplements

None known.

Interactions with Drugs

None known.

Interactions with Foods

None known.

Interactions with Lab Tests

None known.

Interactions with Diseases or Conditions

None known.

Dosage and Administration

No typical dosage.

Comments
Avoid confusion with lemongrass (Cymbopogon citratus). Citronella oil is the essential oil produced by steam distillation of other Cymbopogon species. Ceylon or Lenabatu citronella oil is produced from Cymbopogon nardus, and Java or Maha Pengiri citronella oil is produced from Cymbopogon winterianus.

CIVET

Also Known As
African Civet, Large Indian Civet, Zibeth.

Scientific Names
Viverra civetta (African Civet), synonym Civettictis civetta.
Viverra zibetha (Indian Civet).
Family: Viverridae.

Comments
At the date of publication, this product was not a common ingredient used in brand name supplements marketed to consumers. Details about this product are available at the online version of *Natural Medicines Comprehensive Database*. See www.naturaldatabase.com.

CLARY SAGE

Also Known As
Clary, Clary Wort, Clear Eye, Eyebright, Muscatel Sage, See Bright.
CAUTION: See separate listings for Sage and Eyebright.

Scientific Names
Salvia sclarea.
Family: Lamiaceae/Labiatae.

People Use This For
Orally, clary sage is used for upset stomach, digestive disorders, and kidney diseases.
Topically, clary sage mucilage is used to remove foreign objects from the eye, to remove thorns and splinters from the skin, and for treating tumors.
In foods and beverages, the oil from clary sage is used as a flavoring agent.
In manufacturing, the oil from clary sage is used as a fragrance in soaps and cosmetics.

Safety
LIKELY SAFE ...when used orally in amounts commonly found in foods. Clary sage has Generally Recognized As Safe (GRAS) status in the US (4912).
There is insufficient reliable information available about the safety of medicinal uses of clary sage.
PREGNANCY AND LACTATION: Insufficient reliable information available; avoid using.

Effectiveness
There is insufficient reliable information available about the effectiveness of clary sage.

Mechanism of Action
The applicable parts of clary sage are the flowering top and leaf. The oil has some anticonvulsant activity in animals (11), and it seems to potentiate the effects of hexobarbitone and chloral hydrate (11).

Adverse Reactions
None reported.

Interactions with Herbs & Other Dietary Supplements
None known.

Interactions with Drugs
CHLORAL HYDRATE: Reportedly potentiates narcotic effects (9,11).
HEXOBARBITONE: Reportedly potentiates narcotic effects (9,11).

Interactions with Foods
None known.

Interactions with Lab Tests
None known.

Interactions with Diseases or Conditions
None known.

Dosage and Administration
No typical dosage.

Comments
Avoid confusion with sage leaf (Salvia officinalis).

CLEMATIS

Also Known As
Upright Virgin's Bower.
CAUTION: See separate listings for Traveler's Joy and Woodbine.

Scientific Names
Clematis recta.
Family: Ranunculaceae.

People Use This For
Orally, clematis is used for treatment of rheumatic pains, headaches, varicose veins, syphilis, gout, rheumatism, bone disorders, chronic skin conditions, and as a diuretic.
Topically, clematis is used for blisters and as a poultice to treat purulent wounds and ulcers.

Safety
POSSIBLY UNSAFE ...when the fresh plant is used topically (18).
LIKELY UNSAFE ...when the fresh plant is used orally because it is severely irritating to mucous membranes and the gastrointestinal tract (18).
There is insufficient reliable information available about the safety of the oral or topical use of dried clematis.
PREGNANCY AND LACTATION: LIKELY UNSAFE ...when the fresh plant is used orally. There is insufficient reliable information available for the safety of the dried plant; avoid using.

Effectiveness
There is insufficient reliable information available about the effectiveness of clematis.

Mechanism of Action
When the fresh plant is crushed or cut into small pieces, the glycoside ranunculin is enzymatically changed into a severely irritating protoanemonin, which, in turn, rapidly degrades into the non-toxic anemonin (18). Both protoanemonin and ranunculin are destroyed to an unknown extent during the drying process (2), and both have fungicidal activity (4). Since Clematis recta contains low levels of protoanemonin-forming agents, the adverse effects and toxicity may not be as severe as compared to other species of Ranunculaceae. Clematis also contains saponins (18).

Adverse Reactions
Orally, freshly harvested clematis can cause colic, diarrhea, and severe irritation to the gastrointestinal and urinary tracts (18).
Topically, prolonged skin contact can cause slow-healing blisters and burns (18).

Interactions with Herbs & Other Dietary Supplements
None known.

Interactions with Drugs
None known.

Interactions with Foods
None known.

Interactions with Lab Tests
None known.

Interactions with Diseases or Conditions
None known.

Dosage and Administration
ORAL: Clematis recta is available as drops, extracts, and tea (18).
TOPICAL: The tea is used for poultices (18).

Comments
Avoid confusion with other Clematis species (6). Clematis recta is considered a poisonous plant and is rarely used today (18). Plants that are grown in the sun have a higher ranunculin content than those grown in the shade, and therefore have stronger effects (18).

CLIVERS

Also Known As
Barweed, Bedstraw, Catchweed, Cleavers, Cleaverwort, Coachweed, Eriffe, Everlasting Friendship, Gallium, Gosling Weed, Goose Grass, Goosebill, Grip Grass, Hayriffe, Hayruff, Hedge-Burs, Hedgeheriff, Love-Man, Mutton Chops, Robin-Run-in-the-Grass, Scratchweed, Stick-a-Back, Sweethearts.
CAUTION: See separate listing for Potentilla.

Scientific Names
Galium aparine.
Family: Rubiaceae.

People Use This For
Orally, clivers is used as a diuretic, a mild astringent, for dysuria, lymphadenitis, psoriasis, and specifically for enlarged lymph nodes.
Topically, clivers is used for ulcers, festering glands, breast lumps, and skin rashes.

Safety
POSSIBLY SAFE ...when used orally and appropriately (12). There is no documented toxicity (4).
There is insufficient reliable information available about the safety of the topical use of clivers.
PREGNANCY AND LACTATION: Insufficient reliable information available; avoid using.

Effectiveness
There is insufficient reliable information available about the effectiveness of clivers.

Mechanism of Action
The applicable parts of clivers are the dried or fresh above ground parts. Clivers contain tannins, which are reported to have astringent properties (4).

Adverse Reactions
None reported.

Interactions with Herbs & Other Dietary Supplements
None known.

Interactions with Drugs
None known.

Interactions with Foods
None known.

Interactions with Lab Tests
None known.

Interactions with Diseases or Conditions

DIABETES: Use expressed juice with caution (4).

Dosage and Administration

ORAL: Typical doses are 2-4 grams dried above ground parts three times daily, or one cup tea (steep 2-4 grams herb in 150 mL boiling water 5-10 minutes, strain) three times daily (4). Liquid extract (1:1 in 25% alcohol) 2-4 mL three times daily (4). Expressed juice, 3-15 mL three times daily (4).
TOPICAL: No typical dosage.

CLOVE dried flowerbud, leaf, stem

Also Known As

Caryophylli, Caryophyllus, Clous de Girolfe, Clove Flower, Cloves, Flores Caryophyllum, Gewurznelken Nagelein, Lavanga.
CAUTION: See separate listing for Clove Oil.

Scientific Names

Syzygium aromaticum, synonyms Caryophyllus aromaticus, Eugenia aromatica, Eugenia caryophyllata, Eugenia caryophyllus.
Family: Myrtaceae.

People Use This For

Orally, clove is used for gastrointestinal upset, including flatulence, nausea, and vomiting. It is also used orally as an expectorant.
Topically, clove is used for toothache, as a counterirritant for pain, and for mouth and throat inflammation. It is also used topically as part of a multi-ingredient preparation for treating premature ejaculation.
In manufacturing, clove is used as a flavoring in foods, beverages, and cigarettes.

Safety

LIKELY SAFE ...when used orally in amounts commonly found in foods. Clove extract has Generally Recognized As Safe (GRAS) status in the US (4912).
POSSIBLY SAFE ...when used orally and appropriately for medicinal purposes (12). ...when used topically, short-term as part of a multi-ingredient preparation (SS Cream). This preparation was used safely for premature ejaculation in a clinical trial where the cream was applied and left on the glans penis for 1-hour (2537). Further evaluation is needed to determine its safety after prolonged, repetitive use.
LIKELY UNSAFE ...when inhaled due to its harmful effects. Smoking clove cigarettes can cause respiratory injury (17). Clove cigarettes contain more tar, nicotine, and carbon monoxide than tobacco cigarettes (6,17).
There is insufficient reliable information available about the safety of clove for its other uses.
PREGNANCY AND LACTATION: POSSIBLY SAFE ...when used orally in the amounts found in foods. Avoid amounts that greatly exceed those in foods (4).

Effectiveness

POSSIBLY EFFECTIVE

Premature ejaculation. In one controlled clinical trial, a multi-ingredient cream preparation containing Panax ginseng root, Angelica root, Cistanches deserticola, Zanthoxyl species, Torlidis seed, clove flower, Asiasari root, cinnamon bark, and toad venom (SS Cream) was applied to the glans penis one hour prior to intercourse and washed off immediately before intercourse. Men suffering from premature ejaculation who were treated with the cream had significantly improved ejaculatory latency compared to placebo (2537).

There is insufficient reliable information available about the effectiveness of clove dried flowerbud, leaf, or stem for its other uses.

Mechanism of Action

Cloves contain a volatile oil that can be up to 90% eugenol (11). The mild anesthetic and analgesic properties of clove are attributed to eugenol (4,512). Applied topically, eugenol depresses sensory receptors involved in pain perception by inhibiting prostaglandin biosynthesis (512). Eugenol inhibits platelet activity (4). Some evidence suggests the sesquiterpene constituents might have anticancer activity (838). Other evidence suggests whole cloves might have chemoprotective activity against liver and bone marrow toxicity (6). The multi-ingredient preparation containing clove flower is thought to work in premature ejaculation by increasing the penile vibratory threshold and reducing the amplitude of penile somatosensory evoked potentials (2537).

Adverse Reactions

The inhalation of clove can cause respiratory injury including hemoptysis, bronchospasm, hemorrhagic and nonhemorrhagic pulmonary edema, pleural effusion, respiratory insufficiency, respiratory infection, and aspiration of foreign material. There have been two deaths associated with the smoking of the clove cigarettes (17).
Used topically on the oral mucosa, it can cause oral tissue sensitivity, local tissue irritation, and damage to dental pulp or the supporting periodontium (6002). When the multi-ingredient cream preparation containing clove flower (SS Cream) has been applied topically to the glans penis, sporadic erectile dysfunction, excessively delayed ejaculation, mild pain, and local irritation and burning has occurred (2537).

Interactions with Herbs & Other Dietary Supplements

HERBS WITH ANTICOAGULANT/ANTIPLATELET POTENTIAL: Concomitant use of herbs that have constituents that might affect platelet aggregation could theoretically increase the risk of bleeding in some people. These herbs include angelica, danshen, garlic, ginger, ginkgo, red clover, turmeric, willow, and others (4,19).

Interactions with Drugs

ANTICOAGULANT/ANTIPLATELET DRUGS: Theoretically, clove can potentiate the effects of these drugs.

Interactions with Foods

None known.

Interactions with Lab Tests

None known.

Interactions with Diseases or Conditions

None known.

Dosage and Administration

ORAL: A typical dose of cloves is 120-300 mg (4). Limit clove ingestion to the equivalent of 3.6 mg/kg clove oil per day (4). The buds yield 15-18% volatile oil, The stems yield 4-6% (11).
TOPICAL: Clove is commonly used as a mouthwash, and products usually contain 1-5% clove essential oil (8). A 15% clove tincture can be effective in treating athletes foot (4).

Comments

Clove cigarettes, also called kreteks, generally contain 60% tobacco and 40% ground clove (6). Eugenol in clove cigarettes acts as a topical anesthetic to the posterior oropharynx. It reduces the noxious elements of smoking and can facilitate learning of smoking techniques (17).

CLOVE OIL

Also Known As

Caryophyllum, Caryophyllus, Clous de Girolfe, Flores Caryophylli, Gewurznelken Nagelein, Lavanga, Oil of Clove.
CAUTION: See separate listing for Clove.

Scientific Names

Syzygium aromaticum, synonyms Caryophyllus aromaticus, Eugenia aromatica, Eugenia caryophyllata, Eugenia caryophyllus.
Family: Myrtaceae.

People Use This For

Orally, clove oil is used as an antiemetic, antiflatulent, to manage diarrhea, hernia, and halitosis.
In dentistry, clove oil is used topically for toothache, as a dental anesthetic, for treating postextraction alveolitis (dry socket), and for mouth and throat inflammation. It is sometimes used as a counterirritant. It is also used a component in dental cements and fillings.
In foods and beverages, clove oil is used as a flavoring.
In manufacturing, clove oil is used for fragrance in toothpaste, soaps, cosmetics, and perfumes.

Safety

LIKELY SAFE ...when used orally in amounts commonly found in foods. Clove oil has Generally Recognized As Safe (GRAS) status in the US (4912).
POSSIBLY SAFE ...when applied topically (272,512). Clove oil should not be used for self-medication, especially when undiluted. Repeated oral application can cause gingival damage and skin and mucous membrane

irritation (4,272).
LIKELY UNSAFE ...when taken orally undiluted. 5-15 mL may induce high anion gap acidosis, seizures, coagulopathy, acute liver damage, behavioral changes, and coma (17).
PREGNANCY AND LACTATION: LIKELY UNSAFE ...when used orally; avoid in amounts greater than those commonly found in foods (4).

Effectiveness

INSUFFICIENT RELIABLE EVIDENCE to RATE

Toothache. Clove oil and its constituent eugenol have long been used topically for toothache, but the FDA reclassified eugenol from Category I, meaning that it was safe and effective as it was labeled, to category III, meaning there is insufficient data to support efficacy (272). More evidence is needed to rate clove oil for this use.

Mechanism of Action

Mild anesthetic and analgesic properties of clove oil is attributed to eugenol (3,4). On contact, eugenol acts to depress sensory receptors involved in pain perception by inhibition of prostaglandin biosynthesis (3). It is also a powerful inhibitor of platelet activity (6). Clove bud oil contains 60-90% eugenol, clove leaf oil contains 82-88% eugenol, clove stem oil contains 90-95% eugenol (11). Clove oil has antihistaminic and antispasmodic properties, most likely due to eugenyl acetate (6). Clove oil inhibits gram-positive and gram-negative bacteria. It also has fungistatic action, anthelmintic and larvicidal properties. One report suggests it suppresses aflatoxin production (6). Another suggests eugenol from clove oil may counter some effects of environmental mutagens found in foods (6).

Adverse Reactions

Orally, clove oil can cause nervous system depression, seizures, lactic acidosis, disseminated intravascular coagulation, hepatic dysfunction (17), and irritation to mucosal tissues (2,4,6,512). This is one report of disseminated intravascular coagulation and liver failure following clove ingestion by a two-year-old (6). There is one report of depression and electrolyte imbalance following accidental ingestion by a seven-month-old (6).
Topically, clove oil can be irritating to mucosal tissues and skin (2,4,6,512). There is one report of permanent local facial anesthesia and absence of sweating after clove spilled on an individual's face (6). Used topically to the oral mucosa, it can cause oral tissue sensitivity, local tissue irritation, and damage to dental pulp or the supporting periodontium (6002).

Interactions with Herbs & Other Dietary Supplements

HERBS WITH ANTICOAGULANT/ANTIPLATELET POTENTIAL: Concomitant use of herbs that have constituents that might affect platelet aggregation could theoretically increase the risk of bleeding in some people. These herbs include angelica, danshen, garlic, ginger, ginkgo, red clover, turmeric, willow, and others (4,19).

Interactions with Drugs

ANTICOAGULANT/ANTIPLATELET DRUGS: Theoretically, concomitant use may enhance antiplatelet or anticoagulant effects and adverse effects, due to eugenol content of clove oil (6).

Interactions with Foods

None known.

Interactions with Lab Tests

None known.

Interactions with Diseases or Conditions

PLATELET ABNORMALITIES: Theoretically, clove oil is contraindicated in people with reduced platelet counts or platelet function abnormalities (6).

Dosage and Administration

ORAL: Typical dosages for products containing clove oil include 5-30 drops of the fluid extract, 1-5 drops of the oil extract, and 0.5-1 ounce of a mouth rinse containing clove oil (6002).
TOPICAL: As mouthwash, products equivalent to 1-5% clove oil have been used (8).

Comments

Undiluted clove oil is unsafe for self-use, requires application by a trained professional (512). Clove bud oil is considered more valuable than clove leaf and clove stem oils (11). Clove oil is obtained by distillation of the bud, leaf, or stem of the Clove Tree (Syzygium aromaticum).

CLOWN'S MUSTARD PLANT

Also Known As
Bitter Candy Tuft, Bitter Candytuft, Candytuft, Clowns Mustard Plant.
CAUTION: See separate listings for Black Mustard Oil, Black Mustard Seed, Hedge Mustard, and White Mustard.

Scientific Names
Iberis amara, synonym Iberis coronaria.
Family: Brassicaceae/Cruciferae.

People Use This For
Orally, clown's mustard plant is used for gastrointestinal conditions such as dyspepsia, irritable bowel syndrome (IBS), gastritis, and bloating. It is also used for gout, musculoskeletal aches and pains (rheumatism), tachycardia, asthma, bronchitis, and edema (dropsy).

Safety
POSSIBLY SAFE ...when used orally, short-term. There is some evidence that clown's mustard plant extract can be used safely for up to 7 days (7049).
PREGNANCY AND LACTATION: Insufficient reliable information available; avoid using.

Effectiveness
INSUFFICIENT RELIABLE EVIDENCE to RATE

Dyspepsia. There is some preliminary evidence that a specific combination product containing clown's mustard plant extract as a primary ingredient (Ibergast, Phytopharmica) might be helpful for some patients with dyspepsia (7049). More evidence is needed to rate clown's mustard plant for this use.

Mechanism of Action
The applicable parts of clown's mustard plant are the leaves, stem, root, and seeds. The active ingredients and how it might work for gastrointestinal conditions are not known. Some people think it may contain glycosides or flavonoids that could be responsible for any pharmacological effect. However, this has not been verified by scientific studies. Clown's mustard plant does contain the constituent sinapic acid, which has antioxidant properties (7050).

Adverse Reactions
Orally, clown's mustard plant can cause nausea and diarrhea in some patients. Some patients might be hypersensitive to clown's mustard plant. There is one case of a facial rash following oral use (7051).

Interactions with Herbs & Other Dietary Supplements
None known.

Interactions with Drugs
None known.

Interactions with Foods
None known.

Interactions with Lab Tests
None known.

Interactions with Diseases or Conditions
None known.

Dosage and Administration
No typical dosage.

Comments
There is very little scientific information about this product. Our staff is continually analyzing the available information on natural medicines and will add data here as it becomes available.

CLUB MOSS

Also Known As
Lycopodium, Stag's Horn, Vegetable Sulfur, Witch Meal, Wolfs Claw.
CAUTION: See separate listings for Chinese Club Moss and Huperzine A.

Scientific Names
Lycopodium clavatum.
Family: Lycopodiaceae.

People Use This For
Orally, club moss is used for bladder and kidney disorders, and as a diuretic.

Safety
POSSIBLY UNSAFE ...when used orally. Club moss contains toxic alkaloids but no poisonings have been reported (18).
PREGNANCY AND LACTATION: POSSIBLY UNSAFE ...when used orally; avoid using.

Effectiveness
There is insufficient reliable information available about the effectiveness of club moss.

Mechanism of Action
The applicable parts of club moss are the plant and spores. Club moss contains potentially toxic alkaloids, including lycopodine, dihydrolycopodine, and traces of nicotine (18).

Adverse Reactions
None reported.

Interactions with Herbs & Other Dietary Supplements
None known.

Interactions with Drugs
None known.

Interactions with Foods
None known.

Interactions with Lab Tests
None known.

Interactions with Diseases or Conditions
None known.

Dosage and Administration
No typical dosage.

Comments
Avoid confusion with Chinese club moss. Only Chinese club moss contains huperzine A.

COCA

Also Known As
Bolivian Coca, Cocaine Plant, Health Inca Tea, Huanuco Coca, Inca Health Tea, Inca Tea, Java Coca, Mate-de-Coca, Mate de Coca, Peruvian Coca, Spadic, Truxillo Coca.
CAUTION: See separate listing for Cocoa.

Scientific Names
Erythroxylum coca; Erythroxylum novogranatense.
Family: Erythroxylaceae.

People Use This For

Orally, coca is chewed for relief of hunger and fatigue, and enhancing physical performance. Coca extracts are used for stimulating stomach function, causing sedation, and treating asthma, colds, and other ailments.
Coca is the source of cocaine, which is used nasally, injected, or smoked, for mind-altering effects.
Topically, people use the prescription drug cocaine for corneal, nasal, and throat mucosa anesthesia; severe ophthalmologic pain; and local vasoconstriction.
In manufacturing, decocainized coca extract is used to flavor cola drinks and food products.

Safety

LIKELY SAFE ...when decocainized coca leaf extract is used in amounts commonly found in foods. It has Generally Recognized As Safe (GRAS) status in the US (4912). ...when the constituent, cocaine, is used as an FDA-approved product for topical use.
UNSAFE ...when the constituent, cocaine, is ingested or inhaled as a recreational when the constituent, cocaine, is used orally for medicinal purposes (17). 20 mg of cocaine can cause severe side effects and 1.2 grams can be fatal. Cocaine is a Schedule II controlled substance in the US due to extremely high potential for addiction (17).
PREGNANCY: UNSAFE ...when inhaled or used orally. Coca, and the constituent cocaine, are contraindicated due to abortifacient and teratogenic effects (17,6187). Coca use is also associated with a high incidence of Sudden Infant Death Syndrome (SIDS) (17).
LACTATION: UNSAFE ...when inhaled. Coca and the constituent, cocaine, are contraindicated. Cocaine is excreted into breast milk and intoxication can occur in infants breast-fed by mothers recently exposed to cocaine (17,18).

Effectiveness

LIKELY INEFFECTIVE

Athletic performance. Chewing coca leaves doesn't seem to improve physical performance. Coca increases heart rate, but does not appear to improve cardiac output or other physiologic responses to physical exercise (9455,9456).

There is insufficient reliable information available about the effectiveness of coca for its other uses.

Mechanism of Action

The applicable part of coca is the leaf. The major active constituent of coca leaves is the alkaloid cocaine. The leaves also contain essential oils that have not been well identified. The concentration of cocaine is higher in coca grown at lower altitudes and in coca grown under drought conditions (9457). Cocaine has local anesthetic, beta-1, beta-2, and alpha-adrenergic stimulating properties (17). Preliminary evidence suggests that other active constituents in coca leaves, besides cocaine, contribute to the stimulatory effects (9461,9462).
When coca leaves are chewed to improve physical performance, heart rate increases, but cardiac output is not increased. Coca leaves appear to cause a decrease in plasma volume, which blunts cardiac output resulting from increased heart rate. Coca leaves do not improve glucose or fat utilization or other physiologic responses to exercise (9455,9456).
Coca paste is made by mashing coca leaves with alkali, kerosene, and sulfuric acid. The concentration of cocaine in coca paste is over 75%. Coca paste is sometimes used by smoking after it is added to tobacco, but only about 6% of the cocaine survives the heat of smoking (9460).

Adverse Reactions

Adverse effects of coca generally pertain to the cocaine constituent. Initially, these effects can include euphoria, hyperactivity, and restlessness. Later tremors, hyperreflexia, and seizures can develop. Finally, coma, hyporeflexia, respiratory depression, cardiovascular depression, and death may occur. In the central nervous system (CNS), cocaine can also cause migraine headaches, stroke, and intracranial and intracerebral hemorrhage (17,5092). Chewing coca leaves commonly causes anorexia, which often leads to malnutrition. Poor eating habits may contribute to anemia in people that chew coca leaves (9458). Cocaine use is associated with a high incidence of coronary artery disease or other myocardial disease. Up to 38% of cocaine users may have a defect in left ventricular filling (9459). Other cardiovascular adverse effects include extreme elevations of heart rate and blood pressure, vasoconstriction, myocardial ischemia, myocardial infarction, cardiac arrhythmias, cardiomyopathies, myocarditis, endocarditis, aortic rupture, and diffuse micro-aneurysms (17). There is also some evidence that cocaine use can cause platelet activation, platelet microaggregate formation and platelet alpha granule release, which might increase the risk of thrombosis and accelerate the development of atherosclerosis (6374). Cocaine use may cause mesenteric ischemia and rhabdomyolysis-induced renal failure (17). Liver adverse effects include hepatic necrosis, and elevation of serum transaminase and serum creatinine phosphokinase (17). Metabolic adverse effects include lactic acidosis, hyperthermia, hypoglycemia, and hypoxia (17). Use during pregnancy might cause spontaneous abortion, abruptio placentae, and fetal malformation (17). Fetal exposure to cocaine, a constituent of coca, is associated with impaired auditory information processing in newborns (6187). Psychiatric adverse effects include paranoia, depression, and violence (17). Respiratory adverse effects include exacerbation of asthma, thermal airway injury, adult respiratory distress syndrome, pneumothorax, pneumomediastinum, pulmonary thrombosis, bronchiolitis obliterans, pulmonary edema, pulmonary infiltrates, pulmonary vascular disease, and pulmonary hemorrhage (17). Chronic intranasal cocaine abuse is associated with orbital wall (bone) destruction, acquired nasolacrimal duct obstruction, and orbital cellulitis (1258).

Interactions with Herbs & Other Dietary Supplements
CAPSICUM: Theoretically, concomitant use of coca and capsicum (including exposure to pepper spray which contains capsicum) might increase the effects and risk of adverse effects of the cocaine in coca (1394).
MARIJUANA: Concomitant use can have additive effects, including increased heart rate (17).

Interactions with Drugs
ALCOHOL (Ethanol): Concomitant use of alcohol and coca or the cocaine constituent may have additive negative effects on neurocognitive functioning in the brain (6373).
NIFEDIPINE: Nifedipine (Adalat, Procardia) use just prior to cocaine use increases the likelihood of seizures and death (17).

Interactions with Foods
None known.

Interactions with Lab Tests
URINE DRUG TEST: Using coca preparations can cause a positive urine drug test for cocaine. Even some "decocainized" tea preparations can contain 5 mg of cocaine per bag.

Interactions with Diseases or Conditions
ASTHMA: Cocaine use is associated with more severe exacerbations in people with asthma. One study found exacerbations were more severe among cocaine users, compared to non-users, who presented to an emergency room during an asthma attack (6186).
CARDIOVASCULAR DISORDERS: People with cardiovascular disorders might be at increased risk for cocaine-induced cardiovascular side effects (17).
INTRACEREBRAL HEMORRHAGE: Cocaine use is associated with increased morbidity and mortality in patients who sustain intracerebral hemorrhage (5092).
PLASMA PSEUDOCHOLINESTERASE DEFICIENCY (PPD): People with PPD are at increased risk for cocaine-induced cardiovascular side effects, including seizures and death (17).

Dosage and Administration
No typical dosage.

Comments
Coca is considered unsafe and illegal for self-use. Cocaine, a constituent of coca, is an FDA-approved Schedule C-II drug.
Avoid confusion with cocoa seed (Theobroma cacao). A type of tea, known as Inca tea, health Inca tea, or mate de coca, is made from the leaves of Erythroxylum novogranatense. After preparation in boiling water, the tea contains 0.04% cocaine (9460,9484). This tea is illegal in the US.

COCILLANA

Also Known As
Grape Bark, Guapi, Trompillo, Upas.

Scientific Names
Guarea guidonia, synonym Guarea rusbyi, Sycocarpus rusbyi, Guarea guara, Guarea trichilioides; Guarea spiciflora; related Guarea species.
Family: Meliaceae.

People Use This For
Orally, cocillana is used as an ingredient in cough syrups as an expectorant.
Topically, the root bark of Guarea spiciflora is used for skin indurations, and the leaf of Guarea guidonia is used for skin tumors.

Safety
There is insufficient reliable information available about the safety of cocillana.
Pregnancy and Lactation: Insufficient reliable information available; avoid using.

Effectiveness
There is insufficient reliable information available about the effectiveness of cocillana.

Mechanism of Action
The applicable part of cocillana is the bark. Reported (in the late 1800s) to have expectorant and emetic properties; no recent pharmacological or toxicological data is available (11).

Adverse Reactions
None reported.

Interactions with Herbs & Other Dietary Supplements
None known.

Interactions with Drugs
None known.

Interactions with Foods
None known.

Interactions with Lab Tests
None known.

Interactions with Diseases or Conditions
None known.

Dosage and Administration
ORAL: People typically use 0.5 to 1 gram of the powdered bark. In liquid extract form, the dose is 0.5 to 1 mL (223).

COCOA

Also Known As
Cacao, Chocola, Cocoa Bean, Cocoa Butter, Cocoa Oleum, Cocoa Seed, Cocoa Semen, Cocoa Testae, Theobroma, Theobromine.
CAUTION: See separate listings for Coca, Black Tea, Caffeine, Coffee, Cola Nut, Green Tea, Guarana, and Mate.

Scientific Names
Theobroma cacao, synonyms Theobroma sativum.
Family: Malvaceae or Sterculiaceae.

People Use This For
Orally, cocoa seed is used for infectious intestinal diseases and diarrhea, asthma, bronchitis, and as an expectorant for lung congestion. The seed coat is used for liver, bladder and kidney ailments, diabetes, as a tonic, and as a general remedy. Cocoa powder, enriched with flavonoid constituents, is used for prevention of cardiovascular disease.
Topically, cocoa butter has been used to treat wrinkles on the skin and to prevent stretch marks during pregnancy.
In foods, cocoa seed is used as a flavoring agent. Chocolate is produced from cocoa powder.
In manufacturing, cocoa butter is used as a compounding base for various pharmaceutical preparations.

Safety
LIKELY SAFE ...when used orally in amounts commonly found in foods (6). ...when used orally in moderate amounts for medicinal purposes (6). ...when used topically. Cocoa butter is used extensively as a base for ointments and suppositories and is generally considered safe (11).
POSSIBLY UNSAFE ...when used in large amounts. Due to the caffeine content, when used in excessive doses, significant adverse effects may occur, including tachyarrhythmias and sleep disturbances (18).
PREGNANCY: POSSIBLY SAFE ...when used in moderate amounts or in amounts commonly found in foods. Due to the caffeine content of cocoa preparations, mothers should closely monitor their intake to ensure moderate consumption. Fetal blood concentrations of caffeine approximate maternal concentrations (4260). Use of caffeine in pregnancy is controversial; however, moderate consumption has not been associated with clinically important adverse fetal effects (2708,2709,2710,2711,9606). Some sources suggest keeping caffeine consumption below 200 mg per day (2078). Chocolate products provide 2-35 mg caffeine per serving (2078) and a cup of hot chocolate provides approximately 10 mg (3900). POSSIBLY UNSAFE ...when used orally in large amounts. Caffeine found in cocoa crosses the placenta producing fetal blood concentrations similar to maternal levels (4260). Although controversial, some evidence suggests that high doses of caffeine might be associated with premature delivery, low birth weight, and loss of the fetus (6). Some sources suggest keeping caffeine consumption below 200 mg per day (2078). Excessive

use of cocoa in pregnancy should be avoided.
LACTATION: POSSIBLY SAFE ...when used in moderate amounts or in amounts commonly found in foods. Due to the caffeine content of cocoa preparations, mothers should closely monitor their intake to ensure moderate consumption. Breast milk concentrations of caffeine are thought to be approximately 50% of maternal serum concentrations. Moderate consumption of cocoa would likely result in very small amounts of caffeine exposure to a nursing infant (6). POSSIBLY UNSAFE ...when used orally in large amounts. Consumption of excess chocolate (16 oz per day) may cause irritability and increased bowel activity in the infant (6026). Large doses or excessive intake of cocoa should be avoided during lactation.

Effectiveness

There is insufficient reliable information available about the effectiveness of cocoa.

Mechanism of Action

The applicable parts of cocoa are the seed, seed coat, cocoa powder, and butter. Cocoa seed contains oils, tannins, and alkaloids, including theobromine 1-4%, caffeine 0.07-0.36%, trigonelline, and others. Cocoa butter, also referred to as theobroma oil, is the fat obtained from roasted cocoa seeds. It contains oleic acid 37%, stearic acid 34%, palmitic acid 26%, and linoleic acid 2% (13). Cocoa also contains flavonoids, tyramine, phenylethylamine (PEA), magnesium, and possibly N-acylethanolamines (6018,6019). Cocoa has CNS stimulant, cardiac stimulant, coronary dilatory, and diuretic actions (6). Theobromine is the major methylxanthine found in cocoa and has only one-tenth of the cardiac activity of caffeine. In one study, consumption of 1.5 g/kg body weight of chocolate had no acute hemodynamic or physiologic effects on the hearts of healthy, young adults (1373). There has been recent analyses of the health effects of stearic acid, which is found in substantial amounts in cocoa. Unlike other saturated fatty acids, stearic acid does not increase total and low-density lipoprotein (LDL) cholesterol. However, it has been shown that stearic acid can lower high-density lipoprotein (HDL) levels and increase lipoprotein(a). Because of this, the stearic acid content in cocoa products is not thought to provide a reduction in the risk for coronary heart disease as was once proposed (6017,6027). However, preliminary research indicates that flavonoid constituents found in cocoa might be beneficial in cardiovascular disease, much like aspirin. In vitro data has shown that cocoa can stimulate the formation of nitric oxide and inhibit cyclooxygenase formation. In a human trial, patients receiving cocoa powder enriched with flavonoids had decreased epinephrine- or ADP-stimulated expression of fibrinogen-binding glycoprotein IIb-IIIa, indicating that it might inhibit platelet aggregation (6085). Dark chocolate contains higher amounts of flavonoids than milk chocolate (6018). Preliminary evidence suggests a defatted-cocoa extract might also prevent arteries from constricting in the presence of cholesterol. It has been suggested that stearic acid might activate coagulation factor VII and impair fibrinolysis (6027). In contrast, one study concluded that diets high in stearic acid do not increase the tendency toward thrombosis (6020). PEA found in cocoa is structurally and pharmacologically similar to catecholamines and amphetamine. PEA may be a modulator of mood. N-acylethanolamines are pharmacologically related to anandamide, which activates cannabinoid receptors in the brain (6019).

Adverse Reactions

Orally, cocoa can cause allergic skin reactions, shakiness, increased urination, rapid pulse, constipation, and might trigger migraine headaches (6,18). The cocoa in chocolate can cause nausea, gastrointestinal discomfort, borborygmi, and flatus (1373). Topically, cocoa butter has occasionally caused a rash. In animals, it has been shown to be comedogenic; however, this has not been found in humans (11).

Interactions with Herbs & Other Dietary Supplements

CAFFEINE CONTAINING HERBS/SUPPLEMENTS: The caffeine in cocoa may have an additive effect with other caffeine-containing products, and increase the risk of adverse effects. Natural products that contain caffeine include coffee, tea (black or green), guarana, mate, and cola.
EPHEDRA (Ma Huang): The caffeine in cocoa may potentiate stimulant effects of ephedra and increase risk of adverse effects (1275,1380,6486,10307).

Interactions with Drugs

ADENOSINE (Adenocard): The caffeine in cocoa is a competitive inhibitor of adenosine at the cellular level. However, caffeine doesn't seem to affect supplemental adenosine because high interstitial levels of adenosine overcome the antagonistic effects of caffeine (11771).
ANTIDIABETES DRUGS: Concomitant use might interfere with blood glucose control. Cocoa is reported to have hyperglycemic effects (19).
BETA-ADRENERGIC AGONISTS: Theoretically, concomitant use of large amounts of cocoa might increase cardiac inotropic effects of beta-agonists, due to cocoa's caffeine content (15). Beta-adrenergic agonists include albuterol (Ventolin, Proventil), metaproterenol (Alupent), terbutaline (Brethine, Bricanyl), and isoproterenol (Isuprel).
CIMETIDINE (Tagamet): Theoretically, concomitant use might increase the effects of caffeine found in cocoa. Cimetidine decreases caffeine clearance by 30-50% (15,506).
CLOZAPINE (Clozaril): Theoretically, co-administration of clozapine and large amounts of cocoa might acutely exacerbate psychotic symptoms, due to cocoa's caffeine content. Caffeine increases the effects and toxicity of

clozapine (151). Caffeine doses of 400-1000 mg per day inhibit clozapine metabolism (5051).
CONTRACEPTIVE DRUGS: Theoretically, concomitant use might increase the effects of caffeine found in cocoa. Oral contraceptives reduce caffeine clearance by 40-65% (2714,11737).
DIPYRIDAMOLE (Persantine): Theoretically the caffeine in cocoa might inhibit dipyridamole-induced vasodilation (11770,11772).
DISULFIRAM (Antabuse): Theoretically, concomitant use of disulfiram and large amounts of cocoa might increase the effects of caffeine found in cocoa. Disulfiram reduces caffeine clearance (15).
ERGOTAMINE (Ergomar): Theoretically, concomitant use of ergotamine and large amounts of cocoa might increase the GI absorption of ergotamine, due to cocoa's caffeine content (15).
ESTROGENS: Concomitant use can increase serum caffeine concentrations and the risk of caffeine adverse effects. Estrogen inhibits caffeine metabolism (2714).
FLUCONAZOLE (Diflucan): Concomitant use might increase the effects of caffeine in cocoa. Fluconazole decreases caffeine clearance by approximately 25% (11022).
LITHIUM: Theoretically, abrupt withdrawal of large amounts of cocoa might cause lithium toxicity, due to cocoa's caffeine content. Abrupt caffeine withdrawal reportedly increases serum lithium levels (609).
MEXILETINE (Mexitil): Concomitant use might increase the effects and adverse effects of caffeine in cocoa. Mexiletine can decrease caffeine elimination by 50% (1260,11741).
MONOAMINE OXIDASE INHIBITORS (MAOIs): Theoretically, concomitant use of MAOIs with large amounts of cocoa might precipitate a hypertensive crisis due to cocoa's tyramine content (19).
PHENYLPROPANOLAMINE: Concomitant use of phenylpropanolamine and cocoa might cause an additive increase in blood pressure due to the caffeine in cocoa (11738).
QUINOLONE ANTIBIOTICS: Theoretically, concomitant use might increase the effects of caffeine found in cocoa. Quinolones decrease caffeine clearance (606,607,608). Quinolones (fluoroquinolones) include ciprofloxacin (Cipro), enoxacin (Penetrex), norfloxacin (Chibroxin, Noroxin), sparfloxacin (Zagam), trovafloxacin (Trovan), and grepafloxacin (Raxar).
THEOPHYLLINE: Theoretically, concomitant use of theophylline and large amounts of cocoa might increase the risk of theophylline toxicity, due to cocoa's caffeine content. Caffeine decreases theophylline clearance by 23% to 29% (506).
VERAPAMIL (Calan, Covera, Isoptin, Verelan): Theoretically, concomitant use might increase the effects of caffeine found in cocoa. Verapamil can increase plasma caffeine levels by 25% (15,506).

Interactions with Foods

GRAPEFRUIT JUICE: Theoretically, concomitant use might increase the caffeine effects of cocoa. Grapefruit might decrease caffeine clearance (4300).

Interactions with Lab Tests

5-HYDROXYINDOLEACETIC ACID: Theoretically, large amounts of cocoa might increase urine 5-hydroxyindoleacetic acid concentrations and test results, due to its caffeine content. Caffeine can increase urine catecholamine concentrations (15).
BLEEDING TIME: Theoretically, large amounts of cocoa might prolong bleeding time and increase test results, due to its caffeine content (1701).
BLOOD PRESSURE: Theoretically, large amounts of cocoa might increase blood pressure and blood pressure readings, due to its caffeine content (4).
CATECHOLAMINES: Theoretically, large amounts of cocoa might increase urine catecholamine concentrations and test results, due to its caffeine content (15).
CREATINE: Theoretically, large amounts of cocoa might increase urine creatine concentrations and test results, due to its caffeine content (1701).
PHARMACOLOGICAL STRESS TESTS: The caffeine in cocoa is a competitive antagonist for adenosine receptors (11771). It is recommended that caffeine and caffeine-containing products be stopped 24 hours prior to pharmacological stress tests (11770). However, caffeine appears more likely to interfere with dipyridamole (Persantine) than adenosine (Adenocard) stress testing (11771). The interaction between caffeine and dipyridamole is unlikely to be significant in stress testing if the heart rate increase is greater than 5% after dipyridamole infusion (11772).
URATE: Theoretically, large amounts of cocoa might falsely increase serum urate test results determined by the Bittner method, due to its caffeine content (15).
VANILLYLMANDELIC ACID (VMA): Theoretically, large amounts of cocoa might increase urine VMA concentrations and test results, due to its caffeine content (15).

Interactions with Diseases or Conditions

ANXIETY: Theoretically, large amounts of cocoa might aggravate anxiety disorders, due to its caffeine content (506).
DIABETES: Cocoa might interfere with blood glucose control. Cocoa is reported to have hyperglycemic effects (19).
DEPRESSION: Theoretically, large amounts of cocoa might aggravate depression disorders, due to its caffeine content (506).

GASTRIC ULCERS, DUODENAL ULCERS: Theoretically, large amounts of cocoa might aggravate ulcers, due to its caffeine content (506).
GASTROESOPHAGEAL REFLUX DISEASE (GERD): Cocoa reduces lower esophageal sphincter pressure (1374).
HEART CONDITIONS: Theoretically, large amounts of cocoa might induce cardiac arrhythmias in sensitive individuals, due to its caffeine content (506).
IRRITABLE BOWEL SYNDROME (IBS): Avoid cocoa-containing products including chocolate which might aggravate irritable bowel syndrome (6).
MIGRAINE HEADACHES: Theoretically, cocoa might trigger migraines in sensitive individuals (18).

Dosage and Administration

No typical dosage.

Comments

Avoid confusion with coca leaf (Erythroxylon coca). Bitter chocolate is produced by pressing roasted cocoa kernels between hot rollers. Cocoa powder is produced by expressing the cocoa butter from bitter chocolate and powdering the remaining residue. Sweet chocolate is produced by adding sugar and vanilla to bitter chocolate (13).
The candy company, Mars, Inc., plans to seek a health claim for chocolate from the Food and Drug Administration in the next few years based on preliminary research they sponsored regarding the potential role of cocoa flavonoids in cardiovascular health (1329).

COCONUT OIL

Also Known As

Coconut Palm, Coco Palm.

Scientific Names

Cocos nucifera.
Family: Arecaceae/Palmae.

People Use This For

Orally, coconut oil is used for weight loss, heart disease, hypercholesterolemia, diabetes, chronic fatigue, Crohn's disease, irritable bowel syndrome, disease prevention, thyroid conditions, energy, and boosting the immune system.
Topically, coconut oil is used for psoriasis, as a skin emollient.

Safety

LIKELY SAFE ...when used orally and appropriately in food amounts (4912).
POSSIBLY SAFE ...when used topically and appropriately (12356).
There is insufficient reliable information about the safety of coconut oil when used orally in medicinal amounts.
PREGNANCY AND LACTATION: LIKELY SAFE ...when used orally and appropriately in food amounts (4912).
There is insufficient reliable information about the safety of coconut oil when used orally or topically in medicinal amounts.

Effectiveness

INSUFFICIENT RELIABLE EVIDENCE to RATE

Psoriasis. Applying coconut oil to the skin before treatment of psoriasis with ultra violet-B (UVB) or psoralen and ultraviolet A (PUVA) phototherapy doesn't seem to improve efficacy (12356). More evidence is needed to rate coconut oil for this use.

Mechanism of Action

Coconut oil is obtained from the dried nut (fruit) of the coconut palm. About half of coconut oil is made up of medium-chain fatty acids. Lauric acid is the major constituent, followed by myristic and palmitic acids. Coconut oil is the most saturated oil compared with palm, soybean, and corn oils; and animal fats such as butter and lard. It contains 76 grams of saturated fatty acids per 100 grams of fat (12357,12358).
Although medium-chain fatty acids undergo rapid metabolism, oils such as coconut oil can raise total and low-density lipoprotein (LDL) levels (12358,12361). Animal research suggests that coconut oil has an atherogenic effect, possibly by increasing pro-inflammatory cytokines such as interleukin (IL)-1beta and tumor necrosis factor (TNF)-alpha (12362). However, other preliminary clinical research suggests that coconut oil lowers postprandial tissue plasminogen activator (tPA) antigen and lipoprotein (a) levels, which might have a beneficial effect on cardiovascular disease (12363).
Topically, coconut oil doesn't block ultraviolet A (UVA) or ultraviolet B (UVB) radiation (12356).

Adverse Reactions
Orally, coconut oil can rarely cause allergic reactions (12359,12360). Coconut oil is high in fat, which can cause weight gain. It also can increase cholesterol (12358).

Interactions with Herbs & Other Dietary Supplements
None known.

Interactions with Drugs
None known.

Interactions with Foods
None known.

Interactions with Lab Tests
CHOLESTEROL: Coconut oil can increase total and low-density lipoprotein (LDL) cholesterol levels and test results (12358).

Interactions with Diseases or Conditions
HYPERCHOLESTEROLEMIA: Coconut oil can increase total and low-density lipoprotein (LDL) cholesterol levels and may adversely affect treatment (12358).

Dosage and Administration
No typical dosage.

COD LIVER OIL

Also Known As
Cod Oil, Fish Oil, Liver Oil, N-3 Fatty Acids, Omega-3 Fatty Acids, Polyunsaturated Fatty Acids.
CAUTION: See separate listings for DHA (docosahexaenoic acid), EPA (eicosapentaenoic acid), Fish Oil, and Shark Liver Oil.

Scientific Names
None.

People Use This For
Orally, cod liver oil is used for hyperlipidemia, hypertriglyceridemia, albuminuria associated with diabetic nephropathy, hypertension, coronary heart disease, osteoarthritis, systemic lupus erythematosus (SLE), and otitis media.
Topically, cod liver oil is used to accelerate wound healing.

Safety
LIKELY SAFE ...when used orally and appropriately (3398,3399,4026).
POSSIBLY UNSAFE ...when used orally in excessive doses. Doses greater than 25 mL daily might decrease blood coagulation and increase the risk of bleeding (4025,4026). There is also some concern about vitamin A and vitamin D toxicity. On average 20 mL of cod liver oil provides 15,000 IU vitamin A and 1500 IU vitamin D (4003,4004).
There is insufficient reliable information available about the safety of cod liver oil when used topically.
PREGNANCY AND LACTATION: Insufficient reliable information available; avoid using.

Effectiveness
LIKELY EFFECTIVE

Hypertriglyceridemia. Taking cod liver oil orally can reduce triglyceride levels by 20-50% in patients with hypertriglyceridemia (3399,4026,5705,5706).

POSSIBLY EFFECTIVE

Diabetic nephropathy. There is some evidence that taking cod liver oil orally can reduce albuminuria in type 2 diabetes patients with nephropathy (1025).

Hypertension. Taking cod liver oil orally seems to produce modest, but significant, reductions in systolic and diastolic blood pressure in patients with mild hypertension (1001,1020,3399).

POSSIBLY INEFFECTIVE

Hypercholesterolemia. Taking cod liver oil does not seem to decrease serum total or high-density lipoprotein (HDL) cholesterol or triglycerides in patients with familial hypercholesterolemia (10083).

Osteoarthritis. Taking cod liver oil orally, in combination with nonsteroidal anti-inflammatory drugs (NSAIDs), does not seem to decrease pain or inflammation when compared to NSAID treatment alone (3398).

INSUFFICIENT RELIABLE EVIDENCE to RATE

Otitis media. Preliminary clinical evidence suggests that oral cod liver oil, in combination with a children's multivitamin-mineral preparation containing selenium, might prevent or decrease the frequency of otitis media in young children (10151). More evidence is needed to rate cod liver oil for this use.

Mechanism of Action

Cod liver oil contains high amounts of long-chain, polyunsaturated fats called omega-3 fatty acids. Cod liver oil is especially high in the omega-3 fatty acids docosahexaenoic acid (DHA) and eicosapentaenoic acid (EPA). Cod liver oil also contains a significant amount of vitamins A and D. On average, 20 mL of cod liver oil contains 1.8 grams EPA, 2.2 grams DHA, 15,000 IU vitamin A, and 1500 IU vitamin D (4003,4004,4026). Cod liver oil fatty acids compete with arachidonic acid for the cyclooxygenase and lipoxygenase pathways (4026,10080). Cod liver oil's anti-inflammatory effects are likely due to inhibition of leukotriene synthesis (3392,4026,10080).

Because of this effect, there is interest in cod liver oil for heart disease prevention. Cod liver oil also has antithrombotic effects. It decreases blood viscosity and increases red blood cell deformability, increases prostacyclin synthesis and related vasodilation, reduces thrombogenicity of platelets and monocytes, reduces platelet adhesiveness, and reduces platelet count (3399,4005,4022,4025,10077,10080). Preliminary research suggests cod liver oil may be useful in improving long-term graft patency following arterial bypass reconstruction (10082).

In hypertriglyceridemia, cod liver oil is thought to lower triglycerides by decreasing secretion of very low-density lipoproteins (VLDLs), increasing VLDL apolipoprotein B secretion, possibly by increasing VLDL clearance, decreasing VLDL size, and reducing triglyceride transport (3397,3399,4026).

The DHA and EPA fatty acids found in cod liver oil make up a third of all lipids in the brain's grey matter (425). DHA and EPA play a key role in the structural development of retinal, neural, and synaptic membranes and are thought to be important for normal neural function (424,425). Animals who are deficient in omega-3 fatty acids develop learning and vision disturbances (424).

In patients with non-insulin dependent diabetic neuropathy, cod liver oil is thought to improve albuminuria by reducing microvascular albumin leakage (1025).

Preliminary research suggests concurrent use of cod liver oil with nonsteroidal anti-inflammatory drug (NSAID) administration may play a role in the prevention of NSAID-induced gastropathy (10081).

Some researchers think low levels of EPA, selenium, and vitamin A might predispose some children to acute otitis media (10151).

Adverse Reactions

Orally, cod liver oil can have a fishy taste and might cause belching, nosebleeds, halitosis, and heartburn. High doses can cause nausea and loose stools. Some gastrointestinal side effects can be minimized if cod liver oil is taken with meals and if doses are started low and gradually increased. Doses greater than 25 mL might also decrease blood coagulation and potentially increase the risk of bleeding (1313,4025,4026). Long-term cod liver oil supplementation is associated with an increased risk of cutaneous malignant melanoma in women (3395). There is one case of lipoid pneumonia as a result of long-term cod liver oil use (3396). There is also some concern about vitamin A and vitamin D toxicity in people using cod liver oil long-term. On average, 20 mL of cod liver oil provides 15,000 IU vitamin A and 1500 IU vitamin D (4003,4004).

Interactions with Herbs & Other Dietary Supplements

HERBS & SUPPLEMENTS WITH ANTICOAGULANT/ANTIPLATELET POTENTIAL: Concomitant use of herbs that constituents that might affect platelet aggregation could theoretically increase the risk of bleeding in some people. These herbs include angelica, borage seed oil, clove, danshen, garlic, ginger, ginkgo, red clover, turmeric, willow, and others.

Interactions with Drugs

ANTICOAGULANT/ANTIPLATELET DRUGS: Concomitant use with anticoagulant or antiplatelet drugs can increase the risk of bleeding (3399,4005,4022,4025,10077,10080). Some of these drugs include aspirin, clopidogrel (Plavix), dalteparin (Fragmin), dipyridamole (Persantine), enoxaparin (Lovenox), heparin, ticlopidine (Ticlid), warfarin (Coumadin), and others.

ANTIHYPERTENSIVE DRUGS: Cod liver oil can lower blood pressure and might have additive effects in patients treated with antihypertensives (1001,1020,3399); use with caution.

Interactions with Foods

None known.

Interactions with Lab Tests

BLOOD PRESSURE: Cod liver oil might moderately lower blood pressure and reduce blood pressure readings (1001,1020,3399,4026).

INTERNATIONAL NORMALIZED RATIO (INR), PROTHROMBIN TIME (PT): High doses of greater than 25 mL per day might decrease blood coagulation, increase INR and PT, and increase the risk

of bleeding (1313,4025,4026).
TRIGLYCERIDES: Cod liver oil can reduce serum triglyceride concentrations and test results in patients with hypercholesterolemia (3399,4026,5705,5706).

Interactions with Diseases or Conditions

DIABETES: Cod liver oil should be used with caution because omega-3 fatty acids in cod liver oil might increase blood glucose levels (3397). Monitor blood glucose levels closely. Dose adjustments may be necessary.
HYPERTENSION: Cod liver oil can lower blood pressure and might have additive effects in patients treated with antihypertensives (1001,1020,3399,4026); use with caution.

Dosage and Administration

ORAL: For lowering triglycerides, 20 mL of cod liver oil per day has been used (3399,4026). For familial hypercholesterolemia, 30 ml of cod liver oil per day has been used (10083). For lowering blood pressure, 20 mL of cod liver oil per day has been used (3399,4026).

CODONOPSIS

Also Known As

Bastard Ginseng, Bellflower, Bonnet Bellflower, Chuan Dang, Codonopsis Pilosula Modesta, Dangshen, Radix Codonopsis.
CAUTION: See separate listings for Ashwaganda, Blue Cohosh, Canaigre, Ginseng American, Ginseng Panax, and Ginseng Siberian.

Scientific Names

Codonopsis pilosula; Codonopsis tangshen; Codonopsis tubulosa; other Codonopsis species.
Family: Campanulaceae.

People Use This For

Orally, codonopsis is used to treat HIV infection and as a protective adjuvant to radiotherapy in cancer treatment. It is used orally as a substitute for ginseng in general tonic formulas, as an immune tonic, for weakness, anorexia, chronic diarrhea, dyspnea, palpitations, asthma, cough, thirst, and diabetes.

Safety

POSSIBLY SAFE ...when used orally and appropriately (12).
PREGNANCY AND LACTATION: Insufficient reliable information available; avoid using.

Effectiveness

There is insufficient reliable information available about the effectiveness of codonopsis.

Mechanism of Action

Codonopsis seems to be able to stimulate the central nervous system (CNS). It seems to promote weight gain, increase endurance, increase tolerance to anoxia, elevate temperature, increase macrophage activity, increase red and white blood cell counts, and promote peripheral vasodilation (11). Codonopsis also has hypotensive, adrenergic blocking, radioprotective and ulcer-protective effects (11).

Adverse Reactions

None reported.

Interactions with Herbs & Other Dietary Supplements

None known.

Interactions with Drugs

None known.

Interactions with Foods

None known.

Interactions with Lab Tests

None known.

Interactions with Diseases or Conditions

None known.

Dosage and Administration

ORAL: People typically use 12 to 15 grams codonopsis added to 3 to 4 cups water and boiled until the volume is reduced by one-half. The cooled liquid is taken in 2 doses on an empty stomach (5251).

Comments

No ginseng saponins have been found in codonopsis (11).

COENZYME Q-10

Also Known As

Coenzyme Q10, Co Q10.

Scientific Names

Ubiquinol; Ubiquinone; Ubidecarenone; Mitoquinone.

People Use This For

Orally, coenzyme Q-10 is used for congestive heart failure (CHF), angina, diabetes, hypertension, periodontal disease, cardiotoxicity associated with doxorubicin (Adriamycin) chemotherapy, and breast cancer. It is also used orally for Huntington's disease, Parkinson's disease, muscular dystrophy, increasing exercise tolerance, chronic fatigue syndrome (CFS), and warfarin-induced alopecia. Coenzyme Q-10 is also used orally for stimulating the immune systems of people with HIV/AIDS, life extension, male infertility, idiopathic asthenozoospermia, migraine headache, quinone-responsive mitochondrial encephalomyelopathy, and for preventing "statin"-induced myopathy. Topically, coenzyme Q-10 is used for treating periodontal disease.

Safety

LIKELY SAFE ...when used orally and appropriately. There have been no reports of significant toxicity associated with coenzyme Q-10 in studies lasting up to 30 months (2134,6037,6038,6407,8163,8938,8939,8940). ...when used topically on the gums (2107).

PREGNANCY AND LACTATION: Insufficient reliable information available; avoid using.

Effectiveness

EFFECTIVE

Huntington's disease. Ubiquinol, a reduced form of coenzyme Q-10, has FDA Orphan Drug status for Huntington's disease (11873). Taking coenzyme Q-10 orally in doses of 600 mg per day or less doesn't seem to be effective for slowing the progression or functional decline in patients with Huntington's disease (1357,8940).

Mitochondrial encephalomyopathies. Taking coenzyme Q-10 orally seems to reduce symptoms in some patients with genetic and acquired disorders of mitochondrial dysfunction (8159,8162,8163,8912). The onset of effect is slow, with maximal effect at six months (8163). A specific coenzyme Q-10 formulation (UbiQGel) has FDA Orphan Drug status for mitochondrial encephalomyopathies, including MELAS (myoclonic epilepsy with lactic acidosis and stroke-like episodes) syndrome, Kearns-Sayre syndrome, and MERRF (myoclonus epilepsy with ragged red fibers).

Pediatric congestive heart failure. Ubiquinol, a reduced form of coenzyme Q-10, has FDA Orphan Drug status for pediatric congestive heart failure (11873).

LIKELY EFFECTIVE

Coenzyme Q-10 deficiency. Taking coenzyme Q-10 orally seems to improve symptoms of coenzyme Q-10 deficiency (8160,8161). Rare cases of documented coenzyme Q-10 deficiency with symptoms of weakness, fatigue, and seizures have been reported.

POSSIBLY EFFECTIVE

Congestive heart failure (CHF). Adding oral coenzyme Q-10 to conventional treatments seems to improve quality of life, improve New York Heart Association classification, decrease hospitalization rates, and decrease symptoms of heart failure such as dyspnea, peripheral edema, enlarged liver, and insomnia in patients with mild to severe (New York Heart Association Class II-IV) CHF (6407,6408,6409,8909,11893,12170). However, the effectiveness of coenzyme Q-10 for heart failure is controversial (8910). Some research suggests that coenzyme Q-10 does not improve objective measures of CHF including ejection fraction or exercise tolerance (5090,6037,6038). Tell patients there's no evidence that coenzyme Q-10 can help heart failure when taken alone, but it might be helpful when taken with other heart failure drugs.

HIV/AIDS. Taking coenzyme Q-10 orally seems to improve immune function in people with HIV/AIDS (2123,2124).

Hypertension. Taking coenzyme Q-10 orally with other antihypertensives seems to provide an additional blood pressure lowering effect and might allow dosage reduction or discontinuation of some antihypertensive medications (2122,3365,9890).

Ischemic reperfusion injury. Taking coenzyme Q-10 orally for a week before cardiac bypass or vascular surgery might lessen hypoxic damage during surgery (11902,11903). But other research suggests no effect (11904).

Isolated systolic hypertension. Taking coenzyme Q-10 orally appears to lower systolic blood pressure by about 26% in some people with isolated systolic hypertension after 12 weeks of therapy (8907).

Migraine headache. Taking coenzyme Q-10 orally might be useful for preventing migraine headaches. It seems to reduce migraine attacks by about a third (8135,11872).

Muscular dystrophy. Taking coenzyme Q-10 orally seems to improve physical performance in some patients with muscular dystrophies (2127).

Myocardial infarction (MI). Taking coenzyme Q-10 orally seems to decrease the risk of cardiac events in patients with recent MI who are at risk of atherothrombosis. When started in patients within 72 hours of MI and administered for 1 year, coenzyme Q-10 appears to significantly lower the risk of cardiac events including non-fatal MI and cardiac death (10152).

Parkinson's disease. Taking high doses of coenzyme Q-10, 300-1200 mg orally per day, seems to slow functional decline in people with early Parkinson's disease. The effect appears to be dose dependent (8938).

LIKELY INEFFECTIVE

Athletic performance. Taking coenzyme Q-10 orally doesn't improve aerobic power in athletes (2109,2110,8911). Some evidence suggests coenzyme Q-10 might slightly improve tolerance to higher workloads, but more research is needed to tell if coenzyme Q-10 is effective for this purpose (8911).

Periodontal disease. Coenzyme Q-10 applied topically isn't effective for treating periodontal disease (2107,2108). However, preliminary research suggests that taking coenzyme Q-10 orally might be helpful for periodontal disease (8916,8917,8918); more evidence is needed.

INSUFFICIENT RELIABLE EVIDENCE to RATE

Angina. Some preliminary clinical research suggests that taking coenzyme Q-10 orally might improve exercise tolerance in patients with angina (2121). Breast cancer. There is preliminary evidence that taking coenzyme Q-10 orally might be helpful in advanced breast cancer along with surgery and conventional therapy plus other antioxidants and omega-3 and omega-6 fatty acids (3993,3995).

Diabetes. There is conflicting evidence about the effectiveness of coenzyme Q-10 for diabetes. Some research suggests that taking 200 mg coenzyme Q-10 per day reduces hemoglobin A1c in people with type 2 diabetes (9890,11877). However, other research in type 2 diabetes using the same dose shows no effect on hemoglobin A1c (492). Some research in people with type 1 diabetes also shows no effect (456,2126). In patients with hypertension and coronary artery disease, there is evidence that coenzyme Q-10 might reduce insulin resistance (3365).

Infertility. Preliminary evidence suggests that infertile men with idiopathic asthenozoospermia who take coenzyme Q-10 200 mg/day have increased sperm motility after 6 months of treatment (12169).

Maternally inherited diabetes mellitus and deafness (MIDD). There is some preliminary evidence that taking coenzyme Q-10 orally might prevent progressive insulin secretory defect, exercise intolerance, and hearing loss in people with a rare form of diabetes called maternally inherited diabetes mellitus and deafness (MIDD) (2125).

Statin-induced myopathy. There is some preliminary evidence that coenzyme Q-10 might lessen muscular adverse effects caused by high-dose HMG-CoA reductase inhibitors ("satins"). In people taking high-dose lovastatin investigationally for cancer treatment, coenzyme Q-10 seems to lessen the effect of statins on muscles (11899,11900). But there are no clinical trials of the effect of coenzyme Q-10 in hypercholesterolemic people taking statins at usual doses.

Warfarin-induced hair loss. There is some preliminary evidence that coenzyme Q-10 might be helpful for preventing warfarin-induced hair loss (455).

More evidence is needed to rate coenzyme Q-10 for these uses.

Mechanism of Action

Coenzyme Q-10 is a vitamin-like compound present in virtually all cells and in especially high concentrations in the heart, liver, kidney, and pancreas. Within the cell, 25-30% of total coenzyme Q-10 is found in the nucleus, 40-50% in the mitochondria, 15-20% in the microsomes, and 5-10% in the cytosol. Coenzyme Q-10 is fat soluble and acts similar to a vitamin (2134,11892). Its primary functions include activity as an antioxidant, a membrane stabilizer, and as a cofactor in many metabolic pathways, particularly in the production of adenosine triphosphate (ATP) in oxidative respiration (2134,6037,6048,6410,11892).

The body produces adequate amounts of coenzyme Q-10, so it's not considered a vitamin (11893). It's also ingested in small amounts from dietary sources, including meats and seafood. However, the amounts ingested in foods do not approach therapeutic doses. Coenzyme Q-10 formulated in soy bean oil appears to have superior bioavailability compared to other formulations (457). Peak levels of coenzyme Q-10 after oral administration occur in 5-10 hours, and the half-life is approximately 34 hours (2134,8907).

Many of the therapeutic benefits of coenzyme Q-10 are primarily attributed to its antioxidant effects and its role in the generation of ATP. Genetic or acquired disorders of mitochondrial function cause increases in serum lactate and the lactate/pyruvate ratio, due to impaired oxidative metabolism. Supplementation with coenzyme Q-10 seems to reduce these levels and improve exercise tolerance and function in people with these disorders (8159,8162,8163).

In addition, coenzyme Q-10 may be helpful for people with diseases for which coenzyme Q-10 levels are often lower, including congestive heart failure (CHF), hypertension, periodontal disease, certain muscular diseases, and AIDS (2134,6410).

In the treatment of CHF, the mechanism is thought to involve prevention of oxidative damage. The greatest benefit seems to occur in people with the largest deficiency of coenzyme Q-10 (2134). The effect in the treatment of angina may be due to increased ATP synthesis, reduction of free radicals, or membrane protection (2134). Preliminary evidence suggests that coenzyme Q-10 might enhance endothelium-independent arterial relaxation and improve endothelium-dependent vasodilation, which can lower total peripheral resistance and systolic blood pressure. This effect seems to be caused by increased endothelial production of prostacyclin (PGI2) or increased sensitivity of arterial smooth muscle to PGI2, or both (8908).

Coenzyme Q-10 increases plasma levels of high density lipoprotein (HDL) cholesterol, vitamin E, and vitamin C; and decreases levels of total cholesterol, low density lipoprotein (LDL) cholesterol, and products of lipid peroxidation such as thiobarbituric acid reactive substances (TBARS), malondialdehyde, and diene conjugates. In patients at risk for future coronary events, coenzyme Q-10 may prevent thrombosis and have protective effects on vascular and myocardial remodeling and endothelial function (10152).

Coenzyme Q-10 levels are highest during the first 20 years of life and decline with age. At age 80, coenzyme Q-10 levels may be lower than at birth. In some kinds of bacteria, coenzyme Q-10 supplements seem to prolong life (11895). However, life-long administration of coenzyme Q-10 to rodents doesn't affect lifespan (11896).

Coenzyme Q-10 can undergo oxidation/reduction reactions in various cell membranes such as lysosomes, Golgi, or plasma membranes. The proton gradient caused by the redox ability of coenzyme Q-10 provides a basis for antioxidant action either directly or by regeneration of vitamin E (tocopherol) and ascorbate (8913). Preliminary research suggests that decreased redox status of coenzyme Q-10 might indicate a higher risk for coronary heart disease in people with familial hyperlipidemia (8914). Fenofibrate (Tricor) and coenzyme Q-10 seem to improve endothelial and non-endothelial forearm vasodilator function in dyslipidemic type 2 diabetic patients (11877).

Coenzyme Q-10 appears to be a factor in Parkinson's disease. Parkinson's disease might be caused by impaired function of the mitochondrial electron transport chain, and particularly the mitochondrial enzymes, complex I and complex II. Coenzyme Q-10 is the electron acceptor for these complexes. People with Parkinson's disease seem to have lower levels of coenzyme Q-10 in platelet mitochondria. Preclinical research suggests that supplementation increases cerebral concentrations of coenzyme Q-10 and reduces the loss of dopamine and dopaminergic axons in experimental models of Parkinson's disease (8938,8939).

There is also interest in using coenzyme Q-10 for Huntington's disease, which is also thought to be a mitochondrial disorder. In animal models of Huntington's disease, orally administered coenzyme Q-10 extends survival and delays development of motor deficits, weight loss, cerebral atrophy, and neuronal changes (8941). Usefulness in humans hasn't been demonstrated at doses of 600 mg per day or less (8940). Some researchers suggest that L-carnitine and coenzyme Q-10 might have an additive or synergistic effect. Both coenzyme Q-10 and L-carnitine are involved with maintaining mitochondrial energy production in cells and may help protect against oxidative and toxin-induced damage (3653,9603), but it isn't known whether this has any clinical significance.

As a potential prophylactic treatment for migraine headaches, coenzyme Q-10 might work by improving mitochondrial oxidative phosphorylation, which appears to be impaired in some patients with migraines (8135,11897).

HMG-CoA reductase inhibitors ("statins") may reduce serum coenzyme Q-10 levels. Intramuscular levels don't appear to be affected. Some researchers think statin-induced myopathy may be related to mitochondrial dysfunction. Coenzyme Q-10 and cholesterol share common synthetic pathways. Some evidence suggests that statins may block the synthesis of both. But coenzyme Q-10 does not affect the cholesterol lowering effect of statins (11898).

Some drugs inhibit coenzyme Q-10 activity. Preliminary evidence suggests that the negative inotropic effect of some beta-blockers, particularly propranolol (Inderal), and to a lesser extent metoprolol (Lopressor, Toprol), is caused by inhibition of coenzyme Q-10 dependent enzymes in the myocardium (3368,3369,8958). Preliminary in-vitro evidence suggests coenzyme Q-10 might prevent cardiotoxicity caused by phenothiazines and tricyclic antidepressants. It seems to block mitochondrial dysfunction induced by these drugs (8959).

Coenzyme Q-10 also seems to protect against doxorubicin (Adriamycin) cardiotoxicity, possibly through correction of coenzyme Q-10 deficiencies and scavenging of free radicals (2134). Researchers are also interested in coenzyme Q-10's possible anticancer effects related to its antioxidant properties. Coenzyme Q-10 might also have immunostimulatory activity (3993). There is also some evidence that coenzyme Q-10 concentrations are lower in cancerous breast tissue than healthy tissue (4846,5158). Some researchers speculate that very low levels of coenzyme Q-10 might be an indicator of a poor prognosis (4846).

Adverse Reactions

Orally, coenzyme Q-10 is generally well tolerated. In clinical studies, there have been no reports of significant adverse effects (2134,6037,6038,6047,8135,8938,8939,8940). Coenzyme Q-10 can cause gastrointestinal side effects such as nausea, vomiting, diarrhea, appetite suppression, heartburn, and epigastric discomfort in less than 1% of patients (2134,3370,8135,8938,8939,8940,10152). Some of these adverse effects can be minimized if total daily doses exceeding 100 mg are divided and administered two to three times per day (3370). Allergic rash has been reported (11872).

Interactions with Herbs & Other Dietary Supplements

L-CARNITINE: Some researchers suggest that L-carnitine and coenzyme Q-10 might have an additive or synergistic effect. Both coenzyme Q-10 and L-carnitine are involved with maintaining mitochondrial energy production cells and may help protect against oxidative and toxin-induced damage (3653,9603).

RED YEAST: Theoretically, since red yeast has HMG-CoA reductase inhibitor ("statin") constituents (512), it might reduce coenzyme Q-10 levels.

Interactions with Drugs

ANTIHYPERTENSIVE DRUGS: Coenzyme Q-10 can decrease blood pressure and might have additive blood pressure lowering effects when used with antihypertensive drugs (2122,9890); use with caution.
CHEMOTHERAPY: Preliminary evidence suggests that inhibition of coenzyme Q-10 dependent enzymes contributes to the cardiotoxicity associated with doxorubicin (Adriamycin). Theoretically, CoQ-10 supplements might prevent this toxicity, but might also lower effectiveness (3368). There is some concern that taking antioxidants such as coenzyme Q-10 might protect tumor cells from chemotherapeutic agents that work by inducing oxidative stress, such as the alkylating agents (e.g., cyclophosphamide, Cytoxan) and radiation therapy (5158,5159). Consider potential risk versus potential benefit before using coenzyme Q-10.
WARFARIN (Coumadin): Concomitant use might reduce the anticoagulation effects of warfarin (2128,6048,6199). Coenzyme Q-10 is chemically similar to menaquinone and may have vitamin K-like procoagulant effects. Four cases of decreased warfarin efficacy thought to be due to coenzyme Q-10 have been reported (2128,6048). However, clinical research suggests that coenzyme Q-10 does not affect the anticoagulative effects of warfarin (11905). Closely monitor patients taking warfarin and coenzyme Q-10. Dose adjustment may be necessary.

Drug Influences on Nutrient Levels and Depletion

SOME DRUGS CAN AFFECT COENZYME Q-10 LEVELS:
HMG CoA REDUCTASE INHIBITORS ("Statins"): HMG CoA reductase inhibitors can reduce serum coenzyme Q-10 levels (4404,4405,4406,4407,4408,4409,4410). They block the synthesis of mevalonic acid, which is a precursor of coenzyme Q-10 (3370).
Statins' effect on coenzyme Q-10 appear to be dose-related. Taking atorvastatin (Lipitor) 10 mg/day or pravastatin (Pravachol) 20 mg/day doesn't seem to decrease levels of circulating coenzyme Q-10 in healthy people (8915). But taking atorvastatin 80 mg/day for 30 days reduces coenzyme Q-10 levels by 52% (12099).
The clinical significance of statins' effect on coenzyme Q-10 levels is unclear. For example, taking simvastatin 20 mg/day for 4 weeks reduces serum coenzyme Q-10 levels about 32%, but levels in muscle may actually increase, up to 47% according to one study (3367).
Some researchers suspect that depletion of coenzyme Q-10 levels might result in statin-related side effects such as myopathy. But so far there is no reliable evidence that coenzyme Q-10 depletion is the cause of statin side effects. There is also no proof that taking coenzyme Q-10 supplements reduces statin side effects.
Other "statin" drugs include lovastatin (Mevacor), simvastatin (Zocor), and fluvastatin (Lescol).

Interactions with Foods

None known.

Interactions with Lab Tests

GLYCOSYLATED HEMOGLOBIN (Hemoglobin A1C, Hg A1C): Some clinical research suggests that coenzyme Q-10 can reduce glycosylated hemoglobin in people with type 2 diabetes (9890,11877). However, other research suggests no effect (456,492). Coenzyme Q-10 doesn't seem to affect fasting blood glucose (9890,11877).
LIVER ENZYMES: Coenzyme Q-10 does not seem to adversely affect liver function. Despite earlier concern that doses greater than 300 mg per day might cause increases in SGOT (Serum Glutamic-Oxaloacetic Transaminase) and LDH (Lactic Dehydrogenase) (2134), doses greater than 600 mg per day given for 30 months have not caused changes in liver function (8938,8939,8940).
T4/T8 RATIO: Coenzyme Q-10 can increase the T4/T8 ratio in normal patients and some HIV-positive patients (2123).

Interactions with Diseases or Conditions

HYPOTENSION, HYPERTENSION: Coenzyme Q-10 might lower blood pressure. It can have additive effects with medications used for hypertension (2122,3365,9890); use with caution.
SMOKING: Cigarette smoking depletes body stores of coenzyme Q-10 (7722).

Dosage and Administration

ORAL: For mitochondrial encephalomyopathies, 150 to 160 mg, or 2 mg/kg/day has been used (8159,8162,8163). In some cases, doses have been gradually increased to 3000 mg per day (8912). For heart failure, most studies have used 100 mg per day divided into 2 or 3 doses (6037,6038,6047,8909). Benefits have also been found with 60 mg/day (12170). For angina, 50 mg three times per day has been used (2121). For reducing the risk of future cardiac events in patients with recent myocardial infarction, 120 mg daily in 2 divided doses has been used (10152). For isolated systolic hypertension, 60 mg twice daily has been used (8907). For HIV/AIDS, 200 mg per day has been used (2123,2124). For diabetes, 100 mg once or twice daily has been used (456,492,9890). For Parkinson's disease, 300, 600, and 1200 mg per day in 4 divided doses has been used (8938). For preventing migraine headache, 100 mg three times daily has been used (11872). For muscular dystrophy, 100 mg per day has been used (2127). For hypertension, 120 to 200 mg per day divided into two doses has been used (3365,9890). For quinone-responsive mitochondrial encephalomyopathy, 5 mg/kg/day has been used (3366). To minimize adverse effects, divided daily doses of coenzyme Q-10 are generally recommended when doses exceed 100 mg/day (3370). For documented coenzyme Q-10 deficiency, 150 mg daily has

been used (8160). For male infertility, coenzyme Q-10 200 mg/day has been used (12169).
TOPICAL: No typical dosage.

Comments

Coenzyme Q-10 was first identified in 1957. The "Q-10" refers to the five-carbon isoprenoid units that are attached to the quinone ring. In humans, coenzyme Q-10 is most prevalent; in other species, coenzymes Q-6, Q-7, Q-8, and Q-9 dominate (11892,11894).
Coenzyme Q-10 is widely used in Japan. Millions of Japanese patients receive coenzyme Q-10 as part of their treatment for cardiovascular disease. The Japanese government approved coenzyme Q-10 for the treatment of congestive heart failure in 1974. Coenzyme Q-10 is also used extensively in Europe and Russia. Most of the coenzyme Q-10 used in the US and Canada is supplied by Japanese companies. Coenzyme Q-10 is manufactured by fermenting beets and sugar cane with special strains of yeast.

COFFEE

Also Known As

Cafe, Espresso, Java, Mocha.
CAUTION: See separate listings for Caffeine and Coffee Charcoal.

Scientific Names

Coffea arabica; Coffea canephora, synonyms Coffea robusta, Coffea bukobensis; Coffea liberica, synonym Coffea arnoldiana; other Coffea species.
Family: Rubiaceae.

People Use This For

Orally, coffee is used for short-term relief of mental and physical fatigue, and to increase performance capabilities and mental alertness. Coffee is also used orally to prevent Parkinson's disease, symptomatic gallstone disease, type 2 diabetes, gastrointestinal cancer, and breast cancer. Other uses include headache, hypotension, weight loss, and attention deficit-hyperactivity disorder (ADHD).
Rectally, coffee is used as an enema to treat cancer.

Safety

LIKELY SAFE ...when used orally and appropriately. Drinking decaffeinated coffee or coffee containing caffeine in low to moderate amounts is safe (15).
POSSIBLY UNSAFE ...when used orally in excessive amounts. Drinking caffeinated coffee in amounts greater than 6 cups per day (about 600 mg caffeine) short-term or long-term can cause caffeinism with symptoms of anxiety possibly progressing to delirium and agitation. Chronic use of caffeine, especially in large amounts, can sometimes produce tolerance, habituation, and psychological dependence. Abrupt discontinuance of caffeine can cause physical withdrawal symptoms (11733).
LIKELY UNSAFE ...when used rectally as an enema. Coffee enemas can cause severe electrolyte abnormalities and sometimes septicemia leading to severe side effects including death (3026,3349).
CHILDREN: POSSIBLY UNSAFE ...when coffee containing caffeine is used orally. The adverse effects are usually more severe in children than adults (11733).
PREGNANCY: POSSIBLY SAFE ...when used orally in small amounts. Three cups of coffee (approx. 300 mg caffeine) consumed throughout the day seems to be safe (11733). Caffeine crosses the human placenta but is not considered a teratogen. Fetal blood and tissue levels are similar to maternal concentrations (4260).
POSSIBLY UNSAFE ...when used orally in large amounts. More than 3 cups of coffee (300 mg caffeine) consumed daily may be harmful to the fetus (4260). Drinking more than 6 cups of coffee per day increases the risk of spontaneous abortion (2709). Drinking 8 or more cups of coffee per day doubles the risk of stillbirth, when compared to women who do not drink coffee during pregnancy (10621).
LACTATION: POSSIBLY SAFE ...when used orally. Drinking one or two caffeine-containing beverages per day during lactation is not associated with unacceptable levels of caffeine in human milk (11734). POSSIBLY UNSAFE ...when used orally in large amounts. Caffeine from coffee can cause wakefulness or irritability in breast-fed infants.

Effectiveness

LIKELY EFFECTIVE

Mental alertness. Consumption of coffee and other caffeinated beverages seems to prevent a decline in alertness and cognitive capacity when consumed throughout the day (4221,4224).Caffeine can improve mental performance and alertness following prolonged sleep deprivation (10205).

POSSIBLY EFFECTIVE

Colorectal cancer. Epidemiological evidence suggests that drinking more than 3 cups of coffee daily may significantly reduce the risk of rectal cancer (9222).

Diabetes. Long-term consumption of caffeinated coffee seems to significantly reduce the risk of developing type 2 diabetes. This effect seems to be dose-dependent (11353,11731). Population research suggests drinking 5 to 6 cups of coffee per day reduces diabetes risk by 61% in women and 30% in men. Drinking 10 or more cups of coffee per day reduces diabetes risk by 79% in women and 55% in men. This relationship persists regardless of age, weight, and tobacco or alcohol use (11731).

Gallbladder disease. Consumption of caffeinated beverages including coffee, that provide 400 mg or greater of caffeine per day, is associated with significantly reducing the risk of developing symptomatic gallstone disease (3345,8032). The effect seems to be dose-dependent. Consumption of 800 mg caffeine per day (four or more cups of coffee) has the greatest reduction in risk (3345).

Hypotension. Consuming caffeinated beverages like coffee seems to increase blood pressure in elderly people with postprandial hypotension (11834,11835).

Parkinson's disease. There is evidence that people who consume caffeinated beverages such as coffee, tea, and cola have a decreased risk of Parkinson's disease. For men, the effects seem to be dose related. Men consuming the greatest amount of caffeinated coffee, 28 ounces (three to four cups) per day, or a total of 421 to 2716 mg of caffeine from any source daily, seem to have the greatest reduction in risk. However, a significant reduction in risk exists even with consumption of as little as 124 to 208 mg caffeine per day, approximately 1-2 cups of coffee (6022). In women, the effects do not seem to be dose related. Moderate consumption of caffeinated coffee, one to three cups daily, provides the most reduction in risk (1238). Coffee does not appear to provide additional protection from Parkinson's disease in cigarette smokers (9236).

POSSIBLY INEFFECTIVE

Breast cancer. Consumption of coffee doesn't seem to affect breast cancer incidence (9235).

Digestive tract cancers. Drinking coffee doesn't seem to help prevent esophageal cancer, stomach cancer, or colon cancer. Epidemiological research suggests that coffee intake doesn't affect the risk for developing these digestive tract cancers (9222,9223).

INSUFFICIENT RELIABLE EVIDENCE to RATE

Cognitive function. There is preliminary evidence that suggests that higher lifetime coffee consumption might positively affect cognitive function among elderly women aged 80 or more years (10620). More evidence is needed to rate coffee for this use.

Mechanism of Action

Coffee contains 1% to 2.6% caffeine (7,12,13), which is the primary active ingredient. One cup (six ounces) of coffee contains approximately 60-120 mg of caffeine (8042). Other active constituents include chlorogenic acid, caffeol, and diterpenes. Caffeine acts as a central nervous system (CNS) stimulant, increases heart rate and contractility, increases blood pressure, stimulates gastric acid secretion, causes diuresis, relaxes extracerebral vascular and bronchial smooth muscle, and stimulates the release of catecholamines (8033).

Coffee has properties that might be beneficial in preventing cardiovascular disease and others that might increase risk. There is evidence that caffeine prevents platelet aggregation and that coffee containing caffeine increases the fibrinolytic activity in blood (8029,8030). However, diterpene constituents in unfiltered coffee such as cafestol and kahweol are believed to increase serum cholesterol, which may increase cardiovascular disease risk (1353). Cafestol is also thought to increase triglyceride levels by increasing the production of very-low-density lipoprotein (VLDL) particles which subsequently can cause a rise in low-density lipoprotein (LDL) cholesterol levels (8037). There is also evidence the constituent chlorogenic acid in coffee raises homocysteine levels (8035).

Green coffee beans contain high levels of antioxidant polyphenols, which are thought to be antitumorigenic. Most of these polyphenols are destroyed during the roasting process. Some researchers have reported that a new roasting process maintains higher levels of polyphenols without affecting the flavor. They theorize that such coffee might be healthier to drink (6601); however, this has not been demonstrated.

Epidemiological research suggests that drinking coffee might reduce the risk of type 2 diabetes. The mechanism for this observed effect is unknown, but several constituents of coffee might have an effect on glucose regulation. Chlorogenic acid in coffee might inhibit glucose-6-phosphatase, which might lower hepatic glucose production. Antioxidants in coffee might improve insulin sensitivity. Caffeine seems to stimulate pancreatic beta cells to secrete insulin. Coffee also contains magnesium and phytoestrogens, both of which have been associated with a beneficial effect on diabetes risk (11731,11732). However, some research suggests that the caffeine in coffee might have an adverse effect on diabetes. In people with type 2 diabetes, acute administration of caffeine impairs postprandial glucose metabolism, while acute abstention from caffeine reduces postprandial glucose levels by 21%. Whether these effects also occur with caffeinated beverages and herbs is unknown (12374). Other research in obese people suggests that caffeine ingestion may contribute to insulin resistance (12375).

For prevention of Parkinson's disease, caffeine may prevent the inhibition of dopaminergic transmission by adenosine. This may result in a reduction in the clinical expression of Parkinsonism (6022).

Coffee might also have a protective effect on the gallbladder. It seems to enhance gallbladder contractility, stimulate cholecystokinin (CCK) release, and increase colonic motility, which might lower the risk of gallstone disease (3345).

Proponents of caffeinated coffee enemas believe that caffeine is absorbed into the portal circulation, causing dilation of the bile ducts and stimulation of hepatocellular function to detoxify tumor cell metabolism products. However, these claims have not been substantiated (3026,3346,3347,6653).

Adverse Reactions

Orally, coffee containing caffeine can cause headache, diuresis, gastric distress, nervousness, vomiting, insomnia, anxiety, agitation, ringing in the ears, and heart arrhythmias. Coffee containing caffeine increases intraocular pressure, starting about 30 minutes after consumption and persisting for at least 90 minutes. Decaffeinated coffee does not appear to affect intraocular pressure (8540). Insomnia is a frequent adverse effect in children (10755). Caffeine may cause feeding intolerance and gastrointestinal irritation in infants (6026). Caffeine may exacerbate sleep disturbances in patients with acquired immunodeficiency syndrome (AIDS) (10204).

Although acute administration of caffeine can cause increased blood pressure, regular consumption does not seem to increase either blood pressure or pulse, even in mildly hypertensive patients (1451,1452,2722). Caffeinated coffee consumption consisting of one or more cups per day doesn't seem to increase the risk of developing hypertension in habitual coffee drinkers (8033).

Tolerance to caffeine is a widely held belief, but there is little supportive clinical evidence. If it exists, it appears to be of little clinical significance (11839). Withdrawal symptoms such as irritability, sleepiness, delirium, nausea, vomiting, rhinorrhea, nervousness, restlessness, anxiety, muscle tension, muscle pains, and flushed face have been described. However, these symptoms may be from nonpharmacological factors related to knowledge and expectation of effects. Clinically significant symptoms caused by caffeine withdrawal may be uncommon (2723,11839).

Boiled coffee that is prepared without a filter appears to increase serum cholesterol and triglyceride levels and increase liver aminotransferase enzymes (1353,4200,8036,8539). Drinking one liter of strong, unfiltered coffee daily for two weeks can raise serum cholesterol by 10% and serum triglyceride by 36% (1353). Tell patients to use coffee filters since these effects do not seem to occur with filtered coffee (4200,8036,8539).

Coffee can adversely affect homocysteine levels. Higher homocysteine levels have been associated with cardiovascular disease. One liter of unfiltered strong coffee daily for two weeks can increase plasma homocysteine levels by 10% (1353). The same amount of filtered strong coffee appears to raise plasma homocysteine levels by 20%, although there have been no head-to-head comparisons of filtered versus unfiltered coffee (3344).

A J-shaped association between regular coffee consumption and the risk of developing acute coronary syndromes has been suggested. Moderate consumption of less than 300 mL per day has been associated with a lower risk of developing acute coronary syndromes. However, regular coffee consumption of 300 mL per day or more is associated with an increase in the risk of developing acute coronary syndromes (11318). More than five cups of coffee daily is also associated with myocardial infarction (MI) and unstable angina in patients with existing coronary heart disease (8533).

The association between consumption of coffee and pancreatic cancer is controversial. Coffee may increase the incidence of some types of pancreatic cancers, but it may decrease other types (8535,8536,8537). Some studies do not support this association at all (8038,8040). Patients who are at risk for pancreatic cancer (pancreatitis) should limit their consumption of coffee.

Coffee consumption has also been associated at various times with an increased risk for breast cancer, bladder cancer, colon cancer, and other types of cancers, but there's no good evidence that coffee consumption increases cancer risk (8039,8040,8041).

Some evidence shows caffeine is associated with fibrocystic breast conditions in women, but caffeine restriction doesn't seem to affect breast nodularity, swelling, or pain (8996). Caffeine is associated with endometriosis in women; however, this is controversial since findings are conflicting (8043).

There is preliminary evidence that use of greater than four cups of coffee per day can increase the risk of rheumatoid factor positive rheumatoid arthritis, but this association has not been confirmed (6482).

Combining ephedra with coffee can increase the risk of adverse effects, due to the caffeine contained in coffee. Jitteriness, hypertension, seizures, temporary loss of consciousness, and hospitalization requiring life support has been associated with the combined use of ephedra and caffeine (2729). There is also a report of ischemic stroke in an athlete who consumed ephedra 40-60 mg, creatine monohydrate 6 grams, caffeine 400-600 mg, and a variety of other supplements daily for six weeks (1275).

Rectally, coffee enemas have been associated with three deaths. Two of these deaths are related to severe electrolyte imbalance, and a third is associated with polymicrobial septicemia following use of coffee enema (3026,3347,3349,6652).

There is evidence coffee containing caffeine shortens whole blood fibrinolysis time (8030). There is also some evidence that consumption of three or more cups of caffeinated coffee might increase the risk of Helicobacter pylori infection (8034).

Epidemiological evidence regarding the relationship between caffeine use and the risk for osteoporosis is contradictory. Caffeine can increase urinary excretion of calcium (2669,10202,11317). Women identified with a genetic variant of the vitamin D receptor appear to be at an increased risk for the detrimental effect of caffeine on bone mass (2669). However, moderate caffeine intake, less than 300 mg per day, does not seem to significantly increase osteoporosis risk in most postmenopausal women with normal calcium intake (2669,6025,10202,11317).

Caffeine can cause anaphylaxis in sensitive individuals, although true IgE-mediated caffeine allergy seems to be relatively rare (11315).

Interactions with Herbs & Other Dietary Supplements

CAFFEINE CONTAINING HERBS/SUPPLEMENTS: Concomitant use of coffee and caffeine-containing herbs/supplements constitutes therapeutic duplication (due to the caffeine contained in coffee) which increases the risk of caffeine-related adverse effects. Other natural products which contain caffeine include black tea, cocoa, cola

nut, green tea, guarana, and mate.
CALCIUM: High caffeine intake from foods and beverages including coffee increases urinary calcium excretion (2570).
CREATINE: There is some concern that combining caffeine or caffeine containing beverages and herbs with ephedra, and creatine might increase the risk of serious adverse effects. There is a report of ischemic stroke in an athlete who consumed creatine monohydrate 6 grams, caffeine 400-600 mg, ephedra 40-60 mg, and a variety of other supplements daily for 6 weeks (1275). Caffeine might also decrease creatine's possible beneficial effects on athletic performance. Some researchers think caffeine can inhibit phosphocreatine resynthesis (2117,4575).
EPHEDRA (Ma Huang): Use of ephedra with coffee can increase the risk of caffeine stimulatory adverse effects. There is evidence that using ephedra with caffeine might increase the risk of serious life-threatening or debilitating adverse effects such as hypertension, myocardial infarction, stroke, seizures, and death (1275,6486,10307). Tell patients to avoid taking coffee with ephedra and other stimulants.
MAGNESIUM: Consuming large amounts of coffee can increase excretion of magnesium (11939).

Interactions with Drugs

ADENOSINE (Adenocard): The caffeine in coffee is a competitive inhibitor of adenosine at the cellular level. However, caffeine doesn't seem to affect supplemental adenosine because high interstitial levels of adenosine overcome the antagonistic effects of caffeine (11771). It is recommended that methylxanthines and methylxanthine-containing products be stopped 24 hours prior to pharmacological stress tests (11770). However, methylxanthines appear more likely to interfere with dipyridamole (Persantine) than adenosine-induced stress testing (11771).
ALCOHOL (Ethanol): Concomitant use of alcohol can increase caffeine serum concentrations and the risk of caffeine adverse effects. Alcohol reduces caffeine metabolism (6370).
ALENDRONATE (Fosamax): Separate coffee ingestion and alendronate administration by two hours. Coffee reduces alendronate bioavailability by 60% (11735).
ANTICOAGULANT/ANTIPLATELET DRUGS: Theoretically, caffeine in coffee might increase the risk of bleeding when used concomitantly with these agents. Caffeine is reported to have antiplatelet activity (8028,8029); however, this interaction has not been reported in humans. There is some evidence that caffeinated coffee might increase the fibrinolytic activity in blood (8030). Antiplatelet agents include aspirin, clopidogrel (Plavix), dipyridamole (Persantine), ticlopidine (Ticlid), and others. Anticoagulant agents include ardeparin (Normiflo), dalteparin (Fragmin), enoxaparin (Lovenox), heparin, and warfarin (Coumadin).
ANTIDIABETES DRUGS: Theoretically, concomitant use of coffee and diabetes drugs might interfere with blood glucose control due to the caffeine in coffee. However, data are conflicting. Reports claim that caffeine might increase or decrease blood sugar (6024,8646).
CIMETIDINE (Tagamet): Theoretically, concomitant use might increase serum caffeine concentrations and the risk of adverse effects, due to the caffeine contained in coffee. Cimetidine decreases the rate of caffeine clearance by 30% (11736).
CLOZAPINE (Clozaril): Theoretically, co-administration might acutely exacerbate psychotic symptoms, due to the caffeine contained in coffee. Caffeine can increase the effects and toxicity of clozapine. Caffeine doses of 400-1000 mg per day inhibit clozapine metabolism (5051).
CONTRACEPTIVE DRUGS: Theoretically, concomitant use might increase caffeine concentrations and the risk adverse effects, due to the caffeine contained in coffee. Oral contraceptives decrease the rate of caffeine clearance by 40% to 65% (2714,11737).
DIPYRIDAMOLE (Persantine): The caffeine in coffee inhibits dipyridamole-induced vasodilation (11770,11772). It is recommended that methylxanthines and methylxanthine-containing products be stopped 24 hours prior to pharmacological stress tests (11770). Methylxanthines appear more likely to interfere with dipyridamole (Persantine) than adenosine-induced stress testing (11771).
DISULFIRAM (Antabuse): Coffee contains caffeine. Concomitant use can increase caffeine serum concentrations, and the risk of adverse effects. Disulfiram decreases the rate of caffeine clearance (11840).
EPHEDRINE: Use of ephedrine with coffee can increase the risk of stimulatory adverse effects of caffeine. There is evidence that using ephedrine with caffeine might increase the risk of serious life-threatening or debilitating adverse effects such as hypertension, myocardial infarction, stroke, seizures, and death (1275,6486,10307). Tell patients to avoid taking coffee with ephedrine and other stimulants.
ESTROGENS: Theoretically, concomitant use might increase serum caffeine concentrations and the risk of adverse effects, due to the caffeine contained in coffee. Estrogen inhibits caffeine metabolism (2714).
FLUCONAZOLE (Diflucan): Concomitant use might increase the effects of caffeine. Fluconazole decreases caffeine clearance by approximately 25% (11022).
FLUVOXAMINE (Luvox): Coffee contains caffeine. Concomitant use of fluvoxamine can increase caffeine serum concentrations, and the risk of caffeine adverse effects. Fluvoxamine reduces caffeine metabolism (6370).
LITHIUM: Theoretically, abrupt coffee withdrawal might increase serum lithium levels, due to the caffeine contained in coffee. There are two case reports of lithium tremor that worsened upon abrupt coffee withdrawal (609,610).
MEXILETINE (Mexitil): Concomitant use might increase the effects and adverse effects of caffeine in coffee. Mexiletine can decrease caffeine elimination by 50% (1260,11741).
MONOAMINE OXIDASE INHIBITORS (MAOIs): Theoretically, concomitant intake of large amounts of coffee

with MAOIs might precipitate a hypertensive crisis, due to the caffeine contained in coffee. This is based on the claim that intake of large amounts of caffeine with MAOIs might precipitate a hypertensive crisis (15).

PHENOTHIAZINES: The tannins in coffee might cause precipitation of solutions of fluphenazine (Permitil, Prolixin), chlorpromazine (Thorazine), haloperidol (Haldol), prochlorperazine (Compazine), thioridazine (Mellaril), and trifluoperazine (Stelazine) (626,627).

PHENYLPROPANOLAMINE: Concomitant use of phenylpropanolamine and coffee might cause an additive increase in blood pressure due to the caffeine in coffee (11738).

QUINOLONE ANTIBIOTICS: Theoretically, concomitant use might increase serum caffeine concentrations and the risk of adverse effects, due to the caffeine contained in coffee. Quinolones decrease caffeine clearance (606,607,608). Quinolones (also referred to as fluoroquinolones) include ciprofloxacin (Cipro), enoxacin (Penetrex), gatifloxacin (Tequin), levofloxacin (Levaquin), lomefloxacin (Maxaquin), moxifloxacin (Avelox), norfloxacin (Noroxin), ofloxacin (Floxin), sparfloxacin (Zagam), and trovafloxacin (Trovan).

RILUZOLE (Rilutek): Theoretically, concomitant use might increase serum caffeine and riluzole concentrations and the risk of adverse effects of both caffeine and riluzole, due to the caffeine contained in coffee. Caffeine and riluzole are both metabolized by cytochrome P450 1A2, and concomitant use might reduce metabolism of one or both agents (11739).

STIMULANT DRUGS: Concomitant use might increase the risk of stimulant adverse effects, due to the caffeine contained in coffee (11832). CNS stimulants include nicotine, cocaine, sympathomimetic amines, and amphetamines.

TERBINAFINE (Lamisil): Theoretically, concomitant use might increase serum caffeine concentrations and the risk of adverse effects, due to the caffeine contained in coffee. Terbinafine decreases the rate of caffeine clearance (11740).

THEOPHYLLINE: Theoretically, concomitant use might increase serum theophylline concentrations and the risk of adverse effects, due to the caffeine contained in coffee. Large amounts of caffeine might inhibit theophylline metabolism (11741).

TRICYCLIC ANTIDEPRESSANTS (TCAs): The tannins in coffee might cause precipitation of solutions of amitriptyline (Elavil) or imipramine (Tofranil, Janimine) (626,627).

VERAPAMIL (Calan, Covera, Isoptin, Verelan): Theoretically, concomitant use might increase plasma caffeine concentrations and the risk of adverse effects, due to the caffeine contained in coffee. Verapamil increases plasma caffeine concentrations by 25% (11741).

Interactions with Foods

None known.

Interactions with Lab Tests

5-HYDROXYINDOLEACETIC ACID: Coffee might increase urine 5-hydroxyindoleacetic acid concentrations and test results, due to its caffeine content. Caffeine can increase urine catecholamine concentrations (15).

BLEEDING TIME: Theoretically, coffee might increase bleeding time. Caffeine can prolong bleeding time and increase the results of a bleeding time test (1701). Caffeine is reported to have antiplatelet activity (8028,8029). There is some evidence that caffeinated coffee increases fibrinolytic activity in blood (8030). However, the significance of these effects in humans is not known.

CATECHOLAMINES: Coffee might increase urine catecholamine concentrations and test results, due to its caffeine content. Caffeine can increase urine catecholamine concentrations (8646).

CREATINE: Coffee might increase urine creatine concentrations and test results, due to its caffeine content (1701).

DIPYRIDAMOLE THALLIUM IMAGING: Coffee might interfere with dipyridamole thallium imaging studies, due to its caffeine content. Caffeine attenuates the characteristic cardiovascular responses to dipyridamole and has altered test results (11742).

GLUCOSE: Caffeine, a constituent of coffee, has been reported to cause increases and decreases in blood glucose (8646).

LACTATE: The combination of ephedrine, a constituent of ephedra, and the caffeine in coffee can increase blood lactate levels (8646).

NEUROBLASTOMA TESTS: Coffee (due to its caffeine content) might cause false-positive diagnosis of neuroblastoma, when diagnosis is based on tests of urine vanillylmandelic acid (VMA) or catecholamine concentrations. Caffeine can increase urine catecholamine and VMA concentrations (15).

PHARMACOLOGICAL STRESS TESTS: The caffeine in coffee is a competitive antagonist for adenosine receptors (11771). Caffeine attenuates the characteristic cardiovascular responses to dipyridamole and has altered test results (11742). It is recommended that caffeine and caffeine-containing products be stopped 24 hours prior to pharmacological stress tests (11770). However, caffeine appears more likely to interfere with dipyridamole (Persantine) than adenosine (Adenocard) stress testing (11771). The interaction between caffeine and dipyridamole is unlikely to be significant in stress testing if the heart rate increase is greater than 5% after dipyridamole infusion (11772).

PHEOCHROMOCYTOMA TESTS: Coffee (due to its caffeine content) might cause false-positive diagnosis of pheochromocytoma, when diagnosis is based on tests of urine vanillylmandelic acid (VMA) or catecholamine concentrations. Caffeine can increase urine catecholamine and VMA concentrations (15).

PULMONARY FUNCTION TESTS: People may need to avoid caffeine and caffeinated beverages for at least four

hours prior to lung function testing. Forced expiratory volume in one minute (FEV1) seems to show a small improvement up to two hours after caffeine use. Mid-expiratory flow rates may also improve with caffeine for up to four hours (9607).
URATE: Coffee might falsely increase serum urate test results determined by the Bittner method, due to its caffeine content. Caffeine causes false elevations in serum urate test results determined by the Bittner method (11844).
URINARY CALCIUM: Caffeine, a constituent of coffee, can increase urinary calcium levels (11317).
VANILLYLMANDELIC ACID (VMA): Coffee might increase urine VMA concentrations and test results, due to its caffeine content. Caffeine can increase urine VMA concentrations (15).
WHOLE BLOOD FIBRINOLYSIS TIME (Fearnley method): There is evidence caffeinated coffee may increase the whole blood fibrinolysis time (8030).

Interactions with Diseases or Conditions

ANXIETY DISORDERS: The caffeine in coffee might aggravate anxiety disorders (11743).
BLEEDING DISORDERS: Theoretically, caffeine in coffee might aggravate bleeding conditions. Caffeine is reported to have antiplatelet activity (8028,8029); however, this interaction has not been reported in humans. There is some evidence caffeinated coffee may increase fibrinolytic activity in blood (8030). Caffeine can prolong bleeding time and increase the results of a bleeding time test (1701).
CARDIAC CONDITIONS: The caffeine in coffee can induce cardiac arrhythmias in sensitive individuals (16); use with caution.
DIABETES: Some research suggests that caffeine, a constituent of coffee, may impair postprandial glucose metabolism in people with diabetes and contribute to insulin resistance. The effect of caffeinated beverages and herbs has not been studied (12374,12375). The caffeine in coffee may enhance the frequency and intensity of hypoglycemic warning symptoms in type 1 diabetics. This may increase the ability of diabetics to detect and treat hypoglycemia early. However, it might also increase the frequency of hypoglycemic events (6024); use with caution. Caffeine has been reported to cause increases and decreases in blood glucose (8646); use with caution.
GLAUCOMA: Drinking caffeinated coffee increases intraocular pressure. The increase occurs within 30 minutes and persists for at least 90 minutes (8540).
HEART DISEASE: Consumption of unfiltered (boiled) coffee increases plasma homocysteine levels, serum cholesterol, and triglycerides, which are associated with an increased risk of cardiovascular disease (1353,4200,8036,8539). Some research suggests an association between heart attacks and coffee consumption. Regular coffee consumption of 300 ml per day or more is associated with an increase in the risk of developing acute coronary syndromes (11318). Heavy coffee consumption also seems to increase risk in people with existing coronary heart disease (8042,8533,8538). More than 5 cups of coffee on a regular basis is associated with myocardial infarction and unstable angina in patients with coronary heart disease (CHD) (8533).
HYPERTENSION: Consuming caffeinated coffee might increase blood pressure in people with high blood pressure. However, this effect might be less in habitual caffeine users (2722).
OSTEOPOROSIS: Consuming caffeinated coffee can increase urinary excretion of calcium. Caffeine consumption should be limited to less than 300 mg per day (approximately 2-3 cups of coffee). Adequate calcium supplementation may partially compensate for calcium losses (2669,10202,11317). Postmenopausal women identified with a genetic variant of the vitamin D receptor should use caffeine with caution (2669).

Dosage and Administration

ORAL: The typical dose of caffeine for headache or restoring mental alertness is up to 250 mg per day, about 2 cups of coffee (2718,11743). For preventing Parkinson's disease, consumption of three to four cups (28 oz) of caffeinated coffee per day or 421 mg to 2716 mg total caffeine has been used to reduce the risk of developing Parkinson's disease. However, a significantly lower risk has also been associated with consumption of as little as 124 mg to 208 mg of caffeine (approximately one to two cups of coffee) (6022). In women, more moderate caffeinated coffee consumption seems to be best; one to three cups per day (1238). For preventing symptomatic gallstone disease, consumption of 400 mg or greater of caffeine per day (two or more cups of coffee) has been used for risk reduction (3345,8032). However, consumption of at least 800 mg caffeine per day (four or more cups of coffee) seems to be associated with the greatest reduction in risk (3345). For preventing type 2 diabetes, long-term consumption of about 900 mg caffeine per day (6 or more cups of coffee per day) has been used (11353). Use filtered coffee to avoid some adverse effects. Choice of coffee, grind, ratio of coffee to water, and other factors determine flavor and strength of the beverage. Caffeine content of coffee (per average cup): percolated, 100-150 mg caffeine; instant, 85-100 mg caffeine; and decaffeinated, approximately 8 mg caffeine (13). Darker roasts contain less caffeine due to sublimation during roasting (13).

Comments

Coffee enemas are used as a part of the "Gerson Therapy." Cancer patients are treated with caffeinated coffee, in the form of four-hourly enemas on a daily basis. The enemas are combined with a diet of liver, vegetables, and a variety of oral medications, including potassium, pepsin, Lugol's solution, niacin, pancreatin, and thyroid extracts (3348,6653). The Gerson Therapy is considered an unacceptable medical practice in the US, but continues to be used at The Hospital of the Baja California in Tijuana, Mexico, one mile from the US (3346,3347,3348,6652,6653).

COFFEE CHARCOAL

Also Known As
None.
CAUTION: See separate listings for Activated Charcoal and Coffee.

Scientific Names
Coffea arabica; Coffea canephora; Coffea liberica.
Family: Rubiaceae.

People Use This For
Orally, coffee charcoal is used for nonspecific, acute diarrhea.
Topically, coffee charcoal is used for inflammation of the oral and pharyngeal mucosa, and for festering wounds.

Safety
POSSIBLY SAFE ...when used orally or topically (2).
PREGNANCY AND LACTATION: Insufficient reliable information available; avoid using.

Effectiveness
There is insufficient reliable information available about the effectiveness of coffee charcoal.

Mechanism of Action
Coffee charcoal can have adsorbent and astringent properties (2).

Adverse Reactions
None reported.

Interactions with Herbs & Other Dietary Supplements
None known.

Interactions with Drugs
ORAL DRUGS: Coffee charcoal can reduce the absorption of orally administered drugs (2) and should be separated from oral drug administration by at least two hours.

Interactions with Foods
None known.

Interactions with Lab Tests
None known.

Interactions with Diseases or Conditions
None known.

Dosage and Administration
ORAL: The average single dose of coffee charcoal is 3 grams (18), and the total daily dose is 9 grams per day (2). Store coffee charcoal in a well-sealed container (18). Diarrhea persisting beyond 3 to 4 days should be evaluated by a health care professional (2).
TOPICAL: No typical dosage.

Comments
Coffee charcoal is produced by roasting the outer portion of the coffee beans until blackened or charred. Avoid confusion with coffee seed or activated charcoal.

COLA NUT

Also Known As

Bissy Nut, Guru Nut, Gworo, Kola Nut, Soudan Coffee.
CAUTION: See separate listings for Caffeine and Gotu Kola.

Scientific Names

Cola acuminata, synonym Sterculia acuminata; Cola nitida, synonym Sterculia nitida; and related species.
Family: Sterculiaceae or Malvaceae.

People Use This For

Orally, cola nut is used for short-term relief of mental and physical fatigue and depressive states, especially those associated with general muscle weakness. It is also used orally for melancholy, atony, exhaustion, dysentery, atonic diarrhea, anorexia, and migraines.
In foods and beverages, cola nut is used as a flavoring ingredient.

Safety

LIKELY SAFE ...when used in amounts commonly found in foods. Cola nut extract has Generally Recognized As Safe (GRAS) status in the US (4912).
POSSIBLY SAFE ...when used orally and appropriately (12).
POSSIBLY UNSAFE ...when cola nut is used orally in large amounts or for prolonged periods of time. Chewing cola nut is associated with an increased risk of mouth cancer and gastrointestinal cancer (11963).
LIKELY UNSAFE ...when used orally in very high doses. Cola nut contains caffeine. The fatal acute oral dose of caffeine is estimated to be 10-14 grams (150-200 mg per kilogram). Serious toxicity can occur at lower doses depending on variables in caffeine sensitivity such as smoking, age, prior caffeine use, etc (11832).
CHILDREN: LIKELY SAFE ...when used orally in amounts found in foods (4912,11833).
PREGNANCY: POSSIBLY SAFE ...when used orally in amounts found in foods. Due to the caffeine content of cola nut, mothers should closely monitor their intake to ensure moderate consumption. Fetal blood concentrations of caffeine approximate maternal concentrations (4260). Use of caffeine in pregnancy is controversial; however, moderate consumption has not been associated with clinically important adverse fetal effects (2708,2709,2710,2711,9606). Caffeine crosses the human placenta, but is not considered a teratogen. Mothers should keep caffeine consumption below 200 mg per day. This is similar to the amount of caffeine found in 1-2 cups of coffee or tea (2708).
POSSIBLY UNSAFE ...when used orally in large amounts. Caffeine crosses the placenta, producing fetal blood concentrations similar to maternal levels (4260). Mothers should avoid consuming more than 200 mg of caffeine daily (2708). Maternal doses of greater than 200 mg per day throughout pregnancy have resulted in symptoms of caffeine withdrawal in newborn infants (9891). High doses of caffeine have been associated with spontaneous abortion, premature delivery, and low birth weight (2709,2711). Fetal birth weight is reduced by 28 grams for every 100 mg per day of caffeine consumed during pregnancy. But this is unlikely to be clinically important except for women consuming more than 600 mg of caffeine daily (9606). Teratogenicity studies have not been performed.
LACTATION: POSSIBLY SAFE ...when used orally in amounts found in foods. Due to the caffeine content of cola nut, nursing mothers should closely monitor caffeine intake. Breast milk concentrations of caffeine are thought to be approximately 50% of maternal serum concentrations. Minimal consumption would likely result in limited exposure to a nursing infant (9892). POSSIBLY UNSAFE ...when used orally in large amounts. Consumption of cola nut might cause irritability and increased bowel activity in nursing infants (6026). Large doses or excessive intake of cola nut should be avoided during lactation. Whether potentially carcinogenic constituents of cola nut are transferred via breast milk is unknown.

Effectiveness

There is insufficient reliable information available about the effectiveness of cola nut.

Mechanism of Action

The applicable part of cola nut is the seed (nut). Cola nut contains 1% to 2.5% caffeine (12). Cola nut also contains high concentrations of tannins and N-nitroso compounds that are potential carcinogens (11963).
Caffeine is responsible for most of the pharmacologic effects of cola nut. Caffeine is a methylxanthine compound and is structurally related to theophylline, theobromine, and uric acid (6372). It is 100% bioavailable after oral administration and is metabolized principally in the liver to paraxanthine, theophylline, and theobromine (6370). The half-life of caffeine is about six hours (8644).
Caffeine stimulates the central nervous system (CNS), heart, muscles, and possibly the pressor centers that control blood pressure (2722). Possible mechanisms include adenosine receptor blockade and phosphodiesterase inhibition (2722). By blocking adenosine receptors, caffeine is thought to increase the release of neurotransmitters such as dopamine (6370). Caffeine also decreases airway resistance and stimulates respiration, via adenosine receptor blockade and phosphodiesterase inhibition (11836). It has also been proposed that caffeine may decrease GABA and serotonin signaling (6370). Caffeine stimulates gastric acid secretion, and increases plasma catecholamine

levels (11837). Caffeine can have positive inotropic and chronotropic effects on the heart (11836). Caffeine can also acutely elevate both diastolic and systolic blood pressure, but might not have this effect in habitual users (2722). Caffeine exerts a diuretic effect, with water losses estimated at 1.17 mL per milligram of caffeine (2712). Tachyphylaxis to the diuretic effect develops rapidly, diminishing fluid losses associated with caffeine intake (10206). Caffeine-containing beverages consumed during moderate endurance exercise do not appear to compromise bodily hydration status (2713). Caffeine does not substantially affect the fluid status of people who drink caffeinated beverages on a regular basis (10206). Caffeine's CNS stimulant effects are thought to improve vigilance and psychomotor performance (2720,10205). For improving athletic performance, caffeine has been shown to decrease perceived levels of exertion, which enables the athlete to feel less tired and increase their performance (6370). Caffeine alone or in combination with ephedrine can improve anaerobic exercise performance. Caffeine seems to enhance muscle metabolism and increases time to exhaustion and oxygen deficit, which may lead to better performance (8646). Studies have also suggested caffeine possibly influences cardiovascular stress reactivity, either by potentiating the stress response itself or adding to the level reached during stress (6372). Caffeine may cause a slight decrease in heart rate after consumption and appears to raise blood pressure during psychological stress (6372). Large amounts of caffeine, >10 mg/kg/day, can also produce tachycardia and premature ventricular contractions (6372). Caffeine, a constituent of cola nut, has been reported to cause increases and decreases in blood glucose. In people with type 2 diabetes, acute administration of caffeine impairs postprandial glucose metabolism, while acute abstention from caffeine reduces postprandial glucose levels by 21%. Whether these effects also occur with caffeinated beverages and herbs is unknown (12374). Other research in obese people suggests that caffeine ingestion may contribute to insulin resistance (12375). However, one study found that type 1 diabetics taking 200 mg of caffeine twice daily had increased frequency and intensity of warning signs of hypoglycemia. This may be due to a reduction in blood flow to the brain and an increase in glucose utilization by the brain (6024). For preventing Parkinson's disease, caffeine may protect dopaminergic neurons in the brain. This effect appears to be related to modulation of adenosine receptors (10201). This may result in a reduction in the clinical expression of Parkinsonism (6022). Evidence suggests that tolerance to caffeine's neuroendocrine and cardiovascular effects may develop during consumption throughout the day, but tolerance appears to be lost during overnight abstinence of caffeine (6372). Preliminary evidence also suggests caffeine may increase plasma levels of cortisol and adrenocorticotrophic hormone (ACTH), decrease levels of extracellular potassium, and increase levels of intracellular calcium in skeletal muscle; but the mechanisms are poorly understood (6370). Caffeine may be beneficial in the prevention of cardiovascular disease. There is evidence caffeine inhibits platelet aggregation and suppresses thromboxane formation during blood clotting (8028,8029). There is also evidence caffeine might be associated with decreased levels of testosterone and increased levels of estrone and sex-hormone binding globulin. These findings might explain why some studies have reported associations between caffeine and hormone-dependent conditions such as fibrocystic disease, osteoporosis, breast cancer, and endometriosis (8043). Caffeine is often used in combination with ephedra for weight loss and seems to have additive pharmacodynamic effects. A single dose of ephedra in combination with caffeine can increase heart rate from 67 beats per minute to 82 beats per minute in young, healthy people. The combination also increases systolic blood pressure and to a lesser extent, diastolic pressure (8644). Caffeine in combination with ephedra also increases oxygen consumption. Whether the increased oxygen consumption is an indication of a significant increase in metabolism and contributes to weight loss is unknown (8645).

Adverse Reactions

Orally, cola nut can cause symptoms of caffeine toxicity. Caffeine can cause insomnia, nervousness, restlessness, gastric irritation, nausea, vomiting, tachycardia, quickened respiration, tremors, delirium, convulsions, and diuresis. Large doses can produce headache, anxiety, agitation, ringing in the ears, premature heartbeat, and arrhythmia (11832,11838). In fatal caffeine overdose, the cause of death is usually ventricular fibrillation (11838,11845). Insomnia is a frequent adverse effect in children (10755). Caffeine may cause feeding intolerance and gastrointestinal irritation in infants (6023). Caffeine may exacerbate sleep disturbances in patients with acquired immunodeficiency syndrome (AIDS) (10204).

Some evidence shows caffeine is associated with fibrocystic breast disease, breast cancer, and endometriosis in women; however, this is controversial since findings are conflicting (8043). Restricting caffeine in women with fibrocystic breast conditions doesn't seem to affect breast nodularity, swelling, or pain (8996).

Although acute administration of caffeine can cause increased blood pressure, regular consumption does not seem to increase either blood pressure or pulse, even in mildly hypertensive patients (1451,1452,2722).

Tolerance to caffeine is a widely held belief, but there is little supportive clinical evidence. If it exists, it appears to be of little clinical significance (11839). Withdrawal symptoms such as irritability, sleepiness, delirium, nausea, vomiting, rhinorrhea, nervousness, restlessness, anxiety, muscle tension, muscle pains, and flushed face have been described. However, these symptoms may be from nonpharmacological factors related to knowledge and expectation of effects. Clinically significant symptoms caused by caffeine withdrawal may be uncommon (2723,11839).

Epidemiological evidence regarding the relationship between caffeine use and the risk for osteoporosis is contradictory. Caffeine can increase urinary excretion of calcium (2669,10202,11317). Women identified with a genetic variant of the vitamin D receptor appear to be at an increased risk for the detrimental effect of caffeine on bone mass (2669). However, moderate caffeine intake, less than 300 mg per day, does not seem to significantly increase osteoporosis risk in most postmenopausal women with normal calcium intake (2669,6025,10202,11317).

Combining ephedra with caffeine can increase the risk of adverse effects. Jitteriness, hypertension, seizures,

temporary loss of consciousness, and hospitalization requiring life support has been associated with the combined use of ephedra and caffeine (2729). There is also a report of ischemic stroke in an athlete who consumed ephedra 40-60 mg, creatine monohydrate 6 grams, caffeine 400-600 mg, and a variety of other supplements daily for six weeks (1275).
Caffeine can cause anaphylaxis in sensitive individuals, although true IgE-mediated caffeine allergy seems to be relatively rare (11315).
Preliminary research suggests that chewing cola nut could increase the risk of oral and gastrointestinal cancer. Cola nut contains high amounts of tannins and N-nitroso compounds, which are carcinogenic. Chewing cola nuts is practiced widely in Nigeria, which has a high incidence of oral and gastrointestinal cancer. The risk may be even higher in smokers (11963).

Interactions with Herbs & Other Dietary Supplements

CAFFEINE CONTAINING HERBS/SUPPLEMENTS: Concomitant use of cola nut and caffeine-containing herbs/supplements constitutes therapeutic duplication (due to the caffeine contained in cola nut) which increases the risk of caffeine-related adverse effects. Other natural products which contain caffeine include black tea, cocoa, coffee, green tea, guarana, and mate.
CALCIUM: High caffeine intake from foods, beverages, and herbs including cola nut increases urinary calcium excretion (2570).
CREATINE: There is some concern that combining caffeine, ephedra, and creatine might increase the risk of serious adverse effects. There is a report of ischemic stroke in an athlete who consumed creatine monohydrate 6 grams, caffeine 400-600 mg, ephedra 40-60 mg, and a variety of other supplements daily for six weeks (1275). Caffeine might also decrease creatine's possible beneficial effects on athletic performance. Some researchers think caffeine can inhibit phosphocreatine resynthesis (2117,4575).
EPHEDRA (ma huang): Use of ephedra with cola nut can increase the risk of stimulatory adverse effects due to its caffeine content. There is evidence that using ephedra with caffeine might increase the risk of serious life-threatening or debilitating adverse effects such as hypertension, myocardial infarction, stroke, seizures, and death (6486,10307). Tell patients to avoid taking cola nut with ephedra and other stimulants.

Interactions with Drugs

ADENOSINE (Adenocard): The caffeine in cola nut is a competitive inhibitor of adenosine at the cellular level. However, caffeine doesn't seem to affect supplemental adenosine because high interstitial levels of adenosine overcome the antagonistic effects of caffeine (11771).
ALCOHOL (Ethanol): Concomitant use of alcohol can increase caffeine serum concentrations and the risk of caffeine adverse effects. Alcohol reduces caffeine metabolism (6370).
AMPHETAMINES: Theoretically, the caffeine in cola nut might increase the risk of additive CNS effects (2719).
ANTIDIABETES DRUGS: Theoretically, concomitant use of caffeine and diabetes drugs might interfere with blood glucose control. Data are conflicting. Reports claim that caffeine might increase or decrease blood sugar (6024,8646).
CIMETIDINE (Tagamet): Theoretically, concomitant use might increase serum caffeine concentrations and the risk of adverse effects, due to the caffeine contained in cola nut. Cimetidine decreases the rate of caffeine clearance by 30% to 50% (11736).
CLOZAPINE (Clozaril): Theoretically, co-administration might acutely exacerbate psychotic symptoms, due to the caffeine contained in cola nut. Caffeine can increase the effects and toxicity of clozapine (151). Caffeine doses of 400-1000 mg per day inhibit clozapine metabolism (5051).
COCAINE: Theoretically, the caffeine in cola nut might increase the risk of additive CNS effects (2719).
CONTRACEPTIVE DRUGS: Theoretically, concomitant use might increase caffeine concentrations and the risk adverse effects, due to the caffeine contained in cola nut. Oral contraceptives decrease the rate of caffeine clearance by 40% to 65% (2714,11737).
DIPYRIDAMOLE (Persantine): The caffeine in cola nut might inhibit dipyridamole-induced vasodilation (11770,11772).
DISULFIRAM (Antabuse): Theoretically, concomitant use might increase serum caffeine concentrations and the risk of adverse effects, due to the caffeine contained in cola nut. Disulfiram decreases the rate of caffeine clearance (15).
EPHEDRINE: Use of ephedrine with caffeine can increase the risk of stimulatory adverse effects. There is evidence that using ephedrine with caffeine might increase the risk of serious life-threatening or debilitating adverse effects such as hypertension, myocardial infarction, stroke, seizures, and death (1275,6486,10307). Tell patients to avoid taking caffeine with ephedrine and other stimulants.
ESTROGENS: Theoretically, concomitant use might increase serum caffeine concentrations and the risk of adverse effects, due to the caffeine contained in cola nut. Estrogen inhibits caffeine metabolism (2714).
FLUCONAZOLE (Diflucan): Concomitant use might increase the effects of caffeine in cola nut. Fluconazole decreases caffeine clearance by approximately 25% (11022).
FLUVOXAMINE (Luvox): Concomitant use can increase caffeine serum concentrations, and the risk of caffeine adverse effects. Fluvoxamine reduces caffeine metabolism (6370).
LITHIUM: Theoretically, abrupt cola nut withdrawal might increase serum lithium levels, due to the caffeine

contained in cola nut. There are two case reports of lithium tremor that worsened upon abrupt coffee withdrawal (609,610).
MEXILETINE (Mexitil): Theoretically, concomitant use might increase serum caffeine concentrations and the risk of adverse effects, due to the caffeine contained in cola nut. Mexiletine reduces caffeine metabolism (11741).
MONOAMINE OXIDASE INHIBITORS (MAOIs): Theoretically, concomitant intake of large amounts of cola nut with MAOIs might precipitate a hypertensive crisis, due to the caffeine contained in cola nut. This is based on the claim that intake of large amounts of caffeine with MAOIs might precipitate a hypertensive crisis (15).
NICOTINE: Theoretically, the caffeine in cola nut might increase the risk of additive CNS effects (2719).
PHENYLPROPANOLAMINE: Concomitant use of phenylpropanolamine and cola nut might cause an additive increase in blood pressure due to the caffeine in cola nut (11738).
QUINOLONE ANTIBIOTICS: Theoretically, concomitant use might increase serum caffeine concentrations and the risk of adverse effects, due to the caffeine contained in cola nut. Quinolones decrease caffeine clearance (606,607,608). Quinolones (also referred to as fluoroquinolones) include ciprofloxacin (Cipro), enoxacin (Penetrex), gatifloxacin (Tequin), levofloxacin (Levaquin), lomefloxacin (Maxaquin), moxifloxacin (Avelox), norfloxacin (Noroxin), ofloxacin (Floxin), sparfloxacin (Zagam), and trovafloxacin (Trovan).
RILUZOLE (Rilutek): Theoretically, concomitant use of riluzole and caffeinated products such as cola nut might increase serum caffeine and riluzole concentrations and the risk of adverse effects of both caffeine and riluzole, due to the caffeine contained in cola nut. Caffeine and riluzole are both metabolized by cytochrome P450 1A2, and concomitant use might reduce metabolism of one or both agents (11739).
TERBINAFINE (Lamisil): Theoretically, concomitant use might increase serum caffeine concentrations and the risk of adverse effects, due to the caffeine contained in cola nut. Terbinafine decreases the rate of caffeine clearance (11740).
THEOPHYLLINE: Theoretically, concomitant use of theophylline and large amounts of cola nut might increase the risk of theophylline toxicity, due to cola nut's caffeine content. Caffeine decreases theophylline clearance 23% to 29% (11741).
VERAPAMIL (Calan, Covera, Isoptin, Verelan): Theoretically, concomitant use might increase plasma caffeine concentrations and the risk of adverse effects, due to the caffeine contained in cola nut. Verapamil increases plasma caffeine concentrations by 25% (11741). Some of these drugs include Calan, Isoptin, and Verelan.

Interactions with Foods

CAFFEINE-CONTAINING BEVERAGES: Concomitant use can have additive therapeutic and adverse effects due to the caffeine content.
GRAPEFRUIT JUICE: Grapefruit juice interacts with the caffeine in cola nut and can increase caffeine levels, its activity, and the risk of adverse effects (504).

Interactions with Lab Tests

5-HYDROXYINDOLEACETIC ACID: Cola nut might increase urine 5-hydroxyindoleacetic acid concentrations and test results, due to its caffeine content. Caffeine can increase urine catecholamine concentrations (15).
BLEEDING TIME: Cola nut might prolong bleeding time and increase test results, due to its caffeine content (1701).
CATECHOLAMINES: Cola nut might increase urine catecholamine concentrations and test results, due to its caffeine content (15).
CREATINE: Cola nut might increase urine creatine concentrations and test results, due to its caffeine content (1701).
DIPYRIDAMOLE THALLIUM IMAGING: Cola nut might interfere with dipyridamole thallium imaging studies, due to its caffeine content. Caffeine attenuates the characteristic cardiovascular responses to dipyridamole and has altered test results (11742).
GLUCOSE: Caffeine has been reported to cause increases and decreases in blood glucose (8646).
LACTATE: The combination of ephedrine, a constituent of ephedra, and caffeine, a constituent of cola nut, can increase blood lactate levels (8646).
NEUROBLASTOMA TESTS: Cola nut (due to its caffeine content) might cause false-positive diagnosis of neuroblastoma, when diagnosis is based on tests of urine vanillylmandelic acid (VMA) or catecholamine concentrations. Caffeine can increase urine catecholamine and VMA concentrations (15).
PHARMACOLOGICAL STRESS TESTS: The caffeine in cola nut is a competitive antagonist for adenosine receptors (11771). It is recommended that caffeine and caffeine-containing products be stopped 24 hours prior to pharmacological stress tests (11770). However, caffeine appears more likely to interfere with dipyridamole (Persantine) than adenosine (Adenocard) stress testing (11771). The interaction between caffeine and dipyridamole is unlikely to be significant in stress testing if the heart rate increase is greater than 5% after dipyridamole infusion (11772).
PHEOCHROMOCYTOMA TESTS: Cola nut (due to its caffeine content) might cause false-positive diagnosis of pheochromocytoma, when diagnosis is based on tests of urine vanillylmandelic acid (VMA) or catecholamine concentrations. Caffeine can increase urine catecholamine and VMA concentrations (15).
PULMONARY FUNCTION TESTS: People may need to avoid caffeine and caffeine-containing beverages and products such as cola nut for at least four hours prior to lung function testing. Forced expiratory volume in one minute (FEV1) seems to show a small improvement up to two hours after caffeine use. Mid-expiratory flow rates may also improve with caffeine for up to four hours (9607).

URATE: Cola nut might falsely increase serum urate test results determined by the Bittner method, due to its caffeine content. Caffeine causes false elevations in serum urate test results determined by the Bittner method (15).
URINARY CALCIUM: Caffeine, a constituent of cola nut, can increase urinary calcium levels (11317).
VANILLYLMANDELIC ACID (VMA): Cola nut might increase urine VMA concentrations and test results, due to its caffeine content (15).

Interactions with Diseases or Conditions

ANXIETY DISORDERS: The caffeine in cola nut might aggravate anxiety disorders (11743).
BLEEDING DISORDERS: Theoretically, caffeine in cola nut might aggravate these conditions. Caffeine is reported to have antiplatelet activity (8028,8029); however, this interaction has not been reported in humans (1701). Caffeine can prolong bleeding time and increase the results of a bleeding time test (1701).
CARDIAC CONDITIONS: Caffeine in cola nut can induce cardiac arrhythmias in sensitive individuals (11845); use with caution.
DIABETES: Caffeine in cola nut may enhance the frequency and intensity of hypoglycemic warning symptoms in type 1 diabetics. This may increase the ability of diabetics to detect and treat hypoglycemia early. However, it might also increase the frequency of hypoglycemic events (6024); use with caution. Caffeine has been reported to cause increases and decreases in blood glucose (8646); use with caution.
GLAUCOMA: Consuming cola nut increases intraocular pressure due to its caffeine content. The increase occurs within 30 minutes and persists for at least 90 minutes (8540).
HYPERTENSION: The caffeine in cola nut might increase blood pressure in people with high blood pressure. However, this doesn't seem to occur in people who regularly consume cola nut or other caffeinated products (1451,1452,2722).
OSTEOPOROSIS: Consuming cola nut can increase urinary excretion of calcium due to its caffeine content. Caffeine consumption should be limited to less than 300 mg per day. Adequate calcium supplementation may partially compensate for calcium losses (2669,10202,11317). Postmenopausal women identified with a genetic variant of the vitamin D receptor should use caffeine with caution (2669).

Dosage and Administration

No typical dosage.

Comments

Cola nut is used widely in Nigeria and many West African countries as part of traditional hospitality and cultural and social ceremonies (11963).

COLLOIDAL MINERALS

Also Known As

Bioelectrical Minerals, Clay Suspension Products, Colloidal Trace Minerals, Humic Shale, Plant-Derived Liquid Minerals.

Scientific Names

Anhydrous aluminum silicates.

People Use This For

Orally, colloidal minerals are used as a supplemental source of trace minerals, a dietary supplement to increase energy, for improving blood sugar levels in diabetes, arthritis symptoms, reducing blood cell clumping, reversing early cataracts, turning gray hair dark again, flushing poisonous heavy metals from the body, improving general well being, reducing aches and pains.

Safety

POSSIBLY UNSAFE ...when used orally. These products contain varying amounts of aluminum, arsenic, lead, barium, nickel and titanium. Some products contain as much as 1800-4400 ppm aluminum and 20 ppm arsenic (1159); generally, foods do not contain more than 10 ppm of aluminum (1159). While no cases of toxicity have been reported, there are concerns about colloidal mineral supplements containing unsafe levels of radioactive metals (1161).
PREGNANCY AND LACTATION: POSSIBLY UNSAFE ...when used orally (1159); avoid using.

Effectiveness

There is insufficient reliable information available about the effectiveness of colloidal minerals.

Mechanism of Action

Commercial colloidal mineral products are derived from clay or humic shale deposits (1159). Clay minerals are layer type aluminosilicates that figure in terrestrial biogeochemical cycles, in the buffering capacity of the oceans, and in the containment of toxic waste materials (1160). Humic shale is a common source of plant-derived colloidal minerals (1157). When mixed with water, the surfaces of clay particles become negatively charged. This allows the particles to bind with ionic minerals, such as magnesium, sodium, calcium, and potassium (1159). The content of trace minerals in individual products depends upon the rock source used (1159). Proponents claim that, due to mineral depletion of soil, many people do not take in the dietary trace minerals once plentiful in the human diet (1158). However, there is no evidence that there is increased bioavailability of ingested minerals in this form (1159).

Adverse Reactions
None reported.

Interactions with Herbs & Other Dietary Supplements
None known.

Interactions with Drugs
None known.

Interactions with Foods
None known.

Interactions with Lab Tests
None known.

Interactions with Diseases or Conditions
HEMOCHROMATOSIS, WILSON'S DISEASE: Theoretically, colloidal minerals could exacerbate conditions in which metal accumulation is a problem.

Dosage and Administration
No typical dosage.

Comments
The medicinal use of clay-based products in modern days was first encouraged by a southern Utah rancher. Historically, some Native American tribes used clay medicinally (1157). There is a tremendous amount of promotional claims for colloidal mineral products. There is no reliable medical evidence to support using these products. Commercial colloidal mineral products are derived from clay or humic shale deposits (1159).

COLLOIDAL SILVER

Also Known As
Colloidal Silver Protein, Silver Protein.

Scientific Names
Silver in suspending agent.

People Use This For
Orally, colloidal silver is used to treat ear infections, emphysema, bronchitis, fungal infections, Lyme disease, Rosacea, sinus infections, stomach ulcers, yeast infections, chronic fatigue syndrome, AIDS, and tuberculosis. It is used orally for antibacterial properties, for food poisoning, to promote rapid healing and subdue inflammation, and to treat gum disease. It is used to improve digestion, and to prevent flu and colds. Colloidal silver is also used for allergies, appendicitis, arthritis, blood parasites, bubonic plague, cancer, cholera, colitis, cystitis, conjunctivitis, atopic dermatitis (cradle cap), diabetes, dysentery, eczema, gastritis, and gonorrhea. Other uses include impetigo; hay fever; herpes; leprosy; leukemia; lupus; lymphangitis; malaria; meningitis; parasitic infections; pneumonia; pneumococci; psoriasis; prostatitis; rhinitis; ringworm; scarlet fever; and septic conditions of the eyes, ears, mouth, and throat. It is also used for Salmonella, septicemia, shingles, skin cancer, syphilis, tonsillitis, toxemia, trench foot, viruses, warts, and yeast infections. Colloidal silver is used during pregnancy to aid the baby's growth and health as well as the mother's delivery and recovery.
Topically, colloidal silver is used for acne, burns, eye infections, fungal infections, throat infections, skin infections, and Staphylococcus infections.

Safety
POSSIBLY SAFE ...when used orally in amounts that do not exceed a total intake (including food and water) of 14 mcg/kg/day of silver (350 microgram/day/70kg person). Two liters of water meeting EPA standards could contain up to 200 mcg, plus a regular diet could contain 90 mcg (5525) for a total of 290 mcg without any additional oral or

topical silver use. It is likely that taking colloidal silver supplements on top of regular dietary consumption would increase silver intake to an unsafe level.
LIKELY UNSAFE ...when used orally or topically for medicinal purposes. Silver accumulates in the body and can lead to an irreversible bluish skin discoloration known as argyria. Neurological deficits, diffuse silver deposition in visceral organs, renal damage, and metal flume fever can occur (5525,5526,8148,8149,10647,10648,12092).
PREGNANCY AND LACTATION: POSSIBLY UNSAFE ...when used orally. Epidemiological evidence links increased silver levels to babies born with developmental anomalies of the ear, face, and neck (5525).

Effectiveness

There is insufficient reliable information available about the effectiveness of colloidal silver.

Mechanism of Action

Compounds that contain inorganic silver are germicidal. Silver binds to the reactive groups of proteins, causing denaturation and precipitation. Silver can also inactivate enzymes by binding to sulfhydryl, amino, carboxyl, phosphate, and imidazole groups. When absorbed, silver is most concentrated in the skin, liver, spleen, and adrenals with lesser amounts in the muscle and brain. The half-life depends on the silver salt used. Half-life can range from days to months. Silver deposited in the skin has a much longer half-life. Silver primarily leaves the body via fecal elimination with active biliary excretion (5525).

Adverse Reactions

Orally or topically, colloidal silver can lead to an irreversible bluish deposition of silver in the mucous and skin membranes known as argyria (5525,8148,8149,10647,10648,12092). Argyria typically first appears in the gingiva with a slate-blue silver line (5525). Toxicity may also present as blueish-gray discoloration of the fingernails (8149,10648). Colloidal silver can also stimulate melanin production in skin. Areas exposed to the sun will become increasingly discolored. Colloidal silver can also cause neurological deficits, diffuse silver deposition in visceral organs, renal damage, and metal flume fever (5525,8148,10647).

Interactions with Herbs & Other Dietary Supplements

None known.

Interactions with Drugs

LEVOTHYROXINE: Theoretically, levothyroxine might have reduced absorption if given with colloidal silver.
PENICILLAMINE: Theoretically, drugs such as penicillamine (Cuprimine) might have reduced absorption if given with colloidal silver.
QUINOLONE ANTIBIOTICS: Theoretically, quinolones such as ciprofloxacin (Cipro), norfloxacin (Noroxin), ofloxacin and others might have reduced absorption if given with colloidal silver.
TETRACYCLINE ANTIBIOTICS: Theoretically, drugs such as tetracycline might have reduced absorption if given with colloidal silver.

Interactions with Foods

None known.

Interactions with Lab Tests

None known.

Interactions with Diseases or Conditions

None known.

Dosage and Administration

No typical dosage.

Comments

Interestingly, there are many internet ads for the components of a generator to produce colloidal silver at home. Those who produce colloidal silver at home will likely have no means to assay the product to assure any standard potency. There are many products that are far safer and more effective than colloidal silver. Silver has no known physiological function and is not an essential mineral supplement, contrary to promoters' claims.

COLOCYNTH

Also Known As
Alhandal, Bitter Apple, Bitter Cucumber, Colocynth Pulp, Colocynthidis Fructus, Koloquinthen, Tumba, Vine-of-Sodom, Wild Gourd.

Scientific Names
Citrullus colocynthis, synonyms Colocynthis vulgaris, Cucumis colocynthis.
Family: Cucurbitaceae.

People Use This For
Orally, colocynth is used in combination products for acute and chronic constipation, and for liver and gallbladder ailments.

Safety
UNSAFE ...when used orally. Colocynth was banned by the FDA in 1991, due to toxicity (17).
PREGNANCY AND LACTATION: UNSAFE ...when used orally (17); avoid using.

Effectiveness
There is insufficient reliable information available about the effectiveness of colocynth.

Mechanism of Action
The applicable part of colocynth is the ripe fruit. It contains up to 3% cucurbitacin, a poisonous constituent that irritates mucous membranes, including GI mucosa (2) .

Adverse Reactions
Orally, ingestion of 0.6-1 grams of colocynth can cause severe irritation of the gastric mucosa, bloody diarrhea, kidney damage, hemorrhagic cystitis, and diuresis leading to anuria (2,18). Colocynth ingestion can also cause acute toxic colitis (10653). Doses of 2 grams or more can cause convulsions; paralysis; and if untreated, death from circulatory collapse (18).

Interactions with Herbs & Other Dietary Supplements
POTASSIUM DEPLETING HERBS: Theoretically, concomitant use with horsetail plant or licorice rhizome increases the risk of potassium depletion.
STIMULANT LAXATIVE HERBS: Theoretically, concomitant use with other stimulant laxative herbs may increase the risk of potassium depletion. Stimulant laxative herbs include aloe dried leaf sap, wild cucumber fruit (Ecballium elaterium), blue flag rhizome, alder buckthorn, European buckthorn, butternut bark, cascara bark, castor oil, gamboge bark exudate, jalap root, black root, manna bark exudate, podophyllum root, rhubarb root, senna leaves and pods, and yellow dock root (19).

Interactions with Drugs
DIGOXIN (Lanoxin): Theoretically, overuse/abuse of this product increases the risk of adverse effects of cardiac glycoside drugs.
DIURETIC DRUGS: Colocynth might compound diuretic-induced potassium loss (19). People taking colocynth along with potassium depleting diuretics might have an increased risk for hypokalemia. Some diuretics that can deplete potassium include chlorothiazide (Diuril), chlorthalidone (Thalitone), furosemide (Lasix), hydrochlorothiazide (HCTZ, HydroDIURIL, Microzide), and others.

Interactions with Foods
None known.

Interactions with Lab Tests
POTASSIUM: Excessive use of colocynth might cause potassium depletion, reducing serum potassium concentrations and test results (19).
URINE OUTPUT: Excessive use of colocynth might lead to cessation of urine output (anuria) (18).

Interactions with Diseases or Conditions
GASTROINTESTINAL (GI) CONDITIONS: Colocynth can irritate gastrointestinal tract. It is contraindicated in individuals with infectious or inflammatory gastrointestinal conditions (19).

Dosage and Administration
No typical dosage.

Comments
Colocynth is considered unsafe; avoid using. The use of colocynth is not justified due to significant risks (2). Death has resulted from the consumption of as little as 1 1/2 teaspoons of the powder. In the management of poisoning, a dilute tannic acid solution should be taken, followed by large quantities of albuminous drinks (215).

COLOMBO

Also Known As
Calomba Root, Calumba, Calumbo Root.

Scientific Names
Jateorhiza palmata, synonyms Wateorhiza palmata, Cocculus palmatus, Jateorhiza columba, Jateorhiza miersii, Menispermum columba, Menispermum palmatum.
Family: Menispermaceae.

People Use This For
Orally, colombo is used to treat gastritis, dyspepsia, chronic enterocolitis, and diarrhea.

Safety
There is insufficient reliable information available about the safety of colombo.
Pregnancy and Lactation: Insufficient reliable information; avoid using.

Effectiveness
There is insufficient reliable information available about the effectiveness of colombo.

Mechanism of Action
The applicable part of colombo is the root. Colombo contains alkaloids that have narcotic properties and side effects similar to morphine (7,18). Colombo might increase the resting tone of smooth muscle in the intestinal tract (7,18). In frogs, the alkaloids appear to act as a central nervous system (CNS) paralyzing agent (18). Palmatine, the main alkaloid component, has a similar effect in mammals (18). Colombo's use as a digestive aid is empirically based upon the bitter content, which is believed to increase stomach acid secretion via vagal nerve stimulation (19).

Adverse Reactions
Orally, large doses of colombo may cause vomiting and epigastric pain (18). Overdose can lead to paralysis and unconsciousness (18).

Interactions with Herbs & Other Dietary Supplements
None known.

Interactions with Drugs
ANTACIDS: Theoretically, due to reports that colombo increases stomach acid, colombo might decrease the effectiveness of antacids (19).
H2-BLOCKERS: Theoretically, due to reports that colombo increases stomach acid, colombo might decrease the effectiveness of H2-blockers (19). The H2 blockers include cimetidine (Tagamet), ranitidine (Zantac), nizatidine (Axid), and famotidine (Pepcid).
PROTON PUMP INHIBITORS (PPIs): Theoretically, due to reports that colombo increases stomach acid, colombo might decrease the effectiveness of PPIs (19). PPIs include omeprazole (Prilosec), lansoprazole (Prevacid), rabeprazole (Aciphex), pantoprazole (Protonix), and esomeprazole (Nexium).

Interactions with Foods
None known.

Interactions with Lab Tests
None known.

Interactions with Diseases or Conditions
None known.

Dosage and Administration
ORAL: A typical dose is 2 teaspoons of the boiled root as tea taken every hour (18). For single use, 20 drops of the extract or 2.5 grams of the tincture has been used (18). The root should be stored in a dry area (18).

Comments
Colombo is no longer used as a digestive aid and is rarely used as an antidiarrheal agent because of its morphine-like effects (18).

COLOSTRUM

Also Known As
Bovine Colostrum, Bovine Immunoglobulin, Cow Milk Colostrum, Goat Colostrum, Hyperimmune Bovine Colostrum.

Scientific Names
None.

People Use This For
Orally, bovine colostrum is used for stimulating the immune system, healing injuries, repairing nervous system damage, burning fat, building lean muscle, increasing stamina and vitality, elevating mood and sense of well being, slowing and reversing aging, and as an antibacterial and antifungal agent. Orally, hyperimmune bovine colostrum is also used in treating AIDS-related diarrhea (FDA Orphan Drug Status), diarrhea associated with graft versus host disease following bone marrow transplant, and rotavirus diarrhea in children.
Rectally, bovine colostrum is used for treating colitis.

Safety
LIKELY SAFE ...when used orally and appropriately. There are no reports of significant toxicity in multiple human trials (4901,4903,4904,4905,4906,4907,4908,4909). Bovine colostrum seems to be safe, however, it is derived from animals, and there is some concern about contamination with diseased animal parts (1825). So far, there are no reports of disease transmission to humans due to use of contaminated bovine colostrum.
POSSIBLY SAFE ...when used rectally and appropriately as a 10% enema (9730).
PREGNANCY AND LACTATION: Insufficient reliable information available; avoid using.

Effectiveness
POSSIBLY EFFECTIVE

Infectious diarrhea. Taking bovine colostrum orally seems to reduce infectious diarrhea in children and immunocompromised patients including patients with HIV/AIDS and bone marrow transplant recipients. It seems to be effective against rotaviral diarrhea in children (4903,4904,4909), cryptosporidium-related diarrhea in immunocompromised patients (4905,4906,4907,4908,10659), and diarrhea caused enterotoxigenic Escherichia coli (2067,2068,2069) or Shigella flexneri (2070). Hyperimmune bovine colostrum has FDA orphan status for AIDS-related diarrhea (9840).
Most clinical trials have used colostrum from pregnant cows which have been immunized against specific pathogens. The hyperimmune colostrum provides high antibody titers against organisms for which the cow has been immunized (4905).

INSUFFICIENT RELIABLE EVIDENCE to RATE

Athletic performance. Preliminary evidence suggests oral bovine colostrum may increase athletic performance in events that rely on peak anaerobic power, such as vertical jumping and bicycle sprints, after 8 weeks of supplementation (11453).
Distal colitis. There is some preliminary evidence that a 10% rectal enema of bovine colostrum might be helpful for treating distal colitis (9730).
More evidence is needed to rate bovine colostrum for these uses.

Mechanism of Action
Colostrum is the milky fluid produced by mammals within the first few days after giving birth. Most nutritional colostrum preparations come from cows (3567). Bovine colostrum contains proteins, carbohydrates, fat, vitamins, minerals, and immunoglobulin A (IgA) and immunoglobulin G (IgG) in concentrations approximately 100 times higher than dairy milk (4901). Because of the antibody content, bovine colostrum was thought to offer passive immunotherapy to people with enteric infections; however, bovine colostrum contains only low concentrations of antibodies against enteric pathogens and does not provide high enough titers to prevent disease. Hyperimmune bovine colostrum can be produced by immunizing pregnant cows against specific pathogens (e.g. cryptosporidium or rotavirus) resulting in increased specific colostrum antibody titers (4903). Hyperimmune bovine colostrum has been primarily used in clinical trials; however, the small amounts of antibodies that have been recovered from people who ingested hyperimmune colostrum were nonreactive (2072).
Taking bovine colostrum might increase peak anaerobic power and improve exercise performance; however, the mechanism of action is not yet understood. Animals fed bovine colostrum have shown an increase in skeletal muscle protein synthesis, creating an interest in the use of bovine colostrum for improvement in exercise performance (11453).

Oral bovine colostrum supplementation does not appear to affect insulin response or the plasma nutrient absorptive capacity of alanine or glucose, once suggested as possible mechanisms (11454). Some evidence suggests bovine colostrum contains insulin-like growth factors (IGF), and appears to increase serum insulin-like growth factor I (IGF-I) and insulin in athletes (4901). However, separate evidence suggests bovine colostrum does not alter plasma IGF-I (11453).
Bovine colostrum contains growth factors, cytokines, hormones, and other factors biologically active components that might improve growth and repair of the gastrointestinal system (9731). Preliminary data indicates that bovine colostrum reduces indomethacin-induced gastrointestinal injury and addition of colostrum to drinking water prevents experimental small intestinal injury (4911). Some evidence suggests that bovine colostrum promotes small intestinal growth (4901). The phosphatidylethanolamine in hyperimmune bovine colostrum may prevent Helicobacter pylori from binding to the gastric mucosa (2065). The effectiveness of hyperimmune bovine colostrum may decrease when it is taken with a meal (2070), possibly due to stomach acid and digestive enzymes (2071).

Adverse Reactions

Orally, bovine colostrum has caused nausea and vomiting in an individual with HIV-related cryptosporidiosis. Elevated liver function tests and decreased serum hematocrit have also been reported in HIV patients treated for infectious diarrhea (4905). It may cause allergic reaction in individuals allergic to bovine milk products. There is also some concern that bovine colostrum that is obtained from cows in countries where bovine spongiform encephalitis (BSE) has been reported might be unsafe, however, there is no research indicating that colostrum can be contaminated with the BSE-causing prion. Countries where BSE has been reported include Great Britain, France, The Netherlands, Portugal, Luxembourg, Ireland, Switzerland, Oman, and Belgium (1825). Until more is known, tell patients to avoid these products unless country of origin can be determined. Patients should avoid products that are produced in countries where BSE has been found.

Interactions with Herbs & Other Dietary Supplements

None known.

Interactions with Drugs

None known.

Interactions with Foods

MEALS: Taking hyperimmune bovine colostrum with food may decrease antibody activity due to the increase in stomach acid and digestive enzyme secretion (2070,2071,2072).

Interactions with Lab Tests

None known.

Interactions with Diseases or Conditions

BOVINE MILK ALLERGY: Avoid using.

Dosage and Administration

ORAL: For enhanced athletic performance, 125 mL colostrum whey product twice daily or 60 grams bovine colostrum protein powder daily has been used; however, these products are not available in the US (11453,11454,4901). For AIDS-related Cryptosporidium parvum diarrhea, 10 grams powder four times daily for 21 days has been used (4905). For AIDS-related cryptosporidial and other infectious diarrhea, 10-20 grams daily for 10 days has been used (4906). For graft versus host disease following bone marrow transplant, 10 grams per day for 10 days has been used (4907). For rotavirus diarrhea in children 10 grams, equivalent to 3.6 grams antirotavirus antibodies, per day for 4 days has been used (4903). 100 mL four times per day for 4 days has also been used (4904).
RECTAL: For treating distal colitis, 100 mL of a 10% enema of bovine colostrum two times daily has been used for 4 weeks (9730).

Comments

Bovine colostrum is the milk secreted by cows during the first few days after calving (4901). Hyperimmune bovine colostrum is produced by cows immunized against specific pathogens. Bovine colostrum is not on the banned drug list of the International Olympic Committee (4901).

COLTSFOOT

Also Known As

Ass's Foot, Brandlattich, British Tobacco, Bullsfoot, Colts Foot, Coughwort, Farfarae Folium leaf, Fieldhove, Filuis Ante Patrem, Flower Velure, Foal's Foot, Foalswort, Guflatich, Hallfoot, Horsefoot, Horsehoof, Kuandong Hua, Pas d'Ane, Pas Diane, Pferdefut, Tussilage.

Scientific Names

Tussilago farfara.
Family: Asteraceae/Compositae.

People Use This For

Orally, coltsfoot is used for bronchitis, asthma, laryngitis, pertussis, acute respiratory tract mucous membrane inflammation with cough and hoarseness, acute or mild inflammation of the oral and pharyngeal mucosa, and sore throat.
As an inhalant, coltsfoot is used for coughs and wheezing.

Safety

UNSAFE ...when used orally (7,12,515). All parts of coltsfoot contain unsaturated pyrrolizidine alkaloids (UPAs) in varying amounts (7). The unsaturated pyrrolizidine alkaloids are considered to be hepatotoxic and hepatocarcinogenic (7,515). UPAs are extracted into teas when prepared from coltsfoot leaves (7). Repeated exposure to low concentrations of UPAs has been linked to veno-occlusive disease (4,12,515). UPAs might also be mutagenic (12). Dietary supplement products sold in the United States are not required to include the amount of UPAs they may contain; therefore, all preparations used orally containing coltsfoot should be considered potentially unsafe (3484).
PREGNANCY AND LACTATION: UNSAFE ...when used orally; contraindicated due to its potential to be abortifacient (4,19) and hepatotoxic (4,12,575). Hepatotoxic UPAs may be excreted in breast milk (4,12,18).

Effectiveness

There is insufficient reliable information available about the effectiveness of coltsfoot.

Mechanism of Action

The applicable part of coltsfoot is the leaf. Coltsfoot has been documented to have expectorant, antitussive, demulcent, and anti-inflammatory effects on mucous membranes (4). The mucilage content of coltsfoot has a soothing effect on the throat (6,515). Coltsfoot contains the unsaturated pyrrolizidine alkaloids (UPAs) senkirkirine and senecionine (4,7,515). UPAs are known to be hepatotoxic in animals and humans (4,7,515). UPAs destroy and damage centrilobular hepatocytes of the liver and also destroy small branches of the hepatic vein (7). Animals fed various amounts of coltsfoot have been reported to develop cancerous tumors in the liver (515,3484). In animals, coltsfoot has anti-inflammatory and antibacterial activity against gram negative bacteria (4). It also contains an inhibitor of the platelet activating factor (PAF). PAF is known to play a key role in the inflammatory cascade. The presence of a PAF inhibitor in coltsfoot can account for the effect of coltsfoot in asthma (4). The constituent tusilagone has respiratory stimulant and cardiovascular (including pressor) activities (4). Cardiovascular effects are thought to be mediated by peripheral mechanisms and the respiratory effects by central mechanisms (4). An isolated coltsfoot constituent interacts with the cardiac calcium channel blocker receptor complex (dihydropyridine receptor), but it also has calcium channel blocking activity (4). In animals, coltsfoot is reported to have a pressor effect similar to dopamine but without tachyphylaxis and to be phototoxic (4).

Adverse Reactions

Nonspecific symptoms such as anorexia, lethargy and abdominal pain can result after chronic use of coltsfoot (7). Further use can lead to hepatotoxicity (4,7). There is one case report of fatal hepatic veno-occlusive disease in a neonate associated with regular maternal consumption during pregnancy of an herb tea containing several pyrrolizidine alkaloid herbs, including coltsfoot (575). Coltsfoot may cause an allergic reaction in individuals sensitive to the Asteraceae/Compositae family. Members of this family include ragweed, chrysanthemums, marigolds, daisies, and many other herbs.

Interactions with Herbs & Other Dietary Supplements

EUCALYPTUS: Theoretically, concomitant use can increase the toxicity of coltsfoot due to enzyme induction by eucalyptus (19).
UNSATURATED PYRROLIZIDINE ALKALOID (UPA)-CONTAINING HERBS: Concomitant use is contraindicated due to the risk of additive toxicity. Herbs containing UPAs include alkanna; borage; gravel root; hemp agrimony; hound's tongue; petasites; comfrey; and the Senecio species dusty miller, alpine ragwort, groundsel, golden ragwort, and tansy ragwort (4,12,19,271).

Interactions with Drugs
ANTIHYPERTENSIVE DRUGS: Theoretically, excessive doses of coltsfoot may interfere with antihypertensive or cardiovascular therapy (4).

Interactions with Foods
None known.

Interactions with Lab Tests
None known.

Interactions with Diseases or Conditions
CROSS-ALLERGENICITY: Coltsfoot may cause an allergic reaction in individuals sensitive to the Asteraceae/Compositae family. Members of this family include ragweed, chrysanthemums, marigolds, daisies, and many other herbs.
HYPERTENSION, CARDIOVASCULAR DISEASE: Excessive amounts of coltsfoot may interfere with therapy for hypertension or cardiovascular disease (4).
LIVER DISEASE: Coltsfoot is contraindicated due to its hepatotoxic potential (19).

Dosage and Administration
No typical dosage.

COLUMBINE

Also Known As
Culverwort.

Scientific Names
Aquilegia vulgaris.
Family: Ranunculaceae.

Comments
At the date of publication, there was very little scientific information about this product. Our staff is continually analyzing the available information on natural medicines and will add data to the online version of *Natural Medicines Comprehensive Database* as it becomes available. See www.naturaldatabase.com.

COMFREY

Also Known As
Ass Ear, Black Root, Blackwort, Bruisewort, Common Comfrey, Consolidae Radix, Consound, Gum Plant, Healing Herb, Knitback, Knitbone, Salsify, Slippery Root, Symphytum Radix, Wallwort.

Scientific Names
Symphytum officinale.
Family: Boraginaceae.

People Use This For
Orally, comfrey is used as a tea for gastritis, ulcers, excessive menstrual flow, diarrhea, bloody urine, persistent cough, rheumatoid arthritis, pleuritis, bronchitis, cancer, angina, as a gargle for gum disease, and pharyngitis. Topically, comfrey is used for ulcers, wounds, joint inflammation, bruises, phlebitis, gout, and fractures.

Safety
POSSIBLY SAFE ...when used topically short-term on unbroken skin at or below a daily dosage of 100 mcg of the hepatotoxic pyrrolizidine alkaloids. Externally applied pyrrolizidine alkaloids are absorbed through the skin (11990,11992).
UNSAFE ...when used orally because of its potential for acute or chronic liver toxicity. Comfrey contains pyrrolizidine alkaloids. Chronic ingestion of more than 1 mg per day for 2 weeks or more than 0.1 mg per day for longer periods can cause liver disease. Pyrrolizidine alkaloids may also be carcinogenic (11987). The FDA has recommended removal of oral comfrey products from the market (11988).

PREGNANCY AND LACTATION: UNSAFE ...when used orally or topically. In addition to hepatotoxicity and possibly carcinogenicity, the pyrrolizidine alkaloids in comfrey might be teratogenic. Pyrrolizidine alkaloids are absorbed through the skin (11987,11988,11990).

Effectiveness

INSUFFICIENT RELIABLE EVIDENCE to RATE

Bruises and sprains. Preliminary clinical research suggests that applying comfrey topically might improve pain and tenderness of bruises, sprains, and painful conditions of the muscles and joints (11991). More evidence is needed to rate comfrey for this use.

Mechanism of Action

The applicable parts of comfrey are the leaf, rhizome, and root. Comfrey contains symphytine, lasiocarpine and other pyrrolizidine alkaloids that are hepatotoxic and possibly carcinogenic, mutagenic, and teratogenic. Pyrrolizidine alkaloids cause veno-occlusive liver disease. They destroy and damage centrilobular hepatocytes of the liver and also destroy small branches of the hepatic vein. Pyrrolizidine alkaloids can also damage the lungs, resulting in pulmonary hypertension (11987,11988,11990). The pyrrolizidine alkaloid content of comfrey varies with time of harvesting and plant age. The roots have 10 times higher concentrations of pyrrolizidine alkaloids than the leaves (11990,11991). Pyrrolizidine alkaloids are metabolized in the liver by the cytochrome P450 enzyme system to toxic dehydroalkaloids and pyrroles. Enzyme inducers such as phenobarbital seem to enhance toxicity (11990). Pyrroles are excreted as N-acetyl cysteine conjugates. Some researchers speculate that early administration of N-acetylcysteine might reduce toxicity (11988).

Adverse Reactions

Orally, comfrey can cause acute veno-occlusive disease characterized by sudden abdominal pain, vomiting, ascites, and hepatomegaly. In subacute disease, comfrey can cause ascites, hepatomegaly, abdominal pain, diarrhea, vomiting, and abdominal swelling. Chronic toxicity appears as asthenia and progressive ascites. Hepatic fibrosis and inflammation may resolve, but hepatic failure is common with more severe disease. This may occur as late as 2 years after the initial ingestion. Other signs and symptoms of pyrrolizidine toxicity include bile duct proliferation, fatty changes of the liver, fibrosis, cirrhosis, and vascular lesions (11988). The mortality of comfrey toxicity is 50%. However, toxicity seems to vary among individuals (11990).

Topically, pyrrolizidine alkaloids can be absorbed in quantities sufficient to cause toxicity with extended use or in high concentrations (11990).

Interactions with Herbs & Other Dietary Supplements

HEPATOTOXIC HERBS: Theoretically, comfrey might have additive effects with herbs that cause hepatotoxicity (11988,11990). Other products that might affect the liver include chaparral, bishop's weed, borage, kava, uva ursi, and others.

HERBS THAT INDUCE CYTOCHROME P450 3A4 (CYP3A4): Theoretically, herbs that induce CYP3A4 might increase the conversion of comfrey to toxic metabolites, enhancing toxicity (11990). Herbs that induce CYP3A4 include St. John's wort and garlic.

PYRROLIZIDINE ALKALOID-CONTAINING HERBS: Concomitant use is contraindicated due to the risk of additive toxicity. Herbs containing pyrrolizidine alkaloids include alkanna, borage, butterbur, coltsfoot, forget-me-not, gravel root, hemp agrimony, hound's tongue, lungwort, and the Senecio species dusty miller, alpine ragwort, groundsel, golden ragwort, and tansy ragwort (11988,11990).

Interactions with Drugs

CYTOCHROME P450 3A4 (CYP3A4) INDUCERS: Theoretically, drugs that induce CYP3A4 might increase the conversion of comfrey to toxic metabolites, enhancing toxicity (11990). Some drugs that induce CYP3A4 include carbamazepine (Tegretol), phenobarbital, phenytoin (Dilantin), rifampin, rifabutin (Mycobutin), and others.

HEPATOTOXIC DRUGS: Theoretically, comfrey might have additive adverse effects on the liver when used with hepatotoxic drugs (11988,11990). Some drugs that can adversely affect the liver include acetaminophen (Tylenol), amiodarone (Cordarone), carbamazepine (Tegretol), isoniazid (INH), methotrexate (Rheumatrex), methyldopa (Aldomet), and many others.

Interactions with Foods

None known.

Interactions with Lab Tests

LIVER FUNCTION TESTS: The pyrrolizidine alkaloids in comfrey might increase liver function tests including alkaline phosphatase, aspartic acid transaminase (AST,SGOT) alanine aminotransferase (ALT, SGPT), total bilirubin, gamma-glutamyltransferase, and lactate dehydrogenase (11988).

Interactions with Diseases or Conditions

BROKEN, DAMAGED SKIN: Contraindicated. Apply only to unbroken skin. Broken skin might result in exposure to high concentrations of pyrrolizidine alkaloids (11990).
LIVER DISEASE: Theoretically, comfrey might exacerbate liver dysfunction in patients with liver disease (11988,11990).

Dosage and Administration

No typical dosage.

Comments

Some products labeled common comfrey or Symphytum officinale actually contain the more toxic prickly comfrey (Symphytum asperum) or Russian comfrey (Symphytum x uplandicum) species (11991).

COMMON STONECROP

Also Known As

Bird Bread, Creeping Tom, Gold Chain, Golden Moss, Jack-of-the-Buttery, Mousetail, Prick Madam, Wall Ginger, Wallpepper.

Scientific Names

Sedum acre. Family: Crassulaceae.

People Use This For

Orally, common stonecrop is used for coughs and hypertension.
Topically, common stonecrop is used for wounds, burns, hemorrhoids, warts, eczema, and mouth ulcers.

Safety

There is insufficient reliable information available about the safety of common stonecrop.
Pregnancy and Lactation: Insufficient reliable information available; avoid using.

Effectiveness

There is insufficient reliable information available about the effectiveness of common stonecrop.

Mechanism of Action

There is insufficient reliable information available about the possible mechanism of action and active ingredients.

Adverse Reactions

Orally, common stonecrop can cause vomiting and diarrhea if consumed in greater then medicinal amounts (18).

Interactions with Herbs & Other Dietary Supplements

None known.

Interactions with Drugs

None known.

Interactions with Foods

None known.

Interactions with Lab Tests

None known.

Interactions with Diseases or Conditions

GI AND LOWER URINARY TRACT INFLAMMATION: Contraindicated (18).

Dosage and Administration

ORAL: Typically, one cup tea (simmer 1 teaspoon or 1.5 grams in 150 mL boiling water for 10-15 minutes, strain) twice daily (18).
TOPICAL: Crush fresh plant and place on eczematous skin or warts.

CONDURANGO

Also Known As
Common Condorvine, Condurango Cortex, Eagle-Vine Bark.

Scientific Names
Marsdenia cundurango, synonym Marsdenia reichenbachii; Gonolobus condurango.
Family: Apocynaceae or Asclepiadaceae.

People Use This For
Orally, condurango is used as an appetite stimulant and for dyspeptic complaints, and for stomach cancer.

Safety
LIKELY SAFE ...when used orally and appropriately (2).
PREGNANCY AND LACTATION: Insufficient reliable information available; avoid using.

Effectiveness
There is insufficient reliable information available about the effectiveness of condurango.

Mechanism of Action
The applicable part of condurango is the bark. The condurango alkaloid constituents, which as a group are referred to as condurangin, stimulate salivation and the secretion of gastric juices (8).

Adverse Reactions
Orally, anaphylaxis can occur with the use of condurango bark (1501).

Interactions with Herbs & Other Dietary Supplements
None known.

Interactions with Drugs
None known.

Interactions with Foods
None known.

Interactions with Lab Tests
None known.

Interactions with Diseases or Conditions
LATEX ALLERGY: Cross-sensitivity to condurango can occur in individuals allergic to natural rubber latex (1500), including anaphylaxis (1501). Avoid the use of condurango in these individuals.

Dosage and Administration
ORAL: The typical dose of the bark is 2-4 grams per day (2). The usual dose of the water extract is 200-500 mg per day (2). The common dose of the liquid extract is 2-4 grams per day (2), and the tincture is usually given as 2-5 grams per day (2).

CONJUGATED LINOLEIC ACID

Also Known As
CLA, CLA-Free Fatty Acid, CLA-FFA, CLA-Triacylglycerol, Linoleic Acid.

Scientific Names
cis-9,trans-11 conjugated linoleic acid; Trans-10,cis-12 conjugated linoleic acid.

People Use This For
Orally, conjugated linoleic acid (CLA) is used for cancer, obesity, cachexia, bodybuilding, for limiting food allergy reactions, and for atherosclerosis.

Safety

LIKELY SAFE ...when used orally in amounts found in foods. Conjugated linoleic acid occurs naturally in milk fat, beef, and meat of other ruminant animals (5924,5925,5932,5933).
POSSIBLY SAFE ...when used orally and appropriately in medicinal amounts (2819,2821,3153,4947,10410,11327).
PREGNANCY AND LACTATION: LIKELY SAFE ...when used orally in amounts found in foods (5924,5932,5933). There is insufficient reliable information available about the safety of conjugated linoleic acid when used in medicinal amounts during pregnancy or lactation; avoid using.

Effectiveness

POSSIBLY EFFECTIVE

Obesity. Taking conjugated linoleic acid (CLA) orally seems to improve body composition in patients who are overweight or obese. Taking 0.7 to 4.5 grams/day seems to significantly decrease body fat mass (BFM) and might increase lean body mass (LBM) in some patients. But CLA does not seem to reduce total body weight (2819,2821,3153,4947,10410). CLA also seems to reduce hunger and improve satiety and feeling of fullness, but this appetite suppression does not necessarily result in a lower energy intake or improved body weight maintenance (11327).

INSUFFICIENT RELIABLE EVIDENCE to RATE

Breast cancer. There is preliminary evidence that CLA might help reduce the risk of breast cancer. Postmenopausal women who have a higher intake of CLA in foods, particularly cheese, seem to have a lower risk of developing breast cancer (5058). More evidence is needed to rate CLA for this use.

Mechanism of Action

Conjugated linoleic acid (CLA) refers to a group of conjugated dienoic isomers of linoleic acid, including cis-9, trans-11 linoleic acid and trans-10, cis-12 linoleic acid. Different isomeric forms might have different physiological effects (3158). Dairy products and beef are the major dietary sources. These primarily contain the cis-9, trans-11 isomer. Plant oils contain only small amounts of CLA. Plant oils are good sources of linoleic acid, but in humans linoleic acid does not seem to be converted to CLA in significant amounts (5933). Conjugated linoleic acid can also be produced synthetically by exposing oils rich in linoleic acid, such as safflower and soybean, to a base and heat. This CLA product is high in both the cis-9, trans-11 and the trans-10, cis-12 isomers (3001). There's a lot of interest in using CLA for weight loss in obesity. Researchers think that CLA might reduce body fat deposits by promoting apoptosis in adipose tissue (3070,5928). There is some evidence that only the trans-10, cis-12 isomer has an effect on body fat mass (3001). Additional evidence, however, shows the trans-10, cis-12 isomer may also increase insulin resistance and glycemia, and reduce HDL cholesterol (2821). There is also interest in using CLA for cancer prevention. Preliminary evidence suggests CLA may be cytotoxic to human breast cancer cells. It may also inhibit the proliferation of human malignant melanoma and colorectal cancer cells (8997). CLA appears to enhance immune function (5926,5934), increase peripheral blood mononuclear cell production (2810), and inhibit cyclooxygenase and lipoxygenase pathways in tumor cells (5926,5934). CLA might also modulate cellular response to tumor necrosis factor-alpha (TNF-alpha) (5924).

Adverse Reactions

Orally, the most common adverse effect of conjugated linoleic acid is gastrointestinal upset including diarrhea, nausea, loose stools, and dyspepsia (3153,4947). In some cases patients can experience fatigue (3153).

Interactions with Herbs & Other Dietary Supplements

VITAMIN A: Some evidence suggests conjugated linoleic acid might increase vitamin A (retinol) storage in liver and breast tissues (5931).

Interactions with Drugs

None known.

Interactions with Foods

None known.

Interactions with Lab Tests

CHOLESTEROL: Conjugated linoleic acid appears to reduce total, low-density lipoprotein (LDL), and high-density lipoprotein (HDL) cholesterol levels (3153).

Interactions with Diseases or Conditions

DIABETES: Conjugated linoleic acid (CLA) may increase insulin resistance and glycemia. Monitor blood glucose level closely (2821).

Dosage and Administration
ORAL: For weight loss in obese patients, a dose of 2 to 7 grams per day has been used. However, doses greater than 3.4 grams per day do not seem to offer any additional benefit (3153,11327).

Comments
An average diet supplies 15-174 mg of conjugated linoleic acid (CLA) daily (2820).

CONTRAYERVA

Also Known As
Contrayerba, Herbe-Chapeau.

Scientific Names
Dorstenia contrayerva; Dorstenia contrajerva.
Family: Moraceae.

Comments
At the date of publication, this product was not a common ingredient used in brand name supplements marketed to consumers. Details about this product are available at the online version of *Natural Medicines Comprehensive Database*. See www.naturaldatabase.com.

COOLWORT

Also Known As
Foam Flower, Mitrewort.

Scientific Names
Tiarella cordifolia.
Family: Saxifragaceae.

Comments
At the date of publication, this product was not a common ingredient used in brand name supplements marketed to consumers. Details about this product are available at the online version of *Natural Medicines Comprehensive Database*. See www.naturaldatabase.com.

COPAIBA BALSAM

Also Known As
Balsam, Copaiba, Copaiba Oleoresin, Copaiva, Jesuit's Balsam.

Scientific Names
Copaifera officinalis; Copaifera langsdorffii; Copaifera reticulata; and other Copaifera species.
Family: Fabaceae/Leguminosae.

People Use This For
Orally, copaiba balsam is used for chronic bronchitis, hemorrhoids, chronic diarrhea, chronic cystitis, urinary tract infections, as a stimulant, and a laxative.
In foods and beverages, copaiba balsam oleoresin is used as an ingredient.
In manufacturing, copaiba balsam oleoresin and oil are used in soaps, cosmetics, and perfumes.
In pharmaceutical preparations, both the oleoresin and oil are used in cough medicines and diuretics.

Safety
LIKELY SAFE ...when used orally in amounts commonly found in foods. Copaiba has Generally Recognized As Safe (GRAS) status in the US (4912). ...when used topically (11).
POSSIBLY UNSAFE ...when used orally for medicinal purposes. Copaiba balsam can irritate mucous membranes. Ingesting 5 grams can cause stomach pains (18).
PREGNANCY AND LACTATION: POSSIBLY UNSAFE ...when used orally for medicinal purposes; avoid using.

Effectiveness
There is insufficient reliable information available about the effectiveness of copaiba balsam.

Mechanism of Action
Copaiba balsam contains a volatile oil consisting of alpha and beta-caryophyllene, L-cadinenes, and copene. It also has resins, including diterpenoid oleoresins. Some evidence suggests copaiba balsam might have bacteriostatic (18), diuretic, expectorant, disinfectant, and stimulant activity (11). In addition to these properties, the oil exhibits antibacterial activity (11). Some evidence suggests the oleoresin of the Brazilian Copaifera species might have anti-inflammatory effects (11).

Adverse Reactions
Orally, ingesting 5 grams of copaiba balsam orally can cause stomach pains (18); repeated doses can cause shivers, tremor, groin pain, and insomnia (18). Large amounts may cause vomiting, diarrhea, and measles-like rash (11). Topically, copaiba balsam can cause contact dermatitis with erythema, papular or vesicular rash, urticaria, petechiae, and the rash may leave brown spots after healing (18).

Interactions with Herbs & Other Dietary Supplements
None known.

Interactions with Drugs
None known.

Interactions with Foods
None known.

Interactions with Lab Tests
None known.

Interactions with Diseases or Conditions
None known.

Dosage and Administration
No typical dosage.

Comments
Copaiba balsam is an oleoresin rather than a true balsam collected from the trunk of Copaifera species trees (11). Copaiba oil is distilled from the oleoresin (11). Copaiba balsam is considered obsolete for medicinal purposes (18).

COPPER

Also Known As
Cuivre, Cupric Oxide, Elemental Copper.

Scientific Names
Copper; Cu; atomic number 29.

People Use This For
Orally, copper is used for treating copper deficiency, anemia due to copper deficiency, zinc-induced copper deficiency, improving wound healing, osteoarthritis, and osteoporosis.

Safety
LIKELY SAFE ...when used orally and appropriately. Copper is safe in amounts that do not exceed 10 mg per day, the Tolerable Upper Intake Level (UL) (7135).
POSSIBLY UNSAFE ...when used orally in high doses. Tell patients to avoid exceeding the UL of 10 mg per day. Higher intake can cause liver damage (7135). Renal failure and death can occur with ingestion of as little as 1 gram of copper sulfate (17).
CHILDREN: LIKELY SAFE ...when used orally and appropriately. Copper is safe in amounts that do not exceed the UL of 1 mg per day for children 1 to 3 years, 3 mg per day for children 4 to 8 years, 5 mg per day for children 9 to 13 years, and 8 mg per day for adolescents (7135). POSSIBLY UNSAFE ...when used orally in high doses. Tell patients to avoid exceeding the UL of 1 mg per day for children 1 to 3 years, 3 mg per day for children 4 to 8 years, 5 mg per day for children 9 to 13 years, and 8 mg per day for adolescents (7135). Higher intake can

cause liver damage (7135).

PREGNANCY: LIKELY SAFE ...when used orally and appropriately. Copper is safe in amounts that do not exceed the UL of 8 mg per day for women 14 to 18 years, or 10 mg per day for women 19 and older (7135). POSSIBLY UNSAFE ...when used orally in high doses. Tell patients to avoid exceeding the UL of 8 mg per day for women 14 to 18 years, or 10 mg per day for women 19 and older. Higher intake can cause liver damage (7135).

LACTATION: LIKELY SAFE ...when used orally and appropriately. Copper is safe in amounts that do not exceed the UL of 10 mg per day for breast-feeding women 19 or older, or 8 mg per day for breast-feeding women ages 14 to 18 years (7135). POSSIBLY UNSAFE ...when used orally in high doses. Tell patients to avoid exceeding the UL of 10 mg per day for breast-feeding women 19 or older, or 8 mg per day for breast-feeding women ages 14 to 18 years. Higher intake can cause liver damage (7135).

Effectiveness

LIKELY EFFECTIVE

Copper deficiency. Taking copper orally or intravenously is effective for treating copper deficiency and anemia due to copper deficiency. Copper deficiency is rare. It is seen most commonly in people receiving prolonged parenteral nutrition (7135).

There is insufficient reliable information available about the effectiveness of copper for its other uses.

Mechanism of Action

Copper is an essential trace mineral. It is widely distributed in foods particularly in organ meats, seafood, nuts, seeds, wheat bran cereals, grain products, and cocoa products (7135). Absorption occurs primarily in the small intestine with lesser absorption in the stomach (7135). The majority of copper in the body is in the skeleton and muscles; the liver maintains plasma copper concentrations. Excretion of copper into the gastrointestinal tract regulates copper homeostasis; greater excretion is the result of increased absorption (7135). Biochemically, copper acts as a catalytic agent via the many copper metalloenzymes which act as oxidases (7135). Amine oxidases are important in a variety of processes including allergic reactions, serotonin and catecholamine degradation, and connective tissue development. Ferroxidases, copper enzymes in the plasma, are required for ferrous iron oxidation and binding of iron to transferrin. The main copper protein in plasma Ferroxidase I, also called ceruloplasmin, might have antioxidant functions. Another copper enzyme, cytochrome-c oxidase, is a mitochondrial enzyme that catalyzes the reduction of oxygen to water to fuel ATP synthesis. Cytochrome-c oxidase is most abundant in highly metabolic tissues, including the heart, brain, and liver. Other copper enzymes are responsible for precursors of dopa and melatonin formation, conversion of dopamine to norepinephrine, production of amides, and protection from free radical damage (7135). The activity of copper enzymes decreases with copper depletion (7135). Copper deficiency in humans is rare, but has been associated with excessive zinc intake, intestinal bypass surgery, parenteral nutrition, and malnourished infants (706,707,708). Copper deficiency is manifested by normocytic hypochromic anemia, leukopenia, and neutropenia (7135). In infants and children, osteoporosis may be seen (7135). No single lab test is available to determine copper deficiency. Diagnosis of copper deficiency is made by several indicators, including serum or plasma copper concentration, ceruloplasmin concentration, and erythrocyte superoxide dismutase activity (7135).

Adverse Reactions

Orally, copper is most commonly associated with gastrointestinal side effects including abdominal pain, cramps, nausea, diarrhea, and vomiting. Copper toxicity is rare in humans, except in those people with a hereditary defect in copper homeostasis. Acute hepatic failure has been reported in a patient taking 30 to 60 mg of copper daily for more than 4 years (7135). Renal failure and death can occur with ingestion of as little as 1 gram of copper sulfate (17). Symptoms of acute copper poisoning include nausea, vomiting, bloody diarrhea, hypotension, hemolytic anemia, uremia, and cardiovascular collapse (159). Chronic exposure symptoms include sporadic fever, vomiting, epigastric pain, diarrhea, and jaundice (159).

Interactions with Herbs & Other Dietary Supplements

IRON: In infants, high iron concentrations in formula can reduce absorption of copper and reduce copper status (7135). It isn't known if this is clinically significant, or if it occurs in adults who take iron supplements.

VITAMIN C (ascorbic acid): 1500 mg of vitamin C taken daily decreases serum levels of copper and the copper transport protein, ceruloplasmin, in young men (710). The acidity of vitamin C may convert copper in the gut to a less absorbable form. It's unlikely that this is clinically significant unless dietary copper intake is low (710).

ZINC: Large amounts of zinc can inhibit copper absorption, due to competition for absorption from the gut (706,707,708). Toxic levels of zinc intake can cause significant copper deficiency and associated anemia (706). It's unlikely that normal supplemental doses of zinc would affect copper levels.

Interactions with Drugs

PENICILLAMINE: Copper chelates penicillamine, decreasing its absorption. Separate dose times by at least 2 hours (4412,4453,4531,4535,9630).

Drug Influences on Nutrient Levels and Depletion

SOME DRUGS CAN AFFECT COPPER LEVELS:
ETHAMBUTOL (Myambutol): Ethambutol, and to a greater extent its metabolite, chelates copper (8971). Tissue depletion of copper can occur (8971). It's suggested that copper chelation in the retina might contribute to ethambutol-induced optic neuropathy (4453,4535). Chelation of copper ions in cytochrome-c oxidase may inhibit mitochondrial activity in optic nerve axons (4535). Whether supplemental copper can prevent this side effect isn't known. Preliminary evidence suggests that copper supplements do not inhibit the antimicrobial action of ethambutol (4535).
PENICILLAMINE (Cuprimine, Depen): Penicillamine chelates copper in the gastrointestinal tract and decreases absorption. The need for copper supplementation in diseases such as rheumatoid arthritis (RA) has not been adequately studied. If used, copper supplements should be separated from penicillamine by at least 2 hours (4453,4531,4535,9630).
ZIDOVUDINE (Retrovir, AZT): Decreased plasma copper levels are found in some people with HIV infection treated with zidovudine (4531). However, preliminary evidence suggests this is beneficial; AIDS patients with lower copper levels appear to have a slight survival advantage (8970). Advise patients on zidovudine not to take copper supplements unless recommended by their physician.

Interactions with Foods

None known.

Interactions with Lab Tests

None known.

Interactions with Diseases or Conditions

IDIOPATHIC COPPER TOXICOSIS: Copper supplementation can worsen this genetic condition (7135).
INDIAN CHILDHOOD CIRRHOSIS: Copper supplementation can worsen this genetic condition (7135).
WILSON'S DISEASE: Copper supplementation can worsen this condition or interfere with penicillamine therapy (7135).

Dosage and Administration

ORAL: For copper deficiency, doses up to 0.1 mg/kg cupric sulfate per day have been used. The National Institute of Medicine has determined Adequate Intake (AI) of copper for infants: 0 to 6 months, 200 mcg (30 mcg/kg/day); 7 to 12 months, 220 mcg (24 mcg/kg/day) (7135).
For children, a Recommended Dietary Allowance (RDA) has been set: 1 to 3 years, 340 mcg/day; 4 to 8 years, -440 mcg/day; 9 to 13, 700 mcg/day; 14 to 18 years, 890 mcg/day. For men and women age 19 years and older, the RDA is 900 mcg/day. For pregnancy, the RDA is 1000 mcg/day, and lactation 1300 mcg/day for women of all ages (7135).
The average dietary intake of copper by US women is 1.0 to 1.1 mg/day, men consume 1.2 to 1.6 mg/day (7135).
Tolerable Upper Intake Levels (UL) have been established for children and adults. All copper intake by infants should be from food or formula, unless under medical supervision (7135). The ULs for copper are: children 1 to 3 years, 1 mg/day; 4 to 8 years, 3 mg/day; 9 to 13 years, 5 mg/day; 14 to 18 years (including pregnancy and lactation) 8 mg/day; adults age 19 and older (including lactation), 10 mg/day; pregnancy age 19 and older, 8 mg/day (7135).
INTRAVENOUS: For copper deficiency, 1 to 2 mg per day is added to the parenteral nutrition solution (505).

Comments

There is no evidence that copper supplementation is needed or beneficial for people eating a normal diet, including athletes (703,704,705,709).

CORAL

Also Known As

Calcium Carbonate Matrix, Coral Calcium, Coralline Hydroxyapatite, Sea Coral.
CAUTION: See separate listing for Calcium, Coral Root.

Scientific Names

Goniopora species; Madrepora species; Porites species.

People Use This For

Orally, coral is used as a calcium supplement; to treat multiple sclerosis; and to treat and prevent cancer, heart disease, and other chronic health problems.
Orthopedically, coral is used as a substrate for growing new bone in areas damaged by trauma, maxillofacial reconstruction, cosmetic facial surgery, and damaged weight-bearing bones.

Safety

LIKELY SAFE ...when used surgically as a bone substitute (10736,10737,10738,10739,10741). There is insufficient reliable information available about the safety of the oral use of coral.
PREGNANCY AND LACTATION: Insufficient reliable information available; avoid using.

Effectiveness

LIKELY EFFECTIVE

Bone substitute. Coral can be used in place of allographic or autographic bone for spinal fusions and bone tumors; as well as in periodontal, craniofacial, orthopedic, and neurosurgery surgery (10736,10737,10738,10739,10741).

There is insufficient reliable information available about the effectiveness of coral for its other uses.

Mechanism of Action

Coral (calcium carbonate matrix) is derived form coral exoskeletons. The structure of coral is similar to that of cancellous (spongy) bone. Coral is advantageous over bone autographs because it causes less trauma. It is also advantageous over human bone allographs because it doesn't carry the risk of transmitting infections such as Acquired Immunodeficiency Syndrome (AIDS), Hepatitis C, and Creutzfeldt-Jakob disease. The local infection rate was 4% for coral grafts as compared to the bone allograph infection rate of 20%. Coral seems to act as an adequate carrier for bone growth factors. It seems to allow osteocyte attachment, growth, spreading, and differentiation (10741). New bone and fibrovascular tissue grow within the implanted coral. Over time, the calcium carbonate framework is resorbed (10737).

Adverse Reactions

Surgically, coral can cause infections (10741).

Interactions with Herbs & Other Dietary Supplements

None known.

Interactions with Drugs

None known.

Interactions with Foods

None known.

Interactions with Lab Tests

None known.

Interactions with Diseases or Conditions

None known.

Dosage and Administration

No typical dosage.

Comments

The Federal Trade Commission has charged the marketers of a coral supplement called "Coral Calcium Supreme" with making unsubstantiated health and medical claims about the product's ability to cure cancer or other diseases such as multiple sclerosis and heart disease (10742). There's no evidence that calcium from a coral source has any advantages over calcium from other sources. Some coral calcium products contain excess lead. In one independent laboratory analysis a coral calcium product contained 2.5 mcg of lead per 1 gram of calcium (9598). Avoid confusion with coral root (Corallorhiza odontorhiza).

CORAL ROOT

Also Known As

Chicken Toe, Crawley, Crawley Root, Fever Root, Scaley Dragon's Claw, Turkey Claw.
CAUTION: See separate listing for Coral.

Scientific Names

Corallorhiza odontorhiza, synonym Cymbidium odontorhizum.
Family: Orchidaceae.

People Use This For
Orally, coral root is used for colds and inducing perspiration.

Safety
There is insufficient reliable information available about the safety of coral root.
Pregnancy and Lactation: Insufficient reliable information available; avoid using.

Effectiveness
There is insufficient reliable information available about the effectiveness of coral root.

Mechanism of Action
The applicable part of coral root is the rhizome and root. Reported to have diaphoretic, antipyretic, and sedative effects (18).

Adverse Reactions
None reported.

Interactions with Herbs & Other Dietary Supplements
None known.

Interactions with Drugs
None known.

Interactions with Foods
None known.

Interactions with Lab Tests
None known.

Interactions with Diseases or Conditions
None known.

Dosage and Administration
ORAL: People typically prepare coral root as a tea, adding 1 teaspoon of root to 1 cup of water. The tea is taken hot or cold, 1 to 2 cups per day. In tincture form, the coral root dose is 10 to 20 drops (5263).

Comments
Avoid confusion with coral. Scarcity of this plant limits use (18).

CORDYCEPS

Also Known As
Caterpillar Fungus, Cs-4, Dong Chong Xia Cao, Dong Chong Zia Cao, Hsia Ts'Ao Tung Ch'Ung, Vegetable Caterpillar.

Scientific Names
Cordyceps sinensis.
Family: Ascomycetes or Clavicipitaceae.

People Use This For
Orally, cordyceps is used for strengthening the immune system, improving athletic performance, reducing the effects of aging, promoting longevity, treating lethargy, and improving liver function in people with hepatitis B. It is also used to treat coughs, chronic bronchitis, respiratory disorders, kidney disorders, frequent nocturia, male sexual dysfunction, anemia, heart arrhythmias, high cholesterol, liver disorders, dizziness, weakness, tinnitus, wasting, and opium addiction. It is also used as a stimulant, a tonic, and an adaptogen which is used to increase energy, enhance stamina, and reduce fatigue.

Safety
POSSIBLY SAFE ...when used orally and appropriately. Cordyceps and a specific cordyceps preparation (CordyMax Cs-4) appear to be safe when used orally, short-term (12,3417,3418,3419,3435,12095).
PREGNANCY AND LACTATION: Insufficient reliable information available; avoid using.

Effectiveness

POSSIBLY INEFFECTIVE

Athletic performance. Taking cordyceps orally doesn't seem to be effective for improving athletic performance. Endurance-trained cyclists who take a specific cordyceps preparation (CordyMax Cs-4) 3.15 grams/day for 5 weeks do not seem to have improved endurance time trials or improved aerobic capacity (VO2-peak) (12095).

INSUFFICIENT RELIABLE EVIDENCE to RATE

Aminoglycoside-induced nephrotoxicity. There is preliminary evidence that using cordyceps with amikacin might reduce amikacin-induced nephrotoxicity in older people (3419). It's not known if cordyceps helps for nephrotoxicity related to other aminoglycosides.

Chemotherapy. There is preliminary evidence that taking cordyceps orally following cancer chemotherapy might improve quality of life and cellular immunity (3417).

Cyclosporine-induced nephrotoxicity. There is preliminary evidence that taking cordyceps with cyclosporine can reduce cyclosporine-related nephrotoxicity in kidney-transplant recipients (3418).

Hepatitis B. There's preliminary evidence that taking cordyceps orally might improve liver function in hepatitis B patients (3435).

More evidence is needed to rate cordyceps for these uses.

Mechanism of Action

Cordyceps seems to have a beneficial effects on the immune, endocrine, cardiovascular, respiratory, renal, sexual, hepatic, immunologic, and nervous systems (3403,3404). Preliminary studies suggest cordyceps might stimulate immune function by increasing the number of T helper cells (3431); increasing the natural killer cell activity (3425,3427); stimulating the blood mononuclear cells (3414); increasing the levels of interferon-gamma, tumor necrosis factor-alpha, and interleukin-1 (3414); and prolonging the survival of lymphocytes (3432). Studies in animals with cancer suggest cordyceps improves immune response, reduces tumor size (3409,3431,3434), and lengthens survival time (3434,3437). Some evidence suggests cordyceps might be cytotoxic to cancer cells (3410,3416,3420), particularly lung carcinoma (3407) and melanoma (3427). Other evidence suggests that cordyceps might reduce the risk of renal toxicity from cyclosporine or aminoglycoside drugs (3411,3418,3419), and prove beneficial in chronic renal failure (3428). Cordyceps shows evidence that it can inhibit platelet aggregation and thrombus formation (3429). Other information suggests it might counteract or prevent arrhythmias, while decreasing heart rate and contractility (3436). Cordyceps polysaccharides show evidence that they might increase corticosterone production (3412). Other studies suggest they might reduce blood glucose (3415) without reducing plasma insulin levels (3415,3421), as well as reduce plasma triglycerides and cholesterol (3415). Preliminary animal studies suggest cordyceps could possibly be beneficial in treating systemic lupus erythematosus (3424). Limited human evidence suggests cordyceps can improve liver function in patients with chronic hepatitis B (3435).

Adverse Reactions

None reported.

Interactions with Herbs & Other Dietary Supplements

None known.

Interactions with Drugs

CYCLOPHOSPHAMIDE: Theoretically, cordyceps might reduce the immunosuppressive effects of cyclophosphamide (3427,3431).

PREDNISOLONE: Theoretically, cordyceps might reduce the immunosuppressive effects of prednisolone (3431,3437).

Interactions with Foods

None known.

Interactions with Lab Tests

LIVER FUNCTION TESTS: Cordyceps might improve liver function and test results in people with chronic hepatitis B (3435).

Interactions with Diseases or Conditions

HEPATITIS B: Based on limited human evidence, cordyceps might improve liver function and provide other benefits for people with chronic hepatitis B (3435).

Dosage and Administration

ORAL: A typical dosage of fermented Cordyceps sinensis is 3 grams per day (3403,3404).

Comments

Cordyceps sinensis is a fungus parasite that lives on caterpillars in high mountain regions of China (512). For commercial purposes, the cordyceps cells (Cs-4 strain) can be artificially propagated in the laboratory (512). Jinshuibao capsules are the commercially available form of fermented Cordyceps sinensis Cs-4 (3403).

CORIANDER

Also Known As

Chinese Parsley, Cilantro, Coriandri Fructus, Dhanyaka, Koriander, Kustumburi.

Scientific Names

Coriandrum sativum.
Family: Apiaceae/Umbelliferae.

People Use This For

Orally, coriander is used for dyspepsia, loss of appetite, nausea, diarrhea, as a stomach function stimulant, spasmolytic, antiflatulent, bactericide, fungicide, and to augment lactation. Coriander is also used to treat measles, hernia, hemorrhoids, toothaches, worms, rheumatism, and joint pain.
In foods, coriander is used as a culinary spice and to prevent food poisoning.
In manufacturing, coriander is used as a flavoring agent in pharmaceutical preparations, as a fragrance component in cosmetics and soaps, and for flavoring tobacco.

Safety

LIKELY SAFE ...when used orally in amounts commonly found in foods. Coriander and coriander oil have Generally Recognized As Safe (GRAS) status in the US (4912).
POSSIBLY SAFE ...when used orally and appropriately for medicinal purposes (12).
PREGNANCY AND LACTATION: Insufficient reliable information available; avoid amounts in excess of those found in foods.

Effectiveness

There is insufficient reliable information available about the effectiveness of coriander.

Mechanism of Action

The applicable parts of coriander are the seed and leaves. Coriander is a rich source of vitamin C, calcium, magnesium, potassium, and iron (19). The odor and taste of coriander are due to the volatile oil, which consists mainly of linalool (60-70%) (7). In animals, coriander seems to have hypoglycemic activity (11). Coriander oil also has larvicidal properties (11).
There is interest in coriander to prevent food poisoning because constituents in coriander leaves seem to have bacteriocidal activity against the food-borne pathogen, salmonella (12031).

Adverse Reactions

Powdered coriander and especially the oil can cause allergic reactions and photosensitivity (8). Like other members of the Apiaceae/Umbelliferae (carrot family), coriander can cause contact dermatitis (19). Coriander has been associated with endocrine toxicity. A case report describes severe diarrhea, stomach pain, skin darkness, depressed mood, amenorrhea, and dehydration following consumption of 200 mL of a 10% coriander extract for 7 days (10635).

Interactions with Herbs & Other Dietary Supplements

None known.

Interactions with Drugs

None known.

Interactions with Foods

None known.

Interactions with Lab Tests

None known.

Interactions with Diseases or Conditions

None known.

Dosage and Administration
No typical dosage.

CORIOLUS MUSHROOM

Also Known As
Boletus Versicolor, Coriolus, Kawaratake, Krestin, Polyporus Versicolor, Polysaccharide-K, Polysaccharide Krestin, Polysaccharide Peptide, Polystictus Versicolor, PSK, PSP, Turkey Tail, Yun-Zhi (cloud mushroom).

Scientific Names
Coriolus versicolor, synonyms Trametes versicolor, Polyporus versicolor, Boletus versicolor, Polystictus versicolor. Family: Polyporaceae.

People Use This For
Orally, coriolus mushroom or its derivatives are used for stimulating the immune system; treating herpes, chronic fatigue syndrome, hepatitis, and pulmonary disorders; reducing phlegm; improving body building; increasing energy; curing ringworm and impetigo; treating upper respiratory, urinary, and digestive tract infections; curing liver disorders including hepatitis; ameliorating the toxic effects and pain of chemotherapy and radiation therapy; promoting curative effect of chemotherapy; prolonging life and raising the quality of life; increasing appetite; and improving the effectiveness of cancer chemotherapy.

Safety
POSSIBLY SAFE ...when coriolus mushroom is used orally and appropriately (5477). ...when isolated PSK and PSP are used orally and appropriately (1635,1636,1640,1641,1648,1649,1650,1651,1652,1653,1654,1655,1656,1657,1658,1659,1660,1661,1662).
PREGNANCY AND LACTATION: Insufficient reliable information available; avoid using.

Effectiveness
POSSIBLY EFFECTIVE

Cancer. Taking polysaccharide krestin (PSK), a constituent of coriolus mushroom, orally may improve response and survival in some patients with cancer. It is given as a biologic response modifier (such as interferon or interleukin-2) as an adjunct to standard chemotherapy. It has been used in Japan for several decades for breast cancer, esophageal cancer, gastric cancer, lung cancer, hepatic cancer, colorectal cancer, and nasopharyngeal cancer (1640,1648,1649,1650,1651,1652,1653,1654,1655,1656,1657,1658,1659,1660,1661).

There is insufficient reliable information available about the effectiveness of coriolus mushroom for its other uses.

Mechanism of Action
The applicable parts of coriolus mushroom are the fruiting body and mycelium (5494). Coriolus mushrooms have a long history in folk medicine, but researchers are just beginning to isolate and identify substances in coriolus that have pharmacological activity (5477,1635). Coriolus contains several polysaccharides, including polysaccharide peptide (PSP) and polysaccharide krestin (PSK), shown to have antitumor and immunomodulating effects (1600,1635,1636,1637,1638,1639,1640,1641,1642,1648,1649,1650,5484,5494). PSK has been used in Japan as a biological response modifier in cancer chemotherapy regimens with varying results (1640,1641,1651,1652,1653,1654,1655,1656,1657,1658,1659,1660,1661,1662).

Early evidence suggests that PSP may have activity against lung cancers, leukemia, and gastric cancers (1635).

When given with cyclophosphamide, PSP seems to improve immune function by increasing white cell, natural killer cell, and antibody levels (10291). These effects suggest that PSP might be a useful adjuvant in cancer therapy.

Coriolus might also have activity against the human immunodeficiency virus (HIV) (1643,1644).

Preliminary evidence suggests that coriolus might have analgesic activity and protect against acetaminophen-induced hepatotoxicity (1645,1646,1647).

Adverse Reactions
There have been no adverse reports for coriolus mushroom (1635,1636). Patients receiving PSK as an adjunct to chemotherapy experienced nausea, leukopenia, and liver function impairment (1651); however, this may have been due to the chemotherapy.

Interactions with Herbs & Other Dietary Supplements
None known.

Interactions with Drugs
None known.

Interactions with Foods
None known.

Interactions with Lab Tests
None known.

Interactions with Diseases or Conditions
None known.

Dosage and Administration
ORAL: A typical dose of tea is prepared from 20 grams of dried coriolus fruiting bodies three times daily, or take capsules containing up to 5 grams per day of the dried fruiting bodies. As an adjuvant to cancer chemotherapy, 3 grams of PSK is taken daily (1650,1654,1656,1658).

CORKWOOD TREE

Also Known As
Pituri.

Scientific Names
Duboisia myoporoides.
Family: Solanaceae.

People Use This For
Orally, corkwood quids (cured and rolled leaves) are chewed to ward off hunger, pain, and tiredness. Alkaloids derived from the plant are used as a therapeutic substitute for atropine.

Safety
LIKELY UNSAFE ...when used orally. Corkwood tree leaves contain tropane alkaloids that are potent anticholinergics (6). Large doses of scopolamine and related alkaloids can be fatal (6).
PREGNANCY AND LACTATION: LIKELY UNSAFE ...when used orally (6); avoid using.

Effectiveness
There is insufficient reliable information available about the effectiveness of corkwood tree.

Mechanism of Action
The applicable part of corkwood tree is the leaf. Researchers document tropane alkaloids (atropine, scopolamine, etc.) as constituents (6). Stimulant and hallucinogenic properties are due to anticholinergic effects (6).

Adverse Reactions
Orally, corkwood tree can cause central nervous system disturbances (6).

Interactions with Herbs & Other Dietary Supplements
None known.

Interactions with Drugs
None known.

Interactions with Foods
None known.

Interactions with Lab Tests
None known.

Interactions with Diseases or Conditions
None known.

Dosage and Administration
ORAL: Leaves are cured and rolled into a quid which Australian natives chew (6).

Comments
Although at one time used as a source of scopolamine, other sources are more commercially viable (6).

CORN COCKLE

Also Known As
Cockle, Corn Campion, Corn Rose, Crown-of-the-Field, Purple Cockle.

Scientific Names
Agrostemma githago.
Family: Caryophyllaceae.

People Use This For
Orally, corn cockle has also been used as a diuretic, expectorant, menstrual stimulant, poison, vermifuge, and for jaundice.
Topically, corn cockle seeds are used for treating cancers, hard tumors, warts, hard swelling of the uterus, and to induce inflammation of the conjunctiva and cornea. The root is used for exanthemata (acute skin eruptions signifying a viral or coccal infection), and hemorrhoids.

Safety
LIKELY UNSAFE ...when used orally, due to toxicity (6).
There is insufficient reliable information available about the safety of the topical use of corn cockle.
PREGNANCY AND LACTATION: LIKELY UNSAFE ...when used orally (6); avoid using.

Effectiveness
There is insufficient reliable information available about the effectiveness of corn cockle.

Mechanism of Action
The applicable parts of corn cockle are the root and seed. Poisonous constituents, githagin and agrostemmic acid, are reportedly absorbed from the GI tract causing GI irritation, severe muscle pain and twitching, depression, and coma (6).

Adverse Reactions
Orally, corn cockle can cause GI irritation, severe muscle pain and twitching, depression, and coma (6). Acute poisoning symptoms include: diarrhea, salivation, vertigo, vomiting, paralysis, and respiratory depression (6). Repeated poisoning by small doses is referred to as "githagism" (6).

Interactions with Herbs & Other Dietary Supplements
None known.

Interactions with Drugs
None known.

Interactions with Foods
None known.

Interactions with Lab Tests
None known.

Interactions with Diseases or Conditions
None known.

Dosage and Administration
No typical dosage.

CORN POPPY

Also Known As

Copperose, Corn Rose, Cup-Puppy, Headache, Headwark, Rakta-Posta, Rakta Khakasa, Red Poppy, Rhoeados Flos. CAUTION: See separate listing for California Poppy.

Scientific Names

Papaver rhoeas.
Family: Papaveraceae.

People Use This For

Orally, corn poppy is used for respiratory tract diseases and discomforts, cough, disturbed sleep, and pain relief.
For food uses, corn poppy is an ingredient in some "metabolic" teas. In other teas, it is used as a brightening agent.

Safety

POSSIBLY SAFE ...when the dried corn poppy flower petals are used orally and appropriately in medicinal amounts (2,18).
CHILDREN: POSSIBLY UNSAFE ...when the fresh leaves or blossoms are eaten because this can cause poisoning (18). There is insufficient reliable information available for the safety of dried corn poppy flower petals used in children.
PREGNANCY AND LACTATION: Insufficient reliable information available; avoid using.

Effectiveness

There is insufficient reliable information available about the effectiveness of corn poppy.

Mechanism of Action

The applicable part of corn poppy is the flower. There is insufficient reliable information available about the possible mechanism of action and active ingredients.

Adverse Reactions

No adverse effects in adults have been reported (2). However, poisonings have been reported in children who consumed the fresh leaves and blossoms. Symptoms include vomiting and stomach pain (18).

Interactions with Herbs & Other Dietary Supplements

None known.

Interactions with Drugs

None known.

Interactions with Foods

None known.

Interactions with Lab Tests

None known.

Interactions with Diseases or Conditions

None known.

Dosage and Administration

ORAL: For bronchial irritation, one cup tea (steep 2 teaspoons dried petals in boiling water 5-10 minutes, strain) 2 to 3 times daily (may be sweetened with honey) has been used (18).

CORN SILK

Also Known As

Cornsilk, Indian Corn, Maidis Stigma, Maize Silk, Stigma Maydis, Zea.

Scientific Names

Zea mays.
Family: Poaceae/Gramineae.

People Use This For

Orally, corn silk is used for cystitis, urethritis, nocturnal enuresis, prostatitis, acute chronic inflammation of the urinary system, as a diuretic for congestive heart failure, to treat diabetes, and for hypertension.

Safety

LIKELY SAFE ...when used orally in amounts commonly found in foods. Corn silk, corn silk extract, and corn silk oil has Generally Recognized As Safe (GRAS) status in the US (4912).
POSSIBLY SAFE ...when used orally and appropriately in medicinal amounts (12).
PREGNANCY: POSSIBLY SAFE ...when consumed in food. LIKELY UNSAFE ...when used orally in larger amounts because it might have uterine stimulant effects (4); avoid using.
LACTATION: Insufficient reliable information available; avoid using.

Effectiveness

There is insufficient reliable information available about the effectiveness of corn silk.

Mechanism of Action

Corn silk contains tannins, which are astringent; and cryptoxanthin, which has vitamin A activity (4).

Adverse Reactions

Orally, prolonged use may cause hypokalemia (4).
Topically, allergy to cornsilk, corn pollen, or cornstarch may result in contact dermatitis or urticaria (4).

Interactions with Herbs & Other Dietary Supplements

None known.

Interactions with Drugs

ANTIDIABETES DRUGS: Theoretically, because some evidence suggests corn silk can reduce blood glucose levels, excessive amounts might interfere with diabetes therapy (4).
ANTIHYPERTENSIVE DRUGS: Theoretically, excessive doses of corn silk might cause hypotension and interfere with drugs used to treat hypertension or hypotension (4).
CORTICOSTEROIDS: Theoretically, prolonged use of corn silk might have additive effects with drugs that deplete potassium, including corticosteroids (4).
DIURETIC DRUGS: Overuse of corn silk might compound diuretic-induced potassium loss (4). There is some concern that people taking corn silk along with potassium depleting diuretics might have an increased risk for hypokalemia. Initiation of potassium supplementation or an increase in potassium supplement dose may be necessary for some patients. Some diuretics that can deplete potassium include chlorothiazide (Diuril), chlorthalidone (Thalitone), furosemide (Lasix), hydrochlorothiazide (HCTZ, HydroDIURIL, Microzide), and others.
WARFARIN (Coumadin): Corn silk contains vitamin K. Individuals taking warfarin should consume a consistent daily amount to maintain consistent anticoagulation (19).

Interactions with Foods

None known.

Interactions with Lab Tests

None known.

Interactions with Diseases or Conditions

DIABETES: Theoretically, excessive doses might reduce blood glucose level (4), interfering with control.
HYPERTENSION, HYPOTENSION: Theoretically, excessive doses might interfere with control of these conditions (4).
POTASSIUM DEPLETION: Theoretically, excessive doses might exacerbate this condition (4).

Dosage and Administration

ORAL: 4-8 grams dried style/stigma three times daily, or one cup tea (steep 0.5 grams dried corn silk in 150 mL boiling water 5-10 minutes, strain) several times daily (4,8). Liquid extract of maize stigmas, 4-8 mL (4). Tincture (1:5 in 25% alcohol), 5-15 mL three times daily (4). Syrup of maize stigmas, 8-15 mL (4).

Comments

Corn silk is the so-called "silk" of an ear of ordinary Indian corn or maize.

CORNFLOWER

Also Known As

Batchelor's Buttons, Blue Cap, Blue Centaury, Bluebonnet, Bluebottle, Bluebow, Corn Flower, Cyani Blossoms, Cyani Flos, Cyani Flowers, Cyani Petals, Hurtsickle.
CAUTION: See separate listings for Buttercup and Feverfew.

Scientific Names

Centaurea cyanus, synonym Centaurea segetum.
Family: Asteraceae/Compositae.

People Use This For

Orally, cornflower is used for fever, menstrual disorders, vaginal candidiasis; and as a laxative, diuretic, expectorant, tonic, bitter, and as a liver and gallbladder stimulant.
Topically, cornflower is used for eye irritation or discomfort.
In foods, cornflower is utilized in herbal teas as a coloring agent.

Safety

LIKELY SAFE ...when used as a coloring agent in herbal teas (2).
There is insufficient reliable information available about the safety of cornflower for its other uses.
PREGNANCY AND LACTATION: Insufficient reliable information available; avoid using.

Effectiveness

There is insufficient reliable information available about the effectiveness of cornflower.

Mechanism of Action

The applicable part of cornflower is the dried flower. The color is due to anthocyanin constituents (1502).

Adverse Reactions

Cornflower may cause an allergic reaction in individuals sensitive to the Asteraceae/Compositae family. Members of this family include ragweed, chrysanthemums, marigolds, daisies, and many other herbs.

Interactions with Herbs & Other Dietary Supplements

None known.

Interactions with Drugs

None known.

Interactions with Foods

None known.

Interactions with Lab Tests

None known.

Interactions with Diseases or Conditions

CROSS-ALLERGENICITY: Cornflower may cause an allergic reaction in individuals sensitive to the Asteraceae/Compositae family. Members of this family include ragweed, chrysanthemums, marigolds, daisies, and many other herbs.

Dosage and Administration

ORAL: People typically use the crushed dried flowers as a tea. The tea is prepared by adding 1 gram of cornflower per cup of water (5252).
TOPICAL: No typical dosage.

CORYDALIS

Also Known As
Early Fumitory, Squirrel Corn.

Scientific Names
Corydalis cava, synonym Corydalis tuberosa.
Family: Fumariaceae.

Comments
At the date of publication, there was very little scientific information about this product. Our staff is continually analyzing the available information on natural medicines and will add data to the online version of *Natural Medicines Comprehensive Database* as it becomes available. See www.naturaldatabase.com.

COSTUS OIL

Also Known As
Auckland Costus, Kushta, Kushtha, Kuth, Mokko, Mokkou, Mu Xiang, Yun Mu Xiang.
CAUTION: See separate listing for Costus root.

Scientific Names
Saussurea costus, synonyms Saussurea lappa, Aucklandia costus, Aplotaxis lappa.
Family: Asteraceae/Compositae.

People Use This For
Orally, costus oil is used as a tonic; gastric stimulant; antiflatulent; and for treating asthma, cough, dysentery, and cholera.
In foods and beverages, costus oil is used as a flavoring component.
In manufacturing, costus oil is used as a fixative and fragrance in cosmetics.

Safety
LIKELY SAFE ...when used in amounts commonly found in foods. Costus oil has Generally Recognized As Safe (GRAS) status in the US (4912).
UNSAFE ...when aristolochic acid-contaminated costus oil is used orally. Costus oil is commonly contaminated with aristolochic acid, which is nephrotoxic and carcinogenic. The FDA considers all products containing aristolochic acid to be unsafe and adulterated. Only products analytically verified to be aristolochic acid-free should be used (6118).
There is insufficient reliable information available about the safety of costus oil when used for medicinal purposes.
PREGNANCY AND LACTATION: Insufficient reliable information available; avoid using.

Effectiveness
There is insufficient reliable information available about the effectiveness of costus oil.

Mechanism of Action
Costus oil is reported to inhibit bronchospasm and lower blood pressure in animals (11).

Adverse Reactions
Orally, costus oil might cause allergic reactions, including contact dermatitis (11). Costus oil can cause an allergic reaction in individuals sensitive to the Asteraceae/Compositae family. Members of this family include ragweed, chrysanthemums, marigolds, daisies, and many other herbs.
Costus oil is commonly contaminated with aristolochic acid, which is nephrotoxic and carcinogenic (6118).

Interactions with Herbs & Other Dietary Supplements
None known.

Interactions with Drugs
None known.

Interactions with Foods
None known.

Interactions with Lab Tests
None known.

Interactions with Diseases or Conditions
CROSS-ALLERGENICITY: Costus oil can cause an allergic reaction in individuals sensitive to the Asteraceae/Compositae family. Members of this family include ragweed, chrysanthemums, marigolds, daisies, and many other herbs.

Dosage and Administration
No typical dosage.

Comments
Costus oil is the distilled, extracted oil from the root of Saussurea costus. Avoid confusion with costus root. Costus oil is frequently contaminated with aristolochic acid, which is nephrotoxic and carcinogenic. The FDA considers all products containing aristolochic acid to be unsafe and adulterated (6118). The FDA intends to automatically detain, without physical examination, any product which contains plants known or suspected to contain aristolochic acid, or which might be adulterated with plants known to contain aristolochic acid. Each detained product will be released only after the responsible party provides direct analytical evidence that it is free of aristolochic acid (6118).

COSTUS root

Also Known As
Auckland Costus, Kushta, Kushtha, Kuth, Mokko, Mokkou, Mu Xiang, Yun Mu Xiang.
CAUTION: See separate listing for Costus Oil.

Scientific Names
Saussurea costus, synonyms Saussurea lappa, Aucklandia costus, Aplotaxis lappa.
Family: Asteraceae/Compositae.

People Use This For
Orally, costus root is used as an antinematode therapy.

Safety
POSSIBLY SAFE ...when used orally and appropriately (12).
UNSAFE ...when aristolochic acid-contaminated costus root is used orally. Costus root is commonly contaminated with aristolochic acid, which is nephrotoxic and carcinogenic. The FDA considers all products containing aristolochic acid to be unsafe and adulterated. Only products analytically verified to be aristolochic acid-free should be used (6118).
PREGNANCY AND LACTATION: Insufficient reliable information available; avoid using.

Effectiveness
POSSIBLY EFFECTIVE

Nematodes. Taking costus root orally seems to be effective against nematodes when the root or methanol extract of root is taken (1516).

Mechanism of Action
In children, costus root reduces the number of fecal eggs per gram similarly to treatment with pyrantel pamoate (1516).

Adverse Reactions
Orally, costus root can cause an allergic reaction in individuals sensitive to the Asteraceae/Compositae family. Members of this family include ragweed, chrysanthemums, marigolds, daisies, and many other herbs. Costus root is commonly contaminated with aristolochic acid which is nephrotoxic and carcinogenic (6118).

Interactions with Herbs & Other Dietary Supplements
None known.

Interactions with Drugs
None known.

Interactions with Foods
None known.

Interactions with Lab Tests
None known.

Interactions with Diseases or Conditions
CROSS-ALLERGENICITY: Costus root can cause an allergic reaction in individuals sensitive to the Asteraceae/Compositae family. Members of this family include ragweed, chrysanthemums, marigolds, daisies, and many other herbs.

Dosage and Administration
ORAL: As an antinematodal, 50 mg/kg root (or equivalent amount of methanol extract of root) as a single dose has been used (1516).

Comments
Avoid confusion with costus oil.
Costus root is frequently contaminated with aristolochic acid, which is nephrotoxic and carcinogenic. The FDA considers all products containing aristolochic acid to be unsafe and adulterated (6118). The FDA intends to automatically detain, without physical examination, any product which contains plants known or suspected to contain aristolochic acid, or which might be adulterated with plants known to contain aristolochic acid. Each detained product will be released only after the responsible party provides direct analytical evidence that it is free of aristolochic acid (6118).

COTTON

Also Known As
Cotton Root, Karpasa.
CAUTION: See separate listing for Gossypol.

Scientific Names
Gossypium herbaceum; Gossypium hirsutum; other Gossypium species.
Family: Malvaceae.

People Use This For
Orally, cotton is used for amenorrhea; dysmenorrhea; irregular, painful, or profuse menstrual bleeding; climacteric complaints; poor lactation; nausea; fever; headache; diarrhea; dysentery; urethritis; nerve inflammation; hemorrhage; as an oxytocic; and to expel afterbirth.
Cotton has been used as an anti-fertility drug in males, as well as in topical, vaginal contraceptive preparations.

Safety
POSSIBLY SAFE ...when used orally in medicinal amounts (12). ...when preparations of the root bark are used in amounts found in foods. Canadian regulations limit use to less than 450 ppm of free gossypol (including cotton seed meal and oil) (12).
PREGNANCY: LIKELY UNSAFE ...when used orally because it is a possible abortifacient and uterine stimulant (12).
LACTATION: Insufficient reliable information available; avoid using.

Effectiveness
There is insufficient reliable information available about the effectiveness of cotton.

Mechanism of Action
The applicable part of cotton is the root bark. It is believed to stimulate menstrual flow, act as an oxytocic, and male contraceptive (18). Some evidence suggests cotton root can cause histamine release (18). The constituent, gossypol that is extracted from cotton seed is used as a male contraceptive (6).

Adverse Reactions
None reported. However, in animals, long-term feeding with cotton seed cakes has been linked to poisonings and deaths (18).

Interactions with Herbs & Other Dietary Supplements
None known.

Interactions with Drugs
None known.

Interactions with Foods
None known.

Interactions with Lab Tests
None known.

Interactions with Diseases or Conditions
UROGENITAL IRRITATION OR SENSITIVITY: Contraindicated (12).

Dosage and Administration
ORAL: People typically prepare cotton root bark using one teaspoon boiled in a covered container with 3 cups of water for 30 minutes. The liquid is cooled slowly in the closed container and taken cold, 1 to 2 cups per day (5254).

Comments
Avoid confusion with gossypol (cotton seed extract).
Cotton's use as a male contraceptive agent is in question because it may potentially cause irreversible sterility (6002).

COUNTRY MALLOW

Also Known As
Bala, Bariar, Heartleaf, Khareti, Vatya.
CAUTION: See separate listings for Mallow flower, Mallow leaf, and Marshmallow.

Scientific Names
Sida cordifolia.
Family: Malvaceae.

People Use This For
In herbal combinations country mallow is used orally for weight loss, to burn fat, to increase energy, for impotence, sinus, allergy, throat diseases, asthma and bronchitis, and to promote a strong skeletal system. In combination with ginger, country mallow root is used orally for intermittent fever. In combination with milk and sugar, country mallow root is used for urinary urgency and leukorrhea.
Traditionally, country mallow is used orally to treat bronchial asthma, colds, flu, chills, lack of perspiration, headaches, nasal congestion, cough and wheezing, urinary infections, and edema. It is also traditionally used orally for heart disease, facial paralysis, healing chronic tissue inflammation, sciatica, insanity, neuralgia, nerve inflammation, chronic rheumatism, and emaciation. Country mallow is also traditionally used orally as a stimulant, analgesic, diuretic, tonic, aphrodisiac, and before and after cancer chemotherapy to aid recovery. Country mallow is traditionally used topically for numbness, nerve pain, muscle cramps, skin disorders, tumors, joint diseases, wounds, ulcers, and as a massage oil.

Safety
LIKELY UNSAFE ...when used orally. Country mallow contains the constituent ephedrine, similar to the herb ephedra. Ephedra, country mallow and other ephedrine-containing herbs are banned in the US due to several case reports that have linked ephedra to serious side effects including hypertension, myocardial infarction (MI), seizure, stroke, psychosis, and others (1276,2729,6486,6998,9167,10689). Tell patients to avoid this and other products that contain ephedrine.
PREGNANCY: LIKELY UNSAFE ...when used orally; avoid using. The ephedrine constituent can stimulate uterine contractions (12).
LACTATION: Insufficient reliable information available; avoid using.

Effectiveness
There is insufficient reliable information available about the effectiveness of country mallow.

Mechanism of Action

The applicable parts of country mallow are the root, leaves, and seeds. Country mallow contains 0.8%-1.2% ephedrine (4304,4310), but ephedrine is most concentrated in the seeds (4314). Some evidence suggests country mallow has anticonvulsant, antipyretic, antibacterial, antifungal, and antiviral activity (4310). Other information suggests the extracts of the aerial and root parts have analgesic, anti-inflammatory, and hypoglycemic properties (4299). An aqueous extract shows evidence that it limits the virulence of dental bacteria, reducing the rate of plaque formation (4303).

Adverse Reactions

Orally, the country mallow ephedrine constituent can cause dizziness, motor restlessness, irritability, insomnia, headache, anorexia, nausea, vomiting, flushing, tingling, difficulty urinating, tachycardia, and heart palpitations (2,6,7,13). Use of botanical sources of ephedrine such as country mallow have been associated with muscle conditions including myalgia, cardiomyopathy, rhabdomyolysis, eosinophilia myalgia syndrome (1270), and hypersensitivity myocarditis (1271). Botanical sources of ephedrine such as country mallow have also been associated with kidney stones (1272), acute hepatitis, (1273), psychosis (1276), and sudden death (1274). The country mallow constituent ephedrine can also cause a drastic increase in blood pressure, cardiac arrhythmias (2), heart failure, asphyxia, and hyperthermia (18).

Interactions with Herbs & Other Dietary Supplements

CAFFEINE: Concomitant use with the country mallow constituent ephedrine can cause increased stimulatory adverse effects (7).
COFFEE, GUARANA, TEA: Theoretically, concomitant use with the country mallow constituent ephedrine can cause additive stimulatory adverse effects (7).
DIGITALIS: Theoretically, using digitalis with the country mallow constituent ephedrine can cause cardiac arrhythmias (2).
SECALE ALKALOID DERIVATIVES (Ergot): Concomitant use with the country mallow constituent ephedrine can cause hypertension (2).

Interactions with Drugs

ANTIDIABETES DRUGS: The country mallow constituent ephedrine can raise blood glucose levels. Monitor closely (19).
DEXAMETHASONE (Decadron): The country mallow constituent ephedrine can increase the clearance and reduce the effectiveness of dexamethasone (19).
ERGOT DERIVATIVES: Concomitant use with the country mallow constituent ephedrine might cause hypertension (15).
METHYLXANTHINES: Concomitant use with the country mallow constituent ephedrine can cause increased stimulatory adverse effects (7,19).
MONOAMINE OXIDASE INHIBITORS (MAOIs): Contraindicated; concomitant use of the country mallow ephedrine constituent with MAOIs might increase the risk of hypertension (15).
QT INTERVAL-PROLONGING DRUGS: Theoretically, country mallow may have an additive effect with drugs that prolong the QT interval. This may increase the risk of ventricular arrhythmias. This has been reported for another ephedrine containing herb, ephedra (11355). Drugs that prolong the QT interval include amiodarone (Cordarone), disopyramide (Norpace), dofetilide (Tikosyn), ibutilide (Corvert), procainamide (Pronestyl), quinidine, sotalol (Betapace), thioridazine (Mellaril), and many others.
RESERPINE: Theoretically, concomitant use of reserpine along with the country mallow constituent ephedrine can antagonize the sympathomimetic effects of reserpine (19). The significance of this interaction is not clear.

Interactions with Foods

COFFEE, TEA: Theoretically, concomitant use of the country mallow constituent ephedrine and large amounts of caffeinated coffee or tea might increase the stimulatory effects and adverse effects of caffeine and ephedrine.

Interactions with Lab Tests

BLOOD GLUCOSE: The country mallow ephedrine constituent might increase blood glucose levels (19), or other constituents of country mallow might reduce blood glucose levels (4299).
URINE: The country mallow ephedrine constituent can cause positive urine tests for ephedrine, a substance banned by many athletic organizations.

Interactions with Diseases or Conditions

ANGINA: Contraindicated; the country mallow ephedrine constituent might induce or exacerbate angina due to its cardiac stimulant effects (15,512).
ANOREXIA: Contraindicated; the country mallow ephedrine constituent might suppress the appetite (12,19).
ANXIETY: Large doses of the country mallow ephedrine constituent might cause or exacerbate anxiety due to its CNS stimulant effects (2,12,15,512).

BENIGN PROSTATIC HYPERTROPHY (BPH): The country mallow ephedrine constituent might exacerbate urinary retention in patients with BPH due to its effects on the detrusor muscle (15,512).
BULIMIA: Contraindicated; bulimic patients might be at increased risk for the adverse effects of the country mallow ephedrine constituent due to inadequate nutritional status (12,19).
CEREBRAL INSUFFICIENCY: Contraindicated; the country mallow ephedrine constituent might further decrease cerebral blood flow because it has vasoconstrictive effects (2,12,512).
DIABETES: The country mallow ephedrine constituent might interfere with blood sugar control, and exacerbate high blood pressure and circulatory problems in people with diabetes (15,19,512). However, extract of country mallow shows evidence of hypoglycemic effect (4299). Monitor closely.
ESSENTIAL TREMOR: The country mallow ephedrine constituent could exacerbate tremor (1715).
HEART DISEASE: Contraindicated; the country mallow ephedrine constituent might cause tachycardia, arrhythmias, or induce angina in patients with heart disease due to its cardiac stimulant effects (15,512).
HYPERTENSION: The country mallow ephedrine constituent might exacerbate hypertension (2,12,15,512); contraindicated in uncontrolled hypertension.
HYPERTHYROID, THYROTOXICOSIS: Contraindicated; the country mallow ephedrine constituent might stimulate the thyroid and exacerbate hyperthyroid symptoms (2,12,15,512).
KIDNEY STONES: The country mallow ephedrine constituent can cause kidney stones (1272).
MYASTHENIA GRAVIS: Large doses of the country mallow ephedrine constituent might increase muscle strength in patients with myasthenia gravis (15).
NARROW-ANGLE GLAUCOMA: The country mallow ephedrine constituent might exacerbate narrow-angle (angle-closure) glaucoma by causing mydriasis (2,12,15,512).
PHEOCHROMOCYTOMA: Contraindicated; the country mallow ephedrine constituent might exacerbate the symptoms of pheochromocytoma (2).
URINARY RETENTION: Large doses of the country mallow ephedrine constituent might exacerbate urinary retention due to its effects on the detrusor muscle (2,12,15,512).

Dosage and Administration

ORAL: A typical dose of powder (root, leaves, seeds) is 0.5 -1 gram twice daily. A typical dose of the fresh juice is 15-30 mL twice daily (4310).
TOPICAL: No typical dosage.

Comments

Country mallow is used extensively in Ayurvedic medicine because it is reported to simultaneously balance the three laws of physiology (Vata, Pitta, Kapha) (4321).
On December 30, 2003, the FDA announced that it will ban ephedra, country mallow, and other ephedrine-containing products in the US (10055). The ban went into effect in April 2004.

COWHAGE

Also Known As

Atmagupta, Couhage, Cowitch, Feijao macaco, HP 200, HP-200, Kapikachchhu, Kaunch, Kawanch, Kiwach, Mucuna, Mucuna prurient, Pica Pica, Pica-Pica, Velvet Bean.

Scientific Names

Mucuna pruriens; Mucuna pruriens var. hirsuta, synonyms Mucuna hirsuta, Stizolobium hirsutum.
Family: Fabaceae/Leguminosae.

People Use This For

Orally, cowhage is used for Parkinson's disease, anxiety, arthritis, hyperprolactinemia, and for parasitic infections. It's also used as an analgesic for pain, for fever, to induce vomiting, and as an aphrodisiac. Cowhage is also used prophylactically as snakebite remedy.
Topically, cowhage is used as a rubefacient or counterirritant for rheumatic conditions, myalgias, to stimulate cutaneous blood flow in paralytic conditions, and to treat scorpion stings.

Safety

POSSIBLY SAFE ...when used orally and appropriately. Powdered formulations of cowhage seed have been used safely for up to 20 weeks (6899,7020,7203).
POSSIBLY UNSAFE ...when the hair of the cowhage bean pod is used orally or topically. The bean pod hairs are strong irritants and can cause severe itching, burning, and inflammation (18).
PREGNANCY AND LACTATION: Insufficient reliable information available; avoid using.

Effectiveness

INSUFFICIENT RELIABLE EVIDENCE to RATE

Hyperprolactinemia. There is some evidence that cowhage might be useful for chlorpromazine-induced hyperprolactinemia in men (7207), but it does not appear to be effective for hyperprolactinemia of unknown cause in women (7206).

Parkinson's disease. There is preliminary evidence that some cowhage preparations might help improve symptoms of Parkinson's disease when used in combination with conventional drugs such as amantadine, selegiline, and anticholinergic agents. Cowhage contains 3-6% levodopa (L-dopa). Specific cowhage extracts standardized to 3.3% L-dopa (HP-200) and other powdered formulations providing 75 to 220 mg per day of L-dopa are being used for patients with Parkinson's (6899,7020,7203).

More evidence is needed to rate cowhage for these uses.

Mechanism of Action

The applicable parts of cowhage are the bean or seed and the hair on the bean pod. Cowhage is thought to work for Parkinson's disease because it contains a significant amount of levodopa (L-dopa). The whole cowhage bean contains about 3-6% L-dopa (7020,7021). The inner layer (endocarp) of the pericarp, which has also been studied in patients with Parkinson's disease, usually contains the highest amount of L-dopa, about 5.3% (7020). Symptoms of Parkinson's disease occur in patients due to a depletion of the neurotransmitter dopamine. L-dopa is a precursor to dopamine. To be effective for Parkinson's disease, L-dopa must cross the blood-brain barrier where it is then decarboxylated to dopamine. However, the majority of L-dopa is metabolized peripherally and probably less than 1% actually reaches the brain (15). Some powdered cowhage seed preparations containing L-dopa seem to lessen symptoms of Parkinson's disease at a relatively low dose, compared to conventional L-dopa products. So there is some speculation that constituents other than levodopa might have antiparkinson activity (7203).

Cowhage also contains prurieninin, which might slow heart rate, decrease blood pressure, and stimulate intestinal peristalsis (18). Cowhage has also been reported to have anthelmintic, antiflatulent, and cholesterol lowering properties (18), but these effects have not been verified in humans.

Animal studies show that cowhage might lower blood glucose levels (7221) and possibly slow the development of diabetic nephropathy (7220). Cowhage contains significant amounts of minerals, including calcium, magnesium, phosphorus, iron, manganese, zinc, and copper. Some researchers speculate that cowhage might exert its hypoglycemic effect due to trace element stimulation of insulin or possibly because of orally active insulin-like compounds in cowhage (7221).

There is interest in using cowhage for snakebite. Cowhage extract seems to have a procoagulant effect against the venom of the saw scaled viper (Echis carinatus), when given at least 24 hours prior to laboratory exposure to the venom (7222).

Cowhage also possesses counterirritant and rubefacient properties (18). The hairs (spicules) of the bean pod or seed cause severe itching, burning, and inflammation when they penetrate the epidermis (18,6898). Serotonin and protein constituents such as mucunain are released into the skin, causing blood vessel dilation, redness, and inflammation (18,6898). Repeated boiling of the bean is sometimes used to eliminate the pharmacologically and toxicologically active principles so that the bean can be consumed as food (7021,7205).

Adverse Reactions

Orally, cowhage seems to be fairly well tolerated when a standardized powdered formulation, known as HP-200, made from the inner portion (endocarp) of the bean wall (pericarp) is used. The most common side effects reported are nausea and a sensation of abdominal distention. Other side effects less frequently reported are vomiting, dyskinesias, and insomnia (7020). Adverse effects reported with other cowhage bean preparations include headache; palpitations; sweating; flatulence; diarrhea; dry mouth; rash and pruritus; changes in urine color; and symptoms of psychosis including confusion, giddiness, agitation, hallucinations, and paranoid delusions (7203,7021). Cowhage-induced psychosis has been successfully treated with intravenous chlorpromazine (Thorazine) (7021). Theoretically, due to the levodopa (L-dopa) constituent, cowhage is likely to cause the same adverse effects that have been attributed to the purified L-dopa prescription drug. Some of these side effects include elevated liver enzymes, respiratory disturbances, urinary retention, darkening of bodily fluids, muscle cramps, headache, and priapism (15). However, these effects have not yet been reported for cowhage. Ingestion of hairs from the bean pod or seed can result in significant mucosal irritation and should be avoided.

Topically, hairs from the cowhage bean pod or seed can cause severe itching, burning, inflammation, and erythematous macular rashes (18,6898). Symptoms resolve spontaneously within several hours, but may also be relieved with antihistamines (6898). The hairs can be removed from the skin by washing, but the hairs can also be retained, and transferred to other people, in fabrics and carpets. Clothing and other materials that come in contact with the cowhage hairs should also be thoroughly washed (6898).

Interactions with Herbs & Other Dietary Supplements

HERBS AND SUPPLEMENTS WITH HYPOGLYCEMIC EFFECTS: There is some evidence that cowhage might have hypoglycemic effects (7221). Theoretically, concomitant use with other herbs and supplements that decrease blood glucose levels might increase the risk of hypoglycemia. Some of these products include bitter melon, ginger, goat's rue, fenugreek, kudzu, willow bark, and others.

KAVA: Theoretically, kava might reduce the effectiveness of cowhage. There is some evidence that kava might have antidopaminergic effects and possibly decrease the effects of levodopa (L-dopa) in cowhage (19).
VITAMIN B6 (Pyridoxine): Vitamin B6 can decrease the effectiveness of the cowhage constituent levodopa (L-dopa) in patients with Parkinson's disease. Vitamin B6 increases peripheral decarboxylation of L-dopa to dopamine (15). Tell patients taking cowhage for Parkinson's disease to avoid taking vitamin B6 supplements.

Interactions with Drugs

ANESTHESIA: Concomitant use of some anesthetics and the cowhage constituent, levodopa (L-dopa) has resulted in cardiac arrhythmia. This effect has only been associated with cyclopropane and the halogenated hydrocarbons. Other anesthetics have not been implicated (15). Use other anesthetics in patients taking cowhage or tell patients to stop taking cowhage at least 2 weeks before surgery.
ANTIDIABETES DRUGS: There is some evidence that cowhage might have hypoglycemic effects (7221). Theoretically, concomitant use with drugs that decrease blood glucose levels might increase the risk of hypoglycemia. Dosing adjustments for insulin or oral hypoglycemic agents may be necessary. Oral hypoglycemic drugs include glimepiride (Amaryl), glipizide (Glucotrol), glyburide (Diabeta, Micronase), tolazamide (Tolinase), tolbutamide (Orinase), and others.
ANTIPSYCHOTIC DRUGS: Due to the antidopaminergic effects of antipsychotic medications, concomitant use of cowhage and these drugs might decrease the effectiveness of some antipsychotics (15). Some of these drugs include chlorpromazine (Thorazine), clozapine (Clozaril), fluphenazine (Prolixin), haloperidol (Haldol), olanzapine (Zyprexa), perphenazine (Trilafon), prochlorperazine (Compazine), quetiapine (Seroquel), risperidone (Risperdal), thioridazine (Mellaril), and thiothixene (Navane).
GUANETHIDINE (Ismelin): Cowhage might have additive hypotensive effects when used concomitantly with guanethidine (15); avoid using.
METHYLDOPA (Aldomet): Cowhage might have additive hypotensive effects when used concomitantly with methyldopa. Furthermore, methyldopa can inhibit peripheral decarboxylation of the cowhage constituent levodopa (L-dopa). This could increase the amount of L-dopa reaching the central nervous system and potentially lead to toxicity (15).
MONOAMINE OXIDASE INHIBITORS (MAOIs): Due to the levodopa (L-dopa) content of cowhage, it should not be given with non-selective MAOIs such as phenelzine (Nardil) and tranylcypromine (Parnate). Concomitant use can cause hypertensive crisis. However, cowhage can be used concurrently with the MAO-B selective inhibitor selegiline (Deprenyl) (15).
TRICYCLIC ANTIDEPRESSANTS (TCAs): There is some concern that TCAs might decrease absorption of the active cowhage constituent, levodopa (L-dopa). TCAs can slow gastric emptying which can prevent L-dopa from being fully absorbed. There have also been rare reports of hypertension and dyskinesias in some patients taking both TCAs and L-dopa (15). Concomitant use of cowhage and TCAs should be done cautiously or avoided. Some TCAs include amitriptyline (Elavil), clomipramine (Anafranil), desipramine (Norpramin), doxepin (Sinequan), imipramine (Tofranil), nortriptyline (Pamelor), and protriptyline (Vivactil).

Interactions with Foods

None known.

Interactions with Lab Tests

GLUCOSE: Due to the levodopa (L-dopa) content, cowhage might cause false-positive urine glucose tests when cupric sulfate reagents, such as Benedict's reagent or Clinitest tablets, are used. Cowhage might cause false-negatives when glucose oxidase tests such as Clinistix and Tes-Tape are used (15).
KETONES: Due to the levodopa (L-dopa) content, cowhage might cause a false positive urine ketones reaction when sodium nitroprusside reagents such as Acetest, Ketostix, and Labstix are used (15).
LIVER FUNCTION TESTS: Due to the levodopa content, cowhage might cause elevated liver function tests. L-dopa has caused transiently increased liver function tests including alkaline phosphatase, aspartate aminotransferase (AST or SGOT), alanine aminotransferase (ALT or SGPT), lactate dehydrogenase (LDH), and bilirubin (15). However, this effect has not yet been reported for cowhage.
URIC ACID: Due to the levodopa (L-dopa) content of cowhage, serum and urine uric acid levels might appear elevated when colorimetric tests are used. However, cowhage does not effect tests using uricase (15).

Interactions with Diseases or Conditions

CARDIOVASCULAR DISEASE: Due to the levodopa (L-dopa) content of cowhage, it should be avoided or used cautiously in patients with cardiovascular disease. L-dopa can frequently cause orthostatic hypotension, dizziness, and syncope. Much less frequently, L-dopa can also cause palpitations and cardiac arrhythmias (15).
DIABETES: There is some evidence that cowhage can lower blood glucose levels and might cause hypoglycemia (7221). Advise patients to increase blood glucose monitoring. Dosing adjustments to diabetes medications may be necessary.
HEPATIC DISEASE: Due to the levodopa (L-dopa) content of cowhage, use cautiously in patients with liver disease. L-dopa has been reported to cause increased liver function tests (15).
HYPOGLYCEMIA: There is some evidence that cowhage can lower blood glucose levels and might exacerbate

hypoglycemia (7221).
MELANOMA: Since levodopa (L-dopa) in cowhage is a precursor to the skin pigment melanin, there is some concern that it might worsen melanoma (15). Tell patients with malignant melanoma, history of melanoma or a suspicious undiagnosed skin lesions to avoid cowhage.
PEPTIC ULCER DISEASE (PUD): Since cowhage contains levodopa (L-dopa), there is some concern that it might induce gastrointestinal bleeding in patients with peptic ulcer disease. L-dopa has been reported to cause gastrointestinal bleeding in patients with PUD (15). However, this has not yet been reported with cowhage.
PSYCHIATRIC DISEASE: Due to the levodopa (L-dopa) content, cowhage might worsen psychiatric disease in patients with an existing condition (15). Furthermore, patients with a history of mental illness might be more likely to experience a cowhage-induced psychiatric disturbance.

Dosage and Administration

ORAL: For Parkinson's disease, a powdered cowhage extract known as HP-200, standardized to contain 3.3% levodopa (L-dopa) has been used. Dosages ranged from 22.5 to 67.5 grams divided into 2 to 5 doses per day (7020). Nonstandardized ground cowhage preparations have also been used. These contain 4.5% to 5.5% levodopa (L-dopa) and have been taken in doses of 40 to 60 grams per day in 4 divided doses (7203).

Comments

Cowhage is a legume that grows wild in the tropics, including India and the Bahamas, and its range may extend to southern Florida (6898). It has been used since ancient times in Ayurvedic medicine for the treatment of Parkinson's disease (7223). Prior to commercial synthesis of levodopa from vanillin, cowhage was investigated as a potential source of the drug with efforts to increase the yield of levodopa from the seeds and leaves (7203,7204). The barbed spicules detach easily from the fruiting pods and have been sold commercially as itching powder (6898).

COWSLIP

Also Known As

Arthritica, Buckels, Butter Rose, Crewel, English Cowslip, Fairy Caps, Herb Perter, Key Flower, Key of Heaven, Mayflower, Our Lady's Keys, Paigle, Paigle Peggle, Palsywort, Password, Peagle, Peagles, Petty Mulleins, Plumrocks, Primrose, Primula.
CAUTION: See separate listing for Marsh Marigold.

Scientific Names

Primula veris, synonym Primula officinalis; Primula elatior.
Family: Primulaceae.

People Use This For

Orally, cowslip flower is used for respiratory tract mucous membrane inflammation, cough, bronchitis, insomnia, nervous excitability, headache, hysteria, neuralgia, tremors, hydroticum, as a diuretic, antispasmodic, as a heart tonic for sensations of dizziness and cardiac insufficiency, whooping cough, asthma, gout, and neurologic complaints.
In combination with gentian root, European elder flower, verbena, and sorrel, cowslip is used orally for maintaining healthy sinuses and treating sinusitis.

Safety

POSSIBLY SAFE ...when used orally and appropriately (2,12). ...when used orally with gentian root, European elder flower, verbena, and sorrel (Quanterra Sinus Defense, Sinupret) (7,374,379).
PREGNANCY AND LACTATION: Insufficient reliable information available; avoid using.

Effectiveness

POSSIBLY EFFECTIVE

Sinusitis. Taking cowslip orally in combination with gentian root, European elder flower, verbena, and sorrel (Quanterra Sinus Defense, Sinupret), seems to help improve symptoms and resolve acute or chronic sinusitis (7,374,379).

There is insufficient reliable information available about the effectiveness of cowslip for its other uses.

Mechanism of Action

The applicable parts of cowslip are the flower and root. Cowslip is a rich source of beta-carotene and vitamin C (19). Cowslip is reported to have antispasmodic, diuretic, expectorant, hypnotic, laxative, secretion-reducing, and sedative activities (2,4). Evidence suggests the saponin fraction might initially cause hypotension followed by long-lasting hypertension (4). Flavonoid constituents might have anti-inflammatory and antispasmodic effects. The tannin constituents have astringent effects (4).

Adverse Reactions
Orally, cowslip can cause gastric discomfort and nausea (2,4,12). It may cause an allergic reaction in sensitive individuals (4). Toxicity, when it occurs, seems to be associated with saponin constituents of the underground parts of the plant (4).

Interactions with Herbs & Other Dietary Supplements
None known.

Interactions with Drugs
CNS DEPRESSANTS: Cowslip may potentiate effects of sedatives (6002).
DIURETIC DRUGS: Cowslip may potentiate effects of diuretics (6002).

Interactions with Foods
None known.

Interactions with Lab Tests
None known.

Interactions with Diseases or Conditions
HYPERTENSION, HYPOTENSION: Theoretically, excessive doses may interfere with control of these conditions (4).

Dosage and Administration
ORAL (flower): One cup tea (1-2 grams dried flowers steeped in 150 mL of boiling water 5-10 minutes, strain) three times daily (4). Liquid extract (1:1 in 25% alcohol), 1-2 mL three times daily (4). Tincture, 2.5-7.5 grams per day (2). For acute or chronic sinusitis, two Sinupret tablets three times daily for up to two weeks has been used in clinical trials (7,374,379), equivalent to gentian root 12 mg, European elder flower 36 mg, verbena 36 mg, cowslip flower 36 mg, and sorrel 36 mg three times daily.
ORAL (root): 0.5-1.5 grams dried root per day, or as prepared tea. Tincture, 1.5-3 grams per day (2).

CRAMP BARK

Also Known As
Common Guelder-Rose, Crampbark, European Cranberry-Bush, Guelder Rose, Guelder-Rose, High-Bush Cranberry, Snowball Bush.
CAUTION: See separate listings for Alpine Cranberry, Black Haw, Cranberry, and Uva Ursi.

Scientific Names
Viburnum opulus.
Family: Adoxaceae/Viburnaceae or Caprifoliaceae.

People Use This For
Orally, cramp bark is used to relieve cramps, including muscle spasms, menstrual cramps, and cramps during pregnancy. It is also used orally as a kidney stimulant in painful or spasmodic urinary conditions, cancer, hysteria, infection, nervous disorders, scurvy, and uteritis. It has also been used as a diuretic, emetic, purgative, and sedative.

Safety
POSSIBLY SAFE ...when used orally and appropriately (12).
PREGNANCY AND LACTATION: Insufficient reliable information available; avoid using.

Effectiveness
There is insufficient reliable information available about the effectiveness of cramp bark.

Mechanism of Action
The applicable parts of cramp bark are the bark and root bark. There is insufficient reliable information available about the possible mechanism of action and active ingredients.

Adverse Reactions
None reported.

Interactions with Herbs & Other Dietary Supplements
None known.

Interactions with Drugs
None known.

Interactions with Foods
None known.

Interactions with Lab Tests
None known.

Interactions with Diseases or Conditions
None known.

Dosage and Administration
ORAL: No typical dosage. However, a dose of 2-4 grams of the dried bark, 2-4 mL of a liquid extract (1:1 in 25% alcohol), or 5-10 mL of a tincture (1:5 in 45% alcohol), three times daily (2822) has been used.

Comments
Canadian regulations prohibit cramp bark as a non-medicinal ingredient for oral use products (12). Avoid confusion with black haw (Vibernum prunifolium), which is sometimes referred to as cramp bark.

CRANBERRY

Also Known As
American Cranberry, Arandano Americano, Arandano Trepador, Cranberries, European Cranberry, Grosse Moosbeere, Kranbeere, Large Cranberry, Moosebeere, Mossberry, Ronce d'Amerique, Small Cranberry, Trailing Swamp Cranberry, Tsuru-kokemomo.
CAUTION: See separate listings for Alpine Cranberry, Cramp Bark (European Cranberry-Bush), and Uva Ursi (Mountain Cranberry).

Scientific Names
Vaccinium macrocarpon, synonym Oxycoccus macrocarpos; Vaccinium oxycoccos, synonyms Oxycoccus hagerupii, Oxycoccus microcarpus, Oxycoccus palustris, Oxycoccus quadripetalus, Vaccinium hagerupii, Vaccinium microcarpum, Vaccinium palustre.
Family: Ericaceae.

People Use This For
Orally, cranberry is used for prevention and treatment of urinary tract infections, neurogenic bladder, as a urinary deodorizer for people with incontinence, prevention of urinary catheter blockage, and to heal skin around urostomy stomas. Cranberry is also used for type 2 diabetes, scurvy, pleurisy, as a diuretic, antiseptic, antipyretic, and for cancer.
In foods, cranberry fruit is used in fruit juice, jelly, and sauce.

Safety
LIKELY SAFE ...when used orally and appropriately (6758,7008,8253,8995).
CHILDREN: LIKELY SAFE ...when used orally and appropriately (2811,6759).
PREGNANCY AND LACTATION: LIKELY SAFE ...when used orally in amounts commonly found in food (5). There is insufficient reliable information about the safety of cranberry when used therapeutically during pregnancy or lactation; avoid using.

Effectiveness
POSSIBLY EFFECTIVE

Urinary odor. Cranberry juice appears to reduce urinary odors when given orally on a regular basis to patients with urinary incontinence (3333,3334,8254).
Urinary tract infections (UTIs). Daily consumption of cranberry juice 10 oz (300 mL) seems to prevent recurrent UTIs in some young and elderly women (6758,7008,8253). A combination product containing cranberry juice plus alpine cranberry (Vaccinium vitis-idaea) also seems to be helpful for prevention (8253). But neither cranberry juice nor cranberry extract seem to prevent UTI in adults or children related to neurogenic bladder (2811,6759,11980).

Tell patients not to try cranberry juice for treating UTIs. There's not enough evidence it works (8252,8995).
Some patients are trying encapsulated forms of concentrated cranberry. So far, there is little reliable evidence that these preparations offer the same benefits as the juice (6760). Tell women interested in trying cranberry for UTI prevention to stick with the juice.

POSSIBLY INEFFECTIVE

Diabetes. Taking cranberry supplements orally doesn't seem to improve fasting serum glucose, glycosylated hemoglobin (HbA1c), fructosamine, triglyceride, high-density lipoprotein (HDL) cholesterol, or low-density lipoprotein (LDL) cholesterol levels in patients with type 2 diabetes (11328).

There is insufficient reliable information available about the effectiveness of cranberry for its other uses.

Mechanism of Action

The applicable part of the cranberry plant is the fruit. The cranberry is acidic, but does not acidify the urine as previously thought. Cranberries contain proanthocyanidins, also known as condensed tannins, and a high-molecular weight compound that has not yet been identified. These constituents seem to interfere with bacterial adherence to the urinary tract epithelial cells (2812,2814,3335,3337,3339,6753,6755,6757). For example, proanthocyanidins seem to be capable of "wrapping" around Escherichia coli (E. coli), which is the cause of most urinary tract infections (UTIs), and preventing it from adhering to the urinary tract wall (3333,3338,6690). It probably also has this effect against other urinary tract pathogens (2815). Cranberry, however, does not seem to have the ability to release bacteria which are already adhered to the urinary tract epithelial cells (8252). Laboratory evidence suggests that fructose in cranberries might also contribute to the anti-infective activity (2813,3333,6757). Cranberry juice has shown antibacterial activity in culture medium against E. coli, Staphylococcus aureus, Klebsiella pneumoniae, Pseudomonas aeruginosa, and Proteus mirabilis (3333,3338,6753). Whether urinary concentrations of the active constituents reach bactericidal levels is currently a topic of research (6753).

Preliminary data suggest that a high molecular weight cranberry constituent might prevent adhesion of plaque bacteria that cause periodontal disease (2816). Cranberry compounds might also prevent adhesion of Helicobacter pylori (H. pylori) in the stomach (6690). Early evidence shows that cranberry juice might increase the antioxidant capacity of plasma (6754). There is also preliminary evidence that the proanthocyanidin fraction of cranberry might have anticarcinogenic activity (888).

Adverse Reactions

Orally, cranberry is usually well tolerated (6758,7008,8253,8995). However, in very large doses, for example 3-4 L per day of juice, cranberry can cause gastrointestinal upset and diarrhea. Consuming more than 1 L per day over a prolonged period of time might also increase the risk of uric acid kidney stone formation (3334).

Interactions with Herbs & Other Dietary Supplements

None known.

Interactions with Drugs

CYTOCHROME P450 2C9 (CYP2C9) SUBSTRATES: There's preliminary evidence that flavonoids in cranberry might inhibit cytochrome P450 2C9 (CYP2C9) enzymes (10452,11115). Some drugs metabolized by CYP2C9 include amitriptyline (Elavil), diazepam (Valium), zileuton (Zyflo), and others.

WARFARIN (Coumadin): Cranberry juice can cause increases in the international normalized ratio (INR) in patients taking warfarin, which has been associated with severe bleeding (10452). Flavonoids in cranberry might inhibit cytochrome P450 2C9 (CYP2C9) isoenzyme, which could reduce the metabolism of warfarin and increase the anticoagulant effect (11115).

Interactions with Foods

None known.

Interactions with Lab Tests

None known.

Interactions with Diseases or Conditions

ATROPHIC GASTRITIS: Cranberry juice might increase absorption of dietary vitamin B12 in people with atrophic gastritis due to its acidity (4485).

DIABETES: Caution patients with diabetes to avoid cranberry juice cocktail products sweetened with sugar and instead to use cranberry juice cocktail products sweetened with artificial sweeteners.

HYPOCHLORHYDRIA: Cranberry juice might increase absorption of dietary vitamin B12 in people with hypochlorhydria due to its acidity (4485).

KIDNEY STONES (Nephrolithiasis): There is some concern that cranberry juice and cranberry extracts might increase the risk of kidney stones because of its high oxalate content. Drinking cranberry juice 30 mL typically provides approximately 1.9 mg of oxalate. Concentrated cranberry extracts might contain higher amounts of oxalate. There is some evidence that some cranberry extract tablets can boost urinary oxalate concentration by as much as

43% (7074). Tell patients with a history of kidney stones to avoid cranberry extract products or excessive consumption of cranberry juice.

Dosage and Administration

ORAL: For preventing urinary tract infections (UTIs), cranberry juice 1-10 oz per day has been used (6758,7008,8995). However, the ideal dose has not yet been determined. Some people drink up to 10-32 oz per day of cranberry juice for treating UTIs (515). For preventing UTIs in children a dose of 15ml/kg daily as 30% cranberry concentrate has been used (6759). For use as a urinary deodorizer for incontinent patients, 3-6 oz per day of cranberry juice has been used (8254). For type 2 diabetes, six capsules (equivalent to 240 ml cranberry juice cocktail) daily for 12 weeks has been used (11328). Encapsulated formulations are often taken in doses of 300-400 mg twice daily (7010).
Approximately 1500 grams of fresh fruit produces 1 L of juice. Cranberry juice cocktail is approximately 26%-33% pure cranberry juice, sweetened with fructose or artificial sweetener (515,3335).

CREATINE

Also Known As

Cr, Creatine Monohydrate.

Scientific Names

N-amidinosarcosine; N-(aminoiminomethyl)-N methyl glycine.

People Use This For

Orally, creatine is used for improving exercise performance and increasing muscle mass in athletes and older adults. Creatine is also used orally for congestive heart failure (CHF), neuromuscular disease, mitochondrial cytopathies, gyrate atrophy of the choroid and retina, and hyperlipidemia. It is also used orally for slowing the progression of amyotrophic lateral sclerosis (ALS, Lou Gehrig's disease), rheumatoid arthritis, McArdle disease, and for various muscular dystrophies.
Intravenously, creatine is used in cardiac surgery and for congestive heart failure.

Safety

POSSIBLY SAFE ...when used orally and appropriately. Creatine supplementation appears generally to be safe when used in appropriate doses in healthy adults (1367,2100,2101,2103,3996,4569,6052,10062,10064). Creatine has been safely used daily for up to 5 years (3996).
POSSIBLY UNSAFE ...when used orally in high doses. There is some concern that very high doses of creatine might adversely affect renal, hepatic, or cardiac function and have other adverse effects, such as hypertension (1367,6052); however, a clear association between high dose creatine and significant adverse effects has not yet been established.
PREGNANCY AND LACTATION: Insufficient reliable information available; avoid using.

Effectiveness

POSSIBLY EFFECTIVE

Athletic performance. Taking creatine orally seems to enhance muscle performance during repeated bouts of brief, high-intensity exercise. Numerous studies suggest that creatine is beneficial for certain types of high-intensity exercises (2100,2101,2102,4591,4592,4593,4594,4601,4602,4604,4605,6015,10064,11331); however, for other exercises, creatine appears to offer no benefit (4582,4595,4596,4597,4606,6183). Creatine seems to be more effective for increasing muscular power in healthy young adults during repeated, short, maximal energy bursts than for single event performances (4593,4598,4599,4600,6052,10064,11331). It might also be beneficial for exercise of longer duration with the intensity alternating between anaerobic and aerobic metabolism (6926). Many variables seem to determine the effect of creatine on performance, including the subject's training status, the type of sport being tested, diet, age of the subject, and the dose regimen of creatine. Creatine does not seem to improve performance in aerobic exercises, or benefit older individuals. Additionally, creatine doesn't increase endurance or improve performance in highly trained athletes (2103,2105,2106,4607). It is possible that the benefit in certain sports is offset by weight gain from creatine supplementation (2106,4576,4601,4604,4605,6015,6052). Acute creatine loading may be more effective than chronic continuous use (4603). Most studies have used 20 grams daily for 5 days for creatine loading; however, various other regimens have been studied. One study used 9 grams daily for 5 days and was beneficial in weight lifters, while another study used 20 grams daily for 3 days and was not beneficial for single sprints in cyclists (4576,4599,6015). Due to the variety of study methodologies and some conflicting findings, it has yet to be determined exactly who can benefit from creatine supplementation and what dosing schedule might be most effective. All studies have been limited by small sample size; all have involved fewer than 40 subjects and most fewer than 25.

Congestive heart failure (CHF). Taking creatine orally seems to improve exercise tolerance, but does not affect ejection fraction in people with CHF (4562,4563). Intravenous creatine improves cardiac function, including ejection fraction, even in the presence of conventional pharmacologic therapy. Following an infusion of 6 grams of IV creatine, improvements in ejection fraction persist for more than 12 hours (1369).

Gyrate atrophy of the choroid and retina. Creatine supplementation seems to slow visual deterioration in patients with gyrate atrophy (4577,4578).

McArdle's disease. There is some preliminary clinical evidence that daily high-dose creatine supplementation can increase exercise capacity and decreases exercise-induced muscle pain in some patients with McArdle's disease (70).

Muscular dystrophy. Taking creatine orally short-term seems to improve muscle strength and daily-life activity in adults and children with various muscular dystrophies (6182). Creatine monohydrate daily for eight weeks seems to mildly improve muscle strength and daily-life activity in children and adults with facioscapulohumeral dystrophy, Becker dystrophy, Duchenne dystrophy, or sarcoglycan-deficient limb girdle muscular dystrophy (6182). Taking creatine orally also seems to improve refractory muscle pain in patients with myotonic dystrophy type 2/proximal myotonic myopathy (DM2/PROMM). Muscle strength and performance might also improve in these patients after three months of treatment (10654).

POSSIBLY INEFFECTIVE

Amyotrophic lateral sclerosis (ALS, Lou Gehrig's disease). Taking creatine orally doesn't seem to have any beneficial effect on disease progression or survival in patients with ALS (11332).

Rheumatoid arthritis (RA). Taking creatine orally doesn't seem to help symptoms of RA. Creatine supplementation can increase muscle creatine content and muscle strength, but has no significant effect on physical functional ability or disease activity (6929).

LIKELY INEFFECTIVE

Athletic conditioning. Taking creatine orally doesn't seem to improve isometric strength and body composition in adults over age 60 (4570,4571,4572). Creatine dosed at 20 grams per day for 5 days followed by lower maintenance doses has no beneficial effect on exercise except reducing muscle fatigue (4570,4571,4572). In one study it had no effect on quadriceps fatigue after repeated sets of explosive work (6183).

Mechanism of Action

Creatine is found primarily in skeletal muscle (95%), but is also found in heart, brain, testes, retina, and other tissues (3997,3998). The body synthesizes 1 to 2 grams of creatine a day, primarily in the liver, kidneys, and pancreas (3997). Dietary sources, such as fish and meats, supply an additional 1 to 2 grams. For example, one pound of fresh uncooked steak contains about 2 grams of creatine (4575). Intestinal absorption of creatine is nearly 100% (6052). Creatine is irreversibly converted to creatinine and excreted by the kidneys (3997). Creatine in skeletal muscles exists in dynamic equilibrium with phosphocreatine (3997). Body stores of phosphocreatine in skeletal muscle serve as a precursor to the energy molecule, adenosine triphosphate (ATP). Higher levels of creatine are thought to enhance the ability to renew ATP for short 10-20 second energy bursts and improve resynthesis of phosphocreatine during recovery from intense exercise. Creatine supplementation enhances both creatine and phosphocreatine concentrations, providing a larger total creatine pool in the skeletal muscle. Creatine hinders the creatine-creatine kinase-phosphocreatine circuit. However, there is some debate about whether increased phosphocreatine resynthesis actually occurs (2103,3997,4574,4576,4580,4583,6925,6927,11330).

People who have lower initial total creatine, such as vegetarians, are more likely to respond to supplemental creatine, while people with higher initial levels may not respond (4574). Repeated creatine dosing causes a reduction in creatine clearance. Skeletal muscle has a saturation point at which additional supplemental creatine will not increase intracellular creatine levels. This reduction may result from skeletal muscle saturation (10065), which occurs within the first few days of loading (3999,6052,10065). Excess supplementation increases urinary creatine and creatinine (4576). Exogenous creatine supplementation also appears to reduce endogenous creatine production; whether this has any clinically significant negative effect on metabolic regulation within the liver is unknown (6052). After discontinuing supplementation, endogenous creatine production and creatine levels typically return to baseline within 28 days (2101,4582,6052).

Although some laboratory evidence identifies creatine as a potential lean body mass builder, most clinical evidence supports increased cellular water retention as the primary cause of creatine-induced muscle gain (4569,4575,4576,4579,4588,6061,10062). The muscle enlargement due to increased water retention is short term. This is compared to the muscle enlargement from strength training, which results in an increase in contractile and structural muscle proteins (6052). Creatine may allow athletes to train harder due to increased phosphocreatine resynthesis and subsequent energy production (6061). Creatine might also reduce lactate production (4604); however, this has not been consistently found in studies (4592). In patients with congestive heart failure (CHF), the cardiac creatine phosphate/adenosine triphosphate is lower than in people with normal cardiac function and correlates with the severity of heart failure (1369). Creatine phosphate appears to improve CHF by preserving intracellular high-energy phosphates in the myocardium, stabilizing the sarcolemma, preventing peroxidative damage, and improving microcirculation (1369). In patients with gyrate atrophy, an inherited metabolic disease in which phosphocreatine is depleted, supplemental creatine increased myofibrillar protein synthesis resulting in muscle accretion (4576,4587). In myophosphorylase deficiency, known as McArdle disease, a rare genetic metabolic disease in which ATP cannot be formed from glycogen in skeletal muscle, supplemental creatine is thought to serve as a source of energy (70).

Creatine appears to also affect lipid metabolism. There is some preliminary evidence that it can modestly reduce total cholesterol and very low-density lipoprotein (VLDL) cholesterol (4573). Early laboratory evidence also suggests that creatine might be useful in diseases such as amyotrophic lateral sclerosis, Huntington's disease, and Parkinson's disease, possibly due to neuroprotective effects (4566,4567,4568). There is conflicting evidence on creatine and cancer. Some research suggests that creatine and its analogs, such as cyclocreatine, inhibit tumor growth (1393,1406,1432,1481). Creatine might alter energy production by the creatine kinase system, which appears to play a role in controlling some types of tumors such as breast tumors and neuroblastomas (1393,1406). Other research suggests that creatine or its metabolites can form mutagenic substances when combined at room temperature with sugars or heated (1486,1487), but this has not been verified.

Adverse Reactions

Orally, creatine can cause gastrointestinal pain, nausea, and diarrhea (2103,4576,6052). Case reports have found that 25% of male collegiate athletes taking creatine have muscle cramping (4584). A theoretical increase in risk of dehydration due to intracellular fluid shifts has led most creatine manufacturers to caution about adequate hydration with creatine supplementation (4576). Tell patients who are controlling their weight and engaging in strenuous exercise and/or exercising in hot environments to avoid creatine supplementation (6052). Creatine typically causes a weight gain of 0.5 to 1.6 kg that increases with prolonged supplementation (3997). This weight gain, most likely due to water retention, has been thought to also increase the risk for high blood pressure. However, a recent study showed no effect of 20 grams daily of creatine for 5 days on blood pressure (4569). Creatine might also cause renal dysfunction (184,2118), but this appears to be rare in people with healthy kidneys (1368,2120,3996). Most studies have not found alterations in renal function in people taking 5-20 grams of creatine daily for up to 5 years (3996,4569). However, there is one report of acute interstitial nephritis and focal tubular injury after four weeks of creatine at 5 grams four times daily (184). In another case, supplemental creatine, loaded at 15 grams per day for one week, then 2 grams per day, caused a significant decline in creatinine clearance in a man receiving cyclosporine for steroid-resistant focal segmental glomerulosclerosis (2118). Medical supervision is suggested for people who have kidney disease or have a high risk of kidney disease and use creatine (4569,6052). There is one report of ischemic stroke in an athlete who consumed a combination of 6 grams of creatine monohydrate, 400-600 mg of caffeine, 40-60 mg of ephedra, and a variety of other supplements daily for six weeks (1275).

Interactions with Herbs & Other Dietary Supplements

CAFFEINE: There is some concern that combining caffeine, ephedra, and creatine might increase the risk of serious adverse effects. There is a report of ischemic stroke in an athlete who consumed creatine monohydrate 6 grams, caffeine 400-600 mg, ephedra 40-60 mg, and a variety of other supplements daily for 6 weeks (1275). Caffeine might also decrease creatine's beneficial effects on athletic performance. Some researchers think caffeine can inhibit phosphocreatine resynthesis (2117,4575).

EPHEDRA: There is some concern that combining ephedra, caffeine, and creatine might increase the risk of serious adverse effects. There is a report of ischemic stroke in an athlete who consumed creatine monohydrate 6 grams, caffeine 400-600 mg, ephedra 40-60 mg, and a variety of other supplements daily for 6 weeks (1275).

Interactions with Drugs

NEPHROTOXIC DRUGS: There is some concern about using creatine with drugs that can be nephrotoxic. Since high doses of creatine might adversely affect renal function (6052), combining creatine with potentially nephrotoxic drugs might have additive harmful effects on kidney function. However, this effect has not yet been reported. Some potentially nephrotoxic drugs include cyclosporine (Neoral, Sandimmune); aminoglycosides including amikacin (Amikin), gentamicin (Garamycin, Gentak, others), and tobramycin (Nebcin, others); nonsteroidal anti-inflammatory drugs (NSAIDs) including ibuprofen (Advil, Motrin, Nuprin, others), indomethacin (Indocin), naproxen (Aleve, Anaprox, Naprelan, Naprosyn), piroxicam (Feldene); and numerous others.

Interactions with Foods

CARBOHYDRATES: Combining carbohydrates with creatine can increase muscle creatine levels more than creatine alone. Supplementing 5 grams of creatine with 93 grams of simple carbohydrates four times daily for 5 days can increase muscle creatine levels as much as 60% more than creatine alone (10063).

Interactions with Lab Tests

SERUM CREATININE (SCr): Creatine is metabolized to creatinine. Higher than normal serum creatinine levels can result in patients taking creatine, despite normal renal function (2100,2103).

Interactions with Diseases or Conditions

KIDNEY DYSFUNCTION: Creatine should be avoided by people with pre-existing renal disease or by people with diseases such as diabetes that increase the risk for renal dysfunction (4576). There is some concern that creatine might exacerbate renal dysfunction in these patients.

Dosage and Administration

ORAL: For improving physical performance, several dosing regimens have been tried. Creatine is typically acutely loaded with 20 grams per day (or 0.3 grams per kg) for 5 days followed by a maintenance dose of 2 or more grams (0.03 grams per kg) daily (4576,11331). Although 5 day loading is typical, 2 days of loading has also been used (4576).

A loading dose of 9 grams per day for 6 days has also been used (6015). Some sources suggest that, instead of acutely loading, similar results can be obtained with 3 grams per day for 28 days (2104). During creatine supplementation, the water intake should be 64 ounces per day (2103,2104). For heart failure, 20 grams per day for 5-10 days has been used in clinical trials (4562,4563). For gyrate atrophy, 1.5 grams per day has been used (4577,4578). For McArdle disease, 150mg/kg daily for 5 days followed by 60 mg/kg per day has been used (70). For muscular dystrophies, 10 grams per day has been used by adults and 5 grams per day has been used by children (6182). For myotonic dystrophy type 2/proximal myotonic myopathy, 10 grams per day has been used (10654). For amyotrophic lateral sclerosis (ALS, Lou Gehrig's disease), 10 grams daily for 12-16 months has been used (11332).

Comments
Creatine is allowed by the International Olympic Committee, National Collegiate Athletic Association (NCAA), and professional sports (3998,4575,4576). However, the NCAA no longer allows colleges and universities to supply creatine to their students with school funds. Students are permitted to buy creatine on their own and the NCAA has no plans to ban creatine unless sufficient medical evidence indicates that it is harmful (6140). With current testing methods, detection of supplemental creatine use would not be possible (4575). Creatine use is widespread among professional and amateur athletes and has been acknowledged by well-known athletes such as Mark McGuire, Sammy Sosa, and John Elway (3998). Following the finding that carbohydrate solution further increased muscle creatine levels more than creatine alone, creatine sports drinks have become popular (4576,4589). Annual consumption of creatine in the US is estimated to exceed 4 million kg (3998). California is considering legislation that would ban the sale of creatine and other supplements frequently used in sports performance-enhancing products to anyone under the age of 18. The bill, which received Senate approval and is now in the Assembly, would also require warning labels about the adverse effects of creatine (8639).

CROTON SEEDS

Also Known As
Croton, Tiglium, Tiglium Seeds.

Scientific Names
Croton tiglium.
Family: Euphorbiaceae.

People Use This For
Orally, croton seeds are used as a purgative, treat gallbladder colic, bowel obstruction, and malaria.
Topically croton seeds are used for rheumatism, gout, neuralgia, and bronchitis.

Safety
LIKELY UNSAFE ...when used orally. One drop of the oil can be toxic, and one mL (20 drops) of oil is considered lethal (18). Also, the phorbol esters in the oil are co-carcinogens (18). ...when used topically; avoid using (18).
PREGNANCY: UNSAFE ...when used orally due to abortifacient properties (19); avoid using.
LACTATION: UNSAFE ...when used orally (18); avoid using.

Effectiveness
There is insufficient reliable information available about the effectiveness of croton seeds.

Mechanism of Action
The applicable part of croton seeds is the oil from the seed. Croton seeds possess powerful, irritant, cathartic properties due to phorbol esters (3800). The diterpene, TPA, is carcinogenic, affecting prostaglandin metabolism (18).

Adverse Reactions
Orally, croton seeds can cause burning of mouth, vomiting, dizziness, stupor, painful bowel movements, and collapse (18).
Topically, croton seeds can cause itching, burning and blistering of skin (18).

Interactions with Herbs & Other Dietary Supplements
None known.

Interactions with Drugs
None known.

Interactions with Foods
None known.

Interactions with Lab Tests
None known.

Interactions with Diseases or Conditions
None known.

Dosage and Administration
No typical dosage.

CUBEBS

Also Known As
Cubeb, Cubeb Berries, Cubeba, Cubeba officinalis, Java Pepper, Tailed Chubebs, Tailed Pepper.

Scientific Names
Piper cubeba.
Family: Piperaceae.

People Use This For
Orally, cubebs is used as a diuretic, urinary antiseptic, for amoebic dysentery, as an antiflatulent, stimulating expectorant, for gonorrhea, and cancer.
In foods, cubebs oil is used as a flavoring ingredient.

Safety
LIKELY SAFE ...when used orally in amounts commonly found in foods. Cubebs has Generally Recognized As Safe (GRAS) status in the US (4912).
POSSIBLY SAFE ...when used orally and appropriately in medicinal amounts (12).
PREGNANCY AND LACTATION: Insufficient reliable information available; avoid using.

Effectiveness
There is insufficient reliable information available about the effectiveness of cubebs.

Mechanism of Action
The applicable part of cubebs is the dried, fully grown but unripe fruit. Researchers think that the constituent cubebic acid is responsible for the stimulant effect on urinary and respiratory tract (11).

Adverse Reactions
None reported.

Interactions with Herbs & Other Dietary Supplements
None known.

Interactions with Drugs
ANTACIDS: Theoretically, due to reports that cubebs increases stomach acid, cubebs might decrease the effectiveness of antacids (19).
H2-BLOCKERS: Theoretically, due to reports that cubebs increases stomach acid, cubebs might decrease the effectiveness of H2-blockers (19). The H2 blockers include cimetidine (Tagamet), ranitidine (Zantac), nizatidine (Axid), and famotidine (Pepcid).
PROTON PUMP INHIBITORS (PPIs): Theoretically, due to reports that cubebs increases stomach acid, cubebs might decrease the effectiveness of PPIs (19). PPIs include omeprazole (Prilosec), lansoprazole (Prevacid), rabeprazole (Aciphex), pantoprazole (Protonix), and esomeprazole (Nexium).

Interactions with Foods
None known.

Interactions with Lab Tests
None known.

Interactions with Diseases or Conditions

GASTROINTESTINAL (GI) CONDITIONS: Cubebs may irritate the GI tract; contraindicated in individuals with infectious or inflammatory GI conditions (19).
NEPHRITIS: Cubebs is contraindicated in individuals with nephritis (12).

Dosage and Administration

ORAL: People typically use 2 to 4 grams of the powdered fruit or 2 to 4 mL of the liquid extract (223).

CUDWEED

Also Known As

Cotton Dawes, Cotton Weed, Dysentery Weed, Everlasting, Mouse Ear, Wartwort.
CAUTION: See separate listings for Cat's Foot and Mouse Ear.

Scientific Names

Gnaphalium uliginosum, synonym Filaginella uliginosa
Family: Asteraceae/Compositae.

People Use This For

Topically, cudweed is used as a gargle or rinse for diseases of the mouth or throat.

Safety

There is insufficient reliable information available about the safety of cudweed.
Pregnancy and Lactation: Insufficient reliable information available; avoid using.

Effectiveness

There is insufficient reliable information available about the effectiveness of cudweed.

Mechanism of Action

The applicable parts of cudweed are the above ground parts. Cudweed has astringent effects, and promotes and improves appetite (18). Unsubstantiated sources report it has antidepressant, aphrodisiac, and hypotensive effects (18).

Adverse Reactions

Topically, cudweed can cause an allergic reaction in individuals sensitive to the Asteraceae/Compositae family. Members of this family include ragweed, chrysanthemums, marigolds, daisies, and many other herbs.

Interactions with Herbs & Other Dietary Supplements

None known.

Interactions with Drugs

None known.

Interactions with Foods

None known.

Interactions with Lab Tests

None known.

Interactions with Diseases or Conditions

CROSS-ALLERGENICITY: Cudweed may cause an allergic reaction in individuals sensitive to the Asteraceae/Compositae family. Members of this family include ragweed, chrysanthemums, marigolds, daisies, and many other herbs.

Dosage and Administration

ORAL: People typically use 2 to 4 mL of the liquid extract (223).

Comments

Avoid confusion with Antennaria dioica, which is also referred to as cudweed. Avoid confusion with Pilosella officinarum, also known as mouse ear.

CUMIN

Also Known As
Cummin, Jeeraka, Svetajiraka, Zira.

Scientific Names
Cuminum cyminum, synonym Cuminum odorum.
Family: Apiaceae/Umbelliferae.

People Use This For
Orally, cumin is used as an antiflatulent, stimulant, antispasmodic, diuretic, aphrodisiac, for stimulating menstrual flow, treating diarrhea, colic, and flatulence.
In spices, foods, and beverages, cumin is used as a flavoring component.
In other manufacturing processes, cumin oil is used as a fragrance component in cosmetics (maximum use level 0.4% in perfumes).

Safety
LIKELY SAFE ...when used orally in amounts commonly found in foods. Cumin and cumin oil have Generally Recognized As Safe (GRAS) status in the US (4912).
POSSIBLY SAFE ...when used orally and appropriately in medicinal amounts (12).
PREGNANCY AND LACTATION: Insufficient reliable information available; avoid using in excess of food amounts.

Effectiveness
There is insufficient reliable information available about the effectiveness of cumin.

Mechanism of Action
The applicable part of cumin is the fruit/seed. Cumin is a rich source of iron (19). Cumin oil and constituent, cuminaldehyde, have been reported to exhibit strong larvicidal and antibacterial activity (6). Demonstrated phototoxic effects are reportedly not due to cuminaldehyde (11).

Adverse Reactions
Orally, use of undiluted cumin oil has phototoxic effects (6).

Interactions with Herbs & Other Dietary Supplements
None known.

Interactions with Drugs
ANTIDIABETES DRUGS: Monitor blood glucose levels closely due to claims that cumin has hypoglycemic effects (19).

Interactions with Foods
None known.

Interactions with Lab Tests
None known.

Interactions with Diseases or Conditions
None known.

Dosage and Administration
ORAL: The average single amount used is 5-10 fruits (18).

Comments
Fine grinding of the seed can cause loss of 50% of volatile oil, most within 1 hour (6).

CUP PLANT

Also Known As
Indian Gum, Pilot Plant, Polar Plant, Prairie Dock, Ragged Cup, Rosinweed, Turpentine Weed.
CAUTION: See separate listing for Rosinweed.

Scientific Names
Silphium perfoliatum.
Family: Asteraceae/Compositae.

Comments
At the date of publication, this product was not a common ingredient used in brand name supplements marketed to consumers. Details about this product are available at the online version of *Natural Medicines Comprehensive Database*. See www.naturaldatabase.com.

CUPMOSS

Also Known As
Chin Cups.

Scientific Names
Cladonia pyxidata.
Famly: Cladoniaceae.

Comments
At the date of publication, this product was not a common ingredient used in brand name supplements marketed to consumers. Details about this product are available at the online version of *Natural Medicines Comprehensive Database*. See www.naturaldatabase.com.

CYCLAMEN

Also Known As
Groundbread, Ivy-Leafed Cyclamen, Sowbread, Swinebread.

Scientific Names
Cyclamen purpurascens, synonym Cyclamen europaeum.
Family: Primulaceae

People Use This For
Orally, cyclamen is used for menstrual complaints, "nervous emotional states," and digestive problems.

Safety
LIKELY UNSAFE ...when used orally. Doses as low as 300 mg can cause poisoning (18).
PREGNANCY AND LACTATION: LIKELY UNSAFE ...when used orally (18); avoid using.

Effectiveness
There is insufficient reliable information available about the effectiveness of cyclamen.

Mechanism of Action
The applicable parts of cyclamen are the rhizome and root. There is insufficient reliable information available about the possible mechanism of action and active ingredients.

Adverse Reactions
Orally, poisoning has been reported with doses as low as 300 mg; symptoms include stomach pain, nausea, vomiting, and diarrhea (18). High doses can cause severe poisoning; symptoms include spasm and asphyxiation (18,553).

Interactions with Herbs & Other Dietary Supplements
None known.

Interactions with Drugs
None known.

Interactions with Foods
None known.

Interactions with Lab Tests
None known.

Interactions with Diseases or Conditions
None known.

Dosage and Administration
ORAL: People typically use 20 to 40 grains (1300 to 2600 mg) of powdered cyclamen root (5267). Cyclamen should not be used without medical supervision (5263).

CYPRESS

Also Known As
None.

Scientific Names
Cupressus sempervirens.
Family: Cupressaceae.

Comments
At the date of publication, this product was not a common ingredient used in brand name supplements marketed to consumers. There was also very little scientific information available about this product. Our staff is continually analyzing the available information on natural medicines and will add data to the online version of *Natural Medicines Comprehensive Database* as it becomes available. See www.naturaldatabase.com.

CYPRESS SPURGE

Also Known As
None.

Scientific Names
Euphorbia cyparissias.
Family: Euphorbiaceae.

People Use This For
Orally, cypress spurge is used for diseases of the respiratory organs, diarrhea, and skin diseases.

Safety
UNSAFE ...when used orally. The plant contains poisonous white latex (milky liquid) and cocarcinogenic agents (18). Both the fresh and dried latex are toxic (18).
PREGNANCY AND LACTATION: UNSAFE ...when used orally due to toxicity (18); avoid using.

Effectiveness
There is insufficient reliable information available about the effectiveness of cypress spurge.

Mechanism of Action
The applicable parts of cypress spurge are the flowering plant and root. Cypress spurge contains varied diterpenes and triterpenes. The ingenan esters are potent inflammatory and cocarcinogenic agents (18). Euphorbia species have topical irritant, GI irritant, emetic, and purgative effects (19).

Adverse Reactions
Orally, cypress spurge, which is part of the Euphorbia species, may cause GI irritation, nausea, vomiting, and diarrhea (19). Ingestion of the latex can cause burning of the mouth, vomiting, mydriasis, dizziness, painful bowel

movements, stupor, cardiac arrhythmias, and collapse (18).
Topically, Euphorbia species may cause contact dermatitis (19). Skin contact with the latex causes reddening, itching, burning, and blisters (18). Eye contact can cause eyelid swelling, conjunctival inflammation, and corneal defects (18).

Interactions with Herbs & Other Dietary Supplements
None known.

Interactions with Drugs
None known.

Interactions with Foods
None known.

Interactions with Lab Tests
None known.

Interactions with Diseases or Conditions
DIARRHEA: Euphorbia species have purgative effects (19); avoid using.
GASTROINTESTINAL (GI) IRRITATION, INFLAMMATION: Euphorbia species have GI irritant effects (19); avoid using.
NAUSEA, VOMITING: Euphorbia species have emetic effects (19); avoid using.

Dosage and Administration
No typical dosage.

DA QING YE

Also Known As
Dyer's Woad, Farberwaid (Färberwaid), Hierba Pastel, Pastel Des Teinturiers, Quing Dai.

Scientific Names
Isatis tinctoria, synonym Isatis indigotica.
Family: Brassicaceae/Cruciferae.

People Use This For
Orally, da qing ye is used to treat acute parotitis, upper respiratory infection, encephalitis, hepatitis, lung abscess, dysentery, acute gastroenteritis, and HIV.
In combination with other herbs, da qing ye is used to treat prostate cancer.

Safety
There is insufficient reliable information available about the safety of da qing ye.
PREGNANCY AND LACTATION: LIKELY UNSAFE ...when used orally. It is reported to cause uterine contractions (5541); avoid using.

Effectiveness
There is insufficient reliable information available about the effectiveness of da qing ye.

Mechanism of Action
The applicable part of da qing ye is the dried leaf. The dried leaf appears to have antibacterial and antiviral activity and can increase the phagocytic activity of leukocytes. It also shows evidence of antipyretic, anti-inflammatory, and biliary stimulant properties. Da qing ye seems to relax smooth muscles but contracts the uterine muscle. The dried leaf of da qing ye contains the glycosides indican and isatin B. Of the ingested dose of da qing ye, 90% is excreted in the urine (5541).

Adverse Reactions
Orally, da qing ye can cause nausea and vomiting (5541).
Intramuscularly, da qing ye can cause blood in the urine (5541).

Interactions with Herbs & Other Dietary Supplements
None known.

Interactions with Drugs
None known.

Interactions with Foods
None known.

Interactions with Lab Tests
None known.

Interactions with Diseases or Conditions
None known.

Dosage and Administration
No typical dosage.

Comments
Other herbs considered to be da qing ye include Isatis tinctoria, Baphicacanthus cusia, Clerodendron cyrtophyllum, and Polyconum tinctorium (5541).

DAFFODIL

Also Known As
Lent Lily.

Scientific Names
Narcissus pseudonarcissus.
Family: Amaryllidaceae.

People Use This For
Orally, daffodil is used to soothe mucous membrane irritation resulting from whooping cough, colds, asthma, bronchial catarrh, and as an emetic.
Topically, a plaster made from daffodil bulbs is used for wounds, burns, strains, and joint pain.

Safety
POSSIBLY UNSAFE ...when used topically. Severe cases of dermatitis have been reported (5004).
LIKELY UNSAFE ...when used orally (19). Merely chewing on the stem may be enough to cause a chill, shivering, and fainting. The constituent lycorine can cause salivation, vomiting, diarrhea at low doses, and paralysis and collapse at higher doses (271).
PREGNANCY AND LACTATION: LIKELY UNSAFE ...when used orally or topically (19); avoid using.

Effectiveness
There is insufficient reliable information available about the effectiveness of daffodil.

Mechanism of Action
The applicable parts of daffodil are the bulb, leaf, and flower. Daffodil contains numerous active constituents including alkaloids (lycorine and galanthamine) and chelidonic acid (18). In small amounts, lycorine causes salivation, vomiting, and diarrhea. At higher doses, it causes paralysis and collapse. Galanthamine is a cholinesterase inhibitor and analgesic (271), and it is being investigated for use in the treatment of Alzheimer's disease (5007). Lycorine, narciclasine, and other constituents are cytotoxic (271). The mucus and sap of daffodil plants and bulbs contain calcium oxalate crystals, which are most likely responsible for the skin irritation (5004). "Micro trauma" to the skin from the oxylate crystals allows penetration of other irritants and worsens dermatitis (5004).

Adverse Reactions
Orally, daffodil can cause irritation and swelling of the mouth, tongue, and throat (19), as well as vomiting, salivation, diarrhea, central nervous disorders, and respiratory or cardiovascular collapse and subsequent death (18). This is due to the lycorine component (6002).
Topically, daffodil use can cause dermatitis (5004,5005). People who simply handle daffodil plants or bulbs can get "Lily rash" or "daffodil itch" (18,5004).

Interactions with Herbs & Other Dietary Supplements
CALCIUM, IRON, ZINC: Concurrent use might decrease mineral absorption. Daffodil contains oxalate (5004), which can bind multivalent metal ions in the gastrointestinal tract and decrease mineral absorption.

Interactions with Drugs
None known.

Interactions with Foods
CALCIUM, IRON, ZINC: Concurrent use might decrease mineral absorption from foods. Daffodil contains oxalate (5004), which can bind multivalent metal ions in the gastrointestinal tract and decrease mineral absorption.

Interactions with Lab Tests
None known.

Interactions with Diseases or Conditions
None known.

Dosage and Administration
ORAL: Typically used as a powder and an extract (amount unspecified) (18).

DAMIANA

Also Known As
Damiana Aphrodisiaca, Damiana Herb, Damiana Leaf, Herba de la Pastora, Mexican Damiana, Mizibcoc, Old Woman's Broom, Turnerae diffusae folium, Turnerae Diffusae Herba.

Scientific Names
Turnera diffusa, synonym Turnera microphylla; Turnera diffusa var. aphrodisiaca.
Family: Turneraceae.

People Use This For
Orally, damiana is used to treat headache, bedwetting, depression, nervous dyspepsia, atonic constipation, for prophylaxis and treatment of sexual disturbances, strengthening and stimulation during exertion (overwork), boosting and maintaining mental and physical capacity, and as an aphrodisiac.
By inhalation, damiana is used for a subtle "high."

Safety
LIKELY SAFE ...when used orally in amounts commonly found in foods. Damiana has Generally Recognized As Safe (GRAS) status in the US (4912).
POSSIBLY SAFE ...when used orally and appropriately in medicinal amounts (12).
PREGNANCY AND LACTATION: Insufficient reliable information available; avoid using.

Effectiveness
There is insufficient reliable information available about the effectiveness of damiana.

Mechanism of Action
The applicable parts of damiana are the leaf and stem. Ethanolic extracts are reported to exhibit CNS depressant activity (4). The quinone arbutin may be responsible for antibacterial properties (4).

Adverse Reactions
Orally, 200 grams of damiana extract has caused tetanus-like convulsions and paroxysms resulting in symptoms similar to rabies or strychnine poisoning (4).

Interactions with Herbs & Other Dietary Supplements
None known.

Interactions with Drugs
ANTIDIABETES DRUGS: Theoretically, damiana may interfere with diabetes therapy due to hypoglycemic activity (4).

Interactions with Foods
None known.

Interactions with Lab Tests
None known.

Interactions with Diseases or Conditions
DIABETES: Theoretically, damiana may interfere with blood glucose control (4).

Dosage and Administration
ORAL: Typical dosages are 2-4 grams dried leaf three times daily, or one cup tea (steep 2-4 grams dried leaf in 150 mL boiling water 5-10 minutes, strain) three times a day (4). Liquid extract of damiana, 2-4 mL has also been used (4).

DANDELION above ground parts

Also Known As
Blowball, Cankerwort, Common Dandelion, Dandelion Herb, Lion's Tooth, Pissenlit, Priest's Crown, Swine Snout, Taraxaci herba, Taraxacum, Wild Endive.
CAUTION: See separate listing for Dandelion entire plant.

Scientific Names
Taraxacum officinale, synonyms Taraxacum vulgare, Leontodon taraxacum, Taraxacum dens-leonis.
Family: Asteraceae/Compositae.

People Use This For
Orally, dandelion above ground parts are used for loss of appetite and dyspepsia, diuretic, flatulence, and feelings of fullness. They are also used as a laxative, promoter of healthy circulation, skin toner, blood vessel cleanser and strengthener, for rheumatism, arthritic joints, and as a tonic.
In foods, dandelion above ground parts are used in salad greens, soups, and wine.

Safety
LIKELY SAFE ...when used orally and appropriately in medicinal amounts (12). ...when used orally in amounts commonly found in foods. Dandelion has Generally Recognized As Safe (GRAS) status in the US (4912).
PREGNANCY AND LACTATION: Insufficient reliable information available; avoid using amounts greater than those in foods.

Effectiveness
There is insufficient reliable information available about the effectiveness of dandelion above ground parts.

Mechanism of Action
The sesquiterpene lactones are responsible for the diuretic effects and can contribute to dandelion's mild anti-inflammatory activity. Dandelion also contains an appetite-stimulating bitter identified as eudesmanolides, which was previously called taraxacin (6). Dandelion can have a slight laxative effect (5).

Adverse Reactions
Topically, dandelion can cause contact dermatitis in sensitive individuals (6). Dandelion can cause an allergic reaction in individuals sensitive to the Asteraceae/Compositae family. Members of this family include ragweed, chrysanthemums, marigolds, daisies, and many other herbs.

Interactions with Herbs & Other Dietary Supplements
None known.

Interactions with Drugs
POTASSIUM-SPARING DIURETICS: Dandelion contains large amounts of potassium (4). Concomitant use of these drugs along with dandelion might increase the risk of hyperkalemia. Potassium-sparing diuretics include amiloride (Midamor), spironolactone (Aldactone), and triamterene (Dyrenium).

Interactions with Foods
None known.

Interactions with Lab Tests
None known.

Interactions with Diseases or Conditions
CROSS-ALLERGENICITY: Dandelion may cause an allergic reaction in individuals sensitive to the Asteraceae/Compositae family. Members of this family include ragweed, chrysanthemums, marigolds, daisies, and many other herbs.
OBSTRUCTION: The use of dandelion is contraindicated in patients with obstruction of bile ducts or the gallbladder. If gallstones are present, physician consultation is necessary before the use of dandelion (2).

Dosage and Administration
ORAL: The typical dose of dandelion is 4-10 grams of the dried above ground parts three times daily. The common dose of the liquid extract (1:1 in 25% alcohol) is 4-10 mL three times daily (2).

Comments
Dandelions contain more vitamin A than carrots (6002). Avoid confusion with dandelion as a whole plant.

DANDELION entire plant

Also Known As
Blowball, Cankerwort, Common Dandelion, Dandelion Root, Lion's Tooth, Pissenlit, Priest's Crown, Swine Snout, Taraxacum, Wild Endive.
CAUTION: See separate listing for Dandelion above ground parts.

Scientific Names
Taraxacum officinale, synonyms Leontodon taraxacum, Taraxacum vulgare.
Family: Asteraceae/Compositae.

People Use This For
Orally, dandelion plant is used for gallstones, bile stimulation, muscle aches, breast cancer, low urine output, indigestion, constipation, flatulence, as a tonic, and in anti-smoking preparations. It is also used orally for diabetes, rheumatic conditions, heartburn, bruises, gout, stiff joints, eczema, and cancer.
In foods, dandelion leaves are added to salads. The roasted root and extract are used as coffee substitutes.
In food manufacturing, dandelion plant is a flavoring component for foods as well as beverages.

Safety
LIKELY SAFE ...when used orally in amounts commonly found in foods. Dandelion has Generally Recognized As Safe (GRAS) status in the US (4912).
POSSIBLY SAFE ...when used orally and appropriately in medicinal amounts (12).
PREGNANCY: POSSIBLY SAFE ...when consumed in food amounts; avoid amounts greater than those found in foods (4).
LACTATION: Insufficient reliable information available; avoid using.

Effectiveness
POSSIBLY EFFECTIVE

Urinary tract infections (UTIs). A specific oral combination of dandelion root and uva ursi leaf extracts seems to help reduce the recurrence rate of UTIs in women (1932). In this combination uva ursi is used for its antibacterial properties and dandelion is used to increase urination. However, this combination should not be used long-term against recurrent UTIs because uva ursi is thought not to be safe for extended use.

There is insufficient reliable information available about the effectiveness of dandelion entire plant for its other uses.

Mechanism of Action
The dandelion constituent taraxacin favorably effects digestion. The bitter constituents in dandelion root are responsible for increasing bile flow (7). The extracts demonstrate diuretic effects in animals and antitumor activity in vitro (4). The root extract has anti-inflammatory activity in animals (4). Hypoglycemic activity can also occur with the use of dandelion in animals (4). The sesquiterpene lactone constituents can be responsible for allergic reactions (4).

Adverse Reactions
Orally, dandelion plant can cause gastric hyperacidity (2).Topically, dandelion can cause contact dermatitis (4). It can cause an allergic reaction in individuals sensitive to the Asteraceae/Compositae family. Members of this family include ragweed, chrysanthemums, marigolds, daisies, and many other herbs.

Interactions with Herbs & Other Dietary Supplements

DIURETIC HERBS: Theoretically, dandelion can have additive effects with herbs having diuretic properties. Herbs thought to have diuretic properties include agrimony, artichoke, broom, buchu, burdock, celery, cornsilk, couch grass, elder, guaiacum, juniper, pokeroot, shepherd's purse, squill, uva ursi, and yarrow.
HYPOGLYCEMIC HERBS: Theoretically, dandelion can have additive effects with herbs having hypoglycemic effects.

Interactions with Drugs

ANTACIDS: Theoretically, due to reports that dandelion increases stomach acid, dandelion might decrease the effectiveness of antacids (19).
ANTIDIABETES DRUGS: Monitor blood glucose levels closely because dandelion can exhibit hypoglycemic effects (19).
H2-BLOCKERS: Theoretically, due to reports that dandelion increases stomach acid, dandelion might decrease the effectiveness of H2-blockers (19). The H2 blockers include cimetidine (Tagamet), ranitidine (Zantac), nizatidine (Axid), and famotidine (Pepcid).
LITHIUM: Theoretically, concomitant use can cause lithium toxicity due to sodium loss brought about by dandelion (19).
POTASSIUM-SPARING DIURETICS: Dandelion contains large amounts of potassium (4). Concomitant use of these drugs along with dandelion might increase the risk of hyperkalemia. Potassium-sparing diuretics include amiloride (Midamor), spironolactone (Aldactone), and triamterene (Dyrenium).
PROTON PUMP INHIBITORS (PPIs): Theoretically, due to reports that dandelion increases stomach acid, dandelion might decrease the effectiveness of PPIs (19). PPIs include omeprazole (Prilosec), lansoprazole (Prevacid), rabeprazole (Aciphex), pantoprazole (Protonix), and esomeprazole (Nexium).

Interactions with Foods

None known.

Interactions with Lab Tests

None known.

Interactions with Diseases or Conditions

CROSS-ALLERGENICITY: Dandelion may cause an allergic reaction in individuals sensitive to the Asteraceae/Compositae family. Members of this family include ragweed, chrysanthemums, marigolds, daisies, and many other herbs.
DIABETES: Monitor blood glucose levels closely because dandelion can exhibit hypoglycemic effects (19).
GALLSTONES: Professional evaluation is needed before the use of the dandelion plant in individuals with gallstones (2).
GASTROINTESTINAL CONDITIONS: Dandelion plant is contraindicated in cases of acute gallbladder inflammation, bile duct obstruction, and intestinal blockage (2).

Dosage and Administration

ORAL: The typical dose of the dandelion leaf is 4-10 grams of the dried leaf or one cup of the tea three times daily (4). The tea is prepared by steeping 4-10 grams of the dried leaf in 150 mL boiling water for 5-10 minutes and then straining. The usual dose of the liquid leaf extract (1:1 in 25% alcohol) is 4-10 mL three times a day (4). The typical dose of the dandelion root is 2-8 grams of the dried root or one cup of the tea three times daily (4). The tea is prepared by steeping 3-8 grams of the dried root in 150 mL boiling water for 5-10 minutes and then straining (4). The usual dose of the root tincture (1:5 in 45% alcohol) is 5-10 mL three times daily (4). The common dose of the whole plant is as a tea, which is prepared by steeping 3-4 grams of the powdered whole plant in 150 mL boiling water for 5-10 minutes and then straining (2). The dose of the liquid extract of taraxacum is typically 2-8 mL (4). The juice of taraxacum is given as 4-8 mL (4).

Comments

The dandelion plant contains more vitamin A than carrots (6002). Avoid confusion with the above ground parts of dandelion.

DANSHEN

Also Known As

Ch'ih Shen, Dan Shen, Dan-Shen, Huang Ken, Pin-Ma Ts'ao, Red Rooted Sage, Red Sage, Salvia Root, Shu-Wei Ts'ao, Tan-Shen, Tzu Tan-Ken.
CAUTION: See separate listing for Sage.

Scientific Names

Salvia bowleyana; Salvia miltiorrhiza; Salvia przewalskii; Salvia yunnanensis.
Family: Labiatae/Lamiaceae.

People Use This For

Orally, danshen is used for circulation problems, ischemic stroke, angina pectoris, and other cardiovascular diseases. It is also used orally for menstrual problems, chronic hepatitis, abdominal masses, insomnia due to palpitations and tight chest, acne, psoriasis, eczema, and other skin conditions. Danshen is also used orally to relieve bruising and to aid in wound healing.

Safety

POSSIBLY SAFE ...when used orally and appropriately (12).
PREGNANCY AND LACTATION: Insufficient reliable information available; avoid using.

Effectiveness

There is insufficient reliable information available about the effectiveness of danshen.

Mechanism of Action

The applicable part of danshen is the root. The constituents protocatechualdehyde and 3,4-dihydroxyphenyl-lactic acid may play a role in vasoactivity (6048). Other constituents, including the diterpenoids miltirone, Ro090680, and salvinone, as well as tanshinone derivatives, seem to have anticoagulant properties (7162,10649). Danshen appears to interfere with hemostasis by inhibiting platelet aggregation, interfering with extrinsic blood coagulation, mimicking the activity of antithrombin III, and promoting fibrinolytic activity (2237).
Danshen constituents and digoxin have some structural and pharmacological similarities. The tanshinone constituents of danshen have an aglycon ring that contains a common phenanthrene ring structure like digoxin and other cardiac glycosides (7311). Danshen is thought to work for cardiovascular diseases by dilating coronary arteries and affecting cardiac function. It appears to produce dose-dependent hypotensive effects, positive inotropic effects, and negative chronotropic effects (5884,6048,7311).

Adverse Reactions

Orally, danshen can cause pruritus, upset stomach, and reduced appetite (12).

Interactions with Herbs & Other Dietary Supplements

CARDIAC GLYCOSIDE-CONTAINING HERBS: Theoretically, using danshen with herbs containing cardiac glycosides might increase the risk cardiovascular effects and side effects such as arrhythmia. Danshen has structural and pharmacological similarities to cardiac glycosides (5884,6048,7311). Cardiac glycoside containing herbs include black hellebore, Canadian hemp roots, digitalis leaf, hedge mustard, figwort, lily of the valley roots, motherwort, oleander leaf, pheasant's eye plant, pleurisy root, squill bulb leaf scales, and strophanthus seeds.
HERBS WITH ANTICOAGULANT/ANTIPLATELET POTENTIAL: Taking danshen with herbs that affect platelet aggregation could theoretically increase the risk of bleeding in some people (7162). These herbs include angelica, clove, feverfew, garlic, ginger, ginkgo, Panax ginseng, horse chestnut, red clover, turmeric, and others.
METHYL SALICYLATE OIL: There is one case report of increased international normalized ratio (INR) with concomitant use of topical methyl salicylate oil, oral danshen, and warfarin (612).

Interactions with Drugs

ANTICOAGULANT/ANTIPLATELET DRUGS: Concomitant use might increase the risk of bleeding due to decreased platelet aggregation. Danshen has been reported to have antithrombotic effects (6048); avoid concomitant use. Some of these drugs include aspirin, clopidogrel (Plavix), dalteparin (Fragmin), enoxaparin (Lovenox), heparin, ticlopidine (Ticlid), warfarin (Coumadin), and others.
DIGOXIN (Lanoxin): Theoretically, using danshen with digoxin might increase cardiovascular effects and side effects such as arrhythmia. Danshen has structural and pharmacological similarities to cardiac glycosides (5884,6048,7311).
WARFARIN (Coumadin): Concomitant use increases the anticoagulant effects of warfarin and the risk of bleeding (611,612). There have been several case reports of increased international normalized ratio (INR) after concomitant use of danshen and warfarin (611,612,2237,5883,5884). Elevations in INR have occurred as early as 3-5 days after start of danshen. Danshen might increase the rate of absorption and decrease the elimination rate of warfarin (5884,6048). Avoid concomitant use.

Interactions with Foods

None known.

Interactions with Lab Tests

DIGOXIN: Danshen can interfere with serum digoxin measurements. It falsely elevates serum digoxin concentrations when fluorescence polarization immunoassay (FPIA) is used. It falsely lowers digoxin concentrations when microparticle enzyme immunoassay (MEIA) is used. This interference is likely related to the structural similarity of danshen to digoxin. Danshen interference can be eliminated by monitoring the free digoxin concentration. This assay takes advantage of the stronger plasma protein binding of danshen than digoxin (7311).

Interactions with Diseases or Conditions

BLEEDING DISORDERS: Theoretically, danshen may increase the risk of bleeding (2237); avoid using.

Dosage and Administration

No typical dosage.

DATE PALM

Also Known As

Kharjura.

Scientific Names

Phoenix dactylifera.
Family: Arecaceae/Palmae.

Comments

At the date of publication, there was very little scientific information about this product. Our staff is continually analyzing the available information on natural medicines and will add data to the online version of *Natural Medicines Comprehensive Database* as it becomes available. See www.naturaldatabase.com.

DEANOL

Also Known As

2-Dimethyl Aminoethanol, Deanol aceglumate, Deanol acetamidobenzoate, Deanol benzilate, Deanol bisorcate, Deanol cyclohexylpropionate, Deanol hemisuccinate, Deanol pidolate, Deanol tartrate, Dimethylaminoethanol, Dimethylethanolamine, DMAE.

Scientific Names

2-Dimethylaminoethanol.

People Use This For

Orally, deanol is used for treating attention deficit-hyperactivity disorder (ADHD), enhancing memory and mood, boosting cognitive function, treating Alzheimer's disease, increasing intelligence and physical energy, and improving athletic performance. It is also used for preventing aging or liver spots, improving red blood cell function, improving muscle reflexes, increasing oxygen efficiency, extending life span, treating autism, and treating tardive dyskinesia. Topically, deanol is used for signs of aging skin, particularly loose or sagging skin.

Safety

POSSIBLY SAFE ...when used orally or topically and appropriately (1668,1671,1672,1673,1674,1675,1676,1679,1680,1681,12023).

PREGNANCY AND LACTATION: Insufficient reliable information available; avoid using.

Effectiveness

POSSIBLY EFFECTIVE

Athletic performance. Taking deanol orally in combination with ginseng, vitamins, and minerals seems to improve exercise performance by increasing total work load and maximal oxygen consumption during exercise (1671).

LIKELY INEFFECTIVE

Alzheimer's disease. Taking deanol orally doesn't seem to improve symptoms of Alzheimer's disease (1680,1681).

Tardive dyskinesia. Taking deanol orally doesn't seem to improve tardive dyskinesia (1672,1673,1674,1675,1676,1803,1804).

INSUFFICIENT RELIABLE EVIDENCE to RATE

Aging skin. There's preliminary evidence that applying a 3% deanol gel to facial skin can decrease sagging skin

by increasing skin tension (12023).
Attention deficit-hyperactivity disorder (ADHD). Clinical studies using deanol for treating ADHD have produced inconclusive results (1669,1677,1679).
More evidence is needed to rate deanol for these uses.

Mechanism of Action
Deanol is a precursor to choline and might enhance central acetylcholine formation (1669).
There is interest in deanol for Alzheimer's disease because it is thought to increase acetylcholine levels in the brain and potentially improve memory and cognitive function (1680,1681).
Deanol is also theorized to increase acetylcholine in tissues and therefore possible increase skin tone (12023). However, there is no reliable evidence that deanol increases acetylcholine levels in tissues when applied topically.
Deanol is often used in anti-aging preparations. But preliminary animal research suggests that it does not increase life span (1682,1683).
Deanol has been formulated in a variety of salts and esters including deanol aceglumate, deanol acetamidobenzoate, deanol bisorcate, deanol cyclohexylpropionate (cyprodenate, cyprodemanol), deanol hemisuccinate, deanol pidolate, and deanol tartrate. The hydrochloride salt of deanol benzilate (deanol diphenylglycoate, benzacine) has been included in antispasmodic preparations (9).

Adverse Reactions
Orally, deanol can cause constipation, urticaria, headache, drowsiness, insomnia, overstimulation, vivid dreams, confusion, depression, blood pressure elevation, hypomania, an increase in schizophrenia symptoms, and orofacial and respiratory tardive dyskinesia (1674,1680,1684,1685,1686,2706).

Interactions with Herbs & Other Dietary Supplements
None known.

Interactions with Drugs
ANTICHOLINERGIC DRUGS: Theoretically, concomitant use might decrease the effect of drugs with anticholinergic activity, due to the potential cholinergic activity of deanol (1669).

Interactions with Foods
None known.

Interactions with Lab Tests
None known.

Interactions with Diseases or Conditions
CLONIC-TONIC SEIZURES: Deanol is relatively contraindicated in people with clonic-tonic seizure disorders (2706).
DEPRESSION: Deanol might worsen depression. It is reported to cause depression as an adverse effect (1685).
SCHIZOPHRENIA: Deanol can worsen schizophrenia symptoms (1674); avoid using in patients with schizophrenia.

Dosage and Administration
ORAL: Doses have ranged from 300 to 2000 mg per day in clinical studies (1669,1672,1673).
TOPICAL: For aging skin, a 3% deanol gel has been used (12023).

Comments
Deanol was previously marketed as the prescription drug, Deaner, by Riker Laboratories for the management of children with behavior problems and learning difficulties (1669,2706). Deanol is not an approved food additive in the US, nor is it an orphan drug, as some supplement advertising suggests.

DEER VELVET

Also Known As
Cornu Cervi Parvum, Deer Antler, Deer Antler Velvet, Elk Antler, Elk Antler Velvet, Horns of Gold, Lu Rong, Nokyong, Rokujo, Velvet Antler, Velvet of Young Deer Horn.

Scientific Names
Cervus nippon; Cervus elaphus.

People Use This For

Orally, deer velvet is used to boost strength and endurance, for muscle aches and pains, to promote youthfulness, increase mental clarity, as an aphrodisiac, to treat sexual dysfunction, to boost estrogen and testosterone levels, to counter the effects of stress, to improve immune system functioning, and to promote rapid recovery from illness. It is used to improve fertility, for menstrual and menopause problems, to reduce hormone replacement therapy dose, to reduce cholesterol and high blood pressure, for liver and kidney disorders, to protect the liver from toxins, for migraines, asthma, indigestion, osteoporosis, and acne. It is also used for its anticancer and anti-inflammatory properties, as a source of growth factors IGR-1 & IGF-2, to stimulate production and circulation of blood, to increase blood count, and lower the level of free radicals.

In herbal combinations, deer velvet is used to improve athletic performance, for an anti-aging effect, arthritis and osteoporosis, anemia, gonadotropic disorders, gynecological disorders, skin conditions, tissue and bone rejuvenation. It is also used to increase mental capacity and performance, increase blood circulation to the brain, reduce early stages of muscular degeneration, to improve eyesight and hearing, to help PMS, impotence, and reduce stress.

In Chinese medicine, deer velvet is used to treat symptoms of impotence; cold extremities; soreness and weakness in the lower back and knees; leukorrhea; uterine bleeding; chronic skin ulcers; and frequent, copious, clear urination. It has also been used as a tonic for children with failure to thrive, mental retardation, learning disabilities, insufficient growth, or skeletal deformities including rickets.

In Korean medicine, deer velvet is used at the onset of winter to ward off infections.

Safety

There is insufficient reliable information available about the safety of deer velvet.

Pregnancy and Lactation: Insufficient reliable information available; avoid using.

Effectiveness

There is insufficient reliable information available about the effectiveness of deer velvet.

Mechanism of Action

By weight, deer velvet is approximately 50% amino acids (5502). Deer velvet also contains vitamin A, estrone and estradiol, sphingomyelin, ganglioside, some prostaglandins (5502), and epidermal growth factor (5518). Deer velvet is believed to stimulate the growth of body tissues, particularly the reticuloendothelial cells and leukocytes. It also appears to stimulate wound healing. Deer velvet seems to reduce fatigue by improving sleep and stimulating appetite. It is believed to improve health, especially in children and the elderly (5502). Preliminary evidence suggests that athletes taking deer velvet experience increased muscular strength and endurance in training. They also seem to recover faster from muscle tissue damage that results from exercise (5505). Other evidence suggests deer velvet extract might counteract certain effects of repeated doses of morphine, such as the development of tolerance (5503).

Adverse Reactions

None reported.

Interactions with Herbs & Other Dietary Supplements

None known.

Interactions with Drugs

None known.

Interactions with Foods

None known.

Interactions with Lab Tests

None known.

Interactions with Diseases or Conditions

ESTROGEN-SENSITIVE CONDITIONS: Theoretically, women with conditions sensitive to estrogen, i.e. history of breast or cervical cancer, should avoid using deer velvet.

Dosage and Administration

ORAL: A typical dose for treatment is 0.9-2.4 grams. Double-boiled, 3-4.5 grams are used. Alternately, it can be soaked in wine (5501) or prepared as a 20% tincture in wine (5502).

Comments

Deer velvet is the epidermis that covers the inner structure of the growing bone and cartilage that will become deer antlers (5504).

DEERTONGUE

Also Known As
Carolina Vanilla, Deer's Tongue, Hound's Tongue, Liatris, Vanilla Leaf, Vanilla Plant, Vanilla Trilisa, Wild Vanilla.
CAUTION: See separate listing for Hound's Tongue (Cyonglossum officinale).

Scientific Names
Trilisa odoratissima, synonyms Carphephorus odoratissimus.
Family: Asteraceae/Compositae.

People Use This For
Orally, deertongue is used for malaria.
In manufacturing, deertongue extracts are used to flavor tobacco, as a fragrance in cosmetics and soaps, and as a fixative in some products.

Safety
LIKELY UNSAFE ...when used orally for medicinal purposes. ...when used in amounts commonly found in foods. The use of deertongue is not permitted in foods in the US (11).
PREGNANCY AND LACTATION: LIKELY UNSAFE ...when used orally due to potential effects of coumarin constituents (11); avoid using.

Effectiveness
There is insufficient reliable information available about the effectiveness of deertongue.

Mechanism of Action
The applicable part of deertongue is the dried leaf. Coumarin constituents are reported to cause liver injury and hemorrhage (11).

Adverse Reactions
Liver injury and hemorrhage are possible due to coumarin content (11). Deertongue can cause an allergic reaction in individuals sensitive to the Asteraceae/Compositae family. Members of this family include ragweed, chrysanthemums, marigolds, daisies, and many other herbs.

Interactions with Herbs & Other Dietary Supplements
HERBS THAT AFFECT BLOOD CLOTTING: Theoretically, deertongue may enhance effects of other herbs that might also affect blood clotting. Some of these herbs include alfalfa, angelica, clove, feverfew, garlic, ginger, Panax ginseng, quassia, and red clover.

Interactions with Drugs
ANTICOAGULANT/ANTIPLATELET DRUGS: Theoretically, concomitant use may increase risk of bleeding.

Interactions with Foods
None known.

Interactions with Lab Tests
None known.

Interactions with Diseases or Conditions
CROSS-ALLERGENICITY: Deertongue may cause an allergic reaction in individuals sensitive to the Asteraceae/Compositae family. Members of this family include ragweed, chrysanthemums, marigolds, daisies, and many other herbs.

Dosage and Administration
No typical dosage.

DELPHINIUM

Also Known As
Delphinii Flos, Knight's Spur, Lark Heel, Larkspur, Lark's Claw, Lark's Toe, Rittersspornblüten, Staggerweed.

Scientific Names
Consolida regalis, synonym Delphinium consolida.
Family: Ranunculaceae.

People Use This For
Orally, delphinium is used as an anthelmintic, diuretic, sedative, and appetite stimulant.

Safety
LIKELY UNSAFE ...when used orally. Delphinium can be toxic to the heart and respiratory systems (17).
PREGNANCY AND LACTATION: LIKELY UNSAFE ...when used orally (17); avoid using.

Effectiveness
There is insufficient reliable information available about the effectiveness of delphinium.

Mechanism of Action
The applicable part of delphinium is the flower. Delphinium has a paralyzing effect on peripheral and motor nerve endings (18). The alkaloid constituents are thought to be cardiotoxic and seem to be responsible for the curare-like paralysis of the respiratory system (2).

Adverse Reactions
Orally, delphinium can cause bradycardia, hypotension, cardiac arrest, and respiratory failure (2). Animal deaths from poisoning are common (18).

Interactions with Herbs & Other Dietary Supplements
None known.

Interactions with Drugs
None known.

Interactions with Foods
None known.

Interactions with Lab Tests
None known.

Interactions with Diseases or Conditions
None known.

Dosage and Administration
No typical dosage.

Comments
Avoid confusion with Consolida orientalis (Delphinium orientale).

DEVIL'S CLAW

Also Known As
Devil's Claw Root, Grapple Plant, Griffe Du Diable, Harpagophyti Radix, Harpagophytum, Wood Spider.

Scientific Names
Harpagophytum procumbens, synonym Uncaria procumbens.
Family: Pedaliaceae.

People Use This For
Orally, devil's claw is used for arteriosclerosis, osteoarthritis, rheumatoid arthritis, gout, myalgia, fibrositis, lumbago, tendonitis, pleuritic chest pain, gastrointestinal (GI) upset or dyspepsia, fever, and migraine headache. It is also used for difficulties in childbirth, menstrual problems, allergic reactions, loss of appetite, kidney and bladder disease, and degenerative disorders of the locomotor system.
Topically, devil's claw is used for skin injuries and disorders.

Safety
POSSIBLY SAFE ...when used orally and appropriately, short-term. Devil's claw seems to be well tolerated when used daily for up to 16 weeks (6472).
There is insufficient reliable information available about the safety of topical or long-term oral use of devil's claw.
PREGNANCY: LIKELY UNSAFE ...when used orally. Devil's claw seems to have oxytocic effects (4); avoid using.
LACTATION: Insufficient reliable information available; avoid using.

Effectiveness
POSSIBLY EFFECTIVE

Osteoarthritis. Taking devil's claw orally in conjunction with nonsteroidal anti-inflammatory drugs (NSAIDs) seems to help decrease osteoarthritis-related pain (6472,8608). Devil's claw seems to be comparable to diacerhein (a slow-acting drug for osteoarthritis; not available in the US) for improving osteoarthritis pain in the hip and knee after 16 weeks of treatment. Patients taking devil's claw also seem to be able to decrease use of NSAIDs for pain relief (6472). This study used a specific powdered devil's claw root product (Harpadol) containing 2% of the constituent harpagoside (9.5 mg per capsule) and 3% total iridoid glycosides (14.5 mg per capsule) (6472). Another specific devil's claw extract (Doleteffin) has been used in a dose of 60 mg harpagoside per day (8608).

INSUFFICIENT RELIABLE EVIDENCE to RATE

Back pain. Preliminary evidence suggests that a specific devil's claw extract (Doleteffin) might decrease non-specific low back pain (8608).

Rheumatoid arthritis (RA). Preliminary evidence suggests that oral devil's claw extract might not improve RA (8613).

More evidence is needed to rate devil's claw for these uses.

Mechanism of Action
The applicable part of devil's claw is the tuber. Devil's claw contains iridoid glycoside constituents primarily harpagoside, but also including harpagide, and procumbide; it appears that other compounds besides harpagoside contribute to its effect (8614,8616). It also contains the phenylethanol derivatives acteoside (verbascoside) and isoaceteoside, and the oligosaccharide stachyose (8616). People use devil's claw for osteoarthritis and other inflammatory conditions because the iridoid glycoside constituents seem to have an anti-inflammatory effect (6472). Some research suggests that harpagoside inhibits both the cyclooxygenase and lipoxygenase inflammatory pathways (8612); however, other research shows no effect of devil's claw on the arachidonic acid pathway (10642). Some evidence suggests that the anti-inflammatory effect is due to increased synthesis and release of tumor necrosis factor (TNF)-alpha by compounds other than harpagoside (8616).
There is also some evidence that devil's claw products might be cardioactive due to a harpagide constituent. Low doses seem to slow the heart rate and increase the strength of contraction. High doses seem to weaken heart contraction and coronary blood flow (8609). Devil's claw extract and isolated harpagoside appear to have antiarrhythmic effects (8609,8610). Preliminary evidence suggests that devil's claw extract might be inactivated by stomach acid and might be more effective with parenteral or sublingual administration (8611,8614,8615,8617). However, this is somewhat controversial. Other researchers describe little effect of gastric pH on devil's claw (8612). There also seems to be variability in harpagoside content among various commercial extracts, possibly because some products are prepared from a mixture of Harpagophytum procumbens and Harpagophytum zeyheri. These species are similar pharmacologically, but may have differing concentrations of harpagoside and related compounds (8615).

Adverse Reactions
Orally, devil's claw is generally well tolerated. The most common adverse effect is diarrhea, occurring in approximately 8% of patients in one study (6472). Other gastrointestinal complaints include nausea, vomiting, and abdominal pain. Devil's claw can cause allergic skin reactions. It might also cause dysmenorrhea and hemodynamic instability (8608). There is also a report of throbbing frontal headache, tinnitus, anorexia, and loss of taste associated with devil's claw (8613).

Interactions with Herbs & Other Dietary Supplements
None known.

Interactions with Drugs

ANTACIDS: Theoretically, due to reports that devil's claw increases stomach acid, devil's claw might decrease the effectiveness of antacids (19).
ANTIDIABETES DRUGS: Devil's claw might decrease blood glucose levels (4) and have additive effects with medications used for diabetes. Monitor blood glucose levels closely. Dose adjustments may be necessary.
ANTIHYPERTENSIVE DRUGS: Devil's claw might decrease blood pressure (4); use cautiously.
H2-BLOCKERS: Theoretically, due to reports that devil's claw increases stomach acid, devil's claw might decrease the effectiveness of H2-blockers (19). The H2 blockers include cimetidine (Tagamet), ranitidine (Zantac), nizatidine (Axid), and famotidine (Pepcid).
PROTON PUMP INHIBITORS (PPIs): Theoretically, due to reports that devil's claw increases stomach acid, devil's claw might decrease the effectiveness of PPIs (19). PPIs include omeprazole (Prilosec), lansoprazole (Prevacid), rabeprazole (Aciphex), pantoprazole (Protonix), and esomeprazole (Nexium).
WARFARIN (Coumadin): Purpura has occurred in a patient taking warfarin and devil's claw concurrently, suggesting over-anticoagulation (613). Devil's claw should be avoided or used cautiously in patients taking warfarin. Warfarin dose adjustments may be necessary.

Interactions with Foods

None known.

Interactions with Lab Tests

None known.

Interactions with Diseases or Conditions

CARDIAC DISORDERS, HYPERTENSION, HYPOTENSION: Since devil's claw can affect heart rate, contractility of the heart, and blood pressure (4), it might adversely affect people with cardiovascular conditions; use cautiously.
DIABETES: Devil's claw might decrease blood glucose levels (4) and have additive effects with medications used for diabetes. Monitor blood glucose levels closely. Dose adjustments may be necessary.
GALLSTONES: Devil's claw might increase bile production and adversely affect people with gallstones (8); avoid using.
PEPTIC ULCER DISEASE (PUD): Since devil's claw might increase gastric acid secretion (19), it might adversely effect people with gastric or duodenal ulcer; avoid using

Dosage and Administration

ORAL: For osteoarthritis, one clinical study used a specific powdered devil's claw root product (Harpadol) dosed at 2.6 grams per day. This dose provided a total of 57 mg of the harpagoside constituent and 87 mg of total iridoid glycosides daily. Each 435 mg capsule contained 2% harpagoside (9.5 mg per capsule) and 3% total iridoid glycosides (14.5 mg per capsule) (6472). For other uses, the usual dose is from 1-4.5 grams of the root per day (6472).

Comments

The botanical name Harpagophytum means "hook plant" in Greek. The plant, which is native to Africa, gets its name from the appearance of its fruit, which is covered with hooks meant to attach onto animals in order to spread the seeds (6002,8611).

DEVIL'S CLUB

Also Known As

Cukilanarpak, Devils Club, Fatsia, Panax horridum.

Scientific Names

Oplopanax horridus; synonyms Echinopanax horridus, Fatsia horrida.
Family: Araliaceae.

People Use This For

Orally, devil's club is used for arthritis, as a purgative, an emetic, for wound healing, fever, tuberculosis, stomach trouble, coughs, colds, diabetes, hypoglycemia, and pneumonia.
Topically, devil's club is used as a treatment for swollen glands, boils, sores, and skin infections. The ashes have been used to treat burns.

Safety
POSSIBLY SAFE ...when used orally (12).
There is insufficient reliable information available about the safety of devil's club for its other uses.
PREGNANCY AND LACTATION: Insufficient reliable information available; avoid using.

Effectiveness
There is insufficient reliable information available about the effectiveness of devil's club.

Mechanism of Action
The applicable part of devil's club is the root bark. Several animal studies found no evidence of activity (6).

Adverse Reactions
Orally, devil's club may have a hypoglycemic effect (6).

Interactions with Herbs & Other Dietary Supplements
None known.

Interactions with Drugs
ANTIDIABETES DRUGS: Monitor blood glucose levels closely due to claims that devil's club has hypoglycemic effects (19).

Interactions with Foods
None known.

Interactions with Lab Tests
None known.

Interactions with Diseases or Conditions
DIABETES: Devil's club might reduce blood sugar levels. There are repeated anecdotal reports of hypoglycemic activity in individuals with diabetes (6).

Dosage and Administration
ORAL: People typically use 15 to 30 drops of the extract mixed in warm water three times daily between meals. The alcohol content is 55 to 65% (6006).
TOPICAL: The inner bark is baked slowly until it is very dry, then rubbed between the hands until broken and soft. The pulp is placed on the affected area to draw out infection (4215).

Comments
Devil's club is a common plant in southeastern Alaska. It is considered the most important medicinal and magical plant of the Yakutat Tlingit. Both the shaman and the layman chew the stem bark (with the thorns removed) for its effects as an emetic, a purgative, and a general cure all (4215).

DHA (DOCOSAHEXAENOIC ACID)

Also Known As
DHA, Docosahexaenoic, Fish Oil Fatty Acid, N-3 Fatty Acid, Neuromins, Omega 3 Fatty Acid, W-3 Fatty Acid.
CAUTION: See separate listings for Cod Liver Oil, EPA (eicosapentaenoic acid), and Fish Oils.

Scientific Names
Docosahexaenoic acid.

People Use This For
Orally, docosahexanoic acid (DHA) is used as a supplement for preterm infants, as an ingredient in infant formula, during the first four months of life to enhance mental development. It is also used for treating type 2 diabetes, coronary artery disease (CAD), dementia, and attention deficit-hyperactivity disorder (ADHD). DHA is also used for enhancing vision, preventing age-related macular degeneration (AMD), preventing and treating depression, and reducing aggressive behavior in people under stressful situations.
In combination with eicosapentaenoic acid (EPA), DHA is used for a variety of conditions, including the prevention and reversal of heart disease, decreasing ectopic ventricular beats, asthma, cancer, painful menses, hay fever, lung diseases, lupus erythematosus, lupus nephritis, and IgA nephropathy. EPA and DHA are also used in combination for migraine headache prophylaxis in adolescents, atopic dermatitis, Behcet's syndrome, hyperlipidemia, hypertension,

psoriasis, Raynaud's syndrome, rheumatoid arthritis, bipolar disorder, and ulcerative colitis. DHA is also used in combination with arachidonic acid during the first four to six months of life to enhance mental development of infants. It is also used orally in combination with evening primrose oil, thyme oil, and vitamin E (Efalex) to improve movement disorders in children with dyspraxia.

Safety

LIKELY SAFE ...when used orally and appropriately (1016,1043,11333). DHA has been used safely for four years (11333). Fish oil supplements containing DHA have been used safely for seven years (1016).
POSSIBLY SAFE ...when used intravenously and appropriately, short-term (1004).
POSSIBLY UNSAFE ...when used orally in high doses. Doses greater than 3 grams daily might decrease blood coagulation and increase the risk of bleeding (1313).
CHILDREN: POSSIBLY SAFE ...when used orally and appropriately (424,1045,5708,5941,7599).
PREGNANCY AND LACTATION: Insufficient reliable information available; avoid using.

Effectiveness

POSSIBLY EFFECTIVE

Age-related macular degeneration (AMD). Increased dietary consumption of DHA is associated with a decreased risk of AMD (10324).

Coronary artery disease. Increased dietary consumption of DHA may reduce the risk of death in patients with coronary artery disease (10322).

Psoriasis. DHA given intravenously in combination with eicosapentaenoic acid (EPA) appears to improve psoriatic lesions better than omega-6-lipid emulsion (1004).

POSSIBLY INEFFECTIVE

Attention deficit-hyperactivity disorder (ADHD). Low plasma levels of DHA are associated with ADHD in children (7599). However, taking DHA 345 mg orally per day doesn't seem to improve objective or subjective measures of ADHD symptoms (7599).

Depression. Taking DHA orally as monotherapy, does not seem to relieve symptoms of depression (10869).

Diabetes. Taking DHA orally does not substantially improve serum cholesterol or other lipids in patients with type 2 diabetes. DHA may worsen control of blood glucose (10321).

INSUFFICIENT RELIABLE EVIDENCE to RATE

Dyslexia. Taking DHA orally seems to improve night vision in children with dyslexia. Dyslexic children, who receive fish oils rich in DHA, developed significantly better dark adaptation when compared with controls (5708).

Dyspraxia. Taking DHA orally, in combination with evening primrose oil, thyme oil, and vitamin E (Efalex), seems to improve movement disorders in children with dyspraxia. One small clinical trial has shown that this combination significantly decreases movement disorders as determined by objective measures (5708).

More evidence is needed to rate DHA for these uses.

Mechanism of Action

DHA (docosahexanoic acid) is a long-chain n-3 polyunsaturated fatty acid that is found in the tissues of marine mammals and oily fish. DHA is also found in fish liver oils and in commercial fish oil products. DHA can be converted into EPA (eicosapentaenoic acid) in humans (1044). DHA competes with arachidonic acid for inclusion in cyclooxygenase and lipoxygenase pathways (8696). This may have an anti-inflammatory effect in diseases such as psoriasis (1004).

DHA may reduce cardiovascular mortality risk by several mechanisms. Its effects on lipids are mixed. Pure DHA reduces serum triglycerides in adults, and increases serum high-density lipoprotein (HDL) 2 cholesterol (1014,6143). It also increases low-density lipoprotein (LDL) cholesterol and LDL particle size, but has no effect on total cholesterol or fasting glucose in mildly hypercholesterolemic men (6143). DHA decreases blood viscosity and increases red blood cell deformability, which may protect against thrombosis (11111,11112). However, DHA does not significantly affect platelet function, clotting factors, fibrinogen concentrations, plasminogen activator inhibitor-1 or tissue plasminogen activator activity (10323,11112,11113).

Long-chain polyunsaturated fatty acids make up a third of all lipids in brain grey matter (425). DHA is thought to be important for normal neural function and might play a key role in the structural development of neural and synaptic membranes (424,425,8704,8705). There is preliminary evidence DHA might affect retinal, visual, learning, and memory function (8704,8705,8715). DHA accrues rapidly in the human brain during the third trimester of pregnancy and during the early postnatal period (8705). DHA is present in human breast milk, but not in standard infant formulas. Formula-fed infants have lower plasma and cerebral cortex DHA levels than breast milk-fed infants; the clinical significance of this, if any, is unknown. There is also concern pregnancy might cause long-term effects on the DHA stores in women. However, there is evidence that maternal DHA status probably normalizes within one year after pregnancy, and there is no evidence to suggest an association with the number of completed pregnancies and DHA stores (8716).

Adverse Reactions

Orally, DHA may cause nausea, flatulence, bruising, and prolonged bleeding (11333). Adverse reactions, however, are not commonly reported for DHA alone. For fish oils containing EPA and DHA, side effects can include fishy taste, belching, nosebleeds, nausea, and loose stools. High doses of fish oils might also decrease blood coagulation and increase the risk of bleeding (1313,8699,10007). Three people with pre-existing familial adenomatous polyposis were diagnosed with malignant lesions during the course of long-term fish oil use (999). There is also some evidence that increased serum levels of DHA might be associated with an increased risk for atrophic gastritis associated with Helicobacter pylori infection, but further research is needed to clarify this finding (8709).

Interactions with Herbs & Other Dietary Supplements

HERBS WITH ANTICOAGULANT/ANTIPLATELET POTENTIAL: DHA alone does not seem to affect blood clotting (11112,11113). However, when given in combination with EPA as fish oil, concomitant use with herbs that constituents that might affect platelet aggregation could theoretically increase the risk of bleeding in some people. These herbs include angelica, danshen, garlic, ginger, ginkgo, red clover, turmeric, willow, and others.

Interactions with Drugs

ANTICOAGULANT/ANTIPLATELET DRUGS: DHA alone does not seem to affect blood clotting (11112,11113). However, theoretically, when given in combination with EPA as fish oil, concomitant use with anticoagulant or antiplatelet drugs (including aspirin) might increase risk of bleeding.
ANTIHYPERTENSIVE DRUGS: Fish oils containing DHA can lower blood pressure and might have additive effects in patients treated with antihypertensives (1001,1020,1030,1033); use with caution.

Interactions with Foods

None known.

Interactions with Lab Tests

CHOLESTEROL: DHA can increase serum HDL2 cholesterol concentrations, LDL cholesterol concentrations, LDL particle size, and test results in mildly hypercholesterolemic patients (6143).
GLUCOSE: In people with type 2 diabetes, DHA seems to increase fasting blood glucose levels (10321).
INSULIN: DHA can increase fasting insulin concentrations and test results in mildly hypercholesterolemic patients (6143).
INTERNATIONAL NORMALIZED RATIO (INR)/PROTHROMBIN TIME (PT): DHA alone does not seem to affect blood clotting (11112,11113). However, when given in combination with EPA as fish oil, doses greater than 3 grams per day might decrease blood coagulation, increase INR and PT, and increase the risk of bleeding (1313).
PULMONARY FUNCTION TESTS: DHA might cause a decline in pulmonary function tests in aspirin-sensitive individuals (11869).
TRIGLYCERIDES: DHA can reduce serum triglyceride concentrations and test results in patients with hypercholesterolemia (6143).

Interactions with Diseases or Conditions

ASPIRIN-SENSITIVITY: Fish oils and other omega-3 fatty acids can lower pulmonary function tests in some aspirin-sensitive patients (10869).
DIABETES: Fish oils containing EPA and DHA can interfere with blood glucose control (10321). Monitor blood glucose levels closely. Dose adjustments may be necessary.
HYPERTENSION: Fish oils containing DHA can lower blood pressure and might have additive effects in patients with high blood pressure who are treated with antihypertensives (1001,1020,1030,1033).

Dosage and Administration

ORAL: As a supplement in infant formula, 0.32% DHA has been used (424). For improving dark adaptation of vision in dyslexic individuals, a daily oral fish oil dose containing 480 mg DHA has been used (5708). For improving movement disorders in children with dyspraxia, a daily oral tuna fish oil dose containing 480 mg DHA, combined with 35 mg arachidonic acid, 96 mg gamma-alpha linoleic acid from evening primrose oil, 24 mg thyme oil, and 80 mg vitamin E (Efalex) has been used (5708).
INTRAVENOUS: For plaque psoriasis, DHA 4.2 grams and eicosapentaenoic acid (EPA) 4.2 grams per day has been used (1004).

Comments

Avoid confusing DHA with EPA (eicosapentaenoic acid).

DHEA

Also Known As
Dehydroepiandrosterone, GL701, Prasterone.
CAUTION: See separate listing for 7-Keto-DHEA.

Scientific Names
Dehydroepiandrosterone; Prasterone.

People Use This For
Orally, DHEA is used for slowing or reversing aging; promoting weight loss; stimulating immunity; and increasing strength, energy, and muscle mass. It is also used for treating systemic lupus erythematosus (SLE), multiple sclerosis, Addison's disease, depression, schizophrenia, chronic fatigue syndrome (CFS), menopausal symptoms, and atrichia pubis. It is also used orally for improving cognitive function, and slowing the progression of Parkinson's disease and Alzheimer's disease. For people with HIV disease, DHEA is used to improve depressed mood and fatigue. It is also used orally by men for erectile dysfunction and by healthy women and women who have adrenal or androgen insufficiency to improve well-being and sexuality. It is also used for preventing heart disease, breast cancer, and diabetes.
Vaginally, DHEA is used in postmenopausal women for vaginal atrophy and increasing bone mineral density.
Intravenously, DHEA is being investigated for improving skin graft-site healing.

Safety
POSSIBLY SAFE ...when used orally and appropriately, short-term. Most studies have been small and lasted from a few weeks to 6 months (793,2133,3231,4249,4251,4252,4253,4254,4255,9691,9692,10986). Some studies have also used oral DHEA with apparent safety for up to 12 months (2113,6446,10406,11464). ...when used intravaginally and appropriately. DHEA has been safely used intravaginally by postmenopausal women in a study lasting 12 months (4242).
POSSIBLY UNSAFE ...when used orally, long-term or in high doses. There is concern that long-term use or use of amounts that cause higher than normal physiological DHEA levels might increase the risk of prostate cancer (2111,2116), breast cancer, or other hormone-sensitive cancers (6445). In some cases, 50-100 mg daily can produce slightly higher than normal physiological DHEA levels (4249,4251).
PREGNANCY AND LACTATION: POSSIBLY UNSAFE ...when used orally. DHEA can cause higher than normal androgen levels (2133,4249,4251,4253), which might adversely affect pregnancy or a nursing infant.

Effectiveness
POSSIBLY EFFECTIVE

Adrenal insufficiency. Taking low-dose DHEA orally, 20-50 mg per day, seems to improve feelings of well-being, skin and hair, and sexuality in women with adrenal insufficiency or androgen deficiency due to hypopituitarism (3231,8593).

Aging skin. Taking DHEA orally seems to increase epidermal thickness, sebum production, skin hydration, and decrease facial skin pigmentation in elderly men and women (6446).

Erectile dysfunction (ED). Taking DHEA orally for 24 weeks seems to improve ED, orgasmic function, sexual desire, and overall sexual satisfaction in men with erectile dysfunction. DHEA seems to help men with erectile dysfunction secondary to hypertension or idiopathic erectile dysfunction, but doesn't seem to improve erectile dysfunction related to diabetes or neurological disorders (793,8596).

Schizophrenia. Taking DHEA orally seems to improve both negative and positive symptoms in patients with schizophrenia. It may be more effective in women than in men (9692).

Menopausal symptoms. Taking DHEA orally 25 mg per day seems to improve subjective vasomotor symptoms such as hot flashes, as well as psychological symptoms throughout 12 months of therapy (11464).

Systemic lupus erythematosus (SLE). Taking DHEA orally in conjunction with conventional treatment may help reduce SLE disease activity, frequency of flare-ups, and corticosteroid doses needed (2113,2114,2136,6447,6068). DHEA also seems to improve bone mineral density in SLE patients being treated with high dose corticosteroids (6068,6097,6447).

POSSIBLY INEFFECTIVE

Alzheimer's disease. Taking DHEA orally for 6 months does not appear to be any more effective than placebo for improving symptoms of Alzheimer's disease (11334).

Cognitive function. Taking DHEA orally doesn't seem to improve cognitive function in healthy elderly people (3893).

Muscle strength. Taking DHEA orally doesn't seem to improve muscle mass or muscle strength in elderly patients (10406).

Sexual arousal. Taking DHEA orally doesn't seem to influence response to sexual stimuli in sexually functional premenopausal women (8594). However, there is preliminary clinical evidence that suggests that a single 300 mg dose of DHEA might improve sexual response in postmenopausal women (9906). More evidence is needed.

INSUFFICIENT RELIABLE EVIDENCE to RATE

Addison's disease. Preliminary clinical evidence suggests that oral DHEA might improve symptoms of Addison's disease (8595).

Atrichia pubis. Preliminary clinical research suggests treatment with oral DHEA might stimulate growth of pubic hair and stimulate body growth in adolescent girls and young women with atrichia pubis (9691).

Chronic fatigue syndrome (CFS). Preliminary clinical evidence suggests that oral DHEA might improve symptoms of CFS (7559).

Depression. Some clinical research suggests that taking DHEA orally might improve symptoms of depression and dysthymia (3270,3892,4233).

HIV-Lipodystrophy. Supplemental DHEA given sublingually might help lipodystrophy in people with advanced HIV infection (8598).

Vaginal atrophy. Applying DHEA vaginally seems to be effective for treating vaginal atrophy in elderly postmenopausal women (4242). It might also increase bone mineral density in these patients.

More evidence is needed to rate DHEA for these uses.

Mechanism of Action

DHEA is endogenously produced in the adrenal glands and liver in humans. In men, DHEA is also secreted by the testes. Additionally, the brain synthesizes minute quantities. DHEA and its sulfate ester, dehydroepiandrosterone sulfate (DHEA-S), are interconvertible. DHEA is initially converted to DHEA-S, which is considered the storage form of DHEA (5874,8592). Peripheral tissues and target organs convert DHEA-S back to DHEA, which is then metabolized to androstenedione, the major human precursor to androgens and estrogens (3232,6098). DHEA and DHEA-S levels are higher in men than in women, and naturally decline with age in both sexes in most people. However, in about one-third of the population, DHEA-S levels increase with age (4248,6013,6014,8597). DHEA-S levels don't seem to correlate with mortality in women. Mortality risk appears to be higher in men under 70 years old with very low DHEA-S levels. Men who smoke and have low DHEA-S levels seem to have a mortality risk more than 6 times greater than nonsmokers with high DHEA-S levels (8597). The cause of this increased risk and whether DHEA supplementation can lower mortality risk in men are unknown.

DHEA supplementation seems to change the circulating androgen/estrogen ratio in a gender-specific manner. That is, there appears to be significant increases in the levels of estrogens, but not as much of an increase in the amount of androgens in the blood of men given DHEA. Conversely, women given DHEA develop significant increases in the levels of androgens, but not as much of an increase in estrogen levels (6010,6011,9694,11465). For example, in elderly men, administration of DHEA 50 mg daily for 12 months increases DHEA-S to levels comparable with young adults; and testosterone levels don't significantly increase, but estradiol levels do significantly increase. In elderly women, administration of the same dose initially increases DHEA-S levels above those of young adults, but after 12 months of use levels fall back to the young adult range. Also, testosterone levels increase to levels comparable with young adults and estradiol levels increase, but not to levels as high as in young adults (6446). In both men and women, extended use seems to result in increased elimination of DHEA-S. After continuous oral administration of DHEA, DHEA-S levels seem to significantly increase after 6 months of use, but after 12 months of use, DHEA-S levels fall back some; however, DHEA-S levels remain higher than before supplementation began (6446). This suggests that the human body might have an adaptive mechanism, which limits the accumulation of DHEA-S and androgenic compounds (6446). The androgen-like or estrogen-like effects might be responsible for some of the benefits of DHEA (2115).

Researchers speculate that DHEA might have similar therapeutic benefits to estrogen-progestin hormone replacement therapy (HRT). In a low-estrogen environment such as menopause, DHEA has estrogenic effects. Some of the effects in postmenopausal women are similar to HRT including increasing estradiol, estrone, osteocalcin, growth hormone, and insulin-like growth factor 1 (IGF-1); however, unlike HRT, DHEA also increases androstenedione and testosterone (7327,11464). Conversion to estrogen doesn't seem to be necessary for its estrogenic activity. DHEA-S stimulates the growth of estrogen receptor-positive breast cancer cells. It can overcome the estrogen receptor blocking activity of drugs such as tamoxifen (Nolvadex) and fulvestrant (Faslodex). Some researchers think controlling DHEA-S serum levels may be useful in the treatment of breast cancer (10370).

Researchers have also suggested that replacing DHEA by supplementation might prevent some of the diseases and conditions associated with aging (6446). However, people whose DHEA-S levels increase with age don't seem to age any differently than people with declining DHEA-S levels. There does not appear to be an association between prematurely low DHEA-S levels and increased risk for diseases commonly seen with old age (6013,6014,8597). A correlation between DHEA-S levels and cognitive status or cognitive decline in elderly men has not been demonstrated (5874); however, it has been shown that endogenous DHEA levels are affected by certain activities and disease states. For example, exercising at maximal and submaximal levels and consuming food naturally increases endogenous DHEA levels. DHEA is decreased in anorexia nervosa, depression, end-stage renal disease, type 2 diabetes mellitus, schizophrenia, chronic fatigue syndrome (CFS), and systemic lupus erythematosus (SLE) (4248,5872,7558). Because decreased serum DHEA-S levels have been reported in men under age 60 with erectile dysfunction (5868), DHEA supplements are being used for erectile dysfunction. DHEA-S levels are also decreased in men with congestive heart failure (CHF), in proportion to its severity, possibly due to the effects of oxidative stress on electron transport required for DHEA synthesis (5871). DHEA is used for SLE because endogenous DHEA levels are decreased in SLE patients. It is thought that a high-estrogen, low-androgen state may contribute to the presence or activity of SLE, and that an increase in the level of androgens could help patients with this disease. DHEA has also been reported to correct defective interleukin-2 production in T-lymphocytes in people with SLE (5872,6098). The effects of DHEA on stimulation of bone formation in SLE patients has been attributed to the androgenic properties of DHEA (6447); however, the reduction in corticosteroid dose that DHEA permits might also be responsible for this effect. In women with adrenal insufficiency, DHEA does not seem to significantly affect measures of body composition including weight and bone mineral composition. The minor increase in osteocalcin in these patients does not appear to be clinically significant (9601).

In the brain, DHEA is concentrated in the limbic regions, and may function as an excitatory neuroregulator, antagonizing gamma-aminobutyric acid (GABA) transmission (5870). Low serum DHEA levels seem to be predictors of progression to AIDS in people with HIV infection (8598). DHEA has been used for HIV disease because of reports of modest antiviral effects of DHEA, possible immunomodulating effects, and findings that DHEA decreases with declining CD4 lymphocyte counts (3865,3866,3867); however, DHEA does not affect CD4 counts, even at doses as high as 2.25 grams per day (3865).

Research also suggests that DHEA might have beneficial effects on microvascular circulation and cardiovascular risk. Supplemental DHEA seems to inhibit synthesis of thromboxane A2 in platelets, increase serum levels of insulin-like growth factor 1 (IGF-1), and increase levels of cyclic guanosine monophosphate (GMP) and nitric oxide synthesis (8592). Some research also suggests DHEA might have a beneficial on lipid levels in postmenopausal women (10985). Endogenous DHEA is increased in some individuals taking diltiazem and alprazolam. Danazol, insulin, and morphine decrease DHEA levels (4248). Exogenous glucocorticoids also seem to suppress DHEA production. In vivo, glucocorticoids and DHEA are secreted concomitantly. Some researchers speculate that concurrent administration of DHEA with exogenous glucocorticoids might help combat the adverse effects of glucocorticoids (7328). Male sex hormones appear to have a harmful effect on organ function after trauma hemorrhage. DHEA attenuates depressed cardiac and hepatic function secondary to trauma hemorrhage in male rats, possibly due to estrogenic activity (6101). Estrogenic activity, together with nitric oxide release, may also be responsible for an antiatherosclerotic effect of DHEA observed in animal models (5869). Some preliminary animal research suggests that DHEA might have an additive anorexic effect when used with dexfenfluramine (Redux, no longer marketed in the US) (8599). The pharmacokinetics of DHEA are well defined. It has excellent absorption by the oral route. The elimination half-life of DHEA is 15 to 38 minutes; the half-life of DHEA-S is 7 to 22 hours. The kidneys eliminate 51 to 73% of DHEA-S and its metabolites (8592).

Adverse Reactions

Orally, DHEA can cause acne, hair loss, hirsutism, voice deepening, insulin resistance, decreased HDL cholesterol, changes in menstrual pattern, hepatic dysfunction, abdominal pain, and hypertension (2111,2116,6098). When used in very high doses it can cause mild insomnia (4248). In individuals with HIV, it is associated with nasal congestion, fatigue, and headache (4248). Doses up to 2.25 grams taken for four months were well tolerated with no serious adverse effects in people with mild HIV (3865). There are three cases of mania in men taking DHEA (5870,6102,7023). This has occurred in people with no history of psychiatric disease (6102) and in those with a history of mania (5870) and bipolar disorder (7023). Mania can occur with doses ranging from 50-300 mg per day. However, mania may not occur for 2-6 months after starting DHEA (6102,7023).

Interactions with Herbs & Other Dietary Supplements

SOY: Theoretically, soy might decrease the effects of DHEA. Soy consumption seems to decrease serum DHEA-S levels in premenopausal women (6445).

Interactions with Drugs

ANASTROZOLE (Arimidex): DHEA is a potent estrogen agonist. It may interfere with the anti-estrogen effects of anastrozole and other aromatase inhibitors (10401).

CORTICOSTEROIDS: Corticosteroid drugs can suppress endogenous DHEA production (7328). Some corticosteroid drugs include dexamethasone (Decadron), hydrocortisone (Cortef), methylprednisolone (Medrol), and prednisone (Deltasone). DHEA does not affect the pharmacokinetics of prednisolone or additively suppress excretion of endogenous corticosteroids when given with prednisolone (9693).

CYTOCHROME P450 3A4 (CYP3A4) SUBSTRATES: DHEA may increase levels of drugs metabolized by cytochrome P450 3A4 (CYP3A4) due to enzyme inhibition (1389); however, the clinical significance of these potential interactions is not known. Drugs that are substrates of CYP3A4 include alfentanil (Alfenta), alprazolam (Xanax), amitriptyline (Elavil), amiodarone (Cordarone), buspirone (BuSpar), cerivastatin (Baycol), citalopram (Celexa), felodipine (Plendil), fexofenadine (Allegra), itraconazole (Sporanox), ketoconazole (Nizoral), lansoprazole (Prevacid), losartan (Cozaar), lovastatin (Mevacor), midazolam (Versed), ondansetron (Zofran), prednisone (Deltasone, Orasone), sertraline (Zoloft), sibutramine (Meridia), sildenafil (Viagra), simvastatin (Zocor), verapamil (Calan, Covera-HS, Isoptin), and many others.

EXEMESTANE (Aromasin): DHEA is a potent estrogen agonist. It may interfere with the anti-estrogen effects of exemestane and other aromatase inhibitors (10401).

FULVESTRANT (Faslodex): DHEA is a potent estrogen agonist. It can overcome the estrogen receptor antagonist action of fulvestrant in estrogen-receptor positive cancer cells (10370). Patients with estrogen receptor positive cancers such as breast cancer, uterine cancer, and ovarian cancer should not take DHEA, even if they are

being treated with fulvestrant.
INSULIN: Insulin can decrease levels of endogenous DHEA-S. Therefore, taking insulin might decrease the effectiveness of DHEA supplements which are converted to DHEA-S in the body (8592).
LETROZOLE (Femara): DHEA is a potent estrogen agonist. It may interfere with the anti-estrogen effects of letrozole and other aromatase inhibitors (10401).
TAMOXIFEN (Nolvadex): DHEA is a potent estrogen agonist. It can overcome the estrogen receptor antagonist activity of tamoxifen in estrogen-receptor positive cancer cells (10370,10403). Patients with estrogen receptor-positive cancers such as breast cancer, uterine cancer, and ovarian cancer should not take DHEA, even if they are being treated with tamoxifen.
TRIAZOLAM (Halcion): DHEA can increase plasma triazolam concentrations. Administration of DHEA 200 mg/day for two weeks was shown to inhibit cytochrome P450 3A4 (CYP3A4) metabolism of triazolam and is due to DHEA-S, rather than DHEA (1389).

Interactions with Foods

VEGETARIAN DIET: Strict vegetarians and lactovegetarians have higher serum DHEA levels than non-vegetarians. However, this difference is not apparent in postmenopausal vegetarians (6445). The clinical significance of these findings is not known.

Interactions with Lab Tests

TRIAZOLAM: DHEA can increase plasma triazolam concentrations and test results. DHEA-S, the activated form of DHEA, inhibits triazolam metabolism (1389).

Interactions with Diseases or Conditions

DIABETES: DHEA can increase insulin resistance or sensitivity. Monitor blood glucose level closely (2112,4249,4250).
HORMONE SENSITIVE CANCERS/HORMONE SENSITIVE CONDITIONS: DHEA is a potent estrogen receptor agonist. Theoretically, it might increase the risk of breast cancer and other hormone sensitive conditions. DHEA should be avoided in patients with hormone sensitive conditions such as breast cancer, uterine cancer, ovarian cancer, endometriosis, and uterine fibroids (6445,10370,10401,10403).
HYPERLIPIDEMIA: Theoretically, DHEA may adversely affect lipid levels. Preliminary research shows that DHEA may increase macrophage foam cell formation, a pro-atherogenic effect. This formation seems to involve the upregulation of lipoprotein-processing enzymes via the androgen receptor (11345).
LIVER DYSFUNCTION: DHEA can exacerbate liver dysfunction (2111,2116).
MOOD DISORDERS: There is some concern that patients with a history of depression and bipolar disorder might be at an increased risk of psychiatric adverse events associated with DHEA. DHEA has been found to cause hypomania, mania, irritability, sexual inappropriateness and psychosis in some patients with suspected mood disorders (4233,5870,7023).

Dosage and Administration

ORAL: In postmenopausal women and in elderly men, doses of 25-50 mg daily are commonly used (4249,4251,4252,4254,4255,11464). For depression, doses of DHEA 30-90 mg daily have been used, either alone or in combination with conventional antidepressant therapy (3270,4233). For treatment of schizophrenia, increasing doses of DHEA of 25 mg daily for 2 weeks, 25 mg two times daily for 2 weeks, and 50 mg two times daily for 2 weeks have been used (9692). For replacement therapy in individuals with adrenal suppression, clinical trials have used 25-50 mg, given daily as a single dose (2133,3231,4253,6012,11465). For systemic lupus erythematosus (SLE), the typical dose is 200 mg per day as an adjunct to conventional medical treatment (2113,2114), but doses up to 600 mg per day have been used (5872). For erectile dysfunction, 50 mg per day has been used (793). For treatment of atrichia pubis in adolescent girls and young women, DHEA 15 to 30 mg per meter squared has been used (9691). For Alzheimer's disease, 50 mg twice daily has been used (11334).
VAGINAL: A 10% cream applied daily has been used (4242).

Comments

DHEA is manufactured from constituents of wild yam extract. The wild yam constituents, such as diosgenin, are converted in the laboratory to DHEA. However, diosgenin from ingested wild yam cannot be converted to DHEA in the human body, as has been reported. So taking wild yam extract will not increase DHEA levels in humans (2112). People interested in taking DHEA should avoid wild yam products labeled as "natural DHEA."
DHEA is banned by the National Collegiate Athletic Association (NCAA) (5041).

DIACYLGLYCEROL

Also Known As

DAG, Diglyceride, Diacylglycerol Oil, Dicylglycerol Oil.

Scientific Names

Diacylglycerol; 1,2-diglyceride; 1,3-diglyceride.

People Use This For

Orally, diacylglycerol is used for weight loss and hypertriglyceridemia.
In manufacturing, it is used as an emulsifier, stabilizer, thickener, and texturizer.

Safety

POSSIBLY SAFE ...when used orally and appropriately. Diacylglycerol seems to be safe when used orally for up to 24 weeks (9142,9143,9144).
PREGNANCY AND LACTATION: Insufficient reliable information available; avoid using.

Effectiveness

POSSIBLY EFFECTIVE

Obesity. Diacylglycerol incorporated into food products such as muffins, crackers, soup, cookies and granola bars might help modest weight loss when it is consumed as an alternative to dietary fat. Eating 2 to 5 servings per day with each serving containing 8 to 9 grams of diacylglycerol oil seems to cause a modest weight loss of 3.6% and body fat reduction of 8.3% in overweight and obese adults when used for 6 months (9142,9144).

INSUFFICIENT RELIABLE EVIDENCE to RATE

Diabetes. Some research suggests that diacylglycerol might be helpful in people with type 2 diabetes and hypertriglyceridemia. Diacylglycerol 10 grams per day in place of triglyceride fats seems to reduce triglycerides by about 40% and reduce hemoglobin A1C by about 10% (9143). More evidence is needed to rate diacylglycerol for this use.

Mechanism of Action

Diacylglycerol is a minor component of various edible oils and fats. It is synthesized commercially by enzyme-catalyzed esterification of glycerol with fatty acids from oils such as canola, soybean, corn, and olive oil to produce an 80% mixture of 1,3-diglyceride and 1,2-diglyceride in a 7 to 3 ratio. The main fatty acid constituents of diacylglycerol are oleic, linoleic, and linolenic acids (9142).

Diacylglycerol seems to induce weight loss by increasing fat oxidation and energy expenditure. Diacylglycerol contains approximately the same number of calories as triglyceride oils and seems to be digested to the same extent. However, the structural differences in diacylglycerol result in differences in metabolism. In the intestine, diacylglycerol is readily hydrolyzed to monoglycerides and fatty acids. Unlike triglyceride fats, diacylglycerol is not resynthesized and assembled into chylomicrons (9146). Triglyceride serum levels rise after ingestion of triglyceride fats, but not after ingestion of diacylglycerol (9142,9145). Diacylglycerol doesn't seem to affect fat-soluble vitamin absorption or serum lipid levels (9146).

Adverse Reactions

Orally, diacylglycerol can cause mild adverse effects such as gastrointestinal complaints, headache, taste disturbances, acne, and rash (9142).

Interactions with Herbs & Other Dietary Supplements

None known.

Interactions with Drugs

None known.

Interactions with Foods

None known.

Interactions with Lab Tests

None known.

Interactions with Diseases or Conditions

None known.

Dosage and Administration

ORAL: For weight loss and body fat reduction, 10 to 45 grams of diacylglycerol per day in foods in place of other fats has been used. Typically, each serving contains 8 to 9 grams of diacylglycerol oil, used in place of other dietary fats, in 2 to 5 servings per day (9142).

Comments

The FDA is reviewing the manufacturer's (Kao Corporation) application for Generally Recognized As Safe (GRAS) status for diacylglycerol. Currently, plant-derived oils that contain up to 15 percent diglycerides (compared with 80 percent in diacylglycerol) are considered GRAS (9140).

DIBENCOZIDE

Also Known As

Adenosylcobalamin, Cobalamin Enzyme, Cobamamide, Coenzyme B12, Co-enzyme B12, Coenzyme B-12, Co-enzyme B-12.
CAUTION: See separate listing for Vitamin B12.

Scientific Names

None.

People Use This For

Orally or sublingually, dibencozide is used as a preparation to stimulate protein metabolism; increase muscle mass and strength; increase mental concentration, and to treat depression, anxiety, and panic attacks.

Safety

LIKELY SAFE ...when used orally. There are no reports of toxicity from excessive amounts of cobalamins (272,5133). When tissue binding sites are saturated, excessive dibencozide is excreted in urine and bile (5133).
PREGNANCY AND LACTATION: Insufficient reliable information available; avoid using.

Effectiveness

There is insufficient reliable information available about the effectiveness of dibencozide.

Mechanism of Action

The term vitamin B12 refers to all cobalamins that are active as coenzymes in humans, including dibencozide (adenosylcobalamin), methylcobalamin, and hydroxocobalamin (5133). Cyanocobalamin, the most stable of the cobalamins, is metabolized in the body to an active coenzyme (5133). Vitamin B12 is involved in fat, protein, and carbohydrate metabolism. It is active in all cells, particularly in the bone marrow, CNS, and GI tract (272). Produced almost exclusively by microorganisms, vitamin B12 is found in animal protein and in some legumes in small amounts (272). Adults who eat meat in their diet usually ingest more than the RDA of 2.4 mcg (6243). Vitamin B12 is conserved by enterohepatic circulation. Deficiency takes about three years to develop in people with normal absorption (272). No benefit has been shown from taking large quantities of cobalamins unless an individual is deficient (272).

Adverse Reactions

None reported.

Interactions with Herbs & Other Dietary Supplements

VITAMIN C: Preliminary evidence suggests that vitamin C supplements can destroy dietary vitamin B12. However, other components of food, such as iron and nitrates, might counteract this effect (9511). It isn't clear whether this interaction is clinically significant, and it can likely be avoided if vitamin C supplements are taken at least 2 hours after meals.

Interactions with Drugs

CHLORAMPHENICOL: May impair hematopoietic response to vitamin B12 (15).

Drug Influences on Nutrient Levels and Depletion

SOME DRUGS CAN AFFECT DIBENCOZIDE LEVELS:
AMINOSALICYLIC ACID (para-aminosalicylic acid, PAS, Paser): Aminosalicylic acid can reduce oral vitamin B12 absorption, possibly by as much as 55%, as part of a general malabsorption syndrome (9574). Megaloblastic changes, and occasional cases of symptomatic anemia have occurred, usually after doses of 8 to 12 grams/day for several months (4558,9395,9397). Monitor vitamin B12 levels in people taking aminosalicylic

acid for more than one month.
ANTIBIOTICS: Disruption of the normal gastrointestinal (GI) flora may interrupt enterohepatic recirculation of vitamin B12 and increase fecal excretion (4436). Vitamin B12 is also synthesized by the GI flora, but mainly in the colon where absorption is poor. The majority of bacterially synthesized vitamin B12 is therefore excreted in the feces and does not significantly contribute to the body's store of vitamin B12 (4437,9502). The effects of antibiotics on gastrointestinal bacteria are unlikely to have clinically significant effects on vitamin B12 levels. In people with bacterial overgrowth of the small bowel, antibiotics such as metronidazole (Flagyl) can actually improve vitamin B12 status. An increased bacterial load can bind significant amounts of vitamin B12 in the gut, preventing its absorption (4437,9502).
COBALT IRRADIATION: Cobalt irradiation of the small bowel can decrease gastrointestinal (GI) absorption of vitamin B12 (15).
COLCHICINE: Colchicine in doses of 1.9 to 3.9 mg/day can disrupt normal intestinal mucosal function, leading to malabsorption of several nutrients, including vitamin B12 (4543,4544,4545). Lower doses don't seem to have a significant effect on vitamin B12 absorption after 3 years of colchicine therapy (5921). The significance of this interaction isn't clear. Monitor vitamin B12 levels in people taking large doses of colchicine for prolonged periods.
COLESTIPOL (Colestid), CHOLESTYRAMINE (Questran): These resins can decrease gastrointestinal (GI) absorption of vitamin B12 by binding intrinsic factor and vitamin B12-intrinsic factor complexes (10542,10543). However, absorption isn't completely prevented (10542). It's unlikely that this interaction will deplete body stores of vitamin B12 unless there are other factors contributing to deficiency. In a group of children treated with cholestyramine for up to 2.5 years there wasn't any change in serum vitamin B12 levels (4455). Routine supplements aren't necessary.
H2-BLOCKERS: Reduced secretion of gastric acid and pepsin produced by H2-blockers can reduce absorption of protein-bound (dietary) vitamin B12, but not supplemental vitamin B12 (4539,4540,4541,9513,9514,9528). Gastric acid is needed to release vitamin B12 from protein for absorption (4541,9513,9514,9528). Clinically significant vitamin B12 deficiency and megaloblastic anemia are unlikely, unless H2-blocker therapy is prolonged (2 years or more), or the person's diet is poor (4539,9513,9514). It is also more likely if the person is rendered achlorhydric (4483), which occurs more frequently with proton pump inhibitors than H2-blockers. Monitor vitamin B12 levels in people taking high doses of H2 blockers for prolonged periods. The H2-blockers include cimetidine (Tagamet), ranitidine (Zantac), nizatidine (Axid), and famotidine (Pepcid).
METFORMIN (Glucophage): Metformin may reduce serum folic acid and vitamin B12 levels (32,4490,8834). These changes can lead to hyperhomocysteinemia, adding to the risk of cardiovascular disease in people with diabetes (32,4490,7839). There are also rare reports of megaloblastic anemia in people who have taken metformin for 5 years or more (9520,9521,9522). Possible mechanisms for lowered vitamin B12 levels are decreased intrinsic factor secretion, reduced uptake of vitamin B12-intrinsic factor complexes, altered bowel motility, and bacterial overgrowth (32,9521). Reduced absorption of vitamin B12 can be measured with the Schilling test after a few weeks of metformin therapy (7841). Reduced serum levels of vitamin B12 occur in up to 30% of people taking metformin chronically (4490,9520,9521,9523). However, clinically significant deficiency isn't likely to develop if dietary intake of vitamin B12 is adequate (9521). Deficiency can be corrected with vitamin B12 supplements even if metformin is continued (9520,9522). The metformin-induced malabsorption of vitamin B12 is reversible by oral calcium supplementation (8834,9523). A multivitamin preparation may also be valuable for some patients. Monitor for signs and symptoms of vitamin B12 and folic acid deficiency. Advise people taking metformin chronically to include adequate amounts of vitamin B12 in their diet, and have their serum vitamin B12 and homocysteine levels checked annually.
NEOMYCIN: Absorption of vitamin B12 can be reduced by neomycin, but prolonged use of large doses is needed to induce pernicious anemia (3046,8434). Supplements aren't needed with normal doses.
NITROUS OXIDE: Nitrous oxide inactivates the cobalamin form of vitamin B12 by oxidation. Symptoms of vitamin B12 deficiency, including sensory neuropathy, myelopathy, and encephalopathy, can occur within days or weeks of exposure to nitrous oxide anesthesia in people with subclinical vitamin B12 deficiency. Symptoms are treated with high doses of vitamin B12, but recovery can be slow and incomplete. People with normal vitamin B12 levels have sufficient vitamin B12 stores to make the effects of nitrous oxide insignificant, unless exposure is repeated and prolonged (nitrous oxide abuse) (9527,9532). In people with risk factors for vitamin B12 deficiency, check vitamin B12 levels prior to using nitrous oxide anesthesia.
ORAL CONTRACEPTIVES: The data regarding the effects of oral contraceptives on vitamin B12 serum levels are conflicting. Some studies have found reduced serum levels in oral contraceptive users (4547,9371,9373,9505), but others have found no effect despite use of oral contraceptives for up to 6 months (4498,7843,9372). When reduced serum levels are detected, vitamin B12 absorption, urinary excretion, tissue and erythrocyte levels, methylmalonic acid levels, and homocysteine are normal (9371,9373,9505,10123). When oral contraceptive use is stopped, normalization of vitamin B12 levels usually occurs (10123). It's suggested that oral contraceptives reduce production of transcobalamin I, the protein which transports vitamin B12 in the blood (4547,9373,9505). Thus more of the vitamin is available for tissue uptake and serum levels may be reduced. Vitamin B12 supplements don't seem to increase serum levels of vitamin B12 (9373). Lower vitamin B12 serum levels seen with oral contraceptives probably aren't clinically significant.
PHENYTOIN (Dilantin), PHENOBARBITAL, PRIMIDONE (Mysoline): These anticonvulsants have been associated with reduced vitamin B12 absorption, and reduced serum and cerebrospinal fluid levels in some patients. This may contribute to the megaloblastic anemia, primarily caused by folate deficiency, associated with

these drugs (7843,10502,10503,10504). It's also suggested that reduced vitamin B12 levels may contribute to the neuropsychiatric side effects of these drugs (10504,10505). Encourage patients to maintain adequate dietary vitamin B12 intake, and check folate and vitamin B12 status if symptoms of anemia develop.
PROTON PUMP INHIBITORS (PPIs): The reduced secretion of gastric acid and pepsin produced by PPIs can reduce absorption of protein-bound (dietary) vitamin B12, but not supplemental vitamin B12 (4483,4484,4485,4486,9513,9528). Gastric acid is needed to release vitamin B12 from protein for absorption (4484,4486,9513,9528). Reduced vitamin B12 levels may be more common with PPIs than with H2-blockers, because they are more likely to produce achlorhydria (complete absence of gastric acid secretion) (4483,4486). However, clinically significant vitamin B12 deficiency is unlikely, unless PPI therapy is prolonged (2 years or more) or dietary vitamin intake is low (4483,4484,9513). Monitor vitamin B12 levels in people taking high doses of PPIs for prolonged periods. The PPIs include omeprazole (Prilosec, Losec), lansoprazole (Prevacid), rabeprazole (Aciphex), pantoprazole (Protonix, Pantoloc), and esomeprazole (Nexium).
ZIDOVUDINE (AZT, Combivir, Retrovir): Reduced serum vitamin B12 levels may occur when zidovudine therapy is started (30,10531). This adds to other factors that cause low vitamin B12 levels in people with HIV, and might contribute to the hematological toxicity associated with zidovudine (10531,10532). However, data suggests vitamin B12 supplements aren't helpful for people taking zidovudine (10532,10533).

Interactions with Foods

ALCOHOL (Ethanol): Excessive alcohol intake lasting longer than two weeks can decrease vitamin B12 absorption from the gastrointestinal tract (15).

Interactions with Lab Tests

None known.

Interactions with Diseases or Conditions

GI CONDITIONS: Ileal disease or resection, intrinsic factor deficiency can cause vitamin B12 malabsorption (272).

Dosage and Administration

No typical dosage.

Comments

Cyanocobalamin and hydroxocobalamin are the only forms of vitamin B12 stable for storage (5139).

DIGITALIS

Also Known As

Dead Man's Bells, Digitalis purpurea, Fairy Cap, Fairy Finger, Foxglove, Lady's Thimble, Lion's Mouth, Purple Foxglove, Scotch Mercury, Throatwort, Witch's Bells, Wolly Foxglove.

Scientific Names

Digitalis purpurea; Digitalis lanata.
Family: Scrophulariaceae.

People Use This For

Orally, digitalis is used for congestive heart failure, atrial fibrillation or flutter, for diureses in edema, asthma, as an emetic, for epilepsy, tuberculosis, constipation, headache, spasm, and wound and burn healing.

Safety

UNSAFE ...when used orally for self-medication. Use requires monitoring by a medical professional (12). Can cause heart arrhythmias and death (17). All parts of the plant are toxic (501). US regulations require labeling to inform consumers that digitalis is inappropriate for use as an anti-obesity agent (12). Canadian regulations prohibit digitalis in foods (12). Deaths have occurred when digitalis was mistaken for comfrey (501).
CHILDREN: LIKELY UNSAFE ...when used orally. Sucking on the flowers, ingesting seeds, or parts of the leaves has caused children to become ill (6).
PREGNANCY AND LACTATION: UNSAFE ...when used orally for self-medication (12); avoid using.

Effectiveness

LIKELY EFFECTIVE

Atrial fibrillation. Taking digitalis orally is effective for treating atrial fibrillation or flutter (6).

Congestive heart failure (CHF). Taking digitalis orally is effective for treating CHF and CHF-related edema (6).

There is insufficient reliable information available about the effectiveness of digitalis for its other uses.

Mechanism of Action

The applicable part of digitalis is the leaf. Digitalis contains varied glycosides, primarily glycoside A and glycoside B, which are precursors to digitoxin and gitoxin, respectively. Digitalis lanata contains lanatosides A,B,C,D, and E that yield digitoxin, gitoxin, digoxin, digitalin, and gitaloxin, respectively (6). Cardiac glycosides increase cardiac contractility, decrease heart rate and reduce AV node conduction, stabilize the heart rate, increase cardiac output, and relieve pulmonary congestion and peripheral edema (6).

Adverse Reactions

Orally, chronic use of digitalis can lead to intoxication symptoms including visual halos, yellow-green vision, and GI upset (6). Acute poisoning of digitalis includes GI upset, contracted pupils, blurred vision, strong slow pulse, nausea, vomiting, dizziness, excessive urination, fatigue, muscle weakness and tremors, stupor, confusion, convulsions, atrial arrhythmias, AV block, and death (6,159,501).

Interactions with Herbs & Other Dietary Supplements

CARDIAC GLYCOSIDE-CONTAINING HERBS: Contraindicated; concomitant use can increase the risk of cardiac glycoside toxicity. Cardiac glycoside containing herbs, including black hellebore, Canadian hemp roots, digitalis leaf, hedge mustard, figwort, lily of the valley roots, motherwort, oleander leaf, pheasant's eye plant, pleurisy root, squill bulb leaf scales, and strophanthus seeds (19).
LICORICE/HORSETAIL: Theoretically, overuse/misuse of licorice rhizome or horsetail plant with cardiac glycoside-containing herbs increases the risk of toxicity due to potassium depletion (19).
OTHER CARDIOACTIVE HERBS: Avoid concomitant use with other cardioactive herbs due to unpredictability of effects and adverse effects. Other cardioactive herbs include calamus, cereus, cola, coltsfoot, devil's claw, European mistletoe, fenugreek, fumitory, ginger, Panax ginseng, hawthorn, white horehound, mate, parsley, quassia, scotch broom flower, shepherd's purse, and wild carrot (4).
STIMULANT LAXATIVE HERBS: Theoretically, overuse/misuse of stimulant laxatives with cardiac glycoside-containing herbs increases the risk of cardiac toxicity due to potassium depletion (19). Stimulant laxative herbs include aloe dried leaf sap, blue flag rhizome, alder buckthorn, European buckthorn, butternut bark, cascara bark, castor oil, colocynth fruit pulp, gamboge bark exudate, jalap root, black root, manna bark exudate, podophyllum root, rhubarb root, senna leaves and pods, wild cucumber fruit (Ecballium elaterium), and yellow dock root.

Interactions with Drugs

DIGOXIN (Lanoxin): Contraindicated; therapeutic duplication increases the risk of cardiac glycoside toxicity (2).
DIURETIC DRUGS: Theoretically, concomitant use of potassium depleting diuretics and digitalis can increase the risk of cardiac glycoside toxicity due to potassium depletion (506). Some diuretics that can deplete potassium include chlorothiazide (Diuril), chlorthalidone (Thalitone), furosemide (Lasix), hydrochlorothiazide (HCTZ, HydroDIURIL, Microzide), and others.
MACROLIDE ANTIBIOTICS: Theoretically, concomitant use may increase risk of cardiac glycoside toxicity (17).
QUININE: Use of quinine can with digitalis can increase the risk of digitalis toxicity (506).
STIMULANT LAXATIVES: Theoretically, overuse or misuse of stimulant laxative can increase risk of cardiac glycoside toxicity due to potassium depletion (506).
TETRACYCLINE ANTIBIOTICS: Theoretically, concomitant use may increase risk of cardiac glycoside toxicity (17).

Interactions with Foods

None known.

Interactions with Lab Tests

ELECTROCARDIOGRAM (ECG): Digitalis can normalize arrhythmias, and ECG readings, associated with atrial fibrillation or flutter in patients with congestive heart failure (15).

Interactions with Diseases or Conditions

HEART DISEASE: Self-use contraindicated; requires diagnosis, treatment, and monitoring (515,150).
RENAL DISEASE: May reduce excretion of digitalis, increasing the potential for toxicity (150).

Dosage and Administration

No typical dosage.

Comments

Digitalis is unsafe for self-medication. Digitalis lanata is the major source of digoxin in the US (6).

DIINDOLYLMETHANE

Also Known As
DIM.
CAUTION: See separate listing for Indole-3-Carbinol.

Scientific Names
3,3'-Diindolylmethane.

People Use This For
Orally, diindolylmethane is used for preventing breast and uterine cancer. It is also used orally to prevent benign prostatic hypertrophy (BPH) and treat premenstrual syndrome (PMS).

Safety
LIKELY SAFE ...when used orally in amounts typically found in foods. The typical diet supplies 2-24 mg of diindolylmethane (7170,7176,7664).
CHILDREN: LIKELY SAFE ...when used orally in amounts typically found in foods (7170,7176,7664).
PREGNANCY AND LACTATION: LIKELY SAFE ...when used orally in amounts typically consumed in foods (7170,7176,7664). There is insufficient reliable information available about the safety of diindolylmethane when used in amounts greater than those found in foods during pregnancy and lactation; avoid using.

Effectiveness
There is insufficient information available about the effectiveness of diindolylmethane.

Mechanism of Action
Diindolylmethane is a major active metabolite of indole-3-carbinol (7664), which is a constituent of Cruciferous vegetables such as cabbage, Brussels sprouts, cauliflower, and broccoli. Indole-3-carbinol is thought to be one of the agents responsible for the cancer-protective properties of these vegetables (7664,7668). In stomach acid, indole-3-carbinol is unstable and readily converted to a variety of compounds including diindolylmethane (7669). A typical diet provides 20-120 mg of indole-3-carbinol per day. Approximately 10-20% is converted to diindolylmethane, providing 2-24 mg daily (7170,7176,7664).
Researchers are interested in diindolylmethane due to potential activity against breast cancer cells (7664,7665,7666,7668,7669). Diindolylmethane has partial estrogen receptor agonist and antagonistic activity (7664,7669). There is preliminary evidence that diindolylmethane can inhibit the growth of mammary tumors in animal models (7666). Diindolylmethane induces apoptosis (programmed cell death) in human breast cancer cells in vitro (7668).

Adverse Reactions
None reported.

Interactions with Herbs & Other Dietary Supplements
None known.

Interactions with Drugs
CYTOCHROME P450 1A2 (CYP1A2) SUBSTRATES: There is some preliminary evidence that diindolylmethane can induce CYP1A2 (7667). Theoretically, diindolylmethane might increase metabolism of CYP1A2 substrates and lower serum concentrations. Some CYP1A2 substrates include clozapine (Clozaril), cyclobenzaprine (Flexeril), fluvoxamine (Luvox), haloperidol (Haldol), imipramine (Tofranil), mexilitine (Mexitil), olanzapine (Zyprexa), pentazocine (Talwin), propranolol (Inderal), tacrin (Cognex), theophylline, zileuton (Zyflo), zolmitriptan (Zomig), and others.

Interactions with Foods
None known.

Interactions with Lab Tests
None known.

Interactions with Diseases or Conditions
None known.

Dosage and Administration
No typical dosage.

DILL above ground parts

Also Known As
American Dill, Anethi herba, Dill Herb, Dillweed, Dill Weed, Dilly, European Dill, Madhura, Satahva, Sotapa, Sowa.
CAUTION: See separate listing for Dill seed.

Scientific Names
Anethum graveolens, synonyms Anethum sowa, Peucedanum graveolens.
Family: Apiaceae/Umbelliferae.

People Use This For
Orally, dill above ground parts are used for diseases and disorders of the gastrointestinal tract, kidney, and urinary tract. Dill is also used for spasms, flatulence, and sleep disorders.
In foods, dill and dill oil are used as flavoring agents.
In manufacturing, dill oil is used as a fragrance component in cosmetics, soaps, and perfumes.

Safety
LIKELY SAFE ...when used orally in amounts commonly found in foods. Dill has Generally Recognized As Safe (GRAS) status in the US (4912).
POSSIBLY SAFE ...when used orally and appropriately for medicinal purposes (12).
PREGNANCY AND LACTATION: Insufficient reliable information available; avoid using amounts greater than those found in foods.

Effectiveness
There is insufficient reliable information available about the effectiveness of dill above ground parts.

Mechanism of Action
An aqueous dill extract administered intravenously lowers blood pressure, dilates blood vessels, stimulates respiration, and slows heart rate in animals (11). The dill leaf is reported to be a rich source of beta-carotene, iron, and potassium (19).

Adverse Reactions
Topically, photodermatosis is possible after contact with juice from the freshly harvested plants (18,19). Dill can also cause contact dermatitis (19).

Interactions with Herbs & Other Dietary Supplements
None known.

Interactions with Drugs
None known.

Interactions with Foods
None known.

Interactions with Lab Tests
None known.

Interactions with Diseases or Conditions
CROSS REACTIVITY: The use of dill above ground parts can cause allergic reactions in people with allergies to the carrot family plants, which include asafoetida, caraway, celery, coriander, and fennel (19).

Dosage and Administration
ORAL: The common dose of the dried fruits is 1 to 4 grams three times daily (6002). The usual dose of the dill oil is 0.05-2 mL three times daily (6002).

Comments
Dill oil (dillweed oil, dill herb oil) is distilled from freshly harvested dill (Anetheum graveolens). During the Middle Ages, people sometimes used dill as a charm against witchcraft and enchantments (6002). Avoid confusion with dill seed.

DILL seed

Also Known As
American Dill, Anethi fructus, Dilly, European Dill, Madhura, Satahva, Sotapa, Sowa.
CAUTION: See separate listing for Dill above ground parts.

Scientific Names
Anethum graveolens, synonyms Anethum sowa, Peucedanum graveolens.
Family: Apiaceae/Umbelliferae.

People Use This For
Orally, dill seed is used for loss of appetite, fever and colds, cough, bronchitis, tendency towards infection, liver and gallbladder complaints, as a digestive aid, for flatulence, hemorrhoids, bronchial asthma, neuralgias, renal colic, dysuria, genital ulcers, and dysmenorrhea.
Topically, dill seed is used for mouth and throat inflammation.
In foods, dill seed is used as a culinary spice.

Safety
LIKELY SAFE ...when dill seed is used orally in amounts commonly found in foods. Dill seed has Generally Recognized As Safe (GRAS) status in the US (4912).
POSSIBLY SAFE ...when used orally and appropriately in medicinal amounts (12).
PREGNANCY: LIKELY UNSAFE ...when used in amounts greater than those found in foods. Dill seed might stimulate menstrual flow (19).
LACTATION: Insufficient reliable information available; avoid amounts greater than those found in foods.

Effectiveness
There is insufficient reliable information available about the effectiveness of dill seed.

Mechanism of Action
Dill seed contains an essential oil rich in carvone (2). Dill seed has antibacterial, antispasmodic, sedative, and diuretic effects. They also think it stimulates lactation (2,11) and is a urinary irritant (19). Dill seed oil has spasmolytic effects on smooth muscle (11). Some evidence suggests an intravenous emulsion might increase respiratory volume and lower blood pressure (2,11).

Adverse Reactions
Topically, photodermatosis is possible after contact with juice from freshly harvested plants (18,19).

Interactions with Herbs & Other Dietary Supplements
None known.

Interactions with Drugs
None known.

Interactions with Foods
None known.

Interactions with Lab Tests
None known.

Interactions with Diseases or Conditions
URINARY TRACT INFLAMMATION: Avoid due to claims that dill seed is a urinary irritant (19).

Dosage and Administration
ORAL: People typically use 3 grams of dill seed daily. People also add 2 teaspoons bruised seeds to a cup of boiling water and drink up to 3 cups per day. As a tincture, dill is taken up to 1 teaspoon up to 3 times daily. As a breath freshener, up to 1 teaspoon is chewed. Oil of dill is taken 100 to 300 mg (2 to 6 drops) daily (5250,5252).

Comments
Avoid confusion with dill above ground parts. Dill seed oil is distilled from the crushed, dried fruit (seed) of the dill plant (Anetheum graveolens).

DIMETHYLGLYCINE

Also Known As
Dimethyl Glycine, (Dimethylamino) acetic Acid, DMG, N,N-dimethylaminoacetic Acid, N-methylsarcosine.
CAUTION: Dimethylglycine is one of the compounds found in pangamic acid formulations. See separate listing for Pangamic Acid.

Scientific Names
N,N-dimethylglycine.

People Use This For
Orally, dimethylglycine is used to improve speech and behavior in autism, for attention deficit-hyperactivity disorder (ADHD), to improve neurological function, and for epilepsy. It is also used to reduce physical and environmental stress, improve oxygen utilization, enhance liver function, and optimize athletic performance. Other uses include as an anti-inflammatory and for anti-aging effects. Dimethylglycine is used to improve the immune response; to treat tumors; and to enhance anti-viral, anti-bacterial, and anti-tumor defenses. It is also used for chronic fatigue syndrome, allergies, respiratory disorders, alcoholism, and drug addiction. Dimethylglycine is also used to lower blood cholesterol and triglycerides, and to help normalize blood pressure and blood glucose.

Safety
POSSIBLY UNSAFE ...when used orally. Dimethylglycine may react with nitrites in the gastrointestinal tract to form the potent carcinogen, dimethylnitrosamine (5827), although this has been questioned (5830).
PREGNANCY AND LACTATION: POSSIBLY UNSAFE ...when used orally (5827); avoid using.

Effectiveness
POSSIBLY INEFFECTIVE

Autism. Taking dimethylglycine orally doesn't seem to improve autism (5819).

Epilepsy. Taking dimethylglycine orally doesn't seem to be effective for the treatment of epilepsy (5823).

There is insufficient reliable information available about the effectiveness of dimethylglycine for its other uses.

Mechanism of Action
Dimethylglycine is the dimethylated form of the amino acid glycine, but it only exists in the body for seconds at a time, and in very small quantities (5827). It is formed from betaine during the methylation of homocysteine (5828). The effects of supplemental doses in excess of naturally occurring amounts are unknown. Preliminary evidence suggests that dimethylglycine enhances humoral and cell-mediated immune responses in humans and in some, but not all, animals (5820,5822,5825). Dimethylglycine has been reported to have anticonvulsant effects in animals (5828), including antagonizing strychnine- and penicillin-induced seizures (5824,5829). A single case report described a dramatic improvement in a person with mixed complex partial and grand mal seizures (5826), but a small study in people with generalized or akinetic/myoclonic seizures found no benefit with dimethylglycine 300 to 600 mg per day (5823). Several small studies in athletes have not found any benefit of dimethylglycine on athletic performance (5821); including maximal treadmill performance measured by maximal and recovery heart rates, treadmill time, and pre-test and post-test blood glucose and lactate levels (2645). A small study using low-dose dimethylglycine did not find any benefit in children with autism (5819).

Adverse Reactions
Orally, dimethylglycine may react with nitrites in the gastrointestinal tract to form carcinogenic substances (5827).

Interactions with Herbs & Other Dietary Supplements
None known.

Interactions with Drugs
None known.

Interactions with Foods
None known.

Interactions with Lab Tests
None known.

Interactions with Diseases or Conditions
None known.

Dosage and Administration
No typical dosage.

Comments
In the 1980s, a federal court in Chicago forbade interstate sale of a brand of dimethylglycine stating that it was an unsafe food additive (5827).

DIOSMIN

Also Known As
Citrus Bioflavonoid, Citrus Bioflavonoids, Diosmetin, Flavonoid.
CAUTION: See separate listings for Chrysin, Hesperidin, Methoxylated Flavones, Quercetin, Rue, and Rutin.

Scientific Names
Diosmetin, Diosmin.

People Use This For
Orally, diosmin is used for treating acute internal hemorrhoids, preventing relapse of acute internal hemorrhoids, treating varicose veins, venous stasis, subconjunctival and retinal hemorrhage, lymphedema following breast cancer surgery, venous stasis, and gingival bleeding. Diosmin has also been used to protect against liver toxicity.

Safety
POSSIBLY SAFE ...when used orally and appropriately, short-term. Diosmin seems to be safe when used for up to 6 months (4861,4898,10227,10229).
There is insufficient reliable information available about the safety of diosmin when used for greater than 6 months.
PREGNANCY AND LACTATION: Insufficient reliable information available; avoid using.

Effectiveness
POSSIBLY EFFECTIVE

Hemorrhoids. The combination of diosmin 1350 mg plus hesperidin 150 mg twice daily for 4 days followed by diosmin 900 mg and hesperidin 100 mg twice daily for 3 days seems to significantly improve signs and symptoms of internal hemorrhoids. The combination can stop acute bleeding in up to 92% of patients after 4 days of treatment. It can also reduce symptoms such as anal discomfort, pain, discharge, and local lesions. Subjective symptoms can be relieved within 2 days of treatment. The combination also seems to reduce the duration and intensity of hemorrhoidal flare-ups (4861,4900). Some clinicians use diosmin in lower doses and in combination with bulk laxatives instead of hesperidin. Diosmin 600 mg three times daily for 4 days, then 300 mg twice daily for 10 more days plus the bulk laxative psyllium 11 grams daily does seem to slightly help after 4 days of treatment (4898). However, this combination does not seem to be as effective as the higher dose of diosmin plus hesperidin combination. Maintenance use of diosmin 450 mg plus hesperidin 50 mg twice daily for 3 months in patients following acute treatment for internal hemorrhoids seems to significantly decrease the relapse rate (4861).

Venous stasis ulcers. Diosmin, in combination with hesperidin and compression dressing, seems to improve healing of venous stasis ulcers less than 10 cm in size (10229).

POSSIBLY INEFFECTIVE

Lymphedema. Diosmin, in combination with hesperidin, may improve drainage of lymph from the arms of women after breast cancer surgery, but it does not reduce arm swelling or other clinical signs of lymphedema (10227).

Clinical trials have used specific brand name formulations of diosmin (Daflon 500 and Daflon, Les Laboratoires Servier, France). Each tablet of Daflon 500 contains a micronized formulation of diosmin 450 mg and hesperidin 50 mg extracted from rutaceae species. Each tablet of Daflon contains only diosmin 150 mg.

There is insufficient reliable information available about the effectiveness of diosmin for its other uses.

Mechanism of Action
Diosmin is one of over 4,000 flavonoids found in plants (4919,4959,5006). Diosmin is in a class of flavonoids primarily derived from citrus fruits and is known as a citrus bioflavonoid. It is closely related to other citrus bioflavonoids such as quercetin, rutin, and hesperidin. Diosmin alone, or in combination with other citrus bioflavonoids, is most often used for vascular conditions such as hemorrhoids and varicose veins. Diosmin seems to work by improving venous tone, reducing stasis, restoring normal capillary permeability, and improving lymphatic drainage. Diosmin might improve venous tone and reduce stasis by improving vasculature response to adrenergic stimulation. Diosmin's anti-inflammatory effects seem to help restore normal capillary permeability. Diosmin inhibits phosphodiesterase and increases intracellular cyclic adenosine monophosphate (cAMP), which causes decreased production of inflammatory prostaglandins E2 and F2 and thromboxane B2. Diosmin can also reduce the generation of free radicals (4861,4898,4900,4954). Some diosmin preparations use a micronized formulation. The smaller particle size seems

to help increase absorption (4900). There is preliminary evidence that a diosmin metabolite, diosmetin, might also be hepatoprotective. Diosmetin might have direct antioxidant effects, increase glutathione (GSH) levels, and decrease lipid peroxidation (4954).

Adverse Reactions

Orally, diosmin can cause gastrointestinal side effects, including abdominal pain, diarrhea, and gastritis. Headache can also occur in some patients (4861,4898,4900).

Interactions with Herbs & Other Dietary Supplements

None known.

Interactions with Drugs

None known.

Interactions with Foods

None known.

Interactions with Lab Tests

None known.

Interactions with Diseases or Conditions

None known.

Dosage and Administration

ORAL: For the treatment of internal hemorrhoids, diosmin 1350 mg plus hesperidin 150 mg twice daily for 4 days followed by diosmin 900 mg and hesperidin 100 mg twice daily for 3 days has been used (4861,4900). Some clinicians also try diosmin 600 mg three times daily for 4 days, followed by 300 mg twice daily for 10 days, in combination with psyllium 11 grams daily (4898). However, this lower diosmin dose does not seem to be as effective. For prevention of relapse internal hemorrhoids, diosmin 450 mg plus hesperidin 50 mg twice daily for 3 months of therapy has been used (4861). For treating lymphedema following surgery for breast cancer, the combination of 900 mg diosmin and 100 mg hesperidin daily has been used for up to 6 months (10227). For the treatment of venous stasis ulcers, the combination of 900 mg diosmin and 100 mg hesperidin daily has been used for up to 2 months (10229).

DIVI-DIVI

Also Known As

Bonduc, Divi Divi, Gray Nicker, Nichol Seeds, Nikkar Nuts, Putikaranja, Udakiryaka.

Scientific Names

Caesalpinia bonduc, synonyms Caesalpinia bonducella, Caesalpinia crista, Guilandina bonduc, Guilandina bonducella.
Family: Fabaceae/Leguminosae.

Comments

At the date of publication, this product was not a common ingredient used in brand name supplements marketed to consumers. Details about this product are available at the online version of *Natural Medicines Comprehensive Database*. See www.naturaldatabase.com.

DIVINER'S SAGE

Also Known As

Divine Mexican Mint, Diviner's Mint, Diviners Sage, Divinorin, Divinorin A, Herb-of-the-Virgin, Herba de María, Hierba de la Virgen, Hojas de la Pastora, La Hembra, Leaves of the Virgin Shepherdess, Mexican Sage, Mexican Sage Incense, Pipiltzintzintli, Sadi, Salvia, Salvinorin, Salvinorin A, Sage of the Seers, Ska Maria, Ska Maria Pastora, Yerba de Maria.
CAUTION: See separate listings for Boneset, Clary Sage, Danshen, German Sarsaparilla, Purple Loosestrife, Sage, Spearmint, and Wood Sage.

Scientific Names

Salvia divinorum. Family: Lamiaceae/Labiatae.

People Use This For
Orally and by inhalation, diviner's sage is used as a hallucinogen.
Orally, diviner's sage is used for diarrhea, headache, rheumatism, abdominal distension, and as a tonic and end-of-life remedy. It is also used orally to regulate urination and defecation.

Safety
There is insufficient reliable information available about the safety of diviner's sage.

Effectiveness
There is insufficient reliable information available about the effectiveness of diviner's sage.

Mechanism of Action
The applicable part of diviner's sage is the leaf. The leaves are chewed and swallowed, made into an infusion (tea), or smoked for hallucinogenic effects. The active constituent is the diterpene salvinorin A, which is also called divinorin A. Unlike other hallucinogens, salvinorin A is not an alkaloid (7350,7351,7352). Salvinorin A is the most potent hallucinogen known. It causes hallucinations in doses of 200 mcg to 500 mcg when vaporized and inhaled (7351). Salvinorin A is absorbed by the oral mucosa when chewed, but is inactivated by the gastrointestinal system when swallowed. It is absorbed and produces pharmacological activity when it is heated and the vapors are inhaled (7352). The onset of hallucinogenic activity occurs within 5 to 10 minutes when chewed and within 30 seconds when inhaled. The effects last about an hour when chewed and 20 to 30 minutes via inhalation (7352). However, the duration of effect appears to be dose-dependent (7351).
It's not clear how diviner's sage constituents cause hallucinations. Diviner's sage does not appear to affect receptor sites such as serotonin, dopamine, or monoamine oxidase that are often affected by other hallucinogens (7352).

Adverse Reactions
Orally, diviner's sage can cause nausea, dizziness, and slurred speech. It can also cause confusion and hallucinations (7350,7351).

Interactions with Herbs & Other Dietary Supplements
None known.

Interactions with Drugs
None known.

Interactions with Foods
None known.

Interactions with Lab Tests
None known.

Interactions with Diseases or Conditions
None known.

Dosage and Administration
No typical dosage.

Comments
Diviner's sage has been used for centuries in religious ceremonies by the Mazatec Indians, a native people who live in Oaxaca, Mexico. The Mazatecs believe it is an incarnation of the Virgin Mary (7350). Diviner's sage is widely available on the Internet. Its possession and use is legal in the US, but the Drug Enforcement Agency (DEA) is reviewing it for possible controlled substance regulation (7349).

DMSO (DIMETHYLSULFOXIDE)

Also Known As
Dimethyl Sulfoxide, Dimethyl Sulphoxide, Dimethylis sulfoxidum, Methyl sulphoxide, NSC-763, SQ-9453, Sulphinybismethane.

Scientific Names
Dimethylsulfoxide.

People Use This For

Orally, DMSO is used for the management of amyloidosis and related symptoms.
Topically, DMSO is used to decrease pain and speed the healing of wounds, burns, and acute musculoskeletal injuries. DMSO is also used topically to treat headache, inflammation, arthritis, tic douloureux, cataracts, glaucoma, retinal degeneration, bunions, calluses, fungus toenails, asthma, to flatten raised keloid scars, and for cancer. It is also used topically to prevent tissue necrosis after extravasation with antineoplastic agents, to treat osteoarthritis, rheumatoid arthritis, scleroderma, and amyloidosis. It is also used topically for reducing skin flap ischemia following surgery, complex regional pain syndromes, as a vehicle in combination with idoxuridine to decrease the development of inflammatory reactions and lesions associated with herpes zoster infection, and decrease the pain associated with postherpetic neuralgia.
Intravenously, DMSO is used to manage symptoms associated with secondary amyloidosis and to lower intracranial hypertension. DMSO is administered by intravesical instillation to treat symptoms of interstitial cystitis such as urinary frequency, urgency, nocturia and suprapubic pain. It is also used by intravesical instillation to treat symptoms associated with chronic inflammatory bladder disease. DMSO is infused alternatively with methyl-tert-butyl ether and a buffer solution of EDTA and sodium deoxycholate through a nasobiliary catheter for the dissolution of bile duct stones. DMSO is used for the cryopreservation of hematopoietic stem cells to be infused and transplanted at a later date.
In manufacturing, DMSO is used as an industrial solvent for herbicides, fungicides, antibiotics, and plant hormones.

Safety

LIKELY SAFE ...when used by intravesical instillation (5692,5694,5695,5696,5697). An aqueous 50% solution of DMSO is FDA approved for intravesical use in the treatment of interstitial cystitis (5692,5694).
POSSIBLY UNSAFE ...when used topically. It has been reported that industrial grade DMSO is being used topically for self-treatment of several disease conditions. Industrial grade DMSO is not of the same quality of that used for drug research purposes since it may contain impurities. DMSO readily penetrates the skin and enhances the absorption of impurities and other substances, which may be hazardous to health (6326).
PREGNANCY AND LACTATION: Insufficient reliable information available; avoid using.

Effectiveness

EFFECTIVE

Interstitial cystitis. Intravesical instillation of DMSO is effective for treatment of interstitial cystitis (5692,5694).

POSSIBLY EFFECTIVE

Amyloidosis. Applying DMSO topically seems to help treat amyloidosis (6304,6306).
Biliary stones. DMSO infused alternatively with methyl-tert-butyl ether and a buffer solution of EDTA and sodium deoxycholate through a nasobiliary catheter seems to dissolve bile duct stones (6315).
Extravasation. Applying DMSO topically seems to help prevent tissue necrosis after extravasation with antineoplastic agents (5698,5699).
Herpes zoster (shingles). Applying DMSO topically as a vehicle in combination with idoxuridine (40% idoxuridine in DMSO) seems to reduce the number of lesions and decrease the inflammatory reaction associated with herpes zoster infection (6308,6309,6311,6312).
Inflammatory bladder disease. DMSO used by intravesical instillation seems to decrease symptoms associated with chronic inflammatory bladder disease (5695,5696,5697).
Intracranial pressure. DMSO used intravenously seems to lower intracranial pressure (6300,6301).
Osteoarthritis. Applying DMSO topically seems to help decrease symptoms associated with osteoarthritis (6303,6304).
Postherpetic neuralgia. DMSO used topically as a vehicle in combination with idoxuridine (40% idoxuridine in DMSO) seems to decrease the pain associated with postherpetic neuralgia (6310,6311,6312). Trigeminal herpes zoster seems most responsive (6312).
Rheumatoid arthritis (RA). Applying DMSO topically seems to help decrease symptoms associated with RA (6303,6304).
Skin flap ischemia. Applying DMSO topically seems to reduce skin flap ischemia after surgery (6307).

POSSIBLY INEFFECTIVE

Scleroderma. Applying 2% or 70% DMSO topically does not seem to help treat symptoms of scleroderma such as open ulcers (6313). Open studies on DMSO for scleroderma have been conflicting (6304,6313,6314).

LIKELY INEFFECTIVE

Cancer. Applying DMSO topically is not effective for treating cancer (6327).

There is insufficient reliable information available about the effectiveness of DMSO for its other uses.

Mechanism of Action

DMSO is a highly polar solvent used for many organic and inorganic substances. It also interacts with other molecules such as proteins, carbohydrates, lipids, water and ethanol (6331).
DMSO easily penetrates the skin (6326), and distributes widely into body fluids and tissues after administration. DMSO is metabolized to dimethyl sulfone and dimethyl sulfide in the body. The dimethyl sulfide metabolite is thought to cause the distinctive odor associated with DMSO use.

Concentrated DMSO (80-100%) penetrates more effectively than concentrations of less than 70%. This is thought to be due to DMSOs ability to exchange and interchange water molecules in cell membranes (6326), and also its ability to interfere with and cause conformational changes in cell membrane phospholipids (6331,6330). DMSO facilitates topical penetration of many medications (6326,6330).
DMSO has been found to decrease skin adhesions by possibly dissolving collagen fibers and not elastic fibers (6330). DMSO also stabilizes lysosomal membranes and causes vasodilation (6330).
DMSO has free hydroxyl radical scavenging properties (6326,6330) which might contribute to DMSOs anti-inflammatory, cryopreservative, cryoprotective, anti-ischemic, and possible radioprotective activity (6326).
DMSO also demonstrates antimicrobial activity (6326,6330), possibly by changing the RNA structure necessary for bacterial protein synthesis (6330). Cardiovascular and vasoactive effects of DMSO such as lowered vagal threshold and increased response to nerve and muscle stimulation on skeletal, smooth, and cardiac muscle are thought to be due to inhibition of anticholinesterase activity (6326,6330).
In vitro, DMSO appears to protect against ischemic injury by increasing levels of prostaglandin-E1 (PGE1) which in turn increases cyclic-AMP levels and reduces platelet aggregation. DMSO also appears to protect against ischemic injury by decreasing the secretion of vasoactive substances such as fibrinogen and thromboxane A2 from platelets that can cause vasoconstriction, vasospasm, or obstruction of vessels (6302,6330). Evidence also suggests DMSO slows the conduction of C-type nerve fibers which might explain its analgesic effects (6329).
DMSO also causes histamine release from mast cells, which is thought to be responsible for the eosinophilia and hypersensitivity reactions associated with its use (6324).
DMSO might affect sensory nerves during bladder instillations by stimulating bladder afferent pathways, causing release of nitrogen oxide from afferent neurons (9,5693). Nitrogen oxide is thought to act as a peripheral neurotransmitter controlling the lower urinary tract function (5693). Some data suggests DMSO could help antineoplastic agents cross the blood-brain barrier (6327), but other results show DMSO doesn't significantly increase uptake of these compounds (6330).
There is also evidence that suggests DMSO may induce differentiation of tumor cells present in frozen cryopreserved marrow (6328). Preliminary evidence suggests DMSO may be effective in treating duodenal ulceration in patients infected with Helicobacter pylori (6321).

Adverse Reactions
Topically, DMSO can cause sedation, headache, dizziness, drowsiness, nausea, vomiting, diarrhea, constipation, anorexia, and eosinophilia, erythema, pruritus, burning, blistering, drying and scaling skin, dry or sore throat, cough, dry nasal passages, dyspnea, worsening of bronchial asthma, and an influenza-like syndrome (6303,6304,6306,6308,6309,6311,6312,6313).
Intravenously, DMSO can cause facial flushing, fluid overload, hypernatremia, electrolyte disturbances, diuresis, increased serum osmolality, eosinophilia, hemolysis, hematuria, weakness, confusion, lethargy, disorientation, agitation, dysarthria, hypoactive reflexes, decreased consciousness, vasodilation, hypotension, chest pains, sinus tachycardia, increased serum creatinine, and encephalopathy (6300,6301,6315,6325).
Intravesical instillation of DMSO may cause a chemical cystitis, bladder discomfort, and spasm (9). Infusion of hematopoietic stem cells cryopreserved with DMSO can cause rigors, nausea, vomiting (6318), hypertension with tachycardia, bradycardia, chest tightness, fever, chills, abdominal cramps, ventricular extrasystoles (6320), electrolyte disturbances, and decreased hemoglobin (5695,5696,5697). Garlic-like taste, breath, and garlic-onion-oyster body odor may be experienced with all routes of administration. Hypersensitivity reactions may be experienced by all routes of administration, rarely causing anaphylaxis. Headache and transient eye, nose, and throat irritations have been reported by individuals caring for patients with DMSO body odor (6323).

Interactions with Herbs & Other Dietary Supplements
None known.

Interactions with Drugs
INJECTABLE DRUGS: Evidence from animal studies suggest DMSO may potentiate the action of numerous medications (6330).
ORAL DRUGS: Evidence from animal studies suggest DMSO may potentiate the action of numerous medications (6330).
TOPICAL DRUGS: Evidence from animal studies suggest DMSO may potentiate the action of numerous medications (6330).

Interactions with Foods
None known.

Interactions with Lab Tests
None known.

Interactions with Diseases or Conditions

DIABETES: Topical administration of DMSO has been reported to potentiate the effects of insulin (6326); use with caution. Increased monitoring of blood glucose and insulin dosing adjustments may be necessary.
HEMATOLOGIC CONDITIONS: Hemolysis with intravenous use has been reported (9); use with caution.
INTRACRANIAL PRESSURE: Extreme serum hyperosmolality has been reported in patients with elevated intracranial pressure who were treated with DMSO (6325).
LIVER CONDITIONS: Liver function tests are recommended every 6 months (9). Hepatotoxicity with infusion of DMSO has been reported (9); use with caution.
RENAL CONDITIONS: Renal function tests are recommended every 6 months (9). Acute tubular necrosis has been reported (9); use with caution.

Dosage and Administration

ORAL: For symptoms of amyloidosis, 7-15 grams of DMSO daily has been used (6304).
TOPICAL: For prevention of tissue necrosis after extravasation with antineoplastic agents, 77-90% DMSO is typically applied every 3-8 hours for 10-14 days. For acute musculoskeletal injuries and inflammation, 60-90% DMSO solution or gel is typically applied to the affected area 1-3 times daily for 1-3 weeks (6304). For osteoarthritis, 60-90% DMSO is typically applied to the affected area daily (6304). For rheumatoid arthritis, 60-90% DMSO solution is typically applied to the affected area 2-4 times daily (6304,6313). For scleroderma, 50-90% DMSO solution is typically applied to the affected area or the affected area is immersed in solution twice daily (6304). For amyloidosis, 50-100% DMSO solution is typically applied twice weekly to the affected area (6304). For amyloid-produced itching, 50-100% DMSO solution has been applied to the affected area daily (6304). For surgical flaps, 60% DMSO has been applied to the flaps every 4 hours for 10 days (6307). For herpes zoster, 5-40% idoxuridine in DMSO has been started within 48 hours after the appearance of a rash and applied every 4 hours for 4 days (6308). For neuropathic pain, 50% DMSO solution has been used 4 times daily for up to 3 weeks (6317).
INTRAVENOUS: For intracranial hypertension, a 10% solution of DMSO has been infused rapidly at a dose of 1 g/kg or a 20% DMSO solution is infused and titrated against the intracranial pressure (6300). A 28% solution of DMSO has also been used by infusing rapidly at a dose of 1.12 g/kg (6301).
INTRAVESICAL INSTILLATION: For interstitial cystitis, typically 50 mL of aqueous 50% DMSO solution is instilled into the bladder, the catheter is removed and the patient is instructed to hold the medication in the bladder for 15-20 minutes before voiding (5692). 100 mg of hydrocortisone has been added to the solution before instillation for added anti-inflammatory action in patients who do not respond favorably (5694). For chronic inflammatory bladder disease, 50 mL of aqueous 50% DMSO solution is typically instilled every 2 weeks for 3 treatments and then once every 4 weeks until symptoms decrease or patient is symptom free. Patients are usually instructed to hold in the medication for 30 minutes after instillation before voiding (5695).
NASOBILIARY CATHETER: For dissolution of bile duct stones, a mixture of 70/30 DMSO/methyl tert-butyl ether and a mixture of 26 mM ethylene diamine tetraacetic acid with 40 mM sodium deoxycholate and 30% DMSO has been infused alternatively and continuously for 2 hours via a nasobiliary catheter in the common bile duct until disappearance of stones (6315).

DODDER

Also Known As

Beggarweed, Cuscutae, Devil's Guts, Dodder Of Thyme, Hellweed, Lesser Dodder, Scaldweed, Strangle Tare, Tu Si Zi, Tu Sizi.

Scientific Names

Cuscuta epithymum; Cuscuta chinensis.
Family: Convolvulaceae.

Comments

At the date of publication, there was very little scientific information about this product. Our staff is continually analyzing the available information on natural medicines and will add data to the online version of *Natural Medicines Comprehensive Database* as it becomes available. See www.naturaldatabase.com.

DOLOMITE

Also Known As
Dolomitic Limestone.
CAUTION: See separate listings for Calcium and Magnesium.

Scientific Names
None.

People Use This For
Orally, dolomite is used as a mineral supplement of calcium and magnesium.

Safety
POSSIBLY UNSAFE ...when used orally. Dolomite supplements may contain lead; safer supplements are available (997,11719).
CHILDREN: POSSIBLY UNSAFE ...when used orally long-term due to the presence of lead in some products. Children are more sensitive to lead than adults (152).
PREGNANCY AND LACTATION: POSSIBLY UNSAFE ...when used orally (997,11719); avoid using.

Effectiveness
There is insufficient reliable information available about the effectiveness of dolomite.

Mechanism of Action
Dolomite is a type of limestone. It is rich in magnesium and calcium carbonate, and has smaller amounts of several other minerals. Dolomite can be contaminated with heavy metals such as lead (997,11719).

Adverse Reactions
Orally, some dolomite products are contaminated with heavy metals including aluminum, arsenic, lead, mercury, nickel, and others that may cause heavy metal poisoning (997,11719). Contaminated products have induced seizure activity in otherwise well-controlled patients who have seizure disorders (997). Calcium used orally can cause gastrointestinal irritation and constipation (9). Calcium carbonate can cause acid rebound (9). Large amounts of calcium carbonate can cause hypercalcemia and alkalosis (9). Magnesium can cause gastrointestinal irritation, nausea, vomiting, and diarrhea (9,15). Larger amounts may cause hypermagnesemia (9) with symptoms including thirst, hypotension, drowsiness, confusion, loss of tendon reflexes, muscle weakness, respiratory depression, cardiac arrhythmias, coma, cardiac arrest, and death (9).

Interactions with Herbs & Other Dietary Supplements
BORON: Can increase serum magnesium levels (940).
CALCIUM: Theoretically, concomitant use with other calcium containing supplements can cause constipation.
MAGNESIUM: Theoretically, concomitant use with other magnesium containing supplements can cause diarrhea.
VITAMIN D: Concomitant use can increase active absorption of oral calcium (945).

Interactions with Drugs
BISPHOSPHONATES: Cations, including calcium and magnesium decrease absorption of bisphosphonates. Advise patients to take bisphosphonates at least 30 minutes before dolomite, but preferably at a different time of day (15). The bisphosphonates include alendronate (Fosamax), etidronate (Didronel), risedronate (Actonel), and tiludronate (Skelid).
ESTROGENS: Concomitant use of estrogen increases calcium absorption in postmenopausal women (995).
LEVOTHYROXINE (Synthroid, Levothroid, Levoxyl, and others): The calcium in dolomite reduces levothyroxine absorption, probably by forming insoluble complexes (5082). Calcium carbonate supplements reduce effectiveness of levothyroxine in patients with hypothyroid (5081,5082,6137). Advise patients to take levothyroxine and dolomite at least four hours apart.
POTASSIUM-SPARING DIURETICS: Potassium-sparing diuretics also have magnesium-sparing properties, which can counteract the magnesium losses associated with loop and thiazide diuretics (9613,9614,9622). Theoretically, dolomite might cause increased magnesium levels with concomitant use of potassium-sparing diuretics. Potassium-sparing diuretics include amiloride (Midamor), triamterene (Dyrenium), and spironolactone (Aldactone).
QUINOLONE ANTIBIOTICS: Taking dolomite at the same time as quinolones reduces quinolone absorption. Multivalent cations such as calcium and magnesium form insoluble complexes with quinolones (4412,10339). Advise patients to take these drugs at least 2 hours before, or four to six hours after dolomite (10339). Quinolones include ciprofloxacin (Cipro), levofloxacin (Levaquin), ofloxacin (Floxin), moxifloxacin (Avelox), gatifloxacin (Tequin), gemifloxacin (Factive), and others.
SOTALOL (Betapace): The calcium in dolomite appears to reduce the absorption of sotalol, probably by forming insoluble complexes (10018). Advise patients to separate doses by at least 2 hours before or four

to six hours after dolomite.
TETRACYCLINE ANTIBIOTICS: Multivalent cations such as calcium and magnesium decrease the absorption of tetracyclines by forming insoluble complexes (9). Advise patients to take these drugs at least two hours before, or four to six hours after dolomite. Tetracyclines include demeclocycline (Declomycin), doxycycline (Vibramycin), and minocycline (Minocin).
THIAZIDE DIURETICS: Thiazides reduce calcium excretion by the kidneys (1902). Using thiazides along with moderately large amounts of dolomite increases the risk of milk-alkali syndrome (hypercalcemia, metabolic alkalosis, renal failure). These diuretics include chlorothiazide (Diuril), hydrochlorothiazide (HydroDIURIL, Esidrix), indapamide (Lozol), metolazone (Zaroxolyn), chlorthalidone (Hygroton), etc.

Drug Influences on Nutrient Levels and Depletion

SOME DRUGS CAN AFFECT DOLOMITE LEVELS:
CORTICOSTEROIDS: Concomitant use can decrease calcium absorption (15).

Interactions with Foods

DIETARY FIBER: Certain constituents of dietary fiber inhibit calcium absorption, including uronic acid and phytic acid, which is found in wheat bran (945).
FOOD: Concomitant ingestion with food, and food high in vitamin D, increases absorption of supplemental calcium (945).
IRON: Calcium carbonate taken with iron supplements and food might decrease supplemental iron absorption. Calcium carbonate taken with iron supplements on an empty stomach appears to have little effect on supplemental iron absorption (945).

Interactions with Lab Tests

ALKALINE PHOSPHATASE: The magnesium component might cause a false increase in serum alkaline phosphatase test results due to enzyme activation (275).
ANGIOTENSIN-CONVERTING ENZYME: The magnesium component might decrease serum ACE levels and test results (275).
CALCIUM: The magnesium component might cause a false increase in serum calcium test results in some procedures using edetate disodium (EDTA) (275).
DIAGNEX BLUE: The magnesium component might increase urine Diagnex blue excretion due to heavy metal displacement of Diagnex blue (275).
GASTRIN: The calcium component might cause a physiological increase in serum levels 30-75 minutes after using (275).
LIPASE: The calcium component might cause an analytical decrease in serum concentrations above 5 mmol/L on method of Tietz (275).

Interactions with Diseases or Conditions

HEART BLOCK: Magnesium is contraindicated in people with heart block (9).
HYPERPARATHYROIDISM: Primary hyperparathyroidism predisposes individuals to increased calcium absorption (945).
HYPOPARATHYROIDISM: Hypoparathyroidism predisposes individuals to reduced calcium absorption (945).
RENAL INSUFFICIENCY: Magnesium is contraindicated in people with severe renal disease. Use cautiously in individuals with reduced kidney function due to increased risk of hypermagnesemia (9). Calcium supplementation increases the risk of hypercalcemia and alkalosis in people with renal disease (9). Renal insufficiency predisposes individuals to reduced calcium absorption (945).
SARCOIDOSIS: Increases the risk of excessive calcium absorption and hypercalcemia (945).

Dosage and Administration

No typical dosage.

DONG QUAI

Also Known As

Chinese Angelica, Dang Gui, Danggui, Dong Qua, Dong-Quai, Ligustilides, Phytoestrogen, Tan Kue Bai Zhi, Tang Kuei.
CAUTION: See separate listings for Angelica root and Angelica herb, seed.

Scientific Names

Angelica sinensis, synonym Angelica polymorpha var. sinensis.
Family: Apiaceae/Umbelliferae.

People Use This For

Orally, dong quai is used for gynecological ailments including menstrual cramps, irregularity, retarded flow, weakness during the menstrual period, and symptoms of menopause. It is also used orally as a "blood purifier"; to manage hypertension, rheumatism, ulcers, anemia, and constipation; and in the prevention and treatment of allergic attacks. Dong quai is also used orally is for the treatment of skin depigmentation and psoriasis.

Safety

POSSIBLY SAFE ...when used orally and appropriately (10054).
POSSIBLY UNSAFE ...when used orally in large amounts. Dong quai contains several constituents that are carcinogenic (7162).
PREGNANCY: UNSAFE ...when used orally due to uterine stimulant and relaxant effects (8142).
LACTATION: Insufficient reliable information available; avoid using.

Effectiveness

POSSIBLY INEFFECTIVE

Menopausal symptoms. Dong quai does not seem to have any effect on endometrial wall thickness or menopausal symptoms (738).

There is insufficient reliable information available about the effectiveness of dong quai for its other uses.

Mechanism of Action

The applicable part of dong quai is the root. Dong quai root has several coumarin constituents including osthol, psoralen, and bergapten, and contains 0.4-0.7% volatile oil (10054). Some coumarins can act as vasodilators and antispasmodics. Osthol appears to inhibit platelet aggregation and smooth muscle contraction, and cause hypotension (10057). Psoralen and bergapten are photosensitizing and can cause severe photodermatitis (10057,10071). Bergapten and other dong quai constituents, such as safrole and isosafrole, are carcinogenic (7162). Dong quai also contains a low molecular weight polysaccharide that shows anti-tumor activity in animals (10056).

Limited research suggests that dong quai does not have estrogenic effects and therefore is not a phytoestrogen (736,738). However, other research suggests that suggests estrogenic effects (6180). Dong quai might stimulate the growth of breast cancer cells (7860,10979).

A dong quai extract competitively inhibits estradiol binding to estrogen receptors and induces transcription activity in estrogen-responsive cells (6180).

Preliminary research suggests dong quai might protect against ischemia- reperfusion injury (9985).

Adverse Reactions

Orally, dong quai is well-tolerated (738). Dong quai contains constituents that are carcinogenic (7162). Whether these constituents are present in concentrations large enough to cause cancer with long-term or high-dose use is unknown. Dong quai also contains psoralens that may cause photosensitivity and photodermatitis (10054,10071).

Interactions with Herbs & Other Dietary Supplements

HERBS WITH ANTICOAGULANT/ANTIPLATELET POTENTIAL: Concomitant use of herbs that have antiplatelet/anticoagulant effects could theoretically increase the risk of bleeding in some people (3526). These herbs include angelica, clove, danshen, garlic, ginger, ginkgo, Panax ginseng, poplar, red clover, willow, and others.

Interactions with Drugs

ANTICOAGULANT/ANTIPLATELET DRUGS: Theoretically, dong quai might potentiate the therapeutic and adverse effects of these drugs. Dong quai has been reported to inhibit platelet aggregation (6048).
WARFARIN (Coumadin): Concomitant use increases the anticoagulant effects of warfarin and the risk of bleeding (3526,6048). In one case, after 4 weeks of dong quai 565 mg once or twice daily, INR increased to 4.9. INR normalized 4 weeks after discontinuation of dong quai. Dong quai is thought to inhibit platelet activation and aggregation (6048).

Interactions with Foods

None known.

Interactions with Lab Tests

PROTHROMBIN TIME (PT), INTERNATIONAL NORMALIZATION RATIO (INR): Dong quai can enhance the effects of warfarin, resulting in increased PT and INR test results (3526).

Interactions with Diseases or Conditions

HORMONE SENSITIVE CANCERS/CONDITIONS: Because dong quai has estrogenic effects, women with hormone sensitive conditions including breast cancer, uterine cancer, ovarian cancer, endometriosis, and uterine fibroids should avoid using dong quai (6180,7860).

Dosage and Administration
ORAL: For menopausal symptoms, 4.5 g of powdered Dong Quai root has been used daily (738).

DRAGON'S BLOOD

Also Known As
Draconis Resina, Dracorubin, Dragons Blood, Dragon's-Blood Palm, Sanguis Draconis, Xue Jie.
CAUTION: See separate listings for Herb Robert and Sangre de Grado.

Scientific Names
Daemonorops draco, synonym Calamus draco.
Family: Arecaceae/Palmae.

People Use This For
Orally, dragon's blood is used for diarrhea, digestive disorders and as a coloring agent.
Topically, dragon's blood is used as an astringent.

Safety
POSSIBLY SAFE ...when used orally (12). There is insufficient reliable information available about the safety of the topical use of dragon's blood.
PREGNANCY AND LACTATION: Insufficient reliable information available; avoid using.

Effectiveness
There is insufficient reliable information available about the effectiveness of dragon's blood.

Mechanism of Action
The applicable part of dragon's blood is the fruit. There is insufficient reliable information available about the possible mechanism of action and active ingredients.

Adverse Reactions
None reported.

Interactions with Herbs & Other Dietary Supplements
None known.

Interactions with Drugs
None known.

Interactions with Foods
None known.

Interactions with Lab Tests
None known.

Interactions with Diseases or Conditions
None known.

Dosage and Administration
ORAL: Dragon's blood has been used as a powder (18).
TOPICAL: No typical dosage.

Comments
Dragon's blood is the red resin extracted from the fruit of Daemonorops draco (18).

DUCKWEED

Also Known As
None.

Scientific Names
Lemna minor.
Family: Lemnaceae.

Comments
At the date of publication, there was very little scientific information about this product. Our staff is continually analyzing the available information on natural medicines and will add data to the online version of *Natural Medicines Comprehensive Database* as it becomes available. See www.naturaldatabase.com.

DUSTY MILLER

Also Known As
None.

Scientific Names
Senecio cineraria, synonym Cineraria maritima.
Family: Asteraceae/Compositae.

People Use This For
Orally, dusty miller is used in preparations for eyesight problems (spots before the eyes), migraine, and to promote menstrual flow.

Safety
LIKELY UNSAFE ...when any part of the plant is used orally. Dusty miller contains hepatotoxic unsaturated pyrrolizidine alkaloids (UPAs) (18,19). Repeated exposure to low concentrations of UPAs are linked to veno-occlusive disease (4,12). UPAs may also be carcinogenic and mutagenic (12). ...when used topically on abraded or broken skin because it might be absorbed systemically (12,19).
PREGNANCY AND LACTATION: LIKELY UNSAFE ...when used orally because it contains UPA constituents (12). There is insufficient reliable information available about the safety of the topical use of dusty miller during pregnancy and lactation; avoid using.

Effectiveness
There is insufficient reliable information available about the effectiveness of dusty miller.

Mechanism of Action
Some unsaturated pyrrolizidine alkaloids (UPAs) have shown carcinogenic and mutagenic properties, and there are reports of renal toxicity. However, the primary concern is veno-occlusive disease (12). UPAs are known to be hepatotoxic in animals and humans (4).

Adverse Reactions
Orally, dusty miller may cause acute toxicity which may result in hepatic necrosis; chronic toxicity may cause veno-occlusive liver disease. The potential for hepatotoxicity, due to the presence of unsaturated pyrrolizidine alkaloids (UPAs), increases with larger doses and longer periods of use (4,12). Dusty miller may cause an allergic reaction in individuals sensitive to the Asteraceae/Compositae family. Members of this family include ragweed, chrysanthemums, marigolds, daisies, and many other herbs.

Interactions with Herbs & Other Dietary Supplements
EUCALYPTUS: Theoretically, concomitant use with dusty miller might increase the risk of unsaturated pyrrolizidine alkaloid (UPA) toxicity due to enzyme induction by eucalyptus (19).
UNSATURATED PYRROLIZIDINE ALKALOID (UPA)-CONTAINING HERBS: Concomitant use with dusty miller is contraindicated due to the risk of additive toxicity (4,12,19). Herbs containing UPAs include alkanna, borage, gravel root, hemp agrimony, hound's tongue, petasites, comfrey, coltsfoot, and the other Senecio species including alpine ragwort, groundsel, golden ragwort, and tansy ragwort.

Interactions with Drugs
None known.

Interactions with Foods
None known.

Interactions with Lab Tests
None known.

Interactions with Diseases or Conditions
CROSS-ALLERGENICITY: Dusty miller may cause an allergic reaction in individuals sensitive to the Asteraceae/Compositae family. Members of this family include ragweed, chrysanthemums, marigolds, daisies, and many other herbs.
LIVER DISEASE: Contraindicated.

Dosage and Administration
No typical dosage.

Comments
American Herbal Products Association recommends labeling all botanical products that contain toxic pyrrolizidine alkaloids "For external use only. Do not apply to broken or abraded skin; do not use when nursing" (12).

DWARF ELDER

Also Known As
Blood Elder, Blood Hilder, Danewort, Walewort.
CAUTION: See separate listings for American Elder, Elderberry, and Elderflower.

Scientific Names
Sambucus ebulus.
Family: Adoxaceae/Sambucaceae or Caprifoliaceae.

People Use This For
Orally, dwarf elder is used for arthritis, weight reduction, and as a diuretic.

Safety
LIKELY UNSAFE ...when large quantities of any part of the plant are used orally. It can cause loss of consciousness and death (18).
There is insufficient reliable information available about the safety of the oral use of dwarf elder in small amounts.
PREGNANCY AND LACTATION: LIKELY UNSAFE ...when used orally in large quantities (18).

Effectiveness
There is insufficient reliable information available about the effectiveness of dwarf elder.

Mechanism of Action
Dwarf elder contains iridoide monoterpene glycosides. The constituents that cause nausea or purgative effects have not been identified (18).

Adverse Reactions
Orally, ingestion of large quantities of any plant part of dwarf elder may cause vomiting, bloody diarrhea, cyanosis, dizziness, headache and unconsciousness. Death has been reported (18). Cyanide poisoning can be caused by any plant part of dwarf elder. Sambunigrine, a cyanogenic glycoside, is present in the plant.

Interactions with Herbs & Other Dietary Supplements
None known.

Interactions with Drugs
None known.

Interactions with Foods
None known.

Interactions with Lab Tests
None known.

Interactions with Diseases or Conditions
None known.

Dosage and Administration
No typical dosage.

Comments
Dwarf elder is considered unsafe; avoid using. Dwarf elder is considered obsolete as a medicinal herb in many countries (18). Avoid confusion with Elderberry and American Elder, which are also members of the Sambucus genus (6002).

DWARF PINE NEEDLE

Also Known As
None.
CAUTION: See separate listings for Fir, Fir Needle Oil, Pine, Poplar, and Scotch Pine Needle Oil.

Scientific Names
Pinus mugo, synonym Pinus montana; Pinus mugo var. pumilio, synonym Pinus pumilio.
Family: Pinaceae.

People Use This For
Orally, dwarf pine needle is used as an expectorant.
Topically, dwarf pine needle is used in liniments and as an antiseptic.
In foods and beverages, dwarf pine needle is used as a flavoring agent.
In other manufacturing processes, dwarf pine needle is used as a flavoring and fragrance component in pharmaceutical preparations (cough and cold medicines, vaporizer fluids, nasal decongestants, analgesic ointments), and as a fragrance ingredient in soaps and cosmetics (maximum use level 1.2% in perfumes).

Safety
LIKELY SAFE ...when used orally in amounts commonly found in foods. Dwarf pine needle has Generally Recognized As Safe (GRAS) status in the US (4912).
POSSIBLY SAFE ...when used topically. There is possible human skin irritation and demonstrated sensitizing in some individuals (11).
PREGNANCY AND LACTATION: Insufficient reliable information available; avoid using.

Effectiveness
There is insufficient reliable information available about the effectiveness of dwarf pine needle.

Mechanism of Action
The applicable part of dwarf pine needle is the oil. Constituents bornyl acetate, dipentene, and limonene are believed to have antibacterial and antiviral properties (11).

Adverse Reactions
Topically, dwarf pine needle can cause skin irritation (11). It also may be sensitizing in some individuals (11).

Interactions with Herbs & Other Dietary Supplements
None known.

Interactions with Drugs
None known.

Interactions with Foods
None known.

Interactions with Lab Tests
None known.

Interactions with Diseases or Conditions
ALLERGY: Avoid dwarf pine needle if allergic or sensitive to pine oil.

Dosage and Administration
No typical dosage.

Comments
Dwarf pine needle oil is produced by distillation of dwarf pine (Pinus mugo) needles and twigs. Avoid confusion with fir needle oil and scotch pine needle oil.

DYER'S BROOM

Also Known As
Broom Flower, Dyers Broom, Dyer's Greenwood, Dyer's Weed, Dyer's Whin, Furze, Green Broom, Greenweed, Wood Waxen.

Scientific Names
Genista tinctoria.
Family: Leguminosae or Fabaceae.

People Use This For
Orally, dyer's broom is used for digestive disorders, gout, as an emetic or purgative, and to remove bladder stones. It is also used orally to "detoxify" blood, to increase heart rate, strengthen blood vessels, stimulate blood flow to the kidneys, and to alter metabolism. It has been used to deepen breathing and alleviate pain in the lower back and pelvis.

Safety
POSSIBLY UNSAFE ...when above ground parts are used orally (12).
PREGNANCY: LIKELY UNSAFE ...when used orally because it could have uterine-stimulant activity (12).
LACTATION: POSSIBLY UNSAFE ...when used orally; avoid using.

Effectiveness
There is insufficient reliable information available about the effectiveness of dyer's broom.

Mechanism of Action
Dyer's broom contains quinolizidine alkaloids, including methylcytisine, anagyrine, isopsparteine, lupanine, tinctorin, and cysisine. It also contains flavonoids (including luteolin glycosides), isoflavonoids (including genistein and genistin), and lectins (18).

Adverse Reactions
Orally, dyer's broom may cause nausea and vomiting. Overuse of dyer's broom can lead to diarrhea (18).

Interactions with Herbs & Other Dietary Supplements
None known.

Interactions with Drugs
None known.

Interactions with Foods
None known.

Interactions with Lab Tests
None known.

Interactions with Diseases or Conditions
None known.

Dosage and Administration
No typical dosage.

ECDYSTERONE

Also Known As
Alfa-ecdysone, Beta-ecdysone, Ecdisten, Ecdysone, Hydroxyecdysterone, Isoinokosterone, Suma.
CAUTION: See separate listing for Suma.

Scientific Names
None.

People Use This For
Orally, ecdysterone is used to increase muscle mass and improve athletic performance.

Safety
There is insufficient reliable information available about the safety of ecdysterone.
Pregnancy and Lactation: Insufficient reliable information available.

Effectiveness
There is insufficient reliable information available about the effectiveness of ecdysterone.

Mechanism of Action
Ecdysterone is a chemical found in insects, some aquatic animals, and some plants. In insects and arthropods, ecdysterone promotes the act of molting (9903,10389).
Ecdysterone is chemically similar to testosterone, which has lead to the belief that it might possess anabolic properties. Animal research suggests that ecdysterone affects steroid receptors. It is unclear whether this effect is mediated by receptor or feedback loop regulation rather than bioconversion into steroids. Possible mechanisms include anticatabolic effects from blocking cortisol receptors and stimulation of anabolic or androgenic steroid receptors (9904,9905,10390). However, there is no research in humans demonstrating androgenic or myotrophic effect.
After oral administration, ecdysterone and its metabolites appear in the urine for approximately 68 hours. The primary metabolites are deoxyecdysterone and dexoyecdysone (9903).

Adverse Reactions
None reported.

Interactions with Herbs & Other Dietary Supplements
None known.

Interactions with Drugs
None known.

Interactions with Foods
None known.

Interactions with Lab Tests
None known.

Interactions with Diseases or Conditions
None known.

Dosage and Administration
No typical dosage.

ECHINACEA

Also Known As
American Cone Flower, Black Sampson, Black Susans, Brauneria Angustifolia, Brauneria Pallida, Comb Flower, Coneflower, Echinaceawurzel, Hedgehog, Igelkopfwurzel, Indian Head, Kansas Snakeroot, Narrow-leaved Purple Cone Flower, Pale Coneflower, Purple Cone Flower, Purpursonnenhutkraut, Purpursonnenhutwurzel, Racine d'echininacea, Red Sunflower, Rock-Up-Hat, Roter Sonnenhut, Schmallblaettrige Kegelblumenwurzel, Schmallblaettriger Sonnenhut, Scurvy Root, Snakeroot, Sonnenhutwurzel.

Scientific Names
Echinacea angustifolia; Echinacea pallida; Echinacea purpurea.
Family: Asteraceae/Compositae.

People Use This For
Orally, echinacea is used for treating and preventing the common cold and other upper respiratory infections. Echinacea is also used orally as an immunostimulant for fighting a variety of other infections, including urinary tract infections (UTIs), vaginal candidiasis (yeast infections), and genital herpes (HSV Type 1 and 2). Echinacea is also used orally for septicemia, nasopharyngeal catarrh, allergic rhinitis, pyorrhea, tonsillitis, streptococcus infections, syphilis, typhoid, malaria, and diphtheria. Other uses include rheumatism, migraines, dyspepsia, pain, dizziness, rattlesnake bites, and attention deficit-hyperactivity disorder (ADHD).
Topically, echinacea is used for boils, abscesses, skin wounds and ulcers, eczema, psoriasis, UV radiation skin damage, herpes simplex, bee stings, and hemorrhoids.
Intravenously, echinacea is used for recurrent vaginal candidiasis (yeast infections), and urinary tract infections (UTIs).
Intravenously and intramuscularly, echinacea is used to prolong survival time in patients with advanced hepatocellular carcinoma and colorectal cancer.

Safety
LIKELY SAFE ...when used orally and appropriately, short-term. Echinacea has been used safely in trials lasting up to 12 weeks (1412,3279,3280,3281,3282,6417). ...when used topically and appropriately (12).
There is insufficient reliable information available about the safety of echinacea when used orally, long-term.
PREGNANCY: POSSIBLY SAFE ...when used orally, short-term. There is some evidence that mothers can safely use echinacea for 5-7 days during the first trimester of pregnancy without adversely affecting the fetus (7056). However, this evidence is preliminary. Tell pregnant patients not to use echinacea without the supervision of their healthcare provider.
LACTATION: Insufficient reliable information available; avoid using.

Effectiveness
POSSIBLY EFFECTIVE

Common cold. Taking echinacea orally might help treat the common cold. Although some studies show no benefit (3282,10800,11970), most evidence suggests that echinacea modestly reduces symptom severity and duration, ranging from about 10% to 30% (1412,3281,6384,6385,6392,6417,10782,10802,12355). Tell patients that echinacea seems to be most effective if started when symptoms are first noticed and continued for 7-10 days. However, echinacea does not seem to help when taken prophylactically to prevent the common cold (3281,3282,6386,6417,8228,10782,12354). Most studies have used Echinacea purpurea species, but several other preparations have also been used including extracts of the herb, combination root and herb extracts, extracts of the root, as well as root extracts of Echinacea pallida and Echinacea angustifolia (1412,3280,3281,6417,8226). Echinacea teas and fixed combination herbal preparations containing echinacea have also been used (3281,6384,6392).

Vaginal candidiasis. Taking echinacea orally in combination with a topical antifungal cream seems to be effective for preventing recurrent vaginal yeast infection. Herb juice of Echinacea purpurea in combination with topical econazole (Spectazole) lowers recurrence rate to 16.7% compared to 60.5% with econazole alone (4800).

POSSIBLY INEFFECTIVE

Herpes simplex virus (HSV). Taking echinacea orally doesn't seem to prevent or treat recurrent genital herpes infection. A specific Echinacea purpurea extract (Echinaforce by Bioforce AG) 800 mg twice daily for six months does not seem to prevent or reduce frequency or duration of recurrent genital herpes in patients with herpes simplex virus (HSV) type 1 or 2 (7087).

Clinical studies have used a wide variety of specific extracts and dosage forms of echinacea. Some of these include a Echinacea purpurea 95% herb and 5% root extract (Echinaforce, Bioforce); a fixed combination of Echinacea purpurea plus cedar and wild indigo extracts (Esberitox N, Enzymatic Therapy); and a tea containing a blend of Echinacea purpurea and Echinacea angustifolia leaves, stems, and flowers plus a dry extract of Echinacea purpurea root (Echinacea Plus, Traditional Medicinals).

INSUFFICIENT RELIABLE EVIDENCE to RATE

Influenza. Taking echinacea orally might modestly reduce some influenza symptoms. However, there is not

enough specific evidence to know if echinacea is effective for influenza (3281,6384,6385,6386).
Leukopenia. An isolated polysaccharide fraction of Echinacea purpurea given intravenously might reduce leukopenia caused by chemotherapy (8523).
More evidence is needed to rate echinacea for these uses.

Mechanism of Action

The applicable parts of echinacea are the roots and the above ground parts. Echinacea is used for upper respiratory tract infections such as the common cold and influenza infections because it is reported to have antiviral and immune system stimulatory effects (3279). Echinacea increases phagocytosis and increases lymphocyte activity, possibly by promoting the release of tumor necrosis factor (TNF), interleukin-1 (IL-1), and interferon (3279,6388,6389). Several constituents of echinacea seem to be involved in stimulating this non-specific immune response. Some of these include high-molecular weight polysaccharides, such as heteroxylan and arabinogalactan; and lower molecular weight compounds, including alkylamides and caffeoyl conjugates such as chicoric acid and echinacosides (3279). Heteroxylan might activate phagocytosis, and arabinogalactan seems to induce macrophages to produce the cytokines TNF, IL-1, and interferon beta-2 (3279). Macrophages activated by arabinogalactan have been found to be cytotoxic against tumor cells and micro-organisms (6388). The chicoric acid and echinacosides constituents are thought to also play a role in enhancing phagocytosis (3279). Polysaccharides in echinacea also seem to have moderate effects on B-lymphocytes, but no apparent activity on T-lymphocytes (6389). However, echinacea doesn't seem to have any effect on the immune system of healthy volunteers (10797). Some researchers suggest that when echinacea is used for greater than eight weeks, the immunostimulatory effects might decline, making it less effective (6417,6418). To prevent this decline in activity, it is often recommended that a one-week drug holiday be taken after each eight-week treatment period (6418). However, there is no reliable evidence to support either of these claims.
Echinacea's effect on cold symptoms might result from anti-inflammatory activity. In vitro research suggests constituents of echinacea might inhibit cyclooxygenase and 5-lipogenase (10798,10799). Clinical research also suggests and anti-inflammatory effect. Serum ferritin, which appears to be an indicator of inflammatory cytokines, is lowered in people treated with echinacea (10797).
Echinacea is also reported to have antifungal properties, so people use it for yeast infections (vaginal candidiasis). Polyacetylenic compounds in echinacea, including ketoalkenes and ketoalkynes, seem to have antifungal activity, including activity against Candida yeast (6390).
For wound healing, echinacea seems to promote the formation of mesenchymal mucopolysaccharides, stimulate histogenic and hematogenic phagocytes, promote differentiation of fibrocytes from fibroblasts; and it also stimulates the anterior pituitary-adrenal cortex (11). Several conjugates isolated from echinacea have also been reported to inhibit tissue, and bacterial hyaluronidase and have anti-inflammatory activity (3279). The constituent echinacin has also been found to promote tissue granulation (3279). Preliminary information suggests that the caffeoyl constituents of echinacea might help treat or prevent UV radiation skin damage by protecting collagen from free radical damage (8227).
Preliminary research also suggests that high concentrations of Echinacea purpurea might reduce sperm and ova fertility (4239,4240). Initial research also shows that very high doses of echinacea do not seem to have genotoxic or carcinogenic effects (1413).

Adverse Reactions

Orally, echinacea is usually very well tolerated (1412,3279,3280,3282,6387,11970); however, some patients may experience allergic reactions, fever, nausea, vomiting, heartburn, constipation, abdominal pain, diarrhea, unpleasant taste, dry mouth, sore throat, burning sensation and numbness of the tongue, mouth ulcers, headache, dizziness, insomnia, and disorientation (8225,11970,12354,12355). Allergic reactions can include urticaria; erythema nodosum (7057); itchy, watery eyes; runny nose (8225); chest tightness; dyspnea; bronchospasm; acute asthma; facial and upper airway angioedema; and anaphylaxis (638,1358,8225). Allergic reactions seem to be relatively uncommon, but some people are more likely to be sensitive. For example, atopic individuals, people with a genetic tendency toward allergic conditions, are at increased risk for allergic reactions to echinacea (1358,8225). Individuals sensitive to the Asteraceae/Compositae plant family might also be more likely to experience an allergic reaction to echinacea (4239,4240,8225). Members of this family include ragweed, chrysanthemums, marigolds, daisies, and many other herbs.
Sjogren's syndrome has occurred in a patient taking herbal supplements including echinacea, St. John's wort, and kava. Laboratory, but not clinical, research suggests that echinacea has immunostimulant effects. Because Sjogren's syndrome is an autoimmune disorder, echinacea was suspected as the causative agent. However, the role of echinacea and the other herbal products in developing this syndrome is unclear (10319).
There is some preliminary evidence that suggests that high doses of echinacea might reduce male and female fertility (4239,4240). However, this effect has not yet been demonstrated in humans.
Parenterally, echinacea has been associated with shivering, muscle weakness, and slight reddening with transient pain at the injection site (6387).

Interactions with Herbs & Other Dietary Supplements

None known.

Interactions with Drugs

CYTOCHROME P450 3A4 (CYP3A4) SUBSTRATES: There's preliminary evidence that suggests that echinacea can inhibit the cytochrome P450 3A4 (CYP3A4) isoenzymes (6450,12155). Theoretically, echinacea might increase levels of drugs metabolized by CYP3A4. However, so far, this interaction has not been reported in humans. Some drugs metabolized by CYP3A4 include lovastatin (Mevacor), ketoconazole (Nizoral), itraconazole (Sporanox), fexofenadine (Allegra), triazolam (Halcion), and numerous others. Use echinacea cautiously or avoid in patients taking these drugs.

IMMUNOSUPPRESSANTS: Theoretically, echinacea may interfere with immunosuppressant therapy (3279) because of its immunostimulating activity. Echinacea stimulates phagocytosis and increases respiratory cellular activity and the mobility of leukocytes. Immunosuppressant drugs include azathioprine (Imuran), basiliximab (Simulect), cyclosporine (Neoral, Sandimmune), daclizumab (Zenapax), muromonab-CD3 (OKT3, Orthoclone OKT3), mycophenolate (CellCept), tacrolimus (FK506, Prograf), sirolimus (Rapamune), prednisone (Deltasone, Orasone), and other corticosteroids (glucocorticoids).

MIDAZOLAM (Versed): Taking midazolam and echinacea together seems to increase midazolam availability. This suggests that echinacea inhibits cytochrome P450 3A4 (CYP3A4) (12155).

Interactions with Foods

None known.

Interactions with Lab Tests

None known.

Interactions with Diseases or Conditions

ATOPY: Individuals with atopy (a genetic tendency toward allergic conditions) may be more likely to experience an allergic reaction when taking echinacea. Case reports describe 23 cases of allergic reactions to echinacea consistent with IgE mediated hypersensitivity. Thirty-four percent of the reactions were in patients with atopy (1358). In a related study, 20% of 100 atopic patients tested who had never taken echinacea had positive skin test reactions to echinacea, indicating hypersensitivity without previous exposure (1358,8225).

PEMPHIGUS VULGARIS: In one case, a patient with well-controlled pemphigus vulgaris took echinacea and within 1 week developed a disease flare including blisters on his trunk, head, and oral mucosa. When echinacea was discontinued, symptoms decreased, but did not entirely resolve (12171). The immunostimulatory effects of echinacea are thought to exacerbate this and other autoimmune disorders.

Dosage and Administration

ORAL: For treatment of upper respiratory infections including the common cold and influenza, a wide variety of doses have been used depending on the formulation. A tablet containing 6.78 mg of Echinacea purpurea crude extract based on 95% herb and 5% root (Echinaforce, Bioforce AG) is dosed as two tablets given 3 times daily (1412). Freeze-dried echinacea juice extract capsules 100 mg three times daily have been used (11970). Echinacea purpurea herb juice has been used in a daily dose of 6-9 mL for up to a maximum of 8 weeks (3282). Echinacea purpurea herb juice has also been used in a dose of 20 drops every 2 hours for the first day followed by 20 drops three times daily until symptoms resolve. An echinacea pallida root tincture, equivalent to 900 mg herb daily, has also been used (3281). An echinacea herbal compound tea (Echinacea Plus, Traditional Medicinals), consisting of leaves, flowers, and stems of Echinacea purpurea and Echinacea angustifolia plus dried extract of Echinacea purpurea root, has been used by drinking 5-6 cups of tea on the first day of symptoms and titrating down to 1 cup per day over the next 5 days (6384). The tea is prepared by pouring 8 ounces of boiling water over one tea bag and steeping, covered, for 10-15 minutes (6384). Echinacea liquid (Echinagard) 20 drops every 2 hours for the first day of symptoms, then 3 times daily for up to 10 days has been used to decrease the duration of symptoms of the common cold (10320).

TOPICAL: No typical dosage.

INTRAVENOUS: No typical dosage.

Comments

There are three main Echinacea species of medicinal interest: Echinacea angustifolia, Echinacea pallida, and Echinacea purpurea. Echinacea species are native to North America and were used as traditional herbal remedies by the Great Plains Indian tribes, and were adopted for medicinal use by settlers (3279). Echinacea angustifolia and Echinacea pallida were official in the US National Formulary from 1916 to 1950 (11). Conventional use of echinacea fell out of favor in the United States with the discovery of antibiotics and due to the lack of scientific data supporting its use, but it continued to be widely used in Europe (3279). The development of antibiotic resistance has contributed to the renewed interest in echinacea. Echinacea products have been commonly adulterated. The results from clinical studies performed prior to 1991 might be unreliable unless the plant material used was positively confirmed (1414,3279). Identification of Echinacea is now confirmed by HPLC analysis (1414). Although some echinacea extract products are standardized for their echinacoside content, echinacoside is not a specific marker for Echinacea purpurea, Echinacea angustifolia or Echinacea pallida (11). It has been suggested that Echinacea preparations could be standardized according to their alkamide content because alkamides levels have been found to vary significantly between the parts and commercial products of Echinacea purpurea (6391).

EDTA

Also Known As

Calcium Disodium Edathamil, Calcium Disodium Edetate, Calcium Disodium EDTA, Calcium Disodium Versenate, Calcium Edetate, Calcium EDTA, Disodium Edathamil, Disodium Edetate, Disodium EDTA, Disodium Tetraacetate, Iron EDTA, Sodium Edetate.

Scientific Names

Ethylenediamine tetraacetic acid; Disodium ethylenediamine tetraacetic acid; Trisodium ethylenediamine tetraacetic acid.

People Use This For

Topically, EDTA has been used as an ointment for skin irritations produced by metals such as chromium, nickel and copper.
Intravenously and intramuscularly, EDTA is used for acute and chronic lead poisoning and lead encephalopathy. Intravenous EDTA is also used in the calcium EDTA mobilization test which is used to evaluate a patient's response to chelation therapy for suspected lead poisoning. EDTA is also used intravenously to treat poisonings by radioactive products such as plutonium, thorium, uranium, and strontium. It is also used intravenously for removing copper in patients with Wilson's disease, hypercalcemia, cardiac glycoside-induced arrhythmias, atherosclerotic vascular disease, scleroderma, porphyria, hypercholesterolemia, and in the diagnosis of hypoparathyroidism. EDTA has also been used intravenously to treat essential hypertension, Raynaud's syndrome, intermittent claudication, gangrene, cancer, rheumatoid arthritis, osteoarthritis, decreased vision due to macular degeneration, diabetes, Alzheimer's disease, multiple sclerosis, Parkinson's disease, psoriasis, and angina.
Ophthalmically, EDTA is used for corneal calcium deposits in the eye.
In foods, EDTA is used as iron EDTA to fortify grain-based products such as breakfast cereals and cereal bars. EDTA is also used as calcium disodium EDTA and disodium EDTA as an additive to preserve food; and to promote the color, texture, and flavor of food.
In manufacturing, EDTA is used as disodium EDTA and trisodium EDTA to improve stability in pharmaceutical preparations, detergents, liquid soaps, shampoos, agricultural chemical sprays, oil emulsion devices, contact lens cleaners and cosmetics. It is also used in manufactured clinical laboratory evacuated blood collection tubes to anticoagulate blood specimens.

Safety

LIKELY SAFE ...when used orally in amounts commonly found in foods. EDTA has Generally Recognized As Safe (GRAS) status in the US (4912,10266). ...when used intravenously or intramuscularly and appropriately, short-term. Parenteral EDTA in the disodium and calcium disodium forms are FDA-approved prescription products (15).
POSSIBLY SAFE ...when used ophthalmically and appropriately (5774). Solutions of 0.35-1.85% EDTA in the disodium form seem to be safe (5774).
LIKELY UNSAFE ...when used intravenously or intramuscularly in excessive doses or long-term. Doses exceeding 50 mg/kg/day or greater than 3 grams per day, or used longer than 5-7 days per treatment course are associated with severe toxicity including nephrotoxicity (5733). ...when used intravenously and infused at an excessive rate. Infusion of the disodium form of EDTA over less than 3 hours can cause severe, life-threatening adverse effects including hypocalcemia and death (5737).
PREGNANCY AND LACTATION ...when used orally and appropriately in amounts commonly found in foods (7705,10266). There is insufficient reliable information available for other forms of EDTA; avoid using.

Effectiveness

EFFECTIVE

Lead toxicity. Administering EDTA intravenously and intramuscularly is effective for treating acute and chronic lead poisoning and lead encephalopathy (15,5730,5731,5734,5735,5736). The calcium disodium form of EDTA is FDA approved for these uses (15). Calcium disodium EDTA is used when blood lead concentrations are 45 ug/dL or greater or when patients are symptomatic. Treatment of 3-5 days is usually required to lower blood lead levels below 40 ug/dL (15,5730,5733). A second treatment course can be required if blood lead concentrations rebound to 45 ug/dL or greater within 5-7 days after the initial treatment (15). Treatment with calcium disodium EDTA improves symptoms of lead poisoning such as abdominal pain, fatigue, constipation, and anorexia (5730). It also seems slow progression of renal dysfunction in patients who have had chronic lead poisoning (5732). Calcium disodium EDTA is preferred to disodium EDTA for lead poisoning because unlike calcium disodium EDTA, disodium EDTA can significantly lower serum calcium levels and cause hypocalcemia when used in doses necessary to treat lead poisoning (15). However, EDTA does not seem to be effective for diagnosing lead poisoning. Some clinicians use a diagnostic test known as the calcium EDTA mobilization test. Many experts consider the test obsolete due to technical inconsistencies in administering and interpreting the test (5733). Treatment of lead poisoning should not be delayed for performance of this test if blood lead levels are 45 mcg/dL or greater (15).

LIKELY EFFECTIVE

Cardiac glycoside-induced ventricular arrhythmias. Administering EDTA intravenously is effective for emergency treatment of cardiac glycoside-induced ventricular arrhythmias. The disodium form of EDTA is approved by the FDA for this use. Disodium EDTA works rapidly to control ventricular arrhythmias, but it is very short acting (15,5761,5762). Clinicians do not consider it the preferred treatment (15). Other agents such as lidocaine or phenytoin (Dilantin) (505) are typically used because they are safer and more effective (15).

Hypercalcemia. Administering EDTA intravenously is effective for emergency treatment of hypercalcemia. The disodium form of EDTA is approved by the FDA for this use (15). Disodium EDTA can temporarily lower serum calcium to safe levels (15). However, clinicians generally prefer other methods of treatment such as forced diuresis with saline or use of pamidronate (Aredia), calcitonin (Miacalcin, others), or glucocorticoids (5775). These treatments more effectively lower serum calcium concentrations over longer periods of time than would be achieved with disodium EDTA and are less likely to cause renal side effects (15).

POSSIBLY EFFECTIVE

Corneal calcium deposits. A single ophthalmic application of the disodium form of EDTA can clear corneal calcium deposits, and improve eyesight (5773,5774). However, debridement of the corneal epithelium prior to application of EDTA is required (5773,5774).

POSSIBLY INEFFECTIVE

Scleroderma. Administering EDTA intravenously doesn't seem to be effective for treating localized and systemic scleroderma. Although there have been some anecdotal reports showing benefit (5757,5760), clinical studies show no significant changes or improvements in the skin or joints of scleroderma patients treated with disodium EDTA (5757,5758,5759,5760).

LIKELY INEFFECTIVE

Coronary heart disease. Administering EDTA intravenously isn't effective for treating coronary heart disease or peripheral arterial occlusive disease. The effectiveness of EDTA in chelation therapy is highly debated (5738,5739). Proponents often cite anecdotal reports or poorly controlled studies as evidence to support EDTA chelation therapy (5737,5738,5739,5740,5742,5743,5751,5770), but well-designed research shows that EDTA offers no significant benefit for these conditions (5737,5740,5742,5750,5752,5753,5754).

Mechanism of Action

Ethylenediaminetetraacetic acid (EDTA) is known as a chelating agent. It is a complex molecule with a claw-like structure, which binds and seizes divalent and trivalent metal ions such as calcium and aluminum to form a stable ring structure (5729,5749). EDTA binds and chelates metal ions in the following decreasing order: chromium, iron (ferric ion), mercury, copper, aluminum, nickel, zinc, calcium, cobalt, iron (ferrous ion), manganese, calcium, and magnesium (5737). After intravenous administration, accessible metal ions are chelated forming stable soluble complexes, which are then excreted in the urine (505). EDTA is not metabolized, but elimination is decreased with renal dysfunction (5737). Calcium disodium EDTA and disodium EDTA are the two forms of EDTA available for clinical use (15). Calcium disodium EDTA is the form of EDTA used primarily for lead poisoning (5730,5731,5732,5733,5734,5735,5736). The calcium in calcium disodium EDTA is displaced by metal ions such as lead to form a soluble complex that is then excreted in the urine (15). Unlike disodium EDTA, calcium disodium EDTA can be administered in large quantities without causing substantial changes in serum or total body calcium concentrations (15). Radioactive isotopes such as uranium and plutonium can also be chelated to a limited extent by calcium disodium EDTA (15).

Disodium EDTA antagonizes the ventricular inotropic and chronotropic effects of cardiac glycosides on the heart by decreasing the amount of extracellular calcium in the blood (5761,5762). Some researchers think that decreased extracellular calcium can increase potassium re-entry into myocardial cells which then counteracts with the intracellular potassium depletion caused by cardiac glycosides (5762).

Ophthalmically, disodium EDTA is used to dissolve corneal calcium deposits by binding with calcium in the eye (5774). EDTA can also disorganize the outer membrane of gram-negative bacteria, inhibit the coaggregation between pairs of microorganisms and is possibly an effective inhibitor of bacterial adhesins (5764).

Chelation therapy using disodium EDTA has been purported by many as being efficacious in the treatment of many disease conditions, including atherosclerosis (5738,5739,5743,5751,5768). Many biochemical mechanisms have been proposed to justify the use of disodium EDTA in the treatment of atherosclerotic vascular disease (5738,5741,5743). Mechanisms claimed include that EDTA chelation therapy can extract calcium out of atherosclerotic plaques and clear atherosclerotic arteries (5742,5749) or that calcium removed by chelation is replaced by calcium from the bone, causing secretion of parathyroid hormone (PTH) which then promotes a transfer of calcium from hardened arterial tissue and plaque to bone (5749).

Other mechanisms claimed also include that EDTA blocks production of free radicals involved in reactions causing atherosclerosis by reducing iron loads (5738), by binding toxic metals released when blood clots in occluded arteries (5749), or that disodium EDTA prevents damage and mutation of arterial cells caused by free radicals (5749). None of these proposed mechanisms have been scientifically proven (5749,5756), and controlled scientific clinical studies have been unable to confirm that EDTA can reverse peripheral arterial occlusive disease (5740,5742) or atherosclerotic vascular disease (5746,5750,5752,5753,5754,5769).

Severe nephrotoxicity is the major toxicity that can result when disodium EDTA and calcium disodium EDTA is used in excessively large doses (15). The degeneration of proximal tubular cells that results is proposed to be due to an interaction between EDTA and endogenous metals in the tubular cells (505). EDTA can also chelate and cause increased urinary excretion of magnesium (15), which may also result in decreased serum concentrations and increased excretion of potassium (15). Sudden decreases in calcium can occur if disodium EDTA is administered too rapidly, resulting in tetany, cardiac arrhythmias, and respiratory arrest (5763).

Disodium EDTA inhibits the growth of Candida albicans in vitro. EDTA binds the calcium that is required for growth of this fungal species (4621).

Adverse Reactions

Intravenously, EDTA can commonly cause abdominal cramps, anorexia, nausea, vomiting, diarrhea, headache (15), hypotension (5737), exfoliative dermatitis (15), and a burning sensation and pain at the site of infusion (5744). EDTA can also sometimes cause fever, chills, fatigue, malaise, thirst, sneezing and nasal congestion (15), arrhythmias (5771,5772), thrombophlebitis (15), anemia (15), prolonged prothrombin time (PT) (5737), transient bone marrow depression (5737,5772), and urinary urgency and frequency (5772).

The calcium disodium form of EDTA can also cause zinc deficiency (5771,5772), hypercalcemia (5771,5772), mild elevations of serum alanine aminotransferase (ALT) and aspartate aminotransferase (AST) and decreased alkaline phosphatase levels (15).

The disodium form of EDTA can occasionally cause muscle cramps, back pains, muscle weakness, tremors, tingling, myalgias, paresthesias (15), decreased magnesium and potassium serum concentrations (5771,5772), and rarely cause histamine-like reactions and insulin shock (5737).

The most serious adverse effect of both forms of EDTA is nephrotoxicity (5772), which is dose dependent of greater than 3 grams per day (15). Both forms of EDTA can cause nocturia, hyperuricemia, polyuria, dysuria, oliguria, proteinuria, glycosuria, hematuria and distal tubule and glomeruli changes (15). Both forms of EDTA can also cause acute renal tubular necrosis, and renal insufficiency and failure (5772). Rapid infusion of disodium EDTA or when given in too concentrated a solution can cause hypocalcemia, tetany, convulsions, severe cardiac arrhythmias, respiratory arrest, and death (15). When used ophthalmically, disodium EDTA can cause transient chemosis and stromal edema (15). Inhalation of disodium EDTA contained in nebulizer solutions has been reported to cause dose-related bronchoconstriction (5765).

Interactions with Herbs & Other Dietary Supplements

MAGNESIUM: EDTA can bind to and cause increased urinary excretion of magnesium (15).

TRACE METALS (copper, iron, zinc, etc.): EDTA can bind to and cause increased urinary excretion of trace metals (15,5733).

Interactions with Drugs

DIURETIC DRUGS: EDTA can decrease serum potassium levels and increase excretion of potassium (15). There is some concern that people receiving EDTA along with potassium depleting diuretics might be at an increased risk for hypokalemia. Initiation of potassium supplementation or an increase in potassium supplement dose may be necessary for some patients. Some diuretics that can deplete potassium include chlorothiazide (Diuril), furosemide (Lasix), and hydrochlorothiazide (HCTZ, HydroDIURIL, Microzide).

INSULIN: Concomitant use of disodium EDTA with insulin can cause severe decreases in blood glucose concentrations (5737,5771). EDTA chelates zinc in insulin products (15) and might interfere with the designed onset and duration of activity of various insulin preparations.

WARFARIN (Coumadin): There is some concern that disodium EDTA can decrease the anticoagulant effects of warfarin. Disodium EDTA has been reported to decrease international normalized ratio (INR) in a patient taking warfarin (4611).

Interactions with Foods

None known.

Interactions with Lab Tests

ALANINE AMINOTRANSFERASE (ALT, SGPT): Calcium disodium EDTA can cause mild increases in serum ALT (15).

ALKALINE PHOSPHATASE: Disodium EDTA can decrease serum alkaline phosphatase concentrations (15,3314). Disodium EDTA can cause low magnesium serum concentrations, which decreases the activity of alkaline phosphatase (15).

ASPARTATE AMINOTRANSFERASE (AST, SGOT): Calcium disodium EDTA can cause mild increases in AST (15).

CALCIUM: Calcium serum concentrations cannot be determined by colorimetric methods in patients receiving disodium EDTA due to chelation of a calcium disodium complex.

Oxalate and other precipitation methods may also give falsely decreased levels when disodium

EDTA is present (15).
PROTHROMBIN TIME (PT): Disodium EDTA can increase prothrombin time (PT) in some patients (5737).

Interactions with Diseases or Conditions

ASTHMA: Nebulizer solutions containing disodium EDTA as a preservative can produce dose-related bronchoconstriction in some asthmatics (5765).
CARDIAC RHYTHM IRREGULARITIES: Calcium disodium EDTA can cause ECG changes such as T wave inversions (15). Disodium EDTA can have negative inotropic effects on the heart (15). Use with caution in patients with pre-existing cardiac rhythm irregularity conditions.
DIABETES: Use of disodium EDTA may result in poor control of glucose levels in diabetic patients due to disodium EDTA's interactions with insulin preparations and serum glucose lowering effect (15).
HYPOCALCEMIA: Disodium EDTA can decrease serum calcium levels. Disodium EDTA may exacerbate hypocalcemia in patients with existing low calcium levels (15); avoid using.
HYPOKALEMIA: EDTA can increase urinary excretion of potassium and reduce serum potassium concentrations (15). EDTA might exacerbate hypokalemia in patients with existing potassium deficiency; avoid using.
HYPOMAGNESEMIA: EDTA can chelate magnesium and cause increased urinary excretion of magnesium resulting in depletion of serum magnesium concentrations (15). EDTA might exacerbate hypomagnesemia in patients with existing magnesium depletion; avoid using.
LIVER DYSFUNCTION AND HEPATITIS: Calcium disodium EDTA can cause mild increases in serum ALT (SGPT) and AST (SGOT) (15). Theoretically, EDTA might exacerbate liver dysfunction in patients with liver dysfunction or hepatitis; avoid using.
RENAL DYSFUNCTION: EDTA is nephrotoxic and might exacerbate existing renal disease. Avoid using in patients with severe renal disease and renal failure. EDTA doses should be reduced in patients with renal insufficiency (15).
SEIZURE DISORDERS: There is some concern that disodium EDTA might increase the risk of seizure in people with epilepsy or those prone to seizure (15). Disodium can cause severe decreases in serum calcium which can induce seizure (15).
TUBERCULOSIS: Use of disodium EDTA is contraindicated in people with active tuberculosis or healed calcified tubercular lesions (15). Theoretically, use of EDTA may cause the chelation of calcium from calcified tubercular lesions, resulting in possible reactivation of the tuberculosis disease process.

Dosage and Administration

TOPICAL: For corneal calcium deposits, a 0.35% to 1.85% solution is prepared with sterile 0.9% sodium chloride and commercially available disodium EDTA preparations for injection (15). Debridement of the corneal epithelium must be done before application of the solution since EDTA does not penetrate the epithelium (5773,5774). The solution is applied as a corneal bath one time for 15-20 minutes (15) followed by debridement of the calcium (5774), or a cellulose sponge is soaked in disodium EDTA solution and wiped over the deposits until the calcium is removed (5774). The eye should be irrigated with 0.9% sodium chloride following application of disodium EDTA solution (15).
INTRAVENOUS: For acute and chronic lead poisoning and lead encephalopathy, a dose of calcium disodium EDTA 50 mg per kilogram body weight to a maximum daily dose of 3 grams (15) is diluted with 5% dextrose or 9% sodium chloride to a concentration of 2-4 mg/mL and given as a single infusion over 8-24 hours for up to 5 days (15). A minimal 2-day waiting period is suggested before starting a second 5-day course of chelation therapy to further minimize development of nephrotoxicity (15). For blood lead levels greater than 70 mcg/dL, it is recommended that dimercaprol (BAL, British Anti-Lewisite) be used in conjunction with calcium disodium EDTA (5731). For people exposed long-term to low levels of lead and with decreased renal function, 1 gram of calcium disodium EDTA has been used and mixed with 200 mL of 5% dextrose and infused over 2 hours once weekly for 2 months (5732). For hypercalcemia, a dose of disodium EDTA 50 mg/kg body weight up to a maximum daily dosage of 3 grams is diluted with 5% dextrose or 0.9 % sodium chloride to a concentration of 2-4 mg/mL and infused over 3 hours or more (15). For cardiac glycoside-induced ventricular arrhythmias, disodium EDTA is given in a dose of 15 mg/kg per hour to a maximum of 60 mg/kg infused in 5% dextrose (15). For the treatment of atherosclerotic vascular disease, people have used disodium EDTA in a dose of 50 mg/kg up to a maximum of 5 grams diluted in 500-1000 mL of a 150-osmolar carrier (5737). Heparin, sodium ascorbate, elemental magnesium, lidocaine, pyridoxine, and sodium bicarbonate is often added to the infusion with optional additives of adrenal cortex extract, cyanocobalamin, niacin, pantothenic acid, and vitamin-B complex (5737). People usually eat before treatment and bring snacks to eat during a 3-hour infusion (5738).
INTRAMUSCULAR: For acute and chronic lead poisoning and lead encephalopathy, the dosage of calcium disodium EDTA is the same as intravenous administration in divided doses every 8-12 hours (15). When given in conjunction with dimercaprol, the daily dosage is given in equally divided doses every 4 hours. To decrease pain at the injection site, 1 mL of 1% lidocaine HCl or 1 mL of 1% procaine HCl is added to each mL of calcium disodium EDTA to obtain a final lidocaine or procaine HCl concentration of 5 mg/mL (15).

Comments

The American College for Advancement of Medicine (ACAM) strongly supports using EDTA chelation therapy for cardiovascular conditions. ACAM has a standard chelation therapy protocol and has trained more than 6000 practitioners to administer chelation treatments for various conditions (5768). However, the majority of the medical community does not support chelation therapy due to the lack of supporting evidence (5747,5749,5756). An iron-EDTA chelate is also used for iron fortification of grain-based foods. The established acceptable daily intake (ADI) for iron EDTA is 2.5 mg/kg/day. Iron EDTA has Generally Recognized As Safe (GRAS) status in the US (5728).

ELDERBERRY

Also Known As

Baccae, Baises De Sureau, Black-Berried Alder, Black Elder, Black Elderberry, Boor Tree, Bountry, Elder, Elder Berry, Elderberries, Ellanwood, Ellhorn, European Alder, European Elder Fruit, European Elderberry, Holunderbeeren, Sambuci Sambucus.
CAUTION: See separate listings for Elderflower, Dwarf Elder, and American Elder.

Scientific Names

Sambucus nigra.
Family: Adoxacaea/Sambucaceae or Caprifoliaceae.

People Use This For

Orally, elderberry fruit juice-containing syrup is used for treating the flu.
Elderberry fruit is also used as a laxative, diuretic, diaphoretic, to treat allergic rhinitis, sinusitis, sciatica, neuralgia, and cancer.
In manufacturing, elderberry fruit is used for making wine and as a food flavoring.

Safety

POSSIBLY SAFE ...when the cooked fruit is used orally (4,6,12).
POSSIBLY UNSAFE ...when the fruit is not cooked sufficiently, it can cause nausea and vomiting (8,12).
PREGNANCY AND LACTATION: Insufficient reliable information available; avoid using.

Effectiveness

POSSIBLY EFFECTIVE

Influenza. Elderberry juice syrup taken orally seems to reduce the symptoms and duration of influenza infection. Symptom relief occurs within 2 to 3 days. The brand Sambucol (JB Harris) has been used in clinical research (5260).

There is insufficient reliable information available about the effectiveness of elderberry fruit for its other uses.

Mechanism of Action

Elderberries contain the flavonoids rutin, isoquertin, and hyperoside (4,8). They also contain 3% tannins, as well as anthocyan glycosides, an essential oil, cyanogenic glycosides including sambunigrin, and a lectin (4,8,12,4151). Elderberry has both antiviral and immunomodulating effects. Elderberry extract inhibits hemagglutinin activity and replication of several strains of influenza viruses A and B (5260). Elderberry also seems to increase production of inflammatory cytokines, such as interleukins and tumor necrosis factor (10796).

Adverse Reactions

Orally, raw and unripe fruit might cause nausea, vomiting, or severe diarrhea (4,12). Weakness, dizziness, numbness, and stupor are reported following ingestion of elderberry juice (6). No adverse effects were reported in a clinical trial of elderberry syrup in children and adults (5260).

Interactions with Herbs & Other Dietary Supplements

None known.

Interactions with Drugs

None known.

Interactions with Foods

None known.

Interactions with Lab Tests

None known.

Interactions with Diseases or Conditions

None known.

Dosage and Administration

ORAL: For treating influenza, an adult dose of four tablespoons of elderberry juice-containing syrup (Sambucol) daily for three days has been used (5260); a dose of two tablespoons of Sambucol daily for three days has been used in children (5260).

Comments

Avoid confusion with American elder (Sambucus canadensis).

ELDERFLOWER

Also Known As

Black-Berried Alder, Black Elder, Boor Tree, Bountry, Common Elder, Elder Flowers, Ellanwood, Ellhorn, European Alder, European Elder Flower, Sambucus, Sweet Elder.
CAUTION: See separate listings for American Elder, Dwarf Elder, and Elderberry.

Scientific Names

Sambucus nigra.
Family: Adoxaceae/Sambucaceae or Caprifoliaceae.

People Use This For

Orally, elderflower is used as a diuretic, laxative, and diaphoretic. It is also used orally to treat colds, flu, cough, and bronchitis.
Topically, elderflower preparations are used as a gargle and mouthwash for coughs, headcolds, laryngitis, flu, and shortness of breath. It is used on the skin as an astringent for rheumatism, swelling, and inflammation.
In combination with gentian root, verbena, cowslip flower, and sorrel, elderflower is used orally for maintaining healthy sinuses and treating sinusitis.
In foods and beverages, elderflowers are used as a flavoring component.
In manufacturing, elderflower extracts are used in perfumes. Elderflower water is used as a vehicle in eye and skin lotions.

Safety

LIKELY SAFE ...when used orally in amounts commonly found in foods. Elderflower has Generally Recognized As Safe (GRAS) status in the US (4912). ...when used orally and appropriately (2,4,12) in therapeutic amounts; no adverse effects have been reported (2,4,6,12).
POSSIBLY SAFE ...when used orally with gentian root, verbena, cowslip flower, and sorrel (Quanterra Sinus Defense, Sinupret) (7,374,379).
There is insufficient reliable information available about the safety of the topical use of elderflower.
PREGNANCY AND LACTATION: Insufficient reliable information available; avoid using.

Effectiveness

POSSIBLY EFFECTIVE

Sinusitis. Taking elderflower orally with gentian root, verbena, cowslip flower, and sorrel (Quanterra Sinus Defense, Sinupret) seems to be effective for treating acute or chronic sinusitis (7,374,379).

There is insufficient reliable information available about the effectiveness of elderflower for its other uses.

Mechanism of Action

Elderflower may have sweat-inducing, diuretic, and laxative effects. It also soothes mucous membranes and stimulates bronchial secretions (2,4,11). Compounds responsible for diuretic and laxative properties have not yet been isolated. Elderflower has demonstrated anti-inflammatory, antiviral, and diuretic effects in animals (4). Constituents of a related species, Sambucus formosana, appear to have a hepatoprotective activity against liver damage (6).

Adverse Reactions

None reported.

Interactions with Herbs & Other Dietary Supplements

None known.

Interactions with Drugs

None known.

Interactions with Foods
None known.

Interactions with Lab Tests
None known.

Interactions with Diseases or Conditions
None known.

Dosage and Administration
ORAL: People typically use one cup tea (steep 2-4 grams dried flowers in 250 mL boiling water 10-15 minutes, strain) three times daily (4); average daily dose 10-15 grams dried flowers (2). Liquid extract (1:1 in 25% alcohol), 2-4 mL three times daily has also been used (4). For acute or chronic sinusitis, two Sinupret tablets three times daily for up to two weeks has been used in clinical trials (7,374,379), equivalent to gentian root 12 mg, elderflower 36 mg, verbena 36 mg, cowslip flower 36 mg, and sorrel 36 mg three times daily.
TOPICAL: No typical dosage.

Comments
Avoid confusion with American elder (Sambucus canadensis). American elder (sambucus candadensis) and European elder (sambucus nigra), are discussed together despite the fact most of the information available pertains to American elder (11).

ELECAMPANE

Also Known As
Alant, Elfdock, Elfwort, Horse-Elder, Horseheal, Inula, Scabwort, Velvet Dock, Wild Sunflower, Yellow Starwort.

Scientific Names
Inula helenium, synonyms Helenium grandiflorum, Aster officinalis, Aster helenium.
Family: Asteraceae/Compositae.

People Use This For
Orally, elecampane is used as an expectorant, antitussive, and diaphoretic, for diseases of the respiratory tract, as an anthelmintic, for improving stomach function, as a diuretic, asthma, bronchitis, whooping cough, cough associated with tuberculosis, nausea, and diarrhea.
In foods and beverages, elecampane is used as a flavoring ingredient.
In other manufacturing processes, elecampane is used as a fragrance component in cosmetics and soaps.

Safety
LIKELY SAFE ...when used orally in amounts commonly found in foods. Elecampane has Generally Recognized As Safe (GRAS) status in the US (4912).
POSSIBLY SAFE ...when the root and rhizome are used orally and appropriately in medicinal amounts (12).
POSSIBLY UNSAFE ...when used orally in large amounts. Elecampane can cause gastrointestinal upset and symptoms of paralysis (12).
PREGNANCY AND LACTATION: LIKELY UNSAFE ...when used orally (12); avoid using

Effectiveness
There is insufficient reliable information available about the effectiveness of elecampane.

Mechanism of Action
The applicable parts of elecampane are the rhizome/root. Alantolactone and isoalantolactone, sesquiterpene alkaloids found in elecampane, show antibacterial and antifungal (11) activity in vitro and anthelmintic activity in humans (11). Alantolactone is used as an anthelmintic in Europe and the UK (11).

Adverse Reactions
Orally, large doses may cause vomiting, diarrhea, spasms, and symptoms of paralysis (12).
Topically, elecampane may cause allergic contact dermatitis (4).
It can cause an allergic reaction in individuals sensitive to the Asteraceae/Compositae family. Members of this family include ragweed, chrysanthemums, marigolds, daisies, and many other herbs.

Interactions with Herbs & Other Dietary Supplements
HERBS WITH SEDATIVE PROPERTIES: Theoretically, concomitant use with herbs that have sedative properties might enhance therapeutic and adverse effects. Some of these supplements include 5-HTP, calamus, California poppy, catnip, hops, Jamaican dogwood, kava, St. John's wort, scullcap, valerian, yerba mansa, and others.

Interactions with Drugs
CNS DEPRESSANTS: Theoretically, concomitant use with drugs with sedative properties may cause additive effects (4).

Interactions with Foods
None known.

Interactions with Lab Tests
None known.

Interactions with Diseases or Conditions
CROSS-ALLERGENICITY: Can cause an allergic reaction in individuals sensitive to the Asteraceae/Compositae family. Members of this family include ragweed, chrysanthemums, marigolds, daisies, and many other herbs.
DIABETES: Theoretically, elecampane may interfere with blood glucose control (4).
HYPERTENSION, HYPOTENSION: Theoretically, elecampane may interfere with blood pressure control (4).

Dosage and Administration
ORAL: Typically, 1.5-4 grams of rhizome/root three times daily, or one cup tea (simmer 1.5-4 grams of rhizome/root in 150 mL boiling water 5-10 minutes, strain) three times daily is used (4). Liquid extract (1:1 in 25% alcohol) 1.5-4 mL three times daily is also used (4). As an anthelmintic for adults, alantolactone 300 mg daily for 2 courses of 5 days, with an interval of 10 days, is used. For children, alantolactone 50-200 mg daily is used (4).

ELEMI

Also Known As
Elemi Oleoresin, Elemi Resin, Manila Elemi.

Scientific Names
Canarium luzonicum, synonym Pimela luzonica; Canarium indicum, synonym Canarium commune.
Family: Burseraceae.

People Use This For
Orally, elemi is used for improving stomach function, as an expectorant, and as a local stimulant.
In foods and beverages, elemi is used as a flavoring agent.
In other manufacturing processes, elemi is used as a fixative and fragrance in cosmetics and soaps.

Safety
LIKELY SAFE ...when used orally in amounts commonly found in foods. Elemi is has Generally Recognized As Safe (GRAS) status in the US (4912).
There is insufficient reliable information available about the safety of the oral use of elemi in amounts greater than those found in foods.
PREGNANCY AND LACTATION: Insufficient reliable information available; avoid using.

Effectiveness
There is insufficient reliable information available about the effectiveness of elemi.

Mechanism of Action
The applicable parts of elemi are the gum and oil. There is insufficient reliable information available about the possible mechanism of action and active ingredients.

Adverse Reactions
None reported.

Interactions with Herbs & Other Dietary Supplements
None known.

Interactions with Drugs
None known.

Interactions with Foods
None known.

Interactions with Lab Tests
None known.

Interactions with Diseases or Conditions
None known.

Dosage and Administration
No typical dosage.

Comments
Elemi gum is resin exuded by the elemi tree (Canarium luzonicum). Elemi oil is produced by distillation of elemi gum resin.

ELLAGIC ACID

Also Known As
None.

Scientific Names
3,4,3',4'-hydroxyl-benzopyranol[5,4,3-c,d,e][1]benzopyrn-6-6'-dione.

People Use This For
Orally, ellagic acid is used to prevent cancer, and as an antiviral and antibacterial.

Safety
There is insufficient reliable information available about the safety of ellagic acid.
Pregnancy and Lactation: Insufficient reliable information available.

Effectiveness
There is insufficient reliable information available about the effectiveness of ellagic acid.

Mechanism of Action
Ellagic acid is a naturally occurring complex hydrocarbon. The best dietary sources of ellagic acid are raspberries, blackberries, strawberries, and walnuts (8955). Researchers are interested in potential anticancer activity of ellagic acid. Ellagic acid has lipophilic antioxidant activity, free radical scavenging capability, and the ability to inhibit DNA topoisomerases (8955,10342,11335). These characteristics support the observation that ellagic acid inhibits lipid peroxidation at lower concentrations than vitamin E (11335). Ellagic acid also seems to have anti-inflammatory and antimutagenic activity (11335). Derivatives of ellagic acid have the ability to induce DNA damage and inhibit the growth of yeast cells that model the growth of cancer cells (10343). Some researchers have suggested that the hydroxyl groups and lactone rings in the chemical structure of ellagic acid may bind or inactivate carcinogens (10340). Preliminary evidence also suggests ellagic acid may have potential use against malaria, due to its antiplasmodial activity (11460). However, the clinical usefulness of ellagic acid may be limited by its poor absorption and rapid elimination from the body. Because the ability to inhibit carcinogenesis appears to be highly dependent upon its functional groups, alterations in the molecule to improve absorption or decrease the rate of elimination often decrease the activity of ellagic acid (10340,10342). However, short-term freezing and storage does not appear to decrease the activity of ellagic acid and related compounds in red raspberries (10344).

Adverse Reactions
None reported.

Interactions with Herbs & Other Dietary Supplements
None known.

Interactions with Drugs
None known.

Interactions with Foods
None known.

Interactions with Lab Tests
None known.

Interactions with Diseases or Conditions
None known.

Dosage and Administration
No typical dosage.

ELM BARK

Also Known As
Smooth-Leaved Elm.

Scientific Names
Ulmus minor.
Family: Ulmaceae.

Comments
At the date of publication, this product was not a common ingredient used in brand name supplements marketed to consumers. Details about this product are available at the online version of *Natural Medicines Comprehensive Database*. See www.naturaldatabase.com.

EMU OIL

Also Known As
Emu.

Scientific Names
Dromiceius novahollandiae (Emu).

People Use This For
Orally, emu oil is used for improving cholesterol levels, as a source of polyunsaturated and monounsaturated fatty acids, for weight loss, and as a cough syrup for colds and flu.
Topically, emu oil is used for relief from sore muscles; aching joints, pain or inflammation; carpal tunnel syndrome; sciatica, shin splints; and gout. It is also used topically to improve healing of wounds, incisions, and burns from radiation therapy; to reduce bruises and stretch marks; to reduce scarring and keloids; to heal the donor site of skin grafting; to diminish acne inflammation; to soften dry cuticles and promote healthy nails; for skin cancers; athlete's foot; diaper rash; canker sores; chapped lips; circulation; dry skin, eczema, psoriasis, wrinkles or age spots; dry or damaged hair; dandruff; in massage therapy; for its anti-aging properties; to protect skin from sun damage; and to promote skin rejuvenation. Emu oil is also used topically to reduce pain and irritation from shingles, bedsores, hemorrhoids, diabetic neuropathy, insect bites, earaches, eye irritation, "growing pains", and frostbite. It is used for rashes, razor burn and nicks, rosacea, and roseola.
Intranasally, emu oil is used to treat colds and flu.
In combination, emu oil (7%) is used with glycolic acid (10%) for lowering cholesterol, triglycerides, and low density lipoprotein; preventing and treating allergies; preventing scarring; treating headaches, especially migraines; preventing nosebleeds; treating and preventing cold and flu symptoms; and relieving discomfort associated with menstruation.
In veterinary practice, emu oil is used to reduce swelling in joints, prevent cracked or peeling paws, calm "hot spots," and reduce irritation of flea bites.
In manufacturing, emu oil is used to sharpen and oil industrial machinery, for polishing timber and leather, and for conditioning and waterproofing.

Safety
There is insufficient reliable information available about the safety of emu oil.
Pregnancy and Lactation: Insufficient reliable information available; avoid using.

Effectiveness
There is insufficient reliable information available about the effectiveness of emu oil.

Mechanism of Action
Emu oil is obtained from the fat of the emu, a large flightless bird native to Australia. Though not standardized, emu oil typically contains myristic, palmitic, palmitoleic, stearic, oleic, linoleic, and linolenic fatty acids (8278). Topical emu oil has moisturizing, cosmetic, and texture properties similar to those of topical mineral oil. It appears to penetrate the stratum corneum barrier of the skin (10643). Preliminary animal evidence suggests that a topical emu lotion (a combination of emu oil, vitamin E and botanical oil) has the ability to promote wound healing by exerting both anti-inflammatory and anti-catalytic effects on soft tissue (8277). Additional animal evidence suggests topical emu oil is more effective in acute inflammation than in chronic inflammation (5923).

Adverse Reactions
None reported.

Interactions with Herbs & Other Dietary Supplements
HERBS WITH ANTICOAGULANT/ANTIPLATELET POTENTIAL: Theoretically, concomitant use of herbs that have constituents or affect platelet aggregation could theoretically increase the risk of bleeding in some people. These herbs include angelica, clove, danshen, garlic, ginger, ginkgo, Panax ginseng, red clover, turmeric, and others.

Interactions with Drugs
None known.

Interactions with Foods
None known.

Interactions with Lab Tests
None known.

Interactions with Diseases or Conditions
None known.

Dosage and Administration
No typical dosage.

ENGLISH ADDER'S TONGUE

Also Known As
Christs Spear, Christ's Spear, English Adders Tongue, Green Oil of Charity, Serpents Tongue, Serpent's Tongue.
CAUTION: See separate listing for American Adder's Tongue.

Scientific Names
Ophioglossum vulgatum.
Family: Ophioglossaceae.

People Use This For
Topically, English adder's tongue is used to treat ulcers.

Safety
There is insufficient reliable information available about the safety of English adder's tongue.
Pregnancy and Lactation: Insufficient reliable information available; avoid using.

Effectiveness
There is insufficient reliable information available about the effectiveness of English adder's tongue.

Mechanism of Action
The applicable parts of English adder's tongue are the root and leaf. English adder's tongue is stated to have emollient properties when applied. When used orally, it is has emetic properties (18).

Adverse Reactions
None reported.

Interactions with Herbs & Other Dietary Supplements
None known.

Interactions with Drugs
None known.

Interactions with Foods
None known.

Interactions with Lab Tests
None known.

Interactions with Diseases or Conditions
None known.

Dosage and Administration
TOPICAL: Fresh English adder's tongue leaves are applied as a poultice.

Comments
Avoid confusion with American adder's tongue (Erythronium americanum).

ENGLISH HORSEMINT

Also Known As
Biblical Mint, Wild Mint.

Scientific Names
Mentha longifolia, synonym Mentha sylvestris.
Family: Lamiaceae/Labiatae.

Comments
At the date of publication, this product was not a common ingredient used in brand name supplements marketed to consumers. Details about this product are available at the online version of *Natural Medicines Comprehensive Database*. See www.naturaldatabase.com.

ENGLISH IVY

Also Known As
Gum Ivy, Hederae helicis folium, Ivy, True Ivy, Woodbind.

Scientific Names
Hedera helix, synonym Hedera taurica.
Family: Araliaceae.

People Use This For
Orally, English ivy is used for inflammation of mucous membranes in respiratory passages, symptomatic treatment of chronic inflammatory bronchial conditions, as an expectorant, as an antispasmodic, to improve lung function in children with chronic obstructive bronchitis, liver disorders, spleen disorders, gallbladder disorders, gout, rheumatism, and scrofulosis.
Topically, English ivy is used for burn wounds, calluses, cellulitis, inflammations, neuralgia, parasitic disorders, ulcers, rheumatic complaints, and for phlebitis.

Safety
POSSIBLY SAFE ...when used orally and appropriately (2).
There is insufficient reliable information available about the safety of English ivy for its other uses.
PREGNANCY AND LACTATION: Insufficient reliable information available; avoid using.

Effectiveness

POSSIBLY EFFECTIVE

Chronic obstructive bronchitis. There is some evidence that taking English ivy orally might help improve lung function in children with chronic obstructive bronchitis (3471).

There is insufficient reliable information available about the effectiveness of English ivy for its other uses.

Mechanism of Action

The applicable part of English ivy is the leaf. English ivy has expectorant and antispasmodic actions. It irritates skin and mucosa (2). Researchers think the ivy leaf acts on the gastric mucosa to cause stimulation of mucous glands in the bronchi via parasympathetic sensory pathways (7). Fresh leaves contain the contact allergen falcarinol (7). Preliminary evidence suggests ivy leaf dried extract may improve lung function (measured as forced expiratory volume in one second) in children with chronic obstructive bronchitis due to its secretolytic and spasmolytic effects (3471). Human studies are needed to determine whether ivy leaf dried extract is as effective or beneficial as conventional agents used prophylactically to improve and maintain lung function such as bronchodilators and corticosteroids.

Adverse Reactions

Orally, fresh English ivy leaves can cause skin irritation (7). Saponin constituents, hederacosides, and hederin monodesmosides have acrid and/or bitter taste (7).

Interactions with Herbs & Other Dietary Supplements

None known.

Interactions with Drugs

None known.

Interactions with Foods

None known.

Interactions with Lab Tests

None known.

Interactions with Diseases or Conditions

None known.

Dosage and Administration

ORAL: People have used 300-800 mg dried leaf per day (2,18), or one cup tea, steep 1 heaping teaspoon of dried leaf in 1/4 cup boiling water 10 minutes, strain, up to three times daily (18). For chronic obstructive bronchitis in children, 35 mg dried leaf extract three times a day or 14 mg dried leaf alcohol-based extract three times a day has been used (3471).

TOPICAL: Fresh leaves placed on festering wounds and burns have been used (18). For rheumatism, prepare tea, simmer 200 grams of fresh leaves in 1 L boiling water 5-10 minutes, strain (18).

Comments

English ivy is most often used in the form of an extract and seldom used as a prepared tea (7).

ENGLISH WALNUT

Also Known As

Akschota, Fructus Cortex, Juglans, Juglandis, Juglandis Folium, Walnussblätter, Walnussfrüchtschalen, Walnut, Walnut Fruit, Walnut Hull, Walnut Leaf.

CAUTION: See separate listing for Black Walnut.

Scientific Names

Juglans regia.

Family: Juglandaceae.

People Use This For

Orally, English walnut fruit is used as a part of the diet for lowering cholesterol. The hull of English walnut is used to treat gastrointestinal mucous membrane inflammation. The leaf is used orally for treating diarrhea.

Topically, English walnut hull is used for skin diseases, abscesses, and eye lid inflammation. The leaf is used

topically for superficial inflammation of the skin; excessive hand and/or foot perspiration; and for skin conditions such as acne, eczema, scrophula, pyodermia, and ulcers.
In combination with other herbs, English walnut hull is used to treat diabetes mellitus, gastritis, and anemia.
Traditionally, English walnut hull has been used to treat "blood poisoning" and as a "blood purifier" to remove undesirable agents from the blood. The leaf is used traditionally for gastrointestinal mucous membrane inflammation, as an anthelmintic, and "blood-purifying" agent.
In foods, English walnut is commonly consumed, usually as a snack, in baking, and in salads.

Safety

LIKELY SAFE ...when the fruit is consumed in amounts normally found in foods (6431,8476,8477).
POSSIBLY SAFE ...when the leaf is used topically and appropriately, short-term (2,18,4800).
POSSIBLY UNSAFE ...when the hull is used topically. English walnut hulls might contain the carcinogenic constituent juglone; however, the amount of juglone contained in hulls is not clear. Daily topical use of walnut preparations known to contain juglone has been associated with skin discoloration and increased risk of cancer of the tongue and lip leukoplakia (2,4800).
There is insufficient reliable information available about the safety of the oral use of English walnut for medicinal purposes.
PREGNANCY AND LACTATION: POSSIBLY UNSAFE ...when the hull is used topically. English walnut hulls might contain the carcinogenic constituent juglone (2,4800); avoid using. There is insufficient reliable information available about the safety of the oral use of English walnut leaf during pregnancy and lactation; avoid using.

Effectiveness

POSSIBLY EFFECTIVE

Coronary heart disease. There is some evidence that people who increase dietary consumption of walnuts and other nuts might have a lower risk of coronary heart disease and death due to coronary events (8477,8478).
Hypercholesterolemia. Consuming walnuts as part of a low fat diet seems to lower cholesterol. Total cholesterol and lipoproteins are decreased when walnuts are substituted for other fatty foods and constitute up to 20% of the calories in the diet. When English walnuts are added to a low fat diet, total cholesterol may be decreased by 4-12% and low-density lipoprotein (LDL) may be decreased by 8-16% (6431,8476,8477).

There is insufficient reliable information available about the effectiveness of English walnut for its other uses.

Mechanism of Action

The applicable parts of English walnut are the fruit, hull, and leaf. English walnut hull contains the tannins, galloylglucose and ellagitannins; naphthalene derivatives including juglone; and flavonoids including hyperoside and quercitrin (8,18). The leaf of the English walnut also contains tannins (2,4800). The astringent properties of English walnut hull and leaf can be attributed to the tannins (2,8,18,4800). Juglone and the essential juglone oil from the leaves have antifungal effects. The juglone component of the leaves may quickly break down when leaves are handled or dried (8,18). Compared with most other nuts, which contain monounsaturated fatty acids, English walnuts are unique because they are rich in n-6 (linoleate) and n-3 (linolenate) polyunsaturated fatty acids (6431,8476,8478). This might explain the beneficial effect of English walnut on lipids. English walnut also contains antioxidants, including ellagic acid. This effect may reduce oxidation of circulating lipids (8955).

Adverse Reactions

Orally, the fruit of English walnut is well tolerated (8476,8477); however, it can cause softening of stools, and mild bloating (6431). Oral allergy syndrome may occur in people who are allergic to English walnuts. This is characterized by itching of the oral cavity immediately after consumption. Rarely this syndrome may cause swelling of the lips and tongue (angioedema) (8479).
No adverse reactions with English walnut leaf have been reported. Daily use of juglone-containing preparations is associated with tongue cancer and lip leukoplakia (2). Juglone is reported to have mutagenic effects in animals (12). English walnut hull is thought to contain juglone, but it is not clear what concentration of juglone it contains (2) and the extent of the risk.
Topically, walnut preparations containing the juglone constituent leads to yellow or brown discoloration of skin and mucous membranes (2).

Interactions with Herbs & Other Dietary Supplements

None known.

Interactions with Drugs

None known.

Interactions with Foods

None known.

Interactions with Lab Tests
None known.

Interactions with Diseases or Conditions
None known.

Dosage and Administration
ORAL: For lowering cholesterol, the fruit of approximately 8-11 English walnuts were consumed per day with the diet in one study (6431). For English walnut leaf, as an adjuvant for skin conditions, one cup tea (simmer 1.5 grams of finely chopped dried leaf in 150 mL boiling water 3-5 minutes, steep) one to three times daily (8).
TOPICAL: For dressing, lotion, poultice or hip bath, simmer 2-3 grams of finely chopped dried English walnut leaf per 100 mL boiling water (2,8). Average daily amount is 3-6 grams of dried leaf (18).

EPA (EICOSAPENTAENOIC ACID)

Also Known As
EPA, Eicosapentaenoic Acid, Ethyl Eicosapentaenoic Acid, Fish Oil Fatty Acid, N-3 Fatty Acid, Omega Fatty Acid, Omega-3 Fatty Acid, W-3 Fatty Acid.
CAUTION: See separate listings for Cod Liver Oil, DHA (docosahexaenoic acid), and Fish Oils.

Scientific Names
Eicosapentaenoic acid.

People Use This For
Orally, eicosapentaenoic acid (EPA) is used for treating the symptoms of cystic fibrosis, reducing the risk of intrauterine growth retardation, treating depression, treating pregnancy-induced hypertension in high-risk pregnancies, preventing age-related macular degeneration (AMD), treating coronary artery disease, treating schizophrenia, personality disorder, and treating diabetes.
In combination, EPA is used with docosahexaenoic acid (DHA) in fish oil preparations for a variety of conditions, including preventing and reversing heart disease, decreasing ectopic ventricular beats, asthma, cancer, dysmenorrhea, hay fever, lung diseases, lupus erythematosus, lupus nephritis, and IgA nephropathy. They are also used in combination for migraine headache prophylaxis in adolescents, atopic dermatitis, Behcet's syndrome, hyperlipidemia, hypertension, psoriasis, Raynaud's syndrome, rheumatoid arthritis, Crohn's disease, and ulcerative colitis. EPA is also used in combination with RNA and L-arginine in the perioperative period to reduce infections, improve wound healing, and shorten recovery time.

Safety
LIKELY SAFE ...when used orally or intravenously, and appropriately (1004,1016,7819).
POSSIBLY UNSAFE ...when used orally in high doses. Doses greater than 3 grams daily might decrease blood coagulation and increase the risk of bleeding (1313).
PREGNANCY AND LACTATION: Insufficient reliable information available; avoid using.

Effectiveness
POSSIBLY EFFECTIVE

Coronary artery disease. Increased dietary consumption of EPA may slightly decrease the risk of death in patients with coronary artery disease (10322).

Depression. Taking eicosapentaenoic acid (EPA) orally 1 gram twice daily with standard therapy seems to improve symptoms of recurrent major depression, such as depressed mood, guilt feelings, worthlessness, and insomnia after two weeks of treatment (10872). Some research suggests that the ethyl form of EPA, ethyl-eicosapentaenoate (ethyl-EPA), might also be helpful for treating depression. It appears that 1 gram per day of ethyl-EPA may be more effective for depression than 2 or 4 grams per day (10215). Personality disorder. Taking EPA (as ethyl eicosapentaenoic acid) orally provides modest improvement in aggressive behavior and depression in women with moderately severe borderline personality disorder (10348).

Psoriasis. Taking EPA in combination with low-dose (20 mg per day) etretinate (Tegison, no longer available in the US) seems to be more effective than etretinate alone for plaque psoriasis (1000). EPA given intravenously in combination with docosahexaenoic acid (DHA) appears to improve psoriatic lesions better than omega-6-lipid emulsion (1004).

Surgery. Supplementing the diet with EPA in combination with RNA and L-arginine before surgery or in the postoperative period appears to reduce the number of perioperative infections, improves wound healing, and shortens recovery time (5531,5532,5533,7819).

POSSIBLY INEFFECTIVE

Age-related macular degeneration (AMD). Increased dietary consumption of EPA does not appear

to prevent AMD (10324).
Allergic rhinitis (hayfever). Taking EPA orally doesn't appear to relieve hayfever symptoms, including wheezing, cough, and nasal symptoms (1036).
Asthma. Taking EPA orally doesn't seem to have any effect on asthma symptoms when given for four weeks (1023).
Cystic fibrosis. Taking EPA orally as a single agent doesn't seem to improve symptoms of cystic fibrosis (1006,1027).
Diabetes. Taking EPA orally does not seem to substantially improve cholesterol or other serum lipids, and may worsen blood glucose control in people with type 2 diabetes (10321).
Intrauterine growth. Taking EPA orally doesn't seem to reduce the risk of intrauterine growth (1027).
Pregnancy-induced hypertension. Taking EPA orally doesn't seem to improve pregnancy-induced hypertension in women with high-risk pregnancies (1027).
Schizophrenia. Taking EPA orally does not consistently improve positive or negative symptoms of schizophrenia when used in conjunction with standard antipsychotic therapy (8720,10347).

There is insufficient reliable information available about the effectiveness of EPA for its other uses.

Mechanism of Action

Eicosapentaenoic acid (EPA) is a long-chain n-3 polyunsaturated fatty acid that is found in the tissues of marine mammals and oily fish. EPA is also found in fish liver oils and in commercial fish oil products. EPA competes with arachidonic acid for inclusion in cyclooxygenase and lipoxygenase pathways (8696). This may have an anti-inflammatory effect in diseases such as psoriasis (1004).

EPA decreases blood viscosity and increases red blood cell deformability. It also decreases platelet aggregation (9930). However, EPA does not significantly affect clotting factors, fibrinogen concentrations, plasminogen activator inhibitor-1 or tissue plasminogen activator activity (10323). Pure EPA reduces serum triglyceride concentrations, increases fasting insulin and glucose concentrations, but has no effect on total and low-density lipoprotein (LDL) cholesterol in mildly hypercholesterolemic men (6143,10322). There is some evidence that higher ratios of EPA to arachidonic acid are associated with lower ratios of total to high-density lipoprotein (HDL) cholesterol. EPA can increase HDL cholesterol by approximately 12% (10321). There is preliminary evidence that EPA decreases natural killer (NK) cell activity. Researchers think this effect might be beneficial in preventing rejection after bone marrow and organ transplantation, but further research is needed (8718).

There is evidence EPA might have an additive effect to standard treatment on symptoms associated with schizophrenia and recurrent unipolar depressive disorder, but it is unknown if EPA has any antipsychotic and antidepressant activity of its own (8720,10872). Some evidence suggests that supplemental EPA might slow weight loss in cachectic cancer patients, possibly by inhibiting lipolysis. Other research suggests EPA does not inhibit lipolysis or lipid oxidation, suggesting a different mechanism might be responsible for this effect (8717).

Adverse Reactions

Orally, adverse reactions have not been reported for eicosapentaenoic acid (EPA) alone. However, for fish oils containing EPA and DHA, side effects can include fishy taste, belching, nosebleeds, nausea, and loose stools (10007). Three people with pre-existing familial adenomatous polyposis were diagnosed with malignant lesions during the course of long-term fish oil use (999). High doses of fish oils might also decrease blood coagulation and increase the risk of bleeding (1313). There is preliminary evidence that EPA in fish oil decreases natural killer (NK) cell activity. Due to this effect, there is concern that increased intake of EPA might have some adverse immunologic effects and possibly increase the risk for viral infections and some cancers (8718).

Interactions with Herbs & Other Dietary Supplements

HERBS WITH ANTICOAGULANT/ANTIPLATELET POTENTIAL: Concomitant use of herbs that have constituents that might affect platelet aggregation could theoretically increase the risk of bleeding in some people (9930). These herbs include angelica, clove, danshen, garlic, ginger, ginkgo, Panax ginseng, red clover, turmeric, and others.

Interactions with Drugs

ANTICOAGULANT/ANTIPLATELET DRUGS: Theoretically, concomitant use of EPA with anticoagulant or antiplatelet drugs, including aspirin, can increase the risk of bleeding (9930).
ANTIHYPERTENSIVE DRUGS: Fish oils containing EPA can lower blood pressure and might have additive effects in patients treated with antihypertensives (1001,1020,1030,1033); use with caution.

Interactions with Foods

None known.

Interactions with Lab Tests

INSULIN: EPA can increase fasting insulin concentrations and test results in mildly hypercholesterolemic patients (6143).
INTERNATIONAL NORMALIZED RATIO (INR), PROTHROMBIN TIME (PT): High doses of greater than

3 grams per day might decrease blood coagulation, increase INR and PT, and increase the risk of bleeding (1313).
PULMONARY FUNCTION TESTS: EPA might cause a decline in pulmonary function tests in aspirin-sensitive individuals (11869).
TRIGLYCERIDES: EPA can reduce serum triglyceride concentrations and test results in patients with hypercholesterolemia (6143).

Interactions with Diseases or Conditions

ASPIRIN-SENSITIVITY: Fish oils and other omega-3 fatty acids can lower pulmonary function tests in some aspirin-sensitive patients (11869).
DIABETES: EPA may interfere with blood glucose control in patients with type 2 diabetes (10322). Monitor blood glucose levels closely. Dose adjustments may be necessary.
HYPERTENSION: Fish oils including EPA can lower blood pressure and might have additive effects in patients with high blood pressure who are treated with antihypertensives (1001,1020,1030,1033).

Dosage and Administration

ORAL: Eicosapentaenoic acid (EPA) is usually administered with DHA (docosahexaenoic acid) as fish oil. A wide range of doses has been used. A typical dose is 5 grams of fish oil containing 169-563 mg of EPA and 72-312 mg of DHA. As an adjunct to standard antidepressant therapy for recurrent unipolar depressive disorder, 1 gram EPA twice daily has been used (10872). As an adjunct to standard antipsychotic therapy for schizophrenia, a dose of 3 grams EPA daily, in 2 to 3 divided doses (as ethyl eicosapentaenoic acid), has been used for 12-16 weeks (8720). For treatment of borderline personality disorder, 1 gram of EPA daily (as ethyl eicosapentaenoic acid) has been used for up to 8 weeks (10348). For plaque psoriasis, EPA ethyl ester 1800 mg daily has been used (1000). Many fish oil preparations also contain small amounts of vitamin E as an antioxidant.
INTRAVENOUS: For plaque psoriasis, EPA 4.2 grams and docosahexaenoic acid (DHA) 4.2 grams per day has been used (1004).

Comments

Avoid confusion with DHA (docosahexaenoic acid) and fish oils, which contain EPA and DHA. Most available data involving EPA are from research and clinical experience with fish oil products containing variable combinations of EPA and DHA. For more information, see the separate listing for Fish Oils.
Researchers are investigating oils containing stearidonic acid (SDA) from genetically modified plants as an alternative source of omega-3 fatty acids. SDA is metabolized to EPA and DHA in animals. However, further research is needed on the effects and safety of SDA in humans.

EPHEDRA

Also Known As

Cao Mahuang, Chinese ephedra, Chinese joint-fir, Cao Ma-Huang, Desert Herb, Ephedrae herba, Ephedra sinensis, Herbal Ecstasy, Indian Jointfir, Joint Fir, Ma Huang, Mahuanggen (ma huang root), Mongolian Ephedra, Muzei Ma Huang, Pakistani ephedra, Popotillo, Sea Grape, Shuang Sui Ma Huang, Teamster's Tea, Yellow Astringent, Yellow Horse, Zhong Mahuang.
CAUTION: See separate listing for Mormon Tea.

Scientific Names

Ephedra distachya, synonym Ephedra vulgaris; Ephedra equisetina, synonym Ephedra shennungiana; Ephedra gerardiana; Ephedra intermedia; Ephedra sinica; and other Ephedra species.
Family: Ephedraceae.

People Use This For

Orally, ephedra is used for weight loss and obesity and to enhance athletic performance. It is also used for allergies and allergic rhinitis; nasal congestion; and respiratory tract conditions such as bronchospasm, asthma, and bronchitis. It is also used orally for colds, flu, fever, chills, headache, anhidrosis, joint and bone pain, and as a diuretic for edema.

Safety

LIKELY UNSAFE ...when used orally. Ephedra can cause severe life-threatening or disabling adverse effects in some people. Ephedra is banned in the US. Several case reports have linked ephedra to serious side effects including hypertension, myocardial infarction (MI), seizure, stroke, psychosis, and others (1276,2729,6486,6998,9167,10689). Prolonged use or use of high doses might increase the risk of serious adverse effects (2729). Some suggest that ephedra is only harmful when used inappropriately in excessive doses or for prolonged periods. However, there are several cases of significant adverse events in patients who used ephedra short-term in relatively low doses ranging from 20-60 mg of ephedra alkaloids (2729,6486). There is some evidence that people who take doses greater than

32 mg per day might have more than triple the risk of hemorrhagic stroke, including subarachnoid hemorrhage and intracerebral hemorrhage (9167). It is not possible to determine who is at the greatest risk. However, people with existing conditions such as cardiovascular disease or those using ephedra products in combination with other stimulants such as caffeine, might be at increased risk. Tell patients to avoid ephedra-containing products.
CHILDREN: LIKELY UNSAFE ...when used orally. Children can be more susceptible to the adverse effects of ephedra (12).
PREGNANCY: LIKELY UNSAFE ...when used orally. Ephedra can stimulate uterine contraction (12); contraindicated.
LACTATION: Insufficient reliable information available; avoid using.

Effectiveness

POSSIBLY EFFECTIVE

Obesity. Taking ephedra orally may produce weight loss of approximately 0.9 kg per month for up to 6 months. It is not known if weight loss can be sustained beyond this timeframe or if weight returns after ephedra is discontinued. Caffeine may provide additional weight loss (9740,9741). There is preliminary evidence that a specific combination product containing ephedra, guarana, and 17 other vitamins, minerals, and supplements (Metabolife-356) might help reduce weight by approximately 2.7 kg over eight weeks when used with a low-fat diet and exercise (3719). Ephedra 90 mg in combination with caffeine from kola nut 192 mg per day for six months seems to cause a modest weight reduction (5.3 kg) in people with a body mass index (BMI) between 25 and 40 kg per meter squared. This combination, along with limiting fat intake to 30 percent of calories and moderate exercise, also seems to reduce body fat, decrease low-density lipoprotein (LDL) cholesterol, and increase high-density lipoprotein (HDL) cholesterol. Even in carefully screened and monitored otherwise healthy adults, ephedra combinations can cause small changes in blood pressure and heart rate (8647). There are serious concerns about the safety of these products since they combine significant amounts of the stimulants ephedra and caffeine and are often taken without monitoring for adverse effects. Tell patients to avoid using combination ephedra/caffeine products without medical supervision.

There is insufficient reliable information available about the effectiveness of ephedra for its other uses.

Mechanism of Action

The applicable part of ephedra is primarily the dried, young branch. Less commonly, the root or whole plant is used (18). Ephedra in dietary supplements is usually either a formulation of powdered stems and aerial portions or a dried extract (6488). Dried extracts contain more ephedra alkaloids per unit weight of material, due to the extraction process. The principal alkaloid constituents are ephedrine, pseudoephedrine, and sometimes small amounts of phenylpropanolamine (6008,6009). Other constituents that have been isolated include norpseudoephedrine, methylephedrine, and norephedrine (8644).

Ephedrine and pseudoephedrine are both non-selective alpha- and beta-receptor agonists. The ephedrine and pseudoephedrine constituents can directly and indirectly stimulate the sympathetic nervous system (9). Ephedrine and pseudoephedrine can increase systolic and diastolic blood pressure, heart rate, and cardiac contractility, and cause peripheral vasoconstriction, bronchodilation, and central nervous system stimulation (8644). Ephedrine, which was used in combination with theophylline and phenobarbital (Tedral) for many years to treat asthma, causes bronchodilation and increased oxygen consumption. Whether the increased oxygen consumption is an indication of a significant increase in metabolism and contributes to weight loss is unknown (8645). A single dose of ephedra in combination with caffeine can increase heart rate from 67 beats per minute to 82 beats per minute in young, healthy people. The combination also increases systolic blood pressure and to a lesser extent, diastolic pressure (8644,11355). Ephedrine seems to cause thermogenesis and modest short-term weight loss, possibly by stimulating norepinephrine release. Some evidence suggests that aspirin and caffeine might act synergistically with ephedrine for weight loss by inhibiting prostaglandin, which increases norepinephrine release (314,729,10003).

Ephedra alkaloids have been linked to myocarditis and myocardial infarction. This has been attributed to coronary artery vasoconstriction and possibly vasospasm caused by ephedra. Ephedra might also cause cardiac arrhythmia due to adrenergic effects that shorten the cardiac refractory period, causing re-entrant arrhythmias (6468). The weight loss product Metabolife 356, which contains ephedra and caffeine in addition to 17 other ingredients, prolongs the QT interval by an average of 27 milliseconds in healthy volunteers (11355). As an indicator of ventricular depolarization and repolarization, a prolonged QT interval increases the risk of potentially serious ventricular arrhythmias such as torsades de pointes. Atrial premature contractions have been demonstrated in healthy volunteers taking recommended doses of Metabolife 356 for 14 days (11708).

Cerebral hemorrhage associated with ephedra has been attributed primarily to hypertensive effects and possibly due to cerebral vasculitis, which has been reported with other adrenergic drugs. Ischemic stroke has been attributed to ephedra's vasoconstrictive effects on cerebral vasculature and possibly platelet aggregation effects due to adrenergic stimulation (6486).

Ephedrine also seems to have antitussive (7), bacteriostatic (2), and anti-inflammatory (11) activity. Ephedrine can have diuretic effects, but can also exacerbate urinary retention (512). Ephedra can have either hypoglycemic or hyperglycemic effects. It can also stimulate uterine contraction, and theoretically can be catabolized to mutagenic nitrosamines (11). Ephedrine causes relaxation of the smooth muscle in the gastrointestinal tract, urinary retention by relaxing the detrusor muscle, and diminishes contraction of the bladder sphincter (15). There's some evidence that ephedrine alone or in combination with caffeine can improve anaerobic exercise performance. Ephedrine causes catecholamine release and increases CNS stimulation, which may lead to better performance (8646). Above ground parts of ephedra seem to cause sweating, but the root seems to inhibit sweating (11). Ephedrine is absorbed faster if it is consumed as the powdered extract. However, onset of action and extent of absorption does not differ greatly between the powdered extract and the powdered herb (6008,6009). Some sources claim ephedra is safer than pure ephedrine and pseudoephedrine because ephedrine from ephedra is absorbed more slowly. However, pharmacokinetic studies have found no differences in the pharmacokinetics of ephedrine from ephedra versus the purified form (6488). The time to maximum concentration (t max) for ephedra is 2.4 hours. The half-life is 6.1 hours (8644).

Adverse Reactions

Orally, ephedra is frequently associated with adverse reactions. In some cases, adverse effects can be severe or life-threatening. Ephedra is banned in the US Poison control center data indicates ephedra is the herb most frequently associated with reports of adverse effects. It is 100 times more likely than other herbs to generate an adverse reaction report. Ephedra accounts for less than 1% of herbal product sales, but causes 64% of herbal adverse reaction reports to poison control centers (9170).

Ephedra most commonly causes dizziness, restlessness, anxiety, irritability, personality changes, difficulty concentrating, insomnia, headache, increased thirst, dry mouth, anorexia, nausea, vomiting, heartburn, flushing, tingling, difficulty urinating, tachycardia, heart palpitations, hyperthermia, and increased blood pressure (1276,3719,6008,6486,8647,10004,10382). Psychosis can occur in some people and in some cases it is prolonged for several months after discontinuation (1276,6998,10689). Long-term use or use in high doses has also been associated with dependence and tolerance (1381).

There are also several reports of serious life-threatening or debilitating adverse effects associated with ephedra products. Ephedra use has been associated with cardiomyopathy (1270), hypersensitivity myocarditis (1271,6487), chest tightness, myocardial infarction (6486), cardiac arrest and sudden death (1274,6486), and cardiac arrhythmias. In healthy volunteers, EKG changes including prolonged QT interval and premature atrial contractions can occur with ingestion of recommended doses of ephedra containing products (11135,11708). Other reported events include stroke, transient ischemic attack, cerebral hemorrhage, seizure, and loss of consciousness (1275,1380,1381,2729,6486,8643). In a review of 926 cases reported to the FDA of possible adverse effects of ephedra, 37 patients had serious or fatal adverse reactions. Ephedra use was temporally related to 16 strokes, 10 myocardial infarctions, and 11 sudden deaths. These effects occurred in people aged 30 to 56 years. There is some evidence that people who take doses greater than 32 mg per day might have more than triple the risk of hemorrhagic stroke, including subarachnoid hemorrhage and intracerebral hemorrhage (9167).

There are also reports of myopathies, including myalgia, rhabdomyolysis, eosinophilia-myalgia syndrome (1270), nephrolithiasis (1272), and acute hepatitis (1273). However, the single case of hepatitis is more likely the result of product contamination than due to ephedra itself (1273). Other reported events include sudden hearing loss (10005). Adverse effects are consistent with catecholamine excess (8643). The use of ephedra causes a 2.2- to 3.6-fold increase in the risk of developing psychiatric, autonomic, or gastrointestinal (GI) symptoms; and cardiac palpitations (9740). Large studies looking at the safety of ephedra have not been performed. Since most of the adverse effect data are from case reports, it is impossible to determine the overall incidence of these adverse effects. It is also difficult to determine which patient groups might be most likely to experience an adverse event. Patients with a history of cardiovascular disease would be expected to be at a higher risk. However, there have been several reports of serious events in patients with no known pre-existing medical condition. In many of these cases, ephedra was used in combination with another stimulant such as caffeine (10307). However, there are also reports of serious adverse effects when ephedra has been used alone. The safety of ephedra is controversial and highly debated. Some claim that ephedra is only unsafe when it is used inappropriately and in excessive doses. The supplement industry maintains that ephedra is safe when taken in doses recommended on labeling. However, there are several cases where severe life-threatening or debilitating effects occurred with short-term use of relatively low doses ranging from 20-60 mg ephedra alkaloids per day (6486). There is also considerable inter- and intra-product variability in labeled ephedra content, which adds to concern about ephedra toxicity (8643,11336). Contaminants such as norpseudoephedrine, a schedule 4 controlled substance, are also present in some products (8643). Until more is known, warn patients that the potential risks of using ephedra outweigh any potential benefit. Advise patients against using products containing ephedra, especially in combination with other stimulants such as caffeine, or if they have a pre-existing condition such as cardiovascular disease.

Interactions with Herbs & Other Dietary Supplements

ERGOT ALKALOID DERIVATIVES: Theoretically, concomitant use might cause excessive vasoconstriction and hypertension due to the ephedrine contained in ephedra (6009).

HERBS AND SUPPLEMENTS WITH STIMULANT PROPERTIES: Use of ephedra and other stimulant herbs, such as those containing caffeine, can increase the risk of common side effects such as insomnia, jitteriness, tremulousness, dizziness, etc. Using ephedra with other stimulants might also increase the risk of more serious adverse effects such as hypertension, myocardial infarction (MI), stroke, and death. There are several reports of serious life-threatening or debilitating adverse events in patients taking ephedra in combination with caffeine and other stimulants (1275,1380,6486,10307). Some herbs and supplements with significant caffeine content include black tea,

coffee, cola nut, green tea, guarana, mate, and others.
PANAX GINSENG: Panax ginseng can cause prolonged QT interval with initial use. It might have an additive effect with ephedra on the QT interval, increasing the risk for arrhythmias (4322,11355).

Interactions with Drugs

ANTIDIABETES DRUGS: Ephedra can raise blood glucose levels and might decrease the effectiveness of drug therapy. Monitor blood glucose concentrations closely (19).
DEXAMETHASONE (Decadron): Theoretically, concomitant use might reduce the effectiveness of dexamethasone, due to the ephedrine contained in ephedra. Ephedrine increases the clearance rate of dexamethasone (11462).
ERGOT DERIVATIVES: Theoretically, concomitant use of ephedra and ergot alkaloids might cause hypertension, due to the ephedrine contained in ephedra (6009).
METHYLXANTHINES: Use of ephedra with caffeine or other methylxanthines such as theophylline might increase the risk of stimulatory adverse effects (8641). There is also some evidence that using ephedra with caffeine might increase the risk of serious life-threatening or debilitating adverse effects such as hypertension, myocardial infarction (MI), stroke, seizures, and death (1275,1380,6486,10307). Tell patients to avoid taking ephedra with caffeine and other stimulants.
MONOAMINE OXIDASE INHIBITORS (MAOIs): Concomitant use of ephedra with MAOIs might increase the risk of hypertension (6009).
QT INTERVAL-PROLONGING DRUGS: Ephedra may have an additive effect with drugs that prolong the QT interval. This may increase the risk of ventricular arrhythmias (11355). Drugs that prolong the QT interval include amiodarone (Cordarone), disopyramide (Norpace), dofetilide (Tikosyn), ibutilide (Corvert), procainamide (Pronestyl), quinidine, sotalol (Betapace), thioridazine (Mellaril), and many others.
RESERPINE: Theoretically, concomitant use with reserpine might antagonize the indirect sympathomimetic effects of the ephedrine contained in ephedra (19). The significance of this interaction is not clear.

Interactions with Foods

COFFEE, TEA: Theoretically, concomitant use of large amounts of caffeinated coffee or tea might increase the stimulatory effects and adverse effects of caffeine and the ephedrine-associated adverse effects of ephedra.

Interactions with Lab Tests

AMPHETAMINE/METHAMPHETAMINE: Ephedra might cause false-positive urine amphetamine or methamphetamine test results. False-positive urine methamphetamine assays have been attributed to the use of herbal supplements containing ephedra (1381,10688).
CATECHOLAMINE: Ephedrine, a constituent of ephedra, can increase plasma catecholamine levels (8646).
EPHEDRINE: Ephedra can cause a positive urine ephedrine test due to its ephedrine content. A case of an athlete whose urine tested positive for norpseudoephedrine was attributed to the use of an herbal supplement labeled to contain ephedra. However, the product might also have contained added norpseudoephedrine as an unlabeled ingredient (1259).
GLUCOSE: Ephedra can increase blood glucose levels and test results (8646). Monitor blood glucose levels in diabetes patients closely.
LACTATE: Ephedrine, a constituent of ephedra, can increase blood lactate levels (8646).

Interactions with Diseases or Conditions

ANGINA: Ephedra is contraindicated in people with angina; it might induce or exacerbate angina due its cardiac stimulant effects (512).
ANOREXIA: Ephedra is contraindicated in people with anorexia due to the purported appetite suppressant effects of ephedra. Anorexic patients might be at increased risk for the adverse effects of ephedra due to inadequate nutritional status (19).
ANXIETY: Large doses of ephedra might cause or exacerbate anxiety due to central nervous system (CNS) stimulant effects (512).
BENIGN PROSTATIC HYPERPLASIA (BPH): Ephedra might exacerbate urinary retention in patients with BPH due to effects on the detrusor muscle (512).
BULIMIA: Ephedra is contraindicated in cases of bulimia; bulimic patients might be at increased risk for the adverse effects of ephedra due to inadequate nutritional status (19).
CEREBRAL INSUFFICIENCY: Ephedra might further decrease cerebral blood flow due to its vasoconstrictive effects (512).
DIABETES: Ephedra might interfere with blood sugar control, and exacerbate high blood pressure and circulatory problems in people with diabetes (512).
ESSENTIAL TREMOR: Ephedra might exacerbate essential tremor (1715).
HEART DISEASE: Ephedra might cause tachycardia, arrhythmias, or induce angina in patients with heart disease due to its cardiac stimulant effects (11355,11708).
HYPERTENSION: Ephedra might exacerbate hypertension (11355); contraindicated in uncontrolled hypertension.
HYPERTHYROID, THYROTOXICOSIS: Ephedra might stimulate the thyroid and exacerbate hyperthyroid

symptoms; contraindicated (512).
KIDNEY STONES: Ephedra and ephedrine can cause kidney stones (1272).
LONG QT INTERVAL SYNDROME: Ephedra appears to prolong the QT interval (11355). It might increase the risk of ventricular arrhythmias in patients with long QT interval syndrome.
NARROW-ANGLE GLAUCOMA: Ephedra might exacerbate narrow-angle (angle-closure) glaucoma by causing mydriasis (512).
PHEOCHROMOCYTOMA: Ephedra might exacerbate the symptoms of pheochromocytoma; contraindicated (2).
URINARY RETENTION: Large doses of ephedra might exacerbate urinary retention due effects on the detrusor muscle (512).

Dosage and Administration

ORAL: For reducing weight in obese patients, ephedra 12 mg in combination with guarana 40 mg three times daily plus 17 other vitamins, minerals, and supplements (Metabolife 356) has been used (3719). Ephedra 90 mg plus caffeine 192 mg per day has also been used for weight loss (8647). The typical dose of ephedra is 15-20 mg of the ephedra alkaloids calculated as ephedrine taken up to three times daily (6486). Doses up to 300 mg per day have been used (12). However, doses as low as 12-36 mg per day have been associated with severe adverse effects. One cup of ephedra tea is also commonly taken three times per day. The tea is prepared by steeping 1-4 grams in 150 mL boiling water for 5-10 minutes and then straining. The tincture (1:1) is usually given as 5 grams per dose. Another tincture (1:4) is given 6-8 mL three times per day. The typical dose of the extract is 1-3 mL three times per day (18). For children over the age of 6 years, some sources suggest a dose of 0.5 mg/kg up to a maximum of 2 mg/kg per day (12), but due to safety concerns, ephedra should not be used in children.

Comments

On December 30, 2003, the FDA announced that it will ban ephedra products in the US (10055). The ban went into effect in April 2004. There has been a lot of debate about the safety of ephedra and legal wrangling over its status (8640,8641). In June of 1997, the FDA proposed restrictions on the ephedrine content of dietary supplements, new warning labels for ephedra alkaloid-containing products, and a prohibition on combination products containing ephedra and other natural stimulants, such as guarana and cola nut, both of which contain significant amounts of caffeine (2729). These proposals were dropped after the link between ephedra use and serious adverse effects was challenged by the General Accounting Office (GAO) and the dietary supplement industry (1381). According to the Dietary Supplement Health and Education Act of 1994, FDA must prove a supplement is unsafe before it can be withdrawn from the market (8642). The FDA reviewed numerous adverse event reports involving ephedra alkaloid-containing products, with 140 of the reports receiving in-depth clinical review by FDA and outside experts (1381,5047,6486). Findings from experts outside the FDA support the FDA's initial finding that ephedra is likely the cause of many of the reports (6486).
Ephedra use is banned by the National Collegiate Athletic Association, International Olympic Committee, and National Football League (8642).
Ephedra is sometimes marketed as a recreational drug "herbal ecstasy." The FDA has announced that ephedra products marketed as recreational drugs are unapproved and misbranded drugs subject to seizure and injunction (5047).
Mormon tea and ephedra are often confused. Mormon tea or American ephedra comes from Ephedra nevadensis and ephedra or ma huang comes primarily from Ephedra sinica. Mormon tea is alkaloid-free and lacks both the therapeutic effects and the toxicity of ephedrine (12).

EPIMEDIUM

Also Known As

Barrenwort, Herba Epimedii, Horny Goat Weed, Japanese Epimedium, Xian Ling Pi, Yin Yang Huo.

Scientific Names

Epimedium grandiflorum; Epimedium brevicornum; Epimedium sagittatum; Epimedium acuminatum; Epimedium grandiflorum f. flavescens, synonym Epimedium koreanum; Epimedium pubescens; Epimedium wushanense; other Epimedium species.
Family: Berberidaceae.

People Use This For

Orally, epimedium is used for impotence, involuntary ejaculation, weak back and knees, arthralgia, mental and physical fatigue, memory loss, hypertension, coronary heart disease, bronchitis, chronic hepatitis, polio, chronic leukopenia, viral myocarditis, and as a tonic and aphrodisiac.
Epimedium is included in some personal care products for its antimicrobial effects.

Safety

POSSIBLY SAFE ...when preparations of the leaf are taken orally, short-term (12).
POSSIBLY UNSAFE ...when used orally, long-term (12).
LIKELY UNSAFE ...when large amounts are used orally. Some species of epimedium can cause respiratory arrest (10346).
PREGNANCY: POSSIBLY UNSAFE ...when used orally; avoid using. Epimedium might have androgenic activity (10346).
LACTATION: Insufficient reliable information available; avoid using.

Effectiveness

There is insufficient reliable information available about the effectiveness of epimedium.

Mechanism of Action

The applicable part of epimedium is the leaf. Researchers think flavonoids, icariin, polysaccharides, glycosides, ceryl alcohol, essential oils, and fatty acids are the active constituents. Epimedium causes vasodilation, possibly by blocking calcium channels. It also seems to have hypotensive effects, possibly by catecholamine blockade (10346). The glycosides in epimedium might have hormonal effects. Animal research suggests that epimedium promotes semen secretion and stimulates growth of prostate, testes, and anus rector muscles. Some researchers think it might increase testosterone secretion (10346). Preliminary research suggests epimedium increases coronary blood flow and decreases platelet aggregation. It may also have immunostimulatory activity and activity against HIV (1512,10346).

Adverse Reactions

Orally, extended use of epimedium may result in dizziness, vomiting, dry mouth, thirst, and nosebleed. Large doses of epimedium may cause respiratory arrest and exaggeration of tendon reflexes to the point of spasm (10346).

Interactions with Herbs & Other Dietary Supplements

HERBS AND SUPPLEMENTS WITH HYPOTENSIVE EFFECTS: Epimedium might have hypotensive effects (10346). Theoretically, concurrent use of epimedium with other herbs and supplements that decrease blood pressure might increase risk of hypotension. Some of these products include danshen, ginger, Panax ginseng, turmeric, valerian, and others.
HERBS WITH ANTICOAGULANT/ANTIPLATELET POTENTIAL: Concomitant use of herbs that constituents that might affect platelet aggregation could theoretically increase the risk of bleeding in some people when taken with epimedium (10346). These herbs include angelica, clove, danshen, garlic, ginger, ginkgo, quassia, red clover, turmeric, willow, and others.

Interactions with Drugs

ANTICOAGULANT/ANTIPLATELET DRUGS: Theoretically, epimedium might potentiate the effects of anticoagulant and antiplatelet drugs and possibly increase the risk of bleeding (10346). However, this effect has not yet been demonstrated in humans. Until more is known, use cautiously in patients taking anticoagulant or antiplatelet drugs. Some of these drugs include aspirin, clopidogrel (Plavix), dalteparin (Fragmin), enoxaparin (Lovenox), heparin, ticlopidine (Ticlid), warfarin (Coumadin), and others.
ANTIHYPERTENSIVE DRUGS: Epimedium might have hypotensive effects (10346). Theoretically, concomitant use with antihypertensives might have additive effects on blood pressure and increase the risk of hypotension.

Interactions with Foods

None known.

Interactions with Lab Tests

None known.

Interactions with Diseases or Conditions

HYPOTENSION: Epimedium might have hypotensive effects (10346). Theoretically, use in people with existing low blood pressure might exacerbate hypotension and possibly lead to syncope.

Dosage and Administration

No typical dosage.

Comments

The leaf of Japanese epimedium (Epimedium grandiflora) is generally used (12). Leaf, petiole, and stem of other Epimedium species are also sometimes used (11). As many as 15 Epimedium species are interchangeable as "yin yang huo" (11).

ERGOT

Also Known As
Cockspur Rye, Hornseed, Mother of Rye, Secale cornutum, Smut Rye, Spurred Rye.

Scientific Names
Claviceps purpurea. Plant host: Rye (Secale cereale).
Family: Clavicipitaceae.

People Use This For
Orally, ergot is used for obstetric and gynecologic conditions, including hemorrhage, climacteric hemorrhage, menorrhagia, metrorrhagia (before and after miscarriage), expulsion of placenta, shortening of afterbirth period, and atonia of the uterus.

Safety
UNSAFE ...when used orally due to poisoning risk and interactions with many disease states (11163,11164).
PREGNANCY AND LACTATION: UNSAFE ...when used orally due to high level of risk (11163,11164); avoid using.

Effectiveness
There is insufficient reliable information available about the effectiveness of ergot.

Mechanism of Action
Ergot is a fungal growth that occurs on rye (Secale cereale), and to a lesser extent, other grasses such as wheat (Triticum aestivum). The fungus contains ergot alkaloids (ergolines). Derivatives of ergot including lysergic acid, ergocristine, ergotamine, ergonovine (ergometrine), and many others have been isolated. Ergot alkaloids have various pharmacologic activities. They act as serotonin agonists, which can cause arterial vasoconstriction. Ergot alkaloids also act as dopamine agonists. For example, bromocriptine (Parlodel) is an ergot derivative. Some act as alpha-adrenergic antagonists and cause vasoconstriction. Ergot alkaloids, particularly ergonovine, also cause uterine smooth-muscle contraction. Ergot also contains histamine, tyramine, and acetylcholine, but these are probably not significantly absorbed when ergot is taken orally (11163).

Adverse Reactions
Orally, ergot can cause gastrointestinal (GI) symptoms such as nausea and abdominal pain. Weakness, muscle pain of the extremities, and numbness and tingling of the fingers and toes may also occur (9). Symptoms of acute overdose include nausea, vomiting, diarrhea, extreme thirst, coldness, tingling and itching of the skin, a rapid and weak pulse, hypotension, shock, confusion, seizures, unconsciousness, and death (9). Chronic toxicity or ergotism rarely occurs after a single oral dose. It usually results from cumulative doses over a short period of time (11163). Symptoms of ergotism are related to circulatory disturbances. Numbness, coldness, and tingling of the extremities, particularly the feet and legs occur along with paleness or cyanosis. There may be no pulse in the affected area. This may develop into gangrene, especially in the toes (9,11163). A convulsive form of ergotism may also occur. Symptoms include muscle spasms in the trunk and limbs, painful involuntary flexion of the fingers and wrists, and either flexion or extension of the ankles. Central nervous system (CNS) adverse effects such as drowsiness, delirium, lethargy, mental changes, and visual disturbances can also occur. Sweating, fever, muscle stiffness, twitching and seizures have also been reported (9,11163). Ergotism from food is rare today. It is more common from overdoses of prescription ergot alkaloids (11164).

Interactions with Herbs & Other Dietary Supplements
HERBS AND SUPPLEMENTS WITH SEROTONERGIC PROPERTIES: Theoretically, ergot might increase the effects and adverse effects of products that increase serotonin levels, including 5-hydroxytryptophan, Hawaiian baby woodrose, l-tryptophan S-adenosylmethionine (SAMe), and St. John's wort (11163).
HERBS AND PLEMENTS WITH SYMPATHOMIMETIC ACTIVITY: Theoretically, ergot might enhance the effects and adverse effects of herbs and supplements that have sympathomimetic activity, including bitter orange, caffeine, country mallow, guarana, and ephedra (11163).

Interactions with Drugs
ANTIDEPRESSANT DRUGS: Combining serotonergic antidepressants with ergot might increase the risk of serotonergic side effects including serotonin syndrome and cerebral vasoconstrictive disorders such as Call-Fleming syndrome (8056,11163). These drugs include the selective serotonin reuptake inhibitors (SSRIs) such as fluoxetine (Prozac), paroxetine (Paxil), sertraline (Zoloft), and others; and tricyclic and atypical antidepressants such as amitriptyline (Elavil), clomipramine (Anafranil), imipramine (Tofranil), and others.
CYTOCHROME P450 3A4 (CYP3A4) INHIBITORS: Ergotamine, a constituent of ergot, is a substrate of cytochrome P450 3A4 (CYP3A4) (11163). Theoretically, drugs that inhibit CYP3A4 might increase the risk of ergot

toxicity. Some of these drugs include amiodarone (Cordarone), clarithromycin (Biaxin), diltiazem (Cardizem), erythromycin (E-mycin, Erythrocin), indinavir (Crixivan), ritonavir (Norvir), saquinavir (Fortovase, Invirase), and many others.
DEXTROMETHORPHAN (Robitussin DM, and others): Combining serotonergic drugs such as dextromethorphan with ergot might increase the risk of serotonergic side effects including serotonin syndrome and cerebral vasoconstrictive disorders such as Call-Fleming syndrome (8056,11163).
ERGOT DERIVATIVES: Ergot alkaloids or derivatives may increase the risk of adverse effects (11163). Some of these include bromocriptine (Parlodel), dihydroergotamine (Migranal, DHE-45), ergotamine (Cafergot), and pergolide (Permax).
MEPERIDINE (Demerol): Combining serotonergic drugs such as meperidine with ergot might increase the risk of serotonergic side effects including serotonin syndrome and cerebral vasoconstrictive disorders such as Call-Fleming syndrome (8056,11163).
MONOAMINE OXIDASE INHIBITORS (MAOIs): Combining serotonergic drugs such as one of the MAOIs with ergot might increase the risk of serotonergic side effects including serotonin syndrome and cerebral vasoconstrictive disorders such as Call-Fleming syndrome (8056,11163).
PENTAZOCINE (Talwin): Combining serotonergic drugs such as pentazocin with ergot might increase the risk of serotonergic side effects including serotonin syndrome and cerebral vasoconstrictive disorders such as Call-Fleming syndrome (8056,11163).
STIMULANT DRUGS: Co-administration with ergot may increase the risk of vasoconstriction. Some sympathomimetics include albuterol (Proventil, Ventolin), diethylpropion (Tenuate), dopamine, epinephrine, phentermine (Ionamin), pseudoephedrine (Sudafed), and many others (11163).
TRAMADOL (Ultram): Combining serotonergic drugs such as tramadol with ergot might increase the risk of serotonergic side effects including serotonin syndrome and cerebral vasoconstrictive disorders such as Call-Fleming syndrome (8056,11163).

Interactions with Foods
None known.

Interactions with Lab Tests
None known.

Interactions with Diseases or Conditions
HEART DISEASE: Ergot can cause arterial constriction and may worsen coronary insufficiency (11163).
HEPATIC DISEASE: Reduced hepatic clearance of ergot may increase the risk of ergot poisoning (9).
KIDNEY DISEASE: Reduced renal clearance of ergot may increase the risk of ergot poisoning (9).
PERIPHERAL VASCULAR DISEASE: Ergot can cause vasoconstriction and may worsen peripheral vascular disease (9).

Dosage and Administration
No typical dosage.

Comments
Historically, ergot was used to speed labor, but its use was abandoned when increased risk of stillbirth was recognized (11163).
During the Middle Ages, ergotism was common from food contamination (such as rye bread) and was known as St. Anthony's fire. It was often cured by visiting the shrine of St. Anthony, which happened to be in an ergot-free region of France. Some historians think the Salem witchcraft trials of 1692 might have resulted from a convulsive form of ergotism (11164).

ERYNGO above ground parts

Also Known As
Eringo, Eryngii Herba, Sea Holly, Sea Holme, Sea Hulver.
CAUTION: See separate listing for Eryngo root.

Scientific Names
Eryngium campestre, synonyms Eryngium maritimum, Eyrnigium planum, Eryngium yuccifolium.
Family: Apiaceae/Umbelliferae.

People Use This For
Orally, people use eryngo above ground parts for urinary tract infections, inflammation of the urinary tract, prostatitis, and mucous membrane inflammation of the bronchi.

Safety
There is insufficient reliable information available about the safety of eryngo above ground parts.
Pregnancy and Lactation: Insufficient reliable information available; avoid using.

Effectiveness
There is insufficient reliable information available about the effectiveness of eryngo above ground parts.

Mechanism of Action
Eryngo above ground parts are stated to have a diuretic effect (18).

Adverse Reactions
None reported.

Interactions with Herbs & Other Dietary Supplements
None known.

Interactions with Drugs
None known.

Interactions with Foods
None known.

Interactions with Lab Tests
None known.

Interactions with Diseases or Conditions
None known.

Dosage and Administration
ORAL: Eryngo above ground parts are typically administered as an extract (amount used unspecified) (18).

ERYNGO root

Also Known As
Eringo, Eryngii Radix, Sea Holly, Sea Holme, Sea Hulver.
CAUTION: See separate listing for Eryngo above ground parts.

Scientific Names
Eryngium campestre, synonyms Eryngium maritimum, Eyrnigium planum, Eryngium yuccifolium.
Family: Apiaceae/Umbelliferae.

People Use This For
Orally, eryngo root is used for kidney and bladder stones, renal colic, kidney and urinary tract inflammation, urinary retention, edema, coughs, bronchitis, and skin and respiratory disorders.

Safety
POSSIBLY SAFE ...when used orally and appropriately (12).
PREGNANCY AND LACTATION: Insufficient reliable information available; avoid using.

Effectiveness
There is insufficient reliable information available about the effectiveness of eryngo root.

Mechanism of Action
Eryngo root is reported to have mild expectorant and antispasmodic properties (18).

Adverse Reactions
None reported.

Interactions with Herbs & Other Dietary Supplements
None known.

Interactions with Drugs
None known.

Interactions with Foods
None known.

Interactions with Lab Tests
None known.

Interactions with Diseases or Conditions
None known.

Dosage and Administration
ORAL: Typical dose is 3 to 4 cups of tea (steep 1 teaspoon ground root in 150 mL of boiling water until cold; strain) daily (18). Alternatively, 2-3 cups decoction (boil 4 teaspoons of ground root in 1 L water for 10 minutes, steep for 15 minutes, strain) daily (18); or 50-60 drops tincture (soak 20 grams powdered root in 80 grams of 60% alcohol for 10 days) divided into 3 or 4 doses daily have been used.

EUCALYPTUS dried leaf

Also Known As
Blue Gum, Blue Mallee, Eucalypti Folium, Eucalyptusblatter, Fever Tree, Fevertree, Fieberbaumblatter, Gully Gum, Gum Tree, Red Gum, Stringy Bark Tree, Sugandhapatra, Tailapatra, Tasmanian Blue Gum.
CAUTION: See separate listing for Eucalyptus Oil.

Scientific Names
Eucalyptus globulus; Eucalyptus bicostata; Eucalyptus smithii; Eucalyptus odorata, synonym Eucalyptus fruticetorum; Eucalyptus polybractea.
Family: Myrtaceae.

People Use This For
Orally, dried eucalyptus leaf is used as an antiseptic, antipyretic, expectorant, gastrointestinal (GI) remedy, and as a stimulant for respiratory ailments. It is also used orally for treating respiratory tract mucous membrane inflammation, whooping cough, asthma, pulmonary tuberculosis, aching joints, rheumatism, acne, wounds, poorly healing ulcers, burns, bacterial dysentery, ringworms, liver and gallbladder complaints, loss of appetite, stomatitis, bleeding gums, bladder diseases, gonorrhea, fever, flu, diabetes, neuralgia, and cancer.
In foods, dried eucalyptus leaf is used as a flavoring agent.

Safety
LIKELY SAFE ...when used orally in amounts commonly found in foods. Eucalyptus has Generally Recognized As Safe (GRAS) status in the US (4912).
POSSIBLY SAFE ...when the dried leaf is used orally and appropriately (12). ...when preparations of the dried leaf are used topically.
CHILDREN: LIKELY UNSAFE ...when applied topically to the face or in the nose of infants and young children (2,12). It can cause bronchospasm. There is insufficient reliable information available about the safety of oral use in young children; avoid using.
PREGNANCY AND LACTATION: Insufficient reliable information available; avoid using.

Effectiveness
POSSIBLY EFFECTIVE

Respiratory congestion. Taking eucalyptus dried leaf orally seems to be effective when used as an expectorant (3). Depending on the species, the product must contain 70-85% eucalyptol or cineole (3).

There is insufficient reliable information available about the effectiveness of dried eucalyptus leaf for its other uses.

Mechanism of Action
The leaf can have secretion-stimulating, expectorant, antiseptic, and weakly antispasmodic properties (2,4). The antiseptic and expectorant properties of the leaf are due to its volatile oils, particularly eucalyptol (4). Other evidence suggests eucalyptus can be a urinary irritant.

Adverse Reactions

Orally, eucalyptus dried leaf rarely can cause nausea, vomiting, and diarrhea (2). Signs of eucalyptus poisoning include epigastric burning, nausea, vomiting, diarrhea, dizziness, muscular weakness, miosis, feeling of suffocation, cyanosis, delirium, convulsions, and death (4). The ingestion of 3.5 mL of the eucalyptus oil can be fatal (11).

Interactions with Herbs & Other Dietary Supplements

None known.

Interactions with Drugs

ANTIDIABETES DRUGS: Eucalyptus leaf extract may have hypoglycemic activity due to phenolic glycoside constituents (4). Monitor blood glucose levels closely.

Interactions with Foods

None known.

Interactions with Lab Tests

None known.

Interactions with Diseases or Conditions

DIABETES: Theoretically, eucalyptus can interfere with blood glucose control (4).
OTHER CONDITIONS: Contraindicated in cases of gastrointestinal (GI) tract and bile duct inflammation, liver disease (2), hypotension, and kidney inflammation (500).

Dosage and Administration

ORAL: The typical dose of the eucalyptus leaf is one cup of the freshly prepared tea 3 times daily (3). The tea is made by steeping 2 grams of the dried leaf in 150 mL boiling water and then straining. Limit the daily intake to 4-6 grams per day of the dried leaf or equivalent preparations (2). The usual dose of the tincture is 3-9 grams per day (2), and the fluid extract is dosed 2-4 grams per day (4).

EUCALYPTUS OIL

Also Known As

Blue Mallee Oil, Gully Gum Oil.
CAUTION: See separate listing for Eucalyptus dried leaf.

Scientific Names

Eucalyptus odorata, synonym Eucalyptus fruticetorum; Eucalyptus polybractea; Eucalyptus globulus, synonym Eucalyptus bicostata; Eucalyptus smithii.
Family: Myrtaceae.

People Use This For

Orally, eucalyptus oil is used for inflammation of respiratory tract mucous membranes, for suppressing coughs, as an expectorant, antiseptic, antipyretic; and for wounds, burns, ulcers, cancer, and in vaporizer fluids.
Topically, eucalyptus oil is used for inflammation of respiratory tract mucous membranes, rheumatic complaints, and nasal stuffiness.
In dentistry, eucalyptus oil is a component of sealers and solvents for root canal fillings.
In manufacturing, eucalyptus oil is utilized as a flavoring and a fragrance component in perfumes. It is also used as a mouthwash; antiseptic; liniment; ointment; and in toothpaste, cough drops, and gum lozenges.

Safety

LIKELY SAFE ...when used orally in amounts commonly found in foods. Eucalyptus oil has Generally Recognized As Safe (GRAS) status in the US (4912).
POSSIBLY SAFE ...when used orally and appropriately in medicinal amounts (2,12). It must be used in very small amounts or diluted (2,12).
POSSIBLY UNSAFE ...when the undiluted oil is used topically (4).
LIKELY UNSAFE ...when undiluted oil is ingested orally. Ingesting 3.5 mL of undiluted oil can be fatal (4).
CHILDREN: LIKELY UNSAFE ...when used topically on the face, especially the nose, of infants and young children (2) because it can cause bronchospasm. ...when the oil is used orally (4).
PREGNANCY: LIKELY UNSAFE ...when used orally in medicinal amounts; contraindicated (4).
LACTATION: Insufficient reliable information available; avoid using in amounts greater than found in foods (4).

Effectiveness

There is insufficient reliable information available about the effectiveness of eucalyptus oil.

Mechanism of Action

Eucalyptus oil contains 70-85% eucalyptol (1,8-cineole), which stimulates production and secretion of saliva (11). This, in turn, activates the swallowing reflex. Voluntary swallowing can suppress an impending cough (7). Taken by mouth, eucalyptus oil aids in expectorating secretions (2,4), has mild antibacterial action (4), and is mildly antispasmodic (2). In vitro, it has antibacterial and fungicidal effects.
Topically, it acts as a mild counterirritant (2) and may inhibit prostaglandin synthesis (18). The crude eucalyptus leaf extract has demonstrated hypoglycemic activity in rabbits (4). Eucalyptus can be a urinary irritant (19). Eucalyptus oil might also induce liver enzymes (2).

Adverse Reactions

Orally, eucalyptus oil can cause nausea, vomiting, and diarrhea (2). Signs of eucalyptus oil poisoning include epigastric burning, nausea, vomiting, dizziness, muscular weakness, constricted pupils of eyes, feeling of suffocation, cyanosis, delirium, and convulsions. The ingestion of 3.5 mL of the oil can be fatal (4).

Interactions with Herbs & Other Dietary Supplements

UNSATURATED PYRROLIZIDINE ALKALOID (UPA)-CONTAINING PLANTS: Eucalyptus oil can potentiate the toxicity of borage, coltsfoot, comfrey, hound's tooth, and Senecio species (500).

Interactions with Drugs

None known.

Interactions with Foods

None known.

Interactions with Lab Tests

None known.

Interactions with Diseases or Conditions

DIABETES: Theoretically, eucalyptus oil can interfere with blood sugar control (4).
OTHER CONDITIONS: Eucalyptus oil is contraindicated in cases of gastrointestinal (GI) tract and bile duct inflammation, severe liver disease (2), hypotension, kidney inflammation, and low blood pressure (500).

Dosage and Administration

ORAL: The typical dose is 300-600 mg of the eucalyptus oil per day (2), and about 0.05-0.2 mL per dose (4).
TOPICAL: Semi-solid or vegetable oil preparations usually contain 5%-20% eucalyptus oil (2,4), and aqueous-alcoholic preparations contain 5%-10% eucalyptus oil (2). The oil is also typically used for local application by diluting 30 mL oil to 500 mL lukewarm water (4). Avoid the use of the undiluted essential oil. The essential oil diluted in vegetable oil is preferred for applications on the skin (4). Avoid use on areas of the face, especially the nose, of infants and young children (2).

Comments

Eucalyptus oil is the steam distilled volatile oil from fresh leaves and branch tops of various species of Eucalyptus.

EUPHORBIA

Also Known As

Asthmaplant, Pillbearing Spurge, Snakeweed.

Scientific Names

Chamaesyce hirta, synonyms Euphorbia hirta, Euphorbia pilulifera; Euphorbia capitulata.
Family: Euphorbiaceae.

People Use This For

Orally, euphorbia is used for respiratory disorders including asthma, bronchitis, catarrh, laryngeal spasm, hay fever, and tumors, and as an expectorant and an emetic. It is also used orally for treating worms, dysentery, gonorrhea, and digestive problems in India.

Safety
There is insufficient reliable information available about the safety of euphorbia.
PREGNANCY AND LACTATION: POSSIBLY UNSAFE ...when used orally; avoid using. Euphorbia is reported to cause smooth muscle contraction and relaxation (4).

Effectiveness
There is insufficient reliable information available about the effectiveness of euphorbia.

Mechanism of Action
The applicable parts of euphorbia are the above ground parts. It is reported to have antispasmodic, histamine potentiator, antitumor, and antibacterial activity against gram positive and gram negative organisms in animals (4). The constituent choline is reported to produce contraction of isolated pig ileum. The constituent shikimic acid produces relaxation (11).

Adverse Reactions
Orally, euphorbia may cause nausea and vomiting (12). Skin contact with fresh euphorbia can cause irritation or contact dermatitis (19).

Interactions with Herbs & Other Dietary Supplements
None known.

Interactions with Drugs
None known.

Interactions with Foods
None known.

Interactions with Lab Tests
None known.

Interactions with Diseases or Conditions
GI CONDITIONS: Euphorbia can irritate the gastrointestinal tract. Contraindicated in individuals with infectious or inflammatory gastrointestinal conditions (19).

Dosage and Administration
ORAL: Typical dose is one cup tea prepared by steeping 120-300 mg above ground parts in 150 mL boiling water 5-10 minutes and then straining (4). Liquid extract, concentration unspecified, 0.12-0.3 mL, and tincture, concentration unspecified, 0.6-2 mL have also been used (4). As and expectorant, 2 grams above ground parts has been used; emetic dose may be similar.

EUROPEAN BARBERRY

Also Known As
Agracejo, Berberidis cortex, Berberidis fructus, Berberidis radicis cortex, Berberidis radix, Berberitze, Berberry, Berbis, Common Barberry, Epine-Vinette, Espino Cambrón, Jaundice Berry, Mountain Grape, Oregon Grape, Pipperidge, Piprage, Sauerdorn, Sow Berry, Vinettier.
CAUTION: See separate listing for Oregon Grape.

Scientific Names
Berberis vulgaris, synonyms Berberis jacquinii, Berberis sanguinea.
Family: Berberidaceae.

People Use This For
Orally, the fruit of European barberry is used for kidney, urinary tract, and gastrointestinal tract discomforts such as heartburn, stomach cramps, constipation, lack of appetite, liver and spleen disease, for bronchial and lung discomforts, spasms, as a stimulant for circulation, for people susceptible to infection, and as a supplemental source of vitamin C. The bark, root, and root bark of European barberry are also used orally for ailments and complaints of the GI tract, liver, gallbladder, kidney and urinary tract, respiratory tract, heart and circulatory system, as an antipyretic, "blood purifier", and for narcotic withdrawal. European barberry root bark is used for liver dysfunction, gallbladder disease, jaundice, splenopathy, diarrhea, indigestion, hemorrhoids, renal and urinary tract diseases, gout, rheumatism, arthritis, mid and low back pain, malaria, and leishmaniasis.

In foods, European barberry fruit is used in making jam, jellies, and wine.
In manufacturing, the fruit syrup is used for masking tastes in pharmaceutical preparations.

Safety

LIKELY SAFE ...when the fruit is consumed in food amounts. The fruit is considered to contain only trace amounts of berberine (2,12).
POSSIBLY SAFE ...when the fruit, root, bark, or root bark are used orally and appropriately for medicinal uses. Amounts of less than 500 mg of berberine are usually considered safe (2,12,18).
LIKELY UNSAFE ...when more than 500 mg of berberine is consumed. Berberine is considered moderately toxic (12). The LD50 in humans is reported to be 27.5 mg/kg (12).
PREGNANCY: LIKELY UNSAFE ...when used orally because it can have uterine stimulant properties (11,12).
LACTATION: Insufficient reliable information is available; avoid using.

Effectiveness

There is insufficient reliable information available about the effectiveness of European barberry.

Mechanism of Action

The applicable parts of European barberry are the bark, fruit, root, and root bark. European barberry fruit contains vitamin C (18). Researchers think it has mild diuretic activity due to the acid content (18). The bark, root, and root bark of European barberry contain isoquinolone alkaloid constituents, including berberine, berbamine, columbamine, jatorrhizine, palmatine, and oxyacanthine (11,19). The constituents berberine, columbamine, and oxyacanthine show evidence of antibacterial activity (11). Berberine has anticonvulsant, sedative, hypotensive, antifibrillatory, and bile-stimulating effects. In low doses, it is a cardiac and respiratory stimulant. In high doses it is a depressant (11,12,515). Some evidence suggests berberine sulfate might be amebicidal and trypanocidal (11). Other information suggests the constituent berbamine might have antiarrhythmic, hypotensive, spasmolytic, and immunostimulating activity (11,515).

Adverse Reactions

Orally, ingestion of greater than 500 mg berberine, which is found in European barberry, can cause lethargy, nose bleed, skin and eye irritation, nephritis and kidney irritation (2). It might also cause dyspnea, hypotension, cardiac damage (12), nausea, vomiting, diarrhea, hemorrhagic nephritis, respiratory spasms and arrest, and death (2).

Interactions with Herbs & Other Dietary Supplements

BERBERINE-CONTAINING HERBS: Concomitant use can increase the risk of berberine toxicity. Berberine-containing herbs include: bloodroot, goldenseal, celandine, Chinese goldthread, goldthread, Oregon grape (Mahonia species), amur cork tree, and Chinese corktree (12).

Interactions with Drugs

None known.

Interactions with Foods

None known.

Interactions with Lab Tests

None known.

Interactions with Diseases or Conditions

GI IRRITATION: European barberry can irritate gastrointestinal tract. It is contraindicated in individuals with infectious or inflammatory gastrointestinal conditions (19).
KIDNEY DISEASE: Berberine, which is found in European barberry, can cause kidney irritation and nephritis (2).

Dosage and Administration

ORAL :A typical dose is one cup tea. To make tea, steep 1-2 teaspoons of whole or squashed berries in 150 mL boiling water 10-15 minutes and strain (18) or steep 2 grams of root bark in 250 mL boiling water 5-10 minutes and strain (18). Root bark is typically used as a tincture (1:10), 20-40 drops per day (18). Root tea is not recommended (2,18).

EUROPEAN BUCKTHORN

Also Known As
Buckthorn, Buckthorn Berry, Hartshorn, Highwaythorn, Kreuzdornbeeren, Ramsthorn, Rhamni cathartica fructus, Waythorn.
CAUTION: See separate listings for Alder Buckthorn, Sea Buckthorn, and Cascara (California Buckthorn).

Scientific Names
Rhamnus cathartica.
Family: Rhamnaceae.

People Use This For
Orally, European buckthorn is used for constipation.

Safety
POSSIBLY SAFE ...when the standardized preparations of the berry are used orally and appropriately for less than eight to ten days (12). It is important not to exceed recommended amounts (12).
POSSIBLY UNSAFE ...when standardized preparations are used more than ten days (12).
LIKELY UNSAFE ...when nonstandardized preparations are used orally (12).
CHILDREN: LIKELY UNSAFE ...when used orally in children younger than 12 years of age (12).
PREGNANCY AND LACTATION: LIKELY UNSAFE ...when used orally (12); avoid using.

Effectiveness
LIKELY EFFECTIVE

Constipation. Taking European buckthorn orally is effective as a stimulant laxative for constipation (3,4,7,12) and is comparable to the gentle, laxative effects of cascara (3).

Mechanism of Action
The applicable part of European buckthorn is the berry. The anthraquinones in the European buckthorn berry can increase intestinal GI motility by inhibiting stationary contractions and stimulating propulsive contractions (2). Stimulation of active chloride secretion increases the water and electrolytes in intestinal contents, increasing the risk of electrolyte loss with overuse or misuse of the berry (2). Anthroid laxative use is not associated with an increased risk of developing colorectal adenoma or carcinoma (6138).

Adverse Reactions
Orally, European buckthorn can cause abdominal pain, cramps, or watery diarrhea (12). Chronic use or abuse of the berry can lead to potassium depletion, albuminuria, and hematuria. Potassium depletion can lead to disturbed heart function and muscle weakness (2). Chronic use can cause pseudomelanosis coli (pigment spots in intestinal mucosa) which is harmless, usually reverses with discontinuation (2), and is not associated with an increased risk of developing colorectal adenoma or carcinoma (6138).

Interactions with Herbs & Other Dietary Supplements
CARDIAC GLYCOSIDE-CONTAINING HERBS: Theoretically, overuse or abuse of European buckthorn can increase the risk of cardiac glycoside toxicity. Cardiac glycoside containing herbs include black hellebore, Canadian hemp roots, digitalis leaf, hedge mustard, figwort, lily of the valley root, motherwort, oleander leaf, pheasant's eye plant, pleurisy root, squill bulb leaf scales, and strophanthus seeds (19).
HORSETAIL/LICORICE: Theoretically, concomitant use of European buckthorn berry with horsetail plant or licorice rhizome increases the risk of potassium depletion (19).
STIMULANT LAXATIVE HERBS: Theoretically, concomitant use of European buckthorn with other stimulant laxative herbs can increase the risk of potassium depletion (19). Stimulant laxative herbs include aloe dried leaf sap, wild cucumber fruit (Ecballium elaterium), blue flag rhizome, alder buckthorn, butternut bark, cascara bark, castor oil, colocynth fruit pulp, gamboge bark exudate, jalap root, black root, manna bark exudate, podophyllum root, rhubarb root, senna leaves and pods, and yellow dock root.

Interactions with Drugs
DIGOXIN (Lanoxin): The overuse or abuse of European buckthorn can increase the toxicity of cardiac glycoside drugs (19).
DIURETIC DRUGS: Overuse of European buckthorn might compound diuretic-induced potassium loss (19). There is some concern that people taking European buckthorn along with potassium depleting diuretics might have an increased risk for hypokalemia. Initiation of potassium supplementation or an increase in potassium supplement dose may be necessary for some patients. Some diuretics that can deplete potassium include chlorothiazide (Diuril), chlorthalidone (Thalitone), furosemide (Lasix), hydrochlorothiazide (HCTZ, HydroDIURIL, Microzide), and others.
ORAL DRUGS: European buckthorn can decrease bowel transit time, reducing absorption of oral drugs (19).

Interactions with Foods
None known.

Interactions with Lab Tests
COLORIMETRIC TESTS: Due to its anthraquinone content, European buckthorn can discolor urine (pink, red, purple, orange, rust), interfering with diagnostic tests that depend on a color change (12,275).
POTASSIUM: Excessive use of European buckthorn can cause potassium depletion, reducing serum potassium concentrations and test results (12,19).

Interactions with Diseases or Conditions
GASTROINTESTINAL (GI) CONDITIONS: European buckthorn is contraindicated in individuals with intestinal obstruction; abdominal pain of unknown origin; and intestinal inflammation, including appendicitis, Crohn's disease, irritable bowel syndrome (IBS), and ulcerative colitis (12).

Dosage and Administration
ORAL: The typical dose of European buckthorn berry is 20-30 mg of the hydroxyanthracene derivative per day calculated as glucofrangulin A (2). One cup of the tea is commonly taken in the evening, and if needed, in the morning and afternoon (8,12). The tea is prepared by steeping 2-4 grams of the fruit in 150 mL boiling water for 10-15 minutes and then straining (8,12). Use the smallest amount necessary to achieve a soft stool (2) and discontinue in the event of diarrhea or watery stools (12). Limit the use of European buckthorn to a maximum of 8 to 10 days (12). This preparation should be used only if no effect can be obtained through a change of diet or use of bulk-forming laxative products (2).

Comments
Avoid confusion with alder buckthorn (Rhamus frangula). The American Herbal Products Association (AHPA) recommends the following label statement: "Do not use this product if you have abdominal pain or diarrhea. Consult a healthcare provider prior to use if you are pregnant or nursing. Discontinue use in the event of diarrhea or watery stools. Do not exceed dose. Not for long-term use." (12). Today, European buckthorn is primarily used as a dye.

EUROPEAN CHESTNUT

Also Known As
Castaneae Folium, Husked Nut, Jupiter's Nut, Kastanienblaetter, Sardian Nut, Spanish Chestnut, Sweet Chestnut.
CAUTION: See separate listing for American Chestnut leaf.

Scientific Names
Castanea sativa, synonyms Castanea vesca, Castanea vulgaris, Fagus castanea, Fagus procera.
Family: Fagaceae.

People Use This For
Orally, European chestnut is used for respiratory tract complaints including bronchitis and whooping cough, disorders affecting the legs and circulation, diarrhea, fever, the passage of bloody stools, hydrocele, infection, inflammation, kidney disorders, myalgias, nausea, paroxysm, sclerosis, inflammation of the lymph nodes due to tuberculosis infection, and stomach disorders.
Topically, European chestnut is used as a gargle for sore throat and for wounds.

Safety
POSSIBLY SAFE ...when used orally and appropriately (12).
There is insufficient reliable information available about the safety of European chestnut for its other uses.
PREGNANCY AND LACTATION: Insufficient reliable information available; avoid using.

Effectiveness
There is insufficient reliable information available about the effectiveness of European chestnut.

Mechanism of Action
The applicable part of European chestnut is the leaf. European chestnut contains 9% tannins, which exert an astringent effect on the mucosal tissue. This effect causes localized dehydration that turns the external cells into a protective layer (12). Plants with 10% tannins or more may cause gastrointestinal disturbances, kidney damage, and necrotic conditions of the liver (12). Some animal experiments show that tannins may cause cancer; others show that they may prevent it (12). Regular consumption of herbs with high tannin concentrations correlates with increased incidence of esophageal or nasal cancer (12).

Adverse Reactions
None reported.

Interactions with Herbs & Other Dietary Supplements
TANNIN-CONTAINING HERBS: Theoretically, herbs that contain high percentages of tannins (such as European chestnut) may cause precipitation of constituents of other herbs.

Interactions with Drugs
ORAL DRUGS: Theoretically, concomitant oral administration may cause precipitation of some drugs due to the high tannin content of European chestnut (19). Separate administration of oral drugs and tannin-containing herbs by the longest period of time practical (19).

Interactions with Foods
None known.

Interactions with Lab Tests
None known.

Interactions with Diseases or Conditions
None known.

Dosage and Administration
ORAL: People typically prepare European chestnut as a tea with 1 teaspoon of leaves and bark boiled in a covered container with 2 cups of water for 30 minutes. The liquid is cooled slowly in the closed container and taken cold, 1 to 2 cups per day (5254).

EUROPEAN FIVE-FINGER GRASS

Also Known As
Cinquefoil, European Five Finger Grass, Five-Finger Blossom, Five Fingers, Sunkfield, Synkfoyle.

Scientific Names
Potentilla reptans.
Family: Rosaceae.

People Use This For
Orally, European five-finger grass is used for diarrhea and fever.
Topically, European five-finger grass is used for inflammation of the mucous membranes of the mouth and gums, toothache, and heartburn. It is also used as an astringent and to treat open wounds.

Safety
There is insufficient reliable information available about the safety of European five-finger grass.
Pregnancy and Lactation: Insufficient reliable information available; avoid using.

Effectiveness
There is insufficient reliable information available about the effectiveness of European five-finger grass.

Mechanism of Action
The astringent effects of European five-finger grass are most likely secondary to tannin content (18).

Adverse Reactions
None reported.

Interactions with Herbs & Other Dietary Supplements
None known.

Interactions with Drugs
None known.

Interactions with Foods
None known.

Interactions with Lab Tests
None known.

Interactions with Diseases or Conditions
None known.

Dosage and Administration
ORAL: Typically, one cup of tea is taken 2-3 times daily. The tea is prepared by simmering 3 grams of dried plant in 100 mL of boiling water for 10-15 minutes and straining.
TOPICAL: A tea is made by simmering 6 grams of dried plant in 100 mL of boiling water for 10-15 minutes and strained before use. It is also used in baths as one handful of dried plant to a bathful of water (18).

Comments
European five-finger grass is easily confused with Potentilla canadensis (18).

EUROPEAN MANDRAKE

Also Known As
Alraunwurzel, Mandragora, Mandragore, Mandrake, Satan's Apple.
CAUTION: See separate listings for Bryonia (English Mandrake) and Podophyllum (American Mandrake).

Scientific Names
Mandragora officinarum, synonym Mandragora vernalis.
Family: Solanaceae.

People Use This For
European mandrake root is used orally as an emetic, purgative, sedative, anesthetic, pain killer, and aphrodisiac. It has also been used orally for treating stomach ulcers, colic, asthma, hay fever, convulsions, rheumatism, and whooping cough.
Topically, European mandrake fresh leaves and leaf extracts are used for treating skin ulcers.

Safety
POSSIBLY UNSAFE ...when used orally. European mandrake contains several anticholinergic alkaloids, which can cause significant side effects when used in therapeutic doses (12). Excessive doses of anticholinergic alkaloids can cause respiratory and cardiac arrest and death (15,17).
CHILDREN: LIKELY UNSAFE ...when used orally. Children can be more susceptible to the adverse effects of anticholinergic alkaloid constituents of European mandrake (15); avoid using.
PREGNANCY AND LACTATION: LIKELY UNSAFE ...when used orally. European mandrake contains anticholinergic alkaloids that can cross the placenta and adversely effect the fetus (15); avoid using.

Effectiveness
There is insufficient reliable information available about the effectiveness of European mandrake.

Mechanism of Action
The applicable parts of European mandrake are the root and leaf. European mandrake contains atropine, belladonnine, hyoscyamine, mandragorine, scopolamine, and scopoletin (513,816). The root contains 0.4% tropane alkaloids, principally hyoscyamine (18). All plant parts contain tropane alkaloids, principally hyoscyamine and scopolamine (17). The tropane alkaloids have anticholinergic effects, which inhibit the actions of acetylcholine at muscarinic receptors (15). They reduce saliva and gastric acid production; inhibit gastrointestinal motility; decrease the tone and amplitude of contractions of the ureters and bladder; reduce bronchial secretions; produce bronchodilation; inhibit sweat gland secretions reducing the volume of perspiration; reduce the movement disorders associated with Parkinsonism; prevent motion-induced nausea and vomiting; and block the responses of the sphincter muscle of the iris and the ciliary muscle of the lens, producing mydriasis and cycloplegia (15). In large doses tropane alkaloids cause tachycardia (15).

Adverse Reactions
Orally, European mandrake most commonly causes anticholinergic side effects including confusion, drowsiness, dry mouth, tachycardia, mydriasis, blurred vision, photophobia, decreased urination, decreased sweating and overheating, and flushing (15,17,18). Although some adverse reactions can occur even with low doses, adverse effects are dose related. Large doses can cause severe adverse reactions including somnolence, central excitation (restlessness, hallucinations, delirium, manic episodes), exhaustion, respiratory and cardiac arrest, and death (17,18).

All parts of the European mandrake plant including the root, leaves, and fruit contain anticholinergic alkaloids and can cause these effects (17). Elderly patients and children can be more susceptible to the adverse effects of anticholinergic constituents of European mandrake (15).
There is some evidence that subcutaneous injection may cause anaphylactic shock including swelling of lips and eyelids, nausea, tingling in palms and scalp, abdominal cramping, stool incontinence, and loss of consciousness. This reaction has occurred with a very low dose of 2 mL of a 3 mcg/mL solution of European mandrake extract. Although Immunoglobulin E (IgE) antibodies to European mandrake may not be detected, in vitro evaluation may find strong T lymphocyte proliferation. Skin patch tests with European mandrake root powder in sensitive individuals is likely to produce a delayed-type reaction with erythema resembling acute dermatitis (7022). Skin patch tests should be performed to rule-out hypersensitivity before administration of subcutaneous European mandrake.

Interactions with Herbs & Other Dietary Supplements

HERBS WITH ANTICHOLINERGIC EFFECTS: Theoretically, concurrent use might have additive effects and adverse effects. Anticholinergic herbs include belladonna, henbane, scopolia, and bittersweet nightshade (2).

Interactions with Drugs

ANTICHOLINERGIC DRUGS: Concurrent use may cause additive anticholinergic effects and adverse effects. Anticholinergic drugs include conventional medications containing tropane alkaloids such as atropine, as well as phenothiazines, amantadine, some antiparkinson drugs, glutethimide, meperidine, tricyclic antidepressants, antiarrhythmic agents, and antihistamines (15).
ORAL DRUGS: Theoretically, concurrent use might increase absorption of some drugs because of inhibited gastrointestinal (GI) motility caused by European mandrake (15).

Interactions with Foods

None known.

Interactions with Lab Tests

None known.

Interactions with Diseases or Conditions

CONGESTIVE HEART FAILURE: Avoid using European mandrake due to anticholinergic effects (12,513).
CORONARY ARTERY DISEASE: Avoid using European mandrake due to anticholinergic effects (12,513).
DOWN SYNDROME: Avoid using European mandrake in people with Down syndrome. They may be hypersensitive to antimuscarinic effects of anticholinergics (12,513).
GASTRIC ULCER: Avoid using European mandrake due to anticholinergic effects (12,513).
GI INFECTIONS: Avoid using European mandrake due to anticholinergic effects (12,513).
HEPATIC OR RENAL DYSFUNCTION: Avoid using European mandrake due to anticholinergic effects (12,513).
HIATAL HERNIA: Avoid using European mandrake due to anticholinergic effects (12,513).
HYPERTENSION: Avoid using European mandrake due to anticholinergic effects (12,513).
HYPERTHYROIDISM: Avoid using European mandrake due to anticholinergic effects (12,513).
MYASTHENIA GRAVIS: Contraindicated due to the anticholinergic effects of European mandrake (12,513).
NARROW/CLOSED-ANGLE GLAUCOMA: Contraindicated due to the anticholinergic effects of European mandrake (12,513).
OBSTRUCTIVE GASTROINTESTINAL DISEASE: Contraindicated due to the anticholinergic effects of European mandrake (12,513).
OBSTRUCTIVE UROPATHY: Contraindicated due to the anticholinergic effects of European mandrake (12,513).
PARALYTIC ILEUS or INTESTINAL ATONY: Contraindicated due to the anticholinergic effects of European mandrake (12,513).
PROSTATIC HYPERTROPHY: Avoid using European mandrake due to anticholinergic effects (12,513).
REFLUX ESOPHAGITIS: Contraindicated due to the anticholinergic effects of European mandrake (12,513).
SPASTIC PARALYSIS/BRAIN DAMAGE: Avoid using European mandrake in children with spastic paralysis or brain damage. They may be hypersensitive to antimuscarinic effects of anticholinergics (12,513).
TACHYARRHYTHMIAS: Avoid using European mandrake due to anticholinergic effects (12,513).
ULCERATIVE COLITIS OR TOXIC MEGACOLON: Contraindicated due to the anticholinergic effects of European mandrake (12,513).
UNSTABLE CARDIOVASCULAR STATUS IN ACUTE HEMORRHAGE OR THYROTOXICOSIS: Contraindicated due to the anticholinergic effects of European mandrake (12,513).

Dosage and Administration

No typical dosage.

Comments

European mandrake has had many superstitions associated with it and has been claimed to have magical properties.

EUROPEAN MISTLETOE

Also Known As

All-Heal, Birdlime Mistletoe, Devil's Fuge, Drudenfuss, Eurixor, Helixor, Hexenbesen, Iscador, Isorel, Leimmistel, Mistlekraut, Mistletein, Mistletoe, Mystyldene, Visci, Visci albi folia, Visci albi fructus, Visci albi herba, Visci albi stipites, Vogelmistel, Vysorel.
CAUTION: See separate listing for American Mistletoe.

Scientific Names

Viscum album.
Family: Viscaceae.

People Use This For

Orally, European mistletoe is used for cancer; reducing side effects of chemotherapy and radiation therapy; cardiovascular conditions including high blood pressure, internal bleeding, hemorrhoids, epilepsy and infantile convulsions; arteriosclerosis; gout; psychiatric conditions such as depression; sleep disorders; headache; amenorrhea; symptoms of menopause; and for "blood purifying". It is also used orally for treating mental and physical exhaustion, as a tranquilizer, for whooping cough, asthma, vertigo, diarrhea, chorea, and liver and gallbladder conditions.
Subcutaneously, European mistletoe injections are used for cancer and for degenerative joint disease.

Safety

POSSIBLY SAFE ...when used orally or subcutaneously and appropriately. There is some evidence that European mistletoe extracts can be used safely (7039,9769). However, they have a narrow therapeutic range; high doses are not safe. Tell patients not to consume more than 3 mistletoe berries or 2 leaves (12). Advise patients not to use European mistletoe for self-medication.
LIKELY UNSAFE ...when used orally in high doses. Ingestion of high doses of mistletoe berry or leaf can cause serious adverse reactions. More than 3 berries or 2 leaves can cause seizures, slow heart rate, low blood pressure, and death in some patients (7039).
PREGNANCY: LIKELY UNSAFE ...when used orally or subcutaneously. European mistletoe might have uterine stimulant and abortifacient activity (19).
LACTATION: Insufficient reliable information available; avoid using.

Effectiveness

LIKELY INEFFECTIVE

Cancer. Administering European mistletoe subcutaneously doesn't improve survival in patients with any form of cancer. Most cancer studies have been poorly designed and have produced inconsistent results. Discourage patients from relying on European mistletoe for treating cancer (10672). European mistletoe extract doesn't seem to significantly improve rates of partial or complete remission in patients with stage IV pancreatic cancer (3707,7039,8848). European mistletoe doesn't seem to improve survival in patients with stage IV kidney cancer (7039). Combining European mistletoe extract plus surgery or radiation for glioma doesn't improve overall survival or disease-free survival (7039). European mistletoe extract does not seem to improve overall survival or disease-free survival in patients with stage I or stage IIB melanoma (7039). Combining European mistletoe extract with surgery or radiation for head and neck squamous cell carcinoma doesn't improve overall survival or disease-free survival (8842).

INSUFFICIENT RELIABLE EVIDENCE to RATE

Breast cancer, colorectal cancer, and gastric cancer. There is some preliminary clinical research that indicates European mistletoe extracts might improve survival in patients with solid tumors of the breast, colon, and stomach (7039,7044,7045), but more research with better-designed studies is needed. Tell patients there isn't enough reliable research to support using European mistletoe to improve survival in any type of cancer.
Hepatitis C. Subcutaneous injection of an aqueous extract of European mistletoe may decrease viral load and improve quality of life in some patients with chronic hepatitis C (9769).
More evidence is needed to rate European mistletoe for these uses.

Mechanism of Action

The applicable parts of European mistletoe are the berries, leaf, and stem. European mistletoe is a parasitic plant that grows on several different trees, including pine, oak, apple, maple, and numerous others. So, the chemical composition of mistletoe preparations can vary depending on the species of tree it grows on, the time of harvest, and other factors (7039,7106). European mistletoe has several active constituents, including the three main glycoprotein lectins: MLI, also known as viscumin, MLII, and MLIII; as well as viscotoxins, alkaloids, and monoterpene glucosides (7039,8840,8841,8849,9770).
European mistletoe is best known as a potential anticancer agent. Researchers think it might work as a biological response modifier that both stimulates the immune system and exerts cytotoxic effects (7039). There is good evidence that European mistletoe can stimulate the immune system in both animal models and humans. It seems to cause

leukocytosis, increasing both the number and activity of neutrophils and natural killer cells (8843,8844). European mistletoe also seems to increase white blood cell (WBC) secretion of cytokines interleukin-1 (IL-1), IL-6, and tumor necrosis factor-alpha (TNF-alpha) (7039,8843,8844). Additional evidence suggests European mistletoe might possess a DNA stabilizing effect, restricted primarily to the mononuclear cells of the peripheral blood in vitro (8844). There is also some evidence that European mistletoe can be cytotoxic to tumor cells in vitro and in animals, possibly by inhibiting cellular protein synthesis (8841,8849). Some researchers think it might induce apoptosis in tumor cells (7039). The toxicity appears to be specific to tumor cells, sparing normal lymphocytes (8845,8846,8847). The toxic glycoprotein lectin, viscumin, known also as ML-I seems to be primarily responsible for many of these immune stimulating and cytotoxic effects (8840,8841,8846,8847,8849). However, there is some evidence that viscotoxins and alkaloids might also play a role (7039,8840). So far, evidence for cytotoxic or antitumor effects of these has been conflicting.

Although European mistletoe does seem to affect the immune system in humans and possibly has cytotoxic effects, the clinical benefits in humans are unproven. Clinical studies show that European mistletoe does not improve survival in patients with a variety of cancers. Researchers theorize that it might not work in humans for several reasons. Mistletoe lectins may not be able to bind to certain human cells. Human plasma proteins might interfere or break down active components of mistletoe; or humans may produce antibodies that destroy active constituents of mistletoe (7039). In addition to potential anticancer effects, European mistletoe might also have hypotensive, cardiac depressant, anti-inflammatory, and sedative effects (11).

Adverse Reactions

Orally, European mistletoe can be well tolerated when used in small amounts. Consumption of 3 berries or 2 leaves or less does not seem to cause significant adverse effects. Larger amounts can cause significant toxicity. Oral use can cause vomiting, diarrhea, intestinal cramps, hepatitis, hypotension, contraction of the pupil, uncontrollable eye movement, seizures, coma, and death (18).

European mistletoe was once associated with hepatitis in a patient taking a combination herbal product (3932). However, it is unlikely that mistletoe actually caused this adverse effect. It was most likely attributable to another ingredient, or product contamination. There have never been additional reports of hepatitis from European mistletoe.

Subcutaneously, European mistletoe can cause pain at the injection site, chills, high fever, headaches, angina, orthostatic circulatory disturbances, eosinophilia, and allergic reaction (2).

Intraperitoneal injection and injection directly into a tumor can cause pain at the injection site, nausea, and eosinophilia (7106). Necrosis can also occur at the site of injection (8).

Interactions with Herbs & Other Dietary Supplements

HAWTHORN: There is some evidence that European mistletoe might have cardiotoxic and negative inotropic effects (4). Theoretically, European mistletoe might decrease the effectiveness of positive inotropic agents such as hawthorn.

Interactions with Drugs

ANTIHYPERTENSIVE DRUGS: There is some evidence that European mistletoe can cause hypotension (4). Theoretically, it might have additive blood pressure lowering effects and increase the risk of hypotension; use cautiously.

IMMUNOSUPPRESSANTS: There is some concern that European mistletoe might decrease the effectiveness of immunosuppressants (4). European mistletoe has immunostimulant effects and might counteract the effects of immunosuppressants. Immunosuppressant drugs include azathioprine (Imuran), basiliximab (Simulect), cyclosporine (Neoral, Sandimmune), daclizumab (Zenapax), muromonab-CD3 (OKT3, Orthoclone OKT3), mycophenolate (CellCept), tacrolimus (FK506, Prograf), sirolimus (Rapamune), prednisone (Deltasone, Orasone), and other corticosteroids (glucocorticoids).

Interactions with Foods

None known.

Interactions with Lab Tests

EOSINOPHILIA: Subcutaneous, intraperitoneal, and intratumoral administration has been associated with eosinophilia. Intratumoral administration has caused hypereosinophilia, up to 43% of the white blood cell count (7106).

Interactions with Diseases or Conditions

CARDIOVASCULAR DISEASE: There is some evidence European mistletoe can have cardiotoxic and negative inotropic effects and might worsen cardiovascular conditions (4).

ORGAN TRANSPLANT: There is some concern that European mistletoe might decrease the effectiveness of immunosuppressants in organ transplant patients (4). European mistletoe has immunostimulant effects and might potentially contribute to transplant rejection.

Dosage and Administration
SUBCUTANEOUS: Aqueous extract of European mistletoe 1 mL, containing 5 mg of viscum album, given 3 times weekly, has been used to treat chronic hepatitis C (9769).

Comments
Interest in mistletoe for cancer is growing in North America. A lot of patients are asking about it since Suzanne Somers announced on Larry King Live that she is using it to treat her breast cancer. European mistletoe has been used for treating cancer since the 1920s, especially in Europe. Several brand name mistletoe extracts are available there: Iscador, Eurixor, Helixor, Isorel, Vysorel, and ABNOBAviscum (7039). So far these products are not readily available in North America. There is no proof they work for breast or other cancers. Advise patients to avoid these and stick with proven cancer treatments.

EVENING PRIMROSE OIL

Also Known As
EPO, Evening Primrose, Fever Plant, Huile D'Onagre, King's Cureall, Gamma Linolenic Acid (GLA), Linoleic Acid, Night Willow-Herb, Primrose, Scabish, Sun Drop.
CAUTION: See separate listings for Black Currant, Borage Seed Oil, Flaxseed Oil, Gamma Linolenic Acid, and Omega-6 Fatty Acids.

Scientific Names
Oenothera biennis, synonyms Oenothera muricata, Oenothera purpurata, Oenothera rubricaulis, Oenothera suaveolens, Onagra biennis; and other Oenothera species.
Family: Onagraceae.

People Use This For
Orally, evening primrose oil is used for premenstrual syndrome (PMS), mastalgia, endometriosis, and symptoms of menopause such as hot flashes. It is also used orally for atopic eczema, psoriasis, acne, rheumatoid arthritis, osteoporosis, Raynaud's syndrome, multiple sclerosis, and Sjogren's syndrome. Evening primrose oil is also used orally for cancer, hypercholesterolemia and coronary heart disease, dyspraxia in children, intermittent claudication, alcoholism, Alzheimer's disease, and schizophrenia. It is also used orally for chronic fatigue syndrome (CFS); asthma; diabetic neuropathy; neurodermatitis; hyperactivity in children and attention deficit-hyperactivity disorder (ADHD); obesity and weight loss; whooping cough; and gastrointestinal disorders including ulcerative colitis, irritable bowel syndrome, and peptic ulcer disease. Evening primrose oil has also been used orally in pregnancy for preventing pre-eclampsia, shortening the duration of labor, stimulating labor, and preventing post-date deliveries.
In foods, evening primrose oil is used as a dietary source of essential fatty acids.
In manufacturing, evening primrose oil is used in soaps and cosmetics.

Safety
LIKELY SAFE ...when used orally and appropriately. Evening primrose oil is generally considered safe and has been used in several studies without reports of significant side effects (1106,6034,6036,6406,6847,7565,7566,7567,9794).
CHILDREN: POSSIBLY SAFE ...when used orally and appropriately. Doses of 3 grams per day for 16 weeks have been used in children with apparent safety (6443,6462,7565,7568,7570).
PREGNANCY: POSSIBLY UNSAFE ...when used orally. Evening primrose oil might increase the risk for pregnancy complications, including delayed rupture of membranes, oxytocin augmentation, arrest of descent, and vacuum extraction (1411); avoid using.
LACTATION: POSSIBLY SAFE ...when used orally. Nursing mothers who supplement their diets with evening primrose oil secrete high levels of the constituent gamma linolenic acid into breast milk (1982); however, gamma linolenic acid is a fatty acid that is normally present in significant proportions in breast milk (11884).

Effectiveness
POSSIBLY EFFECTIVE

Mastalgia. There is some evidence that taking evening primrose oil orally can relieve cyclic mastalgia in 45% of patients and non-cyclic mastalgia in 27% of patients (6406,9794). It may not be effective for chronic severe breast pain (9156). Evening primrose oil seems to be less effective than danazol, but similarly effective as bromocriptine (6406).

Osteoporosis. Taking evening primrose oil orally, in combination with fish oils and calcium, seems to decrease bone turnover and increase spinal and femoral bone mineral density in elderly people with osteoporosis (7611).

POSSIBLY INEFFECTIVE

Atopic dermatitis (eczema). Taking evening primrose oil orally for 16 to 24 weeks doesn't seem to improve symptoms of atopic eczema in adults or children (7565,7566,7567). Most studies have used the brand product Epogam (Scotia Pharmaceuticals). Earlier studies, which lasted 12 weeks or less, showed effectiveness, but the positive results appear to be due to flawed study designs (2039,7568,7569,7570).

Attention deficit-hyperactivity disorder (ADHD). Taking evening primrose oil orally doesn't improve symptoms of ADHD in children. Evening primrose oil is comparable to placebo for most measures of improvement (6443,6462).

Menopausal symptoms. Taking evening primrose oil orally doesn't seem to improve menopausal vasomotor symptoms. Evening primrose oil 4 grams daily for 6 months doesn't seem to help hot flashes or night sweats (274).

Premenstrual syndrome (PMS). Taking evening primrose oil orally doesn't seem to relieve symptoms associated with PMS (1105,1106,6034,6847). Multiple small-scale studies have not demonstrated significant benefit when compared to placebo (1105,1106). However, some researchers suggest that studies should last at least six months to allow the placebo effect to wear off and the benefit of evening primrose oil to become apparent (8129); most studies published have lasted no more than four months (1105).

Most clinical studies have used Epogam (Scotia Pharmaceuticals), which contains 40 mg of gamma-linolenic acid and 10 mg of vitamin E. It is sold as a prescription product in some countries and is not available in the US.

INSUFFICIENT RELIABLE EVIDENCE to RATE

Chronic fatigue syndrome (CFS). There is preliminary evidence that a specific combination of evening primrose oil and fish oils (Efamol Marine) might reduce the symptoms of CFS; however, study results have not been consistent (7563,7564).

Pregnancy-related complications. Taking evening primrose oil doesn't seem to shorten the duration of labor (1409,1411), prevent pre-eclampsia (1409), or prevent post-date deliveries in pregnant women (1411).

Rheumatoid arthritis (RA). There is some preliminary evidence that suggests taking evening primrose oil supplements might reduce subjective symptoms of pain in patients with rheumatoid arthritis (6036,12036). However, there is also evidence that suggests no benefit (12035).

Sjogren's syndrome. There is preliminary evidence that taking evening primrose oil supplements does not improve symptoms of Sjogren's syndrome (12037,12038).

More evidence is needed to rate evening primrose oil for these uses.

Mechanism of Action

Evening primrose oil is obtained from the seed of Oenothera biennis. It contains 2-16% gamma-linolenic acid (GLA), 65-80% linoleic acid, and vitamin E (3908,6036).

Evening primrose oil is thought to help for rheumatoid arthritis, eczema, and other inflammatory conditions due its potential anti-inflammatory effects. GLA seems to be responsible for the anti-inflammatory effects of evening primrose oil. GLA is rapidly metabolized to dihomogammalinolenic acid (DGLA). DGLA is a precursor of the prostaglandin-1 series (PGE1), which inhibits the inflammatory polymorphonuclear leukocyte cells. DGLA is also converted to 15-hydroxy-DGLA, which blocks the transformation of arachidonic acid into inflammatory leukotrienes. GLA and DGLA seem to improve the ratio of inflammatory and non-inflammatory prostaglandins and leukotrienes (2039,6036).

There is also interest in using evening primrose oil for conditions that might result from metabolic deficiencies. For example, patients with premenstrual syndrome (PMS) are thought to have lower levels of GLA, possibly due to a defect in the conversion of linoleic acid to GLA (6034). Some children with attention deficit-hyperactivity disorder (ADHD) might also have deficiencies in certain essential fatty acids, including DGLA (6462).

Evening primrose oil might have other pharmacological effects related to its GLA content. There is some evidence it might lower elevated plasma lipids and inhibit platelet aggregation (1979). There is also preliminary evidence from animal models that evening primrose oil might improve neuronal blood supply and possibly play a role in preventing diabetic neuropathy (3909).

Preliminary evidence suggests GLA might have an antiestrogenic effect and might hasten the response to tamoxifen (Nolvadex) in women with estrogen-sensitive breast cancer (5902). GLA also seems to modulate the sensitivity of breast cancer cells to paclitaxel (Taxol) and fulvestrant (Faslodex), enhancing malignant cell killing without adverse effects on normal cells (8133,11791). However, other research suggests that taking GLA alone might stimulate the growth of breast cancer cells at low concentrations and inhibit growth at higher concentrations (11339).

Adverse Reactions

Orally, evening primrose oil is generally well tolerated (1106,6034,6036,6847). There is one case report of nocturnal seizures associated with the use of evening primrose oil, black cohosh, and chasteberry (588). Evening primrose oil might increase the risk for pregnancy complications, including prolonged rupture of membranes, oxytocin augmentation, arrest of descent, and vacuum extraction (1411).

Interactions with Herbs & Other Dietary Supplements

HERBS WITH ANTICOAGULANT/ANTIPLATELET POTENTIAL: Concomitant use of herbs that have constituents that might affect platelet aggregation could theoretically increase the risk of bleeding in some people (1979). These herbs include angelica, clove, danshen, garlic, ginger, ginkgo, red clover, turmeric, and others.

Interactions with Drugs

ANESTHESIA: There is a report of seizure in a patient taking evening primrose oil and receiving anesthesia; however, the patient was also taking other drugs. It is unclear if evening primrose or the other

drugs were the cause (613).
ANTICOAGULANT/ANTIPLATELET DRUGS: Evening primrose oil, which contains gamma-linolenic acid (GLA), could have anticoagulant effects (1979). Theoretically, taking evening primrose oil with other anticoagulant or antiplatelet drugs might increase the risk of bruising and bleeding. Some of these drugs include aspirin, clopidogrel (Plavix), nonsteroidal anti-inflammatory drugs (NSAIDs) such as diclofenac (Voltaren, Cataflam, others), ibuprofen (Advil, Motrin, others), naproxen (Anaprox, Naprosyn, others), dalteparin (Fragmin), enoxaparin (Lovenox), heparin, warfarin (Coumadin), and others.
PHENOTHIAZINES: Theoretically, products containing gamma linolenic acid (GLA) and vitamin E might increase the risk of seizures in people being treat concomitantly with phenothiazine drugs (11021); use with caution.

Interactions with Foods

None known.

Interactions with Lab Tests

BLEEDING TIME: There is some concern that evening primrose oil might prolong bleeding time. Evening primrose oil contains gamma linolenic acid (GLA), which can inhibit platelet aggregation (1979).
LIPID PROFILE: Evening primrose oil might affect cholesterol levels. Evening primrose oil contains gamma-linolenic acid (GLA), which can lower plasma triglycerides and increase high-density lipoprotein (HDL) cholesterol (1979).

Interactions with Diseases or Conditions

BLEEDING DISORDERS: There is some concern that evening primrose oil might prolong bleeding time and increase the risk of bruising and bleeding. Evening primrose oil contains gamma-linolenic acid (GLA), which can inhibit platelet aggregation (1979).
EPILEPSY/SEIZURE DISORDER: There is concern that evening primrose oil might lower the seizure threshold or unmask undiagnosed temporal lobe epilepsy. However, current reports have only identified seizure in association with phenothiazine (11021).
SCHIZOPHRENIA: Seizures have been reported in people with schizophrenia treated concomitantly with phenothiazine drugs, GLA, and vitamin E (11021); use with caution.

Dosage and Administration

ORAL: For mastalgia, 3-4 grams daily has been used (6034,6406,9156). For premenstrual syndrome (PMS), 2-4 grams daily has been used (6034). For rheumatoid arthritis, doses ranging from 540 mg daily to 2.8 grams daily have been used (6036). For improving movement disorders in children with dyspraxia, 24 mg thyme oil combined with fish oils providing DHA 480 mg and 35 mg arachidonic acid, 96 mg gamma-alpha linoleic acid from evening primrose oil, and 80 mg vitamin E (Efalex) have been used (5708). For atopic eczema, 4-6 grams daily has been used in adults (2039,7569) and 3 grams in children (7565,7568).

Comments

The Medicines Control Agency (MCA), the British equivalent of the Food and Drug Administration, recently withdrew the licenses for evening primrose oil products marketed as prescription drug products under the brand names of Epogam and Efamast. Epogam was authorized for the symptomatic relief of atopic eczema in children and adults and Efamast was licensed to treat mastalgia. The licenses were withdrawn because the agency concluded that there is not enough evidence that they are effective (9882). The manufacturer claims to have data to support the use of evening primrose oil for atopic eczema, but it has not been published. Studies using borage seed oil, which also contains gamma-linolenic acid, have found no effect on atopic dermatitis (11341,11342).

EYEBRIGHT

Also Known As

Augentrostkraut, Euphraisia Eye Bright, Euphrasiae herba, Eye Bright, Herbe d'Euphraise.
CAUTION: See separate listing for Clary Sage.

Scientific Names

Eurphrasia rostkoviana; Euphrasia officinalis.
Family: Scrophulariaceae.

People Use This For

Orally, eyebright is used to treat nasal mucous membrane inflammation, allergies, allergic rhinitis, common cold, bronchial conditions, and sinusitis. It is also used orally for cancers, coughs, conjunctivitis, earaches, epilepsy, headaches, hoarseness, inflammation, jaundice, ophthalmia, rhinitis, skin ailments, and sore throat.
Topically, eyebright is used as an ophthalmic in the form of a lotion, poultice, or eyebath for a variety of conditions

including conjunctivitis; blepharitis; eye fatigue; inflammation of the blood vessels, eyelids and conjunctiva; and for "glued" and inflamed eyes. Eyebright is also used topically to prevent mucous and mucous membrane inflammation of the eyes.
In foods, eyebright is used as a flavoring ingredient.

Safety

POSSIBLY SAFE ...when used orally and appropriately (12). ...when used orally in amounts commonly found in foods. Eyebright is listed by the Council of Europe as a natural source of food flavoring (4).
POSSIBLY UNSAFE ...when used as an ophthalmic; avoid using due to hygienic concerns. Eye products may be subject to contamination (8,11).
PREGNANCY AND LACTATION: Insufficient reliable information available; avoid using.

Effectiveness

There is insufficient reliable information available about the effectiveness of eyebright.

Mechanism of Action

Tannin constituents may be responsible for astringent properties (4). The constituent caffeic acid has bacteriostatic activity (4). Constituents, aucubin and iridoid glycosides, have purgative activity (4).

Adverse Reactions

Orally or topically, 10-60 drops eyebright tincture may induce mental confusion, headache, increased eye pressure with lacrimation, itching, redness, swelling of eyelid margins, dim vision, photophobia, weakness, sneezing, nausea, toothache, constipation, cough, dyspnea, insomnia, polyuria, and sweating (4).

Interactions with Herbs & Other Dietary Supplements

None known.

Interactions with Drugs

None known.

Interactions with Foods

None known.

Interactions with Lab Tests

None known.

Interactions with Diseases or Conditions

None known.

Dosage and Administration

ORAL: 2-4 grams dried above ground parts three times daily (4), or one cup tea (steep 2-4 grams dried above ground parts in 150 mL boiling water 5-10 minutes, strain) three times daily (4). Liquid extract (1:1 in 25% alcohol), 2-4 mL three times daily (4). Tincture (1:5 in 45% alcohol), 2-6 mL three times daily (4).
TOPICAL: No typical dosage.

Comments

Avoid use of nonsterile solutions (including homemade products) in the eye(s), due to high risk of infection. Ophthalmic application of eyebright is not recommended. Historically, eyebright has been used in British Herbal Tobacco, which was smoked for chronic bronchial conditions and colds (5).

FALSE UNICORN

Also Known As

Blazing Star, Fairywand, Helonias, Starwort.

Scientific Names

Chamaelirium luteum, synonyms Chamaelirium carolianum, Helonias dioica, Helonias lutea, Veratrum luteum.
Family: Liliaceae or Melanthiaceae.

People Use This For
Orally, false unicorn is used for ovarian cysts, menstrual problems, menopause, threatened miscarriage, vomiting from pregnancy, infertility, digestive problems, and to normalize hormones after oral contraceptive use. It is also used orally as a diuretic and to rid the intestines of worms.

Safety
POSSIBLY SAFE ...when the root preparations are used orally and appropriately (12).
PREGNANCY: LIKELY UNSAFE ...when used orally because it is a potential uterine stimulant (12,18).
LACTATION: Insufficient reliable information available; avoid using.

Effectiveness
There is insufficient reliable information available about the effectiveness of false unicorn.

Mechanism of Action
The applicable parts of false unicorn are the rhizome and root. False unicorn reportedly has anthelmintic, diuretic (18), uterine stimulant, and menstruation stimulant activity (12).

Adverse Reactions
Orally, large doses of false unicorn may cause nausea and vomiting (4).

Interactions with Herbs & Other Dietary Supplements
None known.

Interactions with Drugs
None known.

Interactions with Foods
None known.

Interactions with Lab Tests
None known.

Interactions with Diseases or Conditions
GI CONDITIONS: Can irritate the gastrointestinal tract. Contraindicated in individuals with infectious or inflammatory gastrointestinal conditions (19).

Dosage and Administration
ORAL: 1-2 grams dried root 3 times per day, or one cup tea (steep 1-2 grams dried root in 150 mL boiling water 5-10 minutes, strain) 3 times daily (4) has been used. As a liquid extract (1:1 in 45% alcohol), 1-2 mL has been used 3 times daily (4). As a tincture (1:5 in 45% alcohol), 2-5 mL 3 times daily has been used (4).

FENNEL fruit, seed

Also Known As
Bari-Sanuf, Bitter Fennel, Carosella, Common Fennel, Finnochio, Florence Fennel, Garden Fennel, Large Fennel, Phytoestrogen, Sanuf, Shatapuspha, Sweet Fennel, Wild Fennel.
CAUTION: See separate listing for Fennel Oil.

Scientific Names
Foeniculum vulgare, synonyms Anethum piperitum and Foeniculum piperitum; Foeniculum officinale; Foeniculum capillaceum; Anethum foeniculum.
Family: Apiaceae/Umbelliferae.

People Use This For
Orally, fennel fruit/seed is used to enhance lactation, promote menstruation, facilitate birth, increase libido, and to treat indigestion. It is also used for upper respiratory tract mucous membrane inflammation, coughs, bronchitis, cholera, backache, bedwetting, loss of appetite, visual problems, and for colic in infants.
Topically, fennel powder is used as a poultice for hard-to-heal snake bites.

Safety

LIKELY SAFE ...when the seed is used orally in food amounts (11,12).
POSSIBLY SAFE ...when used orally and appropriately for short periods of time (2,12).
POSSIBLY UNSAFE ...when used orally in medicinal amounts for prolonged periods of time. The constituent, estragole, is a procarcinogen (12).
PREGNANCY: LIKELY UNSAFE ...when used orally (2); avoid using.
LACTATION: Insufficient reliable information available; avoid using.

Effectiveness

There is insufficient reliable information available about the effectiveness of fennel fruit or seed.

Mechanism of Action

Fennel is a rich source of beta-carotene and vitamin C (19). The seed contains a volatile oil composed largely of trans-anethole, but also contains fenchone, estragole, and other constituents. It also contains significant amounts of calcium, magnesium, and iron, and lesser amounts of other metal cations (6135). Fennel seed can promote GI motility, and in higher concentrations, it can act as an antispasmodic (2). The constituents, anethole and fenchone, reduce upper respiratory tract secretions (11). Some evidence suggests the aqueous fennel extract might also increase mucociliary activity (11). The constituent anethole appears to be allergenic, insecticidal, and toxic. Polymers of anethole have estrogenic activity (11). The constituent estragole is a procarcinogen but the carcinogenic risk is minimal. It is not directly hepatotoxic or hepatocarcinogenic but requires activation by liver enzymes to reach full toxicity. In the liver, other enzymes inactivate the carcinogenic metabolites, limiting possible damage to the liver (12).

Adverse Reactions

Orally, fennel can cause allergic reactions affecting the skin and respiratory system (2). It can also cause photodermatitis. Avoid excessive sunlight or ultraviolet light exposure while using this product (19). Allergic cross-sensitivity is possible in people with allergies to carrot, celery, mugwort, or other Apiaceae family plants (6,18).

Interactions with Herbs & Other Dietary Supplements

None known.

Interactions with Drugs

CIPROFLOXACIN (Cipro): Concomitant administration might reduce the effectiveness of ciprofloxacin therapy. Preliminary evidence suggests that fennel reduces ciprofloxacin bioavailability by nearly 50%, possibly due to interaction with the metal cations contained in fennel. Evidence also suggests that fennel increases tissue distribution and slows elimination of ciprofloxacin (6135).
CONTRACEPTIVE DRUGS: Theoretically, concomitant use of large amounts of fennel might interfere with contraceptive drugs through competition for estrogen receptors (11).
ESTROGENS: Theoretically, concomitant use of large amounts of fennel might interfere with hormone replacement therapy through competition for estrogen receptors (11).
TAMOXIFEN (Nolvadex): Theoretically, large doses of fennel might interfere with tamoxifen because of its potential estrogenic effects (11).

Interactions with Foods

None known.

Interactions with Lab Tests

None known.

Interactions with Diseases or Conditions

CELERY, CARROT, MUGWORT ALLERGY: Allergic cross-sensitivity to fennel possible (6,18).
HORMONE SENSITIVE CANCERS/CONDITIONS: Because fennel oil might have estrogenic effects (11), women with hormone sensitive conditions should avoid fennel oil. Some of these conditions include breast, uterine, and ovarian cancer, and endometriosis and uterine fibroids.

Dosage and Administration

ORAL: The typical dose of fennel is 5-7 grams of the dried fruit or seed per day or one cup of the tea three times daily (2,18). The tea is prepared by steeping 1-2 grams of the crushed or ground fruit or seed in 150 mL boiling water for 5-10 minutes and then straining. The common dose of the tincture compound is 5-7.5 grams per day (2). Fennel should be used on a short-term basis (2).

FENNEL OIL

Also Known As
Foeniculi antheroleum, Phytoestrogen.
CAUTION: See separate listing for Fennel fruit, seed.

Scientific Names
Foeniculum vulgare, synonyms Foeniculum officinale, Foeniculum capillaceum, Anethum foeniculum.
Family: Apiaceae/Umbelliferae.

People Use This For
Orally, fennel oil is used for mild spastic disorders of the gastrointestinal (GI) tract, the feeling of fullness, flatulence, improving appetite and digestion, and other stomach complaints.
It is also used to treat upper respiratory tract mucous membrane inflammation, coughs, and bronchitis.
The honey syrup is used for upper respiratory tract mucous membrane inflammation in children.
In foods and beverages, fennel oil is used as a flavoring agent.
In other manufacturing processes, fennel oil is used as a flavoring agent in certain laxatives, and as a fragrance component in soaps and cosmetics.

Safety
LIKELY SAFE ...when used orally in amounts commonly found in foods. Fennel oil has Generally Recognized As Safe (GRAS) status in the US (4912).
POSSIBLY SAFE ...when used orally in medicinal amounts for less than 2 weeks (18).
POSSIBLY UNSAFE ...when used orally, long-term.
CHILDREN: LIKELY UNSAFE ...when used orally. Contraindicated for oral use in infants and toddlers (2).
PREGNANCY: LIKELY UNSAFE ...when used orally in medicinal amounts (2).
LACTATION: Insufficient reliable information available; avoid using amounts larger than those found in foods.

Effectiveness
There is insufficient reliable information available about the effectiveness of fennel oil.

Mechanism of Action
Fennel oil is composed largely of trans-anethole, with lesser amounts of fenchone, estragole, and other constituents. The oil can promote GI motility, and in higher concentrations, it can act as an antispasmodic (2). The constituents, anethole and fenchone, reduce upper respiratory tract secretions (11). The constituent anethole appears to be allergenic, insecticidal, and toxic. Polymers of anethole have estrogenic activity (11). The constituent estragole is a procarcinogen, but the carcinogenic risk is minimal. It is not directly hepatotoxic or hepatocarcinogenic but requires activation by liver enzymes to reach full toxicity. In the liver other enzymes inactivate the carcinogenic metabolites, limiting possible damage to the liver (12).
Preliminary evidence suggests that fennel oil can inhibit contractions of uterine tissue induced by prostaglandin E2. However, it does not inhibit uterine contractions induced by oxytocin (10349).

Adverse Reactions
Allergic cross-sensitivity is possible in people with allergies to carrot, celery, mugwort, or other Apiaceae family plants (18). Allergic reactions that affect the skin and respiratory system are rare (2).

Interactions with Herbs & Other Dietary Supplements
None known.

Interactions with Drugs
None known.

Interactions with Foods
None known.

Interactions with Lab Tests
None known.

Interactions with Diseases or Conditions
CELERY, CARROT, MUGWORT ALLERGY: Allergic cross sensitivity to fennel is possible (18).
DIABETES: Use caution with the fennel honey syrup in diabetics due to its carbohydrate content (2).
HORMONE SENSITIVE CANCERS/CONDITIONS: Fennel oil might have estrogenic effects (11), women with

hormone sensitive conditions should avoid fennel oil. Some of these conditions include breast cancer, uterine cancer, ovarian cancer, endometriosis, and uterine fibroids.

Dosage and Administration

ORAL: The typical daily dose of fennel oil is 0.1-0.6 mL, which is equivalent to 100-600 mg of the dried fruit or seed. It should only be used up to two weeks without professional evaluation (2). The fennel honey syrup, which contains 500 mg fennel oil/kg, is usually dosed 10-20 grams per day (2).

Comments

Fennel oil is the distilled essential oil of the fennel (Foeniculum vulgare) fruit or seed.

FENUGREEK

Also Known As

Alholva, Bird's Foot, Bockshornklee, Bockshornsame, Chandrika, Foenugraeci Semen, Foenugreek, Greek Clover, Greek Hay, Greek Hay Seed, Hu Lu Ba, Methi, Medhika, Trigonella.

Scientific Names

Trigonella foenum-graecum; Trigonella foenugraecum.
Family: Fabaceae/Leguminosae

People Use This For

Orally, fenugreek is used for lowering blood glucose in people with diabetes, loss of appetite, dyspepsia, gastritis, constipation, atherosclerosis, high serum cholesterol and triglycerides, and for promoting lactation. Fenugreek is used orally for kidney ailments, beriberi, hernia, impotence, and other male problems. Fenugreek is also used orally for fever, mouth ulcers, boils, bronchitis, cellulitis, tuberculosis, chronic coughs, chapped lips, baldness, and cancer. Topically, fenugreek is used as a poultice for local inflammation, myalgia, lymphadenitis, gout, wounds, leg ulcers, and eczema.

For food use, fenugreek is included as an ingredient in spice blends. It is also used as a flavoring agent in imitation maple syrup, foods, beverages, and tobacco. In other manufacturing processes, fenugreek extracts are used in soaps and cosmetics.

Safety

LIKELY SAFE ...when used orally in amounts commonly found in foods. Fenugreek has Generally Recognized As Safe (GRAS) status in the US (4912).
POSSIBLY SAFE ...when used orally in medicinal amounts (4).
POSSIBLY UNSAFE ...when used topically. The repeated use of fenugreek can result in skin sensitization (18).
CHILDREN: POSSIBLY UNSAFE ...when used orally; avoid using. Fenugreek tea has caused loss of consciousness and unusual body odor in children. The body odor may be confused with maple syrup disease (9782).
PREGNANCY: LIKELY UNSAFE ...when used orally in amounts greater than those found in foods because of its potential oxytocic and uterine stimulant activity (4). Consumption of fenugreek just before delivery may cause the neonate to have an unusual body odor, which could be confused with maple syrup disease. It does not appear to cause long-term sequelae (9781).
LACTATION: Insufficient reliable information available; avoid using.

Effectiveness

POSSIBLY EFFECTIVE

Diabetes. Consuming fenugreek, mixed with food during a meal, seems to reduce postprandial blood glucose levels in patients with diabetes. It may be given in combination with guar gum or by itself (10283,10284). Muffins made from a batter consisting of foxtail and barnyard millet, in combination with legumes and fenugreek, do not produce a substantial increase in postprandial blood glucose in diabetic patients (9784).

INSUFFICIENT RELIABLE EVIDENCE to RATE

Hypercholesterolemia. There is conflicting evidence about the use of fenugreek for lowering serum cholesterol (7389,9783,10284). More evidence is needed to rate fenugreek for this use.

Mechanism of Action

The applicable part of fenugreek is the seed. The active constituents include trigonelline, 4-hydroxyisoleucine, and fenugreekine (4). Fenugreek seeds have a distinctive bitter taste and odor, which is why they are used as a spice in food. Soaking fenugreek seeds overnight and washing the seeds in water can decrease some of the taste and odor (9783).

Fenugreek affects gastrointestinal transit, slowing glucose absorption (8112). In healthy individuals, whole seed extracts, gum isolate, extracted seeds, cooked seeds, and the constituent, trigonelline, show evidence of a hypoglycemic effect (4). About 80% of the total content of free amino acids in the seeds is present as 4-hydroxyisoleucine, which appears to directly stimulate insulin (8112). This effect is glucose dependent and only occurs in the presence of moderate to high glucose concentrations. In people with noninsulin-dependent diabetes, the ingestion of the extracted seeds can improve plasma glucose and insulin response (4). In people with insulin-dependent diabetes, the ingestion of the seed powder can reduce plasma glucose, glycosuria, and the daily insulin requirement (4).

Some studies suggest the seed powder can reduce serum cholesterol in people with diabetes (4). Other evidence suggests the seed consumption might decrease calcium oxalate deposition in the kidneys (720).

Fenugreek contains coumarins and other constituents that might affect platelet aggregation, but this might not be significant clinically (7162). The fenugreekine constituent shows evidence of cardiotonic, hypoglycemic, diuretic, anti-inflammatory, antihypertensive, and antiviral properties (4).

Adverse Reactions

Orally, fenugreek can cause diarrhea and flatulence (622). With large doses, hypoglycemia is possible (164). Fenugreek can cause allergic reactions including nasal congestion, hoarseness, persistent coughing, wheezing, facial angioedema, and shock (719). The paste of fenugreek applied to the scalp can cause allergic symptoms, including head numbness, facial swelling, and wheezing (719). Consumption of fenugreek by pregnant women just before delivery may cause the neonate to have an unusual body odor, which may be confused with maple syrup disease. It does not appear to cause long-term sequelae (9781). This unusual body odor may occur in children drinking fenugreek tea. Loss of consciousness may also occur in children drinking tea made from fenugreek (9782).

Interactions with Herbs & Other Dietary Supplements

HERBS WITH ANTICOAGULANT/ANTIPLATELET POTENTIAL: Concomitant use of herbs that have constituents that might affect platelet aggregation could theoretically increase the risk of bleeding in some people (5191,7162,7389). These herbs include angelica, clove, danshen, garlic, ginger, ginkgo, red clover, turmeric, and others.

HERBS WITH HYPOGLYCEMIC POTENTIAL: Theoretically, fenugreek might have additive effects with herbs that decrease blood glucose levels (10283,10284). Herbs with hypoglycemic potential include devil's claw, fenugreek, guar gum, Panax ginseng, and Siberian ginseng.

Interactions with Drugs

ANTICOAGULANT/ANTIPLATELET DRUGS: There is some concern that fenugreek might have additive effects when used with anticoagulant or antiplatelet drugs, resulting in increased risk of bruising and bleeding. Some of the constituents in fenugreek have antiplatelet effects, although these might not be present in concentrations that are clinically significant (5191,7162,7389). Some drugs with anticoagulant or antiplatelet effects include aspirin, clopidogrel (Plavix), nonsteroidal anti-inflammatory drugs (NSAIDs) such as diclofenac (Voltaren, Cataflam, others), ibuprofen (Advil, Motrin, others), naproxen (Anaprox, Naprosyn, others), dalteparin (Fragmin), enoxaparin (Lovenox), heparin, and others.

ANTIDIABETES DRUGS: Fenugreek may reduce blood glucose levels (10283,10284) and might have additive effects on glucose levels when used with antidiabetes drugs. Monitor blood glucose levels closely. Medication dose adjustments may be necessary. Some antidiabetes drugs include glimepiride (Amaryl), glyburide (DiaBeta, Glynase PresTab, Micronase), insulin, pioglitazone (Actos), rosiglitazone (Avandia), and others.

ORAL DRUGS: Theoretically, the high mucilage content of fenugreek can decrease or delay the absorption of oral drugs (4).

WARFARIN (Coumadin): Fenugreek might have additive effects with warfarin and increase the international normalized ratio (INR). Some fenugreek constituents have antiplatelet effects, although these might not be present in concentrations that are clinically significant (7162,7389). Fenugreek in combination with boldo has been associated with increased INR in a patient taking warfarin (5191).

Interactions with Foods

ALLERGY TO FABACEAE: Chickpea, also a member of the Fabaceae family, has shown cross-reactivity in patients allergic to fenugreek. Theoretically, patients who are allergic to other Fabaceae plants including soybeans, peanuts, and green peas might also be allergic to fenugreek (719).

Interactions with Lab Tests

BLOOD GLUCOSE: Fenugreek can lower blood glucose and test results (10283,10284).

URINE ODOR: Fenugreek can cause a maple syrup odor in urine. Avoid confusion with "maple syrup urine" disease (8111).

Interactions with Diseases or Conditions

DIABETES: Fenugreek can alter blood sugar control in people with diabetes (10283,10284). Blood glucose levels should be monitored closely.

KIDNEY STONES: Theoretically, fenugreek can decrease calcium oxalate deposition and stone formation (720).

Dosage and Administration

ORAL: For reducing postprandial blood glucose in patients with diabetes, fenugreek 10 to 15 grams per day, as a single dose or in divided doses, with meals has been used (10283,10284). For treating hyperlipidemia, 0.6 to 2.5 grams of fenugreek 2 times daily with meals has been used. It may be used alone or in combination with guar gum and other plant fibers (7389,10284).

Comments

The taste and odor of fenugreek resembles maple syrup, and it has been used to mask the taste of medicines (8111). Fenugreek leaves are eaten in India as a vegetable (719).

FEVER BARK

Also Known As

Alstonia Bark, Australian Febrifuge, Australian Fever Bush, Australian Quinine, Bitterbark, Devil's Bit, Devil Tree, Dita Bark, Pale Mara, Pali-Mara.

Scientific Names

Alstonia constricta.
Family: Apocynaceae.

People Use This For

Orally, fever bark is used for treating fever, hypertension, diarrhea, rheumatism, and malaria. It is also used as a stimulant and a uterine stimulant.

Safety

POSSIBLY UNSAFE ...when used orally. Fever bark contains reserpine and yohimbine constituents (18), which can cause severe adverse effects including depression, psychosis, and acute renal failure (5,6,11,17,18,19).
PREGNANCY AND LACTATION: Insufficient reliable information available; avoid using.

Effectiveness

There is insufficient reliable information available about the effectiveness of fever bark.

Mechanism of Action

Fever bark contains various alkaloids including yohimbe. The constituents reserpine and deserpidine are likely responsible for its antihypertensive effects. Fever bark might also have antipyretic and antispasmodic properties (18).

Adverse Reactions

Orally, the reserpine constituent of fever bark can cause lethargy, nasal congestion, or depression (17). The yohimbine constituent of fever bark can cause salivation, irritability, fluid retention, skin eruptions, eye dilation, allergy, acute renal failure, and lupus-like syndrome (2,5,6,11,18,19). Yohimbine is reported to trigger psychosis in people predisposed to it (2,5,6,11,18). Symptoms of yohimbine toxicity include paralysis, severe hypotension, cardiac conduction disorders, cardiac failure, and death (6,18).

Interactions with Herbs & Other Dietary Supplements

INDIAN SNAKEROOT: Theoretically, concomitant use of Indian snakeroot with fever root can cause additive effects and side effects due to reserpine and deserpidine content of both herbs.
ST. JOHN'S WORT: Theoretically, concomitant use of St. John's wort extract might antagonize effects of reserpine, a constituent of fever bark (19).
TURMERIC: Theoretically, concomitant use of tumeric might reduce the frequency of gastric and duodenal ulcers associated with reserpine, a constituent of fever bark (19).
YOHIMBE: Theoretically, concomitant use of fever bark with yohimbe can cause additive effects or adverse effects.

Interactions with Drugs

ANESTHESIA: Reserpine, a constituent of fever bark, can increase the risk of cardiovascular instability in individuals receiving general anesthesia (151).
NALOXONE (Narcan): Concomitant use of the fever bark constituent yohimbine and naloxone can cause synergistic effects and adverse reactions (19).
PHENOTHIAZINES: Theoretically, phenothiazines might increase the toxicity of yohimbine, a constituent of fever bark, due to alpha-two adrenoreceptor antagonism (19).

STIMULANT DRUGS: Reserpine, a constituent of fever bark, might increase or decrease effects of sympathomimetics (151).

Interactions with Foods

None known.

Interactions with Lab Tests

5-HYDROXYINDOLEACETIC ACID (5-HIAA): Reserpine can increase test results (275).
17-HYDROXYCORTICOSTEROIDS: Reserpine can decrease urine levels (275).
FFA: Reserpine can increase serum free fatty acids (275).
GUAIACOLS SPOT TEST: Reserpine can cause a false reading with urine screening test of Rogers (275).
HOMOVANILLIC ACID: Reserpine can increase urine levels of homovanillic acid; maximum on second day (275).
HYDROCHLORIC ACID: Reserpine can increase gastric hydrochloric acid levels (275).
NOREPINEPHRINE: Reserpine can decrease urine levels of norepinephrine (275). Yohimbine can increase plasma and cerebrospinal fluid norepinephrine levels and test results (275).
PEPSIN: Reserpine can increase gastric pepsin levels and test results (275).
PLATELETS: Reserpine can decrease blood platelet levels and test results (275).
PROLACTIN: Reserpine can increase plasma prolactin levels and test results (275).
PROTHROMBIN TIME: Reserpine can decrease plasma prothrombin time (275).
SEROTONIN: Reserpine can decrease plasma 5-HT and test results (275).
T-4: Reserpine can decrease thyroxine (T-4) serum levels and test results (275).
TYRAMINE: Reserpine can cause a false positive response to tyramine test (275).
VANILLYLMANDELIC ACID: Reserpine can decrease urine levels and test results (275).

Interactions with Diseases or Conditions

MENTAL DEPRESSION: Theoretically, contraindicated in individuals with a history of mental depression due to reserpine constituent (17,18).
PEPTIC ULCER: Theoretically, contraindicated in individuals with active peptic ulcer due to reserpine constituent (17).
SCHIZOPHRENIA: Theoretically, contraindicated in individuals with schizophrenia because yohimbine constituent might induce psychotic episodes (19).

Dosage and Administration

ORAL: A typical dose is 15 to 20 mL of tea daily. Tea can be made by steeping one part ground bark to 20 parts boiling water for 10-15 minutes, strain. Alternatively, 2-4 mL tincture (1:8 or 1:10) daily; or 4-8 mL of liquid extract (1:1) daily has also been used (18).

Comments

Most of the information available for fever bark concerns its constituents.

FEVERFEW

Also Known As

Altamisa, Bachelor's Buttons, Featerfoiul, Featherfew, Featherfoil, Flirtwort Midsummer Daisy, Santa Maria, Tanaceti parthenii.
CAUTION: See separate listings for Buttercup and Cornflower.

Scientific Names

Tanacetum parthenium, synonyms Chrysanthemum parthenium, Chrysanthemum praealtum Leucanthemum parthenium, Matricaria eximia, Matricaria parthenium, Pyrethrum parthenium.
Family: Asteraceae/Compositae.

People Use This For

Orally, feverfew is used for fever, headaches, prevention of migraines, and menstrual irregularities. It is also used orally for arthritis, psoriasis, allergies, asthma, tinnitus, vertigo, nausea and vomiting. Feverfew is also used for infertility, anemia, cancer, common cold, earache, liver disease, prevention of miscarriage, muscular tension, orthopedic disorders, swollen feet, diarrhea, and dyspepsia including indigestion and flatulence.
Topically, feverfew is used for toothaches and as an antiseptic and insecticide. It is also used as a general stimulant and tonic and for intestinal parasites.

Safety

LIKELY SAFE ...when used orally and appropriately, short-term. Feverfew has been used safely in studies lasting up to 4 months (6959,6960,6961).

There is insufficient reliable information available about the safety of the long-term use of feverfew. Although no significant adverse effects have been reported with long-term use (6711,6959); long-term safety has not been sufficiently evaluated (6711).

PREGNANCY: LIKELY UNSAFE ...when used orally. Feverfew might cause uterine contractions and abortion (4); avoid using.

LACTATION: Insufficient reliable information available; avoid using.

Effectiveness

POSSIBLY INEFFECTIVE

Rheumatoid arthritis (RA). Taking feverfew orally doesn't seem to reduce the symptoms of RA (6933).

INSUFFICIENT RELIABLE EVIDENCE to RATE

Migraine headache. There is some evidence that taking feverfew orally can reduce the frequency of migraine headaches and reduce symptoms of pain, nausea, vomiting, and sensitivity to light and noise (5080,6959,6960,6961,6965). But there is also evidence that feverfew does not improve migraine symptoms or reduce the occurrence of migraine headache (6711,12153). More evidence is needed to rate feverfew for this use.

Most studies have used feverfew products standardized to contain 0.2% to 0.35% of the parthenolide constituent, but this standardization does not seem necessary for effectiveness (726,6935,6938).

Mechanism of Action

The applicable part of feverfew is the leaf. At least 39 constituents of feverfew have been identified (724). However, there has been controversy ragarding which constituents were responsible for feverfew's pharmacological effects. It used to be widely believed that the sesquiterpene lactone, parthenolide, was the active constituent (6935). It was suggested that at least 0.2% of parthenolide was required for efficacy (21,6935,6937). However, a study using an alcoholic extract of feverfew standardized to 0.35% parthenolide was found ineffective for preventing migraine (6938), suggesting that parthenolide may not be the active ingredient and that other constituents are necessary for benefit in the prevention of migraine (49,512,6935,6938). It's not yet clear how feverfew works in the prevention of migraine. Laboratory evidence suggests that feverfew extracts might inhibit platelet aggregation and inhibit serotonin release from platelets and leucocytes (6935,6936,6942,6943,6944,6945); however, platelet studies in people have not found this effect (6951). Feverfew might also inhibit serum proteases and leukotrienes (6939,6946). Feverfew also appears to block prostaglandin synthesis by inhibiting phospholipase, which prevents the release of arachidonic acid (6943,6953,6954). Preliminary research shows that extracts of fresh feverfew leaves and parthenolide might cause irreversible inhibition of vascular muscle contraction (6948,6950). Chrysanthenyl acetate, an essential oil of feverfew, has been suggested as one active component (6938). Chrysanthenyl acetate inhibits prostaglandin synthetase and might have analgesic properties (6711,6713). Feverfew also contains melatonin which might contribute to its pharmacological effect (50). Fresh or dried leaves contain significantly more melatonin than commercially prepared standardized feverfew tablets (50). Migraine attacks have been associated with decreased melatonin excretion (6712). Other pharmacological effects of feverfew include cytostatic effect on tumor cell growth (6957), inhibition of inflammation and pain transmission (6947), and anti-inflammatory effects (6941).

Adverse Reactions

Orally, feverfew in excessive doses can cause abdominal pain, indigestion, diarrhea, flatulence, nausea, and vomiting (1). The traditional method of feverfew administration, chewing fresh feverfew leaves, can result in mouth ulceration, inflamed oral mucosa and tongue, swelling of the lips, and occasionally, loss of taste (6935,6959). Mouth ulceration might result from direct contact with feverfew leaves during chewing, possibly attributable to the sesquiterpene lactone constituent (6959). Some researchers suggest that mouth ulceration is a systemic effect, but one study using dried feverfew capsules reported a higher incidence of mouth ulcers in subjects taking placebo than feverfew (6935,6959,6960). "Post-feverfew syndrome," including anxiety, headaches, insomnia, and muscle and joint stiffness, has been described in people who have taken feverfew over long periods of time (6959).

Topically, allergic contact dermatitis can occur (6958).

Overall, feverfew might be better tolerated than some conventional migraine drugs used for prophylaxis. For example, in clinical trials, feverfew did not affect blood pressure, heart rate, body weight, blood chemistry, or cytology; like some conventional drugs do such as ergot derivatives, serotonin agonists ("triptans"), beta-blockers, valproic acid, and analgesics (6959,6960,6961,6965,6711). Feverfew may cause an allergic reaction in individuals sensitive to the Asteraceae/Compositae family. Members of this family include ragweed, chrysanthemums, marigolds, daisies, and many other herbs.

Interactions with Herbs & Other Dietary Supplements

HERBS WITH ANTICOAGULANT/ANTIPLATELET POTENTIAL: Some evidence suggests that feverfew may inhibit platelet aggregation. However, this has not been demonstrated in humans (6935,6936,6942,6943,6944,6945,6951). Theoretically, concomitant use of feverfew and herbs that affect platelet aggregation could increase the risk of bleeding in some people. Some of these herbs include angelica, clove, danshen, garlic, ginger, ginkgo, Panax ginseng, horse chestnut, red clover, turmeric, and others.

Interactions with Drugs

ANTICOAGULANT/ANTIPLATELET DRUGS: Some evidence suggests that feverfew may inhibit platelet aggregation. However, this has not been demonstrated in humans (6935,6936,6942,6943,6944,6945,6951). Theoretically, feverfew might have additive effects and increase the risk of bleeding when used with these drugs.
NONSTEROIDAL ANTI-INFLAMMATORY DRUGS (NSAIDs): Theoretically, NSAIDs might decrease the effectiveness of feverfew (6). This potential interaction might be mediated through NSAIDs' effects on prostaglandins (21).

Interactions with Foods

None known.

Interactions with Lab Tests

None known.

Interactions with Diseases or Conditions

CROSS-ALLERGENICITY: Feverfew may cause an allergic reaction in individuals sensitive to the Asteraceae/Compositae family. Members of this family include ragweed, chrysanthemums, marigolds, daisies, and many other herbs.

Dosage and Administration

ORAL: For migraine headache prophylaxis, clinical studies have used 50 to 100 mg of feverfew extract daily. Although most extracts used in clinical studies were standardized to 0.2% to 0.35% parthenolide content, this standardization does not appear to be necessary for effectiveness (6935,6938,6959,6960,6961). The typical dose of the fresh leaf is 2.5 leaves daily with or after food (4). The freeze-dried leaf is taken at 50-125 mg per day with or after food (4,6,724,725).
TOPICAL: No typical dosage.

Comments

Some feverfew tablet products can contain little or no feverfew. The Therapeutic Products Directorate of the Health Products and Food Branch of Health Canada issued a Drug Identification Number (DIN) to a feverfew leaf (capsules) product standardized to 0.2% parthenolide, with the labeling claim "used as a prophylactic against migraines" (724).

FICIN

Also Known As

Doctor Oje, Leche de Higueron, Leche de Oje, Oje.

Scientific Names

Ficus insipida, synonyms Ficus anthelminthica, Ficus glabrata, and Ficus laurfolia.
Family: Moraceae.

People Use This For

Orally, ficin is used as a digestive aid, and as an anthelmintic.
In medical procedures, ficin is used to clean and prepare intestinal submucosa for the production of sutures, to clean and prepare animal arteries for human implantation, and in serologic testing (e.g., for Rh factor determination).
In manufacturing, ficin is used in European anti-inflammatory preparations, cheese manufacturing, chillproofing beer, preparation of protein hydrolysates, edible collagen films, and sausage casings. Ficin is sometimes included in meat tenderizers, usually in combination with papain and/or bromelain.

Safety

LIKELY UNSAFE ...when used topically. Crude ficin is corrosive to skin and prolonged contact can cause bleeding (11).
There is insufficient reliable information available about the safety of the oral use of ficin.

PREGNANCY AND LACTATION: LIKELY UNSAFE ...when used topically (11). There is insufficient reliable information available about the safety of ficin for oral use during pregnancy or lactation; avoid using.

Effectiveness

There is insufficient reliable information available about the effectiveness of ficin.

Mechanism of Action

Ficin is a sulfhydryl proteinase and can hydrolyze proteins, amides, esters, and small peptides (11). Some evidence suggests ficin might be useful in treating helminthiasis (11,3766). Other evidence suggests ficin has anti-inflammatory activity (11).

Adverse Reactions

Orally, large amounts of ficin can cause catharsis (11).
Topically, crude ficin is corrosive to skin and can cause bleeding with prolonged contact (11). Ficin can also cause contact allergies (11).

Interactions with Herbs & Other Dietary Supplements

None known.

Interactions with Drugs

None known.

Interactions with Foods

None known.

Interactions with Lab Tests

None known.

Interactions with Diseases or Conditions

None known.

Dosage and Administration

ORAL: As an anthelmintic, 1.0 cc of prepared latex/kg per day for 3 days to be repeated every 3 months has been used (3766).

Comments

Ficin is the latex harvested from the trunk of felled Ficus insipida trees. Crude ficin consists of the latex combined with acetic acid to prevent coagulation and sodium benzoate as a preservative (11). Purified ficin is not pure ficin. Rather, it is a mixture of several proteases and small amounts of other enzymes and other constituents (11).

FIELD SCABIOUS

Also Known As

Bluebuttons, Gypsy's-Rose.

Scientific Names

Knautia arvensis, synonym Scabiosa arvensis.
Family: Dipsacaceae.

People Use This For

Orally, field scabious is used for cough and throat complaints.
Topically, field scabious is used for chronic skin conditions; eczema; anal fissures; anal itching; urticaria; scabies; favus (roundworm); and cleansing and healing ulcers, bruises, and inflammation.

Safety

There is insufficient reliable information available about the safety of field scabious.
Pregnancy and Lactation: Insufficient reliable information available; avoid using.

Effectiveness

There is insufficient reliable information available about the effectiveness of field scabious.

Mechanism of Action

The applicable parts of field scabious are the above ground parts. Field scabious contains triterpene saponins including knatioside, knautioside A and B, iridoide monoterpenes including dipsacan, flavonoids, and tannins. It is reported to have astringent, antiseptic, expectorant, and purgative properties (18).

Adverse Reactions

None reported.

Interactions with Herbs & Other Dietary Supplements

None known.

Interactions with Drugs

None known.

Interactions with Foods

None known.

Interactions with Lab Tests

None known.

Interactions with Diseases or Conditions

None known.

Dosage and Administration

ORAL: For chronic eczema, people typically drink 2 glasses tea (add 4 teaspoons to 240 mL boiling water, steep for 10 minutes and strain) throughout the day (18).
TOPICAL: It is typically used as an alcoholic extract and tea.

FIG

Also Known As

Caricae Fructus, Feigen.

Scientific Names

Ficus carica.
Family: Moraceae.

People Use This For

Orally, fig is used as a laxative.

Safety

LIKELY SAFE ...when used orally in food amounts as fresh or dried fruit.
PREGNANCY AND LACTATION: LIKELY SAFE ...when used orally in food amounts as fresh or dried fruit.

Effectiveness

There is insufficient reliable information available about the effectiveness of fig.

Mechanism of Action

The applicable parts of fig are the fruit and leaf. However, very little is known about pharmacological effects of fig. An aqueous leaf extract can cause hypoglycemic activity in animals (6625).

Adverse Reactions

Orally, fig use can cause photodermatitis. Avoid excessive sunlight or ultraviolet light exposure while using this product (19). There has been one report of anaphylaxis following consumption of a dried fig (8815).

Interactions with Herbs & Other Dietary Supplements

None known.

Interactions with Drugs

None known.

Interactions with Foods
None known.

Interactions with Lab Tests
None known.

Interactions with Diseases or Conditions
None known.

Dosage and Administration
No typical dosage.

FIGWORT

Also Known As
Carpenter's Square, Common Figwort, Heal-all, Rosenoble, Scrophula Plant, Scrophularia, Throatwort.

Scientific Names
Scrophularia marilandica; Scrophularia nodosa.
Family: Scrophulariaceae.

People Use This For
Orally, figwort is used as a diuretic.
Topically, figwort is used for chronic skin diseases such as eczema, itching, and psoriasis, and hemorrhoids, swelling, and eruptions.

Safety
There is insufficient reliable information available about the safety of figwort.
Pregnancy and Lactation: Insufficient reliable information available; avoid using.

Effectiveness
There is insufficient reliable information available about the effectiveness of figwort.

Mechanism of Action
The applicable parts of figwort are the above ground parts and root. It is reported to have diuretic and laxative effects (18). Constituents, aucubin and catalpol, exert purgative action in mice; harpagide may have cardioactive and anti-inflammatory activity (4).

Adverse Reactions
None reported.

Interactions with Herbs & Other Dietary Supplements
CARDIAC GLYCOSIDE-CONTAINING HERBS: Contraindicated, and concomitant use can increase the risk of cardiac glycoside toxicity. Cardiac glycoside-containing herbs include black hellebore, Canadian hemp roots, digitalis leaf, hedge mustard, lily of the valley roots, motherwort, oleander leaf, pheasant's eye plant, pleurisy root, squill bulb leaf scales, strophanthus seeds, and uzara (19).

Interactions with Drugs
DIURETIC DRUGS: Theoretically, overuse of figwort might compound diuretic-induced potassium loss. There is some concern that people taking figwort along with potassium depleting diuretics might have an increased risk for hypokalemia. Initiation of potassium supplementation or an increase in potassium supplement dose may be necessary for some patients. Some diuretics that can deplete potassium include chlorothiazide (Diuril), chlorthalidone (Thalitone), furosemide (Lasix), hydrochlorothiazide (HCTZ, HydroDIURIL, Microzide), and others.

Interactions with Foods
None known.

Interactions with Lab Tests
None known.

Interactions with Diseases or Conditions
DIABETES: Theoretically, figwort may alter blood glucose control (4); monitor closely.
VENTRICULAR TACHYCARDIA: Contraindicated (4,12).

Dosage and Administration
ORAL: As a tea, use 2-8 grams dried above ground parts in 150 mL boiling water 5-10 minutes, steep (4). As a liquid extract (1:1 in 25% alcohol), 2-8 mL has been used (4). As a tincture (1:10 in 45% alcohol), 2-4 mL has been used (4).
TOPICAL: No typical dosage.

Comments
Figwort is stated to be a suitable substitute for devil's claw (due to similar chemical composition) (4).

FIR

Also Known As
Fir Tree, Norway Spruce, Piceae turiones recentes, Spruce, Spruce Fir.
CAUTION: See separate listings for Dwarf Pine Needle, Fir Needle Oil, Pine Needle Oil, Pine, Poplar, and Scotch Pine Needle.

Scientific Names
Abies alba, synonyms Abies alba f. pendula, Abies alba f. pyramidalis; Picea abies, synonyms Picea excelsa, Pinus abies, Pinus viminalis.
Family: Pinaceae.

People Use This For
Orally, fir is used for respiratory tract inflammation, colds, cough, bronchitis, fever, inflammation of the mouth and pharynx, muscle and nerve pain, tendency toward infection, and tuberculosis.
Topically, fir is used for mild myalgia, neuralgia, rheumatic pain, and applied externally as a bath additive for mental illness.

Safety
POSSIBLY SAFE ...when used orally or topically and appropriately (2).
PREGNANCY AND LACTATION: Insufficient reliable information available; avoid using.

Effectiveness
There is insufficient reliable information available about the effectiveness of fir.

Mechanism of Action
The applicable part of fir is the shoot. Fir shoot can reduce secretions, enhance local circulation, and act as a mild antiseptic (2). The essential oil can have secretory and antibacterial effects on bronchial mucous membranes (18). The essential oil also acts as a rubefacient (counterirritant) and improves circulation when applied externally (18).

Adverse Reactions
None reported.

Interactions with Herbs & Other Dietary Supplements
None known.

Interactions with Drugs
None known.

Interactions with Foods
None known.

Interactions with Lab Tests
None known.

Interactions with Diseases or Conditions
ASTHMA, PERTUSSIS (whooping cough): The fir shoot can exacerbate these conditions (18).
Contraindicated for use as a bath additive for individuals with extensive skin injuries, acute skin diseases, feverish or infectious diseases, cardiac insufficiency, or hypertonia (18).

Dosage and Administration
ORAL: The typical dose is 5-6 grams of the fresh fir shoots per day (2,18). The essential oil is usually given as 4 drops in water or on a sugar lump three times daily (18).
TOPICAL: Boil 200-300 grams of the shoots in 1 L water, steep for 5 minutes, strain, and add to a full bath (2,18).
INHALATION: Inhale the vapor of 2 grams of the essential oil in hot water several times per day (18).

Comments
Avoid confusion with fir needle oil.

FIR NEEDLE OIL

Also Known As
Fichtennadelöl, Piceae aetheroleum, White Spruce Oil.
CAUTION: See separate listing for Dwarf Pine Needle, Scotch Pine Needle Oil, Poplar, Fir, and Pine.

Scientific Names
Picea abies, synonyms Picea excelsa, Pinus abies, Pinus viminalis; Picea aetheroleum; Abies alba, synonyms Abies alba f. pendula, Abies alba f. pyramidalis; Abies sachalinensis; Abies sibirica.
Family: Pinaceae.

People Use This For
Orally, fir needle oil is used for upper and lower respiratory tract infections and conditions.
Topically, fir needle oil is used for upper and lower respiratory tract infections and conditions. It is also used topically for rheumatic, neuralgic, and muscle pains. Fir needle oil is commonly used as a liniment in alcoholic solutions, ointments, gels, emulsions, and oils. It is also used topically as a bath additive.
Fir needle oil is also used as an inhalant.

Safety
POSSIBLY SAFE ...when used orally or topically (2).
PREGNANCY AND LACTATION: Insufficient reliable information available; avoid using.

Effectiveness
There is insufficient reliable information available about the effectiveness of fir needle oil.

Mechanism of Action
Fir needle oil is made from the tips of branches or twigs. Fir needle oil has mild antiseptic and counterirritant properties. It also breaks up respiratory secretions (2).

Adverse Reactions
Orally, fir needle oil can increase bronchospasms (2).
Topically, fir needle oil increases skin and mucous membrane irritation (2).

Interactions with Herbs & Other Dietary Supplements
None known.

Interactions with Drugs
None known.

Interactions with Foods
None known.

Interactions with Lab Tests
None known.

Interactions with Diseases or Conditions
ASTHMA, PERTUSSIS (whooping cough): Fir needle oil is contraindicated in individuals with these conditions because it can increase bronchospasms (2).

Dosage and Administration
No typical dosage.

FIREWEED

Also Known As
Blood Vine, Blooming Sally, Flowering Willow, French Willow, French-Willow, Great Willowherb, Persian Willow, Purple Rocket, Rose Bay Willow, Rosebay Willow, Tame Withy, Wickup, Wicopy, Willow Herb, Willowherb.

Scientific Names
Epilobium angustifolium, synonyms Chamaenerion angustifolium, Chamerion angustifolium, Epilobium spicatum. Family: Onagraceae.

People Use This For
Orally, fireweed is used for inflammation, fevers, tumors, wounds, as an astringent, and as a tonic.

Safety
POSSIBLY SAFE ...when used orally (12).
PREGNANCY AND LACTATION: Insufficient reliable information available; avoid using.

Effectiveness
There is insufficient reliable information available about the effectiveness of fireweed.

Mechanism of Action
The applicable parts of fireweed are the above ground parts. Preliminary evidence suggests that aqueous extracts of fireweed might affect reproduction (858) and have anti-inflammatory effects (859,860).

Adverse Reactions
None reported.

Interactions with Herbs & Other Dietary Supplements
None known.

Interactions with Drugs
None known.

Interactions with Foods
None known.

Interactions with Lab Tests
None known.

Interactions with Diseases or Conditions
None known.

Dosage and Administration
No typical dosage.

Comments
Other Epilobium species are also referred to as willow herb (18).

FISH OILS

Also Known As
Cod Liver Oil, Marine Oils, Menhaden Oil, N-3 Fatty Acids, N3-polyunsaturated Fatty Acids, Omega-3 Fatty Acids, PUFA, Salmon Oil, W-3 Fatty Acids.
CAUTION: See separate listings for Cod Liver Oil, DHA, EPA, and Shark Liver Oil.

Scientific Names
None.

People Use This For

Orally, fish oils are used for hyperlipidemia, hypertriglyceridemia, coronary heart disease, hypertension, stroke, bipolar disorder, depression, rheumatoid arthritis (RA), osteoporosis, psoriasis, atopic dermatitis, ulcerative colitis, Behcet's syndrome, and Raynaud's syndrome. Fish oils are also used orally for weight loss, asthma, cancer, painful menses, lung diseases, allergic rhinitis, Crohn's disease, chronic fatigue syndrome, albuminuria associated with diabetic neuropathy, restenosis after angioplasty, miscarriage, preeclampsia, preterm labor, and intrauterine growth retardation. Fish oils are used for systemic lupus erythematosus, cystic fibrosis, gingivitis, renal impairment associated with cirrhosis, hyperglycemia associated with type 2 diabetes, and claudication. Fish oils are also used to treat attention deficit-hyperactivity disorder (ADHD), dyslexia, and dyspraxia. Other uses include preventing muscular soreness after exercise, preventing thrombosis after placement of a hemodialysis graft, renal impairment associated with IgA nephropathy; and high blood pressure and renal impairment associated with heart transplantation.

In combination with linoleic and gamma-linoleic acid, fish oils are used orally for treating post-viral fatigue syndrome. Fish oils are also used orally in combination with garlic to treat hypercholesterolemia.

Intravenously, fish oils are used to treat psoriasis.

Safety

LIKELY SAFE ...when used orally and appropriately. Doses of 3 grams per day and less can be safely used by most people. Fish oils have Generally Recognized As Safe (GRAS) status in the US (1313,4912).

POSSIBLY UNSAFE ...when used orally in large amounts. Doses greater than 3 grams per day can inhibit blood coagulation and potentially increase the risk of bleeding. Doses greater than 3 grams per day might also suppress immune response (1313,7384).

CHILDREN: POSSIBLY SAFE ...when used orally and appropriately (5708,5711).

PREGNANCY AND LACTATION: There is insufficient reliable information available about the safety of fish oils when used in medicinal amounts during pregnancy and breast-feeding.

Effectiveness

LIKELY EFFECTIVE

Hypertriglyceridemia. Fish oils from supplements or from dietary sources can reduce triglyceride levels by 20% to 50% (1024,2299,2300,2301,2302,2315,2317,5702,5705,5706,6394,6399,7368,7369,7380). This effect appears to be dose-dependent (5706,7380). However, fish oil supplements in doses of 4 grams per day do not seem to be as effective as gemfibrozil (Lopid) 1200 mg per day (7377). For patients with hypertriglyceridemia associated with the atherogenic lipoprotein phenotype (ALP), which is thought to be a marker for cardiovascular disease, 6 grams of supplemental fish oils taken daily might reduce triglyceride levels by 35% (8683).

POSSIBLY EFFECTIVE

Age-related maculopathy. There is some evidence that people who ingest fish oils from dietary fish sources more than once per week have a reduced risk of developing age-related maculopathy (6260).

Angioplasty. Taking fish oils orally seems to prevent restenosis after percutaneous transluminal coronary angioplasty (PTCA) (8680). Fish oils appear to decrease restenosis rate (up to 26% reduction) when given for one month before PTCA and continued for one month thereafter. When given for less than one month before PTCA, fish oils don't seem to have any effect on restenosis (1028,1038,2320).

Antiphospholipid syndrome-associated miscarriage. Taking fish oils orally seems to prevent recurrent miscarriage and increase live birth rate in pregnant women with antiphospholipid syndrome (1032).

Atherosclerosis. Fish oil supplements 6 grams per day for three months and then 3 grams per day for 21 months might modestly slow the progression, or cause mild to moderate regression of atherosclerosis as measured by angiography in people with coronary artery disease. However, fish oils don't seem to improve luminal diameter (1022,2311) or decrease intima-media thickness of the carotid arteries in people with coronary artery disease (8681).

Atrial fibrillation. People aged 65 years and older who regularly consume tuna or other broiled or baked fish providing omega-3 fatty acids (fish oils) seem to have a lower risk of atrial fibrillation compared to those who eat fish less than once per month. People who consume fish 5 or more times per week have a 31% lower risk. People who consume fish 1 to 4 times per week have a 28% lower risk. However, consuming fried fish or fish sandwiches is not associated with a decreased risk of atrial fibrillation (12055).

Bipolar disorder. Taking fish oils orally, with conventional therapies, seems to improve symptoms of depression and increase length of remission (7202). However, fish oils do not seem to have beneficial effects on manic symptoms in bipolar patients (5713,7202).

Cachexia. Taking a high-dose (7.5 grams per day) fish oil supplement seems to slow weight loss in some patients with cancer-related cachexia (11979). Lower doses (3 grams per day) don't seem to have any effect (10008). There is some preliminary evidence that a protein product supplemented with fish oils might help to improve appetite and increase lean body mass in patients with advanced pancreatic cancer (5701).

Cancer. Fish oils from dietary sources seems to decrease the general risk of cancer. Intake of 1 gram per week of omega-3 fatty acids from fish seems to significantly lower the risk of several cancers including oral cancer, pharyngeal cancer, esophageal cancer, colon cancer, rectal cancer, breast cancer, and ovarian cancer (10153).

Coronary artery bypass. Taking supplemental fish oils orally seems to decrease the incidence of coronary artery bypass graft occlusion following coronary artery bypass grafting (2314).

Coronary heart disease. Consuming dietary fish oils seems to reduce the risk of death from coronary heart disease (primary prevention). Epidemiological research suggests that long-term consumption of a diet that regularly includes fish reduces the risk of death from coronary heart disease in healthy people, regardless of age. Fish oils might lower mortality risk by decreasing ventricular ectopic beats (7360,10006). Consumption of one to two servings per week of fish oils from dietary sources appears to reduce the risk of coronary heart disease death by 25%. Higher fish intake doesn't appear to provide additional benefit (2309,8672). There is also some epidemiological evidence that consumption of omega-3 fatty acids and fish might decrease the risk of acute myocardial infarction (MI). However, further study in populations at high risk for MI is needed to confirm this finding (8675). Additionally, fish oils from dietary sources or oral supplements also seems to reduce the risk of cardiovascular events and death in patients with existing coronary heart disease (secondary prevention). Fish oils 1 gram daily starting within three months after MI and continued for at least a year appears to reduce the risk of total cardiac events, non-fatal MI, and total cardiac mortality by 15% (1007,2307). There is also some evidence that consuming 2-3 servings of fish each week can reduce the risk of death after MI (7359). Population studies also suggest that fish oils from dietary sources or supplements may reduce overall mortality, mortality due to MI, and sudden death in people with coronary heart disease, possibly by beneficial effects on heart rate variability and antiarrhythmic effects (8673,8676). However, fish oil supplements do not appear to have antiarrhythmic effects in survivors of ventricular tachyarrhythmias (11344). Fish oil supplements also do not seem to reduce the risk of post-MI cardiovascular events in people whose diet already includes fish (7361).

Cyclosporine-induced hypertension. Taking fish oils orally seems to prevent cyclosporine-induced hypertension following cardiac transplant. There is also some evidence that fish oils can maintain pre-cyclosporine blood pressures in patients taking cyclosporine (1012).

Cyclosporine-induced nephrotoxicity. Taking fish oils orally seems to prevent cyclosporine-induced nephrotoxicity, and significantly improve glomerular filtration rate (GFR) and renal blood flow in individuals taking cyclosporine (1021).

Depression. Taking fish oils orally seems to improve response to conventional antidepressants (10871). Low omega-3 levels in plasma and red blood cells are associated with depression (10859,10860). Epidemiological research suggests eating fish lowers the risk of depression and suicide (10867), and the prevalence of depression is lower in countries with higher fish consumption (10868).

Diabetic nephropathy. Taking fish oils orally seems to reduce albuminuria in individuals with diabetic nephropathy (1025).

Dyslexia. Taking fish oils orally seems to improve night vision in children with dyslexia. Dyslexic children who take fish oils seem to develop significantly better dark adaptation (5708).

Dyslipidemia. Taking 12 grams of fish oils orally in combination with garlic 900 mg daily seems to lower total cholesterol, triglycerides and the ratios of total cholesterol to high-density lipoprotein (HDL) and low-density lipoprotein (LDL) to HDL in patients with hypercholesterolemia (2318,2319). There is also some evidence that taking fish oils can decrease elevated triglyceride levels, decrease secretion of very low-density lipoproteins (VLDLs), increase VLDL apolipoprotein B secretion, and increase levels of HDL cholesterol in people with type 2 diabetes and dyslipidemia (8714,8807). However, elevated levels of small, dense LDL cholesterol particles, are unaffected by fish oils in patients with type 2 diabetes (8714). There's also preliminary data that suggests fish oils, combined with pravastatin, might be helpful when used orally to correct the dyslipidemia associated with post-renal transplantation (8805).

Dysmenorrhea. Taking fish oils, alone or in combination with vitamin B12, seems to decrease pain and interference with daily activities in adolescent girls and women with dysmenorrhea (7574,7575).

Dyspraxia. Taking fish oils orally, in combination with evening primrose oil, thyme oil, and vitamin E (Efalex), seems to improve movement disorders in children with dyspraxia. One small clinical trial has shown that this combination significantly decreases movement disorders as determined by objective measures (5708).

Endometrial cancer. There is some evidence that women who regularly consume approximately two servings per week of fatty fish have a reduced risk for endometrial cancer (8690,9774).

Heart transplant. Taking fish oils orally seems to preserve renal function and reduce the long-term continuous rise in blood pressure after heart transplantation. There is evidence a dose of 4 grams of fish oils daily (46.5% EPA and 37.8% DHA) after heart transplantation prevents changes in systolic and diastolic blood pressures, glomerular filtration rate, and serum creatinine (8687).

Hemodialysis grafts. Taking fish oils orally seems to help prevent thrombosis in hemodialysis grafts. Fish oil supplements 4 grams daily started within two weeks of graft placement seems to prevent the development of access thrombosis in hemodialysis patients (8684).

Hypertension. Taking fish oils orally seems to produce modest, but significant reductions in systolic and diastolic blood pressure in patients with mild hypertension with or without type 2 diabetes (1001,1020,2301).

IgA nephropathy. Long-term use (two years) of fish oils 4-8 grams daily can slow the rate of renal function loss in high-risk patients with IgA nephropathy (8686,8711).

Obesity. There is some evidence that fish oils from dietary fish sources can improve weight loss and decrease blood glucose and insulin concentrations in overweight and hypertensive patients (2049).

Osteoporosis. Taking fish oils orally, in combination with evening primrose oil and calcium, seems to decrease bone turnover and increase spinal and femoral bone mineral density in elderly people with osteoporosis (7611).

Prostate cancer. Population studies indicate that prostate cancer risk is significantly lower in men who regularly include fish oils in the diet. It appears that to significantly reduce the risk of prostate cancer at least 3 meals per week containing fish oil should be consumed (7378,9773,9774). Men who have higher serum levels of eicosapentaenoic acid (EPA) and docosahexaenoic acid (DHA), fatty acids that are in fish, seem to have a lower risk of developing prostate cancer (6395).

Psoriasis. There is some evidence that administering fish oils intravenously can decrease severity of symptoms in patients with acute, extended guttate psoriasis and chronic plaque psoriasis. Fish oils seem to be superior to omega-6 fatty acids for this use (1004,1034). However, fish oils taken orally do not seem to have any effect on psoriasis despite promising preliminary research (1035,8708).

Raynaud's syndrome. There's some evidence that taking fish oils orally can improve tolerance to cold and delay the onset of vasospasm in people with primary Raynaud's syndrome. People with Raynaud's syndrome caused by progressive systemic sclerosis don't seem to respond to fish oil supplements (7573).

Rheumatoid arthritis (RA). Taking fish oils orally, alone or in combination with naproxen (Naprosyn), seems to significantly decrease the duration of morning stiffness in patients with RA (1017,1039,1041). Use of fish oils might also allow reduction of nonsteroidal anti-inflammatory drug (NSAID) requirements when used concomitantly (1031).

Stroke. Taking fish oils orally seems to reduce the risk of ischemic stroke, specifically thrombotic infarction. Consuming fish oils from dietary sources at least once a week seems to reduce the risk of ischemic stroke by 27% (7373). Higher serum levels of fish oils are also associated with a decreased risk of stroke (7372). Consumption of very high amounts of fish oils from dietary sources seems to increase the risk of stroke. People who eat more than 46 grams per day of fish or more than 660 mg per day of n-3 fatty acids appear to be nearly twice as likely to have an ischemic or hemorrhagic stroke. Tell patients that moderate consumption of fish (once or twice a week) is probably a good idea, but very high consumption of fish oils might be harmful (1313,7603,7610,8699). Dietary fish oils don't seem to further reduce ischemic stroke risk in people who already take aspirin (7373).

POSSIBLY INEFFECTIVE

Cirrhosis. Taking fish oils orally doesn't seem to help renal impairment associated with advanced cirrhosis (1013).

Claudication. Taking fish oils orally appears to have no effect on walking distance in patients with stable claudication (1002).

Gingivitis. Taking fish oils orally doesn't seem to improve gingivitis (1005).

Helicobacter pylori (H pylori). Taking fish oils orally, in combination with pantoprazole and clarithromycin (Biaxin), is inferior for eradicating H. pylori infection when compared with a combination of pantoprazole, clarithromycin, and metronidazole (8710).

Mastalgia. Taking fish oils orally aren't any more effective than placebo when 3 grams daily are taken for 6 months for severe chronic breast pain (9156).

Migraine headache. Taking fish oils orally doesn't appear to have any effect in decreasing the frequency or severity of migraine headaches in adolescents and adults (8712,8713).

Myalgia. Taking fish oils 1.8 grams per day taken orally for a month prior to and during physical exercise doesn't seem to prevent muscle soreness (8524).

Systemic lupus erythematosus (SLE). Taking fish oils orally doesn't seem to reduce disease activity or improve renal function when taken for a year in patients with SLE (7571). There's some weak evidence that fish oils plus a low-fat diet might reduce lupus symptoms, but it's too preliminary to recommend this combination (7572).

LIKELY INEFFECTIVE

Diabetes. Taking fish oils orally has no effect on fasting plasma glucose levels or serum hemoglobin A1c levels at doses less than 6 grams per day in people with type 2 diabetes (2299,2300,2302,7368,7369).

Several clinical studies have used fish oil products containing specific proportions of the fatty acids eicosapentaenoic acid (EPA) and docosahexanoic acid (DHA). Most commonly used products have contained 35% EPA and 25% DHA.

INSUFFICIENT RELIABLE EVIDENCE to RATE

Attention deficit-hyperactivity disorder (ADHD). There is preliminary evidence that taking fish oils orally might be helpful for ADHD (8800).

Chronic fatigue syndrome (CFS). There is some conflicting evidence about the use of a proprietary combination of fish oils and evening primrose oil (Efamol Marine) to reduce the symptoms CFS (7563,7564).

Chronic renal insufficiency. Preliminary clinical evidence suggests fish oils might reduce elevated levels of C-reactive protein (CRP) and increase hemoglobin, albumin levels, and urine output in patients on chronic hemodialysis (8685). However, fish oils don't appear to have any effect in healthy people with low CRP levels. Whether fish oils have any beneficial effects in patients with elevated CRP levels and conditions such as coronary artery disease is unknown (10155).

Inflammatory bowel disease (IBD). There is some conflicting evidence suggesting fish oils might be helpful for IBD, but more evidence is needed (1037,1040,5709,6257,6258,6259).

Pregnancy-associated complications. There is controversial evidence that suggests the use of fish oils with or without evening primrose oil may be effective for preventing pre-eclampsia, preterm labor, and intrauterine growth retardation in pregnant women. Some researchers suggest fish oils can prevent premature delivery when given during the third trimester of pregnancy (30 weeks and after) (8706). Other researchers have found no effect (1026,1027,1042).

Schizophrenia. There is a case report of daily fish oils monotherapy (4 grams EPA and 2 grams DHA) improving

symptoms of schizophrenia in a pregnant female (8702).
More information is needed to rate fish oils for these uses.

Mechanism of Action

Fish such as herring, kipper, mackerel, menhaden, pilchard, salmon, sardine, and trout contain oils with high amounts of long-chain, polyunsaturated fats called omega-3 fatty acids. These fish oils are especially high in the omega-3 fatty acids eicosapentaenoic acid (EPA) and docosahexaenoic acid (DHA). EPA and DHA seem to have different physiologic effects than their precursor alpha linolenic acid, a plant-derived omega-3 fatty acid (10323).
Omega-3 fatty acids from fish oils have anti-inflammatory and antithrombotic effects because they compete with arachidonic acid in the cyclooxygenase and lipoxygenase pathways. Fish oils inhibit the arachidonic acid synthesis of thromboxane A2, which causes platelet aggregation and vasoconstriction. Fish oils can also cause increased production of prostacyclin, a prostaglandin that causes vasoconstriction and reduces platelet aggregation (8671,8679,8696). Preliminary clinical evidence suggests that fish oils might have an additive or synergistic effect with aspirin on inhibiting synthesis of thromboxane A2 and the highly inflammatory leukotriene B4 (8701), but it's too early to recommend this combination. Fish oils are used for cardiovascular conditions, including stroke and heart disease, due to anti-inflammatory and antithrombotic effects.
Fish oils decrease blood viscosity, increase red blood cell deformability, and possibly provide protection against red cell hemolysis. Vasodilatory effects of omega-3 fatty acids in fish oils may also prevent increases in blood pressure and maintain renal function. Fish oils may have an antiarrhythmic effect. There is some evidence prostaglandins derived from arachidonic acid are proarrhythmic, whereas equivalent prostaglandins derived from EPA are not. Fish oils also might regulate calcium movement through calcium channels in the heart and suppress intracellular calcium activity, which has been associated with arrhythmias. Increased dietary intake of omega-3 fatty acids increases the amount of EPA and DHA in cell membranes, which is thought to cause changes in enzyme and receptor function that secondarily leads to changes in calcium fluxes across cell membranes (8676). There's also some evidence fish oils might affect sodium channels and inhibit ischemia-induced arrhythmias (7360,7362,7363,8671,8676,8677,8687). Regular consumption of fish also seems to decrease heart rate, which might further protect against cardiovascular events. Omega-3 fatty acids in fish oil, especially DHA, are associated with decreased heart rate (10154).
In hypertriglyceridemia, fish oils are thought to lower triglycerides by decreasing secretion of very low-density lipoproteins (VLDLs), increasing VLDL apolipoprotein B secretion, possibly by increasing VLDL clearance, and reducing triglyceride transport (5707). In addition, fish oils appear to decrease synthesis of VLDL by inhibiting 1,2-diacylglycerol-sterol o-acyltransferase or phosphatidate phosphatase (6394). Fish oils may decrease chylomicron concentrations. More lipoprotein lipase becomes available due to decreased VLDL levels, which causes increased hydrolysis of chylomicrons (6394). Fish oils also increase fatty acid oxidation by peroxisomal and mitochondrial routes, reduce fatty acid synthesis, divert fatty acids into phospholipid synthesis, increase hepatic uptake of triglycerides, and down-regulate fatty acid esterifying enzymes (5707).
Fish oils may decrease cholesterol absorption from the gut and decrease cholesterol synthesis (5707). There is evidence fish and fish oils increase high-density lipoproteins (HDL) and decrease the total cholesterol to HDL ratio (2318,5707,8674,8678,8698). Fish oils may increase low-density lipoprotein (LDL) concentrations (2299,2318,8678,8698) by increasing the size of LDL particles (9771). It is thought that fish oils might cause a more buoyant LDL to be formed, which might be less atherogenic (2299,8678). There is some evidence that vitamin B12 used with fish oils might have additive effects in lowering cholesterol, but the mechanism for this effect is unknown (8894). Fish oils also improve flow-mediated arterial dilation in people with hypercholesterolemia (5702). Oxidation of LDL cholesterol in macrophages seems to be increased by fish oil. This detrimental effect on atherosclerosis might decrease the benefit of fish oil in atherosclerosis (9771).
Unlike some other kinds of dietary fat, omega-3 fatty acids from fish oils do not seem to impair endothelial function, which is thought to be a precursor to atherogenesis (5702,7382). In some patients, fish oils appears to improve arterial compliance (1029,5707).
Fish oil can change the way dietary fatty acids are utilized. Omega-3 fatty acids found in fish oil compete metabolically with omega-6 fatty acids and omega-3 fatty acids in vegetable oils. Alpha linolenic acid and gamma linolenic acid are the primary omega-3 and omega-6 (respectively) fatty acids found in vegetable oils. Fish oil can modify the way these dietary fatty acids are incorporated into fatty acid chains and cell membranes and how they are used in other metabolic processes (7381,8693,9772). Omega-6 fatty acids, from fish oil, seem to inhibit the incorporation of omega-3 fatty acids into tissue lipids. In addition, omega-3 fatty acids inhibit the conversion of the omega-6 fatty acids into arachidonic acid. There is some concern that dietary vegetable oils in the diet might negate the beneficial cardiovascular effects of fish oils, but omega-3 fatty acids from fish oils seem to reduce cardiovascular risk factors despite concurrent omega-6 fatty acid ingestion (7381,8693). By increasing the intake of omega-3 fatty acids EPA and DHA, a corresponding increase of these fatty acids seems to occur in cell membranes and circulatory lipids along with a simultaneous reduction of omega-6 fatty acids (8677). The efficacy of omega-3 fatty acid containing products such as fish oils seems to be determined by an increased intake of omega-3 fatty-acids, a decreased intake of omega-6 fatty acids, and a decreased ratio of arachidonic acid to EPA and DHA (8671,8694).
Fish oils can suppress mediators of immune function by reducing the production of cytokines such as interleukin-1(IL-1), interleukin-2 (IL-2), and tumor necrosis factor (TNF). Some researchers think fish oils might prevent weight loss in cancer patients by inhibiting cytokines, which cause muscle catabolism. Fish oils also suppress T- and B-cell proliferation and decrease delayed-type hypersensitivity skin response (DTH). They also decrease antibody

production and increase free radical activity (1313,7383,7384,11979).

Due to fish oils' anti-inflammatory effects, they are tried for a variety of inflammatory conditions, including psoriasis, systemic lupus erythematosus (SLE), inflammatory bowel disease, and others. Fish oils seem to be beneficial in rheumatoid arthritis due to anti-inflammatory effects, and epidemiological data that suggests EPA levels are decreased in total plasma fatty acids and synovial fluid, and DHA is decreased in the synovial fluid of patients with rheumatoid arthritis (5710).

Preliminary clinical evidence suggest fish oil supplements might prolong pregnancy and depress levels of thromboxane A2 which is thought to cause vasoconstriction, platelet aggregation, and reduced uteroplacental blood flow associated with preeclampsia (8707).

Fish oils have been proposed as a treatment for attention deficit-hyperactivity disorder (ADHD) due to epidemiological data that suggests symptoms of ADHD might be inversely related to the omega 3-fatty acid phospholipid content (5711). In individuals with bipolar disorder, the fatty acids in fish oils are thought to have an effect similar to lithium or valproate, slowing nerve signaling (7202). In depression, omega-3s might normalize altered neuronal membrane microstructure and faulty neurotransmission in patients with depression. Omega-3s might also play a role in correcting defects in the arachidonic acid cascade, which is involved in second messenger processes that affect neurotransmitter uptake (10871). A diet deficient in omega-3 fatty acids may affect the fatty acid composition of cells in the central nervous system and alter neural function, including intellectual or cognitive development. DHA is thought to be important for normal neural function and might play a key role in the structural development of neural and synaptic membranes (8704,8705,8803). There is preliminary evidence that low levels of omega-3 fatty acids, especially DHA, might affect retinal, visual, learning, and memory function (8704,8705,8715).

Some researchers think fish oils might also help prevent some forms of cancer. People with high EPA and DHA levels in their erythrocytes seem to have decreased rates of prostate cancer (6395). EPA and DHA might compete with arachidonic acid as substrates for cyclooxygenases that produce prostaglandins that can enhance tumor growth (6385,7378). There is evidence fish oil supplementation decreases the expression of the enzyme cyclooxygenase-2 (COX-2) which has been found in prostate cancer tissue and is thought to play a role in promoting the growth of cancer cells (8689). There is also preliminary evidence that high levels of EPA and DHA can be beneficial for prolonging cancer remission. Fish oils might decrease production of lactic acid by tumor cells. Lactic acidosis is a marker of unfavorable metabolic conditions associated with many cancers (6398). There is also some evidence that fish oils might be cytotoxic to some cancer cells (1008). Preliminary evidence suggests that omega-3 fatty acids are first oxidized and then accumulate in tumor cell membranes, resulting in cell membrane perforation and eventually tumor cell death (8691).

Adverse Reactions

Orally, fish oils are generally well-tolerated at doses of 3 grams or less per day. Fish oils sometimes have a fishy taste and can cause belching, halitosis, heartburn, and gastrointestinal upset (6258,10007). High doses can cause nausea and loose stools. Some gastrointestinal side effects can be minimized if fish oils are taken with meals and if doses are started low and gradually increased.

Doses greater than 3 grams per day of fish oil or high dietary intake of fish can inhibit platelet aggregation, cause bleeding, and potentially increase the risk for hemorrhagic stroke (1313,8699). Very high consumption of fish (more than 46 grams per day) seems to increase the risk of both ischemic and hemorrhagic stroke (7603).

There's also some evidence that fish oils in doses greater than 3 grams per day might adversely affect immune function. Fish oils appear to suppress T- and B-cell function and to reduce the production of cytokines, which might be detrimental to elderly people and people with suppressed immune function such as patients with human immunodeficiency virus (HIV) infection (1313,7383,7384).

In patients with diabetes or impaired glucose tolerance, fish oil doses greater than 3 grams per day might worsen glycemia (10007).

Fish oils don't seem to adversely affect low-density lipoprotein (LDL) cholesterol or cause development of atherosclerosis, despite earlier concerns that polyunsaturated fatty acids, such as omega-3 fatty acids, might increase the oxidation of LDL (1011,2322,2323,7366). Supplemental fish oils do not seem to increase the susceptibility of LDL to oxidation (8695,8700). Although thiobarbituric acid reacting substances (TBARS) rise during fish oil supplementation, TBARS is now thought to inaccurately reflect LDL oxidation. More specific indicators of lipid peroxidation, such as F2-isoprostanes and malondialdehyde (MDA), suggest that fish oils are unlikely to have a negative effect on LDL and the risk for atherosclerosis (2323). There is also some evidence that fish oil supplements do not alter the serum concentrations of growth factors such as platelet-derived growth factor or transforming growth factor beta, which are also thought to play a role in the development of atherosclerotic plaques (8697).

Some fish oil preparations (e.g., cod liver oil) contain large amounts of vitamin A and vitamin D. If these preparations are used long-term or in large doses, there is a risk of vitamin A and D toxicity (see separate listing for cod liver oil) (6874).

Preliminary evidence suggests that increased serum levels of omega-3 fatty acids, especially DHA, might increase the risk for atrophic gastritis (8709).

There is some concern that fish oil products might be contaminated with toxins or pesticides if the fish were caught in contaminated waters (6875). Heavy metals, especially mercury, are a particular concern (259). However, laboratory analysis of some fish oil supplements found no detectable levels of mercury in the 20 products tested. Fish typically contain 10 to 1000 parts per billion of mercury. Mercury accumulates in fish meat much more so than fish oils,

which might explain the lack of detectable mercury in fish oil supplements (7379).
Fish oils also contribute to caloric intake and may cause weight gain if used long-term. One gram of fat or oil provides 9 kcal (6871). Fish oil capsules containing 500 mg omega-3 fatty acids in 1 gram of oil would supply about 13.5 kcal per capsule (6871,6874). Fish oil supplements also contain cholesterol in amounts from 1 to 6 mg per gram of fish oils (3022,6871).

Interactions with Herbs & Other Dietary Supplements

HERBS WITH ANTICOAGULANT/ANTIPLATELET POTENTIAL: Concomitant use of herbs that have antiplatelet/anticoagulant constituents could theoretically increase the risk of bleeding in some people (8671,8679,8696). These herbs include angelica, clove, danshen, garlic, ginger, ginkgo, Panax ginseng, red clover, turmeric, willow, and others.
VITAMIN E: Fish oils can reduce vitamin E levels. The mechanism is unknown, but might result from reduced vitamin E absorption or increased vitamin E utilization by tissues to reduce free radicals and prevent peroxidative damage (7384).

Interactions with Drugs

ANTICOAGULANT/ANTIPLATELET DRUGS: Concomitant use with anticoagulant or antiplatelet drugs may increase the risk of bleeding (8671,8679,8696,11343). However, conflicting research suggests that 3 to 6 grams of fish oils per day does not significantly affect the INRs of patients taking warfarin (8801). Monitor INRs of patients taking fish oils and drugs that affect bleeding. Some of these drugs include aspirin, clopidogrel (Plavix), dalteparin (Fragmin), dipyridamole (Persantine), enoxaparin (Lovenox), heparin, ticlopidine (Ticlid), warfarin (Coumadin), and others.
ANTIHYPERTENSIVE DRUGS: Fish oils can lower blood pressure and might have additive effects in patients treated with antihypertensives (1001,1020,1030,1033); use with caution.
CONTRACEPTIVE DRUGS: There is some evidence that contraceptive drugs might interfere with the triglyceride lowering effects of fish oils (8694). Some of these drugs include ethinyl estradiol and levonorgestrel (Triphasil), ethinyl estradiol and norethindrone (Ortho-Novum 1/35, Ortho-Novum 7/7/7), and others.

Interactions with Foods

None known.

Interactions with Lab Tests

BLOOD PRESSURE: Fish oils can moderately lower blood pressure and reduce blood pressure readings in patients with hypertension (1001,1020,1030,1033).
INTERNATIONAL NORMALIZED RATIO (INR), PROTHROMBIN TIME (PT): High doses of fish oils, greater than 3 grams per day, might decrease blood coagulation, increase INR and PT, and increase the risk of bleeding (1313).
TRIGLYCERIDES: Fish oils can reduce serum triglyceride concentrations and test results by 20% to 50% in patients with elevated triglycerides (1003,1009,1014,1024).

Interactions with Diseases or Conditions

BIPOLAR DISORDER and DEPRESSION: Symptoms of hypomania can develop in patients taking fish oils who have bipolar (5713,7202) or major depressive disorders (6396).
CIRRHOSIS: Theoretically, use of fish oils may lower mean arterial pressure (MAP) to hypotensive levels, and may increase risk of bleeding (1013); use with caution.
DIABETES: Fish oils in doses greater than 3 grams per day can increase blood glucose levels. However, lower doses don't seem to affect blood glucose. Tell patients with diabetes to avoid exceeding a dose of 3 grams per day (7368,7369,10007).
FAMILIAL ADENOMATOUS POLYPOSIS: Fish oils might further increase the risk of cancer in people with familial adenomatous polyposis. Three people, who had pre-existing familial adenomatous polyposis, were diagnosed with malignant lesions during the course of long-term use of fish oils (999).
HYPERTENSION: Fish oils can lower blood pressure and might have additive effects in patients treated with antihypertensives (1001,1020,1030,1033).
IMMUNODEFICIENCY: Higher doses of fish oils might cause suppression of immune and inflammatory response (1313,7383,7384). Tell immunocompromised patients (e.g., patients with HIV/AIDS) to avoid exceeding a dose of 3 grams per day.

Dosage and Administration

ORAL: For lowering triglycerides, studies have used 1 to 4 grams of fish oils per day (5707,6394,6399). To lower triglycerides in patients with the atherogenic lipoprotein phenotype (ALP), 6 grams per day has been used (8683).
For lowering blood pressure, studies have used either 4 grams of fish oils or fish oils providing eicosapentaenoic acid (EPA) 2.04 grams and docosahexaenoic acid (DHA) 1.4 grams daily (1001,1020).
For hypertension secondary to cyclosporine in heart transplant patients, 4 grams per day has been used (1012).
For atrial fibrillation, consuming tuna or baked or broiled fish providing omega-3 fatty acids (fish oils) one or more times per week seems to reduce the risk of atrial fibrillation in patients aged 65 or older compared to consuming fish

once per month or less (12055). However, this benefit is not found with fried fish or fish sandwiches.
For cyclosporine nephrotoxicity, 12 grams per day containing 2.2 grams EPA and 1.4 grams DHA has been used (1021). For reducing mortality after a myocardial infarction, a daily oral dose of fish oils providing EPA 850 mg to 1.08 grams with or without 882 mg DHA, or a daily serving of 1.25 ounces or more of fish has been used (1007,2307).
For reducing overall mortality and sudden death in patients with coronary heart disease, a daily dose of fish oils providing EPA 0.3 to 6 grams with 0.6 to 3.7 grams DHA has been used (8673).
For preventing and reversing the progression of atherosclerosis in the coronary arteries, 6 grams of fish oil for the first three months, followed by 3 grams daily thereafter, has been used (2311).
For improving endothelial function in individuals with hypercholesterolemia, 4 grams per day has been used (5702).
For decreasing duration of morning stiffness secondary to rheumatoid arthritis, fish oils providing EPA 3.8 grams and DHA 2 grams per day have been used (1039).
For preventing miscarriage in women with antiphospholipid antibody syndrome and a history of recurrent miscarriage, 5.1 grams fish oils with a 1.5 EPA:DHA ratio has been used (1032).
For treating dysmenorrhea, a daily dose of EPA 1080 mg and DHA 720 mg has been (7574).
For treating primary Raynaud's syndrome, a total daily dose of 3.96 grams EPA and 2.64 grams DHA has been used (7573).
As an adjunct to standard therapy for bipolar disorder, fish oils providing EPA 6.2 grams and DHA 3.4 grams daily have been used (7202).
For weight loss, a daily serving of 2-7 ounces of fish containing approximately 3.65 grams omega-3 fatty acids (0.66 gram from EPA and 0.60 gram from DHA) has been used (2049).
For slowing weight loss in patients with cancer, 7.5 grams fish oils providing EPA 4.7 grams and DHA 2.8 grams daily have been used (11979).
For improving dark vision adaptation in dyslexic individuals, fish oils providing DHA 480 mg daily have been used (5708).
For improving movement disorders in children with dyspraxia, fish oils providing DHA 480 mg combined with 35 mg arachidonic acid and 96 mg gamma-alpha linoleic acid from evening primrose oil, 24 mg thyme oil, and 80 mg vitamin E (Efalex) have been used (5708).
For treatment of depression along with conventional antidepressants, fish oils 9.6 grams per day have been used (10871).
For decreasing the frequency of vein graft occlusion after coronary bypass grafting, 4 grams of fish oil per day containing EPA 2.04 grams and DHA 1.3 grams has been used (2314).
For preventing restenosis after percutaneous transluminal coronary angioplasty (PTCA), 6 grams daily of fish oil starting one month before PTCA and continuing one month after PTCA, followed by 3 grams of fish oil daily thereafter for six months, has been used (8680).
For reducing and preventing the long-term continuous rise in blood pressure and to preserve renal function after heart transplantation, 4 grams daily of fish oils (46.5% EPA and 37.8% DHA) has been used (8687).
For preventing thrombosis after placement of a hemodialysis graft, 6 grams of fish oils has been used daily (8684).
For preserving renal function in patients with severe IgA nephropathy, 4-8 grams daily of fish oil has been used (8686,8711).
For combined hypertriglyceridemia and hypercholesterolemia, fish oils providing EPA 1800-2160 mg and DHA 1200-1440 mg combined with garlic powder 900-1200 mg daily has been used to lower total cholesterol, LDL, triglycerides, and the ratios of total cholesterol to HDL, and LDL to HDL (2318,2319).
For preventing muscle soreness after physical exercise, fish oil 1.8 grams per day has been used (8524).
Fish oil supplements often contain small amounts of vitamin E as an antioxidant to prevent spoilage. They might also be combined with calcium, iron, or vitamins A, B1, B2, B3, C, or D. Fish that are good sources of omega-3 fatty acids, including mackerel, tuna, salmon, sturgeon, mullet, bluefish, anchovy, sardines, herring, trout, and menhaden, provide about 1 gram of omega-3 fatty acids per 3.5 ounces of fish.
INTRAVENOUS: For chronic plaque psoriasis, a daily 200 mL intravenous dose of parenteral fish oil-based lipid emulsion (Omegavenous), containing 4.2 grams EPA and 4.2 grams DHA, has been used for 14 days (1004). For acute, extended guttate psoriasis, a daily intravenous dose of a parenteral fish oil product, containing 2.1 grams EPA and 21 grams DHA, has been used for 10 days (1034).

Comments

Fish oils come from a variety of marine life including mackerel, herring, tuna, halibut, salmon cod liver, whale blubber, and seal blubber. Products that are commercially available contain varying amounts and ratios of docosahexaenoic acid (DHA) and eicosapentaenoic acid (EPA).

FLAXSEED

Also Known As

Atasi, Flax Seed, Graine De Lin, Leinsamen, Lini Semen, Linseed, Lint Bells, Linum, Phytoestrogen, Winterlien.
CAUTION: See separate listings for Alpha Linolenic Acid, Conjugated Linoleic Acid (CLA), Decosahexaenoic Acid (DHA), Eicosapentaenoic Acid (EPA), Fish Oils, and Flaxseed Oil.

Scientific Names

Linum usitatissimum, synonyms Linum crepitans, Linum humile.
Family: Linaceae.

People Use This For

Orally, flaxseed is used for chronic constipation, colon damage due to laxative abuse, diverticulitis, irritable bowel syndrome (IBS) or irritable colon, gastritis, and enteritis. It is also used for menopausal symptoms, bladder inflammation, hypercholesterolemia, hypertriglyceridemia, atherosclerosis, protection against cancer, osteoporosis, attention deficit-hyperactivity disorder (ADHD), and systemic lupus erythematosus (SLE) nephritis.
Topically, flaxseed is used as a poultice for skin inflammation.
Ophthalmically, flaxseed is used for the removal of foreign bodies from the eye.

Safety

LIKELY SAFE ...when used orally and appropriately (5899,6800,6802,6803,6808,8020). Flaxseed is well tolerated when taken with sufficient fluid. Tell patients to consume at least 150 mL of liquid for every 10 grams of whole or cracked flaxseed (12).
PREGNANCY AND LACTATION: Insufficient reliable information available.

Effectiveness

LIKELY EFFECTIVE

Constipation. Taking flaxseed orally as a bulk forming laxative is effective for relieving constipation (6803).

Hypercholesterolemia. Various flaxseed preparations, including raw, ground, partially defatted, and flaxseed bread and muffins seem to significantly reduce total cholesterol and low-density lipoprotein (LDL) cholesterol in people with normal cholesterol levels (5899,6803) and in people with hypercholesterolemia (6800,6808). Preparations providing flaxseed 40 to 50 grams per day seem to reduce total cholesterol by 5-9% and LDL cholesterol by 8-18% (5899,6800,6803,6808,10952), but flaxseed doesn't seem to have much effect on LDL in hypercholesteremic postmenopausal women (10952,10978). However, flaxseed does not affect high-density lipoprotein (HDL) cholesterol. Apolipoprotein A-1 and apolipoprotein B, which are indicators of the risk for coronary heart disease, may be decreased by 6 and 7.5%, respectively (10952). Most flaxseed preparations also do not affect triglyceride levels, but partially defatted flaxseed (flaxseed without as much alpha-linolenic acid content) can increase triglycerides by approximately 10% (6808).

POSSIBLY EFFECTIVE

Menopausal symptoms. Taking flaxseed orally 40 grams per day seems to be similar to hormone therapy for improving mild menopausal symptoms (10978). Whether flaxseed is effective for moderate to severe menopausal symptoms is unknown.

Systemic lupus erythematosus (SLE) nephritis. Taking flaxseed orally seems to improve renal function in people with systemic lupus erythematosus (SLE) nephritis. There is evidence that daily use of flaxseed can lower serum creatinine (6802,8021).

POSSIBLY INEFFECTIVE

Osteoporosis. Taking flaxseed orally doesn't seem to prevent osteoporosis in postmenopausal women. Flaxseed 40 grams per day doesn't seem to affect markers of bone metabolism (10952).

There is insufficient reliable information available about the effectiveness of flaxseed for its other uses.

Mechanism of Action

Flaxseed is a bulk-forming fibrous product that stimulates intestinal peristalsis, producing a laxative effect (18). The soluble fiber in flaxseed is found primarily in the seed coat gum, which is a mixture of polysaccharides including glucuronic acids, rhamnose, arabinose, xylose, and galactose (6808). Ten grams of flaxseed typically provides approximately 44 kilocalories energy, 2 grams protein, 4 grams fat and 4 grams dietary fiber (6801). Flaxseed is a rich source of alpha-linolenic acid and long-chain n-3 polyunsaturated fatty acids. Supplementation with flaxseed significantly increases n-3 polyunsaturated fatty acids in plasma and erythrocytes (5899,6803). Flaxseed is used for atherosclerosis because it can reduce platelet aggregation and serum cholesterol and thereby might lower atherogenic risks (6,6808). In animal models, flaxseed supplementation seems to significantly reduce the risk of developing aortic atherosclerosis (6806,6807). The fiber content of flaxseed is thought to be important for flaxseed's lipid lowering effects. High fiber diets increase fecal elimination of bile acids, which increases primary bile acid synthesis (6800,6808). The alpha-linolenic acid content of flaxseed might also help lower serum cholesterol (6800). However, because partially defatted flaxseed also seems to lower cholesterol, other mechanisms are likely involved (6807,6808).

Alpha-linolenic acid may also be involved in the beneficial effects on platelets (6800).
Flaxseed might also have hypoglycemic effects. The postprandial glucose response to a 50 gram carbohydrate load given as flaxseed bread is 27% lower compared with regular white bread (5899). Flaxseed also seems to lower insulin levels in postmenopausal women (10978).
Flaxseed is also the most abundant indirect food source of lignans (5897,8026). Secoisolariciresinol diglycoside (SDG), a major lignan precursor, is found in high concentrations in flaxseed. SDG is converted by bacteria in the colon to the lignans enterolactone and enterodiol, which undergo enterohepatic circulation and then are excreted in the urine as glucuronide conjugates (5897,8022,8023,9592). The lignan precursor content of flaxseed can vary significantly depending on growing location and harvest year (5897). Serum concentrations and urinary excretion of lignans can increase in variable amounts when people consume large amounts of flaxseed and other lignan-containing foods (5894,6801,6803,8026). Lignans might have some beneficial effects. Lignans have weak estrogenic effects and possibly anti-estrogenic effects. There is preliminary evidence that flaxseed supplementation may decrease cellular proliferation in mammary glands (8022,8867,9593). Inhibition of mammary tumor growth by the lignans enterolactone and enterodiol has been reported in vitro (5895,8867). Preliminary evidence shows enterolactone and estradiol inhibit each other's proliferative effect on estrogen-dependent breast cancer cells. This competition might reduce endogenous estrogen binding to estrogen receptors, resulting in an anti-estrogen effect (8868,9593). Lignans have also been shown to stimulate sex hormone binding globulin production in the liver, and inhibit aromatase enzyme activity in preadipose cells. These effects may inhibit growth of hormone-dependent cancer cells such as breast cancer cells (6801,8024,9591,9592). In postmenopausal women, the urinary excretion of enterolactone and enterodiol seems to be lower in women with breast cancer than in women without breast cancer (8025,9592,9593). Supplementation with flaxseed also increases urinary excretion of certain estrogen metabolites, especially 2-hydroxyestrogen. This metabolite has been hypothesized to confer protective effects against breast cancer in premenopausal and postmenopausal women since it has little estrogenic activity and may even have antiestrogenic activity (5893,8020). There is preliminary evidence that flaxseed may also reduce insulin-like growth factor I (IGF-I) plasma level concentrations, a factor associated with increased breast cancer risk (8023).
Flaxseed and the constituent secoisolariciresinol diglycoside have also been reported to be protective against chemical-induced carcinogenesis in animal models (5897). Preliminary evidence shows secoisolariciresinol diglycoside seems to be effective against new tumor development and alpha-linolenic acid seems to be effective in reducing growth of established tumors (6805). Alpha-linolenic acid also seems to suppress the production of interleukin-1 (IL-1), tumor necrosis factor (TNF) and leukotriene B4, and production of oxygen free radicals by polymorphonuclear (PMN) leukocytes and monocytes (6806). Although both alpha-linolenic acid and lignans constituents have been reported to have antioxidant effects (6806), there is some evidence that partially defatted flaxseed might actually have pro-oxidant activity (6808). There is some evidence lignans may have platelet activating factor (PAF) receptor antagonist effects (6802,6806), stimulate production of sex-hormone binding globulin in the liver (6801), and inhibit angiogenesis (6803). Inhibition of colon tumor growth by the lignans enterolactone and enterodiol has also been reported in vitro (5895).
For systemic lupus erythematosus (SLE), flaxseed is thought to improve renal function by decreasing blood viscosity, reducing serum cholesterol, and reducing inflammatory response (6802).
Preliminary evidence suggests that flaxseed constituents such as alpha-linolenic acid and lignans might have a beneficial effect on bone, but thus far, clinical evidence does not support this (8504,10952).
Flaxseed also contains cyanogenic glycosides (linustatin, neolinustatin, and linamarin), which can increase blood levels and urinary excretion of thiocyanate in humans consuming raw flaxseed, and can cause toxicity in grazing animals (5899); however, these glycosides have not been detected after flaxseed is baked in muffins (5899).

Adverse Reactions

Orally, flaxseed can significantly increase the number of bowel movements and the risk for diarrhea (6803,8021). Doses greater than 45 grams per day may not be tolerated for this reason (6802). For every 10 grams of whole or cracked flaxseed, 150 mL or greater of liquid should be consumed to prevent intestinal blockage (12). Occasionally, allergic and anaphylactic reactions have been reported after ingestion of flaxseed and flaxseed oil. Individuals handling and processing flax products can develop a positive antigen test to flaxseed and may be more likely to be hypersensitive (6,6809).

Interactions with Herbs & Other Dietary Supplements

None known.

Interactions with Drugs

ANTICOAGULANT/ANTIPLATELET DRUGS: There is some evidence that flaxseed oil can decrease platelet aggregation and increase bleeding time (5898). Theoretically, using flaxseed oil in combination with anticoagulant or antiplatelet drugs might have additive effects and increase the risk of bleeding. Some of these drugs include aspirin, clopidogrel (Plavix), dalteparin (Fragmin), enoxaparin (Lovenox), heparin, ticlopidine (Ticlid), warfarin (Coumadin), and others.
ANTIDIABETES DRUGS: Flaxseed can lower blood glucose levels (5899,10978) and might have additive effects when used with antidiabetes drugs. This might increase the risk of hypoglycemia in some patients. Monitor blood glucose levels closely. Some antidiabetes drugs include glimepiride (Amaryl), glyburide (DiaBeta, Glynase PresTab,

Micronase), insulin, metformin (Glucophage), pioglitazone (Actos), rosiglitazone (Avandia), and others.
ORAL DRUGS: The fiber in flaxseed can impair absorption of oral drugs (19).

Interactions with Foods

None known.

Interactions with Lab Tests

CHOLESTEROL: Flaxseed can lower total serum cholesterol and low-density lipoprotein cholesterol levels, and test results (5899,6800,6803).
GLUCOSE: Flaxseed might lower blood glucose concentrations (5899,10978).
TRIGLYCERIDES: Partially defatted flaxseed (flaxseed without as much alpha-linolenic acid content) can increase triglyceride levels, and test results (6808).

Interactions with Diseases or Conditions

BLEEDING DISORDERS: There is some evidence that flaxseed can decrease platelet aggregation and increase bleeding time (5898). Theoretically, flaxseed might increase the risk of severe bleeding in patients with bleeding disorders; use with caution.
DIABETES: Flaxseed can lower blood glucose levels and might have additive effects when used with antidiabetes drugs (5899,10978). This might increase the risk of hypoglycemia in some patients. Monitor blood glucose levels closely.
GASTROINTESTINAL OBSTRUCTION: People with bowel obstruction, esophageal stricture, and acute intestinal inflammation should avoid flaxseed. Flaxseed is a bulk forming laxative and might further contribute to obstruction (12).
HORMONE SENSITIVE CANCERS/CONDITIONS: Because flaxseed might have estrogenic effects (5893,8020), women with hormone sensitive conditions should avoid flaxseed. Some of these conditions include breast, uterine, and ovarian cancer; endometriosis; and uterine fibroids.
HYPERTRIGLYCERIDEMIA: Partially defatted flaxseed (flaxseed with less alpha linolenic acid content) might increase triglyceride levels (6808) and should be avoided in patients with hypertriglyceridemia.

Dosage and Administration

ORAL: For hypercholesterolemia, baked goods such as muffins containing flaxseed have been used to provide a daily dose of 50 grams of flaxseed per day (6803,6808). For improving renal function in patients with systemic lupus erythematosus (SLE) nephritis, 15 grams of ground flaxseed has been used twice daily with cereal, or tomato or orange juice (8021). For improving mild menopausal symptoms, 40 grams of crushed flaxseed daily has been used (10978).

FLAXSEED OIL

Also Known As

Atasi, Flax Oil, Flax Seed Oil, Graine De Lin, Linoleic Acid, Linseed Oil.
CAUTION: See separate listings for Alpha Linolenic Acid (ALA), Conjugated Linoleic Acid (CLA), Decosahexaenoic Acid (DHA), Eicosapentaenoic Acid (EPA), Evening Primrose Oil (EPO), Fish Oils, and Flaxseed.

Scientific Names

Linum usitatissimum, synonyms Linum crepitans, Linum humile.
Family: Linaceae.

People Use This For

Orally, flaxseed oil is used as a laxative for constipation, for arthritis, cancer, anxiety, benign prostatic hyperplasia (BPH), vaginitis, weight loss, hypertriglyceridemia, hypercholesterolemia, dry eyes, and to prevent heart attacks. Flaxseed oil is also used as a supplemental source of dietary alpha-linolenic acid.
Topically, flaxseed oil is used for its demulcent and emollient properties.
In foods, flaxseed oil is used as a cooking oil and in margarines.
In manufacturing, flaxseed oil is used as a component in paints, varnishes, linoleum, and soap; and as a waterproofing agent.

Safety

LIKELY SAFE ...when used orally in amounts found in foods.
POSSIBLY SAFE ...when used orally and appropriately for medicinal purposes, short-term. Flaxseed oil has been used safely in studies lasting up to 3 months (845,3912,5898).
There is insufficient reliable information available about the safety of topical use of flaxseed oil.
PREGNANCY: LIKELY SAFE ...when used orally in amounts found in foods. LIKELY UNSAFE ...when used

orally in medicinal amounts. Flaxseed oil might affect menstruation (19); contraindicated.
LACTATION: LIKELY SAFE ...when used orally in amounts found in foods. There is insufficient reliable information available about the safety of flaxseed oil in breast-feeding women when used in medicinal amounts; avoid using.

Effectiveness

POSSIBLY INEFFECTIVE

Rheumatoid arthritis (RA). Taking flaxseed oil daily for 3 months does not seem to improve symptoms of pain and stiffness, and has no effect on laboratory measures of RA, such as C-reactive protein and erythrocyte sedimentation rate (ESR) (5898).

There is insufficient reliable information available about the effectiveness of flaxseed oil for its other uses.

Mechanism of Action

Flaxseed oil contains linolenic, linoleic, and oleic acids (6). It is among the best sources of alpha-linolenic acid (6). Linoleic acid and alpha-linolenic acid are required for the structural integrity of all cell membranes. Alpha-linolenic acid raises serum omega-3 polyunsaturated fatty acids, including eicosapentaenoic acid (EPA) and docosahexaenoic acid (DHA) (845,6803).
There is some evidence that flaxseed oil can lower triglyceride levels (3911). Flaxseed oil seems to have other potentially beneficial cardiovascular effects. There is also some preliminary evidence that a low fat diet plus the flaxseed oil can increase systemic arterial elasticity, which might improve circulatory function (5896).
Some researchers think flaxseed oil can also decrease platelet aggregation (845,6806), and increase the bleeding time (5898), but data are conflicting (3912). Higher serum levels of linoleic acid, an omega-6 fatty acid contained in flaxseed oil, seems to protect against ischemic stroke and lacunar infarction, possibly by lowering blood pressure and improving blood flow by reducing platelet aggregation and enhancing erythrocyte deformability (9562).
Flaxseed oil is used for rheumatoid arthritis because it might have anti-inflammatory effects. Alpha-linolenic acid contained in flaxseed oil is a precursor of eicosapentaenoic acid (EPA) and docosahexaenoic acid (DHA) which are converted to non- or anti-inflammatory prostaglandins and leukotrienes in the body. Supplementation with flaxseed oil or alpha-linolenic acid increases the ratio of EPA and DHA to the pro-inflammatory arachidonic acid (5898). Alpha-linolenic acid has also been reported to suppress the production of interleukin-1 (IL-1), tumor necrosis factor (TNF), leukotriene B4, and oxygen free radicals by polymorphonuclear (PMN) leukocytes and monocytes (6806).
There is some evidence that alpha-linolenic acid from flaxseed oil might have anti-tumor effects, possibly by increasing peroxidation of fatty acids in tumor cell membranes, or by altering the balance of prostaglandin production away from tumor promoting prostaglandins of the E2 series (6805). Flaxseed oil seems to reduce the volume of chemically-induced mammary tumors in animal models (6805).

Adverse Reactions

Orally, flaxseed oil is typically well-tolerated. However, doses of flaxseed oil of 30 grams per day and higher have been associated with loose stools and diarrhea (5898). Allergic and anaphylactic reactions have been reported with flaxseed oil ingestion and also in workers processing flaxseed products (6809).

Interactions with Herbs & Other Dietary Supplements

None known.

Interactions with Drugs

ANTICOAGULANT/ANTIPLATELET DRUGS: There is some evidence that flaxseed oil can decrease platelet aggregation and increase bleeding time (5898). Theoretically, using flaxseed oil in combination with anticoagulant or antiplatelet drugs might have additive effects and increase the risk of bleeding. Some of these drugs include aspirin, clopidogrel (Plavix), dalteparin (Fragmin), enoxaparin (Lovenox), heparin, ticlopidine (Ticlid), warfarin (Coumadin), and others.

Interactions with Foods

None known.

Interactions with Lab Tests

PROTHROMBIN TIME (PT): Flaxseed oil may affect platelet aggregation and prolong bleeding time and test results (5898).
TRIGLYCERIDES: Flaxseed oil might decrease serum triglyceride concentrations and test results in some patients with hyperlipoproteinemia (3911).

Interactions with Diseases or Conditions

BLEEDING DISORDERS: There is some evidence that flaxseed oil can decrease platelet aggregation and increase bleeding time (5898). Theoretically, flaxseed oil might increase the risk of severe bleeding in patients with bleeding disorders; use with caution.

Dosage and Administration

ORAL: A typical dose is 15-30 mL daily (3912).
TOPICAL: No typical dosage.

Comments

Specific deficiencies from inadequate intakes of essential fatty acids are rare except in individuals with severe, untreated fat malabsorption or those suffering from famine. Symptoms include dry, cracked, scaly and bleeding skin, excessive water loss from the skin, and impaired liver function resulting from the accumulation of lipid in the liver (i.e. fatty liver) (298).

FLUORIDE

Also Known As

Acidulated Phosphate Fluoride, Fluorophosphate, Hydrogen Fluoride, Monofluorophosphate, MFP, Sodium Fluoride, Sodium Monofluorophosphate, Stannous Fluoride.

Scientific Names

F; atomic number 9.

People Use This For

Orally, fluoride is used for treating osteoporosis and preventing dental caries. It is also used orally to prevent bone loss in people with rheumatoid arthritis and Crohn's disease.
Topically, fluoride is used for preventing dental caries.

Safety

LIKELY SAFE ...when used orally and appropriately. Fluoride is safe when used in doses below the tolerable upper intake level (UL) of 10 mg per day of elemental fluoride (7555). ...when used topically and appropriately. Fluoride is safe when used in quantities typically found in toothpastes, mouth rinses, and professionally applied fluoride dental treatments (8950).
POSSIBLY SAFE ...when used orally in higher doses of up to 20 mg per day of elemental fluoride. Monofluorophosphate containing 20 mg elemental fluoride taken daily has been used safely for up to 4 years (9124,9125). Sustained release sodium fluoride 11.3 mg containing elemental fluoride has been used safely for 42 weeks using a 12 months on, 3 months off cyclic regimen (9103).
POSSIBLY UNSAFE ...when used orally in high doses, long term. Doses greater than 20 mg elemental fluoride for 9 months are associated with increased risk of fractures (8949). Long-term exposure to high doses above the daily upper intake level (UL) of 10 mg for greater than 10 years can cause skeletal fluorosis (7555).
CHILDREN: LIKELY SAFE ...when used orally and appropriately. Fluoride is safe when used in doses below the tolerable upper intake level (UL) of 10 mg per day of elemental fluoride for children age 8 years and older, 2.2 mg per day for children 4 to 8 years, 1.3 mg per day for children 1 to 3 years, 0.9 mg for infants 7 through 12 months, and 0.7 mg for infants 6 months and younger (7555). ...when used topically and appropriately. Fluoride is safe in quantities typically found in toothpastes, mouth rinses, and professionally applied fluoride dental treatments (8950,9100). POSSIBLY UNSAFE ...when used orally in high doses, long term. Long-term exposure for greater than ten years to high doses above the daily upper intake level (UL) can cause skeletal fluorosis (7555).
PREGNANCY AND LACTATION: LIKELY SAFE ...when used orally and appropriately. Fluoride is safe when used in doses below the tolerable upper intake level (UL) of 10 mg per day of elemental fluoride (7555). ...when used topically and appropriately. Fluoride is safe in quantities typically found in toothpastes, mouth rinses, and professionally applied fluoride dental treatments (8950). POSSIBLY UNSAFE ...when used orally at high doses above the daily upper intake level (UL) of 10 mg for prolonged periods. Long-term exposure to high doses can cause skeletal fluorosis, but pregnancy or lactation doesn't seem to affect susceptibility to skeletal fluorosis (7555).

Effectiveness

EFFECTIVE

Dental caries. Fluoride added to drinking water and fluoride in toothpastes, mouthwashes, and other dental products can reduce dental caries (tooth decay) (7555,8950,9102,9128).

POSSIBLY EFFECTIVE

Osteoporosis. Elemental fluoride taken orally in daily doses, 11.3 mg to 20 mg, continuously or cyclicly might increase bone mineral density. Monofluorophosphate containing 20 mg elemental fluoride taken daily on a continuous basis for 96 weeks by postmenopausal women with osteopenia appears to increase spinal bone mineral density by 2.4%. In combination with hormone replacement therapy, monofluorophosphate may increase spinal bone mineral density by 11.8% (9125). In postmenopausal women with osteoporosis, monofluorophosphate containing 20 mg elemental fluoride taken daily for 4 years seems to increase spinal bone mineral density by 10% (9124). Monofluorophosphate containing 15 mg elemental fluoride taken daily on a cyclical basis (three months on, one month off) for 3 years by men with osteoporosis seems to spinal bone mineral density by 9% (8948). The effect on fractures is less clear. Sustained-release sodium fluoride 25 mg daily (equivalent to 11.3 mg elemental fluoride) given cyclicly for 12 months on followed by 2 months off for 42 months seems to reduce the risk for vertebral fracture by 32% in postmenopausal women with osteoporosis (9103). In postmenopausal women with osteoporosis, monofluorophosphate appears to reduce the risk of vertebral fracture from 10% in women taking only calcium to 2.4% in women taking fluoride plus calcium (9124). In men with osteoporosis, fluoride treatment seems to reduce the risk of vertebral fracture by 30% and also to reduce back pain (8948). Other studies have found no effect on fractures (9132,9133). Studies have generally been small and have used various fluoride preparations including sodium fluoride, enteric-coated sodium fluoride, sustained-release sodium fluoride, and sodium monofluorophosphate (8948,8949,9103,9124,9125,9129,9132,9133). Some researchers suggest that staring fluoride early in the course of osteoarthritis and treating with 20 mg per day along with 800 to 1000 mg per day of calcium for at least 3 years is necessary for efficacy (9162). Long-term (20 years) exposure to fluorinated water seems to reduce the risk of hip fracture in older women by 31% and the risk of vertebral fracture by 27% (9102).

INSUFFICIENT RELIABLE EVIDENCE to RATE

Crohn's disease. Preliminary clinical evidence suggests fluoride might increase vertebral bone mass in Crohn's disease patients who have low bone mass (9134).

Rheumatoid arthritis (RA). Preliminary clinical evidence suggests fluoride might increase vertebral bone mass in RA patients who have low bone mass (9130).

More evidence is needed to rate fluoride for these uses.

Mechanism of Action

Fluoride is the ionic form of fluorine, a halogen and the most electronegative of the elements on the periodic table. Fluoride combines reversibly with hydrogen to form hydrogen fluoride. Diffusion of hydrogen fluoride accounts for much of its physiological behavior, including absorption from the stomach, distribution between extra- and intracellular-fluid compartments, and renal clearance (7555). Fluoride has a high affinity for calcium; more than 99% of calcium in the body is in calcified tissue.

Fluoride exerts a cariostatic (decay preventing) effect on the teeth by interfering with metabolism of bacteria in dental plaque and preserving tooth enamel. The fluoride concentration in plaque is dependent on exposure to fluoride concentrations in water, beverages, foods, and dental products, and the frequency of their use. Plaque is affected by topical exposure to fluoride and as well as fluoride secreted in saliva and gingival crevicular fluid after oral ingestion. Fluoride protects dental enamel by inhibiting bacterial enzymes that produce acid in plaque. It also reduces acid solubility of enamel, promotes remineralization of early enamel lesions, and prevents demineralization of plaque (7555).

Unlike most other drugs used for osteoporosis which prevent bone resorption, fluoride stimulates osteoblast activity. Fluoride has been used on and off again for over 30 years as a treatment for osteoporosis. Although fluoride increases bone mineral density (BMD), there is a corresponding decrease in elasticity and strength of bone. Fluoride is also thought to alter the crystalline structure of bone (9129).

Preliminary evidence suggests that fluoride can inhibit the calcification of soft tissues, including the aorta. This suggests that adequate fluoridation of the water supply might reduce the risk of ischemic heart disease, but more research is needed (7555).

Most fluoride in the diet comes from fluorinated water, beverages, and dental products, but some foods and beverages such as marine fish and tea contain significant amounts of fluorine. Up to 80% of ingested fluoride is absorbed from gastrointestinal tract. Elimination is almost entirely via the kidneys with a variable degree of tubular resorption, depending on urinary pH (7555).

Adverse Reactions

Orally, fluoride can cause gastric pain and nausea, and lower extremity pain, particularly with long term use (9129). Enteric-coated and sustained-release dosage forms of sodium phosphate and sodium monofluorophosphate may cause fewer adverse effects than plain sodium fluoride (9127,9129). Adverse effects appear to be dose related. Daily doses of 40 to 65 mg sodium fluoride can cause nausea, vomiting, GI bleeding, and stress fractures (15,9127). Fluoride at high doses for prolonged periods, over 10 mg per day for 10 or more years, can cause skeletal fluorosis. Skeletal fluorosis is characterized by joint stiffness and pain initially, followed by crippling due to calcification of ligaments, osteosclerosis, muscle wasting, and neurological defects due to hypercalcification of the vertebra. Crippling skeletal fluorosis is extremely rare in the US (7555).

Fluoride can cause enamel fluorosis, a condition in which the teeth of children who ingest excessive amounts of fluoride during development of permanent teeth may be discolored and pitted. This is a cosmetic adverse effect; tooth enamel may be stronger and more resistant to caries with enamel fluorosis (7555).

Fluoride can cause allergic reactions including urticaria, exfoliative dermatitis, atopic dermatitis, stomatitis, and gastrointestinal allergic reactions. Respiratory allergic reactions occur rarely (15).

Interactions with Herbs & Other Dietary Supplements

CALCIUM: Calcium can decrease the bioavailability of fluoride. Calcium can form insoluble compounds with fluoride and reduce absorption by 10 to 25% (7555).

Interactions with Drugs

None known.

Interactions with Foods

INFANT FORMULA: Infant formula rich in calcium and other divalent or trivalent ions can form insoluble compounds and reduce fluoride bioavailability by up to 25% (7555,9161).
MILK, CALCIUM-RICH FOODS: Foods rich in calcium can decrease the bioavailability of fluoride by up to 25% (7555,9161).

Interactions with Lab Tests

None known.

Interactions with Diseases or Conditions

None known.

Dosage and Administration

ORAL: In the US, municipal water is fluorinated to a concentration of 0.7 to 1.2 parts per million (ppm) (8950). To prevent dental caries in areas where the fluoride ion level in drinking water is less than 0.3 ppm (such as in well water), children 6 months to 3 years should receive a fluoride supplement of 0.25 mg per day; children 3 to 6 years, 0.5 mg per day; and children 6 to 16 years, 1 mg per day. For children living in areas where the fluoride level is 0.3 to 0.6 ppm, children 3 to 6 years should receive 0.25 mg per day, and children 6 to 16 years, 0.5 mg per day. No supplement is needed in areas where the fluoride in drinking water exceeds 0.6 ppm (9101).
For treating osteoporosis, 15 to 20 mg per day of elemental fluoride has been used (8948,8949,9103,9125).
The daily Adequate Intakes (AI) for elemental fluoride from all sources including drinking water are: infants birth through 6 months, 0.01 mg; babies age 7 through 12 months, 0.5 mg; children 1 through 3 years, 0.7 mg; 4 through 8 years, 1 mg; 9 through 13 years, 2 mg; 14 through 18 years, 3 mg; men 19 years and older, 4 mg; women 14 years and older, including those pregnant or lactating, 3 mg.
The daily upper intake levels (UL) for fluoride are 0.7 mg for infants birth through 6 months; 0.9 mg for infants 7 through 12 months; 1.3 mg for children 1 through 3 years; 2.2 mg for children 4 through 8 years and 10 mg for children older than 8 years, adults, and pregnant and lactating women (7555).
Sodium fluoride contains 45% elemental fluoride. Monofluorophosphate contains 19% elemental fluoride (8948,8949).

Comments

Currently, the FDA requires this warning on all fluoride toothpastes: "If you accidentally swallow more than used for brushing, seek professional help or contact a poison control center." The warning is intended to reduce the risk of dental fluorosis, in which light spots form on developing permanent teeth. However, fluorosis is develops with extended use, rather than following a single dose, causing some experts to question this warning (7555,9100).
Toothpaste and fluoride rinses should not be routinely swallowed, particularly by children. Recommend limiting use of toothpaste to a pea-sized amount for children under six in case of accidental swallowing (9100).

FO-TI

Also Known As

Chinese Cornbind, Chinese Knotweed, Climbing Knotweed, Flowery Knotweed, Fo Ti, Fo-Ti-Tient, Foti, He Shou Wu, He-Shou-Wu, Heshouwu, Ho Shou Wu, Ho-Shou-Wu, Hoshouwu, Multiflora Preparata, Polygonum, Radix Polygoni Multiflori, Radix Polygoni Shen Min, Shen Min, Shou Wu, Shou-Wu, Shouwu, Shou-Wu-Pian, Zhihe Shou Wu, Zhihe-Shou-Wu, Zhiheshouwu, Zi Shou Wu, Zi-Shou-Wu, Zishouwu.

Scientific Names

Polygonum multiflorum.
Family: Polygonaceae.

People Use This For

Orally, fo-ti is used for treating lymph node tuberculosis, cancer, and constipation. It is also used orally as a liver and kidney tonic; as a blood and vital essence toner; and to fortify muscles, tendons, and bones. Fo-ti is also used orally for hyperlipidemia, insomnia, limb numbness, lower back and knee soreness or weakness, premature graying, and dizziness with tinnitus.
Topically, fo-ti is used for sores, carbuncles, skin eruptions, and itching.
In manufacturing, fo-ti extract is used as an ingredient in hair and skin care products.

Safety

POSSIBLY UNSAFE ...when used orally. Fo-ti may cause hepatitis in some patients (7626,7627). There is insufficient reliable information available about the topical use of fo-ti.

PREGNANCY: POSSIBLY UNSAFE ...when used orally. Fo-ti contains anthraquinone constituents, which can exert a stimulant laxative effect. Bulk-forming or emollient laxatives are preferred in pregnancy (272). There is insufficient reliable information available about the topical use of fo-ti during pregnancy.

LACTATION: POSSIBLY UNSAFE ...when used orally. Anthraquinone constituents can cross into breast milk and might cause loose stools in some breast-fed infants (272). There is insufficient reliable information available about the topical use of fo-ti while nursing.

Effectiveness

There is insufficient reliable information available about the effectiveness of fo-ti.

Mechanism of Action

The applicable part of fo-ti is the rhizome. Fo-ti is either used raw (uncured) or processed (cured) by repeated steaming and sun drying. Raw fo-ti root contains the anthraquinone derivatives, chrysophanol and emodin, along with a small amount of rhein. These constituents have stimulant laxative effects, which probably accounts for fo-ti's use in constipation. Curing fo-ti reduces these constituents by 42-96% (5). Some evidence suggests that isolated stilbene glycoside constituents in the raw fo-ti root might have liver protectant effects, including inhibition of alanine aminotransferase (ALT, formerly SGOT) and aspartate aminotransferase (AST) (11). However, the anthraquinones in fo-ti are converted to highly reactive anthrones in the gastrointestinal tract, which may cause hepatitis (7626,7627). Fo-ti reportedly has hypoglycemic effects (5,19). Cured fo-ti shows evidence it might increase the levels of superoxide dismutase (SOD), serotonin, norepinephrine, dopamine, and decrease levels of monoamine oxidase-B (MAO-B), lipid peroxide, and malonyl dialdehyde (MDA) (11); these are believed to be markers for anti-aging effects. Some evidence suggests fo-ti might also increase serum ceruloplasmin levels, reduce thymus gland atrophy, and inhibit atrophy of adrenal glands; enhancing nonspecific and cellular immunity, and antagonizing the immunosuppressive effects of prednisolone or hydrocortisone (11). Other evidence suggests the alcoholic extract might increase high-density lipoprotein (HDL) cholesterol, reduce total cholesterol, free cholesterol, triglycerides, and retard atherosclerosis (11). The aqueous extract appears to inhibit the replication of hepatitis B (11). Some evidence suggests fo-ti has approximately 0.3% of the estrogen activity of 17-beta-estradiol itself and is approximately equivalent to the estrogen activity found in soy and red clover (10143).

Adverse Reactions

Orally, fo-ti, particularly the raw root, may cause catharsis, diarrhea, abdominal pain, nausea, and vomiting (12). There is some concern that fo-ti can cause hepatitis in some patients. There have been 2 cases of hepatitis occurring 2 weeks after starting fo-ti in the usual recommended doses. It was characterized by symptoms including jaundice, dark urine, malaise, and increased liver function tests (LFT). The symptoms and increased LFTs resolved within a month after discontinuing fo-ti (7626,7627).

Interactions with Herbs & Other Dietary Supplements

None known.

Interactions with Drugs

ANTIDIABETES DRUGS: Theoretically, concomitant use of fo-ti with antidiabetic agents might increase the risk of hypoglycemia. Fo-ti reportedly has hypoglycemic effects (5,19). Dosing adjustments for insulin or oral hypoglycemic agents may be necessary. Oral hypoglycemic drugs include glimepiride (Amaryl), glipizide (Glucotrol), glyburide (Diabeta, Micronase), tolazamide (Tolinase), tolbutamide (Orinase), and others. Monitor blood glucose levels closely.

DIGOXIN (Lanoxin): Theoretically, overuse of anthraquinone laxatives (e.g., fo-ti) might increase the risk of hypokalemia and digoxin cardiotoxicity (151,272).

DIURETIC DRUGS: Overuse of fo-ti might compound diuretic-induced potassium loss (151,272). There is some concern that people taking fo-ti along with potassium depleting diuretics might have an increased risk for hypokalemia. Initiation of potassium supplementation or an increase in potassium supplement dose may be necessary for some patients. Some diuretics that can deplete potassium include chlorothiazide (Diuril), chlorthalidone (Thalitone), furosemide (Lasix), hydrochlorothiazide (HCTZ, HydroDIURIL, Microzide), and others.

STIMULANT LAXATIVES: Theoretically, concomitant use of fo-ti with other laxatives can increase the risk of fluid and electrolyte depletion (151,272).

Interactions with Foods

None known.

Interactions with Lab Tests

CHOLESTEROL: Theoretically, cured fo-ti might reduce serum total cholesterol concentrations and test results (11).
COLORIMETRIC TESTS: Fo-ti might discolor urine (pink, red, purple, orange, rust), interfering with diagnostic tests that depend on a color change, due to its anthraquinone content (11,275).
GLUCOSE: Theoretically, fo-ti might decrease blood glucose concentrations and test results (5,6,19).
POTASSIUM: Excessive use of fo-ti might cause hypokalemia, reducing serum potassium concentrations and test results due to its anthraquinone content (11).
TRIGLYCERIDES: Theoretically, cured fo-ti might reduce serum triglyceride concentrations and test results (11).

Interactions with Diseases or Conditions

GASTROINTESTINAL DISEASE: Fo-ti exerts a stimulant effect on the intestinal tract (5). Avoid its use in diarrhea, intestinal obstruction, acute intestinal inflammation (Crohn's disease, ulcerative colitis, appendicitis), ulcer, abdominal pain of unknown origin, nausea, and vomiting.
HEART CONDITIONS: Theoretically, the laxative effect of fo-ti might cause hypokalemia with overuse/misuse, potentially decreasing cardiac function (15).
LIVER DISEASE: Fo-ti should be avoided in patients with a history of liver disease, because it has been associated with hepatitis in isolated cases (7626,7627).

Dosage and Administration

No typical dosage.

Comments

Avoid confusion with the commercial product Fo-ti-Teng which contains no fo-ti (6).

FOLIC ACID

Also Known As

B Complex Vitamin, Folacin, Folate, Vitamin B9.

Scientific Names

Pteroylglutamic acid; Pteroylmonoglutamic acid; Pteroylpolyglutamate.

People Use This For

Orally, folic acid is used for preventing and treating folate deficiency, megaloblastic anemia resulting from folate or vitamin B12 deficiency, megaloblastic anemia in sickle cell disease, and for folate deficiency in intestinal malabsorption or sprue. It is also used for preventing neural tube defects, reducing the risk of colorectal cancer, and preventing pregnancy loss. Folic acid is also used for hyperhomocysteinemia, coronary artery disease, fragile-X syndrome, gingival hyperplasia, memory deficit, Alzheimer's disease, vitiligo, osteoporosis, restless leg syndrome, insomnia, depression, peripheral neuropathy, myelopathy, and AIDS. It is also used for reducing lometrexol and methotrexate toxicity; and for preventing signs of aging, heart attack, and stroke. Folic acid is also used for other conditions commonly associated with folate deficiency, including ulcerative colitis; liver disease; alcoholism; renal dialysis; and drug-induced deficiency related to phenytoin, primidone, barbiturates, oral contraceptives, and nitrofurantoin.
Topically, folic acid is used for treating gingival hyperplasia and gingivitis.
Parenterally, folic acid is used intramuscularly, subcutaneously, or intravenously for treating folate deficiency, particularly in patients with malabsorption or those who cannot take oral treatment. Folic acid has also been used parenterally to treat chronic fatigue syndrome.

Safety

LIKELY SAFE ...when used orally or parenterally and appropriately. Folic acid is safe when used in doses less than 1000 mcg per day (6241). In cases of megaloblastic anemia resulting from folate deficiency or malabsorption disorders such as sprue, oral doses of 1-5 mg per day can also be used safely until hematologic recovery is documented if vitamin B12 levels are routinely measured (6241,7725,8739).
POSSIBLY UNSAFE ...when used orally in large doses. Doses above 1000 mcg per day should be avoided if possible to prevent precipitation or exacerbation of neuropathy related to vitamin B12 deficiency (6241,6242,6245). However, there is some evidence that doses of 5 mg per day orally for up to 4 months can be used safely if vitamin B12 levels are routinely measured (7725). Very high doses of 15 mg per day can cause significant central nervous system (CNS) and gastrointestinal side effects (505).
PREGNANCY AND LACTATION: LIKELY SAFE ...when used orally and appropriately. Folic acid 300-400 mcg is commonly used during pregnancy for prevention of neural tube defects (8739).

Effectiveness

EFFECTIVE

Folate deficiency. Administering folic acid orally or parenterally improves folate deficiency (505,8739).

LIKELY EFFECTIVE

End-stage renal disease (ESRD). Taking folic acid orally reduces homocysteine levels in people with ESRD, including those on hemodialysis. Over 85% of people with ESRD have hyperhomocysteinemia. Treatment of hyperhomocysteinemia in people with ESRD is often more difficult than in people with normal renal function (1489,3324,7289,9409,9413,9414,9416). The reasons for this aren't fully understood; renal uptake and metabolism of homocysteine may be reduced in severe renal failure, and hemodialysis may contribute to vitamin deficiencies (6884,9414,9417). Doses of 0.8 to 15 mg folic acid/day are generally used, but the degree of homocysteine reduction is very variable (between 12-50%), and normal homocysteine levels (<12 micromoles/L) cannot always be achieved (1489,6884,7289,7881,9322,9413,9414,9415,9416). Folic acid 2.5 to 5 mg three times weekly also reduces homocysteine levels in ESRD patients on dialysis (9417). Doses greater than 15 mg per day don't provide additional benefit. Doses of 30 to 60 mg seem to cause a rebound in homocysteine levels when treatment is stopped (9219). Folic acid supplementation also doesn't appear to improve endothelial function, suggesting folic acid does not prevent or treat vascular disease in patients with ESRD (9322). In most studies vitamin B12 (0.4 to 1 mg/day) and pyridoxine (20 to 50 mg/day) were taken with the folic acid (3324,6884,7881,9414,9415,9416). As in people with normal renal function, vitamin B12 probably has an additional homocysteine-lowering effect over folic acid alone, especially in people with low vitamin B12 levels (7289), and pyridoxine helps reduce post-methionine load homocysteine levels (1489).

Hyperhomocysteinemia. Taking folic acid orally 0.4 to 5 mg/day lowers fasting homocysteine levels by about 20-30% in people with normal renal function (3047,6366,9307,9400,9401,9405,9408,9409,9410,10350,11337,11338). However, 0.8-1 mg/day seems to provide maximal reduction of homocysteine levels (9307,9408). Doses greater than 1 mg/day do not seem to produce any greater benefit (2147,9307,9410), except in some people with certain gene mutations that cause homocysteine levels of 20 micromoles/L or higher (9408). In people with asymptomatic atherosclerosis, lowering homocysteine levels with folic acid reduces progression of the atherosclerosis and improves arterial blood flow (412,3886,3887,6236,7725). In patients with high coronary risk or atherosclerotic disease, there is preliminary evidence that 10 mg per day of folic acid for 2 months improves coagulation status, oxidative stress, and endothelial dysfunction (9319). The effects of folic acid increase with increasing pretreatment of homocysteine levels, and decreasing pretreatment of folate levels (2149,9400,9405,9409). Taking folic acid orally also seems to reduce increased homocysteine concentrations associated with nitrous oxide general anesthesia. A supplement containing 25 mg pyridoxine, with 2.5 mg of folic acid and 500 mcg of vitamin B12, taken daily was used (9481). Additional evidence suggests that the higher the initial homocysteine levels, the lower the folic acid dose needed to attain maximum reduction of homocysteine levels (9307). However, some reduction in the fasting homocysteine levels is seen when dietary folate and supplemental folic acid (including multivitamins) are increased in people who are not folate deficient and have normal homocysteine levels (<12 micromoles/L) (412,2146,2147,9302,9303,9304,9305,9306,9401). Increasing folic acid intake by supplements or folate-fortified cereal products is more effective for reducing homocysteine levels than increasing intake of folate-rich foods (6367). However, initial data suggest that the US Government-mandated fortification of cereals and flour with 140 mcg folic acid per 100 grams is reducing the mean homocysteine level in the general population by about 7% (7881,9404,9407). Consumption of at least 300 mcg per day of dietary folate seems to be associated with a 20% lower risk of stroke and a 13% lower risk of cardiovascular disease when compared with consumption of less than 136 mcg of folate per day (9318). Taking folic acid orally, in combination with pyridoxine, seems to reduce post-prandial hyperhomocysteinemia (indicated by elevated homocysteine levels after consuming a methionine load). Folic acid 0.5 to 5 mg/day alone reduces homocysteine levels by 27-30%, but addition of pyridoxine (50 to 250 mg/day) produces greater reductions and is generally recommended (1489,9406,9408). Adding vitamin B12 (mean dose, 0.5 mg/day) to folic acid therapy produces an additional decrease in homocysteine levels of about 7% on average (9400,9405,9409), but probably only in people with vitamin B12 deficiency (2147,3047). Some people recommend routine use of vitamin B12 in homocysteine-lowering regimens, to avoid the risk of neuropathy in people with undetected vitamin B12 deficiency (9405). Adding pyridoxine (vitamin B6) to the regimen doesn't produce any additional lowering of fasting homocysteine levels (2148,3047,9405). Elevated homocysteine levels are an independent risk factor for vascular disease. But elevated homocysteine levels may be a marker instead of a cause of vascular disease (11387,11388). Although folic acid lowers homocysteine levels, it's not yet known whether this reduces the risk of vascular disease (cardiac, peripheral, or cerebral). Preliminary data suggest it might. Large-scale clinical trials are currently underway to determine whether homocysteine-lowering therapy is of any benefit (9306,9308). However, folic acid supplementation alone or in combination with pyridoxine and vitamin B12 doesn't seem to help with secondary prevention of death or cardiovascular events such as stroke or myocardial infarction in people with existing coronary artery disease or prior stroke (11337,11387). There is also conflicting evidence that suggests supplemental folic acid might improve endothelial function, prevent nitric oxide synthase dysfunction induced by continuous nitroglycerin, and nitrate tolerance in patients with hyperhomocysteinemia (9313,9314,9315,9316). Large randomized controlled trials are needed to confirm or refute these findings. Until definitive data are available, the current recommendation is screening of 40 year old men and 50 year old women for hyperhomocysteinemia. For patients with homocysteine levels greater than 11 micromoles/L, supplement with folic acid and vitamin B12 (9308).

Methotrexate toxicity. Taking folic acid orally seems to reduce methotrexate toxicity symptoms such as nausea and vomiting in the treatment of rheumatoid arthritis (RA) and psoriasis (768,2162,2163,2164,4492,4493,4494,9369,9419).

Neural tube birth defects. Consuming a high dietary intake of folate and taking folic acid supplements orally reduces the risk of neural tube birth defects (3325,9309). High dietary intake of vegetables during pregnancy improves plasma and red blood cell folate concentrations and reduces the risk of folate deficiency (9309).

POSSIBLY EFFECTIVE

Breast cancer. Consuming dietary folate seems to decrease the risk of breast cancer, especially in women who also consume high amounts of dietary methionine, vitamin B12, or pyridoxine (vitamin B6) (9328).

Colorectal cancer. Taking folic acid orally from dietary and supplemental sources seems to reduce the risk of colon cancer (505,2140,2141,2142,2143,2144,2145,2250,9325,9326). Dietary intake of folate greater than 249 mcg per day in men and 400 mcg per day in women is associated with a reduced risk of colon cancer, especially in women with a family history of the disease (9325,9326). There is also evidence daily use of folic acid-containing multivitamins for greater than 5 years can decrease the risk of colon cancer by almost 50% in women with a family history of colon cancer (9326).

Depression. Taking folic acid orally with conventional antidepressants might improve treatment response (3657,10884,10887). However, limited clinical research suggests that folic acid is not effective as a replacement for conventional antidepressant therapy (10886).

Pancreatic cancer. Consuming greater than 280 mcg per day of dietary folate is associated with a decreased risk of exocrine pancreatic cancer (9327).

Phenytoin-induced gingival hyperplasia. Applying folic acid topically seems to inhibit gingival hyperplasia secondary to phenytoin therapy (2151). However, taking folic acid orally doesn't seem to improve gingival hyperplasia secondary to phenytoin therapy (2150,2151,2152).

Pregnancy-related gingivitis. Applying folic acid topically seems to improve gingivitis in pregnancy (2152).

Vitiligo. Taking folic acid orally seems to improve symptoms of vitiligo (2153,2154).

POSSIBLY INEFFECTIVE

Chronic fatigue syndrome (CFS). Daily injections of a combination of folic acid, bovine liver extract, and vitamin B12 for three weeks appear to have no effect on CFS symptoms (7561).

Coronary artery disease. Taking folic acid orally doesn't seem to be useful for secondary prevention in people with existing coronary artery disease. Supplementation with 0.5 mg folic acid daily, in addition to statin therapy, doesn't seem to affect risk for death or cardiovascular events such as stroke or myocardial infarction in people with existing CAD (11337).

Lometrexol toxicity. Taking folic acid orally doesn't seem to reduce lometrexol toxicity (2161).

Stroke. Taking folic acid orally doesn't seem to be useful for preventing stroke recurrence. In people with a history of stroke, neither high dose folic acid combinations containing 25 mg of pyridoxine, 0.4 mg of vitamin B12, and 2.5 mg of folic acid nor low dose combinations containing 200 mcg of pyridoxine, 6 mcg of vitamin B12, and 20 mcg of folic acid seem to affect risk of recurring stroke (11387).

LIKELY INEFFECTIVE

Fragile-X syndrome. Taking folic acid orally doesn't improve symptoms of fragile-X syndrome (2155,2156,2157,2158,2159,2160).

INSUFFICIENT RELIABLE EVIDENCE to RATE

Angioplasty. There are conflicting findings about the benefits of taking folic acid plus vitamin B6 and vitamin B12 following angioplasty. Some evidence suggests that folic acid 1 mg plus vitamin B12 400 mcg and pyridoxine 10 mg daily can decrease the rate of restenosis in patients treated with balloon angioplasty (8009,9412). But this combination does not seem to be as effective for reducing restenosis in patients after coronary stenting (8009). An intravenous loading dose of folic acid, vitamin B6, and vitamin B12 followed by oral administration of folic acid 1.2 mg plus vitamin B6 48 mg and vitamin B12 60 mcg taken daily after coronary stenting also does not seem to reduce restenosis and might actually increase restenosis (12150,12151). Due to the lack of evidence of benefit and potential for harm, this combination of vitamins should not be recommended for patients receiving coronary stents (12151).

Fenofibrate (Tricor)-associated hyperhomocysteinemia. There is some evidence 10 mg of folic acid taken every other day might reduce elevated plasma homocysteine levels (up to 59%) associated with fenofibrate (Tricor) administration (9321).

Infertility. Some research suggests that daily consumption of folic acid 5 mg plus zinc sulfate 66 mg can increase sperm count in subfertile men. Further study is required to determine the effect of this combination on infertility (9334).

Lung cancer. There does not appear to be a relationship between deficiency of folic acid and lung cancer (9454).

Restless leg syndrome. There are reports of folic acid reducing symptoms associated with restless leg syndrome such as numbness, cramps, and paresthesias. Whether restless leg syndrome is due to acquired or familial folate deficiency is unknown and requires further study (9332).

Sickle cell disease. Daily intake of 700 mcg of folic acid in combination with 4.2-6 mcg of vitamin B12 and 4.2-6.0 mg of pyridoxine (vitamin B6) might lower homocysteine levels, but it is unknown if this effect will reduce the risk of endothelial damage in patients with sickle cell disease (9324).

Ulcerative colitis-associated cancer. Preliminary clinical evidence suggests folate supplementation might protect against cancer in people with ulcerative colitis (6271). More evidence is needed to rate folic acid for these uses.

Mechanism of Action

Folate is the general term that refers to a variety of chemical forms folic acid. Folic acid, or pteroylmonoglutamic acid, is the form used in vitamin supplements and fortified foods. Folate in food is pteroylpolyglutamate, which has a polyglutamate side chain with peptide linkages (6241). Folic acid is distributed in a wide variety of foods, but it is most abundant in green leafy vegetables (9518).

Folate in food is about 40-50% less bioavailable than synthetic folic acid, which is almost 100% bioavailable. Before folate from food can be absorbed, the polyglutamate side chain must undergo enzymatic deconjugation in the small intestine to form the absorbable monoglutamate form (6241,9300). Folate deconjugation occurs maximally at a pH of 6-7 (6241,9300). After folic acid is absorbed, it is reduced to tetrahydrofolate and then enters a methylation cycle (9317).

In humans, tetrahydrofolate-based coenzymes play a major role in intracellular metabolism. Tetrahydrofolate plays an indirect role in the rate-limiting step of DNA synthesis. Abnormalities in this process that occur with folic acid deficiency can cause megaloblastic anemia. Folic acid reduces damage to DNA and prevents replication errors (2139,2144). Folic acid deficiency disturbs cell cycling, induces cell apoptosis, and increases the rate of cell death (9329).

In the bone marrow, abnormal cellular maturation and division caused by folic acid deficiency leads to the development of abnormal red blood cell precursors, which are known as megaloblasts. Megaloblasts are unable to mature into red blood cells properly and many of them are phagocytosed by macrophages in the bone marrow, which contributes to the development of megaloblastic anemia (9518).

Folic acid is also involved in the metabolism of homocysteine. Low folate levels are associated with increased plasma homocysteine levels. Hyperhomocysteinemia is a risk factor for coronary, cerebral, and peripheral atherosclerosis; recurrent thromboembolism; deep vein thrombosis; myocardial infarction; and ischemic stroke (1899,2147,3047,3323,9402,9405,9408,9409). Low serum folate levels (less than 9.9 nmol/L) and low dietary folate intake (less than 211 mcg per day) are also associated with an increased risk for acute coronary events and cardiovascular disease mortality (9311,9312). A 5 micromole increase in plasma homocysteine increases the risk of cerebrovascular disease by 50%, and the risk of coronary heart disease by 60% in men and 80% women (9407,9411). The best predictor of response to folic acid therapy is the baseline homocysteine plasma concentration. The higher the homocysteine level, the better the response is to folic acid therapy. Folic acid has little effect on normal homocysteine levels. Genetic variations in the enzyme 5,10-methylenetetrahydrofolate reductase can influence the effectiveness of folate in reducing homocysteine levels (9219). The mechanisms of the adverse effects of homocysteine isn't fully understood, but might include vascular endothelial cell damage, impaired endothelium dependent vasodilation due to reduced nitric oxide activity, arterial stiffening due to increased oxidation and arterial deposition of low-density lipoproteins (LDL), increased platelet adhesiveness, and activation of the clotting cascade (2147,3047,9310,9403,9408).

Homocysteine is metabolized via two pathways: remethylation or trans-sulfuration. Remethylation of homocysteine to methionine requires folate and vitamin B12 as cofactors (3047,9310,9320,9407,9409). The methyl donor is 5-methyltetrahydrofolate, and the enzymes involved are 5,10-methyltetrahydrofolate reductase (MTHFR), and 5-methyltetrahydrofolate-homocysteine-methyltransferase, which is vitamin B12-dependent (2148,9310). Impairment of this pathway leads to increased fasting homocysteine levels, and can occur in people with folate deficiency, vitamin B12 deficiency, or who are homozygous for the mutations of the gene for MTHFR (TT genotype) (1489,9301,9315,9409). Mutation of the MTHFR gene produces a variant of the enzyme that is thermolabile, less active, and it impairs the formation of 5-methyltetrahydrofolate (9301,9320). Folic acid supplements increase the activity of this pathway, which lowers homocysteine levels (412,2146,2147,2148,2149,3886,9301). Trans-sulfuration of homocysteine results in degradation to cystathionine and then to cysteine by the pyridoxine (vitamin B6) dependent enzymes cystathionine-beta-synthase and cystathionine-gamma-synthase (2148,3047,9310,9407,9409). This pathway is primarily active after ingesting a methionine load (animal protein). Deficiencies of pyridoxine or cystathionine-beta-synthase impair this pathway, raising post-methionine load homocysteine levels (1489,2148,9408). Elevation of these levels is a risk factor for cardiovascular disease, independent of elevated fasting homocysteine levels (1489).

Folic acid might also improve endothelial dysfunction and the coagulation and oxidative status in individuals with high coronary risk and atherosclerotic disease. There is preliminary evidence folic acid can decrease concentrations of von Willebrand factor, which is associated with endothelial dysfunction. Folic acid might also decrease fibrinogen concentrations, while increasing plasminogen, antithrombin III, glutathione peroxidase, red cell glutathione, and red cell superoxide dismutase concentrations (9319).

Folic acid might also prevent nitroglycerin-induced nitrate tolerance and cross tolerance to endothelial nitric oxide. Nitrate tolerance is associated with an increased vascular production of superoxide anions by NADPH oxidase and endothelial nitric oxide synthase. Folic acid is thought to deplete NADPH and decrease the activity of these enzymes (9317).

Folic acid also plays an important role in pregnancy. Low folate levels are associated with recurrent spontaneous pregnancy loss (6237). Folic acid supplementation also prevents neural tube defects in the fetus, but the exact role of folic acid in this process is not completely understood.

Folic acid might play a role in Alzheimer's disease. Preliminary evidence indicates that low folate concentrations might be related to atrophy of the cerebral cortex, particularly in people with neocortical lesions related to Alzheimer's disease (6234). Homocysteine is thought to be neurotoxic, causing DNA damage and cell apoptosis (9331). Low serum folate levels are strongly correlated with cerebral atrophy on autopsy (6234). Functional and mental deterioration is also sometimes associated with low folate levels and low intake of folate in elderly people (6238,9330).

Folic acid deficiency is common among people with depression (10879,10880,10881). Low folate levels have been linked to poor response to antidepressant treatment (6239,10880). In the general population, people with low folate status or

lower dietary folate intake have a higher risk for depression (10882,10883). The exact role of folic acid in depression is unknown. It is required for the remethylation of homocysteine to methionine and for s-adenosylmethionine (SAMe) conversion (5232). Folate is also required for the methylation of tetrahydrobiopterin, an essential cofactor for the hydroxylase enzymes involved in the production of neurotransmitters such as serotonin (10884,10885).
Some patients with chronic fatigue syndrome (CFS) also have decreased folic acid levels (6082,6083), so some people try folic acid supplements for chronic fatigue.
Crohn's disease has also been associated with decreased folate levels (6269). Folic acid is thought to prevent carcinogenesis. Folate and methionine are important factors in the methylation of DNA. There is evidence that folate deficiency might cause massive misincorporation of uracil into DNA and increased chromosomal breaks (9325,9236,9327,9328). Low red blood cell folate levels have been associated with the development of dysplasia and cancer in ulcerative colitis (6270).

Adverse Reactions

Orally, folic acid is well tolerated in amounts found in fortified foods and supplements in doses less than 1000 mcg per day (6243). Doses of 5 mg per day can cause abdominal cramps, diarrhea, and rash (7225). Folic acid 15 mg per day can sometimes cause altered sleep patterns, vivid dreaming, irritability, excitability, overactivity, confusion, impaired judgment, exacerbation of seizure frequency and psychotic behavior, nausea, abdominal distention, flatulence, bitter taste in the mouth, allergic skin reactions, and zinc depletion (15). Large doses of folic acid can also precipitate or exacerbate neuropathy in people deficient in vitamin B12 (6243).
Allergic reactions only rarely occur. Symptoms can include rash, erythema, itching, malaise, and bronchospasm. An anaphylactic reaction has been reported in one patient receiving intravenous folic acid. Use of folic acid for undiagnosed anemia has masked the symptoms of pernicious anemia, resulting in lack of treatment and eventual neurological damage (15). Patients should be warned not to self-treat suspected anemia.

Interactions with Herbs & Other Dietary Supplements

None known.

Interactions with Drugs

FOSPHENYTOIN (Cerebyx): Folic acid may be a cofactor in phenytoin metabolism (4471). Folic acid, in doses of 1 mg per day or more, can reduce serum levels of phenytoin in some patients (4471,4477,4531,4536). Increases in seizure frequency have been reported. If folic acid supplements are added to established phenytoin therapy, monitor serum phenytoin levels closely. If phenytoin and folic acid are started at the same time and continued together, adverse changes in phenytoin pharmacokinetics are avoided (4471,4472,4473,4531). Note that phenytoin also reduces serum folate levels.
METHOTREXATE (MTX, Rheumatrex): Methotrexate exerts its cytotoxic effects by preventing conversion of folic acid to the active form needed by cells. There is some evidence that folic acid supplements reduce the efficacy of methotrexate in the treatment of acute lymphoblastic leukemia, and theoretically they could reduce its efficacy in the treatment of other cancers (9420). Advise cancer patients to consult their oncologist before using folic acid supplements. In patients treated with long-term, low-dose methotrexate for rheumatoid arthritis (RA) or psoriasis, folic acid supplements can reduce the incidence of side effects, without reducing efficacy (768,2162,4492,4493,4494,4546,9369). Note that methotrexate can reduce serum folate levels.
PHENOBARBITAL (Luminal): Folic acid can have direct convulsant activity in some people, reversing the effects of phenobarbital and worsening seizure control (4427,9357,9358). Monitor closely for increased seizure activity. Note that phenobarbital also reduces serum folate levels.
PHENYTOIN (Dilantin): Folic acid may be a cofactor in phenytoin metabolism (4471). Folic acid, in doses of 1 mg per day or more, can reduce serum levels of phenytoin in some patients (4471,4477,4531,4536). Increases in seizure frequency have been reported. If folic acid supplements are added to established phenytoin therapy, monitor serum phenytoin levels closely. If phenytoin and folic acid are started at the same time and continued together, adverse changes in phenytoin pharmacokinetics are avoided (4471,4472,4473,4531). Note that phenytoin also reduces serum folate levels.
PRIMIDONE (Mysoline): Folic acid can have direct convulsant activity in some people, reversing the effects of primidone and worsening seizure control (4427,9357,9358). Monitor closely for increased seizure activity. Note that primidone also reduces serum folate levels.
PYRIMETHAMINE (Daraprim): Folic acid can antagonize the antiparasitic effects of pyrimethamine against Toxoplasmosis and Pneumocystis carinii pneumonia. Folic acid doesn't antagonize the effects of pyrimethamine in the treatment of malaria, because malarial parasites cannot use exogenous folic acid. Use folinic acid as an alternative to folic acid when indicated (9380). Note that pyrimethamine also reduces serum folate levels.

Drug Influences on Nutrient Levels and Depletion

SOME DRUGS CAN AFFECT FOLIC ACID LEVELS:
AMINOSALICYLIC ACID (para-aminosalicylic acid, PAS, Paser): Aminosalicylic acid can reduce dietary folate absorption, worsening the folate deficiency often seen with active tuberculosis, or preventing its reversal during treatment (9363,9388,9395,9396,9397). Megaloblastic anemia occurs rarely, and usually when there are other contributing factors such as concurrent vitamin B12 malabsorption (4559). Advise patients being treated for

tuberculosis to take folic acid supplements if their dietary folate intake is low.
ANTACIDS: Folic acid absorption in the small intestine is optimal at pH 5.5 to 6 (8441). Chronic use of large doses of antacids can reduce folic acid absorption, but this is likely only significant if dietary folate intake is very low (2677,8441). Advise patients to maintain the recommended daily intake of folic acid in their diet.
ANTIBIOTICS: Antibiotic therapy can disrupt the normal gastrointestinal (GI) flora, interfering with enterohepatic recirculation (reabsorption) of folic acid (4436). The normal GI flora also synthesizes and consumes folic acid, which may also be disrupted by antibiotics (2677,4437,6243). The contribution of bacterially synthesized is uncertain. Folic acid synthesized by GI bacteria can be absorbed in the large intestine, but the amount synthesized and absorbed is variable (4437,6243). For instance, it can depend on dietary fiber intake and gastric pH; hypochlorhydria causes bacterial overgrowth and increased folate synthesis (4437,9364). In most people it's unlikely that a course of antibiotics will reduce folic acid levels significantly, and therefore supplements are unnecessary.
ASPIRIN: Aspirin may decrease serum folate levels by reducing the amount bound to plasma proteins, especially when large doses are taken regularly (e.g., for treatment of rheumatoid arthritis, RA). But there doesn't seem to be an increase in urinary folate losses and red blood cell levels are normal (9351,9360). This suggests folate is just being redistributed in the body and deficiency isn't likely.
CARBAMAZEPINE (Tegretol): Carbamazepine can reduce serum folate levels, but megaloblastic anemia has not been reported (4426,4427,4428,4429,9359). Reduced folate levels might contribute to mild, asymptomatic reductions in nerve conduction velocities, and mental changes seen with carbamazepine (4427,4429). Possible mechanisms include reduced folic acid absorption, and increased metabolism by induced hepatic enzymes (4426,4428,4429). Pregnant women taking carbamazepine may be especially at risk from reduced folate levels (9355). Low folate levels during pregnancy may contribute to birth defects and pregnancy loss (9355,9356). However, folic acid supplements have worsened seizure control in some people with epilepsy (4427). Advise patients taking carbamazepine chronically to consult their physician before starting folic acid supplements.
CHOLESTYRAMINE (Questran): Cholestyramine reduces folic acid absorption. It can lower serum and red blood cell folate levels in children taking large doses (0.2 to 1.1 grams/kg/day) for several months (4455). There aren't any reports of deficiency in adults. Encourage patients to maintain a good dietary intake of folic acid.
COLESTIPOL (Colestid): Colestipol can interfere with absorption of folic acid, and reduced serum folate levels may occur (4461). Encourage patients to maintain a good dietary intake of folic acid.
CYCLOSERINE (Seromycin Pulvules): Cycloserine can reduce serum folate levels, rare cases of megaloblastic anemia have occurred (4531,4536,9363). The mechanism is uncertain, but may involve absorption and metabolism of folate (4531,4536). Advise patients receiving long-term treatment to maintain a good dietary intake of folic acid.
DIURETICS: Limited data suggests these drugs may increase excretion of folic acid. Reduced red blood cell folate levels, possibly contributing to increased homocysteine levels, a risk factor for cardiovascular disease, were found in one group of people taking diuretics for six months or longer (1898). The need for folic acid supplementation during diuretic therapy hasn't been adequately studied. Advise patients to maintain a good dietary intake of folic acid.
ESTROGENS: Reduced serum and red blood cell folate levels can occur in some women taking conjugated estrogens (Premarin) or oral contraceptives, but this is unlikely in women with adequate dietary folate intake (4459,4498,7843,7844,9371,9373). There are rare reports of megaloblastic anemia associated with oral contraceptive use, usually in women with other conditions contributing to folate deficiency (9371,9372). Possible mechanisms by which estrogens contribute to folate deficiency include reduced absorption of dietary folate, increased excretion, induction of liver enzymes which use folate, and increased protein binding of folate in serum (4459,9371). There is some evidence that oral contraceptives can increase the rate of progression of cervical dysplasia to cervical cancer, and that folic acid can slow or reverse this dysplasia (9352,9370). Advise women taking oral contraceptives or other estrogens to maintain a good dietary intake of folate. Recommend supplements only for those women with inadequate dietary intake or other conditions that contribute to folate deficiency (4459,9371,9373), and for those diagnosed with, or at increased risk for, cervical dysplasia (e.g., due to family history).
H2 BLOCKERS: Folic acid absorption from the small intestine is optimal at pH 5.5 to 6 (8441). The increased pH associated with use of H2 blockers may therefore reduce folic acid absorption, but this is probably only significant if dietary folate intake is very low (4483,8441). Advise patients to maintain the recommended daily dietary intake of folic acid. The H2 blockers include cimetidine (Tagamet), ranitidine (Zantac), nizatidine (Axid), and famotidine (Pepcid).
METFORMIN (Glucophage): Reduced vitamin B12 and, to a lesser extent, folate levels occur in some people with diabetes and can contribute to hyperhomocysteinemia, which adds to their already increased risk of cardiovascular disease (32,4490,9366,9367). The reduced folate levels seen in diabetics have been linked to metformin use in some cases, possibly as a result of reduced folic acid absorption (32,9367,9368). Symptomatic folate deficiency is unlikely to occur with metformin, but people with diabetes may need folic acid supplements to reduce hyperhomocysteinemia (9367).
METHOTREXATE: Methotrexate is a folate antagonist which prevents conversion of folic acid to its active form, and lowers plasma and red blood cell folate levels (4492,4493,4494,4546). In patients treated with long-term, low-dose methotrexate for rheumatoid arthritis (RA) or psoriasis development of folate deficiency is associated with increased risk of certain side effects. These include gastrointestinal effects, stomatitis, alopecia, abnormal liver function tests, myelosuppression, megaloblastic anemia, and increased homocysteine levels (768,4492,4493,4494,4546). Folic acid supplements (1 to 5 mg/day) reduce these side effects without reducing the efficacy of methotrexate in treating RA or psoriasis (768,2162,4492,4493,4494,9369,9418). Advise patients taking methotrexate for these conditions to take a folic acid supplement (1 mg/day is probably sufficient), especially if their dietary folate intake is low and they are experiencing the side effects described (4494,4546,9369,9419). It's likely that people who have experienced side effects

will need to continue taking folic acid for the duration of methotrexate therapy (9418). Advise patients being treated with methotrexate for cancer to avoid folic acid supplements, unless recommended by their oncologist. Folic acid could interfere with the anticancer effects of methotrexate (9420).

METHYLPREDNISOLONE: Reduced serum folate levels were noted in people with multiple sclerosis (MS) after treatment with methylprednisolone sodium succinate (Solu-Medrol) 1 gram daily for 10 days. The clinical significance of this change isn't known (9362).

NONSTEROIDAL ANTI-INFLAMMATORY DRUGS (NSAIDs): Folate-dependent enzymes are inhibited in vitro by NSAIDs with carboxylic acid-containing side chains (e.g., ibuprofen [Advil, Motrin], naproxen [Anaprox, Aleve], indomethacin [Indocin], and sulindac [Clinoril]). The clinical significance of this isn't clear (2677,9361).

PANCREATIC ENZYMES, PANCRELIPASE, PANCREATIN: Reduced folate levels can occur in some people taking pancreatic extracts. This may be due to reduced absorption, since folate can form insoluble complexes with pancreatic extracts (9374). Advise patients to have their folate levels checked if they take pancreatic enzymes for prolonged periods, and to take a supplement if the level is low. These drugs include Pancrease, Cotazym, Viokase, Creon, Ultrase, and others.

PENTAMIDINE: Pentamidine is a weak folate antagonist which prevents conversion of folic acid to its active form, although this isn't thought to contribute significantly to its antiprotozoal activity (9378). Decreased serum folate levels and megaloblastic bone marrow changes can occur rarely with prolonged parenteral pentamidine therapy (9378). Most patients are unlikely to need folic acid supplements. These drugs include Pentacarinat, and Pentam 300.

PHENOBARBITAL (Luminal), PRIMIDONE (Mysoline): These drugs can reduce serum folate levels, occasionally leading to megaloblastic anemia (usually in people with low dietary folate intake), and possibly contributing to neurological side effects, mental changes, and cerebral atrophy (4427,4530,4536,9333,9357,9358,9359). Possible mechanisms include reduced folic acid absorption, increased metabolism, increased demand for folic acid as a coenzyme for induced hepatic enzymes, or competitive interaction between folate coenzymes and phenobarbital (9357). Pregnant women taking phenobarbital or primidone may be especially at risk from reduced folate levels (9354,9355). Low folate levels during pregnancy may contribute to birth defects and pregnancy loss (9355,9356). Folic acid therapy seems to reverse these neurological effects (9333). However, folic acid can worsen seizure control. Advise patients taking phenobarbital or primidone chronically to consult their physician before taking folic acid supplements.

PHENYTOIN (Dilantin), FOSPHENYTOIN (Cerebyx): Phenytoin can reduce serum folate levels, occasionally leading to megaloblastic anemia, and possibly contributing to neurological side effects and mental changes (4427,4536,9357,9358,9359). Possible mechanisms include reduced folic acid absorption, increased metabolism, increased demand for folic acid as a coenzyme for induced hepatic enzymes, or competitive interaction between folate coenzymes and phenytoin (9357). Folic acid supplements may reduce phenytoin side effects (4471,4477). Pregnant women taking phenytoin may be especially at risk from reduced folate levels (9354,9355). Low folate levels during pregnancy may contribute to birth defects and pregnancy loss (9355,9356). However, folic acid can reduce phenytoin serum levels and increase seizure frequency. Advise patients taking phenytoin chronically to consult their physician before taking folic acid supplements.

PROTON PUMP INHIBITORS (PPIs): Folic acid absorption in the small intestine is optimal at pH 5.5 to 6 (8441). The increased pH associated with use of PPIs could theoretically reduce folic acid absorption (8441), but preliminary data suggests use of PPIs for several years doesn't cause folate deficiency (4483). Advise patients to maintain the recommended dietary intake of folic acid. PPIs include omeprazole (Prilosec), lansoprazole (Prevacid), rabeprazole (Aciphex), pantoprazole (Protonix), and esomeprazole (Nexium).

PYRIMETHAMINE (Daraprim): Pyrimethamine is a folate antagonist that prevents conversion of folic acid to its active form (4425,4532). At high doses used to treat toxoplasmosis (50 to 75 mg/day), megaloblastic anemia may occur due to deficiency of active folate, and it's recommended that all patients receive folinic acid (leucovorin calcium, Wellcovorin, an active form of folic acid) to prevent this (4532). Folinic acid doesn't antagonize the therapeutic effect of pyrimethamine because Toxoplasma does not have a membrane transport system for exogenous folinic acid (9380). Advise patients to avoid folic acid supplements since they can antagonize the therapeutic effect of pyrimethamine against Toxoplasma and Pneumocystis carinii. Advise patients taking lower doses of pyrimethamine for prolonged periods to maintain the recommended dietary folate intake. Monitor for folate deficiency.

SULFASALAZINE (Azulfidine): Sulfasalazine competitively inhibits absorption of folic acid in the intestine (2677,4515,4560,9353). It also interferes with the breakdown of dietary folate to its absorbable form, and can cause hemolysis, which increases folate requirements for formation of new red blood cells (4515,4560). Long-term sulfasalazine therapy can cause reduced serum and red blood cell folate levels and hyperhomocysteinemia, which is a risk factor for cardiovascular disease (4515,9377). Occasionally, megaloblastic anemia develops, usually with higher doses of sulfasalazine (e.g., >2 grams/day), and when there are other factors contributing to folate deficiency (4515,4516,4517,4536,9376,9377). Reduced folate levels are often found in people with severe chronic ulcerative colitis, due both to the disease and sulfasalazine therapy. Reduced folate levels might contribute to the increased risk of colon cancer and its precursor, colonic mucosal dysplasia, seen in people with ulcerative colitis. Preliminary evidence suggests that folate supplements can reduce this risk (9379). Advise patients on chronic sulfasalazine therapy to increase their dietary folate intake, and to take a supplement if they have any other condition which could also contribute to deficiency (2677,9353,9379).

TRIAMTERENE (Dyrenium): Triamterene is a folate antagonist that prevents conversion of folic acid to its active form, and also reduces folate absorption (4425,4536,4537,9375). Reduced serum and red blood cell folate levels have occurred, and occasional cases of megaloblastic anemia, usually in people with other conditions contributing to folate deficiency (4537,9375). Advise patients on chronic triamterene therapy to maintain the recommended dietary folate intake, or to take a supplement if this is not possible.

TRIMETHOPRIM (Trimpex): Trimethoprim, including trimethoprim contained in the combination antibiotic trimethoprim/sulfamethoxazole (TMP/SMX, co-trimoxazole, Bactrim, Septra), inhibits the enzyme involved in conversion of folic acid to its active form (4468,4531). The bacterial and protozoal enzymes are 1000 to 10,000 times more sensitive to trimethoprim than human enzymes (2677,4468,9382). Therefore, low doses of trimethoprim (e.g., 100 to 200 mg/day, 10 mg/kg/day) don't affect human enzymes and symptoms of folate deficiency aren't seen (9381,9383,9394). However, at high doses, trimethoprim inhibits the enzyme in human bone marrow and megaloblastic anemia can occur in people taking 1 gram or more daily (20 mg/kg/day) for 2 to 4 weeks, or 500 mg daily for several months (4468,9383,9384). The risk is higher if the person has other conditions contributing to folate deficiency or megaloblastic anemia (9382,9394). Its generally agreed that if megaloblastic anemia occurs, trimethoprim should be stopped and treatment with folinic acid (an active form of folic acid) should be given (9382). This can be followed by treatment with folic acid if necessary, once the activating enzymes have had time to recover from the effects of trimethoprim (9382). Whether folic acid or folinic acid can be given concurrently with trimethoprim to prevent megaloblastic anemia is controversial. The practice may not be effective, especially in people with AIDS in whom immunologic reactions, as well as folate deficiency, probably contribute to hematologic changes (9385,9386,9398). There is a general belief that folic/folinic acid supplements don't interfere with the therapeutic effects of trimethoprim, because infecting organisms can't utilize exogenous folate sources (2677,9382,9384). However, this view has been challenged (4468,9386), and failure of trimethoprim therapy has occurred rarely when folinic acid is given concurrently (9387,9399). Advise patients taking low doses of trimethoprim (e.g., 100 to 200 mg/day) for treatment or prophylaxis of urinary tract infections that they are unlikely to need folate supplements. Advise patients taking high doses of trimethoprim (e.g., 20 mg/kg/day) to maintain good dietary folate intake, but to avoid folate supplements unless prescribed by their physician.

VALPROIC ACID, SODIUM VALPROATE, DIVALPROEX SODIUM (Depakene, Depakote): Valproate may reduce folate levels in some people, but symptomatic deficiency has not been reported (4428,9356,9359). Pregnant women taking valproate may be especially at risk from reduced folate levels (9355). Low folate levels during pregnancy may contribute to birth defects and pregnancy loss (9355,9356). However, folic acid supplements have worsened seizure control in some people with epilepsy (4427). Advise patients taking valproate chronically to consult their physician before taking folic acid supplements.

Interactions with Foods

FOOD: The absorption of supplemental folic acid is reduced slightly when taken with food (6241,6243). Bioavailability is around 85% with food, compared with nearly 100% when taken on an empty stomach, this difference is not clinically significant (6241,6243).

ZINC: The data on the effects of supplemental folic acid on dietary zinc absorption is conflicting (9389,9390,9391,9392,9393,9421). However, normal supplemental doses of folic acid are unlikely to have an adverse effect on zinc balance in people with adequate dietary zinc intake (7135,9391).

Interactions with Lab Tests

MEAN CORPUSCULAR VOLUME (MCV): Folic acid supplementation can normalize megaloblastic anemia in cases of folic acid and vitamin B12 deficiencies. In cases of vitamin B12 deficiency or pernicious anemia, treatment with folic acid will normalize hematological findings, but will not prevent neurological damage (7725).

Interactions with Diseases or Conditions

ANGIOPLASTY: An intravenous loading dose of folic acid, vitamin B6, and vitamin B12 followed by oral administration of folic acid 1.2 mg plus vitamin B6 48 mg and vitamin B12 60 mcg taken daily after coronary stenting might actually increase restenosis rates (12150). Due to the potential for harm this combination of vitamins should not be recommended for patients receiving coronary stents (12151).

PERNICIOUS ANEMIA: Folic acid can mask pernicious anemia by decreasing megaloblastic anemia. This can prevent appropriate treatment with vitamin B12 and result in neurological damage (6241,7725,8739). Patients should be warned to avoid treating undiagnosed anemia with folic acid.

SEIZURE DISORDERS: Supplemental folic acid might exacerbate seizures in people with seizure disorders, particularly in very high doses. Doses less than 1000 mcg have rarely been associated with increased seizure activity (9901).

Dosage and Administration

ORAL: For folate deficiency, the typical dose is 250-1000 mcg per day. For severe folate deficiency, such as in cases of megaloblastic anemia and malabsorption disorders, 1-5 mg per day is used until hematologic recovery is documented (8739). For preventing neural tube defects, at least 400 mcg folic acid per day from supplements or fortified food should be taken by women capable of becoming pregnant and continued through the first month of pregnancy (3325,6241,6243,8739). Women with a history of previous pregnancy complicated by such neural tube defects usually take 4 mg per day beginning one month before and continuing for three months after conception (8739). For reducing colon cancer risk, 400 mcg per day has been used (2250,9326). For treating hyperhomocysteinemia, 0.5 to

5 mg/day has been used (3047,6366,9307,9400,9401,9405,9408,9409,9410,10350), although 0.8 to 1 mg/day is appears to provide maximal reduction of homocysteine levels (9307,9408). In patients with high coronary risk or atherosclerotic disease, 10 mg per day of folic acid has been used to improve coagulation status, oxidative stress, and endothelial dysfunction (9319). In people with end-stage renal disease, hyperhomocysteinemia may be more resistant to treatment, and doses of 0.8 to 15 mg/day have been used (1489,6884,7289,7881,9322,9413,9414,9415,9416). Other regimens such as 2.5 to 5 mg three times weekly have also been used (9417). Doses higher than 15 mg daily do not seem provide additional homocysteine-lowering effect (9219). For preventing increases in homocysteine levels after nitrous oxide anesthesia, folate 2.5 mg in combination with pyridoxine 25 mg and vitamin B12 500 mcg has been used daily for 1 wk before surgery (9481). As adjunct treatment with conventional antidepressants, 200 to 500 mcg per day has been used (10884). For enhancing response to antidepressants, 500 mcg daily has been used (3657). For vitiligo, 5 mg is typically taken twice daily (2153). For reduction of toxicity associated with methotrexate therapy for rheumatoid arthritis (RA) or psoriasis, 1 mg/day is probably sufficient, but up to 5 mg/day may be used (768,2162,4492,4493,4494,9369,9418). The adequate intakes (AI) for infants are 65 mcg for infants 0-6 months and 80 mcg for infants 7-12 months of age (6243). The recommended dietary allowances (RDAs) for folate in DFE, including both food folate and folic acid from fortified foods and supplements are: Children 1-3 years, 150 mcg; Children 4-8 years, 200 mcg; Children 9-13 years, 300 mcg; Adults over 13 years, 400 mcg; Pregnant women 600 mcg; and Lactating women, 500 mcg (6243). The tolerable upper intake levels (UL) of folate are 300 mcg for children 1-3 years of age, 400 mcg for children 4-8 years, 600 mcg for children 9-13 years, 800 mcg for adolescents 14-18 years, and 1000 mcg for everyone over 18 years of age (6243).
TOPICAL: No typical dosage.

Comments

Beginning in 1998, the US government required folic acid fortification of all cold cereals and baking flour, which extends to breads, pastas, bakery items, cookies, crackers, etc (6241). Foods that are naturally high in folate content with 60-90% folic acid bioavailability include leafy vegetables (such as spinach, broccoli, and lettuce), okra, asparagus, fruits (such as bananas, melons, and lemons) legumes, yeast, mushrooms, animal protein (such as beef liver and kidney), orange juice, and tomato juice (6241,8739,9300). Folic acid is frequently used in combination with other B vitamins in vitamin B complex formulations. Vitamin B complex generally includes vitamin B1 (thiamine), vitamin B2 (riboflavin), vitamin B3 (niacin/niacinamide), vitamin B5 (pantothenic acid), vitamin B6 (pyridoxine), vitamin B12 (cyanocobalamin), and folic acid. However, some products do not contain all of these ingredients and some may include others, such as biotin, para-aminobenzoic acid (PABA), choline bitartrate, and inositol (3022).

FOOL'S PARSLEY

Also Known As

Dog Parsley, Dog Poison, Fool's-Cicely, Fools Parsley, Lesser Hemlock, Small Hemlock.
CAUTION: See separate listings for Parsley leaf, root; Parsley seed; and Parsley Piert.

Scientific Names

Aethusa cynapium.
Family: Apiaceae/Umbelliferae.

People Use This For

Orally, fool's parsley is used for gastrointestinal complaints in children, infantile cholera, Summer diarrhea, and convulsions.

Safety

LIKELY UNSAFE ...when used orally; avoid using. Plant parts are considered poisonous and are associated with serious, potentially life-threatening poisonings (18).
PREGNANCY AND LACTATION: UNSAFE ...when used orally; contraindicated, due to potential for poisoning (18).

Effectiveness

There is insufficient reliable information available about the effectiveness of fool's parsley.

Mechanism of Action

Fool's parsley contains varied flavone glycosides (rutoside, narcissine, camphor oil-3-glucorhamnoside). Freshly harvested leaves (only) contain polyenes aethusin, aethusanol A, and asthusanol B (18).

Adverse Reactions

Orally, there are reports that fool's parsley caused deaths when it was mistaken for garden parsley; however, there is some evidence that the botanical to blame was actually spotted hemlock (18). Nevertheless, caution is warranted.

Interactions with Herbs & Other Dietary Supplements
None known.

Interactions with Drugs
None known.

Interactions with Foods
None known.

Interactions with Lab Tests
None known.

Interactions with Diseases or Conditions
None known.

Dosage and Administration
No typical dosage.

Comments
Fool's parsley is considered unsafe; avoid using. Fool's parsley looks a lot like young garden parsley; hence its name. Be careful not to confuse the two, since fool's parsley is poisonous (18).

FORGET-ME-NOT

Also Known As
Field Scorpion Grass, Forget Me Not.

Scientific Names
Myosotis arvensis.
Family: Boraginaceae.

People Use This For
Orally, forget-me-not is used for respiratory disorders and nose bleeds.

Safety
LIKELY UNSAFE ...when used orally. The flowering plant preparations contain hepatotoxic unsaturated pyrrolizidine alkaloids (UPAs) (18). Repeated exposure to low concentrations of UPAs is linked to serious liver toxicity. UPAs are also thought to be carcinogenic and mutagenic (12).
PREGNANCY AND LACTATION: LIKELY UNSAFE ...when used orally. It contains toxic UPAs (12,19).

Effectiveness
There is insufficient reliable information available about the effectiveness of forget-me-not.

Mechanism of Action
The applicable part of forget-me-not is the whole flowering plant. Forget-me-not contains unsaturated pyrrolizidine alkaloids (UPAs) that can cause toxicity (18).

Adverse Reactions
Orally, acute toxicity may result in hepatic necrosis; chronic toxicity may cause veno-occlusive liver disease. The potential for hepatotoxicity increases with larger doses and longer periods of use (4,12).

Interactions with Herbs & Other Dietary Supplements
None known.

Interactions with Drugs
None known.

Interactions with Foods
None known.

Interactions with Lab Tests
None known.

Interactions with Diseases or Conditions
None known.

Dosage and Administration
No typical dosage.

FORSKOLIN

Also Known As
Borforsin, Coleus barbatus, Coleus Forskohlii, Colforsin, Forskohlii, HL-362, L-75-1362B, Plectranthus barbatus.

Scientific Names
17beta-acetoxy-8,13-epoxy-1alpha,6beta,9alpha-trihydroxylabd-14-en-11-one.

People Use This For
Orally, forskolin is used for asthma, allergies, eczema, psoriasis, obesity, dysmenorrhea, irritable bowel syndrome (IBS), urinary tract infections (UTI), bladder infections, hypertension, angina, metastatic cancer, thrombosis, impotence, insomnia, and convulsions.
Intravenously, forskolin is used for idiopathic congestive cardiomyopathy and congestive heart failure (CHF).
By inhalation, forskolin is used for asthma and bronchospasm.
Ophthalmologically, forskolin is used for glaucoma.

Safety
POSSIBLY SAFE ...when used intravenously and appropriately, short term. Intravenous forskolin seems to be safe and well tolerated when given at an appropriate rate of 0.5 mcg/kg/minute and increased at 15 minute intervals to 1.0, 2.0, and 3.0 mcg/kg/minute up to 1 hour (7278,7279). ...when used by inhalation and appropriately. Single-dose inhalation of forskolin powder (10 mg) from a Spinhaler inhalator seems to be safe and well tolerated (7281). ...when used ophthalmologically and appropriately. Forskolin suspension eye drops (1%) seem and well-tolerated (7282,7283,7284,7402,7403,7405).
PREGNANCY AND LACTATION: Insufficient reliable information available; avoid using.

Effectiveness
POSSIBLY EFFECTIVE

Asthma. There is some evidence that a single-dose inhalation of forskolin powder 10 mg from a Spinhaler inhaler can significantly increase forced expiratory volume in 1 second (FEV1) in patients with asthma (7281).

Idiopathic congestive cardiomyopathy. There is some evidence that intravenous forskolin, starting at 0.5 mcg/kg/minute, increasing at 15 minute intervals to 1.0, 2.0, and 3.0 mcg/kg/minute, is effective in improving cardiac output and pulmonary vascular pressures in patients with idiopathic congestive cardiomyopathy (7278).

INSUFFICIENT RELIABLE EVIDENCE to RATE

Intraocular pressure. There is some preliminary evidence that forskolin suspension eye drops (1%) can significantly decrease intraocular pressure in healthy people without eye disease (7282,7283,7284,7402,7403,7405). Forskolin has not yet been tested in patients with glaucoma. More evidence is needed to rate forskolin for this use.

Mechanism of Action
Forskolin is a diterpene and the major active constituent found in the roots of the plant Plectranthus barbatus (Coleus forskohlii) (7277). Forskolin stimulates and activates the enzyme adenylate cyclase in the heart and smooth muscle. This causes increased production of cyclic AMP (cAMP), which causes calcium channels to open and intracellular calcium concentrations to increase, resulting in increased contractility of heart muscle and relaxation of smooth muscle (7277,7406,7407,7408,7409). Researchers speculate that forskolin might also activate adenylate cyclase in other cells of the body such as platelet cells and cells in the thyroid, pancreas, adrenal, or pituitary glands (7277). There is preliminary evidence that forskolin prevents platelet aggregation and adhesion (7410,7411); and may also block tumor cell-induced human platelet aggregation, prevent tumor cell growth, and prevent cancer metastasis (7412,7413).

Adverse Reactions
Intravenously, forskolin can cause flushing and hypotension (7279).
Inhalation of forskolin can cause throat and upper respiratory tract irritation, mild to moderate cough, tremor, and restlessness (7281). Ophthalmologically, forskolin can cause stinging of the eyes and conjunctival hyperemia (7283).

Interactions with Herbs & Other Dietary Supplements

CARDIOACTIVE HERBS: Theoretically, concomitant use of forskolin and cardioactive herbs could potentiate the cardiac effects and adverse effects (7278,7279). Some cardioactive herbs include calamus, cereus, cola, coltsfoot, devil's claw, European mistletoe, fenugreek, fumitory, ginger, Panax ginseng, white horehound, mate, parsley, quassia, scotch broom flower, shepherd's purse, wild carrot, and some cardiac glycoside-containing herbs such as digitalis leaf or lily-of-the-valley roots.

HERBS WITH ANTICOAGULANT/ANTIPLATELET POTENTIAL: Theoretically, concomitant use of forskolin with herbs that affect platelet aggregation could potentially increase the risk of bruising and bleeding. Some of these herbs include angelica, anise, arnica, asafetida, bogbean, boldo, capsicum, celery, chamomile, clove, danshen, fenugreek, feverfew, garlic, ginger, ginkgo, Panax ginseng, horseradish, licorice, meadowsweet, prickly ash, onion, papain, passionflower, poplar, quassia, red clover, turmeric, wild carrot, wild lettuce, willow, and others.

Interactions with Drugs

ANTICOAGULANT/ANTIPLATELET DRUGS: Theoretically, concomitant use of forskolin and anticoagulant or antiplatelet agents might increase the risk of bruising and bleeding. There is some evidence forskolin can inhibit platelet aggregation and adhesion (7410,7411). Some anticoagulant and antiplatelet drugs include abciximab (ReoPro), anagrelide (Agrylin), antithrombin III (Thrombate III), ardeparin (Normiflo), cilostazol (Pletal), clopidogrel (Plavix), dalteparin (Fragmin), danaparoid (Orgaran), dicumarol, dipyridamole (Persantine), enoxaparin (Lovenox), eptifibatide (Integrilin), heparin, lepirudin (Refludan), tirofiban (Aggrastat), and warfarin (Coumadin).

CALCIUM CHANNEL BLOCKERS: Using forskolin with calcium channel blockers such as verapamil (Calan, Covera-HS, Verelan), nifedipine (Procardia), and diltiazem (Cardizem, Dilacor, Tiazac) might cause additive coronary vasodilatory effects (7278,7279).

NITRATES: Using forskolin with nitrates such as nitroglycerin (Nitro-Bid, Nitro-Dur, Nitrostat) and isosorbide (Imdur, Isordil, Sorbitrate) might cause additive coronary vasodilatory effects (7278,7279).

Interactions with Foods

None known.

Interactions with Lab Tests

BLEEDING TIME: Theoretically, forskolin might increase measures of bleeding time and increase tests results for prothrombin time (PT) and international normalized ratio (INR). There is some evidence that forskolin inhibits platelet aggregation and adhesion (7410,7411).

Interactions with Diseases or Conditions

BLEEDING DISORDERS: Theoretically, forskolin may increase the risk of bleeding. There is some evidence that forskolin inhibits platelet aggregation and adhesion (7278,7279).

CARDIOVASCULAR DISEASE: There is some concern that forskolin might interfere with treatment for cardiovascular disease and potentially worsen cardiovascular conditions. Forskolin can cause vasodilation and significantly lower blood pressure (7278,7279). Use forskolin with caution in patients with cardiovascular conditions.

Dosage and Administration

INTRAVENOUS: For idiopathic congestive cardiomyopathy, intravenous forskolin has been infused at 0.5 mcg/kg/min and increased at 15 minute intervals as tolerated up to 1.0, 2.0, and 3.0 mcg/kg/minute for up to 1 hour (7278,7279).

INHALATION: For asthma, 10 mg of forskolin powder, using a Spinhaler inhalator, has been used (7281).

OPHTHALMIC: For lowering intraocular pressure, 50 microliters of forskolin suspension eye drops (1%), applied topically to the cornea, has been used in healthy people (7282,7283,7284,7402,7403,7405). An appropriate dose for patients with glaucoma is not known.

ORAL: No typical dosage.

Comments

Forskolin comes from Coleus forskohlii, an herb that has been used since ancient times to treat heart and respiratory disorders. Herbal product manufacturers are now producing Coleus forskohlii extracts with elevated levels of the constituent forskolin. These preparations are being promoted for the same conditions for which forskolin has been used. However, there is no reliable scientific information that shows Coleus forskohlii extracts offer any therapeutic benefit.

FRANKINCENSE

Also Known As
Bible Frankincense, Olibanum.
CAUTION: See separate listing for Indian Frankincense.

Scientific Names
Boswellia sacra, synonym Boswellia carteri.
Family: Burseraceae.

People Use This For
Orally, frankincense is used for colic and flatulence.
Topically, frankincense is used in hand cream. The essential oil of frankincense is used topically and by inhalation as an analgesic.

Safety
POSSIBLY SAFE ...when used orally (12). ...when the frankincense essential oil is used topically and by inhalation (7107).
PREGNANCY AND LACTATION: Insufficient reliable information available; avoid using.

Effectiveness
There is insufficient reliable information available about the effectiveness of frankincense.

Mechanism of Action
The applicable part of frankincense is the resin. There is insufficient reliable information available about the possible mechanism of action and active ingredients.

Adverse Reactions
Topically, frankincense can cause mild irritation (18).

Interactions with Herbs & Other Dietary Supplements
None known.

Interactions with Drugs
None known.

Interactions with Foods
None known.

Interactions with Lab Tests
None known.

Interactions with Diseases or Conditions
None known.

Dosage and Administration
No typical dosage.

Comments
Frankincense is the hardened gum resin extruded from incisions made in the trunk of Boswellia carteri. Olibanum is a term which refers to the oleogum resin exuded from incisions in the bark of several Boswellia species, including Boswellia serrata (Indian frankincense), Boswellia sacra (Bible frankincense), Boswellia frereana (African elemi), and Boswellia bhau-dajiana (11). The black kohl used by Egyptian women to paint their eyelids is an ingredient from charred frankincense. Frankincense is considered obsolete as a medicinal herb (18).

FRINGETREE

Also Known As
Chionanthus, Fringe Tree, Gray Beard Tree, Old Man's Beard, Poison Ash, Snowdrop Tree, Snowflower, White Fringe.
CAUTION: See separate listings for Traveler's Joy, Usnea, and Woodbine.

Scientific Names
Chionanthus virginicus.
Family: Oleaceae.

Comments
At the date of publication, there was very little scientific information available about this product. Our staff is continually analyzing the available information on natural medicines and will add data to the online version of *Natural Medicines Comprehensive Database* as it becomes available. See www.naturaldatabase.com.

FROSTWORT

Also Known As
Frost Plant, Frostweed, Rock-Rose, Sun Rose.

Scientific Names
Helianthemum canadense, synonym Cistus canadensis.
Family: Cistaceae.

Comments
At the date of publication, there was very little scientific information about this product. Our staff is continually analyzing the available information on natural medicines and will add data to the online version of *Natural Medicines Comprehensive Database* as it becomes available. See www.naturaldatabase.com.

FRUCTO-OLIGOSACCHARIDES

Also Known As
Beta-D-fructofuranosidase, Chicory Inulin Hydrolysate, FOS, Fructo Oligo Saccharides, Fructooligosaccharides, Inulin Hydrolysate, Oligofructose, Oligosaccharides, Prebiotic, SC-FOS, Short Chain Fructo-Oligosaccharides.
CAUTION: See separate listing for Inulin.

Scientific Names
Beta-D-fructofuranosidase.

People Use This For
Orally, fructo-oligosaccharides are used for constipation, traveler's diarrhea, increasing fecal mass, and reducing serum cholesterol. Fructo-oligosaccharides are also used as prebiotics.
In foods, fructo-oligosaccharides are used as a sweetener.

Safety
POSSIBLY SAFE ...when used orally and appropriately in amounts less than 30 grams per day (741,745,8505).
PREGNANCY AND LACTATION: Insufficient reliable information available; avoid using.

Effectiveness
POSSIBLY INEFFECTIVE

Traveler's diarrhea. Taking fructo-oligosaccharides orally doesn't seem to reduce the incidence of traveler's diarrhea (10373).

INSUFFICIENT RELIABLE EVIDENCE to RATE

Constipation. Some evidence suggests that fructo-oligosaccharides may relieve constipation by increasing fecal mass (8505). More evidence is needed to rate fructo-oligosaccharides for this use.

Mechanism of Action

Fructo-oligosaccharides (FOS) are plant sugars that occur in a wide variety of fruits, vegetables, and cereals. Chemically, fructo-oligosaccharides are made up of a glucose molecule joined to fructose molecules. They are produced commercially from sucrose using an enzymatic process, or they can be produced by partial hydrolysis of chicory inulin (750,8507,8563).

Fructo-oligosaccharides have prebiotic activity. Prebiotics are substances that selectively promote the growth and activity of specific species of bacteria in the gut. Fructo-oligosaccharides pass undigested through the small intestine. Colonic bacteria that produce acids, such as bifidobacteria and lactobacilli, are symbiotic with fructo-oligosaccharides. In the colon, fructo-oligosaccharides specifically promote the growth of beneficial bacteria, which in turn produce enzymes that metabolize fructo-oligosaccharides (750,8505,8507,8508,8509,8563). Fructo-oligosaccharides are not hydrolyzed by human digestive enzymes (746), and they are not recoverable in the feces. This suggests complete metabolism by colonic microflora (747).

Colonic fermentation leads to increased fecal biomass, decreased ceco-colonic pH, and production of short chain fatty acids. The short chain fatty acids exert systemic effects on lipid metabolism similarly to dietary fiber (744).

Preliminary evidence suggests that fructo-oligosaccharides might protect against colon cancer (748). In experimental models of colon cancer, fructo-oligosaccharides seem to stimulate local immune surveillance to inhibit tumor formation (8506).

FOS are derived from asparagus, Jerusalem artichokes, and soybeans, or produced synthetically (746,8563). FOS pass undigested through the small intestine and are fermented in the colon.

Adverse Reactions

Orally, the use of fructo-oligosaccharides can cause flatulence, belching, abdominal pain, intestinal sounds, and bloating (740,750,8609). These symptoms occur commonly but are generally mild at lower doses (less than 10 grams per day) (745,750,8509).

Interactions with Herbs & Other Dietary Supplements

BIFIDOBACTERIA: Concomitant use of fructo-oligosaccharides can promote the growth of supplemental bifidobacteria.

Interactions with Drugs

None known.

Interactions with Foods

None known.

Interactions with Lab Tests

None known.

Interactions with Diseases or Conditions

None known.

Dosage and Administration

ORAL: For treating constipation, a dose of 10 grams per day has been used (8505). For prebiotic effect (to increase fecal bifidobacteria), the typical dose is 4 to 10 grams per day (749,750).

Comments

Fructo-oligosaccharides are used as prebiotics, food constituents that increase the number of beneficial bacteria in the intestine. Don't confuse prebiotics with probiotics such as lactobacillus, bifidobacteria, and saccharomyces, which are live organisms used to re-colonize beneficial intestinal microorganisms (8509).

FUMITORY

Also Known As

Beggary, Earth Smoke, Fumiterry, Fumus, Hedge Fumitory, Herba fumariae, Vapor, Wax Dolls.

Scientific Names

Fumaria officinalis.
Family: Fumariaceae.

People Use This For

Orally, fumitory is used for GI spasms and as a bile flow stimulant.
Historically, fumitory has been used for skin eruptions, eczema, conjunctivitis, cardiovascular disorders, as a diuretic, and a laxative.

Safety

POSSIBLY SAFE ...when above ground parts are used orally and appropriately. No significant toxicity usually occurs in standard doses (4,6).
POSSIBLY UNSAFE ...when used orally in large amounts because it contains the alkaloid protopine. Other Fumariaceae species that contain alkaloids including protopine can cause convulsions and death when large amounts are ingested (6). ...when homemade, non-sterile products are used for ophthalmic use (4).
PREGNANCY AND LACTATION: Insufficient reliable information available; avoid using (4).

Effectiveness

INSUFFICIENT RELIABLE EVIDENCE to RATE

Biliary disorders. There's anecdotal evidence that fumitory might help reduce colicky pain associated with biliary disorders (280). More evidence is needed to rate fumitory for this use.

Mechanism of Action

The applicable parts of fumitory are the above ground parts. Fumitory can have weak antispasmodic effects on the smooth muscle of the bile duct and upper GI tract (2,4,18). The major alkaloid constituent, protopine, has antihistamine, hypotensive, bradycardic, and sedative activity in small doses, and it causes excitation and convulsions in large doses (4). Fumitory can exhibit bactericidal activity against gram-positive organisms, including Bacillus anthracis and Staphylococcus (4).

Adverse Reactions

Orally, adverse reactions to fumitory are not common; however, large quantities of alkaloids in other members of this family (Fumariaceae) have caused trembling, convulsions, and death (2).

Interactions with Herbs & Other Dietary Supplements

None known.

Interactions with Drugs

None known.

Interactions with Foods

None known.

Interactions with Lab Tests

None known.

Interactions with Diseases or Conditions

None known.

Dosage and Administration

ORAL: The typical dose of fumitory is 2-4 grams of the above ground parts per day or as a tea 3 times daily (4). The tea is prepared by steeping the herb in 150 mL boiling water for 5-10 minutes and then straining. The usual dose of the liquid extract (1:1 in 25% alcohol) is 2-4 mL 3 times daily, and the tincture (1:5 in 45% alcohol) is commonly dosed 1-4 mL 3 times daily (4).
INHALATION: Nebulizers have been used to administer the extract; no typical dosage (6).

Comments

The fumitory plant is a low shrub with gray pointed leaves, and from a distance the plant can have the wispy appearance of smoke, because of this it received the name "earth smoke" (6).

GABA (GAMMA-AMINOBUTYRIC ACID)

Also Known As
GABA, Gamma Amino Butyric Acid.

Scientific Names
Gamma-aminobutyric acid.

People Use This For
Orally, GABA is used for relieving anxiety, elevating mood, relieving premenstrual syndrome (PMS), and treating attention deficit-hyperactivity disorder (ADHD). It is also used for promoting lean muscle growth, burning fat, stabilizing blood pressure, and relieving pain.
Sublingually, GABA is used for increasing feeling of well being, relieving injuries, improving exercise tolerance, decreasing body fat, and increasing lean body weight.

Safety
There is insufficient reliable information available about the safety of GABA.
Pregnancy and Lactation: Insufficient reliable information available; avoid using.

Effectiveness
There is insufficient reliable information available about the effectiveness of GABA.

Mechanism of Action
In the central nervous system, GABA is the primary inhibitory neurotransmitter. It is synthesized in the brain by the decarboxylation of glutamate (5109,5110). GABA exerts anticonvulsant, sedative, and anxiolytic effects at the cellular level (5109,5110). Single, oral doses of GABA given to people with photo-convulsant epilepsy had no effect (5113). Single, oral doses of 5 or 10 grams of GABA caused a rise in C-peptide, insulin, and glucagon; but did not effect serum glucose in healthy people (5114). GABA given intravenously can cause dysphoria and dose-related increases in blood pressure and pulse (5116). In healthy volunteers, a single 5 gram dose of GABA increased growth hormone, but chronic four-day administration of 18 grams of GABA decreased growth hormone and increased serum prolactin (5115).

Adverse Reactions
Intravenously GABA can cause dysphoria and dose-related increases in blood pressure and pulse (5116).

Interactions with Herbs & Other Dietary Supplements
None known.

Interactions with Drugs
None known.

Interactions with Foods
None known.

Interactions with Lab Tests
None known.

Interactions with Diseases or Conditions
None known.

Dosage and Administration
No typical dosage.

GALBANUM

Also Known As
Galbanum Gum, Galbanum Gum Resin, Galbanum Oleogum Resin, Galbanum Oleoresin, Galbanum Resin.

Scientific Names
Ferula gummosa, synonym Ferula galbaniflua. Family: Apiaceae/Umbelliferae.

People Use This For
Orally, galbanum is used for digestive disorders and flatulence, as an appetite stimulant, expectorant, and antispasmodic.
Topically, galbanum is used for wound treatment.
In food and beverages, galbanum oil and resin are used as flavor components.
In manufacturing, galbanum oil and resin are used as fragrance components in cosmetics. Galbanum is rarely used in pharmaceuticals.

Safety
LIKELY SAFE ...when used orally in amounts commonly found in foods. Galbanum has Generally Recognized As Safe (GRAS) status in the US (4912). POSSIBLY SAFE ...when used topically (11).
There is insufficient reliable information available about the safety of the oral use of galbanum in medicinal amounts.
PREGNANCY AND LACTATION: There is insufficient reliable information available about the safety of the oral use of galbanum in medicinal amounts during pregnancy and lactation.

Effectiveness
There is insufficient reliable information available about the effectiveness of galbanum.

Mechanism of Action
The applicable part of galbanum is the gum resin from the roots and trunk. In vitro data suggest antimicrobial activity, particularly against Staphylococcus aureus. Galbanum may also be effective as an emulsion preservative. Emulsions containing galbanum were stable for up to 6 months (11).

Adverse Reactions
None reported.

Interactions with Herbs & Other Dietary Supplements
None known.

Interactions with Drugs
None known.

Interactions with Foods
None known.

Interactions with Lab Tests
None known.

Interactions with Diseases or Conditions
None known.

Dosage and Administration
No typical dosage.

GAMBOGE

Also Known As
Camboge, Gambodia, Gummigutta, Gutta Cambodia, Gutta Gamba, Guttagamba, Tom Rong.
CAUTION: See separate listing for Garcinia.

Scientific Names
Garcinia hanburyi.
Family: Clusiaceae.

People Use This For
Orally, gamboge is used for constipation, generally in combination with other laxatives, and for the evacuation of intestinal worms.

Safety

POSSIBLY UNSAFE ...when used orally. Deaths have been reported with ingestion of 4 grams (18).
PREGNANCY AND LACTATION: POSSIBLY UNSAFE ...when used orally (18); avoid using.

Effectiveness

There is insufficient reliable information available about the effectiveness of gamboge.

Mechanism of Action

The applicable part of gamboge is the resin. It contains resins (benzophenones and xanthones) and mucilages. Gamboge reportedly has strong laxative effect (18).

Adverse Reactions

Orally, abdominal pain and vomiting has been reported with as little as 200 mg; deaths were reported with ingestion of 4 grams (18).

Interactions with Herbs & Other Dietary Supplements

DIGITALIS: Theoretically, overuse/misuse may cause potassium depletion and increase risk of cardiotoxicity (19).
POTASSIUM DEPLETING HERBS: Theoretically, concomitant use with horsetail plant or licorice rhizome increases the risk of potassium depletion (19).
STIMULANT LAXATIVE HERBS: Theoretically, concomitant use with other stimulant laxative herbs may increase the risk of potassium depletion (19). Stimulant laxative herbs include aloe dried leaf sap, wild cucumber fruit (Ecballium elaterium), blue flag rhizome, alder buckthorn, European buckthorn, butternut bark, cascara bark, castor oil, colocynth fruit pulp, jalap root, black root, manna bark exudate, podophyllum root, rhubarb root, senna leaves and pods, and yellow dock root.

Interactions with Drugs

CORTICOSTEROIDS: Theoretically, prolonged use might have additive effects with drugs that deplete potassium, including corticosteroids (18,19).
DIGOXIN (Lanoxin): Theoretically, overuse of gamboge could decrease potassium levels, increasing the risk of toxicity for cardiac glycoside drugs such as digoxin (Lanoxin) (19).
DIURETIC DRUGS: Overuse of gamboge might compound diuretic-induced potassium loss (19). There is some concern that people taking gamboge along with potassium depleting diuretics might have an increased risk for hypokalemia. Initiation of potassium supplementation or an increase in potassium supplement dose may be necessary for some patients. Some diuretics that can deplete potassium include chlorothiazide (Diuril), chlorthalidone (Thalitone), furosemide (Lasix), and hydrochlorothiazide (HCTZ, HydroDIURIL, Microzide), and others.
STIMULANT LAXATIVES: Concomitant use of gamboge with stimulant laxatives may increase the risk of fluid and electrolyte loss (19).

Interactions with Foods

None known.

Interactions with Lab Tests

None known.

Interactions with Diseases or Conditions

HEART CONDITIONS: Theoretically, overuse/misuse may cause potassium depletion and exacerbate condition. Gamboge is contraindicated in intestinal obstruction, acute intestinal inflammation (Crohn's disease, ulcerative colitis, appendicitis), ulcer, abdominal pain of unknown origin, nausea, and vomiting.

Dosage and Administration

No typical dosage.

Comments

The resin is extracted from Garcinia hanburyi. Avoid confusion with garcinia (Garcinia cambogia).
Gamboge may be adulterated with rice and wheat starches, sand, and vegetable fragments. These adulterated products are usually coarser and hard (215).

GAMMA BUTYROLACTONE (GBL)

Also Known As

1,2-Butanolide, 2(3H)-Furanone Dihydro, 3-Hydroxybutyric Acid Lactone, 4-Butanolide, 4-Butyrolactone, 4-Hydroxybutanoic Acid Lactone, Butyrolactone, Butyrolactone Gamma, Dihydro-2(3H)-Furanone, Gamma Butyrolactone, Gamma Hydroxybutyric Acid Lactone, GBL, Tetrahydro-2-Furanone.
CAUTION: See separate listings for Gamma Hydroxybutyrate (GHB) and Butanediol (BD).

Scientific Names

2,3 dihydro furanone; synonyms 2(3H) furanone dihydro, butyrolactone gamma, 2(3H)-furanone dihydro, butyrolactone, 4-butyrolactone, dihydro-2(3H)-furanone, 4-butanolide, tetrahydro-2-furanone.

People Use This For

Orally, gamma butyrolactone is used for relaxation, calming, increased mental clarity, fat loss, as a body or muscle "builder", recreational drug, for releasing growth hormone, improving athletic performance, inducing and improving sleep, relieving depression and stress, prolonging life, and improving sexual performance and pleasure.

Safety

UNSAFE ...when used orally. The use of GBL or the closely related substances gamma hydroxybutyrate (GHB) and butanediol (BD) has been linked to at least 3 deaths and 122 serious adverse effects (3678,3679). GBL can cause dangerously low respiratory rates and heart rates, seizures, and coma (4259).
PREGNANCY AND LACTATION: UNSAFE ...when used orally (3678,3679); avoid using.

Effectiveness

There is insufficient reliable information available about the effectiveness of gamma butyrolactone (GBL).

Mechanism of Action

Gamma butyrolactone (GBL) is metabolized in the body to gamma hydroxybutyrate (GHB) (see separate listing for GHB) (1430). However, it is more rapidly absorbed than GHB, has greater lipid solubility, and may avoid first-pass metabolism due to its lactone structure (5813). This can lead to higher serum concentrations and more marked hypnotic activity than with similar doses of GHB (5813). GHB can be converted in the brain to the neurotransmitter gamma aminobutyric acid (GABA) (3699), and specific GHB uptake systems, transport systems and receptors have also been identified (713,3699,5800,5801). Stimulation of GHB receptors reduces dopamine release in the brain (713,3699,5801), which may be the mechanism for GBL-induced reductions in dopamine neuronal impulse flow (5811). GBL has been reported to inhibit stereotyped behavior induced by dopamine agonists (5810,5811). The indirect dopamine agonist amphetamine has been reported to partially reverse effects of GBL (5810). GBL may also have some direct GABA agonist activity (5802), although the GABA antagonist bicuculline only partially reverses GBL-induced inhibition of apomorphine activity (5810). GBL, possibly through conversion to GHB, also affects the endogenous opioid system, and the opiate antagonists naloxone and naltrexone attenuate or abolish the electrical seizure activity, behavioral abnormalities, and increased striatal dopamine content produced by GBL (5812). GHB induces REM and non-REM sleep, hypothermia, abnormalities on the EEG similar to those seen in petit mal epilepsy (5800,5803), and it stimulates growth hormone secretion (5804).

Adverse Reactions

Orally, GBL has been associated with a minimum of 55 cases of adverse effects (at least five cases involving children), including involuntary muscle movements, fainting and seizures, bowel incontinence, vomiting, slow breathing, respiratory depression, apnea, slow heart rate, mental changes, severe central nervous system depression, agitation, combativeness, and amnesia. One death, two cases of respiratory arrest, and one case of cardiac arrest have been reported. Nineteen of the 55 cases involved unconsciousness or coma, and in some cases intubation was required for assisted breathing (665,682,1430). Withdrawal symptoms, including insomnia, tremor, anxiety, tachycardia, hypertension, hallucinations, and delirium can occur in chronic users of GBL and GHB (1430,10375,10376).

Interactions with Herbs & Other Dietary Supplements

HERBS AND SUPPLEMENTS WITH SEDATIVE PROPERTIES: Concomitant use is likely to cause additive sedation with GBL, increasing the risk of serious adverse effects.

Interactions with Drugs

ALCOHOL (Ethanol): Concomitant use with GBL and its metabolite GHB may increase the risk of serious CNS and respiratory depression (1430,3678).
AMPHETAMINE: Concomitant use with GHB (a metabolite of GBL) has been associated with severe side effects. Theoretically, concomitant use may also antagonize the effects of GHB (3682).
ANTICONVULSANTS: Theoretically, GHB (a metabolite of GBL) may antagonize the effects of GHB (3682).
ANTIPSYCHOTIC DRUGS: Concomitant use with GHB (a metabolite of GBL) has been associated with severe

side effects. Antipsychotics can potentiate the effects of GHB (3682).
BENZODIAZEPINES: Concomitant use with GHB (a metabolite of GBL) has been associated with severe side effects Benzodiazepines can potentiate the effects of GHB (3682).
CNS DEPRESSANTS: Concomitant use with GHB (a metabolite of GBL) has been associated with severe side effects. Additive sedative effects with GBL may occur (3682,3679).
HALOPERIDOL (Haldol): Theoretically, Haloperidol may antagonize the effects of GHB (a metabolite of GBL) (3682).
NALOXONE (Narcan): Theoretically, concomitant use with GHB (a metabolite of GBL) may antagonize the effects of GHB (3682).
NARCOTIC DRUGS: Concomitant use with GHB (a metabolite of GBL) has been associated with severe side effects. Concomitant use of GHB with narcotic drugs can potentiate the therapeutic and adverse effects of narcotic analgesics (3682,3679).
RITONAVIR (Norvir): Concomitant use of the protease inhibitor-type antiretroviral drugs ritonavir and saquinavir with GHB (a metabolite of GBL) reportedly caused a near-fatal reaction, probably due to inhibition of GHB metabolism (1431).
SAQUINAVIR (Fortovase, Invirase): Concomitant use of the protease inhibitor-type antiretroviral drugs ritonavir and saquinavir with GHB (a metabolite of GBL) reportedly caused a near-fatal reaction, probably due to inhibition of GHB metabolism (1431).
SKELETAL MUSCLE RELAXANTS: Concomitant use with GHB (a metabolite of GBL) has been associated with severe side effects. Concomitant use with GHB can potentiate the therapeutic and adverse effects of skeletal muscle relaxants (3682).

Interactions with Foods

ALCOHOL: GHB (a metabolite of GBL) acts synergistically with alcohol to produce CNS and respiratory depression (1430).

Interactions with Lab Tests

None known.

Interactions with Diseases or Conditions

BRADYCARDIA: GHB and GBL should be avoided since they can cause bradycardia (4259).
EPILEPSY: GHB and GBL should be avoided due to their possible capacity to induce seizures (10658).
HYPERTENSION: GHB and GBL should be avoided since they may increase blood pressure (10658).

Dosage and Administration

No typical dosage.

Comments

FDA WARNING: Avoid all gamma butyrolactone containing products due to safety concerns (682). GBL has been marketed as an alternative to gamma hydroxybutyrate (GHB), but it is illegal to manufacture or market GBL or the related products GHB and butanediol (BD) (3678). Publication of a Federal Register notice on 3/13/00 brought into effect the Hillory J. Farias and Samantha Reid Date-Rape Drug Prohibition Act of 2000, which effected changes to the Controlled Substances Act, making GHB a schedule 1 controlled substance (like heroin), and GBL a list 1 chemical (3681). GBL, GHB and BD are associated with at least 122 reports of serious adverse effects including dangerously low respiratory rates (intubation might be required), unconsciousness/coma, vomiting, seizures, slowed heart rate, and death (4259).

GAMMA-HYDROXYBUTYRATE (GHB)

Also Known As

4-Hydroxy Butyrate, Gamma Hydrate, Gamma Hydroxybutyrate Sodium, Gamma Hydroxybutyric Acid, Gamma-OH, GHB, Sodium Gamma-Hydroxybutyrate, Sodium Oxybate, Sodium Oxybutyrate.
CAUTION: See separate listings for Gamma Butyrolactone (GBL) and Butanediol (BD).

Scientific Names

Gamma hydroxybutyrate; 4-hydroxybutyric acid; Sodium 4-hydroxybutyrate.

People Use This For

Orally, gamma hydroxybutyrate (GHB) is used for reducing weight, enhancing muscle growth, as an aphrodisiac, as an hypnotic, for management of opiate withdrawal and alcohol dependence and withdrawal, and for posthypoxic cerebral edema. It is also used for improving pain, fatigue, and the alpha sleep anomaly in patients with fibromyalgia. GHB is also used orally as a sedative alternative to the dietary supplement L-tryptophan.

As an orphan drug, GHB has been approved by the FDA for treatment of narcolepsy (improving nighttime sleep, and the auxiliary symptoms of cataplexy, sleep paralysis, hypnagogic hallucinations, and automatic behavior). Intravenously, GHB has been used as part of an anesthetic regimen, and to reduce intracranial pressure associated with trauma.

Safety

POSSIBLY SAFE ...when used orally and appropriately. GHB has FDA orphan drug status (4261).
UNSAFE ...when used orally without medical supervision. GHB can cause serious side effects including dangerously low respiratory rates, tonic-clonic seizure, coma, and death if used inappropriately (3678,3679,3680,3688,4259,10657,10658). GHB can also cause dependence requiring in-patient detoxification (6612,6613,10656). There is insufficient reliable information available about the safety of GHB for its other uses.
PREGNANCY AND LACTATION: UNSAFE ...when used orally. GHB has been associated with life-threatening toxicities (3678,3679,3680,3688,4259); contraindicated.

Effectiveness

EFFECTIVE

Narcolepsy. Taking GHB orally is effective for improving overnight sleep quality and reducing cataplexy in people with narcolepsy (3683,3689,3690,3691,3692). GHB has FDA orphan drug status for treatment of narcolepsy and associated symptoms (4261).

POSSIBLY EFFECTIVE

Alcoholism. Taking GHB orally might reduce alcohol withdrawal symptoms in alcoholics. It also appears to be useful for treating alcohol dependence (3684,3686,3696).

Fibromyalgia. Taking GHB orally seems to help reduce fibromyalgia-associated pain, fatigue, and alpha sleep anomaly (711).

Opiate withdrawal. Taking GHB orally seems to suppress withdrawal symptoms in heroin addicted and methadone-maintained patients (3694,3695).

There is insufficient reliable information available about the effectiveness of GHB for its other uses.

Mechanism of Action

GHB occurs naturally in several areas of the brain, with the highest concentrations found in the basal ganglia. It is also found in other tissues including kidneys, liver, heart, and skeletal muscle and brown fat (3699,3682,10658). In the brain, it is formed as a metabolite of the neurotransmitter gamma aminobutyric acid (GABA), and can also be converted back to GABA during metabolism (3699,10658). Specific uptake and transport systems have been identified for GHB in the brain (3699,5800), and specific GHB receptors have been identified. Stimulation of GHB receptors results in a reduction in dopamine release in the basal ganglia (713,5801,10658), and it also influences dopamine release in the substantia nigra (3699). Some authors suggest that GHB interacts with GABA(B) receptors (713), but others report that GABA formed from GHB is likely involved and that GHB itself is not a GABA agonist (5801,5802). Another GHB metabolite, gamma butyrolactone (GBL) may have some GABA agonist activity (5802). GHB has also been reported to affect the endogenous opioid system, raising dynorphin levels (3682,5803).

GHB induces REM and non-REM sleep, hypothermia, and abnormalities on the EEG similar to those seen in petit mal epilepsy (5800,5803). It stimulates growth hormone secretion which occurs during slow wave sleep (5804); this has led to claims of anabolic effects (3688). It is also involved in preventing the production of, and scavenging, oxygen-derived free radicals in the brain (3682,5805). It decreases brain glucose utilization (3683), lowers cerebral energy requirements, and it may play a neuroprotective role, protecting against the effects of anoxia or excessive metabolic demand (3682,5800,5803). It has been suggested that the natural function of GHB may be to induce and maintain physiological states such as sleep and hibernation in which energy utilization is depressed (5803). Some of the effects of GHB are antagonized by the opiate antagonist, naloxone and anticonvulsant drugs (5800); but the stimulation of growth hormone release is antagonized by flumazenil (a benzodiazepine antagonist) and metergoline (a serotonin receptor antagonist) (5806).

The effects of GHB on sleep have been used to improve nighttime sleep quality, sleep continuity, stage 3 and 4 sleep, and cataplexy in people with narcolepsy, with some studies also reporting a reduction in the number of daytime sleep attacks (3689,3690,3691,3692).

Studies in rats indicate that a cross-tolerance can develop between GHB and ethanol with chronic exposure, leading to investigations of GHB for management of ethanol dependence and withdrawal (3686). Efficacy has also been reported in the management of opiate withdrawal (3694,3695).

Adverse Reactions

Orally, GHB can cause headaches, hallucinations, dizziness, confusion, nausea, vomiting, drowsiness, agitation, and diarrhea. It can also cause sexual arousal, numbing of legs, loss of peripheral vision, tightness of chest, slowed heart rate, depressed respiration, nystagmus, ataxia, eosinophilia-myalgia syndrome, and seizure-like activity (6016,10658). The symptoms usually occur within 15 to 60 minutes and subside within 2 to 96 hours (6016,10658), although dizziness can continue for up to 14 days. Doses of GHB greater than 10 mg/kg can cause amnesia and reduced muscle tone (6016). GHB and the chemically-related products, gamma butyrolactone (GBL) and 1,4 butanediol, have been associated with at least 122 reports of serious adverse reactions including dangerously low respiratory rates, some requiring intubation; unconsciousness and coma; vomiting, seizures; bradycardia; and multiple deaths (3680,4259,10657,10658). At least two deaths involved the use of GHB and alcohol. Death occurred in less than 24 hours after ingestion and was due to circulatory and respiratory collapse. The amount of GHB consumed in these two cases is not known; however, the GHB levels in blood and urine were significantly elevated (6016). GHB can cause dependence requiring in-patient detoxification. Withdrawal syndrome symptoms include nausea, vomiting, diarrhea, diaphoresis, tachycardia, hypertension, delirium with auditory and visual hallucinations; insomnia, panic, terror, anxiety, and tremor (6612,6613,10656,10658).

Interactions with Herbs & Other Dietary Supplements

PRODUCTS WITH SEDATIVE PROPERTIES: Theoretically, concomitant use with herbs that have sedative properties might enhance therapeutic and adverse effects. Some of these supplements include 5-HTP, calamus, California poppy, catnip, hops, Jamaican dogwood, kava, melatonin, St. John's wort, scullcap, valerian, yerba mansa, and others.

Interactions with Drugs

ALCOHOL (Ethanol): Concomitant use may increase the risk of serious CNS and respiratory depression (3678).
AMPHETAMINE: Concomitant use with GHB has been associated with severe side effects. Theoretically, concomitant use may also antagonize the effects of GHB (3682).
ANTICONVULSANTS: Theoretically, GHB may antagonize the effects of GHB (3682).
ANTIPSYCHOTIC DRUGS: Concomitant use with GHB has been associated with severe side effects. Antipsychotics can potentiate the effects of GHB (3682).
BENZODIAZEPINES: Concomitant use with GHB has been associated with severe side effects. Benzodiazepines can potentiate the effects of GHB (3682).
CNS DEPRESSANTS: Concomitant use with GHB has been associated with severe side effects. Additive sedative effects with GBL may occur (3682,3679).
HALOPERIDOL (Haldol): Theoretically, Haloperidol may antagonize the effects of GHB (3682).
NALOXONE (Narcan): Theoretically, concomitant use with GHB may antagonize the effects of GHB (3682).
NARCOTIC DRUGS: Concomitant use with GHB can potentiate the therapeutic and adverse effects of narcotic analgesics. Although GHB has been used with apparent safety to treat narcotic addiction, there is a case report of a fatality with concurrent use of GHB and heroin (3694,3695,5807).
RITONAVIR (Norvir): Concomitant use of the protease inhibitor-type antiretroviral drugs ritonavir and saquinavir with GHB reportedly caused a near-fatal reaction, probably due to inhibition of GHB metabolism (1431).
SAQUINAVIR (Fortovase, Invirase): Concomitant use of the protease inhibitor-type antiretroviral drugs ritonavir and saquinavir with GHB reportedly caused a near-fatal reaction, probably due to inhibition of GHB metabolism (1431).
SKELETAL MUSCLE RELAXANTS: Concomitant use with GHB has been associated with severe side effects. Concomitant use with GHB can potentiate the therapeutic and adverse effects of skeletal muscle relaxants (3682).

Interactions with Foods

ALCOHOL: Concomitant use with GHB can potentiate the CNS and respiratory depression effects of alcohol and GHB (3682).

Interactions with Lab Tests

None known.

Interactions with Diseases or Conditions

BRADYCARDIA: GHB should be avoided since they can cause bradycardia (4259).
EPILEPSY: GHB should be avoided due to their possible capacity to induce seizures (10658).
HYPERTENSION: GHB should be avoided since they may increase blood pressure (10658).

Dosage and Administration

ORAL: For narcolepsy and associate symptoms, a dose of 25 mg/kg at bedtime, repeated 3 hours later has been used (3689,3690). For treating alcohol dependence, 50 to 150 mg/kg divided into 3 to 6 doses per day has been used (3684,3696). As a hypnotic, 75-100 mg/kg has been used (3693).

Comments

Gamma butyrolactone (GBL) and butanediol (BD) are closely related to GHB and produce similar adverse effects (3678,3679). Due to reports of serious adverse effects, the FDA removed GHB from the market in 1990, but clandestine manufacture continued, with the drug being widely available on the Internet, and being implicated as a date rape agent (3687). Publication of a Federal Register notice on 3/13/00 brought into effect the Hillory J. Farias and Samantha Reid Date-Rape Drug Prohibition Act of 2000, which effected changes to the Controlled Substances Act, making GHB a schedule I controlled substance (like heroin), which it is illegal to produce, sell or possess, except for medical use (3680,3681). GHB is available under the generic name sodium oxybate and trade name Xyrem (Orphan Medical), for the treatment of cataplexy associated with narcolepsy. It is a Schedule III Controlled Substance (4261).

GAMMA LINOLENIC ACID

Also Known As
Gamma-Linolenic Acid, Gamolenic Acid, GLA.
CAUTION: See separate listings for Black Currant, Borage Seed Oil, Evening Primrose Oil, and Omega-6 Oils.

Scientific Names
(Z,Z,Z)-Octadeca-6,9,12-trienoic acid.

People Use This For
Orally, gamma linolenic acid (GLA) is used for rheumatoid arthritis, oral mucoceles (mucous polyps), hyperlipidemia, heart disease, Syndrome-X, systemic sclerosis, diabetic neuropathy, cancer prevention, and to hasten the response to tamoxifen in people with breast cancer. It is also used for attention deficit-hyperactivity disorder (ADHD), depression, postpartum depression, chronic fatigue syndrome, allergic rhinitis, psoriasis, and eczema.

Safety
POSSIBLY SAFE ...when used orally and appropriately. Gamma linolenic acid appears to be safe when taken in oral doses of 2.8 grams per day or less for up to a year (1983,7701,7702,8926).
PREGNANCY AND LACTATION: Insufficient reliable information available; avoid using.

Effectiveness
POSSIBLY EFFECTIVE

Diabetic neuropathy. Taking gamma linolenic acid orally for 6 months to 1 year seems to reduce symptoms and prevent neurological deterioration in neuropathy patients who have type 1 or type 2 diabetes (1980,1981,1984,8926). It seems to be more effective in patients with better glucose control compared to patients with poor glucose control (8926).

POSSIBLY INEFFECTIVE

Scleroderma. Taking gamma linolenic acid orally doesn't seem to be effective for reducing symptoms of scleroderma (1977).

INSUFFICIENT RELIABLE EVIDENCE to RATE

Breast cancer. There is preliminary evidence that taking gamma linolenic acid orally seems to improve the response to tamoxifen in patients with breast cancer (5902). More evidence is needed to rate gamma linolenic acid for this use.

Mechanism of Action
Gamma linolenic acid (GLA) is an omega-6 fatty acid, derived from the seeds of plants such as evening primrose and borage (7701). GLA can be converted to compounds that have anti-inflammatory and antiproliferative properties (1975), including prostaglandins with vasoactive properties. Some research suggests that dihomogammalinolenic acid, a metabolite of GLA and precursor of prostaglandin E1, might act directly on T-cells to modulate immune response in diseases such as rheumatoid arthritis (RA) (7701). There is also some evidence that GLA might reduce interleukin-1-beta (IL-1-beta) auto induction, which is thought to be the cause of synovitis in patients with RA (8134). Preliminary evidence suggests GLA can hasten the response to tamoxifen (Nolvadex) in individuals with estrogen-sensitive primary breast cancer (5902). GLA might have an antiestrogenic effect. It seems to modulate the sensitivity of breast cancer cells to paclitaxel (Taxol) and fulvestrant (Faslodex), enhancing malignant cell killing without adverse effects on normal cells (8133,11791). However, other research suggests that GLA alone can stimulate the growth of breast cancer cells at low concentrations and inhibit growth at higher concentrations (11339).
GLA is believed to benefit individuals who have ischemic lesions associated with systemic sclerosis (1977) and individuals with diabetic neuropathy (1980,1981). Some evidence suggests that gamma linolenic acid might lower plasma triglycerides, increase HDL cholesterol, and prolong bleeding time (1979). Epidemiological research suggests that increased serum levels of GLA might be related to decreased risk for atrophic gastritis associated with Helicobacter pylori (H. pylori) infection. Further study is needed to confirm this observation and to determine a mechanism of action (8709).

Adverse Reactions
Orally, gamma linolenic acid (GLA) can cause mild gastrointestinal effects such as nausea, vomiting, soft stools, diarrhea, flatulence, and belching (7701,7702,8926). GLA might prolong bleeding time (1979).

Interactions with Herbs & Other Dietary Supplements
None known.

Interactions with Drugs
ANTICOAGULANT/ANTIPLATELET DRUGS: Gamma-linolenic acid (GLA) appears to have anticoagulant effects (1979). Theoretically, taking GLA with other anticoagulant or antiplatelet drugs might increase the risk of

bruising and bleeding. Some of these drugs include aspirin, clopidogrel (Plavix), nonsteroidal anti-inflammatory drugs (NSAIDs) such as diclofenac (Voltaren, Cataflam, others), ibuprofen (Advil, Motrin, others), naproxen (Anaprox, Naprosyn, others), dalteparin (Fragmin), enoxaparin (Lovenox), heparin, warfarin (Coumadin), and others.

PHENOTHIAZINES: Theoretically, products containing gamma linolenic acid (GLA) and vitamin E might increase the risk of seizures in people being treat concomitantly with phenothiazine drugs (11021); use with caution.

Interactions with Foods

None known.

Interactions with Lab Tests

BLEEDING TIME: Gamma linolenic acid inhibits platelet aggregation and prolongs bleeding time and lab assay results (1979).

LIPID PROFILE: Gamma linolenic acid might lower plasma triglycerides and increase high-density lipoprotein (HDL) cholesterol (1979).

Interactions with Diseases or Conditions

BLEEDING DISORDERS: There is some concern that gamma linolenic acid (GLA) might prolong bleeding time and increase the risk of bruising and bleeding. GLA has platelet inhibiting effects (1979).

Dosage and Administration

ORAL: For rheumatoid arthritis, gamma linolenic acid (GLA) 1.1 grams per day has been used (1985).
For diabetic neuropathy, 360 to 480 mg per day has been used (1984,8926). For hyperlipidemia, 1.5-6 grams per day has been used (1976,1979).

GAMMA ORYZANOL

Also Known As

Gamma-Oryzanol, Gamma-OZ, Oryzanol.

Scientific Names

Gamma oryzanol.

People Use This For

Orally, gamma oryzanol is used for hypercholesterolemia and dyslipidemia, increasing testosterone and human growth hormone levels, improving strength during resistance exercise training, and for treating symptoms associated with menopause and aging.

Safety

POSSIBLY SAFE ...when used orally and appropriately (751,752,753,754,755).
PREGNANCY AND LACTATION: Insufficient reliable information available; avoid using.

Effectiveness

POSSIBLY EFFECTIVE

Dyslipidemia. There is some preliminary clinical evidence that gamma oryzanol can significantly decrease total cholesterol, low-density lipoprotein (LDL) cholesterol, and triglyceride levels. Effects on high-density lipoprotein (HDL) cholesterol levels are conflicting (752,757).

There is insufficient reliable information available about the effectiveness of gamma oryzanol for its other uses.

Mechanism of Action

Gamma oryzanol is a group of constituents derived primarily from rice bran oil. It is also found in wheat bran and some fruits and vegetables. Gamma oryzanol itself is poorly absorbed from the gut (755). Researchers think it might help lower cholesterol by decreasing cholesterol absorption from the gut (756). Gamma oryzanol is also often promoted for treating menopause, but it is unclear how it would work for this use. Some researchers suspect it might be helpful due to effects on luteinizing hormone (LH) (755). However, this effect has not been verified in humans. Some people use gamma oryzanol for increasing testosterone and growth hormone levels. However, gamma oryzanol appears to have no effect on these hormone levels (751). Animal studies using parenteral administration actually show gamma oryzanol can be anti-anabolic by suppressing the release of LH and increasing the release of catecholamines, dopamine, and norepinephrine in the brain (755). If this occurs in humans, gamma oryzanol might actually reduce testosterone production (755). There is some evidence gamma oryzanol can reduce elevated serum TSH levels in hypothyroid patients. Some researchers think gamma-oryzanol inhibits serum TSH levels by a direct action at the hypothalamus rather than the pituitary (753).

Adverse Reactions
None reported.

Interactions with Herbs & Other Dietary Supplements
None known.

Interactions with Drugs
None known.

Interactions with Foods
None known.

Interactions with Lab Tests
CHOLESTEROL: Gamma oryzanol can reduce serum total cholesterol (752,757) and low-density lipoprotein (LDL) cholesterol (752) concentrations and test results. Gamma oryzanol might also increase serum high-density lipoprotein (HDL) cholesterol concentrations in some patients (757).
THYROID STIMULATING HORMONE (TSH): Gamma oryzanol can reduce serum TSH concentrations in patients with hypothyroidism (753).
TRIGLYCERIDES: Gamma oryzanol can reduce serum triglyceride concentrations and test results (757).

Interactions with Diseases or Conditions
PRIMARY HYPOTHYROIDISM: Gamma oryzanol can decrease TSH serum levels (753).

Dosage and Administration
ORAL: For reducing serum cholesterol, the usual dose of gamma oryzanol is 300 mg daily (752,757). In one study, 100 mg three times daily was used (752).

Comments
Gamma oryzanol is an extraction product from rice bran oil.

GARCINIA

Also Known As
Brindal Berry, Brindle Berry, Garcinia Cambogia, Gorikapuli, HCA, Hydroxycitrate, Hydroxycitric Acid, Kankusta, Malabar Tamarind, Vrikshamla.
CAUTION: See separate listings for Gamboge, Malabar Nut, Mangosteen, and Tamarind.

Scientific Names
Garcinia gummi-guta, synonyms Cambogia gummi-guta, Garcinia cambogia, Mangostana cambogia.
Family: Clusiaceae/Guttiferae.

People Use This For
Orally, garcinia is used for weight loss, rheumatism, dysentery, as a purgative, and for treating worms and parasites. In foods, garcinia is used as a condiment in Thai and Indian cuisine.

Safety
POSSIBLY SAFE ...when used orally and appropriately for 12 weeks or less (728,11977).
There is insufficient reliable information available about the safety of the long-term use of garcinia.
PREGNANCY AND LACTATION: Insufficient reliable information available; avoid using.

Effectiveness
POSSIBLY INEFFECTIVE

Obesity. Taking garcinia fruit rind extract orally doesn't seem to help decrease weight, satiety, fat oxidation, or energy expenditure in obese people (728,8572,11407). There is some mixed evidence that garcinia might reduce food intake while sustaining satiety, but it's too early to recommend it for this use (8572).

There is insufficient reliable information available about the effectiveness of garcinia for its other uses.

Mechanism of Action
The applicable parts of garcinia are the fruit and rind. Garcinia fruit rind extract, reported to contain 50% hydroxycitrate acid (HCA), is theorized to interfere with lipogenesis (728). The active ingredient HCA is believed to be a competitive inhibitor of ATP-citrate-lyase, the enzyme responsible for converting citrate into

acetyl-coenzyme A (acetyl-CoA). This conversion into acetyl-CoA occurs when the energy consumed exceeds the energy requirements of the body (4476,4478,4480). Other researchers think that garcinia inhibits the supply of fatty acids without affecting adipose conversion. Preliminary research suggests that garcinia inhibits the accumulation of lipid droplets in fat cells and thereby reduces lipid levels and decreases lipid accumulation in the liver (8571). The HCA found in garcinia is also theorized to improve exercise endurance by increasing lipid oxidation and decreasing carbohydrate utilization (4487). Some animal research suggests that HCA might suppress appetite (11977).

Adverse Reactions
Orally, garcinia can cause nausea, GI discomfort, and headache (11977).

Interactions with Herbs & Other Dietary Supplements
None known.

Interactions with Drugs
None known.

Interactions with Foods
None known.

Interactions with Lab Tests
None known.

Interactions with Diseases or Conditions
None known.

Dosage and Administration
ORAL: For weight loss, an extract containing 50% hydroxycitric acid, 1000 mg three times daily has been used (728). Hydroxycitric acid, 500 mg four times daily has also been used for weight loss (11407).

Comments
Avoid confusion with gamboge resin (Garcinia hanburyi).

GARDEN CRESS

Also Known As
None.

Scientific Names
Lepidium sativum.
Family: Brassicaceae/Cruciferae.

People Use This For
Orally, garden cress is used for coughs, vitamin C deficiency, constipation, poor immunity, and as a diuretic.

Safety
There is insufficient reliable information available about the safety of garden cress.
Pregnancy and Lactation: Insufficient reliable information available; avoid using.

Effectiveness
There is insufficient reliable information available about the effectiveness of garden cress.

Mechanism of Action
The applicable parts of garden cress are the above ground parts. Garden cress may have in vitro antibacterial activity, but the activity appears to be dependent on the age of the plant at harvest. It also appears to have antiviral activity against the encephalitis virus Columbia SH (animal data) (18).

Adverse Reactions
Orally, ingesting large amounts of garden cress may cause gastrointestinal irritation (18).

Interactions with Herbs & Other Dietary Supplements
None known.

Interactions with Drugs
None known.

Interactions with Foods
None known.

Interactions with Lab Tests
None known.

Interactions with Diseases or Conditions
None known.

Dosage and Administration
ORAL: Garden cress is used as a fresh use herb in oral preparations (18).

Comments
Garden cress is rarely adulterated because it is usually cultivated rather than harvested (18).

GARDEN VIOLET

Also Known As
None.
CAUTION: See separate listing for Sweet Violet.

Scientific Names
Viola odorata.
Family: Violaceae.

Comments
At the date of publication, there was very little scientific information about this product. Our staff is continually analyzing the available information on natural medicines and will add data to the online version of *Natural Medicines Comprehensive Database* as it becomes available. See www.naturaldatabase.com.

GARLIC

Also Known As
Aged Garlic Extract, Ail, Ajo, Allii Sativi Bulbus, Allium, Camphor of the Poor, Clove Garlic, Garlic Clove, Lasuna, Nectar of the Gods, Poor Man's Treacle, Rust Treacle, Stinking Rose.

Scientific Names
Allium sativum.
Family: Alliaceae or Liliaceae.

People Use This For
Orally, garlic is used for hypertension, hyperlipidemia, preventing coronary heart disease, preventing age-related vascular changes and atherosclerosis, reducing reinfarction and mortality rate post-myocardial infarction, earaches, and menstrual disorders. Garlic is also used orally for HIV-drug induced lipid disorders, and to treat Helicobacter pylori infection. Garlic is used to prevent colorectal cancer, gastric cancer, breast cancer, lung cancer, to treat and prevent prostate cancer, and to treat bladder cancer. Other uses include treatment of benign prostatic hyperplasia (BPH), diabetes, arthritis, allergies, traveler's diarrhea, colds and flu. It is also used for immune system stimulation, prevention of tick bites, and prevention and treatment of bacterial and fungal infections. Garlic is also used for diarrhea, amoebic and bacterial dysentery, tuberculosis, bloody urine, diphtheria, whooping cough, scalp ringworm, hypersensitive teeth, and vaginal trichomoniasis. Other uses include treatment of fever, coughs, headache, stomachache, sinus congestion, athlete's foot, gout, rheumatism, hemorrhoids, asthma, bronchitis, shortness of breath, arteriosclerosis, low blood pressure, hypoglycemia, hyperglycemia, and snakebites. It is also used as a diuretic, stimulant, cathartic, aphrodisiac, for enhancing circulation, fighting stress and fatigue, and maintaining healthy liver function.
Topically, garlic oil is used for tinea pedis, tinea corporis, tinea cruris, and onychomycosis.
Intravaginally, garlic is used alone or in combination with yogurt for vaginitis.
In foods and beverages, fresh garlic, garlic powder, and garlic oil are used as flavor components.

Safety

LIKELY SAFE ...when used orally and appropriately. Garlic has been used safely in clinical studies lasting up to four years without reports of significant toxicity (1873,4782,4783,4784,4785,4786,4787,4789,4790,4797,4798,6457,6897).
POSSIBLY UNSAFE ...when used topically (585). Garlic applied topically might cause severe skin irritation.
CHILDREN: POSSIBLY SAFE ...when used orally and appropriately, short-term. In one study, garlic extract 300 mg three times daily had side effects comparable to placebo when used in children ages 8-18 years for eight weeks (4796). POSSIBLY UNSAFE ...when used orally in large amounts. Some sources suggest that high doses of garlic could be dangerous or even fatal to children (12); however, the reason for this warning is not known. There are no case reports available of significant adverse events or mortality in children associated with ingestion of garlic.
PREGNANCY: LIKELY SAFE ...when used orally in amounts commonly found in foods (3319). POSSIBLY UNSAFE ...when used orally in medicinal amounts. Garlic is reported to have abortifacient activity (11020). One study also suggests that garlic constituents are distributed to the amniotic fluid after a single dose of garlic (4828). However, there are no published reports of garlic adversely affecting pregnancy. In one study, garlic 800 mg daily was used during the third trimester of pregnancy with no reported adverse outcomes (9201). There is insufficient reliable information available about the safety of topical garlic use during pregnancy.
LACTATION: POSSIBLY UNSAFE ...when used orally in amounts greater than those commonly found in foods. Several small studies suggest that garlic constituents are secreted in breast milk, and that nursing infants of mothers consuming garlic are prone to extended nursing and an altered flavor in breast milk (3319,4829,4830). There is insufficient reliable information available about the safety of topical garlic use during lactation.

Effectiveness

POSSIBLY EFFECTIVE

Atherosclerosis. Taking low doses of garlic powder orally, 300 mg per day, seems to lessen age-related decreases in aortic elasticity. Higher doses of 900 mg per day seem to slow development of atherosclerosis in both aortic and femoral arteries when used over a four-year period (3315,4797,4798).

Colorectal cancer. Several population studies suggest that increased dietary garlic consumption can decrease risk of developing colorectal cancer (3320,4770,4771,4772). However, garlic supplements do not seem to offer this benefit (4773).

Gastric cancer. There is some evidence from population studies that increasing dietary garlic consumption can decrease risk of developing stomach cancer (3320,4775,4776). It's not known if garlic supplements have this same benefit.

Hyperlipidemia. There is controversy over the effectiveness of taking garlic orally for hyperlipidemia. Some studies show no significant benefit (731,732,4792,4793,4794,4795,4807), but the majority of evidence suggests that garlic has modest benefit. It seems to decrease total cholesterol, low-density lipoprotein (LDL) cholesterol, and triglyceride levels (279,4782,4783,4784,4785,4786,4787,6457,6465,6897,9209). When used for 4-25 weeks, garlic seems to lower total cholesterol levels by about 4-12% (4786,6457). As a comparison, conventional "statin" drugs typically decrease cholesterol levels by 17-55% (6457). Garlic does not seem to affect high-density lipoprotein (HDL) cholesterol (6897). Because of the relatively minor cholesterol level reductions possible with garlic, some clinicians question its value in reducing cardiovascular disease. There is also some concern that garlic may not produce long-term benefits. Some studies show no significant benefit when used for 6 months or longer (6465,6897). Garlic alone is probably not appropriate for patients that require significant reductions in cholesterol levels. Most garlic preparations used in clinical studies were standardized based on the alliin constituent or the allicin yield. But there is also some evidence that aged garlic extracts (odorless garlic) standardized based on the S-allyl-L-cysteine constituent might also be beneficial (1873,1875,1876). Garlic is sometimes given in combination with fish oils (4789,4790) and ginkgo (4791); however, these combinations do not add substantially to the beneficial plasma lipid effects.

Hypertension. There is some evidence that taking garlic orally can modestly reduce blood pressure by 2-7% after 4 weeks of treatment (277,278,279,1873,6897).

Prostate cancer. Men who eat 2.14 grams of garlic (about one clove) per day seem to have a 50% decrease in the risk of developing prostate cancer (9876). There is preliminary evidence that suggests garlic supplements can also decrease the risk of developing prostate cancer (4777). There is also preliminary evidence that suggests a garlic extract might help improve urinary flow, decrease urinary frequency, and reduce other symptoms associated with prostate cancer (10374).

Tick bites. People consuming high doses of garlic (1200 mg daily) over a 20-week period seem to have a reduced number of tick bites when compared to controls (3318,8027).

Tinea corporis. Applying a garlic gel containing 0.6% ajoene seems to be as effective as terbinafine 1% cream for tinea corporis (4767).

Tinea cruris. Applying a garlic gel containing 0.6% ajoene seems to be as effective as terbinafine 1% cream for tinea cruris (4767).

Tinea pedis (athlete's foot). Applying a garlic gel containing 1% ajoene seems to be more effective than 0.6% ajoene gel, and seems to be as effective as 1% terbinafine (Lamisil) for tinea pedis infections. Sixty days after completing one week of treatment 1% ajoene produces 100% mycologic cure, 0.6 % produces 72% mycologic cure, and 1% terbinafine produces 94% mycologic cure (4766,8019).

POSSIBLY INEFFECTIVE

Breast cancer. Taking garlic orally does not seem to decrease the risk of developing breast cancer (4779).

Diabetes. Taking garlic orally has no significant effect on glucose in persons with or without diabetes (6465,6897).

Familial hypercholesterolemia. In children with familial hyperlipidemia, taking garlic powdered extract, standardized based on alliin content, orally does not seem to significantly improve total serum cholesterol, low-density lipoprotein (LDL) or high-density lipoprotein (HDL) cholesterol levels, triglycerides, lipoprotein (a), apolipoprotein B-100, homocysteine, fibrinogen, or blood pressure (4796).

Helicobacter pylori (H pylori). Taking garlic orally for H. pylori infection used to look promising due to laboratory and epidemiological evidence showing potential activity against H. pylori. However, when garlic cloves, powder, or oil is used in humans, it doesn't seem to have any beneficial effect for treating patients infected with H. pylori (3316,3322,4761,4762,4763,4764,4765,4774).

Lung cancer. Taking garlic orally does not seem to decrease the risk of developing lung cancer (4778).

Peripheral arterial disease. After 12 weeks of treatment, taking garlic orally does not seem to improve walking distance in patients with stage II peripheral arterial occlusive disease (4801,4809).

Most clinical studies have used the brand name product Kwai (Lichtwer Pharma), a dried garlic powder preparation standardized to contain 1.3% alliin. Some studies have used the brand name product Kyolic (Wakunaga of America), an aged garlic extract standardized based on the S-allyl-L-cysteine constituent.

INSUFFICIENT RELIABLE EVIDENCE to RATE

Benign prostatic hyperplasia (BPH). There is some preliminary evidence that taking garlic orally might be helpful for improving urinary flow, decreasing urinary frequency, and other symptoms associated with BPH (10374).

Common cold. Preliminary clinical research suggests garlic might reduce the frequency and number of colds when taken prophylactically (10787).

More evidence is needed to rate garlic for these uses.

Mechanism of Action

The applicable part of garlic is the bulb. Garlic is mostly used for its antihyperlipidemic, antihypertensive, and antifungal effects. However, it is also reported to have antibacterial, anthelmintic, antiviral, antispasmodic, diaphoretic, expectorant, immunostimulant, and antithrombotic effects (3234,4366,4768,8017,8018). Many of the pharmacological effects of garlic are attributed to the allicin, ajoene, and other organosulfur constituents such as S-allyl-L-cysteine (8017).

It's thought that the effectiveness of garlic products might to be determined by their ability to yield allicin, which in turn triggers production of other active constituents (3251). Intact garlic cells in fresh garlic contain the odorless amino acid, alliin. When intact cells are broken, alliin comes into contact with the enzyme allinase in garlic, producing allicin, an unstable, odiferous compound (3251,4768). Fresh garlic contains approximately 1% alliin. One milligram of alliin is converted to 0.458 mg allicin (4800). Further conversion yields ajoene. The amount of allicin in garlic preparations is dependent upon the method of preparation. Processes that involve maceration of the garlic clove increase the activity of allicinase. Freeze-dried garlic may contain little or no allicin. To improve effectiveness, garlic preparations may be enteric coated to protect the active constituents from degeneration by stomach acid (9203). Heat and steam distillation used to produce garlic oil from crushed garlic converts allicin to allyl sulfides which are also thought to have biological activity (3251). Garlic is aged to reduce the content of other sulfur compounds and the odor commonly associated with garlic. The process to produce odorless aged garlic extract reduces the alliin content to only 3% of what is typically contained in fresh garlic (4800). Aged garlic extract is usually standardized to S-allyl-L-cysteine, another major organosulfur constituent in garlic (3234).

In patients with hyperlipidemia, garlic might lower cholesterol levels by acting as a HMG-CoA reductase inhibitor (statin) (4810,4811). There is some evidence the constituent S-allyl-L-cysteine may be a potent inhibitor of hepatic cholesterol synthesis (8407).

For age-related vascular changes and atherosclerosis, garlic is thought to be beneficial and protect vascular endothelial cells from injury by reducing oxidative stress, inhibiting low-density lipoprotein (LDL) oxidation, and through antithrombotic effects (1880,4813,8017,8408). There is evidence that LDL oxidation may be inhibited by the constituents S-allyl cysteine, S-allyl mercaptocysteine, alliin, allixin, and by N-acetyl-S-allyl cysteine, a metabolite of S-allyl cysteine (8408). Garlic appears to prevent endothelial cell depletion of glutathione, which may be responsible for its antioxidant effects (1880). Garlic powder and aged garlic preparations have been shown to have antiplatelet properties in both patients with cardiovascular disease and in healthy volunteers (1874,3234,4366,4802,4803). Garlic has been found to have antithrombotic properties and can increase fibrinolytic activity, decrease platelet aggregation and adhesion, increase the prothrombin time (PT), and inhibit metabolic enzymes in platelets responsible for the conversion of arachidonic acid into prostaglandins and other products (3234,4366,8017). Raw garlic seems to have more potent antiplatelet properties than cooked garlic (4799,4804). Garlic oil does not appear to affect platelet aggregation (4805).

For hypertension, garlic is thought to reduce blood pressure by causing smooth muscle relaxation and vasodilation by activating production of endothelium-derived relaxation factor (EDRF, nitric oxide) (4812).

There is preliminary evidence that suggests garlic and aged garlic extract may have pharmacological effects that are similar to Bacillus Calmette-Guerin (BCG) vaccine in the treatment of bladder cancer (8018). Garlic also seems to have humoral and cellular immunostimulant activity. There is evidence garlic and aged garlic extract might stimulate

T-cell proliferation; restore suppressed antibody responses; stimulate macrophage cytotoxicity and phagocytosis of tumor cells; and induce the release of interleukin-2 (IL-2), tumor necrosis factor-alpha (TNF-alpha), and gamma interferon (8018). The constituents in garlic S-allyl cysteine and S-allyl mercaptocysteine have been shown to have radical scavenging activity. S-allyl mercaptocysteine has also been shown to have activity against erythroleukemic cancer cells, breast cancer cells, and prostate cancer cells (1871,1877,1878,1879,1880,1881,1882). The constituent ajoene has been observed to induce apoptosis in human leukemia cells (8017). Laboratory evidence suggests garlic may induce detoxifying enzymes such as glutathione-S-transferase to remove harmful electrophiles from carcinogens (8017). Additionally, garlic might enhance selenium absorption and protect against tumorigenesis (4815).

The constituents allicin and ajoene are thought to be responsible for garlic's antifungal activity against tinea infections (8017,8019). Fresh garlic, but not aged garlic, has shown activity against Escherichia coli, methicillin-resistant Staph aureus, salmonella enteritidis, and Candida albicans in the laboratory; it has been suggested as a food additive to prevent food poisoning (4808). Preliminary evidence suggests that garlic compounds might have activity against viruses such as herpes simplex virus type 1, herpes simplex virus type 2, parainfluenza virus type 3, vaccinia virus, vesicular stomatitis virus, and human rhinovirus type 2 (4769).

S-allyl cysteine and S-allyl mercaptocysteine might protect the liver against acetaminophen and carbon tetrachloride, according to laboratory studies (9873). Other preliminary evidence suggests S-allyl cysteine might ameliorate doxorubicin-induced cardiac and hepatic toxicity (4780). Preliminary reports regarding possible hepatoprotective effects of aged garlic extract have been conflicting (1883,1884). Early evidence suggests a possible protective effect of aged garlic on intestinal toxicity induced by methotrexate (MTX) and fluorouracil (5FU) (1885,9208). Preliminary evidence suggests that garlic might interfere with the oral absorption of lead; the sulfur containing amino acids might chelate lead in the gastrointestinal tract (9202).

Preliminary clinical research suggests some compounds in garlic, such as S-methylcysteine sulfoxide and S-allylcysteine sulfoxide, might have some antidiabetic activity (9875). However, garlic doesn't seem to affect blood glucose in people without diabetes (9874). There are no reports of garlic affecting blood glucose in patients with diabetes.

There is some evidence that garlic might affect the cytochrome P450 enzyme system. Some findings indicate that garlic might mildly inhibit cytochrome P450 2D6 (CYP2D6) activity by about 9% in humans (1303). This limited inhibition is not likely to produce clinically significant increases in drugs that are metabolized by the CYP2D6 isoenzyme. However, researchers suspect that garlic supplements containing allicin induce the cytochrome P450 3A4 (CYP3A4) isoenzyme and can produce clinical significant decreases in levels of drugs metabolized by this enzyme (7027). An extract, containing alliin and alliinase, does not affect the activity of CYP2D6 or CYP3A4 (10335). The ability of garlic to induce or inhibit cytochrome P450 enzymes may depend upon the presence of other constituents in the preparation that is being used.

Samgyetang, a soup made from chicken, jujube, panax ginseng, garlic, and chestnuts, appears to offer protection from experimentally induced peptic ulcers (10249).

Adverse Reactions

Orally, garlic has dose-related adverse effects, which most commonly include breath and body odor, mouth and gastrointestinal burning or irritation, heartburn, flatulence, nausea, vomiting, and diarrhea. These effects can be more pronounced with consumption of raw garlic or in patients unaccustomed to eating garlic (3319,4783,4800). Oral use of garlic can also cause changes to the intestinal flora (3319,4800), which might result in gastrointestinal upset. Garlic's effect on platelet function is well known, and can possibly increase the risk of bleeding. Consumption of dietary garlic has caused platelet dysfunction, prolonged bleeding time, retrobulbar hemorrhage (bleeding behind the eye) postoperative bleeding, and spinal epidural hematoma (586,587,11325). Asthma has been reported in people working with garlic (4816,8017). Other allergic reactions associated with garlic include rhinitis, conjunctivitis, urticaria, anaphylaxis, and angioedema (6897). True IgE-mediated garlic allergy seems to be relatively rare, but can occur more often in young people with pollen allergy (4816).

Topically, exposure and application of fresh garlic has caused dermatitis, eczema, blisters, and scarring (3317,4832,4833,8017). Application of a garlic poultice has caused ulcernecrotic lesions and burns that are similar in appearance to a second or third degree burn. Lesions usually heal without scarring within 3 weeks after discontinuation of the poultice (8017).

Interactions with Herbs & Other Dietary Supplements

EICOSAPENTAENOIC ACID (EPA, Fish Oils): Concomitant use of garlic can theoretically enhance antithrombotic effects (3234,4366,8017).

HERBS WITH ANTICOAGULANT/ANTIPLATELET POTENTIAL: Concomitant use of herbs that have constituents that might affect platelet aggregation could theoretically increase the risk of bleeding in some people. These herbs include angelica, clove, danshen, ginger, ginkgo, red clover, turmeric, vitamin E, willow, and others (1874,3234,4366,4802,4803).

Interactions with Drugs

ANTICOAGULANT/ANTIPLATELET DRUGS: Garlic might enhance the effects of warfarin (Coumadin) as measured by the International Normalized Ratio (INR) (616). Theoretically, garlic might also enhance the effects and adverse effects of other anticoagulant and antiplatelet drugs, including aspirin, clopidogrel (Plavix),

enoxaparin (Lovenox), and others.
CONTRACEPTIVE DRUGS: The effect of garlic preparations on the metabolism of contraceptive drugs may vary. Some garlic preparations containing allicin might decrease the effectiveness of contraceptive drugs by increasing the activity of the cytochrome P450 3A4 (CYP3A4) isoenzyme (7027). However, other extracts, containing alliin and alliinase may not affect the activity of CYP3A4 (10335). Until more is known about this potential interaction, advise women taking garlic supplements and contraceptive drugs concurrently to use an additional or alternative form of birth control.
CYCLOSPORINE (Neoral, Sandimmune): The affect of garlic preparations on the metabolism of cyclosporine may vary. Some garlic preparations containing allicin might decrease the effectiveness of cyclosporine by increasing the activity of the cytochrome P450 3A4 (CYP3A4) isoenzyme (7027). However, other extracts, containing alliin and alliinase may not affect the activity of CYP3A4 (10335). Until more is known about this potential interaction, patients that are taking cyclosporine should avoid using garlic preparations.
CYTOCHROME P450 3A4 (CYP3A4) SUBSTRATES: It appears that some garlic preparations containing allicin may increase the activity of the cytochrome P450 3A4 (CYP3A4) isoenzymes (7027). However, other extracts, containing alliin and alliinase may not affect the activity of CYP3A4 (10335). Until more is known about this potential interaction, use caution when considering concomitant use of garlic and other drugs affected by this system. Drugs that might be affected include some calcium channel blockers (diltiazem, nicardipine, verapamil), chemotherapeutic agents (etoposide, paclitaxel, vinblastine, vincristine, vindesine), antifungals (ketoconazole, itraconazole), glucocorticoids, alfentanil (Alfenta), cisapride (Propulsid), fentanyl (Sublimaze), lidocaine (Xylocaine), losartan (Cozaar), fexofenadine (Allegra), midazolam (Versed), and others.
NON-NUCLEOSIDE REVERSE TRANSCRIPTASE INHIBITORS (NNRTIs): Some garlic preparations containing allicin may decrease plasma concentrations of the protease inhibitor saquinavir (Fortovase, Invirase) (7027). However, other extracts, containing alliin and alliinase may not affect the activity of CYP3A4 (10335). NNRTIs and protease inhibitors are metabolized through similar routes. Until more is known about this potential interaction, patients taking these medications should avoid using garlic. NNRTI-type antiretroviral drugs include nevirapine (Viramune), delavirdine (Rescriptor), and efavirenz (Sustiva).
SAQUINAVIR (Fortovase, Invirase): The effect of garlic preparations on the metabolism of saquinavir may vary. Some garlic preparations containing allicin might decrease area under the curve (AUC) of saquinavir by 51%. Peak concentrations of saquinavir might be decreased by 54% and mean levels decreased by 49%. These decreases are thought to be due to induction of the cytochrome P450 3A4 (CYP3A4) isoenzyme (7027). These subtherapeutic concentrations might cause therapeutic failure, increase development of viral resistance, and development of drug class resistance. However, other extracts, containing alliin and alliinase may not affect the activity of CYP3A4 (10335). Prolonged use (e.g., 10 days) of garlic supplements seems to be necessary for significant enzyme induction. Therefore, even occasional moderate to high consumption of garlic from dietary sources is not expected to cause a significant interaction. So far, this interaction has only been shown for saquinavir, but other protease inhibitors are also likely to be affected. Until more is known about this potential interaction, patients taking these medications should avoid taking garlic. Other protease inhibitors include amprenavir (Agenerase), nelfinavir (Viracept), and ritonavir (Norvir).
WARFARIN (Coumadin): Garlic might enhance the effects of warfarin (Coumadin) as measured by the International Normalized Ratio (INR) (616). Monitor patients using this combination closely. Dose adjustment may be necessary.

Interactions with Foods

None known.

Interactions with Lab Tests

BLOOD PRESSURE: Garlic can lower blood pressure and blood pressure readings (277,278,279).
CHOLESTEROL: Garlic can lower serum cholesterol concentrations and test results (277,278,279).
INTERNATIONAL NORMALIZED RATIO (INR), PROTHROMBIN TIME (PT): Garlic can increase INR in patients anticoagulated with warfarin (Coumadin). There are two case reports of increased INR associated with concomitant use of garlic products and warfarin (616).

Interactions with Diseases or Conditions

BLEEDING DISORDERS: Theoretically, garlic might increase the risk of bleeding (3234,4366,8017); contraindicated.
GASTROINTESTINAL (GI) IRRITATION: Garlic can irritate the GI tract; use with caution in individuals with infectious or inflammatory GI conditions (3319,4783,4800).
SURGERY: Garlic can prolong bleeding time and should be discontinued one to two weeks prior to scheduled surgery (587,4800,11325).

Dosage and Administration

ORAL: For hyperlipidemia and hypertension, garlic extract 600-1200 mg divided and given three times daily has been used in clinical trials. Most clinical studies have used a standardized garlic powder extract containing 1.3% alliin content (279,3321,4782,4783,4784,4785,4786,4787,4788,4789,4790) (4791,6457,6465,6897). Aged garlic extract 600 mg to 7.2 grams per day has also been used. Aged garlic typically contains only 0.03% alliin (1874,1875,3319,3321).

Fresh garlic 4 grams (approximately one clove) once daily has also been used. Fresh garlic typically contains 1% alliin (3319,4800). For prevention of colorectal and stomach cancer, fresh or cooked garlic 3.5-29 grams weekly has been used (3320). Garlic preparations are sometimes dosed based on the allicin constituent. For every milligram of alliin, 0.458 mg of allicin is typically generated. Therefore, a dose of garlic extract 600 mg that contains 1.3% alliin typically produces 3600 mcg allicin. A dose of fresh garlic 4 grams containing 1% alliin typically produces approximately 18,300 mcg of allicin.
TOPICAL: For tinea infections, clinical studies have used the garlic constituent ajoene as a 0.4% cream, 0.6% gel, and 1% gel applied twice daily for 1 week (4766,4767,8019).

Comments

There is some concern than marketed garlic preparations may not generate an adequate amount of the active ingredient allicin to be effective. There is a lot of variation among garlic products (9203). Some odorless garlic preparations may not contain active compounds at all (1877).

GELATIN

Also Known As

Collagen Hydrolysate, Denatured Collagen, Gelatine, Hydrolyzed Collagen Protein, Hydrolyzed Gelatin.

Scientific Names

Gelatin.

People Use This For

Orally, gelatin is used for osteoarthritis; osteoporosis; rheumatoid arthritis; weight loss; and strengthening bones, joints, and fingernails. It is also used for improving the quality of scalp hair and to shorten recovery after exercise and sports-related injury.
In manufacturing, gelatin is used for preparation of foods, cosmetics, and pharmaceuticals.

Safety

LIKELY SAFE ...when used orally in amounts commonly found in foods. Gelatin has Generally Recognized As Safe (GRAS) status in the US (4912).
POSSIBLY SAFE ...when used orally and appropriately in medicinal amounts (7704). There's some evidence that gelatin in doses up to 10 grams daily can be safely used for up to 6 months (7704). However, since gelatin is often derived from bovine bones and skin, there is some concern about contamination with diseased animal parts (1825). So far, there are no reports of disease transmission to humans due to use of contaminated gelatin preparations.
PREGNANCY AND LACTATION: There is insufficient reliable information available about the safety of gelatin during pregnancy and lactation when used in medicinal amounts.

Effectiveness

INSUFFICIENT RELIABLE EVIDENCE to RATE

Osteoarthritis. There is some clinical evidence that gelatin might relieve pain and improve joint function in patients with osteoarthritis (7704). More evidence is needed to rate gelatin for this use.

Mechanism of Action

Gelatin is a purified protein formed by hydrolysis of collagen obtained from the bones and hides of pigs and cows (7704). There is preliminary research in animal models of rheumatoid arthritis that suggests gelatin in combination with the antioxidant enzyme superoxide dismutase (SOD) might suppress joint inflammation. Oxygen radicals are thought to play a role in the joint damage caused by rheumatoid arthritis (7707).
There is preliminary research that gelatin might inhibit bone collagen breakdown in people with osteoporosis (7704). Gelatin may also cause increased production of collagen by chondrocytes. Chondrocytes are the cells responsible for maintenance of the connective tissue in the joints (10345).

Adverse Reactions

Orally, gelatin can cause unpleasant taste, sensation of heaviness in the stomach, bloating, dyspepsia, and belching (7704).
Gelatin can cause allergic reactions. Gelatin in foods can cause initial sensitization (7703).
Gelatin-containing medicines including oral medications, suppositories, vaccines, and injectable products can cause IgE-medicated allergic reactions, including urticaria, angioedema, wheezing, hypotension, and anaphylaxis (7708,7709,7710). In the US, gelatin is used as a stabilizer in some vaccines such as measles, mumps, and rubella (MMR), and diphtheria, pertussis, tetanus (DPT) (7711). Since gelatin is sometimes produced from bovine bones and skin, there is some concern about the potential risk of contamination with diseased animals and transmission of bovine spongiform encephalopathy (BSE, mad cow disease) and other diseases. Although bovine

hide and bone tissue do not seem to carry a high risk of BSE disease infectivity, in some cases manufacturing methods might lead to contamination with other diseased animal tissues. So far there are no reports of BSE or other disease transmission to humans from dietary supplements containing animal materials and the risk of potential disease transmission is thought to be low. Although many manufacturers 'guarantee' the safety of their gelatin products, most manufacturers do not seem to take adequate measures to eliminate the risk of contamination.

Interactions with Herbs & Other Dietary Supplements
None known.

Interactions with Drugs
None known.

Interactions with Foods
None known.

Interactions with Lab Tests
None known.

Interactions with Diseases or Conditions
None known.

Dosage and Administration
ORAL: For osteoporosis, 10 grams daily has been used (7704).

Comments
Gelatin-chondroitin complexes have been investigated as intra-articular drug delivery systems to treat osteoporosis and rheumatoid arthritis (7706).

GELSEMIUM

Also Known As
Caroline Jasmine, Evening Trumpet Flower, False Jasmin, Gelsemii Rhizoma, Gelsemin, Gelsemiumwurzelstock Jessamine, Trumpet Flower, Woodbine, Yellow Jasmine, Yellow Jessamine Root.
CAUTION: See separate listings for Jasmine, American Ivy, Honeysuckle, and Woodbine.

Scientific Names
Gelsemium sempervirens, synonyms Gelsemium nitidum, Bignonia sempervirens.
Family: Loganiaceae or Gelsemiaceae.

People Use This For
Orally, gelsemium is used as an analgesic for trigeminal neuralgia and migraine headaches, and for asthma and in respiratory ailments.

Safety
UNSAFE ...when the rhizome or root are used orally. All parts of the plant contain toxic alkaloids. The adult lethal dose is 2-3 grams or 4 mL of the fluid extract (18).
CHILDREN: UNSAFE ...when used orally. The lethal dose is 500 mg (18).
PREGNANCY AND LACTATION: UNSAFE ...when used orally due to toxicity (6).

Effectiveness
There is insufficient reliable information available about the effectiveness of gelsemium.

Mechanism of Action
The applicable parts of gelsemium are the rhizome and root. Researchers think the active components in gelsemium are gelsamine alkaloids and related compounds (gelsemine, gelsemicine, gelsedine) (6). Gelsemium and the principal alkaloid, gelsemine, are reported to have CNS stimulant (6), CNS depressant (9) and analgesic effects (6).

Adverse Reactions
Orally, gelsemium can cause headache, drooping of the eyelid, double vision, difficulty swallowing, dizziness, muscle weakness or rigidity, seizures, dyspnea and bradycardia. Death due to failure of respiratory muscles can occur (18).

Interactions with Herbs & Other Dietary Supplements
None known.

Interactions with Drugs
None known.

Interactions with Foods
None known.

Interactions with Lab Tests
None known.

Interactions with Diseases or Conditions
HEART DISEASE and WEAKNESS: Use of gelsemium is contraindicated in people with heart disease or weakness (18).

Dosage and Administration
ORAL: People typically use 0.3 to 1 mL gelsemium tincture (223).

Comments
There is a very narrow safety margin and medicinal preparations are considered obsolete (18). Avoid confusion with jasmine or woodbine (Clematis virginiana). Also, avoid confusing gelsemium with American ivy or honeysuckle, which are also known as woodbine.

GENISTEIN COMBINED POLYSACCHARIDE

Also Known As
Basidiomycetes Polysaccharide, Fermented Genistein, Fermented Isoflavone, Genistein Polysaccharide, GCP, Isoflavone Combined Polysaccharide, Soy Isoflavone Polysaccharide.
CAUTION: See separate listing for Soy.

Scientific Names
Genistein Combined Polysaccharide.

People Use This For
Orally, genistein combined polysaccharide is used for prostate cancer and breast cancer.

Safety
There is insufficient reliable information available about the safety of genistein combined polysaccharide.
Pregnancy and Lactation: Insufficient reliable information; avoid using.

Effectiveness
INSUFFICIENT RELIABLE EVIDENCE to RATE

Prostate cancer. There is anecdotal evidence that a patient with prostate cancer who took genistein combined polysaccharide had reduced prostate size and decreased PSA levels from 19.7 to 4.2 ng/mL after 6 weeks of treatment (12110). More evidence is needed to rate genistein combined polysaccharide for this use.

Mechanism of Action
Genistein combined polysaccharide is a soy-based product. It consists of a mixture of the soy isoflavone genistein and polysaccharide from the basidiomycetes, which are a variety of mushrooms. It is prepared by a fermentation in which a soy extract is fermented with basidiomycetes mushrooms (12110).
The fermentation process deglycosylates existing soy isoflavones in addition to forming novel isoflavones specific to this process (12110).
Both the genistein and polysaccharide components are thought to have pharmacological activity. Genistein is a phytoestrogen. It binds to beta-estrogen receptor more strongly that alpha-estrogen receptor. The beta-estrogen receptor predominates in the heart, vasculature, bone, and bladder. This might account for some of the beneficial effects attributed to phytoestrogens (3983).
Genistein seems to decrease expression of aromatase and 5-alpha reductase (12110). Some researchers suspect this might give genistein antiproliferative effects against hormone-dependent cancers such as breast cancer and prostate cancer. Genistein also seems to have antioxidant and antiangiogenic effects (3983).
Genistein is also an inhibitor of epidermal growth factor receptor tyrosine kinase (12110).

Polysaccharides from basidiomycetes are thought to have antiviral, antibacterial, antitumor, and immune modulating effects (12110).

Adverse Reactions
None reported.

Interactions with Herbs & Other Dietary Supplements
None known.

Interactions with Drugs
None known.

Interactions with Foods
None known.

Interactions with Lab Tests
None known.

Interactions with Diseases or Conditions
ESTROGEN SENSITIVE CANCERS/CONDITIONS: Genistein combined polysaccharide might have mild estrogenic effects (3983). Women with estrogen-sensitive conditions should avoid genistein combined polysaccharide. Some estrogen-sensitive conditions include breast cancer, uterine cancer, ovarian cancer, endometriosis, and uterine fibroids.

Dosage and Administration
ORAL: For prostate cancer, 1.5 grams/day has been used (12110).

GENTIAN

Also Known As
Bitter Root, Bitterwort, Gall Weed, Gentiana, Gentianae radix, Pale Gentian, Stemless Gentian, Yellow Gentian, Wild Gentian.
CAUTION: See separate listing for Canadian Hemp.

Scientific Names
Gentiana lutea; Gentiana acaulis, synonym Gentiana kochiana.
Family: Gentianaceae.

People Use This For
Orally, gentian is used for digestive disorders, such as loss of appetite, fullness, flatulence, diarrhea, gastritis, heartburn, and vomiting. It is used orally for fever, for hysteria, to stimulate menstrual flow, as an anthelmintic, and antiseptic.
Topically, gentian is used for treating wounds and cancer.
In combination with European elder flower, verbena, cowslip flower, and sorrel, gentian is used orally for maintaining healthy sinuses and treating sinusitis. It is used in combination with other products for malaria.
In foods and beverages, gentian is used as an ingredient.
In manufacturing, gentian is used in cosmetics.

Safety
LIKELY SAFE ...when the root preparations are used in amounts commonly found in foods. Gentian root has Generally Recognized As Safe (GRAS) status in the US (4912).
POSSIBLY SAFE ...when used orally in therapeutic amounts (2). ...when gentian root is used orally with European elder flower, verbena, cowslip flower, and sorrel (Quanterra Sinus Defense, Sinupret) (7,374,379).
There is insufficient reliable information available about the safety of the topical use of gentian.
PREGNANCY: LIKELY UNSAFE ...when used orally; gentian is a potential mutagen and may effect the menstrual cycle (4).
LACTATION: Insufficient reliable information available; avoid using.

Effectiveness

POSSIBLY EFFECTIVE

Sinusitis. Taking gentian orally in a specific combination product that also contains elderflower, verbena, cowslip flower, and sorrel (Quanterra Sinus Defense, Sinupret) seems help treat acute or chronic sinusitis (374,379).

There is insufficient reliable information available about the effectiveness of gentian for its other uses.

Mechanism of Action

The applicable part of gentian is the root. The bitter constituents, gentiamarin, gentiopicrin, amarogentin, and swertiamarin, seem to increase saliva and digestive juice secretion (2,4). Some evidence suggests the constituent gentianine has anti-inflammatory activity (11). The constituents, gentisin and isogentisin, are both mutagenic (4). The constituent gentiopicrin is lethal to mosquito larvae (11).

Adverse Reactions

Orally, gentian root can cause gastrointestinal (GI) irritation, nausea, and vomiting (6). It can also cause headaches in individuals sensitive to bitter substances (12).

Interactions with Herbs & Other Dietary Supplements

None known.

Interactions with Drugs

ANTACIDS: Theoretically, due to reports that gentian increases stomach acid, gentian might decrease the effectiveness of antacids (19).

H2-BLOCKERS: Theoretically, due to reports that gentian increases stomach acid, gentian might decrease the effectiveness of H2-blockers (19). The H2 blockers include cimetidine (Tagamet), ranitidine (Zantac), nizatidine (Axid), and famotidine (Pepcid).

PROTON PUMP INHIBITORS (PPIs): Theoretically, due to reports that gentian increases stomach acid, gentian might decrease the effectiveness of PPIs (19). PPIs include omeprazole (Prilosec), lansoprazole (Prevacid), rabeprazole (Aciphex), pantoprazole (Protonix), and esomeprazole (Nexium).

Interactions with Foods

None known.

Interactions with Lab Tests

None known.

Interactions with Diseases or Conditions

DUODENAL AND GASTRIC ULCERS: Contraindicated due to bitter constituents (2).

GASTRIC IRRITATION OR INFLAMMATION: Contraindicated due to bitter constituents (12).

HYPERTENSION: Gentian root may not be well-tolerated in hypertensive individuals (5).

Dosage and Administration

ORAL: The typical dose of gentian is 0.6-2 grams of the dried root three times daily with a maximum of 4 grams per day. One cup of the tea is also taken three times daily (2,4,18). The tea is prepared by steeping 0.6-2 grams of the dried root in 150 mL boiling water for 5-10 minutes and then straining (2,4,18). The tea can be sweetened with honey. The common dose of the tincture (1:5 in 45% alcohol) is 1-3 grams daily (2) or 1-4 mL three times daily (4). The usual dose of the fluid extract is 2-4 grams daily (2). The irritating qualities of the gentian root are minimized in the tea and maximized in the tincture form (12).

For acute or chronic sinusitis, two Sinupret tablets three times daily for up to two weeks has been used in clinical trials (7,374,379), equivalent to gentian root 12 mg, European elder flower 36 mg, verbena 36 mg, cowslip flower 36 mg, and sorrel 36 mg three times daily.

TOPICAL: No typical dosage.

Comments

The highly toxic white hellebore (Veratrum album) can grow in proximity to gentian and has caused accidental poisoning when used in home-made preparations (11). A related Gentiana species is used in Chinese medicine for treating jaundice, headache, sores, inflammation, and rheumatoid arthritis (11). The gentian root is unrelated to the gentian violet dye.

GERMAN CHAMOMILE

Also Known As

Blue Chamomile, Camomilla, Camomille Allemande, Chamomilla, Chamomile, Echte Kamille, Feldkamille, Fleur de Camomile, Hungarian Chamomile, Kamillen, Kleine Kamille, Manzanilla, Matricaire, Matricariae Flos, Pin Heads, Sweet False Chamomile, True Chamomile, Wild Chamomile.
CAUTION: See separate listing for Roman Chamomile.

Scientific Names

Matricaria recutita, synonyms Chamomilla recutita, Matricaria chamomilla.
Family: Asteraceae/Compositae.

People Use This For

Orally, German chamomile is used for flatulence, travel sickness, nasal mucous membrane inflammation, allergic rhinitis, nervous diarrhea, attention deficit-hyperactivity disorder (ADHD), restlessness, and insomnia. It is also used for gastrointestinal (GI) spasms, inflammatory diseases of the GI tract, GI ulcers associated with nonsteroidal anti-inflammatory drugs (NSAIDs) and alcohol consumption, and as an antispasmodic for menstrual cramps.
Topically, German chamomile is used for hemorrhoids; mastitis; leg ulcers; skin, anogenital, and mucous membrane inflammation; and bacterial skin diseases, including those of the mouth and gums. It is also used topically for treating or preventing chemotherapy- or radiation-induced oral mucositis.
As an inhalant, German chamomile is used to treat inflammation and irritation of the respiratory tract.
In foods and beverages, German chamomile is used as flavor components.
In manufacturing, German chamomile is used in cosmetics, soaps, and mouthwashes.

Safety

LIKELY SAFE ...when used orally in amounts commonly found in foods. German chamomile has Generally Recognized As Safe (GRAS) status in the US (4912).
POSSIBLY SAFE ...when preparations of the flower are used orally in medicinal amounts short-term (12).
POSSIBLY UNSAFE ...when used orally as highly concentrated hot tea because it can cause vomiting (12).
...when used topically; avoid applying it near the eyes (10377).
PREGNANCY AND LACTATION: Insufficient reliable information available; avoid using.

Effectiveness

POSSIBLY EFFECTIVE

Oral mucositis. Using a German chamomile oral rinse (Kamillosan Liquidum) might help prevent or treat mucositis induced by radiation therapy and some types of chemotherapy (6655). German chamomile oral rinse seems to prevent or treat mucositis secondary to radiation therapy and some types of chemotherapy including asparaginase (Elspar), cisplatin (CDDP, Platinol-AQ), cyclophosphamide (Cytoxan, Neosar), daunorubicin (DaunoXome), doxorubicin (Adriamycin, Rubex), etoposide (VP-16, Etopophos, VePesid, Toposar), hydroxyurea (Hydrea), mercaptopurine (6-MP, Purinethol), methotrexate (MTX, Rheumatrex), procarbazine (MIH, Mutlane), and vincristine (VCR, Oncovin, Vincasar) (6655). However, the rinse doesn't seem to be better than placebo for preventing fluorouracil (5-FU)-induced oral mucositis (6656).

POSSIBLY INEFFECTIVE

Dermatitis. Applying German chamomile cream topically does not seem to prevent dermatitis induced by cancer radiation therapy (9767).

Some clinical studies have used German chamomile extracts and flowers standardized to 1.2% apigenin.

Mechanism of Action

The applicable part of German chamomile is the flowerhead. Active constituents of German chamomile include quercetin, apigenin, and coumarins, and the essential oils matricin, chamazulene, alpha bisaboloid, and bisaboloid oxides (10377).
Chamomile extract can inhibit the enzymes cyclooxygenase and lipooxygenase, which reduces the production of prostaglandins and leukotrienes. Quercetin and apigenin can inhibit histamine release from mast cells that are antigen stimulated (10377).
Apigenin can bind to gamma-aminobutyric acid (GABA) receptors. GABA receptors are the primary receptor sites of benzodiazepines in the central nervous system. Preliminary evidence suggests that apigenin can exert sedative action by binding to GABA receptors (9765).

Adverse Reactions

Orally, highly concentrated German chamomile tea can cause vomiting (12). It can cause allergic reactions including severe hypersensitivity reactions and anaphylaxis (567). Animal studies suggest no toxicity or teratogenicity of bisabolol, the main active constituent of German chamomile (8178). German chamomile can cause an allergic reaction in individuals sensitive to the Asteraceae/Compositae family. Members of this family include ragweed,

chrysanthemums, marigolds, daisies, and many other herbs.
Topically, German chamomile may cause allergic dermatitis and eczema (9766,9768,10377). If used near the eyes, it can be irritating (10377).

Interactions with Herbs & Other Dietary Supplements

HERBS WITH SEDATIVE PROPERTIES: Theoretically, concomitant use with herbs that have sedative properties might enhance therapeutic and adverse effects. Some of these supplements include 5-HTP, calamus, California poppy, catnip, hops, Jamaican dogwood, kava, St. John's wort, scullcap, valerian, yerba mansa, and others.

Interactions with Drugs

BENZODIAZEPINES: Theoretically, concomitant use with benzodiazepines might cause additive effects and side effects (19).
CNS DEPRESSANTS: Theoretically, concomitant use with drugs with sedative properties can cause additive effects and side effects (19).
CYTOCHROME P450 3A4 (CYP3A4) SUBSTRATES: There's preliminary evidence that suggests that German chamomile might inhibit the cytochrome P450 3A4 (CYP3A4) isoenzymes (6450). Theoretically, German chamomile might increase levels of drugs metabolized by CYP3A4. However, so far, this interaction has not been reported in humans. Some drugs metabolized by CYP3A4 include lovastatin (Mevacor), ketoconazole (Nizoral), itraconazole (Sporanox), fexofenadine (Allegra), triazolam (Halcion), and numerous others. Use German chamomile cautiously or avoid in patients taking these drugs.

Interactions with Foods

None known.

Interactions with Lab Tests

None known.

Interactions with Diseases or Conditions

ASTHMA: German chamomile may exacerbate this condition (4).
CROSS-ALLERGENICITY: German chamomile may cause an allergic reaction in individuals sensitive to the Asteraceae/Compositae family. Members of this family include ragweed, chrysanthemums, marigolds, daisies, and many other herbs.

Dosage and Administration

ORAL: The typical dose of German chamomile is 2-8 grams of the dried flower heads three times daily (4) or one cup of the tea three to four times daily. The tea is prepared by steeping 3 grams of the dried flower heads in 150 mL boiling water for 5-10 minutes and then straining (2). The liquid extract (1:1 in 45% alcohol) is commonly dosed as 1-4 mL three times daily (4). Clinical studies on the effectiveness of German chamomile have used extracts and flowers standardized to 1.2% apigenin.
TOPICAL: German chamomile is used as a poultice and as a rinse. The freshly prepared tea (steep 4 teaspoons of the dried flower heads in 1.5 cups boiling water for 15 minutes and then strain) is commonly used topically as well (18). The 3-10% ointments and gels are for external use only (18). Avoid topical use near the eyes (12). For inflammation of mucous membranes of the mouth and throat, the freshly prepared tea is commonly used as a mouthwash or gargle (2). For chemotherapy- or radiation-induced oral mucositis, an oral rinse made with 10-15 drops of German chamomile liquid extract in 100 ml warm water has been used three times daily (6655).
INHALATION: No typical dosage.

Comments

Avoid confusion with Roman chamomile. Although ointments, creams, and lotions containing the volatile oil of chamomile are intended for the treatment of various skin conditions and are used in Europe, they have not been approved in the US (3).

GERMAN IPECAC

Also Known As

Swallow wort.
CAUTION: See separate listing for Pleurisy Root.

Scientific Names

Vincetoxicum hirundinaria, synonyms Cynanchum vincetoxicum, Asclepias vincetoxicum, Vincetoxicum officinale.
Family: Apocynaceae or Asclepiadaceae.

People Use This For
Orally, German ipecac is used for digestive and kidney disorders, dysmenorrhea, edema, the plague, snake bite, as a diuretic, emetic, and diaphoretic.
Topically, German ipecac is used in poultices for healing swelling and bruising.

Safety
POSSIBLY UNSAFE ...when used orally (18).
There is insufficient reliable information available about the safety of German ipecac for its other uses.
PREGNANCY AND LACTATION: POSSIBLY UNSAFE ...when used orally (18); avoid using.

Effectiveness
There is insufficient reliable information available about the effectiveness of German ipecac.

Mechanism of Action
The applicable parts of German ipecac are the leaf and root/rhizome. There is insufficient reliable information available about the possible mechanism of action and active ingredients.

Adverse Reactions
Orally, high doses of German ipecac may cause vomiting, apnea, and cardiac arrest. Seed extracts may cause advancing paralysis of the central nervous system (18).

Interactions with Herbs & Other Dietary Supplements
None known.

Interactions with Drugs
None known.

Interactions with Foods
None known.

Interactions with Lab Tests
None known.

Interactions with Diseases or Conditions
None known.

Dosage and Administration
No typical dosage.

GERMAN SARSAPARILLA

Also Known As
Caricis rhizoma, Red Wheatgrass, Red Sage, Sandriedgraswurzelstock, Sand Sedge, Sea Sedge.
CAUTION: See separate listings for Sarsaparilla, Sage, and Wheatgrass.

Scientific Names
Carex arenaria.
Family: Cyperaceae.

Comments
At the date of publication, this product was not a common ingredient used in brand name supplements marketed to consumers. Details about this product are available at the online version of *Natural Medicines Comprehensive Database*. See www.naturaldatabase.com.

GERMANDER

Also Known As
Wall Germander, Wild Germander.

Scientific Names
Teucrium chamaedrys.
Family: Lamiaceae/Labiatae.

People Use This For
Orally, germander is used orally for treating gallbladder conditions, fever, stomachaches, mild diarrhea, as a digestive aid, an adjunct for weight loss, an antiseptic, and as "a rinse for gout."
Topically, germander is used as a mouthwash for oral hygiene.
In manufacturing, germander is used as a flavoring agent in alcoholic beverages.

Safety
LIKELY UNSAFE ...when used orally. Germander is associated with multiple cases of hepatitis and death (271,3741,3742,3743,3744). France has banned its sale (17). Canada does not allow germander to be included in oral products as a non-medicinal ingredient (12). However, the US still allows germander to be used in small amounts as a flavoring agent in alcoholic beverages (12).
PREGNANCY AND LACTATION: LIKELY UNSAFE ...when used orally (271,3741,3742,3743,3744).

Effectiveness
There is insufficient reliable information available about the effectiveness of germander.

Mechanism of Action
The applicable parts of germander are the above ground parts. Germander contains teucrin A, a diterpene, which causes hepatic necrosis in mice (3740).

Adverse Reactions
Orally, germander has been associated with hepatitis, liver cell necrosis, and death (271,3741,3742,3743,3744).

Interactions with Herbs & Other Dietary Supplements
None known.

Interactions with Drugs
None known.

Interactions with Foods
None known.

Interactions with Lab Tests
None known.

Interactions with Diseases or Conditions
None known.

Dosage and Administration
No typical dosage.

GERMANIUM

Also Known As
Bis-Carboxyethyl Germanium Sesquioxide, Carboxyethylgermanium Sesquioxide, Ge-132, GE-132, Ge-Oxy 132, Germanium Lactate Citrate, Inorganic Germanium, Organic Germanium, Spirogermanium.

Scientific Names
Germanium; Ge; atomic number 32; Bis-carboxyethyl germanium sesquioxide; Germanium lactate citrate.

People Use This For

Orally, germanium is used for osteoarthritis, pain relief, osteoporosis, low energy, AIDS, cancer, high blood pressure, high cholesterol, heart disease, glaucoma, and cataracts. It is used orally for rheumatoid arthritis (RA), depression, hepatitis, cirrhosis, food allergies, candidiasis, chronic viral infections, and heavy metal poisoning (including mercury, cadmium). Germanium is also used orally for increasing circulation of blood to the brain, supporting the immune system, and as an antioxidant.

Safety

LIKELY UNSAFE ...when used orally; avoid using. There have been more than 30 reports of renal failure, hepatic steatosis, myopathy, lactic acidosis, or death caused by ingestion of 15-300 grams over 2 to 36 months (2360,10040,10041,10042,10043,10044,10052,10072,10073,10074).
PREGNANCY AND LACTATION: LIKELY UNSAFE ...when used orally due to reported toxicity (2360,10051); avoid using.

Effectiveness

INSUFFICIENT RELIABLE EVIDENCE to RATE

Cancer. Researchers are interested in germanium as an alternative or palliative treatment for various kinds of cancer including breast cancer, colon cancer, prostate cancer, ovary cancer, head and neck cancer, and lung cancer (10035,10037,10038,10039,10049,10050). One case report showed complete remission of pulmonary spindle cell carcinoma after treatment with oral germanium sesquioxide (10037). However, the majority of research in phase I and phase II trials suggests that germanium is unsafe for use due to various life-threatening side-effects (10035,10038,10039,10072,10073,10074). More evidence is needed to rate the effectiveness of germanium for this use.

Mechanism of Action

Germanium is considered an ultra-trace element, with an atomic number of 32. Preliminary research suggests that germanium might have anti-viral, anti-inflammatory, and immunological properties. It may also have antioxidant properties. However, the exact mechanisms are poorly understood (10046,10048,10051). Animal studies indicate that germanium accumulates in the tissues of the body, especially in the nerves and kidneys, after long-term exposure (10034). Germanium deficiency might be a contributing factor in the etiology of Kashin-Beck disease (10047).

Adverse Reactions

Orally, germanium can cause renal tubular degeneration, renal failure, anemia, muscle weakness, myopathy, hepatic steatosis, peripheral neuropathy, lactic acidosis, and death (2360,10040,10041,10042,10043,10044,10045,10052,10072,10073,10074).

Interactions with Herbs & Other Dietary Supplements

None known.

Interactions with Drugs

FUROSEMIDE (Lasix): There is one case report of furosemide resistance associated with a ginseng product containing germanium (770).

Interactions with Foods

None known.

Interactions with Lab Tests

None known.

Interactions with Diseases or Conditions

None known.

Dosage and Administration

No typical dosage.

GINGER

Also Known As

African Ginger, Black Ginger, Cochin Ginger, Gingembre, Ginger Root, Imber, Jamaica Ginger, Jiang, Race Ginger, Shoga, Sunthi, Zingiber officinalis, Zingiberis rhizoma.

Scientific Names

Zingiber officinale, synonym Amomum zingiber. Family: Zingiberaceae.

People Use This For

Orally, ginger is used for motion sickness, morning sickness, colic, dyspepsia, flatulence, chemotherapy-induced nausea, rheumatoid arthritis (RA), osteoarthritis, loss of appetite, post-surgical nausea and vomiting, migraine headache, and for discontinuing selective serotonin reuptake inhibitor (SSRI) drug therapy. It is also used orally for anorexia, upper respiratory tract infections, cough, bronchitis, as a galactagogue, diaphoretic, diuretic, as a stimulant; and for treating stomachache, diarrhea, nausea, cholera, and bleeding. Fresh ginger is used orally for treating acute bacterial dysentery, baldness, malaria, orchitis, poisonous snake bites, rheumatism, and toothaches.
Topically, the fresh juice of ginger is used for treating thermal burns. The essential oil of ginger is used topically as an analgesic.
In foods and beverages, ginger is used as a flavoring agent.
In manufacturing, ginger is used as a fragrance component in soaps and cosmetics. The oleoresin of ginger is also used as an ingredient in digestive, laxative, antitussive, antiflatulent, and antacid preparations.

Safety

LIKELY SAFE ...when used orally in amounts commonly found in foods. Ginger, ginger extract, and ginger oil have Generally Recognized As Safe (GRAS) status in the US (4912). ...when used topically (4,11).
POSSIBLY SAFE ...when used orally and appropriately in medicinal amounts (721,722,723,5343,7048,7400).
PREGNANCY: POSSIBLY SAFE ...when used orally for medicinal purposes. Using ginger during pregnancy is controversial (1921,7083). There is concern due to preliminary evidence that ginger might affect fetal sex hormones (7083), and an anecdotal report of spontaneous abortion during the twelfth week of pregnancy in a patient who used ginger for morning sickness (721). However, studies in pregnant women suggest that ginger can be used safely for morning sickness without harm to the fetus. The risk for major malformations in infants of women taking ginger does not appear to be higher than the baseline rate of 1-3% (721,1922,5343,11346). As with any medication given during pregnancy, the potential benefit to risk must be weighed.
LACTATION: Insufficient reliable information available: avoid using amounts greater than those found in foods.

Effectiveness

POSSIBLY EFFECTIVE

Chemotherapy-induced nausea. There is some evidence that taking ginger orally might help prevent chemotherapy-induced nausea when given following administration of intravenous (IV) prochlorperazine (Compazine) (1919).
Morning sickness. Ginger taken orally seems to reduce feelings of nausea in some pregnant patients with morning sickness (721,1922,5343,11346). The decision to use ginger (or any drug) during pregnancy should be based on possible benefit compared to potential risk.
Postoperative nausea and vomiting. Taking ginger orally seems to be effective for preventing postoperative nausea and vomiting in the absence of narcotic anesthesia or analgesia (722,723,1919). There is some evidence that ginger might be as effective as metoclopramide (Reglan) for reducing postsurgical nausea and vomiting in patients not concurrently receiving anesthesia or narcotic analgesia (722,723,1919). However, taking ginger orally doesn't prevent postoperative nausea and vomiting in the presence of narcotic anesthesia or analgesia (3452,3453).
Vertigo. One gram of ginger taken orally may reduce symptoms of vertigo, including nausea; however, nystagmus is not reduced (7623).

POSSIBLY INEFFECTIVE

Motion sickness. Taking ginger orally, 500 mg to 1000 mg, up to 4 hours prior to travel does not seem to prevent motion sickness (7624,7625). Some patients report subjective feelings of improvement, but objective measures are not significantly affected by ginger (7400).

INSUFFICIENT RELIABLE EVIDENCE to RATE

Migraine headache. Anecdotal evidence suggests that ginger might reduce the severity and duration of migraine headache (7623).
Osteoarthritis. There is preliminary evidence that ginger might offer very modest benefits in osteoarthritis. Two studies have evaluated a specific ginger extract (Eurovita Extract 33; EV ext-33) taken orally 170 mg three times daily or 255 mg twice daily (510 mg total daily dose) for 3-6 weeks (7048,7084). Ginger might modestly improve pain after standing or walking and joint stiffness in some patients, but it does not seem to significantly improve functionality, quality of life, or use of relief analgesics (7084,7085). Ginger does reduce pain as well as ibuprofen 400 mg three times daily (7048).
Rheumatoid arthritis (RA). There is some preliminary evidence that ginger might be helpful for decreasing joint pain in patients with RA (7401).
More evidence is needed to rate ginger for these uses.

Mechanism of Action

The applicable parts of ginger are the rhizome and root. Ginger contains active constituents known as gingerols and gingerdione. These constituents seem to have a variety of pharmacological properties including antipyretic, analgesic, antitussive, cardiac inotropic, sedative, antibiotic, weak antifungal, and other properties (7628). However, all of these pharmacological effects may not occur when whole ginger preparations are used. For example, whole ginger-containing products do not seem to have antipyretic effects (6131).

The mechanism by which ginger reduces nausea and vomiting might be due to the 6-gingerol constituent (1924). It was once thought that ginger might work by increasing gastrointestinal (GI) motility (1923), but more recent evidence shows that ginger does not influence GI emptying time (7621,7624). Other ginger constituents such as 6-shogaol and galanolactone seem to act on serotonin receptors (1924). Galanolactone seems to act primarily on 5-HT3 receptors in the ileum, which are the same receptors affected by some prescription antiemetics such as ondansetron (Zofran). The predominant antiemetic action of ginger is localized in the GI tract, but there is some evidence that ginger constituents may also have central nervous system (CNS) activity (1924).

Ginger is sometimes used for inflammatory conditions such as rheumatoid arthritis (RA). Some researchers speculate that certain constituents of ginger might inhibit cyclooxygenase (COX) and lipoxygenase pathways (7401). The ginger constituent 6-gingerol, does seem to have anti-inflammatory effects, but the whole ginger preparation may not (6131).

There is preliminary evidence that ginger may also have hypoglycemic, hypotensive or hypertensive, hypocholesterolemic, anthelmintic, gastroprotective, and antiplatelet effects (11). The antiplatelet effect of ginger is exerted by its ability to inhibit platelet thromboxane (7622).

There is very preliminary evidence that some extracts and constituents of ginger might have mutagenic properties. However, these constituents may only be mutagenic when in the presence of other mutagens. Other ginger constituents such as zingerone have the opposite effect and are antimutagenic. Whole ginger preparations may not have mutagenic effects (11299). Animal research hasn't shown any evidence of teratogenicity (11297,11298). However, one study did find evidence of embryo mortality (11298).

Ginger inhibits thromboxane synthetase. This could affect testosterone receptor binding in the fetus and theoretically affect sex steroid differentiation of the fetal brain (7083). However, this has not been seen in animals or humans.

Adverse Reactions

Orally, ginger is usually well tolerated when used in typical doses. However, higher doses of 5 grams per day increase the risk of side effects and decrease tolerability (7622). Common side effects of ginger include abdominal discomfort, heartburn, diarrhea, and a pepper-like irritant effect in the mouth and throat (5343,7400). Large overdoses can cause central nervous system (CNS) depression and cardiac arrhythmias (5).

Topically, ginger can cause dermatitis in sensitive individuals (4).

Interactions with Herbs & Other Dietary Supplements

HERBS WITH ANTICOAGULANT/ANTIPLATELET POTENTIAL: Concomitant use of herbs that have constituents that might affect platelet aggregation could theoretically increase the risk of bleeding in some people. These herbs include angelica, clove, danshen, garlic, ginkgo, Panax ginseng, red clover, turmeric, and others.

Interactions with Drugs

ANTACIDS: Theoretically, due to reports that ginger increases stomach acid, ginger might decrease the effectiveness of antacids (19).

ANTICOAGULANT/ANTIPLATELET DRUGS: Theoretically, excessive amounts of ginger might increase the risk of bleeding. Ginger is thought to inhibit thromboxane synthetase and decrease in platelet aggregation (4,6048).

ANTIDIABETES DRUGS: Theoretically, ginger might interfere with diabetes therapy due to hypoglycemic effects (4).

ANTIHYPERTENSIVE DRUGS: Theoretically, ginger might interfere with antihypertensive blood pressure therapy due to the cardiac stimulant effects of ginger (7628).

BARBITURATES: Theoretically, ginger might enhance barbiturate effects (6). Some of these sedative medications include pentobarbital (Nembutal), phenobarbital (Luminal), secobarbital (Seconal), and others.

H2-BLOCKERS: Theoretically, due to reports that ginger increases stomach acid, ginger might decrease the effectiveness of H2-blockers (19). The H2 blockers include cimetidine (Tagamet), ranitidine (Zantac), nizatidine (Axid), and famotidine (Pepcid).

PROTON PUMP INHIBITORS (PPIs): Theoretically, due to reports that ginger increases stomach acid, ginger might decrease the effectiveness of PPIs (19). PPIs include omeprazole (Prilosec), lansoprazole (Prevacid), rabeprazole (Aciphex), pantoprazole (Protonix), and esomeprazole (Nexium).

Interactions with Foods

None known.

Interactions with Lab Tests

None known.

Interactions with Diseases or Conditions

BLEEDING CONDITIONS: Theoretically, excessive doses of ginger can interfere with these conditions and increase risk of bleeding (4).

DIABETES: Theoretically, excessive doses of ginger can cause hypoglycemia, necessitating a change in dose of diabetes medication (4).

GALLSTONES: Individuals with gallstones should not use ginger except after medical evaluation determines ginger will not make gallstone symptoms worse (12).

HEART CONDITIONS: Theoretically, excessive doses of ginger might have cardiotonic activity that can interfere with therapy for heart conditions (4).
HIGH BLOOD PRESSURE, LOW BLOOD PRESSURE: Theoretically, excessive doses of ginger might increase or reduce blood pressure, interfering with blood pressure control (4).

Dosage and Administration

ORAL: For morning sickness, 250 mg ginger 4 times daily has been used in studies (721,5343). For motion sickness, 1 gram of dried powdered ginger root 30 minutes to 4 hours before travel has been used (1919,7400). For osteoarthritis, a specific ginger extract (Eurovita Extract 33; EV ext-33), 170 mg three times daily or 255 mg twice daily has been used (7048,7084). For nausea and disequilibrium resulting from selective serotonin reuptake inhibitor (SSRI) discontinuation or tapering, 550-1100 mg ginger 3 times daily has been used (3451). For preventing postoperative nausea and vomiting, 1 gram powdered ginger root 1 hour before induction of anesthesia has been used (722,723). For migraine headache, ginger 500 mg at the onset and repeated every 4 hours up to 1.5 to 2 grams per day for 3 to 4 days has been used (7623). For chemotherapy-induced nausea, powdered ginger 2-4 grams daily has been used (1920). A ginger tea has also been used and is typically prepared and taken on the day of chemotherapy and continued for as long as needed (1920). As a general anti-emetic, powdered root 2 grams daily is typically used (1920).
It is generally recommended that doses not exceed 4 grams per day (1920). Ginger tea is prepared by steeping 0.5-1 gram dried root in 150 mL boiling water for 5-10 minutes and then straining (4,18). Tinctures are typically taken in doses of 0.25-3 mL (4).
TOPICAL: No typical dosage.

Comments

Ginger is commonly found in the warmer climates, including India, Jamaica, and China. Its flowers are similar to orchids. The rhizome is used as the source for the dried, powder spice.

GINKGO leaf (GINKGO leaf extract)

Also Known As

Adiantifolia, Bai Guo Ye, Fossil Tree, Ginkgo Folium, Japanese Silver Apricot, Kew Tree, Maidenhair Tree, Salisburia Adiantifolia, Yinhsing.
CAUTION: See separate listing for Ginkgo seed.

Scientific Names

Ginkgo biloba.
Family: Ginkgoaceae.

People Use This For

Orally, ginkgo leaf is used for dementia, including Alzheimer's, vascular, and mixed dementia. Ginkgo leaf is also used orally for conditions associated with cerebral vascular insufficiency, especially in the elderly, including memory loss, headache, tinnitus, vertigo, dizziness, difficulty concentrating, mood disturbances, and hearing disorders. It is also used orally for relief of walking pain associated with intermittent claudication, particularly in patients with Fontaine's stage IIa or IIb peripheral arterial occlusive disease. Ginkgo leaf is also used orally to treat sexual dysfunction and to reverse sexual dysfunction caused by SSRI antidepressants. It is also used orally for cognitive disorders secondary to depression; eye problems, including macular degeneration and glaucoma; attention deficit-hyperactivity disorder (ADHD); thrombosis; heart disease; arteriosclerosis; angina pectoris; hypercholesterolemia; cardiac reperfusion injury; premenstrual syndrome (PMS); dysentery and filariasis; and diabetic retinopathy. Ginkgo leaf is also used orally to improve cognitive behavior and sleep patterns in patients with depression, and for the prevention of winter depression. Ginkgo leaf is also used orally for preventing acute mountain sickness and aging, regulating gastric acidity, improving liver and gallbladder function, regulating bacterial flora, controlling blood pressure, and treating Raynaud's disease. It is also used orally to treat asthma, allergies, bronchitis, and for various disorders of the central nervous system.
In combination with Panax ginseng, ginkgo leaf is used orally to enhance memory and improve symptoms of attention deficit-hyperactivity disorder (ADHD).
Topically, ginkgo leaf is used to wash chilblains, which are lesions on the fingers, toes, heels, ears, and nose caused by exposure to extreme cold. It is also used topically in wound dressings to improve circulation in the skin.
Intravenously, ginkgo leaf is used to increase cerebral blood flow, improve cognition, for psychiatric conditions in the elderly, and for metastatic colorectal cancer.
In manufacturing, ginkgo leaf extract has been used in cosmetics.

Safety

LIKELY SAFE ...when used orally and appropriately. Standardized ginkgo leaf extracts have been used safely in trials lasting from several weeks to a year (1514,1515,3461,5717,5718,6211,6212,6213,6214,6215,6216,6222,6223,6224,6225,6490). Tell

patients to avoid crude ginkgo plant parts; which can exceed concentrations of 5 ppm of the toxic ginkgolic acid constituents, and can cause severe allergic reactions (5714).
POSSIBLY SAFE ...when used intravenously. Ginkgo extract EGb 761 given intravenously seems to be safe for short-term use for up to 10 days (9871,9872).
There is insufficient reliable information available about the safety of ginkgo leaf when used topically.
PREGNANCY AND LACTATION: Insufficient reliable information available; avoid using.

Effectiveness

POSSIBLY EFFECTIVE

Age-related memory impairment. Taking ginkgo leaf extract orally seems to improve cognitive function in some elderly people with mild to moderate age-related memory impairment. Ginkgo leaf extract might modestly improve some measures of cognitive function, particularly short-term visual memory and possibly speed of cognitive processing, in non-demented patients with age-related memory impairment (5717,6216). But taking ginkgo leaf extract doesn't seem to improve memory in people over the age of 60 with normal mental function (5718,8586,8587,8588). Tell cognitively healthy older patients ginkgo probably won't help forgetfulness.

Altitude sickness. In mountain climbers, taking ginkgo leaf extract orally 80 mg twice daily seems to significantly reduce the occurrence of symptoms of acute altitude sickness including headache, fatigue, dyspnea, nausea, and vomiting. Ginkgo leaf extract also seems to improve cold tolerance by approximately 23% (6230).

Cognitive function. Taking ginkgo leaf extract orally seems to improve some measures of cognitive function in healthy young to middle-aged people. Ginkgo might modestly improve memory and speed of cognitive processing, including increasing speed of performance on factors assessing attention in people with no complaints of memory impairment (6214,6215,8236,8544,8588,9759). Lower doses of 120-240 mg per day seem to be as effective or more effective than higher doses up to 600 mg per day (6214,8236,8588). Some evidence suggests a combination of Panax ginseng and ginkgo is effective for enhancing memory and that the combination might be more effective than either product alone (1903,8591).

Dementia. Taking ginkgo leaf orally seems to modestly improve symptoms of Alzheimer's, vascular, or mixed dementias. Studies lasting from 3 months to a year show that ginkgo leaf extract can stabilize or improve some measures of cognitive function and social functioning in patients with multiple types of dementia (1514,1515,2665,2666,6222,6223,6225). Although there is one report with conflicting findings (5720), the majority of evidence indicates that ginkgo leaf extract can be modestly helpful. Some researchers suggest that the improvement with ginkgo leaf extract is roughly equivalent to a six-month delay in disease progression (1514). However, outcome studies have not yet verified ginkgo's effects on disease progression. Doses ranging from 120 mg to 240 mg daily have been beneficial after six to eight weeks of treatment. German practitioners consider ginkgo leaf extract the treatment of choice for dementia (6491). However, ginkgo leaf extract has not been directly compared to conventional medicines for dementia. Improvement appears to be less than that found with the prescription drugs donepezil (Aricept), tacrine (Cognex), and other cholinesterase inhibitors. Reserve ginkgo for patients who cannot take cholinesterase inhibitors (1514,1515,6224,6490,11981).

Diabetic retinopathy. There is some evidence that taking ginkgo leaf extract orally for six months can significantly improve measures of color vision in patients with early diabetic retinopathy (6175).

Glaucoma. Taking ginkgo leaf extract orally seems to improve pre-existing damage to the visual field in patients with normal tension glaucoma (10378).

Intermittent claudication. Taking ginkgo leaf orally seems to increase pain-free walking distance in patients with Fontaine's IIb peripheral arterial occlusive disease and intermittent claudication (3461,6211,6212,6213). Although significant benefit has been found with doses as low as 120-160 mg per day (6211), there is some evidence that a higher dose of 240 mg per day might be more beneficial in some patients (3461,6212).

Premenstrual syndrome (PMS). Taking ginkgo leaf extract orally seems to produce significant relief in breast tenderness and neuropsychological symptoms associated with PMS when started during the 16th day of the menstrual cycle and continued until the 5th day of the following cycle (6229).

Raynaud's syndrome. Taking ginkgo leaf extract orally seems to decrease the number of painful attacks per week in patients with Raynaud's syndrome (11363).

Vertigo. Taking ginkgo leaf orally seems to improve symptoms of vertigo and equilibrium disorders (6208,6220,6221). There is evidence from two clinical studies that ginkgo leaf extract is significantly more effective than placebo (6220) and possibly as effective as betahistine for improving vertigo and dizziness caused by vascular vestibular disorders and vestibular disorders of unknown origin (6220,6221).

POSSIBLY INEFFECTIVE

Antidepressant-induced sexual dysfunction. Although some preliminary clinical research suggests taking ginkgo leaf extract orally might help sexual dysfunction caused by antidepressant therapy (3965,3967), subsequent research indicates that it is probably ineffective (207,3966,3969,10893).

Seasonal affective disorder (SAD). Taking ginkgo leaf extract orally doesn't seem to prevent winter depression symptoms in patients with SAD (8233).

Tinnitus. Taking ginkgo leaf extract orally doesn't seem to improve symptoms of tinnitus. Some studies have shown benefit, but the majority of evidence indicates that ginkgo leaf extract is not consistently effective for patients with tinnitus (221,910,6208,6218,6219,9871).

Most of the clinical studies on the effectiveness of ginkgo leaf have used the standardized extracts Egb 761

(Tanakan) and LI 1370 (Lichtwer Pharma). These two extracts are similar and prepared to contain approximately 24% to 25% flavone glycosides and 6% terpene lactones. Products with similar ingredients include Ginkai (Lichtwer Pharma), Ginkgo 5 (Pharmline), Ginkgold and Ginkgo (Nature's Way), and Quanterra Mental Sharpness (Warner-Lambert).

INSUFFICIENT RELIABLE EVIDENCE to RATE

Age-related macular degeneration (AMD). Preliminary clinical research suggests that taking ginkgo leaf extract orally might improve symptoms of AMD (6227,6228,11797). There is limited evidence that ginkgo leaf extract might significantly improve distance vision in patients with AMD (6227).

Attention deficit-hyperactivity disorder (ADHD). There is preliminary evidence that ginkgo leaf extract, in combination with American ginseng (Panax quinquefolius), might help improve symptoms in children with ADHD (8235).

Colorectal cancer. Preliminary clinical research suggests the intravenous ginkgo extract (Egb 761) in combination with 5-fluorouracil might be useful for metastatic colorectal cancer (9872).

Hearing loss. There is preliminary evidence that ginkgo leaf extract 120 mg twice daily might help short-term idiopathic hearing loss (8543), but because many of these patients recover spontaneously, evaluating its effectiveness for this use is difficult.

More evidence is needed to rate ginkgo leaf for these uses.

Mechanism of Action

Ginkgo leaf and its extracts contain several active constituents including flavonoids, terpenoids, and organic acids. Many ginkgo leaf extracts are standardized to contain 24% to 25% flavonoid glycosides and 6% of the terpenoids. The major flavonoids are primarily derived from the flavonol rutin and include isorhamnetin, quercetin, kaempferol, and proanthocyanidins. The primary terpenoids are ginkgolides A, B, C, M, and J, and bilobalide (1515). Although many of ginkgo's constituents have intrinsic pharmacological effects individually, there is some evidence that the constituents work synergistically to produce more potent pharmacological effects than any individual constituent (1514,6494).

Although the mechanism of action of ginkgo leaf is only partially understood, there are several theories about how it might work for various disease states. One theory is that ginkgo leaf might work by protecting tissues from oxidative damage. Ginkgo leaf flavonoids have antioxidant and free radical scavenging properties (2660,5715,5717,5719). The flavonoids seem to prevent or reduce cell membrane lipid peroxidation (1515) and decrease oxidative damage to erythrocytes (5717). Ginkgo's flavonoids also protect neurons and retinal tissue from oxidative stress (1515,5719) and injury following ischemic episodes (1515,2660). Protecting neurons and other tissues from oxidative damage might prevent progression of tissue degeneration in patients with dementia and other conditions. Central nervous system (CNS) disorders, such as dementia, and other conditions including peripheral arterial disease, hypersensitivity disorders, allergies, asthma, and bronchitis might benefit from ginkgo's anti-inflammatory effects.

Ginkgolides in the leaf competitively inhibit platelet activating factor (PAF) binding at the membrane receptors of numerous cells (5719,9760). PAF inhibition decreases platelet aggregation (5717), decreases phagocyte chemotaxis, decreases smooth muscle contraction (1515), prevents degranulation of neutrophils, decreases free radical production (5716,5717), decreases damaging glycine production after brain injury, and reduces excitatory amino acid receptor function (2660). Inhibition of PAF might increase cardiac contractility and coronary blood flow. Preliminary research suggests that ginkgo leaf extract might also inhibit formation of platelet thromboxane A2, further reducing platelet aggregation (8583).

However, there is contradictory, but questionable, evidence that ginkgo leaf does not reduce platelet aggregation and blood clotting. In this study, healthy men who took the specific ginkgo leaf extract (EGb 761) 160 mg twice daily for 7 days did not have reduced prothrombin times (12114).

Ginkgo leaf products might benefit CNS and vascular conditions by improving circulation. Ginkgo leaf seems to improve blood flow to capillaries throughout the body including in the CNS, eyes, ears, extremities, and other tissues. Ginkgo leaf likely improves circulation by both decreasing blood viscosity and affecting vascular smooth muscle. Ginkgo leaf seems to restore the balance between prostacyclin and thromboxane A2, resulting in improved vasoregulation. Therefore, ginkgo leaf relaxes spasmodic contracting vasculature and contracts abnormally dilated vessels. It is not clear exactly how ginkgo causes vascular contraction and improves venous tone, but these effects might be due to phosphodiesterase inhibition, resulting in increased cAMP levels and release of catecholamines (6492). Some ginkgo constituents may also have a potent relaxing effect on vascular smooth muscle and improve blood flow to the corpus cavernosum; which is thought to be helpful for erectile dysfunction (213). Overall, ginkgo leaf seems to increase cerebral and peripheral blood flow microcirculation, and reduce vascular permeability (5721,6492).

Ginkgo leaf extract might be helpful for Alzheimer's disease due to effects on beta-amyloid proteins. There is preliminary evidence that ginkgo leaf extract can inhibit toxicity and cell death induced by beta-amyloid peptides (6494). However, this has not yet been demonstrated in vivo. Ginkgo might also influence certain neurotransmitter systems, such as the cholinergic system (6490), and seems to produce EEG changes similar to the acetylcholinesterase inhibitor tacrine (Cognex) (6067). There has been some speculation that ginkgo leaf inhibits monoamine oxidase A and B (5721), but so far studies have found conflicting results (6231,6232,6233). It is suggested that ginkgo leaf inhibits catechol-O-methyl transferase (COMT, an enzyme which breaks down adrenergic transmitters) and increases the number of alpha-adrenoreceptors in the brain; which would help reverse the decline in brain alpha-adrenoceptor

activity that occurs with aging (2660).
There is some evidence that ginkgo flavonoids have GABA-ergic effects and might directly affect benzodiazepine receptors (6423). However, the clinical significance of this effect is not known.
The ginkgolides A and B seem to decrease glucocorticoid biosynthesis, which might also play a role in ginkgo's proposed anti-stress and neuroprotective effects (5723,5724,8236).
Ginkgo leaf might have some antimicrobial activity, including activity against Pneumocystis carinii and possibly some gram-positive bacteria and yeast (6069). There is also some preliminary evidence that ginkgo might have a role in fighting syndrome X.
In healthy volunteers, ginkgo leaf extract can increase pancreatic beta-cell function in response to glucose loading and seems to reduce blood pressure. Some researchers think it might decrease development of hyperinsulinemia associated with hypertension, which often precedes development of type 2 diabetes and atherosclerotic cardiovascular disease (5719).
Some crude extracts from ginkgo leaves contain the constituent ginkgolic acid. This constituent can have strong allergenic properties and might have possible mutagenic and carcinogenic properties. Standardized ginkgo leaf extracts such as EGb761 contain no greater than 5 ppm in concentration of ginkgolic acids (5714,8584).
Ginkgo leaves and ginkgo leaf extracts also contain the neurotoxin ginkgotoxin (4'-O-methylpyridoxine). Ginkgotoxin antagonizes the activity of pyridoxine, possibly by inhibiting enzymes such as pyridoxal kinase or glutamate decarboxylase in the brain. Ginkgotoxin is present in much higher amounts in ginkgo seeds than leaves. It is unlikely to be present in ginkgo leaf extracts in high enough concentrations to cause toxicity (11296).
There is some preliminary evidence that ginkgo leaf extract can inhibit cytochrome P450 1A2 (CYP1A2) activity by approximately 13% and CYP2D6 by approximately 9%. Ginkgo leaf extract seems to inhibit CYP2D6 more in males than females (1303). The effects of ginkgo leaf extract on CYP3A4 are unclear. There is some in vitro evidence that ginkgo leaf extract might inhibit CYP3A4 (6450); while in vivo, ginkgo leaf extract does not seem to inhibit CYP3A4 activity (1303). In addition, there is anecdotal evidence that suggests ginkgo leaf extract might actually induce CYP3A4 (6423), but this effect has not yet been verified. The ginkgo leaf extract EGb761, which is the most common extract used in clinical studies, also seems to strongly inhibit CYP2C9 in vitro. The terpenoidic fraction (ginkgolides) only inhibits CYP2C9. The flavonoidic fraction (quercetin, keampferol, etc) seems to inhibit CYP2C9, CYP1A2, CYP3A4, and CYP2E1 (12061).

Adverse Reactions

Orally, ginkgo leaf extract in typical doses can cause mild gastrointestinal (GI) upset, headache, dizziness, palpitations, constipation, and allergic skin reactions (5719,5721,6220). Large doses can cause restlessness, diarrhea, nausea, vomiting, lack of muscle tone, and weakness.
Spontaneous bleeding is one of the most concerning potential side effects. There are several case reports of subdural hematoma and spontaneous hyphema (bleeding from the iris into the anterior part of the eye) associated with ginkgo use (579,8581). Retrobulbar hemorrhage (bleeding behind the eye) during cataract surgery has been associated with ginkgo (10450). Excessive postoperative bleeding requiring transfusion has also occurred following laparoscopic surgery in a patient who had been taking ginkgo leaf extract (887).
Ginkgo leaf extract can cause serious allergic skin reactions in some patients. There is one case of Stevens-Johnson syndrome following a second administration of a preparation containing ginkgo leaf extract, choline, vitamin B6, and vitamin B12 (208).
There is some concern that ginkgo might be associated with seizures in some patients. Ginkgo leaf and ginkgo leaf extract contain trace amounts of ginkgotoxin, which can cause seizures and death in high doses. The antidote for ginkgotoxin poisoning is pyridoxine. Ginkgotoxin is present in much higher amounts in ginkgo seeds. The small amount in the leaves and leaf extract is unlikely to cause toxicity (11296). However, there are anecdotal reports of seizure occurring after use of ginkgo leaf preparations both in patients without a history seizure disorder and in those with previously well-controlled epilepsy (7030,7090). There is not enough evidence to prove that ginkgo leaf is the sole cause of seizure in these patients. Until more is known, advise patients with a seizure disorder and those patients taking drugs that lower the seizure threshold to avoid ginkgo leaf products. There is some in vitro evidence that suggests high concentrations of ginkgo might reduce male and female fertility (4239,4240); however, this has not been demonstrated in humans.

Interactions with Herbs & Other Dietary Supplements

ANTICOAGULANT, ANTIPLATELET HERBS AND SUPPLEMENTS: Concomitant use of herbs and supplements that affect platelet aggregation could theoretically increase the risk of bleeding in some people due to ginkgo's effects on platelet aggregation (5717,5719). Some of these herbs and supplements include angelica, anise, arnica, asafoetida, bogbean, boldo, capsicum, celery, chamomile, clove, danshen, fenugreek, feverfew, fish oil, garlic, ginger, horse chestnut, horseradish, licorice, meadowsweet, onion, Panax ginseng, papain, passionflower, poplar, prickly ash, quassia, red clover, turmeric, vitamin E, wild carrot, wild lettuce, willow, and others.
SEIZURE THRESHOLD LOWERING HERBS AND SUPPLEMENTS: There is some concern that ginkgo leaf might induce seizures in some patients. Ginkgo leaf and ginkgo leaf extract contain trace amounts of ginkgotoxin, which can cause seizures in high doses, but the amount of ginkgotoxin in ginkgo leaf and leaf extract is unlikely to cause toxicity (11296). However, there are anecdotal reports of seizure occurring after use of ginkgo leaf both in patients without a history seizure disorder and in those with previously well-controlled epilepsy (7030,7090).

Theoretically, patients taking supplements that lower the seizure threshold might be at greater risk. Advise patients taking these supplements to avoid ginkgo leaf products. Some of these supplements include borage seed oil, butanediol (BD), cedar leaf, Chinese club moss, EDTA, evening primrose oil, folic acid, gamma butyrolactone (GBL), gamma hydroxybutyrate (GHB), ginkgo seed, glutamine, huperzine A, hydrazine sulfate, hyssop, juniper, L-carnitine, melatonin, rosemary, sage, wormwood above ground parts, and others.
ST. JOHN'S WORT: Ginkgo in combination with buspirone (BuSpar), fluoxetine (Prozac), melatonin, and St. John's wort might cause hypomania in patients with depression (8582). Whether Ginkgo alone, or in combination with St. John's wort, can cause hypomania is unknown.

Interactions with Drugs

ANTICOAGULANT/ANTIPLATELET DRUGS: Concomitant administration can increase the risk of bleeding. Ginkgo leaf has been shown to decrease platelet aggregation. It is thought that the ginkgo constituent, ginkgolide B, displaces platelet-activating factor (PAF) from its binding sites, decreasing blood coagulation (6048,9760). Some of these drugs include aspirin, clopidogrel (Plavix), dalteparin (Fragmin), enoxaparin (Lovenox), heparin, indomethacin (Indocin), ticlopidine (Ticlid), warfarin (Coumadin), and others.
BUSPIRONE (BuSpar): Ginkgo in combination with fluoxetine (Prozac), St. John's wort, melatonin, and buspirone might cause hypomania in patients with depression (8582). Whether ginkgo alone or in combination with buspirone can cause hypomania is unknown.
CYTOCHROME P450 1A2 (CYP1A2) SUBSTRATES: There is preliminary evidence that ginkgo leaf extract can mildly affect cytochrome P450 1A2 (CYP1A2) enzymes (1303,6423,6450). Since ginkgo leaf extract seems to only mildly affect these enzymes, it is not likely to produce clinically significant interactions; however, it might slightly increase levels of some drugs metabolized by these enzymes. Until more is known, use ginkgo cautiously in patients taking drugs metabolized by these enzymes. Some drugs metabolized by CYP1A2 include acetaminophen (Tylenol), amitriptyline (Elavil), clopidogrel (Plavix), clozapine (Clozaril), diazepam (Valium), estradiol, olanzapine (Zyprexa), ondansetron (Zofran), propranolol (Inderal), ropinirole (Requip), tacrine (Cognex), theophylline, verapamil (Calan, Covera-HS, Isoptin, Verelan), warfarin (Coumadin), and others.
CYTOCHROME P450 2C9 (CYP2C9) SUBSTRATES: There is preliminary evidence that a specific standardized extract of ginkgo leaf (EGb761) can strongly inhibit CYP2C9 (12061). The terpenoid (ginkgolides) and flavonoid (quercetin, keampferol, etc) constituents seem to be responsible for the enzyme inhibition. Most ginkgo extracts contain some amount of these constituents. Therefore, other ginkgo leaf extracts likely also inhibit the CYP2C9 enzyme. Ginkgo leaf extracts might increase levels of drugs metabolized by CYP2C9. Advise patients not to take ginkgo leaf or use it cautiously if they take any CYP2C9 substrate. Some of these drugs include warfarin (Coumadin), glyburide, glipizide, amitriptyline valdecoxib (Bextra), phenytoin (Dilantin), and many others.
CYTOCHROME P450 2D6 (CYP2D6) SUBSTRATES: There is preliminary evidence that ginkgo leaf extract can mildly affect cytochrome P450 2D6 enzymes (CYP2D6) (1303,6423,6450). Since ginkgo leaf extract seems to only mildly affect these enzymes, it is not likely to produce clinically significant interactions; however, it might slightly increase levels of some drugs metabolized by these enzymes. Some drugs metabolized by CYP2D6 include amitriptyline (Elavil), clozapine (Clozaril), codeine, desipramine (Norpramin), donepezil (Aricept), fentanyl (Duragesic), flecainide (Tambocor), fluoxetine (Prozac), meperidine (Demerol), methadone (Dolophine), metoprolol (Lopressor, Toprol XL), olanzapine (Zyprexa), ondansetron (Zofran), tramadol (Ultram), trazodone (Desyrel), and others.
CYTOCHROME P450 3A4 (CYP3A4) SUBSTRATES: There is preliminary evidence that ginkgo leaf extract can affect cytochrome P450 3A4 enzymes (CYP3A4). However, there is conflicting evidence about whether it induces or inhibits CYP3A4 (1303,6423,6450). Until more is known, use ginkgo cautiously in patients taking drugs metabolized by these enzymes. Some drugs metabolized by CYP3A4 include lovastatin (Mevacor), ketoconazole (Nizoral), itraconazole (Sporanox), fexofenadine (Allegra), triazolam (Halcion), and others.
FLUOXETINE (Prozac): Ginkgo in combination with buspirone (BuSpar), St. John's wort, melatonin, and fluoxetine might cause hypomania in patients with depression (8582). Whether ginkgo alone or in combination with fluoxetine can cause hypomania is unknown.
INSULIN: Ginkgo leaf extract can alter insulin secretion and metabolism, and might affect blood glucose levels (5719). People taking insulin should monitor glucose levels closely. Insulin dose adjustments might be necessary.
SEIZURE THRESHOLD LOWERING DRUGS: There is some concern that ginkgo leaf might induce seizures in some patients. Ginkgo leaf and ginkgo leaf extract contain trace amounts of ginkgotoxin, which can cause seizures in high doses. But the amount of ginkgotoxin in ginkgo leaf and leaf extract is unlikely to cause toxicity (11296). However, there are anecdotal reports of seizure occurring after use of ginkgo leaf both in patients without a history of seizure disorder and in those with previously well-controlled epilepsy (7030,7090). Theoretically, patients taking drugs that lower the seizure threshold might be at greater risk. Advise patients taking these drugs to avoid ginkgo leaf products. Some drugs that lower the seizure threshold include anesthetics (propofol, others), antiarrhythmics (mexiletine), antibiotics (amphotericin, penicillin, cephalosporins, imipenem), antidepressants (bupropion, others), antihistamines (cyproheptadine, others), immunosuppressants (cyclosporin), narcotics (fentanyl, others), stimulants (methylphenidate), theophylline, and others.
THIAZIDE DIURETICS: Ginkgo leaf can increase blood pressure when used concomitantly with thiazide diuretics (613).
TRAZODONE (Desyrel): Use of ginkgo leaf extract with trazodone has been associated with coma. In one case, an

Alzheimer's patient taking trazodone 20 mg twice daily and ginkgo leaf extract 80 mg twice daily for four doses became comatose. The coma was reversed by administration of flumazenil (Romazicon). Coma might have been induced by excessive GABA-ergic activity. Ginkgo flavonoids are thought to have GABA-ergic activity and act directly on benzodiazepine receptors. Ginkgo might also increase metabolism of trazodone to active GABA-ergic metabolites, possibly by inducing cytochrome P450 3A4 (CYP3A4) metabolism (6423).
WARFARIN (Coumadin): Ginkgo leaf can increase the anticoagulant effects of warfarin and risk of bleeding (576). Ginkgo is thought to have antiplatelet effects and might have additive effects when used with warfarin. There is also some evidence that ginkgo leaf extract can inhibit cytochrome P450 2C9, the enzyme that metabolizes warfarin, and therefore might increase warfarin levels (12061). Advise patients on warfarin not to take ginkgo. Warfarin dose adjustment may be necessary.

Interactions with Foods
None known.

Interactions with Lab Tests
None known.

Interactions with Diseases or Conditions
BLEEDING DISORDERS: Ginkgo leaf can decrease platelet aggregation by inhibiting platelet-activating factor (PAF) and may exacerbate bleeding disorders (6048,9760); use with caution.
DIABETES: Theoretically, ginkgo may interfere with the management of diabetes. Ginkgo has been reported to increase pancreatic beta-cell function in response to glucose and may also increase the metabolic clearance of insulin (5719). Monitor blood glucose levels closely. Diabetes medications might require dose adjustment.
EPILEPSY: There is some concern that ginkgo use might be associated with seizure. Ginkgo leaf and ginkgo leaf extract contain trace amounts of ginkgotoxin, which can cause seizures in high doses, but the amount of ginkgotoxin in ginkgo leaf and leaf extract is unlikely to cause toxicity (11296). However, there are several anecdotal reports of seizure occurring in patients taking combination products containing ginkgo and single ingredient ginkgo products. However, there is not yet enough evidence to prove that ginkgo can actually cause seizure in certain patients (7030). Until more is known, use cautiously or avoid in epileptic patients or patients prone to seizure.
INFERTILITY: Some evidence suggests that ginkgo biloba might inhibit oocyte fertilization and should be avoided in couples attempting to conceive (4239,4240). This effect has not yet been demonstrated in humans; however, until more is known, use with caution in couples attempting to conceive and avoid use in couples having difficulty conceiving.
SURGERY: Ginkgo leaf extract has antiplatelet effects and can cause excessive bleeding if used prior to surgery (887). Tell patients to discontinue ginkgo at least 2 weeks before elective surgical procedures.

Dosage and Administration
ORAL: For dementia syndromes, a dosage of 120-240 mg per day of ginkgo leaf extract, divided in two or three doses, has been used (1514,1515). To relieve walking pain in patients with intermittent claudication, a dosage of 120-240 mg per day of ginkgo leaf extract, divided into two or three doses, has been used; however, the higher dose may be more effective (3461). For reversing sexual dysfunction due to SSRIs, the typical starting dose is 60 mg twice daily of ginkgo leaf extract. This dose can be titrated up to 240 mg twice daily (212). For cognitive function improvement in healthy young people, dosages of 120-600 mg per day have been used (6214,6215,8236). For vertigo or tinnitus, dosages of 120-160 mg per day of ginkgo leaf extract, divided into two or three doses, have been used (221). For prevention of altitude sickness, 80 mg of ginkgo leaf extract twice daily has been used (6230). For premenstrual syndrome (PMS), 80 mg twice daily, starting on the sixteenth day of the menstrual cycle until the fifth day of the next cycle has been used (6229). For the treatment of attention deficit-hyperactivity disorder (ADHD), a dosage of 50 mg ginkgo leaf extract combined with 200 mg American ginseng twice daily has been used (8235). For the treatment of normal tension glaucoma, ginkgo leaf extract 40 mg 3 times daily has been used for up to 4 weeks (10378). For Raynaud's disease, a dosage of 360 mg per day of ginkgo leaf extract, divided into three doses, has been used (11363). For all indications, start at a lower dose of not more 120 mg per day to avoid adverse gastrointestinal (GI) effects. Titrate to higher doses as needed. Dosing may vary depending on the specific formulation used. Most trials used specific standardized Ginkgo biloba leaf extracts. Some people take 0.5 mL of a standard 1:5 tincture of the crude ginkgo leaf three times daily (5011). Tell patients to avoid crude ginkgo plant parts; which can exceed concentrations of 5 ppm of the toxic ginkgolic acid constituents, and can cause severe allergic reactions (5714).

Comments
When people talk about Ginkgo biloba, they usually mean ginkgo leaf extract. However, traditionally only Ginkgo biloba fruit was used. "Ginkgo biloba" comes from the Chinese term Yin-Kuo, meaning "silver apricot," and biloba also describes its two-lobed, fan shaped leaves (6208). Ginkgo biloba is the oldest living tree species in the world. Ginkgo trees can live as long as a thousand years. Using ginkgo for asthma and bronchitis was described in the first pharmacopoeia, Chen Noung Pen T'sao, dating to 2600 BC (6208). Ginkgo is the most frequently prescribed herbal medicine in Germany (6208) and is the preferred treatment for dementia (6491). Some ginkgo products have problems with dissolution (8584). The National Center for Complementary and Alternative Medicine (NCCAM) is conducting a

5-year study of 3000 people aged 75 and older to determine if ginkgo, 240 mg daily, prevents dementia or Alzheimer's disease (6226). In isolated cases ginkgo has been contaminated with colchicine (8541). However, follow-up studies indicate that this contamination is not widespread (8542).

GINKGO seed

Also Known As

Baiguo, Fossil Tree, Japanese Silver Apricot, Kew Tree, Maidenhair Tree, Yinhsing.
CAUTION: See separate listing for Ginkgo leaf (Ginkgo leaf extract). Ginkgo leaf is the most commonly used form of Ginkgo.

Scientific Names

Ginkgo biloba.
Family: Ginkgoaceae.

People Use This For

Orally, ginkgo seed is used as an antitussive, expectorant, to treat asthma, bronchitis, genitourinary complaints, to aid digestion, and to prevent drunkenness.
Topically, ginkgo seed is used for scabies and skin sores.
In foods, roasted ginkgo seed, which has the pulp removed, is an edible delicacy in Japan and China.

Safety

POSSIBLY SAFE ...when the boiled seed is consumed as food (11296).
POSSIBLY UNSAFE ...when the roasted seed is used orally for medicinal purposes. High doses of roasted seeds, more than 10 per day, can cause difficulty breathing, weak pulse, seizures, loss of consciousness, and shock (8231,8232).
UNSAFE ...when the fresh seed is used orally. Fresh seeds are toxic and potentially deadly (11296).
There is insufficient reliable information available about the safety of the topical use of ginkgo seed.
CHILDREN: LIKELY UNSAFE ...when used orally. The fresh seeds have caused seizures and death in children (8231,11296).
PREGNANCY AND LACTATION: POSSIBLY SAFE ...when the boiled seed is eaten as food (11296).
POSSIBLY UNSAFE ...when used orally for medicinal purposes; avoid using (8231,8232).

Effectiveness

There is insufficient reliable information available about the effectiveness of ginkgo seed.

Mechanism of Action

Ginkgo seeds seem to have antibacterial and antifungal effects (11701,11702). Ginkgo seeds also contain the neurotoxin ginkgotoxin (4'-O-methylpyridoxine). Ginkgotoxin can cause seizures and death in high doses. It antagonizes the activity of pyridoxine, possibly by inhibiting enzymes such as pyridoxal kinase or glutamate decarboxylase in the brain. Ginkgotoxin is present in much larger amounts in ginkgo seeds than leaves. Boiling ginkgo seeds seems to reduce the ginkgotoxin content to safe levels (11296).

Adverse Reactions

Orally, fresh seeds can cause stomachache, nausea, vomiting, diarrhea, restlessness, difficulty breathing, weak pulse, seizures, loss of consciousness, and shock. Ingesting roasted seeds in amounts larger than the normal food amounts of 8-10 seeds per day, or long-term, can also cause these same adverse reactions (8231,8232). The fresh seeds contain ginkgotoxin, which can cause seizures and death. The antidote for ginkgotoxin poisoning is pyridoxine (11296).
Topically, ginkgo fruit and pulp can cause severe allergic skin reactions and irritation of mucous membranes and the gastrointestinal tract (12). Cross-reactivity is possible with ginkgo fruit in individuals allergic to poison ivy, poison oak, poison sumac, mango rind, and cashew shell oil (380).

Interactions with Herbs & Other Dietary Supplements

SEIZURE THRESHOLD LOWERING HERBS AND SUPPLEMENTS: Ginkgo seeds contain ginkgotoxin, which can cause seizures in high doses (11296). Theoretically, patients taking supplements that lower the seizure threshold might be at greater risk. Advise patients taking these supplements to avoid ginkgo leaf products. Some of these supplements include borage seed oil, butanediol (BD), cedar leaf, Chinese club moss, EDTA, evening primrose oil, folic acid, gamma butyrolactone (GBL), gamma hydroxybutyrate (GHB), glutamine, huperzine A, hydrazine sulfate, hyssop, juniper, L-carnitine, melatonin, rosemary, sage, wormwood above ground parts, and others.

Interactions with Drugs

ANTICONVULSANTS: Theoretically, raw ginkgo seeds, which contain ginkgotoxin might antagonize the anticonvulsant effects of medications taken for epilepsy (11296). Some anti-epileptic drugs include phenobarbital, primidone (Mysoline), valproic acid (Depakene), gabapentin (Neurontin), carbamazepine (Tegretol), phenytoin (Dilantin), and others.
SEIZURE THRESHOLD LOWERING DRUGS: Consumption of raw ginkgo seeds can cause seizures (8232). Ginkgo seed extract contain trace amounts of ginkgotoxin, which can cause seizures in high doses (11296). Theoretically, patients taking drugs that lower the seizure threshold might be at greater risk. Advise patients taking these drugs to avoid ginkgo leaf products. Some drugs that lower the seizure threshold include anesthetics (propofol, others), antiarrhythmics (mexiletine), antibiotics (amphotericin, penicillin, cephalosporins, imipenem), antidepressants (bupropion, others), antihistamines (cyproheptadine, others), immunosuppressants (cyclosporin), narcotics (fentanyl, others), stimulants (methylphenidate), theophylline, and others.

Interactions with Foods

None known.

Interactions with Lab Tests

None known.

Interactions with Diseases or Conditions

SEIZURE DISORDERS: Ginkgo seed extract contain trace amounts of ginkgotoxin, which can cause seizures in high doses (11296). Consumption of raw ginkgo seeds can cause seizures (8232).

Dosage and Administration

ORAL: People typically use 120-240 mg ginkgo tablets or capsules daily in two or three divided doses (6002).

GINSENG, AMERICAN

Also Known As

American Ginseng, Anchi Ginseng, Canadian Ginseng, Ginseng, Ginseng Root, North American Ginseng, Occidental Ginseng, Ontario Ginseng, Red Berry, Ren Shen, Sang, Shang, Wisconsin Ginseng, Xi Yang Shen.
CAUTION: See separate listings for Blue Cohosh, Canaigre, Codonopsis, Ginseng Siberian, Ginseng Panax, Panax Pseudoginseng, and Ashwaganda.

Scientific Names

Panax quinquefolius.
Family: Araliaceae.

People Use This For

Orally, American ginseng is used as an adaptogen, for increasing resistance to environmental stress, as a general tonic, stimulant, diuretic, and digestive aid. It is also used for anemia, diabetes, insomnia, neurasthenia, gastritis, impotence, fever, hangover symptoms, stimulating immune function, attention deficit-hyperactivity disorder (ADHD), and for eradicating Pseudomonas infection in cystic fibrosis. American ginseng is also used for acute respiratory illness, improving stress resistance, preventing the effects of aging, improving stamina, blood and bleeding disorders, atherosclerosis, loss of appetite, vomiting, colitis, dysentery, cancer, insomnia, neuralgia, rheumatism, memory loss, dizziness, headaches, convulsions, and disorders of pregnancy and childbirth.
In food manufacturing, American ginseng is used in soft drinks.
In other manufacturing processes, American ginseng oil and extracts are used in soaps and cosmetics.

Safety

POSSIBLY SAFE ...when used orally and appropriately, short-term (8235,11351).
PREGNANCY: POSSIBLY UNSAFE ...when used orally. Ginsenoside Rb1, an active constituent of American ginseng, has teratogenic effects in animal models (10447); avoid using.
LACTATION: Insufficient reliable information available; avoid using.

Effectiveness

POSSIBLY EFFECTIVE

Acute respiratory illness (ARI). Taking American ginseng orally seems to protect against ARI in elderly patients in long-term care. American ginseng extract, 200 mg twice daily for 8-12 weeks, may reduce the relative risk of ARI by 89% when administered during the influenza season (11351).
Diabetes. Taking American ginseng 3 grams orally, up to two hours before a meal, can significantly reduce

postprandial glucose levels in patients with type 2 diabetes (1018,6461). However, doses greater than 3 grams do not seem to offer any additional benefit (6461). The glucose lowering effect may vary among preparations because of variations in the concentration of ginsenosides (9732).

INSUFFICIENT RELIABLE EVIDENCE to RATE

Attention deficit-hyperactivity disorder (ADHD). There is preliminary evidence that American ginseng in combination with Ginkgo biloba leaf extract might help improve symptoms in children with ADHD (8235). More evidence is needed to rate American ginseng for this use.

Mechanism of Action

The applicable part of American ginseng is the root. The principle constituents of American ginseng are known as ginsenosides, panaxosides, or saponins (11). American ginseng contains primarily ginsenoside Rb-1, which reportedly lowers blood pressure; has antihemolytic, antipyretic, antipsychotic, CNS depressant, and ulcer protective activity; increases GI motility; and decreases islet insulin concentrations (4,11). At least 11 chemical forms of ginsenosides are known to exist in varying concentrations in the assorted species of ginseng (9735). Most research has focused on the related species, Panax ginseng, which contains ginsenosides Rb-1, Rc, and Rg-1 (4).

An American ginseng extract decreases LH (luteinizing hormone) levels and increases serum ceruloplasmin oxidase activity (a measure of estrogenic activity in the liver) in an animal model (6180). Preliminary research suggests that American ginseng extract might reduce breast cancer cell growth (389); however, this effect may be outweighed by its estrogenic action, which might increase the growth of breast cancer cells (7860). American ginseng might have immunomodulating activity. It seems to activate monocytes and induce tumor necrosis factor (TNF)-alpha (7602). Ginsenosides might improve memory by influencing the effect of acetylcholine in the central nervous system by an unknown mechanism. Ginsenosides do not appear to change metabolism, release, or reuptake of acetylcholine (9736). There's also some evidence that ginsenosides might cause an increase in sexual drive (11162).

Preliminary evidence suggests that saponins found in the stems and leaves of American ginseng can reduce oxidation of low density lipoprotein (LDL) cholesterol. These saponins might reverse the decrease in venous relaxation in response to acetylcholine that occurs in the presence of oxidized LDL (9733). A hot water extract of American ginseng root seems to decrease endothelial constriction by promoting the release of nitric oxide (9734).

Adverse Reactions

Orally, American ginseng can cause gastrointestinal, nervous and cardiovascular system adverse effects; however, these are similar to placebo (11351). Adverse reactions reported for the related species Panax ginseng include insomnia, mastalgia, vaginal bleeding, tachycardia, mania, cerebral arteritis, Stevens Johnson syndrome, cholestatic hepatitis (associated with a panax-containing, multi-ingredient product, Prostata), amenorrhea, decreased appetite, edema, hyperpyrexia, pruritus, rose spots, hypotension, palpitations, headache, vertigo, euphoria, and neonatal death (589,590,591,592,594,595,596,598). Diarrhea or allergic skin reactions can occur, especially with large amounts or prolonged use. There are reports of ginseng abuse syndrome, which includes hypertension, nervousness, insomnia, and increased libido; however, this is controversial and has not been verified by other reports (515).

Interactions with Herbs & Other Dietary Supplements

CAFFEINE, COFFEE, GUARANA, MATE, TEA: Concomitant use of American ginseng can potentiate the stimulant effects of these drugs (4,12).

Interactions with Drugs

ANTIDIABETES DRUGS: American ginseng may lower blood glucose (1018,6461). Theoretically, concomitant use with antidiabetes drugs might enhance blood glucose lowering effects and possibly cause hypoglycemia. Monitor blood glucose levels closely. Some antidiabetes drugs include glimepiride (Amaryl), glyburide (Diabeta, Glynase PresTab, Micronase), insulin, pioglitazone (Actos), rosiglitazone (Avandia), and others.

ANTIPSYCHOTIC DRUGS: Theoretically, American ginseng may interfere with antipsychotic drugs. Ginsenoside fractions of Panax ginseng seem to inhibit the uptake of several neurotransmitters in animals.

MONOAMINE OXIDASE INHIBITORS (MAOIs): Theoretically, American ginseng may interfere with MAOI therapy. There is one case report of insomnia, headache, and tremors with concomitant phenelzine (Nardil) and unspecified ginseng use (617). There is also one case report of hypomania with concomitant phenelzine (Nardil) and unspecified ginseng use (618).

STIMULANT DRUGS: Theoretically, concomitant use of American ginseng may potentiate the activity of stimulant drugs (4,12).

WARFARIN (Coumadin): American ginseng can decrease the effectiveness of warfarin therapy. Healthy patients receiving warfarin 5 mg daily, who also take American ginseng 1 gram twice daily, seem to have a significantly reduced international normalized ratio (INR) (619,12032). To avoid this potential interaction, advise patients who take warfarin not to take American ginseng.

Interactions with Foods

COFFEE, TEA: Theoretically, concomitant use of ginseng can potentiate the stimulant effects of coffee or tea (4,12).

Interactions with Lab Tests

BLOOD GLUCOSE: American ginseng may decrease postprandial blood glucose levels and test results (1018,6461).
PROTHROMBIN TIME (PT): Theoretically, American ginseng may prolong thrombin time (TT) and activated partial thromboplastin time (aPTT), which is based on in vitro studies with the related species, Panax ginseng (1522).

Interactions with Diseases or Conditions

BLEEDING CONDITIONS: American ginseng has been reported to decrease blood coagulation (4); contraindicated in cases of hemorrhage or thrombosis.
CARDIAC CONDITIONS: American ginseng is reported to have negative inotropic and chronotropic activity and hypotensive effects. Ginseng might adversely affect patients with cardiac disorders (4); use with caution.
DIABETES: American ginseng has hypoglycemic activity (4,1018,6461). Use in diabetics might increase the risk of hypoglycemic episodes; use with caution.
HORMONE SENSITIVE CANCERS OR CONDITIONS: Because American ginseng might have estrogenic effects, women with hormone sensitive conditions should avoid American ginseng. Some of these conditions include breast cancer, uterine cancer, ovarian cancer, endometriosis, and uterine fibroids (6180,7860).
INSOMNIA: High doses of American ginseng have been associated with insomnia (597). Theoretically, use in patients with insomnia might worsen the condition; use with caution.
SCHIZOPHRENIA: High doses of American ginseng have been associated with insomnia and agitation in schizophrenic patients (597); use with caution.

Dosage and Administration

ORAL: For reducing postprandial glucose levels in patients with type 2 diabetes, 3-9 grams up to two hours before a meal has been used (1018,6461). However, there is no added benefit to taking more than 3 grams (6461). American ginseng should be taken within two hours of a meal to avoid potential hypoglycemia (1018,6461). For preventing acute respiratory illness (ARI) in elderly patients, American ginseng extract 200 mg twice daily for 8-12 weeks has been used (11351). In children with attention deficit-hyperactivity disorder (ADHD), American ginseng 200 mg two times daily has been used for four weeks, in combination with Ginkgo biloba (8235).

Comments

Avoid confusion with Eleutherococcus senticosus, referred to as Siberian ginseng; and Panax ginseng, referred to as Asian ginseng. Wild American ginseng is so extensively sought that it has been declared an endangered species in the US (515).

GINSENG, PANAX

Also Known As

Asian Ginseng, Asiatic Ginseng, Chinese Ginseng, Ginseng, Ginseng Asiatique, Ginseng Radix, Ginseng Root, Guigai, Hong Shen, Japanese Ginseng, Jen-Shen, Jinsao, Jintsam, Insam, Korean Ginseng, Korean Panax Ginseng, Korean Red Ginseng, Ninjin, Oriental Ginseng, Panax Ginseng, Radix Ginseng Rubra, Red Ginseng, Ren Shen, Renshen, Renxian, Sang, Seng, Sheng Shai Shen, White Ginseng.
CAUTION: See separate listings for Blue Cohosh, Canaigre, Codonopsis, Ginseng American, Ginseng Siberian, Panax Pseudoginseng, and Ashwaganda.

Scientific Names

Panax ginseng, synonym Panax schinseng.
Family: Araliaceae.

People Use This For

Orally, Panax ginseng is used as a so-called "adaptogen" for increasing resistance to environmental stress and as a general tonic for improving well-being. It is also used for stimulating immune function, improving physical and athletic stamina, improving cognitive function, concentration, memory, and work efficiency. It is also used orally for depression, anxiety, Pseudomonas infection in cystic fibrosis, chronic bronchitis, irritated or inflamed tissues, and as a diuretic. Panax ginseng is also used orally for anemia, diabetes, gastritis, neurasthenia, erectile dysfunction, impotence and male fertility, fever, hangover, and asthma. It is also used orally for bleeding disorders, loss of appetite, vomiting, colitis, dysentery, cancer, insomnia, neuralgia, rheumatism, dizziness, headache, convulsions, disorders of pregnancy and childbirth, hot flashes due to menopause, and to slow the aging process.
Topically, Panax ginseng is used as part of a multi-ingredient preparation for treating premature ejaculation.
In manufacturing, Panax ginseng is used to make soaps, cosmetics, and as a flavoring in beverages.

Safety

POSSIBLY SAFE ...when used orally and appropriately, short-term. Panax ginseng seems to be safe when used for less than 3 months (8813,8814). ...when used topically, short-term as part of a multi-ingredient preparation (SS Cream).

This preparation seems to be safe when applied and left on the glans penis for one hour (2537). Further evaluation is needed to determine its safety after prolonged, repetitive topical use.
POSSIBLY UNSAFE ...when used orally, long-term. There is some concern about the long-term safety due to potential hormone-like effects, which might cause adverse effects with prolonged use (7). Tell patients to limit continuous use to less than 3 months.
CHILDREN: LIKELY UNSAFE ...when used orally in infants. Use of Panax ginseng in newborns is associated with intoxication that can lead to death (12). There is insufficient reliable information about use in older children; avoid using.
PREGNANCY: POSSIBLY UNSAFE ...when used orally. Ginsenoside Rb1, an active constituent of Panax ginseng, has teratogenic effects in animal models (10447); avoid using.
LACTATION: Insufficient reliable information available; avoid using.

Effectiveness

POSSIBLY EFFECTIVE

Cognitive function. Taking Panax ginseng orally might improve abstract thinking, mental arithmetic skills, and reaction times in healthy, middle-aged people (2064). Panax ginseng alone does not seem to improve memory (2064), but there is some evidence that a combination of Panax ginseng and ginkgo leaf extract can improve memory in otherwise healthy people ages 38 to 66 years (1903,8591).

Diabetes. There is some evidence that taking Panax ginseng orally, 200 mg daily, can decrease fasting blood glucose levels and hemoglobin A1c (HbA1c) in patients with type 2 diabetes (4225).

Erectile dysfunction (ED). Taking Panax ginseng orally seems to improve sexual function in men with erectile dysfunction (8813).

Premature ejaculation. Applying a multi-ingredient cream preparation containing Panax ginseng, angelica root, Cistanches deserticola, Zanthoxyl species, torlidis seed, clove flower, asiasari root, cinnamon bark, and toad venom (SS Cream) to the glans penis one hour prior to intercourse and washing off immediately before intercourse seems to improve ejaculatory latency in men with premature ejaculation (2537).

POSSIBLY INEFFECTIVE

Athletic performance. Taking Panax ginseng orally doesn't seem to improve aerobic exercise performance (1427,4230,4231,4236).

Menopausal symptoms. Taking Panax ginseng orally doesn't seem to help vasomotor symptoms such as hot flashes in postmenopausal women (10981). In postmenopausal women, some preliminary clinical research suggests that panax ginseng might improve quality of life, and menopausal symptoms such as fatigue, insomnia, and depression (3863,10981).

Quality of life. Taking Panax ginseng orally doesn't seem to be helpful for improving mood, sense of well being and overall quality of life. Although some research suggests that Panax ginseng might improve self-rated quality of life (6254), other studies show no benefit (8601,10314). Tell patients not to rely on Panax ginseng to improve mood or sense of well being.

INSUFFICIENT RELIABLE EVIDENCE to RATE

Bronchitis. Taking a specific Panax ginseng extract (G115) orally might be beneficial when used adjunctively for treating acute exacerbations of chronic bronchitis. Panax ginseng, combined with antibiotic therapy, might reduce bronchial bacterial counts more than antibiotic therapy alone (8814).

Cancer. Epidemiological data suggests that taking ginseng orally might decrease the incidence of cancer, specifically stomach cancer, lung cancer, liver cancer, ovarian cancer, and skin cancer (2063,3122).

Common cold. There is some evidence that taking a specific Panax ginseng extract (G115) orally can decrease the chance of catching a cold (589).

Congestive heart failure (CHF). An intravenous formulation of ginseng seems to increase ejection fraction in patients with congestive heart failure. Ginseng might improve hemodynamics and might work synergistically with digoxin (4243,8604).

Influenza. There is some preliminary evidence that suggests taking a specific Panax ginseng extract (G115) orally four weeks prior to influenza vaccination and continued for eight more weeks can decrease the risk of getting the flu (589).

More evidence is needed to rate Panax ginseng for these uses.

Mechanism of Action

The applicable part of Panax ginseng is the root. Panax ginseng contains several active constituents. The constituents thought to be of most importance are triterpenoid saponins referred to collectively as ginsenosides or panaxosides. Ginsenosides is the term developed by Asian researchers, and the term panaxosides was developed by early Russian researchers. Numerous subtypes of ginsenosides have been identified. Other constituents include pectin, B vitamins, and various flavonoids (11).
The ginsenosides have a wide range of pharmacological activity and effects. In some cases, these isolated constituents seem to counteract each other's activity. For example, ginsenoside Rg1, raises blood pressure and acts as a central nervous system (CNS) stimulant. Ginsenoside Rb1 lowers blood pressure and acts as a CNS depressant (11). They also seem to interfere with platelet aggregation and coagulation (1522). They also have papaverine-like effects on smooth muscle, as well as analgesic and anti-inflammatory effects (6). Ginsenosides also potentiate nerve growth

factor (11) and might confer neuroprotection through nicotinic activity (3109). There is also evidence that ginsenosides can relax human bronchial smooth muscle by stimulating the release of nitrous oxide from airway epithelium which may account for the potential anti-asthmatic effect of Panax ginseng (11007). However, research on related ginseng species, Panax pseudoginseng, suggests these ginsenosides may not be pharmacologically significant. Rb1 has a low oral bioavailability, and Rg1 is rapidly eliminated from the blood in animal models (11153).

Ginseng is widely used as a general tonic or "adaptogen" for fighting stress. There is some evidence that it might work against stress by affecting the hypothalamic-pituitary-adrenal (HPA) axis. Panax ginseng saponins seem to increase serum cortisol concentrations (3256,3257) and stimulate adrenal function (13). Panax ginseng might also increase dehydroepiandrosterone sulfate (DHEA-S) levels in women (3863).

Panax ginseng might affect immune function and might have anticancer effects. Panax ginseng appears to stimulate natural-killer cell activity and possibly other immune-system activity. It might also have some antitumor activity (3122). Extracts of Panax ginseng decrease the production of tumor necrosis factor (TNF), diminish DNA strand breakage, and inhibit the formation of induced skin tumors (11006). There is conflicting research about the antioxidant and free radical scavenging activity of panax ginseng (4227,8602). Ginsenosides have been shown to inhibit tumor cell invasion and suppress sister chromatid exchanges in human lymphocytes (11006). Panax ginseng also contains water insoluble polyacetylenic constituents such as panaxynol, panaxydol, and panaxytriol. Panaxydol seems to have antiproliferative effects on various types of cancer cells by inhibiting cancer cell growth at the cell cycle G1 to S transition phase (11005).

In peptic ulceration, Panax ginseng has shown inhibitory activity on Helicobacter pylori-induced hemagglutination (3121). Samgyetang, a soup made from chicken, panax ginseng, garlic, jujube, and chestnuts, appears to offer protection from experimentally induced peptic ulcers (10249).

Panax ginseng also seems to promote growth of normal intestinal flora while inhibiting Clostridial species (7). Panax ginseng may also lower serum cholesterol and triglycerides (6). However, panax ginseng appears to have negligible effects on cardiovascular function (4322). Preliminary evidence suggests that Panax ginseng might prevent insulin resistance and changes in gene expression in Type II diabetes (8605).

The estrogenic effects of ginseng are controversial. Some clinical evidence suggests it doesn't have estrogen-mediated effects such as increasing follicle-stimulating hormone (FSH), estradiol levels, or endometrial thickness (10981). However, case reports of ginseng side effects such as postmenopausal vaginal bleeding suggest estrogen activity (590,591,592,10982,10983). Panax ginseng extract has been shown to increase serum ceruloplasmin oxidase activity (a measure of estrogenic activity in the liver) in animal models when ovaries are removed (6180). In vitro research also shows estrogen activity. Studies on human breast cancer cells indicate that ginseng, specifically its constituent ginsonside-Rb1, acts as a phytoestrogen (10984).

Panaxagin, a protein isolated from unprocessed ginseng root, seems to have antiviral and antifungal activity, according to preliminary research. It appears to inhibit HIV reverse transcriptase and ribosomal activity of some fungi (8603).

A multi-ingredient cream preparation containing Panax ginseng is thought to work in premature ejaculation by increasing the penile vibratory threshold and reducing the amplitude of penile somatosensory evoked potentials (2537). Some people try ginseng for cystic fibrosis because there is preliminary evidence that it has activity against Pseudomonas aeruginosa lung infections, but this effect has not yet been demonstrated in humans (3095,3096). There is some evidence that a Panax ginseng root extract can mildly inhibit cytochrome P450 2D6 (CYP2D6) activity by approximately 6% in humans. However, it appears to have no effect on CYP3A4 activity (1303).

Adverse Reactions

Orally, Panax ginseng is usually well tolerated, but some patients can experience side effects. The most common side effect is insomnia (589). Less commonly patients can experience mastalgia (590), vaginal bleeding (591,592,3354), amenorrhea, tachycardia and palpitations, hypertension, hypotension, edema, decreased appetite, diarrhea, hyperpyrexia, pruritus, rose spots, headache, vertigo, euphoria, and mania (594). Uncommon side effects can include cerebral arteritis (595), Stevens-Johnson syndrome (596), cholestatic hepatitis (associated with a Panax ginseng-containing, multi-ingredient product, Prostata) (598), and anaphylaxis (11971).

When the multi-ingredient cream preparation (SS Cream) has been applied topically to the glans penis, sporadic erectile dysfunction, excessively delayed ejaculation, mild pain, and local irritation and burning has occurred (2537).

There is a lot of controversy about the existence of a "ginseng abuse syndrome". In the late 1970s one author reported the existence of this syndrome that occurred after long-term use of ginseng. Symptoms included one or more of the following: hypertension, nervousness, insomnia, increased libido, estrogenic effects, skin eruptions, edema, and diarrhea (3353). Experts now agree there is not a ginseng abuse syndrome (515). However, many of these individual side effects can occur in some patients, even after short-term use of Panax ginseng.

Interactions with Herbs & Other Dietary Supplements

COFFEE, GUARANA, TEA: Concomitant use may potentiate therapeutic and adverse effects due to the caffeine content of coffee, guarana, or tea (12).

EPHEDRA: Ephedra-containing supplements may prolong the QT interval. This might have an additive effect with Panax ginseng and increase the risk of life-threatening ventricular arrhythmias (4322,11355).

HERBS AND SUPPLEMENTS WITH HYPOGLYCEMIC EFFECTS: There is some evidence that Panax ginseng might lower blood glucose (4225). Theoretically, concomitant use with other herbs and supplements that decrease blood glucose levels might increase the risk of hypoglycemia. Some of these products include bitter melon, ginger, goat's rue, fenugreek, kudzu, willow bark, and others.

Interactions with Drugs

ANTICOAGULANT/ANTIPLATELET DRUGS: In vitro evidence suggests that ginsenoside constituents in Panax ginseng might decrease platelet aggregation (1522,11891). However, research in humans suggests that ginseng does not affect platelet aggregation (11890). Animal research indicates low oral bioavailability of Rb1 and rapid elimination of Rg1, which might explain the discrepancy between in vitro and human research (11153). Until more is known, use with caution in patients concurrently taking anticoagulant or antiplatelet drugs. Some antiplatelet and anticoagulant drugs include aspirin, cilostazol (Pletal), clopidogrel (Plavix), dalteparin (Fragmin), enoxaparin (Lovenox), heparin, ticlopidine (Ticlid), and others.
ANTIDIABETES DRUGS: Theoretically, concomitant use might enhance blood glucose lowering effects (4225). Monitor blood glucose levels closely. Some antidiabetes drugs include glimepiride (Amaryl), glyburide (DiaBeta, Glynase PresTab, Micronase), insulin, pioglitazone (Actos), rosiglitazone (Avandia), and others.
ANTIPSYCHOTIC DRUGS: Ginsenoside fractions of Panax ginseng seem to inhibit the uptake of several neurotransmitters in animals. Theoretically, Panax ginseng may interfere with antipsychotic drugs (4).
CAFFEINE: There is some concern that long-term use of 3 grams of Panax ginseng daily in combination with caffeine might lead to hypertension in some patients (19).
CYTOCHROME P450 2D6 (CYP2D6) SUBSTRATES: There is some evidence that Panax ginseng can inhibit the cytochrome P450 2D6 (CYP2D6) enzyme by approximately 6% (1303). Although this effect is unlikely to produce clinically significant interactions, it might cause slightly elevated levels of drugs metabolized by the CYP2D6 enzyme. Some of these drugs include amitriptyline (Elavil), clozapine (Clozaril), codeine, desipramine (Norpramin), donepezil (Aricept), fentanyl (Duragesic), flecainide (Tambocor), fluoxetine (Prozac), meperidine (Demerol), methadone (Dolophine), metoprolol (Lopressor, Toprol XL), olanzapine (Zyprexa), ondansetron (Zofran), tramadol (Ultram), trazodone (Desyrel), and others.
FUROSEMIDE (Lasix): There is some concern that Panax ginseng might contribute to diuretic resistance. There is one case of resistance to furosemide diuresis in a patient taking a germanium-containing ginseng product (770).
IMMUNOSUPPRESSANTS: Theoretically, concurrent use might interfere with immunosuppressive therapy. Panax ginseng might have immune system stimulating properties (3122). Immunosuppressant drugs include azathioprine (Imuran), basiliximab (Simulect), cyclosporine (Neoral, Sandimmune), daclizumab (Zenapax), muromonab-CD3 (OKT3, Orthoclone OKT3), mycophenolate (CellCept), tacrolimus (FK506, Prograf), sirolimus (Rapamune), prednisone (Deltasone, Orasone), and other corticosteroids (glucocorticoids).
INSULIN: There is some concern that Panax ginseng might have additive hypoglycemic effects when used with insulin. Insulin dose adjustments might be necessary in patients taking Panax ginseng (19); use with caution.
MONOAMINE OXIDASE INHIBITORS (MAOIs): Theoretically, Panax ginseng can interfere with MAOI therapy. Concomitant use with phenelzine (Nardil) is associated with insomnia, headache, tremors (617), and hypomania (618).
STIMULANT DRUGS: Panax ginseng can potentiate stimulant drug effects (12).
WARFARIN (Coumadin): There has been a single case report of decreased effectiveness of warfarin in a patient who also took Panax ginseng (619). However, it's questionable whether Panax ginseng was the cause of this decrease in warfarin effectiveness. Research in humans and animals suggests that Panax ginseng does not affect the pharmacokinetics of warfarin (2531,11890).

Interactions with Foods

COFFEE, TEA: Concomitant use may potentiate effects due to the caffeine content of coffee or tea (12).

Interactions with Lab Tests

ACTIVATED PARTIAL THROMBOPLASTIN TIME (aPTT), THROMBIN TIME (TT): Theoretically, Panax ginseng might prolong aPTT, TT, and increase test results (1522).
GLUCOSE: Panax ginseng might reduce fasting blood glucose concentrations and test results (4225).
GLYCOSYLATED HEMOGLOBIN (HbA1c): Panax ginseng might improve glucose control and reduce HbA1c values in patients with type 2 diabetes (4225).

Interactions with Diseases or Conditions

BLEEDING CONDITIONS: Ginseng has been reported to decrease blood coagulation (3122); contraindicated in cases of hemorrhage or thrombosis.
CARDIAC CONDITIONS: Ginseng can slightly increase the QT interval and slightly decrease diastolic blood pressure in healthy adults on the first day of therapy. However, there are no changes with prolonged use (4322). Ginseng has not been studied in people with cardiovascular disease. Use with caution.
DIABETES: Ginseng is reported to have hypoglycemic activity (4225). Use in diabetics might increase the risk of hypoglycemic episodes; use with caution.
HORMONE SENSITIVE CANCERS/CONDITIONS: Because ginseng seems to have estrogenic effects (6180,10984), women with hormone sensitive conditions should avoid ginseng. Some of these conditions include breast cancer, uterine cancer, ovarian cancer, endometriosis, and uterine fibroids.

INSOMNIA: High doses of ginseng have been associated with insomnia (597). Theoretically, use in patients with insomnia might worsen the condition; use with caution.
ORGAN TRANSPLANT RECIPIENTS: Theoretically, concurrent use might interfere with immunosuppressive therapy. Panax ginseng might have immune system stimulating properties (3122); avoid concurrent use.
SCHIZOPHRENIA: High doses of ginseng have been associated with insomnia and agitation in schizophrenic patients (597); use with caution.

Dosage and Administration

ORAL: For reducing the risk of getting the common cold or flu, Panax ginseng 100 mg daily started four weeks prior to influenza vaccination and continued for eight weeks thereafter has been used (589). For use in an acute attack of chronic bronchitis, Panax ginseng 100 mg twice daily for 9 days combined with antibiotic therapy has been used (8814). For erectile dysfunction, Panax ginseng 900 mg three times daily has been used (8813). For treating type 2 diabetes, 200 mg daily has been used (4225).
TOPICAL: For premature ejaculation, a cream containing panax ginseng and other ingredients has been applied to the glans penis 1 hour before intercourse and washed off before intercourse (2537).

Comments

Ginseng has been used for medicinal purposes for over two thousand years. Approximately six million Americans use it regularly. Some consider the age of the ginseng roots important. In 1976, a four hundred year old root of Manchurian ginseng from the mountains of China reportedly sold for $10,000 per ounce. The contents of commercial preparations labeled as containing Panax ginseng can vary greatly; many contain little or no Panax ginseng (6,13). Sometimes you will hear people refer to ginseng as red or white ginseng. This distinguishes how some ginseng roots are prepared. For example, red ginseng is produced by steam-curing the root. Heat treatment of ginseng at a temperature and pressure higher than what is conventionally used to prepare red ginseng has been found to cause increased production of the ginsenosides Rg3, Rg5, Rg6, Rh2, Rh3, Rh4, and Rs3 which are usually absent or present in only small amounts in preparations of white or red ginseng (11006). In contrast to the usual promotion of ginseng as a stimulant, ginseng is used in Traditional Chinese Medicine (TCM) as a calming and sedative agent. It is also widely used in China as a cardiovascular agent. Typically, higher doses are used in TCM than Western medicine (8600,8604).

GINSENG, SIBERIAN

Also Known As

Ci Wu Jia, Ciwujia, Devil's Bush, Devil's Shrub, Eleuthero Ginseng, Eleutherococci Radix, Eleutherococcus, Ginseng, Ginseng Root, Phytoestrogen, Prickly Eleutherococcus, Russian Root, Shigoka, Siberian Ginseng, Thorny Bearer of Free Berries, Touch-Me-Not, Untouchable, Ussuri, Ussurian Thorny Pepperbrush, Wild Pepper, Wu Jia Pi, Wu-jia.
CAUTION: See separate listings for American Ginseng, Ashwaganda, Blue Cohosh, Canaigre, Codonopsis, Panax Ginseng, and Panax Pseudoginseng.

Scientific Names

Eleutherococcus senticosus, synonym Acanthopanax senticosus, Hedera senticosa.
Family: Araliaceae.

People Use This For

Orally, people use Siberian ginseng as an adaptogen, for increasing resistance to environmental stress. It is also used orally for normalizing high or low blood pressure, atherosclerosis, pyelonephritis, craniocerebral trauma, rheumatic heart disease, neuroses, insomnia, and increasing work capacity. Other oral uses include Alzheimer's disease, attention deficit-hyperactivity disorder (ADHD), chronic fatigue syndrome, diabetes, fibromyalgia, rheumatoid arthritis, influenza, chronic bronchitis, tuberculosis, improving athletic performance, reducing toxicity of chemotherapy, and symptomatic treatment of herpes simplex type II infections. It is also used orally as a general stimulant, diuretic, appetite stimulant, immune system stimulant, and for preventing colds and flu. In manufacturing, Siberian ginseng is added to skin care products.

Safety

POSSIBLY SAFE ...when used orally and appropriately, short-term. Siberian ginseng root extract has been used safely for up to 6 weeks (7522).
PREGNANCY AND LACTATION: Insufficient reliable information available; avoid using.

Effectiveness

POSSIBLY EFFECTIVE

Herpes simplex virus type 2 (HSV-2). Taking a specific Siberian ginseng extract, standardized to contain eleutheroside 0.3% (Elagen), orally seems to reduce the frequency, severity, and duration of herpes simplex type II infections (730,1427).

POSSIBLY INEFFECTIVE

Athletic performance. Taking Siberian ginseng orally doesn't seem to increase speed, quality, and capacity for physical work. A specific Siberian ginseng root liquid extract standardized to eleutherosides B and E content 3.4 mL daily doesn't seem to have any effect on endurance; performance; or psychological, cardiac, or respiratory parameters in trained distance runners (7522,7593). In trained endurance cyclists, Siberian ginseng 1200 mg per day (Endurox) doesn't seem to have any effect on glycogen, fat utilization, or cycling performance time (2335). It also doesn't seem to improve respiration; reduce lactate production; or hasten heart rate recovery during stair-stepping exercise, treadmill, or cyclic ergometry (7600,7601,8994).

INSUFFICIENT RELIABLE EVIDENCE to RATE

Cognitive performance. There is preliminary evidence that suggests Siberian ginseng might improve memory and feelings of well-being in middle-aged people (2574).

Heart disease. There is preliminary evidence that suggests administering Siberian ginseng intravenously might be useful for hyperlipidemia, and arrhythmias (7523,7524).

Ischemic stroke. There is preliminary evidence that suggests administering Siberian ginseng intravenously might be useful for treating acute cerebral infarction (7529).

More evidence is needed to rate Siberian ginseng for these uses.

Mechanism of Action

The applicable parts of Siberian ginseng are the root and leaf. The root, which is most commonly used, contains active compounds referred to as eleutherosides A through M (1954). Eleutheroside B (syringin) and eleutheroside E (syringaresinol) are the most plentiful and are used as marker compounds for Siberian ginseng products (7533). The eleutherosides include a variety of diverse compounds including saponins (daucosterol, beta-sitosterol, hederasaponin B), coumarins (isofraxidin), lignans (sesamin, syringaresinol), phenylpropanoids (syringin, caffeic acid, sinapyl alcohol, coniferyl aldehyde, protocatechuic acid), betulinic acid, vitamin E, and provitamins like beta-carotene (1954). Several constituents including syringin, syringoresinol, sesamin, beta sitosterol, caffeic acid, and coniferyl aldehyde are thought to have antioxidant and possible anticancer effects (1954). In addition, there is some evidence that the constituent coniferyl aldehyde protects DNA against breakage caused by ultraviolet light (1954). Siberian ginseng root extracts seem to have an antiproliferative effect on leukemia cells and appear to potentiate the effect of antimetabolites such as cytarabine (7525). There's also preliminary evidence that suggests it might act as an antioxidant and prevent damage in ischemic stroke (7529). Siberian ginseng root, the lignan constituent sesamin, and the phenylpropanoid syringin seem to have immunostimulatory effects (1954). Siberian ginseng increases lymphocyte counts and phagocyte activity (6206).

Siberian ginseng constituents have a variety of other pharmacological effects. Protocatechuic acid seems to inhibit platelet aggregation (7592). Siberian ginseng constituents have a variety of other pharmacological effects. Eleutherosides A through G, particularly eleutheroside G, appears to have hypoglycemic activity (7591). Other constituents are also thought to be anti-inflammatory, sedative, diuretic, gonadotropic, estrogenic, protein-anabolic, and stimulate the pituitary-adrenocortical system (7531). Siberian ginseng root extract seems to inhibit RNA-type viruses including human rhinovirus, respiratory syncytial virus (RSV), and influenza A virus, but has no effect on DNA viruses such as adenovirus or herpes simplex type 1 virus (HSV-1) (7526). Polysaccharide derivatives of Siberian ginseng appear to inhibit growth of the tuberculosis bacterium (7530).

The possible pharmacologic effects of Siberian ginseng leaves are also a current area of research. The leaves contain saponins that might have hypoglycemic effects and antihistaminic effects (7527,7592). There's also preliminary evidence that leaf saponins, given intravenously, might reduce myocardial infarct (MI) size (7528).

Whole plant extracts, as well as root extracts, seem to have an inhibitory effect on cytochrome P450 (CYP450) enzymes. Preliminary evidence suggests that Siberian ginseng might inhibit CYP1A2, CYP2C9, CYP2D6, and CYP3A4 (7531,7532). However, Siberian ginseng does not appear to inhibit drug metabolism by CYP2D6 and CYP3A4 in humans (7532,10400).

Adverse Reactions

Orally, Siberian ginseng can cause slight drowsiness, anxiety, irritability, and melancholy. Mastalgia can also occur. These adverse effects are more likely with higher than normal doses. Siberian ginseng should be used cautiously in patients with cardiovascular disorders (e.g., atherosclerotic or rheumatic heart disease), because it can cause palpitations, tachycardia, and hypertension (6500). Headache and pericardial pain can also occur in patients with rheumatic heart disease. Long term use of Siberian ginseng is associated with inflamed nerves, often the sciatic nerve, which can then cause muscle spasms. There is one case report of neonatal androgenization following maternal use of Siberian ginseng (593,6500). However, it was later discovered that the androgenization was not due to Siberian ginseng, but due to silk vine (Periploca sepium) bark contamination (850,6500).

Interactions with Herbs & Other Dietary Supplements

ANTICOAGULANT, ANTIPLATELET HERBS AND SUPPLEMENTS: Concomitant use with herbs and supplements that affect platelet aggregation could theoretically increase the risk of bleeding in some people due to Siberian ginseng's possible effect on platelet aggregation (7592). Some of these herbs and supplements include angelica, clove, danshen, fish oil, garlic, ginger, Panax ginseng, red clover, turmeric, vitamin E, others.

HERBS AND SUPPLEMENTS WITH HYPOGLYCEMIC EFFECTS: There is preliminary evidence that suggests Siberian ginseng might have hypoglycemic effects (7591). Theoretically, concomitant use with other herbs and supplements that decrease blood glucose levels might increase the risk of hypoglycemia. Some of these products include bitter melon, ginger, goat's rue, fenugreek, kudzu, gymnema, and others.

HERBS WITH SEDATIVE PROPERTIES: There is preliminary evidence that Siberian ginseng root extract might cause dose-dependent sedation (7531). Theoretically, concomitant use with herbs that have sedative properties might enhance therapeutic and adverse effects. These include calamus, California poppy, catnip, German chamomile, gotu kola, hops, Jamaican dogwood, kava, lemon balm, sage, St. John's wort, sassafras, scullcap, valerian, wild carrot, wild lettuce, and others.

Interactions with Drugs

ALCOHOL (Ethanol): There is preliminary evidence that suggests that Siberian ginseng root extract might have sedative effects (7531). Theoretically, it might have an additive sedative effect with alcohol.

ANTICOAGULANT/ANTIPLATELET DRUGS: A constituent of Siberian ginseng, dihydroxybenzoic acid, appears to inhibit platelet aggregation (7592). Concomitant use with anticoagulant or antiplatelet drugs might increase the risk of bleeding.

ANTIDIABETES DRUGS: Certain constituents of Siberian ginseng appear to have hypoglycemic activity (7591). Monitor blood glucose levels closely. Some antidiabetes drugs include glimepiride (Amaryl), glyburide (DiaBeta, Glynase PresTab, Micronase), insulin, pioglitazone (Actos), rosiglitazone (Avandia), and others.

CNS DEPRESSANTS: There is preliminary evidence that suggests that Siberian ginseng root extract may have sedative properties (7531). Theoretically, concomitant use with drugs with sedative properties may cause additive effects and side effects.

CYTOCHROME P450 1A2 (CYP1A2) SUBSTRATES: Preliminary evidence suggests that standardized extracts of Siberian ginseng might inhibit cytochrome P450 1A2 (CYP1A2) in vitro and in animal models (7532). Until more is known about the effect on CYP1A2 Siberian ginseng should be used cautiously in patients taking drugs that are metabolized by these CYP450 enzymes. Some drugs metabolized by CYP1A2 include clozapine (Clozaril), cyclobenzaprine (Flexeril), fluvoxamine (Luvox), haloperidol (Haldol), imipramine (Tofranil), mexiletine (Mexitil), olanzapine (Zyprexa), Pentazocine (Talwin), propranolol (Inderal), tacrine (Cognex), theophylline (Slo-bid, Theo-Dur, others), zileuton (Zyflo), Zolmitriptan (Zomig), and others.

CYTOCHROME P450 2C9 (CYP2C9) SUBSTRATES: Preliminary evidence suggests that standardized extracts of Siberian ginseng might inhibit cytochrome P450 2C9 (CYP2C9) in vitro and in animal models (7532). Until more is known about the effect on CYP2C9, Siberian ginseng should be used cautiously in patients taking drugs that are metabolized by these CYP450 enzymes. Some drugs metabolized by CYP2C9 include amitriptyline (Elavil), diazepam (Valium), estradiol (Estrace), tacrine (Cognex), verapamil (Calan), warfarin (Coumadin), zileuton (Zyflo), and others.

CYTOCHROME P450 2D6 (CYP2D6) SUBSTRATES: Preliminary evidence suggests that standardized extracts of Siberian ginseng might inhibit cytochrome P450 2D6 (CYP2D6) in vitro and in animal models. However, Siberian ginseng does not appear to inhibit drug metabolism by CYP2D6 in humans (7532,10400).

CYTOCHROME P450 3A4 (CYP3A4) SUBSTRATES: Preliminary evidence suggests that standardized extracts of Siberian ginseng might inhibit cytochrome P450 3A4 (CYP3A4) in vitro and in animal models. However, Siberian ginseng does not appear to inhibit drug metabolism by CYP3A4 in humans (7532,10400).

DIGOXIN (Lanoxin): One case report associated Siberian ginseng with elevated serum digoxin levels, without symptoms of toxicity (543). However, it is not clear if this was due to an interaction or whether the product ingested in this case actually contained cardiac glycoside-like constituents. The product was found to be free of digoxin and digitoxin (543), but was not tested for the presence of eleutherosides (797). It is unclear whether the product actually contained Eleutherococcus. It has been postulated that it may have contained silk vine (Periploca sepium) which is reported to contain cardiac glycosides, and silk vine is a common adulterant of Eleutherococcus senticosus (797).

Interactions with Foods

None known.

Interactions with Lab Tests

BLOOD GLUCOSE: Theoretically, Siberian ginseng might lower blood glucose levels. Eleutheroside constituents of Siberian ginseng appear to have hypoglycemic activity (7591).

Interactions with Diseases or Conditions

CARDIOVASCULAR CONDITIONS: Siberian ginseng can cause palpitations, tachycardia, and hypertension and should be used cautiously in patients with cardiovascular disorders (e.g. atherosclerotic or rheumatic heart disease). It can also cause headache and pericardial pain in patients with rheumatic heart disease (6500).

HORMONE SENSITIVE CANCERS/CONDITIONS: Because Siberian ginseng might have estrogenic effects (6180), women with hormone sensitive conditions should avoid Siberian ginseng. Some of these conditions include breast cancer, uterine cancer, ovarian cancer, endometriosis, and uterine fibroids.
HYPERTENSION: Siberian ginseng is contraindicated in individuals with blood pressure exceeding 180/90. Siberian ginseng can potentially exacerbate hypertension (12).
MYOCARDIAL INFARCTION (MI): Theoretically, Siberian ginseng may exacerbate MI (4); use with caution.
PSYCHIATRIC CONDITIONS: Theoretically, Siberian ginseng may exacerbate some psychiatric conditions including hysteria, mania, and schizophrenia (4); use with caution.

Dosage and Administration

ORAL: For herpes simplex type II infections, Siberian ginseng extract standardized to contain eleutheroside E 0.3% in doses of 400 mg per day has been used (1427).

Comments

"Adaptogen" is a non-medical term used to suggest that a substance can act to strengthen the body and increase general resistance. It is often used to describe the purported activity of Siberian ginseng (1954). The chemical content and potency of various Siberian ginseng products can vary (7533). Siberian ginseng is often misidentified or adulterated. Siberian ginseng is a completely different herb than American or Panax ginseng. American and Panax ginseng can be considerably more expensive. It is said that the Soviet Union wanted to provide its athletes with the advantage offered by ginseng but wanted a less expensive version. Therefore Siberian ginseng became popular, and this is why most studies on Siberian ginseng have been done in Russia. Exercise caution in differentiating ginseng products. Silk vine is a common adulterant of Siberian ginseng (797).

GLOBE FLOWER

Also Known As

Globe Crowfoot, Globe Ranunculus, Globe Trollius.

Scientific Names

Trollius europaeus.
Family: Ranunculaceae.

People Use This For

Orally, globe flower is used for scurvy.

Safety

LIKELY UNSAFE ...when any part of the fresh plant is used orally or topically because it can cause severe local irritation (18).
There is insufficient reliable information available about the safety of the dried, cut globe flower plant.
PREGNANCY AND LACTATION: LIKELY UNSAFE ...when any part of the fresh plant is used orally or topically (18). There is insufficient reliable information available about the safety of the dried, cut globe flower plant during pregnancy and lactation.

Effectiveness

There is insufficient reliable information available about the effectiveness of globe flower.

Mechanism of Action

The applicable part is the whole fresh plant. When the fresh plant is crushed or cut into small pieces, the glycoside ranunculin is enzymatically changed into a severely irritating protoanemonin, which, in turn, rapidly degrades into the less toxic anemonin (18). Both protoanemonin and ranunculin are destroyed to an unknown extent during the drying process (2).

Adverse Reactions

Orally, ingestion of globe flower can cause severe irritation of the gastrointestinal tract, with colic and diarrhea. Irritation of the urinary tract can also occur.
Topically, skin contact can cause blisters and burns that are difficult to heal (18).

Interactions with Herbs & Other Dietary Supplements

None known.

Interactions with Drugs

None known.

Interactions with Foods
None known.

Interactions with Lab Tests
None known.

Interactions with Diseases or Conditions
None known.

Dosage and Administration
No typical dosage.

GLOSSY PRIVET

Also Known As
Chinese Privet, Dongqingzi, Ligustro, Ligustrum, Ligustrum Fruit, Nu Zhen, Nu Zhen Zi, Nuzhenzi, Privet, To-Nezumimochi, Troène De Chine, Trueno, White Waxtree.

Scientific Names
Ligustrum lucidum.
Family: Oleaceae.

People Use This For
Orally, glossy privet is used for promoting growth and darkening of hair, reducing facial dark spots, palpitations, rheumatism, swelling, tumors, vertigo, common cold, congestion, constipation, deafness, debility, fever, headache, hepatitis, insomnia, rejuvenation and longevity. It is also used as a diaphoretic and tonic, for improving immune function, and reducing the side effects of chemotherapy. Glossy privet is also used for blurred vision, invigorating the liver and kidney, for dizziness, tinnitus, and for sore back and knees.

Safety
POSSIBLY SAFE ...when used orally and appropriately (12).
PREGNANCY AND LACTATION: Insufficient reliable information available; avoid using.

Effectiveness
There is insufficient reliable information available about the effectiveness of glossy privet.

Mechanism of Action
The applicable part of glossy privet is the ripe fruit (11). It contains triterpenoids, including oleanolic acid (ligustrin), acetyloleanolic acid, and ursolic acid; glycosides (including ligustroside, oleuropein, 4-hydroxy-beta-phenylethyl-beta-D-glucoside); mannitol; fatty oil, consisting mainly of linoleic, linolenic, oleic and palmitic acids; and a volatile oil consisting primarily of esters, alcohols, thioketones and hydrocarbons (11). Ligustrum is used clinically in China for treating leukopenia, although data involving experimentally-induced leukopenia did not show any effect (418). Ligustrum might also have immunomodulatory and antitumor effects (11). Preliminary evidence suggests that glossy privet fruit might inhibit growth of renal cell carcinoma, possibly via augmentation of phagocyte and lymphokine-activated killer cell activity (419). Glossy privet extracts inhibit mutagenicity in bacteria (420), stimulate T-cell function in cancer tissue (423), and reverse tumor-induced macrophage suppression (421). Preliminary evidence suggests that glossy privet fruit, and the ingredient ligustrin, might have anti-inflammatory, anti-allergic, mild cardiotonic, diuretic, sedative, lipid-lowering, blood flow enhancing, blood glucose lowering, and liver protectant effects (11).

Adverse Reactions
None reported. However, respiratory allergies (allergic rhinitis, asthma) and cross-allergenicity have been reported with the pollen of other Oleaceae species including common privet (Ligustrum vulgare), olive, ash, and lilac (416,417).

Interactions with Herbs & Other Dietary Supplements
None known.

Interactions with Drugs
None known.

Interactions with Foods
None known.

Interactions with Lab Tests
None known.

Interactions with Diseases or Conditions
None known.

Dosage and Administration
No typical dosage.

Comments
Avoid confusion with other species of privet such as Japanese privet (Ligustrum japonicum), border privet (Ligustrum obtusifolium), Chinese privet (Ligustrum sinense), privet (Ligustrum tschonoskii), common privet (Ligustrum vulgare), and golden privet (Ligustrum x vicaryi). The fruits of glossy privet (Ligustrum lucidum) and Ilex chinensis are both referred to by the Chinese name dongqingzi (11).

GLUCOMANNAN

Also Known As
Konjac, Konjac Mannan.

Scientific Names
Amorphophallus konjac, synonym Amorphophallus rivieri.
Family: Araceae.

People Use This For
Orally, glucomannan is used for constipation, weight loss in adults and children, type 2 diabetes, blood glucose control, and reducing serum cholesterol.
In foods, glucomannan is used in food preparation.

Safety
POSSIBLY SAFE ...when used orally in powdered or encapsulated form (180,182,11357,11358,11359).
LIKELY UNSAFE ...when used orally in tablet form. There have been reports of esophageal and gastrointestinal obstruction (11293).
CHILDREN: POSSIBLY SAFE ...when used orally and appropriately in powdered or encapsulated form for up to 4 months (179,180). LIKELY UNSAFE ...when used orally in tablet form. There have been reports of esophageal and gastrointestinal obstruction (11293).
PREGNANCY AND LACTATION: Insufficient reliable information available; avoid using.

Effectiveness
POSSIBLY EFFECTIVE

Diabetes. Taking glucomannan orally seems to reduce serum cholesterol and blood glucose levels in patients with type 2 diabetes (183,11357,11359). Glucomannan may improve serum total cholesterol, low-density lipoprotein (LDL) levels, glycemic control, and systolic blood pressure in patients with type 2 diabetes and hyperlipidemia. Glucomannan also seems to improve insulin resistance syndrome, a prediabetic metabolic condition. The positive effect on insulin resistance syndrome appears to occur when glucomannan is mixed and consumed with carbohydrate foods (11358).

INSUFFICIENT RELIABLE EVIDENCE to RATE

Constipation. Preliminary clinical research suggests that taking glucomannan orally might relieve constipation. As a nonabsorbable dietary fiber, glucomannan may have a bulk laxative effect (11294,11295).

Obesity. There is preliminary evidence that taking glucomannan orally might help reduce weight in obese children and adults (180,181,182,183). But some research shows no effect (179).

More evidence is needed to rate glucomannan for these uses.

Mechanism of Action
Glucomannan is an unabsorbable polysaccharide composed of glucose and mannose that is derived from konjac (Amorphophallus konjac) root (11361). Glucomannan contains insoluble fiber that may increase water absorption by the stools (11294,11295).
Glucomannan seems to reduce serum total cholesterol and low-density lipoprotein (LDL) cholesterol levels in

healthy men (178) and in adults with type 2 diabetes (11357). Glucomannan appears to improve lipid profiles by enhancing fecal excretion of cholesterol and bile acid (11357). Glucomannan may improve glycemic control in people with type 2 diabetes (11357,11359), possibly by slowing gastric emptying and increasing the viscosity of gastrointestinal contents (11361). Glucomannan also seems to improve systolic blood pressure in people with type 2 diabetes (11359).

Adverse Reactions
Orally, esophageal and gastrointestinal obstructions have been reported when the tablet form has been used (11293).

Interactions with Herbs & Other Dietary Supplements
HERBS AND SUPPLEMENTS WITH HYPOGLYCEMIC EFFECTS: There is some evidence that glucomannan might have hypoglycemic effects (183,11357,11359). Theoretically, concomitant use with other herbs and supplements that decrease blood glucose levels might increase the risk of hypoglycemia. Some of these products include bitter melon, cowhage, ginger, goat's rue, fenugreek, kudzu, willow bark, and others.

Interactions with Drugs
ANTIDIABETES DRUGS: Glucomannan can reduce blood glucose levels in patients with type 2 diabetes (11357,11359) and might have additive effects on glucose levels when used with antidiabetes drug therapy. Monitor blood glucose levels closely. Medication dose adjustments may be necessary. Some antidiabetes drugs include glimepiride (Amaryl), glyburide (DiaBeta, Glynase PresTab, Micronase), insulin, pioglitazone (Actos), rosiglitazone (Avandia), and others.
ORAL DRUGS: Glucomannan may decrease absorption of drugs taken orally, including sulfonylurea medications (11360). Some sulfonylurea drugs include chlorpropamide (Diabinese), glimepiride (Amaryl), glipizide (Glucotrol), glyburide (DiaBeta, Glynase PresTab, Micronase), and others. Take oral drugs one hour before or four hours after glucomannan to avoid decreased or delayed absorption.

Interactions with Foods
None known.

Interactions with Lab Tests
CHOLESTEROL: Glucomannan might reduce serum total cholesterol, LDL cholesterol, and test results in obese adults and adults with type 2 diabetes (181,182,183,11357,11359).
GLUCOSE: Glucomannan might reduce blood glucose concentrations and test results in patients with type 2 diabetes (11357,11359).
TRIGLYCERIDES: Glucomannan might reduce serum triglycerides and test results in obese adults (181,182)

Interactions with Diseases or Conditions
DIABETES: Glucomannan may interfere with blood sugar control (11357,11359), monitor closely.

Dosage and Administration
ORAL: For adult weight loss, 1 gram three times daily (1 hour before each meal) (182), has been used. For child weight loss, 2 to 3 grams per day has been used (180). For type 2 diabetes with hyperlipidemia, 3.6 to 10.6 grams per day has been used (11357,11359). For insulin resistance syndrome, 8 to 13 grams per day has been used (11358).

GLUCOSAMINE HYDROCHLORIDE

Also Known As
2-amino-2-deoxy-beta-D-glucopyranose, Amino Monosaccharide, Chitosamine, D-Glucosamine HCL, Glucosamine HCL, Glucose-6-Phosphate.
CAUTION: See separate listings for Glucosamine Sulfate and N-Acetyl Glucosamine.

Scientific Names
2-amino-2-deoxyglucose hydrochloride.

People Use This For
Orally, glucosamine hydrochloride is used for osteoarthritis and glaucoma.

Safety
POSSIBLY SAFE ...when used orally and appropriately, short-term. Glucosamine hydrochloride has been used safely in studies lasting up to 16 weeks (1520,4237).
There is insufficient reliable information available about the safety of long-term use of glucosamine hydrochloride.
PREGNANCY AND LACTATION: Insufficient reliable information available; avoid using.

Effectiveness

POSSIBLY EFFECTIVE

Osteoarthritis. Glucosamine hydrochloride seems to reduce subjective pain levels in some patients with osteoarthritis of the knee (1520,10312). The majority of evidence supporting glucosamine hydrochloride involves a specific combination product, which contains glucosamine hydrochloride, chondroitin sulfate, and manganese ascorbate (CosaminDS). This combination seems to improve both objective and subjective measures of pain in patients with osteoarthritis of the knee (4237,7169). It is not known if this benefit is due to glucosamine hydrochloride or the other ingredients. There is significantly more evidence supporting glucosamine sulfate for osteoarthritis. Encourage patients interested in trying glucosamine to use the glucosamine sulfate formulation.

There is insufficient reliable information available about the effectiveness of glucosamine hydrochloride for its other uses.

Mechanism of Action

Glucosamine hydrochloride is one of the salt forms of the amino sugar glucosamine, which is a constituent of cartilage proteoglycans. Other salt forms are also available including glucosamine sulfate and N-acetyl glucosamine. Although glucosamine is administered in a salt form, the salt is likely cleaved off in the stomach. Glucosamine base is completely ionized in the stomach. Laboratory data suggests that glucosamine base, glucosamine hydrochloride, and glucosamine sulfate may be equally active, but there are no head-to-head clinical studies (8128). Glucosamine is usually derived from marine exoskeletons or produced synthetically. Glucosamine is required for the synthesis of glycoproteins, glycolipids, and glycosaminoglycans (also known as mucopolysaccharides); these carbohydrate-containing compounds are found in tendons, ligaments, cartilage, synovial fluid, mucous membranes, structures in the eye, blood vessels, and heart valves. Glucosamine stimulates metabolism of chondrocytes in the articular cartilage and synovial cells in the synovial tissues. Glucosamine is also a component of biologically active compounds such as heparin, but it does not react with heparin-induced thrombocytopenia (HIT) antibodies (7640,7641,11831).

There has been a lot of concern about the effect of glucosamine on glucose metabolism. Preliminary evidence suggests glucosamine might decrease glucose-induced insulin secretion by inhibiting pancreatic glucokinase in the beta cells of the islet of Langerhans (371,372,3406). Other preliminary research suggests that glucosamine might also impair insulin-mediated glucose uptake and metabolism in skeletal muscle (372,3406). Animal research suggests glucosamine might increase glucose metabolism through the hexosamine pathway, a pattern of change in glucose metabolism similar to that seen in type 2 diabetes (3405,3406). However, animals may handle glucosamine differently than humans. Most of the research in humans suggests that glucosamine doesn't affect the pharmacokinetics of glucose. Research in people with normal glucose metabolism suggests glucosamine doesn't affect insulin sensitivity or plasma glucose (7637,7638). Clinical research in people with type 2 diabetes and people without diabetes suggests that glucosamine doesn't have any significant effect on blood glucose when given for up to 3 years (7026,10311,10317). Preliminary clinical research suggests that endogenous glucosamine and insulin levels are elevated in nondiabetic patients with ischemic heart disease (7640,7641). Some researchers think that increased glucosamine production might contribute to endothelial cell dysfunction (8944). Some glucosamine preparations are provided as topical creams. It is not known if glucosamine is absorbed transdermally.

Some researchers think the sulfate moiety in glucosamine sulfate might be responsible for its effect on osteoarthritis. Sulfate is required for articular cartilage glycosaminoglycan synthesis. Glucosamine might increase the absorption of sulfate. Glucosamine sulfate increases serum and synovial sulfate levels. Acetaminophen given concurrently with glucosamine sulfate, decreases sulfate levels, suggesting that use of acetaminophen in clinical trials might alter results. If the sulfate is the active moiety of glucosamine sulfate, theoretically glucosamine hydrochloride would be less effective (10313), but there are no head-to-head clinical studies of the sulfate and hydrochloride salts of glucosamine. More research is needed to determine the role of sulfate in the efficacy of glucosamine sulfate.

Adverse Reactions

Orally, glucosamine hydrochloride can cause mild gastrointestinal (GI) symptoms such as gas, abdominal bloating, and cramps (1520). Anecdotal reports have associated glucosamine with renal toxicity, but changes in renal function have not been reported in long-term studies (7026,8942,10408,10409).

Elevated blood glucose levels in patients with diabetes have been reported (22). However, 90 days of glucosamine therapy does not seem to affect hemoglobin A1C levels in people with type 2 diabetes (10311,10317). There is some concern that it might increase the risk of metabolic disturbances resulting in increased cholesterol levels and blood pressure. However, glucosamine hydrochloride does not appear to increase the risk of these adverse effects (7075). In people older than 45, who have taken glucosamine for 3 years, there doesn't seem to be any adverse effects on blood glucose metabolism, lipid metabolism, or any other disturbances in metabolism (7026,8942).

Tell patients to look out for glucosamine plus chondroitin combination products that also contain manganese (e.g., CosaminDS). Remind patients to adhere to product directions. When taken at doses slightly higher than the recommended dose, these products can sometimes supply greater than the tolerable upper limit (UL) for manganese (11 mg per day). Ingestion of more than 11 mg per day of manganese might cause significant central nervous system toxicity (7135).

Interactions with Herbs & Other Dietary Supplements

None known.

Interactions with Drugs

ANTIDIABETES DRUGS: Preliminary research suggests that glucosamine might increase insulin resistance, or decrease insulin production, and potentially worsen diabetes control (371,372,3406,7637,7638). But there is some clinical evidence that suggests that taking glucosamine for 3 months does not increase hemoglobin A1c (HbA1c) in people with type 2 diabetes who have well-controlled glucose levels (10311,10317). Until more is known, advise patients with diabetes who take glucosamine to monitor their blood glucose levels closely. Some antidiabetes drugs include glimepiride (Amaryl), glyburide (DiaBeta, Glynase PresTab, Micronase), insulin, pioglitazone (Actos), rosiglitazone (Avandia), and others.
ANTIMITOTIC CHEMOTHERAPY: Theoretically, glucosamine might induce resistance to etoposide (VP16, VePesid) and doxorubicin (Adriamycin) by reducing the drugs' inhibition of topoisomerase II, an enzyme required for DNA replication in tumor cells (7639).
WARFARIN (Coumadin): There's some concern that high-dose glucosamine (3000 mg per day), combined with high-dose chondroitin sulfate (2400 mg per day), may enhance the effects of warfarin (Coumadin) as measured by the INR (11389). Chondroitin is a small component of a heparinoid and might have weak anticoagulant activity. Glucosamine is also a small component of heparin, but is does not seem to have anticoagulant activity. It's not known if glucosamine contributes to this potential interaction. Interactions with warfarin have not been reported at recommended dosages of glucosamine or chondroitin.

Interactions with Foods

None known.

Interactions with Lab Tests

BLOOD GLUCOSE: Glucosamine doesn't seem to adversely affect blood glucose control in people with type 2 diabetes, as measured by hemoglobin A1C (10311,10317). It also doesn't seem to affect blood glucose in nondiabetic people older than 45, who have taken glucosamine for osteoarthritis for 3 years (7026,8942). Some preliminary research raised concerns that glucosamine might exacerbate diabetes by increasing insulin resistance and/or decreasing insulin production, resulting in elevated blood glucose levels (5059). However, other research has shown no effect (7637,7638). There are also anecdotal reports of reduced blood glucose control in people with diabetes who take glucosamine (22,1203,1204,3405,3406). However, clinical studies indicate that glucosamine has little or no effect blood glucose (7026,8942,10311,10317).
INTERNATIONAL NORMALIZED RATIO (INR)/PROTHROMBIN TIME (PT): High dose glucosamine (3000 mg per day), combined with high dose chondroitin sulfate (2400 mg per day), may increase the INR in patients taking warfarin (Coumadin). There is one case report of an increased INR associated with concomitant use of warfarin a glucosamine-chondroitin supplement taken above recommended dosages (11389).

Interactions with Diseases or Conditions

ASTHMA: Glucosamine might exacerbate asthma by an unidentified allergic mechanism. Use glucosamine hydrochloride cautiously in patients with asthma (10002).
DIABETES: Glucosamine doesn't seem to adversely affect blood glucose control in people with type 2 diabetes, as measured by hemoglobin A1C (10311,10317). Some preliminary research raised concerns that glucosamine might exacerbate diabetes by increasing insulin resistance and/or decreasing insulin production, resulting in elevated blood glucose levels (5059). However, other research has shown no effect on insulin sensitivity or plasma glucose (7637,7638). There are also anecdotal reports of reduced blood glucose control in people with diabetes who take glucosamine (22,1203,1204,3405,3406). However, clinical studies indicate that glucosamine seems to be safe in people with type 2 diabetes (10311,10317).
SHELLFISH ALLERGY: There is concern that glucosamine hydrochloride products derived from marine exoskeletons might cause reactions in people allergic to shellfish, although no reactions have been reported. Until more is known, and because the source of glucosamine hydrochloride products is not required to be listed on product labels, use glucosamine hydrochloride with caution in people with shellfish allergy.

Dosage and Administration

ORAL: For osteoarthritis, one study used glucosamine hydrochloride 500 mg three times daily (1520).
A combination of glucosamine hydrochloride, 1500 mg/day, chondroitin sulfate, 1200 mg/day, and manganese ascorbate, 228 mg/day (Cosamin-DS, Nutramax Laboratories) has also been used (4237).

Comments

Read glucosamine product labels carefully for content. Avoid confusion with glucosamine sulfate and N-acetyl glucosamine. These products may not be interchangeable. Glucosamine sulfate has been studied the most for osteoarthritis. However, there is no clinical evidence to support the use of N-acetyl glucosamine for osteoarthritis. There is great variability among glucosamine and glucosamine plus chondroitin products. Actual content versus label claim varies from 25% to 115% (8128).

GLUCOSAMINE SULFATE

Also Known As

2-amino-2-deoxy-beta-D-glucopyranose, Amino Monosaccharide, Chitosamine, D-Glucosamine, G6S, Glucosamine, Glucosamine Sulphate, Glucose-6-phosphate, Glucose-6-sulfate, Glucose-6-sulphate, GS, Mono-Sulfated Saccharide, Sulfated Monosaccharide, Sulfated Saccharide, Sulphated Monosaccharide.
CAUTION: See separate listings for Glucosamine Hydrochloride and N-Acetyl Glucosamine.

Scientific Names

2-amino-2-deoxyglucose sulfate.

People Use This For

Orally, glucosamine sulfate is used for osteoarthritis, glaucoma, temporomandibular joint (TMJ) arthritis, and weight loss. Glucosamine sulfate is also used orally in combination with other products, including chondroitin sulfate, glucosamine hydrochloride, or N-acetyl glucosamine.
Topically, glucosamine sulfate is used in combination with chondroitin sulfate, shark cartilage, and camphor for osteoarthritis.
Parenterally, glucosamine sulfate is used short-term for reducing the symptoms of osteoarthritis.

Safety

LIKELY SAFE ...when used orally and appropriately. Glucosamine has been used safely in multiple clinical trials lasting from 4 weeks to 3 years (2533,2600,2602,2603,2604,2606,7026,8942,11340).
POSSIBLY SAFE ...when used intramuscularly and appropriately, short-term. Intramuscular glucosamine seems to be well tolerated when given twice weekly for up to six weeks (2605). ...when used topically and appropriately, short term. Glucosamine sulfate in combination with chondroitin sulfate, shark cartilage, and camphor appears to be safe when applied topically on an as-needed basis for up to eight weeks (10327).
PREGNANCY AND LACTATION: Insufficient reliable information available; avoid using.

Effectiveness

LIKELY EFFECTIVE

Osteoarthritis. Taking glucosamine sulfate orally can significantly improve symptoms of pain and functionality indices in patients with osteoarthritis of the knee. These benefits have been consistently demonstrated in studies lasting from a few weeks to three years (2533,2600,2602,2603,2604,2606,7026,8942,10310,10312). There is evidence that suggests that glucosamine sulfate is comparable to the nonsteroidal anti-inflammatory drugs (NSAIDs) ibuprofen (2602,2604) and piroxicam (Feldene) for symptom relief (2606); however, NSAIDs appear to relieve symptoms within 2 weeks compared to 4 to 8 weeks with glucosamine sulfate (2602,2604,2606). Unlike NSAIDs and analgesics, glucosamine might have disease-modifying activity, slowing joint degeneration in patients with osteoarthritis. There is evidence that patients taking glucosamine for up to 3 years have significantly less knee joint degeneration, less joint space narrowing, and significant symptom improvement when compared with placebo (7026,8942). However, preliminary evidence suggests that glucosamine might not prevent disease flare-ups (9118). It might also not be very effective for more severe, long-standing osteoarthritis (1330,11459); and osteoarthritis in older and heavier patients (1330).
So far, most studies have only evaluated glucosamine sulfate for osteoarthritis of the knee. However, there is preliminary clinical evidence that suggests that glucosamine sulfate might also be helpful for osteoarthritis of the lumbar spine (1316). Intramuscular glucosamine sulfate also seems to help. When given twice per week for 6 weeks it reduces the severity of symptoms of knee osteoarthritis in patients with mild to moderately severe disease (radiological stage I-III) compared to placebo (2605). There is also a report that a topical preparation of glucosamine sulfate in combination with chondroitin sulfate, shark cartilage, and camphor reduces osteoarthritis symptoms. But any symptom relief is most likely due to the counterirritant effect of camphor and not the other ingredients (10327). There's no research showing that glucosamine is absorbed topically. Don't recommend topical glucosamine products. Most clinical trials have used a specific patented oral formulation of glucosamine sulfate (Dona, Viartril-S, Rottapharm, Italy) (11340). Glucosamine sulfate is often combined with chondroitin, but it's not known if this combination is any more effective than the individual ingredients.

POSSIBLY EFFECTIVE

Temporomandibular joint (TMJ) arthritis. Taking glucosamine sulfate orally appears to be at least as effective as analgesic doses of ibuprofen for relieving pain and improving TMJ function such as chewing, yawning, talking, and laughing. In some patients pain relief persists for up to 90 days after glucosamine sulfate is discontinued (3714).

There is insufficient reliable information available about the effectiveness of glucosamine sulfate for its other uses.

Mechanism of Action

Glucosamine is an amino sugar, which is a constituent of cartilage proteoglycans. It is derived from marine exoskeletons or produced synthetically. Glucosamine is required for the synthesis of glycoproteins, glycolipids, and glycosaminoglycans (also known as mucopolysaccharides). These carbohydrate-containing compounds are found in tendons, ligaments, cartilage, synovial fluid, mucous membranes, structures in the eye, blood vessels, and heart valves. Glucosamine is also a component of biologically active compounds such as heparin, but it does not react with heparin-induced thrombocytopenia (HIT) antibodies (7640,7641,11831).

In osteoarthritis, glucosamine stimulates metabolism of chondrocytes in the articular cartilage and of synovial cells in the synovial tissues. There is evidence that suggests that glucosamine might have a disease-modifying effect, stopping or slowing the progression of osteoarthritis (7026). Preliminary research suggests that glucosamine inhibits protein N-glycosylation and cytokine-stimulated production of mediators of inflammation and cartilage degradation (9119). Glucosamine seems to inhibit interleukin 1-beta, IL-1beta, which stimulates the gene expression and protein synthesis of cyclooxygenase-2, COX-2 (9121). Glucosamine doesn't seem to directly affect cyclooxygenase, which is responsible for anti-inflammatory and analgesic effects of nonsteroidal anti-inflammatory drugs (NSAIDs), as well as adverse gastrointestinal effects (2604).

Glucosamine might have activity against human immunodeficiency virus (HIV). Preliminary evidence suggests that it might inhibit the intracellular viral movement and block viral replication (7642).

There has been a lot of concern about the effect of glucosamine on glucose metabolism. Preliminary evidence suggests glucosamine might decrease glucose-induced insulin secretion by inhibiting pancreatic glucokinase in the beta cells of the islet of Langerhans (371,372,3406). Other preliminary research suggests that glucosamine might also impair insulin-mediated glucose uptake and metabolism in skeletal muscle (372,3406). Animal research suggests glucosamine might increase glucose metabolism through the hexosamine pathway, a pattern of change in glucose metabolism similar to that seen in type 2 diabetes (3405,3406). However, animals may handle glucosamine differently than humans. Most of the research in humans suggests that glucosamine doesn't affect the pharmacokinetics of glucose. Research in people with normal glucose metabolism suggests glucosamine doesn't affect insulin sensitivity or plasma glucose (7637,7638). Clinical research in people with type 2 diabetes and people without diabetes suggests glucosamine doesn't have any significant effect on blood glucose when given for up to 3 years (7026,8942,10311,10317). Preliminary clinical research suggests that endogenous glucosamine and insulin levels are elevated in nondiabetic patients with ischemic heart disease (7640,7641). Some researchers think that increased glucosamine production might contribute to endothelial cell dysfunction (8944). However, preliminary evidence suggests that glucosamine might have a protective effect against atherosclerosis. It seems to prevent oxidation of lipoproteins by scavenging reactive carbonyl intermediates produced by oxidized lipoproteins (9122).

Glucosamine sulfate is absorbed 90% after oral administration. The bioavailability is approximately 26% to 44% after first-pass metabolism (2608,10316). Although the plasma concentration of glucosamine doesn't increase substantially after oral glucosamine sulfate, radiolabeling techniques demonstrate that it is significantly absorbed. The plasma half-life of glucosamine is about one hour. However, glucosamine is incorporated into plasma proteins and tissues and therefor stays in the body much longer. The half-life of elimination is about 95 hours (2607,10316). Although glucosamine is administered in a salt form, most commonly as the hydrochloride or sulfate, the salt is likely cleaved off in the stomach. Glucosamine base is completely ionized in the stomach. Some glucosamine preparations are provided as topical creams. It is not known if glucosamine is absorbed transdermally; however, preliminary research suggests that topical glucosamine in combination with chondroitin sulfate, shark cartilage, and camphor might relieve osteoarthritic pain (10327).

Some researchers think the sulfate moiety in glucosamine sulfate might be responsible for its effect on osteoarthritis. Sulfate is required for articular cartilage glycosaminoglycan synthesis. Glucosamine might increase the absorption of sulfate. Glucosamine sulfate increases serum and synovial sulfate levels. Acetaminophen given concurrently with glucosamine sulfate, decreases sulfate levels, suggesting that use of acetaminophen in clinical trials might alter results. If the sulfate is the active moiety of glucosamine sulfate, theoretically glucosamine hydrochloride would be less effective (10313). However, there are no head-to-head clinical studies of the sulfate and hydrochloride salts of glucosamine. More research is needed to determine the role of sulfate in the efficacy of glucosamine sulfate.

Adverse Reactions

Orally, glucosamine sulfate can commonly cause mild gastrointestinal (GI) problems including nausea, heartburn, diarrhea, and constipation. Drowsiness, skin reactions, and headache have also been reported (2608). However, adverse effects in clinical studies have generally been comparable to placebo (7026). Glucosamine sulfate 1500 mg per day is tolerated at least as well as the nonsteroidal anti-inflammatory drug (NSAID) ibuprofen 1200 mg per day, and it is better tolerated than piroxicam (Feldene) 20 mg daily (2602,2604,2606).

Anecdotal reports have associated glucosamine with renal toxicity, but changes in renal function have not been reported in long-term studies (7026,8942,10408,10409).

Elevated blood glucose levels in patients with diabetes have also been reported (22). However, 80-90 days of

glucosamine therapy does not seem to affect hemoglobin A1C or blood glucose levels in people with type 2 diabetes or healthy people (10311,10317,12107).
There is some concern that it might increase the risk of metabolic disturbances resulting in increased cholesterol levels and blood pressure. However, glucosamine does not appear to increase the risk of these adverse effects (7075).
In people older than 45, taking glucosamine sulfate for 3 years doesn't seem to have any adverse effects on blood glucose metabolism, lipid metabolism, or any other disturbances in metabolism (7026,8942).
There is concern that glucosamine sulfate products derived from marine exoskeletons might cause reactions in people allergic to shellfish, although no reactions have been reported. Some manufacturers claim that their glucosamine sulfate products are so purified, shellfish allergies should not be a concern. However, since preparation methods and quality standards can vary significantly, use glucosamine sulfate with caution, or avoid using in patients with shellfish allergy.

Interactions with Herbs & Other Dietary Supplements

None known.

Interactions with Drugs

ACETAMINOPHEN (Tylenol, Others): Very preliminary research suggests that the sulfate portion of glucosamine sulfate may contribute to its effect in osteoarthritis. Since acetaminophen metabolism requires sulfur and reduces serum sulfate concentrations, it may theoretically interfere with the action of glucosamine sulfate. Conversely, the administration of sulfate may theoretically decrease the effectiveness of acetaminophen in sulfate-deficient people by increasing its clearance (10313).
ANTIDIABETES DRUGS: Glucosamine sulfate seems to have little or no effect on control of blood glucose in patients with type 2 diabetes (10311,10317). Preliminary research suggests that glucosamine might increase insulin resistance or decrease insulin production (371,372,3406,7637,7638). However, clinical research suggests that glucosamine doesn't adversely affect diabetes treatment (10311,10317). Some antidiabetes drugs include glimepiride (Amaryl), glyburide (DiaBeta, Glynase PresTab, Micronase), insulin, pioglitazone (Actos), rosiglitazone (Avandia), and others.
ANTIMITOTIC CHEMOTHERAPY: Theoretically, glucosamine might induce resistance to etoposide (VP16, VePesid), teniposide (VM26), and doxorubicin (Adriamycin). Glucosamine sulfate might contribute to the development of chemotherapeutic resistance by reducing the drugs' inhibition of topoisomerase II, an enzyme required for DNA replication in tumor cells (7639,9559).
WARFARIN (Coumadin): There's some concern that high-dose glucosamine (3000 mg per day), combined with high-dose chondroitin sulfate (2400 mg per day), may enhance the effects of warfarin (Coumadin) as measured by the INR (11389). Chondroitin is a small component of a heparinoid and might have weak anticoagulant activity. Glucosamine is also a small component of heparin, but it does not seem to have anticoagulant activity. It's not known if glucosamine contributes to this potential interaction. Interactions with warfarin have not been reported at recommended dosages of glucosamine or chondroitin.

Interactions with Foods

None known.

Interactions with Lab Tests

BLOOD GLUCOSE: Glucosamine doesn't seem to adversely affect blood glucose control in people with type 2 diabetes, as measured by hemoglobin A1C (10311,10317). It also doesn't seem to affect blood glucose in nondiabetic people older than 45, taking glucosamine for osteoarthritis for 3 years (7026,8942). Some preliminary research raised concerns that glucosamine sulfate might exacerbate diabetes by increasing insulin resistance and/or decreasing insulin production, resulting in elevated blood glucose levels (5059), but other research has shown no effect (7637,7638). There are also anecdotal reports of reduced blood glucose control in people with diabetes who take glucosamine (22,1203,1204,3405,3406). However, clinical studies indicate that glucosamine sulfate has little or no effect blood glucose (7026,8942,10311,10317).
INTERNATIONAL NORMALIZED RATIO (INR)/PROTHROMBIN TIME (PT): High dose glucosamine (3000 mg per day), combined with high dose chondroitin sulfate (2400 mg per day), may increase the INR in patients taking warfarin (Coumadin). There is one case report of an increased INR associated with concomitant use of warfarin a glucosamine-chondroitin supplement taken above recommended dosages (11389).

Interactions with Diseases or Conditions

ASTHMA: Glucosamine might exacerbate asthma by an unidentified allergic mechanism. Use cautiously in patients with asthma (10002).
DIABETES: Glucosamine doesn't seem to adversely affect blood glucose control in people with type 2 diabetes, as measured by hemoglobin A1C (10311,10317). Some preliminary research raised concerns that glucosamine sulfate might exacerbate diabetes by increasing insulin resistance and/or decreasing insulin production, resulting in elevated blood glucose levels (5059), but other research has shown no effect on insulin sensitivity or plasma glucose (7637,7638,12107). There are also anecdotal reports of reduced blood glucose control in people with diabetes who take glucosamine (22,1203,1204,3405,3406). However, clinical studies indicate that glucosamine sulfate seems to be safe in people with type 2 diabetes (10311,10317).

HYPERLIPIDEMIA: Glucosamine doesn't seem to adversely affect lipid levels in people over age 45 who have taken glucosamine sulfate for 3 years (7026,8942). There was some concern that glucosamine sulfate might increase cholesterol and triglyceride levels. There is preliminary evidence that glucosamine sulfate can increase insulin levels. Hyperinsulinemia is associated with elevated triglycerides and cholesterol (5059,7075). However, glucosamine appears to have little or no effect on insulin, lipids, or triglycerides in humans (7026,8942).
HYPERTENSION: Glucosamine doesn't seem to adversely affect blood pressure in people older than 45 who have taken glucosamine sulfate for 3 years (7026,8942). There is some concern that glucosamine sulfate might increase blood pressure. Preliminary evidence suggested that glucosamine sulfate might increase insulin levels. Hyperinsulinemia is associated with increased blood pressure levels (7075). However, glucosamine appears to have little or no effect on insulin or blood pressure in humans (7026,8942).
SHELLFISH ALLERGY: Glucosamine sulfate products derived from marine exoskeletons might cause reactions in people allergic to shellfish, although no reactions have been reported. Some manufacturers claim that their glucosamine sulfate products are so purified, shellfish allergies should not be a concern. However, since preparation methods and quality standards can vary significantly, use glucosamine sulfate with caution or avoid using in patients with shellfish allergy.

Dosage and Administration

ORAL: For osteoarthritis, the typical dose is 1500 mg once daily or in 3 divided doses (2600,2602,2603,2606,7026,8942). For temporomandibular joint (TMJ) osteoarthritis, 500 mg 3 times daily has been used (3714).
TOPICAL: For osteoarthritis, topical administration of a cream containing glucosamine sulfate, 30 mg/g; chondroitin sulfate, 50 mg/g; shark cartilage, 140 mg/g; and camphor, 32 mg/g; has been used as needed on sore joints for up to 8 weeks (10327).
PARENTERAL: In other countries, intravenous, intramuscular, and intra-articular products are used (2601); however, these products are not available in the US. In one trial, glucosamine sulfate 400 mg intramuscularly twice per week was used (2605).

Comments

Although chondroitin sulfate and glucosamine sulfate are frequently marketed together in combination products, there is no evidence that the combination has greater benefit than either product alone. There is great variability among glucosamine and glucosamine plus chondroitin products. Actual content versus label claim varies from 0% to 115% (11340). The National Institutes of Health (NIH) is sponsoring its first clinical trial of glucosamine sulfate in combination with chondroitin sulfate. The 24 week, parallel group, double-blind randomized controlled trial (RCT) includes five separate treatment arms, in which patients will ingest: placebo, glucosamine sulfate 500 mg three times per day, chondroitin 400 mg three times per day, a combination of glucosamine sulfate and chondroitin, or celecoxib (Celebrex) (11012).

GLUTAMINE

Also Known As

GLN, Glutamate, Glutamic Acid, Glutaminate, Levoglutamide, Levoglutamine, L-Glutamic Acid, L-Glutamic Acid 5-Amide, l-Glutamine, L-Glutamine, Q.

Scientific Names

L-(+)-2-Aminoglutaramic acid.

People Use This For

Orally, glutamine is used for depression, moodiness, irritability, anxiety, insomnia, short bowel syndrome, Crohn's disease, and enhancing exercise performance. Glutamine is also used orally for HIV wasting, abnormal intestinal permeability in people with HIV, chemotherapy-induced mucositis, chemotherapy-induced diarrhea, chemotherapy-induced neuropathy, and protection of immune and gut barrier function in people with esophageal cancer undergoing radiochemotherapy. It is also used for attention deficit-hyperactivity disorder (ADHD), cystinuria, peptic ulcer, ulcerative colitis, sickle cell anemia, improving recovery after bone marrow transplant, and for alcohol withdrawal support. It is also used orally as enteral nutrition, for preventing morbidity in trauma patients, preventing infectious complications in critically ill patients, and for paclitaxel-induced myalgia and arthralgia.
Intravenously, glutamine is administered for improving recovery after surgery and after bone marrow transplant, and preventing chemotherapy-induced mucositis.

Safety

POSSIBLY SAFE ...when used orally and appropriately. Glutamine seems to be safe in doses up to 40 grams per day (2334,2337,2338,2364,2365,5029,5462,7233,7288,7293). ...when used intravenously. Glutamine seems to be safe in doses up to 570 mg/kg/day when incorporated into parenteral nutrition (2363,2366,5448,5452,5453,5454,5458,7293).
CHILDREN: POSSIBLY SAFE ...when used orally and appropriately. Glutamine seems safe in amounts that do not

exceed 0.65 grams per kg per day in children 3 to 18 years (11364). There is insufficient reliable information available about the safety of glutamine in higher amounts when used in children.

PREGNANCY AND LACTATION: Insufficient reliable information available; avoid using.

Effectiveness

POSSIBLY EFFECTIVE

Critical illness (trauma). Administering glutamine enterally in nutrition formulas seems to help prevent morbidity in trauma patients and infectious complications in critically ill patients. Glutamine seems to improve nutritional and immunologic status, and to reduce complications in critically ill (5450) and multiple-trauma patients (5449,7309). Preliminary evidence suggests glutamine might help prevent bacterial translocation from the intestine and subsequent infection when administered enterally after trauma or major surgery (7731,8184). There is also some preliminary evidence that suggests parenteral glutamine might lessen protein breakdown and branched-chain amino acid catabolism in critical illness such as sepsis, cancer, trauma, and burn injury (8182). Additionally, some preliminary research suggests that glutamine administered in parenteral nutrition with growth hormone and insulin-like growth factor might improve nitrogen balance in critically ill patients (8186).

HIV/AIDS-related wasting. Taking glutamine orally seems to enhance intestinal absorption of nutrients, decrease intestinal permeability, and increase weight gain in people with HIV/AIDS. Doses of 40 grams per day seem to produce the best effect (2337,2702,5461,7729). Lower doses (14 grams per day) might also be effective when used in combination with arginine and beta-hydroxy-beta-methylbutyrate (a leucine metabolite) (7310).

Oral mucositis. Taking glutamine orally seems to help reduce chemotherapy-induced mucositis (stomatitis). Glutamine appears to decrease the incidence, severity, and duration of mouth pain in some patients undergoing cancer chemotherapy or bone marrow transplant (2336,2364,2368,2704,5029), but glutamine is not effective for all patients (2365,5451,5462,7296). It's not clear which patients are most likely to benefit. However, some researchers speculate that those cancer patients with glutamine deficiency may benefit most (2368). Upcoming clinical trials will help clarify the best way to use glutamine and which patients are most likely to benefit (7288).

Surgery. Administering glutamine intravenously seems to improve recovery after bone marrow transplant and abdominal surgery. Most patients receiving glutamine-supplemented parenteral nutrition after bone marrow transplantation seem to have improved nitrogen balance, a diminished incidence of clinical infection, lower rates of microbial colonization, shortened hospital stay, and increased hepatic function and lymphocyte recovery compared with patients receiving standard parenteral nutrition (2366,5452,5453,5454). However, not all bone marrow transplant patients seem to benefit (5451). Glutamine-fortified parenteral nutrition appears to preserve intestinal mucosal structure and permeability, improve nitrogen balance, improve immune function, and shorten hospital stay in patients recovering from major abdominal surgery and other major surgeries (2363,5448,7299,7300,7732).

POSSIBLY INEFFECTIVE

Athletic performance. Taking glutamine orally doesn't seem to enhance exercise performance (2341,2342,5455,5456,5464,5465,5466).

Crohn's disease. Taking glutamine orally doesn't seem to improve symptoms of Crohn's disease (2338,6256). Neither supplemental glutamine 7 grams three times daily nor a glutamine-enriched diet seems to have any benefit in patients with Crohn's disease (2338,6256,7297).

Cystinuria. Taking glutamine orally doesn't seem to help improve cystinuria (2339).

Diarrhea. Taking glutamine orally doesn't seem to help improve acute diarrhea in infants. Glutamine administered in the standard World Health Organization (WHO) glucose-electrolyte solution doesn't seem to have any effect on diarrheal stool output, duration of diarrhea, or volume of rehydration solution required to achieve and maintain hydration (7298).

INSUFFICIENT RELIABLE EVIDENCE to RATE

Chemotherapy-induced diarrhea. There is preliminary evidence that glutamine might reduce the occurrence of chemotherapy-induced diarrhea (7235,7285), but so far research findings have been inconsistent (7233,7295).

Chemotherapy-induced lymphocytopenia. There is conflicting evidence regarding the potential benefits of glutamine for preventing chemotherapy-induced reduction of lymphocytes (2705,7295).

Paclitaxel-induced myalgia and arthralgia. There is early evidence that glutamine might help reduce paclitaxel-induced myalgia and arthralgia (6433).

Short bowel syndrome. Research findings are inconsistent for the combination of glutamine and growth hormone in the treatment of short bowel syndrome (8185). Glutamine plus growth hormone seems to decrease dependence on parenteral nutrition in some patients (2334,2361,2362,2703), but glutamine alone doesn't appear to be effective (7730). Glutamine currently has orphan drug status for this use (1691).

More evidence is needed to rate glutamine for these uses.

Mechanism of Action

Glutamine is the most abundant free amino acid in the body (7739). It is produced primarily in skeletal muscle and then released into the circulation. Tissues that require glutamine such as the immune system, gastrointestinal tract, kidneys, and liver obtain glutamine as needed from the blood (7729). Glutamine acts as an inter-organ nitrogen and carbon transporter (5467). Although traditionally classified as a non-essential amino acid, glutamine is essential for maintaining intestinal function, immune response, and amino acid homeostasis during times of severe stress, suggesting that it is more appropriately called a conditionally essential amino acid (5468,7736).

The rapidly growing fetus and premature infant seem to require glutamine for growth and normal physiologic functions (7740). Glutamine is metabolized in the mitochondria and is important for providing metabolic fuel to lymphocytes, macrophages, and fibroblasts (5468,5469,7739).

Glutamine can enhance the function of stimulated immune cells. It seems to affect lymphocyte proliferation, cytokine production, bacterial killing by neutrophils, and phagocytic and secretory activities of macrophages (7734). In patients with cancer, some research suggests it might restore natural killer cell function in healthy cells and improve protein metabolism (7739). Neutrophils and monocytes are dependent upon glutamine to maintain phagocytic action (10225).

Glutamine also functions as a precursor for other amino acids, glucose, purines and pyrimidines, glutathione, and glutamate (5468,5469,5470,7292,7740).

Following surgery or accidental injury, about one third of the nitrogen mobilized for wound repair and vital organ function is from glutamine (7735). During physical stress the body consumes more glutamine than the skeletal muscle can produce. Progressive muscle breakdown (wasting) can occur as the body tries to meet glutamine requirements (7729). Decreased glutamine concentrations following surgery seems to impair the function of neutrophils and monocytes, which might increase the risk of infection (10225).

The intestinal mucosa can also synthesize glutamine, but not enough to compensate for the body's needs during severe physiologic stress (7733). There's some evidence suggesting that glutamine, in addition to serving as a metabolic fuel for enterocytes, might play a regulatory role in the intestine, affecting cell proliferation and differentiation (7733). The gastrointestinal tract is one of the largest utilizers of glutamine in the body (5469). Depletion of glutamine can result in atrophy, ulceration and necrosis of intestinal epithelium.

Some cancer patients may have reduced levels of glutamine (2368). Since gastrointestinal cells are rapidly dividing, they are highly susceptible to the cytotoxic effects of chemotherapy. Glutamine treatment is thought to help prevent chemotherapy and radiation-induced gastrointestinal toxicity by maintaining viability of gastrointestinal tissues (2368).

Some preliminary evidence suggests that glutamine might protect the heart from ischemia and EKG changes in patients with chronic stable angina (8183).

Adverse Reactions

Orally and intravenously glutamine seems to be well tolerated (7293). Some patients find the grittiness of glutamine administered in water unacceptable (11364). Significant side effects have not been reported in clinical studies (2336,2364,2365,2368,2704,5029,5451,5462,7233,7235,7285,7288). However, glutamine is metabolized to glutamate and ammonia, both of which might have neurological effects in people with neurological and psychiatric diseases (7293). Mania has been reported in people with bipolar disorder and supplementation with glutamine (7291).

There is also some concern that glutamine might be used by rapidly growing tumors and possibly stimulate tumor growth. Although tumors may utilize glutamine and other amino acids, preliminary research shows that glutamine supplementation does not increase tumor growth (5469,7233,7738). In fact, there is preliminary evidence that glutamine might actually reduce tumor growth (5469).

Interactions with Herbs & Other Dietary Supplements

None known.

Interactions with Drugs

ANTICONVULSANTS: Theoretically, glutamine, which is metabolized to the excitatory neurotransmitter glutamate, might antagonize the anticonvulsant effects of medications taken for epilepsy (7292,7293,7294). Some anti-epileptic drugs include phenobarbital, primidone (Mysoline), valproic acid (Depakene), gabapentin (Neurontin), carbamazepine (Tegretol), phenytoin (Dilantin), and others.

CHEMOTHERAPY: There has been concern that glutamine might alter the pharmacokinetics of chemotherapeutic drugs or reduce effectiveness by enhancing tumor growth. However, available clinical data suggests that glutamine does not adversely affect outcomes when used concurrently with chemotherapy (7738).

LACTULOSE: Theoretically, glutamine might antagonize the anti-ammonia effects of lactulose. Glutamine is metabolized to ammonia (7293).

Interactions with Foods

None known.

Interactions with Lab Tests

AMMONIA SERUM LEVELS: Glutamine is partially metabolized to ammonia. In higher doses, it can increase serum ammonia levels (7293,11364).

GLUTAMATE SERUM LEVELS: Glutamine is partially metabolized to glutamate. In higher doses, it can increase serum glutamate levels (7293,11364).

Interactions with Diseases or Conditions

HEPATIC ENCEPHALOPATHY: Theoretically, glutamine, which is metabolized to ammonia, might worsen hepatic encephalopathy (7293).

MANIA, HYPOMANIA: Glutamine might cause affective changes in people with mania or hypomania (7291). Glutamine is a precursor of the excitatory neurotransmitter glutamate (7292).
MONOSODIUM GLUTAMATE (MSG) HYPERSENSITIVITY: People who are sensitive to MSG, also known as "Chinese Restaurant Syndrome," might be sensitive to glutamine. Glutamine is metabolized to glutamate in the body (5469,7291).
SEIZURE DISORDERS: Theoretically excess amounts of glutamine and its metabolite, glutamate, might lower the seizure threshold (7292,7293).

Dosage and Administration

ORAL: For reducing chemotherapy-induced mucositis (stomatitis), a variety of dosage regimens have been used. Most often glutamine suspension 4 grams swish and swallow every four hours around the clock starting with the first dose of chemotherapy and continued until discharge or resolution of symptoms has been used (5029). In some cases, 4 grams swish and swallow twice daily from day one of chemotherapy for 28 days, or for four days past the resolution of symptoms, has been used (2364). Other successful regimens include 2 grams per meter squared swish and swallow twice daily (2336) or 1 gram per meter squared swish and swallow 4 times daily (2368) on days of chemotherapy administration and for at least 14 additional days, or 500 mg/kg per day (2704). For children receiving chemotherapy, 0.35 to 0.65 grams per kilogram per day has been used (11364). For chemotherapy-induced diarrhea, 6 grams mixed in water three times daily beginning five days before chemotherapy for 15 consecutive days has been used (7285). For short bowel syndrome, 630 mg/kg per day has been used (2334). For HIV wasting, 8-40 grams per day has been used. However, 40 grams daily may be the most beneficial (2335,2702,5461). For preventing drops in lymphocyte counts and attenuating gut permeability in people with esophageal cancer during radiochemotherapy, 30 grams per day has been used (2705). For Crohn's disease, 7 grams three times daily has been used (2338). For treating paclitaxel-induced myalgia and arthralgia, 10 grams three times daily starting 24 hours after paclitaxel infusion has been used (6433).
INTRAVENOUS: For improving recovery after bone marrow transplantation, 570 mg/kg/day has been used (2366). For improving recovery after major surgery, doses of 20 grams and 300 mg/kg/day have been added to parenteral nutrition (2363,5448). When glutamine dipeptide is used following major surgery, 18 to 30 grams of glutamine dipeptides per day (equivalent to 13 to 20 grams of glutamine) is typically used in a 60 to 70 kg patient. Higher doses are used for severely stressed patients with multiple injuries, burns, sepsis, and immune deficiency (7737).

Comments

Glutamine powder can be ordered through most wholesale drug suppliers. Glutamine for commercial use is produced by a fermentation process with glutamine-producing bacteria (7736). Glutamine has low solubility and limited stability in parenteral amino acid solutions. Synthetic glutamine dipeptides, such as l-alanyl-l-glutamine, are sometimes used to overcome these problems. The glutamine dipeptide is cleaved in vivo (7732,7737).

GLUTATHIONE

Also Known As

gamma-Glutamylcysteinylglycine, gamma-L-Glutamyl-L-cysteinylglycine, L-Glutathione, GSH.

Scientific Names

N-(N-L-gamma-Glutamyl-L-cysteinyl)glycine.

People Use This For

Orally, glutathione is used for treating cataracts, glaucoma, preventing aging, treating or preventing alcoholism, asthma, cancer, heart disease (atherosclerosis and hypercholesterolemia), hepatitis, liver disease, immunosuppression (including AIDS and chronic fatigue syndrome), maintaining immune function, memory loss, Alzheimer's disease, osteoarthritis, Parkinson's disease, and detoxifying metal and drugs.
Inhaled, glutathione is used for treating lung diseases, including idiopathic pulmonary fibrosis, cystic fibrosis, and lung disease in individuals with HIV disease.
Intramuscularly, glutathione is used for preventing toxicity of chemotherapy and for treating male infertility.
Intravenously, glutathione is used for preventing anemia in patients undergoing hemodialysis, preventing renal dysfunction after coronary bypass surgery, treating Parkinson's disease, improving blood flow and decreasing clotting in individuals with atherosclerosis, treating diabetes, and preventing toxicity of chemotherapy.

Safety

POSSIBLY SAFE ...when used orally (5361,5362). ...when used by inhalation (9,5367,5368,5369). ...when used intramuscularly (5374,5375,5384). ...when used as an intravenous injection (5344,5354,5357,5358,5359,5360,5373,5374,5375,5376,5377,5378,5379,5380,5381,5382,5383).
PREGNANCY AND LACTATION: Insufficient reliable information available; avoid using.

Effectiveness

POSSIBLY EFFECTIVE

Chemotherapy toxicity. Administering glutathione by intravenous injection seems to help prevent chemotherapy toxicity (5373,5374,5375,5376,5377,5378,5379,5380,5381,5382,5383).

There is insufficient reliable information available about the effectiveness of glutathione for its other uses.

Mechanism of Action

Glutathione is primarily synthesized in the liver (5387,5388). It is involved in DNA synthesis and repair, protein and prostaglandin synthesis, amino acid transport, metabolism of toxins and carcinogens, immune system function, prevention of oxidative cell damage, and enzyme activation (5344,5386). Cellular glutathione levels increase during exercise (5398,5386). Glutathione deficiency is associated with aging, age-related macular degeneration (AMD), diabetes, lung and gastrointestinal disease, pre-eclampsia, Parkinson's disease and other neurodegenerative disorders, and poor prognosis in AIDS (5344,5346,5347,5348,5349,5350,5351,5352,5353,5354,5393,5394,5395,5396,5397). Although glutathione is present in fruits, vegetables, and meats, the levels in the body do not seem to correlate to dietary intake. This suggests that oral glutathione might be inactivated by peptidases in the gut (5344). Despite evidence that suggests that glutathione is bioavailable in rodents (5363,5364), oral doses of 3 grams cause negligible increases in human plasma levels (5362). Preliminary evidence suggests glutathione intake from fruits and vegetables might be associated with a reduced risk of pharyngeal cancer (5345). In individuals with cirrhosis, oral glutathione has no effect on liver function tests (5361).

Glutathione may inhibit the activity of enzymes that help the flu virus colonize cells lining the mouth and throat. Flu-infected mice fed glutathione-enriched drinking water have lower tissue virus levels than untreated mice. Human studies are needed to determine the effects of glutathione on flu infection (5061).

Currently, researchers are investigating whether administering glutathione precursors, such as glutamine and n-acetylcysteine might increase glutathione levels (5344,5389,5392).

Adverse Reactions

None reported.

Interactions with Herbs & Other Dietary Supplements

None known.

Interactions with Drugs

None known.

Drug Influences on Nutrient Levels and Depletion

SOME DRUGS CAN AFFECT GLUTATHIONE LEVELS:

ACETAMINOPHEN: Drugs that deplete glutathione, such as acetaminophen, might decrease the therapeutic effects of glutathione (5394).

ALCOHOL (Ethanol): Drugs that deplete glutathione, such as alcohol, might decrease the therapeutic effects of glutathione (5394).

Interactions with Foods

None known.

Interactions with Lab Tests

None known.

Interactions with Diseases or Conditions

ASTHMA: Inhaled (nebulized) glutathione can cause bronchospasm in individuals with asthma (5372).

Dosage and Administration

ORAL: Supplemental doses range from 50-600 mg per day, with a typical dose of 250 mg daily; however, orally administered glutathione is probably not bioavailable (5362).

INHALATION: A common dose is 600 mg, aerosolized twice daily (5367,5368,5369).

INTRAMUSCULAR: For infertility, 600 mg every other day for 2 months has been used (5384). As a chemotherapy adjunct, 600 mg on days 2 through 5 of chemotherapy has been used (5374,5375).

INTRAVENOUS: As a chemotherapy adjunct, 2.5 grams or 1.5 grams/meter squared immediately prior to chemotherapy has been used (5373,5374,5375,5376,5377,5378,5379,5380,5381,5382,5383).

Comments

The role of glutathione is being studied in the wasting of AIDS, heavy metal poisoning, sepsis, myocardial ischemia, renal dysfunction and nephrotoxicity, liver disorders, corneal disorders, and eczema (9,5344,5345).

GLYCEROL

Also Known As
Glicerol, Glucerite, Glycerin, Glycerolum, Glyceryl Alcohol.

Scientific Names
Glycerol; 1,2,3-propanetriol.

People Use This For
Orally, glycerol is used for weight loss, enhancing exercise performance, improving rehydration during acute gastrointestinal disease, and reducing intraocular pressure. Glycerol is also used by athletes as an aid to hydration.
Intravenously, glycerol is used for reducing intra-cranial pressure in various conditions including stroke, meningitis, encephalitis, Reye's syndrome, pseudotumor cerebri, central nervous system (CNS) trauma, and CNS tumors or space-occupying lesions; for reducing brain volume for neurosurgical procedures; and for postural syncope.
Topically, glycerol is used as a humectant to moisturize the skin.
Ophthalmically, glycerol is an ingredient for reducing corneal edema to facilitate ophthalmic exams.
Rectally, glycerol is used as a laxative.

Safety
LIKELY SAFE ...when used rectally, ophthalmically, or topically and appropriately (15,272). ...when used orally for glaucoma; glycerol is an FDA-approved prescription product for this use.
POSSIBLY SAFE ...when used orally (2474,2475).
POSSIBLY UNSAFE ...when used intravenously. In one study, hemolysis was reported in 98% of people treated for acute ischemic stroke (2482).
There is insufficient reliable information available about the safety of glycerol for its other uses.
PREGNANCY AND LACTATION: Insufficient reliable information available; avoid using.

Effectiveness
LIKELY EFFECTIVE
Constipation. Use of glycerol rectal suppositories have a laxative effect and decrease constipation (15).
POSSIBLY INEFFECTIVE
Weight loss. Taking glycerol orally doesn't seem to be effective for losing weight (2485).
LIKELY INEFFECTIVE
Athletic performance. Taking glycerol orally doesn't seem to improve physical exercise performance (2474,2475).
Stroke. Intravenous use of glycerol doesn't seem to improve symptoms of acute stroke (2480,2481,2482,2484,2486).
There is insufficient reliable information available about the effectiveness of glycerol for its other uses.

Mechanism of Action
Supplemental glycerol increases serum osmolality (2477). It also has hyperosmotic laxative activity (15). Glycerol consumption failed to enhance human exercise performance (2476,2492) or reduce water loss in underwater divers (2478). However, one study reported that following glycerol ingestion, participants had improved exercise tolerance and reduced heart rate during stationary cycling (2479). Intravenous glycerol failed to improve acute ischemic stroke survival in several clinical trials (2480,2481,2482,2484,2486). However, one study of elderly people with acute ischemic stroke found glycerol improved initial survival (2483).

Adverse Reactions
Orally, the use of glycerol can cause mild headache, dizziness, bloating, nausea, vomiting, thirst, and diarrhea (15,2475).
Intravenously, the use of glycerol has caused hemolysis in people treated for acute ischemic stroke (2480,2482).

Interactions with Herbs & Other Dietary Supplements
None known.

Interactions with Drugs
None known.

Interactions with Foods
None known.

Interactions with Lab Tests
None known.

Interactions with Diseases or Conditions
None known.

Dosage and Administration
ORAL: For enhancing exercise performance, the usual dose of glycerol is 1 gram/kg with 1.5 L fluid 60-120 minutes before competition (2475). For weight loss, 7.5 grams in a 25% solution is typically taken before meals (2485).
RECTAL: As an adult laxative, the common dose is a 2-3 grams suppository or a 5-15 mL enema (15). For children younger than six years old, the dose is a 1-1.7 grams suppository or a 2-5 mL enema (15).
OPHTHALMIC: Glycerol is an FDA-approved prescription product for reducing intraocular pressure.
INTRAVENOUS: No typical dosage.

GLYCINE

Also Known As
Athenon, G Salt, Free Base Glycine, Glycocoll, Glycosthene, Iconyl, L-Glycine, Monazol.

Scientific Names
Aminoacetic Acid.

People Use This For
Orally, glycine is used for schizophrenia, strokes, memory enhancement, benign prostatic hyperplasia (BPH), protection of the liver and kidneys, and cancer prevention. It is also used for 3-phosphoglycerate dehydrogenase deficiency and isovaleric acidemia.
Topically, glycine is used to treat leg ulcers and for wound healing.

Safety
POSSIBLY SAFE ...when used orally and appropriately (10250,10251,10252). ...when used topically and appropriately (10255).
PREGNANCY AND LACTATION: Insufficient information available; avoid using.

Effectiveness
POSSIBLY EFFECTIVE

Leg ulcers. Applying a cream containing glycine, l-cysteine, and dl-threonine seems to reduce pain and slightly improve healing of leg ulcers (10255).

Schizophrenia. Taking glycine orally in addition to conventional treatment seems to reduce negative symptoms of schizophrenia in patients that are resistant to monotherapy with conventional antipsychotics such as thioridazine (Mellaril), haloperidol (Haldol), and perphenazine (Trilafon). However, when used with the atypical neuroleptic agent clozapine (Clozaril), glycine appears to have a negligible effect or worsen symptoms of schizophrenia (10253,11321). Additionally, glycine does not seem to improve positive symptoms of schizophrenia (10250,10251,10252).

Stroke. Taking glycine sublingually may have neuroprotective effects if started within 6 hours after the onset of acute ischemic stroke (11320).

INSUFFICIENT RELIABLE EVIDENCE to RATE

3-phosphoglycerate dehydrogenase (3-PGDH) deficiency. There is preliminary evidence that suggests that oral glycine might reduce seizures in patients with 3-PGDH deficiency. 3-PGDH deficiency is a rare condition in which serine is not synthesized properly (10254).

Cognitive performance. Preliminary evidence suggests oral glycine may improve memory (11322).

Isovaleric acidemia. Glycine has been used orally with l-carnitine to treat isovaleric acidemia, which is caused by a defective enzyme needed for metabolism of leucine (10256).

More evidence is needed to rate glycine for these uses.

Mechanism of Action
Glycine is an amino acid. It is not considered an essential amino acid because the body makes glycine from serine. A typical diet contains about 2 grams of glycine daily. The primary sources are protein rich foods including meat, fish, dairy, and legumes (10252).
In the central nervous system (CNS) glycine acts as an agonist at the glutamate receptor N-methyl-D-aspartate (NMDA). NMDA receptors are associated with negative and positive symptoms of schizophrenia (10257). NMDA receptors also seem to be associated with memory and learning processes (11322). The concentration of glycine in the brain is fairly stable due to the dietary consumption of glycine. However, addition of supplements can increase CNS concentrations of glycine (10252).
Preliminary evidence suggests that glycine can protect the kidneys from damage induced by cyclosporine, possibly by reducing cyclosporine-induced hypoxia and free radicals (10258,10259).

Glycine may also help improve recovery of the liver after alcohol-induced damage. Glycine might reduce the production of tumor necrosis factor-alpha (TNF-alpha) by Kupffer cells. This effect leads to a reduction in inflammation, necrosis, and steatosis in alcohol-induced hepatitis (10260).
There is also evidence that glycine may inhibit the growth of certain types of cancer. It may decrease the growth of melanoma cells by inhibiting vascularization (10261). A similar effect may inhibit the growth of liver tumors (10262).

Adverse Reactions

Orally and topically, glycine is generally well tolerated. Nausea, vomiting, upper gastrointestinal (GI) tract discomfort, and mild sedation have occurred rarely with oral use of glycine. These symptoms resolve rapidly with discontinuation of glycine (10252,11320).

Interactions with Herbs & Other Dietary Supplements

None known.

Interactions with Drugs

CLOZAPINE (Clozaril): Glycine can make symptoms worse when given with clozapine (Clozaril) in patients with schizophrenia (10253). Although this effect has not been reported with other atypical antipsychotic agents, glycine should be used cautiously with all atypical antipsychotics.

Interactions with Foods

None known.

Interactions with Lab Tests

None known.

Interactions with Diseases or Conditions

None known.

Dosage and Administration

ORAL: In the treatment of schizophrenia, glycine has been used in doses ranging from 0.4 to 0.8 g/kg daily in divided doses. It is usually started at 4 g daily and increased by 4 g per day until the therapeutic dosage is obtained (10250,10251,10252,10253). For treating seizures induced by 3-PGDH deficiency, glycine 200 mg/kg daily has been used in combination with serine supplements (10254). In the treatment of isovaleric acidemia, glycine 250 mg/kg daily has been used; it may be given with or without l-carnitine (10256).
SUBLINGUAL: For neuroprotection after the onset of acute ischemic stroke, 1 to 2 g per day glycine started within 6 hours after stroke onset has been used (11320).
TOPICAL: For treating leg ulcers a cream containing 10 mg glycine, 2 mg l-cysteine, and 1 mg dl-threonine per gram of cream has been used. The cream was applied at each wound cleaning and dressing change once daily, every other day, or twice daily (10255).

GOA POWDER

Also Known As

Araoba, Bahia Powder, Brazil Powder, Chrysatobine, Crude Chrysarobin, Ringworm Powder.

Scientific Names

Vataireopsis araroba, synonym Andira araroba.
Family: Fabaceae/Leguminosae.

People Use This For

Topically, goa powder is used for psoriasis and fungal infections of the skin.

Safety

POSSIBLY UNSAFE ...when used topically. Goa powder is severely irritating to skin and mucous membranes. It can also be absorbed through the skin with adverse effects. As little as 10 mg absorbed is associated with vomiting, diarrhea, and kidney inflammation (18).
PREGNANCY AND LACTATION: Insufficient reliable information available; avoid using.

Effectiveness

There is insufficient reliable information available about the effectiveness of goa powder.

Mechanism of Action
The applicable part of goa powder is the latex. Goa powder contains anthrone derivatives including chrysophanolanthrone. The powder is a strong reducing agent and inhibits glucose-6-phosphated-dehydrogenization in psoriatic skin conditions. It is considered a potent irritant to skin and mucous membranes and is easily absorbed through the skin (18).

Adverse Reactions
Orally, vomiting, diarrhea, and kidney inflammation can follow if ingested (18).
Topically, application of goa powder can cause redness, swelling, pustules, and conjunctivitis.

Interactions with Herbs & Other Dietary Supplements
None known.

Interactions with Drugs
None known.

Interactions with Foods
None known.

Interactions with Lab Tests
None known.

Interactions with Diseases or Conditions
None known.

Dosage and Administration
TOPICAL: People typically use a 2% goa powder ointment.

Comments
Goa powder has been replaced by synthetic anthranol (18). Goa should not be used internally (223).

GOAT'S RUE

Also Known As
French Honeysuckle, French Lilac, Galegae officinalis herba, Geissrautenkraut, Goats Rue, Goat's Rue Herb, Italian Fitch.
CAUTION: See separate listing for Rue.

Scientific Names
Galega officinalis, synonyms Galega bicolor, Galega patula.
Family: Fabaceae/Leguminosae.

People Use This For
Orally, goat's rue is used as supportive therapy for diabetes and as a diuretic.
In combination with other herbs, goat's rue is used for adrenal gland and pancreas stimulation, for glandular disturbances, blood purification, purifying the mesenchyma, digestive fluid secretion disturbances, fermentative dyspepsia, Roemheld syndrome, diarrhea, abnormal colonic bacterial flora, status lymphaticus and exudative diathesis, for stimulating lactation, as a tonic, and as a liver-protectant.

Safety
There is insufficient reliable information available about the safety of goat's rue.
Pregnancy and Lactation: Insufficient reliable information available; avoid using.

Effectiveness
There is insufficient reliable information available about the effectiveness of goat's rue.

Mechanism of Action
The applicable parts of goat's rue are the above ground parts. In vitro, the constituent galegine has hypoglycemic effects (2,18,4006), but these effects have not been demonstrated with goat's rue (2,18). In experimental rats, an intravenously administered aqueous extract suppresses platelet aggregation (4007). Fatal poisonings have been reported in grazing animals. Toxicity may involve galegine (4008).

Adverse Reactions
None reported in humans. However, fatal poisonings have been reported in grazing animals following ingestion of large amounts of goat's rue (2,18); poisoning symptoms in sheep, include salivation, spasms, paralysis, and asphyxiation (2,18).

Interactions with Herbs & Other Dietary Supplements
HYPOGLYCEMIC HERBS: Theoretically, concomitant use could potentiate effects of other herbs that cause hypoglycemia (2,4006).

Interactions with Drugs
ANTIDIABETES DRUGS: Theoretically, concomitant use could potentiate hypoglycemic drug effects. Monitor closely (2,4006).

Interactions with Foods
None known.

Interactions with Lab Tests
BLOOD GLUCOSE: Theoretically, could cause a true decrease in blood glucose levels and test results (2,4006).

Interactions with Diseases or Conditions
DIABETES: Goat's rue may interfere with effective diabetes treatment; avoid using.

Dosage and Administration
ORAL: As prepared tea (steep 2 grams finely cut above ground parts in 150 mL boiling water 5-10 minutes, strain); frequency of use not specified (18).

Comments
Avoid confusion with rue (Ruta graveolens). Goat's rue is not recommended for diabetes mellitus therapy because its effectiveness is uncertain.

GOLDEN RAGWORT

Also Known As
Cocash Weed, Coughweed, False Valerian, Female Regulator, Golden Groundsel, Golden Senecio, Grundy Swallow, Life Root, Liferoot, Ragwort, Squaw Weed, Squawweed.
CAUTION: See separate listings for Alpine Ragwort and Tansy Ragwort.

Scientific Names
Senecio aureus.
Family: Asteraceae/Compositae.

People Use This For
Orally, golden ragwort is used for diabetes mellitus, high blood pressure, spasms, as a uterine stimulant, to minimize bleeding, and as a diuretic and mild expectorant.
Golden ragwort is also used orally for treating conditions involving the female reproductive tract, including functional amenorrhea, menopausal neurosis, dysmenorrhea, pain associated with childbirth, and for inducing uterine contractions.
Topically, golden ragwort is used to treat bleeding after tooth extraction and as a douche for leukorrhea.

Safety
LIKELY UNSAFE ...when used orally. Golden ragwort contains hepatotoxic unsaturated pyrrolizidine alkaloids (UPAs) (12,19). Repeated exposure to low concentrations of UPAs has been linked to veno-occlusive disease, a serious condition (4,12). UPAs may also be carcinogenic and mutagenic (12). ...when used topically on abraded or broken skin, due to the potential for systemic absorption of UPAs (12,19).
PREGNANCY: UNSAFE ...when used orally due to the possibility that it might stimulate menstruation, have oxytocic activity, or cause teratogenic effects (19).
LACTATION: UNSAFE ...when used orally due to UPA content (19).

Effectiveness
There is insufficient reliable information available about the effectiveness of golden ragwort.

Mechanism of Action

Some unsaturated pyrrolizidine alkaloids (UPAs) have shown carcinogenic and mutagenic properties, and there are reports of associated renal toxicity. However, the primary concern is veno-occlusive disease (12). UPAs are known to be hepatotoxic in animals and humans (4).

Adverse Reactions

Orally, acute toxicity may result in hepatic necrosis; chronic toxicity may cause veno-occlusive liver disease. The potential for hepatotoxicity, due to presence of unsaturated pyrrolizidine alkaloids (UPAs), increases with larger doses and longer periods of use (4,12). Golden ragwort may cause an allergic reaction in individuals sensitive to the Asteraceae/Compositae family. Members of this family include ragweed, chrysanthemums, marigolds, daisies, and many other herbs.

Interactions with Herbs & Other Dietary Supplements

EUCALYPTUS: Theoretically, concomitant use might increase the risk of unsaturated pyrrolizidine alkaloid toxicity due to enzyme induction by eucalyptus (19).
UNSATURATED PYRROLIZIDINE ALKALOID (UPA)-CONTAINING HERBS: Concomitant use is contraindicated due to the risk of additive toxicity. Herbs containing UPAs include alkanna (12), borage (271), gravel root (4), hemp agrimony (271), hound's tongue (19), petasites (19), comfrey (271), coltsfoot, and the Senecio species plants; dusty miller (19), alpine ragwort (19), groundsel (271), golden ragwort (19), and tansy ragwort (271).

Interactions with Drugs

None known.

Interactions with Foods

None known.

Interactions with Lab Tests

None known.

Interactions with Diseases or Conditions

CROSS-ALLERGENICITY: Golden ragwort may cause an allergic reaction in individuals sensitive to the Asteraceae/Compositae family. Members of this family include ragweed, chrysanthemums, marigolds, daisies, and many other herbs.
LIVER DISEASE: Golden ragwort is hepatotoxic and may exacerbate liver conditions; contraindicated (6).

Dosage and Administration

No typical dosage.

Comments

Even though golden ragwort is considered unsafe for oral use (12,18), it is still included in some herbal preparations designed to treat irregular menses and other gynecological disorders. Golden ragwort is sometimes confused with other plants credited with broad healing powers, such as mandrake and ginseng (6).

GOLDENROD

Also Known As

Aaron's Rod, Canadian Goldenrod, Early Goldenrod, European Goldenrod, Woundwort.

Scientific Names

Solidago virgaurea (European goldenrod); Solidago canadensis (Canadian goldenrod), synonym Solidago longifolia; Solidago gigantea (Early goldenrod), synonym Solidago serotina.
Family: Asteraceae/Compositae.

People Use This For

Orally, goldenrod is used as a diuretic, anti-inflammatory, and antispasmodic. It is also used orally for gout, rheumatism, arthritis, eczema, and other skin conditions. Goldenrod is also used for acute exacerbations of pulmonary tuberculosis, diabetes, enlargement of the liver, hemorrhoids, internal bleeding, allergic rhinitis, asthma, and prostatic hypertrophy. It is also used as "irrigation therapy" where it is taken with copious amounts of fluids to increase urine flow to treat inflammatory diseases of the lower urinary tract, urinary calculi, and kidney gravel. As "irrigation therapy," it is also used as prophylaxis for urinary calculi and kidney gravel.

Topically, goldenrod is used as a mouth rinse for inflammation of the mouth and throat and externally for poorly healing wounds.

Safety

LIKELY SAFE ...when above ground parts are used orally and appropriately (2).
There is insufficient reliable information available about the safety of the topical use of goldenrod.
PREGNANCY AND LACTATION: Insufficient reliable information available; avoid using.

Effectiveness

There is insufficient reliable information available about the effectiveness of goldenrod.

Mechanism of Action

The applicable parts of goldenrod are the above ground parts. Goldenrod is classified as an aquaretic, a compound that increases urine volume (water loss) but not electrolyte excretion (512). The anti-inflammatory and aquaretic effects of goldenrod may be due to the saponin and flavonoid constituents (8,512). Goldenrod may also has bacteriostatic activity (512).

Adverse Reactions

Orally, goldenrod may cause an allergic reaction in individuals sensitive to the Asteraceae/Compositae family. Members of this family include ragweed, chrysanthemums, marigolds, daisies, and many other herbs.

Interactions with Herbs & Other Dietary Supplements

None known.

Interactions with Drugs

DIURETIC DRUGS: Theoretically, goldenrod might interfere with diuretic therapy (512).

Interactions with Foods

None known.

Interactions with Lab Tests

None known.

Interactions with Diseases or Conditions

CROSS-ALLERGENICITY: Goldenrod may cause an allergic reaction in individuals sensitive to the Asteraceae/Compositae family. Members of this family include ragweed, chrysanthemums, marigolds, daisies, and many other herbs.
EDEMA DUE TO HEART OR KIDNEY CONDITIONS: "Irrigation therapy," where goldenrod is taken with copious amounts of fluids to increase urine flow, is contraindicated in these conditions with edema (2).
HYPERTENSION: Theoretically, goldenrod might increase sodium retention and worsen hypertension (512).
URINARY TRACT INFECTIONS (UTIs): Herbal "irrigation therapy" can be insufficient and require the addition of antibacterial agent. "Irrigation therapy" should be monitored closely (8).

Dosage and Administration

ORAL: The typical dose of goldenrod is one cup of the tea two to four times daily between meals (18). The tea is prepared by steeping 1-2 teaspoons, 3-5 grams, of the dried herb in 150 mL boiling water for 5-10 minutes and then straining. The usual dose ranges from 6-12 grams of the herb per day (2). The common dose of the liquid extract, 1:1 in 25% ethanol, is 0.5-2 mL two to three times daily (18). The typical dose of the tincture, 1:5 in 45% ethanol, is 0.5-1 mL two to three times daily (18). Drink plenty of water, at least 2 liters per day, with the use of goldenrod (18).

Comments

Avoid confusion with mullein (Verbascum densiflorum; also referred to as goldenrod). Early goldenrod, European goldenrod, and Canadian goldenrod are used interchangeably.

GOLDENSEAL

Also Known As

Eye Balm, Eye Root, Golden Seal, Goldenroot, Goldsiegel, Ground Raspberry, Hydrastis, Hydrastis Canadensis, Indian Dye, Indian Plant, Indian Tumeric, Jaundice Root, Orange Root, Sceau D'Or, Turmeric Root, Warnera, Wild Curcuma, Yellow Indian Paint, Yellow Paint, Yellow Puccoon, Yellow Root.
CAUTION: See separate listings for Barberry, Goldthread, Javanese Turmeric, Oregon Grape, Ox-Eye Daisy, and Turmeric.

Scientific Names

Hydrastis canadensis.
Family: Ranunculaceae.

People Use This For

Orally, goldenseal is used for the common cold and other upper respiratory tract infections, nasal congestion, allergic rhinitis, gastritis, peptic ulcers, colitis, diarrhea, constipation, flatulence, inflammation of vaginal and uretal mucous membranes, urinary tract infections (UTIs), menorrhagia, and dysmenorrhea. It is also used orally for hemorrhoids, anal fissures, internal hemorrhage, liver disorders, cancer, to mask urine tests for illicit drugs, jaundice, gonorrhea, child birth, post-partum hemorrhage, fever, pneumonia, malaria, whooping cough, and anorexia.
Topically, goldenseal is used as a mouthwash for sore gums and mouth. It is also used topically for skin rashes, skin ulcers, wound infections, itching, eczema, acne, dandruff, ringworm, herpes blisters, and herpes labialis.
Ophthalmically, goldenseal is used as an eyewash for eye inflammation and conjunctivitis.
Otologically, goldenseal is used for ringing of the ears, earache, and catarrhal deafness.

Safety

POSSIBLY SAFE ...when used orally and appropriately, short-term (12).
LIKELY UNSAFE ...when used orally in high doses or long-term. Doses providing more than 500 mg of the constituent berberine can cause significant toxicity. This may correspond to 8-100 grams of dry root, depending on the concentration of berberine (12). Overdoses of goldenseal can cause cardiac damage, spasms, and death (4). The LD50 of the berberine constituent in humans is thought to be 27.5 mg/kg (12). Prolonged use has also been associated with significant side effects, including digestive disorders and hallucinations (18).
CHILDREN: LIKELY UNSAFE ...when used orally in newborns. The berberine constituent of goldenseal can cause kernicterus in newborns, particularly preterm neonates with hyperbilirubinemia (2589).
PREGNANCY: LIKELY UNSAFE ...when used orally. Goldenseal is thought to affect menstruation and have oxytocic effects (4,12). Berberine and other constituents are also thought to cross the placenta and may cause harm to the fetus. Kernicterus has developed in newborn infants exposed to goldenseal (2589).
LACTATION: LIKELY UNSAFE ...when used orally. Berberine and other harmful constituents can be transferred to the infant through breast milk (2589).

Effectiveness

POSSIBLY INEFFECTIVE

Urine drug tests. Goldenseal is often promoted to mask illicit drugs in the urine, but taking goldenseal orally doesn't seem to cause a false negative immunoassay (EMIT and TDx) for marijuana, cocaine, or for Microgenics CEDIA DAU assay for amphetamines, barbiturates, benzodiazepines, cocaine, opiates, phencyclidine, and tetrahydrocannabinol. Drinking one gallon of water with goldenseal didn't increase the number of false negatives over water alone (260,261). Some people also claim that goldenseal can cause a false positive on a drug screen. But goldenseal does not seem to cause false positives for the fluorescent polarization immunoassay (FPIA) or thin-layer chromatography (TLC) assays for amphetamines, opiates, cocaine metabolites, methadone, or their metabolites (2590).

There is insufficient reliable information available about the effectiveness of goldenseal for its other uses.

Mechanism of Action

The applicable parts of goldenseal are the dried rhizome and root. The alkaloids hydrastine, berberine, canadine, and canadaline are the principle active constituents in goldenseal (7265,8012). However, these alkaloids are poorly absorbed when given orally (2591) and might not reach adequate concentrations to have significant pharmacological activity in humans. The isolated constituents have a variety of pharmacological effects. The berberine constituent has antimicrobial effects including antibacterial, antifungal, and some antimycobacterial and antiprotozoal activity (7258,7259). Berberine has activity against Staphylococcus aureus, Streptococcus pyogenes, Eschericha coli, Shigella boydii, Vibrio cholerae, Mycobacterium tuberculosis, Candida albicans, Candida tropicalis, Trichophyton mentagrophytes, Microsporum gypseum, Cryptococcus neoformans, Sporotrichum schenkii, Entamoeba histolytica, and Giardia lamblia (2530,2587,2588,7258,7259,8012). The constituents canadine and canadaline have activity against Pseudomonas aeruginosa. Both berberine and canadaline have similar activity against Escherichia coli, but canadaline has been shown to have more activity against gram-positive organisms than berberine (8012). These effects have not been demonstrated specifically for goldenseal. Due to the poor oral absorption of these alkaloids, goldenseal preparations might not be capable of achieving alkaloid serum concentrations high enough to be effective in humans. However, berberine from goldenseal is thought to concentrate in the bladder. Theoretically, goldenseal could potentially have activity against the binding of urinary tract pathogens, such as Escherichia coli, to bladder walls (2583). There is also preliminary evidence that the berberine constituent might have antitumor properties (7260). Isolated berberine and hydrastine seem to have cardiovascular effects. Berberine seems to increase coronary blood flow and stimulates the heart; although higher doses or long-term use are thought to inhibit cardiac activity (4,12). Berberine has antimuscarinic and antihistaminic activity (4). Hydrastine, in low doses, has hypotensive effects (4); however, at higher doses, hydrastine constricts peripheral blood vessels, potentially leading to hypertensive effects (4). There is preliminary evidence goldenseal might stimulate immunoglobulin M (IgM) antibody production (2530).

Adverse Reactions

Orally, prolonged use of goldenseal can cause digestive disorders, constipation, excitatory states, hallucinations, and occasionally delirium (18). Overdoses can cause stomach upset, nausea, vomiting, nervousness, depression, dyspnea, bradycardia, cardiac damage, hypotension, seizures, paralysis, spasms, and death (4,6). High doses of the constituent hydrastine can cause exaggerated reflexes, convulsions, paralysis, and death from respiratory failure (4). The fresh plant can cause mucosal irritation (12). Using goldenseal vaginally as a douche can cause ulceration (4). Use of goldenseal during pregnancy, lactation or in newborn infants can cause kernicterus, and several resulting fatalities have been reported (2589). The LD50 of the berberine constituent in humans is reported to be 27.5 mg/kg (12).

Interactions with Herbs & Other Dietary Supplements

B VITAMINS: Theoretically, prolonged use of goldenseal can decrease B vitamin absorption (4).
HERBS WITH SEDATIVE PROPERTIES: Theoretically, concomitant use with herbs that have sedative properties might enhance therapeutic and adverse effects. Some of these supplements include 5-HTP, calamus, California poppy, catnip, hops, Jamaican dogwood, kava, St. John's wort, sculIcap, valerian, yerba mansa, and others.

Interactions with Drugs

ANTACIDS: Theoretically, due to reports that goldenseal increases stomach acid, goldenseal might decrease the effectiveness of antacids (19).
ANTIHYPERTENSIVE DRUGS: Theoretically, large amounts of goldenseal might interfere with blood pressure control due to vasoconstrictive action of constituent hydrastine (4).
CNS DEPRESSANTS: Theoretically, concomitant use with drugs with sedative properties might cause additive effects and side effects (4).
CYTOCHROME P450 3A4 (CYP3A4) SUBSTRATES: There's conflicting research on the effect of goldenseal on cytochrome P450 3A4 (CYP3A4) enzymes (6450). Preliminary research suggests that goldenseal might inhibit CYP3A4 and increase levels of CYP3A4 substrates. However, goldenseal given in combination with indinavir (Crixivan), which is metabolized by CYP3A4, doesn't seem to affect peak concentration or oral clearance of indinavir in healthy volunteers (10690). Use goldenseal cautiously in patients taking drugs metabolized by CYP3A4. Some drugs metabolized by CYP3A4 include lovastatin (Mevacor), ketoconazole (Nizoral), itraconazole (Sporanox), fexofenadine (Allegra), triazolam (Halcion), and numerous others.
H2-BLOCKERS: Theoretically, due to reports that goldenseal increases stomach acid, goldenseal might decrease the effectiveness of H2-blockers (19). The H2 blockers include cimetidine (Tagamet), ranitidine (Zantac), nizatidine (Axid), and famotidine (Pepcid).
PROTON PUMP INHIBITORS (PPIs): Theoretically, due to reports that goldenseal increases stomach acid, goldenseal might decrease the effectiveness of PPIs (19). PPIs include omeprazole (Prilosec), lansoprazole (Prevacid), rabeprazole (Aciphex), pantoprazole (Protonix), and esomeprazole (Nexium).

Interactions with Foods

None known.

Interactions with Lab Tests

BILIRUBIN: Theoretically, goldenseal might increase bilirubin levels. This has been demonstrated with isolated berberine constituent, but not specifically with goldenseal. Berberine can cause a true increase in total and unbound bilirubin concentrations because it displaces bilirubin from albumin (2589).

Interactions with Diseases or Conditions

CARDIOVASCULAR DISEASE: Theoretically, low doses can increase coronary blood flow and stimulate the heart, while large doses can inhibit cardiac function (4).
GASTROINTESTINAL IRRITATION: Might irritate gastrointestinal tract. Contraindicated in individuals with infectious or inflammatory gastrointestinal conditions (19).
HYPERBILIRUBINEMIA: The berberine in goldenseal can cause kernicterus in newborns, particularly preterm neonates with hyperbilirubinemia (2589); contraindicated in newborns.
HYPERTENSION: Vasoconstrictive action of the constituent hydrastine might interfere with blood pressure control (4); use with caution.

Dosage and Administration

ORAL: Doses of 0.5-1 gram three times daily of the dried root or rhizome or as a tea have been used. The tea is prepared by simmering 0.5-1 gram dried root or rhizome in 150 mL of boiling water for 5-10 minutes and then straining (4, 12). 0.3-1.0 mL of the liquid extract, 1:1 in 60% ethanol, has been used three times daily (12). 2-4 mL of the tincture, 1:10 in 60% ethanol, has been used times daily (12).
TOPICAL: Goldenseal is used as a mouthwash 3-4 times daily. The mouthwash is prepared by steeping 2 teaspoons, 6 grams, of dried herb in 150 mL boiling water for 5-10 minutes, strain and allow to cool (3).

Comments
Goldenseal is commonly found in the deep woods from Vermont to Arkansas and received its name from the golden-yellow scars on the base of the stem. When the stem is broken, the scar resembles a gold wax letter seal. In the 1900s, goldenseal was immensely popular and has become endangered due to over-harvesting (13). In 1997, goldenseal became listed under Appendix II of the Convention on International Trade in Endangered Species of Wild Flora and Fauna (CITIES), which controls export of the root to other countries. Goldenseal is now being cultivated in many states as cash crop. Because it is so expensive, it is often adulterated. Common adulterants include Coptis and Xanthorrhiza (6). The concept of using goldenseal as an adulterant in drug screens came from the novel Stringtown on the Pike by the pharmacist John Uri Lloyd, but goldenseal caused a false positive for strychnine poisoning in this fictional situation (6).

GOLDTHREAD

Also Known As
Cankerroot, Chinese Goldthread, Coptide, Coptis, Coptis Chinesis, Gold Thread, Goldenthread, Huang Lian, Mouth Root, Yellowroot.

Scientific Names
Coptis chinensis; Coptis deltoidea; Coptis teeta, synonym Coptis teetoides; Coptis trifolia, synonyms Coptis groenlandica, Anemone groenlandica.
Family: Ranunculaceae.

People Use This For
Orally, goldthread is used for digestive disorders.

Safety
POSSIBLY SAFE ...when used orally and appropriately (12).
PREGNANCY: LIKELY UNSAFE ...when used orally; avoid using. Goldthread may induce menstruation and uterine contractions (12,19).
LACTATION: Insufficient reliable information available; avoid using.

Effectiveness
There is insufficient reliable information available about the effectiveness of goldthread.

Mechanism of Action
The applicable part of goldthread is the rhizome. Goldthread contains the bitter berberine, which stimulates bile secretion (12). Berberine also has antimicrobial, diuretic, smooth muscle relaxant, and cardiac depressant activities (12). Small doses stimulate the cardiac and respiratory systems and decrease intestinal peristalsis (12). High doses stimulate smooth muscle in the intestines and uterus, and depress respiration and cardiac function (12). In animal studies, berberine depresses cardiac function by dilating blood vessels and stimulating the vagal nerve (12).

Adverse Reactions
Orally, purified berberine can cause lethargy, nosebleed, dyspnea, skin and eye irritation, kidney irritation, nephritis, nausea, vomiting, and diarrhea (2).

Interactions with Herbs & Other Dietary Supplements
None known.

Interactions with Drugs
ANTACIDS: Theoretically, due to reports that goldthread increases stomach acid, goldthread might decrease the effectiveness of antacids (19).
H2-BLOCKERS: Theoretically, due to reports that goldthread increases stomach acid, goldthread might decrease the effectiveness of H2-blockers (19). The H2 blockers include cimetidine (Tagamet), ranitidine (Zantac), nizatidine (Axid), and famotidine (Pepcid).
PROTON PUMP INHIBITORS (PPIs): Theoretically, due to reports that goldthread increases stomach acid, goldthread might decrease the effectiveness of PPIs (19). PPIs include omeprazole (Prilosec), lansoprazole (Prevacid), rabeprazole (Aciphex), pantoprazole (Protonix), and esomeprazole (Nexium).

Interactions with Foods
None known.

Interactions with Lab Tests
None known.

Interactions with Diseases or Conditions
PEPTIC ULCER DISEASE: Contraindicated. Goldthread might increase stomach acid (19).

Dosage and Administration
ORAL: People typically use 0.5 to 1.2 grams of the powdered rhizome (223). As a liquid, 1 teaspoon is boiled with 1 cup water, and dosed 1 tablespoon 3 to 6 times daily. The liquid is sometimes used as a mouthwash or gargle. The tincture is taken 5 to 10 drops at a time (5263).

GOSSYPOL

Also Known As
Cottonseed Oil, Karpasa.
CAUTION: See separate listing for Cotton.

Scientific Names
Gossypium hirsutum; Gossypium herbaceum; other Gossypium species.
Family: Malvaceae.

People Use This For
Orally, gossypol is used as a male contraceptive. Gossypol is also used in treating uterine myoma, endometriosis, dysfunctional uterine bleeding, metastatic carcinoma of the endometrium or ovary, and HIV disease.
Topically, gossypol is used as a spermicidal cream or gel.

Safety
POSSIBLY UNSAFE ...when used orally (5914,8290,8463). The inhibitory effects on spermatogenesis are not predictably reversible, although sperm counts usually return to normal within three months to two years after discontinuation. In approximately 10% of men, the sperm counts remain suppressed for more than 4.5 years, following chronic use (8463). Gossypol might also be cytotoxic to endometrial cells (6).
There is insufficient reliable information available about the safety of the topical use of gossypol.
PREGNANCY: LIKELY UNSAFE ...when used orally; gossypol seems to have abortifacient and uterine stimulant effects, avoid using (6,12).
LACTATION: POSSIBLY UNSAFE ...when used orally; avoid using.

Effectiveness
POSSIBLY EFFECTIVE

Contraception. Taking gossypol orally seems to effectively inhibit sperm motility and production after 12-16 weeks of treatment in about 60% of men. A dose of 15 mg per day is given for 12-16 weeks to achieve spermatogenesis suppression, followed by a maintenance dose of 7.5-10 mg per day. Normalization of sperm function returns within three months to two years after discontinuation of treatment in about 50% of men (8290). There is also preliminary evidence that a topical gossypol preparation might also be effective as a spermicide (8906).

There is insufficient reliable information available about the effectiveness of gossypol for its other uses.

Mechanism of Action
Gossypol is an polyphenolic extract of the seed of the cotton plant. The cottonseed oil, stem, and roots of the cotton plant are extracted (5914).
Gossypol seems to suppress sperm independent of serum concentration, but recovery of spermatogenesis seems to be concentration dependent (8290). During continued treatment, sperm counts drop dramatically in the first two months and continue to be suppressed for at least six months (8463). The contraceptive action of gossypol results from the reduction of total cellular and microtubular tubulin content in sperm and spermatogenetic cells. Although the exact molecular mechanism of this reduction is not completely understood, evidence suggests that it is a result of inhibition of the enzyme lactate dehydrogenase X. This enzyme is crucial to energy metabolism in sperm and spermatogenic cells (8287,8290). Gossypol might also reduce the rate of tubulin synthesis or prevent the tubulin from assembling into microtubules (8287). Other research suggests that gossypol might damage spermatozoa by decreasing glucose uptake and increasing peroxidation of the cell membrane (7877). The contraceptive effect might also be mediated through inhibition of prostaglandin synthesis (17).
Gossypol is not toxic to genetic material and doesn't cause DNA changes (8464).
When used topically as a spermicidal agent, gossypol significantly reduces sperm motility, by decreasing intracellular concentration of cyclic adenosine monophosphate (cAMP) by decreasing its formation or increasing its

breakdown. It also promotes damage to the cell membrane of spermatocytes. Topical gossypol concentrations of at least 20 mcg/mL reduce sperm motility (3586).

In women who consume gossypol, the uterus may decrease in size and amenorrhea may occur. During gossypol therapy, estrogen and progesterone levels drop and follicle stimulating hormone (FSH) and leuteinizing hormone (LH) levels increase. This is the basis for the use of gossypol in uterine myoma, endometriosis, dysfunctional uterine bleeding and other gynecologic disorders. However, the effects are not long lasting, requiring hysterectomy following gossypol (8463).

There is also interest in using gossypol to treat cancer. Early evidence suggests gossypol exhibits cytotoxic and anti-tumor properties on a large number of cytosolic and mitochondrial enzyme systems. These enzyme systems are necessary for tumor cell growth in preliminary studies using cellular and animal models. Gossypol is cytotoxic toward a variety of tumor cell lines including melanoma, endometrial, colon, lung, prostate, breast, brain, and adrenocortical cancer cells (5915,8289,8291,8292,8294,8295,8463).

Gossypol might have antiviral activity. It has shown activity against herpes simplex type 2 viruses and the human immunodeficiency virus (HIV) (8462). Gossypol also seems to increase interferon levels (8463).

The average half-life of gossypol is 286 hours (8463). The serum concentration of gossypol needed to reduce the sperm count is about 132 ng/mL (5914).

Adverse Reactions

Orally, gossypol can cause fatigue, changes in appetite, and gastrointestinal effects including diarrhea, mucosal sloughing, mucosal necrosis, ileus, and intestinal hemorrhage (6,9,17,21,8290).

Gossypol can cause persistent oligospermia. It can also cause a reduction in testicular volume, which is usually reversible (5914). The inhibitory effects on spermatogenesis are not predictably reversible, although reversibility seems to be better at lower doses. Sperm counts usually return to normal within 12 months after discontinuation (8290). In approximately 10% of men, the sperm counts remain suppressed for over 4.5 years, following chronic use (8463). Chronic use can cause sterility (12). Animal data suggest that gossypol might reduce libido in males, but this has not been observed in humans (8466,8290).

Gossypol can cause hypokalemia, which is more common in people with potassium deficient diets (5914,8288,8290). This hypokalemia can be caused by renal loss of potassium and may be resistant to potassium supplementation or potassium-sparing diuretics (9,21,8463).

High doses (100 to 700 times the contraceptive dose) may cause, hair discoloration, malnutrition, circulatory problems, and heart failure (6). Gossypol can cause amenorrhea and decreased uterine size. Gossypol can cause a photosensitivity reaction known as "burning fever," in which skin that is exposed to the sun develops a burning sensation, accompanied by generalized fatigue (8463).

Topically, gossypol might cause a burning sensation on the face and hands (9,17).

Interactions with Herbs & Other Dietary Supplements

CARDIAC GLYCOSIDE-CONTAINING HERBS: Theoretically, concomitant use might increase the risk of cardiac glycoside toxicity due to the potassium depleting effects of gossypol. Cardiac glycoside-containing herbs include black hellebore, Canadian hemp roots, digitalis leaf, hedge mustard, figwort, lily of the valley roots, motherwort, oleander leaf, pheasant's eye plant, pleurisy root, squill bulb leaf scales, and strophanthus seeds (19).

LICORICE/HORSETAIL: Theoretically, overuse/misuse of licorice rhizome or horsetail plant with gossypol might increase the risk of potassium depletion (19).

STIMULANT LAXATIVE HERBS: Theoretically, overuse or misuse of stimulant laxatives with gossypol might increase the risk of potassium depletion. Stimulant laxative herbs include aloe dried leaf sap, blue flag rhizome, alder buckthorn, European buckthorn, butternut bark, cascara bark, castor oil, colocynth fruit pulp, gamboge bark exudate, jalap root, black root, manna bark exudate, podophyllum root, rhubarb root, senna leaves and pods, wild cucumber fruit (Ecballium elaterium), and yellow dock root (19).

Interactions with Drugs

DIGOXIN (Lanoxin): Theoretically, concomitant use with gossypol might increase the risk of cardiac glycoside drug toxicity due to the potassium-depleting effects of gossypol (9).

DIURETIC DRUGS: Overuse of gossypol might compound diuretic-induced potassium loss (9). There is some concern that people taking gossypol along with potassium depleting diuretics might have an increased risk for hypokalemia. Initiation of potassium supplementation or an increase in potassium supplement dose may be necessary for some patients. Some diuretics that can deplete potassium include chlorothiazide (Diuril), chlorthalidone (Thalitone), furosemide (Lasix), and hydrochlorothiazide (HCTZ, HydroDIURIL, Microzide), and others.

NONSTEROIDAL ANTI-INFLAMMATORY DRUGS (NSAIDs): Concomitant use might increase the risk of gastrointestinal side effects (21). Some of these drugs include diclofenac (Voltaren, Cataflam, others), ibuprofen (Advil, Motrin, others), and naproxen (Anaprox, Naprosyn).

STIMULANT LAXATIVES: Theoretically, overuse or misuse of stimulant laxatives with gossypol might increase the risk of potassium depletion (19). Some of these drugs include cascara, bisacodyl (Dulcolax), and senna (Senkot).

THEOPHYLLINE: Theoretically, concomitant use might reduce the ability of gossypol to decrease sperm motility (3586).

Interactions with Foods

ALCOHOL: Preliminary evidence indicates that gossypol can inhibit alcohol dehydrogenase and aldehyde dehydrogenase, which may permit blood levels of ethanol and acetaldehyde to accumulate. Patients should avoid alcoholic beverages while taking gossypol (8461).

Interactions with Lab Tests

None known.

Interactions with Diseases or Conditions

HYPOKALEMIA: Gossypol may induce or exacerbate hypokalemia (8288).
UROGENITAL IRRITATION OR SENSITIVITY: Contraindicated (12).

Dosage and Administration

ORAL: For male contraception, 15-20 mg is typically used daily for 12-16 weeks, followed by a maintenance dose of 7.5-10 mg per day (8290).
TOPICAL: No typical dosage.

Comments

Gossypol is considered unsafe for self-medication due to toxic potential; administration requires monitoring. Gossypol is found in cotton root, root bark, seed, and stem, but is commercially extracted from cotton seed (6).

GOTU KOLA

Also Known As

Brahma-Buti, Brahma-Manduki, Brahmi, Centella, Centellase, Gota Kola, Gotu Cola, Gotu-Kola, Hydrocotyle, Hydrocotyle Asiatique, Indischer Wassernabel, Idrocotyle, Indian Pennywort, Indian Water Navelwort, Luei Gong Gen, Madecassol, Mandukaparni, Manduk Parani, Marsh Penny, Talepetrako, Thick-Leaved Pennywort, Tsubo-kusa, Tungchian, White Rot.
CAUTION: See separate listings for Brahmi and Cola Nut.

Scientific Names

Centella asiatica, synonym Hydrocotyle asiatica; Centella coriacea.
Family: Apiaceae/Umbelliferae.

People Use This For

Orally, gotu kola is used for reducing fatigue, improving memory and intelligence, venous insufficiency including varicose veins, wound healing, and increasing longevity. It is also used for the common cold and influenza (flu), sunstroke, tonsillitis, pleurisy, urinary tract infection (UTI), hepatitis, jaundice, abdominal pain, diarrhea, indigestion, gastritis, peptic ulcer disease, dysentery, trauma, shingles, leprosy, cholera, syphilis, psychiatric disorders, epilepsy, asthma, anemia, diabetes, and hypertension. Gotu kola is also used for contraception, amenorrhea, elephantiasis, systemic lupus erythematosus (SLE), tuberculosis, memory loss, and as an aphrodisiac.
Topically, gotu kola is used for wound healing and reducing scars.
Parenterally, gotu kola is used for bladder lesions associated with schistosomiasis.

Safety

POSSIBLY SAFE ...when used orally or topically and appropriately (6887).
PREGNANCY: POSSIBLY UNSAFE ...when used orally. Gotu kola might be an abortifacient (4); avoid using.
LACTATION: Insufficient reliable information available; avoid using.

Effectiveness

POSSIBLY EFFECTIVE

Schistosomiasis. Using gotu kola parenterally seems to help bladder lesions of schistosomiasis (bilharzial infections) (9785).

Venous insufficiency. Taking gotu kola orally seems to help treat chronic venous insufficiency (6887). Triterpenes from gotu kola may reduce ankle edema and improve lower leg circulation in venous insufficiency (9786).

INSUFFICIENT RELIABLE EVIDENCE to RATE

Keloids. There is some evidence that applying gotu kola topically can help prevent keloids and hypertrophic scarring (4).

Psoriasis. Applying gotu kola topically seems to help treat psoriasis (6887).

Wound healing. Applying gotu kola topically seems to help improve wound healing (6887).

More evidence is needed to rate gotu kola for these uses.

Mechanism of Action

The applicable parts of gotu kola are the above ground parts. The primary constituents responsible for the pharmacological effects are thought to be the saponin-containing triterpene acids, 1% to 8%, and their sugar esters, including asiatic acid, madecassic acid, asiaticoside, asiaticoside A (madecassoside), and asiaticoside B. Gotu kola also contains essential oils, flavonoids, flavone derivatives including quercetin and kaempferol, sesquiterpenes, stigmasterol, sitosterol and isothankuniside (6887,10276).

The triterpenoid saponins (e.g., asiaticoside, madecassoside) seem to be involved in wound healing and decreasing venous pressure in venous insufficiency (780,2700,9786); asiaticoside and madecassoside have anti-inflammatory activity (11). There is also some evidence that asiaticosides might promote wound healing by stimulating collagen and glycosaminoglycan synthesis (1890,2700).

Topical application of gotu kola extracts increase collagen synthesis, intracellular fibronectin content, and mitotic activity in the germ layer, and enlarges kerato-hyaline granules in scar tissue.

There's preliminary evidence that asiaticosides might also have preventive and therapeutic effects on gastrointestinal ulcers (6887,7691). Anti-ulcer mechanisms may be due to strengthening action on gastric mucosal lining and suppression of damaging effects of free radicals (7691).

The asiaticosides have several other pharmacological effects, including elevating blood glucose, triglycerides, and cholesterol levels. They also seem to decrease blood urea nitrogen (BUN) and acid phosphatase levels.

Early evidence suggests that purified isothankuniside may decrease fertility. However, a crude extract of Centella asiatica does not reduce fertility (10276).

Some researchers think the asiaticoside derivatives, asiatic acid, asiaticoside 6, and SM2, might have a role in Alzheimer's disease. There is some early evidence that they might protect neurons from beta-amyloid toxicity (1889).

There is preliminary evidence that gotu kola extracts might have sedative, anticonvulsant, and analgesic effects, possibly mediated in part via increased levels of the inhibitory transmitter, GABA (6887). The terpenoid constituents brahmoside and brahminoside might be responsible for sedative effects (4).

Gotu kola extracts also seem to have antibacterial activity in vitro against Pseudomonas pyocyaneus, Trichoderma mentagrophytes, and Entamoeba histolytica, and antiviral activity against Herpes simplex type II (6887).

There is some interest in using gotu kola to treat cancer. Dried powder extracts of gotu kola exhibit cytotoxic and anti-tumor properties in preliminary studies. Normal lymphocytes are not harmed, which suggests gotu kola exerts selective toxicity towards tumor cells (7692).

Adverse Reactions

Orally, gotu kola is usually well tolerated when used in typical doses. However, in some patients it can cause gastrointestinal upset and nausea (6887), widespread pruritus and photosensitivity (4). Caution patients using gotu kola to use sunscreen and wear adequate clothing to prevent sunburn. Large doses of gotu kola might increase blood pressure, glucose, and cholesterol levels (4). There is also some concern that large doses of gotu kola might cause sedation and drowsiness (4).

Topically, gotu kola can cause allergic contact dermatitis, characterized by erythema, itching, papules, and a burning sensation (4,6887,9789). Gotu kola may also cause eczema when applied topically (10277,10278).

Subcutaneous injection of gotu kola can cause pain and discoloration at injection site (6). This can be prevented by using intramuscular injections (6).

Interactions with Herbs & Other Dietary Supplements

HERBS WITH SEDATIVE PROPERTIES: Theoretically, concomitant use with herbs that have sedative properties might enhance therapeutic and adverse effects. Some of these supplements include 5-HTP, calamus, California poppy, catnip, hops, Jamaican dogwood, kava, St. John's wort, scullcap, valerian, yerba mansa, and others.

Interactions with Drugs

CNS DEPRESSANTS: Theoretically, concomitant use with drugs with sedative properties might cause additive effects and side effects (4). The constituents brahmoside and brahminoside might have CNS depressant action (4).

Interactions with Foods

None known.

Interactions with Lab Tests

None known.

Interactions with Diseases or Conditions

DIABETES: The asiaticoside constituent of Gotu kola might elevate blood glucose levels (4).

HYPERLIPIDEMIA: The asiaticoside constituent of Gotu kola might elevate triglyceride and cholesterol levels (4).

Dosage and Administration

ORAL: Typical dosages are 600 mg dried leaves three times per day (18), or one cup tea (steep 600 mg dried leaves in 150 mL boiling water 5-10 minutes, strain) three times per day (18). Clinical trials for venous insufficiency used 60-120 mg titrated extract per day for two months (780).
TOPICAL: For wound healing, 1% gotu kola creams have been used (6887).
PARENTERAL: No typical dosage.

Comments

Avoid confusion with cola nut (Cola acuminata). Also avoid confusion with swamp pennywort (Centella cordifolia). Centella cordifolia is often misidentified as Centella asiatica (gotu kola).

GOUTWEED

Also Known As

Achweed, Ashweed, Bishop's Elder, Bishopsweed, Bishopswort, Eltroot, English Goatweed, Gout Herb, Goutwort, Ground Elder, Herb Gerard, Jack-Jump-About, Masterwort, Pigweed, Weyl Ash, White Ash.
CAUTION: See separate listings for Bishop's Weed and Masterwort.

Scientific Names

Aegopodium podagraria.
Family: Apiaceae/Umbelliferae.

People Use This For

Orally, goutweed is used for gout and rheumatic disease. It is also used for hemorrhoids, kidney, bladder, and intestinal disorders.

Safety

There is insufficient reliable information available about the safety of goutweed.
Pregnancy and Lactation: Insufficient reliable information available.

Effectiveness

There is insufficient reliable information available about the effectiveness of goutweed.

Mechanism of Action

The applicable parts of goutweed are the above ground parts. Goutweed contains a volatile oil, flavonol glycosides (hyperoside, isoquercitrin), and caffeic acid derivatives including chlorogenic acid (18).

Adverse Reactions

None reported.

Interactions with Herbs & Other Dietary Supplements

None known.

Interactions with Drugs

None known.

Interactions with Foods

None known.

Interactions with Lab Tests

None known.

Interactions with Diseases or Conditions

None known.

Dosage and Administration

ORAL: People typically use 2 to 4 mL of liquid goutweed extract (223).
TOPICAL: The fresh herb is squeezed or softened by soaking in water for poultices (18).

Comments

Avoid confusion with bishop's weed (Ammi majus) and masterwort (Heracleum sphondylium).

GRAINS OF PARADISE

Also Known As
Guinea Grains, Mallaguetta Pepper, Melegueta Pepper.
CAUTION: See separate listing for Capsicum.

Scientific Names
Aframomum melegueta, synonym Amomum melegueta.
Family: Zingiberaceae.

People Use This For
Orally, grains of paradise fruit and seeds are used as a stimulant.

Safety
POSSIBLY SAFE ...when used orally and appropriately (12).
PREGNANCY AND LACTATION: Insufficient reliable information available; avoid using.

Effectiveness
There is insufficient reliable information available about the effectiveness of grains of paradise.

Mechanism of Action
The applicable parts of grains of paradise are the fruit and seed. Grains of paradise contains a volatile oil and the constituents hydroxyphenylalkanones and hydroxyphenylalkanoles. The seed is said to be a stimulant (18).

Adverse Reactions
Theoretically, grains of paradise may cause GI and lower urinary tract irritation when taken orally (18).

Interactions with Herbs & Other Dietary Supplements
None known.

Interactions with Drugs
None known.

Interactions with Foods
None known.

Interactions with Lab Tests
None known.

Interactions with Diseases or Conditions
None known.

Dosage and Administration
ORAL: People typically use 4 to 6 grams added to 3 to 4 cups of water and boiled until the volume is reduced by one-half. The cooled liquid is taken in 3 doses on an empty stomach (5251).

Comments
Avoid confusion with capsicum (Capsicum annuum), also known as grains of paradise.

GRAPE fruit, skin

Also Known As
Black Grape Raisins, Cabernet Franc, Cabernet Sauvignon, Calzin, Chardonnay, Draksha, Emperor, Enocianina, Flame Seedless, Grape, Grapes, Grape Fruit, Grape Fruit Skin, Grape Juice, Grape Skin, Grape Skin Extract, Merlot, Petite Sirah, Raisins, Red Globe, Red Malaga, Sauvignon Blanc, Sultanas, Table Grapes, Thompson Seedless, Wine Grapes.
CAUTION: See separate listings for Grape leaf, Grape seed, Grapefruit, Resveratrol, and Wine.

Scientific Names
Vitis vinifera. Family: Vitaceae.

People Use This For

Orally, grapes and grape preparations, including grape skin and grape juice are used to prevent coronary heart disease. They are also used as a dietary source of antioxidants. Grapes have also been used for varicose veins, hemorrhoids, capillary fragility, and as a mild laxative for constipation. Grape fasts have been used for "detoxification." Dried grapes, raisins or sultanas, have been used as an expectorant for cough.
In beverages and drink mixes, including wine, grape skin extract is used as a coloring agent.

Safety

LIKELY SAFE ...when used orally in amounts commonly found in foods. Grape skin extracts have Generally Recognized As Safe (GRAS) status in the US (4912).
There is insufficient reliable information available about the safety of grape fruit or skin for its other uses.
PREGNANCY AND LACTATION: There is insufficient reliable information about the safety of medicinal amounts of grape skin during pregnancy and breast-feeding; avoid using.

Effectiveness

INSUFFICIENT RELIABLE EVIDENCE to RATE

Cardiovascular disease. There is preliminary evidence that consumption of purple grape products, such as purple grape juice and red wine, might improve endothelium-dependent vasodilation, prevent LDL oxidation, and suppress platelet-mediated thrombosis. Chronic ingestion of these products might reduce the risk of cardiovascular disease (8745,8746). More evidence is needed to rate grape fruit and skin for this use.

Mechanism of Action

Grapes and grape preparations provide a variety of constituents that are thought to be pharmacologically active. Grape products contain phenolic compounds belonging to 4 major classes, cinnamates and 3 types of flavonoids: anthocyanins, flavonols, and polyflavan-3-ols. Flavonoids have antioxidant, vasorelaxant, and other properties that might prevent heart disease (8745). Red grape varieties provide more oxidation protection than white or blush grape varieties (3579). Red wine contains approximately 10 times the amount flavonoids of white wine (8745). A significant correlation appears to exist between total phenol content, anthocyanin content, and the antioxidant activity of grape products (3579,8745). The phenol content in red grapes is primarily from anthocyanins, which are responsible for producing the color in red grapes (3579). Flavonoids with antioxidant, vasodilating, and antiplatelet properties; including quercetin, catechin, myricetin, kaemforal, and tannins, are abundant in red grape products such as purple grape juice and red wine. Preliminary evidence suggests that quercetin is a powerful antioxidant, catechin can inhibit low-density lipoprotein (LDL) oxidation, and tannins have endothelium-dependent vasodilating activity. Intake of myricetin, kaemferol, and quercetin has been associated with reduced rates of coronary heart disease (8746). There is also evidence that flavonoids in red grape products decrease platelet aggregation, decrease superoxide production, increase nitric oxide release from platelets, and modestly increase the levels of antioxidants such as alpha-tocopherol. Flavonoids seem to be primarily responsible, due to a direct effect on platelets and partially due to flavonoids inhibiting or decreasing platelet protein-kinase C (PKC) activity (8745). It is unknown, however, if the vasorelaxing and antioxidant properties of red grape products persist with chronic ingestion (8746).
Grapes are also reported to have laxative and expectorant properties (4201). Black grape raisins are thought to have similar antioxidant potential as red wine (2540). Grape skin extract also contains anthocyanin pigments (11). Some evidence suggests that anthocyanins might strengthen capillaries and have antifungal and antibacterial activity (11). The anthocyanidins delphinidin and delphinidin/cyanidin dimer show some evidence that they might induce chromosomal damage (4074).

Adverse Reactions

Excessive consumption of grapes, dried grapes, raisins, or sultanas, might cause diarrhea due to laxative effects (4201). There is one report of an anaphylactic reaction to grape skin extract, which included urticaria and angioedema (4073).

Interactions with Herbs & Other Dietary Supplements

LACTOBACILLUS ACIDOPHILUS: Grape anthocyanins can inhibit the growth of Lactobacillus acidophilus. Concurrent administration might prevent Lactobacillus acidophilus colonization of the gastrointestinal tract (11); avoid concurrent use.

Interactions with Drugs

CYTOCHROME P450 1A2 (CYP1A2) SUBSTRATES: Grape juice is thought to induce cytochrome P450 1A2 (CYP1A2) metabolism and may decrease plasma levels of substrates of CYP1A2 (2539). Drugs metabolized by CYP1A2 include amitriptyline (Elavil), caffeine, chlordiazepoxide (Librium), clomipramine (Anafranil), clopidogrel (Plavix), clozapine (Clozaril), cyclobenzaprine (Flexaril), desipramine (Norpramin), diazepam (Valium), estradiol (Estrace, others), flutamide (Eulexin), fluvoxamine (Luvox), grepafloxacin (Raxar), haloperidol (Haldol), imipramine (Tofranil), mexiletine (Mexitil), mirtazapine (Remeron), naproxen (Naprosyn), nortriptyline (Pamelor), olanzapine (Zyprexa), ondansetron (Zofran), propafenone (Rythmol), propranolol (Inderal), riluzole (Rilutek),

ropinirole (Requip), ropivacaine (Naropin), tacrine (Cognex), theophylline (Theo-Dur, others), verapamil (Calan, Covera-HS, others), warfarin (Coumadin), and zileuton (Zyflo).
PHENACETIN: Grape juice decreases phenactin, but not acetaminophen plasma levels. It may decrease levels by inducing cytochrome P450 1A2 (CYP1A2) metabolism (2539).

Interactions with Foods
None known.

Interactions with Lab Tests
None known.

Interactions with Diseases or Conditions
None known.

Dosage and Administration
No typical dosage.

GRAPE leaf

Also Known As
Folia Vitis Viniferae, Grape Leaf Extract, Red Vine Leaf Extract, Red Vine Leaf AS 195.
CAUTION: See separate listings for Grape seed; Grape fruit, skin; Resveratrol; and Grapefruit.

Scientific Names
Vitis vinifera.
Family: Vitaceae.

People Use This For
Orally, grape leaf is used for vascular or circulatory disorders, especially venous diseases such as chronic venous insufficiency, varicose veins, and edema. It is also used for attention deficit-hyperactivity disorder (ADHD), diarrhea, heavy menstrual bleeding, uterine hemorrhage, hemorrhoids, and canker sores.
Intravaginally, grape leaf infusions are used as a douche.
Grape leaf is used as a food, particularly in Greek cooking.

Safety
LIKELY SAFE ...when used orally in amounts found in foods (18).
POSSIBLY SAFE ...when used orally and appropriately for medicinal purposes. Significant adverse effects have not been reported (18). In one study using a grape leaf extract, no significant adverse events were reported during 12 weeks of treatment (2538).
PREGNANCY AND LACTATION: Insufficient reliable information available; avoid using.

Effectiveness
POSSIBLY EFFECTIVE

Chronic venous insufficiency. In one clinical trial, a specific grape leaf extract, known as red vine leaf extract AS 195 (Antistax, Boehringer Ingelheim), was given orally to patients with stage I and stage II chronic venous insufficiency. Leg edema significantly decreased after 6 weeks of treatment compared to placebo. Doses of 360 mg and 720 mg daily were both effective, but the higher dose produced a slightly greater effect. Patients also reported significant decreases in subjective complaints such as tired or heavy legs, tension, and tingling and pain after 12 weeks of treatment (2538).

There is insufficient reliable information available about the effectiveness of grape leaf for its other uses.

Mechanism of Action
Grape leaf preparations contain flavonoids that are thought to be responsible for its pharmacological effects (18). The red vine grape extract AS 195 (Antistax, Boehringer Ingelheim) used in one clinical trial primarily contains the flavonoids quercetin-3-O-beta-glucuronide and isoquercitrin (2538). However, its mechanism of action in chronic venous insufficiency is not clearly understood. Grape leaf is reported to have anti-inflammatory and astringent properties (18,4201). These properties are reported to be greatest in the red leaves (4201).

Adverse Reactions
In one study, the most common adverse effects were gastrointestinal and included abdominal discomfort, diarrhea, dyspepsia, dry mouth, and retching. Other adverse effects included infections, headache and musculoskeletal disorders. One case of leg hematoma following a minor trauma was also reported in a person using grape leaf extract (2538).

Interactions with Herbs & Other Dietary Supplements
None known.

Interactions with Drugs
None known.

Interactions with Foods
None known.

Interactions with Lab Tests
None known.

Interactions with Diseases or Conditions
None known.

Dosage and Administration
ORAL: For chronic venous insufficiency, one clinical trial used a standardized red vine grape extract AS 195 (Antistax, Boehringer Ingelheim). The dose used was 360 mg or 720 mg once daily (2538).

GRAPE seed

Also Known As
Activin, Extrait De Pepins De Raisin, Grape Seed Extract, Grape Seed Oil, Grapeseed, Leucoanthocyanin, Muskat, Oligomeric Proanthocyanidins, Oligomeric Procyanidins, OPC, OPCs, PCO, PCOs, Proanthodyn, Procyanidolic Oligomers.
CAUTION: See separate listings for Grape leaf; Grape fruit, skin; Grapefruit Seed Extract; Pycnogenol; and Resveratrol.

Scientific Names
Vitis vinifera; Vitis coignetiae.
Family: Vitaceae.

People Use This For
Orally, grape seed is used for treating and preventing vascular or circulatory disorders including venous insufficiency, varicose veins, atherosclerosis, hypertension, peripheral vascular disease, edema associated with injury or surgery, and myocardial or cerebral infarction. It is also used orally for hemorrhoids, strengthening blood vessels, inflammation, diabetic complications such as neuropathy or retinopathy, improving wound healing, preventing dental caries, cancer prevention, macular degeneration, poor night vision, liver cirrhosis, allergic rhinitis, and prevention of collagen breakdown associated with collagen diseases and aging. Grape seed oil is used orally as a supplemental dietary source of essential fatty acids and tocopherols.

Safety
LIKELY SAFE ...when used orally in the amounts commonly found in foods (272).
POSSIBLY SAFE ...when used orally and appropriately in medicinal doses for up to 8 weeks (9182).
PREGNANCY AND LACTATION: Insufficient reliable information available; avoid using amounts greater than those found in foods.

Effectiveness
POSSIBLY EFFECTIVE

Chronic venous insufficiency. Taking grape seed extract or its procyanidin constituents orally seems to reduce subjective symptoms of chronic venous insufficiency and improves venous tone (2541).

Ocular stress. Taking grape seed extract containing procyanidin constituents orally might help decrease ocular stress from glare (2541).

POSSIBLY INEFFECTIVE

Allergic rhinitis (hayfever). Grape seed extract taken for 8 weeks before ragweed pollen season doesn't seem to decrease seasonal allergic rhinitis symptoms or antihistamine usage (9182).

INSUFFICIENT RELIABLE EVIDENCE to RATE

Night vision. Preliminary research suggests grape seed extract containing procyanidins might also be beneficial for improving night vision (3580). More evidence is needed to rate grape seed for this use.

Mechanism of Action

Grape seeds are typically obtained as a by-product of the manufacturing of wine. Constituents called oligomeric proanthocyanidins (OPCs) or procyanidins may have pharmacological effects. OPCs from grape seed might help prevent and treat cardiovascular and circulatory conditions due to antioxidant and potential anti-lipoperoxidant activity (10156). Grape seed extract (Leucoselect) containing an equivalent of 300 mg of grape seed procyanidins seems to increase serum total antioxidant activity in healthy people (10156). Some evidence suggests that proanthocyanidins from grape seeds can decrease reperfusion injury after cardiac ischemia because of their ability to remove free radicals. This might also decrease the incidence of cardiac arrhythmias that sometimes occurs in cardiac reperfusion injury (10223). Preliminary evidence also suggests grape seed proanthocyanidins may provide greater protection against reactive oxygen species, free radical-induced lipid peroxidation, and DNA damage than the combination of vitamin E, vitamin C, and beta-carotene or a combination of vitamin E and vitamin C (10157).

Grape seed proanthocyanidins seem to inhibit the cytochrome P450 2E1 (CYP2E1) enzyme, which might protect normal cells against drug and chemical-induced toxicity (10157). There is preliminary evidence that grape seed proanthocyanidins might protect against tobacco-induced and chemotherapy drug-induced damage to normal cells. It may also minimize damage to the liver and kidneys after overdosage of acetaminophen (10157).

Grape seed proanthocyanidins seem to decrease the proliferation of gastric adenocarcinoma, breast cancer, lung cancer, prostate cancer cells by inhibiting cell growth and increasing cell death (10224,10157).

OPCs are also thought to inhibit the proteolytic enzymes collagenase, elastase, hyaluronidase, and beta glucuronidase, which are involved in the breakdown of structural components of the vasculature and skin (3900).

Grape seeds also contain catechin, which preclinical research suggests might inhibit allergen-induced histamine release from mast cells (9182).

Adverse Reactions

Orally, grape seed extract is well tolerated. In patients with allergic rhinitis, it has caused headache, abdominal pain, sore throat, nausea, and cough, but these effects were similarly frequent in patients taking placebo (9182).

Interactions with Herbs & Other Dietary Supplements

None known.

Interactions with Drugs

WARFARIN (Coumadin): Theoretically, due to the tocopherol content of grape seed oil, concomitant use with warfarin might increase warfarin's effects and the risk of bleeding (272); use with caution.

Interactions with Foods

None known.

Interactions with Lab Tests

None known.

Interactions with Diseases or Conditions

None known.

Dosage and Administration

ORAL: Grape seed extract as tablets or capsules dosed at 75-300 mg daily for three weeks followed by a maintenance dose of 40-80 mg daily has been suggested by some sources (3900). For chronic venous insufficiency, grape seed extract procyanidin doses of 150-300 mg per day have been used (2541). For reducing ocular stress due to glare, grape seed extract procyanidin doses of 200-300 mg per day have been used (2541).

Comments

Pycnogenol (pinebark extract) is similar to the grape seed extract in active ingredients and medicinal uses (272). Both pycnogenol and grape seed contain oligomeric proanthocyanidins (OPCs). Several other natural medicines contain constituents that are similar to the OPCs, including wine, cranberries, bilberries, green and black teas, black currant, onions, legumes, parsley, and hawthorn.

GRAPEFRUIT

Also Known As

Paradisapfel, Pomelo, Toronja.
CAUTION: See separate listings for Grapefruit Seed Extract and Grapefruit Oil.

Scientific Names

Citrus paradisi; Citrus maxima, synonym Citrus decumana.
Family: Rutaceae.

People Use This For

Orally, grapefruit is used for reducing cholesterol and reversing atherosclerosis; as a supplemental source of potassium, vitamin C, and fiber; for reducing hematocrit counts; as an anti-cancer agent; for psoriasis; and as an aid in weight reduction.
In foods, grapefruit is consumed as fruit and juice.

Safety

LIKELY SAFE ...when used orally in amounts commonly found in foods. Grapefruit has Generally Recognized As Safe (GRAS) status in the US (4912).
There is insufficient reliable information available about the safety of medicinal amounts of grapefruit.
PREGNANCY AND LACTATION: There is insufficient reliable information about the safety of medicinal amounts of grapefruit during pregnancy and breast-feeding; avoid using.

Effectiveness

INSUFFICIENT RELIABLE EVIDENCE to RATE

Asthma. There is some evidence that consumption of vitamin C-rich citrus fruits, including grapefruit and others, might improve lung function in people with asthma. Intake of citrus fruits 1-2 times per week has produced this benefit in some studies (6049,6055,6056). However, other studies have not found this benefit (6057,6058). More evidence is needed to rate the effectiveness of grapefruit for this use.

Mechanism of Action

The applicable parts of grapefruit are the fruit and juice. Whole grapefruit is high in water and fiber. It is a good dietary source of potassium, vitamin C, pectin, and other nutrients. The potential benefits of grapefruit in asthma might be due to antioxidant properties of vitamin C or other fruit constituents (6049,6054,6055).
Grapefruit juice contains furanocoumarins, including bergamottin and dihydroxybergamottin, which inhibit cytochrome P450 3A4 (CYP3A4) (3769,5070,5071,11273). In addition, bergamottin inhibits CYP1A2, CYP2A6, CYP2C9, CYP2C19, CYP2D6, and CYP2E1 (5072). Grapefruit juice also contains naringin, naringenin, limonin, quercetin, kaempferol, and obacunone, which are known to inhibit human hepatic microsomes (7778). It is likely that multiple constituents of grapefruit juice are responsible for its inhibition of CYP3A4 (11276).
Grapefruit juice selectively inhibits gut wall CYP3A4 and increases bioavailability and plasma concentrations of numerous drugs (1386). In higher doses, it may also inhibit hepatic CYP3A4 (7776,11275). Human research indicates that blended grapefruit segments, and an extract of grapefruit core and peel, also inhibit CYP3A4 activity (1388). Research on triazolam suggests that single doses of grapefruit juice increase plasma concentrations by inhibiting intestinal CYP3A4 during first pass metabolism. Repeated consumption of grapefruit juice inhibits hepatic CYP3A4 and prolongs elimination half-life (7776). Grapefruit juice appears to irreversibly inhibit CYP3A4, possibly leading to a down-regulation of CYP3A4. Within 4 hours, grapefruit juice reduces intestinal CYP3A4 by 47% (11273). The maximum effect on drug metabolism appears to be within 24 hours of grapefruit consumption, but reduced drug metabolism can occur to a lesser degree for 3 to 7 days (7778,7782,11362). Research on midazolam suggests that recovery of gut wall CYP3A4 function occurs in 3 days after single exposure of grapefruit juice (10159). For some drugs, such as felodipine and nisoldipine, it may be necessary to allow a 3 day interval between grapefruit juice and drug administration to avoid interactions (5068,5069).
The effect of grapefruit juice on drugs is difficult to predict because the uptake of compounds such as naringenin varies greatly among individuals. The chemical constituents of grapefruit such as dihydroxybergamottin also vary (3775,7777,7779,11273).
There is conflicting research about the effect of grapefruit on the drug transporter P-glucoprotein (1390,11270,11278,11362). However, research in humans using digoxin as a specific probe for P-glycoprotein activity suggests that grapefruit juice has little effect on P-glycoprotein (11277,11282). Preliminary research suggests that grapefruit juice inhibits organic anion transporting polypeptides (OATPs), which could reduce the bioavailability of some oral drugs (11278).

Adverse Reactions

Orally, grapefruit causes few adverse reactions. One study shows it can reduce hematocrit counts (531).

Interactions with Herbs & Other Dietary Supplements

RED YEAST (Cholestin): Concomitant use of grapefruit with red yeast increases the serum levels of lovastatin, a constituent of red yeast (527).

Interactions with Drugs

ARTEMETHER (Artenam, Paluther): Grapefruit juice increases the oral bioavailability of artemether in healthy men by 90% to 250% (5065,5066).

BENZODIAZEPINES: Grapefruit juice can increase plasma triazolam (Halcion) concentrations. Repeated consumption of grapefruit juice greatly increases triazolam concentrations and prolongs the half-life, probably due to inhibition of cytochrome P450 3A4 (CYP3A4) (7776). Some studies suggest that grapefruit juice reduces the clearance and increases the maximum blood levels, area under the plasma concentration curve (AUC), and duration of effect of midazolam (Versed). Other studies suggest there is no effect (4300,10159). Grapefruit juice increases the maximum blood levels and duration of effect of diazepam (Valium), but the clinical significance of this is not known (3228). Grapefruit juice, particularly when taken in large quantities, can increase the AUC, and maximum blood levels of midazolam (Versed) (11275).

BUSPIRONE (BuSpar): Grapefruit juice increases absorption and plasma concentrations of buspirone (3771).

CAFFEINE: Some studies suggest grapefruit juice decreases caffeine clearance, possibly increasing the effects or adverse effects (4300).

CALCIUM CHANNEL BLOCKERS: Grapefruit juice increases absorption and plasma concentrations of amlodipine (Norvasc) (523), nifedipine (Procardia, Adalat) (528), nisoldipine (Sular) (529), felodipine (Plendil), nimodipine (Nimotop), nicardipine (Cardene), diltiazem (Cardizem) (524,528,1388,4300,7780), and verapamil (Calan, Isoptin, Verelan) (7779,8285). This interaction is likely the result of the inhibition of intestinal metabolism by CYP3A4 (7779,7780). Extensive intake of grapefruit juice (1 liter per day) can increase steady state concentrations of verapamil by as much as 50% (8285). Some references dispute the clinical relevance of the interactions with amlodipine, diltiazem, and verapamil (3230,4300). However, there is considerable interindividual variability in the effect of grapefruit juice on drug metabolism, which might account for inconsistent study results (7777,7779,8285). In healthy older adults, the hemodynamic response to felodipine (Plendil) plus grapefruit juice might be influenced by altered autonomic regulation. In older healthy adults, a single dose of grapefruit juice and felodipine enhanced the blood pressure lowering effects of felodipine. However, after a week of grapefruit juice and felodipine (steady state), the hypotensive activity was reduced, possibly due to compensatory tachycardia (1392). Research indicates it is necessary to withhold grapefruit juice for three days to avoid interactions with felodipine and nisoldipine (5068,5069,6453).

CARBAMAZEPINE (Tegretol): Grapefruit juice increases absorption and plasma concentrations of carbamazepine (524).

CARVEDILOL (Coreg): Grapefruit juice is reported to increase the bioavailability of a single dose of carvedilol by 16% (5071).

CISAPRIDE (Propulsid): Grapefruit juice increases absorption and plasma concentrations of cisapride (1383,3226).

CLOMIPRAMINE (Anafranil): Grapefruit juice increases blood levels of clomipramine. Two cases are reported in which trough clomipramine blood levels increased significantly after adding grapefruit juice to the therapeutic regimen (5064).

CYCLOSPORINE (Neoral, Sandimmune): Grapefruit juice increases absorption and plasma concentrations of cyclosporine (522,11270). The mechanism of action is unclear. Advise patients taking cyclosporine to avoid grapefruit.

CYTOCHROME P450 3A4 (CYP3A4) SUBSTRATES: Grapefruit juice can inhibit CYP3A4 metabolism of drugs, causing increased drug levels and potentially increasing the risk of adverse effects (3227,3774,8283,8285,8286). Some drugs metabolized by CYP3A4 that might be affected include amitriptyline (Elavil), amiodarone (Cordarone), citalopram (Celexa), felodipine (Plendil), lansoprazole (Prevacid), ondansetron (Zofran), prednisone (Deltasone, Orasone), sertraline (Zoloft), sibutramine (Meridia), and many others.

DEXTROMETHORPHAN (Robitussin DM, and others): Grapefruit juice can inhibit cytochrome P450 3A4 (CYP3A4) metabolism (11362), causing increased dextromethorphan levels and potentially increasing the risk of adverse effects.

ERYTHROMYCIN: Concomitant use of erythromycin with grapefruit can inhibit CYP3A4 metabolism of erythromycin, increasing absorption and plasma concentrations (8286). Plasma concentrations of erythromycin can increase by 35% when administered with grapefruit juice.

ESTROGENS: Grapefruit juice increases absorption and plasma concentrations of 17-beta-estradiol (526) and ethinyl-estradiol (525).

ETOPOSIDE (VePesid): Grapefruit juice may decrease the absorption and plasma concentrations of etoposide. There is some evidence that grapefruit juice coadministered with oral etoposide can reduce the area under the concentration-time curve (AUC) of etoposide on average by 26.2% (8744).

FEXOFENADINE (Allegra): Grapefruit juice can significantly decrease oral absorption and blood levels of fexofenadine when taken together. Quarter-strength grapefruit juice decreases bioavailability of fexofenadine by about 24% and full strength by 67%. Grapefruit juice seems to inhibit organic anion transporting polypeptide (OATP), which is a drug transporter in the gut, liver, and kidney (7046). It's not yet known how long grapefruit juice inhibits OATP. Separating administration times might not prevent this interaction. Tell patients it's best to take their medications with a plain glass of water.

HMG-CoA REDUCTASE INHIBITORS ("Statins"): Grapefruit juice inhibits metabolism and increases absorption and plasma concentrations of lovastatin (Mevacor) (527,11274), simvastatin (Zocor) (3774,7782), and atorvastatin (Lipitor) (3227,12179). It does not affect pravastatin (3227,12179). There is considerable interindividual variability in the effect of grapefruit juice on drug metabolism, so individual patient response is difficult to predict (7777,7781).

ITRACONAZOLE (Sporanox): Grapefruit juice impairs itraconazole absorption (310).

LOSARTAN (Cozaar): Concomitant use of grapefruit juice and losartan might reduce losartan effectiveness, but this requires further study. Losartan is an inactive prodrug which must be metabolized to its active form, E-3174, to be effective. In one human study, grapefruit juice reduced losartan metabolism, increased losartan AUC, and reduced the AUC of the major active losartan metabolite, E-3174 (1391).

METHYLPREDNISOLONE: Grapefruit juice can increase plasma concentration of orally administered methylprednisolone. Grapefruit juice 200 mL three times daily given with methylprednisolone 16 mg increased methylprednisolone half-life by 35%, peak plasma concentration by 27%, and total area under the curve by 75% (3123). In some patients, consumption of large amounts of grapefruit juice with methylprednisolone might increase the risk of adverse effects; use cautiously. Some of these drugs include Adlone, A-Methapred, depMedalone, Depoject, Medrol, and Solu-Medrol.

PRAZIQUANTEL (Biltricide): Grapefruit juice can inhibit CYP3A4 metabolism of praziquantel, increasing plasma concentrations (8282). Plasma concentrations of praziquantel can increase by as much as 160% when administered with 250 mL of commercially squeezed grapefruit juice.

QUINIDINE: Grapefruit juice decreases quinidine clearance and prolongs the half-life by about 20% (5067). The clinical effect of this interaction is unknown.

SAQUINAVIR (Fortovase, Invirase): Grapefruit juice increases absorption and plasma concentrations of the protease inhibitor (PI)-type antiretroviral drug saquinavir (3773). However, grapefruit juice does not seem to significantly affect indinavir (Crixivan) pharmacokinetics (11269,11280).

SCOPOLAMINE: Grapefruit juice can inhibit CYP3A4 metabolism of scopolamine, increasing absorption and plasma concentrations (8284). Oral bioavailability of scopolamine can increase by 30% when administered with 150 mL of grapefruit juice.

SILDENAFIL (Viagra): Grapefruit juice can inhibit CYP3A4 metabolism of sildenafil, increasing absorption and plasma concentrations (8283). Oral bioavailability of sildenafil can increase by 23% when administered with 500 mL of commercial grapefruit juice.

TERFENADINE (Seldane): Grapefruit juice increases absorption and plasma concentrations of terfenadine (530).

THEOPHYLLINE: Grapefruit juice seems to modestly decrease theophylline levels when given concurrently with sustained-release theophylline (11013). The mechanism of this interaction is unknown.

WARFARIN (Coumadin): Grapefruit juice might increase warfarin effects. One case is reported of significantly increased international normalized ratio (INR) associated with consumption of 50 ounces of grapefruit juice daily (12061). But smaller amounts of grapefruit juice might not be a problem. In a small clinical trial, consumption of 24 ounces of grapefruit juice daily for one week had no effect on INR in a group of men anticoagulated with warfarin (12063).

Interactions with Foods

TONIC WATER: Grapefruit's inhibitory effect on cytochrome P450 (CYP450) isoenzymes may interfere with the metabolism of quinine in tonic water. Grapefruit in combination with tonic water containing quinine should be avoided in people with rhythm disorders such as long QT syndrome that may worsen with quinine (10158).

WINE: Red wine in combination with grapefruit juice appears to have an additive inhibitory effect on CYP3A4, theoretically increasing the risk for interactions with other drugs. White wine does not appear to affect CYP3A4 (7778).

Interactions with Lab Tests

DRUG ASSAYS: Grapefruit juice decreases metabolism, and increases plasma concentrations and test results of amlodipine (Norvasc) (523), nifedipine (Procardia, Adalat) (528), nisoldipine (Sular) (529), felodipine (Plendil), nimodipine (Nimotop), nicardipine (Cardene), diltiazem (Cardizem, Dilacor XR, Tiazac) (524,528,1388,4300), verapamil (Calan, Isoptin, Verelan) (3229), buspirone (BuSpar) (3771), losartan (Cozaar) (1391), midazolam (Versed) and triazolam (Halcion) (4300), diazepam (Valium) (3228), carbamazepine (Tegretol) (524), cisapride (Propulsid) (3226), cyclosporine (Sandimmune, Neoral) (522), 17-beta-estradiol (526), ethinyl-estradiol (525), lovastatin (Mevacor) (527), saquinavir (Fortovase, Invirase) (3773), simvastatin (Zocor) (3774), atorvastatin (Lipitor) (3227), and terfenadine (530).

HEMATOCRIT: Some clinical research suggests that grapefruit may lower hematocrit count in people with an elevated hematocrit. However, in people with a low hematocrit, it may increase hematocrit. The effect appears to be the same with one-half or a whole grapefruit daily. The grapefruit constituent naringin may be responsible for this effect (531).

Interactions with Diseases or Conditions

SMOKING: Smoking can have an antagonistic effect on grapefruit-drug interactions. Smokers taking calcium channel blockers and grapefruit juice, or other drugs that interact with grapefruit juice, require special dosing considerations (8285).

Dosage and Administration
No typical dosage.

Comments
Drug interactions with grapefruit juice are well documented. The chemistry of the grapefruit varies by the species, the growing conditions, and the process used to extract the juice. Because grapefruit juice is not standardized, use as an adjunct to drug therapy is not recommended (3775).

GRAPEFRUIT OIL

Also Known As
Cold-Pressed Grapefruit Oil, Expressed Grapefruit Oil, Pomelo, Shaddock Oil.
CAUTION: See separate listings for Grapefruit and Grapefruit Seed Extract.

Scientific Names
Citrus paradisi; Citrus maxima, synonym Citrus decumana.
Family: Rutaceae.

People Use This For
Topically, grapefruit oil is used to relieve muscle fatigue, to promote hair growth, for toning the skin, and for reducing acne and oily skin. It is also used to aid with the common cold and flu.
Inhaled, the vapors are used to help the body retain water and to relieve headache and stress. The aroma is used to relieve depression.
In food and beverages, grapefruit oil is used as a flavoring component.
In manufacturing, grapefruit oil is used as a fragrance component in soaps and cosmetics.

Safety
LIKELY SAFE ...when used in amounts commonly found in foods. Grapefruit oil Generally Recognized As Safe (GRAS) status in the US (4912).
There is insufficient reliable information available about the safety grapefruit oil for its other uses.
PREGNANCY AND LACTATION: There is insufficient reliable information available about the safety of larger amounts used during pregnancy and lactation; avoid using.

Effectiveness
There is insufficient reliable information available about the effectiveness of grapefruit oil.

Mechanism of Action
Grapefruit oil is obtained by cold expression from the fruit peel of the Citrus X paradisi tree (11).
Antibacterial activity has been suggested. Grapefruit oil contains furocoumarins, including bergaptens, which are photosensitizing, phototoxic, and mutagenic (2). They are responsible for adverse dermatological reactions in other plants that contain them (see separate listings for Angelica and Rue) (11,515). Animal data suggests that 9,10-dimethyl-1,2-benzanthracene, the primary carcinogen, promoted tumor formation when grapefruit oil was applied directly to the skin. Dermatological studies have suggested that grapefruit oil is nonirritating, nonsensitizing, and nonphototoxic to human skin (11).

Adverse Reactions
Contact dermatitis and phototoxic reactions, including skin blisters, have occurred with other furocoumarin-containing herbs following topical exposure and exposure to sunlight (11).

Interactions with Herbs & Other Dietary Supplements
None known.

Interactions with Drugs
None known.

Interactions with Foods
None known.

Interactions with Lab Tests
None known.

Interactions with Diseases or Conditions
None known.

Dosage and Administration
No typical dosage.

GRAPEFRUIT SEED EXTRACT

Also Known As
Bioflavonoid Concentrate, Citrus Grandis Extract, Citrus Seed Extract, CSE, Grapefruit Extract, Grapefruit Seed Glycerate, GSE, Standardized Extract of Grapefruit.
Caution: See separate listings for Grapefruit; Grapefruit Oil; Grape fruit, seed; and Grape seed.

Scientific Names
Citrus paradisi; Citrus maxima, synonym Citrus decumana.
Family: Rutaceae.

People Use This For
Orally, grapefruit seed extract is used for preventing and treating infections due to bacteria, viruses, fungi, and parasites. It is particularly promoted for yeast infections, and intestinal parasites such as Giardia lamblia and Entamoeba histolytica, including intestinal infections associated with travel.
Topically, grapefruit seed extract is used as a facial cleanser, first-aid treatment, and treatment for mild skin irritations. It is also used as an ear or nasal rinse for prevention and treatment of infections, a throat gargle for sore throat, a dental rinse to prevent gingivitis and to promote healthy gums and fresh breath, and a vaginal douche for candidiasis. It has also been nebulized for the treatment of lung infections.
In manufacturing, grapefruit seed extract is used in soaps and cosmetics; and as a household cleaner for fruits, vegetables, meats, kitchen surfaces, dishes, etc.
In agriculture, grapefruit seed extract is used as a bactericide and fungicide, a mold inhibitor and antiparasitic for animal feeds, a food preservative and antioxidant, and a water disinfectant.

Safety
POSSIBLY SAFE ...when preservative-free products are used orally as a food additive. Grapefruit seed has Generally Recognized As Safe (GRAS) status in the US (4912).
POSSIBLY UNSAFE ...when products with preservatives are used orally. The preservative benzethonium chloride has been detected in some commercial grapefruit seed extracts. This substance is restricted to use in rinse-off cosmetics and is not permitted for use in drugs or foods in Germany (5867). It can cause vomiting, collapse, convulsions and coma when ingested (3082).
There is insufficient reliable information about the safety of grapefruit seed extract for its other uses.
PREGNANCY AND LACTATION: Insufficient reliable information available; avoid using.

Effectiveness
INSUFFICIENT RELIABLE EVIDENCE to RATE

Atopic dermatitis (eczema). There is preliminary evidence that suggests citrus seed extract (ParaMycrocidin) can decrease complaints of constipation, flatulence, and abdominal discomfort possibly due to changes in intestinal microflora, in people with atopic eczema (5866). More evidence is needed to rate grapefruit seed extract for this use.

Mechanism of Action
Grapefruit seeds contain numerous constituents including naringin, nomilin, deacetyl-nomilin, nomilinic-acid-17-O-beta-D-glucoside, deacetyl-nomilinic-acid-17-O-beta-D-glucoside, limonol, deoxy-limonol, 7-obacunol, obacunone, epi-iso-obacunoic-acid-17-O-beta-D-glucoside, iso-obacunoic-acid-17-O-beta-D-glucoside, and trans-obacunoic-acid-17-O-beta-D-glucoside (513). However, the role these play in any potential therapeutic actions of grapefruit seed extract is unknown. Naringin has been reported to induce red blood cell aggregation in vitro (6). Naringin and obacunone have been reported to have inhibitory effects on liver enzymes (6).
A commercial citrus seed extract used at a concentration of 0.5% has been reported to inhibit the in vitro growth of some bacteria, yeasts and molds (Streptococcus species, Staph. aureus, enterococci, Enterobacter, E. coli, Candida, Geotrichum, Aspergillus and Penicillium species) (5866). Grapefruit seed extracts have been reported to reduce counts of Salmonella Typhimurium when sprayed on chicken skins (5862), but to have no effect in controlling fungal growth on unshelled peanuts (5864,5865).
When examined by HPLC, a commercial grapefruit seed extract was found to contain significant amounts of the preservatives methyl-p-hydroxybenzoate and triclosan, which were not present in an ethanol extract of grapefruit seeds (5863). In another study, five of six commercial grapefruit seed extracts tested contained significant amounts of

the preservative benzethonium chloride, and three of these also contained triclosan and methyl-p-hydroxybenzoate. These five extracts had significant antibacterial activity, as measured by in vitro tests, but a sixth commercial extract which was preservative-free had no in vitro antibacterial activity (5867). It has therefore been hypothesized that the reported antimicrobial activity of grapefruit seed extract products is due to the preservative content (5867).

Adverse Reactions

When preservative-containing products are used vomiting, collapse, convulsions and coma can occur (3082).

Interactions with Herbs & Other Dietary Supplements

RED YEAST (Cholestin): Theoretically, concomitant use of grapefruit seed extract with red yeast can increase the serum levels of lovastatin, a constituent of red yeast (527). Grapefruit seed extract products can contain grapefruit pulp and the naringin constituent, which can inhibit cytochrome P450 metabolism of lovastatin (6).

Interactions with Drugs

ARTEMETHER (Artenam, Paluther): Theoretically, grapefruit seed extract can increase the oral bioavailability of artemether (5065,5066). Grapefruit seed extract contains grapefruit pulp and the constituent naringin, which can inhibit cytochrome P450 (CYP450) metabolism of this and other drugs (6).

BENZODIAZEPINES: Theoretically, grapefruit seed extract might increase blood levels of some benzodiazepines, such as diazepam (Valium), midazolam (Versed), and triazolam (Halcion) (3228,4300). Grapefruit seed extract contains grapefruit pulp and the constituent naringin, which can inhibit cytochrome P450 (CYP450) metabolism of these and other drugs (6).

BUSPIRONE (BuSpar): Theoretically, grapefruit seed extract can increase plasma concentrations of buspirone (3771). Grapefruit seed extract contains grapefruit pulp and the constituent naringin, which can inhibit cytochrome P450 (CYP450) metabolism of this and other drugs (6).

CAFFEINE: Theoretically, grapefruit seed extract can increase caffeine levels and adverse effects (4300). Grapefruit seed extract contains grapefruit pulp and the constituent naringin, which can inhibit cytochrome P450 (CYP450) metabolism of this and other drugs (6).

CALCIUM CHANNEL BLOCKERS: Theoretically, grapefruit seed extract can increase plasma concentrations of amlodipine (Norvasc) (523), nifedipine (Procardia, Adalat) (528), nisoldipine (Sular) (529), felodipine (Plendil), nimodipine (Nimotop), nicardipine (Cardene), diltiazem (Cardizem) (524,528,1388,4300), and verapamil (Calan, Isoptin, Verelan) (3229). Grapefruit seed extract contains grapefruit pulp and the constituent naringin, which can inhibit cytochrome P450 (CYP450) metabolism of these and other drugs (6).

CARBAMAZEPINE (Tegretol): Theoretically, grapefruit seed extract can increase plasma concentrations of carbamazepine (524). Grapefruit seed extract contains grapefruit pulp and the constituent naringin, which can inhibit cytochrome P450 (CYP450) metabolism of this and other drugs (6).

CARVEDILOL (Coreg): Theoretically, grapefruit seed extract might increase plasma concentration of carvedilol (5071). Grapefruit seed extract contains grapefruit pulp and the constituent naringin, which can inhibit cytochrome P450 (CYP450) metabolism of this and other drugs (6).

CISAPRIDE (Propulsid): Theoretically, grapefruit seed extract can increase plasma concentrations of cisapride (1383,3226). Grapefruit seed extract contains grapefruit pulp and the constituent naringin, which can inhibit cytochrome P450 (CYP450) metabolism of this and other drugs (6).

CLOMIPRAMINE (Anafranil): Theoretically, grapefruit seed extract can increase blood levels of clomipramine (5064). Grapefruit seed extract contains grapefruit pulp and the constituent naringin, which can inhibit cytochrome P450 (CYP450) metabolism of this and other drugs (6).

CYCLOSPORINE (Neoral, Sandimmune): Theoretically, grapefruit seed extract can increase plasma concentrations of cyclosporine (522). Grapefruit seed extract contains grapefruit pulp and the constituent naringin, which can inhibit cytochrome P450 (CYP450) metabolism of this and other drugs (6).

CYTOCHROME P450 3A4 (CYP3A4) SUBSTRATES: Theoretically, grapefruit seed extract can inhibit the cytochrome P450 3A4 (CYP3A4) enzyme (522,3226, 3771). Some drugs metabolized by CYP3A4 include lovastatin (Mevacor), ketoconazole (Nizoral), itraconazole (Sporanox), fexofenadine (Allegra), triazolam (Halcion), and numerous others.

ESTROGENS: Theoretically, grapefruit seed extract can increase plasma concentrations of 17-beta-estradiol (526) and ethinyl-estradiol (525). Grapefruit seed extract contains grapefruit pulp and the constituent naringin, which can inhibit cytochrome P450 (CYP450) metabolism of this and other drugs (6).

HMG-CoA REDUCTASE INHIBITORS ("Statins"): Theoretically, grapefruit seed extract can increase plasma concentrations of lovastatin (Mevacor) (527), simvastatin (Zocor) (3774), and atorvastatin (Lipitor) (3227). Grapefruit seed extract contains grapefruit pulp and the constituent naringin, which can inhibit cytochrome P450 (CYP450) metabolism of these and other drugs (6).

QUINIDINE: Theoretically, grapefruit seed extract can increase plasma levels (5067). Grapefruit seed extract contains grapefruit pulp and the constituent naringin, which can inhibit cytochrome P450 (CYP450) metabolism of this and other drugs (6).

SAQUINAVIR (Fortovase, Invirase): Theoretically, grapefruit seed extract might increases absorption and plasma concentrations of the protease inhibitor (PI)-type antiretroviral drug saquinavir (3773).

TERFENADINE (Seldane): Theoretically, grapefruit seed extract can increase plasma concentrations of

terfenadine (530). Grapefruit seed extract contains grapefruit pulp and the constituent naringin, which can inhibit cytochrome P450 (CYP450) metabolism of this and other drugs (6).
WARFARIN (Coumadin): Theoretically, grapefruit seed extract might increase warfarin effects. Grapefruit seed extract contains grapefruit pulp and the constituent naringin, which can inhibit cytochrome P450 (CYP450) metabolism of this and other drugs (6).

Interactions with Foods
None known.

Interactions with Lab Tests
None known.

Interactions with Diseases or Conditions
None known.

Dosage and Administration
No typical dosage.

Comments
Grapefruit seed extract is processed from grapefruit seeds and pulp obtained as a byproduct from grapefruit juice production. Vegetable glycerin is added to the final product to reduce acidity and bitterness.

GRAVEL ROOT

Also Known As
Joe Pye, Joe-Pye Weed, Kidney Root, Kydney Root, Purple Boneset, Queen of the Meadow, Roter Wasserhanf, Trumpet Weed.
CAUTION: See separate listing for Boneset.

Scientific Names
Eupatorium purpureum, synonym Eupatoriadelphus purpureus.
Family: Asteraceae/Compositae.

People Use This For
Orally, gravel root is used for urinary calculus, renal or vesicular calculi, cystitis, painful urination, urethritis, prostatitis, rheumatism, and gout. It is also used orally for fever from malaria, dengue virus, fever, typhus; and as an antacid, aperitif, diuretic, emetic, stimulant, tonic, and for inducing sweating.

Safety
UNSAFE ...when used orally. Gravel root contains hepatotoxic unsaturated pyrrolizidine alkaloids (UPAs) (12,19). Repeated exposure to low concentrations of UPAs is linked to veno-occlusive disease, a serious condition (4,12). UPAs may also be carcinogenic and mutagenic (12). Topical use on abraded or broken skin might be unsafe due to potential for systemic absorption (12,19).
PREGNANCY: UNSAFE ...when used orally (12,19). Gravel root might be an abortifacient (19).
LACTATION: UNSAFE ...when used orally due to concern that UPAs might be excreted into breast milk (4,12,18,19).

Effectiveness
There is insufficient reliable information available about the effectiveness of gravel root.

Mechanism of Action
The applicable parts of gravel root are the above ground parts, rhizome, and roots. Although people think gravel root has antilithic, diuretic, and antirheumatic properties (4), this has not been studied. Some evidence suggests an ethanolic extract might have anti-inflammatory activity (4020). The above ground parts of gravel root contain echinatine, an unsaturated pyrrolizidine alkaloid (UPA) (4). Pyrrolizidine alkaloids with an unsaturated pyrrolizidine nucleus can be hepatotoxic in animals and humans (4). Herbs containing UPAs have shown carcinogenic, mutagenic, and renal toxic effects. However, the primary concern regarding UPAs is veno-occlusive disease (12).

Adverse Reactions
Although no adverse effects are reported for gravel root, chronic exposure to other plants containing UPA constituents has been associated with veno-occlusive disease (4021). Symptoms of acute veno-occlusive disease are characterized by a dull, dragging ache in the right upper abdomen and marked distention of the abdomen. These symptoms are sometimes accompanied by reduced urine output. Subacute veno-occlusive disease is associated with

vague symptoms and persistent liver enlargement (4021). Gravel root can cause an allergic reaction in individuals sensitive to the Asteraceae/Compositae family. Members of this family include ragweed, chrysanthemums, marigolds, daisies, and many other herbs.

Interactions with Herbs & Other Dietary Supplements

EUCALYPTUS: Theoretically, concomitant use might increase the risk of unsaturated pyrrolizidine alkaloid (UPA) toxicity due to enzyme induction by eucalyptus (19).
UNSATURATED PYRROLIZIDINE ALKALOID-CONTAINING HERBS (UPAs): Concomitant use is contraindicated due to the risk of additive toxicity. Herbs containing UPAs include alkanna (12), borage (271), hemp agrimony (271), hound's tongue (19), petasites (19), comfrey (271), coltsfoot, and the Senecio species plants dusty miller (19), alpine ragwort (19), groundsel (271), golden ragwort (19), and tansy ragwort (271).

Interactions with Drugs

None known.

Interactions with Foods

None known.

Interactions with Lab Tests

None known.

Interactions with Diseases or Conditions

CROSS-ALLERGENICITY: Gravel root may cause an allergic reaction in individuals sensitive to the Asteraceae/Compositae family. Members of this family include ragweed, chrysanthemums, marigolds, daisies, and many other herbs.
LIVER DISEASE: Gravel root is contraindicated due to the potential for hepatotoxicity (19).

Dosage and Administration

No typical dosage.

GRAVIOLA

Also Known As

Brazilian Cherimoya, Brazilian Paw Paw, Corossolier, Corossol epineux, Durian Benggala, Guanabana, Guanavana, Nangka Blanda, Nangka Londa, Soursop, Sour Sop, Toge-Banreisi.

Scientific Names

Annona muricata, synonym Annona macrocarpa; Annona cherimola.
Family: Annonaceae.

People Use This For

Orally, graviola is used as an antibiotic, sedative, antiparasitic, cathartic, emetic; and for coughs, catarrh, herpes, leshmaniasis, and cancer.
Topically, graviola is used for arthritis.
In foods, graviola is used in cooking and beverages.

Safety

LIKELY UNSAFE ...when used orally. Consumption of graviola fruit may cause movement disorders, similar to Parkinson's disease (7854). Tea made from the leaves and stems of graviola is associated with neurotoxicity (7856).

Effectiveness

There is insufficient reliable information available about the effectiveness of graviola.

Mechanism of Action

The applicable parts of graviola are the fruit, seeds, leaves, and bark. Many active constituents have been identified, with acetogenins being the most important class of chemicals. Over 220 types of acetogenins have been isolated from graviola (7857). In vitro, the acetogenins have antimicrobial activity against Leishmania species (7858).
Graviola also contains isoquinolone compounds which contribute to the neurotoxicity caused by preparations containing this plant (7856).
The alkaloids contained in graviola are toxic to dopaminergic and GABAnergic neurons in extremely low concentrations. The chloroform extract, which contains all of the alkaloids found in graviola, is toxic to dopaminergic neurons at a concentration of 10mcg/mL. This is the mechanism by which graviola causes

movement disorders (7876).
In multidrug resistant (MDR) cancer cells, acetogenins block the production of adenosine triphosphate (ATP), which inhibits the pump that removes cancer drugs from the cell. This permits chemotherapy to be more effective. Certain types of acetogenins are directly cytotoxic to cancer cells, by lowering the concentration of ATP (7857).
The ethanol extract of the bark of the graviola plant has in vitro activity against Herpes simplex virus-1 (HSV1) with a minimum inhibitory concentration of 1 mg/mL. This extract does not exhibit toxicity toward uninfected cells in culture (7855). Extracts of the leaf, root, stem, and bark of graviola are toxic to snails in concentrations of 60 to 100 parts per million. This action may be useful for controlling a vector for schistosomiasis (10379).

Adverse Reactions
Orally, graviola may cause movement disorders and myeloneuropathy. The symptoms of these disorders are similar to Parkinson's disease (7854). Consumption of tea made from the leaves of graviola may cause myeloneuropathy of the optic nerve (7856).

Interactions with Herbs & Other Dietary Supplements
None known.

Interactions with Drugs
None known.

Interactions with Foods
None known.

Interactions with Lab Tests
None known.

Interactions with Diseases or Conditions
PARKINSON'S DISEASE: There is some concern that graviola might exacerbate Parkinson's symptoms because acetogenin constituents are neurotoxins (7854,7856).

Dosage and Administration
No typical dosage.

GREAT PLANTAIN

Also Known As
Common Plantain, General Plantain, Greater Plantain.
CAUTION: See separate listings for Black Psyllium, Blond Psyllium, Buckhorn Plantain, and Water Plantain.

Scientific Names
Plantago major.
Family: Plantaginaceae.

People Use This For
Orally, great plantain has been used for cystitis with hematuria, bronchitis, colds, and for irritated or bleeding hemorrhoids. Topically, great plantain is used for dermatological conditions, and eye irritation or discomfort.

Safety
POSSIBLY SAFE ...when the leaf is used orally and appropriately (12).
POSSIBLY UNSAFE ...when used topically. Great plantain can cause allergic contact dermatitis (4).
PREGNANCY: LIKELY UNSAFE ...when used orally because it can increase uterine tone (4).
LACTATION: Insufficient reliable information available; avoid using.

Effectiveness
INSUFFICIENT RELIABLE EVIDENCE to RATE

Bronchitis. There is preliminary evidence that suggests taking great plantain orally might be beneficial for treating chronic bronchitis (4).
Common cold. There is preliminary evidence that suggests taking great plantain orally might help reduce the symptoms of the common cold (4).
More evidence is needed to rate great plantain for these uses.

Mechanism of Action
The applicable part of great plantain is the leaf. Great plantain contains low levels of tannins (4), and relatively high concentrations of vitamin K, beta-carotene, and calcium (19). It also contains a variety of acids, amino acids, carbohydrates, and iridoids (4). The anti-inflammatory and wound-healing effects demonstrated in animal studies are attributed to the constituents chlorogenic acid and neochlorogenic acid (4). Studies in humans show great plantain is beneficial in treating chronic bronchitis and the common cold (4). In guinea pigs, an aqueous extract had bronchodilator effects; however, effects were less and had shorter duration than salbutamol or atropine (4). In animals, great plantain extract also lowers blood pressure, and decreases total plasma lipids, cholesterol, and triglycerides (4). In vitro, an aqueous extract increases animal uterine tissue tone (4), and fresh juice has antibacterial activity (4). Great plantain inhibits carcinogenesis and mammary tumor formation in experimental animals (6).

Adverse Reactions
Orally, excessive amounts of great plantain may have laxative and hypotensive effects (4).
Topically, application can cause allergic contact dermatitis (4).

Interactions with Herbs & Other Dietary Supplements
HERBS WITH CLOTTING POTENTIAL: Excessive use of herbs that contain vitamin K, an essential coagulation factor, can increase the risk of clotting in people using anticoagulants. These herbs include alfalfa, parsley, nettle, plantain, and others.

Interactions with Drugs
WARFARIN (Coumadin): Theoretically, consumption of large amounts of great plantain may antagonize drug effects due to vitamin K content. Individuals using anticoagulants should consume a consistent daily amount to maintain effect of anticoagulation therapy (19).

Interactions with Foods
None known.

Interactions with Lab Tests
BLOOD CLOTTING TESTS: Theoretically, consumption of large amounts of great plantain may reduce clotting time and test results due to vitamin K content (19).

Interactions with Diseases or Conditions
MELON ALLERGY: Plantago species pollen may cause cross-reactivity in people allergic to melon (4075).
PLANTAIN HYPERSENSITIVITY: Contraindicated.

Dosage and Administration
ORAL: People typically used 2-4 grams dried leaf three times daily, or one cup tea (steep 2-4 grams dried leaf in 150 mL boiling water 5-10 minutes, strain) three times daily (4). Liquid extract (1:1 in 25% in ethanol) 2-4 mL three times daily. Tincture (1:5 in 45% in ethanol) 2-4 mL three times daily (4).

Comments
Avoid confusion with Buckhorn plantain (Plantago lanceolata), Blond psyllium (Plantago ovata), and Black psyllium (Plantago psyllium).

GREATER BINDWEED

Also Known As
Bearbind, Bear's-Bind, Devil's Vine, Hedge Bindweed, Hedge Convolvulus, Hedge Lily, Lady's Nightcap, Old Man's Night Cap, Rutland Beauty.

Scientific Names
Calystegia sepium.
Family: Convolvulaceae.

People Use This For
Orally, greater bindweed is used for fever, urinary tract diseases, as a purgative for constipation, and for increasing bile production.

Safety
POSSIBLY UNSAFE ...when the whole plant is used orally because it has strong contact cathartic effects (271).
PREGNANCY AND LACTATION: POSSIBLY UNSAFE ...when used orally (271); avoid using.

Effectiveness
There is insufficient reliable information available about the effectiveness of greater bindweed.

Mechanism of Action
Greater bindweed is said to be a potent smooth muscle stimulant and to increase bile production (18). Constituent gluco-resins (glycoretins) are contact cathartics which cause an increase in water elimination and peristalsis (271).

Adverse Reactions
Theoretically, large amounts of greater bindweed may cause intestinal and stomach pain (18).

Interactions with Herbs & Other Dietary Supplements
CARDIAC GLYCOSIDE-CONTAINING HERBS: Concomitant use may increase the risk of cardiac glycoside toxicity. Cardiac glycoside-containing herbs include black hellebore, Canadian hemp roots, digitalis leaf, hedge mustard, figwort, lily-of-the-valley roots, motherwort, oleander leaf, pheasant's eye plant, pleurisy root, squill bulb leaf scales, and strophanthus seeds (19).
LICORICE/HORSETAIL: Theoretically, overuse/misuse of licorice rhizome or horsetail plant with cardiac glycoside-containing herbs increases the risk of cardiac toxicity due to potassium depletion (19).
STIMULANT LAXATIVE HERBS: Theoretically, concomitant use with other stimulant laxative herbs may increase the risk of potassium depletion. Stimulant laxative herbs include aloe dried leaf sap, blue flag rhizome, alder buckthorn, European buckthorn, butternut bark, cascara bark, castor oil, colocynth fruit pulp, gamboge bark exudate, jalap root, black root, manna bark exudate, podophyllum root, rhubarb root, senna leaves and pods, wild cucumber fruit (Ecballium elaterium), and yellow dock root (19).

Interactions with Drugs
DIGOXIN (Lanoxin): Theoretically, overuse or abuse of greater bindweed might increase the risk of adverse effects of cardiac glycoside drugs.
DIURETIC DRUGS: Overuse of Greater bindweed might compound diuretic-induced potassium loss (271). There is some concern that people taking greater bindweed along with potassium depleting diuretics might have an increased risk for hypokalemia. Initiation of potassium supplementation or an increase in potassium supplement dose may be necessary for some patients. Some diuretics that can deplete potassium include chlorothiazide (Diuril), chlorthalidone (Thalitone), furosemide (Lasix), hydrochlorothiazide (HCTZ, HydroDIURIL, Microzide), and others.

Interactions with Foods
None known.

Interactions with Lab Tests
None known.

Interactions with Diseases or Conditions
GI CONDITIONS: Contraindicated in individuals with intestinal obstruction, abdominal pain of unknown origin, or any inflammatory condition of intestines including appendicitis, colitis, Crohn's disease, irritable bowel syndrome (IBS), and others (12).

Dosage and Administration
ORAL: People typically use one level teaspoon of the powdered root once or twice daily. A liquid is prepared by boiling 1 teaspoon of the flowering plant in 1 cup of water. This is taken 1 tablespoon at a time, as needed.

GREATER BURNET

Also Known As
Garden Burnet, Sanguisorba.

Scientific Names
Sanguisorba officinalis, synonyms Poterium officinale, Sanguisorba carnea, Sanguisorba polygama.
Family: Rosaceae.

People Use This For
Orally, greater burnet is used for heavy menstrual flow during menopause, hot flashes, irregular menstrual flow, ulcerative colitis, diarrhea, dysentery, enteritis, bladder restraint, hemorrhoids, phlebitis, and varicose veins.
Topically, greater burnet is used in a plaster for wounds and boils.

Safety
There is insufficient reliable information available about the safety of greater burnet.
Pregnancy and Lactation: Insufficient reliable information available; avoid using.

Effectiveness
There is insufficient reliable information available about the effectiveness of greater burnet.

Mechanism of Action
The applicable parts of greater burnet are the flowering above ground parts. Greater burnet appears to have antihemorrhagic, antihemorrhoidal, astringent, and styptic properties (4).

Adverse Reactions
None reported.

Interactions with Herbs & Other Dietary Supplements
None known.

Interactions with Drugs
None known.

Interactions with Foods
None known.

Interactions with Lab Tests
None known.

Interactions with Diseases or Conditions
None known.

Dosage and Administration
ORAL: People typically use 2-6 grams dried above ground parts three times daily (4), or one cup tea (steep 2-6 grams herb in 150 mL boiling water 5-10 minutes, strain) three times daily (4). Liquid extract (1:1 in 25% alcohol) 2-6 mL three times daily (4). Tincture (1:5 in 45% alcohol) 2-8 mL three times daily (4).
TOPICAL: Used as plasters, no additional dosing or administration available (18).

GREATER CELANDINE dried above ground parts

Also Known As
Bai Qu Cai, Celandine, Celandine Herb, Chelidonii, Chelidonii Herba, Schollkraut, Tetterwort.
CAUTION: See separate listings for Greater Celandine root, Jewelweed, and Lesser Celandine.

Scientific Names
Chelidonium majus.
Family: Papaveraceae.

People Use This For
Orally, greater celandine is for spastic discomfort of bile ducts and the gastrointestinal tract, as an analgesic, antitussive, anti-inflammatory, detoxicant, liver and gallbladder complaints, loss of appetite, gastroenteritis, stomach cancer, cramps, intestinal polyps, breast lumps, angina, edema, arteriosclerosis, hypertension, asthma, gout, and arthritis.
Topically, greater celandine dried above ground parts are used for warts, blister rashes, scabies, tooth pain, and to ease tooth extraction.

Safety
POSSIBLY SAFE ...when used orally. Greater celandine are considered safe when used orally and appropriately (2,7,12); however, greater celandine has been implicated in ten cases of hepatitis involving five different brand

products manufactured in Germany (363).
There is insufficient reliable information available about the safety of the topical use of greater celandine dried above ground parts.
CHILDREN: UNSAFE ...when used orally (12); avoid using.
PREGNANCY: UNSAFE ...when used orally; the berberine content might stimulate uterine contractions (12).
LACTATION: Insufficient reliable information available; avoid using.

Effectiveness
There is insufficient reliable information available about the effectiveness of greater celandine dried above ground parts.

Mechanism of Action
Greater celandine dried above ground parts contain 0.1-1% isoquinoline alkaloids (7,12), including chelidonine, which reportedly acts as an antispasmodic and weak central analgesic (7,8). This product is thought to have a papaverine-like effect on the upper gastrointestinal tract (2). In animal studies, an alcoholic extract increased bile flow (7), caused non-specific immune stimulation (2), and acted as a hepatoprotectant (8). The above ground parts of greater celandine also contain small amounts of berberine, which is a uterine stimulant and in large amounts can depress cardiac function (12).

Adverse Reactions
Orally, greater celandine dried above ground parts have been strongly implicated in at least ten cases of hepatitis (363). Large amounts can cause stomach pain, intestinal colic, urinary urgency, and hematuria accompanied by dizziness and stupor (7).

Interactions with Herbs & Other Dietary Supplements
None known.

Interactions with Drugs
None known.

Interactions with Foods
None known.

Interactions with Lab Tests
LIVER FUNCTION TESTS: Greater celandine-induced hepatitis can increase liver enzyme serum levels and results of liver function tests (363).

Interactions with Diseases or Conditions
BILE TRACT OBSTRUCTION: Use of greater celandine dried above ground parts may exacerbate condition (2).
GLAUCOMA: Use of greater celandine dried above ground parts may affect treatment (12).
HEPATITIS/LIVER DISEASE: Greater celandine taken orally has been implicated in causing hepatitis (363); avoid using in people with liver disease.

Dosage and Administration
ORAL: Dried herb or herb powder 2-5 grams per day (equivalent to 12-30 mg total alkaloids calculated as chelidonine) has been used (2). Fluid extract: 1-2 mL three times daily has also been used (18). Do not use in children. Greater celandine tea preparations are difficult to dose properly and are not recommended (7).
TOPICAL: No typical dosage.

Comments
Recently, greater celandine dried above ground parts have been strongly implicated in at least ten cases of hepatitis involving five different brand products manufactured in Germany (363). Until more is known, avoid using products containing greater celandine dried above ground parts. Avoid confusion with greater celandine rhizome, root and lesser celandine (Family: Ranunculus ficaria).

GREATER CELANDINE rhizome, root

Also Known As
Celandine Root.
CAUTION: See separate listings for Greater Celandine dried above ground parts, Jewelweed, and Lesser Celandine.

Scientific Names
Chelidonium majus.
Family: Papaveraceae.

Comments
At the date of publication, there was very little scientific information about this product. Our staff is continually analyzing the available information on natural medicines and will add data to the online version of *Natural Medicines Comprehensive Database* as it becomes available. See www.naturaldatabase.com.

GREEK SAGE

Also Known As
Greek Oregano, Three-Lobe Sage.

Scientific Names
Salvia fruticosa, synonym Salvia triloba.
Family: Lamiaceae/Labiatae.

People Use This For
Orally, Greek sage is used for inflammation of the mouth and throat.

Safety
There is insufficient reliable information available about the safety of Greek sage.
Pregnancy and Lactation: Insufficient reliable information available; avoid using.

Effectiveness
There is insufficient reliable information available about the effectiveness of Greek sage.

Mechanism of Action
Greek sage contains 2-3% volatile oil. Of the volatile oil, 60% is cineole, 5% is thujone (8). Greek sage can inhibit smooth-muscle contractions induced by acetylcholine, histamine, serotonin and BaCl2 (4152). Constituents of the leaf can prolong hexobarbital sleep (4152). Some evidence suggests an aqueous extract of Greek sage might have a blood pressure-lowering effect (4152).

Adverse Reactions
None reported.

Interactions with Herbs & Other Dietary Supplements
None known.

Interactions with Drugs
HEXOBARBITAL: Greek sage can prolong the effects of hexobarbital (4152).

Interactions with Foods
None known.

Interactions with Lab Tests
None known.

Interactions with Diseases or Conditions
None known.

Dosage and Administration

ORAL: Greek sage is used as a tea. The tea is prepared by pouring boiling water over 3 grams of finely chopped leaf. After 10 minutes, strain (8).

Comments

Greek sage is very rare but sometimes it is found as an adulterant of Salvia officinalis (4,5).

GREEN TEA

Also Known As

Chinese Tea, EGCG, Epigallo Catechin Gallate, Epigallocatechin Gallate, Japanese Tea, Tea, Tea Green.
CAUTION: See separate listings for Black Tea and Caffeine.

Scientific Names

Camellia sinensis, synonyms Camellia thea, Camellia theifera, Thea bohea, Thea sinensis, Thea viridis.
Family: Theaceae.

People Use This For

Orally, green tea is used to improve cognitive performance, and to improve mental alertness. It is also used to treat stomach disorders, vomiting, diarrhea, and headaches. Green tea is also used as a diuretic and in combination products for weight loss. Green tea is also used to treat solid tumor cancers, and to reduce the risk of breast cancer, prostate cancer, colon cancer, gastric cancer, cancer related to ultraviolet (UV) radiation (e.g., sunburn), and other environmental causes. It is also used to maintain remission in people with Crohn's disease, to prevent Parkinson's disease, heart disease, hypotension, dental caries, kidney stones, and skin damage.

Topically, green tea bags are used as a wash to soothe sunburn, as a poultice for bags under the eyes, as a compress for headache or tired eyes, and to stop the bleeding of tooth sockets. Green tea in chewable candy is used for gingivitis. Green tea is also used topically to prevent skin damage and cancer related to ultraviolet (UV) radiation (e.g., sunburn) and other environmental causes.

In foods, green tea is consumed as a beverage.

Safety

LIKELY SAFE ...when used orally in moderate amounts (733,6031,9222,9223,9225,9226,9227,9228). Green tea is often consumed daily in Asian cultures and has not been associated with significant adverse effects (6031).

POSSIBLY SAFE ...when green tea extract is used orally. Green tea extract containing 7% caffeine has been used safely for six months (8117). ...when used topically and appropriately (6065,11310).

POSSIBLY UNSAFE ...when used orally long term in high doses. Green tea contains a significant amount of caffeine. Chronic use, especially in large amounts, can produce tolerance, habituation, psychological dependence, and other significant adverse effects. Doses greater than 250-300 mg per day have been associated with significant adverse effects such as tachyarrhythmias and sleep disturbances (11832). These effects would not be expected to occur with the consumption of decaffeinated green tea.

LIKELY UNSAFE ...when used orally in very high doses. The fatal acute oral dose of caffeine in green tea is estimated to be 10-14 grams (150-200 mg per kilogram). Serious toxicity can occur at lower doses depending on variables in caffeine sensitivity such as smoking, age, prior caffeine use, etc (11832).

CHILDREN: POSSIBLY SAFE ...when used in amounts commonly found in foods and beverages (7705,11833).

PREGNANCY: POSSIBLY SAFE ...when used orally in moderate amounts. Due to the caffeine content of green tea, mothers should closely monitor their intake to ensure moderate consumption. Fetal blood concentrations of caffeine approximate maternal concentrations (4260). Use of caffeine in pregnancy is controversial; however, moderate consumption has not been associated with clinically important adverse fetal effects (2708,2709,2710,2711,9606). Caffeine crosses the human placenta, but is not considered a teratogen. Mothers should keep caffeine consumption below 200 mg per day. This is similar to the amount of caffeine found in 1-2 cups of coffee or tea (2708).

POSSIBLY UNSAFE ...when used orally in large amounts. Caffeine crosses the placenta, producing fetal blood concentrations similar to maternal levels (4260). Mothers should avoid consuming more than 200 mg of caffeine daily or more than 1-2 cups of tea or coffee per day (2708). Maternal doses of greater than 200 mg per day throughout pregnancy have resulted in symptoms of caffeine withdrawal in newborn infants (9891). High doses of caffeine have been associated with spontaneous abortion, premature delivery, and low birth weight (2709,2711). Fetal birth weight is reduced by 28 grams for every 100 mg per day of caffeine consumed during pregnancy. But this is unlikely to be clinically important except for women consuming more than 600 mg of caffeine daily (9606).

LACTATION: POSSIBLY SAFE ...when used orally in moderate amounts. Due to the caffeine content of green tea, nursing mothers should closely monitor caffeine intake. Breast milk concentrations of caffeine are thought to be approximately 50% of maternal serum concentrations. Minimal consumption would likely result in limited exposure to a nursing infant (9892).

POSSIBLY UNSAFE ...when used orally in large amounts. Consumption of green tea might cause irritability and increased bowel activity in nursing infants (6026). Large doses or excessive intake of green tea should be avoided during lactation.

Effectiveness

LIKELY EFFECTIVE

Mental alertness. Consumption of green tea and other caffeinated beverages seems to prevent a decline in alertness and cognitive capacity when consumed throughout the day (4221,4224).

POSSIBLY EFFECTIVE

Bladder cancer, esophageal cancer, and pancreatic cancer. Drinking green tea seems to reduce the risk of bladder cancer, esophageal cancer, and pancreatic cancer (733,1457,1458,1459,6031).

Breast cancer. Drinking green tea seems to help reduce the risk of recurrence of breast cancer (3926,4218).

Cervical dysplasia. Green tea as an oral or topical preparation seems to reduce cervical dysplasia caused by human papilloma virus (HPV) infection (11310).

Gastric cancer. Drinking green tea seems to reduce the risk of stomach cancer. This effect appears to be dose related, with the most protection occurring in people drinking 10 or more cups of green tea daily (8903,9222,9225,9226,9227). Consuming less that 10 cups daily doesn't consistently provide protection (7033,9223).

Hyperlipidemia. Green tea taken orally seems to lower cholesterol and triglycerides. A theaflavin-enriched green tea extract, 375 mg daily for 12 weeks, seems to cause mild reductions in low-density lipoprotein (LDL) levels (11308). Epidemiological evidence suggests that higher consumption of green tea is associated with significantly lowered serum total cholesterol, triglycerides, LDL, and increased high-density lipoprotein (HDL) levels (6403).

Hypotension. Consuming caffeinated beverages seems to increase blood pressure in elderly people with postprandial hypotension (11834,11835).

Oral leukoplakia. Drinking green tea orally seems to decrease the size of lesions in patients with oral leukoplakia (4213).

Ovarian cancer. Drinking at least 1 cup of green tea each week seems to reduce the risk of ovarian cancer (9228).

Parkinson's disease. Consuming green tea orally seems to help prevent or delay the onset of Parkinson's disease. There is some evidence from large-scale epidemiological studies that people who consume caffeinated beverages such as coffee, tea, and cola have a decreased risk of Parkinson's disease. For men, the effects seem to be dose related. Men consuming a total of 421 mg to 2716 mg of caffeine (approximately 5-33 cups of tea) from any source daily seem to have the greatest reduction in risk. However, there seems to be a significant reduction in risk even with consumption of as little as 124 mg to 208 mg caffeine per day (approximately one to three cups tea) (6022). In women, the effects do not seem to be dose related. Moderate consumption of approximately one to four cups daily, seems to provide the most reduction in risk (1238).

POSSIBLY INEFFECTIVE

Colorectal cancer. Epidemiological evidence suggests that consuming green tea doesn't have any effect on colon cancer risk (9222,9223).

INSUFFICIENT RELIABLE EVIDENCE to RATE

Cardiovascular disease. Epidemiological studies suggest that consuming green tea might protect against ischemic heart disease and death after myocardial infarction; however, most of the tea drinkers consumed black tea. Whether green tea has a similar beneficial effect is unknown (8119,8120,8121).

Gingivitis. Green tea extract in chewable candy appears to reduce plaque accumulation and gingival inflammation (7594).

Obesity. Preliminary clinical information suggests that a specific green tea extract (AR25, Exolise) standardized to 25% epigallocatechin gallate (EGCG) might help reduce weight in moderately obese patients (8114).

Prostate cancer. Preliminary clinical research suggests that green tea doesn't have any effect on androgen-independent prostate cancer (11366).

More information is needed to rate green tea extract for these uses.

Mechanism of Action

The applicable parts of green tea are the leaf bud, leaf, and stem. Green tea is different than black and oolong teas because it is not fermented. Black tea is fully fermented and oolong tea is partially fermented. Green tea is produced by steaming fresh leaves at high temperatures. This process inactivates certain oxidizing enzymes, but does not decrease polyphenols. Polyphenols such as flavanols, flavandiols, flavonoids, and phenolic acids are abundant in green tea. Flavanols including epigallocatechin gallate (EGCG), epigallocatechin (EGC), epicatechin gallate (ECG), and epicatechin (EC), are all referred to as catechins. These seem to be responsible for many of the proposed benefits of green tea (6031,8118,11310).

It's often thought that green tea has more polyphenols, and therefore greater potential health benefits, than black tea. But there is some evidence that suggests there is no difference in quantity and quality of polyphenols between green and black teas (12087).

Black tea also contains 2% to 4% caffeine (519) or 10-80 mg caffeine per cup (4218). The caffeine in green tea stimulates the central nervous system (CNS), heart, muscles, and possibly the pressor centers that control blood pressure (2722). Possible mechanisms include adenosine receptor blockade and phosphodiesterase inhibition (2722). By blocking adenosine receptors, caffeine is thought to increase the release of neurotransmitters such as dopamine (6370).

Caffeine also decreases airway resistance and stimulates respiration, via adenosine receptor blockade and phosphodiesterase inhibition (11836). It has also been proposed that caffeine may decrease GABA and serotonin signaling (6370). Caffeine stimulates gastric acid secretion, and increases plasma catecholamine levels (11837). Caffeine can have positive inotropic and chronotropic effects on the heart (11836). Caffeine can also acutely elevate both diastolic and systolic blood pressure, but might not have this effect in habitual users (2722).

Caffeine exerts a diuretic effect, with water losses estimated at 1.17 mL per milligram of caffeine (2712). Tachyphylaxis to the diuretic effect develops rapidly, diminishing fluid losses associated with caffeine intake (10206). Caffeine-containing beverages consumed during moderate endurance exercise do not appear to compromise bodily hydration status (2713). Caffeine does not substantially affect the fluid status of people who drink caffeinated beverages on a regular basis (10206). The caffeine content is also thought to be responsible for green tea's effects on cognitive performance (4221).

Some preliminary studies show that flavonoids found in green tea might reduce lipoprotein oxidation (6032,6033,9232). In vitro tests indicate that catechins in green tea reduce proliferation of vascular smooth muscle that occurs with high concentrations of low-density lipoproteins (9229). There is some evidence green tea suppresses thromboxane formation during blood clotting by inhibiting the release of arachidonic acid from platelets (8028). However, when used in humans, green tea does not consistently exhibit useful effects on cardiovascular risk factors. Green tea does not reduce inflammation, vascular reactivity, or lipid oxidation. This may be due to low bioavailability of polyphenols (9230,9231).

Caffeine, a constituent of green tea, has been reported to cause increases and decreases in blood glucose. In people with type 2 diabetes, acute administration of caffeine impairs postprandial glucose metabolism, while acute abstention from caffeine reduces postprandial glucose levels by 21%. Whether these effects also occur with caffeinated beverages and herbs is unknown (12374). Other research in obese people suggests that caffeine ingestion may contribute to insulin resistance (12375). However, one study found that type 1 diabetics taking 200 mg of caffeine twice daily had increased frequency and intensity of warning signs of hypoglycemia. This may be due to a reduction in blood flow to the brain and an increase in glucose utilization by the brain (6024).

It remains unclear exactly how green tea might reduce the risk of some cancers, but preliminary animal research suggests EGCG might prevent new blood vessel growth (angiogenesis) in tumors. EGCG may also inhibit tumor cell proliferation, causing cell cycle arrest or apoptosis (1454,1455,1456,8117,11309). ECG appears to induce apoptosis in cancer cells by reactive oxygen species formation and mitochondrial depolarization (8118). Green tea may also reduce oxidative DNA damage, lipid peroxidation, and free radical generation (4212); and might reduce mutagenic activity in smokers (4217). There is preliminary evidence that green tea might enhance the effects of doxorubicin (Adriamycin) on tumor cells (3940). Some research suggests that constituents of green tea may increase the activity of doxorubicin (Adriamycin). Caffeine, theanine, and EGCG appear to increase the concentration of doxorubicin inside tumor cells by inhibiting the efflux mechanisms that remove doxorubicin from the cell (7690).

The polyphenols in green tea appear to reduce the cellular adhesiveness of bacteria associated with dental disease (7594). Some evidence suggests that EGCG and EGC might inhibit 5 alpha-reductase and might potentially be useful in androgen-mediated skin disorders such as androgenic alopecia, hirsutism, and acne (8113).

Green tea is thought to be beneficial for preventing skin damage and cancer from ultraviolet (UV) radiation due to the antioxidant effects of polyphenols in green tea. Polyphenolic extracts of green tea, specifically EGCG and epicatechin-3-gallate, seem to produce dose-dependent topical protection against UVA and UVB sunburn. Areas of skin where green tea extracts were applied had fewer sunburned cells and less damage to epidermal Langerhans cells, which are responsible for cutaneous immune response. Green tea extracts also seem to prevent UV radiation-induced DNA damage (1359). Animal models indicate that green tea extracts reduce oxidative skin damage, skin inflammation, and epidermal hyperplasia due to UV radiation and other causes (6065). Unlike conventional sunscreens, green tea extracts do not absorb significant amounts of light in the UV range (1359).

Green tea is also used for weight loss. Early evidence indicates that a green tea extract rich in EGCG can increase calorie and fat metabolism. The caffeine, catechin, and theanine constituents of green tea might contribute to this effect (1453,8115,11960). There is also some evidence that EGCG might suppress appetite. However, there is some question about how well EGCG is absorbed orally (3922). The impact of EGCG and green tea on weight loss remains to be determined with well-designed studies in obese people.

Tannins in green tea can produce antidiarrheal effects. The polyphenols in green tea might increase the level of lactobacilli and bifidobacteria and reduce the population of enterobacteria (3941).

For prevention of Parkinson's disease, caffeine in green tea may prevent adenosine's inhibition of dopaminergic transmission. This may result in a reduction in the clinical expression of Parkinsonism (6022). Preliminary evidence suggests that EGCG may prevent oxidation and apoptosis of neurons, which may protect people from developing Alzheimer's disease (9224). Epidemiological research suggests that drinking green tea for at least ten years increases bone mineral density. The exact mechanism for the effects on bone is unknown, but several possibilities have been suggested. Tea leaves contain fluoride, which might slow osteoporosis. Tea also contains flavonoids and phytoestrogens, which might affect bone mineral density. Other proposed mechanisms include inhibition of bone resorption and effects on mineral metabolism by polyphenols and tannins (8116).

Adverse Reactions

Orally, green tea can cause nausea, vomiting, abdominal bloating and pain, dyspepsia, flatulence, and diarrhea. It can also cause central nervous system stimulation and adverse effects such as dizziness, insomnia, fatigue, agitation, tremors, restlessness and confusion. These effects are more common with higher doses of green tea or green tea extract, equivalent to 5 to 6 liters of tea per day (8117,11366). Although acute administration of green tea can cause increased blood pressure, regular consumption does not seem to increase either blood pressure or pulse when consumed on a regular basis, even in mildly hypertensive patients (1451,1452). Caffeine in green tea may exacerbate sleep disturbances in patients with acquired immunodeficiency syndrome (AIDS) (10204).

Allergic reactions to green tea include cough, dyspnea, loss of consciousness, and asthma. Occupational exposure to green tea dust can also cause sensitization, which may include nasal and asthmatic symptoms (11365). Caffeine in green tea can cause anaphylaxis in sensitive individuals, although true IgE-mediated caffeine allergy seems to be relatively rare (11315).

Although tolerance to caffeine is a widely held belief, there is little supportive clinical evidence. If it exists, it appears to be of little clinical significance (11839). Withdrawal symptoms such as irritability, sleepiness, delirium, nausea, vomiting, rhinorrhea, nervousness, restlessness, anxiety, muscle tension, muscle pains, and flushed face have been described. However, these symptoms may be from nonpharmacological factors related to knowledge and expectation of effects. Clinically significant symptoms caused by caffeine withdrawal may be uncommon (2723,11839).

Some evidence shows caffeine in green tea is associated with fibrocystic breast disease, breast cancer, and endometriosis in women; however, this is controversial since findings are conflicting (8043). Restricting caffeine in women with fibrocystic breast conditions doesn't seem to affect breast nodularity, swelling, or pain (8996).

Epidemiological evidence regarding the relationship between caffeinated beverages such as green tea and the risk for osteoporosis is contradictory. Caffeine can increase urinary excretion of calcium (2669,10202,11317). Women identified with a genetic variant of the vitamin D receptor appear to be at an increased risk for the detrimental effect of caffeine on bone mass (2669). However, moderate caffeine intake, less than 300 mg per day, does not seem to significantly increase osteoporosis risk in most postmenopausal women with normal calcium intake (2669,6025,10202,11317).

Combining ephedra with caffeine can increase the risk of adverse effects. Jitteriness, hypertension, seizures, temporary loss of consciousness, and hospitalization requiring life support has been associated with the combined use of ephedra and caffeine (2729). There is also a report of ischemic stroke in an athlete who consumed ephedra 40-60 mg, creatine monohydrate 6 grams, caffeine 400-600 mg, and a variety of other supplements daily for six weeks (1275).

Topically, green tea ointment can cause cervical and vaginal inflammation, vaginal irritation, and vulval burning (11310).

Interactions with Herbs & Other Dietary Supplements

CAFFEINE-CONTAINING HERBS/SUPPLEMENTS: Concomitant use can have additive effects with the caffeine in green tea, and can increase the risk of adverse effects Some natural products that contain caffeine include coffee, black tea, guarana, mate, cola, and others.

CREATINE: There is some concern that combining caffeine, ephedra, and creatine might increase the risk of serious adverse effects. There is a report of ischemic stroke in an athlete who consumed creatine monohydrate 6 grams, caffeine 400-600 mg, ephedra 40-60 mg, and a variety of other supplements daily for 6 weeks (1275). Caffeine might also decrease creatine's possible beneficial effects on athletic performance. Some researchers think caffeine can inhibit phosphocreatine resynthesis (2117,4575).

EPHEDRA (Ma Huang): Use of ephedra with green tea can increase the risk of stimulatory adverse effects due to its caffeine content. There is evidence that using ephedra with caffeine might increase the risk of serious life-threatening or debilitating adverse effects such as hypertension, myocardial infarction, stroke, seizures, and death (6486,10307). Tell patients to avoid taking green tea with ephedra and other stimulants.

IRON: Green tea appears to reduce absorption of non-heme iron from foods (8110,8904). Infants given tea to drink seem to have an increased risk of microcytic anemia (631). However, a study of iron-deficient elderly patients suggests that concomitant use does not alter iron absorption in this population (185). Theoretically, green tea might reduce the absorption of iron supplements. For most patients, this effect will not be clinically significant. Advise patients with iron deficiency to consume tea between meals rather than with meals to lessen this interaction (8904).

Interactions with Drugs

ADENOSINE (Adenocard): The caffeine in green tea is a competitive inhibitor of adenosine at the cellular level. However, caffeine doesn't seem to affect supplemental adenosine because high interstitial levels of adenosine overcome the antagonistic effects of caffeine (11771). It is recommended that methylxanthines and methylxanthine-containing products be stopped 24 hours prior to pharmacological stress tests (11770). However, methylxanthines appear more likely to interfere with dipyridamole (Persantine) than adenosine-induced stress testing (11771).

ALCOHOL (Ethanol): Concomitant use of alcohol can increase caffeine serum concentrations and the risk of caffeine adverse effects. Alcohol reduces caffeine metabolism (6370).

AMPHETAMINES: Theoretically, the caffeine in green tea might increase the risk of additive CNS effects (2719).

ANTICOAGULANT/ANTIPLATELET DRUGS: Theoretically, green tea might increase the risk of bleeding when used concomitantly with these agents. Green tea and caffeine are reported to have antiplatelet activity (733,8028,8029); however, this interaction has not been reported in humans. Antiplatelet agents include aspirin, clopidogrel (Plavix), dipyridamole (Persantine), ticlopidine (Ticlid), and others. Anticoagulant agents include ardeparin (Normiflo), dalteparin (Fragmin), enoxaparin (Lovenox), heparin, and warfarin (Coumadin).

ANTIDIABETES DRUGS: Theoretically, concomitant use of green tea and diabetes drugs might interfere with

blood glucose control due to the caffeine in green tea. The data are conflicting. Reports claim that caffeine might increase or decrease blood sugar (6024,8646).
ANTIPSYCHOTIC DRUGS: Theoretically, green tea might cause precipitation of fluphenazine (Permitil, Prolixin), chlorpromazine (Thorazine), haloperidol (Haldol), prochlorperazine (Compazine), thioridazine (Mellaril), and trifluoperazine (Stelazine) (626,627).
CIMETIDINE (Tagamet): Concomitant use might increase the effects and adverse effects of caffeine in green tea. Cimetidine can reduce caffeine clearance by 31% to 42% (11736).
CLOZAPINE (Clozaril): Theoretically, concomitant administration might cause acute exacerbation of psychotic symptoms due to the caffeine in green tea. Caffeine can increase the effects and toxicity of clozapine. Caffeine doses of 400-1000 mg per day inhibit clozapine metabolism (5051).
COCAINE: Theoretically, the caffeine in green tea might increase the risk of additive CNS effects (2719).
CONTRACEPTIVE DRUGS: Concomitant use might increase the effects and adverse effects of caffeine in green tea. Oral contraceptives can decrease caffeine clearance by 40-65% (8644).
DIPYRIDAMOLE (Persantine): The caffeine in green tea might inhibit dipyridamole-induced vasodilation (11770,11772). It is recommended that methylxanthines and methylxanthine-containing products be stopped 24 hours prior to pharmacological stress tests (11770). Methylxanthines appear more likely to interfere with dipyridamole (Persantine) than adenosine-induced stress testing (11771).
DISULFIRAM (Antabuse): Concomitant use might increase the risk of adverse effects of caffeine in green tea. Disulfiram decreases the clearance and increases the half-life of caffeine (11840).
EPHEDRINE: Use of ephedrine with caffeine-containing products can increase the risk of stimulatory adverse effects. There is evidence that using ephedrine with caffeine might increase the risk of serious life-threatening or debilitating adverse effects such as hypertension, myocardial infarction, stroke, seizures, and death (6486,10307). Tell patients to avoid taking caffeine with ephedrine or other stimulants.
ESTROGENS: Concomitant use can increase serum concentrations of caffeine, a constituent of green tea, and the risk of caffeine adverse effects. Estrogen inhibits caffeine metabolism (2714).
FLUCONAZOLE (Diflucan): Concomitant use might increase the effects of caffeine in green tea. Fluconazole decreases caffeine clearance by approximately 25% (11022).
FLUVOXAMINE (Luvox): Concomitant use can increase serum concentrations of caffeine, a constituent of green tea, and the risk of caffeine adverse effects. Fluvoxamine reduces caffeine metabolism (6370).
LITHIUM: Theoretically, abrupt caffeine withdrawal can increase serum lithium levels (609). Two cases of lithium tremor which worsened with abrupt coffee withdrawal have been reported (610).
MEXILETINE (Mexitil): Concomitant use might increase the effects and adverse effects of caffeine in green tea. Mexiletine can decrease caffeine elimination by 50% (1260).
MONOAMINE OXIDASE INHIBITORS (MAOIs): Theoretically, concomitant intake of large amounts of green tea with MAOIs might precipitate a hypertensive crisis, due to the caffeine contained in green tea. This is based on the claim that intake of large amounts of caffeine with MAOIs might precipitate a hypertensive crisis (15).
NICOTINE: Theoretically, the caffeine in green tea might increase the risk of additive CNS effects (2719).
PHENYLPROPANOLAMINE: Concomitant use of phenylpropanolamine and green tea might cause an additive increase in blood pressure due to the caffeine in green tea (11738).
QUINOLONE ANTIBIOTICS: Concomitant use might increase the effects and risk of adverse effects of caffeine in green tea. Quinolones decrease caffeine clearance (606,607,608). Quinolones include ciprofloxacin (Cipro), enoxacin (Penetrex), norfloxacin (Chibroxin, Noroxin), sparfloxacin (Zagam), trovafloxacin (Trovan), and grepafloxacin (Raxar).
RILUZOLE (Rilutek): Theoretically, concomitant use of riluzole and caffeinated beverages such as green tea might increase serum caffeine and riluzole concentrations and the risk of adverse effects of both caffeine and riluzole, due to the caffeine contained in green tea. Caffeine and riluzole are both metabolized by cytochrome P450 1A2, and concomitant use might reduce metabolism of one or both agents (11739).
TERBINAFINE (Lamisil): Concomitant use can increase serum caffeine concentrations and the risk of caffeine adverse effects. Terbinafine decreases the clearance of intravenous caffeine by 19% (11740).
THEOPHYLLINE: Concomitant use might increase the effects and adverse effects of theophylline due to the caffeine in green tea. Caffeine can reduce theophylline clearance, increase elimination half-life, and increase serum levels (11862).
VERAPAMIL (Calan, Covera, Isoptin, Verelan): Theoretically, concomitant use of verapamil and caffeinated beverages such as green tea might increase plasma caffeine concentrations and the risk of adverse effects, due to the caffeine contained in green tea. Verapamil increases plasma caffeine concentrations by 25% (11741).
WARFARIN (Coumadin): Consumption of large amounts of green tea is reported to antagonize the effects of warfarin. This has been attributed to the vitamin K1 in green tea (4211). However, there is so little vitamin K1 in green tea (0.03 +/- 0.1 mcg/mL) that the interaction is more likely due to other constituents (1460,1461,1462,1463).

Interactions with Foods

IRON: Green tea appears to reduce absorption of non-heme iron from foods (631,8110,9237).
MILK: When taken together, milk might bind the antioxidants in tea and reduce their beneficial effects (220); however, in one study this interaction did not occur (6032).

Interactions with Lab Tests

5-HYDROXYINDOLEACETIC ACID: Green tea might increase urine 5-hydroxyindoleacetic acid concentrations and test results, due to its caffeine content. Caffeine can increase urine catecholamine concentrations (15).
BLEEDING TIME: Theoretically, green tea might increase the bleeding time. Caffeine theoretically can prolong bleeding time and increase the results of a bleeding time test, but this has not been reported in humans (1701). Caffeine is reported to have antiplatelet activity (8028,8029).
CATECHOLAMINE: The caffeine in green tea can increase plasma catecholamine levels (8646).
CREATINE: The caffeine in green tea can increase urine creatine levels (1701).
DIPYRIDAMOLE THALLIUM IMAGING: Green tea might interfere with dipyridamole thallium imaging studies, due to its caffeine content. Caffeine attenuates the characteristic cardiovascular responses to dipyridamole and has altered test results (11742).
FERRITIN: Drinking green tea may cause a reduction in serum ferritin in iron-deficient people (9237).
GLUCOSE: Caffeine, a constituent of green tea, has been reported to cause increases and decreases in blood glucose (8646).
HEMOGLOBIN: Drinking green tea may cause a reduction in hemoglobin in iron-deficient people (9237).
IRON: In people with iron deficiency, green tea may further reduce the concentration of serum iron (9237).
LACTATE: The combination of ephedrine, a constituent of ephedra, and the caffeine in green tea can increase blood lactate levels (8646).
NEUROBLASTOMA TESTS: Green tea (due to its caffeine content) might cause false-positive diagnosis of neuroblastoma, when diagnosis is based on tests of urine vanillylmandelic acid (VMA) or catecholamine concentrations. Caffeine can increase urine catecholamine and VMA concentrations (15).
PHARMACOLOGICAL STRESS TESTS: The caffeine in green tea is a competitive antagonist for adenosine receptors (11771). It is recommended that caffeine and caffeine-containing products be stopped 24 hours prior to pharmacological stress tests (11770). However, caffeine appears more likely to interfere with dipyridamole (Persantine) than adenosine (Adenocard) stress testing (11771). The interaction between caffeine and dipyridamole is unlikely to be significant in stress testing if the heart rate increase is greater than 5% after dipyridamole infusion (11772).
PHEOCHROMOCYTOMA TESTS: Green tea (due to its caffeine content) might cause false-positive diagnosis of pheochromocytoma, when diagnosis is based on tests of urine vanillylmandelic acid (VMA) or catecholamine concentrations. Caffeine can increase urine catecholamine and VMA concentrations (15).
PULMONARY FUNCTION TESTS: People may need to avoid caffeine and caffeinated beverages such as green tea for at least four hours prior to lung function testing. Forced expiratory volume in one minute (FEV1) seems to show a small improvement up to two hours after caffeine use. Mid-expiratory flow rates may also improve with caffeine for up to four hours (9607).
URATE: Green tea might falsely increase serum urate test results determined by the Bittner method, due to its caffeine content. Caffeine causes false elevations in serum urate test results determined by the Bittner method (11844).
URINARY CALCIUM: The caffeine in green tea can increase urinary calcium levels (11317).
VANILLYLMANDELIC ACID (VMA): Green tea might increase urine VMA concentrations and test results, due to its caffeine content. Caffeine can increase urine VMA concentrations (15).

Interactions with Diseases or Conditions

ANEMIA: Drinking green tea may worsen anemia in people with iron deficiency (9237).
ANXIETY DISORDERS: The caffeine in green tea might aggravate anxiety disorders (11743).
BLEEDING DISORDERS: Theoretically, caffeine in green tea might aggravate these conditions. Caffeine is reported to have antiplatelet activity (8028,8029); however, this interaction has not been reported in humans (1701). Caffeine can prolong bleeding time and increase the results of a bleeding time test (1701).
CARDIAC CONDITIONS: Caffeine in green tea can induce cardiac arrhythmias in sensitive individuals (11845); use with caution.
DIABETES: Some research suggests that caffeine, a constituent of green tea, may impair postprandial glucose metabolism in people with diabetes and contribute to insulin resistance. The effect of caffeinated beverages and herbs has not been studied (12374,12375). Caffeine in green tea may enhance the frequency and intensity of hypoglycemic warning symptoms in type 1 diabetics. This may increase the ability of diabetics to detect and treat hypoglycemia early. However, it might also increase the frequency of hypoglycemic events (6024). Caffeine has been reported to cause increases and decreases in blood glucose (8646); use with caution.
GLAUCOMA: Drinking caffeinated green tea increases intraocular pressure. The increase occurs within 30 minutes and persists for at least 90 minutes (8540).
HYPERTENSION: The caffeine in green tea might increase blood pressure in people with high blood pressure. However, this doesn't seem to occur in people who regularly consume green tea or other caffeinated products (1451,1452,2722).
OSTEOPOROSIS: Consuming caffeinated green tea can increase urinary excretion of calcium. Caffeine consumption should be limited to less than 300 mg per day (approximately 2-3 cups of green tea). Adequate calcium supplementation may partially compensate for calcium losses (2669,10202,11317). Postmenopausal women identified with a genetic variant of the vitamin D receptor should use caffeine with caution (2669).

Dosage and Administration

ORAL: Doses of green tea vary significantly, but usually range between 1-10 cups daily. The commonly used dose of green tea is based on the amount typically consumed in Asian countries, which is about 3 cups per day, providing 240-320 mg of polyphenols. The typical dose of caffeine for headache or restoring mental alertness is up to 250 mg per day (2718,11743). For improving cognitive performance, tea providing 60 mg of caffeine, or approximately 1 cup, has been used (4221). For reducing cholesterol, 10 or greater cups per day has been associated with decreased cholesterol levels (6403). Theaflavin-enriched green tea extract, 375 mg daily for 12 weeks, has also been used for cholesterol reduction (11308). For preventing breast cancer or breast cancer recurrence, three or more cups of green tea per day have been used (3926). For human papilloma virus (HPV) infected cervical lesions, green tea extract, 200 mg daily alone or in combination with topical green tea ointment, for 8-12 weeks has been used (11310). For preventing Parkinson's disease, men consuming 421-2716 mg total caffeine (approximately 5-33 cups of green tea) daily have the lowest risk of developing Parkinson's disease. However, a significantly lower risk is also associated with consumption of as little as 124-208 mg of caffeine (approximately 1-3 cups of green tea) daily (6022). In women, more moderate caffeine consumption seems to be best; equivalent to approximately 1-4 cups of green tea per day (1238). To make tea, people typically use 1 teaspoon of tea leaves in 8 ounces boiling water.
TOPICAL: For human papillomavirus (HPV)-infected cervical lesions, green tea ointment in an unspecified concentration has been used alone or in combination with oral green tea extract, twice weekly for 8-12 weeks (11310).

Comments

Camellia sinensis leaves and stems are used to manufacture green tea (non-fermented), oolong tea (partially fermented), and black tea (fermented) (4218). Leaves used for green tea are prepared immediately after harvest to limit enzymatic changes.

GROUND IVY

Also Known As

Alehoof, Catsfoot, Cat's-Paw, Creeping Charlie, Gill-Go-By-The-Hedge, Gill-Go-Over-The-Ground, Haymaids, Hedgemaids, Lizzy-Run-Up-The-Hedge, Nepeta hederacea, Robin-Run-In-The-Hedge, Tun-Hoof, Turnhoof.
CAUTION: See separate listing for Cat's Foot.

Scientific Names

Glechoma hederacea.
Family: Lamiaceae/Labiatae.

People Use This For

Orally, ground ivy is used for mild upper respiratory complaints, coughs, arthritis, rheumatism, as a diuretic in individuals with bladder and kidney stones, for menstrual irregularities, bronchitis, chronic bronchial inflammation, tinnitus, diarrhea, intestinal inflammation, hemorrhoids, cystitis, and gastritis.
Topically ground ivy is used for poorly healing wounds, ulcers, and other skin conditions.
In food manufacturing, ground ivy is used as a flavoring agent.

Safety

POSSIBLY SAFE ...when preparations of the above ground parts are consumed in amounts found in foods; listed by the Council of Europe as natural source of food flavoring (4). ...when used orally in medicinal amounts (4,18).
PREGNANCY: LIKELY UNSAFE ...when used orally because of abortifacient activity (4); avoid using.
LACTATION: Insufficient reliable information available; avoid using.

Effectiveness

There is insufficient reliable information available about the effectiveness of ground ivy.

Mechanism of Action

Ground ivy contains rosmarinic acid, which may be an astringent (4). It also contains the volatile oil pulegone, which has hepatotoxic, abortifacient, and irritant properties. The concentration of pulegone in ground ivy is low (4). Fatal poisonings have occurred in animals (18).

Adverse Reactions

Orally, ground ivy in excessive doses may irritate the GI mucosa and kidneys (4).

Interactions with Herbs & Other Dietary Supplements

PENNYROYAL: Avoid concomitant use, both herbs contain potentially hepatotoxic constituent, pulegone (4).

Interactions with Drugs
None known.

Interactions with Foods
None known.

Interactions with Lab Tests
None known.

Interactions with Diseases or Conditions
KIDNEY DISEASE: The volatile oil is contraindicated due to potential for kidney irritation (4).
LIVER DISEASE: Contraindicated, due to presence of hepatotoxic pulegone (4).
SEIZURE DISORDERS: Contraindicated (4).

Dosage and Administration
ORAL: 2-4 grams dried plant three times daily (4), or, one cup tea (steep 2-4 grams dried plant in 150 mL boiling water 5-10 minutes, strain) three times daily (4). Liquid extract (1:1 in 25% alcohol), 2-4 mL three times daily (4).
TOPICAL: Apply crushed leaves to affected area(s) (18).

Comments
Ground ivy is a rich plant source of potassium and iron (19).

GROUND PINE

Also Known As
Bugle, Yellow Bugle.

Scientific Names
Ajuga chamaepitys, synonym Teucrium chamaepitys.
Family: Lamiaceae/Labiatae.

Comments
At the date of publication, this product was not a common ingredient used in brand name supplements marketed to consumers. Details about this product are available at the online version of *Natural Medicines Comprehensive Database*. See www.naturaldatabase.com.

GROUNDSEL

Also Known As
Common Groundsel, Ground Glutton, Grundy Swallow, Simson.

Scientific Names
Senecio vulgaris.
Family: Asteraceae/Compositae.

People Use This For
Orally, groundsel is used for worm infestations and colic. The pressed juice is used orally in the treatment of dysmenorrhea and epilepsy.
Topically, groundsel pressed juice is used as a dental styptic.

Safety
UNSAFE ...when used orally (2,18). Excessive doses or long-term use increases risk of adverse effects due to unsaturated pyrrolizidine alkaloids (UPAs) (4,12). UPAs are linked to veno-occlusive disease (4,12) and are considered to be hepatotoxic and hepatocarcinogenic (7,515). They might also be mutagenic (12). Dietary supplements sold in the US are not required to include the amount of UPAs they contain (3484); therefore, all preparations used orally containing groundsel should be considered potentially unsafe.
PREGNANCY AND LACTATION: UNSAFE ...when used orally due to unsaturated pyrrolizidine alkaloid (UPA) content (12).

Effectiveness

There is insufficient reliable information available about the effectiveness of groundsel.

Mechanism of Action

The applicable part of groundsel is the whole flowering plant. Some pyrrolizidine alkaloids have shown carcinogenic and mutagenic properties, and there are reports of renal toxicity. However, the primary concern is veno-occlusive disease (12). Unsaturated pyrrolizidine alkaloids are known to be hepatotoxic and hepatocarcinogenic in animals and humans (4,7). UPAs destroy and damage centrilobular hepatocytes of the liver and also destroy small branches of the hepatic vein (7).

Adverse Reactions

Chronic exposure to other plants containing UPA constituents has been associated with veno-occlusive disease (4021). Symptoms of acute veno-occlusive disease are characterized by nausea, vomiting (5606), anorexia, lethargy (7), a dull, dragging ache in the right upper abdomen and marked distention of the abdomen (4021). These symptoms are sometimes accompanied by reduced urine output. Subacute veno-occlusive disease is associated with vague symptoms and persistent liver enlargement (4021). There is one case report of fatal hepatic veno-occlusive disease in an infant resulting from groundsel tea consumption (5606). It can cause an allergic reaction in individuals sensitive to the Asteraceae/Compositae family. Members of this family include ragweed, chrysanthemums, marigolds, daisies, and many other herbs.

Interactions with Herbs & Other Dietary Supplements

EUCALYPTUS: Theoretically, concomitant use might increase the risk of unsaturated pyrrolizidine alkaloid toxicity due to enzyme induction by eucalyptus (19).
UNSATURATED PYRROLIZIDINE ALKALOID (UPA)-CONTAINING HERBS: Concomitant use is contraindicated due to the risk of additive toxicity. Herbs containing UPAs include alkanna, borage, gravel root, hemp agrimony, hound's tongue, petasites, comfrey, coltsfoot; and the Senecio species plants dusty miller, alpine ragwort, golden ragwort, and tansy ragwort (4,12,19,271).

Interactions with Drugs

None known.

Interactions with Foods

None known.

Interactions with Lab Tests

None known.

Interactions with Diseases or Conditions

CROSS-ALLERGENICITY: Groundsel may cause an allergic reaction in individuals sensitive to the Asteraceae/Compositae family (19). Members of this family include ragweed, chrysanthemums, marigolds, daisies, and many other herbs.
LIVER DISEASE: Theoretically, use of groundsel is contraindicated (19).

Dosage and Administration

No typical dosage.

GUAIAC WOOD resin, wood

Also Known As

Guaiac, Guaiac Heartwood, Guaiacum, Guajaci Lignum, Lingum Vitae, Pockwood.
CAUTION: See separate listing for Guaiac Wood Oil.

Scientific Names

Guaiacum officinale; Guaiacum sanctum, synonym Guaiacum guatemalense.
Family: Zygophyllaceae.

People Use This For

Orally, guaiac wood is used for subacute and chronic rheumatism, chronic rheumatoid arthritis, preventing gout, respiratory complaints, skin disorders, and syphilis. Topically, guaiac wood is used as a bacteriostatic agent in mouthwashes. In lab tests, guaiac resin is used as a diagnostic reagent in tests for occult blood. As a flavoring agent, guaiac wood is used in foods and in edible oils and fats.

Safety
POSSIBLY SAFE ...when used orally in amounts commonly found in foods. Guaiac wood has Generally Recognized As Safe (GRAS) status in the US (4912). ...when used orally and appropriately for medicinal purposes. The resin can have low toxicity (4).
There is insufficient reliable information available about the safety of guaiac wood/resin for its other uses.
PREGNANCY AND LACTATION: Insufficient reliable information available; avoid using.

Effectiveness
There is insufficient reliable information available about the effectiveness of guaiac wood/resin.

Mechanism of Action
Guaiac wood/resin can have antirheumatic, anti-inflammatory, diuretic, mild laxative, diaphoretic, and fungistatic activity (4,18).

Adverse Reactions
Orally, guaiac wood/resin can cause skin rashes (18). High doses can cause diarrhea, gastroenteritis, or intestinal colic (18).

Interactions with Herbs & Other Dietary Supplements
None known.

Interactions with Drugs
None known.

Interactions with Foods
None known.

Interactions with Lab Tests
None known.

Interactions with Diseases or Conditions
ACUTE INFLAMMATORY CONDITIONS: The use of guaiac wood/resin is contraindicated in acute inflammatory conditions and individuals allergic or hypersensitive to the product (4).

Dosage and Administration
ORAL: The typical dose of guaiac wood is one cup of the tea three times daily (2,4,18). The tea is prepared by simmering 1.5 grams of the wood or resin in 150 mL boiling water for 5-10 minutes and then straining. The usual dose of the liquid extract (1:1 in 80% alcohol) is 1-2 mL per dose. The common dose of the tincture of is 1-4 mL, which is about 20-40 drops (4,18).
TOPICAL: No typical dosage.

Comments
Avoid confusion with guaiac wood oil.

GUAR GUM

Also Known As
Dietary Fiber, Guar Flour, Indian Cluster Bean, Indian Guar Plant, Jaguar Gum.
CAUTION: See separate listing for Guarana.

Scientific Names
Cyamopsis tetragonoloba, synonyms Cyamopsis psoraloides, Dolichos psoraloides, Psoralea tetragonoloba.
Family: Fabaceae/Leguminosae.

People Use This For
Orally, guar gum is used as a bulk laxative. It is also used for treating diarrhea, irritable bowel syndrome (IBS), obesity, and diabetes; and for reducing serum cholesterol and preventing atherosclerosis.
In foods and beverages, guar gum is used as a thickening, stabilizing, suspending, and binding agent.
In manufacturing, guar gum is used as a binding and disintegrating agent in tablets, and as a thickening agent in lotions and creams.

Safety

LIKELY SAFE ...when used orally and appropriately (8305,10325,10326). Guar gum has Generally Recognized As Safe (GRAS) status in the US (4912).
PREGNANCY: POSSIBLY SAFE ...when used orally and appropriately in medicinal amounts (10895).
LACTATION: There is insufficient reliable information available about the safety of using medicinal amounts of guar gum in breast-feeding women; avoid using.

Effectiveness

POSSIBLY EFFECTIVE

Constipation. Taking guar gum orally seems to relieve constipation due to its bulk laxative effects (7).
Diabetes. Taking guar gum orally with meals seems to lower post-prandial glucose levels in patients with type 1 diabetes (10896).
Diarrhea. Adding guar gum to the enteral feeding formula may decrease the duration of diarrhea from about 30 days to about 8 days in critical care patients (10325).
Hypertriglyceridemia. Taking guar gum orally seems to lower triglycerides levels in people with hypertriglyceridemia (10897).
Irritable bowel syndrome (IBS). Taking guar gum orally might reduce abdominal pain and improve bowel function in some patients with mild to moderate IBS. It may be more effective than wheat bran (10326).

POSSIBLY INEFFECTIVE

Weight loss. Taking guar gum orally doesn't seem to be beneficial for losing weight (8305).

There is insufficient reliable information available about the effectiveness of guar gum for its other uses.

Mechanism of Action

Guar gum is a soluble dietary fiber produced from the seed of the guar plant. It works as a bulk laxative. When ingested, it expands in the presence of water and tends to normalize bowel function. Like other fibers, it adsorbs glucose and lipids in the gut and decreases their absorption. The bulk forming properties may also cause a sense of fullness and cause decreased appetite (8305,10898).

Adverse Reactions

Orally, guar gum can cause flatulence, diarrhea, nausea, gastrointestinal discomfort (12). Gastrointestinal side effects can be minimized be starting with small doses and titrating up. When guar gum is consumed with inadequate amounts of fluids, it can also cause severe esophageal and small bowel obstruction (602). Tell patients to take guar gum with at least 8 ounces (250 mL) of water (12).
Topically, asthma may result from occupational exposure (600,601).

Interactions with Herbs & Other Dietary Supplements

VITAMIN/MINERAL SUPPLEMENTS: Guar gum can reduce vitamin and mineral absorption (12). Tell patients to take supplements one hour before or several hours after guar gum.

Interactions with Drugs

ANTIDIABETES DRUGS: There is some concern that guar gum can decrease glucose levels and might have additive effects with insulin and other diabetes medications (10897). Monitor blood glucose levels closely. Dose adjustments may be necessary.
ORAL DRUGS: Guar gum can decrease absorption of orally administered drugs (12), including aspirin, anticoagulants, digoxin, metformin, penicillin, and numerous others (532,533). Tell patients to take drugs one hour before or several hours after guar gum.

Interactions with Foods

NUTRIENT ABSORPTION: Long term use with meals may reduce nutrient absorption (12) requiring vitamin/mineral supplementation.

Interactions with Lab Tests

CHOLESTEROL: Guar gum can reduce serum total cholesterol and low-density lipoprotein (LDL) cholesterol levels and test results (10897).
GLUCOSE: Guar gum can reduce postprandial serum glucose concentrations and test results (10896).

Interactions with Diseases or Conditions

GASTROINTESTINAL (GI) OBSTRUCTION: Guar gum is contraindicated in cases of GI obstruction or narrowing, anatomical predisposition to luminal obstruction (12).

Dosage and Administration

ORAL: Typically, 5 grams three times per day just before or with meals is used. Tell patients to take each dose with at least 8 ounces (250 mL) of fluid to prevent esophageal obstruction (12). Recommend starting with a small dose of 3 grams per day and titrating to reduce occurrence of gastrointestinal side effects. Adding 22 grams of guar gum per liter of enteral feeding formula has been used to treat diarrhea in critical care patients (10325).

GUARANA

Also Known As

Brazilian Cocoa, Paullinia, Zoom.
CAUTION: See separate listings for Caffeine and Guar Gum.

Scientific Names

Paullinia cupana, synonym Paullinia sorbilis.
Family: Sapindaceae.

People Use This For

Orally, guarana is used for weight loss, to enhance athletic performance, to reduce mental and physical fatigue, as a stimulant, tonic, aphrodisiac, diuretic, and astringent. It is also used orally to prevent malaria and dysentery, and for chronic diarrhea, fever, heart problems, headache, rheumatism, lumbago, and heat stress.
In food manufacturing, guarana has been used as a flavoring ingredient in beverages and candy.

Safety

LIKELY SAFE ...when consumed in amounts typically found in foods. Guarana's usage in foods is approved in the US (4912).
POSSIBLY SAFE ...when used orally and appropriately short-term (12).
POSSIBLY UNSAFE ...when used orally long-term in high doses. Guarana contains a significant amount of caffeine. Chronic use, especially in large amounts, can produce tolerance, habituation, psychological dependence, and other significant adverse effects. Doses greater than 250-300 mg per day have been associated with significant adverse effects such as tachyarrhythmias and sleep disturbances (11832).
These effects would not be expected to occur with the consumption of decaffeinated guarana.
LIKELY UNSAFE ...when used orally in very high doses. The fatal acute oral dose of caffeine is estimated to be 10-14 grams (150-200 mg per kilogram). Serious toxicity can occur at lower doses depending on variables in caffeine sensitivity such as smoking, age, prior caffeine use, etc (11832).
CHILDREN: POSSIBLY SAFE ...when consumed in amounts commonly found in foods (4912,11833).
PREGNANCY: POSSIBLY SAFE ...when consumed in amounts commonly found in foods. Due to the caffeine content of guarana, mothers should closely monitor their intake to ensure moderate consumption. Fetal blood concentrations of caffeine approximate maternal concentrations (4260). Use of caffeine in pregnancy is controversial; however, moderate consumption has not been associated with clinically important adverse fetal effects (2708,2709,2710,2711,9606). Caffeine crosses the human placenta, but is not considered a teratogen. Mothers should keep caffeine consumption below 200 mg per day. This is similar to the amount of caffeine found in 1-2 cups of coffee or tea (2708). POSSIBLY UNSAFE ...when used orally in large amounts. Caffeine crosses the placenta, producing fetal blood concentrations similar to maternal levels (4260). Mothers should avoid consuming more than 200 mg of caffeine daily or more than 1-2 cups of tea or coffee per day (2708). Maternal doses of greater than 200 mg per day throughout pregnancy have resulted in symptoms of caffeine withdrawal in newborn infants (9891). High doses of caffeine have been associated with spontaneous abortion, premature delivery, and low birth weight (2709,2711). Fetal birth weight is reduced by 28 grams for every 100 mg per day of caffeine consumed during pregnancy. But this is unlikely to be clinically important except for women consuming more than 600 mg of caffeine daily (9606).
LACTATION: POSSIBLY SAFE ...when used orally in amounts commonly found in foods. Due to the caffeine content of guarana, nursing mothers should closely monitor caffeine intake. Breast milk concentrations of caffeine are thought to be approximately 50% of maternal serum concentrations. Minimal consumption would likely result in limited exposure to a nursing infant (9892). POSSIBLY UNSAFE ...when used orally in large amounts. Consumption of guarana might cause irritability and increased bowel activity in nursing infants (6026). Large doses or excessive intake of guarana should be avoided during lactation.

Effectiveness

INSUFFICIENT RELIABLE EVIDENCE to RATE

Obesity. Guarana taken orally might cause weight loss when used in combination with mate and damiana (11866). There is also preliminary evidence that a specific combination product containing guarana, ephedra, and 17 other vitamins, minerals, and supplements (Metabolife-356) might help reduce weight by approximately 2.7 kg over eight weeks when used with a low-fat diet and exercise (3719). More evidence is needed to rate guarana for this use.

Mechanism of Action

The applicable part of guarana is the seed. Guarana contains 3.6% to 5.8% caffeine (compared to 1% to 2% in coffee) (11845). Guarana contains tannins with possible carcinogenic and hepatotoxic properties (12). Caffeine is responsible for the pharmacologic effects of guarana.

Caffeine is a methylxanthine compound and is structurally related to theophylline, theobromine, and uric acid (6372). It is 100% bioavailable after oral administration and is metabolized principally in the liver to paraxanthine, theophylline, and theobromine (6370). The half-life of caffeine is about six hours (8644).

Caffeine stimulates the central nervous system (CNS), heart, muscles, and possibly the pressor centers that control blood pressure (2722). Possible mechanisms include adenosine receptor blockade and phosphodiesterase inhibition (2722). By blocking adenosine receptors, caffeine is thought to increase the release of neurotransmitters such as dopamine (6370). Caffeine also decreases airway resistance and stimulates respiration, via adenosine receptor blockade and phosphodiesterase inhibition (11836). It has also been proposed that caffeine may decrease GABA and serotonin signaling (6370). Caffeine stimulates gastric acid secretion, and increases plasma catecholamine levels (11837). Caffeine can have positive inotropic and chronotropic effects on the heart (11836). Caffeine can also acutely elevate both diastolic and systolic blood pressure, but might not have this effect in habitual users (2722).

Caffeine exerts a diuretic effect, with water losses estimated at 1.17 mL per milligram of caffeine (2712). Tachyphylaxis to the diuretic effect develops rapidly, diminishing fluid losses associated with caffeine intake (10206). Caffeine-containing beverages consumed during moderate endurance exercise do not appear to compromise bodily hydration status (2713). Caffeine does not substantially affect the fluid status of people who drink caffeinated beverages on a regular basis (10206). Caffeine's CNS stimulant effects are thought to improve vigilance and psychomotor performance (2720,10205). For improving athletic performance, caffeine has been shown to decrease perceived levels of exertion, which enables the athlete to feel less tired and increase their performance (6370). Caffeine alone or in combination with ephedrine can improve anaerobic exercise performance. Caffeine seems to enhance muscle metabolism and increases time to exhaustion and oxygen deficit, which may lead to better performance (8646). Studies have also suggested caffeine possibly influences cardiovascular stress reactivity, either by potentiating the stress response itself or adding to the level reached during stress (6372). Caffeine may cause a slight decrease in heart rate after consumption and appears to raise blood pressure during psychological stress (6372). Large amounts of caffeine, >10 mg/kg/day, can also produce tachycardia and premature ventricular contractions (6372). Caffeine has been reported to cause increases and decreases in blood glucose. In people with type 2 diabetes, acute administration of caffeine impairs postprandial glucose metabolism, while acute abstention from caffeine reduces postprandial glucose levels by 21%. Whether these effects also occur with caffeinated beverages and herbs is unknown (12374). Other research in obese people suggests that caffeine ingestion may contribute to insulin resistance (12375). However, one study found that type 1 diabetics taking 200 mg of caffeine twice daily had increased frequency and intensity of warning signs of hypoglycemia. This may be due to a reduction in blood flow to the brain and an increase in glucose utilization by the brain (6024). For preventing Parkinson's disease, caffeine may protect dopaminergic neurons in the brain. This effect appears to be related to modulation of adenosine receptors (10201). This may result in a reduction in the clinical expression of Parkinsonism (6022). Evidence suggests that tolerance to caffeine's neuroendocrine and cardiovascular effects may develop during consumption throughout the day, but tolerance appears to be lost during overnight abstinence of caffeine (6372). Preliminary evidence also suggests caffeine may increase plasma levels of cortisol and adrenocorticotrophic hormone (ACTH), decrease levels of extracellular potassium, and increase levels of intracellular calcium in skeletal muscle; but the mechanisms are poorly understood (6370). Caffeine may be beneficial in the prevention of cardiovascular disease. There is evidence caffeine inhibits platelet aggregation and suppresses thromboxane formation during blood clotting (8028,8029). There is also evidence caffeine might be associated with decreased levels of testosterone and increased levels of estrone and sex-hormone binding globulin. These findings might explain why some studies have reported associations between caffeine and hormone-dependent conditions such as fibrocystic disease, osteoporosis, breast cancer, and endometriosis (8043). Caffeine is often used in combination with ephedra for weight loss and seems to have additive pharmacodynamic effects. A single dose of ephedra in combination with caffeine can increase heart rate from 67 beats per minute to 82 beats per minute in young, healthy people. The combination also increases systolic blood pressure and to a lesser extent, diastolic pressure (8644). Caffeine in combination with ephedra also increases oxygen consumption. Whether the increased oxygen consumption is an indication of a significant increase in metabolism and contributes to weight loss is unknown (8645).

Adverse Reactions

Orally, guarana can cause symptoms of caffeine toxicity. Caffeine can cause insomnia, nervousness, restlessness, gastric irritation, nausea, vomiting, tachycardia, quickened respiration, tremors, delirium, convulsions, and diuresis. Large doses can produce headache, anxiety, agitation, ringing in the ears, premature heartbeat, and arrhythmia (11832,11838). In fatal caffeine overdose, the cause of death is usually ventricular fibrillation (11838,11845). Insomnia is a frequent adverse effect in children (10755). Caffeine may cause feeding intolerance and gastrointestinal irritation in infants (6023). Caffeine may exacerbate sleep disturbances in patients with acquired immunodeficiency syndrome (AIDS) (10204).

Some evidence shows caffeine is associated with fibrocystic breast disease, breast cancer, and endometriosis in women; however, this is controversial since findings are conflicting (8043). Restricting caffeine in women with fibrocystic breast conditions doesn't seem to affect breast nodularity, swelling, or pain (8996).

Although acute administration of caffeine can cause increased blood pressure, regular consumption does not seem to increase either blood pressure or pulse, even in mildly hypertensive patients (1451,1452,2722).
Tolerance to caffeine is a widely held belief, but there is little supportive clinical evidence. If it exists, it appears to be of little clinical significance (11839). Withdrawal symptoms such as irritability, sleepiness, delirium, nausea, vomiting, rhinorrhea, nervousness, restlessness, anxiety, muscle tension, muscle pains, and flushed face have been described. However, these symptoms may be from nonpharmacological factors related to knowledge and expectation of effects. Clinically significant symptoms caused by caffeine withdrawal may be uncommon (2723,11839).
Epidemiological evidence regarding the relationship between caffeine use and the risk for osteoporosis is contradictory. Caffeine can increase urinary excretion of calcium (2669,10202,11317). Women identified with a genetic variant of the vitamin D receptor appear to be at an increased risk for the detrimental effect of caffeine on bone mass (2669). However, moderate caffeine intake, less than 300 mg per day, does not seem to significantly increase osteoporosis risk in most postmenopausal women with normal calcium intake (2669,6025,10202,11317).
Combining ephedra with caffeine can increase the risk of adverse effects. Jitteriness, hypertension, seizures, temporary loss of consciousness, and hospitalization requiring life support has been associated with the combined use of ephedra and caffeine (2729). There is also a report of ischemic stroke in an athlete who consumed ephedra 40-60 mg, creatine monohydrate 6 grams, caffeine 400-600 mg, and a variety of other supplements daily for six weeks (1275).
Caffeine can cause anaphylaxis in sensitive individuals, although true IgE-mediated caffeine allergy seems to be relatively rare (11315).

Interactions with Herbs & Other Dietary Supplements

CAFFEINE CONTAINING HERBS/SUPPLEMENTS: Concomitant use of guarana and caffeine-containing herbs/supplements constitutes therapeutic duplication (due to the caffeine contained in guarana) which increases the risk of caffeine-related adverse effects. Other natural products which contain caffeine include black tea, cocoa, coffee, cola nut, and mate.
CALCIUM: High caffeine intake from foods, beverages, and herbs including guarana increases urinary calcium excretion (2570).
CREATINE: There is some concern that combining caffeine, ephedra, and creatine might increase the risk of serious adverse effects. There is a report of ischemic stroke in an athlete who consumed creatine monohydrate 6 grams, caffeine 400-600 mg, ephedra 40-60 mg, and a variety of other supplements daily for 6 weeks (1275). Caffeine might also decrease creatine's possible beneficial effects on athletic performance. Some researchers think caffeine can inhibit phosphocreatine resynthesis (2117,4575).
EPHEDRA (Ma Huang): Concomitant use can increase the risk of stimulatory adverse effects, due to the caffeine contained in guarana (7). One unpublished report associated jitteriness, hypertension, seizures, temporary loss of consciousness, and hospitalization requiring life support with the use of a combination ephedra and guarana (caffeine) product (1380).

Interactions with Drugs

ADENOSINE (Adenocard): The caffeine in guarana is a competitive inhibitor of adenosine at the cellular level. However, caffeine doesn't seem to affect supplemental adenosine because high interstitial levels of adenosine overcome the antagonistic effects of caffeine (11771).
ALCOHOL (Ethanol): Concomitant use of alcohol can increase caffeine serum concentrations and the risk of caffeine adverse effects. Alcohol reduces caffeine metabolism (6370).
AMPHETAMINES: Theoretically, the caffeine in guarana might increase the risk of additive CNS effects (2719).
ANTICOAGULANT/ANTIPLATELET DRUGS: Theoretically, the caffeine in guarana might increase the risk of bleeding when used concomitantly with these agents. Caffeine is reported to have antiplatelet activity (8028,8029); however, this interaction has not been reported in humans. Antiplatelet agents include aspirin, clopidogrel (Plavix), dipyridamole (Persantine), ticlopidine (Ticlid), and others. Anticoagulant agents include heparin and warfarin (Coumadin).
ANTIDIABETES DRUGS: Theoretically, concomitant use of caffeine, a constituent of guarana, and diabetes drugs might interfere with blood glucose control. Data are conflicting. Reports claim that caffeine might increase or decrease blood sugar (6024,8646).
CIMETIDINE (Tagamet): Theoretically, concomitant use might increase serum caffeine concentrations and the risk of adverse effects, due to the caffeine contained in guarana. Cimetidine decreases the rate of caffeine clearance by 30% to 50% (11736).
CLOZAPINE (Clozaril): Theoretically, co-administration might acutely exacerbate psychotic symptoms, due to the caffeine contained in guarana. Caffeine can increase the effects and toxicity of clozapine (151). Caffeine doses of 400-1000 mg per day inhibit clozapine metabolism (5051).
COCAINE: Theoretically, the caffeine in guarana might increase the risk of additive CNS effects (2719).
CONTRACEPTIVE DRUGS: Theoretically, concomitant use might increase caffeine concentrations and the risk adverse effects, due to the caffeine contained in guarana. Oral contraceptives decrease the rate of caffeine clearance by 40-65% (2714,11737).
DIPYRIDAMOLE (Persantine): The caffeine in guarana might inhibit dipyridamole-induced vasodilation (11770,11772).

DISULFIRAM (Antabuse): Theoretically, concomitant use might increase serum caffeine concentrations and the risk of adverse effects, due to the caffeine contained in guarana. Disulfiram decreases the rate of caffeine clearance (15).
EPHEDRINE: Use of ephedrine with caffeine, a constituent of guarana, can increase the risk of stimulatory adverse effects. There is evidence that using ephedrine with caffeine might increase the risk of serious life-threatening or debilitating adverse effects such as hypertension, myocardial infarction, stroke, seizures, and death (1275,6486,10307). Tell patients to avoid taking caffeine with ephedrine and other stimulants.
ESTROGENS: Theoretically, concomitant use might increase serum caffeine concentrations and the risk of adverse effects, due to the caffeine contained in guarana. Estrogen inhibits caffeine metabolism (2714).
FLUCONAZOLE (Diflucan): Concomitant use might increase the effects of caffeine in guarana. Fluconazole decreases caffeine clearance by approximately 25% (11022).
FLUVOXAMINE (Luvox): Concomitant use of fluvoxamine with caffeine or caffeine-containing herbs such as guarana can increase caffeine serum concentrations, and the risk of caffeine adverse effects. Fluvoxamine reduces caffeine metabolism (6370).
LITHIUM: Theoretically, abrupt guarana withdrawal might increase serum lithium levels, due to the caffeine contained in guarana. There are two case reports of lithium tremor that worsened upon abrupt coffee withdrawal (609,610).
MEXILETINE (Mexitil): Concomitant use might increase the effects and adverse effects of caffeine in guarana. Mexiletine can decrease caffeine elimination by 50% (1260,11741).
MONOAMINE OXIDASE INHIBITORS (MAOIs): Theoretically, concomitant intake of large amounts of guarana with MAOIs might precipitate a hypertensive crisis, due to the caffeine contained in guarana. This is based on the claim that intake of large amounts of caffeine with MAOIs might precipitate a hypertensive crisis (15).
NICOTINE: Theoretically, the caffeine in guarana might increase the risk of additive CNS effects (2719).
PHENYLPROPANOLAMINE: Concomitant use of phenylpropanolamine and guarana might cause an additive increase in blood pressure due to the caffeine in guarana (11738).
QUINOLONE ANTIBIOTICS: Theoretically, concomitant use might increase serum caffeine concentrations and the risk of adverse effects, due to the caffeine contained in guarana. Quinolones decrease caffeine clearance (606,607,608). Quinolones (also referred to as fluoroquinolones) include ciprofloxacin (Cipro), enoxacin (Penetrex), gatifloxacin (Tequin), levofloxacin (Levaquin), lomefloxacin (Maxaquin), moxifloxacin (Avelox), norfloxacin (Noroxin), ofloxacin (Floxin), sparfloxacin (Zagam), and trovafloxacin (Trovan).
RILUZOLE (Rilutek): Theoretically, concomitant use of riluzole with caffeine or caffeine-containing herbs such as guarana might increase serum caffeine and riluzole concentrations and the risk of adverse effects of both caffeine and riluzole, due to the caffeine contained in guarana. Caffeine and riluzole are both metabolized by cytochrome P450 1A2, and concomitant use might reduce metabolism of one or both agents (11739).
TERBINAFINE (Lamisil): Theoretically, concomitant use might increase serum caffeine concentrations and the risk of adverse effects, due to the caffeine contained in guarana. Terbinafine decreases the rate of caffeine clearance (11740).
THEOPHYLLINE: Theoretically, concomitant use of theophylline and large amounts of guarana might increase the risk of theophylline toxicity, due to guarana's caffeine content. Caffeine decreases theophylline clearance 23-29% (11741).
VERAPAMIL (Calan, Covera, Isoptin, Verelan): Theoretically, concomitant use might increase plasma caffeine concentrations and the risk of adverse effects, due to the caffeine contained in guarana. Verapamil increases plasma caffeine concentrations by 25% (11741).

Interactions with Foods

None known.

Interactions with Lab Tests

5-HYDROXYINDOLEACETIC ACID: Guarana might increase urine 5-hydroxyindoleacetic acid concentrations and test results, due to its caffeine content. Caffeine can increase urine catecholamine concentrations (15).
BLEEDING TIME: Guarana might prolong bleeding time and increase test results, due to its caffeine content (1701).
CATECHOLAMINES: Guarana might increase urine catecholamine concentrations and test results, due to its caffeine content. Caffeine can increase urine catecholamine concentrations (15).
CREATINE: Guarana might increase urine creatine concentrations and test results, due to its caffeine content (1701).
DIPYRIDAMOLE THALLIUM IMAGING: Guarana might interfere with dipyridamole thallium imaging studies, due to its caffeine content. Caffeine attenuates the characteristic cardiovascular responses to dipyridamole and has altered test results (11742).
GLUCOSE: Caffeine has been reported to cause increases and decreases in blood glucose (8646).
LACTATE: The combination of ephedrine, a constituent of ephedra, and caffeine, a constituent of guarana, can increase blood lactate levels (8646).
NEUROBLASTOMA TESTS: Guarana (due to its caffeine content) might cause false-positive diagnosis of neuroblastoma, when diagnosis is based on tests of urine vanillylmandelic acid (VMA) or catecholamine concentrations. Caffeine can increase urine catecholamine and VMA concentrations (15).
PHARMACOLOGICAL STRESS TESTS: The caffeine in guarana is a competitive antagonist for adenosine

receptors (11771). It is recommended that caffeine and caffeine-containing products be stopped 24 hours prior to pharmacological stress tests (11770). However, caffeine appears more likely to interfere with dipyridamole (Persantine) than adenosine (Adenocard) stress testing (11771). The interaction between caffeine and dipyridamole is unlikely to be significant in stress testing if the heart rate increase is greater than 5% after dipyridamole infusion (11772).
PHEOCHROMOCYTOMA TESTS: Guarana (due to its caffeine content) might cause false-positive diagnosis of pheochromocytoma, when diagnosis is based on tests of urine vanillylmandelic acid (VMA) or catecholamine concentrations. Caffeine can increase urine catecholamine and VMA concentrations (15).
PULMONARY FUNCTION TESTS: People may need to avoid caffeine and caffeine containing beverages and herbs for at least four hours prior to lung function testing. Forced expiratory volume in one minute (FEV1) seems to show a small improvement up to two hours after caffeine use. Mid-expiratory flow rates may also improve with caffeine for up to four hours (9607).
URATE: Guarana might falsely increase serum urate test results determined by the Bittner method, due to its caffeine content. Caffeine causes false elevations in serum urate test results determined by the Bittner method (15).
URINARY CALCIUM: Caffeine, a constituent of guarana, can increase urinary calcium levels (11317).
VANILLYLMANDELIC ACID (VMA): Guarana might increase urine VMA concentrations and test results, due to its caffeine content. Caffeine can increase urine VMA concentrations (15).

Interactions with Diseases or Conditions
ANXIETY DISORDERS: The caffeine in guarana might aggravate anxiety disorders (11743).
BLEEDING DISORDERS: Theoretically, caffeine in guarana might aggravate these conditions. Caffeine is reported to have antiplatelet activity (8028,8029); however, this interaction has not been reported in humans (1701). Caffeine can prolong bleeding time and increase the results of a bleeding time test (1701).
CARDIAC CONDITIONS: Caffeine in guarana can induce cardiac arrhythmias in sensitive individuals (11845); use with caution.
DIABETES: Some research suggests that caffeine, a constituent of guarana, may impair postprandial glucose metabolism in people with diabetes and contribute to insulin resistance. The effect of caffeinated beverages and herbs has not been studied (12374,12375). Caffeine in guarana may enhance the frequency and intensity of hypoglycemic warning symptoms in type 1 diabetics. This may increase the ability of diabetics to detect and treat hypoglycemia early. However, it might also increase the frequency of hypoglycemic events (6024). Caffeine has been reported to cause increases and decreases in blood glucose (8646); use with caution.
GLAUCOMA: Consuming guarana increases intraocular pressure due to its caffeine content. The increase occurs within 30 minutes and persists for at least 90 minutes (8540).
HYPERTENSION: The caffeine in guarana might increase blood pressure in people with high blood pressure. However, this doesn't seem to occur in people who regularly consume guarana or other caffeinated products (1451,1452,2722).
OSTEOPOROSIS: Consuming guarana can increase urinary excretion of calcium due to its caffeine content. Caffeine consumption should be limited to less than 300 mg per day. Adequate calcium supplementation may partially compensate for calcium losses (2669,10202,11317). Postmenopausal women identified with a genetic variant of the vitamin D receptor should use caffeine with caution (2669).

Dosage and Administration
ORAL: Guarana is often used along with other ingredients in weight loss products.

Comments
Guarana is named for the Guarani tribe in the Amazon, who used the seeds to brew a drink. Guarana is a frequent addition to energy and weight loss products (11845).

GUGGUL

Also Known As
Guggal, Guggul Gum Resin, Guggulipid, Guggulu, Guggulu Suddha, Guggulsterone, Gum Guggal, Gum Guggulu, Indian Bdellium-Tree, Mukul Myrrh Tree.
CAUTION: See separate listing for Indian Frankincense and Myrrh.

Scientific Names
Commiphora wightii, synonyms Commiphora mukul, Balsamodendrum wightii, Balsamodendrum mukul.
Family: Burseracaea.

People Use This For
Orally, guggul gum resin is used for arthritis, lowering high cholesterol, atherosclerosis, nodulocystic acne, skin diseases, and weight loss.

Safety

POSSIBLY SAFE ...when the prepared gum resin is used orally and appropriately. It has been used safely in clinical trials for up to 24 weeks (3267,3268,10371). Some evidence also suggests that long-term use up to 75 weeks may be safe (8158).
PREGNANCY: LIKELY UNSAFE ...when used orally; avoid using. Guggul gum resin appears to stimulate menstrual flow and the uterus (12).
LACTATION: Insufficient reliable information available; avoid using.

Effectiveness

POSSIBLY EFFECTIVE

Nodulocystic acne. Taking guggul orally is comparable to oral tetracycline in the treatment of nodulocystic acne. Both treatments decreased inflammation and the number of relapses (3268).

POSSIBLY INEFFECTIVE

Hypercholesterolemia. Taking guggul orally in doses of 3000 or 6000 mg per day doesn't seem to lower total cholesterol or triglycerides, or raise high density lipoprotein (HDL) cholesterol in people on Western diets. It seems to increase low density lipoprotein (LDL) cholesterol by 9% to 10% (10371). This is in contrast to studies of guggul in Indian populations, where guggul seems to lower total cholesterol, LDL, and triglycerides (366,3267,8158).

INSUFFICIENT RELIABLE EVIDENCE to RATE

Obesity. There's some clinical evidence that suggests that guggul in combination with phosphate, hydroxycitric acid, and L-tyrosine plus exercise and calorie restriction might result in modest weight loss (8152).
Osteoarthritis. Preliminary clinical evidence suggests that guggul (containing 3.5% guggulsterones) 500 mg three times daily might improve osteoarthritis pain (8150,8151).
More evidence is needed to rate guggul for these uses.

Mechanism of Action

Guggul is the extract of the gum resin of the Commiphora mukul tree, which is native to India. The ketonic steroids Z-guggulsterone and E-guggulsterone are found in guggul extracts. Guggulipid is the ethyl acetate extract of the gum resin and contains Z- and E-guggulsterones (3267). Guggulsterones can inhibit the synthesis of cholesterol in the liver and seem to have an antioxidant effect on lipids (3267,8156). The constituent, guggulsterone has thyroid-stimulating activity (8152,8153,8156). It seems to increase T3 synthesis by increasing conversion of T4 to T3 (8156). Preliminary evidence suggests that it has protective effects against drug-induced myocardial necrosis (8154). Guggulipid might reduce secretion of sebum and inhibit bacterial metabolism of triglycerides which induces acne (3268). Other evidence suggests guggul extracts might have anti-inflammatory activity (8150). Guggul might also lower lipoprotein (a) and C-reactive protein (10371). Preliminary evidence also suggests guggul might have antiplatelet and anticoagulant activity (3267,9557).

Adverse Reactions

Orally, guggul can cause headaches, nausea, vomiting, loose stools, diarrhea, belching, bloating, and hiccups (3267,8155,8158,10371). Guggul can also cause hypersensitivity reactions including rash and pruritus (10371).

Interactions with Herbs & Other Dietary Supplements

HERBS WITH ANTICOAGULANT/ANTIPLATELET POTENTIAL: Preliminary research suggests that guggul might have antiplatelet and anticoagulant activity (3267,9557). Concomitant use of herbs that have constituents that might affect platelet aggregation could theoretically increase the risk of bleeding in some people. These herbs include angelica, clove, danshen, garlic, ginger, ginkgo, red clover, turmeric, and others.

Interactions with Drugs

ANTICOAGULANT/ANTIPLATELET DRUGS: Guggul might have antiplatelet and anticoagulant effects (3267,9557). Theoretically, taking guggul with other antiplatelet or anticoagulant drugs might increase the risk of bruising and bleeding. Some of these drugs include aspirin; clopidogrel (Plavix); nonsteroidal anti-inflammatory drugs (NSAIDs) such as diclofenac (Voltaren, Cataflam, others), ibuprofen (Advil, Motrin, others), and naproxen (Anaprox, Naprosyn, others); dalteparin (Fragmin); enoxaparin (Lovenox); heparin; warfarin (Coumadin), and others.
DILTIAZEM (Cardizem): Concomitant oral administration can reduce diltiazem bioavailability and might reduce therapeutic effects (383).
PROPRANOLOL (Inderal): Concomitant oral administration can reduce propranolol bioavailability and might reduce therapeutic effects (383).
THYROID HORMONE: Theoretically, concomitant use might interfere with therapy to normalize thyroid function; monitor (8152,8153).

Interactions with Foods

None known.

Interactions with Lab Tests

SERUM CHOLESTEROL: Guggul can reduce serum total cholesterol and low-density lipoprotein (LDL) cholesterol concentrations and test results (366,3267).
SERUM TRIGLYCERIDES: Guggul can reduce serum triglycerides and test results (366,3267).
THYROID STIMULATING HORMONE (TSH): Theoretically, guggul can lower TSH by feedback from increased triiodothyronine (T3) (8156).
TRIIODOTHYRONINE (T3): Theoretically, guggul can increase T3 levels by stimulating T3 production (8156).

Interactions with Diseases or Conditions

THYROID DISORDERS: Theoretically, concomitant use might interfere with therapy for hyperthyroid or hypothyroid conditions; monitor use (8152,8153).

Dosage and Administration

ORAL: For hypercholesterolemia, a guggul extract (guggulipid), providing 75 to 150 mg of guggulsterones daily, has been given as 1000 to 2000 mg doses 2 to 3 times daily for up to 8 weeks (366,3267,10371). For nodulocystic acne, a dose of the guggulipid equivalent up to 25 mg guggulsterones twice a day has been used (3268).

Comments

Guggul is of the same genus as Commiphora myrrha, the myrrh of the bible. The plant has been used in Ayurvedic medicine for centuries (7161). It was cited in the Ayurvedic texts dating back to 600 BC for treating atherosclerosis. Gugulipid is commercially manufactured in India (3267).

GUMWEED

Also Known As

August Flower, Grindelia, Grindeliae herba, Gum Weed, Gumweed Herb, Rosin Weed, Tar Weed.

Scientific Names

Grindelia camporum, synonym Grindelia robusta; Grindelia squarrosa.
Family: Asteraceae/Compositae.

People Use This For

Orally, gumweed is used for cough, bronchitis, and inflammation of the upper respiratory tract mucous membrane.

Safety

POSSIBLY SAFE ...when used orally and appropriately (2,12).
PREGNANCY AND LACTATION: Insufficient reliable information; avoid using.

Effectiveness

There is insufficient reliable information available about the effectiveness of gumweed.

Mechanism of Action

The applicable parts of gumweed are the dried top and leaf. Gumweed can have antibacterial effects in vitro (2).

Adverse Reactions

Orally, gumweed can cause gastric mucosa irritation (2,12), diarrhea (18), and kidney irritation (12). Gumweed can cause an allergic reaction in individuals sensitive to the Asteraceae/Compositae family. Members of this family include ragweed, chrysanthemums, marigolds, daisies, and many other herbs.

Interactions with Herbs & Other Dietary Supplements

None known.

Interactions with Drugs

None known.

Interactions with Foods

None known.

Interactions with Lab Tests

None known.

Interactions with Diseases or Conditions

CROSS-ALLERGENICITY: Can cause an allergic reaction in individuals sensitive to the Asteraceae/Compositae family. Members of this family include ragweed, chrysanthemums, marigolds, daisies, and many other herbs.

Dosage and Administration

ORAL: The typical dose of gumweed is 4-6 grams of the dried top or leaf per day (2). The usual dose of the fluid extract is 3-6 grams per day (2). The common dose of the 1:10 tincture (60-80% ethanol) is 1.5-3 mL per day, and the usual dose of the 1:5 tincture (60-80% ethanol) is 1.5-3 mL per day (2).

GYMNEMA

Also Known As

Gur-Mar, Gurmar, Gurmarbooti, Gemnema melicida, Madhunashini, Merasingi, Meshashringi, Miracle Plant, Vishani.

Scientific Names

Gymnema sylvestre, synonym Periploca sylvestris.
Family: Apocynaceae.

People Use This For

Orally, gymnema is used to treat diabetes and coughs; and as a snake bite antidote, antimalarial, digestive stimulant, laxative, and diuretic.
In combination with other products, gymnema is used for metabolic control.

Safety

POSSIBLY SAFE ...when used orally and appropriately. Gymnema appears to be safe when used for up to 20 months (45,46).
PREGNANCY AND LACTATION: Insufficient reliable information available; avoid using.

Effectiveness

INSUFFICIENT RELIABLE EVIDENCE to RATE

Diabetes. Preliminary clinical research suggests that taking a specific gymnema extract (GS4) orally in combination with insulin or oral hypoglycemics can further reduce blood glucose and glycosylated hemoglobin in patients with type 1 or type 2 diabetes (45,46). More evidence is needed to rate gymnema for this use.

Mechanism of Action

The applicable part of gymnema is the leaf. For diabetes, gymnema may affect blood glucose in several ways. Gymnemic acids seem to reduce intestinal absorption of glucose and may stimulate pancreatic beta cell growth (47,48,11367). Gymnema can increase serum C-peptide levels, suggesting an increase in endogenous insulin secretion (45).
The constituents, gymnemic acid and gurmarin, inhibit the ability to taste bitter (quinine) or sweet (sugar) without affecting the ability to taste sour, astringent, or pungent flavors (11292).

Adverse Reactions

None reported.

Interactions with Herbs & Other Dietary Supplements

None known.

Interactions with Drugs

ANTIDIABETES DRUGS: Gymnema can enhance the blood glucose lowering effects of hypoglycemic drugs (46). Monitor blood glucose levels closely.
INSULIN: Gymnema can enhance the blood glucose lowering effects of insulin (45); blood glucose levels should be monitored closely.

Interactions with Foods

None known.

Interactions with Lab Tests

BLOOD GLUCOSE: Gymnema can lower blood sugar resulting in lower blood glucose test results (45,46).

Interactions with Diseases or Conditions

DIABETES: Gymnema can affect blood sugar control, and blood glucose levels should be monitored closely (45,46).

Dosage and Administration

ORAL: For diabetes, the gymnema extract GS4 400 mg daily has been used (45,46).

HARONGA

Also Known As

Harongablädder leaf, Harongarinde bark, Harunganae madagascariensis cortex bark, Harunganae madagascariensis folium leaf.

Scientific Names

Harungana madagascariensis, synonym Haronga madagascariensis.
Family: Clusiaceae/Guttiferae or Hypericaceae.

People Use This For

Orally, haronga is used for dyspepsia, mild exocrine pancreatic insufficiency, liver and gallbladder complaints, and loss of appetite.

Safety

POSSIBLY SAFE ...when used orally and appropriately (2). The recommended maximum safe duration of use is two months (2).
PREGNANCY AND LACTATION: Insufficient reliable information available; avoid using.

Effectiveness

There is insufficient reliable information available about the effectiveness of haronga.

Mechanism of Action

The applicable parts of haronga are the bark and leaf. Haronga can have gallbladder stimulating (2), liver protectant, pancreas stimulating, gastric juice secretion stimulating, and antimicrobial effects (18). It can also have possible anti-amoebic activity (1519).

Adverse Reactions

Photosensitivity is possible with the use of haronga, especially in fair-skinned people (2). Phototoxicity is theoretically possible with large doses (18).

Interactions with Herbs & Other Dietary Supplements

None known.

Interactions with Drugs

None known.

Interactions with Foods

None known.

Interactions with Lab Tests

None known.

Interactions with Diseases or Conditions

CONTRAINDICATIONS: The use of haronga is contraindicated in acute pancreatitis and exacerbations of chronic pancreatitis, severe liver dysfunction, gallstones, biliary obstruction, gallbladder empyema, or obstruction of the bowels (2,18).
FAIR-SKINNED INDIVIDUALS: Haronga can cause photosensitivity in fair-skinned individuals (2).

Dosage and Administration

ORAL: The typical dose of the haronga dry extract is 7.5-15 mg per day, which corresponds to 25-50 mg of the herb (2,18). The recommended maximum safe duration of use is two months (2).

HARTSTONGUE

Also Known As
Buttonhole, God's-Hair, Hind's Tongue, Horse Tongue.

Scientific Names
Asplenium scolopendrium, synonym Scolopendrium vulgare.
Family: Aspleniaceae.

Comments
At the date of publication, this product was not a common ingredient used in brand name supplements marketed to consumers. Details about this product are available at the online version of *Natural Medicines Comprehensive Database*. See www.naturaldatabase.com.

HAWAIIAN BABY WOODROSE

Also Known As
Baby Hawaiian Woodrose, Baby Woodrose, Elephant-Climber, Elephant Creeper, Silver-Morning-Glory, Vidhara, Vriddadaru, Wood-Rose, Woolly Morning Glory.

Scientific Names
Argyreia nervosa, synonyms, Argyreia speciosa, Convolvulus nervosus, Convolvulus speciosus, Lettsomia nervosa.
Family: Convolvulaceae.

People Use This For
Orally, Hawaiian baby woodrose is used for pain relief, promoting sweating, for sacramental rituals, and as a hallucinogen.

Safety
LIKELY UNSAFE ...when used orally (17,5301). The seeds of Hawaiian baby woodrose have effects similar to the hallucinogen lysergic acid diethylamide (LSD), including flashbacks (5301).
PREGNANCY AND LACTATION: LIKELY UNSAFE ...when used orally (17,5301); avoid using.

Effectiveness
There is insufficient reliable information available about the effectiveness of Hawaiian baby woodrose.

Mechanism of Action
The applicable part of Hawaiian baby woodrose is the seeds. Hawaiian baby woodrose, an ornamental plant, has seeds that contain hallucinogens including ergonovine, isoergine (isolysergic acid amide), and ergine (lysergic acid amide) (17,5301,5304). Four to eight seeds are equivalent to 10 to 100 mcg of lysergic acid diethylamide (LSD) (5301), a potent serotonin-1A (5-HT1A) agonist (17). The hallucinatory effects of Hawaiian baby woodrose are similar to alcohol intoxication with psychedelic visual effects such as enhanced colors. The effects last 6-8 hours (5301,5304).

Adverse Reactions
Orally, ingestion can cause nausea and vomiting, dizziness, auditory hallucinations, blurred vision, dilated pupils, involuntary, rapid, rhythmic movement of eyeballs, sweating, fast heart rate, and hypertension (5301).

Interactions with Herbs & Other Dietary Supplements
ST. JOHN'S WORT: Theoretically, Hawaiian baby woodrose might increase the effects and adverse effects of products that increase serotonin levels, including St. John's wort (17).

Interactions with Drugs
ANTIDEPRESSANT DRUGS: Theoretically, because Hawaiian baby woodrose contains chemicals related to LSD, it might interact with drugs that increase serotonin including sertraline (Zoloft), paroxetine (Paxil), fluoxetine (Prozac), and other antidepressants. Seizures have occurred in people taking the related compound, LSD, with fluoxetine (Prozac) (17). Individuals who have previously used LSD have developed flashbacks and hallucinations when treated with serotonin reuptake inhibitors (17). Combining serotonergic antidepressants with Hawaiian baby woodrose might increase the risk of serotonergic side effects including serotonin syndrome and cerebral vasoconstrictive disorders such as Call-Fleming syndrome (8056).
CLOZAPINE (Clozaril): Theoretically, because selective 5-HT2 receptor antagonists such as clozapine antagonize the effect of LSD, they might also decrease the effect of Hawaiian baby woodrose (17).

CYPROHEPTADINE: Theoretically, because selective 5-HT2 receptor antagonists such as cyproheptadine antagonize the effect of LSD, they might also decrease the effect of Hawaiian baby woodrose (17).
DEXTROMETHORPHAN (Robitussin DM, and others): Theoretically, concurrent use might cause additive serotonergenic effects and increase the risk of serotonin syndrome. Also, concurrent use might also cause cerebral vasoconstriction disorders such as Call-Fleming syndrome (8056).
MEPERIDINE (Demerol): Combining serotonergic drugs such as meperidine with Hawaiian baby woodrose might increase the risk of serotonergic side effects including serotonin syndrome and cerebral vasoconstrictive disorders such as Call-Fleming syndrome (8056).
MONOAMINE OXIDASE INHIBITORS (MAOIs): Combining serotonergic drugs such as one of the MAOIs with Hawaiian baby woodrose might increase the risk of serotonergic side effects including serotonin syndrome and cerebral vasoconstrictive disorders such as Call-Fleming syndrome (8056).
PENTAZOCINE (Talwin): Combining serotonergic drugs such as pentazocin with Hawaiian baby woodrose might increase the risk of serotonergic side effects including serotonin syndrome and cerebral vasoconstrictive disorders such as Call-Fleming syndrome (8056).
RISPERIDONE (Risperdal): Theoretically, because selective 5-HT2 receptor antagonists such as risperidone antagonize the effect of LSD, they might also decrease the effect of Hawaiian baby woodrose (17).
TRAMADOL (Ultram): Combining serotonergic drugs such as tramadol with Hawaiian baby woodrose might increase the risk of serotonergic side effects including serotonin syndrome and cerebral vasoconstrictive disorders such as Call-Fleming syndrome (8056).

Interactions with Foods
None known.

Interactions with Lab Tests
None known.

Interactions with Diseases or Conditions
PSYCHOSIS: Theoretically, because Hawaiian baby woodrose has effects similar to LSD, individuals with psychotic tendencies might experience prolonged psychotic reactions (17).

Dosage and Administration
No typical dosage.

Comments
Hawaiian baby woodrose is likely unsafe for oral use; avoid using. Hawaiian baby woodrose, a relative of the morning glory, grows in Florida, California, and Hawaii (17). Touted as a "natural LSD" in Internet advertising, the seeds are legal, and easily purchased from Internet sources (5301).

HAWTHORN

Also Known As
Aubepine, Bianco spino, Crataegi Flos, Crataegi Folium, Crataegi Folium Cum Flore, Crataegi Fructus, English Hawthorn, Epine Blanche, Epine de Mai, Haagdorn, Hagedorn, Harthorne, Haw, Hawthorn Extract, Hawthorn Flower, Hawthorn Fruit, Hawthorn Leaf, Hawthorne, Hedgethorn, LI 132, LI132, May, Maybush, Maythorn, Mehlbeebaum, Meidorn, Nan Shanzha, Oneseed Hawthorn, Shanzha, Weissdorn, Whitehorn, WS 1442, WS1442.

Scientific Names
Crataegus monogyna; Crataegus laevigata, synonyms Crataegus oxyacantha, Mespilus laevigata; Crataegus cuneata, synonym Crataegus kulingensis; Crataegus pinnatifida.
Family: Rosaceae.

People Use This For
Orally, hawthorn is used for cardiovascular conditions such as congestive heart failure (CHF), coronary circulation problems, and arrhythmias. It is also used to increase cardiac output reduced by hypertension or pulmonary disease, to treat both hypotension and hypertension, atherosclerosis, hyperlipidemia, and Buerger's disease. Hawthorn is also used as a sedative, antispasmodic, astringent, and diuretic. It is also used for gastrointestinal conditions such as indigestion, enteritis, epigastric distension, diarrhea, and abdominal pain. Hawthorn fruit is also used orally to treat tapeworm infections, acute bacillary dysentery, and amenorrhea.
Topically, hawthorn leaf is used as a poultice for boils, sores, and ulcers. Hawthorn fruit preparations are used as a wash for sores, itching, and frost bite.
In manufacturing, hawthorn fruit is used for making candied fruit slices, jam, jelly, and wine.

Safety

POSSIBLY SAFE ...when used orally and appropriately, short-term. Hawthorn preparations seem to be safe when used for up to 16 weeks. Although hawthorn might be safe for long-term use, current studies have not extended past 16 weeks (406,8279,8280,8281,10144).

There is insufficient reliable information about the safety of hawthorn for its other uses.

PREGNANCY: UNSAFE ...when used orally. Hawthorn has potential uterine activity (4).

LACTATION: Insufficient reliable information available; avoid using.

Effectiveness

POSSIBLY EFFECTIVE

Congestive heart failure (CHF). Taking hawthorn orally, as specific standardized leaf and flower extract (LI 132 or WS 1442), seems to improve ejection fraction, exercise tolerance, and reduce subjective symptoms associated with New York Heart Association stage II heart failure. Maximum effect is usually seen after 6-12 weeks of treatment with 240-600 mg per day of a standardized hawthorn extract (8279,8280,10144,11449). In addition, hawthorn extract WS 1442 combined with pre-existing diuretic therapy can improve exercise tolerance and reduce subjective symptoms associated with New York Heart Association stage III heart failure. Maximum effect is usually seen after 16 weeks of combined diuretic therapy and 1800 mg per day standardized hawthorn extract WS1442 (8281).

There is insufficient reliable information available about the effectiveness of hawthorn for its other uses.

Mechanism of Action

The applicable parts of hawthorn are the leaf, fruit, and flower. The constituents responsible for the pharmacological effects of hawthorn preparations include flavonoids and procyanidins. Other active compounds include the cardiac glycoside vitexin, and the flavonols rutin and hyperoside (406). Hawthorn preparations act on the myocardium by increasing force of contraction and lengthening the refractory period (406,10144,11450), reducing peripheral vascular resistance (406), reducing oxygen consumption (406), and increasing nerve conductivity (406). Hawthorn's cardiotrophic properties are attributed to increased membrane permeability for calcium (150,11450), and phosphodiesterase inhibition, which increases intracellular cAMP. Increased cAMP leads to increased coronary blood flow, vasodilation, and positive inotropic effects (150,11450). Animal evidence suggests that hawthorn might have hypoglycemic activity in individuals with diabetes (11451). Hawthorn has been reported to decrease uterine tone and motility, and reduce lipid levels. It also has antibacterial, spasmolytic, and analgesic effects (11).

Adverse Reactions

Orally, hawthorn preparations can cause nausea, gastrointestinal complaints, fatigue, sweating, and a rash on hands. Hawthorn can also cause palpitations, headache, dizziness, vertigo, dyspnea, nosebleeds, sleeplessness, agitation, and circulatory disturbances (406,8281,10144).

Interactions with Herbs & Other Dietary Supplements

OTHER CARDIOACTIVE HERBS: Avoid concomitant use with other cardioactive herbs due to unpredictability of effects and adverse effects. Other cardioactive herbs include calamus, cereus, cola, coltsfoot, devil's claw, European mistletoe, fenugreek, fumitory, ginger, Panax ginseng, white horehound, mate, parsley, quassia, scotch broom flower, shepherd's purse, and wild carrot (4).

Interactions with Drugs

CALCIUM CHANNEL BLOCKERS: Using hawthorn with calcium channel blockers such as verapamil (Calan, Covera-HS, Verelan), nifedipine (Procardia), and diltiazem (Cardizem, Dilacor, Tiazac) might cause additive coronary vasodilatory effects (406).

CNS DEPRESSANTS: Concomitant use of hawthorn and CNS depressants might have additive depressant effects on the CNS (4,406).

DIGOXIN (Lanoxin): Concomitant use of hawthorn and digoxin might potentiate the effects of digoxin requiring digoxin dose reduction (12,406).

NITRATES: Using hawthorn with nitrates such as nitroglycerin (Nitro-Bid, Nitro-Dur, Nitrostat) and isosorbide (Imdur, Isordil, Sorbitrate) might cause additive coronary vasodilatory effects (406).

Interactions with Foods

None known.

Interactions with Lab Tests

None known.

Interactions with Diseases or Conditions

CARDIOVASCULAR CONDITIONS: Concomitant use of hawthorn with conventional cardiovascular drug therapy might potentiate or interfere with the treatment of these conditions (4,12).

Dosage and Administration
ORAL: For heart failure, standardized hawthorn leaf with flower extract (LI 132 or WS 1442) 160 to 1800 mg (3.5-39.6 mg of total flavonoids calculated as hyperoside or 30-338 mg of procyanidins) has been used in 2-3 divided doses daily (406,8279,8280,8281,10144,11449).

HAZELNUT

Also Known As
Aveleira, Avelinier, Avellano, Cobnut, Coudrier, European Filbert, European Hazel, Haselnuss, Haselstrauch, Hazel, Hazel Nut, Noisetier.

Scientific Names
Corylus avellana; Corylus heterophylla.
Family: Betulaceae or Corylaceae.

People Use This For
Orally, hazelnut oil is used to reduce cholesterol and as an antioxidant.
Hazelnuts are commonly consumed as food.

Safety
LIKELY SAFE ...when used in amounts commonly found in foods.
PREGNANCY AND LACTATION: LIKELY SAFE ...when used in amounts commonly found in foods. There is insufficient reliable information available about the safety of the use of hazelnut in larger amounts; avoid using.

Effectiveness
There is insufficient reliable information available about the effectiveness of hazelnut.

Mechanism of Action
Hazelnuts contain 54.6-63.2% oil, 14.3-18.2% protein, and 9.8%-13.2% fiber (5995). Preliminary information suggests hazelnut oil and beta-carotene together might increase aminopyrine-N-dimethylase activity in the cytochrome P-450 system (5599).

Adverse Reactions
Orally, hazelnut can cause an allergic reaction in sensitive individuals (5991). Hazelnut has been associated with exercise-induced anaphylactic reaction (5998) and one outbreak of botulism from contaminated yogurt (5999).

Interactions with Herbs & Other Dietary Supplements
None known.

Interactions with Drugs
None known.

Interactions with Foods
None known.

Interactions with Lab Tests
None known.

Interactions with Diseases or Conditions
CROSS-ALLERGENICITY:Hazelnut is believed to be cross reactive with peanuts (5991), mugwort pollen (5993), brazil nut (5994), birch pollen (5996), and macadamia nut (5997).

Dosage and Administration
No typical dosage.

HEART'S EASE

Also Known As
European Wild Pansy, Field Pansy, Hearts Ease, Heartsease, Johnny-Jump-Up, Ladies' Delight, Pansy, Pensee Sauvage, Viola, Violae Tricoloris Herba, Wild Pansy.

Scientific Names
Viola tricolor.
Family: Violaceae.

People Use This For
Orally, heart's ease is used for promoting metabolism, as a demulcent for respiratory disorders such as throat inflammation and whooping cough, and as a laxative.
Topically, heart's ease is used for mild seborrheic skin disorders, milk scall (seborrhea of the scalp) in children, warts, mild skin inflammation, acne, exanthema (skin eruption), eczema, impetigo, and itching of the female external genitalia.

Safety
POSSIBLY SAFE ...when orally and appropriately (12). ...when used topically and appropriately (12).
PREGNANCY AND LACTATION: Insufficient reliable information; avoid using.

Effectiveness
There is insufficient reliable information available about the effectiveness of heart's ease.

Mechanism of Action
The applicable parts of heart's ease are the above ground parts. Heart's ease can have anti-inflammatory and antioxidant properties (18).

Adverse Reactions
Orally, heart's ease has caused hemolysis in a nine-month-old infant with glucose-6-phosphate-dehydrogenase (G6PD) deficiency (11324).

Interactions with Herbs & Other Dietary Supplements
None known.

Interactions with Drugs
None known.

Interactions with Foods
None known.

Interactions with Lab Tests
None known.

Interactions with Diseases or Conditions
None known.

Dosage and Administration
ORAL: The typical dose of heart's ease is one cup of the tea three times per day (18). The tea is prepared by steeping 1.5 grams of the above ground parts in 150 mL boiling water for 5-10 minutes and then straining.
TOPICAL: Heart's ease is commonly applied externally three times per day as a poultice or the prepared tea (18).

Comments
Store heart's ease in a well-sealed container and away from light (18).

HEATHER

Also Known As
Callunae vulgaris herba, Calluna vulgaris flos, Ling, Scotch Heather.

Scientific Names
Calluna vulgaris, synonyms Erica vulgaris.
Family: Ericaceae.

People Use This For
Orally, heather is taken for ailments of the kidney and lower urinary tract, prostate enlargement, diuresis, gastrointestinal ailments and diseases, diarrhea, gastrointestinal spasm, colic, disease of the liver and gallbladder, gout, arthritis, sleep disorders, respiratory disorders, cough, colds, and diaphoresis.
Topically, heather is used for wounds and inflamed eyes.
In combination with other herbs, heather is used for diabetes, menstrual discomfort, menopause, stimulation of digestion, nervous exhaustion, and regulation of the circulatory system.

Safety
POSSIBLY SAFE ...when used orally or topically and appropriately (12).
PREGNANCY AND LACTATION: Insufficient reliable information available; avoid using.

Effectiveness
There is insufficient reliable information available about the effectiveness of heather.

Mechanism of Action
The applicable parts of heather are the flower, leaf, and plant top. There is insufficient reliable information available about the possible mechanism of action and active ingredients.

Adverse Reactions
None reported.

Interactions with Herbs & Other Dietary Supplements
None known.

Interactions with Drugs
None known.

Interactions with Foods
None known.

Interactions with Lab Tests
None known.

Interactions with Diseases or Conditions
None known.

Dosage and Administration
ORAL: A typical dosage is one cup of tea (simmer 1.5 grams of flower/leaf/plant top in 250 mL boiling water 3 minutes, strain) three times daily between meals (18).
TOPICAL: As a bath, 500 grams of flower/leaf/plant top has been used in a few liters of water; strain and add to full bath (18).

HEDGE-HYSSOP

Also Known As
Gratiola, Hedge Hyssop.

Scientific Names
Gratiola officinalis.
Family: Scrophulariaceae.

People Use This For
Orally, hedge-hyssop is used orally for treating the liver, as an emetic, and to induce bowel evacuation. It is also used in the elimination of intestinal parasites, and to increase urination.

Safety
UNSAFE ...when used orally (18).
PREGNANCY AND LACTATION: UNSAFE ...when used orally due to toxic potential (18).

Effectiveness
There is insufficient reliable information available about the effectiveness of hedge-hyssop.

Mechanism of Action
The applicable parts of hedge-hyssop are the above ground parts. Hedge-hyssop contains cucurbitacin glycosides which are released in aqueous environments and are extremely irritating to mucous membranes (18).

Adverse Reactions
Orally, taken in toxic doses, hedge-hyssop may cause vomiting, bloody diarrhea, colic, and kidney irritation characterized by initial diuresis followed by anuria. When people ingest very large amounts, spasms, paralysis, and circulatory collapse occur. Death occurs rarely (18).

Interactions with Herbs & Other Dietary Supplements
None known.

Interactions with Drugs
None known.

Interactions with Foods
None known.

Interactions with Lab Tests
None known.

Interactions with Diseases or Conditions
None known.

Dosage and Administration
No typical dosage.

Comments
Hedge-hyssop is considered unsafe for oral use; avoid using (18).

HEDGE MUSTARD

Also Known As
English Watercress, Erysimum, Singer's Plant, St. Barbara's Hedge Mustard, Thalictroc.
CAUTION: See separate listings for Black Mustard Oil, Black Mustard seed, and White Mustard.

Scientific Names
Sisymbrium officinale, synonym Erysimum officinale.
Family: Brassicaceae/Cruciferae.

People Use This For
Orally, hedge mustard is taken to treat urinary tract diseases, coughs, chronic bronchitis, and inflammation of the gallbladder.
Topically, hedge mustard is used as a gargle or mouthwash.

Safety
LIKELY UNSAFE ...when the flowering above ground parts are used orally since they contain cardioactive glycosides (18).
There is insufficient reliable information available about the safety of hedge mustard for its other uses.
PREGNANCY AND LACTATION: LIKELY UNSAFE ...when used orally; avoid using.

Effectiveness
There is insufficient reliable information available about the effectiveness of hedge mustard.

Mechanism of Action
The applicable parts of hedge mustard are the above ground parts. The foliage contains vitamin C and 0.05% cardenolides (cardioactive glycosides) including sinigrin and gluconapin. Hedge mustard also contains the volatile mustard oil allyl isothiocyanate and 3-butenylisothiocyanate (18).

Adverse Reactions
Theoretically, digitalis-like effects are possible (vomiting, diarrhea, headache, and cardiac rhythm disorders) (18).

Interactions with Herbs & Other Dietary Supplements
CARDIAC GLYCOSIDE-CONTAINING HERBS: Contraindicated, and concomitant use can increase the risk of cardiac glycoside toxicity. Cardiac glycoside-containing herbs include black hellebore, Canadian hemp root, digitalis leaf, figwort, lily of the valley root, motherwort, oleander leaf, pheasant's eye plant, pleurisy root, squill bulb leaf scale, strophanthus seed, and uzara (19).
LICORICE/HORSETAIL: Theoretically, overuse/misuse of licorice rhizome or horsetail plant with cardiac glycoside-containing herbs increases the risk of cardiac toxicity due to potassium depletion (19).
OTHER CARDIOACTIVE HERBS: Avoid concomitant use with other cardioactive herbs due to unpredictability of effects (4).
STIMULANT LAXATIVE HERBS: Theoretically, overuse or misuse of stimulant laxatives with cardiac glycoside-containing herbs increases the risk of cardiac toxicity due to potassium depletion (19).

Interactions with Drugs
DIGOXIN (Lanoxin): Contraindicated due to therapeutic duplication and an increased risk of cardiac glycoside toxicity (2).
DIURETIC DRUGS: Theoretically, concomitant use of potassium depleting diuretics and hedge mustard can increase the risk of cardiac glycoside toxicity due to potassium depletion (506). Some diuretics that can deplete potassium include chlorothiazide (Diuril), chlorthalidone (Thalitone), furosemide (Lasix), hydrochlorothiazide (HCTZ, HydroDIURIL, Microzide), and others.
MACROLIDE ANTIBIOTICS: Theoretically, concomitant use may increase risk of cardiac glycoside toxicity (17).
QUININE: Theoretically, concomitant use of hedge mustard with quinine may increase risk of cardiac toxicity (506).
STIMULANT LAXATIVES: Theoretically, overuse or misuse of stimulant laxatives may increase the risk of cardiac glycoside toxicity due to potassium depletion (2).
TETRACYCLINE ANTIBIOTICS: Theoretically, concomitant use with hedge mustard may increase risk of cardiac glycoside toxicity (17).

Interactions with Foods
None known.

Interactions with Lab Tests
None known.

Interactions with Diseases or Conditions
HEART DISEASE: Theoretically, cardiac glycosides contained in hedge mustard may exacerbate condition or interfere with existing drug therapy; contraindicated.

Dosage and Administration
ORAL: A typical dosage is one cup tea (preparation unspecified) 3-4 times daily (18); average amount is 0.5-1 grams above ground parts per day (18).
TOPICAL: Tea is commonly used as a mouthwash or gargle, several times daily (18).

Comments
Avoid confusion with black mustard (Brassica nigra) and white mustard (Sinapis alba).

HEMLOCK

Also Known As

California Fern, Carrot Weed, Conium, Conium maculata, Nebraska Fern, Poison Fool's Parsley, Poison-Hemlock, Spotted Hemlock, Wild Carrot.
CAUTION: See separate listings for Water Hemlock and Hemlock Water Dropwort.

Scientific Names

Conium maculatum.
Family: Apiaceae/Umbelliferae.

People Use This For

Orally, hemlock is used as a sedative, antispasmodic, and paralyzer. It is also used orally for nervous motor excitability, teething in children, cramps, spasms of the larynx and gullet, acute mania, bronchitis, whooping cough, asthma, and as an antidote to strychnine poisoning. It is also used orally for indolent tumors, swollen and painful joints, skin infections, epilepsy, Parkinson's disease, Sydenham's chorea, and acute cystitis.

Safety

UNSAFE ...when used orally (6338). All parts of hemlock including seeds, flowers, and fruits are considered poisonous (6338,6339). Death has resulted after ingestion of hemlock (6340). Prompt medical attention is advised after ingestion of hemlock (6341).
CHILDREN: UNSAFE ...when used orally (6340). Acute, sometimes lethal poisoning has resulted after ingestion of leaf material (6340) or when hollow stems are used as peashooters, flutes, or whistles (6338).
PREGNANCY AND LACTATION: UNSAFE ...when used orally because ingestion can be lethal (6338); avoid using.

Effectiveness

There is insufficient reliable information available about the effectiveness of hemlock.

Mechanism of Action

All plant parts of hemlock can cause toxicity. Coniceine and coniine are the alkaloids in hemlock which account for its toxicity (6338,6340,6341). The amount of poisonous alkaloids in hemlock increase as the plant and fruit ripens and is also dependent on the amount of solar exposure and soil moisture (6338). It is most toxic during early stages of growth in the spring (6338,6339). Green fruit contains larger amounts of toxic alkaloids than mature fruit and seeds. The amount of toxic alkaloids in hemlock decreases as the plant reaches maturity (6338). Coniine predominates in the plant during sunny dry weather. During cloudy and rainy weather, coniine and coniceine are produced in equal amounts in hemlock (6339). Coniceine predominates during early growth periods of hemlock and coniine predominates in mature hemlock plants and seeds (6339). The alkaloid's effects occur at the neuromuscular junction of the autonomic ganglia (6341), stimulating and then paralyzing nicotinic receptors (6340). Larger doses of the alkaloids produce narcotic-like depressant activity (6340). Death usually occurs by respiratory failure (6341).

Adverse Reactions

Orally, hemlock can cause salivation, drowsiness, mydriasis, muscle pain, rapid swelling and stiffening of muscles, tachycardia followed by bradycardia, loss of speech, paralysis, rhabdomyolysis, unconsciousness, cardiovascular collapse, and death (6340,6341). It also causes burning of the mouth, throat, and abdomen (6341).

Interactions with Herbs & Other Dietary Supplements

None known.

Interactions with Drugs

None known.

Interactions with Foods

None known.

Interactions with Lab Tests

None known.

Interactions with Diseases or Conditions

None known.

Dosage and Administration
No typical dosage.

Comments
Hemlock is native to Europe and western Asia and was introduced into North America as an ornamental plant (6338,6339,6341). It is frequently found in the United States and southern Canada (6338). Hemlock is found along fences, in modified soils, roadsides, ditches, abandoned construction sites, pastures, crops, and fields (6338,6341). Hemlock can remain in a vegetative state throughout the winter (6338,6339) and accidental ingestion occurs after mistaking the root for parsnip, leaves for parsley, and seeds for anise (6338,6344). Poisoning and death have been reported after human consumption of migratory wild birds that have eaten hemlock seeds (6338,6340).

HEMLOCK SPRUCE

Also Known As
Balm of Gilead Fir, Balsam Fir, Canada Balsam, Fir Tree, Norway Pine, Norway Spruce, Picea aetheroleum, Picea turiones recentes, Spruce, Spruce Fir.
CAUTION: See separate listings for Hemlock, Hemlock Water Dropwort, and Water Hemlock.

Scientific Names
Picea abies, synonym Picea excelsa, Pinus abies, Pinus viminalis; Abies excelsa.
Family: Pinaceae.

People Use This For
Orally, hemlock spruce is used for coughs, the common cold, bronchitis, fever, inflammation of the mouth and pharynx, muscular and nerve pain, arthritis, as an antibacterial, and for tuberculosis.
Topically, hemlock spruce is used for inflammation of the respiratory tract, arthritis pain, nerve pain, and for feelings of tension. It is also used topically as a counterirritant and to improve circulation, and as a bath additive for individuals who are mentally ill.

Safety
There is insufficient reliable information available about the safety of hemlock spruce.
Pregnancy and Lactation: Insufficient reliable information available; avoid using.

Effectiveness
There is insufficient reliable information available about the effectiveness of hemlock spruce.

Mechanism of Action
The applicable part of hemlock spruce is the oil obtained by steam distillation from the needles, branch tips or branches and the fresh fir shoots of Picea abies (18). There is insufficient reliable information available about the possible mechanism of action and active ingredients.

Adverse Reactions
None reported.

Interactions with Herbs & Other Dietary Supplements
None known.

Interactions with Drugs
None known.

Interactions with Foods
None known.

Interactions with Lab Tests
None known.

Interactions with Diseases or Conditions
ASTHMA and WHOOPING COUGH: Hemlock spruce may theoretically worsen asthma and whooping cough(18).
CARDIAC INSUFFICIENCY: Avoid using of hemlock spruce (18).
EXTENSIVE SKIN INJURIES, ACUTE SKIN DISEASES: Hemlock spruce should not be applied to broken skin (18).

Dosage and Administration

ORAL: The typical daily dose is 4 drops of oil on a lump of sugar taken three times daily. Alternately, 2 grams of oil can be added to hot water and inhaled several times daily (18).
TOPICAL: Hemlock spruce is used as a 10-50% semi-solid preparation. Several drops of this oil are rubbed into the affected area (18).

Comments

Hemlock spruce is very similar sounding to water hemlock and European water hemlock, which are entirely different plants. Be careful not to confuse hemlock spruce with either form of water hemlock, because the water hemlocks are very toxic (18).

HEMLOCK WATER DROPWORT

Also Known As

Dead Tongue, Five-Fingered Root, Horsebane, Yellow Water Dropwort.
CAUTION: See separate listings for Hemlock, Hemlock Spruce, and Water Hemlock.

Scientific Names

Oenanthe crocata.
Family: Apiaceae/Umbelliferae.

People Use This For

Topically, hemlock water dropwort is used as a poultice for skin eruptions.

Safety

UNSAFE ...when used orally (6334). Ingestion of very small amounts of root may be fatal (6335,6337). Accidental ingestion requires prompt medical attention (6334).
There is insufficient reliable information available about the safety of hemlock water dropwort when used topically.
CHILDREN: UNSAFE ...when used orally (6334). Poisoning has occurred after accidental ingestion of roots or tubers (6334).
PREGNANCY AND LACTATION: UNSAFE ...when used orally. Ingestion can be lethal (6334); avoid using.

Effectiveness

There is insufficient reliable information available about the effectiveness of hemlock water dropwort.

Mechanism of Action

The applicable part of hemlock water dropwort is the root. Oenanthetoxin, a highly unsaturated alcohol (6334), is the active principle toxin found in hemlock water dropwort (6332). The roots of hemlock water dropwort are considered to be the most poisonous part of the plant and the toxin is contained in a yellowish staining juice of the root (6334). The toxin is unstable when exposed to air and is chemically similar to cicutoxin found in water hemlock (Cicuta virosa) (6334). The exact mechanism of action of the toxin is unknown, but animal studies suggest that oenanthetoxin has an antagonizing effect on nerve impulses in the brain stem (6334).

Adverse Reactions

Orally, hemlock water dropwort can cause nausea, dizziness, (6334), abdominal pain (6335), vomiting, sweating (6332), salivation, weakness, confusion, slurred speech, muscle spasms, tonic-clonic movements, glycosuria, hematuria, hyperventilation, cyanosis, exhaustion (6334), seizures, metabolic acidosis (6335), generalized convulsions (6332), unconsciousness (6334), dilated pupils, and death (6332).

Interactions with Herbs & Other Dietary Supplements

None known.

Interactions with Drugs

None known.

Interactions with Foods

None known.

Interactions with Lab Tests

None known.

Interactions with Diseases or Conditions

None known.

Dosage and Administration

No typical dosage.

Comments

Hemlock water dropwort is commonly found in ditches, watering places, and marshy areas and banks (6334,6337). It is considered to be the most poisonous plant in the British Isles (6334). Hemlock water dropwort has been accidentally ingested after mistaking the tuber for wild parsnip, sweet flag, or pignut (6334,6337).

HEMP AGRIMONY

Also Known As

Alpenkraut, Chanvrin, Donnerkraut, Dostenkraut, Drachenkraut, Dutch Agrimony, Dutch Eupatoire Commune, Eupatorium, Gemeiner Wasswedost, Herbe de Sainte Cunegonde, Hirshklee, Holy Rope, Kunigundendraut, Leberkraut, Origan De Marais, St. John's Herb, Sweet Mandulin, Sweet-Smelling Trefoil, Thoroughwort, Wasshanf, Waterhemp, Water Maudlin.

Scientific Names

Eupatorium cannabinum.
Family: Asteraceae/Compositae.

People Use This For

Orally, hemp agrimony is used for liver and gallbladder disorders, colds, and fever.

Safety

LIKELY UNSAFE ...when used orally. Hemp agrimony contains hepatotoxic unsaturated pyrrolizidine alkaloids (UPAs) (12,19). Repeated exposure to low concentrations of UPAs are linked to veno-occlusive disease, a serious condition (4,12). UPAs may also be carcinogenic and mutagenic (12). ...when used topically on abraded or broken skin due to potential for systemic absorption (12,19).
PREGNANCY: UNSAFE ...when used orally due to possible menstrual stimulant and abortifacient activities (19); avoid using.
LACTATION: LIKELY UNSAFE ...when used orally due to concern that UPAs might be excreted into breast milk (19).

Effectiveness

There is insufficient reliable information available about the effectiveness of hemp agrimony.

Mechanism of Action

The applicable part of hemp agrimony is the flowering herb. Some pyrrolizidine alkaloids have shown carcinogenic and mutagenic properties, and there are reports of renal toxicity. However, the primary concern is veno-occlusive disease (12). Unsaturated pyrrolizidine alkaloids are known to be hepatotoxic in animals and humans (4).

Adverse Reactions

Orally, acute toxicity may result in hepatic necrosis; chronic toxicity may cause veno-occlusive liver disease. The potential for hepatotoxicity (due to presence of pyrrolizidine alkaloids) increases with larger doses and longer periods of use (4,12). It can cause an allergic reaction in individuals sensitive to the Asteraceae/Compositae family. Members of this family include ragweed, chrysanthemums, marigolds, daisies, and many other herbs.

Interactions with Herbs & Other Dietary Supplements

EUCALYPTUS: Theoretically, concomitant use might increase the risk of unsaturated pyrrolizidine alkaloid toxicity due to enzyme induction by eucalyptus (19).
PYRROLIZIDINE ALKALOID-CONTAINING HERBS: Concomitant use is contraindicated due to the risk of additive toxicity. Herbs containing unsaturated pyrrolizidine alkaloids include alkanna (12), borage (271), gravel root (4), hound's tongue (19), petasites (19), comfrey (271), coltsfoot, and the Senecio species plants; dusty miller (19), alpine ragwort (19), groundsel (271), golden ragwort (19), and tansy ragwort (271).

Interactions with Drugs

None known.

Interactions with Foods
None known.

Interactions with Lab Tests
None known.

Interactions with Diseases or Conditions
CROSS-ALLERGENICITY: Can cause an allergic reaction in individuals sensitive to the Asteraceae/Compositae family. Members of this family include ragweed, chrysanthemums, marigolds, daisies, and many other herbs.

Dosage and Administration
No typical dosage.

HEMPNETTLE

Also Known As
Galeopsidis Herba.

Scientific Names
Galeopsis segetum, synonym Galeopsis ochroleuca.
Family: Lamiaceae/Labiatae.

People Use This For
Orally, hempnettle is used for mild respiratory tract inflammation, cough, bronchitis, and as a diuretic.

Safety
POSSIBLY SAFE ...when used orally and appropriately (2).
PREGNANCY AND LACTATION: Insufficient reliable information available; avoid using.

Effectiveness
There is insufficient reliable information available about the effectiveness of hempnettle.

Mechanism of Action
The applicable parts of hempnettle are the above ground parts. Hempnettle can have astringent and expectorant effects (18).

Adverse Reactions
None reported.

Interactions with Herbs & Other Dietary Supplements
None known.

Interactions with Drugs
None known.

Interactions with Foods
None known.

Interactions with Lab Tests
None known.

Interactions with Diseases or Conditions
None known.

Dosage and Administration
ORAL: The typical dose of hempnettle is 6 grams of the above ground parts per day or one cup of the tea up to three times daily. The tea is prepared by steeping 2 grams of the above ground parts in 150 mL boiling water for 5-10 minutes and then straining (18). The use of hempnettle in children requires a dosing adjustment; however, no additional information is available on the exact dosing adjustments (510).

HENBANE

Also Known As
Devil's Eye, Fetid Nightshade, Hen Bell, Hog Bean, Hyoscyami Folium, Jupiter's Bean, Khurasani-Ajavayan, Parasigaya, Poison Tobacco, Stinking Nightshade.
CAUTION: See separate listings for Belladonna and Bittersweet Nightshade.

Scientific Names
Hyoscyamus niger.
Family: Solanaceae.

People Use This For
Orally, henbane leaf is used for spasms of the gastrointestinal tract.
Topically, henbane leaf oil is used for treating scar tissue.

Safety
POSSIBLY SAFE ...when the leaf is used orally and appropriately short-term under medical supervision (2). Henbane contains hyoscyamine and scopolamine alkaloids (2).
LIKELY UNSAFE ...when used orally for self-medication. Hyoscyamine and scopolamine have a narrow range of safe use. Excessive doses can cause poisoning and death (18).
There is insufficient reliable information available about the safety of henbane for its other uses.
PREGNANCY AND LACTATION: LIKELY UNSAFE ...when used orally because of its risk of poisoning (18).

Effectiveness
There is insufficient reliable information available about the effectiveness of henbane.

Mechanism of Action
The applicable part of henbane is the leaf. The alkaloid constituents, which include hyoscyamine and scopolamine, competitively inhibit acetylcholine, causing anticholinergic and parasympathetic effects (18). With storage, hyoscyamine converts to atropine. The inhibition of acetylcholine affects the muscarinic action but not the nicotinic effects of acetylcholine on ganglia and motor endplates. Henbane causes smooth muscle relaxation particularly in the GI tract, relieves muscle tremors of CNS origin, and has a sedative effect (2).

Adverse Reactions
Orally, henbane can cause dry mouth, red skin, constipation, overheating, reduced sweating, vision disturbances, tachycardia, and difficulty with urinating (2,18). Overdose poisoning symptoms include somnolence followed by CNS stimulation described as restlessness, hallucinations, delirium, and manic episodes followed by exhaustion and sleep. Henbane can cause death by asphyxiation (18).

Interactions with Herbs & Other Dietary Supplements
ANTICHOLINERGIC CONTAINING HERBS: Theoretically, concomitant use of henbane with other anticholinergic alkaloid-containing herbs, including belladonna, deadly nightshade, and jimson weed, can have additive therapeutic and adverse effects.

Interactions with Drugs
ANTICHOLINERGIC DRUGS: Concomitant use of henbane can have additive anticholinergic effects and adverse effects with amantadine, antihistamines, atropine, belladonna alkaloids, hyoscyamine, phenothiazines, procainamide, scopolamine, and tricyclic antidepressants (2).

Interactions with Foods
None known.

Interactions with Lab Tests
None known.

Interactions with Diseases or Conditions
CONGESTIVE HEART FAILURE (CHF): Contraindicated; henbane might cause tachycardia and exacerbate CHF due to its hyoscyamine (atropine) and scopolamine content (15).
CONSTIPATION: Contraindicated; henbane might cause constipation due to its hyoscyamine (atropine) and scopolamine content (15).
DOWN SYNDROME: Caution, patients with Down syndrome might be hypersensitive to the antimuscarinic effects (mydriasis, positive chronotropic heart effects, etc.) of hyoscyamine (atropine) and scopolamine contained

in henbane (15).
ESOPHAGEAL REFLUX: Contraindicated; henbane might delay gastric emptying and decrease lower esophageal pressure, promoting gastric retention and exacerbating reflux due to its hyoscyamine (atropine) and scopolamine content (15).
FEVER: Contraindicated; henbane might increase the risk of hyperthermia in patients with fever due to its hyoscyamine (atropine) and scopolamine content (15).
GASTRIC ULCER: Contraindicated; henbane might delay gastric emptying and exacerbate gastric ulcers due to its hyoscyamine (atropine) and scopolamine content (15).
GI INFECTIONS: Contraindicated; henbane might suppress GI motility causing retention of infecting organisms or toxins due to its hyoscyamine (atropine) and scopolamine content (15).
HIATAL HERNIA: Contraindicated; henbane might delay gastric emptying and decrease lower esophageal pressure, promoting gastric retention and exacerbating hiatal hernia due to its hyoscyamine (atropine) and scopolamine content (15).
NARROW-ANGLE GLAUCOMA: Contraindicated; henbane might increase ocular tension in patients with narrow-angle (angle-closure) glaucoma due to its hyoscyamine (atropine) and scopolamine content (2,15).
OBSTRUCTIVE GI TRACT DISEASE: Contraindicated; henbane might exacerbate obstructive GI tract diseases (including atony, paralytic ileus, and stenosis) due to its hyoscyamine (atropine) and scopolamine content (15).
TACHYARRHYTHMIAS: Contraindicated; henbane might cause tachycardia due to its hyoscyamine (atropine) and scopolamine content (2,15).
TOXIC MEGACOLON: Contraindicated; henbane might suppress intestinal motility, which might produce paralytic ileus and exacerbate toxic megacolon, due to its hyoscyamine (atropine) and scopolamine content (2,15).
ULCERATIVE COLITIS: Contraindicated; henbane might suppress intestinal motility, which might produce paralytic ileus and precipitate toxic megacolon, due to its hyoscyamine (atropine) and scopolamine content (15).
URINARY RETENTION: Contraindicated; henbane might increase urinary retention due to its hyoscyamine (atropine) and scopolamine content (2,15).

Dosage and Administration

ORAL: The average single dose of the standardized henbane powder is 500 mg, which corresponds to 250-350 mg of the total alkaloid (2). The maximum single dose of henbane is 1 gram, which corresponds to 500-700 mg of the total alkaloid (2). The maximum daily dosage is 3 grams, which corresponds to 1.5-2.1 grams of the total alkaloid calculated as hyoscyamine (2).
TOPICAL: No typical dosage.

Comments

Avoid confusion with bittersweet nightshade (Solanum dulcamara) and belladonna (deadly nightshade). The flowering branches, dried seeds, and whole, fresh flowering plant of henbane may have medicinal uses (18).

HENNA

Also Known As

Alcanna, Egyptian Privet, Hennae folium, Henne, Jamaica Mignonette, Mehndi, Mendee, Mignonette Tree, Reseda, Smooth Lawsonia.
CAUTION: See separate listing for Alkanna (Alkanna tinctoria).

Scientific Names

Lawsonia inermis, synonym Lawsonia alba.
Family: Lythraceae.

People Use This For

Orally, henna is used for gastrointestinal ulcers.
Topically, henna is used for dandruff, eczema, scabies, fungal infections, and ulcers. It is also used topically for applying decorative henna "tattoos."
Traditionally, henna has been used for amebic dysentery, cancer, enlarged spleen, headache, jaundice, and skin conditions.
In manufacturing, henna is used in cosmetics; hair dyes and hair care products; and as a dye for nails, hands, and clothing. Lawsone, a constituent, can be used as an indicator for titration of strong acids with weak bases.

Safety

LIKELY SAFE ...when the leaf is applied topically. It is approved for topical use as a color additive in hair cosmetics in the US (11). However, contact dermatitis and hypersensitivity reactions have been reported with topical use (1370,4146,4148,6144,6145,6146,6147,6148,6149,6150,6151).
UNSAFE ...when used orally (12).

CHILDREN: POSSIBLY UNSAFE ...when applied topically on children, and especially on infants (4147,6144,6149,6150,10381). Use is associated with hemolysis in infants deficient in glucose-6-phosphate dehydrogenase (G6PD) (4147,10381). UNSAFE ...when used orally (12).
PREGNANCY: UNSAFE ...when used orally. Henna is believed to have abortifacient properties (12).
LACTATION: UNSAFE ...when used orally (12).

Effectiveness

There is insufficient reliable information available about the effectiveness of henna.

Mechanism of Action

The applicable part of henna is the leaf. Henna leaf contains lawsone, gallic acid, and 5-10% tannin (11). It is thought to have astringent and diuretic properties (18). Some evidence suggests henna might have activity against Mycobacterium tuberculosis (4150). In female rats, henna leaves inhibit fertility (11). The constituents, lawsone and gallic acid, have antibacterial properties (11). Studies suggest that lawsone might also have antifungal, antitumor, antispasmodic and weak vitamin K activity (11). Evidence shows it might be able to decrease the formation of sickled cells in individuals with sickle cell anemia (4149). An ethanol extract containing luteolin, beta-sitosterol, and lawsone was claimed to have anti-inflammatory, antihyaluronidase, and analgesic activity (11).

Adverse Reactions

Orally, henna can cause an upset stomach, possibly due to tannin content (18).
Topically, henna can cause contact dermatitis, including redness, itching, burning, swelling, scaling, fissuring, papules, blisters, and scarring (1370,4146,6144,6145,6146,6147,6148,6149,6150). There are two reports of occupational exposure associated with immediate-type hypersensitivity involving urticaria, rhinitis, wheezing, and bronchial asthma (4148,6151). In infants with glucose 6-phosphate dehydrogenase (G6PD) deficiency, topical henna use has been associated with hemolysis, anemia, reticulocytosis, and indirect hyperbilirubinemia (4147,10381). Prolonged use on hair may turn the hair orange-red, unless mixed with other dyes to get different shades (11).

Interactions with Herbs & Other Dietary Supplements

None known.

Interactions with Drugs

None known.

Interactions with Foods

None known.

Interactions with Lab Tests

None known.

Interactions with Diseases or Conditions

GLUCOSE-6-PHOSPHATE DEHYDROGENASE (G6PD) DEFICIENCY: There are reports of hemolysis in infants with G6PD deficiency after topical exposure to henna (4147,10381).
HENNA HYPERSENSITIVITY: Avoid topical exposure by individuals with henna hypersensitivity.

Dosage and Administration

No typical dosage.

Comments

Henna should not be confused with henna root (Alkanna tinctoria), also referred to as alkanna root (6).

HERB PARIS

Also Known As

Einbeere, Herb-Paris, One Berry, Oneberry, Tilki Uzumu, Uva De Raposa, Wang Sun.

Scientific Names

Paris quadrifolia.
Family: Trilliaceae.

People Use This For

Traditionally, Herb Paris is used for headache; longevity; neuralgia; rheumatism; genital tumors; palpitation; spasms; and as an emetic, narcotic, poison, and purgative.

Safety
LIKELY UNSAFE ...when used orally. The plant and berry are poisonous (18).
PREGNANCY AND LACTATION: UNSAFE ...when used orally (18).

Effectiveness
There is insufficient reliable information available about the effectiveness of Herb Paris.

Mechanism of Action
The applicable part of Herb Paris is the whole plant with ripe fruit. Herb Paris contains triterpene saponins (pennogenintetra glycosides), also referred to as parissaponins, which cause local irritation, increasing absorption of the toxic constituent, paristyphnin (18). Paristyphnin causes miosis and respiratory paralysis (18).

Adverse Reactions
Orally, Herb Paris can cause nausea, vomiting, diarrhea, headache, miosis, and respiratory paralysis (18).

Interactions with Herbs & Other Dietary Supplements
None known.

Interactions with Drugs
None known.

Interactions with Foods
None known.

Interactions with Lab Tests
None known.

Interactions with Diseases or Conditions
None known.

Dosage and Administration
No typical dosage.

HERB ROBERT

Also Known As
Dragon's Blood, Mountain Geranium, Stinky Bob, Storkbill, Wild Crane's-Bill.
CAUTION: See separate listings for Dragon's Blood (Daemonorops draco) and Sangre de Grado.

Scientific Names
Geranium robertianum.
Family: Geraniaceae.

People Use This For
Orally, Herb Robert is used for diarrhea; to improve functioning of the liver and gallbladder; to reduce inflammation of the kidney, bladder, and gallbladder; and to prevent the formation of calculi.
Topically, Herb Robert is used as a mouthwash or gargle. The fresh leaves are chewed to relieve inflammation of the mouth and throat.

Safety
There is insufficient reliable information available about the safety of Herb Robert.
Pregnancy and Lactation: Insufficient reliable information is available; avoid using.

Effectiveness
There is insufficient reliable information available about the effectiveness of Herb Robert.

Mechanism of Action
The applicable parts of Herb Robert are the above ground parts. Herb Robert contains several flavonoids including rutin. Some evidence suggests an ethanolic extract can inhibit the growth of E. coli, P. aeruginosa, and S. aureus. Other evidence indicates the extract of the fresh herb, including the root, has a mild antiviral effect against the vesicular stomatitis virus (18). Although general reviews report Herb Robert has hypotensive

effects, no specific information is available (18). Some data show a crystalline fraction can protect the tobacco plant from pathogenic viruses (18).

Adverse Reactions
None reported.

Interactions with Herbs & Other Dietary Supplements
None known.

Interactions with Drugs
None known.

Interactions with Foods
None known.

Interactions with Lab Tests
None known.

Interactions with Diseases or Conditions
None known.

Dosage and Administration
ORAL: Herb Robert is used as tea, 2 to 3 cups daily between meals (18). To make tea, 1 teaspoon of herb is added to 500 mL of cold water, brought to a boil, allowed to draw, and strained.
TOPICAL: The prepared tea is used as mouthwash or gargle (18). Fresh leaves are chewed to relieve mouth or throat inflammation (18).

Comments
Herb Robert is characterized by an unpleasant smell of goats or bugs (18).

HESPERIDIN

Also Known As
Citrus Bioflavonoid, Citrus Bioflavonoids, Flavonoid.
CAUTION: See separate listings for Chrysin, Diosmin, Methoxylated Flavones, Quercetin, Rue, and Rutin.

Scientific Names
Hesperidin.

People Use This For
Orally, hesperidin is used for treating acute internal hemorrhoids, preventing relapse of acute internal hemorrhoids, lymphedema following breast cancer surgery, and for treating varicose veins and venous stasis.

Safety
POSSIBLY SAFE ...when used orally and appropriately, short-term. Hesperidin seems to be safe when used for up to 6 months (4861,10227,10229). There is insufficient reliable information available about the safety of hesperidin when used for longer than 6 months.
PREGNANCY AND LACTATION: Insufficient reliable information available; avoid using.

Effectiveness
POSSIBLY EFFECTIVE

Internal hemorrhoids. The combination of hesperidin 150 mg plus diosmin 1350 mg twice daily for 4 days, followed by hesperidin 100 mg and diosmin 900 mg twice daily for 3 days, seems to significantly improve signs and symptoms of internal hemorrhoids. The combination can stop acute bleeding in up to 92% of patients after 4 days of treatment. It can also reduce symptoms such as anal discomfort, pain, discharge, and local lesions. Subjective symptoms can be relieved within 2 days of treatment. The combination also seems to reduce the duration and intensity of hemorrhoidal flare-ups (4861,4900). Maintenance use of hesperidin 50 mg plus diosmin 450 mg twice daily for 3 months in patients following acute treatment for hemorrhoids seems to significantly decrease the relapse rate (4861).

Venous stasis ulcers. Hesperidin, in combination with diosmin and compression dressing, seems to improve healing of venous stasis ulcers less than 10 cm in size (10229).

POSSIBLY INEFFECTIVE

Lymphedema. Hesperidin, in combination with diosmin, may improve drainage of lymph from the arms of women after breast cancer surgery, but it does not reduce arm swelling or other clinical signs of lymphedema (10227).

Clinical trials have used specific brand name formulations of hesperidin (Daflon 500, Les Laboratoires Servier, France). Each tablet of Daflon 500 contains hesperidin 50 mg and a micronized formulation of diosmin 450 mg extracted from rutaceae species.

There is insufficient reliable information available about the effectiveness of hesperidin for its other uses.

Mechanism of Action

Hesperidin is one of over 4,000 flavonoids found in plants (4919,4959,5006). Hesperidin is in a class of flavonoids primarily derived from citrus fruits and is known as a citrus bioflavonoid. It is closely related to other citrus bioflavonoids such as quercetin, rutin, and diosmin. Hesperidin alone, or in combination with other citrus bioflavonoids, is most often used for vascular conditions such as hemorrhoids and varicose veins. Hesperidin seems to work by improving venous tone, reducing stasis, restoring normal capillary permeability, and improving lymphatic drainage. Hesperidin might improve venous tone and reduce stasis by improving vasculature response to adrenergic stimulation. Hesperidin's anti-inflammatory effects seem to help restore normal capillary permeability. Hesperidin inhibits phosphodiesterase and increases intracellular cyclic adenosine monophosphate (cAMP), which causes decreased production of inflammatory prostaglandins E2 and F2 and thromboxane B2. Hesperidin's analgesic effect seems to work through peripheral rather than central mechanisms. Hesperidin can also reduce the generation of free radicals and inhibit tumor growth (4861,4900,4919,4956).

Adverse Reactions

Orally, hesperidin can cause gastrointestinal side effects, including abdominal pain, diarrhea, and gastritis. Headache can also occur in some patients (4861,4900).

Interactions with Herbs & Other Dietary Supplements

None known.

Interactions with Drugs

None known.

Interactions with Foods

None known.

Interactions with Lab Tests

None known.

Interactions with Diseases or Conditions

None known.

Dosage and Administration

ORAL: For the treatment of internal hemorrhoids, hesperidin 150 mg plus diosmin 1350 mg twice daily for 4 days, followed by hesperidin 100 mg and diosmin 900 mg twice daily for 3 days, has been used (4861,4900). For prevention of relapse internal hemorrhoids, hesperidin 50 mg plus diosmin 450 mg twice daily for 3 months of therapy has been used (4861). For the treatment of venous stasis ulcers, a combination of 100 mg hesperidin and 900 mg diosmin daily has been used for up to 2 months (10229). For treating lymphedema following surgery for breast cancer, a combination of 100 mg hesperidin and 900 mg diosmin daily has been used for up to 6 months (10227).

HIBISCUS

Also Known As

Guinea Sorrel, Jamaica Sorrel, Karkade, Red Tea, Roselle, Sudanese Tea.

Scientific Names

Hibiscus sabdariffa.
Family: Malvaceae.

People Use This For

Orally, hibiscus is used for loss of appetite, colds, upper respiratory tract and stomach mucous membrane inflammation, disorders of circulation, for dissolving phlegm, and as a gentle laxative and diuretic. Historically, hibiscus was used for treating heart and nerve diseases.

In foods and beverages, hibiscus is used as a flavoring. It is also used to improve the odor, flavor, or appearance of tea mixtures.

Safety

LIKELY SAFE ...when used orally in amounts commonly found in foods. Hibiscus has Generally Recognized As Safe (GRAS) status in the US (4912).
POSSIBLY SAFE ...when used orally in medicinal amounts (2,12); there are no known risks (2).
PREGNANCY: LIKELY UNSAFE ...when used orally. Hibiscus is thought to be a menstrual stimulant, and might have abortifacient effects (19).
LACTATION: Insufficient reliable information available; avoid using.

Effectiveness

There is insufficient reliable information available about the effectiveness of hibiscus.

Mechanism of Action

The applicable part of hibiscus is the flower and calyx. People think the laxative effects of hibiscus are due to high content of poorly absorbable fruit acids (18). Extracts have intestinal and uterine muscle antispasmodic activity (11,18), hypotensive effects (11,18), anthelmintic properties (11), and in vitro antibacterial activity (11).

Adverse Reactions

None reported.

Interactions with Herbs & Other Dietary Supplements

None known.

Interactions with Drugs

None known.

Interactions with Foods

None known.

Interactions with Lab Tests

None known.

Interactions with Diseases or Conditions

None known.

Dosage and Administration

ORAL: To prepare tea, steep 1.5 grams of flowers in 150 mL boiling water 5-10 minutes, strain (18).

HISTIDINE

Also Known As

Levo-Histidine, L-Histidine.

Scientific Names

L-2-Amino-3-(1H-imidazol-4-yl) propionic acid; alpha-amino-4-imidazole propanoic acid.

People Use This For

Orally, histidine is used for rheumatoid arthritis, allergic diseases, ulcers, and anemia.

Safety

POSSIBLY SAFE ...when used orally and appropriately. Clinical studies note the absence of side effects at doses up to 4 grams per day (2347,2353).
PREGNANCY AND LACTATION: Insufficient reliable information available; avoid using.

Effectiveness

POSSIBLY INEFFECTIVE

Anemia. Taking histidine orally doesn't seem to be effective for treating anemia of uremia or anemia associated with chronic dialysis (2352,2353).

Rheumatoid arthritis (RA). Taking histidine orally doesn't seem to be effective for treating RA (2350,2351).

There is insufficient reliable information available about the effectiveness of histidine for its other uses.

Mechanism of Action
Histidine is an essential amino acid involved in a wide range of metabolic processes (2354).

Adverse Reactions
None reported.

Interactions with Herbs & Other Dietary Supplements
None known.

Interactions with Drugs
None known.

Interactions with Foods
None known.

Interactions with Lab Tests
URINE FORMIMINOGLUTAMIC ACID (FIGLU): Use of histidine in people with folic acid deficiency can cause accumulation of the metabolite formiminoglutamic (2355).

Interactions with Diseases or Conditions
FOLIC ACID DEFICIENCY: Use of histidine in individuals with folic acid deficiency can cause accumulation of the metabolite formiminoglutamic acid (FIGLU) (2355).

Dosage and Administration
ORAL: For rheumatoid arthritis, the usual dose of histidine is 3.7-4.5 grams daily (2347,2350,2351). For anemia of uremia or anemia associated with maintenance dialysis, the typical dose is 1-4 grams daily (2352,2353).

HOLLY

Also Known As
Christ's Thorn, Holm, Holme Chase, Holy Tree, Hulm, Hulver Bush, Hulver Tree.

Scientific Names
Ilex aquifolium; Ilex opaca; Ilex vomitoria.
Family: Aquifoliaceae.

People Use This For
Orally, preparations of holly leaf are used as a diuretic, for coughs, digestive disorders, and jaundice. Ilex aquifolium leaves are used orally for treating intermittent fevers and rheumatism, as an antipyretic, astringent, diuretic, and expectorant. Ilex opaca leaves are used as a diuretic, tonic, purgative, and cardiac stimulant. Other Ilex species are used for treating coronary heart disease, dizziness, and hypertension.
Historically, Ilex opaca fruit tea was used as a cardiac stimulant by American Indians. Ilex vomitoria was used as an emetic, and Youpon tea (mixed leaves of Ilex cassine, Ilex vomitoria, and Ilex dahoon) was used as a ceremonial "cleanser" in South America.

Safety
UNSAFE ...when the berries are ingested. Eating berries can be fatal (18).
There is insufficient reliable information available about the safety of holly leaves.
CHILDREN: UNSAFE ...when the berries are ingested. Eating berries can be fatal (6).
PREGNANCY AND LACTATION: UNSAFE ...when berries are ingested (6). There is insufficient reliable information available about the safety of holly leaves; avoid using.

Effectiveness
There is insufficient reliable information available about the effectiveness of holly.

Mechanism of Action
The applicable parts of holly are the leaf and berry. The constituent saponins are thought to cause GI irritation and emetic effects (6). Holly also contains a cyanogenic glycoside (4).

Adverse Reactions
Orally, ingestion of the leaf can cause GI irritation, diarrhea, nausea, and vomiting (6,18). Leaf spines may tear or puncture skin or mucous membranes (6). Ingestion of as few as 2 berries can cause vomiting and diarrhea in small children (6). Ingestion of more than 5 berries can cause nausea, vomiting, diarrhea, and stupor (6,18). Ingestion of 20-30 berries can cause death (18).

Interactions with Herbs & Other Dietary Supplements
None known.

Interactions with Drugs
None known.

Interactions with Foods
None known.

Interactions with Lab Tests
None known.

Interactions with Diseases or Conditions
DEHYDRATION: In addition to toxic effects, berry ingestion may cause or exacerbate dehydration by inducing vomiting and diarrhea (6).
ELECTROLYTE IMBALANCE: Berry ingestion may cause or exacerbate electrolyte imbalance by inducing vomiting and diarrhea (6).

Dosage and Administration
ORAL: People typically use 3.9 grams of powdered leaves in a tea, taken to reduce the effects of intermittent fevers (5254).

Comments
Many other Ilex species are referred to as holly. English holly, Oregon holly, American holly are used as ornamental Christmas holly (6). Yaupon, Appalachian tea, cassena, deer berry, Indian holly and Indian black drink may be included in discussions of holly (6). Leaf spines may tear or puncture skin or mucous membranes (6).

HOLLYHOCK

Also Known As
Althea Rose, Hollyhock Flower, Malvae arboreae flos, Malva, Malva Flower, Rose Mallow.

Scientific Names
Alcea rosea, synonym Althaea rosea, Althaea ficifolia.
Family: Malvaceae.

Comments
At the date of publication, there was very little scientific information about this product. Our staff is continually analyzing the available information on natural medicines and will add data to the online version of *Natural Medicines Comprehensive Database* as it becomes available. See www.naturaldatabase.com.

HONEY

Also Known As
Clarified Honey, Honig, Mel, Miel Blanc, Purified Honey, Strained Honey.
CAUTION: See separate listings for Bee Pollen, Bee Venom, and Royal Jelly.

Scientific Names
Apis mellifera (honey bee).
Family: Apidae.

People Use This For

Orally, honey is used for cough, asthma, and as an expectorant. It is also used orally for diarrhea and gastric ulcer associated with Helicobacter pylori. Honey is also used orally as a source of carbohydrate during vigorous exercise.
Topically, honey is used to speed healing in mild sores, wounds, skin ulcerations, and burns; and for treating cataracts and postherpetic corneal opacities.
In foods, honey is used as a sweetening agent.
In manufacturing, honey is used as a fragrance and a moisturizer in soaps and cosmetics.

Safety

POSSIBLY SAFE ...when used topically (395,396,397,398,399,7847,7849).
CHILDREN: POSSIBLY UNSAFE ...when used orally in infants and young children. Ingestion of honey contaminated with Clostridium botulinum spores may cause botulism poisoning in infants and young children (6,11). This is not a danger for older children or adults.
PREGNANCY AND LACTATION: Insufficient reliable information.

Effectiveness

POSSIBLY EFFECTIVE

Burns. Honey applied directly in gauze applications seems to improve formation of granulation tissue and healing time in partial thickness burns. It appears to compare favorably with silver sulfadiazine and moisture permeable polyurethane dressing (OpSite) (395,396,397,398,399). However, surgical intervention with tangential excision and skin grafting is more effective than honey for moderate burns (7848).

Skin ulceration. Applying honey topically seems to improve healing of skin ulceration, wounds, and mild sores (7847,7849).

INSUFFICIENT RELIABLE EVIDENCE to RATE

Athletic performance. Some preliminary clinical evidence suggests that honey might normalize blood sugar following exercise and improve performance when given during exercise (7851). More evidence is needed to rate honey for this use.

Mechanism of Action

Honey is produced by bees (Apis mellifera) from the nectar of several varieties of plants. Pharmacological activity can vary depending on the type of plant from which the nectar is obtained. For example, honey produced from poisonous plants can be poisonous (6). Honey improves wound healing by promoting the formation of granulation tissue. It promotes the growth of epithelial cells by providing a barrier to moisture which helps keep the wound hydrated. Enzymes and hydrogen peroxide in honey can aid in debridement (395,396,399,7849). In surgery for some types of malignant cancer, cells from the tumor can become seeded in the wound margins during excision, resulting in growth of the cancer in the wound. Preliminary evidence indicates that honey can reduce the growth of these tumors, by impeding the seeding or inhibiting the growth of these cancer cells (7852).
Honey has antibacterial and antifungal activity, which might offer benefit in preventing wound infection and Helicobacter pylori infection in peptic ulcer disease. Honey inhibits the growth of Pseudomonas pyocyanea, Pseudomonas aeruginosa, Escherichia coli, Staphylococcus aureus, Proteus mirabilis, coliform species, Klebsiella species, Streptococcus faecalis, and Streptococcus pyogenes (7847,7849). Antibacterial peptides (apidaecins and abaecin) have been isolated in honeybees (6). The high osmolality, low pH, and hydrogen peroxide in honey also contribute to antimicrobial activity. High osmolality causes shrinkage of microbes, because of intracellular water loss. Hydrogen peroxide is formed by the action of glucose oxidase (396,1261,1428,7850).
Honey and solutions with similar sugar content (15% w/v) demonstrate similar effectiveness at inhibiting Helicobacter pylori (1428), and 2-4% v/v dilutions of various types of honey inhibit the growth of coagulase-positive Staphylococcus aureus isolated from infected wounds (1261).

Adverse Reactions

Orally, honey can cause allergic reactions. Some honey is contaminated with Clostridium botulinum spores, which poses a risk to infants, but not older children or adults (6,11). Botulinum spores can proliferate in the intestines of infants and cause botulism poisoning.
Topically, honey may cause excessive dryness of wounds, which could delay healing. This can be managed by application of saline packs as needed (7850).

Interactions with Herbs & Other Dietary Supplements

None known.

Interactions with Drugs

None known.

Interactions with Foods

None known.

Interactions with Lab Tests
None known.

Interactions with Diseases or Conditions
POLLEN ALLERGIES: Honey may cause allergic reactions (6).

Dosage and Administration
TOPICAL: For the treatment of burns, honey has been applied directly or as a dressing made from gauze impregnated with honey. The dressings have been left in place for up to 25 days, with wound inspection every 2 days (397,398). When used directly, 15 to 30 mL of honey has been applied every 1 to 2 days, and covered with a dry sterile gauze and bandage (396,399).

Comments
Avoid confusion with bee pollen, bee venom, and royal jelly. Honey for medicinal use should be collected from hives that are free from pathogens and not treated with antibiotics. The nectar should be from plants that have not been treated with pesticides (7847).

HONEYSUCKLE

Also Known As
Goat's Leaf, Honey Suckle, Japanese Honeysuckle, Jinyinhua, Lonicera, Madreselva, Nindo, Ren Dong, Suikazura, Woodbine.
CAUTION: See separate listings for American Ivy, Gelsemium, and Woodbine.

Scientific Names
Lonicera caprifolia; Lonicera japonica, synonym Lonicera aureoreticulata; and other Lonicera sp.
Family: Caprifoliaceae.

People Use This For
Orally, honeysuckle is used for digestive disorders, malignant tumors, and to promote sweating. It is also used orally as a laxative, for colds, fever, inflammation, swelling, boils, sores, and viral and bacterial infections.
Topically, honeysuckle is used for inflammation, itching, and as an astringent and antimicrobial.

Safety
There is insufficient reliable information available about the safety of honeysuckle.
Pregnancy and Lactation: Insufficient reliable information available; avoid using.

Effectiveness
There is insufficient reliable information available about the effectiveness of honeysuckle.

Mechanism of Action
The applicable parts of honeysuckle are the flower, seed, and leaf. In vitro data suggests antimicrobial activity against Staphylococcus aureus, Salmonella typhi, Mycobacterium tuberculosis, and bacilli which cause dysentery. It may also have antiviral activity against HIV and influenza virus. It is active, but less so, against dermatophytes. Animal data suggest anti-inflammatory effects, with possible increased resistance to infection, inhibited tumor formation, and decreased intestinal cholesterol absorption. Animal data also suggest that honeysuckle has stimulant effects at about one-sixth the activity of caffeine. Some of these biological activities are attributed to the saponin and chlorogenic acid content of honeysuckle. The LD50 of honeysuckle is low, approximately 53 g/kg when given subcutaneously to mice (11).

Adverse Reactions
Orally, honeysuckle may cause irritation of the gastrointestinal tract, kidneys, and urinary tract (18).

Interactions with Herbs & Other Dietary Supplements
None known.

Interactions with Drugs
None known.

Interactions with Foods
None known.

Interactions with Lab Tests
None known.

Interactions with Diseases or Conditions
None known.

Dosage and Administration
No typical dosage.

Comments
Avoid confusion with woodbine (Clematis virginiana). Also, avoid confusing honeysuckle with American ivy or gelsemium, which are also known as woodbine.

HOODIA

Also Known As
Hoodia Cactus, Hoodia Extract, Hoodia Gordonii Cactus, Hoodia P57, Kalahari Cactus, Kalahari Diet, P57, Xhoba.

Scientific Names
Hoodia gordonii.
Family: Apocynaceae.

People Use This For
Orally, hoodia is used as an appetite suppressant for obesity and weight loss.

Safety
There is insufficient reliable information available about the safety of hoodia.
Pregnancy and Lactation: Insufficient reliable information available; avoid using.

Effectiveness
There is insufficient reliable information available about the effectiveness of hoodia.

Mechanism of Action
The applicable parts of hoodia are the stems and roots. Hoodia is a cactus that grows in the Kalahari Desert. It is claimed that the San bushmen eat the cactus to stave off hunger during long hunts.
A specific component of hoodia extract is thought to be responsible for appetite suppressant properties. This constituent has been dubbed P57 (12002). This substance is thought to act centrally to stimulate sensations of satiety. The precise mechanism is not known.
Preliminary unpublished evidence suggests that overweight men who consume P57 have significantly lower calorie intake than those on placebo (12004). More evidence is needed to determine if hoodia is effective for any clinical condition.

Adverse Reactions
None reported.

Interactions with Herbs & Other Dietary Supplements
None known.

Interactions with Drugs
None known.

Interactions with Foods
None known.

Interactions with Lab Tests
None known.

Interactions with Diseases or Conditions
None known.

Dosage and Administration

No typical dosage.

Comments

The constituent of the hoodia extract called P57 is under development by Phytopharm. The company indicates that it has completed a positive study on the benefits of P57 for weight loss, but this study has not yet been published (12004).

P57 was at one time licensed to Pfizer for development. Pfizer discontinued clinical development of P57 in 2003 (12003).

News reports suggest that some samples of hoodia products sold on the Internet show no evidence of containing actual hoodia (12002). Advise patients that they might not be getting what's listed on the label.

HOPS

Also Known As

Common Hops, European Hops, Hop Strobile, Hop Strobili, Hopfenzapfen, Houblon, Lupuli Strobulus.

Scientific Names

Humulus lupulus.

Family: Cannabaceae.

People Use This For

Orally, hops are used for restlessness, anxiety, sleep disorders, tension, excitability, attention deficit-hyperactivity disorder (ADHD), nervousness, and irritability. It is also used orally as an appetite stimulant, diuretic, a bitter tonic, and for indigestion. Other uses include tuberculosis, cystitis, intestinal cramps, mucous colitis, neuralgia, and priapism.

Topically, hops are used for leg ulcers and as an anti-bacterial.

In foods and beverages, the extracts and oil are used as flavor components. The strobile is often used for brewing beer.

In manufacturing, the extract is used in skin creams and lotions.

Safety

LIKELY SAFE ...when consumed in amounts commonly found in foods. Hops and hops oil have Generally Recognized As Safe (GRAS) status in the US (4912).

POSSIBLY SAFE ...when used orally and appropriately for medicinal purposes (12).

PREGNANCY AND LACTATION: Insufficient reliable information available; avoid using.

Effectiveness

There is insufficient reliable information available about the effectiveness of hops.

Mechanism of Action

The applicable part of hops is the dried, female flowering part (strobile). Nine flavonoids have been isolated from hops (10683). Hops contains a potent flavonoid phytoestrogen, 8-prenylnaringenin (10684). The flavonoid is structurally similar to estradiol and selective estrogen-receptor modulators (SERMs). The phenolic ring allows hops to bind to both the alpha and beta estrogen receptors, but with a higher affinity for the beta estrogen receptor. An extract of hops competitively inhibits estradiol binding to estrogen receptors and induces transcription activity in estrogen-responsive cells (6180). The weak endocrine activity of hops is believed to be primarily due to the high estrogenic activity of 8-prenylnaringenin (10685). Preliminary evidence suggests hops may possess antiproliferative properties, indicating potential chemoprevention against breast cancer and ovarian cancer (10683). One mechanism suggested includes the inhibition of the P450 enzymes that activate carcinogens (10686). Hops can also decrease LH (luteinizing hormone) levels in female rats that have had their ovaries removed (6180).

Adverse Reactions

Topically, allergic reactions are possible through contact with the fresh plant and plant dust. Contact dermatitis is attributed to the pollen (4).

Interactions with Herbs & Other Dietary Supplements

HERBS WITH SEDATIVE PROPERTIES: Theoretically, concomitant use with herbs that have sedative properties might enhance therapeutic and adverse effects. Some of these supplements include 5-HTP, calamus, California poppy, catnip, Jamaican dogwood, kava, St. John's wort, scullcap, valerian, yerba mansa, and others.

Interactions with Drugs

ALCOHOL (Ethanol): Concomitant use of hops can potentiate the sedative effects of alcohol (4).
CNS DEPRESSANTS: Theoretically, concomitant use with drugs having sedative properties can cause additive therapeutic and adverse effects (4,19).

Interactions with Foods

ALCOHOL (Ethanol): Concomitant use of hops with alcohol can potentiate the sedative effects (4).

Interactions with Lab Tests

None known.

Interactions with Diseases or Conditions

DEPRESSION: Hops may contribute to depression (12).

Dosage and Administration

No typical dosage.

HORSE CHESTNUT

Also Known As

Buckeye, Chestnut, Escine, Hippocastani Cortex, Hippocastani Flos, Hippocastani folium, Hippocastani Semen, Marron Europeen, Spanish Chestnut, Venastat, Venostat, Venostasin Retard.

Scientific Names

Aesculus hippocastanum.
Family: Hippocastanaceae.

People Use This For

Orally, horse chestnut seed and leaf are used for the treatment of varicose veins, hemorrhoids, and phlebitis. Horse chestnut seed is used for diarrhea, fever, and enlarged prostate. Standardized horse chestnut seed extract products are used orally for the treatment of chronic venous insufficiency. A specially prepared product made from horse chestnut seed is used orally for the treatment of varicose veins, hemorrhoids, phlebitis, diarrhea, fever, and enlarged prostate. Horse chestnut branch bark is used for malaria and dysentery. Horse chestnut leaf is used for eczema, menstrual spastic pain, soft tissue swelling from bone fracture and sprains, complaints after concussion, cough, arthritis, and rheumatism.
Topically, horse chestnut branch bark is used for lupus and skin ulcers.

Safety

LIKELY SAFE ...when used orally and appropriately, short-term. Standardized horse chestnut seed extracts seem to be safe when used for 2-12 weeks (281,282,283,284,285,12113). These extracts have removed the primary toxic constituent, esculin (6420).
UNSAFE ...when the raw seed, bark, flower, or leaf is used orally. Horse chestnut contains significant amounts of the toxin esculin, and can be lethal (17).
CHILDREN: UNSAFE ...when the raw seeds, bark, flower, or leaves are used orally. Poisoning has been reported from children drinking tea made with twigs and leaves (9).
PREGNANCY AND LACTATION: UNSAFE ...when used orally as the raw seed, bark, flower, or leaf. Horse chestnut preparations can be lethal (17); avoid using. There is insufficient reliable information available about the safety of horse chestnut seed extract when used during pregnancy and lactation; avoid using.

Effectiveness

LIKELY EFFECTIVE

Chronic venous insufficiency. Taking horse chestnut seed extract orally can reduce some symptoms of chronic venous insufficiency, such as varicose veins, pain, tiredness, tension, swelling in the legs, itching, and edema (281,282,283,284,285,12113).
Clinical studies investigating the effectiveness of horse chestnut seed have used extracts standardized to 16-20% aescin.

There is insufficient reliable information available about the effectiveness of horse chestnut for its other uses.

Mechanism of Action

The applicable parts of horse chestnut are the seed, bark, flower, and leaf. An extract of horse chestnut seed is most commonly used. Horse chestnut contains triterpene saponins referred to as aescin (escin) and the toxic glycoside aesculin (esculin) (11). Aesculin is a hydroxycoumarin which may increase bleeding time due to antithrombin activity (19). Aescin decreases the permeability of venous capillaries. In vitro, aescin constricts veins and reduces the capillary permeability induced by histamine or serotonin (7162). These properties of the saponin components are the basis for the cosmetic applications of horse chestnut seed extract (4). In some countries, an intravenous mixture containing aescin is used after surgery (9). Aescin also seems to have a weak diuretic activity (7162). Aescin binds to plasma proteins (4). Horse chestnut branch bark and flower also contains sterols, stigmasterol, alpha-spinasterol, and beta-sitosterol (11).

Adverse Reactions

Orally, horse chestnut seed extract with the toxic constituent esculin removed, seems to be well-tolerated.
Some people who take this extract can experience dizziness, nausea, headache, and pruritis (12113).
The horse chestnut seed and bark can cause GI irritation and toxic nephropathy (4).
Horse chestnut contains esculin which has antithrombotic effects and might increase the risk of bleeding or bruising (19).
Symptoms of horse chestnut poisoning include muscle twitching, weakness, loss of coordination, dilated pupils, vomiting, diarrhea, depression, paralysis, and stupor (9).
Pollen from the horse chestnut flower can cause allergic reactions in children (7775). Horse chestnut can also cause hypersensitivity reactions, which occur more commonly in people who are allergic to latex (7853,8418).
Rectally, horse chestnut may cause severe allergic contact dermatitis and proctitis (10383).
Intramuscularly, horse chestnut leaf extract has been associated with cholestatic liver damage (2).
Intravenously, administration of aescin can cause anaphylaxis (18). Isolated cases of kidney and liver toxicity have occurred after intravenous administration (512).

Interactions with Herbs & Other Dietary Supplements

HERBS WITH ANTICOAGULANT/ANTIPLATELET POTENTIAL: Concomitant use of herbs that have constituents that might affect platelet aggregation could theoretically increase the risk of bleeding in some people. These herbs include angelica, clove, danshen, garlic, ginger, ginkgo, Panax ginseng, red clover, and others.
HERBS WITH HYPOGLYCEMIC ACTIVITY: Theoretically, concomitant use with herbs having hypoglycemic activity could have additive effects and adverse effects. Some herbs and supplements with hypoglycemic effects include alpha-lipoic acid, chromium, devil's claw, fenugreek, garlic, guar gum, Panax ginseng, psyllium, Siberian ginseng, and others.

Interactions with Drugs

ANTICOAGULANT/ANTIPLATELET DRUGS: Horse chestnut might have antiplatelet effects (19). Theoretically, taking horse chestnut with other antiplatelet or anticoagulant drugs might increase the risk of bruising and bleeding. Some of these drugs include aspirin, clopidogrel (Plavix), nonsteroidal anti-inflammatory drugs (NSAIDs) such as diclofenac (Voltaren, Cataflam, others), ibuprofen (Advil, Motrin, others), naproxen (Anaprox, Naprosyn, others), dalteparin (Fragmin), enoxaparin (Lovenox), heparin, warfarin (Coumadin), and others.
ANTIDIABETES DRUGS: Monitor blood glucose levels closely due to claims that horse chestnut seeds and bark can have hypoglycemic effects (19).

Interactions with Foods

None known.

Interactions with Lab Tests

None known.

Interactions with Diseases or Conditions

DIABETES: Monitor blood glucose levels closely due to claims that horse chestnut seeds can have hypoglycemic effects (19).
GI IRRITATION: Horse chestnut seeds and bark can irritate gastrointestinal tract; contraindicated in individuals with infectious or inflammatory gastrointestinal conditions (19).
HEPATIC IMPAIRMENT: There is one report of liver injury associated with horse chestnut (4); avoid using.
LATEX ALLERGY: People that are allergic to latex should not take horse chestnut because cross hypersensitivity may occur (7853,8418).
RENAL IMPAIRMENT: Toxic nephropathy has been reported as an adverse effect (4); avoid using.

Dosage and Administration

ORAL: For chronic venous insufficiency, horse chestnut seed extract 300 mg containing 50 mg aescin has been used twice daily (281,283).

Comments

Sometimes buckeye is referred to as horse chestnut. Do not confuse horse chestnut with the related species, Aesculus californica and Aesculus glabra, known respectively as the California and Ohio buckeye.

HORSEMINT

Also Known As
Monarda Lutea, Spotted Monarda, Wild Bergamot.

Scientific Names
Monarda punctata.
Family: Lamiaceae/Labitae.

People Use This For
Orally, horsemint is used for digestive disorders, flatulence, and dysmenorrhea. It is also used orally to promote menstruation and as a stimulant.

Safety
There is insufficient reliable information available about the safety of horsemint.
PREGNANCY: UNSAFE ...when used orally due to menstruation promoting and uterine stimulant effects (12).
LACTATION: Insufficient reliable information available; avoid using.

Effectiveness
There is insufficient reliable information available about the effectiveness of horsemint.

Mechanism of Action
There is insufficient reliable information available about the possible mechanism of action and active ingredients.

Adverse Reactions
None reported.

Interactions with Herbs & Other Dietary Supplements
None known.

Interactions with Drugs
None known.

Interactions with Foods
None known.

Interactions with Lab Tests
None known.

Interactions with Diseases or Conditions
None known.

Dosage and Administration
ORAL: The average daily dose is 2-4 mL of syrup prepared from the herb (18).

Comments
Horsemint has a pungent, bitter taste, and has a scent reminiscent of thyme (18).

HORSERADISH

Also Known As
Amoraciae Rusticanae Radix, Great Raifort, Meerrettich, Mountain Radish, Pepperrot, Red Cole.

Scientific Names
Armoracia rusticana, synonyms Armoracia lopathifolia, Cochlearia armoracia, Nasturtium armoracia, Rorippa armoracia.
Family: Brassicaceae/Cruciferae.

People Use This For
Orally, horseradish is used for urinary tract infection, urinary stones, edematous conditions, cough, bronchitis, for expelling afterbirth, treating gout, rheumatism, gallbladder disorders, sciatica pain, relief of colic, increasing urination, and intestinal worms in children.
Topically, horseradish is used for inflamed joints or tissues and minor muscle aches.
In foods, horseradish is used as a flavoring agent.

Safety
LIKELY SAFE ...when the root is used orally in amounts commonly found in foods. Horseradish has Generally Recognized As Safe (GRAS) status in the US (4912).
POSSIBLY SAFE ...when used orally and appropriately in larger amounts (2,4,6,12,18). ...when topical preparations containing 2% mustard oil, or less are used (2). Mustard oil is a constituent of horseradish.
CHILDREN: LIKELY UNSAFE ...when used orally in children less than 4 years of age because it can cause gastrointestinal problems (2,12,19).
PREGNANCY AND LACTATION: LIKELY UNSAFE ...when used orally in excessive amounts. Horseradish contains toxic and irritating mustard oil constituents (4). ...when the tincture is used regularly and in large amounts, it is considered an abortifacient (19).

Effectiveness
There is insufficient reliable information available about the effectiveness of horseradish.

Mechanism of Action
The applicable part of horseradish is the root. Researchers state horseradish has antimicrobial efficacy against gram negative and gram positive bacteria. It also has antispasmodic properties. Horseradish shows evidence that it can stimulate local blood flow; it might also be carcinostatic (2,18). The toxic mustard oil constituents of horseradish are extremely irritating to mucous membranes (2,4) and the urinary tract (19).

Adverse Reactions
Orally, consuming large amounts of horseradish can cause gastrointestinal upset, bloody vomiting and diarrhea (2,6), and irritation of mucous membranes (2,4) and the urinary tract (19). Horseradish, and other members of the cabbage and mustard family are associated with depressed thyroid function (4).
Topically, skin contact with fresh horseradish can cause irritation (4,19) or allergic reaction (4).

Interactions with Herbs & Other Dietary Supplements
HERBS WITH ANTICOAGULANT/ANTIPLATELET POTENTIAL: Concomitant use of herbs that have constituents that might affect platelet aggregation could theoretically increase the risk of bleeding in some people. These herbs include angelica, clove, danshen, garlic, ginger, ginkgo, Panax ginseng, red clover, turmeric, and others.

Interactions with Drugs
LEVOTHYROXINE (Synthroid, Levothroid, Levoxyl, others): Theoretically, concomitant use of horseradish can interfere with levothyroxine or hypothyroid therapy (4).

Interactions with Foods
None known.

Interactions with Lab Tests
None known.

Interactions with Diseases or Conditions
GI CONDITIONS: Horseradish can irritate gastrointestinal tract. Contraindicated in individuals with infectious or inflammatory gastrointestinal conditions, or stomach or intestinal ulcers (19).
HYPOTHYROIDISM: Theoretically, horseradish might exacerbate hypothyroidism or interfere with therapy (19).
KIDNEY DISORDERS: Theoretically, because it has a strong diuretic effect (19), horseradish is contraindicated in individuals with kidney inflammation (2,18,19).

Dosage and Administration
ORAL: The typical dose of horseradish is 6-20 grams per day of the root or equivalent preparations (4,6,18).
TOPICAL: Ointments with a maximum of 2% mustard oil content are commonly used (6,18).

Comments
Horseradish has been cultivated for more than two thousand years (6) and is sometimes added to toxic substances as a taste repellent for animals (6002).

HORSETAIL

Also Known As
Bottle Brush, Corn Horsetail, Dutch Rushes, Equisetum, Field Horsetail, Horse Willow, Paddock-Pipes, Pewterwort, Prele, Scouring Rush, Souring Rush, Shave Grass, Toadpipe.

Scientific Names
Equisetum arvense; Equisetum telmateia.
Family: Equisetaceae.

People Use This For
Orally, horsetail is used for diuresis, edema, kidney and bladder stones, urinary tract infections, and general disturbances of the kidney and bladder. It is also used for alopecia, tuberculosis, brittle fingernails, rheumatic diseases, gout, frostbite, profuse menstruation, and nasal, pulmonary, and gastric hemorrhage.
Topically, horsetail is used for supportive treatment of wounds and burns.

Safety
POSSIBLY UNSAFE ...when used orally and appropriately short-term (6,12).
LIKELY UNSAFE ...when used orally long-term. It can cause thiamine deficiency. The inorganic silica content can cause toxicity similar to nicotine poisoning (12).
CHILDREN: LIKELY UNSAFE ...when used orally. Horsetail contains inorganic silica and the powdered herb can cause toxicity similar to nicotine poisonings. Poisoning has been reported in children who chewed on the stem (12).
PREGNANCY AND LACTATION: Insufficient reliable information available; avoid using.

Effectiveness
There is insufficient reliable information available about the effectiveness of horsetail.

Mechanism of Action
The applicable parts of horsetail are above ground parts. Evidence suggests horsetail has a mild diuretic action (18), which is likely due to the constituents, equisetonin and flavone glycosides (6). It also contains minute amounts of nicotine (6).

Adverse Reactions
Orally, horsetail may lead to thiamine deficiency, and Canadian products are required to be certified as free from thiaminase-like effect (12). Toxicity has occurred in children who chewed the stems and is similar to nicotine poisoning (12).
Topically, horsetail can cause seborrheic dermatitis (6).

Interactions with Herbs & Other Dietary Supplements
CARDIAC GLYCOSIDE-CONTAINING HERBS: Concomitant use may increase the risk of cardiac glycoside toxicity due to potassium depletion. Cardiac glycoside-containing herbs, include black hellebore, Canadian hemp roots, digitalis leaf, hedge mustard, figwort, lily of the valley roots, motherwort, oleander leaf, pheasant's eye plant, pleurisy root, squill bulb leaf scales, and strophanthus seeds (18,500).
CHROMIUM-CONTAINING SUPPLEMENTS: Horsetail contains chromium (0.0006%) and could increase the risk of chromium toxicity when taken with chromium supplements or chromium-containing herbs such as cascara (Rhamus purshiana) (9141).
LICORICE: Theoretically, overuse/misuse of licorice rhizome with horsetail increases the risk of cardiac toxicity due to potassium depletion (19).
STIMULANT LAXATIVE HERBS: Theoretically, concomitant use increases the risk of potassium depletion. Stimulant laxative herbs include aloe dried leaf sap, blue flag rhizome, alder buckthorn, European buckthorn, butternut bark, cascara bark, castor oil, colocynth fruit pulp, gamboge bark exudate, jalap root, black root, manna bark exudate, podophyllum root, rhubarb root, senna leaves and pods, wild cucumber fruit (Ecballium elaterium), and yellow dock root (19).

Interactions with Drugs
CORTICOSTEROIDS: Theoretically, concomitant use of horsetail with corticosteroids with mineral corticoid activity increases the risk of hypokalemia (4,13).
DIGOXIN (Lanoxin): Increased digoxin toxicity might occur due to the loss of potassium associated with the diuretic effect of horsetail (19).
DIURETIC DRUGS: Overuse of horsetail might compound diuretic-induced potassium loss (4,13). There is some concern that people taking horsetail along with potassium depleting diuretics might have an increased risk for hypokalemia. Initiation of potassium supplementation or an increase in potassium supplement dose may be necessary for some patients. Some diuretics that can deplete potassium include

chlorothiazide (Diuril), chlorthalidone (Thalitone), furosemide (Lasix), hydrochlorothiazide (HCTZ, HydroDIURIL, Microzide), and others.

Interactions with Foods

REGULAR DIET: Horsetail can breakdown thiamine and theoretically increases the risk of thiamine deficiency (19).

Interactions with Lab Tests

None known.

Interactions with Diseases or Conditions

IMPAIRED HEART OR KIDNEY FUNCTION: The diuretic effect of horsetail can cause an increased excretion of potassium (19); avoid using.
THIAMINE DEFICIENCY: Theoretically, the horsetail stem can cause or exacerbate thiamine deficiency (12).

Dosage and Administration

ORAL: The typical dose of horsetail is 6 grams of the dried stem per day with ample fluid intake (18). One cup of the tea is commonly taken several times per day between meals. The tea is prepared by steeping 1.5 grams of the dried stem in 150 mL boiling water for 10-15 minutes and then straining (18). The powdered stem should be used only on a short-term basis in adults. Avoid the use of the powdered stem in children due to its inorganic silica content (12). The usual dose of the liquid extract (1:1 in 25% alcohol) is 1-4 mL three times per day (18). Do not exceed 2 grams of the powdered extract per day (12).
TOPICAL: Horsetail is commonly used as a compress containing 10 grams of the dried stem per L of water (18).

Comments

Adulteration with Equisetum palustre, which contains the toxic alkaloid palustrine, has occurred. Palustrine can be toxic in cattle, but toxicity in humans has not yet been established (12).

HOUND'S TONGUE

Also Known As

Cynoglossi herba, Cynoglossi radix, Dog-Bur, Dog's Tongue, Dogs Tongue, Gypsy Flower, Hounds Tongue, Sheep-Lice, Woolmat.
CAUTION: See separate listing for Deertongue (Trilisa odoratissima).

Scientific Names

Cynoglossum officinale.
Family: Boraginaceae.

People Use This For

Orally, hound's tongue is used for diarrhea and other GI tract complaints, infections, skin diseases, and bronchitis. It is also used orally as an analgesic, expectorant, and cough sedative.
Topically, hound's tongue is used for painful discomfort of extremities, myalgia, neuralgia, trauma, nervous diseases, wound healing, and for care of scar tissue.

Safety

LIKELY UNSAFE ...when used orally (2,18) due to significant amounts of unsaturated pyrrolizidine alkaloids (UPAs) (2,19). Repeated exposure to low concentrations of UPAs has been linked to serious liver toxicity (4,12). UPAs may also be carcinogenic and mutagenic (12).
There is insufficient reliable information available about the safety of hound's tongue for topical use; avoid using.
PREGNANCY AND LACTATION: LIKELY UNSAFE ...when used orally due to UPA content (2,18).

Effectiveness

There is insufficient reliable information available about the effectiveness of hound's tongue.

Mechanism of Action

Researchers think the constituent cynoglossin paralyzes peripheral nerve endings (18). Hound's tongue contains significant amounts of hepatotoxic and hepatocarcinogenic pyrrolizidine alkaloids (2,18). Unsaturated pyrrolizidine alkaloids are known to be hepatotoxic in animals and humans (4).

Adverse Reactions
Chronic exposure to plants containing UPA constituents has been associated with veno-occlusive disease (4021). Symptoms of acute veno-occlusive disease are characterized by a dull, dragging ache in the right upper abdomen and marked distention of the abdomen. These symptoms are sometimes accompanied by reduced urine output. Subacute veno-occlusive disease is associated with vague symptoms and persistent liver enlargement (4021).

Interactions with Herbs & Other Dietary Supplements
EUCALYPTUS: Theoretically, concomitant use may increase the risk of unsaturated pyrrolizidine alkaloid toxicity due to enzyme induction by eucalyptus (19).
PYRROLIZIDINE ALKALOID-CONTAINING HERBS: Concomitant use is contraindicated due to the risk of additive toxicity. Herbs containing unsaturated pyrrolizidine alkaloids include alkanna (12), borage (271), gravel root (4), hemp agrimony (271), hound's tongue (19), petasites (19), comfrey (271), coltsfoot, and the Senecio species plants; dusty miller (19), alpine ragwort (19), groundsel (271), golden ragwort (19), and tansy ragwort (271).

Interactions with Drugs
None known.

Interactions with Foods
None known.

Interactions with Lab Tests
None known.

Interactions with Diseases or Conditions
LIVER DISEASE: Contraindicated due to hepatotoxic potential (19).

Dosage and Administration
No typical dosage.

HOUSELEEK

Also Known As
Aaron's Rod, Ayegreen, Ayron, Bullock's Eye, Hens and Chickens, Jupiter's Beard, Jupiter's Eye, Liveforever, Sengreen, Thor's Beard, Thunder Plant.

Scientific Names
Sempervivum tectorum.
Family: Crassulaceae.

People Use This For
Orally, houseleek is used for severe diarrhea.
Topically, houseleek is used for burns, ulcers, warts, and itchy, burning skin and swelling associated with insect bites. The diluted juice is used as a gargle for stomatitis.

Safety
There is insufficient reliable information available about safety of houseleek.
Pregnancy and Lactation: Insufficient reliable information available; avoid using.

Effectiveness
There is insufficient reliable information available about the effectiveness of houseleek.

Mechanism of Action
The applicable part of houseleek is the leaf of the nonflowering plant. There is insufficient reliable information available about the possible mechanism of action and active ingredients.

Adverse Reactions
None reported.

Interactions with Herbs & Other Dietary Supplements
None known.

Interactions with Drugs
None known.

Interactions with Foods
None known.

Interactions with Lab Tests
None known.

Interactions with Diseases or Conditions
None known.

Dosage and Administration
ORAL: Houseleek is used as a tea (18).
TOPICAL: Houseleek is used as freshly pressed leaves and juice (18).

HUPERZINE A

Also Known As
HupA, Huperzine, Huperzine-A, Selagine.
CAUTION: See separate listing for Chinese Club Moss.

Scientific Names
Huperzine A.

People Use This For
Orally, huperzine A is used for Alzheimer's disease, memory and learning enhancement, age-related memory impairment, increasing alertness and energy, protection from neurotoxic agents including organophosphate nerve gases, glutamate toxicity, and for treating myasthenia gravis.

Safety
POSSIBLY SAFE ...when used orally and appropriately, short-term. Huperzine A has been used safely in clinical trials lasting from 1-3 months (3138,3140,3171,3561,4624,4626).
PREGNANCY AND LACTATION: Insufficient reliable information available; avoid using.

Effectiveness
POSSIBLY EFFECTIVE

Cognitive function. Taking huperzine A orally seems to improve memory function for healthy adolescents. In a small-scale, placebo controlled trial, Chinese middle school children complaining of poor memory had significant improvement in memory quotient scores after taking huperzine A for 4 weeks compared to placebo (4626).

Dementia. Taking huperzine A orally seems to improve memory, cognitive function, and behavioral function in patients with Alzheimer's, multi-infarct, and senile dementia (3138,3140,3171,4624). In one clinical trial, patients with Alzheimer's disease treated with huperzine A had significant improvement in memory, cognitive, and behavioral function scales compared to placebo after 8 weeks of treatment (3138). In a small-scale, placebo-controlled trial, multi-infarct and senile dementia patients treated with huperzine A had significant improvement in memory function after 2-4 weeks of treatment (3140). Long-term, large scale trials are necessary to confirm these findings and determine huperzine A's potential role in dementia.

Myasthenia gravis. Administering huperzine A intramuscularly seems to prevent muscle weakness in patients with myasthenia gravis. In a short-term, small-scale, open-label trial, stabilized patients with myasthenia gravis given huperzine A intramuscularly for 10 days maintained muscle strength as well as patients treated with intramuscular neostigmine alternating with intramuscular huperzine A. Huperzine A was reported to have a 7 hour duration of effect compared to 4 hours for neostigmine (3561). Well-controlled, large-scale trials are necessary to confirm huperzine A's potential benefit in myasthenia gravis.

There is insufficient reliable information available about the effectiveness of huperzine A for its other uses.

Mechanism of Action
Huperzine A is an alkaloid isolated from Chinese club moss, Huperzia serrata and from Lycopodium selago. It is an optically active stereoisomer. Only the levorotatory-isomer is pharmacologically active (3561). Huperzine A is thought to be beneficial in dementia, memory impairment, and myasthenia gravis due to its effects on acetylcholine levels (3133,3134,3135,3136,3172). It is a reversible inhibitor of acetylcholinesterase (AChE) for up to three hours, and crosses the blood-brain barrier. It produces a variable degree of acetylcholine elevation in different areas of the brain, with

maximal values in the frontal and parietal cortex (125% and 105% respectively), and 22-65% in other brain regions (3141). It might be more specific for AChE and have a longer duration of action than AChE inhibitors such as tacrine (Cognex) or donepezil (Aricept), which are marketed as prescription drugs for Alzheimer's disease (3131,3132). In animal studies, huperzine A was found to be 64 times more potent than tacrine. It also is more bioavailable and penetrates the blood-brain barrier better than tacrine (3561). Huperzine A protects neurons against toxic levels of glutamate by blocking glutamate-induce neuronal calcium influx and cell death (3131,3561). Although it has low affinity, huperzine A is also a cerebral cortex N-methyl-D-aspartate (NMDA) receptor antagonist (3129,3137). It might also protect against seizures and neuropathological changes caused by exposure to organophosphate nerve agents such as soman, by protecting peripheral and central stores of acetylcholine (3137,3139).

Adverse Reactions

Orally, huperzine A can cause nausea, sweating, blurred vision, hyperactivity, anorexia, decreased heart rate, and fasciculations (3140,3172,3561,4625). It has been suggested that huperzine A might have fewer cholinergic side effects than tacrine (Cognex) and donepezil (Aricept), but this has not been confirmed in human trials (3131).

Interactions with Herbs & Other Dietary Supplements

None known.

Interactions with Drugs

ACETYLCHOLINESTERASE (AChE) INHIBITORS: Theoretically, concurrent use might have additive effects with drugs that promote acetylcholine activity because huperzine A has AChE inhibitor properties (3131). AChE inhibitors and cholinergic drugs include bethanechol (Urecholine), donepezil (Aricept), echothiophate (Phospholine Iodide), edrophonium (Enoln, Reversol, Tensilon), neostigmine (Prostigmin), physostigmine (Antilirium), pyridostigmine (Mestinon, Regonol), succinylcholine (Anectine, Quelicin), and tacrine (Cognex).

ANTICHOLINERGIC DRUGS: Theoretically, concurrent use of anticholinergic drugs and huperzine A might decrease the effectiveness of huperzine A or the anticholinergic agent. In an animal model, huperzine A reversed cognitive deficits induced by scopolamine (3135). Other anticholinergic drugs include atropine, benztropine (Cogentin), biperiden (Akineton), procyclidine (Kemadrin), and trihexyphenidyl (Artane).

CHOLINERGIC DRUGS: Theoretically, concurrent use might have additive effects with drugs that promote acetylcholine activity because huperzine A has AChE inhibitor properties (3131). AChE inhibitors and cholinergic drugs include bethanechol (Urecholine), donepezil (Aricept), echothiophate (Phospholine Iodide), edrophonium (Enoln, Reversol, Tensilon), neostigmine (Prostigmin), physostigmine (Antilirium), pyridostigmine (Mestinon, Regonol), succinylcholine (Anectine, Quelicin), and tacrine (Cognex).

Interactions with Foods

None known.

Interactions with Lab Tests

None known.

Interactions with Diseases or Conditions

BRADYCARDIA/CARDIOVASCULAR DISEASE: Huperzine A can cause decreased heart rate and might exacerbate bradycardia and other cardiac conditions sensitive to decreased heart rate (3561); use with caution.

EPILEPSY: Theoretically, huperzine A might exacerbate seizure disorders (3561); use with caution.

GASTROINTESTINAL TRACT OBSTRUCTION: Theoretically, huperzine A might exacerbate gastrointestinal obstruction due to its pro-secretory effects (3561); use with caution.

PEPTIC ULCER DISEASE: Theoretically, huperzine A might exacerbate peptic ulcer disease due to its pro-secretory effects (3561); use with caution.

PULMONARY CONDITIONS: Theoretically, huperzine A might exacerbate pulmonary conditions such as asthma and chronic obstructive pulmonary disease due to its pro-secretory effects (3561); use with caution.

UROGENITAL TRACT OBSTRUCTION: Theoretically, huperzine A might exacerbate urogenital tract obstruction due to its pro-secretory effects (3561); use with caution.

Dosage and Administration

ORAL: For Alzheimer's disease and multi-infarct dementia, doses of 50-200 mcg twice daily have been used (3138,3140,4625). For senile or presenile dementia, doses of 30 mcg twice daily have been used (3140). For improving memory in adolescents, doses of 100 mcg twice daily have been used (4626).

INTRAMUSCULAR: For prevention of muscle weakness in myasthenia gravis, doses of 400 mcg daily have been used (3561).

Comments

The Cerebra brand name used for huperzine A has been confused with the prescription drugs Celebrex, Celexa, and Cerebyx (3142). Huperzine A is also referred to as selagine. Avoid confusion with the prescription drug selegiline (Eldepryl). Huperzine A is a drug that stretches the guidelines of the Dietary Supplement Health and Education Act

(DSHEA). Although derived from a plant, huperzine A is a laboratory-manipulated, highly purified drug, unlike herbs which typically contain hundreds of constituents. Chemical hybrids of huperzine A plus tacrine and huperzine A plus donepezil are being investigated (4625). The hybrid of huperzine A plus donepezil has been referred to as huprine X (4625). Laboratory studies indicate that these hybrids have substantially greater affinity for AChE than tacrine or donepezil and show potential for enhanced efficacy at lower doses, with fewer side effects (4625).

HYALURONIC ACID

Also Known As

Hyaluran, Hyaluronan, Hyaluronate, Hyaluronate Sodium, Sodium Hyaluronate.
CAUTION: See separate listings for Glucosamine Hydrochloride, Glucosamine Sulfate, and N-Acetyl Glucosamine.

Scientific Names

Glycoaminoglycan.

People Use This For

Orally, hyaluronic acid is used for various joint disorders, including osteoarthritis and preventing the effects of aging.
By injection, hyaluronic acid is used as an adjunct in cataract surgery, detached retina, corneal transplantation, and eye trauma. It is also used for treating osteoarthritis and as a lip filler in plastic surgery.
Topically, hyaluronic acid is used for healing wounds, burns, skin ulcers, stomatitis, and moisturizing the skin.
In the ear, hyaluronic acid is used in tympanostomy tubes (ear tubes).

Safety

LIKELY SAFE ...when used topically and appropriately (7889,9126). ...when used parenterally and appropriately (7885,7886,7887,9319). There is insufficient reliable information about the safety of oral use of hyaluronic acid.
PREGNANCY: POSSIBLY SAFE ...when used parenterally and appropriately (7890). There is insufficient reliable information about the safety of oral and topical use of hyaluronic acid; avoid using.
LACTATION: POSSIBLY UNSAFE ...when used parenterally. There is insufficient reliable information about the safety of oral and topical use of hyaluronic acid. It is not known if hyaluronic acid is excreted in breast milk, avoid using (7890).

Effectiveness

LIKELY EFFECTIVE

Cataracts. Injecting hyaluronic acid into the eye is effective as an adjunct to cataract surgery (9139). Hyaluronic acid is approved by the FDA for use as an adjunct to cataract surgery, corneal transplantation, lens implantation, and glaucoma filtering surgery (8923).

Oral mucositis. Applying hyaluronic acid topically is an effective treatment for oral mucositis (stomatitis) (7889). An oral gel preparation of hyaluronic acid is approved by the FDA for treating oral mucositis (7892).

POSSIBLY EFFECTIVE

Osteoarthritis. Despite being approved by the FDA for treatment of osteoarthritis by intra-articular injection, hyaluronic acid seems to be variably effective (7887,7888,7890,7891). Subjective symptoms of stiffness and joint pain decrease modestly with hyaluronic acid treatment, but the effect of treatment is often not clinically significant (7887,7888). Whether hyaluronic acid might delay or lessen progressive joint damage with long-term use is unknown (7886).

INSUFFICIENT RELIABLE EVIDENCE to RATE

Eye trauma. In ophthalmology, some research suggests hyaluronic acid might be used as an intraocular injection in detached retina and eye trauma (9126).

Wound healing. Preliminary evidence suggests topical hyaluronic acid might be useful for treating burns, wounds, and skin ulcers (8497,9126,9139).

More evidence is needed to rate hyaluronic acid for these uses.

Mechanism of Action

Hyaluronic acid is a polysaccharide chain of repeating disaccharide units. It is found throughout the body where it serves as part of the supporting structure in the extracellular space. It is found most abundantly in cartilage, synovial fluid, skin, and the aqueous humor in the eye (9139). The disaccharide moiety consists of sodium acetyl glucosamine and sodium glucuronate (8498). Hyaluronic acid is obtained from rooster combs and from bacterial fermentation. The source and preparation method determine the molecular weight, which varies between 90,000 and 5,000,000 daltons. The primary therapeutic effects of hyaluronic acid are physical lubricating and cushioning. The viscosity of hyaluronic acid increases as the concentration, molecular weight, and polysaccharide chain length increase (9139).
In addition to its physiochemical properties, hyaluronic acid might act as an antioxidant and modulate the immune system. Some research suggests it might prevent the breakdown of natural cushioning barriers in joint (9134,9139).
Hyaluronic acid seems to bind to cellular receptors on located on the surface membrane of cartilage and other cell

types, possibly modulating immune response and improving wound healing (7883,9126). In osteoarthritis, hyaluronic acid might inhibit the release of enzymes that contribute to the breakdown of cartilage. It seems to inhibit chemotactic factors and phagocytosis by mononuclear leukocytes. High molecular weight hyaluronic acid (greater than 500,000 daltons) is used for treating osteoarthritis. After intraarticular injection, hyaluronic acid is present for only a few days, but its effects last for about six months (7883,7884). In promoting wound healing, hyaluronic acid might improve blood flow, regulate inflammatory processes, and promote formation of granulation tissue (9126). In addition, hyaluronic acid improves hydration of the wound margins (8497).

Preliminary evidence indicates that hyaluronic acid can decrease adhesions to devices implanted during surgical procedures (7882). It does not improve healing in experimental models of tympanostomy tube (ear tube) placement (8493).

The half-life of hyaluronic acid in serum is 2.5 to 5.5 minutes. It is eliminated from circulation through uptake and biotransformation in the liver and spleen (9139). No information is available about the behavior of hyaluronic acid after oral administration. However, because of its pharmacokinetic characteristics, it would not be expected to achieve significant blood concentrations after oral administration.

Adverse Reactions

Injected intra-articularly, hyaluronic acid can cause redness and soreness at the site of injection. Hyaluronic acid may rarely cause allergic reactions. Anaphylaxis occurs extremely rarely (7884,7885,7894).

After intraocular injection during eye surgery, hyaluronic acid commonly causes increased intraocular pressure. Increased intraocular pressure peaks approximately 24 hours after injection and resolves within 48 to 72 hours (8494,8495,9139). Aspiration of residual hyaluronic acid following surgery does not completely prevent this increased pressure (8496). Timolol drops 0.5% may be used to reduce the intraocular pressure (7893).

Interactions with Herbs & Other Dietary Supplements

None known.

Interactions with Drugs

None known.

Interactions with Foods

None known.

Interactions with Lab Tests

None known.

Interactions with Diseases or Conditions

None known.

Dosage and Administration

INTRA-ARTICULAR INJECTION: For treating osteoarthritis, hyaluronic acid 20 mg once per week for three to five weeks has been used (7886,7887).

Comments

Hyaluronic acid has been touted as a "fountain of youth." However, there is no evidence to support the claim that oral or topical use can prevent changes associated with aging.

HYDRANGEA

Also Known As

Mountain Hydrangea, Seven Barks, Smooth Hydrangea, Wild Hydrangea.

Scientific Names

Hydrangea arborescens, synonyms Viburnum alnifolium, Viburnum americanum.
Family: Hydrangeaceae.

People Use This For

Orally, hydrangea is used for conditions of the urinary tract, such as cystitis, urethritis, prostatitis, enlarged prostate, and urinary calculi. It is also used orally for allergic rhinitis.

Safety
POSSIBLY SAFE ...when used orally and appropriately, short-term (12).
LIKELY UNSAFE ...when used orally in excessive amounts (over 2 grams of dried rhizome/root per dose) (4,12).
...when used orally long-term (4,12).
PREGNANCY AND LACTATION: Insufficient reliable information available; avoid using.

Effectiveness
There is insufficient reliable information available about the effectiveness of hydrangea.

Mechanism of Action
The applicable parts of hydrangea are the rhizome and root. Researchers think hydrangea possesses mild diuretic activity and properties that prevent the formation of stones or calculus (4). The cyanogenic glycoside constituent, hydrangin, may be responsible for some of the potential adverse effects (12).

Adverse Reactions
Orally, hydrangea can cause gastroenteritis (4). Overdose symptoms include vertigo and a feeling of tightness in the chest (4). There is one case report of cholestatic hepatitis associated with Prostata, a multi-ingredient product containing hydrangea (598).

Interactions with Herbs & Other Dietary Supplements
None known.

Interactions with Drugs
None known.

Interactions with Foods
None known.

Interactions with Lab Tests
None known.

Interactions with Diseases or Conditions
None known.

Dosage and Administration
ORAL: A typical dose is 2-4 grams dried rhizome and root three times daily or one cup tea (steep 2-4 grams dried rhizome and root in 150 mL boiling water 5-10 minutes, strain) three times daily (4,12). Liquid extract (1:1 in 25% alcohol), 2-4 mL three times daily has been used (4,12). Tincture (1:5 in 45% alcohol), 2-10 mL three times daily is commonly used (4).

HYDRAZINE SULFATE

Also Known As
Hydrazine, Sehydrin.

Scientific Names
Hydrazine sulfate.

People Use This For
Orally, hydrazine sulfate is used for treating colorectal cancer, lung cancer, neuroblastoma, Hodgkin's disease, and other cancers. It is also used for the general weight loss and wasting (cachexia) associated with cancer.

Safety
POSSIBLY UNSAFE ...when used orally (8005,10384,10385).
PREGNANCY: POSSIBLY UNSAFE ...when used orally (8005,10384,10385).
LACTATION: Insufficient reliable information available; avoid using.

Effectiveness
POSSIBLY INEFFECTIVE

Colorectal cancer. Taking hydrazine sulfate orally as a single agent doesn't seem to improve metastatic colorectal cancer (8002).

LIKELY INEFFECTIVE

Lung cancer. Taking hydrazine sulfate orally as an adjunct to chemotherapy is not helpful for treating non-small cell lung cancer. Hydrazine doesn't significantly improve quality of life, tumor response, weight gain, or survival in these patients (8001,8003,11368).

INSUFFICIENT RELIABLE EVIDENCE to RATE

Cachexia. There is preliminary evidence that hydrazine sulfate might slow weight loss in some cancer patients (8004).

Cancer. Preliminary clinical research suggests hydrazine sulfate is ineffective for treating ovarian cancer, colorectal cancer, breast cancer, lung cancer, pancreatic cancer, endocervical cancer, prostate cancer, uterine cancer, melanoma, and other kinds of cancer (11767).

Neuroblastoma and Hodgkin's disease. There is some evidence that hydrazine sulfate might prevent the growth of neuroblastoma and advanced Hodgkin's disease (10385).

More evidence is needed to rate hydrazine sulfate for these uses.

Mechanism of Action

Hydrazine sulfate is an organic compound used in various industrial processes and as jet fuel. Hydrazine sulfate inhibits phosphoenolpyruvate kinase (8000), an enzyme involved in gluconeogenesis. Some researchers theorize that excessive gluconeogenesis might be partially responsible for the cachexia that occurs in cancer patients (8000,8005). By blocking gluconeogenesis, hydrazine sulfate might reduce cachexia (8000).

Adverse Reactions

Orally, hydrazine sulfate can cause gastrointestinal adverse effects including nausea, vomiting, anorexia, heartburn, and diarrhea or constipation. It also frequently causes neurologic adverse effects including paresthesias, dizziness, drowsiness, peripheral neuropathies, mood stimulation, excitement, weakness, confusion, headache, blurred vision, and taste disturbances. Other adverse effects include irregular breathing, hypoglycemia or hyperglycemia, and diaphoresis. It can also cause lethargy, violent behavior, restlessness, seizures, coma, renal toxicity, and hepatotoxicity (8005,10384,10385,11767).

Interactions with Herbs & Other Dietary Supplements

HERBS AND SUPPLEMENTS WITH HYPOGLYCEMIC EFFECTS: There is some evidence that hydrazine sulfate might have hypoglycemic effects (11767). Theoretically, concomitant use with other herbs and supplements that decrease blood glucose levels might increase the risk of hypoglycemia. Some of these products include bitter melon, cowhage, ginger, goat's rue, fenugreek, kudzu, willow bark, and others.

PYRIDOXINE (Vitamin B6): Hydrazine may antagonize the action of pyridoxine (10384).

Interactions with Drugs

ANTIDIABETES DRUGS: Hydrazine sulfate can reduce blood glucose levels and might have additive effects on glucose levels when used with antidiabetes drug therapy (11767). Monitor blood glucose levels closely. Medication dose adjustments may be necessary. Some antidiabetes drugs include glimepiride (Amaryl), glyburide (DiaBeta, Glynase PresTab, Micronase), insulin, pioglitazone (Actos), rosiglitazone (Avandia), and others.

CNS DEPRESSANTS: Concomitant use with alcohol, barbiturates, or benzodiazepines can increase the toxicity and decrease the effectiveness of hydrazine (8005).

MONOAMINE OXIDASE INHIBITORS (MAOIs): Theoretically, concomitant use might increase the effects and adverse effects associated with MAOIs (8005).

Interactions with Foods

TYRAMINE-CONTAINING FOODS: Avoid concomitant use, hydrazine sulfate may have monoamine oxidase inhibiting activity (8005). Tyramine-containing foods, include avocado, banana, brewer's yeast, broad beans, caviar, aged cheese, aged red wine, herring, liver, and pickled meats.

Interactions with Lab Tests

5-HYDROXYINDOLACETIC ACID (5-HIAA): Hydrazine sulfate can decrease urine levels and test results (275).

ALANINE AMINOTRANSFERASE (ALT): Hydrazine sulfate can increase serum levels and test results secondary to hepatotoxicity (275).

ALKALINE PHOSPHATASE (Alk Phos): Hydrazine sulfate can increase serum levels and test results secondary to hepatotoxicity (11767).

ASPARTATE AMINOTRANSFERASE (AST): Hydrazine sulfate can increase serum levels and test results secondary to hepatotoxicity (11767).

BILE: Hydrazine sulfate can increase urine levels and test results secondary to hepatotoxicity (275).

BILIRUBIN: Hydrazine sulfate can increase serum levels and test results secondary to hepatotoxicity (11767).

BROMOSULFOPHTHALEIN (BSP) RETENTION: Hydrazine sulfate can increase serum levels and test results secondary to hepatotoxicity (275).

ERYTHROCYTE SEDIMENTATION RATE (ESR): Hydrazine sulfate can increase sedimentation rate results secondary to a SLE-type syndrome (275).

GLUCOSE: Hydrazine sulfate can decrease serum glucose and test results by potentiating insulin effects (11767).
LACTATE DEHYDROGENASE (LDH): Hydrazine sulfate can increase LDH levels (11767).
LUPUS ERYTHEMATOSUS (LE) CELLS: Hydrazine sulfate can cause a positive blood test result by activating LE (275).
LYMPHOCYTES: Hydrazine sulfate can decrease blood levels and test results with megadose supplementation (275).
METANEPHRINES (total): Hydrazine sulfate can increase urine levels and test results (275).
NORMETANEPHRINE: Hydrazine sulfate can increase urine levels and test results (275).
VANILLYLMANDELIC ACID: Hydrazine sulfate can increase urine levels and test results (275).

Interactions with Diseases or Conditions

DIABETES: Hydrazine sulfate might interfere with blood glucose control due to effects on gluconeogenesis (8000).

Dosage and Administration

ORAL: For cachexia in people with cancer on a chemotherapy regimen, a typical dose used is 60 mg three times daily for a cycle of 30-45 days followed by a rest period of 2-6 weeks (8004,8005,10385).

Comments

Although some information shows hydrazine sulfate might be useful in the general weight loss and wasting associated with cancer, information is very limited and inconclusive.

HYDROXYMETHYLBUTYRATE (HMB)

Also Known As

B-Hydroxy B-Methylbutyrate Monohydrate, Beta-Hydroxy-Beta-Methylbutyric Acid, Beta-Hydroxy Beta-Methylbutyric Acid, HMB, Hydroxymethyl Butyrate.

Scientific Names

Beta-hydroxy-beta-methylbutyrate.

People Use This For

Orally, HMB is used for increasing the benefits from weight training and exercise, and treating cardiovascular disease, hypercholesterolemia, and hypertension. In combination with arginine and glutamine, HMB is also used orally for treating weight loss in people with AIDS.

Safety

POSSIBLY SAFE ...when used orally and appropriately, short-term. Doses of 3 grams per day or less for up to eight weeks seem to be safe (1909,2167,2168,3374).
PREGNANCY AND LACTATION: Insufficient reliable information available; avoid using.

Effectiveness

POSSIBLY EFFECTIVE

AIDS-related wasting. Taking HMB orally in combination with arginine and glutamine seems to increase body weight and lean body mass, and possibly improve immune function when used over eight weeks to prevent wasting in patients with Acquired Immunodeficiency Syndrome (AIDS) (1909).

INSUFFICIENT RELIABLE EVIDENCE to RATE

Athletic conditioning. There is conflicting evidence about the usefulness of HMB for weight training. Some research suggests HMB might increase muscular strength and body composition, and reduce muscle damage; other research shows no effect (1929,2167,2168,8968). Additionally, there are data that suggest that HMB may be more effective in people who have not previously trained, than in well-trained individuals (11003).
Hypercholesterolemia. There is preliminary clinical evidence that HMB can lower cholesterol (3374).
Hypertension. There is preliminary clinical evidence that HMB can lower blood pressure (3374).
More evidence is needed to rate HMB for these uses.

Mechanism of Action

Hydroxymethylbutyrate (HMB) is a byproduct of metabolism of the amino acid leucine (2168). HMB is also a precursor to cholesterol. HMB found in the cytosol of liver and muscle cells is converted to beta-hydroxy-beta-methylglutarate-Co-A (HMG-CoA). HMG-CoA is used for the cellular synthesis of cholesterol, and might also promote muscle growth by reducing the catabolism of muscle protein (2168,3374). There is also some evidence that HMB lowers levels of creatine phosphokine (CK) and lactate dehydrogenase (LDH), and decreases the excretion of 3-methylhistidine (3-MH). This suggests that HMB might also prevent or decrease muscle membrane inflammation or injury, and prevent increased proteolysis that is often associated with intense exercise (1929,2168).

Adverse Reactions
None reported.

Interactions with Herbs & Other Dietary Supplements
None known.

Interactions with Drugs
None known.

Interactions with Foods
None known.

Interactions with Lab Tests
None known.

Interactions with Diseases or Conditions
None known.

Dosage and Administration
ORAL: For treatment of AIDS-related wasting, 3 grams HMB in combination with 14 grams each of arginine and glutamine administered in two divided doses daily has been used (1909). For lowering cholesterol and blood pressure, 3 grams daily has been used (3374). For muscle building and increasing body strength during weight training, doses of 1 gram three times daily (1929,2167) or 1.5 grams once or twice daily has been used (3374).

HYSSOP

Also Known As
Hissopo, Hysope Officinale, Jufa, Rabo De Gato, Ysop.

Scientific Names
Hyssopus officinalis.
Family: Lamiaceae/Labiatae.

People Use This For
Orally, hyssop is used for liver and gallbladder complaints, intestinal inflammation, coughs, colds, respiratory and chest ailments, sore throats, asthma, urinary tract inflammation, gas and colic, to stimulate appetite and circulation, as an expectorant, for menstrual complaints, and for digestive and intestinal problems.
Topically, hyssop is used as a gargle; in baths to induce sweating; and for treating skin irritations, burns, bruises, and frostbite.
In foods, hyssop oil and extract are used as a flavoring.
In manufacturing, hyssop oil is used as a fragrance in soaps and cosmetics.

Safety
LIKELY SAFE ...when used orally in amounts commonly found in foods. Hyssop, hyssop oil, and hyssop extract have Generally Recognized As Safe (GRAS) status in the US (4912).
POSSIBLY SAFE ...when used orally and appropriately in medicinal amounts (12).
POSSIBLY UNSAFE ...when the oil is used orally for medicinal purposes. There are reports that associate ingestion of the oil with tonic-clonic convulsions (2,18).
There is insufficient reliable information available about the safety of hyssop for its other uses.
CHILDREN: LIKELY UNSAFE ...when used orally because of a report that 2-3 drops of oil over several days caused tonic-clonic convulsions (2,18); avoid using.
PREGNANCY: LIKELY UNSAFE ...when used orally because it might cause uterine stimulant and menstrual stimulant effects (12).
LACTATION: Insufficient reliable information available; avoid using.

Effectiveness
There is insufficient reliable information available about the effectiveness of hyssop.

Mechanism of Action
The applicable parts of hyssop are the above ground parts. Constituent marrubiin (11) has cardioactive effects and stimulates bronchial secretions (4). Caffeic acid and tannins may be responsible for the effect of extracts of dried

leaves. Extracts show antiviral activity against herpes simplex virus and HIV in vitro (6,11). Hyssop oil causes convulsions (of CNS origin) and death in experimental rats (6), thought due to constituents pincamphone and isopincamphone (6). Hyssop oil is associated with tonic-clonic convulsions in adults and children (2,18).

Adverse Reactions
Orally, hyssop was associated with tonic-clonic convulsions in two adults (10-30 drops) and in one child (2-3 drops for several days) (2,18).

Interactions with Herbs & Other Dietary Supplements
None known.

Interactions with Drugs
None known.

Interactions with Foods
None known.

Interactions with Lab Tests
None known.

Interactions with Diseases or Conditions
SEIZURE DISORDERS: Theoretically, hyssop oil may exacerbate seizure disorders.

Dosage and Administration
ORAL: Typically people take two 445 mg capsules containing the hyssop herb three times daily (5019). Some people take 10-15 drops of the hyssop extract (12-14% by volume) in water two to three times daily (5023). People also consume or gargle the hyssop tea three times daily (6002). The tea is prepared by steeping 1-2 teaspoons of the dried hyssop flower tops in 150 mL boiling water for 10-15 minutes and then straining. Avoid internal use of hyssop oil due to possible neurotoxicity.
TOPICAL: No typical dosage.

IBOGA

Also Known As
None.

Scientific Names
Tabernanthe iboga.
Family: Apocyanceae.

People Use This For
Orally, iboga is used as an aperitif, aphrodisiac, tonic, for convalescence, debility, fever, flu, hypertension, neurasthenia, and preventing fatigue and drowsiness.

Safety
There is insufficient reliable information available about the safety of iboga.
Pregnancy and Lactation: Insufficient reliable information available; avoid using.

Effectiveness
There is insufficient reliable information available about the effectiveness of iboga.

Mechanism of Action
The applicable part of iboga is the root. The hallucinogenic properties of iboga are due to the indole alkaloids, ibogaine, ibogamone, iboluteine, and tabernanthine (6,271). Ibogaine inhibits cholinesterase, leading to synaptic acetylcholine accumulation (6). The associated dose-dependent CNS stimulation ranges from mild excitation and euphoria to visual and auditory hallucinations (6,271). Ibogaine has kappa agonist effects; it is serotonergic; and it exhibits nicotinic and N-methyl-D-aspartate (NMDA) antagonism (813). Animal experiments suggest these effects may have value in treating human addictions to alcohol, nicotine, opioids, cocaine, and other stimulants (812,813). The constituent tabernanthine demonstrates cardiac conduction effects similar to those of calcium channel antagonists (6).

Adverse Reactions
Iboga taken orally may cause bradycardia, hypotension, convulsions, paralysis, and respiratory arrest (6). Amounts large enough to induce hallucinations may also cause anxiety, apprehension, and death (6).

Interactions with Herbs & Other Dietary Supplements
None known.

Interactions with Drugs
ANTICHOLINERGIC DRUGS: Theoretically, concomitant use can antagonize anticholinergic effects.
CHOLINERGIC DRUGS: Theoretically, concomitant use may enhance effects and adverse effects.

Interactions with Foods
None known.

Interactions with Lab Tests
None known.

Interactions with Diseases or Conditions
None known.

Dosage and Administration
ORAL: Dry root bark powder or root is chewed (6).

Comments
Iboga is used for ritual and ceremonial purposes in some African cultures (6,271,812).

ICELAND MOSS

Also Known As
Centraria, Eryngo-leaved Liverwort, Iceland Lichen, Lichen Islandicus.

Scientific Names
Cetraria islandica.
Family: Parmeliaceae.

People Use This For
Orally, Iceland moss is used for irritation of the oral and pharyngeal mucous membranes and associated dry cough, for loss of appetite, common cold, cough and bronchitis, dyspeptic complaints, fevers, and the tendency toward infection, lung disease, and kidney and bladder complaints.
Topically Iceland moss is used for poorly healing wounds.
In foods, Iceland moss is utilized as an emergency food source in Iceland.
In manufacturing, Iceland moss is utilized as a flavoring agent in alcoholic beverages.

Safety
POSSIBLY SAFE ...when the dried plant is used orally, short-term for medicinal use (3,12). The dried plant can be contaminated with lead (3).
POSSIBLY UNSAFE ...when consumed in larger amounts as a food source because lead contamination can occur in amounts of up to 30 mg/kg of its dry weight (3). It is regulated in the US and allowable only as a flavoring agent in alcoholic beverages (12).
PREGNANCY AND LACTATION: POSSIBLY UNSAFE ...when used orally; avoid Iceland moss due to the potential for lead contamination (3).

Effectiveness
There is insufficient reliable information available about the effectiveness of Iceland moss.

Mechanism of Action
The applicable part of Iceland moss is the dried plant body. Iceland moss has soothing and mild antimicrobial action (2). The mucilage constituents, lichenin and isolichenin, and the bitter principles can be responsible for its effects (2,3). The bitter organic acid constituents can be responsible for an antibiotic effect (18).

Adverse Reactions
Orally, Iceland moss can cause GI irritation (12). Sensitization to Iceland moss is rare (18). It can be contaminated with lead up to 30 mg/kg of its dry weight (3).

Interactions with Herbs & Other Dietary Supplements
None known.

Interactions with Drugs
ORAL DRUGS: The mucilage in Iceland moss can impair absorption of oral drugs (19).

Interactions with Foods
None known.

Interactions with Lab Tests
None known.

Interactions with Diseases or Conditions
GASTRODUODENAL ULCERS: The alcohol extract and powder of Iceland moss is contraindicated due to the potential for mucosal irritation (12).

Dosage and Administration
ORAL: The typical dose of Iceland moss is one cup of tea several times daily. The tea is prepared by steeping or simmering 1.5-3 grams of the dried plant in 150 mL boiling water for 5-10 minutes and then straining (3,7). The maximum dose of the moss is 4-6 grams per day of the dried plant or equivalent preparations (2).

Comments
Iceland moss is a lichen, or an algae and a fungus growing together in a symbiotic relationship (3). Iceland is one the least polluted countries in the world, which is important for lichens. Lichens derive their nutrients from the environment and are easily contaminated with radioactive or heavy metals. Most of the lichens in Europe were contaminated by the fallout from the Chernobyl accident, but Iceland only received negligible radioactive levels (6002).

IDEBENONE

Also Known As
Hydroxydecyl benzoquinone.

Scientific Names
2,3-dimethoxy-5-methyl-6-(10-hydroxydecyl)-1,4-benzoquinone.

People Use This For
Orally, idebenone is used for Alzheimer's disease, Leber's disease, liver disease, cerebrovascular disease, mitochondrial encephalomyopathies, and Friedreich's ataxia.

Safety
POSSIBLY SAFE ...when used orally and appropriately. Idebenone seems to be safe when used for up to 2 years (11410,11413,11421,11427).
PREGNANCY AND LACTATION: Insufficient reliable information available; avoid using.

Effectiveness
POSSIBLY EFFECTIVE

Alzheimer's disease. There's some evidence that taking idebenone orally slows cognitive function decline in patients with Alzheimer's disease. Idebenone appears most effective in patients with moderately severe Alzheimer's disease, based on standard Alzheimer's disease rating scales (11421,11427).

INSUFFICIENT RELIABLE EVIDENCE to RATE

Friedreich's ataxia. Some preliminary clinical evidence suggests that taking idebenone orally may help control cardiac hypertrophy associated with Friedreich's ataxia, a genetic degenerative neurological disorder (11410,11413,11416,11418). Other research has failed to show an effect (11415). However, idebenone does not appear to slow the progression of ataxia (11410,11411).

Mitochondrial encephalomyopathies. There is preliminary clinical research that suggests idebenone given orally might reduce symptoms in patients with mitochondrial dysfunction such as MELAS (myoclonic

epilepsy with lactic acidosis and stroke-like episodes) syndrome (11422,11424,11426).
More evidence is needed to rate idebenone for these uses.

Mechanism of Action

Idebenone is a synthetic quinone, similar to coenzyme Q-10. It diffuses across cell membranes more readily than coenzyme Q-10 and reaches concentrations in the brain similar to the plasma. Idebenone also distributes into tissues, with highest concentrations found in the kidney, gut, and liver. After oral administration, the half-life of idebenone is approximately 18 hours (11414,11417).
Many of the therapeutic benefits of idebenone are attributed to its antioxidant effects. As an antioxidant, idebenone appears to protect a wide variety of cell membranes and mitochondria from oxidative stress by inhibiting lipid peroxidation. Idebenone also seems to maintain ATP formation in ischemic sites, possibly by functioning as a carrier within the electron transport chain. These properties seem to protect the central nervous system from nerve damage and ischemia (11412,11417,11419,11420,11423,11425). Idebenone may also slow cognitive function decline in patients with Alzheimer's disease, possibly by stimulating nerve growth factor (11417).

Adverse Reactions

Orally, idebenone is well tolerated. In clinical studies, there have been no reports of significant adverse effects (11410,11413,11416,11418,11421,11422,11424,11426,11427).

Interactions with Herbs & Other Dietary Supplements

None known.

Interactions with Drugs

None known.

Interactions with Foods

None known.

Interactions with Lab Tests

None known.

Interactions with Diseases or Conditions

None known.

Dosage and Administration

ORAL: For Alzheimer's disease, idebenone 90 to 120 mg three times daily has been used (11421,11427). For Friedreich's ataxia, 5 to 10 mg per kg divided three times daily has been used (11409,11413). For mitochondrial encephalomyopathies, 90 to 270 mg divided three times daily has been used (11422,11424,11426).

IGNATIUS BEAN

Also Known As

Lu Song Guo, Saint Ignatius-beans.

Scientific Names

Strychnos ignatii, synonym Strychnos tieute.
Family: Loganiaceae.

People Use This For

Orally, ignatius bean is used for faintness; as a bitter or tonic; and as an agent to invigorate, refresh, or restore body function.

Safety

UNSAFE ...when used orally due to its strychnine content (18). The FDA banned strychnine from nonprescription drug products in 1989.
PREGNANCY AND LACTATION: UNSAFE ...when used orally due to toxic effects (18).

Effectiveness

There is insufficient reliable information available about the effectiveness of ignatius bean.

Mechanism of Action
Ignatius bean contains the centrally-acting neurotoxins strychnine and brucine (18). Strychnine competitively antagonizes post-synaptic binding of the inhibitory transmitter glycine, leading to heightened reflex excitability of muscles and convulsions (505). Strychnine can selectively inhibit the spinal cord in subconvulsive amounts (2). However, strychnine accumulates with extended administration, particularly in individuals with liver damage. Chronic use of subconvulsive amounts can cause death after a period of weeks (18).

Adverse Reactions
Orally, 30-50 mg ignatius bean (5 mg strychnine) can cause restlessness, feelings of anxiety, heightening of sense perception, enhanced reflexes, equilibrium disorders, painful neck and back stiffness, followed later by twitching, tonic spasms of jaw and neck muscles, painful convulsions of the entire body triggered by visual or tactile stimulation with possible opisthotonos, muscle hypertonicity, and agitation. Dyspnea may follow spasm of respiratory muscles (18). Seizures occur within 15 minutes of ingestion (or 5 minutes of inhalation) and may result in hyperthermia, metabolic and respiratory acidosis, rhabdomyolysis, and myoglobinuric renal failure (17). 1-2 grams of ignatius bean (50 mg strychnine) can be fatal (18); most deaths occur 3-6 hours post-ingestion from respiratory and subsequent cardiac arrest, anoxic brain damage, or multiple organ failure secondary to hyperthermia (18,505). Strychnine accumulates with extended administration, particularly in individuals with liver damage. Chronic use of subconvulsive amounts can cause death after a period of weeks (18).

Interactions with Herbs & Other Dietary Supplements
None known.

Interactions with Drugs
None known.

Interactions with Foods
None known.

Interactions with Lab Tests
None known.

Interactions with Diseases or Conditions
LIVER DISEASE: Contraindicated; strychnine accumulates in individuals with liver damage. Also, strychnine accumulation can cause liver damage (18).

Dosage and Administration
No typical dose.

Comments
Strychnine may be detected by thin-layer chromatography (qualitative analysis) and high performance liquid chromatography (quantitative analysis). Urine and gastric aspirate are most useful in confirming poisoning (17).

IMMORTELLE

Also Known As
Common Shrubby Everlasting, Eternal Flower, Goldilocks, Yellow Chaste Weed.
CAUTION: See separate listing for Sandy Everlasting.

Scientific Names
Helichrysum arenarium.
Family: Asteraceae/Compositae.

People Use This For
Orally, immortelle is used for liver and gallbladder disorders, including chronic gallstones with accompanying cramps. It is also used orally for dyspepsia, loss of appetite, to stimulate bile flow, as a diuretic, and as an antimicrobial.

Safety
There is insufficient reliable information available about the safety of immortelle.
Pregnancy and Lactation: Insufficient reliable information available; avoid using.

Effectiveness
There is insufficient reliable information available about the effectiveness of immortelle.

Mechanism of Action
The applicable part of immortelle is the dried flower. There is insufficient reliable information available about the possible mechanism of action and active ingredients.

Adverse Reactions
When immortelle is used in people with gallstones, it may cause colic (18). Immortelle can cause an allergic reaction in individuals sensitive to the Asteraceae/Compositae family. Members of this family include ragweed, chrysanthemums, marigolds, daisies, and many other herbs.

Interactions with Herbs & Other Dietary Supplements
None known.

Interactions with Drugs
None known.

Interactions with Foods
None known.

Interactions with Lab Tests
None known.

Interactions with Diseases or Conditions
BILIARY OBSTRUCTION: Immortelle is contraindicated during biliary obstruction secondary to its possible stimulation of biliary flow.
CROSS-ALLERGENICITY: Can cause an allergic reaction in individuals sensitive to the Asteraceae/Compositae family. Members of this family include ragweed, chrysanthemums, marigolds, daisies, and many other herbs.

Dosage and Administration
ORAL: One cup of tea daily. The tea is prepared by steeping 3-4 grams dried flower in 150 mL of boiling water for 10 minutes and straining. The tea is sometimes drunk throughout the day, but must be made fresh each time. The average daily dose is 3 grams of immortelle (18).

Comments
Immortelle is a protected species. It can easily be confused with sandy everlasting (Helichrysum augustifolium, synonym Helichrysum italicum), or Helichrysum stoechas (18). Avoid confusion with immortal (Asclepias asperula) (11).

INDIAN FRANKINCENSE

Also Known As
Boswellia, Boswellin, Boswellin Serrata Resin, Indian Olibanum, Salai Guggal, Shallaki.
CAUTION: See separate listings for Frankincense and Guggul.

Scientific Names
Boswellia serrata.
Family: Burseraceae.

People Use This For
Orally, Indian frankincense is used for arthritis, as an anti-inflammatory agent, and for ulcerative colitis. It is also used orally for rheumatism, syphilis, painful menstruation, pimples, sores, tumors, cancers, asthma, allergic rhinitis, sore throat, abdominal pain, stomach troubles, nervous problems, as a stimulant, respiratory antiseptic, diuretic, and for stimulating menstrual flow.
In manufacturing, Indian frankincense resin oil and extracts are used in soaps, cosmetics, foods, and beverages.

Safety
POSSIBLY SAFE ...when used orally and appropriately in medicinal amounts (6,12).
There is insufficient reliable information available about the safety of Indian frankincense for its other uses.
PREGNANCY AND LACTATION: Insufficient reliable information available.

Effectiveness

INSUFFICIENT RELIABLE EVIDENCE to RATE

Osteoarthritis. There is some preliminary evidence that taking Indian frankincense orally might reduce the symptoms of osteoarthritis (11).

Ulcerative colitis. There is preliminary evidence that taking Indian frankincense orally might reduce symptoms of ulcerative colitis (6).

More evidence is needed to rate Indian frankincense for these uses.

Mechanism of Action

The applicable part of Indian frankincense is the resin. The principle constituents of Indian frankincense are boswellic acid and alpha-boswellic acid, which have anti-inflammatory properties (6,11,1706). In preliminary research, Indian frankincense extracts show anti-inflammatory and antiarthritis effects, but various Indian frankincense-containing products fail to show antiarthritis, anti-inflammatory, or antipyretic effects (6131). However, an Indian frankincense resin-containing herb/mineral combination product reduces pain and disability in people with arthritis symptoms (6). Indian frankincense resin might improve ulcerative colitis (1709), bronchial asthma symptoms, and indices of respiratory function (1708).

Adverse Reactions

None reported.

Interactions with Herbs & Other Dietary Supplements

None known.

Interactions with Drugs

None known.

Interactions with Foods

None known.

Interactions with Lab Tests

None known.

Interactions with Diseases or Conditions

None known.

Dosage and Administration

ORAL: For ulcerative colitis, a gum resin preparation of 350 mg three times daily has been used (1709). For bronchial asthma, a dosage of 300 mg three times daily has been used (1708).

Comments

Olibanum is a term which refers to the oleogum resin exuded from incisions in the bark of several Boswellia species, including Boswellia serrata (Indian frankincense), Boswellia carterii (Bible frankincense), Boswellia frereana (African elemi), and Boswellia bhau-dajiana.

INDIAN GOOSEBERRY

Also Known As

Aamalaki, Amalaki, Amblabaum, Amla, Aonla, Emblic, Emblic Myrobalan, Emblica, Groseillier de Ceylan, Indian-Gooseberry, Mirobalano, Myrobalan Emblic, Neli.

Scientific Names

Phyllanthus emblica, synonyms Emblica officinalis, Mirobalanus embilica.
Family: Euphorbiaceae.

People Use This For

Orally, Indian gooseberry is used for lowering cholesterol, treating atherosclerosis, diabetes, pancreatitis cancer, dyspepsia, eye problems, joint pain, diarrhea, dysentery, "organ restoration", and as an anti-inflammatory and antimicrobial. It is also used orally for obesity.

Safety

LIKELY SAFE ...when consumed in amounts commonly found in foods (6,2076).
There is insufficient reliable information available about the safety of Indian gooseberry when used medicinally.
PREGNANCY AND LACTATION: Insufficient reliable information available; avoid using.

Effectiveness

There is insufficient reliable information available about the effectiveness of Indian gooseberry.

Mechanism of Action

The applicable part of Indian gooseberry is primarily the fruit (2075), but extracts from the leaves have also been used (2078,2079). Preliminary evidence suggests that Indian gooseberry fruit and juice may lower total serum cholesterol, low-density lipoprotein (LDL), triglycerides, and phospholipids without affecting high-density lipoprotein (HDL) levels; and it may have positive effects on atherosclerosis (2077,8180). Indian gooseberry fruit juice may also have antimicrobial, antimutagenic, and antioxidant activity (2080,2081). The leaf extract might have anti-inflammatory activity (2078,2079).

Adverse Reactions

None reported.

Interactions with Herbs & Other Dietary Supplements

None known.

Interactions with Drugs

None known.

Interactions with Foods

None known.

Interactions with Lab Tests

None known.

Interactions with Diseases or Conditions

None known.

Dosage and Administration

No typical dosage.

Comments

Indian gooseberry is a native deciduous tree in India and the Middle East. Indian gooseberry has been used in Ayurvedic medicine for thousands of years. Reference to Indian gooseberry appeared in an Ayurvedic medicine text in the seventh century (3563).

INDIAN LONG PEPPER

Also Known As

Bi Bo, Jaborandi Pepper, Kana, Langer Pfeffer, Long Pepper, Magadhi, Pimenta-Longa, Pippali, Poivre Long, Ushana.
CAUTION: See separate listings for Black Pepper and White Pepper, and Capsicum.

Scientific Names

Piper longum.
Family: Piperaceae.

People Use This For

Orally, Indian long pepper is used to treat headache, toothache, asthma, beri-beri, bronchitis, mucous membrane inflammation, cholera, coma, cough, diarrhea, dysentery, epilepsy, fever, frigidity, stomachache, stroke, heartburn, indigestion, insomnia, leprosy, lethargy, enlarged spleen, muscle pain, nasal discharge, painful menses, paralysis, psoriasis, sterility in women, snake bites, tetanus, thirst, tuberculosis, and tumors. It is also used during childbirth, and during the 3-6 weeks following childbirth while the uterus returns to normal size. The fruit is used orally to stimulate menstrual flow, appetite, and bile flow; to improve digestion; induce sweating; and as an abortifacient, analgesic, antiflatulent, aphrodisiac, astringent, bactericide, diuretic,

larvicide, sedative, stimulant, tonic, and vermifuge.
In foods, the fruit is used in cooking, both as an ingredient and a spice. It is used in fresh or dried form.

Safety
There is insufficient reliable information available about the safety of Indian long pepper.

Effectiveness
There is insufficient reliable information available about the effectiveness of Indian long pepper.

Mechanism of Action
The applicable part of Indian long pepper is the fruit. Piper longum contains piperine which can increase oral absorption of drugs and other substances, possibly by modulating intestinal membrane dynamics (3757). Some evidence suggests an ethanolic extract and isolated piperine might have amoebicidal activity (3758). An Ayurvedic herbal preparation containing Piper longum and Butea monosperma (Pippali rasayana) shows evidence that it is useful for managing giardiasis (3754,3755). In mice, an ethanolic extract of piper longum administered chronically increased weights of lung, spleen, and reproductive organs. It also increased sperm count and motility without demonstrating acute or chronic toxicity (3756).

Adverse Reactions
None reported.

Interactions with Herbs & Other Dietary Supplements
SCOTCH BROOM: Piperine increases the bioavailability of sparteine, a constituent of scotch broom (19).

Interactions with Drugs
PHENYTOIN (Dilantin): Concomitant administration speeds absorption and slows elimination of phenytoin (Dilantin) (537).
PROPRANOLOL (Inderal): Concomitant administration speeds and increases absorption, and increases serum concentrations of propranolol (538).
THEOPHYLLINE: Concomitant administration increases absorption and serum concentrations of theophylline (538).

Interactions with Foods
None known.

Interactions with Lab Tests
SERUM DRUG ASSAYS: Indian long pepper can increase phenytoin, propranolol, and theophylline serum concentrations and test results (537,538).

Interactions with Diseases or Conditions
None known.

Dosage and Administration
No typical dosage.

Comments
Piper nigrum, the source of black pepper and white pepper, also contains the constituent piperine. However, red pepper and cayenne do not.

INDIAN PHYSIC

Also Known As
American Ipecacuanha, Bowman's Root, Gillenia, Indian Hippo.
CAUTION: See separate listings for Black Root and Canadian Hemp.

Scientific Names
Gillenia trifoliata, synonyms Porteranthus trifoliatus, Spiraea trifoliata.
Family: Rosaceae.

People Use This For
Orally, Indian physic is used for digestive disorders and as an emetic.

Safety
There is insufficient reliable information available about the safety of Indian physic.
Pregnancy and Lactation: Insufficient reliable information available; avoid using.

Effectiveness
There is insufficient reliable information available about the effectiveness of Indian physic.

Mechanism of Action
The applicable parts of Indian physic are the dried root and root bark. Indian physic is stated to have expectorant, emetic, and "blood purification" properties (18).

Adverse Reactions
None reported.

Interactions with Herbs & Other Dietary Supplements
None known.

Interactions with Drugs
None known.

Interactions with Foods
None known.

Interactions with Lab Tests
None known.

Interactions with Diseases or Conditions
None known.

Dosage and Administration
ORAL: Used as a powder in tea or tonic (18).

Comments
Avoid confusion with Canadian hemp (Apocynum cannabinum), also known as Indian physic (12). Avoid confusion with black root (Leptandra virginica), also known as bowman's root.

INDIAN SNAKEROOT

Also Known As
Ajmaline, Chandrika, Chota-Chand, Covanamilpori, Dhanburua, Pagla-Ka-Dawa, Patalagandhi, Rauwolfae radix, Rauwolfia, Rauwolfia Serpentina, Rauwolfiawurzel, Sarpagandha, Serpentine-Wood, She Gen Mu.

Scientific Names
Rauvolfia serpentina, synonym Ophioxylon serpentinum.
Family: Apocynaceae.

People Use This For
Orally, Indian snakeroot is used for mild essential hypertension, symptomatic relief in individuals with agitated psychosis unable to tolerate other agents, for nervousness, and insomnia. Indian snakeroot is also used orally for snake and reptile bites, insanity, fever, constipation, feverish intestinal diseases, liver ailments, rheumatism, dropsy (edema), as a tonic for general debilities, for mental illness, and epilepsy.
As a prescription product, it is used to treat mild to moderate hypertension, schizophrenia, and vasospastic attacks due to peripheral vascular disorders.

Safety
POSSIBLY SAFE ...when the prescription product is used orally (15). ...when the standardized extract is used orally under the supervision of a medical professional trained in the use of Indian snakeroot (18).
POSSIBLY UNSAFE ...when used orally for self-medication. Appropriate use of Indian snakeroot requires medical diagnosis and treatment. Large amounts or overdose can lead to CNS depression, convulsions, extrapyramidal effects, and coma (15). ...when used by individuals operating motor vehicles or machinery. Indian snakeroot can alter reaction time (2,15).

PREGNANCY: LIKELY UNSAFE ...when used orally (2,18); the reserpine alkaloid constituents cross the placenta and can be potentially teratogenic (15,4260).
LACTATION: POSSIBLY UNSAFE ...when used orally. The reserpine alkaloids are excreted in breast milk (4260); avoid using.

Effectiveness

INSUFFICIENT RELIABLE EVIDENCE to RATE

Insomnia. Early evidence indicates that Indian snakeroot in a specific combination with two other herbs might offer some benefit for insomnia (6051). More evidence is needed to rate the effectiveness for this use.

Mechanism of Action

The applicable part of Indian snakeroot is the root. The properties of the whole root of rauwolfia serpentina differ from those of reserpine. The whole root contains over 50 alkaloids (13). Rauwolfia serpentina demonstrates hypotensive, sedative, and tranquilizing effects (15). It also reduces heart rate (13), has anti-arrhythmic effects (18), and causes a general sense of euphoria (13). The active constituents of the whole root include the rauwolfia alkaloids, reserpine, rescinnamine, and deserpidine (11-desmethoxyreseroine) (13). Hypotensive effects are believed to be due to the depletion of both catecholamine and serotonin stores and to the prevention of reabsorption (13,18). The greater the proportion of alkaloids present, the greater the hypotensive activity (13). The sedative effects of Indian snakeroot can result from the depletion of amine stores in the central nervous system (CNS) (13).

Adverse Reactions

Orally, low amounts of Indian snakeroot may cause adverse reactions including nasal congestion, abdominal cramps, diarrhea, nausea, vomiting, anorexia, increased gastric acid secretion, drowsiness, fatigue, lethargy, slowed reflexes, sexual dysfunction, and bradycardia. In larger amounts, mental depression may slowly develop. After discontinuation of Indian snakeroot, mental depression may persist for several months. In extremely large amounts, Parkinson-like symptoms, extrapyramidal reactions, and convulsions may occur. Allergic reactions from the use of Indian snakeroot are rare, but it may precipitate asthma (15).

Interactions with Herbs & Other Dietary Supplements

CARDIOACTIVE GLYCOSIDE-CONTAINING HERBS: Theoretically, concomitant use of Indian snakeroot may increase the risk of bradycardia (2,18), angina-like symptoms, and arrhythmias (15). Cardioactive glycoside containing herbs include black hellebore, digitalis, lily of the valley, oleander leaf, pheasant's eye, and squill (19).
EPHEDRA: Theoretically, concomitant use of ephedra with Indian snakeroot may decrease ephedrine effects (15).

Interactions with Drugs

ALCOHOL (Ethanol): Use Indian snakeroot and ethanol with caution; concomitant use may increase the risk of additive CNS-depressant effects (15).
ANTIPSYCHOTIC DRUGS: Concomitant use of neuroleptics with Indian snakeroot may potentiate the effects of these drugs and the rauwolfia alkaloids (2,18).
BARBITURATES: Concomitant use of barbiturates with Indian snakeroot may potentiate the effects of these drugs and the rauwolfia alkaloids (2,18). Some of these sedative medications include pentobarbital (Nembutal), phenobarbital (Luminal), secobarbital (Seconal), and others.
DIGOXIN (Lanoxin): Concomitant use of digoxin with Indian snakeroot may cause bradycardia (2,18), angina-like symptoms, and arrhythmias (15). Avoid large amounts of the rauwolfia alkaloids together with digitalis cardiac glycosides (15).
DIURETIC DRUGS: Concomitant use of diuretics with Indian snakeroot may potentiate the hypotensive effects of rauwolfia alkaloids (15).
EPHEDRINE: Concomitant use of ephedrine with Indian snakeroot may reduce indirect-sympathomimetic drug activity (15).
LEVODOPA: Avoid using Indian snakeroot with levodopa; concomitant use may reduce drug effectiveness and increase extrapyramidal motor symptoms (15,18).
MONOAMINE OXIDASE INHIBITORS (MAOIs): Avoid concomitant or overlapping use of Indian snakeroot and MAOIs within several days. The overlap may increase the risk of excitation and hypertension (15).
PROPRANOLOL (Inderal): Concomitant use of propranolol with Indian snakeroot may enhance beta-blockade due to the rauwolfia alkaloid catecholamine-depleting effects (15).
STIMULANT DRUGS: Concomitant use of sympathomimetic drugs with Indian snakeroot may cause an initial increase in blood pressure and enhance or prolong the pressor effects (15,18).
TRICYCLIC ANTIDEPRESSANTS (TCAs): Concomitant use of tricyclic antidepressants with Indian snakeroot may decrease the effectiveness of rauwolfia alkaloids (15).

Interactions with Foods

ALCOHOL (Ethanol): Concomitant use of Indian snakeroot with ethanol should be used with caution; concomitant use with alcohol may increase the risk of additive CNS-depressant effects (15).

Interactions with Lab Tests

4-HYDROXY-3-METHOXY PHENYLETHYLENE GLYCOL (HMPG): Theoretically, Indian snakeroot might increase or decrease urinary HMPG concentrations and test results, due to its reserpine content. Reserpine can increase urinary HMPG concentrations by causing release of stored norepinephrine. Long-term reserpine administration can decrease urinary HMPG concentrations (275).
5-HYDROXYINDOLEACETIC ACID (5-HIAA): Large doses of Indian snakeroot might increase urinary 5-HIAA excretion and test results. Large doses of rauwolfia alkaloids may release serotonin (5-HT) from brain tissues, resulting in increased urinary 5-HIAA excretion (15,275).
17-HYDROXYCORTICOSTEROIDS: Indian snakeroot might reduce urinary 17-hydroxycorticosteroid concentrations and test results, possibly due to suppression of central 17-hydroxycorticosteroid synthesis by its rauwolfia alkaloid content. Indian snakeroot might interfere with colorimetric assays of urinary 17-hydroxycorticosteroid concentrations by the Glenn-Nelson technique, due to its rauwolfia alkaloid content. Theoretically, Indian snakeroot might interfere with colorimetric assays of urinary 17-hydroxycorticosteroid concentrations which rely on the Porter-Silber reaction, due to its reserpine content (15,275).
17-KETOSTEROIDS: Indian snakeroot might interfere with colorimetric assays of urinary 17-ketosteroids by the Holtorff Koch modification of the Zimmerman reaction, due to its rauwolfia alkaloid content (15).
BILIRUBIN: Theoretically, large doses of Indian snakeroot might cause falsely high serum bilirubin test results, due to the reserpine content. Reserpine concentrations greater than 61 mg/L can cause falsely high serum bilirubin test results when measured by the Jendrassik and Grof method (275).
BLOOD PRESSURE: Indian snakeroot might lower blood pressure and blood pressure readings in patients with mild to moderate hypertension, due to the alkaloids (2,15).
CATECHOLAMINES: Overdose of Indian snakeroot might initially increase urinary catecholamine excretion and test results. Rauwolfia alkaloids release stored norepinephrine, resulting in increased urinary catecholamine excretion. Chronic use of Indian snakeroot might decrease urinary catecholamine excretion, due to its rauwolfia alkaloid content. Chronic use of rauwolfia alkaloids decreases urinary catecholamine excretion (15,275).
GLUCOSE: Theoretically, Indian snakeroot might increase blood glucose concentrations and test results, due to its reserpine content. Reserpine might increase blood glucose concentrations following administration (275).
GUAIACOLS SPOT TEST: Theoretically, Indian snakeroot might cause false-positive urine guaiacols spot test results, due to the reserpine content. Reserpine can cause a false-positive reaction for urinary guaiacols with the screening test of Rogers (275).
LUPUS ERYTHEMATOSUS (LE) CELLS: Theoretically, Indian snakeroot might trigger the presence of LE cells in the blood and positive LE cell test results, due to the reserpine content. Reserpine might cause systemic lupus erythematosus (SLE) and the presence of LE cells in the blood; however, this usually normalizes when reserpine is discontinued (275).
NOREPINEPHRINE: Theoretically, Indian snakeroot might decrease urinary norepinephrine concentrations, due to the reserpine content.
OCCULT BLOOD: Theoretically, Indian snakeroot might activate peptic ulcers, resulting in bleeding and positive fecal occult blood tests, due to the reserpine content (275).
PLATELETS: Theoretically, Indian snakeroot might cause thrombocytopenia, decreasing blood platelets and platelet counts. Reserpine might cause thrombocytopenia (275).
PROLACTIN: Theoretically, large doses of Indian snakeroot might increase plasma prolactin levels and test results in patients with hypertension, due to the reserpine content. Reserpine, in daily doses greater than 0.25 mg, may increase plasma prolactin levels in patients with hypertension (275).
THYROXINE (T4): Theoretically, Indian snakeroot might decrease serum T4 concentrations and test results, due to the reserpine content. Reserpine may decrease serum T4 concentrations by increasing hepatic T4 metabolism (275).
TYRAMINE: Theoretically, Indian snakeroot might cause false-negative tyramine test results, due to the reserpine content. Reserpine may inhibit patient responsiveness to tyramine tests (275).
VANILLYLMANDELIC ACID (VMA): Overdose of Indian snakeroot might initially increase urinary VMA excretion and test results. Rauwolfia alkaloids release stored norepinephrine, resulting in increased urinary VMA excretion. Chronic use of Indian snakeroot might decrease urinary VMA excretion, due to its rauwolfia alkaloid content. Chronic use of rauwolfia alkaloids decreases urinary VMA excretion (15,275).

Interactions with Diseases or Conditions

ELECTROCONVULSIVE THERAPY (ECT): Indian snakeroot is contraindicated during ECT (15), and one week should elapse between cessation of rauwolfia alkaloids and initiation of ECT (15).
GALLBLADDER DISEASE: Use cautiously in individuals with a history of gallstones; Indian snakeroot may precipitate biliary colic (15).
GASTROINTESTINAL (GI) CONDITIONS: Indian snakeroot is contraindicated in individuals with active peptic ulcer disease or ulcerative colitis (15). Use Indian snake root cautiously in individuals with a history of these diseases.
HYPERSENSITIVITY: Indian Snakeroot is contraindicated in individuals hypersensitive to rauwolfia alkaloids (15).
MENTAL DEPRESSION: Indian snakeroot is contraindicated, especially in individuals with a past history of depression or suicidal tendencies (15).
PHEOCHROMOCYTOMA: Contraindicated (18).

Dosage and Administration

ORAL: The average daily amount of Indian snakeroot is 600 mg of the powdered whole root, which is equivalent to 6 mg total alkaloids (2,18). Rauwolfia serpentina, deserpidine, and reserpine are available as an FDA-approved prescription drugs (15).

Comments

Reserpine is commercially obtained from Rauvolfia serpentina and the related species, Rauvolfia micrantha, Rauvolfia tetraphylla, and Rauvolfia vomitoria (13). Spelling note: The genus, Rauvolfia, is correctly spelled with a "v", while Rauwolfia or Rauwolfia serpentina (names for the dried root of Rauvolfia serpentina) are correctly spelled with a "w" (2,13).

INDOLE-3-CARBINOL

Also Known As

I3C, 3-Hydroxymethyl Indole, 3 Hydroxymethyl Indole, Indole 3 Carbinol, 3-(hydroxymethyl), 3 (hydroxymethyl) Indole, 3-Indolylcarbinol, 3 Indolylcarbinol, 3-Indolylmethanol, 3 Indolylmethanol, Indole.

Scientific Names

Indole-3-methanol.

People Use This For

Orally, indole-3-carbinol is used for prevention of breast cancer, colon cancer, and other types of cancer. Indole-3-carbinol is also used orally for fibromyalgia, laryngeal papillomatosis, cervical dysplasia, and systemic lupus erythematosus (SLE). It is also used to balance hormone levels, detoxify the intestines and liver, and to support the immune system.

Safety

LIKELY SAFE ...when used orally in amounts typically found in the diet. Dietary consumption of indole-3-carbinol is typically 20-120 mg per day (7170,7176).
POSSIBLY SAFE ...when used orally and appropriately in medicinal amounts. Doses of 200-400 mg per day seem to be safe and well tolerated when used for up to 3 months (7173,7174,7175). There is also some evidence that lower doses of 100-200 mg per day can be used safely for up to 15 months (7172).
CHILDREN: LIKELY SAFE ...when used orally in amounts typically found in the diet (7170,7176). POSSIBLY SAFE ...when used orally and appropriately in medicinal amounts. There is some evidence that indole-3-carbinol can be safely used in children ages 2 to 12 years. Doses of 100-200 mg, based on body weight, seem to be safe and well tolerated when used for up to 15 months (7172).
PREGNANCY AND LACTATION: LIKELY SAFE ...when used in amounts typically consumed in foods (7170). There is insufficient reliable information available about the safety of indole-3-carbinol when used in amounts greater than those found in the diet during pregnancy and lactation; avoid using.

Effectiveness

POSSIBLY EFFECTIVE

Cervical dysplasia (cervical intraepithelial neoplasia, CIN). Treatment with indole-3-carbinol for 12 weeks seems to cause complete regression of CIN in 45-50% of patients with stage II-III CIN. Lower doses of 200 mg per day seem to be just as effective as higher doses of 400 mg per day (7173).

INSUFFICIENT RELIABLE EVIDENCE to RATE

Respiratory papillomatosis. There is some preliminary clinical evidence that long-term use of indole-3-carbinol might reduce papilloma growth in patients with recurrent respiratory papillomatosis (7172). More evidence is needed to rate indole-3-carbinol for this use.

Mechanism of Action

Indole-3-carbinol is a constituent of cruciferous vegetables of the Brassica genus. Some of these vegetables include broccoli, Brussels sprouts, cabbage, collards, cauliflower, kale, kohlrabi, mustard greens, rapeseed, and root vegetables such as turnips and rutabagas (7170,7176). One head of cabbage contains approximately 1200 mg of indole-3-carbinol (7173). Daily dietary intake of indole-3-carbinol is typically 20-120 mg (7170,7176). In plant cells, indole-3-carbinol exists in the form of 3-indolylmethyl glucosinolate, which is then converted to indole-3-carbinol when the plant is cut or chewed (7170). However, indole-3-carbinol is also produced synthetically (7170). Indole-3-carbinol itself is not active. When indole-3-carbinol comes in contact with stomach acid it is converted to active metabolites, diindoylmethane and indolylcarbazole. Therefore, parenterally administered indole-3-carbinol does not produce active metabolites (7188). Researchers are interested in indole-3-carbinol for cancer prevention, particularly breast, cervical and endometrial, and colorectal cancer. Their reason is that diets with higher amounts of fruit and vegetable consumption are associated with a decreased risk of developing cancer. Researchers suspect indole-3-carbinol is one of several vegetable components that might be cancer protective (7174,7180,7181,7182,7187). However, researchers are finding that indole-3-carbinol has a variety of effects on liver metabolism of toxins. Some effects on metabolism seem to be cancer protective while others might potentially increase cancer risk. Some researchers think indole-3-carbinol might be particularly helpful against hormone-dependent cancers such as breast cancer. Indole-3-carbinol induces cytochrome P450 1A1 (CYP1A1) and 1A2 (CYP1A2), which alters estrogen metabolism. Estradiol is normally metabolized to both 16-alpha-hydroxyestrone and 2-alpha-hydroxyestrone. The 16-alpha-hydroxysestrone metabolite has both genotoxic and tumorigenic effects and is thought to increase the risk of breast and cervical cancers. Indole-3-carbinol shifts metabolism of estradiol from 16-alpha-hydroxyestrone to the weaker estrogen and more benign 2-alpha-hydroxyestrone metabolite, possibly producing a protective effect against hormone-mediated cancers (7175,7177,7179,7180,7181,7182). Indole-3-carbinol also induces cytochrome P450 2B1, 2B2, 3A1, and 3A2, as well as phase II enzymes including glutathione S-transferase (GST), quinone reductase, and uridine diphosphate glucuronide transferase (7176,7187). The phase II enzyme induction seems to have a detoxifying effect by increasing water solubility and increasing excretion of carcinogenic toxins (7176). There is some evidence that indole-3-carbinol might have other protective effects including antioxidant properties (7178,7188) and might also cause cancer cell apoptosis and cell cycle arrest (7176,7188). The majority of evidence seems to indicate that indole-3-carbinol has a protective effect against cancer. However, there is some concern that it might enhance carcinogenicity in some cases (7170,7171,7184,7185,7186). Some of the effects of indole-3-carbinol on metabolism actually seem to increase carcinogenicity of certain toxins. Since indole-3-carbinol induces CYP1A1 metabolism, it can also increase conversion of procarcinogens to their active carcinogenic form (7170). Ultimately, whether indole-3-carbinol has a cancer preventive effect or increases cancer risk in humans probably depends on several factors, including dietary factors, and duration and timing of exposure to indole-3-carbinol. For example, in animal models, there is some evidence that indole-3-carbinol has a protective role if administered before or in conjunction with a carcinogenic agent. If indole-3-carbinol is given after carcinogen exposure during the initiation phase of tumor induction, it might act as a tumor promoting agent and increase the risk of developing a tumor (7184,7185,7186). However, there is some conflicting evidence (7189). Indole-3-carbinol seems be active against diseases that are related to the human papilloma virus, including cervical cancer and laryngeal papillomatosis (7172,7173,7183). Indole-3-carbinol also seems to have immune modulating effects. In animal models, high doses of indole-3-carbinol seem to depress natural killer cell activity, but enhance delayed-type hypersensitivity in laboratory models (7190). Whether these immune system effects contribute to the effects of indole-3-carbinol on carcinogenicity is unknown (7190).

Adverse Reactions

Orally, indole-3-carbinol is usually well tolerated. However, some patients can experience skin rash and small increases in the liver enzyme alanine aminotransferase (ALT, SGPT) (7170,7174). However, this seems to rarely occur. In very high doses, greater than 400 mg per day, dysequilibrium symptoms, tremor, and nausea can occur (7172). There is some concern that certain patients might be at risk for tumor promoting effects of indole-3-carbinol. There is some preliminary evidence that indole-3-carbinol might promote tumorigenesis in patients who are in the initiation phase of tumor induction due to carcinogen exposure (7171). However, this potential risk is controversial and has never been documented in humans. Until more is known, it is not possible to determine if there is a real risk to humans or who might be susceptible to this risk.

Interactions with Herbs & Other Dietary Supplements

None known.

Interactions with Drugs

CYTOCHROME P450 1A2 (CYP1A2) SUBSTRATES: There is some evidence that indole-3-carbinol induces CYP1A2 isozymes (7187). Theoretically, indole-3-carbinol might increase the metabolism of CYP1A2 substrates and lower serum concentrations. Some substrates of CYP1A2 include clozapine (Clozaril), cyclobenzaprine (Flexeril), fluvoxamine (Luvox), haloperidol (Haldol), imipramine (Tofranil), mexiletine (Mexitil), olanzapine (Zyprexa), pentazocine (Talwin), propranolol (Inderal), tacrine (Cognex), theophylline, zileuton (Zyflo), zolmitriptan (Zomig), and others.

Interactions with Foods

None known.

Interactions with Lab Tests

ALANINE AMINOTRANSFERASE (ALT, SGPT): A mild increase in ALT can occur in some patients taking indole-3-carbinol (7174). However, this effect seems to rarely occur. Routine liver function tests are probably not necessary.

Interactions with Diseases or Conditions

None known.

Dosage and Administration

ORAL: For cervical dysplasia, 200-400 mg per day has been used. However, 200 mg seems to be as effective as the higher dose (7173). For breast cancer prevention, 300 mg per day has been used (7174). For adults with recurrent respiratory papillomatosis, 200 mg twice daily has been used (7172). For children with respiratory papillomatosis, dosing is weight based. For children weighing 6-10 kg, 50 mg twice daily has been used. For children weighing 11-19 kg, 75 mg twice daily has been used. For children weighing 20-29 kg, 100 mg twice daily has been used, etc. Children 60 kg and above have used the adult dose of 200 mg twice daily (7172).

Comments

Indole-3-carbinol is becoming a very popular dietary supplement. Usage of indole-3-carbinol is expected to grow by 3000% between the year 2000 and 2002 (7170,7176). The National Institutes of Health (NIH) has reviewed indole-3-carbinol as a possible cancer preventive agent and is now sponsoring clinical research for breast cancer prevention (7170).

INOSINE

Also Known As

Hypoxanthine Riboside, Hypoxanthosine.

Scientific Names

2,3-Diphosphoglycerate; 6,9-Dihydro-9-B-D-ribofuranosyl-1H-puin-6-one; 9-B-D-ribofuranosylhypoxanthine.

People Use This For

Orally, inosine is used for enhancing athletic performance.

Safety

There is insufficient reliable information available about the safety of inosine.
Pregnancy And Lactation: Insufficient reliable information available; avoid using.

Effectiveness

LIKELY INEFFECTIVE

Athletic performance. Taking inosine orally does not improve athletic performance (2369,2370).

Mechanism of Action

Preliminary evidence suggests inosine might stimulate axon growth from uninjured nerve cells to injured nerve cells of the central nervous system. Further studies in humans are needed to establish whether this finding has significance in restoring function after spinal cord injuries (370).

Adverse Reactions

None reported.

Interactions with Herbs & Other Dietary Supplements

None known.

Interactions with Drugs

None known.

Interactions with Foods

None known.

Interactions with Lab Tests

None known.

Interactions with Diseases or Conditions

GOUT: Excess purinesm such as inosine, can aggravate gout.

Dosage and Administration

ORAL: 5 to 6 grams per day have been used in clinical studies of effects on athletic performance (2369,2370).

INOSITOL

Also Known As

Antialopecia Factor, Cyclohexitol, D-chiro-inositol, Dambrose, Inose, Inosite, Inositol Monophosphate, Lipositol, Meso-inositol, Mouse Antialopecia Factor, Myo-inositol, Vitamin B8.
CAUTION: See separate listings for Inositol Nicotinate and IP-6.

Scientific Names

Hexahydroxycyclohexane, synonyms 1,2,3,4,5,6-Cyclohexanehexol, cis-1,2,3,5-trans-4,6-Cyclohexanehexol; D-chiro-inositol, synonym (+)-chiroinositol, 1,2,5/3,4,6-inositol, (1S)-inositol, (1S)-1,2,4/3,5,6-inositol.

People Use This For

Orally, inositol is used for diabetic neuropathy, conditions associated with disorders of fat transport and metabolism, panic disorder, high cholesterol, insomnia, cancer, depression, schizophrenia, Alzheimer's disease, attention deficit-hyperactivity disorder (ADHD), autism, treating lithium-induced side effects, psoriasis, and promoting hair growth. Inositol is also used orally for treating conditions associated with polycystic ovary syndrome, including anovulation, hypertension, hypertriglyceridemia, and elevated serum concentrations of testosterone.
Parenterally, inositol is used for treating respiratory distress syndrome in premature infants.

Safety

POSSIBLY SAFE ...when used orally and appropriately. Inositol has been used in amounts up to 12 grams per day for up to 4 weeks, and 6 grams daily for 10 weeks with no significant adverse effects (2184,2185,2187).
CHILDREN: POSSIBLY SAFE ...when used parenterally and appropriately for treating respiratory distress syndrome in premature infants (2191,2192).
PREGNANCY: Insufficient reliable information available; avoid using.
LACTATION: Insufficient reliable information available; avoid using. Breast milk is rich in endogenous inositol (2138); however, the effects of exogenously administered inositol are not known.

Effectiveness

POSSIBLY EFFECTIVE

Lithium-induced side effects. Taking inositol orally seems to improve psoriasis associated with lithium. But it doesn't seem to help psoriasis in patients who aren't taking lithium (11972). Additionally, preliminary evidence suggests that taking inositol orally is not beneficial for reducing lithium-induced adverse effects, including tremor, thirst, and thyroid and adrenal function (2027).

Obsessive-compulsive disorder (OCD). There is some evidence that OCD patients who receive inositol orally for 6 weeks have significant improvement, based on Yale-Brown Obsessive Compulsive Scale scores, compared to placebo (2186).

Panic disorder. Taking inositol orally seems to be helpful for treating panic disorder with or without agoraphobia. Inositol seems to significantly reduce the severity and rate of panic attacks and the severity of agoraphobia over 4 weeks of treatment (2184). Some research suggests that it may be as effective as fluvoxamine (Luvox) for treatment of panic disorder (10387). Large scale, long-term trials are needed to confirm inositol's potential benefit in panic disorders.

Polycystic ovary syndrome. Taking the inositol isomer D-chiro-inositol orally seems to decrease serum triglyceride and testosterone levels, modestly decreases blood pressure, and induces ovulation in obese women with polycystic ovary syndrome (2028).

Respiratory distress syndrome. Administering inositol parenterally as a nutritional supplement seems to improve survival and symptoms in premature infants with respiratory distress syndrome. Inositol seems to lower inspiratory oxygen requirements, mean airway pressure, and the incidence of bronchopulmonary dysplasia in premature infants not receiving surfactant when compared to placebo and glucose (2191,2192).

POSSIBLY INEFFECTIVE

Alzheimer's disease. Taking inositol orally doesn't seem to improve symptoms of Alzheimer's disease (2189).

Autism. Taking inositol orally doesn't seem to improve symptoms of autism (2190).

Depression. Although limited research suggests that depressed patients receiving inositol for 4 weeks may improve, patients initially responding to inositol seem to relapse rapidly upon discontinuation of treatment (2026,2185). Inositol given in combination with SSRIs doesn't improve the effectiveness of SSRIs or improve depression in SSRI treatment failures (2025,10851).

Schizophrenia. Taking inositol orally doesn't seem to improve symptoms of schizophrenia (2188).

LIKELY INEFFECTIVE

Diabetic neuropathy. Taking inositol orally doesn't improve the symptoms of diabetic neuropathy (2193,2194,2195).

INSUFFICIENT RELIABLE EVIDENCE to RATE

Attention deficit-hyperactivity disorder (ADHD). Preliminary evidence suggests inositol might not help improve ADHD symptoms (2187). More evidence is needed to rate inositol for this use.

Mechanism of Action
Endogenous inositol is an essential component of cell membrane phospholipids. It has weak lipotropic activity, and can move fat out of liver and intestine cells (2187). Inositol is a constituent of the intracellular phosphatidyl inositol second messenger system, which is linked to serotonin, norepinephrine, and cholinergic receptors (10850,11972). Inositol has a variety of stereoisomers, including myo-inositol and D-chiro-inositol. Myo-inositol is the most abundant form in the central nervous system (CNS). Biological function varies among the isomers (2047,2048). Inositol might reverse desensitization of serotonin receptors (2187). Limited clinical evidence suggests exogenous inositol may have benefits similar to selective-serotonin-reuptake inhibitors (SSRIs) in conditions such as panic disorder, depression, and obsessive-compulsive disorder. Researchers think that D-chiro-inositol isomer induces ovulation in women with polycystic ovary syndrome by improving insulin sensitivity. Reduced insulin resistance is also thought to be responsible for improving other symptoms associated with polycystic ovary syndrome, including hypertension, hyperlipidemia, type 2 diabetes, obesity, and increased serum testosterone concentrations (2028). Additionally, patients with insulin resistance, including those with impaired glucose tolerance and type 2 diabetes, might have D-chiro-inositol deficiency (2028).
Supplemental inositol seems to help psoriasis that is made worse or triggered by lithium. The mechanism is unknown, but lithium seems to cause a reduction of inositol in both the brain and other tissues. Supplementation with inositol doesn't seem to adversely affect the efficacy of lithium for bipolar disorder (11972).

Adverse Reactions
Orally, inositol is generally well tolerated. It can cause nausea, tiredness, headache, and dizziness (10387,11972).

Interactions with Herbs & Other Dietary Supplements
None known.

Interactions with Drugs
None known.

Interactions with Foods
MINERALS: Phytic acid, the form of inositol found in foods, may interfere with absorption of minerals, especially calcium, zinc, and iron (16).

Interactions with Lab Tests
None known.

Interactions with Diseases or Conditions
None known.

Dosage and Administration
ORAL: For depression, inositol 12 grams per day has been used (2185). For panic disorder, 12 to 18 grams per day has been used (2184,10387). For obsessive-compulsive disorder, inositol 18 grams per day has been used (2186). For treating symptoms associated with polycystic ovary syndrome, D-chiro-inositol 1200 mg per day has been used (2028). For treating lithium-related psoriasis, 6 grams daily has been used (11972).
PARENTERAL: For respiratory distress syndrome in premature infants, inositol 80 mg/kg parenterally per day has been used (2191).

INOSITOL NICOTINATE

Also Known As
Hexanicotinoyl Inositol, Inositol Hexaniacinate, Inositol Hexanicotinate, Inositol Niacinate, Meso-Inositol Hexanicotinate, No-Flush Niacin.
CAUTION: See separate listings for Inositol and Niacin and Niacinamide (Vitamin B3).

Scientific Names
Hexanicotinyl cis-1,2,3-5-trans-4,6-cyclohexane; Myo-inositol hexa-3-pyridine-carboxylate.

People Use This For
Orally, inositol nicotinate is used for improving circulation and for treating peripheral vascular disease, cerebral vascular disease, intermittent claudication, stasis dermatitis, and Raynaud's disease. It is also used for hypercholesterolemia, atherosclerosis-related migraines, scleroderma, supporting nervous system and brain function, improving sleep, lowering blood pressure, calming effects, restless leg syndrome, acne, dermatitis herpetiformis, exfoliative glossitis, psoriasis, and schizophrenia and other mental illnesses.

Safety
POSSIBLY SAFE ...when used orally and appropriately (496).
PREGNANCY AND LACTATION: Insufficient reliable information available; avoid using.

Effectiveness
POSSIBLY EFFECTIVE

Hyperlipidemia. Taking inositol nicotinate orally seems reduce serum lipid levels, especially in combination with clofibrate (496,499,1546).

Peripheral vascular disease. Taking inositol nicotinate orally seems to be effective for improving symptoms of peripheral vascular disorders, including intermittent claudication and Raynaud's syndrome (496,498,1544,1545). Several weeks of treatment may be necessary before the full beneficial effects are seen (1544,1545).

There is insufficient reliable information available about inositol nicotinate for its other uses.

Mechanism of Action
Inositol nicotinate consists of six molecules of niacin (nicotinic acid) chemically linked to an inositol molecule. It is hydrolyzed in the body to free niacin and inositol, although this occurs slowly, with peak serum levels not occurring until approximately 10 hours after ingestion (496). It is theoretically possible that this slow conversion might reduce peak plasma levels and thereby reduce the incidence of side effects that have been associated with niacin such as flushing. The mechanism of action of inositol nicotinate is believed to be the same as that of niacin (496). Several weeks of treatment may be necessary before the full beneficial effects of inositol nicotinate are seen in peripheral vascular disorders such as Raynaud's disease, suggesting that fibrinolysis, lipid lowering, and vasodilatory action contribute to its beneficial effects (1544,1545).

Adverse Reactions
Adverse effects from the use of inositol nicotinate in usual doses appear to be rare (496). However, inositol nicotinate is metabolized to niacin which is associated with numerous side effects including flushing, pruritus, GI complaints, hepatotoxicity, hyperuricemia, and impaired glucose tolerance (496).

Interactions with Herbs & Other Dietary Supplements
None known.

Interactions with Drugs
ANTICOAGULANT/ANTIPLATELET DRUGS: Theoretically, concomitant use might increase the risk of bleeding, due to the fibrinolytic effects of inositol nicotinate (496).
ANTIDIABETES DRUGS: Concomitant use might interfere with blood glucose control. Inositol nicotinate is metabolized to niacin in the body (496). Niacin and niacinamide can interfere with blood glucose control requiring dosing adjustment of antidiabetic agents. Niacin and niacinamide can cause hyperglycemia, abnormal glucose tolerance, and glycosuria. Increased blood glucose monitoring may be necessary, particularly early in the course of treatment (4859,4860,12033).
HMG-CoA REDUCTASE INHIBITORS ("Statins"): Concomitant use of niacin and HMG-CoA reductase inhibitors increases the risk of myopathy. Inositol nicotinate is metabolized to niacin in the body (496). HMG-CoA reductase inhibitors include cerivastatin (Baycol), atorvastatin (Lipitor), lovastatin (Mevacor), pravastatin (Pravachol), and simvastatin (Zocor).
TRANSDERMAL NICOTINE (Nicoderm, Nicotrol): Concomitant use of niacin and transdermal nicotine increases the risk of flushing and dizziness. Inositol nicotinate is metabolized to niacin in the body (496).

Interactions with Foods
HOT DRINKS: Niacin-induced flushing can be magnified by concomitant ingestion of hot drinks. Inositol nicotinate is metabolized to niacin (6243).

Interactions with Lab Tests
CATECHOLAMINES: Niacin, a metabolite of inositol nicotinate, can produce fluorescent substances in the urine, which cause false elevations in some fluorometric tests of urinary catecholamines (15).
LIVER FUNCTION TESTS: Inositol nicotinate may increase levels of liver enzymes. Liver function should be monitored periodically when using doses of 2000 mg per day or more (496).

Interactions with Diseases or Conditions
ALLERGIES: Niacin, a metabolite of inositol nicotinate, might exacerbate allergies by causing histamine release (15,496).
CORONARY ARTERY DISEASE/UNSTABLE ANGINA: Large amounts of niacin, a metabolite of inositol nicotinate, can increase the risk of cardiac arrhythmias (15,496). One study showed an increased incidence of cardiac arrhythmias when niacin was used in patients with coronary artery disease (15); use with caution.
DIABETES: Niacin, a metabolite of inositol nicotinate, can interfere with blood glucose control requiring dosing

adjustment of antidiabetic agents. Niacin and niacinamide can cause hyperglycemia, abnormal glucose tolerance, and glycosuria. Increased blood glucose monitoring may be necessary, particularly early in the course of treatment (4859,4860,12033).
GALLBLADDER DISEASE: Niacin, a metabolite of inositol nicotinate, might exacerbate gallbladder disease (15,496); use with caution.
GOUT: Large amounts of niacin or niacinamide might precipitate gout. Niacin and niacinamide can cause hyperuricemia (12033); use with caution.
HYPOTENSION: Niacin, a metabolite of inositol nicotinate, can cause hypotension (15,496).
KIDNEY DISEASE: Niacin, a metabolite of inositol nicotinate, is excreted unchanged in the urine and might accumulate in patients with kidney disease (15,496); use with caution.
LIVER DISEASE: Inositol nicotinate should be avoided in people with liver disease. Niacin and niacinamide have been associated with liver damage (12033).
NIACIN HYPERSENSITIVITY: Inositol nicotinate is metabolized to niacin (15,496).
PEPTIC ULCER DISEASE: Large amounts of niacin, a metabolite of inositol nicotinate, might activate peptic ulcer disease (15,496).

Dosage and Administration

ORAL: For hyperlipoproteinemia, the typical dosing range is 1500-4000 mg daily given in 2-4 divided doses (496). For peripheral vascular disorders, the typical dosing range is 1500-4000 mg daily given in 2-4 divided doses (496).

Comments

Inositol nicotinate has been used in conventional medical practice in Great Britain for improving symptoms of peripheral vascular disorders and treating hyperlipidemia for many years, although it is not considered an agent of first choice.

INULIN

Also Known As

Chicory Extract, Chicory Inulin, Dahlia Extract, Dahlia Inulin, Fructo-Oligosaccharides, Fructooligosaccharides, Long-chain Oligosaccharides, Oligosaccharides, Prebiotic.
CAUTION: See separate listings for Chicory and Fructo-Oligosaccharides.

Scientific Names

Beta(2-1)fructans.

People Use This For

Orally, inulin is used for hypercholesterolemia, hypertriglyceridemia, hyperlipidemia, obesity and weight loss, improving gastrointestinal function, and as a food additive.

Safety

POSSIBLY SAFE ...when used orally and appropriately, short-term. Doses of 8 to 14 grams daily have been safely used for up to eight weeks (7604,7605,7606,7607,8451).
PREGNANCY AND LACTATION: Insufficient reliable information available; avoid using.

Effectiveness

POSSIBLY EFFECTIVE

Constipation. Taking inulin orally seems to increase the number of stools from 1-2 per week to 8-9 per week in elderly patients (10415).

Hypertriglyceridemia. Taking inulin orally seems to reduce triglycerides by up to 19% after eight weeks of treatment (7604).

POSSIBLY INEFFECTIVE

Hypercholesterolemia. Taking inulin orally as a supplement does not seem to significantly decrease serum cholesterol (7604,8450,10412,10413).

Obesity. Taking inulin orally, in combination with chromium picolinate, capsicum, L-phenylalanine, and other nutrients, doesn't seem to significantly reduce weight in moderately obese patients (7607).

Mechanism of Action

Inulin is an oligosaccharide, composed of chains of 2 to 60 glucose and fructose molecules. The major source of inulin in the diet is in wheat, onions, bananas, leaks, artichokes, and asparagus (10412,10414). Although inulin is found in many fruits, vegetables, and herbs, it is usually obtained by hot water extraction from chicory root (7606). Because it contributes very little in dietary calories, inulin is used as a food additive to increase bulk and palatability (8449). Inulin is related to short-chain oligosaccharides (SCO), which are often referred to as fructo-oligosaccharides. Partial hydrolysis of chicory inulin yields SCO, which are usually 2 to 7 sugar molecules in length and have many of the same effects as inulin (7606).

Inulin has a prebiotic effect, meaning that it is not digested or absorbed, and it promotes the growth of specific types of bacteria in the large intestine. Inulin preferentially promotes the growth of bifidobacteria. Fermentation of inulin decreases fecal pH and increases fecal volume (7605,8447,10414). The products of fermentation are short-chain fatty acids that are absorbed and metabolized (8449).

Inulin decreases serum triglycerides by decreasing fatty acid synthesis and reducing production of very low density lipoproteins (VLDL) (7604). Preliminary evidence indicates that SCO can reduce the formation of very low density lipoproteins (VLDL) (8448).

Adverse Reactions

Orally, inulin can commonly cause flatulence, bloating, gastrointestinal cramps, and intestinal noises. These symptoms become more bothersome at doses over 30 grams (7604,8450,8509). Some people can experience severe allergic reactions to inulin-containing foods. There is one report of anaphylaxis following consumption of foods with a high concentration of inulin including salsify, artichoke leaves, and margarine with inulin as a food additive (7608).

Interactions with Herbs & Other Dietary Supplements

None known.

Interactions with Drugs

None known.

Interactions with Foods

CALCIUM: Inulin appears to have no clinically significant effect on the absorption of dietary calcium. Inulin does not seem to affect ionized calcium, parathyroid hormone levels, or calcium excretion (8451,10274).

Interactions with Lab Tests

None known.

Interactions with Diseases or Conditions

None known.

Dosage and Administration

ORAL: For hypertriglyceridemia, the typical dose of inulin is 10 to 14 grams daily (7604). For treatment of hypercholesterolemia, inulin 6 grams three times daily has been used for up to 6 weeks (10412). For treatment of constipation in elderly, 20 to 40 grams per day for 19 days has been used (10415).

Comments

Inulin is used as an additive in many food products because it improves their palatability (7605).

IODINE

Also Known As

Potassium Iodide, Povidone Iodine.

Scientific Names

Iodine; I; atomic number 53.

People Use This For

Orally, iodine is used as an expectorant, for treating endemic goiter, thyroid storm, hyperthyroidism, treating radiation emergency associated with radioactive iodides, cutaneous sporotrichosis, and fibrocystic breast disease. Topically it is used as an antiseptic, for preventing mucositis from chemotherapy, and treating diabetic ulcers. Iodine is also used for water purification.

Safety

LIKELY SAFE ...when used orally and appropriately. Iodine is safe in amounts that do not exceed 1100 mcg per day, the Tolerable Upper Intake Level (UL) (7135). Higher doses can be safely used therapeutically with appropriate medical monitoring (2197,7080). Advise patients not to use doses greater than the UL without medical supervision.
...when used topically as a 2% solution (15). Iodine is an FDA-approved prescription product.

POSSIBLY UNSAFE ...when used orally in high doses. Tell patients to avoid prolonged use of doses exceeding the UL of 1100 mcg per day without proper medical supervision. Higher intake can increase the risk of side effects such as thyroid dysfunction (7135).

CHILDREN: LIKELY SAFE ...when used orally and appropriately (7135). Iodine is safe in amounts that do not exceed the UL of 200 mcg per day for children 1 to 3 years, 300 mcg per day for children 4 to 8 years, 600 mcg per day for children 9 to 13 years, and 900 mcg per day for adolescents (7135). ...when used topically as a 2% solution (15). Iodine is an FDA-approved prescription product. POSSIBLY UNSAFE ...when used orally in high doses. Tell patients to avoid prolonged use of doses exceeding the UL of 200 mcg per day for children 1 to 3 years, 300 mcg per day for children 4 to 8 years, 600 mcg per day for children 9 to 13 years, and 900 mcg per day for adolescents (7135). Higher intake can cause thyroid dysfunction (7135).

PREGNANCY AND LACTATION: LIKELY SAFE ...when used orally and appropriately. Iodine is safe in amounts that do not exceed the UL of 1100 mcg per day (7135). ...when used topically as a 2% solution (15). Iodine is an FDA-approved prescription product. POSSIBLY UNSAFE ...when used orally in high doses. Tell patients to avoid exceeding the UL of 1100 mcg per day or 900 mcg per day for pregnant women ages 14 to 18. Higher intake can cause thyroid dysfunction (7135).

Effectiveness

EFFECTIVE

Cutaneous sporotrichosis. Taking iodine orally improves cutaneous sporotrichosis (15).

Radiation. Iodine taken orally is effective for radiation emergency associated with radioactive iodides (7517,7518).

Respiratory congestion. Iodine taken orally is effective as an expectorant (15).

Skin infection. Iodine used topically is an effective antiseptic (15).

Thyroid conditions. Taking iodine orally can improve thyroid storm, hyperthyroidism, and endemic goiter (15).

Water purification. Adding iodine to water is effective for purification (15,16).

POSSIBLY EFFECTIVE

Diabetic foot ulcers. Topical use of iodine may be useful for treating diabetic foot ulcers (2200).

Fibrocystic breast disease. Taking iodine orally may improve fibrocystic breast disease (2197).

Oral mucositis. Topical use of iodine may prevent oral mucositis caused by chemotherapy (2198,2199).

There is insufficient reliable information available about the effectiveness of iodine for its other uses.

Mechanism of Action

Iodine is an essential nutrient in humans. About 90% of iodine, which is ingested in a variety of chemical forms, is absorbed (7135). The iodine content of most foods is low and is affected by agricultural factors such as soil quality and climate. Marine animals concentrate iodine from seawater and have a higher content than most other foods (7135). Processed foods may add to dietary iodine due to the addition of iodate to salt. The thyroid gland in humans concentrates iodine for thyroid synthesis. Lesser amounts of iodine are found in the salivary glands, breast, choroid plexus, and gastric mucosa. Iodine is excreted by the kidney (7135). Iodine comprises 65% of thyroxine (T4) and 59% of triiodothyronine (T3). These iodine-rich thyroid hormones control many biochemical reactions, particularly protein synthesis and enzymatic processes. In people with hyperthyroidism, iodine inhibits the release and synthesis of thyroid hormone (15). Iodine in the form of potassium iodide can block or reduce the accumulation of radioactive iodine and damage to the thyroid gland if taken prior to or immediately following exposure to radioactive iodine (7517,7518).

Iodine deficiency is most devastating on the developing brain (7135). Thyroid hormone is responsible for myelination of the developing central nervous system. Iodine deficiency is associated with mental retardation, and in extreme cases, cretinism (7135). Most developed countries, including the US and Canada, screen for hypothyroidism at birth (7135). The earliest clinical symptom of iodine deficiency is thyroid enlargement (goiter) (7135). Iodide salts, such as potassium iodide, might increase respiratory tract secretions and thereby decrease mucus viscosity, but there is limited supporting evidence for this effect (15). When used topically, iodine oxidizes organic substrates, killing microorganisms (15).

Adverse Reactions

Orally, iodine can cause marked sensitivity. Symptoms of iodine hypersensitivity are angioedema, cutaneous and mucosal hemorrhage, fever, arthralgia, lymph node enlargement, eosinophilia, urticaria, thrombotic thrombocytopenic purpura, and fatal periarteritis (15). Large amounts or chronic use of iodine can cause metallic taste; soreness in teeth and gums; burning in mouth and throat; increased salivation; coryza; sneezing; eye irritation and eyelid swelling; headache; cough; pulmonary edema; swelling of parotid and submaxillary glands; inflammation of the pharynx, larynx and tonsils; acneform skin lesions; gastric upset; diarrhea; anorexia; and depression (15,2138). Prolonged use of iodides can cause thyroid gland hyperplasia, thyroid adenoma, goiter, and severe hypothyroidism (15).

Topically, iodine may stain skin, irritate tissues, and cause sensitization in some individuals (15). Iodine burns are associated with application of 7% hydroalcoholic solution (15).

Interactions with Herbs & Other Dietary Supplements

None known.

Interactions with Drugs

ACE INHIBITORS (ACEIs): Concomitant use of these drugs with potassium iodide increases the risk of hyperkalemia (15). The ACE inhibitors include benazepril (Lotensin), captopril (Capoten), enalapril (Vasotec), fosinopril (Monopril), lisinopril (Prinivil, Zestril), moexipril (Univasc), perindopril (Aceon), quinapril (Accupril), ramipril (Altace), and trandolapril (Mavik).
AMIODARONE (Cordarone): Amiodarone contains 37.3% iodine. Plasma iodide levels may be increased and additive with iodine supplements (15,7135). Monitor thyroid function.
ANGIOTENSIN RECEPTOR BLOCKERS (ARBs): Concomitant use of these drugs with potassium iodide increases the risk of hyperkalemia (15). The ARBs include losartan (Cozaar), valsartan (Diovan), irbesartan (Avapro), candesartan (Atacand), telmisartan (Micardis), and eprosartan (Teveten).
ANTITHYROID DRUGS: Concomitant use may result in additive hypothyroid activity, and may cause hypothyroidism (2138).
LITHIUM: Concomitant use may have additive or synergistic hypothyroid effects (15).
POTASSIUM-SPARING DIURETICS: Concomitant use of potassium iodide with potassium sparing diuretics increases the risk of hyperkalemia (15). Potassium-sparing diuretics include spironolactone (Aldactone), Triamterene (Dyrenium), and amiloride (Midamor).

Interactions with Foods

None known.

Interactions with Lab Tests

THYROID HORMONES: Excess iodine intake can lower serum thyroid hormone and result in elevated thyroid stimulating hormone (TSH) levels (7135).

Interactions with Diseases or Conditions

AUTOIMMUNE THYROID DISEASE (AITD): People with AITD may have increased sensitivity to adverse effects of iodine (7135).
THYROID DYSFUNCTION: Prolonged use or excessive amounts of iodides may cause or exacerbate thyroid gland hyperplasia, thyroid adenoma, goiter, and hypothyroidism (15).

Dosage and Administration

ORAL: For fibrocystic breast disease, 80 mcg/kg molecular iodine has been used (2197). For radiation emergencies, potassium iodide (KI) should be taken just prior to, or as soon as possible after, exposure. Radiation is most toxic to pregnant or lactating women and children, so KI is dosed according to amount of radiation exposure and age. For infants, babies, children, adolescents, and pregnant or lactating women, KI is given if radiation exposure is 5 centigrays (cGy) or more. For birth through 1 month, the dose is KI 16 mg; for babies and children over 1 month through 3 years, 32 mg; for children 3 to 12 years, 65 mg; for adolescents 12 through 18 years, 65 mg or 120 mg if the adolescent is approaching adult size; and pregnant or lactating women, 120 mg. For adults 18 to 40 years with exposure to 10 cGy or more, KI 130 mg is given. For adults over 40 years with exposure to 500 cGy or more, KI 130 mg is given (7518). Tablets can be crushed and mixed with fruit juice, jam, milk, etc (7517). The National Institute of Medicine has set Adequate Intake (AI) of iodine for infants: 0 to 6 months, 110 mcg/day; 7 to 12 months, 130 mcg/day (7135). For children and adults, Recommended Dietary Amounts (RDA) have been set: children 1 to 8 years, 90 mcg/day; 9 to 13 years, 120 mcg/day; people age 14 and older, 150 mcg/day (7135). For pregnant women, the RDA is 209 mcg/day, and breast-feeding women, 290 mcg/day (7135). Tolerable Upper Intake Levels (UL) for iodine intake have been set: children 1 to 3 years, 200 mcg/day; 4 to 8 years, 300 mcg/day; 9 to 13 years, 600 mcg/day; 14 to 18 years (including pregnancy and lactation), 900 mcg/day. For adults older than age 19 including pregnant and breast-feeding women, the UL is 1100 mcg/day (7135).
TOPICAL: As an antiseptic, 2% aqueous solution applied to affected skin areas (15). For preventing mucositis from chemotherapy, rinse mouth with povidone iodine solution 4 times daily (2198,2199). To treat diabetic foot ulcers, 0.9% iodine ointment (2200) has been used. Avoid occluding skin areas treated with iodine to reduce risk of iodine burn (15).

Comments

Iodine deficiency is a common world health problem (7135). Early in the twentieth century, iodine deficiency was common in the US and Canada, but the addition of iodine to salt has improved public health. The addition of potassium iodide at 100 ppm, or 76 mg of iodine per kg of salt, is mandatory in Canada, and iodized salt is used optionally by half of the US population (7135). Potassium iodide tablets for use in a radiation emergency are available as FDA-approved products (Thyro-Block, Iostat) and on the Internet as food supplements. Tell patients that potassium iodide should only be used in a radiation emergency, not as prophylaxis in case of a radiation emergency.

IP-6

Also Known As

Fytic Acid, Inositol Hexaphosphate, IP6, Phytic Acid.
Caution: See separate listings for Inositol, Inositol Nicotinate, and Vitamin B3.

Scientific Names

Inositol hexaphosphate.

People Use This For

Orally, IP-6 is used to treat and prevent cancer, increase white blood cell production, prevent heart attacks, prevent and treat kidney stones, enhance the immune system, and as an antioxidant.

Safety

LIKELY SAFE ...when consumed in amounts commonly found in foods (1854).
There is insufficient reliable information available about the safety of IP-6 when used in supplemental doses in amounts greater than those found in foods.
PREGNANCY AND LACTATION: LIKELY SAFE ...when consumed in amounts commonly found in foods (1854). There is insufficient reliable information available about the safety of IP-6 when used in amounts greater than those found in foods; avoid using.

Effectiveness

POSSIBLY EFFECTIVE

Kidney stones (nephrolithiasis). There is some evidence that people with high dietary intake of IP-6 have a decreased risk of developing kidney stones (10296).

There is insufficient reliable information available about the effectiveness of IP-6 for its other uses.

Mechanism of Action

Inositol hexaphosphate (IP-6), the hexaphosphate ester of inositol, is the major phosphorus storage compound in plants, comprising from 1-7% of the dry weight of most cereals, nuts, and legumes (1855,1858). IP-6 and other less phosphorylated forms (e.g., inositol triphosphate) are also endogenous to most mammalian cells in much smaller amounts (1857). Cellular functions include signal transduction and cellular proliferation and differentiation (1857).
IP-6 chelates multivalent metal ions (particularly zinc, calcium, and iron) forming insoluble salts in the gastrointestinal (GI) tract and decreasing mineral bioavailability (1858,1869,1870). Preliminary evidence suggests that the ability of IP-6 to chelate minerals might decrease iron-mediated colon cancer risk, and lower serum cholesterol and triglycerides (1858).
In the urine, IP-6 can reduce the formation of calcium and oxalate crystals (10297). IP-6 appears to reduce the concentration of calcium and the formation of calcium crystals in renal papillary tissue (10298).
As a natural antioxidant, IP-6 added to food reduces lipid peroxidation and retards spoilage (1855,1858). In preliminary research, IP-6 inhibits cancer cell proliferation and increases cancer cell differentiation, sometimes resulting in reversion to a normal phenotype (1859). IP-6 has shown anticancer activity in breast tissue, colon tissue, liver tissue, prostate tissue, and experimental tumors (1860,1861,1862,1863,1864,1865). IP-6 might also inhibit platelet aggregation and lower serum cholesterol and triglycerides, according to preliminary studies (1867,1868).

Adverse Reactions

None reported.

Interactions with Herbs & Other Dietary Supplements

CALCIUM, IRON, ZINC: Concurrent use of IP-6 may decrease mineral absorption. IP-6 can chelate multivalent metal ions in the gastrointestinal tract, forming insoluble salts and decreasing mineral absorption (1858).
HERBS WITH ANTICOAGULANT/ANTIPLATELET POTENTIAL: Theoretically, concomitant use of IP-6 with herbs that affect platelet aggregation might increase the risk of bleeding. In vitro IP-6 can inhibit platelet aggregation (1867). This effect has not been demonstrated in humans. Herbs with potential anticoagulant or antiplatelet properties include angelica, clove, danshen, garlic, ginger, ginkgo, Panax ginseng, red clover, turmeric, and others.

Interactions with Drugs

ANTICOAGULANT/ANTIPLATELET DRUGS: Theoretically, concomitant use of IP-6 with drugs that affect platelet aggregation may increase the risk of bleeding. In vitro IP-6 can inhibit platelet aggregation (1867). This effect has not been demonstrated in humans.

Interactions with Foods

None known.

Interactions with Lab Tests

CHOLESTEROL/TRIGLYCERIDES: Theoretically, IP-6 may reduce serum cholesterol and triglyceride levels. Preliminary research suggests that IP-6 can lower cholesterol and triglyceride levels (1868). This effect has not been demonstrated in humans.

Interactions with Diseases or Conditions

CLOTTING DISORDERS: Theoretically, IP-6 may increase risk of bleeding (1867). In vitro, IP-6 can inhibit platelet aggregation (1867). This effect has not been demonstrated in humans.
IRON-DEFICIENCY ANEMIA: IP-6 might decrease dietary and supplemental iron absorption. IP-6 chelates multivalent metal ions in the gastrointestinal tract, preventing absorption (1858).
OSTEOPOROSIS/OSTEOPENIA (Paget's Disease): IP-6 may decrease dietary and supplemental calcium absorption. IP-6 chelates multivalent metal ions in the gastrointestinal tract, preventing absorption (1858).

Dosage and Administration

No typical dosage.

Comments

Preliminary studies of inositol hexaphosphate in cancer have been ongoing since 1988; however, to date, no studies in humans with cancer have been performed (1866). "IP-6, Nature's Revolutionary Cancer-Fighter," a book by prominent inositol hexaphosphate researcher, Abulkalam M. Shamsuddin, MD, PhD, has popularized inositol hexaphosphate (1854).

IPECAC

Also Known As

Brazil Root, Brazilian Ipecac, Cartagena Ipecac, Ipecacuanha, Matto Grosso Ipecac, Nicaragua Ipecac, Panama Ipecac, Rio Ipecac.

Scientific Names

Psychotria ipecacuanha, synonyms Callicocca ipecacuanha, Cephaelis acuminata, Cephaelis ipecacuanha; Uragoga ipecacuanha; Uragoga granatensis.
Family: Rubiaceae.

People Use This For

Orally, ipecac is used as an expectorant and emetic, for croupous bronchitis in children, amebic dysentery, as an appetite stimulant (small doses), and for treating cancer.
Intravenously, ipecac is used for amebic abscesses and hepatitis.

Safety

POSSIBLY SAFE ...when the rhizome or syrup of ipecac is used orally and appropriately short-term (12).
POSSIBLY UNSAFE ...when used orally long-term. Theoretically, prolonged use might blunt the emetic reflex (19). ...when in contact with skin or when inhaled. The constituent emetine is a skin irritant, and ipecac powder is a respiratory irritant (6,18).
LIKELY UNSAFE ...when used orally in large amounts. Misuse can lead to serious toxicity or death (6,12). ...when a total dose of more than 1 gram is injected, it can cause nervous system symptoms, blood in the urine, and circulatory collapse (6).
CHILDREN: LIKELY SAFE ...when used orally and appropriately as an emetic (272,11349).
LIKELY UNSAFE ...when used orally in large doses and in infants under 1 year old (12,19). Children are more sensitive to large doses and effects on the nervous system than adults (19).
PREGNANCY: LIKELY UNSAFE ...when used orally; ipecac is a potential uterine stimulant (12,19).
LACTATION: Insufficient reliable information available; avoid using.

Effectiveness

POSSIBLY EFFECTIVE

Poisoning. Taking syrup of ipecac orally is an effective emetic (15). Ipecac is an FDA-approved prescription product. However, the efficacy in preventing pediatric deaths with routine use of ipecac at home has never been proven. The American Academy of Pediatrics recommended in 1983 that all households keep a 1-ounce bottle of syrup of ipecac at home. Ipecac could then be used on the advice of a physician, emergency department, or poison control center to induce vomiting. This recommendation has recently been reversed stating, "Syrup of ipecac should no longer be routinely used as a poison treatment intervention in the home" (11349).

There is insufficient reliable information available about the effectiveness of ipecac for its other uses.

Mechanism of Action
Ipecac contains the alkaloids, emetine and cephaeline (13). Ipecac produces emesis by irritating the GI mucosa and by stimulating the chemoreceptor trigger zone in the brain (6,13).

Adverse Reactions
Orally, ipecac causes nausea, vomiting (3,6,13,15,18), GI irritation, dizziness, hypotension, dyspnea, and tachycardia (11). Chronic use is associated with myopathies and death (6,18). Overdose is associated with erosion of GI tract mucous membranes, cardiac arrhythmias, disorders of respiratory function, convulsions, shock, and coma (18).
Topically, emetine is a skin irritant (6). Ipecac powder is a respiratory irritant.
Intravenously, emetine may cause inflammation of the muscle tissue at the injection site with chronic administration. In total doses over 1 gram, it can lead to gastrointestinal and nervous system symptoms, hematuria and circulatory collapse (6).

Interactions with Herbs & Other Dietary Supplements
PODOPHYLLUM: Ipecac reduces the intensity of the cathartic effect of podophyllum (19).

Interactions with Drugs
ACTIVATED CHARCOAL: Activated charcoal adsorbs and inactivates syrup of ipecac; avoid co-administration (506).

Interactions with Foods
None known.

Interactions with Lab Tests
None known.

Interactions with Diseases or Conditions
GI CONDITIONS: Ipecac can irritate gastrointestinal tract. Contraindicated in individuals with infectious or inflammatory gastrointestinal conditions (19).
HEART DISEASES: Use of ipecac is contraindicated (12), due to cardiotoxic potential of emetine (6), and its depressive effect on the heart (19).
POISONINGS: Ipecac is contraindicated in individuals poisoned with corrosives (risks re-exposure of esophageal tissue), petroleum distillates (risks aspiration pneumonia), strychnine (risk of convulsions) (12,19).
UNCONSCIOUSNESS: Contraindicated (12).

Dosage and Administration
ORAL: Expectorant (adults), 0.4-1.4 mL ipecac syrup (USP) (12). Emetic, 15 mL ipecac syrup (USP) followed by 1-2 glasses of water (12); may repeat once in 20 minutes if no results (12,13). Before using ipecac syrup to treat poisoning, call poison control for recommendation. Ipecac syrup is available both as a nonprescription product and as an FDA-approved prescription product.

IPORURU

Also Known As
Iporoni, Iporuro, Ipurosa, Ipururo, Macochihua, Niando.

Scientific Names
Alchornea castaneifolia.
Family: Euphorbiaceae.

People Use This For
Orally, iporuru is used for coughs; rheumatism; impotence; lowering blood sugar levels in individuals with diabetes; diarrhea; headache; toothache; snakebite; bronchitis; chancre; chills; conjunctivitis; dysentery; dysmenorrhea; gonorrhea; hemorrhoids; jaundice; leprosy; malaria; ophthalmia; ringworm; stimulating digestion; thrush; urethritis, and as a cathartic, diuretic, emetic, and aphrodisiac.
Topically, iporuru is used for arthritis, colds, muscle pain, rheumatism, and for stingray wounds.

Safety
There is insufficient reliable information available about the safety of iporuru.
Pregnancy and Lactation: Insufficient reliable information available; avoid using.

Effectiveness
There is insufficient reliable information available about the effectiveness of iporuru.

Mechanism of Action
The applicable parts of iporuru are the bark, leaf, and root. There is insufficient reliable information available about the possible mechanism of action and active ingredients.

Adverse Reactions
None reported.

Interactions with Herbs & Other Dietary Supplements
None known.

Interactions with Drugs
None known.

Interactions with Foods
None known.

Interactions with Lab Tests
None known.

Interactions with Diseases or Conditions
None known.

Dosage and Administration
ORAL: Iporuru is typically prepared as a tea with 1 teaspoon of dried leaf added to 4 ounces of boiling water and taken 1 to 3 times daily. A 4:1 tincture is taken in a dose of 2 to 3 mL twice daily (5255).

IPRIFLAVONE

Also Known As
7-Isopropoxy-Isoflavone, 7-Isopropoxy Isoflavone, FL-113, TC-80.
CAUTION: See separate listings for Red Clover and Soy.

Scientific Names
7-isopropoxyisoflavone.

People Use This For
Orally, ipriflavone is used for preventing and treating postmenopausal and senile osteoporosis, preventing drug-induced osteoporosis, relieving osteoporotic pain, treating Paget's disease and renal osteodystrophy, and for reducing bone loss in hemiplegic stroke patients. Ipriflavone is also used by bodybuilders as an anabolic agent.

Safety
LIKELY SAFE ...when used orally and appropriately. Ipriflavone seems to be safe when used for up to 3 years (427,428,430,431,432,433,1196,2169,2170,2171,2172,2173,2174,2175,4749,10228). However, there is concern that ipriflavone can cause subclinical (asymptomatic) lymphocytopenia in some patients taking it for greater than 6 months (see Adverse Reactions) (1196). Monitor white blood cell (WBC) count in patients taking ipriflavone long-term. Tell patients not to take ipriflavone without proper medical supervision and monitoring.
PREGNANCY AND LACTATION: Insufficient reliable information available; avoid using.

Effectiveness
LIKELY EFFECTIVE

Osteoporosis. Taking ipriflavone orally in combination with calcium 1000 mg daily can prevent loss of bone mineral density (BMD) in postmenopausal women with osteoporosis or low bone mass (430,432,433,2169,2170,2175). There is some evidence that it might actually increase BMD in some of these patients (428,2173,2175,4756). Concurrent use of calcium in doses of at least 1000 mg per day might be necessary for greatest benefit. One study using ipriflavone with only 500 mg per day of calcium found no effect on BMD (1196). Ipriflavone can also significantly reduce osteoporotic pain and seems to be as effective as inhaled calcitonin (432,2175,4756,4757). Taking Ipriflavone plus calcium or vitamin D prophylactically also seems to help prevent osteoporosis in postmenopausal women (2171,2174). However, using ipriflavone in combination with low-dose estrogen seems to be more beneficial than ipriflavone alone for preventing osteoporosis. Ipriflavone plus conjugated estrogen 0.3 mg per day and calcium 500-1000 mg daily seems to consistently increase BMD in postmenopausal women (427,2171,2172). Ipriflavone in combination with conjugated estrogen 0.625 mg per day can also decreases loss of bone mineral density (BMD) better than estrogen or ipriflavone alone in oophorectomized women (4749). Ipriflavone also seems to prevent loss of bone mineral density (BMD) induced by the gonadotropin hormone-releasing hormone agonist, leuprolide (Lupron) (10228). Adding calcium provides further benefit (4746). Ipriflavone in combination with vitamin D, seems to prevent BMD loss significantly better than vitamin D alone in hemiplegic stroke patients with vitamin D deficiency (429).

POSSIBLY EFFECTIVE

Paget's disease. There is some evidence that ipriflavone 600 mg or 1200 mg given orally for 30 days can reduce serum alkaline phosphatase and hydroxyproline/creatinine excretion and decrease bone pain in patients with Paget's disease (2176).

Renal osteodystrophy. Taking ipriflavone orally seems to be beneficial for people with renal osteodystrophy (2177).

There is insufficient reliable information available about the effectiveness of ipriflavone for its other uses.

Mechanism of Action

Ipriflavone is a semisynthetic isoflavone manufactured in the laboratory from daidzein, a compound derived from soy (431). Ipriflavone enhances osteoblast function and inhibits bone resorption, mainly by inhibiting recruitment of osteoclasts (2173,2176,2179). Preliminary evidence suggests that ipriflavone prevents bone density loss without suppressing the rate of bone formation (unlike 17-beta-estradiol which suppresses the rate of bone formation) (426). Ipriflavone has no direct estrogenic activity in postmenopausal women, but might potentiate the effects of estrogen on bone, increase uterotropic activity of estrogen, and stimulate estrogen-induced calcitonin secretion (434,2179). Clinical evidence suggests that using ipriflavone in combination with conjugated estrogens for postmenopausal osteoporosis might allow for use of a lower estrogen dose (427,2171,2172). Ipriflavone, or its metabolite 7-hydroxy-isoflavone, might inhibit cytochrome P450 (CYP450) enzymes CYP1A2 and CYP2C9 (2178). Laboratory evidence suggests that isoflavones can inhibit oxidative and conjugative metabolism (4736). Isoflavones might also affect drug absorption and biliary excretion by interacting with drug transporters such as P-glycoprotein and the canalicular multispecific organic anion transporter (4736). Whether ipriflavone has similar activity is unknown.

Adverse Reactions

Orally, ipriflavone is usually well-tolerated. However, some patients taking ipriflavone can experience epigastric pain, diarrhea, and dizziness (432). There is some concern about ipriflavone causing lymphocytopenia. In one study, subclinical (asymptomatic) lymphocytopenia occurred in about 13% of patients. Decreased lymphocytes (less than 500/microliter) seems to be most likely to occur after 6 months of treatment, but may not occur until much later (1196). The clinical significance of this effect on lymphocytes is not known. Monitor white blood cell (WBC) counts in patients taking ipriflavone long-term. Consider discontinuing ipriflavone if lymphocytes drop below 1000 per microliter. Lymphocyte counts seem to normalize in most patients within 12 months after discontinuing ipriflavone (1196). Tell patients not to take ipriflavone without proper medical supervision and monitoring.

Interactions with Herbs & Other Dietary Supplements

CALCIUM: Concomitant use may enhance effects in preventing osteoporosis (2169,2170,2171,2173,2175).

VITAMIN D: Concomitant use may enhance effects in preventing osteoporosis (2174).

Interactions with Drugs

CYTOCHROME P450 1A2 (CYP1A2) SUBSTRATES: Ipriflavone is thought to competitively inhibit cytochrome P450 1A2 (CYP1A2) (2178). Theoretically, concurrent use of ipriflavone and drugs metabolized by these enzymes might result in decreased drug elimination, increased serum levels, and potential toxicity. Some drugs metabolized by CYP1A2 include clozapine (Clozaril), cyclobenzaprine (Flexeril), fluvoxamine (Luvox), haloperidol (Haldol), imipramine (Tofranil), mexiletine (Mexitil), olanzapine (Zyprexa), Pentazocine (Talwin), propranolol (Inderal), tacrine (Cognex), theophylline (Slo-bid, Theo-Dur, others), zileuton (Zyflo), Zolmitriptan (Zomig), and others.

CYTOCHROME P450 2C9 (CYP2C9) SUBSTRATES: Ipriflavone is thought to competitively inhibit cytochrome P450 2C9 (CYP2C9) (2178). Theoretically, concurrent use of ipriflavone and drugs metabolized by these enzymes might result in decreased drug elimination, increased serum levels, and potential toxicity. Some drugs metabolized by CYP2C9 include amitriptyline (Elavil), diazepam (Valium), estradiol (Estrace), tacrine (Cognex), verapamil (Calan), warfarin (Coumadin), zileuton (Zyflo), and others.

IMMUNOSUPPRESSANTS: Concurrent use of ipriflavone and immunosuppressant drugs might have additive effects on inhibiting immune function. Some patients taking ipriflavone experience subclinical (asymptomatic) lymphocytopenia (1196); avoid concurrent use. Immunosuppressant drugs include azathioprine (Imuran), basiliximab (Simulect), cyclosporine (Neoral, Sandimmune), daclizumab (Zenapax), muromonab-CD3 (OKT3, Orthoclone OKT3), mycophenolate (CellCept), tacrolimus (FK506, Prograf), sirolimus (Rapamune), prednisone (Deltasone, Orasone), and other corticosteroids (glucocorticoids).

THEOPHYLLINE: Concomitant use of theophylline and ipriflavone can increase serum theophylline levels.

Increased theophylline levels have occurred in two cases after patients started taking ipriflavone (2178,6604). Ipriflavone is thought to decrease theophylline metabolism through competitive inhibition of the cytochrome P450 1A2 (CYP1A2) enzyme (2178,6604).

Interactions with Foods

None known.

Interactions with Lab Tests

LYMPHOCYTES: Ipriflavone can decrease lymphocytes in some patients. Lymphocytes can often decrease by about 27% in patients after 6 months of use and then they stabilize. However, in a smaller number of patients, about 13% in one study, subclinical (asymptomatic) lymphocytopenia (less than 500/microliter) can occur (1196). White blood cell (WBC) count should be monitored in patients using ipriflavone long-term. Consider discontinuing ipriflavone if lymphocytes drop below 1000 per microliter. Lymphocyte counts seem to normalize in most patients within 12 months after discontinuing ipriflavone (1196).

Interactions with Diseases or Conditions

IMMUNOSUPPRESSION: Theoretically, ipriflavone might have additive immunosuppressive effects in patients with a compromised immune system. Ipriflavone can cause lymphocytopenia in some patients (1196); use with caution.

LYMPHOCYTOPENIA: Since ipriflavone has been reported to cause lymphocytopenia in some patients (1196), it might further decrease lymphocyte counts when used in patients with pre-existing lymphocytopenia; use with caution.

Dosage and Administration

ORAL: The typical dose for postmenopausal osteoporosis is 200 mg three times daily (2169,2170,2171,2172,2173,2175). For Paget's disease, ipriflavone 600-1200 mg daily has been used (2176). For treating renal osteodystrophy, 400-600 mg ipriflavone daily has been used (2177). For reducing drug-induced bone mineral loss, ipriflavone 600 mg daily has been used (10228).

Comments

Ipriflavone is used in Italy and Japan in the treatment of osteoporosis.

IRON

Also Known As

Elemental Iron, Fer, Ferrous Carbonate Anhydrous, Ferrous Fumarate, Ferrous Gluconate, Ferrous Pyrophosphate, Ferrous Sulfate.

Scientific Names

Iron; Fe; atomic number 26.

People Use This For

Orally, iron salts are used for preventing and treating iron deficiency and iron deficiency anemia. It is also used for attention deficit-hyperactivity disorder (ADHD), improving athletic performance, treating oral canker sores, Crohn's disease, depression, fatigue, female infertility, and menorrhagia.

Safety

LIKELY SAFE ...when used orally and appropriately. For people age 14 and older with adequate iron stores, iron supplements are safe when used in doses below the tolerable upper intake level (UL) of 45 mg per day of elemental iron. The UL is not meant to apply to those who receive iron under medical supervision (7135). To treat iron deficiency, most people can safely take up to 300 mg elemental iron per day (15).

LIKELY UNSAFE ...when used orally in excessive doses. Doses greater than the UL of 45 mg frequently cause gastrointestinal side effects such as constipation and nausea (7135). Doses of 30 mg/kg are associated with acute toxicity. Long-term use of high doses of iron can cause hemosiderosis and multiple organ damage. The estimated lethal dose of iron is 180-300 mg/kg; however, doses as low as 60 mg/kg have also been lethal (15).

CHILDREN: LIKELY SAFE ...when used orally and appropriately (7135). LIKELY UNSAFE ...when used orally in excessive amounts. Tell patients who are not iron-deficient not to use doses above the tolerable upper intake level (UL) of 40 mg per day of elemental iron for infants and children. Higher doses frequently cause gastrointestinal side effects such as constipation and nausea (7135). Iron is the most common cause of pediatric poisoning deaths. Doses as low as 60 mg/kg can be fatal (15).

PREGNANCY AND LACTATION: LIKELY SAFE ...when used orally and appropriately. Iron is safe for pregnant and breast-feeding women with adequate iron stores when used in doses below the tolerable upper intake level (UL) of 45 mg per day of elemental iron (7135). LIKELY UNSAFE ...when used orally in high doses. Tell patients who are not iron deficient to avoid exceeding the tolerable upper intake level (UL) of 45 mg per day of elemental iron. Higher doses frequently cause gastrointestinal side effects such as nausea and vomiting. High hemoglobin concentrations at the time of delivery are associated with adverse pregnancy outcomes (7135).

Effectiveness

EFFECTIVE

Anemia of chronic disease. Taking iron orally with epoetin alfa (erythropoietin, EPO, Epogen, Procrit) is effective for treating anemia associated with chronic renal failure and chemotherapy. Epoetin alfa is needed to ensure that the response is not limited by lack of iron for erythropoiesis (1087,1091).

Iron deficiency anemia. Taking iron orally is effective for treating iron deficiency anemia (1089,7135).

POSSIBLY EFFECTIVE

ACE inhibitor-associated cough. Taking iron orally seems to inhibit cough associated with angiotensin converting enzyme (ACE) inhibitors. Ferrous sulfate 256 mg daily might reduce or eliminate cough associated with ACE inhibitors such as captopril (Capoten), enalapril (Vasotec), Lisinopril (Prinivil, Zestril), and others (7307).

Cognitive function. Taking iron orally seems to improve cognitive function in iron-deficient children and adolescents. Supplemental iron seems to improve verbal learning and memory in non-anemic iron-deficient adolescent girls (1095). It might also reverse developmental and learning deficits in iron-deficient children (1104).

INSUFFICIENT RELIABLE EVIDENCE to RATE

Attention deficit-hyperactivity disorder (ADHD). Taking iron orally might improve symptoms of attention deficit-hyperactivity disorder (ADHD) (1093).

Fatigue. There is preliminary evidence that iron supplementation might improve unexplained fatigue in non-anemic women. Ferrous sulfate 80 mg daily may improve fatigue primarily in women with borderline or low serum ferritin concentrations (11406).

More evidence is needed to rate iron for these uses.

Mechanism of Action

Iron is a trace mineral found in two ionic forms in the body. It exists in a reduced state as ferrous iron and in an oxidized state as ferric iron. Most of the iron in the body is found in the hemoglobin of red blood cells and in the myoglobin of muscle cells where it is required for oxygen and carbon dioxide transport (1093). Iron also functions in the electron transport chain as an electron carrier in cytochromes. It is also found in the functional groups of most enzymes in the Krebs cycle (945). Iron is an essential cofactor in the synthesis of neurotransmitters such as dopamine, norepinephrine, and serotonin.

Iron deficiency anemia in early life seems to negatively affect behavioral and neural development (1093,9962). Signs and symptoms of deficiency include microcytic and hypochromic anemia, lethargy, cognitive impairment, developmental delay, amenorrhea, hair loss, enlarged liver, and others (7135). Iron deficiency in pregnancy has been associated with adverse pregnancy outcomes and increased perinatal maternal mortality (7135). The rate of iron absorption from food and supplements is variable. Absorption of iron from foods depends on the source. Meats, such as red meat, poultry, and fish provide iron in heme and non-heme forms. Meats contain about 40% heme iron and 60% non-heme iron. Heme iron is absorbed at a rate of 23% compared to 2-20% for non-heme iron. Iron from plant sources is only in the non-heme form. Iron bioavailability from a vegetarian diet is estimated to be 5 to 10%. Meats and fish seem to enhance the absorption of non-heme iron (7135). Boiling, steaming, or stir-frying appears to enhance the bioavailability of iron contained in many vegetables including asparagus, broccoli, cabbage, red and green peppers, and tomatoes; but cold storage of cooked vegetables might greatly reduce the increases in iron bioavailability gained from cooking (5044). Overall, dietary iron absorption is only 10-15%. However, this varies significantly depending on the person and the iron demand of the body (403). Vegetarians and people who engage in intense physical exercise, particularly female athletes, may have increased iron requirements (7135). Blood loss and rapid growth also increase gastrointestinal absorption (1101). Iron is stored as ferritin or hemosiderin (7135). Body iron is highly conserved. In the absence of bleeding (including menstruation) or pregnancy, the body loses only a small quantity of iron each day, mostly through the feces (7135). Iron also seems to reduce nitric oxide production. This effect might be clinically useful in the suppression of cough associated with angiotensin converting enzyme (ACE) inhibitors. Iron might reduce the generation of nitric oxide, which is thought to be increased by ACE inhibitors (7303).

Adverse Reactions

Orally, iron can cause gastrointestinal irritation, abdominal pain, constipation or diarrhea, nausea, and vomiting. At doses below the tolerable upper intake level (UL) of 45 mg per day of elemental iron in adults with normal iron stores, gastrointestinal adverse effects are uncommon (7135). Higher doses can be taken safely in adults with iron deficiency, but gastrointestinal side effects may occur. Taking iron supplements with food seems to reduce gastrointestinal side effects (7135). Liquid oral preparations can blacken teeth (9). Long-term use of high doses of iron can cause hemosiderosis that clinically resembles hemochromatosis (15). Acute overdosage, 60 mg/kg and more, can cause vomiting and diarrhea, followed by cardiovascular or metabolic toxicity, and death (7135). There is a debate regarding the potential association between high levels of iron stores and cancer. So far, data are conflicting and inconclusive (1098,1099,1100,1102). There is also a debate regarding a potential association between coronary heart disease or myocardial infarction (MI) and high iron intake or high body iron stores; some studies have reported associations (1492,7135,9542,9544,9545). Some studies only found an association with high heme iron intake (1492,9546). However, the majority of research has found no association (1097,1099,9543,9547,9548,9549,9550). The currently available data doesn't support a recommendation to reduce iron intake to reduce cardiovascular risks, especially considering the potential problems associated with iron deficiency (9543).

Interactions with Herbs & Other Dietary Supplements

ACACIA: Acacia forms an insoluble gel with ferric iron (16). It isn't known whether this leads to a significant interaction when the two are ingested together.

CALCIUM: Calcium inhibits the absorption of dietary heme- and non-heme iron (7135,7308,9573). However, in people with adequate iron stores, this doesn't appear to be clinically significant (1848,1849,1850,7135,7308). Advise people at risk for iron deficiency to take calcium supplements at bedtime, instead of with meals, to avoid inhibiting dietary iron absorption (7308). Calcium supplements can also inhibit absorption of iron supplements. However, the effect is very variable and depends on the salt form used, presence or absence of food, and the type of food (9586). The clinical significance is unclear, but advise patients to take calcium and iron supplements at different times of the day if possible.

RIBOFLAVIN (Vitamin B2): Riboflavin supplements may improve the hematological response to iron supplements in some people with anemia (9518). Riboflavin is thought to be involved in mobilization of iron for heme synthesis from the storage form, ferritin, and in globin synthesis (9518). This effect is probably only significant in people with riboflavin deficiency.

SOY: Soy protein reduces absorption of dietary non-heme (plant-derived) iron, probably due to binding of iron by phytate and calcium present in soy (5053,9573). Fermented soy products seem to inhibit of iron absorption less (9586). The clinical significance of these effects hasn't been determined.

VITAMIN A, BETA-CAROTENE: Vitamin A appears to be involved in mobilizing iron from tissue stores for delivery to developing red blood cells in the bone marrow. Improvements in hemoglobin levels can occur in people with anemia and low serum retinol levels when they are given vitamin A supplements (9586). Vitamin A may also be involved in the differentiation and proliferation of blood stem cells in the bone marrow, and in the synthesis of erythropoietin (9518). Preliminary evidence also suggests that vitamin A and beta-carotene may enhance non-heme iron absorption from iron-fortified wheat and corn flour, and rice. It's suggested that these vitamins bind to iron in the gut, improving its solubility and preventing binding by dietary polyphenols and phytate, which reduce iron absorption (9569). It's unlikely that vitamin A supplements would have significant effects on iron status in people without vitamin A deficiency.

VITAMIN C (Ascorbic acid): Supplemental or dietary vitamin C improves absorption of supplemental or dietary non-heme (plant-derived) iron ingested at the same time (9518,9571,9586). The amount of vitamin C in the diet is a factor in dietary iron absorption and iron status (9570,9572). Vitamin C can counteract the effects of substances which inhibit iron absorption such as dietary phytates, polyphenols, and tannins possibly by chemically reducing iron and preventing the formation of less soluble ferric compounds (9518,9573,9586). Taking a vitamin C supplement to improve absorption of dietary or supplemental iron probably isn't necessary for most people, especially if their diet contains plenty of vitamin C (9571).

ZINC: Under some circumstances iron and zinc can interfere with each other's absorption. When high supplemental doses of zinc are taken on an empty stomach there is a measurable reduction in iron absorption, and high supplemental doses of non-heme iron taken on an empty stomach can reduce zinc absorption, especially when dietary mineral intake is low (8856,9579,9580,9581,9582,9583,9584). This is probably because the carriers for iron and zinc in the gut become saturated at high doses, and the ions then compete for non-specific carriers. If one of the ions is present in excess, absorption of the other will be decreased (9580). When food is present, the ions become complexed with food components and don't compete for absorption (9579). Therefore, there isn't a significant interaction between dietary iron and zinc, or between supplemental iron and zinc when taken with food (8866,9579,9581). Advise patients to take these supplements with food.

Interactions with Drugs

BISPHOSPHONATES: Divalent cations, including iron, can decrease absorption of bisphosphonates by forming insoluble complexes (15). Advise patients that doses of bisphosphonates should be separated by at least two hours from doses of all other medications, including supplements such as iron. The bisphosphonates include alendronate (Fosamax), etidronate (Didronel), risedronate (Actonel), and tiludronate (Skelid).

CHLORAMPHENICOL: Chloramphenicol can reduce the response to iron therapy in iron deficiency anemia, because it interferes with erythrocyte maturation (15,3046). Since chloramphenicol isn't usually taken for prolonged periods, this isn't likely to be clinically significant.

LEVODOPA: There is some evidence in healthy people that iron forms chelates with levodopa, reducing the amount of levodopa absorbed by around 50% (9567). The clinical significance of this hasn't been determined. Advise patients to separate doses of levodopa and iron as much as possible.

LEVOTHYROXINE (Levothroid, Levoxyl, Synthroid, and others): Iron can decrease the absorption and efficacy of levothyroxine by forming insoluble complexes in the gastrointestinal tract (9568). Advise patients to separate levothyroxine and iron doses by at least two hours.

METHYLDOPA (Aldomet): Concomitant use can decrease absorption of methyldopa, resulting in increases in

blood pressure (7900). Advise patients to separate iron and methyldopa doses by at least two hours.
MYCOPHENOLATE MOFETIL (CellCept): Oral iron supplements markedly reduce absorption of mycophenolate mofetil, probably by forming nonabsorbable chelates. If concurrent therapy is essential, advise patients to take iron four to six hours before, or two hours after mycophenolate mofetil (3046).
PENICILLAMINE: Oral iron supplements can reduce absorption of penicillamine by 30% to 70%, probably due to chelate formation. Efficacy of penicillamine is reduced in Wilson's Disease; the clinical significance in people with rheumatoid arthritis (RA) hasn't been determined (3046,3072). Advise patients to take penicillamine at least two hours before or after iron-containing supplements.
QUINOLONE ANTIBIOTICS: Iron decreases the absorption of quinolones due to formation of insoluble complexes (15). Advise patients to take these antibiotics at least 2 hours before or 2 hours after iron-containing supplements (3072). Quinolones include ciprofloxacin (Cipro), levofloxacin (Levaquin), ofloxacin (Floxin), and others.
TETRACYCLINE ANTIBIOTICS: Concomitant use can decrease absorption of tetracyclines by 50-90% (15). Advise patients to take tetracyclines at least two hours before or after iron-containing supplements. Some of these drugs include doxycycline (Vibramycin), minocycline (Minocin), tetracycline (Achromycin), and others.

Drug Influences on Nutrient Levels and Depletion

SOME DRUGS CAN AFFECT IRON LEVELS:
AMINOSALICYLIC ACID: Aminosalicylic acid sometimes causes a malabsorption syndrome, resulting in weight loss, iron and vitamin depletion, and excessive fat in the stools (steatorrhea) (9574). Advise patients to consult their physician if these symptoms occur. Some of these drugs include para-aminosalicylic acid, PAS, and Paser.
ANTACIDS: Gastric acid is important for absorption of dietary, non-heme (plant-derived) iron (4539). Antacids may therefore reduce iron absorption by increasing gastric pH and reducing iron solubility (3072). This isn't likely to be clinically significant in most people with adequate dietary iron intake. However, antacids can reduce absorption of iron from supplements by 30% to 40%, and reduced efficacy has occurred occasionally (3046). Advise patients who need iron supplements to avoid antacids or separate the doses as much as possible.
ASPIRIN, NONSTEROIDAL ANTI-INFLAMMATORY DRUGS (NSAIDs): Aspirin and NSAIDs can cause mucosal damage and bleeding throughout the gastrointestinal (GI) tract. This may be asymptomatic and undetected. In people taking these drugs for prolonged periods, including those taking low-dose aspirin for cardiovascular protection, this chronic blood loss may contribute to iron deficiency anemia (8888,9515,9576,9577). Advise patients to consult their physician promptly if they have symptoms of anemia, GI irritation, or blood in the stools. Since iron supplements may also irritate the GI tract, patients should not use them concurrently with NSAIDs unless recommended by a physician. Encourage patients to include iron-rich foods in their diet.
CHOLESTYRAMINE (Questran), COLESTIPOL (Colestid): Cholestyramine and colestipol may bind iron in the gut, reducing its absorption (9566). Clinically significant iron deficiency induced by these drugs hasn't been reported, and supplements aren't likely to be needed. If patients are taking iron supplements for other causes of deficiency, recommend they separate the iron and cholestyramine or colestipol doses by at least four hours.
H2-BLOCKERS: Gastric acid is important for the absorption of iron, particularly dietary non-heme (plant-derived) iron (4539). Dose-dependent reductions in dietary iron absorption have been noted with cimetidine, ranging from 28% to 65% with single doses of 300 to 900 mg (8876). However, long-term treatment, up to 18 years, with H2-blockers isn't associated with iron depletion or anemia in people with normal iron stores (4483,4539,9578). Advise people to maintain adequate dietary iron intake. Supplements aren't necessary unless people have other factors contributing to iron deficiency. The H2-blockers include cimetidine (Tagamet), ranitidine (Zantac), famotidine (Pepcid), and nizatidine (Axid).
QUINOLONES: Fluoroquinolones form complexes with iron in the GI tract, which could reduce absorption of both the fluoroquinolone and iron if taken at the same time (2682). Significant effects on iron levels are unlikely when quinolones are taken at least two hours before, or four to six hours after iron supplements or iron-containing foods. Quinolones include ciprofloxacin (Cipro), levofloxacin (Levaquin), ofloxacin (Floxin), moxifloxacin (Avelox), gatifloxacin (Tequin), and others.
PANCREATIC ENZYMES, PANCRELIPASE, PANCREATIN: There is some evidence that pancreatic enzyme supplements can reduce iron absorption, possibly by binding iron or altering pH (9575,9585). It's unlikely that this will be clinically significant, except in people with cystic fibrosis who need pancreatic enzyme supplements for prolonged periods, and have other factors contributing to iron deficiency (9575). Advise these patients to have their iron status checked regularly. Some of these drugs include Pancrease, Cotazym, Viokase, Creon, and Ultrase.
PENICILLAMINE (Cuprimine, Depen): Penicillamine chelates iron in the gastrointestinal tract and decreases absorption. If iron supplements are used, separate from penicillamine by at least 2 hours (9630).
PROTON PUMP INHIBITORS: Gastric acid is important for the absorption of iron, particularly dietary non-heme (plant-derived) iron (4539). However, long-term treatment, up to 12.5 years, with proton pump inhibitors isn't associated with iron depletion or anemia in people with normal iron stores (4483,8850,9578). Advise people to maintain adequate dietary iron intake. Supplements aren't necessary unless people have other factors contributing to iron deficiency. Proton pump inhibitors include lansoprazole (Prevacid), omeprazole (Prilosec), rabeprazole (Aciphex), pantoprazole (Protonix, Pantoloc), and others.
TETRACYCLINES: Tetracyclines form complexes with iron in the GI tract, reducing absorption of both the tetracycline and iron if taken at the same time (4412). Significant effects on iron levels are unlikely when tetracyclines

are taken at least two hours before or after iron supplements or iron-containing foods. Tetracyclines include demeclocycline (Declomycin), doxycycline (Vibramycin and others), and minocycline (Minocin and others).

Interactions with Foods

COFFEE AND TEA: These beverages can reduce absorption of both dietary and supplemental iron when taken at the same time. This is likely due to binding of iron in the gut by polyphenols and tannins in tea and coffee (8887,9570,9571,9573). Body iron stores (measured by serum ferritin) are inversely related to coffee and tea intake (9571). These effects could potentially contribute to iron deficiency anemia, especially in people with other risk factors.
DAIRY PRODUCTS: Calcium in dairy products such as milk and cheese can reduce the absorption of dietary and supplemental iron (8875). This is unlikely to be clinically significant in people with adequate iron stores. Advise patients who need iron supplements to take them with a meal that is relatively low in dairy products whenever possible. Maximal absorption of iron supplements would occur when they are taken on an empty stomach, but this increases the risk of gastric irritation and shouldn't be recommended.

Interactions with Lab Tests

GUAIAC TEST: Iron may cause a false-positive reading for occult fecal blood. However, the benzidine test for occult fecal blood is not likely to be affected (15).

Interactions with Diseases or Conditions

ACHLORHYDRIA: Decreased stomach acidity may impair iron absorption (7135).
CHRONIC UNDERNUTRITION, MICRONUTRIENT DEFICIENCY: Supplemental iron can normalize serum ferritin, but may not raise low hemoglobin in chronic undernutrition and multiple micronutrient deficiency (6923).
HEMODIALYSIS: Supplemental iron absorption is decreased in people requiring chronic hemodialysis (1088,1090).
HEMOGLOBIN DISEASES: Iron overload is likely to occur in people with hemoglobinopathies or other refractory anemias erroneously diagnosed as iron deficiency anemia (15).
IRON DEFICIENCY: Iron absorption is increased (945).
MALABSORPTION SYNDROMES: Oral iron therapy may be ineffective in individuals with diarrhea, post-gastrectomy, or other malabsorption syndromes (945).
PEPTIC ULCER DISEASE, REGIONAL ENTERITIS, ULCERATIVE COLITIS: Iron can exacerbate these conditions (15); contraindicated.
PREMATURE INFANTS: Use of oral iron preparations in premature infants with low serum vitamin E levels may cause hemolysis and hemolytic anemia (15); vitamin E deficiency should be corrected before administering supplemental iron (15).

Dosage and Administration

ORAL: For treating iron deficiency anemia in adults, 50-100 mg elemental iron is given three times daily. For children with iron deficiency anemia, the dose is 4-6 mg/kg per day divided into three doses (15). Treatment is usually continued 6 months to replenish iron stores (15). Two to three months of treatment may reverse anemia without replenishing iron stores (945). Iron deficiency due to chronic, uncontrolled bleeding requires continuous iron therapy (945). For preventing iron deficiency in menstruating women who have undergone gastric bypass surgery, 320 mg twice daily has been used (1089). For improving unexplained fatigue in non-anemic women, ferrous sulfate 80 mg daily has been used (11406). For improving cognitive function in iron-deficient adolescents, 650 mg ferrous sulfate twice daily has been used (1095). For reducing angiotensin converting enzyme (ACE) inhibitor cough, 256 mg ferrous sulfate has been given daily (7307).
The adequate intake (AI) of iron for infants 6 months of age and less is 0.27 mg/day (7135).
For older infants and children, the recommended daily allowances (RDAs) for iron are: Infants 7 to 12 months, 11 mg/day; children 1 to 3 years, 7mg/day; 4 to 8 years, 10 mg/day; 9 to 13 years, 8 mg/day; boys 14 to 18 years, 11 mg/day; girls 14 to 18 years, 15 mg/day. For adults, the RDA for iron is 8 mg/day for men ages 19 and older, and women ages 51 and older. For women 19 to 50 years, the RDA is 18 mg/day. For pregnant women, the RDA is 27 mg/day. For lactating women, the RDA is 10 mg/day for ages 14 to 18 years, and 9 mg/day for ages 19 to 50 (7135).
Tolerable upper intake levels (UL) for iron are: infants and children birth to age 13, 40 mg/day; people age 14 and older (including pregnancy and lactation), 45 mg/day (7135). UL recommendations do not apply to people under medical supervision for iron deficiency (7135). All forms of iron are not equivalent; 1 gram of ferrous gluconate = 120 mg elemental iron (12% iron); 1 gram of ferrous sulfate = 200 mg elemental iron (20% iron); 1 gram of ferrous fumarate = 330 mg elemental iron (33% iron) (15).

Comments

Premenopausal women who have asymptomatic iron deficiency can improve their iron status by altering their diet to include more iron-rich foods, although changes are generally less than with iron supplements (9540,9541). High iron foods include beef, liver, and lamb. Medium iron foods include pork, ham, chicken, fish, and beans (9540).

JABORANDI

Also Known As

Arruda Bravam, Arruda Do Mato, Jamguarandi, Juarandi, Maranhao Jaborandi.

Scientific Names

Pilocarpus microphyllus.
Family: Rutaceae.

People Use This For

Orally, jaborandi is used to treat diarrhea, and as a diaphoretic.
Topically, jaborandi is used for glaucoma.

Safety

UNSAFE ...when the leaf is used orally or topically, because it contains pilocarpine. The lethal dose of jaborandi is estimated to be 5-10 grams of leaf (18).
PREGNANCY: UNSAFE ...when used orally or topically because it has teratogenic and uterine stimulant effects and contains pilocarpine (19).
LACTATION: UNSAFE ...when used orally or topically because it contains pilocarpine(18).

Effectiveness

There is insufficient reliable information available about the effectiveness of jaborandi.

Mechanism of Action

The applicable part of jaborandi is the leaf. Jaborandi contains the parasympathetic system stimulant pilocarpine. Among its cholinergic effects are the stimulation of saliva secretion, sweat, and smooth muscle contraction in the gastrointestinal tract (18). It also causes ocular miosis (15).

Adverse Reactions

The lethal oral dose of the pilocarpine constituent in jaborandi is approximately 60 mg, corresponding to approximately 5-10 grams of jaborandi leaf. Symptoms of poisoning include bradycardia, bronchospasm, colic, cardiac collapse and possible arrest, convulsions, hypotension, dyspnea, nausea, severe salivation, strong secretion of sweat, and vomiting (18).

Interactions with Herbs & Other Dietary Supplements

None known.

Interactions with Drugs

None known.

Interactions with Foods

None known.

Interactions with Lab Tests

INTRAOCULAR PRESSURE: Jaborandi might reduce intraocular pressure due to its pilocarpine content (15,18).

Interactions with Diseases or Conditions

None known.

Dosage and Administration

TOPICAL: Pharmaceutical pilocarpine eye drops are a prescription only medication (15,18).

Comments

Jaborandi itself is obsolete as a medicinal herb, but it is used in the production of pilocarpine (18). Avoid confusing jaborandi with Pilocarpus jaborandi (Pernambuco jaborandi) (19) and Pilocarpus pennatifolius (Paraguay jaborandi).

JACOB'S LADDER

Also Known As
Charity, English Green Valerian, Jacobs Ladder.
CAUTION: See separate listings for Abscess Root and Lily-of-the-Valley.

Scientific Names
Polemonium caeruleum.
Family: Polemoniaceae.

Comments
At the date of publication, this product was not a common ingredient used in brand name supplements marketed to consumers. Details about this product are available at the online version of *Natural Medicines Comprehensive Database*. See www.naturaldatabase.com.

JALAP

Also Known As
Jalapa, Jalape, Mechoacán.
CAUTION: See separate listings for Mexican Scammony Root, Pokeweed berry, and Pokeweed root.

Scientific Names
Ipomoea purga, synonym Exogonium purga; Convolvulus purga.
Family: Convolvulaceae.

People Use This For
Orally, jalap is used as a cathartic, purgative, and diuretic.

Safety
UNSAFE ...when used orally. Jalap has potent purgative effects (12).
PREGNANCY AND LACTATION: UNSAFE ...when used orally. Jalap can be a menstrual stimulant (19); avoid using.

Effectiveness
There is insufficient reliable information available about the effectiveness of jalap.

Mechanism of Action
The applicable part of jalap is the root. The roots of the jalap (ipomoea purga) plant contain gluco-resins that act as a cathartic. They increase water elimination and cause peristalsis (271).

Adverse Reactions
Orally, jalap has potent purgative effects (12).

Interactions with Herbs & Other Dietary Supplements
CARDIAC GLYCOSIDE-CONTAINING HERBS: Overuse/abuse of jalap may increase the risk of cardiac glycoside toxicity. Cardiac glycoside-containing herbs include black hellebore, Canadian hemp roots, digitalis leaf, hedge mustard, figwort, lily of the valley roots, motherwort, oleander leaf, pheasant's eye plant, pleurisy root, squill bulb leaf scales, and strophanthus seeds (19). Jalap may increase risk of cardioglycoside toxicity due to increase risk of potassium loss.
HORSETAIL/LICORICE: Theoretically, concomitant use with horsetail plant or licorice rhizome increases the risk of potassium depletion (19).
STIMULANT LAXATIVE HERBS: Theoretically, concomitant use with other stimulant laxative herbs may increase the risk of potassium depletion. Stimulant laxative herbs include aloe dried leaf sap, blue flag rhizome, alder buckthorn, European buckthorn, butternut bark, cascara bark, castor oil, colocynth fruit pulp, gamboge bark exudate, black root, manna bark exudate, podophyllum root, rhubarb root, senna leaves and pods, wild cucumber fruit (Ecballium elaterium), and yellow dock root (19).

Interactions with Drugs
DIGOXIN (Lanoxin): Theoretically, overuse or abuse of jalap might increase the toxicity of cardiac glycoside drugs due to possible potassium loss.
DIURETIC DRUGS: Overuse of jalap might compound diuretic-induced potassium loss (19). There is some concern

that people taking jalap along with potassium depleting diuretics might have an increased risk for hypokalemia. Initiation of potassium supplementation or an increase in potassium supplement dose may be necessary for some patients. Some diuretics that can deplete potassium include chlorothiazide (Diuril), chlorthalidone (Thalitone), furosemide (Lasix), hydrochlorothiazide (HCTZ, HydroDIURIL, Microzide), and others.
ORAL DRUGS: Theoretically, jalap may reduce absorption of drugs due to reduced transit time (19).
STIMULANT LAXATIVES: Concomitant use of jalap with other laxatives may lead to electrolyte and fluid depletion (19).

Interactions with Foods
None known.

Interactions with Lab Tests
None known.

Interactions with Diseases or Conditions
GASTROINTESTINAL (GI) CONDITIONS: Jalap may have GI irritant effects (19). Contraindicated in individuals with infectious or inflammatory gastrointestinal conditions (19). Stimulant laxatives are contraindicated in individuals with symptoms of appendicitis (abdominal pain, nausea, and vomiting) (272).

Dosage and Administration
ORAL: Jalap is typically prepared as a liquid, using 1 teaspoon root to 1 cup of water. The dose is 1 cup daily, a mouthful at a time (5263). The usual dose of the powdered root is 3 to 20 grains (195 to 1300 mg) (5267). The resin from the root is dosed 60 to 300 mg, and the tincture is taken 2 to 4 mL (223).

Comments
Avoid confusion with pokeweed (Phytolacca americana) or Mexican scammony root (Ipomoea orizabensis), also known as jalap.

JAMAICAN DOGWOOD

Also Known As
Fishfudle, Fish Poison Bark, Fish-Poison Tree, Jamaica Dogwood, West Indian Dogwood.
CAUTION: See separate listing for American Dogwood.

Scientific Names
Piscidia piscipula, synonyms Erythrina piscipula, Ichthyomethia piscipula, Piscidia erythrina; Piscidia communis.
Family: Fabaceae/Leguminosae.

People Use This For
Orally, Jamaican dogwood is used for anxiety and fear, as a daytime sedative, for neuralgia, migraine, insomnia (especially sleeplessness due to nervous tension), and dysmenorrhea.

Safety
LIKELY UNSAFE ...when the root bark is used orally for self-medication because it is considered toxic (4). The elderly are particularly sensitive to potent neuro-muscular depressant effects (19).
CHILDREN: LIKELY UNSAFE ...when used orally; avoid using. Children are particularly sensitive to potent, neuro-muscular depressant effects (19).
PREGNANCY: LIKELY UNSAFE ...when used orally; avoid using due to possible uterine depressant effects (4).
LACTATION: LIKELY UNSAFE ...when used orally (4); avoid using.

Effectiveness
There is insufficient reliable information available about the effectiveness of Jamaican dogwood.

Mechanism of Action
The applicable part of Jamaican dogwood is the root bark. Animal studies have shown that an extract of Jamaican dogwood has sedative effects, marked antitussive and antipyretic activities, and also anti-inflammatory and antispasmodic action on smooth muscles (4,11). In some in vitro tests, the extract's antispasmodic effects have been at least as strong as papaverine's (4). The constituent rotenone has shown some anticancer activity towards lymphocytic leukemia and human epidermoid carcinoma of the nasopharynx; yet, paradoxically, rotenone is also documented to be carcinogenic (4). Rotenone is toxic to fish and insects, and to animals when administered parenterally, but non-toxic when administered orally (4). Another constituent, ichtynone, is toxic to fish (4).

Adverse Reactions
Orally, Jamaican dogwood is an irritant and toxic to humans (4). Overdose symptoms include numbness, tremors, salivation, and sweating (4).

Interactions with Herbs & Other Dietary Supplements
HERBS WITH SEDATIVE PROPERTIES: Theoretically, concomitant use with herbs that have sedative properties might enhance therapeutic and adverse effects. Some of these supplements include 5-HTP, calamus, California poppy, catnip, hops, kava, St. John's wort, scullcap, valerian, yerba mansa, and others.

Interactions with Drugs
CNS DEPRESSANTS: Jamaican dogwood may potentiate sedative effects (4).

Interactions with Foods
None known.

Interactions with Lab Tests
None known.

Interactions with Diseases or Conditions
None known.

Dosage and Administration
No typical dosage.

Comments
Jamaican dogwood is likely unsafe and without any documented effectiveness; avoid using. Root bark and liquid extract are reportedly no longer used (18). Avoid confusion with American dogwood (Cornus florida).

JAMBOLAN bark

Also Known As
Badijamun, Jambu, Jambul, Jamum, Java Plum, Jumbul, Mahajambu, Phadena, Rajajambu, Rose Apple, Syxygii cumini cortex.
CAUTION: See separate listing for Jambolan seed.

Scientific Names
Syzygium cumini, synonyms Eugenia cumini, Eugenia jambolana, Syzygium jambolanum.
Family: Mytraceae.

People Use This For
Orally, jambolan bark is used for nonspecific, acute diarrhea, bronchitis, asthma, and dysentery.
Topically, jambolan bark is used for mild inflammation of the oral-pharyngeal mucosa and of the skin, and for ulcers.

Safety
POSSIBLY SAFE ...when used orally or topically, and appropriately (2,12).
PREGNANCY AND LACTATION: Insufficient reliable information available; avoid using.

Effectiveness
There is insufficient reliable information available about the effectiveness of jambolan bark.

Mechanism of Action
The astringent effects of jambolan bark can result from the tannin constituents (2). Jambolan bark also possesses antibacterial, hypoglycemic, and CNS-depressant activities (4).

Adverse Reactions
None reported.

Interactions with Herbs & Other Dietary Supplements
None known.

Interactions with Drugs
None known.

Interactions with Foods
None known.

Interactions with Lab Tests
None known.

Interactions with Diseases or Conditions
None known.

Dosage and Administration
ORAL: The typical dose of jambolan is 3-6 grams of the dried bark per day (2,18). It can also be taken as a tea, which is prepared by simmering 1-2 teaspoons of the dried bark in 150 mL boiling water for 5-10 minutes and then straining (18).
TOPICAL: Jambolan bark is commonly used as a compress made from the tea (18).

Comments
Avoid confusion with jambolan seed.

JAMBOLAN seed

Also Known As
Jambul, Jamum, Java Plum, Jumbul, Rose Apple, Syxygii cumini semen.
CAUTION: See separate listing for Jambolan bark.

Scientific Names
Syzygium cumini, synonyms Eugenia cumini, Eugenia jambolana, Syzygium jambolanum.
Family: Myrtaceae.

Comments
At the date of publication, there was very little scientific information about this product. Our staff is continually analyzing the available information on natural medicines and will add data to the online version of *Natural Medicines Comprehensive Database* as it becomes available. See www.naturaldatabase.com.

JAPANESE MINT

Also Known As
American Corn Mint, Brook Mint, Canadian Mint, Chinese Mint, Chinese Mint Oil, Corn Mint, Cornmint Oil, Field Mint Oil, Mentha arvensis aetheroleum, Mint Oil, Minzol, Poleo, Pudina, Putiha.

Scientific Names
Mentha canadensis, synonym Mentha arvensis var. piperascens.
Family: Lamiaceae/Labiatae.

People Use This For
Orally, Japanese mint is used for flatulence, improving gastrointestinal and gallbladder function, for gallstones, and irritable bowel syndrome (IBS) common cold, cough, bronchitis, fever, mouth and pharynx inflammation, pain, liver and gallbladder complaints, tendency to infection, for improving appetite and digestion, indigestion, nausea, sore throat, diarrhea, headaches, toothaches, cramps, earache, tumors, sores, cancer, a stimulant, an antiseptic, a local anesthetic, and an antispasmodic. Japanese mint is also used for functional cardiac complaints, breathing difficulties, and sensitivity to weather changes.
Topically, Japanese mint is used for myalgia, neuralgic ailments, pruritus, urticaria, oral mucosal inflammation, and rheumatic conditions.
When inhaled, Japanese mint is used for mucous membrane inflammation of the upper respiratory tract.
In manufacturing, Japanese mint is also used as a fragrance in toothpaste, mouthwash, gargles, soaps, detergents, creams, lotions, and perfumes. Commercially it is used as a source of menthol.

Safety

POSSIBLY SAFE ...when the oil is used orally and appropriately (2). ...when used topically and appropriately (2). There is insufficient reliable information available about the safety of Japanese mint for its other uses.
CHILDREN: LIKELY UNSAFE ...when the oil is used topically on the faces of infants and children, particularly in the nasal area, it can trigger glottal or bronchial spasm, asthma-like attacks, or even respiratory failure (2). There is insufficient reliable information about Japanese mint used for medicinal purposes; avoid using.
PREGNANCY AND LACTATION: Insufficient reliable information available; avoid using.

Effectiveness

There is insufficient reliable information available about the effectiveness of Japanese mint.

Mechanism of Action

Japanese mint oil is thought to have antiflatulent and cooling effects (2). It might also stimulate bile flow (2). Some evidence demonstrates that Japanese mint oil has cytotoxic properties. Other evidence suggests it might have antimicrobial activity (11). Japanese mint oil contains up to 95% menthol (11). Used topically it has the potential to cause sensitization (18). Processing removes some of the menthol in the Japanese mint oil that is commercially available (2,11).

Adverse Reactions

Orally, Japanese mint oil can cause stomach upset when taken orally (2).
Topically, contact dermatitis can result from use (11). In children, topical use on the face can trigger glottal or bronchial spasm, asthma-like attacks, or even respiratory failure (18).
By inhalation, the menthol content of Japanese mint oil can worsen bronchial asthma spasms (18). Menthol can also cause allergic reactions including flushing or headache (11).

Interactions with Herbs & Other Dietary Supplements

None known.

Interactions with Drugs

None known.

Interactions with Foods

None known.

Interactions with Lab Tests

None known.

Interactions with Diseases or Conditions

BRONCHIAL SPASMS: Theoretically, the menthol content of Japanese mint oil might worsen bronchial asthma spasms (18).
GALLBLADDER CONDITIONS: Use of Japanese mint is contraindicated in individuals with bile duct obstruction or gallbladder inflammation (2). Individuals with gallstones may experience pain and spasms (18).
LIVER DISEASE: Use of Japanese mint is contraindicated in individuals with severe liver damage (2).

Dosage and Administration

ORAL: A typical dose is 3-6 drops of oil daily (2).
TOPICAL: Rub several drops of oil or equivalent preparations into affected areas of skin (2). Japanese mint oil is also available as 5-20% oil and semi-solid preparations, in hydroalcoholic preparations of 5-10%, and as 1-5% essential oil in nasal ointments (2).
INHALATION: A typical dose is 3-4 drops of oil in hot water (2).

Comments

Japanese mint oil is the partially dementholated, distilled oil of the above ground parts of Japanese mint (Mentha canadensis) (2,11). There are more than 20 different species of Mentha with as many as 2300 named variations. Commercial varieties of mint oil can be distinguished by the relative amounts of menthol and carvone (11).

JASMINE

Also Known As

Catalonina Jasmine, Common Jasmine, Italian Jasmine, Jati, Poet's Jessamine, Royal Jasmine, Spanish Jasmine.
CAUTION: See separate listing for Gelsemium.

Scientific Names

Jasminum grandiflorum, synonym Jasminum officinale.
Family: Oleaceae.

People Use This For

Orally, jasmine has been used for hepatitis, hepatic pain due to cirrhosis, and abdominal pain due to dysentery. Many Jasminum species have been used as a sedative, aphrodisiac, or in cancer treatment.
In foods, jasmine is utilized to flavor beverages, frozen dairy desserts, candy, baked goods, gelatins, and puddings.
In manufacturing, jasmine is used to add fragrance to creams, lotions, and perfumes.

Safety

LIKELY SAFE ...when used orally in the amounts commonly found in foods. Jasmine has Generally Recognized As Safe (GRAS) status in the US (4912).
There is insufficient reliable information available about the safety jasmine in medicinal amounts.
PREGNANCY AND LACTATION: Insufficient reliable information available; avoid using in amounts greater than those found in food.

Effectiveness

There is insufficient reliable information available about the effectiveness of jasmine.

Mechanism of Action

The applicable part of jasmine is the flower. There is insufficient reliable information available about the possible mechanism of action and active ingredients.

Adverse Reactions

Jasmine may possibly cause hypersensitivity (11).

Interactions with Herbs & Other Dietary Supplements

None known.

Interactions with Drugs

None known.

Interactions with Foods

None known.

Interactions with Lab Tests

None known.

Interactions with Diseases or Conditions

None known.

Dosage and Administration

ORAL: People typically prepare jasmine as a tea, adding 1 to 2 teaspoons of jasmine flowers to 1 cup of water. The dose is 1 cup daily (5263).

Comments

Concrétes are the fat-soluble abstracts of the flower. Absolutes, the alcoholic extracts of concrétes, are more commonly used as a fragrance (11).

JAVA TEA

Also Known As

Orthosiphon, Orthosiphonis folium.

Scientific Names

Orthosiphon aristatus, synonyms Orthosiphon stamineus, Clerodendranthus spicatus, Clerodendrum spicatum, Ocimum aristatum.
Family: Lamiaceae/Labiatae.

People Use This For
Orally, java tea is taken as "irrigation therapy" (where it is used as a mild diuretic along with copious fluid intake to increase urine flow), for bacterial and inflammatory diseases of the lower urinary tract, renal gravel, and liver and gallbladder complaints. It is also used orally for bladder and kidney disorders, gallstones, gout, and rheumatism.

Safety
POSSIBLY SAFE ...when used orally and appropriately (2).
PREGNANCY AND LACTATION: Insufficient reliable information available; avoid using.

Effectiveness
There is insufficient reliable information available about the effectiveness of java tea.

Mechanism of Action
The applicable parts of java tea are the leaf and stem tip. Java tea is stated to have diuretic, weak antispasmodic, and antimicrobial effects (2,18).

Adverse Reactions
None reported.

Interactions with Herbs & Other Dietary Supplements
None known.

Interactions with Drugs
None known.

Interactions with Foods
None known.

Interactions with Lab Tests
None known.

Interactions with Diseases or Conditions
EDEMA: Java tea is contraindicated for use as "irrigation therapy" in cases of edema due to limited heart or kidney function (2).

Dosage and Administration
ORAL: The typical dose of java tea is 6-12 grams of the dried leaf or stem tips per day or equivalent preparations, including the prepared tea (2,18). Adequate fluid intake is essential, at least 2 L per day (18).

JAVANESE TURMERIC

Also Known As
Curcuma, Curcumae xanthorrhizae rhizoma, Java Turmeric, Temu Lawak, Temu Lawas, Tewon Lawa.
CAUTION: See separate listings for Goldenseal, Turmeric, and Zedoary.

Scientific Names
Curcuma xanthorrhiza.
Family: Zingiberaceae.

People Use This For
Orally, Javanese turmeric is used for indigestion, feelings of fullness, bloating after meals, flatulence, peptic disorders, for improving appetite and digestion, and for liver and gallbladder complaints.

Safety
POSSIBLY SAFE ...when the dried rhizome is used orally and appropriately for short periods of time (2,8).
POSSIBLY UNSAFE ...when used orally in large amounts or for prolonged use. It can cause gastric irritation and nausea (2,8).
PREGNANCY AND LACTATION: Insufficient reliable information available; avoid using.

Effectiveness
There is insufficient reliable information available about the effectiveness of Javanese turmeric.

Mechanism of Action
The applicable part of Javanese turmeric is the root. Javanese turmeric root contains a volatile oil with the chief components of alpha-curcumene, xanthorrhizole, beta-curcumene, germacrene, furanodien, and furanodienone. The root also contains curcumin, demethoxycurcumin, and non-phenolic diarylheptanoids (18). Javanese turmeric is thought to stimulate bile production (2). It might also have antitumor effects (18).

Adverse Reactions
Orally, use of large amounts or for prolonged periods of time can cause gastric irritation and nausea (2,8).

Interactions with Herbs & Other Dietary Supplements
None known.

Interactions with Drugs
None known.

Interactions with Foods
None known.

Interactions with Lab Tests
None known.

Interactions with Diseases or Conditions
LIVER OR GALLBLADDER DISEASE: Javanese turmeric is contraindicated in people with acute bile duct inflammation, biliary tree inflammation (8), bile duct obstruction (2,8), or jaundice (8) due to bile stimulating effects (2). Individuals with gallstones should have medical evaluation before using (2).

Dosage and Administration
ORAL: To stimulate bile production, a typical oral dose is one cup tea several times daily between meals. To make tea, steep 0.5-1 grams coarsely powdered root in 150 mL boiling water for 5-10 minutes, and strain. The average daily amount used is 2 grams root or equivalent preparations (2). For improving appetite, digestion, or for flatulence, a typical dose is one cup tea before or during meals. To make tea, steep 0.5-1 grams coarsely powdered root in 150 mL boiling water for 5-10 minutes, and strain (8). The average daily amount used is 2 grams root or equivalent preparations (2).

Comments
Javanese turmeric is indigenous to the forests of Indonesia and the Malaysian peninsula (18).

JEWELWEED

Also Known As
Balsam-Weed, Garden Balsam, Impatiens, Jewel Balsam Weed, Jewel Weed, Quick-In-The-Hand, Silverweed, Slipper Weed, Speckled Jewels, Spotted Touch-Me-Not, Touch-Me-Not, Wild Balsam, Wild Celandine, Wild Lady's Slipper.
CAUTION: See separate listings for Greater Celandine above ground parts, Greater Celandine rhizome/root, Lesser Celandine, and Potentilla.

Scientific Names
Impatiens pallida; Impatiens balsamina, synonyms Balsamina foemina, Impatiens giorgii; Impatiens capensis, synonym Impatiens biflora.
Family: Balsaminaceae.

People Use This For
Orally, jewelweed is used for mild digestive disorders.
Orally and topically, jewelweed is used for poison ivy dermatitis.

Safety
POSSIBLY SAFE ...when used orally. ...when used topically. There are no published reports of significant toxicity for either route of administration (18).
PREGNANCY AND LACTATION: Insufficient reliable information available; avoid using.

Effectiveness
There is insufficient reliable information available about the effectiveness of jewelweed.

Mechanism of Action
The applicable parts of jewelweed are the above ground parts. Impatiens balsamina has digestive and diuretic effects (18). One constituent, 2-methoxynaphthoquinone, has antifungal activity (6).

Adverse Reactions
None reported.

Interactions with Herbs & Other Dietary Supplements
None known.

Interactions with Drugs
None known.

Interactions with Foods
None known.

Interactions with Lab Tests
None known.

Interactions with Diseases or Conditions
None known.

Dosage and Administration
No typical dosage.

Comments
Avoid confusion with potentilla (Potentillae anserinae), also known as silverweed.

JIAOGULAN

Also Known As
Adaptogen, Amachazuru, Dungkulcha, Fairy Herb, Gynostemma, Immortality Herb, Jiao Gu Lan, Miracle Grass, Penta Tea, Southern Ginseng, Xianxao.
CAUTION: See separate listings for Blue Cohosh, Canaigre, Codonopsis, Ginseng American, Ginseng Siberian, Ginseng Panax, Panax Pseudoginseng, and Ashwaganda.

Scientific Names
Gynostemma pentaphyllum, synonyms Gynostemma pedatum, Vitis pentaphylla.
Family: Cucurbitaceae.

People Use This For
Orally, jiaogulan is used for hyperlipidemia, hypertension, strengthening immune function, and increasing stamina and endurance. It is also used orally for appetite stimulation, chronic bronchitis, chronic gastritis, ulcers, constipation, gallstones, obesity, cancer, diabetes, insomnia, backache, and pain. Jiaogulan is also used orally for improving memory, improving coronary and cardiovascular functions, stress, preventing hair loss, and as an anti-aging agent. It is also used orally as an anti-inflammatory agent, antioxidant, detoxifying agent, decongestant and cough suppressant, and as an "adaptogen" for increasing resistance to environmental stress.

Safety
POSSIBLY SAFE ...when used orally and appropriately, short-term. There is preliminary evidence that jiaogulan can be safely used for up to 30 days (7069,7070).
PREGNANCY: POSSIBLY UNSAFE ...when used orally. Ginsenoside Rb1, which is identical to the jiaogulan constituent gypenoside 3, has teratogenic effects in animal models; avoid using (10447).
LACTATION: Insufficient reliable information available; avoid using.

Effectiveness

POSSIBLY EFFECTIVE

Hypercholesterolemia. There is some evidence that taking jiaogulan orally can decrease total cholesterol and increase the high-density lipoprotein (HDL)/total cholesterol ratio in patients with high cholesterol levels (7069,7070).

There is insufficient reliable information available about the effectiveness of jiaogulan for its other uses.

Mechanism of Action

The applicable part of jiaogulan is the leaf. The leaves of jiaogulan contain a large number of triterpene saponins referred to as gypenosides. Many of the gypenosides are identical to the ginsenosides found in Panax ginseng. For example, gypenoside 3 is identical to ginsenoside Rb1, gypenoside 4 is the same as ginsenoside Rb3, and gypenoside 8 is the same as ginsenoside Rd. The amount of saponins in the leaves of jiaogulan is similar to the amount found in ginseng roots. Due to the similar chemical make up between jiaogulan and ginseng, jiaogulan is often assumed to have the same effects as ginseng. Most jiaogulan products are standardized by the amount of saponins they contain. However, jiaogulan contains a wide variation of gypenosides which makes standardizing according to specific gypenosides difficult. Most of the evidence about the pharmacological effects of jiaogulan comes from preliminary animal or in vitro research (6).

There is some evidence that jiaogulan has antioxidant activity. There is also some evidence that the gypenoside constituents have several cardiovascular effects and may prevent the development of atherosclerosis and slow the aging process (9349).

Preliminary evidence suggests the gypenosides in jiaogulan have antilipid peroxidation activity and protect vascular endothelial cells and their membranes from oxidative damage (9349). In animal research, jiaogulan seems to lower blood pressure, heart rate, blood vessel resistance, increase coronary blood flow, inhibit platelet aggregation, and possibly protect against cerebral ischemic damage (7071). Evidence from human studies suggest that jiaogulan has cholesterol lowering effects (7069,7070).

There is also preliminary evidence a combination of jiaogulan with Nelumbo nucifera (Lotus flower or seed) and Crataegus cuneata (Hawthorn) might have both a cholesterol- and triglyceride-lowering effect. It is unclear whether these effects are due to an interaction among these agents or if one of the agents is primarily responsible (9348). There is preliminary evidence that jiaogulan may have immunostimulatory effects and possible anti-cancer activity (6).

Some research suggests that hot water extracts of jiaogulan contain a factor that induces platelet aggregation, but the effect occurs only with washed platelets and is not observed in platelet-rich plasma. This suggests the factor is unlikely to cause thrombosis in vivo. It is unknown if this factor might affect other cells or tissues. However, its discovery might help investigators better understand the mechanism of platelet activation (9350).

Adverse Reactions

Orally, use of jiaogulan might cause severe nausea and increased bowel movements (6).

Interactions with Herbs & Other Dietary Supplements

HERBS WITH ANTICOAGULANT/ANTIPLATELET POTENTIAL: Concomitant use of jiaogulan with herbs that inhibit platelet aggregation might increase the risk of bleeding in some people (7071). Some of these herbs include angelica, clove, danshen, garlic, ginger, ginkgo, Panax ginseng, horse chestnut, red clover, turmeric, and others.

Interactions with Drugs

ANTICOAGULANT/ANTIPLATELET DRUGS: Theoretically, using jiaogulan with drugs that have anticoagulant or antiplatelet effects might increase the risk of bruising and bleeding. Jiaogulan also seems to have antiplatelet effects (7071). Some of these drugs with anticoagulant or antiplatelet effects include aspirin, dalteparin (Fragmin), enoxaparin (Lovenox), heparin, indomethacin (Indocin), ticlopidine (Ticlid), warfarin (Coumadin), and others.

IMMUNOSUPPRESSANTS: Theoretically, concurrent use might interfere with immunosuppressive therapy (6); avoid concurrent use. Immunosuppressant drugs include azathioprine (Imuran), basiliximab (Simulect), cyclosporine (Neoral, Sandimmune), daclizumab (Zenapax), muromonab-CD3 (OKT3, Orthoclone OKT3), mycophenolate (CellCept), tacrolimus (FK506, Prograf), sirolimus (Rapamune), prednisone (Deltasone, Orasone), and other corticosteroids (glucocorticoids).

Interactions with Foods

None known.

Interactions with Lab Tests

BLEEDING TIME: Theoretically, jiaogulan might increase measures of bleeding time such as prothrombin time (PT) or international normalize ratio (INR) (7071).

BLOOD PRESSURE: Theoretically, jiaogulan might reduce blood pressure and blood pressure readings (6).

CHOLESTEROL: Jiaogulan might reduce serum total cholesterol concentrations and test results (6).

Interactions with Diseases or Conditions

BLEEDING DISORDERS: Theoretically, jiaogulan might increase the risk of bleeding due to its antiplatelet effects (7071).

Dosage and Administration

ORAL: For hypercholesterolemia, jiaogulan extract 10 mg three times daily has been used (7069).

Comments

Jiaogulan grows wild in China. It is sometimes referred to as Southern Ginseng because it grows in south central China and is used in similar ways as ginseng. Jiaogulan is a newcomer to traditional Chinese medicine. Jiaogulan has reportedly been adulterated with Cayratia japonica.

JIMSON WEED

Also Known As

Angel Tulip, Datura, Devil's Apple, Devil's Trumpet, Jamestown Weed, Locoweed, Mad-Apple, Nightshade, Peru-Apple, Stinkweed, Stinkwort, Stramonium, Thorn-Apple.

Scientific Names

Datura stramonium, synonyms Datura inermis, Datura tatula.
Family: Solanaceae.

People Use This For

Orally, jimson weed is used to treat asthma, spastic or convulsive cough, pertussis during bronchitis and influenza, and as basic therapy for diseases of the autonomic nervous system. It is also used orally to induce hallucinations and euphoria.

Safety

UNSAFE ...when the leaf or seed are used orally, inhaled (13,5622). Although all parts of the plant contain belladonna alkaloids and are poisonous, the seeds contain the most (5623). Ingestion of jimson weed can cause acute anticholinergic poisoning and death (17,5621,5622). The lethal dose for adults is 15-100 grams of leaf or 15-25 grams of the seeds (equivalent to 100 mg atropine) (18).
CHILDREN: UNSAFE ...when the seed or leaf are used orally or inhaled. Children are more sensitive to the effects than adults, and the lethal dose is less (18).
PREGNANCY AND LACTATION: UNSAFE ...when used orally (2); avoid using.

Effectiveness

There is insufficient reliable information available about the effectiveness of jimson weed.

Mechanism of Action

The applicable parts of jimson weed are the leaf and seed. Jimson weed contains 0.1-0.6% alkaloids including atropine, l-hyoscyamine and l-scopolamine which are responsible for anticholinergic action and toxicity (2).

Adverse Reactions

Orally, ingestion of jimson weed can cause dilated pupils, dry mouth, dry skin, extreme thirst, dry mucous membranes, tachycardia, blurred vision, nausea and vomiting, decreased bowel sounds, difficulty swallowing and speaking, auditory and visual hallucinations, hyperthermia, hypertension, seizure, loss of consciousness, and coma (13,18,5623). Potential adverse effects also include confusion, emotional lability, reduced coordination, and headache (636). Death may result from central nervous system depression, circulatory collapse, and hypotension (18). Edema of the lungs and petechial hemorrhages of the endocardium have been reported at autopsy (5622).

Interactions with Herbs & Other Dietary Supplements

None known.

Interactions with Drugs

ANTICHOLINERGIC DRUGS: Concomitant use with jimson weed may increase anticholinergic effects and adverse effects. Anticholinergic drugs include amantadine, atropine, belladonna alkaloids, phenothiazines, scopolamine, tricyclic antidepressants (506); avoid using.

Interactions with Foods

None known.

Interactions with Lab Tests
None known.

Interactions with Diseases or Conditions
CONGESTIVE HEART FAILURE (CHF): Contraindicated; jimson weed might cause tachycardia and exacerbate CHF due to its hyoscyamine (atropine) and scopolamine content (15).
CONSTIPATION: Contraindicated; jimson weed might cause constipation due to its hyoscyamine (atropine) and scopolamine content (15).
DOWN SYNDROME: Caution, patients with Down syndrome might be hypersensitive to the antimuscarinic effects (mydriasis, positive chronotropic heart effects, etc.) of hyoscyamine (atropine) and scopolamine contained in jimson weed (15).
ESOPHAGEAL REFLUX: Contraindicated; jimson weed might delay gastric emptying and decrease lower esophageal pressure, promoting gastric retention and exacerbating reflux due to its hyoscyamine (atropine) and scopolamine content (15).
FEVER: Contraindicated; jimson weed might increase the risk of hyperthermia in patients with fever due to its hyoscyamine (atropine) and scopolamine content (15).
GASTRIC ULCER: Contraindicated; jimson weed might delay gastric emptying and exacerbate gastric ulcers due to its hyoscyamine (atropine) and scopolamine content (15).
GASTROINTESTINAL (GI) INFECTIONS: Contraindicated; jimson weed might suppress GI motility causing retention of infecting organisms or toxins due to its hyoscyamine (atropine) and scopolamine content (15).
HIATAL HERNIA: Contraindicated; jimson weed might delay gastric emptying and decrease lower esophageal pressure, promoting gastric retention and exacerbating reflux due to its hyoscyamine (atropine) and scopolamine content (15).
NARROW-ANGLE GLAUCOMA: Contraindicated; jimson weed might increase ocular tension in patients with narrow-angle (angle-closure) glaucoma due to its hyoscyamine (atropine) and scopolamine content (2,15).
OBSTRUCTIVE GASTROINTESTINAL (GI) TRACT DISEASE: Contraindicated; jimson weed might exacerbate obstructive GI tract diseases (including atony, paralytic ileus, and stenosis) due to its hyoscyamine (atropine) and scopolamine content (15).
TACHYARRHYTHMIAS: Contraindicated; jimson weed might cause tachycardia due to its hyoscyamine (atropine) and scopolamine content (2,15).
TOXIC MEGACOLON: Contraindicated; jimson weed might suppress intestinal motility, which might produce paralytic ileus and exacerbate toxic megacolon, due to its hyoscyamine (atropine) and scopolamine content (2,15).
ULCERATIVE COLITIS: Contraindicated; jimson weed might suppress intestinal motility, which might produce paralytic ileus and precipitate toxic megacolon, due to its hyoscyamine (atropine) and scopolamine content (15).
URINARY RETENTION: Contraindicated; jimson weed might increase urinary retention due to its hyoscyamine (atropine) and scopolamine content (2,15).

Dosage and Administration
No typical dosage.

JOJOBA

Also Known As
Deernut, Goatnut, Pignut.

Scientific Names
Simmondsia chinensis, synonyms Buxus chinensis, Simmondsia californica.
Family: Simmondsiaceae.

People Use This For
Topically, jojoba is used for acne, psoriasis, sunburn, and chapped skin. It is also used topically as a hair restorer.
In manufacturing, jojoba is used as a component in shampoo; lipstick; makeup; cleansing products; and in face, hand, and body lotions.
In foods, roasted jojoba seeds are used as a coffee substitute.

Safety
LIKELY SAFE ...when used topically (6).
LIKELY UNSAFE ...when used orally because it contains 14% erucic acid, which can cause myocardial fibrosis (6); avoid using.
PREGNANCY AND LACTATION: LIKELY SAFE ...when used topically for hygienic uses (6).
LIKELY UNSAFE ...when used orally (6).

Effectiveness
There is insufficient reliable information available about the effectiveness of jojoba.

Mechanism of Action
The applicable parts of jojoba are the oil and wax. Jojoba seeds yield a colorless, odorless oil that is an emollient (11). Jojoba oil penetrates skin and skin oils easily, unclogging hair follicles and preventing sebum build up, which could lead to hair loss (6). Taken by mouth, jojoba wax passes through the body without being digested, but is stored in intestinal cells and the liver (18).

Adverse Reactions
Topically, contact dermatitis occurs with use of shampoos and hair conditioners containing jojoba oil (6). Hypoallergenic sensitivity to jojoba wax may occur (6).

Interactions with Herbs & Other Dietary Supplements
None known.

Interactions with Drugs
None known.

Interactions with Foods
None known.

Interactions with Lab Tests
None known.

Interactions with Diseases or Conditions
None known.

Dosage and Administration
TOPICAL: Jojoba oil ingredient levels vary. In skin care products 5-10%; shampoos and conditioners 1-2%; bar soaps 0.5-3% (6).

Comments
Jojoba oil and wax are produced from the seeds of jojoba, a shrub native to arid regions of northern Mexico and the southwestern US (3901). Jojoba wax is unsuitable for food use (18).

JUJUBE

Also Known As
Black Date, Chinese Date, Chinese Jujube, Da Zao, Hei Zao, Hong Zao, Jujube Plum, Jujubi, Red Date, Zao, Zizyphus, Zyzyphus Jujube.

Scientific Names
Ziziphus jujuba, synonyms Ziziphus sativa, Ziziphus spinosa, Ziziphus vulgaris, Ziziphus zizyphus, Rhamnus zizyphus.
Family: Rhamnaceae.

People Use This For
Orally, jujube is used for improving muscular strength, as a prophylaxis for liver diseases and stress ulcers, as a sedative, and to neutralizing drug toxicities. Jujube is also used for dry and itchy skin, lack of appetite, fatigue, diarrhea, hysteria, anemia, hypertension, purpura, fever, wounds, ulcers, inflammation, asthma, and eye diseases.
In foods, jujube is used in a variety of recipes.
In manufacturing, jujube extracts are used in skin care products as an anti-inflammatory, antiwrinkle, moisturizer, and for relief from sunburn.

Safety
There is insufficient reliable information available about the safety of jujube.
Pregnancy and Lactation: Insufficient reliable information available; avoid using.

Effectiveness
There is insufficient reliable information available about the effectiveness of jujube.

Mechanism of Action
The applicable part of jujube is the fruit. Animal data suggests that jujube increases body weight, increases swimming endurance and protects against carbon tetrachloride-induced liver damage. Animal data also suggests that an ethanolic extract may have anti-inflammatory effects and inhibit growth of Bacillus subtilis. A methanolic extract containing oleanolic acid and ursolic acid inhibits dental cavity-producing activity of Streptococcus mutans in vitro (11).
Samgyetang, a soup made from chicken, jujube, panax ginseng, garlic, and chestnuts, appears to offer protection from experimentally induced peptic ulcers (10249).

Adverse Reactions
None reported.

Interactions with Herbs & Other Dietary Supplements
None known.

Interactions with Drugs
None known.

Interactions with Foods
None known.

Interactions with Lab Tests
None known.

Interactions with Diseases or Conditions
None known.

Dosage and Administration
No typical dosage.

Comments
Jujube is no longer used medicinally (18).

JUNIPER

Also Known As
Common Juniper Berry, Enebro, Geniévre, Ginepro, Juniperi fructus, Wacholderbeeren, Zimbro.
CAUTION: See separate listing for Cade Oil.

Scientific Names
Juniperus communis.
Family: Cupressaceae.

People Use This For
Orally, juniper is used for dyspepsia, flatulence, heartburn, bloating, loss of appetite, urinary tract infections (UTIs), kidney and bladder stones, snakebite, intestinal worms, gastrointestinal infections, and cancer.
Topically, juniper is used for rheumatic pains in joints and muscles, inflammatory diseases, and wounds.
As an inhalant, the essential oil of juniper is used as an analgesic for pain and for bronchitis as an inhaled vapor.
In foods, the juniper berry is often used as a culinary condiment, a flavor component in gin and bitter preparations, and the extract and oil are used as a flavoring agent in foods and beverages.
In manufacturing, the juniper oil is used as a fragrance component in soaps and cosmetics.

Safety
LIKELY SAFE ...when used orally in amounts commonly found in foods. Juniper, juniper berry, and juniper extract have Generally Recognized As Safe (GRAS) status in the US (4912).
POSSIBLY SAFE ...when used orally and appropriately in medicinal amounts short-term (12). ...when used topically on limited areas of skin (12,18). ...when the oil is used by inhalation and appropriately as aromatherapy (7107).
LIKELY UNSAFE ...when used orally in excessive amounts, long-term. Prolonged use of high doses can increase the potential for severe side effects such as convulsions or kidney damage (8,19). ...when used topically on large skin wounds or in individuals with acute skin conditions (18).
PREGNANCY: UNSAFE ...when used orally. Juniper can increase uterine tone, interfere with fertility and

implantation, and cause abortion (4,19).
LACTATION: Insufficient reliable information available; avoid using.

Effectiveness
There is insufficient reliable information available about the effectiveness of juniper.

Mechanism of Action
The applicable part of juniper is the berry. Juniper berry has aquaretic, antiseptic, antiflatulent, and antirheumatic effects. It also stimulates stomach function (4,512). Aquaretics increase urine volume (water loss) but not electrolyte excretion (512). The constituent terpinen-4-ol increases the glomerular filtration rate, but it can also irritate the kidneys (4). In vitro, juniper berry exhibits antiviral activity against the herpes simplex virus and has antifungal activity (4). In experimental animals, the juniper berry extract shows abortifacient, antifertility, anti-inflammatory, anti-implantation, hypotensive, hypertensive, and hypoglycemic effects (4). The juniper berry oil stimulates uterine activity (4). It has diuretic, GI antiseptic, and irritant effects (11). The oil prevents antispasmodic effects in smooth muscle (11).

Adverse Reactions
Orally, excessive amounts of the juniper berry oil can cause kidney irritation (4). Overdose symptoms include kidney pain, diuresis, albuminuria, hematuria, purplish urine, tachycardia, hypertension, convulsions, metrorrhagia, and abortion (4).
Topically, juniper can cause skin irritation (4). Signs of topical poisoning include burning, erythema, inflammation with blisters, and edema (4). Repeated exposure to the juniper pollen can cause occupational allergies that affect the skin and respiratory tract (6).

Interactions with Herbs & Other Dietary Supplements
None known.

Interactions with Drugs
ANTIDIABETES DRUGS: Theoretically, juniper berry might potentiate diabetes therapy due to hypoglycemic activity (4).
DIURETIC DRUGS: Theoretically, juniper berry might interfere with diuretic therapy (4,512).

Interactions with Foods
None known.

Interactions with Lab Tests
URINE TESTS: The juniper berry can interfere with urine assays, and large amounts can cause purplish urine (4).

Interactions with Diseases or Conditions
DIABETES: Monitor blood glucose level closely due to claims that juniper has hypoglycemic effects (4,19).
GI CONDITIONS: Juniper berry can irritate the gastrointestinal tract (19). It is contraindicated in individuals with infectious or inflammatory gastrointestinal conditions (19).
HYPERTENSION, HYPOTENSION: Theoretically, juniper berry might interfere with blood pressure control (4,512).
KIDNEY DISEASE: Contraindicated (4,12).
SEIZURE DISORDERS: Theoretically, the juniper berry might exacerbate these conditions.
OTHER: Individuals with cardiac insufficiency, hypertonia, fever, acute skin disease, or large skin wounds should not use juniper berry (18).

Dosage and Administration
ORAL: The typical dose of juniper is 1-2 grams of the berry three times daily (4) or one cup of the tea three to four times daily (8). The tea is prepared by steeping 1 teaspoon of the crushed juniper berry, about 2-3 grams, in 150 mL boiling water for 10 minutes and then straining. Juniper should be used up to a maximum of 10 grams of the dried berry per day, corresponding to 20-100 mg of the essential oil (2). This dose should not be used longer than four weeks without physician consultation (8). The usual dose of the liquid extract (1:1 in 25% alcohol) is 2-4 mL three times daily (4). The common dose of the tincture (1:5 in 45% alcohol) is 1-2 mL three times daily (4). The berry oil (1:5 in 45% alcohol) is typically taken as 0.03-0.2 mL three times daily (4). CAUTION: The juniper berry oil should only be used under supervision (4).
TOPICAL: The juniper berry is commonly used in bath salts for treating rheumatism (18).

Comments
Avoid confusion with cade oil, which is distilled from juniper wood (Juniperus oxycedrus). Turpentine oil has been used to adulterate juniper berry oil (512).

KAMALA

Also Known As
Kamcela, Kameela, Rottlera Tinctoria, Spoonwood.

Scientific Names
Mallotus philippensis.
Family: Euphorbiaceae.

Comments
At the date of publication, there was very little scientific information about this product. Our staff is continually analyzing the available information on natural medicines and will add data to the online version of *Natural Medicines Comprehensive Database* as it becomes available. See www.naturaldatabase.com.

KAOLIN

Also Known As
Argilla, Bolus Alba, China Clay, Heavy Kaolin, Light Kaolin, Porcelain Clay, White Bole.

Scientific Names
Hydrated aluminum silicate.

People Use This For
Orally, kaolin is used for mild to moderate acute diarrhea, cholera, enteritis, and dysentery.
Topically, kaolin is used as a poultice, dusting powder, drying agent, and emollient.
In combination products, kaolin is used for symptomatic diarrhea control, in relief of radiation-induced mucositis, in the treatment of chronic ulcerative colitis, and to treat spontaneous pneumothorax.
Diagnostic uses of kaolin include, as a contrast media agent (C,D), automated testing for activated coagulation time (ACT), serodiagnosis of tuberculosis, and the kaolin agglutination test (KAT).
In manufacturing, kaolin is used as a diluent in tablet preparation, and a filtering or decolorizing agent.
Kaolin is also a food additive.

Safety
LIKELY SAFE ...when used orally in appropriate amounts. Kaolin is not absorbed systemically and is generally nontoxic (6). ...when sterile products are used topically with appropriately (9,16). Kaolin is an FDA-approved prescription product.
PREGNANCY AND LACTATION: Insufficient reliable information available.

Effectiveness
POSSIBLY EFFECTIVE

Diarrhea. Taking kaolin orally, alone or in combination with pectin and other drugs, may help symptomatic control of mild to moderate acute diarrhea (excluding pseudomembranous enterocolitis) (15). Kaolin is an FDA-approved prescription product.

Oral mucositis. Kaolin taken orally seems to decrease the pain and severity of radiation-induced mucositis (186,187).

There is insufficient reliable information available about the effectiveness of kaolin for its other uses.

Mechanism of Action
Kaolin may absorb bacteria and toxins in the GI tract, increase fecal bulk, and restore stool consistency (6,9,15,16).
In radiation-induced mucositis, kaolin may act as a protective coating to decrease the severity of pain (186).
Topically, kaolin acts as a drying agent adsorbing a wide variety of substances (6,9,16).

Adverse Reactions
Orally, kaolin can cause constipation, particularly in children and the elderly (15).
Occupational kalinosis (pulmonary disease) is reported in miners following inhalation (6,195,196,197).

Interactions with Herbs & Other Dietary Supplements
None known.

Interactions with Drugs
ORAL DRUGS: Kaolin actively adsorbs a wide variety of substances (6,9). Concomitant use of kaolin or kaolin/pectin could decrease systemic absorption of digoxin, quinidine, lincomycin, clindamycin, phenothiazines, chloroquine, and trimethoprim (6,198,199,250,251,252,253). Separate doses of chloroquine and kaolin by at least four hours.

Interactions with Foods
None known.

Interactions with Lab Tests
None known.

Interactions with Diseases or Conditions
None known.

Dosage and Administration
ORAL: For diarrhea, the dose varies ranging between 15-60 grams (6,9) and 50-100 grams at three hour intervals (16). Kaolin is usually taken at the first sign of diarrhea and after each loose bowel movement. Doses of 15-60 grams (6,9) and doses of 50-100 grams at 3 hours intervals reported (16). For relief of radiation-induced mucositis, 15 ml (50% kaolin/pectin, a 50% diphenhydramine) solution is used as a rinse four times a day (186). Kaolin is an FDA-approved prescription product.

Comments
Kaolin is hydrated aluminum silicate (16) purified for pharmaceutical use by treatment with hydrochloric acid or sulfuric acid, or both, then washed with water (6,9,16). Heavy kaolin (Kaolinum ponderosum) is the purified natural form of variable composition (9,16), and light kaolin is prepared from heavy kaolin by elutriation (separation of finer from coarser particles by suspension in water) (9,16).

KARAYA GUM

Also Known As
Bassora Tragacanth, Indian Tragacanth, Kadaya, Kadira, Karaya, Katila, Kullo, Mucara, Sterculia Gum.

Scientific Names
Sterculia urens; Sterculia villosa; Sterculia tragacantha; other Sterculia species.
Family: Malvaceae or Sterculiaceae.

People Use This For
Orally, karaya gum is used as a bulk laxative and as an aphrodisiac.
In manufacturing, karaya gum is used as a thickener in pharmaceuticals and cosmetics; denture and ostomy adhesives; and a binder and stabilizer in foods and beverages.

Safety
LIKELY SAFE ...when used orally in amounts commonly found in foods. Karaya gum has Generally Recognized As Safe (GRAS) status in the US (4912). ...when used orally in medicinal amounts (6).
PREGNANCY AND LACTATION: Insufficient reliable information available.

Effectiveness
POSSIBLY EFFECTIVE

Constipation. Taking karaya gum orally seems to be effective for treating constipation when used as a bulk-forming laxative (6,11).

There is insufficient reliable information available about the effectiveness of karaya gum for its other uses.

Mechanism of Action
Karaya gum is not digested or absorbed but swells in the presence of water, forming a viscous colloidal solution that stimulates peristalsis in the GI tract (6,11).

Adverse Reactions
None reported.

Interactions with Herbs & Other Dietary Supplements
None known.

Interactions with Drugs
ORAL DRUGS: Co-administration of oral drugs with bulk forming laxatives may decrease the absorption of the drugs (12).

Interactions with Foods
None known.

Interactions with Lab Tests
None known.

Interactions with Diseases or Conditions
BOWEL OBSTRUCTION: In general, bulk laxatives are contraindicated in individuals with bowel obstruction (12).

Dosage and Administration
No typical dosage.

Comments
Karaya gum is exuded from Sterculia species trees, that are native to India, when charred or scarred (6,3901). Adequate fluid intake is important with bulk forming laxatives.

KAVA

Also Known As
Ava, Ava Pepper, Ava Root, Awa, Gea, Gi, Intoxicating Long Pepper, Intoxicating Pepper, Kao, Kava Pepper, Kava Root, Kavain, Kavapipar, Kawa Kawa, Kawa Pepper, Kawapfeffer, Kew, Long Pepper, Maori Kava, Malohu, Maluk, Meruk, Milik, Rauschpfeffer, Rhizome Di Kava-Kava, Sakau, Tonga, Wurzelstock, Yagona, Yangona, Yaqona, Yongona.
CAUTION: See separate listing for Indian Long Pepper.

Scientific Names
Piper methysticum.
Family: Piperaceae.

People Use This For
Orally, kava is used to treat anxiety disorders, stress, attention deficit-hyperactivity disorder (ADHD), insomnia, and restlessness. It is also used orally for epilepsy, psychosis, depression, headaches including migraines, common cold and other respiratory tract infections, tuberculosis, cancer prevention, musculoskeletal pain, and bladder cancer. Kava is also used orally for urinary tract infection (UTI), uterine inflammation, venereal disease, menstrual discomfort, vaginal prolapse, and as an aphrodisiac.
Topically, kava is used for skin diseases including leprosy, to promote wound healing, and as an analgesic. It is also used topically as a poultice for otitis and abscesses, and as a mouthwash for canker sores and toothaches.
Ceremonially, kava is used as a beverage to induce relaxation.

Safety
POSSIBLY UNSAFE ...when used orally. There is concern that kava preparations can induce hepatotoxicity and liver failure in patients taking relatively normal doses, short-term. Kava extracts have been safely used under medical supervision for up to six months (2092,2093,2094,2095,4032,7325). However, there are at least 68 reported cases of liver toxicity following kava use. The use of kava for as little as one to three months has resulted in the need for liver transplants, and even death (7024,7068,7086,7096). However, some experts question the clinical validity of several of these cases (11369,11371). Kava has been banned from the market in Switzerland, Germany, Canada, and several other countries are considering similar action. Some patients may be more at risk than others. Patients who are "poor metabolizers" might be at greatest risk, but this has not been verified (7068). Until more is known, tell patients to avoid kava. Recommend routine liver function tests for patients who continue to use kava.
PREGNANCY: POSSIBLY UNSAFE ...when used orally. There is some concern that pyrone constituents in kava can cause loss of uterine tone (19); avoid using.
LACTATION: POSSIBLY UNSAFE ...when used orally. There is concern that the toxic pyrone constituents of kava can pass into breast milk (19); avoid using.

Effectiveness

LIKELY EFFECTIVE

Anxiety. Kava extracts standardized to 70% kava-lactones are superior to placebo (2093,2094,2095,7325,11372), and possibly comparable to low-dose benzodiazepines (2092). Treatment for 1-8 weeks may be necessary for significant improvement (2094,2095). Most clinical studies on the effectiveness of kava for anxiety disorders have used the standardized extract WS 1490 (W. Schwabe). This extract is standardized to contain 70% kava-lactones (also known as kavapyrones). This extract is more than twice as concentrated as most products that are commercially available.

POSSIBLY EFFECTIVE

Benzodiazepine withdrawal. There is some evidence that upwardly titrating kava over one week while tapering the benzodiazepine over two weeks can prevent withdrawal symptoms in some people with non-psychotic anxiety (7325).

Menopausal anxiety. Two small trials have shown that kava standardized to 15% or 70% kava-lactones is superior to placebo taken orally for short-term treatment of neurovegetative and anxiety symptoms related to climacteric. Significant improvement occurred after one week of treatment (2096).

INSUFFICIENT RELIABLE EVIDENCE to RATE

Cancer. Epidemiological evidence suggests that increasing kava consumption might lower incidence of cancer (8175).

Social anxiety. Preliminary clinical research in healthy volunteers suggests that taking kava orally might reduce physiological reactivity during stressful situations (9893).

More evidence is needed to rate kava for these uses.

Mechanism of Action

The applicable parts of kava are the rhizome, root, and stem. Pharmacological activity has largely been attributed to the kava-lactones (also known as kavapyrones), kawain (kavain), dihydrokawain, methysticin, dihydromethysticin, yangonin, and others (9920,9923). The dried herb typically contains at least 3.5% kava-lactones. Kava is traditionally prepared by water extraction from the fresh root. Kava is prepared commercially with ethanol, yielding 30% kava-lactones or acetone, yielding 70% kava-lactones (9920,9921).

Kava has been found to have a variety of pharmacological effects, including anxiolytic, sedative, anti-convulsant, local anesthetic, spasmolytic, anti-inflammatory, and analgesic activities; however, the exact mechanism for these effects is not known. Some evidence suggests the sedative effects may be due to an increase in the number of GABA binding sites (4037,8440,9923). Other preliminary evidence suggests the sedative effects might be the result of dopamine antagonism, particularly by the vangonin constituent (4055,7727,8415,8740). There is some evidence the kava pyrones (+)-methycystine, (+)-kavain, and (±)-kavain also inhibit the uptake of noradrenaline which might also contribute to the psychotropic actions of kava (8740). Kava is not, however, thought to affect benzodiazepine receptors (6401,4038,11373). Analgesia is not believed to occur by the opiate pathway because naloxone does not reverse the effects of kava. Furthermore, kava is thought to produce motor sedation without affecting respiratory processes (2095). Kava doesn't seem to impair cognitive function (2097,2098,11373). Even at intoxicating doses, the only cognitive impairment observed with kava is a decline in accuracy of visual attention (11373).

Some research suggests that kava can produce muscle paralysis by a mechanism similar to local anesthetics such as cocaine (9924). When chewed, kava root reportedly numbs the mouth similar to cocaine (1740). Some evidence suggests kava may affect the limbic system (6002). People consuming kava have reported feeling more sociable, tranquil, and generally happy (1740). The kavapyrones desmethoxyyangonin and methysticin appear to competitively inhibit monoamine oxidase B (MAO-B) (2500). Kava is thought to work for a variety of inflammatory conditions by inhibiting both COX-1 and COX-2 enzymes, the enzymes responsible for converting arachidonic acid to prostaglandins (8413).

There is some evidence the kavapyrone (+)-kavain has antithrombotic activity. By inhibiting cyclooxygenase and decreasing the synthesis of thromboxane A2, (+)-kavain appears to decrease the aggregation of platelets (2501).

Adverse Reactions

Orally, kava can cause gastrointestinal (GI) upset, headache, dizziness, drowsiness, enlarged pupils and disturbances of oculomotor equilibrium and accommodation, dry mouth, and allergic skin reactions (4032,11370). It may also cause extrapyramidal side effects such as involuntary oral and lingual reflexes, and twisting movements of the head and trunk, possibly due to dopamine antagonism (4055,8415). Unlike benzodiazepines, kava is not thought to be associated with impaired cognitive function (2097,2098,11373). Use of normal doses of kava may affect the ability to drive or operate machinery. Driving under the influence (DUI) citations have been issued to individuals observed driving erratically after drinking large amounts of kava tea (535).

Hepatoxicity is a particular concern with kava. There are at least 68 reported cases of hepatotoxicity following use of kava products (7024,7068,7086,7096,11795). However, some experts question the clinical validity of several of these cases (11369,11371). In susceptible patients, symptoms can show up after as little as 3-4 weeks of kava use, including yellowed skin (jaundice), fatigue, and dark urine (7024,7068). Liver function tests can be elevated after 3-8 weeks of use, possibly followed by hepatomegaly and onset of encephalopathy (7024). Kava can also exacerbate hepatitis in patients with a history of recurrent hepatitis. Symptoms seem to resolve spontaneously after discontinuation of kava (390). Liver toxicity is more frequently associated with prolonged use of very high doses (6401). But there is some

concern that even short-term use of kava in typical doses might cause acute hepatitis in some patients, including severe hepatocellular necrosis. Death or liver transplant has been required after as little as 1-3 months of kava use (7024,7068,7086,11795). Symptoms of liver toxicity may occur following a single occasion of alcohol consumption while taking kava (7068). Kava supplements have been banned in Switzerland, Germany, and Canada. Several other countries are considering removing kava from the market (7086).
Most patients taking kava have not experienced such severe adverse effects. Kava mixed with water is used in the Pacific Islands as a ceremonial and social beverage without reported hepatotoxicity (11794). It is unclear which patients might be susceptible to adverse liver effects. There is some speculation that so-called "poor metabolizers" or those patients with deficiency in the cytochrome P450 2D6 (CYP2D6) isoenzyme may be at increased risk for hepatotoxic effects of kava (7068). Up to 10% of people of European descent have a genetic deficiency of CYP2D6. This deficiency has not been found in Pacific Islanders. Some people speculate that the type of extraction method could be responsible. Alcohol and acetone extracts of kava have been linked to liver toxicity; water extracts have not. But there is no research to support the contention that water-extracted kava is safe(11794).Until more is known, tell patients to avoid kava. Advise patients who continue to use kava to routinely monitor liver function. In patients who develop symptoms, discontinue kava and monitor liver function tests. Liver function tests may normalize within eight weeks following discontinuation (7068).
Long-term use of very large amounts of kava, especially in high doses (400 mg kava pyrones daily) is also associated with overall poor health including symptoms of low body weight, reduced protein levels, puffy face, hematuria, increased red blood cell volume, decreased platelets and lymphocytes, and possibly pulmonary hypertension (4032,6402). Chronic use of high doses of kava has also been associated with kava dermopathy, which consists of reddened eyes; dry, scaly, flaky skin; and temporary yellow discoloration of the skin, hair, and nails (6401,8414,8417,11370). This pellagra-like syndrome is unresponsive to niacinamide treatment (6240,7728,11370). The cause is unknown, but may relate to interference with cholesterol metabolism (6240). Kava's adverse effects on liver function might also contribute to kava dermopathy (6401,8417). Kava dermopathy usually occurs within three months to one year of regular kava use, and resolves when the kava dose is decreased or discontinued (6401,8414). Kava dose should be decreased or discontinued if kava dermopathy occurs (6401).
Kava has been associated with severe, rapidly progressive, persistent Parkinsonism. In a previously healthy 45-year-old woman with a family history of essential tremor, Parkinsonian symptoms developed following ten days of taking 65 mg kava per day. Parkinsonian symptoms improved with administration of anticholinergics, but residual symptoms required chronic medication (7727).
Sjogren's syndrome has been associated with a herbal supplement containing kava, echinacea, and St. John's wort. Echinacea may have been the primary cause, because Sjogren's syndrome is an autoimmune disorder. The role of kava in this syndrome is unclear (10319).

Interactions with Herbs & Other Dietary Supplements

HEPATOTOXIC HERBS AND SUPPLEMENTS: There is some concern that kava can adversely affect the liver (7024,7068). Theoretically, concomitant use with other potentially hepatotoxic products might increase the risk of developing liver damage. Some of these products include androstenedione, chaparral, coenzyme Q10 (only in high doses), comfrey, DHEA, germander, niacin, pennyroyal oil, red yeast, and others.
HERBS AND SUPPLEMENTS WITH SEDATIVE PROPERTIES: Theoretically, concomitant use with herbs and supplements that have sedative properties might increase the risk of excessive drowsiness. Some of these supplements include 5-HTP, calamus, California poppy, catnip, hops, Jamaican dogwood, kava, St. John's wort, scullcap, valerian, yerba mansa, and others.

Interactions with Drugs

ALPRAZOLAM (Xanax): There is one report of an individual who was hospitalized due to lethargy and disorientation that occurred when alprazolam, cimetidine, terazosin, and kava were used concomitantly (536).
CNS DEPRESSANTS: Concomitant use of kava and alcohol, barbiturates, benzodiazepines, or other CNS depressants can increase the risk of drowsiness and motor reflex depression (2093,2098).
CYTOCHROME P450 1A2 (CYP1A2) SUBSTRATES: Preliminary evidence suggests that kava significantly inhibits cytochrome P450 1A2 (CYP1A2) (8743). Some substrates of CYP1A2 include clozapine (Clozaril), cyclobenzaprine (Flexeril), fluvoxamine (Luvox), haloperidol (Haldol), imipramine (Tofranil), mexiletine (Mexitil), olanzapine (Zyprexa), pentazocine (Talwin), propranolol (Inderal), tacrine (Cognex), theophylline, zileuton (Zyflo), zolmitriptan (Zomig), and others. Use kava cautiously or avoid in patients taking these drugs.
CYTOCHROME P450 2C9 (CYP2C9) SUBSTRATES: Preliminary evidence suggests that kava significantly inhibits cytochrome P450 2C9 (CYP2C9) (8743). Some substrates of CYP2C9 include celecoxib (Celebrex), diclofenac (Voltaren), fluvastatin (Lescol), glipizide (Glucotrol), ibuprofen (Advil, Motrin), irbesartan (Avapro), losartan (Cozaar), phenytoin (Dilantin), piroxicam (Feldene), tamoxifen (Nolvadex), tolbutamide (Tolinase), torsemide (Demadex), and warfarin (Coumadin). Use kava cautiously or avoid in patients taking these drugs.
CYTOCHROME P450 2C19 (CYP2C19) SUBSTRATES: Preliminary evidence suggests that kava significantly inhibits cytochrome P450 2C19 (CYP2C19) (8743). Some substrates of CYP2C19 include amitriptyline (Elavil), clomipramine (Anafranil), cyclophosphamide (Cytoxan), diazepam (Valium), lansoprazole (Prevacid), omeprazole (Prilosec), lansoprazole (Protonix), phenytoin (Dilantin), phenobarbital (Luminal), progesterone, and others. Use kava cautiously or avoid in patients taking these drugs.

CYTOCHROME P450 2D6 (CYP2D6) SUBSTRATES: Preliminary evidence suggests that kava significantly inhibits cytochrome P450 2D6 (CYP2D6) (8743). Some drugs metabolized by CYP2D6 include amitriptyline (Elavil), codeine, desipramine (Norpramin), flecainide (Tambocor), haloperidol (Haldol), imipramine (Tofranil), metoprolol (Lopressor, Toprol XL), ondansetron (Zofran), paroxetine (Paxil), risperidone (Risperdal), tramadol (Ultram), venlafaxine (Effexor), and others. Use kava cautiously or avoid in patients taking these drugs.
CYTOCHROME P450 3A4 (CYP3A4) SUBSTRATES: Preliminary evidence suggests that kava significantly inhibits cytochrome P450 3A4 (CYP3A4) (8743). Some drugs metabolized by CYP3A4 include alprazolam (Xanax), amlodipine (Norvasc), clarithromycin (Biaxin), cyclosporine (Sandimmune), erythromycin, lovastatin (Mevacor), ketoconazole (Nizoral), itraconazole (Sporanox), fexofenadine (Allegra), triazolam (Halcion), verapamil (Calan, Isoptin) and many others. Use kava cautiously or avoid in patients taking these drugs.
HEPATOTOXIC DRUGS: There is some concern that kava can adversely affect the liver (7024,7068). Theoretically, concomitant use with other potentially hepatotoxic drugs might increase the risk of developing liver damage. Some of these drugs include acarbose (Precose, Prandase), amiodarone (Cordarone), atorvastatin (Lipitor), azathioprine (Imuran), carbamazepine (Tegretol), cerivastatin (Baycol), diclofenac (Voltaren), felbamate (Felbatol), fenofibrate (Tricor), fluvastatin (Lescol), gemfibrozil (Lopid), isoniazid, itraconazole, (Sporanox), ketoconazole (Nizoral), leflunomide (Arava), lovastatin (Mevacor), methotrexate (Rheumatrex), nevirapine (Viramune), niacin, nitrofurantoin (Macrodantin), pioglitazone (Actos), pravastatin (Pravachol), pyrazinamide, rifampin (Rifadin), ritonavir (Norvir), rosiglitazone (Avandia), simvastatin (Zocor), tacrine (Cognex), tamoxifen, terbinafine (Lamisil), valproic acid, and zileuton (Zyflo).
LEVODOPA: There is some concern that kava might decrease the effectiveness of levodopa. In one case, kava seemed to reduce efficacy of levodopa. This effect might be due to dopamine antagonism by kava (19).

Interactions with Foods

ALCOHOL: Concomitant use of kava with alcohol can increase the risk of side effects such as drowsiness and motor reflex depression (19). There is also some concern that concomitant use of kava and alcohol can increase the risk of developing hepatotoxicity (7068).

Interactions with Lab Tests

LIVER FUNCTION TESTS: There is some concern that kava can cause liver damage and increase liver function tests (LFTs) in some patients. Liver toxicity is primarily associated with prolonged use of high doses (6401). However, in some patients, short-term use (3-8 weeks) of typical doses might result in liver damage and increase liver function tests (390,7024,7068). Liver function tests affected include aspartate aminotransferase (AST), alanine aminotransferase (ALT), alkaline phosphatase, gamma-glutamyltransferase, lactate dehydrogenase (LDH), and total and conjugated bilirubin (7024,7068). Consider monitoring liver function tests in patients taking kava for more than one month or in patients symptoms of liver problems such as fatigue, yellowing of the skin (jaundice), or dark urine.

Interactions with Diseases or Conditions

DEPRESSION: There is some concern about using kava in depressed patients. Kava seems to have CNS depressant effects and theoretically might exacerbate depression in some patients (19); use with caution.
HEPATITIS: Kava might adversely affect the liver, especially when taken for prolonged periods or in high doses. Even when used short-term in typical doses, kava might exacerbate hepatitis in patients with a history of recurrent hepatitis (390). Tell patients with active hepatitis or a history of hepatitis to avoid kava.
PARKINSON'S DISEASE: There is some concern about using kava in patients with Parkinson's disease. Dopamine antagonism has been reported even when used in typical doses. Tell patients with Parkinson's Disease to avoid kava (4032,8134,8415).

Dosage and Administration

ORAL: For anxiety disorders, most clinical trials have used kava extract standardized to 70% kava-lactone content. Doses of the kava extract were most commonly 100 mg (70 mg kava-lactones) three times daily (2092,2093,2094,2095,2096). For preventing benzodiazepine withdrawal, the 70% kava-lactone standardized extract has been used in doses increasing from 50 mg to 300 mg per day over one week, while the benzodiazepine is tapered over 2 weeks (7325). Because kava-lactone content varies substantially among products, appropriate dosing will also vary.

Comments

Kava was discovered by Captain Cook who named the plant, "intoxicating pepper" (6240). In the South Pacific, kava is a popular social drink, similar to alcohol in Western societies (9921). Kava is also prepared in a defined ritual manner and used for ceremonial purposes and has been used for thousands of years by Pacific Islanders (782,6240). The ban of kava in some countries has had a detrimental effect on the economies of Pacific Island countries that export kava (11794).

KEFIR

Also Known As
Fermented Dairy Product, Fermented Milk, Kefir Cheese, Kefir Grains, Kefir Yogurt.

Scientific Names
None.

People Use This For
Orally, kefir is used for improving digestion, lactose intolerance, and hyperlipidemia.

Safety
POSSIBLY SAFE ...when used orally and appropriately. Kefir appears safe when used for up to 6 months (7636,8452,8457,8480).
PREGNANCY AND LACTATION: ...Insufficient reliable information available; avoid using.

Effectiveness
LIKELY INEFFECTIVE

Hyperlipidemia. Taking kefir orally appears to have very little or no effect on total cholesterol and low-density lipoprotein (LDL) cholesterol (7636,8452,8457,8480).

There is insufficient reliable information available about the effectiveness of kefir for its other uses.

Mechanism of Action
Kefir consists of milk that has been fermented for 18 to 48 hours following the addition of kefir grain. After fermentation, kefir may have a pH as low as 4.5. It has a sour or effervescent taste and consistency. The primary active constituents of kefir include the polysaccharide, kefiran, and beta-galactosidase. Kefir grain is made up of a mixture of lactic acid bacteria, acetic acid bacteria, and yeast which is held together, in clumps, by polysaccharide links. When properly prepared, kefir grains resemble cooked cauliflower in color and texture. The composition of kefir grain varies with its origin, and as a result, there is considerable variation in the microbial content of the kefir after fermentation.

During fermentation, kefir becomes increasingly viscous due to the formation of additional kefiran polysaccharides by the lactic acid bacteria (8481,8482,8483,8484). Lactobacillus lactis, Lactobacillus casei, Lactobacillus helveticus, and other Lactobacillus species may be present in kefir. In addition, Streptococcus thermophilus and yeast species, including Kluyveromyces marxianus, Saccharomyces cerevisiae, and Candida species may be isolated (8485). Many of these species can survive transit through the stomach and inoculate the intestinal tract (8487).

The beta-galactosidase in kefir can facilitate the breakdown of lactose in the gastrointestinal tract, according to preliminary evidence. This action may increase the absorption of galactose and glucose after consuming milk (8485). The lactose found in milk decreases from 5% to about 3.6% during fermentation of kefir (8486).

Early evidence indicates that oral kefiran polysaccharide may increase both the intestinal and systemic immune response (8488,8489). This immune response may decrease the growth of carcinoma and sarcoma cells (8481,8482,8489).

Adverse Reactions
Orally, kefir can cause intestinal cramping and constipation, especially with initial use. These symptoms usually resolve after continued consumption of kefir (7636). Otherwise kefir appears to be well tolerated (7636,8452,8457,8480).

Interactions with Herbs & Other Dietary Supplements
None known.

Interactions with Drugs
IMMUNOSUPPRESSANTS: Kefir contains actively growing bacteria and yeast (8481,8482,8483,8484). Theoretically, patients taking immunosuppressant therapy might be more likely to develop an infection from the organisms. Use with caution in patients taking cyclosporine (Sandimmune, Neoral), azathioprine (Imuran), tacrolimus (FK506, Prograf), and others.

Interactions with Foods
None known.

Interactions with Lab Tests
None known.

Interactions with Diseases or Conditions

AIDS: Kefir contains actively growing bacteria and yeast (8481,8482,8483,8484). Theoretically, patients with an impaired immune system might be more likely to develop infections from these bacteria or yeast.
IMMUNOSUPPRESSION: There is some concern that immunocompromised patients taking kefir might be at an increased risk for fungemia or bacteriemia (8481,8482,8483,8484).

Dosage and Administration

ORAL: For hyperlipidemia, kefir 125 to 500 mL daily has been used for up to six months (7636,8452,8457,8480).

KHAT

Also Known As

Abyssinian Tea, Arabian-Tea, Chaat, Gat, Kat, Kus es Salahin, Miraa, Qut, Tchaad, Tohai, Tohat, Tschut.

Scientific Names

Catha edulis, synonym Celastrus edulis.
Family: Celastraceae.

People Use This For

Orally, khat leaf is used for depression, fatigue, obesity, gastric ulcers, and male infertility. The leaf and stem are chewed by people in East Africa and the Arabian countries as a euphoriant. It is also used to suppress the need for food and sleep, decrease sexual desires, and increase aggression.

Safety

POSSIBLY UNSAFE ...when used orally. Khat leaf is not physically addicting but is associated with psychological dependence (6). High doses of khat can cause paranoia, psychosis, and aggression (10120).
PREGNANCY: POSSIBLY UNSAFE ...when used orally. Khat may reduce infant birth weight (6).
LACTATION: POSSIBLY UNSAFE ...when used orally. Khat contains norpseudoephedrine, which passes into mother's milk (6); avoid using.

Effectiveness

There is insufficient reliable information available about the effectiveness of khat.

Mechanism of Action

The applicable parts of khat are the leaf and stem. Khat contains cathine, which has 1/10 the stimulant effect of d-amphetamine. It also contains cathinone, which is a more powerful stimulant than cathine and closely resembles ephedrine and amphetamine in chemical structure (10120). Both khat constituents decrease food intake and increase locomotor activity (6).

Adverse Reactions

Orally, consumption of Khat results in central stimulation including euphoria, increased alertness, excessive talkativeness, hyperactivity, excitement, aggressiveness, anxiety, elevated blood pressure, and manic behavior. Insomnia, malaise, and lack of concentration usually follow (6). Increased consumption can cause users to become paranoid and psychotic (10120). True psychotic reactions occur much less often than with amphetamines (6). Cardiovascular effects include tachycardia, palpitations, and increased blood pressure. Other effects include increased respiratory rate, hyperthermia, sweating, pupil dilation and decreased intraocular pressure, stomatitis, esophagitis, gastritis, periodontal disease, temporomandibular joint dysfunction and keratosis of buccal mucosa, and constipation (6). Chronic use in young people is linked to hypertension.
Severe adverse effects include migraine, cerebral hemorrhage, myocardial infarction (MI), pulmonary edema, and hepatic cirrhosis. Khat causes initial increase in men's libido followed by loss of sexual drive, spermatorrhea, and impotence (6). Females report increased sexual desire and improved performance (6).
There are also cases of infection with Fasciola hepatica following chewing khat leaves. Fasciola hepatica contamination might be most likely with freshly picked, damp leaves. Signs of Fasciola hepatica infection can include pain below the ribs, leukocytosis with eosinophilia, and large liver mass on CT examination (6464).

Interactions with Herbs & Other Dietary Supplements

None known.

Interactions with Drugs

None known.

Interactions with Foods
None known.

Interactions with Lab Tests
None known.

Interactions with Diseases or Conditions
DIABETES: Khat use suppresses appetite causing people to skip meals, decrease adherence to dietary advice, and increase consumption of sweetened beverages aggravating hyperglycemia (6).

Dosage and Administration
No typical dosage.

Comments
Khat is considered to be a dependence producing drug by the World Health Organization (WHO). In Somalia, civilian and military use of khat has been blamed for fueling civil conflict, draining the nation's economy, and thwarting international relief efforts (10120).

KHELLA

Also Known As
Ammi, Bischofskrautfruchte, Bishop's Weed, Bishop's Weed Fruit, Bishops Weed, Fruits de Khella, Khella Fruit, Khellin, Toothpick Ammi, Toothpick Plant, Visnaga, Visnagae, Visnagafruchte, Visnaga Fruit, Visnagin.
CAUTION: See separate listings for Goutweed and Bishop's Weed.

Scientific Names
Ammi visnaga, synonyms Ammi daucoides, Daucus visagna.
Family: Apiaceae/Umbelliferae.

People Use This For
Orally, khella is used for colic and abdominal cramps, kidney stones, menstrual pain, and premenstrual syndrome (PMS). Khella is also used for respiratory conditions including asthma, bronchitis, cough, and whooping cough. It is also used for cardiovascular disorders including hypertension, cardiac arrhythmias, congestive heart failure (CHF), angina, atherosclerosis, and hypercholesterolemia. It is also used for liver and gall bladder disorders, diabetes, and as a diuretic.
Topically, khella is used for vitiligo, psoriasis, wound healing, inflammation conditions, and poisonous bites.

Safety
POSSIBLY UNSAFE ...when used orally in high doses. High doses of khella can cause increases in liver enzymes and possible liver damage (2).
PREGNANCY: LIKELY UNSAFE ...when used orally. The active constituent, khellin, has uterine stimulant activity (19); contraindicated.
LACTATION: Insufficient reliable information available; avoid using.

Effectiveness
There is insufficient reliable information available about the effectiveness of khella.

Mechanism of Action
The applicable parts of khella are the dried, ripe fruits (7161). Khella has several constituents with known pharmacological activity, including visnadin, visnagin, and khellin. All of these constituents seem to have cardiovascular effects due to calcium channel blocking actions (8,2525). Visnadin is the most active. It can inhibit vascular smooth muscle contraction and seems to dilate peripheral and coronary vessels and increase coronary circulation (8,9,2523,2524). Visnagin also has negative chronotropic and inotropic effects and reduces peripheral vascular resistance (869). The khellin constituent also acts as a vasodilator and has bronchodilatory activity (9). There is some preliminary evidence that khellin might also increase high-density lipoprotein (HDL) levels without affecting total cholesterol or triglyceride concentrations (2522). A khella extract seems to have some antimicrobial activity. This might be attributable to both the khellin and visnagin constituents, which both seem to have antifungal, antibacterial, and antiviral activity (1907). Researchers are interested in khella for use in psoriasis. The khellin constituent is structurally similar to the psoralen nucleus and might be useful as a photosensitizer in patients with psoriasis (1908).

Adverse Reactions
Orally, prolonged use or use of high doses of khella can cause nausea, dizziness, constipation, lack of appetite, headache, itching, and insomnia. In some patients, khella can cause elevated liver transaminase and gamma-glutamyltransferase (GGT) levels (2), probably due to the khellin constituent, which is known to affect liver enzymes (6,2522). Liver dysfunction and jaundice is typically reversible when khella is discontinued (2). There is also some concern that khella might cause photosensitivity because of the constituents khellin and furocoumarin (2,7162).

Interactions with Herbs & Other Dietary Supplements
DIGITALIS: Theoretically, khella might decrease the effectiveness of digitalis. The visnagin constituent of khella has negative inotropic effects, which might counter the effects of digitalis (869).
HEPATOTOXIC HERBS: Khella might have additive effects with herbs that cause hepatotoxicity. Khella can cause increase liver enzymes and liver dysfunction in some patients. Other products that might affect the liver include borage, chaparral, uva ursi, and others (2,2522).
PHOTOSENSITIZING HERBS: Theoretically, khella might have an additive effects with products that increase sun sensitivity, such as St. John's wort (7162).

Interactions with Drugs
DIGOXIN (Lanoxin): Theoretically, khella might decrease the effectiveness of cardiac glycosides like digoxin. The khella constituent visnadin has negative inotropic effects that might counter the effects of cardiac glycosides (19,869).
HEPATOTOXIC DRUGS: Theoretically, khella might have additive adverse effects on the liver when used with hepatotoxic drugs. Khella can increase liver transaminases (2,2522). Some drugs that can adversely effect the liver include acetaminophen (Tylenol), amiodarone (Cordarone), carbamazepine (Tegretol), isoniazid (INH), methotrexate (Rheumatrex), methyldopa (Aldomet) and many others.
PHOTOSENSITIZING DRUGS: Theoretically, concomitant use might result in increased photosensitivity. Khella constituents can cause photosensitivity (2521,7162). Some drugs that cause photosensitivity include amitriptyline (Elavil), quinolones (Ciprofloxacin, others), sulfa drugs (Septra, Bactrim, others), and tetracycline.

Interactions with Foods
None known.

Interactions with Lab Tests
HIGH-DENSITY LIPOPROTEIN (HDL): Theoretically, khella might increase HDL levels. The isolated khella constituent khellin seems to increase in HDL levels without affecting total cholesterol or triglycerides (2522).
LIVER FUNCTION TESTS: In some patients, khella can cause elevated liver transaminase and gamma-glutamyltransferase (GGT) levels (2), probably due to the khellin constituent, which is known to affect liver enzymes (6,2522). Liver dysfunction is typically reversible when khella is discontinued (2).

Interactions with Diseases or Conditions
LIVER DISEASE: Khella might exacerbate liver dysfunction in patients with liver disease. Khella can increase liver enzymes in some patients, probably due to the khellin constituent (2,2522).

Dosage and Administration
ORAL: Khella is typically given as an extract standardized based on khellin content. Extracts are usually standardized to 12% khellin (6002). A typical dose of khella is an amount that provides 20 mg of the khellin constituent per day (8). For angina, khella in an amount providing doses of 30-300 mg of the khellin constituent has also been used (6002). Khella is sometimes used as a tea. The tea is usually prepared by pouring boiling water over powdered fruit, steeping 10-15 minutes, and straining (8).

Comments
Several conventional drugs including amiodarone, nifedipine, and cromolyn, have been developed from khella (9,7161). Khella is sometimes confused with its less used relative, bishop's weed (Ammi majus). The two species have some common chemical constituents and pharmacological effects, but khella is more commonly used for cardiac and pulmonary conditions, and bishop's weed is more commonly used for dermatological conditions (7161). Isolated khellin, a constituent of khella and bishop's weed, is used for angina pectoris; asthma; and in conjunction with phototherapy for vitiligo, psoriasis, and alopecia areata (9,560,849,868).

KINETIN

Also Known As
Kinerase, Kinetase, Kn.

Scientific Names
N-(2-furanylmethyl)-1H-purin-6-amine; N(6)furfuryladenine; 6-furfurylaminopurine.

People Use This For
Topically, kinetin is used to reduce the effects of skin aging; to reduce skin roughness; fine wrinkles; telangiectasias; and mottled, excessive pigmentation.
In combination, kinetin is used topically with retinol palmitate to treat signs of aging.

Safety
There is insufficient reliable information about the safety of kinetin.
Pregnancy and Lactation: Insufficient reliable information available; avoid using.

Effectiveness
There is insufficient reliable information available about the effectiveness of kinetin.

Mechanism of Action
Kinetin is a cytokinin, a plant growth factor. In plants, it seems to work to prevent or slow the aging process (12022). Effects in animals are not well understood. There is some evidence that kinetin acts as an antioxidant and might protect DNA from oxidative damage (4278). There is also some in vitro evidence kinetin might decrease some of the morphological changes that normally occur in human fibroblast cells as they age. However, kinetin doesn't not seem to increase the overall lifespan of these fibroblasts (12022).

Adverse Reactions
None reported.

Interactions with Herbs & Other Dietary Supplements
None known.

Interactions with Drugs
None known.

Interactions with Foods
None known.

Interactions with Lab Tests
None known.

Interactions with Diseases or Conditions
None known.

Dosage and Administration
TOPICAL: A typical dose is 0.05% cream or lotion or 0.1% cream or lotion applied twice daily (4284).

KIWI

Also Known As
China Gooseberry, Chinese Gooseberry, Kiwi Fruit.

Scientific Names
Actinidia chinensis.
Family: Actinidiaceae.

People Use This For
For food use, kiwi is eaten as a food, used as a meat tenderizer, and is a component in some sports drinks.

Safety
LIKELY SAFE ...when used in food amounts (6).
PREGNANCY AND LACTATION: LIKELY SAFE ...when used in food amounts (6).

Effectiveness
INSUFFICIENT RELIABLE EVIDENCE to RATE

Asthma. There is some evidence that consumption of vitamin C-rich citrus fruits, including kiwi and others, might improve lung function in people with asthma. Intake of citrus fruits 1-2 times per week has produced this benefit in some studies (6049,6055,6056). However, other studies have not found this benefit (6057,6058). More evidence is needed to rate kiwi for this use.

Mechanism of Action
The applicable part of kiwi is the fruit. Kiwi fruit contains high concentrations of vitamin C and serotonin (6). The potential benefits of kiwi in asthma might be due to antioxidant properties of vitamin C or other fruit constituents (6049,6054,6055). The constituent, actinidin, is an enzyme with proteolytic activity similar to papain (6). Enzymatic components may be responsible for adverse effects (6).

Adverse Reactions
Orally, eating kiwi fruit or drinking the juice can lead to hypersensitivity reactions of the mouth, including dysphagia, urticaria, and vomiting immediately following ingestion (6).
Topically, use can cause contact urticaria (6). Kiwi may cause hypersensitivity reactions, which are more common in patients who are allergic to latex (6197,7853).

Interactions with Herbs & Other Dietary Supplements
None known.

Interactions with Drugs
None known.

Interactions with Foods
None known.

Interactions with Lab Tests
URINE TESTS: Kiwi may elevate urine levels of 5-hydroxyindoleacetic acid and interfere with lab tests for this serotonin metabolite (6).

Interactions with Diseases or Conditions
LATEX ALLERGY: People who are allergic to latex should avoid eating kiwi or taking products containing kiwi because of the possibility of cross hypersensitivity between kiwi and latex (6197,7853).

Dosage and Administration
No typical dosage.

KNOTWEED

Also Known As
Allseed Nine-Joints, Armstrong, Beggarweed, Bird's Tongue, Birdweed, Centinode, Cow Grass, Crawlgrass, Doorweed, Hogweed, Knot Grass, Knotgrass, Knotweed Herb, Mexican Sanguinaria, Ninety-Knot, Pigrush, Pigweed, Polygoni Avicularis Herba, Red Robin, Sparrow Tongue, Swine's Grass, Swynel Grass, Vogelknoeterichkraut.

Scientific Names
Polygonum aviculare.
Family: Polygonaceae.

People Use This For
Orally, knotweed is used for bronchitis, cough, gingivitis, and inflammation of the mouth and pharynx. It is also used for supportive treatment of pulmonary diseases, skin disorders, to suppress perspiration associated with tuberculosis, as a diuretic, and to stop bleeding.

Safety

POSSIBLY SAFE ...when used orally or topically (2,18,9347).
PREGNANCY AND LACTATION: Insufficient reliable information available; avoid using.

Effectiveness

INSUFFICIENT RELIABLE EVIDENCE to RATE

Gingivitis. Preliminary clinical research suggests a root extract of knotweed might be useful as a mouth rinse to treat gingivitis. It seems to decrease bleeding and inflammation of the gums associated with gingivitis. Some evidence suggests it might also interfere with the aggregation and adherence of plaque to teeth (9347). More evidence is needed to rate knotweed for this use.

Mechanism of Action

The applicable part of knotweed is the whole flowering plant. Knotweed might have astringent, anti-inflammatory, antihemorrhagic, antiglycolytic, and anticholinergic activity (2,18,9347). Knotweed contains flavonoids (avicularin, kaempferol, quercetin, myrecitin) and gallic acid. In addition to the astringent properties of knotweed, the flavonoids it contains might decrease capillary fragility and have a cortisone-like effect on gingival tissues. Its antiglycolytic activity might disrupt the aggregation and adherence of dental plaque to teeth (9347).

Adverse Reactions

None reported.

Interactions with Herbs & Other Dietary Supplements

None known.

Interactions with Drugs

None known.

Interactions with Foods

None known.

Interactions with Lab Tests

None known.

Interactions with Diseases or Conditions

None known.

Dosage and Administration

ORAL: One cup of tea (simmer 1.4 grams dried ground herb in 150 mL of boiling water for 10-15 minutes, strain) is typically taken orally 3 to 5 times daily. A daily oral dose of 4-6 grams dried ground herb has also been used (2,18). For gingivitis, twice daily use of an oral rinse containing sterilized water and root extract of knotweed (1mg/mL) has been used (9347).

KOMBUCHA TEA

Also Known As

Champagne Of Life, Combucha Tea, Dr. Sklenar's Kombucha Mushroom Infusion, Fungus Japonicus, Kargasok Tea, Kombucha Mushroom Tea, Kwassan, Manchurian Fungus, Manchurian Mushroom Tea, Spumonto, T'Chai from the Sea, Tschambucco.

Scientific Names

None.

People Use This For

Orally, kombucha tea is used for memory loss, premenstrual syndrome, rheumatism, aging, anorexia, AIDS, cancer, hypertension, increasing T-cell counts, strengthening the immune system and metabolism, constipation, arthritis, and hair regrowth.
Topically, it is used for analgesia.

Safety

POSSIBLY UNSAFE ...when used orally because non-sterile home preparations have a high risk of contamination (2650,2651,2652,2653).

LIKELY UNSAFE ...when used orally by individuals with compromised immunity, including HIV/AIDS, due to the risk of transmission of opportunistic pathogens (2652,2653), including Aspergillus (2652,2653) and anthrax (Bacillus anthracis) (2651). ...when kombucha tea prepared in a lead-glazed ceramic container is used orally. Lead poisoning was reported in two people who consumed kombucha tea prepared in a lead-glazed ceramic pot for six months (1366).
PREGNANCY AND LACTATION: POSSIBLY UNSAFE ...when used orally; avoid using.

Effectiveness

There is insufficient reliable information available about the effectiveness of kombucha tea.

Mechanism of Action

Kombucha tea can contain up to 1.5% alcohol, vinegar (acetic acid), and a variety of other metabolites (2655). The product contains high levels of B vitamins (2653). No clinically relevant pharmacology has been defined for the kombucha symbiot or its products (6). Caffeine (black tea) and sugar are theorized to account for the increased energy claimed by some tea users (2654). Kombucha tea has the potential to incubate pathogenic organisms, including Aspergillus and anthrax, during its preparation, which is commonly ten days of fermentation at room temperature (2651,2652,2653). Due to the vinegar and ethanol content, it also has the potential to leach lead and other toxic chemicals from the walls of the preparation and storage containers (2650).

Adverse Reactions

Orally, use of kombucha tea can cause stomach problems, yeast infections (2652), allergic reactions, jaundice, nausea, vomiting, head and neck pain (2656), anthrax (2651), and possibly death (2655). Symptomatic lead poisoning requiring chelation decontamination therapy was reported in two people who consumed kombucha tea prepared in a lead-glazed ceramic pot for six months (1366).

Interactions with Herbs & Other Dietary Supplements

None known.

Interactions with Drugs

DISULFIRAM (Antabuse): Theoretically, concomitant use with kombucha tea can cause a disulfiram reaction due to the alcohol contained in the fermented tea (2650).

Interactions with Foods

None known.

Interactions with Lab Tests

LIVER FUNCTION TESTS: There is one report of increased liver function tests after three weeks of consumption of kombucha tea (6).

Interactions with Diseases or Conditions

ALCOHOLISM: Kombucha tea is contraindicated in people with stabilized or therapeutically-controlled alcoholism, because the alcohol content of the tea can aggravate this condition (2650).
COMPROMISED IMMUNITY: Contraindicated because kombucha tea can harbor or culture organisms that cause opportunistic infections (2652,2653).

Dosage and Administration

No typical dosage.

Comments

The kombucha "mushroom" is a yeast or bacteria fungal symbiot and not an actual mushroom. It is derived from the fermentation of yeasts and bacteria with black tea, sugar, and other ingredients (6,2650). The resulting liquid is called kombucha tea. Although advocates of kombucha tea have attributed many therapeutic effects to the drink in the popular press, there is no scientific evidence to support any therapeutic claims (6,2650,2652,2654,2655). An outbreak of anthrax in twenty people in Iran confirmed the tea is a good culture medium for Bacillus anthracis (2651).

KOUSSO

Also Known As

Cossoo, Kooso, Kosso.

Scientific Names

Hagenia abyssinica, synonym Banksia abyssinica; Brayera anthelmintica.
Family: Rosaceae.

People Use This For
Orally, kousso is used orally for tapeworm infestations.

Safety
LIKELY UNSAFE ...when used orally (18).
PREGNANCY: UNSAFE ...when used orally due to abortifacient activity (19).
LACTATION: UNSAFE ...when used orally due to its potential for toxicity (18).

Effectiveness
There is insufficient reliable information available about the effectiveness of kousso.

Mechanism of Action
There is insufficient reliable information available about the possible mechanism of action or active ingredients.

Adverse Reactions
Orally, kousso can cause gastrointestinal irritation with accompanying salivation, headache, and general weakness. With overdose, people experience syncope and vision disorders. It can also cause colic, spasms, acidosis, and shock (18).

Interactions with Herbs & Other Dietary Supplements
None known.

Interactions with Drugs
None known.

Interactions with Foods
None known.

Interactions with Lab Tests
None known.

Interactions with Diseases or Conditions
GASTROINTESTINAL (GI) CONDITIONS: Kousso can irritate the GI tract. Contraindicated in individuals with infectious or inflammatory GI conditions (19).

Dosage and Administration
No typical dosage.

KUDZU

Also Known As
Daidzein, Fen Ke, Fenge, Gange, Ge Gen, Gegen, Isoflavone, Isoflavones, Japanese Arrowroot, Kudsu, Kudzu Vine, Kwaao Khruea, Mealy Kudzu, Pueraria, Pueraria Root, Radix Puerariae, Yege.

Scientific Names
Pueraria montana var. lobata, synonyms Pueraria lobata, Pueraria thunbergiana, Pueraria pseudohirsuta, Dolichos lobatus, Dolichos hirsutus, Neustanthus chinensis, Pachyrhizus thunbergianus, Pueraria hirsuta, Pueraria lobata var. chinensis; Pueraria montana var. thomsonii, synonym Pueraria thomsonii; Pueraria candollei, synonym Pueraria mirifica; Pueraria tuberosa, synonym Hedysarum tuberosum.
Family: Fabaceae/Leguminosae.

People Use This For
Orally, kudzu is used alone or in combination with other products for symptoms of alcohol hangover, such as headache, upset stomach, dizziness, and vomiting, and for managing alcoholism and drunkenness. Kudzu is also used orally for menopause, myalgia, measles, dysentery, gastritis, fever, diarrhea, thirst, cold, flu, neck stiffness, and as a diaphoretic. Other oral uses include for hypertension, angina pectoris, arrhythmia, migraine, deafness, diabetes, traumatic injuries, sinusitis, urticaria, pruritus, and psoriasis.
Kudzu root is consumed as food.

Safety

POSSIBLY SAFE ...when used orally and appropriately. Kudzu appears to be safe for up to 4 months (10386,11386). The long-term safety of kudzu is unknown.
PREGNANCY AND LACTATION: Insufficient reliable information available; avoid using.

Effectiveness

INSUFFICIENT RELIABLE EVIDENCE to RATE

Alcoholism. Preliminary clinical research suggests kudzu does not reduce craving for alcohol or improve sobriety in chronic alcoholics (10386).

Menopausal symptoms. Preliminary clinical research suggests kudzu taken orally does not affect menopausal changes. It doesn't significantly change lipid profiles, sex hormone levels, menopausal symptoms, or bone turnover markers. Kudzu may, however, have a positive effect on cognitive function in postmenopausal women (11386).

More evidence is needed to rate kudzu for these uses.

Mechanism of Action

The applicable parts of kudzu are the root and flower. Kudzu contains isoflavone constituents including daidzin, daidzein, and puerarin (11711). Kudzu extract, daidzein, and daidzin decrease alcohol consumption and peak blood alcohol levels, and shorten alcohol-induced sleep in alcohol-craving animals. Decreased peak blood alcohol levels might be due to delayed gastric emptying (1523,1524).

Preliminary research suggests that the isoflavone constituents have both estrogenic and antiestrogenic activity, similar to selective estrogen receptor modulators (11386).

There is also some evidence that suggests puerarin might decrease heart rate, plasma renin activity, capillary permeability, and platelet aggregation (11). Puerarin might have hypoglycemic, hypocholesterolemic, antiarrhythmic, antipyretic, and antioxidant activity (11). Kudzu root extracts dilate coronary and cerebral blood vessels; increase myocardial and cerebral blood flow; decrease vascular resistance, myocardial oxygen demand, and lactic acid production in anaerobic myocardial tissues; and increase the blood oxygen supply (11).

Adverse Reactions

None reported.

Interactions with Herbs & Other Dietary Supplements

HERBS WITH ESTROGENIC ACTIVITY: Theoretically, kudzu might have additive or antagonistic effects with other herbs that have estrogenic activity (11386). These herbs include alfalfa, black cohosh, chasteberry, flaxseed, hops, ipriflavone, licorice, red clover, and soy.

Interactions with Drugs

ANTICOAGULANT/ANTIPLATELET DRUGS: Theoretically, kudzu might potentiate the effects of anticoagulants. A constituent of kudzu inhibits platelet activating factor (11).
ANTIDIABETES DRUGS: Theoretically, concomitant use might have additive hypoglycemic effects. A constituent of kudzu has hypoglycemic activity in animals (11).
ASPIRIN: Theoretically, concomitant use might increase the potential for hypoglycemic effects of kudzu. Aspirin increases the hypoglycemic effects of a kudzu constituent in diabetic mice (11).
CONTRACEPTIVE DRUGS: Theoretically, kudzu might competitively inhibit the effects of oral contraceptives (11386).
ESTROGENS: Theoretically, kudzu might competitively inhibit the effects of estrogen therapy (11386).
TAMOXIFEN (Nolvadex): Theoretically, kudzu might interfere with tamoxifen because of its potential estrogenic effects. Tell patients taking tamoxifen to avoid kudzu (11386).

Interactions with Foods

None known.

Interactions with Lab Tests

BLOOD GLUCOSE: Theoretically, kudzu might decrease blood glucose levels and test results. A constituent of kudzu has hypoglycemic activity in animals (11).
SERUM CHOLESTEROL: Theoretically, kudzu might decrease serum cholesterol levels and test results. A constituent of kudzu reduces serum cholesterol levels in animals (11).

Interactions with Diseases or Conditions

CARDIOVASCULAR CONDITIONS: Theoretically, kudzu might interfere with cardiovascular treatments. Kudzu extracts decrease heart rate and have vasodilatory and antiarrhythmic effects in animals (11).
CLOTTING DISORDERS: Theoretically, kudzu might interfere with anticoagulant therapies. A constituent of kudzu inhibits platelet activating factor (11).

DIABETES: Theoretically, kudzu might interfere with blood glucose control requiring dosing adjustment of diabetes drug therapy. A constituent of kudzu has hypoglycemic activity in animals (11).
HORMONE SENSITIVE CANCERS/CONDITIONS: Kudzu might have estrogenic effects (11386). Women with hormone sensitive conditions should avoid kudzu. Some of these conditions include breast cancer, uterine cancer, ovarian cancer, endometriosis, and uterine fibroids.

Dosage and Administration

ORAL: For treatment of chronic alcoholism, kudzu root extract 1.2 grams 2 times daily has been used for 4 months (10386). For hormone replacement therapy (HRT), kudzu powder (containing 100 mg isoflavones) dissolved in water once daily has been used for 3 months (11386).

L-ARGININE

Also Known As

Arg, Arginine, Arginine HCl, Arginine Hydrochloride, L Arginine, L-Arginine HCl, L-Arginine-HCl, L-Arginine Hydrochloride.

Scientific Names

2-Amino-5-guanidinopentanoic acid.

People Use This For

Orally, L-arginine is used for cardiovascular conditions including congestive heart failure (CHF), angina pectoris, hypertension, and coronary artery disease. L-arginine is also used for intermittent claudication, senile dementia, erectile dysfunction, and male infertility. Furthermore, L-arginine is used for prevention of the common cold, interstitial cystitis, cyclosporine nephrotoxicity, pre-eclampsia, improving athletic performance, improving immune function, and preventing necrotizing enterocolitis in premature infants

In combination with ibuprofen, L-arginine is used orally for migraine headaches, and as an adjunct to chemotherapy in breast cancer. In combination with hydroxymethylbutyrate (HMB) and glutamine, L-arginine is used orally for treating weight loss in people with AIDS. In the perioperative period, to reduce infections, improve wound healing, and shorten recovery time, L-arginine is used orally in combination with RNA and EPA.

Topically, L-arginine is used as an aid in wound healing, for treating cold hands and feet, and for male and female sexual dysfunction.

Intravenously, L-arginine is used for intermittent claudication, for detecting growth hormone deficiency, nutritional supplementation for the critically ill, metabolic acidosis, and persistent pulmonary hypertension in newborns.

Safety

LIKELY SAFE ...when used orally and appropriately. L-arginine is generally considered safe and has only been associated with minor side effects in clinical studies lasting a few days to six months (114,3330,3331,3460,3593,3595,3596,5531,5532,5533,6028,7813,7815,7816,7819,7822,8014,8473). ...when used intravenously and appropriately. Parenteral L-arginine is an FDA-approved prescription product (15).

There is insufficient reliable information available about the safety of the topical use of L-arginine.

CHILDREN: POSSIBLY SAFE ...when used orally in premature infants (8474).

PREGNANCY: POSSIBLY SAFE ...when used orally and appropriately, short-term. L-arginine 12 grams per day for 2 days has been used with apparent safety in women with gestational length of 28 to 36 weeks (11828). There is insufficient reliable information available about the safety of L-arginine for longer-term use in pregnant women.

LACTATION: Insufficient reliable information available; avoid using.

Effectiveness

POSSIBLY EFFECTIVE

AIDS-related wasting. Taking L-arginine orally, in combination with hydroxymethylbutyrate (HMB) and glutamine, seems to increase body weight, particularly lean body mass, and positively affect immune status when used for 8 weeks in patients with HIV/AIDS (1909).

Angina. Taking L-arginine orally seems to decrease symptoms and improve exercise tolerance and quality of life in patients with class II, III, and IV angina (3593,7815,7816). Some patients with class IV angina who have frequent attacks at rest despite treatment with standard antianginal agents might also benefit from L-arginine (3593). However, L-arginine does not seem to improve objective measures of blood vessel dilation or increase circulating concentrations of nitric oxide (7817).

Congestive heart failure (CHF). Taking L-arginine orally, in combination with conventional treatment, seems to improve glomerular filtration rate (GFR), creatinine clearance, and sodium and water elimination after saline loading (3596). However, improvements in exercise tolerance, quality of life, and peripheral vascular resistance are not consistently obtained (3595,6028,7813,8014). Tell patients that L-arginine should not be substituted for conventional treatment.

Erectile dysfunction (ED). Taking L-arginine orally in high doses, 5 grams daily, might improve subjective assessment of sexual function in men with organic ED caused by decreased nitric oxide excretion production (222). But taking lower doses, 500 mg L-arginine 3 times daily, in men with mixed-type impotence doesn't seem to be beneficial (2038). Some preliminary clinical evidence suggests that adding pycnogenol might improve the effectiveness of L-arginine for ED (10416).

Interstitial cystitis. Taking L-arginine orally seems to reduce symptoms, especially pain associated with interstitial cystitis (107,114,3460). Evidence suggests that patients with interstitial cystitis having a bladder capacity greater than 800 mL and/or a history of recurrent genitourinary infections might respond more favorably to L-arginine than patients with bladder capacity less than 800 mL and/or no history of recurrent genitourinary infections. Three months of treatment may be necessary before significant improvement occurs (3460).

Migraine headache. Taking L-arginine orally, in combination with ibuprofen, seems to be effective for treating migraine headache (109).

Necrotizing enterocolitis (NEC). Taking L-arginine orally seems to be effective for preventing NEC in premature infants. L-arginine supplements added to formula may reduce the incidence of NEC by about 75% (8474).

Nitrate tolerance. Taking L-arginine orally 700 mg four times daily seems to prevent tolerance to transdermal nitrate, and theoretically to other nitrates, in patients with angina (8475).

Peripheral arterial disease. Using L-arginine intravenously or orally seems to improve symptoms of intermittent claudication associated with peripheral arterial disease (3465,7822).

Post-surgery recovery. Taking L-arginine enterally or orally, with RNA and eicosapentaenoic acid (EPA), seems to help reduce the recovery time after surgery or serious illness. Supplementing the diet of patients after surgery with RNA, L-arginine, and EPA appears to reduce the number of perioperative infections, improve wound healing, and shorten recovery time. Dietary supplementation may take place before surgery or in the postoperative period (5531,5532,5533,7819).

Renal transplant. Taking L-arginine orally seems to improve renal vasodilation and sodium excretion in renal transplant patients treated with cyclosporine (112).

POSSIBLY INEFFECTIVE

Pre-eclampsia. Taking L-arginine orally doesn't seem to lower diastolic blood pressure in women with pre-eclampsia at a gestational length of 28 to 36 weeks (11828).

LIKELY INEFFECTIVE

Coronary heart disease. Population studies indicate that intake of L-arginine does not reduce acute coronary events such as myocardial infarction or coronary heart disease-related mortality (3332,6896,7821,7822,10637).

INSUFFICIENT RELIABLE EVIDENCE to RATE

Dementia. Preliminary research suggests that L-arginine might improve senile dementia (8473).

Head and neck cancer. There is some interest in using L-arginine to enhance immune function in patients undergoing surgery for head and neck cancer. However, enteral nutrition supplemented with L-arginine does not seem to have any beneficial effects on markers of immune function such as interleukin-6 (IL-6) and tumor necrosis factor-alpha (TNF-alpha) (10160).

Hypertension. There is some preliminary evidence that oral administration of L-arginine can slightly reduce systolic and diastolic blood pressure in healthy people and mildly hypertensive patients with type 2 diabetes (7818,10636). It may also improve the effect of angiotensin converting enzyme (ACE) inhibitors in treating hypertension (7822).

Sickle cell disease. Preliminary research suggests that L-arginine, 0.1 grams per kg three times daily for five days, might be useful for patients with pulmonary hypertension in sickle cell disease (11428).

More evidence is needed to rate L-arginine for these uses.

Mechanism of Action

L-arginine is an amino acid necessary for protein synthesis. It is found naturally in foods such as red meat, poultry, fish, and dairy products (3330). L-arginine is best known for its effects on the vascular system. L-arginine is a substrate for the nitric oxide synthase (NOS) enzyme. NOS in vascular endothelial cells converts L-arginine to nitric oxide (NO), also known as endothelium-derived relaxation factor (EDRF), which causes vasodilation. L-arginine can improve coronary endothelial function and brachial artery endothelium-dependent dilation and reduce monocyte/endothelial cell adhesion in patients with coronary artery disease (CAD) or hypercholesterolemia, resulting in increased coronary blood flow (110,116,1362,1363,3330). The production of NO from L-arginine may be responsible for mildly reducing blood pressure (10636). Some evidence is available indicating the effect on coronary blood flow is larger in African-Americans than in Caucasians (8472). L-arginine seems to prevent nitrate tolerance by improving nitric acid bioavailability and may act as an antioxidant, decreasing production of vascular superoxide (8475). Intravenous L-arginine can have many beneficial hemodynamic effects in heart failure, including decreased heart rate (8 beats/minute), decreased mean arterial pressure (14 mmHg), increased cardiac output (0.7 l/minute), and increased stroke volume (14 mL) (8444). The production of NO from L-arginine substrate is impaired in patients with severe congestive heart failure (CHF) (8016). The beneficial effect of L-arginine on NO may help patients with pulmonary hypertension secondary to sickle cell disease. During times of sickle cell crisis, NO, a potent vasodilator, is deficient, and pulmonary hypertension may occur. L-arginine donates nitrogen for NO synthesis. L-arginine also decreases levels of circulating plasma endothelin-1, a potent vasoconstrictor (11428). In most people with a normal diet, the concentration of L-arginine inside the cells of the body is adequate to ensure that the NOS enzyme is producing NO at maximal capacity. As a result, L-arginine supplementation is likely to be more effective in patients who have a deficiency of L-arginine (7820,7822).

Besides its effect on the systemic cardiovascular system, NO also increases the relaxation of urinary tract smooth muscle (3259,3460) and is involved in erectile function. Although L-arginine appears to be helpful for erectile dysfunction, L-arginine may not affect the hemodynamics of the corpus cavernosum (222).

Nitric oxide might also be involved in host inflammatory and microbial killing responses (3460). L-arginine is a precursor for collagen synthesis and together with fibroblast NO production might be important for wound healing (3259,3260).

L-arginine has actions on the cardiovascular system and other systems that are independent of the conversion to NO. Among other actions, L-arginine can directly reduce blood viscosity, reduce the activity of angiotensin converting enzyme, and reduce lipid peroxidation. Other physiologic actions include stimulating the release of growth hormone (GH), prolactin, glucagon, and insulin (7820). L-arginine also increases gastrin concentrations and inhibits tubular reabsorption of protein (3331,3460,8015).

There is interest in L-arginine for adjunctive use in treating breast cancer. There is some evidence that L-arginine modifies immune system function and might potentiate tumor cell response to anti-cancer drugs and possibly reduce the immunosuppressive effects of chemotherapy agents. L-arginine seems to increase lymphocyte reactivity to polyclonal mitogenic agents and might also enhance natural cytotoxicity (3331). However, L-arginine also promotes the growth of tumors by providing a source of nitrogen. In some situations the nutritional value of L-arginine may outweigh its antitumor effects (7814).

L-arginine has an oral bioavailability of 68% and an elimination half-life of approximately 80 minutes (108).

Adverse Reactions

Orally, L-arginine can cause abdominal pain and bloating, diarrhea, and gout (3331,3595). It can also cause allergic response or airway inflammation and exacerbation of airway inflammation in asthma (117,121).

Intravenous administration can cause allergic reactions including urticaria, periorbital edema, and pruritus (11830). Excessively rapid infusion of L-arginine has caused flushing, nausea and vomiting, local venous irritation, numbness, and headache. Extravasation has caused necrosis and superficial phlebitis (3330).

Interactions with Herbs & Other Dietary Supplements

XYLITOL: Concomitant use can reduce the glucagon response to L-arginine (15).

Interactions with Drugs

ANTIHYPERTENSIVE DRUGS: Theoretically, concomitant use might cause additive hypotensive effects; use with caution (7822,10636).

NITRATES: Theoretically, concomitant use might cause additive vasodilation and have a hypotensive effect; use with caution (7822,10636).

SILDENAFIL (Viagra): Theoretically, concurrent use of sildenafil and L-arginine might result in additive vasodilation and cause hypotension (7822,10636). However, this interaction has not been reported. Until more is known, use with caution or avoid using in combination.

Interactions with Foods

None known.

Interactions with Lab Tests

None known.

Interactions with Diseases or Conditions

ALLERGIC TENDENCIES/ASTHMA: L-arginine can cause an allergic response or aggravate airway inflammation (117), and inhaled L-arginine can amplify the inflammatory airway response in people with asthma (121); use with caution.

CIRRHOSIS OF THE LIVER: L-arginine-containing infusions can lead to a hyperdynamic circulatory state related to an elevation of the plasma level of nitrous oxide by L-arginine (122); use with caution.

HERPES VIRUS: Theoretically, L-arginine might exacerbate this condition. Preliminary evidence suggests that L-arginine may be necessary for viral replication (118,119).

HYPOTENSION: Theoretically, L-arginine might exacerbate hypotension (7822,10636).

Dosage and Administration

ORAL: For congestive heart failure, doses ranging from 6-20 grams per day, often as three divided doses, have been used in clinical studies (3595,3596,6028). For angina pectoris associated with coronary artery disease, 3-6 grams three times per day has been used for up to one month (110,3593,7816,7817). For preventing nitrate tolerance in angina patients, 700 mg four times daily has been used (8475). For hypertension, hyperlipidemia, and congestive heart failure, L-arginine 6 grams daily has been given in combination with protein, vitamin C, vitamin E, folic acid, and other vitamins and minerals (7815,7822). In patients with diabetes, to reduce low density lipoprotein (LDL) cholesterol,

7 grams 2 times a day for six weeks has been used (7821). For interstitial cystitis, 500 mg-1.5 grams per day has been used (114,3330,3460). For organic erectile dysfunction, 5 grams per day has been used (222). For senile dementia, 1.6 grams daily for three months has been used (8473). For stimulation of host defenses in breast cancer patients undergoing chemotherapy, an oral dose of 10 grams three times per day for three days has been used (3331). For preventing necrotizing enterocolitis in premature infants, 261 mg/kg has been added to oral feedings daily for the first 28 days of life (8474).
INTRAVENOUS: For intermittent claudication associated with peripheral arterial occlusive disease, 8 grams two times a day for three weeks has been used (3465).

Comments

Arginine butyrate has orphan drug status for beta-hemoglobinopathy, beta-thalassemia, and sickle cell disease (1691).

L-CARNITINE

Also Known As

B(t) Factor, Carnitine, Carnitor, D-Carnitine, DL-Carnitine, Levocarnitine, Vitacarn, Vitamin B(t).
CAUTION: See separate listings for Acetyl-L-Carnitine and Propionyl-L-Carnitine.

Scientific Names

3-carboxy-2-hydroxy-N,N,N-trimethyl-1-propanaminium inner salt; (3-carboxy2-hydroxypropyl) trimethylammonium hydroxide inner salt; B-hydroxy-N-trimethyl aminobutyric acid; beta-hydroxy-gamma-trimethylammonium butyrate; L-3-hydroxy-4-(trimethylammonium)-butyrate; (R)-(3-carboxy-2-hydroxypropyl) trimethylammonium hydroxide; (R)-3-hydroxy-4-trimethylammonio-butyrate; 3-hydroxy-4-N-trimethylaminobutyrate.

People Use This For

Orally, L-carnitine is used for treating primary L-carnitine deficiency, secondary L-carnitine deficiency due to inborn errors of metabolism, and L-carnitine deficiency in people requiring hemodialysis. It is also used orally for treating drug-induced L-carnitine deficiency and for treating valproate-induced toxicity. L-carnitine is also used orally for myopathies associated with zidovudine and isotretinoin, myocarditis associated with diphtheria, male infertility, Rett Syndrome, chronic stable angina pectoris, congestive heart failure (CHF), and myocardial infarction. It is also used orally as a supplement in low birthweight and preterm infants, in strict vegetarians or vegans, and in dieters.
L-carnitine is also used for anorexia, chronic fatigue syndrome, diabetes, hyperlipidemia, hyperthyroidism, attention deficit-hyperactivity disorder (ADHD), peripheral vascular disease and intermittent claudication, leg ulcers, and to enhance athletic performance and endurance.
Intravenously, L-carnitine is used to treat secondary L-carnitine deficiencies in people with inborn errors of metabolism who require hemodialysis; and to treat severe valproic acid-induced hepatotoxicity, especially in patients treated for overdose or accidental ingestion of valproic acid. It is also used intravenously for increasing CD4 cell counts in people with HIV/AIDS, acute myocardial infarction, and as a supplement in people receiving total parenteral nutrition.

Safety

LIKELY SAFE ...when used orally and appropriately (8047). ...when used parenterally as an FDA-approved prescription medicine. Avoid using D-carnitine and DL-carnitine, because they can act as competitive inhibitors of L-carnitine and cause symptoms of L-carnitine deficiency (1946).
PREGNANCY: Insufficient reliable information available; avoid using.
LACTATION: POSSIBLY SAFE ...when used orally. Supplemental doses of L-carnitine have been given to infants in breast milk and formula with no reported adverse effects. The effects of large doses used while nursing are unknown, but L-carnitine is secreted in the breast milk (9,3616).

Effectiveness

EFFECTIVE

End-stage renal disease (ESRD). Administering L-carnitine orally or intravenously can improve red blood cell count and hemoglobin during hemodialysis. However, it does not improve serum lipids or cholesterol (9790). Use of intravenous L-carnitine for prevention and treatment of L-carnitine deficiency in people with ESRD who are undergoing hemodialysis is an FDA-approved indication for L-carnitine.

L-carnitine deficiency. Administering L-carnitine orally or intravenously is effective for acute or chronic treatment of primary L-carnitine deficiency or secondary L-carnitine deficiency due to inborn errors of metabolism. This is an FDA-approved indication for L-carnitine (4949).

POSSIBLY EFFECTIVE

Angina. Taking L-carnitine orally seems to improve exercise tolerance in people with chronic stable angina (3623,3624).

Congestive heart failure (CHF). Taking L-carnitine orally seems to improve symptoms in people with congestive heart failure (3625,3626).

Hyperthyroidism. Taking 2-4 grams per day of L-carnitine seems to significantly improve symptoms associated with hyperthyroidism such as palpitations, nervousness, and asthenia. It also seems to reduce elevated serum levels of alanine aminotransferase (ALT), aspartate aminotransferase (AST), gamma-glutamyl transpeptidase (GGT), and ferritin elicited by thyroid hormone (8047).

Infertility. Taking L-carnitine orally, in combination with acetyl-L-carnitine for 6 months seems to increase sperm motility in men with infertility (12352). Taking L-carnitine orally, in combination with acetyl-L-carnitine and nonsteroidal anti-inflammatory drugs, seems to increase sperm count and motility in men with infertility caused by abacterial prostatovesiculoepididymitis; an inflammation of the prostate gland, seminal vesicles, and epididymis. L-carnitine supplementation should follow 2 months of treatment with nonsteroidal anti-inflammatory drugs (9791).

Low birth weight. Administering L-carnitine orally or intravenously seems to improve fat utilization in preterm infants on total parenteral nutrition (3633,3634,3635,3636,3637).

Myocardial infarction (MI). Taking L-carnitine orally after MI seems to reduce complications and mortality (3627,3628,3629).

Myocarditis. Taking L-carnitine orally seems to reduce the morbidity and mortality of myocarditis associated with diphtheria (3620,3621).

Valproic acid-induced toxicities. There is evidence that patients taking valproic acid orally or intravenously, who have neurologic or hepatic deterioration or hyperammonemia, seem to have improved neurologic and hepatic function and plasma ammonia levels within normal limits when L-carnitine is supplemented (1438,1914,1915,1916,1917,4523,5798,5799). Valproic acid toxicities are often associated with L-carnitine deficiency. There is also some evidence that intravenous L-carnitine can prevent the development of severe valproic acid-induced hepatotoxicity when given to patients being treated for overdose and accidental ingestion of valproic acid (1438,4528,5798,5799), especially if treatment is initiated early (4528).

LIKELY INEFFECTIVE

Athletic performance. Taking L-carnitine orally doesn't enhance athletic performance or endurance (1947,3639). Maximal exercise in trained athletes has been associated with a fall in plasma L-carnitine levels (3648). Although increases in maximum oxygen uptake and power output have been reported with L-carnitine supplements in some studies (3649,3650), there is no evidence that L-carnitine supplementation will improve exercise performance in individuals including trained athletes (1947,3639).

INSUFFICIENT RELIABLE EVIDENCE to RATE

Attention deficit-hyperactivity disorder (ADHD). Preliminary clinical research suggests L-carnitine might reduce ADHD symptoms (9956).

Peripheral vascular disease. Preliminary evidence suggests that L-carnitine may improve walking distances in people with peripheral vascular disease (3631).

Rett syndrome. Preliminary clinical research suggests that L-carnitine might improve well-being and motor skills in girls with Rett syndrome (1433,3622).

More evidence is needed to rate L-carnitine for these uses.

Mechanism of Action

L-carnitine is naturally found in the body. About 25% of L-carnitine is synthesized in the liver, kidneys, and brain from the amino acids lysine and methionine. The remaining 75% is obtained from the diet. L-carnitine is found in the diet in meat and dairy products. Most L-carnitine in the body is found in cardiac and skeletal muscle. The highest concentration of L-carnitine is in the epididymal fluid (12352).

L-carnitine plays a key role in cellular energy production. It is essential for beta-oxidation of long-chain fatty acids in the mitochondria. To enter the mitochondria, fatty acids must bind to coenzyme A, forming acyl-CoA. Long-chain acyl-CoA molecules are too large to cross the internal mitochondrial membrane and rely on enzymatic transportation that requires L-carnitine. In the mitochondria, fatty acids undergo beta-oxidation to adenosine triphosphate (ATP) and L-acetyl-carnitine is excreted to begin a new transport cycle (12352).

L-carnitine may also have antioxidant properties (12352).

Primary tissue deficiency of L-carnitine can arise from hepatic synthesis failure, membrane transport failure, or disorders of reabsorption by the kidney. It is characterized by low concentrations of L-carnitine in plasma, red blood cells and tissues (3616). L-carnitine deficiency can also occur due to other disorders, such as inborn errors of metabolism, cirrhosis, and hypopituitarism.

Muscle L-carnitine deficiency has been reported in children with Duchenne muscular dystrophy (3640), and in people with myopathies due to zidovudine (3618) or isotretinoin (3619). Increased urinary losses of L-carnitine have been reported with ifosfamide and cisplatin therapy (3641,3642). Low serum L-carnitine levels can occur in patients taking valproic acid therapy (1910,1911,1912,1913,4526,4528), in pregnant women (3643), in people with chronic fatigue syndrome (3630), HIV-AIDS (3617), and in patients with hyperthyroidism (8047). However, the relationship between serum and tissue L-carnitine levels is not fully understood, and it is not known whether or not low serum levels necessarily lead to symptomatic deficiency (4528,4529,5798).

Symptomatic deficiency is unlikely to arise from insufficient dietary intake since the body is usually able to synthesize adequate quantities. However, preterm neonates have a reduced capacity to synthesize L-carnitine and they may become deficient, especially if receiving total parenteral nutrition without L-carnitine supplements (3633). Breast milk and some formulas contain L-carnitine; those that do not, generally do not induce symptomatic deficiencies in healthy full-term infants unless a metabolic disorder is also present, although utilization of fats may be impaired (3644).

Hemodialysis is associated with significant losses of L-carnitine (3616,3645); which may contribute to malaise, muscle weakness, cardiomyopathy, and cardiac arrhythmias (3616). L-carnitine supplements, usually given intravenously after dialysis may improve exercise performance, reduce muscle cramps and hypotension, improve erythrocyte survival time, and decrease dose requirements for erythropoietin used to treat anemia (3645,3646,3647).

In people with angina, a reduction in tissue L-carnitine levels has been observed during myocardial ischemia. L-carnitine can be decreased by as much as 50% in failing myocardium (8048). Preliminary studies have reported that daily infusions of L-carnitine may improve CD4 cell counts in people with HIV infection and reduce the percentage of CD4 and CD8 cells undergoing apoptosis. There is some evidence L-carnitine inhibits the enzyme activity of acidic sphingomyelinase and prevents sphingomyelin breakdown in these cells (798,3632,8049).

Preliminary studies also suggest that intravenous infusions of L-carnitine may produce short-term improvements in insulin sensitivity in people with type 2 diabetes (3651,3652).

In hyperthyroidism, L-carnitine seems to reduce symptoms by blocking entry of thyroid hormone into the nucleus of hepatocytes, neurons, and fibroblasts (8047).

L-carnitine and acetyl-L-carnitine are present in human sperm and seminal fluid (3607). Their levels increase in sperm during the maturation process in the epididymis and coincide with the acquisition of progressive motility (3608,3609). An increase in sperm motility is seen in vitro when L-carnitine or acetyl-L-carnitine is added to the semen sample (3612).

Adverse Reactions

L-carnitine used orally or intravenously has been associated with nausea, vomiting, abdominal cramps, heartburn, gastritis, diarrhea, body odor, and seizures (3616).

DL-carnitine, but not L-carnitine, has been associated with myasthenia syndrome with severe weakness, muscle wasting, and discolored urine possibly due to myoglobinuria. This may be due to competitive inhibition of L-carnitine by D-carnitine, leading to symptoms of L-carnitine deficiency (1946).

Interactions with Herbs & Other Dietary Supplements

D-CARNITINE: Taking D-carnitine may cause symptoms of L-carnitine deficiency (1946); avoid using.

Interactions with Drugs

ACENOCOUMAROL (Sintrom): Taking L-carnitine 1 gram/day seems to significantly increase the anticoagulant effects of acenocoumarol. This drug is an oral anticoagulant similar to warfarin, but shorter-acting (9878,12165). In one case, INR was stable in the normal range of 1.99-2.94 and then increased to 4.65 after L-carnitine was started and continued for 10 weeks. INR normalized after discontinuation of L-carnitine (12165).

WARFARIN (Coumadin): Taking L-carnitine 1 gram/day seems to potentiate an anticoagulant drug similar to warfarin called acenocoumarol. This drug is an anticoagulant that is shorter acting than warfarin (9878,12165). There isn't enough information to know whether this interaction is significant for warfarin.

Drug Influences on Nutrient Levels and Depletion

SOME DRUGS CAN AFFECT L-CARNITINE LEVELS:

VALPROIC ACID (VPA, valproate, Depakene, Depakote): Valproic acid can induce L-carnitine deficiency by altering carnitine metabolism and synthesis (4528,4529,5798). However, carnitine blood levels seem to be more dependent on nutritional status than valproic acid concentration. L-carnitine supplementation is not necessary for patients who have adequate nutritional intake (9612).

ZIDOVUDINE (AZT, azidothymidine, Retrovir): Zidovudine appears to inhibit cellular transport of L-carnitine (9885). Low serum carnitine levels are found in some people with HIV infection (3617). Consider zidovudine supplementation as the clinical situation warrants.

Interactions with Foods

None known.

Interactions with Lab Tests

CD4/CD8 COUNTS: L-carnitine infusions can increase CD4 and CD8 lymphocyte counts in some individuals with HIV-1 infection who have not been treated with antiretroviral therapy (798,8049).

HIGH-DENSITY LIPOPROTEIN (HDL) CHOLESTEROL: Intravenous L-carnitine supplementation can increase serum HDL cholesterol concentrations and test results in children on hemodialysis with type IV hyperlipoproteinemia (275).

TRIGLYCERIDES: Intravenous L-carnitine supplementation can decrease serum triglyceride concentrations and test results in children on hemodialysis with type IV hyperlipoproteinemia (275).

Interactions with Diseases or Conditions

CHRONIC LIVER DISEASE: Avoid due to impaired L-carnitine metabolism or increased L-carnitine biosynthesis, and potential for intrinsically high L-carnitine levels (1931,1948).
HEMODIALYSIS/ANURIA/UREMIA: Avoid DL-carnitine; it is reported to cause myasthenia-like symptoms when administered by IV after dialysis (L-carnitine has not been reported to have this effect) (1946).
SEIZURES: An increase in seizure frequency or severity has been reported in people with a history of seizures who have used L-carnitine orally or intravenously (3616).

Dosage and Administration

ORAL: For primary or secondary L-carnitine deficiencies in adults, 990 mg two to three times per day in tablets or as an oral solution is used (3616). For valproate-induced toxicities often associated with L-carnitine deficiency, 50 to 100 mg/kg/day in three or four divided doses, to a maximum of 3 grams/day is used (3616,4528,5798). For chronic stable angina and congestive heart failure (CHF), 1 gram twice daily has been used (3623,3624,3625,3626). Following myocardial infarction, 2 to 6 grams daily have been used (3627,3628,3629). For peripheral vascular disease, a dose of 2 grams of L-carnitine twice daily has been used (3631). People on hemodialysis have used 2 to 4 grams per day in divided doses (1933). For Rett syndrome, 100 mg/kg/day L-carnitine in three divided doses has been used (1433). For myocarditis associated with diphtheria, DL-carnitine 100 mg/kg/day for 4 days has been used (3620,3621). For hyperthyroidism, 1-2 grams twice daily has been used (8047). For male infertility, 2 grams of L-carnitine plus 1 gram of L-acetyl-carnitine daily has been used (12352). For male infertility secondary to abacterial prostatovesiculoepididymitis, carnitine 1 gram plus acetyl-L-carnitine 500 mg every 12 hours has been used following 2 months of treatment with nonsteroidal anti-inflammatory drugs (9791).
INTRAVENOUS: For inborn error of metabolism resulting in secondary L-carnitine deficiency, 50 mg/kg given as a slow (2 to 3 minute) bolus injection or by infusion followed by 50 mg/kg administered in divided doses every 3 to 4 hours over the next 24 hours is used. Subsequent daily maintenance doses are usually in the range of 50 mg/kg (3616). For people with L-carnitine deficiency secondary to hemodialysis, 10 to 20 mg/kg adjusted according to plasma L-carnitine levels is used (3616). For treating and preventing valproic acid-induced hepatotoxicity in patients being treated for accidental ingestion or overdose of valproic acid, 150-500 mg/kg/day up to 3 grams/day is used (4528,5798). A dose of 10 mg/kg has been used to improve fat utilization in premature infants on total parenteral nutrition (3637).

L-TRYPTOPHAN

Also Known As

L-trypt, Tryptophan.
CAUTION: See separate listing for 5-HTP.

Scientific Names

L-2-amino-3-(indole-3-yl) propionic acid.

People Use This For

Orally, L-tryptophan is used for insomnia, depression, myofascial pain, premenstrual syndrome (PMS), smoking cessation, bruxism, grinding teeth during sleep, attention deficit-hyperactivity disorder (ADHD), Tourette's syndrome, and to improve athletic performance.

Safety

UNSAFE ...when used orally due to the risk of eosinophilia-myalgia syndrome (EMS) and death (7067,8053,10085,11474,11478). In 1990, L-tryptophan was removed from the market due to these safety concerns (7067).
PREGNANCY: UNSAFE ...when used orally because it can cause respiratory depression in utero (1142); avoid using.
LACTATION: Insufficient reliable information available; avoid using.

Effectiveness

POSSIBLY EFFECTIVE

Premenstrual dysphoric disorder (PMDD). Taking L-tryptophan orally 6 grams per day seems to decrease mood swings, tension, and irritability in women with PMDD (6246).
Smoking cessation. Taking L-tryptophan orally seems to help as adjunct treatment for smoking cessation (1138).

POSSIBLY INEFFECTIVE

Athletic performance. Taking L-tryptophan orally doesn't seem to improve athletic performance (1135).
Bruxism. Taking L-tryptophan orally doesn't seem help treat bruxism (1139).
Myofascial pain. Taking L-tryptophan orally doesn't seem to reduce myofascial pain (1140,1145).

INSUFFICIENT RELIABLE EVIDENCE to RATE

Attention deficit-hyperactivity disorder (ADHD). Preliminary clinical research suggests L-tryptophan levels

are lower in children with ADHD, but oral L-tryptophan supplements don't appear to help ADHD symptoms (9948,9952).
Depression. Some preliminary clinical research suggests that L-tryptophan might improve the effectiveness of conventional antidepressants (6245,10856).
Seasonal affective disorder (SAD). Preliminary clinical evidence suggests L-tryptophan might be helpful in SAD (6247).
Sleep apnea. There is preliminary evidence that taking L-tryptophan orally might improve sleep in patients with obstructive sleep apnea. It does not appear to be beneficial in patients with central sleep apnea (1144,1146).
More evidence is needed to rate L-tryptophan for these uses.

Mechanism of Action

L-tryptophan is an essential amino acid present in concentrations of 1-2% in many plant and animal proteins (5). The body absorbs tryptophan from dietary protein sources, converts it to 5-hyrdoxytryptophan (5-HTP), then to serotonin (5-hydroxytryptamine). Both L-tryptophan and 5-HTP can penetrate the blood-brain barrier (10853,10857).
L-tryptophan has sedative effects (1143).
Tryptophan depletion can cause a relapse in treated depression and precipitate depressive symptoms in patients with a history or family history of depression, as well as in healthy volunteers (10854,10855). Additionally, dietary tryptophan depletion has been associated with bulimia relapse (1133) and deterioration of schizophrenia symptoms (1134), but it does not seem to worsen symptoms in people with untreated depression (1136).

Adverse Reactions

Orally, L-tryptophan can cause gastrointestinal (GI) side effects such as heartburn, stomach pain, belching and flatulence, nausea, vomiting, diarrhea, headache, lightheadedness, dry mouth, visual blurring, ataxia, drowsiness, and anorexia (10853).
In 1989, more than 1500 cases of eosinophilia-myalgia syndrome (EMS) and 37 deaths were associated with L-tryptophan use in the US. Ninety-five percent of all EMS cases were traced to L-tryptophan produced by a single manufacturer in Japan. In 1990, an FDA alert was put into force limiting the importation of all over-the-counter L-tryptophan products (7067,11477,11478). After the limitation of L-tryptophan products, the incidence of EMS dropped abruptly (11474). Symptoms of EMS associated with L-tryptophan use include intense eosinophilia; fatigue; incapacitating myalgia; neuropathy; sclerodermiform skin changes; alopecia; rash; and inflammatory disorders affecting the joints, connective tissue, lungs, heart, and liver (8053,11477). Symptoms tend to improve over time; however some individuals may still experience symptoms up to 2 years after the onset of EMS and complete resolution of symptoms may not occur (8053,10287). There is some evidence suggesting that daily use of a multivitamin or B-complex vitamin supplement prior to the onset of EMS may have decreased the severity of symptoms in some cases (8052). The exact cause of EMS in patients taking L-tryptophan is unknown, but some evidence suggests it may be due to contaminated L-tryptophan products (8050,8051,11477,11478). Some experts disagree with the hypothesis that contaminated L-tryptophan products are the cause of EMS. These experts suggest the true cause of EMS has not yet been identified (11475,11476). There are 5 contaminants that have been associated with EMS after taking L-tryptophan, but other causal factors cannot be ruled out (8054,10288,10289). There are also cases of EMS following L-tryptophan use that have not been linked to apparent contamination. There is also some evidence of an association between L-tryptophan-related EMS and the occurrence of chronic B-cell lymphocytic leukemia (8055).

Interactions with Herbs & Other Dietary Supplements

HERBS AND SUPPLEMENTS WITH SEDATIVE PROPERTIES: L-tryptophan can cause drowsiness and sedation (1143). Theoretically, concomitant use with herbs that have sedative properties might enhance therapeutic and adverse effects. Some of these supplements include 5-HTP, calamus, California poppy, catnip, hops, Jamaican dogwood, kava, St. John's wort, scullcap, valerian, yerba mansa, and others.
HERBS AND SUPPLEMENTS WITH SEROTONERGIC PROPERTIES: Theoretically, l-tryptophan might increase the effects and adverse effects of products that increase serotonin levels, including 5-hydroxytryptophan, Hawaiian baby woodrose, S-adenosylmethionine (SAMe), and St. John's wort (1141).

Interactions with Drugs

ANTIDEPRESSANT DRUGS: Combining serotonergic antidepressants with L-tryptophan might increase the risk of serotonergic side effects including serotonin syndrome, and cerebral vasoconstrictive disorders such as Call-Fleming syndrome (1141,8056). These drugs include the selective serotonin reuptake inhibitors (SSRIs) such as fluoxetine (Prozac), paroxetine (Paxil), sertraline (Zoloft), and others; and tricyclic and atypical antidepressants such as amitriptyline (Elavil), clomipramine (Anafranil), imipramine (Tofranil), and others.
BENZODIAZEPINES: Concomitant use of L-tryptophan with benzodiazepines can cause sexual disinhibition, reversible dyskinesias, and reversible Parkinsonian-like rigidity (9). Benzodiazepines include clonazepam (Klonopin), diazepam (Valium), lorazepam (Ativan), and others.
CNS DEPRESSANTS: Theoretically, concomitant use with medications that cause sedation may have additive effects when taken with medications that cause sedation such as clonazepam (Klonopin), lorazepam (Ativan), phenobarbital (Donnatal), zolpidem (Ambien), and others. L-tryptophan can cause fatigue and drowsiness (1143).
DEXTROMETHORPHAN (Robitussin DM, and others): Theoretically, concurrent use might cause additive

serotonergic effects and increase the risk of serotonin syndrome (1141). Also, concurrent use might theoretically cause cerebral vasoconstriction disorders such as Call-Fleming syndrome (8056).
MEPERIDINE (Demerol): Theoretically, concurrent use with meperidine might cause additive serotonergic effects, and increase the risk of serotonin syndrome (1141). Also, concurrent use might theoretically cause cerebral vasoconstriction disorders such as Call-Fleming syndrome (8056).
MONOAMINE OXIDASE INHIBITORS (MAOIs): Combining serotonergic drugs such as MAOIs with L-tryptophan might increase the risk of serotonergic side effects including serotonin syndrome and cerebral vasoconstrictive disorders such as Call-Fleming syndrome (8056).
PENTAZOCINE (Talwin): Theoretically, concurrent use with pentazocine might cause additive serotonergic effects and increase the risk of serotonin syndrome (1141). Also, concurrent use might theoretically cause cerebral vasoconstriction disorders such as Call-Fleming syndrome (8056).
PHENOTHIAZINES: Concomitant use of L-tryptophan with phenothiazines can cause sexual disinhibition, reversible dyskinesias, and reversible Parkinsonian-like rigidity (9). Phenothiazines include chlorpromazine (Thorazine), prochlorperazine (Compazine), and others.
TRAMADOL (Ultram): Theoretically, concurrent with use tramadol might cause additive serotonergic effects and increase the risk of serotonin syndrome (1141). Also, concurrent use might theoretically cause cerebral vasoconstriction disorders such as Call-Fleming syndrome (8056).

Interactions with Foods
None known.

Interactions with Lab Tests
EOSINOPHIL COUNT: In cases of eosinophilia myalgia syndrome, L-tryptophan can increase serum eosinophil counts and test results (8053).
LIVER FUNCTION TESTS: In cases of eosinophilia myalgia syndrome, L-tryptophan can increase serum liver enzyme levels and test results (8053).

Interactions with Diseases or Conditions
EOSINOPHILIA: Theoretically, L-tryptophan may exacerbate this condition. L-tryptophan use has been associated with the development of eosinophilia-myalgia syndrome (EMS) (7067).
KIDNEY OR LIVER DYSFUNCTION: Theoretically, L-tryptophan may exacerbate these conditions since its use has been associated with the development of eosinophilia-myalgia syndrome (EMS) (7067).

Dosage and Administration
ORAL: Clinical studies for sleep disorders have used doses from 1 to 2.5 grams (1144,1146). For depression, 300 mg daily in combination with antidepressants has been used (6245). For premenstrual syndrome, 6 grams daily was used in one study (6246). High dose L-tryptophan (50 mg/kg/day) has been used as adjunct therapy for smoking cessation (1138).

Comments
L-tryptophan is not available as a dietary supplement in the US. It is unclear whether supplement manufacturers are able to produce contaminant-free, pure L-tryptophan products (7067). L-tryptophan in the United States is limited for use under medical supervision in special dietary products such as infant formulas, enteral products, and approved parenteral drug products (7067). Older people may require lower amounts (9).

LABDANUM

Also Known As
Ambreine, Ciste, Cyste, Rockrose.

Scientific Names
Cistus ladanifer, synonym Cistus ladaniferus; Cistus creticus, synonyms Cistus incanus, Cistus villosus; Cistus polymorphus; and other Cistus species.
Family: Cistaceae.

People Use This For
Orally, labdanum is used for inflammation of the respiratory tract mucous membrane, bronchitis, diarrhea, edema, hernia, tumors, leprosy, and spleen sclerosis. Labdanum is also used orally for its expectorant, stimulant, purgative, and cleansing properties. Topically, labdanum is used for its astringent and hemostatic properties.
In foods and beverages, the absolute, oleoresin, and oil are used as flavoring agents.
In cosmetics, labdanum absolute and oil are used as fixative and fragrance components.
In addition, people use labdanum as a fumigant and insecticide.

Safety

LIKELY SAFE ...when used orally in amounts commonly found in foods. Labdanum has Generally Recognized As Safe (GRAS) status in the US (4912).
POSSIBLY SAFE ...when used topically for medicinal purposes. It is nontoxic and nonirritating to human skin (11). There is insufficient reliable information available about the safety of labdanum for its other uses.
PREGNANCY AND LACTATION: Insufficient reliable information available; avoid using.

Effectiveness

There is insufficient reliable information available about the effectiveness of labdanum.

Mechanism of Action

The applicable parts of labdanum are the above ground parts. Beta-pinene, eugenol, eucalyptol (cineole), and benzaldehyde are thought to be the most active constituents of labdanum (11). Some evidence suggests the essential oil of labdanum and resin might have antibacterial and antifungal activity (11). Other evidence indicates an aqueous extract of Cistus incanus might protect against gastric lesions (4050). One study in experimental animals found that a non-alkaloid substance extracted by alcohol but not water caused liver changes (11), which might indicate some safety risks.

Adverse Reactions

None reported.

Interactions with Herbs & Other Dietary Supplements

None known.

Interactions with Drugs

None known.

Interactions with Foods

None known.

Interactions with Lab Tests

None known.

Interactions with Diseases or Conditions

None known.

Dosage and Administration

No typical dosage.

Comments

Labdanum oleoresin (gum, gum cistus) is obtained by boiling the above ground parts of labdanum (Cistus ladanifer) in water and separating the resin layer (11). Labdanum oil is distilled from the above ground parts of labdanum (Cistus ladanifer). Labdanum absolute (cyste absolute) is obtained by evaporation of the alcohol extract of fat soluble portions of labdanum (Cistus ladanifer) after removal of alcohol insoluble substances (11).

LABRADOR TEA

Also Known As

Continental Tea, St. James' Tea.
CAUTION: See separate listing for Marsh Tea.

Scientific Names

Rhododendron groenlandicum, synonyms Ledum groenlandicum, Ledum latifolium.
Family: Ericaceae.

People Use This For

Orally, labrador tea is used as an expectorant, abortifacient, for "female disorders", sore throats, coughs, pulmonary infections and other chest ailments, dysentery, diarrhea, kidney problems, rheumatism, headache, and cancer.
Topically or in a bath, labrador tea is used for skin problems.
As a beverage, labrador tea is used as beverage or to make beer more intoxicating by adding leaves.

Safety
POSSIBLY SAFE ...when the leaves or flowering shoots are used orally as weak tea or in small amounts (6).
LIKELY UNSAFE ...when used orally in concentrated solutions or in large amounts. It can cause delirium, paralysis, and death (6).
PREGNANCY: UNSAFE ...when used orally because it might induce abortion (18).
LACTATION: Insufficient reliable information available; avoid using.

Effectiveness
There is insufficient reliable information available about the effectiveness of labrador tea.

Mechanism of Action
The applicable parts of labrador tea are the leaf and flowering shoots. Labrador tea has expectorant activity (18) and narcotic properties (6). The constituent ledol (ledum camphor) can cause gastrointestinal (GI) irritation (vomiting, gastroenteritis, diarrhea) and central nervous system (CNS) excitation, spasms, and paralysis (18). The constituent grayanotoxin (andromedotoxin), can cause bradycardia, hypotension, loss of coordination, convulsions, paralysis, and death (6).

Adverse Reactions
Orally, labrador tea can cause gastrointestinal irritation (vomiting, gastroenteritis, diarrhea); and central nervous system excitation, spasms, paralysis, and death (6,18).

Interactions with Herbs & Other Dietary Supplements
None known.

Interactions with Drugs
None known.

Interactions with Foods
None known.

Interactions with Lab Tests
None known.

Interactions with Diseases or Conditions
None known.

Dosage and Administration
No typical dosage.

Comments
Medicinal uses of labrador tea are now largely obsolete (18).

LABURNUM

Also Known As
Bean Trifoil, Golden Chain, Legume, Pea Tree.

Scientific Names
Laburnum anagyroides, synonyms Cytisus laburnum, Cytisus alschingeri.
Family: Fabaceae/Leguminosae.

People Use This For
Orally, laburnum is used as an emetic and purgative.
In manufacturing, laburnum is used as a pesticide.

Safety
UNSAFE ...when used orally (18).
PREGNANCY AND LACTATION: UNSAFE ...when used orally (18).

Effectiveness
There is insufficient reliable information available about the effectiveness of laburnum.

Mechanism of Action
The applicable part of laburnum is the seed. There is insufficient reliable information available about the possible mechanism of action and active ingredients.

Adverse Reactions
Orally, the fatal adult dose of laburnum is 20 seeds or 3-4 unripe berries. Symptoms of laburnum poisoning include nausea, dizziness, salivation, and pain in the mouth, throat and stomach. This is accompanied by sweating, headaches, and extended, severe, and occasionally bloody vomiting. The centrally-stimulating effects of laburnum lead to tonic-clonic spasms followed by paralysis. Some patients experience anuria or uremia. Death occurs by asphyxiation (18).

Interactions with Herbs & Other Dietary Supplements
None known.

Interactions with Drugs
None known.

Interactions with Foods
None known.

Interactions with Lab Tests
None known.

Interactions with Diseases or Conditions
None known.

Dosage and Administration
No typical dosage.

Comments
Laburnum is spelled very similarly to labdanum, but they are very different plants. The similar spelling could cause confusion.

LACTASE

Also Known As
None.

Scientific Names
Beta-galactosidase.

People Use This For
Orally, lactase is used for preventing symptoms of lactose intolerance, of which symptoms include cramps, diarrhea, and gas.

Safety
LIKELY SAFE ...when used orally and appropriately. There is an absence of adverse effects up to 9,900 IU of lactase (2371,2372,2373). It is an FDA-approved, nonprescription product available in the US.
PREGNANCY AND LACTATION: Insufficient reliable information available; avoid using.

Effectiveness
LIKELY EFFECTIVE

Lactose intolerance. Taking lactase orally is effective for reducing GI symptoms in lactose-intolerant people when used before the consumption of lactose or when added to milk prior to consumption (2371,2372,2373).

Mechanism of Action
Lactase is a sugar-splitting enzyme that hydrolyzes lactose, a milk sugar, to produce glucose and galactose (9,511).

Adverse Reactions
None reported.

Interactions with Herbs & Other Dietary Supplements
None known.

Interactions with Drugs
None known.

Interactions with Foods
None known.

Interactions with Lab Tests
None known.

Interactions with Diseases or Conditions
None known.

Dosage and Administration
ORAL: The typical dose of lactase is 6000-9000 IU tablets chewed and swallowed at the start of a lactose-containing meal (2374) or 2000 IU of the solution added to 500 mL of milk immediately before consumption (2375).

Comments
Lactase deficiency can be one of several factors that predispose an individual to the development of osteoporosis, possibly through diminished calcium intake (2376,2377).

LACTOBACILLUS

Also Known As
Acidophilus, L. Acidophilus, L. amylovorus, L. brevis, L. bulgaricus, L. casei, L. crispatus, L. delbrueckii, L. fermentum, L. gallinarum, L. johnsonii, L. johnsonii LC-1, L. plantarum, L. reuteri, L. sporogenes, LC-1, Lacto Bacillus, Lactobacilli, Lactobacillus GG, Lactobacillus rhamnosus GG, Probiotics.
CAUTION: See separate listings for Bifidobacteria, Saccharomyces Boulardii, and Yogurt.

Scientific Names
Lactobacillus acidophilus; Lactobacillus amylovorus; Lactobacillus brevis; Lactobacillus bulgaricus; Lactobacillus casei; Lactobacillus casei sp. rhamnosus; Lactobacillus crispatus; Lactobacillus delbrueckii; Lactobacillus fermentum; Lactobacillus gallinarum; Lactobacillus johnsonii; Lactobacillus plantarum; Lactobacillus reuteri; Lactobacillus rhamnosus; Lactobacillus sporogenes.
Family: Lactobacillaceae.

People Use This For
Orally, lactobacillus is used for treating and preventing diarrhea, including infectious types such as rotaviral diarrhea in children and traveler's diarrhea. It is used orally to prevent and treat antibiotic-associated diarrhea. It is used to prevent respiratory infections in children attending day-care centers. Lactobacillus is also used orally for general digestion problems, irritable bowel syndrome (IBS), inflammatory bowel syndrome (IBD, Crohn's disease, ulcerative colitis), relapsing Clostridium difficile colitis, bacterial overgrowth in short bowel syndrome, and Helicobacter pylori infection. It is also used orally for lactose intolerance, urinary tract infections, vaginal and Candida-related (yeast) infections, high cholesterol levels, hives, fever blisters, canker sores, and adolescent acne. Lactobacillus is used to treat and prevent atopic allergy in infants. It is also used orally to prevent cancer or the formation of carcinogens, to stimulate the immune system, and as a vaccine adjuvant.
Intravaginally, lactobacillus is used to treat vaginitis and urinary tract infections.

Safety
LIKELY SAFE ...when used orally and appropriately. Several species of lactobacillus, including Lactobacillus acidophilus, Lactobacillus bulgaricus, Lactobacillus casei, Lactobacillus delbrueckii, Lactobacillus rhamnosus, and Lactobacillus plantarum have been safely used in studies lasting up to nine months (4367,4380,6087,12108).
POSSIBLY SAFE ...when used intravaginally and appropriately. Several species of lactobacillus including Lactobacillus casei sp. rhamnosus and Lactobacillus fermentum have been used safely in studies lasting from ten weeks to six months (4397,6094,6095,12108).
CHILDREN: LIKELY SAFE ...when used orally and appropriately. Lactobacillus GG, a specific strain of Lactobacillus rhamnosus, has been used safely in studies lasting from seven days to 15 months (4369,4372,4373,4377,7741,8565,8566,8567,8568). Lactobacillus reuteri has been used safely for up to five days (7751,8566,8567). Lactobacillus sporogenes has been used safely in newborn infants for 12 months (7742,8515). The safety of other

Lactobacillus species in children is not known.
PREGNANCY: POSSIBLY SAFE ...when used orally and appropriately. Lactobacillus GG, a specific strain of Lactobacillus rhamnosus, has been used with apparent safety during pregnancy starting 2 to 4 weeks before delivery (7743,8515). The safety of other Lactobacillus species in pregnant women is not known.
LACTATION: POSSIBLY SAFE ...when used orally and appropriately. Lactobacillus GG, a specific strain of Lactobacillus rhamnosus, has been used with apparent safety in lactating women for up to six months (7743,8515). The safety of other Lactobacillus species in lactating women is not known.

Effectiveness

LIKELY EFFECTIVE

Rotaviral diarrhea. Lactobacillus GG, a specific strain of Lactobacillus rhamnosus, can reduce the duration of the diarrheal phase of rotavirus infection by 1-3 days in infants and young children (4369,4377). Lactobacillus reuteri also seems to reduce the duration of acute diarrhea (mostly rotavirus) in hospitalized infants and young children (7751). Lactobacillus casei also seems to shorten the course of acute diarrhea in infants and young children (1253). For babies and children ages 6 to 36 months, a daily dose of 10 billion live, freeze-dried Lactobacillus reuteri reduces the duration of diarrhea (7753). A combination of Lactobacillus rhamnosus and Lactobacillus reuteri seems to reduce the diarrhea phase of rotaviral infection in hospitalized babies and children ages 6 to 36 months by 20% and also seems to reduce the duration of rotavirus excretion. Combination treatment seems to be similarly effective to single-strain Lactobacillus treatments. In patients with diarrhea for less than 60 hours before the start of treatment (early intervention), probiotic treatment can reduce hospital stay by 48% (8567). The combination of Lactobacillus rhamnosus and Lactobacillus reuteri also seems to reduce the duration of diarrhea in babies and children ages 9 to 44 months attending day-care centers. Early intervention reduces recovery time by about 43% (8566). Overall, Lactobacillus seems to reduce the duration of diarrhea by 0.7 days and diarrheal stools by 1.6 stools on day 2 of treatment (8568). Effectiveness appears to be dose dependent, at least 10 billion colony-forming units during the first 48 hours should be used.

POSSIBLY EFFECTIVE

Antibiotic-associated diarrhea. Concurrent oral treatment with Lactobacillus GG, a specific strain of Lactobacillus rhamnosus, and antibiotics significantly decreases stool frequency and improves stool consistency compared to treatment with antibiotics alone in children (4371,8511). Lactobacillus GG seems to reduce the rate of antibiotic-associated diarrhea by approximately 11% (4372). However, Lactobacillus GG does not seem to reduce the occurrence of antibiotic-associated diarrhea in hospitalized adults (7306).

Atopic dermatitis (eczema). There is some evidence that taking Lactobacillus GG orally can reduce symptoms of atopic eczema in infants allergic to cow's milk. Lactobacillus seems to decrease markers of hypersensitivity reactions and intestinal inflammation, such as tumor necrosis factor (TNF), and alpha 1-antitrypsin (4369,11383). Lactobacilli also seem to stimulate the production of transforming growth factor-beta (TGF-beta), which protects against allergy (7743).

Atopic disease. Lactobacillus GG taken orally two to four weeks before delivery and continued for the first three to six months of breast-feeding seems to prevent atopic allergies (asthma, allergic rhinitis, and eczema) in infants with a family history of atopy. It appears to be equally effective when taken by the breast-feeding woman or by the bottle-feeding infant (7743,8515,11381). This preventive effect of lactobacillus in at-risk infants appears to extend up to 4 years of age (11381).

Chronic pouchitis. There is some evidence that continuous oral treatment for nine months with a specific concentrated formulation of Lactobacillus, Bifidobacterium, and Streptococcus can maintain remission in 85% of patients (6087).

Clostridium difficile diarrhea. Patients treated with metronidazole and vancomycin for Clostridium difficile diarrhea have a 20% chance for developing a secondary or recurring Clostridium difficile infection when antibiotic therapy is stopped. Taking Lactobacillus GG, a specific strain of Lactobacillus rhamnosus, orally during conventional antibiotic therapy seems to reduce the recurrence rate of Clostridium difficile diarrhea after antibiotics are stopped; and also seems to improve some symptoms of an active Clostridium difficile infection, including cramping and diarrhea (4392,4394). Preliminary evidence suggests another strain, Lactobacillus plantarum 299v, may also prevent recurrent episodes of Clostridium difficile diarrhea (11378).

Diarrhea. Lactobacillus GG given prophylactically on hospital admission seems to reduce the risk of non-rotaviral diarrhea and nosocomial rotavirus gastroenteritis in infants and children ages 1 to 36 months (7741). Lactobacillus GG, a specific strain of Lactobacillus rhamnosus, can significantly reduce the occurrence of diarrhea from all causes in undernourished children (4373). Lactobacillus sporogenes seems to reduce the incidence and duration of diarrhea in newborns in rural areas of developing countries (7742).

Helicobacter pylori (H pylori). Taking Lactobacillus acidophilus orally, in a lyophilized and inactivated form, seems to increase the effectiveness of rabeprazole (Aciphex), clarithromycin (Biaxin), and amoxicillin (Amoxil, others) for treating H. pylori (8562).

Irritable bowel syndrome (IBS). Heat-killed Lactobacillus acidophilus given in capsule form or as a Lactobacillus plantarum beverage seems to improve abdominal pain, bloating, number and quality of stools, and general physical state (7744,10419). A lactobacillus combination probiotic including strains of viable lyophilized bacteria species, called VSL#3, also appears to improve IBS symptoms (11379). However, substitution of Lactobacillus acidophilus milk for regular cow's milk seems to have no effect on symptoms of IBS (123).

Respiratory infections. Children ages 1 to 6 years who attend day-care centers seem to get fewer and less severe respiratory infections when given milk with Lactobacillus GG. Children receiving milk with lactobacilli also seem to have fewer days of illness-related absence (8565).

Travelers' diarrhea. Taking Lactobacillus GG orally seems to reduce the occurrence of diarrhea in travelers (4374,10216). The effectiveness of Lactobacillus GG can vary significantly based upon the destination of travel. Destinations in the same country can have different results, probably because of differences in bacteria and other microorganisms at different locations (10216).

POSSIBLY INEFFECTIVE

Intestinal bacterial overgrowth. Lactobacillus fermentum 100 to 300 billion cells given orally twice daily for two weeks doesn't seem to improve symptoms such as abdominal pain and bloating, or stool frequency in adults with overgrowth of intestinal bacteria such as Klebsiella, Bacteroides, Escherichia coli, Enterococcus, or Proteus mirabilis. It also doesn't lower breath hydrogen concentration, a measure of intestinal bacterial overgrowth (8514).

Lactose intolerance. Consuming Lactobacillus acidophilus milk seems to produce the same symptoms of intolerance as regular cow's milk in people with lactose intolerance (123).

Vulvovaginitis. A combination of Lactobacillus rhamnosus plus Bifidobacterium longum (Lactobac) given orally or a combination of Lactobacillus rhamnosus, Lactobacillus delbruekii, Lactobacillus acidophilus, and Streptococcus thermophilus (Femilac) given vaginally doesn't seem to reduce the chance of vaginal candidiasis infection following use of antibiotics (12108).

INSUFFICIENT RELIABLE EVIDENCE to RATE

Bacterial vaginosis. Preliminary clinical evidence suggests that eating yogurt enriched with lactobacillus acidophilus daily may slightly decrease the incidence of bacterial vaginosis. However, it does not appear to reduce candidal vaginitis (1245).

Urinary tract infections (UTIs). There is some preliminary evidence that intravaginal use of some Lactobacillus species might be helpful for preventing UTIs, but there have been some conflicting findings in studies (4581,6094,6095).

More evidence is needed to rate lactobacillus for these uses.

Mechanism of Action

Lactobacillus refers to a group of lactic acid producing, gram-positive rods that are obligate and facultative anaerobes (7755,7760). Most are non-spore-forming with the exception of Lactobacillus sporogenes (8563). Lactobacilli are symbiotic and make up some of the 400 normal flora in the human gastrointestinal and genitourinary tracts (6089,6094,6096,7754,7755). They are also found in some fermented food products such as yogurt as well as in capsule form (6099). Some of the specific lactobacillus species include Lactobacillus acidophilus, Lactobacillus bulgaricus, Lactobacillus casei sp. rhamnosus, Lactobacillus delbrueckii, Lactobacillus fermentum, Lactobacillus plantarum, Lactobacillus reuteri, Lactobacillus rhamnosus, and Lactobacillus sporogenes. Of these, Lactobacillus reuteri is the most commonly occurring species in the gastrointestinal tract. It is also found in breast milk (7751,7755). Lactobacilli are used therapeutically as probiotics, the opposite of antibiotics. They are considered "friendly" bacteria and are taken for the purpose of re-colonizing areas of the body where they normally would occur. The human body relies on the normal flora for several functions including metabolizing foods and certain drugs, absorbing nutrients, and preventing colonization by pathogenic bacteria. Lactobacilli seem to provide nutritional benefits including inducing growth factors and increasing the bioavailability of minerals (7754). Lactobacilli also stabilize the mucosal barrier and decrease intestinal permeability (7751,7755). Probiotics such as lactobacillus are typically used in cases when a disease occurs or might occur due to depleted normal flora. For example, treatment with antibiotics can kill off pathogenic bacteria and also the normal flora of the gastrointestinal and genitourinary tracts. Altering the normal flora allows for potential colonization by pathogenic organisms (6088), which can result in side effects such as diarrhea, cramping, and less commonly pseudomembranous colitis caused by Clostridium difficile. The theory is that taking lactobacillus probiotics during antibiotic treatment can prevent or minimize normal flora depletion and pathogenic bacteria colonization. There is some evidence to support this theory (5500,11382). When taken orally, lactobacilli pass through the gut and attach to the intestinal mucosa where they can persist for at least one week (5500). When probiotic lactobacilli latch on to and colonize the intestinal and urogenital mucosa, it seems to prevent epithelial attachment by pathogenic bacteria (4369,4378,6086,6089,6091,6092). Lactobacilli seem to have this effect by increasing epithelial mucus production and competing with pathogens for mucosal binding sites, possibly through steric hindrance (4388,6086,6089,6091,6092,7755,8562). Lactobacilli also inhibit bacterial pathogens by producing lactic acid, and many lactobacilli also produce hydrogen peroxide (6089,6090,6096). Hydrogen-peroxide producing lactobacilli are bacteriocidal to the vaginal pathogen Gardnerella vaginalis, and their presence in the vagina has been associated with decreased frequencies of bacterial vaginosis and trichomoniasis (7745). In the vagina, lactic acid from lactobacilli lowers vaginal pH, which can prevent pathogen growth. Lactobacilli might also produce substances called bacteriocins that can inhibit growth of some bacteria and fungi, and biosurfactants that can prevent some bacteria from adhering to the epithelium (6089,6090,6091,6096,8514). Lactobacilli might also inhibit the translocation of bacteria across the intestinal mucosa by strengthening the epithelial barrier and by promoting accelerated epithelial repair (8516). Some researchers think lactobacilli and other probiotics might have immunomodulating effects (4368,4369,8512). Lactobacilli seem to modulate non-specific cellular and humoral immunity possibly by stimulating lymphocyte and macrophage activity (6089,8565) and modulating cytokine production by mononuclear cells (4379,8512). They also appear to enhance synthesis of antibodies in response to microbial pathogens, particularly secretory immunoglobulin A (7754). However, the way lactobacilli affect immune function may differ depending on the health status of the patient. In people with an immune system hypersensitivity, lactobacilli seem to down-regulate immune function. In healthy people without an immune system hypersensitivity, lactobacilli seem to stimulate the immune system (4399). In healthy children attending day-care centers, lactobacilli seem to have an immunostimulatory effect (8565). Due to these immunomodulating effects, some researchers think lactobacillus and other probiotics might not only fight intestinal and urogenital pathogens, but might also be helpful for conditions such as inflammatory bowel disease, pouchitis, food allergy, and for use as an adjuvant to vaccination (4368,4379,4393,4399).

Clinical research suggests that Lactobacillus rhamnosus taken orally might enhance natural immunity in healthy adults. It appears to increase the phagocytic activity in polymorphonuclear cells and monocytes, and enhance natural killer cell tumor killing activity (7756,7757). Orally administered lactobacillus brevis seems to increase the production of interferon-alpha (7758). Whether lactobacilli administration can increase resistance to disease is unknown. Some preliminary research suggests that lactobacilli and other probiotics might inhibit pathogens such as Candida albicans and prolong survival in immune deficiency states (7746). Other preliminary research suggests that Lactobacillus reuteri might prevent infection with Cryptosporidium parvum in immunodeficient patients. Lactobacillus reuteri is known to secrete reuterin, which has activity against Salmonella, Listeria, Clostridium, and Escherichia species and other pathogens (7749,7755). Fermentation of milk products with lactobacilli might increase the content of vitamins such as folic acid, niacin, riboflavin, thiamine, pyridoxine, and cyanocobalamin (8564). There is also some preliminary evidence that lactobacilli and other probiotics might help protect against cancer. In animal models, lactobacillus has been shown to bind dietary carcinogens (4376) and decrease development of tumors in the colon after carcinogen challenge (4382,4387,8564). Preliminary research also suggests that lactobacilli, especially Lactobacillus plantarum, can reduce the severity of chemotherapy-induced enterocolitis. There is also some preliminary research that suggests the ability of lactobacilli to reduce adherence of pathogenic bacteria to the colonic mucosa, and to reduce bacterial translocation, which might make it useful in the treatment of conditions such as Crohn's disease (7747,7750,7754). Additional preliminary evidence suggests lactobacillus GG milk products might be useful as a vehicle for antibodies against human cariogenic bacteria (11380). Other preliminary research suggests that Lactobacillus bulgaricus and Lactobacillus sporogenes might have hypolipidemic and antiatherosclerotic effects. Limited clinical evidence suggests that it can reduce total and low-density lipoprotein (LDL) cholesterol with no effect on high-density lipoprotein (HDL) (7759,8563). Fermented dairy products, such as yogurt and acidophilus milk also seem to have a beneficial effect on cholesterol. Lactobacilli and other probiotic bacteria seem to bind bile acids to cholesterol, resulting in increased bile acid-cholesterol excretion. They also seem to increase fatty acid production in the intestine, which decreases circulatory fatty acid concentrations either by inhibiting hepatic cholesterol synthesis or redistributing cholesterol from the plasma to the liver. To be clinically useful, fermented dairy products would likely have to be taken daily (8559).

Most researchers agree that the effectiveness of lactobacilli and other probiotics for all indications depends on their ability to colonize an area of tissue. To do this, lactobacillus preparations must contain live and viable organisms. Products stored for long periods of time or stored improperly may contain few live and active organisms. For oral preparations, bacteria must also remain viable after passing through the gut and then they must be able to latch on to the intestinal epithelium. Lactobacilli strains might vary in their effectiveness due to differences in their ability to adhere to the epithelial cells (4373,6091,6094). Some strains might also have differing activity against specific pathogens (6094). Host factors such as hormone levels can also influence adherence and effectiveness. The ability of lactobacilli to attach to epithelial cells can change during a woman's menstrual cycle in response to changing hormone levels. In post-menopausal women, correcting low estrogen levels can help restore lactobacillus colonization without supplementation (6089,6094). There is some evidence that Lactobacillus GG, a strain of Lactobacillus rhamnosus, attaches to intestinal epithelial cells better than Lactobacillus acidophilus (4373). Lactobacillus casei may adhere better to urogenital cells than other lactobacillus species (6091). Lactobacilli, even strains of the same species, might not act similarly at the same site. Lactobacillus rhamnosus GR-1 seems to have anti-yeast and antiviral effects in the vagina that persist for at least 14 days after vaginal administration, while the effects of Lactobacillus rhamnosus GG diminish quickly (8560). Probiotic strains may also differ in specific metabolic activities, and not all lactobacilli species inhibit a wide range of pathogenic bacteria (6093). Therefore, some researchers theorize that probiotic preparations containing several species might offer more benefit than a single species (6087,6094). However, this theory has not yet been evaluated in studies.

Adverse Reactions

Orally, lactobacillus species are usually well tolerated (6087,8565,8566,8567,8568). The most common side effect is flatulence; however; it is usually mild and subsides as therapy continues. Since lactobacillus preparations contain live and active microorganisms, there is some concern that they might cause pathological infection in some patients. Lactobacillus bacteremia has been reported in severely ill and immunocompromised patients (4380). Fatal Lactobacillus rhamnosus septicemia has been reported in an immunocompromised patient consuming yogurt and taking prolonged courses of multiple broad spectrum antibiotics (8561). There are no reports of pathogenic colonization in relatively healthy patients with intact immune systems (4380,4389,4390,4391,4393,4398). Adults infected with HIV have taken 10 billion live Lactobacillus reuteri orally daily for 21 days without safety or tolerance problems (7752).

Intravaginally, lactobacillus species is usually well tolerated (6094).

Interactions with Herbs & Other Dietary Supplements
None known.

Interactions with Drugs
ANTIBIOTIC DRUGS: There is some concern that concomitant administration of antibiotics might decrease the effectiveness of lactobacillus. Since lactobacillus preparations usually contain live and active organisms, simultaneously taking antibiotics might kill a significant number of the organisms (1740). Tell patients to separate administration of antibiotics and lactobacillus preparations by at least two hours.
IMMUNOSUPPRESSANTS: Theoretically, lactobacillus could cause infection in patients taking medications that suppress the immune system. These include cyclosporine (Neoral, Sandimmune), tacrolimus (Prograf), azathioprine (Imuran), and cancer chemotherapeutic agents like cyclophosphamide (Cytoxan) and cisplatin (Platinol) (4380,4391,4393,4398).

Interactions with Foods
None known.

Interactions with Lab Tests
None known.

Interactions with Diseases or Conditions
IMMUNODEFICIENCY: There is some concern that lactobacillus preparations might cause pathogenic colonization, especially in patients who are immunocompromised. Although lactobacilli have caused bacteremia and other pathogenic infections, it rarely occurs. Pathogenic colonization is more likely to occur in severely immunocompromised patients (4380,4391,4393,4398). Adults infected with HIV have taken 10 billion live Lactobacillus reuteri orally daily for 21 days without safety or tolerance problems (7752). The risk of longer-term treatment or in very severely compromised patients is unknown.

Dosage and Administration
ORAL: The strength of lactobacillus preparations is usually quantified by the number of living organisms per capsule. Typical doses usually range from 1 to 10 billion viable organisms taken daily in 3-4 divided doses (6002). For children with diarrhea, 5-10 billion live Lactobacillus GG in a rehydrating solution has been used (4369,4370). For babies and children with diarrhea, 10 to100 billion live Lactobacillus reuteri daily for up to 5 days has been used (7751,7753). Lower doses may not be effective (7753). Also, combination of Lactobacillus rhamnosus and Lactobacillus reuteri, 10 billion live cells of each strain, has been used twice daily for 5 days for babies and children with diarrhea (8567). For preventing antibiotic-associated diarrhea in children, 20 billion live Lactobacillus GG daily was used throughout the conventional antimicrobial treatment period (4372). For preventing diarrhea in hospitalized infants and children ages 1 to 36 months, 6 billion live Lactobacillus GG has been used twice daily (7741). For preventing and shortening the duration of diarrhea in newborns within the first year of life in rural areas of developing countries, 100 million live Lactobacillus sporogenes have been given daily for one year (7742). For preventing respiratory infections in children attending day-care centers, milk with 500,000 to 1 million colony-forming units of Lactobacillus GG per ml has been used; average milk consumption was 260 ml (8565). For recurrent Clostridium difficile, 1.25 billion live Lactobacillus GG in two divided doses for 2 weeks has been used (4394). For milk hypersensitivity, 2600 million Lactobacillus GG daily has been used (4399). For preventing atopic allergies in infants with a family history of atopy, 20 billion live Lactobacillus GG daily has been given to pregnant women for 2 to 4 weeks prior to delivery, and then for the first 3 to 6 months to the breast-feeding women or bottle-feeding infants (7743,8515). For chronic pouchitis, 3 grams twice daily of a specific concentrated formula containing 300 billion viable bacteria per gram of several strains of Lactobacillus, Bifidobacterium, and Streptococcus has been used (6087). For preventing traveler's diarrhea Lactobacillus GG, 2 billion organisms daily, has been used (10216). For treating irritable bowel syndrome (IBS), 10 billion heat-killed Lactobacillus acidophilus given orally twice daily in capsule form, 450 billion viable lyophilized Lactobacillus (VSL#3) powder divided twice daily in capsule form, or 20 billion colony-forming units of Lactobacillus plantarum given daily as a beverage have been used for 4 to 6 weeks (7744,10419,11379).
INTRAVAGINAL: For bacterial vaginitis, vaginal suppositories containing 1 billion live Lactobacillus GG twice daily for 7 days has been used (4397). For reducing the risk of recurrent urinary tract infection's (UTI's), lactobacillus suppositories containing 0.5 gram (1.6 billion organisms) of L. casei var rhamnosus and L. fermentum has been used twice weekly for two weeks, then once a month for two months (6095). A vaginal solution containing 100 billion viable bacteria/mL in a dose of 1 mL twice weekly has also been used (6094).

Comments
Some products labeled to contain Lactobacillus acidophilus have been found to actually contain little or no Lactobacillus acidophilus. Products may also contain other strains of lactobacillus, including Lactobacillus bulgaricus. Some products have been found to also contain contaminants, including Enterococcus faecium, Clostridium sporogenes, and Pseudomonas species. Lactobacilli, when prepared properly, seem to be stable in pharmaceutical preparations. Various strains of Lactobacillus remain viable after freeze-drying and 1 year of storage

when anaerobic conditions are maintained (7745,7755). Cultivation at a pH of 5 seems in improve survival of Lactobacillus reuteri when subjected to freeze-drying (7748). Lactobacillus products are used as functional foods (7755).

LACTOFERRIN

Also Known As
Bovine lactoferrin, lactoferrins.

Scientific Names
Lactoferrin.

Comments
At the date of publication, there was very little scientific information about this product. Our staff is continually analyzing the available information on natural medicines and will add data to the online version of *Natural Medicines Comprehensive Database* as it becomes available. See www.naturaldatabase.com.

LADY FERN

Also Known As
Brake Root, Common Polypod, Oak Fern, Rock Brake, Rock of Polypody.

Scientific Names
Athyrium filix-femina, synonym Polypodium filix-femina.
Family: Dryopteridaceae.

Comments
At the date of publication, this product was not a common ingredient used in brand name supplements marketed to consumers. Details about this product are available at the online version of *Natural Medicines Comprehensive Database*. See www.naturaldatabase.com.

LADY'S BEDSTRAW

Also Known As
Cheese Rennet, Cheese Renning, Curdwort, Ladys Bedstraw, Maid's Hair, Petty Mugget, Yellow Cleavers, Yellow Galium.

Scientific Names
Galium verum.
Family: Rubiaceae.

People Use This For
Orally, lady's bedstraw is used for treating swollen ankles, as a diuretic for bladder and kidney mucous discharge, for cancer, epilepsy, hysteria, spasms, tumors, and for relief of chest and lung ailments. It is also used orally to induce sweating; as a tonic; to stimulate appetite; as an aphrodisiac; and for astringent, cleansing, and purgative effects. Topically, lady's bedstraw is used for poorly healing wounds and to stop bleeding.

Safety
There is insufficient reliable information available about the safety of lady's bedstraw.
Pregnancy and Lactation: Insufficient reliable information available; avoid using.

Effectiveness
There is insufficient reliable information available about the effectiveness of lady's bedstraw.

Mechanism of Action
The applicable parts of lady's bedstraw are the above ground parts. There is insufficient reliable information available about the possible mechanism of action and active ingredients.

Adverse Reactions
None reported.

Interactions with Herbs & Other Dietary Supplements
None known.

Interactions with Drugs
None known.

Interactions with Foods
None known.

Interactions with Lab Tests
None known.

Interactions with Diseases or Conditions
None known.

Dosage and Administration
ORAL: Typically, lady's bedstraw is used as a tea (18).
TOPICAL: Lady's bedstraw is used as a poultice. To prepare, pour 250 mL cold water over 2 heaping teaspoons of above ground parts, bring to simmer, and allow to steep (18).

LAMINARIA

Also Known As
Brown Algae, Kelp, Kombu, Makombu Thallus, Sea Girdles, Seagirdle Thallus.
CAUTION: See separate listings for Algin and Bladderwrack.

Scientific Names
Laminaria digitata; Laminaria japonica.
Family: Laminariaceae.

People Use This For
Orally, laminaria is used for weight loss, preventing cancer, hypertension, as a bulk laxative for constipation, and for treating radioactive intoxication.
Topically, laminaria is used as a "tent" placed into the cervix to cause cervical dilation prior to D & C, for removal of intrauterine devices, diagnostic procedures, for relief of cervical stenosis, and to facilitate uterine placement of therapeutic radium. Laminaria tents are also used in pregnancy for near-term or term cervical ripening particularly for a first pregnancy, to facilitate labor, alone or as adjunct to prostaglandins, and for inducing first-trimester abortions.

Safety
POSSIBLY UNSAFE ...when used orally. The average laminaria-based supplement might contain as much as 1000 mcg iodine. Ingesting more than 150 mcg iodine per day can cause hypothyroidism, hyperthyroidism, or exacerbate existing hyperthyroidism (9556). In addition, some laminaria supplements may contain arsenic (645,10275). There is insufficient reliable information available about the safety of laminaria for its other uses.
PREGNANCY: POSSIBLY UNSAFE ...when used topically for cervical ripening; there is an increased risk of maternal and neonatal infection (8945). LIKELY UNSAFE ...when used topically to induce labor because use is associated with maternal endometriosis, neonatal sepsis, fetal hypoxia, and intrauterine death (6). UNSAFE ...when used orally because of potential hormonal effects (19); avoid using.
LACTATION: LIKELY UNSAFE ...when used orally because of potential toxicity (19).

Effectiveness
POSSIBLY INEFFECTIVE

Parturition. Applying laminaria topically doesn't seem to be effective for cervical ripening. Although laminaria might reduce the duration of induction, it doesn't seem to reduce the incidence of birth by cesarian section. It also increases maternal and fetal infectious complications (8945).

There is insufficient reliable information available about the effectiveness of laminaria for its other uses.

Mechanism of Action

Laminaria is a seaweed that is native to Japan (8945). Laminaria contains iodine (9556), and is considered to be a rich source of iron and potassium (19). Iodine, which is the essential substrate for the thyroid hormone, is present in concentrations from 0.03-1.0% in laminaria (18). The constituents of laminaria include alginate, lamine, and laminarin (6).

Much of the utility of laminaria relates to its ability to form a viscous colloidal solution of gel in water. This allows laminaria to function as a bulk laxative. It also allows laminaria to be used to dilate the cervix for procedures or to ripen the cervix and hasten the onset of labor. For these uses, laminaria "tents" are inserted cervically. They absorb ambient moisture, gradually swelling to a diameter of 1/2 inch over 4-6 hours. This swelling causes cervical dilation that can induce labor (6).

The mechanism of cervical "ripening" might be similar to that of a foreign body that disrupts the normal chorioamniotic balance and initiates prostaglandin synthesis. That, in turn, causes myometrial contractions and cervical ripening. An alternative theory is that laminaria causes ripening because it contains high levels of the prostaglandin precursor, arachidonic acid. Still another theory is that laminaria causes partial detachment of the placenta and induces cervical dilation. Although laminaria can reduce the duration of labor induction, it is associated with an increased risk for maternal endometritis and neonatal sepsis (6).

Some other laminaria constituents might also have medical uses. The polysaccharide constituent of laminaria, laminarin, has antilipemic activity when partially sulfated and anticoagulant activity similar to heparin when more extensively sulfated. The basal portion of the blades is used as a hypotensive agent; the constituents histamine and lamine may be responsible for hypotensive effects (6). The constituent algin (sodium alginate) has bulk laxative and demulcent (soothing) effects (272). Alginate-containing kelp reduces absorption of radioactive strontium in animals and humans and it has been used for managing radioactive intoxication (6). Preliminary evidence also suggests that alginate-containing kelp extracts might have antiviral effects, possibly by inhibiting viral enzyme activity (9554). However, the risk of adverse effects resulting from laminaria's iodine content may outweigh the benefits of its use as a routine preventative measure (515).

Adverse Reactions

Orally, laminaria can induce or exacerbate acne (9555). Oral use may also cause hypothyroidism or hyperthyroidism, or exacerbate existing hyperthyroidism (9556). Iodine can cause idiosyncratic or allergic reactions (18). Arsenic poisoning is a risk with laminaria, because the plant concentrates arsenic from the ocean. The concentration of arsenic in laminaria may vary depending upon the part of the world where it was harvested. The concentration of arsenic has been reported to be higher in laminaria preparations in Australia than in Great Britain (645,10275).

Topically, laminaria used for cervical ripening can cause pelvic cramps and cervical bleeding. Its use for cervical ripening is associated with neonatal and maternal infection (8945); however, in a small study of "tent" use (see People Use This For) with manufacturer recommended procedures, no infection occurred. Manufacturer recommendation included prior swabbing of the cervical canal with a suitable lubricant and antibacterial agent, then packing the canal with antibacterial gel. Uterine contractions associated with laminaria use have been implicated in fetal hypoxia and subsequent intrauterine death. Tent use is also associated with possible rupture of the cervical wall and subsequent infection (6).

Interactions with Herbs & Other Dietary Supplements

POTASSIUM SUPPLEMENTS: Theoretically, due to the potassium content of laminaria, concomitant use can increase the risk of hyperkalemia (19).

Interactions with Drugs

ACE INHIBITORS (ACEIs): Theoretically, due to the potassium content of laminaria, concomitant use might increase the risk of hyperkalemia (19).

DIGOXIN (Lanoxin): Theoretically, due to the potassium content laminaria may cause hyperkalemia in susceptible individuals and potentiate digoxin effects and adverse effects (19). Use with caution.

POTASSIUM-SPARING DIURETICS: Theoretically, due to the potassium content of laminaria, concomitant use may cause hyperkalemia (19).

THYROID HORMONE: Theoretically, due to the significant iodine content laminaria might interfere with drugs for hyper or hypothyroidism (9556).

Interactions with Foods

None known.

Interactions with Lab Tests

POTASSIUM: Theoretically, laminaria may increase serum potassium levels and test results (19).

THYROID HORMONES: Theoretically, the iodine in laminaria might elevate thyroid stimulating hormone (TSH) levels (9556).

Interactions with Diseases or Conditions

RENAL INSUFFICIENCY: Theoretically, laminaria may induce hyperkalemia in people with renal insufficiency on a potassium restricted diet (19). Laminaria also contains significant amounts of iodine (9556). Use with caution.
THYROID DISEASE: Laminaria contains significant amounts of iodine, which might exacerbate hyper- or hypothyroidism (9556).

Dosage and Administration

ORAL: People typically use capsules or tablets containing 500 to 650 mg of ground laminaria once daily (6002).
TOPICAL: No typical dosage.

LARCH ARABINOGALACTAN

Also Known As

AG, Ara-6, Arabinogalactan, Dietary Fiber, Larch, Larch Gum, Larix, Mongolian Larch, Mongolian Larchwood, Stractan, Western Larch, Wood Gum, Wood Sugar.
CAUTION: See separate listing for Larch Turpentine.

Scientific Names

Larix occidentalis; Larix gmelinii var. gmelinii, synonyms Larix dahurica, Abies gmelinii.
Family: Pinaceae.

People Use This For

Orally, larch arabinogalactan is used for the common cold, flu, metastatic liver disease, pediatric otitis media, HIV/AIDS, adjunctive therapy during cancer chemotherapy, as a dietary fiber supplement, immunostimulant, anti-inflammatory agent, and for hepatic encephalopathy.
In foods, Larch arabinogalactan is used as a stabilizer, emulsifier, binder, and sweetener.

Safety

LIKELY SAFE ...when used in amounts found in foods. Larch arabinogalactan is approved by the FDA for use in foods (3529).
POSSIBLY SAFE ...when used orally, appropriately, and short-term in therapeutic amounts (6,3529,3530).
There is insufficient reliable information available about the safety of the long-term use of larch arabinogalactan.
PREGNANCY AND LACTATION: Insufficient reliable information available; avoid using.

Effectiveness

There is insufficient reliable information available about the effectiveness of larch arabinogalactan.

Mechanism of Action

Larch arabinogalactan is a polysaccharide produced from the bark of the Larch tree. Arabinogalactans are found throughout nature and are found in other plants with immunostimulatory activity, including echinacea. Larch arabinogalactan is thought to have immunostimulatory effects by increasing release of interferon gamma, tumor necrosis fact alpha, interleukin-1 and interleukin-6 and stimulating phagocytosis and natural killer cell activity. Larch arabinogalactan is a fibrous product which ferments in the gut. It increases gut microflora, e.g., Lactobacillus, increases short-chain fatty acid production, and minimizes ammonia production and absorption. These effects suggest it may be beneficial as a dietary fiber supplement for improving gastrointestinal health and as an adjunct for treating hepatic encephalopathy. Larch arabinogalactan has been shown to concentrate in the liver. Some people think it might block hepatic receptors for metastatic cells and decrease liver metastases (3529,3530).

Adverse Reactions

Orally, bloating and flatulence have been reported (3530).

Interactions with Herbs & Other Dietary Supplements

None known.

Interactions with Drugs

IMMUNOSUPPRESSANTS: Theoretically, larch arabinogalactan might interfere with immunosuppression therapy due its immunostimulatory activity (3529,3560). Immunosuppressant drugs include azathioprine (Imuran), basiliximab (Simulect), cyclosporine (Neoral, Sandimmune), daclizumab (Zenapax), muromonab-CD3 (OKT3, Orthoclone OKT3), mycophenolate (CellCept), tacrolimus (FK506, Prograf), sirolimus (Rapamune), prednisone (Deltasone, Orasone), and other corticosteroids (glucocorticoids).

ORAL DRUGS: Theoretically, concurrent administration might decrease the absorption of some oral drugs due to the fibrous nature of larch arabinogalactan.

Interactions with Foods
None known.

Interactions with Lab Tests
None known.

Interactions with Diseases or Conditions
TRANSPLANT RECIPIENTS: Theoretically, larch arabinogalactan might interfere with immunosuppression therapy.

Dosage and Administration
ORAL: For colds and the flu, one teaspoon of larch arabinogalactan powder in juice or water is usually taken 2-3 times daily until symptoms are relieved (3531).

Comments
Larch arabinogalactan specifically concentrates in hepatocytes and might have future application as a diagnostic tool or as a vehicle for delivering drugs to the liver (3529,3530).

LARCH TURPENTINE

Also Known As
Terebinthina Laricina, Terebinthina Veneta, Venetian Turpentine.
CAUTION: See separate listing for Larch Arabinogalactan.

Scientific Names
Larix decidua, synonyms Larix europaea, Pinus larix.
Family: Pinaceae.

People Use This For
Topically, larch turpentine is used for treating neuralgia, rheumatic discomfort, furuncles, fevers, colds, cough, bronchitis, tendency toward infection, blood pressure problems, and inflammation of the mouth and pharynx.

Safety
POSSIBLY SAFE ...when used topically and appropriately on intact skin (2).
POSSIBLY UNSAFE ...when used orally (18). ...when used topically on damaged skin, particularly if used on large areas (18). Skin damage allows systemic absorption, which can cause kidney and central nervous system toxicity (18). ...when inhaled, because it can cause acute airway inflammation (18).
PREGNANCY AND LACTATION: Insufficient reliable information available; avoid using.

Effectiveness
There is insufficient reliable information available about the effectiveness of larch turpentine.

Mechanism of Action
Larch turpentine is an oily exudate obtained by drilling into the trunks of Larix decidua trees. It contains up to 20% volatile oil (2). When topically applied, it increases local blood flow and can have an antiseptic effect (2).

Adverse Reactions
Topically, larch turpentine can cause allergic skin reactions (2).
When taken orally or applied to large areas of skin or damaged skin, it can cause kidney and central nervous system damage (18).
Inhalation can cause acute respiratory tract inflammation (18).

Interactions with Herbs & Other Dietary Supplements
None known.

Interactions with Drugs
None known.

Interactions with Foods
None known.

Interactions with Lab Tests
None known.

Interactions with Diseases or Conditions
BRONCHITIS: Inhalation of larch turpentine is contraindicated because it may worsen respiratory tract inflammation (2).

Dosage and Administration
TOPICAL: The ointments, gels, emulsions, and oils commonly contain 10 to 20 percent larch turpentine as liniments for external application (2).

LATHYRUS

Also Known As
Caley Pea, Chickling Vetch, Chick-Pea, Everlasting Pea, Flat-Podded Vetch, Singletary Pea, Spanish Vetchling, Sweet Pea, Wild Pea.

Scientific Names
Lathyrus cicera; Lathyrus clymenum; Lathyrus hirsutus; Lathyrus incanus; Lathyrus odoratus; Lathyrus pusillus; Lathyrus sativus; Lathyrus sylvestris.
Family: Fabaceae/Leguminosae.

People Use This For
In foods, Lathyrus sativus is used in unleavened Indian bread. Lathyrus seeds are eaten as food and used as animal fodder throughout the world.
The flowers of sweet pea (Lathyrus odoratus) are cultivated for their color and fragrance.

Safety
LIKELY UNSAFE ...when used orally. The seeds of Lathyrus can be neurotoxic (6).
PREGNANCY AND LACTATION: LIKELY UNSAFE ...when used orally (6); avoid using.

Effectiveness
There is insufficient reliable information available about the effectiveness of lathyrus.

Mechanism of Action
Lathyrus seeds contain multiple constituents including phytates, divicine, and a mixture of alkaloids (6). The toxicity of lathyrus results from several compounds. The neurotoxic effects are linked to constituent beta-N-oxalyl-L-alpha, beta-diaminopropionic acid (ODAP). Constituent beta-aminopropionitrile (BAPN) causes skeletal abnormalities and damage to blood vessels (6).

Adverse Reactions
Orally, lathyrus can cause neurotoxic manifestations including muscular rigidity, spasticity, weakness, paralysis of leg muscles, weak pulse, shallow breathing, convulsions, or death (6). Prolonged neurotoxicity is characterized by poor central motor coordination and reduced nerve conduction in the lower limbs (6).

Interactions with Herbs & Other Dietary Supplements
None known.

Interactions with Drugs
None known.

Interactions with Foods
None known.

Interactions with Lab Tests
None known.

Interactions with Diseases or Conditions
None known.

Dosage and Administration
No typical dosage.

Comments
Neurolathyrism and its complications are rare in western countries, yet they have been documented for more than a century in Europe, Africa, and Asia. Despite the attempt to ban the sale of Lathyrus sativus in several states of India, distribution continues. To deactivate the toxin, several methods have been tried. Typically they involve soaking the seeds in water followed by steaming or sun drying. Roasting the seeds at high temperatures for twenty minutes also helps to destroy the neurotoxic constituent. However, these methods are only 80-85% effective (6).

LAURELWOOD

Also Known As
Alexandrian-laurel, Alexandrinischer Lorbeer, Borneo-mahogany, Calanolide, Caulophyllum Tree, Indian-laurel, Kamani Punna, Mahogany, Palo de Santa Maria, Palo Maria, Punnanga, Undi.

Scientific Names
Calophyllum inophyllum.
Family: Clusiaceae/Guttiferae.

People Use This For
Orally, the laurelwood constituent (+)-calanolide A is used for HIV infection. Laurelwood is also used orally for leprosy, piles, scabies, gonorrhea, vaginitis, and chicken pox.
Topically, tamanu oil from the nut of the laurelwood is used for skin ailments including sunburn, rashes, burns, psoriasis, dermatitis, scratches, skin blemishes, acne, skin allergies, bedsores, rosacea, and hemorrhoids; and for infant skin care.

Safety
POSSIBLY SAFE ...when the laurelwood constituent (+)-calanolide A is used orally by HIV-negative individuals (4290).
There is insufficient reliable information available about the safety of laurelwood for its other uses.
PREGNANCY AND LACTATION: Insufficient reliable information available; avoid using.

Effectiveness
There is insufficient reliable information available about the effectiveness of laurelwood.

Mechanism of Action
Laurelwood is one of many species of Calophyllum that contains constituents that seem to have activity against the HIV virus. Recent interest has centered on the calanolide compounds, particularly (+)-calanolide A. This constituent, now in phase I testing, appears to be a unique and specific non-nucleoside inhibitor of the reverse transcriptase of the HIV-1 virus (4292,4293). It does not appear to have activity against HIV-2 (4295). Some evidence suggests calanolide A might have synergistic effects with zidovudine (Retrovir), lamivudine (Epivir), nelfinavir (Viracept) (4290), and nevirapine (Viramune) (4294). At least two isomers of calanolide A known as costatolide and dihydrocostatolide possess similar properties (4291,4292). Calanolide A also shows evidence of antituberculosis effects (4290).

Adverse Reactions
Orally, the use of the laurelwood constituent, (+)- calanolide A, by healthy individuals can cause dizziness, oily aftertaste, headache, and nausea (4290).
Topically, there are no reported adverse reactions when tamanu oil from the nut of laurelwood is used.

Interactions with Herbs & Other Dietary Supplements
None known.

Interactions with Drugs
None known.

Interactions with Foods
None known.

Interactions with Lab Tests
None known.

Interactions with Diseases or Conditions
None known.

Dosage and Administration
No typical dosage.

Comments
The laurelwood constituent (+)-canolide A is in Phase IB testing as an anti-HIV agent. The purpose of the current study is to determine its safety and its effect on development of resistance, CD4 count and viral load (4289). Phase IA testing in 94 healthy HIV-negative individuals showed it was well tolerated (4290). Sarawak MediChem Pharmaceuticals Inc. (Lemont, Illinois) is the agency supporting testing (4289). Avoid confusing laurelwood (Caulophyllum inophyllum) with blue cohosh (Caulophyllum thalictroides).

LAVENDER

Also Known As
Alhucema, Common Lavender, English Lavender, French Lavender, Garden Lavender, Spanish Lavender, Spike Lavender, True Lavender.
CAUTION: See separate listing for Lavender Cotton.

Scientific Names
Lavandula angustifolia, synonyms Lavandula officinalis, Lavandula vera, Lavandula spica; Lavandula dentata; Lavandula latifolia; Lavandula pubescens; Lavandula stoechas.
Family: Lamiaceae/Labiatae.

People Use This For
Orally, lavender is used for restlessness, insomnia, nervousness, depression, meteorism (abdominal swelling from gas in the intestinal or peritoneal cavity), and loss of appetite. Lavender is also used orally for flatulence, upset stomach, giddiness, migraine headaches, toothaches, sprains, neuralgia, rheumatism, acne, sores, nausea, vomiting, to promote menstruation, and to treat cancer.
Topically, lavender is used for alopecia areata, pain, and in baths for circulation disorders.
By inhalation, lavender is used as aromatherapy for insomnia and pain.
In foods and beverages, lavender is used as a flavor component.
In manufacturing, lavender is utilized in pharmaceutical products and as a fragrance ingredient in soaps and cosmetics. Lavender is also used as an insect repellent.

Safety
LIKELY SAFE ...when used orally in amounts commonly found in foods. Lavender has Generally Recognized As Safe (GRAS) status for food use in the US (4912).
POSSIBLY SAFE ...when used orally and appropriately (9792). ...when used topically and appropriately (5177). Lavender oil has been used safely for up to 7 months (5177). ...when the essential oil is inhaled as a part of aromatherapy (7107).
PREGNANCY AND LACTATION: Insufficient reliable information available; avoid using.

Effectiveness
POSSIBLY EFFECTIVE

Alopecia areata. There is some evidence that applying lavender oil in combination with the essential oils from thyme, rosemary, and cedarwood might improve hair growth by as much as 44% after 7 months of treatment (5177).

INSUFFICIENT RELIABLE EVIDENCE to RATE

Depression. In mild to moderate depression, tincture of lavender appears to be slightly less effective than imipramine (Tofranil). Lavender might have some additive antidepressant effect with imipramine (9792). More evidence is needed to rate lavender for this use.

Mechanism of Action
The applicable parts of lavender are the flower and oil. Lavender preparations and the isolated constituents seem to have several pharmacological effects in vitro and in animals. However, effects in humans are less well known. Lavender seems to induce relaxation and sedation. Lavender decreases EEG potentials and decreases alertness in

humans (7). Lavender might also have stimulant effects on hair growth (5177); however, the mechanism of this effect is not known. There is some evidence that lavender has spasmolytic effects on smooth muscle (6) and might have analgesic effects (7107). There is some interest in lavender as an anticancer agent. The constituent perillyl alcohol seems to have some anticancer activity in vitro and in animal models (6). Theoretically, lavender can potentiate the effects of HMG CoA reductase inhibitors due to the perillyl alcohol content (6). There is also some evidence from animal models that lavender might have anticonvulsant effects and possibly potentiate chloral hydrate and pentobarbital effects (7).

Adverse Reactions

Orally, tincture of lavender may cause constipation, headache, and increased appetite (9792).
Topically, use of lavender rarely can cause contact dermatitis (6).

Interactions with Herbs & Other Dietary Supplements

None known.

Interactions with Drugs

BARBITURATES: Theoretically, lavender can potentiate the therapeutic effects of barbiturates (7). Some of these sedative medications include pentobarbital (Nembutal), phenobarbital (Luminal), secobarbital (Seconal), and others.
CHLORAL HYDRATE: Theoretically, lavender can potentiate the therapeutic effects of chloral hydrate (7).
CNS DEPRESSANTS: Theoretically, lavender can enhance the therapeutic and adverse effects of CNS depressants (7).

Interactions with Foods

None known.

Interactions with Lab Tests

SERUM CHOLESTEROL: Theoretically, lavender can decrease serum cholesterol levels and test results (6).

Interactions with Diseases or Conditions

None known.

Dosage and Administration

ORAL: For depression, tincture of lavender (1:5 in 50% alcohol) 60 drops per day has been used for 4 weeks (9792).
TOPICAL: For alopecia areata, one study used a combination of essential oils including lavender 3 drops (108 mg), rosemary 3 drops (114 mg), thyme 2 drops (88 mg), and cedarwood 2 drops (94 mg), all mixed with 3 mL jojoba oil and 20 mL grapeseed oil. Each night, the mixture is massaged into the scalp for 2 minutes with a warm towel placed around the head to increase absorption (5177).

Comments

Lavender is a popular component in perfumes, potpourri, and decorations (6002). Lavender is commonly adulterated with related species, including Lavandula hybrida, which is a cross between Lavandula angustifolia and Lavandula latifolia, from which lavandin oil is obtained (8).

LAVENDER COTTON

Also Known As

Santolina.
CAUTION: See separate listing for Lavender.

Scientific Names

Santolina chamaecyparissus.
Family: Asteraceae/Compositae.

People Use This For

Orally, lavender cotton is used for digestive disorders, premenstrual syndrome (PMS), worm infestations, jaundice, and as a spasmolytic. It is also used as an anti-inflammatory.
Topically, lavender cotton is used as an insect repellent.

Safety

There is insufficient reliable information available about the safety of lavender cotton.
Pregnancy and Lactation: Insufficient reliable information available; avoid using.

Effectiveness
There is insufficient reliable information available about the effectiveness of lavender cotton.

Mechanism of Action
The applicable parts of lavender cotton are the above ground parts and root bark. There is insufficient reliable information available about the possible mechanism of action and active ingredients.

Adverse Reactions
Lavender cotton may cause an allergic reaction in individuals sensitive to the Asteraceae/Compositae family. Members of this family include ragweed, chrysanthemums, marigolds, daisies, and many other herbs.

Interactions with Herbs & Other Dietary Supplements
None known.

Interactions with Drugs
None known.

Interactions with Foods
None known.

Interactions with Lab Tests
None known.

Interactions with Diseases or Conditions
CROSS-ALLERGENICITY: Lavender cotton may cause an allergic reaction in individuals sensitive to the Asteraceae/Compositae family. Members of this family include ragweed, chrysanthemums, marigolds, daisies, and many other herbs.

Dosage and Administration
ORAL: People typically prepare lavender cotton root bark using one teaspoon boiled in a covered container with 3 cups of water for 30 minutes. The liquid is cooled slowly in the closed container and taken cold, 1 to 2 cups per day (5254).

Comments
The whole lavender cotton plant is used externally as a moth and insect repellent due to its strong smell (18). Lavender cotton is unrelated to lavender and its scent is distinctly different from that of lavender (513).

LECITHIN

Also Known As
Egg Lecithin, Ovolecithin, Soy Bean Lecithin, Soy Lecithin, Soya Lecithin, Soybean Lecithin, Vegilecithin, Vitellin.
CAUTION: See separate listings for Alpha-GPC, Choline, Phosphatidylcholine, Phosphatidylserine, and Soy.

Scientific Names
None.

People Use This For
Orally, lecithin is used for treating dementia and Alzheimer's disease, for extrapyramidal disorders, reducing hepatic steatosis (fat accumulation) in long-term parenteral nutrition patients, treating gallbladder disease, aiding ultrafiltration in peritoneal dialysis, treating liver disease, treating manic-depressive illness, improving memory, treating hypercholesterolemia, for anxiety, and eczema. It is also used as a source of choline, inositol, phosphorus, and linoleic and linolenic acids.
Topically, lecithin is used as a moisturizing agent for dermatitis and dry skin.
As a pharmaceutical and food additive, lecithin is used for emulsifying and stabilizing water-based products, and as an antioxidant in foods and pharmaceutical preparations. In the manufacture of preparations for intravenous and subcutaneous use, lecithin is used both as an emulsifying agent and a stabilizing agent.

Safety
LIKELY SAFE ...when used orally in amounts found in foods. Lecithin has Generally Recognized As Safe (GRAS) status in the US (4912). ...when used orally and appropriately for medicinal purposes (2619,4914). ...when used topically (4914). ...when used intravenously or subcutaneously and appropriately (16,4914).

PREGNANCY AND LACTATION: Insufficient reliable information available; avoid using in amounts greater than found in foods.

Effectiveness

LIKELY EFFECTIVE

Dermatitis. Applying lecithin topically seems to improve dermatitis (272).

Dry skin. Applying lecithin topically seems to reduce dry skin (272).

POSSIBLY EFFECTIVE

Hepatic steatosis. Taking lecithin orally seems to reduce hepatic steatosis in patients on long-term parenteral nutrition (5140).

POSSIBLY INEFFECTIVE

Gallbladder disease. Taking lecithin orally doesn't seem to resolve gallbladder disease (5142,5155).

Hypercholesterolemia. Taking lecithin orally doesn't seem to lower cholesterol levels (5147,5148).

LIKELY INEFFECTIVE

Alzheimer's disease and dementia. Taking lecithin orally doesn't improve symptoms of dementia and Alzheimer's disease (5149,5150,5151,5152).

Extrapyramidal disorders. Taking lecithin orally doesn't help extrapyramidal disorders (5139,6243).

There is insufficient reliable information available about the effectiveness of lecithin for its other uses.

Mechanism of Action

Lecithin is a phospholipid composed of phosphatidyl esters (phosphatides), chiefly consisting of phosphatidylcholine, phosphatidylethanolamine, phosphatidylserine and phosphatidylinositol, and varying amounts of other substances such as triglycerides, fatty acids, and carbohydrates, depending on source (9). For example, egg lecithin contains 69% phosphatidylcholine and 24% phosphatidylethanolamine, while soybean lecithin contains 24% phosphatidylcholine, 22% phosphatidylethanolamine, and 19% phosphatidylinositol. Lecithin is a precursor to acetylcholine (5156).

Adverse Reactions

Orally, lecithin can cause diarrhea, nausea, abdominal pain, or fullness (5140,6243).

Interactions with Herbs & Other Dietary Supplements

None known.

Interactions with Drugs

None known.

Interactions with Foods

None known.

Interactions with Lab Tests

None known.

Interactions with Diseases or Conditions

None known.

Dosage and Administration

ORAL: A typical oral dose is 1.2-2.4 grams/day (5153). for reducing cholesterol 20-30 grams daily has been used in studies (5147,5148). For improving memory and Alzheimer's disease, 20-45 grams daily has been tried (5146,5149,5151,5152).

Comments

Unlike choline, lecithin does not cause unpleasant body and breath odor (5153). Lecithin contains phosphatidylcholine, which contains choline (16). Although closely related, these terms are not synonymous.

LEMON

Also Known As

Limon, Nimbaka, Nimbuka.

Scientific Names

Citrus limon, synonym Citrus limonum.
Family: Rutaceae.

People Use This For

Orally, lemon is used as a source of vitamin C in the treatment of scurvy, low resistance, and colds. It is also used as a digestive aid, an anti-inflammatory, diuretic, and to improve vascular permeability.
In foods, lemon is used as a food and flavoring agent.

Safety

LIKELY SAFE ...when used in amounts commonly found in foods. Lemon has Generally Recognized As Safe (GRAS) status in the US (4912).
POSSIBLY SAFE ...when used orally in medicinal amounts (12).
PREGNANCY AND LACTATION: Avoid using in amounts greater than those typically found in foods.

Effectiveness

There is insufficient reliable information available about the effectiveness of lemon.

Mechanism of Action

The applicable parts of lemon are the fruit, juice, and peel. Limonene is the most abundant monoterpene in lemon juice (4946). The furocoumarins bergapten and oxypeucedanin in lemon oil are photosensitizing (11019).

Adverse Reactions

Topically, photosensitivity can occur especially in fair-skinned people (11909).

Interactions with Herbs & Other Dietary Supplements

None known.

Interactions with Drugs

None known.

Interactions with Foods

None known.

Interactions with Lab Tests

None known.

Interactions with Diseases or Conditions

None known.

Dosage and Administration

ORAL: Lemon is taken as an oil, tincture, or fresh fruit (18).

LEMON BALM

Also Known As

Balm, Cure-All, Dropsy Plant, Honey Plant, Melissa, Melissae folium, Melissenblatt, Sweet Balm, Sweet Mary.

Scientific Names

Melissa officinalis.
Family: Lamiaceae/Labiatae.

People Use This For

Orally, lemon balm is used for promoting digestion, as a mild tranquilizer, for stimulating appetite, as an antispasmodic, for Graves' disease, and for functional gastrointestinal disorders with distention and gas. Lemon balm is also used for promoting sweating, promoting menstrual flow, female discomforts, nervous problems, insomnia, cramps, headache, toothache, sores, tumors, and insect bites. It is also used for attention deficit-hyperactivity disorder (ADHD), Alzheimer's disease, nervous stomach, hysteria and melancholia, chronic bronchial mucous membrane inflammation, nervous palpitations, vomiting, and high blood pressure.
As an inhalant, lemon balm is used as aroma therapy for Alzheimer's disease.
Topically, lemon balm is used for cold sores (herpes labialis).
In foods and beverages, the extract and oil of lemon balm are used for flavoring.

Safety

LIKELY SAFE ...when used orally in amounts commonly found in foods. Lemon balm has Generally Recognized As Safe (GRAS) status in the US (4912).

POSSIBLY SAFE ...when used appropriately for oral or topical medicinal purposes on a short-term basis (790,9993,9994,9995). Oral lemon balm has been used with apparent safety for up to 4 months (9993). The safety of long-term use is unknown.

PREGNANCY AND LACTATION: Insufficient reliable information available; avoid using.

Effectiveness

POSSIBLY EFFECTIVE

Alzheimer's disease. Taking a standardized extract of lemon balm orally, daily for 4 months, seems to reduce agitation and improve symptoms of mild to moderate Alzheimer's disease on standard Alzheimer's disease rating scales (9993).

Herpes labialis (cold sores). Applying a lip balm containing 1% lemon balm extract seems to shorten healing time, prevent infection spread, and reduce symptoms of recurring herpes labialis (790,9995).

Sleep. Taking lemon balm orally, in combination with valerian, appears to improve the quality and quantity of sleep (10423).

There is insufficient reliable information available about the effectiveness of lemon balm for its other uses.

Mechanism of Action

The applicable part of lemon balm is the leaf and leaf oil. Lemon balm seems to have sedative, antioxidant, and antiviral effects (790,9993,9994,9995). Lemon balm contains citronellal, neral, and geranial monoterpenoid aldehydes; flavonoids and polyphenolic compounds (including rosmarinic acid); and monoterpene glycosides. These substances may contribute to the behavioral effects of lemon balm dried leaf and essential oil (9994). Some research suggests lemon balm might have acetylcholine receptor activity with both nicotinic and muscarinic binding properties (9994). Clinical research suggests that lemon balm induces a calming effect and reduces alertness (9994).

Lemon balm is used in aroma therapy. The essential oil of lemon balm contains terpenes, which are rapidly absorbed through the lungs and cross the blood-brain barrier. In addition, these may possess cholinergic activity or act on gamma-aminobutyric acid (GABA) receptors (10422).

Adverse Reactions

Orally, lemon balm is well tolerated. It can cause nausea, vomiting, abdominal pain, dizziness, and wheezing (9993). Topically, there is one report of irritation and one report of exacerbation of herpes symptoms when lemon balm was applied (790).

Interactions with Herbs & Other Dietary Supplements

HERBS WITH SEDATIVE PROPERTIES: Theoretically, concomitant use with herbs that have sedative properties might enhance therapeutic and adverse effects (9994). Some of these supplements include 5-HTP, calamus, California poppy, catnip, hops, Jamaican dogwood, kava, St. John's wort, scullcap, valerian, yerba mansa, and others.

Interactions with Drugs

CNS DEPRESSANTS: Theoretically, concomitant use of lemon balm with drugs with sedative properties may cause additive effects and side effects (9994).

Interactions with Foods

ETHANOL: Theoretically, lemon balm might increase the sedative effects of ethanol (9994).

Interactions with Lab Tests

None known.

Interactions with Diseases or Conditions

None known.

Dosage and Administration

ORAL: For mild to moderate Alzheimer's disease, 60 drops per day of a standardized lemon balm extract, prepared 1:1 in 45% alcohol, has been used (9993). For sleep, lemon balm extract 80 mg, with valerian extract 120 mg 3 times daily, has been used for up to 30 days (10423).

TOPICAL: For herpes labialis (cold sores), the cream or ointment containing 1% of a 70:1 lyophilized aqueous extract is usually applied two to four times daily from first sign of prodrome to a few days after the lesions have healed (790,9995).

LEMON VERBENA

Also Known As
Herb Louisa, Lemon-Scented Verbena, Louisa, Verveine Citronelle.
CAUTION: See separate listing for Verbena.

Scientific Names
Aloysia citrodora, synonyms Aloysia triphylla, Lippia citrodora, Lippia triphylla, Verbena triphylla, Zappania citrodora.
Family: Verbenaceae.

People Use This For
Orally, lemon verbena is used for digestive disorders, agitation, insomnia, asthma, cold, fever, flatulence, colic, diarrhea, indigestion, febrile hemorrhoids, varicose veins, skin conditions, chills, and constipation.
In foods and manufacturing, lemon verbena is used as an ingredient in herbal teas, as a fragrance component in perfumes, and also as an ingredient in alcoholic beverages.

Safety
LIKELY SAFE ...when used orally in amounts commonly found in foods. Lemon verbena has Generally Recognized As Safe (GRAS) status in the US (4912).
POSSIBLY SAFE ...when used orally and appropriately in medicinal amounts (12).
There is insufficient reliable information available about the safety of lemon verbena when used topically.
PREGNANCY AND LACTATION: Insufficient reliable information available; avoid using.

Effectiveness
There is insufficient reliable information available about the effectiveness of lemon verbena.

Mechanism of Action
The applicable parts of lemon verbena are the leaf and flowering tops. Oil of verbena (the essential oil distilled from lemon verbena leaf) may be acaricidal and bactericidal (6). Terpene-rich volatile oils in the plant are considered irritants (4).

Adverse Reactions
Orally, volatile oils may irritate the kidneys during excretion (4).
Topically, contact dermatitis may occur (6).

Interactions with Herbs & Other Dietary Supplements
None known.

Interactions with Drugs
None known.

Interactions with Foods
None known.

Interactions with Lab Tests
None known.

Interactions with Diseases or Conditions
KIDNEY DISEASE: Avoid excessive amounts due to possible kidney irritation (4).

Dosage and Administration
ORAL: One cup tea has been used two to five times daily (18). The tea is prepared by steeping 5-29 grams of the leaf in 1 L of boiling water for 10-15 minutes then straining (18).
TOPICAL: No typical dosage.

LEMONGRASS

Also Known As
British Indian Lemongrass, Capim-Cidrao, Ceylon Citronella Grass, Citronella, Cochin Lemongrass, East Indian Lemongrass, Fever Grass, Guatemala Lemongrass, Lemon Grass, Madagascar Lemongrass, West Indian Lemongrass.
CAUTION: See separate listings for Citronella Oil and Stone Root.

Scientific Names
Cymbopogon citratus, synonym Andropogon citratus; Cymbopogon flexuosus, synonym Andropogon flexuosus.
Family: Poaceae/Gramineae.

People Use This For
Orally, lemongrass is used for treating gastrointestinal spasms, stomachache, hypertension, convulsions, pain and neuralgia, vomiting, cough, rheumatism, fever, common cold, and exhaustion. It is also used orally as an antiseptic and as a mild astringent.
Topically, lemongrass and its essential oil are used for headache, stomachache, abdominal pain, and musculoskeletal pain.
By inhalation, the essential oil of lemongrass is used as aromatherapy for musculoskeletal pain.
In food and beverages, lemongrass is used as a flavoring.
In manufacturing, lemongrass is used as a fragrance in soaps and cosmetics. Lemongrass is also used in synthesizing vitamin A and natural citral.

Safety
LIKELY SAFE ...when used orally in amounts commonly found in foods. Lemongrass has Generally Recognized As Safe (GRAS) status in the US (4912).
POSSIBLY SAFE ...when used orally or topically, short-term for medicinal purposes. Lemongrass has been safely used in studies lasting up to 2 weeks (6,12,2612,7107). ...when the essential oil of lemongrass is used by inhalation as a component of aromatherapy (7107).
PREGNANCY: LIKELY UNSAFE ...when used orally. Lemongrass seems to have uterine and menstrual flow stimulating effects (12); avoid using.
LACTATION: Insufficient reliable information available; avoid using.

Effectiveness
There is insufficient reliable information available about the effectiveness of lemongrass.

Mechanism of Action
The applicable part of lemongrass is the leaf and oil. The lemongrass leaves are commonly used as "lemon" flavoring in herbal teas. The essential oil from lemongrass contains geraniol, limonene, alpha-pinene, and alpha-terpineole, which have antimicrobial properties (2130,7162). The oil has in vitro antimicrobial activity against a variety of common gram positive and gram negative organisms, including Acinetobacter calcoacetica, Enterococcus faecalis, Escherichia coli, Klebsiella pneumoniae, Pseudomonas aeruginosa, Salmonella species, Serratia marcescens, Staphylococcus aureus, and the yeast Candida albicans (2131). Lemongrass oil also contains citral, 65-85%. Although citral is a central nervous system (CNS) depressant (11,7162), lemongrass does not seem to have significant CNS effects (2612). Lemongrass is also thought to have analgesic, antipyretic, and antioxidant properties (11), as well as uterine and menstrual flow stimulating effects (12).

Adverse Reactions
Orally, there is a single report of fatal poisoning after a child ingested a lemongrass oil-based insect repellent (2).
Topically, rare allergic reactions have occurred following use (2,18).
By inhalation, there have been two cases of toxic alveolitis associated with an unknown quantity of lemongrass oil (2).

Interactions with Herbs & Other Dietary Supplements
None known.

Interactions with Drugs
None known.

Interactions with Foods
None known.

Interactions with Lab Tests
AMYLASE, BILIRUBIN: Lemongrass may cause elevations in serum bilirubin (direct) and amylase levels (2612).

Interactions with Diseases or Conditions
None known.

Dosage and Administration
ORAL: People typically use 1 to 2 teaspoons of lemongrass in 6 oz boiling water as a tea (6006).
TOPICAL: No typical dosage.

Comments
Avoid confusion with citronella oil (Cymbopogon nardus).

LENTINAN

Also Known As
None.
CAUTION: See separate listing for Shiitake Mushroom.

Scientific Names
Polysaccharide derived from Lentinus edodes, synonyms Lenticus edodes, Lentinan edodes, Lentinula edodes, Tricholomopsis edodes.
Family: Polyporaceae.

People Use This For
Lentinan is given by intravenous, intramuscular, and intraperitoneal injection as an adjunctive treatment for cancer and HIV infection.

Safety
There is insufficient reliable information available about the safety of lentinan.
Pregnancy and Lactation: Insufficient reliable information available; avoid using.

Effectiveness
POSSIBLY EFFECTIVE

Breast cancer. Administering lentinan by injection as adjunctive treatment seems to help improve response in patients being treated for breast cancer (1112).

Gastric cancer. Administering lentinan by injection as adjunctive treatment seems to help improve response in patients being treated for gastric cancer (1108,1113).

HIV/AIDS. Administering lentinan by injection as adjunctive treatment in combination with didanosine (ddI) seems to increase CD4 counts compared to ddI alone (1107).

Prostate cancer. Administering lentinan by injection as adjunctive treatment seems to help improve response in patients being treated for prostate cancer (1109).

Mechanism of Action
Lentinan is not directly cytotoxic, but may augment natural killer cell activity, activate macrophages and may enhance T-helper cell function (6). It may enhance the anti-HIV effects of zidovudine (6).

Adverse Reactions
Mild thrombocytopenia (6); minor adverse effects (unspecified) were reported in clinical trials (one case report) (6). Rapid intravenous infusion of lentinan is reported to cause "oppression" of the anterior chest and dryness of the throat; these symptoms disappeared with slow drip infusion (1111).

Interactions with Herbs & Other Dietary Supplements
None known.

Interactions with Drugs
None known.

Interactions with Foods
None known.

Interactions with Lab Tests
CD4 COUNTS: Intravenously administered lentinan, combined with didanosine (ddI, Videx), might enhance drug-induced increases in CD4 concentrations and test results in some HIV+ patients with low CD4 counts (1107).

Interactions with Diseases or Conditions
MALNUTRITION: In one clinical trial, gastric cancer patients with low serum protein levels (consistent with poor nutritional status) did not respond to lentinan therapy, while patients with normal serum protein levels (consistent with adequate nutritional status) had favorable responses to lentinan (1110).

Dosage and Administration
ORAL: No typical dosage.
INJECTION: 1-4 mg per week have been used in clinical trials (6,1108,1111).

Comments
Lentinan is a polysaccharide derived from shiitake mushroom (Lenticus edode).

LESSER CELANDINE

Also Known As
Ficaria, Figwort, Pilewort, Ranunculus, Smallwort.
CAUTION: See separate listings for Amaranth, Bulbous Buttercup, Greater Celandine, and Jewelweed.

Scientific Names
Ranunculus ficaria.
Family: Ranunculaceae.

People Use This For
Orally, lesser celandine is used for scurvy.
Topically, lesser celandine is used for bleeding wounds and gums, swollen joints, warts, scratches, and hemorrhoids (internal or prolapsed piles, with or without hemorrhage).
For food uses, fresh leaf sheaths of lesser celandine are sometimes used in salads.

Safety
POSSIBLY SAFE ...when small amounts of fresh leaf sheaths are eaten (18).
POSSIBLY UNSAFE ...when used topically (4,18). Extended contact with the fresh, bruised plant can cause blisters (18).
LIKELY UNSAFE ...when used orally (4,18); avoid using.
PREGNANCY AND LACTATION: LIKELY UNSAFE ...when used orally (4); avoid using.

Effectiveness
There is insufficient reliable information available about the effectiveness of lesser celandine.

Mechanism of Action
The applicable parts of lesser celandine are the above ground parts. Lesser celandine contains large amounts of vitamin C (18). It also has astringent and demulcent effects (4). Protoanemonin, a constituent, is believed to be an acrid skin irritant (4). However, when the above ground parts are dried or prepared, protoanemonin changes into a pungent, volatile intermediate that quickly dimerizes to a form that does not irritate the mucous membrane (18). Some studies suggest the constituents, anemonin and protoanemonin, might have antibacterial and antifungal activity (4). The saponin constituents show some evidence of antihemorrhoidal activity (4). Large amounts of protoanemonin-forming plants have caused death of experimental animals by asphyxiation (18).

Adverse Reactions
Orally, use is associated with severe GI irritation, colic, diarrhea, and irritation of the urinary tract (18). One report associates the use of lesser celandine with a case of recurrent, acute hepatitis (390).
Topically, use can cause mucous membrane and skin irritation (18). Extended contact with fresh, bruised plant can cause blisters (18). Some Ranunculus species also cause photodermatitis (19).

Interactions with Herbs & Other Dietary Supplements
None known.

Interactions with Drugs
None known.

Interactions with Foods
None known.

Interactions with Lab Tests
None known.

Interactions with Diseases or Conditions
GI CONDITIONS: Lesser celandine can irritate gastrointestinal tract. Contraindicated in individuals with infectious or inflammatory gastrointestinal conditions (19).

Dosage and Administration
ORAL: No typical dosage.
TOPICAL: Liquid extract (1:1 in 25% alcohol), 2-5 mL 3 times daily (4). Ointment (3%) or Pilewort Ointment (30% fresh herb in benzoinated lard) (4). Liquid extract can be added to baths for hemorrhoids, warts, or scratches (18).

Comments
Avoid confusion with greater celandine (Chelidonium majus). Scrophularia nodosa (Family: Scrophulariaceae) is also referred to as figwort (4). Amaranth and bulbous buttercup are also referred to as pilewort.

LEVANT BERRY

Also Known As
Cocculus, Cocculus Indicus, Coculus Fructus, Fish Berries, Fish Killer, Hockle Elderberry, Indian Berry, Levant Nut, Louseberry, Poisonberry.
CAUTION: See separate listings for Chenopodium Oil, Mugwort, Wormseed, Wormwood, and Wormwood Oil.

Scientific Names
Anamirta cocculus, synonyms Anamirta paniculata, Menispermum cocculus, Menispermum lacunosum; Cocculus suberosus; Cocculus lacunosus.
Family: Menispermaceae.

People Use This For
Orally, levant berry is used for peripheral and vestibular nystagmus and peripherally-based dizziness. The constituent, picrotoxin, is used orally for treating epilepsy, night sweats, and as a stimulant for barbituric acid poisoning.
Topically, it is used as a powder to treat scabies.
In India, the leaves are inhaled as snuff to relieve malaria; whole fruits are used for paralyzing fish and killing birds or dogs; picrotoxin is applied to arrow tips for hunting by jungle tribes, and was formerly used to paralyze fish in the fishing industry; extracts are applied topically for lice.

Safety
POSSIBLY UNSAFE ...when used topically; avoid application to broken skin (6).
LIKELY UNSAFE ...when used orally due to toxic potential (6). Picrotoxin 30 mg/kg or 2-3 cocculus kernels can cause death (6,18).
PREGNANCY AND LACTATION: LIKELY UNSAFE ...when used orally or topically (6); avoid using.

Effectiveness
There is insufficient reliable information available about the effectiveness of levant berry.

Mechanism of Action
The applicable parts of levant berry are the dried fruit and seed. The seed contains highly toxic picrotoxin (6,18), which stimulates the central nervous system via parasympathetic nerves, is a GI irritant, stimulates the medulla oblongata resulting in changes in respiration rate, slows heart rate due to vagal nerve stimulation, and increases blood pressure (6,18).

Adverse Reactions
Picrotoxin is a GI irritant and central nervous system stimulant (6). Mild poisoning can lead to headache, dizziness, nausea, coordination disturbances, depression, and spasms or twitching (18). Larger amounts can cause salivation,

vomiting, purging, rapid shallow breathing, drowsiness, palpitations or bradycardia, tonic-clonic spasms, stupor, loss of consciousness, and death (6). The lethal dose is stated to be 30 mg/kg (6) or 2-3 Cocculus kernels (seeds) (18).

Interactions with Herbs & Other Dietary Supplements
None known.

Interactions with Drugs
None known.

Interactions with Foods
None known.

Interactions with Lab Tests
None known.

Interactions with Diseases or Conditions
None known.

Dosage and Administration
No typical dosage.

Comments
Although picrotoxin is used experimentally, medicinal use has been abandoned in the US and Europe (6).

LICORICE

Also Known As
Alcacuz, Alcazuz, Chinese Licorice, Gan Cao, Gan Zao, Glycyrrhiza, Glycyrrhiza glabra typica, Glycyrrhiza glabra violacea, Isoflavone, Isoflavones, Jethi-Madh, Mulhathi, Lakritze, Licorice Root, Liquiritiae radix, Liquirizia, Liquorice, Orozuz, Phytoestrogen, Reglisse, Regliz, Russian Licorice, Spanish Licorice, Subholz, Sweet Root, Yashtimadhu, Yashti-Madhu, Yashti-Madhuka.

Scientific Names
Glycyrrhiza glabra; Glycyrrhiza glabra var. glandulifera; Glycyrrhiza uralensis.
Family: Fabaceae/Leguminosae.

People Use This For
Orally, licorice is used for gastric and duodenal ulcers, sore throat, bronchitis, chronic gastritis, colic, primary adrenocortical insufficiency, dry cough, arthritis, systemic lupus erythematosus (SLE), and for bacterial and viral infections. It is also used orally for cholestatic liver disorders, hypokalemia, hypertonia, malaria, tuberculosis, abscesses, food poisoning, diabetes insipidus, and contact dermatitis.

In combination with Panax ginseng and Bupleurum falcatum, licorice is used orally to help stimulate adrenal gland function, particularly in patients with a history of long-term corticosteroid use. As a component of the herbal formula, Shakuyaku-Kanzo-To, licorice is used to increase fertility in women with polycystic ovary syndrome. In combination with other herbs, licorice is used to treat prostate cancer.

Topically, licorice is used as a shampoo to reduce sebum secretion.

Intravenously, licorice components are used for treating hepatitis B and C.

Licorice is used as a flavoring in foods, beverages, and tobacco.

Safety
LIKELY SAFE ...when used orally in amounts commonly found in foods. Licorice has Generally Recognized As Safe (GRAS) status in the US (4912). The maximum safe daily intake of licorice is equivalent to 100 mg glycyrrhizin (2).

POSSIBLY SAFE ...when used orally and appropriately for medicinal purposes, short-term. Advise patients to avoid using licorice for more than 4-6 weeks or in large amounts without medical supervision (12).

PREGNANCY: UNSAFE ...when used orally. Licorice has abortifacient, estrogenic, and steroid effects; and can cause uterine stimulation. Heavy consumption of licorice, 500 mg per week or more, during pregnancy seems to increase the risk of delivering before gestational age of 38 weeks (7619,10618); avoid using.

LACTATION: Insufficient reliable information available; avoid using.

Effectiveness

INSUFFICIENT RELIABLE EVIDENCE to RATE

Hepatitis. Preliminary evidence suggests that isolated constituents of licorice may be effective for treating hepatitis B and C. Glycyrrhizin- and glycyrrhizic acid-containing intravenous preparations (Stronger Neominophagen C and Remefa S) show activity against hepatitis B and hepatitis C in humans, but the trials are too small to draw any definitive conclusions (3247,3250,3251).

Peptic ulcers. There is some evidence that deglycyrrhizinated licorice (DGL) might accelerate the healing of peptic ulcers (11312,11313).

Weight loss. There is conflicting information about the use of licorice for weight loss. Licorice has been shown to reduce body fat, however accompanying fluid retention offsets any change in body weight (6196).

More evidence is needed to rate licorice for these uses.

Mechanism of Action

The applicable part of licorice is the root. Licorice has antispasmodic, anti-inflammatory, laxative, and soothing properties. The constituents glycyrrhizin and glycyrrhetinic acid inhibit 11-beta-hydroxysteroid dehydrogenase, an enzyme located in the aldosterone receptor cells of the cortical collecting duct (4,10619). Glycyrrhizin may contribute to licorice-associated mineralocorticoid side effects, including hypertension and hypokalemia, by both binding directly to mineralocorticoid receptors and by decreasing the conversion of active cortisol to inactive cortisone (3252,3253,6600,7620,10619). Panax ginseng appears to compliment licorice by increasing serum cortisol concentrations (3257).

Licorice appears to block metabolism of prostaglandins E and F2 alpha, which suggests a possible beneficial effect on peptic ulcer. Concomitant use of licorice and nonsteroidal anti-inflammatory drugs (NSAIDs) might compound sodium and water retention (504), and protect against NSAID-induced damage to the gastrointestinal (GI) mucosa (19). Preliminary information suggests deglycyrrhizinated licorice (DGL) may accelerate the healing of peptic ulcers. DGL seems to be similar to carbenoxolone for ulcer reduction without the fluid retention or electrolyte imbalance of carbenoxolone. Carbenoxolone is a semisynthetic derivative of glycyrrhetic acid that is used outside the US for treating gastric and duodenal ulcer disease (11311,11312,11313).

Licorice appears to have anti-estrogenic and estrogenic action. Preliminary research indicates that licorice does not stimulate the growth of estrogen dependent breast cancer cells (7860). However, the estrogenic effects of licorice might be concentration dependent. Glabridin, an isoflavone constituent of licorice, seems to have an estrogen receptor-dependent growth-promoting effect at low concentrations. At higher concentrations, it seems to have an estrogen receptor-independent antiproliferative effect (10617).

Licorice has been shown to reduce body fat, however accompanying fluid retention offsets any change in body weight (6196). Licorice also decreases testosterone production, which might account for the decreased serum testosterone concentrations in young healthy men who eat licorice (3246). Glycyrrhizin- and glycyrrhizic acid-containing intravenous preparations (Stronger Neominophagen C and Remefa S) show activity against hepatitis B and C in humans, but the trials are too small to draw any definitive conclusions (3247,3250,3251). In vitro data suggests that glycyrrhizin suppresses the production and expression of hepatitis B surface antigen (HbS-Ag) (3248,3249). Preliminary evidence suggests that glycyrrhizin may inhibit the growth of the coronavirus, which is associated with severe acute respiratory syndrome (SARS). The exact mechanism of the antiviral effect of glycyrrhizin is not known (10299).

Adverse Reactions

Orally, licorice may cause hypertension, sodium and water retention, edema, lethargy, amenorrhea, and headache with consumption of 50 grams per day or chronic use longer than six weeks. Higher levels of consumption may cause hypokalemia, hypokalemic myopathy, rhabdomyolysis, myoglobinuria, severe congestive heart failure (CHF), pulmonary edema, lower extremity weakness, hypertensive encephalopathy, and quadriplegia due to pseudoaldosteronism and hypermineralocorticoidism (781,6600,7620,10619,10393). Hypokalemia caused by licorice can cause muscle weakness and dropped head syndrome (DHS) (10393). Because licorice can decrease serum testosterone and increase 17-hydroxyprogesterone, it might cause decreased libido and sexual dysfunction in men (3246). Chewing tobacco flavored with licorice has also been associated with toxicity (6).

Interactions with Herbs & Other Dietary Supplements

HERBS WITH CARDIAC ACTIVITY: Theoretically, the overuse or misuse of licorice can increase the risk of cardiotoxicity due to potassium depletion (10393). Cardioactive herbs include digitalis, lily-of-the-valley, pheasant's eye, and squill.

STIMULANT LAXATIVE HERBS: Theoretically, concomitant overuse or misuse of licorice with stimulant laxatives can increase the risk of potassium depletion (10393). Stimulant laxative herbs include aloe vera, alder buckthorn, European buckthorn, cascara sagrada, castor oil, rhubarb, and senna.

Interactions with Drugs

ANTIHYPERTENSIVE DRUGS: Theoretically, licorice might reduce the effect of antihypertensive drug therapy. Large amounts of licorice can cause sodium and water retention, and hypertension (515).

CORTICOSTEROIDS: Theoretically, concomitant use might potentiate the duration of activity of corticosteroids,

e.g., hydrocortisone (19). Concomitant use of licorice and corticosteroids might also increase potassium loss and increase the risk of potassium depletion. Overuse or misuse of licorice can cause potassium depletion (10393).
CYTOCHROME P450 2B6 (CYP2B6) SUBSTRATES: There's preliminary evidence that licorice can inhibit the cytochrome P450 2B6 (CYP2B6) isoenzymes (10300). Theoretically, licorice might increase levels of drugs metabolized by CYP2B6; however, as of yet, these interactions have not been reported in humans. Some drugs that are metabolized by CYP2B6 include ketamine (Ketalar), phenobarbital, orphenadrine (Norflex), secobarbital (Seconal), and dexamethasone (Decadron). Use licorice cautiously or avoid in patients taking these drugs.
CYTOCHROME P450 3A4 (CYP3A4) SUBSTRATES: There's preliminary evidence that licorice can inhibit the cytochrome P450 3A4 (CYP3A4) isoenzymes (6450,10300). Theoretically, licorice might increase levels of drugs metabolized by CYP3A4; however, as of yet, these interactions have not been reported in humans. Some drugs metabolized by CYP3A4 include lovastatin (Mevacor), ketoconazole (Nizoral), itraconazole (Sporanox), fexofenadine (Allegra), triazolam (Halcion), and numerous others.
DIGOXIN (Lanoxin): Overuse or misuse of licorice with cardiac glycoside therapy might increase the risk of cardiac toxicity due to potassium loss (19).
DIURETIC DRUGS: Overuse of licorice might compound diuretic-induced potassium loss (10393). There is some concern that people taking licorice along with potassium depleting diuretics might have an increased risk for hypokalemia. Initiation of potassium supplementation or an increase in potassium supplement dose may be necessary for some patients. Some diuretics that can deplete potassium include chlorothiazide (Diuril), chlorthalidone (Thalitone), furosemide (Lasix), hydrochlorothiazide (HCTZ, HydroDIURIL, Microzide), and others.
ESTROGENS: Theoretically, licorice might interfere with hormone therapy due to estrogenic and anti-estrogenic effects (4).
ETHACRYNIC ACID (Edecrin): Theoretically, ethacrynic acid might enhance the mineralocorticoid effects of licorice by inhibiting the enzyme that converts cortisol to cortisone; however, bumetanide (Bumex) does not appear to have this effect (3255).
FUROSEMIDE (Lasix): Theoretically, furosemide might enhance the mineralocorticoid effects of licorice by inhibiting the enzyme that converts cortisol to cortisone; however, bumetanide (Bumex) does not appear to have this effect (3255).
INSULIN: Theoretically, concomitant use might cause hypokalemia and sodium retention (19).

Interactions with Foods

GRAPEFRUIT JUICE: Theoretically, grapefruit juice and its component naringenin might enhance the mineralocorticoid activities of licorice, by blocking the conversion of cortisol to cortisone (3254,3255).

Interactions with Lab Tests

17-HYDROXYPROGESTERONE: Licorice can increase serum 17-hydroxyprogesterone concentrations and test results (3246).
BLOOD PRESSURE: Excessive use of licorice can cause hypertension and increase blood pressure readings (1372).
POTASSIUM: Excessive use of licorice can cause hypokalemia, reducing serum potassium levels and test results (10393).
TESTOSTERONE: Licorice can decrease serum testosterone concentrations and test results (3246).

Interactions with Diseases or Conditions

DIABETES: The mineralocorticoid effects of licorice may interfere with blood glucose control (12). Advise patients with diabetes to avoid licorice.
HEART DISEASE: The mineralocorticoid effects of licorice can induce fluid retention and worsen congestive heart failure (4). Licorice can also cause hypokalemia and increase the risk of arrhythmias. Advise patients with heart disease to avoid licorice.
HORMONE SENSITIVE CANCERS/CONDITIONS: Licorice might have estrogenic effects (6180). Women with hormone sensitive conditions should avoid using licorice. Some of these conditions include breast cancer, uterine cancer, ovarian cancer, endometriosis, and uterine fibroids.
HYPERTENSION: The mineralocorticoid effects of licorice increase blood pressure. Advise patients with hypertension to avoid licorice (1372).
HYPERTONIA: Licorice-induced hypokalemia may worsen hypertonia (2).
HYPOKALEMIA: Licorice can cause hypokalemia (10393).
KIDNEY INSUFFICIENCY: The mineralocorticoid effects of licorice may worsen renal function. Advise patients with severe renal insufficiency to avoid licorice (2).
LIVER DISEASE: Licorice is contraindicated in cholestatic liver disorders and liver cirrhosis (2). Patients with liver disease might be more sensitive to the mineralocorticoid effects of licorice (4).
SEXUAL DYSFUNCTION: Theoretically, licorice might decrease libido and worsen erectile dysfunction by decreasing testosterone and increasing 17-hydroxyprogesterone serum concentrations (3246).

Dosage and Administration

ORAL: The typical dose of licorice is 1-4 grams of the powdered root or one cup of the tea three times daily (4). The tea is prepared by simmering 1-4 grams of the powdered root in 150 mL boiling water for 5-10 minutes and then

straining. The usual dose of Succus liquiritiae is 0.5-1 gram for upper respiratory tract mucous membrane inflammation and 1.5-3 grams for gastric and duodenal ulcers.
TOPICAL: No typical dosage.
INTRAVENOUS: No typical dosage.

Comments
Many "licorice" products manufactured in the US actually don't contain any licorice. Instead, they contain anise oil, which has the characteristic smell and taste of the flavor black licorice.

LILY-OF-THE-VALLEY

Also Known As
Constancy, Convallaria, Convallaria herba, Convall-Lily, Jacob's Ladder, Ladder-To-Heaven, Lily, Lily of the Valley, May Bells, May Lily, Muguet, Our Lady's Tears.
CAUTION: See separate listings for Abscess Root and Jacob's Ladder.

Scientific Names
Convallaria majalis.
Family: Liliaceae or Convallariaceae.

People Use This For
Orally, lily-of-the-valley is used for mild cardiac insufficiency, heart insufficiency due to old age, chronic cor pulmonale, arrhythmias, urinary tract infections (UTIs), kidney stones, weak contractions in labor, epilepsy, edema, strokes and ensuing paralysis, conjunctivitis, and leprosy.

Safety
POSSIBLY SAFE ...when the standardized extract is used orally under medical supervision (2,12). Poor oral absorption of its cardiac glycosides can reduce the risk of poisoning (18), but the number of glycosides and their varied properties makes controlled use difficult (7).
LIKELY UNSAFE ...when the standardized extract is used orally for self-medication (12).
PREGNANCY AND LACTATION: UNSAFE ...when used orally for self-medication (12).

Effectiveness
There is insufficient reliable information available about the effectiveness of lily-of-the-valley.

Mechanism of Action
The applicable parts of lily-of-the-valley are the root, rhizome, and dried flowering tops. Lily-of-the-valley contains over 40 cardioactive glycosides, principally convallatoxin; and other minor glycosides, including canvallatoxol and convalloside (13). The cardiac glycosides exert positive inotropic, negative chronotropic, negative dromotropic (conduction), and positive bathmotropic (excitability) effects (7). They can lower elevated left-ventricular diastolic pressure as well as pathologically elevated venous pressure (2). Diuretic, natriuretic, and dose-dependent vasoconstrictive effects have been observed in experimental animals (18).

Adverse Reactions
Orally, lily-of-the-valley can cause nausea, vomiting, cardiac arrhythmias (2), headache, and stupor (18). Visual color disturbances can also occur (18).

Interactions with Herbs & Other Dietary Supplements
CARDIAC GLYCOSIDE-CONTAINING HERBS: Contraindicated. Concomitant use can increase the risk of cardiac glycoside toxicity. Cardiac glycoside-containing herbs include black hellebore, Canadian hemp root, digitalis leaf, hedge mustard, figwort, motherwort, oleander leaf, pheasant's eye plant, pleurisy root, squill bulb leaf scales, strophanthus seeds, and uzara (2,18,19,500).
LICORICE/HORSETAIL: Theoretically, the overuse or misuse of licorice rhizomes or horsetail plant with cardiac glycoside-containing herbs increases the risk of cardiac toxicity due to potassium depletion (19).
OTHER CARDIOACTIVE HERBS: Avoid concomitant use with other cardioactive herbs due to the unpredictability of therapeutic and adverse effects. Other cardioactive herbs include calamus, cereus, cola, coltsfoot, devil's claw, European mistletoe, fenugreek, fumitory, ginger, Panax ginseng, hawthorn, white horehound, mate, parsley, quassia, scotch broom flower, shepherd's purse, and wild carrot (4).
STIMULANT LAXATIVE HERBS: Theoretically, the overuse or misuse of stimulant laxatives with cardiac glycoside-containing herbs increases the risk of cardiac toxicity due to potassium depletion. Stimulant laxative herbs include aloe dried leaf sap, blue flag rhizome, alder buckthorn, European buckthorn, butternut bark, cascara bark, castor oil, colocynth fruit pulp, gamboge bark exudate, jalap root,

black root, manna bark exudate, podophyllum root, rhubarb root, senna leaves and pods, wild cucumber fruit (Ecballium elaterium), and yellow dock root (19).

Interactions with Drugs

CALCIUM SUPPLEMENTS: Calcium salts can enhance the therapeutic and adverse effects of lily-of-the-valley (18).
CORTICOSTEROIDS: Theoretically, concomitant, long-term corticosteroid use can increase the risk of cardiac glycoside toxicity due to potassium depletion (2).
DIGOXIN (Lanoxin): Contraindicated; therapeutic duplication increases the risk of cardiac glycoside toxicity (2).
DIURETIC DRUGS: Concomitant use of potassium depleting diuretics and lily-of-the-valley can increase the risk of cardiac glycoside toxicity due to potassium depletion (506). Some diuretics that can deplete potassium include chlorothiazide (Diuril), chlorthalidone (Thalitone), furosemide (Lasix), hydrochlorothiazide (HCTZ, HydroDIURIL, Microzide), and others.
MACROLIDE ANTIBIOTICS: Theoretically, concomitant use may increase risk of cardiac glycoside toxicity (17).
QUININE: Theoretically, concomitant use of lily-of-the-valley and quinine can increase the risk of cardiac toxicity (506).
STIMULANT LAXATIVES: Theoretically, the overuse or misuse of stimulant laxatives can increase the risk of cardiac glycoside toxicity due to potassium depletion (19).
TETRACYCLINE ANTIBIOTICS: Theoretically, concomitant use may increase the risk of cardiac glycoside toxicity (17).

Interactions with Foods

None known.

Interactions with Lab Tests

None known.

Interactions with Diseases or Conditions

HEART DISEASE: Self-medication with lily-of-the-valley is contraindicated; treatment requires diagnosis, treatment, and monitoring (515).
POTASSIUM DEFICIENCY: Contraindicated (2).

Dosage and Administration

ORAL: The average daily amount is 600 mg of the standardized lily-of-the-valley powder (0.2% to 0.3% cardioactive glycosides) or equivalent preparations (2).

Comments

The large number of cardiac glycosides in lily-of-the-valley makes monitoring and therapeutic control more difficult than digitalis or digoxin therapy (7). Lily-of-the-valley has a short duration of action. This correlates with lower absorption rates and makes treatment more difficult to control than with isolated cardiac glycosides, especially due to the narrow therapeutic range of these constituents (7). When indicated, digoxin of standard potency and purity is a safer alternative than nonstandardized lily-of-the-valley (7). Store lily-of-the-valley in well-sealed containers and protect from light (18).

LIME fruit, peel

Also Known As

Adam's Apple, Bara Nimbu, Bijapura, Italian Limetta, Limette, Turanj.
CAUTION: See separate listing for Lime Oil.

Scientific Names

Citrus aurantifolia, synonyms Citrus medica var. acida, Citrus acida, Citrus lima, Citrus limetta var. aromatica, Limonia aurantiifolia.
Family: Rutaceae.

People Use This For

Orally, lime is used as a source of vitamin C for treating scurvy and low resistance.

Safety

LIKELY SAFE ...when used orally in amounts commonly found in foods. Lime has Generally Recognized As Safe (GRAS) status in the US (4912).
POSSIBLY SAFE ...when used orally in medicinal amounts (12).

PREGNANCY AND LACTATION: Insufficient reliable information available; avoid using in amounts greater than those typically found in foods.

Effectiveness

There is insufficient reliable information available about the effectiveness of lime fruit, peel.

Mechanism of Action

The applicable parts of lime are the peel, fruit, and juice from the fruit. Lime juice contains bergamottin. Bergamottin competitively inhibits cytochrome P450 3A4 (CYP3A4) activity (11976).

Adverse Reactions

None reported.

Interactions with Herbs & Other Dietary Supplements

None known.

Interactions with Drugs

CYTOCHROME P450 3A4 (CYP3A4) SUBSTRATES: Lime juice inhibits cytochrome P450 3A4, causing increased drug levels and potentially increasing the risk of adverse effects (11976).
Some drugs metabolized by CYP3A4 that might be affected are some benzodiazepines such as alprazolam (Xanax), diazepam (Valium), midazolam (Versed), triazolam (Halcion); calcium channel blockers such as amlodipine (Norvasc), diltiazem (Cardizem, Dilacor, others), felodipine (Plendil), verapamil (Calan, Verelan, others); cyclosporine (Neoral, Sandimmune); some HIV antivirals such as indinavir (Crixivan), ritonavir (Norvir), saquinavir (Fortovase, Invirase); some HMG CoA reductase inhibitors such as atorvastatin (Lipitor), lovastatin (Mevacor); some macrolide antibiotics such as erythromycin and clarithromycin (Biaxin); quinidine; and many others.

Interactions with Foods

None known.

Interactions with Lab Tests

None known.

Interactions with Diseases or Conditions

None known.

Dosage and Administration

No typical dosage.

LIME OIL

Also Known As

Adam's Apple, Bara Nimbu, Bijapura, Italian Limetta, Key Lime, Limette Turanj.
CAUTION: See separate listing for Lime fruit, peel.

Scientific Names

Citrus aurantifolia, synonyms Citrus medica var. acida, Citrus acida, Citrus lima, Citrus limetta var. aromatica, Limonia aurantiifolia.
Family: Rutaceae.

People Use This For

Topically, lime oil is used as a stimulant, antiseptic, and for nausea.
In cosmetics, expressed lime oil is used as a fragrance component. Distilled lime oil is used as a fixative in cosmetics.
In foods, lime oil is used as flavor component in foods and beverages.

Safety

LIKELY SAFE ...when used in amounts commonly found in foods. Lime oil has Generally Recognized As Safe (GRAS) status in the US (4912).
POSSIBLY UNSAFE ...when used topically. Lime oil contains photosensitizing constituents (11909).
PREGNANCY AND LACTATION: There is insufficient reliable information available about the safety of lime oil in medicinal amounts during pregnancy and lactation; avoid using.

Effectiveness
There is insufficient reliable information available about the effectiveness of lime oil.

Mechanism of Action
The furocoumarins bergapten and oxypeucedanin in lime oil are photosensitizing (11019). Some evidence suggests expressed and distilled lime oils might promote tumors in the presence of carcinogenic chemicals (11).

Adverse Reactions
Topically, use is associated with hypersensitivity (4058). Photosensitivity might occur, especially in fair-skinned people (11909).

Interactions with Herbs & Other Dietary Supplements
None known.

Interactions with Drugs
PHOTOSENSITIZING DRUGS: Theoretically, concomitant use with photosensitizing drugs may increase the risk of phototoxicity (11909).

Interactions with Foods
None known.

Interactions with Lab Tests
None known.

Interactions with Diseases or Conditions
None known.

Dosage and Administration
No typical dosage.

Comments
Distilled lime oil is the distilled essential oil of the whole crushed fruit of the lime tree. Expressed lime oil is obtained from unripe lime peel.

LINDEN CHARCOAL

Also Known As
Basswood, European Linden, Lime Tree, Tiliae carbo.
CAUTION: See separate listings for Linden dried flower, Linden dried leaf, Linden dried sapwood, and Silver Linden.

Scientific Names
Tilia cordata, synonyms Tilia parvifolia, Tilia ulmifolia; Tilia platyphyllos, synonyms Tilia grandifolia, Tilia rubra.
Family: Malvaceae or Tiliaceae.

Comments
At the date of publication, this product was not a common ingredient used in brand name supplements marketed to consumers. Details about this product are available at the online version of *Natural Medicines Comprehensive Database*. See www.naturaldatabase.com.

LINDEN dried flower

Also Known As
Basswood, European Linden, Lime Blossom, Lime Flower, Lime Tree, Linden Tree, Tiliae flos.
CAUTION: See separate listings for Linden Charcoal, Linden dried leaf, Linden dried sapwood, and Silver Linden.

Scientific Names
Tilia cordata, synonyms Tilia parvifolia, Tilia ulmifolia; Tilia platyphyllos, synonyms Tilia grandifolia, Tilia rubra.
Family: Malvaceae or Tiliaceae.

People Use This For
Orally, linden dried flower is used for coughs, colds, nasal congestion, throat irritation, nervous palpitations, hypertension, headaches, insomnia, sinus headache, migraines, incontinence, hemorrhage, hysteria, arteriosclerotic hypertension, feverish colds, nervous tension, and as a diuretic.
Topically, linden dried flower is used for itchy skin and rheumatism.

Safety
POSSIBLY SAFE ...when used orally and appropriately (12).
PREGNANCY AND LACTATION: Insufficient reliable information available; avoid using.

Effectiveness
There is insufficient reliable information available about the effectiveness of linden dried flower.

Mechanism of Action
The linden dried flower has antispasmodic, diaphoretic, diuretic, sedative, and mild astringent properties (4), and antifungal activity (6). In vitro, its antispasmodic activity is attributed to p-coumaric acid and the flavonoid constituents (4). Diaphoretic effects can be due to kaempferol, p-coumaric acid, and quercetin (6), or perhaps due to the heat of the liquid as a tea combined with warm bed rest (7). The volatile oils, including citral, citronellal, citronellol, eugenol, and limonene, exert sedative and antispasmodic effects (4,6). A diuretic effect can be due to the irritant action of terpenoid on the kidneys (4).

Adverse Reactions
Orally, frequent use of the linden dried flower tea is associated with cardiac damage, but this is rare (6).
Topically, linden dried flower can cause contact urticaria (6).

Interactions with Herbs & Other Dietary Supplements
None known.

Interactions with Drugs
None known.

Interactions with Foods
None known.

Interactions with Lab Tests
None known.

Interactions with Diseases or Conditions
HEART DISEASE: Frequent use of linden dried flower tea is associated with cardiac damage and should be used with caution in individuals with heart disease (6).

Dosage and Administration
ORAL: The typical dose of linden dried flower is one to two cups of the tea used as hot as possible (8). The tea is prepared by steeping 2 grams of the flowers in 150 mL boiling water for 5-10 minutes and then straining. The linden dried flower should only be used up to 2-4 grams daily (2). The usual dose of the tincture (1:5 in 45% alcohol) is 2-4 mL (4). The common dose of the liquid extract (1:1 in 25% alcohol) is 1-2 mL (4).

Comments
Tilia sylvestris, a related species, has been reported to possess anti-inflammatory and wound healing effects (6).

LINDEN dried leaf

Also Known As
Basswood, European Linden, Lime Tree, Tiliae folium.
CAUTION: See separate listings for Linden Charcoal, Linden dried flower, Linden dried sapwood, and Silver Linden.

Scientific Names
Tilia cordata, synonyms Tilia parvifolia, Tilia ulmifolia; Tilia platyphyllos, synonyms Tilia grandifolia, Tilia rubra.
Family: Malvaceae or Tiliaceae.

Comments
At the date of publication, there was very little scientific information about this product. Our staff is continually analyzing the available information on natural medicines and will add data to the online version of *Natural Medicines Comprehensive Database* as it becomes available. See www.naturaldatabase.com.

LINDEN dried sapwood

Also Known As
Basswood, European Linden, Lime Tree, Linden Wood, Tiliae lignum.
CAUTION: See separate listings for Linden Charcoal, Linden dried flower, Linden dried leaf, and Silver Linden.

Scientific Names
Tilia cordata, synonyms Tilia parvifolia, Tilia ulmifolia; Tilia platyphyllos, synonyms Tilia grandifolia, Tilia rubra.
Family: Malvaceae or Tiliaceae.

Comments
At the date of publication, there was very little scientific information about this product. Our staff is continually analyzing the available information on natural medicines and will add data to the online version of *Natural Medicines Comprehensive Database* as it becomes available. See www.naturaldatabase.com.

LIPASE

Also Known As
None.

Scientific Names
Triacylglycerol lipase.

People Use This For
Orally, lipase is used for indigestion, heartburn, celiac disease, Crohn's disease, and cystic fibrosis.

Safety
LIKELY SAFE ...when used orally (15).
PREGNANCY AND LACTATION: Insufficient reliable information available; avoid using.

Effectiveness
There is insufficient reliable information available about the effectiveness of lipase.

Mechanism of Action
Lipase is a digestive enzyme that is widely distributed in the plant world, in milk, milk products, bacteria, molds, and animal tissues (2383). Lipase aids in fat digestion by hydrolyzing fat to yield fatty acids and glycerol (9). Castor beans and dehulled oats are also plant sources of acid-stable lipases (2383). Lipase is included in many prescription and OTC combination pancreatic enzyme products. Most clinical studies use combination pancreatic enzyme products, rather than lipase-only products, although pancreatic enzyme dosing is often expressed in units of lipase (2384).

Adverse Reactions
Orally, taking large amounts of lipase can cause nausea, cramping, and/or diarrhea (15).

Interactions with Herbs & Other Dietary Supplements
None known.

Interactions with Drugs
None known.

Interactions with Foods
None known.

Interactions with Lab Tests
None known.

Interactions with Diseases or Conditions

CYSTIC FIBROSIS: High doses of lipase appear to increase the risk of fibrosing colonopathy and colonic strictures in individuals with cystic fibrosis (2379,2380,2381,2382).

Dosage and Administration

No typical dosage.

LITHIUM

Also Known As

Lithium Carbonate, Lithium Citrate, Lithium Orotate.

Scientific Names

Lithium; Li; atomic number 3.

People Use This For

Orally, lithium is used for bipolar disorder, depression, schizophrenia, anorexia nervosa, bulimia, headache and alcoholism. Other uses include neutropenia, epilepsy anemia, diabetes, liver disease, kidney disorders, arthritis, seborrhea, and hyperthyroidism. It is also used for syndrome of inappropriate antidiuretic hormone (SIADH), asthma, Huntington chorea, Graves' disease, herpes simplex, drug-induced tardive dyskinesia, Tourette syndrome, cyclical vomiting, Meniere's disease, paresthesias, control of levodopa side effects, and ulcerative colitis in patients with affective disorders.

Safety

LIKELY SAFE ...when used orally and appropriately. Lithium carbonate and lithium citrate are FDA-approved drugs (15).
CHILDREN: POSSIBLY SAFE ...when lithium carbonate and lithium citrate are used orally and appropriately (15).
PREGNANCY: POSSIBLY SAFE ...when lithium carbonate and lithium citrate are used orally (15). Lithium can cause fetal toxicity and increases the risk for cardiac and other abnormalities, but it may be given with careful monitoring when the potential maternal benefits outweigh the possible risk to the fetus (15,9166).
LACTATION: UNSAFE ...when used orally. Lithium is secreted into breast milk and may cause adverse effects in the nursing infant (15).
There is insufficient reliable information about the safety of lithium orotate.

Effectiveness

EFFECTIVE

Bipolar disorder. Taking lithium orally is FDA-approved for treatment of mania in mixed bipolar disorder and prevention of recurrence of bipolar episodes (15).

LIKELY EFFECTIVE

Depression. Taking lithium orally appears to be effective in some patients with major depression (15).

POSSIBLY EFFECTIVE

Attention deficit-hyperactivity disorder (ADHD). Preliminary evidence suggests that lithium might be effective for impulsive aggressive behavior, aggression associated with ADHD (15).

Schizophrenia. Lithium is typically used in combination with antipsychotic drugs when it is used for schizophrenia or schizoaffective disorders. In some cases, lithium is beneficial as monotherapy for these patients (15).

There is insufficient reliable information available about the effectiveness of lithium for its other uses.

Mechanism of Action

Lithium is the lightest of the alkali metal elements. It is a monovalent cation and has some chemical properties of calcium and magnesium (15). Lithium is normally present in all organs and tissues with highest concentrations in the brain and kidneys. Lithium is uniformly distributed in body water; there is only a small difference between extracellular and intracellular levels. It does not bind to plasma proteins (15,9163). Lithium salts are virtually 100% absorbed from the small intestine via the sodium channels and are excreted primarily by the kidneys. Lithium appears to be an essential micronutrient; however, defined human lithium deficiency diseases have not been observed. Primary dietary sources include grains and vegetables with smaller amounts obtained from animal-derived foods. The average daily intake of an American 70 kg adult ranges from 650 to 3100 mcg. In some geographical areas, drinking water may contribute significantly to lithium intake (9163). Epidemiological evidence suggests that areas with lower lithium content in tap water have higher rates of mental hospital admissions, suicides, homicides, and other crimes, suggesting that lithium intake might affect behavior (9163). Animal studies suggest that lithium deficiency can adversely affect mortality and reproduction. Lithium appears to be essential for fetal development, particularly during the first trimester of gestation. It appears to have a role in fetal blood cell development.

Lithium is involved with many physiological functions. It works with other elements, drugs, enzymes, hormones, vitamins, and growth and transforming factors. Theoretically, many of the biological actions of lithium are caused by the powerful polarizing effect caused by its small atomic radius, allowing it to displace sodium, potassium, magnesium, and calcium from membrane or enzyme binding sites (9163).

The exact mechanism of action of lithium in psychological and behavioral disorders is unknown. It appears to affect dopamine and serotonin activity (15). Lithium might increase monoamine oxidase (MAO) activity. It also enhances folate and vitamin B12 transport into brain cells, which might affect mood (9163).

Lithium stimulates the production of colony-stimulating factor by monocytes. It produces neutrophilia and may also increase erythrocyte and platelet counts, and decrease lymphocyte counts. The increase in neutrophils is usually seen 3 to 7 days after initial of lithium and rapidly reverses 1 to 2 weeks after lithium is discontinued (15).

Lithium causes changes in renal function, often producing a mild nephrogenic diabetes insipidus. The drug decreases renal concentrating ability and water reabsorption. Initially, sodium and potassium excretion increases. Some of these effects improve with physiologic compensation; others may persist. Glomerular filtration rate (GFR) may decrease with prolonged therapy (15).

Lithium is excreted unchanged, predominately in the urine. The elimination half-life is 20 to 24 hours with normal renal function, but increases with decreasing renal function. The half-life in elderly patients may increase to 36 hours. In renal impairment, the half-life can increase to 40 to 50 hours.

Lithium has a narrow therapeutic window and must be monitored to avoid toxicity. Lithium levels should be drawn 12 hours after the last dose of lithium after steady state concentrations have been attained (4 to 7 days). For depression and schizoaffective disorders, therapeutic levels are 0.4 to 1.3 mEq/L. For acute mania, therapeutic levels are 1.0 to 1.3 mEq/L. Toxicity is most common at levels of 1.5 mEq/L, although some patients develop toxicity at levels less than 1 mEq/L, especially children and older patients (15).

The onset of activity is slow, often requiring 10 to 21 days to achieve full therapeutic effect (15).

Adverse Reactions

Orally, lithium can cause nausea, diarrhea, vertigo, muscle weakness, lethargy, fatigue, and a dazed feeling. These adverse effects often improve with continued use. Fine tremor, polyuria, and polydipsia can occur and may persist with continued use. Weight gain and edema, which should not be treated with diuretics, are also seen. Lithium can also cause or exacerbate skin disorders such as acne, psoriasis, and rashes. Long-term effects include hypothyroidism, goiter, (rarely hyperthyroidism), and mild cognitive and memory impairment (9,15).

Signs of lithium toxicity include increasing diarrhea, vomiting, anorexia, muscle weakness, lethargy, giddiness with ataxia, lack of coordination, choreoathetosis, tinnitus, blurred vision, coarse tremor of the extremities and lower jaw, muscle hyperirritability, dysarthria, and drowsiness. Severe toxicity can cause toxic psychosis, syncope, renal failure, dehydration, circulatory failure, coma, and occasionally death (9).

Abrupt drops in serum lithium levels can precipitate recurrence of bipolar symptoms (9165).

Preclinical studies suggest that lithium orotate might be more likely to cause nephrotoxicity than lithium carbonate (9164).

Interactions with Herbs & Other Dietary Supplements

CAFFEINE CONTAINING HERBS/SUPPLEMENTS: Concomitant use can increase lithium clearance (9,15). Natural products that contain caffeine include black tea, coffee, green tea, guarana, mate, and cola nut.

DIURETIC HERBS: Theoretically, herbs having diuretic properties might reduce the clearance of lithium (9,15). Herbs thought to have diuretic properties include agrimony, artichoke, broom, buchu, burdock, celery, cornsilk, couch grass, elder, guaiac wood, juniper, pokeroot, shepherd's purse, squill, uva ursi, and yarrow.

HERBS/SUPPLEMENTS WITH SEROTONERGIC ACTIVITY: Theoretically, lithium might increase the effects and adverse effects of products that increase serotonin levels, including 5-hydroxytryptophan, Hawaiian baby woodrose, L-tryptophan, S-adenosylmethionine, and St. John's wort (9,15).

Interactions with Drugs

ACE INHIBITORS (ACEIs): Concomitant administration may increase lithium concentrations. Lithium dosage reductions may be necessary (9,15). Some ACE inhibitors are captopril (Capoten), enalapril (Vasotec), lisinopril (Prinivil, Zestril), ramipril (Altace), and others.

ANTICONVULSANTS: Drugs such as carbamazepine (Tegretol) and phenytoin (Dilantin) might increase the risk of neurotoxicity (9,15).

ANTIDEPRESSANT DRUGS: Combining serotonergic antidepressants with lithium might increase the risk of serotonergic side effects including serotonin syndrome and cerebral vasoconstrictive disorders such as Call-Fleming syndrome (8056). These drugs include the selective serotonin reuptake inhibitors (SSRIs) such as fluoxetine (Prozac), paroxetine (Paxil), sertraline (Zoloft), and others; and tricyclic and atypical antidepressants such as amitriptyline (Elavil), clomipramine (Anafranil), imipramine (Tofranil), and others.

CALCIUM CHANNEL BLOCKERS: Calcium channel blockers might reduce lithium concentrations. Monitor lithium levels with concurrent use. Calcium channel blockers might also increase adverse neurological and gastrointestinal adverse effects (9,15). Calcium channel blockers include nifedipine (Adalat, Procardia), verapamil (Calan, Isoptin, Verelan), diltiazem (Cardizem), isradipine (DynaCirc), felodipine (Plendil), amlodipine (Norvasc), and others.

DEXTROMETHORPHAN (Robitussin DM, and others): Combining serotonergic drugs such as dextromethorphan with lithium might increase the risk of serotonergic side effects including serotonin syndrome and cerebral vasoconstrictive disorders such as Call-Fleming syndrome (8056).
LOOP DIURETICS: Loop diuretics might reduce lithium excretion, particularly in sodium-restricted patients. Monitor lithium levels (9,15). Loop diuretics include bumetanide (Bumex), ethacrynic acid (Edecrin), and furosemide (Lasix).
MEPERIDINE (Demerol): Combining serotonergic drugs such as meperidine with lithium might increase the risk of serotonergic side effects including serotonin syndrome and cerebral vasoconstrictive disorders such as Call-Fleming syndrome (8056).
METHYLDOPA (Aldomet): Concurrent use of methyldopa increases the risk of lithium toxicity (9).
METHYLXANTHINES: Xanthines such as aminophylline, caffeine, and theophylline (Theo-Dur, Theo-24, others) might increase the clearance of lithium. Monitor lithium levels (9,15).
MONOAMINE OXIDASE INHIBITORS (MAOIs): Combining serotonergic drugs such as one of the MAOIs with lithium might increase the risk of serotonergic side effects including serotonin syndrome and cerebral vasoconstrictive disorders such as Call-Fleming syndrome (8056).
NONSTEROIDAL ANTI-INFLAMMATORY DRUGS (NSAIDs): NSAIDs can decrease the renal clearance of lithium levels and increase lithium levels (9,15). NSAIDs include diclofenac (Voltaren, Cataflam, others), ibuprofen (Advil, Motrin, others), naproxen (Anaprox, Naprosyn, others), and others.
PENTAZOCINE (Talwin): Combining serotonergic drugs such as pentazocine with lithium might increase the risk of serotonergic side effects including serotonin syndrome and cerebral vasoconstrictive disorders such as Call-Fleming syndrome (8056).
PHENOTHIAZINES: Concomitant use of lithium with phenothiazines might reduce lithium concentrations. Lithium might also reduce phenothiazine concentrations, making the pharmacokinetic effect unpredictable (9,15). Some phenothiazines are fluphenazine (Permitil, Prolixin), chlorpromazine (Thorazine), prochlorperazine (Compazine), thioridazine (Mellaril), trifluoperazine (Stelazine), and others.
SKELETAL MUSCLE RELAXANTS: Lithium might prolong neuromuscular blockade. Monitor carefully with concurrent use (9,15). Neuromuscular blockers include atracurium (Tracrium), pancuronium (Pavulon), succinylcholine (Anectine), and others.
THIAZIDE DIURETICS: Thiazide diuretics reduce lithium excretion and increase lithium levels. Reduce lithium dose by 50 per cent and monitor lithium levels (9,15). Thiazides include chlorothiazide (Diuril), hydrochlorothiazide (HydroDIURIL, Esidrix), indapamide (Lozol), metolazone (Zaroxolyn), and chlorthalidone (Hygroton).
TRAMADOL (Ultram): Combining serotonergic drugs such as tramadol with lithium might increase the risk of serotonergic side effects including serotonin syndrome and cerebral vasoconstrictive disorders such as Call-Fleming syndrome (8056).

Interactions with Foods
None known.

Interactions with Lab Tests
ERYTHROCYTES: Lithium can increase erythrocyte counts (15).
LEUKOCYTES: Lithium usually causes a reversible leukocytosis with leukocyte counts of 10,000 to 15,000 per cubic millimeter (15).
PLATELETS: Lithium can increase platelet counts (15).
THYROID FUNCTION TESTS (LFTs): Lithium can cause hypothyroidism, and less frequently, hyperthyroidism (15).

Interactions with Diseases or Conditions
CARDIOVASCULAR DISEASE: Lithium may cause arrhythmias. Cardiovascular disease may increase the risk for toxicity (15).
RENAL IMPAIRMENT: Lithium is excreted renally. Dosage reductions may be required depending on the severity of renal dysfunction (9).
THYROID DISEASE: Lithium may worsen thyroid disease (15).

Dosage and Administration
ORAL: For acute manic episodes, lithium carbonate 1.8 g or 20 to 30 mg per kg per day in 2 to 3 divided doses is used. Some clinicians begin therapy at 600 to 900 mg per day and titrate up. For bipolar disorder and other psychiatric conditions, the usual adult maintenance dose is 900 mg to 1.2 g per day in 2 to 4 divided doses. Lithium citrate solution 24 to 32 mEq given in 2 to 4 divided doses daily has also been used. Maintenance doses usually should not exceed 2.4 g of lithium carbonate or 65 mEq lithium citrate daily. For children, 15 to 60 mg per kg (0.4 to 1.6 mEq per kg) per day in divided doses has been used (9,15).
Lithium may be administered as a single daily dose, but is usually given in divided doses to lessen side effects (15). Abrupt discontinuation of lithium therapy increases the risk for relapse of bipolar disorder. Lithium should be tapered gradually over at least 14 days (9165).

There is no recommended dietary allowance (RDA) for lithium. A provisional RDA of 1 mg per day for a 70 kg adult has been suggested (9163).

Comments
Lithium gets its name from the Greek word for stone, lithos, because it is present in trace amounts in virtually all rocks (9163).

LIVER EXTRACT

Also Known As
Aqueous Liver Extract, Hydrolyzed Liver Extract, Liquid Liver Extract, Liver, Liver Concentrate, Liver Factors, Liver Fractions, Liver Hydrolysate, Liver Substance, Raw Liver.
CAUTION: See separate listing for Shark Liver Oil.

Scientific Names
None.

People Use This For
Orally, liver extract is used for improving liver function, treating chronic liver diseases, preventing liver damage, and regenerating liver tissue. It is also used for allergies; enhancing muscle development in bodybuilders; improving stamina, strength, and physical endurance; enhancing detoxification; and as an aid to recovery from chemical addiction or poisoning.

Safety
There is insufficient reliable information available about the safety of liver extract. However, since some preparations are derived from animals, there is concern about contamination with diseased animal parts (1825). So far, there are no reports of disease transmission to humans due to use of contaminated liver extract.
Pregnancy and Lactation: Insufficient reliable information available; avoid using.

Effectiveness
There is insufficient reliable information available about the effectiveness of liver extract.

Mechanism of Action
Liver extract is a concentrated product derived from animal liver, most commonly from cattle. It contains vitamin B12, folic acid, and up to 3-4 mg of heme iron per gram of product (6614). Liver extract increases liver weight and shows evidence of stimulating liver cell proliferation in experimental animals after partial hepatectomy (6650). However, information about pharmacological effects in humans is not available.

Adverse Reactions
Adverse reactions have not been reported. However, there is some concern about the possibility of contamination. Liver extract is derived from raw animal liver gathered from slaughterhouses, possibly from sick or diseased animals (6616). Products made from contaminated or diseased organs might present a human health hazard. There is also concern that liver extracts produced from cows in countries where bovine spongiform encephalitis (BSE) has been reported might be contaminated with diseased tissue. Countries where BSE has been reported include Great Britain, France, The Netherlands, Portugal, Luxembourg, Ireland, Switzerland, Oman, and Belgium (1825). However, there have been no reports of BSE transfer to humans from contaminated liver extract products. Until more is known, tell patients to avoid these products unless the country of origin can be determined. Patients should avoid products that are produced in countries where BSE has been found.

Interactions with Herbs & Other Dietary Supplements
IRON: Concomitant use might increase the risk of iron overload. Liver extract can contain 3-4 mg heme iron per gram of product (6614).

Interactions with Drugs
None known.

Interactions with Foods
None known.

Interactions with Lab Tests

HEMOGLOBIN: Liver extract might increase hemoglobin concentrations and test results due to its iron content (6614).
IRON: Liver extract might increase iron concentrations and test results due to its iron content (6614).

Interactions with Diseases or Conditions

IRON METABOLISM DISORDERS: Liver extract contains 3-4 mg of heme iron and might adversely affect people with iron metabolism disorders, including hemochromatosis (6614); contraindicated.

Dosage and Administration

No typical dosage.

LIVERWORT

Also Known As

American Liverleaf, Anémone à Lobes Aigus, Anémone d'Amérique, Hepatici noblis herba, Hépatique à Lobes Aigus, Hépatique d'Amérique, Herb Trinity, Kidney Wort, Leberbluemchenkraut, Liverleaf, Liverweed, Liverwort-Leaf, Round-Leaved Hepatica, Round-Lobe Hepatica, Sharp-Lobe Hepatica, Trefoil.
CAUTION: See separate listings for Agrimony and Red Clover.

Scientific Names

Anemone acutiloba, synonym Hepatica nobilis var. acuta; Anemone americana, synonym Hepatica nobilis var. obtusa; Anemone hepatica.
Family: Ranunculaceae.

People Use This For

Orally, liverwort is used for liver diseases, jaundice, liver enlargement, congestion, portal vein problems, hepatitis, and liver cirrhosis. It is also used orally for gastric and digestive discomfort, stimulating appetite, relieving sensation of fullness, for treating gallstones and gravel, for regulating bowel function, stimulating pancreatic function, regulating blood lipid levels, for varicose veins, stimulating systemic and cardiac circulation, increasing myocardium blood supply, strengthening nerves, "purifying" blood, stimulating metabolism, relief of menopausal symptoms, and as a general tonic or sedative.
Topically, liverwort is used for hemorrhoids or as an external rinse.

Safety

LIKELY UNSAFE ...when the fresh above ground parts are used orally or topically (2).
There is insufficient reliable information available about the safety of dried liverwort.
PREGNANCY: LIKELY UNSAFE ...when used orally or topically (2).
LACTATION: LIKELY UNSAFE ...when the fresh above ground parts are used orally or topically (2). There is insufficient reliable information available about the safety of dried liverwort while breast-feeding; avoid using.

Effectiveness

There is insufficient reliable information available about the effectiveness of liverwort.

Mechanism of Action

The applicable parts of liverwort are the fresh or dried above ground parts (2). Liverwort contains ranunculin (18), which hydrolyzes to toxic, unstable protoanemonin, which readily dimerizes to nontoxic anemonin (4). Some evidence suggests anemonin might be cytotoxic (4). Other evidence indicates anemonin and protoanemonin might have sedative and antipyretic activity (4). Protoanemonin has antimicrobial activity (2). It causes central nervous system stimulation, then paralysis in experimental animals (2). Kidney and urinary tract irritation might be due to the alkylating action of protoanemonin (2).

Adverse Reactions

Orally, fresh liverwort can cause colic, diarrhea, gastrointestinal irritation (18), and kidney and urinary tract irritation (2).
Topically, skin contact with fresh liverwort can cause irritation, mucous membrane irritation, itching, and pustule formation known a ranunculus dermatitis (2).
Inhalation of protoanemonin-containing volatile oil can cause nasal mucosal and conjunctival irritation (4).

Interactions with Herbs & Other Dietary Supplements

None known.

Interactions with Drugs
None known.

Interactions with Foods
None known.

Interactions with Lab Tests
None known.

Interactions with Diseases or Conditions
None known.

Dosage and Administration
No typical dosage.

LOBELIA

Also Known As
Asthma Weed, Bladderpod, Emetic Herb, Gagroot, Lobelie, Indian Tobacco, Pukeweed, Vomit Wort, Wild Tobacco.

Scientific Names
Lobelia inflata.
Family: Campanulaceae or Lobeliaceae.

People Use This For
Orally, lobelia is used for asthma, bronchitis, whooping cough, inducing sweating, and as a sedative. Lobelia is also used as an ingredient in smoking cessation products and for treating apnea in newborn infants.
Topically, lobelia is used for muscle inflammation, rheumatic nodules, bruises, sprains, insect bites, poison ivy, and ringworm.
In manufacturing, lobelia is used in cough preparations and counterirritant products.

Safety
LIKELY UNSAFE ...when used orally (3,11). 0.6-1 gram of the leaf is said to be toxic and 4 grams may be fatal (18). There is insufficient reliable information available about the safety of the topical use of lobelia.
PREGNANCY AND LACTATION: LIKELY UNSAFE ...when used orally because it has emetic effects (4,12). There is insufficient reliable information available about the safety of lobelia for topical use during pregnancy and lactation.

Effectiveness
LIKELY INEFFECTIVE

Smoking cessation. Taking lobeline, a constituent of lobelia, is not effective when used orally for smoking cessation (13).

There is insufficient reliable information available about the effectiveness of lobelia for its other uses.

Mechanism of Action
The applicable parts of lobelia are the above ground parts. Lobelia has some anti-asthmatic, antispasmodic, emetic, expectorant, and respiratory stimulant effects (4,13). The primary constituent, (-)-lobeline, is known as alpha lobeline, to distinguish it from the mixture of lobelia alkaloids formerly called lobeline. Like nicotine but weaker, alpha lobeline exhibits effects on the peripheral circulation, neuromuscular system and central nervous system (CNS) (4,13). Small amounts of lobeline stimulate respiration and have expectorant activity (11,18). Larger amounts have emetic, purgative, and diuretic effects (11). Lobeline first causes CNS stimulation then CNS and respiratory depression (505).

Adverse Reactions
Orally, lobelia can cause nausea, vomiting, diarrhea, coughing, dizziness, and tremors (4). Overdose may cause sweating, tachycardia, convulsions, hypothermia, hypotension, coma, and possibly death (4,11).

Interactions with Herbs & Other Dietary Supplements
TOBACCO: Concomitant use with lobelia may enhance nicotine effects and adverse effects (505).

Interactions with Drugs
None known.

Interactions with Foods
None known.

Interactions with Lab Tests
None known.

Interactions with Diseases or Conditions
GASTROINTESTINAL (GI) CONDITIONS: Lobelia can irritate the GI tract. It is contraindicated in individuals with infectious or inflammatory GI conditions (19).
HEART DISEASE: Caution; dose-dependent cardiac activity is reported with lobelia (12).

Dosage and Administration
ORAL: A typical dose as an expectorant is 100 mg of leaf, 0.6-2.0 mL of the tincture (12). The dosage of specific products varies widely from 375 mg once daily to 820 mg three times daily. One supplier warns not to exceed 50 mg of the dried lobelia. An extract of lobelia is used in a dose of 2 to 5 drops three to four times daily. The extract contains alcohol (6006).

Comments
Clinical research was unable to demonstrate lobeline efficacy greater than placebo in smoking cessation (13) and it was disallowed as an ingredient in anti-smoking products in the US in 1993 (11).

LOGWOOD

Also Known As
Bloodwood, Peachwood.

Scientific Names
Haematoxylum campechianum; Haematoxylum lignum.
Family: Fabaceae/Leguminosae.

Comments
At the date of publication, this product was not a common ingredient used in brand name supplements marketed to consumers. Details about this product are available at the online version of *Natural Medicines Comprehensive Database*. See www.naturaldatabase.com.

LOOSESTRIFE

Also Known As
Yellow Willowherb.
CAUTION: See separate listing for Purple Loosestrife.

Scientific Names
Lysimachia vulgaris.
Family: Primulaceae.

Comments
At the date of publication, this product was not a common ingredient used in brand name supplements marketed to consumers. Details about this product are available at the online version of *Natural Medicines Comprehensive Database*. See www.naturaldatabase.com.

LORENZO'S OIL

Also Known As
Lorenzos Oil, Glycerol Trierucate Oil, Glycerol Trioleate Oil.

Scientific Names
13-Docosenoic acid (erucic acid); cis-9-Octadecenoic acid (oleic acid).

People Use This For
Orally, Lorenzo's oil is used as a treatment for two related genetic neurological syndromes: adrenoleukodystrophy, which occurs in children, and adrenomyeloneuropathy, which occurs in adults.

Safety
There is insufficient reliable information available about the safety of Lorenzo's oil.
Pregnancy and Lactation: Insufficient reliable information available; avoid using.

Effectiveness
LIKELY INEFFECTIVE

Adrenoleukodystrophy and adrenomyeloneuropathy. Taking Lorenzo's oil orally doesn't seem to be effective for treating adrenoleukodystrophy and adrenomyeloneuropathy (920,921,922,923,924,930). There is one case report of modest clinical benefit in a child with symptomatic adrenoleukodystrophy (929).

Mechanism of Action
Adrenoleukodystrophy and adrenomyeloneuropathy are rare genetic disorders that result in an impaired ability to oxidize saturated, very-long chain fatty acids. Buildup of these acids is thought to cause neurologic symptoms associated with the disorder (6). Monounsaturated fatty acids have been shown to inhibit production of very-long-chain fatty acids (6). However, when Lorenzo's oil is given to patients with adrenoleukodystrophy, eruric acid does not enter the brain in a significant quantity, which may be a factor in the negative results (931).

Adverse Reactions
Orally, Lorenzo's oil can cause asymptomatic thrombocytopenia (924,927) and asymptomatic neutropenia (6). One case report of purpura, petechia, and bleeding (926). May cause decrease in plasma docosahexanoic acid levels without essential fatty acid deficiency (individuals studied were also taking supplemental safflower and fish oils) (6).

Interactions with Herbs & Other Dietary Supplements
ESSENTIAL FATTY ACIDS: Supplemental essential fatty acids taken concomitantly may not prevent decreased plasma levels of docosahexaenoic acid (6).

Interactions with Drugs
None known.

Interactions with Foods
None known.

Interactions with Lab Tests
PLATELET COUNTS: Lorenzo's oil may cause false low platelet counts (927). High monounsaturated fat diets may cause true thrombocytopenia (925,927). A hand-count of platelets is recommended in individuals taking Lorenzo's oil (927).

Interactions with Diseases or Conditions
THROMBOCYTOPENIA and NEUTROPENIA: Theoretically, Lorenzo's oil may worsen existing conditions.

Dosage and Administration
ORAL: People typically use a mixture of approximately 20% erucic acid and 80% oleic acid (5278). One clinical study used 0.3 gram per kg per day of erucic acid and 1.7 grams per kg of oleic acid per day (5277).

Comments
Lorenzo's oil is a combination of erucic acid and oleic acid in a 1:4 ratio.

LOTUS flower

Also Known As
Lian Fang, Lian Xu.
CAUTION: See separate listing for Lotus seed.

Scientific Names
Nelumbo nucifera, synonyms Nelumbo caspica, Nelumbo komarovii, Nelumbo nelumbo, Nelumbo speciosum, Nymphaea nelumbo.
Family: Nelumbonaceae.

Comments
At the date of publication, this product was not a common ingredient used in brand name supplements marketed to consumers. Details about this product are available at the online version of *Natural Medicines Comprehensive Database*. See www.naturaldatabase.com.

LOTUS seed

Also Known As
Lian Zi, Semen Nelumbinis.
CAUTION: See separate listing for Lotus flower.

Scientific Names
Nelumbo nucifera, synonyms Nelumbo caspica, Nelumbo komarovii, Nelumbo nelumbo, Nelumbo speciosum, Nymphaea nelumbo.
Family: Nelumbonaceae.

Comments
At the date of publication, there was very little scientific information about this product. Our staff is continually analyzing the available information on natural medicines and will add data to the online version of *Natural Medicines Comprehensive Database* as it becomes available. See www.naturaldatabase.com.

LOVAGE

Also Known As
Lavose, Levistici radix, Love Parsley, Maggi Plant, Sea Parsley, Smallage, Smellage.

Scientific Names
Levisticum officinale, synonyms Angelica levisticum, Hipposelinum levisticum, Ligusticum levisticum.
Family: Apiaceae/Umbelliferae.

People Use This For
Orally, lovage is used as "irrigation therapy" for inflammation of the lower urinary tract, for prevention of kidney gravel, and as a diuretic for urinary tract infections or pedal edema. Lovage is also used orally for indigestion, heartburn, stomach distention, flatulence, as an expectorant, to loosen secretions in respiratory conditions, for menstrual irregularities, sore throat, boils, jaundice, malaria, pleurisy, gout, rheumatism, and migraines.
In foods and beverages, lovage is used as a flavor component.
In manufacturing, lovage is used as a fragrance component in soaps and cosmetics.

Safety
LIKELY SAFE ...when used orally in amounts commonly found in foods. Lovage has Generally Recognized As Safe (GRAS) status in the US (4912).
POSSIBLY SAFE ...when used orally and appropriately (12).
PREGNANCY: LIKELY UNSAFE ...when used orally; lovage is reported to have uterine and menstrual stimulant effects (12).
LACTATION: Insufficient reliable information available; avoid using.

Effectiveness
There is insufficient reliable information available about the effectiveness of lovage.

Mechanism of Action
The applicable parts of lovage are the rhizome and root. Lovage contains 0.2-2% volatile oil (5,6,8,11). Its principal constituents are lactone derivatives known as phthalides. Of these, ligustilide has sedative (6,8,11), antispasmodic (6,8,11), and aquaretic (5,6,8,11,512) effects in experimental animals. Aquaretics increase urine volume (water loss) but not electrolyte excretion (512). It can also have varied actions including cholinergic and antimicrobial activity (18), increased uterine tone (12), and increased gastrointestinal blood flow (6). The bitter taste and aroma of lovage can increase the production of saliva and gastric juices (6,8,18). The furanocoumarin constituents might cause phototoxic reactions including photosensitivity dermatitis (2,5,6,8,11,12).

Adverse Reactions
Orally, long term use may result in an increased risk of phototoxic reactions, including photosensitivity dermatitis (2,5,6,8,11,12). Avoid excessive exposure to the sun or UV light if using lovage (2,12).

Interactions with Herbs & Other Dietary Supplements
None known.

Interactions with Drugs
DIURETIC DRUGS: Theoretically, lovage root might interfere with diuretic therapy due to the aquaretic effects of lovage (512).

Interactions with Foods
None known.

Interactions with Lab Tests
None known.

Interactions with Diseases or Conditions
EDEMA: "Irrigation therapy," which is the use of a mild diuretic and copious fluid intake to increase urine flow, is contraindicated in cases of edema that are due to limited heart or kidney function (2).
HYPERTENSION: Theoretically, lovage root might increase sodium retention and worsen hypertension (512).
RENAL DISEASE: Lovage is contraindicated in acute kidney inflammation (2,8,12) or impaired kidney function (2,12).

Dosage and Administration
ORAL: The typical dose of lovage is one cup of the tea two to three times per day (8). The tea is prepared by steeping 1.5-3 grams of the dried root in 150 mL boiling water for 10-15 minutes and then straining. Lovage should only be used up to 4-8 grams of the dried root per day (2,7). Ample fluid intake is essential when used for "irrigation therapy" (18). For stomach complaints, one cup of the tea is commonly taken 30 minutes before meals (8). Avoid excessive sun or UV light exposure with prolonged use of lovage due to its phototoxic adverse effects.

LUFFA

Also Known As
Angled Loofah, Dishcloth Sponge, Loofa, Loofah, Luffaschwamm, Sigualuo, Silky Loofah, Smooth Loofah, Sponge Cucumber, Vegetable Sponge, Water Gourd.

Scientific Names
Luffa aegyptiaca; Luffa acutangula; Luffa cylindrica.
Family: Cucurbitaceae.

People Use This For
Orally, luffa is used for treating and preventing colds, nasal inflammation, sinusitis, suppuration of the sinuses, for arthritis pain, muscle pain, chest pain, amenorrhea, and to promote lactation.
Topically, luffa sponge is used to remove dead skin and stimulate the skin. Luffa charcoal is used topically for shingles in the face and eye region.
In foods, young luffa fruits are eaten as vegetables.
In cosmetics, powdered luffa is used in skin care products as an anti-inflammatory and detoxicant.

Safety
LIKELY SAFE ...when used topically as a sponge for exfoliation (11).
POSSIBLY SAFE ...when used orally in amounts found in foods (11).
There is insufficient reliable information available about the safety of luffa for its other uses.
PREGNANCY AND LACTATION: POSSIBLY SAFE ...when used orally in amounts found in foods (11).

Effectiveness
There is insufficient reliable information available about the effectiveness of luffa.

Mechanism of Action
The applicable part of luffa is the dried fiber structure from the ripe fruit. The toxicity of luffa is low.

Adverse Reactions
None reported.

Interactions with Herbs & Other Dietary Supplements
None known.

Interactions with Drugs
None known.

Interactions with Foods
None known.

Interactions with Lab Tests
None known.

Interactions with Diseases or Conditions
None known.

Dosage and Administration
ORAL: No typical dosage.
TOPICAL: Luffa is powdered and used in skin care products. The intact sponge is also used to remove dead skin (11).

LUNGMOSS

Also Known As
Lungwort, Oak Lungs.
CAUTION: See separate listing for Lungwort.

Scientific Names
Lobaria pulmonaria.
Family: Lobariaceae.

Comments
At the date of publication, this product was not a common ingredient used in brand name supplements marketed to consumers. Details about this product are available at the online version of *Natural Medicines Comprehensive Database*. See www.naturaldatabase.com.

LUNGWORT

Also Known As
Dage of Jerusalem, Lungenkraut, Pulmonariae herba.
CAUTION: See separate listing for Lungmoss.

Scientific Names
Pulmonaria officinalis.
Family: Boraginaceae.

People Use This For
Orally, lungwort is used to treat conditions of the respiratory tract, gastrointestinal (GI) tract, kidney tract, and urinary tract. Lungwort is also used orally in irritant-relieving cough medicines, as a diuretic, and to treat lung diseases such as tuberculosis.
Topically, it is used as an astringent and to treat wounds.

Safety
There is insufficient reliable information available about the safety of lungwort.
Pregnancy and Lactation: Insufficient reliable information available; avoid using.

Effectiveness
There is insufficient reliable information available about the effectiveness of lungwort.

Mechanism of Action
The applicable parts of lungwort are the above ground parts. Lungwort was thought to contain hepatotoxic unsaturated pyrrolizidine alkaloids (UPAs), but gas chromatography analysis of multiple samples failed to detect these compounds (12).

Adverse Reactions
None reported.

Interactions with Herbs & Other Dietary Supplements
None known.

Interactions with Drugs
None known.

Interactions with Foods
None known.

Interactions with Lab Tests
None known.

Interactions with Diseases or Conditions
None known.

Dosage and Administration
ORAL: One cup of tea has been taken as sips repeatedly with honey throughout the day. The tea is prepared by heating or scalding 1.5 grams dried herb rapidly in 150 mL of boiling water, then straining for 5-10 minutes (18).

Comments
The taste of lungwort is described as dry and slimy. Pulmonaria officinalis and lungmoss (Lobaria pulmonaria) are both known as lungwort, but are physically distinct. Pulmonaria officinalis is a plant and lungmoss is a lichen (18).

LUTEIN

Also Known As
Xanthophyll, Zeaxanthin.

Scientific Names
Beta,epsilon-carotene-3,3'-diol.

People Use This For
Orally, lutein is used for preventing age-related macular degeneration (AMD), cataracts, retinitis pigmentosa, and colon cancer.

Safety
LIKELY SAFE ...when used orally (219,3219,3220).
PREGNANCY AND LACTATION: LIKELY SAFE ...when used orally (219,3219,3220).

Effectiveness
POSSIBLY EFFECTIVE

Age-related macular degeneration (AMD). There is some epidemiological evidence that people who consume higher amounts of lutein in their diet have a reduced risk of developing AMD (219,2394). Preliminary clinical research suggests that taking lutein supplements 10 mg per day for 12 months can improve some symptoms of AMD such as macular pigment optical density and glare recovery, near vision acuity, and contrast sensitivity. But lutein supplements don't seem to affect the progression of AMD. It's not known whether lutein supplements can decrease the risk of AMD as effectively as dietary lutein (11798).

Cataracts. There are epidemiological studies that suggest a reduced risk of developing severe cataracts that require surgical removal in people consuming higher amounts of lutein in their diet (2395,3219,3220). It is not known if supplemental lutein offers the same benefit.

Colorectal cancer. There is epidemiological evidence that suggests a reduced risk of developing colon cancer in people consuming higher amounts of lutein in their diet (3962). It is not known if supplemental lutein offers the same benefit.

INSUFFICIENT RELIABLE EVIDENCE to RATE

Retinitis pigmentosa. Preliminary clinical evidence suggests that oral lutein might be helpful in the treatment of retinitis pigmentosa (10279). More evidence is needed to rate lutein for this use.

Mechanism of Action

Lutein is a carotenoid that is typically found in combination with its stereoisomer, zeaxanthin. Lutein makes up about 11% of the total carotenoids in serum and about 20% of the carotenoids in adipose tissue. Serum and adipose tissue levels are affected by dietary intake. Lutein levels in breast adipose tissue seem to be affected by diet, which could explain the lower incidence of breast cancer with increased fruit and vegetable intake (10243). Additionally, there is some evidence of an inverse association between serum lutein levels and breast cancer risk (10132). Lutein and zeaxanthin are the two major carotenoid pigments in the human macula and retina (2388,3225). They are thought to function as antioxidants and as blue light filters, protecting underlying ocular tissues from photodamage. Epidemiological evidence has associated high dietary lutein intake with reduced risk of developing age-related macular degeneration (AMD) and cataracts (2394,2395,3219,3220). Increasing dietary lutein intake increases serum lutein levels and macular pigment density (2389,10245). Low dietary lutein intake is associated with males, smokers, and people who drink alcohol (more than 2 drinks per week); while higher dietary lutein intake is associated with females, increasing age, and people with hypertension (2398). Foods containing high concentrations of lutein such as broccoli, spinach, and kale, are associated with the greatest eye health benefits (3219,3220). Other carotenoids and antioxidants such as vitamin A, lycopene, alpha- or beta-carotene, vitamin C, and vitamin E have not been associated with this benefit (3219,3220,3221,3222,3223). Epidemiologic studies have shown that carotenoids might be inversely associated with cancer (3963,3964).

Adverse Reactions

None reported.

Interactions with Herbs & Other Dietary Supplements

BETA-CAROTENE: Concomitant administration may reduce bioavailability of lutein and may reduce or increase bioavailability of beta-carotene (2390,2391).

Interactions with Drugs

None known.

Interactions with Foods

OLESTRA: Theoretically, use of Olestra may interfere with supplemental lutein activity. Olestra (fat substitute) lowers serum lutein concentrations in healthy people (2392).

Interactions with Lab Tests

None known.

Interactions with Diseases or Conditions

None known.

Dosage and Administration

ORAL: For reducing the risk of cataracts and age-related macular degeneration (AMD), 6 mg of lutein per day, either through diet or supplementation has been suggested. People consuming 6.9-11.7 mg of lutein per day through diet had the lowest risk of developing AMD and cataracts (3219,3220). For reducing symptoms of AMD, 10 mg per day of lutein supplements have been used (11797). There is 44 mg of lutein per cup of cooked kale, 26 mg/cup of cooked spinach, and 3 mg/cup of broccoli (219,3219,3220). Commercial products containing 6 mg or 20 mg of lutein are available (5020). Supplemental esterified lutein is better absorbed when taken with high fat (36 grams fat) meals compared to low-fat (3 grams fat) meals (6133).

Comments

Centrum and Centrum Silver now contain lutein 0.25 mg per tablet, but probably not enough to provide much benefit (219,3219,3220). Avoid confusion with lutein extract (dried powdered hog corpora lutea) formerly used as a source of progesterone (511). Although dark green leafy vegetables contain 15-47% lutein, they have a very low zeaxanthin content (0-3%). Corn is richest in lutein (60% of total carotenoids), and orange pepper is richest in zeaxanthin (37% of total). Substantial amounts of lutein and zeaxanthin (30-50%) are also present in kiwi fruit, grapes, spinach, orange juice, zucchini, and different kinds of squash (3224).

LYCIUM

Also Known As
Barberry Matrimony Vine, Chinese Boxthorn, Chinese Wolfberry, Di Gu Pi, Digupi, Fructus Lycii, Fructus Lycii Berry, Goji, Goji Berry, Goji Juice, Gou Qi Zi, Gouqizi, Lycii Berries, Matrimony Vine, Ning Xia Gou Qi, Wolfberry.

Scientific Names
Lycium chinense; Lycium barbarum.
Family: Solanaceae.

People Use This For
Orally, lycium is used for diabetes, hypertension, fever, malaria, and cancer. It's also used for improving circulation, erectile dysfunction, dizziness, tinnitus; and as an eye tonic for blurred vision, macular degeneration, and other ophthalmic disorders. Lycium is also used orally to strengthen muscles and bone, and as a blood, liver, and kidney tonic. It is used orally to reduce fever, sweating, irritability, thirst, nosebleeds, hemoptysis, cough, and wheezing. In foods, the berries are eaten raw and used in cooking.

Safety
POSSIBLY SAFE ...when used orally and appropriately (12,7126).
PREGNANCY AND LACTATION: LIKELY UNSAFE ...when used orally. Lycium contains betaine, which is an emmenagogue and abortifacient (12,7123); avoid using.

Effectiveness
There is insufficient reliable information available about the effectiveness of lycium.

Mechanism of Action
The applicable parts of lycium are the dried berries and root bark. Both the root bark and berries contain pharmacologically active constituents. Both contain beta-sitosterol which can reduce cholesterol levels by preventing cholesterol absorption in the gastrointestinal tract (5814,7123,7126). The root bark also contains the constituent kukoamine, which might also have cholesterol lowering effects and antihypertensive effects (7123,7126). Lycium root bark also seems to have hypoglycemic effects. Peak blood glucose lowering effects are thought to occur after 3-4 hours and last for 7-8 hours. Lycium root bark is also thought to have antibacterial, antipyretic, and antihypersensitivity properties (7126). Both the root bark and berry contain betaine, which has uterine stimulant properties (7123,7126). The berries also contain beta-carotene, niacin, pyridoxine, and ascorbic acid (7123). There is some preliminary evidence that a cerebroside constituent found in lycium berry might also have hepatoprotective properties (7125).

Adverse Reactions
Orally, the dried root bark has been associated with nausea and vomiting (7126).

Interactions with Herbs & Other Dietary Supplements
HERBS AND SUPPLEMENTS WITH HYPOGLYCEMIC EFFECTS: Lycium root bark might have hypoglycemic effects (7126). Theoretically, concomitant use with other herbs and supplements that decrease blood glucose levels might increase the risk of hypoglycemia. Some of these products include bitter melon, ginger, goat's rue, fenugreek, kudzu, willow bark, and others.
HERBS AND SUPPLEMENTS WITH HYPOTENSIVE EFFECTS: Lycium root bark might have antihypertensive effects (7126). Theoretically, concurrent use of lycium root bark with other herbs and supplements that decrease blood pressure might increase risk of hypotension. Some of these products include danshen, ginger, Panax ginseng, turmeric, valerian, and others.

Interactions with Drugs
ANTIDIABETES DRUGS: Lycium root bark might have hypoglycemic effects (7126). Theoretically, concomitant use with drugs used for diabetes might enhance blood glucose lowering effects and increase the risk of hypoglycemia. Monitor blood glucose levels closely. Some antidiabetes drugs include glimepiride (Amaryl), glyburide (Diabeta, Glynase PresTab, Micronase), insulin, pioglitazone (Actos), rosiglitazone (Avandia), and others.
ANTIHYPERTENSIVE DRUGS: Lycium root bark might have hypotensive effects (7126). Theoretically, concomitant use with antihypertensives might have additive effects on blood pressure and increase the risk of hypotension.
CYTOCHROME P450 2C9 (CYP2C9) SUBSTRATES: There is some evidence that lycium can inhibit CYP2C9 (7158). Watch for an increase in the levels of drugs metabolized by CYP2C9 in patients taking lycium. Some drugs metabolized by CYP2C9 include amitriptyline (Elavil), diazepam (Valium), estradiol (Estrace), tacrine (Cognex), verapamil (Calan), warfarin (Coumadin), zileuton (Zyflo), and others.

WARFARIN (Coumadin): There is some evidence that lycium can increase the effects of warfarin and possibly increase the risk of bleeding. International normalized ratio (INR) can increase in patients stabilized on warfarin who begin taking lycium. Researchers think that lycium inhibits cytochrome P450 2C9 (CYP2C9) metabolism of warfarin and increases warfarin levels (7158). Use with caution. Warfarin dose adjustments may be necessary.

Interactions with Foods
None known.

Interactions with Lab Tests
BLOOD GLUCOSE: Lycium root bark might lower blood glucose levels in some patients (7126).
WHITE BLOOD CELL COUNT (WBC): Lycium berries might increase leukocyte and lymphocyte counts in some patients (7126).

Interactions with Diseases or Conditions
DIABETES: Lycium root bark might have hypoglycemic effects (7126). Theoretically, use in patients treated with antidiabetes medications might enhance blood glucose lowering effects and increase the risk of hypoglycemia. Monitor blood glucose levels closely (7126).
HYPERTENSION: Lycium root bark might have hypotensive effects (7126). Theoretically, concomitant use in patients treated with antihypertensives might have additive effects on blood pressure and potentially increase the risk of hypotension.
HYPOTENSION: Lycium root bark might have hypotensive effects (7126). Theoretically, use in people with existing low blood pressure might exacerbate hypotension and possibly lead to syncope.

Dosage and Administration
ORAL: Lycium is usually taken as a tea. A typical dose is one or more cups of tea daily; however, the strength of the tea can vary depending on the condition being treated. Typically the tea is made by boiling 20 grams of berries or root bark in 3 cups of water and simmered until the volume is reduced to 2 cups. For fever, one cup daily of this preparation is commonly used (7122). For diabetes, 6 to 12 grams is commonly boiled and consumed as a tea. For hypertension, 30 grams of the root bark boiled in 100 mL is commonly used. For treating malaria, 30 grams of the root bark is commonly boiled and consumed as a tea (7126).

Comments
Lycium is a native Chinese deciduous shrub with bright red berries. The use of lycium was first described in the first century AD in Chinese literature. Traditionally, lycium has been used to promote longevity. Legend reports that one herbalist who used lycium in combination with other tonic herbs lived 252 years (7122).

LYCOPENE

Also Known As
All-Trans Lycopene, Lycopenes.

Scientific Names
All-Trans-Lycopene, Psi-Psi-Carotene.

People Use This For
Orally, lycopene is used for preventing atherosclerosis, cardiovascular disease, and cancer. Lycopene is also used to treat prostate cancer, human papilloma virus (HPV) infection, and asthma.

Safety
LIKELY SAFE ...when consumed in amounts commonly found in foods (2406,7772,7773).
POSSIBLY SAFE ...when used orally in medicinal amounts. Lycopene supplements 30 mg daily have been used safely for eight weeks (7771,7898,7899).
PREGNANCY AND LACTATION: LIKELY SAFE ...when consumed in amounts commonly found in foods. There is insufficient reliable information available about the safety of lycopene supplements used during pregnancy and lactation; avoid using in amounts greater than those typically found in foods.

Effectiveness
POSSIBLY EFFECTIVE

Asthma. Taking a specific tomato extract containing lycopene (Lyc-o-mato) orally seems to reduce exercise-induced asthma. Lycopene seems to prevent decreases in forced expiratory volume (FEV1) in response to exercise in some people with exercise-induced asthma (7898).

Lung cancer. There is epidemiological evidence that consuming lycopene from foods (12 mg per day or more for men, and 6.5 mg per day or more for women) decreases the risk of lung cancer in nonsmoking men aged 40 to 75, and non-smoking women aged 30 to 55 (2595).

Ovarian cancer. There is some evidence a diet rich in carotenoids, including lycopene, can decrease the risk of ovarian cancer in premenopausal women (10133).

Prostate cancer. Men who consume 6 mg per day or more of lycopene from foods such as tomatoes and tomato products seem to have a significantly reduced risk of developing prostate cancer (2406,7772,7773,7895). Men with high lycopene plasma levels seem to have an 83% lower risk of prostate cancer compared to men with low plasma lycopene levels (7773). Lycopene supplements haven't been studied for prostate cancer prevention. Recommend a diet high in tomatoes and tomato products, particularly tomato sauce, to men concerned about prostate cancer prevention (7772). However, there is preliminary evidence that lycopene supplements might help for prostate cancer treatment. Taking lycopene supplements, 15 mg twice daily, for three weeks before radical prostatectomy might decrease tumor growth (7771).

POSSIBLY INEFFECTIVE

Bladder cancer. Consuming dietary lycopene doesn't seem to reduce the risk of bladder cancer. Epidemiological research shows no association between dietary lycopene intake or serum lycopene levels and the risk of bladder cancer (2407).

Cardiovascular disease. Epidemiologic evidence in women without heart disease suggests that there is no association between dietary lycopene intake and the risk of myocardial infarction, stroke, and other cardiovascular events (10418). Epidemiologic evidence in men at low risk for heart disease suggests dietary intake of lycopene doesn't prevent myocardial infarction (9594).

Colorectal cancer. Epidemiological research shows no association between dietary lycopene intake and the risk of colon cancer (3962).

INSUFFICIENT RELIABLE EVIDENCE to RATE

Atherosclerosis. Epidemiological studies of dietary lycopene intake and prevention of atherosclerosis are inconclusive (1446,1449).

Breast cancer. Preliminary research suggests that higher serum levels of lycopene might be protective against breast cancer (10132).

Human papilloma virus (HPV). Preliminary evidence suggests that women with higher plasma levels of lycopene have a faster rate of oncogenic HPV clearance compared to women with lower levels of plasma lycopene. Women with higher levels of lycopene cleared oncogenic HPV in an average of 8.5 months compared to 11-12 months in women with lower levels (12177).

More evidence is needed to rate lycopene for these uses.

Mechanism of Action

Lycopene is a carotenoid, but contains no vitamin A activity (1928,7771,7895,7896). It is the pigment that gives some fruits and vegetables, such as tomatoes, their red color (1928,2401). It is also found in watermelons, pink grapefruits, apricots, and pink guavas.

In North America, 85% of dietary lycopene comes from tomato-derived products such as tomato juice or paste. One cup (240 mL) of tomato juice provides about 23 mg of lycopene (1499). Lycopene exists naturally in fresh fruits and vegetables in the trans configuration, which is poorly absorbed (1928). Heat processing of raw foods into products such as tomato paste, juice, ketchup, and others induces the isomerization of lycopene from the trans- to the cis-configuration. The cis isomer has better bioavailability (1928,1497). Serum concentrations and adipose tissue concentrations of lycopene are influenced by dietary intake (10243). Lycopene supplements seem to have a similar bioavailability to foods; lycopene supplements can provide serum lycopene levels similar to tomato juice when ingested in equivalent amounts (1498).

Lycopene is a predominant carotenoid in blood and tissues (7773,10243). It is highly lipophilic and is commonly found within cellular membranes. Lycopene has the most potent antioxidant activity of any common carotenoid; it might reduce cancer risk by scavenging free radicals and quenching singlet oxygen, which prevents oxidative damage to DNA (2401,7773). Some researchers are interested in lycopene as a prevention of cancer, atherosclerosis, and other conditions. In vitro, lycopene seems to inhibit the oxidation of low density lipoproteins (LDL) (1928). Like other carotenoid substances, lycopene is transported in the blood and on LDL cholesterol, making it readily available to act as an antioxidant. Preliminary evidence suggests that lycopene may decrease cholesterol synthesis and increase removal of LDL cholesterol from circulation (7896). Lower tissue levels of lycopene have been associated with increased risk of myocardial infarction (MI), but epidemiological studies have found no correlation between lycopene intake and MI risk (7897,9594,10418).

In vitro, lycopene inhibits the proliferation of breast cancer, lung cancer, and prostate cancer (1928). There is also some evidence that decreased serum or tissue lycopene concentrations might increase the risk of developing prostate cancer (1447,1496,2405,2406,2407). Lycopene seems to have some direct effects within the prostate, specifically up-regulating tumor suppressor genes (7771). Animal research suggests lycopene alone might not affect prostate cancer risk. Tomato products, which contain lycopene, inhibit experimentally induced prostate cancer; lycopene alone does not (11304,11305). Lycopene supplements for prostate cancer have not been studied in humans.

Lycopene seems to reduce proliferation of prostatic epithelial cells (11237). But there's no credible clinical research to support using lycopene supplements to treat or prevent benign prostatic hyperplasia (BPH).

Adverse Reactions
None reported.

Interactions with Herbs & Other Dietary Supplements
BETA-CAROTENE: Concomitant ingestion may increase lycopene absorption (2403).

Interactions with Drugs
None known.

Interactions with Foods
None known.

Interactions with Lab Tests
PROSTATE-SPECIFIC ANTIGEN (PSA): Lycopene seems to reduce plasma PSA levels in men with prostate cancer (7771,7774).

Interactions with Diseases or Conditions
None known.

Dosage and Administration
ORAL: For decreasing the growth of prostate cancer, lycopene 15 mg twice daily has been used (7771). For reducing the risk of prostate cancer, at least 6 mg of lycopene per day from foods is needed (2406). For reducing the risk of lung cancer in non-smoking men, at least 12 mg of lycopene per day from foods is needed (2595). For reducing the risk of lung cancer in non-smoking women, at least 6.5 mg of lycopene per day from foods is needed (2595). For preventing exercise-induced asthma, lycopene 30 mg daily has been used (7898).

LYSINE

Also Known As
L-Lysine, Lys, Lysine Hydrochloride, Lysine Monohydrochloride.

Scientific Names
L-2,6-diaminohexanoic acid.

People Use This For
Orally, lysine is used for preventing and treating clinical symptoms of recurrent herpes simplex labialis. It is also used as an aid to improving athletic performance.
Lysine monohydrochloride is used to treat metabolic alkalosis.

Safety
POSSIBLY SAFE ...when used orally and appropriately for up to one year (1114,1120).
PREGNANCY AND LACTATION: Insufficient reliable information available; avoid using.

Effectiveness
POSSIBLY EFFECTIVE

Herpes labialis (cold sores). Taking lysine orally seems to reduce recurrences of herpes simplex labialis infections (1114,1115,1116,1118,1120), and reduce the severity and healing time of herpes simplex labialis infections (1119,1120).

There is insufficient reliable information available about the effectiveness of lysine for its other uses.

Mechanism of Action
Lysine is required for collagen synthesis and it may be important to bone health (1124,1130). Lysine antagonizes herpes simplex virus (HSV) growth in vitro and this effect may be important clinically (119).

Adverse Reactions
Orally, diarrhea and abdominal pain occur have been reported (1114,1115,1116,1118,1120). There is one case report of supplemental lysine use associated with tubulointerstitial nephritis progressing to chronic renal failure (1121).

Interactions with Herbs & Other Dietary Supplements
CALCIUM SUPPLEMENTS: Concomitant use may increase supplemental calcium absorption and decrease urine calcium loss (1131).

Interactions with Drugs

CALCIUM SUPPLEMENTS: Concomitant use may increase supplemental calcium absorption and decrease urine calcium loss (1131).

Interactions with Foods

None known.

Interactions with Lab Tests

None known.

Interactions with Diseases or Conditions

KIDNEY DISEASES: There is one case report of supplemental lysine associated with tubulointerstitial nephritis progressing to chronic renal failure (1121).
OSTEOPOROSIS: Concomitant use of lysine and calcium supplements may increase supplemental calcium absorption and decrease urine calcium loss (1131).

Dosage and Administration

ORAL: Recurrent herpes simplex labialis infections, 1000 mg daily for twelve months and 1000 mg three times daily for six months reported in clinical trials (1114,1120).

MACA

Also Known As

Ayak Chichira, Ayuk Willku, Maca Maca, Maino, Maka, Peruvian Ginseng.

Scientific Names

Lepidium meyenii, synonym Lepidium peruvianum.
Family: Brassicaceae/Cruciferae.

People Use This For

Orally, maca is used for anemia; chronic fatigue syndrome; and enhancing energy, stamina, athletic performance, and memory. It is also used for female hormone imbalance, menstrual irregularities, enhancing fertility, menopause symptoms, depression, stomach cancer, leukemia, AIDS, tuberculosis, as an aphrodisiac, for impotence, and as an immunostimulant.
In foods, maca is eaten baked or roasted, prepared as a soup, and used for making a fermented drink, maca chicha.

Safety

LIKELY SAFE ...when maca is consumed in food amounts (9926).
POSSIBLY SAFE ...when used orally and appropriately, short term. Maca appears to be safe in doses up to 3 grams daily for 12 weeks (10218).
PREGNANCY AND LACTATION: There is insufficient reliable information available about the safety of maca in medicinal amounts during pregnancy and lactation; avoid using.

Effectiveness

POSSIBLY EFFECTIVE

Sexual desire. Taking maca orally 1.5 to 3 grams per day seems to increase subjective feelings of sexual desire in healthy men (9928).

There is insufficient reliable information available about the effectiveness of maca for its other uses.

Mechanism of Action

The applicable part of maca is the root. Dried maca root contains 59% carbohydrates; 10.2% protein; 8.5% fiber; and 2.2% lipids including linolenic, palmitic, and oleic acids. It contains sterols such as campesterol, stigmasterol, and beta-sitosterol. It also contains significant amounts of minerals including iron, calcium, and copper (9929). Two polyunsaturated fatty acids, macaene and macamide, are used as marker compounds for maca (9926). Lipid extracts of macaene and macamide seem to increase sexual activity and correct erectile dysfunction in experimental animals. The mechanism for this activity is unknown (10218). Maca does not appear to significantly affect serum concentrations of reproductive hormones including testosterone, estradiol, and 17-hydroxyprogesterone in healthy men (10219).
Maca also contains glucosinolates, which might have cancer-protecting properties and central nervous system effects (9927,9929).

Adverse Reactions
None reported.

Interactions with Herbs & Other Dietary Supplements
None known.

Interactions with Drugs
None known.

Interactions with Foods
None known.

Interactions with Lab Tests
None known.

Interactions with Diseases or Conditions
None known.

Dosage and Administration
ORAL: For enhancing sexual desire in men, 1500 to 3000 mg daily in 3 divided doses has been used. The 1500 mg dose appears to be as effective as the 3000 mg dose (9928).

Comments
Maca grows in central Peru in the high plateaus of the Andes mountains. It has been cultivated as a vegetable crop in the Andes mountains of Peru for at least 3000 years. Maca is a relative of the radish and has an odor similar to butterscotch. It was also used to enhance the fertility of humans and livestock (9925,9926).

MADAGASCAR PERIWINKLE

Also Known As
Cape Periwinkle, Catharanthus, Church-Flower, Magdalena, Myrtle, Old Maid, Periwinkle, Ram-Goat Rose, Red Periwinkle.
CAUTION: See separate listing for Periwinkle.

Scientific Names
Catharanthus roseus, synonyms Vinca rosea, Lochnera rosea, Ammocallis rosea.
Family: Apocynaceae.

People Use This For
Orally, Madagascar periwinkle is used for diabetes, cancer, as a cough remedy, for easing lung congestion, throat inflammation, and as a diuretic.
Topically, it is used as a hemostatic, for insect bites, wasp stings, eye irritation, infection, and inflammation.

Safety
LIKELY UNSAFE ...when the plant or root are used orally. Madagascar periwinkle contains vinca alkaloids which can cause death (6).
There is insufficient reliable information available about the safety of the topical use of Madagascar periwinkle.
PREGNANCY: LIKELY UNSAFE ...when used orally because it has abortifacient and teratogenic properties (19).
LACTATION: LIKELY UNSAFE ...when used orally (6); avoid using.

Effectiveness
There is insufficient reliable information available about the effectiveness of Madagascar periwinkle.

Mechanism of Action
The applicable parts of Madagascar periwinkle are the above ground parts. The vinca alkaloids, vincristine and vinblastine, block cell mitosis, have immunosuppressive effects, and in high concentrations, exert effects on nucleic acid and protein synthesis (6,15). The constituent, catharanthine, demonstrates diuretic properties (6). Hypotensive constituents, reserpine and alstonine, have also been isolated from Madagascar periwinkle root (6). The constituent, ajmalicine, may improve cerebral blood flow; it has been combined with rauwolfia alkaloids for treating high blood pressure (6). Concentrated extracts are reported to lower blood glucose (6), but studies by one pharmaceutical company found the plant had no effect on blood glucose levels (6).

Adverse Reactions
Orally, the plant is an hallucinogen, and has caused seizures, GI upset, hepatotoxicity, and alopecia (17). Adverse effects of Vinca alkaloids include nausea, vomiting, alopecia, dizziness, nystagmus, vertigo, hearing impairment, leukopenia, thrombocytopenia, bleeding, hyperuricemia, neurotoxicity, and possibly death (6,15).

Interactions with Herbs & Other Dietary Supplements
None known.

Interactions with Drugs
ANTIDIABETES DRUGS: Madagascar periwinkle may cause hypoglycemia (6,19); monitor blood glucose control closely.

Interactions with Foods
None known.

Interactions with Lab Tests
BLOOD GLUCOSE: Madagascar periwinkle may lower blood glucose. There is conflicting information about possible hypoglycemic activity (6,19).

Interactions with Diseases or Conditions
DIABETES: Madagascar periwinkle may cause hypoglycemia (6,19).

Dosage and Administration
No typical dosage.

Comments
Madagascar periwinkle is considered likely unsafe; avoid, due to presence of toxic vinca alkaloids. The vinca alkaloids, vinblastine and vincristine, isolated from Madagascar periwinkle, are FDA approved for use as chemotherapeutic agents to treat cancers, including Hodgkin's disease, leukemia, Kaposi's sarcoma, malignant lymphomas, mycosis fungoides neuroblastoma, and Wilm's tumor (6).

MADDER

Also Known As
Dyer's Madder, Farberrote, Garance, Robbia, Rubia, Rubiae tinctorum radix.

Scientific Names
Rubia tinctorum.
Family: Rubiaceae.

People Use This For
Orally, madder is used for preventing kidney stones, for disintegrating kidney stones, and for general menstrual and urinary disorders.

Safety
LIKELY UNSAFE ...when used orally. It is potentially carcinogenic and mutagenic (2,18,19).
PREGNANCY: UNSAFE ...when used orally because it may be a potential menstrual stimulant and a genotoxin (2,19).
LACTATION: UNSAFE ...when used orally because it is a potential genotoxin (2,19). It also can cause red-colored breast milk (2).

Effectiveness
There is insufficient reliable information available about the effectiveness of madder.

Mechanism of Action
The applicable part of madder is the root. Madder contains lucidin, which is an anthracene derivative. The Ames test shows that anthracene has genotoxic activity, and causes dose-dependent increases in benign and malignant liver and kidney tumors in experimental rats (3718). Madder also seems to decrease calcium oxalate crystallization in the kidney, which potentially could induce kidney or bladder stones (2).

Adverse Reactions
Orally, madder can cause red colored urine, saliva, perspiration, and breast milk (2). There is some concern that madder can stain contact lenses. Advise patients to be cautious (6002).

Interactions with Herbs & Other Dietary Supplements
None known.

Interactions with Drugs
None known.

Interactions with Foods
None known.

Interactions with Lab Tests
COLORIMETRIC TESTS: Theoretically, madder might interfere with colorimetric tests involving urine, saliva, perspiration, and breast milk due to red coloring of these body fluids (2).

Interactions with Diseases or Conditions
None known.

Dosage and Administration
ORAL: People typically prepare madder bark using one teaspoon boiled in a covered container with 3 cups of water for 30 minutes. The liquid is cooled slowly in the closed container and taken cold, 1 to 2 cups per day (5254).

MAGNESIUM

Also Known As
Chelated Magnesium, Epsom Salts, Magnesia, Magnesium Aspartate, Magnesium Carbonate, Magnesium Chloride, Magnesium Citrate, Magnesium Gluconate, Magnesium Hydroxide, Magnesium Lactate, Magnesium Orotate, Magnesium Oxide, Magnesium Sulfate, Magnesium Trisilicate, Milk of Magnesia.
CAUTION: See separate listings for Chelated Minerals and Dolomite.

Scientific Names
Magnesium; Mg; atomic number 12.

People Use This For
Orally, magnesium is used for treating and preventing hypomagnesemia. It is also used orally as a laxative for constipation and for preparation of the bowel for surgical or diagnostic procedures. Magnesium is also used orally for treating symptoms of asthma and allergic rhinitis; for cardiovascular diseases including angina, arrhythmias, hypertension, coronary heart disease and hyperlipidemia, low high-density lipoprotein (HDL) levels, mitral valve prolapse, vasospastic angina, myocardial infarction, multiple sclerosis; and as an antacid for symptoms of gastric hyperacidity. It is also used orally for treating attention deficit-hyperactivity disorder (ADHD), chronic fatigue syndrome (CFS), fibromyalgia, pregnancy-induced leg cramps, diabetes, kidney stones, migraine headaches, osteoporosis, premenstrual syndrome, altitude sickness, urinary incontinence, kidney stones, erythromelalgia, restless leg syndrome, and for preventing hearing loss. Magnesium is also used orally by athletes to increase energy and endurance.
Topically, magnesium is used for treating infected skin ulcers, boils, and carbuncles; and for speeding wound healing. It is also used topically as a cold compress in the treatment of erysipelas and as a hot compress for deep-seated skin infections.
Parenterally, magnesium is used for acute hypomagnesemia occurring in conditions such as pancreatitis, malabsorption disorders, and cirrhosis, and for treating pre-eclampsia and eclampsia. It is also used as an additive to total parenteral nutrition (TPN) for prevention of hypomagnesemia. Intravenously, magnesium is used for controlling seizures associated with epilepsy, glomerulonephritis, or hypothyroidism when low serum magnesium levels are present. It is also used intravenously in the treatment of atrial and ventricular arrhythmias, including torsades de pointes, for preventing arrhythmias after myocardial infarction, and for cardiac arrest. Magnesium is also used intravenously for treating acute exacerbations of asthma and chronic obstructive pulmonary disease (COPD), for migraine headaches, neuropathic pain and postoperative pain, as an osmotic agent for cerebral edema, and for tetanus.

Safety

LIKELY SAFE ...when used orally and appropriately. Oral magnesium is safe when used in doses below the tolerable upper intake level (UL) of 350 mg per day (7555). ...when used parenterally and appropriately. Parenteral magnesium sulfate is an FDA-approved prescription product (9495).

POSSIBLY UNSAFE ...when used orally in excessive doses. Doses greater than the tolerable upper intake level (UL) of 350 mg frequently cause loose stools and diarrhea (7555). ...when magnesium sulfate is used topically, long-term. Prolonged use may damage the skin (9).

CHILDREN: LIKELY SAFE ...when used orally and appropriately. Magnesium is safe when used in doses below the tolerable upper intake level (UL) of 65 mg per day for children 1 to 3 years, 110 mg per day for children 4 to 8 years, and 350 mg per day for children older than 8 years (7555). ...when used parenterally and appropriately (9496). LIKELY UNSAFE ...when used orally in excessive doses. Tell patients not to use doses above the tolerable upper intake level (UL). Higher doses can cause diarrhea and symptomatic hypermagnesemia including hypotension, nausea, vomiting, and bradycardia (7555,8095).

PREGNANCY AND LACTATION: LIKELY SAFE ...when used orally and appropriately. Magnesium is safe for pregnant and breast-feeding women when used in doses below the tolerable upper intake level (UL) of 350 mg per day (7555). POSSIBLY SAFE ...when given intramuscularly prior to delivery (15). POSSIBLY UNSAFE ...when used orally in excessive doses. Tell patients to avoid exceeding the tolerable upper intake level (UL) of 350 mg per day. Higher doses frequently can cause diarrhea (7555). LIKELY UNSAFE ...when used intravenously less than two hours before delivery. Intravenous infusions of magnesium sulfate can cause neonatal respiratory depression when given to toxemic mothers (15).

Effectiveness

EFFECTIVE

Constipation. Taking magnesium orally is helpful as a laxative for constipation and for preparation of the bowel for surgical or diagnostic procedures. Magnesium citrate, sulfate, and hydroxide salts are typically used for this indication. The magnesium sulfate salt is the most potent (6430).

Gastroesophageal reflux disease (GERD). Taking magnesium orally as an antacid reduces symptoms of gastric hyperacidity or GERD. Typically, magnesium carbonate, hydroxide, oxide, or trisilicate salts are used. Magnesium hydroxide has the fastest onset of action. Magnesium carbonate is slower due to its crystal structure. Magnesium trisilicate has the slowest onset and longest duration due to poor solubility (6844).

Hypomagnesemia. Taking magnesium orally or parenterally is helpful for treating and preventing hypomagnesemia. Magnesium deficiency typically occurs in certain disease states such as alcoholism and cirrhosis of the liver, congestive heart failure, severe or prolonged diarrhea or vomiting, kidney dysfunction, inflammatory bowel disease (IBS), pancreatitis, and various malabsorption syndromes (6280,6281,8088,8089). Hypomagnesemia is often associated with other electrolyte disorders such as hypokalemia, hyponatremia, hypophosphatemia, and hypocalcemia (8088). Magnesium deficiency can also negatively affect insulin sensitivity and metabolic control in type 2 diabetes (10664). There is some controversy regarding whether parenteral or oral magnesium replacement is better. Because higher oral doses of magnesium might result in diarrhea, some suggest parenteral administration is better. However, oral magnesium can be used carefully in adequate doses for replacement without causing diarrhea. Magnesium gluconate or chloride are preferred for oral replacement because they cause diarrhea less often (6430). Oral magnesium chloride solution has also been used for replacement purposes (10664). Magnesium oxide should be avoided due to greater risk of diarrhea. Magnesium carbonate may not be soluble enough to adequately replace magnesium levels and should also be avoided. Magnesium-rich mineral water (Hepar) has also been used for dietary supplementation (8099).

LIKELY EFFECTIVE

Pre-eclampsia and eclampsia. Administering magnesium parenterally is helpful for preventing and managing pre-eclampsia and eclampsia (9473). Intravenous or intramuscular magnesium sulfate is considered the agent of choice for pre-eclampsia and eclampsia (15).

Torsade de pointes. Administering magnesium intravenously is helpful for treating torsade de pointes. Magnesium sulfate is first-line therapy for torsade de pointes (6844).

POSSIBLY EFFECTIVE

Acute myocardial infarction (MI). Administering magnesium intravenously seems to reduce arrhythmia and mortality after an acute MI. Intravenous magnesium appears to reduce the incidence of complex ventricular arrhythmias after myocardial infarction (9497). However, intravenous magnesium therapy in an acute MI is controversial (8999), and oral magnesium supplementation seems to be ineffective for this use (1198,6844).

Arrhythmias. Administering magnesium intravenously seems to be helpful for treating atrial tachycardia, ventricular fibrillation and tachycardia, and supraventricular tachycardia (15).

Asthma. Administering magnesium intravenously seems to improve acute asthma attacks. A single dose of magnesium seems to improve pulmonary function in asthma exacerbation (9495,9496). However, magnesium supplementation doesn't seem to improve forced expiratory volume in one second (FEV1) or reduce the need for bronchodilator use in patients with chronic asthma (1173).

Cancer-associated neuropathic pain. Administering magnesium intravenously seems to relieve neuropathic pain associated with cancer. Single 500 mg to 1 gram doses of magnesium sulfate seem to relieve neuropathic pain for up to four hours (6846).

Chronic fatigue syndrome (CFS). Administering magnesium intramuscularly seems to improve symptoms for CFS. There is some controversy about the clinical benefits of magnesium for CFS. In people with low red blood cell magnesium, there is some evidence that weekly intramuscular injections of 1 gram magnesium sulfate might improve CFS symptoms (7556). However, there is additional evidence that most patients with CFS have normal magnesium stores (7557,8084,8086,8087). Also, measurement of red cell magnesium is considered to be a poor indicator of body magnesium (8085).
Chronic obstructive pulmonary disease (COPD). Administering magnesium intravenously seems to be helpful for treating acute exacerbation of COPD (1208).
Cluster headache. Administering magnesium intravenously seems to improve cluster headaches (1184,1185).
Coronary artery disease. Taking magnesium orally seems to reduce anginal attacks in people with coronary artery disease (1181).
Diabetes. Higher dietary magnesium intake seems to lower the risk of developing type 2 diabetes, especially in overweight middle-aged women (11352). However, magnesium doesn't seem to improve glycemic control in type 2 diabetes (1171,1172).
Fibromyalgia. Taking magnesium hydroxide plus malic acid (Super Malic tablets) orally seems to decrease fibromyalgia-related pain and tenderness in some patients (3262).
Hearing loss. Taking magnesium orally seems to prevent hearing loss in individuals exposed to loud noise (1205).
Hypercholesterolemia. There is some evidence that taking magnesium chloride and magnesium oxide orally can produce small decreases in low-density lipoprotein (LDL) and total cholesterol levels, and small increases in high-density lipoprotein (HDL) levels. However, magnesium does not seem to improve lipoprotein (a) levels (1193).
Hypertension. Taking magnesium orally can reduce blood pressure to a small extent in people with mild to moderate hypertension. The effect appears to be dose related, requiring doses of 600 to 1000 mg daily (1192,1199,9465). However, significantly lower doses do not seem to have this effect (1180,1195,1197,8098).
Kidney stones (nephrolithiasis). Taking magnesium orally seems to prevent the recurrence of kidney stones. Prophylactic treatment with magnesium hydroxide might decrease the recurrence rate of calcium stone formation (2007). Magnesium in combination with pyridoxine (vitamin B6) also seems to decrease urinary oxalate levels in people with hyperoxaluria who have previously had kidney stones (1201). However, it's unclear if this effect on urinary oxalate levels translates into a reduced incidence of kidney stones. There is also evidence that treatment with other medications such as chlorthalidone (Hygroton) may be more effective than magnesium hydroxide in preventing kidney stone formation (8097).
Migraine headache. Taking high-dose magnesium citrate or trimagnesium dicitrate orally seems to reduce the frequency and severity of migraine headaches (4891,9498). In children, treatment with magnesium oxide may also reduce the frequency and severity of migraine headaches (10663). Although some patients with normal magnesium levels can respond to intravenous magnesium for acute migraine, most patients who benefit seem to have low magnesium levels (6844).
Mitral valve prolapse. Taking magnesium orally seems to reduce symptoms of mitral valve prolapse in people with low serum magnesium levels (1191).
Osteoporosis. There is preliminary evidence that suggests taking magnesium orally might prevent bone loss in postmenopausal osteoporosis (9104).
Post-hysterectomy pain. Administering magnesium intravenously seems to be helpful for pain control after hysterectomy. There is some evidence that a high magnesium dose of 3 grams followed by a 500 mg per hour infusion can reduce discomfort and analgesic requirements in patients post-hysterectomy. However, lower doses of 200 mg followed by an infusion of 200 mg per hour are not effective and might actually increase pain in some patients (6846).
Pregnancy-induced leg cramps. Taking magnesium orally seems to be helpful for treating pregnancy-induced leg cramps (1194).
Premenstrual syndrome (PMS). Taking magnesium orally seems to relieve symptoms of PMS. There is some evidence that magnesium supplementation can improve symptoms including mood changes and fluid retention in some patients with PMS (1187,1188,6847). Taking magnesium orally also seems to prevent premenstrual migraine (1186,6847).
Stroke. There is some evidence that increasing dietary magnesium intake might decrease the relative risk of stroke in men. However, there is no proof that taking magnesium supplements has this same effect (9001,9002). There is also preliminary clinical evidence that suggests intravenous magnesium may act as a neuroprotective agent in patients diagnosed with acute stroke (9000,9003).
Preterm labor. Administering magnesium intravenously seems to be helpful for acute prevention of uterine contractions in preterm labor (tocolysis) (9,15). The use of magnesium for tocolysis is controversial. Not all experts agree it is beneficial (6844). However, most clinicians consider magnesium and beta-adrenergic agonists first-line therapy when tocolysis is indicated. Intravenous magnesium sulfate seems to be effective for delaying delivery for 24 to 48 hours (9,15). Oral magnesium therapy is not effective because it cannot achieve sufficiently high magnesium plasma levels (15).
Vasospastic angina. Administering magnesium intravenously seems to prevent coronary spasm in patients with vasospastic angina. There is evidence that administration of intravenous magnesium (0.27 mmol/kg body weight over 20 minutes) dilates coronary arteries and suppresses acetylcholine-induced coronary spasms in patients with

vasospastic angina (8091).

Wound healing. Applying magnesium topically seems to speed wound healing including skin ulcers and inflammatory conditions such as boils and carbuncles (9).

POSSIBLY INEFFECTIVE

Athletic performance. Taking magnesium orally doesn't seem to increase energy and endurance during athletic activity. Magnesium oxide, aspartate, and orotate salts don't seem to improve exercise performance when used alone or in combination with potassium (2825,2826,2827,2828,2829,2830).

Cardiac arrest. Administering magnesium intravenously doesn't seem to improve successful resuscitation in people with cardiac arrest (1190).

Cerebral palsy. Administering magnesium intravenously doesn't seem to decrease the risk of cerebral palsy in premature infants. Earlier evidence suggested that treatment with magnesium sulfate for tocolysis might also be protective against cerebral palsy. However, there is no additional evidence to confirm that such an association exists (8093).

INSUFFICIENT RELIABLE EVIDENCE to RATE

Attention deficit-hyperactivity disorder (ADHD). Children with ADHD seem to have lower magnesium levels (9969); preliminary clinical research suggests that magnesium might be useful for ADHD in children with low magnesium levels (1189).

Multiple sclerosis (MS). There is some evidence that magnesium may reduce the spasticity associated with MS (9499).

Restless leg syndrome. Preliminary clinical research suggests that taking magnesium orally might be useful for treating restless leg syndrome (periodic limb movement during sleep). In some patients, magnesium treatment may decrease the amount of movement and increase the amount of sleep in patients with restless leg syndrome or periodic limb movement during sleep (9466). However, both magnesium deficiency and high magnesium blood levels have been observed in patients with restless leg syndrome (8096,9472).

More evidence is needed to rate magnesium for these uses.

Mechanism of Action

Magnesium is the second most plentiful cation in the intracellular fluid and the most plentiful cation in the body. Up to 50% of the magnesium in the body is found in bone. Magnesium is important for normal bone structure (272), and plays an essential role in more than 300 cellular reactions (945). Magnesium is required for the formation of cyclic AMP (cAMP) and is involved in ion movements across cell membranes (945). It is involved in protein synthesis and carbohydrate metabolism (272). Extracellular magnesium is critical to both maintaining nerve and muscle electrical potentials and transmitting impulses across neuromuscular junctions (272).

Dietary sources of magnesium include legumes, green leafy vegetables, animal proteins, and nuts (8088). Aging and stress are thought to increase magnesium requirements. Low intake and impaired absorption of magnesium have also been associated with the development of various disease states such as osteoporosis, hypertension, atherosclerotic vascular disease, cardiomyopathy, diabetes, and stroke (8088,8099,8998,9001). Symptoms of severe magnesium deficiency include convulsions, confusion, muscle weakness, abnormal muscle movements, and others (403).

As antacids, magnesium salts work by reacting with gastric acid to form magnesium chloride. Magnesium hydroxide has the fastest onset of action, magnesium carbonate is slower due to its crystal structure, and magnesium trisilicate has the slowest onset and longest duration due to its poor solubility (6844).

The laxative effects and diarrhea produced by magnesium salts are due to the osmotic effects of unabsorbed salts in the intestine and colon, and stimulation of gastric motility due to the release of gastrin and cholecystokinin (6844). The inhibitory effect of magnesium on preterm labor contractions (tocolysis) is attributed to antagonism of calcium-mediated myometrial contractions (6844).

The mechanism of action for magnesium in pre-eclampsia and eclampsia is not clear. There is some evidence that magnesium dilates blood vessels in the central nervous system (CNS) to reduce ischemia. Contrary to this view are indications that magnesium may decrease CNS blood flow (9473). Additionally, magnesium may have anticonvulsant actions in eclampsia due to depression of neuromuscular transmission, direct depressant effect on smooth muscle, and CNS depression (6844). There is some evidence that magnesium is important in regulating blood pressure (1170,1182). Magnesium deficiency has been found to cause intracellular concentrations of sodium and potassium to increase, which can lead to increased peripheral resistance and vasospasm (8088). In cell membranes, a decreased concentration of magnesium and increased calcium to magnesium ratio has also been associated with hypertension (8092). There is also some evidence that hypertensive patients with hypomagnesemia usually require more antihypertensive medications than hypertensive patients with normal magnesium levels (8088).

There is some evidence that serum magnesium deficiency might play a role in both ischemic and hemorrhagic stroke (8998). Preliminary information shows magnesium may act as a neuroprotective agent in patients diagnosed with acute stroke. Several possible mechanisms of neuroprotection exist, including noncompetitive N-methyl-D-aspartate (NMDA) antagonism and calcium channel antagonism (9000,9003).

In patients with congestive heart failure, there is evidence magnesium reduces coronary vascular resistance, increases coronary artery blood flow, has antiarrhythmic effects, and improves cardiac indexes (8088).

There is some evidence that low magnesium levels play a role in diabetes and migraine headaches (1168,1183,6844). Magnesium seems to affect glucose control and insulin homeostasis. Magnesium blood levels might play a role in insulin resistance (1168,6844,11352). There is also some evidence that low dietary intake of magnesium increases the risk

of developing type 2 diabetes (6845,11352).
Magnesium deficiency might be a risk factor for postmenopausal osteoporosis, but its exact role is unknown. Magnesium is involved in calcium transport and seems to affect bone resorption and mineralization (7555).
Intracellular levels of magnesium, measured in erythrocytes and leukocytes, have been found to be lower in women with premenstrual syndrome (PMS), leading to the use of magnesium supplements for PMS (6847). Magnesium is reported to be an antagonist at N-methyl-D-aspartate (NMDA) receptors, which are involved in the potentiation of pain. This effect and magnesium's depressant effects on nerves and smooth muscle are thought to contribute to the possible effects of magnesium in relieving symptoms associated with migraine headaches, postoperative pain, neuropathic pain, erythromelalgia, Raynaud's Phenomenon, and other vascular disorders and pain syndromes (6846,6848,8094).
There is some evidence that magnesium metabolism is a factor in renal stone formation and prevention (2006,2007).
There is preliminary evidence that magnesium can reduce hypertension and nephrotoxicity induced by cyclosporine. Magnesium supplementation appears to reduce the thickening of the renal vascular walls that may occur with cyclosporine therapy; potassium supplementation may increase the effectiveness of magnesium for this use (9500).
In asthma, intravenous administration of magnesium might cause bronchodilation (2003).

Adverse Reactions

Orally, magnesium can cause gastrointestinal irritation, nausea, vomiting, and diarrhea (4891,10661,10663). Although rare, larger amounts might cause hypermagnesemia with symptoms including thirst, hypotension, drowsiness, confusion, loss of tendon reflexes, muscle weakness, respiratory depression, cardiac arrhythmias, coma, cardiac arrest, and death (8095). There are two reports of fatal hypermagnesemia. One report involved a 28 month-old child treated with 800 mg of oral magnesium oxide per day for constipation, then given 2400 mg magnesium oxide for several days before hospital admission (serum magnesium 20.3 mg/dL) (1360). Another report involved a patient who gargled with Epsom salts over several weeks. Epsom salts are almost 100% magnesium sulfate. The patient used an entire box two days prior to hospital admission (serum magnesium 23.6 mg/dL) (8095).
Topically, prolonged use of magnesium sulfate in the treatment of boils and carbuncles can cause damage to surrounding skin (9). Intravenously, urticaria has been reported (9). Chronic use of magnesium-containing antacids, especially those that do not contain aluminum, can cause diarrhea leading to fluid and electrolyte imbalances (15).

Interactions with Herbs & Other Dietary Supplements

BORON: Boron supplements can reduce urinary excretion of magnesium and increase serum levels in women (940,9623,9529). In young women, age 18 to 25 years, the effect appears to be greater in sedentary than athletic women (940). In postmenopausal women, the effect is more marked in women with low dietary magnesium intake (9623). The clinical significance of these effects, and whether they occur in men, isn't known.
CALCIUM: Calcium supplements can decrease the absorption of dietary magnesium. However, in people with adequate magnesium stores, calcium doesn't have any clinically significant effect on long-term magnesium balance. Advise patients at high risk for magnesium deficiency to take calcium supplements at bedtime, instead of with meals, to avoid inhibiting dietary magnesium absorption (4623,11159).
MALIC ACID: Malic acid is used with magnesium hydroxide for reducing pain and tenderness associated with fibromyalgia (3262). The mechanism of the effect and any interactions between the two isn't known.
VITAMIN D: One intestinal route of magnesium absorption is thought to be vitamin D dependent (9634). Various forms of vitamin D, including ergocalciferol, 25-hydroxyergocalciferol, 25-hydroxycholecalciferol (calcifediol), and 1,25-dihydroxycholecalciferol (calcitriol) increase magnesium absorption; especially when taken in high doses (9634,9635,9636,9637). This effect has been used to treat hypomagnesemia in people with malabsorption syndromes (9635,9636,9516).
ZINC: Supplementation with high doses of zinc, 142 mg/day, appears to decrease magnesium absorption and magnesium balance in healthy adult males (9624). The clinical significance of this isn't clear.

Interactions with Drugs

AMINOGLYCOSIDE ANTIBIOTICS: Use of an aminoglycoside antibiotic and magnesium concurrently can lead to neuromuscular weakness and possible paralysis. Both agents reduce presynaptic acetylcholine release, which can lead to neuromuscular blockade. This is most likely to occur with high doses of magnesium given intravenously (15). The aminoglycosides include amikacin (Amikin), gentamicin (Garamycin), kanamycin (Kantrex), streptomycin, and tobramycin (Nebcin).
BISPHOSPHONATES: Cations, including magnesium, can decrease bisphosphonate absorption. Advise patients to separate doses of magnesium and these drugs by at least 2 hours (9). The bisphosphonates include alendronate (Fosamax), etidronate (Didronel), tiludronate (Skelid), and risedronate (Actonel).
CALCIUM CHANNEL BLOCKERS: Magnesium inhibits calcium entry into smooth muscle cells and may therefore have additive effects with calcium channel blockers. Severe hypotension and neuromuscular blockades can occur when nifedipine is used with intravenous magnesium (3046). High doses of magnesium could theoretically have additive effects with other calcium channel blockers. These drugs include nifedipine (Adalat, Procardia), nicardipine (Cardene), isradipine (DynaCirc), amlodipine (Norvasc), and others.
POTASSIUM-SPARING DIURETICS: Potassium-sparing diuretics also have magnesium-sparing properties, which can counteract the magnesium losses associated with loop and thiazide diuretics (9613,9614,9622). Theoretically,

increased magnesium levels could result from concomitant use of potassium-sparing diuretics and magnesium supplements. The potassium-sparing diuretics include amiloride (Midamor), triamterene (Dyrenium), and spironolactone (Aldactone).
QUINOLONE ANTIBIOTICS: Magnesium can form insoluble complexes with quinolones and decrease their absorption (3046). Advise patients to take these drugs at least 2 hours before, or 4 to 6 hours after, magnesium supplements. Quinolones include ciprofloxacin (Cipro), levofloxacin (Levaquin), ofloxacin (Floxin), moxifloxacin (Avelox), gatifloxacin (Tequin), and others.
SKELETAL MUSCLE RELAXANTS: Parenteral magnesium can potentiate the effects of skeletal muscle relaxants by decreasing acetylcholine release from motor nerve terminals (3046). These drugs include atracurium (Tracrium), cisatracurium (Nimbex), mivacurium (Mivacron), rapacuronium (Raplon), rocuronium (Zemuron), pancuronium (Pavulon), vecuronium (Norcuron), and others.
TETRACYCLINE ANTIBIOTICS: Magnesium can form insoluble complexes with tetracyclines and decrease their absorption (9). Advise patients to take these drugs at least 2 hours before, or 4 to 6 hours after, magnesium supplements. Tetracyclines include demeclocycline (Declomycin), doxycycline (Vibramycin), minocycline (Minocin), and tetracycline (Achromycin, Sumycin).

Drug Influences on Nutrient Levels and Depletion

SOME DRUGS CAN AFFECT MAGNESIUM LEVELS:
ALDESLEUKIN (interleukin-2, IL-2, Proleukin): Asymptomatic hypomagnesemia can occur with aldesleukin therapy, probably due to an intracellular shift of magnesium. There isn't any increase in urinary magnesium, and serum levels normalize a few days after the drug is stopped (8874).
AMIFOSTINE (Ethyol, WR-2721): Amifostine reduces serum magnesium levels by reducing renal tubular reabsorption of magnesium and increasing urinary losses (9625). This effect seems to occur acutely after a single dose, and levels may return to normal within 24 hours (9625). The clinical significance therefore isn't clear.
AMINOGLYCOSIDES: Nephrotoxicity caused by aminoglycosides may lead to increased urinary losses of various electrolytes, including magnesium. Monitor patients closely to detect declining renal function and electrolyte disturbances. The aminoglycoside may need to be discontinued and intravenous electrolyte replacement given (15). Some aminoglycosides include amikacin (Amikin), gentamicin (Garamycin), kanamycin (Kantrex), streptomycin, and tobramycin (Nebcin).
AMPHOTERICIN-B (Abelcet, Amphotec, AmBisome, Amphocin, Fungizone): Electrolyte disturbances, including low serum magnesium levels, develop in a large proportion of patients receiving amphotericin-B. Lipid-based formulations might have a lesser effect than the conventional formulations (15). This disturbance has been association with nephrotoxicity, and may necessitate stopping the drug and giving intravenous electrolyte replacement.
BETA-2 AGONISTS: Beta-2 agonists promote movement of magnesium from the extracellular to the intracellular space, and increase magnesium excretion in the urine (2644,9517,9641). Reduced serum magnesium levels occur after a single dose of albuterol or terbutaline orally, by IV infusion, SC injection, or by inhalation (2644,6203,6205,6209,6217,8882,9517). The reductions are generally small, about 4.5-9%, or 0.04 to 0.06 mmol/L compared with the normal serum magnesium range of 0.65 to 1.1 mmol/L (6205,6217). However, it's been suggested that these acute changes could contribute to ECG changes, including prolonged QT intervals (2644,8882). With chronic use of beta-2 agonists, it appears that serum magnesium levels return to normal, but muscle magnesium levels remain low (6209,6210,9507). The clinical significance of this is not clear. It's unlikely that people using regular doses of beta-2 agonists for treatment of asthma will need magnesium supplements, unless they have other factors contributing to magnesium deficiency. The beta-2 agonists include albuterol (salbutamol, Proventil, Ventolin), bitolterol (Tornalate), isoetharine, levalbuterol (Xopenex), metaproterenol (Alupent), pirbuterol (Maxair), salmeterol (Serevent), and terbutaline (Brethine).
CARBOPLATIN (Paraplatin), CISPLATIN (Platinol-AQ): Carboplatin and cisplatin can cause hypomagnesemia due to renal tubular damage, which increases urinary magnesium losses (9626). With carboplatin, hypomagnesemia is rarely symptomatic and usually doesn't require magnesium supplements. Hypomagnesemia is usually more severe with cisplatin and worsens with progressive courses of treatment. Most patients who receive cumulative doses of cisplatin above 400 mg/m2 will develop hypomagnesemia (9626). Intravenous or oral magnesium supplements reduce the severity of this hypomagnesemia (9626). Monitor patients closely.
CHOLESTYRAMINE (Questran): Preliminary evidence suggests that cholestyramine may slightly increase urinary magnesium excretion, possibly by binding vitamin D and leading to reduced magnesium absorption (9566,9627). Clinically significant magnesium deficiency hasn't been reported, and supplements aren't likely to be needed.
CORTICOSTEROIDS (glucocorticoids): Chronic use of corticosteroids increases the amount of magnesium excreted in the urine. This is thought to be due to catabolism of bone which releases magnesium and increases the amount available for excretion (9628,9629). However, there doesn't seem to be a significant effect on serum levels (9507,9508,9509). Monitor magnesium levels in patients with other conditions that could contribute to magnesium deficiency.
CYCLOSPORINE (Neoral, Sandimmune): Cyclosporine can cause significant loss of magnesium in the urine, probably by reducing tubular reabsorption and causing tubular damage (9117,9632,9633). Hypomagnesemia may contribute to seizures and neurotoxicity associated with cyclosporine (9117,9632). Monitor magnesium levels carefully.

If hypomagnesemia occurs magnesium supplements may be needed, and/or dosage reduction or discontinuation of cyclosporine.

DIGOXIN (Lanoxin, Lanoxicaps): Digoxin decreases renal tubular reabsorption of magnesium, increasing excretion in the urine (4556,9631). People taking digoxin for heart failure may also be taking loop or thiazide diuretics, increasing the potential for hypomagnesemia (9613,9631). Low magnesium levels increase the risk of arrhythmias associated with high digoxin levels (9631). Monitor patients carefully.

DIURETICS: Loop diuretics and, to a lesser extent thiazide diuretics, interfere with magnesium reabsorption in the kidneys, which increases urinary losses and reduces serum magnesium levels (4412,9613,9614,9622). Some patients taking these diuretics chronically may also be taking digoxin, and may be at risk for cardiac arrhythmias. Low serum magnesium levels increases the risk of digoxin toxicity and arrhythmias (9613,9614). Potassium-sparing diuretics, such as amiloride, triamterene, or spironolactone, are also magnesium-sparing, and can therefore counteract the magnesium losses seen with loop diuretics and thiazides (9613,9614,9622). Monitor patients closely and use magnesium supplements or potassium-sparing diuretics when needed. The loop diuretics include furosemide (Lasix), bumetanide (Bumex), ethacrynic acid (Edecrin), and torsemide (Demadex). The thiazides include hydrochlorothiazide (Esidrix, HydroDIURIL), chlorothiazide (Diuril), and others.

ESTROGENS and ESTROGEN-CONTAINING ORAL CONTRACEPTIVES: Estrogens enhance magnesium uptake by soft tissues and bones, lowering serum levels (9621,9639). There appears to be an inverse relationship between estrogen levels and magnesium serum levels (9638,9639,9640). Estrogen therapy, including the use of oral contraceptives, lowers serum magnesium levels and can cause hypomagnesemia, especially in people with low dietary magnesium intake or other factors contributing to magnesium loss (9639,9640). It's likely that hypomagnesemia can contribute to the thromboembolic complications associated with estrogens (9621,9639). Monitor magnesium levels in patients.

FLUOROQUINOLONES: Fluoroquinolones form complexes with magnesium in the GI tract (3046). This could theoretically reduce absorption of both the fluoroquinolone and magnesium if taken at the same time. Significant effects on magnesium levels are unlikely when fluoroquinolones are taken at least 2 hours before, or 4 to 6 hours after magnesium supplements. Fluoroquinolones include ciprofloxacin (Cipro), levofloxacin (Levaquin), ofloxacin (Floxin), moxifloxacin (Avelox), gatifloxacin (Tequin), and others.

FOSCARNET (Foscavir): Foscarnet can cause various electrolyte disturbances, including symptomatic hypomagnesemia (8869,9617). This may be due to chelation of magnesium and increased elimination (8869). Monitor magnesium levels. Magnesium supplements may be needed, especially if foscarnet can't be discontinued (8869,9617).

PENICILLAMINE (Cuprimine): Penicillamine chelates magnesium, although with lower affinity than other metals such as copper, iron, and zinc (9630). It can potentially contribute to hypomagnesemia, especially in people with other factors which lower serum magnesium (4534). Magnesium supplements should be taken several hours apart from penicillamine to avoid forming nonabsorbable chelates in the gut.

PENTAMIDINE (NebuPent, Pentacarinat, Pentam 300): Symptomatic hypomagnesemia can occur with pentamidine, especially when given intravenously. This is likely due to renal tubular injury, leading to increased urinary losses of magnesium. Hypomagnesemia usually requires treatment with intravenous, followed by oral, magnesium supplements. Supplementation may need to be continued after pentamidine is stopped since the drug effects remain for six to eight weeks (8872,9618,9619). It isn't known whether magnesium given prophylactically with pentamidine can prevent hypomagnesemia. Monitor patients closely.

SODIUM PHOSPHATES (monobasic sodium phosphate and dibasic sodium phosphate, Fleet Phospho-soda): Use of high doses of sodium phosphates, such as those used for bowel cleansing before surgery, can cause hypomagnesemia (9615,9616). Advise people to avoid using high doses of these products for self-treatment of constipation.

TACROLIMUS (FK506, Prograf): Tacrolimus reduces renal tubular reabsorption of magnesium, producing increased magnesium wasting (8900,9620). This leads to hypomagnesemia in a significant proportion of people treated with tacrolimus (9620). Monitor magnesium levels.

TETRACYCLINES: Tetracyclines form complexes with magnesium in the GI tract, which could reduce absorption of both the tetracycline and magnesium when taken at the same time (9). Significant effects on calcium levels are unlikely when tetracyclines are taken at least 2 hours before, or 4 to 6 hours after, magnesium supplements. Tetracyclines include demeclocycline (Declomycin), doxycycline (Vibramycin), minocycline (Minocin), and tetracycline (Achromycin, Sumycin).

Interactions with Foods

None known.

Interactions with Lab Tests

ALKALINE PHOSPHATASE (ALK PHOS): Magnesium salts can cause a false increase in serum alkaline phosphatase test results due to the activation of enzymes used in lab procedures (275).

ANGIOTENSIN-CONVERTING ENZYME (ACE): Magnesium sulfate can reduce serum ACE concentrations and test results (275).

BLOOD PRESSURE: Orally, magnesium can lower blood pressure and reduce blood pressure readings in patients with mild to moderate hypertension (1192,1199).

CALCIUM: Magnesium salts can cause a false increase in serum calcium test results in some procedures using edetate disodium (EDTA) (275).
CORTISOL: Intravenous magnesium sulfate can decrease plasma cortisol concentrations and test results (275).
DIAGNEX BLUE: Magnesium salts can increase urine diagnex blue concentrations and test results by heavy metal displacement of diagnex blue (275).
ELECTROCARDIOGRAM (ECG): Orally, magnesium can normalize arrhythmias and ECG readings in some patients with angina (1181). Intravenous magnesium can normalize arrhythmias and ECG readings in some people with atrial fibrillation or ventricular tachydysrhythmias (1202,3314).
PARATHYROID HORMONE: Intravenous magnesium sulfate can reduce plasma parathyroid hormone concentrations and test results (275).
TESTOSTERONE: Intravenous magnesium sulfate can reduce serum testosterone concentrations and test results (275).

Interactions with Diseases or Conditions

ELDERLY: The elderly are at an increased risk for hypomagnesemia. They are more prone to decreased magnesium absorption, increased urinary loss, and disease states associated with abnormal magnesium status (1167).
HEART BLOCK: Hypermagnesemia can cause heart block. Intravenous magnesium is contraindicated in people with heart block (9,15).
MALABSORPTION SYNDROMES: Intestinal magnesium absorption can be decreased in bile insufficiency states, gastrointestinal infections, gluten enteropathy, immune diseases with villous atrophy, inflammatory bowel disease, intestinal fistulas, lymphectasia, primary idiopathic hypomagnesemia, radiation enteritis, sprue, and others (6280,6281).
RENAL DISEASE: Use cautiously in individuals with reduced kidney function due to an increased risk of hypermagnesemia (9).
RESTLESS LEG SYNDROME: High magnesium levels were reported in association with restless leg syndrome, but a causal relationship was not established (8096). Magnesium deficiency may also be associated with restless leg syndrome (9472).

Dosage and Administration

ORAL: For reducing the frequency and severity of migraine headaches, magnesium citrate 1830 mg in 3 divided doses has been used for up to 3 months (9498). Trimagnesium dicitrate 600 mg (24 mmol) daily for up to 3 months has also been used (4891). For reducing the frequency and severity of migraine headaches in children, magnesium oxide 9 mg per kg in 3 divided doses has been used for up to 16 weeks (10663). For treatment of hypomagnesemia in patients with type 2 diabetes, a dose of 50 ml magnesium chloride solution (containing 50 g magnesium chloride per 1000 ml of solution) daily for 16 weeks has been used (10664).
PARENTERAL: For treatment of hypomagnesemia, doses must be individualized according to serum magnesium levels, but a typical starting dose for mild deficiency is 1 gram intramuscularly (IM) every 6 hours for 4 doses. For more severe deficiency, 5 grams may be given in a 1 liter intravenous (IV) infusion over 3 hours (15). As part of total parenteral nutrition (TPN), adults typically receive 500 mg to 3 grams magnesium sulfate daily (15). For treatment of severe pre-eclampsia or eclampsia, a typical initial dose is 4 grams by IV infusion, followed by 4 to 5 grams IM every 4 hours, or 1 to 3 grams per hour by constant IV infusion. Doses should be adjusted according to serum levels and urinary excretion, and should not exceed 30 to 40 grams daily (15). As a tocolytic in preterm labor, an initial dose of 4 to 6 grams infused IV over 20 minutes has been used, followed by a maintenance infusion of 2 to 4 grams per hour, adjusted according to the response (15). For treatment of life-threatening ventricular arrhythmias such as torsades de pointes, 1 to 6 grams is given IV over several minutes, followed by an IV infusion, and for atrial tachycardia, 3 to 4 grams is given over 30 seconds. These IV push doses should be given with extreme caution (15). For vasospastic angina, a dose of 0.27 mmol/kg body weight infused over 20 minutes has been used to reduce coronary spasm (8091). For reducing cardiovascular morbidity and mortality after a myocardial infarction, magnesium is started within 6 hours of symptoms. A dose of 2 grams IV over 5 to 15 minutes has been used, followed by an IV infusion of 18 grams over 24 hours (15). For reducing the frequency of ventricular arrhythmias after myocardial infarction, 8 grams of magnesium sulfate infused IV over 12 hours has been used (9497). For treatment of acute stroke, 8-16 mmol magnesium sulfate in 100 ml normal saline, given IV over 15 minutes, has been used. This is followed by 65 mmol magnesium sulfate in 100 ml normal saline IV over 24 hours (9000,9003). In the treatment of neuropathic pain associated with cancer, single 500 mg or 1 gram doses have been used (6846). For cluster headaches and acute migraine, 1 gram IV doses have been used (6844). As an adjunct to analgesics for pain after hysterectomy, a 3 gram bolus dose followed by an infusion of 0.5 grams/hour has been used (6848). For adjunctive treatment of acute asthmatic attacks, doses of 1 to 2 grams infused IV over 15 to 30 minutes have been used (6844). For treatment of acute asthma in children, magnesium sulfate 40 mg/kg infused IV over 20 minutes has been used (9496). Acute exacerbations of COPD have also been treated with 1.2 grams magnesium sulfate IV (6844). For treatment of chronic fatigue syndrome (CFS) in patients with low red blood cell magnesium levels, weekly 1 gram intramuscular injections have been used (7556).

Comments

The serum magnesium level is the most commonly used test to assess magnesium status. However, it is also known that the serum magnesium level is depressed only in cases of severe magnesium deficiency and that it poorly correlates with body magnesium (8089). Red cell and urine magnesium levels also have been used but they are also poor indicators of body magnesium (8085,8089). The intravenous magnesium loading test is considered to be a more reliable test to measure magnesium status; but the test is cumbersome and requires full participation from the patient. It is known that serum magnesium actually consists of three fractions: protein-bound, complexed, and free ionic magnesium. It is the free ionic magnesium that is biologically active. Despite whether the serum magnesium level is low or normal, free ionic magnesium levels have been shown to vary consistently with many disorders such as cardiac disease, stroke, diabetes, and migraines. In recent years, instruments have become available that measure free ionic magnesium. It is hoped that by measuring free ionic magnesium, a more accurate assessment of body magnesium can be made (8090).

MAGNOLIA

Also Known As

Beaver Tree, Flos Magnoliae, Holly Bay, Ho-No-Ki, Hou Po, Houpu, Hou Po Hua, Indian Bark, Japanese Whitebark Magnolia, Red Bay, Swamp Laurel, Swamp Sassafras, Sweet Bay, White Bay, White Laurel.

Scientific Names

Magnolia biondii, synonym Magnolia fargesii; Magnolia denudata, synonyms Magnolia conspicua, Magnolia yulan; Magnolia heptaperta; Magnolia virginiana, synonym Magnolia glauca; Magnolia obovata, synonym Magnolia hypoleuca; Magnolia officinalis; Magnolia sprengeri; Magnolia sargentiana; Magnolia emargenata; Magnolia wilsonii, synonyms Magnolia nicholsoniana, Magnolia taliensis; Magnolia salicifolia, synonyms Buergeria salicifolia, Magnolia proctoriana; other Magnolia species.
Family: Magnoliaceae.

People Use This For

Orally, magnolia bark is used for digestive disorders, as a laxative, an anti-inflammatory, a stimulant, and to promote sweating. It is also used for anxiety, stress, depression, weight loss, fever, headache, stroke, and asthma. Magnolia flower bud is used orally for nasal congestion, runny nose, common cold, sinusitis, allergic rhinitis, headache, and facial dark spots.
Topically, magnolia flower bud is used for toothaches.
In skin care products, magnolia flower bud extract is used topically as a skin whitener and to minimize or counteract irritant effects of other ingredients.

Safety

POSSIBLY SAFE ...when the bark or flower bud is used orally and appropriately (12). There is insufficient reliable information available about the topical use of magnolia.
PREGNANCY: UNSAFE ...when the flower bud is used orally due to reports of uterine stimulant activity (11953). There is insufficient reliable information available about the safety of using magnolia bark; avoid using.
LACTATION: Insufficient reliable information available; avoid using.

Effectiveness

There is insufficient reliable information available about the effectiveness of magnolia.

Mechanism of Action

The applicable parts of magnolia are the bark and flower bud. Magnolia bark contains the active constituents magnolol, dihydroxydihdromagnolol, honokiol, and dihydrohonokiol (11945,11946,11947,11948).
Magnolol seems to have central nervous system effects, antiplatelet effects, anti-inflammatory effects, and smooth muscle relaxant effects. Magnolol also suppresses the conversion of cortisol to cortisone by blocking hydroxysteroid dehydrogenase. It increases the production of corticosterone, a glucocorticoid similar to cortisol. This may explain magnolia's use for asthma. Magnolol may also lower cholesterol production (11945). Other preliminary research suggests that magnolol might have anti-leukemic properties (11949). Magnolol and dihydroxydihydromagnolol seem to have antidepressant effects (11950).
Honokiol and dihydrohonokiol seem to have anxiolytic effects in animals, possibly by interacting with gamma-aminobutyric acid-A (GABA-A) receptors (11946,11947). However, dihydrohonokiol doesn't seem to cause motor dysfunction, CNS depression, amnesia, or physical dependence at doses that produce an anxiolytic effect (11948).
At high doses, magnolia bark seems to have CNS depressant effects. Honokiol seems to inhibit catecholamine secretion (11952).
Magnolol and honokiol might enhance cholinergic function, which could be useful in diseases such as Alzheimer's. At high doses, these compounds increase acetylcholine release in the hippocampus of the brain and have a

neurotrophic effect, theoretically improving neuronal function (11951).
Magnolia flower bud seems to have uterine stimulating, hypotensive, antifungal, and skeletal muscle contracting effects. Its constituents, especially magnone, may also have platelet-activating factor antagonist activity, which might explain its use in nasal congestion and rhinitis (11953).

Adverse Reactions

Theoretically, magnolia bark might cause central nervous system depressant effects at high doses (11952).

Interactions with Herbs & Other Dietary Supplements

HERBS AND SUPPLEMENTS WITH SEDATIVE PROPERTIES: Theoretically, concomitant use with herbs and supplements that have sedative properties might increase the risk of excessive drowsiness. Some of these supplements include 5-HTP, calamus, California poppy, catnip, hops, Jamaican dogwood, kava, St. John's wort, scullcap, valerian, yerba mansa, and others (11952).

Interactions with Drugs

ALCOHOL (Ethanol): Theoretically, concomitant use of large doses of magnolia bark and alcohol might increase the risk of drowsiness and motor reflex depression (11952).
BARBITURATES: Theoretically, concomitant use of large doses of magnolia bark and barbiturates might increase the risk of drowsiness and motor reflex depression (11952). Some of these sedative medications include pentobarbital (Nembutal), phenobarbital (Luminal), secobarbital (Seconal), and others.
BENZODIAZEPINES: Theoretically, concomitant use of large doses of magnolia bark and benzodiazepines might increase the risk of drowsiness and motor reflex depression (11952).
CNS DEPRESSANTS: Theoretically, concomitant use of large doses of magnolia bark and CNS depressants might increase the risk of drowsiness and motor reflex depression (11952).

Interactions with Foods

None known.

Interactions with Lab Tests

None known.

Interactions with Diseases or Conditions

None known.

Dosage and Administration

No typical dosage.

Comments

Magnolia bark is an ingredient in the traditional Chinese and Japanese (Kampo) medicines Hange-koboku-to, which is composed of 5 plant extracts, and Saiboku-to, which is composed of 10 plant extracts. These are used to decrease anxiety and nervous tension and to improve sleep. Honokiol, a constituent of magnolia bark, appears to cause these effects (11946).
Some weight loss products include magnolia bark with claims that it reduces cortisol levels. There is no evidence that magnolia bark causes weight loss or reduces cortisol levels. In fact, it appears to increase levels of corticosterone, a glucocorticoid similar to cortisol (11945).

MAIDENHAIR FERN

Also Known As

Five-Finger Fern, Hair of Venus, Maiden Fern, Rock Fern, Venus Hair.

Scientific Names

Adiantum pedatum; Adiantum capillus-veneris.
Family: Adiantiaceae or Pteridaceae.

People Use This For

Orally, maidenhair fern is used for bronchitis, coughs, whooping cough, and painful and excessive menstruation. It is also used orally as an expectorant, demulcent, severe coughs.
Topically, maidenhair fern is used for hair loss and to promote dark hair color.

Safety
POSSIBLY SAFE ...when used orally in amounts found in foods.
There is insufficient reliable information available about the safety of maidenhair fern for its other uses.
PREGNANCY: UNSAFE ...when used orally; contraindicated, most likely due to its emetic effects at higher doses (12).
LACTATION: Insufficient reliable information available; avoid using.

Effectiveness
There is insufficient reliable information available about the effectiveness of maidenhair fern.

Mechanism of Action
There is insufficient reliable information available about the possible mechanism of action and active ingredients.

Adverse Reactions
Orally, people using large amounts may experience emesis (12).

Interactions with Herbs & Other Dietary Supplements
None known.

Interactions with Drugs
None known.

Interactions with Foods
None known.

Interactions with Lab Tests
None known.

Interactions with Diseases or Conditions
None known.

Dosage and Administration
ORAL: Maidenhair fern is usually taken as a tea. A single dose is equivalent to 1.5 grams ground or powdered herb. The tea is prepared by steeping 1.5 grams dried herb in 150 mL of boiling water for 10-15 minutes and straining (18).

Comments
Maidenhair tree is another name for Ginkgo biloba, and is distinct from maidenhair fern (18).

MAITAKE MUSHROOM

Also Known As
Dancing Mushroom, Grifola, Hen Of The Woods, King Of Mushrooms, Maitake, Monkey's Bench, Shelf Fungi.

Scientific Names
Grifola frondosa.
Family: Polyporaceae.

People Use This For
Orally, maitake mushroom is used for cancer, HIV/AIDS, chronic fatigue syndrome (CFS), hepatitis, hay fever, diabetes, high blood pressure, hyperlipidemia, weight loss or control, and chemotherapy support.
For food uses, maitake mushroom is edible and has been consumed in Asia for thousands of years.

Safety
POSSIBLY SAFE ...when used orally and appropriately (12).
PREGNANCY AND LACTATION: Insufficient reliable information available; avoid using.

Effectiveness
INSUFFICIENT RELIABLE EVIDENCE to RATE

Diabetes. Preliminary clinical evidence suggests that maitake mushroom polysaccharides (MMP) might lower blood glucose in people with type 2 diabetes (8188). More evidence is needed to rate maitake mushroom for this use.

Mechanism of Action
The applicable parts of maitake mushroom are the fruiting body and mycelium. Maitake mushroom contains beta-glucan, which has been shown to possess antitumor activity. The "D-fraction" of beta-glucan appears to be the most active and potent form. Maitake mushroom has immunostimulant effects and activates natural killer cells, cytotoxic T-cells, interleukin-1, and superoxide anions. Preliminary research suggests that maitake mushroom can prevent metastasis of experimentally induced tumors as well as prevent tumor occurrence in normal cells. Researchers are particularly interested in maitake mushroom and its extracts because they appear to be active orally (8189,8190,8191). Other research suggests that maitake mushroom can lower blood pressure (1213,1214), and improve the lipid profile in experimental hyperlipidemia (1211). Polysaccharides from the fruiting bodies in maitake mushroom appear to have a hypoglycemic effect, possibly by activating insulin receptors (1212,8188). Maitake mushroom also appears to cause weight loss (8188).

Adverse Reactions
None reported.

Interactions with Herbs & Other Dietary Supplements
HERBS & SUPPLEMENTS WITH HYPOGLYCEMIC POTENTIAL: Maitake mushroom might lower blood glucose levels and might have additive effects when used with other herbs and supplements that also lower glucose levels (19,1212,8188). This might increase the risk of hypoglycemia in some patients. Some herbs and supplements with hypoglycemic effects include alpha-lipoic acid, bitter melon, chromium, devil's claw, fenugreek, garlic, guar gum, horse chestnut, Panax ginseng, psyllium, Siberian ginseng, and others.

Interactions with Drugs
ANTIDIABETES DRUGS: Monitor blood glucose levels closely. Maitake mushroom appears to have hypoglycemic effects (19,1212,8188).

Interactions with Foods
None known.

Interactions with Lab Tests
BLOOD GLUCOSE: Maitake mushroom might lower blood glucose and test results in patients with type 2 diabetes (19,1212,8188).

Interactions with Diseases or Conditions
None known.

Dosage and Administration
No typical dosage.

Comments
Warn patients about the importance of positive identification of maitake mushroom to avoid confusion with poisonous mushrooms.

MALABAR NUT

Also Known As
Adulsa, Arusa.
CAUTION: See separate listing for Garcinia.

Scientific Names
Justicia Adhatoda.
Family: Acanthaceae.

People Use This For
Orally, malabar nut is used as an expectorant and secretory agent. It is also used as a bronchodilatory agent and mild spasmolytic.

Safety
There is insufficient reliable information available about the safety of malabar nut.
PREGNANCY: UNSAFE ...when used orally; contraindicated (18).
LACTATION: Insufficient reliable information available; avoid using.

Effectiveness
There is insufficient reliable information available about the effectiveness of malabar nut.

Mechanism of Action
The applicable part of malabar nut is the leaf. The quinazoline alkaloid vasicine has excitatory activity when taken in large amounts (18).

Adverse Reactions
None reported.

Interactions with Herbs & Other Dietary Supplements
None known.

Interactions with Drugs
None known.

Interactions with Foods
None known.

Interactions with Lab Tests
None known.

Interactions with Diseases or Conditions
None known.

Dosage and Administration
No typical dosage.

Comments
Vasicine was formerly used as the starting substance for production of mucolytics Bromhexin and Ambroxol. Neither of these products are available in the US (18).

MALE FERN

Also Known As
American Aspidium, Bear's Paw, European Aspidium, Knotty Brake, Marginal Fern, Shield Fern.

Scientific Names
Dryopteris Filix-Mas.
Family: Dryopteridaceae.

People Use This For
Orally, male fern is used to treat recurrent nose bleeds, heavy menstrual bleeding, wounds, tumors, and as an anthelmintic.
In veterinary medicine, male fern is used as an anthelmintic.

Safety
LIKELY UNSAFE ...when used orally. Male fern can be a violent poison (2,11). For this reason, it should no longer be used internally (2). Canada requires that it be labeled "For external use only" (12).
There is insufficient reliable information available about the safety of male fern for its other uses.
PREGNANCY AND LACTATION: LIKELY UNSAFE ...when used orally; contraindicated (12). There is insufficient reliable information available about the safety of male fern used topically; avoid using.

Effectiveness
There is insufficient reliable information available about the effectiveness of male fern.

Mechanism of Action
The applicable parts of male fern are the above ground parts, leaf, and rhizome. Male fern contains filicin and filmarone. These are active anthelmintics and act as a vermifuge to kill worms. Active constituents are soluble derivatives of phloroglucinol. These constituents are inactivated in an alkaline environment. Male fern also contains volatile oils, tannin, albaspidin, and desaspidin. All of these compounds together are called filicin, and work together

to kill tapeworms. It is important to remember that once the tapeworm has been killed, a simultaneously administered saline laxative is used expel the worm (6).

Adverse Reactions
Orally, male fern may cause headaches, dyspnea, nausea, diarrhea, vertigo, tremors, convulsions, cardiac and respiratory failure, and optic neuritis (6). Death has occurred with severe poisoning. Symptoms of toxicity include muscular weakness, coma, temporary or permanent blindness (11).

Interactions with Herbs & Other Dietary Supplements
CASTOR OIL: Taking castor oil enhances the absorption and toxic potential of male fern (6).

Interactions with Drugs
None known.

Interactions with Foods
FATS, OILS, AND ALCOHOL: Increases absorption and side effects (2).

Interactions with Lab Tests
None known.

Interactions with Diseases or Conditions
GASTROINTESTINAL (GI) CONDITIONS: Theoretically, damaged GI mucosa or conditions which prolong GI transit may increase absorption and the risk of side effects.

Dosage and Administration
ORAL: Adults in a fasting state usually receive 3-6 mL orally. Children up to age two receive up to 2 mL in divided doses. Children over age two are given 0.25-0.5 mL per year of age up to a total of 4 mL in divided doses. The dose is typically given with a purgative (saline laxative) to aid expulsion of tapeworms (6,11).

Comments
High toxicity potential precludes use (2,6). Treatment of overdose consists of giving saline cathartic followed by demulcent fluids. It is important to avoid fats and oils. If seizures occur, benzodiazepines may be used, and assisting respiration may be required. Since there are other products available that are effective and safer than male fern, it should not be used (6002).

MALLOW flower

Also Known As
Blue Mallow Flower, Cheeseflower, Gul-Khair, High Mallow, Malvae flos, Mauls.
CAUTION: See separate listings for Mallow leaf, Country Mallow, and Marshmallow.

Scientific Names
Malva sylvestris, synonym Malva mauritiana.
Family: Malvaceae.

People Use This For
Orally, mallow flower is used for irritation of the mucosa of the mouth and throat and the associated dry cough, bronchitis, as a mild astringent for gastroenteritis, and for bladder complaints.
Topically, mallow flower has been used as a poultice or bath additive for wounds.
In foods, it is used as a food-coloring agent.

Safety
POSSIBLY SAFE ...when used orally and appropriately (12).
PREGNANCY AND LACTATION: Insufficient reliable information available; avoid using.

Effectiveness
There is insufficient reliable information available about the effectiveness of mallow flower.

Mechanism of Action
Mallow flower contains mucilage, which protects and soothes mucous membranes (2,18). The anthocyanins constituents are a source of color (8).

Adverse Reactions
None reported.

Interactions with Herbs & Other Dietary Supplements
None known.

Interactions with Drugs
None known.

Interactions with Foods
None known.

Interactions with Lab Tests
None known.

Interactions with Diseases or Conditions
None known.

Dosage and Administration
ORAL: The typical dose of mallow flower is one cup of the tea several times daily (6,18). The tea is prepared by steeping 1.5-2 grams of the dried flowers in 150 mL boiling water for 10 minutes and then straining. Up to 5 grams of the dried flowers should be ingested per day (2,8,18).

Comments
Avoid confusion with mallow leaf, other malvae varieties, and marshmallow (Althaea officinalis).

MALLOW leaf

Also Known As
Blue Mallow, Dwarf Mallow, Gul-Khair, High Mallow, Malvae folium.
CAUTION: See separate listings for Mallow flower, Country Mallow, and Marshmallow.

Scientific Names
Malva sylvestris, synonym Malva mauritiana; Malva neglecta, synonym Malva rotundifolia.
Family: Malvaceae.

People Use This For
Orally, mallow leaf is used for irritation of the oral and pharyngeal mucosa, dry cough, colds, upper respiratory mucous membrane inflammation, and as a mild astringent for gastroenteritis. Topically, mallow leaf is used as a poultice for wounds.

Safety
POSSIBLY SAFE ...when used orally and appropriately (2).
PREGNANCY AND LACTATION: Insufficient reliable information available; avoid using.

Effectiveness
There is insufficient reliable information available about the effectiveness of mallow leaf.

Mechanism of Action
Mallow leaf contains mucilage which protects and soothes mucous membranes (2,18). The mucilage has been shown in vitro to inactivate the serum complement, which is a component in the host defense system (1526).

Adverse Reactions
None reported.

Interactions with Herbs & Other Dietary Supplements
None known.

Interactions with Drugs
None known.

Interactions with Foods
None known.

Interactions with Lab Tests
None known.

Interactions with Diseases or Conditions
None known.

Dosage and Administration
ORAL: The typical dose of mallow leaf is one cup of the tea several times per day and in the evening before going to sleep (6). It can be sweetened with honey (6). The tea is prepared by steeping 3-5 grams of the dried leaves in 150 mL boiling water for 10-15 minutes and then straining (6). The maximum use of mallow is 5 grams of the dried leaves per day (2).

Comments
Mallow leaf is a rich plant source of vitamin C (19).

MANACA

Also Known As
Pohl, Vegetable Mercury.

Scientific Names
Brunfelsia uniflora, synonym Brunfelsia hopeana.
Family: Solanaceae.

Comments
At the date of publication, there was very little scientific information about this product. Our staff is continually analyzing the available information on natural medicines and will add data to the online version of *Natural Medicines Comprehensive Database* as it becomes available. See www.naturaldatabase.com.

MANGANESE

Also Known As
Manganese Amino Acid Chelate, Manganese Aminoate, Manganese Ascorbate, Manganese Aspartate Complex, Manganese Chloride, Manganese Chloridetetrahydrate, Manganese Dioxide, Manganese Gluconate, Manganese Sulfate, Manganese Sulfate Monohydrate, Manganese Sulfate Tetrahydrate, Manganum.

Scientific Names
Manganese; Mn; atomic number 25.

People Use This For
Orally, manganese is used for prevention and treatment of manganese deficiency, osteoporosis, microcytic anemia, and symptoms of premenstrual syndrome (PMS).
In combination, Manganese is used with chondroitin sulfate and glucosamine hydrochloride for osteoarthritis.
Intravenously, manganese is used as a trace element in total parenteral nutrition (TPN) preparations.

Safety
LIKELY SAFE ...when used orally and appropriately. Manganese is usually safe in doses up to 11 mg per day for adults 19 years and older (7135).
POSSIBLY UNSAFE ...when used orally in high doses. Doses exceeding 11 mg per day can cause significant adverse effects (7135).
CHILDREN: LIKELY SAFE ...when used orally and appropriately. Manganese is usually safe in children when used in daily doses less than the tolerable upper intake level (UL) of 2 mg in children 1 to 3 years, 3 mg in children 4 to 8 years, 6 mg in children 9 to 13 years, 9 mg in children 14 to 18 years (7135). POSSIBLY UNSAFE ...when used orally in excessive doses. Daily doses greater than the tolerable upper intake level (UL) are associated with a greater risk of toxicity (7135).
PREGNANCY AND LACTATION: LIKELY SAFE ...when used orally and appropriately. Manganese is usually safe in pregnant or lactating adult women aged 19 or older when used in doses of less than 11 mg per day. However,

pregnant and lactating women under age 19 should limit doses to less than 9 mg per day (7135).
POSSIBLY UNSAFE ...when used orally in excessive doses. Doses over 11 mg per day are associated with a greater risk of toxicity (7135).

Effectiveness

EFFECTIVE

Manganese deficiency. Taking manganese orally or intravenously is effective for preventing or treating manganese deficiency (15).

POSSIBLY EFFECTIVE

Osteoporosis. Taking manganese orally in combination with calcium, zinc, and copper seems to help reduce spinal bone loss in postmenopausal women (1994).

Premenstrual syndrome (PMS). Taking manganese orally in combination with calcium seems to help improve symptoms of crying, loneliness, anxiety, restlessness, irritability, mood swings, depression, and tension (2004).

There is insufficient reliable information available about the effectiveness of manganese for its other uses.

Mechanism of Action

Manganese is an essential nutrient that acts as a cofactor in several metabolic and enzymatic reactions (2003,7135). Manganese is found in several foods including nuts, legumes, seeds, tea, whole grains, and leafy green vegetables (2005,2008,7135). However, typically less than 5% of dietary manganese is absorbed. It's not known if absorption of manganese from supplements is better or worse than manganese from dietary sources. Men seem to absorb less manganese than women. The reason for this is not known, but it might be due to higher serum ferritin concentrations in men. Ferritin is associated with decreased manganese absorption (7135). Manganese is involved in amino acid, cholesterol, and carbohydrate metabolism (7135). Manganese metalloenzymes include arginase, glutamine synthetase, phosphoenolpyruvate decarboxylase, and manganese superoxide (7135).

Researchers think manganese might have a role in osteoporosis. Decreased plasma manganese concentrations have been linked to osteoporosis, and bone mineral density seems to improve when trace minerals including manganese are added to calcium supplementation (7135). In patients with premenstrual syndrome (PMS), low dietary manganese has been associated with altered mood and increased pain (7135). Some researchers think that supplementing manganese in women with PMS might improve symptoms. Manganese is cleared hepatically and chronic liver disease can cause manganese accumulation and toxicity (1992). Manganese accumulation seems to play a role in Parkinsonian symptoms and encephalopathy associated with chronic liver disease (1992,10666). Researchers believe neurotoxicity of manganese may result from the depletion of dopamine and production of dopamine quinone and hydrogen peroxide (10665). Manganese is transported by transferrin. The globus pallidus and substantia nigra, areas of the brain associated with the extrapyramidal system, are high in transferrin receptor density, which may result in concentration of manganese (7135).

Adverse Reactions

Orally, manganese is usually well tolerated when used in doses below 11 mg per day (7135). There is some concern that higher doses might increase risk of neurotoxicity, including Parkinsonian-like extrapyramidal symptoms (7135,10665,10666). People with impaired manganese excretion can also experience these effects even with very low manganese intake. Manganese accumulation due to chronic liver disease seems to cause Parkinsonian-like extrapyramidal symptoms, encephalopathy, and psychosis (1992,7135).

Chronic occupational exposure to manganese dust or fumes can also cause extrapyramidal reactions, orthostatic hypotension, decreased heart rate, mood disturbance, and dementia (1990,7135).

Interactions with Herbs & Other Dietary Supplements

CALCIUM: Concomitant administration can decrease manganese absorption (2000).

IP-6 (Phytic Acid): IP-6 found in foods, such as cereals, nuts, and beans, and in supplements can decrease manganese absorption (7135). IP-6 chelates multivalent metal ions in the gastrointestinal tract and prevents absorption (1858). Suggest that patients separate intake of manganese and IP-6 by at least two hours.

IRON: Concomitant administration can decrease manganese absorption (2004).

ZINC: Concomitant administration can increase manganese absorption and plasma levels (2000).

Interactions with Drugs

QUINOLONE ANTIBIOTICS: Theoretically, manganese might reduce the absorption of quinolones. Interactions occur with other multivalent cations, such as calcium and iron (488). quinolones include ciprofloxacin (Cipro), levofloxacin (Levaquin), gatifloxacin (Tequin), sparfloxacin (Zagam), and others.

TETRACYCLINE ANTIBIOTICS: Theoretically, manganese might reduce the absorption of tetracyclines. Interactions occur with other multivalent cations, such as calcium and iron (488). Tetracyclines include demeclocycline (Declomycin), minocycline (Minocin), and tetracycline (Achromycin).

Interactions with Foods

None known.

Interactions with Lab Tests

ALKALINE PHOSPHATASE: Manganese salts can cause a false increase in serum alkaline phosphatase test results due to enzyme activation in the laboratory procedure (275).
BONE MINERAL DENSITY (BMD): Manganese (in combination with calcium, zinc, and copper) might improve BMD and BMD test results in patients with osteoporosis (1994).
STOOL COLOR: Manganese dioxide might cause stool to turn dark brown to black (275).

Interactions with Diseases or Conditions

CHRONIC LIVER DISEASE: Chronic liver disease can lead to manganese accumulation and toxicity (1992,2001); use manganese cautiously.
IRON-DEFICIENCY ANEMIA: Individuals with iron-deficiency anemia might have enhanced manganese absorption (2002).

Dosage and Administration

ORAL: For osteoporosis, 5 mg per day combined with 1000 mg elemental calcium, 15 mg zinc, and 2.5 mg copper has been used (1994).
No recommended dietary allowances (RDA) for manganese have been established. The daily Adequate Intake (AI) levels for manganese are: infants birth to 6 months, 3 mcg; 7 to 12 months, 600 mcg; children 1 to 3 years, 1.2 mg; 4 to 8 years 1.5 mg; boys 9 to 13 years, 1.9 mg; 14 to 18 years, 2.2 mg; girls 9 to 18 years, 1.6 mg; men age 19 and older 2.3 mg; women 19 and older 1.8 mg; pregnancy age 14 to 50, 2 mg; lactation 2.6 mg (7135). Tolerable Upper Intake Levels (UL) for manganese have been established (7135). The daily ULs for manganese are: children 1 to 3 years, 2 mg; 4 to 8 years, 3 mg; 9 to 13 years, 6 mg; 14 to 18 years (including pregnancy and lactation) 9 mg; for adults 19 years and older (including pregnancy and lactation), 11 mg (7135).
INTRAVENOUS: In parenteral nutrition, manganese is administered in doses of 150 to 800 mcg per day for adults and 2 to 10 mcg/kg per day for children (157).

Comments

Tell patients to look out for manganese hidden in some supplements. Certain supplements, including those commonly used for osteoarthritis (e.g., CosaminDS), contain manganese. Remind patients to adhere to product directions. When taken at doses slightly higher than the recommended dose, these products provide more than the tolerable upper limit (UL) of 11 mg per day.

MANGOSTEEN

Also Known As

Amibiasine, Mang Cut, Manggis, Manggistan, Mangosta, Mangostan, Mangostana, Mangostanier, Mangostao, Mangoustanier, Mangouste, Mangostier, Manguita, Meseter, Queen of Fruits, Sementah, Semetah, Xango, Xango Juice.
CAUTION: See separate listing for Garcinia.

Scientific Names

Garcinia mangostana.
Family: Clusiaceae.

People Use This For

Orally, mangosteen is used for dysentery, diarrhea, urinary tract infections (UTI), gonorrhea, thrush, tuberculosis, menstrual disorders, stimulating the immune system, cancer, osteoarthritis, and improving mental health.
Topically, mangosteen is used for eczema and other skin conditions.

Safety

There is insufficient reliable information available about the safety of mangosteen.
Pregnancy and Lactation: Insufficient reliable information available; avoid using.

Effectiveness

There is insufficient reliable information available about the effectiveness of mangosteen.

Mechanism of Action

The applicable parts of mangosteen are the fruit, juice, rind, bark, and twigs. The fruit and juice are consumed as a healthful and medicinal food and drink. The dried and powdered rind is most commonly used for medicinal purposes. The bark extract, called Amibiasine, is used for amebic dysentery.
Mangosteen fruit, rind, and bark seem to contain several pharmacologically active constituents. The activity of some

of these isolated constituents has been characterized. But there is no reliable information about the effects of eating the whole fruit or taking the powdered rind or bark extracts.

The mangosteen rind reportedly contains tannins. Tannins can have an astringent effect on mucosal tissue and can reduce secretions. This astringent effect might reduce diarrhea.

Mangosteen also contains xanthones that have antioxidant and other effects. The specific xanthones include alpha-mangostins, beta-mangostins, and gamma-mangostins (12016). Alpha- and beta-mangostins appear to have in vitro activity against the human leukemia cell line HL60 (12013) and Mycobacterium tuberculosis (12014). Mangosteen also contains the xanthone derivatives garcinone B and garcinone E. These constituents also appear to have in vitro activity against Mycobacterium tuberculosis (12014). Garcinone E also has in vitro cytotoxic activity against hepatocellular carcinomas (12015).

The alpha- and gamma-mangostins also appear to have serotonin and histamine receptor blocking effects (12017).

Adverse Reactions
None reported.

Interactions with Herbs & Other Dietary Supplements
None known.

Interactions with Drugs
None known.

Interactions with Foods
None known.

Interactions with Lab Tests
None known.

Interactions with Diseases or Conditions
None known.

Dosage and Administration
No typical dosage.

Comments
Mangosteen is a tropical fruit. Its fruit is sourly sweet. It's often consumed as a dessert fruit or made into jams. It was thought to be Queen Victoria's favorite fruit.

Mangosteen juice is becoming a popular healthful and medicinal drink. It is usually marketed with the name xango juice. Some marketers claim that xango juice can treat diarrhea, menstrual problems, urinary tract infections, tuberculosis, and a variety of other conditions. There is no reliable scientific evidence to support these claims.

MANNA

Also Known As
Flake Manna, Flowering Ash, Manna Ash.

Scientific Names
Fraxinus ornus.

Family: Oleaceae.

People Use This For
Orally, the dried sap of manna is used as a laxative for constipation and a stool softener for anal fissure, hemorrhoids, and after anorectal surgery.

Safety
POSSIBLY SAFE ...when used orally and appropriately on a short-term basis (2); avoid extended use of manna (2,18).

PREGNANCY AND LACTATION: Insufficient reliable information available; avoid using.

Effectiveness
There is insufficient reliable information available about the effectiveness of manna.

Mechanism of Action

Manna consists of the dried sap collected from the splits in branches and trunk of Fraxinus ornus. The manna bark contains coumarins which can inactivate the serum complement, a component in the host defense system (1527). Manna contains 40-90% mannitol (9,18), which acts as an osmotic laxative (2,18).

Adverse Reactions

Orally, manna can cause nausea or flatulence (2,18).

Interactions with Herbs & Other Dietary Supplements

POTASSIUM DEPLETING HERBS: Theoretically, due to manna's laxative effect concomitant use of manna with horsetail plant or the licorice rhizome increases the risk of potassium depletion.
STIMULANT LAXATIVE HERBS: Theoretically, concomitant use of manna with stimulant laxatives might increase the risk of potassium depletion. Stimulant laxative herbs include aloe latex, wild cucumber fruit (Ecballium elaterium), blue flag rhizome, alder buckthorn, European buckthorn, butternut bark, cascara bark, castor oil, colocynth fruit pulp, gamboge bark exudate, jalap root, black root, podophyllum root, rhubarb root, senna leaves and pods, and yellow dock root (19).

Interactions with Drugs

DIGOXIN (Lanoxin): Theoretically, the overuse or abuse of manna might increases the risk of adverse effects of cardiac glycoside drugs. Manna contains mannitol, which acts as an osmotic laxative (19).
DIURETIC DRUGS: Overuse of manna might compound diuretic-induced potassium loss (19). There is some concern that people taking manna along with potassium depleting diuretics might have an increased risk for hypokalemia. Initiation of potassium supplementation or an increase in potassium supplement dose may be necessary for some patients. Some diuretics that can deplete potassium include chlorothiazide (Diuril), chlorthalidone (Thalitone), furosemide (Lasix), hydrochlorothiazide (HCTZ, HydroDIURIL, Microzide), and others.

Interactions with Foods

None known.

Interactions with Lab Tests

None known.

Interactions with Diseases or Conditions

GI OBSTRUCTION: Manna is contraindicated in cases of bowel obstruction or ileus (2,18).

Dosage and Administration

ORAL: For adults, the typical dose of manna is 20-30 grams per day or equivalent preparations (2,18). For children, the common dose is 2-16 grams per day (2,18). Manna should not be taken for prolonged use (2,18).

MARIJUANA

Also Known As

Anashca, Banji, Bhang, Blunt, Bud, Cannabis, Charas, Dope, Esrar, Gaga, Ganga, Grass, Hash, Hashish, Hemp, Joint, Kif, Mariguana, Marihuana, Mary Jane, Pot, Sawi, Sinsemilla, Weed.

Scientific Names

Cannabis sativa.
Family: Cannabaceae.

People Use This For

Orally, marijuana is used recreationally as a euphoriant. A cannabinoid from marijuana is used in the prescription-only product dronabinol (Marinol) for the treatment of anorexia or appetite loss associated with AIDS and for cancer chemotherapy induced nausea and vomiting unresponsive to traditional medications. Cannabinoid constituents from marijuana have also been used orally to treat pain and multiple sclerosis (MS).
As an inhalant, marijuana is smoked for nausea, glaucoma, appetite stimulation, and recreationally for altering senses (psychoactivity) and euphoria. Marijuana is also smoked for mucous membrane inflammation, leprosy, fever, dandruff, hemorrhoids, obesity, asthma, urinary tract infections, cough, anorexia associated with weight loss in AIDS patients, pain, multiple sclerosis, and for producing immunosuppression after renal transplantation.

Safety

LIKELY SAFE ...when the cannabinoid constituent dronabinol is used orally and appropriately. Dronabinol (Marinol) is an FDA-approved prescription product (6606,10241).
POSSIBLY UNSAFE ...when marijuana is used orally or inhaled (1395,1396).
PREGNANCY: UNSAFE ...when used orally or inhaled; marijuana passes through the placenta and can reduce fetal growth. Marijuana use during pregnancy is also associated with childhood leukemia (4260).
LACTATION: LIKELY UNSAFE ...when used orally or inhaled because dronabinol (THC) is concentrated and excreted in breast milk (2619,2620).

Effectiveness

POSSIBLY EFFECTIVE

Glaucoma. Smoking marijuana seems to reduce intraocular pressure in patients with glaucoma (1268). There is some evidence marijuana can decrease intraocular pressure, but it also seems to decrease blood flow to the optic nerve. So far, it is not known if it can improve visual function (1268).

HIV/AIDS-related weight loss. Smoking marijuana seems to stimulate the appetite of patients with AIDS. Marijuana cigarettes can increase caloric intake and weight gain in HIV positive patients also taking indinavir (Crixivan) or nelfinavir (Viracept) without affecting viral load (6606,11166).

Multiple sclerosis (MS). Marijuana seems to be effective when smoked, or when the cannabinoids are taken orally for the treatment of spasticity and tremor associated with MS (11167,11168).

There is insufficient reliable information available about the effectiveness of marijuana for its other uses.

Mechanism of Action

The applicable parts of marijuana are the flower and leaf. Marijuana contains cannabinoids, including tetrahydrocannabinol (THC, dronabinol), that act on the central nervous system (CNS) (13). The THC concentration is highest in the flowers and leaves and lowest in the stems, roots, and seeds (6). THC can interact with cell-wall lipids or affect prostaglandin biosynthesis (18). It can act via cannabinoid receptors in neural tissues (2619) or opiate receptors in the forebrain, leading to indirect inhibition of the emetic center in the medulla oblongata (13).

Two types of cannabinoid receptors have been identified in animals: CB1, which is found predominantly in the CNS and is thought to be responsible for the psychoactive effects, and CB2 which is found in high levels on immune system cells including leukocytes, and to a lesser extent in the brain (5887,5888,5889). Endogenous substances which bind to these receptors have been identified (5887,5888).

Tetrahydrocannabinol is a partial CB1 receptor agonist and has limited CB2 agonist activity (5889). While short-term inhalation increases bronchodilation and reduces bronchospasm, long-term use impairs lung function, which can result in constrictive lung disease. The cannabinoids in marijuana are allergenic in animal models (6).

THC is absorbed orally or by inhalation, is rapidly distributed throughout the body, and has a high affinity for fat tissues (6). The metabolites appear in the urine for ten days or more after a single exposure and for several weeks after chronic exposure (6). In an animal model of multiple sclerosis, tetrahydrocannabinol has been reported to reduce tremor and spasticity, possibly through its activity at CB1 receptors in the brain (5889).

THC seems to suppress the immune function by its action at the CB2 receptors. It increases the activity of interleukin-10 (IL-10) and IL-4, and other cytokines that inhibit immune function. This effect might reduce resistance to infections (10239,10240).

Research on the effect of cannabinoids on cancer is conflicting. The effect of THC on IL-10, IL-4, and other cytokines suggests it might promote the growth of cancer cells (10239,10240). However, cannabinoids seem to inhibit human breast cancer cell proliferation in vitro. When THC is infused directly into the tumor mass, it seems to produce tumor eradication or improvements in survival in animals with experimentally induced malignant gliomas (a type of brain tumor). THC induces tumor cell apoptosis via CB1 and CB2 receptors expressed on the glioma cells (5887).

Adverse Reactions

The use of marijuana can cause xerostomia (dry mouth), nausea, vomiting, and a characteristic reddening of the eyes. Cardiovascular effects can include tachycardia, hypotension or hypertension, syncope, palpitations, and vasodilation (13,2619).

Intoxicating doses of marijuana impair reaction time, motor coordination, and visual perceptions, and can also produce panic reactions, hallucinations, flashbacks, depression and other emotional disturbances. An individual's driving ability can be impaired up to 8 hours (18). Long-term use of marijuana can cause cognitive impairment that lasts longer than the period of acute intoxication. These cognitive impairments develop slowly and worsen as the years of marijuana use increase, becoming clinically significant after about 2 decades of use (10242).

The chronic use of marijuana can cause laryngitis, bronchitis, apathy, psychic decline, sexual dysfunction, and abnormal menstruation (18), and has been associated with several cases of an unusual pattern of bullous emphysema (1395). Signs of acute poisoning from marijuana include nausea, vomiting, lacrimation, hacking cough, disturbed cardiac function, and limb numbness (18). Marijuana has a high abuse potential (6). Regular smoking of 3-4 marijuana cigarettes per day is reported to produce as many symptoms as an average of 22 tobacco cigarettes per day, and comparable airway histological effects as 20 tobacco cigarettes per day (1395).

Regular use of marijuana in middle-aged persons has been associated with an increased risk of myocardial infarction.

Unpublished evidence indicates that there is a 4.8 fold increase in relative risk of myocardial infarction within the first hour following smoking marijuana. Regular marijuana smoking was defined as smoking marijuana less than once a month to daily (1356).

Interactions with Herbs & Other Dietary Supplements

SUPPLEMENTS WITH SEDATIVE PROPERTIES: Theoretically, concomitant use of marijuana with supplements that have sedative properties might increase the risk of excessive drowsiness (2619). Some of these supplements include 5-HTP, calamus, California poppy, catnip, hops, Jamaican dogwood, kava, St. John's wort, scullcap, valerian, yerba mansa, and others.

Interactions with Drugs

BARBITURATES: Marijuana can decrease barbiturate clearance rate (2619). Some of these sedative medications include pentobarbital (Nembutal), phenobarbital (Luminal), secobarbital (Seconal), and others.
CNS DEPRESSANTS: Use of dronabinol can have additive or synergistic effects drugs such as narcotics, antihistamines, benzodiazepines and other CNS depressants (2619).
DISULFIRAM (Antabuse): Concomitant use with marijuana can cause transient hypomanic episodes (2619).
FLUOXETINE (Prozac): Concomitant use with marijuana can cause transient hypomanic episodes (2619).
THEOPHYLLINE : Concomitant use with marijuana can increase theophylline metabolism (2619).

Interactions with Foods

ALCOHOL: Concomitant use of alcohol with dronabinol can have additive or synergistic CNS effects (2619).

Interactions with Lab Tests

INTRAOCULAR PRESSURE: Marijuana smoking reduces intraocular pressure and test results in some patients with glaucoma (1268).

Interactions with Diseases or Conditions

CARDIOVASCULAR DISEASES: Marijuana has the potential to cause tachycardia and transient hypertension (6).
COMPROMISED IMMUNE FUNCTION: Cannabinoids in marijuana can decrease immune function, which might reduce resistance to infections (10239,10240).
RESPIRATORY DISEASES: Long-term use of marijuana can exacerbate respiratory conditions (6). Chronic marijuana use has been associated with several cases of an unusual pattern of bullous emphysema (1395).
SEIZURE DISORDERS: Marijuana might exacerbate, or help control, seizure disorders in some individuals (6).

Dosage and Administration

ORAL: People typically use 5 to 15 drops of marijuana tincture or 1 to 3 drops of fluid extract. The prescription product dronabinol (Marinol) is used in doses of 5 to 15 mg/m2 every 2 for 4 hours for cancer chemotherapy-induced nausea and vomiting, and 2.5 to 10 mg twice daily for appetite stimulation in people with AIDS (6606,11166).
INHALATION: People typically use 1 to 3 grains (65 to 195 mg) of cannabis for smoking. Hashish, the plant resin, is smoked in a dose of up to 1 grain (16 to 65 mg). Potency may vary. The drug deteriorates rapidly, requiring ascending doses to produce its effect (5267).

Comments

Avoid confusion with hemp, a distinct variety of Cannabis sativa cultivated for its fiber and seeds, which contains less than 1% THC. Marijuana is classified as a Schedule I controlled substance, making possession illegal. The cannabinoid constituent of marijuana, dronabinol (Marinol), is an FDA-approved prescription product. It's approved for AIDS-related anorexia and chemotherapy induced nausea and vomiting (6606,10241,11166). Cannabinoids are at least as effective as prochlorperazine (Compazine), metoclopramide (Reglan), chlorpromazine (Compazine), thiethylperazine (Torecan), and other conventional antiemetic drugs (6606,10241).
Cannabinoids from marijuana also appear to be similar to codeine for treatment of pain. However, excessive sedation and other central nervous system effects make cannabinoids undesirable as analgesics (10235).

MARJORAM

Also Known As

Garden Marjoram, Gartenmajoran, Knotted Marjoram, Majoran, Majorana Aetheroleum Oil, Majorana Herb, Marjolaine, Mejorana, Sweet Marjoram.
CAUTION: See separate listing for Oregano.

Scientific Names

Origanum majorana, synonyms Majorana hortensis, Majorana majorana.
Family: Lamiaceae/Labiatae.

People Use This For

Orally, marjoram is used for rhinitis and colds in infants and toddlers, gastritis, stimulating appetite, as a digestive aid, antispasmodic, antiflatulent, astringent, ulcus ventriculi, to promote circulation, healthy sleep, and treat mood swings. Marjoram is also used orally for liver disease, gallstones, dry and irritating coughs, swellings of the nasal and pharyngeal mucosa, inflammation of the ears, headaches, reducing blood glucose levels, promoting lactation, urogenital bleeding, climacteric complaints, as a nerve tonic, heart tonic, and sprains, bruises, lumbago.
Marjoram oil is used for coughs, gall bladder complaints, gastrointestinal cramps and disorders, depression, dizziness, migraines, nervous headaches, neurasthenia, paralysis, paroxysmal coughs, rhinitis, and as a diuretic.
In foods, marjoram is a culinary spice and commonly used in foods. The oil and oleoresin are used as flavor ingredients in foods and beverages.
In manufacturing, the oil is used as a fragrance component in soaps and cosmetics.

Safety

LIKELY SAFE ...when used in amounts commonly found in foods. Marjoram has Generally Recognized As Safe (GRAS) status in the US (4912).
POSSIBLY SAFE ...when the leaf is used orally for medicinal purposes (12) on a short-term basis (2). ...when marjoram oil is used orally and appropriately (11).
POSSIBLY UNSAFE ...when the flower, leaf, and oil are used long-term because marjoram contains arbutin and hydroxyquinone. Some information suggests hydroxyquinone might cause cancer (2). ...when using fresh marjoram topically because it can cause eye and skin inflammation (11).
CHILDREN: POSSIBLY UNSAFE ...when excessive amounts are used in children; avoid using (2).
PREGNANCY: POSSIBLY UNSAFE ...when used in medicinal amounts; marjoram has the potential for stimulating menstruation (19).
LACTATION: Insufficient reliable information available; avoid using in amounts larger than those found in foods.

Effectiveness

There is insufficient reliable information available about the effectiveness of marjoram.

Mechanism of Action

The applicable parts of marjoram are the flower, leaf and oil. Marjoram has antiflatulent, antispasmodic, diaphoretic, and diuretic properties (11). The volatile oil demonstrates antimicrobial and insecticidal activity (18). There is some evidence that marjoram has antibacterial activity and antiviral activity against the herpes simplex virus (11). The constituents of marjoram include small amounts of arbutin and hydroxyquinone (2). Arbutin, an antibacterial principle, is poorly absorbed from the gastrointestinal tract (7). Marjoram is a rich source of calcium and iron (19).

Adverse Reactions

Topically, fresh marjoram can cause eye and skin inflammation (11). Hydroxyquinone can cause skin depigmentation (2); however, this adverse effect has not been reported with the use of the marjoram ointment (2).

Interactions with Herbs & Other Dietary Supplements

None known.

Interactions with Drugs

None known.

Interactions with Foods

None known.

Interactions with Lab Tests

None known.

Interactions with Diseases or Conditions

CROSS-ALLERGENICITY: Marjoram can cause allergic reactions in people allergic to the Lamiaceae family plants, which include basil, hyssop, lavender, mint, oregano, and sage (3705).

Dosage and Administration

ORAL: The typical dose of marjoram is one to two cups of the tea throughout the day (18). The tea is prepared by steeping 1-2 teaspoons of the flower or leaf in 250 mL boiling water for 5 minutes and then straining.
TOPICAL: Marjoram is commonly used as a poultice or mouthwash (18).

Comments

In early Greek mythology, the goddess of love, Aphrodite, was believed to have grown marjoram, and marjoram has since been used in various love potions (6002). Avoid confusion with oregano (Origanum vulgare), also referred to as wild marjoram and winter marjoram (2,18).

MARSH BLAZING STAR

Also Known As

Backache Root, Blazing-Star, Button Snakeroot, Colic Root, Devil's Bite Prairie-Pine, Gayfeather, Gay-Feather.

Scientific Names

Liatris spicata, synonyms Laciniaria spicata, Liatris callilepis, Serratula spicata.
Family: Asteraceae/Compositae.

People Use This For

Orally, marsh blazing star is used for kidney disorders, dysmenorrhea, gonorrhea, and as a diuretic.

Safety

There is insufficient reliable information available about the safety of marsh blazing star.
Pregnancy and Lactation: Insufficient reliable information available; avoid using.

Effectiveness

There is insufficient reliable information available about the effectiveness of marsh blazing star.

Mechanism of Action

The applicable part of marsh blazing star is the root. Marsh blazing star contains coumarin as its active principle (18). However, coumarin itself is not an anticoagulant. It has only 0.1%-0.02% of the anticoagulant effect of bishydroxycoumarin (295). Some studies suggest coumarin might be effective in reducing edemas and inflammations by increasing venous and lymphatic return (295).

Adverse Reactions

Orally, marsh blazing star, which contains coumarin, can be associated with nausea and vomiting (286), diarrhea, dizziness, insomnia (287), asymptomatic SGOT elevations (286), and liver toxicity (6,18).
Topically, handling the plant can cause contact dermatitis (3837).
Marsh blazing star can cause an allergic reaction in individuals sensitive to the Asteraceae/Compositae family. Members of this family include ragweed, chrysanthemums, marigolds, daisies, and many other herbs.

Interactions with Herbs & Other Dietary Supplements

None known.

Interactions with Drugs

None known.

Interactions with Foods

None known.

Interactions with Lab Tests

None known.

Interactions with Diseases or Conditions

CROSS-ALLERGENICITY: Can cause an allergic reaction in individuals sensitive to the Asteraceae/Compositae family. Members of this family include ragweed, chrysanthemums, marigolds, daisies, and many other herbs.

Dosage and Administration

ORAL: The ground root is used as tea (6).

MARSH MARIGOLD

Also Known As

Bull's Eyes, Cowslip, Horse Blobs, Kingcups, Leopard's Foot, Meadow Routs, Palsy Root, Solsequia, Sponsa Solis, Verrucaria, Water Blobs, Water Dragon.
CAUTION: See separate listing for Cowslip.

Scientific Names

Caltha palustris, synonym Caltha palustris.
Family: Ranunculaceae.

People Use This For

Orally, marsh marigold is used to stop pain and cramps, for menstrual disorders, bronchial inflammation, jaundice, and liver and biliary disorders. Marsh marigold is also used orally as a laxative, diuretic, and to lower cholesterol levels and raise blood sugar.
Topically, marsh marigold is used for cleaning skin lesions and sores.

Safety

LIKELY UNSAFE ...when the fresh above ground parts are used orally or topically because they cause severe local irritation (18).
There is insufficient reliable information about the safety of the medicinal use of the dried above ground parts.
PREGNANCY AND LACTATION: LIKELY UNSAFE ...when the fresh above ground parts are used orally or topically (18). There is insufficient reliable information available about the safety of the dried above ground parts during pregnancy and lactation.

Effectiveness

There is insufficient reliable information available about the effectiveness of marsh marigold.

Mechanism of Action

The applicable parts of marsh marigold are the above ground parts of the flowering plant. When the fresh plant is crushed or cut into small pieces, the glycoside ranunculin is enzymatically changed into a severely irritating protoanemonin, which, in turn, rapidly degrades into the less toxic anemonin (18). Both protoanemonin and ranunculin are destroyed to an unknown extent during the drying process (2).

Adverse Reactions

Orally, ingestion of marsh marigold can cause severe irritation of the gastrointestinal tract, with colic and diarrhea. Irritation of the urinary tract can also occur.
Topically, skin contact with the fresh plant can cause blisters and burns that are difficult to heal (18).

Interactions with Herbs & Other Dietary Supplements

None known.

Interactions with Drugs

None known.

Interactions with Foods

None known.

Interactions with Lab Tests

None known.

Interactions with Diseases or Conditions

None known.

Dosage and Administration

No typical dosage.

MARSH TEA

Also Known As

James' Tea, Ledi palustris herba, Marsh Citrus, Moth Herb, Romarin Sauvage, Sumpfporst, Swamp Tea, Wild Rosemary.
CAUTION: See separate listing for Labrador Tea.

Scientific Names

Rhododendron tomentosum var. tomentosum, synonyms Ledum palustre, Rhododendron palustre.
Family: Ericaceae

People Use This For

Orally, marsh tea is used for rheumatic discomforts, whooping cough, for bronchitis, cold, cough, whitlow (herpes infection of the finger), relieving chest and lung ailments, stimulating milk flow, as a diaphoretic, diuretic, abortifacient, expectorant, and narcotic.

Safety

LIKELY UNSAFE ...when large amounts are used orally to try to cause abortion (2). The essential oil of marsh tea causes severe gastrointestinal (GI) tract irritation, kidneys and urinary tract damage, and central nervous system (CNS) excitation followed by paralysis (2).
There is insufficient reliable information available about the safety of marsh tea for its other uses.
PREGNANCY: LIKELY UNSAFE ...when used orally; avoid using (2,19). Marsh tea is considered to be a potential uterine stimulant (19).
LACTATION: Insufficient reliable information available; avoid using.

Effectiveness

There is insufficient reliable information available about the effectiveness of marsh tea.

Mechanism of Action

Some evidence suggests marsh tea might have antitussive and anti-inflammatory activity. It might also inhibit motility (2) and stimulate uterine activity (19).

Adverse Reactions

Orally, ingestion of large amounts of marsh tea can cause poisoning (2). The essential oil of marsh tea can cause severe irritation of the gastrointestinal (GI) tract, vomiting, diarrhea, irritation and damage to the kidneys and urinary tract, heavy perspiration, myalgias, arthralgias, and central nervous system excitation with narcotic intoxication, followed by paralysis (2).

Interactions with Herbs & Other Dietary Supplements

None known.

Interactions with Drugs

CNS DEPRESSANTS: Marsh tea can potentiate effects of barbiturates and alcohol (2).

Interactions with Foods

None known.

Interactions with Lab Tests

None known.

Interactions with Diseases or Conditions

GASTROINTESTINAL (GI) IRRITATION: Theoretically, might exacerbate gastrointestinal tract inflammation or irritation (2).
KIDNEY DYSFUNCTION: Contraindicated in individuals with kidney dysfunction (2).
URINARY TRACT IRRITATION: Theoretically, might exacerbate urinary tract irritation and inflammation (2).

Dosage and Administration

No typical dosage.

MARSHMALLOW

Also Known As
Alteia, Althaeae folium, Althaeae radi, Althea, Herba Malvae , Mallards, Mortification Root, Racine De Guimauve, Sweet Weed, Wymote.
CAUTION: See separate listings for Mallow flower and Mallow leaf.

Scientific Names
Althaea officinalis, synonym Althaea taurinensis.
Family: Malvaceae.

People Use This For
Orally, marshmallow leaf and root are used for respiratory tract mucous membrane inflammation, dry cough, inflammation of the gastric mucosa, diarrhea, peptic ulcers, constipation, urinary tract inflammation, and urinary calculus.
Topically, marshmallow leaf and root are used for abscesses, for varicose and thrombotic ulcers, as a poultice for skin inflammation or burns, and for other wounds. Marshmallow leaf is used topically as a poultice for insect bites. Marshmallow root is used topically in ointments for chapped skin and chilblains.
For foods, marshmallow leaf is used as a flavoring agent.
In manufacturing, the marshmallow root is used in foods and beverages.

Safety
LIKELY SAFE ...when used in amounts commonly found in foods. Marshmallow root has Generally Recognized As Safe (GRAS) status in the US (4912). ...when taken orally in medicinal amounts (4,12).
POSSIBLY SAFE ...when used topically (4).
PREGNANCY AND LACTATION: Insufficient reliable information available.

Effectiveness
There is insufficient reliable information available about the effectiveness of marshmallow.

Mechanism of Action
The applicable parts of marshmallow are the leaves and the root. Marshmallow leaf and root contain mucilage polysaccharides that can soothe and protect mucous membranes from local irritation by forming a protective layer (1,4,6,7,9,18). The mucilage can inhibit mucociliary transport (1,6,18), stimulate phagocytosis (1,18), suppress cough (1,6,8,11), increase the anti-inflammatory effects of topical dexamethasone (1,6,18), and have hypoglycemic activity (1,4). The mucilage can also have antimicrobial, spasmolytic, antisecretory, diuretic, antilithic, and wound-healing effects (4,6).

Adverse Reactions
Orally, marshmallow can cause hypoglycemia (4,11,18).

Interactions with Herbs & Other Dietary Supplements
HERBS AND SUPPLEMENTS: Concomitant use of marshmallow can retard the absorption of other herbs or supplements (1,11,12).

Interactions with Drugs
ANTIDIABETES DRUGS: Theoretically, due to claims of hypoglycemic effects, marshmallow might interfere with hypoglycemic therapy (4).
ORAL DRUGS: The mucilage in marshmallow might impair absorption of oral drugs (1,11,12,19).

Interactions with Foods
None known.

Interactions with Lab Tests
BLOOD GLUCOSE: Theoretically, marshmallow could lower blood glucose and test results (4,11,18).

Interactions with Diseases or Conditions
DIABETES: Theoretically, marshmallow could interfere with blood sugar control (4).

Dosage and Administration
ORAL: For irritation of the mouth or pharynx and associated dry cough, the typical dose of marshmallow is 2-5 grams of the dried leaf, 5 grams of the dried root or one cup of either leaf or root tea three times daily (4). The leaf

tea is prepared by steeping 2-5 grams of the dried leaf in 150 mL boiling water for 5-10 minutes and then straining. The root tea is prepared by steeping 2-5 grams of the dried root in 150 mL cold water for 1-1.5 hours, straining, and then warming before consumption. The usual dose of the liquid leaf or root extract (1:1 in 25% alcohol) is 2-5 mL three times daily (4). For irritation of oral or pharyngeal mucosa and the associated cough, the common dose of the marshmallow root syrup is 2-10 mL up to three times daily (1,4).
TOPICAL: The 5% powdered leaf in an ointment base is commonly applied three times daily (4).

Comments
Avoid confusion with the mallow (Malva sylvestris) flower and leaf.

MARTAGON

Also Known As
Purple Turk's Cap Lily, Turk's Cap.

Scientific Names
Lilium martagon.
Family: Liliaceae

Comments
At the date of publication, this product was not a common ingredient used in brand name supplements marketed to consumers. Details about this product are available at the online version of *Natural Medicines Comprehensive Database*. See www.naturaldatabase.com.

MASTERWORT

Also Known As
Cow Cabbage, Cow Parsnip, Hogweed, Madnep, Radix Pimpinelle Franconiae, Woolly Parsnip, Youthwort.
CAUTION: See separate listing for Goutweed (Aegopodium podagraria).

Scientific Names
Heracleum sphondylium, Heracleum sphondylium subsp. montanum, synonyms Heracleum lanatum, Heracleum maximum, Heracleum montanum.
Family: Apiaceae/Umbelliferae.

People Use This For
Orally, masterwort is used for relief of muscle cramps, stomach disorders, digestive problems, diarrhea, and mucous membrane inflammation of the GI tract.

Safety
POSSIBLY UNSAFE ...when used orally. Masterwort can cause phototoxicity (19), and some of the furocoumarin constituents can be carcinogenic (4).
PREGNANCY: LIKELY UNSAFE ...when used orally; contraindicated for use in early pregnancy, due to the reported ability to stimulate menstruation (19).
LACTATION: POSSIBLY UNSAFE ...when used orally (4); avoid using.

Effectiveness
There is insufficient reliable information available about the effectiveness of masterwort.

Mechanism of Action
Masterwort is considered to be a mild expectorant, although this effect remains unproven (18). It contains furocoumarins (bergapten, isopimpinellin, pimpinellin, isoberapten, spondin) and a volatile oil containing n-octylacetate (18). Bergapten, also known as 5-methoxypysoralen, is phototoxic and may also be carcinogenic (4).

Adverse Reactions
Orally, use increases skin sensitivity to UV light and can lead to phototoxicity (19).
Topically, application of the fresh plant can cause photodermatitis (3835).
Masterwort may also be carcinogenic.

Interactions with Herbs & Other Dietary Supplements
None known.

Interactions with Drugs
PHOTOSENSITIZING DRUGS: Contraindicated due to additive photosensitizing effect (19).

Interactions with Foods
None known.

Interactions with Lab Tests
None known.

Interactions with Diseases or Conditions
ULTRAVIOLET LIGHT THERAPY: Contraindicated due to photosensitizing effect (19); avoid excessive periods in sun (19).

Dosage and Administration
No typical dosage.

Comments
Masterwort is reportedly used as a replacement/adulterant for greater burnet-saxifrage (Pimpinella major) (7).

MASTIC

Also Known As
Lentisk, Mastich, Mastix.

Scientific Names
Pistacia lentiscus.
Family: Anacardiaceae.

People Use This For
Orally, mastic is used for gastric and duodenal ulcers, respiratory conditions, muscle aches, and to improve circulation. It is also used for bacterial and fungal infections.
Topically, mastic is used as skin care for cuts, as an insect repellent, to improve adhesive strength in surgical tapes, and as a drug releasing vehicle.
In dentistry, mastic resin is used as a material for fillings. The masticated resin releases substances that freshen the breath and tighten the gums.
In manufacturing, mastic resin is used in the food and drink industries and in the production of chewing gum.

Safety
POSSIBLY SAFE ...when used orally (18).
PREGNANCY AND LACTATION: Insufficient reliable information available; avoid using.

Effectiveness
There is insufficient reliable information available about the effectiveness of mastic.

Mechanism of Action
The applicable part of mastic is the resin. Mastic tree contains resins including the triterpenes mastic acid, isomastic acid, oleanlic acid, and tirucallol. It also contains a volatile oil containing alpha-pinene as a constituent. The volatile oil and the resin are both thought to have astringent and aromatic effects (18). For prevention of gastric and duodenal ulcers, some researchers think mastic might have antisecretory and possibly cytoprotective effects. Animal models show that it seems to help protect the gastric mucosa during aspirin, phenylbutazone, or reserpine therapy (4142). This effect has not yet been found in humans. There is some in vitro evidence that mastic extract has antimicrobial and antifungal activity (4141). There is also preliminary evidence that mastic might have hypotensive and antioxidant effects (6).

Adverse Reactions
Children who ingest mastic tree resin might develop diarrhea (18). The pollen of mastic tree is allergenic (4140). Exposure to mastic tree can cause allergic reactions in individuals allergic to Schinus terebintifolious and other Pistacia species (4140).

Interactions with Herbs & Other Dietary Supplements
CROSS-ALLERGENICITY: Individuals allergic to mastic tree might also have an allergic reaction to Schinus terebintifolious and other Pistacia species (4140).

Interactions with Drugs
None known.

Interactions with Foods
None known.

Interactions with Lab Tests
None known.

Interactions with Diseases or Conditions
None known.

Dosage and Administration
No typical dosage.

Comments
Mastic resin is the resin from the trunk of Pistacia lentiscus.

MATE

Also Known As
Chimarrao, Hervea, Ilex, Jesuit's Tea, Maté Folium, Paraguay Tea, St. Bartholemew's Tea, Yerba Maté.
CAUTION: See separate listing for Caffeine.

Scientific Names
Ilex paraguariensis.
Family: Aquifoliaceae.

People Use This For
Orally, mate is used as a stimulant to relieve mental and physical fatigue. It's also used as a diuretic, for modifying mood or affective disorders, as a mild analgesic for headache and rheumatic pains, and as a laxative in large amounts. It is also used orally for depression, weight loss, urinary tract infection, cardiac insufficiency, arrhythmias, hypotension, nervous heart complaints, kidney and bladder stones, and to promote cleansing and excretion of waste. In foods, the use of mate includes a tea-like beverage.

Safety
POSSIBLY SAFE ...when used orally and appropriately on a short-term basis (11866).
POSSIBLY UNSAFE ...when mate is used orally in large amounts or for prolonged periods of time. Mate is associated with an increased risk of mouth cancer, esophageal cancer, laryngeal cancer, kidney cancer, bladder cancer, and lung cancer (1528,1529,1530,1531,11863,11864).
LIKELY UNSAFE ...when used orally in very high doses. Mate contains caffeine. The fatal acute oral dose of caffeine is estimated to be 10-14 grams (150-200 mg per kilogram). Serious toxicity can occur at lower doses depending on variables in caffeine sensitivity such as smoking, age, prior caffeine use, etc (11832).
CHILDREN: POSSIBLY UNSAFE ...when used orally. Mate is associated with an increased risk of mouth cancer, esophageal cancer, laryngeal cancer, kidney cancer, bladder cancer, and lung cancer (1528,1529,1530,1531,11863,11864).
PREGNANCY: POSSIBLY UNSAFE ...when used orally. Mate is associated with an increased risk of mouth cancer, esophageal cancer, laryngeal cancer, kidney cancer, bladder cancer, and lung cancer (1528,1529,1530,1531,11863,11864). Teratogenic studies have not been performed. Mate contains caffeine. Caffeine crosses the placenta, producing fetal blood concentrations similar to maternal levels. Maternal doses of greater than 200 mg per day throughout pregnancy have resulted in symptoms of caffeine withdrawal in newborn infants (9891).
High doses of caffeine have been associated with spontaneous abortion, premature delivery, and low birth weight (2709,2711).
LACTATION: POSSIBLY UNSAFE ...when used orally. Mate is associated with an increased risk of mouth cancer, esophageal cancer, laryngeal cancer, kidney cancer, bladder cancer, and lung cancer (1528,1529,1530,1531,11863,11864). Whether carcinogenic constituents of mate are transferred via breast milk is unknown. Mate contains caffeine. Consumption of mate might cause irritability and increased bowel activity in nursing infants (6026).

Effectiveness

INSUFFICIENT RELIABLE EVIDENCE to RATE

Obesity. Mate taken orally might cause weight loss when used in combination with guarana and damiana (11866). More evidence is needed to rate mate for this use.

Mechanism of Action

The applicable parts of mate are the leaf and leaf stem. It contains caffeine, theobromine, theophylline, phytol, stigmasterol, and squalene. The concentrations of these constituents vary with growing conditions, harvesting, and preparation methods (11865,11867). Mate also contains various minerals including phosphorus, iron, calcium, thiamine, riboflavin, vitamin C, and vitamin E. Other constituents include tannins and N-nitroso compounds that are potential carcinogens (11863,11865).

The usual concentration of caffeine in mate is 0.5% to 0.8% (compared to 1-2% in coffee) (11865,11867). The caffeine in mate stimulates the central nervous system (CNS), heart, muscles, and possibly the pressor centers that control blood pressure (2722). Possible mechanisms include adenosine receptor blockade and phosphodiesterase inhibition (2722). By blocking adenosine receptors, caffeine is thought to increase the release of neurotransmitters such as dopamine (6370). Caffeine also decreases airway resistance and stimulates respiration, via adenosine receptor blockade and phosphodiesterase inhibition (11836). It has also been proposed that caffeine may decrease GABA and serotonin signaling (6370). Caffeine stimulates gastric acid secretion, and increases plasma catecholamine levels (11837). Caffeine can have positive inotropic and chronotropic effects on the heart (11836). Caffeine can also acutely elevate both diastolic and systolic blood pressure, but might not have this effect in habitual users (2722).

Caffeine exerts a diuretic effect, with water losses estimated at 1.17 mL per milligram of caffeine (2712). Tachyphylaxis to the diuretic effect develops rapidly, diminishing fluid losses associated with caffeine intake (10206). Caffeine-containing beverages consumed during moderate endurance exercise do not appear to compromise bodily hydration status (2713). Caffeine does not substantially affect the fluid status of people who drink caffeinated beverages on a regular basis (10206).

Caffeine, a constituent of mate, has been reported to cause increases and decreases in blood glucose. In people with type 2 diabetes, acute administration of caffeine impairs postprandial glucose metabolism, while acute abstention from caffeine reduces postprandial glucose levels by 21%. Whether these effects also occur with caffeinated beverages and herbs is unknown (12374). Other research in obese people suggests that caffeine ingestion may contribute to insulin resistance (12375). However, one study found that type 1 diabetics taking 200 mg of caffeine twice daily had increased frequency and intensity of warning signs of hypoglycemia. This may be due to a reduction in blood flow to the brain and an increase in glucose utilization by the brain (6024).

In vitro and epidemiological research suggests that mate may be carcinogenic. Carcinogenesis may result from thermal injury; mate is consumed as a hot beverage in South America. Because smoking in combination with mate greatly increases cancer risk, some researchers think that mate might act as a solvent for carcinogens in tobacco.

Adverse Reactions

Orally, the prolonged use of mate is associated with an increased risk of mouth cancer, esophageal cancer, laryngeal cancer, kidney cancer, bladder cancer, and lung cancer (1528,1529,1530,1531,11863,11864). The effect seems to be cumulative-dose dependent. The risk of cancer with mate use seems to increase if it is taken as a warm beverage. Tobacco and alcohol use can increase risk 7-fold (11863). There is one report of venous occlusive disease associated with excessive, long-term mate consumption (5614).

The caffeine constituent of mate can cause insomnia, nervousness, restlessness, gastric irritation, nausea and vomiting, as well as tachycardia, quickened respiration, tremors, delirium, convulsions, and diuresis (11832,11838). Caffeine may exacerbate sleep disturbances in patients with acquired immunodeficiency syndrome (AIDS) (10204). Caffeine can cause anaphylaxis in sensitive individuals, although true IgE-mediated caffeine allergy seems to be relatively rare (11315).

Large doses of caffeine can produce headache, anxiety, agitation, ringing in the ears, premature heartbeat, and arrhythmia (11832,11838). In fatal overdose, the cause of death is usually ventricular fibrillation (11838). High doses of mate providing 250 mg of caffeine can also increase blood pressure. This doesn't seem to occur in people who habitually consume caffeine products (2722). Although tolerance to caffeine is a widely held belief, there is little supportive clinical evidence. If it exists, it appears to be of little clinical significance (11839). Withdrawal symptoms such as irritability, sleepiness, delirium, nausea, vomiting, rhinorrhea, nervousness, restlessness, anxiety, muscle tension, muscle pains, and flushed face have been described. However, these symptoms may be from nonpharmacological factors related to knowledge and expectation of effects. Clinically significant symptoms caused by caffeine withdrawal may be uncommon (2723,11839).

Some evidence shows caffeine is associated with fibrocystic breast disease, breast cancer, and endometriosis in women; however, this is controversial since findings are conflicting (8043). Restricting caffeine in women with fibrocystic breast conditions doesn't seem to affect breast nodularity, swelling, or pain (8996).

Epidemiological evidence regarding the relationship between caffeine use and the risk for osteoporosis is contradictory. Caffeine can increase urinary excretion of calcium (2669,10202,11317). Women identified with a genetic variant of the vitamin D receptor appear to be at an increased risk for the detrimental effect of caffeine on bone mass (2669). However, moderate caffeine intake, less than 300 mg per day, does not seem to significantly increase osteoporosis risk in most postmenopausal women with normal calcium intake (2669,6025,10202,11317).

Combining ephedra with mate increases the risk of adverse effects, due to the caffeine contained in mate (2729). One unpublished report associated jitteriness, hypertension, seizures, temporary loss of consciousness, and hospitalization requiring life support with the use of a combination ephedra and guarana (caffeine) product (1380). There is one report of ischemic stroke in an athlete who consumed ephedra 40-60 mg, creatine monohydrate 6 grams, caffeine 400-600 mg, and a variety of other supplements daily for six weeks (1275). Some evidence shows caffeine is associated with fibrocystic breast disease, breast cancer, and endometriosis in women; however, this is controversial since findings are conflicting (8043).

Interactions with Herbs & Other Dietary Supplements

CAFFEINE-CONTAINING HERBS/SUPPLEMENTS: Concomitant use of mate and caffeine-containing herbs/supplements constitutes therapeutic duplication (due to the caffeine contained in mate) which increases the risk of caffeine-related adverse effects. Other natural products which contain caffeine include cocoa, coffee, cola nut, black tea, and guarana.

CALCIUM: High caffeine intake from foods and beverages including mate increases urinary calcium excretion (2570).

CREATINE: There is some concern that combining caffeine, a constituent of mate, with ephedra and creatine might increase the risk of serious adverse effects. There is a report of ischemic stroke in an athlete who consumed creatine monohydrate 6 grams, caffeine 400-600 mg, ephedra 40-60 mg, and a variety of other supplements daily for 6 weeks (1275). Caffeine might also decrease creatine's possible beneficial effects on athletic performance. Some researchers think caffeine can inhibit phosphocreatine resynthesis (2117,4575).

EPHEDRA (Ma Huang): Use of ephedra with mate can increase the risk of stimulatory adverse effects due to its caffeine content. There is evidence that using ephedra with caffeine might increase the risk of serious life-threatening or debilitating adverse effects such as hypertension, myocardial infarction, stroke, seizures, and death (6486,10307). Tell patients to avoid taking mate with ephedra and other stimulants such as bitter orange.

Interactions with Drugs

ADENOSINE (Adenocard): The caffeine in mate is a competitive inhibitor of adenosine at the cellular level. However, caffeine doesn't seem to affect supplemental adenosine because high interstitial levels of adenosine overcome the antagonistic effects of caffeine (11771).

ALCOHOL (Ethanol): Concomitant use of alcohol can increase caffeine serum concentrations and the risk of caffeine adverse effects. Alcohol reduces caffeine metabolism (6370).

AMPHETAMINES: Theoretically, the caffeine in mate might increase the risk of additive CNS effects (2719).

ANTICOAGULANT/ANTIPLATELET DRUGS: Theoretically, the caffeine in mate might increase the risk of bleeding when used concomitantly with these agents. Caffeine is reported to have antiplatelet activity (8028,8029); however, this interaction has not been reported in humans. Antiplatelet agents include aspirin, clopidogrel (Plavix), dipyridamole (Persantine), ticlopidine (Ticlid), and others. Anticoagulant agents include heparin and warfarin (Coumadin).

ANTIDIABETES DRUGS: Theoretically, concomitant use of caffeine, a constituent of mate, and diabetes drugs might interfere with blood glucose control. Data are conflicting. Reports claim that caffeine might increase or decrease blood sugar (6024,8646).

CIMETIDINE (Tagamet): Theoretically, concomitant use might increase serum caffeine concentrations and the risk of adverse effects, due to the caffeine contained in mate. Cimetidine decreases the rate of caffeine clearance by 30% to 50% (11736).

CLOZAPINE (Clozaril): Theoretically, co-administration might acutely exacerbate psychotic symptoms, due to the caffeine contained in mate. Caffeine can increase the effects and toxicity of clozapine (151). Caffeine doses of 400-1000 mg per day inhibit clozapine metabolism (5051).

COCAINE: Theoretically, the caffeine in mate might increase the risk of additive CNS effects (2719).

CONTRACEPTIVE DRUGS: Theoretically, concomitant use might increase caffeine concentrations and the risk adverse effects, due to the caffeine contained in mate. Oral contraceptives decrease the rate of caffeine clearance by 40% to 65% (2714,11737).

DIPYRIDAMOLE (Persantine): The caffeine in mate might inhibit dipyridamole-induced vasodilation (11770,11772).

DISULFIRAM (Antabuse): Theoretically, concomitant use might increase serum caffeine concentrations and the risk of adverse effects, due to the caffeine contained in mate. Disulfiram decreases the rate of caffeine clearance (15).

EPHEDRINE: Use of ephedrine with caffeine, a constituent of mate, can increase the risk of stimulatory adverse effects. There is evidence that using ephedrine with caffeine might increase the risk of serious life-threatening or debilitating adverse effects such as hypertension, myocardial infarction, stroke, seizures, and death (1275,6486,10307). Tell patients to avoid taking caffeine with ephedrine and other stimulants.

ESTROGENS: Theoretically, concomitant use might increase serum caffeine concentrations and the risk of adverse effects, due to the caffeine contained in mate. Estrogen inhibits caffeine metabolism (2714).

FLUCONAZOLE (Diflucan): Concomitant use might increase the effects of caffeine in mate. Fluconazole decreases caffeine clearance by approximately 25% (11022).

FLUVOXAMINE (Luvox): Concomitant use of fluvoxamine with caffeine or caffeine-containing herbs such as mate can increase caffeine serum concentrations, and the risk of caffeine adverse effects. Fluvoxamine reduces caffeine metabolism (6370).

LITHIUM (Eskalith): Theoretically, abrupt mate withdrawal might increase serum lithium levels, due to the caffeine contained in mate. There are two case reports of lithium tremor that worsened upon abrupt coffee withdrawal (609,610).
MEXILETINE (Mexitil): Concomitant use might increase the effects and adverse effects of caffeine in mate. Mexiletine can decrease caffeine elimination by 50% (1260,11741).
MONOAMINE OXIDASE INHIBITORS (MAOIs): Theoretically, concomitant intake of large amounts of mate with MAOIs might precipitate a hypertensive crisis, due to the caffeine contained in mate. This is based on the claim that intake of large amounts of caffeine with MAOIs might precipitate a hypertensive crisis (15).
NICOTINE: Theoretically, the caffeine in mate might increase the risk of additive CNS effects (2719).
PHENYLPROPANOLAMINE: Concomitant use of phenylpropanolamine and mate might cause an additive increase in blood pressure due to the caffeine in mate (11738).
QUINOLONE ANTIBIOTICS: Theoretically, concomitant use might increase serum caffeine concentrations and the risk of adverse effects, due to the caffeine contained in mate. Quinolones decrease caffeine clearance (606,607,608). Quinolones (also referred to as fluoroquinolones) include ciprofloxacin (Cipro), enoxacin (Penetrex), gatifloxacin (Tequin), levofloxacin (Levaquin), lomefloxacin (Maxaquin), moxifloxacin (Avelox), norfloxacin (Noroxin), ofloxacin (Floxin), sparfloxacin (Zagam), and trovafloxacin (Trovan).
RILUZOLE (Rilutek): Theoretically, concomitant use might increase serum caffeine and riluzole concentrations and the risk of adverse effects of both caffeine and riluzole, due to the caffeine contained in mate. Caffeine and riluzole are both metabolized by cytochrome P450 1A2, and concomitant use might reduce metabolism of one or both agents (11739).
TERBINAFINE (Lamisil): Theoretically, concomitant use might increase serum caffeine concentrations and the risk of adverse effects, due to the caffeine contained in mate. Terbinafine decreases the rate of caffeine clearance (11740).
THEOPHYLLINE: Theoretically, concomitant use of theophylline and large amounts of mate might increase the risk of theophylline toxicity, due to mate's caffeine content. Caffeine decreases theophylline clearance 23% to 29% (11741).
VERAPAMIL (Calan, Covera, Isoptin, Verelan): Theoretically, concomitant use might increase plasma caffeine concentrations and the risk of adverse effects, due to the caffeine contained in mate. Verapamil increases plasma caffeine concentrations by 25% (11741).

Interactions with Foods

None known.

Interactions with Lab Tests

5-HYDROXYINDOLEACETIC ACID: Mate might increase urine 5-hydroxyindoleacetic acid concentrations and test results, due to its caffeine content. Caffeine can increase urine catecholamine concentrations (15).
BLEEDING TIME: Mate might prolong bleeding time and increase test results, due to its caffeine content (1701).
CATECHOLAMINES: Mate might increase urine catecholamine concentrations and test results, due to its caffeine content. Caffeine can increase urine catecholamine concentrations (8646).
CREATINE: Mate might increase urine creatine concentrations and test results, due to its caffeine content (1701).
DIPYRIDAMOLE THALLIUM IMAGING: Mate might interfere with dipyridamole thallium imaging studies, due to its caffeine content. Caffeine attenuates the characteristic cardiovascular responses to dipyridamole and has altered test results (11742).
GLUCOSE: Caffeine, a constituent of mate, has been reported to cause increases and decreases in blood glucose (8646).
LACTATE: The combination of ephedrine, a constituent of ephedra, and caffeine, a constituent of mate, can increase blood lactate levels (8646).
NEUROBLASTOMA TESTS: Mate (due to its caffeine content) might cause false-positive diagnosis of neuroblastoma, when diagnosis is based on tests of urine vanillylmandelic acid (VMA) or catecholamine concentrations. Caffeine can increase urine catecholamine and VMA concentrations (15).
PHARMACOLOGICAL STRESS TESTS: The caffeine in mate is a competitive antagonist for adenosine receptors (11771). It is recommended that caffeine and caffeine-containing products be stopped 24 hours prior to pharmacological stress tests (11770). However, caffeine appears more likely to interfere with dipyridamole (Persantine) than adenosine (Adenocard) stress testing (11771). The interaction between caffeine and dipyridamole is unlikely to be significant in stress testing if the heart rate increase is greater than 5% after dipyridamole infusion (11772).
PHEOCHROMOCYTOMA TESTS: Mate (due to its caffeine content) might cause false-positive diagnosis of pheochromocytoma, when diagnosis is based on tests of urine vanillylmandelic acid (VMA) or catecholamine concentrations. Caffeine can increase urine catecholamine and VMA concentrations (15).
PULMONARY FUNCTION TESTS: People may need to avoid caffeine and caffeine containing herbs such as mate for at least four hours prior to lung function testing. Forced expiratory volume in one minute (FEV1) seems to show a small improvement up to two hours after caffeine use. Mid-expiratory flow rates may also improve with caffeine for up to four hours (9607).
URATE: Mate might falsely increase serum urate test results determined by the Bittner method, due to its caffeine

content. Caffeine causes false elevations in serum urate test results determined by the Bittner method (11844).
URINARY CALCIUM: Caffeine, a constituent of mate, can increase urinary calcium levels (11317).
VANILLYLMANDELIC ACID (VMA): Mate might increase urine VMA concentrations and test results, due to its caffeine content. Caffeine can increase urine VMA concentrations (15).

Interactions with Diseases or Conditions

ALCOHOLISM: Heavy alcohol with long-time mate consumption increases the risk of cancer from 3-fold to 7-fold (11864).
ANXIETY DISORDERS: The caffeine in mate might aggravate anxiety disorders (11743).
BLEEDING DISORDERS: Theoretically, caffeine in mate might aggravate these conditions. Caffeine is reported to have antiplatelet activity (8028,8029); however, this interaction has not been reported in humans.
CARDIAC CONDITIONS: Caffeine in mate can induce cardiac arrhythmias in sensitive individuals (11845); use with caution.
DIABETES: Some research suggests that caffeine, a constituent of mate, may impair postprandial glucose metabolism in people with diabetes and contribute to insulin resistance. The effect of caffeinated beverages and herbs has not been studied (12374,12375). Caffeine in mate may enhance the frequency and intensity of hypoglycemic warning symptoms in type 1 diabetics. This may increase the ability of diabetics to detect and treat hypoglycemia early. However, it might also increase the frequency of hypoglycemic events (6024); use with caution. Caffeine has been reported to cause increases and decreases in blood glucose (8646); use with caution.
GLAUCOMA: Consuming mate increases intraocular pressure due to the caffeine content. The increase occurs within 30 minutes and persists for at least 90 minutes (8540).
HYPERTENSION: The caffeine in mate might increase blood pressure in people with high blood pressure. Consumption of 250 mg caffeine can increase blood pressure in healthy people, but this doesn't seem to occur in people who habitually consume caffeine products (2722).
OSTEOPOROSIS: Consuming mate can increase urinary excretion of calcium due to its caffeine content. Caffeine consumption should be limited to less than 300 mg per day (approximately 2-3 cups of mate). Adequate calcium supplementation may partially compensate for calcium losses (2669,10202,11317). Postmenopausal women identified with a genetic variant of the vitamin D receptor should use caffeine with caution (2669).
SMOKING: The risk of cancer increases from 3-fold to 7-fold in people who smoke and consume mate for extended periods of time (11864).

Dosage and Administration

No typical dosage.

Comments

Mate, also known as Yerba Maté, is a popular beverage, much like coffee or tea, in Brazil, Paraguay, and Argentina (6002). The beverage is often prepared from leaves of Ilex paraguariensis, also referred to as Jesuit's tea, Jesuit's Brazil tea, Paraguay tea, and St. Bartholemew's tea. The herbal tea has caused multiple anticholinergic poisonings. However, belladonna alkaloids were identified and the poisonings were traced to a single contaminated lot of imported herbs (785).

MEADOWSWEET

Also Known As

Bridewort, Dolloff, Dropwort, Filipendula, Lady Of The Meadow, Meadow Queen, Meadow-Wart, Queen Of The Meadow, Spiraeae flos, Spireae herba.

Scientific Names

Filipendula ulmaria, synonym Spiraea ulmaria.
Family: Rosaceae.

People Use This For

Orally, meadowsweet is used for colds, bronchitis, dyspepsia, heartburn, peptic ulcer disease, and rheumatic disorders including gout. It is also used orally as a diuretic and urinary antiseptic for acute cystitis.

Safety

POSSIBLY SAFE ...when used orally and appropriately (12).
POSSIBLY UNSAFE ...when an aqueous extract (tea) is used in large amounts or for prolonged periods of time because meadowsweet contains high amounts of tannins (4).
PREGNANCY: LIKELY UNSAFE ...when used orally. Some evidence suggests meadowsweet might stimulate uterine activity (4).
LACTATION: Insufficient reliable information available; avoid using.

Effectiveness
There is insufficient reliable information available about the effectiveness of meadowsweet.

Mechanism of Action
The applicable parts of meadowsweet are the above ground parts. Meadowsweet has stomachic, mild urinary antiseptic, antirheumatic, astringent, and antacid activities (4). It contains tannins and salicin, a plant salicylate (7,12). In animals, the above ground parts of meadowsweet decrease motor activity, lower temperature, induce muscle relaxation, and potentiate the effect of narcotics (4). In animals, the flower extract increases life expectancy; decreases vascular permeability; increases bronchial, intestinal, and uterine tone; and promotes uric acid excretion. In vitro, it has bacteriostatic activity (4). Meadowsweet aqueous extracts contain high concentrations of tannins with strong astringent effects (4).

Adverse Reactions
Orally, meadowsweet can cause nausea and other stomach complaints (18). Bronchospastic activity has occurred with use (4). Meadowsweet contains salicylate constituents. There is insufficient reliable information available to know if the side effects and toxicity normally associated with salicylates could occur. The adverse reactions associated with salicylates include gastric and renal irritation, hypersensitivity, blood in stool, tinnitus, nausea, and vomiting. Salicin has been associated with skin rashes (4).

Interactions with Herbs & Other Dietary Supplements
None known.

Interactions with Drugs
ASPIRIN: Meadowsweet contains salicin, a plant salicylate. Theoretically, meadowsweet might have an additive effect with other salicylate-containing drugs such as aspirin. Salicin doesn't seem to have the antiplatelet effects of aspirin (12).
CHOLINE MAGNESIUM TRISALICYLATE (Trilisate): Meadowsweet contains salicin, a plant salicylate. Theoretically, meadowsweet might have an additive effect with other salicylate-containing drugs such as choline magnesium trisalicylate (12).
NARCOTIC DRUGS: Theoretically, meadowsweet can potentiate narcotic effects (4).
SALSALATE (Disalcid): Meadowsweet contains salicin, a plant salicylate. Theoretically, meadowsweet might have an additive effect with other salicylate-containing drugs such as salsalate (12).

Interactions with Foods
None known.

Interactions with Lab Tests
None known.

Interactions with Diseases or Conditions
ASPIRIN ALLERGY: Use meadowsweet cautiously in individuals with aspirin allergy; it contains salicylate constituents.
ASTHMA: Theoretically, meadowsweet might exacerbate asthma due to bronchospastic effects. Use cautiously in individuals with asthma (4).

Dosage and Administration
ORAL: For adults, the typical dose is one cup of the tea several times per day (8). The tea is prepared by steeping 2.5-3.5 grams of the dried flower or 4-5 grams of the above ground parts in 150 mL boiling water for 10 minutes and then straining. The usual dose of the liquid extract (1:1 in 25% alcohol) is 1.5-6 mL three times per day (4). The common dose of the tincture (1:5 in 45% alcohol) is 2-4 mL three times per day (4).

MEDIUM CHAIN TRIGLYCERIDES (MCT)

Also Known As
MCT, MCT's, MCTs, Medium-Chain Triglycerides.

Scientific Names
Medium chain triglycerides.

People Use This For

Orally, medium chain triglycerides (MCTs) are used as adjunctive therapy for malabsorption syndromes including diarrhea, steatorrhea (fat indigestion), gastrectomy, lymphatic abnormalities, celiac disease, hepatic disease, and intestinal resection (short bowel syndrome). MCTs are also used for chyluria and chylothorax; gallbladder disease; AIDS; cystic fibrosis; and for seizures in children, including akinetic, clonic, and petit mal. MCTs are also used for nutritional support of athletic training, and decreasing body fat and increasing lean muscle mass.
Intravenously, MCTs are used as a source of fat in total parenteral nutrition.

Safety

LIKELY SAFE ...when used orally and appropriately (2273,2274). ...when used parenterally and appropriately (2275,2276,2278).
PREGNANCY AND LACTATION: LIKELY SAFE ...when used orally and appropriately (15).

Effectiveness

POSSIBLY EFFECTIVE

Cachexia. Intravenous MCTs can provide calories in critically ill patients, but don't seem to offer any advantages over long chain triglycerides (2275,2276,2278).

Seizures. Using MCTs orally seems to help reduce seizures in children, including akinetic, clonic, and petit mal types (2273,2274).

POSSIBLY INEFFECTIVE

AIDS-related wasting. Using MCTs orally doesn't seem to be any better than multivitamins and minerals alone for prevention of weight loss associated with AIDS (11730).

INSUFFICIENT RELIABLE EVIDENCE to RATE

Chylothorax. Using MCTs orally or in parenteral nutrition might prevent malnutrition and immunocompromise in pediatric and adult patients with chylothorax, according to preliminary clinical research (11726,11727,11728,11729). More evidence is needed to rate MCTs for this use.

Mechanism of Action

Medium chain triglycerides (MCTs) are semi-synthetic lipids composed of fatty acids, mostly lauric acid, with a chain length of six to twelve carbon atoms. MCTs are made from hydrolyzed coconut oil or palm kernel oils. The resulting fatty acids are fractionated and esterified to produce MCTs (11724,11725).
MCTs are efficiently absorbed. At physiological pH, MCTs are weak electrolytes and highly ionized, which increases their solubility (11724). Unlike long chain triglycerides (dietary fat), MCTs don't require the intestinal lymphatic system or bile salts for absorption (11723). They are usually used in patients who can't absorb conventional long chain fatty acids. MCTs do not contain essential fatty acids, and therefore they are normally only substituted for 50-70% of dietary fat. Some evidence suggests that absorption of long chain triglycerides may improve if combined with MCTs (11723). MCTs are metabolized primarily in the liver (11724).
MCTs are absorbed by the portal system rather than by the intestinal lymph system. MCTs have been tried for chylothorax, an effusion of a milky fluid (chyle) into the pleural space, due to trauma or a defect of the thoracic duct. Administering MCTs may decrease lymph flow in the thoracic duct will diminish and allow the thoracic duct defect to heal (11726,11727,11728,11729).
There has been some interest in using MCTs for injured and stressed patients since it causes mild ketosis and may decrease skeletal muscle catabolism (11725). However, clinical trials have not shown any clear advantage of MCTs over long chain triglycerides (2275,2276,2278).
In healthy people, single doses of MCT oil can reduce blood triglyceride levels (834). Some preliminary evidence suggests that MCT may increase metabolic rate and energy expenditures by the body when substituted in the diet for other types of fat. MCT may induce satiety, leading to decreased consumption of calories. Increased metabolic rate and decreased caloric intake may lead to a slight decrease in body fat; however, these effects have not been rigorously tested in humans (10421,11724). MCTs contain 6 to 8.5 kcal per gram (11724).

Adverse Reactions

Orally, MCTs can cause diarrhea, vomiting, irritability, nausea, abdominal discomfort, intestinal gas noises, and essential fatty acid deficiency (2274,11723). MCT oil contains 6 to 8.5 calories per gram, and one tablespoon provides about 14 grams and about 115 calories (11724). Excessive consumption could result in weight gain.

Interactions with Herbs & Other Dietary Supplements

None known.

Interactions with Drugs

None known.

Interactions with Foods

FOOD: Co-administration of MCTs with food can reduce the adverse effects associated with MCTs (2273).

Interactions with Lab Tests

TRIGLYCERIDES: MCTs can lower blood triglyceride levels and test results (834).

Interactions with Diseases or Conditions

DIABETES: MCTs can cause ketosis; use with caution (11724).
HEPATIC ENCEPHALOPATHY, CIRRHOSIS: MCTs are primarily metabolized in the liver. MCTs can cause narcosis and coma in patients with hepatic cirrhosis; use with caution (11724).

Dosage and Administration

ORAL: For improving seizure control in children, MCT oil is used as 60% of the caloric intake (2274).
INTRAVENOUS (IV): As a fat source in total parenteral nutrition formulations, a fat mixture containing 50% MCT and 50% long chain triglycerides is commonly used (2275,2276,2278).

Comments

Ingesting MCTs with food reduces the adverse effects (2273).

MELANOTAN-II

Also Known As

Melanotan II, MT-II.
CAUTION: See separate listing for Melatonin.

Scientific Names

Melanotan-II.

People Use This For

Subcutaneously, melanotan-II has been used to evaluate its effects on psychogenic erectile dysfunction, organic erectile dysfunction, and its effects after unilateral nerve-sparing radical prostatectomy. It has also been used subcutaneously to evaluate its effects on tanning of the skin and for the prevention of sunlight-induced skin cancers.

Safety

POSSIBLY SAFE ...when used subcutaneously to initiate penile erections in men with psychogenic or organic erectile dysfunction (5687,5688). Controlled clinical studies suggest mild to moderate adverse effects such as decreased appetite, facial flushing and nausea might occur with a dosage of 0.025 mg/kg (5685,5687,5688).
There is insufficient reliable information available about the safety of melanotan-II for its other uses or at other dosages.
PREGNANCY AND LACTATION: Insufficient reliable information available; avoid using.

Effectiveness

POSSIBLY EFFECTIVE

Erectile dysfunction (ED). Preliminary clinical trials have shown melanotan-II used subcutaneously is superior to placebo in men with psychogenic or organic erectile dysfunction for initiating spontaneous sustained penile erections (5685,5687,5688).

Tanning skin. Using melanotan-II subcutaneously seems to be effective for visible tanning of the skin (5685). A controlled clinical pilot study demonstrated melanotan-II caused increased pigmentation in the face, upper body, and buttocks (5685).

There is insufficient reliable information available about the effectiveness of melanotan-II for its other uses.

Mechanism of Action

Melanotan-I and Melanotan-II are two alpha-melanocyte-stimulating-hormone analogues currently being extensively studied (5686). Both analogues have the ability to darken and tan the skin (5686) and were developed to not only promote skin pigmentation but also to possibly prevent sunlight-induced skin cancers (5683,5686). Compared to alpha-melanocyte-stimulating-hormone, melanotan-I and melanotan-II have increased melanotropic potency (26-100-fold) and increased resistance to degradation by plasma enzymes due to two amino acid substitutions (norleucine for methionine at position 4 and racemization of D-phenylalanine at position 7) in the alpha-melanocyte-stimulating-hormone peptide sequence (5685,5686). Melanotan-II is a cyclic heptapeptide containing a lactam bridge between the amino acids lysine and aspartic acid, enabling it to have even greater melanotropic potency than melanotan-I, a linear tridecapeptide (5685,5686). During a pilot phase-I clinical study, it was discovered by observers that melanotan-II not only caused increased visible tanning but also spontaneous penile erections with use (5685). Subsequent controlled clinical trials have shown melanotan-II initiates erections in men with psychogenic and organic dysfunction (5687,5688). The exact mechanism of action is unknown, but it is hypothesized that melanotan-II acts on pro-erectile pathways at the level of the central nervous system (5687). There are distinct melanocortin receptors found primarily in the brain (5686) and animal data suggests melanotropic peptides act in the hypothalamic regions surrounding the third ventricle (5687). Since dopamine agonists also induce penile erections (and yawning), evidence suggests the central mechanism involves a dopamine-oxytocin pathway (5687).

Adverse Reactions

Subcutaneously, melanotan-II can cause gastrointestinal cramping (5685), nausea (5685,5687,5688), decreased appetite (5687), facial flushing (5685,5688), fatigue, somnolence (5685), yawning, stretching, and spontaneous penile erections (5685,5687,5688). It can also cause increased pigmentation of the face, upper body, and buttocks (5685).

Interactions with Herbs & Other Dietary Supplements

None known.

Interactions with Drugs

None known.

Interactions with Foods

None known.

Interactions with Lab Tests

None known.

Interactions with Diseases or Conditions

None known.

Dosage and Administration

SUBCUTANEOUS: The typical dosage is 0.025 mg/kg (5685,5687,5688).

Comments

Commercial dosage forms of melanotan-II such as a nasal spray or as an eyedrop are being investigated (5684,5687).

MELATONIN

Also Known As

MEL, MLT, Pineal Hormone.
CAUTION: See separate listing for Melanotan-II.

Scientific Names

N-acetyl-5-methoxytryptamine.

People Use This For

Orally, melatonin is used for jet lag, insomnia, shift-work disorder, circadian rhythm disorders in the blind, and benzodiazepine and nicotine withdrawal. Melatonin is also used orally for Alzheimer's disease, tinnitus, depression, delayed sleep phase syndrome (DSPS), chronic fatigue syndrome (CFS), fibromyalgia, migraine and cluster headaches, idiopathic stabbing headache, and insomnia associated with attention deficit-hyperactivity disorder (ADHD). Other uses include hypertension, hyperpigmentation, osteoporosis, breast cancer, brain cancer, lung cancer, prostate cancer, head cancer, neck cancer, and gastrointestinal cancer. It is also used for thrombocytopenia, cachexia, neuropathy, and asthenia associated with cancer chemotherapy. Melatonin is also used orally for epilepsy, as an antiaging agent, for menopause, as preanesthetic medication, and for birth control.
Transbuccal and sublingual forms of melatonin are also used for insomnia, shift-work disorder, and as preanesthetic medication.
Topically, melatonin is used as a skin protectant against ultraviolet (UV) light and sunburn.
Intramuscularly, melatonin is used for treating cancer.

Safety

LIKELY SAFE ...when used orally or parenterally and appropriately, short-term. Melatonin seems to be safe when used for up to two months (1049,1068,1077,1085,1738,1754,5854,5855,5857). ...when used topically and appropriately (1066,1768,1769,4713,4714).
POSSIBLY SAFE ...when used orally and appropriately, long-term. There is some evidence melatonin can be used safely for up to nine months in some patients (7040,7043).
CHILDREN: POSSIBLY UNSAFE ...when used orally or parenterally. Melatonin supplementation might adversely

affect children. Young people up to the age of 20 years produce melatonin endogenously in high levels (1740). Melatonin levels are inversely related to gonadal development (1739,1742,1743). Theoretically, exogenously administered melatonin might adversely affect gonadal development; use with caution.

PREGNANCY: POSSIBLY UNSAFE ...when used orally or parenterally. High doses might inhibit ovulation, causing a contraceptive effect (1740,6002,8271). It is not known if lower doses cause this effect. Until more is known about the safety of melatonin, advise pregnant patients and patients wishing to become pregnant to avoid using melatonin at any dose.

LACTATION: Insufficient reliable information available; avoid using.

Effectiveness

LIKELY EFFECTIVE

Circadian rhythm sleep disorders. Taking melatonin orally helps improve circadian rhythm sleep disorders in blind children and adults. Melatonin has FDA orphan drug status for this indication (1082,1691,1744,1749,6585).

Sleep-wake cycle disturbances. Taking melatonin orally is helpful for sleep-wake cycle disturbances in children and adolescents with mental retardation, autism, and other central nervous system disorders (1056,1745,1746,1747,1771). Melatonin also appears to improve the time to fall asleep in children with developmental disabilities, including cerebral palsy, autism, and mental retardation (9707). Melatonin treatment seems to subjectively improve secondary insomnia associated with various sleep-wake cycle disturbances (1053,1729,8240,8245).

POSSIBLY EFFECTIVE

Benzodiazepine withdrawal. Taking melatonin orally seems to be beneficial for facilitating benzodiazepine withdrawal in elderly people with insomnia. This benefit has only been demonstrated with a controlled-release formulation of melatonin (349,1751).

Cluster headache. Taking melatonin orally 10 mg every evening might reduce the frequency of episodic cluster headaches (1127). However, 2 mg at bedtime doesn't seem to be effective (9702).

Delayed sleep phase syndrome (DSPS). Taking melatonin orally seems to improve insomnia and other quality of life factors such as mental health, vitality, and bodily pain in young adults with DSPS (8244).

Insomnia. Melatonin supplementation seems to be most beneficial for elderly patients with insomnia related to melatonin deficiency (1072,1729,1738,1754,7081). Melatonin might also improve subjective quality of sleep in non-elderly patients, but probably will not improve objective measures such as the time it takes to fall asleep (sleep latency) or total sleep time (1068,1070,1083). In children with insomnia due to delayed onset of sleep, melatonin seems to shorten the time that it takes to fall asleep and increase the duration of sleep (9708). Melatonin also seems to improve secondary insomnia related to depression (1053,1729), schizophrenia (8245), Alzheimer's disease (1729), hospitalization (9709), and insomnia termed "ICU syndrome" referring to sleep disturbances while in the intensive care unit (8240). Sustained-release melatonin preparations seem to be better for improving sleep maintenance (1738,1754), and immediate-release preparations seem to be more beneficial for decreasing sleep latency (1738).

Jet lag. Taking melatonin orally seems to reduce symptoms of jet lag, although some researchers have found no effect (6496). However, the majority of evidence shows that melatonin can modestly improve certain symptoms of jet lag such as alertness and psychomotor performance. Melatonin can also improve, to a lesser extent, other jet lag symptoms such as daytime sleepiness and fatigue. Doses between 0.5 mg and 5 mg appear to be equally effective, but higher doses produce a greater hypnotic effect. Travelers traveling eastward through five or more time zones may find 2 mg to 3 mg of melatonin useful when taken at local bedtime on the day of arrival and for 2-5 nights thereafter. Taking melatonin in advance of travel doesn't help prevent jet lag. The usefulness of melatonin for westward travel or over fewer time zones is less clear (1049,1077,1079,1085,1722,8273,9181,9750). Taking melatonin in advance of travel doesn't help prevent jet lag.

Nicotine withdrawal. A single oral dose of melatonin 0.3 mg 3.5 hours after nicotine withdrawal in smokers seems to reduce subjective symptoms of anxiety, restlessness, irritability, depression, and cigarette craving over the next 10 hours (2424).

Preoperative anxiety and sedation. Melatonin used sublingually seems to help reduce preoperative anxiety and improve sedation. Sublingual melatonin in doses of 0.05, 0.1, or 0.2 mg per kilogram appears to be as effective as comparable doses of midazolam as a preanesthetic agent (1125). In some cases, melatonin might be preferable to midazolam because melatonin doesn't seem to cause anterograde amnesia or impair cognitive and psychomotor skills (1125).

Prostate cancer. Taking melatonin orally, in combination with the luteinizing hormone-releasing hormone (LHRH) analogue triptorelin, might be beneficial for metastatic prostate cancer. There is evidence that 20 mg of oral melatonin used daily in combination with 37.5 mg of intramuscular triptorelin injected every 28 days can significantly decrease levels of prostate-specific antigen (PSA) and growth factors for prostate cancer, prolactin (PRL), and insulin-like growth factor-1 (IGF-1) (7255).

Solid tumors. There is some evidence that taking combined high-dose melatonin with conventional chemotherapy or with interleukin-2 (IL-2) might improve tumor regression rate in patients with breast cancer, lung cancer, kidney cancer, liver cancer, pancreatic cancer, stomach cancer, or colon cancer (1692,5854,5855,5857,7040,7043,8268). Melatonin plus chemotherapy in patients with metastatic solid tumors seems to increase regression rate and one-year survival rate by approximately 50% compared to chemotherapy alone (7040). The addition of melatonin also seems to help reduce chemotherapy toxicities, including hematologic complications, cachexia, asthenia, and neuropathy (8268). There is also some preliminary evidence that melatonin alone, orally or intramuscularly, might improve stabilization rate and possibly one-year survival rate in patients with resistant or untreatable lung neoplasms, liver neoplasms, pancreas neoplasms, colon neoplasms, breast neoplasms, and brain neoplasms (1080,1688,1693,2566).

Sunburn. Applying melatonin topically seems to prevent erythema (sunburn) from ultraviolet (UV) light exposure. When applied prior to UV light exposure, melatonin seems to significantly decrease erythema (1066,1768,1769). In one study, topically applied vitamin E in combination with vitamin C and melatonin, provided modest photoprotective effect when used prior to UV exposure, but had no effect when used during or after UV exposure (4713,4714)

Tardive dyskinesia. Taking melatonin orally 10 mg daily seems to decrease symptoms by 24-30% in some patients with TD after six weeks of treatment (7082).

Thrombocytopenia. There is some evidence that taking melatonin orally can improve thrombocytopenia associated with cancer, cancer treatment, and other disorders. There is also some evidence melatonin can prevent thrombocytopenia induced by chemotherapy or interleukin-2 (IL-2) (1694,1695,1696,1697,2564,8268).

POSSIBLY INEFFECTIVE

Chronic fatigue syndrome (CFS). Taking melatonin orally 5 mg every evening doesn't seem to relieve CFS symptoms (9705).

Rotating shift work. Taking melatonin orally doesn't seem to improve sleep and adjustment to rotating shift work (1052,1054,1721).

LIKELY INEFFECTIVE

Depression. Although melatonin might help improve insomnia in some patients with depression, it does not seem to improve objective measures of depression (1053,1764,1766). There is also some concern that oral melatonin can worsen symptoms in some patients (1764). Some preliminary clinical research suggests melatonin may decrease winter depression symptoms in patients with seasonal affective disorder (SAD) (10670). Until more is known, tell patients with depression to avoid melatonin.

INSUFFICIENT RELIABLE EVIDENCE to RATE

Attention deficit-hyperactivity disorder (ADHD). Preliminary clinical research suggests melatonin might be useful for treating insomnia in children with ADHD (9980).

Beta-blocker-induced insomnia. Beta-blockers such as atenolol and propranolol seem to decrease endogenous melatonin levels. This might result in insomnia as a side effect. There is preliminary evidence that taking a melatonin supplement might decrease the insomnia caused by beta-blockers (1062,1780).

Fibromyalgia. Melatonin may decrease the severity of pain and the number of painful joints in people with fibromyalgia (9701).

Menopausal symptoms. Preliminary clinical research suggests that taking melatonin orally is ineffective for relieving menopausal symptoms. Melatonin in combination with soy isoflavones might help psychological symptoms associated with menopause (11806).

Migraine headache. There is preliminary evidence that patients with episodic migraine headache who take melatonin prophylactically, 3 mg every evening before bed, have significantly reduced migraine frequency, decreased migraine intensity, and decreased migraine duration (12149).

Seizures. There is some evidence that melatonin 3 mg at bedtime may reduce the frequency and duration of both nocturnal and daytime seizures in children with epilepsy (9699,9745,9746). It should be used cautiously, because melatonin may increase the frequency of seizures in some patients (8248,9744).

Stabbing headache. Case reports suggest that melatonin 3 to12 mg per day may prevent idiopathic stabbing headache (11806).

More evidence is needed to rate melatonin for these uses.

Mechanism of Action

Melatonin is a hormone synthesized endogenously in the pineal gland (1123), collected by the venous capillary system, then secreted into the cerebrospinal fluid and the venous systemic circulation (1123,8239). It is produced from tryptophan, which is converted to 5-hydroxytryptophan, then to serotonin, then to N-acetylserotonin, and finally to melatonin (1773). In the brain, melatonin appears to increase the binding of gamma-aminobenzoic acid (GABA) to its receptors, by affecting membrane characteristics, not by increasing the number of receptors. Melatonin may decrease neurotransmission by a direct effect on nerve cells (9695).

Melatonin's primary role seems to be regulation of the body's circadian rhythm, endocrine secretions, and sleep patterns (1773,7043). Melatonin production is influenced by day/night cycles. Light inhibits melatonin secretion and darkness stimulates secretion (1773). For example, people who suffer from an insufficient amount of environmental light often have decreased endogenous melatonin secretion (8247). Endogenous melatonin is involved in several other functions including growth hormone secretion and sexual maturation (1776,1777,1778,6497,8246), pain control, balance, and sexual activity (1776,1777,1778,6497). However, it does not appear to directly affect heart function or blood pressure (9714). Excretion of melatonin is similar in males and females (9747). Some research suggests that meditation techniques might increase endogenous melatonin concentrations (9748). Melatonin release peaks between one to three years of age. Nocturnal serum melatonin levels naturally decline with increasing pubertal stages (1781,8246,8263). Recent evidence also indicates that melatonin suppression by light is not affected by age (1775). However, there is good evidence that melatonin levels can be abnormally low in certain conditions or disease states. For example, infants with low melatonin production are more likely to experience a life-threatening event (ALTE) (8262). Insomniacs of all ages can also have decreased melatonin levels. Patients with sleep disorders related to other conditions, such as fibromyalgia and depression, can also have low levels (6498). Recent information also shows that music therapy can improve endogenous serum melatonin levels in patients with Alzheimer's disease, possibly a contributing factor to patients' relaxed and calm mood (8241). In other conditions, melatonin's response to light can be altered. For example, in patients with bipolar I disorder, melatonin response to light appears to be abnormal, but is not affected in less severe bipolar II disorder or unipolar depression (1123).

When exogenous melatonin is administered, it has a rapid, transient, and mild sleep-inducing effect. Orally administered melatonin has the ability to shift the circadian rhythm. Taking melatonin can delay the rhythm when given in the morning and advance the rhythm when administered in the evening (8274). It can lower alertness, body temperature, blood pressure, and performance for three to four hours after oral administration. However, there is not usually a "hangover" effect the following day (1068,1132,1753,1756,1757,1758,1759,1774,8272). People with jet lag and insomnia use melatonin primarily for its effects on circadian rhythm (8272,8274).

People use melatonin for cluster headache due to its effects on body temperature. Those with cluster headache seem to have a rise in body heat, and melatonin can lower core body temperature (1128,1129,1132). However, there is no clear relationship between pain perception and urinary concentrations of melatonin metabolites (9700).

Melatonin has been tried for idiopathic stabbing headache due to its structural similarity to indomethacin (Indocin), one of the few effective treatments for this condition. The mechanism of action for both melatonin and indomethacin for idiopathic stabbing headache is unknown (11806).

The production of melatonin is increased in patients with uncontrolled epilepsy. This observation may be explained in two, contradictory ways. The brain may be attempting to reduce epileptic nerve transmissions by increasing the concentration of melatonin (9696). In contrast, it may be that melatonin has proconvulsant activity. Concentrations of melatonin are increased at night and there is also an increased incidence of seizures during the night (9697). It is thought that melatonin might increase seizure activity by affecting the activity of dopamine in the brain (9744). However, many people with seizures have low endogenous melatonin levels, which increase after a seizure occurs. This suggests that melatonin levels increase to compensate for the increased nerve activity that occurs during a seizure (8249). In addition, some anticonvulsant medications increase concentrations of endogenous melatonin (9698), and exogenous melatonin may be used to treat some types of epilepsy (9699). Until more is known about the potential for melatonin to increase seizure activity, it should be avoided in people with seizure disorders (9744).

Melatonin is a potent antioxidant. It is thought to be 6-10 times more active than vitamin E as an antioxidant (7082). It may act as an oxygen free radical scavenger and by preventing several enzymatic reactions that generate reactive oxygen species (ROS). The antioxidant activity of melatonin may be useful in preventing oxidative injury in shock, inflammation, and reperfusion damage following coronary revascularization procedures (9712).

There is a lot of interest in using melatonin for patients with cancer. This area of research started due to the "Melatonin Hypothesis" which suggests that people with decreased pineal gland function are at an increased risk for developing cancer. Some researchers predicted that increased exposure to light would lower melatonin production and increase risk for some cancers (7042). Population studies have in fact found that blind patients and people living in arctic regions have relatively lower rates of breast cancer (7041,7042). There is also evidence that patients with advanced cancer have pineal gland hypofunction and low melatonin levels. Researchers now think supplemental melatonin might help prevent and treat certain cancers due to several pharmacological effects including antioxidant, immunomodulatory, and oncostatic effects. Cancer prevention may be the result of reduced cell proliferation, reduced cellular transformation, and DNA synthesis changes (8238). Melatonin seems to have very potent antioxidant effects. It might reduce chemotherapy toxicity by scavenging free radicals produced by treatment. Preliminary data suggest that melatonin may decrease oxidative renal damage caused by cisplatin (9749). Melatonin seems to also affect immune function by activating monocytes and increasing interleukin 2 (IL-2) activity. It appears to enhance IL-2-induced lymphocytosis (2568). Melatonin might improve survival in patients with cancer by preventing the immunosuppression caused by chemotherapy (7040). It may also help prevent thrombocytopenia associated with cancer chemotherapy by preventing chemotherapy-induced apoptosis of bone marrow cells, and acting synergistically with cytokines to stimulate platelet generation (2564). Other pineal hormones, such as 5-methoxytryptamine, may also contribute to the thrombopoietic effects of melatonin (2565). Melatonin also seems to have oncostatic effects. Melatonin slows growth of breast cancer cells in vitro and inhibits melanoma cell growth in vitro and in animal models (1064,5856,9751). Researchers think it has direct oncostatic effects, possibly by controlling oncogene expression and inducing cancer cell apoptosis (7040). Melatonin can also affect hormones that influence cancer cell growth. For example, it seems to reduce levels of insulin-like growth factor 1 (IGF-1) and prolactin (PRL), which have a role in breast cancer and prostate cell proliferation (1064,5854,5855,5857,7043,7255). In breast cancer cells, melatonin seems to reduce the number and activity of estrogen receptors (9711).

Melatonin has a variety of other effects. Melatonin is thought to be 6-10 times more effective than vitamin E as an antioxidant. Some researchers are interested in using melatonin for tardive dyskinesia (TD). Melatonin is theorized to work in TD due to a potential antioxidant effect on dopaminergic neurons. There is also some evidence that patients with TD have pineal gland calcification and low endogenous melatonin levels (7082).

Animal research suggests melatonin may reduce the volume of cerebral infarction when used within 2 hours of stroke onset (10671).

Melatonin seems to promote osteoblast differentiation and matrix mineralization in bone (3265). There is preliminary evidence that very high melatonin doses plus norethisterone can have additive or synergistic effects on inhibiting

ovarian function in women and possibly act as a contraceptive (769,1740).
There is also interest in using melatonin for menopausal symptoms. Melatonin seems to reverse or reduce menopause related changes in thyroid hormone, luteinizing hormone (LH), and follicle stimulating hormone (FSH) in menopausal women (2425). However, it does not significantly alter catecholamine levels or cardiovascular responses in postmenopausal women (9704).
In vitro evidence suggests that melatonin may inhibit the biochemical processes involved with the development of myeloid plaques found in the brains of patients with Alzheimer's disease. The clinical significance of these findings is not established (9710). There is some interest in melatonin for its antimicrobial effects. Preliminary evidence shows that melatonin alone or in combination with isoniazid (INH) is active against some Mycobacterium species (330).
Some people use melatonin for improving sexual performance. In animal models, melatonin has dose dependent effects on sexual function. Repeated high doses seem to decrease sexual behavior. However, a single low dose of melatonin does seem to increase sexual behavior (6497).
Exogenous melatonin undergoes extensive and rapid first-pass metabolism (1773,6498,8239). After a typical oral dosage, an average of 30-60 % of the melatonin is rapidly metabolized by this first pass effect (8239). It is first hydroxylated and then undergoes sulphate conjugation (1773,6498). There is also some evidence that cytochrome P450 1A2 and 2C19 catalyze melatonin hydroxylation (6498).
Orally, melatonin has an absolute bioavailability of 15% for doses of 2 and 4 mg (1126). Half-life is about 30-60 minutes in humans (1385,1772). Melatonin can be absorbed transdermally, but time to peak levels is delayed (1058).
The timing of melatonin administration is important for best therapeutic effect. For jet lag and insomnia, evening doses are best because melatonin has the ability to advance the circadian rhythm (7081,8269,8273,8274). For cancer, researchers theorize that evening doses are best because melatonin might have the greatest activity in the evening (1064). In otherwise healthy people, melatonin given at bedtime doesn't seem to affect nocturnal sleep. When given in the early evening (presumably in the absence of endogenous melatonin), it appears to be similar to temazepam (Restoril) in hypnotic effect (9706).

Adverse Reactions

Orally, melatonin can cause headache, transient depressive symptoms, daytime fatigue and drowsiness, mild tremor, mild anxiety, dizziness, abdominal cramps, irritability (169,1078,8272,8273,9701), reduced alertness (1078), confusion, nausea, vomiting (8273), and hypotension (8272). In perimenopausal women, melatonin may cause a resumption of spotting or menstrual flow (11806).
People should not drive or use machinery for 4 to 5 hours after taking melatonin (1772). Aircraft crew undergoing multiple time zone travel might experience further disruption in circadian rhythms (1722). Melatonin has exacerbated dysphoria in depressed patients (1764). Whether chronic administration of melatonin suppresses endogenous production of melatonin by the pineal gland is unknown (1772).
Not all melatonin products are safe. Some preparations of melatonin contain contaminants that are associated with eosinophilia-myalgia syndrome (9715,9716). Most commercial melatonin is synthesized in the laboratory. However, in rare cases it can be derived from animal pineal gland. Melatonin from animal sources should be avoided due to the possibility of contamination (1772,8266).

Interactions with Herbs & Other Dietary Supplements

HERBS/SUPPLEMENTS WITH SEDATIVE PROPERTIES: Theoretically, concomitant use with herbs that have sedative properties might enhance therapeutic and adverse effects (1772). Some of these supplements include 5-HTP, calamus, California poppy, catnip, hops, Jamaican dogwood, kava, St. John's wort, scullcap, valerian, yerba mansa, and others.
HERBS WITH ANTICOAGULANT/ANTIPLATELET POTENTIAL: Theoretically, melatonin might increase the effect of herbs that have antiplatelet/anticoagulant constituents might theoretically increase the risk of bleeding in some people (9181). These herbs include angelica, clove, danshen, garlic, ginger, ginkgo, Panax ginseng, red clover, willow, and others.

Interactions with Drugs

ANTICOAGULANT/ANTIPLATELET DRUGS: There are isolated case reports of minor bleeding and decreased prothrombin activity in people taking melatonin with warfarin (Coumadin). The mechanism, if any, of this interaction is unknown. Theoretically, melatonin might increase the effect of anticoagulant or antiplatelet drugs (9181). Some drugs with anticoagulant or antiplatelet effects include aspirin, clopidogrel (Plavix), nonsteroidal anti-inflammatory drugs (NSAIDs) such as diclofenac (Voltaren, Cataflam, others), ibuprofen (Advil, Motrin, others), naproxen (Anaprox, Naprosyn, others), dalteparin (Fragmin), enoxaparin (Lovenox), heparin, and others.
ANTIDIABETES DRUGS: Melatonin might impair glucose utilization and increase insulin resistance (9713). Although the clinical significance is not known, melatonin may theoretically decrease the ability of hypoglycemic drugs to reduce blood glucose. Hypoglycemic drugs include insulin, glyburide (Micronase, DiaBeta), glipizide (Glucotrol), chlorpropamide (Diabinese), and tolbutamide (Orinase).
BENZODIAZEPINES: Theoretically, chronic benzodiazepine administration might decrease endogenous melatonin levels (8270).
CAFFEINE: Caffeine consumption can decrease endogenous melatonin levels. Theoretically, caffeine use may decrease the effectiveness of oral melatonin (8265).

CNS DEPRESSANTS: Theoretically, concomitant use of melatonin with alcohol, benzodiazepines, or other sedative drugs might cause additive sedation.
CONTRACEPTIVE DRUGS: Contraceptive drugs can increase the levels of endogenous melatonin. Theoretically, it may increase the effects and adverse effects of oral melatonin use (8265).
FLUMAZENIL (Romazicon): Preliminary evidence suggests that flumazenil may inhibit the effect of melatonin (9703).
FLUVOXAMINE (Luvox): Fluvoxamine can significantly increase melatonin levels. In some cases, fluvoxamine might increase bioavailability of exogenously administered melatonin by up to 20 times (5038,6499,8251). Some researchers think this might be a beneficial interaction and be potentially useful for cases of refractory insomnia (6499). However, this interaction might also cause unwanted excessive drowsiness and possibly other adverse effects. Fluvoxamine is known to increase endogenous melatonin secretion (6498). It seems to increase serum levels of exogenously administered melatonin possibly by decreasing melatonin metabolism by inhibiting cytochrome P450 (CYP450) 1A2 and 2C19 or by inhibiting melatonin elimination. This effect has been found in healthy people taking fluvoxamine 50-75 mg and melatonin 5 mg (5038,6498,6499,8251).
IMMUNOSUPPRESSANTS: Melatonin can stimulate immune function and might interfere with immunosuppressive therapy (7040); avoid using. Immunosuppressant drugs include azathioprine (Imuran), basiliximab (Simulect), cyclosporine (Neoral, Sandimmune), daclizumab (Zenapax), muromonab-CD3 (OKT3, Orthoclone OKT3), mycophenolate (CellCept), tacrolimus (FK506, Prograf), sirolimus (Rapamune), prednisone (Deltasone, Orasone), and other corticosteroids (glucocorticoids).
NIFEDIPINE GITS (Procardia XL): Melatonin can decrease the effectiveness of nifedipine GITS. Immediate-release melatonin 5 mg at night in combination with nifedipine GITS 30-60 mg daily increases systolic blood pressure an average of 6.5 mmHg and diastolic by an average of 4.9 mmHg. Concomitant use with melatonin also increases heart rate by 3.9 bpm (6436). The mechanism of this interaction is not known.
VERAPAMIL (Calan, Covera, Isoptin, Verelan): Concomitant use can increase melatonin excretion (1063).

Interactions with Foods

None known.

Interactions with Lab Tests

BLOOD PRESSURE: Melatonin can increase blood pressure in patients treated with antihypertensive medications. Immediate-release melatonin 5 mg at night in combination with nifedipine GITS (Procardia XL) increases systolic blood pressure an average of 6.5 mmHg and diastolic by an average of 4.9 mmHg (6436).
HEART RATE: Melatonin in combination with antihypertensive medications can increase heart rate. Immediate-release melatonin 5 mg at night in combination with nifedipine GITS (Procardia XL) increases heart rate by an average of 3.9 bpm (6436).
HUMAN GROWTH HORMONE: Melatonin supplementation can increase human growth hormone serum levels and test results (1076,1779).
LUTEINIZING HORMONE: Melatonin supplementation can decrease serum luteinizing hormone levels and test results (1741).
OXYTOCIN: Melatonin can produce dose-dependent changes in plasma oxytocin concentrations and test results. A 500 mcg melatonin dose increases oxytocin levels; a 5 mg melatonin dose reduces oxytocin levels (1779).
VASOPRESSIN: Melatonin can produce dose-dependent changes in plasma vasopressin concentrations and test results. A 500 mcg melatonin dose increases vasopressin levels; a 5 mg melatonin dose reduces vasopressin levels (1779).

Interactions with Diseases or Conditions

CANCER: Melatonin can decrease the incidence of cytokine (interleukin II and tumor necrosis factor) induced hypotension in cancer patients (1069).
DEPRESSION: Melatonin can worsen dysphoria in some people with depression (1764).
DIABETES: Melatonin may decrease glucose utilization and increase insulin resistance (9713). It may theoretically increase blood glucose concentrations in people with diabetes.
HYPERTENSION: Melatonin can worsen blood pressure in patients who are taking antihypertensive medications. Immediate-release melatonin 5 mg at night in combination with nifedipine GITS (Procardia XL) increases systolic blood pressure an average of 6.5 mmHg, diastolic blood pressure by an average of 4.9 mmHg, and. increases heart rate by 3.9 bpm (6436). The mechanism of this interaction is not known.
SEIZURE DISORDERS: Exogenous melatonin may increase the incidence of seizures (9744). Children with multiple neurological disorders, including seizure activity, might have an increase in seizure activity after treatment with oral melatonin for sleep disorders (8248); use with caution.

Dosage and Administration

ORAL: For insomnia, a typical dose of 0.3-5 mg at bedtime has been used (1072,1729,1738,1754,7081). In children with insomnia due to delayed sleep onset, melatonin 5 mg at 6:00 PM daily has been used (9708). Melatonin 5 mg at 8:00 PM daily has been used to treat insomnia in children with developmental disorders, including cerebral palsy, autism, and mental retardation (9707). Both immediate-release and sustained-release preparations have been used.

For jet lag, 0.5-5 mg at bedtime is commonly taken on the arrival day at the destination, continuing for 2-5 days. Low doses of 0.5-3 mg are often used to avoid the hypnotic properties of the higher 4-5 mg doses (1049,1077,1079,1085,1722,8269,8273).
For tardive dyskinesia, 10 mg daily of a controlled-release formulation has been used (7082). As adjunctive treatment for solid tumors, 10-50 mg in combination with radiotherapy, chemotherapy, or interleukin 2 (IL-2) has been used in clinical studies. Melatonin is typically started 7 days prior to start of chemotherapy and continued throughout full treatment course (1773,7040,7043,8268).
For treatment of metastatic prostate cancer resistant to triptorelin used alone, 20 mg taken daily has been used in combination with 3.75 mg of triptorelin injected intramuscularly every 28 days (7255).
For prevention and treatment of thrombocytopenia associated with cancer chemotherapy, a dose of 20 mg each evening has been used (2564).
For benzodiazepine withdrawal in elderly people with insomnia, 2 mg of controlled-release melatonin taken at bedtime for 6 weeks (the benzodiazepine dosage is reduced 50% during the second week, 75% during weeks 3 and 4, and stopped during weeks 5 and 6) and continued up to 6 months, has been used (349).
For treatment of winter depression, 0.125 mg twice daily has been used (10670).
For prevention of cluster headache, an evening dose of 10 mg has been used (1127).
For preventing migraine headaches, 3 mg every evening before bed has been used (12149).
For prevention of idiopathic stabbing headache, 3 to 12 mg at bedtime has been used (11806). As premedication for surgery in adults, 0.05 mg/kg sublingually has been used (1125,1768,1769). For reducing the symptoms of acute nicotine withdrawal, 0.3 mg orally 3.5 hours after stopping smoking has been used (2424).
TOPICAL: No typical dosage.

Comments

The controlled-released product, Circadin (not available in the US), is undergoing a multi-center Phase III clinical study in France for the indication of sleep. The manufacturer, Neurim Pharmaceutical Labs (Israel), has applied for approval of Circadin as a prescription drug in Canada and Europe.

MENTZELIA

Also Known As

Anguraté.

Scientific Names

Mentzelia cordifolia.
Family: Loasaceae.

Comments

At the date of publication, this product was not a common ingredient used in brand name supplements marketed to consumers. Details about this product are available at the online version of *Natural Medicines Comprehensive Database*. See www.naturaldatabase.com.

MERCURY HERB

Also Known As

None.

Scientific Names

Mercurialis annua.
Family: Euphorbiaceae.

People Use This For

Orally, mercury herb is used for inflammation with pus, as a laxative, a diuretic, and as an adjuvant treatment for gastrointestinal and urinary tract disease.

Safety

LIKELY UNSAFE ...when the fresh plant, particularly the root and rhizome are used orally (18). Small amounts might cause symptoms no worse than diarrhea.
PREGNANCY AND LACTATION: LIKELY UNSAFE ...when used orally (18); avoid using.

Effectiveness
There is insufficient reliable information available about the effectiveness of mercury herb.

Mechanism of Action
Mercury herb contains saponins, a small amount of cyanogenic glycosides, pyridone derivatives including hermidin, amines including methylamine, and flavonoids including rutin, narcissin, and isorhamnetin (18). The root and stock of mercury herb act as strong laxatives (18). There is no information regarding the toxic compound in the plant (18). The insignificant amount of cyanogenic glycosides cannot account for the plant's toxicity (18).

Adverse Reactions
Orally, ingestion might cause diarrhea and overactive bladder (18). Symptoms of poisoning might include nerve paralysis, liver and kidney failure, as well as death (18). The pollen has shown to be allergenic (4143,4144), and may be responsible for rhinitis and asthmatic symptoms (4143). Mercury herb might also cause allergic reactions in individuals allergic to Olea europaea, Fraxinus elatior, Ricinus communis, Salsola kali, Parietaria judaica, and Artemisia vulgaris (4143).

Interactions with Herbs & Other Dietary Supplements
CROSS-ALLERGENICITY: Individuals allergic to mercury herb might also be allergic to Mercurialis annua and Olea europaea, Fraxinus elatior, Ricinus communis, Salsola kali, Parietaria judaica, and Artemisia vulgaris (4143).

Interactions with Drugs
None known.

Interactions with Foods
None known.

Interactions with Lab Tests
None known.

Interactions with Diseases or Conditions
None known.

Dosage and Administration
ORAL: Mercury herb is typically administered as an extract or in juice (18).

MESOGLYCAN

Also Known As
Aortic Glycosaminoglycans, Aortic GAGs, Glycosaminoglycans, Heparinoid Fraction, Heparinoids, Mucopolysaccharide, Sulfomucopolysaccharide.
CAUTION: See separate listing for Chondroitin Sulfate.

Scientific Names
None.

People Use This For
Orally, mesoglycan is used for treating atherosclerosis, varicose veins, hemorrhoids, phlebitis, thrombophlebitis, lower limb ischemia, deep vein thrombosis, hyperlipidemia, peripheral obliterative arterial disease, venous insufficiency, venous stasis ulcers, cerebrovascular disease, and stroke.
Topically, mesoglycan is used for treating leg ulcers.
Intramuscularly, mesoglycan is used for treating venous insufficiency, venous stasis ulcers, cerebrovascular disease, stroke, and cutaneous necrotizing venulitis.
Intravenously, mesoglycan is used for treating lower limb ischemia.

Safety
POSSIBLY SAFE ...when used orally or parenterally and appropriately (6630,6635,6637,6638,6639,6644,6645). Since these products are derived from animals there are concerns about contamination with diseased animal parts (1825). However, there are no reports of disease transmission to humans due to use of contaminated mesoglycan.
There is insufficient information available about the safety of mesoglycan when used topically or intravenously.
PREGNANCY AND LACTATION: Insufficient reliable information available; avoid using.

Effectiveness

POSSIBLY EFFECTIVE

Cerebrovascular disease. Taking mesoglycan orally seems to reduce ischemic events, improved quality of life, and provide subjective improvement when used over a 6 month period in patients with cerebrovascular disease (6635,6637,6639). There is some evidence that mesoglycan might be comparable to standard antiplatelet drug therapy (6639).

Hypertriglyceridemia. There is some evidence that taking mesoglycan orally seems to reduce total and VLDL triglycerides in patients with hypertriglyceridemia (6646).

Peripheral arterial disease. Alternating intravenous and oral mesoglycan seems to improve walking distance in patients with intermittent claudication due to peripheral arterial disease (6629).

Venous insufficiency. There is some evidence from uncontrolled trials that administering mesoglycan orally or parenterally may improve the subjective and objective symptoms associated with various venous conditions including varicose syndromes, post-phlebitic syndromes, and thrombophlebitis when used over a 1-3 month period (6630,6638,6644,6645). Applying mesoglycan topically also seems to be helpful for treating leg ulcers in patients with chronic venous insufficiency (6627).

Venous stasis ulcers. Administering a combination of intramuscular and oral mesoglycan as an adjunct to traditional chronic venous stasis ulcer therapy seems to improve the rate of healing compared to traditional therapy alone (11479).

POSSIBLY INEFFECTIVE

Deep vein thrombosis (DVT). Oral mesoglycan plus compression stockings appears to be no better than placebo, following standard DVT therapy, for preventing recurrent DVT and/or pulmonary embolism during a follow-up period ranging from 5 to 48 months (6640).

Stroke. There seems to be no difference in outcome in patients treated for acute ischemic stroke with intravenous dexamethasone alone, or in combination with intramuscular mesoglycan for 5 days followed by 25 days of oral mesoglycan (6641).

INSUFFICIENT RELIABLE EVIDENCE to RATE

Atherosclerosis. There is some early evidence that mesoglycan might slow the progression of atherosclerosis by decreasing the rate of carotid and femoral artery intima-media thickening (6628).

Cutaneous necrotizing venulitis. There is some preliminary evidence that intramuscular mesoglycan might be useful for treating cutaneous necrotizing venulitis in patients with reduced fibrinolytic activity (6634).

More evidence is needed to rate mesoglycan for these uses.

Mechanism of Action

Mesoglycan belongs to a broad class of compounds called glycosaminoglycans (GAG). GAGs, also called mucopolysaccharides, are amino hexose polysaccharides contained in mucoproteins, glycoproteins, and blood group substances. GAGs are a heparinoid (non-heparin) byproduct of heparin extraction from cow lung tissue or aorta, and pig intestinal mucosa (15). Mesoglycan specifically is composed of dermatan sulfate and heparan sulfate, with smaller concentrations of chondroitin sulfate, hyaluronic acid, and related hexosaminoglycans (6614). The concentrations of these substances can vary depending on the origin of the product. People try it for vascular conditions because it seems to have numerous pharmacological effects on the vascular system. Mesoglycan exhibits profibrinolytic activity without influencing hemaglutination in humans after oral administration (6631,6642). It seems to also decrease plasma fibrinogen concentrations without affecting prothrombin time, partial thromboplastin time, or antithrombin III (6633). Mesoglycan might restore normal fibrinolysis in patients with reduced cutaneous fibrinolytic activity (6634). However, mesoglycan has been shown to prolong activated partial thromboplastin time (aPTT) (6629). Mesoglycan seems to reduce pericapillary connective tissue edema, and capillary and venule dilation, in patients with primary venous insufficiency (6630). It also improves arterial wall elasticity, transcutaneous oxygen perfusion, and blood flow (6643,6644). Mesoglycan reduces total and VLDL triglyceride concentrations and increases lipoprotein lipase activity in patients with hypertriglyceridemia (6646). It reduces total cholesterol and triglyceride concentrations, and increases HDL cholesterol concentrations in patients recovering from cerebral ischemic episode (6633).

Adverse Reactions

Orally, nausea, vomiting, epigastric pain, heartburn, headache, diarrhea, and local cutaneous reactions have been reported (6629).

There is some concern about potential contamination. Mesoglycan is derived from raw animal tissues gathered from slaughterhouses, possibly from sick or diseased animals. Products made from contaminated or diseased organs might present a human health hazard. There is also concern that mesoglycan produced from cows in countries where bovine spongiform encephalitis (BSE) has been reported might be contaminated with diseased tissue. Countries where BSE has been reported include Great Britain, France, The Netherlands, Portugal, Luxembourg, Ireland, Switzerland, Oman, and Belgium (1825). However, there have been no reports of BSE transfer to humans from contaminated mesoglycan products. Until more is known, tell patients to avoid these products unless country of origin can be determined. Patients should avoid products that are produced in countries where BSE has been found.

Interactions with Herbs & Other Dietary Supplements

None known.

Interactions with Drugs

ANTICOAGULANT/ANTIPLATELET DRUGS: Theoretically, combined use might increase bleeding risk. However, human evidence suggests that mesoglycan has profibrinolytic activity without affecting coagulation (6631,6642). These agents include aspirin, clopidogrel (Plavix), dalteparin (Fragmin), enoxaparin (Lovenox), heparin, ticlopidine (Ticlid), warfarin (Coumadin), and others.
THROMBOLYTIC DRUGS: Theoretically, combined use might increase bleeding risk (6629). These drugs include alteplase (Activase), anistreplase (Eminase), reteplase (Retavase), streptokinase (Streptase), and urokinase (Abbokinase).

Interactions with Foods

None known.

Interactions with Lab Tests

ACTIVATED PARTIAL THROMBOPLASTIN TIME (aPTT): Intravenous mesoglycan prolongs activated partial thromboplastin time (6629).
CHOLESTEROL: Intramuscular mesoglycan reduces total cholesterol and increases HDL cholesterol concentrations and test results (6633).
FIBRINOGEN: Intramuscular mesoglycan decreases plasma fibrinogen concentrations and test results (6633).
TRIGLYCERIDES: Intramuscular mesoglycan decreases plasma triglyceride concentrations and test results (6633).

Interactions with Diseases or Conditions

COAGULATION DISORDERS: Mesoglycan might cause bleeding in people with coagulation disorders (6633).
HEPARINOID HYPERSENSITIVITY: Mesoglycan might cause allergic reactions in people hypersensitive to heparin or heparinoid derivatives (15).

Dosage and Administration

ORAL: A typical dose is 100 mg per day (6614). For cerebrovascular disease, 100-144 mg per day has been used (6635,6639,6641). For deep vein thrombosis (DVT), 72 mg per day has been used (6640). For hypertriglyceridemia, 96 mg per day has been used (6646). For venous insufficiency, 50 mg three times daily has been used (6638).
INTRAMUSCULAR: For cerebrovascular disease, 30 mg once or twice daily has been used (6635,6637,6639). For venous insufficiency, 30 mg per day has been used (6630,6638,6644,6645). For venous stasis ulcers, as an adjunct to traditional chronic venous ulcer therapy, 30 mg intramuscular mesoglycan per day has been used for three weeks followed by 100 mg oral mesoglycan per day for up to 21 weeks (11479).
TOPICAL: No typical dosage.

METHIONINE

Also Known As

DL-Methionine, DL Methionine, L-Methionine.

Scientific Names

L-2-amino-4-(methylthio)butyric acid.

People Use This For

Orally, methionine is used to prevent liver damage in acetaminophen poisoning and to test individuals for hyperhomocysteinemia. It is also used orally for lowering urinary pH, treating liver disorders, and improving wound healing. Methionine is also used orally for treating depression, alcoholism, allergies, asthma, copper toxicity, radiation side effects, schizophrenia, drug withdrawal, and Parkinson's disease.

Safety

POSSIBLY SAFE ...when used orally or intravenously, and appropriately (2410,2411,2413).
POSSIBLY UNSAFE ...when used orally or intravenously in excessive doses. Doses larger than 100 mg/kg should be avoided to prevent severe and potentially lethal cerebral effects (9339).
CHILDREN: POSSIBLY SAFE ...when used orally or intravenously, and appropriately. POSSIBLY UNSAFE ...when used intravenously in infants receiving parenteral nutrition. In infants, blood methionine concentration can increase due to lower enzyme activity and inability to metabolize methionine. High levels of methionine can cause liver toxicity (9338).
PREGNANCY AND LACTATION: Insufficient reliable information available; avoid using.

Effectiveness

POSSIBLY EFFECTIVE

Acetaminophen poisoning. Taking methionine orally or intravenously seems to be effective for treating acetaminophen poisoning (2413). Methionine 2.5 grams every 4 hours for 4 doses seems to be as effective as acetylcysteine in preventing liver damage and death after an acetaminophen overdose if methionine is given within 10 hours of acetaminophen ingestion (2413).

INSUFFICIENT RELIABLE EVIDENCE to RATE

Cobalamin deficiency. There is some evidence methionine administered preoperatively might prevent the adverse effects mimicking those of cobalamin deficiency due to prolonged exposure to nitrous oxide (2414).

Colorectal cancer. There is some evidence a high dietary intake of methionine and folate might have a synergistic effect in decreasing the risk of colon cancer, especially in individuals with a family history of colon cancer and those who consume large amounts of alcohol (9325,9326).

More evidence is needed to rate methionine for these uses.

Mechanism of Action

Methionine is a sulfur-containing essential amino acid found in animal protein (9,9343). Methionine plays a role in many cellular functions. It is used for protein synthesis, and methylation of DNA, RNA, and other molecules (9336,9342).

To be metabolized, methionine enters the methionine cycle and is transformed into S-adenosylmethionine (SAMe). After donating its methyl group, SAMe is hydrolyzed to homocysteine, and then either remethylated to methionine or transsulfurated, which leads to the formation of cysteine, taurine, and glutathione (9336,9338). As an antioxidant, glutathione prevents free radical injury to the liver and taurine plays a role in bile acid conjugation (9338).

Failure to maintain the homeostasis of the methionine cycle is thought to result in liver injury. Patients with alcohol-induced liver disease often exhibit hypermethioninemia, which is thought to be caused by decreased metabolism of methionine to SAMe. With low levels of glutathione, the liver is at an increased risk of damage from free radicals (9336,9338).

Toxic levels of methionine can be corrected with glycine. Glycine seems to enhance the degradation of methionine through transsulfuration by acting as a receptor for methyl groups. Excessive methionine competes for glycine and limits the availability of glycine for other metabolic interactions, such as the synthesis of glutathione (2415).

In acetaminophen poisoning, methionine seems to prevent liver damage and necrosis by promoting glutathione synthesis. The toxic metabolite of acetaminophen (N-acetyl-p-benzquinoneimine) will then bind to glutathione instead of liver cells (9340).

Dietary methionine usually has no effect on homocysteine levels. Levels can increase and possibly cause hyperhomocysteinemia if enzymes used for the metabolism of homocysteine are defective and/or there is a deficiency in folate, vitamin B12, or vitamin B6 (9343). Hyperhomocysteinemia might cause endothelial damage and increase the risk for vascular disease (2410,2411). Hyperhomocysteinemia that is unresponsive to vitamin supplementation sometimes responds to dietary restriction of methionine (9345).

Methionine might play a role in preventing adverse effects caused by prolonged nitrous oxide exposure. Nitrous oxide toxicity resembles cobalamin deficiency. Preliminary evidence suggests nitrous oxide can selectively impair the function of cobalamin-dependent methionine synthase. Administering methionine preoperatively might prevent the inactivation of methionine synthase and prevent cobalamin inactivation in patients undergoing nitrous oxide anesthesia (2414).

Many amino acids are known to stimulate growth hormone. There is preliminary evidence that methionine also potentiates the secretion of basal growth hormone and growth hormone induced by growth hormone releasing hormone (GHRH) (2412).

Methionine might act synergistically with folate to decrease the risk of colon cancer (9325,9326). However, there is also evidence a high dietary intake of methionine with salt and nitrates might increase the risk of gastric cancer (2409). Rates of methylation are much higher in tumor than in normal tissue (9342). Most tumors are dependent on exogenous, preformed methionine for growth (9341). Preliminary clinical evidence suggests restriction of dietary methionine in cancer patients might inhibit tumor growth and improve cancer treatment outcomes (9341,9342).

Adverse Reactions

Orally or intravenously, methionine can cause nausea, vomiting, dizziness, drowsiness, hypotension, and irritability (9339,9340). Methionine may aggravate existing liver damage and should be used with caution in patients with severe liver disease (9336,9338,9340). A single dose of 8 grams methionine can cause hepatic encephalopathy to occur in patients with cirrhosis (9340). Methionine may cause decreased serum folate levels, leucocytosis, and increased urinary calcium excretion at dosages of 8 to13.9 g/day for 4 to 5 days (9340). Methionine can cause changes in the serum pH and should not be used in patients with acidosis (9340). Cerebral effects such as cerebral edema can occur when plasma methionine levels rise above 3000 umol/L (9339). In schizophrenic patients, large doses of methionine (e.g., 20 g/day for 5 days) can cause confusion, disorientation, delirium, agitation, listlessness, and other similar symptoms (9339,9340).

Long-term use of methionine-containing parenteral nutrition solution has been linked to liver toxicity in infants (9338).

Interactions with Herbs & Other Dietary Supplements
None known.

Interactions with Drugs
None known.

Interactions with Foods
SALT and NITRITE: Some evidence suggests that a diet rich in methionine, salt, and nitrite might increase the risk of gastric cancer (2409).

Interactions with Lab Tests
BLOOD pH: Methionine can lower serum pH by increasing sulfuric acid formation (9344).
HOMOCYSTEINE: Methionine might increase plasma homocysteine levels and test results (2410,2411). Patients who are deficient in folate, vitamin B12, or vitamin B6; or patients who have disorders of homocysteine metabolism are particularly sensitive to methionine (2410,9343).

Interactions with Diseases or Conditions
ACIDOSIS: Methionine can cause changes in the serum pH and should not be used in patients with acidosis (9340). Metabolism of methionine can result in the formation of sulfuric acid (9344).
ATHEROSCLEROSIS: Theoretically, methionine might promote or exacerbate atherosclerosis (2410). Dietary or supplemental methionine can increase homocysteine levels (2410,2411), especially in patients who are deficient in folate, vitamin B12, or B6, or patients who have disorders of homocysteine metabolism (9343). Hyperhomocysteinemia is associated with an increased risk for vascular disease (2410,2411).
CANCER: Most tumors are dependent on exogenous, preformed methionine for growth (9341). There is some evidence restriction of dietary methionine in cancer patients might inhibit tumor growth and improve cancer treatment outcomes (9341,9342).
LIVER DISEASE AND CIRRHOSIS: Methionine may aggravate existing damage in the liver in patients with liver disease (9).
METHYLENETETRAHYDROFOLATE REDUCTASE (MTHFR) DEFICIENCY: Patients with a genetic mutation, MTHFR C677T, which results in homocysteine metabolic deficiency, should avoid methionine supplements. Theoretically, methionine in patients with this genotype could increase the risk for the adverse vascular effects of hyperhomocysteinemia (11014,11709).
SCHIZOPHRENIA: Large doses of methionine (e.g., 20 g/day for 5 days) might cause confusion, disorientation, delirium, agitation, listlessness, and other similar symptoms in patients with schizophrenia (9339,9340).

Dosage and Administration
ORAL: For acetaminophen poisoning, methionine 2.5 grams every 4 hours for 4 doses has been used to prevent liver damage and death (2413). For testing for hyperhomocysteinemia, an oral loading dose of 50-100 mg/kg is usually used (2410,2411).

Comments
Methionine is possibly unsafe, and should only be used by emergency room personnel for medical emergencies.

METHOXYLATED FLAVONES

Also Known As
Citrus Bioflavones, Citrus Bioflavonoids, Citrus Flavones, Citrus Flavonoids, Citrus Polymethoxylated Flavones, Flavonoids, Gardenin D, Heptamethoxyflavones, Hexamethoxyflavones, Methoxyflavones, Nobiletin, Pentamethoxyflavones, PMF, Polymethoxylated Flavones, Sinensetin, Tangeretin, Tetramethoxyflavones.
CAUTION: See separate listings for Chrysin, Diosmin, Hesperidin, Quercetin, and Rutin.

Scientific Names
5,6,7,8,4'-pentamethoxyflavone (Tangeretin); 5,6,7,3',4'-pentamethoxyflavone (Sinensetin); 5,6,7,8,3',4'-hexamethoxyflavone (nobiletin); 3,5,6,7,8,3',4'-heptamethoxyflavone (heptamethoxyflavone).

People Use This For
Orally, methoxylated flavones are used for venous insufficiency, varicose veins, cardiovascular disease, hyperlipidemia, and cancer.

Safety

LIKELY SAFE ...when consumed orally in amounts typically found in foods (12078).
There is insufficient reliable information available about the safety of methoxylated flavones when used in amounts greater than those in foods or when taken as a dietary supplement.
PREGNANCY AND LACTATION: LIKELY SAFE ...when consumed orally in amounts typically found in foods (12078). There is insufficient reliable information about the safety of methoxylated flavones when used in amounts greater than those found in foods during pregnancy or breast-feeding; avoid using.

Effectiveness

There is insufficient reliable information available about the effectiveness of methoxylated flavones.

Mechanism of Action

Methoxylated flavones are one group in the huge class of flavonoids. Flavonoids are plant pigments found in every vascular plant. These pigments give flowers and foods there yellow, orange, or red color (12078).
Methoxylated flavones occur in many foods. Citrus foods are a predominant source. Orange juice contains 2-7 ppm of the methoxylated flavones sinensetin, tangeretin, nobiletin, and heptamethoxylated flavone (12079).
Methoxylated flavones might be more stable than some other flavonoids. For example, quercetin is readily broken down through oxidative metabolism. Due to the methylation of phenolic groups of methoxylated flavones, they are thought to resist oxidative breakdown (12078).
Flavonoids, including the methoxylated flavones, are thought to be beneficial for cardiovascular disease. There is some evidence that methoxylated flavones can decrease platelet aggregation and erythrocyte sedimentation rate in animals and in vitro (12079,12080,12082,12083). There is also evidence that nobiletin can prevent experimentally induced thrombosis to a greater extent than heparin (12081). The antiplatelet effects of the methoxylated flavones seem to be greater than the flavonoids quercetin, rutin or hesperidin. Within the methoxylated flavone group, tangeretin seems to have the least antiplatelet effect and sinensetin has the greatest effect. Nobiletin and heptamethoxyflavone fall in the middle (12079,12082). These effects on platelet adhesion could theoretically play a role in prevention cardiovascular disease.
Dietary consumption of methoxylated flavones might reduce lipid levels. In animal models of hyperlipidemia, a diet consisting of 1% tangeretin or 1% tangeretin plus nobiletin significantly reduces total cholesterol, low-density lipoprotein (LDL) cholesterol, and triglycerides. But a diet consisting of a smaller concentration of these methoxylated flavones, 0.25%, does not seem to significantly reduce cholesterol levels. It's thought that methoxylated flavones might alter lipid metabolism in the liver (12112).
Methoxylated flavones seem to have some effect on immune function. Tangeretin, a polymethoxylated flavonoid, seems to reduce expression of class II histocompatibility antigens in human blood monocytes. But neither tangeretin nor another polymethoxylated flavone, nobiletin, seem to decrease antigen-induced histamine release (12078).
Methoxylated flavones, like many other flavonoids, have antioxidant capabilities and seem to decrease lipid peroxidation (12078).
There is interest in flavonoids including methoxylated flavones for preventing cancer due to their antioxidant effects and other potential protective effects. Tangeretin seems to induce apoptosis of HL-60 cells. Nobiletin and tangeretin seem to induce liver metabolism and detoxification of some hydrocarbon carcinogens. They also inhibit growth of squamous cell carcinoma and gliosarcoma cells in culture. But these flavonoids don't seem to inhibit proliferation of normal cells, which suggests that they have a specific action against tumor cells (12078). Methoxylated flavones have also been shown to have in vitro activity against six human cancer cell lines including melanoma, prostate, colon, and lung cancer cells (12084).
Nobiletin has anti-inflammatory effects which are estimated to have a potency of about 68% of hydrocortisone (12081). Tetramethoxyflavones seem to have antiviral activity against the rhinovirus in vitro (12081).
Tangeretin is thought to be demethoxylated via cytochrome P450 (CYP450) metabolism. Tangeretin might also induce cytochrome P450 1A2 (CYP1A2), possibly by increasing gene transcription (12078).

Adverse Reactions

None reported.

Interactions with Herbs & Other Dietary Supplements

None known.

Interactions with Drugs

CYTOCHROME P450 1A2 (CYP1A2) SUBSTRATES: There is preliminary evidence that methoxylated flavones might induce CYP1A2 (12078). Theoretically, concurrent use of methoxylated flavones and drugs metabolized by these enzymes might result in increased drug elimination, decreased serum levels, and decreased effectiveness. Some drugs metabolized by CYP1A2 include clozapine (Clozaril), cyclobenzaprine (Flexeril), fluvoxamine (Luvox), haloperidol (Haldol), imipramine (Tofranil), mexiletine (Mexitil), olanzapine (Zyprexa), Pentazocine (Talwin), propranolol (Inderal), tacrine (Cognex), theophylline (Slo-bid, Theo-Dur, others), zileuton (Zyflo), Zolmitriptan (Zomig), and others.

Interactions with Foods
None known.

Interactions with Lab Tests
None known.

Interactions with Diseases or Conditions
None known.

Dosage and Administration
No typical dosage.

Comments
In 1936, it was proposed that flavonoids be recognized as vitamins. It was thought that they were necessary to prevent abnormal capillary permeability and capillary fragility. But there was not adequate evidence to establish flavonoids as vitamins (12079).
Flavonoids are plant pigments found in all vascular plants. They are responsible for many of the yellow, red, and orange colors in plants. Common food sources include red wine, stems, flowers, fruits, vegetables, nuts, seeds, herbs, spices, coffee, and teas. They are prominent components of citrus fruits (12078). Flavonoids are grouped based on slight differences in structure. These subdivisions include flavonols, anthocyanidins, flavones, flavanones, and chalcones (12078).
There have been over 4000 unique flavonoids identified from plant sources (12078).

MEXICAN SCAMMONY ROOT

Also Known As
Ipomoea, Orizaba Jalap.
CAUTION: See separate listings for Jalap, Pokeweed berry, and Pokeweed root.

Scientific Names
Ipomoea orizabensis, synonyms Convolvulus orizabensis, Convolvulus superbus, Ipomoea superba, Ipomoea tyrianthina.
Family: Convolvulaceae.

People Use This For
Orally, Mexican scammony root is used as a purgative.

Safety
There is insufficient reliable information available about the safety of Mexican scammony root.
PREGNANCY: LIKELY UNSAFE ...when used orally (18); avoid using.
LACTATION: There is insufficient reliable information available about the safety of Mexican scammony root during pregnancy; avoid using.

Effectiveness
There is insufficient reliable information available about the effectiveness of Mexican scammony root.

Mechanism of Action
Mexican scammony root exerts a potent stimulant laxative effect on the intestines. It contains 12-15% resinous polymeric ester glycosides (18).

Adverse Reactions
Orally, it can cause intestinal colic, and in large amounts, vomiting (18).

Interactions with Herbs & Other Dietary Supplements
CARDIAC GLYCOSIDE-CONTAINING HERBS: Overuse or abuse of Mexican scammony root may increase the risk of cardiac glycoside toxicity (19).
HORSETAIL/LICORICE: Theoretically, concomitant use of Mexican scammony root with horsetail plant or licorice rhizome increases the risk of potassium depletion (19).
STIMULANT LAXATIVE HERBS: Theoretically, concomitant use with other stimulant laxative herbs may increase the risk of potassium depletion (19).

Interactions with Drugs

DIGOXIN (Lanoxin): Theoretically, overuse or abuse of Mexican scammony root might increase the risk of adverse effects of cardiac glycoside drugs.
DIURETIC DRUGS: Overuse of Mexican scammony might compound diuretic-induced potassium loss (18). There is some concern that people taking Mexican scammony along with potassium depleting diuretics might have an increased risk for hypokalemia. Initiation of potassium supplementation or an increase in potassium supplement dose may be necessary for some patients. Some diuretics that can deplete potassium include chlorothiazide (Diuril), chlorthalidone (Thalitone), furosemide (Lasix), hydrochlorothiazide (HCTZ, HydroDIURIL, Microzide), and others.
ORAL DRUGS: Theoretically, Mexican scammony may reduce absorption of drugs due to reduced transit time (19).
STIMULANT LAXATIVES: Concomitant use of Mexican scammony and laxatives may lead to electrolyte and fluid depletion (19).

Interactions with Foods

None known.

Interactions with Lab Tests

None known.

Interactions with Diseases or Conditions

GI CONDITIONS: Contraindicated; may have GI irritant effects (19). Stimulant laxatives are contraindicated in individuals with symptoms of appendicitis (abdominal pain, nausea and vomiting) (272).

Dosage and Administration

ORAL: People typically take 3 to 12 grains (195 to 780 mg) of the powdered root. The powdered resin from the root is dosed 3 to 8 grains (195 to 520 mg) (5267).

Comments

Ipomoea orizabensis is no longer used as a purgative because of the adverse effect of vomiting.

MEZEREON

Also Known As

Camolea, Daphne, Dwarf Bay, Spurge Flax, Spurge Laurel, Spurge Olive, Wild Pepper.

Scientific Names

Daphne mezereum.
Family: Thymelaeaceae.

People Use This For

Orally, mezereon is used to relieve headaches and toothaches.
Topically, mezereon is used for joint pains and to increase circulation in rheumatic conditions.

Safety

POSSIBLY UNSAFE ...when used topically (18). Prolonged skin contact can lead to necrosis (18).
LIKELY UNSAFE ...when used orally. The plant is poisonous and can cause death (18).
PREGNANCY AND LACTATION: LIKELY UNSAFE ...when used orally or topically (18); avoid using.

Effectiveness

There is insufficient reliable information available about the effectiveness of mezereon.

Mechanism of Action

The applicable part of mezereon is the bark. Mezereon contains diterpenes including mezerein and daphnetoxin. It possesses powerful skin stimulating effects and can be hallucinogenic (18).

Adverse Reactions

Orally, mezereon can cause reddening and swelling of the oral mucous membranes, salivation, thirst, stomach pains, vomiting, and severe diarrhea (18). Symptoms can also include headache, dizziness, stupor, tachycardia, spasms, and death through circulatory collapse (18).
Topically, mezereon can cause red, painful swelling of the skin, blister formation, and shedding of the epidermis (18). Extended exposure can cause necrosis (18). Contact with the eyes can cause severe conjunctivitis (18).

Interactions with Herbs & Other Dietary Supplements
None known.

Interactions with Drugs
None known.

Interactions with Foods
None known.

Interactions with Lab Tests
None known.

Interactions with Diseases or Conditions
None known.

Dosage and Administration
TOPICAL: Mezereon was typically used as a 20% ointment (18).

Comments
Mezereon is a protected species (18). It is seldom used medicinally today (18).

MGN-3

Also Known As
Biobran, Hemicellulose Complex with Arabinoxylane.

Scientific Names
None.

People Use This For
Orally, MGN-3 is used for boosting immune function, preventing and treating cancer, treating AIDS, hepatitis, diabetes, chronic fatigue syndrome and other immunodeficiency disorders.

Safety
There is insufficient reliable information available about the safety of MGN-3.
Pregnancy and Lactation: Insufficient reliable information available; avoid using.

Effectiveness
There is insufficient reliable information available about the effectiveness of MGN-3.

Mechanism of Action
MGN-3 is a hemicellulose complex containing arabinoxylane as a major component. It is produced by hydrolyzing rice bran using enzymes from mycelia of Shiitake, Kawaratake, and Suehirotake mushrooms. Some studies suggest it might improve immunity by enhancing natural killer cell activity, increasing interferon-gamma production by peripheral blood mononuclear cells, and acting synergistically with interleukin-2 (aldesleukin) to increase natural killer cell activity and production of tumor necrosis factor alpha (3116,3117). Other evidence suggests that MGN-3 has activity against HIV (3113). Results from three small studies of healthy individuals and individuals with cancer suggest that MGN-3 also enhances natural killer cell activity (3118,3119,3120).

Adverse Reactions
None reported.

Interactions with Herbs & Other Dietary Supplements
None known.

Interactions with Drugs
None known.

Interactions with Foods
None known.

Interactions with Lab Tests
None known.

Interactions with Diseases or Conditions
None known.

Dosage and Administration
ORAL: A dose of 3 grams per day has been used in cancer patients (3119,3120).

Comments
The FDA is seeking a permanent injunction against the marketing of MGN-3 by Lane Labs. The complaint charges that MGN-3 is an unapproved drug product promoted as treatment for cancer and HIV infection (387).

MILK THISTLE

Also Known As
Blessed Milk Thistle, Cardui mariae fructus, Cardui Mariae Herba, Holy Thistle, Lady's Thistle, Legalon, Marian Thistle, Mariendistel, Mary Thistle, Milk Thistle Above Ground Parts, Milk Thistle Fruit, Milk Thistle Seed, Our Lady's Thistle, St. Mary Thistle, Silybin, Silybum, Silymarin.
CAUTION: See separate listing for Blessed Thistle.

Scientific Names
Silybum marianum, synonym Carduus marianus.
Family: Asteraceae/Compositae.

People Use This For
Orally, milk thistle is used as a liver protectant to lessen damage from potentially hepatotoxic drugs, and for treating liver disorders including toxic liver damage caused by chemicals, Amanita phalloides mushroom poisoning, jaundice, chronic inflammatory liver disease, hepatic cirrhosis, and chronic hepatitis. It is also used orally for loss of appetite, dyspeptic and gallbladder complaints, hangover, and diseases of the spleen. Milk thistle is used orally for prostate cancer, pleurisy, malaria, depression, uterine complaints, stimulating breast milk flow, and stimulating menstrual flow.
Intravenously, milk thistle is used as a supportive treatment for Amanita phalloides mushroom poisoning.
In foods, the milk thistle leaves and flowers are eaten as a vegetable and seeds are roasted for use as a coffee substitute.

Safety
POSSIBLY SAFE ...when used orally and appropriately. Milk thistle extracts standardized to contain 70-80% of the silymarin constituent seems to be safe when used for up to 41 months (2614,2616).
There is insufficient reliable information available about the safety of intravenous formulations of milk thistle and its constituents.
PREGNANCY AND LACTATION: Insufficient reliable information available; avoid using.

Effectiveness
INSUFFICIENT RELIABLE EVIDENCE to RATE

Alcohol-related liver disease. Preliminary clinical research suggests that milk thistle taken orally might be helpful for treating alcoholic liver disease (2613,2616,2618,7321,7322,7355).
Amanita mushroom poisoning. Administering silibinin, a constituent of milk thistle, intravenously (IV) may lessen liver damage due to Amanita phalloides mushroom (death cap) poisoning (2615). Silibinin is not readily available in the US.
Diabetes. Preliminary clinical evidence suggests that the milk thistle constituent silymarin can reduce insulin resistance in people with coexisting diabetes and alcoholic cirrhosis (2617).
Hepatitis B or Hepatitis C. Preliminary clinical research suggests a specific oral preparation of silibinin, an active constituent extracted from milk thistle, complexed with phosphatidylcholine (Silipide), may improve liver function tests (LFTs) in patients with chronic active hepatitis. Silibinin is complexed with phosphatidylcholine to theoretically improve the bioavailability of silibinin (7356).
Toxin-induced liver damage. Some research suggests milk thistle may limit liver damage after exposure to industrial toxicants such as toluene and xylene (2614).
Most clinical studies of milk thistle's effectiveness have used a specific extract standardized to 70-80% silymarin (Legalon). In the US, this formulation is found in the brand name product Thisilyn (Nature's Way).
More evidence is needed to rate milk thistle for these uses.

Mechanism of Action

The applicable parts of milk thistle are the seed and above ground parts. The seed is most commonly used medicinally. Silymarin, the active constituent of the milk thistle seed, consists of four flavonolignans called silibinin (silybin), isosilybinin, silichristin (silychristin), and silidianin. Silibinin makes up about 70% of silymarin (7318,8956). When ingested, silymarin undergoes enterohepatic recirculation and has higher concentrations in liver cells.
Silymarin is a potent inhibitor of tumor necrosis factor (TNF). The cytotoxicity, inflammation, and apoptosis induced by TNF are effectively blocked by silymarin. Although the mechanism of this effect is not clear, it probably involves intracellular signaling (7859). Silybin is an antioxidant, a free radical scavenger, and an inhibitor of lipid peroxidation (8957). In vitro silybin has shown an affinity for binding to p-glycoprotein, a transporter thought to be involved in the drug resistance of cancer cells (11481).
Several activities seem to contribute to the therapeutic effect of silymarin in liver disease. Silymarin seems to cause an alteration of the outer hepatocyte cell membrane that prevents toxin penetration. It also stimulates nucleolar polymerase A, resulting in increased ribosomal protein synthesis, which can stimulate liver regeneration and the formation of new hepatocytes. There is also some evidence that suggests that silymarin might have antifibriotic, anti-inflammatory, and immunomodulating effects that could also be beneficial in liver disease (6879). Silymarin and silybin inhibit beta-glucuronidase, which might help protect against hepatic injury and possibly colon cancer. Inhibition of beta-glucuronidase is thought to reduce the hydrolysis of glucuronides into toxic metabolites in the liver and intestine (7354).
Preliminary evidence indicates that milk thistle constituents might protect against kidney damage. In vitro, silibinin and silicristin can protect the kidney cells from nephrotoxic drugs such as acetaminophen, cisplatin, and vincristine. Silibinin and silicristin also appear to have a regenerative effect on kidney cells, similar to the effects on hepatic cells (7320).
There is some interest in using milk thistle for prostate cancer. In vitro research shows that silymarin and silibinin have antiproliferative effects on androgen-responsive prostate cancer cells (7319).
The above ground parts seem to have some estrogenic activity. A milk thistle plant extract appears to enhance estradiol binding to estrogen receptors, induce transcription activity in estrogen-responsive cells, and enhance estradiol-induced transcription activity in estrogen-responsive cells (6180). There is also preliminary evidence that suggests that milk thistle might affect drug metabolism. In vitro, silymarin and its flavonolignan, silibinin, inhibit cytochrome P450 2C9 (CYP2C9) and cytochrome P450 3A4 (CYP3A4), the major phase 1 hepatic enzyme. However, silymarin does not seem to affect the metabolism of indinavir (Crixivan), a CYP3A4 substrate, in healthy volunteers (10427). In vitro, silymarin and silibinin also inhibit uridine diphosphoglucuronosyl transferase (UGT), the major phase 2 enzyme that is responsible for glucuronidation (6450,7089,7318).

Adverse Reactions

Orally, milk thistle is usually well-tolerated (6879,8956). It can cause an occasional laxative effect (8956). Other less common gastrointestinal (GI) effects include nausea, diarrhea, dyspepsia, flatulence, abdominal bloating, fullness or pain, and anorexia (6879). There is one case of a woman who experienced intermittent episodes of sweating, nausea, abdominal pain, vomiting, diarrhea, weakness, and collapse, requiring hospitalization (3525).
Some patients may have allergic reactions to milk thistle including pruritus, rash, urticaria, eczema, and anaphylaxis (6879,8956). Allergic reactions may be more likely to occur in patients sensitive to the Asteraceae/Compositae family. Members of this family include ragweed, chrysanthemums, marigolds, daisies, and many other herbs.

Interactions with Herbs & Other Dietary Supplements

None known.

Interactions with Drugs

CYTOCHROME P450 2C9 (CYP2C9) SUBSTRATES: There's preliminary evidence that milk thistle might inhibit cytochrome P450 2C9 (CYP2C9) (7089,8234). So far, this interaction has not been reported in humans. However, watch for an increase in the levels of drugs metabolized by CYP2C9 in patients taking milk thistle. Some drugs metabolized by CYP2C9 include amitriptyline (Elavil), diazepam (Valium), verapamil (Calan), warfarin (Coumadin), zileuton (Zyflo), and others. Use milk thistle cautiously or avoid in patients taking these drugs.
CYTOCHROME P450 3A4 (CYP3A4) SUBSTRATES: There's preliminary evidence that milk thistle might inhibit cytochrome P450 3A4 (CYP3A4) enzyme (6450,7089,7318,8234). So far, this interaction has not been reported in humans. Milk thistle does not affect plasma concentrations of the CYP3A4 substrate indinavir in healthy volunteers, so interactions with drugs metabolized by CYP3A4 are not likely clinically significant (10427).
ESTROGENS: Theoretically, silymarin, an active constituent of milk thistle, might increase the clearance of estrogen by inhibiting beta-glucuronidase (6879).
GLUCURONIDATED DRUGS: Theoretically, silymarin, an active constituent of milk thistle, might increase the clearance of drugs that undergo glucuronidation. Some of these drugs include acetaminophen, atorvastatin (Lipitor), diazepam (Valium), digoxin, entacapone (Comtan), irinotecan (Camptosar), lamotrigine (Lamictal), lorazepam (Ativan), lovastatin (Mevacor), meprobamate, morphine, oxazepam (Serax), and others (7318,7354).
INDINAVIR (Crixivan): Milk thistle does not appear to affect the metabolism of indinavir in healthy volunteers (10427). Although preclinical research suggested milk thistle might inhibit CYP3A4 and potentially increase indinavir levels (7318), milk thistle does not appear to affect the pharmacokinetics of indinavir in humans.

Interactions with Foods
None known.

Interactions with Lab Tests
None known.

Interactions with Diseases or Conditions
CROSS-ALLERGENICITY: Milk thistle may cause an allergic reaction in individuals sensitive to the Asteraceae/Compositae family. Members of this family include ragweed, chrysanthemums, marigolds, daisies, and many other herbs.
HORMONE SENSITIVE CANCERS/CONDITIONS: Because milk thistle plant extract might have estrogenic effects (6180), women with hormone sensitive conditions should avoid milk thistle above ground parts. Some of these conditions include breast cancer, uterine cancer, ovarian cancer, endometriosis, and uterine fibroids. The more commonly used milk thistle seed extracts are not known to have estrogenic effects.

Dosage and Administration
ORAL: For hepatic cirrhosis, a milk thistle extract containing 70-80% silymarin (Legalon), 420 mg per day has been used (2616). For chronic active hepatitis, a milk thistle constituent, silibinin (Silibide), 240 mg twice daily as been used (7356). Some people make a milk thistle tea, but the active ingredients are not very soluble in water (515).
INTRAVENOUS: For Amanita phalloides mushroom poisoning, the common dose is 20-50 mg/kg over 24 hours, divided into four infusions, each administered over a two hour period. This is usually started within 48 hours after mushroom ingestion (2615). Intravenous silibinin is not available in the US.

Comments
The broken leaves of the milk thistle plant exude a milky sap. The leaves have distinctive white markings which, according to legend, were the Virgin Mary's milk (7161). Milk thistle is grown as a vegetable for salads and as a substitute for spinach. Avoid confusion with blessed thistle (Cnicus benedictus).

MONEYWORT

Also Known As
Creeping Jenny, Creeping Joan, Herb Two-Pence, Meadow Runagates, Running Jenny, Serpentaria, String Of Sovereigns, Twopenny Grass, Wandering Jenny, Wandering Tailor.

Scientific Names
Lysimachia nummularia.
Family: Primulaceae.

Comments
At the date of publication, this product was not a common ingredient used in brand name supplements marketed to consumers. Details about this product are available at the online version of *Natural Medicines Comprehensive Database*. See www.naturaldatabase.com.

MORINDA

Also Known As
Ba Ji Tian, Bois Douleur, Canarywood, Cheese Fruit, Hai Ba Ji, Hog Apple, Indian Mulberry, Luoling, Mengkudu, Menkoedoe, Mora De La India, Mulberry, Nhau, Noni, Nono, Nonu, Pau-Azeitona, Rotten Cheese Fruit, Ruibarbo Caribe, Tahitian Noni Juice, Ura, Wild Pine, Wu Ning.
CAUTION: See separate listing for Ba Ji Tian.

Scientific Names
Morinda citrifolia.
Family: Rubiaceae.

People Use This For
Orally, morinda is used for colic, convulsions, cough, diabetes, dysuria, stimulating menstrual flow, fever, hepatosis, constipation, leukorrhea, malarial fever, and nausea. It is also used for smallpox, splenomegaly, swelling, asthma, arthritis and other bone and joint problems, cancer, cataracts, colds, depression, digestive problems, and gastric ulcers. Other uses include high blood pressure, infections, kidney disorders, migraine, premenstrual syndrome,

stroke, pain, and sedation. The fruit juice is used for arthritis, diabetes, high blood pressure, muscle aches and pains, menstrual difficulties, headaches, heart disease, AIDS, cancers, gastric ulcers, sprains, depression, senility, poor digestion, atherosclerosis, circulation problems, and drug addiction. The leaves have been used in medicines for rheumatic aches and swelling of the joints, stomachache, dysentery, and swelling caused filariasis. The bark has been used in a preparation to aid childbirth.

Topically, morinda is used as an emollient and to reduce signs of aging. The leaves are used topically for arthritis by wrapping around the affected joint, for headache by applying to the forehead, and for direct application to burns, sores, wounds, and leprotic lesions. A mixture of leaves and fruit is applied to abscesses, and preparations of the root are used on stonefish and sting-ray wounds, and as a smallpox salve.

In foods, the fruits, leaves, roots, seeds, and bark are eaten.

Safety

POSSIBLY SAFE ...when used orally or topically and appropriately for medicinal purposes (11944). ...when the fruit is consumed as food (11944).

PREGNANCY: POSSIBLY UNSAFE ...when used orally. Historically, morinda has been used as an abortifacient (11964).

LACTATION: Insufficient reliable information available; avoid using.

Effectiveness

There is insufficient reliable information available about the effectiveness of morinda.

Mechanism of Action

The applicable parts of morinda are the fruits, leaves, flowers, stems, bark, and roots. Morinda contains potassium, vitamin C, anthraquinones, beta-sitosterol, carotene, vitamin A, flavone glycosides, linoleic acid, caproic acid (which may explain its foul odor), ursolic acid, rutin, and other constituents (11944). The fruit juice also contains a significant amount of potassium, approximately 56 mEq/L (1298).

Preliminary research suggests that constituents in the fruit and roots of morinda might have antibacterial, antiviral (including HIV), and antihelmintic effects. Other preliminary research suggests that morinda might have analgesic, hypotensive, and immunological activity (11944,11964).

The fruit juice contains a polysaccharide-rich substance which increases survival in mice with Lewis lung carcinoma, possibly by activating the host immune system (441). Damnacanthal, an anthraquinone isolated from the roots of morinda, may affect second messenger signaling and reverse mutagenicity of cancer cells (442,443). It also seems to promote capillary degeneration and death in experimental tumor tissue (11965). Other very preliminary research suggests that morinda may inhibit cancer cell proliferation (11964). In mice, lyophilized aqueous extracts of morinda roots have sedative and central analgesic effects, the latter blocked by naloxone (444). Animal research suggests morinda root extract might have antidepressant activity (11966).

A report has been published in a botanical journal about 2 constituents of morinda, xeronine and proxeronine, that are touted in advertising about morinda. However, these compounds have not been chemically identified or described in medical literature and are currently regarded as questionable (11964).

There is no reliable published clinical research on morinda.

Adverse Reactions

None reported.

Interactions with Herbs & Other Dietary Supplements

None known.

Interactions with Drugs

POTASSIUM-SPARING DIURETICS: Theoretically, concomitant use of morinda fruit juice and potassium sparing diuretics might increase the risk of hyperkalemia. Morinda fruit juice contains approximately 56 mEq/L of potassium (1298).

Interactions with Foods

None known.

Interactions with Lab Tests

URINE COLOR: The anthraquinone constituents can discolor urine from pink to rust and interfere with diagnostic tests, due to anthraquinone content (275).

Interactions with Diseases or Conditions

CHRONIC RENAL INSUFFICIENCY: Use of morinda fruit juice may increase the risk of hyperkalemia; use with caution. One reported case associates the use on morinda fruit juice with hyperkalemia in a patient with chronic renal insufficiency (1298). Morinda fruit juice contains approximately 56 mEq/L of potassium (1298).

HYPERKALEMIA: Caution, use of morinda fruit juice may contribute to elevated potassium levels; contraindicated. Morinda fruit juice contains approximately 56 mEq/L of potassium (1298).

Dosage and Administration

No typical dosage.

Comments

Morinda is a small evergreen tree in the Pacific Islands, Southeast Asia, Australia, and India that often grows among lava flows. Morinda's most common traditional use is topical. Morinda roots and bark have been used to make a red or yellow dye for clothing. The smell and taste of some Morinda citrifolia fruit and juice (noni juice) are unpleasant. The FDA has issued multiple warnings to morinda manufacturers about unsubstantiated claims (11944,11964).
The National Center for Complimentary and Alternative Medicine is sponsoring a Phase I study on the use of morinda freeze-dried noni fruit extract. Study results have not been published (11967).

MORMON TEA

Also Known As

Brigham Tea, Desert Tea, Gray Ephedra, Nevada Ephedra, Popotillo, Teamster's Tea, Squaw Tea.
CAUTION: See separate listing for Ephedra.

Scientific Names

Ephedra nevadensis.
Family: Ephedraceae.

People Use This For

Orally, Mormon tea is used for syphilis, gonorrhea, colds, kidney disorders, and as a "spring" tonic. It is also used as a beverage.

Safety

LIKELY SAFE ...when consumed in food amounts (12).
There is insufficient reliable information about the safety of Mormon tea for medicinal use.
PREGNANCY AND LACTATION: Insufficient reliable information available; avoid using in amounts greater than those commonly found in foods.

Effectiveness

There is insufficient reliable information available about the effectiveness of Mormon tea.

Mechanism of Action

Mormon tea contains large amounts of tannins (515). Tannin constituents exert an astringent effect on the mucosal tissue. This effect dehydrates the tissue, reducing internal secretions, and binding external cells into a protective layer (12). Plants with at least 10% tannins can cause gastrointestinal disturbances, kidney damage, and necrotic conditions of the liver (12). Some animal experiments show that tannins might cause cancer. Others show they might prevent it (12). Regular consumption of herbs with high tannin concentrations correlates to an increase in esophageal or nasal cancer (12). Despite being in the Ephedra genus, Mormon tea contains no ephedrine or other alkaloids (515). An aqueous extract demonstrates mild diuresis and constipation (515).

Adverse Reactions

None reported.

Interactions with Herbs & Other Dietary Supplements

TANNIN-CONTAINING HERBS: Theoretically, herbs that contain high percentages of tannins might cause precipitation of constituents of other herbs (19).

Interactions with Drugs

ORAL DRUGS: Theoretically, concomitant oral administration may cause precipitation of some drugs due to the high tannin content of Mormon tea (19). Separate administration of oral drugs and tannin-containing herbs by the longest period of time practical (19).

Interactions with Foods

None known.

Interactions with Lab Tests
None known.

Interactions with Diseases or Conditions
None known.

Dosage and Administration
ORAL: Mormon tea is typically prepared by steeping the dried branches in 150 mL boiling water for five to ten minutes and then straining (6002).

MOTHERWORT

Also Known As
Leonuri cardiacae herba, Leonurus, Lion's Ear, Lion's Tail, Roman Motherwort, Throw-Wort.

Scientific Names
Leonurus cardiaca.
Family: Lamiaceae/Labiatae.

People Use This For
Orally, motherwort is used for cardiac symptoms of neurosis, cardiac insufficiency, fast heart rate or other arrhythmias, amenorrhea, flatulence, and hyperthyroidism.
Topically, motherwort is used for itching and shingles. The seeds of Leonurus artemisia or Leonurus heterophyllus are used to improve eyesight and as a general tonic.

Safety
POSSIBLY SAFE ...when used orally and appropriately (12).
PREGNANCY: LIKELY UNSAFE ...when used orally because it might have uterine-stimulating effects (4,12,19).
LACTATION: Insufficient reliable information available; avoid using.

Effectiveness
There is insufficient reliable information available about the effectiveness of motherwort.

Mechanism of Action
The applicable parts of motherwort are the above ground parts. Motherwort has sedative (4,18), negative chronotropic, hypotonic (18), cardiac-inhibitory, and antispasmodic effects (4). Constituents include leonurine and stachydrine, which can stimulate uterine tone and blood flow (4,12,19). Ursolic acid can have antiviral, tumor-inhibiting, and cytotoxic activity (4). The intravenous administration of a Leonurus heterophyllus extract can decrease blood viscosity by decreasing platelet aggregation, decreasing fibrinogen, and increasing erythrocyte deformability (1533).

Adverse Reactions
Orally, use of motherwort in amounts greater than 3 grams can cause diarrhea, stomach irritation, and uterine bleeding (12). The leaves can cause contact dermatitis, and the oil can cause photosensitivity (4). Motherwort can also cause allergic reactions in sensitive individuals (4).

Interactions with Herbs & Other Dietary Supplements
CARDIAC GLYCOSIDE-CONTAINING HERBS: Contraindicated; concomitant use can increase the risk of cardiac glycoside toxicity (19). Cardiac glycoside-containing herbs include black hellebore, Canadian hemp roots, digitalis leaf, hedge mustard, figwort, lily of the valley roots, oleander leaf, pheasant's eye plant, pleurisy root, squill bulb leaf scales, strophanthus seeds, and uzara.

Interactions with Drugs
CNS DEPRESSANTS: Concomitant use of motherwort can potentiate the sedative and tranquilizing effects of these drugs, including the sedative effects of antihistamines (19).

Interactions with Foods
None known.

Interactions with Lab Tests
THYROID FUNCTION: Motherwort might improve thyroid function and thyroid function test results in patients with thyroid hyperfunction (2).

Interactions with Diseases or Conditions

CARDIAC DISORDERS: Excessive use of motherwort can interfere with the treatment of cardiac disorders (4).
UTERINE BLEEDING CONDITIONS: Theoretically, it can exacerbate uterine bleeding due to its possible stimulation of uterine blood flow (4,12,19).

Dosage and Administration

ORAL: The typical dose of motherwort is 2 grams of the dried above ground parts or 1 cup of the tea 3 times per day (4). To prepare tea steep 2 grams of the dried above ground parts in 150 mL boiling water for 5-10 minutes, then strain. The average amount used is 4.5 grams per day (2).

MOUNTAIN ASH

Also Known As

Eberesche, Ebereschenbeeren, European Mountain-Ash, Quickbeam, Rowan Tree, Sorb Apple, Sorbi acupariae fructus, Witchen.

Scientific Names

Sorbus aucuparia, synonym Pyrus aucuparia.
Family: Rosaceae.

People Use This For

Orally, mountain ash is used for kidney diseases, diabetes, arthritis, disorders of uric acid metabolism, dissolution of uric acid deposits, mucous membrane inflammation, internal inflammations, vitamin C deficiency, alkalizing the blood, increasing metabolism, purifying the blood, and for menstrual complaints. It is also used orally for diarrhea and lung conditions, especially those associated with fever.
In manufacturing, mountain ash is used as an ingredient in marmalade, stewed fruit, juice, liqueur, vinegar, and in tea mixtures.

Safety

POSSIBLY UNSAFE ...when large amounts of fresh berries are ingested. The constituent, parasorbic acid is an irritant and large amounts can cause gastric irritation and kidney damage (18).
There is insufficient reliable information available about the safety of the oral use of dried or cooked berries.
PREGNANCY AND LACTATION: POSSIBLY UNSAFE ...when large amounts of fresh berries are ingested (18).
There is insufficient reliable information available about the safety of dried or cooked berries; avoid using.

Effectiveness

There is insufficient reliable information available about the effectiveness of mountain ash.

Mechanism of Action

The applicable part of mountain ash is the berry used fresh, dried, or cooked then dried. Mountain ash berry contains parasorbic acid, cyanogenic glycosides, fruit acids (malic acid, tartaric acid), tannins, and vitamin C (18). The parasorbic acid that is contained in the fresh berry can cause local irritation. However, the compound is partially degraded by drying and completely destroyed by cooking (2).

Adverse Reactions

Orally, large amounts of fresh berries may cause gastroenteritis, vomiting, queasiness, gastric pain, diarrhea, kidney damage (albuminuria, glycosuria), and polymorphic xanthomas due to parasorbic acid (18).

Interactions with Herbs & Other Dietary Supplements

None known.

Interactions with Drugs

None known.

Interactions with Foods

None known.

Interactions with Lab Tests

None known.

Interactions with Diseases or Conditions
None known.

Dosage and Administration
No typical dosage.

MOUNTAIN FLAX

Also Known As
Dwarf Flax, Fairy Flax, Mill Mountain, Purging Flax.

Scientific Names
Linum catharticum.
Family: Linaceae.

People Use This For
Orally, mountain flax is used as an emetic and purgative to cause bowel elimination.

Safety
POSSIBLY UNSAFE ...when used orally, particularly with long-term use (18).
PREGNANCY AND LACTATION: UNSAFE ...when used orally due to possible emetic effects (18).

Effectiveness
There is insufficient reliable information available about the effectiveness of mountain flax.

Mechanism of Action
The applicable parts of mountain flax are the above ground flowering parts. Mountain flax is thought to have laxative effects at 0.5 grams. It contains the lignan achromatin, tannins and a volatile oil (18).

Adverse Reactions
Orally, mountain flax can cause vomiting, gastrointestinal tract inflammation and diarrhea (18).

Interactions with Herbs & Other Dietary Supplements
None known.

Interactions with Drugs
None known.

Interactions with Foods
None known.

Interactions with Lab Tests
None known.

Interactions with Diseases or Conditions
None known.

Dosage and Administration
No typical dosage.

MOUNTAIN LAUREL

Also Known As
Broad-Leafed Laurel, Calico Bush, Lambkill, Laurel, Mountain Ivy, Rose Laurel, Sheep Laurel, Spoon Laurel.

Scientific Names
Kalmia latifolia.
Family: Ericaceae.

People Use This For

Topically, mountain laurel is used for tinea capitis, psoriasis, herpes, and secondary syphilis.

Safety

UNSAFE ...when used orally. Mountain laurel leaf is not only an irritant, but can also lead to cardiac arrest, respiratory failure and death (18).
There is insufficient reliable information available about safety of the topical use of mountain laurel.
PREGNANCY AND LACTATION: UNSAFE ...when used orally (18). There is insufficient reliable information available about safety of mountain laurel for topical use; avoid using.

Effectiveness

There is insufficient reliable information available about the effectiveness of mountain laurel.

Mechanism of Action

The applicable part of mountain laurel is the fresh or dried leaf. Mountain laurel contains andromedan derivatives, flavonoids, and acylphloroglucinols (18). Andromedan derivatives act on the sodium channels, inhibiting conduction by preventing closure of the excitable cells (18). The andromedan derivative Grayanotoxin I and the acylphloroglucinol constituents can be cytotoxic (4145).

Adverse Reactions

Orally, mountain laurel can result in painful oral and gastric mucous membranes, increased salivation, cold sweat, nausea, vomiting, diarrhea, and paresthesias (18). Dizziness; headache; fever attacks; and intoxicated states with temporary loss of vision, muscle weakness, coordination disorders, and spasms can also develop. Bradycardia, cardiac arrhythmias, drop in blood pressure, eventual cardiac arrest, and respiratory failure can lead to death (18).

Interactions with Herbs & Other Dietary Supplements

None known.

Interactions with Drugs

None known.

Interactions with Foods

None known.

Interactions with Lab Tests

None known.

Interactions with Diseases or Conditions

None known.

Dosage and Administration

TOPICAL: Mountain laurel is only available in homeopathic preparations (18).

MOUSE EAR

Also Known As

None.
CAUTION: See separate listing for Cudweed.

Scientific Names

Hieracium pilosella, synonym Pilosella officinarum.
Family: Asteraceae/Compositae.

People Use This For

Orally, mouse ear is used for asthma, bronchitis, coughs and whooping cough. It is also used orally as a diuretic, to promote sweating, and to relieve flatulence and colic.
Topically, mouse ear is used for wounds.

Safety

There is insufficient reliable information available about the safety of mouse ear.
Pregnancy and Lactation: Insufficient reliable information available; avoid using.

Effectiveness
There is insufficient reliable information available about the effectiveness of mouse ear.

Mechanism of Action
The applicable parts of mouse ear are the above ground flowering plant parts. There is insufficient reliable information available about the possible mechanism of action and active ingredients.

Adverse Reactions
Mouse ear can cause an allergic reaction in individuals sensitive to the Asteraceae/Compositae family. Members of this family include ragweed, chrysanthemums, marigolds, daisies, and many other herbs.

Interactions with Herbs & Other Dietary Supplements
None known.

Interactions with Drugs
None known.

Interactions with Foods
None known.

Interactions with Lab Tests
None known.

Interactions with Diseases or Conditions
CROSS-ALLERGENICITY: Can cause an allergic reaction in individuals sensitive to the Asteraceae/Compositae family. Members of this family include ragweed, chrysanthemums, marigolds, daisies, and many other herbs.

Dosage and Administration
ORAL: Mouse ear is used as a liquid extract (18).
TOPICAL: It is used as a liquid extract (18).

MSM (METHYLSULFONYLMETHANE)

Also Known As
Crystalline DMSO, Dimethyl Sulfone, DMSO2, Methyl-Sulfonyl-Methane, Methyl Sulfone, MSM, Sulfonyl Sulfur.

Scientific Names
Methylsulfonylmethane; Dimethylsulfone.

People Use This For
Orally and topically, MSM is used for chronic pain, arthritis, joint inflammation, rheumatoid arthritis, osteoporosis, bursitis, tendinitis, tenosynovitis, musculoskeletal pain, muscle cramps, scleroderma, scar tissue, stretch marks, wrinkles, protection against sun/wind burn, eye inflammation, oral hygiene, periodontal disease, wounds, cuts, and abrasions/accelerated wound healing. Orally, MSM is also used for relief of allergies (allergic rhinitis, allergic sinusitis, allergy-induced asthma, inhalant allergens, environmental allergens), drug hypersensitivity, gastrointestinal upset, chronic constipation, gastric hyperacidity, ulcers, diverticulosis, premenstrual syndrome (PMS), mood elevation, obesity, poor circulation, hypertension, and elevated serum cholesterol. It is also used orally for diabetes mellitus type 2 (NIDDM), interstitial cystitis, hepatic dysfunction, Alzheimer's disease, snoring, lung dysfunction including emphysema and pneumonia, chronic fatigue syndrome, auto-immune disorders (systemic lupus erythematous), HIV infection and AIDS, and cancer (breast cancer and colon cancer). Other oral uses of MSM include eye inflammation, mucous membrane inflammation, myositis ossificans generalis, temporomandibular joint dysfunction, leg cramps, connective tissue disorders, migraine, headaches, hangover, parasitic infections of the intestinal and urogenital tracts including Trichomonas vaginalis and Giardia, Candida albicans and other yeast infections, insect bites, radiation poisoning, and as an immunostimulant.

Safety
POSSIBLY SAFE ...when used orally and appropriately short term. MSM 2600 mg per day has been used safely for up to 30 days (8574).
There is insufficient reliable information available about the safety of topical use of MSM.
PREGNANCY AND LACTATION: Insufficient reliable information available; avoid using.

Effectiveness

INSUFFICIENT RELIABLE EVIDENCE to RATE

Allergic rhinitis (hayfever). Preliminary clinical evidence suggests MSM given orally might relieve some symptoms of seasonal allergic rhinitis (8574). However, this study has been criticized for lack of information on pollen counts and severity of symptoms (12000). More evidence is needed to rate MSM for this use.

Mechanism of Action

MSM is a naturally occurring compound found in green plants such as field horsetail (Equisetum arvense), certain species of algae, fruits, vegetables, grains, and both bovine and human adrenal glands, milk, and urine (8574). It is an odorless metabolite of dimethyl sulfoxide (DMSO) (10625). MSM is a source of sulfur for cysteine and methionine. Incorporation of MSM-derived sulfur into methionine is regulated by a limiting step involving micro-organisms in the intestinal lumen (3501). MSM supplements cross the blood-brain barrier (12351).

Preliminary research suggests MSM might inhibit degenerative changes in arthritis (8576). MSM delays chemically-induced colon cancer tumor onset in animals (3502). A 4% MSM solution delays the latency period between induction and onset of chemically-induced mammary tumors or cancers in rats (3503). MSM does not affect expression of autoimmune diabetes in spontaneously diabetic mice (3504).

There is little reliable clinical research on the use of MSM in humans.

Adverse Reactions

Orally, MSM can cause nausea, diarrhea, and headache in some patients. It can also cause pruritus and increased allergy symptoms (8574).

Interactions with Herbs & Other Dietary Supplements

None known.

Interactions with Drugs

None known.

Interactions with Foods

None known.

Interactions with Lab Tests

None known.

Interactions with Diseases or Conditions

None known.

Dosage and Administration

ORAL: For allergic rhinitis, 2600 mg per day has been used (8574).

TOPICAL: No typical dosage.

Comments

MSM has been popularized by the book, The Miracle of MSM: The Natural Solution for Pain (8575). There is little published scientific research to support its use. Contrary to some MSM promotional literature, there is no Recommended Dietary Allowance (RDA) for sulfur or MSM. Sulfur deficiency has not been described in the medical literature. Directions for compounding MSM nose drops for snoring have been published, but there's no evidence that MSM has any effect on snoring (8577).

MUGWORT

Also Known As

Armoise Commune, Artemisia, Artemisiae vulgaris herba, Artemisiae vulgaris radix, Carline Thistle, Felon Herb, Gemeiner Beifuss, Hierba de San Juan, Nagadamni, Sailor's Tobacco, St. John's Plant, Wild Wormwood.

CAUTION: See separate listings for Tarragon, Wormseed, and Wormwood.

Scientific Names

Artemisia vulgaris.

Family: Asteraceae/Compositae.

People Use This For

Orally, mugwort above ground parts are used for gastrointestinal (GI) problems such as colic, diarrhea, constipation, cramps, weak digestion, worm infestations, and persistent vomiting. It is also used to stimulate gastric juice and bile secretion, as a laxative in cases of obesity, as a liver tonic; and for hysteria, epilepsy, convulsions in children, menstrual problems, irregular periods, to promote circulation, and as a sedative.
Orally, mugwort root is used as a tonic in individuals with diminished strength and energy.
In combination with other ingredients, mugwort root is used for psychoneuroses, neurasthenia, depression, hypochondria, autonomic neuroses, general irritability, restlessness, insomnia, and anxiety.

Safety

There is insufficient reliable information available about the safety of mugwort.
PREGNANCY: LIKELY UNSAFE ...when used orally. Mugwort is said to be an abortifacient and a menstrual and uterine stimulant (2,12).
LACTATION: Insufficient reliable information available; avoid using.

Effectiveness

There is insufficient reliable information available about the effectiveness of mugwort.

Mechanism of Action

The applicable parts of mugwort are the above ground parts and root. Mugwort contains sesquiterpene lactones, lipophilic flavonoids, polyenes, umbelliferone and aesculetin. It also contains a complex volatile oil with constituents of 1,8 cineole, camphor, linalool or thujone (18). Some evidence suggests mugwort can stimulate uterine activity (19), possibly due to the thujone content (19). Other evidence suggests the aqueous extract and the volatile oil have antimicrobial properties (18).

Adverse Reactions

Orally, mugwort may cause an allergic reaction in individuals sensitive to the Asteraceae/Compositae family. Members of this family include ragweed, chrysanthemums, marigolds, daisies, and many other herbs. Mugwort pollen may cause reactions in people who are allergic to tobacco (3716). Theoretically, mugwort might cause allergic reaction in people allergic to honey or royal jelly (3717).

Interactions with Herbs & Other Dietary Supplements

None known.

Interactions with Drugs

None known.

Interactions with Foods

None known.

Interactions with Lab Tests

None known.

Interactions with Diseases or Conditions

CROSS-ALLERGENICITY: Mugwort may cause an allergic reaction in individuals sensitive to the Asteraceae/Compositae family. Members of this family include ragweed, chrysanthemums, marigolds, daisies, and many other herbs.
Theoretically, mugwort might cause allergic reactions in individuals with allergies to honey or royal jelly (3717). Mugwort pollen might cause reactions in people allergic to tobacco (3716).

Dosage and Administration

ORAL: People use 5 mL of mugwort tincture 30 minutes before bedtime or 1-4 mL of the tincture up to three times daily (6002). Some people use 10 to 25 drops of the tincture, 1:5, 50% alcohol (5013). Two to three cups of tea is taken daily before meals (6002). The tea is prepared by steeping 15 grams of the dried herb in 500 mL of boiling water and straining (6002).

Comments

Mugwort has a pleasant, tangy taste. The plant is indigenous to Asia, North America, and Northern Europe (18).

MUIRA PUAMA

Also Known As
Muira-Puama, Muirapuama, Potency Wood, Ptychopetali lignum.

Scientific Names
Ptychopetalum olacoides; Ptychopetalum uncinatum.
Family: Olacaceae.

People Use This For
Orally, muira puama is used for preventing sexual disorders, and as an aphrodisiac. It is also used orally as a nerve stimulant, for dyspepsia, menstrual irregularities, rheumatism, paralysis caused by poliomyelitis, a general tonic, and as an appetite stimulant.
Topically, it is used as an aphrodisiac, for rheumatism, and muscle paralysis.
In combination with other herbs, muira puama is used as a remedy for sexual impotence.

Safety
There is insufficient reliable information available about the safety of muira puama.
Pregnancy and Lactation: Insufficient reliable information available; avoid using.

Effectiveness
There is insufficient reliable information available about the effectiveness of muira puama.

Mechanism of Action
The applicable parts of muira puama are the wood and root. No constituents in muira puama are known to exhibit any pronounced physiological activity (5).

Adverse Reactions
None reported.

Interactions with Herbs & Other Dietary Supplements
None known.

Interactions with Drugs
None known.

Interactions with Foods
None known.

Interactions with Lab Tests
None known.

Interactions with Diseases or Conditions
None known.

Dosage and Administration
ORAL: People typically use 1 to 2 mL of the muira puama extract in water two to three times daily. The number of drops recommended varies among products. The labeling on one product says one dropperful equals 1 mL and contains 500 mg muira puama. Other products do not specify the concentration of the active ingredient. Shake well before using; contains alcohol (6006).
TOPICAL: No typical dosage.

Comments
Previously, Liriosma ovata and Acanthea virilis were each thought to be the source of muira puama. They continue to be sold as muira puama in the herb trade (5).

MULLEIN

Also Known As
Aaron's Rod, Adam's Flannel, American Mullein, Beggar's Blanket, Blanket Herb, Blanket Leaf, Bouuillon Blanc, Candleflower, Candlewick, Clot-Bur, Clown's Lungwort, Cuddy's Lungs, Duffle, European Mullein, Feltwort, Flannelflower, Fluffweed, Hag's Taper, Hare's Beard, Hedge Taper, Higtaper, Jacob's Staff, Longwort, Orange Mullein, Our Lady's Flannel, Rag Paper, Shepherd's Club, Shepherd's Staff, Torches, Torch Weed, Velvet Plant, Verbasci flos, Wild Ice Leaf, Woolen.

Scientific Names
Verbascum densiflorum; Verbascum phlomides; Verbascum thapiforme; Verbascum thapsus.
Family: Scrophulariaceae.

People Use This For
Orally, mullein is used for respiratory tract mucous membrane inflammation, cough, earaches, colds, chills and flu, tracheitis, asthma, diarrhea, gastrointestinal bleeding, migraines, gout, tuberculosis, as a sedative, narcotic, diuretic, and antirheumatic. The root is used for croup.
Topically, mullein is used for wounds, burns, hemorrhoids, bruises, frostbite, erysipelas, and inflamed mucosa. The leaves are used topically to soften and protect the skin.
In manufacturing, mullein is used as a flavoring component in alcoholic beverages.

Safety
POSSIBLY SAFE ...when used orally and appropriately (5,12).
There is insufficient reliable information available about the safety of the topical use of mullein.
PREGNANCY AND LACTATION: Insufficient reliable information available; avoid using.

Effectiveness
There is insufficient reliable information available about the effectiveness of mullein.

Mechanism of Action
The applicable part of mullein is the flower. Mullein contains mucilage which alleviates local irritation (5,6,18). The saponins in mullein have an expectorant effect (5,8,18), and the extract may have activity against influenza and herpes simplex viruses (1534).

Adverse Reactions
None reported.

Interactions with Herbs & Other Dietary Supplements
None known.

Interactions with Drugs
None known.

Interactions with Foods
None known.

Interactions with Lab Tests
None known.

Interactions with Diseases or Conditions
None known.

Dosage and Administration
ORAL: The typical dose of mullein is 1.5-2 grams of the dry petals or one cup of tea. up to 3-4 grams dry petals per day (7,8,18). The tea is prepared by steeping 1.5-2 grams of the finely chopped, dry petals in 150 mL boiling water for 10-15 minutes and then strain.
TOPICAL: No typical dosage.

Comments
Avoid confusion with goldenrod (Solidago species), also known as Aaron's rod. There is confusion as to which Verbascum species are associated with the name American mullein and which are associated with the name European mullein.

MUSK

Also Known As
Deer Musk, Tonquin Musk.

Scientific Names
Moschus moschiferus (Musk Deer).
Family: Moschidae.

People Use This For
Orally, musk is used for stroke, coma, neurasthenia, convulsions, heart pains, and ulcerous sores.
In foods, musk is often used with nut, caramel, and fruit-type flavors.
In manufacturing, musk is used as a constituent of fragrances and a fixative in perfumes.

Safety
There is insufficient reliable information available about the safety of musk.
Pregnancy and Lactation: Insufficient reliable information available; avoid using.

Effectiveness
There is insufficient reliable information available about the effectiveness of musk.

Mechanism of Action
Musk is the secretion from the musk gland of the male musk deer. Musk contains muscone (0.3%-2%) and normuscone, steroids, paraffins, triglycerides, waxes, mucopyridine, and fatty acids, which may have anti-inflammatory and antihistaminic activity (6).

Adverse Reactions
Musk components are known to cause a variety of dermal hypersensitivity reactions (6).

Interactions with Herbs & Other Dietary Supplements
None known.

Interactions with Drugs
None known.

Interactions with Foods
None known.

Interactions with Lab Tests
None known.

Interactions with Diseases or Conditions
None known.

Dosage and Administration
No typical dosage.

Comments
Avoid confusion with sumbul, which is also known as musk root (Ferula sumbul, Family: Apiaceae), which is sometimes substituted for musk (6).

MYRRH

Also Known As
Abyssinian Myrrh, African Myrrh, Arabian Myrrh, Bal, Balsamodendron Myrrha, Bdellium, Bol, Bola, Commiphora, Didin, Didthin, Gum Myrrh, Heerabol, Opopanax, Somalien Myrrh, Yemen Myrrh.

Scientific Names
Commiphora myrrha, synonyms Commiphora molmol, Balsamodendrum myrrha; Commiphora habessinica, synonyms Commiphora abyssinica, Balsamodendrum habessinicum; Commiphora madagascariensis; Commiphora kataf, synonyms Commiphora erythraea, Amyris kataf, Hemprichia erythraea; other Commiphora species.
Family: Burseraceae.

People Use This For
Orally, myrrh is used for indigestion, ulcers, colds, cough, asthma, bronchial congestion, arthritic pain, cancer, leprosy, and syphilis. It is also used orally as a stimulant, antispasmodic, and to increase menstrual flow.
Topically, myrrh is used for mild inflammation of the oral and pharyngeal mucosa, aphthous ulcers, gingivitis, chapped lips, hemorrhoids, bedsores, wounds, abrasions, furunculosis, bad breath, and loose teeth.
In foods and beverages, myrrh is used as a flavoring component.
In manufacturing, myrrh is used as a fragrance and fixative in cosmetics.
It is also used in embalming and as incense.

Safety
LIKELY SAFE ...when consumed in amounts commonly found in food (11). Myrrh is approved for use in foods in the US (11).
POSSIBLY SAFE ...when used orally and appropriately (12). ...when used topically and appropriately (2,4,5,11,18).
POSSIBLY UNSAFE ...when used orally in excessive doses (12).
PREGNANCY: LIKELY UNSAFE ...when used orally because myrrh stimulates uterine tone and blood flow, and possibly has an abortifacient effect (4,12,19). There is insufficient reliable information available about the safety of the topical use of myrrh during pregnancy.
LACTATION: Insufficient reliable information available; avoid using.

Effectiveness
There is insufficient reliable information available about the effectiveness of myrrh.

Mechanism of Action
The applicable part of myrrh is resin. Myrrh resin contains a volatile oil and mucilage that have antimicrobial (4,6), deodorizing (8), anti-inflammatory (4,8), antitumor (1536), and astringent effects (4,6). In animals, it exhibits antipyretic and hypoglycemic effects (4), as well as protects against the development of gastric ulcers (1535). Myrrh can stimulate smooth muscle (6,12) and possibly peristalsis (6). It stimulates uterine tone (6,12) and promotes uterine blood flow (12,19).

Adverse Reactions
Topically, dermatitis has been reported with the use of myrrh (6).
Orally, amounts greater than 2-4 grams can cause kidney irritation and diarrhea (12). Large amounts can affect the heart rate (19).

Interactions with Herbs & Other Dietary Supplements
None known.

Interactions with Drugs
ANTIDIABETES DRUGS: Myrrh extract might interfere with diabetic therapy due to hypoglycemic effects (4).

Interactions with Foods
None known.

Interactions with Lab Tests
BLOOD GLUCOSE: Theoretically, myrrh can lower blood glucose and test results.

Interactions with Diseases or Conditions
DIABETES: Theoretically, myrrh can interfere with diabetes therapy (4).
HEART CONDITIONS: Use myrrh with caution in individuals with heart conditions, because large amounts can affect the heart rate (19).
OTHER: Use myrrh with caution because it can exacerbate uterine bleeding (12,19), fever, and systemic inflammation (19).

Dosage and Administration
TOPICAL: For mild mouth and throat irritation, dab the undiluted tincture of myrrh on affected areas two to three times daily. Myrrh is also commonly used as a rinse or gargle with 5-10 drops in a glass of water (2,8). A typical mouthwash can contain 30-60 drops in a glass of water also (8). The tooth powder contains 10% powdered resin (2,18).

Comments
Myrrh is the oleo-gum resin exuded from fissures or cuts in the bark of Commiphora species trees. Commiphora mukul, a related species, is not a source of myrrh (8).

MYRTLE

Also Known As
Myrti aetherolum, Myrti folium.

Scientific Names
Myrtus communis.
Family: Myrtaceae.

People Use This For
Orally, myrtle is used for treating acute and chronic respiratory infections including bronchitis, whooping cough, tuberculosis, bladder conditions, diarrhea, and worm infestation.

Safety
LIKELY UNSAFE ...when the undiluted oil is used orally because it contains cineole. Ingesting more than 10 grams of cineole can result in respiratory failure and collapse (18).
There is insufficient reliable information available about the safety of myrtle leaf and branch.
CHILDREN: LIKELY UNSAFE ...when used orally. Avoid facial contact with myrtle oil preparations which may cause glottal spasm, bronchospasm, asthma-like attacks, or respiratory failure in infants or small children (18).
PREGNANCY AND LACTATION: LIKELY UNSAFE ...when used orally (18); avoid using.

Effectiveness
There is insufficient reliable information available about the effectiveness of myrtle.

Mechanism of Action
The applicable parts of myrtle are the leaf and branch. Myrtle contains a volatile oil, tannins, and acylphloroglucinols. Myrtol, a volatile oil, stimulates mucous membranes of the stomach and deodorizes the breath. It might also have fungicidal, disinfectant, and antibacterial properties (18). The volatile oil contains between 15-45% of 1,8-cineole, a constituent responsible for toxicity (18).

Adverse Reactions
Orally, myrtle can cause nausea, vomiting, and diarrhea (18). Consumption of large amounts might lead to low blood pressure, circulatory disorders, respiratory failure, and collapse (18).
Topically, facial contact with myrtle oil preparations may cause glottal or bronchial spasm, asthma-like attacks, or respiratory failure in infants and children (18).

Interactions with Herbs & Other Dietary Supplements
None known.

Interactions with Drugs
None known.

Interactions with Foods
None known.

Interactions with Lab Tests
None known.

Interactions with Diseases or Conditions
None known.

Dosage and Administration
ORAL: A typical dose is 200 mg one time only (18).

Comments
Myrtle leaves resemble the leaves of Bux semper-virens and Vaccinium vitisidaea (18).

N-ACETYL CYSTEINE

Also Known As
Acetylcysteine, L-Cysteine, NAC, N-Acetylcysteine, N-Acetyl-B-Cysteine, N-Acetyl L-Cysteine, N-Acetyl-Cysteine.

Scientific Names
N-acetyl-L-cysteine.

People Use This For
Orally, N-acetyl cysteine is used as an antidote for acetaminophen and carbon monoxide poisoning. It is also used for unstable angina, common bile duct obstruction in infants, lysosomal storage disorders, amyotrophic lateral sclerosis (ALS, Lou Gehrig's disease), Alzheimer's disease, phenytoin-induced hypersensitivity, and keratoconjunctivitis. It is also used for reducing lipoprotein (a) levels, reducing homocysteine levels, reducing risk of cardiovascular events in patients with end-stage renal disease, chronic bronchitis, chronic obstructive pulmonary disease (COPD), allergic rhinitis, fibrosing alveolitis, head and neck cancer, and lung cancer. N-acetyl cysteine is also used orally for myoclonus epilepsy; otitis media; hemodialysis-related pseudoporphyria; Sjogren's syndrome; preventing sports injury complications; radiation therapy; increasing immunity to flu; and for detoxifying heavy metals such as mercury, lead, and cadmium. It is also used orally for preventing alcoholic liver damage; for protecting against environmental pollutants including carbon monoxide, chloroform, urethanes and certain herbicides; for reducing toxicity of ifosfamide and doxorubicin; as a hangover remedy; for preventing nonionic low-osmolality contrast agent-induced reduction of renal function in patients with renal insufficiency; and for human immunodeficiency virus (HIV).

Topically, N-acetyl cysteine is used for reducing dental plaque.

Intravenously, N-acetyl cysteine is used for acetaminophen overdose, acrylonitrile poisoning, amyotrophic lateral sclerosis (ALS, Lou Gehrig's disease), for hepatorenal syndrome, for decreasing mortality rate due to multisystem organ failure, for unstable angina in combination with nitroglycerin, and for acute myocardial infarction with nitroglycerin and streptokinase.

Rectally, N-acetyl cysteine is used for meconium ileus and meconium ileus equivalent.

By inhalation or intratracheal installation, N-acetyl cysteine is used as a mucolytic agent in acute and chronic lung disorders such as pneumonia, bronchitis, emphysema, cystic fibrosis, and others.

Safety
LIKELY SAFE ...when used orally, intravenously, intratracheally, by inhalation, and appropriately. N-acetyl cysteine is an FDA-approved prescription drug (832,1539,1705,1710,2245,2246,2252,2253,2254,2256,2258,2259,2260) (5808,6176,6611,7868,10270,10271).

PREGNANCY: POSSIBLY SAFE ...when used orally, intratracheally, or by inhalation. N-acetyl cysteine crosses the placenta, but has not been associated with adverse effects to the fetus or mothers (1711). However, N-acetyl cysteine should only be used in pregnant women when clearly indicated, such as in cases of acetaminophen toxicity.

LACTATION: Insufficient reliable information available; avoid using.

Effectiveness
EFFECTIVE

Acetaminophen poisoning. Administering N-acetyl cysteine orally or intravenously is equally effective in decreasing mortality rate and preventing the permanent sequelae of acetaminophen poisoning (17).

Atelectasis. N-acetyl cysteine is helpful for atelectasis caused by mucus obstruction (15).

Bronchial diagnostic studies. N-acetyl cysteine is helpful when used for preparing people for bronchial diagnostic studies (15).

Bronchopulmonary disorders. Administering N-acetyl cysteine by inhalation is effective as a mucolytic for adjunctive treatment of acute and chronic bronchopulmonary disorders (15).

Cystic fibrosis. N-acetyl cysteine is effective for cystic fibrosis (15).

Tracheostomy care. N-acetyl cysteine is effective when used as an adjunct for preventing endotracheal crusting in tracheostomy care (15).

POSSIBLY EFFECTIVE

Angina. Administering N-acetyl cysteine orally or intravenously seems to improve unstable angina pectoris in combination with nitroglycerin (2245,2246). Concurrent intravenous administration of N-acetyl cysteine also seems to reduce development of nitroglycerin tolerance (832,2245). However, severe headache can occur when N-acetyl cysteine and nitroglycerin are administered together and may limit feasibility of concomitant use (2245).

Bronchitis. Taking N-acetyl cysteine orally seems to reduce the risk of acute exacerbations of chronic bronchitis when used over a three to six month period (6176).

Chronic obstructive pulmonary disease (COPD). In patients with moderate to severe COPD, taking N-acetyl cysteine orally can decrease the number of acute exacerbations by about 40% when used in addition to standard therapy (10429).

Contrast agent-induced nephropathy. Taking N-acetyl cysteine orally seems to prevent nonionic low-osmolality contrast agent-induced nephropathy in patients with renal insufficiency. Oral N-acetyl cysteine, with hydration with intravenous saline, seems to prevent acute renal damage in patients with chronic renal insufficiency (serum creatinine greater than 2.4 mg/dL) receiving iopromide (Ultravist-300) administration for elective computed tomography (CT) or coronary angiography (6611,10428). However, in patients with reduced renal function (serum creatinine greater than 1.2 ml/dL, but less than 2.4 ml/dL), oral N-acetyl cysteine doesn't seem to reduce the risk of contrast agent-induced renal damage after coronary angiography (11430).

End-stage renal disease (ESRD). Taking N-acetyl cysteine orally seems to reduce the incidence of cardiovascular events such as ischemic stroke and myocardial infarction by about 40% in patients with ESRD. However, the risk of total mortality or mortality from cardiovascular causes is not decreased (10430).

Epilepsy. Taking N-acetyl cysteine orally seems to be helpful for treating myoclonus epilepsy (2259).

Fibrosing alveolitis. Taking N-acetyl cysteine orally seems to improve pulmonary function tests and decrease biochemical markers of disease in patients with fibrosing alveolitis (7868).

Hyperhomocysteinemia. Taking N-acetyl cysteine orally seems to reduce homocysteine levels (2256,2258).

Ifosfamide (Ifex) toxicity. Taking N-acetyl cysteine orally seems to reduce ifosfamide-induced bladder toxicity (5808,10270). However, mesna (Mesnex) seems to be more effective for preventing ifosfamide toxicity than N-acetyl cysteine (10748).

Influenza. Taking N-acetyl cysteine orally seems to reduce symptoms of influenza (2260).

POSSIBLY INEFFECTIVE

Amyotrophic lateral sclerosis (ALS, Lou Gehrig's disease). Administering N-acetyl cysteine intravenously doesn't seem to improve symptoms of ALS (2254).

Doxorubicin-induced cardiac toxicity. Taking N-acetyl cysteine orally doesn't seem to prevent or reverse doxorubicin-induced cardiac toxicity (2252,2253).

LIKELY INEFFECTIVE

Alzheimer's disease. Taking N-acetyl cysteine orally doesn't improve symptoms of Alzheimer's disease (7870).

Head and neck cancer or lung cancer. Taking N-acetyl cysteine orally in patients with head and neck cancer or lung cancer doesn't prevent second primary tumors (1710). N-acetyl cysteine alone, or in combination with retinyl palmitate, has no effect on mortality or event-free survival in patients with head and neck cancer or lung cancer (1705,1710).

Multisystem organ failure. Administering N-acetyl cysteine intravenously, greater than 24 hours after hospital admission, might increase mortality rate due to multisystem organ failure. The effect of N-acetyl cysteine given within 24 hours of hospital admission requires further study (7871).

Nitrate tolerance. Taking N-acetyl cysteine orally doesn't reduce nitroglycerin tolerance (2281,2282).

INSUFFICIENT RELIABLE EVIDENCE to RATE

Colorectal cancer. Oral N-acetyl cysteine may reduce the likelihood of colorectal cancer in patients with a history of adenomatous colon polyps (7873).

Hepatorenal syndrome. There is some preliminary clinical evidence that intravenous N-acetyl cysteine might improve renal function in hepatorenal syndrome (1752).

Lamellar ichthyosis. There is some evidence that topical N-acetyl cysteine might be useful for lamellar ichthyosis, a congenital skin disease (3974,3975).

Myocardial infarction (MI). Early evidence shows that intravenous N-acetyl cysteine, when given with nitroglycerin and streptokinase, in patients with evolving MI, may preserve left ventricular function and reduce oxidative stress (7872).

More evidence is needed to rate N-acetyl cysteine for these uses.

Mechanism of Action

N-acetyl cysteine is the N-acetyl derivative of the amino acid L-cysteine (1705). N-acetyl cysteine is a precursor of glutathione, which is a potent antioxidant. Glutathione can not cross the cell membrane, but N-acetyl cysteine easily crosses the cell membrane where it is converted to cysteine and, subsequently, glutathione. Reactive oxygen species (ROS) such as hydrogen peroxide and hydroxyl-free radicals reduce intracellular and extracellular concentrations of glutathione. N-acetyl cysteine is a very efficient way to replenish glutathione and reduce damage caused by ROS (7874,1761).

The antioxidant effects of N-acetyl cysteine may explain its apparent ability to prevent adverse effects caused by toxic chemicals, drug reactions, and nonionic low-osmolality contrast agents (1762,6611). The antioxidant and free radical properties might also make N-acetyl cysteine useful in the treatment of pulmonary and cardiac disease (1705,1765). N-acetyl cysteine also appears to reduce cellular production of pro-inflammatory mediators such as tumor necrosis factor-alpha, TNF-alpha, and interleukin 1, IL-1 (1763).

N-acetyl cysteine is effective for acetaminophen hepatotoxicity because it restores glutathione levels in the liver and acts as an alternative substrate for conjugation of toxic acetaminophen metabolites (15). N-acetyl cysteine might be helpful in the congenital skin disease lamellar ichthyosis due to antiproliferative effects on skin cells (3975). N-acetyl cysteine may also have anticarcinogenic properties by inhibiting the invasive activity of tumor cells and angiogenesis of tumor cells (1767).

N-acetyl cysteine might decrease bladder toxicity caused by ifosfamide. The exact mechanism is not understood, but it probably involves binding of the thiol-sulfhydryl groups in N-acetyl cysteine to ifosfamide and its metabolite acrolein. N-acetyl cysteine does not appear to affect the anticancer activity of ifosfamide (10269,10268).

Preliminary evidence indicates that N-acetyl cysteine can impair platelet aggregation. N-acetyl cysteine appears to increase synthesis of nitric oxide, a potent inhibitor of platelet function (10272).

In patients with human immunodeficiency virus (HIV) disease, N-acetyl cysteine can increase levels of glutathione. Increased concentration of glutathione seems to reduce oxidative stress associated with HIV disease and to improve the number and activity of CD4 T-lymphocytes (1539).

Assessing the pharmacokinetics of N-acetyl cysteine is difficult because it binds to cysteine and other sulfhydryl molecules. Because these compounds are widely available in tissues, N-acetyl cysteine is rapidly removed from plasma. After oral administration of N-acetyl cysteine, the time to maximum plasma concentration (Tmax) is approximately 0.72 hours. With a dose of 250 mg/m2, the maximum plasma concentration (Cmax) is about 1.75 mcg/mL. The half life (T1/2) of N-acetyl cysteine is about 2 hours (10268).

Adverse Reactions

Orally, N-acetyl cysteine can cause gastrointestinal adverse effects including nausea, abdominal pain, vomiting, constipation, and diarrhea, particularly when used in high doses (1539,10270,10271,11430). N-acetyl cysteine has an unpleasant odor that sometimes makes it difficult for patients to take orally. Using a straw to drink N-acetyl cysteine solutions can improve tolerability (17). In some cases, placement of a nasogastric or duodenal tube and administration of metoclopramide or ondansetron can also be helpful for patients unable to tolerate oral N-acetyl cysteine (17). Rarely, generalized urticaria with mild fever, sulfhemoglobinemia, headache, hypotension, rash, and hepatotoxicity has occurred (17).

Intravenously, N-acetyl cysteine can sometimes cause allergic reactions including anaphylactoid reactions (1716). For less severe allergic reactions, diphenhydramine can be administered and the N-acetyl cysteine infusion can be continued. For more severe reactions (e.g., angioedema, respiratory symptoms), the infusion should be temporarily discontinued and resumed an hour after diphenhydramine administration (1716).

By inhalation, N-acetyl cysteine has been associated with stomatitis, nausea, vomiting, drowsiness, clamminess, and severe rhinorrhea (15). Fever, chills, chest tightness, and bronchoconstriction have been reported rarely (15). Sensitization and dermal eruptions have also been reported. However, sensitization has not been confirmed by patch testing (15).

In cases of N-acetyl cysteine overdose, symptoms typically resemble a severe anaphylactoid reaction (17).

Interactions with Herbs & Other Dietary Supplements

None known.

Interactions with Drugs

ACTIVATED CHARCOAL: N-acetyl cysteine appears to reduce the capacity of charcoal to adsorb acetaminophen and salicylic acid (7869). But concomitant use of activated charcoal does not seem to reduce the effectiveness of N-acetyl cysteine (1755).

NITROGLYCERIN: Concomitant administration of N-acetyl cysteine and intravenous nitroglycerin can cause severe hypotension (2246) and intolerable headaches (2245,2280).

Interactions with Foods

None known.

Interactions with Lab Tests

BLOOD PRESSURE: Concomitant administration of intravenous NAC and nitroglycerin can lower blood pressure and reduce blood pressure readings (2246).

CHLORIDE: NAC can cause false-positive serum chloride test results measured with the Beckman Synchron CX3 analyzer (275).

CREATININE: Intravenous NAC can cause falsely low serum creatinine test results when measured by single-slide method on Kodak Ektachem systems (275).

CYSTEINE (FREE): Intravenous NAC can increase free cysteine plasma concentrations and test results (275).

GOLD: Intravenous NAC can increase urinary gold excretion (concentration) and test results in patients previously given gold (275).
KETONES: NAC can cause false-positive urine ketone test results when measured with Chemstrips (Boehringer Mannheim) or Multistix (Miles) (275).
LIPOPROTEIN A: Used orally, NAC might reduce serum lipoprotein A concentrations and test results in some patients (275).
LITHIUM: Very high serum NAC concentrations might cause falsely low serum lithium test results when measured with Kodak Ektachem systems (275).
LIVER FUNCTION TESTS: NAC might increase liver enzyme (AST, ALT) concentrations and test results. Liver function tests were markedly elevated on two occasions in a child with cystic fibrosis after receiving large NAC doses by rectal and naso-gastric tube administration (15).
PROTHROMBIN TIME (PT): Intravenous NAC can decrease PT and test results (1341).
SALICYLATE: Serum NAC concentrations of 50 mg/dL (occurring with intravenous NAC administration) can cause falsely low serum salicylate test results when measured with Kodak Ektachem systems. Serum NAC concentrations of 10 mg/dL (occurring with oral NAC administration) do not interfere with serum salicylate results measured with Kodak Ektachem systems (275).

Interactions with Diseases or Conditions

ALLERGY: Contraindicated in individuals with acetylcysteine allergy (15).
ASTHMA: Oral NAC inhalation or intratracheal administration might cause bronchospasm, monitor closely (15).
HEMODIALYSIS-ASSOCIATED PSEUDOPORPHYRIA: NAC might improve pseudoporphyria skin lesions associated with hemodialysis. Two cases are reported in which pseudoporphyria skin lesions healed with oral NAC administration in patients on chronic hemodialysis (5052).

Dosage and Administration

ORAL: For acetaminophen overdose, an oral loading dose of 140 mg/kg of a 5% solution should be administered. The commercially available 10% and 20% solutions may be diluted with water, carbonated, or non-carbonated beverages, and administered through a straw to lessen the disagreeable odor of N-acetyl cysteine. Seventeen additional doses of 70 mg/kg as a 5% solution should be given every 4 hours, for a total dose of 1330 mg/kg over 72 hours (17). A typical dose for unstable angina is 600 mg three times daily with transdermal nitroglycerin (2245). For preventing acute exacerbations of chronic bronchitis, doses of 200 mg twice daily, 200 mg three times daily, 300 mg slow-release twice daily, and 600 mg controlled-release twice daily have been used (6176). For treating chronic obstructive pulmonary disease (COPD), N-acetyl cysteine 600 mg once daily, in addition to standard care, has been used for up to 6 months (10429). For treating fibrosing alveolitis, N-acetyl cysteine 600 mg 3 times daily has been used (7868). For prophylaxis of urinary bladder toxicity due to ifosfamide, 1 to 2 grams every 6 hours has been used (5808,10268,10269,10270,10271). For reducing plasma homocysteine levels, 1.2 grams daily has been used (2258). For myoclonus epilepsy, 4-6 grams daily has been used (2259). For reducing symptoms of influenza, 600 mg twice daily has been used (2260). For reducing the risk of cardiovascular events in patients with end-stage renal disease, 600 mg twice daily has been used (10430). For hemodialysis-associated pseudoporphyria skin lesions, 200 mg four times daily or 600 mg twice daily has been used (5052). For preventing iopromide (Ultravist-300)-induced reduction of renal function in patients with chronic renal insufficiency, 400 to 600 mg N-acetyl cysteine twice daily on the day before and on the day of iopromide administration, with IV saline (0.45%) 1 mL/kg body weight per hour for 12 hours before and 12 hours after iopromide administration, has been used (6611,10428). In Alzheimer's disease, N-acetyl cysteine 50 mg/kg/day has been used (7870).
INTRAVENOUS: There are 2 dosage regimens for intravenous N-acetyl cysteine. For patients presenting 10 to 24 hours after acetaminophen ingestion, particularly if large doses were taken, the following 48-hour regimen should be used (17). Administer a loading dose of 140 mg IV N-acetyl cysteine as a 3% solution over 1 hour. The 3% solution is prepared by diluting the 20% IV solution with 5% dextrose. Twelve additional doses of 70 mg/kg IV N-acetyl cysteine should be administered over 1 hour every 4 hours thereafter. The alternative 20-hour regimen consists of IV administration of 150 mg/kg N-acetyl cysteine in 200 ml of 5% dextrose solution, administered over 15 minutes. Follow this dose with 50 mg/kg N-acetyl cysteine in 500 mL 5% dextrose over 4 hours and 100 mg/kg in 1 liter 5% dextrose over 16 hours. The total dose is 300 mg/kg over 20 hours. This regimen is most effective if begun within 8 hours of acetaminophen ingestion (17). In evolving acute myocardial infarction (MI), N-acetyl cysteine 20 mg/minute for 1 hour followed by 10 mg/minute for 23 hours, for a total of 15 grams/24 hours, has been used. Intravenous nitroglycerin and streptokinase were also given (7872). For reducing mortality rate due to multisystem organ disease, N-acetyl cysteine 150 mg/kg bolus, followed by a continuous infusion of 12 mg/kg/hr for 3 to 5 days has been used; however, mortality rate was not significantly reduced (7871).

N-ACETYL GLUCOSAMINE

Also Known As

Acetylglucosamine, Glucosamine N-Acetyl, N-Acetyl D-Glucosamine, N-Acetyl-D-Glucosamine, NAG, N-A-G, Poly-NAG.
CAUTION: See separate listings for Glucosamine Sulfate and Glucosamine Hydrochloride.

Scientific Names

2-acetamido-2-deoxyglucose.

People Use This For

Orally, N-acetyl glucosamine is used for osteoarthritis and inflammatory bowel disease (IBD), including ulcerative colitis and Crohn's disease.

Safety

There is insufficient reliable information available about the safety of N-acetyl glucosamine.
Pregnancy and Lactation: Insufficient reliable information available; avoid using.

Effectiveness

INSUFFICIENT RELIABLE EVIDENCE to RATE
Inflammatory bowel disease (IBD). There is preliminary evidence that oral or rectal N-acetyl glucosamine might decrease symptoms of IBD in children with Crohn's disease or ulcerative colitis (10234). More evidence is needed to rate N-acetyl glucosamine for this use.

Mechanism of Action

N-acetyl glucosamine is the acetylated derivative of the amino sugar glucosamine, which is a constituent of cartilage proteoglycans. It is derived from marine exoskeletons or produced synthetically. Glucosamine is required for the synthesis of glycoproteins, glycolipids, and glycosaminoglycans (also known as mucopolysaccharides); these carbohydrate-containing compounds are found in tendons, ligaments, cartilage, synovial fluid, mucous membranes, structures in the eye, blood vessels, and heart valves. Glucosamine is also a component of biologically active compounds such as heparin, but it does not react with heparin-induced thrombocytopenia (HIT) antibodies (7640,7641,11831). In osteoarthritis, glucosamine stimulates metabolism of chondrocytes in the articular cartilage and synovial cells in the synovial tissues. There is some evidence that suggests that glucosamine might have a disease-modifying effect, therefor stopping or slowing the progression of osteoarthritis (7026). Glucosamine doesn't seem to directly affect cyclooxygenase, which is responsible for anti-inflammatory and analgesic effects of nonsteroidal anti-inflammatory drugs (NSAIDs), as well as adverse gastrointestinal (GI) effects (2604). In inflammatory bowel disease (IBD), N-acetylation of glucosamine is relatively deficient, possibly reducing the synthesis of the gastric and intestinal mucosa's protective glycoprotein cover (2609). Theoretically, supplementation with N-acetyl glucosamine could remedy this deficiency and restore the glycoprotein cover (2609). However, aren't any human studies that have evaluated this claim.
There has been a lot of concern about the effect of glucosamine on glucose metabolism. Preliminary evidence suggests that glucosamine might decrease glucose-induced insulin secretion by inhibiting pancreatic glucokinase in the beta cells of the islet of Langerhans (371,372,3406). Other preliminary research suggests that glucosamine might also impair insulin-mediated glucose uptake and metabolism in skeletal muscle (372,3406). Animal research suggests glucosamine might increase glucose metabolism through the hexosamine pathway, a pattern of change in glucose metabolism similar to that seen in type 2 diabetes (3405,3406). However, animals may handle glucosamine differently than humans. Most of the research in humans suggests that glucosamine doesn't affect the pharmacokinetics of glucose. Research in people with normal glucose metabolism suggests glucosamine doesn't affect insulin sensitivity or plasma glucose (7637,7638). Clinical research in people with type 2 diabetes and people without diabetes suggests glucosamine doesn't have any significant effect on blood glucose when given for up to 3 years (7026,8942,10311,10317). Preliminary clinical research suggests that endogenous glucosamine and insulin levels are elevated in nondiabetic patients with ischemic heart disease (7640,7641). Some researchers think that increased glucosamine production might contribute to endothelial cell dysfunction (8944). Glucosamine is absorbed 90% after oral administration. The bioavailability is approximately 26% after first pass metabolism (2608). Glucosamine is incorporated into plasma proteins during first-pass metabolism, and unbound glucosamine is concentrated in the articular cartilage (2608). Free glucosamine is undetectable in the plasma (2607).

Adverse Reactions

Orally, N-acetyl glucosamine might cause mild gastrointestinal (GI) problems, including nausea, heartburn, diarrhea, and constipation; similar to the effects seen with glucosamine sulfate. Drowsiness, skin reactions, and headache have also been reported (2608). Anecdotal reports have associated glucosamine with renal toxicity, but changes in renal function have not been reported in long-term studies (7026,8942,10408,10409).
Elevated blood glucose levels in patients with diabetes have also been reported (22). Some research suggests that

glucosamine sulfate can also increase insulin levels in non-diabetic people, but glucosamine doesn't seem to cause hyperglycemia or diabetes in otherwise healthy patients taking 1500 mg per day for three years. Also, glucosamine doesn't seem to cause any adverse effects on blood glucose metabolism, lipid metabolism, or any other disturbances in metabolism (3406,5059,7026,8942).
There is concern that use of N-acetyl glucosamine products derived from marine exoskeletons might cause reactions in people allergic to shellfish, although no reactions have been reported. Until more is known, and because the source of N-acetyl glucosamine products is not listed on product labels, use N-acetyl glucosamine with caution in people with shellfish allergy.

Interactions with Herbs & Other Dietary Supplements

None known.

Interactions with Drugs

ANTIDIABETES DRUGS: Preliminary research suggests that glucosamine might increase insulin resistance, or decrease insulin production, and potentially worsen diabetes control (371,372,3406,7637,7638). But there is some clinical evidence that suggests that taking glucosamine for 3 months does not increase hemoglobin A1c (HbA1c) in people with type 2 diabetes who have well-controlled glucose levels (10311,10317). Until more is known, advise patients with diabetes who take glucosamine to monitor their blood glucose levels closely. Some antidiabetes drugs include glimepiride (Amaryl), glyburide (DiaBeta, Glynase PresTab, Micronase), insulin, pioglitazone (Actos), rosiglitazone (Avandia), and others.
CHEMOTHERAPY: Theoretically, glucosamine might induce resistance to etoposide (VP16, VePesid) and doxorubicin (Adriamycin) by reducing the drugs' inhibition of topoisomerase II, an enzyme required for DNA replication in tumor cells (7639).
WARFARIN (Coumadin): There's some concern that high-dose glucosamine (3000 mg per day), combined with high-dose chondroitin sulfate (2400 mg per day), may enhance the effects of warfarin (Coumadin) as measured by the INR (11389). Chondroitin is a small component of a heparinoid and might have weak anticoagulant activity. Glucosamine is also a small component of heparin, but is does not seem to have anticoagulant activity. It's not known if glucosamine contributes to this potential interaction. Interactions with warfarin have not been reported at recommended dosages of glucosamine or chondroitin.

Interactions with Foods

None known.

Interactions with Lab Tests

BLOOD GLUCOSE: Glucosamine doesn't seem to adversely affect blood glucose control in people with type 2 diabetes, as measured by hemoglobin A1C (10311,10317). It also doesn't seem to affect blood glucose in nondiabetic people older than 45 who have taken glucosamine for osteoarthritis for 3 years (7026,8942). Some preliminary research raised concerns that glucosamine might exacerbate diabetes by increasing insulin resistance and/or decreasing insulin production, resulting in elevated blood glucose levels (5059), but other research showed no effect (7637,7638). There are also anecdotal reports of reduced blood glucose control in people with diabetes who take glucosamine (22,1203,1204,3405,3406). However, clinical studies indicate that glucosamine has little or no effect blood glucose (7026,8942,10311,10317).
INTERNATIONAL NORMALIZED RATIO (INR)/PROTHROMBIN TIME (PT): High dose glucosamine (3000 mg per day), combined with high dose chondroitin sulfate (2400 mg per day), may increase the INR in patients taking warfarin (Coumadin). There is one case report of an increased INR associated with concomitant use of warfarin a glucosamine-chondroitin supplement taken above recommended dosages (11389).

Interactions with Diseases or Conditions

ASTHMA: Glucosamine might exacerbate asthma by an unidentified mechanism. Use N-acetyl glucosamine cautiously in patients with asthma (10002).
DIABETES: Glucosamine doesn't seem to adversely affect blood glucose control in people with type 2 diabetes, as measured by hemoglobin A1C (10311,10317). Some preliminary research raised concerns that glucosamine might exacerbate diabetes by increasing insulin resistance and/or decreasing insulin production, resulting in elevated blood glucose levels (5059), but other research showed no effect on insulin sensitivity or plasma glucose (7637,7638). There are also anecdotal reports of reduced blood glucose control in people with diabetes who take glucosamine (22,1203,1204,3405,3406). However, clinical studies indicate that glucosamine seems to be safe in people with type 2 diabetes (10311,10317).
SHELLFISH ALLERGY: There is concern that N-acetyl glucosamine products derived from marine exoskeletons might cause reactions in people allergic to shellfish, although no reactions have been reported. Until more is known, and because the source of N-acetyl glucosamine products is not listed on product labels, use N-acetyl glucosamine with caution in people with shellfish allergy.

Dosage and Administration

ORAL: For inflammatory bowel disease in children, N-acetyl glucosamine 3 to 6 grams per day in 3 divided doses has been used (10234).
RECTAL: For inflammatory bowel disease in children, N-acetyl glucosamine 3 to 4 grams per day in 2 divided doses has been used (10234).

Comments

Avoid confusion with glucosamine sulfate and glucosamine hydrochloride. Read glucosamine product labels carefully for their content. Although glucosamine sulfate and glucosamine hydrochloride are marketed together in combination products with N-acetyl glucosamine, there haven't been any human studies that have evaluated these combinations for treating osteoarthritis. Chitosan is the deacylated polymer of N-acetyl glucosamine.

NADH

Also Known As

B-DPNH, BNADH, Coenzyme 1, Enada, NAD, Reduced DPN, Reduced Nicotinamide Adenine Dinucleotide.

Scientific Names

NADH.

People Use This For

Orally, NADH is used for improving mental clarity, alertness, and concentration; improving memory; cellular energy; for antioxidant effects; chronic fatigue syndrome (CFS); depression; jet lag; hypertension; Alzheimer's disease; Parkinson's disease; improving athletic endurance; enhancing energy; improving DNA repair; enhancing immune function; reducing aging; protecting the liver from alcohol damage; preventing alcohol-induced inhibition of testosterone; lowering cholesterol levels; and protecting against zidovudine (AZT) toxicity.
Intravenously, NADH is used as an IM or IV injection for Parkinson's disease and depression.

Safety

POSSIBLY SAFE ...when used orally and appropriately (8267,8275). NADH is generally considered safe and has been used for up to 12 weeks without reports of side effects.
PREGNANCY AND LACTATION: Insufficient reliable information available; avoid using.

Effectiveness

POSSIBLY INEFFECTIVE

Dementia. Taking NADH orally seems to be ineffective for mild to moderate dementia of the Alzheimer's, vascular, or fronto-temporal type (8275). Dementia patients treated with 10 mg per day NADH had no significant improvement in memory, cognitive, and behavioral function scales after 12 weeks of treatment.

INSUFFICIENT RELIABLE EVIDENCE to RATE

Chronic fatigue syndrome (CFS). There is preliminary clinical evidence that NADH might reduce the symptoms of CFS when used as an adjunctive therapy to traditional medications (8267).

Parkinson's disease. There is conflicting preliminary research about the usefulness of NADH for Parkinson's disease (3086,3089,3090).

More evidence is needed to rate NADH for these uses.

Mechanism of Action

NADH is the reduced form of NAD (nicotinamide adenine dinucleotide), a coenzyme necessary to dehydrogenate primary and secondary alcohols (3082). In dehydrogenation, NAD acts as a hydrogen acceptor, forming NADH. NADH, in turn, serves as a hydrogen donor in the respiratory chain. NADH is an essential intermediate in the cellular processes that generate energy from glucose in the form of ATP. Some evidence suggests oral NADH reduces blood pressure, total cholesterol, and low-density lipoprotein (LDL) (3083). Preliminary evidence suggests that NADH might help people with chronic fatigue syndrome (CFS) by triggering energy production through ATP generation (8267). Preliminary research suggests that NADH might protect against age-related hypertension, possibly by lowering lipid peroxidation and free radical formation (8260). NADH has been proposed as a therapeutic agent for people with Parkinson's disease because evidence suggests it might increase tyrosine hydroxylase activity and dopamine production (3085,3086,3088,3091).

Adverse Reactions

None reported.

Interactions with Herbs & Other Dietary Supplements
None known.

Interactions with Drugs
None known.

Interactions with Foods
None known.

Interactions with Lab Tests
None known.

Interactions with Diseases or Conditions
None known.

Dosage and Administration
ORAL: For nutrition and energy enhancement, a typical dose is 2.5-5 mg daily or every other day (3462). For therapeutic support of Alzheimer's disease (3462,8275), Parkinson's disease and chronic fatigue syndrome (CFS) (3462,8267), a typical dose is 10-15 mg daily or every other day. Some people recommend the disodium salt form of NADH, taken with water either 30 minutes before or two hours after meals (3462).

NASTURTIUM

Also Known As
Indian Cress.
CAUTION: See separate listing for Watercress.

Scientific Names
Tropaeolum majus.
Family: Tropaeolaceae.

People Use This For
Orally and in combination with other herbs, nasturtium is used for urinary tract infection, respiratory tract mucous membrane inflammation, and cough and bronchitis.
Topically, nasturtium is used in combination with other herbs for mild muscular pain.

Safety
POSSIBLY SAFE ...when used topically (2). ...when used orally in combination with other herbs (2).
There is insufficient reliable information available about the safety of nasturtium used orally as a single entity.
CHILDREN: LIKELY UNSAFE ...when used orally in combination with other herbs. Contraindicated (2,18).
There is insufficient reliable information about the safety of the topical use of nasturtium by children.
PREGNANCY AND LACTATION: Insufficient reliable information available; avoid using nasturtium by itself or in combination with other herbs.

Effectiveness
There is insufficient reliable information available about the effectiveness of nasturtium.

Mechanism of Action
The applicable parts of nasturtium are the above ground parts. Nasturtium contains 300 mg vitamin C per 100 grams of fresh plant (18). Benzyl mustard oil (benzyl isothiocyanate), the principal active constituent of nasturtium, may have bacteriostatic, virustatic, antimycotic (2,18), and antitumor (1537) activity. It is accumulated and excreted mainly in the respiratory and the urinary tracts (2,18). Applied topically, benzyl mustard oil has rubefacient activity (2,18).

Adverse Reactions
Orally, large amounts of nasturtium or benzyl mustard oil can cause GI tract irritation (2,18); one case of urticarial exanthema is reported (2). Large amounts of nasturtium can cause albuminuria due to glomerular and tubular damage (2).
Topically, long term intensive contact with the plant can cause skin irritation (18); benzyl mustard oil can cause skin and mucosal irritation (2). Benzyl mustard oil is a contact allergen if applied to the skin (2).

Interactions with Herbs & Other Dietary Supplements
None known.

Interactions with Drugs
None known.

Interactions with Foods
None known.

Interactions with Lab Tests
None known.

Interactions with Diseases or Conditions
GI ULCERS: Contraindicated in individuals with gastric or intestinal ulcers (2,18).
KIDNEY DISEASE: Contraindicated in individuals with kidney disease.

Dosage and Administration
No typical dosage.

NATTOKINASE

Also Known As
BSP, Natto Extract, NK, Fermented Soybeans, Subtilisin NAT.
CAUTION: See separate listing for Soy.

Scientific Names
Nattokinase.

People Use This For
Orally, nattokinase is used for cardiovascular disease, stroke, angina, deep vein thrombosis (DVT), atherosclerosis, hemorrhoids, venous stasis, varicose veins, peripheral vascular disease, claudication, pain, fibromyalgia, chronic fatigue syndrome, endometriosis, uterine fibroids, muscle spasms, hypertension, infertility, cancer, and beriberi.

Safety
LIKELY SAFE ...when used orally in amounts commonly found in foods. Nattokinase is a natural component of the soy food natto. It has been routinely consumed in Japanese cultures for hundreds of years (12072,12073).
POSSIBLY SAFE ...when used orally in two doses. There is preliminary evidence that taking two doses separated by 6 hours of a specific combination product containing nattokinase (Flite Tabs) seems to be safe (12075). There is not enough evidence to know if taking multiple doses of nattokinase supplements is safe.
PREGNANCY AND LACTATION: Insufficient information available; avoid using.

Effectiveness
INSUFFICIENT RELIABLE EVIDENCE to RATE

Deep vein thrombosis (DVT). There is some evidence that taking a specific combination product (Flite Tabs) might decrease the risk of DVT during long-haul plane flights. The product combines a blend of 150 mg of nattokinase plus pycnogenol. Two capsules are taken 2 hours before the flight and then again 6 hours later (12075). More evidence is needed to rate nattokinase for this use.

Mechanism of Action
Nattokinase is a fibrinolytic enzyme derived from a Japanese food called natto. Natto is boiled soybeans fermented with the bacteria Bacillus natto (12072,12090). Nattokinase is thought to be produced through this specific fermentation process. Therefore, nattokinase isn't a component of other soy foods.

Nattokinase works by inactivating plasminogen activator inhibitor 1 (PAI-1) (12070,12091). Nattokinase has fibrinolytic activity that is 4-times more potent than plasmin (12074). Its average activity is about 40 CU (plasmin units) /gram (12072).

Nattokinase is thought to help for atherosclerosis due to its fibrinolytic activity at the blood vessel wall. There is preliminary evidence from animal models that taking a natto extract containing nattokinase can reduce vessel wall thickening following endothelial injury. Nattokinase also seems to cause lysis of thrombi that form at the vessel wall (12070,12071).

Nattokinase seems to be orally available when administered to humans. Taking enteric-coated nattokinase capsules 1.3 grams three times daily seems to significantly increase measures of fibrinolytic activity for 2 to 8 hours (12073).

Adverse Reactions
None reported.

Interactions with Herbs & Other Dietary Supplements
SUPPLEMENTS WITH ANTICOAGULANT/ANTIPLATELET POTENTIAL: Nattokinase has thrombolytic activity (12070). Taking nattokinase along with other supplements that might have antiplatelet or anticoagulant effects might increase the risk of bruising and bleeding. Some supplements that might have antiplatelet or anticoagulant activity include angelica, clove, danshen, garlic, ginger, ginkgo, fish oil, turmeric, vitamin E, willow, and others.

Interactions with Drugs
ANTICOAGULANT/ANTIPLATELET DRUGS: Nattokinase has thrombolytic activity (12070). Theoretically, taking nattokinase with drugs that have antiplatelet or anticoagulant effects might increase the risk of bruising and bleeding. Some of these drugs include aspirin, clopidogrel (Plavix), diclofenac (Voltaren, Cataflam, others), ibuprofen (Advil, Motrin, others), naproxen (Anaprox, Naprosyn, others), dalteparin (Fragmin), enoxaparin (Lovenox), heparin, warfarin (Coumadin), and others.

Interactions with Foods
None known.

Interactions with Lab Tests
None known.

Interactions with Diseases or Conditions
BLEEDING DISORDERS: Nattokinase has thrombolytic effects (12070) and may exacerbate bleeding disorders; use with caution.

Dosage and Administration
ORAL: For preventing deep vein thrombosis (DVT) during long-haul flights, a specific product (Flite Tabs) containing a 150 mg blend of nattokinase plus pycnogenol has been used. Two capsules are taken 2 hours before the flight and 2 capsules are taken 6 hours later (12075).

Comments
Nattokinase was discovered by a University of Chicago researcher, Dr. Hiroyuki Sumi. He referred to it as "The Enzyme of Enzymes." Natto, which nattokinase is derived from, has been a popular food in the Japanese culture for hundreds of years. It has also been used as a folk remedy for cardiovascular diseases.

NEEM

Also Known As
Arishta, Bead Tree, Holy Tree, Indian Lilac, Margosa, Nim, Nimb, Nimba, Persian Lilac, Pride of China.

Scientific Names
Azadirachta indica, synonyms Antelaea azadirachta, Melia azadirachta.
Family: Meliaceae.

People Use This For
Orally, neem is used for fever, dyspepsia, respiratory conditions, and infectious diseases. The bark is used for malaria and skin diseases. The leaves are used for worm infections, ulcers, cardiovascular disease, diabetes and gingivitis. The stem, root bark, and fruit are used as a tonic and astringent.
Topically, neem is used to treat head lice, for skin diseases, and as a mosquito repellent.
Intravaginally, neem is used as a contraceptive.
Neem is also used as an insecticide.

Safety
POSSIBLY SAFE ...when the oil is used orally (6).
LIKELY UNSAFE ...when large amounts of seeds are used orally because it can cause poisoning (6).
There is insufficient reliable information available about the safety of the above ground parts of neem.
CHILDREN: LIKELY UNSAFE ...when the oil or seeds are taken orally. There are reports of infants who were severely poisoned and died (3473,3474,3476).
PREGNANCY AND LACTATION: Insufficient reliable information available; avoid using.

Effectiveness
There is insufficient reliable information available about the effectiveness of neem.

Mechanism of Action
The applicable parts of neem are the above ground parts. Neem has varied constituents and pharmacological activity. Neem bark and leaves contain tannin and oil (18). Neem seeds yield a fixed oil composed primarily of glycerides and bitter compounds including nimbin, nimbinin and nimbidol (6). A small study in women demonstrated neem oil has spermicidal and contraceptive properties when used intravaginally (6). In animals, oral administration of oil reduced blood glucose levels by up to 48%, which lends some credence to the folk use for diabetes (6). In vitro studies suggest neem oil possesses antibacterial activity against varied organisms (6). A toothpaste containing neem extract exhibited antimicrobial activity and low levels of abrasiveness (6). Leaves of neem may be useful in preventing plaque formation (3). Constituents gedunin and nimbolide show in vitro antimalarial activity (6). Though neem oil is toxic to infants and children, the toxic constituent is unknown (3473,3475). Researchers speculate that a long-chain monounsaturated free acid may be responsible (3475).

Adverse Reactions
Orally, severe poisoning in infants and small children characterized by vomiting, loose stools, drowsiness, metabolic acidosis, anemia, polymorphonuclear leukocytosis, seizure, loss of consciousness, coma, cerebral edema, Reye-like syndrome symptoms and death have been reported to occur within hours after ingestion of neem oil (3473,3474,3476). Liver and renal biopsy reports have revealed pathologic findings seen typically in Reye's syndrome (3473,3474,3475).

Interactions with Herbs & Other Dietary Supplements
None known.

Interactions with Drugs
None known.

Interactions with Foods
None known.

Interactions with Lab Tests
None known.

Interactions with Diseases or Conditions
None known.

Dosage and Administration
ORAL: Neem is typically used as a tincture (18).
TOPICAL: No typical dosage.

Comments
Azadirachtin, the insecticide constituent of seeds, is effective in concentrations as low as 0.1 ppm. It is biodegradable, non-mutagenic and nontoxic to fish, birds and "warm-blooded animals" (6). The Environmental Protection Agency has approved the use of a neem formulation (Margosan-O) as a pesticide for limited use on nonfood crops (6).

NERVE ROOT

Also Known As
American Valerian, Bleeding Heart, Cypripedium, Lady's Slipper, Moccasin Flower, Monkey Flower, Noah's Ark, Shoe, Slipper Root, Venus Shoe, Yellows.

Scientific Names
Cypripedium parviflorum, synonym Cypripedium pubescens; Cypripedium calceolus.
Family: Orchidaceae.

People Use This For
Orally, nerve root is used for menorrhagia and diarrhea. Nerve root is also used orally for insomnia; emotional tension; hysteria; anxiety states; agitation; nervousness; and specifically, anxiety states associated with insomnia. Topically, nerve root is used to treat pruritus vulvae.

Safety
POSSIBLY UNSAFE ...when the root or rhizome is used orally. Nerve root is reported to cause hallucinations (4).
PREGNANCY AND LACTATION: POSSIBLY UNSAFE ...when used orally (4); avoid using.

Effectiveness
There is insufficient reliable information available about the effectiveness of nerve root.

Mechanism of Action
The applicable parts of nerve root are the rhizome and root. Nerve root contains tannins, glycosides, resins, quinones and a volatile oil (4,18), and is said to have astringent and styptic properties (18). The quinone constituent of nerve root is thought to be responsible for its sensitizing properties (4).

Adverse Reactions
Orally, nerve root can cause hallucinations (4). Large doses are associated with giddiness, restlessness, headache, mental excitement and visual hallucinations (4).
Topically, it can cause contact dermatitis (4).

Interactions with Herbs & Other Dietary Supplements
None known.

Interactions with Drugs
None known.

Interactions with Foods
None known.

Interactions with Lab Tests
None known.

Interactions with Diseases or Conditions
None known.

Dosage and Administration
ORAL: A typical dose is 2-4 grams dried rhizome/root or as tea (steep 2-4 grams dried rhizome/root in 150 mL of boiling water for 5-10 minutes, strain), three times daily (4). A liquid extract (1:1 in 45% alcohol) 2-4 mL is typically used three times daily (4).

Comments
Avoid confusion with Calypso bulbosa (Cypripedium bulbosum) and Cypripedium parviflorum, related species also known as lady's slipper.

NEW JERSEY TEA

Also Known As
Jersey Tea, Mountain-Sweet, Redroot, Red Root, Walpole Tea, Wild Snowball.

Scientific Names
Ceanothus americanus, synonym Ceanothus intermedius.
Family: Rhamnaceae.

People Use This For
Orally, New Jersey tea has been used orally as an expectorant, antispasmodic, clotting agent, an astringent, to treat gonorrhea, syphilis, colds, fever, chills, pelvic cysts, and as a lymphagogue.

Safety
LIKELY SAFE ...when used as an oral medicinal (12,18).
PREGNANCY AND LACTATION: Insufficient reliable information available; avoid using.

Effectiveness
There is insufficient reliable information available about the effectiveness of New Jersey tea.

Mechanism of Action
The applicable parts of New Jersey tea are the root, root bark, and leaf. New Jersey tea contains cyclic peptide alkaloids and triterpenes (18). An aqueous-ethanol extract of New Jersey tea is said to reduce the blood-clotting time by 25% in blood taken from young rats (18).

Adverse Reactions
None reported.

Interactions with Herbs & Other Dietary Supplements
None known.

Interactions with Drugs
None known.

Interactions with Foods
None known.

Interactions with Lab Tests
None known.

Interactions with Diseases or Conditions
None known.

Dosage and Administration
ORAL: New Jersey tea is typically used as an extract (18).

NEW ZEALAND GREEN-LIPPED MUSSEL

Also Known As
Green Lipped Mussel, New Zealand Green Lipped Mussel, NZGLM.

Scientific Names
Perna canaliculus.
Family: Mytilidae.

People Use This For
Orally, New Zealand green-lipped mussel is used for symptoms of rheumatoid arthritis and osteoarthritis.

Safety
POSSIBLY SAFE ...when used orally. There is only limited information available (6).
PREGNANCY: POSSIBLY UNSAFE ...when used orally; avoid using. It may cause retarded fetal development and delay in parturition (936).
LACTATION: Insufficient reliable information available; avoid using.

Effectiveness
POSSIBLY INEFFECTIVE

Rheumatoid arthritis (RA). Taking New Zealand green-lipped mussel orally doesn't seem to help RA (6,935).

There is insufficient reliable information available about the effectiveness of New Zealand green-lipped mussel for its other uses.

Mechanism of Action
The dried New Zealand green-lipped mussels may contain a prostaglandin inhibitor that exerts an anti-inflammatory effect (932,933). Researchers report that an extract of New Zealand green-lipped mussel reduced symptoms in dogs with advanced arthritis. The results of this unpublished study were presented at the Experimental Biology 2000 conference (5055).

Adverse Reactions
Orally, New Zealand green-lipped mussel can cause diarrhea, nausea, and flatulence (6). One case was reported of reversible, granulomatous hepatitis associated with New Zealand green-lipped mussel (6).

Interactions with Herbs & Other Dietary Supplements
None known.

Interactions with Drugs
None known.

Interactions with Foods
None known.

Interactions with Lab Tests
None known.

Interactions with Diseases or Conditions
None known.

Dosage and Administration
ORAL: New Zealand green-lipped mussel extract 300-350 mg three times per day was used in human studies for rheumatoid arthritis; except for one early trial, studies found New Zealand green-lipped mussels ineffective (6,935).

Comments
New Zealand green-lipped mussels are available commercially as a freeze dried, ground, and encapsulated product.

NIACIN AND NIACINAMIDE (VITAMIN B3)

Also Known As
3-Pyridine Carboxamide, Anti-Blacktongue Factor, Antipellagra Factor, B Complex Vitamin, Niacin-Niacinamide, Niacin/Niacinamide, Nicamid, Nicosedine, Nicotinamide, Nicotinic Acid Amide, Nicotylamidum, Pellagra Preventing Factor, Vitamin B-3, Vitamin PP.
CAUTION: See separate listings for Inositol Nicotinate (Inositol Hexaniacinate) and Tryptophan.

Scientific Names
Niacin; Niacinamide; Nicotinic acid; Vitamin B3.

People Use This For
Orally, niacin is used for hyperlipidemia. It is also used in conjunction with other therapies for peripheral vascular disease, vascular spasm, migraine headache, Meniere's syndrome, vertigo, and to reduce the diarrhea associated with cholera. Orally, niacin or niacinamide is also used for preventing vitamin B3 deficiency, treating pellagra, schizophrenia, drug-induced hallucinations, Alzheimer's disease and age-related cognitive decline, chronic brain syndrome, hyperkinesis, depression, motion sickness, alcohol dependence, vasculitis associated with skin lesions, and edema. Niacin or niacinamide is also used for acne, leprosy, attention deficit-hyperactivity disorder (ADHD), preventing premenstrual headache, improving digestion, for protection from toxins and pollutants, for reducing the effects of aging, memory loss, arthritis, lowering blood pressure, improving circulation, promoting relaxation, improving orgasm, and preventing cataracts. Niacinamide is also used orally treating diabetes, and the skin conditions bullous pemphigoid and granuloma annulare.
Topically, niacinamide is used for treating inflammatory acne vulgaris.

Safety
LIKELY SAFE ...when used orally and appropriately. Niacin and niacinamide are FDA-approved products (12033).
POSSIBLY SAFE ...when niacinamide is used topically and appropriately up to 12 weeks (5940).
PREGNANCY AND LACTATION: LIKELY SAFE ...when used orally in amounts that do not exceed the recommended dietary allowance (RDA). The RDA for pregnant and lactating women, 14-18 years is 30 mg. For pregnant and lactating women older than 18 years the RDA is 35 mg (6243). There is insufficient reliable information available about the safety of larger oral doses of niacin, niacinamide, or topical niacinamide when used during pregnancy or lactation; avoid using.

Effectiveness
EFFECTIVE

Hyperlipidemia. Some niacin products are FDA-approved prescription products for treating hyperlipidemia. These prescription niacin products typically come in high strengths of 500 mg or higher. Dietary supplement forms of niacin usually come in strengths of 250 mg or less. Since very high doses of niacin are required for hyperlipidemia, dietary supplement niacin usually isn't appropriate.

Prescription niacin is generally considered a second-line therapy for patients who mainly need to decrease low-density lipoprotein (LDL) cholesterol. But niacin is often considered first-line for patients with mixed hyperlipidemia or patients who need to increase high-density lipoprotein (HDL) cholesterol. Niacin only reduces LDL cholesterol by about 5% to 25%, compared to 18% to 55% with statins. But niacin can decrease triglycerides by 20% to 50% and increase HDL by 15% to 35% (4818,4867,4886,4887,4888,4889,4890,12033). Niacin is also commonly combined with other cholesterol-lowering drugs when diet and single-drug therapy are not adequately effective (4867). Concurrent use of statins with 1 or 2 grams of sustained release niacin daily can additionally reduce total cholesterol by 8% or 21%, LDL by 8% or 31%, triglycerides by 24% or 27%, and increase HDL by 23% or 27% (8545).

The effects of niacin are dose-dependent. The most pronounce increases in HDL and decreases in triglycerides occur at 1200-1500 mg/day. Niacin's greatest effects on LDL occur at 2000-3000 mg/day (12033). A very low dose of niacin, 50 mg daily, can modestly increase HDL cholesterol by 2.1 mg/dL, but appears to have no effect on total cholesterol, LDL cholesterol, or triglycerides when added to statin therapy (8546). Niacin also seems to be effective for isolated hypoalphalipoproteinemia (4817). Niacinamide has no effect on lipid levels in patients with hyperlipidemia.

Niacin deficiency and pellagra. Both niacin and niacinamide are FDA-approved for the prevention and treatment of niacin deficiency and pellagra. Niacinamide is sometimes preferred for this indication because it lacks the vasodilating effects of niacin (15,6243).

POSSIBLY EFFECTIVE

Alzheimer's disease. There is some evidence that people who consume higher amounts of niacin (17-45 mg/day) from food and multivitamin sources have a lower risk of developing Alzheimer's disease compared to people who consume less niacin (14 mg/day) (12077). Food sources high in niacin include meat, fish, beans, nuts, coffee, and fortified grains and cereals. Explain to patients that there is no reliable evidence that taking a stand-alone niacin supplement is beneficial for reducing the risk of Alzheimer's disease.

Atherosclerosis. Taking niacin orally, in combination with a bile acid sequestrant, seems to reduce atherosclerosis in high-risk men with existing cardiovascular disease. In a large-scale trial, niacin plus colestipol significantly decreased coronary atherosclerosis progression; increased frequency of atherosclerosis regression; and decreased incidence of cardiovascular events including death, myocardial infarction, and revascularization procedures (4848).

Cardiovascular disease. Taking niacin orally, in combination with simvastatin (Zocor), seems to reduce cardiovascular disease risk in people with coronary disease and low high-density lipoprotein (HDL) cholesterol. Patients titrated up to 2-4 grams of sustained-release niacin and 10-20 mg simvastatin daily seem to have a reduced risk of a first cardiovascular event such as death, myocardial infarction (MIs), or stroke. This combination also seems to cause regression of coronary stenosis (7388). Taking niacin alone also seems to reduce the risk of secondary MIs. In a large scale, long-term study, high-dose niacin significantly reduced the risk of a second heart attack in men; however, there was not a significant decrease in overall or cause-specific mortality (4847).

Cataracts. Taking niacin orally seems to reduce the occurrence of cataracts. A large-scale population-based study found high dietary intake of niacin is associated with a reduced risk of nuclear cataracts (6378).

Cholera. Taking niacin orally seems to control fluid loss due to cholera (4868). In a randomized controlled study, divided doses of 2 grams of nicotinic acid daily reduced diarrhea in adults with cholera (4868). Laboratory evidence supports the use of nicotinic acid, but not niacinamide, to reduce intestinal secretion induced by cholera toxin (4869).

Diabetes. Taking high-dose niacinamide orally seems to help reduce the risk of type 1 diabetes in high-risk children (4874). Following the success of this trial, a very large, multinational, long-term study was begun to determine whether regular use of niacinamide can prevent diabetes (4876). Preliminary results released by a German group found no protective effect, but the authors cautioned that their findings did not exclude the possibility that niacinamide might be effective (4875). There is also evidence that suggests niacinamide might reserve residual beta-cell function in newly diagnosed type 1 diabetes (4877,4878,4879,4880). Clinical trials, including one placebo-controlled trial and one vitamin E-comparison study showed niacinamide might prolong the "honeymoon period" in newly-diagnosed type 1 diabetes when the pancreas is still capable of producing some insulin (4877,4878,4879,4880). The clinical studies to date have been performed by one group of Italian investigators. Concerns about potential concurrent induction of insulin resistance have been raised (4881). Niacinamide is also useful when used orally for protecting residual beta-cell function and improving glycemic control in adults with type 2 diabetes (4882). In a small, placebo-controlled, single-blind study, niacinamide increased C-peptide release and improved insulin secretion in lean diabetics who had failed sulfonylurea therapy (4882).

Osteoarthritis. Taking niacinamide orally, 3 grams daily in divided doses, seems to improve joint flexibility and reduce inflammation, and might allow for a reduction in standard anti-inflammatory drug doses (4883).

INSUFFICIENT RELIABLE EVIDENCE to RATE

Attention deficit-hyperactivity disorder (ADHD). There is conflicting preliminary clinical evidence regarding the usefulness of niacinamide in combination with other megadose vitamins for the treatment of ADHD (3351,9957). More evidence is needed to rate niacinamide for this use.

Mechanism of Action

Vitamin B3 includes niacin (nicotinic acid) and niacinamide (nicotinamide) (6243). The term niacin refers specifically to nicotinic acid, but is also used collectively to refer to both nicotinic acid and nicotinamide (niacinamide). Niacin is converted to niacinamide when ingested in amounts that do not exceed physiological requirements. The pharmacological effects of niacin and niacinamide are indistinguishable. Niacin is a water-soluble vitamin which is well absorbed when used orally (6243). Dietary sources include meats, beans, and various niacin-fortified foods. In addition, dietary tryptophan is biosynthetically converted to niacin (60 mg tryptophan equals 1 mg of niacin or one niacin equivalent) (6243). Niacinamide is required for lipid metabolism, tissue respiration, and glycogenolysis. Niacinamide is incorporated into the coenzymes, nicotinamide adenine dinucleotide (NAD), and nicotinamide adenine dinucleotide phosphate (NADP). These coenzymes act as hydrogen-carrier molecules.

Niacin deficiency causes pellagra, a condition that affects the gastrointestinal tract, skin, and central nervous system (6243). Pellagra was common in the early twentieth century, but niacin-fortified foods have virtually eliminated this deficiency disease except in conditions such as chronic alcoholism (4850). Some researchers think that sleep deprivation-induced dermatitis might be caused by niacin depletion because of similarities between this condition and pellagra (1350). Causes of niacin deficiency include poor diet, isoniazid therapy, carcinoid tumors that decrease endogenous production, and Hartnup disease, an autosomal recessive disorder that interferes with tryptophan absorption (6243). Conditions that increase niacin requirements, such as hyperthyroidism, diabetes mellitus, liver cirrhosis, pregnancy, and lactation, rarely cause deficiency (4969).

When doses of niacin or niacinamide greater than 300-800 mg daily are administered different pharmacological effects occur. Niacin 1000 mg or more per day can decrease total cholesterol by 8 to 21%, low-density lipoprotein (LDL) cholesterol by 8 to 25%, triglycerides by 20 to 50%, and increase high-density lipoprotein (HDL) concentrations by 15 to 35% (4867,8545). The exact mechanism for the beneficial effects on serum lipids is unknown, but niacin inhibits free fatty acid release from adipose tissue; and inhibits cyclic AMP accumulation which controls the activity of triglyceride lipase and hence lipolysis. It also decreases the rate of liver synthesis of LDL and VLDL; and increases the rate of chylomicron triglyceride removal from plasma secondary to increased lipoprotein lipase activity (6243). Niacin produces vasodilation of cutaneous blood vessels of the face, neck, and chest, probably mediated by prostaglandins, such as prostacyclin. In most individuals, tolerance to these effects occurs within two weeks (15). Preliminary clinical data suggest that some people with schizophrenia do not experience the characteristic vasodilatory response to niacin, suggesting an impaired response to phospholipid-dependent signaling (4870). Niacin also causes the release of histamine, which increases gastric motility and acid secretion (15). Niacin in combination with riboflavin might reduce the incidence of cataract development in older people (4885). Niacin might have beneficial effects on coagulation in people at risk for cardiovascular disease. Preliminary clinical research indicates that niacin reduces fibrinogen concentrations in plasma and stimulates fibrinolysis in hyperlipidemic men (4871). In patients with peripheral arterial disease niacin lowers fibrinogen and F1.2, a marker of thrombin conversion (8547). Large amounts of niacin can decrease uric acid excretion (15).

Niacinamide has no beneficial effect on lipids and should not be used for treating hyperlipidemia (6243). Niacinamide does not cause the vasodilation associated with niacin (6243). High-dose niacinamide prevents or delays insulin deficiency in laboratory models of type 1 diabetes and protects islet cells from cytotoxic actions (4872,4873). Niacinamide is a free radical scavenger and might alter the auto-immune processes in type 1 diabetes that cause beta-cell destruction (4872,4873). Niacinamide is hypothesized to inhibit induction of nitric oxide synthase by interleukin 1 in chondrocytes, leading researchers to speculate about its potential use in destructive joint diseases (4884).

Adverse Reactions

Orally, small amounts of niacin and niacinamide typically found in dietary supplements are well-tolerated and cause minor adverse reactions. But doses of niacin as low as 30 mg/day can sometimes cause flushing, burning, tingling, and itching sensations as well as erythema on the face, arms, and chest (6243). Flushing may be accompanied by itching, headache, increased intracranial blood flow, and occasionally, pain (6243). Onset is highly variable, from within 30 minutes to as long as 6 weeks after the initial dose (6243). Higher doses of niacin are more likely to cause these side effects. Slow dose titration, pretreatment with 325 mg aspirin, and taking niacin with meals or the sustained release product at bedtime may reduce flushing (4852,4853,4854,4858). Flushing tends to decrease over time, despite dosage elevation (4864).

At higher doses, side effects distinguish niacin and niacinamide (6243). Niacinamide in large amounts is associated with headache, dizziness, nausea and vomiting, diarrhea, blurred vision, hepatotoxicity, hyperglycemia, abnormal prothrombin times, and hypoalbuminemia (15).

Niacin in large amounts is associated with flushing, pruritus, burning sensations, stinging or tingling of the skin, nausea, bloating, flatulence, hunger pains, vomiting, heartburn, diarrhea, increased sebaceous gland activity, hypotension, dizziness, tachycardia, arrhythmias, syncope, vasovagal attacks, headache, and blurred vision (15). Dental and gingival pain have also been reported (4862). In most people taking niacin, flushing and other skin sensations, increased sebaceous gland activity, and increased gastrointestinal motility disappear within two weeks; however, adverse effects have been reported to appear up to 2 years after initiation of therapy (4851).

Immediate-release niacin products are more likely to cause flushing and other vasodilatory side effects. Extended-release formulations may reduce the occurrence of these side effects (4857). But extended release or sustained release niacin products seem to increase the risk of hepatotoxicity (4855,4856,12026).

Niacin, particularly at doses of 3 to 9 grams per day, might cause jaundice and elevated serum transaminases (6243).

The drug should be discontinued if liver function tests rise to three times the upper limit of normal (4863). Severe hepatotoxicity with fulminant hepatitis and subsequent liver transplant has been reported (6243).
Chronic use of large amounts of niacin have been associated with rash, hyperpigmentation resembling acanthosis nigricans, dry skin, xerostomia, hyperuricemia, gout, peptic ulcer, amblyopia, proptosis, loss of central vision secondary to an atypical form of cystoid macular edema, nervousness, panic, hyperglycemia, abnormal glucose tolerance and glycosuria, hepatotoxicity, abnormal prothrombin times and hypoalbuminemia (15). Niacin in higher doses can significantly raise homocysteine levels; 17% increase with 1000 mg niacin per day and 55% with 3000 mg per day (1733). Elevated homocysteine levels are an independent risk factor for arterial occlusive disease (490); however, the clinical significance of the effect of niacin on homocysteine is not yet known.

Interactions with Herbs & Other Dietary Supplements

ANTIOXIDANTS: Concurrent use of the antioxidants vitamins C and E, beta-carotene, and selenium seems to blunt the positive effect of niacin on high-density lipoprotein (HDL) cholesterol. Antioxidant supplements also appear to antagonize the beneficial effect of the combination of simvastatin (Zocor) and sustained-release niacin on cardiovascular disease risk (7388). This combination of antioxidants reduces the HDL-2-raising effects of niacin and HMG-CoA reductase inhibitors by more than 50% in people with heart disease (7388).
HEPATOTOXIC HERBS AND SUPPLEMENTS: Niacin can adversely affect the liver (4863). Theoretically, concomitant use with other potentially hepatotoxic products might increase the risk of developing liver damage. Some of these products include androstenedione, borage leaf, chaparral, coenzyme Q-10 (only in high doses), comfrey, dehydroepiandrosterone (DHEA), germander, pennyroyal oil, red yeast, and others.

Interactions with Drugs

ANTIDIABETES DRUGS: Niacin and niacinamide can interfere with blood glucose control requiring dosing adjustment of antidiabetic agents. Niacin and niacinamide can cause hyperglycemia, abnormal glucose tolerance, and glycosuria. Increased blood glucose monitoring may be necessary, particularly early in the course of treatment (4859,4860,12033). Monitor blood glucose levels carefully.
HMG-CoA REDUCTASE INHIBITORS ("Statins"): Concomitant use of niacin with HMG-CoA reductase inhibitors can increase the risk of myopathy. HMG-CoA reductase inhibitors include atorvastatin (Lipitor), cerivastatin (Baycol), fluvastatin (Lescol), lovastatin (Mevacor), pravastatin (Pravachol), and simvastatin (Zocor). NCEP guidelines suggest combination therapy only when diet and single drug therapy is not sufficiently effective (4867).
TRANSDERMAL NICOTINE (Nicoderm, Nicotrol): Concomitant use with niacin can increase the risk of flushing and dizziness (15).

Drug Influences on Nutrient Levels and Depletion

SOME DRUGS CAN AFFECT NIACIN AND NIACINAMIDE LEVELS:
ANTIBIOTICS: Destruction of normal gastrointestinal flora by antibiotics can cause decreased production of B vitamins. The clinical significance of this decreased production is not known. Consider supplementation only if clinical judgment warrants it (4434,4435,4436,4437,4438,4439,4440,4441,4442,4443).
BILE ACID SEQUESTRANTS: Cholestyramine (Questran) and colestipol (Colestid) reduce niacin absorption (15).
ISONIAZID (INH): Isoniazid inhibits the conversion of tryptophan to niacin and might induce pellagra, particularly in poorly nourished patients (4865,4866).

Interactions with Foods

HOT DRINKS: Concomitant ingestion of niacin and hot drinks can magnify niacin-induced flushing (6243).

Interactions with Lab Tests

CATECHOLAMINES: Niacin can falsely increase some urinary catecholamine fluorometric assay results. Niacin produces fluorescent substances in the urine, which can falsely elevate test results (15).
GLUCOSE: Niacin can cause a false-positive reactions with urine glucose tests which rely on cupric sulfate solution (Benedict's reagent) (15).
HOMOCYSTEINE: At higher doses, niacin can increase homocysteine levels. Doses of 1000 mg and 3000 mg per day reportedly increase homocysteine levels by 17% and 55% respectively (1733).
LIVER FUNCTION TESTS: Both niacin and niacinamide can increase serum bilirubin, alanine aminotransferase (ALT), aspartate aminotransferase (AST), and lactate dehydrogenase (LDH) concentrations and test results. Liver function tests should be monitored regularly, particularly early in the course of therapy and in patients receiving long-term treatment with high doses of niacin or niacinamide. Niacin should be discontinued if liver function tests rise to three times the upper limit of normal (4863).

Interactions with Diseases or Conditions

ALLERGIES: Niacin and niacinamide might exacerbate allergies by causing histamine release (15).
CORONARY ARTERY DISEASE/UNSTABLE ANGINA: Large amounts of niacin can increase the risk of cardiac arrhythmias. One study showed an increased incidence of cardiac arrhythmias when niacin was used in patients with coronary artery disease (15); use with caution.

CROHN'S DISEASE: Nicotinic acid (niacin) serum levels decrease with increases in the Crohn's disease activity index in patients who do not receive nutritional treatments (6269).
DIABETES: Niacin and niacinamide can interfere with blood glucose control requiring dosing adjustment of antidiabetic agents. Niacin and niacinamide can cause hyperglycemia, abnormal glucose tolerance, and glycosuria. Increased blood glucose monitoring may be necessary, particularly early in the course of treatment (4859,4860,12033).
GALLBLADDER DISEASE: Niacin or niacinamide might exacerbate gallbladder disease (15); use with caution.
GOUT: Large amounts of niacin or niacinamide might precipitate gout. Niacin and niacinamide can cause hyperuricemia (12033); use with caution.
KIDNEY DISEASE: Niacin is excreted unchanged in the urine and might accumulate in patients with kidney disease (15); use with caution.
LIVER DISEASE: Contraindicated; niacin and niacinamide have been associated with liver damage. Avoid large amounts in patients with a history of liver disease (12026,12033).
PEPTIC ULCER DISEASE: Contraindicated in patients with active peptic ulcer disease. Large amounts of niacin or niacinamide might activate peptic ulcer disease (15); use with caution in patients with a history of peptic ulcer disease.
SEVERE HYPOTENSION: Contraindicated; niacin can cause hypotension (15).

Dosage and Administration

ORAL: For hyperlipidemia the effects of niacin are dose-dependent. The most pronounce increases in HDL and decreases in triglycerides occur at 1200-1500 mg/day. Niacin's greatest effects on LDL occur at 2000-3000 mg/day (12033). To prevent coronary events in people with hyperlipidemia, niacin 4 grams daily has been used (4848). For preventing and treating vitamin B3 deficiency, doses of nicotinic acid and niacinamide are considered equivalent. For mild vitamin B3 deficiency, niacin or niacinamide 50-100 mg per day is used. For pellagra in adults, niacin or niacinamide 300-500 mg daily is given in divided doses. For pellagra in children, niacin or niacinamide 100-300 mg daily is given in divided doses. For Hartnup disease, niacin or niacinamide 50-200 mg daily is used (15). For reducing fluid loss induced by cholera toxin, niacin 2 grams daily has been used (4868). To prevent type 1 diabetes in high-risk children, sustained-release niacinamide 1.2 grams/m2 (body surface area) per day has been used (4875). To slow disease progression of newly diagnosed type 1 diabetes, niacinamide 25 mg/kg daily has been used (4878). For treating osteoarthritis, niacinamide 3 grams per day in divided doses has been used (4883). A daily dietary intake of approximately 44 mg of niacin has been associated with reduced risk of nuclear cataracts (6378).
The daily recommended dietary allowances (RDAs) of niacin are: Infants 0-6 months, 2 mg; Infants 7-12 months, 4 mg; Children 1-3 years, 6 mg; Children 4-8 years, 8 mg; Children 9-13 years, 12 mg; Men 14 years and older, 16 mg; Women 14 years and older, 14 mg; Pregnant women, 18 mg; and Lactating women, 17 mg (6243). The maximum daily dose of niacin is: Children 1-3 years, 10 mg; Children 4-8 years, 15 mg; Children 9-13 years, 20 mg; Adults, including Pregnant and Lactating women, 14-18 years, 30 mg; and Adults, including pregnant and lactating women, older than 18 years, 35 mg (6243).

Comments

Vitamin B3 is present in many foods including yeast, meat, fish, milk, eggs, green vegetables, and cereal grains. The term niacin is used to refer specifically to nicotinic acid, but is also used collectively to refer to both nicotinic acid and nicotinamide (niacinamide). Niacin and niacinamide are frequently used in combination with other B vitamins in vitamin B complex formulations. Vitamin B complex generally includes vitamin B1 (Thiamine), vitamin B2 (Riboflavin), vitamin B3 (Niacin/Niacinamide), vitamin B5 (pantothenic acid), vitamin B6 (pyridoxine), vitamin B12 (cyanocobalamin), and folic acid. However, some products do not contain all of these ingredients and some may include others, such as biotin para-aminobenzoic acid (PABA), choline bitartrate, and inositol.

NIAULI OIL

Also Known As

Caje Oil, Niauli Aetheroleum.
CAUTION: See separate listings for Cajeput Oil and Tea Tree Oil.

Scientific Names

Melaleuca viridiflora.
Family: Myrtaceae.

People Use This For

Orally and topically, niauli oil is used for upper respiratory tract mucous membrane inflammation, cough, and bronchitis.

Safety
POSSIBLY SAFE ...when used orally and appropriately (2,18). ...when used topically and appropriately (12,18).
LIKELY UNSAFE ...when greater than 10 grams of oil is ingested orally. Can cause hypotension, circulatory disorders, and respiratory failure (18).
CHILDREN: LIKELY UNSAFE ...when used topically in the nasal and facial areas because it could cause bronchospasm, asthma-like symptoms, and respiratory failure (2,18).
PREGNANCY AND LACTATION: Insufficient reliable information available; avoid using.

Effectiveness
There is insufficient reliable information available about the effectiveness of niauli oil.

Mechanism of Action
Niauli oil contains cineole (7,9), which has in vitro antibacterial activity and stimulates circulation (2,18). Cineole has actions similar to that of eucalyptus oil (9). Cineole induces liver enzymes involved with drug metabolism (18).

Adverse Reactions
Orally, niauli oil can cause nausea, vomiting, and diarrhea (2). The consumption of amounts greater than 10 grams can cause hypotension, circulatory disorders, collapse, and respiratory failure (18).
Topically, it can cause glottal spasm, bronchospasm, and respiratory failure when applied to facial and nasal areas of infants and small children (2,18).

Interactions with Herbs & Other Dietary Supplements
None known.

Interactions with Drugs
None known.

Interactions with Foods
None known.

Interactions with Lab Tests
None known.

Interactions with Diseases or Conditions
GI TRACT DISEASE: Niauli oil is contraindicated in individuals with inflammatory diseases of the GI tract.
LIVER DISEASE: Contraindicated in individuals with severe liver disease or bile duct inflammation (2,18).

Dosage and Administration
ORAL: The typical dose of niauli oil is 200 mg per administration, up to 2 grams per day (2,18).
TOPICAL: Niauli oil is commonly used as oily nose drops, consisting of 2-5% niauli oil in vegetable oil (2,18). Other topical preparations contain 10-30% niauli oil in an oil base (2,18).

Comments
Niauli oil consists of the essential oil distilled from leaves of Melaleuca viridiflora. Avoid confusion with tea tree oil (Maleleuca alternifolia) and cajeput oil (Melaleuca leucodendra and Melaleuca quinquenervia).

NORTHERN PRICKLY ASH

Also Known As
Angelica Tree, Pepper Wood, Prickly Ash, Toothache Bark, Xanthoxylum, Yellow Wood, Zanthoxylum.
CAUTION: See separate listings for Ash and Southern Prickly Ash.

Scientific Names
Zanthoxylum americanum.
Family: Rutaceae.

People Use This For
Orally, northern prickly ash is used for cramps, intermittent claudication, Raynaud's syndrome, chronic rheumatic conditions, peripheral circulatory insufficiency associated with rheumatic symptoms, for low blood pressure, fever, inflammation, as a tonic, stimulant, for toothache, sores, ulcers, as a diaphoretic in fever, and cancer (as an ingredient in Hoxsey cure). In manufacturing, northern prickly ash is used as a flavoring agent in foods and beverages.

Safety
POSSIBLY SAFE ...when the bark is used orally and appropriately in medicinal amounts (12).
There is insufficient reliable information available about the safety of the oral use of northern prickly ash berry.
PREGNANCY: POSSIBLY UNSAFE ...when the bark is used orally (12); avoid using. There is insufficient reliable information available about the safety of the berry during pregnancy; avoid using.
LACTATION: insufficient reliable information available; avoid using.

Effectiveness
There is insufficient reliable information available about the effectiveness of northern prickly ash.

Mechanism of Action
The applicable parts of northern prickly ash are the bark and berry. There is insufficient reliable information available about the possible mechanism of action and active ingredients. Northern prickley ash contains alkaloids, coumarins, resin, acid volatile oil, and tannins which may be pharmacologically active (4).

Adverse Reactions
None reported.

Interactions with Herbs & Other Dietary Supplements
HERBS WITH ANTICOAGULANT/ANTIPLATELET POTENTIAL: Concomitant use of herbs that have constituents that might affect platelet aggregation could theoretically increase the risk of bleeding in some people. These herbs include angelica, danshen, garlic, ginger, ginkgo, Panax ginseng, horse chestnut, red clover, turmeric, and others.

Interactions with Drugs
ANTACIDS: Theoretically, due to reports that northern prickly ash increases stomach acid, northern prickly ash might decrease the effectiveness of antacids (19).
H2-BLOCKERS: Theoretically, due to reports that northern prickly ash increases stomach acid, northern prickly ash might decrease the effectiveness of H2-blockers (19). The H2 blockers include cimetidine (Tagamet), ranitidine (Zantac), nizatidine (Axid), and famotidine (Pepcid).
PROTON PUMP INHIBITORS (PPIs): Theoretically, due to reports that northern prickly ash increases stomach acid, northern prickly ash might decrease the effectiveness of PPIs (19). PPIs include omeprazole (Prilosec), lansoprazole (Prevacid), rabeprazole (Aciphex), pantoprazole (Protonix), and esomeprazole (Nexium).

Interactions with Foods
None known.

Interactions with Lab Tests
None known.

Interactions with Diseases or Conditions
GASTROINTESTINAL ULCERS: Contraindicated. Northern prickly ash can stimulate gastrointestinal secretions (19).
GI CONDITIONS: Northern prickly ash can irritate the gastrointestinal tract. It is contraindicated in individuals with infectious or inflammatory gastrointestinal conditions (19).

Dosage and Administration
ORAL, Bark: 1-3 grams dried bark, or drink as decoction (boil 1-3 grams dry bark 10-15 minutes, strain), three times daily; liquid bark extract (1:1 in 45% alcohol) 1-3 mL three times daily; bark tincture (1:5 in 45% alcohol) 2-5 mL three times daily (4).
ORAL, Berry: Liquid berry extract (1:1 in 45% alcohol) 0.5-1.5 mL (4).

NUTMEG AND MACE

Also Known As
Jaatipatree, Jatikosha, Jatipatra, Jatipatri, Jatiphala, Jatiphalam, Mace, Macis, Muscadier, Muskatbuam, Muskatnuss, Myristica, Myristicae Aril, Myristicae Semen, Noix Muscade, Nuez Moscada, Nutmeg, Nux Moschata.

Scientific Names
Myristica fragrans, synonym Myristica officinalis.
Family: Myristicaceae.

People Use This For

Orally, nutmeg and mace are used for diarrhea, nausea, gastric spasms, flatulence, and gastric mucosal inflammation. They are also used for cancer, kidney disease, insomnia, increasing menstrual flow, inducing abortion, as a hallucinogen, and a general tonic.
Topically, nutmeg and mace are used as an analgesic, especially for rheumatism, mouth sores, and toothache.
In foods, nutmeg and mace are used as culinary spices. In foods and beverages, nutmeg, nutmeg oil, mace, and mace oil are used as flavor components.
In manufacturing, nutmeg oil is used as a fragrance component in soaps and cosmetics.

Safety

LIKELY SAFE ...when used orally in amounts commonly found in foods. Nutmeg, mace, nutmeg oil and mace oil have Generally Recognized As Safe (GRAS) status in the US (4912).
LIKELY UNSAFE ...when used orally for self-medication in medicinal amounts (12). There is insufficient reliable information available about the safety of the topical use of nutmeg and mace.
PREGNANCY: POSSIBLY UNSAFE ...when used orally in medicinal amounts. Nutmeg and mace might have abortifacient activity, and safrole content might be mutagenic (12).
LACTATION: There is insufficient reliable information available about the safety of nutmeg and mace during lactation; avoid using.

Effectiveness

There is insufficient reliable information available for the effectiveness of nutmeg and mace.

Mechanism of Action

Both nutmeg and mace contain volatile oils with constituents that include myristicin, elemicin, eugenol, isoeugenol, gerinol, pinese, cineole, borneol, and safrole (2563). Volatile oil constituents of nutmeg and mace have a variety of individual pharmacological effects, some of which oppose others. For example, the volatile oil borneol is thought to be responsible for CNS stimulant effects, whereas several others such as methyleugenol, isoeugenol, safrole, myristicin, 1,8-cineole, geranyl acetate, and 1,8-p-methadiene seem to have sedative effects (2563). Alpha- and beta-pinene, and 1,8-cineole seem to have convulsant activity, whereas safrole, eugenol, and methyleugenol have anticonvulsant activity (2563). Nutmeg also has psychoactive effects and can cause hallucinations, feelings of unreality, euphoria, and delusions (2563). The constituents myristicin and elemicin are thought to be metabolized to amphetamine-related compounds (6), but this has not yet been verified (2563). Myristicin and elemicin might also have effects on serotonergic systems and possibly have an antidepressant effect (2563). Some constituents have anesthetic activity such as myristicin, methyleugenol, methylisoeugenol, safrole, and 1,8-cineole (2563). Antihistaminic effects have been found with elemicin and methylisoeugenol (2563). High doses of nutmeg can cause anticholinergic side effects, but the constituents 1,8-cineole and alpha-terpinene are reported to have anticholinesterase activity (2563). Nutmeg and mace and their oils have a variety of other effects including antispasmodic (2,6), antioxidant (11), hypotensive (2563), emetic (6), antibacterial, antifungal (6) and larvicidal effects (11). Calcium antagonist activity has been reported with myristicin, eugenol, and safrole (2563). Myristicin, eugenol, and isoeugenol inhibit prostaglandin activity and might have anti-inflammatory properties (6). Safrole found in nutmeg oil promotes liver carcinomas in mice (6). Animal studies suggest myristicin acts as an inducer of cytochrome P-450 enzyme systems (3492,3493) and may inhibit tumor formation (3492).

Adverse Reactions

Orally, nutmeg and mace can cause significant side effects when used in amounts greater than those found in foods. Anticholinergic effects can occur with doses of 9 teaspoons of nutmeg powder such as flushing, tachycardia, and dry mouth (2563). Higher doses can cause more significant side effects. For example, ingestion of 5 grams or more of powdered nutmeg or mace can cause thirst, dry mouth, nausea and vomiting, burning epigastric pain, urgency, weak pulse, tachycardia, hypotension, flushing, feeling of pressure in the chest or lower abdomen, hot and cold sensations, sweating, hypothermia, dizziness, blurred vision, double and triple vision, miosis, nystagmus, headache, numbness, weakness, unsteady gait, drowsiness, stupor, disorientation, euphoria, anxiety, panic, mild to intense visual hallucinations, often with sensation of limb loss and fear of impending death, auditory hallucinations, agitation, hyperactivity, aimless wandering, incoherent and irrelevant speech, combativeness, seizures, shock, coma, and occasionally death (9,12,2492,2563,3492,3494). Many of these symptoms are attributed to excessive anticholinergic activity. Symptoms generally occur 2-6 hours after ingestion and recovery usually occurs within 24 hours, but can take several days, depending on the dose used (3492).
In pregnant women, large amounts can also cause abortion (2).
Topically, nutmeg can cause allergic dermatitis (6,18).

Interactions with Herbs & Other Dietary Supplements

SAFROLE-CONTAINING HERBS: Avoid concomitant use with other safrole-containing herbs due to potential for additive toxicity (12). Other herbs that contain safrole include basil, camphor, and cinnamon (12).

Interactions with Drugs

CYTOCHROME P450 1A1 (CYP1A1) SUBSTRATES: Theoretically, concomitant use may affect drugs metabolized by cytochrome P450 1A1(CYP1A1) enzyme system (3493). Some of these drugs include chlorzoxazone, theophylline, and bufuralol.
CYTOCHROME P450 1A2 (CYP1A2) SUBSTRATES: Theoretically, concomitant use may affect drugs metabolized by cytochrome P450 1A2 (CYP1A2) enzyme system (3493).
CYTOCHROME P450 2B1 (CYP2B1) SUBSTRATES: Theoretically, concomitant use may affect drugs metabolized by cytochrome P450 2B1 (CPY2B1) enzyme system (3493).
CYTOCHROME P450 2B2 (CYP2B2) SUBSTRATES: Theoretically, concomitant use may affect drugs metabolized by cytochrome P450 2B2 (CYP2B2) enzyme system (3493).
PHENOBARBITAL (Luminal): Theoretically, concomitant use may decrease the therapeutic effects of phenobarbital (3492). Studies suggest myristicin, a constituent of nutmeg and mace, acts as an inducer of cytochrome P450 enzyme systems (3492,3493).

Interactions with Foods

None known.

Interactions with Lab Tests

None known.

Interactions with Diseases or Conditions

None known.

Dosage and Administration

ORAL: Typical dose for antiflatulent effect is 0.03 mL nutmeg oil (17). For nausea, gastric upset, or chronic diarrhea, the common dose is 3-5 drops of the essential oil on a sugar lump or in honey (6002). For diarrhea, 4-6 tablespoons of the powder has been used daily (6002).
TOPICAL: For toothache, 1 to 2 drops of essential oil are applied to the surrounding gum (6002).

Comments

Nutmeg is the shelled, dried seed of Myristica fragrans (11). Nutmeg oil is distilled from worm-eaten nutmeg seeds; the worms remove much of the starch and fat leaving portions of the seed rich in volatile oil (11). Mace is the dried aril (netlike covering) surrounding the shell of the seed of Myristica fragrans (11). Ingestion of 5-20 grams of nutmeg powder (1-3 whole seeds) might cause psychoactive effects (6). Because nutmeg and mace are so similar, high doses of mace might also have psychoactive effects but as yet this has not been proven (6).

NUX VOMICA

Also Known As

Brechnusssamen, Poison Nut, Quaker Buttons, Shudha Kupilu, Strychni Semen, Strychnos Seed, Vishamushti.

Scientific Names

Strychnos nux-vomica.
Family: Loganiaceae.

People Use This For

Orally, nux vomica is used for impotence and for glycine encephalopathy. It is also used in combination for diseases of the gastrointestinal tract, organic and functional disorders of the heart and circulatory system, diseases of the eye, nervous conditions, depression, migraine, climacteric complaints, facial neuralgias (Sympatalgien), and Raynaud's disease.
Historically, nux vomica has been thought of as an oral tonic, and used as an appetite-stimulant. It has also been used for diseases of the respiratory tract, anemia, and geriatric complaints. Nux vomica contains strychnine and brucine and has, therefore, been used in manufacturing. It is used as a rodenticide.

Safety

UNSAFE ...when used orally (2,13,18,505). Nux vomica in doses of 30-50 mg contains approximately 5 mg of strychnine, and can cause severe adverse effects. 1-2 grams of nux vomica contains 60-90 mg of strychnine, and can be fatal (13,18). Chronic ingestion of lesser amounts can cause death after a period of weeks (18).
PREGNANCY AND LACTATION: UNSAFE ...when used orally (2,13,18,505); avoid using.

Effectiveness
There is insufficient reliable information available about the effectiveness of nux vomica.

Mechanism of Action
The applicable part of nux vomica is the seed. Nux vomica contains strychnine and brucine (13). These are centrally-acting neurotoxins. Strychnine competitively antagonizes post-synaptic binding of the inhibitory transmitter glycine, which leads to heightened reflex excitability of muscles. External irritations or centrally-acting stimulants can trigger convulsions (2,505). Nux vomica can selectively inhibit the spinal cord in subconvulsive amounts (2). However, strychnine accumulates with extended administration, particularly in individuals with liver damage (2). Chronic use of subconvulsive amounts can cause death after a period of weeks (18). Strychnine causes convulsions by leading to a full contraction of all voluntary muscles. Death is secondary to impaired respiration or exhaustion (13,18,505).

Adverse Reactions
Orally, 30-50 mg nux vomica (5 mg strychnine) can cause restlessness, feelings of anxiety, heightening of sense perception, enhanced reflexes, equilibrium disorders, painful neck and back stiffness, followed later by twitching, tonic spasms of jaw and neck muscles, painful convulsions of the entire body triggered by visual or tactile stimulation with possible opisthotonos, muscle hypertonicity and agitation. Dyspnea may follow spasm of the respiratory muscles (18). Seizures occur within 15 minutes of ingestion (or 5 minutes of inhalation) and may result in hyperthermia, metabolic and respiratory acidosis, rhabdomyolysis, and myoglobinuric renal failure (17). 1-2 grams of nux vomica (60-90 mg strychnine) can be fatal (13,505); most deaths occur 3-6 hours post-ingestion from respiratory and subsequent cardiac arrest, anoxic brain damage, or multiple organ failure secondary to hyperthermia (18,505). Strychnine accumulates with extended administration, particularly in individuals with liver damage (2). Chronic use of subconvulsive amounts can cause death after a period of weeks (18).

Interactions with Herbs & Other Dietary Supplements
None known.

Interactions with Drugs
None known.

Interactions with Foods
None known.

Interactions with Lab Tests
None known.

Interactions with Diseases or Conditions
LIVER DISEASE: Contraindicated. Strychnine accumulates in individuals with liver damage (2). Also, strychnine accumulation can cause liver damage (18).

Dosage and Administration
Toxic, avoid using.

Comments
Strychnine may be detected by thin-layer chromatography (qualitative analysis) and high performance liquid chromatography (quantitative analysis). Urine and gastric aspirate are most useful in confirming poisoning (17). Nux vomica powder may be confused with the powder of date nuts, olive stones, and by-products of stone-nut processing (18).

OAK bark

Also Known As
Common Oak, Durmast Oak, Eichenrinde, English Oak, Pedunculate Oak, Quercus cortex, Sessile Oak, Stave Oak, Stone Oak, Tanner's Bark, Tanner's Oak.

Scientific Names
Quercus robur, synonym Quercus pedunculata; Quercus petraea, synonym Quercus sessiliflora; Quercus alba. Family: Fagaceae.

People Use This For

Orally, oak bark is used for diarrhea, colds, fever, cough and bronchitis, and for stimulating appetite and improving digestion.
Topically, oak bark is used for inflammatory skin conditions; mild inflammation of the mouth, throat, genital, and anal region; and for chilblains.

Safety

POSSIBLY SAFE ...when used orally (2,12) for up to 3-4 days for treating diarrhea (7). ...when used topically up to 2-3 weeks on intact skin (2).
LIKELY UNSAFE ...when used topically on extensive areas of damaged skin or for longer than 2-3 weeks (2).
PREGNANCY AND LACTATION: Insufficient reliable information available; avoid using.

Effectiveness

There is insufficient reliable information about the effectiveness of oak bark.

Mechanism of Action

Oak bark contains 8-20% tannins, including gallotannins (7,8). Gallotannins are extensively hydrolyzed in the upper small intestine and are unlikely to produce astringent activity in the colon (7,3901). Some studies suggest tannins might have antiviral and antimicrobial effects, and CNS depressant and cariostatic effects (11). Other studies suggest they can depress growth. Tannins exert an astringent effect on mucosal tissue. This effect dehydrates the tissue, internally reducing secretions, and externally forming a protective layer of harder, constricted cells (12). Plants with at least 10% tannins can cause gastrointestinal disturbances, kidney damage, and necrotic conditions of the liver (12). Some evidence suggests that tannins might cause cancer. Others information suggests they might prevent it (12). Regular consumption of herbs with high tannin concentrations correlates to an increased incidence of esophageal or nasal cancer (12).

Adverse Reactions

Orally, oak bark can cause gastrointestinal disturbances, kidney damage, and necrotic conditions of the liver (12).

Interactions with Herbs & Other Dietary Supplements

IRON: Theoretically, concomitant administration might precipitate iron salts due to tannin content (19).
TANNIN-CONTAINING HERBS: Theoretically, herbs that contain high percentages of tannins such as oak bark may cause precipitation of alkaloids and other constituents of herbs (19).

Interactions with Drugs

None known.

Interactions with Foods

None known.

Interactions with Lab Tests

None known.

Interactions with Diseases or Conditions

CARDIAC CONDITIONS: Oak bark baths are contraindicated in individuals with cardiac insufficiency (2).
ECZEMA: Oak bark baths are contraindicated in individuals with weeping eczema or large areas of skin damage (2).
HYPERTONIA: Oak bark baths are contraindicated in individuals with hypertonia (2).
INFECTION: Oak bark baths are contraindicated in individuals with febrile or infectious diseases (2).
KIDNEY DYSFUNCTION: Theoretically, oral use of oak bark might worsen kidney dysfunction (12).
LIVER DYSFUNCTION: Theoretically, oral use of oak bark might worsen liver dysfunction (12).

Dosage and Administration

ORAL: A typical dose of oak bark for diarrhea is one cup tea up to three times a day for up to 3-4 days. To make tea, add 1 gram coarsely powdered bark to 150 mL cold water, boil for a short period of time, strain (8).
TOPICAL: For rinses, compresses, poultices, and gargles, prepare with 20 grams bark in 1 L of water (18). For baths, prepare with 5 grams of bark in 1 L of water, added to bath water (18). Oak bark should not be used topically longer than 2-3 weeks (2).

OAK MOSS

Also Known As
Lichen Oak Moss, Tree Moss.
CAUTION: See separate listing for Usnea.

Scientific Names
Evernia prunastri.
Family: Usneaceae.

People Use This For
Orally, oak moss is used as an intestinal tonic.
In manufacturing, it is used as a fragrance component in perfumes.

Safety
POSSIBLY SAFE ...when used orally in prepared teas or aqueous forms for short periods of time (12). Although water extracts of oak moss contain the constituent thujone that is known to cause adverse effects, the amount of thujone is low (2).
LIKELY UNSAFE ...when used orally long-term, in large amounts of tea, or as a hot alcoholic extract (12) because enough thujone might be consumed to cause renal damage (4,12).
There is insufficient reliable information available about the safety of oak moss for its other uses.
PREGNANCY AND LACTATION: POSSIBLY UNSAFE ...when used orally. The constituent thujone shows evidence of uterine stimulant activity (19).

Effectiveness
There is insufficient reliable information available about the effectiveness of oak moss.

Mechanism of Action
Oak moss contains thujone, a ketone that shows evidence of neurotoxicity. Thujone intoxication causes psychoactivity resembling that of cannabinoid intoxication (12). Some data suggest thujone-containing volatile oils have uterine stimulant effects (19). Other information suggests thujone might exacerbate liver conditions, e.g., porphyria (12).

Adverse Reactions
Orally, large amounts or long-term use of thujone-containing products can cause restlessness, vomiting, vertigo, tremors, renal damage, and convulsions (12).
Topically, use of oak moss can cause contact sensitivity (4034,4039) and allergic reaction in people with lichen and moss allergy (4023,4033).

Interactions with Herbs & Other Dietary Supplements
THUJONE CONTAINING HERBS: Avoid; concomitant use may increase the risk of thujone toxicity. Thujone-containing herbs include oriental arborvitae, sage, tansy, thuja (cedar), tree moss, and wormwood (2,4,11,12).

Interactions with Drugs
None known.

Interactions with Foods
None known.

Interactions with Lab Tests
None known.

Interactions with Diseases or Conditions
CROSS-ALLERGENICITY: Oak moss may cause reaction in people allergic to lichens and mosses (4023,4033).
PORPHYRIA: Oak moss may exacerbate porphyria in patients with underlying defects in hepatic heme synthesis (12).
RENAL DYSFUNCTION: Oak moss may exacerbate renal dysfunction (12).

Dosage and Administration
No typical dosage.

Comments
Avoid confusing oak moss (Evernia prunastri) with other usnea species. Many, including oak moss, are referred to as tree moss.

OAT above ground parts

Also Known As
Avenae herba, Oat Herb, Wild Oat Herb.
CAUTION: See separate listings for Oat Bran, Oat Straw, and Oats.

Scientific Names
Avena sativa, synonyms Avena byzantina, Avena orientalis, Avena volgensis.
Family: Poaceae/Gramineae.

People Use This For
Orally, the above ground parts of oats are used for acute or chronic anxiety, excitation and stress, neurasthenia and pseudoneurasthenia syndromes, weak bladder, connective tissue disorders, for gout, kidney ailments, old age syndromes, opium and nicotine withdrawal, rheumatism, skin diseases, and as a tonic.
In combination with other herbs, oat above ground parts are used orally for cardiovascular, respiratory, and metabolic diseases, diseases and discomforts of old age, anemia, hypothyroidism, neuralgias and neuritis, hematoma, pulled muscles, sexual disorders, tobacco abuse, spasms, increasing milk production, and for increasing performance capacity.

Safety
POSSIBLY SAFE ...when the spikelet, the top of the herb, is used orally or topically (12).
PREGNANCY AND LACTATION: Insufficient reliable information available; avoid using.

Effectiveness
There is insufficient reliable information available about effectiveness of oat above ground parts.

Mechanism of Action
The above ground parts of oat contain soluble oligosaccharides and polysaccharides including saccharose, kestose, neokestose, beta-glucans, galactoarabinoxylans, silicic acid, steroid saponins, avenic acid A and B and flavonoids (18).

Adverse Reactions
None reported.

Interactions with Herbs & Other Dietary Supplements
None known.

Interactions with Drugs
MORPHINE: Theoretically, concomitant use might antagonize morphine (19).

Interactions with Foods
None known.

Interactions with Lab Tests
None known.

Interactions with Diseases or Conditions
None known.

Dosage and Administration
ORAL: A typical oral dose is 1 cup tea used repeatedly throughout the day and shortly before bedtime. To make tea, boil 3 grams above ground parts in 250 mL water, and strain (18).

OAT BRAN

Also Known As

Cereal Fiber, Dietary Fiber.
CAUTION: See separate listings for Oat above ground parts, Oat Straw, Oats, and Wheat Bran.

Scientific Names

Avena sativa, synonyms Avena byzantina, Avena orientalis, Avena volgensis. Family: Poaceae/Gramineae.

People Use This For

Orally, oat bran is used for reducing the risk of heart disease as part of a diet low in saturated fat and cholesterol; lowering blood cholesterol; reducing postprandial blood glucose in people with diabetes; blocking fat absorption; preventing gallstones; reducing risk of colon cancer; preventing gastric cancer; and treating irritable bowel syndrome (IBS), diverticulosis, and inflammatory bowel disease.

Safety

LIKELY SAFE ...when used orally and appropriately (4960,4969). Oat bran has Generally Recognized As Safe (GRAS) status in the US (4912).
PREGNANCY AND LACTATION: Insufficient reliable information available; avoid using in amounts greater than found in foods.

Effectiveness

EFFECTIVE

Cardiovascular disease. A diet that includes foods high in fiber, such as oat bran, reduces the risk of heart disease and death from cardiovascular disease when consumed as part of a diet low in saturated fat and cholesterol (2737,4960,4962,4963,4964,4965,4966,4967,4968).

Hypercholesterolemia. Oat bran and other soluble fibers can modestly reduce total and low-density lipoprotein (LDL) cholesterol when used orally as part of a diet low in saturated fat. Eating 3 bowls of oatmeal (28 gram servings) daily can decrease total cholesterol by about 5 mg/dL (4972,4973,4974,4975,4976,4977,5786,5788,6188). Oat bran products (oat bran muffins, oat bran flakes, oat bran Os, etc.) may vary in their ability to lower cholesterol, depending on the total soluble fiber content and other dietary variables (6188). Whole oat products might be more effective in lowering LDL and total cholesterol than foods containing oat bran plus beta-glucan soluble fiber (10145).

POSSIBLY EFFECTIVE

Diabetes. Taking oat bran orally seems to reduce postprandial blood glucose in people with diabetes (4960,4980,4982,6266). In a randomized crossover study of 13 people with type 2 diabetes, a high fiber diet that included oat bran was more effective than the standard ADA diet in lowering preprandial blood glucose and the area under the curve for 24-hour plasma glucose and glucose (measured every 2 hours), and improving cholesterol and triglyceride levels (6266).

Gastric cancer. Consuming a diet that includes dietary cereal fiber might reduce the incidence of stomach cancer (10435).

POSSIBLY INEFFECTIVE

Colorectal cancer. Taking oat bran orally doesn't reduce the risk of colon cancer. Fiber, including oat-bran fiber, does not prevent the recurrence of colorectal adenomas (4820,5104).

There is insufficient reliable information available about the effectiveness of oat bran for its other uses.

Mechanism of Action

Oat bran decreases serum cholesterol and dependent cardiovascular risk by decreasing absorption of cholesterol or fatty acids and decreasing absorption of biliary cholesterol or bile acids (4974,4960,4963). Dietary fiber, including oat bran, is also thought to decrease the risk of cardiovascular disease by decreasing fasting insulin levels, resulting in decreased obesity, hypertension, and improved lipid profile (2737). Beta-glucan (oat gum), a constituent of oat bran, increases the viscosity of food in the small intestine and delays absorption, thereby reducing peak postprandial plasma glucose and insulin levels both in people with diabetes and normal people (4961,4980,4981,4982,4983). Oat bran combines with intestinal water which forms a gum (4961), increases stool weight, and stool fat excretion (4970). Beta-glucan may help control appetite by slowing stomach emptying, prolonging the feeling of fullness and stabilizing blood sugar (11135). Oat bran alters the metabolism of bile acids (4984). Although earlier studies did not differentiate between types of fiber (5105,5106,5108), later studies indicate that oat bran, unlike wheat bran, does not protect against colon cancer (5104,5107).

Adverse Reactions

Oat bran may cause bezoars (concretions) and intestinal obstruction, especially in people who have difficulty chewing or swallowing food, or have conditions that decrease small bowel motility (4979,4985). Oat bran can cause reactions in people with gluten allergy, due to its gluten content (2).

Interactions with Herbs & Other Dietary Supplements

CHOLESTEROL-REDUCING HERBS: Theoretically, concomitant use might cause additive cholesterol-lowering effects.

Interactions with Drugs

None known.

Interactions with Foods

FATTY FOODS: Concomitant use of foods high in saturated fats or cholesterol can interfere with the cholesterol-lowering effect of oat bran (4960).

Interactions with Lab Tests

BLOOD GLUCOSE: Oat bran lowers postprandial blood glucose and test results (4961).
CHOLESTEROL: Oat bran lowers blood levels total and low density lipoprotein (LDL) cholesterol and test results (5788).
INSULIN: Oat bran lowers postprandial insulin levels and test results (4961).

Interactions with Diseases or Conditions

CELIAC DISEASE: Contraindicated in individuals with celiac disease due to gluten content (6).
GI CONDITIONS: Contraindicated in people with intestinal ulcerations, stenosis, disabling adhesions, cathartic colon or other conditions that may result in intestinal or esophageal obstruction (272). Use with caution or avoid in people with difficulty chewing or swallowing food, or conditions that decrease small bowel motility (272).

Dosage and Administration

ORAL: A typical dose for lowering plasma cholesterol, cardiovascular risk and post-prandial glucose is 3 grams of soluble fiber per day (4960). 38 grams of oat bran or 75 grams of dry oatmeal contains about 3 grams of beta-glucan (4961,5788).

Comments

Oat bran is milled from the outer layer of hulled whole oats and is made up of both soluble and insoluble fiber (4960,4961,4970). Oat bran contains oat gum or beta-glucan, a soluble polysaccharide (4961,4981). The FDA allows medical claims for foods containing over 51% whole grains. Therefore, certain breads and cereals, etc., can claim to reduce the risk of certain medical conditions such as heart disease.

OAT STRAW

Also Known As

Avenae stramentum, Oatstraw, Straw.
CAUTION: See separate listings for Oat above ground parts, Oat Bran, and Oats.

Scientific Names

Avena sativa, synonyms Avena byzantina, Avena orientalis, Avena volgensis.
Family: Poaceae/Gramineae.

People Use This For

Orally, oat straw is used as a tea for flu and coughs, abdominal fatigue, bladder and rheumatic disorders, eye ailments, frostbite, gout, impetigo, and metabolic diseases.
Topically, oat straw is used for skin inflammation, irritation, injury, pruritus, seborrhea, warts, arthritis, paralysis, liver disorders, and in foot baths for chronically cold or tired feet.

Safety

POSSIBLY SAFE ...when used topically and appropriately (2).
There is insufficient reliable information available about the safety of oat straw for its other uses.
PREGNANCY AND LACTATION: Insufficient reliable information available.

Effectiveness

There is insufficient reliable information available about the effectiveness of oat straw.

Mechanism of Action

There is insufficient reliable information available about the possible mechanism of action and active ingredients.

Adverse Reactions
None reported.

Interactions with Herbs & Other Dietary Supplements
None known.

Interactions with Drugs
None known.

Interactions with Foods
None known.

Interactions with Lab Tests
None known.

Interactions with Diseases or Conditions
None known.

Dosage and Administration
TOPICAL: To use as a bath additive, simmer 100 grams of chopped straw in 3 liters of water for 20 minutes, strain, and add to bath water (2,18).

Comments
Oat straw consists of the dried threshed, leaf and stem of the oat plant (Avena sativa).

OATS

Also Known As
Avena Fructus, Cereal Fiber, Dietary Fiber, Groats, Oat Fruit, Oat Grain, Oatmeal.
CAUTION: See separate listings for Beta-Glucans, Oat above ground parts, Oat Bran, and Oat Straw.

Scientific Names
Avena sativa, synonyms Avena byzantina, Avena orientalis, Avena volgensis. Family: Poaceae/Gramineae.

People Use This For
Orally, oat fruit is used for hypercholesterolemia and for disorders of the gastrointestinal tract, gallbladder, kidney, and cardiovascular systems. It is used for constipation, diarrhea, rheumatism, throat and chest complaints, physical fatigue, diabetes, neurasthenia and neurasthenia syndrome, colon cancer prevention, stomach cancer prevention, nicotine withdrawal, lowering uric acid levels, hypertension, and in tonics. It is also used as a sedative, a diuretic, and as an aid in opium withdrawal.
Topically, oats are used for managing dry, itchy skin; weeping eczema; contact dermatitis; chickenpox; and to enhance skin hydration.
In foods, oats are used as a grain or cereal.
In manufacturing, oats are a component of bath products and soaps.

Safety
LIKELY SAFE ...when used orally in food or medicinal amounts (6).
PREGNANCY AND LACTATION: LIKELY SAFE ...when used orally.

Effectiveness
LIKELY EFFECTIVE

Hypercholesterolemia. Consuming 56-150 grams of whole oat products such as oatmeal and oat bran, containing 3.6-10 grams of soluble fiber, can significantly lower total and low density lipoprotein (LDL) cholesterol levels 1.42 mg/dL (0.037 mmol/L) and 1.23 mg/dL (0.032 mmol/L) respectively per gram of soluble fiber (5786,5787,5788,5792,5794,5795,5796,8521). Doses of soluble fiber greater than 10 grams per day don't seem to increase effectiveness (5788). Whole oat products seem to be more effective in lowering LDL and total cholesterol than foods containing oat bran and beta-glucan soluble fiber (10145).

POSSIBLY EFFECTIVE

Diabetes. Consuming a high fiber diet for six weeks significantly decreases preprandial blood glucose, 24-hour plasma glucose, and insulin levels in people with type 2 diabetes (6266). There is some evidence that consuming 50 grams daily, containing 25 grams of soluble fiber, might be more effective than the moderate fiber diet of

24 grams daily recommended by the American Diabetes Association (ADA).

Gastric cancer. Epidemiologic evidence suggests that dietary cereal fiber, including oats, might reduce the incidence of stomach cancer (10435).

POSSIBLY INEFFECTIVE

Colorectal cancer. Increasing dietary fiber intake does not seem to reduce the risk of colorectal adenomas, which are precursors to cancer (4820).

Hypertension. Consumption of oats as oat meal and oat cereal does not seem to reduce diastolic or systolic blood pressure in men with minor elevations in blood pressure (2956).

There is insufficient reliable information available about the effectiveness of oats for other uses.

Mechanism of Action

The applicable part of oats is the fruit or seed. Oats are consumed as part of the diet and are a good source of protein, fat, and fiber. Oats contain fibers which are both water-soluble and insoluble, but oats contain a greater proportion of water-soluble fiber than any other grain (4963).

Oats are a good source for beta-glucan, which is a water-soluble fiber that seems to be responsible for many of oats' beneficial effects. Beta-glucan is thought to be responsible for the cholesterol-lowering effects of oats. Soluble fibers such as beta-glucan lower cholesterol levels by binding with bile acids in the gut and increasing fecal bile acid excretion (4974,5786,5787,5789). This decreases enterohepatic circulation of bile acids, which increases hepatic conversion of cholesterol to bile acids, increases up-regulation of low-density lipoprotein (LDL)-receptors, and increases clearance of LDL cholesterol (5786,5787).

There are several other theories about how beta-glucan might affect cholesterol levels. Beta-glucan might also decrease cholesterol absorption by inhibiting formation of micelles, which are necessary for fat absorption (5786). There is also some evidence that soluble fibers, such as beta-glucan, ferment to short-chain fatty acids in the gut, such as acetate, propionate, and butyrate. Absorption of these short-chain fatty acids then might inhibit cholesterol synthesis in the liver (5786,5787,5788).

Oats also contain alpha-tocotrienols. There is some preliminary evidence that alpha-tocotrienols can inhibit hepatic hydroxymethylglutaryl coenzyme A (HMG-CoA) reductase, which is the rate-limiting enzyme required for cholesterol synthesis (5786).

Because of the high fiber content, oats also seem to affect bowel movement regularity. Oats can act as a bulk-forming laxative in patients with constipation by stretching the intestinal walls and stimulating increased peristalsis (6).

Adverse Reactions

Orally, oats are usually very well tolerated. However, because of the high fiber content, they cause increased frequency of defecation, anal irritation, gaseous distention, and flatulence (6). To minimize side effects, doses should be slowly titrated to the desired level. Adverse effects usually subside with continued use.

Topically, oat flour can cause contact dermatitis in some patients (6).

Interactions with Herbs & Other Dietary Supplements

None known.

Interactions with Drugs

MORPHINE: Theoretically, oats extract might decrease the analgesic effect of morphine (19).

ORAL DRUGS: Oats might interfere with absorption of orally administered drugs because of its high fiber content (19). Advise patients to take medications either one hour before or four hours after oats.

Interactions with Foods

None known.

Interactions with Lab Tests

None known.

Interactions with Diseases or Conditions

CELIAC DISEASE: Contraindicated due to gluten content (6).

Dosage and Administration

ORAL: For hypercholesterolemia, 56-150 grams of whole oat products such as oat bran or oatmeal, containing 3.6-10 grams of soluble fiber, is used daily as part of a low-fat diet (5786,5787,5788,5792,5794,5795,5796,10145). For lowering blood glucose levels in patients with type 2 diabetes, high fiber foods such as whole oat products containing 25 grams of soluble fiber are used daily (6266).

TOPICAL: No typical dosage.

Comments

Current FDA regulations and guidelines allow food products containing whole oats to be labeled with the health claim that the product may reduce the risk of heart disease if they contain at least 750 mg of soluble fiber per serving, when included as part of a diet low in saturated fat and cholesterol (5792,5797). The FDA also recommends that approximately 3 grams of soluble fiber taken daily is needed to lower blood cholesterol levels (5792,5797); however, evidence from controlled clinical studies show at least 3.6 grams of soluble fiber daily is needed (5786,5787,5788,5794,5795,5796).

OCTACOSANOL

Also Known As

Hexacosanol (26-C), Tetracosanol (24-C), Triacontanol (30-C).
CAUTION: See separate listing for Policosanol.

Scientific Names

1-Octacosanol; N-octacosanol; Octacosyl alcohol.

People Use This For

Orally, octacosanol is used for exercise performance including strength, stamina and reaction time; for herpes; inflammatory skin diseases; Parkinson's disease; amyotrophic lateral sclerosis (ALS, Lou Gehrig's disease); hyperlipidemia; and atherosclerosis.

Safety

There is insufficient reliable information available about the safety of octacosanol.
Pregnancy and Lactation: Insufficient reliable information available; avoid using.

Effectiveness

INSUFFICIENT RELIABLE EVIDENCE to RATE

Amyotrophic lateral sclerosis (ALS, Lou Gehrig's disease). Preliminary evidence suggests that octacosanol does not improve objective symptoms of ALS (12156).

Parkinson's disease. Preliminary evidence suggests that some patients with Parkinson's disease who take octacosanol might have improved symptoms (11901).

More evidence is needed to rate octacosanol for these uses.

Mechanism of Action

Octacosanol is a 28-carbon alcohol that can be extracted from a variety of plant sources including sugar cane and wheat germ oil. It is related in structure to vitamin E. Octacosanol products are sometimes a mixture of 24- to 36-carbon alcohols, including tetracosanol (24-C), hexacosanol (26-C), and triacontanol (30-C). Octacosanol is not a normal component of the diet (12156).

It is hypothesized that octacosanol could improve oxygen utilization during anaerobic glycolysis and aid in lactic acid removal by increasing the efficiency of the tricarboxylic acid cycle (17).

In rats, octacosanol suppresses lipid accumulation in adipose tissue and increases the mobilization of free fatty acids from the fat cells in muscle (2924,2925).

There is interest in using octacosanol for various central nervous system disorders. Even though octacosanol is not a typical component of the diet, it is present in the central nervous system (12156).

Adverse Reactions

None reported.

Interactions with Herbs & Other Dietary Supplements

None known.

Interactions with Drugs

LEVODOPA/CARBIDOPA (Sinemet): Octacosanol might worsen dyskinesias and increase nervous tension in patients being treated with levodopa/carbidopa (11901).

Interactions with Foods

None known.

Interactions with Lab Tests

None known.

Interactions with Diseases or Conditions

PARKINSON'S DISEASE: Octacosanol might worsen dyskinesias associated with the levodopa/carbidopa treatment of Parkinson's disease (11901).

Dosage and Administration

ORAL: For Parkinson's disease, the typical dose of octacosanol is 5 mg three times a day with meals (11901). For amyotrophic lateral sclerosis (ALS, Lou Gehrig's disease), the usual dose is 40 mg per day (2921,12156).

Comments

Avoid confusion with policosanol.

OLEANDER

Also Known As

Common Oleander, Oleanderblatter, Oleandri folium, Rose Bay, Rose Laurel, Yellow Oleander.

Scientific Names

Nerium oleander, synonyms Nerium indicum, Nerium odorum; Thevetia peruviana, synonyms Cascabela thevetia, Cerbera thevetia, Thevetia neriifolia.
Family: Apocynaceae.

People Use This For

Orally, oleander is used for cardiac conditions, asthma, epilepsy, cancer, dysmenorrhea, leprosy, malaria, ringworm, indigestion, venereal disease, and as an abortifacient. A fixed combination of oleander leaf powdered extract, pheasant's eye fluid extract, lily-of-the-valley fluid extract, and squill powdered extract has been used for treating mild limited heart failure with circulatory instability.
Topically, oleander is used to treat skin eruptions and warts.

Safety

LIKELY UNSAFE ...when used orally. Ingestion of oleander leaf, oleander leaf tea, and oleander seeds has led to fatal poisonings (9,3495).
There is insufficient reliable information available about the safety of the topical use of oleander.
PREGNANCY AND LACTATION: LIKELY UNSAFE ...when used orally. Oleander has been reported to have abortifacient properties (5000). There is insufficient reliable information available about the safety of topical use of oleander during pregnancy and lactation; avoid using.

Effectiveness

There is insufficient reliable information available about the effectiveness of oleander.

Mechanism of Action

All parts of the oleander plant contain the cardiac glycosides oleandrin, oleandroside, nerioside, digitoxigenin, which have positive inotropic and negative chronotropic actions (3495). They bind to sodium- and potassium-sensitive membrane-bound enzymes called ATPases and inhibit enzyme activities, resulting in increased intracellular sodium ions and calcium ions and increased extracellular potassium levels (3477,5000). At toxic levels, the sodium and calcium ions depolarize the cell after repolarization, causing late afterdepolarization and increased automaticity. Severe toxicity produces bradycardia and heart block (3477). Oleander leaf also contains other biologically active constituents that have antimitotic and insecticidal properties (5000). Oleander is also reported to have emetogenic, cathartic, insecticidic, parasiticidic, anthelmintic, menstrual stimulant, and abortifacient activities (6002).

Adverse Reactions

Orally, oleander can cause bitter taste, burning sensation in mouth, nausea, vomiting, diarrhea, weakness, headache, stupor (17,18,3495), mucus membrane irritation, increased salivation, abdominal pain, buccal erythema, visual disturbances, mydriasis, peripheral neuritis (3495,5000), malignant dysrhythmias, ventricular ectopy, cardiovascular collapse, cardiac arrest (17), hyperkalemia (2532,3495) and death (3495). Oleander poisoning resembles digitoxin poisoning. Predominant symptoms are nausea and vomiting (onset in several hours), and cardiac toxicity, with conduction delays lasting for 3-6 days (17). Yellow oleander toxicity has been reported to be reversed with anti-digoxin Fab fragments. The majority of patients with yellow oleander toxicity who received anti-digoxin Fab fragments converted from an oleander-induced arrhythmia to normal sinus rhythm within 8 hours. A dose of 800 mg anti-digoxin Fab fragments was used intravenously. Associated hyperkalemia reversed within the first two hours (2532). A recurrence of arrhythmia can occur 48 hours post-exposure from any seed fragments remaining in the gastrointestinal tract (2532).

Interactions with Herbs & Other Dietary Supplements

CALCIUM: Calcium supplements may enhance the therapeutic effects of oleander (18).
CARDIAC GLYCOSIDE-CONTAINING HERBS: Contraindicated, and concomitant use can increase the risk of cardiac glycoside toxicity. Cardiac glycoside-containing herbs include black hellebore, Canadian hemp roots, digitalis leaf, hedge mustard, figwort, lily of the valley roots, motherwort, pheasant's eye plant, pleurisy root, squill bulb leaf scales, strophanthus seeds, and uzara (19).
LICORICE/HORSETAIL: Theoretically, overuse/misuse of licorice rhizome or horsetail plant with cardiac glycoside-containing herbs increases the risk of cardiac toxicity due to potassium depletion (19).
OTHER CARDIOACTIVE HERBS: Avoid concomitant use with other cardioactive herbs due to unpredictability of effects (4).
STIMULANT LAXATIVE HERBS: Theoretically, overuse or misuse of stimulant laxatives with cardiac glycoside-containing herbs increases the risk of cardiac toxicity due to potassium depletion (19).

Interactions with Drugs

CALCIUM SUPPLEMENTS: Calcium salts may enhance the therapeutic effects of oleander (18).
DIGOXIN (Lanoxin): Contraindicated; therapeutic duplication increases risk of cardiac glycoside toxicity (2).
DIURETIC DRUGS: Theoretically, concomitant use of potassium depleting diuretics and oleander can increase the risk of cardiac glycoside toxicity due to potassium depletion (506). Some diuretics that can deplete potassium include chlorothiazide (Diuril), chlorthalidone (Thalitone), furosemide (Lasix), hydrochlorothiazide (HCTZ, HydroDIURIL, Microzide), and others.
MACROLIDE ANTIBIOTICS: Theoretically, concomitant use may increase risk of cardiac glycoside toxicity (17).
QUININE: Theoretically, concomitant use of quinine and oleander may increase the risk of cardiac toxicity (506).
STIMULANT LAXATIVES: Theoretically, overuse or misuse or stimulant laxatives may increase the risk of cardiac glycoside toxicity due to potassium depletion (2).
TETRACYCLINE ANTIBIOTICS: Theoretically, concomitant use may increase risk of cardiac glycoside toxicity (17).

Interactions with Foods

None known.

Interactions with Lab Tests

None known.

Interactions with Diseases or Conditions

ELECTROLYTE IMBALANCE: Theoretically, based on digitalis glycosides (15), contraindicated in individuals with potassium deficiency states and hypercalcemia.
HEART DISEASE: Self-use contraindicated; requires diagnosis, treatment, and monitoring (515).

Dosage and Administration

No typical dosage.

Comments

The annual incidence of oleander poisoning in Sri Lanka exceeds 150 per 100,000. Approximately 10% of these ingestions are fatal (2532). Abbott TDx Digoxin II assay can be used for rapid confirmation of the ingestion of oleander (17).

OLIVE leaf

Also Known As

Oleae folium, Olivier.
CAUTION: See separate listing for Olive Oil.

Scientific Names

Olea europaea.
Family: Oleaceae.

People Use This For

Orally, olive leaf is used for treatment of conditions caused by, or associated with, a virus, retrovirus, bacterium, or protozoan including influenza, the common cold, meningitis, Epstein-Barr Virus (EBV), encephalitis, herpes I and II, human herpes virus 6 and 7, shingles, HIV/ARC/AIDS, chronic fatigue, and hepatitis B. It is also used for pneumonia; tuberculosis; gonorrhea; malaria; dengue; bacteremia; severe diarrhea; blood poisoning; and dental, ear, urinary tract, and surgical infections. Other uses include hypertension, diabetes, allergic rhinitis, improving renal and digestive function, and as a diuretic and antipyretic.

Safety

There is insufficient reliable information available about the safety of olive leaf.
Pregnancy and Lactation: Insufficient reliable information available; avoid using.

Effectiveness

POSSIBLY EFFECTIVE

Hypertension. Taking olive leaf extract orally seems to lower blood pressure in patients with hypertension (1540).
There is insufficient reliable information available about the effectiveness of olive leaf for its other uses.

Mechanism of Action

In animal experiments, olive leaf preparations demonstrate multiple properties including antispasmodic, hypotensive, antiarrhythmic and arrhythmogenic (2,18), hypoglycemic (810), bronchodilator, coronary dilator, antipyretic, and diuretic (2). The constituent, oleuropein, has bacteriostatic (1541) and antioxidant (271) activity. Constituent flavonoids have serum complement-inactivating activity (1542). An aqueous olive leaf extract reduced blood pressure in one small, uncontrolled trial of people with hypertension (1540).

Adverse Reactions

Orally, olive leaf hasn't been associated with adverse effects (1540). Olive tree pollen causes seasonal respiratory allergy (1543).

Interactions with Herbs & Other Dietary Supplements

HERBS WITH HYPOGLYCEMIC POTENTIAL: Theoretically, olive leaf might have additive effects with herbs that decrease blood glucose levels (1540). Herbs with hypoglycemic potential include devil's claw, fenugreek, garlic, guar gum, horse chestnut, Panax ginseng, psyllium, and Siberian ginseng.

Interactions with Drugs

ANTIDIABETES DRUGS: Theoretically, concomitant use might enhance blood glucose lowering effects (1540). Monitor blood glucose levels closely. Some antidiabetes drugs include glimepiride (Amaryl), glyburide (DiaBeta, Glynase PresTab, Micronase), insulin, pioglitazone (Actos), rosiglitazone (Avandia), and others.
ANTIHYPERTENSIVE DRUGS: Theoretically, concomitant use may enhance blood pressure-lowering effects (1540).

Interactions with Foods

None known.

Interactions with Lab Tests

BLOOD PRESSURE: Olive leaf might reduce blood pressure and blood pressure readings (1540).
CALCIUM: Olive leaf might reduce serum calcium levels and test results (1540).
GLUCOSE: Olive leaf might reduce blood glucose levels and test results (1540).

Interactions with Diseases or Conditions

DIABETES: Olive leaf might lower blood glucose (1540). Monitor glucose levels and adjust therapy accordingly.
HYPOTENSION: Theoretically, may exacerbate this condition due to blood pressure-reducing effects (1540).

Dosage and Administration

ORAL: For hypertension, olive leaf extract 400 mg four times daily has been used (1540). A typical dose is one cup of tea (steep 2 teaspoons dried leaf in 150 mL boiling water 30 minutes, strain) three to four times per day (18).

OLIVE OIL

Also Known As

Monounsaturated Fatty Acid, n-9 Fatty Acid, Olivae oleum, Omega-9, Omega-9 Fatty Acid, Omega-9 Fatty Acids, Salad Oil, Sweet Oil, Unsaturated Fatty Acid.
CAUTION: See separate listing for Olive leaf.

Scientific Names

Olea europaea.
Family: Oleaceae.

People Use This For

Orally, olive oil is commonly used for preventing cardiovascular disease, hypertension, hypercholesterolemia, and diabetes. It is also used orally for breast cancer and rheumatoid arthritis. Olive oil is also used orally for migraine headache in adolescents; firming the breasts; treating bile duct and gallbladder inflammation, gallstones, jaundice, flatulence, and meteorism (swelling of the abdomen due to intestinal or peritoneal gas); prevention of colorectal cancer; as a mild laxative for constipation; and Roemheld syndrome. Some people also use olive oil to boost bacteria in the gut and as a "cleanser" or "purifier."

Topically, olive oil is used for softening earwax, treating ringing and pain in the ears, as nose drops, for wound dressing, treating minor burns and psoriasis, preventing and treating stretch marks due to pregnancy, and for protecting the skin from ultraviolet (UV) damage after sun exposure.

For food use, olive oil is used as a cooking and salad oil.

In manufacturing, olive oil is used to make soaps, in commercial plasters and liniments, and as a setting-retardant in dental cements.

Safety

LIKELY SAFE ...when used orally in the amounts found in foods.

There is insufficient reliable information available about the safety of olive oil used in amounts greater than those used in food preparation.

PREGNANCY AND LACTATION: LIKELY SAFE ...when consumed in food amounts; avoid using in amounts greater than those found in foods (18).

Effectiveness

LIKELY EFFECTIVE

Constipation. Taking olive oil orally is effective as a mild laxative for reducing constipation (16).

POSSIBLY EFFECTIVE

Breast cancer. People who have higher dietary intake of olive oil seem to have a lower risk of developing breast cancer (2221,2222,2223).

Colorectal cancer. There is some evidence that people with higher intakes of dietary olive oil have a decreased risk of developing colorectal cancer. Olive oil intake also seems to reduce colorectal mucosal changes and polyp formation, which are two factors involved in the sequence of developing colorectal cancer (3362).

Hypercholesterolemia. Increasing dietary olive oil consumption can significantly reduce total serum cholesterol levels (2219,2220,3285,3286,3287,3288,3289,3290). However, some research suggests other dietary oils such as sunflower and rapeseed (canola) might reduce low-density lipoprotein (LDL) cholesterol and apolipoprotein B better than olive oil (9780).

Hypertension. Consuming a modified diet including high amounts of extra virgin olive oil over 6 months, in conjunction with conventional treatments for hypertension, can significantly improve blood pressure. In some cases, patients with mild to moderate hypertension can decrease doses or discontinue use of antihypertensive medications (2219,2220,3289,5091).

Migraine headache. Taking olive oil preparations containing oleic acid (1,382 mg daily over a 2 month period) seems to reduce frequency, duration, and severity of migraine headaches in adolescents (5097).

Myocardial infarction (MI). Epidemiological research suggests that including olive oil in the diet might reduce the risk of first MI. A high dietary intake of olive oil (54 grams per day) was shown to cause an 82% relative reduction in risk of first MI compared with a low intake of 7 grams or less per day (8131).

Rheumatoid arthritis (RA). There is some evidence that people consuming high amounts of dietary olive oil have a decreased risk of developing RA (3454).

POSSIBLY INEFFECTIVE

Earwax. Applying olive oil topically doesn't seem to soften earwax (3274).

Otitis media. Applying olive oil topically doesn't seem to be effective for treating ear pain in children with acute otitis media (3276).

INSUFFICIENT RELIABLE EVIDENCE to RATE

Diabetes. Olive oil in a Mediterranean-type diet seems to reduce chylomicron remnant particles compared with a polyunsaturated diet in diabetes patients, suggesting that it might reduce the risk of atherosclerosis (8132). Olive oil rather than polyunsaturated oils such as sunflower oil might be a better choice for patients with diabetes. More evidence is needed to rate olive oil for this use.

Mechanism of Action

Olive oil contains the monounsaturated fatty acid oleic acid (56-83%), palmitic acid (8-20%), and linoleic acid (4-20%) (18). People use olive oil to prevent coronary heart disease and atherogenesis because it seems to lower certain cardiac risk factors (2219,2220,2224,10673). Phenolic compounds present in olive oil seem to possess antioxidant, vasodilating, and antiplatelet properties. The compounds act as free radical scavengers, inhibiting platelet aggregation and thromboxane release (10673). Olive oil seems to increase low-density lipoprotein (LDL) cholesterol resistance to oxidation and therefore possibly decreases its contribution to atherogenesis (2219,2220,2224). It also seems to improve the function of endothelial tissue in patients with hypercholesterolemia. Olive oil seems to lower blood pressure and decrease postprandial factor VII clotting activity (8131). Olive oil might also have anti-inflammatory effects by decreasing pro-inflammatory omega-6 fatty acid concentrations and increasing anti-inflammatory omega-3 fatty acid concentrations (3289). The metabolites of oleic acid, an omega-9 monounsaturated fatty acid, in olive oil seem to competitively inhibit the production of inflammatory omega-6 fatty acid prostaglandins and leukotrienes. Oleic acid metabolites might also suppress production of inflammatory cytokines (3454). Some researchers think olive oil might have a role in preventing colon cancer. Consumption of olive oil seems to reduce production of deoxycholic acid, a bile acid thought to be involved in the development of mucosal changes and polyp formation preceding colorectal cancer (3362). Other compounds in olive oil called secoiridoides (oleuropein and derivatives) have broad-spectrum antimicrobial activity in vitro (3284).

Adverse Reactions

Orally, olive oil may cause biliary colic in people with gallstones (2,18,19).
Topically, olive oil may cause allergic reactions (rare) (2), and may irritate eyes; avoid eye contact (19).
Delayed hypersensitivity and contact dermatitis are reported with topical use (289,3275).

Interactions with Herbs & Other Dietary Supplements

None known.

Interactions with Drugs

ANTIDIABETES DRUGS: Monitor blood glucose levels closely due to claims that olive oil has hypoglycemic effects (19).

Interactions with Foods

None known.

Interactions with Lab Tests

None known.

Interactions with Diseases or Conditions

GALLSTONES: Contraindicated; may trigger gallbladder colic (2,18,19).

Dosage and Administration

ORAL: As adjunctive therapy in hypertension, 30-40 grams per day of extra-virgin olive oil has been used as part of the diet (5091). As a laxative, 30 mL has been used (16). For reducing the risk of myocardial infarction, 54 grams per day has been associated with a reduced risk of first myocardial infarction (8132).
TOPICAL: No typical dosage.

Comments

Olive oil consists of the fatty oil pressed from the drupes (fruit) of olive trees (Olea europaea). It is classified, in part, according to oleic acid content. Extra virgin olive oil contains a maximum of 1% free oleic acid, virgin olive oil contains 2%, and ordinary olive oil contains 3.3%. Unrefined olive oils with more than 3.3% free oleic acid are considered "unfit for human consumption" (3273). The American Heart Association recommends a maximum 30% of dietary calories from fat (2224). Some studies show beneficial effects when olive oil is the main source of dietary fat intake (2224).

Ozonated olive oil is promoted for everything from bee stings and insect bites to bacterial and fungal skin infections to cancer. The Food and Drug Administration allows the use of ozone as an antimicrobial agent on food, including meat and poultry, but the food industry has been slow to adopt it (8187). Ozone is extremely unstable and must be produced on site. Topical olive oil products purported to contain ozone are unlikely to remain stable during shipping. There are no clinically proven medical uses of ozone or ozonated olive oil. Tell patients other topical anti-infectives are a better choice.

OMEGA-6 FATTY ACIDS

Also Known As

N-6, N-6 EFAs, N-6 Essential Fatty Acids, Omega 6 Fatty Acids, Omega 6 Oils, Omega-6 Fatty Acid, Omega-6 Oils, Polyunsaturated Fatty Acids, PUFAs.
CAUTION: See separate listings for Gamma Linolenic Acid, Evening Primrose Oil, Borage Seed Oil, and Black Currant.

Scientific Names

Omega-6 polyunsaturated fatty acids.

People Use This For

Orally, omega-6 fatty acids are used for reducing the risk of coronary heart disease, lowering total cholesterol and LDL cholesterol levels, increasing HDL cholesterol levels, and reducing cancer risk.
Arachidonic acid, an omega-6 fatty acid, is used as a supplement in infant formulas.

Safety

There is insufficient reliable information available about the safety of omega-6 fatty acids.
Pregnancy and Lactation: Insufficient reliable information available; avoid using.

Effectiveness

POSSIBLY INEFFECTIVE

Enhancing infant development. Taking arachidonic acid (an omega-6 fatty acid) orally as a supplement in infant formula doesn't seem to be effective for improving cognitive and mental development or growth up to 18 months of age (424).

There is insufficient reliable information available about the effectiveness of omega-6 fatty acids for its other uses.

Mechanism of Action

Omega-6 fatty acids are essential polyunsaturated fatty acids (PUFA) with a double bond at the 6 position of the carbon chain. Some omega-6 fatty acids include linoleic acid, gamma-linolenic acid and arachidonic acid. Linoleic acid is found in vegetable oils, including corn, evening primrose seed, safflower, and soybean oils. Gamma-linolenic acid is found in black currant seed, borage seed, and evening primrose oils (7701).
Omega-6 fatty acids are components of cell membrane structure and play a role in cell signaling pathways and epithelial cell function (11120). Preliminary studies suggest that omega-6 fatty acids might play a role in breast cancer development (3508); however, it is unclear whether omega-6 fatty acids are associated with breast cancer in humans (3508,3511). A low-fat diet with reduced omega-6 fatty acid content can decrease sex steroid hormone levels, alter eicosanoid biosynthesis, and play a role in preventing and treating breast and prostate cancers (3510). Long-chain polyunsaturated fatty acids, such as arachidonic acid, make up a third of all lipids in the brain's grey matter (425). Arachidonic acid is a membrane component in the central nervous system, and may have a role as a neurotransmitter (424,425). Arachidonic acid is present in human breast milk but not in standard infant formulas. Formula-fed infants have lower plasma arachidonic acid levels than breast milk-fed infants; the clinical significance of this, if any, is unknown (424).

Adverse Reactions

Orally, omega-6 fatty acids can elevate triglycerides (3509).

Interactions with Herbs & Other Dietary Supplements

None known.

Interactions with Drugs

None known.

Interactions with Foods

None known.

Interactions with Lab Tests

None known.

Interactions with Diseases or Conditions

HYPERTRIGLYCERIDEMIA: Omega-6 fatty acids can elevate triglyceride levels (3509); avoid using.

Dosage and Administration

No typical dosage.

Comments

Information on omega-6 fatty acid dietary supplementation derives from studies using specific omega-6 fatty acids or plant oils containing omega-6 fatty acids. See separate listings for black currant seed oil, borage seed oil, and evening primrose oil.

ONION

Also Known As
Allii cepae bulbus, Green Onion, Onions, Shallot.

Scientific Names
Allium cepa.
Family: Alliaceae or Liliaceae.

People Use This For
Orally, onion is used for loss of appetite, preventing atherosclerosis, for treating dyspepsia, fever, colds, cough, bronchitis, hypertension, tendency toward infection, inflammation of the mouth and pharynx, whooping cough, asthma, angina, stimulation of gallbladder, dehydration, and as a menstruation aid. Onion is also used for hypertension, diabetes, and as an antiflatulent, anthelmintic, and diuretic.
Topically, onion is used for insect bites, wounds, light burns, furuncles, warts, and bruises
In foods, onion is considered a culinary food and condiment.
In manufacturing, the oil is used as a flavoring agent in foods.

Safety
LIKELY SAFE ...when consumed in amounts commonly found in foods. Onion has Generally Recognized As Safe (GRAS) status in the US (4912).
POSSIBLY SAFE ...when used orally and appropriately (2). A maximum of 35 mg of the diphenylamine constituent is recommended per day if onion preparations are used over several months (2).
There is insufficient reliable information available about the safety of onion for its other uses.
PREGNANCY AND LACTATION: Insufficient reliable information available; avoid amounts greater than used in foods.

Effectiveness
There is insufficient reliable information available about the effectiveness of onion.

Mechanism of Action
The applicable part of the onion is the bulb. Onion contains essential oils (2), sulfur compounds, and cysteine sulfoxide compounds. One of the sulfur compounds, thiosulphinate, exhibits antimicrobial effects (18). The methyl and propyl compounds of cysteine sulfoxide are primarily responsible for onion flavor and lacrimation (7,11). Diphenylamine is also a constituent of onion (513). Diphenylamine is referred to as a dose standard (2). The mechanism of the diuretic effect of onion is unknown. In people with asthma, an ethanolic onion extract significantly reduced bronchial constriction (18). In sensitized guinea pigs, onion juice provided protection from asthma attacks (18). In humans, eating onions reversed the effect of a fatty meal, restoring fibrinolytic activity (7). In humans, onion also inhibits platelet aggregation (7). Onions show hypoglycemic actions, and in animals, both cholesterol lowering effects and antifungal activities have been noted (11).

Adverse Reactions
The consumption of large quantities of onions can cause stomach distress (18). Hand eczema can occur with frequent contact (18).

Interactions with Herbs & Other Dietary Supplements
HERBS WITH ANTICOAGULANT/ANTIPLATELET POTENTIAL: Concomitant use of herbs that have constituents that might affect platelet aggregation could theoretically increase the risk of bleeding in some people. These herbs include angelica, clove, danshen, garlic, ginger, ginkgo, Panax ginseng, horse chestnut, red clover, turmeric, and others.

Interactions with Drugs
ANTICOAGULANT/ANTIPLATELET DRUGS: Theoretically, concomitant use with onion might enhance antiplatelet drug activity and increase bleeding risk (19).
ANTIDIABETES DRUGS: Theoretically, concomitant use with onion might enhance antidiabetes drug effects and alter blood sugar control (19).
ASPIRIN: Concomitant intake might augment onion allergy. One case is reported of severe urticaria and swelling in a person with a known mild onion allergy after consuming onion and aspirin (5054).

Interactions with Foods
None known.

Interactions with Lab Tests
BLOOD GLUCOSE: Onions can decrease blood glucose levels and test results (19).

Interactions with Diseases or Conditions
DIABETES: Theoretically, therapeutic amounts of onions can interfere with blood sugar control. Monitor blood sugar carefully when using onion for medicinal purposes (19).

Dosage and Administration
ORAL: The typical dose is 50 grams of fresh onion per day. The juice of 50 grams fresh onion or 20 grams dried onion is also used per day (2). A maximum of 35 mg diphenylamine per day is recommended if onion preparations are used over several months (2).
TOPICAL: An onion slice is typically placed on the skin, or the juice is used as a poultice (18).

Comments
Onions are rich in vitamin C (19) and in folk medicine, were cooked in milk and used as a mucolytic to clear congested airways (7).

OPIUM ANTIDOTE

Also Known As
Combretum, Jungle Weed.

Scientific Names
Combretum micranthum.
Family: Combretaceae.

Comments
At the date of publication, this product was not a common ingredient used in brand name supplements marketed to consumers. Details about this product are available at the online version of *Natural Medicines Comprehensive Database*. See www.naturaldatabase.com.

ORCHIC EXTRACT

Also Known As
Bovine Orchic Extract, Bovine Testicle Extract, Bull Balls Extract, Orchic, Orchic Concentrate, Orchic Factors, Orchic Substance.

Scientific Names
None.

People Use This For
Orally, men use orchic extract to maintain healthy testicular function.

Safety
There is insufficient reliable information available about the safety of orchic extract. However, since orchic extract preparations are derived from animals, there is concern about contamination with diseased animal parts (1825). So far, there are no reports of disease transmission to humans due to use of contaminated orchic extract.
Pregnancy and Lactation: Insufficient reliable information available; avoid using.

Effectiveness
There is insufficient reliable information available about the effectiveness of orchic extract.

Mechanism of Action
Orchic extract is obtained from bovine testicles (1319). Marketers imply that orchic extracts are a good source of testosterone. However, there is no evidence to support this claim.

Adverse Reactions
Adverse effects for orchic extract have not been reported. However, there are concerns about possible product contamination. Orchic extract is derived from raw bovine testes gathered from slaughterhouses, possibly from sick or

diseased animals (1319). Products made from contaminated or diseased organs might present a human health hazard. There is also concern that orchic extracts produced from cows in countries where bovine spongiform encephalitis (BSE) has been reported might be contaminated with diseased tissue. Countries where BSE has been reported include Great Britain, France, The Netherlands, Portugal, Luxembourg, Ireland, Switzerland, Oman, and Belgium (1825). However, there have been no reports of BSE transfer to humans from contaminated orchic extract products. Until more is known, tell patients to avoid these products unless country of origin can be determined. Patients should avoid products that are produced in countries where BSE has been found.

Interactions with Herbs & Other Dietary Supplements
None known.

Interactions with Drugs
None known.

Interactions with Foods
None known.

Interactions with Lab Tests
ANABOLIC STEROIDS: Theoretically, orchic extract might cause a positive anabolic steroid screening test result (1320). However, this effect has not been demonstrated.

Interactions with Diseases or Conditions
None known.

Dosage and Administration
No typical dosage.

OREGANO

Also Known As
Carvacrol, Dostenkraut, European Oregano, Mediterranean Oregano, Mountain Mint, Oil of Oregano, Oregano Oil, Organy, Origani vulgaris herba, Origano, Origanum, Phytoprogestin, Wild Marjoram, Winter Marjoram, Wintersweet.
CAUTION: See separate listing for Marjoram.

Scientific Names
Origanum vulgare.
Family: Lamiaceae/Labiatae.

People Use This For
Orally, oregano is used for respiratory tract disorders such as coughs, asthma, croup, and bronchitis. Oregano is also used orally for gastrointestinal disorders, such as dyspepsia and bloating. It is also used orally for dysmenorrhea, rheumatoid arthritis, urinary tract disorders including urinary tract infections (UTIs), headaches, and heart conditions. The oil of oregano is also used orally for intestinal parasites, allergies, sinusitis, arthritis, cold and flu, earaches, and fatigue.
Topically, oregano oil is used for acne, athlete's foot, dandruff, insect and spider bites, canker sores, gum disease, toothaches, psoriasis, seborrhea, ringworm, rosacea, muscle pain, varicose veins, and warts. It is also used topically as an insect repellent.
In foods and beverages, oregano is used as a culinary spice and a food preservative.

Safety
LIKELY SAFE ...when used orally in amounts commonly found in foods. Oregano leaf and oil have Generally Recognized As Safe (GRAS) status in the US (4912).
POSSIBLY SAFE ...when used orally or topically and appropriately in medicinal amounts (12).
There is insufficient reliable information available about the safety of oregano oil when used in medicinal amounts.
PREGNANCY: POSSIBLY UNSAFE ...when used orally in medicinal amounts. Oregano is thought to have abortifacient and emmenagogue effects (19,7122).
LACTATION: There is insufficient reliable information available about the safety of oregano when used in medicinal amounts while nursing.

Effectiveness

POSSIBLY EFFECTIVE

Intestinal parasitic infection. Taking the emulsified oil of oregano orally 200 mg three times daily for 6 weeks can eradicate the parasites Blastocystis hominis, Entamoeba hartmanni, and Endolimax nana from the stools of infected patients (6878).

There is insufficient reliable information available about the effectiveness of oregano for its other uses.

Mechanism of Action

The applicable part of oregano is the leaf and oil. Oregano contains the constituents carvacrol and thymol which have anthelmintic, fungicidal, and irritant properties (2129). The essential oil is thought to have diuretic, expectorant, and antispasmodic properties. It might also stimulate bile production (11). Oregano oil also has in vitro activity against a variety of common gram positive and gram negative organisms, including Acinetobacter calcoacetica, Enterococcus faecalis, Escherichia coli, Klebsiella pneumoniae, Pseudomonas aeruginosa, Salmonella species, Serratia marcescens, Staphylococcus aureus, and the yeast Candida albicans (316,2129,2130,3702,3703,3704). The carvacrol and thymol constituents also inhibit bacterial growth, with additive or possibly synergistic activity in oregano oil (2130). Carvacrol has a bacteriocidal effect on Bacillus cereus, a common food pathogen, by altering bacterial membrane permeability (165). Oregano oil seems to inhibit the growth intestinal parasites in vivo (6878). There is preliminary evidence that oregano may contain phytoprogestins that bind the progesterone receptor (3701).

Adverse Reactions

Orally, large amounts of oregano can cause gastrointestinal upset. Concentrated, non-emulsified oil of oregano can cause localized irritation of the gastrointestinal tract (6878). Oregano might also cause systemic allergic reactions (3705). Individuals allergic to Lamiaceae family plants including basil, hyssop, lavender, marjoram, mint, and sage, might also demonstrate an allergic reaction to oregano (3705).

Interactions with Herbs & Other Dietary Supplements

None known.

Interactions with Drugs

None known.

Interactions with Foods

None known.

Interactions with Lab Tests

None known.

Interactions with Diseases or Conditions

CROSS-ALLERGENICITY: Oregano can cause reactions in people allergic to Lamiaceae family plants, including basil, hyssop, lavender, marjoram, mint, and sage (3705).

Dosage and Administration

ORAL: For intestinal parasitic infection, emulsified oil of oregano has been used in a dose of 200 mg three times daily for 6 weeks (6878). Traditionally, a typical dose is one cup of tea. To make tea, steep 1 heaping teaspoon of leaf in 250 mL boiling water 10 minutes, strain. Tea may be sweetened with honey (18).

TOPICAL: No typical dosage. Traditionally, unsweetened tea is used as a gargle or mouthwash (18). To use oregano as a bath additive, steep 100 grams dried leaf in 1 L water for 10 minutes, strain, and add to a full bath (18).

Comments

Oregano oil has been tested as an insect repellent for Culicodoides imicola, a pathogen-bearing species of insects commonly known as no-see-ums or biting midges. Oregano oil is not as effective as DEET for protecting horses (and presumably, people) from C. imicola (2119).

OREGON FIR BALSAM

Also Known As

Balsam, Balsam Fir Oregon, Balsam Oregon, Coastal Douglas Fir, Douglas Fir, Douglas Spruce, Oregon Balsam, Red Fir.

Scientific Names

Pseudotsuga menziesii, synonym Pseudotsuga douglasii; Pseudotsuga mucronata; Pseudotsuga taxifolia.
Family: Pinaceae.

Comments

At the date of publication, there was very little scientific information about this product. Our staff is continually analyzing the available information on natural medicines and will add data to the online version of *Natural Medicines Comprehensive Database* as it becomes available. See www.naturaldatabase.com.

OREGON GRAPE

Also Known As

Barberry, Blue Barberry, Creeping Barberry, Holly Barberry, Holly-Leaved Berberis, Holly Mahonia, Mountain-Grape, Oregon Barberry, Oregon-Grape, Oregon Grape-Holly, Scraperoot, Trailing Mahonia, Water-Holly.
CAUTION: See separate listing for European Barberry.

Scientific Names

Mahonia aquifolium, synonyms Berberis aquifolium, Berberis diversifolia, Mahonia diversifolia; Mahonia nervosa, synonym Berberis nervosa; Mahonia repens, synonyms Berberis repens, Berberis sonnei, Mahonia sonnei.
Family: Beberidaceae.

People Use This For

Orally, Oregon grape is used for ulcers, heartburn, stomach problems, as a bitter tonic, as a cathartic, and to treat infections. The American Indians used Oregon grape for general debility and as an appetite stimulant.
Topically, Oregon grape is used for psoriasis, as a disinfectant.

Safety

POSSIBLY SAFE ...when used topically and appropriately (854,857). Canada has approved a Mahonia aquifolium product for topical use based on safety data (856). ...when used orally. Amounts of less than 500 mg per day of berberine, a constituent of Oregon grape, are usually considered safe (12).
LIKELY UNSAFE ...when more than 500 mg per day berberine is consumed (12). Berberine is considered moderately toxic (12). The human LD50 for berberine is reported to be 27.5 mg/kg (12).
PREGNANCY: LIKELY UNSAFE ...when used orally (12) due to potential uterine stimulant activity of berberine (19).
LACTATION: Insufficient reliable information available; avoid using.

Effectiveness

INSUFFICIENT RELIABLE EVIDENCE to RATE

Psoriasis. There is some evidence that Oregon grape, applied topically, may be useful for treating psoriasis (854,857). More evidence is needed to rate Oregon grape for this use.

Mechanism of Action

The applicable parts of Oregon grape are the rhizome and root. Oregon grape root contains 2.4-4.5% of isoquinoline alkaloid constituents including berberine, berbamine, and oxyacanthine (515). Berberine and oxyacanthine show evidence of antibacterial activity (11). Berberine has anticonvulsant, sedative, hypotensive, antifibrillatory, bile-stimulating, and anti-inflammatory effects. In low doses, it is a cardiac and respiratory stimulant. In high doses it is a depressant (515,10377). Some evidence suggests berberine sulfate might be amebicidal and trypanocidal (11). Other information suggests the constituent berbamine might have antiarrhythmic, hypotensive, spasmolytic, and immunostimulating activity (515).

Adverse Reactions

No reports of adverse effects associated with Oregon grape. Ingesting more than 500 mg berberine, a constituent of Oregon grape, can cause lethargy, nosebleed, skin and eye irritation, kidney irritation (12), hemorrhagic nephritis (2), dyspnea, hypotension, cardiac damage (12), nausea, vomiting, diarrhea, respiratory spasms and arrest, and death (2). When used topically, Oregon grape can cause itching, burning, skin irritation, and allergic reactions (854).

Interactions with Herbs & Other Dietary Supplements

BERBERINE-CONTAINING HERBS: Concomitant use can increase the risk of berberine toxicity. Berberine-containing herbs include bloodroot, goldenseal, celandine, Chinese goldthread, goldthread, amur cork tree, Chinese corktree (12).

Interactions with Drugs

None known.

Interactions with Foods

None known.

Interactions with Lab Tests

None known.

Interactions with Diseases or Conditions

KIDNEY IRRITATION: CAUTION, berberine may exacerbate kidney irritation. It can cause kidney irritation and nephritis (2).

Dosage and Administration

ORAL: The common dose of the tincture is 2-4 mL three times daily, and the usual dose of the powder is 0.5 to 1 gram three times daily (6002).
TOPICAL: For psoriasis, 10% Mahonia aquifolium bark extract ointment is typically applied to affected areas two to three times daily. Mahonia aquifolium 10% root extract cream is typically massaged into affected areas three times daily or as directed by physician (854).

Comments

A Mahonia aquifolium root extract product, Prime Relief, received a Drug Identification Number (DIN) from Health Canada. The DIN allows this product to be labeled and marketed for treating psoriasis in Canada (856).

ORIENTAL ARBORVITAE

Also Known As

Biota orientalis, Ce Bai, Chinese Arborvitae.

Scientific Names

Platycladus orientalis, synonyms Retinispora juniperoides, Thuja orientalis.
Family: Cupressaceae.

People Use This For

Orally, oriental arborvitae is used orally for headache, apprehension, calming nervous disorders and excitement, for cancer, constipation, convulsions, dysmenorrhea, ejaculation problems, narrowing of intestine, fever, vomiting blood, bloody stools, blood in urine, hemorrhage, insomnia, painful menses, heavy menstrual flow, irregular and variable menstrual bleeding, nausea, neurasthenia, palpitation, perspiration, rheumatism, tumors, and as a tonic. It is also used orally for diuretic, laxative, menstrual-stimulant, pain-reliever, parasiticide, and sedative effects.
Topically, oriental arborvitae is used for nosebleed, piles, for burns and scalds, and as a hair tonic. It is also used topically for its astringent and antiperspirant properties.

Safety

POSSIBLY SAFE ...when the seed is used orally (12). ...when the leafy twigs are used orally in tea. It is important to use it short-term and not to exceed the usual dose (12).There is insufficient reliable information available about the safety of oriental arborvitae for its other uses.
PREGNANCY AND LACTATION: POSSIBLY UNSAFE ...when used orally because it contains thujone (12) which shows some evidence of uterine stimulant activity (19); avoid using.

Effectiveness

There is insufficient reliable information is available about the effectiveness of oriental arborvitae.

Mechanism of Action

The applicable parts of oriental arborvitae are the seed and the cacumen (leafy twigs) (12). Oriental arborvitae contains thujone in the volatile oil. Alcoholic extracts and essential oils containing thujone can cause neurotoxicity including convulsions and hallucinations (12). Some evidence suggests Thuja orientalis might have antibacterial activity (4041).

Adverse Reactions

Thujone intoxication can cause psychoactivity similar to tetrahydrocannabinol, the active constituent in marijuana. Long-term or high dosages of plants containing thujone can cause restlessness, vomiting, dizziness, tremors, renal damage, and convulsions (12).

Interactions with Herbs & Other Dietary Supplements

THUJONE CONTAINING HERBS: Concomitant use may increase the risk of thujone toxicity. Thujone-containing herbs include oak moss (12), sage (2,4,12), tansy (2,4,12), thuja (cedar) (11,12), tree moss (12), and wormwood (2,12); avoid using.

Interactions with Drugs

None known.

Interactions with Foods

None known.

Interactions with Lab Tests

None known.

Interactions with Diseases or Conditions

PORPHYRIA: Can exacerbate porphyria in patients with underlying defects in hepatic heme synthesis (12).
RENAL DYSFUNCTION: Can exacerbate this condition (12).

Dosage and Administration

ORAL: A standard dose for the leafy twigs is 5-15 grams of raw or charred, daily as tea (12).
TOPICAL: No typical dosage.

ORNITHINE

Also Known As

L-Ornithine.
CAUTION: See separate listing for Ornithine Ketoglutarate.

Scientific Names

L-5-aminorvaline; L-2,5-diaminovaleric acid.

People Use This For

Orally, ornithine is used for improving athletic performance, reducing glutamine toxicity in the treatment of hepatic encephalopathy, and for wound healing.

Safety

There is insufficient reliable information available about the safety of ornithine.
Pregnancy and Lactation: Insufficient reliable information available; avoid using.

Effectiveness

POSSIBLY INEFFECTIVE

Athletic performance. Taking ornithine orally doesn't seem to enhance athletic performance (2417,2418).

INSUFFICIENT RELIABLE EVIDENCE to RATE

Hepatic encephalopathy. Preliminary clinical research suggests an L-ornithine-L-aspartate infusion might reduce the harmful effects of glutamine in the treatment of hepatic encephalopathy (10655). More evidence is needed to rate ornithine for this use.

Mechanism of Action

Ornithine is a non-essential amino acid produced in the body by hydrolysis of arginine. By supplementing ornithine, people believe they can increase their anabolic hormone levels, reducing skeletal muscle hypertrophy (2417).

However, supplemental ornithine has no effect on insulin secretion (2417,2418) or serum human growth hormone (hGH) levels in bodybuilders (2418).

Adverse Reactions
None reported.

Interactions with Herbs & Other Dietary Supplements
None known.

Interactions with Drugs
None known.

Interactions with Foods
None known.

Interactions with Lab Tests
None known.

Interactions with Diseases or Conditions
None known.

Dosage and Administration
ORAL: The typical dose is one 500 mg capsule containing L-ornithine daily on an empty stomach before bedtime (5020).

Comments
Avoid confusion with ornithine alpha-ketoglutarate (OKG).
There is very little scientific information about this product. Our staff is continually analyzing the available information on natural medicines and will add data here as it becomes available.

ORNITHINE KETOGLUTARATE

Also Known As
OKG, Ornicetil, Ornithine Alphaketoglutarate, L-Ornithine Alpha-Ketoglutarate, Ornithine Alpha Ketoglutarate.
CAUTION: See separate listing for Ornithine.

Scientific Names
L(+)-ornithine alpha-ketoglutarate.

People Use This For
Orally, ornithine ketoglutarate is used for enhancing athletic performance and wound healing.
Intravenously, it is used as a component in total parenteral nutrition for preventing growth retardation in children receiving long-term total parenteral nutrition. It is also used intravenously for improving skeletal muscle protein synthesis after surgery, preventing decreases in muscle free glutamine concentrations, and preserving protein synthesis after total hip replacement or stroke.

Safety
POSSIBLY SAFE ...when use intravenously and appropriately (2444,2445,2446,2448).
There is insufficient reliable information available about the safety of the oral use of ornithine ketoglutarate.
PREGNANCY AND LACTATION: Insufficient reliable information available; avoid using.

Effectiveness
POSSIBLY EFFECTIVE

Burns. Taking ornithine ketoglutarate orally seems to improve wound healing in burn patients (2443).

POSSIBLY INEFFECTIVE

Athletic performance. Taking ornithine ketoglutarate orally doesn't seem to enhance athletic performance (2452).

LIKELY INEFFECTIVE

Hepatic encephalopathy. Administering ornithine ketoglutarate intravenously isn't effective for treating encephalopathy in patients with acute and chronic liver disease (2449,2450).

INSUFFICIENT RELIABLE EVIDENCE to RATE

Growth retardation. Preliminary clinical research suggests ornithine ketoglutarate might prevent growth retardation in children receiving long-term total parenteral nutrition (2444).

Surgery related myoatrophy. Preliminary clinical research suggests ornithine ketoglutarate might improve skeletal muscle protein synthesis after surgery (2446,2448).
More evidence is needed to rate ornithine ketoglutarate for these uses.

Mechanism of Action

Ornithine ketoglutarate modifies amino acid metabolism and increases blood insulin and glucagon levels in healthy people (2415).

Adverse Reactions

None reported.

Interactions with Herbs & Other Dietary Supplements

None known.

Interactions with Drugs

None known.

Interactions with Foods

None known.

Interactions with Lab Tests

None known.

Interactions with Diseases or Conditions

None known.

Dosage and Administration

ORAL: For the healing of burn wounds, 30 grams is taken daily as an enteral bolus (2443).
INTRAVENOUS: For preventing growth retardation in children receiving long-term total parenteral nutrition (TPN), 15 grams of ornithine ketoglutarate is typically added to the daily TPN (2444). For improving skeletal muscle protein synthesis after surgery, 350 mg/kg per day is added to the TPN (2446). For preventing decreases in muscle free glutamine concentrations and preserving protein synthesis after total hip replacement, 280 mg/kg per day is added to the TPN (2448).

Comments

Avoid confusion with ornithine.

ORRIS

Also Known As

Blue Flag, Daggers, Flaggon, Flag Lily, Fliggers, Florentine Iris, Gladyne, Iris, Jacob's Sword, Liver Lily, Myrtle Flower, Poison Flag, Rhizoma Iridis, Segg, Sheggs, Snake Lily, Water Flag, White Dragon Flower, Wild Iris, Yellow Flag, Yellow Iris.
CAUTION: See separate listing for Blue Flag.

Scientific Names

Iris pallida, synonym Iris junonia; Iris germanica; Iris germanica var. florentina, synonym Iris florentina.
Family: Iridaceae.

People Use This For

Orally, orris root is used for "blood-purifying", "gland-stimulating", increasing kidney activity, skin diseases, bronchitis, cold, cancer, stimulating appetite and digestion, stimulating bile flow, sciatica, sclerosis, splenitis. It is also used as a diuretic, emetic, laxative, purgative, and sedative. Orris root is also used orally for headache, toothache, muscle and joint pain, migraine, bowel sluggishness, bloating, diabetes, urinary tract inflammation, and skin diseases.
Topically, orris root is used for halitosis, nasal polyps, teething, tumors, uric acid sedimentation, kyphosis, keloid formation, rheumatic disorders, burns, and cuts.

Safety
POSSIBLY SAFE ...when used orally (12). Orris root must be carefully peeled and dried before using (2). Fresh root and juice can cause severe mucosal and skin irritation (12).
There is insufficient reliable information available about the safety of the topical use of orris.
PREGNANCY AND LACTATION: Insufficient reliable information available; avoid using.

Effectiveness
There is insufficient reliable information available about the effectiveness of orris.

Mechanism of Action
The applicable parts of orris are the rhizome and root. Orris root contains triterpenes, including irigermanal, and isoflavonoids, including irilon, irisolone, irigenine, and tectoridine. It also contains C-glucosylxanthones and a volatile oil. The chief constituents of the volatile oil are irones, particularly alpha-, beta-, and gamma-irone. Some think orris root has mild expectorant effects (18).

Adverse Reactions
No adverse effects are reported when orris root has been carefully peeled and dried. However, taken orally the fresh plant juice or root can cause severe mucosal irritation, abdominal pain, vomiting, and bloody diarrhea (18). Topically, the fresh plant juice or root can cause severe skin and mucosal irritation (12,18).

Interactions with Herbs & Other Dietary Supplements
None known.

Interactions with Drugs
None known.

Interactions with Foods
None known.

Interactions with Lab Tests
None known.

Interactions with Diseases or Conditions
None known.

Dosage and Administration
No typical dosage.

Comments
Orris root is generally used in combination with other herbs and can be found in homeopathic dilutions and tea preparations (18). Historically, orris root was highly prized in the perfume industry. Upon drying, the root develops a pleasant violet-like scent. This scent continues to improve in storage, reaching its peak in about three years. Orris root was widely used in face powders and other cosmetics until it was determined to cause allergic reactions. Orris root powder is still used extensively in potpourris, sachets, and pomanders. It is one of the most effective fixatives and it prolongs the scent of the more transient volatile oils. Of the two orris species, Iris germanica var. florentina root is considered superior to Iris pallida (4081).

OSCILLOCOCCINUM

Also Known As
Anas Barbariae, Avian Heart and Liver, Avian Liver Extract, Canard de Barbarie, Duck Liver Extract, Muscovy Duck, Oscillo.

Scientific Names
Cairina moschata; Anas barbaria; Anas moschata.

People Use This For
Orally, oscillococcinum is used for symptoms of influenza infections ("the flu").

Safety

POSSIBLY SAFE ...when used orally. Oscillococcinum has been safely used in clinical trials (10804). This is a homeopathic product and contains no measurable amount of active ingredient. Therefore this product is not expected to cause any beneficial or adverse effect.

PREGNANCY AND LACTATION: Insufficient reliable information available. This product has not been studied in these patients. However, it is a homeopathic product and contains no measurable amount of active ingredient. Therefore this product is not expected to cause any beneficial or adverse effect.

Effectiveness

INSUFFICIENT RELIABLE EVIDENCE to RATE

Influenza. Oscillococcinum does not seem to help prevent influenza illness. However, there is preliminary evidence that oscillococcinum might reduce the duration of influenza symptoms by 0.28 days (10804). This small decrease in duration may not be clinically meaningful. The credibility of this finding is questioned due to the methodological flaws of the study. More evidence is needed to rate oscillococcinum for this use.

Mechanism of Action

Oscillococcinum is a homeopathic dilution of duck liver and heart extract. Homeopathy is a system of medicine established in the 19th century by a German physician named Samuel Hahnemann. Its basic principles are that "like treats like" and "potentiation through dilution." For example, in homeopathy, influenza would be treated with an extreme dilution of a substance that normally causes influenza when taken in high doses.

A French physician discovered a substance he called "oscillococci" while investigating the Spanish flu in 1917. But he was mistaken that his oscillococci were the cause of the flu (12011).

Practitioners of homeopathy believe that more dilute preparations are more potent. Many homeopathic preparations are so diluted that they contain little or no active ingredient. Therefore, most homeopathic products are not expected to have any pharmacological effects, drug interactions, or other harmful effects. Any beneficial effects are controversial and cannot be explained by current scientific methods.

Dilutions of 1 to 10 are designated by an "X." So, a 1X dilution = 1:10; 3X = 1:1000; 6X = 1:1,000,000. Dilutions of 1 to 100 are designated by a "C." A 1C dilution = 1:100; 3C = 1:1,000,000. Dilutions of 24X or 12C or more contain zero molecules of the original active ingredient. Oscillococcinum is usually diluted from 9C to 200C and therefore usually contains no measurable active ingredient (12011).

Adverse Reactions

None reported. Oscillococcinum is a homeopathic product and contains no active ingredient. Therefore, it is not expected to cause any adverse effects.

Interactions with Herbs & Other Dietary Supplements

None known.

Interactions with Drugs

None known.

Interactions with Foods

None known.

Interactions with Lab Tests

None known.

Interactions with Diseases or Conditions

None known.

Dosage and Administration

ORAL: For influenza, one manufacturer (Boiron) recommends taking the contents of one tube up to 3 times per day.

Comments

Oscillococcinum is a brand name homeopathic product manufactured by Boiron. Similar homeopathic products are found in other brands. Boiron claims that their Oscillococcinum is the number one over-the-counter medicine for flu in France and the number one homeopathic remedy for flu in the US.

Homeopathic products are permitted for sale in the US due to legislation passed in 1938 sponsored by a homeopathic physician who was also a Senator. The law still requires that the FDA allow the sale of products listed in the Homeopathic Pharmacopeia of the United States. However, homeopathic preparations are not held to the same safety and effectiveness standards as conventional medicines.

OSHA

Also Known As

Bear Root, Chuchupate, Colorado Cough Root, Indian Parsley, Mountain Lovage, Porter's Licorice Root, Wild Celery Root.
CAUTION: See separate listings for Lovage and Licorice.

Scientific Names

Ligusticum porteri.
Family: Apiaceae/Umbelliferae.

People Use This For

Orally, osha is used for sore throat, bronchitis, cough, common cold, influenza, pneumonia, and indigestion. It is also used orally to treat other viral infections including herpes and AIDS/HIV.
Topically, osha is used to prevent infections of skin wounds.
Traditionally, osha has also been used by Native American and Hispanic cultures for pneumonia, colds, bronchitis, influenza, tuberculosis, hay fever, and coughs.

Safety

POSSIBLY SAFE ...when used orally and appropriately (12).
PREGNANCY: LIKELY UNSAFE ...when used orally. Osha has been used to stimulate menstruation and is reported to have abortifacient activity (12,19); contraindicated.
LACTATION: Insufficient reliable information available; avoid using.

Effectiveness

There is insufficient reliable information available about the effectiveness of osha.

Mechanism of Action

The applicable part of osha is the root (12). Osha contains the compound ligustilide, which might have antimicrobial and antiviral activities (6734,6736). Preliminary evidence indicates that osha might have viral protease inhibitory effects. It might also inhibit the influenza virus (6733). To date, there are no studies published of osha use in humans or animals.

Adverse Reactions

None reported.

Interactions with Herbs & Other Dietary Supplements

None known.

Interactions with Drugs

None known.

Interactions with Foods

None known.

Interactions with Lab Tests

None known.

Interactions with Diseases or Conditions

None known.

Dosage and Administration

ORAL: As a tincture, osha is commonly taken as 20-60 drops up to 5 times daily. These are usually prepared as a 1:2 tincture with the fresh root or 1:5 tincture with the dried root (6729). Osha is often combined with other herbs and supplements and sold as a multi-ingredient product.

Comments

The leaves of osha are similar in appearance to the very toxic poison hemlock. Osha must be identified by the root, which is described as malodorous with a strong celery-like odor, or should be obtained from reputable commercial sources. Osha, which grows at higher elevations in the western US, is difficult to cultivate. The popularity of Osha has led to over harvesting of the wild plant (6735). Osha has been designated an endangered plant by conservationists (6735).

OSTRICH FERN

Also Known As
Fiddlehead Fern, Garden Fern, Hardy Fern.

Scientific Names
Matteuccia struthiopteris, synonym Osmunda struthiopteris.
Family: Dryopteridaceae.

People Use This For
Orally, ostrich fern is used as a gargle for sore throat.
Topically, ostrich fern is used for wounds and boils.
Ostrich fern is used for food. It is regarded as a seasonal delicacy.

Safety
LIKELY SAFE ...when used as a food if prepared appropriately (6,5002).
LIKELY UNSAFE ...when not cooked properly (6); may cause severe food poisoning.
PREGNANCY AND LACTATION: Insufficient reliable information available; avoid using.

Effectiveness
There is insufficient reliable information available about the effectiveness of ostrich fern.

Mechanism of Action
The applicable part of ostrich fern is the young shoot top. One field guide states wild ostrich fern greens have laxative properties (6). Toxins responsible for poisonings have not been identified, but they are believed deactivated by boiling. The CDC recommends thorough cooking (e.g., boiling for 10 minutes) before eating (5002).

Adverse Reactions
Centers for Disease Control and Prevention (CDC) links outbreaks of severe food poisoning to consumption of raw or lightly cooked ostrich ferns (6,5002). Ostrich fern can cause nausea, vomiting, abdominal cramping (6), diarrhea, and headaches after ingestion (5002).

Interactions with Herbs & Other Dietary Supplements
None known.

Interactions with Drugs
None known.

Interactions with Foods
None known.

Interactions with Lab Tests
None known.

Interactions with Diseases or Conditions
None known.

Dosage and Administration
ORAL: Cook young shoots of ostrich fern (fiddleheads) thoroughly (e.g., boiling for 10 minutes) before eating (5002).

Comments
The tops of the young shoots of ostrich fern, known as fiddleheads, are regarded as a seasonal delicacy. They are available canned, frozen or fresh (6). Boil at least 10 minutes before eating.

OSWEGO TEA

Also Known As

Bee Balm, Blue Balm, High Balm, Low Balm, Monarda, Mountain Balm, Mountain Mint, Scarlet Monarda.
CAUTION: See separate listing for Horsemint.

Scientific Names

Monarda didyma.
Family: Lamiaceae/Labiatae.

People Use This For

Orally, oswego tea is used for digestive disorders including flatulence and premenstrual syndrome. It is also used as an antispasmodic and diuretic.
In Europe, oswego tea is used for decreasing fever and as a fragrance.

Safety

There is insufficient reliable information available about the safety of oswego tea.
PREGNANCY: UNSAFE ...when used orally because it may possibly promote menstruation and stimulate menstrual flow (12).
LACTATION: Insufficient reliable information available; avoid using.

Effectiveness

There is insufficient reliable information available about the effectiveness of oswego tea.

Mechanism of Action

There is insufficient reliable information available about the possible mechanism of action and active ingredients.

Adverse Reactions

None reported.

Interactions with Herbs & Other Dietary Supplements

None known.

Interactions with Drugs

None known.

Interactions with Foods

None known.

Interactions with Lab Tests

None known.

Interactions with Diseases or Conditions

None known.

Dosage and Administration

ORAL: Oswego tea is taken as tea prepared from the powdered herb (18).

Comments

Oswego tea got the alternate name bergamot because of the similarity of its pleasant scent to that of the oil of bergamot oranges (see separate listing). During the period of the Boston tea party, it was drunk in place of black tea. Lemon balm is also known as bee balm, a common name for oswego tea, and may be confused with it.

OX-EYE DAISY

Also Known As

Butter Daisy, Dun Daisy, Golden Daisy, Goldenseal, Great Ox-Eye, Herb Margaret, Horse Daisy, Horse Gowan, Marguerite, Maudlin Daisy, Maudlinwort, Moon Daisy, Moon Flower, Moon Penny, Ox Eye Daisy, Poverty Weed, White Daisy, White Weed.
CAUTION: See separate listing for Goldenseal (Hydrastis canadensis).

Scientific Names

Chrysanthemum leucanthemum.
Family: Compositae.

People Use This For

Orally, ox-eye daisy is used for indications similar to German chamomile. These uses include the common cold, cough, bronchitis, fever, mouth and pharynx inflammation, liver and gallbladder complaints, loss of appetite, and susceptibility to infection. It is also used as an antispasmodic, diuretic, and tonic.
Topically, ox-eye daisy is used for skin inflammation, wounds, and burns.

Safety

There is insufficient reliable information available about the safety of ox-eye daisy.
Pregnancy and Lactation: Insufficient reliable information available; avoid using.

Effectiveness

There is insufficient reliable information available about the effectiveness of ox-eye daisy.

Mechanism of Action

The applicable parts of ox-eye daisy are the above ground flowering parts. There is insufficient reliable information available about the possible mechanism of action and active ingredients.

Adverse Reactions

Ox-eye daisy can cause an allergic reaction in individuals sensitive to the Asteraceae/Compositae family. Members of this family include ragweed, chrysanthemums, marigolds, daisies, and many other herbs.

Interactions with Herbs & Other Dietary Supplements

None known.

Interactions with Drugs

None known.

Interactions with Foods

None known.

Interactions with Lab Tests

None known.

Interactions with Diseases or Conditions

CROSS-ALLERGENICITY: Can cause an allergic reaction in individuals sensitive to the Asteraceae/Compositae family. Members of this family include ragweed, chrysanthemums, marigolds, daisies, and many other herbs.

Dosage and Administration

ORAL: The daily dose is equivalent to 10-15 grams dried herb, taken as tea. The tea is prepared by steeping 3 grams dried leaf in 150 mL of boiling water for 10-15 minutes and straining (18).
TOPICAL: A tea is prepared by steeping 2 teaspoons of dried leaf in 1 cup of boiling water for 15 minutes, straining and applied topically. As a bath additive, 50 grams of dried herb is added to 1 L bath water (18).

Comments

Ox-eye daisy is alternately known as goldenseal, but it is unrelated to the more commonly known goldenseal (Hydrastis canadensis).

PAGODA TREE

Also Known As
Chinese Scholartree, Japanese Pagoda Tree.

Scientific Names
Styphnolobium japonicum, synonym Sophora japonica.
Family: Fabaceae/Leguminosae.

People Use This For
Orally, pagoda tree is used in dilutions for dysentery.

Safety
POSSIBLY UNSAFE ...when the seeds are used orally (18). Regular use of seed meal can cause facial edema or even death. High doses could cause cystine poisoning (18).
PREGNANCY AND LACTATION: POSSIBLY UNSAFE ...when used orally (18); avoid using.

Effectiveness
There is insufficient reliable information available about the effectiveness of pagoda tree.

Mechanism of Action
The applicable parts of the pagoda tree are the seeds. Cystine poisoning may occur with high dosages (18).

Adverse Reactions
None reported with short-term use. Using pagoda tree seed long-term may cause edema and death (18).

Interactions with Herbs & Other Dietary Supplements
None known.

Interactions with Drugs
None known.

Interactions with Foods
None known.

Interactions with Lab Tests
None known.

Interactions with Diseases or Conditions
None known.

Dosage and Administration
No typical dosage.

PANAX PSEUDOGINSENG

Also Known As
Chai-Jen-Shen, Field Seven, Himalayan Ginseng, Jia Renshen, Nepal Ginseng, Pseudoginseng Root, Samch'il, San Qi, San-Qi Ginseng, San Qui, Sanshichi, Three Seven, Tian Qi.
CAUTION: See separate listing for Ginseng, Panax.

Scientific Names
Panax pseudoginseng, synonyms Panax notoginseng, Aralia pseuodoginseng.
Family: Araliaceae

People Use This For
Orally, panax pseudoginseng is used as a hemostatic for conditions including vomiting and coughing up blood, blood in the urine or stool, nosebleed, and hemorrhagic disease. It is also used to relieve pain; and to reduce swelling, blood cholesterol, and blood pressure. Panax pseudoginseng is also used for angina, dizziness, and acute sore throat.

Topically, Panax pseudoginseng is used to stop bleeding.
In combination with seven other herbs (PC-SPES), Panax pseudoginseng is used to treat prostate cancer.

Safety

There is insufficient reliable information available about the safety of Panax pseudoginseng.
PREGNANCY AND LACTATION: LIKELY UNSAFE ...when used orally; contraindicated (5559). Ginsenoside Rb1, an active constituent of Panax pseudoginseng, has teratogenic effects in animal models (10447).

Effectiveness

There is insufficient reliable information available about the effectiveness of Panax pseudoginseng.

Mechanism of Action

Panax pseudoginseng root contains 12% saponins; the most important are triterpenoid saponins referred to collectively as ginsenosides or panaxosides. Ginsenosides is the term developed by Asian researchers, and the term panaxosides was developed by Russian researchers. Numerous subtypes of ginsenosides have been identified. Like Panax ginseng, Panax pseudoginseng contains the ginsenosides Rb1 and Rg1. Rb1 has a low oral bioavailability, and Rg1 is rapidly eliminated from the blood in animal models, which limits its pharmacologic effects (11153).
Panax pseudoginseng is believed to dilate the coronary vessels, reduce vascular resistance, and improve the coronary collateral circulation. This could increase blood flow while reducing blood pressure. It would also reduce the heart metabolic rate and oxygen consumption. Evidence also suggests Panax pseudoginseng has an antiarrhythmic effect (5558). Animal evidence suggests orally administered Panax pseudoginseng root can reduce fibrinogenemia, an increased level of fibrinogen in the blood (11487). Evidence also suggests oral administration can decrease plasma lipid levels by reducing total cholesterol and triglycerides (11487). Trilinolein, a triacylglycerol purified from Panax pseudoginseng, might have antioxidant activity (6289). When applied topically, however, preliminary information suggests the dried root of panax pseudoginseng may be useful as a hemostatic agent because it appears to shorten bleeding time (4056).
In vitro research shows estrogen-like activity. Studies on human breast cancer cells indicate that Panax pseudoginseng root, specifically its constituent ginsenonside-Rg1, acts as a phytoestrogen by stimulating human breast cancer cell proliferation (11488).
Pananotin, a protein isolated from Panax pseudoginseng root, seems to have antiviral and antifungal activity, according to preliminary research. It appears to inhibit HIV reverse transcriptase in vitro (11485,11486).

Adverse Reactions

Orally, Panax pseudoginseng can cause dry mouth, flushed skin, nervousness, insomnia, nausea, and vomiting (5558).

Interactions with Herbs & Other Dietary Supplements

None Known.

Interactions with Drugs

None Known.

Interactions with Foods

None known.

Interactions with Lab Tests

CARDIAC FUNCTION: Panax pseudoginseng might improve tests of cardiovascular function.

Interactions with Diseases or Conditions

HORMONE SENSITIVE CANCERS/CONDITIONS: Because Panax pseudoginseng seems to have estrogenic effects, women with hormone sensitive conditions including breast cancer, uterine cancer, ovarian cancer, endometriosis, and uterine fibroids should avoid using panax pseudoginseng (11488).

Dosage and Administration

ORAL: A typical dose is 1-1.5 grams divided into three doses per day (5558).
TOPICAL: No typical dosage.

PANCREATIN

Also Known As
Pancreatinum, Pancreatis pulvis.

Scientific Names
Pancreatin.

People Use This For
Orally, pancreatin is used to treat malabsorption syndromes associated with pancreatic insufficiency in cystic fibrosis, chronic pancreatitis, or pancreas removal. It is also used orally for flatulence or as a digestive aid.

Safety
LIKELY SAFE ...when used orally and appropriately for replacement therapy by individuals with pancreatic insufficiency (15). Some pancreatin products contaminated by Salmonella have caused illness (9). Use only products from reputable manufacturers.
PREGNANCY AND LACTATION: Insufficient reliable information available; avoid using unless essential for replacement therapy (15).

Effectiveness
EFFECTIVE

Pancreatic insufficiency. Taking pancreatin orally is effective as replacement therapy in pancreatic insufficiency due to cystic fibrosis, chronic pancreatitis, or pancreas removal (15).

LIKELY INEFFECTIVE

Digestive disorders. Taking pancreatin orally isn't effective for treating digestive disorders not related to pancreatic insufficiency, including flatulence (15,16).

Mechanism of Action
Pancreatin contains digestive enzymes, including lipase, protease, and amylase. These enzymes are usually obtained from pork or beef pancreas (15). These enzymes catalyze the hydrolysis of fats, peptides, and starches in the small intestine. Pancreatin is inactivated when acid, including gastric acid, is present in more than trace amounts (15,506).

Adverse Reactions
Orally, excessive doses of pancreatin can cause nausea, vomiting, diarrhea, or other transient intestinal upset, and perianal soreness. Extremely high doses have been associated with high uric acid level in blood and urine, and colon strictures (15).
Topically, pancreatin preparations that are held in the mouth prior to swallowing can cause irritation of the mucosa, including ulceration and stomatitis (15). Pancreatin powder is irritating to the skin, eyes, mucus membranes, and respiratory tract. Hypersensitivity reactions, e.g., sneezing, lacrimation, and skin rash, have been reported (15).
Inhalation of dust containing pancreatin has been associated with pulmonary hypersensitivity reactions, allergic rhinitis, bronchospasm, and asthma (11768,11769).

Interactions with Herbs & Other Dietary Supplements
FOLIC ACID: Pancreatin can decrease absorption of folic acid (9).

Interactions with Drugs
ACARBOSE (Precose, Prandase): Enzymes present in pancreatin can decrease the efficacy of acarbose (9).

Interactions with Foods
ACIDIC FOODS: Concomitant intake of acidic foods or fruit juices can break down pancreatin enzymes, reducing the activity of pancreatin preparations that are not enteric-coated (15).
ALKALINE FOODS: Mixing enteric-coated granules into alkaline foods, e.g., chicken, veal, or green beans, might destroy the coating (15).

Interactions with Lab Tests
URIC ACID: Pancreatin, particularly at high doses, can cause an increase in serum and urine uric acid levels (15).

Interactions with Diseases or Conditions
None known.

Dosage and Administration

ORAL: For pancreatic replacement therapy, the initial dose of pancreatin is usually 8,000 to 24,000 USP units of lipase activity taken before or with each meal or snack. To control steatorrhea, dose can be increased as needed or until nausea, vomiting or diarrhea occurs (15). Pancreatin is available as enteric-coated tablets, powder, or capsules containing the powder or enteric-coated granules (506).

Comments

Each mg of pancreatin contains not less than 25 USP units of amylase activity, not less than 2 USP units of lipase activity, and not less than 25 USP units of protease activity (15,16). Pancreatin that is more potent is labeled as a multiple of these three minimum activities, e.g., pancreatin 4X (10,16).

PANGAMIC ACID

Also Known As

Calcium Pangamate, Calgam, Di-isopropylamine Dichloroacetate, Vitamin B15.
CAUTION: See separate listing for Dimethylglycine.

Scientific Names

None.

People Use This For

Orally, pangamic acid is used for detoxifying the body; treating asthma and allied diseases; conditions of the skin and respiratory tract; painful nerve and joint afflictions; cell proliferation like cancer; eczema; arthritis; neuritis; and improving the oxygenation of the heart, brain, and other vital organs. It is also used orally for alcoholism, hangovers, fatigue, protecting against urban air pollutants, extending cell life, stimulating increased immune system response, lowering blood cholesterol levels, and assisting in hormone regulation.

Safety

POSSIBLY UNSAFE ...when used orally (5,2623). There is no standard chemical identity for pangamic acid. Dichloroacetate, present in some formulations, is mutagenic, possibly carcinogenic. Dimethylglycine, present in some formulations, can react with nitrites in the intestines to form the potent carcinogen, dimethylnitrosamine (5).
PREGNANCY AND LACTATION: POSSIBLY UNSAFE ...when used orally; avoid using because it is difficult to know what constituents are present. Dichloroacetate, present in some formulations, is mutagenic according to the Ames test (5).

Effectiveness

POSSIBLY INEFFECTIVE

Athletic performance. Taking pangamic acid orally doesn't seem to improve exercise endurance (2645).

There is insufficient reliable information available about the effectiveness of pangamic acid for its other uses.

Mechanism of Action

There is no standard chemical identity for pangamic acid. Formulations can include one or more of the following: sodium gluconate, calcium gluconate, glycine, diisopropylamine dichloroacetate, dimethylglycine, calcium chloride, dicalcium phosphate, stearic acid, cellulose, or other constituents (5). Diisopropylamine acts on the smooth muscle to reduce blood pressure (5). In the intestines, dimethylglycine reacts with nitrates to form the potent carcinogen, dimethylnitrosamine (5).

Adverse Reactions

Orally, use of pangamic acid can be potentially carcinogenic (2623).

Interactions with Herbs & Other Dietary Supplements

CARDIAC GLYCOSIDE-CONTAINING HERBS: Theoretically, concomitant use of these herbs with large amounts of calcium salts, including calcium chloride and dicalcium phosphate, can increase the inotropic effects of cardiac glycosides and the risk of arrhythmias. Cardiac glycoside-containing herbs include black hellebore, Canadian hemp, digitalis, figwort, lily of the valley, motherwort, oleander, pheasant's eye, pleurisy root, squill, and strophanthus (4,19).

Interactions with Drugs

CALCIUM CHANNEL BLOCKERS: Theoretically, concomitant use of calcium channel blockers with calcium salts, including calcium chloride and dicalcium phosphate, can decrease the drug's effects (506). Calcium channel blockers include nifedipine (Adalat, Procardia), verapamil (Calan, Isoptin, Verelan), diltiazem (Cardizem),

isradipine (DynaCirc), felodipine (Plendil), amlodipine (Norvasc), and others.
DIGOXIN (Lanoxin): Theoretically, concomitant use of digoxin with large amounts of calcium salts, such as calcium chloride and dicalcium phosphate, can increase the inotropic effects of digoxin and the risk of arrhythmias (15).
THIAZIDE DIURETICS: Theoretically, concomitant use of these diuretics with calcium salts like calcium chloride and dicalcium phosphate can result in hypercalcemia (15).

Interactions with Foods
None known.

Interactions with Lab Tests
None known.

Interactions with Diseases or Conditions
KIDNEY DYSFUNCTION: Use pangamic acid with caution, because it can cause oxalate stones and other kidney problems (5).

Dosage and Administration
No typical dosage.

Comments
There is no standard chemical identity for pangamic acid. Pangamic acid is the name given to a product originally claimed to contain D-gluconodimethyl aminoacetic acid, which was obtained from apricot kernels and later from rice bran (5). It is also referred to as vitamin B15, but pangamic acid is not generally recognized as a vitamin (2623). Research by Soviet sports scientists focused attention on pangamic acid, but little, if any, research has been conducted in the US. The claims of pangamic acid's effectiveness are controversial (5). Natural sources for D-gluconodimethyl aminoacetic acid include brewer's yeast, whole brown rice, sesame seeds, and pumpkin seeds.

PANTETHINE

Also Known As
Bis (pantothenamidoethyl) Disulfide, D-Pantethine, Pantetina, Pantomin, Pantosin.
CAUTION: See separate listings for Pantothenic Acid and Coenzyme Q10.

Scientific Names
D-bis-(N-Pantothenyl-B-aminoethyl)-disulfide.

People Use This For
Orally, pantethine is used for lowering cholesterol, preventing inflammation, boosting immune function, treating cystinosis, treating gastrointestinal diseases, and improving athletic performance. It is also used orally for improving energy, lowering cardiovascular risk, improving adrenal function, protecting against mental and physical stress, and preventing allergy symptoms in people allergic to formaldehyde.

Safety
POSSIBLY SAFE ...when used orally and appropriately. Pantethine appears to be safe for up to 12 months (8313,8314,8315,10237,10238).
PREGNANCY AND LACTATION: Insufficient reliable information available; avoid using.

Effectiveness
POSSIBLY EFFECTIVE

Hyperlipoproteinemia. A clinically significant effect of pantethine on hyperlipoproteinemia appears to be modest. Taking pantethine orally might slightly lower triglycerides, total cholesterol, and low-density lipoprotein (LDL) cholesterol; and raise high-density lipoprotein (HDL) cholesterol (8313,8314,8317,8318,8319,9123,10238). The lipoprotein lowering effect seems to be maintained with continued treatment for up to one year (10238). Pantethine also appears to correct lipoprotein abnormalities that often occur in patients with renal failure undergoing hemodialysis (10237). Other investigators have found no effect (8315,8316). Pantethine seems to be less effective than gemfibrozil (Lopid) for lowering lipids and triglycerides (9123).

INSUFFICIENT RELIABLE EVIDENCE to RATE

Athletic performance. Some clinical research suggests that pantethine in combination with pantothenic acid and thiamine (given as allithiamin) does not improve muscular strength or endurance in well-trained athletes (10432).
Cystinosis. Preliminary evidence suggests that pantethine might be beneficial for cystinosis, an autosomal recessive genetic disease (8860). More evidence is needed to rate pantethine for these uses.

Mechanism of Action

Pantethine is a vitamin-like dietary supplement. In the body, it is converted to pantetheine, which is a precursor and component of coenzyme A. Pantethine is related to pantothenic acid (vitamin B5), but seems to have different physiological effects (8318,8320). Pantethine seems to have a beneficial effect on triglyceride and lipoprotein levels by producing cystamine. The hydrolysis product cystamine inhibits acetyl-CoA carboxylase, which in turn reduces triglyceride synthesis. Pantethine might also reduce cholesterol synthesis by inhibiting HMG-CoA reductase (8320,8321,8861,8863), by inhibiting the conversion of lanosterol to cholesterol (8865), and by inhibiting the lipid peroxidation of low-density lipoproteins (LDL) (8861,8864). Preliminary research suggests that pantethine might reduce atherosclerosis (8322). Some clinical evidence indicates pantethine might decrease platelet aggregation (9123). By producing cystamine that can deplete the cystinotic fibroblasts of cystine, pantethine might be beneficial for cystinosis, an autosomal recessive genetic disease (8860). Preliminary evidence also suggests pantethine might prevent the hypersecretion of cortisol associated with high mental and physical stress conditions, but the mechanisms are poorly understood (8859).

Pantethine seems to slow formation of experimentally induced cataracts, but in mice that develop age-related cataracts, pantethine doesn't seem to provide any protective effect (8323,8324,8325).

Adverse Reactions

Orally, pantethine seems to be well-tolerated (8313,8314,8316,8317,8318,8319). It can cause minor gastrointestinal complaints such as nausea, diarrhea, and epigastric discomfort (8315).

Interactions with Herbs & Other Dietary Supplements

ANTICOAGULANT, ANTIPLATELET HERBS AND SUPPLEMENTS: Concomitant use of herbs and supplements that affect platelet aggregation could theoretically increase the risk of bleeding in some people due to the possible effects of pantethine on platelet aggregation (9123). Some of these herbs and supplements include angelica, clove, danshen, fenugreek, feverfew, fish oils, garlic, ginger, horse chestnut, Panax ginseng, red clover, turmeric, vitamin E, and others.

Interactions with Drugs

ANTICOAGULANT/ANTIPLATELET DRUGS: Concomitant administration might increase the risk of bleeding. Some evidence suggests that pantethine reduces platelet aggregation (9123). When taken concurrently with drugs that affect platelets or coagulation, it might have an additive effect. Some of these drugs include aspirin, clopidogrel (Plavix), dalteparin (Fragmin), enoxaparin (Lovenox), heparin, indomethacin (Indocin), ticlopidine (Ticlid), warfarin (Coumadin), and others.

Interactions with Foods

None known.

Interactions with Lab Tests

None known.

Interactions with Diseases or Conditions

BLEEDING DISORDERS: There is some evidence that pantethine can decrease platelet aggregation (9123). Theoretically, pantethine might increase the risk of severe bleeding in patients with bleeding disorders; use with caution.

Dosage and Administration

ORAL: For treating hyperlipoproteinemia, 300 mg has been used 3 to 4 times daily (8313,8314,8315,8316,8317,8318,8319,8862,9123). For treating lipoprotein abnormalities in patients with renal failure undergoing hemodialysis, 600 to 1200 mg pantethine daily has been used (10237).

PANTOTHENIC ACID (VITAMIN B5)

Also Known As

B Complex Vitamin, Calcii Pantothenas, Calcium Pantothenate, D-Calcium Pantothenate, D-Panthenol, D-Pantothenyl Alcohol, Dexpanthenol, Dexpanthenolum, Panthenol, Pantothenic, Pantothenol, Pantothenylol, Vitamin B-5, Vitamin B5.

CAUTION: See separate listing for Pantethine.

Scientific Names

D-pantothenic acid; Pantothenic acid.

People Use This For

Orally, pantothenic acid is used for treating dietary deficiencies, acne, alcoholism, allergies, alopecia, asthma, attention deficit-hyperactivity disorder (ADHD), autism, burning feet syndrome, candidiasis, cardiac failure, carpal tunnel syndrome, respiratory disorders, celiac disease, colitis, conjunctivitis, convulsions, and cystitis. It is also used orally for dandruff, depression, diabetic neuropathy, enhancing immune function, improving athletic performance, glossitis, gray hair, headache, hyperactivity, hypoglycemia, insomnia, irritability, low blood pressure, multiple sclerosis, muscular dystrophy, muscular cramps in the legs associated with pregnancy or alcoholism, neuralgia, and obesity. Pantothenic acid is also used orally for osteoarthritis, rheumatoid arthritis, Parkinson's disease, peripheral neuritis, premenstrual syndrome (PMS), prostatitis, protection against mental and physical stress and anxiety, reducing adverse effects of thyroid therapy in congenital hypothyroidism, reducing signs of aging, reducing susceptibility to colds and other infections, retarded growth, shingles, skin disorders, stimulating adrenal glands, stomatitis, chronic fatigue syndrome, salicylate toxicity, streptomycin neurotoxicity, vertigo, and wound healing.
Topically, dexpanthenol, an analog of pantothenic acid, is used for itching, promoting healing of mild eczemas and dermatoses, insect stings, bites, poison ivy, diaper rash, acne, and preventing and treating acute radiotherapy skin reactions.
Intramuscularly or by intravenous infusion, dexpanthenol is used for stimulating intestinal peristalsis, to minimize the possibility of paralytic ileus after major abdominal surgery, for intestinal atony causing abdominal distension, postoperative or postpartum flatus, for postoperative delay in resumption of intestinal motility, and for treating paralytic ileus.

Safety

LIKELY SAFE ...when used orally and appropriately. Amounts up to 10 grams have been ingested without significant adverse effects (15).
PREGNANCY: LIKELY SAFE ...when used orally in amounts not exceeding the recommended daily allowance (RDA). The RDA during pregnancy is 6 mg (3094). There is insufficient reliable information about the safety of using pantothenic acid in amounts exceeding the RDA during pregnancy; avoid using.
LACTATION: LIKELY SAFE ...when used orally in amounts not exceeding the recommended daily allowance (RDA). The RDA during lactation is 7 mg (3094). There is insufficient reliable information available about the safety of using pantothenic acid in amounts exceeding the RDA during lactation; avoid using.

Effectiveness

EFFECTIVE

Pantothenic acid deficiency. Taking pantothenic acid orally is effective for treating and preventing pantothenic acid deficiency (15).

POSSIBLY INEFFECTIVE

Irradiated skin. Twice daily topical application of dexpanthenol, an analog of pantothenic acid, to areas of irradiated skin does not seem to reduce erythema, desquamation, itching, or pain following radiation treatment (7192).

INSUFFICIENT RELIABLE EVIDENCE to RATE

Athletic performance. Some clinical research suggests that pantothenic acid in combination with pantethine and thiamine (given as allithiamin) does not improve muscular strength or endurance in well-trained athletes (10432).
Attention deficit-hyperactivity disorder (ADHD). There is conflicting preliminary clinical evidence regarding the usefulness of pantothenic acid in combination with other megadose vitamins for the treatment of ADHD (3351,9957).
Osteoarthritis and rheumatoid arthritis. Preliminary clinical research suggests pantothenic acid (given as calcium pantothenate) does not significantly reduce the symptoms of arthritis in patients with rheumatoid arthritis, osteoarthritis, or other forms of arthritis (10433).
More evidence is needed to rate pantothenic acid for these uses.

Mechanism of Action

Pantothenic acid is required for intermediary metabolism of carbohydrates, proteins, and lipids (15). Dexpanthenol is converted in the body to pantothenic acid. Pantothenic acid is a precursor of coenzyme A, which is required in the acetylation reactions in gluconeogenesis; in the release of energy from carbohydrates; in the synthesis and degradation of fatty acids; and in the synthesis of sterols, steroid hormones, porphyrins, acetylcholine, and other compounds (15). Pantothenic acid also appears to be essential to normal epithelial function (15). Dietary deficiency of pantothenic acid has not been identified, but experimentally-induced deficiency has been associated with somnolence, fatigue, headache, paresthesia of the hands and feet followed by hyperreflexia and muscle weakness in the legs, cardiovascular instability, gastrointestinal (GI) complaints, changes in disposition, and increased susceptibility to infections (15). In large parenteral doses, dexpanthenol has been reported to increase GI peristalsis by stimulating acetylation of choline to acetylcholine, but efficacy has not been proven (15).

Adverse Reactions

Orally, large amounts of pantothenic acid can cause diarrhea. There is also one case of eosinophilic pleuropericardial effusion in a patient taking pantothenic acid 300 mg per day in combination with biotin 10 mg per day for 2 months (3914).

Interactions with Herbs & Other Dietary Supplements

None known.

Interactions with Drugs

None known.

Drug Influences on Nutrient Levels and Depletion

SOME DRUGS CAN AFFECT PANTOTHENIC ACID LEVELS:
ANTIBIOTICS: Destruction of normal gastrointestinal flora by antibiotics can cause decreased production of B vitamins. The clinical significance of this decreased production is not known. Consider supplementation only if clinical judgment warrants it (4434,4435,4436,4437,4438,4439,4440,4441,4442,4443).

Interactions with Foods

None known.

Interactions with Lab Tests

None known.

Interactions with Diseases or Conditions

GI OBSTRUCTION: Dexpanthenol, an alcohol analog of pantothenic acid, injection is contraindicated in individuals with gastrointestinal obstruction (15).
HEMOPHILIA: Dexpanthenol may prolong bleeding time (15).

Dosage and Administration

ORAL: As a dietary supplement, 5-10 mg pantothenic acid has been used (15) Recommended daily intakes for vitamin B5 are as follows: Infants 0-6 months, 1.7 mg; Infants 7-12 months, 1.8 mg; Children 1-3 years, 2 mg; Children 4-8 years, 3 mg; Children 9-13 years, 4 mg; Men and women 14 years and older, 5 mg (3094); Pregnant women, 6 mg; and Lactating women, 7 mg (3094).
TOPICAL: Dexpanthenol 2% is cream applied to the affected areas once or twice daily (15).
INJECTION: Dexpanthenol as an injection is an FDA-approved prescription drug.

Comments

Only the dextrorotatory isomer of pantothenic acid has biologic activity (15). Vitamin B5 is commercially available as D-pantothenic acid and the synthetic derivatives, dexpanthenol and calcium pantothenate (15). Pantothenic acid is widely distributed in plant and animal tissues; rich sources include meat, vegetables, cereal grains, legumes, eggs, and milk (15). Calcium pantothenate 10 mg is equivalent to pantothenic acid 9.2 mg (15). Pantothenic acid is frequently used in combination with other B vitamins in vitamin B complex formulations. Vitamin B complex generally includes vitamin B1 (thiamine), vitamin B2 (riboflavin), vitamin B3 (niacin/niacinamide), vitamin B5 (pantothenic acid), vitamin B6 (pyridoxine), vitamin B12 (cyanocobalamin), and folic acid. However, some products do not contain all of these ingredients and some may include others, such as biotin, para-aminobenzoic acid (PABA), choline bitartrate, and inositol (3022).

PAPAIN

Also Known As

Papainum Crudum, Plant Protease Concentrate, Vegetable Pepsin.
CAUTION: See separate listings for Bromelain, Papaya, and American Pawpaw.

Scientific Names

Carica papaya.
Family: Caricacea.

People Use This For

Orally, papain is used for inflammation and edema following trauma and surgery, as a digestive aid, for treating parasitic worms, inflammation of the throat and pharynx, herpes zoster symptoms, chronic diarrhea, hay fever, nasal drainage, and psoriasis. Papain is also used as an adjuvant treatment for tumors.

Topically, it is used to treat infected wounds, sores, and ulcers.
In manufacturing, papain is a component of cosmetics, dentifrices, enzymatic soft contact lens cleaners, meat tenderizers, and meat products. It is also used for stabilizing and chillproofing beer.

Safety

LIKELY SAFE ...when used orally in amounts commonly found in foods. Papain has Generally Recognized As Safe (GRAS) status in the US (4912).
POSSIBLY SAFE ...when used orally and appropriately for medicinal purposes (964,968,969).
POSSIBLY UNSAFE ...when used orally in large amounts. In excessive doses, papain can cause significant side effects including esophageal perforation (6) ...when raw papain is used topically. Raw papain or papaya latex is a severe irritant and vesicant (6).
PREGNANCY: POSSIBLY UNSAFE ...when used orally. There is some concern that crude papain is teratogenic and embryotoxic (6).
LACTATION: Insufficient reliable information available; avoid using.

Effectiveness

POSSIBLY EFFECTIVE

Herpes zoster (shingles). Taking papain orally may improve the symptoms of herpes zoster (965).
Pharyngitis. Taking papain orally, in combination with other agents, may relieve pharyngeal inflammation and swelling (964,968,969).

There is insufficient reliable information available about the effectiveness of papain for its other uses.

Mechanism of Action

Papain is actually a mixture of the proteolytic enzymes papain, chymopapain A, chymopapain B, and papaya peptidase A isolated from the fruit of Carica papaya. Chymopapain A and B have a similar proteolytic spectrum to papain but are less potent (6). There is some evidence that a multi-enzyme preparation containing papain can increase the release of reactive oxygen species (ROS) by polymorphonuclear cells (PMNs). ROS are thought to have tumoricidal effects (962). The multi-enzyme preparation also seems to induce the cytokines tumor necrosis factor (TNF)-alpha, interleukin-1 (IL-1)-beta, and interleukin-6 (IL-6) in a time and dose dependent manner (1364).

Adverse Reactions

Orally, large amounts of papain can cause esophageal perforation (6). Ingestion of papaya latex (raw papain) can cause severe gastritis.
Topically, papaya latex can cause severe irritation and blisters (6). Topical use of papain can cause itching (966). Severe allergic reactions have been reported in sensitive individuals (6,967). One case report suggests that there may be cross-sensitivity between papain, fig, and kiwi (963).

Interactions with Herbs & Other Dietary Supplements

HERBS WITH ANTICOAGULANT/ANTIPLATELET POTENTIAL: Concomitant use of herbs that have constituents that might affect platelet aggregation could theoretically increase the risk of bleeding in some people. These herbs include angelica, clove, danshen, garlic, ginger, ginkgo, Panax ginseng, red clover, turmeric, and others.

Interactions with Drugs

None known.

Interactions with Foods

FIG, KIWI: Cross sensitivity to papain may occur in individuals sensitive to fig and kiwi (963).
POTATO PROTEIN: May inhibit papain proteolytic activity (958).

Interactions with Lab Tests

INTERNATIONAL NORMALIZATION RATIO (INR): Concomitant use of papaya extract (papain) and warfarin may increase INR (613).

Interactions with Diseases or Conditions

CLOTTING DISORDERS: Theoretically, may increase bleeding risk (2); avoid using.

Dosage and Administration

ORAL: 1500 mg (2520 FIP units) per day have been used in clinical trials to treat inflammation and swelling following trauma and surgery (2).
TOPICAL: No typical dosage.

PAPAYA

Also Known As

Caricae papayae folium, Chirbhita, Erandachirbhita, Mamaerie, Melon Tree, Melonenbaumblaetter, Papaw, Papayas.
CAUTION: See separate listings for Papain and American Pawpaw.

Scientific Names

Carica papaya, synonyms Papaya carica, Carica peltata, Carica posoposa.
Family: Caricaceae.

People Use This For

Orally, papaya is used orally for preventing and treating gastrointestinal tract disorders, intestinal parasite infections, and as sedative and diuretic.
Topically, papaya is used for nervous pains and elephantoid growths.

Safety

LIKELY SAFE ...when used orally in amounts commonly found in foods. Papaya has Generally Recognized As Safe (GRAS) status in the US (4912).
POSSIBLY SAFE ...when used orally and appropriately in medicinal amounts (6).
POSSIBLY UNSAFE ...when used orally in excessive amounts; papaya may cause esophageal perforation (6).
...when used topically; papaya latex (raw papain) is a severe irritant and vesicant (6).
PREGNANCY: POSSIBLY UNSAFE ...when used orally; avoid using. Crude papain shows evidence that it is teratogenic and embryotoxic (6); however, this might be due to extraneous substances rather than papain (11).
LACTATION: Insufficient reliable information available; avoid using.

Effectiveness

There is insufficient reliable information available about the effectiveness of papaya.

Mechanism of Action

The applicable part of papaya is the leaf. Papaya leaf contains 2% papain and carpain (6). Papain is a mixture of enzymes that degrade protein, carbohydrates, and fats (515). Papain is unstable in digestive juices, which raises questions about whether it can be effective when used orally (515). Carpain is thought to be amebicidal. It might cause bradycardia (4009) or have central nervous system depressant or paralytic effects.

Adverse Reactions

Ingestion of large amounts of papain might cause esophageal perforation. Severe allergic reactions can occur in individuals sensitive to papain (6,515). Papaya may cause hypersensitivity reactions, which occur more commonly in people who are allergic to latex (6197,7853).

Interactions with Herbs & Other Dietary Supplements

PAPAIN: Concomitant use of papain and papaya can increase the effects and adverse effects of papain.

Interactions with Drugs

WARFARIN (Coumadin): Concomitant use might potentiate the effects of warfarin increasing the international normalization ratio (INR) (613).

Interactions with Foods

None known.

Interactions with Lab Tests

INTERNATIONAL NORMALIZATION RATIO (INR): Papain, which is in papaya leaf, can increase INR in people maintained on warfarin (Coumadin) (613).

Interactions with Diseases or Conditions

LATEX ALLERGY: People who are allergic to latex should avoid eating papaya or taking papaya-containing products because of the possibility of cross hypersensitivity between latex and papaya (6197,7853).

Dosage and Administration

ORAL: People typically use papaya with enzyme chewable tablets which contain 250 mg of papaya powder, 150 mg of dried pineapple juice powder, and 10 mg of papain (5024). One tablet is chewed up to three times daily, preferably after a meal (5024).
TOPICAL: No typical dosage.

Comments
Fermenting papaya leaves may make more potent, richer brewed teas (515).

PARA-AMINOBENZOIC ACID (PABA)

Also Known As
4-Aminobenzoic Acid, ABA, Aminobenzoate Potassium, Aminobenzoic Acid, Ethyl Dihydroxypropyl Aminobenzoate, Glyceryl Paraaminobenzoate, Octyl Diemthyl PABA, PABA, Padamate O, P-Aminobenzoic Acid, Para Amino Benzoic Acid, Para Aminobenzoic Acid, Paraaminobenzoic Acid, Vitamin B10, Vitamin H.

Scientific Names
Para-aminobenzoic acid; 4-aminobenzoic acid.

People Use This For
Orally, PABA is used for vitiligo, pemphigus, dermatomyositis, morphea, scleroderma, and Peyronie's disease. PABA is also used orally to treat female infertility, arthritis, anemia, rheumatic fever, constipation, disseminated systemic lupus erythematosus, lymphoblastoma cutis, and headaches. It is also used orally to darken gray hair, prevent hair loss, rejuvenate the skin, and prevent phototoxic reactions.
Topically, PABA is used as a sunscreen.

Safety
LIKELY SAFE ...when used topically and appropriately. PABA is FDA approved for topical use and there have not been reports of significant toxicity (266,272).
POSSIBLY SAFE ...when used orally and appropriately (10). PABA is an FDA-approved drug, but some potentially serious side effects have been reported (10).
POSSIBLY UNSAFE ...when used orally in high doses. Doses greater than 12 grams per day have been associated with leukopenia (1061).
CHILDREN: LIKELY SAFE ...when used topically and appropriately (266,272). POSSIBLY SAFE ...when used orally and appropriately (10). PABA is an FDA-approved drug for use in children, but serious side effects have been reported (10). POSSIBLY UNSAFE ...when used orally in high doses. Doses greater than 220 mg/kg/day have been associated with fatal toxic effects (1061).
PREGNANCY AND LACTATION: LIKELY SAFE ...when used topically and appropriately (266,272). There is insufficient reliable information available about the safety of the oral use of PABA during pregnancy and breast-feeding; avoid using.

Effectiveness
EFFECTIVE

Sunburn. PABA is an FDA-approved sunscreen (266,8952). PABA seems to be effective during sweating, but not when skin is immersed in water (272).

POSSIBLY INEFFECTIVE

Scleroderma. Although PABA is FDA-approved for scleroderma, evidence supporting using PABA orally for scleroderma is limited. Some retrospective studies suggest it might help for some symptoms of scleroderma, but the most convincing evidence shows that it does not help (1071,1073,1074,1075).

INSUFFICIENT RELIABLE EVIDENCE to RATE

Dermatomyositis. PABA is FDA-approved for use in dermatomyositis, but there is limited evidence to support these uses (10).
Morphea. PABA is FDA-approved for use in morphea, but there is limited evidence to support these uses (10).
Pemphigus. PABA is FDA-approved for use in pemphigus, but there is limited evidence to support these uses (10).
Peyronie's disease. PABA is FDA-approved for use in Peyronie's disease, but there is very limited evidence to support this use (1067,8951).
Vitiligo. PABA is FDA-approved for use in vitiligo, but, there is limited evidence to support these uses (10).
More evidence is needed to rate PABA for these uses.

Mechanism of Action
Para-aminobenzoic Acid (PABA) is a part of the folic acid molecule (16) and is found naturally in several foods including grains, eggs, milk, and meat (266). PABA was once considered to be a B vitamin, but is now considered a nonessential nutrient (16,8954). Interestingly, pathogenic bacteria require PABA to synthesize folic acid. Sulfonamide antibiotics exert their antibacterial effect by inhibiting folic acid synthesis from PABA (16). Although blood, urine, sweat, and spinal fluid contain detectable amounts of PABA, deficiency of PABA has not been described in humans (266). Endogenous PABA seems to be involved in a number of biologic processes, but its precise role is not known (10,266).

PABA is exogenously administered for fibrotic diseases such as dermatomyositis, morphea, pemphigus, Peyronie's disease, and scleroderma. Fibrosis might be caused by a long-term imbalance of serotonin and monoamine oxidase (MAO) activity at the tissue level. MAO requires significant tissue oxygenation to function properly. PABA may enhance MAO activity by increasing tissue oxygenation (10,266,8951).

PABA is also taken orally to darken gray hair. Although the exact mechanism is unknown, PABA appears to have an effect on melanin metabolism (8953,8954). PABA may act synergistically with cortisone in the treatment of rheumatoid arthritis. Although the mechanism is not completely understood, it is theorized that the metabolism of cortisone by the liver is decreased when oral PABA and intramuscular cortisone are given simultaneously (4488).

Topically, PABA is used as a sunscreen because it can act as a filter to block the penetration of ultraviolet (UV) radiation to the cells of the epidermis. PABA primarily blocks UVB sunlight, but may give some protection against UVA radiation at higher concentrations (272,8952).

Adverse Reactions

Orally, nausea, vomiting, dyspepsia, diarrhea, and anorexia are the most common side effects of PABA (10,1074). PABA should be discontinued if adverse effects prevent the patient from eating (10). In one report up to 25% of patients discontinued PABA due to intolerance of side effects (1074). Allergic reactions including fever and skin rash have also occurred (10,1074). Liver toxicity, including fatal hepatitis has been reported in patients taking high doses (12-48 grams per day) (1061,1094). In one case 12 grams per day for 2 months caused liver toxicity (1094). Although PABA is sometimes used to treat vitiligo, it has also been reported to cause vitiligo (1086). High dose PABA (up to 48 grams per day) can also cause decreased white blood count below 4,000 mm3 in approximately 30% of patients (1061). Death has also been reported in 3 children treated with 24 grams of PABA per day for rheumatic fever or arthritis. At autopsy, all had fatty changes in the liver, kidney, and myocardium (1061).

Topically, PABA can cause contact dermatitis and sometimes paradoxical photosensitivity (272). Some forms of PABA may stain clothing with a yellow discoloration (266).

Interactions with Herbs & Other Dietary Supplements

None known.

Interactions with Drugs

CORTISONE (Cortisone Acetate): PABA might decrease the metabolism of cortisone when oral PABA and intramuscular cortisone are given simultaneously, possibly increasing both the effects and side-effects of cortisone (4488). Dosage adjustments of cortisone may be necessary.

DAPSONE (Avlosulfon): PABA might inhibit the antibacterial effects of dapsone; avoid concurrent use (266).

SULFONAMIDE ANTIBIOTICS: PABA inhibits the antimicrobial activity of sulfonamide antibiotics. Sulfonamide antibiotics exert antibacterial effect by competitively inhibiting folic acid synthesis from PABA. Excess PABA may overcome the folate depleting effect of the sulfonamides (10). Avoid using PABA concurrently with sulfonamide antibiotics. Sulfonamide antibiotics include sulfadiazine, sulfisoxazole (Gantrisin), sulfamethoxazole (Gantanol), sulfamethizole (Thiosulfil Forte), sulfasalazine (Azulfidine), and co-trimoxazole (trimethoprim-sulfamethoxazole, Bactrim, Septra).

Interactions with Foods

None known.

Interactions with Lab Tests

LEUKOPENIA: White blood cell count might be transiently reduced when PABA is initiated, especially with high doses, but normalizes with continued administration (10).

LIVER FUNCTION TESTS: PABA has been reported to elevate liver function tests (1084). Monitor liver function tests at baseline, one month after initiating PABA therapy, and every 3 to 6 months thereafter (1084).

Interactions with Diseases or Conditions

RENAL DISEASE: PABA is renally excreted and might accumulate in patients with renal dysfunction (10); use cautiously. Dose adjustments may be necessary.

Dosage and Administration

ORAL: For vitiligo, pemphigus, dermatomyositis, morphea, scleroderma, and Peyronie's disease, the FDA approved dose for adults is 12 grams daily in 4 to 6 divided doses of the potassium salt of PABA (10). In children, the FDA approved dose is 220 mg/kg per day in 4 to 6 divided doses. PABA should be taken with meals or a snack to avoid stomach upset (10). Since PABA is renally excreted, dosage adjustments might be necessary in renal dysfunction.

TOPICAL: PABA sunscreens come in concentrations of 1% to 15% (272).

Comments

PABA appears to have fallen into disuse due to lack of proven efficacy and fears of significant toxicity (1061,1065,1084).

PAREIRA

Also Known As
Ice Vine, Pereira Brava, Velvet Leaf.
CAUTION: See separate listing for Abuta.

Scientific Names
Chondrodendron tomentosum.
Family: Menispermaceae.

People Use This For
Orally, pareira is used as a diuretic and to promote menstruation.
Parenterally, the component tubocurarine is used as a neuromuscular blocking agent.

Safety
There is insufficient reliable information available about the safety of pareira.
PREGNANCY: UNSAFE ...when used orally or parenterally because it may promote menstruation (19).
LACTATION: Insufficient reliable information available; avoid using.

Effectiveness
There is insufficient reliable information available about the effectiveness of pareira.

Mechanism of Action
The applicable part of pareira is the root. Pareira contains tubocurarine, which is used in modern anesthetics. It competitively inhibits acetylcholine binding at the nicotinic receptors at the neuromuscular junction, resulting in skeletal muscle paralysis. Tubocurarine and the other curare-like alkaloids contained in pareira are quaternary alkaloids and carry a positive charge that is not altered by pH. For this reason, they are poorly absorbed when taken orally and therefore have little neuromuscular blocking activity (505).

Adverse Reactions
None reported when pareira is used orally (18). Tubocurarine can cause hypotension due to histamine release and ganglionic blockade if IV administration is too rapid. The histamine release can also cause increased salivation, and bronchospasm. The ganglionic blockade can cause decreased GI motility and tone. Tubocurarine can also cause allergic reactions in susceptible patients (15).

Interactions with Herbs & Other Dietary Supplements
None known.

Interactions with Drugs
None known.

Interactions with Foods
None known.

Interactions with Lab Tests
None known.

Interactions with Diseases or Conditions
None known.

Dosage and Administration
No typical dosage.

Comments
Tubocurarine, a constituent of pareira, is unsafe for parenteral self-medication (15,505).

PARSLEY leaf, root

Also Known As
Common Parsley, Garden Parsley, Hamburg Parsley, Persely, Persil, Petersylinge, Petroselini herba, Petrosilini radix, Rock Parsley.
CAUTION: See separate listings for Fool's Parsley, Parsley Piert, and Parsley seed.

Scientific Names
Petroselinum crispum, synonyms Apium petroselinum, Apium crispum, Carum petroselinum, Petroselinum hortense, Petroselinum sativum, Petroselinum vulgare.
Family: Apiaceae/Umbelliferae.

People Use This For
Orally, parsley leaf and root are used as a breath freshener, for urinary tract infections, kidney stones, gastrointestinal disorders, constipation, jaundice, flatulence, indigestion, colic, bronchitic cough, asthma, general edema, rheumatism, anemia, hypotension, prostate conditions, and spleen conditions, and to promote menstrual flow. It is also used as an aphrodisiac.
Topically, parsley leaf and root are used for cracked or chapped skin, bruises, tumors, insect bites, lice, parasites, and to stimulate hair growth.
In foods and beverages, parsley leaf and root are widely used as a garnish, condiment, food, and as a flavoring.

Safety
LIKELY SAFE ...when used orally in amounts commonly found in foods. Parsley has Generally Recognized As Safe (GRAS) status in the US (4912).
POSSIBLY SAFE ...when used orally and appropriately in medicinal amounts (12).
LIKELY UNSAFE ...when used orally in very large doses (i.e., 200 grams); the apiole constituent could cause toxicity. Apiole can cause blood dyscrasias, kidney toxicity, and liver toxicity (4). ...when parsley oil is used orally due to the amount of the potentially toxic constituents, apiole and myristicin, in the oil (11). Myristicin can cause giddiness and hallucinations (4).
There is insufficient reliable information available about the safety of the topical use of parsley leaf/root.
PREGNANCY: LIKELY UNSAFE ...when medicinal amounts are used orally due to potential abortifacient, uterine or menstrual flow stimulant effects (4,12,515).
LACTATION: Insufficient reliable information available; avoid using.

Effectiveness
There is insufficient reliable information available about the effectiveness of parsley leaf and root.

Mechanism of Action
Parsley leaf and root contain volatile oils, carotene, vitamin B1, vitamin B2, and vitamin C (515). Parsley leaf also contains significant amounts of vitamin K (11285). The volatile oil contains apiole, myristicin, and photosensitizing furanocoumarins (psoralens) (512); however, the amounts vary significantly among varieties of parsley (512). Parsley has antiflatulent, antispasmodic, antirheumatic, expectorant, antimicrobial, and aquaretic effects (4,6,18,512). Aquaretics increase urine volume (water loss) but not electrolyte excretion (512). The constituent apiole appears to be associated with antispasmodic, vasodilation, and menstrual flow-stimulant effects. Apiole can also increase smooth muscle contractibility in the bladder and intestines (11). Both the apiole and myristicin constituents are believed to have aquaretic and uterine stimulant effects (512). The mechanism of aquaresis is thought to be that parsley irritates the kidney epithelium which increases renal blood flow and glomerular filtration rate (512). Apiole and myristicin have a structure similar to safrole. Safrole is considered carcinogenic and hepatotoxic (4).

Adverse Reactions
Orally, adverse effects specifically associated with more than 10 grams of the constituent, apiole, include hemolytic anemia, thrombocytopenia purpura, nephrosis, hepatic dysfunction, and kidney irritation (4). Adverse effects specifically associated with the constituent myristicin, include giddiness, deafness, hallucinations, hypotension, bradycardia, paralysis, and fatty degeneration of the liver and kidneys (4). Parsley oil can cause contact photodermatitis with sun exposure (4).
Topically, parsley leaf and root can occasionally cause allergic skin or mucous membrane reactions (2).

Interactions with Herbs & Other Dietary Supplements
None known.

Interactions with Drugs
ANTICOAGULANT/ANTIPLATELET DRUGS: Theoretically, large amounts of parsley leaf and root might interfere with oral anticoagulant therapy, due to vitamin K contained in parsley (19).

ASPIRIN: Concomitant intake with parsley might augment parsley allergy. There is one case report of severe urticaria and swelling in a person with a known mild parsley allergy after consuming parsley and aspirin (5054).
DIURETIC DRUGS: Theoretically, parsley leaf and root might interfere with diuretic therapy (512).

Interactions with Foods
None known.

Interactions with Lab Tests
INTERNATIONAL NORMALIZED RATIO (INR)/PROTHROMBIN TIME (PT): Theoretically, parsley leaf might decrease coagulation test results due to high vitamin K content (11285).

Interactions with Diseases or Conditions
EDEMA: Theoretically, parsley leaf and root might increase sodium retention and worsen edema (512).
HYPERTENSION: Theoretically, parsley leaf and root might increase sodium retention and worsen hypertension (512).
KIDNEY DISEASE: Parsley is contraindicated in individuals with kidney disease or inflammation. Parsley leaf and root can aggravate these conditions (4,19).

Dosage and Administration
No typical dosage.

PARSLEY PIERT

Also Known As
Field Lady's Mantle, Parsley Breakstone, Parsley Piercestone.
CAUTION: See separate listings for Fool's Parsley; Parsley leaf, root, and seed; Alpine lady's mantle; and Alchemilla.

Scientific Names
Aphanes arvensis, synonyms Alchemilla arvensis, Alchemilla occidentalis.
Family: Rosaceae.

Comments
At the date of publication, this product was not a common ingredient used in brand name supplements marketed to consumers. Details about this product are available at the online version of *Natural Medicines Comprehensive Database*. See www.naturaldatabase.com.

PARSLEY seed

Also Known As
Common Parsley, Garden Parsley, Parsley Fruit, Persil, Petroselini fructus.
CAUTION: See separate listings for Fool's Parsley; Parsley leaf, root; and Parsley Piert.

Scientific Names
Petroselinum crispum, synonyms Apium petroselinum, Carum petroselinum, Petroselinum hortense, Petroselinum sativum.
Family: Apiaceae/Umbelliferae.

People Use This For
Orally, parsley seed is used for ailments of the gastrointestinal tract and urinary tract, stimulating appetite and improving digestion, treating flatulence, and stimulating menstrual flow. It is also used orally for inducing abortion, treating jaundice, menstrual difficulties, asthma, cough, indigestion, and edema.
In foods, parsley seed oil is used as a flavoring.
In manufacturing, parsley seed oil is used as a fragrance in soaps, cosmetics, and perfumes.

Safety
LIKELY SAFE ...when used orally in amounts commonly found in foods.
POSSIBLY UNSAFE ...when parsley seed is used orally in tea. The volatile oil of parsley has toxic constituents, and the tea might have a low volatile oil content (2).
LIKELY UNSAFE ...when parsley seed or seed oil is used orally in amounts greater than found in foods.

The volatile oil constituent has been associated with renal epithelium irritation and cardiac arrhythmias (2). ...when parsley seed oil is used topically, it can cause photodermatitis upon sun exposure (4).
PREGNANCY: LIKELY UNSAFE ...when used orally (2,19) because it might have abortifacient, uterine, and menstrual flow-stimulating effects (4,515).
LACTATION: Insufficient reliable information available; avoid using.

Effectiveness
There is insufficient reliable information available about the effectiveness of parsley seed.

Mechanism of Action
Parsley seed might stimulate appetite and improve digestion as a result of its volatile oil content (515). The volatile oil is also believed to have mild aquaretic and laxative properties (515,8812). The volatile oil contains apiole, myristicin, and photosensitizing furanocoumarins (psoralens); however, the amounts vary significantly among varieties of parsley (512).
Aquaretics increase urine volume (water loss) but not electrolyte excretion. Researchers think aquaretic effects of parsley result from irritation of the kidney epithelium, which increases renal blood flow and glomerular filtration rate (512). Parsley seed might cause a laxative effect by inhibition of the Na-K pump and by stimulation of the NaKCL2 transporter (8812).
The constituent apiole is thought to be responsible for antispasmodic, vasodilator, and menstrual flow-stimulant effects. Apiole can increase smooth muscle contractibility in the bladder and intestines (11). Both the apiole and myristicin constituents are believed to have aquaretic and uterine stimulant effects (512). Apiole and myristicin are documented to have a structure similar to safrole, which is known to be carcinogenic and hepatotoxic (4). Parsley seed oil is reported to stimulate hepatic regeneration (4).

Adverse Reactions
Orally, parsley seed oil can cause renal damage and cardiac arrhythmias (2). Adverse effects specifically associated greater than 10 grams of the constituent apiole include hemolytic anemia, thrombocytopenia purpura, nephrosis, hepatic dysfunction, and kidney irritation (4). Adverse effects specifically associated with the constituent myristicin include giddiness, deafness, hallucinations, hypotension, bradycardia, paralysis, and fatty degeneration of the liver and kidneys (4).
Topically, parsley seed oil can cause contact photodermatitis upon exposure to the sun (4).

Interactions with Herbs & Other Dietary Supplements
None known.

Interactions with Drugs
DIURETIC DRUGS: Theoretically, parsley seed might interfere with diuretic therapy (512).

Interactions with Foods
None known.

Interactions with Lab Tests
None known.

Interactions with Diseases or Conditions
EDEMA: Theoretically, parsley seed might increase sodium retention and worsen edema (512).
HYPERTENSION: Theoretically, parsley seed might increase sodium retention and worsen hypertension (512).
KIDNEY DISEASE: Contraindicated in individuals with kidney disease or inflammation. Parsley seed can aggravate these conditions (4,19).

Dosage and Administration
ORAL: A typical oral dose is one cup tea up to 2-3 times per day. To make tea, steep 1 gram of fresh crushed seed in 150 mL boiling water for 10 minutes, strain (18).

Comments
Parsley seed oil is distilled from the seeds of parsley (Petroselinum crispum).

PARSNIP above ground parts

Also Known As
Pastinacae herba.
CAUTION: See separate listing for Parsnip root.

Scientific Names
Pastinaca sativa.
Family: Apiaceae/Umbelliferae.

Comments
At the date of publication, this product was not a common ingredient used in brand name supplements marketed to consumers. Details about this product are available at the online version of *Natural Medicines Comprehensive Database*. See www.naturaldatabase.com.

PARSNIP root

Also Known As
Pastinacae Radix.
CAUTION: See separate listing for Parsnip above ground parts.

Scientific Names
Pastinaca sativa.
Family: Apiaceae/Umbelliferae.

People Use This For
Orally, parsnip root is used for kidney complaints, fever, and as an analgesic and a diuretic.

Safety
LIKELY SAFE ...when used orally in food amounts (18).
There is insufficient reliable information available about the safety of parsnip root in medicinal amounts.
PREGNANCY AND LACTATION: LIKELY SAFE ...when used orally in food amounts. There is insufficient reliable information available about the safety of using medicinal amounts during pregnancy and breast-feeding; avoid using.

Effectiveness
There is insufficient reliable information available about the effectiveness of parsnip root.

Mechanism of Action
Parsnip root contains several furocoumarins including bergapten, xanthotoxin, and psoralen. Furocoumarins are phototoxic, mutagenic, photosensitizing, and are responsible for adverse dermatological reactions (10071).

Adverse Reactions
Topically, contact dermatitis and phototoxic reactions (including skin blisters) are possible following exposure to fresh parsnip root and exposure to sunlight. Light-skinned people may be particularly susceptible to these reactions (10071).

Interactions with Herbs & Other Dietary Supplements
None known.

Interactions with Drugs
None known.

Interactions with Foods
None known.

Interactions with Lab Tests
None known.

Interactions with Diseases or Conditions
None known.

Dosage and Administration
ORAL: One teaspoon of freshly grated parsnip root taken three times daily (18).

Comments
Parsnip root closely resembles and can be confused with the parsley root. Avoid confusing parsnip root with similar appearing hemlock and bear's breech (or hogweed) root, both of which are toxic (18).

PASSIONFLOWER

Also Known As
Apricot Vine, Corona De Cristo, Fleischfarbige, Fleur De La Passion, Flor De Passion, Madre Selva, Maracuja, Maypop, Maypop Passion Flower, Passiflora, Passiflorae herba, Passiflore, Passiflorina, Passion Flower, Passion Vine, Passionaria, Passionblume, Passionflower Herb, Passionsblumenkraut, Purple Passion Flower, Water Lemon, Wild Passion Flower.

Scientific Names
Passiflora incarnata.
Family: Passifloraceae.

People Use This For
Orally, passionflower is used for insomnia, gastrointestinal (GI) upset related to anxiety or nervousness, generalized anxiety disorder (GAD), and symptoms of opiate withdrawal. Passionflower is also used orally for neuralgia, generalized seizures, hysteria, spasmodic asthma, climacteric (menopausal) symptoms, attention deficit-hyperactivity disorder (ADHD), nervousness and excitability, palpitations, cardiac rhythm abnormalities, high blood pressure, and pain relief.
Topically, passionflower is used in bath preparations, for hemorrhoids, burns, and inflammation.
In foods and beverages, passionflower extract is used as a flavoring.

Safety
LIKELY SAFE ...when used orally in amounts commonly found in foods. Passionflower has Generally Recognized As Safe (GRAS) status in the US (4912).
POSSIBLY SAFE ...when used orally and appropriately, short-term for medicinal purposes. There is some evidence that passionflower liquid extracts can be safely used for up to one month (12,2303,8007).
POSSIBLY UNSAFE ...when used orally in excessive amounts (4).
There is insufficient reliable information available about the safety of the topical use of passionflower.
PREGNANCY: UNSAFE ...when used orally. Some passionflower constituents show evidence of uterine stimulation (4,6).
LACTATION: Insufficient reliable information available; avoid using.

Effectiveness
POSSIBLY EFFECTIVE

Adjustment disorder with anxious mood. A specific six-ingredient combination product (Euphytose, EUP) that includes passionflower seems to relieve some symptoms of adjustment disorder with anxious mood. However, it's not known which ingredient or ingredients are responsible for the beneficial effects. Other herbs in the product are crataegus, ballota, and valerian, which have mild sedative effects, and cola and paullinia with stimulant properties (6250).

Generalized anxiety disorder (GAD). There is some evidence that passionflower liquid extract 45 drops can be comparable to oxazepam (Serax) 30 mg for treating symptoms of GAD in some patients (8007).

Insomnia. Taking passionflower orally seems to be effective for mild insomnia (1).

Opiate withdrawal. Passionflower liquid extract 60 drops in combination with clonidine 0.8 mg daily seems to be significantly better than clonidine alone when used for reducing symptoms such as anxiety, irritability, insomnia, and agitation. However, the combination is no better than clonidine alone for physical symptoms such as tremor and nausea (2303).

There is insufficient reliable information available about the effectiveness of passionflower for its other uses.

Mechanism of Action
The applicable parts of passionflower are the above ground parts. Passionflower contains several active constituents, including the flavonoids apigenin, luteolin, quercetin, kaempferol, and vitexin. The harman (harmala) alkaloids identified in passionflower include harmine, harmaline, harmalol, harman, and harmin (8811,9558). Experts do not

agree about whether passionflower contains the cyanogenic glycoside gynocardine (11,19,9558). Passionflower has sedative, hypnotic, anxiolytic, and antispasmodic effects (8811,9558). It also relieves pain (4). Some evidence suggests the passionflower constituent apigenin binds to central benzodiazepine receptors (4001), possibly causing anxiolytic effects without impairing memory or motor skills (4001). Other evidence suggests passionflower extracts might reduce amphetamine-induced hypermotility, aggressiveness, and restlessness; and raise the pain threshold (1,4,11). Although animal data suggest the constituents maltol and ethylmaltol can reduce spontaneous motor activity, prolong barbiturate-induced sleep time, and show anticonvulsant activity (1,4), not enough maltol is found in passionflower preparations to cause these effects (1). Some evidence suggests the harman alkaloids have central nervous system (CNS) stimulant activity via a monoamine oxidase mechanism (4,4002); however, the sedative effects of maltol and ethylmaltol can mask these effects. The constituent passicol shows some evidence of antibacterial and antifungal activity (4).

Adverse Reactions

Orally, passionflower can cause dizziness, confusion, and ataxia in some patients (8007).

There are some reports of more severe side effects. Vasculitis and altered consciousness have been reported with use of a specific herbal product (Relaxir) produced mainly from the fruits of passionflower (6). There is also a case report involving a 34-year-old woman who developed severe nausea, vomiting, drowsiness, prolonged QT interval, and episodes of nonsustained ventricular tachycardia, requiring hospitalization for IV hydration and cardiac monitoring following use of therapeutic doses of passionflower (6251).

There is some debate about whether passionflower contains cyanogenic glycosides. Several related Passiflora species do contain them (3), including Passiflora edulis, which is associated with liver and pancreas toxicity (7).

Interactions with Herbs & Other Dietary Supplements

HERBS WITH ANTICOAGULANT/ANTIPLATELET POTENTIAL: Concomitant use of herbs that have constituents that might affect platelet aggregation could theoretically increase the risk of bleeding in some people. These herbs include angelica, clove, danshen, garlic, ginger, ginkgo, Panax ginseng, horse chestnut, red clover, turmeric, and others.

HERBS WITH SEDATIVE PROPERTIES: Theoretically, concomitant use with herbs that have sedative properties might enhance therapeutic and adverse effects. Some of these supplements include 5-HTP, calamus, California poppy, catnip, hops, Jamaican dogwood, kava, St. John's wort, scullcap, valerian, yerba mansa, and others.

Interactions with Drugs

BARBITURATES: Theoretically, concomitant use can increase drug-induced sleep time (1). Some of these sedative medications include pentobarbital (Nembutal), phenobarbital (Luminal), secobarbital (Seconal), and others.

CNS DEPRESSANTS: Theoretically, concomitant use can potentiate the effects of these drugs, including the sedative effects of antihistamines (19).

Interactions with Foods

None known.

Interactions with Lab Tests

None known.

Interactions with Diseases or Conditions

None known.

Dosage and Administration

ORAL: For generalized anxiety disorder (GAD), 45 drops of passionflower liquid extract has been used daily (8007). For reducing symptoms associated with opiate withdrawal, 60 drops of passionflower liquid extract in combination with 0.8 mg of clonidine has been used daily (2303).

The typical dose of crude passionflower herb is 0.25-2 grams of the dried above ground parts three times daily or one cup of the tea two to three times daily and 30 minutes before bedtime (1,4). The tea is prepared by steeping 0.25-2 grams of the dried above ground parts in 150 mL boiling water for 10-15 minutes and then straining. The average amount of passionflower is 4-8 grams per day. The usual dose of the liquid extract (1:1 in 25% alcohol) is 0.5-1.0 mL three times daily. The common dose of the tincture (1:8 in 45% alcohol) is 0.5-2 mL three times daily (4).

TOPICAL: Passionflower is typically used as a hemorrhoid rinse, which is prepared by simmering 20 grams of the dried above ground parts in 200 mL water, straining, and cooling before use (18).

Comments

In 1569, Spanish explorers discovered passionflower in Peru. They believed the flowers symbolized Christ's passion and indicated his approval for their exploration (6). Passionflower is found in combination herbal sedative products, some of which include German chamomile, hops, kava, scullcap, and valerian. Passionflower was formerly approved as an OTC sedative and sleep aid in the US, but it was taken off the market in 1978 because safety and effectiveness had not been proven (11,515).

PATCHOULY OIL

Also Known As
Huo xiang, Patchouli, Patchouly, Putcha-Pat.

Scientific Names
Pogostemon cablin, synonyms Mentha cablin, Pogostemon patchouly; Pogostemon heyneanus.
Family: Lamiaceae/Labiatae.

People Use This For
Orally, patchouly oil is used for colds, tumors, headaches, nausea, vomiting, diarrhea, and abdominal pain. It is also used to treat bad breath, particularly when it is associated with alcohol ingestion.
In foods and beverages, patchouly oil is used as a flavor ingredient.
In manufacturing, patchouly oil is used in perfumes and cosmetics.

Safety
LIKELY SAFE ...when used orally in amounts commonly found in foods. Patchouly has Generally Recognized As Safe (GRAS) status in the US (4912). There is insufficient reliable information available about the safety of patchouly oil in medicinal amounts.
PREGNANCY AND LACTATION: Insufficient reliable information available; avoid using.

Effectiveness
There is insufficient reliable information available about the effectiveness of patchouly oil.

Mechanism of Action
Patchouly oil is the oil distilled from the dried leaf, young leaves, and shoots. Animal data suggests that patchouly oil is nontoxic with short term oral use. Patchouly oil may have bactericidal activity, and the component pogostone appears to have antibacterial and antifungal activities. The components eugenol, cinnamaldehyde, and benzaldehyde may have insecticidal activity against insects in stored grain (11).

Adverse Reactions
None reported.

Interactions with Herbs & Other Dietary Supplements
None known.

Interactions with Drugs
None known.

Interactions with Foods
None known.

Interactions with Lab Tests
None known.

Interactions with Diseases or Conditions
None known.

Dosage and Administration
No typical dosage.

Comments
Patchouly oil can be adulterated with other oils, including gurjun balsam oil, copaiba balsam oil, and cedarwood oil (11).

PAU D'ARCO

Also Known As
Ipe, Ipe Roxo, Ipes, Lapacho, Lapacho Colorado, Lapacho Morado, Pau dArco, Pau de Arco, Purple Lapacho, Red Lapacho, Taheebo, Taheebo Tea, Trumpet Bush.

Scientific Names
Tabebuia impetiginosa, synonyms Tabebuia avellanedae, Tabebuia palmeri, Tecoma impetiginosa;
Tabebuia heptaphylla, synonyms Bignonia heptaphylla, Tabebuia ipe, Tecoma ipe.
Family: Bignoniaceae.

People Use This For
Orally, pau d'arco is used for Candida yeast infections, infectious diarrhea, bladder infections, parasitic infections, cancer, diabetes, ulcers, gastritis, liver ailments, asthma, bronchitis, cystitis, prostatitis, ringworm, rheumatism, hernias, gonorrhea, syphilis, chlorosis, boils, wounds, as a "tonic and blood builder", and for viral respiratory infections including the common cold and flu
Topically, pau d'arco is used for Candida infections.

Safety
POSSIBLY UNSAFE ...when used orally in typical doses. Significant evaluation of the safety of pau d'arco in typical doses has not been conducted; however, serious toxicities have been found with higher doses (6,515). Pau d'arco should be used with caution.
LIKELY UNSAFE ...when used orally in large doses. In studies in cancer patients, when doses were elevated to provide therapeutic plasma levels of the active constituent lapachol, patients experienced significant toxicities, including increased risk of bleeding (6,515). Doses of pau d'arco providing greater than 1.5 grams per day of the lapachol constituent have been associated with the most risk (6).
There is insufficient reliable information available about the safety of pau d'arco for its other uses.
PREGNANCY: POSSIBLY UNSAFE ...when used orally in typical doses; avoid using. LIKELY UNSAFE ...when used orally in large doses; contraindicated. Significant evaluation of the safety of pau d'arco in typical doses has not been conducted; however, serious toxicities have been found with higher doses (6,515).
There is insufficient reliable information available about the safety of pau d'arco used topically in pregnancy.
LACTATION: Insufficient reliable information; avoid using.

Effectiveness
There is insufficient reliable information available about the effectiveness of pau d'arco.

Mechanism of Action
The applicable parts of pau d'arco are the bark and the wood. The active constituents are thought to be a naphthoquinone derivative, lapachol, and its derivatives. The wood contains lapachol and the bark contains mostly lapachol derivatives. Lapachol and its derivatives are thought to have similar pharmacological activities (515). Lapachol is thought to be responsible for increasing the risk of bleeding by prolonging prothrombin time. Its effects on clotting are reversible by vitamin K (6). Preliminary data suggests that lapachol also has anti-inflammatory, antimalarial, antibacterial, antifungal, antiparasitic, and immunomodulatory activity (6,515). Some evidence suggests that lapachol is active against sarcomas, but at potentially effective levels, adverse effects are severe enough to prevent its use for that indication (515).

Adverse Reactions
Orally, pau d'arco causes severe nausea, vomiting, diarrhea, dizziness, anemia, and increases the risk of bleeding when used in high doses (515). Doses of pau d'arco providing greater than 1.5 grams per day of the lapachol constituent have been associated with the most risk (6).

Interactions with Herbs & Other Dietary Supplements
HERBS WITH ANTICOAGULANT/ANTIPLATELET POTENTIAL: Theoretically, concomitant use with herbs that have constituents that might affect platelet aggregation could theoretically increase the chance of bleeding in some people. These herbs include alfalfa, angelica, clove, danshen, horse chestnut, red clover, turmeric, and others.

Interactions with Drugs
ANTICOAGULANT/ANTIPLATELET DRUGS: Theoretically, concomitant use with pau d'arco might increase clotting time and increase the risk for bleeding (515).

Interactions with Foods
None known.

Interactions with Lab Tests
PROTHROMBIN TIME (PT)/INTERNATIONAL NORMALIZED RATION (INR): Pau d'arco can increase PT and INR test results and increase the risk of bleeding (6,515).

Interactions with Diseases or Conditions
COAGULATION DISORDERS: Pau d'arco can increase bleeding time and might interfere with therapy in patients with coagulation disorders (6,515); use with caution.

Dosage and Administration
ORAL: People typically use 1 to 4 grams daily in 2 to 3 divided doses. One manufacturer warns that the product should not be used for more than 7 days; however, the reason for this warning is not known. The contents of pau d'arco capsules may also be emptied and prepared as a tea. A tincture in the amount of 0.5 to 1 mL and a glycerin-based liquid in the amount of 1 to 3 mL, are used 3 times daily (6006).

Comments
Pau d'arco wood is extremely hard and almost indestructible (515). In South America, the Indians used the tree to make bows for hunting. Pau d'arco is the Spanish name for "bow stick" (6002). Teas, labeled as pau d'arco or lapacho, do not always contain the Tabebuia species; in some cases they have contained the related species, Tecoma curialis (515). Some report that the inner-bark preparations of pau d'arco are preferred because they are the most effective. Some products may use the outer-bark and mislabel the product as true inner-bark pau d'arco (3564). The anticancer activity of the pau d'arco constituent lapachol was extensively researched in the 1960s. The research was abandoned due to its toxicity (6).

PEANUT OIL

Also Known As
Arachis, Earth-Nut, Groundnuts, Monkey Nuts.

Scientific Names
Arachis hypogaea.
Family: Fabaceae/Leguminosae.

People Use This For
Orally, peanut oil is used to lower cholesterol and prevent heart disease. It is also used orally to aid in weight loss and decrease appetite, and to help prevent cancer.
Topically, peanut oil is used for arthritis and joint pain, scalp crusting and scaling without hair loss, dry skin, eczema, and ichthyosis (noninflammatory skin disorders that cause scaling).
Rectally, peanut oil is used in ointments and medicinal oils for treating constipation.
It is also used as a vehicle for external, enteral, and parenteral pharmaceutical formulations.
In manufacturing, peanut oil is used in skin care products and baby care products.

Safety
LIKELY SAFE ...when used orally in amounts commonly found in foods. Peanut oil has Generally Recognized As Safe (GRAS) status in the US (4912). ...when used orally, topically, or rectally in medicinal amounts.
PREGNANCY AND LACTATION: There is insufficient reliable information about the safety of medicinal amounts of peanut oil during pregnancy and breast-feeding; avoid using.

Effectiveness
There is insufficient reliable information available about the effectiveness of peanut oil.

Mechanism of Action
Peanuts contain beta-sitosterol and resveratrol, which may contribute to cardioprotective and cancer protective activity (4263,4267). The high monounsaturated, low saturated fat content of peanut oil is thought to prevent heart disease and lower cholesterol. Population studies suggest people who eat nuts have a lower risk of developing heart disease (4264). This benefit must be weighed against animal evidence that suggests peanut oil is atherogenic, perhaps due to the triglyceride content or the presence of a lectin (4265,4266).

Adverse Reactions
Peanut oil can cause a severe allergic reaction in individuals allergic to the Fabaceae family. Members of this family include peanuts and soybeans (4079,4080).

Interactions with Herbs & Other Dietary Supplements

None known.

Interactions with Drugs

None known.

Interactions with Foods

None known.

Interactions with Lab Tests

None known.

Interactions with Diseases or Conditions

CROSS-ALLERGENICITY: Peanut oil can cause a severe allergic reaction in individuals sensitive to the Fabaceae family. Members of this family include peanuts and soybeans (4079,4080).

Dosage and Administration

ORAL: No typical dosage.
TOPICAL: For bath use, 4 mL peanut oil is added to 10 L water. Adults bathe for 15-20 minutes 2-3 times daily. Children bathe for a few minutes 2-3 times weekly (18).
RECTAL: As an enema, 130 mL of room temperature peanut oil has been used.

Comments

Sometimes the less expensive soya oil is added to peanut oil (18).

PEAR

Also Known As

Pears.

Scientific Names

Pyrus communis, synonyms Pyrus asiae-mediae, Pyrus balansae, Pyrus bourgaeana, Pyrus domestica, Pyrus elata, Pyrus medvedevii.
Family: Rosaceae.

People Use This For

Orally, pear fruit is used for mild digestive disorders, cholera, colic, diarrhea, nausea, liver sclerosis, spasms, tumors, and for reducing fevers. It is used orally for its laxative, bactericidal, calmative, and diuretic properties.
Topically, pear fruit is used as an astringent.
In foods, pears are eaten as fresh fruit, preserved fruit, and used in cooking.

Safety

LIKELY SAFE ...when used orally (18).
There is insufficient reliable information available about the safety of pear fruit for its other uses.
PREGNANCY AND LACTATION: LIKELY SAFE ...when consumed in amounts commonly found in foods (18).

Effectiveness

There is insufficient reliable information available about the effectiveness of pear.

Mechanism of Action

The applicable part of the pear is the fruit. Pear fruit contains pectin (18) that might contribute to antidiarrheal activity (7).

Adverse Reactions

None reported.

Interactions with Herbs & Other Dietary Supplements

None known.

Interactions with Drugs

None known.

Interactions with Foods
None known.

Interactions with Lab Tests
None known.

Interactions with Diseases or Conditions
None known.

Dosage and Administration
No typical dosage.

PECTIN

Also Known As
Pectinic Acid.

Scientific Names
Pectin.

People Use This For
Orally, pectin is used as an adsorbent, for reducing high cholesterol and triglycerides, for reducing the risk of colon cancer, for reducing damage from radiation, for treating diabetes, for treating gastroesophageal reflux disease (GERD), and as an antibacterial.
Topically, pectin is used for protecting raw or ulcerated mouth and throat sores.
In combination with kaolin (Kaopectate) or paregoric (Parepectolin), pectin is used to treat diarrhea.
In food manufacturing, pectin is used as a thickening agent in cooking and baking.
In manufacturing, pectin is used as a denture adhesive component.

Safety
LIKELY SAFE ...when used in amounts commonly found in foods. Pectin has Generally Recognized As Safe (GRAS) status in the US (4912). ...when used orally in medicinal amounts (16).
PREGNANCY AND LACTATION: Insufficient reliable information; avoid using.

Effectiveness
EFFECTIVE

Diarrhea. Taking pectin orally is an effective adsorbent for treating diarrhea, usually in combination with kaolin or other ingredients (15).

POSSIBLY EFFECTIVE

Hypercholesterolemia. Taking pectin orally seems to lower cholesterol (2214,2215,2216,2217).

There is insufficient reliable information available about the effectiveness of pectin for its other uses.

Mechanism of Action
Pectin is a soluble fiber (polysaccharide) obtained from the inner portion of the rind of citrus fruits and apple pomace. It is found in the cell walls of plant tissue and helps give plants rigidity (6). Pectin acts as an adsorbent and bulk-forming agent and can interfere with drug and nutrient absorption (19).
Pectin might be able to reduce the amount of stomach contents refluxed into the esophagus. Like alginic acid (Gaviscon), it floats on top of the stomach contents and may serve as a barrier between the stomach acid and the esophagus. Pectin does not affect the pH in the stomach. It might be useful for treating gastroesophageal reflux disease (GERD), but more clinical research is needed before pectin can be recommended for this use (10431).

Adverse Reactions
The occupational inhalation of pectin dust can cause asthma (580,581,582,583,584).

Interactions with Herbs & Other Dietary Supplements
BETA-CAROTENE: Concomitant use of pectin can significantly reduce beta-carotene absorption (2225).
NUTRITIONAL SUPPLEMENTS: Concomitant use of pectin can interfere with the absorption of nutritional supplements (6).

Interactions with Drugs
BETA-CAROTENE: Concomitant use of pectin can significantly reduce beta-carotene absorption (2225).
DIGOXIN (Lanoxin): Concomitant use of pectin can interfere with the intestinal absorption of digoxin (2212).
LOVASTATIN (Mevacor): Concomitant use of pectin can interfere with the intestinal absorption of lovastatin (615).
TETRACYCLINE ANTIBIOTICS: Concomitant use of pectin can interfere with the intestinal absorption of tetracyclines (2213).

Interactions with Foods
NUTRIENTS: Pectin can interfere with the absorption of dietary nutrients (6).

Interactions with Lab Tests
CHOLESTEROL: Pectin can decrease serum cholesterol and test results (275).

Interactions with Diseases or Conditions
PECTIN HYPERSENSITIVITY: Contraindicated.

Dosage and Administration
ORAL: As an adsorbent, 30 mL of 10% pectin in a mixture with kaolin is taken as needed (16). As an antihyperlipidemic, 15 grams per day was used in one study (2214).
TOPICAL: No typical dosage.

Comments
Commercial pectin can contain sugars of organic acids and other additives, but pharmaceutical grade pectin contains no impurities or additives (13). The FDA is currently reevaluating the effectiveness of pectin combinations for diarrhea (272).

PELLITORY

Also Known As
Akarakarabha.
CAUTION: See separate listing for Pellitory-of-the-Wall.

Scientific Names
Anacyclus pyrethrum, synonym Anthemis pyrethrum.
Family: Asteraceae/Compositae.

People Use This For
Orally, pellitory is used for arthritis and as a digestive aid.
Topically, pellitory is used for toothaches and as an insecticide.

Safety
There is insufficient reliable information available about the safety of pellitory.
Pregnancy and Lactation: Insufficient reliable information available; avoid using.

Effectiveness
There is insufficient reliable information available about the effectiveness of pellitory.

Mechanism of Action
The applicable part of pellitory is the root. Application of pellitory to skin may stimulate nerve endings and result in redness and irritation, which is felt as a hot, burning sensation. Alkylamines may possibly contribute, since they may stimulate mucous membranes (18).

Adverse Reactions
Signs of skin irritation may occur with overuse (18). Pellitory can cause an allergic reaction in individuals sensitive to the Asteraceae/Compositae family. Members of this family include ragweed, chrysanthemums, marigolds, daisies, and many other herbs.

Interactions with Herbs & Other Dietary Supplements
None known.

Interactions with Drugs
None known.

Interactions with Foods
None known.

Interactions with Lab Tests
None known.

Interactions with Diseases or Conditions
CROSS-ALLERGENICITY: Can cause an allergic reaction in individuals sensitive to the Asteraceae/Compositae family. Members of this family include ragweed, chrysanthemums, marigolds, daisies, and many other herbs.

Dosage and Administration
No typical dosage.

Comments
Avoid confusing with the similar sounding pellitory-of-the-wall.

PELLITORY-OF-THE-WALL

Also Known As
Lichwort, Pellitory of the Wall.
CAUTION: See separate listing for Pellitory.

Scientific Names
Parietaria officinalis.
Family: Urticaceae.

People Use This For
Orally, pellitory-of-the-wall is used as a diuretic, laxative, and as a demulcent. It is also used for chronic cough and for a variety of kidney disorders including urinary tract infections (UTIs) and pyelonephritis, renal pain, and kidney stones.
Topically, pellitory-of-the-wall is used for treating burns and wounds.

Safety
POSSIBLY SAFE ...when used orally (12).
PREGNANCY AND LACTATION: Insufficient reliable information available; avoid using.

Effectiveness
There is insufficient reliable information available about the effectiveness of pellitory-of-the-wall.

Mechanism of Action
The applicable parts of pellitory-of-the-wall are the aerial parts. It contains flavonoids and tannins (7161).

Adverse Reactions
Pellitory-of-the-wall pollen has been associated with seasonal allergy (7161).

Interactions with Herbs & Other Dietary Supplements
None known.

Interactions with Drugs
None known.

Interactions with Foods
None known.

Interactions with Lab Tests
None known.

Interactions with Diseases or Conditions
None known.

Dosage and Administration
No typical dosage.

Comments
The name pellitory-of-the-wall comes from its habit of growing in old walls and dry, stony areas (7161). Avoid confusion between pellitory-of-the-wall and the similar sounding pellitory.

PENNYROYAL leaf

Also Known As
American Pennyroyal, European Pennyroyal, Lurk-In-The-Ditch, Mosquito Plant, Penny Royal, Piliolerial, Pudding Grass, Pulegium, Run-By-The-Ground, Squaw Balm, Squawmint, Stinking Balm, Tickweed.
CAUTION: See separate listing for Pennyroyal Oil.

Scientific Names
Mentha pulegium, synonym Pulegium vulgare; Hedeoma pulegioides, synonym Melissa pulegioides.
Family: Lamiaceae/Labiatae.

People Use This For
Orally, pennyroyal leaf is used as an antispasmodic, antiflatulent, diaphoretic, stimulant, for bowel disorders, pneumonia, stomach pains, weakness, and as a diuretic. It is also used orally as an abortifacient, menstrual stimulant or regulator, for intestinal disorders, colds, digestive disorders, liver and gall bladder disorders, and respiratory ailments.

Safety
LIKELY UNSAFE ...when the alcoholic extract is used orally. Repeated use of the alcoholic extract over a period of two weeks was linked to a death (650).
There is insufficient reliable information available about the safety of the oral use of pennyroyal leaf as tea.
CHILDREN: UNSAFE ...when used orally. Two infants developed severe hepatic and neurologic injuries and one infant died (4,291).
PREGNANCY: LIKELY UNSAFE ...when used orally as pennyroyal leaf tea which is reported to cause onset of menses (650). UNSAFE ...when the oil is used orally because it is considered to be an abortifacient and can cause death (4).
LACTATION: LIKELY UNSAFE ...when used orally as an alcoholic extract or oil (650). There is insufficient reliable information available for oral use of pennyroyal leaf tea; avoid using.

Effectiveness
There is insufficient reliable information available about the effectiveness of pennyroyal leaf.

Mechanism of Action
Both American and European pennyroyal leaves contain 1-2% of essential oils, tannins, and flavonoids (12,18). The volatile oil, pulegone and its metabolite, menthofuran, or methofuran's metabolites might be responsible for hepatotoxicity, neurotoxicity, and bronchiolar epithelial cell destruction (6,650). The oxidative metabolites of pulegone and menthofuran are thought to cause cell damage by binding to target proteins (650). Some metabolites of pulegone also extensively deplete hepatic glutathione levels (650,291), which allows metabolite accumulation and direct cellular damage similar to acetaminophen toxicity (291). Pulegone is less concentrated in the American species (30%) than in European species (62-97%) (12).

Adverse Reactions
Orally, pennyroyal leaf can cause abdominal cramping and pain, fever, nausea (4,6,650), vomiting (possibly bloody), lethargy alternating with agitation, confusion, delirium, restlessness, seizures, dizziness, weakness, syncope (650), auditory and visual hallucinations (6), elevated blood pressure and pulse rate, bilateral lung congestion, hepatic failure, renal failure, acidosis, disseminated intravascular coagulation, abortion, respiratory failure, shock, and death (6,18,650). Topically, it can cause an urticarial rash (4) and dermatitis (6).

Interactions with Herbs & Other Dietary Supplements
None known.

Interactions with Drugs
None known.

Interactions with Foods
None known.

Interactions with Lab Tests
None known.

Interactions with Diseases or Conditions
KIDNEY DISEASE: The volatile oil can cause kidney irritation (19).

Dosage and Administration
No typical dosage.

Comments
American pennyroyal and European pennyroyal are historically interchangeable as a source of pennyroyal oil (12). About 50-100 grams of leaves are required to produce 1 ml of pennyroyal oil (4).

PENNYROYAL OIL

Also Known As
American Pennyroyal, European Pennyroyal, Lurk-In-The-Ditch, Mosquito Plant, Penny Royal, Piliolerial, Pudding Grass, Pulegium, Run-By-The-Ground, Squaw Balm, Squawmint, Stinking Balm, Tickweed.
CAUTION: See separate listing for Pennyroyal leaf.

Scientific Names
Hedeoma pulegioides, synonym Melissa pulegioides; Mentha pulegium, synonym Pulegium vulgare.
Family: Lamiaceae/Labiatae.

People Use This For
Orally, pennyroyal oil is used as an antispasmodic, antiflatulent, diaphoretic, stimulant, and as a diuretic. It is also used for pneumonia, stomach pains, and weakness. It is also used orally as an abortifacient; as a menstrual stimulant or regulator; and for intestinal disorders, colds, respiratory ailments, digestive disorders, and liver and gallbladder disorders.
Topically, pennyroyal oil is used as an antiseptic, insect repellent, and for skin diseases. It is also used topically for tactile hallucinations, gout, venomous bites, mouth sores, as a flea-killing bath, and as a counterirritant.
In foods, pennyroyal oil is used as a flavoring agent.
In manufacturing, pennyroyal oil is used as a dog and cat flea repellent, and a fragrance for detergents, perfumes, and soaps.

Safety
POSSIBLY SAFE ...when used orally as a food flavoring. Pulegone-free American pennyroyal is allowed only in alcoholic beverages in Canada (4). The Council of Europe lists pennyroyal as a natural source of food flavoring, without assessment of toxicity (4).
LIKELY UNSAFE ...when used orally or topically (4). Neurologic injury has been reported in adults consuming 2.5-5.0 mL of pennyroyal oil (5,6,9). Nephrotoxicity, hepatotoxicity, and death have been reported after ingestion of 15-30 mL (4,5,6,12,5601). Some evidence suggests that the oil can be absorbed systemically (6,292).
PREGNANCY: LIKELY UNSAFE ...when used orally or topically. Pennyroyal oil is an abortifacient (4).
LACTATION: LIKELY UNSAFE ...when used orally or topically (4); avoid using.

Effectiveness
There is insufficient reliable information available about the effectiveness of pennyroyal oil.

Mechanism of Action
Pennyroyal oil contains pulegone, which may cause hepatotoxicity, neurotoxicity, and bronchiolar epithelial cell destruction (6). The oxidative metabolites of pulegone and menthofuran may cause cell damage by binding to target proteins (650), depleting hepatic glutathione levels (650,292), and by direct cellular damage similar to acetaminophen toxicity (291). Its abortifacient effect might be due to uterine contractions triggered by genitourinary tract irritation (4,6,19). Large doses required for the abortifacient effect can cause irreversible kidney damage, hepatic damage, and death (6). In the American species, pulegone is 30% less concentrated than in the European species (62-97%) (12).

Adverse Reactions
Orally, pennyroyal oil can cause abdominal pain and tenderness, nausea, vomiting (possibly bloody), burning of the throat, fever, lethargy alternating with agitation, confusion, delirium, restlessness, seizures, dizziness, auditory and visual hallucinations, elevated blood pressure and pulse rate, bilateral lung congestion, acidosis, disseminated intravascular coagulation, abortion, hepatic failure, renal failure, respiratory failure, shock, and death (4,6,17,5601).
Topically, it can cause a urticarial rash (4,5601) and dermatitis (6).

Interactions with Herbs & Other Dietary Supplements
None known.

Interactions with Drugs
None known.

Interactions with Foods
None known.

Interactions with Lab Tests
None known.

Interactions with Diseases or Conditions
KIDNEY DISEASE: The volatile oil can cause kidney irritation (19).

Dosage and Administration
No typical dosage.

Comments
Historically, American pennyroyal and European pennyroyal are interchangeable as sources of pennyroyal oil (12).

PEONY flower

Also Known As
Common Peony, Coral Peony, European Peony, Paeonia, Paeoniae flos, Piney.
CAUTION: See separate listing for Peony root.

Scientific Names
Paeonia mascula, synonym Paeonia caucasica; Paeonia officinalis.
Family: Paeoniaceae.

People Use This For
Orally, peony flowers are used for gout, arthritis, respiratory tract ailments, and as a cough remedy. Peony flowers are also used orally for epilepsy, bowel complaints, as an emetic, and for inducing menstruation or miscarriage.
Topically, peony flowers are used for skin and mucous membrane diseases, and for healing fissures, especially anal fissures associated with hemorrhoids.
In herb combinations, peony flowers are used orally for heart trouble and gastritis.
In manufacturing, peony flowers are used commercially to color cough syrups. They are used in herbal teas to improve their appearance.

Safety
There is insufficient reliable information available about the safety of peony flower.
PREGNANCY: LIKELY UNSAFE ...when used orally due to historical use as an abortifacient and menstruation-inducing agent (18).
LACTATION: Insufficient reliable information available; avoid using.

Effectiveness
There is insufficient reliable information available about the effectiveness of peony flower.

Mechanism of Action
Hypertonia has been reported in animal tests, but the peony part(s)/product used were not specified (18).

Adverse Reactions
Orally, overdose has reportedly led to gastroenteritis with vomiting, colic, and diarrhea (8,18).

Interactions with Herbs & Other Dietary Supplements
None known.

Interactions with Drugs
None known.

Interactions with Foods
None known.

Interactions with Lab Tests
None known.

Interactions with Diseases or Conditions
None known.

Dosage and Administration
ORAL: A typical dosage is one cup of tea (steep 1 gram flowers in 150 mL boiling water 5-10 minutes, strain) daily (8,18).
TOPICAL: No typical dosage.

Comments
Avoid confusion with peony root.

PEONY root

Also Known As
Common Peony, Coral Peony, European Peony, Paeonia, Paeoniae Radix, Piney.
CAUTION: See separate listing for Peony flower.

Scientific Names
Paeonia mascula, synonym Paeonia caucasica; Paeonia officinalis.
Family: Paeoniaceae.

People Use This For
Orally, peony root is used for spasms. It is also used for epilepsy, excitability, whooping cough, arthritis, bowel complaints, as an emetic, and for inducing menstruation.
In herbal combinations, peony root is used for arthritis, gastrointestinal (GI) tract diseases, conditions of the heart and circulatory system, neuralgia, migraines, as a tonic, and for chronic fatigue syndrome (CFS).

Safety
There is insufficient reliable information available about the safety of peony root.
PREGNANCY: LIKELY UNSAFE ...when used orally. Historically, it has been used to induce menstruation (18,19).
LACTATION: Insufficient reliable information available; avoid using.

Effectiveness
There is insufficient reliable information available about the effectiveness of peony root.

Mechanism of Action
Peony root extract exhibits neuroprotective activity and prevents experimentally induced brain neuron spike discharges in rats (3818). Researchers attribute neuroprotection to the gallotannin and paeoniflorin constituents (3818).

Adverse Reactions
Orally, peony root overdose can result in gastroenteritis with vomiting, colic, and diarrhea (8,18).

Interactions with Herbs & Other Dietary Supplements
None known.

Interactions with Drugs
PHENYTOIN (Dilantin): Peony root might reduce levels of phenytoin and potentially reduce the therapeutic effectiveness of phenytoin (8657). It's theorized that peony root might affect cytochrome P450 2C9 (CYP2C) enzymes, which metabolizes phenytoin. But there is evidence that peony root does not alter levels of losartan, which

is also metabolized by CYP2C9 (11480). More evidence is needed to determine if peony root affects other drugs metabolized by CYP2C9.

Interactions with Foods
None known.

Interactions with Lab Tests
None known.

Interactions with Diseases or Conditions
None known.

Dosage and Administration
No typical dosage.

Comments
Avoid confusion with peony flower.

PEPPERMINT leaf

Also Known As
Brandy Mint, Lamb Mint, Menthae piperitae folium, Menthe poivree, Paparaminta.
CAUTION: See separate listing for Peppermint Oil.

Scientific Names
Mentha piperita, synonym Mentha lavanduliodora.
Family: Lamiaceae/Labiatae.

People Use This For
Orally, peppermint leaf is used for loss of appetite; spasms of the gastrointestinal tract, gallbladder, and bile ducts; and for flatulence, gastritis, enteritis, nausea, vomiting, morning sickness, respiratory infections, and dysmenorrhea. In foods, peppermint leaf is used as a culinary spice.

Safety
LIKELY SAFE ...when used orally in amounts commonly found in foods. Peppermint has Generally Recognized As Safe (GRAS) status for food use in the US (4912).
POSSIBLY SAFE ...when used orally and appropriately for medicinal purposes (1,12).
CHILDREN: POSSIBLY UNSAFE ...when used orally in infants and small children; peppermints menthol content can cause unpleasant choking sensations (512).
PREGNANCY: POSSIBLY UNSAFE ...when used orally in medicinal amounts due to its potential to induce menstrual bleeding (19).
LACTATION: Insufficient reliable information available; avoid using in medicinal amounts.

Effectiveness
There is insufficient reliable information available about the effectiveness of peppermint leaf.

Mechanism of Action
Peppermint leaf has spasmolytic and antiflatulent activities. It also stimulates bile production (2,18). The constituents include the volatile oil menthol (7,11,18), flavonoids (11,18), and azulene (11). In vitro and in animals, menthol's antispasmodic effects result from a direct action on the digestive tract smooth muscle that is characteristic of calcium antagonist activity (1,7). Flavonoids have bile-stimulating effects. In animals, azulene has anti-inflammatory and anti-ulcer effects (11). Peppermint's soothing effect in coughs or colds results from the stimulation of salivation, which increases the swallowing reflex and suppresses cough (3).

Adverse Reactions
Orally, peppermint leaf can increase colic in people with gallstones (2,19). It can also cause an unpleasant choking sensation in infants and small children (512).

Interactions with Herbs & Other Dietary Supplements
None known.

Interactions with Drugs
None known.

Interactions with Foods
None known.

Interactions with Lab Tests
None known.

Interactions with Diseases or Conditions
GALLSTONES: Physician consultation is advised before the use of the peppermint leaf in individuals with gallstones (2), because it can increase symptoms of colic (18).
HIATAL HERNIA: Theoretically, peppermint leaf can exacerbate hernia symptoms due to its relaxation of the lower esophageal sphincter (500).

Dosage and Administration
ORAL: For upset stomach, the typical dose of peppermint leaf is one cup of the tea three to four times daily between meals (1,512). The tea is prepared by steeping 1 tablespoon of the dried leaf in 150 mL boiling water for 10 minutes and then straining. It can also be consumed at meal times or as needed (7). The average daily amount of the peppermint leaf is 3-6 grams (18). Peppermint tea is contraindicated in infants and small children because its menthol content can cause an unpleasant choking sensation (512). The usual dose of the tincture (1:5 in 45% ethanol) is 2-3 mL three times daily (1).

PEPPERMINT OIL

Also Known As
Menthae piperitae Aetheroleum, Menthe Poivree, Paparaminta.
CAUTION: See separate listing for Peppermint leaf.

Scientific Names
Mentha piperita, synonym Mentha lavanduliodora.
Family: Lamiaceae/Labiatae.

People Use This For
Orally, peppermint oil is used for colds, coughs, inflammation of the mouth and pharynx, liver and gallbladder complaints, irritable bowel syndrome (IBS), cramps of the upper gastrointestinal (GI) tract and bile ducts, dyspepsia, as an antipyretic and antiflatulent, and for tension headache. It is also used orally for nausea, vomiting, morning sickness, respiratory infections, dysmenorrhea, indigestion, diarrhea, and as a stimulant.
Topically, peppermint oil is used for headache, myalgias, neuralgias, toothache, oral mucosa inflammation, rheumatic conditions, pruritus, urticaria, as an antibacterial and antiviral agent, as an antispasmodic in barium enemas, and for repelling mosquitoes.
As an inhalant, peppermint oil is used as an aromatic, for symptomatic treatment of cough and colds, and as an analgesic for pain.
In foods and beverages, peppermint oil is a common flavoring agent.
In manufacturing, peppermint oil is used as a fragrance component in soaps and cosmetics, and as a flavoring agent in pharmaceuticals.

Safety
LIKELY SAFE ...when used orally in amounts commonly found in foods. Peppermint oil has Generally Recognized As Safe (GRAS) status in the US (4912).
POSSIBLY SAFE ...when used orally, topically, or rectally and appropriately for medicinal purposes (3801,3804,6190,6740,6741,10075,12009). ...when used by inhalation as aromatherapy (7107).
LIKELY UNSAFE ...when used orally in large amounts. High doses of peppermint oil have been associated with interstitial nephritis and acute renal failure (7). Menthol, a major constituent, is considered lethal at a dose of 2-9 grams (7).
CHILDREN: POSSIBLY SAFE ...when used orally in medicinal amounts in children 8 years of age and older. Enteric-coated peppermint oil capsules seem to be safe when used under medical supervision in children 8 years of age and older (4469). LIKELY UNSAFE ...when used orally in medicinal amounts in infants and small children. Oral peppermint oil has caused tongue spasms and respiratory arrest in infants and small children (4800). ...when applied topically to the facial, nasal, and chest areas of infants and small children. Peppermint oil can cause bronchospasm, spasms of the tongue, or respiratory arrest (4800). ...when inhaled for medicinal purposes by small children (502).
PREGNANCY: LIKELY UNSAFE ...when used orally in medicinal amounts. High doses of peppermint oil can

induce menstruation (19).
LACTATION: Insufficient reliable information available; avoid using.

Effectiveness

POSSIBLY EFFECTIVE

Barium enema-related colonic spasm. Rectal use of peppermint oil, added as an ingredient in barium enema preparations, seems to relax the colon during barium enema radiologic examination (6739,6749,12009). Adding peppermint oil to the barium enema seems to be at least as effective as using systemic scopolamine (Buscopan) for decreasing colon spasms. Adding peppermint oil to the barium solution does not seem to impair image quality (12009).

Dyspepsia. Taking peppermint oil orally in combination with caraway oil seems to reduce symptoms of non-ulcerative dyspepsia including feelings of fullness and mild gastrointestinal (GI) spasms (6740,6741,10075). The combination of enteric-coated peppermint oil 90 mg and caraway oil 50 mg, which is not available in the US, appears to be similar to cisapride for relieving dyspepsia.

Postoperative nausea. Taking peppermint oil orally seems to help reduce postoperative nausea (3804).

Tension headache. Applying peppermint oil topically seems to help relieve tension headaches (3801,6190).

INSUFFICIENT RELIABLE EVIDENCE to RATE

Irritable bowel syndrome (IBS). Taking enteric-coated peppermint oil capsules orally seems to reduce abdominal pain, distention, flatulence, and bowel movements in some patients with IBS (3802,3804,4469,11778,11779). However, other research using equal doses of enteric-coated peppermint oil has shown no effect (3803,11777,11789).

Postherpetic neuralgia. Preliminary clinical information suggests that peppermint oil applied topically might provide temporary relief from postherpetic pain (11781).

More evidence is needed to rate peppermint oil for these uses.

Mechanism of Action

Peppermint oil is obtained by steam distilling the fresh above ground parts of the flowering peppermint plant (4800). Peppermint oil is a complex mixture of compounds, including 28-29% menthol, 20-31% menthone, and 3-10% menthyl acetate (3582). However, pharmaceutical grade peppermint oil is typically standardized to contain at least 44% menthol.

Peppermint oil is thought to be helpful for respiratory tract symptoms associated with the common cold by increasing salivation; which increases the swallowing reflex, suppresses the cough reflex (3,7), reduces bronchial secretions, and can have nasal decongestant activity (1).

Peppermint oil is used for irritable bowel syndrome (IBS) due to its antispasmodic effects. The antispasmodic activity appears to results from direct relaxing effects on the gastrointestinal (GI) tract smooth muscle, characteristic of calcium antagonist action. Peppermint oil may also inhibit potassium depolarization-induced responses in the intestine (6744,11775). This is thought to prevent the hypercontractility that is commonly found in patients with IBS.

Peppermint oil is thought to be helpful for gaseousness and flatulence by relaxing the lower esophageal sphincter and equalizing the intraluminal pressures between the stomach and esophagus (3582), which increases belching (512).

Preliminary evidence suggests that peppermint oil in combination with caraway oil can reduce gastroduodenal motility when administered orally in enteric-coated capsules (6742).

Menthol and other peppermint oil constituents are rapidly absorbed in the proximal intestine, and upper gastrointestinal effects such as relaxing the lower esophageal sphincter results. For peppermint oil to exert effects on the lower intestine, it must pass through the upper gastrointestinal tract unmetabolized. Enteric coated peppermint oil formulations prevent upper gastrointestinal tract metabolism (11780). Preliminary research suggests that administering menthol-beta-D-glucuronide orally as a prodrug might deliver menthol to the large intestine. In the intestine, menthol-beta-D-glucuronide is hydrolyzed by bacterial beta-D-glucuronidases to menthol, possibly increasing its usefulness in treating diseases such as ulcerative colitis and Crohn's disease (11776).

For pain in myalgias and neuralgias, topical peppermint oil is thought to have counterirritant effects (3582).

Peppermint oil has antimicrobial and antiviral activities in vitro (11).

Adverse Reactions

Orally, peppermint oil can cause heartburn; nausea and vomiting; and allergic reactions, including flushing and headache. Enteric-coated capsules help reduce the incidence of heartburn (3582,3802,4469,6740,11777). Enteric-coated capsules can cause anal burning in conditions where bowel transit time is decreased (11782). Oral peppermint oil has also been associated with burning mouth syndrome and chronic mouth ulceration in people with contact sensitivity to peppermint (6743). Peppermint oil, when used in combination with caraway oil, may cause a substernal burning sensation, belching, heartburn, nausea, vomiting, and diarrhea (6740,6741,6742,10075). Theoretically, the oil can worsen the symptoms of a hiatal hernia due to its relaxation of gastrointestinal (GI) smooth muscle (6).

Topically, peppermint oil can cause skin irritation and contact dermatitis (11781). Application of the oil to facial, nasal, or chest areas of babies and small children can cause laryngeal and bronchial spasms and instant respiratory collapse (1,6,11). When inhaled, peppermint oil can cause allergic reactions including flushing and headache (6).

Interactions with Herbs & Other Dietary Supplements

None known.

Interactions with Drugs

ANTACIDS: Drugs that decrease stomach acid and raise gastric pH can cause premature dissolution of enteric-coated peppermint oil (787). Separate dose administration times by at least 2 hours.
CYCLOSPORINE (Neoral, Sandimmune): Preliminary research suggests that peppermint oil inhibits cyclosporine metabolism and may increase cyclosporine levels. Inhibition of CYP3A4 may be partially responsible for this interaction (11784). An interaction between peppermint oil and cyclosporin has not been reported in humans.
CYTOCHROME P450 3A4 (CYP3A4) SUBSTRATES: There's preliminary evidence that peppermint oil can inhibit cytochrome P450 3A4 (CYP3A4) enzymes (11783). Peppermint oil might increase levels of drugs metabolized by CYP3A4. Some drugs metabolized by CYP3A4 include lovastatin (Mevacor), ketoconazole (Nizoral), itraconazole (Sporanox), fexofenadine (Allegra), triazolam (Halcion), and numerous others. Use peppermint oil cautiously or avoid in patients taking these drugs.
H2-BLOCKERS: Drugs that decrease stomach acid and raise gastric pH can cause premature dissolution of enteric-coated peppermint oil (787). The H2 blockers include cimetidine (Tagamet), ranitidine (Zantac), nizatidine (Axid), and famotidine (Pepcid).
PROTON PUMP INHIBITORS (PPIs): Drugs that decrease stomach acid and raise gastric pH can cause premature dissolution of enteric-coated peppermint oil (787). PPIs include omeprazole (Prilosec), lansoprazole (Prevacid), rabeprazole (Aciphex), pantoprazole (Protonix), and esomeprazole (Nexium).

Interactions with Foods

FOOD: Enteric-coated peppermint oil capsules used for treating irritable bowel syndrome (IBS) should be taken between meals (787).

Interactions with Lab Tests

None known.

Interactions with Diseases or Conditions

ACHLORHYDRIA: Enteric-coated peppermint oil should not be used when the stomach is not producing hydrochloric acid. Achlorhydria increases gastric pH and may cause premature dissolution of the enteric coating (787).
DIARRHEA: Conditions that greatly increase intestinal motility interfere with the absorption of enteric coated peppermint formulations. Insufficient absorption may cause high concentrations of unabsorbed menthol in anal mucosa and cause anal burning (11782).

Dosage and Administration

ORAL: For irritable bowel syndrome (IBS), the usual dose is 0.2-0.4 mL three times daily in enteric-coated capsules (3802,11778,11779). For children 8 years of age and older with IBS, the usual dose is 0.1-0.2 mL three times daily in enteric-coated capsules (4469). For non-ulcerative dyspepsia, peppermint oil 90 mg per day has been used in combination with caraway oil (6740,6741,10075). It's usually taken between meals (787).
TOPICAL: For tension headaches, 10% peppermint oil in ethanol solution applied across the forehead and temples, repeated after 15 and 30 minutes, has been used (6190). To decrease colonic spams during barium enema, 8 mL of peppermint oil was added 100 mL water along with a surface active agent, Tween 80. The insoluble fract was removed, then 30 mL of the remaining peppermint solution was added to 300 mL of the barium solution (12009).
INHALATION: A typical dose is 3-4 drops of the oil in hot water. A lozenge containing 2-10 mg is also used (1,2).

Comments

Avoid confusion with peppermint leaf and rectified mint oil (18). In 1990, the FDA banned the sale of peppermint oil as an over-the-counter drug for use as a digestive aid due to lack of proof of efficacy (512).

PERILLA

Also Known As

Beefsteak Plant, Wild Coleus.
CAUTION: See separate listing for Alpha-Linolenic Acid.

Scientific Names

Perilla frutescens, synonyms Dentidia nankinensis, Ocimum frutescens, Perilla arguta, Perilla nankinensis, Perilla ocymoides.
Family: Lamiaceae/Labiatae.

People Use This For

Orally, perilla is used for treating asthma. It is also used orally for nausea, sunstroke, inducing sweating, and as an antispasmodic.

In foods, perilla is used as a flavoring.
In manufacturing, perilla seed oil is used commercially in the production of varnishes, dyes, and inks.

Safety

POSSIBLY SAFE ...when used orally and appropriately. There is some evidence perilla can be safely used for up to 4 weeks (1338).
PREGNANCY AND LACTATION: Insufficient reliable information available; avoid using.

Effectiveness

INSUFFICIENT RELIABLE EVIDENCE to RATE

Asthma. There is preliminary evidence that perilla seed oil might improve pulmonary function in people with asthma (1338). More evidence is needed to rate perilla for this use.

Mechanism of Action

The applicable parts of perilla are the leaf and seed. Perilla contains multiple flavones. The major flavones apigenin and luteolin are found in the leaves and seeds, along with other flavones including shishonin (6). Perilla seed oil is also high in the fatty acid alpha-linolenic acid. Alpha-linolenic acid is thought decrease serum cholesterol and triglyceride levels, increase the concentration of the fatty acids eicosapentaenoic acid and arachidonic acid and inhibit production of inflammatory leukotrienes. Perilla seed oil is thought to help asthma because of the alpha-linolenic acid effects on leukotrienes (1338). Animal and in vitro studies suggest perilla oil may have antitumor effects (6). Perilla extract may have an immunosuppressant effect by preferentially attenuating IgE production (6). Patch testing suggests 1-perillaldehyde and perillalcohol contained in perilla oil are responsible for the occurrence of dermatitis (6). Cell studies have shown luteolin to have anti-proliferative activity (5003). Animals grazing on perilla have developed pulmonary edema and respiratory distress. Animal studies show the oil constituent, perilla ketone, induces pulmonary edema. Aldehyde antioxide contained in perilla oil may be toxic (6).

Adverse Reactions

Topically, perilla may cause contact dermatitis (6).

Interactions with Herbs & Other Dietary Supplements

None known.

Interactions with Drugs

None known.

Interactions with Foods

None known.

Interactions with Lab Tests

None known.

Interactions with Diseases or Conditions

None known.

Dosage and Administration

ORAL: For asthma, perilla seed oil 10 to 20 grams per day has been used (1338).

PERIWINKLE

Also Known As

Common Periwinkle, Earlyflowering, Evergreen, Lesser Periwinkle, Myrtle, Periwinkle, Small Periwinkle, Vincae minoris herba, Wintergreen.
CAUTION: See separate listing for Madagascar Periwinkle.

Scientific Names

Vinca minor.
Family: Apocynaceae.

People Use This For

Orally, periwinkle is used for "brain health" (increasing cerebral circulation, supporting brain metabolism, increasing mental productivity, preventing memory and concentration impairment and feebleness, improving memory and thinking capacity, preventing premature aging of brain cells, and geriatric support). It also is used orally for mucous membrane inflammation, diarrhea, vaginal discharge, "blood-purification", throat ailments, tonsillitis, angina, sore throat, intestinal inflammation, toothache, edema, promoting wound healing, improving immune function, as a diuretic, sedative, antihypertensive, and hemostatic remedy.

Safety

UNSAFE ...when used orally (2,17). Periwinkle contains pharmacologically active toxic alkaloids that can cause nerve, liver, and kidney damage (17).
PREGNANCY AND LACTATION: UNSAFE ...when used orally (2,17); avoid using.

Effectiveness

There is insufficient reliable information available about the effectiveness of periwinkle.

Mechanism of Action

The applicable parts of periwinkle are the above ground parts. Periwinkle contains pharmacologically active, toxic alkaloids including vincristine which have cytotoxic and neurological actions and can injure liver and kidneys (513). Periwinkle may have astringent activity (19). The constituent, vincamine, has hypotensive activity (19). In animals, periwinkle causes leukocytopenia, lymphocytopenia, and lowers alpha-1, alpha-2, and gamma-globulin levels presumably due to immune suppression (2).

Adverse Reactions

Orally, periwinkle may cause cytotoxic, neurologic, liver, and kidney damage due to vinca alkaloid constituents (17). Periwinkle may also potentially cause GI complaints and skin flushing (18). Consuming large amounts may cause severe drop in blood pressure (18).

Interactions with Herbs & Other Dietary Supplements

None known.

Interactions with Drugs

ANTIHYPERTENSIVE DRUGS: Theoretically, concomitant use may increase therapeutic effects of antihypertensive therapy due to hypotensive activity of vincamine, a constituent of periwinkle (12,19).

Interactions with Foods

None known.

Interactions with Lab Tests

None known.

Interactions with Diseases or Conditions

CONSTIPATION: Use of periwinkle is contraindicated due to astringent activity (12,19).
HYPOTENSION: Use of periwinkle is contraindicated due to potential hypotensive effects (12,19).

Dosage and Administration

ORAL: People typically add 3 to 10 drops of the extract to water and use two to three times daily. Periwinkle extract contains glycerin and alcohol (6006).

Comments

The periwinkle constituent, vincamine, can be converted in the laboratory to the compound vinpocetine which is marketed as a dietary supplement (1799) (see separate listing for Vinpocetine). Avoid confusing periwinkle with Madagascar periwinkle (Catharanthus roseus).

PERU BALSAM

Also Known As

Balsam, Balsam of Peru, Balsam Peru, Balsamum Peruvianum, Black Balsam, Indian Balsam, Peruvian Balsam.
CAUTION: See separate listing for Tolu Balsam.

Scientific Names

Myroxylon balsamum var. pereirae, synonyms Myrospermum pereirae, Myroxylon pereirae, Toluifera pereirae.
Family: Fabaceae/Leguminosae.

People Use This For

Orally, Peru balsam is used for cancer, as a diuretic, and to expel worms.
Topically, Peru balsam is used for infected and poorly healing wounds, burns, decubitus ulcers (bed sores), frost bite, ulcus cruris, bruises caused by prosthetics, hemorrhoids, anal pruritus, diaper rash, intertrigo, and bleeding.
In dentistry, Peru balsam is a component of dental preparations for treating dry socket and as an ingredient in some dental impression materials. It is also used in toothpaste and toothpowder.
In manufacturing, Peru balsam is utilized as a fixative or fragrance in soaps and cosmetics and as a food flavoring agent.

Safety

POSSIBLY SAFE ...when Peru balsam preparations are used topically for less than 1 week (2). In some individuals, peru balsam is a contact allergen (11).
LIKELY UNSAFE ...when used orally; avoid using. Peru balsam is for external use only (2,6). Kidney damage can occur with internal consumption of large doses (18).
PREGNANCY: Insufficient reliable information available; avoid using.
LACTATION: POSSIBLY UNSAFE ...when used topically because systemic toxicity to babies can occur following application of Peru balsam to the nipples of nursing mothers (6).

Effectiveness

There is insufficient reliable information available about the effectiveness of Peru balsam.

Mechanism of Action

The applicable part of peru balsam is the oleo resin. Peru balsam's volatile oil consists mainly of benzoic and cinnamic acid esters, including benzyl benzoate (11). Benzyl benzoate is an effective scabicide (19). Peru balsam also has mild antiseptic and antibacterial properties and is believed to promote epithelial cell growth (11).

Adverse Reactions

Orally, Peru balsam can cause kidney damage with consumption of large amounts (18).
Topically, Peru balsam can cause allergic skin reactions and contact dermatitis, including urticaria, recurring aphthoid oral ulcers, Quincke's disease, and diffuse purpurea (2,18). It has the potential to cause photodermatitis and phototoxicity (18). Kidney damage can also occur with the external use of large amounts (18).

Interactions with Herbs & Other Dietary Supplements

None known.

Interactions with Drugs

None known.

Interactions with Foods

None known.

Interactions with Lab Tests

None known.

Interactions with Diseases or Conditions

KIDNEY DISEASE: Use Peru balsam with caution or avoid due to its potential to cause kidney damage.

Dosage and Administration

TOPICAL: Preparations of Peru balsam usually contain 5-20% Peruvian balsam (2). The maximum concentration for extensive surface application is 10% Peruvian balsam (2).

Comments

Avoid confusion with tolu balsam, which is the oleo resin exuded from scorched tree stems of Myroxylon balsamum.

PEYOTE

Also Known As

Devil's Root, Dumpling Cactus, Mescal Buttons, Mescaline, Pellote, Sacred Mushroom.

Scientific Names

Lophophora williamsii. Family: Cactaceae.

People Use This For
Orally, peyote is used for treating fevers, rheumatism, and paralysis.
Topically, peyote is used for treating fractures, wounds, and snake bite.
Recreationally, peyote is used as a hallucinogen.

Safety
UNSAFE ...when used orally. Peyote is illegal in the US. It is an FDA schedule I controlled substance (9,17,11757).
PREGNANCY AND LACTATION: UNSAFE ...when used orally. The active constituent of peyote, mescaline, may be teratogenic (11758).

Effectiveness
There is insufficient reliable information available about the effectiveness of peyote.

Mechanism of Action
The applicable parts of peyote, which is a small cactus, are the above ground parts. The cactus crown has disc-shaped buttons that are cut from the plant, sliced, and dried. The dried buttons may be chewed, or soaked in water and the resulting liquid used (11757).
The clinical effects of peyote are due to mescaline. Mescaline has sympathomimetic and hallucinogenic activity similar to LSD. Mescaline is less potent than LSD. Its effects last up to 12 hours (9).

Adverse Reactions
Orally, ingestion of peyote can cause mild gastrointestinal effects, nausea, vomiting, and rarely diarrhea, which may occur during the first 30 to 60 minutes of ingestion. Sympathomimetic effects including mydriasis, mild tachycardia and hypertension, sweating, and tremor may follow. Psychic effects and visual hallucinations similar to LSD peak between 4 to 6 hours of ingestion. An average mescaline dose of 5 mg per kilogram causes psychic effects and visual hallucinations. Anxiety, paranoia, fear, and emotional instability can cause self-inflicted or accidental injury. At high doses (greater than 20 mg per kilogram of mescaline), hypertension, bradycardia, respiratory depression, and rarely death can occur. Symptoms usually subside in about 12 hours after ingestion (9,17).

Interactions with Herbs & Other Dietary Supplements
None known.

Interactions with Drugs
STIMULANT DRUGS: Concomitant use may increase the risk of adverse CNS effects (9,17). Some CNS stimulants include nicotine, cocaine, sympathomimetic amines, and amphetamines.

Interactions with Foods
None known.

Interactions with Lab Tests
None known.

Interactions with Diseases or Conditions
None known.

Dosage and Administration
No typical dosage.

PHEASANT'S EYE

Also Known As
Adonis herba, False Hellebore, Oxeye, Red Morocco, Rose-A-Rubie, Sweet Vernal, Yellow Pheasant's Eye, Yellow Pheasants Eye.
CAUTION: See separate listings for American Hellebore, Black Hellebore, and White Hellebore.

Scientific Names
Adonis vernalis.
Family: Ranunculaceae.

People Use This For

Orally, pheasant's eye is used for mild heart failure, arrhythmia, nervous heart complaints, cramps, fever, and menstrual disorders.

Safety

POSSIBLY SAFE ...when the standardized extract is used orally under the supervision of a medical professional trained in the appropriate use of pheasant's eye (2).
LIKELY UNSAFE ...when the standardized extract is used orally without appropriate medical supervision (18,512). Pheasant's eye contains cardiac glycosides and monitoring is required to minimize serious adverse effects.
UNSAFE ...when the plant is ingested. Pheasant's eye is highly poisonous (18).
PREGNANCY AND LACTATION: LIKELY UNSAFE ...when used orally for self-medication (512).

Effectiveness

There is insufficient reliable information available about the effectiveness of pheasant's eye.

Mechanism of Action

The applicable parts of pheasant's eye are the above ground parts. Pheasant's eye contains cardioactive glycosides (7,18). It has cardiac effects similar to digoxin, including positive inotropic and negative chronotropic effects (7). In experimental animals, pheasant's eye demonstrates a tonic effect on veins (2).

Adverse Reactions

Orally, symptoms of pheasant's eye overdose include nausea, vomiting, and arrhythmias (2).

Interactions with Herbs & Other Dietary Supplements

CALCIUM: Concomitant use with calcium can increase the risk of cardiac toxicity (3805).
CARDIAC GLYCOSIDE-CONTAINING HERBS: Contraindicated. Concomitant use can increase the risk of cardiac glycoside toxicity. Cardiac glycoside-containing herbs include black hellebore, Canadian hemp roots, digitalis leaf, hedge mustard, figwort, lily of the valley roots, motherwort, oleander leaf, pleurisy root, squill bulb leaf scales, strophanthus seeds, and uzara (19).
CARDIOACTIVE HERBS: Avoid concomitant use with cardioactive herbs due to unpredictability of effects and adverse effects. These include calamus, cereus, cola, coltsfoot, devil's claw, European mistletoe, fenugreek, fumitory, ginger, Panax ginseng, hawthorn, white horehound, mate, parsley, quassia, scotch broom flower, shepherd's purse, and wild carrot (4).
LICORICE/HORSETAIL: The overuse or misuse of licorice rhizome or horsetail plant increases the risk of cardiac toxicity due to potassium depletion (19).
STIMULANT LAXATIVE HERBS: The overuse or misuse of stimulant laxatives increases the risk of cardiac toxicity due to potassium depletion. Stimulant laxative herbs include aloe dried leaf sap, blue flag rhizome, alder buckthorn, European buckthorn, butternut bark, cascara bark, castor oil, colocynth fruit pulp, gamboge bark exudate, jalap root, black root, manna bark exudate, podophyllum root, rhubarb root, senna leaves and pods, wild cucumber fruit (Ecballium elaterium), and yellow dock root (19).

Interactions with Drugs

CALCIUM SUPPLEMENTS: Concomitant use of pheasant's eye with calcium can increase the risk of cardiac glycoside arrhythmias (3805).
CORTICOSTEROIDS: Concomitant use with pheasant's eye can increase the therapeutic and adverse effects of long-term corticosteroid use (2).
DIGOXIN (Lanoxin): Concomitant use of pheasant's eye is contraindicated due to an increased risk of cardiac glycoside toxicity (4).
DIURETIC DRUGS: Theoretically, concomitant use of potassium depleting diuretics and pheasant's eye can increase the risk of cardiac glycoside toxicity due to potassium depletion (506). Some diuretics that can deplete potassium include chlorothiazide (Diuril), chlorthalidone (Thalitone), furosemide (Lasix), hydrochlorothiazide (HCTZ, HydroDIURIL, Microzide), and others.
QUINIDINE: Concomitant use with pheasant's eye can increase cardiac effects and adverse effects (2).
STIMULANT LAXATIVES: Concomitant use of stimulant laxatives with pheasant's eye can increase the risk of cardiac glycoside toxicity due to potassium loss (2).

Interactions with Foods

None known.

Interactions with Lab Tests

None known.

Interactions with Diseases or Conditions

HYPERCALCEMIA: Using pheasant's eye in people with hypercalcemia is contraindicated (3805).
HYPOKALEMIA: Using pheasant's eye in people with hypokalemia is contraindicated (3805).

Dosage and Administration

No typical dosage.

Comments

Pheasant's eye is considered a poisonous plant (18).

PHENYLALANINE

Also Known As

DLPA, D-Phenylalanine, DL-Phenylalanine, L-Phenylalanine.

Scientific Names

Alpha-aminohydrocinnamic acid; Beta-phenyl-alanine.

People Use This For

Orally, phenylalanine is used for depression, attention deficit-hyperactivity disorder (ADHD), Parkinson's disease, chronic pain, osteoarthritis, rheumatoid arthritis, alcohol withdrawal symptoms, and vitiligo.
Topically, it is used for vitiligo.

Safety

LIKELY SAFE ...when L-phenylalanine is consumed in amounts typically found in foods (11120).
POSSIBLY SAFE ...when L-phenylalanine is used orally for therapeutic purposes (2455,2456,2461,2463,2465,2466,2467,2468,2469).
There is insufficient reliable information available about the safety of D-phenylalanine.
PREGNANCY: LIKELY SAFE ...when L-phenylalanine is consumed in amounts typically found in foods by pregnant women with normal phenylalanine metabolism and serum levels (2020,11120).
UNSAFE ...when L-phenylalanine is consumed in amounts typically found in foods by pregnant women with high serum phenylalanine concentrations or when L-phenylalanine is taken in high doses. Serum levels of phenylalanine greater than 360 micromol/L increases the risk of birth defects (1402,11468). The risk for facial defects is highest at gestation weeks 10-14, neurological and growth abnormalities between 3-16 weeks, and cardiovascular defects at 3-8 weeks. Experts recommend that women with high phenylalanine serum concentrations follow a low phenylalanine diet for at least 20 weeks prior to conception to decrease the risk for birth defects (1402). In addition, some experts recommend screening in women not tested for phenylketonuria (PKU) at birth (1401).
There is insufficient reliable information available about the safety of oral, therapeutic amounts of L-phenylalanine in pregnant women with normal phenylalanine metabolism and serum concentrations; avoid using.
There is insufficient reliable information available about the safety of oral D-phenylalanine in pregnant women; avoid using.
LACTATION: LIKELY SAFE ...when L-phenylalanine is consumed in amounts typically found in foods by breast-feeding women with normal phenylalanine metabolism (2020,11120). There is insufficient reliable information available about the safety of oral, therapeutic amounts of L-phenylalanine in breast-feeding women with normal phenylalanine metabolism; avoid using. There is insufficient reliable information available about the safety of oral D-phenylalanine during lactation; avoid using.

Effectiveness

POSSIBLY EFFECTIVE

Vitiligo. Taking L-phenylalanine orally in combination with UVA exposure or applying L-phenylalanine topically in combination with UVA exposure seems to be effective for treating vitiligo in adults (2461,2463,2464,2466) and in children (2467).

POSSIBLY INEFFECTIVE

Attention deficit-hyperactivity disorder (ADHD). Taking phenylalanine orally doesn't seem to have any effect on ADHD. Some research suggests that patients with ADHD have lower levels of amino acids such as phenylalanine (9948), but neither D-phenylalanine nor DL-phenylalanine appears to have any sustained effect on ADHD symptoms (9950,9951).

Pain. Taking D-phenylalanine orally doesn't seem to improve chronic pain of varied etiology (2459).

INSUFFICIENT RELIABLE EVIDENCE to RATE

Acupuncture anesthesia. Preliminary clinical research suggests that oral D-phenylalanine might enhance acupuncture anesthesia during tooth extraction (2456). However, it doesn't seem to enhance acupuncture anesthesia for chronic low back pain (2456).

Depression. Limited clinical research performed over 2 decades ago suggests L-phenylalanine or DL-phenylalanine might be useful for depression (2468,2469), but this research needs to be replicated with up-to-date study methods.
Parkinson's disease. Limited clinical research suggests taking D-phenylalanine orally might decrease symptoms of Parkinson's disease (2455). However, taking DL-phenylalanine orally doesn't seem to be effective for treating Parkinson's disease (2454).
Phenylalanine deficiency. Preliminary clinical research suggests administering phenylalanine orally might improve phenylalanine deficiency in children who have tyrosinemia, while maintaining tyrosine levels at less than 600 micromol/L. Phenylalanine deficiency is a necessary consequence of an effective treatment regimen for tyrosinemia (11469).
More evidence is needed to rate phenylalanine for these uses.

Mechanism of Action

Phenylalanine exists as two enantiomers, D-phenylalanine and L-phenylalanine. The racemic mix DL-phenylalanine (50% D-, 50% L-phenylalanine) is produced by laboratory synthesis. D-phenylalanine is non-nutritive (not an essential human amino acid), and its role in humans is not currently understood. Human data suggests that about one-third of a 25 mg/kg dose of D-phenylalanine is converted to L-phenylalanine (2052). L-phenylalanine is an essential human amino acid, and is the only form of phenylalanine found in proteins. Major dietary sources of L-phenylalanine include meat, fish, eggs, cheese, and milk (2023). L-phenylalanine is normally metabolized to tyrosine (2052,9949).
L-phenylalanine exacerbates tardive dyskinesia in people with schizophrenia (2457) and can contribute to the development and severity of tardive dyskinesia in people with unipolar depression treated with neuroleptics (2458). L-phenylalanine does not alter pain tolerance to burns in healthy people (2460). D-phenylalanine increases the pain threshold in animals, inducing a naloxone-reversible analgesia by blocking enzymatic degradation of enkephalin (2459). Large neutral amino acids (LNAAs) including DL-phenylalanine, leucine, and isoleucine can exacerbate tremor, rigidity, and the "on-off" syndrome in people with Parkinson's disease who have used levodopa for more than 5-10 years (2454,3291). The amount of dietary LNAAs appears to affect the severity of "on-off" symptoms and may be independent of dietary protein-induced alterations in oral levodopa bioavailability (3291,3292,3293,3294). DL-phenylalanine and other LNAAs might worsen symptoms by decreasing the amount of levodopa that crosses the blood-brain barrier (3291,3294). Preliminary evidence suggests that L-phenylalanine, given with the non-selective monoamine oxidase (MAO-A/MOA-B) inhibitor pargyline, might prevent the elimination of tyramine, increasing the risk of hypertensive crisis (2021). However, hypertensive crisis was not reported in a small number of patients who used L-phenylalanine with the partially selective monoamine oxidase B (MAO-B) inhibitor, selegiline (Eldepryl) (2469).

Adverse Reactions

Orally, L-phenylalanine can exacerbate tardive dyskinesia in people with schizophrenia (2457). Large neutral amino acids (LNAAs; including DL-phenylalanine, leucine and isoleucine) exacerbate tremor, rigidity, and the "on-off" syndrome in patients with Parkinson's disease using levodopa (2454,3291,3292,3293,3294).

Interactions with Herbs & Other Dietary Supplements

None known.

Interactions with Drugs

ANTIPSYCHOTIC DRUGS: Concomitant use of L-phenylalanine and neuroleptics can contribute to the development and severity of tardive dyskinesia in patients with neuroleptic-treated unipolar depression (2458).
LEVODOPA: Concomitant use of DL-phenylalanine and levodopa can exacerbate tremor, rigidity, and the "on-off" syndrome in patients with Parkinson's disease (2454,3291,3292,3293,3294).
MONOAMINE OXIDASE INHIBTORS (MAOIs): Theoretically, concomitant use of L-phenylalanine and non-selective MAOI drugs might increase the risk of hypertensive crisis. Some evidence suggests that L-phenylalanine, given with the non-selective MAOI drug pargyline, might prevent the elimination of tyramine, increasing the risk of hypertensive crisis (2021).

Interactions with Foods

None known.

Interactions with Lab Tests

None known.

Interactions with Diseases or Conditions

HYPERPHENYLALANINEMIA: Phenylalanine should be avoided in people with inherited disorders of phenylalanine metabolism. Hyperphenylalaninemia is the result of impaired metabolism of phenylalanine due to a deficiency of the liver enzyme phenylalanine hydroxylase. People with the genetic disorder known as phenylketonuria (PKU) have an absence or lack of this enzyme activity, and normally show high levels of blood

phenylalanine, and build up phenylketones (10754,11468). Warn patients that phenylalanine consumption may cause mental retardation, hypertension, stroke, and many other adverse effects in people with an inability to properly metabolize phenylalanine (2084,10754,11468).
SCHIZOPHRENIA: Use with caution. L-phenylalanine can exacerbate tardive dyskinesia in people with schizophrenia (2457).

Dosage and Administration

ORAL: For Parkinson's disease, the dose of D-phenylalanine is typically 200 to 500 mg per day (2455). As an adjunct to acupuncture anesthesia or analgesia in tooth extraction, 4 grams of D-phenylalanine is usually taken 30 minutes before acupuncture (2456). For unipolar depression, the usual dose of L-phenylalanine is 250 mg with 5-10 mg L-deprenyl per day (2469), and the common dose of DL-phenylalanine is 150 to 200 mg per day (2468). For vitiligo in adults, 50-100 mg/kg of L-phenylalanine is typically used per day along with UVA exposure (2461,2463,2464,2465,2466). For phenylalanine deficiency in tyrosinemia, phenylalanine 30-40 mg/kg per day has been used in children (11469).
TOPICAL: A 10% L-phenylalanine cream along with UVA exposure is commonly used for vitiligo (2461).

PHOSPHATE SALTS

Also Known As

Aluminum Phosphate; Calcium Phosphate- Bone Ash, Bone Phosphate, Calcium Orthophosphate, Calcium Phosphate Dibasic Anhydrous, Calcium Phosphate Dibasic Dihydrate, Calcium Phosphate Tribasic, Di-Calcium Phosphate, Dicalcium Phosphate, Dicalcium Phosphates, Neutral Calcium Phosphate, Precipitated Calcium Phosphate, Tertiary Calcium Phosphate, Tricalcium Phosphate, Whitlockite; Potassium Phosphate: Dipotassium Hydrogen Orthophosphate, Dipotassium Monophosphate, Dipotassium Phosphate, Monobasic Potassium Phosphate, Potassium Acid Phosphate, Potassium Biphosphate, Potassium Dihydrogen Orthophosphate. Sodium Phosphate: Anhydrous Sodium Phosphate, Dibasic Sodium Phosphate, Disodium Hydrogen Orthophosphate, Disodium Hydrogen Orthophosphate Dodecahydrate, Disodium Hydrogen Phosphate, Disodium Phosphate, Phosphate of Soda, Sodium Orthophosphate.
CAUTION: Do not confuse Phosphate Salts with toxic substances such as Organophosphates, or with Tribasic Sodium Phosphates and Tribasic Potassium Phosphates which are strongly alkaline.

Scientific Names

Aluminum phosphate; Calcium phosphate; Potassium phosphate; Sodium phosphate.

People Use This For

Orally, phosphate salts are used for treating hypophosphatemia and hypercalcemia, hypophosphatemic rickets or osteomalacia, and for prevention of recurrent nephrolithiasis (kidney stones). Phosphate salts are also used orally for enhancing exercise performance, as an antacid for gastroesophageal reflux disease (GERD), and as a laxative for presurgical bowel preparation.
Topically, phosphate salts are used with calcium in dentistry for sensitive teeth.
Rectally, phosphate salts are used as a laxative for presurgical bowel preparation.
Intravenously, potassium phosphate is used for hypophosphatemia and hypokalemia, preventing hypophosphatemia in people receiving parenteral nutrition, and treating hypercalcemia.

Safety

LIKELY SAFE ...when sodium, potassium, aluminum, and calcium phosphates are used orally and appropriately short-term (15). ...when sodium phosphate is used rectally and appropriately short-term (15). Long-term use or high doses used orally or rectally require monitoring of serum electrolytes (2494,2495,2496,2497,2498,3092). ...when used intravenously, potassium phosphate is an FDA-approved prescription drug (15).
POSSIBLY UNSAFE ...when phosphate (expressed as phosphorus) intake exceeds the tolerable upper intake level (UL). Hyperphosphatemia, resulting in electrolyte disturbances, alterations in calcium homeostasis, and calcification of nonskeletal tissues, may occur. The UL for adults under age 70 is 4 grams per day. For adults older than age 70, the UL is 3 grams per day (7555).
CHILDREN: LIKELY SAFE ...when used orally and appropriately at recommended dietary allowances (RDAs). The daily RDAs are: children 1-3 years, 460 mg; children 4-8 years, 500 mg; males and females 9-18 years, 1250 mg (7555). ...when sodium phosphate is used rectally and appropriately short-term (15). ...when used intravenously, potassium phosphate is an FDA-approved prescription drug (15). POSSIBLY UNSAFE ...when phosphate (expressed as phosphorus) intake exceeds the tolerable upper intake level (UL). Hyperphosphatemia, resulting in electrolyte disturbances, alterations in calcium homeostasis, and calcification of nonskeletal tissues, may occur.
The ULs are: children 1-8 years, 3 grams per day; children 9 years and older, 4 grams per day (7555).
PREGNANCY AND LACTATION: LIKELY SAFE ...when used orally and appropriately at recommended dietary allowances (RDAs) of 1250 mg daily for women 14-18 years of age and 700 mg daily for those over 18 years of age (7555). ...when sodium phosphate is used rectally and appropriately short-term (15). ...when used intravenously,

potassium phosphate is an FDA-approved prescription drug (15). POSSIBLY UNSAFE ...when phosphate (expressed as phosphorus) intake exceeds the tolerable upper intake level (UL). Hyperphosphatemia, resulting in electrolyte disturbances, alterations in calcium homeostasis, and calcification of nonskeletal tissues, may occur. The UL for pregnant women age 14-50 is 3.5 grams per day. For lactating women age 14-50, the UL is 4 grams per day (7555).

Effectiveness

EFFECTIVE

Hypophosphatemia. Taking sodium and potassium phosphates orally is effective for preventing and treating hypophosphatemia (15). The FDA-approved IV product is also used for the correction of hypophosphatemia (8302,8303).

LIKELY EFFECTIVE

Hypercalcemia. Taking sodium and calcium phosphates orally is effective for treating hypercalcemia (15).

POSSIBLY EFFECTIVE

Kidney stones (nephrolithiasis). Taking potassium and sodium phosphate salts orally may help prevent kidney stones in patients with hypercalciuria (2209,6470).

LIKELY INEFFECTIVE

Athletic performance. Taking phosphates orally doesn't improve exercise performance (2499,8300,8301).

There is insufficient information available to about the effectiveness of phosphate salts for their other uses.

Mechanism of Action

Phosphate is the most common form of phosphorus (7555). It is the most abundant intracellular anion in the body. It is critical for membrane structure, transport, and energy storage (3092). In adults, phosphorus makes up from 0.65 % to 1.1% of the body. Eighty-five per cent is in bone. Normal plasma concentrations range from 0.8-1.6 mmol/L, or 2.5-5 mg/dL (0.032 mmol phosphate = 1 mg). Phosphate plays an important role in buffering body fluids, and plays a primary role in the renal excretion of hydrogen ions. It is present in carbohydrates, proteins, lipids and various enzymes involved in energy transfer (7555). Vitamin D3 and its metabolites influence phosphate absorption from the gut and also affect renal tubular reabsorption of phosphate (3092,3372,8821). Inadequate dietary phosphate lowers serum phosphate levels, which are inversely related to serum calcium levels (3372,8821). Hypophosphatemia causes an increase in intestinal calcium absorption and increased calcium in the blood, which can inhibit formation of new bone (3372,8821), and potentially lead to a greater risk of renal calcium stone formation (3372). Hyperphosphatemia can occur with excessive intake of vitamin D (3092). Sodium phosphates are used as saline laxatives. They cause influx of fluids in the intestine by an osmotic action and increase peristalsis (15). Aluminum phosphate used orally neutralizes gastric acid (15). Oral ingestion of large amounts of sodium dihydrogen phosphate can lower urine pH (1).

Adverse Reactions

Orally, phosphate salts can cause gastrointestinal irritation, fluid and electrolyte disturbances including hyperphosphatemia and hypocalcemia, and extraskeletal calcification. Potassium phosphates can cause hyperkalemia. Sodium phosphates can cause hypernatremia and hypokalemia (15,2494,2495,2496,2497). Sodium and potassium phosphates can cause diarrhea (15). Aluminum phosphate can cause constipation (15). Rectally, phosphate salts can cause fluid and electrolyte disturbances including hyperphosphatemia and hypocalcemia (15).

Interactions with Herbs & Other Dietary Supplements

None known.

Interactions with Drugs

ANTACIDS: Antacids containing aluminum, calcium, or magnesium can bind phosphate in the gut and prevent its absorption (3371). Some patients with phosphate depletion due to chronic antacid abuse might also present with recurrent nephrolithiasis and ureter obstruction (3371).

CHOLESTYRAMINE (Questran): Concomitant administration of bile acid sequestrants and phosphate can decrease oral absorption of phosphate supplements (15).

COLESTIPOL (Colestid): Concomitant administration of bile acid sequestrants and phosphate can decrease oral absorption of phosphate supplements (15).

Drug Influences on Nutrient Levels and Depletion

SOME DRUGS CAN AFFECT PHOSPHATE LEVELS:

ALUMINUM SALTS: Use of aluminum salts can bind phosphate in the gut and reduce serum phosphate levels. Avoid prolonged administration of large doses of aluminum-containing drugs, which might lead to hypophosphatemia (3371,4400).

Interactions with Foods

None known.

Interactions with Lab Tests

ACID PHOSPHATASE: Phosphates can cause a false-decrease in serum test results. High substrate concentrations can inhibit the analytic reaction (275).
ALKALINE PHOSPHATASE: Phosphates can cause a false-decrease in serum test results. High substrate concentrations can inhibit the analytic reaction (275).
AMMONIA: Phosphates can cause a false-decrease in plasma test results by inhibiting formation of indophenol color in Berthelot reaction (275).
CALCIUM: Phosphates can increase fecal levels and test results (275). Phosphates can cause a false-decrease in serum and urine test results by inhibiting emission in some flame methods and by competing with EDTA for calcium (275).
LIPID GLYCEROL: Phosphates can cause a false-decrease in serum test results by inhibiting phospholipase with method of Horney (275).
MAGNESIUM: Phosphates can decrease urine levels and test results by reducing increased excretion with bed rest (275).
PARATHYROID HORMONE: Phosphates can increase plasma levels and test results (275).
PHOSPHATE: Phosphates increase fecal, serum, and urine levels and test results (275).
POTASSIUM: Phosphates (except potassium phosphate) can decrease serum levels and test results (275).
PYRUVATE KINASE: Phosphates can cause a false-increase in red blood cell test results by activating analytic enzyme (275).

Interactions with Diseases or Conditions

CARDIAC DISEASE: Use sodium-containing phosphates cautiously in people with cardiac disease (15).
EDEMA: Use sodium-containing phosphates with caution in people with cirrhosis, heart failure, or other edematous conditions (15).
HYPERCALCEMIA: Use cautiously in individuals with high serum calcium levels. The product of serum phosphate and calcium levels should not exceed 60 to prevent precipitation of calcium phosphate and soft tissue calcification (6479).
HYPERPHOSPHATEMIA: People with Addison's disease, severe cardiopulmonary, renal disease, or hepatic disease are at risk for hyperphosphatemia and hypocalcemia when taking phosphates (2497). Hyperphosphatemia might also occur in people with renal insufficiency, hypoparathyroidism, severe hyperthyroidism, untreated adrenal insufficiency (due to volume contraction, metabolic acidosis and reduced glomerular permeability), metabolic, lactic or respiratory acidosis, rhabdomyolysis, infarction, hemolysis, or tumor lysis syndrome (3092).
HYPOPHOSPHATEMIA: Low phosphate levels can be associated with many conditions, including poor oral intake or absorption, reduced renal tubular reabsorption, respiratory alkalosis, excessive insulin use, certain malignancies, diabetic ketoacidosis, and chronic alcoholism (3092).
KIDNEY DYSFUNCTION: Closely monitor serum electrolytes when phosphates are used by people with mild to moderate renal impairment (15).

Dosage and Administration

ORAL: For bowel preparation for diagnostic tests, a typical dose is dibasic sodium phosphate 3.42 to 7.56 grams and monobasic sodium phosphate 9.1-20.2 grams daily given as a single dose (15). Phosphate laxative preparations should be taken with plenty of water (15). Treating hypophosphatemia or hypercalcemia with oral phosphates requires monitoring of serum electrolyte levels (15). For kidney stones, potassium and sodium phosphate salts providing 1200-1500 mg of elemental phosphate have been used (2209,6470).
As a supplement, the recommended daily dietary allowances (RDAs) of phosphate (expressed as phosphorus) are: Children 1-3 years, 460 mg; Children 4-8 years, 500 mg; Males and females 9-18 years, 1250 mg; Males and females over 18 years, 700 mg (3094). The adequate intakes (AI) for infants are: 100 mg for infants 0-6 months old and 275 mg for infants 7-12 months of age (7555). Tolerable upper intake levels for phosphate (expressed as phosphorus) per day are: children 1-8 years, 3 grams per day; children and adults 9-70 years, 4 grams; adults older than 70 years, 3 grams; pregnant 14-50 years, 3.5 grams; and lactating women 14-50 years, 4 grams (7555).
RECTAL: For bowel preparation for diagnostic tests, a typical dose is dibasic sodium phosphate 6.84-7.56 grams and monobasic sodium phosphate 18.24-20.16 grams daily, administered as a single dose. Treating hypophosphatemia with rectal phosphates requires monitoring of serum electrolyte levels (15).
INTRAVENOUS: Injectable potassium phosphate is an FDA-approved prescription product.

Comments

Foods high in phosphate include daily products, whole grain cereals, nuts, and some meats (7555). Phosphates present in dairy products and meats are soluble and readily absorbed, whereas those in cereal grains are bound and insoluble, and may be poorly absorbed (3092). Cola drinks contain significant amounts of phosphate, and excessive intake can result in hyperphosphatemia and hypocalcemia (7555).

PHOSPHATIDYLCHOLINE

Also Known As
Phosphatidyl Choline.
CAUTION: See separate listings for Alpha-GPC, Choline, Lecithin, Phosphatidylserine, and Soy.

Scientific Names
None.

People Use This For
Orally, phosphatidylcholine is used for treating anxiety, eczema, gallbladder disease, hepatitis, manic-depressive illness, peripheral vascular disorders, hyperlipidemias, improving ultrafiltration in peritoneal dialysis, tardive dyskinesia, premenstrual syndrome, memory loss, Alzheimer's disease, immunodepression, and preventing aging.

Safety
POSSIBLY SAFE ...when used orally and appropriately. Large doses up to 30 grams per day for 6 weeks, have been well tolerated (5223). Lecithin, which contains a substantial amount of phosphatidylcholine, has Generally Recognized As Safe (GRAS) status in the US (4912).
PREGNANCY AND LACTATION: Insufficient reliable information available; avoid using.

Effectiveness
POSSIBLY EFFECTIVE

Hepatitis C. Taking the polyunsaturated form of phosphatidylcholine orally, in combination with interferon, seems to help reduce liver enzymes in patients with chronic hepatitis C (5226).

POSSIBLY INEFFECTIVE

Hepatitis A. Taking phosphatidylcholine orally doesn't seem to reduce serum bilirubin or liver enzyme levels in patients with hepatitis A (5225).

Peritoneal dialysis. Taking phosphatidylcholine orally doesn't seem to improve ultrafiltration in peritoneal dialysis (5222).

Tardive dyskinesia. Taking phosphatidylcholine orally doesn't seem to improve tardive dyskinesia (5223).

INSUFFICIENT RELIABLE EVIDENCE to RATE

Hepatitis B. Studies regarding hepatitis B show conflicting results (5224,5226).

Memory. There is preliminary evidence that taking a single dose of phosphatidylcholine 25 grams (PC-55, TwinLab) can improve some measures of memory in healthy college students (5228).

More evidence is needed to rate phosphatidylcholine for these uses.

Mechanism of Action
Phosphatidylcholine is a phospholipid and a major constituent of lecithin. Egg lecithin contains 69% phosphatidylcholine, while soybean lecithin contains 24% phosphatidylcholine (4914).
Choline is a component of phosphatidylcholine. Choline is a precursor to acetylcholine (5228).
Acetylcholine is thought to be involved in memory. Since phosphatidylcholine might increase acetylcholine, there is interest in using it for improving memory and for conditions such as Alzheimer's disease.
The hydrolysis of phosphatidylcholine by pancreatic phospholipase A2 appears to play a direct role in regulating the absorption of certain lipids and lipid-soluble vitamins (8808). Polyunsaturated phosphatidylcholine may also provide protection against liver fibrosis and alcohol induced oxidative stress, although the exact mechanisms are not completely understood (8809).

Adverse Reactions
Orally, phosphatidylcholine can increase sweating (5229). Ingesting large amounts (30 grams per day) can cause gastrointestinal upset and diarrhea (5223).

Interactions with Herbs & Other Dietary Supplements
None known.

Interactions with Drugs
None known.

Interactions with Foods
None known.

Interactions with Lab Tests
None known.

Interactions with Diseases or Conditions

None known.

Dosage and Administration

ORAL: For hepatitis C, 1.8 grams of lecithin used daily with hepatitis C interferon (5226).

Comments

The term "phosphatidylcholine" is sometimes used interchangeably with "lecithin" although the two are different. Choline is a component of phosphatidylcholine, which is a component of lecithin. Although closely related, these terms are not synonymous. However, in the clinical literature, they are often confused.

PHOSPHATIDYLSERINE

Also Known As

BC-PS, Bovine Cortex Phosphatidylserine, Bovine Phosphatidylserine, Cephalin, Kephalin, LECI-PS, Lecithin Phosphatidylserine, PS, PtdSer, Soy-PS, Soy Phosphatidylserine.
CAUTION: See separate listings for Choline, Lecithin, Phosphatidylcholine, and Soy.

Scientific Names

Phosphatidylserine.

People Use This For

Orally, phosphatidylserine is used for Alzheimer's disease and other dementias, age-related decline in mental function, improving cognitive function in young people, attention deficit-hyperactivity disorder (ADHD), depression, preventing exercise-induced stress, and improving athletic performance.

Safety

POSSIBLY SAFE ...when used orally and appropriately. Phosphatidylserine seems to be safe when used for up to 6 months (2255,2437,2438,2439,2440,2441,7118). Most studies have used bovine cortex derived phosphatidylserine. Since these preparations are derived from animals, there is some concern about contamination with diseased animal parts (1825). So far, there are no reports of disease transmission to humans due to use of contaminated phosphatidylserine preparations. Most manufacturers now only produce soy or cabbage derived phosphatidylserine (1825,7115).
CHILDREN: POSSIBLY SAFE ...when used orally and appropriately (7117).
PREGNANCY AND LACTATION: Insufficient reliable information available; avoid using.

Effectiveness

POSSIBLY EFFECTIVE

Age-related cognitive impairment. Phosphatidylserine seems to improve attention, arousal, verbal fluency, and memory in aging people with cognitive deterioration (2440,2441,7119,7120).
Alzheimer's disease. Taking phosphatidylserine orally can increase cognitive function, global improvement rating scales, and improve behavioral rating scales over 6-12 weeks of treatment (2255,2437,2438,2439,7114,7118). Phosphatidylserine seems to be most effective in patients with less severe symptoms (2437,2439). Phosphatidylserine might lose its effectiveness with extended use. After 16 weeks of treatment, progression of Alzheimer's disease seems to overcome any benefit of phosphatidylserine (2255).
Most clinical studies have used phosphatidylserine derived from bovine cortex. However, most supplements now use soy or cabbage derived phosphatidylserine. Clinical studies have not yet evaluated phosphatidylserine from soy or other sources. It is not known if phosphatidylserine from soy and other sources is as effective as bovine-derived products.

INSUFFICIENT RELIABLE EVIDENCE to RATE

Depression. There is some preliminary evidence that phosphatidylserine might improve depression in geriatric patients (7113).
Exercise-induced stress. There is some evidence that athletes taking phosphatidylserine orally during over-training might have the perception of well being and reduced muscle soreness (2264). Some research also suggests that non-athletically trained healthy men might benefit from both acute and chronic phosphatidylserine administration (8851,8852).
More evidence is needed to rate phosphatidylserine for these uses.

Mechanism of Action

Phosphatidylserine is a fat-soluble phospholipid that occurs endogenously in humans. It is the most abundant phospholipid in the human brain and is important in neuronal membrane functions such as maintenance of the cell's internal environment, signal transduction, secretory vesicle release, cell-to-cell communication, and cell growth regulation (2437,7115). Phosphatidylserine is also a component of the mitochondrial membrane, where it might function as a metabolic reservoir for other phospholipids (7121). Although the body is able to synthesize phosphatidylserine through an elaborate series of reactions and substantial energy expenditure, the body obtains most phosphatidylserine from dietary sources. Phosphatidylserine is present in small quantities in most foods (7116).

It is not clear how phosphatidylserine works for dementia such as Alzheimer's disease and age-related memory impairment. However, one theory is that patients with dementia or age-related memory impairment have structural or functional abnormalities in neuronal membranes that cause changes in neurotransmitter functioning. People with cognitive dysfunction often have changes in acetylcholine, norepinephrine, and serotonin levels. Some researchers think the abnormal neuronal function can be attributed to changes in lipid composition of the brain. It is thought that exogenous administration of phosphatidylserine might then normalize brain lipid content and return neuronal function to normal (2441). Phosphatidylserine has been shown to increase acetylcholine, norepinephrine, serotonin, and dopamine levels in animal models and patients with Alzheimer's disease (2437,8857,8858). In animal models, phosphatidylserine improves spatial memory and passive avoidance (8858). It also appears to minimize age-related neuronal dendrite loss and atrophy of cholinergic neurons (2437,8857). The fatty acid docosahexaenoic acid (DHA), which is readily present in neuronal cells, appears to further promote the accumulation of phosphatidylserine in cell membranes, which in turn prevents apoptotic cell death (8857).

Evidence shows that high levels of procoagulant endothelial particles containing phosphatidylserine are present in patients with acute coronary syndromes. Although these increased levels are hypothesized to contribute to plaque disruption and thrombosis, the exact mechanisms are not yet understood (8855).

There is also interest in phosphatidylserine for decreasing exercise-induced stress. Some preliminary evidence shows that phosphatidylserine might blunt the rise in cortisol and adrenocorticotropin following strenuous training (2264,8851,8852). Very preliminary clinical laboratory research suggests that phosphatidylserine 300 mg per day might improve mood and subjective feelings of stress (11963).

In animal models of multiple sclerosis, phosphatidylserine reduces tremor, spasticity, and urinary incontinence, possibly by suppressing the release of the cytokine tumor necrosis factor (8853,8854).

Adverse Reactions

Orally, phosphatidylserine is typically well tolerated. Some patients can experience gastrointestinal upset or insomnia. These side effects are more likely to occur with higher doses, 300 mg for gastrointestinal upset and 600 mg for insomnia (7116,7121). Most phosphatidylserine supplements used to be derived from bovine cortex, so there has been some concern about possible contamination from sick or diseased animals, including those harboring bovine spongiform encephalopathy (BSE, mad cow disease). Using supplements produced from diseased animals might present a human health hazard. So far there are no reports of BSE or other disease transmission to humans from dietary supplements containing animal materials and the risk of potential disease transmission is thought to be low. However, because of this concern most manufacturers now only produce soy or cabbage derived phosphatidylserine.

Interactions with Herbs & Other Dietary Supplements

None known.

Interactions with Drugs

None known.

Interactions with Foods

None known.

Interactions with Lab Tests

ALANINE AMINOTRANSFERASE (ALT, SGPT): Phosphatidylserine 300 mg daily can reduce alanine aminotransferase levels (7116).

URIC ACID: Phosphatidylserine 300 mg daily can reduce uric acid levels (7116).

Interactions with Diseases or Conditions

None known.

Dosage and Administration

ORAL: For Alzheimer's disease, senile dementia, and age-related cognitive or memory impairment, 100 mg three times daily has been used in clinical studies (2437,2438,2440,2441). For treatment of attention deficit-hyperactivity disorder (ADHD) in children, people typically use 200 to 300 mg daily (7117).

Comments

Cephalin (synonym kephalin) is the term formerly used to refer to what are now known as phosphatidylserine and phosphatidylethanolamine.

PICRORHIZA

Also Known As
Hu Huang Lian, Katki, Katuka, Katuko, Katurohini, Katvi, Kuru, Kutki, Xi Zang Hu Huang Lian.

Scientific Names
Picrorhiza kurroa; Neopicrorhiza scrophulariiflora, synonym Picrorhiza scrophulariiflora.
Family: Scrophulariacae.

People Use This For
Orally, picrorhiza is used for jaundice, acute viral hepatitis, indigestion, constipation, fever, allergy, and asthma. Other uses include vitiligo, eczema, infection, scorpion stings, chronic diarrhea, epilepsy, malaria, and rheumatoid arthritis.

Safety
POSSIBLY SAFE ...when used orally and appropriately. Picrorhiza seems to be safe when used for up to 1 year (11493,11848,11858).
PREGNANCY AND LACTATION: Insufficient reliable information available; avoid using.

Effectiveness
POSSIBLY EFFECTIVE

Vitiligo. Taking picrorhiza orally for up to 1 year, in combination with oral and topical methoxsalen, seems to help treat vitiligo in adults and children (11493).

POSSIBLY INEFFECTIVE

Asthma. Taking picrorhiza orally for up to 12 weeks doesn't seem to help asthma symptoms or improve measurements of lung function (11858).

INSUFFICIENT RELIABLE EVIDENCE to RATE

Viral hepatitis. Preliminary clinical research suggests that picrorhiza given orally for 2 weeks might help acute viral hepatitis. It seems to improve symptoms such as anorexia, nausea, malaise, and lower bilirubin and transaminase levels (11848). Picrorhiza has not been tested in patients with hepatitis B. More evidence is needed to rate picrorhiza for this use.

Mechanism of Action
The applicable parts of picrorhiza are the leaves and rhizome. There is preliminary evidence that the constituent picroside might protect against liver injury (11848). Picroliv, a combination of picroside, kutkoside, cucurbitacin glycosides, and other unidentified constituents, also appears to have hepatoprotective activity. Picroliv seems to protect the liver from hepatotoxic agents, such as ethanol and the Amanita mushroom (11850,11852,11856). This protective effect against liver damage might be due to the prevention of lipid peroxidation and generation of free radicals, decreasing the formation of reactive metabolites (11491,11494).

Picroliv also appears to have anticarcinogenic activity when used orally or topically in experimentally-induced liver and skin cancer. Picroliv might also inhibit topoisomerase I and II, which might inhibit cancer cell proliferation (11849,11851).

Picrorhiza has been used traditionally for asthma, but human research has been negative (11858). Picroliv might have immunostimulant and antiallergic activity, possibly by stabilizing mast cells (11853). The picrorhiza constituent androsin may contribute to the antiallergic effect by inhibiting platelet-activating factor (11857).

Animal data suggests both the leaves and rhizomes of picrorhiza have immunostimulatory activity (11492).

The immunostimulatory actions of picrorhiza might also be involved in improving vitiligo (11493). The picrorhiza constituent apocynin may have anti-inflammatory activity. Research in animals suggests it may have anti-arthritic activity (11847,11859,11860).

Picroliv also appears to have activity against parasites such as Leishmania donovani, which causes leishmaniasis, and Plasmodium berghei, which causes malaria (11854,11855).

Adverse Reactions
Orally, picrorhiza can cause vomiting, rash, anorexia, diarrhea, itching, and giddiness (11858).

Interactions with Herbs & Other Dietary Supplements
None known.

Interactions with Drugs
IMMUNOSUPPRESSANTS: Theoretically, picrorhiza may interfere with immunosuppressant therapy. Picrorhiza seems to have immunostimulating activity (11492,11853). Immunosuppressant drugs include azathioprine (Imuran), basiliximab (Simulect), cyclosporine (Neoral, Sandimmune), daclizumab (Zenapax), muromonab-CD3 (OKT3, Orthoclone OKT3), mycophenolate (CellCept),

tacrolimus (FK506, Prograf), sirolimus (Rapamune), prednisone (Deltasone, Orasone), and other corticosteroids (glucocorticoids).

Interactions with Foods
None known.

Interactions with Lab Tests
None known.

Interactions with Diseases or Conditions
AUTOIMMUNE DISEASES: There is some concern that picrorhiza might adversely affect patients with autoimmune disorders because of its immune stimulating effects (11492,11853). Avoid using in patients with multiple sclerosis (MS), systemic lupus erythematosus (SLE), rheumatoid arthritis (RA), or other autoimmune disorders.

Dosage and Administration
ORAL: For vitiligo, picrorhiza rhizome powder 200 mg orally two times a day has been used, in combination with oral and topical methoxsalen therapy (11493). For acute viral hepatitis, picrorhiza root powder 375 mg orally three times a day has been used (11848).

Comments
Picrorhiza grows in the Himalayan mountains. It has been harvested to near extinction. It is a constituent of many Ayurvedic medicines (11848).

PIMPINELLA above ground parts

Also Known As
Bibernellkraut, Burnet Saxifrage, Pimpernell, Pimpinellae herba, Saxifrage.
CAUTION: See separate listing for Pimpinella root.

Scientific Names
Pimpinella saxifraga; Pimpinella major, synonyms Pimpinella magna.
Family: Apiaceae/Umbelliferae.

Comments
At the date of publication, there was very little scientific information about this product. Our staff is continually analyzing the available information on natural medicines and will add data to the online version of *Natural Medicines Comprehensive Database* as it becomes available. See www.naturaldatabase.com.

PIMPINELLA root

Also Known As
Burnet Saxifrage, Greater Burnet-Saxifrage, Pimpernell, Pimpinellae radix, Saxifrage.
CAUTION: See separate listing for Pimpinella above ground parts.

Scientific Names
Pimpinella saxifraga; Pimpinella major, synonyms Pimpinella magna.
Family: Apiaceae/Umbelliferae.

People Use This For
Orally, pimpinella root is used for upper respiratory tract mucous membrane inflammation, urinary tract disorders and inflammation, bladder and kidney stones, edema, and "flushing out" therapy for urinary tract bacterial inflammation.
Topically, pimpinella root is used for inflammation of the oral and pharyngeal mucous membranes, and as a bath additive for poorly healing wounds.

Safety
POSSIBLY SAFE ...when used orally and appropriately (2).
There is insufficient reliable information available about the safety of the topical use of pimpinella root.
PREGNANCY AND LACTATION: Insufficient reliable information available; avoid using.

Effectiveness
There is insufficient reliable information available about the effectiveness of pimpinella root.

Mechanism of Action
Pimpinella root is reported to loosen and aid in moving bronchial secretions (18).

Adverse Reactions
None reported. However, it may cause photosensitivity in fair-skinned individuals (18).

Interactions with Herbs & Other Dietary Supplements
None known.

Interactions with Drugs
None known.

Interactions with Foods
None known.

Interactions with Lab Tests
None known.

Interactions with Diseases or Conditions
None known.

Dosage and Administration
ORAL: People typically use one cup tea (briefly steep 3 grams finely cut root in 150 mL boiling water, strain) 3 to 4 times daily (8); up to 6-12 grams root per day (2). Tincture (1:5), 6-15 mL per day (8).
TOPICAL: No typical dosage.

Comments
Pimpinella root is often adulterated with other herbs including Hercaleum sphondylium, Heracleum mantegazianum, and Pastinaca sativa (8,18).

PINE

Also Known As
Dwarf-Pine, Pini Turiones, Pix Liquida, Pumilio Pine, Scotch Fir, Scotch Pine, Swiss Mountain Pine.
CAUTION: See separate listings for Dwarf Pine Needle, Fir, Fir Needle Oil, Poplar, and Scotch Pine Needle.

Scientific Names
Pinus sylvestris.
Family: Pinaceae.

People Use This For
Orally, pine is used for upper and lower respiratory tract mucous membrane inflammation, blood pressure problems, common cold, cough or bronchitis, fevers, tendency towards infection, to treat uncomplicated coughs and acute bronchial disease, nasal congestion, and hoarseness.
Topically, pine is used for mild muscular pain and neuralgia.

Safety
POSSIBLY SAFE ...when used orally and appropriately (2). ...when used topically and appropriately (2).
PREGNANCY AND LACTATION: Insufficient reliable information available; avoid using.

Effectiveness
There is insufficient reliable information available about the effectiveness of pine.

Mechanism of Action
The applicable part of pine is the sprout. Pine sprouts can dry secretions. They demonstrate mild antiseptic effects and stimulate peripheral circulation (2,18). Pine sprouts contain an essential oil that can stimulate serous bronchial gland function, suppress mucous gland function (7), and aid with expectoration (7).

Adverse Reactions
None reported.

Interactions with Herbs & Other Dietary Supplements
None known.

Interactions with Drugs
None known.

Interactions with Foods
None known.

Interactions with Lab Tests
None known.

Interactions with Diseases or Conditions
FEVER, INFECTIOUS DISEASE, CARDIAC INSUFFICIENCY, OR HYPERTONIA: Pine extract is contraindicated as a bath additive (18).
RESPIRATORY CONDITIONS: Pine exrtract is contraindicated for oral use in individuals with bronchial asthma or whooping cough (18).
SKIN CONDITIONS: Pine extract is contraindicated as a bath additive in individuals with extensive skin injury or acute skin diseases.

Dosage and Administration
ORAL: The average daily amount of pine sprout is 2-9 grams (2,18) as teas, syrups, or tinctures.
TOPICAL: It is applied topically as a 20-50% pine sprout extract in an alcoholic solution, oil, ointment, liquid, or semi-solid preparation (2,18). As a bath, 100 grams of the alcoholic extract is usually added to the bath water (18).

Comments
Avoid confusion with fir shoots (Picea bies or Abies alba) or pine oil.

PINELLIA TERNATA

Also Known As
Banha, Ban Xia, P. Ternata, Pinellia tuber.

Scientific Names
Pinellia ternata, synonym Pinellia Tubifera.
Family: Araceae.

People Use This For
Orally, Pinellia ternata is used for nausea, morning sickness, cough, birth control, influenza (flu), and inflammation.

Safety
POSSIBLY UNSAFE ...when used orally. Pinellia ternata contains ephedrine alkaloids and is banned in the US (12147). There is no reliable evidence available about the safety of Pinellia ternata in humans. Because it contains ephedrine alkaloids, it is likely that Pinellia ternata might potentially cause the adverse effects reported with ephedra, including heart attack, stroke, seizure, and other serious side effects.
PREGNANCY AND LACTATION: Insufficient reliable information; avoid using.

Effectiveness
There is insufficient reliable information available about the effectiveness of Pinellia ternata.

Mechanism of Action
The applicable part of Pinellia ternata is the tuber. Tuber extracts are thought to have antiemetic, anti-inflammatory, antitussive, sedative, and anti-implantation effects (12143).
The constituent responsible of the antiemetic effect seems to be present in an ethanol extract of the Pinellia ternata tuber (12143).
In an animal model, an aqueous extract of Pinellia ternata seems suppress gastric emptying (12144).
There is interest in Pinellia ternata for the flu (influenza). Pinellic acid from the Pinellia ternata tuber seems to increase IgA and IgG antibody titers in mice when used in conjunction with influenza vaccine (12146).

Pinellia ternata is also a plant source of ephedrine alkaloids (12147). The tuber contains approximately 0.002% L-ephedrine (12172).

Adverse Reactions

Orally, there is no reliable evidence available about the safety or side effects associated with Pinellia ternata in humans. Because it contains ephedrine alkaloids, it is likely that Pinellia ternata might potentially cause the adverse effects reported with ephedra, including heart attack, stroke, seizure, and other serious side effects (12147).
Inhaled, Pinellia ternata can cause IgE-mediated occupational asthma (12145).

Interactions with Herbs & Other Dietary Supplements

None known.

Interactions with Drugs

None known.

Interactions with Foods

None known.

Interactions with Lab Tests

None known.

Interactions with Diseases or Conditions

None known.

Dosage and Administration

No typical dosage.

Comments

On December 30, 2003, the FDA announced that it will ban dietary supplements containing ephedrine alkaloids. This includes Pinellia ternata, ephedra, and heart leaf (country mallow) (10055). The ban went into effect in April 2004 (12147).
Pinellia ternata is a common component in Traditional Chinese Medicine formulations. Many of these formulations are used for morning sickness. Pinellia ternata, along with ginger, is an ingredient in the herbal formulation Xiao-Ban-Xia-Tang (XBXT), which is used as an antiemetic (12144). Pinellia ternata is also used in Japanese Kampo medicine. It is an ingredient in Sho-seiryu-to (SST) (12146), which is used for the flu.

PINK ROOT

Also Known As

American Wormgrass, Carolina Pink, Indian Pink, Maryland Pink, Pinkroot, Starbloom, Wormgrass.

Scientific Names

Spigelia marilandica, synonym Lonicera marilandica.
Family: Loganiaceae.

People Use This For

Orally, pink root is used to treat worm infestation.

Safety

POSSIBLY SAFE ...when used orally and appropriately, short-term (12).
POSSIBLY UNSAFE ...when fresh root is used or when use is not accompanied by catharsis (12).
PREGNANCY: LIKELY UNSAFE ...when used orally. For pink root to be effective, it must be used along with a purgative laxative. However, purgative laxative use is contraindicated during pregnancy (272). For this reason, pink root should not be used in pregnancy.
LACTATION: Insufficient reliable information available; avoid using.

Effectiveness

There is insufficient reliable information available about the effectiveness of pink root.

Mechanism of Action
The applicable parts of pink root are the dried rhizome and root. Pink root has anthelmintic actions (18). Although there has been no recent research involving pink root, older sources identify the chief constituents as acidic resins, volatile oil, tannins, waxes, and a volatile base (presumably identical to isoquinoline) (18).

Adverse Reactions
Pink root allegedly contains a toxin that can paralyze the spinal marrow and lead to death by asphyxiation (18). Theoretically, prolonged use of pink root can cause depressive effects on the heart (19).

Interactions with Herbs & Other Dietary Supplements
None known.

Interactions with Drugs
None known.

Interactions with Foods
None known.

Interactions with Lab Tests
None known.

Interactions with Diseases or Conditions
None known.

Dosage and Administration
ORAL: A typical adult dose is 2-5 grams twice daily (12). A common dose for children over 4 years is 0.5-4 grams twice daily (12). A strong purgative laxative (e.g., senna) should always be used with pink root (12).

Comments
As late as 1955, pink root was commonly used throughout the country as an anthelmintic. Various unpleasant symptoms have been reported from use of the fresh root or when use is not accompanied by catharsis (12).

PINUS BARK

Also Known As
Canada Pitch, Canadian Hemlock, Eastern Hemlock, Hemlock Bark, Hemlock Gum, Hemlock Spruce, Hemlocktanne, Pruche de l'Est.

Scientific Names
Tsuga canadensis.
Family: Pinaceae or Abietaceae.

People Use This For
Orally, pinus bark is used for digestive disorders, diarrhea, and diseases of the mouth and throat. Historically, pinus bark was used to treat scurvy.

Safety
There is insufficient reliable information available about the safety of pinus bark.
Pregnancy and Lactation: Insufficient reliable information available; avoid using.

Effectiveness
There is insufficient reliable information available about the effectiveness of pinus bark.

Mechanism of Action
Pinus bark is reputed to have astringent, anti-inflammatory, and diuretic properties. It is also thought to induce sweating. The astringent effects of pinus bark are attributed to its tannin content (18). Tannins dehydrate the mucous membrane tissue, reducing internal secretions and causing external cells to form a protective layer. Plants with at least 10% tannins may cause gastrointestinal disturbances, kidney damage, and necrotic conditions of the liver. Some animal experiments show that tannins may cause cancer; others show they may prevent it. Regular consumption of herbs with high tannin concentrations correlates with increased incidence of esophageal or nasal cancer (12).

Adverse Reactions
None reported.

Interactions with Herbs & Other Dietary Supplements
TANNIN-CONTAINING HERBS: Theoretically, herbs that contain high percentages of tannins (such as pinus bark) may cause precipitation of constituents of other herbs (19).

Interactions with Drugs
ORAL DRUGS: Theoretically, concomitant oral administration may cause precipitation of some drugs due to the high tannin content of pinus bark (19). Separate administration of oral drugs and tannin-containing herbs by the longest period of time practical (19).

Interactions with Foods
None known.

Interactions with Lab Tests
None known.

Interactions with Diseases or Conditions
None known.

Dosage and Administration
No typical dosage.

Comments
Pinus bark is seldom used (18).

PIPSISSEWA

Also Known As
Bitter Winter, Bitter Wintergreen, Chimaphila, Ground Holly, Holly, King's Cure, King's Cureall, Love in Winter, Prince's Pine, Rheumatism Weed, Spotted Wintergreen, Umbellate Wintergreen.

Scientific Names
Chimaphila umbellata synonym Chimaphila corymbosa.
Family: Ericaceae.

People Use This For
Orally, pipsissewa is used as a urinary antiseptic. It is also used orally as a diuretic, astringent, mild disinfectant, antispasmodic, for bladder stones, epilepsy, nervous disorders, and cancer.
Topically, pipsissewa is used for treating ulcerous sores and blisters.
In food and beverages, pipsissewa extracts are used as flavor components.

Safety
LIKELY SAFE ...when used in amounts commonly found in foods. Pipsissewa leaf extract has Generally Recognized As Safe (GRAS) status in the US (4912).
POSSIBLY SAFE ...when used orally short-term (12).
POSSIBLY UNSAFE ...when used orally long-term because it can cause hydroquinone toxicity (18).
There is insufficient reliable information available about the topical use of pipsissewa.
PREGNANCY AND LACTATION: Insufficient reliable information.

Effectiveness
There is insufficient reliable information available about the effectiveness of pipsissewa.

Mechanism of Action
The applicable parts of pipsissewa are the above ground plant parts. The component chimaphilin has a weak sensitizing effect. It is not suitable for long term use due to its hydroquinone glycoside content (18). Chimaphilin may have urinary antiseptic, bacteriostatic, and astringent activity (11). Animal data suggests pipsissewa may elicit hypoglycemia. Arbutin may have urinary antiseptic properties due to hydrolysis to its hydroquinone by the intestinal flora (7,11).

Adverse Reactions
Orally, chronic use may lead to hydroquinone toxicity. Symptoms of toxicity include tinnitus, vomiting, delirium, convulsions, and collapse (11).

Interactions with Herbs & Other Dietary Supplements
None known.

Interactions with Drugs
None known.

Interactions with Foods
None known.

Interactions with Lab Tests
None known.

Interactions with Diseases or Conditions
None known.

Dosage and Administration
No typical dosage.

Comments
Pipsissewa is used similarly to uva ursi (18).

PITCHER PLANT

Also Known As
Eve's Cups, Fly-Catcher, Fly-Trap, Huntsman's Cup, Pitcher Plant, Purple Pitcher Plant, Purple Side-Saddle Flower, Sarapin, Side-Saddle Plant, Smallpox Plant, Water-cup.

Scientific Names
Sarracenia purpurea.
Family: Sarraceniaceae.

People Use This For
Orally, pitcher plant is used for digestive disorders, particularly constipation, urinary tract diseases, as a diuretic, a cure for smallpox, and to prevent scar formation.
By injection, pitcher plant extract (Sarapin) is used as a trigger point injection to treat pain including sciatic pain, intercostal pain, alcoholic or occipital neuritis, brachial plexus neuralgia, meralgia paresthetica, and lumbar or trigeminal neuralgia. Pitcher plant extract (Sarapin) has been used by injection in combination with bupivacaine hydrochloride 0.5% (Marcaine) and gamma globulin to treat the omohyoideus myofascial pain syndrome. It has been used in combinations by injection (extract triamcinolone and lidocaine with adrenalin) to treat migraine cephalagia, for diagnosis and treatment of forms of sciatic pain including piriformis syndrome (extract and lidocaine), quadratus lumborum syndrome (extract and corticosteroid), and in combination with physiotherapy and an intraoral splint to treat the Ernest Syndrome that is often mistaken for temporomandibular joint problems. It is also used in prolotherapy (phenol and extract) to cause inflammation at the site where the ligaments and tendons attach to the bone to stimulate the body to proliferate stronger, shorter, and less painful ligaments and/or tendons.

Safety
LIKELY SAFE ...when the extract of pitcher plant, Sarapin (a prescription product), is used appropriately by injection by a qualified health professional (5971).
There is insufficient reliable information available about the safety of the oral use of pitcher plant.
POSSIBLY UNSAFE ...when the extract of pitcher plant, Sarapin (a prescription product), is injected in areas of inflammation (5971).
PREGNANCY AND LACTATION: Insufficient reliable information available; avoid using.

Effectiveness
There is insufficient reliable information available about the effectiveness of pitcher plant.

Mechanism of Action

The pitcher plant leaf and root contain sarracenia acid, tannin, resin, and the alkaloid sarracenin (5944). The extract has an effect on sensory nerves without changing skin sensation or affecting motor nerves. Some evidence suggests that pitcher plant extract affects only C nerve fibers, perhaps containing a biological antagonist that potentiates the action of the ammonium ion (5975). This could be beneficial in chronic neuropathic pain.

Adverse Reactions

Used by injection, pitcher plant extract can cause a local sensation of heaviness. Some individuals experience a local sensation of heat or aggravation of symptoms.

Interactions with Herbs & Other Dietary Supplements

None known.

Interactions with Drugs

None known.

Interactions with Foods

None known.

Interactions with Lab Tests

None known.

Interactions with Diseases or Conditions

None known.

Dosage and Administration

INJECTION: Pitcher plant extract (Sarapin) is given by nerve block or local infiltration. Doses are as follows: 2-3 mL cervical, 5-10 mL dorsal, 5-10 mL lumbar, 3-5 mL sacral, 10 mL caudal canal, 10 mL sciatic nerve, 5-10 mL local infiltration. Following injection, patients should be maintained in recumbent position for 15 minutes (5971). For use in migraine, 4 mg triamcinolone, 0.75 mL Sarapin and 0.15 mL lidocaine with adrenalin drawn into a syringe in that order have been administered at the trigger points in both temples using a 28 gauge, 5/8 inch needle (5973). Sarapin is an FDA-approved prescription product. For additional information, contact the manufacturer, High Chemical Company, 1-800-447-8792.

PLEURISY ROOT

Also Known As

Butterfly Weed, Canada Root, Flux Root, Orange Milkweed, Orange Swallow Wort, Pleurisy, Swallow-Wort, Tuber Root, White Root, Wind Root.
CAUTION: See separate listing for Amaranth.

Scientific Names

Asclepias tuberosa.
Family: Asclepiadaceae or Apocynaceae.

People Use This For

Orally, pleurisy root is used for coughs, pleurisy, uterine disorders, to ease breathing, as an analgesic, expectorant, antispasmodic, and to promote sweating. It is also used orally for bronchitis, pneumonitis, and influenza.

Safety

POSSIBLY UNSAFE ...when the root is used orally because it contains digitalis-like cardenolide glycosides (4). It can cause vomiting (12). Canadian regulations do not allow pleurisy root as a non-medicinal ingredient for oral use products (12).
PREGNANCY: UNSAFE ...when used orally (12) because it might have uterine stimulant and estrogenic activity (19).
LACTATION: POSSIBLY UNSAFE ...when used orally (12); avoid using.

Effectiveness

There is insufficient reliable information available about the effectiveness of pleurisy root.

Mechanism of Action

Pleurisy root contains digitalis-like cardenolide glycosides (18). Animal data suggest that pleurisy root does not affect blood pressure, respiration, or heart muscle (4).

Adverse Reactions

Pleurisy root may cause dermatitis. It is also a gastrointestinal irritant and emetic, and can cause nausea and vomiting (19). At higher doses, it may cause digitalis-like poisoning symptoms (18).

Interactions with Herbs & Other Dietary Supplements

CARDIAC GLYCOSIDE-CONTAINING HERBS: Contraindicated. Concomitant use can increase the risk of cardiac glycoside toxicity. Cardiac glycoside-containing herbs include black hellebore, Canadian hemp roots, digitalis leaf, hedge mustard, figwort, lily of the valley roots, motherwort, oleander leaf, pheasant's eye plant, squill bulb leaf scales, strophanthus seeds, and uzara (19).

Interactions with Drugs

DIGOXIN (Lanoxin): Because pleurisy root contains cardenolide glycosides, it could have additive effects with digoxin (19).

DIURETIC DRUGS: Theoretically, concomitant use of potassium-depleting diuretics and pleurisy root can increase the risk of cardiac glycoside toxicity due to potassium depletion (19). Some diuretics that can deplete potassium include chlorothiazide (Diuril), chlorthalidone (Thalitone), furosemide (Lasix), hydrochlorothiazide (HCTZ, HydroDIURIL, Microzide), and others.

ESTROGENS: Theoretically, excessive amounts of pleurisy root might interfere with hormone drug therapy (4).

Interactions with Foods

None known.

Interactions with Lab Tests

None known.

Interactions with Diseases or Conditions

CARDIAC CONDITIONS: Pleurisy root may worsen or interfere with cardiac drug therapy (4).

Dosage and Administration

No typical dosage.

PODOPHYLLUM

Also Known As

American Mandrake, Devil's Apple, Duck's Foot, Ground Lemon, Himalayan Mayapple, Hog Apple, Indian Apple, Indian Podophyllum, Mandrake, Mayapple, Podophylli pelati rhizoma/resina, Raccoon Berry, Vegetable Mercury, Wild Lemon, Wild Mandrake.

CAUTION: See separate listings for Bryonia (English Mandrake) and European Mandrake.

Scientific Names

Podophyllum hexandrum, synonyms Podophyllum emodi, and Sinopodophyllum emodi; Podophyllum peltatum.
Family: Berberidaceae.

People Use This For

Topically, podophyllum resin is used for removal of topical warts, including plantar warts, condyloma acuminata (venereal warts), and other papillomas. Podophyllum resin is also used orally as a cathartic, for jaundice and liver ailments, fever, syphilis, and cancer. The resin has also been used orally as an anthelmintic, antidote for snake bites, and as an abortifacient.

Safety

POSSIBLY SAFE ...when used topically and appropriately (9,12). Podophyllum must be applied in low concentration solutions, 0.5% podophyllotoxin (6,9), to small surface areas, 25 square cm or less (7,18), with protection of adjacent skin (7) and washed off within 1-4 hours (6,9). Contact with skin should not exceed 6 hours (6). Risk of systemic toxicity increases if applied to large areas, open lesions, normal skin or mucous membranes, with prolonged use (9), and use of the ointment form (6).

LIKELY UNSAFE ...when used orally; podophyllum is potentially lethal (6,9,5617). ...when used topically near the eyes (19). ...when used topically on cervical or urethral warts (9). It is contraindicated for use on moles, birthmarks, or inflamed warts because it can cause permanent skin damage (19). Fatalities have been reported from oral ingestion and topical application (6,9,5617).

PREGNANCY: LIKELY UNSAFE ...when used orally or topically for self-medication; avoid using. Podophyllum is considered potentially embryotoxic and teratogenic (7,9,11,12,5618). Fetal intrauterine death and multiple birth deformities associated with oral and topical podophyllum use have been reported (5618).

LACTATION: LIKELY UNSAFE ...when used orally or topically for self-medication (6,9,5617); avoid using.

Effectiveness

LIKELY EFFECTIVE

Constipation. Taking podophyllum orally is an effective laxative for constipation (6,7,9,11,13,15); however, it is unsafe for oral ingestion (6,9).

Epithelial growths. Applying podophyllum resin topically is effective for removal of benign epithelial growths such as keratoses (15).

Genital warts (condylomata acuminata). Applying podophyllum resin topically is effective for removal of anogenital warts caused by human papillomavirus (15).

Mechanism of Action

The applicable parts of podophyllum are the root, rhizome, and resin. The major active constituents in podophyllum are lignan derivatives (6,9,11), including podophyllotoxin (6,7,9,11), which is antimitotic (9,11,13,18) and antineoplastic (6,11). Podophyllum induces catharsis through irritation of the intestinal mucosa (6,9). It also induces lymphocyte activating factor/interleukin 1, stimulates macrophage proliferation, and modulates other cytokines (11). Significant absorption occurs through the skin (6) and gastrointestinal (GI) tract (5617). Etoposide and teniposide, semisynthetic analogs of podophyllotoxin, are active against testicular cancer, small cell lung cancer, leukemia, lymphoma (6,11,13), Kaposi's sarcoma, neuroblastoma (13), rheumatoid arthritis (RA) (6,11), and psoriasis (11). Podophyllotoxin exposure during pregnancy is considered to be highly embryotoxic (6,7,11,5618); teratogenicity has been reported (6,5618) but not confirmed by studies in experimental animals (7,11).

Adverse Reactions

Oral ingestion and topical application can cause severe abdominal pain, nausea, vomiting, bloody-watery diarrhea, vomiting of bile, dizziness, headache, coordination disorders, spasms, nephritis, fever, altered mental status, visual hallucinations, confusion, tachypnea, peripheral neuropathy, muscle paralysis, hypotension, bone marrow suppression, renal failure, coma, respiratory failure, and death (6,18,5617). Chronic use as a cathartic can cause hypokalemia and metabolic alkalosis (6,5617). Oral or topical use of podophyllum in pregnant women can cause fetal congenital malformations and death (6,5618). Podophyllum can cause severe local irritation, especially to eyes and mucous membranes (9,11,18). It might also cause transformation of condyloma to squamous cell carcinoma (9). Symptoms of toxicity usually do not appear for a period of time, ranging from a few to 13 hours after ingestion or absorption (5617). Neurologic changes may progress rapidly after onset of symptoms (6).

Interactions with Herbs & Other Dietary Supplements

CARDIAC GLYCOSIDE-CONTAINING HERBS: Contraindicated; concomitant use with podophyllum may increase the risk of cardiac glycoside toxicity. Cardiac glycoside-containing herbs include black hellebore, Canadian hemp roots, digitalis leaf, hedge mustard, figwort, lily of the valley roots, motherwort, oleander leaf, pheasant's eye plant, pleurisy root, squill bulb leaf scales, and strophanthus seeds (19).

POTASSIUM-DEPLETING HERBS: Theoretically, concomitant use of podophyllum with horsetail (Equisetum arvense) plant or licorice (Glycyrrhiza glabra) rhizome increases the risk of potassium depletion.

STIMULANT LAXATIVE HERBS: Theoretically, concomitant use of podophyllum with other stimulant laxative herbs may increase the risk of potassium depletion. Stimulant laxative herbs include aloe dried leaf sap, wild cucumber fruit (Ecballium elaterium), blue flag rhizome, alder buckthorn, European buckthorn, butternut bark, cascara bark, castor oil, colocynth fruit pulp, gamboge bark exudate, jalap root, black root, manna bark exudate, rhubarb root, senna leaves and pods, and yellow dock root (19).

Interactions with Drugs

DIURETIC DRUGS: Overuse of podophyllum might compound diuretic-induced potassium loss (19). There is some concern that people taking podophyllum along with potassium-depleting diuretics might have an increased risk for hypokalemia. Initiation of potassium supplementation or an increase in potassium supplement dose may be necessary for some patients. Some diuretics that can deplete potassium include chlorothiazide (Diuril), chlorthalidone (Thalitone), furosemide (Lasix), hydrochlorothiazide (HCTZ, HydroDIURIL, Microzide), and others.

Interactions with Foods

None known.

Interactions with Lab Tests

None known.

Interactions with Diseases or Conditions

GALLSTONES: Contraindicated; theoretically, podophyllum can stimulate bile secretion (19).
GASTROINTESTINAL (GI) CONDITIONS: Contraindicated; podophyllum can irritate the GI tract, exacerbating infectious or inflammatory conditions (19).

Dosage and Administration

TOPICAL: 1.5-3 grams root or fluid extract, or 2.5-7.5 grams tincture, 5-25% in benzoin, is typically applied once or twice per week to an area no more than 25 square cm, with protection of surrounding skin (2,6,7,13,18). Alternatively, 0.5% solution after 1-6 hours (6-9), or 0.15% cream applied twice per day for three days (9). Lower concentrations applied twice per day are at least as effective as higher concentrations applied twice per week applied twice per day for three days, washed off (6,7,9). Podophyllum should not be used for self-treatment.

Comments

Podophyllum resin is prepared from the root and rhizome of the plant. Podophyllum toxicity has been successfully treated using charcoal hemoperfusion (6,5617).

POINSETTIA

Also Known As

Christmas Flower, Easter Flower, Lobster Flower Plant, Lobsterplant, Mexican Flame Leaf, Paintedleaf, Papagallo.

Scientific Names

Euphorbia pulcherrima, synonym Poinsettia pulcherrima; Euphorbia poinsettia.
Family: Euphorbiaceae.

People Use This For

Orally, poinsettia is used as an antipyretic, to stimulate milk production, and as an abortifacient. The latex is used orally as an analgesic, antibacterial, and emetic.
Topically, poinsettia latex is used as a depilatory, skin remedy, for warts, and for toothaches.

Safety

POSSIBLY UNSAFE ...when used orally or topically, but toxicity is limited to local irritation, contact dermatitis, mucosal burns, and keratoconjunctivitis (17).
CHILDREN: POSSIBLY UNSAFE ...when used orally or topically. Poinsettia was implicated in the poisoning death of a 2 year old child (6).
PREGNANCY AND LACTATION: POSSIBLY UNSAFE ...when used orally or topically (17); avoid using.

Effectiveness

There is insufficient reliable information available about the effectiveness of poinsettia.

Mechanism of Action

The applicable parts of poinsettia are the whole plant and latex. There is insufficient reliable information available about the possible mechanism of action and active ingredients.

Adverse Reactions

Toxicity is limited to local irritation, contact dermatitis, mucosal burns, and keratoconjunctivitis (17).

Interactions with Herbs & Other Dietary Supplements

None known.

Interactions with Drugs

None known.

Interactions with Foods

None known.

Interactions with Lab Tests

None known.

Interactions with Diseases or Conditions

GI IRRITATION, INFLAMMATION: Euphorbia species are said to have GI irritant effects (19); avoid using.

Dosage and Administration
No typical dosage.

Comments
Recent studies indicate that the plant is less toxic than once believed (6). American Association of Poison Control Centers reported 22,793 cases of poisoning with no fatalities and 92.4% with no toxicity (3838).

POISON IVY

Also Known As
Markweed, Poison Vine, Three-Leafed Ivy.

Scientific Names
Toxicodendron radicans, synonym Rhus radicans; Toxicodendron pubescens, synonyms Rhus toxicodendron, Toxicodendron quercifolium, Toxicodendron toxicarium.
Family: Anacardiaceae.

People Use This For
Orally, poison ivy is used to treat pain.

Safety
LIKELY UNSAFE ...when used orally or topically (6).
PREGNANCY AND LACTATION: LIKELY UNSAFE ...when used orally or topically (6); avoid using.

Effectiveness
There is insufficient reliable information available about the effectiveness of poison ivy.

Mechanism of Action
Poison ivy is a severe skin irritant that stimulates the immune system (18). Contact sensitivity is due to the urushiols, which bind to skin proteins, sensitizing the individual (6). Once sensitized, re-exposure leads to allergic reactions (6).

Adverse Reactions
Orally, the plant can cause severe mucous membrane irritation, nausea, vomiting, intestinal colic, diarrhea, dizziness, stupor, nephritis, hematuria, fever, and unconsciousness (18).
Topically, the plant can cause contact dermatitis, reddening, swelling, herpes-like blisters (18), and erythema multiforme (3839). Eye contact can cause severe conjunctivitis, corneal inflammations, or loss of sight (18).
Inhalation due to burning of the plant can result in fever, major lung infection, and death from throat swelling (6).

Interactions with Herbs & Other Dietary Supplements
GINKGO BILOBA: Fruit pulp can cause cross-reactivity in people allergic to poison ivy (6).

Interactions with Drugs
None known.

Interactions with Foods
CASHEW: Nut shell oil can cause cross-reactivity in people allergic to poison ivy (6,735).
MANGO: Fruit skin can cause cross-reactivity in people allergic to poison ivy (6,735).

Interactions with Lab Tests
None known.

Interactions with Diseases or Conditions
None known.

Dosage and Administration
No typical dosage.

Comments
To prevent poison ivy from causing skin irritation, wash exposed area with water within 5 to 10 minutes (6). Use soap and water first, then ether or alcohol (18).

POISONOUS BUTTERCUP

Also Known As

Celery-Leafed Crowfoot, Cursed Crowfoot.
CAUTION: See separate listings for Buttercup and Bulbous Buttercup.

Scientific Names

Ranunculus sceleratus.
Family: Ranunculaceae.

People Use This For

Topically, poisonous buttercup is used as a stimulant for skin diseases (e.g., scabies) and leucoderma.

Safety

LIKELY UNSAFE ...when the above ground parts are used orally or topically. The fresh plant causes severe local irritation (18).
There is insufficient reliable information about the safety of the oral or topical use of the dried, cut leaf.
PREGNANCY AND LACTATION: LIKELY UNSAFE ...when used orally or topically (18,19). Oral use might possibly stimulate uterine activity (19).

Effectiveness

There is insufficient reliable information available about the effectiveness of poisonous buttercup.

Mechanism of Action

The applicable parts of poisonous buttercup are the above ground parts. Poisonous buttercup contains ranunculin, anemonin, and protoanemonin. Protoanemonin is a potent topical irritant (18). It causes pain and burning sensations, severe tongue inflammation, and increases salivation. When the freshly harvested plant is cut into small pieces or perhaps when it is dried, protoanemonin changes into a pungent, volatile intermediate that quickly dimerizes to a form that does not irritate the mucous membrane. In vitro, leaf extracts have shown a wide fungicidal spectrum of activity (3836).

Adverse Reactions

Topically, extended contact with fresh or bruised plant can lead to blisters and burns that are difficult to heal (18). Some species of Ranunculus can cause photodermatitis. Avoid excessive sunlight or ultraviolet light exposure while using this product (19).

Interactions with Herbs & Other Dietary Supplements

None known.

Interactions with Drugs

None known.

Interactions with Foods

None known.

Interactions with Lab Tests

None known.

Interactions with Diseases or Conditions

None known.

Dosage and Administration

TOPICAL: Poisonous buttercup is used as a tincture (18).

POKEWEED berry

Also Known As

American Nightshade, American Spinach, Bear's Grape, Branching Phytolacca, Cancer Jalap, Chongras, Coakum, Coakum-Chorngras, Cokan, Crowberry, Fitolaca, Garget, Hierba Carmín, Inkberry, Jalap, Kermesbeere, Phytolacca Berry, Pigeonberry, Pocan, Poke, Pokeberry, Raisin d'Amérique, Red-Ink Plant, Red Plant, Red Weed, Scoke, Skoke, Teinturière, Virginian Poke.
CAUTION: See separate listings for Jalap, Mexican Scammony Root, and Pokeweed root.

Scientific Names

Phytolacca americana, synonym Phytolacca decandra.
Family: Phytolaccaceae.

People Use This For

In foods, pokeweed berry is eaten, used as red food coloring, and as a wine coloring agent.
In manufacturing, pokeweed berry is used to make ink and dye.

Safety

LIKELY UNSAFE ...when the fresh berry is ingested. One berry can be toxic to a child; 10 berries to an adult (6,18). Green berries are considered more toxic than mature, red berries (4). ...when pokeweed berry and juice comes in contact with broken skin or is ingested, it can cause hematological changes (4,3477,3481,3482). Protective gloves should be used to handle the plant (6,3477). All parts of the pokeweed plant, especially the root, are considered to be toxic (3477,3479,3483). Severe poisoning has been reported from ingesting tea brewed from pokeweed root (6,3478) and pokeweed leaves (3480). Poisoning also has resulted from ingestion of pokeberry wine and pokeberry pancakes (3479).
CHILDREN: UNSAFE ...when used orally. Consumption of even one berry can be toxic. Children have died after ingesting pokeweed berries (3479,3483).
PREGNANCY AND LACTATION: LIKELY UNSAFE ...when the fresh berry is ingested; avoid using. Evidence suggests the berry has uterine stimulant and abortifacient effects (4,19).

Effectiveness

There is insufficient reliable information available about the effectiveness of pokeweed berry.

Mechanism of Action

Pokeweed contains saponin glycosides, proteinaceous mitogens (3477,3478), tannin, and resin (6). The toxicity of pokeweed is attributed to proteinaceous mitogens and the saponin glycosides which include phytolaccatoxin and phytolaccagenin. The saponin glycosides cause gastrointestinal irritation and the proteinaceous mitogens are thought to affect thymus-dependent (T) cells and thymus-independent (B) lymphocytes (3477,3478).

Adverse Reactions

Orally, all parts of the pokeweed plant can cause nausea, vomiting, cramping, abdominal pain, diarrhea, burning sensation in mouth and throat, weakness, bloody emesis, hypotension, bloody diarrhea, tachycardia, difficulty in breathing, salivation, urinary incontinence, spasm, convulsion (4,3477,3478,3479), severe thirst, somnolence, transient blindness, respiratory failure (18,3477,3479), and death (4,18,3477,3483). Plasmacytosis, mitotic changes in peripheral blood cells, eosinophilia, thrombocytopenia, abnormal platelet morphology, and other hematologic abnormalities may result from topical exposure (especially in individuals with cuts or abrasions on hands or other extremities) and ingestion of pokeweed plant, berries, or root (3477,3478,3481,3482).

Interactions with Herbs & Other Dietary Supplements

None known.

Interactions with Drugs

None known.

Interactions with Foods

None known.

Interactions with Lab Tests

None known.

Interactions with Diseases or Conditions

None known.

Dosage and Administration
No typical dosage.

Comments
Avoid confusion with jalap (Ipomoea orizabensis). All parts of the pokeweed plant are considered toxic except the above ground leaves grown in early spring (6). The immature leaves are canned and marketed as the food product, "poke salad" (6). In folk medicine, the leaves have been used for rheumatism, arthritis, emesis, and purging (6). Ongoing research is investigating the use of pokeweed in flu, HSV-1, and polio (4,18). The United Kingdom allows pokeweed in medicinal products provided toxic constituents are absent and the product adheres to mandated limits (4).

POKEWEED root

Also Known As
American Nightshade, American Spinach, Bear's Grape, Branching Phytolacca, Cancer Jalap, Chongras, Coakum, Coakum-Chorngras, Cokan, Crowberry, Fitolaca, Garget, Hierba Carmín, Inkberry, Jalap, Kermesbeere, Phytolacca Berry, Pigeonberry, Pocan, Poke, Poke Root, Pokeberry, Raisin d'Amérique, Red-Ink Plant, Red Plant, Red Weed, Scoke, Skoke, Teinturière, Virginian Poke.
CAUTION: See separate listings for Jalap, Mexican Scammony Root, and Pokewood berry.

Scientific Names
Phytolacca americana, synonym Phytolacca decandra.
Family: Phytolaccaceae.

People Use This For
Orally, pokeweed root is used as an emetic.
Historically, pokeweed root has been used for rheumatism, mucous membrane inflammation of upper and lower respiratory tract, tonsillitis, laryngitis, adenitis, mastitis, mumps, skin infections (scabies, tinea, sycosis, ringworm, acne), mammary abscesses, edema, skin cancers, dysmenorrhea, and syphilis.

Safety
LIKELY UNSAFE ...when used orally. All parts of the pokeweed plant, especially the root, are considered to be toxic (3477,3479,3483). The Herb Trade Association recommends against selling pokeweed root as an herbal beverage or food (4,3478). Severe poisoning has been reported from ingesting tea brewed from pokeweed root (6,3478) and pokeweed leaves (3480). ...when root comes in contact with broken skin or is ingested, it can cause hematological changes (3477,3481,3482). Protective gloves should be used to handle the plant (6,3477).
PREGNANCY AND LACTATION: LIKELY UNSAFE ...when used orally; avoid using. Evidence suggests it might have uterine stimulant and abortifacient effects (4,19).

Effectiveness
There is insufficient reliable information available about the effectiveness of pokeweed root.

Mechanism of Action
Pokeweed contains saponin glycosides, proteinaceous mitogens (3477,3478), tannin, and resin (6). The toxicity of pokeweed is attributed to proteinaceous mitogens and the saponin glycosides which include phytolaccatoxin and phytolaccagenin. The saponin glycosides cause gastrointestinal irritation and the proteinaceous mitogens are thought to affect thymus-dependent (T) cells and thymus-independent (B) lymphocytes (3477,3478).

Adverse Reactions
Orally, all parts of the pokeweed plant can cause nausea, vomiting, cramping, abdominal pain, diarrhea, burning sensation in mouth and throat, weakness, bloody emesis, hypotension, bloody diarrhea, tachycardia, difficulty in breathing, salivation, urinary incontinence, spasm, convulsion (4,3477,3478,3479), severe thirst, somnolence, transient blindness, respiratory failure (18,3477,3479), and death (4,18,3477,3483). Plasmacytosis, mitotic changes in peripheral blood cells, eosinophilia, thrombocytopenia, abnormal platelet morphology, and other hematologic abnormalities may result from topical exposure (especially in individuals with cuts or abrasions on hands or other extremities) and ingestion of pokeweed plant, berries, or root (3477,3478,3481,3482).

Interactions with Herbs & Other Dietary Supplements
None known.

Interactions with Drugs
None known.

Interactions with Foods
None known.

Interactions with Lab Tests
None known.

Interactions with Diseases or Conditions
None known.

Dosage and Administration
No typical dosage.

Comments
Avoid confusion with jalap (Ipomoea orizabensis). All parts of the pokeweed plant are considered toxic except the above ground leaves grown in early spring (6). The immature leaves are canned and marketed as the food product, "poke salad" (6). In folk medicine, the leaves have been used for rheumatism, arthritis, emesis, and purging (6). Ongoing research is investigating the use of pokeweed in flu, HSV-1, and polio (4,18). The United Kingdom allows pokeweed in medicinal products provided toxic constituents are absent and the product adheres to mandated limits (4).

POLICOSANOL

Also Known As
32-C, Dotriacontanol, Heptacosanol, Hexacosanol, Nonacosanol, Octacosanol, Tetracosanol, Tetratriacontanol, Triacontanol.
CAUTION: See separate listing for Octacosanol.

Scientific Names
Policosanol.

People Use This For
Orally, policosanol is used for hyperlipidemia, intermittent claudication, decreasing myocardial ischemia in patients with coronary heart disease, and as an anti-plaque agent.

Safety
POSSIBLY SAFE ...when used orally and appropriately. Policosanol seems to be safe when used in doses of 10-20 mg per day for up to 2 years (2927,2928,2929,2930,2931,2943,2944,12166).
PREGNANCY AND LACTATION: Insufficient reliable information available; avoid using.

Effectiveness
POSSIBLY EFFECTIVE

Hypercholesterolemia. Taking policosanol orally 10-20 mg/day seems to significantly decrease total cholesterol and low-density lipoprotein (LDL) cholesterol, and increase high-density lipoprotein (HDL) cholesterol (2927,2928,2929,2930,2943,2944). Policosanol 10 mg daily seems to be similar to fluvastatin 20 mg (Lescol) daily in cholesterol-lowering ability (8147). Most of these studies have used policosanol derived from sugarcane. It is not known if policosanol from other plant sources is effective. There is some evidence that wheat germ-derived policosanol 20 mg/day does not significantly lower cholesterol after 4 weeks of treatment (12166). The reason for this potential difference is unclear since wheat germ derived policosanol is almost identical to sugarcane policosanol. More evidence is needed to determine the effectiveness of non-sugarcane derived policosanol.

Intermittent claudication. Taking policosanol orally seems to significantly improve walking distance in patients with intermittent claudication (2931).

Mechanism of Action
Policosanol is a mixture of waxy alcohols derived from a variety of plant sources including sugar cane and wheat germ oil. It refers to a mixture of 24-34 carbon alcohols comprised primarily of octacosanol (28-C) and also including tetracosanol (24-C), hexacosanol (26-C), heptacosanol (27-C), nonacosanol (29-C), triacosanol (30-C), dotriacontanol (32-C), and tetratriacontanol (268,269,270).
Sugarcane derived policosanol contains 66% to 67% octacosanol, 12% to 14% triacosanol, 7% to 8% hexacosanol,

and 11% to 15% of other carbon alcohols. Wheat germ derived policosanol contains about 68% octacosanol, 12.6% triacosanol, 8% hexacosanol, and about 11% of other carbon alcohols (12166).
Policosanol seems to lower cholesterol levels by inhibiting hepatic cholesterol synthesis (2934,2939) and increasing the degradation of low-density lipoprotein (LDL) cholesterol (2939).
Policosanol also decreases arachidonic acid and collagen-induced platelet aggregation (2933,2935,2936,2937,2938).
Policosanol 20 mg per day reduces platelet aggregation about as much as aspirin 100 mg per day (2937), but it does not seem to significantly affect coagulation time (2935,2937).

Adverse Reactions
Orally, policosanol is usually well-tolerated (2927,2928,2929,2930,2931,2943,2944,12166). In some patients it can cause erythema (2929), migraines, insomnia, somnolence, irritability, dizziness, upset stomach, polyphagia, dysuria, weight loss, skin rash, and nose and gum bleeding (2937).

Interactions with Herbs & Other Dietary Supplements
None known.

Interactions with Drugs
ANTICOAGULANT/ANTIPLATELET DRUGS: Policosanol can inhibit platelet aggregation (2936,2937,2938). Theoretically, taking policosanol with other antiplatelet or anticoagulant drugs might increase the risk of bruising and bleeding. Some of these drugs include aspirin, clopidogrel (Plavix), nonsteroidal anti-inflammatory drugs (NSAIDs) such as diclofenac (Voltaren, Cataflam, others), ibuprofen (Advil, Motrin, others), naproxen (Anaprox, Naprosyn, others), dalteparin (Fragmin), enoxaparin (Lovenox), heparin, warfarin (Coumadin), and others.

Interactions with Foods
None known.

Interactions with Lab Tests
CHOLESTEROL: Policosanol can decrease serum total cholesterol and low-density lipoprotein (LDL) cholesterol levels and increase high density lipoprotein (HDL) cholesterol levels (2927,2928,2943).

Interactions with Diseases or Conditions
None known.

Dosage and Administration
ORAL: For hypercholesterolemia, the typical dose of policosanol is 5-10 mg twice daily (2927,2928,2929,2930). For intermittent claudication, 10 mg twice daily has been used (2931).

POMEGRANATE

Also Known As
Dadima, Granada, Grenadier, Shi Liu Gen Pi, Shi Liu Pi.

Scientific Names
Punica granatum.
Family: Lythraceae or Punicaceae.

People Use This For
Orally, pomegranate is used for tapeworm infestations and opportunistic intestinal worms. It is also used as an astringent, for diarrhea and dysentery, and as an abortive.
Topically, pomegranate is used as a gargle for sore throat and to treat hemorrhoids.

Safety
POSSIBLY SAFE ...when the rind (peel), fruit, or seeds are used orally and appropriately (12,8310).
UNSAFE ...when the root is used orally. The root contains the toxic alkaloid pelletierine (12). ...when the fruit rind is used in individuals with diarrhea (12).
There is insufficient reliable information available about the topical safety of pomegranate bark and root.
PREGNANCY: UNSAFE ...when used orally. The bark, root, and fruit rind can stimulate menstruation or uterine contractions (12,19).
LACTATION: UNSAFE ...when the bark or root is used orally (12).
There is insufficient reliable information available about the safety of pomegranate during pregnancy and breast-feeding when used topically; avoid using.

Effectiveness

There is insufficient reliable information available about the effectiveness of pomegranate.

Mechanism of Action

The applicable parts of the pomegranate are the bark, rind, root, seed, and stem (18,1287). The seed oil contains polyphenols and fatty acids, including punicic acid, palmitic acid, stearic acid, oleic acid, and linoleic acid (1287). The active constituents of pomegranate are anthocyanidins, including delphinidin, cyanidin, and pelargonidin.
Preliminary tests indicate that these substances exert antioxidant activity (8308). Antioxidant effects have been demonstrated in fermented pomegranate juice and cold pressed seed oil (1287). Estrone and other nonsteroidal estrogenic substances are found in pomegranate seeds (8311). Pomegranate root and stem contain the piperidine alkaloids isopelletierine, N-methyliospelletierine, and pseudopelletierin. The root contains up to 25% tannins, and the fruit rind contains up to 28% tannins (18). Tannins can exert an astringent effect on mucosal tissues, dehydrating the tissue, reducing internal secretions and forming a hardened, external protective layer of cells. Some preliminary data suggest that tannins might cause cancer; other data suggest tannins may prevent it (12).
Preliminary data suggests pomegranate juice may slow the progression of atherosclerosis. The antioxidant effects may contribute to decreased macrophage activity in atherosclerotic plaques and reduced lipid peroxidation of low-density lipoproteins (LDL) (8309).
Pomegranate juice can reduce the activity of angiotensin converting enzyme (ACE) and reduce blood pressure in patients with hypertension. The serum activity of ACE is reduced approximately 36%, with incremental decreases occurring in patients already taking angiotensin converting enzyme inhibitors (ACEIs). Systolic blood pressure is decreased about 5% (8310).

Adverse Reactions

Orally, pomegranate fruit or seeds may cause allergic reactions. These allergic reactions occur more commonly in people who are allergic to other plants (7674). After oral ingestion of the fruit, pomegranate may rarely cause angioedema. Angioedema seems to occur without warning and in people who have eaten pomegranate for many years. Patients should be told to stop eating pomegranate if swelling of the tongue or face develops (7673).
Pomegranate can cause gastrointestinal disturbances, kidney damage, and necrotic conditions of the liver, due to the high concentration of tannins. Regular consumption of herbs with high tannin concentrations correlates with increased incidence of esophageal or nasal cancer (12).
Pomegranate root and stem contain pelletierine. Orally, overdoses can cause strychnine-like effects in the form of heightened reflex arousal that can escalate to paralysis. At amounts greater than 80 grams, people experience vomiting including bloody emesis, followed by dizziness, chills, vision disorders, collapse, and possibly death due to respiratory failure. Total blindness can occur within a few hours to a few days after ingestion, and resolves after several weeks (18).
Topically, pomegranate may cause contact hypersensitivity characterized by urticaria, angioedema, rhinorrhea, red itchy eyes, and dyspnea arising within a few minutes of exposure (8445).

Interactions with Herbs & Other Dietary Supplements

HERBS AND SUPPLEMENTS WITH HYPOTENSIVE EFFECTS: Pomegranate juice might have antihypertensive effects (8310). Theoretically, concurrent use of pomegranate juice with other herbs and supplements that decrease blood pressure might increase risk of hypotension. Some of these products include danshen, ginger, Panax ginseng, turmeric, valerian, and others.
TANNIN-CONTAINING HERBS: Theoretically, herbs that contain high percentages of tannins (such as pomegranate) may cause precipitation of constituents of other herbs (19).

Interactions with Drugs

ACE INHIBITORS (ACEIs): Pomegranate juice might have additive ACE inhibitor effects (8310). Monitor blood pressure and potassium levels. ACE inhibitors include captopril (Capoten), enalapril (Vasotec), lisinopril (Prinivil, Zestril), ramipril (Altace), and others.
ANTIHYPERTENSIVE DRUGS: Theoretically, concomitant use with pomegranate juice might cause additive hypotensive effects; use with caution (8310).
ORAL DRUGS: Theoretically, concomitant oral administration may cause precipitation of some drugs due to the high tannin content of pomegranate (19). Separate administration of oral drugs and tannin-containing herbs by the longest period of time practical (19).

Interactions with Foods

None known.

Interactions with Lab Tests

None known.

Interactions with Diseases or Conditions

HYPERTENSION: Pomegranate juice might have hypotensive effects (8310). Theoretically, concomitant use in patients treated with antihypertensives might have additive effects on blood pressure and potentially increase the risk of hypotension.
HYPOTENSION: Pomegranate juice might have hypotensive effects (8310). Theoretically, use in people with existing low blood pressure might exacerbate hypotension and possibly lead to syncope.
PLANT ALLERGIES: People with plant allergies seem to be at greater risk for allergic reactions to pomegranate (7674).

Dosage and Administration

No typical dosage.

Comments

The root and stem bark are unsafe for self-medication (12). When used to treat parasites, the fruit rind should not be taken with fats or oils (12).

POPLAR

Also Known As

Balm of Gilead, Balsam Poplar Buds, Jia Yang, Pappelknospen, Populi Gemma.
CAUTION: See separate listings for Dwarf Pine Needle, Fir Needle Oil, Fir, Pine, and Scotch Pine Needle.

Scientific Names

Populus canadensis, synonyms Populus euramericana, Populus marilandica, Populus serotina; Populus balsamifera subsp. balsamifera, synonyms Populus tacamahacca, Populus candicans.
Family: Salicaceae.

People Use This For

Orally, poplar is used as an ingredient in herbal cough preparations. It is also used orally as a stimulant and expectorant.
Topically, poplar is used for sores, bruises, cuts, pimples, external hemorrhoids, frostbite, and sunburn.

Safety

LIKELY SAFE ...when applied topically and used appropriately (2,12).
There is insufficient reliable information available about the safety of poplar for its other uses.
PREGNANCY AND LACTATION: Insufficient reliable information available; avoid using.

Effectiveness

There is insufficient reliable information available about the effectiveness of poplar.

Mechanism of Action

The applicable parts of the poplar are the dried unopened leaf buds. Poplar contains salicin (11).

Adverse Reactions

Topically, occasional allergic skin reactions can occur with the use of poplar (2).
There are no reports of aspirin-type allergic reactions with the use of salicin-rich plants (12).

Interactions with Herbs & Other Dietary Supplements

None known.

Interactions with Drugs

None known.

Interactions with Foods

None known.

Interactions with Lab Tests

None known.

Interactions with Diseases or Conditions

ALLERGIES: Contraindicated in people allergic to poplar buds, propolis, Peru balsam, or salicylates (2,18).

Dosage and Administration

ORAL: No typical dosage.
TOPICAL: The common application of poplar is 5 grams of the dried buds per day or semi-solid preparations equivalent to 20-30% dried buds per day (2,18).

Comments

Available information supports only the external use of poplar. Avoid confusion with spruce (Picea abies) and Canada balsam (Abies balsamea), also known as balm of Gilead.

PORIA MUSHROOM

Also Known As

Fu Ling, FuShen, Hoelen, Indian Bread, Matsuhodo, Polyporus, Poria, Sclerotium Poriae Cocos, Tuckahoe.

Scientific Names

Wolfiporia cocos, synonym Poria cocos.
Family: Polyporaceae.

People Use This For

Traditionally, poria mushroom filaments have been used for amnesia, anxiety, restlessness, fatigue, tension, nervousness, dizziness, dysuria and urination problems, edema, insomnia, splenitis, stomach problems, diarrhea, tumors, and as an antitussive. In herbal combinations, poria filaments have been used as a component of various herbal combinations for treating diarrhea, chronic glomerulonephritis, tinnitus, and for decreasing upper gastrointestinal tract bleeding.

Safety

POSSIBLY SAFE ...when used orally (12).
PREGNANCY AND LACTATION: Insufficient reliable information available; avoid using.

Effectiveness

There is insufficient reliable information available about the effectiveness of poria mushroom.

Mechanism of Action

The applicable part of poria mushroom is the sclerotium (filament). Poria contains pachyman which prevents urinary protein excretion, serum cholesterol elevation, and reduces the degree of histopathological changes in nephritic rats (3727). Some evidence suggests a hydroalcoholic extract (3728) and isolated triterpene constituents (3729,3736,3737) might have anti-inflammatory activity. Other evidence suggests poria extracts might also have immunosuppressive effects (3726). In addition, isolated triterpene constituents show evidence that they might have antitumor (3729) and anti-emetic effects (3730).

Adverse Reactions

None reported.

Interactions with Herbs & Other Dietary Supplements

None known.

Interactions with Drugs

None known.

Interactions with Foods

None known.

Interactions with Lab Tests

None known.

Interactions with Diseases or Conditions

None known.

Dosage and Administration

No typical dosage.

Comments

Various combination herbal mixtures containing poria are reported to be effective for treating diarrhea (3731,3732), chronic glomerulonephritis (3733), tinnitus (3734), and decreasing upper gastrointestinal tract bleeding (3735). Further studies are needed to verify these results.

POTASSIUM

Also Known As

Potassium Acetate, Potassium Bicarbonate, Potassium Chloride, Potassium Citrate, Potassium Gluconate, Potassium Phosphate.

Scientific Names

Potassium; K; atomic number 19.

People Use This For

Orally, potassium is used for treating and preventing hypokalemia, hypertension, Menière's disease, thallium poisoning, hypercalciuria, insulin resistance, myocardial infarction, stroke prevention, symptoms of menopause, and infant colic. It is also used orally for allergies, headaches, acne, alcoholism, Alzheimer's disease, arthritis, blurred vision, cancer, chronic fatigue syndrome, colitis, confusion, constipation, dermatitis, edema, fever, gout, insomnia, irritability, mononucleosis, muscle weakness, muscular dystrophy, stress, and as an adjunct for treating myasthenia gravis.

Intravenously, potassium is used for treating and preventing hypokalemia, cardiac arrhythmias including atrial tachycardia and ventricular arrhythmias, and myocardial infarction.

Safety

LIKELY SAFE ...when used orally in amounts up to 80-90 mEq total potassium (supplements and diet) per day (15,16). Larger amounts increase the risk of hyperkalemia (15). ...when used intravenously (IV). Parental potassium is an FDA-approved prescription product (15).

UNSAFE ...when used in excessive amounts. Doses that increase potassium blood levels above 7 mEq/L are potentially life-threatening (15).

PREGNANCY AND LACTATION: LIKELY SAFE ...when used orally in dietary amounts of 40-80 mEq per day (15).

Effectiveness

EFFECTIVE

Hypokalemia. Administering potassium orally or intravenously is effective for treating and preventing hypokalemia (15).

POSSIBLY EFFECTIVE

Hypercalciuria. Taking potassium orally seems to decrease calcium in the urine (2208,2209).

Hypertension. Taking potassium orally seems to reduce systolic blood pressure by about 2-4 mm Hg and diastolic blood pressure by about 0.5-3.5 mm Hg (3385). Potassium seems to be most effective for people with low potassium levels, high daily sodium intake, and for African Americans (3384,3385,3386). Consuming potassium from dietary sources also seems to decrease the risk of developing hypertension. Foods that provide at least 350 mg of potassium per serving and that are low in sodium, saturated fat, and cholesterol might help reduce the risk of developing high blood pressure (1310,8817). However, there is no proof that taking potassium supplements can help prevent hypertension.

Stroke. Consuming potassium from dietary sources seems to decrease the risk of stroke. There is some evidence that foods providing at least 350 mg of potassium per serving and that are low in sodium, saturated fat, and cholesterol might help reduce the risk stroke (1310,8817). However, there is no proof that taking potassium supplements can decrease the risk of stroke.

There is insufficient reliable information available about the effectiveness of potassium for its other uses.

Mechanism of Action

The potassium mineral plays a role in many body functions including acid-base balance, electrodynamic characteristics of the cell, isotonicity, and various enzymatic reactions (15). It is essential in physiological processes including nerve impulse transmission; cardiac, smooth, and skeletal muscle contraction; gastric secretion; renal function; tissue synthesis; and carbohydrate synthesis (15). Inadequate dietary intake of potassium might play a role in the development of hypertension, stroke, and cardiovascular disease. It is likely that potassium works together with other nutrients to produce beneficial physiological effects (1310,8817).

Adverse Reactions

Orally or intravenously (IV), potassium can cause stomach upset, nausea, diarrhea, vomiting, belching, flatulence, and ulcerations (15,16,3385). Hyperkalemia, typically serum potassium above 5 mEq/L, can cause paresthesia, generalized weakness, flaccid paralysis, listlessness, vertigo, mental confusion, hypotension, blood in the stool, cardiac arrhythmias, heart block, and death (15,16,3385).

Interactions with Herbs & Other Dietary Supplements

VITAMIN B12 (cyanocobalamin, hydroxocobalamin): Transient hypokalemia can occur when severe megaloblastic anemia is treated with parenteral vitamin B12. The increase in red blood cell production creates new intracellular sites that can drain extracellular sites of potassium. The resulting hypokalemia is usually temporary and corrected by normal homeostatic mechanisms (9519). Monitor serum potassium levels in people with other risk factors for hypokalemia.

Interactions with Drugs

ACE INHIBITORS (ACEIs): Concomitant use of these drugs with potassium supplements increases the risk of hyperkalemia (15). The ACE inhibitors include benazepril (Lotensin), captopril (Capoten), enalapril (Vasotec), fosinopril (Monopril), lisinopril (Prinivil, Zestril), moexipril (Univasc), perindopril (Aceon), quinapril (Accupril), ramipril (Altace), and trandolapril (Mavik).

ANGIOTENSIN RECEPTOR BLOCKERS (ARBs): Concomitant use of these drugs with potassium supplements increases the risk of hyperkalemia (15). The ARBs include losartan (Cozaar), valsartan (Diovan), irbesartan (Avapro), candesartan (Atacand), telmisartan (Micardis), and eprosartan (Teveten).

POTASSIUM-SPARING DIURETICS: Concomitant use of these drugs with potassium supplements increases the risk of hyperkalemia (15). Potassium-sparing diuretics include amiloride (Midamor), spironolactone (Aldactone), and triamterene (Dyrenium).

Drug Influences on Nutrient Levels and Depletion

SOME DRUGS CAN AFFECT POTASSIUM LEVELS:

AMINOGLYCOSIDES: Nephrotoxicity caused by aminoglycosides may lead to increased urinary losses of various electrolytes, including potassium (9519). Monitor patients closely for declining renal function and electrolyte disturbances. Aminoglycosides may need to be discontinued, and intravenous electrolyte replacement given (15). Aminoglycosides include amikacin (Amikin), gentamicin (Garamycin), kanamycin (Kantrex), streptomycin, and tobramycin (Nebcin).

AMPHOTERICIN-B (Abelcet, Amphotec, AmBisome, Amphocin, Fungizone): Amphotericin-B increases urinary potassium losses due to toxic effects on renal tubular epithelium. Hypokalemia can occur in up to 50% of patients (9519). Monitor serum potassium and give supplements when necessary. If hypokalemia is associated with worsening renal function, amphotericin-B may need to be discontinued.

BETA-2 AGONISTS: Binding of agonists to beta-2 receptors stimulates adenylate cyclase, increasing intracellular cyclic-AMP and activating membrane Na/K-ATPase pumps. This increases cellular potassium uptake, potentially leading to hypokalemia (8880,8886). Reduced serum potassium levels can occur with oral, parenteral, or inhaled beta-2 agonists, especially during acute use of high doses (6217,7001,8880,8881,8882,8883,8884,8885,8886,8889,8890,9534,9599). Occasionally, ventricular ectopy, prolonged QTc intervals, and arrhythmias have been associated with beta-2 agonists induced hypokalemia (7001,8880,8883,8891,9534). This usually occurs in people with low baseline serum potassium levels, heart disease, digoxin therapy, or concomitant use of other potassium-lowering drugs (8882,8883,8890,9534,9599). Tachyphylaxis to the hypokalemic effect occurs, i.e., serum potassium levels return to baseline despite continued use of the beta-2 agonist (8880,8882,8883,8886,8890,8891). Monitor serum potassium levels in people receiving acute high dose beta-2 agonists (acute asthma attacks or preterm labor), and in those with other risk factors for hypokalemia; potassium supplements may be necessary if symptomatic hypokalemia develops (8880). Beta-2 agonists include albuterol (salbutamol, Proventil, Ventolin), bitolterol (Tornalate), isoetharine, levalbuterol (Xopenex), metaproterenol (Alupent), pirbuterol (Maxair), salmeterol (Serevent), and terbutaline (Brethine).

DIURETICS, LOOP and THIAZIDE: Loop and thiazide diuretics increase urinary potassium excretion. Monitor serum potassium levels and give potassium supplements when necessary (4412,4425,4449). Loop diuretics include furosemide (Lasix), bumetanide (Bumex), ethacrynic acid (Edecrin), and torsemide (Demadex). Thiazide diuretics include chlorothiazide (Diuril), hydrochlorothiazide (Hydrodyuril, Esidrix), indapamide (Lozol), metolazone (Zaroxolyn), chlorthalidone (Hygroton), and others.

FLUCONAZOLE (Diflucan): Fluconazole can increase urinary potassium losses, possibly due to toxic effects on the renal tubular epithelium (9519). Monitor serum potassium in people with additional risk factors for hypokalemia, and those taking fluconazole for prolonged periods.

GLUCOCORTICOIDS, MINERALOCORTICOIDS: Mineralocorticoids and some glucocorticoids (corticosteroids) cause sodium retention, resulting in compensatory renal potassium excretion and hypokalemia. This effect is dose-related and depends on mineralocorticoid potency. It is most common with hydrocortisone (Cortef, Hydrocortone, Solu-Cortef), cortisone (Cortone), and fludrocortisone (Florinef), followed by prednisone (Deltasone) and prednisolone (Delta-Cortef). Glucocorticoids without significant salt-retaining activity include betamethasone (Celestone), dexamethasone (Decadron), methylprednisolone (Medrol, Depo-Medrol, Solu-Medrol), and triamcinolone (Aristocort, Kenalog) (4425,4453). Monitor serum potassium regularly. If levels become low, change to a

glucocorticoid with less mineralocorticoid activity, or give potassium supplements.
LAXATIVES, STIMULANT: Long-term use of stimulant laxatives, or acute use of high doses (e.g., in bowel-cleansing regimens), can result in potassium loss and hypokalemia. Advise people to limit stimulant laxative to short-term use of recommended doses (4411,4412,4425,4453). Some stimulant laxatives include cascara (CitraMax Plus), senna (Senokot), bisacodyl (Dulcolax), and others.
LEVODOPA (L-DOPA, Larodopa, Dopar): Increased urinary potassium losses occur in some people treated with levodopa. The mechanism isn't clear, but the effect doesn't occur when a peripheral decarboxylase inhibitor, such as carbidopa, is used with levodopa (as in Sinemet) (7201). This interaction is therefore unlikely to be clinically significant.
METHYLXANTHINES: Theophylline and related drugs can reduce serum potassium levels, possibly by increasing intracellular uptake of potassium. Hypokalemia is most likely to occur after acute overdose of these drugs (17). However, reduced potassium levels can occur with therapeutic doses, and the incidence and degree of hypokalemia increases with increasing serum theophylline levels (9534,9537,9538,9539). Monitor potassium levels in people with other risk factors for hypokalemia.
PENICILLINS: Penicillins which are formulated as sodium salts present a large sodium load to the kidneys. Increased amounts of sodium are reabsorbed, and the penicillin moiety acts as a non-reabsorbable anion, promoting urinary potassium excretion (9519). Penicillins associated with hypokalemia include penicillin G sodium (Pfizerpen), mezlocillin (Mezlin), carbenicillin (Geocillin), ticarcillin (Ticar), and piperacillin (Pipracil). Monitor serum potassium levels and give potassium supplements, or switch to an alternative antibiotic, as necessary.
SODIUM PHOSPHATES (monobasic sodium phosphate and dibasic sodium phosphate, Fleet Phospho-soda): Use of high doses (> 45 mL in 24 hours), such as those used for bowel cleansing before surgery, can lead to serious electrolyte disturbances, including hypokalemia. Avoid large doses, especially in the elderly and people with other risk factors for electrolyte disturbances (8877,9531). Advise people to avoid using high doses of these products for self-treatment of constipation.
TETRACYCLINES: Use of outdated tetracyclines can lead to nephropathy and electrolyte disturbances, including hypokalemia. This is due to toxic effects of a degradation product (4425). Advise people to complete courses of tetracyclines as prescribed, and not to save them for later use.

Interactions with Foods

POTASSIUM-CONTAINING FOODS: Theoretically, concomitant use can increase potassium levels and the risk of adverse effects, especially in individuals with renal dysfunction, ACE inhibitor or potassium-sparing diuretic therapy. Potassium-containing foods include fruits (especially dried), cereals, beans, milk, and vegetables (16).
POTASSIUM-CONTAINING SALT SUBSTITUTES: Theoretically, concomitant use can increase potassium levels and the risk of adverse effects, especially in individuals with renal dysfunction, ACE inhibitor, or potassium-sparing diuretic therapy.

Interactions with Lab Tests

BLOOD PRESSURE: Potassium taken orally can reduce blood pressure and blood pressure readings (3385).

Interactions with Diseases or Conditions

ASPIRIN OR TARTRAZINE SENSITIVITY: Avoid oral potassium products that contain tartrazine (15).
GI MOTILITY CONDITIONS: Oral potassium tablets and capsules are contraindicated in individuals with gastrointestinal motility conditions (15).

Dosage and Administration

ORAL: Potassium supplementation must be individualized and based on the person's serum potassium level, which should be maintained between 3.5-5 mEq/L. The normal adult daily requirement and usual dietary intake is 40-80 mEq daily (15). For preventing hypokalemia, 20 mEq is typically taken daily (15). The common dose of potassium for treating hypokalemia is 40-100 mEq or more daily, in two to four divided amounts (15). For hypercalciuria, 1 mEq/kg is taken daily (2208,2209) or four tablets of Urophos-K are taken twice a day (2209). The typical dose for hypertension is 48-90 mEq daily (3385). For preventing stroke, dietary intake of approximately 75 mEq (about 3.5 g of elemental potassium) daily may reduce risk. Foods that contain at least 350 mg potassium can be labeled "Diets containing foods that are good sources of potassium and low in sodium may reduce the risk of high blood pressure and stroke (1310,8817).

POTATO

Also Known As
Irish Potato, White Potato.
CAUTION: See separate listing for African Wild Potato.

Scientific Names
Solanum tuberosum.
Family: Solanaceae.

People Use This For
Orally, raw potato juice is used for gastritis, stomach disorders, and edema. A purified protein extract from potato is used as an appetite suppressant for weight loss.
Topically, raw potato is used as a poultice for arthritis, infections, boils, burns, and sore eyes.
Potato is eaten as a food, used as a source of starch, and fermented into alcohol.

Safety
LIKELY SAFE ...when unblemished, ripe potatoes are used as food (6).
POSSIBLY SAFE ...when the purified protein extract from potato is used orally and appropriately (473). ...when unblemished, ripe potatoes are used orally for medicinal purposes (6).
LIKELY UNSAFE ...when damaged, green potatoes and sprouts are consumed. These contain toxic solanum alkaloids that cannot be destroyed by cooking and can cause serious adverse effects (6).
There is insufficient reliable information available about the safety of potato for its other uses.
PREGNANCY AND LACTATION: LIKELY SAFE ...when unblemished, ripe potatoes are used orally in food amounts. There is insufficient reliable information available about the safety of oral or topical use of potato in pregnancy and lactation for medicinal purposes.

Effectiveness
There is insufficient reliable information available about the effectiveness of potato.

Mechanism of Action
The applicable part of the potato is the tuber. Potatoes are a source of vitamin C, iron, riboflavin, and are rich in carbohydrates (6). A proteinase inhibitor isolated from potatoes is claimed to increase the effects of cholecystokinin (CCK), by blocking the effects of the enzymes chymotrypsin and trypsin, which break down CCK (473). CCK produces satiety and has been shown to play a role in the short-term inhibition of food intake (476,477,6255). It has been reported by the manufacturer of a purified protein extract from potato (Satietrol), which contains this proteinase inhibitor and other nutrients and minerals claimed to affect CCK, that the product reduced feelings of hunger by 30-32% 3.5 hours after a fixed calorie meal. These effects were also found in a group of people who lost weight on a calorie-controlled diet (473). Damaged, green potatoes, and sprouts contain toxic solanum alkaloids that cannot be destroyed by cooking. Researchers report that a potato peel extract inhibited bacterial adhesion to host cells without killing the bacteria. They believe this activity might be due to polyphenol oxidase, a compound known to have anti-adhesive properties (6107).

Adverse Reactions
Adverse reactions have not been reported with unblemished, ripe potatoes. Solanum glycosides found in damaged, green potatoes and sprouts can cause headache, flushing, nausea, vomiting, diarrhea, abdominal pain, thirst, and restlessness. Deaths have been reported in malnourished individuals who may not have received adequate medical care (17). Twenty mg solanine per 100 grams potato is the maximum concentration considered safe. Solanum glycosides cannot be destroyed by cooking (6). Exposure to potato dust is associated with a high-incidence of respiratory symptoms due to bacterial and fungal contaminants (6).

Interactions with Herbs & Other Dietary Supplements
None known.

Interactions with Drugs
THROMBOLYTIC DRUGS: Theoretically, concomitant use of potato may enhance thrombolytic effects. A carboxypeptidase inhibitor isolated from potato tubers may have inhibitory effects on thrombin-activatable thrombolysis inhibitor, and thereby enhance the activity of thrombolytic agents (474,475).

Interactions with Foods
None known.

Interactions with Lab Tests
None known.

Interactions with Diseases or Conditions
DIABETES: Potatoes can affect blood sugar control. They should be consumed as appropriate carbohydrate equivalents (6).

Dosage and Administration
ORAL: For appetite suppression and weight loss, a purified protein extract from potato (Satietrol) containing a proteinase inhibitor, is marketed as a powder to be mixed with 8 ounces of water and taken 15 minutes before meals (473). There is no typical dosage of potato juice.
TOPICAL: Raw potato is used as a poultice (6).

Comments
The potato is one of the main food crops of the world (6).

POTENTILLA

Also Known As
Crampweed, Goose Grass, Goose Tansy, Goosewort, Moor Grass, Prince's Feather, Silverweed, Trailing Tansy, Wild Agrimony.
CAUTION: See separate listings for Agrimony, Amaranth, Clivers, Tormentil, and Jewelweed.

Scientific Names
Potentilla anserina.
Family: Rosacea.

People Use This For
Orally, potentilla flower and leaf are used for premenstrual syndrome (PMS), mild dysmenorrhea, and diarrhea. Topically, potentilla flower and leaf are used for the local treatment of oropharyngeal inflammation.

Safety
POSSIBLY SAFE ...when used orally and appropriately (2).
PREGNANCY AND LACTATION: Insufficient reliable information available; avoid using.

Effectiveness
There is insufficient reliable information available about the effectiveness of potentilla.

Mechanism of Action
The applicable parts of potentilla are the flower and leaf. The tannin constituents of potentilla have astringent effects (2) and are likely responsible for antidiarrheal and local anti-inflammatory activity. Potentilla also increases tonus and the contraction frequency of isolated animal uterus (2,7).

Adverse Reactions
Orally, potentilla can cause stomach irritation (7,12).

Interactions with Herbs & Other Dietary Supplements
None known.

Interactions with Drugs
None known.

Interactions with Foods
None known.

Interactions with Lab Tests
None known.

Interactions with Diseases or Conditions
None known.

Dosage and Administration

ORAL: For premenstrual syndrome (PMS), dysmenorrhea, and acute diarrhea, the typical dose is 4-6 grams per day (2,18). Potentilla is often prepared as a tea and given in a dose of one cup 2-3 times daily. The tea is prepared by steeping 2 grams of the finely cut flower or leaf in 150 mL boiling water for 10 minutes and then straining (18).
TOPICAL: No typical dosage.

Comments

Avoid confusion with agrimony (Agrimonia eupatoria) and tormentil (Potentilla erecta), also referred to as potentilla. Avoid confusion with jewelweed, also known as silverweed.

PRECATORY BEAN

Also Known As

Bead Vine, Black-Eyed Susan, Buddhist Rosary Bead, Crab's Eye, Indian Bead, Jequirity Bean, Jequirity Seed, Legume, Love Bean, Lucky Bean, Ojo De Pajaro, Prayer Beads, Prayer Head, Rosary Pea, Seminole Bead, Weather Plant.

Scientific Names

Abrus precatorius, synonym Glycine abrus.
Family: Fabaceae/Leguminosae.

People Use This For

Orally, precatory bean is used orally to quicken labor, as an abortifacient, oral contraceptive, and as an analgesic in terminally-ill patients. The whole plant is used for ophthalmic inflammations.

Safety

LIKELY UNSAFE ...when used orally. Ingesting 5 mg of abrin, a constituent of precatory bean, is toxic to humans (6). Significant precatory bean ingestion causes severe gastroenteritis, followed by diarrhea and vomiting that can become bloody. Symptoms may not appear for several days (3499). Fatalities can occur after 3-4 days of persistent gastroenteritis (17,3499).
CHILDREN: UNSAFE ...when used orally. Ingestion of one seed in young children can be fatal (3499,5607). Older children aged 9-13 years have been reported to experience severe abdominal pain, vomiting, bloody stools (5607,11473), and pulmonary edema after ingesting just one or more seeds (11473).
PREGNANCY AND LACTATION: LIKELY UNSAFE ...when used orally (6); avoid using.

Effectiveness

There is insufficient reliable information available about the effectiveness of precatory bean.

Mechanism of Action

The precatory bean plant contains the indole alkaloids abrine, abrus agglutinin, hyaphorine, and precatorine (6). Abrin, isolated from the seeds, is a potent inhibitor of protein synthesis and moderate inhibitor of DNA synthesis. In vitro, ethanol extracts of the seeds causes irreversible impairment in human sperm motility (3842), and aqueous extracts of the seeds agglutinate human red blood corpuscles (6369). Some isoflavanquinone constituents isolated from the root inhibit platelet aggregation; others possess potent anti-inflammatory and antiallergic effects (3841).

Adverse Reactions

Orally, seeds that are chewed or have cracked shells can cause stomach cramping, nausea, vomiting, severe diarrhea (possibly bloody), cold sweat, fever, drowsiness, weakness, and tachycardia. Pulmonary edema, kidney failure, liver toxicity, coma, circulatory collapse, cerebral edema, and death (3499,5608,11473). Signs of toxicity, including gastroenteritis, may sometimes occur several hours after ingestion of the seeds, followed by the development of bloody diarrhea. More often, however, there can be a latent period of approximately 3-4 days after ingestion of the seeds, prior to the development of toxic symptoms. Symptoms, including death, may occur up to 10-14 days after ingestion of the seeds (11473).
Topically, the seeds can cause dermatitis when used as a necklace (6). Eye contact with the seed's contents can cause necrotizing conjunctivitis (3499).
TOXICITY MANAGEMENT: There is no known antidote. There is no method for enhancing elimination. Patients seen within 4 hours of seed ingestion should be treated with usual decontamination methods including lavage, charcoal, and cathartics. In cases of diarrhea, the need for cathartics may be unnecessary (17).

Interactions with Herbs & Other Dietary Supplements

None known.

Interactions with Drugs
None known.

Interactions with Foods
None known.

Interactions with Lab Tests
None known.

Interactions with Diseases or Conditions
None known.

Dosage and Administration
No typical dosage.

Comments
Children are attracted to the bright colors of the seed (17). The hard coat of a mature seed may resist digestion when swallowed but treatment for suspected poisoning should begin as soon as possible (3499). Abrin, a constituent of precatory bean, is being investigated for the treatment of experimental cancers and is used as a "molecular probe" to investigate cell function (6).

PREGNENOLONE

Also Known As
None.
CAUTION: See separate listings for Progesterone and Wild Yam.

Scientific Names
Pregnenolone; (3 beta)-3-hydroxypregn-5-en-20-one; delta 5-pregnen-3 beta-ol-20-one;
17 beta-(1-ketoethyl)- delta 5-androsten-3 beta-ol.

People Use This For
Orally, pregnenolone is used for slowing or reversing aging, for arthritis, depression, endometriosis, fatigue, fibrocystic breast disease, memory enhancement, menopause, premenstrual syndrome (PMS), stress, increasing energy, and improving immunity. It is also used for strengthening the heart, Alzheimer's disease, allergic reactions, detoxification, lupus, multiple sclerosis (MS), prostate disorders, psoriasis, scleroderma, seizures, trauma, and injuries.

Safety
There is insufficient reliable information available about the safety of pregnenolone.
Pregnancy and Lactation: Insufficient reliable information available; avoid using.

Effectiveness
There is insufficient reliable information available about the effectiveness of pregnenolone.

Mechanism of Action
Pregnenolone is synthesized in the body from cholesterol and is the precursor for all the steroid hormones, including progesterone, aldosterone, cortisol, dehydroepiandrosterone (DHEA), testosterone, and estrogens (3008). Lower cerebrospinal fluid (CSF) pregnenolone levels have been reported in people with affective disorders, particularly episodes of active depression (3005). Pregnenolone has antagonist activity at GABA-A receptors in the brain and induces changes in the sleep EEG by increasing the time spent in slow wave sleep (3007). Higher pregnenolone serum concentrations during the luteal phase are associated with more severe PMS symptoms (3006). Reliable information on the effects of exogenously administered pregnenolone is not available (3005).

Adverse Reactions
Orally, supplemental pregnenolone may cause steroid-related adverse effects (3008).

Interactions with Herbs & Other Dietary Supplements
DEHYDROEPIANDROSTERONE (DHEA): Theoretically, pregnenolone can enhance the effects of steroid hormone drugs including DHEA (3008).

Interactions with Drugs

ESTROGENS: Theoretically, pregnenolone can enhance the effects of steroid hormone drugs including estrogens (3008).
PROGESTIN: Theoretically, pregnenolone can enhance the effects of steroid hormone drugs including progestin (3008).
TESTOSTERONE: Theoretically, pregnenolone can enhance the effects of steroid hormone drugs including testosterone (3008).

Interactions with Foods

None known.

Interactions with Lab Tests

None known.

Interactions with Diseases or Conditions

HORMONE SENSITIVE CANCERS/CONDITIONS: Because pregnenolone is converted to estrogens (3008), women with hormone sensitive conditions should avoid pregnenolone. Some of these conditions include breast cancer, uterine cancer, ovarian cancer, endometriosis, and uterine fibroids.

Dosage and Administration

No typical dosage.

Comments

Pregnenolone was studied for stress, fatigue, and arthritis in the 1940s before synthetic hormones became available.

PREMORSE

Also Known As

Devil's Bit, Ofbit, Premorse Scaboius.

Scientific Names

Scabiosa succisa.
Family: Dipsacaceae.

Comments

At the date of publication, this product was not a common ingredient used in brand name supplements marketed to consumers. Details about this product are available at the online version of *Natural Medicines Comprehensive Database*. See www.naturaldatabase.com.

PRICKLY PEAR CACTUS

Also Known As

Barbary-fig Cactus, Cactus Flowers, Cactus Fruit, Cactus Pear Fruit, Gracemere-Pear, Indian-fig Prickly Pear Cactus, OPI, Opuntia, Opuntia ficus, Nopal, Nopol, Tuna Cardona, Westwood-Pear.

Scientific Names

Opuntia ficus-indica; Opuntia hyptiacantha; Opuntia lasciacantha; Opuntia macrocentra, synonym Opuntia violacea; Opuntia megacantha; Opuntia puberula; Opuntia streptacantha, synonym Opuntia cardona; Opuntia velutina.
Family: Cactaceae.

People Use This For

Orally, prickly pear cactus is used for diabetes, hypercholesterolemia, obesity, alcohol-induced hangover (veisalgia), and as an antiviral agent. It is also used for colitis, diarrhea, and benign prostatic hypertrophy (BPH).
In foods, the prickly pear juice is used in jellies and candies.

Safety

LIKELY SAFE ...when used orally as a food (5969).
POSSIBLY SAFE ...when the leaves, stems, or standardized extracts from the prickly pear cactus are used orally short-term (5959,5960,5963,12085,12086). Single doses of prickly pear cactus extract or fruit seem to be safe (5959,5960,5963,12085). There is also evidence that taking 250 grams of fresh prickly pear cactus fruit pulp twice daily for

2 weeks might be safe (12086). ...when flowers of prickly pear cactus are used orally. Preliminary evidence suggests that powdered prickly pear cactus flowers 1500 mg/day can be safely used for up to 8 months (12175).
PREGNANCY AND LACTATION: Insufficient reliable information available; avoid using.

Effectiveness

POSSIBLY EFFECTIVE

Diabetes. There is some preliminary clinical evidence that prickly pear cactus used orally can decrease blood glucose levels in patients with type 2 diabetes. Single doses can decrease blood glucose levels by 17% to 46% in some patients (5959,5961,5962,5964). However, it is not known if extended daily use can consistently lower blood glucose levels and decrease HbA1c levels. Only the broiled stems of the specific species Opuntia streptacantha seem to be beneficial. Raw or crude stems do not seem to decrease glucose levels (5961). Other prickly pear cactus species do not seem to significantly lower blood glucose levels either (5970,7028).

Hangover. There is some evidence that taking a specific prickly pear cactus fruit extract (Tex-OE, Extracts Plus, Inc.) might reduce symptoms of alcohol-induced hangover. Taking 1600 IU of the extract 5 hours prior to binge alcohol consumption seems to reduce the chance of having a severe hangover the following day by about 50%. It also seems to significantly reduce some specific symptoms of hangover such as nausea, anorexia, and dry mouth. But it does not seem to reduce other symptoms such as headache, dizziness, diarrhea, or soreness (12085).

INSUFFICIENT RELIABLE EVIDENCE to RATE

Benign prostatic hypertrophy (BPH). Preliminary evidence suggests that some patients who take powdered prickly pear cactus flowers 500 mg 3 times daily for 2-8 months have subjective improvements in symptoms such as urgency and feelings of fullness in the bladder (12175). More evidence is needed to rate prickly pear cactus for this use.

Mechanism of Action

The applicable parts of prickly pear cactus are the leaves, flowers, stems, and fruit. Prickly pear cactus is often consumed as part of the diet. Ingesting 500 grams of prickly pear cactus provides 14.3 grams carbohydrate, 8.25 grams protein, 1.05 grams lipids, 18.85 grams cellulose (fibrous polysaccharide), 455.75 grams water, and 99.75 kilocalories (7028).

Some species of prickly pear cactus can lower blood glucose and lipid levels (5958,5959,5960,5963). This effect is often attributed to the high fibrous polysaccharide content, including pectin (5958). Fiber can slow carbohydrate absorption and decrease lipid absorption from the gut. However, some researchers suspect prickly pear might also have an insulin sensitizing effect (7028).

Broiled stems seem to be more effective for reducing blood glucose levels than raw stems (5961,5964). The reason for this difference is not known. The hypoglycemic effects of prickly pear cactus peak 3-4 hours after ingestion and can last for up to 6 hours.

There is also some evidence that the pectin component of prickly pear cactus can also alter the liver metabolism of cholesterol and affect cholesterol levels (5958).

Prickly pear cactus is thought to reduce symptoms of alcohol-induced hangovers by decreasing inflammation. Alcohol-induced hangovers are associated with an inflammatory response. Alcohols containing high amounts of impurities known as congeners (tequila, bourbon, scotch) are associated with increased inflammatory response and increased severity of hangover. People with an alcohol induced hangover have increase levels of the inflammatory markers C-reactive protein (CRP) and cortisol. People who take a specific prickly pear cactus extract seem to have lower CRP and cortisol levels, suggesting that prickly pear cactus might have anti-inflammatory effects (12085).

Prickly pear cactus also has antioxidant effects. Consuming prickly pear cactus fruit pulp for 2 weeks seems to decrease pro-oxidants, decrease oxidation of lipids, and improve antioxidant status. This may be due to the vitamin C and the plant pigments called betanin and indicaxanthin contained in prickly pear cactus (12086).

There is some preliminary evidence that prickly pear cactus has antiviral activity against the herpes simplex virus (HSV), respiratory syncytial virus (RSV), and human immunodeficiency virus (HIV) (5956).

Adverse Reactions

Orally, prickly pear cactus is usually well-tolerated. However, prickly pear cactus can cause some side effects including mild diarrhea, nausea, increased stool volume, increased stool frequency, abdominal fullness, and headache (7028). Although the prickly pear cactus reduces blood glucose levels in people with diabetes, it does not seem to cause hypoglycemia (5959,5960,5963).

Interactions with Herbs & Other Dietary Supplements

None known.

Interactions with Drugs

CHLORPROPAMIDE (Diabinese): Using chlorpropamide and prickly pear cactus together can have additive effects on blood glucose and insulin levels in patients with type 2 diabetes (5968).

There is some concern that people taking both chlorpropamide or other hypoglycemic drugs and prickly pear cactus might be at an increased risk for hypoglycemia.

Advise patients to monitor glucose levels closely. Dose adjustments may be necessary.

Other hypoglycemic drugs include glimepiride (Amaryl), glipizide (Glucotrol), glyburide (Diabeta, Micronase), tolazamide (Tolinase), tolbutamide (Orinase), and others.

Interactions with Foods
None known.

Interactions with Lab Tests
BLOOD GLUCOSE: Prickly pear cactus can reduce blood glucose levels and lab tests (5957).
CHOLESTEROL: There is some evidence that prickly pear cactus might reduce total and low-density lipoprotein (LDL) cholesterol levels (5958).

Interactions with Diseases or Conditions
DIABETES: Prickly pear cactus can reduce blood glucose in patients with type 2 diabetes (5957). Prickly pear cactus might have additive effects with diabetes medications and potentially cause hypoglycemia. Advise patients to closely monitor glucose levels after starting prickly pear cactus. Dose adjustments to diabetes medications may be necessary.

Dosage and Administration
ORAL: For diabetes, broiled stems 100-500 grams daily is typically used (5964). Doses are often divided and given three times daily.
For alcohol-induced hangover, 1600 IU of a specific prickly pear cactus extract (Tex-OE, Extracts Plus, Inc.) taken 5 hours before alcohol ingestion has been used (12085).
For benign prostatic hypertrophy (BPH), powdered flowers of prickly pear cactus, 500 mg three times daily, has been used (12175).

Comments
Prickly pear cactus is primarily used in Mexican and Mexican-American cultures as a part of the diet and as a treatment for type 2 diabetes. Most research on this product has been performed in Mexico. The immature form of prickly pear cactus is used. Mature stems are fibrous and tough and not appropriate for consumption (7028).

PROCAINE

Also Known As
Gero-Vita, Gerovital, Gerovital-H3, GH-3, KH-3, Procaine Hydrochloride.

Scientific Names
2-Diethylaminoethyl p-aminobenzoate monohydrochloride.

People Use This For
Orally or parenterally, procaine is used for arthritis, cerebral atherosclerosis, dementia, depression, hair loss, hypertension, sexual dysfunction, and an overall rejuvenating effect.
Parenterally, prescription-only procaine is used for local anesthesia.

Safety
LIKELY SAFE ...when the prescription-only product is used parenterally as a local anesthetic (15).
There is insufficient reliable information available about the safety of the oral use of procaine.
PREGNANCY: LIKELY UNSAFE ...when used for self-medication; avoid using (6).
LACTATION: There is insufficient reliable information available about the safety of procaine for self-medication; avoid using.

Effectiveness
EFFECTIVE

Pain. Procaine injection is an FDA-approved prescription product used as a local anesthetic (15).

Mechanism of Action
Procaine has poor oral absorption, and there is no evidence that pharmacologic levels are achieved with oral administration (6). Hematoporphyrin is added to some oral preparations to increase procaine absorption (6), although no evidence supports this effect.

Adverse Reactions
Orally, procaine can cause heartburn, migraines, and systemic lupus erythematosus (SLE) (6).

Interactions with Herbs & Other Dietary Supplements

DIGITALIS: Intravenous use of procaine hydrochloride is contraindicated with concurrent use of digitalis (15).

Interactions with Drugs

AMINOSALICYLIC ACID: A metabolite of procaine, aminobenzoic acid, can antagonize the effect of aminosalicylic acid. Theoretically, procaine might also reduce aminosalicylic activity (15).
DIGOXIN (Lanoxin): Intravenous use of procaine hydrochloride is contraindicated (15).
SKELETAL MUSCLE RELAXANTS: Intravenous use of procaine hydrochloride is contraindicated (15).
SUCCINYLCHOLINE: Intravenous use of procaine hydrochloride is contraindicated (15).
SULFONAMIDE ANTIBIOTICS: A metabolite of procaine, aminobenzoic acid, can antagonize the effect of sulfonamides. Theoretically, procaine might also reduce sulfonamide activity (15). Some sulfonamides include sulfamethoxazole (Gantanol), sulfasalazine (Azulfidine), sulfisoxazole (Gantrisin), and trimethoprim/sulfamethoxazole (Bactrim, Septra).

Interactions with Foods

None known.

Interactions with Lab Tests

None known.

Interactions with Diseases or Conditions

MYASTHENIA GRAVIS: The intravenous use of procaine is contraindicated in individuals with myasthenia gravis, which is progressive muscular weakness (15).
PSEUDOCHOLINESTERASE DEFICIENCY: Contraindicated (6).
SYSTEMIC LUPUS ERYTHEMATOSUS (SLE): Contraindicated. Theoretically, procaine might exacerbate this condition (6).

Dosage and Administration

ORAL: People typically take procaine in a cyclical regimen: 200 mg procaine once or twice daily for 25 days, then no drug for 5 days, then repeat the cycle (5274).

PROGESTERONE

Also Known As

Corpus Luteum Hormone, Luteal Hormone, Luteohormone, Lutine, NSC-9704, Pregnancy Hormone, Pregnanedione, Progestational Hormone, Progesteronum.
CAUTION: See separate listings for Pregnenolone and Wild Yam.

Scientific Names

Progesterone; 4-Pregnene-3; 20-Dione.

People Use This For

Orally, progesterone is used for treating secondary amenorrhea, abnormal uterine bleeding associated with hormonal imbalance, treating severe symptoms of premenstrual syndrome (PMS), and treating benzodiazepine dependence and withdrawal. Oral progesterone preparations are also used in combination with estrogens as part of hormone replacement therapy to prevent irregular bleeding and the increased risk of endometrial carcinoma associated with estrogen monotherapy.
Topically, progesterone is used as an alternative to oral treatment as a component of hormone replacement therapy and for treating menopausal vasomotor symptoms. Topical progesterone is also used for treating or preventing hormone-mediated allergies, bloating, breast tenderness, decreased sex drive, depression, fatigue, fibrocystic breasts, headaches, hypoglycemia, increased blood clotting, infertility, irritability, memory loss, miscarriages, osteoporosis, premenopausal bone loss, symptoms of premenstrual syndrome, thyroid dysfunction, unclear thinking, uterine cancer, uterine fibroids, water retention, weight gain, and treating vulval lichen sclerosis.
Intravaginally, progesterone is used for cervical ripening, mastodynia in women with benign breast disease, and to prevent and treat endometrial hyperplasia. Progesterone is also used intravaginally or intramuscularly for treating infertility in women, anovulatory bleeding, and treating symptoms of premenstrual syndrome (PMS).

Safety

LIKELY SAFE ...when used orally and appropriately. Micronized progesterone (Prometrium) is an FDA-approved prescription product. Micronized progesterone (Prometrium) has been safely used in multiple clinical trials lasting up to 3 years (226,228,1216,1220,1221,1224). ...when used intravaginally and appropriately, short-term (1225,2031,2032,2033,2034).

Progesterone intravaginal gel (Crinone) is an FDA-approved prescription product. Progesterone intravaginal gel (Crinone) has been safely used in trials lasting up to 3 months (1225,2031,2033,2034,2041). ...when used intramuscularly and appropriately, short-term (227,1218,1225,2034). Progesterone oil for intramuscular injection is an FDA-approved prescription product (227,1218,1225,2034). ...when used transdermally and appropriately. Transdermal progesterone has been used safely in clinical trials lasting up to a year (224,1229).
There is insufficient reliable information available about the safety of other progesterone preparations.
PREGNANCY: LIKELY SAFE ...when used intravaginally and appropriately as part of infertility treatment. Intravaginal progesterone gel (Crinone 8%) is FDA-approved for use in conjunction with infertility treatment (1225). LIKELY UNSAFE ...when used orally, intramuscularly, intravaginally, or transdermally for purposes other than medically supervised adjunctive treatment for infertility; contraindicated (15).
LACTATION: Insufficient reliable information available; avoid using.

Effectiveness

LIKELY EFFECTIVE

Amenorrhea. Taking progesterone orally and applying progesterone gel intravaginally is effective for treating secondary amenorrhea in premenopausal women. Micronized progesterone is FDA-approved for the treatment of secondary amenorrhea (15). Intravaginal progesterone gel (Crinone 4%) is FDA-approved for the treatment of secondary amenorrhea. Several open-label clinical trials have shown intravaginal progesterone gel (Crinone 4%) to be effective for restoring menses when used in conjunction with estrogen replacement therapy (2041,2091).

Hormone replacement therapy (HRT). Micronized progesterone (Prometrium) is FDA-approved for use with estrogen as a component of HRT. Micronized progesterone (Prometrium) has been shown to provide the same protection against the effects of unopposed estrogen therapy as medroxyprogesterone in women with a uterus (226,228,1216,1217,1226,1230,8144). In one trial, micronized progesterone (Prometrium) did not reduce the beneficial lipid effects of estrogen therapy as much as medroxyprogesterone (226); however, this effect was not seen in another trial (1216).

Infertility. Intravaginal progesterone gel (Crinone 8%) is FDA-approved for use as a component of infertility treatment in women. Clinical trials suggest that both intravaginal and intramuscular progesterone achieves pregnancy rates comparable to oral progesterone in women infertile due to various etiologies (227,1225,2032,2091). Clinical trials comparing intravaginal progesterone to intramuscular progesterone have shown varying relative efficacy results (1218,2086,2089).

POSSIBLY EFFECTIVE

Endometrial hyperplasia. Intravaginal progesterone (Crinone) seems to prevent endometrial hyperplasia in women with an intact uterus taking estrogen replacement therapy (2031). Also, one short-term, open label clinical trial has shown that a specific intravaginal progesterone cream may help reverse endometrial hyperplasia and decrease vaginal bleeding in premenopausal women with benign endometrial hyperplasia (2033).

Mastodynia. Intravaginal progesterone gel (Crinone) seems to reduce breast pain and tenderness in women with benign breast disease (1223).

Menopausal symptoms. One clinical trial has shown that topical progesterone cream (Progest) is superior to placebo for reducing vasomotor symptoms such as hot flashes in menopausal women (224).

POSSIBLY INEFFECTIVE

Benzodiazepine withdrawal. Oral micronized progesterone is comparable to placebo for relieving symptoms of withdrawal and for helping patients remain drug-free from diazepam (1221).

Osteoporosis. Topical progesterone is comparable to placebo for increasing bone mineral density in postmenopausal women (224).

Premenstrual syndrome (PMS). Taking progesterone orally doesn't seem to have any effect on the behavioral or physical symptoms of PMS (1220,10332).

Vulval lichen sclerosis. One clinical trial has shown that topical progesterone is comparable to placebo and inferior to clobetasol (Temovate) for treating the signs and symptoms of vulval lichen sclerosis (225).

INSUFFICIENT RELIABLE EVIDENCE to RATE

Cardiovascular disease. Preliminary evidence suggests that progesterone vaginal gel might be beneficial for cardiovascular disease. It can increase exercise time to myocardial ischemia compared with oral medroxyprogesterone in women with coronary artery disease or previous myocardial infarction (8146). More evidence is needed to rate progesterone for this use.

Mechanism of Action

Progesterone is an endogenous progestin secreted by the corpus luteum. The hormone is not available from any natural source without extraction and synthesis. Products marketed as natural progesterone are those products that are structurally identical to endogenous progesterone. "Natural progesterones," including the prescription products Crinone and Prometrium, are synthesized from the constituent diosgenin, isolated from wild yam or soy. In the laboratory, this constituent is converted to pregnenolone and then to progesterone. The human body is not capable of synthesizing progesterone from diosgenin in vivo (8143).
Progesterone is primarily secreted during the luteal phase of the menstrual cycle, but small amounts are also secreted during the follicular phase (15). The normal physiological effects of progesterone are responsible for its therapeutic benefit when administered exogenously. Progesterone transforms proliferative endometrium into a secreting

endometrium. This effect is beneficial in preventing and treating endometrial hyperplasia. It may also be beneficial in infertility because progesterone is necessary for implantation of the fertilized ovum and for maintaining pregnancy (15). In premenstrual syndrome (PMS), progesterone has been proposed as a therapy because the symptoms of PMS are thought to correlate with physiological fluctuations in endogenous progesterone (1220). It was thought to be beneficial for preventing benzodiazepine withdrawal because metabolites of progesterone have been found to have sedative-hypnotic properties (1221).

Other effects of progesterone include growth of mammary tissue and uterine smooth muscle relaxation. Progesterone also has mild estrogenic and androgenic effects (15). Micronized progesterone seems to have effects similar to medroxyprogesterone on endothelium-dependent vasodilator responsiveness and markers of inflammation, hemostasis, and fibrinolysis inhibition, suggesting a possible protective effect for atherosclerosis (8145). Intravaginal, topical, and intramuscular administration of progesterone may be advantageous over oral dosing because it avoids first-pass effect and may achieve greater concentrations in the uterus (2033,2034).

Adverse Reactions

Orally, progesterone can cause gastrointestinal (GI) disturbances, changes in appetite, weight gain, fluid retention and edema, fatigue acne, drowsiness or insomnia, allergic skin rashes, hives, fever, headache, depression, breast discomfort or enlargement, PMS-like syndrome, altered menstrual cycles, and irregular bleeding (506,1224). Topically, progesterone can cause vaginal spotting (224).

Interactions with Herbs & Other Dietary Supplements

None known.

Interactions with Drugs

ESTROGENS: Concomitant use can cause breast tenderness (228). Use of conjugated equine estrogens with oral micronized progesterone in postmenopausal women may blunt the beneficial effects of estrogen on the lipoprotein profile (1216), although it might not affect estrogen-induced reduction in plasma lipoprotein (a) (1217).

Interactions with Foods

None known.

Interactions with Lab Tests

16-ALPHA-HYDROXYPROGESTERONE: Can cause increase in plasma test results (275).
17-HYDROXYCORTICOSTEROIDS: Can decrease urine level and test results (275).
ALANINE AMINOTRANSFERASE (ALT): Can increase serum levels and test results due to hepatotoxicity (275).
ALBUMIN: May increase serum levels and test results (275).
ALKALINE PHOSPHATASE (Alk Phos): Can increase serum levels and test results due to hepatotoxicity (275).
ASPARTATE AMINOTRANSFERASE (AST): Progesterone can decrease serum levels and test results in healthy people or increase serum levels and test results due to hepatotoxicity (275).
BILE: Can increase urine levels and test results due to hepatotoxicity (275).
BILIRUBIN: Can increase serum levels and test results due to hepatotoxicity (275).
CHOLESTEROL: Might decrease serum levels and test results (275).
GAMMA-GLOBULIN: Can increase serum levels and test results (275).
GLOBULIN: Can decrease serum levels and test results (275).
GLUCARIC ACID: Can increase urine level and test results (275).
LUTEINIZING HORMONE (LH): Can decrease peak plasma level and test results (275).
MAGNESIUM: Can increase serum level and test results (275).
PREGNANEDIOL: Can decrease urine level and test results (275).
PROGESTERONE: Can decrease plasma levels and test results (275).
PROSTAGLANDIN: Can decrease urine levels and test results (275).
PROTEIN: Can increase serum levels and test results (275).
SODIUM: Can increase serum and test results due to sodium retention (275). Large doses of progesterone can increase urine levels and test results (275).
THYROXINE (T4) BINDING GLOBULIN: Can increase serum levels and test results due to increased synthesis (275).

Interactions with Diseases or Conditions

ARTERIAL DISEASE: Contraindicated in individuals with high risk arterial disease (9).
BREAST CANCER: Should be avoided except as part of the management of breast cancer (9).
DEPRESSION: Use cautiously in individuals with a history of major depression (9).
LIVER DISEASE: Contraindicated. Progesterone has been associated with attacks of acute porphyria (9).
VAGINAL BLEEDING: Contraindicated in women who have undiagnosed vaginal bleeding (9).

Dosage and Administration

ORAL: For hormone replacement therapy, 200 mg micronized progesterone (Prometrium) orally per day is typically used for 12 days of a 25 day cycle with 0.625 mg conjugated estrogens (1215,1217).
TOPICAL: For menopausal vasomotor symptoms, 20 mg progesterone cream (equivalent to 1/4 teaspoon Progest cream) is typically applied daily to rotating sites including upper arms, thighs or breasts (224).
INTRAMUSCULAR: As a component of in vitro fertilization, 50 mg is commonly used intramuscularly (227,1218,1225,2034).
INTRAVAGINAL: For mastodynia associated with benign breast disease, a typical dose of 4 grams of vaginal cream containing 2.5% natural progesterone is placed intravaginally from the 19th to the 25th day of a 28 day cycle (1223). As a component of in vitro fertilization, one applicator (90 mg) of progesterone gel (Crinone 8%) is placed intravaginally 1-2 times daily (2032,2036). For secondary amenorrhea, one applicator (90 mg) of progesterone gel (Crinone 4% or 8%) is typically placed intravaginally every other day for 6 days per month (2041). For hormone replacement therapy, one applicator (90 mg) of progesterone gel (Crinone 4% or 8%) is typically placed intravaginally on days 17, 19, 21, 23, 25, and 27 of a 28 day cycle with 0.625 mg conjugated equine estrogens (2031). For reducing intravaginal bleeding and reversal of hyperplasia in premenopausal women with benign endometrial hyperplasia, a dose of 100 mg progesterone cream placed intravaginally daily from day 10 to day 25 of a 28 day cycle has been used (2033).

Comments

Progestin is a general term for a substance that causes some or all of the biologic effects of progesterone. The term "progestin" is sometimes used to specifically refer to the synthetic derivatives of progesterone in oral contraceptives and hormone replacement therapy (8143). However, all progesterone and progestin products are synthetic. The term "natural progesterone" is really a misnomer. OTC progesterone products may not contain progesterone concentrations as labeled. According to a British report, two-ounce jars of Progest cream used in a clinical trial contained 100 mg progesterone per ounce rather than the 465 mg claimed by the manufacturer (1228,1231). Topical progesterone products marketed as cosmetics require no FDA approval prior to marketing. There is currently no limit on the amount of progesterone allowed in cosmetic products. In 1993 the FDA proposed, but never finalized, a rule limiting progesterone-containing cosmetic products to a maximum level of 5 mg/oz with the product label specifying consumer usage not to exceed 2 oz per month (365).

PROPIONYL-L-CARNITINE

Also Known As

L-Carnitine Propionyl, LPC, PLC.
CAUTION: See separate listings for Acetyl-L-Carnitine and L-Carnitine.

Scientific Names

Propionyl-L-carnitine.

People Use This For

Orally, propionyl-L-carnitine is used for treating peripheral vascular disease (PVD), atherosclerotic and diabetic angiopathies, intermittent claudication, and congestive heart failure (CHF).
In combination with acetyl-L-carnitine, propionyl-L-carnitine is used orally for treating chronic fatigue syndrome (CFS) and symptoms of male aging.
Intravenously, propionyl-L-carnitine is used for treating peripheral vascular disease and intermittent claudication; to improve healing of ulcerative lesions in people with peripheral vascular disease; and to treat ischemic heart disease, angina, and congestive heart failure.

Safety

LIKELY SAFE ...when used orally and appropriately (1434,1435,1436,1437). ...when single intravenous doses are used under appropriate medical supervision (1571,1572,1573,1575).
PREGNANCY AND LACTATION: Insufficient reliable information available; avoid using.

Effectiveness

POSSIBLY EFFECTIVE

Angina. Taking propionyl-L-carnitine orally seems to produce small improvements in myocardial ischemia and exercise capacity in patients with chronic, stable angina (1579,1580,1581).
Chronic ischemic heart disease. In patients with chronic myocardial ischemia, intravenous administration of propionyl-L-carnitine may improve left ventricular function and cardiac output, as well as decrease myocardial ischemia (1571,1572,1573).
Congestive heart failure (CHF). Taking propionyl-L-carnitine orally seems to improve left ventricular function and exercise capacity in people with class II or III congestive heart failure (1575,1582,1583).

Intermittent claudication. Administering propionyl-L-carnitine orally or intravenously may help some patients with intermittent claudication and peripheral vascular disease. In patients with peripheral vascular disease and intermittent claudication that restricts walking distance to less than 250 meters, propionyl-L-carnitine may increase walking distance and time. Propionyl-L-carnitine doesn't seem to help milder peripheral vascular disease (1434,1435,1436,1437,1576,10456).

Male aging. Taking propionyl-L-carnitine orally in combination with acetyl-L-carnitine seems to help symptoms of androgen decline in older men. The combination taken for 6 months seems to be similar to testosterone for improving sexual dysfunction, depression, and fatigue (12353).

INSUFFICIENT RELIABLE EVIDENCE to RATE

Chronic fatigue syndrome (CFS). Preliminary clinical research suggests that propionyl-L-carnitine might improve general fatigue in patients with CFS. The combination of propionyl-L-carnitine and acetyl-L-carnitine appears to be less effective than either supplement alone (11788). More evidence is needed to rate the effectiveness of propionyl-L-carnitine for this use.

Mechanism of Action

L-carnitine is an essential cofactor in skeletal muscle and myocardium for transfer of long-chain fatty acids to intramitochondrial beta-oxidation sites where they are transformed into energy. There may be altered homeostasis and reduced levels of L-carnitine in peripheral vascular disease, myocardial ischemia, and heart failure (1572). Within cells, propionyl-L-carnitine helps to maintain mitochondrial acyl-CoA/CoA ratios which are increased in L-carnitine deficiency states, leading to deficient metabolism of fatty acids and urea synthesis (1439). Propionyl-L-carnitine also increases pyruvate flux into the Krebs Cycle, stimulates pyruvate dehydrogenase activity, has free radical scavenging activity, improves homeostasis in the coagulation cascade, and has positive effects on blood viscosity (1578).

Compared with L-carnitine, propionyl-L-carnitine may produce greater increases in cellular L-carnitine concentrations, possibly by being transported more easily into muscle fibers, and may provide additional substrates for muscle-cell energy production. Heart tissues may be able to utilize exogenous propionyl-L-carnitine to stimulate the tricarboxylic acid cycle and protect against ischemia (1439).

Intravenous and oral treatment may improve physical functioning in some people with peripheral vascular disease (1434,1435,1436,1437,1576), but a study suggesting that propionyl-L-carnitine was superior to L-carnitine in this regard used only single intravenous doses, and the clinical significance of the difference was questionable (1437).

Propionyl-L-carnitine improves energy, metabolism, and myocardial contractility in experimental models of heart failure (1577). Small studies suggest that propionyl-L-carnitine may have a positive inotropic effect and improve ventricular function and cardiac output in chronic heart failure (1571,1572,1573). It reduces myocardial ischemia, as measured by ST segment depression, in people with angina (1573,1579).

Carnitines, including propionyl-L-carnitine, are increased by male and female sex hormones (12353).

Adverse Reactions

Orally, nausea, vomiting, gastric pain, asthenia, and angina have been reported (1579,1580,1581,1582,1583).

Interactions with Herbs & Other Dietary Supplements

None known.

Interactions with Drugs

None known.

Interactions with Foods

None known.

Interactions with Lab Tests

None known.

Interactions with Diseases or Conditions

None known.

Dosage and Administration

ORAL: For peripheral vascular disease (PVD), atherosclerotic or diabetic arteriopathies, and intermittent claudication, 500-1500 mg propionyl-L-carnitine twice daily has been used (1434,1435,1436,10456). One study in peripheral vascular disease used 1000 mg three times daily (1576). A dose of 500 mg three times daily has been used in congestive heart failure and stable angina (1579,1580,1581,1583). For symptoms of male aging, 2 grams of acetyl-L-carnitine plus 2 grams of propionyl-L-carnitine daily has been used (12353).

INTRAVENOUS: A 1500 mg bolus followed by 1 mg/kg/minute infused for 30 minutes has been used to restore muscle L-carnitine levels in people with peripheral vascular disease (1434,1435,1436,1437,1576,10456). Single 600 mg bolusdoses have also been tested in people with peripheral vascular disease (1437), and infusions of 2000 mg twice daily have been used to improve healing of ulcerative lesions in people with peripheral vascular disease (1574). Single doses of 15 to 30 mg/kg have been used in people with chronic ischemic heart disease or congestive heart failure (1571,1572,1573,1575).

PROPOLIS

Also Known As

Bee Glue, Bee Propolis, Hive Dross, Propolis Balsam, Propolis Resin, Propolis Wax, Russian Penicillin.

Scientific Names

Propolis.

People Use This For

Orally, propolis is used for tuberculosis, bacterial and fungal infections, protozoal infections, nasopharyngeal carcinoma, treating the common cold, and improving immune response. Propolis is also used orally for treating gastrointestinal disturbances including Helicobacter pylori infection in peptic ulcer disease. It is also used as an antioxidant and anti-inflammatory agent.

Topically, propolis is used for wound cleansing, genital herpes, as a mouth rinse for enhancing healing following oral surgery, and for the treatment of minor burns.

In manufacturing, propolis is used as an ingredient in cosmetics.

Safety

There is insufficient reliable information available about the safety of propolis.

Pregnancy and Lactation: Insufficient reliable information available; avoid using.

Effectiveness

POSSIBLY EFFECTIVE

Herpes simplex virus type 2 (HSV-2). A 3% propolis ointment seems to significantly improve healing of recurrent genital lesions caused by herpes simplex virus type 2 (HSV-2). There is some evidence that it might help heal lesions faster and more completely than 5% acyclovir ointment (1926).

Sulcoplasty. Propolis mouth rinse following sulcoplasty seems to improve healing and reduce pain and inflammation (799).

INSUFFICIENT RELIABLE EVIDENCE to RATE

Common cold. There is some evidence that propolis might be helpful for treating the common cold. Propolis might decrease the duration of cold symptoms by 2.5 times compared with placebo in patients with rhinovirus infection (6602).

Minor burns. Propolis used topically might help in the treatment of minor burns. There is some evidence propolis skin cream compared with silver sulfadiazine might be as effective in preventing infection. It might also be more effective in the re-epithelization and healing of minor burn wounds such as superficial second degree burns (8663).

More evidence is needed to rate propolis for these uses.

Mechanism of Action

Propolis is a resinous material from poplar and conifer buds. Bees use it for maintaining their hives. Since propolis is incorporated into beehives, harvesting the pure product is difficult. Many propolis preparations are frequently contaminated with beehive by-products (3574).

Therapeutic uses of propolis are primarily attributed to antiviral, antibacterial, and antimycotic effects. Propolis contains flavonoids including pinocembrin, galangin, pinobanksin, and pinobanksin-3-acetate which are thought to be responsible for its antimicrobial effects (5,1926). Propolis extracts that contain the constituents pinocembrim and galagin have been shown to inhibit the growth and enzyme activity of Streptococcus mutans, an organism that causes dental caries (2631). Propolis also seems to have in vitro activity against a variety of bacteria that cause periodontal disease such as Porphyromonas gingivalis, Prevotella intermedia, Actinobacillus actinomycetemcomitans, and Fusobacterium nucleatum (8664).

Propolis might also have anti-inflammatory effects. There is preliminary evidence that it might suppress the lipoxygenase pathway of arachidonic acid metabolism and decrease the synthesis of prostaglandins and leukotrienes involved in inflammation (2630).

Topically applied propolis seems to help accelerate epithelial repair in animal models (800). Propolis also contains caffeic acid phenethyl esters (CAPE), which might have cancer chemopreventative properties (2629). These same constituents seem to also be contact allergens (2633). Propolis also has weak free radical scavenging properties (6).

Adverse Reactions

Orally, propolis can cause allergic reactions (6,2632) and acute oral mucositis with ulceration from the use of the propolis-containing lozenges (2632). Patients allergic to bees or bee products may be more likely to experience allergic reactions.

Topically, propolis-containing products, including some cosmetics can cause eczematous contact dermatitis (6,2632).

Interactions with Herbs & Other Dietary Supplements

None known.

Interactions with Drugs

None known.

Interactions with Foods

None known.

Interactions with Lab Tests

None known.

Interactions with Diseases or Conditions

ASTHMA: Some sources suggest allergens in propolis may worsen asthma (3574); avoid using.

HYPERSENSITIVITY: Avoid using propolis in people hypersensitive to bee by-products including honey, conifers, poplars, Peruvian balsam, and salicylates (19).

Dosage and Administration

ORAL: No typical dosage.

TOPICAL: As a mouth rinse after sulcoplasty, a 5% aqueous alcohol solution of propolis is commonly used (799). For herpetic lesions, 3% propolis ointment applied to the lesions 4 times daily has been used (1926).

Comments

Propolis has a long history of medicinal use, dating back to 350 B.C., the time of Aristotle. Greeks have used propolis for abscesses; Assyrians have used it for healing wounds and tumors; and Egyptians have used it for mummification (3574).

PUFF BALL

Also Known As

Bovista, Deer Balls, Hart's Truffle Puffball.

Scientific Names

Lycoperdon sp.

Family: Gasteromycetes.

People Use This For

Orally, puff ball is used for nosebleeds and skin disorders.

For food uses, young puff ball mushrooms are edible.

Safety

LIKELY SAFE ...when young puff ball mushrooms are consumed as food (18).

There is insufficient reliable information available about the safety of the oral use of puff ball for medicinal purposes.

PREGNANCY AND LACTATION: Insufficient reliable information available; avoid using.

Effectiveness

There is insufficient reliable information available about the effectiveness of puff ball.

Mechanism of Action
The applicable parts of puff ball are the aerial parts and spores. Puff ball contains amino acids, glucosamine, sterol, enzymes, and approximately 3% urea (18).

Adverse Reactions
Inhaling the spores can cause respiratory illness, pneumonia-like symptoms, and widespread lung densities (3846,3847).

Interactions with Herbs & Other Dietary Supplements
None known.

Interactions with Drugs
None known.

Interactions with Foods
None known.

Interactions with Lab Tests
None known.

Interactions with Diseases or Conditions
None known.

Dosage and Administration
ORAL: Puff ball is used in pulverized form or in alcoholic extracts (18).

PULSATILLA

Also Known As
Easter Flower, European Pasqueflower, Meadow Anenome, Meadow Windflower, Pasque Flower, Pasqueflower, Passe Flower, Wind Flower.

Scientific Names
Anemone pulsatilla, synonym Pulsatilla vulgaris, Anemone serotina; Anemone pratensis, synonym Anemone nigricans, Pulsatilla nigricans, Pulsatilla pratensis.
Family: Ranunculacaeae.

People Use This For
Orally, pulsatilla is used for painful conditions of the male or female reproductive system, such as dysmenorrhea, orchitis, ovaralgia, or epididymitis. Pulsatilla is also used for tension headache, hyperactive states, insomnia, boils, asthma and pulmonary disease, earache, migraines, neuralgia, general restlessness, diseases and functional disorders of the gastrointestinal GI and urinary tract.
Topically, pulsatilla is used for boils, skin eruptions associated with bacterial infection, and inflammatory and infectious diseases of the skin and mucosa.

Safety
LIKELY UNSAFE ...when fresh above ground parts are used orally or topically; pulsatilla is a severe local irritant (4).
There is insufficient reliable information available about the safety of the use of dried pulsatilla.
PREGNANCY: LIKELY UNSAFE ...when used orally. The fresh or dried above ground parts are contraindicated due to abortifacient and teratogenic effects (2). ...when the fresh above ground parts are used topically. There is insufficient reliable information available about the safety of topical dried pulsatilla during pregnancy.
LACTATION: LIKELY UNSAFE ...when the fresh above ground parts are used for oral or topical use (19). There is insufficient reliable information available about the safety of dried pulsatilla during breast-feeding.

Effectiveness
There is insufficient reliable information available about the effectiveness of pulsatilla.

Mechanism of Action
The applicable parts of pulsatilla are the above ground parts. Pulsatilla has analgesic, antispasmodic, sedative, and antibacterial properties. It exhibits both uterine stimulant and depressant activities. Pulsatilla contains ranunculin. Ranunculin hydrolyzes to a toxic unstable compound called protoanemonin, which readily dimerizes to nontoxic

anemonin (4). Protoanemonin causes central nervous system (CNS) stimulation, then paralysis in experimental animals. It also has antimicrobial activity (2). Both anemonin and protoanemonin show some evidence of sedative and antipyretic activity (4). Irritation of the kidney and urinary tract might be due to the alkylating action of protoanemonin (2). Some evidence suggests anemonin might be cytotoxic (4).

Adverse Reactions
Orally, fresh pulsatilla is a toxic gastrointestinal (GI) irritant (4,19). It can also cause kidney and urinary tract irritation (2).
Topically, contact with the fresh plant can cause skin irritation, mucous membrane irritation, itching, and pustule formation known as ranunculus dermatitis (2).
Inhalation of protoanemonin-containing volatile oil may cause nasal mucosal and conjunctival irritation (4). Allergic reactions have been documented with patch tests (4).

Interactions with Herbs & Other Dietary Supplements
None known.

Interactions with Drugs
None known.

Interactions with Foods
None known.

Interactions with Lab Tests
None known.

Interactions with Diseases or Conditions
None known.

Dosage and Administration
ORAL: A typical oral dose is 120-300 mg dried above ground parts three times daily. Alternatively one cup tea consumed three times daily. To make tea, steep or simmer 120-300 mg dried above ground parts in 150 mL water 5-10 minutes, strain (4). 0.12-0.3 mL of the liquid extract, 1:1 in 25% alcohol, has been used three times daily (4). 0.3-1 mL of the tincture, 1:10 in 40% alcohol, has been used three times daily (4).
TOPICAL: No typical dosage.

PUMPKIN

Also Known As
Cucurbitea peponis semen, Field Pumpkin, Pepo, Pumpkin Seed.

Scientific Names
Cucurbita pepo, synonyms Cucumis pepo, Cucurbita galeottii, Cucurbita mammeata.
Family: Cucurbitaceae.

People Use This For
Orally, pumpkin is used for dysuria secondary to benign prostatic hyperplasia (BPH), bladder irritation, treating intestinal worms, and treating pyelonephritis.
In combination, pumpkin is used in an herbal combination to treat symptoms of BPH.
The roasted pumpkins seeds are considered a snack food.

Safety
POSSIBLY SAFE ...when used orally and appropriately (2,7,18).
PREGNANCY AND LACTATION: Insufficient reliable information available; avoid using amounts greater than those found in food.

Effectiveness

POSSIBLY INEFFECTIVE

Benign prostatic hyperplasia (BPH). Taking pumpkin seed oil extract orally alone, or with saw palmetto, may help BPH symptoms (11231,11232). An herbal product containing pumpkin seed oil extract 160 mg, saw palmetto lipoidal extract 106 mg, nettle root extract 80 mg, lemon bioflavonoid extract 33 mg, and vitamin A (100% as beta-carotene) 190 IU used three times daily for six months may shrink the prostate epithelium, although it may not significantly improve symptoms in some men (5093).

There is insufficient reliable information available about the effectiveness of pumpkin for its other uses.

Mechanism of Action

The applicable part of pumpkin is the seed. Pumpkin seeds contain as much as 35% fatty oil, 38% protein, and 37% carbohydrate content (8257). Pumpkin seeds are also rich in carotenoids, including lutein, carotene, and beta-carotene (515). The seed oil is rich in unsaturated fatty acids, including 47% linoleic acid, 29% oleic acid, 14% palmitic acid, and 8% stearic acid (8257). The oil is also rich in vitamin E, including both gamma-tocopherol and alpha-tocopherol (3 mg/100 g) (8257). The enzyme acyl-coenzyme A oxidase (ACOX) is present in the pumpkin seed. The ACOX enzyme catalyzes fatty acid oxidation, specifically the oxidation of fatty acid CoA esters with 4 to 10 carbon atoms (8256). Pumpkin seed oil can exhibit a diuretic effect, which can relieve bladder discomfort, causing the perception of reduced prostate gland swelling without reducing the gland size. The phytosterol constituents are also believed to affect urine flow (515). Animal research suggests it might improve bladder and urethral function, which might help BPH symptoms (11233).

Another constituent, cucurbitin, has anthelmintic effects. Concentration of cucurbitin varies significantly among Cucurbita species (515).

Adverse Reactions

One case is reported of decreased ejaculatory volume associated with an herbal blend product containing pumpkin seed oil extract, saw palmetto extract, nettle root extract, lemon bioflavonoid extract, and beta-carotene (5093).

Interactions with Herbs & Other Dietary Supplements

None known.

Interactions with Drugs

None known.

Interactions with Foods

None known.

Interactions with Lab Tests

None known.

Interactions with Diseases or Conditions

None known.

Dosage and Administration

ORAL: For benign prostatic hyperplasia, pumpkin seed oil extract 480 mg per day in 3 divided doses in combination with saw palmetto and other herbs has been used (5093,11232).

Comments

Seeds of autumn squash (Cucurbita maxima) and Canadian pumpkin (crooked neck squash, Cucurbita moschata) have properties similar to Cucurbita pepo seed (515).

PUNCTURE VINE

Also Known As

Abrojos, Caltrop, Cat's-Head, Common Dubbletjie, Devil's-Thorn, Devil's-Weed, Espigón, Goathead, Gokhru, Gokshura, Nature's Viagra, Puncturevine, Tribule terrestre, Tribulis, Tribulis Terrestris, Tribulus, Tribulus Terrestris.

Scientific Names

Tribulus terrestris.
Family: Zygophyllaceae.

People Use This For

Orally, puncture vine is used for angina pectoris, male impotence, enhancing athletic performance, treating anemia, Bright's disease, cancer, coughs, improving digestion, treating flatulence, gonorrhea, headache, hepatitis, inflammation, stomatitis, vertigo, leprosy, nasal tumors, neurasthenia, painful urination, childbirth, psoriasis, rheumatism, scabies, sore throat, and spermatorrhea. It is also used as a gentle laxative, for stimulating appetite and milk flow, as an abortifacient, aphrodisiac, astringent, diuretic, tonic, and vermifuge.

Safety

LIKELY UNSAFE ...when the spine-covered fruit is used orally. There has been one report of a bilateral pneumothorax adverse effect (818).
There is insufficient reliable information available about the safety of the parts of puncture vine other than the fruit.
PREGNANCY: POSSIBLY UNSAFE ...when used orally; avoid using. It has been used as an abortifacient (3919).
LACTATION: Insufficient reliable information available; avoid using.

Effectiveness

There is insufficient reliable information available about the effectiveness of puncture vine.

Mechanism of Action

Puncture vine contains diosgenin and other saponins (3929). An unidentified saponin of Tribulus terrestris is reported effective for treating angina pectoris in people with coronary heart disease (3931).

Adverse Reactions

Orally, there is one case report of bilateral pneumothorax following the removal of a puncture vine fruit with sharp spines (818).

Interactions with Herbs & Other Dietary Supplements

None known.

Interactions with Drugs

None known.

Interactions with Foods

None known.

Interactions with Lab Tests

None known.

Interactions with Diseases or Conditions

None known.

Dosage and Administration

ORAL: Puncture vine is used as an extract (817).

Comments

Puncture vine was so named because its sharp seeds can flatten bicycle tires (817).

PURPLE LOOSESTRIFE

Also Known As

Blooming Sally, Flowering Sally, Long Purples, Loosestrife, Lythrum, Milk Willow-Herb, Purple Willow-Herb, Rainbow Weed, Salicare, Soldiers, Spiked Loosestrife, Willow Sage.
CAUTION: See separate listings for Loosestrife and Sage.

Scientific Names

Lythrum salicaria.
Family: Lythraceae.

Comments

At the date of publication, this product was not a common ingredient used in brand name supplements marketed to consumers. Details about this product are available at the online version of *Natural Medicines Comprehensive Database*. See www.naturaldatabase.com.

PYCNOGENOL

Also Known As

Condensed Tannins, French Marine Pine Bark Extract, French Maritime Pine Bark Extract, Leucoanthocyanidins, Oligomeric Proanthocyanidins, OPC, OPCs, Pine Bark, Pine Bark Extract, Pinus marittima, Procyanidin Oligomers, Procyandiol Oligomers, Procyanodolic Oligomers, PCO, PCOs, Pygenol.

Scientific Names

Pinus pinaster, synonym Pinus maritima.
Family: Pinaceae.

People Use This For

Orally, pycnogenol is used for treating chronic venous insufficiency, allergies, hypertension, muscle soreness, pain, arthritis, diabetes, attention deficit-hyperactivity disorder (ADHD), endometriosis, dysmenorrhea, erectile dysfunction, and retinopathy. It is also used orally for preventing stroke, preventing vascular conditions such as heart disease and varicose veins, slowing the aging process, maintaining skin health, improving athletic endurance, and improving sperm morphology in subfertile men.
Topically, pycnogenol is used as a component of "anti-aging" creams.

Safety

POSSIBLY SAFE ...when used orally and appropriately. Pycnogenol has been safely used in doses of 120 to 450 mg daily for up to three months (2435,2451,2462,2553,2554,2556,7693,10214,10416,12012).
There is insufficient reliable information available about the safety of pycnogenol for its other uses.
PREGNANCY AND LACTATION: Insufficient reliable information available; avoid using.

Effectiveness

POSSIBLY EFFECTIVE

Athletic performance. Taking pycnogenol orally 200 mg daily for 30 days seems to improve treadmill exercise capacity in recreational athletes aged 20 to 35 years (2554).

Chronic venous insufficiency. Taking pycnogenol orally seems to significantly reduce symptoms of leg pain and heaviness, and edema in people with chronic venous insufficiency (CVI) when used for 3 to 12 weeks. The dose of pycnogenol used most often is 100-120 mg three times daily (2451,2462,2493,7693), but a lower dose of 45 mg to 90 mg once daily also seems to be effective (2435). Some people also use horse chestnut seed extract to treat CVI, but pycnogenol alone appears to be more effective (7693).

Hypertension. In patients with mild hypertension (systolic 140-159 mm Hg; diastolic 90-99 mm Hg), taking pycnogenol orally may reduce systolic blood pressure to approximately 133 mm Hg. Diastolic blood pressure is not significantly reduced (10214).

Retinopathy. Taking pycnogenol 50 mg three times daily for two months seems to slow or prevent further deterioration of retinal function in patients with retinopathy caused by diabetes, atherosclerosis, or central venous thrombosis. Patients can have some improvement in visual acuity and retinal vascularization (2536).

POSSIBLY INEFFECTIVE

Attention deficit-hyperactivity disorder (ADHD). Taking pycnogenol orally doesn't seem to help ADHD symptoms in adults (9984). There are anecdotal reports that pycnogenol helps ADHD in children, but there isn't any research to support this claim (6558).

INSUFFICIENT RELIABLE EVIDENCE to RATE

Coronary artery disease. There is some evidence that pycnogenol 150 mg three times daily for 4 weeks might improve certain factors such as microcirculation, myocardial ischemia, and the potential for platelet aggregation in patients with coronary artery disease (2553).

Deep vein thrombosis (DVT). There is some evidence that taking a specific combination product (Flite Tabs) might decrease the risk of DVT during long-haul plane flights. The product combines a blend of 150 mg of pycnogenol plus nattokinase. Two capsules are taken 2 hours before the flight and then again 6 hours later (12075).

Erectile dysfunction (ED). Preliminary clinical research suggests pycnogenol, used alone (12012) or in combination with L-arginine (10416), might improve sexual function in men with erectile dysfunction. It seems to take up to 3 months of treatment for significant improvement.

Hypercholesterolemia. There is also some evidence that pycnogenol 120 mg three times daily lowers low-density lipoprotein (LDL) cholesterol (7693).

Pelvic pain. There is preliminary evidence that pycnogenol might help reduce pelvic pain in women with endometriosis or dysmenorrhea (2555).

More evidence is needed to rate pycnogenol for these uses.

Mechanism of Action

Pycnogenol is an extract from the bark of the French maritime pine tree (2431). Pycnogenol contains several active constituents including flavonoid monomers such as catechin, epicatechin, and taxifolin. It also contains condensed procyanidins (also called flavonoids or proanthocyanidins) such as procyanidin B1, B3, B6, and B7 which are dimers, oligomers, and polymers of catechin and epicatechin (2431,2433). Pycnogenol also contains phenolic acids including gallic, ferulic, caffeic, vanillic, p-coumaric, protocatechuic, and p-hydroxybenzoic acids, and their glucosides and glucose esters (2431,2433,2435,2543).

In chronic venous insufficiency (CVI, varicose veins) procyanidins in pycnogenol reduce capillary permeability, which contributes to edema and microbleeding, by cross-linking capillary wall proteins such as collagen and elastin (2435,2544). There is also some evidence that procyanidins make elastin more resistant to degradation by elastase (2451,2635), and that pycnogenol might inhibit elastase and collagenase released by activated macrophages (2462). Pycnogenol might also help prevent capillary permeability due to the antioxidant effects of several of its constituents (2433,2435,2636,2542,2451). Pycnogenol also seems to recycle ascorbyl and tocopheryl radicals, helping to maintain vitamin C and E levels (2542,7698). Benefits for other uses, including diabetic retinopathy and improving athletic performance, are also thought to be due to the antioxidant effects of pycnogenol (2536,2554).

Some research suggests that pycnogenol might be useful in the prevention of cardiovascular disease. In vitro, pycnogenol prevents oxidation of low-density lipoprotein (LDL) cholesterol and protects DNA from damage by free radicals (2433). It also seems to prevent free-radical induced endothelial damage in vitro (2433). Pycnogenol inhibits epinephrine-induced platelet aggregation, such as that seen in smokers (2435,3285), but pycnogenol does not appear to increase bleeding risk or affect smoking-related increases in blood pressure or heart rate (3283). In non-smokers, it decreases serum thromboxane B2 and reduces systolic blood pressure (10214). Pycnogenol inhibits angiotensin converting enzyme (ACE) in vitro, but is unlikely to have clinically significant hypotensive effects when used orally in humans (2435). Pycnogenol might also increase production of nitric oxide from vascular endothelial cells by stimulating nitric oxide synthetase. This can lead to vasodilatation and possibly reduce the potential for atherogenesis and thrombus formation (2433,2451,2545,2637). Increased nitric oxide production might also be the mechanism for the possible benefit of pycnogenol in erectile dysfunction (10416,12012).

Some people think pycnogenol may be beneficial for cardiovascular disease because of its anti-inflammatory effects. However, the anti-inflammatory effects of pycnogenol are controversial. Pycnogenol appears to have no effect on levels of inflammatory markers including C-reactive protein (CRP), interleukin-1 (IL-1), or interleukin-6 (IL-6) (7694). An increased risk of cardiovascular disease may be associated with increases in these inflammatory markers.

There is also interest in using pycnogenol to protect against sunburn. Skin exposure to ultraviolet radiation has been shown to increase levels of free radicals that can damage the skin. It is theorized that pycnogenol may counteract the damaging effects of ultraviolet radiation through its antioxidant effects. Oral supplementation with pycnogenol at doses of 1.10 mg/kg/day for 4 weeks followed by 1.66 mg/kg/day for an additional 4 weeks increases the amount of ultraviolet radiation, both UVA and UVB, required to cause erythema and pinkness of the skin in human volunteers. The higher dose appears more protective than the lower dose since a greater amount of ultraviolet radiation is required to cause erythema when the higher dose is taken (7696). Some research suggests that topical pycnogenol might be useful for skin diseases related to increased cell adhesion and inflammation such as psoriasis, atopic dermatitis, and lupus erythematosus. Preclinical research suggests that it reduces inflammation in keratinocytes (10213).

Preliminary evidence suggests that pycnogenol might stimulate the immune system. It seems to boost natural killer cell activity (2435) and improves T- and B-cell function in animal models (2636). Pycnogenol also increase tumor necrosis factor-alpha (TNF-alpha) secretion and natural factor-KB (NF-KB) activity also increase (7697). Pycnogenol appears to slow the development of immune dysfunction in animal models infected with a retrovirus similar to human immunodeficiency virus (HIV) by restoring imbalanced T-helper 1 and T-helper 2 cytokine secretion (7695).

Pycnogenol might have some activity in Alzheimer's disease. In vitro, pycnogenol protects animal brain cells from the toxic effects of high levels of glutamate, and also from the toxic effects of amyloid-beta-protein, which is found in the plaques characteristic of Alzheimer's Disease (2435,7699).

There is a developing interest in using pycnogenol to prevent obesity. In vitro, pycnogenol appears to inhibit insulin-induced lipogenesis and may stimulate lipolysis (8307).

Constituents of pycnogenol are metabolized through glucuronide and sulfate conjugation. Ferulic acid and taxifolin conjugates are excreted in the urine within 18 to 24 hours. Conjugated metabolites of the procyanidin fraction are excreted within 28 to 34 hours (2431,2543,10212).

Adverse Reactions

None reported.

Interactions with Herbs & Other Dietary Supplements

None known.

Interactions with Drugs

IMMUNOSUPPRESSANTS: Theoretically, pycnogenol may interfere with immunosuppressant therapy because of its immunostimulating activity (2435,2636). Immunosuppressant drugs include azathioprine (Imuran), basiliximab (Simulect), cyclosporine (Neoral, Sandimmune), daclximab (Zenapax), muromonab-CD3 (OKT3, Orthoclone OKT3), mycophenolate (CellCept), tacrolimus (FK506, Prograf), sirolimus (Rapamune), prednisone (Deltasone, Orasone), and other corticosteroids (glucocorticoids).

Interactions with Foods

None known.

Interactions with Lab Tests

None known.

Interactions with Diseases or Conditions

AUTOIMMUNE DISEASES: There is some concern that pycnogenol might adversely affect patients with autoimmune disorders because of its immune stimulating effects (2435,2636). Avoid using in patients with multiple sclerosis, systemic lupus erythematosus (SLE), rheumatoid arthritis, or other autoimmune disorders.

Dosage and Administration

ORAL: For chronic venous insufficiency, 45 to 360 mg daily, or 100 mg three times daily have been used (2435,2451,2462,2493). For diabetic and other retinopathies, 50 mg three times daily has been used (2536). For coronary artery disease, 150 mg three times daily has been used (2553). For erectile dysfunction, 120 mg daily has been used (10416, 12012). For hypercholesterolemia, a dose of 120 mg three times daily has been used (7693). For mild hypertension, 200 mg of pycnogenol daily has been used (10214). To improve exercise capacity in athletes, 200 mg daily has been used (2554). For chronic pelvic pain, dysmenorrhea, and endometriosis in women, 30 to 60 mg daily has been used (2555). To improve sperm morphology in subfertile men, 200 mg daily has been used (2556). For protection against sunburn, doses of 1.10 and 1.66 mg/kg/day have been used (7696).
TOPICAL: No typical dose.

Comments

Pycnogenol is the US registered trademark for an extract derived from French Maritime Pine Bark (Pinus pinaster) which contains procyanidins, a group of bioflavonoids. Originally, the term "pycnogenol" was used as a generic term for procyanidins. Procyanidins are also referred to as condensed tannins, leucoanthocyanidins, proanthocyanidins, oligomeric proanthocyanidins (OPCs), and procyandiol oligomers (PCOs). They are derived from various other sources besides French maritime pine bark, including peanut skins (Arachis hypogaea), grape seed (Vitis vinifera) (515), and witch hazel bark (Hamamelis virginiana) (2641).

PYGEUM

Also Known As

African Plum Tree.

Scientific Names

Prunus africana, synonym Pygeum africanum.
Family: Rosaceae.

People Use This For

Orally, pygeum is used for treating functional symptoms of benign prostatic hyperplasia (BPH) (nocturia, dysuria, pollakiuria micturitional disorders, and bladder fullness) and prostatic adenoma.
Traditionally, pygeum is used orally for inflammation, kidney disease, urinary problems, malaria, stomachache, fever, difficult urination, fever, madness, prostate gland inflammation, and as an aphrodisiac.

Safety

LIKELY SAFE ...when used orally and appropriately (3902,3903,6368,10425,10426).
PREGNANCY AND LACTATION: Insufficient reliable information available; avoid using.

Effectiveness

LIKELY EFFECTIVE

Benign prostatic hyperplasia (BPH). Taking pygeum orally reduces the functional symptoms of BPH. Pygeum decreases nocturia by 19%, increases peak urine flow by 23%, and reduces residual urine volume by 24% in men with BPH (3902,3903,3904,4302,6368,10425,10426).

Mechanism of Action

The applicable part of pygeum is the bark. There is evidence that suggests pygeum extracts have antiproliferative effects on prostatic fibroblasts and epithelial cells. Pygeum might inhibit growth factors such as basic fibroblast growth factor (bFGF), epidermal growth factor (EGF), and insulin-like growth factor (IGF), which might inhibit prostate growth and cellular hyperplasia (4301,6769,11226). Preclinical research suggests that pygeum improves bladder contractility. It seems to affect adrenal androgens and to restore the secretory activity of prostate epithelium. It also decreases production of leukotrienes and other 5-lipoxygenase metabolites, which suggests possible anti-inflammatory activity (6769,10425,10426).

Adverse Reactions

Orally, pygeum bark is generally well tolerated. It can cause nausea and abdominal pain (10425,10426).

Interactions with Herbs & Other Dietary Supplements

None known.

Interactions with Drugs

None known.

Interactions with Foods

None known.

Interactions with Lab Tests

None known.

Interactions with Diseases or Conditions

None known.

Dosage and Administration

ORAL: For functional symptoms of benign prostatic hyperplasia (BPH), 75-200 mg standardized lipophilic extract (14% triterpenes, 0.5% n-docosanol) per day has been used (10425,10426). Some research suggests once or twice daily dosing is equally effective (6368).

PYRETHRUM

Also Known As

Dalmation Insect Flowers, Dalmation Pellitory.

Scientific Names

Tanacetum cinerariifolium, synonyms Chrysanthemum cinerariifolium, Pyrethrum cinerariifolium.
Family: Asteraceae/Compositae.

People Use This For

Topically, pyrethrum is used as an insecticide, particularly for head lice, crablice and their nits, and as an antiscabies agent.

Safety

LIKELY SAFE ...when the commercially available combination of pyrethrins (0.17-0.33%) and piperonyl butoxide (2-4%) are used topically and appropriately in a nonaerosol preparation (272).
POSSIBLY SAFE ...when pyrethrins are used topically in amounts less than 2 grams (18).
CHILDREN: POSSIBLY UNSAFE ...when used in children under the age of 2 years (4084).
PREGNANCY AND LACTATION: Insufficient reliable information available; avoid using.

Effectiveness

EFFECTIVE

Lice. Applying pyrethrins topically and appropriately in concentrations of 0.17-.0.33% for 12-24 hours is effective for treating head lice and crab lice. They are usually combined with piperonyl butoxide (2-4%) (272). Brand names include A-200 Pyrinate, Barc, Lice-Enz, Licetrol, Pronto, R and C, RID, Tisit, Tisit Blue, and Triple X.

INEFFECTIVE

Scabies. Applying pyrethrum flowers topically is not effective for treating scabies (4084).

Mechanism of Action

The applicable part of pyrethrum is the flower head. Pyrethrum is also the name of the crude extract obtained from flowers of Chrysanthemum cinerariifolium. Pyrethrin refers to more refined extract containing several naturally occurring pyrethrins (505). The active constituents, the pyrethrins, are toxic to insect nervous systems (18).

Adverse Reactions

Pyrethrum has limited toxicity. The symptoms of overdose include headache, tinnitus, nausea, tingling of fingers and toes, respiratory disturbances, and other symptoms of neurotoxicity (18). The pyrethrum flower or derivatives of it might cause an allergic reaction in individuals sensitive to the Asteraceae/Compositae family. Members of this family include ragweed, chrysanthemums, marigolds, daisies, and many other herbs.

Interactions with Herbs & Other Dietary Supplements

None known.

Interactions with Drugs

None known.

Interactions with Foods

None known.

Interactions with Lab Tests

None known.

Interactions with Diseases or Conditions

ASTHMA: Exposure to pyrethrin might severely exacerbate asthma; avoid using. There is one case report of fatal asthma in a child with a history of asthma after bathing a pet dog with a 0.2% pyrethrin shampoo. There is speculation that this might have been due to allergenic impurities from the pyrethrin extraction process (6654).
CROSS-ALLERGENICITY: Can cause an allergic reaction in individuals sensitive to the Asteraceae/Compositae family. Members of this family include ragweed, chrysanthemums, marigolds, daisies, and many other herbs.

Dosage and Administration

TOPICAL: Externally as a liquid extract, rinse after use (18). In general, the OTC combination of pyrethrins (0.17-0.33%) and piperonyl butoxide (2-4%) are applied to the infested area and allowed to remain for not less than 10 minutes. It is then thoroughly washed off with warm water (272).

Comments

To treat lice, the OTC combination products with piperonyl butoxide are preferred for safety and effectiveness (272).

PYRIDOXINE (VITAMIN B6)

Also Known As

Adermine Hydrochloride, B Complex Vitamin, B6, Pyridoxal, Pyridoxal Phosphate, Pyridoxal-5-Phosphate, Pyridoxamine, Pyridoxine, Pyridoxine HCl, Pyridoxine Hydrochloride.

Scientific Names

Pyridoxine; Vitamin B6.

People Use This For

Orally, pyridoxine is used most commonly for treating premenstrual syndrome (PMS), vitamin B6 deficiency, "morning sickness" in pregnancy, depression associated with pregnancy or oral contraceptive use, primary homocystinuria, hyperhomocysteinemia, and preventing neuritis associated with isoniazid or penicillamine. Pyridoxine is also used orally for boosting immunity, muscle cramps, protection against cancer, diuresis, conjunctivitis, cystitis, primary hyperoxaluria, preventing kidney stones, carpal tunnel syndrome (CTS), night leg cramps, arthritis, and allergies. It is used for attention deficit-hyperactivity disorder (ADHD), Down syndrome, migraine headaches, asthma, pyridoxine-responsive sideroblastic anemia, sickle cell anemia, preventing anemia due to pyridoxine deficiency, xanthurenic aciduria, primary cystathioninuria, acne, various skin conditions, stimulating appetite, hyperlipidemia, heart disease, radiation sickness, menopausal symptoms, infertility, amenorrhea-galactorrhea syndrome, suppressing postpartum lactation, and to improve dream recall. Pyridoxine is also used orally for dizziness, motion sickness, psychosis, autism, hyperkinesis, acute chorea, chronic progressive hereditary chorea, tardive dyskinesia, absence (petit mal) seizures, febrile convulsions, gyrate atrophy of the choroid and retina, diabetes, diabetic neuropathy, alcohol intoxication, preventing leukopenia secondary to mitomycin, reversing procarbazine neurotoxicity, preventing seizures associated with cycloserine, fluorouracil-induced erythrodysesthesia, and acute hydrazine toxicity. It is also used orally to decrease the rate of restenosis after coronary angioplasty. Intravenously, pyridoxine is used for seizures in infants unresponsive to other therapies, acute toxicity due to isoniazid, cycloserine or hydrazine overdose, and acute poisoning from mushrooms of the genus Gyromitra.

Safety

LIKELY SAFE ...when used orally and appropriately (15). ...when used parenterally and appropriately. Injectable pyridoxine is an FDA-approved prescription product (15).
POSSIBLY SAFE ...when used orally and appropriately in amounts exceeding the recommended dietary allowance (8558).
POSSIBLY UNSAFE ...when used orally in excessive doses, long-term. Doses exceeding 1000 mg daily or total doses of 1000 grams or more pose the most risk, although neuropathy can occur with lower daily or total doses (8195).
CHILDREN: LIKELY SAFE ...when used orally and appropriately (3094). POSSIBLY SAFE ...when used orally and appropriately in amounts exceeding the recommended dietary allowance (5049,8579). POSSIBLY UNSAFE ...when used orally in excessive doses, long-term (3094).
PREGNANCY: LIKELY SAFE ...when used orally in doses not exceeding the recommended dietary allowance (RDA). The RDA for pregnant women is 1.9 mg per day (3094). POSSIBLY SAFE ...when used orally and appropriately in amounts exceeding the recommended dietary allowance. A special sustained-release product providing pyridoxine 75 mg per day is FDA-approved for use in pregnancy. However, it should not be used long-term or without medical supervision and close monitoring. POSSIBLY UNSAFE ...when used orally in excessive doses. There is some concern that high-dose maternal pyridoxine can cause neonatal seizures (4609,6397,8197).
LACTATION: LIKELY SAFE ...when used orally in doses not exceeding the recommended dietary allowance (RDA) (3094). The RDA in lactating women is 2 mg per day. There is insufficient reliable information about the safety of pyridoxine when used in higher doses in lactating women.

Effectiveness

EFFECTIVE

Hereditary sideroblastic anemia. Taking pyridoxine orally is effective for treating hereditary sideroblastic anemia (15).

Pyridoxine-dependent seizures. Refractory seizures in neonates that are caused by pyridoxine dependence are typically controlled within minutes of intravenous administration of pyridoxine. Pyridoxine-dependent seizures can be due to genetic (autosomal recessive) pyridoxine dependency, or more commonly, the result of the use of high-dose pyridoxine in pregnancy (8197,8198).

Pyridoxine deficiency. Taking pyridoxine orally is effective for preventing and treating pyridoxine deficiency (15).

LIKELY EFFECTIVE

Hyperhomocysteinemia. Taking pyridoxine orally alone or in combination with folic acid is effective for treating postprandial hyperhomocysteinemia. Pyridoxine 50 to 200 mg/day reduces postprandial homocysteine levels by 32-35% (9406,10350). Pyridoxine doesn't seem to lower homocysteine concentrations unless folic acid and vitamin B12 are at physiologic levels, but it appears to reduce homocysteine concentrations when given with folic acid and vitamin B12 supplements (3047,9451). A combination of pyridoxine 100 mg and folic acid 0.5 mg/day seems to lower homocysteine levels by about 35% (9406). A combination of these vitamins is generally recommended for people with postprandial hyperhomocysteinemia (1489,9406,9408). Pyridoxine in doses up to 200 mg/day has no effect on fasting homocysteine levels (2149,9406,9408), and doesn't add to the effect of folic acid alone on fasting homocysteine levels in healthy people (9400,9405,9409). However, pyridoxine does seem to reduce homocysteine levels in patients with end-stage renal disease (ESRD), renal transplant patients (1489,6884,9414,9415), and patients who receive general anesthesia with nitrous oxide (9481). Hyperhomocysteinemia is a risk factor for coronary, cerebral and peripheral atherosclerosis; recurrent thromboembolism; deep vein thrombosis; myocardial infarction; and ischemic stroke (1899,2147,3047,3323,9402,9405,9408,9409). But elevated homocysteine levels may be a marker instead of a cause of vascular disease (11387,11388). A 5 micromole increase in plasma homocysteine increases the risk of cerebrovascular disease by 50%, and the risk of coronary heart disease by 60% in women and 80% in men (9407,9411). However, it's not clear if lowering homocysteine levels results in reduced cardiovascular morbidity and mortality (1489,6883,6884,9308,9400,9405,9409). Folic acid, pyridoxine (vitamin B6), and vitamin B12 supplementation can reduce total homocysteine from 13.4 to 11.0 micromoles per liter. However, this reduction doesn't seem to help with secondary prevention of death or cardiovascular events such as stroke or myocardial infarction in people with prior stroke (11387). More evidence is needed to fully explain the association of total homocysteine levels with vascular risk. Until definitive data is available, the current recommendation is screening of 40-year-old men and 50-year-old women for hyperhomocysteinemia (9308).

POSSIBLY EFFECTIVE

Hyperkinetic cerebral dysfunction syndrome. There is preliminary evidence that taking pyridoxine orally may have a beneficial effect on hyperkinetic children who have low levels of blood serotonin (3351).

Kidney stones (nephrolithiasis). There is some evidence that taking pyridoxine orally, alone, or in combination with magnesium, can decrease urinary oxalate levels in people with type I primary hyperoxaluria, a hereditary disorder (1201,6437,6438,6439,6440,8548,8549,8550). However, it doesn't appear to help people with other kinds of kidney stones (8551). There is preliminary evidence that higher pyridoxine intake in women is associated with decreased risk of kidney stone formation in women with no history of stone formation (6441), but this association has not been found in men (6442).

Lung cancer. Taking pyridoxine orally seems to decrease the risk of lung cancer. Epidemiological research suggests that male smokers with higher serum levels of pyridoxine have a lower risk of lung cancer (9454).

Pregnancy-induced nausea and vomiting. Taking pyridoxine orally 25 mg every eight hours for 72 hours decreases vomiting and severe nausea in pregnancy. However, it doesn't seem to improve mild to moderate nausea (6168). Lower doses, pyridoxine 10 mg every eight hours, improves nausea, but not vomiting in pregnancy (6167).

Premenstrual syndrome (PMS). There is some evidence that taking pyridoxine orally can improve symptoms of PMS such as breast pain or tenderness (mastalgia) and PMS-related depression in some patients. Pyridoxine 50 mg per day plus magnesium oxide 200 mg per day seems to relieve PMS-related anxiety (8555). Although some clinicians advocate higher doses of pyridoxine for PMS, such as 200-500 mg per day, lower doses of 50-100 mg per day seem to work just as well. There is no apparent dose-response curve for PMS, so the lowest effective dose should be used. Higher doses might increase the risk of side effects (3093).

Tardive dyskinesia. Pyridoxine 400 mg per day seems to improve Parkinsonian, dystonic, and dyskinetic symptoms in patients taking neuroleptic drugs for schizophrenia (8558).

POSSIBLY INEFFECTIVE

Autism. A moderate dose of 200 mg per day, and a high dose of 600 mg per day, of pyridoxine in combination with magnesium given for ten to 35 weeks doesn't seem to improve autistic behaviors in children (5049,8579).

Carpal tunnel syndrome. Most research suggests that people with carpal tunnel syndrome are not generally pyridoxine deficient and do not benefit from pyridoxine supplements (8203,8937,9448,9450,9453,9478,9482). Although early studies by a single group of researchers, and anecdotal reports, suggest pyridoxine may relieve carpal tunnel symptoms, more reliable research does not support pyridoxine for this use (8200,8201,8202,8204,9445,9446,9447,9449,9483). Some researchers have identified pyridoxine deficiency in people with carpal tunnel syndrome (8199). People who have peripheral neuropathy, as opposed to carpal tunnel syndrome, may benefit from pyridoxine (9453).

Stroke. Taking pyridoxine orally doesn't seem to be useful for preventing stroke recurrence. In people with a history of stroke, neither high dose pyridoxine combinations containing 25 mg of pyridoxine, 0.4 mg of vitamin B12, and 2.5 mg of folic acid nor low dose combinations containing 200 mcg of pyridoxine, 6 mcg of vitamin B12, and 20 mcg of folic acid seem to affect risk of recurring stroke (11387).

INSUFFICIENT RELIABLE EVIDENCE to RATE

Angioplasty. There are conflicting findings about the benefits of taking folic acid plus vitamin B6 and vitamin B12 following angioplasty. Some evidence suggests that folic acid 1 mg plus vitamin B12 400 mcg and pyridoxine 10 mg daily can decrease the rate of restenosis in patients treated with balloon angioplasty (8009,9412). But this combination does not seem to be as effective for reducing restenosis in patients after coronary stenting (8009). An intravenous loading dose of folic acid, vitamin B6 and vitamin B12 followed by oral administration of folic acid 1.2 mcg plus vitamin B6 48 mg and vitamin B12 60 mcg taken daily after coronary stenting also does not seem to reduce restenosis and might actually increase restenosis (12150,12151). Due to the lack of evidence of benefit and potential for harm, this combination of vitamins should not be recommended for patients receiving coronary stents (12151).

Asthma. There is some interest in using pyridoxine for asthma in patients who take theophylline. Some research suggests that children with severe asthma might inadequately metabolize tryptophan, indicating inadequate pyridoxine status (8552). Theophylline seems to lower pyridoxine levels (4522,7066,9503). Some clinicians are trying pyridoxine 200-300 mg daily to see if it improves symptoms, but the effectiveness of supplementation is questionable; many patients don't seem to benefit, and studies show conflicting results (7064,7065).

Attention deficit-hyperactivity disorder (ADHD). Preliminary clinical research suggests oral pyridoxine might help ADHD, alone or in combination with high doses of other B vitamins (41,9960). However, research using megadose pyridoxine in combination with other megadose vitamins seems to have no effect on ADHD symptoms (9957).

More evidence is needed to rate pyridoxine for these uses.

Mechanism of Action

Pyridoxine is required for amino acid metabolism. It is also involved in carbohydrate and lipid metabolism (15). In the body, pyridoxine is converted to coenzymes pyridoxal phosphate and pyridoxamine phosphate, in a wide variety of metabolic reactions. These reactions include transamination of amino acids, conversion of tryptophan to niacin, synthesis of gamma-aminobutyric acid (GABA) in the CNS, metabolism of serotonin, norepinephrine and dopamine, metabolism of polyunsaturated fatty acids and phospholipids, and the synthesis of the heme component of hemoglobin (15). Pyridoxine deficiency in adults principally affects the peripheral nerves, skin, mucous membranes, and hematopoietic system. In children, the CNS is also affected. Deficiency can occur in people with uremia, alcoholism, cirrhosis, hyperthyroidism, malabsorption syndromes, congestive heart failure (CHF), and in those receiving certain drugs (15). Pyridoxine is a cofactor for enzymes involved in one of the two pathways for the metabolism of homocysteine. Remethylation of homocysteine to methionine requires folate and vitamin B12 (3047,9407,9409). Folic acid supplements increase the activity of this pathway, lowering fasting homocysteine levels. Pyridoxine is not involved in this pathway and therefore doesn't affect fasting homocysteine levels (3047,9400,9406). Trans-sulfuration of homocysteine to form cystathionine is catalyzed by cystathione-beta-synthase, which is pyridoxine (vitamin B6) dependent (2148,3047,9407,9409). This pathway is primarily active after ingesting a methionine load (i.e., after a meal). Deficiencies of pyridoxine or cystathione-beta-synthase impair this pathway, raising post-methionine load homocysteine levels (1489,2148,9408). Pyridoxine supplements can lower post-methionine load homocysteine levels (1489,3047,7881). Evidence suggests elevated homocysteine levels might cause vascular endothelial cell damage, impaired endothelium dependent vasodilation due to reduced nitric oxide activity, increased oxidation and arterial deposition of low-density lipoproteins (LDL), increased platelet adhesiveness, and activation of the clotting cascade (2147,3047,9403,9408).

Decreased pyridoxine concentrations are associated with increased plasma levels of C-reactive protein (CRP). CRP is an indicator of inflammation that is implicated in increased cardiovascular morbidity (9452).

Pyridoxine has some antioxidant and free radical scavenging activities, which might explain its beneficial effects on tardive dyskinesia (8558). For kidney stones, pyridoxine is thought to be beneficial by decreasing urinary excretion of oxalate in some patients. Most kidney stones are composed of calcium oxalate, and high urinary oxalate has been associated with development and recurrence of kidney stones. In patients with type I primary hyperoxaluria, pyridoxine seems to reduce stone formation by shifting the breakdown of the oxalic acid precursor, glyoxalic acid, to glycine as opposed to oxalic acid (6437,6438,6439,6440,6441,6442,8205). In attention deficit-hyperactivity disorder (ADHD), some kids can have low serotonin levels (41); however, this is controversial (6444). It's thought that pyridoxine can increase serotonin levels and might improve symptoms in some kids with low serotonin levels (41). Some researchers think pyridoxine supplementation might also be useful for some dysphoric mental states because it increases the production of serotonin and GABA, but the evidence is still preliminary (8554). It has been suggested that large doses of vitamin B6 may be useful in carpal tunnel syndrome, based on an observation of low vitamin B6 tissue levels in autopsy specimens from people who had the syndrome (6885). However, tissue levels decline in dead or infarcted tissue and the existence of vitamin B6 deficiency during life cannot be deduced from these observations (6885).

Adverse Reactions

Orally or by injection, pyridoxine can cause nausea, vomiting, abdominal pain, loss of appetite, headache, paresthesia, somnolence, increased serum aspartate transaminase (AST, SGOT), decreased serum folic acid concentrations, skin and other allergic reactions, breast soreness or enlargement, and photosensitivity (8195,9479).

Pyridoxine can cause sensory neuropathy, which is related to daily dose and duration of intake. Doses exceeding 1000 mg daily or total doses of 1000 grams or more pose the most risk, although neuropathy can occur with lower daily or total doses as well (8195). The mechanism of the neurotoxicity is unknown, but is thought to occur when the liver's capacity to phosphorylate pyridoxine, via the active coenzyme pyridoxal phosphate, is exceeded (8204). Some researchers recommend pyridoxal phosphate to avoid pyridoxine neuropathy, but its safety is unknown (8204).

Pyridoxine neuropathy is characterized by numbness and impairment of the sense of position and vibration of the distal limbs, and a gradual progressive sensory ataxia (8196,10439). The syndrome is usually reversible with discontinuation of pyridoxine at the first appearance of neurologic symptoms. Residual symptoms have been reported in patients taking more than 2 grams daily for extended periods (8195,8196). Tell patients daily doses of 100 mg or less are unlikely to cause problems (3094).

High-dose pyridoxine (80 mg/day) and vitamin B12 (20 micrograms/day) may cause rosacea fulminans characterized by intense erythema with nodules, papules, and pustules. Symptoms may persist for up to 4 months after the supplement is stopped, and may require treatment with systemic corticosteroids and topical therapy (10998).

There is some concern that long-term dietary pyridoxine intake in small amounts ranging from 3.56-6.59 mg daily can increase the risk of developing ulcerative colitis (3350). However, this concern is preliminary. It is too soon to suggest that patients cut back on pyridoxine intake.

Interactions with Herbs & Other Dietary Supplements

None known.

Interactions with Drugs

AMIODARONE (Cordarone): Preliminary research suggests that pyridoxine could exacerbate amiodarone-induced photosensitivity. Other research suggests a protective effect (8892,8893).

LEVODOPA: Pyridoxine enhances the metabolism of levodopa, reducing its anti-parkinsonism effects. However, this interaction doesn't occur when carbidopa is used concurrently with levodopa (Sinemet), therefore it isn't likely to be a problem in most people (3046).

PHENOBARBITAL (Luminal): Preliminary data suggests that pyridoxine 200 mg/day can reduce plasma levels of phenobarbital, possibly by increasing metabolism. It isn't known whether lower doses have any effect. Advise people taking phenobarbital drugs to avoid high doses of pyridoxine (3046,10801).

PHENYTOIN (Dilantin): Preliminary data suggests that pyridoxine 200 mg/day can reduce plasma levels of phenytoin, possibly by increasing metabolism. It isn't known whether lower doses have any effect. Advise people taking phenytoin to avoid high doses of pyridoxine (3046,10801).

Drug Influences on Nutrient Levels and Depletion

SOME DRUGS CAN AFFECT PYRIDOXINE LEVELS:

ANTIBIOTICS: Destruction of normal gastrointestinal flora by antibiotics can cause decreased production of B vitamins. The clinical significance of this decreased production is not known. Consider supplementation only if clinical judgment warrants it (4434,4435,4436,4437,4438,4439,4440,4441,4442,4443).

ESTROGENS and ESTROGEN-CONTAINING ORAL CONTRACEPTIVES: Use of estrogens and estrogen-containing oral contraceptives can interfere with pyridoxine metabolism, reducing serum pyridoxine levels. The need for pyridoxine supplementation has not been adequately studied (4498).

HYDRALAZINE (Apresoline): Hydralazine can increase pyridoxine requirements. The need for pyridoxine supplementation has not been adequately studied (4453,4531,4533).
ISONIAZID (INH, Rifamate): Isoniazid can increase pyridoxine requirements. Patients receiving more than 10 mg/kg/day of INH should be supplemented with 50-100 mg of pyridoxine per day (4481,4482).
PENICILLAMINE (Cuprimine): Penicillamine can increase pyridoxine requirements. The need for pyridoxine supplementation has not been adequately studied (4453,4531).
THEOPHYLLINE (Theo-Dur): Theophylline interferes with pyridoxine metabolism (4522,7066). Theophylline can inhibit pyridoxal kinase, which decreases the conversion of pyridoxine into its physiologically active forms (4522,9480,9503). However, the clinical significance of this is not known. Some clinicians try supplementing with pyridoxine 200-300 mg daily in asthmatic patients taking theophylline (7064,7065), but the effectiveness of supplementation is questionable. Many patients don't seem to benefit, and outcomes with pyridoxine supplementation are not consistent (7064,7065).

Interactions with Foods

None known.

Interactions with Lab Tests

UROBILINOGEN: Pyridoxine can cause a false positive result in the spot test with Ehrlich's reagent (15).

Interactions with Diseases or Conditions

ANGIOPLASTY: An intravenous loading dose of folic acid, vitamin B6 and vitamin B12 followed by oral administration of folic acid 1.2 mcg plus vitamin B6 48 mg and vitamin B12 60 mcg taken daily after coronary stenting might actually increase restenosis rates (12150). Due to the potential for harm this combination of vitamins should not be recommended for patients receiving coronary stents (12151).

Dosage and Administration

ORAL: For vitamin B6 deficiency in adults, the typical dose is 2.5-25 mg daily for three weeks, then 1.5-2.5 mg per day as maintenance therapy (15). For vitamin B6 deficiency in women taking oral contraceptives, the dose is 25-30 mg per day (15). For symptoms associated with premenstrual syndrome (PMS), the daily dose is 50-100 mg. Doses as high as 500 mg per day have been used, but daily doses over 100 mg don't appear to have additional benefit, and may increase the risk for adverse effects (3093). For hereditary sideroblastic anemia, initially 200-600 mg per day is used, decreasing to 30-50 mg daily after an adequate response (15). For metabolic disorders, including xanthurenic aciduria, primary cystathioninuria, or primary homocystinuria, 100-500 mg daily is generally effective (15). For post-prandial hyperhomocysteinemia, 50 to 200 mg of pyridoxine used alone or a combination of pyridoxine 100 mg and folic acid 0.5 mg has been used daily (1489,9406,10350). For kidney stones, 25-500 mg daily has been used (6437,6439). For primary hyperoxaluria, 2 to 200 mg has been used (6439,6440). When used with magnesium for preventing kidney stones, pyridoxine 10 mg daily has been used in combination with magnesium 300 mg daily (1201). For preventing anemia due to pyridoxine deficiency or neuritis in people receiving isoniazid or penicillamine, the typical dose is 10-50 mg daily (15). For treating tardive dyskinesia, 100 mg per day has been titrated weekly up to 400 mg per day, given in two divided doses (8558). For preventing seizures in people receiving cycloserine, 100-300 mg is taken daily in divided doses (15). For nausea during pregnancy, 10-25 mg pyridoxine every eight hours has been used (6167,6168); alternatively, 75 mg of sustained-release pyridoxine combined with 12 mcg vitamin B12 (cyanocobalamin), 1 mg folic acid, and 200 mg calcium (PremesisRx) is used daily as an FDA-approved prescription supplement for nausea during pregnancy (23). For hyperkinetic cerebral dysfunction syndrome in children, 300 mg daily has been used in a clinical trial. However, some children can require larger dosages ranging from 500 mg to 2 grams daily (3351). To decrease the rate of restenosis after coronary angioplasty, a combination of pyridoxine 10 mg plus vitamin B12 400 mcg and folic acid 1 mg taken daily has been used (8008). The daily recommended dietary allowances (RDAs) of vitamin B6 are: Infants 0-6 months, 0.1 mg; Infants 7-12 months, 0.3 mg; Children 1-3 years, 0.5 mg; Children 4-8 years, 0.6 mg; Children 9-13 years, 1 mg; Males 14-50 years, 1.3 mg; Males over 50 years, 1.7 mg; Females 14-18 years, 1.2 mg; Females 19-50 years, 1.3 mg; Females over 50 years, 1.5 mg; Pregnant women, 1.9 mg; and Lactating women, 2 mg (3094). Some researchers think the RDA for women 19-50 years should be increased to 1.5-1.7 mg per day (8556). The recommended maximum daily intake is: Children 1-3 years, 30 mg; Children 4-8 years, 40 mg; Children 9-13 years, 60 mg; Adults, pregnant and lactating women, 14-18 years, 80 mg; and Adults, pregnant and lactating women, over 18 years, 100 mg (3094).
INJECTION: This is an FDA-approved prescription product that is available as a 100 mg/mL injection. For seizures in neonates and infants, 10 to 100 mg pyridoxine IV or IM is recommended (15).

Comments

Pyridoxine is present in many foods including cereal grains, legumes, vegetables, liver, meat, and eggs (15). Pyridoxine is frequently used in combination with other B vitamins in vitamin B complex formulations. Vitamin B complex generally includes vitamin B1 (thiamine), vitamin B2 (riboflavin), vitamin B3 (niacin/niacinamide), vitamin B5 (pantothenic acid), vitamin B6 (pyridoxine), vitamin B12 (cyanocobalamin), and folic acid. However, some products do not contain all of these ingredients and some may include others, such as biotin, para-aminobenzoic acid (PABA), choline bitartrate, and inositol (3022). Pyridoxine and the sedative antihistamine doxylamine were ingredients in Bendectin, a widely-prescribed antinausea product for use in pregnancy. The product was removed from the US market in 1983 due to litigation costs. A similar product, Diclectin, has remained available in Canada. Animal studies have disclosed no teratogenic potential or pyridoxine or Bendectin. Following removal of Bendectin from the market, there was no reduction in birth defects, but a doubling in hospitalization rates for pregnancy-related nausea and vomiting (8195).

PYRUVATE

Also Known As

2-Oxypropanoic Acid, Acetylformic Acid, Alpha-Keto Acid, Alpha-Ketopropionic Acid, Calcium Pyruvate, Magnesium Pyruvate, Potassium Pyruvate, Proacemic Acid, Pyruvic Acid, Sodium Pyruvate.

Scientific Names

2-Oxopropanoate (pyruvate); 2-oxopropanoic acid (pyruvic acid).

People Use This For

Orally, pyruvate is used for weight loss, improving exercise endurance, and inhibiting tumor growth.
Topically, pyruvic acid is used for signs of aging skin such as wrinkles.

Safety

POSSIBLY SAFE ...when used orally and appropriately, short-term. There is some evidence that pyruvate can be safely used for up to 6 weeks (2472,2474). ...when used topically and appropriately. There is some evidence that a 50% pyruvic acid skin peel can be safely applied by a health professional (12020).
PREGNANCY AND LACTATION: Insufficient reliable information available; avoid using.

Effectiveness

POSSIBLY EFFECTIVE

Aging skin. Applying a 50% pyruvic acid skin peel once a week for 4 weeks seems to smooth skin, decrease fine wrinkles, and decrease hyperpigmentation associated with photoaging (12020).

Weight loss. Taking pyruvate orally in place of a portion of dietary carbohydrates and in combination with a low calorie diet seems to help increase weight loss (2472,2474).

Mechanism of Action

Pyruvic acid is an alpha-keto acid which is converted to the alpha-hydroxy acid lactic acid. It seems to be helpful for aging skin by exfoliating the surface layers of skin (12020).
Some evidence suggests that pyruvate reduces free radical production (2487), increases lipid oxidation, and decreases carbohydrate oxidation (2488).
Very small clinical trials suggest dietary supplementation with dihydroxyacetone and pyruvate increases arm and leg exercise endurance (807,808).
Very preliminary evidence also suggests a liquid diet supplemented with pyruvate might inhibit tumor growth (806).

Adverse Reactions

Intravenously, one death was associated with pyruvate use in a child with restrictive cardiomyopathy (2473).
Topically, applying pyruvic acid as a facial peel can cause an intense burning sensation. It should only be applied over small areas. Vapors have been reported to cause respiratory irritation and should only be applied in a room with adequate ventilation (12020).

Interactions with Herbs & Other Dietary Supplements

None known.

Interactions with Drugs

None known.

Interactions with Foods

None known.

Interactions with Lab Tests

None known.

Interactions with Diseases or Conditions

CARDIOMYOPATHY: One death was associated with intravenous use in a child with restrictive cardiomyopathy (2473).

Dosage and Administration

ORAL: For weight loss 22 to 44 grams per day, as an adjunct to a low-cholesterol, low-fat diet has been used (2474).
TOPICAL: For aging skin, a 50% pyruvic acid peel applied once weekly for 4 weeks has been used (12020).

QUASSIA

Also Known As

Amargo, Bitter-Ash, Bitter Wood, Bitterwood, Jamaican Quassia, Picrasma, Quassia Bark, Ruda, Surinam Quassia, Surinam Wood.

Scientific Names

Quassia amara; Picrasma excelsa.
Family: Simaroubaceae.

People Use This For

Orally, quassia is used for anorexia; indigestion; constipation; fever; as an anthelmintic for thread worms, nematodes, and ascaris; as a tonic or purgative; and as a mouthwash.
Topically, quassia is used for pediculosis.
Rectally, quassia is used for nematode infestation.
In manufacturing, quassia is used as a flavoring agent in foods, beverages, pastilles, lozenges, and laxatives. The bark and wood have been used as an insecticide.

Safety

POSSIBLY SAFE ...when used in amounts commonly found in foods. Quassia has Generally Recognized As Safe (GRAS) status in the US (4912).
POSSIBLY UNSAFE ...when used orally in therapeutic amounts. Quassia wood contains cardioactive glycosides (4), but toxicity is likely limited by emetic effects of large doses (4).
There is insufficient reliable information available about the safety of the topical or rectal use of quassia.
PREGNANCY AND LACTATION: LIKELY UNSAFE ...when used orally; avoid using. Quassia has cytotoxic and emetic properties (4,18,19). There is insufficient reliable information available about the safety of rectal or topical use during pregnancy or lactation; avoid using.

Effectiveness

POSSIBLY EFFECTIVE

Lice. Applying quassia tincture topically to the scalp seems to be an effective treatment for head lice (4).
There is insufficient reliable information available about the effectiveness of quassia for its other uses.

Mechanism of Action

The applicable part of quassia is the wood (4,8,11). Quassia leaves are also reportedly used (6). Quassia contains quassinoids that have potent bitter properties (11). Quassia also contains beta-carboline alkaloids, quassin, quassimarin, canthin-6-one (4), and small amounts of the coumarin scopoletin (4). The quassinoid constituents increase gastric acid and bile secretions, perhaps accounting for appetite stimulant and digestive effects (18,19,4). There is evidence that the beta-carboline alkaloids might have positive inotropic activity (4). The constituent canthin-6-one is reported to have antibacterial, antifungal, and cytotoxic activity (4). Quassimarin demonstrates evidence of antileukemic (11) and antitumor effects (18,4). Quassin demonstrates antilarval activity against Culex quinquefasciatus (mosquito) (3302).

Adverse Reactions

Quassia can cause mucous membrane irritation, nausea, and vomiting (4,18). Long-term use can cause vision changes and blindness (18).

Interactions with Herbs & Other Dietary Supplements

CARDIOACTIVE GLYCOSIDE-CONTAINING HERBS: Theoretically, concomitant use with other cardiac glycoside-containing herbs might increase risk of cardiac toxicity. Cardiac glycoside containing herbs include black hellebore, Canadian hemp roots, digitalis leaf, hedge mustard, figwort, lily of the valley roots, motherwort, oleander leaf, pheasant's eye plant, pleurisy root, squill bulb leaf scales, and strophanthus seeds (19).
CARDIOACTIVE HERBS: Avoid concomitant use with other cardioactive herbs due to unpredictability of effects and adverse effects. Other cardioactive herbs include calamus, cereus, cola, coltsfoot, devil's claw, European mistletoe, fenugreek, fumitory, ginger, Panax ginseng, hawthorn, white horehound, mate, parsley, scotch broom flower, shepherd's purse, and wild carrot (4).

STIMULANT LAXATIVE HERBS: Theoretically, abuse might increase risk of cardiac toxicity due to potassium depletion. Stimulant laxative herbs include aloe dried leaf sap, blue flag rhizome, alder buckthorn, European buckthorn, butternut bark, cascara bark, castor oil, colocynth fruit pulp, gamboge bark exudate, jalap root, black root, manna bark exudate, podophyllum root, rhubarb root, senna leaves and pods, wild cucumber fruit (Ecballium elaterium), and yellow dock root (19).

Interactions with Drugs

ANTACIDS: Theoretically, due to reports that quassia increases stomach acid, quassia might decrease the effectiveness of antacids (19).
DIGOXIN (Lanoxin): Theoretically, concomitant use with cardiac medications might increase the risk of therapeutic and adverse effects (4).
DIURETIC DRUGS: Overuse of quassia might compound diuretic-induced potassium loss (13). There is some concern that people taking quassia along with potassium depleting diuretics might have an increased risk for hypokalemia. Initiation of potassium supplementation or an increase in potassium supplement dose may be necessary for some patients. Some diuretics that can deplete potassium include chlorothiazide (Diuril), chlorthalidone (Thalitone), furosemide (Lasix), and hydrochlorothiazide (HCTZ, HydroDIURIL, Microzide), and others.
H2-BLOCKERS: Theoretically, due to reports that quassia increases stomach acid, quassia might decrease the effectiveness of H2-blockers (19). The H2 blockers include cimetidine (Tagamet), ranitidine (Zantac), nizatidine (Axid), and famotidine (Pepcid).
PROTON PUMP INHIBITORS (PPIs): Theoretically, due to reports that quassia increases stomach acid, quassia might decrease the effectiveness of PPIs (19). PPIs include omeprazole (Prilosec), lansoprazole (Prevacid), rabeprazole (Aciphex), pantoprazole (Protonix), and esomeprazole (Nexium).

Interactions with Foods

None known.

Interactions with Lab Tests

None known.

Interactions with Diseases or Conditions

GI IRRITATION AND INFLAMMATION: In large amounts quassia can irritate the gastrointestinal tract; avoid using (8).

Dosage and Administration

ORAL: A typical dose is one cup tea 2-3 times daily (12). To make tea, simmer 1-2 grams of wood in 150 mL boiling water 10-15 minutes, strain (12).
RECTAL: As an enema (1:20), 150 mL is typically used rectally every morning for 3 days with 16 gram magnesium sulfate orally (4).
TOPICAL: No typical dosage.

Comments

Quassia bark has been used as an insecticide (11).

QUEBRACHO

Also Known As

Quebracho Blanco, White Quebracho.

Scientific Names

Aspidosperma quebracho-blanco.
Family: Apocynaceae.

People Use This For

Orally, quebracho is used for asthma and conditions of the lower respiratory tract. It is also used as an expectorant and respiratory tract stimulant. Sometimes it is used to lower blood pressure (particularly arterial hypertension), as a spasmolytic, diuretic, peripheral vasoconstrictor, uterine sedative, local anesthetic, to decrease fever, and as an aphrodisiac.
In foods and beverages, it is used as a flavoring agent.

Safety

LIKELY SAFE ...when used in amounts commonly found in foods. Quebracho has Generally Recognized As Safe (GRAS) status in the US (4912).
There is insufficient reliable information available about the safety of quebracho bark in medicinal amounts.
PREGNANCY AND LACTATION: There is insufficient reliable information about the safety of medicinal amounts of quebracho during pregnancy and breast-feeding; avoid using.

Effectiveness

There is insufficient reliable information available about the effectiveness of quebracho.

Mechanism of Action

The applicable part of quebracho is the bark. There is insufficient reliable information available about the possible mechanism of action and active ingredients.

Adverse Reactions

Orally, people who take quebracho bark may experience side effects including salivation, headache, outbreaks of sweating, vertigo, stupor and sleepiness. In large doses, it can cause nausea and vomiting (18).

Interactions with Herbs & Other Dietary Supplements

None known.

Interactions with Drugs

None known.

Interactions with Foods

None known.

Interactions with Lab Tests

None known.

Interactions with Diseases or Conditions

None known.

Dosage and Administration

ORAL: It is used as an extract or powder and in combination bronchial preparations (18).

Comments

The bark is odorless and has a bitter taste. Quebracho Colorado or red quebracho is also known as quebracho, but is chemically distinct from white quebracho. Be careful not to confuse these two plants (11).

QUEEN'S DELIGHT

Also Known As

Cockup Hat, Marcory, Queens Delight, Queen's Root, Queens Root, Silver Leaf, Stillingia, Yaw Root.

Scientific Names

Stillingia sylvatica, synonym Stillingia tenuis.
Family: Euphorbiaceae.

People Use This For

Orally, queen's delight is used as a "blood purifier"; for digestive disorders; treatment of hepatic, gallbladder, and skin diseases; and as an emetic and laxative. Queen's delight is also used orally for bronchitis, laryngitis, laryngismus stridulus, and constipation.
Topically, queen's delight is used for cutaneous eruptions, hemorrhoids, and exudative skin eruptions with lymphatic involvement.

Safety

POSSIBLY UNSAFE ...when used orally in medicinal amounts; the dried root preparations contain diterpene esters that are highly irritating (4,12). Queen's delight might activate latent viruses, and it might be carcinogenic (18). ...when the dried or fresh root preparations are used topically (4).
LIKELY UNSAFE ...when the fresh root is used orally; it contains a caustic white latex that is highly irritating to

mucous membranes (12).
PREGNANCY: POSSIBLY UNSAFE ...when the dried root preparations are used orally. ...when the dried or fresh root is used topically; avoid using (4). LIKELY UNSAFE ...when the fresh root preparations are used orally (12).
LACTATION: POSSIBLY UNSAFE ...when the dried or fresh root are used topically. LIKELY UNSAFE ...when used orally; contraindicated (4,12,19).

Effectiveness
There is insufficient reliable information available about the effectiveness of queen's delight.

Mechanism of Action
The applicable part of queen's delight is the root. Queen's delight contains a volatile oil and diterpenes including prostatin, gnidilatidin, and others (18). Diterpene esters, isolated in the latex (or milky juice) of the fresh or green root, are potent irritants that cause swelling of the skin and mucous membranes (4,18). Diterpenes may also be carcinogenic agents; they are believed able to activate latent viruses (18).

Adverse Reactions
Orally, queen's delight can cause vomiting, diarrhea, and nausea (18,19). In large amounts, it may cause a burning sensation of the mouth, throat, diarrhea, nausea, vomiting, dysuria, aches and pains, pruritus, skin eruptions, cough, depression, fatigue, and perspiration (4).
Topically, it may cause inflammation, swelling, and contact dermatitis (18,19).

Interactions with Herbs & Other Dietary Supplements
None known.

Interactions with Drugs
None known.

Interactions with Foods
None known.

Interactions with Lab Tests
None known.

Interactions with Diseases or Conditions
GASTROINTESTINAL (GI) CONDITIONS: Queen's delight is contraindicated in individuals with GI irritation, inflammation, nausea or vomiting (19).

Dosage and Administration
ORAL: People typically prepare queen's delight as a liquid, boiling 1 teaspoon of the dried root with one cup of water. The suggested dose is a cup a day, taken a mouthful at a time. As a tincture, queen's delight is taken in a dose of 5 to 20 drops (5263).

QUERCETIN

Also Known As
Citrus Bioflavonoid, Citrus Bioflavonoids, Flavonoid, Meletin, Sophretin.
CAUTION: See separate listings for Chrysin, Diosmin, Hesperidin, Methoxylated Flavones, and Rutin.

Scientific Names
3,3',4'5,7-Penthydroxyflavone.

People Use This For
Orally, quercetin is used for treating atherosclerosis; hypercholesterolemia; coronary heart disease; vascular insufficiency; diabetes; cataracts; allergies; allergic rhinitis; peptic ulcer; schizophrenia; inflammation; asthma; gout; viral infections; preventing cancer; and for treating chronic, bacterial prostatitis.
Intravenously and intraperitoneally, quercetin is used for treating cancer.

Safety
POSSIBLY SAFE ...when used orally in amounts up to 500 mg twice daily for up to one month (481). ...when used intravenously in amounts less than 945 mg/m2 (9564).
LIKELY UNSAFE ...when used intravenously in amounts greater that 945 mg/m2 which are reported to cause nephrotoxicity (9564).

There is insufficient reliable information available about the safety of intraperitoneal quercetin, or quercetin used orally in larger doses or long-term.

PREGNANCY AND LACTATION: Insufficient reliable information available; avoid using.

Effectiveness

POSSIBLY EFFECTIVE

Prostatitis. Taking quercetin orally seems to reduce pain and improve quality of life, but does not seem to affect voiding dysfunction in patients with chronic, nonbacterial prostatitis (481).

INSUFFICIENT RELIABLE EVIDENCE to RATE

Coronary heart disease. There is preliminary evidence that increasing dietary intake of quercetin might reduce the risk of coronary heart disease mortality in elderly men (7726).

Hypercholesterolemia. Short-term use of quercetin supplements for 1 month does not appear to reduce low-density lipoprotein (LDL) cholesterol, total cholesterol, or increase high-density lipoprotein (HDL) cholesterol (1998,1999).

More evidence is needed to rate quercetin for these uses.

Mechanism of Action

Quercetin is a dietary flavonoid found in many plants (481,483,1995). Buckwheat tea has a high concentration of quercetin. The most common form of quercetin is rutin, in which quercetin is bound to a glucose-rhamnose moiety. Quercetin is also found bound to one or two glucose molecules (monoglycoside and diglycoside forms) (9442,9443). Quercetin has antioxidant, anti-inflammatory, nitric oxide inhibitor, and tyrosine kinase inhibitor (leading to inhibition of the division and growth of T-cells and some cancer cells) activity (481,1995). The anti-inflammatory effects of quercetin might be due to inhibition of the production and activity of leukotrienes and prostaglandins, and inhibition of histamine release by basophils and mast cells (483). Preliminary evidence suggests that quercetin might work similarly to cromolyn, inhibiting antigen-stimulated histamine release from mast cells of patients with allergic rhinitis (9176). Quercetin also appears to reduce capillary fragility, and it might offer some protection against diabetic cataracts, possibly by inhibiting aldose reductase in the lens (483,9563). The anti-inflammatory and antioxidant effects might be responsible for the observed benefits in men with chronic, nonbacterial prostatitis (481).

Quercetin might reduce cancer risk by inactivating malignant precursors or by inhibiting carcinogenesis (9563). Preliminary studies suggest it might have inhibitory effects on various cancer types, including breast, leukemia, colon, ovary, oral squamous cell, endometrial, gastric and non-small-cell lung (483,485). Quercetin has antiestrogenic effects in cultures of breast cancer cells (484). It also inhibits estrone sulfatase and estrogen synthesis in liver cells (489). Existing evidence suggests quercetin alters intestinal cell homeostasis of copper, iron, and manganese (1997). Although researchers believe quercetin might protect against heart disease (1995), short term supplementation does not show affect on any of the known risk factors for heart disease (1998,1999). Preliminary evidence suggests that quercetin might inhibit collagen- and ADP-induced platelet aggregation, but at concentrations much higher than those achieved with typical oral dosing (1999). Quercetin seems to inhibit the ability of monocytes to attach to vascular endothelial cells, which may reduce atherosclerosis (9444).

Evidence also suggests that quercetin might benefit some people with schizophrenia when used in combination with other antioxidants, intestinal adsorbents, and conventional therapy (1996). Quercetin demonstrates activity against retroviruses, Herpes simplex, polio, parainfluenza, and respiratory syncytial viruses (483).

The oral absorption of quercetin is highly variable, depending on the source (481,486,487).

These glycoside forms of quercetin are not absorbed from the gastrointestinal tract and must be hydrolyzed, permitting absorption of the aglycone form of quercetin. The hydrolysis of quercetin glycosides occurs efficiently and completely, resulting in 64 to 80% bioavailability of quercetin (9442).

The time to maximum plasma concentration (Tmax) after oral administration of aglycone quercetin is dose-dependent. After an oral dose of 8, 20, or 50 mg, the Tmax is 1.9, 2.7, or 4.9 hours, respectively. The half-life of quercetin is 15 to 17 hours. However, it appears that quercetin is conjugated in the intestine (9174). In plasma, quercetin is found primarily as glucuronide or sulfate form (9175,9442). In vitro research has been done with unconjugated quercetin. It is questionable whether free quercetin absorption is sufficient to exert a pharmacologic effect. Research in humans suggests that quercetin taken orally doesn't reach serum concentrations at which in vitro activity has been seen (9174). Plasma protein binding might also affect the activity of quercetin (481,486,487).

Plasma concentrations of quercetin glucuronide, sulfate, or unconjugated quercetin aglycone from the glycoside rutin appear to be higher in women than men. When administered as quercetin aglycone, however, there are no bioavailability differences between men and women. Quercetin is absorbed from different parts of the intestines when given as quercetin aglycone or rutin, but the sex differences in bioavailability are not completely understood (9442).

Adverse Reactions

Orally, quercetin can cause headache and tingling of the extremities (481).

Intravenous administration of quercetin is associated with flushing, sweating, dyspnea, nausea, and vomiting (9564). Injection pain can be minimized by premedicating patient with 10 mg of morphine and administering amounts greater than 945 mg/m2 over 5 minutes (9564). Nephrotoxicity has been reported with use of amounts greater than 945 mg/m2 (9563,9564).

Interactions with Herbs & Other Dietary Supplements
None known.

Interactions with Drugs
QUINOLONE ANTIBIOTICS: Quercetin might competitively inhibit quinolone antibiotics by binding to the DNA gyrase site on bacteria (481).

Interactions with Foods
None known.

Interactions with Lab Tests
None known.

Interactions with Diseases or Conditions
KIDNEY DYSFUNCTION: Theoretically, intravenous quercetin may exacerbate kidney dysfunction (9563,9564).

Dosage and Administration
ORAL: A common dose is 400-500 mg three times daily (483). For prostatitis, 500 mg twice daily has been used (481).
INTRAVENOUS: For treating cancer, 420-1400 mg/m2 by IV bolus weekly or in 3-week intervals has been used (9564).
INTRAPERITONEAL: No typical dosage.

Comments
Quercetin is a dietary flavonoid that occurs abundantly in red wine, tea, onions, green tea, apples, berries, and brassica vegetables (481,483,1995,7726). Quercetin is also found in Ginkgo biloba, St. John's Wort (Hypericum perforatum) and American Elder (Sambucus canadensis) (483).

QUILLAIA

Also Known As
China Bark, Murillo Bark, Panama Bark, Quillaja, Soapbark, Soap Tree, Soap Tree Bark.

Scientific Names
Quillaja saponaria.
Family: Rosaceae.

People Use This For
Orally, quillaia inner bark is used for cough, bronchitis, and pulmonary ailments.
Topically, quillaia extract is used to treat skin sores, athletes foot, itchy scalp, in shampoos for dandruff, in hair tonic preparations, in douches, and for leukorrhea.
In foods, quillaia is used in frozen dairy desserts, candy, baked goods, gelatins, and puddings.
In manufacturing, quillaia extracts are used in dermatological creams, as foaming agents in root beer, in beverages, and cocktails. Quillaia is also used as a foaming agent in fire extinguishers.

Safety
LIKELY SAFE ...when used in amounts commonly found in foods. Quillaia has Generally Recognized As Safe (GRAS) status in the US (4912).
POSSIBLY UNSAFE ...when used orally in medicinal amounts. Quillaia is a gastrointestinal tract irritant that contains oxalates and tannins. Large amounts can cause liver damage, respiratory failure, convulsions, and coma (12). There is insufficient reliable information available about the safety of the topical or vaginal use of quillaia.
PREGNANCY AND LACTATION: POSSIBLY UNSAFE ...when used in medicinal amounts (12); avoid using.

Effectiveness
There is insufficient reliable information available about the effectiveness of quillaia.

Mechanism of Action
The applicable part of quillaia is the inner bark. Quillaia contains tannins, oxalates, and saponins. Tannins possess strong astringent properties (7,12). Upon contact, they dehydrate the external layer of tissue, reducing internal secretions, and forming external cells into a protective layer (12). Plants with at least 10% tannins, like quillaia (19) can cause gastrointestinal disturbances, kidney damage, and necrotic conditions of the liver (12). Some evidence suggests that tannins might cause cancer; other evidence shows they might prevent it (12). Regular consumption of

herbs with high tannin concentrations correlates with increased incidence of esophageal or nasal cancer (12). When ingested, oxalates combine with calcium in the blood forming insoluble oxalates and depleting available calcium, potentially to deficiency levels. Insoluble calcium oxalate, deposited in the kidneys can cause mechanical damage. Precipitation of calcium oxalate in renal tubules can result in acute renal failure (12). Some evidence suggests saponins might cause red blood cell hemolysis and GI irritation (11). Other evidence suggests they might have anti-inflammatory, antimicrobial, and cytotoxic effects (11). They also possess expectorant properties, can induce sneezing, and can depress cardiac and respiratory activity (6,11). Preliminary information suggests quillaia saponins can reduce the rate of absorption of bile salts (3850), suggesting they might be effective in reducing cholesterol levels (11). QS-21, an isolated saponin from the bark, appears to be a potent immuno-stimulatory complex adjuvant when administered with vaccines (6). It shows evidence that it might augment both antibody and cell-mediated immune responses (3851), significantly increasing antibody levels (6). For this reason it is being evaluated in HIV patients (11). Another purified saponin, DS-1, is being investigated as a pharmaceutical excipient in nasal and ocular delivery of insulin (3852), and also as a transmucosal delivery agent for the aminoglycoside antibiotics (3853).

Adverse Reactions

Orally, large amounts of quillaia are associated with liver damage, diarrhea, respiratory failure, stomach pain, convulsions, coma (12), red blood cell hemolysis (11), and renal failure (12).
If inhaled, the powder can cause sneezing (6). It also can be caustic to mucosa (12).

Interactions with Herbs & Other Dietary Supplements

CALCIUM, IRON, ZINC: Concurrent use might decrease mineral absorption. Quillaia contains oxalate (7,12), which can bind multivalent metal ions in the gastrointestinal tract and decrease mineral absorption.

Interactions with Drugs

METFORMIN (Glucophage): Quillaia might reduce efficacy of metformin (Glucophage) (7). Quillaia contains tannins that might decrease the absorption of metformin by forming insoluble complexes.
ORAL DRUGS: Theoretically, the tannin content might delay absorption of sedatives, hypnotics, antidepressants, and tranquilizers due to tannin content (7,19).

Interactions with Foods

CALCIUM, IRON, ZINC: Concurrent use might decrease mineral absorption from foods. Quillaia contains oxalate (7,12), which can bind multivalent metal ions in the gastrointestinal tract and decrease mineral absorption.

Interactions with Lab Tests

None known.

Interactions with Diseases or Conditions

GI CONDITIONS: Contraindicated in individuals with gastrointestinal inflammation or irritation due to irritant properties (18).
KIDNEY DISEASE: Contraindicated in individuals with kidney disease or a history of kidney stones due to oxalate content (12,19).

Dosage and Administration

ORAL: A typical dose is 200 mg prepared as tea (12).
TOPICAL: No typical dosage.

Comments

In South America, quillaia bark is used to wash clothes (6).

QUINCE

Also Known As

Cognassier, Coing, Marmelo, Membrillo, Quitte, Quittenbaum.

Scientific Names

Cydonia oblongata, synonyms Cydonia vulgaris, Pyrus cydonia.
Family: Rosaceae.

People Use This For

Orally, quince is used for digestive disorders, diarrhea, coughs, and gastrointestinal inflammation.
Topically, quince is used as a compress or poultice for injuries, inflammation of the joints, injuries of the nipples, and gashed or deeply cut fingers. A topical lotion is used to soothe the eyes.

Safety
There is insufficient reliable information available about the safety of quince.
Pregnancy and Lactation: Insufficient reliable information available; avoid using.

Effectiveness
There is insufficient reliable information available about the effectiveness of quince.

Mechanism of Action
The applicable part of quince is the seed. The seeds contain cyanogenic glycosides as amygdalin at 0.4-1.5%, or 27-75 mg cyanide per 100 grams of seeds, suggesting potential toxicity (18).

Adverse Reactions
None reported.

Interactions with Herbs & Other Dietary Supplements
None known.

Interactions with Drugs
ORAL DRUGS: Quince may impair absorption of concomitantly administered medications due to the high mucilage fiber in quince seeds (19).

Interactions with Foods
NUTRIENTS: Quince may reduce serum nutrient levels due to possible binding by the high water-soluble fiber content of quince seed (19).

Interactions with Lab Tests
None known.

Interactions with Diseases or Conditions
None known.

Dosage and Administration
ORAL: Quince seed is taken as a powder, extract, or tea. The tea is prepared by steeping 1 teaspoon of whole seeds in 150 mL of boiling water for 10-15 minutes and straining (18).
TOPICAL: A viscous poultice is prepared from the ground seeds (18).

RADISH

Also Known As
Radis, Raphani sativi radix, Small Radish, Turnip Radish.

Scientific Names
Raphanus sativus.
Family: Brassicaceae/Cruciferae.

People Use This For
Orally, radish is used for peptic disorders, dyskinesia of the bile ducts, loss of appetite, inflammation of the mouth and pharynx, tendency towards infections, inflammation or excessive mucus of the respiratory tract, bronchitis, fever, colds, and cough.

Safety
LIKELY SAFE ...when used orally in moderate amounts (18). Large amounts may lead to gastrointestinal irritation (18).
PREGNANCY AND LACTATION: Insufficient reliable information available; avoid very large doses.

Effectiveness
There is insufficient reliable information available about the effectiveness of radish.

Mechanism of Action
The applicable part of radish is the root. Radish root stimulates secretions in the upper GI tract, promotes motility, stimulates bile flow, and has antimicrobial effects (2,18).

Adverse Reactions
Orally, large amounts of radish may cause irritation of the gastrointestinal mucus membrane (18).

Interactions with Herbs & Other Dietary Supplements
None known.

Interactions with Drugs
None known.

Interactions with Foods
None known.

Interactions with Lab Tests
None known.

Interactions with Diseases or Conditions
CHOLELITHIASIS: Radish is contraindicated, because it might cause biliary colic (18).

Dosage and Administration
ORAL: A typical dosage is 0.5 tablespoons pressed root juice, several times daily; up to 50-100 mL per day (18).

RASPBERRY leaf

Also Known As
Framboise, Red Raspberry, Rubi idaei folium, Rubus.
CAUTION: See separate listing for Blackberry leaf.

Scientific Names
Rubus idaeus, synonym Rubus buschii; Rubus strigosus.
Family: Rosaceae.

People Use This For
Orally, raspberry leaf is used for GI tract disorders, upper and lower respiratory tract disorders, cardiovascular system disorders, influenza, fever, diabetes, vitamin deficiency, as a diaphoretic or diuretic, for stimulating bile production, "purification of skin and blood", diarrhea, dysmenorrhea, menorrhagia, morning sickness associated with pregnancy, preventing miscarriage, and facilitating labor and delivery.
Topically, raspberry leaf is used for inflammation of the mouth and throat, and skin rash and inflammation.
In foods, raspberry leaf in small quantities is a source of natural flavoring in Europe.

Safety
LIKELY SAFE ...when used orally in amounts commonly found in foods.
POSSIBLY SAFE ...when used orally or topically and appropriately in medicinal amounts (12).
PREGNANCY: POSSIBLY SAFE ...when used orally and appropriately in medicinal amounts during late pregnancy and under the supervision of a healthcare provider. Raspberry leaf is commonly used by nurse midwives to facilitate delivery. There is some evidence that raspberry leaf can be safely used for this purpose (6481,9796). Make sure patients do not use raspberry leaf without the guidance of a health care professional. LIKELY UNSAFE ...when used orally in medicinal amounts throughout pregnancy or for self-treatment. Raspberry leaf can cause uterine contractions (19) and might have estrogenic effects (6180). These effects can adversely affect pregnancy. Tell pregnant patients not to use raspberry leaf at any time during pregnancy without the close supervision of a healthcare provider.
LACTATION: There is insufficient reliable information available about the safety of raspberry leaf in medicinal amounts while breast-feeding; avoid using.

Effectiveness
POSSIBLY INEFFECTIVE

Labor facilitation. Taking raspberry leaf orally does not seem to reduce the length of labor or decrease the need for analgesics in the perinatal time period (9796).

There is insufficient reliable information available about the effectiveness of raspberry leaf for its other uses.

Mechanism of Action
Raspberry leaf contains a high tannin content (13-15%), which is responsible for its astringent properties (4). When applied topically to skin or mucous membranes tannins cause capillary vasoconstriction, decreased vascular

permeability, and a local anti-inflammatory effect (7). The effects of raspberry leaf on smooth muscle, such as that found in the uterus seems to be variable. Different constituents found in raspberry leaf seem to either stimulate or contract uterine smooth muscle. When used in humans, raspberry leaf might have either stimulatory or spasmolytic effects. There is some evidence that these effects might be dose and tissue dependent. For example, in low doses raspberry leaf might cause more contraction, while higher doses might have spasmolytic effects and decrease contraction. Also, raspberry might decrease contraction of tonic tissues and increase contraction of relaxed tissues (1096,1122). Raspberry leaf might also have some estrogenic effects. In an animal model, raspberry leaf seems to increase serum ceruloplasmin oxidase activity, which is a measure of estrogenic activity in the liver (6180).

Adverse Reactions

None reported.

Interactions with Herbs & Other Dietary Supplements

IRON, CALCIUM, MAGNESIUM: Theoretically, concomitant use may decrease mineral absorption due to tannin content (7).

Interactions with Drugs

METFORMIN (Glucophage): Raspberry leaf might reduce efficacy of metformin (Glucophage) (7). Raspberry leaf contains tannins that might decrease the absorption of metformin by forming insoluble complexes.
ORAL DRUGS: Theoretically, the tannin content of raspberry leaf may modify absorption of sedatives, hypnotics, antidepressants, and tranquilizers (19).

Interactions with Foods

None known.

Interactions with Lab Tests

None known.

Interactions with Diseases or Conditions

HORMONE SENSITIVE CANCERS/CONDITIONS: Because raspberry leaf might have estrogenic effects (6180), women with hormone sensitive conditions should avoid raspberry leaf. Some of these conditions include breast, uterine, and ovarian cancer, and endometriosis and uterine fibroids.

Dosage and Administration

ORAL: For facilitating labor, midwives typically prescribe raspberry leaf tea prepared by steeping 2 grams dried leaf in 240 mL of boiling water for 5 minutes and then straining (1122). Doses for other uses are typically one cup of tea up to 6 times daily. The tea is prepared by steeping 1.5 grams (approximately 2 teaspoons) of finely cut leaves in 150 mL boiling water 5 minutes and then straining (18). Alternatively, soak finely cut leaves in cold water for 2 hours and then strain (3). A liquid extract (1:1 in 25% alcohol) is also often used and dosed as 4-8 mL three times daily (4). Raspberry leaf tablets 2.4 grams per day have been used for reducing labor pains, starting at 32 weeks gestation through labor (9796).

Comments

Raspberry leaf extract has been used in Europe for centuries. The therapeutic use of raspberry leaf was first described in 1597 in The Herbal, or a General History of Plants (1096).

RED BUSH TEA

Also Known As

Kaffree Tea, Red Bush, Rooibos, Rooibos Tea.

Scientific Names

Aspalathus linearis, synonyms Aspalathus contaminatus, Borbonia pinifolia, Psoralea linearis.
Family: Fabaceae/Leguminosae.

People Use This For

Orally, red bush tea is used for HIV infection, preventing cancer, and improving cognitive function.
In foods, red bush tea is used as a beverage.

Safety

LIKELY SAFE ...when used orally as a beverage (6,4120).
PREGNANCY AND LACTATION: Insufficient reliable information available; avoid using.

Effectiveness
There is insufficient reliable information available for the effectiveness of red bush tea.

Mechanism of Action
Red bush tea contains polysaccharides (4120,4121), flavonoids (6,4122), a low amount of tannins (less than 5%) (5,6), and a relatively high amount of vitamin C (9.4%) (6). Some evidence suggests daily intake of acid polysaccharides found in the extracts of red bush tea might suppress HIV infection (4120,4121). Other information suggests the tea could prevent age-related changes to the central nervous system (4123) or suppress mutagenic activity (6).

Adverse Reactions
Orally, one report of salmonella contamination has occurred, possibly from lizard origin (6).

Interactions with Herbs & Other Dietary Supplements
None known.

Interactions with Drugs
None known.

Interactions with Foods
None known.

Interactions with Lab Tests
None known.

Interactions with Diseases or Conditions
None known.

Dosage and Administration
No typical dosage.

Comments
Tea is made from the branches and twigs of Aspalathus linearis. The fragrant, caffeine-free tea is the national drink of South Africa (5,6,7).

RED CLOVER

Also Known As
Beebread, Clovone, Cow Clover, Daidzein, Genistein, Isoflavone, Isoflavones, Meadow Clover, Phytoestrogen, Phytoestrogens, Purple Clover, Trefoil, Trifolium, Wild Clover.
CAUTION: See separate listings for Liverwort, Soy, and Sweet Clover.

Scientific Names
Trifolium pratense.
Family: Fabaceae/Leguminosae.

People Use This For
Orally, red clover is used for menopausal symptoms and hot flashes, cyclic breast pain or tenderness (mastalgia), cancer prevention, indigestion, whooping cough, cough, asthma, bronchitis, and sexually transmitted diseases (STDs).
Topically, red clover is used for cancerous growths, skin sores, burns, sore eyes, and chronic skin diseases including eczema and psoriasis.
In foods and beverages, the solid extract of red clover is used as a flavoring ingredient.

Safety
LIKELY SAFE ...when used orally in amounts commonly used in foods. Red clover has Generally Recognized As Safe (GRAS) status in the US (4912,9553,10372).
POSSIBLY SAFE ...when used orally and appropriately in medicinal amounts. Red clover extracts seem to be safe when used for up to one year (3375,6127,8925).
There is insufficient reliable information available about the safety of the topical use of red clover.
PREGNANCY AND LACTATION: LIKELY SAFE ...when used orally in amounts commonly used in foods (4912). LIKELY UNSAFE ...when used orally in medicinal amounts. Red clover has estrogenic

activity (9553); avoid using.
There is insufficient reliable information available about the safety of the topical use of red clover during pregnancy and lactation.

Effectiveness

POSSIBLY INEFFECTIVE

Hypercholesterolemia. Taking red clover extract orally for 12 weeks does not seem to significantly lower cholesterol in postmenopausal women with moderately elevated cholesterol levels (3375).

Menopausal symptoms. Taking red clover extract orally for 12 weeks does not seem to reduce menopausal symptoms such as hot flashes (8925,10975,10976,10991). One specific supplement that contains a high proportion of biochanin A and genistein (Promensil) might relieve hot flashes more quickly, but not more frequently that placebo (10991). Tell women red clover is unlikely to have much, if any, effect on hot flashes.

INSUFFICIENT RELIABLE EVIDENCE to RATE

Benign prostatic hyperplasia (BPH). Research suggests that red clover isoflavones 40-80 mg daily for three months might improve BPH. It seems to decrease nocturnal urinary frequency, international prostate symptom scores (IPSS), and to improve the quality of life in men with BPH. However, red clover isoflavones do not seem to affect urine flow rate, prostatic-specific antigen (PSA) values, or prostate size (6128).

Mastalgia. Preliminary evidence suggests that red clover might relieve cyclic mastalgia. Red clover isoflavones 40-80 mg daily seem to reduce breast pain and tenderness in 45% of patients (9552).

Osteoporosis. Preliminary evidence suggests that red clover isoflavones 40 mg daily for one year can significantly reduce the loss of spinal bone mineral density and bone mineral content (BMC) in pre- and perimenopausal women; however, red clover isoflavones don't seem to have this effect in postmenopausal women. Red clover also does not seem to affect hip bone density or mineral content (6127).

More evidence is needed to rate red clover for these uses.

Mechanism of Action

The applicable parts of red clover are the flowering tops. The flowering tops contain more than 100 different chemicals. Red clover contains isoflavones, a class of phytoestrogens, which are structurally similar to estrogens. The principal isoflavones found in red clover are biochanin A and formononetin. When ingested, biochanin A and formononetin are metabolized to the isoflavones genistein and daidzein, respectively (3375,3376). A substantial portion of the isoflavones are hydrolyzed by beta-glucosidases in the jejunum, releasing genistein and daidzein (3982). A small amount of unhydrolyzed isoflavones still in the methyl form remains in circulation. The health effects of these methylated isoflavones have not been evaluated (9346). Red clover isoflavone constituents might act as selective estrogen-receptor modulators (SERMs), although genistein seems to act as a weak estrogen agonist (3376,8192). In premenopausal women with normal endogenous estrogen levels, isoflavones may have an anti-estrogen effect. In postmenopausal women with low endogenous estrogens, isoflavones are likely to act as weak estrogens (3387,3988,3989,3990,3994,6029). Isoflavones have a higher affinity for the beta estrogen receptor than the classical alpha estrogen receptor (3376,3983,3992,6029). The beta estrogen receptor predominates in the heart, vasculature, bone, and bladder, which may account for some of red clover's beneficial effects (7344,9346). Osteoporosis in postmenopausal women is related to declining estrogen levels. Red clover is thought to be beneficial for preventing osteoporosis due to its weak estrogenic effects (3376,6029,6127). The isoflavone genistein also appears to directly inhibit osteoclast activity (9346).

Dietary phytoestrogens are associated with a reduced risk of endometrial cancer. Besides their effects on estrogen, phytoestrogenic substances in red clover might inhibit aromatase, which converts androstenedione to estrone. Increased estrone is associated with endometrial cancer (10372).

Red clover isoflavones might also have anticarcinogenic activity (4740,4742), possibly due to both estrogenic and nonestrogenic mechanisms (4741). The antiproliferative effects of the isoflavone genistein doesn't seem to be mediated by the estrogen receptors (ER) themselves since these effects occur both in ER-positive and ER-negative cell lines (9346).

Dietary intake of phytoestrogens among Western-culture middle-aged women doesn't seem to affect breast cancer risk, positively or negatively (11391).

For lowering cholesterol, the estrogenic effects of red clover isoflavones might be involved in modulating lipid metabolism. Red clover can also increase bile acid excretion and might up-regulate low-density lipoprotein (LDL) receptors (6029,6030,4738). Some researchers think red clover may play a role in preventing cardiovascular disease due to its potential effects on cholesterol levels, and associated preliminary evidence suggests that it might improve systemic arterial compliance (836,3375,9346). Research is conflicting regarding the effects of red clover on high-density lipoprotein (HDL) levels (9346).

Preliminary research suggests that red clover might affect the prostate. Animal research suggests that red clover might reduce prostate size by an anti-androgenic effect (11239). But preliminary clinical research hasn't shown any effect on prostate size (6128). Red clover seems to increase apoptosis (death) of prostate cells rather than affecting cell proliferation (11240). Laboratory research suggests that genistein, a red clover metabolite, decreases the growth of both benign prostatic hyperplasia (BPH) and prostate cancer tissue (11238).

Red clover also contains the constituent coumestrol, which seems to have activity similar to diethylstilbestrol (DES) (4743). The coumarin constituents contained in red clover can have anticoagulant effects (10977).

There is some evidence that red clover isoflavones can inhibit oxidative and conjugative metabolism (4736). Isoflavones might also affect drug absorption and biliary excretion by interacting with multi-drug transporters such as the P-glycoproteins (4736). Given the wide range of drugs and metabolites whose pharmacokinetics depend on these mechanisms, drug interactions with isoflavones might be more common than literature reports suggest. Genistein and daidzein are widely distributed in the body with peak concentrations at four to eight hours after short-term administration and excreted within 24 hours (3982). Chronic administration of supplemental red clover isoflavones results in a half-life of 13 to 16 hours, suggesting once daily dosing (8193). The absorption of isoflavones from food may be saturable, suggesting improved effect if ingested throughout the day (3982). Supplemental isoflavone bioavailability does not seem to be affected by foods source of isoflavones or other foods in the diet (3982).

Adverse Reactions

Orally, red clover is generally well tolerated (8925). It can cause rash-like reactions, myalgia, headache, nausea, and vaginal spotting (8194).
The ingestion of phytoestrogens in dietary amounts, 1 to 3 mg isoflavones per day, doesn't seem to increase the risk of endometrial cancer (10372).

Interactions with Herbs & Other Dietary Supplements

HERBS WITH ANTICOAGULANT/ANTIPLATELET POTENTIAL: Concomitant use of herbs that have constituents that might affect platelet aggregation could theoretically increase the risk of bleeding in some people (10977). Some of these herbs include angelica, clove, danshen, garlic, ginger, ginkgo, Panax ginseng, horse chestnut, turmeric, and others.
HERBS WITH ESTROGENIC ACTIVITY: Theoretically, red clover could be additive or antagonistic with other herbs that have estrogenic activity (3387,3988,3989,3990,3994,6029). These herbs include alfalfa, black cohosh, chasteberry, flaxseed, hops, ipriflavone, kudzu, licorice, and soy.

Interactions with Drugs

ANTICOAGULANT/ANTIPLATELET DRUGS: Theoretically, concomitant use of large amounts of red clover can increase the anticoagulant effects and bleeding risk of these drugs due to its coumarin content (9553).
CONTRACEPTIVE DRUGS: Theoretically, concomitant use of large amounts of red clover might interfere with contraceptive drugs due to competition for estrogen receptors (4737,4743,9553).
CYTOCHROME P450 3A4 (CYP3A4) SUBSTRATES: There's preliminary evidence that suggests that red clover may inhibit the cytochrome P450 3A4 (CYP3A4) isoenzymes (6450,9553). Theoretically, red clover might increase the levels of drugs metabolized by CYP3A4. However, so far, this interaction has not been reported in humans. Some drugs metabolized by CYP3A4 include lovastatin (Mevacor), ketoconazole (Nizoral), itraconazole (Sporanox), fexofenadine (Allegra), triazolam (Halcion), and numerous others. Use red clover cautiously or avoid use in patients taking these drugs.
ESTROGENS: Theoretically, concomitant use of large amounts of red clover might interfere with hormone replacement therapy through competition for estrogen receptors (4737,4743,9553).
TAMOXIFEN (Nolvadex): There is some concern that red clover might interfere with tamoxifen because of its potential estrogenic effects. There is preliminary evidence that genistein, a constituent of red clover, might antagonize the antitumor effects of tamoxifen (8192). Tell patients taking tamoxifen to avoid red clover.

Interactions with Foods

None known.

Interactions with Lab Tests

None known.

Interactions with Diseases or Conditions

COAGULATION DISORDERS: Use red clover with caution and avoid large amounts due to its coumarin content, which might increase the risk of bleeding (9553).
HORMONE SENSITIVE CANCERS/CONDITIONS: Because the isoflavones in red clover have estrogenic effects (4741,8192,9553), women with hormone sensitive conditions should avoid red clover. Some of these conditions include breast cancer, uterine cancer, ovarian cancer, endometriosis, and uterine fibroids.

Dosage and Administration

ORAL: For reducing hot flashes in postmenopausal women, a red clover isoflavone extract (Promensil) 40-160 mg per day has been used (8925,9553). For cyclic mastalgia, red clover isoflavones 40-80 mg daily has been used (9552).
TOPICAL: No typical dosage.

Comments

Red clover in large quantities induces sterility in livestock (4743). The cheetah population in zoos was threatened by reproductive failure and liver disease, thought to be caused by diets high in isoflavones (4735).

RED MAPLE

Also Known As
Bird's Eye Maple, Sugar Maple, Swamp Maple.

Scientific Names
Acer rubrum.
Family: Aceraceae.

Comments
At the date of publication, there was very little scientific information about this product. Our staff is continually analyzing the available information on natural medicines and will add data to the online version of *Natural Medicines Comprehensive Database* as it becomes available. See www.naturaldatabase.com.

RED SANDALWOOD

Also Known As
Red Sanderswood, Red Saunders, Rubywood, Sandalwood Padauk, Santali lignum rubrum, Sappan.
CAUTION: See separate listings for White Sandalwood Oil and White Sandalwood wood.

Scientific Names
Pterocarpus santalinus.
Family: Fabaceae/Leguminosae.

Comments
At the date of publication, there was very little scientific information about this product. Our staff is continually analyzing the available information on natural medicines and will add data to the online version of *Natural Medicines Comprehensive Database* as it becomes available. See www.naturaldatabase.com.

RED SOAPWORT

Also Known As
Bouncing-Bet, Saponariae rubrae radix, Soapwort.
CAUTION: See separate listing for White Soapwort.

Scientific Names
Saponaria officinalis.
Family: Caryophyllaceae.

People Use This For
Orally, red soapwort is used for inflammation of mucous membranes in the upper and lower respiratory tract.
Topically, red soapwort is used as a remedy for poison ivy, acne, psoriasis, eczema, and boils.
In manufacturing, red soapwort is used as an ingredient in soaps, herbal shampoos, and detergents.
It is used as a foaming agent in beer.

Safety
LIKELY SAFE ...when used topically. Red soapwort is widely used in soaps and shampoos (6) without reports of adverse effects.
POSSIBLY SAFE ...when used orally (2).
PREGNANCY AND LACTATION: Insufficient reliable information available; avoid using.

Effectiveness
There is insufficient reliable information available about the effectiveness of red soapwort.

Mechanism of Action
The applicable part of red soapwort is the root. The root contains saponin constituents that have expectorant effects. Saponins irritate the gastric mucosa, which then stimulate bronchial mucous secretion via the parasympathetic sensory pathways (7). In large amounts, red soapwort is cytotoxic (2).

Adverse Reactions
Orally, red soapwort can cause stomach irritation (2), nausea, and vomiting (7).

Interactions with Herbs & Other Dietary Supplements
None known.

Interactions with Drugs
None known.

Interactions with Foods
None known.

Interactions with Lab Tests
None known.

Interactions with Diseases or Conditions
GI MUCOSAL IRRITATION (e.g. ulcers, etc.): Red soapwort is contraindicated, because it can exacerbate existing GI mucosal irritation due to its saponin content (6).

Dosage and Administration
ORAL: The typical dose of red soapwort is 1.5 grams of the dried root per day as a tea or equivalent preparation (2).
TOPICAL: No typical dosage.

Comments
In the Middle Ages, Franciscan and Dominican monks viewed soapwort as a divine gift that was meant to keep them clean (6). Avoid confusion with white soapwort root.

RED-SPUR VALERIAN

Also Known As
Bouncing Bess, Bovis and Soldier, Delicate Bess, Drunken Sailor, Fox's-Brush, Jupiter's Beard, Pretty Betsy, Red Spur Valerian, Red Valerian.

Scientific Names
Centranthus ruber, synonym Valeriana rubra.
Family: Valerianaceae.

Comments
At the date of publication, this product was not a common ingredient used in brand name supplements marketed to consumers. Details about this product are available at the online version of *Natural Medicines Comprehensive Database*. See www.naturaldatabase.com.

RED YEAST

Also Known As
Hong Qu, Monascus, Red Rice Yeast, Red Yeast Rice, Xue Zhi Kang, Zhi Tai.
CAUTION: See separate listing for Beta-Sitosterol.

Scientific Names
Monascus purpureus; other Monascus species.
Family: Monascaceae.

People Use This For
Orally, red yeast is used for maintaining desirable cholesterol levels in healthy people, reducing cholesterol in people with hyperlipidemia, for indigestion, diarrhea, improving blood circulation, and for spleen and stomach health.
In foods, red yeast is used as a food coloring for Peking duck and other foods.

Safety

POSSIBLY SAFE ...when used orally and appropriately, short-term. Red yeast has been safely used in studies lasting up to 12 weeks (512,2624,6988,6990,6995,6996).
There is insufficient reliable information available about the safety of red yeast when used orally, long-term.
CHILDREN: POSSIBLY UNSAFE ...when used orally. Safety has not been established in children under 18 years of age and questions remain about the benefit of lowering cholesterol in children (512).
PREGNANCY: LIKELY UNSAFE ...when used orally. The red yeast constituent, lovastatin, has induced fetal skeletal malformations in animals (2619); avoid using.
LACTATION: Insufficient reliable information available; avoid using.

Effectiveness

LIKELY EFFECTIVE

Hypercholesterolemia. Taking red yeast orally can significantly lower total and low-density lipoprotein (LDL) cholesterol levels, and triglycerides when used for 8-12 weeks (2624,6990). The dose used most commonly is 2.4 grams per day, but a dose of 1.2 grams per day provides some benefit (6988). Some research suggests that red yeast might be as effective as simvastatin (Zocor) for improving lipid profiles (6993). Most studies used a specific proprietary red yeast product (Cholestin, Pharmanex).

POSSIBLY EFFECTIVE

HIV/AIDS. Taking red yeast orally seems to reduce lipids with dyslipidemia related to HIV infection (9475).

There is insufficient reliable information available about the effectiveness of red yeast for its other uses.

Mechanism of Action

Red yeast is the product of rice fermented with Monascus purpureus yeast (512). Red yeast supplements are different than red yeast rice sold in Chinese grocery stores (6994). Supplements are manufactured by culturing M. purpureus on rice at carefully-controlled temperature and growing conditions to increase the concentration of mevinic acids (6994). Red yeast contains ten mevinic acids, also known as monacolins, the highest concentration of which is constituted by lovastatin (also referred to as monacolin K or mevinolin) (512,2624,6988,9588). These compounds, which constitute about 0.4% of red rice, competitively inhibit 3-hydroxy-3-methyl-glutaryl-coenzyme A (HMG-CoA) reductase, blocking cholesterol biosynthesis (512,2624). Red yeast also contains sterols, including beta-sitosterol, campesterol, stigmasterol, and sapogenin; isolfavones and isoflavone glycosides, and monounsaturated fatty acids (2624,6988). Although the cholesterol lowering effect is likely partially caused by the lovastatin content, it is unclear to what extent. The overall cholesterol-lowering effect of red yeast is likely also the result of the combination of lovastatin, mevinic acids, and other constituents.
Red yeast that is not fermented correctly may contain citrinin. Citrinin is a toxin that may cause kidney failure (9588).

Adverse Reactions

Orally, red yeast can cause gastritis, abdominal discomfort, and elevated liver enzymes (512). In clinical studies, heartburn, flatulence, and dizziness were reported infrequently and did not result in study withdrawal (6988). Anaphylaxis following inhalation of red yeast has also been reported (6997).
Like HMG-CoA reductase inhibitor ("statins") drugs, red yeast may cause rhabdomyolysis, which is related to the mevinic acids that it contains (9587).
The contaminant citrinin may be found in some products containing red yeast. Citrinin is a nephrotoxin that results from incorrect rice fermentation processes (9588).

Interactions with Herbs & Other Dietary Supplements

CHOLESTEROL LOWERING HERBS/SUPPLEMENTS: Theoretically, red yeast might enhance the effects of herbs and supplements that also lower cholesterol. Some of these herbs and supplements include chromium, flaxseed, garlic, guar gum, niacin, oat bran, psyllium, and others.
COENZYME Q10 (CoQ10, Ubiquinone): Theoretically, red yeast can lower coenzyme Q10 levels. Red yeast contains the constituent, lovastatin, and related compounds, which can lower coenzyme Q10 levels (6983,6984,6985,6986).
GRAPEFRUIT: Concomitant use of red yeast (Cholestin) and grapefruit products can increase the serum levels of lovastatin, a constituent of red yeast. Grapefruit and grapefruit seed extract products can inhibit cytochrome P450 metabolism of lovastatin (527).
HEPATOTOXIC HERBS & SUPPLEMENTS: Theoretically, red yeast might enhance the adverse effects of potentially hepatotoxic herbs and supplements such as borage, chaparral, niacin, valerian, and uva ursi; avoid concurrent use.
HERBS/SUPPLEMENTS WITH THYROID ACTIVITY: Theoretically, red yeast might interfere with effects of herbs and supplements that affect thyroid function, including bugleweed, balm leaf, tiratricol, and wild thyme. Concomitant use of levothyroxine with the red yeast constituent lovastatin can also cause thyroid function abnormalities (15); avoid concurrent use.
ST. JOHN'S WORT: Theoretically, St. John's wort might reduce serum levels of red yeast. St. John's wort induces cytochrome P450 3A4 enzyme that can lower serum levels of the lovastatin constituent (1290).

Interactions with Drugs

ALCOHOL (Ethanol): Theoretically, alcohol may adversely affect liver function in patients taking red yeast, due to the lovastatin constituent (15).
CYCLOSPORINE (Neoral, Sandimmune): Theoretically, red yeast in combination with cyclosporine might increase the risk of myopathy due to the red yeast lovastatin constituent (15); use with caution.
CYTOCHROME P450 3A4 (CYP3A4) INHIBITORS: Theoretically, drugs that inhibit the cytochrome P450 3A4 (CYP3A4) enzymes might increase serum levels of red yeast constituents, such as lovastatin, and increase the risk of adverse effects. Drugs with this interaction include clarithromycin, erythromycin, itraconazole, ketoconazole, cimetidine, nefazodone, protease inhibitors, and others (6987).
GEMFIBROZIL (Lopid): Theoretically, red yeast in combination with gemfibrozil might increase the risk of myopathy due to the red yeast lovastatin constituent (15).
HMG-CoA REDUCTASE INHIBITORS ("Statins"): Using red yeast with these drugs might increase the risk of adverse effects without necessarily improving therapeutic benefit; avoid concomitant use. HMG-CoA reductase inhibitors include atorvastatin (Lipitor), cerivastatin (Baycol), fluvastatin (Lescol), lovastatin (Mevacor), pravastatin (Pravachol), and simvastatin (Zocor) (15).
LEVOTHYROXINE (Synthroid, Levothroid, Levoxyl, and others): Theoretically, concomitant use of levothyroxine with red yeast might cause thyroid function abnormalities due to the red yeast lovastatin constituent (15).
NIACIN: Theoretically, red yeast in combination with high-dose niacin might increase the risk of myopathy due to the red yeast lovastatin constituent (15).

Interactions with Foods

ALCOHOL: Theoretically, alcohol may adversely affect liver function in patients taking red yeast due to the lovastatin constituent (15).
FOOD: Food enhances the bioavailability of lovastatin (15), a constituent of red yeast.
GRAPEFRUIT JUICE: Concomitant use of grapefruit juice and lovastatin, a constituent of red yeast, can increase serum lovastatin levels and the risk of adverse effects (527).

Interactions with Lab Tests

CREATINE KINASE (CK): Red yeast might increase serum creatine kinase concentrations and test results due its lovastatin content. Lovastatin can increase serum creatine kinase concentrations and test results (15).
LIVER ENZYMES: Red yeast might increase serum liver transaminase concentrations and test results due its lovastatin content. Lovastatin can increase serum liver transaminase concentrations and test results (15).
SERUM CHOLESTEROL: Red yeast can reduce serum cholesterol concentrations and test results. Red yeast contains a mixture of lovastatin and other HMG-CoA reductase inhibitors (2624).

Interactions with Diseases or Conditions

LIVER DYSFUNCTION: Red yeast is contraindicated in people with liver dysfunction, risk of liver dysfunction, or abnormal liver function test results (2619).
THYROID DYSFUNCTION: Concomitant use of lovastatin with levothyroxine can interfere with thyroid therapy (15).

Dosage and Administration

ORAL: Most clinical studies have used a specific brand product (Cholestin). However, most other red yeast brands contain a similar amount of red yeast, 600 mg. For hypercholesterolemia, a typical dose of red yeast is 1200 mg two times daily with food (2624). A total daily dose of 2400 mg red yeast contains approximately 9.6 mg total statins, of which 7.2 mg is lovastatin (2624). For dyslipidemia related to HIV infection, 1200 mg twice daily has been used (9475).

Comments

Red yeast is the product of rice fermented with the Monascus purpureus yeast that contains monacolin K (lovastatin, mevinolin) and other HMG-CoA reductase inhibiting compounds (512). Cholestin (Pharmanex) was one of the most widely studied red yeast products. But the FDA now considers red yeast to be an unapproved drug because it contains a prescription-only statin (6610). Cholestin has been reformulated and now contains policosanol as the active ingredient.
Red yeast should be treated as a HMG-CoA reductase inhibitor, with all the possible side effects, drug interactions, and precautions associated with this drug class. The American Heart Association has cautioned against using red yeast pending the results of long-term studies (6991).
Chemical assay indicates that red yeast products vary considerably in content and concentration of monacolin K and other monocolins (9588).

REED HERB

Also Known As
Common Reed, Ditch Reed, Giant Reed, Phragmites, Reed, Roseau Commun, Schilf.

Scientific Names
Phragmites australis, synonyms Phragmites communis, Arundo phragmites, Arundo vulgaris, Phragmites longivalvis, Phragmites vulgaris.
Family: Poaceae/Gramineae.

People Use This For
Orally, reed herb is used for digestive disorders, diabetes, leukemia, and breast cancer.
Topically, reed herb is used to relieve insect bites.

Safety
There is insufficient reliable information available about the safety of reed herb.
Pregnancy and Lactation: Insufficient reliable information available; avoid using.

Effectiveness
There is insufficient reliable information available about the effectiveness of reed herb.

Mechanism of Action
The applicable parts of reed herb are the stem and rhizome. Reed herb contains vitamin A, vitamin C, and several vitamins of the B-group (18). It also contains triterpenes (beta-amyrin and taraxerol) and several flavonoids including chrysoeriol, isoquercitrin, luteolin, rutin, and tricin (18). The plant is thought to have diuretic effects and stimulate sweating (18).

Adverse Reactions
None reported.

Interactions with Herbs & Other Dietary Supplements
None known.

Interactions with Drugs
None known.

Interactions with Foods
None known.

Interactions with Lab Tests
None known.

Interactions with Diseases or Conditions
None known.

Dosage and Administration
ORAL/TOPICAL: Reed herb is prepared as a tea (18).

REISHI MUSHROOM

Also Known As
Ling Chih, Ling Zhi, Mannentake, Mushroom of Immortality, Mushroom of Spiritual Potency, Rei-Shi, Reishi, Spirit Plant.

Scientific Names
Ganoderma lucidum.
Family: Ganodermataceae.

People Use This For

Orally, reishi mushroom is used for enhancing the immune system, lowering blood pressure and cholesterol, treating and preventing viral infections and tumors, treating inflammatory disease, cardiovascular disease, asthma and bronchial diseases. It is also used orally for reducing stress, as a kidney tonic, treating hepatitis and liver disease, supporting HIV disease, treating or preventing altitude sickness, and supporting chemotherapy. Other oral uses include preventing fatigue, treating insomnia, gastric ulcers, neurasthenia, poisoning, post-herpetic neuralgia, and herpes zoster pain.

In combination with other herbs, reishi mushroom is used to treat prostate cancer.

Safety

POSSIBLY SAFE ...when used orally and appropriately (12).
PREGNANCY AND LACTATION: Insufficient reliable information available; avoid using.

Effectiveness

There is insufficient reliable information available about the effectiveness of reishi mushroom.

Mechanism of Action

The applicable parts of reishi mushrooms are the fruiting body and mycelium (12). Reishi mushrooms have a long history in folk medicine, but researchers are just beginning to isolate and identify medicinal substances in reishi that have antitumor, immune modulating, anti-aging, cardiovascular, anticoagulant, cholesterol lowering, hypoglycemic, hepatoprotective, antiviral, and antibacterial effects (5476,5477,5481,5482,5483,5484,5485,5486,5487,5488,5489) (5490,5491,5492). Protease inhibitors and other anti-HIV substances have been found in reishi mushrooms (5479,5480). Studies of these compounds have not been performed in humans. Reishi mushroom extracts contain high levels of adenosine (5478).

Adverse Reactions

Orally, reishi mushroom can cause dryness of the mouth, throat, and nasal area; itchiness; stomach upset; nosebleed; and bloody stools which have occurred with extended oral use, 3 to 6 months (12). Also, a rash with the consumption of reishi wine and respiratory allergy to reishi spores can occur (12,5479).

Interactions with Herbs & Other Dietary Supplements

HERBS WITH ANTICOAGULANT/ANTIPLATELET POTENTIAL: Concomitant use of with herbs that have anticoagulant or antiplatelet activity could theoretically increase the risk of bleeding in some people (5476). These herbs include angelica, anise, arnica, clove, danshen, garlic, ginger, ginkgo, Panax ginseng, horse chestnut, red clover, turmeric, and others.
HERBS/SUPPLEMENTS WITH HYPOTENSIVE ACTIVITY: Theoretically, concurrent use might increase risk of hypotension with herbs that lower blood pressure (5488), including black cohosh, celery seed, Panax ginseng, and others.

Interactions with Drugs

ANTICOAGULANT/ANTIPLATELET DRUGS: Reishi may have anticoagulant effects (5476). Theoretically, taking reishi with other anticoagulant or antiplatelet drugs might increase the risk of bruising and bleeding. Some of these drugs include aspirin; clopidogrel (Plavix); nonsteroidal anti-inflammatory drugs (NSAIDs) such as diclofenac (Voltaren, Cataflam, others), ibuprofen (Advil, Motrin, others), naproxen (Anaprox, Naprosyn, others); dalteparin (Fragmin); enoxaparin (Lovenox); heparin, warfarin (Coumadin); and others.
ANTIHYPERTENSIVE DRUGS: Theoretically, concurrent use might increase risk of hypotension with drugs that lower blood pressure (5488). These include captopril (Capoten), enalapril (Vasotec), losartan (Cozaar), valsartan (Diovan), diltiazem (Cardizem), Amlodipine (Norvasc), hydrochlorothiazide (HydroDIURIL), furosemide (Lasix), and many others.

Interactions with Foods

None known.

Interactions with Lab Tests

BLEEDING TIME: Theoretically, reishi mushroom use might prolong coagulation and bleeding time results (5476).

Interactions with Diseases or Conditions

HYPOTENSION: Theoretically, reishi mushroom use might worsen hypotension or interfere with drug therapy to increase blood pressure (5488).
THROMBOCYTOPENIA: Theoretically, reishi mushroom use might increase the risk of bleeding in people with thrombocytopenia (5476).

Dosage and Administration

ORAL: People typically use 1.5-9 grams orally per day of the crude dried mushroom, 1-1.5 grams per day of reishi powder, or 1 mL per day of reishi tincture (5473). Reishi tea is also used therapeutically (5473).

Comments

The flesh of Reishi is described as "tough" and "woody" with a bitter taste.

RESVERATROL

Also Known As

Cis-Resveratrol, Kojo-Kon, Phytoestrogen, Protykin, Resveratrols, Trans-Resveratrol.
CAUTION: See separate listings for Grape fruit, skin; Grape seed; Quercetin; and Wine.

Scientific Names

3,4',5-stilbenetriol; 3,5,4' -trihydroxystilbene; 3,4',5-trihydroxystilbene.

People Use This For

Orally, resveratrol is used for atherosclerosis, lowering cholesterol levels, increasing HDL cholesterol levels, and preventing cancer.

Safety

LIKELY SAFE ...when consumed in amounts found in foods (2030).
There is insufficient reliable information available about the safety of resveratrol when used in supplemental doses in amounts greater than those found in foods.
PREGNANCY AND LACTATION: LIKELY SAFE ...when used in amounts found in some foods (2030).
Resveratrol is found in grape skins, grape juice, wine, and other food sources. Wine should not be used as a source of resveratrol during pregnancy and lactation.

Effectiveness

There is insufficient reliable information available about the effectiveness of resveratrol.

Mechanism of Action

Resveratrol is a polyphenolic compound that exists in nature as cis- and trans- stereoisomers. Resveratrol is primarily found in red wine, red grape skins, purple grape juice, mulberries, and in smaller amounts in peanuts (513,2030,2956). Other sources include eucalyptus (Eucalyptus wandoo, Eucalyptus sideroxylon), spruce (Picea excelsa), and Bauhinia racemosa (2030). Polygonum cuspidatum, the roots of which are used in Chinese and Japanese traditional medicine, is considered to be one of the richest sources of trans-resveratrol (2030).
The trans-resveratrol content of wine is highly dependent on grape type, climate, and practices used to make the wine (9). White wines have very low trans-resveratrol concentrations. Pinot Noir consistently has the highest concentrations of trans-resveratrol, regardless of climate. Other red wines, including Cabernet Sauvignon, produced in cold, humid climates, such as Bordeaux and Canada, have higher trans-resveratrol content than those produced in hot, dry climates (2030). Unfermented grape juice does not contain resveratrol. Resveratrol is not found in significant quantities in fermented grape beverages that are stored in oak barrels, such as cognac (7864).
Resveratrol is rapidly absorbed with peak concentrations occurring within 30 minutes. Resveratrol is conjugated in the intestine and absorbed as the conjugated form. In plasma, resveratrol is found primarily as glucuronide or sulfate form. In vitro research has been done with unconjugated resveratrol. It is questionable whether free resveratrol absorption is sufficient to exert a pharmacologic effect. Research in humans suggests that quercetin taken orally doesn't reach serum concentrations at which in vitro activity has been seen (9174).
Resveratrol is a weak phytoestrogen (2960). It binds to both alpha and beta estrogen receptors, but its affinity for these receptors is about 7,000 times less than estrogen (7865). Resveratrol decreases the activity of inflammatory cytokines, which suggests a mechanism for reducing mortality in cardiovascular diseases and cancer (6126). Early research suggests resveratrol might reduce the risk of cancer (2948,2959). Biological activity in humans has not yet been described (2030). Preliminary evidence suggests that trans-resveratrol has antioxidant and antimutagenic activity (2948). It may also inhibit tumor growth and promote apoptosis (2958,2959). Preliminary evidence suggests that trans-resveratrol interferes with blood coagulation by inhibiting cyclooxygenases 1 and 2, hydroperoxidases, 5-lipoxygenase (2030,2948), and platelet aggregation (2949,2950,2951,2952,2961). It also causes blood vessel dilation (2954). Resveratrol inhibits formation of cholesterol in certain strains of bacteria (7863), but it is not known if this contributes significantly to cholesterol lowering in humans. In human colon cancer cells, resveratrol inhibits cell division and function of RNA and DNA. These effects are reversible and cell growth resumes 40 hours after exposure (7861). Preliminary data suggest that resveratrol may prevent liver cancer cells from invading local tissues (7862). Resveratrol inhibits the replication of herpes simplex virus. Although the mechanism of this action is not fully known, exposure to resveratrol within one hour of cellular infection appears to be most effective in arresting viral growth. This

suggests that resveratrol reduces production of proteins needed to regulate viral proliferation (7866).
The activity of cytochrome P450 (CYP450) enzymes is inhibited by resveratrol in hepatocytes (7864). Whether this action interferes with metabolism of drugs in humans is not known.

Adverse Reactions

None reported.

Interactions with Herbs & Other Dietary Supplements

HERBS WITH ANTICOAGULANT/ANTIPLATELET POTENTIAL: Theoretically, concomitant use of resveratrol with herbs that have anticoagulant or antiplatelet activity could increase the risk of bleeding in some people (2949,2950,2951,2952,2961). These herbs include angelica, clove, danshen, feverfew, garlic, ginger, ginkgo, ginseng Panax, horse chestnut, red clover, turmeric, and others.

Interactions with Drugs

ANTICOAGULANT/ANTIPLATELET DRUGS: Resveratrol seems to have antiplatelet effects (2949,2950,2951,2952,2961). Theoretically, taking resveratrol with other antiplatelet or anticoagulant drugs might increase the risk of bruising and bleeding. Some of these drugs include aspirin; clopidogrel (Plavix); nonsteroidal anti-inflammatory drugs (NSAIDs) such as diclofenac (Voltaren, Cataflam, others), ibuprofen (Advil, Motrin, others), naproxen (Anaprox, Naprosyn, others); dalteparin (Fragmin); enoxaparin (Lovenox); heparin; warfarin (Coumadin); and others.
CYTOCHROME P450 3A4 (CYP3A4) SUBSTRATES: Preliminary evidence shows that resveratrol might inhibit the cytochrome P450 enzymes, CYP3A, CYP1A, and CYP2E1 (7864). Theoretically, it might increase levels of drugs metabolized by these enzymes. However, this interaction has not been reported in humans. Some drugs metabolized by CYP3A include lovastatin (Mevacor), ketoconazole (Nizoral), itraconazole (Sporanox), fexofenadine (Allegra), triazolam (Halcion), and numerous others. Use resveratrol cautiously or avoid in patients taking these drugs.

Interactions with Foods

None known.

Interactions with Lab Tests

None known.

Interactions with Diseases or Conditions

HORMONE SENSITIVE CANCERS/CONDITIONS: Because resveratrol might have estrogenic effects (2960), women with hormone sensitive conditions should avoid resveratrol. Some of these conditions include breast, uterine, and ovarian cancer, and endometriosis and uterine fibroids.

Dosage and Administration

No typical dosage.

RHATANY

Also Known As

Brazilian Rhatany, Krameria, Mapato, Peruvian Rhatany, Pumacuchu, Raiz Para Los Dientes, Ratanhiawurzel, Red Rhatany, Rhatanhia, Rhatania, Ratanhiae radix.

Scientific Names

Krameria lappacea, synonyms Krameria triandra, Krameria iluca; Krameria argentea.
Family: Krameriaceae.

People Use This For

Orally, rhatany is used as an antidiarrheal agent for enteritis and angina.
Topically, rhatany is used for mild inflammation of the oral and pharyngeal mucosa, inflammation of the gums, fissures of the tongue, stomatitis, pharyngitis, non-infectious canker sores, chilblains, and leg ulcers.

Safety

POSSIBLY SAFE ...when used topically short-term (2,12). Use should be limited to two weeks unless medical evaluation determines that there is no problem and use can continue (2).
There is insufficient reliable information available about the safety of rhatany for its other uses.
PREGNANCY AND LACTATION: Insufficient reliable information available; avoid using.

Effectiveness

There is insufficient reliable information available about the effectiveness of rhatany.

Mechanism of Action

The applicable part of rhatany is the root. Rhatany contains high concentrations of proanthocyanidin tannins (10-15%), which are responsible for the observed astringent properties (2,3,18,4100). The alcohol in the tincture preparation may enhance astringent effects (272). Astringents precipitate the surface proteins of cells decreasing the cell size (4101) and secretions from the inflamed tissues (272), diminishing inflammation. Astringents also have the ability to alleviate inflammation by constricting the blood vessels and reducing the supply of blood to the affected area (272).

Adverse Reactions

Orally, rhatany can cause digestive complaints (18).
Topically, allergic mucous membrane reactions have occurred rarely with rhatany (2,18).

Interactions with Herbs & Other Dietary Supplements

None known.

Interactions with Drugs

ORAL DRUGS: Theoretically, concomitant oral administration may cause precipitation of some drugs due to the high tannin content of rhatany. Separate administration of oral drugs and tannin-containing herbs by the longest period of time practical (19).

Interactions with Foods

None known.

Interactions with Lab Tests

None known.

Interactions with Diseases or Conditions

ALLERGY: Contraindicated in people with rhatany allergy.

Dosage and Administration

ORAL: Rhatany is sometimes taken as a decoction of 1 gram of the herb in 1 cup of water or as 5-10 drops of the tincture in one glass of water (6002).
TOPICAL: As mouth wash or gargle (simmer 1-1.5 grams of powdered root in 150 mL boiling water 10-15 minutes, strain) two to three times daily (8). As mouth wash or gargle, 5-10 drops of rhatany tincture in one glass of water two to three times daily (8). Undiluted rhatany tincture (oral paint) used directly on the affected area two to three times daily (2). Limit rhatany use to maximum two weeks without medical evaluation (2).

Comments

Avoid confusion with roots of other Krameria species (18). Rhatany (Krameria triandra) root is difficult to find and adulteration is common with other Krameria species (8).

RHUBARB

Also Known As

Chinese Rhubarb, Da Huang, Garden Rhubarb, Himalayan Rhubarb, Indian Rhubarb, Medicinal Rhubarb, Rhei, Rheum, Rhei radix, Turkey Rhubarb.

Scientific Names

Rheum officinale; Rheum palmatum; Rheum tanguticum; Rheum australe, synonym Rheum emodi; Rheum hybridum, synonyms Rheum cultorum, Rheum rhabarbarum, Rheum rhaponticum.
Family: Polygonaceae.

People Use This For

Orally, rhubarb is used for constipation, diarrhea, dyspepsia, gastritis, gastrointestinal (GI) bleeding, preparation for GI diagnostic procedures after recto-anal surgery, for bowel movement relief when anal fissures are present, and for hemorrhoids.
Topically, rhubarb is used for herpes labialis (cold sores).
In foods, rhubarb stems are edible. Rhubarb is also used as a flavoring agent.

Safety

LIKELY SAFE ...when the root is used in amounts commonly found in foods. Chinese and garden rhubarb have Generally Recognized As Safe (GRAS) status in the US (4912).

POSSIBLY SAFE ...when used orally and appropriately in medicinal amounts for less than eight days (10436). ...when used topically, and appropriately (10437).

CHILDREN: POSSIBLY UNSAFE ...when used orally. Rhubarb root or rhizome should not be used in children under age 12 (12). There is one report of a 4-year-old who ingested rhubarb leaves (containing oxalic acid) and died (17).

PREGNANCY AND LACTATION: POSSIBLY UNSAFE ...when used in medicinal amounts, rhubarb is a stimulant laxative; avoid using (12).

Effectiveness

POSSIBLY EFFECTIVE

Herpes labialis (cold sores). Applying rhubarb topically in combination with sage (Salvia officinalis) seems to improve herpes labialis (cold sores). Treatment of herpes labialis with a cream containing rhubarb and sage may be about as effective as acyclovir (Zovirax) cream. Acyclovir cream heals lesions in about 6.3 days; the rhubarb and sage cream heals lesions in about 7.2 days (10437).

INSUFFICIENT RELIABLE EVIDENCE to RATE

Gastrointestinal bleeding. Preliminary clinical evidence suggests that oral rhubarb powder might be useful for treating gastrointestinal bleeding (10436). More evidence is needed to rate rhubarb for this use.

Mechanism of Action

The applicable parts of rhubarb are the rhizome and root. The active constituents include hydroxyanthracene derivatives, anthraquinones, tannins and calcium oxalate (18,10437). At low doses, the tannin effects predominate and have an astringent effect on the gastrointestinal (GI) tract that relieves diarrhea (7). At higher doses, anthraquinone effects seem to predominate, producing a stimulant laxative effect that relieves constipation (7).

Adverse Reactions

Orally, rhubarb can cause cramp-like or spasmodic gastrointestinal (GI) discomfort, watery diarrhea, and uterine contractions; there is also one report of anaphylaxis with short-term use (18). Chronic use or abuse of rhubarb can cause electrolyte loss (especially potassium), hyperaldosteronism, accelerated bone deterioration, albuminuria, hematuria, dehydration, inhibition of gastric motility, pseudomelanosis coli (pigment spots in intestinal mucosa), arrhythmias, muscular weakness, nephropathies, and edema (12). Chronic use of anthroid laxatives can cause pseudomelanosis coli, which is harmless, usually reverses with discontinuation, and is not associated with an increased risk of developing colorectal adenoma or carcinoma (6138).

Interactions with Herbs & Other Dietary Supplements

CALCIUM, IRON, ZINC: Concurrent use might decrease mineral absorption. Rhubarb contains oxalates, which can bind multivalent metal ions in the gastrointestinal (GI) tract and decrease mineral absorption (12).

CARDIAC GLYCOSIDE-CONTAINING HERBS: Overuse of rhubarb might cause potassium depletion, increasing the risk of cardiac toxicity (500). Cardiac glycoside-containing herbs include black hellebore, Canadian hemp root, digitalis leaf, hedge mustard, figwort, lily of the valley roots, motherwort, oleander leaf, pheasant's eye plant, pleurisy root, squill bulb leaf scales, and strophanthus seeds.

CARDIOACTIVE HERBS: Overuse of rhubarb might cause potassium depletion, increasing risk of toxicity of cardioactive herbs (4). These include calamus, cereus, cola, coltsfoot, devil's claw, European mistletoe, fenugreek, fumitory, ginger, Panax ginseng, hawthorn, mate, parsley, quassia, scotch broom flower, shepherd's purse, white horehound, and wild carrot.

LICORICE/HORSETAIL: Theoretically, concomitant use with horsetail plant or licorice rhizome increases the risk of potassium depletion (19).

STIMULANT LAXATIVE HERBS: Theoretically, concomitant use with other stimulant laxative herbs may increase the risk of potassium depletion (19). Stimulant laxative herbs include aloe dried leaf sap, blue flag rhizome, alder buckthorn, European buckthorn, butternut bark, cascara bark, castor oil, colocynth fruit pulp, gamboge bark exudate, jalap root, black root, manna bark exudate, podophyllum root, senna leaves and pods, wild cucumber fruit (Ecballium elaterium), and yellow dock root.

Interactions with Drugs

CORTICOSTEROIDS: Overuse of rhubarb might compound corticosteroid-induced potassium loss (2).

DIGOXIN (Lanoxin): Overuse of rhubarb might cause potassium depletion, increasing the risk of digoxin toxicity (19).

DIURETIC DRUGS: Overuse of rhubarb might compound diuretic-induced potassium loss (19). There is concern that people receiving rhubarb along with potassium depleting diuretics might be at an increased risk for hypokalemia. Initiation of potassium supplementation or an increase in potassium supplement dose may be necessary for some patients. Some diuretics that can deplete potassium include chlorothiazide (Diuril), chlorthalidone (Thalitone),

furosemide (Lasix), and hydrochlorothiazide (HCTZ, HydroDIURIL, Microzide), and others.
ORAL DRUGS: Concomitant use might reduce absorption of drugs due to reduced gastrointestinal transit time (500).
STIMULANT LAXATIVES: Concomitant use might compound fluid and electrolyte loss.

Interactions with Foods

CALCIUM, IRON, ZINC: Concurrent use might decrease mineral absorption from foods. Rhubarb contains oxalates (7,12), which can bind multivalent metal ions in the gastrointestinal tract and decrease mineral absorption.

Interactions with Lab Tests

URINE TESTS: Rhubarb might discolor urine and interfere with diagnostic tests (2).

Interactions with Diseases or Conditions

CONSTIPATION, DIARRHEA: Rhubarb can exacerbate diarrhea or constipation depending on the preparation used (12).
GASTROINTESTINAL (GI) CONDITIONS: Rhubarb is contraindicated in cases of intestinal obstruction; appendicitis; abdominal pain of unknown origin; and inflammatory conditions of the intestines including Crohn's disease, colitis, and irritable bowel syndrome (IBS) (12).
KIDNEY STONES: Rhubarb contains calcium oxalate. Use it with caution in people with a history of kidney stones (12).

Dosage and Administration

ORAL: Rhubarb is used short-term only, ideally for less than eight days (12). For constipation, 1-4 grams of the dried root has been used daily (7). For diarrhea, 100-300 mg of the dried root has been used daily (7).
TOPICAL: For treatment of herpes labialis (cold sores), a cream containing 23 mg/gram each of rhubarb extract and sage extract has been applied every 2 to 4 hours while awake, with treatment starting within one day of symptoms and continuing for 10 to 14 days (10437).

RIBOFLAVIN (VITAMIN B2)

Also Known As

B Complex Vitamin, Flavin, Flavine, Lactoflavin, Riboflavine, Vitamin B-2, Vitamin G.

Scientific Names

Riboflavin; Vitamin B2.

People Use This For

Orally, riboflavin is used for preventing riboflavin deficiency, treating ariboflavinosis, preventing migraine headaches, treating acne, congenital methemoglobinemia, muscle cramps, burning feet syndrome, carpal tunnel syndrome, red blood cell aplasia, multiple acylcoenzyme A dehydrogenase deficiency, eye fatigue, cataracts, and glaucoma. It is also used orally for increasing energy levels; boosting immune system function; maintaining healthy hair, skin, mucous membranes, and nails; for slowing aging; canker sores; memory loss including Alzheimer's disease; ulcers; boosting athletic performance; promoting healthy reproductive function; burns; alcoholism; liver disease; sickle cell anemia; and for treating lactic acidosis induced by nucleoside analog reverse transcriptase inhibitor (NRTI) drugs.

Safety

LIKELY SAFE ...when used orally. No toxic effects have been reported (1396,1397,1398).
PREGNANCY: LIKELY SAFE ...when used orally at the recommended dietary allowance (RDA) of 1.4 mg per day (3094). There is insufficient reliable information about the safety of using larger amounts during pregnancy.
LACTATION: LIKELY SAFE ...when used orally at the recommended dietary allowance (RDA) of 1.6 mg per day (3094). There is insufficient reliable information about the safety of using larger amounts during lactation.

Effectiveness

EFFECTIVE

Ariboflavinosis. Taking riboflavin orally prevents riboflavin deficiency and improves ariboflavinosis (15).

POSSIBLY EFFECTIVE

Cataracts. Taking riboflavin orally seems to reduce the occurrence of cataracts. A large-scale population-based study found that high dietary intake of riboflavin is associated with a reduced risk of nuclear cataracts (6378).

Migraine headache. There is some evidence that taking riboflavin orally might reduce migraine headache frequency similar to the beta-blockers, bisoprolol (Zebeta) and metoprolol (Lopressor) (1396). But riboflavin doesn't appear to reduce the severity or duration of an acute migraine headache (1398).

INSUFFICIENT RELIABLE EVIDENCE to RATE

AIDS-related lactic acidosis. There is preliminary clinical evidence that riboflavin may be useful for treating lactic acidosis in patients with acquired immunodeficiency syndrome (AIDS) caused by nucleoside analog reverse transcriptase inhibitors (NRTI) (2024,10468). More evidence is needed to rate riboflavin for this use.

Mechanism of Action

Riboflavin is an essential B vitamins (vitamin B2). It is required for tissue respiration. It is converted to the coenzyme riboflavin 5-phosphate (flavin mononucleotide, FMN) and then to the coenzyme flavin adenine dinucleotide (FAD). These act as hydrogen carriers for several enzymes known as flavoproteins, which are involved in oxidation-reduction reactions of organic substrates and in intermediary metabolism (15). It is also indirectly involved in maintaining erythrocyte integrity. Riboflavin deficiency, or ariboflavinosis, is characterized by cheilosis, angular stomatitis, glossitis, sore throat, keratitis, scrotal skin changes, neuropathy, and seborrheic dermatitis. In severe cases there is a normocytic and normochromic anemia (15).

Riboflavin deficiency can occur in people with long-standing infections such as HIV, liver disease, alcoholism, and malignancy (15). Researchers think that riboflavin deficiency might contribute to lactic acidosis that can occur in HIV patients taking stavudine (d4T, Zerit), zidovudine (AZT, Retrovir) and similar nucleoside analog reverse transcriptase inhibitor (NRTI) drugs (2024). Although NRTI-induced lactic acidosis has been considered irreversible and fatal, riboflavin reportedly can reverse this condition in some patients (2024).

Adverse Reactions

Orally, large doses of riboflavin (400 mg per day) might cause diarrhea and polyuria (1398). Riboflavin can cause a yellow-orange discoloration of the urine (15).

Interactions with Herbs & Other Dietary Supplements

IRON: Riboflavin supplements may improve the hematological response to iron supplements in some people with anemia. Riboflavin is thought to be involved in mobilizing iron from the storage form ferritin, for heme and globin synthesis (9518). This effect is probably only significant in people with riboflavin deficiency.

Interactions with Drugs

ANTICHOLINERGIC DRUGS: The rate of supplemental riboflavin absorption is decreased, but the total amount of the vitamin absorbed is increased, by drugs with anticholinergic effects. These drugs reduce gut motility, increasing the time the vitamin is present at absorption sites in the intestine (10513,10514). This has been demonstrated with propantheline (Pro-Banthine), but could theoretically occur with any drug that has anticholinergic effects. The clinical significance isn't known.

PROBENECID (Benemid): Probenecid reduces renal tubular secretion and total urinary excretion of both supplemental and dietary riboflavin (10515,10516,10517). It may also reduce the active intestinal absorption mechanism for riboflavin (10516). After single doses of probenecid, the effect on renal excretion predominates and plasma riboflavin levels are increased (10516,10517). The effect of prolonged probenecid therapy on riboflavin balance, and therefore the clinical significance, isn't known.

Drug Influences on Nutrient Levels and Depletion

SOME DRUGS CAN AFFECT RIBOFLAVIN LEVELS:

ANTIBIOTICS: Interference with the normal gastrointestinal flora by antibiotics may reduce bacterial synthesis of riboflavin (4437). However, this synthesis doesn't seem to significantly contribute to the body's supply of riboflavin, which is primarily obtained from dietary sources in the small intestine (6243,9530). Riboflavin supplements aren't necessary during antibiotic therapy.

ANTIDEPRESSANTS, TRICYCLIC: Tricyclic antidepressants have structural similarities to riboflavin and can interfere with its conversion to the active form flavin adenine dinucleotide (FAD) (10518). In rats, very high doses of amitriptyline and imipramine (50 mg/kg/day) decrease FAD levels in the liver, heart and brain. Lower doses (10 mg/kg/day) only affect the heart (10519). Since these doses are higher than those used therapeutically in humans, it's unlikely that the effect is clinically significant, or that supplements are necessary.

BARBITURATES: Phenobarbital induces metabolism of riboflavin in the liver. Levels of the active form of riboflavin, flavin adenine dinucleotide (FAD), are increased in the liver and levels of a hydroxylated metabolite are increased in the urine (10534,10535). The clinical significance of this isn't clear.

CHLORPROMAZINE (Thorazine): Chlorpromazine has structural similarities to riboflavin and can interfere with its conversion to the active form, flavin adenine dinucleotide (FAD) (10518). In rats, chlorpromazine decreases FAD levels in the liver, kidneys, heart and skeletal muscle, increases urinary riboflavin excretion, and produces changes in erythrocyte enzyme activity consistent with riboflavin deficiency (10518,10519,10520,10521). Chlorpromazine also inhibits renal tubular secretion and reabsorption of riboflavin (10515). Although these effects occur in rats at similar doses to those used in humans, data in humans are lacking. There isn't enough evidence to recommend use of riboflavin supplements with chlorpromazine or other phenothiazines.

DOXORUBICIN (Adriamycin, Rubex): Preliminary evidence indicates that doxorubicin interacts with riboflavin by forming complexes, competing for tissue binding sites, reducing conversion to flavin adenine dinucleotide (FAD, the active form of riboflavin), and increasing urinary excretion (9533,10528,10529,10530). These effects may contribute to

cardiac and muscle toxicity associated with doxorubicin, but data in humans are lacking.
ORAL CONTRACEPTIVES: Oral contraceptives may interfere with the absorption of riboflavin, or its conversion to active coenzyme forms (9505,10525). However, studies are conflicting. Some have found reduced levels of flavin adenine dinucleotide (FAD, the active form of riboflavin), reduced urinary riboflavin excretion, or reduced erythrocyte glutathione reductase activity consistent with riboflavin deficiency, in women taking oral contraceptives (4548,10523,10524,10525). However, many of these studies involved women with marginal or deficient dietary riboflavin intake, who used high-dose oral contraceptives (50 mcg ethinyl estradiol/day). When dietary riboflavin intake is adequate, no interaction with oral contraceptives is found (9373,10526,10527,10536). Routine riboflavin supplementation isn't necessary in women taking oral contraceptives.
PSYLLIUM: Psyllium reduces absorption of supplemental riboflavin in healthy women (10094). It isn't clear whether this occurs with dietary riboflavin, or whether it's clinically significant. Products containing psyllium include Metamucil, Konsyl, and Perdiem.
QUINACRINE: Quinacrine has structural similarities to riboflavin and can interfere with its conversion to the active form flavin adenine dinucleotide (FAD) (505,10521). It's suggested that this could lead to riboflavin deficiency in humans, but it may also contribute to the therapeutic effects of quinacrine against malaria (10522). The clinical significance isn't known.

Interactions with Foods

FOOD: Absorption of riboflavin supplements may be increased when taken with food because bile salts facilitate intestinal uptake of riboflavin (9530). However, the absorption mechanism for riboflavin is saturable; therefore, the clinical significance isn't clear.

Interactions with Lab Tests

ACETOACETATE DECARBOXYLASE: Riboflavin can falsely increase serum acetoacetate decarboxylase test results due to enzyme activation (275).
CATECHOLAMINES: Riboflavin can falsely elevate plasma and urine fluorometric catecholamine test results due to fluorescent metabolites in the plasma and urine (275).
COLORIMETRIC TESTS: Large amounts of riboflavin can interfere with urinalysis based on spectrometry or color reactions. Large amounts of riboflavin cause bright yellow urine (275).
DIAGNEX BLUE EXCRETION: Riboflavin can falsely increase urine Diagnex blue excretion test results, by color interference (275).
DRUGS-OF-ABUSE ASSAYS: Large doses of riboflavin (200 mg twice daily) cause errors in Abbott TDx drugs-of-abuse urine assays. Riboflavin produces a fluorophore that competes with the fluorescein-labeled antibody used in the assay (1266).
UROBILINOGEN: Riboflavin can falsely increase plasma and urine fluorometric urobilinogen test results, due to fluorescent metabolites in the plasma and urine (275).

Interactions with Diseases or Conditions

HEPATITIS, CIRRHOSIS, BILIARY OBSTRUCTION: Riboflavin absorption is decreased in these conditions (15).

Dosage and Administration

ORAL: As a dietary supplement, 1-4 mg a day is generally sufficient (15). For riboflavin deficiency in adults, 5-30 mg is taken daily in divided doses (15). For preventing migraine headaches, a dose of 400 mg per day has been used (1396,1397,1398), and maximum benefit might take up to three months to achieve (1398). A daily dietary intake of approximately 2.6 mg of riboflavin has been associated with reduced risk of nuclear cataracts (6378).
The daily recommended dietary allowances (RDAs) of riboflavin are: Infants 0-6 months, 0.3 mg; Infants 7-12 months, 0.4 mg; Children 1-3 years, 0.5 mg; Children 4-8 years, 0.6 mg; Children 9-13 years, 0.9 mg; Men 14 years or older, 1.3 mg; Women 14-18 years, 1 mg; Women over 18 years, 1.1 mg; Pregnant women, 1.4 mg; and Lactating women, 1.6 mg (3094). For treating stavudine or zidovudine-induced lactic acidosis, 50 mg per day has been used (2024,6132).

Comments

Riboflavin is found in many foods including milk, meat, eggs, nuts, enriched flour, and green vegetables (15). Riboflavin is frequently used in combination with other B vitamins in vitamin B complex formulations. Vitamin B complex generally includes vitamin B1 (thiamine), vitamin B2 (riboflavin), vitamin B3 (niacin/niacinamide), vitamin B5 (pantothenic acid), vitamin B6 (pyridoxine), vitamin B12 (cyanocobalamin), and folic acid. However, some products do not contain all of these ingredients and some may include others, such as biotin, para-aminobenzoic acid (PABA), choline bitartrate, and inositol (3022).

RIBOSE

Also Known As
D-ribose.

Scientific Names
Beta-D-ribofuranose.

People Use This For
Orally, ribose is used to increase muscle function, recovery, athletic performance, boost muscle tissue energy, and enhance effectiveness of creatine, maximize ribose production, replenish ATP stores, and improve or maintain nucleotide salvage and/or synthesis in heart and skeletal muscles following high intensity exercise. It has also been used to improve exercise tolerance, maintain or increase energy stores in the heart or muscle cells, and improve quality of life in individuals with reduced myocardial blood flow such as improving the heart's tolerance to ischemia in patients with coronary artery disease. Oral ribose has been used to prevent symptoms such as cramping, pain, and stiffness after exercise in patients with myoadenylate deaminase deficiency (MAD), also known as AMP deaminase deficiency (AMPD deficiency). Ribose has also been used orally to improve exercise tolerance in patients with McArdle's disease.

Intravenously, ribose has been used to facilitate thallium-201 redistribution and improve imaging of ischemic myocardium in patients with coronary artery disease. It has also been used intravenously in patients with MAD to prevent symptoms such as cramping, pain, and stiffness.

Safety
POSSIBLY SAFE ...when used orally or intravenously and appropriately, short-term (5662,5663,5664,5676,5677,5679,5680). There is insufficient reliable information available about the safety of ribose for its other uses.

PREGNANCY AND LACTATION: Insufficient reliable information available; avoid using.

Effectiveness
POSSIBLY EFFECTIVE

Coronary artery disease. Taking ribose orally seems to be effective for improving the heart's tolerance to ischemia in patients with coronary artery disease. A small randomized and placebo controlled study showed increased time to onset of moderate angina and time to ST depression during treadmill walking exercise testing in patients with coronary artery disease (5664).

Myoadenylate deaminase deficiency (MAD). Taking ribose orally or intravenously seems to be effective for preventing symptoms such as cramping, pain and stiffness after exercise in patients with MAD, also known as AMP deaminase deficiency (AMPD deficiency). One case report and a small clinical study suggest symptoms can be prevented with administration of ribose before and during exercise (5677,5679).

LIKELY INEFFECTIVE

McArdle's disease. Taking ribose orally doesn't improve exercise tolerance in patients with McArdle's disease (5678).

There is insufficient reliable information available about the effectiveness of ribose for its other uses.

Mechanism of Action
Ribose, a pentose sugar which is usually supplied by the oxidative pentose phosphate pathway (PPP) (also known as the hexose monophosphate shunt), is rapidly taken up by cells and phosphorylated to ribose-5-phosphate (5653). Ribose is rate-limiting in the production of phosphoribosyl-pyrophosphate (PRPP) (5652,5653,5682), a precursor for the salvage and de-novo adenine nucleotide synthetic pathways which maintain adenine, ADP, and AMP levels for the resynthesis of ATP (5651,5652,5665,5682). High energy bonds of ATP are the direct source for myocardial contractions (5652). During ischemia, the levels of ATP in the myocardium fall as the rate of oxidative phosphorylation decreases (5651,5653) and do not recover if the period of no perfusion is too long (5651). ADP and AMP levels rise transiently during ischemia but decrease as they are dephosphorylated into metabolites (adenine, inosine and hypoxanthine) which easily diffuse through the cell membrane and are washed out of the myocardium during reperfusion (5652,5653). Since the metabolites which use the salvage synthetic pathway are no longer available as precursors for ATP resynthesis, the de-novo synthetic pathway is activated (5652). Restoration of ATP levels via this pathway is slow in comparison to the salvage pathway (5652,5664) due to the short supply of PRPP which is usually supplied by the oxidative pentose phosphate pathway (5664). Studies suggest that this also occurs during ischemic events after high intensity exercise in skeletal muscle (5656,5657,5658). Evidence suggests exogenous ribose bypasses the PPP when it is converted to ribose-5-phosphate, increasing the amount of PRPP available for the de-novo synthetic pathway and ultimately resulting in the repletion of ATP levels in the myocardium (5652). Animal studies suggest exogenous ribose with adenine improves myocardial ATP, ADP and adenine nucleotide recovery after moderate periods of ischemia and improves recovery of contractile myocardial function (5652,5653). Other animal studies suggest exogenous ribose given during both periods of ischemia and reperfusion significantly increases ATP levels (5659) and may shorten ATP recovery time (5654,5659,5660). There have been no human studies done to confirm these findings. Laboratory evidence

also suggests ribose may have a role in preserving hearts for transplantation by maintaining ATP levels (5666). Controlled human studies have established that infusion of ribose facilitates the distribution and accelerates the clearance of thallium-201 from normal (nonischemic) regions of the coronary artery, leaving only thallium-201 in ischemic myocardium (5662,5663). The mechanism of action on how this occurs is unknown (5662). A small, randomized, placebo study controlled reported oral ribose given to patients with coronary artery disease may improve their tolerance to ischemia during exercise (5664). Other studies suggest oral ribose may prevent exercise-induced muscle pain and stiffness in patients with myoadenylate deaminase deficiency (5677,5676,5679,5680). Randomized, prospective controlled human studies are needed to establish the mechanism of action and the effectiveness of exogenous ribose when used to improve tolerance to exercise-induced ischemia in healthy individuals and patients with unstable cardiac condition such as coronary artery disease.

Adverse Reactions

Orally, ribose can cause diarrhea (5676), decreased blood glucose levels (5667), gastrointestinal discomfort, nausea and headache (5664). Hypoglycemia (5650,5662,5676), slightly increased serum insulin levels (5663) and decreased serum phosphate (5650) have been reported after infusion of ribose.

Interactions with Herbs & Other Dietary Supplements

None known.

Interactions with Drugs

ALCOHOL (Ethanol): Theoretically, ribose may increase the hypoglycemic effect of ethanol (5667).
ANTIDIABETES DRUGS: Theoretically, ribose may increase the hypoglycemic effect of oral antihyperglycemic agents such as the sulfonylureas, biguanides, alfa-glucosidase inhibitors, thiazolidinediones, and meglitinides (5667).
ASPIRIN: Theoretically, ribose may enhance the hypoglycemic effects of salicylate drugs such as aspirin (5667).
CHOLINE MAGNESIUM TRISALICYLATE (Trilisate): Theoretically, ribose may enhance the hypoglycemic effects of salicylate-containing drugs such as choline magnesium trisalicylate (5667).
INSULIN: Theoretically, ribose may increase the hypoglycemic effect of insulin and should be avoided by people taking insulin (5667).
PROPRANOLOL (Inderal): Theoretically, ribose may increase the hypoglycemic effect of propranolol (5667).
SALSALATE (Disalcid): Theoretically, ribose may enhance the hypoglycemic effects of salicylate-containing drugs such as salsalate (5667).

Interactions with Foods

None known.

Interactions with Lab Tests

GLUCOSE: Ribose may decrease serum glucose levels (5650,5662,5667,5676).
INSULIN: Ribose may increase serum insulin levels (5663).
PHOSPHATE: Ribose may decrease serum phosphate levels (5650).

Interactions with Diseases or Conditions

DIABETES: Theoretically, ribose should be avoided in patients with diabetes since it may interfere and enhance the glucose lowering effects of insulin or any oral antihyperglycemic agents.
HYPOGLYCEMIA: Theoretically, ribose should be avoided in patients who have hypoglycemia, or diseases or conditions that may increase their risk for hypoglycemia.

Dosage and Administration

ORAL: To improve exercise tolerance in patients with coronary artery disease, 15 grams four times per day has been used (5664). Beginning 1 hour before exercise until the end of the exercise session, 3 grams every 10 minutes has been used to reduce exercise-induced symptoms such as muscle stiffness and cramps associated with myoadenylate deaminase deficiency (5679).
INTRAVENOUS: For imaging of coronary arteries using thallium-201, a 30 minute 3.3 mg/kg/minute infusion of ribose as a 10% solution has been used (5662,5663).

RICE BRAN

Also Known As

Cereal Fiber, Dietary Fiber, Stabilized Rice Bran, Ricebran Oil, Rice Bran Oil.
CAUTION: See separate listings for Oat Bran and Wheat Bran.

Scientific Names

Oryza sativa.

People Use This For

Orally, rice bran is used for diabetes, hypertension, hyperlipidemia, alcoholism, weight loss, AIDS, preventing cancer, strengthening the immune system, increasing energy, enhancing athletic performance, aiding and improving liver function, preventing cardiovascular disease, and as an antioxidant. Rice bran oil is also used orally for hyperlipidemia.
Topically, rice bran is used for ectopic dermatitis.

Safety

LIKELY SAFE ...when used orally and appropriately. Rice bran and rice bran oil have been used safely in studies lasting up to 5 years (865,876,877,880,1354).
POSSIBLY SAFE ...when used as a bath additive. There is some evidence that a therapeutic bath containing rice bran broth can be safely used (872).
PREGNANCY AND LACTATION: LIKELY SAFE ...when used orally in amounts commonly found in foods. There is insufficient reliable information available about the safety of rice brand when used for medicinal purposes during pregnancy and lactation; avoid using.

Effectiveness

POSSIBLY EFFECTIVE

Atopic dermatitis (eczema). Applying rice bran broth topically seems to help reduce atopic dermatitis (872).
Gastric cancer. Consuming dietary cereal fiber, including rice bran, may decrease the incidence of stomach cancer (10435).
Hypercalciuria. Taking rice bran orally seems to reduce kidney stone (nephrolithiasis) recurrence, urine calcium excretion, and stone formation in people with hypercalciuria. Defatted rice bran 10 grams twice daily for 3 to 5 years seems to reduce urine calcium excretion and the incidence of kidney stone recurrence in people with hypercalcemia (876,878,880,881,882).
Hypercholesterolemia. Taking rice bran orally seems to lower cholesterol (865,877). Full-fat rice bran 85 grams per day, when added to a reduced-fat diet, seems to lower total cholesterol by 8% and low-density lipoprotein (LDL) cholesterol by 14%. Rice bran does not seem to affect triglycerides or high-density lipoprotein (HDL) cholesterol (865). Rice bran in a reduced-fat form at 11.8 grams per day appears to produce only a modest effect on cholesterol (877). Both full-fat and reduced-fat rice bran have comparable effects to oat bran for reducing cholesterol (865,877). Rice bran oil also seems to be effective for hypercholesterolemia. There is some evidence that rice bran oil can reduce total cholesterol by 14%, LDL by 20%, triglycerides by 20%, and increase HDL by 41% (1354).

POSSIBLY INEFFECTIVE

Colorectal cancer. Consuming dietary cereal fiber, including rice bran, doesn't seem to reduce the risk of colorectal cancer (160,4819,4820,4821,5104).

There is insufficient reliable information available about the effectiveness of rice bran for its other uses.

Mechanism of Action

Rice bran is obtained from the outer hull of the rice Oryza sativa. It contains 21% fiber, 21% lipids, 13% amino acids, and a wide variety of vitamins and minerals (884,885). It also contains inositol and IP-6 (7598).
Most of the fiber in rice bran is insoluble. Rice bran contains a relatively high percentage of oil compared with most other brans (865). Although whole rice bran seems to have some antihypercholesterolemic properties, rice bran oil is likely responsible for the most significant effect. The oil contains beta-sitosterol and other phytosterols that are used to reduce cholesterol absorption (7520). Defatted rice bran oil does not appear to affect cholesterol (865,7520,7521). It also contains alpha-linolenic acid, which might increase the concentration of fatty acids such as eicosapentaenoic and docosahexaenoic acids (7520,7521).
Other constituents of rice bran oil are gamma oryzanol and tocotrienols, which might lower cholesterol by altering cholesterol absorption and excretion (7521,7598).
Rice bran also contains lipase, which causes a rapid deterioration of rice bran oil unless the lipase is promptly stabilized by heat or other treatments (865).
Rice bran can increase stool size by several mechanisms, including water retention (871,879). Scientists think increased fecal bulk reduces risk of cancer because it dilutes carcinogens, especially tumor promoters such as secondary bile acids (871). Diets high in fiber have resulted in lower insulin levels, less weight gain, and a reduction in cardiovascular disease risk factors such as hypertension (2737). Rice bran reduces the risk of recurrent urinary stone disease, perhaps because the phytin in rice bran reduces calcium absorption (881). Healthy women on a calcium-rich diet, who added rice bran to their diets decreased renal excretion of calcium and increased renal excretion of oxalic acid (874). A rice bran isolate designated as Compound X shows evidence of antihistamine activity. It also inhibits bacterial growth (884). A modified rice bran isolate, MGN-3 (see separate listing), exhibits anti-HIV activity (866).

Adverse Reactions
Orally, increasing the amount of bran in the diet can cause erratic bowel habits, flatulence, and abdominal discomfort during the first few weeks (272).
Topical use of rice bran broth baths can cause itching and skin redness (872). Rash and itching from rice bran has been associated in rare cases from contact infestation with Pyemotes tritici, an arthropod commonly called straw itch mite (2284).

Interactions with Herbs & Other Dietary Supplements
CALCIUM: Rice bran might reduce absorption of calcium in the intestine (881).
HERBS AND SUPPLEMENTS: Theoretically, rice bran might delay or impair the absorption of herbs and supplements due to the fiber contained inn rice bran.
IRON: The fiber in rice bran might inhibit dietary iron absorption (156).

Interactions with Drugs
ORAL DRUGS: Theoretically, a diet high in rice bran might slow or reduce the absorption of some oral drugs.

Interactions with Foods
None known.

Interactions with Lab Tests
None known.

Interactions with Diseases or Conditions
GASTROINTESTINAL CONDITIONS: Contraindicated in people with intestinal ulcerations, stenosis, disabling adhesions, cathartic colon, or other conditions that may result in intestinal or esophageal obstruction due to the fiber contained in rice bran (272). Use with caution or avoid in people with difficulty chewing or swallowing food, or conditions that decrease small bowel motility.

Dosage and Administration
ORAL: For reducing cholesterol, 12-84 grams rice bran per day (865,877), or 4.8 grams rice bran oil (providing 312 mg tocotrienols, 360 mg tocopherols, and 2.4 grams other non-saponifiables) per day has been used (1354). For reducing the risk of kidney stones, 10 grams rice bran twice daily has been used (881,882). For decontamination of ingested polychlorinated biphenyl (PCB) and polychlorinated dibenzofuran (PCDF), 10 grams rice bran with a dietary fiber content 50% and 4 grams cholestyramine (Questran) three times a day has been used (870).

Comments
Rice bran oil is a popular "healthy oil" in Japan, Asia, and particularly India (7521).

RNA AND DNA

Also Known As
DNA, DeoxyNucleic Acid, Nuclei Acids, Nucleic, Nucleic Acid, Nucleic Acids, Nucleotides, Purines, Pyrimidines, RNA, RNA-DNA, RNA/DNA.

Scientific Names
Deoxyribonucleic Acid; Ribonucleic Acid.

People Use This For
Orally, RNA/DNA combinations are used to improve memory and mental sharpness, to treat or prevent Alzheimer's disease, to treat depression, increase energy, tighten skin, increase sex drive, and to counteract the effects of aging.
Enterally, RNA is used in nutrition formulations that include omega-3 fatty acids and arginine for reducing the time needed for recovery after surgery, to boost immune response, and to improve outcomes of burn patients and intensive care patients.
As an injection, RNA is used to treat eczema, psoriasis, hives, and shingles.

Safety
LIKELY SAFE ...when RNA and DNA are consumed in food. ...when RNA is used in enteral nutrition along with omega-3 fatty acids and L-arginine (5531,5533,5534,5535,5536,7819).
POSSIBLY SAFE ...when RNA is injected subcutaneously (5538).
There is insufficient reliable information available about the safety of oral RNA/DNA supplement combinations.
LIKELY SAFE ...when RNA is used in enteral nutrition along with omega-3 fatty acids and L-arginine

(5531,5533,5534,5535,5536,7819).
POSSIBLY SAFE ...when RNA is injected subcutaneously (5538).
CHILDREN: LIKELY SAFE ...when infant formulas contain nucleotide supplements (5900).
PREGNANCY AND LACTATION: POSSIBLY UNSAFE ...when used orally as supplements. Some evidence suggests some orally ingested DNA might cross the placenta and be mutagenic (5539).

Effectiveness

POSSIBLY EFFECTIVE

Surgical recovery. Supplementing the diet of patients undergoing major surgery with enteral or oral RNA, L-arginine, and eicosapentaenoic acid might improve recovery. This combination administered in the perioperative period appears to boost immune response, reduce perioperative infections, improve wound healing, and shorten recovery time (5531,5532,5533,7819).

POSSIBLY INEFFECTIVE

Burns. Taking RNA and DNA enterally doesn't seem to produce a better outcome in burn patients than standard nutritional formulas (5535).

There is insufficient reliable information available about the effectiveness of RNA and DNA for their other uses.

Mechanism of Action

Although most organisms can synthesize nucleotides (5900), dietary nucleotides (derived from DNA and RNA) appear to be essential under conditions of rapid growth such as intestinal development, liver resection or injury and also during challenges to the immune system. When preformed nucleotides are consumed, they are degraded to free bases in the intestine before absorption. Experimental evidence shows they are incorporated into the hepatic pyrimidine nucleotide pool (5900) and that they affect the hepatic RNA content. The hepatic RNA content, in turn, affects the recovery time from liver injury. In protein-deprived animals, dietary nucleotides appear to benefit the intestinal tract. They can also restore immune function, while restoring the nitrogen balance (protein intake) does not (5543). In the absence of nucleotides, normal T-lymphocyte maturation is blocked (5543). A Crohn's disease model in rats shows RNA has a highly significant effect upon the healing intestinal ulcerations (5900). Supplementing an enteral diet with arginine, RNA, and omega-3 fatty acids can reduce concentrations of tumor necrosis factor alpha, and interleukin-6 and accelerate the recovery in the concentration of interleukin-1 beta and interleukin-2 alpha receptor (5532).

Adverse Reactions

Subcutaneously, an injection of RNA can cause itching, redness, and swelling at the injection site (5538).

Interactions with Herbs & Other Dietary Supplements

None known.

Interactions with Drugs

None known.

Interactions with Foods

None known.

Interactions with Lab Tests

None known.

Interactions with Diseases or Conditions

None known.

Dosage and Administration

ORAL: No typical dosage.
ENTERAL: A typical enteral dose of RNA is 30 mg/kg/day along with arginine and omega-3 fatty acids (5533,5534).
INJECTION: A typical dose is 10 mg injectable RNA every other day for 2-4 weeks (5538).

ROMAN CHAMOMILE

Also Known As

Chamomile, Chamomilla, Chamomillae ramane flos, English Chamomile, Fleur De Camomille Romaine, Flores Anthemidis, Garden Chamomile, Grosse Kamille, Ground Apple, Low Chamomile, Manzanilla, Römische Kamille, Sweet Chamomile, Whig Plant.
CAUTION: See separate listing for German Chamomile.

Scientific Names

Chamaemelum nobile, synonyms Athemis nobilis, Ormenis nobilis.
Family: Asteraceae/Compositae.

People Use This For

Orally, Roman chamomile is used for indigestion, nausea and vomiting, anorexia, morning sickness, painful menstrual periods, flatulent indigestion associated with mental stress, mucous membrane inflammation, sinusitis, and rheumatic disorders.
Topically, Roman chamomile is used for eczema, wounds, and inflammation; and as an antiseptic in ointments, creams, and gels to treat cracked nipples, sore gums, and irritation of the skin and mucosa. It is also used topically for wounds, burns, frostbite, diaper rash, decubitus ulcers, and hemorrhoids.
In oral herbal combinations, Roman chamomile is used for liver and gallbladder disease, gallstones, fatty liver, chronic heartburn, loss of appetite, digestive disturbances, Roemheld syndrome, indigestion in infants, and in spastic constipation. It is used as a "blood purifier", general female tonic, a preventative for menstrual discomforts, and for irregular periods.
In herbal inhalation therapy, Roman chamomile is used in steam baths for sinus inflammation, hay fever, pharyngeal swelling, and ear inflammation, and as an analgesic.
In foods and beverages, the essential oil and extract are used as flavor components.
In manufacturing, the volatile oil of Roman chamomile is used as a fragrance component in soaps, cosmetics, and perfumes; and to flavor cigarette tobacco. The extract is also used in cosmetics, and soaps. Teas have been used as a hair tint and conditioner, and to treat parasitic worm infections.

Safety

LIKELY SAFE ...when used orally in amounts commonly found in foods. Roman chamomile has Generally Recognized As Safe (GRAS) status in the US (4912).
POSSIBLY SAFE ...when used orally and appropriately in medicinal amounts (2,12). ...when the essential oil is inhaled or used topically as aromatherapy (7107).
PREGNANCY: LIKELY UNSAFE ...when used orally in medicinal amounts. Roman chamomile is believed to be an abortifacient (4). There is insufficient reliable information available about the safety of the topical use of Roman chamomile during pregnancy; avoid using.
LACTATION: Insufficient reliable information available; avoid using (4).

Effectiveness

There is insufficient reliable information available about the effectiveness of Roman chamomile.

Mechanism of Action

The applicable part of Roman chamomile is the flowerhead. Roman chamomile possesses antiflatulent, antispasmodic, and sedative properties (4). Large amounts of Roman chamomile can act as an emetic while small amounts act as an anti-emetic (4). In cosmetics, Roman chamomile is considered a deodorant and a stimulant to skin metabolism (11). Roman chamomile contains the coumarin scopoletin-7-glucoside and varied flavonoids, their glycosides (including rutin and volatile oils), as well as other constituents (4). Some evidence suggests azulene constituents contained in volatile oils exert anti-allergy and anti-inflammatory effects by inhibiting histamine release. However, the constituent nobilin, a sesquiterpene lactone, is thought to trigger allergy in sensitive individuals (4). Some evidence suggests Roman chamomile acts on the central nervous system, possibly reducing aggressive behavior (18). Experimental evidence suggests the volatile oil could have anti-inflammatory, antidiuretic, and sedative effects (4). The essential oil is active against gram-positive bacteria and dermatomyces (18). The sesquiterpinoids nobilin, 1,10-epoxynobilin, and 3-dehydronobilin show some evidence of antitumor activity (4). Although the constituents of Roman chamomile are not identical to those of German chamomile both plants are similarly used (512).

Adverse Reactions

Orally, large amounts of Roman chamomile might cause vomiting (11), although this is disputed (12).
Topically, Roman chamomile can cause contact dermatitis (4,567). Allergic skin reactions occur in up to 20% of individuals (19). It can cause an allergic reaction in individuals sensitive to the Asteraceae/Compositae family. Members of this family include ragweed, chrysanthemums, marigolds, daisies, and many other herbs.

Interactions with Herbs & Other Dietary Supplements
None known.

Interactions with Drugs
None known.

Interactions with Foods
None known.

Interactions with Lab Tests
None known.

Interactions with Diseases or Conditions
ASTHMA: May exacerbate asthma (4).
CROSS-ALLERGENICITY: Use of Roman chamomile can cause an allergic reaction in individuals sensitive to the Asteraceae/Compositae family. Members of this family include ragweed, chrysanthemums, marigolds, daisies, and many other herbs.

Dosage and Administration
ORAL: A typical dose is 1-4 grams dried flowerheads three times daily, or one cup tea. To make tea, steep 1-4 grams dried flowerheads in 150 mL of boiling water for 5-10 minutes, strain (4). Liquid extract (1:1 in 70% alcohol), 1-4 mL three times daily (4).
TOPICAL: A 3% steeped tea is prepared for topical use (8).

Comments
Most of the existing information on Roman chamomile concerns German chamomile (4,7), but it is extrapolated to Roman chamomile.

ROSE GERANIUM OIL

Also Known As
Aetheroleum Pelargonii, Algerian Geranium Oil, Bourbon Geranium Oil, Moroccan Geranium Oil, Oleum Geranii, Pelargonium Oil.

Scientific Names
Pelargonium graveolens.
Family: Geraniaceae.

People Use This For
Orally, rose geranium oil is used orally for neuropathic pain and diarrhea.
Topically, rose geranium oil is used as an astringent.
In foods and beverages, rose geranium oil is used as a flavoring agent.
In manufacturing, rose geranium oil is used as an inexpensive substitute for rose oil. It is also used as a fragrance component in soaps, cosmetics, and perfumes.

Safety
LIKELY SAFE ...when used in amounts commonly found in foods. Rose geranium oil has Generally Recognized As Safe (GRAS) status in the US (4912).
There is insufficient reliable information available about the safety of rose geranium oil for its other uses.
PREGNANCY AND LACTATION: Insufficient reliable information; avoid amounts greater than those found in foods.

Effectiveness
There is insufficient reliable information available about the effectiveness of rose geranium oil.

Mechanism of Action
The applicable part of rose geranium is the oil that is distilled from the stem and leaf. The geranium oil constituents citronellol, citronellyl acetate, citronellyl formate, and geraniol exhibit marginal antitumor activity (3751). The essential oils from Pelargonium species show some indication of antibacterial and antifungal activity (3752,3753).

Adverse Reactions
Topically, rose geranium oil has been associated with dermatitis in hypersensitive individuals (11); however, rose geranium oil is generally considered to be nonsensitizing, nonirritating, and nonphototoxic to human skin (11).

Interactions with Herbs & Other Dietary Supplements
None known.

Interactions with Drugs
None known.

Interactions with Foods
None known.

Interactions with Lab Tests
None known.

Interactions with Diseases or Conditions
None known.

Dosage and Administration
No typical dosage.

Comments
Avoid confusing rose geranium oil with East Indian or Turkish geranium oil (known as palmorosa oil) that is derived from a different plant (11).

ROSE HIP

Also Known As
Apothecary rose, Cynosbatos, Dog Rose, Heps, Hip, Hip Fruit, Hip Sweet, Hipberry, Hop Fruit, Rosa de castillo, Rosae pseudofructus cum semen, Rose Hip with seed, Rose Hips, Rosehips, Satapatri, Satapatrika, Wild Boar Fruit.
CAUTION: See separate listings for Acerola, Vitamin C, and Cherokee Rosehip.

Scientific Names
Rosa canina, synonym Rosa lutetiana; Rosa alba; Rosa centifolia; Rosa damascena; Rosa gallica, synonym Rosa provincialis; Rosa rugosa; Rosa villosa, synonym Rosa pomifera; other Rosa species.
Family: Rosaceae.

People Use This For
Orally, rose hip is used as a supplemental source of dietary vitamin C, for preventing and treating colds, influenza-like infections, infectious diseases, vitamin C deficiencies, fever, increasing immune function during exhaustion, gastric spasms, gastric acid deficiency, preventing gastric mucosal inflammation and gastric ulcers, and as a "stomach tonic" for intestinal diseases. It is also used orally for diarrhea, gallstones, gallbladder ailments, lower urinary tract and kidney disorders, dropsy (edema), gout, disorders of uric acid metabolism, arthritis, sciatica, diabetes, increasing peripheral circulation, for reducing thirst, as a laxative and diuretic, and to treat chest ailments.
In foods and in manufacturing, it is used for rose hip tea, jam and soup, and as a natural source of vitamin C.

Safety
LIKELY SAFE ...when used in amounts commonly found in foods. Rose hips extract has Generally Recognized As Safe (GRAS) status in the US (4912).
POSSIBLY SAFE ...when used orally and appropriately for medicinal purposes (12).
PREGNANCY AND LACTATION: Insufficient reliable information available; avoid using in amounts greater than those found in foods.

Effectiveness
There is insufficient reliable information available about the effectiveness of rose hip.

Mechanism of Action
Rose hip contains pectin, citric acid, and malic acid, which can have laxative and diuretic activities (5,18). The diuretic activity is controversial (8). Fresh rose hip contains between 0.5-1.7% vitamin C (5,8) and is estimated to contain 1250 mg vitamin C per 100 grams of rose hip (6). However, much of the vitamin C is destroyed during drying and

processing (11), and declines rapidly with storage (2). Vitamin C is required for collagen formation and tissue repair (15). It is an enzyme cofactor in the synthesis of collagen, carnitine, norepinephrine, and peptide hormones, and in tyrosine metabolism (3042). Vitamin C is also involved in oxidation-reduction reactions, conversion of folic acid to folinic acid, carbohydrate metabolism, synthesis of lipids and proteins, iron metabolism, resistance to infections, and cellular respiration (15). It acts as an antioxidant, decreasing oxidants in gastric juice, decreasing lipid peroxidation, and decreasing oxidative DNA and protein damage (3042). Vitamin C deficiency that lasts for three to five months results in symptomatic scurvy that affects collagenous structures, bones, and blood vessels (15). Vitamin C enhances the absorption of soluble non-heme iron, either by reducing it (converting ferric to ferrous) or by preventing chelation by phytates or other food ligands (3042).

Adverse Reactions

Orally, the adverse effects of vitamin C are related to the amount of vitamin C actually contained in the rose hip product. The adverse reactions include nausea; vomiting; esophagitis; heartburn; abdominal cramps; GI obstruction; fatigue; flushing; headache; insomnia; sleepiness; diarrhea; hyperoxaluria; and precipitation of urate, oxalate, or cysteine stones or drugs in the urinary tract (15). Large amounts are associated with deep vein thrombosis (15). The inhalation of the rose hip dust is reportedly a respiratory allergen in production workers. It can cause mild to moderate anaphylaxis (6).

Topically, the rose hip dust ("itching powder") can cause itching by mechanical irritation (6).

Interactions with Herbs & Other Dietary Supplements

IRON: Concomitant use interacts with the vitamin C in rose hip; 200 mg of vitamin C per 30 mg of elemental iron increases oral iron absorption, especially ferric iron (3042).

Interactions with Drugs

ALUMINUM: Concomitant use interacts with the vitamin C in rose hip and can increase aluminum absorption, but the clinical significance of this is unknown (3046). Administer rose hip with vitamin C two hours before or four hours after antacids (3046).

ASPIRIN: The vitamin C in rose hip can increase urinary excretion of ascorbic acid and decrease excretion of salicylates, but this may not have a clinically significant effect on salicylate plasma levels (3046).

CHOLINE MAGNESIUM TRISALICYLATE (Trilisate): The vitamin C in rose hip can increase urinary excretion of ascorbic acid and decrease excretion of salicylates such as choline magnesium trisalicylate. But this may not have a clinically significant effect on salicylate plasma levels (3046).

ESTROGENS: Theoretically, the vitamin C in large amounts of rose hip might increase absorption and effects of estrogen (129,130).

FLUPHENAZINE (Prolixin): Concomitant use with rose hip decreases blood levels due to vitamin C content (15).

SALSALATE (Disalcid): The vitamin C in rose hip can increase urinary excretion of ascorbic acid and decrease excretion of salicylates such as salsalate. But this may not have a clinically significant effect on salicylate plasma levels (3046).

WARFARIN (Coumadin): Concomitant use interacts with the vitamin C in rose hip. Large amounts of vitamin C can impair the warfarin response (3046).

Interactions with Foods

IRON: Concomitant use interacts with the vitamin C in rose hip and can increase the absorption of dietary (ferric) iron (3042).

Interactions with Lab Tests

ACETAMINOPHEN: The vitamin C in rose hip can cause false negative urine results with methods based on hydrolysis and formation of an indophenol blue chromagen (275).

ASPARTATE AMINOTRANSFERASE (AST, SGOT): Large amounts of the vitamin C in rose hip can cause a false increase in results of serum tests relying on color reactions (Redox reactions) and Technicon SMA 12/60 (275).

BILIRUBIN: Large amounts of the vitamin C in rose hip can cause a false increase in serum test results measured by Technicon SMA 12/60 or colorimetric methods (275).

CALCIUM/SODIUM: 3-6 grams of vitamin C daily can cause a true increase in urinary calcium and test results (15) and a true decrease in urinary sodium and test results.

CARBAMAZEPINE (Tegretol): Large amounts of the vitamin C in rose hip can cause falsely increased serum assay results measured by Ames ARIS method (275).

CREATININE: The vitamin C in rose hip can cause a false increase in serum creatinine or urine test results (275).

GLUCOSE: Large amounts of the vitamin C in rose hip can cause false increases in urine test results measured by copper reduction methods (e.g., Clinitest) and false decreases in results measured by glucose oxidase methods (e.g., Clinistix, Tes-Tape) (15).

LDH: The vitamin C in rose hip can cause a false decrease measured by Technicon SMA 12/60 and Abbott 100 methods (275).

OCCULT BLOOD: The vitamin C in rose hip may cause false negative guaiac results to occur with 250 mg or more of vitamin C per day (3042).

THEOPHYLLINE: Large amounts of the vitamin C in rose hip can cause falsely decreased serum assay results when measured by the ARIS system or Ames Seralyzer photometer (275).
URIC ACID: Large amounts of the vitamin C in rose hip can cause a true decrease in serum uric acid concentrations and test results with enzymatic method assays (15).

Interactions with Diseases or Conditions

DIABETES: The vitamin C in rose hip might affect glycogenolysis and the control of diabetes, but not all experts agree on this (15).
GLUCOSE-6-PHOSPHATE DEHYDROGENASE DEFICIENCY: Large amounts of the vitamin C in rose hip might increase the risk of oxalate stone formation (15).
HEMOCHROMATOSIS, THALASSEMIA, SIDEROBLASTIC ANEMIA: Use rose hip with caution, because the vitamin C content can increase iron absorption, which could worsen this condition (15).
INCREASED NEEDS: Vitamin C requirements increase in pregnancy, lactation, hyperthyroidism, stress, fever, infection, trauma, burns, smoking, and cold exposure (15).
SICKLE CELL DISEASE: The vitamin C in rose hip rarely can decrease the blood pH, precipitating sickle cell crisis (15).

Dosage and Administration

ORAL: The typical dose of rose hips is as a tea, which is prepared by steeping 2-2.5 grams of the crushed rose hips in 150 mL boiling water for 10-15 minutes and then straining (8).

Comments

Rose hip with seed is the ripe, dried receptacle (hip) with fruit (seed) of various Rosa species, including dog rose (Rosa canina), white rose (Rosa alba), provence rose (Rosa centifolia), and damask rose (Rosa damascena). Avoid confusion with Cherokee rosehip, rose flower, and vitamin C. CAUTION: Sometimes rose hip seeds or plain rose hip receptacles without seeds are sold. These are different than rose hip with seed. Fresh rose hips contain a high concentration of vitamin C; however, much of the vitamin C is destroyed during drying and processing (11) and declines rapidly with storage (2). Many rose hip-derived "natural" vitamin C products are supplemented with synthetic vitamin C (6,11), but may not be clearly labeled accordingly (6).

ROSEMARY

Also Known As

Compass Plant, Compass Weed, Old Man, Polar Plant, Rusmari.
CAUTION: See separate listing for Rosinweed.

Scientific Names

Rosmarinus officinalis.
Family: Lamiaceae/Labiatae.

People Use This For

Orally, rosemary is used for dyspepsia, flatulence, inducing abortion, increasing menstrual flow, gout, cough, headache, liver and gallbladder complaints, loss of appetite, and for cardiovascular conditions such as high blood pressure.
Topically, rosemary is used for preventing baldness; alopecia areata; circulatory disturbances; toothache; eczema; joint or musculoskeletal pain such as myalgia, sciatica and intercostal neuralgia; balneotherapy; wound healing; and as an insect repellent.
In foods, rosemary is used as a spice. The leaf and oil are used in foods, and the oil in beverages.
In manufacturing, rosemary oil is used as a fragrant component in soaps and perfumes.

Safety

LIKELY SAFE ...when used orally in amounts typically found in foods. Rosemary has Generally Recognized As Safe (GRAS) status in the US (4912).
POSSIBLY SAFE ...when used orally and appropriately in medicinal amounts (18). ...when used topically and appropriately (5177). Rosemary oil has been used safely for up to 7 months (5177). ...when used by inhalation as aromatherapy (7107).
LIKELY UNSAFE ...when the essential oil is ingested. Ingestion of undiluted oil from rosemary can cause significant adverse effects (515).
PREGNANCY: POSSIBLY UNSAFE ...when used orally in medicinal amounts. Rosemary might have uterine and menstrual flow stimulant effects (4,12,18); avoid using. There is insufficient reliable information available about the safety of the topical use of rosemary during pregnancy.

LACTATION: There is insufficient reliable information available about the safety of using rosemary in medicinal amounts during lactation; avoid using.

Effectiveness

POSSIBLY EFFECTIVE

Alopecia areata. Rosemary oil in combination with the essential oils from thyme, lavender, and cedarwood seem to improve hair growth by 44% after 7 months of treatment for alopecia areata (5177).

POSSIBLY INEFFECTIVE

Abortion. Taking rosemary orally doesn't seem to be effective for use as an abortifacient (5,6).

There is insufficient reliable information available about the effectiveness of rosemary for its other uses.

Mechanism of Action

The applicable part of rosemary is the leaf. The active constituent of rosemary leaves is the essential oil. Dried leaves contain from 1-2.5% of the essential oil (4,5). The oil consists primarily of cineole, borneol, camphor, and pinenes (4,6). The essential oil might have a spasmolytic effect on smooth muscle of the gastrointestinal tract and in the ducts of the gallbladder (4). Rosemary might also have a positive inotropic effect on the heart and increases coronary blood flow (2). It's not clear how rosemary oil works in alopecia areata (5177). However, there is some evidence that topical use of rosemary might irritate the skin and increase blood circulation (2). Rosemary also seems to have antibacterial, antifungal (4), and antioxidant properties (4,6).

Adverse Reactions

Orally, large amounts of leaves containing rosemary oil might cause deep coma, spasm, vomiting, gastroenteritis, uterine bleeding, kidney irritation, pulmonary edema, and death (18). Ingestion of undiluted oil might cause stomach and intestinal irritation, kidney damage, and seizures (5,6). The camphor constituent can sometimes lead to seizures (4).

Topically, rosemary use can lead to photosensitivity, erythema, and dermatitis in hypersensitive individuals (4,6). Asthma due to repeated occupational exposure (occupational asthma) can occur (783).

Interactions with Herbs & Other Dietary Supplements

None known.

Interactions with Drugs

None known.

Interactions with Foods

None known.

Interactions with Lab Tests

None known.

Interactions with Diseases or Conditions

SEIZURE DISORDERS: Theoretically, rosemary might potentiate seizure activity (7107); avoid using.

Dosage and Administration

ORAL: A typical dose is 1-2 grams of crude leaf. Rosemary is often prepared as a tea. A typical dose is one cup tea three times daily, prepared by steeping 1-2 grams leaf in 150 mL boiling water for 5-10 minutes then straining (2,4). A liquid extract (1:1 in 45% alcohol) has also been used in a dose of 2-4 mL three times daily (4).

TOPICAL: Typically, semi-solid or liquid preparations containing 6-10% of the essential oil are used (2). For a rosemary bath, 50 grams crude leaf in 1 L hot water is commonly added to bath water (18). For the treatment of alopecia areata, a combination of the essential oils including rosemary 3 drops or 114 mg, thyme 2 drops or 88 mg, lavender 3 drops or 108 mg, and cedarwood 2 drops or 94 mg, all mixed with 3 mL jojoba oil and 20 mL grapeseed oil has been used. Each night, the mixture is massaged into the scalp for 2 minutes with a warm towel placed around the head to increase absorption (5177).

ROSEROOT

Also Known As

Arctic Root, Golden Root, King's Crown, Rhodiola, Rose Root, Rose Root Extract, Rosenroot, Rodia riza, Lignum rhodium.

Scientific Names

Rhodiola rosea, synonyms Sedum rhodiola, Sedum rosea. Family: Crassulaceae.

People Use This For

Orally, roseroot is used for increasing energy, stamina, strength and mental capacity; and as a so-called "adaptogen" to help the body adapt to and resist physical, chemical, and environmental stress. It is also used for improving athletic performance, improving sexual function, depression, cardiac disorders such as arrhythmias, and hyperlipidemia. Roseoot is also used for treating cancer, tuberculosis, and diabetes; preventing cold and flu, aging, and liver damage; improving hearing; strengthening the nervous system; enhancing immunity; and shortening recovery time after prolonged workouts.

Safety

There is insufficient reliable information about the safety of roseroot.
Pregnancy and Lactation: Insufficient reliable information available; avoid using.

Effectiveness

INSUFFICIENT RELIABLE EVIDENCE to RATE

Fatigue. There is preliminary evidence that a standardized roseroot extract 170 mg daily might help for fatigue in night shift workers. Roseroot extract seems to improve cognitive performance after the first treatment, but its effects don't seem to continue after the second treatment (6877). More evidence is needed to rate roseroot for this use.

Mechanism of Action

The applicable part of roseroot is the root. Roseroot contains a phenylpropanoid glycoside called salidroside (synonyms: rhodioloside, rhodosine), which is reported to have stimulant, anti-stress, and adaptogenic actions (increasing resistance to the harmful effects of stressors) (6877). Animal studies are reported to show protection from stressors such as cold and radiation, increased work capacity, decreased fatigue and improved learning and memory (6877). Roseroot extracts demonstrate antiarrhythmic properties and protection against reperfusion injury after ischemia. These effects can be abolished by naloxone infusion, suggesting that the mechanism might involve an increase in endogenous opioids (3191,3192,3195). Roseroot extracts might also prevent stress-induced cardiac damage by preventing rises in cardiac catecholamines and cyclic-AMP (3193). Roseroot extract reduces experimentally induced mutations, possibly by increasing the efficiency of intracellular DNA repair mechanisms (3190). Roseroot extracts also demonstrate hepatoprotective (3196) and myeloprotective effects (3197). Roseroot extracts also demonstrate potential for improving learning and memory (3198,6877). Preliminary research in a small number of patients with superficial bladder cancer suggests that roseroot extract might improve cell characteristics and reduce relapses (3194).

Adverse Reactions

None reported.

Interactions with Herbs & Other Dietary Supplements

None known.

Interactions with Drugs

None known.

Interactions with Foods

None known.

Interactions with Lab Tests

None known.

Interactions with Diseases or Conditions

None known.

Dosage and Administration

ORAL: Typical doses range from 50-250 mg of roseroot extract 1 to 3 times daily (3188,3189). For improving well-being and psychomotor function during stress, roseroot extract 50 mg twice daily has been used (1927).

Comments

Roseroot is native to the arctic regions of eastern Siberia, Scandinavia, Lapland, and Alaska (3187,3189). It has a long history of use as a medicinal plant in Iceland, Sweden, France, Russia, and Greece, where it is mentioned by Dioscorides in the first century A.D. (6877). It is reported that Chinese emperors sent expeditions to Siberia to collect the plant in the hope that it would bring long life or immortality (3187). Roseroot has been used as an ingredient in folk medicine love potions (3189). The green aerial parts of the plant have been used as a food ingredient (6877).

ROSINWEED

Also Known As

Compass Weed, Pilot Weed, Polar Plant.
CAUTION: See separate listings for Cup Plant and Rosemary.

Scientific Names

Silphium laciniatum.
Family: Asteraceae/Compositae.

Comments

At the date of publication, this product was not a common ingredient used in brand name supplements marketed to consumers. Details about this product are available at the online version of *Natural Medicines Comprehensive Database*. See www.naturaldatabase.com.

ROYAL JELLY

Also Known As

Bee Saliva, Bee Spit, Honey Bee Milk, Honey Bee's Milk.
CAUTION: See separate listings for Bee Pollen, Bee Venom, and Honey.

Scientific Names

Apis mellifera (Honey Bee).
Family: Apidae.

People Use This For

Orally, royal jelly is used for asthma, allergic rhinitis, liver disease, pancreatitis, insomnia, premenstrual syndrome (PMS), stomach ulcers, kidney disease, bone fractures, skin disorders, and hyperlipidemia. It is also used as a general health tonic, for rejuvenation, and potentiating the immune system.
Topically, royal jelly is used as a skin tonic and hair growth stimulant.

Safety

POSSIBLY SAFE ...when used orally and appropriately, short-term. Taking 2 tablets twice daily of a specific combination product containing royal jelly 6 mg, bee pollen extract 36 mg, and bee pollen plus pistil extract 120 mg (Femal, Natumin Pharma) per tablet for up to 2 months seems to be safe (12008). It's not known if other royal jelly doses and formulations are safe.
PREGNANCY and LACTATION: Insufficient reliable information available; avoid using.

Effectiveness

INSUFFICIENT RELIABLE EVIDENCE to RATE

Hyperlipidemia. There is preliminary evidence that royal jelly might lower cholesterol levels in people with hyperlipidemia (3515).

Premenstrual syndrome (PMS). Preliminary evidence suggests that a specific combination product (Femal, Natumin Pharma) seems to decrease some symptoms of PMS including irritability, weight increases, and edema when given over a period of 2 menstrual cycles. This product contains royal jelly 6 mg, bee pollen extract 36 mg, and bee pollen plus pistil extract 120 mg per tablet. It is given as 2 tablets twice daily (12008).

More evidence is needed to rate royal jelly for these uses.

Mechanism of Action

Royal jelly is a milky secretion produced by glands in the heads of nurse honey bees (Apis mellifera). The composition of royal jelly varies with geographical areas and climatic conditions. It typically contains about 60% to 70% water, 12% to 15% crude proteins, 10% to16% sugar, 3% to 6% lipids, and 2% to 3% low molecular weight compounds such as vitamins, salts, and free amino acids (7313). Royal jelly is used for the development and nurturing of queen bees (6). There is very little scientific information available about its effects in humans. In animal models, royal jelly seems to have some antitumor activity (6) and antiatherogenic activity (3515).

Adverse Reactions

Orally, royal jelly appears to cause few side effects in nonallergic people (7314). There is one report of dizziness in a patient who took a combination product containing royal jelly, bee pollen extract, and a bee pollen plus pistil extract (12008).
In people with a history of atopy or asthma, royal jelly appears to cause a high rate of allergic symptoms including

pruritus, urticaria, eczema, eyelid and facial edema, conjunctivitis, rhinorrhea, dyspnea, and asthma (7314,7315,7316,10623). In severe cases, royal jelly can cause status asthmaticus, anaphylaxis, and death (792,7315,7316,10623,10624). Allergic symptoms are associated with IgE-mediated hypersensitivity reactions (3513,10623). Tell people with a history of allergy or asthma not to use royal jelly.
There is also one case report of hemorrhagic colitis with abdominal pain, bloody diarrhea with concomitant hemorrhagic and edematous mucosa of the sigmoid colon after ingestion of royal jelly. Symptoms resolved within 2 weeks following discontinuation of royal jelly and conservative treatment (3516).
Topically, skin irritation, exacerbation of dermatitis, or contact dermatitis may occur (791).

Interactions with Herbs & Other Dietary Supplements

None known.

Interactions with Drugs

None known.

Interactions with Foods

None known.

Interactions with Lab Tests

None known.

Interactions with Diseases or Conditions

ASTHMA, ATOPY: In patients with asthma or atopy, royal jelly causes a high rate of allergic symptoms including pruritus, urticaria, eczema, eyelid and facial edema, conjunctivitis, rhinorrhea, dyspnea, and asthma (7314,7315,7316,10623). In severe cases, royal jelly can cause status asthmaticus, anaphylaxis, and death (792,7315,7316,10623,10624). Allergic symptoms have been associated with IgE-mediated hypersensitivity reactions (3513,10623). Advise people with asthma or allergies not to use royal jelly.
DERMATITIS: Royal jelly might exacerbate dermatitis; avoid using (791).

Dosage and Administration

ORAL: For hyperlipidemia, 50-100 mg per day has been used (3515). For premenstrual syndrome (PMS), two tablets twice daily of a specific combination containing royal jelly 6 mg, bee pollen extract 36 mg, and bee pollen plus pistil extract 120 mg (Femal, Natumin Pharma) per tablet for 2 menstrual cycles has been used (12008).

Comments

Avoid confusion with bee pollen and bee venom.

RUE

Also Known As

Common Rue, Garden Rue, German Rue, Herb-of-Grace, Herbygrass, Raute, Ruda, Rue Officinale, Ruta graveolens, Rutae folium, Rutae herba.
CAUTION: See separate listing for Goat's Rue.

Scientific Names

Ruta graveolens.
Family: Rutaceae.

People Use This For

Orally, the above ground parts of rue are used for menstrual disorders and discomforts, as a uterine stimulant and abortifacient, for loss of appetite, dyspepsia, circulatory disorders, arteriosclerosis, heart palpitations, nervousness, hysteria, fever, feverish infectious diseases, cramps, hepatitis, diarrhea, pleurisy, headaches, neuralgic afflictions, and weakness of the eyes. It is also used orally for respiratory complaints, arthritis, intestinal worm infestations, epilepsy, multiple sclerosis, Bell's palsy, and cancer of the mouth. Rue is also used orally as an antispasmodic, diuretic, antibacterial, antifungal, hemostatic, and as a contraceptive agent.
Topically, rue is used for arthritis, dislocations, sprains, injuries of the bone, inflammation of the skin, oral and pharyngeal cavities, earaches, toothaches, headaches, tumors, warts, and as an insect repellent.
In foods and beverages, rue and its oil are used as flavor components.
In manufacturing, rue oil is used as a fragrance ingredient in soaps and cosmetics.

Safety

LIKELY SAFE ...when used orally in amounts commonly found in foods. Rue and rue oil have Generally Recognized As Safe (GRAS) status in the US (4912).

LIKELY UNSAFE ...when fresh rue is used orally for medicinal purposes (2). Fresh rue can cause severe kidney and liver damage (2). ...when more than 120 grams of leaves or 100 mL of oil are ingested. Rue can cause severe gastrointestinal upset, systemic complications, and death (2,6). Dried rue leaves contain less volatile oil than fresh rue, and has milder effects (515). Canadian regulations prohibit the use of rue as a non-medicinal ingredient in oral products (12). ...when fresh rue is applied topically (2); rue can cause contact dermatitis and severe photodermatitis (2,6,11,19).

PREGNANCY: LIKELY UNSAFE ...when used orally. Rue might have uterine stimulant and abortifacient effects (12); avoid using. Deaths have been reported in women who used rue as an abortifacient (2).

LACTATION: LIKELY UNSAFE ...when used orally in medicinal amounts.

Effectiveness

There is insufficient reliable information available about the effectiveness of rue.

Mechanism of Action

The applicable parts of rue are the above ground parts. Rue contains the alkaloids arborine, arborinine, and gamma-fagarine; and the furocoumarins rutamarin, bergapten, and xanthotoxin. The alkaloids and the furocoumarins have shown evidence of reversible spasmolytic activity, and anti-inflammatory and antihistaminic properties (6,11,515). The furocoumarins may also have photosensitizing, phototoxic, and mutagenic effects (2); and are responsible for adverse skin reactions (6,11,19,515). The constituent chalepensin may have antifertility and anti-implantation effects. The rutin constituent may have antispasmodic activity, and it might also decrease capillary permeability and fragility. Rue oil has anthelmintic activities, possibly due to the constituent 2-undecanone; this constituent can also cause abortions (11). Although rue oil has caused fatal adrenal gland, liver, and kidney hemorrhage in animals, 30 mg per day for three months did not affect liver function in humans (11). The effects of rue extract on neuromuscular conditions are thought to result from potassium channel-blocking in myelinated nerve cells (6).

Adverse Reactions

Orally, rue can cause GI irritation (12), melancholic mood, sleep disorders, tiredness, dizziness, spasms, and severe kidney and liver damage (2). The fresh leaf juice can cause painful stomach and intestinal irritation, fainting, lethargy, bradycardia, abortion, swelling of the tongue, and clammy skin (2). Rue oil causes severe stomach pain, vomiting, exhaustion, confusion, and convulsions (11). Large amounts, over 100 mL of the oil or 120 grams of the leaf, can cause vomiting, violent gastric pain, systemic complications, and death (2,6). Contact dermatitis (2) and phototoxic reactions including skin blisters have occurred with topical exposure to the fresh plant and rue-containing products followed by exposure to sunlight (2,6). There is one case report of increased phototoxic response to PUVA (psoralen plus ultraviolet A) therapy associated with ingestion of a rue remedy (6177).

Interactions with Herbs & Other Dietary Supplements

GOLDENSEAL: The reports regarding overcoming the effects of large amounts of rue by administration of goldenseal are unsubstantiated (515).

Interactions with Drugs

PHOTOSENSITIZING DRUGS: Rue might increase the phototoxic response to PUVA therapy due to its 5-methoxypsoralen content. There is one case report of increased phototoxic response to PUVA therapy associated with ingestion of a rue remedy (6177). Drugs used in PUVA therapy include methoxsalen (8-methoxypsoralen, 8-MOP, Oxsoralen) and Trioxsalen (Trisoralen). Rue might also increase of the risk of phototoxicity when used with other drugs that cause photosensitivity. Some other drugs that cause photosensitivity include amitriptyline (Elavil), quinolones (Ciprofloxacin, others), sulfa drugs (Septra, Bactrim, others), and tetracycline.

Interactions with Foods

None known.

Interactions with Lab Tests

None known.

Interactions with Diseases or Conditions

GASTROINTESTINAL TRACT PROBLEMS: Rue can exacerbate pre-existing inflammation or irritation of the gastrointestinal tract (19).

KIDNEY OR LIVER DYSFUNCTION: Contraindicated (2,12).

URINARY TRACT PROBLEMS: Rue can exacerbate kidney inflammation and urinary tract discomfort (19).

Dosage and Administration

ORAL: People typically use 500 mg crushed rue. A maximum dose of 1 gram per day has been recommended. As a tea, 1 cup of boiling water is poured over 1 teaspoon of the herb. The tea is taken cold, 1 cup per day (5252,5254).
TOPICAL: No typical dosage.

Comments

Avoid confusion with goat's rue (Galega officinalis) and meadow rue (Thalictrum species).

RUPTUREWORT

Also Known As

Bruchkraut, Flax weed, Herniariae herba, Herniary.

Scientific Names

Herniaria glabra; Herniaria hirsuta.
Family: Rutaceae.

Comments

At the date of publication, there was very little scientific information about this product. Our staff is continually analyzing the available information on natural medicines and will add data to the online version of *Natural Medicines Comprehensive Database* as it becomes available. See www.naturaldatabase.com.

RUSTY-LEAVED RHODODENDRON

Also Known As

Rhododendri Ferruginei Folium, Rosebay, Rust-Red Rhododendron, Rusty Leaved Rhododendron, Snow Rose.

Scientific Names

Rhododendron ferrugineum.
Family: Ericaceae.

People Use This For

In combination with other herbs, rusty-leaved rhododendron is used for extreme tension of the muscles or arteries (hypertonia), muscle and joint rheumatism, joint disease, hardening of muscles, muscular pain, weak connective tissue, neuralgia, sensitivity to weather change, sciatica, trigeminal neuralgia, migraine, headaches, intercostal neuralgia, gout, biliary or urinary stones, hypertension, and geriatric and aging disorders.

Safety

LIKELY UNSAFE ...when used orally (2). The entire plant is considered poisonous (2,7,18,3477,3496). Hydroquinone toxicity is also a potential risk with long-term use (2). Most poisonings result from the consumption of honey made from rhododendron nectar (3477).
PREGNANCY AND LACTATION: LIKELY UNSAFE ...when used orally; avoid using.

Effectiveness

There is insufficient reliable information available about the effectiveness of rusty-leaved rhododendron.

Mechanism of Action

The applicable part of rusty-leaved rhododendron is the leaf. Rusty-leaved rhododendron contains grayanotoxins and arbutin (2). Grayanotoxins lower blood pressure (7). Grayanotoxins also prevent nerve conduction by inhibiting the closure of sodium channels on cell membranes, which increases sodium conductance and causes cellular depolarization (18,3477). Grayanotoxin toxicity includes muscular and respiratory paralysis (7). Arbutin is hydrolyzed to hydroquinone by the intestinal flora (7). As a result, long-term use may to lead to hydroquinone toxicity (2).

Adverse Reactions

Orally, the adverse effects of rusty-leaved rhododendron include weakness, dizziness, nausea, vomiting, hypotension, bradycardia, transient A-V dissociation and blurred vision (17,3496). Symptoms of poisoning due to the constituent grayanotoxin include sweating, impaired consciousness, chills, fainting, shock, seizure, cardiac and respiratory arrest, severe stupor, and possibly death (2,18,3477,3496).
Chronic use may lead to hydroquinone toxicity (2). Hydroquinone toxicity is characterized by a gastroenteritis-like syndrome (17).

Interactions with Herbs & Other Dietary Supplements
None known.

Interactions with Drugs
None known.

Interactions with Foods
None known.

Interactions with Lab Tests
None known.

Interactions with Diseases or Conditions
None known.

Dosage and Administration
No typical dosage.

Comments
Rusty-leaved rhododendron is considered likely unsafe; avoid using. Rusty-leaved rhododendron is considered a poisonous plant (2,7,18). Rhododendron honey is also known as "mad honey" (3477,3496).

RUTIN

Also Known As
Citrus Bioflavonoid, Citrus Bioflavonoids, Eldrin, Flavonoid, Oxerutin, Quercetin-3-rhamnoglucoside, Quercetin-3-rutinoside, Rutine, Rutinum, Rutosid, Rutosidum, Sclerutin, Sophorin.
CAUTION: See separate listings for Chrysin, Diosmin, Hesperidin, Methoxylated Flavones, and Quercetin.

Scientific Names
Rutin, rutoside.

People Use This For
Orally, rutin is used as a vascular protectant, reducing capillary permeability and fragility, varicose veins, internal bleeding, hemorrhoids, to prevent strokes, and for prophylaxis of mucositis associated with cancer treatments.
In combination with trypsin and bromelain, rutin is used orally for osteoarthritis.

Safety
LIKELY SAFE ...when used orally in amounts present in fruits and vegetables.
POSSIBLY UNSAFE ...when used orally in medicinal amounts. Although rutin is generally considered nontoxic, there are reports of rutin forming an obstructive mass in the gastrointestinal tract (11). There is also concern that flavonoids, including rutin, could become mutagenic and play a role in the etiology of gastric cancer (3106).
PREGNANCY AND LACTATION: Insufficient reliable information available; avoid using amounts greater than those found in foods.

Effectiveness
POSSIBLY EFFECTIVE

Osteoarthritis. Taking rutin orally in combination with trypsin and bromelain seems to be effective for treating osteoarthritis (6252). In a double-blind trial, 73 patients with painful osteoarthritis of the knee were randomly assigned the combination enzyme product (Phlogenzym) or diclofenac (Voltaren) 50 mg three times daily during the first week and then twice daily in weeks 2 and 3. The enzyme product was similar to diclofenac in relieving pain and improving knee function (6252).

There is insufficient reliable information available about the effectiveness of rutin for its other uses.

Mechanism of Action
Rutin is a flavonoid. Rutin is thought to be an antioxidant, a free radical scavenger, and an iron-chelator (209,3100). It has been reported to decrease capillary fragility and permeability, although the existing evidence is inconclusive (11). Some studies suggest rutin might offer protection from damage induced by asbestos (209,3103), cytotoxic effects of oxidized low density lipoproteins (11,3105), and gastric injury from ethanol (3107). Other evidence suggests it might be beneficial in inflammatory bowel disease (3101,3102). When added to the diet, rutin appears to offer some protection against DNA damage caused by hepatocarcinogens (3104). However, limited preliminary evidence suggests rutin

might worsen the progression of melanoma (211).

After oral administration, rutin is hydrolyzed in the gastrointestinal tract to release quercetin, which is responsible for many of the actions of rutin. It appears that quercetin from rutin is absorbed better in women than in men, although the gender related differences in bioavailability are not completely understood (9442).

Adverse Reactions

Orally, rutin may cause headache, flushing, rashes, or mild gastrointestinal disturbance (313).

Interactions with Herbs & Other Dietary Supplements

IRON: Some information suggests that rutin might have iron-chelating properties (209).

Interactions with Drugs

None known.

Interactions with Foods

None known.

Interactions with Lab Tests

None known.

Interactions with Diseases or Conditions

None known.

Dosage and Administration

ORAL: For relieving symptoms of edema associated with chronic venous insufficiency, a typical dose is 500 mg twice daily (313). For osteoarthritis, a combination enzyme product (Phlogenzym), which contains rutin 100 mg, trypsin 48 mg, and bromelain 90 mg, 2 tablets 3 times daily has been used (6252).

Comments

Rutin (rutoside) is a flavonoid present in numerous plants. The major sources of rutin for medical use include buckwheat, Japanese pagoda tree, and Eucalyptus macrorhyncha. Other sources of rutin include the leaves of several species of eucalyptus, lime tree flowers, elder flowers, hawthorn leaves and flowers, rue, St. John's Wort, Ginkgo biloba, apples, and other fruits and vegetables.

RYE GRASS

Also Known As

Grass Pollen, Grass Pollen Extract, Rye, Rye Grass Pollen, Rye Grass Pollen Extract, Rye Pollen Extract.

Scientific Names

Secale cereale.
Family: Poaceae/Gramineae.

People Use This For

Orally, rye grass is used for benign prostatic hyperplasia (BPH), prostate pain, and chronic prostatitis.

Safety

LIKELY SAFE ...when used orally and appropriately. Rye grass pollen extract appears to be safe when used for up to 24 weeks (5292,5293,5294,5296,8176,8177,8520). Long-term effects are unknown.
PREGNANCY AND LACTATION: Insufficient reliable information available; avoid using.

Effectiveness

POSSIBLY EFFECTIVE

Benign prostatic hyperplasia (BPH). Taking rye grass extracts orally seem to improve symptoms such as frequency, nocturia, urgency, decreased urine flow rate, dribbling, and painful urination in patients with mild to moderate BPH (5292,5293,5294). Some researchers report decreased prostate size, improved urinary flow, and decreased residual urine volume (5292,8520); others report no effect on objective BPH measures (8176). Studies have used a specific rye grass pollen extract (Cernilton) (5292,5293,5294,8176,8520). It is not known if rye grass pollen extract is comparable to finasteride (Proscar) or alpha-blockers. However, rye grass is comparable to Pygeum and Paraprost, a Japanese prostate remedy containing L-glutamic acid, L-alanine, and aminoacetic acid (8176,8177).

INSUFFICIENT RELIABLE EVIDENCE to RATE

Prostatitis and prostatodynia. Preliminary clinical evidence suggests that rye grass pollen extract might relieve chronic prostatitis and prostatodynia (5296). More evidence is needed to rate rye grass for these uses.

Mechanism of Action

The applicable part of rye grass is the pollen extract. Some rye grass pollen extracts are prepared by microbial digestion of the pollen, followed by water and acetone extraction (5290,5295). The extract contains beta-sterols. It seems to relax urethral smooth muscle tone and increase bladder muscle contraction. Some evidence suggests that it might affect alpha-adrenergic receptors and relax the internal and external bladder sphincter muscles (8176). The extract does not affect luteinizing hormone, follicle-stimulating hormone, testosterone, or dihydrotestosterone (5292). Some evidence suggests that rye grass pollen extract might inhibit prostate cancer cell growth (5297). Other evidence suggests that it might interfere with inflammation by inhibiting the biosynthesis of prostaglandins and leukotrienes (5298).

Adverse Reactions

Orally, rye grass can cause abdominal distention, heartburn, and nausea (5293).

Interactions with Herbs & Other Dietary Supplements

None known.

Interactions with Drugs

None known.

Interactions with Foods

None known.

Interactions with Lab Tests

None known.

Interactions with Diseases or Conditions

None known.

Dosage and Administration

ORAL: For benign prostatic hyperplasia (BPH), a specific rye grass pollen extract 126 mg three times daily has been used (5294,8176).

Comments

Rye grass pollen extract (Cernilton) is a registered pharmaceutical product in Western Europe, Japan, Korea, and Argentina (8176).

SACCHAROMYCES BOULARDII

Also Known As

Brewer's Yeast (Hansen CBS 5926), Probiotics, Saccharomyces, Saccharomyces cerevisiae Hansen CBS 5926, S. boulardii.

CAUTION: See separate listings for Brewer's Yeast (Saccharomyces cerevisiae), Bifidobacteria, and Lactobacillus..

Scientific Names

Saccharomyces boulardii.

Family: Saccharomycetaceae.

People Use This For

Orally, Saccharomyces boulardii is used for treating and preventing diarrhea, including infectious types such as rotaviral diarrhea in children, diarrhea caused by bacterial overgrowth in adults, traveler's diarrhea, and diarrhea associated with enteral tube feedings. It is also used orally to prevent and treat antibiotic-associated diarrhea. Saccharomyces boulardii is also used orally for general digestion problems, irritable bowel syndrome (IBS), inflammatory bowel syndrome (IBD, Crohn's disease, ulcerative colitis), relapsing Clostridium difficile colitis, and bacterial overgrowth in short bowel syndrome. It is also used orally for lactose intolerance, urinary tract infections (UTIs), vaginal and Candida-related (yeast) infections, high cholesterol levels, hives, fever blisters, canker sores, and adolescent acne.

Safety

LIKELY SAFE ...when used orally and appropriately (4353).
CHILDREN: POSSIBLY SAFE ...when used orally and appropriately (4347,4356).
PREGNANCY AND LACTATION: Insufficient reliable information available; avoid using.

Effectiveness

POSSIBLY EFFECTIVE

Acne. Taking Saccharomyces boulardii orally seems to help reduce chronic acne as adjuvant treatment (7140).
Antibiotic-associated diarrhea. Although there is a conflicting report (4350,4351), the majority of evidence shows that taking Saccharomyces boulardii orally can be useful for preventing antibiotic-associated diarrhea (4353,4355).
Clostridium difficile diarrhea. Taking Saccharomyces boulardii orally in combination with vancomycin or metronidazole, reduces the risk of recurrence of Clostridium difficile diarrhea (4352,4354). However, for people with an initial episode, Saccharomyces boulardii doesn't seem to be any more effective than the antibiotics alone (4352).
Crohn's disease. Taking Saccharomyces boulardii orally seems to reduce the frequency of bowel movements in patients with Crohn's disease (7646).
Diarrhea. Administering Saccharomyces boulardii in tube feedings seems to prevent diarrhea (4349). Taking Saccharomyces boulardii orally seems to be effective for treating acute diarrhea in infants (4347).
HIV-related diarrhea. Taking Saccharomyces boulardii orally seems to help reduce HIV-related diarrhea (4347).
Traveler's diarrhea. Taking Saccharomyces boulardii orally seems to help prevent traveler's diarrhea (155).

INSUFFICIENT RELIABLE EVIDENCE to RATE

Cystic fibrosis. Taking Saccharomyces boulardii orally doesn't seems to decrease Candida albicans gastrointestinal colonization in patients with cystic fibrosis (7652). More evidence is needed to rate Saccharomyces boulardii for this use.

Mechanism of Action

Saccharomyces boulardii is typically a non-pathogenic yeast (4363). Saccharomyces boulardii is used as a probiotic agent to help colonize the gastrointestinal tract. It is used therapeutically in cases where disease is thought to occur due to depleted intestinal normal flora or colonization with pathogenic organisms. Saccharomyces boulardii typically reaches a maximum steady state in 3 days when taken orally. It does not multiply in the gut. Less than 1% of the ingested dose is recovered from stools (4363).
Saccharomyces boulardii is thought to help for Clostridium difficile infection by producing proteases that might decrease the toxicity of Clostridium difficile toxins A and B (4348,4361). Individuals who have low stool concentrations of Saccharomyces boulardii after repeated use are most likely to have Clostridium difficile recurrence (4360). In addition to its effect on Clostridium difficile, Saccharomyces boulardii also shows evidence of interaction with cholera toxin (4363).
In Crohn's disease, Saccharomyces boulardii increases secretory immune globulin A (IgA) in the intestine (7646). Saccharomyces boulardii might cause an increase in the intestinal chloride resorption, which also may play a role in the treatment of Crohn's disease (4362,7646).

Adverse Reactions

Orally, Saccharomyces boulardii can cause flatulence. Elevated sedimentation rate may occur when Saccharomyces boulardii is used to treat Crohn's disease (7646), but this effect may be part of the disease process.
Rarely, oral use has been associated with fungemia in both immunocompromised and immunocompetent people (1247,4357,4358,4360,7329). The true incidence of fungemia is difficult to determine with Saccharomyces boulardii. Most clinical laboratories are unable to differentiate between Saccharomyces boulardii and Saccharomyces cerevisiae which might come from other sources (7353).

Interactions with Herbs & Other Dietary Supplements

None known.

Interactions with Drugs

ANTIFUNGALS: Theoretically, since Saccharomyces boulardii is a yeast, antifungals might decrease its effectiveness (4363).

Interactions with Foods

None known.

Interactions with Lab Tests

SACCHAROMYCES CEREVISIAE: In patients who experience fungemia following use of Saccharomyces boulardii, cultures can indicate fungemia from Saccharomyces cerevisiae (7329). Most laboratories are unable to distinguish between Saccharomyces cerevisiae and Saccharomyces boulardii (7353).

Interactions with Diseases or Conditions

IMMUNODEFICIENCY: There is some concern that immunocompromised patients taking Saccaromyces boulardii might be at an increased risk for fungemia. Although Saccharomyces is generally a nonpathogenic organism, there have been cases of fungemia following its use (1247,4357,4358,4360).
YEAST ALLERGY: Patients with yeast allergy can be allergic to products containing Saccharomyces boulardii (4363).

Dosage and Administration

ORAL: A typical dose to prevent diarrhea is 250-500 mg two to four times a day (4355). A typical dose to treat recurrent diarrhea in adults is 1 gram daily for four weeks along with antibiotic therapy (4352). In the treatment of Crohn's disease, Saccharomyces boulardii 250 mg three times daily, has been used for up to 9 weeks (7646). For infants: 250 mg two to four times a day has been used according to age (4356). To prevent contamination of indwelling catheters, open packets or capsules with gloves, outside the patient's room (4359).

Comments

Saccharomyces boulardii was previously identified as a unique species of yeast, but is now believed to be a strain of Saccharomyces cerevisiae (baker's yeast) (1227,1251,1282,7353).

SAFFLOWER

Also Known As

American Saffron, Bastard Saffron, Benibana flower, Benibana Oil, Dyer's Saffron, Fake Saffron, False Saffron, Hing Hua, Honghua, Zaffer, Zafran.

Scientific Names

Carthamus tinctorius.
Family: Asteraceae/Compositae.

People Use This For

Orally, safflower seed oil is used for reducing the risk of cardiovascular disease and preventing atherosclerosis, hyperemia in women, and to promote hair growth. Safflower is also used orally for fever, tumors, coughs, bronchial conditions, blood stasis, pain, blood invigoration, amenorrhea, painful menses, stimulating menstruation, coronary heart disease, chest pain, traumatic injuries, inducing sweating, as a laxative, purgative, stimulant, antiperspirant, abortifacient, and expectorant.
In foods, safflower seed oil is used as a cooking oil.
In manufacturing, safflower flower is used to color cosmetics and dye fabrics. Safflower seed oil is used as a paint solvent.

Safety

LIKELY SAFE ...when safflower seed oil is used orally (6).
POSSIBLY SAFE ...when safflower flower is used orally and appropriately as safflower flower (6,12,18).
PREGNANCY: LIKELY UNSAFE ...when safflower flower is used because it has abortifacient, menstrual stimulant, and uterine stimulant effects (11,12).
LACTATION: There is insufficient reliable information available about the safety of safflower flower during lactation; avoid using.

Effectiveness

POSSIBLY EFFECTIVE

Hypercholesterolemia. Taking safflower oil orally as a dietary supplement seems to reduce total and low-density lipoprotein (LDL) cholesterol (6). However, it does not seem to lower triglycerides or increase high-density lipoprotein (HDL) cholesterol (6).

There is insufficient reliable information available about the effectiveness of safflower for its other uses.

Mechanism of Action

The applicable parts of safflower are the flower and seed oil. Safflower flower contains a complex mixture of red and yellow pigments (11,18). The constituent, safflower yellow, has immunosuppressive and anticoagulant activity (11). Safflower polysaccharide has immunopotentiating effects (11). Safflower extracts exhibit cardiac stimulant, vasodilating, hypolipemic, hypotensive, and uterine stimulant properties (11). Safflower seed oil is a rich source of the essential unsaturated fatty acid, linoleic acid (6). It also contains linolenic acid (18). Some evidence suggests essential fatty acids are necessary to maintain the integrity of the central nervous system (6). Other evidence suggests that diets high in unsaturated and polyunsaturated fatty acids reduce atherosclerosis and the risk of heart disease (6). A diet rich in safflower oil can increase platelet linoleic acid levels, reduce serum cholesterol, particularly low-density lipoprotein (LDL) cholesterol, and apolipoprotein B levels (6) without affecting serum triglyceride, high-density (HDL) lipoprotein cholesterol or apolipoprotein A-1 levels (6).

Adverse Reactions
Safflower can cause an allergic reaction in individuals sensitive to the Asteraceae/Compositae family. Members of this family include ragweed, chrysanthemums, marigolds, daisies, and many other herbs.

Interactions with Herbs & Other Dietary Supplements
HERBS WITH ANTICOAGULANT/ANTIPLATELET POTENTIAL: Concomitant use with herbs that have constituents that might affect platelet aggregation could theoretically increase the risk of bleeding in some people. These herbs include angelica, clove, danshen, garlic, ginger, ginkgo, ginseng (Panax), red clover, turmeric, and others.

Interactions with Drugs
ANTICOAGULANT/ANTIPLATELET DRUGS: Theoretically, concomitant use with safflower might increase effects and adverse effects of anticoagulants.

Interactions with Foods
None known.

Interactions with Lab Tests
None known.

Interactions with Diseases or Conditions
BLEEDING DISORDERS: Contraindicated in people with hemorrhagic diseases, peptic ulcers, or clotting disorders. Safflower can prolong coagulation time (12).
CROSS-ALLERGENICITY: Safflower can cause an allergic reaction in individuals sensitive to the Asteraceae/Compositae family. Members of this family include ragweed, chrysanthemums, marigolds, daisies, and many other herbs.

Dosage and Administration
ORAL: A typical dose is one cup of tea up to three times daily. To make tea, simmer 1 gram dried flower in 150 mL boiling water, 5-10 minutes, strain (18).

Comments
Although safflower seed oil is a rich source of linoleic acid, some experts contend gamma-linolenic acid might be more useful as a physiologic source of essential fatty acids. To be useful in the body, linoleic acid must be converted to dihomo-gamma-linolenic acid (DHGA) and arachidonic acid (6). Gamma-linolenic acid does not require this conversion before it can be used in the body.

SAFFRON

Also Known As
Autumn Crocus, Azafron, Croci stigma, Indian Saffron, Kumkuma, Saffron Crocus, Safran, Spanish Saffron, True Saffron.

Scientific Names
Crocus sativus.
Family: Iridaceae.

People Use This For
Orally, saffron is used for asthma, insomnia, cancer, atherosclerosis, cough, whooping cough, stomach gas, and as a sedative. Saffron is also used orally for depression, fright, shock, spitting up blood, pain and difficulties in menstruation, after childbirth, as a digestive stimulant, as an aphrodisiac, as a pain reliever, for stimulating menstruation, for dry skin, to induce sweating, and as an expectorant.
In combination with opium and quinine, it is used for premature ejaculation.
In combination with salicylic acid and vegetable oils, an extract of saffron is used topically for treating baldness.
In foods, saffron is used as a culinary spice, yellow food coloring, and as a flavoring agent.
In manufacturing, saffron extracts are used as fragrance in perfumes and as a dye for cloth.

Safety

LIKELY SAFE ...when used orally in amounts commonly found in foods. Saffron has Generally Recognized As Safe (GRAS) status in the US (4912).
POSSIBLY SAFE ...when used orally and appropriately, short-term for medicinal purposes. A specific saffron extract 30 mg/day (Novin Zaferan Co) seems to be safe when used for up to 6 weeks (11024).
LIKELY UNSAFE ...when used orally in high doses. Taking 5 grams or more of saffron can cause severe side effects (12). Doses of 12-20 grams can be lethal (18).
PREGNANCY: LIKELY UNSAFE ...when used orally in amounts exceeding those commonly found in foods. Larger amounts of saffron have uterine stimulant and abortifacient effects (2,18); avoid using.
LACTATION: Insufficient reliable information available; avoid using.

Effectiveness

INSUFFICIENT RELIABLE EVIDENCE to RATE

Depression. Preliminary evidence suggests that taking a specific saffron extract 30 mg/day (Novin Zaferan Co) might improve symptoms of major depression. This saffron extract seems to be as effective as taking the conventional antidepressant imipramine 100 mg/day after 6 weeks of treatment (11024). But this dose of imipramine is considered subtherapeutic. More evidence is needed to rate saffron for this use.

Mechanism of Action

Saffron constituents include crocin, picrocrocin, and crocetin (6,11). Picrocrocin is responsible for the characteristic bitter taste of saffron and crocin for the yellow-red color (11). Preliminary evidence suggests that crocetin may improve atherosclerosis by increasing plasma oxygen diffusion (6,11) and decreasing cholesterol and triglyceride levels (4110). In addition, crocetin binds to albumin (4109), potentially increasing oxygen diffusion and improving atherosclerosis (4109). Small amounts of saffron stimulate gastric secretions (18); larger amounts appear to stimulate uterine smooth muscle, contributing to abortifacient affects (18). Saffron extracts limit the in vitro growth of experimental tumor colony cells by inhibiting cellular nucleic acid synthesis (4104,4105).

Adverse Reactions

Orally, no adverse effects have been reported with up to 1.5 grams of saffron per day (2,11,12). Poisoning can occur with 5 grams (2,11), symptoms include yellow appearance of the skin, sclera, and mucous membranes (mimicking icterus); vomiting; vertigo; bloody diarrhea; hematuria; bleeding from the nose, lips, eyelids or uterus; numbness; uremic collapse; and thrombocytopenic purpura leading to severe necrosis of the nose (2,11). 10 grams can induce abortion (2), 12-20 grams is reportedly lethal (2,12). Rhinoconjunctivitis and allergy induced asthma have been reported (4106). Anaphylactic reactions can occur within minutes of eating food prepared with saffron (4107).

Interactions with Herbs & Other Dietary Supplements

CROSS-SENSITIVITY: Cross-reactivity exists between saffron and Lolium, Olea (includes olive), and Salsola species plants (4106).

Interactions with Drugs

None known.

Interactions with Foods

None known.

Interactions with Lab Tests

None known.

Interactions with Diseases or Conditions

CROSS-ALLERGENICITY: Cross-reactivity reported between saffron and Lolium, Olea (includes olive), and Salsola species plants (4106).

Dosage and Administration

ORAL: For depression a specific ethanol saffron extract 30 mg/day (Novin Zaferan Co) has been used (11024).

SAGE

Also Known As

Common Sage, Dalmatian Sage, Garden Sage, Meadow Sage, Sauge, Scarlet Sage, Spanish Sage, True Sage.
CAUTION: See separate listings for Boneset, Clary Sage, Danshen, German Sarsaparilla, Purple Loosestrife, Spearmint, and Wood Sage.

Scientific Names

Salvia officinalis; Salvia lavandulaefolia.
Family: Lamiaceae/Labiatae.

People Use This For

Orally, sage is used for loss of appetite; excessive perspiration; dysmenorrhea; diarrhea; gastritis; galactorrhea; reduction of saliva secretion; and digestive problems including flatulence, bloating, and dyspepsia. It is also used for depression, cerebral ischemia, memory enhancement, and Alzheimer's disease.
Topically, sage is used for herpes labialis, laryngitis, pharyngitis, stomatitis, gingivitis, glossitis, minor oral injuries, and inflammation of the nasal mucosa.
As an inhalant, sage is used for asthma.
In foods, it is used as a culinary spice.
In manufacturing, sage is used as a fragrance component in soaps and cosmetics.

Safety

LIKELY SAFE ...when used orally in amounts commonly found in foods. Sage is approved for food use in the US (4912).
POSSIBLY SAFE ...when used orally in therapeutic doses, short term. Sage seems to be safe when taken orally for up to 4 months (10334,10810). ...when used topically (10437).
POSSIBLY UNSAFE ...when used orally in high doses, or when used long-term (12). Some species of sage contain a thujone constituent that can be toxic if enough is consumed (12).
PREGNANCY: LIKELY UNSAFE ...when used orally because the constituent, thujone, can have menstrual stimulant and abortifacient effects (19).
LACTATION: POSSIBLY UNSAFE ...when used orally; sage is thought to reduce the mother's milk supply (19).

Effectiveness

POSSIBLY EFFECTIVE

Alzheimer's disease. Taking extracts of Salvia officinalis and Salvia lavandulaefolia orally seem to improve cognitive function in patients with mild to moderate Alzheimer's disease when used for up to 4 months (10334,10810).

Herpes labialis (cold sores). Topical treatment of herpes labialis with a cream containing sage and rhubarb (Rheum officinale and Rheum palmatum) may be about as effective as acyclovir (Zovirax) cream. Acyclovir cream provides healing of lesions in 6.3 days; the sage and rhubarb cream provides healing of lesion in 7.2 days. The combination of sage and rhubarb appears to improve the time to healing and to reduce pain, compared with sage alone (10437).

INSUFFICIENT RELIABLE EVIDENCE to RATE

Memory. Single doses of Salvia lavandulaefolia might enhance memory in a dose-dependent manner in young adults (10811). More evidence is needed to rate sage for this use.

Mechanism of Action

The applicable part of sage is the leaf and volatile oil. Sage contains 1-2.8% of volatile oil that may be responsible for pharmacological activity. The volatile oil contains several active constituents that have in vitro pharmacological activity. Rosmarinic acid, carvacrol, and luteolin have antioxidant properties. Cirsiliol is a central nervous system (CNS) depressant. Linalool and alpha-terpineol have CNS depressant and anticholinesterase activity. Other constituents with anticholinesterase activity are 1,8-cineole, alpha-pinene, and caryophyllene epoxide. The constituent geraniol exerts estrogenic activity. Some constituents also seem to have anti-inflammatory activity. These constituents might act synergistically and be beneficial for Alzheimer's disease. Animal studies of sage show anticholinesterase activity (10334).
Preliminary research suggests that sage might have hypoglycemic activity (10813).
Sage also contains camphor, which has pro-oxidant effects and is associated with hepatotoxicity and neurotoxicity a high doses (10334). Salvia officinalis contains significant amounts of thujone, a convulsant.
The thujone concentration of the volatile oil varies from 17% to 58%, depending on growing conditions, season of harvest, and other variables (10812). Salvia lavandulaefolia contains only trace amounts of thujone (10334).

Adverse Reactions

Orally, sage can cause nausea, vomiting, abdominal pain, dizziness, agitation, and wheezing (10810). It may increase the blood pressure of hypertensive patients (10334). Thujone, which is found in salvia officinalis, is a neurotoxin and can cause seizures (10812). Camphor, which is present in both of these species of sage, can cause hepatotoxicity and neurotoxicity in high doses (10334).

Interactions with Herbs & Other Dietary Supplements

HERBS WITH HYPOGLYCEMIC POTENTIAL: Theoretically, sage may have additive effects with herbs that decrease blood glucose levels (10813). Herbs with hypoglycemic potential include devil's claw, fenugreek, garlic, guar gum, horse chestnut, Panax ginseng, psyllium, and Siberian ginseng.
HERBS WITH SEDATIVE PROPERTIES: Some constituents of sage have CNS depressant activity (10334). Theoretically, concomitant use with herbs that have sedative properties might enhance therapeutic and adverse effects. Some of these supplements include 5-HTP, calamus, California poppy, catnip, hops, Jamaican dogwood, kava, St. John's wort, scullcap, valerian, yerba mansa, and others.

Interactions with Drugs

ANTICONVULSANTS: Some species of sage can cause convulsions. Theoretically, sage might interfere with the effectiveness of anticonvulsant drugs (10812).
ANTIDIABETES DRUGS: Preliminary research suggests sage might have hypoglycemic activity (10813). Theoretically, sage might have additive therapeutic effects and adverse effects with hypoglycemic drugs.
CNS DEPRESSANTS: Some constituents of sage have CNS depressant activity (10334). Theoretically, concomitant use with drugs with sedative properties might cause additive effects and side effects.

Interactions with Foods

None known.

Interactions with Lab Tests

BLOOD GLUCOSE: Preliminary research suggests sage might have hypoglycemic activity (10813).

Interactions with Diseases or Conditions

DIABETES: Preliminary research suggests sage might have hypoglycemic activity (10813). Monitor blood sugar closely.
HYPERTENSION: Sage can increase blood pressure in some people with hypertension (10334). Monitor blood pressure.
SEIZURE DISORDERS: Salvia officinalis contains significant amounts of thujone, a convulsant. Avoid the use of sage in quantities greater than those in food (10812).

Dosage and Administration

ORAL: For treating Alzheimer's disease, a fixed dose of salvia officinalis hydroalcoholic extract, equivalent to 1 gram of sage per day, has been used (10810). An extract of salvia lavandulaefolia, titrated up to 2.5 mg three times daily, has also been used (10334).
TOPICAL: For treatment of herpes labialis (cold sores) a cream containing 23 mg/gram each of sage extract and rhubarb extract has been applied every 2 to 4 hours while awake, with treatment starting within 1 day of the first symptoms and continuing for 10 to 14 days (10437).

Comments

Sage is a rich source of beta-carotene (19).

SALEP

Also Known As

Cuckoo Flower, Levant Salep, Orchid, Sahlep, Saloop, Satyrion.

Scientific Names

Orchis morio.
Family: Orchidaceae.

People Use This For

Orally, salep is used for diarrhea (particularly in children), heartburn, flatulence, and indigestion.

Safety
POSSIBLY SAFE ...when used orally (18).
PREGNANCY AND LACTATION: Insufficient reliable information available; avoid using.

Effectiveness
There is insufficient reliable information available about the effectiveness of salep.

Mechanism of Action
The applicable part of salep is the tuber. Salep contains up to 40% mucilage including glucans, glucomannans, starch, and protein (18).

Adverse Reactions
None reported.

Interactions with Herbs & Other Dietary Supplements
None known.

Interactions with Drugs
None known.

Interactions with Foods
None known.

Interactions with Lab Tests
None known.

Interactions with Diseases or Conditions
None known.

Dosage and Administration
ORAL: It is typically used as a powdered formulation in medicinal preparations; taken in water before or after meals (18).

SAMe

Also Known As
Ademetionine, Adenosylmethionine, S-Adenosyl Methionine, S-Adenosyl-L-Methionine, S-Adenosylmethionine, S-Adenosyl-Methionine, SAM-e, Sammy.

Scientific Names
S-adenosyl-L-methionine.

People Use This For
Orally, SAMe is used for depression, heart disease, fibromyalgia, osteoarthritis, bursitis, tendonitis, chronic low back pain, dementia, Alzheimer's disease, slowing the aging process, improving intellectual performance, and Parkinson's disease. Other uses include attention deficit-hyperactivity disorder (ADHD), multiple sclerosis, spinal cord injury, seizures, migraine headache, chronic lead poisoning, disorders of porphyrin, and bilirubin metabolism.
Intravenously, SAMe is used for treating depression, osteoarthritis, AIDS-related myelopathy, fibromyalgia, liver disease, cirrhosis, and intrahepatic cholestasis.
Intramuscularly, SAMe is injected for fibromyalgia, depression, and Alzheimer's disease.

Safety
LIKELY SAFE ...when used orally, intravenously, or intramuscularly and appropriately (5231,5232). Serious toxicity has not been reported in multiple clinical studies involving as many as 22,000 patients and lasting from a few days to 2 years (5189,5201,5202,5209,5219,5231).
PREGNANCY: POSSIBLY SAFE ...when used intravenously short-term during the third trimester of pregnancy. In two small-scale trials, SAMe 800 mg daily was used intravenously for 14-20 days during the third trimester of pregnancy for intrahepatic cholestasis. No adverse effects in the mother or fetus were observed (5219,5231,5240). Large-scale trials are needed to confirm the safety of SAMe use in pregnancy. Use of SAMe in pregnancy should only be considered when benefits clearly outweigh the potential risks. There is insufficient reliable information available about the use of SAMe at higher doses, for extended

periods of time, or during the earlier trimesters of pregnancy.
LACTATION: Insufficient reliable information available; avoid using.

Effectiveness

LIKELY EFFECTIVE

Depression. Administering SAMe intravenously or intramuscularly, short-term, is helpful for treatment of major depression. Several small-scale clinical trials have shown that parenterally administered SAMe is superior to placebo and possibly as effective as intravenous or oral tricyclic antidepressants in studies lasting up to 30 days (2082,3562,5184,5189,5200,5231,9109). In some trials, the antidepressant effect occurred rapidly, within 1-2 weeks of initiation of treatment (5200). This benefit is likely the result of the parenteral route of administration (3562). Parenteral SAMe has been used successfully in combination with an oral tricyclic antidepressant to speed the onset of antidepressant action (5193).

Taking SAMe orally also seems to reduce symptoms of major depression. Several studies have shown that orally administered SAMe is superior to placebo and possibly as effective as tricyclic antidepressants in trials lasting up to 42 days (2082,2083,5189,5190,5192,5195,5196,5231,9108,9109). But most studies are limited by small numbers of patients, inconsistent diagnostic criteria, short treatment periods, and flawed study designs (3562,5189,5231,9108). Well designed, large scale studies with placebo controls are needed to clarify the benefit of orally administered SAMe in major depression.

Osteoarthritis. Multiple clinical trials show that taking SAMe orally is superior to placebo and comparable to NSAIDs, including the COX-2 inhibitor celecoxib (Celebrex), for decreasing symptoms associated with osteoarthritis. SAMe is associated with fewer adverse effects than NSAIDs and is comparable in reducing pain and improving functional limitation (5188,5199,5203,5204,5205,5206,5207,5208,5209,5215,9108,9111,12054). Significant symptom relief with SAMe may require up to 30 days of treatment compared to only 15 days with NSAIDs. Some evidence suggests that intravenous loading doses of SAMe given over five days, followed by oral treatment, can speed symptom relief to 14 days (5188).

POSSIBLY EFFECTIVE

AIDS-related myelopathy. Administering SAMe intravenously seems to improve AIDS-related myelopathy. SAMe has investigational orphan drug status for this use (1691,5217,5218).

Fibromyalgia. Taking SAMe orally seems to improve fibromyalgia. Two clinical trials demonstrated significant improvement in symptoms of fibromyalgia compared to placebo (5211,5241). But administering SAMe intravenously doesn't seem to improve symptoms of fibromyalgia (5221).

Intrahepatic cholestasis. Administering SAMe orally or intravenously seems to be helpful for treating intrahepatic cholestasis associated with acute or chronic liver disease and pregnancy-related intrahepatic cholestasis. Multiple clinical trials have shown that short-term SAMe therapy is superior to placebo in decreasing pruritus, fatigue, alkaline phosphatase levels, and total and conjugated bilirubin (5219,5238,5239,5240,9108). Trials have more frequently used injectable dosage forms than oral formulations (5219).

Liver disease. Administering SAMe orally or intravenously seems to decrease signs and symptoms of chronic liver disease caused by medications, alcoholism, or lead poisoning. Multiple clinical trials have shown that SAMe can normalize liver enzymes, decrease bilirubin, and decrease symptoms associated with various forms of chronic liver disease. Most trials have enrolled small numbers of patients and have been short duration (1712,5198,5231,5235,5236,5238). Large-scale studies are needed to confirm SAMe's potential benefit in chronic liver disease.

INSUFFICIENT RELIABLE EVIDENCE to RATE

Attention deficit-hyperactivity disorder (ADHD). Preliminary research suggests SAMe might lessen ADHD symptoms in adults (9981). More evidence is needed to rate SAMe for this use.

Mechanism of Action

S-adenosylmethionine (SAMe) is a naturally occurring molecule that is distributed throughout virtually all body tissues and fluids (5231). Concentrations are highest in childhood and decrease with age (9114). SAMe plays an essential role in more than 100 biochemical reactions involving enzymatic transmethylation. It contributes to the synthesis, activation and/or metabolism of hormones, neurotransmitters, nucleic acids, proteins, phospholipids, and some drugs (5231,5232,9110). SAMe is produced endogenously by adenosine triphosphate (ATP) activation of methionine that is synthesized in the body or obtained from metabolism of dietary protein (9110). SAMe synthesis is closely linked to vitamin B12 and folate metabolism (5231). Deficiencies of these vitamins can result in decreased SAMe concentrations in the central nervous system (CNS) (5231).

The mechanism for the antidepressant effect is unknown, but SAMe is associated with increased serotonin turnover and elevated dopamine and norepinephrine levels (5196,5232,9110). SAMe supplementation may also work by altering cellular membrane fluidity. Changes in neuronal membrane fluidity might facilitate signal transduction across membranes and increase the efficiency of receptor-effector coupling (5196,9110). Neuroimaging studies indicate that SAMe affects the brain similarly to conventional antidepressants (9114).

SAMe supplementation may be beneficial in osteoarthritis due to analgesic and anti-inflammatory effects. After oral administration of 400 mg daily for seven days, SAMe levels in synovial fluid increase by 3 to 4 fold (9110). Preliminary evidence suggests SAMe might stimulate articular cartilage growth and repair, specifically chondrocyte proteoglycan synthesis and proliferation rate (5209,9110). SAMe might also protect against cytokine-induced cell damage by antagonizing the activity of tumor necrosis factor-alpha (TNF-alpha) on synovial cell proliferation and fibronectin mRNA expression (9110).

In liver disease, there appears to be a deficiency in hepatic SAMe. Exogenously administered SAMe might act as an essential nutrient by restoring biochemical factors that are depleted in people with liver dysfunction. People with acute or chronic liver disease lose the ability to synthesize SAMe from methionine, possibly due to low activity of methionine adenosyl transferase (MAP), the enzyme that converts methionine to SAMe (9115). This can lead to deficiencies in cysteine and choline. It can also lead to depletion of glutathione, which plays a major role in liver detoxification and antioxidant reactions. This depletion may in turn exacerbate liver disease (5198,5219,5236,9116).

In alcoholic liver disease, among other actions SAMe may restore levels of glutathione, decreasing inflammation, and increasing the methylation of DNA (10465).

SAMe may also be beneficial in AIDS-related myelopathy, by replenishing depleted endogenous SAMe. Epidemiological data suggests that people with AIDS have a deficiency of SAMe in their cerebrospinal fluid (CSF), and this may lead to myelopathy by impairing SAMe dependent myelin and oligodendrocyte repair mechanisms (1691,5217,5218). Some evidence suggests that SAMe might also have a gastric cytoprotective effect (5213).

SAMe is metabolized to s-adenosylhomocysteine, which can be metabolized to homocysteine (5232). Homocysteine is remethylated to form methionine, which can then form more SAMe, or be converted via transsulfuration to the antioxidant glutathione (5232). These reactions require folate, cyanocobalamin (vitamin B12), and pyridoxine (vitamin B6) (5231). Elevated levels of homocysteine have been linked to cardiovascular and renal disease (1698). The long-term effects of SAMe administration on atherosclerotic and thrombotic vascular disorders is unknown, although there was no difference in cardiovascular mortality in a study of people with cirrhosis taking SAMe 1200 mg daily for two years (1712). Low levels of SAMe have been correlated with coronary artery disease (1714). Administration of SAMe to healthy people has shown a positive effect on 5-methyltetrahydrofolate, a key cofactor in homocysteine metabolism. SAMe supplementation has been suggested as a remedy for elevated homocysteine levels (1713).

Some research suggests that adequate intracellular SAMe promotes remethylation and transsulfuration of homocysteine (9112).

Exogenously administered SAMe has low oral bioavailability, which is presumably the result of significant first-pass effect and rapid hepatic metabolism (5231). It achieves peak plasma concentrations 3 to 5 hours after ingestion of an enteric-coated tablet, has a half-life of about 100 minutes and is excreted in urine and feces (5231). SAMe crosses the blood-brain barrier (5231,9110).

SAMe can induce symptoms resembling Parkinson's disease in animal models. This effect may be related to the ability of SAMe to add methyl groups to L-dopa. L-dopa has been shown to deplete the concentration of SAMe, which might explain the depression sometimes seen with Parkinson's disease (10466).

Adverse Reactions

Orally, SAMe can cause flatulence, nausea, vomiting, diarrhea, constipation, dry mouth, headache, mild insomnia, anorexia, sweating, dizziness, and nervousness (347,9113). These side effects are more common with higher doses (5231). Anxiety has occurred in people with depression (5231) and hypomania in people with bipolar disorder (5231). When used as an injection, SAMe has caused mania in people with bipolar disorder (5216,5231).

Interactions with Herbs & Other Dietary Supplements

HERBS AND SUPPLEMENTS WITH SEROTONERGIC PROPERTIES: Theoretically, SAMe might increase the effects and adverse effects of products that increase serotonin levels, including 5-hydroxytryptophan (5-HTP), Hawaiian baby woodrose, L-tryptophan, and St. John's wort (3521,5193).

Interactions with Drugs

ANTIDEPRESSANT DRUGS: Concurrent use might cause additive serotonergic effects and serotonin syndrome-like effects, including agitation, tremors, anxiety, tachycardia, tachypnea, diarrhea, hyperreflexia, shivering, and diaphoresis (3521,5193); or theoretically concurrent use might cause cerebral vasoconstriction disorders such as Call-Fleming syndrome (8056). In one case report, SAMe 100 mg intramuscularly was given daily along with clomipramine (Anafranil) 25 mg per day. The clomipramine dose was later increased to 75 mg per day, and 48-72 hours later the patient experienced side effects similar to serotonin syndrome, requiring hospitalization (3521). Theoretically, this may also occur when SAMe is used with other tricyclic antidepressants and with non-tricyclic antidepressants (5193) such as fluoxetine (Prozac), paroxetine (Paxil), sertraline (Zoloft), amitriptyline (Elavil), clomipramine (Anafranil), and others. Concurrent use of SAMe with imipramine (Tofranil) has resulted in a more rapid onset of antidepressant action (5193,5231).

DEXTROMETHORPHAN (Robitussin DM, and others): Theoretically, concurrent use might cause additive serotonergic effects and increase the risk of serotonin syndrome (3521,5193). Also, concurrent use might theoretically cause cerebral vasoconstriction disorders such as Call-Fleming syndrome (8056).

LEVODOPA: SAMe methylates levodopa, which might worsen Parkinsonian symptoms. Theoretically, SAMe might reduce the effectiveness of levodopa given for Parkinson's disease (10466).

MEPERIDINE (Demerol): Theoretically, concurrent use with meperidine might cause additive serotonergic effects and increase the risk of serotonin syndrome (3521,5193). Also, concurrent use might theoretically cause cerebral vasoconstriction disorders such as Call-Fleming syndrome (8056).

MONOAMINE OXIDASE INHIBITORS (MAOIs): Theoretically, because the effects of SAMe on serotonin and

other neurotransmitters is similar to that of conventional antidepressants (5196,5232); concomitant use might have additive adverse effects including hypertension, hyperthermia, agitation, confusion, coma, etc. SAMe should be avoided in patients taking MAOIs and for 2 weeks after discontinuing an MAOI.
PENTAZOCINE (Talwin): Theoretically, concurrent use with pentazocine might cause additive serotonergic effects and increase the risk of serotonin syndrome (3521,5193). Also, concurrent use might theoretically cause cerebral vasoconstriction disorders such as Call-Fleming syndrome (8056).
TRAMADOL (Ultram): Theoretically, concurrent use with tramadol might cause additive serotonergic effects and increase the risk of serotonin syndrome (3521,5193). Also, concurrent use might theoretically cause cerebral vasoconstriction disorders such as Call-Fleming syndrome (8056).

Interactions with Foods
None known.

Interactions with Lab Tests
None known.

Interactions with Diseases or Conditions
BIPOLAR DISORDER: Use of SAMe can cause patients to convert from a depressed state to a hypomanic or manic state (3523).
PARKINSON'S DISEASE: SAMe methylates levodopa, which could theoretically worsen Parkinsonian symptoms. However, this has not been reported in humans (10466).

Dosage and Administration
ORAL: For depression, an oral dose of 400-1600 mg per day has been used (5231). Doses of 1600 mg per day are the most commonly used in clinical trials (5189). For osteoarthritis, an oral dose of 200 mg three times daily is typically used (5188). For alcoholic liver disease or cirrhosis, oral doses of 1200-1600 mg per day have been used (1712,5231,5238,5241). For intrahepatic cholestasis, an oral dose of 800 mg twice daily is typically used (5219,5231,5239). For fibromyalgia, an oral dose of 800 mg per day is typically used (5241).
PARENTERAL: For depression, an intravenous or intramuscular injection of 200-400 mg per day is typically used (5231). For speeding the onset of antidepressant effect in combination with a tricyclic antidepressant, SAMe 200 mg intramuscularly for the first 2 weeks of tricyclic antidepressant therapy has been used (5193). For osteoarthritis, an intravenous dose of 400 mg per day has been used (5188). For intrahepatic cholestasis, an intravenous dose of 800 mg per day is typically used (5219,5231). For intrahepatic cholestasis of pregnancy (ICP), an intravenous dose of 800 mg per day has been used (5219,5231,5240). For AIDS-related myelopathy, an intravenous dose of 800 mg daily for 14 days has been used (5217).

Comments
Early studies used parenteral SAMe before an oral formulation was available (5231). Currently, several oral salt forms of SAMe are available: sulfate, sulfate-p-toluenesulfonate (also labeled as tosylate), and butanedisulfonate (5231,5444). The oral bioavailability of the tosylate salt is 1%, and the oral bioavailability of the butanedisulfonate salt is 5%, presumably due to a large first pass effect (1896,1897). Concerns about the stability of the tosylate formulation have been expressed (5446). The butanedisulfonate salt is stable for 2 years at room temperature (1896,5444). SAMe has been available as a dietary supplement in the US since 1999, but it has been used as a prescription drug in Italy since 1979, in Spain since 1985, and Germany since 1989. The potential usefulness of SAMe for treating osteoarthritis was discovered when patients in clinical trials of SAMe for depression noted improvement in their osteoarthritis symptoms (9110).

SAMPHIRE

Also Known As
Crest Marine, Peter's Cress, Pierce-Stone, Sampier, Sea Fennel.

Scientific Names
Crithmum maritimum.
Family: Apiaceae/Umbelliferae.

Comments
At the date of publication, there was very little scientific information about this product. Our staff is continually analyzing the available information on natural medicines and will add data to the online version of *Natural Medicines Comprehensive Database* as it becomes available. See www.naturaldatabase.com.

SANDY EVERLASTING

Also Known As
Common Shrubby Everlasting, Eternal Flower, Everlasting, Fleur de Pied de Chat, Goldilocks, Harnblumen, Helichrysum, Katzenpfotchenbluten, Yellow Chaste Weed.
CAUTION: See separate listing for Immortelle.

Scientific Names
Helichrysum italicum, synonyms Helichrysum angustifolium, Gnaphalium angustifolium, Gnaphalium italicum; Helichrysum orientale, synonyms Elichrysum orientale, Gnaphalium orientale; Helichrysum stoechas, synonyms Elichrysum stoechas, Gnaphalium stoechas.
Family: Asteraceae/Compositae.

People Use This For
Orally, sandy everlasting is used for dyspepsia, liver ailments, chronic cholecystitis, and gallbladder complaints with accompanying cramps. Sandy everlasting is also used orally as a diuretic, for chronic bronchitis, asthma, whooping cough, psoriasis, burns, rheumatism, headache, migraine, and allergies.
In foods, beverages, and tobacco, the extract is used as a flavoring component.
In manufacturing, it is used in perfumes, and before- and after-sun products.

Safety
LIKELY SAFE ...when used orally in amounts commonly found in foods. Sandy everlasting has Generally Recognized As Safe (GRAS) status in the US (4912).
POSSIBLY SAFE ...when used orally and appropriately (2).
PREGNANCY AND LACTATION: Insufficient reliable information available; avoid using in amounts greater than those generally found in foods and beverages.

Effectiveness
There is insufficient reliable information available about the effectiveness of sandy everlasting.

Mechanism of Action
The applicable part of sandy everlasting is the dried flower. Sandy everlasting contains flavonoids, quercitrin, kaempferol, naringenin, and isohelichrysin. These components might increase bile secretion. They have been shown to increase bile secretion in animals (11). The flavonoids also absorb UV light (11). Quercitrin increases the detoxifying function of the liver and exhibits anti-inflammatory activity (11). The constituent arenarin has antibacterial activity and promotes gastric and pancreatic secretions (8). The volatile oil of Helichrysum italicum flowers seems to have some antibacterial and antifungal activity (11).

Adverse Reactions
Sandy everlasting can cause an allergic reaction in individuals sensitive to the Asteraceae/Compositae family. Members of this family include ragweed, chrysanthemums, marigolds, daisies, and many other herbs.

Interactions with Herbs & Other Dietary Supplements
None known.

Interactions with Drugs
None known.

Interactions with Foods
None known.

Interactions with Lab Tests
None known.

Interactions with Diseases or Conditions
BILIARY OBSTRUCTION: Sandy everlasting is contraindicated, due to bile stimulating effects (2,18).
CROSS-ALLERGENICITY: Sandy everlasting can cause an allergic reaction in individuals sensitive to the Asteraceae/Compositae family. Members of this family include ragweed, chrysanthemums, marigolds, daisies, and many other herbs.
GALLSTONES: Sandy everlasting might complicate therapy (2,18).

Dosage and Administration

ORAL: One cup fresh tea (made by steeping 1 gram dried flower in 150 mL boiling water 5-10 minutes, strain) is typically taken several times per day (8,18); average amount 3 grams of dried flower per day (2).
TOPICAL: No typical dosage.

SANGRE DE GRADO

Also Known As

Blood of the Dragon, Drago, Dragon's Blood, Lan-Hiqui, Laniqui, Sangre de Drago, Sangre de Dragon, Sangue de Agua, Sangue de Drago, SP 303, SP-303, Taspine.
CAUTION: See also Dragon's Blood (Draconis resina) and Herb Robert (Geranium robertianum).

Scientific Names

Croton lechleri.
Family: Euphorbiaceae.

People Use This For

Orally, sangre de grado or its constituent, SP-303, is used for treating diarrhea associated with cholera, AIDS, traveling, cancer treatment, Clostridium difficile infection, and irritable bowel syndrome (IBS). It is also used orally for supporting the body's tissue repair mechanisms and treating viral respiratory infection. Additionally, sangre de grado is used orally for oropharyngeal and gastrointestinal ulcers, fever, hemorrhage, bleeding gums, fractures, wound healing, hemorrhoids, eczema, insect bites and stings, vaginitis, for vaginal baths before childbirth, and as a general tonic.
Topically, sangre de grado or its constituent, SP-303, is used for treating herpes simplex virus (types 1 and 2).

Safety

POSSIBLY SAFE ...when SP-303, a derivative of sangre de grado, is used orally or topically and appropriately (2784,2787,2788).
There is insufficient reliable information available about the safety of sangre de grado.
PREGNANCY AND LACTATION: Insufficient reliable information available; avoid using.

Effectiveness

POSSIBLY EFFECTIVE

AIDS-related diarrhea. Taking sangre de grado as part of a standardized resin extract containing SP-303 (SB-Normal Stool Formula, ShamanBotanicals.com) orally seems to reduce stool weight and frequency in people with AIDS-related diarrhea (2784).

Herpes simplex virus (HSV). Applying sangre de grado topically as part of a standardized resin extract containing SP-303, seems to be effective for treating genital and anal herpes simplex lesions in people with AIDS (2788). But it doesn't seem to be effective for treating acyclovir-unresponsive mucocutaneous herpes simplex lesions in these patients (2787).

Traveler's diarrhea. Taking sangre de grado as part of a standardized resin extract containing SP-303 seems to be effective for symptomatic treatment of traveler's diarrhea (2806).

INSUFFICIENT RELIABLE EVIDENCE to RATE

Insect bites and plant reactions. Applying sangre de grado resin alleviated the symptoms of insect bites (fire ants, wasps, bees) and plant reactions in a group of pest control workers (6114). More evidence is needed to rate sangre de grado for this use.

Mechanism of Action

Sangre de grado is a tree native to the Amazon regions of South America (2805,2784). The resin, a viscous red latex, and bark have a long history of oral and topical medicinal use (2784,2797). Sangre de grado is reported to have anti-inflammatory (2804,6114), antibacterial, anti-hemorrhagic, antiseptic, anti-tumor properties (2804). Topically, it has been shown to reduce vasodilation, swelling, and secretory response to irritants, promote mucosal healing, and prevent hyperalgesic responses in the laboratory (6114). Several active constituents of sangre de grado have been isolated, including SP-303 and tapsine (2786,2796). Preliminary evidence suggests that the constituent SP-303 might control diarrhea by inhibiting cyclic adenosine monophosphate (cAMP), which causes chloride and fluid secretion (2786). SP-303 shows activity against types 1 and 2 herpes simplex viruses, respiratory syncytial virus (RSV), and influenza A virus, possibly by inhibiting viral penetration of cells (2790,2791,2792,2793,2794). Tapsine demonstrates anti-inflammatory and wound healing properties when applied topically (2795,2796). Sangre de grado does not stimulate cell proliferation and has not shown carcinogenic activity after 17 months of treatment in experimental models (2796,2797,2798). Preliminary evidence suggests that sangre de grado resin is not cytotoxic, and has antibacterial and pro-oxidant activity (2798,2799).

Adverse Reactions
Orally, no serious adverse reactions or lab abnormalities have been reported in clinical studies using the sangre de grado derivative, SP-303 (2784,2806).
Topically, SP-303 can cause local pain and burning (2787).

Interactions with Herbs & Other Dietary Supplements
None known.

Interactions with Drugs
None known.

Interactions with Foods
None known.

Interactions with Lab Tests
None known.

Interactions with Diseases or Conditions
None known.

Dosage and Administration
ORAL: For treating AIDS-related diarrhea, a sangre de grado extract containing 500 mg of SP-303 (SB-Normal Stool Formula) every 6 hours has been used (2784). For treating traveler's diarrhea, a sangre de grado extract containing 125-500 mg SP-303 (SB-Normal Stool Formula) 4 times daily for 2 days has been used (2806).

Comments
SP-303 was in Phase III clinical trials with "fast track" designation for treatment of AIDS-related diarrhea and Phase II trials for traveler's diarrhea (2807). After the FDA rejected a new drug application and requested additional clinical testing, the manufacturer, Shaman Pharmaceuticals, became Shaman Botanicals and elected to market SP-303 as a dietary supplement, SB-Normal Stool Formula (2807).

SANICLE

Also Known As
European Sanicle, Poolroot, Saniculae herba, Self-Heal, Wood Sanicle.
CAUTION: See separate listing for Self-Heal.

Scientific Names
Sanicula europaea.
Family: Apiaceae/Umbelliferae.

People Use This For
Orally, sanicle is used for mild respiratory tract mucous membrane inflammation, cough, and bronchitis.

Safety
POSSIBLY SAFE ...when used orally and appropriately (2,12).
PREGNANCY AND LACTATION: Insufficient reliable information available; avoid using.

Effectiveness
There is insufficient reliable information available about the effectiveness of sanicle.

Mechanism of Action
The applicable parts of sanicle are the above ground parts. Sanicle contains triterpene saponins, caffeine derivatives, and flavonoids such as rutin, isoquercitrin, astragalin. It seems to have astringent and expectorant effects (18). The expectorant effect seems to result from the irritation caused by the saponins on the gastric mucosa that reflexly stimulates the bronchial mucous glands via parasympathetic sensory pathways (7). Large amounts of saponins may cause stomach upset, nausea, and vomiting (7). In animals, sanicle demonstrates edema reduction (18).

Adverse Reactions
Orally, large amounts of sanicle may cause upset stomach, nausea, and vomiting due to saponin content (7).

Interactions with Herbs & Other Dietary Supplements
None known.

Interactions with Drugs
None known.

Interactions with Foods
None known.

Interactions with Lab Tests
None known.

Interactions with Diseases or Conditions
GI MUCOSAL IRRITATION (e.g., ulcers, etc.): Theoretically, sanicle may exacerbate existing GI mucosal irritation due to saponin content (6); contraindicated.

Dosage and Administration
ORAL: A typical dose is 4-6 grams dried above ground parts per day (2).

Comments
Avoid confusion with Prunella vulgaris, also referred to as self-heal. In commerce, sanicle may be mixed with leaves of Cardamine enneaphylos, and Astrantia major is sometimes labeled as sanicle (18).

SARSAPARILLA

Also Known As
Ecuadorian Sarsaparilla, Honduras Sarsaparilla, Jamaican Sarsaparilla, Mexican Sarsaparilla, Salsaparilha, Salsepareille, Sarsa, Sarsaparillae radix, Sarsaparillewurzel, Smilax, Smilax aristolochiaefolii.
CAUTION: See separate listings for German Sarsaparilla.

Scientific Names
Smilax febrifuga; Smilax aristolochiifolia (Mexican Sarsaparilla), synonym Smilax medica; Smilax regelii (Honduran Sarsaparilla), synonym Smilax ornata; Smilax officinalis; other Smilax species.
Family: Smilacaceae.

People Use This For
Orally, sarsaparilla is used for psoriasis and other skin diseases, rheumatoid arthritis (RA), kidney disease, as an anabolic for performance enhancement or body-building in athletes, gout, and as a diuretic and diaphoretic. Sarsaparilla is also used as an adjunct for treating leprosy and for syphilis.
Mexican and Honduran sarsaparilla are used for treating gonorrhea, fevers, and digestive disorders.
In manufacturing, sarsaparilla is used as a flavoring agent in foods, beverages, and pharmaceuticals.

Safety
LIKELY SAFE ...when used orally in amounts commonly found in foods. Sarsaparilla has Generally Recognized As Safe (GRAS) status in the US (4912).
POSSIBLY SAFE ...when used orally and appropriately for medicinal purposes (12).
POSSIBLY UNSAFE ...when used in excessive amounts; gastrointestinal (GI) irritation may occur due to its saponin constituents (4).
PREGNANCY AND LACTATION: Insufficient reliable information available; avoid using.

Effectiveness
There is insufficient reliable information available about the effectiveness of sarsaparilla.

Mechanism of Action
The applicable part of sarsaparilla is the root. Sarsaparilla can have antirheumatic, antiseptic, and antipruritic activity (4). It contains about 2% saponins and other varied constituents, including quercetin and phytosterols (beta-sitosterol, stigmasterol, pollinastanol). The saponins, including sarsasapogenin and smilagenin (3,4,5,11), may have diuretic, diaphoretic, expectorant, and laxative effects (5). The sterols contained in sarsaparilla are not anabolic steroids nor are they converted in vivo to anabolic steroids (3,11). Testosterone has never been detected in any plant, including sarsaparilla (3,5). Sarsaparilla may improve appetite and digestion (4), and its extracts may improve psoriasis symptoms (4). Preliminary evidence suggests that sarsaparilla may have hepatoprotective and anti-inflammatory activity (4).

Adverse Reactions

Orally, sarsaparilla may cause GI irritation or temporary kidney impairment when used in excessive amounts (11). Large doses can lead to European cholera, diuresis, and shock (18). Occupational exposure to sarsaparilla root dust can cause rhinitis and asthma symptoms (4111).

Interactions with Herbs & Other Dietary Supplements

DIGITALIS: Sarsaparilla may increase digitalis glycoside absorption (2,11).
OTHER HERBS: Theoretically, sarsaparilla may alter the absorption or elimination of simultaneously administered herbs (2).

Interactions with Drugs

DIGOXIN (Lanoxin): Sarsaparilla may increase digitalis glycoside absorption (2,11).

Interactions with Foods

None known.

Interactions with Lab Tests

None known.

Interactions with Diseases or Conditions

ASTHMA: Sarsaparilla root dust can cause the symptoms of asthma (4111).
KIDNEY DYSFUNCTION: Theoretically, sarsaparilla can exacerbate kidney impairment (2,11).

Dosage and Administration

ORAL: The typical oral dose of sarsaparilla is 1-4 grams of the dried root or one cup of the tea three times daily. The tea is prepared by simmering 1-4 grams of the dried root in boiling water for 5-10 minutes and then straining (4). The typical dose of the liquid extract, 1:1 in 20% alcohol or 10% glycerol, is 8-15 mL (4).

Comments

In the Old West of the United States, sarsaparilla was the most popular drink of the cowboys (6002). Avoid confusion with Indian or false sarsaparilla (Hemidesmus indicus, Family: Apocyanaceae), reportedly a widespread adulterant of sarsaparilla (3,5,11). False sarsaparilla contains none of the saponins or other principal constituents found in sarsaparilla (5).

SASSAFRAS

Also Known As

Ague Tree, Cinnamon Wood, Common Sassafras, Kuntze Saloop, Sassafrax, Saxifrax.

Scientific Names

Sassafras albidum, synonyms Sassafras officinale, Sassafras variifolium, Laurus albida.
Family: Lauraceae.

People Use This For

Orally, sassafras is used for urinary tract disorders, mucous membrane inflammation, syphilis, bronchitis, geriatric high blood pressure, gout, arthritis, skin problems, kidney disorders, cancers, and as a tonic and "blood purifier". Topically, sassafras is used to treat skin eruptions, rheumatism, eye inflammation, sprains, swelling, and for relief of insect bites or stings. Sassafras oil is also used topically as an antiseptic and pediculicide.
In beverages and candy, a safrole-free bark extract has limited use as a flavoring agent.

Safety

POSSIBLY SAFE ...when used in amounts commonly found in foods. Safrole-free sassafras has Generally Recognized As Safe (GRAS) status in the US (4912).
POSSIBLY UNSAFE ...when safrole-free sassafras is used in medicinal amounts. Some studies link even safrole-free sassafras extracts to tumors (515).
LIKELY UNSAFE ...when used orally as a medicinal agent; avoid using (3,4). Sassafras root bark and oil contain safrole and related compounds that are carcinogenic and hepatotoxic in animals (4,12,17). Consumption of 5 mL sassafras oil can be fatal in adults (4). ...when used topically; avoid external use due to toxic safrole content (4).
CHILDREN: LIKELY UNSAFE ...when used orally. A few drops of sassafras oil can be fatal (4).
PREGNANCY AND LACTATION: LIKELY UNSAFE ...when used orally (12); avoid using. Sassafras oil has abortifacient effects (4).

Effectiveness
There is insufficient reliable information available about the effectiveness of sassafras.

Mechanism of Action
The applicable part of sassafras is the root bark. The major constituent of the volatile oil, safrole, is carcinogenic (causes malignant liver tumors in experimental animals) (6,11). Safrole and its metabolite, L-hydroxysafrole, are neurotoxic (6).

Adverse Reactions
Orally, sassafras can cause diaphoresis and hot flashes (11). Consumption of large amounts of sassafras oil can cause hallucinations lasting for several days (4). In adults, 5 mL sassafras oil can cause shakes, vomiting, dilated pupils, hypertension, tachycardia, stupor, collapse, abortion, paralysis, liver cancer, and death (4,6). A few drops of sassafras oil may be fatal in children (4).
Topically, sassafras can result in contact dermatitis (6).

Interactions with Herbs & Other Dietary Supplements
HERBS WITH SEDATIVE PROPERTIES: Theoretically, concomitant use with herbs that have sedative properties might enhance therapeutic and adverse effects. Some of these supplements include 5-HTP, calamus, California poppy, catnip, hops, Jamaican dogwood, kava, St. John's wort, scullcap, valerian, yerba mansa, and others.
SAFROLE-CONTAINING HERBS: Avoid concomitant use with other safrole-containing herbs due to potential for additive toxicity (12). Other herbs that contain safrole include basil, camphor, cinnamon, and nutmeg (12).

Interactions with Drugs
CNS DEPRESSANTS: Theoretically, concomitant use with drugs with sedative properties may cause additive effects (19).

Interactions with Foods
None known.

Interactions with Lab Tests
PHENYTOIN: Sassafras oil may cause false-positive blood phenytoin test results (6).

Interactions with Diseases or Conditions
URINARY CONDITIONS: Sassafras can aggravate urinary irritation (19).

Dosage and Administration
No typical dosage.

Comments
Use only safrole-free extract and leaves. Sassafras was used in the past to flavor root beer (11). In 1976, the FDA banned marketing of sassafras as sassafras tea (4). One study estimates that safrole 0.66 mg/kg could be toxic. One cup of tea made with 2.5 grams of sassafras is estimated to contain 200 mg of safrole, approximately 3 mg/kg (4).

SAVIN TOPS

Also Known As
Sabina, Savin, Savine.

Scientific Names
Juniperus sabina.
Family: Cupressaceae.

People Use This For
Orally, savin tops are used to induce abortions.
Topically, savin tops are used as a powder to treat fig warts.

Safety
POSSIBLY UNSAFE ...when used topically. Savin tops can cause severe irritation of skin and mucous membranes (18).
UNSAFE ...when used orally. Savin tops may be fatal if ingested as a powder or tea; 6 drops of the volatile oil can cause death (18).

PREGNANCY AND LACTATION: UNSAFE ...when used orally or topically due to overall toxicity as well as ability to induce abortions (19); avoid using.

Effectiveness

There is insufficient reliable information available about the effectiveness of savin tops.

Mechanism of Action

The applicable parts of savin tops are the branches and leaves. Savin tops contains ligans (thujone, podophyllotoxin, and others), hydroxycoumarins, and volatile oil (3-5%) including sabinyl acetate and sabinene (18). The ligans may have antineoplastic and antiviral properties (18). Savin tops has powerful irritant properties that can cause inflammation of the skin and mucous membranes (18,19).

Adverse Reactions

Orally, symptoms of poisoning include queasiness, cardiac rhythm disorders, spasm, kidney damage, hematuria, central paralysis, unconsciousness, and death (18). Ingestion can also cause irritation of the mucous membranes resulting in gastroenteritis, hepatitis, pneumonitis, and nephritis (19).
Topically, the volatile oil can cause skin irritation, blisters, necroses, and resorbent poisoning (18).

Interactions with Herbs & Other Dietary Supplements

None known.

Interactions with Drugs

None known.

Interactions with Foods

None known.

Interactions with Lab Tests

None known.

Interactions with Diseases or Conditions

INFLAMMATION: Components of the essential oil (sabinene and sabinyl acetate) may increase irritation of the skin or mucous membranes (19).

Dosage and Administration

ORAL: No typical dosage.
TOPICAL: The powder is typically applied twice daily (amount unspecified); "put bandages into skin folds" (18).

Comments

Use only safrole-free extract and leaves. The toxicity of the oil depends on how long it has been stored. Toxicity of oil develops over time through terpene peroxide formation (18). The toxicity of fresh branch tips is apparently low.

SAW PALMETTO

Also Known As

American Dwarf Palm Tree, Cabbage Palm, Ju-Zhong, Palmier Nain, Sabal, Sabal Fructus, Saw Palmetto Berry.

Scientific Names

Serenoa repens, synonyms Serenoa serrulata, Sabal serrulata.
Family: Arecaceae/Palmae.

People Use This For

Orally, saw palmetto is used for symptoms of benign prostatic hyperplasia (BPH). It is also used orally as a mild diuretic, a sedative, an anti-inflammatory, and as an antiseptic. Saw palmetto is used to increase breast size, to improve sexual vigor, and as an aphrodisiac. It is also used to treat chronic nonbacterial prostatitis/chronic pelvic pain syndrome, colds, coughs, irritated mucous membranes, sore throat, asthma, chronic bronchitis, migraines, cancer, and to stimulate hair growth.
In combination with other herbs, saw palmetto is used to treat prostate cancer.
Vaginally, the powdered fruit is used as a uterine and vaginal tonic.

Safety

LIKELY SAFE ...when used orally and appropriately. Saw palmetto has been safely used in clinical studies lasting up to 52 weeks (2732,2735,11354).

PREGNANCY AND LACTATION: LIKELY UNSAFE ...when used orally. Saw palmetto has hormonal activity (6766); avoid using.

Effectiveness

LIKELY EFFECTIVE

Benign prostatic hyperplasia (BPH). Multiple clinical studies lasting up to 48 weeks have shown that saw palmetto significantly improves urinary symptoms such as frequent urination, painful urination, hesitancy, urgency, and perineal heaviness. It also decreases nocturia, improves peak and mean urinary flow, and lowers residual urine volume in patients with BPH (2732,5094,6750,6751,6752,6762,6764,6772,6773,6777,6778,8330). Some research suggests that saw palmetto might not be helpful in men with relatively mild BPH (11314). Saw palmetto seems to be comparable in efficacy to finasteride (Proscar), but saw palmetto might be better tolerated (6424). The combination of a specific brand formulation containing saw palmetto and stinging nettle root (PRO 160/120) also seems to be comparable to finasteride (Proscar) for relieving symptoms of BPH (6763). However, saw palmetto does not reduce prostate size or prostate-specific antigen (PSA) levels like finasteride (6424). Alpha-adrenergic blockers such as prazosin (Minipress) seem to be superior to saw palmetto for relieving symptoms of BPH (6775,6776). However, other preliminary research suggests that saw palmetto is similar in efficacy to tamsulosin (Flomax) after 12 months (11243). The addition of saw palmetto to an alpha-blocker such as tamsulosin doesn't seem to relieve symptoms any better than an alpha-blocker alone (8901). Treatment for one to two months with saw palmetto is usually necessary before significant symptomatic improvement occurs (2732,6750,6778). Most clinical studies have used a liposterolic extract of saw palmetto berry containing 80-90% fatty acids. This formulation is similar to Quanterra Prostate (Warner-Lambert), Super Saw Palmetto (Enzymatic Therapy), ProstaPro (Phytopharmica), Saw Palmetto (Centrum), Standardized Saw Palmetto Extract (Nature's Way), and others.

A different formulation which contains saw palmetto lipid extract 106 mg, nettle root extract 80 mg, pumpkin seed oil extract 160 mg, lemon bioflavonoid extract 33 mg, and beta-carotene 190 IU taken three times daily for six months doesn't seem to be beneficial for men with BPH (5093).

INSUFFICIENT RELIABLE EVIDENCE to RATE

Prostatitis and chronic pelvic pain syndrome. Preliminary clinical research suggests that saw palmetto given orally for one year doesn't help nonbacterial prostatitis and chronic pelvic pain syndrome (11354). More evidence is needed to rate saw palmetto for these uses.

Mechanism of Action

The applicable part of saw palmetto is the ripe fruit. The lipid fraction contains volatile oils and fatty oils, which are active in treating benign prostatic hyperplasia (BPH). Many saw palmetto products are standardized based on the fatty acid content. The most effective saw palmetto products seem to be whole berries or berry extracts prepared with lipophilic nonpolar solvents. Water extraction, including brewed tea, probably does not adequately extract fat-soluble active constituents.

Saw palmetto has antiandrogenic, antiproliferative, and anti-inflammatory properties that seem to be responsible for improving symptoms of benign prostatic hyperplasia (BPH). Saw palmetto appears to noncompetitively inhibit 5 alpha-reductase types 1 and 2 and to prevent the conversion of testosterone to dihydrotestosterone (DHT) in vitro, which might reduce prostate growth (6765,6769,6770,6773). However, 5 alpha-reductase levels in prostatic tissue and serum testosterone, DHT, and PSA are not significantly reduced by saw palmetto in vivo (2735,6771). Saw palmetto does not seem to affect overall prostate size, but shrinks the inner prostatic epithelium (2736,5093). Saw palmetto, which appears to exert prostate-specific activity, might slow prostate cell proliferation by inhibiting fibroblast growth factor and epidermal growth factor and stimulating apoptosis (6765,6769,6770).

Inflammatory mediators appear to contribute to the etiology of BPH. In men with BPH, a liposterolic extract of saw palmetto berry seems to lower tumor necrosis factor (TNF)-alpha and interleukin (IL)-1beta, which are markers of inflammation in prostate tissue (11224). Laboratory evidence suggests that saw palmetto inhibits lipoxygenase and cyclooxygenase (Cox), which are involved in inflammation (6769,6779).

Increased Cox-2 expression is also associated with an increased incidence of prostate cancer. Preliminary research indicates that saw palmetto reduces the proliferation of experimental prostate cells, possibly by inhibiting Cox-2 expression (8902).

Saw palmetto also seems to have antiestrogen, antispasmodic, and alpha-adrenergic inhibitory properties (5095,6766,6780). Laboratory fertility studies indicate that saw palmetto has no effect on oocytes or sperm motility, but it might induce metabolic changes in sperm (4239,4240).

Saw palmetto doesn't seem to affect the cytochrome P450 (CYP450) enzymes, 2D6 (CYP2D6) and 3A4 (CYP3A4), in healthy volunteers taking 320 mg per day (11225). Drug interactions involving these enzymes have not been reported.

Adverse Reactions

Orally, the adverse effects of saw palmetto are generally mild and comparable to placebo. Dizziness, headache and gastrointestinal complaints such as nausea, vomiting, constipation, and diarrhea are the most frequently reported adverse effects (6751,6752,6762,11354). There is one case report of cholestatic hepatitis associated with the use of the multi-ingredient product that contains saw palmetto (Prostata) (598). Some clinicians are concerned that saw palmetto might cause erectile dysfunction, ejaculatory disturbance, or altered libido because of saw palmetto's potential effects on 5-alpha-reductase. There is one case report of decreased ejaculatory volume associated with an herbal blend product containing saw palmetto extract, nettle root extract, pumpkin seed oil extract, lemon bioflavonoid extract, and beta-carotene (5093). However, clinical studies indicate that the occurrence of impotence in men taking saw palmetto is similar to placebo and significantly less than finasteride (Proscar) (2732,6424,6762).

Interactions with Herbs & Other Dietary Supplements

None known.

Interactions with Drugs

ANTICOAGULANT/ANTIPLATELET DRUGS: Theoretically, saw palmetto might increase the risk of bleeding when used concomitantly with these agents. Saw palmetto is reported to prolong bleeding time (8659). Some of these drugs include aspirin; clopidogrel (Plavix); nonsteroidal anti-inflammatory drugs (NSAIDs) such as diclofenac (Voltaren, Cataflam, others), ibuprofen (Advil, Motrin, others), naproxen (Anaprox, Naprosyn, others); dalteparin (Fragmin); enoxaparin (Lovenox); heparin; warfarin (Coumadin); and others.
CONTRACEPTIVE DRUGS: Theoretically, concomitant use with saw palmetto might interfere with contraceptive drugs. Saw palmetto might have antiestrogenic effects (6766).
ESTROGENS: Theoretically, concomitant use with saw palmetto might interfere with hormone therapy. Saw palmetto might have antiestrogenic effects (6766).

Interactions with Foods

None known.

Interactions with Lab Tests

BLEEDING TIME: Saw palmetto can prolong bleeding time and increase the results of bleeding time tests (8659).
PROSTATE-SPECIFIC ANTIGEN: Contrary to earlier concerns, saw palmetto extract appears to have no significant effect on serum prostate-specific antigen (PSA) levels (764).

Interactions with Diseases or Conditions

None known.

Dosage and Administration

ORAL: For treating symptoms of benign prostatic hyperplasia (BPH), the recommended daily dose is 1-2 grams of whole berries. Clinical studies have used 160 mg twice daily or 320 mg once daily of a lipophilic extract containing 80-90% fatty acids (2,512). Traditionally, the liquid extract is dosed as 0.6-1.5 mL A tea prepared by simmering 0.5-1 grams of dried berry in 150 mL boiling water for 5-10 minutes and then straining is taken three times daily (4).

Comments

In the first half of the twentieth century, saw palmetto tea was included in the United States Pharmacopeia and the National Formulary.

SCARLET PIMPERNEL

Also Known As

Adder's Eyes, Poor Man's Weatherglass, Red Chickweed, Red Pimpernel, Shepherd's Barometer.

Scientific Names

Anagallis arvensis.
Family: Primulaceae.

People Use This For

Orally, scarlet pimpernel is used for depression, mucous membrane disorders, liver disorders, herpes, and as supportive therapy for carcinomas. It is also used orally for painful kidney disorders, particularly those with inflammation and an increase in urination.
Topically, scarlet pimpernel is used for poorly healing wounds and pruritus.
It is used both orally and topically to treat painful joints.

Safety

POSSIBLY UNSAFE ...when used orally or topically long-term (18).
There is insufficient reliable information available about the safety of scarlet pimpernel for short-term oral

or topical use.
PREGNANCY: LIKELY UNSAFE ...when used orally or topically long-term. Scarlet pimpernel shows evidence of uterine stimulant activity (18).
LACTATION: POSSIBLY UNSAFE ...when used orally or topically long-term; avoid using.

Effectiveness
There is insufficient reliable information available about the effectiveness of scarlet pimpernel.

Mechanism of Action
The applicable parts of scarlet pimpernel are the above ground flowering plant parts. In vitro data suggests that the aqueous extract has fungitoxic activity, and the isolated components triterpenglycoside, anagalloside and aglycon anagalligenone have bacteriostatic activity. Animal and human tissue data suggests uterine contracting activity. Triterepene saponins isolated from scarlet pimpernel may have activity against human sperm and may have estrogenic activity. A methanolic extract has hemolytic activity in human blood, and has activity against herpes simplex I, adenovirus type II, and polio type II. The gastroenteritis and nephritis that occurs with large doses or long-term administration is probably due to the cucurbitacins that are present in scarlet pimpernel (18).

Adverse Reactions
Orally, gastroenteritis and nephritis may occur with large doses or long-term administration (18).

Interactions with Herbs & Other Dietary Supplements
None known.

Interactions with Drugs
None known.

Interactions with Foods
None known.

Interactions with Lab Tests
None known.

Interactions with Diseases or Conditions
HORMONE SENSITIVE CANCERS/CONDITIONS: Because scarlet pimpernel might have estrogenic effects (18), women with hormone sensitive conditions should not use scarlet pimpernel. Some of these conditions include breast, uterine, and ovarian cancer, and endometriosis and uterine fibroids.
INFERTILITY: Scarlet pimpernel might have activity against sperm (18). Use cautiously or avoid in women trying to conceive and in men with fertility problems.

Dosage and Administration
ORAL: One cup of tea is commonly taken throughout the day. The tea is prepared by steeping teaspoons of dried plant in 150 mL of boiling water for 10 minutes and straining. The usual daily dosage can be up to 1.8 grams 4 times daily (18).
TOPICAL: No typical dosage.

SCHISANDRA

Also Known As
Bac Ngu Vi Tu, Bei Wu Wei Zi, Beiwuweizi, Chinesischer Limonenbaum, Chosen-Gomischi, Five-Flavor-Fruit, Five-Flavor-Seed, Gomishi, Hoku-Gomishi, Kita-Gomishi, Limonnik Kitajskij, M Mei Gee, Magnolia Vine, Matsbouza, Nanwuweizi, Ngu Mei Gee, Northern Schisandra, Omicha, Schisandrae, Schisandra Berry, Schizandra, Schizandrae, Shisandra, Southern Schisandra, Wu Wei Zi, Wu-Wei-Zi, Wuweizi, Western Shisandra, Xiwuweizi.

Scientific Names
Schisandra chinensis, synonym Kadsura chinensis; Schisandra splenanthera, synonym Schisandra chinensis var. rubriflora; other Schisandra species.
Family: Schisandraceae.

People Use This For
Orally, schisandra is used as an adaptogen for increasing resistance to disease and stress, increasing energy, and increasing physical performance and endurance. Schisandra is also used orally for improving vision, boosting muscular activity, improving cellular energy, for hepatitis, liver protection, preventing premature aging, increasing

lifespan, for premenstrual syndrome (PMS), stimulating the immune system, speeding recovery after surgery, protecting against radiation, counteracting the effects of sugar, preventing motion sickness, normalizing blood sugar and blood pressure, reducing high cholesterol, preventing infection, improving adrenal health, and energizing RNA-DNA to rebuild cells. Schisandra is also used for coughs, asthma, insomnia, neurasthenia, chronic diarrhea, dysentery, night sweats, spontaneous sweating, involuntary seminal discharge, thirst, impotence, physical exhaustion, excessive urination, depression, irritability, and memory loss.
Schisandra fruit is eaten as a food.

Safety

POSSIBLY SAFE ...when used orally and appropriately (12,3559).
PREGNANCY: POSSIBLY UNSAFE ...when used orally; avoid using. Some evidence suggests schisandra fruit is a uterine stimulant (11,3559).
LACTATION: Insufficient reliable information; avoid using.

Effectiveness

POSSIBLY EFFECTIVE

Concentration, coordination, and endurance. Taking schisandra fruit extract orally seems to improve concentration, coordination, and endurance (3559).

Hepatitis. Taking schisandra fruit extract orally seems to improve liver function in patients with hepatitis. Schisandra fruit extracts reduce serum glutamic-pyruvic transaminase (SGPT) levels in patients with viral or drug-induced hepatitis (3559).

There is insufficient reliable information available about the effectiveness of schisandra for its other uses.

Mechanism of Action

The applicable part of schisandra is the fruit. A variety of active constituents including schizandrins, schizandrols, gomisins, schizandrers, schisantherins, wuweizisus, and many others, collectively known as lignans, have been isolated from schisandra (11,3559). Some schisandra extracts are standardized based on specific lignan content (3559). Schisandra improves liver function by increasing hepatic glutathione, glucose-6-phosphate, and glutathione-reductase activity. It might also have a hepatoprotective effect by inhibiting lipid peroxidation, increasing liver glycogen production, inducing cytochrome P450 (CYP450) enzymes, and promoting hepatocyte growth (11,3559). Schisandra is referred to as an adaptogen; it seems to increase concentration, coordination, and endurance (3559). The mechanisms for these effects is not yet known. Schisandra also seems to have antioxidant and anti-inflammatory properties (3559). Other reported properties of various schisandra lignans include antitussive (6), anticonvulsant, antidepressant, antifatigue, tranquilizing, respiratory stimulant (11), and platelet activating factor (PAF) inhibition (3767). Some evidence suggests that nigranoic acid, isolated from the stem of Schisandra sphaerandra, might be useful in HIV therapy. In vitro it exhibits anti-HIV reverse transcriptase and polymerase activity (3768).

Adverse Reactions

Orally, schisandra can cause heartburn, acid indigestion, decreased appetite, stomach pain, allergic skin rashes, and urticaria in some patients (11,3559).

Interactions with Herbs & Other Dietary Supplements

None known.

Interactions with Drugs

None known.

Interactions with Foods

None known.

Interactions with Lab Tests

SERUM GLUTAMIC-PYRUVIC TRANSAMINASE (SGPT)/ALANINE AMINOTRANSFERASE (ALT): Schisandra might lower serum SGPT/ALT levels and test results (11,3559).

Interactions with Diseases or Conditions

EPILEPSY: One source recommends to avoid use in patients with epilepsy (3559). The reason for this warning is not clear, but it may be due to schisandra's potential CNS stimulating effects (6).
GASTROESOPHAGEAL REFLUX DISEASE (GERD), PEPTIC ULCER DISEASE (PUD): Schisandra might exacerbate GERD or PUD by increasing gastric acidity (3559).
HIGH INTRACRANIAL PRESSURE: One source recommends to avoid use in patients with high intracranial pressure (3559). The reason for this warning is not clear, but it may be due to schisandra's potential CNS stimulating effects (6).

Dosage and Administration

ORAL: For hepatitis, schisandra extract standardized to 20 mg lignan content (equivalent to 1.5 grams crude schisandra) given daily has been used (3559). For improving mental and physical performance, schisandra extract 500 mg to 2 grams daily or crude schisandra 1.5-6 grams daily have been used (3559); Crude schisandra decoction (boiled tea) 5-15 grams daily has also been used (3559). People have also taken schisandra extract 100 mg twice daily (6002). Appropriate dosing may vary depending on extract type and standardization.

Comments

An antihepatotoxic drug known as DBD has been developed in China derived from the schisandra constituent schisandrin C (3559).

SCOPOLIA

Also Known As

Belladonna, Belladonna Scopola, Glockenbilsenkraut, Japanese Belladonna, Russian Krainer Tollkraut, Scopola, Scopoliae Rhizoma.
CAUTION: See separate listing for Belladonna.

Scientific Names

Scopolia carniolica.
Family: Solanaceae.

People Use This For

Orally, scopolia is used for spasms of the gastrointestinal (GI) tract, bile ducts, and urinary tract, and for liver and gallbladder complaints. Scopolia is also used orally as a diuretic, sedative, hypnotic, narcotic, for dilating pupils, and pain relief.

Safety

LIKELY UNSAFE ...when used orally for self-medication (12). Use of scopolia requires monitoring (12). The lethal adult dose is considered to be 100 mg of atropine which is approximately 20-50 grams of scopolia root or rhizome depending on its alkaloid content (18).
PREGNANCY AND LACTATION: LIKELY UNSAFE ...when used orally for self-medication (12); avoid using.

Effectiveness

There is insufficient reliable information available about the effectiveness of scopolia.

Mechanism of Action

The applicable parts of scopolia are the rhizome and root. Scopolia root or rhizome contains 0.3-0.8% alkaloids, primarily L-hyoscyamine and lesser amounts of atropine and scopolamine (2). L-Hyoscyamine, the levorotatory isomer of atropine, is considered the active principle (2). Scopolia root has parasympatholytic activity. It is a competitive antagonist of acetylcholine, acting preferentially at the muscarinic receptors (2). Scopolia has antispasmodic effects, relaxing the smooth muscle of the gastrointestinal tract and bile ducts (2). Scopolia root can eliminate muscular tremors and muscular rigidity caused by central nervous impulses. It also has positive chronotropic and dromotropic effects (2).

Adverse Reactions

Orally, scopolia root can cause dry mouth, dry and reddened skin, hyperthermia, disturbance of ocular accommodation, tachycardia, difficulty urinating, glaucoma attacks (2), and constipation (18). Early symptoms of poisoning include reddened skin, dry mouth, and tachycardiac arrhythmias (18). Ingestion of large amounts can cause central excitation including restlessness, compulsive speech, hallucinations, delirium, manic episodes, followed by exhaustion and sleep, and asphyxiation (18).

Interactions with Herbs & Other Dietary Supplements

ANTICHOLINERGIC HERBS: Scopolia can potentiate the effects and adverse effects of other herbs with anticholinergic activity including belladonna, henbane, mandrake, and jimson weed (12).

Interactions with Drugs

ANTICHOLINERGIC DRUGS: The alkaloid constituents, hyoscyamine, scopolamine, and atropine could potentiate the effects and adverse effects of anticholinergic drugs (15).
QUINIDINE: Concomitant use with scopolia might increase effects (2).
TRICYCLIC ANTIDEPRESSANTS (TCAs): Concomitant use with scopolia can potentiate anticholinergic effects and adverse effects (2).

Interactions with Foods

None known.

Interactions with Lab Tests

None known.

Interactions with Diseases or Conditions

CONGESTIVE HEART FAILURE (CHF): Contraindicated; scopolia might cause tachycardia and exacerbate CHF due to its hyoscyamine (atropine) and scopolamine content (15).
CONSTIPATION: Contraindicated; scopolia might cause constipation due to its hyoscyamine (atropine) and scopolamine content (15).
DOWN SYNDROME: Caution, patients with Down syndrome might be hypersensitive to the antimuscarinic effects (mydriasis, positive chronotropic heart effects, etc.) of hyoscyamine (atropine) and scopolamine contained in scopolia (15).
ESOPHAGEAL REFLUX: Contraindicated; scopolia might delay gastric emptying and decrease lower esophageal pressure, promoting gastric retention and exacerbating reflux due to its hyoscyamine (atropine) and scopolamine content (15).
FEVER: Contraindicated; scopolia might increase the risk of hyperthermia in patients with fever due to its hyoscyamine (atropine) and scopolamine content (15).
GASTRIC ULCER: Contraindicated; scopolia might delay gastric emptying and exacerbate gastric ulcers due to its hyoscyamine (atropine) and scopolamine content (15).
GI INFECTIONS: Contraindicated; scopolia might suppress GI motility causing retention of infecting organisms or toxins due to its hyoscyamine (atropine) and scopolamine content (15).
HIATAL HERNIA: Contraindicated; scopolia might delay gastric emptying and decrease lower esophageal pressure, promoting gastric retention and exacerbating reflux due to its hyoscyamine (atropine) and scopolamine content (15).
NARROW-ANGLE GLAUCOMA: Contraindicated; scopolia might increase ocular tension in patients with narrow-angle (angle-closure) glaucoma due to its hyoscyamine (atropine) and scopolamine content (2,15).
OBSTRUCTIVE GI TRACT DISEASE: Contraindicated; scopolia might exacerbate obstructive GI tract diseases (including atony, paralytic ileus, and stenosis) due to its hyoscyamine (atropine) and scopolamine content (15).
TACHYARRHYTHMIAS: Contraindicated; scopolia might cause tachycardia due to its hyoscyamine (atropine) and scopolamine content (2,15).
TOXIC MEGACOLON: Contraindicated; scopolia might suppress intestinal motility, which might produce paralytic ileus and exacerbate toxic megacolon, due to its hyoscyamine (atropine) and scopolamine content (2,15).
ULCERATIVE COLITIS: Contraindicated; scopolia might suppress intestinal motility, which might produce paralytic ileus and precipitate toxic megacolon, due to its hyoscyamine (atropine) and scopolamine content (15).
URINARY RETENTION: Contraindicated; scopolia might increase urinary retention due to its hyoscyamine (atropine) and scopolamine content (2,15).

Dosage and Administration

ORAL: The average daily dose is 0.25 mg total alkaloids calculated as hyoscyamine (2). The maximum single dose is 1 mg total alkaloids calculated as hyoscyamine (2). The maximum daily dose is 3 mg total alkaloids calculated as hyoscyamine. Scopolia is administered as pulverized root, powder, or other preparations (2).

SCOTCH BROOM flower

Also Known As

Bannal, Besenginaterkraut, Broom Tops, Butcher's-Broom, Cytisi scoparii flos, Genet a Balais, Ginsterkraut, Herbe de Hogweed, Hogweed, Irish Broom Tops, Scoparius.
CAUTION: See separate listings for Butcher's Broom, Scotch Broom herb, and Spanish Broom.

Scientific Names

Cytisus scoparius, synonyms Sarothamnus scoparius, Sarothamnus vulgaris, Spartium scoparium, Genista andreana.
Family: Fabaceae/Leguminosae.

People Use This For

Orally, scotch broom flower is used as a mild diuretic, for improving circulation, as a cathartic and emetic, for cardiac dropsy, tachycardia, and profuse menstruation.
Topically, scotch broom flower is used for sore muscles, abscesses, and swelling. It is used in hair rinses to lighten and brighten hair.

Safety

LIKELY UNSAFE ...when used orally for self-medication (4,12). Scotch broom contains sparteine, an alkaloid with cardiac depressant activities similar to quinidine (4).
There is insufficient reliable information available about the safety of scotch broom flower for topical use.
PREGNANCY: LIKELY UNSAFE ...when used orally; scotch broom appears to be an abortifacient (5,9,12).
LACTATION: LIKELY UNSAFE ...when used orally in amounts commonly found in foods; avoid using (4,12).

Effectiveness

There is insufficient reliable information available about the effectiveness of scotch broom flower.

Mechanism of Action

Scotch broom flower contains sparteine, an alkaloid, which has curare-like properties and mimics quinidine's anti-arrhythmic effect (4). Sparteine extends diastole without a positive inotropic effect (8). The diuretic effect of the herb may be due to the flavone glycoside, scoparoside (5). It also contains tyramine (4,6,11).

Adverse Reactions

Orally, it may cause nausea, diarrhea, vertigo, stupor, tachycardia with circulatory collapse, and respiratory arrest (4). Smoking scotch broom cigarettes may cause headaches and uterine stimulation (6), and may risk contracting pulmonary aspergillosis (5,6).

Interactions with Herbs & Other Dietary Supplements

None known.

Interactions with Drugs

MONOAMINE OXIDASE INHIBITORS (MAOIs): Scotch broom flower contains tyramine. It should not be used with monoamine oxidase inhibitors because it might cause a hypertensive crisis (2).

Interactions with Foods

None known.

Interactions with Lab Tests

None known.

Interactions with Diseases or Conditions

CARDIAC DISEASE: Contraindicated due to negative inotropic and negative chronotropic effects (2,4).
HYPERTENSION: Contraindicated due to vasoconstrictive effect (2,4).
KIDNEY DISORDERS: The component, scoparin, might have diuretic activity which could aggravate kidney disorders (19).
SPLEEN AND LIVER DISORDERS: Contraindicated (19).

Dosage and Administration

ORAL: It is typically used as tea (steep 1-2 grams in boiling water 5-10 minutes, strain) three times daily (4); a liquid extract (1:1 in 25% alcohol), 1-2 mL (4); or a tincture: (1:5 in 45% alcohol) 0.5-2 mL (4).

Comments

Avoid confusion with butcher's broom root, scotch broom herb, and Spanish broom flower. Scotch broom seeds used as a coffee substitute are dangerous (6).

SCOTCH BROOM herb

Also Known As

Bannal, Basam, Besom, Bizzom, Broom, Browme, Breeam, Brum, Cytisi scoparii herba, Hogweed, Irish Broom, Scoparium, Scoparius.
CAUTION: See separate listings for Butcher's Broom, Scotch Broom flower, and Spanish Broom.

Scientific Names

Cytisus scoparius, synonyms Sarothamnus scoparius, Sarothamnus vulgaris, Spartium scoparium, Genista andreana.
Family: Fabaceae/Leguminosae.

People Use This For

Orally, scotch broom herb is used for heart and circulatory disorders including edema, cardiac arrhythmia, racing heartbeat, and low blood pressure. It is also used orally for heavy menstruation, hemorrhaging after birth, as a contraction stimulant, for bleeding gums, hemophilia, gout, rheumatism, sciatica, gallbladder and kidney stones, enlarged spleen, jaundice, bronchial conditions, and snake bites.

Safety

POSSIBLY SAFE ...when the aqueous-ethanolic extract is used orally and appropriately (2).
LIKELY UNSAFE ...when used orally in excessive amounts. Toxicity has been reported with ingestion of more than 300 mg sparteine (30 grams of above ground parts) (18).
PREGNANCY: POSSIBLY UNSAFE ...when used orally due to potential for uterine contractions (6,18).
LACTATION: Insufficient reliable information available; avoid using.

Effectiveness

There is insufficient reliable information available about the effectiveness of scotch broom herb.

Mechanism of Action

The constituent, sparteine, has negative inotropic and chronotropic effects, which are responsible for its cardiac activity. It also seems to stimulate uterine contractions (6). The constituent tyramine, acts as an indirect vasoconstrictor and hypertensive (18).

Adverse Reactions

Orally, sparteine toxicity can occur with doses greater than 300 mg of sparteine, which is roughly equivalent to 30 grams of scotch broom. Symptoms of this toxicity include dizziness, headache, palpitations, prickling in the extremities, feeling of weakness in the legs, sweating, sleepiness, pupil dilation, and ocular palsy (18).

Interactions with Herbs & Other Dietary Supplements

None known.

Interactions with Drugs

HALOPERIDOL (Haldol): Haloperidol (Haldol) inhibits sparteine metabolism, which is found in scotch broom herb, increasing the risk of adverse effects including circulatory collapse (17).
MONOAMINE OXIDASE INHIBITORS (MAOIs): Scotch broom contains tyramine. It should not be used with monoamine oxidase inhibitors because it might cause a hypertensive crisis (18).
QUINIDINE: Quinidine (Quinidex) inhibits sparteine metabolism, which is found in scotch broom herb, increasing the risk of adverse effects including circulatory collapse (17).

Interactions with Foods

None known.

Interactions with Lab Tests

None known.

Interactions with Diseases or Conditions

ATRIOVENTRICULAR BLOCK (A-V block): Contraindicated (18).
HIGH BLOOD PRESSURE: Contraindicated (18).

Dosage and Administration

ORAL: A cup of freshly brewed tea is typically used 3-4 times daily. To make tea, steep 1 level teaspoon (1-2 grams) above ground parts in 150 mL boiling water 5-10 minutes , strain (7). The liquid extract is typically used 1-2 mL daily (18). The tincture is typically used 0.5-2 mL daily (18). Aqueous-ethanolic extracts are typically used as 1-1.5 grams of above ground parts (7).

Comments

Avoid confusion with butcher's broom, scotch broom flower, and Spanish broom.

SCOTCH PINE NEEDLE

Also Known As

Pine Needle Oil, Pine Oils, Pini Atheroleum.
CAUTION: See separate listings for Dwarf Pine Needle, Fir Needle Oil, Poplar, Fir, and Pine.

Scientific Names

Pinus sylvestris.
Family: Pinaceae.

People Use This For

Orally or by inhalation, scotch pine needle is used for the common cold, cough, and bronchitis.
Orally, it is used for fever, inflammation of the mouth and pharynx, and the tendency for infection.
Topically, scotch pine needle is used for rheumatic and neuralgic ailments.

Safety

There is insufficient reliable information available about the safety of scotch pine needle.
Pregnancy and Lactation: Insufficient reliable information available; avoid using.

Effectiveness

There is insufficient reliable information available about the effectiveness of scotch pine needle.

Mechanism of Action

The applicable part of scotch pine needle is the oil. The essential oil includes alpha-pinene, delta3-carene, camphene, beta-pinene, limonene, myrcene, and terpinolene. People think scotch pine needle oil has hyperemic, weak antiseptic, and secretolytic properties (18).

Adverse Reactions

Orally, scotch pine needle oil can worsen bronchospasms (18).
Topically, scotch pine needle oil can be irritating to the skin and mucous membranes (18).

Interactions with Herbs & Other Dietary Supplements

None known.

Interactions with Drugs

None known.

Interactions with Foods

None known.

Interactions with Lab Tests

None known.

Interactions with Diseases or Conditions

CARDIAC DISORDERS: Avoid using as a bath additive in individuals with a history of cardiac insufficiency (18).
HYPERTONIA: Avoid using as a bath additive (18).
INFECTION: Avoid using as a bath additive in individuals with fever or infectious diseases (18).
RESPIRATORY ILLNESS: Contraindicated in individuals with asthma and whooping cough because scotch pine needle oil might cause or worsen bronchospasms (18).
SKIN CONDITIONS: Avoid using as a bath additive when extensive skin injuries or acute skin diseases are present (18).

Dosage and Administration

ORAL: An average daily dose is 5 grams (18).
INHALATION: Place several drops in hot water and breathe in the vapors (18).
TOPICAL: Several drops or semi-solid preparation containing 10-50 % drug may be rubbed onto the affected area (18). As a bath additive 25 mg drug per liter water is used in bubble bath or bath salts (18).
The essential oil is administered in alcoholic solutions, ointments, gels, emulsions, oils, or as an inhalant (18).

Comments

Avoid confusion with "pine oils" that are synthetically produced (18).

SCOTCH THISTLE

Also Known As

Woolly Thistle.

Scientific Names

Onopordum acanthium.
Family: Asteraceae.

Comments

At the date of publication, this product was not a common ingredient used in brand name supplements marketed to consumers. Details about this product are available at the online version of *Natural Medicines Comprehensive Database*. See www.naturaldatabase.com.

SCURVY GRASS

Also Known As

Scrubby Grass, Spoonwort.
CAUTION: See separate listing for Watercress.

Scientific Names

Cochlearia officinalis.
Family: Brassicaceae/Cruciferae.

People Use This For

Orally, scurvy grass is used for vitamin C deficiency, gout, arthritis, stomach ache, as a diuretic, and as a blood purifier.
Topically, scurvy grass is used for skin irritations, canker sores, and gum disease.
Historically, scurvy grass was used to remove undesirable agents from the blood.

Safety

There is insufficient reliable information available about the safety of scurvy grass.
Pregnancy and Lactation: Insufficient reliable information available; avoid using.

Effectiveness

There is insufficient reliable information available about the effectiveness of scurvy grass.

Mechanism of Action

The applicable parts of scurvy grass are the leaves and aerial parts or pressed juice. Alcohol extracts of scurvy grass are used topically. Scurvy grass contains glucosilinates, an unidentified volatile oil and bitter principle, tannin, and vitamin C. It might have antiseptic, diuretic, and mild laxative actions (7122). The mustard oils in scurvy grass can irritate the mucous membranes (18).

Adverse Reactions

Orally, large amounts of scurvy grass can cause symptoms of gastrointestinal irritation.
Topically, skin irritation may occur with topical application.

Interactions with Herbs & Other Dietary Supplements

None known.

Interactions with Drugs
None known.

Interactions with Foods
None known.

Interactions with Lab Tests
None known.

Interactions with Diseases or Conditions
None known.

Dosage and Administration
No typical dosage.

Comments
Scurvy grass was once used by sailors to prevent scurvy (7122). Scurvy grass is also known as watercress (see separate listing). Be careful not to confuse these two plants. The scurvy grass flowers have a strong fragrance and taste when they are rubbed (18).

SEA BUCKTHORN

Also Known As
Argasse, Argousier, Buckthorn, Dhar-Bu, Espino Armarillo, Espino Falso, Finbar, Grisset, Meerdorn, Oblepikha, Purging Thorn, Rokitnik, Sallow Thorn, Sanddorn, Sceitbezien, Sea Buckhorn, Sea-Buckthorn, Seabuckthorn, Seedorn, Star-Bu, Tindved.
CAUTION: See separate listings for Alder Buckthorn, European Buckthorn, and Cascara (California Buckthorn).

Scientific Names
Hippophae rhamnoides.
Family: Elaeagnaceae.

People Use This For
Orally, sea buckthorn leaves and flowers are used for treating arthritis, gastrointestinal ulcers, gout, and exanthemata. A tea containing sea buckthorn leaves is used as a source of vitamins, flavones, amino acids, fatty acids and minerals; for improving blood pressure and blood lipids; preventing and controlling blood vessel diseases; removing free radicals; and boosting immunity.
Orally, sea buckthorn berries are used for preventing infections, improving sight, and inhibiting sclerosis and aging.
Orally, sea buckthorn seed or berry oil is used as an expectorant, for treating asthma, cardiac disorders including angina, for lowering cholesterol, preventing atheroma, and as an antioxidant. It is also used orally for postponing senility; reducing cancer morbidity and the toxicity of chemotherapy; balancing the immune system; stomach and intestinal diseases including ulcers and reflux esophagitis; treating night blindness; and as a supplemental source of vitamins C, A, and E, beta-carotene, flavonoids, superoxide dismutase, minerals, amino acids, and fatty acids.
Topically, sea buckthorn berries, berry concentrate, and berry or seed oil are used as a sunscreen, for treating radiation damage from x-rays and sunburns; healing wounds including bedsores, burns, and cuts; for acne, dermatitis, dry skin, eczema, skin ulcers, postpartum pigmentation, and for protecting mucus membranes.
In foods, sea buckthorn berries are used to make jellies, juices, purees, and sauces.
In manufacturing, sea buckthorn is used in cosmetics and anti-aging preparations.

Safety
LIKELY SAFE ...when consumed in amounts found in foods (9898). There is insufficient reliable information available about the safety of medicinal use of sea buckthorn.
PREGNANCY AND LACTATION: LIKELY SAFE ...when used in amounts commonly found in foods. Insufficient reliable information available about medicinal use; avoid using in amounts greater than those found in foods.

Effectiveness
There is insufficient reliable information available about the effectiveness of sea buckthorn.

Mechanism of Action

The applicable parts of sea buckthorn are the flowers, fruit, seeds, and leaves. Sea buckthorn fruit, which is used to make jams and jellies, contains fruit acids including malic acid, acetic acid, and quinic acid; as well as volatile oil, sitosterol, and flavonoids. It also contains carotenoids including beta-carotene, gamma-carotene, and lycopene; and fatty oils including oleic acid, isolinol acid, linolenic acid, stearic acid, and palmitoleic acid. The fruit also contains vitamins A, B1, B2, B6, C, and tocopherols (4504,9898).

Preliminary evidence suggests that sea buckthorn extract (plant part not specified) and two constituents of the seed oil (beta-sitosterol-beta-D-glucoside and aglycone) might have activity against gastric ulcers (466,472). The fruit juice reduces the incidence and growth of experimentally-induced tumors (468). The seed oil might protect against carbon tetrachloride, ethyl alcohol and acetaminophen-induced liver damage (469,470). Some data suggest that sea buckthorn extract (plant part not specified) might protect cells against lipid peroxidation injury (471) and might increase the rate and extent of wound tissue epithelialization and granulation (467). Preliminary human evidence indicates that sea buckthorn seed oil might reduce the toxicity of chemotherapy on the blood, gastrointestinal tract and immune system (478), improve symptoms of reflux esophagitis (479), and improve the symptoms and cure rate of peptic ulcers (480). Sea buckthorn berry oil can inhibit aggregation of platelets (10208).

Adverse Reactions

None reported.

Interactions with Herbs & Other Dietary Supplements

HERBS WITH ANTICOAGULANT/ANTIPLATELET POTENTIAL: Concomitant use of herbs that effect platelet aggregation could theoretically increase the risk of bleeding because sea buckthorn berry oil can decrease platelet aggregation (10208). Some of these herbs and supplements include angelica, clove, danshen, feverfew, fish oil, garlic, ginger, ginkgo, Panax ginseng, horse chestnut, red clover, turmeric, vitamin E, and others.

Interactions with Drugs

ANTICOAGULANT/ANTIPLATELET DRUGS: Sea buckthorn berry oil can inhibit platelet aggregation (10208). Theoretically, using sea buckthorn berry oil in combination with anticoagulant or antiplatelet drugs might have additive effects and increase the risk of bleeding. Some of these drugs include aspirin, clopidogrel (Plavix), dalteparin (Fragmin), enoxaparin (Lovenox), heparin, ticlopidine (Ticlid), warfarin (Coumadin), and others.

Interactions with Foods

None known.

Interactions with Lab Tests

None known.

Interactions with Diseases or Conditions

None known.

Dosage and Administration

ORAL: 1-2 cups of a tea prepared from the leaves is typically consumed daily (461). 1-3 seed oil capsules (500 mg per capsule) are commonly used three times daily (462). 3-5 mL of the seed oil is commonly used three times daily (478,479). Up to 2 dropperfuls of the berry oil is commonly used three times daily (463).
TOPICAL: The berry or seed oil is typically applied three or four times per day (462,463).

Comments

Avoid confusion with alder buckthorn (Rhamnus frangula). The fatty oil of sea buckthorn seeds and berries is harvested from August until the first snow of December (18). The fruit juices and purees are popular due to their flavor (4504).

SECRETIN

Also Known As

None.

Scientific Names

Secretin; Oxykrinin.

People Use This For

Sublingually, secretin is used for treating autism.
Intravenously, secretin is used for autism and pervasive developmental disorder, diagnosing Zollinger-Ellison syndrome, pancreatic dysfunction, hyperparathyroidism, preventing stress ulcers, treating duodenal ulcers, gastrointestinal bleeding, pancreatitis, and cardiac failure.

Safety

LIKELY SAFE ...when used parenterally and appropriately. Secretin is an FDA-approved, prescription product (2917,6136).
There is insufficient reliable information available about the safety of secretin when used sublingually.
PREGNANCY AND LACTATION: Insufficient reliable information available; avoid using.

Effectiveness

LIKELY INEFFECTIVE

Autism or pervasive developmental disorder. Administering secretin intravenously doesn't improve symptoms of autism or pervasive developmental disorder. The use of secretin for autism is controversial. There have been some anecdotal and preliminary reports showing subjective improvement in gastrointestinal function, social and behavioral function, and language skills after single infusions of secretin (2917,6632). However, the majority of evidence shows that secretin, both synthetic human and porcine-derived preparations, is no better than placebo for any outcome measure when given in single or repeated doses (5247,6136,7052).

INSUFFICIENT RELIABLE EVIDENCE to RATE

Pancreatitis. There is preliminary evidence secretin might help symptoms of chronic recurrent pancreatitis (2918).
Post-surgical stress ulcers. There is some preliminary evidence that secretin might help prevent post-surgical stress ulcers (2912,2913).
More evidence is needed to rate secretin for these uses.

Mechanism of Action

Secretin is an endogenously occurring gastrointestinal hormone in humans. Secretin is in a family of hormones that also includes glucagon, glucose-dependent insulin releasing peptide (GIP), vasoactive intestinal polypeptide (VIP), and others. Normal fasting serum levels are 3-15 pg/mL. Secretin is released from S cells in the duodenum and proximal jejunum when duodenal pH falls below 4.5. Serum levels can increase to 30 pg/mL after stimulation. The primary action of secretin is to stimulate release of bicarbonate and water from the pancreas. Intravenous administration of secretin in physiological doses has the same effect. The concurrent presence of cholecystokinin (CCK) potentiates the action of secretin on the pancreas. Administration in pharmacological doses also causes decreased release of meal-stimulated gastrin and decreases gastric acid secretion (7053). Secretin is given intravenously because orally administered secretin is inactivated by proteolytic enzymes (15). Synthetic secretin appears to be as effective as secretin of porcine origin (10226).
Many people use secretin for autism, but a potential mechanism of action in autism is not known. Secretin began being used for autism based on anecdotal cases showing improvement in symptoms (2917,6632). Some researchers have speculated that certain autistic patients might have abnormally low secretin levels, but this has not been verified. Reliable clinical evidence now shows that secretin probably does not have a viable role in treating autism (5247,6136,7052).

Adverse Reactions

Intravenously, the most common adverse reaction is flushing of the face, neck, and chest immediately after infusion (6007,7052). Less common potential adverse effects are vomiting (6007,7052), diarrhea, fainting, venous thrombosis (15), fever, and tachycardia (7052). Some patients can have allergic reactions including urticaria, erythema, and anaphylaxis (7052). Because of the potential for these hypersensitivity reactions, a 0.1 mL test dose is often administered prior to giving a full dose (7052).

Interactions with Herbs & Other Dietary Supplements

None known.

Interactions with Drugs

None known.

Interactions with Foods

None known.

Interactions with Lab Tests

None known.

Interactions with Diseases or Conditions
None known.

Dosage and Administration
INTRAVENOUS: For autism, a wide variety of doses have been used. Due to the potential for hypersensitivity reactions, a 0.1 CU test dose is often given prior to administration of the full dose. Clinical studies have used either single infusions or repeated infusions for 2 or more doses separated by 6 weeks or more. Doses are most often 2 CU/kg (5247,7052), but clinicians use a wide range of doses (6007). So far, clinical research does not support the use of secretin for autism. No dosage regimen has yet been proven to improve the symptoms of autism.

Comments
Secretin products are available in the forms of purified porcine secretin and synthetic human secretin (6136).

SELENIUM

Also Known As
L-Selenomethionine, Selenite, Selenium Dioxide, Selenized Yeast, Selenomethionine.

Scientific Names
Selenium; Se; atomic number 34.

People Use This For
Orally, selenium is used for treating HIV/AIDS, heart disease, hypothyroidism, osteoarthritis, rheumatoid arthritis (RA), abnormal pap smears, atherosclerosis, macular degeneration, allergic rhinitis, infertility, gray hair, Osgood-Schlatter disease, Keshan disease, mood disorders, preventing cancer, and preventing miscarriage.

Safety
LIKELY SAFE ...when used orally and appropriately. Selenium is safe in amounts that do not exceed the tolerable upper intake level (UL) of 400 mcg per day (4844,7830,7831,7841,7836,9724).
LIKELY UNSAFE ...when used orally in excessive doses. Doses above 400 mcg may cause significant toxicity (4844,7825).
CHILDREN: LIKELY SAFE ...when used orally and appropriately. Selenium is safe when used in doses below the tolerable upper intake level (UL) of 45 mcg per day for infants up to age 6 months, 60 mcg per day for infants 7 to 12 months, 90 mcg per day for children 1 to 3 years, 150 mcg per day for children 4 to 8 years, 280 mcg per day for children 9 to 13 years, and 400 mcg per day for children age 14 years and older (4844). POSSIBLY SAFE ...when used via a nasogastric tube in premature infants (7835,9764).
PREGNANCY: LIKELY SAFE ...when used orally and appropriately. Selenium is safe in amounts that do not exceed the tolerable upper intake level (UL) of 400 mcg per day (4844). LIKELY UNSAFE ...when used orally in excessive doses. Doses above 400 mcg may cause significant toxicity (4844).
LACTATION: LIKELY SAFE ...when used orally and appropriately. Selenium is safe in amounts that do not exceed the tolerable upper intake level (UL) of 400 mcg per day (4844). LIKELY UNSAFE ...when used orally in excessive doses. Doses above 400 mcg may cause significant toxicity (4844,7838).

Effectiveness
POSSIBLY EFFECTIVE

Prostate cancer. Increased intake of dietary selenium seems to reduce the risk of prostate cancer, as measured by selenium levels in serum, plasma, and toenails (2667,8734,8735,8736). Taking selenized yeast supplements might also help decrease the risk of prostate cancer. Selenized yeast is brewer's yeast that has been grown in selenium rich broth and then used as a selenium supplement (7831). The greatest benefit is obtained in patients who have a selenium deficiency before supplementation (9722). There is also some evidence that adequate dietary vitamin E intake might be important along with adequate selenium for prevention of prostate cancer (10263).

POSSIBLY INEFFECTIVE

Cardiovascular disease. In people with coronary heart disease, selenium 100 mcg daily in combination with beta-carotene and vitamin C and vitamin E doesn't seem to protect against cardiovascular disease progression and related events such as myocardial infarction (MI). There is some evidence that this antioxidant combination might lower high-density lipoprotein 2 (HDL2), which is considered to be the most cardioprotective component of HDL (7388).

Lung cancer. Epidemiologic studies suggest no decrease in the risk of lung cancer as dietary selenium increases, although a small benefit may occur in people that are selenium deficient (9722,9798).

Rheumatoid arthritis (RA). Selenized yeast, providing 200 micrograms daily does not seem to improve objective measures of RA. There might be small improvements in quality of life measures (9763).

Skin cancer. Taking selenium orally 200 mcg daily does not seem to protect against the development of basal cell carcinoma (2664,10687). In addition, daily selenium supplementation may increase the risk of squamous cell carcinoma and total nonmelanoma skin cancer (10687).

INSUFFICIENT RELIABLE EVIDENCE to RATE

Arsenic poisoning. Selenized yeast seems to decrease the concentration of arsenic in Chinese people environmentally exposed to high concentrations of arsenic; however, the effect on clinical signs of arsenic toxicity is not known (7831).

Colorectal cancer. Evidence is conflicting about the effect of selenium on colorectal cancer (2664,2667,9722).

Human immunodeficiency virus (HIV). Preliminary evidence suggests that L-selenomethionine, an organic form of selenium, has no effect on clinical outcome in patients infected with HIV (7830).

Hypothyroidism. In areas of the world that are deficient in iodine, selenium can decrease the concentration of thyroid peroxidase autoantibodies; however, the effect on hypothyroidism is not clear (9797).

Stroke and cancer mortality. There is some evidence that selenized yeast 50 mcg in combination with beta-carotene 15 mg and vitamin E (alpha tocopherol) 60 mg used daily might decrease stroke mortality, cancer mortality, and total mortality (2673).

More evidence is needed to rate selenium for these uses.

Mechanism of Action

Selenium is a metallic substance that is available in a variety of chemical compounds. Often selenium is attached to an organic molecule as in selenocysteine, selenomethionine, and kappa-selenocageenan. In broccoli, garlic, onions, and other selenium-accumulating plants it is found as Se-methylselenocysteine or selenocysathionine (7833,7836). In dietary supplements selenium is commonly provided as selenomethionine or in a selenite or selenate salt form (7841). Often selenium is given as selenized yeast, which is common brewer's yeast that has been grown in selenium-rich media (7838). After ingestion as a selenate salt, selenite salt, or as one of the organic forms, selenium must be reduced or metabolized to form hydrogen selenide, an important intermediary form. Selenide is essential for the activity of selenoproteins, such as the glutathione peroxidase enzyme (GSH-Px). The primary organic forms of selenium are the amino acid-based selenocysteine and selenomethionine. Selenomethionine is incorporated directly into proteins, because RNA does not differentiate it from methionine (7832,9718). Selenomethionine serves as a storage form, releasing selenium as the proteins containing it are catabolized (7834,9718). Although the various organic forms of selenium appear to have similar bioavailability after oral consumption (6485), there are substantial differences in the disposition and biologic action of these various forms (7832,7833). Selenomethionine results in high concentrations of selenium in hair and urine, but it does not have the biologic activity of other selenium compounds (7832,7833). Administration of selenomethionine results in plasma selenium concentrations twice as high as equivalent doses of the selenate form (9762). Of the inorganic salt forms, the bioavailability of the selenate salt is 2 to 3 times higher than the selenite salt, but selenate is more rapidly metabolized. The difference in bioavailability doesn't seem to be significant nutritionally (9717,9761).

The dietary content of selenium required for health falls into a narrow range. Diets containing less than 0.1 mcg/gram of food often result in deficiency, whereas diets containing more than 1 mcg/gram of food may cause toxicity. Consumption of plants that are selenium accumulators, such as Astragalus species (loco weed), can cause significant selenium toxicity if they are grown in selenium-rich soil (7832). Approximately 40 to 100 mcg/day of dietary selenium is needed to maintain a selenium plasma concentration of 70 to 135 nanograms/mL. This is the concentration range needed for maximal activity of selenium dependent enzymes (1665,9718). The content of selenium in the diet is primarily dependent upon the concentration of selenium in the soil. Canada, Japan, Norway, and the United States are the only four countries in the world where the dietary content of selenium is adequate (9718). Dietary selenium is superior to supplements in maintaining adequate plasma concentrations (9721).

At plasma concentrations below 1000 mcg/L, selenium activates glutathione peroxidase (GSH-Px), which reduces oxidative stress by handling free radicals and hydrogen peroxide. At concentrations above 2000 mcg/L selenium paradoxically increases cellular oxidation by promoting the formation of reactive oxygen species (ROS), such as hydroxyl free radicals and superoxide. At higher concentrations selenium also promotes the intracellular formation of nitric oxide, which is converted to toxic nitrous oxide (2664,7825,7826,7827,7828,7829). To reduce the effect of ROS formation, selenium is often given with other antioxidants, such as vitamin E or vitamin C. However, vitamin E might actually increase the cytotoxic effects of high selenium levels, whereas vitamin C appears to reduce the cytotoxicity of selenium (7841). Selenium plays a major role in the synthesis and metabolism of thyroid hormones. The thyroid gland has a higher concentration of selenium than any other organ in the body. Iodothyronine dehydrogenase is at least partially dependent upon selenium for its activity (1665,9724). A deficiency of selenium can exacerbate hypothyroidism in iodine deficiency (1664,9724). In addition, selenium may be able to prevent alterations in thyroid hormone levels that are sometimes observed in patients after trauma (9725). Selenium appears to increase cancer cell death by causing apoptosis and by reducing the formation of ROS. The magnitude of the anticancer effects varies substantially among selenium compounds. Selenite has a high potency to cause apoptosis and selenocystamine is lower. Kappa-selenocageenan also has the ability to induce apoptosis. Selenomethionine has almost no effect on apoptosis (7827,7828). Se-methylselenocysteine found in broccoli, garlic, and onions may be better than supplemental selenite in preventing colonic cancer (7833). Epidemiological evidence indicates that lower blood selenium concentrations increases the likelihood of prostate cancer (8734,8735,8736) and colorectal cancer (9726). However, supplementing the diet with selenium does not appear to reduce the risk for colorectal cancer (9722). However, early data suggests that there may be more effective and less toxic forms of organic selenium, for preventing colorectal cancer, than those used previously (9737). Preliminary data suggests that supplementing the diet with selenium can reduce the risk for developing breast cancer, but no benefit has been shown in humans (9690,9723). The urinary excretion of selenium is increased during cervical cancer, but the clinical significance of this observation is not known (9727). Selenium improves immunologic function by increasing the activity of interleukin-2 (IL-2) and promoting the normal growth and development of T helper cells. These actions may be important in treating acquired immunodeficiency syndrome (AIDS) because selenium deficiency is common in this condition (7829). There is preliminary experimental evidence selenium inhibits reverse transcriptase and replication of human immunodeficiency virus (HIV). However, there is also some evidence that selenium may improve subjective feelings of well-being in patients infected with HIV, but it does not appear to affect overall outcomes (3341,7830,9719). Selenium deficiency is associated with increased viral shedding in women infected with HIV. Supplementing the diet of these women with selenium may decrease the transmission of AIDS (9720). In cardiovascular disease, selenium may prevent the oxidative modification of low-density lipoproteins (LDLs). Selenium deficiency has been implicated in the etiology of Keshan disease, an endemic cardiomyopathy observed in China, and congestive cardiomyopathy in people on artificial nutrition (2676,3341). In children with severe deficiency, Keshan disease may also occur (9718). Selenium is used for arthritis due to its antioxidant effects. It may reduce inflammation by reducing the cellular concentration of reactive oxygen species (ROS) (2662). There is also evidence that suggests that deficiency of selenium may increase inflammatory lung damage caused during influenza virus infection (9728). In liver transplant, ROS are generated when the organ is reperfused with blood following a period of extended warm ischemia. Preliminary evidence suggests that the antioxidant action of selenium can decrease liver damage and improve microcirculation (7839). Selenium may act as part of a defense mechanism, decreasing oxidative stress in peptic ulcer disease (7840). Selenium also might protect patients infected with hepatitis B or C from developing liver cancer (3341). Selenium is required for testosterone biosynthesis and the formation and development of sperm. Low selenium levels have been linked to decreased male fertility. Low selenium levels also appear to be associated with first trimester or recurrent miscarriages, suggesting selenium possibly prevents early pregnancy loss (3341). During pregnancy, the concentration of selenium in blood usually increases. Supplementing the diet with low doses of iron seems to prevent this increase (10217). At the start of breast feeding, the concentration of selenium in blood increases, but the concentration in milk decreases as breast feeding continues (1239). Low levels of selenium appear to be associated with a greater incidence of depression, anxiety, confusion, and hostility. Some researchers think a high dietary or supplemental intake of selenium might improve mood (3341). With severe deficiency, Kaschin-Beck disease, a cartilage abnormality (chondrodystrophy) might occur (9718).

Adverse Reactions

Orally, selenium can cause symptoms of acute toxicity including nausea, vomiting, nail changes, fatigue, irritability, and weight loss (7834). At doses above the tolerable upper intake level (UL) of 400 mcg per day for adults, hair and nail brittleness and loss occur (4844). Chronic toxicity resembles arsenic toxicity, with symptoms including hair loss, white horizontal streaking on fingernails, paronychia, fatigue, irritability, hyperreflexia, nausea, vomiting, garlic odor on breath, and a metallic taste. Muscle tenderness, tremor, lightheadedness, and facial flushing are also observed in selenium poisoning (4844). Selenium can cause thrombocytopenia and moderate hepatorenal dysfunction (4844). Blood selenium levels can be used to assess the degree of toxicity. Levels below 1000 mcg/L are not usually associated with serious damage, whereas levels above 2000 mcg/L are predictive of serious damage (4844,7825). Selenium ingestion has been linked to increased incidence of skin cancer, but research is conflicting. Accidental introduction of inorganic selenium (selenite) in a municipal water supply for 11 years has been associated with a quadruple risk of developing melanoma (3343). However, other research suggests higher plasma selenium levels have no effect on skin cancer risk (11114). Selenium supplementation, 200 mcg per day, has been studied as a prophylactic measure in patients with a history of skin cancer. Selenium supplementation for 6 years seems to have no effect on skin cancer risk (2664). But longer-term supplementation for up to 13 years might slightly increase the risk of squamous cell carcinoma and nonmelanoma skin cancer (10687). More research is needed to establish the effect of long-term selenium supplementation on skin cancer recurrence.

Diets that are high in selenium may cause decreased sperm motility. The impact on male fertility is not known (9729).

Interactions with Herbs & Other Dietary Supplements

IRON: Supplementing the diet with iron, 18 mg daily, may prevent the increased selenium serum concentration that occurs during pregnancy (10217).

Interactions with Drugs

HMG-CoA REDUCTASE INHIBITORS ("Statins"): Concomitant use of selenium in combination with beta-carotene and vitamins C and E appears to decrease the effectiveness of the combination of simvastatin (Zocor) and niacin (7388). Theoretically, selenium could reduce the effectiveness of other HMG-CoA reductase inhibitors such as atorvastatin (Lipitor), fluvastatin (Lescol), lovastatin (Mevacor), and pravastatin (Pravachol).

NIACIN: Concomitant use of selenium in combination with beta-carotene, vitamin C, and vitamin E appears to decrease the effectiveness of the combination of niacin and simvastatin (Zocor) (7388).

Interactions with Foods

None known.

Interactions with Lab Tests

BLOOD SELENIUM ASSAYS: Avoid powdered gloves when drawing blood for selenium and other trace element assays due to the potential for sample contamination (2663).
CREATININE KINASE: Selenium toxicity can elevate serum creatinine kinase levels (17).
ELECTROCARDIOGRAM (ECG): Selenium toxicity can elevate the ST segment and cause T-wave changes characteristic of myocardial infarction (MI) (4844).
HIGH-DENSITY LIPOPROTEIN 2 (HDL2): Selenium in combination with beta-carotene, vitamin C, and vitamin E seems to lower HDL2 levels (7388).
SPERM MOTILITY: Diets that are high in selenium may cause a decrease in sperm motility. The impact on male fertility is not known (9729).

Interactions with Diseases or Conditions

HEMODIALYSIS: Blood selenium levels may be low in patients undergoing hemodialysis. Selenium levels may increase somewhat after hemodialysis, but concentrations remain below normal (1805).
HYPOTHYROIDISM: Selenium deficiency can worsen iodine-deficient hypothyroidism (1664,9724).
IMPAIRED MALE FERTILITY: A diet that is high in selenium may decrease the motility of sperm (9729). This effect could theoretically decrease male fertility.
SKIN CANCER: Long-term use of selenium supplements might slightly increase the risk of skin cancer recurrence, but this is controversial (10687). Tell patients with a history of skin cancer that selenium supplements don't protect against skin cancer recurrence. Until more is known about the possible increase in skin cancer risk, patients with a history of skin cancer should avoid long-term use of selenium supplements.

Dosage and Administration

ORAL: For cancer prevention or to reduce the risk of cancer mortality, 200 mcg of selenium supplied as a 0.5 gram high-selenium brewer's yeast tablet taken daily has been used (2664,2667). In humans, 30 mcg per day is considered necessary to prevent Keshan disease, which is associated with selenium deficiency (2671). For patients infected with human immunodeficiency virus (HIV), 250 mcg of L-selenomethionine daily has been used for 12 months (7830). For people environmentally exposed to arsenic, 100 to 200 mcg of selenized yeast daily has been used for 14 months (7831). To treat selenium deficiency in premature infants, 5 mcg per day of selenized yeast has been given by a nasogastric tube (9764).
The daily recommended dietary allowances (RDAs) of selenium are: Children 1-3 years, 20 mcg; Children 4-8 years, 30 mcg; Children 9-13 years, 40 mcg; People over 13 years, 55 mcg; Pregnant women, 60 mcg; and Lactating women, 70 mcg (3341,4844). Due to the demands of the fetus on the mother, the dietary need for selenium increases during pregnancy (7837).
The RDA for infants has not been determined. For infants up to 6 months old, 2.1 mcg/kg is adequate intake (AI). The AI for infants 7-12 months is 2.2 mcg/kg per day (4844).
The tolerable upper limit for adults is 400 mcg per day for adults and adolescents 14 years and older. The tolerable upper intake level (UL) for infants up to age 6 months is 45 mcg per day; for infants 7 to 12 months, 60 mcg per day; for children 1 to 3 years, 90 mcg per day; for children 4 to 8 years, 150 mcg per day; for children 9 to 13 years, 280 mcg per day (4844,7830,7831,7835,7841).

Comments

Most of the selenium in the body is obtained via the diet. The amount of selenium in food depends on where it is grown or raised. Crab, liver, fish, poultry, and wheat are generally good selenium sources; however, natural selenium levels in the soil are highly variable throughout the world (2671,3341,7834,9718). In the US, the Eastern Coastal Plain, and the Pacific Northwest have the lowest selenium levels, and people in these regions naturally ingest about 60 to 90 mcg per day, which is adequate (2671,9718). The average daily intake in the US is 125 mcg, ranging from 60 to 200 mcg (2671,7834,9718).

SELF-HEAL

Also Known As

All-Heal, Blue Curls, Brownwort, Carpenter's Herb, Carpenter's Weed, Heal-All, Heart of the Earth, Hercules Woundwort, Hock-Heal, Prunella, Self Heal, Sicklewort, Siclewort, Slough-Heal, Woundwort.
CAUTION: See other listing for Sanicle.

Scientific Names

Prunella vulgaris.
Family: Labiatae/Lamiaceae.

People Use This For
Orally, self-heal is used for inflammatory bowel disease (Crohn's disease and ulcerative colitis), HIV/AIDS, fever, headache, colic, vertigo, liver disease, spasm, diarrhea, gastroenteritis, as an antiseptic, expectorant, and astringent. It is also used for mouth and throat ulcers, sore throat, and internal hemorrhaging.
Topically, self-heal is used for leukorrhea, gynecological disorders, wounds and bruises.

Safety
POSSIBLY SAFE ...when used orally (12).
PREGNANCY AND LACTATION: Insufficient reliable information available; avoid using.

Effectiveness
There is insufficient reliable information available about the effectiveness of self-heal.

Mechanism of Action
Self-heal contains entacyclic triterpenes, tannins, caffeic and rosmarinic acids, thiamine, and vitamins C and K. It has antioxidant and astringent properties (7122). Laboratory evidence suggests that an aqueous extract of self-heal has activity against HIV and might work synergistically with zidovudine (AZT, Retrovir) and didanosine (ddI, Videx) (7234,7286).

Adverse Reactions
None reported.

Interactions with Herbs & Other Dietary Supplements
None known.

Interactions with Drugs
None known.

Interactions with Foods
None known.

Interactions with Lab Tests
None known.

Interactions with Diseases or Conditions
None known.

Dosage and Administration
ORAL: One cup of tea is commonly used. The tea is prepared by simmering one teaspoon of the dried plant in 150 mL of boiling water for 10-15 minutes and straining. For a gargle, the tea is simmered for 9 minutes (18).

Comments
Sanicle is also less commonly known as self-heal. Be careful not to confuse these two plants.

SENEGA

Also Known As
Chinese Senega, Flax, Klapperschlangen, Milkwort, Mountain Polygala, Polygala glomerata, Polygala reinii, Polygalae radix, Rattlesnake Root, Senaga Snakeroot, Seneca, Seneca Snakeroot, Senega, Senega Snakeroot, Seneka, Snake Root.
CAUTION: See separate listings for Asarabacca and Bitter Milkwort.

Scientific Names
Polygala japonica; Polygala senega; Polygala tenuifolia.
Family: Polygalaceae.

People Use This For
Orally, senega is used for respiratory tract mucous membrane inflammation, bronchial asthma, chronic bronchitis, emphysema, rattlesnake bite, for inducing sweating, increasing saliva, as an expectorant, and an emetic.
Topically, senega is used as a gargle for pharyngitis.

Safety

POSSIBLY SAFE ...when used orally and appropriately short-term (12).
LIKELY UNSAFE ...when used orally, long-term. Prolonged use can cause gastrointestinal (GI) irritation (12). There is insufficient reliable information available about the safety of the topical use of senega.
PREGNANCY: LIKELY UNSAFE ...when used orally; senega appears to have uterine and menstrual flow stimulant effects (12,19). There is insufficient reliable information available about the safety of the topical use of senega during pregnancy.
LACTATION: Insufficient reliable information available; avoid using.

Effectiveness

There is insufficient reliable information available about the effectiveness of senega.

Mechanism of Action

The applicable part of senega is the root. Senega root contains salicylic acid, methyl salicylate, and a saponin mixture referred to as senegin (4). People claim senega has expectorant and emetic activity, and that it can stimulate sweating and saliva (2,4,515). The active expectorant principles are triterpenoid saponins (515). Researchers think the saponins irritate the gastrointestinal (GI) tract mucosa and cause reflex secretion of mucous in the bronchioles (515). A French patent based on human studies states that a triterpenic acid extract has anti-inflammatory activity, and is effective against graft rejection, eczema, psoriasis, and multiple sclerosis (4).

Adverse Reactions

Orally, prolonged use of senega can cause gastrointestinal (GI) irritation (2). Large amounts can cause diarrhea, dizziness (8), queasiness (18), vomiting, and purging (4).

Interactions with Herbs & Other Dietary Supplements

None known.

Interactions with Drugs

None known.

Interactions with Foods

None known.

Interactions with Lab Tests

None known.

Interactions with Diseases or Conditions

FEVER: Contraindicated due to CNS depressant effects (19).
GASTROINTESTINAL (GI) CONDITIONS: Senega is contraindicated in individuals with gastrointestinal (GI) conditions including inflammation and gastritis or gastric ulcers (4,12) due to local stimulant activity and intestinal irritant effects (19).

Dosage and Administration

ORAL: A typical dose is 0.5-1 grams dried root or 1 cup of tea three times daily. To make tea, steep 0.5-1 grams dried root in 150 mL boiling water 5-10 minutes, and strain (4).
TOPICAL: No typical dosage.

Comments

Avoid confusion with Polygala sibirica, also referred to as polygala.

SENNA

Also Known As

Alexandrian Senna, Alexandrinische Senna, Casse, Indian Senna, Khartoum Senna, Sena Alejandrina, Séné d'Egypte, Sennae folium, Sennae fructus, Sennae fructus acutifoliae, Sennae fructus angustifolia, Tinnevelly Senna, True Senna.

Scientific Names

Senna alexandrina, synonyms Cassia acutifolia, Cassia angustifolia, Cassia senna, Cassia lanceolata.
Family: Fabaceae/Leguminosae

People Use This For

Orally, senna used as a laxative for constipation, after anorectal surgery, for hemorrhoids, evacuating the GI tract to facilitate diagnostic tests, evacuation relief in individuals with anal fissures, and in "slimming" and "cleansing" teas.

Safety

LIKELY SAFE ...when used orally and appropriately short-term (12,272).
POSSIBLY UNSAFE ...when used orally for longer than one to two weeks (12). Frequent use causes the colon to function poorly, creating laxative dependence (6,272).
CHILDREN: LIKELY SAFE ...when the standardized nonprescription products are used orally and appropriately (272). If senna is used to treat constipation, only standardized products should be used.
PREGNANCY: POSSIBLY UNSAFE ...when used orally. Constipation in pregnancy should not be self-medicated (6,12).
LACTATION: POSSIBLY UNSAFE ...when used orally. Anthraquinone constituents cross into breast milk and can cause loose stools in some breast-fed infants (272).

Effectiveness

LIKELY EFFECTIVE

Constipation. Taking senna orally is effective as a laxative for reducing constipation (6).

There is insufficient reliable information available about the effectiveness of senna for its other uses.

Mechanism of Action

The applicable parts of senna are the leaf and fruit. Senna leaf and fruit are stimulant laxatives (272). The cathartic properties of the leaf are greater than the fruit (4). Senna contains anthraquinones including dianthrone that consists mostly of sennosides A and B and minor amounts of sennosides C and D (6,11). Senna also contains small amounts of free anthraquinones. The dianthrone glycosides are not present in the fresh leaf, but appear to form during the drying process (11). Although it is not known exactly how the anthraquinone laxatives work, the cathartic action is limited primarily to the colon (272). Sennosides irritate the lining of the large intestine, causing contraction. Sennosides A and B also seem to induce fluid secretion in the colon. Prostaglandins might be involved in the laxative effect (6). Anthraquinone laxatives produce an effect 8-12 hours after administration, though sometimes up to 24 hours can be required (272). Anthroid laxative use is not associated with an increased risk of developing colorectal adenoma or carcinoma (6138).

Adverse Reactions

Orally, senna can cause abdominal discomfort, colic, and cramps (4). Excessive use or abuse is associated with potassium depletion, finger clubbing, development of cachexia, decreased serum globulin concentrations, heart function disorders, muscular weakness, osteomalacia, arthropathy, hepatitis, coma, neuropathy, asthma, allergy symptoms, and rhinoconjunctivitis (4,6). Chronic use can cause pseudomelanosis coli (pigment spots in intestinal mucosa) which is harmless, usually reverses with discontinuation, and is not associated with an increased risk of developing colorectal adenoma or carcinoma (6138). Prolonged senna use can cause "laxative-dependency syndrome" characterized by poor gastric motility, non-functioning colon, and laxative-induced diarrhea (4,6). Occupational exposure has been linked to asthma and allergy symptoms, including rhinoconjunctivitis (6).

Interactions with Herbs & Other Dietary Supplements

HORSETAIL/LICORICE: Theoretically, concomitant use with horsetail plant or licorice rhizome increases the risk of potassium depletion (19).
STIMULANT LAXATIVE HERBS: Theoretically, concomitant use with other stimulant laxative herbs increases the risk of potassium depletion (19). Stimulant laxative herbs include aloe dried leaf sap, wild cucumber fruit (Ecballium elaterium), blue flag rhizome, alder buckthorn, European buckthorn, butternut bark, cascara bark, castor oil, colocynth fruit pulp, gamboge bark exudate, jalap root, black root, manna bark exudate, podophyllum root, rhubarb root, and yellow dock root.

Interactions with Drugs

DIGOXIN (Lanoxin): Theoretically, overuse/abuse of this product increases the risk of adverse effects of cardiac glycoside drugs.
DIURETIC DRUGS: Overuse of senna might compound diuretic-induced potassium loss (19). There is some concern that people taking senna along with potassium depleting diuretics might have an increased risk for hypokalemia. Initiation of potassium supplementation or an increase in potassium supplement dose may be necessary for some patients. Some diuretics that can deplete potassium include chlorothiazide (Diuril), chlorthalidone (Thalitone), furosemide (Lasix), and hydrochlorothiazide (HCTZ, HydroDIURIL, Microzide), and others.

Interactions with Foods

None known.

Interactions with Lab Tests

COLORIMETRIC TESTS: Senna can discolor urine (pink, red, purple, orange, rust), interfering with diagnostic tests that depend on a color change, due to its anthraquinone content (1,4,12,275).
POTASSIUM: Excessive use of senna can cause potassium depletion, reducing serum potassium concentrations and test results (1,4,12,19).

Interactions with Diseases or Conditions

ELECTROLYTE DISTURBANCES, POTASSIUM DEFICIENCY: Overuse of senna can exacerbate these conditions (2).
FLUID DEPLETION: Senna is contraindicated in individuals with dehydration, diarrhea, or loose stools. It can exacerbate these conditions.
GASTROINTESTINAL (GI) CONDITIONS: Senna is contraindicated in people with abdominal pain, intestinal obstruction, and acute intestinal inflammation including Crohn's disease, ulcerative colitis, appendicitis, stomach inflammation, anal prolapse, hemorrhoids, or undiagnosed abdominal pain (4,19).
HEART DISEASE: Senna can cause electrolyte disturbances and exacerbate these conditions (2).

Dosage and Administration

ORAL: A typical dose is 15-30 mg hydroxyanthracene derivatives daily, calculated as sennoside B (1,2). Senna leaf is used as a tea, one cup in the morning and/or at bedtime. To make tea, steep 0.5-2 grams finely chopped leaf in warm but not boiling water for 10 minutes, and strain (8). Alternatively, a cold water tea might have less adverse GI effects. To make cold water tea, steep 0.5-2 grams finely chopped leaf in cold water for 10-12 hours, and strain (8). Liquid leaf extract (1:1 in 25% alcohol), 0.5-2.0 mL (frequency unspecified) (4). One cup of fruit tea is taken in the morning and/or at bedtime. To make tea, steep 1/2 flat teaspoon of senna fruit in 150 mL warm, but not boiling water, for ten minutes, and strain (8). Individualize senna dosing to the smallest amount necessary to maintain a soft stool (2). Senna leaf should not be used continuously for more than one to two weeks (2). Use of standardized OTC senna leaf preparations reduces variability and improves dosing control (4,515).

Comments

Because senna fruit is gentler than senna leaf, the American Herbal Products Association only warns against long-term use for senna leaf, not senna fruit (12). The AHPA recommends that senna leaf products be labeled "Do not use this product if you have abdominal pain or diarrhea. Consult a healthcare provider prior to use if you are pregnant or nursing. Discontinue use in the event of diarrhea or watery stools. Do not exceed recommended dose. Not for long-term use." (12).

SHARK CARTILAGE

Also Known As

AE-941, MSI-1256F, Neovastat, Shark Cartilage Extract, Shark Cartilage Powder.
CAUTION: See separate listings for Bovine Cartilage, Chondroitin, and Squalamine.

Scientific Names

Squalus acanthias.

People Use This For

Orally, shark cartilage is used for preventing and treating cancer, arthritis, psoriasis, and wound healing. It is also used for enteritis, diabetic retinopathy, and cutaneous Kaposi Sarcoma.
Topically, shark cartilage is used for arthritis and psoriasis.
Rectally, shark cartilage is used for cancer.

Safety

POSSIBLY SAFE ...when used orally and appropriately. Shark cartilage has been safely used for up to 20 weeks (2015,4938,6709,6716,6717) in multiple trials and for up to 40 months in a phase II trial (10900). ...when used topically and appropriately short term. Shark cartilage in combination with glucosamine, chondroitin, and camphor appears to be safe when applied topically on an as-needed basis for up to eight weeks (10327).
There is insufficient reliable information available about the safety of shark cartilage for its other uses.
PREGNANCY AND LACTATION: Insufficient reliable information available; avoid using.

Effectiveness

EFFECTIVE

Renal cell carcinoma. Taking AE-941 orally seems to increase survival in patients with advanced renal cell carcinoma (4894,10900). AE-941 (Neovastat), a derivative of shark cartilage, has FDA orphan drug status for renal cell carcinoma (10899).

POSSIBLY INEFFECTIVE

Cancer. Taking shark cartilage orally appears to offer no benefit in people with advanced, previously treated cancer, including breast cancer, colorectal cancer, lung cancer, prostate cancer, and brain cancer; and non-Hodgkin's lymphoma (2015,6716,6717). However, studies of shark cartilage in people with less advanced cancer or in combination with other cancer treatments have not been published.

INSUFFICIENT RELIABLE EVIDENCE to RATE

Kaposi sarcoma. There is anecdotal evidence that shark cartilage might be beneficial for cutaneous Kaposi sarcoma and possibly decrease Kaposi sarcoma lesions and increase histological regression (4938).

Osteoarthritis. A topical preparation of shark cartilage in combination with chondroitin sulfate, glucosamine sulfate, and camphor reportedly reduces arthritis symptoms. However, any symptom relief is most likely due to the counterirritant effect of camphor and not the other ingredients (10327). There's no research showing that shark cartilage is absorbed topically. Don't recommend topical shark cartilage products.

Plaque psoriasis. Preliminary clinical evidence suggests that AE-941 taken orally might improve appearance and decrease itching of plaque psoriasis (10399).

More evidence is needed to rate shark cartilage for these uses.

Mechanism of Action

Shark cartilage is found in the skeletal structure of sharks. It is made up of about 40% proteins, 5-20% glycosaminoglycans, and calcium salts. Chondroitin, a glycosaminoglycan in cartilage, might be an active constituent (6714).

The use of shark cartilage attracted popular attention after some publications suggested that sharks don't get cancer and implied that shark cartilage could prevent cancer in humans (2014,6722). Since then renal cell carcinoma, lymphoma, and cartilage tumors have been identified in sharks (6714). However, there is still some preliminary evidence that shark cartilage might have some potential as an anticancer agent.

Shark cartilage might inhibit angiogenesis and prevent the new vessel growth required for solid tumor proliferation (2013). There is preliminary clinical evidence that shark cartilage given orally inhibits wound angiogenesis (6709). Topical shark cartilage also seems to inhibit local angiogenic activity. Because macrophages and T lymphocytes found at the sites of psoriasis lesions can produce angiogenic activity, shark cartilage might have potential as a treatment for psoriasis (4893). Preliminary laboratory research suggests that shark cartilage might also have antimutagenic, antioxidant, anti-inflammatory, and analgesic activity (6723,6724,6725).

AE-941 (Neovastat) is one of the components of shark cartilage that is well studied. It is a naturally occurring component of cartilage made up of a mixture of proteins with a molecular weight less than 500 kilodaltons. AE-941 inhibits angiogenesis, the outgrowth of new capillaries from pre-existing blood vessels. Angiogenesis is increased in highly vascularized cancers, suggesting possible usefulness of AE-941in treatment of some malignancies. As an antiangiogenic agent, it interferes with binding of cytokines and other enzymes at their receptor sites. AE-941 competes for binding sites with fibroblast growth factor, tumor necrosis factor-alpha, vascular endothelial growth factor, and other cytokines. It also inhibits a matrix metalloproteinase (MMP), an enzyme that facilitates angiogenesis (10397,10398). In addition, AE-941 induces apoptosis of endothelial cells involved with growth of blood vessels. This action is mediated by activation of caspases, which are key mediators of programmed cell death in many types of cells. AE-941 appears to activate caspase-1 and caspase-2 that are specific mediators of apoptosis in blood vessel endothelial cells (10396).

Adverse Reactions

Orally, shark cartilage can cause taste disturbances, nausea, vomiting, dyspepsia, constipation, hypotension, dizziness, hyperglycemia, hypoglycemia, hypercalcemia, altered consciousness, decreased motor strength, decreased sensation, erythema, peripheral edema, generalized weakness, fatigue, and decreased performance (2014,2015,6716,10900). It might also cause signs of acute hepatitis, including low-grade fever, jaundice, yellowing of eyes, right upper quadrant tenderness, and elevated liver enzymes (2012). Some shark cartilage products have an offensive odor and taste (2014).

Interactions with Herbs & Other Dietary Supplements

CALCIUM: Shark cartilage might cause hypercalcemia (2015,6716). Theoretically, concomitant use with supplemental calcium might exacerbate this adverse effect.

Interactions with Drugs

None known.

Interactions with Foods

FRUIT JUICE: Acidic fruit juice such as orange, apple, grape, or tomato, can decrease potency of shark cartilage over time. If shark cartilage is added to a fruit juice, it should be mixed immediately prior to use (2014).

Interactions with Lab Tests

CALCIUM: Shark cartilage might increase serum calcium levels and test results (2015,6716).

Interactions with Diseases or Conditions
HYPERCALCEMIA: Shark cartilage is reported to cause hypercalcemia (2015,6716) and might exacerbate this condition; avoid using.

Dosage and Administration
ORAL: For refractory metastatic renal cell carcinoma, a specific water-soluble shark cartilage extract, AE-941 (Neovastat), 60-240 mL per day has been used (4894,10900). For the treatment of solid tumors, 30 to 240 mL daily has been used (10397). For the treatment of plaque psoriasis, 30 to 240 mL per day has been used for up to 12 weeks (10399). For cutaneous Kaposi Sarcoma, shark cartilage 3750 to 4500 mg per day has been used (4938). Commercial products typically suggest doses ranging from 500 mg to 4.5 grams given in 2-6 divided doses daily (6002).

Comments
Shark cartilage is typically obtained from sharks caught in the Pacific Ocean. The anti-tumor effects of numerous shark cartilage derivatives and extracts, including squalamine lactate, AE-941, and U-995, are currently being investigated in several preclinical and phase I to III clinical trials (6718,6719,6720,6721,6726,6727).

SHARK LIVER OIL

Also Known As
Basking Shark Liver Oil, Deep Sea Shark Liver Oil, Dog Fish Liver Oil.
CAUTION: See separate listings for Cod Liver Oil, Fish Oils, Liver Extract, Shark Cartilage, and Squalamine.

Scientific Names
Cetorhinus maximus; Centroporus squamosus; Squalus acanthias.

People Use This For
Orally, shark liver oil is used as an adjunctive treatment for leukemia and other cancers, to prevent radiation illness from cancer X-ray therapy, to prevent the common cold and flu, and for general immunostimulation. It is also used orally for increasing leukocyte and thrombocyte counts during chemotherapy.
Topically, shark liver oil is used for skin conditions, skin cancer, and as a topical protectant.

Safety
There is insufficient reliable information available about the safety of shark liver oil.
Pregnancy and Lactation: Insufficient reliable information available; avoid using.

Effectiveness
There is insufficient reliable information available about the effectiveness of shark liver oil.

Mechanism of Action
Shark liver oil is a major source of squalene and alkylglycerols. Shark liver oil is classified as a topical protectant (2551). Alkoxyglycerol derived from shark liver oil may decrease irradiation damage in patients undergoing treatment of uterine cancer (2552). It is thought that the radioprotective properties of alkoxyglycerol may stem from its incorporation into a pool of platelet-activating factors, and resulting in biosynthesis (2550). Alkoxyglycerol may also increase leukocyte and thrombocyte counts within specific dose ranges (2552). Shark liver oil has been shown in animals to have antiangiogenesis properties in certain cancers, including cutaneous lesions, kidney cancer and urinary bladder cancer including L-1 syngeneic (2549). However, other findings are contradictory (2552).

Adverse Reactions
Both shark liver oil and the constituent squalene have been associated with cases of aspiration and subsequent lipoid pneumonia (2546,2547,2548).

Interactions with Herbs & Other Dietary Supplements
None known.

Interactions with Drugs
None known.

Interactions with Foods
None known.

Interactions with Lab Tests
None known.

Interactions with Diseases or Conditions
None known.

Dosage and Administration
No typical dosage.

Comments
Shark liver oil is commercially derived from the livers of three species of shark: the deep sea shark (Centrophorus squamosus), the dogfish (Sqaulus acanthias), and the basking shark (Cetorhinus maximus). The liver constitutes 25% of the total shark body weight.

SHELLAC

Also Known As
Gommelaque, Lac, Lacca.

Scientific Names
Laccifer lacca (Scale insect).
Family: Coccidae.

People Use This For
In dentistry, shellac is used as a binding agent for dentures, restorations, moldings, and as a constituent in "artificial calculus" in dental schools.
In the pharmaceutical industry, shellac is used in tablet coating formulations, enteric coating, microencapsulation, matrix formulation, humidity tolerance, and for its binding ability.
In manufacturing, shellac is used as a finish for furniture, an ingredient in hair spray and in other cosmetics.

Safety
LIKELY SAFE ...when used orally in amounts commonly found in foods. Purified shellac and shellac wax have Generally Recognized As Safe (GRAS) status in the US (4912).
PREGNANCY AND LACTATION: Insufficient reliable information available.

Effectiveness
There is insufficient reliable information available about the effectiveness of shellac.

Mechanism of Action
Aleuretic acid, r-butolic acid, shellolic acid, and jalaric acid are the major constituents of shellac (6).

Adverse Reactions
There is one report of contact cheilitis associated with shellac (6).

Interactions with Herbs & Other Dietary Supplements
None known.

Interactions with Drugs
None known.

Interactions with Foods
None known.

Interactions with Lab Tests
None known.

Interactions with Diseases or Conditions
SHELLAC ALLERGY: Contraindicated.

Dosage and Administration
No typical dosage.

Comments
Shellac is derived from the secretions of the insect Laccifer. Although shellac has been used for years in pharmacy, dentistry, and as a finish for furniture, it has fallen into disfavor for some products because it ages over time (6).

SHEPHERD'S PURSE

Also Known As
Blind Weed, Bursae Pastoris Herba, Capsella, Caseweed, Cocowort, Lady's Purse, Mother's-Heart, Pepper-And-Salt, Pick-Pocket, Poor Man's Parmacettie, Rattle Pouches, Sanguinary, Shepherd's Heart, Shepherd's Purse Herb, Shepherd's Scrip, Shepherd's Sprout, Shovelweed, St. James' Weed, Toywort, Witches' Pouches.

Scientific Names
Capsella bursa-pastoris, synonym Thlaspi bursa-pastoris.
Family: Brassicaceae/Cruciferae.

People Use This For
Orally, shepherd's purse is used for headache, mild cardiac insufficiency, hypotension, nervous heart complaints, premenstrual complaints, prolonged or painful menstrual periods, vomiting blood, blood in urine, diarrhea, and acute catarrhal cystitis.
Topically, it is used for nosebleeds, superficial burns, and bleeding skin injuries.

Safety
POSSIBLY SAFE ...when preparations of the above ground parts are used orally and appropriately (4,12). ...when used topically (4).
POSSIBLY UNSAFE ...when large amounts of shepherd's purse are ingested, it can cause heart palpitations (12).
PREGNANCY: LIKELY UNSAFE ...when used orally or topically, due to possible uterine stimulation, menstrual flow stimulation, and miscarriage (12).
LACTATION: Insufficient reliable information available; avoid excessive use (4).

Effectiveness
There is insufficient reliable information available about the effectiveness of shepherd's purse.

Mechanism of Action
The applicable parts of shepherd's purse are the above ground parts. Shepherd's purse has constituents that cause positive and negative inotropic effects, and positive and negative chronotropic effects. It also seems to cause hypertensive and sometimes antihypertensive effects. It stimulates smooth muscle and increases uterine contraction. It also has abortifacient effects, and antihemorrhagic and urinary antiseptic effects (4,18). One constituent in shepherd's purse is sinigrin, which can be broken down to allyl isothiocyanate. Allyl isothiocyanate is associated with abnormal thyroid function and goiter (4).

Adverse Reactions
Orally, shepherd's purse can cause sedation, hypertension, hypotension, abnormal thyroid function, abnormal menstruation (4), palpitations (12). Toxic doses in animals have caused sedation, paralysis, respiratory depression, and death (4).

Interactions with Herbs & Other Dietary Supplements
None known.

Interactions with Drugs
CNS DEPRESSANTS: Theoretically, concomitant use with drugs with sedative properties may cause additive effects and side effects (4).
THYROID HORMONE: Theoretically, concomitant use may interfere with thyroid dysfunction therapy (4).

Interactions with Foods
None known.

Interactions with Lab Tests
None known.

Interactions with Diseases or Conditions

CARDIOVASCULAR CONDITIONS: Use with caution, shepherd's purse may interfere with therapy (4).
KIDNEY STONES: Shepherd's purse contains oxalates, use with caution in people with a history of kidney stones (12).
THYROID CONDITIONS: Use with caution, shepherd's purse may interfere with therapy (4).

Dosage and Administration

ORAL: A typical dosage is 1-4 grams dried above ground parts three times daily, or one cup tea (steep 1-4 grams dried above ground parts in 150 mL boiling water 10-15 minutes, strain) three times daily (4). The liquid extract (1:1 in 25% alcohol), is used in doses of 1-4 mL three times daily (4). Avoid excessive amounts (12).
TOPICAL: The tea is applied topically. The tea is prepared by steeping 3-5 grams dried above ground parts in 180 mL boiling water 10-15 minutes, strain (2).

SHIITAKE MUSHROOM

Also Known As

Forest Mushroom, Hua Gu, Lentinula, Pasania Fungus, Shiitake, Shitake, Snake Butter.
CAUTION: See separate listing for Lentinan.

Scientific Names

Lentinus edodes, synonyms Lenticus edodes, Lentinan edodes, Lentinula edodes, Tricholomopsis edodes.
Family: Polyporaceae.

People Use This For

Orally, shiitake mushroom is used for boosting the immune system, reducing serum cholesterol levels, as an anti-aging agent, and for prostate cancer.

Safety

LIKELY SAFE ...when consumed in food amounts (6).
POSSIBLY UNSAFE ...when used as an oral medicinal; ingestion of 4 grams shiitake powder daily for 10 weeks can cause eosinophilia (1149).
PREGNANCY AND LACTATION: Insufficient reliable information available; avoid consuming greater than food amounts.

Effectiveness

POSSIBLY INEFFECTIVE

Prostate cancer. Shiitake mushroom extract does not seem to prevent disease progression, as determined by prostate-specific antigen (PSA) levels (10451).

There is insufficient reliable information available about the effectiveness of shiitake mushroom for its other uses.

Mechanism of Action

Shiitake contains very low concentrations of lentinan (0.02%), which has antitumor effects (6). Shiitake may reduce plasma levels of free cholesterol, triglycerides, and phospholipids (1155).

Adverse Reactions

Orally, shiitake mushrooms can cause abdominal discomfort, eosinophilia (1149), "shiitake" dermatitis (1148,1152), and possibly photosensitivity (1148). There is one report of abdominal obstruction and death due to ingestion of a whole shiitake mushroom (1147). Ingestion of 4 grams shiitake powder daily for 10 weeks caused eosinophilia in 5 of 10 healthy humans (1149). An allergic contact dermatitis can be induced by shiitake hyphae (filaments) (1153). In mushroom workers, hypersensitivity pneumonitis due to shiitake spore inhalation has occurred (1150,1151).

Interactions with Herbs & Other Dietary Supplements

None known.

Interactions with Drugs

None known.

Interactions with Foods

None known.

Interactions with Lab Tests
None known.

Interactions with Diseases or Conditions
EOSINOPHILIA: Contraindicated, may exacerbate condition (1149).

Dosage and Administration
ORAL: For prostate cancer, shiitake mushroom extract 8g daily has been used for up to 6 months (10451).

SILVER LINDEN

Also Known As
Hungarian Silver Linden, Silver Lime, Tiliae tormentosae flos.
CAUTION: See separate listings for Linden Charcoal, Linden dried flower, Linden dried leaf, and Linden dried sapwood.

Scientific Names
Tilia tomentosa, synonym Tilia argentea.
Family: Tiliaceae.

Comments
At the date of publication, this product was not a common ingredient used in brand name supplements marketed to consumers. Details about this product are available at the online version of *Natural Medicines Comprehensive Database*. See www.naturaldatabase.com.

SIMARUBA

Also Known As
Bitter Damson, Dysentery Bark, Mountain Damson, Simarouba, Slave Wood, Stave Wood, Sumaruba.

Scientific Names
Simarouba amara, synonym Quassia simarouba.
Family: Simaroubaceae.

People Use This For
Orally, simaruba is used to treat diarrhea, dysentery, malaria, water-retention, fever, unspecified gastrointestinal upset, as a tonic, and to cause abortion.

Safety
There is insufficient reliable information available about the safety of simaruba.
PREGNANCY AND LACTATION: LIKELY UNSAFE ...when used orally due to apparent abortifacient effects (18,4500); avoid using.

Effectiveness
There is insufficient reliable information available about the effectiveness of simaruba.

Mechanism of Action
The applicable part of simaruba is the bark. Simaruba contains the following active ingredients: 20-27% tannins, simarubin, essential oil, and fat (18,4500). It also contains the following bitter substances: quassinoids including simarolide, simarubidin, 13,18-dehydro-glaucarubinone; 0.1-0.2% 5-hydroxy-canthin-6-one a volatile oil; and unspecified alkaloids (18).

Adverse Reactions
Orally, ingesting large amounts of simaruba can cause vomiting (18).

Interactions with Herbs & Other Dietary Supplements
None known.

Interactions with Drugs
None known.

Interactions with Foods
None known.

Interactions with Lab Tests
None known.

Interactions with Diseases or Conditions
None known.

Dosage and Administration
ORAL: A typical dose is 1 gram (18).

Comments
Simaruba amara grows in the Caribbean islands and in the northern parts of South America (18).

SITOSTANOL

Also Known As
24-alpha-ethylcholestanol, Beta-sitostanol, Dihydro-beta-sitosterol, Fucostanol, Phytostanol, Plant Stanol, Plant Stanol Esters, Stigmastanol.
CAUTION: See separate listing for Beta-sitosterol.

Scientific Names
3-beta,5-alpha-stigmastan-3-ol.

People Use This For
Orally, sitostanol is used for prevention of heart disease and hypercholesterolemia.

Safety
LIKELY SAFE ...when used orally and appropriately. Sitostanol has been safely used in studies lasting up to one year (5336,5429,5430,5431,5432,5433,5434,5435,5436,5437,5438,5439,5441,5443,5814).
CHILDREN: LIKELY SAFE ...when used orally and appropriately, short-term. Sitostanol has been safely used in children in studies lasting for up to 3 months (3888,3889,5438,7193,7194). There is insufficient reliable information available about the safety of long-term use of sitostanol in children.
PREGNANCY AND LACTATION: Insufficient reliable information available; avoid using.

Effectiveness
LIKELY EFFECTIVE

Hypercholesterolemia. Taking sitostanol orally is effective for reducing cholesterol levels in adults with hypercholesterolemia (1886,3888,5336,5429,5430,5431,5432,5433,5434,5435,5437,5438) (5439,5441,5443,7103). Sitostanol also seems to be effective for reducing cholesterol levels in healthy children (7193,7194). However, treating children is not recommended unless low-density lipoprotein (LDL) levels are greater that 190 mg/dL or greater that 160 mg/dL in the presence of other coronary risk factors. Sitostanol is usually taken as a component of a sitostanol-enriched food such as margarine. It is effective in about 88% of patients when used alone or in combination with a low-fat diet or HMG-CoA reductase inhibitor ("statin") for reducing total and low-density lipoprotein cholesterol (3888,5431,5433,5435,5437,5814,7195). Sitostanol alone can reduce total and LDL cholesterol levels by 10-15% (5443). Peak cholesterol lowering effects occur at about 2 grams per day. Higher doses do not seem to offer any additional benefit (5814,6185,7195). When added to a statin such as pravastatin (Pravachol) or simvastatin (Zocor), sitostanol reduces total cholesterol by an additional 3-11% and LDL cholesterol by another 7-16% (5431,5433). Treatment with sitostanol for 2-3 weeks is usually necessary before cholesterol levels decrease significantly. If sitostanol is discontinued, cholesterol levels tend to rise within 2-3 weeks (7105).

POSSIBLY EFFECTIVE

Familial hypercholesterolemia. Taking sitostanol orally seems to be effective for treating familial hypercholesterolemia in children (3888,3889,5438).

Mechanism of Action
Sitostanol is a saturated form of plant sterols that structurally resembles cholesterol. It is prepared commercially from vegetable oils or the oil from pine tree wood pulp and is then made fat-soluble with canola oil (5435,5430,5814).

Sitostanol is unabsorbable and tasteless. It competitively inhibits both dietary and biliary cholesterol absorption by competing with cholesterol for the limited space in mixed micelles (5435,5439,5443,5814,7196). However, sitostanol doesn't have to be taken with meals to lower cholesterol blood levels. Some researchers think sitostanol remains in the intestinal lumen or in the enterocytes after ingestion. So administration of sitostanol at any time of day seems to be as effective as multiple daily doses with meals (7103). Cholesterol levels decrease within 2 to 3 weeks of initiation of sitostanol, and return to pretreatment levels within 2 to 3 weeks of discontinuation (7105) which also suggests a prolonged effect. Sitostanol may not have the same effect in all people. Preliminary clinical evidence suggests that sitostanol might work better in people with apolipoprotein E4 alleles, a genetic predisposition to hypercholesterolemia (7105,7195). About 12% of patients do not respond to sitostanol. In certain patients, hepatic cholesterol synthesis might increase in response to decreased availability of cholesterol, resulting in no change in cholesterol levels (5430,5443). There is some concern that sitostanol might decrease absorption of some nutrients since it decreases fat absorption. Sitostanol does seem to reduce the absorption of dietary beta-carotene. However, when corrected for lower levels of LDL, the major carrier of beta-carotene, the reduction in beta-carotene levels may not be clinically significant (7103,7104,7105). Sitostanol does not seem to affect retinol, vitamin D, or lycopene (5434,7104,7105).

Adverse Reactions

Orally, sitostanol seems to be very well tolerated. Adverse effects have not been reported in clinical trials in adults or children (5336,5429,5430,5431,5432,5433,5434,5435,5436,5437,5438,5439,5441,5443,7103,7104,7105,7193,7194). However, because sitostanol decreases cholesterol absorption in the gut, it might be expected to produce some gastrointestinal symptoms like diarrhea and excess amounts of fat in the stool (steatorrhea).

Interactions with Herbs & Other Dietary Supplements

BETA-CAROTENE: Sitostanol can reduce absorption and blood levels of beta-carotene (3888,5434,5814,7103,7104,7105). Sitostanol lowers blood levels of low-density lipoprotein (LDL) cholesterol, which is a major carrier of fat-soluble antioxidants (7103,7104,7105). When corrected for lower LDL levels the reduction in beta-carotene levels does not seem to be clinically significant (7103,7104,7105). Supplementation with beta-carotene is probably not necessary. Suggest that concerned patients increase dietary consumption of beta-carotene rich vegetables or take a multivitamin that contains beta-carotene (7104).

CHOLESTEROL LOWERING HERBS/SUPPLEMENTS: Sitostanol might enhance the effects of herbs and supplements that also lower cholesterol levels. Some of these herbs and supplements include chromium, flaxseed, garlic, guar gum, niacin, oat bran, psyllium, red yeast, and others.

Interactions with Drugs

None known.

Interactions with Foods

BETA-CAROTENE: Sitostanol can reduce absorption and blood levels of beta-carotene (3888,5434,5814,7103,7104,7105). Sitostanol lowers blood levels of low-density lipoprotein (LDL) cholesterol, which is a major carrier of fat-soluble antioxidants (7103,7104,7105). When corrected for lower LDL levels the reduction in beta-carotene levels does not seem to be clinically significant (7103,7104,7105). Supplementation with beta-carotene is probably not necessary. Suggest that concerned patients increase dietary consumption of beta-carotene rich vegetables or take a multivitamin that contains beta-carotene (7104).

Interactions with Lab Tests

SERUM CHOLESTEROL: Sitostanol decreases total and low-density lipoprotein (LDL) cholesterol and test results (5336,5429,5431,5432,5433,5435,5437,5438,5439,5441).

Interactions with Diseases or Conditions

None known.

Dosage and Administration

ORAL: For hypercholesterolemia, clinical studies have used from 800 mg to 4 grams per day (5814). However, doses above 2 grams per day do not seem to provide additional benefit (7195). Effectiveness is not dependent on administration schedule. Single daily doses seem to be as effective as divided doses administered twice or three times daily (7195). For familial hypercholesterolemia in children, clinical studies have used 2-6 grams daily initially and then tapered down to 1.5 grams daily (3888,3889,5438).

Comments

Sitostanol is an ingredient in the functional food product Benecol margarine and in some salad dressings. The FDA authorized the use of labeling health claims for foods containing plant stanol esters, including sitostanol, for reducing the risk of coronary heart disease (CHD). This rule is based on the FDA's conclusion that plant stanol esters in conjunction with a diet low in saturated fat and cholesterol might reduce the risk of CHD by lowering blood cholesterol levels (6668). Although there is plenty of evidence that sitostanol does lower cholesterol levels, so far there is no proof that long-term use actually lowers the risk of developing CHD. Do not confuse sitostanol with beta-sitosterol, an unsaturated plant sterol in the cholesterol-lowering margarine Take Control (5443). Both sitostanol and beta-sitosterol are used for lower cholesterol levels in people with hypercholesterolemia and appear to be equally effective (7196).

SKIRRET

Also Known As
Chervis.

Scientific Names
Sium sisarum.
Family: Apiaceae/Umbelliferae.

Comments
At the date of publication, this product was not a common ingredient used in brand name supplements marketed to consumers. Details about this product are available at the online version of *Natural Medicines Comprehensive Database*. See www.naturaldatabase.com.

SKULLCAP

Also Known As
Blue Pimpernel, Blue Skullcap, Helmet Flower, Hoodwort, Mad Weed, Mad-Dog Skullcap, Quaker Bonnet, Scullcap, Scutelluria.
CAUTION: See separate listing for Baikal Skullcap.

Scientific Names
Scutellaria lateriflora.
Family: Lamiaceae/Labiatae.

People Use This For
Orally or by injection, skullcap is used for cerebral thrombosis or embolism and paralysis caused by stroke. It is also used orally as a nerve tonic, as a tranquilizer fever, for treating fever, hyperlipidemia, atherosclerosis, rabies, grand mal seizures, chorea, epilepsy, hysteria, insomnia, nervous tension, allergic conditions, dermatitis, inflammation, and spasms.

Safety
There is insufficient reliable information available about the safety of skullcap.
Pregnancy and Lactation: Insufficient reliable information available; avoid using.

Effectiveness
There is insufficient reliable information available about the effectiveness of skullcap.

Mechanism of Action
The applicable parts of skullcap are the above ground parts. Skullcap contains flavonoids including scutellarin, baicalin, wogonin, methoxyflavone, and catalpol. It also contains lignins, resins, tannins, and volatile oils (4,12104). Constituents of skullcap seem to bind the serotonin receptor 5-HT7. But it's not known if these constituents have agonist or antagonist properties on the receptor (12104). Skullcap's effects on the serotonin receptor may be involved in potential sedative properties.

Adverse Reactions
Orally, large amounts of skullcap can cause giddiness, stupor, confusion, limb twitching, seizures (4,6), "intermission" of the pulse, and other symptoms consistent with epilepsy (6).
There are four reports of hepatotoxicity, one of which led to a fatality, associated with products thought to contain skullcap. However, it is uncertain whether the products actually contained skullcap. It is thought that the products might have been contaminated with an adulterant such as germander (515), which is known to cause liver damage.

Interactions with Herbs & Other Dietary Supplements

HERBS WITH SEDATIVE PROPERTIES: Theoretically, concomitant use with herbs that have sedative properties might enhance therapeutic and adverse effects. Some of these supplements include 5-HTP, calamus, California poppy, catnip, hops, Jamaican dogwood, kava, St. John's wort, valerian, yerba mansa, and others.

Interactions with Drugs

None known.

Interactions with Foods

None known.

Interactions with Lab Tests

None known.

Interactions with Diseases or Conditions

None known.

Dosage and Administration

ORAL: A typical dose is 1-2 grams or as a tea three times daily (4). To make tea, steep 1-2 grams above ground parts in 150 mL of boiling water for 5-10 minutes, strain. The extract is typically used 2-4 mL (1:1 in 25% alcohol) three times daily. The tincture is typically used 1-2 mL (1:5 in 45% alcohol) three times daily (4).

Comments

Skullcap has been commonly adulterated with germander and teucrium (4,5,12).

SKUNK CABBAGE

Also Known As

Dracontium, Meadow Cabbage, Polecatweed, Skunkweed, Spathyema Foetida, Swamp Cabbage.

Scientific Names

Symplocarpus foetidus, synonym Dracontium foetidum.
Family: Araceae.

People Use This For

Orally, skunk cabbage is used to treat bronchitis, asthma, whooping cough, catarrh, cancer, chorea, convulsions, cough, edema, epilepsy, headache, hemorrhage, hysteria, pregnancy, labor, worms, rheumatism, ringworm, scabies, snakebite, skin sores, spasms, splinters, swellings, toothache, and wounds. It is also used as a gastrointestinal (GI) stimulant.
As a food, the young leaves, roots, and stalks have been boiled and eaten.

Safety

POSSIBLY SAFE ...when used orally and appropriately; the young boiled leaves, roots, and stalks are used as food (4500,4502) without reports of serious adverse effects (4).
PREGNANCY AND LACTATION: POSSIBLY UNSAFE ...when used orally; avoid using. It may affect the menstrual cycle (4), and irritant properties may stimulate uterine contractions (4,12).

Effectiveness

There is insufficient reliable information available about the effectiveness of skunk cabbage.

Mechanism of Action

Skunk cabbage contains a variety of constituents, including an acrid principle, unspecified alkaloids, essential oil, fatty oil, phenolic compounds, and tannins (4,4502). The seeds are reported to contain a narcotic (4502). The root contains calcium oxalate which could irritate the kidney or promote kidney stones in sensitive individuals (12,4502). The leaves contain n-hydroxytryptamine (4).

Adverse Reactions

Orally, large amounts of skunk cabbage are reported to cause nausea, vomiting, headache, vertigo, and dimness of vision (18,4502). Excessive use of gastrointestinal (GI) irritants can cause abdominal cramps, burning, blistering in the mouth and throat, nausea, colic, and watery or bloody diarrhea (12).
Topically, the fresh plant can cause severe itching, inflammation, and blistering (4,4502).

Interactions with Herbs & Other Dietary Supplements
CALCIUM, IRON, ZINC: Concurrent use might decrease mineral absorption. Skunk cabbage contains oxalate (7,12), which can bind multivalent metal ions in the gastrointestinal (GI) tract and decrease mineral absorption.

Interactions with Drugs
None known.

Interactions with Foods
CALCIUM, IRON, ZINC: Skunk cabbage might decrease mineral absorption from foods. Skunk cabbage contains oxalates (7,12), which can bind multivalent metal ions in the gastrointestinal (GI) tract and decrease mineral absorption.

Interactions with Lab Tests
None known.

Interactions with Diseases or Conditions
GASTROINTESTINAL (GI) CONDITIONS: Skunk cabbage may aggravate GI ulcers, GI inflammation or cause GI irritation (12,19).
KIDNEY STONES: Individuals with a history of oxalate kidney stones should avoid skunk cabbage or use it cautiously (12,4502).

Dosage and Administration
ORAL: People typically use the powdered rhizome/root, 0.5-1 mg three times daily mixed with honey or by infusion or decoction (4). 0.5-1 mL the liquid extract, 1:1 in 25% alcohol, has been used three times daily (4). 2-4 mL of the tincture, 1:10 in 45% alcohol, has been used three times daily (4).

Comments
Skunk cabbage is also a common name for members of the toxic Veratrum family. Skunk cabbage gets it name from a volatile oil emitted by the plant that has a highly disagreeable odor (18).

SLIPPERY ELM

Also Known As
Indian Elm, Moose Elm, Red Elm, Sweet Elm.

Scientific Names
Ulmus rubra, synonym Ulmus fulva.
Family: Ulmaceae.

People Use This For
Orally, slippery elm is used for coughs, sore throat, colic, diarrhea, constipation, hemorrhoids, irritable bowel syndrome (IBS), cystitis, urinary inflammation, urinary tract infections, syphilis, herpes, and for expelling tapeworms. It is also used orally for protecting against stomach and duodenal ulcers, for colitis, diverticulitis, GI inflammation, and acidity. Slippery elm is used orally as an abortifacient.
Topically, slippery elm is used for wounds, burns, gout, rheumatism, cold sores, boils, abscesses, ulcers, toothaches, sore throat, and as a lubricant to ease labor.
In manufacturing, slippery elm is used in some baby foods and adult nutritionals, and in some oral lozenges used for soothing throat pain.

Safety
LIKELY SAFE ...when used orally and appropriately (4,12,512).
PREGNANCY: POSSIBLY SAFE ...when the inner bark is used orally in amounts used in foods (4).
LIKELY UNSAFE ...when the whole bark is used. Use of the whole bark is contraindicated because it is an abortifacient (4,6).
LACTATION: Insufficient reliable information available; avoid using.

Effectiveness
POSSIBLY EFFECTIVE

Sore throat. Slippery elm has demulcent properties and, added to lozenges, can soothe sore throats (272,512,1740).
There is insufficient reliable information available about the effectiveness of slippery elm for its other uses.

Mechanism of Action
The applicable part of slippery elm is the inner bark rind. The mucilages are considered the principal constituent. They are responsible for slippery elm's demulcent and emollient effects (4,18). Used internally, slippery elm preparations cause reflex stimulation of nerve endings in the GI tract, leading to mucous secretion (6). This induced mucous may protect the GI tract against ulcers, excess acidity, etc. Tannin constituents have astringent properties (4). Oleoresins of some species are responsible for contact dermatitis (6).

Adverse Reactions
Orally, the whole bark is an abortifacient (4).
Topically, slippery elm extracts can cause contract dermatitis (6). The pollen is an allergen (6).

Interactions with Herbs & Other Dietary Supplements
None known.

Interactions with Drugs
ORAL DRUGS: Theoretically, may slow the absorption and reduce serum levels of orally administered drugs due to mucilage content (19).

Interactions with Foods
None known.

Interactions with Lab Tests
None known.

Interactions with Diseases or Conditions
None known.

Dosage and Administration
ORAL: People typically use the powdered inner bark (1:8 as a decoction), 4-16 mL three times daily (4). As a nutritional supplement, 4 grams powdered inner bark in 500 mL boiling water, three times daily (4) has been used. People typically use the alcohol extract (1:1 in 60% alcohol), 5 mL three times daily (4).
TOPICAL: As a poultice, people typically use the coarse powdered inner bark mixed with boiling water (4).

Comments
Avoid confusing whole bark with inner bark. Commercial lozenges containing slippery elm are preferred to the native herb when used for cough and sore throat, because they provide sustained release of mucilage to the throat (3).

SMARTWEED

Also Known As
Arsesmart, Smart Weed, Water Pepper.

Scientific Names
Polygonum hydropiper.

People Use This For
Orally, smartweed is used to treat bleeding of the womb, menstrual bleeding, bleeding hemorrhoids, and diarrhea. Topically, smartweed is used to wash bloody wounds.

Safety
There is insufficient reliable information available about the safety of smartweed.
Pregnancy and Lactation: Insufficient reliable information available; avoid using.

Effectiveness
There is insufficient reliable information available about the effectiveness of smartweed.

Mechanism of Action
The applicable parts of smartweed are the leaf, and the entire plant during flowering season. Smartweed contains tannins, hydropiperoside, sesquiterpenealdehydes, and flavonoids (18). Smartweed is reported to stop bleeding. It is also thought to influence the elimination of urine and to have some effect on rheumatic pain (18).

Adverse Reactions
Orally, smartweed can cause gastrointestinal irritation (19).
Topically, the fresh plant can cause inflammatory reactions due to chemical irritation (18).

Interactions with Herbs & Other Dietary Supplements
None known.

Interactions with Drugs
WARFARIN (Coumadin): Smartweed is high in vitamin K. Concomitant use can decrease the anticoagulant effects of warfarin (Coumadin) (19).

Interactions with Foods
None known.

Interactions with Lab Tests
None known.

Interactions with Diseases or Conditions
GASTROINTESTINAL DISORDERS: Smartweed can exacerbate inflammatory conditions by irritating the mucous membranes (19).

Dosage and Administration
ORAL: A small amount of the powdered drug three times a day or one cup tea (one teaspoon of the drug per cup, boil) three times per day (18).
TOPICAL: No typical dosage.

Comments
Smartweed has an extraordinary hot pepper-like taste (18).

SMOOTH ALDER

Also Known As
Hazel Alder, Tag Alder.

Scientific Names
Alnus serrulata.
Family: Betulaceae.

Comments
At the date of publication, this product was not a common ingredient used in brand name supplements marketed to consumers. Details about this product are available at the online version of *Natural Medicines Comprehensive Database*. See www.naturaldatabase.com.

SNEEZEWORT

Also Known As
Sneezeweed.

Scientific Names
Achillea ptarmica.
Family: Asteraceae/Compositae

People Use This For
Orally, sneezewort is used for rheumatic and painful disorders, toothache, diarrhea, nausea, vomiting, flatulence, tiredness, urinary tract complaints, and as an appetite stimulant.
Topically, sneezewort is used for toothache.

Safety
There is insufficient reliable information available about the safety of sneezewort.
Pregnancy and Lactation: Insufficient reliable information available; avoid using.

Effectiveness
There is insufficient reliable information available about the effectiveness of sneezewort.

Mechanism of Action
The applicable part of sneezewort is the dried root. Sneezewort contains alkamides, polyynes, and volatile oil (18).

Adverse Reactions
Orally, sneezewort may cause an allergic reaction (18).

Interactions with Herbs & Other Dietary Supplements
None known.

Interactions with Drugs
None known.

Interactions with Foods
None known.

Interactions with Lab Tests
None known.

Interactions with Diseases or Conditions
SNEEZEWORT ALLERGY: Contraindicated.

Dosage and Administration
ORAL: A typical dose is two cups of tea daily. To make tea, simmer 2 teaspoons of the cut root in 2 cups of water (18).
TOPICAL: The fresh root can be chewed (18).

SOLOMON'S SEAL

Also Known As
Dropberry, Lady's Seals, Ladys Seals, Sealroot, Sealwort, Solomons Seal, St Marys Seal, St. Mary's Seal.

Scientific Names
Polygonatum multiflorum.
Family: Liliaceae.

People Use This For
Orally, Solomon's seal is used for respiratory and lung disorders, and as an astringent and anti-inflammatory. Topically, Solomon's seal is used for bruises, furuncles, ulcers or boils on the fingers, hemorrhoids, skin redness, edema, and hematoma.

Safety
POSSIBLY SAFE ...when used orally, short-term (12).
PREGNANCY AND LACTATION: Insufficient reliable information available; avoid using.

Effectiveness
There is insufficient reliable information available about the effectiveness of Solomon's seal.

Mechanism of Action
There is insufficient reliable information available about the possible mechanism of action and active ingredients. Solomon's seal may cause hypoglycemia (19).

Adverse Reactions
Long-term use may cause gastrointestinal irritation. Use of large doses or overdoses may cause nausea, diarrhea, gastric complaints, and nausea (18).

Interactions with Herbs & Other Dietary Supplements

HYPOGLYCEMIC HERBS: Theoretically, concomitant use with other hypoglycemic herbs may have additive effects (19).

Interactions with Drugs

ANTIDIABETES DRUGS: Theoretically, concomitant use may enhance hypoglycemic drug effects and alter blood glucose control (19). Monitor blood glucose.
CHLORPROPAMIDE (Diabinese): Concomitant use may cause additive hypoglycemic effects (19).
INSULIN: Insulin dosage adjustments may be necessary, due to the possible hypoglycemic effects of Solomon's seal (19).

Interactions with Foods

None known.

Interactions with Lab Tests

None known.

Interactions with Diseases or Conditions

DIABETES: Theoretically may interfere with blood glucose control (19).

Dosage and Administration

No typical dosage.

Comments

Solomon's seal is obsolete as a medicinal herb.

SORREL

Also Known As

Acedera Común, Azeda-Brava, Garden Sorrel, Sorrel Dock, Sour Dock, Wiesensauerampfer.

Scientific Names

Rumex acetosa.
Family: Polygonaceae.

People Use This For

Orally, sorrel is used for acute and chronic inflammation of the nasal passages and respiratory tract, and as an adjunct to antibacterial therapy. It is also used as a diuretic and to stimulate secretions.
In combination with gentian root, European elder flower, verbena, and cowslip flower, sorrel is used orally for maintaining healthy sinuses and treating sinusitis.

Safety

POSSIBLY SAFE ...when used orally in amounts commonly found in foods. ...when used orally in combination with gentian root, European elder flower, verbena, and cowslip flower (Quanterra Sinus Defense, Sinupret) (374,379).
LIKELY UNSAFE ...when used in large amounts. A 53 year old died after ingesting 500 grams of sorrel in soup (17).
There is insufficient reliable information available about the safety of sorrel used in medicinal amounts.
CHILDREN: POSSIBLY UNSAFE ...when used orally because it contains oxalic acid. A four-year old child died after consuming rhubarb leaves, which are also a source of oxalic acid (17).
PREGNANCY AND LACTATION: There is insufficient reliable information available about the safety of sorrel in medicinal amounts during pregnancy and lactation; avoid using.

Effectiveness

POSSIBLY EFFECTIVE

Sinusitis. Taking sorrel orally in a specific combination product which also contains gentian root, European elder flower, verbena, and cowslip flower (Quanterra Sinus Defense, Sinupret) seems to help treat acute or chronic sinusitis (374,379).

There is insufficient reliable information available about the effectiveness of sorrel for its other uses.

Mechanism of Action

Sorrel contains 7-15% tannins (11), which exert an astringent effect on the mucosal tissue. This effect dehydrates the tissue, reducing internal secretions and forming the external cells into a protective layer. Plants with at least 10% tannins may cause gastrointestinal disturbances, kidney damage, and necrotic conditions of the liver. Some animal data show that tannins may cause cancer; other data show they may prevent it. Regular consumption of herbs with high tannin concentrations correlates with increased incidence of esophageal or nasal cancer (12). Sorrel leaf has a 0.3% oxalate content (12). Once absorbed, the oxalic acid reacts with calcium in plasma and resulting insoluble calcium oxalate may precipitate in the kidneys, blood vessels, heart, lungs, and liver. This may also cause hypocalcemia (12,17). Oxalate crystals damage mucosal tissue, resulting in severe irritation and possible damage. The systemic absorption of oxalates may result in kidney damage, both in people with pre-existing kidney disease and in healthy kidneys (19).

Adverse Reactions

Orally, excessive amounts of sorrel can cause diarrhea, nausea, polyuria (6), dermatitis (4) and gastrointestinal symptoms. Oxalic acid (constituent) poisoning affects skin, eyes, respiratory system, and kidneys. Oral symptoms of oxalate irritation include swelling of the mouth, tongue, and throat, with difficulty in speaking and suffocation. It has a corrosive effect on the digestive tract and can lead to oxalic acid crystals in the kidneys, blood vessels, heart, lungs, liver, and/or hypocalcemia (17).

Interactions with Herbs & Other Dietary Supplements

CALCIUM, IRON, ZINC: Concurrent use might decrease mineral absorption. Sorrel contains oxalate (7,12), which can bind multivalent metal ions in the gastrointestinal tract and decrease mineral absorption.
TANNIN-CONTAINING HERBS: Theoretically, herbs that contain high percentages of tannins (such as sorrel) may cause precipitation of constituents of other herbs (19).

Interactions with Drugs

ORAL DRUGS: Theoretically, concomitant oral administration may cause precipitation of some drugs due to the high tannin content of sorrel (19). Separate administration of oral drugs and tannin-containing herbs by the longest period of time practical (19).

Interactions with Foods

CALCIUM, IRON, ZINC: Concurrent use might decrease mineral absorption from foods. Sorrel contains oxalate (7,12), which can bind multivalent metal ions in the gastrointestinal tract and decrease mineral absorption.

Interactions with Lab Tests

None known.

Interactions with Diseases or Conditions

COAGULATION DISORDERS: Oxalate constituents can alter the calcium concentrations and decrease coagulation time (4,12).
GI CONDITIONS: Theoretically, sorrel can exacerbate stomach and intestinal ulcers due to mucosal irritant effect (19).
KIDNEY DISEASE: Can damage kidneys with formation of insoluble oxalate; use with caution or avoid in individuals with history of kidney stones (12,19).

Dosage and Administration

ORAL: For acute or chronic sinusitis, two Sinupret tablets three times daily for up to two weeks has been used in clinical trials (7,374,379), equivalent to gentian root 12 mg, European elder flower 36 mg, verbena 36 mg cowslip flower 36 mg and sorrel 36 mg three times daily.

Comments

Roselle (Hibiscus sabdariffa) is also known as Jamaica sorrel or Guinea sorrel. It could be confused with sorrel (11,18).

SOUR CHERRY

Also Known As
Cerezo Acido, Cerisier Acide, English Morello, Ginjeira, Griottier, Guindo, Montmorency Cherry, Morello Cherry, Pie Cherry, Red Cherry, Richmond, Sauerkirsche, Sauerkirschenbaum, Tart Cherry.

Scientific Names
Prunus cerasus, synonyms Cerasus vulgaris, Prunus vulgaris.
Family: Rosaceae.

People Use This For
Orally, sour cherry is used for arthritis, gout, to cause diuresis, and to facilitate digestion.
In foods, sour cherries are eaten as a food or flavoring.
In manufacturing, sour cherry is used to make cherry syrup USP for drugs with an unpleasant taste.

Safety
LIKELY SAFE ...when the fruit is used in amounts commonly found in foods. ...when the fruit is used in medicinal amounts (6).
There is insufficient reliable information available about the safety of the oral use of sour cherry stem.
PREGNANCY AND LACTATION: LIKELY SAFE ...when the fruit is consumed in typical food amounts. There is insufficient reliable information available about the safety of sour cherry stem use during pregnancy or lactation.

Effectiveness
There is insufficient reliable information available about the effectiveness of sour cherry.

Mechanism of Action
The applicable parts of sour cherry are the fruit and stem. Sour cherry fruit contains vitamin C, vitamin A, alpha-linolenic acid, and traces of vitamin E, beta-carotene, folacin thiamine, as well as other constituents (4282). It contains varied antioxidants including kaempferol and quercetin (4282,4283). A preliminary study at Michigan State University suggests compounds found in the sour cherry have anti-inflammatory effects that are ten times stronger than aspirin but without aspirin's side effects (6). The stem of the sour cherry contains an isoflavone constituent, prunetin 5-O-beta-D-glycopyranoside (4284).

Adverse Reactions
None reported.

Interactions with Herbs & Other Dietary Supplements
None known.

Interactions with Drugs
None known.

Interactions with Foods
None known.

Interactions with Lab Tests
None known.

Interactions with Diseases or Conditions
None known.

Dosage and Administration
No typical dosage.

Comments
Of the more than 270 varieties of sour cherry, only a few are important commercially. These include the Montmorency, Richmond, and English morello (6).

SOUTHERN PRICKLY ASH

Also Known As
Prickly Ash, Prickly Yellow Wood, Sea Ash, Toothache Tree, Xanthoxylum, Zanthoxylum.
CAUTION: See separate listings for Ash and Northern Prickly Ash.

Scientific Names
Zanthoxylum clava-herculis.
Family: Rutaceae.

People Use This For
Orally, southern prickly ash is used for cramps, intermittent claudication, Raynaud's syndrome, chronic rheumatic conditions, and peripheral circulatory insufficiency associated with rheumatic symptoms, as a tonic, stimulant, for toothache, sores, ulcers, as a diaphoretic in fever, and for cancer (as an ingredient in Hoxsey cure).

Safety
POSSIBLY SAFE ...when the bark is used orally in medicinal amounts (12).
There is insufficient reliable information about the safety of the oral use of the berry.
PREGNANCY: LIKELY UNSAFE ...when used orally (12) because it might have menstrual stimulant effects (19).
There is insufficient reliable information about the safety of the berry during pregnancy; avoid using.
LACTATION: LIKELY UNSAFE ...when used orally because it might cause colic in nursing infants (19).

Effectiveness
There is insufficient reliable information available about the effectiveness of southern prickly ash.

Mechanism of Action
The applicable parts of southern prickly ash are the bark and berry. Southern prickly ash contains nitidine (hypotensive, antileukemic, hepatic enzyme inhibitor), chelerythrine (anti-inflammatory, antibiotic against gram positive bacteria, potentiates barbiturate induced sleep, hepatic enzyme inhibitor), asarinin (antitubercular), and neoherculin (insecticidal, salivation stimulant) (4). Reports of death after ingestion by cattle, chickens, and fish attributed to the neuromuscular blocking properties of the bark (4).

Adverse Reactions
None reported.

Interactions with Herbs & Other Dietary Supplements
DIGITALIS: May interfere with cardiac glycoside therapy (4).

Interactions with Drugs
ANTACIDS: Theoretically, due to reports that southern prickly ash increases stomach acid, southern prickly ash might decrease the effectiveness of antacids (19).
H2-BLOCKERS: Theoretically, due to reports that southern prickly ash increases stomach acid, southern prickly ash might decrease the effectiveness of H2-blockers (19). The H2 blockers include cimetidine (Tagamet), ranitidine (Zantac), nizatidine (Axid), and famotidine (Pepcid).
PROTON PUMP INHIBITORS (PPIs): Theoretically, due to reports that southern prickly ash increases stomach acid, southern prickly ash might decrease the effectiveness of PPIs (19). PPIs include omeprazole (Prilosec), lansoprazole (Prevacid), rabeprazole (Aciphex), pantoprazole (Protonix), and esomeprazole (Nexium).

Interactions with Foods
None known.

Interactions with Lab Tests
None known.

Interactions with Diseases or Conditions
LIVER DISEASE: Theoretically, may inhibit hepatic enzymes.

Dosage and Administration
ORAL: People typically use 1-3 grams dried bark, or drink as decoction (boil 1-3 grams dry bark 10-15 minutes, strain), three times daily; liquid bark extract (1:1 in 45% alcohol) 1-3 mL three times daily; or bark tincture (1:5 in 45% alcohol) 2-5 mL three times daily (4). People typically use 0.5-1.5 grams dried berry or liquid berry extract (1:1 in 45% alcohol) 0.5-1.5 mL (4).

SOY

Also Known As

Daidzein, Edamame, Frijol de Soya, Genistein, Haba Soya, Hydrolyzed Soy Protein, Isoflavones, Legume, Miso, Natto, Phytoestrogen, Plant Estrogen, Shoyu, Soja, Sojabohne, Soy Fiber, Soy Milk, Soy Protein, Soy Protein Extract, Soya, Soybean, Soybean Curd, Tempeh, Texturized Vegetable Protein, Touchi, Tofu.
CAUTION: See separate listings for Alpha-GPC, Nattokinase.

Scientific Names

Glycine max, synonyms Glycine soja, Dolichos soja, Glycine gracilis, Glycine hispida, Phaseolus max Soja hispida, Soja max.
Family: Fabaceae/Leguminosae.

People Use This For

Orally, soy is used for hyperlipidemia, menopausal symptoms, and preventing osteoporosis. It is also used orally for cyclic breast pain, preventing hot flashes in breast cancer survivors, hypertension, type 2 diabetes, constipation, diarrhea, and muscle soreness caused by exercise. Other uses include slowing the progression of kidney disease, decreasing urine protein excretion, improving memory, and preventing breast cancer, endometrial cancer, prostate cancer, and thyroid cancer.
In foods, soy is used as a milk substitute for infant feeding formulas, and as an alternative to cow's milk. Soybeans are eaten boiled or roasted. Soy flour is used as an ingredient in foods, beverages, and condiments.

Safety

LIKELY SAFE ...when soy protein is used orally and appropriately. Soy protein products in doses up to 60 grams per day providing up to 185 mg isoflavones have been safely used in studies lasting up to 16 weeks (842,2293,2294,2296,3025,3402,3977,4755,6412,8530,8531,10372,11805).
POSSIBLY SAFE ...when soy extracts are used orally and appropriately, short-term. Soy extracts containing concentrated isoflavones in doses of 35-110 mg/day seem to be safe when used for up to 6 months (4751,6455,12040,12048).
POSSIBLY UNSAFE ...when soy extracts are used orally in high doses, long-term. Postmenopausal women who consume soy isoflavone tablets 150 mg/day for 5 years seem to have an increased occurrence of endometrial hyperplasia (12105). However, there is no evidence that consuming a diet that is high in soy foods causes this potential adverse effect. People who consume a diet high in soy foods actually seem to have a reduced risk of endometrial cancer (7338,10372).
CHILDREN: LIKELY SAFE ...when consumed in amounts commonly found in foods (4912). Soy in amounts commonly found in food or as a component of infant formula seem to be safe (3400,7331). Exposure to soy formula in infancy does not appear to cause health or reproductive problems later in life (7331). However, soy milk that's not designed for infants is not a substitute for infant formula. Regular soy milk can lead to nutrient deficiencies (12045).
POSSIBLY UNSAFE ...when used orally as an alternative to cow's milk in children with severe milk allergy. Although soy protein-based infant formulas are often promoted for children with milk allergy, children with a severe allergy to cow's milk are also frequently sensitive to soy protein (9883). There is insufficient reliable information available about the safety of soy products when used in amounts higher than typical food quantities for children.
PREGNANCY: LIKELY SAFE ...when used orally in amounts commonly found in foods (4912).
POSSIBLY UNSAFE ...when used orally in medicinal amounts. Soy contains mildly estrogenic constituents (3373,3988,3989,3990,3994,6029). Theoretically, therapeutic use of soy might adversely affect fetal development; avoid using.
LACTATION: LIKELY SAFE ...when used orally in amounts commonly found in foods (4912). A single 20 gram dose of roasted soybeans, containing 37 mg isoflavones, produces four to six times less isoflavones in breast milk than provided in a soy-based infant formula (2290). There is insufficient reliable information available about the safety of long-term use of therapeutic amounts of soy during lactation.

Effectiveness

LIKELY EFFECTIVE

Hyperlipidemia. Taking soy protein preparations orally reduces total cholesterol and low-density lipoprotein (LDL) levels in both hypercholesterolemic and normocholesterolemic men and women (842,2293,2294,2296,2585,3402,4755,6412,7346,7803,8528,8530). Replacement of dietary animal protein with soy protein decreases serum total cholesterol by 9%, LDL cholesterol by 13%, and triglycerides by 11% after one to two months. The effect on high-density lipoprotein (HDL) cholesterol is not consistent (2560,3401,7659,7804). Some of the beneficial effects might be attributed to the isoflavone content of soy protein, since preparations providing higher concentrations of isoflavones seem to produce more significant effects (3402,6413,10459). However, purified soy isoflavone supplements alone do not seem to decrease LDL cholesterol (8502).
The hormonal changes that occur in perimenopausal women might suppress the effect of soy protein on serum lipoproteins (9679). Soy protein may not reduce cholesterol levels in healthy postmenopausal women aged 60

to 75 years (12034).

Tell patients not to rely on concentrated soy extracts or purified isoflavone supplements for lowering lipids. They lack the fiber and beneficial fatty acids of soy protein and don't seem to be as effective as isoflavone rich foods like soy protein for lowering serum cholesterol concentrations (851,4738,7345,8502,10459). The FDA has approved labeling soy products for cholesterol reduction when used in combination with a diet low in saturated fat and cholesterol. To be eligible for this labeling, soy products must provide at least 6.25 grams of soy protein per serving, which is 25% of the effective amount of 25 grams per day (3977).

POSSIBLY EFFECTIVE

Breast cancer. There is some evidence from population studies that Asian women who eat a diet high in soy have a reduced risk of developing breast cancer (5939,7334,7335,7336). Soy food intake during adolescence seems to correlate with decreased incidence of breast cancer among Chinese women. This benefit persists even when Asian women immigrate to the western cultures where soy is less likely to be a regular component of the diet (7335,7336,9674). This suggests that early exposure to soy might be important for protection against breast cancer later in life. The estrogenic effect of soy might also be more pronounced in Asian women, possibly because of an ethnic difference in response (7663). Some epidemiologic research in Japan suggests that miso (fermented soybean paste) soup and dietary isoflavone consumption reduces breast cancer risk, but other soy foods do not (11807). In Western-culture populations, an association between soy and breast cancer risk has not been established. Total dietary intake of phytoestrogens among Western-culture middle-aged women doesn't appear to be related, positively or negatively, to breast cancer risk (11391).

Diabetes. In postmenopausal women with type 2 diabetes, treatment with a soy product containing 30 grams of soy protein and 132 mg isoflavones daily for 12 weeks seems to lower fasting insulin levels, hemoglobin A1c, insulin resistance, and low-density lipoprotein (LDL) cholesterol (8531). Preliminary clinical research suggests that an extract of the fermented soybean product, touchi, acts as an alpha-glucosidase inhibitor. It seems to modestly lower blood glucose, hemoglobin A1c, and triglycerides in patients with type 2 diabetes (11762).

Diarrhea. Giving soy fiber orally seems to reduce the duration of diarrhea in infants (2291,2292).

Galactosemia, hereditary lactase deficiency, or lactose intolerance. Giving isolated soy protein-based formula orally to infants seems to be helpful for treating galactosemia, hereditary lactase deficiency, or lactose intolerance (3400).

Hypertension. Taking isolated soy protein orally may slightly lower blood pressure in perimenopausal women (2296). Soy protein with psyllium fiber may reduce systolic blood pressure by about 8 mmHg and diastolic blood pressure by about 2 mmHg in adult men and women (10458).

Kidney disease. Taking soy protein orally seems to reduce proteinuria in people with kidney disease (2286,2287,2288).

Menopausal symptoms. Consuming a diet high in soy seems to help reduce hot flashes related to menopause. Varying amounts of soy isoflavones ingested seem to have similar effects on vasomotor symptoms. Patient expectations also seem to be linked to the perceived effectiveness of soy (7801,7802,9916). Soy protein 20-60 grams providing 34-76 mg of isoflavones daily seems to modestly decrease the frequency and severity of hot flashes in some menopausal women (2296,2297,3978,3986,3987,7653,9917,11805). However, not all research has found that soy helps hot flashes, possibly due to a high placebo response (11806). Soy extracts, providing 35-100 mg of isoflavones daily, seem to have similar beneficial effects (4751,6455,10460,11805,11993). Genistein, a soy isoflavone, also seems to reduce hot flashes. A dose of 54 mg per day appears to be about half as effective as estrogen-progesterone supplementation (11994). Soy supplements appear to be helpful in about 30% of postmenopausal women (8499). The optimal dose and administration frequency of soy for menopausal symptoms have not been determined (11805). However, taking soy orally doesn't seem to prevent hot flashes in breast cancer survivors. There is also concern about possible stimulation of cancer cells by soy (3991,7658).

Osteoporosis. Most evidence suggests that soy protein can increase bone mineral density (BMD), or slow BMD loss, and improve biochemical markers of bone turnover in peri- and postmenopausal women (842,6449,9775,12044). The effect of soy protein on osteoporosis seems to be dependent upon the content of isoflavones. Taking isoflavones 80-90 mg, in 40 grams of soy protein, seems to be needed to improve BMD (842,6449,9775). Lower doses of isoflavones, between 4-56 mg, do not seem to be as effective in most women. Although, there is evidence that postmenopausal Japanese women who consume 54.3 mg isoflavones per day from dietary soy seem to have higher BMD than women who consume less (7342); this may be due to the increased sensitivity to the effect of soy isoflavones in Asian women.

There is also some conflicting evidence that suggests soy protein does not improve BMD in some postmenopausal women (4952,12034). The reasons for these inconsistent findings are not clear. However, different findings might be due to the variety of formulations of soy used, different age groups studied, and varying study designs (4950,4952). It's also thought that only "equol-producing" patients might have BMD benefits from soy. These are patients who can convert significant quantities of the daidzein isoflavone to equol, which is estrogenic. Only about 50% of people are "equol-producers" (4952).

Preliminary evidence also suggests that soy might have more pronounced effects on bone mineral content (BMC) in women who are in late postmenopause compared to early postmenopause, women with lower bodyweight compared to higher bodyweight, and women who consume less calcium compared to women who consume higher amounts of calcium (4951).

Soy doesn't seem to affect BMD in premenopausal women or bone turnover in adolescents (7660,8532,9684).

So far there is no evidence that taking soy can reduce the risk of fractures in any patient population (4950).

Prostate cancer. Consumption of soymilk at least once a day seems to reduce the risk of prostate cancer (2298).

POSSIBLY INEFFECTIVE

Exercise-induced muscle soreness. Taking soy isoflavone extract orally for 30 days prior to exercise doesn't seem to ameliorate muscle soreness caused by exercise (8524).

INSUFFICIENT RELIABLE EVIDENCE to RATE

Cognitive function. There is conflicting evidence about the effect of soy on cognitive function. Some evidence suggests that college students who increase soy food consumption providing 100 mg/day of isoflavones have improved short- and long-term memory (12039). Postmenopausal women aged 50 to 65 years who take a soy extract supplement providing 60 mg/day of isoflavones also seem to have some improvement in some measures of cognitive function (12048). There is also evidence that older postmenopausal women aged 55 to 75 years that taking a soy extract supplement providing 110 mg/day of isoflavones might improve verbal memory scores (12040). However, another study in this patient population suggests that consuming 25.6 grams/day of soy protein providing 99 mg of isoflavones does not improve cognitive function (12034). Differing study designs and soy formulations used make comparisons of these findings difficult.

Diabetic nephropathy. There is preliminary clinical evidence that soy might improve lipid profiles in patients with diabetes and potentially slow the development of diabetic nephropathy (7348).

Endometrial cancer. There is some epidemiological evidence that increasing soy intake might lower the risk endometrial cancer. Endometrial cancer incidence is lower in Japan, China, and other Asian countries where the typical diet is low in calories and high in soy and whole grain foods, vegetables, and fruits (7338).

Mastalgia. There is some preliminary evidence that soymilk (34 grams soy protein/day) might reduce cyclical breast pain in some women (2428).

Memory. Some research suggests that a high soy diet might slightly improve performance on memory tests (9671).

Thyroid cancer. Epidemiological research suggests that high dietary intake of soy might reduce the risk of thyroid cancer (7662,12041).

More evidence is needed to rate soy for these uses.

Mechanism of Action

The applicable part of soy is the bean. Soybeans are legumes that contain up to 50% protein; 24% carbohydrates; and 25% oil including stearic, linoleic, and palmitic acids. The active constituents of soybeans are the phytoestrogens, known as isoflavones (3387,3978,4753,6029), and phytosterols such as beta-sitosterol, campesterol, and stigmasterol (8528). Soybeans are also rich in calcium, iron, potassium, amino acids, vitamins, and fiber. Soy protein contains all of the essential amino acids in sufficient quantities to support human life (2426). Non-fortified soy beverages such as soymilk contain only about 10 mg of calcium per serving. But calcium-fortified soymilk can contain from 80-500 mg of calcium per serving in the form of tricalcium phosphate (6414). However, calcium from cow's milk is significantly better absorbed than calcium from fortified soymilk (6414). Fermented soy foods, such as soy sauce, miso, tempeh, and natto, have higher amounts of calcium and vitamin K2 (7342).

Soybeans and soy foods are the most significant dietary source of isoflavones (3387,3978,4753,6029). They contain the isoflavone glucosides genistein and daidzein in their inactive conjugated forms. In the gastrointestinal tract, genistein and daidzein are hydrolyzed by beta-glucosidases in the jejunum, releasing the isoflavone aglycone forms of genistein and daidzein (3982,5937,9346). Daidzein is further metabolized by gut flora to the estrogenic compound, equol. The extent of conversion of daidzein to equol varies among people due to differences in gut flora. Theoretically, people who do not convert significant amounts of daidzein to equol ("non-equol producers") might not experience the same pharmacological effects as people who do convert significant amounts ("equol producers") (12049). About 50% of the population does not produce equol (4952).

The amount of isoflavones varies among the forms of soy. Soy milk and soy powder have a lower concentration of isoflavones than other soy products (7655). Soy protein usually contains 1-3 mg of isoflavones per gram of protein (7333).

Soy isoflavones are heterocyclic phenols with structural similarity to estradiol and selective estrogen-receptor modulators (SERMs). Soy isoflavones bind to both the alpha- and beta-estrogen receptors. But they have a higher affinity for the beta-estrogen receptor (3983,3992,6029,7344,7657).

The beta-estrogen receptor predominates in the heart, vasculature, bone, and bladder; and may account for some of soy's beneficial effects. Actions at the cellular level depend on the target tissue, receptor status of the tissue, and the level of endogenous estrogen (7344).

Soy phytoestrogens might act as SERMs (3387,3990). In premenopausal women with normal endogenous estrogen levels, soy phytoestrogens may have an anti-estrogen effect since soy isoflavones can displace endogenous estrogen from receptors. Consuming soy protein might also lower circulating levels of estradiol in premenopausal women over the entire menstrual cycle (7805). In postmenopausal women with low endogenous estrogens, soy phytoestrogens have a weak estrogenic effect (3373,3988,3989,3990,3994,6029,8529).

Soy has several pharmacological effects that might be beneficial for preventing cardiovascular disease (6029).

It may lower homocysteine levels by unknown mechanisms, possibly related to the folic acid found in soy protein. Soy may also inhibit platelet aggregation (3992,8530,9776). Soy seems to lower blood pressure, in particular the diastolic pressure (9346).

Soy might increase bile acid excretion and up-regulate low-density lipoprotein (LDL) receptors

(2426,2594,6029,6030,7344). Phytosterols in soy also contribute to the lowering of LDL cholesterol by competitively inhibiting cholesterol absorption in the small bowel (2594,8528).

Some preliminary evidence suggests that soy might prevent progression of coronary artery atherosclerosis (7333). The isoflavones found in soy, particularly genistein, inhibit oxidation of LDL particles, a process thought to play a role in early atherosclerosis (2586,6029,7347,9560,9561). The isoflavones seem to inhibit LDL oxidation by acting as free radical scavengers and by inhibiting cyclooxygenase (9683). In addition to preventing LDL oxidation, genistein also seems to protect vascular cells from oxidized LDL (8527). Some evidence suggests that genistein may prevent vascular remodeling, which is an important component of atherosclerotic plaque formation (8503). Genistein might produce these effects by inhibiting tyrosine kinase activity, and reducing the production of proteolytic enzymes and the migration of endothelial cells (9346). Soy also seems to improve arterial compliance in perimenopausal women (851). Unlike oral estrogen, phytoestrogens don't seem to elevate C-reactive protein (CRP) levels (9919). However, lipoprotein (a), which has been identified as an independent risk factor for coronary heart disease, does not seem to be affected by soy in postmenopausal women. In men, most research suggests that soy doesn't negatively affect lipoprotein (a) (7347,8530,8963,8964). The effect of soy on endothelial function, an early marker of vascular disease, is variable. In middle-aged men, soy might improve endothelial function. However, soy does not seem to affect endothelial function in postmenopausal women and might worsen endothelial function in older men (8963,8964).

For preventing postmenopausal osteoporosis, soy is thought to work due to its weak estrogenic effects on bone (5598,6029). Like estrogen, soy seems to have the most effect on the bone mineral density of the lumbar spine (7660). Soy seems to increase serum levels of osteocalcin, a marker of bone formation, in postmenopausal women (7659). The soy isoflavone genistein appears to directly inhibit osteoclast activity (9346). High intake of soy also seems to lower parathyroid hormone levels, which might lower bone turnover (7660). In vitro tests suggest that genistein may promote the proliferation of osteoblasts by inhibiting oxidative damage (9682). However, soy proteins and isoflavones do not seem to influence calcium absorption or calcium retention (7343).

Estrogenic effects of soy have also been attributed to benefit menopausal symptoms such as hot flashes. Genistein seems to relieve hot flashes in some women (11994). However, some research suggests that the incidence of hot flashes does not seem to correlate with serum levels of the phytoestrogens genistein, daidzein, and equol. Components of soy in addition to phytoestrogens may be responsible for reduction in hot flashes (4752).

In cancer, soy is thought to be beneficial due to preliminary evidence that suggests soy isoflavones have antioxidant, antiproliferative, and antiangiogenic activity (2296,3983). Soy also contains other anticarcinogenic compounds such as saponins, phytates, protease inhibitors, and phytosterols (9346).

There is a lot of controversy about soy and its potential role in breast cancer. Some researchers think that soy is protective against breast cancer. Asian women who eat a traditional diet high in soy seem to have a lower risk of developing of breast cancer (4590,5939). This benefit persists even when Asian women immigrate to the western cultures where soy is less likely to be a regular component of the diet (9674). This suggests that exposure to soy early in life (i.e., before menopause), provides the most benefit against breast cancer. It is theorized that isoflavones found in soy enhance early cellular differentiation and maturation of mammary glands. More mature mammary glands seem to be less susceptible to carcinogens (4590). Animal models show that soy protein can prevent chemically induced breast cancer (3976). There is also some evidence that the soy isoflavone, genistein, can suppress breast cancer cell growth by stimulating apoptosis (3378). Other research suggests that genistein influences enzymes involved in signal transduction that regulate cell growth and replication (7337). Genistein seems to exert multiple antiproliferative effects on both estrogen receptor positive (ER+) as well as estrogen receptor negative (ER-) human breast cancer cells (9346,10461). The ability of genistein to inhibit the growth of precancerous dysplastic cells in breast tissue may significantly contribute to the prevention of breast cancer (8965).

There is also some evidence that soy isoflavones can prolong the menstrual cycle and suppress midcycle surges of luteinizing hormone (LH) and follicle stimulating hormone (FSH), which may also decrease the risk of breast cancer (9346). Some research suggests that soy consumption alters the ratios of various estrogen metabolites in the urine, reducing excretion of potentially carcinogenic estrogen metabolites. This suggests that soy might cause a shift in estrogen metabolism to produce more benign metabolites (2430). However, some researchers suggest that due to the estrogenic effects of soy, it might actually increase the risk of breast cancer (6030). There is also preliminary in vitro data suggesting that soy can stimulate proliferation of normal human breast tissue (3980,3981). Higher serum estradiol levels are associated with increased risk of breast cancer. There is evidence that drinking soymilk daily can reduce serum 17-beta-estradiol and progesterone levels in premenopausal women. However, other research shows only a very modest effect of a high soy isoflavone diet on plasma hormones (2429,7654,9676). Tell patients the effect of soy on breast cancer is unknown.

"Unopposed estrogen" from the estrogenic activity of soy and its effects on the uterus has been a concern. There doesn't seem to be any significant effects on vaginal cytology or endometrial biopsy in premenstrual or postmenopausal women (2429,7654,9676,9917). Dietary phytoestrogens are associated with a reduced risk of endometrial cancer. Besides their effect on estrogen, isoflavones and other phytoestrogenic substances in soy might inhibit aromatase, which converts androstenedione to estrone, and may in turn increase endometrial cancer risk (7338,10372).

In prostatic diseases, soy phytoestrogens are thought to be potentially beneficial due to estrogenic mechanisms as well as inhibition of 5-alpha-reductase and 17-beta-hydroxysteroid dehydrogenase (3984,3985). A diet high in soy foods seems to reduce serum estradiol levels and testosterone levels (7339,9683). However, soy does not significantly reduce prostate specific antigen (PSA) levels (9777). Laboratory research suggests that genistein decreases the growth of both benign prostatic hyperplasia (BPH) and prostate cancer tissue (11015).

The soy isoflavones, genistein and daidzein, seem to be responsible for the effects on thyroid hormones. These isoflavones seem to block production of thyroid hormone by interfering with thyroid peroxidase catalyzed iodination of thyroglobulin. This can result in increased thyroid stimulating hormone (TSH) and goiter. However, these clinical results appear most likely to occur in people with low iodine levels (6466). The effect on thyroid function is not likely to be clinically significant in patients with an adequate diet (7806).

Soy isoflavones have potential benefits on cognitive function. Preliminary evidence suggests that the effects of soy isoflavones seem to be equivalent to those of 17 beta-estradiol in up-regulating choline acetyl transferase and nerve growth factor. These chemical factors are thought to be essential for learning and memory. Soy also might decrease the phosphorylation of the brain protein tau. Phosphorylation of this protein is associated with the development of Alzheimer's disease (9346).

Tofu, a soybean product, seems to inhibit the absorption of lead and prevent its build up in the body, possibly because of its phytic acid and calcium content (7656).

There is some evidence that isoflavones can inhibit oxidative and conjugative metabolism of drugs (4736). Isoflavones might also affect drug absorption and biliary excretion by interacting with drug transporters such as P-glycoprotein and the canalicular multispecific organic anion transporter (4736). Given the wide range of drugs and metabolites whose pharmacokinetics depends on these mechanisms, drug interactions with isoflavones might be more common than literature reports suggest. Postmenopausal women with high dietary intake of the soy isoflavone genistein seem to have a lower body mass index, waist circumference, and fasting insulin levels than women with lower intake (7804). However, soy supplementation does not significantly increase leptin concentrations in postmenopausal women. Leptin is a protein that is associated with decreased appetite and weight loss (9681).

Touchi, a traditional Chinese food used as a seasoning agent, seems to have alpha-glucosidase activity. Touchi is prepared by steaming and then fermenting soybeans with the fungus Aspergillus. Touchi extract seems to inhibit intestinal alpha-glucosidase and lower postprandial glucose levels in a dose-dependent manner. It may also lower triglyceride levels (11762).

The isoflavones, genistein and daidzein, are widely distributed in the body and undergo enterohepatic recycling (7330). Peak concentrations appear at 4-8 hours after dietary intake, and excretion is within 24 hours (3982). They are found both free in serum and bound to plasma proteins. The elimination half-life of free genistein and free daidzein are 3.2 and 4.2 hours, respectively. The elimination half-life of total genistein and total daidzein are 9.2 and 8.2 hours, respectively (7661). Both genistein and daidzein are conjugated to sulfate and glucuronide compounds. In plasma, 48% of genistein and 33% of daidzein are present as a glucuronide and 8% of genistein and 26% of daidzein are present as a sulfate. The half-lives of genistein glucuronide and daidzein glucuronide are 3.2 and 8.4 hours, respectively. The half-lives of genistein sulfate and daidzein sulfate are 3.1 and 5.7 hours, respectively (9673).The absorption of isoflavones from food may be saturable, suggesting improved effect if ingested throughout the day, but there is considerable variation in absorption from person to person (3380,3982,7344). There is some variation in how isoflavones are absorbed from different soy products. Soy germ products result in higher plasma levels of daidzein and lower levels of genistein. Soy protein products result in higher levels of genistein. Soy foods such as tofu produce less dramatic rises of daidzein and genistein. Genistein from soy food sources appears to be more bioavailable than daidzein (7330). Isoflavone bioavailability is similar for most soy foods (4750).

Adverse Reactions

Orally, soy is very well-tolerated. The most common side effects include gastrointestinal upset, such as constipation, bloating, and nausea (2297). Some people can also experience insomnia (9917).

Use of soy isoflavone supplements may rarely cause migraine headaches. This effect may be related to the estrogen-like activity of the isoflavones (9680).

Soy can cause allergic reactions such as skin rash and itching in some people (2280,6412). But this does not seem to be common.

There is controversy about the role of soy in breast cancer. Population studies suggest that soy is protective against breast cancer. Asian women who eat a traditional diet high in soy seem to have a lower risk of developing of breast cancer (4590,5939,9674). However, some researchers suggest that, due to the estrogenic effects of soy, it might increase the risk of breast cancer (6030). Preliminary research suggests that soy stimulates proliferation of normal human breast tissue (3980,3981). More research is needed to define to role of soy in breast cancer.

There is also some concern that soy might increase the risk of endometrial hyperplasia due to its estrogenic effects. But there is conflicting evidence. Some studies suggest that soy foods do not have a proliferative effect on endometrial cells (7358,2429,7654,9676,9917). Population studies suggest that consuming soy foods and phytoestrogens in the diet might actually reduce the risk of endometrial cancer (7338,10372). But there is clinical evidence that postmenopausal women who take soy isoflavone tablets for 5 years seem to have a higher occurrence of endometrial hyperplasia (12105).

Soy products have been associated with goiter and hypothyroidism in children taking soy formula. However, this seems to only occur in people with iodine deficiency (6466).

Epidemiologic data suggests that soy products may increase the risk for urinary bladder cancer. Total soy intake of greater than 92.5 grams/1000 Kcal seems to cause a 2.3-fold increase in the risk for bladder cancer compared with intake of less than 36.9 grams/1000 Kcal (9677).

Consumption of large amounts of fermented soy products (e.g., miso, tempeh) might increase the risk of stomach cancer. These associations might be confounded by the higher salt and N-nitroso content of some fermented soy

foods or other dietary factors such as fruit and vegetable intake. However, there is also evidence that nonfermented forms of soy may reduce the risk of stomach cancer (7340,7341). More research is required to determine if soy products have any role in stomach cancer.
Some research suggests that dietary consumption of two or more servings per week of tofu during midlife might decrease cognitive function in later years. However, numerous other factors, such as lifestyle and health could be involved (6415,6416). These findings are too preliminary to be used as a basis for clinical recommendations.
The association of isoflavone consumption and infertility in animals has led to concerns about the effect of isoflavones in infants fed soy-based formulas (7332,7344). Reassure parents that adults who received soy formulas as infants do not experience adverse health or reproductive outcomes compared with people who received cow milk formulas as infants (7331).
Inhaled soy dust and soy hull aeroallergen can trigger symptoms of asthma (5084,5085,5086).
Advise patients to use whole soy foods if possible instead of soy supplements. Since these products and supplements contain differing amounts of isoflavones, high consumption and uncontrolled use of soy supplements could increase the risk of adverse effects (9346).

Interactions with Herbs & Other Dietary Supplements
None known.

Interactions with Drugs
ANTIBIOTIC DRUGS: Antibiotics may decrease the action of isoflavones in soy, because intestinal bacteria are responsible in part for converting the isoflavones into their active forms. Antibiotics may decrease the ability of intestinal bacteria to convert the isoflavones (7657).
ESTROGENS: Theoretically, soy might competitively inhibit the effects of estrogen replacement therapy (3860).
TAMOXIFEN (Nolvadex): There is some concern that soy might interfere with tamoxifen because of its potential estrogenic effects. There is preliminary evidence that soy isoflavones might antagonize the antitumor effects of tamoxifen (7072). Tell patients taking tamoxifen to avoid therapeutic use of soy products.
WARFARIN (Coumadin): Soy milk has been reported to decrease the international normalized ratio (INR) in a patient taking warfarin. The mechanism of this interaction is not known. Soy may also inhibit platelet aggregation (3992). Dosing adjustments for warfarin may be necessary (9672).

Interactions with Foods
PLANT-BASED FOODS: Soy protein isolate reduces the absorption of non-heme iron from foods (5053). Non-heme iron is found in plant-based foods.

Interactions with Lab Tests
PARATHYROID HORMONE: High intake of soy seems to lower parathyroid hormone levels in postmenopausal women (7660).
THYROID STIMULATING HORMONE (TSH): Theoretically, soy might increase TSH levels. Soy can inhibit thyroid hormone synthesis resulting in increased secretion of TSH, and might potentially cause goiter. However, this seems to occur primarily in people with low iodine levels (6466,7806).

Interactions with Diseases or Conditions
ALLERGIC RHINITIS: People with allergic rhinitis are at increased risk for soy hull allergy. The risk and severity of symptoms increase with increased exposure (5084).
ASTHMA: People with asthma are at increased risk for soy hull allergy. The risk and severity of symptoms increase with increased exposure (5084).
BREAST CANCER: Soy isoflavones have estrogenic properties. Some experts are concerned about the use of soy in women with breast cancer because estrogens can increase this risk. However, some preclinical studies show that soy may have protective effects for breast cancer (3976), while others suggest soy might increase breast cell proliferation (3980,3981). Because there is insufficient reliable information about the effects of soy preparations in patients with breast cancer, a history of breast cancer, or a family history of breast cancer, therapeutic use of soy should be done with caution in these patients (956,7072,7655,8192).
CYSTIC FIBROSIS: Children with cystic fibrosis may develop hypoproteinemia when fed soymilk (368).
ENDOMETRIAL CANCER: Long-term use of concentrated soy isoflavone tablets 150 mg/day might increase the occurrence of endometrial hyperplasia (12105). Theoretically, taking these supplements might have an adverse effect on patients with endometrial cancer. However, there is no evidence that consuming soy foods adversely effects endometrial tissue. In fact, there is some evidence that consuming a diet high in soy foods might decrease the risk of endometrial cancer (7338,10372). Advise patients with endometrial cancer to avoid taking concentrated soy isoflavone supplements.
HYPOTHYROIDISM: Theoretically, soy might worsen hypothyroidism. Soy can inhibit thyroid hormone synthesis, increase thyroid stimulating hormone (TSH), and possibly cause goiter. However, this seems to occur primarily in people with low iodine levels (6466,7806); use with caution.
KIDNEY STONES (Nephrolithiasis): There is some concern that soy products might increase the risk of kidney stones because of its high oxalate content. Soy products can contain from 0.5 mg to 14 mg oxalate per gram or

approximately 43 mg to 640 mg per soy serving, depending on soy food type (7073). Tell patients with a history of kidney stones to avoid excessive consumption of soy.
MILK ALLERGY: Children who are severely allergic to cow's milk are frequently sensitive to soy as well (9883); use with caution or avoid.
RENAL FAILURE: In patients with end-stage renal disease (ESRD) phytoestrogens in soy may reach higher plasma concentrations, increasing the risk for toxicity (8522).
URINARY BLADDER CANCER: Soy products might increase the risk for urinary bladder cancer. Soy foods should be avoided in patients who are at risk or have a history of bladder cancer (9677).

Dosage and Administration

ORAL: For lowering cholesterol, a typical dose is 20-50 grams per day of soy protein (2293,2295,2296,3401,6412,7346). For preventing osteoporosis, 40 grams per day soy protein containing 2-2.25 mg isoflavones per gram has been used in clinical studies (842,6449). For reducing the severity and number of hot flashes, 20-60 grams per day of soy protein providing 34-76 mg isoflavones has been used in studies (2296,2297); soy extract tablets and capsules providing 50-60 mg soy isoflavones per day have also been used (4751,6455,11993). Genistein, a soy isoflavone, 54 mg per day has also been used for hot flashes (11994). For lowering cholesterol, 2.5 grams of soy phytosterols (sitosterol, campesterol, and stigmasterol) per day with the noon meal have been used for up to 4 weeks (8528). For reducing the risk of prostate cancer, two or more glasses of soymilk daily has been used (2298). For proteinuria, a diet limited to 700-800 mg/kg soy protein daily has been used (2287). For reducing cyclical breast pain in premenopausal women, 34 grams soy protein daily (as soymilk) has been used (2428). For diarrhea in infants, soy fiber fortified formula containing 18-20 grams of soy protein per liter has been used (2291,2292). For type 2 diabetes, touchi extract 300 mg three times daily with meals has been used (11762). Soy foods contain variable amounts of isoflavones. For type 2 diabetes in postmenopausal women, 30 grams of soy protein daily, containing 132 mg of phytoestrogens, has been used daily for up to 12 weeks (8531). Soy flour contains 2.6 mg isoflavones per gram of soy flour, fermented soy beans contain 1.3 mg per gram, boiled soybeans contain 0.6 mg per gram, soymilk contains 0.4 mg per gram, soybean curd contains 0.5 mg per gram, fried soybean curd contains 0.7 mg per gram, soybean paste contains 0.4 mg per gram, and soy sauce contains 0.016 mg per gram (7342).

SOYBEAN OIL

Also Known As

Intralipid, Legume, Soy, Soy Bean Oil, Soya Oil, Soybean, Soybean Oil, Soybeans, Soyca, Travmulsion.

Scientific Names

Glycine max, synonyms Glycine soja, Dolichos soja, Glycine gracilis, Glycine hispida, Phaseolus max Soja hispida, Soja max.
Family: Fabaceae/Leguminosae.

People Use This For

Orally, plant sterols, derived from soybean oil, are used to lower total and LDL cholesterol. Unsaponifiable fractions of soybean oil are used to treat osteoarthritis.
Parenterally, soybean oil is used in nutrient formulas. It is also used as a source of lecithin.

Safety

LIKELY SAFE ...when soybean oil or the plant sterols from soybean oil are used orally and appropriately in margarine. Hydrogenated soybean oil has generally recognized as safe (GRAS) status in the US (4912). ...when soybean oil is used in pharmaceutical grade parenteral formulas. Soybean oil is listed in the United States Pharmacopeia (10).
POSSIBLY SAFE ...when unsaponifiable fractions of soybean oil are used orally and appropriately in medicinal amounts. Unsaponifiable fractions of soybean oil appear to be safe for up to 6 months (10693).
PREGNANCY: LIKELY SAFE ...when used orally in amounts commonly found in foods. Avoid using in amounts greater than those typically found in foods. POSSIBLY SAFE ...when used parenterally. Theoretically, parenteral use of lipids like soybean oil during pregnancy might lead to hypertriglyceridemia, ketonemia, premature labor, and placental infection. However, women have used parenteral nutrition with lipids to treat severe morning sickness without any adverse effects (4084).
LACTATION: LIKELY SAFE ...when used orally in amounts commonly found in foods. Avoid using in amounts greater than those typically found in foods.

Effectiveness

EFFECTIVE

Parenteral nutrition. Soybean oil is effective when used as a parenteral nutrient (16).

POSSIBLY EFFECTIVE

Hypercholesterolemia. Soybean oil plant sterols used in margarine seem to help lower total and LDL cholesterol without affecting HDL (5336). The FDA has approved such labeling for the products Take Control and Benecol as a structure/function claim under the Dietary Supplement Health Education Act, not as a drug (4087).

Osteoarthritis. Taking unsaponifiable fractions of soybean and avocado oils orally appears to significantly improve pain and overall disability. It seems to be more effective for osteoarthritis of the hip than the knee (10693).

Mechanism of Action

Soybean oil is obtained by cold pressing the seeds of the Glycine soja. Soybean oil is used in parenteral nutrition as a source of fatty acids (16). In a comparison between diets with 20% fat from butter or soybean oil, people using soybean oil demonstrated a 12% decrease in LDL and a 3% reduction in HDL (4085). People using a margarine containing plant sterols from soybean oil reduced total and LDL cholesterol by 8-13% compared to a control group (5336).

Unsaponifiable fractions of plant oils, which are the residual matter obtained after hydrolysis of fatty acids, consist of sterols, squalene, terpenes, and vitamins (11785). Unsaponifiable fractions of soybean and avocado oils may reduce the progression of joint space loss in patients with osteoarthritis who have advanced joint space narrowing of the hip (10694). Preliminary evidence suggests this combination can inhibit cartilage degradation and promote cartilage repair in osteoarthritic chondrocytes (10695).

Adverse Reactions

Soybean oil can cause an allergic reaction in individuals allergic to the Fabaceae/Leguminosea family. Members of this family include peanuts, soybeans, and others (4079,4080).

Interactions with Herbs & Other Dietary Supplements

None known.

Interactions with Drugs

None known.

Interactions with Foods

None known.

Interactions with Lab Tests

CHOLESTEROL: Soybean oil sterols reduce serum total cholesterol and LDL cholesterol concentrations, and test results (5336).

Interactions with Diseases or Conditions

CROSS-ALLERGENICITY: Soybean oil may cause an allergic reaction in individuals sensitive to the Fabaceae/Leguminosea family. Members of this family include peanuts and soybeans (4079,4080).

Dosage and Administration

ORAL: In the form of a plant sterol-enriched margarine, such as Take Control, a serving size is one tablespoon, or 14 grams. For osteoarthritis, 300 mg daily (a combination of one-third avocado and two-thirds soybean unsaponifiables) has been used (10693).

PARENTERAL: No typical dosage.

SPANISH BROOM

Also Known As

Genet, Weaver's Broom.

CAUTION: See separate listings for Butcher's Broom, Scotch Broom flower, and Scotch Broom herb.

Scientific Names

Spartium junceum; Genista juncea.

Family: Fabaceae/Leguminosae.

People Use This For

Orally, Spanish broom is used as a laxative and diuretic.
In foods and beverages, Spanish broom extracts are used as flavor components.
In manufacturing, Spanish broom extract is used as a fragrance in soaps and cosmetics.

Safety

LIKELY SAFE ...when used orally in amounts commonly found in foods. Spanish broom has Generally Recognized As Safe (GRAS) status in the US (4912).
PREGNANCY AND LACTATION: POSSIBLY UNSAFE ...when used orally because large amounts of the alkaloid constituent sparteine can stimulate menstrual flow (19). The most common Spanish broom extract, Genet absolute, should not contain alkaloids because of the extraction method used, however, other extracts might (11).

Effectiveness

There is insufficient reliable information available about the effectiveness of Spanish broom.

Mechanism of Action

The applicable part of Spanish broom is the flower. Sparteine seems to hasten childbirth (11).

Adverse Reactions

None reported.

Interactions with Herbs & Other Dietary Supplements

None known.

Interactions with Drugs

None known.

Interactions with Foods

None known.

Interactions with Lab Tests

None known.

Interactions with Diseases or Conditions

None known.

Dosage and Administration

No typical dosage.

Comments

Avoid confusion with butcher's broom, scotch broom flower, and scotch broom herb. Spanish broom stems have appeared as an adulterant to scotch broom (Cytisus scoparius).

SPANISH ORIGANUM OIL

Also Known As

Origanum Oil, Sicilian Thyme, Spanish Origanum, Spanish Thyme.
CAUTION: See separate listings for Thyme Oil, Thyme, and Wild Thyme.

Scientific Names

Coridothymus capitatus, synonyms Satureja capitata, Thymus capitatus.
Family: Lamiaceae/Labiatae.

People Use This For

Topically, Spanish origanum oil is used for burns and to prevent and treat infections.
In foods and beverages, Spanish origanum oil is used as a flavor component.
In manufacturing, it is used as a fragrance component in soaps, cosmetics, and perfumes.

Safety

LIKELY SAFE ...when used orally in amounts commonly found in foods. Spanish origanum oil has Generally Recognized As Safe (GRAS) status in the US (4912).

There is insufficient reliable information available about the safety of Spanish origanum oil in medicinal amounts. **PREGNANCY AND LACTATION**: There is insufficient reliable information available about the safety of Spanish origanum oil in medicinal amounts during pregnancy; avoid using.

Effectiveness

There is insufficient reliable information available about the effectiveness of Spanish origanum oil.

Mechanism of Action

Spanish origanum oil is characterized by its carvacrol content (11). It contains carvacrol and thymol (11) which show some evidence of anthelmintic (11), antifungal (4059,4060,4062,4063), and antibacterial (4064,4065,4066) activity. These constituents also demonstrate some evidence of antioxidant activity, including decreased Fe (III) catalyzed phospholipid liposome peroxidation and peroxy radical scavenging activity (4067).

Adverse Reactions

None reported.

Interactions with Herbs & Other Dietary Supplements

None known.

Interactions with Drugs

None known.

Interactions with Foods

None known.

Interactions with Lab Tests

None known.

Interactions with Diseases or Conditions

None known.

Dosage and Administration

No typical dosage.

Comments

Spanish origanum oil is distilled from the flowering tops of Thymus capitatus and carvacrol-rich Origanum species.

SPEARMINT

Also Known As

Curled Mint, Fish Mint, Garden Mint, Green Mint, Lamb Mint, Mackerel Mint, Our Lady's Mint, Pahari Pudina, Putiha, Sage of Bethlehem, Spire Mint, Yerba Buena.
CAUTION: See separate listing for Sage.

Scientific Names

Mentha spicata, synonyms Mentha viridis, Mentha cordifolia, Mentha crispa.
Family: Lamiaceae/Labiatae.

People Use This For

Orally, spearmint is used for digestive disorders, including flatulence, indigestion, nausea, sore throat, diarrhea, colds, headaches, toothaches, cramps, cancer, bile duct and gallbladder inflammation, gallstones, upper gastrointestinal tract spasms, irritable bowel syndrome (IBS), and inflammation of respiratory tract. It is also used as an aromatic, stimulant, antiseptic, local anesthetic, and antispasmodic.
Topically, spearmint is used for oral mucosal inflammation, arthritis, local muscle and nerve pain, and skin conditions including pruritus and urticaria.
In foods and beverages, spearmint is used as a flavoring agent.
In manufacturing, spearmint is used in health food products, cosmetics, and oral hygiene products such as mouthwash and toothpaste.

Safety

LIKELY SAFE ...when used in amounts commonly found in foods. Spearmint and spearmint oil have Generally Recognized As Safe (GRAS) status (4912).

POSSIBLY SAFE ...when used orally or topically for medicinal reasons (11,12).
PREGNANCY AND LACTATION: Insufficient reliable information available; avoid using in amounts greater than those typically found in foods.

Effectiveness
There is insufficient reliable information available about the effectiveness of spearmint.

Mechanism of Action
The applicable parts of spearmint are the leaf and oil. There is insufficient reliable information available about the possible mechanism of action and active ingredients.

Adverse Reactions
None reported.

Interactions with Herbs & Other Dietary Supplements
None known.

Interactions with Drugs
None known.

Interactions with Foods
None known.

Interactions with Lab Tests
None known.

Interactions with Diseases or Conditions
None known.

Dosage and Administration
ORAL: Spearmint is used in tea, and is also available in tablets, capsules, tinctures and other oral formulations (11).
TOPICAL: No typical dosage.

SPINACH

Also Known As
Spinaciae folium, Spinatblatter.

Scientific Names
Spinacia oleracea, synonyms Spinacia inermis, Spinacia spinosa.
Family: Chenopodiaceae.

People Use This For
Orally, spinach is used for gastrointestinal complaints and fatigue. It is also used as a blood-builder, an appetite stimulant, for stimulating growth in children, and during convalescence.
In foods, spinach is a commonly consumed vegetable.

Safety
LIKELY SAFE ...when used in amounts commonly found in foods.
CHILDREN: LIKELY UNSAFE ...when used orally in infants under 4 months old; the nitrate content can cause methemoglobinemia (18).
PREGNANCY AND LACTATION: LIKELY SAFE ...when used in amounts commonly found in foods; avoid medicinal amounts.

Effectiveness
There is insufficient reliable information available about the effectiveness of spinach.

Mechanism of Action
The applicable part of spinach is the leaf. Spinach contains vitamin C, vitamin E, vitamin K, magnesium, and nitrates (18,19,11285). It also contains triterpene saponins and oxalic acid (18). Spinach is thought to have hypoglycemic effects (19). Consumption of fresh spinach is associated with a decreased risk of stomach cancer in humans (4112). Preliminary research suggests that compounds contained in spinach might slow aging effects on the nervous system (1418,1419).

Adverse Reactions
Orally, spinach may cause methemoglobinemia in infants younger than 4 months old (18).

Interactions with Herbs & Other Dietary Supplements
CALCIUM, IRON, ZINC: Concurrent use might decrease mineral absorption. Spinach contains oxalate (7,12), which can bind multivalent metal ions in the gastrointestinal tract and decrease mineral absorption.

Interactions with Drugs
ANTIDIABETES DRUGS: Monitor blood glucose level closely due to claims that spinach leaves have hypoglycemic effects (19).
WARFARIN (Coumadin): Spinach contains vitamin K. Individuals using anticoagulants should consume a consistent daily amount to maintain the effect of anticoagulant therapy (19).

Interactions with Foods
CALCIUM, IRON, ZINC: Concurrent use might decrease mineral absorption from foods. Spinach contains oxalate (7,12), which can bind multivalent metal ions in the gastrointestinal tract and decrease mineral absorption.

Interactions with Lab Tests
INTERNATIONAL NORMALIZED RATIO (INR)/PROTHROMBIN TIME (PT): Theoretically, spinach might decrease coagulation test results due to high vitamin K content (11285).

Interactions with Diseases or Conditions
DIABETES: Theoretically, spinach may interfere with blood glucose control (19).
KIDNEY DISEASE: Spinach may cause formation of insoluble oxalate crystals in the kidneys causing further damage (19).

Dosage and Administration
No typical dosage.

SPINY RESTHARROW

Also Known As
Cammock, Ground Furze, Hauhechelwurzel, Land Whin, Ononidis radix, Petty Whin, Restharrow, Stay Plough, Stinking Tommy, Wild Liquorice.

Scientific Names
Ononis spinosa.
Family: Fabaceae/Leguminosae.

People Use This For
Orally, spiny restharrow is used for gout, kidney and bladder stones, rheumatic complaints, urinary tract infections, irrigation therapy for inflammatory disease of the lower urinary tract, and prevention and treatment of kidney gravel.

Safety
POSSIBLY SAFE ...when used orally and appropriately (2).
PREGNANCY AND LACTATION: Insufficient reliable information available; avoid using.

Effectiveness
There is insufficient reliable information available about the effectiveness of spiny restharrow.

Mechanism of Action
The applicable part of spiny restharrow is the root. It contains isoflavonoids including ononin (2,18), triterpenes including alphaonoceradiendiol (18), and volatile oil (18). The volatile oil contains anethole, carvone, and menthol (18). Spiny restharrow is reported to have a diuretic effect (2,18).

Adverse Reactions
None reported.

Interactions with Herbs & Other Dietary Supplements
None known.

Interactions with Drugs
None known.

Interactions with Foods
None known.

Interactions with Lab Tests
None known.

Interactions with Diseases or Conditions
EDEMA: Contraindicated in individuals with edema resulting from cardiac or kidney impairment (2,18).

Dosage and Administration
ORAL: A typical oral dose is 6-12 grams daily or as a tea (2,18). To prepare tea, pour boiling water over 2-2.5 grams of ground drug, strain after 20-30 minutes (18). Drink with plenty of liquid (2,18).

SPLEEN EXTRACT

Also Known As
Bovine Spleen, Hydrolyzed Spleen Extract, Predigested Spleen Extract, Raw Spleen, Spleen, Spleen Concentrate, Spleen Factors, Spleen Peptides, Spleen Polypeptides, Splenopentin, Tuftsin.

Scientific Names
None.

People Use This For
Orally, spleen extract is used as replacement therapy after splenectomy or in people with inadequate spleen function. It is also used orally for treating people with low white blood cell counts, enhancing general immune function and immune function in people with cancer, and for treating bacterial infections. Spleen extract is also used orally for treating celiac disease, dermatitis herpetiformis, glomerulonephritis, HIV-related bacterial infections, rheumatoid arthritis, systemic lupus erythematosus, thrombocytopenia, ulcerative colitis, and vasculitis.

Safety
There is insufficient reliable information available about the safety of spleen extract. However, since spleen extract preparations are derived from animals, there is concern about contamination with diseased animal parts (1825). So far, there are no reports of disease transmission to humans due to use of contaminated spleen extract.
Pregnancy and Lactation: Insufficient reliable information available; avoid using.

Effectiveness
There is insufficient reliable information available about the effectiveness of spleen extract.

Mechanism of Action
Spleen extract is derived from fresh animal spleens. Spleen extract contains the peptides tuftsin and splenopentin (6614). Tuftsin stimulates phagocytosis, motility, and immunogenic response of phagocytic cells, and has bactericidal and tumoricidal activities (6660). Tuftsin activity correlates inversely with splenic function (6662). Spleen extracts are tried in people with HIV disease because some patients have significantly lower tuftsin activity than healthy people (6662). There is preliminary evidence that spleen extract might protect against radiation. Spleen extract seems to shorten the time to regain normal immune response in animals exposed to sublethal doses of radiation (6661).

Adverse Reactions
Adverse reactions have not been reported. However, there is some concern about contamination. Spleen extract is derived from raw animal spleens gathered from slaughterhouses, possibly from sick or diseased animals. Products made from contaminated or diseased organs might present a human health hazard. There is also concern that spleen extracts produced from cows in countries where bovine spongiform encephalitis (BSE) has been reported might be contaminated with diseased tissue. Countries where BSE has been reported include Great Britain, France, The

Netherlands, Portugal, Luxembourg, Ireland, Switzerland, Oman, and Belgium (1825). There have been no reports of BSE transfer to humans from contaminated spleen extract products. Until more is known, tell patients to avoid these products unless country of origin can be determined. Patients should avoid products that are produced in countries where BSE has been found.

Interactions with Herbs & Other Dietary Supplements
None known.

Interactions with Drugs
None known.

Interactions with Foods
None known.

Interactions with Lab Tests
None known.

Interactions with Diseases or Conditions
None known.

Dosage and Administration
ORAL: A typical dose is approximately 1.5 grams total spleen peptides (equivalent to 50 mg of tuftsin and splenopentin) per day (6614).

SQUALAMINE

Also Known As
Spiny Dogfish Shark.

Scientific Names
Squalus acanthias (Spiny dogfish).
Family: Squalidae.

People Use This For
Orally, squalamine is used as an antibiotic.
Topically, synthetic squalamine compounds have been used as antibiotics.
In combination with captopril, oral squalamine is being investigated as an anti-angiogenic therapy for diabetic retinopathy.
Squalamine is also being investigated as a possible treatment for pediatric solid tumors.

Safety
There is insufficient reliable information available about the safety of squalamine or its derivative SM-7.
Pregnancy and Lactation: Insufficient reliable information available.

Effectiveness
There is insufficient reliable information available about the effectiveness of squalamine or its derivative SM-7.

Mechanism of Action
Squalamine was first isolated from the spiny dogfish shark and later synthesized synthetically. It shows evidence that it might have fungicidal and antiprotozoal activity (4139). Squalamine has also demonstrated significant activity against gram (-) and gram (+) bacteria (4139). Some compounds that mimic the structure of squalamine show promise in their activity against gram (-) rods, gram (+) cocci including methicillin-resistant Staphylococcus aureus, vancomycin-resistant Enterococcus faecium, and fungi (4138). In addition to antibiotic activity, squalamine also shows promise in inhibiting angiogenesis, and preventing formation and growth of tumors (4137,5043). Squalamine has also demonstrated activity against breast cancer, lung cancer, and neuroblastoma cancer (5043).

Adverse Reactions
None reported.

Interactions with Herbs & Other Dietary Supplements
None known.

Interactions with Drugs
None known.

Interactions with Foods
None known.

Interactions with Lab Tests
None known.

Interactions with Diseases or Conditions
None known.

Dosage and Administration
No typical dosage.

Comments
Avoid confusion with shark cartilage, which is prepared from the cartilage of spiny dogfish shark, hammerhead shark (Sphyrna lewini), and other shark species. Squalamine has been isolated from the stomach and liver tissues of the spiny dogfish shark. Synthetic products that mimic the structure of squalamine appear to be good candidates for further development as topical antimicrobial agents. They have broad spectrum antimicrobial activity, but their potential for systemic toxicity limits their use (4138).
Researchers at Georgetown University Medical Center plan a study of squalamine as an antiangiogenic therapy in combination with captopril for diabetic retinopathy (1269).
Magainin, the manufacturer of an investigational squalamine drug product plans a clinical study of squalamine in the treatment of pediatric solid tumors (5043).

SQUAWVINE

Also Known As
Checkerberry, Deerberry, Hive Vine, Noon Kie Oo Nah Yeah, One-Berry, Partridgeberry, Running Box, Squaw Berry, Squaw Vine, Twinberry, Two-Eyed Berry, Winter Clover.

Scientific Names
Mitchella repens.
Family: Rubiaceae.

People Use This For
Orally, squawvine is used for amenorrhea, anxiety, diarrhea, edema, excessive menstruation, fibrocystic disease of the breast, oliguria, painful menstruation, postpartum depression, varicose veins, to ease childbirth, improving lactation, insomnia, congestive heart failure, kidney failure, liver failure, chronic dysentery, spermatorrhea, as an emmenagogue, as an abortifacient, as an astringent for treating colitis, and to reduce mucous membrane and leukorrheal discharges.
Topically, squawvine is used for treating sore nipples.

Safety
POSSIBLY SAFE ...when used orally and appropriately (12).
There is insufficient reliable information about the safety of squawvine topically.
PREGNANCY: POSSIBLY UNSAFE ...when used orally due to reported abortifacient properties (12).
LACTATION: Insufficient reliable information available; avoid using.

Effectiveness
There is insufficient reliable information available about the effectiveness of squawvine.

Mechanism of Action
The applicable parts of squawvine are the above ground parts. Squawvine is reported to contain resin, wax, mucilages, dextrin, saponins, alkaloids, glycosides, and tannins (410).

Adverse Reactions
None reported.

Interactions with Herbs & Other Dietary Supplements
None known.

Interactions with Drugs
None known.

Interactions with Foods
None known.

Interactions with Lab Tests
None known.

Interactions with Diseases or Conditions
None known.

Dosage and Administration
ORAL: A typical dose is 20-50 mg.

SQUILL

Also Known As
European Squill, Indian Squill, Mediterranean Squill, Red Squill, Scilla, Sea Onion, Sea Squill Bulb, White Squill.

Scientific Names
Urginea indica, synonyms Drimia indica, Scilla indica; Urginea maritima, synonyms Drimia maritima, Scilla maritima, Urginea scilla.
Family: Liliaceae or Hyacinthaceae.

People Use This For
Orally, squill is used for mild heart failure, arrhythmias, nervous heart complaints, some venous conditions, edema, emetic, as an expectorant, for chronic bronchitis, asthma with bronchitis, and whooping cough. Squill is also used orally as a diuretic, abortifacient, heart tonic, and a rat poison.
In manufacturing, squill is used in pest control as a rodenticide (red squill).

Safety
UNSAFE ...when used orally (4,6,18,512). Squill contains cardiac glycosides that can cause adverse effects (512).
PREGNANCY: UNSAFE ...when used orally because it can have an abortifacient effect (4).
LACTATION: UNSAFE ...when used orally (4).

Effectiveness
There is insufficient reliable information available about the effectiveness of squill.

Mechanism of Action
Squill contains cardioactive glycosides, including bufadienolides, scillaren A, and proscillaridin A (4,6,18). Squill seems to have cardiac effects similar to digoxin, including positive inotropic and negative chronotropic effects (4,7). The aglycones in squill are poorly absorbed from the gastrointestinal tract and are therefore less potent than digitalis cardiac glycosides. Squill has additional cardiovascular properties that include reducing left ventricular diastolic pressure, and reducing pathologically elevated venous pressure (18). Large amounts of squill can induce vomiting due to gastric irritation and central action (4). In lesser amounts squill causes an expectorant-like effect (6).

Adverse Reactions
Orally, squill can cause gastric irritation, loss of appetite, diarrhea, vomiting, stomach disorders, headache, irregular pulse (18), and convulsions (6). Skin contact with the fresh bulb can cause dermatitis (18). Signs of overdose include restlessness, nausea, vomiting, life-threatening arrhythmias (ventricular tachycardia, atrial tachycardia with atrioventricular block, ventricular fibrillation), stupor, vision disorders, depression, confusion, hallucinations, psychosis, seizure, cardiac arrest, asphyxiation, and death (18,3488). A fatality has been reported after ingestion of squill bulb (3488).

Interactions with Herbs & Other Dietary Supplements
CARDIAC GLYCOSIDE-CONTAINING HERBS: Contraindicated, and concomitant use can increase the risk of cardiac glycoside toxicity. Cardiac glycoside-containing herbs include black hellebore, Canadian hemp roots,

digitalis leaf, hedge mustard, figwort, lily of the valley roots, motherwort, oleander leaf, pheasant's eye plant, pleurisy root, strophanthus seeds, and uzara (19).
LICORICE/HORSETAIL: Theoretically, overuse/misuse of licorice rhizome or horsetail plant with cardiac glycoside-containing herbs increases the risk of cardiac toxicity due to potassium depletion (19).
OTHER CARDIOACTIVE HERBS: Avoid concomitant use with other cardioactive herbs due to unpredictability of effects and adverse effects. Other cardioactive herbs include calamus, cereus, cola, coltsfoot, devil's claw, European mistletoe, fenugreek, fumitory, ginger, Panax ginseng, hawthorn, white horehound, mate, parsley, quassia, scotch broom flower, shepherd's purse, and wild carrot (4). See individual product listings.
STIMULANT LAXATIVE HERBS: Theoretically, overuse or misuse of stimulant laxatives with cardiac glycoside-containing herbs increases the risk of cardiac toxicity due to potassium depletion (19). Stimulant laxative herbs include aloe dried leaf sap, blue flag rhizome, alder buckthorn, European buckthorn, butternut bark, cascara bark, castor oil, colocynth fruit pulp, gamboge bark exudate, jalap root, black root, manna bark exudate, podophyllum root, rhubarb root, senna leaves and pods, wild cucumber fruit (Ecballium elaterium), and yellow dock root.

Interactions with Drugs
CALCIUM SUPPLEMENTS: Concomitant use of calcium may increase risk of cardiac toxicity (3805).
CORTICOSTEROIDS: Concomitant use may increase effects and adverse effects of long-term corticosteroid use (2).
DIGOXIN (Lanoxin): Concomitant use is contraindicated due to therapeutic duplication and increased risk of cardiac glycoside toxicity (4).
DIURETIC DRUGS: Theoretically, concomitant use of potassium-depleting diuretics and squill can increase the risk of cardiac glycoside toxicity due to potassium depletion (19). Some diuretics that can deplete potassium include chlorothiazide (Diuril), chlorthalidone (Thalitone), furosemide (Lasix), hydrochlorothiazide (HCTZ, HydroDIURIL, Microzide), and others.
QUINIDINE: Concomitant use may increase the risk of cardiac and adverse effects (2).
STIMULANT LAXATIVES: Concomitant use of squill and stimulant laxatives may increase risk of cardiac glycoside toxicity due to potassium loss (19).

Interactions with Foods
None known.

Interactions with Lab Tests
None known.

Interactions with Diseases or Conditions
CARDIAC CONDITIONS: Contraindicated in individuals with second or third degree atrioventricular block, hypertrophic cardiomyopathy, carotid sinus syndrome, ventricular tachycardia, or thoracic aortic aneurysm Wolff-Parkinson-White syndrome (18).
ELECTROLYTE IMBALANCE: Contraindicated in individuals with hypokalemia or hypercalcemia.
GI CONDITIONS: Can irritate gastrointestinal tract. Contraindicated in individuals with infectious or inflammatory gastrointestinal conditions (19).

Dosage and Administration
ORAL: Mild heart failure (NYHA stage I and II heart disease), 100-500 mg standardized squill bulb powder per day (7).

Comments
Squill is unsafe for self-medication (512). New York Heart Association (NYHA) stage I and II heart disease refers to people with heart disease who do not have limitations of physical activity. They are comfortable at rest but ordinary physical activity results in fatigue, palpitation, trouble breathing, or anginal pain (2).

ST. JOHN'S WORT

Also Known As
Amber, Amber Touch-and-Heal, Demon Chaser, Fuga Daemonum, Goatweed, Hardhay, Hypereikon, Hyperici Herba, Hypericum, Klamath Weed, Millepertuis, Rosin Rose, Saynt Johannes Wort, SJW, Tipton Weed.

Scientific Names
Hypericum perforatum.
Family: Hypericaceae or Clusiaceae.

People Use This For

Orally, St. John's wort is used for depression, dysthymia, anxiety, heart palpitations, mood disturbances associated with menopause, attention deficit-hyperactivity disorder (ADHD), obsessive-compulsive disorder (OCD), and seasonal affective disorder (SAD). Other uses include exhaustion, fibrositis, headache, migraine headache, muscle pain, neuralgia, and sciatica. It is also used orally for secondary symptoms associated with depression such as fatigue, loss of appetite, insomnia, and anxiety. It is also used orally for cancer, vitiligo, HIV/AIDS, hepatitis C, and as a diuretic. Oily St. John's wort preparations are used orally for gastric indigestion.
Topically, oily St. John's wort preparations are used for treating bruises and abrasions, inflammation and muscle pain, first degree burns, wound healing, bug bites, hemorrhoids, vitiligo, and neuralgia.
In manufacturing, the hypericin-free extracts of St. John's wort are used in the making of alcoholic beverages.

Safety

LIKELY SAFE ...when used orally and appropriately, short-term. St. John's wort extracts seem to be safe when used for up to 8 weeks (3547,3548,3549,3550,3551,3552,4835,5087,5096,6400,6434,7047).
POSSIBLY UNSAFE ...when used orally in large doses. St. John's wort extract can be unsafe due to the risk of severe phototoxic skin reactions. Taking 2-4 grams St. John's wort extract (5-10 mg hypericin) daily appears to increase the risk of photosensitivity (758,4631,7808).
CHILDREN: POSSIBLY SAFE ...when used orally, and appropriately, short-term. St. John's wort extracts seem to be safe when used in children under 12 years of age for up to 6 weeks (4538).
PREGNANCY: POSSIBLY UNSAFE ...when used orally. Preliminary research suggests that constituents of St. John's wort might have teratogenic effects (9687); avoid using.
LACTATION: POSSIBLY UNSAFE ...when used orally. Nursing infants can experience colic, drowsiness, and lethargy (1377); avoid using.
There is insufficient reliable information available about the safety of the topical use of St. John's wort.

Effectiveness

LIKELY EFFECTIVE

Depression. St. John's wort extracts, standardized based on hypericin content, are superior to placebo (203,204,205,376,3548,3549,3551,3552,4899,6428,9597), likely as effective as low-dose tricyclic antidepressants (3548,3549,3551,6434), and possibly as effective as the selective serotonin reuptake inhibitors (SSRIs) fluoxetine (Prozac) (3550,4897) and sertraline (Zoloft) (6400). Extracts standardized based on hyperforin content also seem to be effective (761,4538,4630). Most studies have evaluated St. John's wort in adults. However, there is also some evidence it might be effective for depression in children 6 to 16 years old (4538,10844). The effectiveness of St. John's wort for depression has been called into question based on equivocal findings of two studies in psychiatric settings (5096,10843). However, the overwhelming majority of evidence in primary care settings shows that St. John's wort is effective for many patients. Patients in primary care settings may have less severe depression than patients seeking psychiatric care (11154). Consider St. John's wort as another option along with conventional antidepressants for treatment of mild to moderate depression (5087,9597). However, St. John's wort is not appropriate for more severely depressed patients.
Most clinical studies on the effectiveness of St. John's wort have used preparations containing the specific standardized extract Lichtwer LI 160, containing 0.3% hypericin (382,4538). LI 160 is contained in the product Kira (Lichtwer Pharma US, Inc.). Lichtwer LI 160 WS is the hyperforin stabilized version of LI 160. LI 160 WS is contained in the product Quanterra Emotional Balance (Warner-Lambert). Some studies have also used the extract ZE 117, containing 0.2% hypericin (4897,6434). ZE 117 is contained in the product Remotiv (Zeller). One study also used the extract WS 5572, containing 5% hyperforin (761,4630). WS 5572 is contained in the product Movana (Pharmaton).

POSSIBLY EFFECTIVE

Anxiety. Taking standardized hypericum extract, LI 160, orally seems to reduce anxiety symptoms and objective measures of anxiety (9476). However, increased anxiety with St. John's wort may also occur (3569).

POSSIBLY INEFFECTIVE

Hepatitis C. Taking St. John's wort orally as an antiretroviral agent doesn't seem to be effective for treating adults with chronic Hepatitis C Virus (HCV) infection. St. John's wort does not appear to have any detectable antiviral activity in patients with chronic HCV infection (4631).

HIV/AIDS. Taking St. John's wort orally as an antiretroviral agent doesn't seem to be effective for treating HIV-infected adults (206).

Polyneuropathy. Taking St. John's wort orally doesn't seem to relieve most measures of pain in diabetic and non-diabetic patients with polyneuropathy (7047).

INSUFFICIENT RELIABLE EVIDENCE to RATE

Obsessive-compulsive disorder (OCD). Early evidence suggests St. John's wort might be useful for OCD. An extended-release formulation of St. John's wort standardized to 0.3% hypericin taken for 12 weeks seems to significantly improve symptoms in some patients with OCD (5075).

Premenstrual syndrome (PMS). There is preliminary clinical evidence that St. John's wort might be beneficial for PMS. St. John's wort extract standardized to 0.3% hypericin seems to improve symptoms of PMS by approximately 50% in some women (6429).

Seasonal affective disorder (SAD). Preliminary clinical research suggests that St. John's wort might help SAD. St. John's wort appears to improve symptoms of anxiety, decreased libido, and sleep disturbances associated with SAD. It is useful alone or in combination with light therapy (9686).
More evidence is needed to rate St. John's wort for these uses.

Mechanism of Action

The applicable parts of St. John's wort are the flowers and to a lesser extent, the leaves. Several active constituents have been isolated. Two constituents that play a significant role are hypericin and hyperforin (761). Although hypericin was formerly thought to be the component of St. John's wort principally responsible for its action, it is now understood that hyperforin, adhyperforin, and several other related compounds are the primary active constituents (762,763,4521,4629,7807,11408). Both hyperforin and adhyperforin appear to modulate the effects of serotonin, dopamine, and noradrenaline (763,3553,4521,6474,11408); and act as serotonergic 5-HT3 and 5-HT4 receptor antagonists (762). This influence on neurotransmission then appears to cause cortisol stimulation in a dose-dependent manner (11408). Hyperforin also inhibits synaptosomal uptake of gamma-butyric acid (GABA) and L-glutamate (3553,4521). Extracts of St. John's wort inhibit reuptake of serotonin, norepinephrine, and dopamine in vitro (763,6427,8936); and down-regulate beta-adrenergic, and serotonergic 5-HT1 and 5-HT2 receptors when used chronically in animals (763,4632).

St. John's wort effects on serotonin may be primarily responsible for its antidepressant activity (8936). Many constituents appear to contribute to the antidepressant action (762,4520,4521). Hypericin inhibits catechol-O-methyl transferase (COMT) and monoamine oxidase (MAO) in vitro. However, hypericin does not reach adequate concentrations in human tissue to achieve these effects (167,759). Hypericin also has affinity for sigma receptors and acts as a receptor antagonist at adenosine, benzodiazepine, GABA-A, GABA-B, and inositol triphosphate receptors (759). Preclinical research suggests that a 50% ethanolic extract of St. John's wort might have anxiolytic activity (8932).

When used in humans, St. John's wort induces some of the cytochrome P450 (CYP450) enzymes. This results in increased metabolism and reduced plasma concentrations of many drugs (1292,1293,1303,3570,3599,4835,6425,7808). It appears that the hyperforin constituent is responsible for interactions. Hypericin doesn't seem to have any effect on drug metabolism (11889). St. John's wort extract increases induction activity of CYP3A4 by 98% (1303). The effect on CYP3A4 seems to be greater in females than males (10830,10847,11889). It also induces CYP2C9 and CYP1A2 (11889,11890). St. John's wort does not affect or has a marginal effect on CYP2D6 (3599,4835,10830,10847,10848,11889). Some discrepancies in reports about the effect of St. John's wort on CYP isozymes may reflect variability in St. John's wort preparations (10849).

The hyperforin constituent in St. John's wort seems to bind to a nuclear receptor called the pregnane X receptor (PXR), which results in increased expression of CYP3A4 (6463,6475). St. John's wort also induces the intestinal P-glycoprotein/multi-drug resistance 1 (MDR-1) drug transporter (1340). Induction of both intestinal P-glycoprotein/MDR-1 and hepatic CYP3A4 decreases the intestinal absorption and increases hepatic first pass clearance of numerous drugs such as cyclosporine, indinavir, and amitriptyline (382,1340,7808,7810).

St. John's wort does not significantly affect N-acetyltransferase (NAT2) (3571). St. John's wort extracts can prolong narcotic-induced sleep time, decrease barbiturate-induced sleep time, and antagonize the effects of reserpine (758).

There is preliminary evidence that St. John's wort can enhance the analgesic effect of morphine, but St. John's wort alone does not have analgesic effects (1279).

Topical preparations are thought to be beneficial for inflammatory skin conditions and superficial wounds by inhibiting epidermal inflammatory response. It is likely that both the hypericin and hyperforin contribute to this effect (6426).

Hypericin is photodynamically active and is thought to be the constituent responsible for phototoxic reactions (3547). However, the flavonoid component of St. John's wort, primarily quercitrin, appears to play a role in controlling the severity of the phototoxic reactions (11490). St. John's wort and its constituents, hypericin and pseudohypericin, have activity against viruses and bacteria, including influenza virus, herpes simplex virus types I and II, Sindbis virus, poliovirus, retrovirus, murine cytomegalovirus (CMV), hepatitis C, and Gram negative and Gram positive bacteria. Hyperforin can inhibit growth of penicillin- and methicillin-resistant Staphylococcus aureus and other Gram positive organisms, but not Gram negative organisms (3554).

Hyperforin might have activity against cancer cells. It seems to inhibit the growth of a variety of cancer cell types by inducing apoptosis (9205). It is not known if these effects will have clinical applicability. Several factors might influence product variability of St. John's wort. The constituents of St. John's wort seem to have seasonal and regional variations (8933,8934). The hyperforin and hypericin constituents appear to be sensitive to light; amber containers or opaque capsules don't seem to completely protect from light degradation. These constituents may also be sensitive to storage temperature and humidity (8935). Preclinical research suggests that hypericin is teratogenic in rat embryos (9687). The effect of hypericin and St. John's wort on the human embryo is unknown.

Adverse Reactions

Orally, St. John's wort is usually well tolerated. Side effects can include insomnia, vivid dreams, restlessness, anxiety, agitation, irritability, gastrointestinal (GI) discomfort, fatigue, dry mouth, dizziness, and headache (394,758,3547,3569,4518,7808,9881,10845). St. John's wort can also cause skin rash, paresthesia, and hypoglycemia (4835,5073,7404). Insomnia can often be alleviated by decreasing the dose or taking St. John's wort in the morning (3569). In clinical trials, the incidence of adverse effects in patients treated with St. John's wort is similar to placebo and less than conventional antidepressants (4899,10845).

St. John's wort can induce hypomania in depressed patients (325,3524,3568) and mania in depressed patients with occult bipolar disorder (3555,10845).
Both topical use and chronic oral use of St. John's wort can cause significant photodermatitis (206,620,758,4631,6477). The average threshold dose range for an increased risk of photosensitivity appears to be 2-4 grams St. John's wort extract or 5-10 mg hypericin, daily. Lower doses might not cause this effect (4542,7808). For example, a single dose of St. John's wort extract 1800 mg, 5.4 mg hypericin, followed by 900 mg (2.7 mg hypericin) daily does not seem to produce skin hypericin concentrations thought to be high enough to cause phototoxicity (3900,4542). Light or fair-skinned people should employ protective measures against direct sunlight when using St. John's wort either topically or orally (628). Total body erythroderma without exposure to sunlight, accompanied by burning sensation of the skin, has also been reported (8930).
In isolated cases, St. John's wort has been associated with a syndrome consisting of extreme anxiety, confusion, nausea, hypertension, and tachycardia. These symptoms may occur within two to three weeks after it is started, in patients with no other predisposing factors. This syndrome has been diagnosed as the serotonin syndrome (6201,7811). In one case, the symptoms began after consuming foods containing tyramine including aged cheese and red wine (7812). Cardiovascular collapse following induction of anesthesia has been reported in an otherwise healthy patient who had been taking St. John's wort for six months (8931).
St. John's wort can cause intermenstrual or abnormal menstrual bleeding (1292). However, this effect has occurred in patients who were also taking an oral contraceptive. Changes in menstrual bleeding might be the result of a drug interaction (1292).
Overall, St. John's wort extracts seem to be better tolerated than tricyclic antidepressants (3548,3549), but similarly or better tolerated than fluoxetine (Prozac) (3550) and sertraline (Zoloft) (4897,6400). Unlike tricyclic antidepressants, research in healthy volunteers suggests that St. John's wort does not affect heart rate variability. It also doesn't appear to affect cognitive function (11800).
Sexual dysfunction can occur with St. John's wort, but less frequently than with SSRIs (10843). There is one report of loss of sexual libido in a man who took St. John's wort for nine months (7312).
Some in vitro evidence suggests that high doses of St. John's wort might reduce male and female fertility (4239,4240). This effect has not been demonstrated in humans, and animal studies suggest that St. John's wort doesn't adversely affect fertility or gestation 10846.
Neuropathy can also occur with use of St. John's wort (621). There is some speculation that St. John's wort might be associated with a higher incidence of cataracts. The hypericin constituent is photoactive and, in the presence of light, may damage lens proteins, leading to cataracts (1296); however, this effect has not been verified in humans.
St. John's wort has been associated with withdrawal effects similar to those found with conventional antidepressants. Headache, nausea, anorexia, dry mouth, thirst, cold chills, weight loss, dizziness, insomnia, paresthesias, confusion, and fatigue have been reported. Withdrawal effects are most likely to occur within two days after discontinuation, but can occur one week or more after stopping treatment in some people. Occurrence of withdrawal symptoms may not be related to dose or duration of use (3569,11801). Photosensitivity might occur in individuals with light or fair skin, diseased or open-wounded skin, or after extended periods of direct sunlight when using St. John's wort topically (206,620,628,758,4628). Sjogren's syndrome has been reported in a patient taking herbal supplements including St. John's wort, echinacea, and kava. Echinacea may have been the primary cause, because Sjogren's syndrome is an autoimmune disorder. The role of St. John's wort in causing this syndrome is unclear (10319).

Interactions with Herbs & Other Dietary Supplements

DIGITALIS: Concomitant use might reduce the therapeutic effects of digitalis. The St. John's wort extract, LI 160, decreases digoxin serum levels in healthy people. St. John's wort seems to lower digoxin serum concentrations by approximately 25%. St. John's wort seems to induces the activity of the carrier protein P-glycoprotein, which increases the clearance of digitalis (382,6473,7808,7810,9204).
HERBS AND SUPPLEMENTS WITH SEROTONERGIC PROPERTIES: Theoretically, St. John's wort might increase the effects and adverse effects of products that increase serotonin levels; including 5-hydroxytryptophan (5-HTP), Hawaiian baby woodrose, L-tryptophan, and SAMe (763,6427,8936,9204).

Interactions with Drugs

5-HT1 AGONISTS (Triptans): Theoretically, concomitant use of St. John's wort with selective serotonin agonists can increase the risk of serotonergic adverse effects and possibly serotonin syndrome. Concomitant use should be avoided (9204). The "triptans" include frovatriptan (Frova), naratriptan (Amerge), rizatriptan (Maxalt), sumatriptan (Imitrex), and zolmitriptan (Zomig). Also, concurrent use might theoretically cause cerebral vasoconstriction disorders such as Call-Fleming syndrome (8056).
ALPRAZOLAM (Xanax): St. John's wort may decrease the effect of alprazolam. Alprazolam, which is used as a probe for cytochrome P450 3A4 (CYP3A4) activity, has a two-fold increase in clearance when given with St. John's wort. St. John's wort reduces the half-life of alprazolam from 12.4 hours to 6 hours (10830).
AMINOLEVULINIC ACID: Concomitant use with St. John's wort extract may cause synergistic phototoxicity. Delta-aminolevulinic acid (an investigational drug used in oncologic diagnostic procedures) can cause a burning erythematous rash and severe swelling of the face, neck, and hands when taken with St. John's wort (9474).
AMITRIPTYLINE (Elavil): Concomitant use can reduce serum concentrations of amitriptyline by 22% and its metabolite, nortriptyline, by 42% (1378,7808). St. John's wort induces intestinal and hepatic CYP3A4 and intestinal

P-glycoprotein/MDR-1, a drug transporter, which increases amitriptyline clearance (1340).
ANTIDEPRESSANT DRUGS: Concomitant use can lead to increased adverse effects and increase the risk of serotonergic side effects, including serotonin syndrome (166,542,3569). Although this effect has only been reported with nefazodone (Serzone), paroxetine (Paxil), and sertraline (Zoloft), it might also occur with other antidepressants. Use of St. John's wort with other antidepressants should only be done with close supervision. Also, concurrent use might theoretically cause cerebral vasoconstriction disorders such as Call-Fleming syndrome (8056).
BARBITURATES: St. John's wort can decrease barbiturate-induced sleep time (758). Some of these sedative medications include pentobarbital (Nembutal), phenobarbital (Luminal), secobarbital (Seconal), and others.
CONTRACEPTIVE DRUGS: Concomitant use can decrease steroid concentrations resulting in breakthrough bleeding, irregular menstrual bleeding, or unwanted pregnancy. St. John's wort increases the clearance of estrogens and progesterones in contraceptive drugs (11886,11887). Bleeding irregularities have usually occurred after one week of starting St. John's wort and regular cycles returned when St. John's wort is discontinued. Unwanted pregnancy has occurred with concurrent use of oral contraceptives and St. John's wort extract (9880). St. John's wort is thought to induce the cytochrome P450 1A2 (CYP1A2), 2C9 (CYP2C9), and 3A4 (CYP3A4) enzymes, which are responsible for metabolism of oral contraceptives (1292,7809,9204). Women taking St. John's wort and oral contraceptives concurrently should use an additional or alternative form of birth control.
CYCLOSPORINE (Neoral, Sandimmune): Concomitant use can decrease plasma cyclosporine levels by 30-70% (1234,4826,4831,4834,7808,9596,10628). Using St. John's wort with cyclosporine in patients with heart, kidney, or liver transplants can cause subtherapeutic cyclosporine levels and acute transplant rejection (1234,1293,1301,6112,6435,7808,9596). This interaction has occurred with a St. John's wort extract standardized to 0.3% hypericin and dosed at 300-600 mg per day (6435,10628). Withdrawal of St. John's wort can result in increased cyclosporine levels by 64% (1234,4513,4826,4831,4834). St. John's wort induces cytochrome P450 3A4 (CYP3A4) and the multi-drug transporter, P-glycoprotein/MDR-1, which increases cyclosporine clearance (1293,1340,9204,9596).
CYTOCHROME P450 1A2 (CYP1A2) SUBSTRATES: St. John's wort induces cytochrome P450 1A2, but to a lesser extent than CYP3A4 (9204,10848). Some substrates of CYP1A2 include clozapine (Clozaril), cyclobenzaprine (Flexeril), fluvoxamine (Luvox), haloperidol (Haldol), imipramine (Tofranil), mexiletine (Mexitil), olanzapine (Zyprexa), pentazocine (Talwin), propranolol (Inderal), tacrine (Cognex), zileuton (Zyflo), zolmitriptan (Zomig), and others.
CYTOCHROME P450 2C9 (CYP2C9) SUBSTRATES: St. John's wort induces cytochrome P450 2C9, but to a lesser extent than CYP3A4 (9204,10848,11889). Some substrates of CYP2C9 include celecoxib (Celebrex), diclofenac (Voltaren), fluvastatin (Lescol), glipizide (Glucotrol), ibuprofen (Advil, Motrin), irbesartan (Avapro), losartan (Cozaar), phenytoin (Dilantin), piroxicam (Feldene), tamoxifen (Nolvadex), tolbutamide (Tolinase), torsemide (Demadex), and warfarin (Coumadin).
CYTOCHROME P450 3A4 (CYP3A4) SUBSTRATES: St. John's wort induces cytochrome P450 3A4 (9204,10830,10847,10848,11889). Use caution when considering concomitant use of St. John's wort and other drugs affected by these enzymes. Drugs that might be affected include some calcium channel blockers (diltiazem, nicardipine, verapamil), chemotherapeutic agents (etoposide, paclitaxel, vinblastine, vincristine, vindesine), antifungals (ketoconazole, itraconazole), glucocorticoids, cisapride (Propulsid), alfentanil (Alfenta), fentanyl (Sublimaze), losartan (Cozaar), fluoxetine (Prozac), midazolam (Versed), omeprazole (Prilosec), ondansetron (Zofran), propranolol (Inderal), fexofenadine (Allegra), and numerous others (1290,1292,1293,4835,6425,6473,7808,7810,9204,10830).
DEXTROMETHORPHAN (Robitussin DM, and others): Theoretically, concurrent use might cause additive serotonergic effects and increase the risk of serotonin syndrome (763,6427,8936). Also, concurrent use might theoretically cause cerebral vasoconstriction disorders such as Call-Fleming syndrome (8056).
DIGOXIN (Lanoxin): Concomitant use can reduce serum levels and the therapeutic effects of digoxin, requiring dosing adjustments when St. John's wort is started or stopped. St. John's wort extract 900 mg daily can reduce serum digoxin levels by 25% after 10 days in healthy people. St. John's wort is thought to affect the multidrug transporter, P-glycoprotein, which mediates the absorption and elimination of digoxin and other drugs (382,6473,7808,7810,9204).
FENFLURAMINE (Pondimin): Concomitant use with St. John's wort can increase the risk of serotonergic side effects and serotonin syndrome-like symptoms. St. John's wort 600 mg per day with fenfluramine can cause nausea, headache, and anxiety (3569).
FEXOFENADINE (Allegra): A single dose of St. John's wort can decrease the clearance of fexofenadine, resulting in increased plasma concentration of fexofenadine. However, with continued dosing, more than 2 weeks, St. John's wort does not appear to affect fexofenadine levels (9685). Patients taking fexofenadine and who start taking St. John's wort should be monitored for possible fexofenadine toxicity.
IMATINIB (Gleevec): St. John's wort decreases serum levels of imatinib by 30%, probably by inducing CYP3A4 (11888). Advise patients not to take St. John's wort if they are taking imatinib.
IRINOTECAN (Camptosar): Concomitant use with St. John's wort can decrease serum levels of irinotecan by at least 50%. Clearance of the active metabolite of irinotecan, SN-38, is increased resulting in a 42% decrease in the area under the concentration curve (9206). St. John's wort is thought to lower drug levels by inducing cytochrome P450 3A4 (CYP3A4) (7092).
MEPERIDINE (Demerol): Theoretically, concurrent use with meperidine might cause additive serotonergic effects and increase the risk of serotonin syndrome (763,6427,8936). Also, concurrent use might theoretically cause cerebral vasoconstriction disorders such as Call-Fleming syndrome (8056).
MONOAMINE OXIDASE INHIBITORS (MAOIs): Theoretically, because St. John's wort might affect serotonin

similar to conventional antidepressants (763,3553). Concurrent use might cause additive adverse effects, including hypertension, hyperthermia, agitation, confusion, coma, etc. St. John's wort should be avoided in patients taking MAOIs and for 14 days after MAOI discontinuation.

NARCOTIC DRUGS: St. John's wort can increase narcotic-induced sleep time (758) and might also increase analgesic effects (1279).

NEFAZODONE (Serzone): Concomitant use has been associated with serotonergic side effects, including nausea, vomiting, and restlessness (5074).

NON-NUCLEOSIDE REVERSE TRANSCRIPTASE INHIBITORS (NNRTIs): Concomitant use can decrease serum levels of NNRTIs. St. John's wort can increase the oral clearance of nevirapine (Viramune) by 35%. Subtherapeutic concentrations are associated with therapeutic failure, development of viral resistance, and development of drug class resistance. St. John's wort induces intestinal and hepatic cytochrome P450 3A4 (CYP3A4) and intestinal P-glycoprotein/MDR-1, a drug transporter (1290,1340,4837). Other NNRTIs include delavirdine (Rescriptor), and efavirenz (Sustiva).

NORTRIPTYLINE (Pamelor, Aventyl): Concomitant use can reduce serum concentrations of amitriptyline by 22% and its metabolite, nortriptyline, by 42% (1378,7808).

P-GLYCOPROTEIN SUBSTRATES: St. John's wort induces P-glycoprotein. P-glycoprotein is a carrier mechanism responsible for transporting drugs and other substances across cell membranes. When P-glycoprotein is induced in the gastrointestinal (GI) tract, it can prevent the absorption of some medications. In addition, induction of p-glycoprotein can decrease entry of drugs into the central nervous system (CNS) and decrease access to other sites of action. Drugs that might be affected include some chemotherapeutic agents (etoposide, paclitaxel, vinblastine, vincristine, vindesine), antifungals (ketoconazole, itraconazole), protease inhibitors (amprenavir, indinavir, nelfinavir, saquinavir), H2 antagonists (cimetidine, ranitidine), some calcium channel blockers (diltiazem, verapamil), corticosteroids, erythromycin, cisapride (Propulsid), fexofenadine (Allegra), cyclosporine, loperamide (Imodium), quinidine, and others (382,1340,7810,11722).

PAROXETINE (Paxil): Concomitant use with St. John's wort might increase the risk of adverse effects and serotonin syndrome-like symptoms. People taking St. John's wort and paroxetine together can experience nervousness, hyperactivity, diaphoresis, nausea, weakness, fatigue, lethargy, and incoherence (542,3569). Also, concurrent use might theoretically cause cerebral vasoconstriction disorders such as Call-Fleming syndrome (8056).

PENTAZOCINE (Talwin): Theoretically, concurrent use with pentazocine might cause additive serotonergic effects and increase the risk of serotonin syndrome (763,6427,8936). Also, concurrent use might theoretically cause cerebral vasoconstriction disorders such as Call-Fleming syndrome (8056).

PHENOBARBITAL (Luminal): St. John's wort may increase the metabolism of phenobarbital, resulting in loss of seizure control. Plasma concentrations of phenobarbital should be monitored carefully. The dose of phenobarbital may need to be increased when St. John's wort is started and decreased when it is stopped (9204).

PHENPROCOUMON: St. John's wort appears to increase the metabolism of phenprocoumon (an anticoagulant that is not available in the US) by increasing the activity of the cytochrome P450 2C9 (CYP2C9) enzyme. This may result in decreases in the anticoagulant effect and international normalized ratio (INR) (9204).

PHENYTOIN (Dilantin): St. John's wort may increase the metabolism of phenytoin, resulting in the loss of seizure control. Plasma concentrations of phenytoin should be monitored carefully. The dose of phenytoin may need to be increased when St. John's wort is started and decreased when it is stopped (9204).

PHOTOSENSITIZING DRUGS: Theoretically, concomitant use might increase the possibility of photosensitivity reactions (166). Some drugs that cause photosensitivity include amitriptyline, quinolones, sulfa drugs, and tetracycline.

PROTEASE INHIBITORS (PIs): Concomitant use can reduce serum concentrations of PIs. In healthy volunteers, St. John's wort can reduce the serum indinavir (Crixivan) area under the curve (AUC) by 57% and the extrapolated trough by 81%. Subtherapeutic concentrations are associated with therapeutic failure, development of viral resistance, and development of drug class resistance. St. John's wort is thought to induce cytochrome P450 enzymes and might also affect other PI-type antiretroviral drugs (1290,7808); including amprenavir (Agenerase), nelfinavir (Viracept), ritonavir (Norvir), and saquinavir (Fortovase, Invirase). St. John's wort also induces P-glycoprotein, which can result in decreased intracellular protease inhibitor concentrations and increased elimination (9204,9204).

RESERPINE: St. John's wort can antagonize the effects of reserpine (758).

SERTRALINE (Zoloft): Concomitant use can cause serotonergic side effects, including dizziness, nausea, vomiting, epigastric pain, headache, anxiety, confusion, and feelings of restlessness and irritability (5074).

SIMVASTATIN (Zocor): Concomitant use can reduce plasma concentrations of the simvastatin metabolite, simvastatin hydroxy acid, by 28%. St. John's wort induces intestinal and hepatic cytochrome P450 3A4 (CYP3A4) and intestinal P-glycoprotein/MDR-1, a drug transporter, which increases simvastatin clearance. St. John's wort does not appear to affect the plasma concentration of pravastatin (Pravachol) and fluvastatin (Lescol), which are not substrates of CYP3A4 or P-glycoprotein. Theoretically, St. John's wort could reduce the effectiveness of other HMG-CoA reductase inhibitors that are CYP3A4 substrates such as atorvastatin (Lipitor) and lovastatin (Mevacor) (10627).

TACROLIMUS (Prograf, Protopic): A St. John's wort extract (Jarsin) 600 mg daily significantly decreases tacrolimus serum levels. Dose increases of 60% may be required to maintain therapeutic tacrolimus levels in patients taking St. John's wort concomitantly. St. John's wort is thought to lower tacrolimus levels due to cytochrome P450 3A4 (CYP3A4) enzyme induction (7095,10329).

THEOPHYLLINE: St. John's wort doesn't seem to significantly affect theophylline pharmacokinetics (11802). There is a single case report of possible interaction with theophylline. A patient who smoked and was taking 11 other drugs experienced an increase in theophylline levels after discontinuation of St. John's wort. This increase has been attributed to a rebounding of theophylline serum levels after St. John's wort was no longer present to induce cytochrome P450 1A2 (CYP1A2) enzyme (3556,7808,9204). However, studies in healthy volunteers suggest that St. John's wort is unlikely to affect theophylline to any clinically significant degree (11802).
TRAMADOL (Ultram): Theoretically, concurrent use with tramadol might cause additive serotonergic effects and increase the risk of serotonin syndrome (763,6427,8936). Also, concurrent use might theoretically cause cerebral vasoconstriction disorders such as Call-Fleming syndrome (8056).
WARFARIN (Coumadin): Concomitant use might decrease the therapeutic effects of warfarin (1292). St. John's wort seems to significantly decrease International Normalized Ratio (INR) (1292). In healthy volunteers, St. John's wort increases the clearance of both S- and R-warfarin. This suggests it might induce CYP1A2 and CYP3A4, which metabolize R-warfarin and CYP2C9, which metabolizes L-warfarin (11890). In addition, warfarin physically interacts with hypericin and pseudohypericin, active constituents of St. John's wort. When the dried extract is mixed with warfarin in an aqueous medium, up to 30% of warfarin is bound to particles, reducing its absorption (10448). Taking warfarin at the same time as St. John's wort might reduce its bioavailability.

Interactions with Foods

None known.

Interactions with Lab Tests

PROTHROMBIN TIME (PT)/INTERNATIONAL NORMALIZED RATIO (INR): St. John's wort can decrease PT/INR test results in patients treated with warfarin (Coumadin) (1292).
THYROID STIMULATING HORMONE (TSH): Some preliminary research suggests that St. John's wort might elevate TSH levels (8569,8570).

Interactions with Diseases or Conditions

ALZHEIMER'S DISEASE: St. John's wort might induce psychosis in patients with Alzheimer's dementia. In one case, psychotic delirium developed in an elderly woman within three weeks of starting a low dose (75 mg per day) of St. John's wort extract standardized to 0.3% hypericin (St. John's wort, Pharmanex). Symptoms resolved within several days after discontinuing St. John's wort and starting medications for treatment of Alzheimer's disease. Although it is not clear if St. John's wort caused the delirium or contributed to the underlying dementia, there is concern that St. John's wort might contribute to dementia in patients with Alzheimer's disease (5249).
ANESTHESIA: St. John's wort might cause cardiovascular collapse during anesthesia. St. John's wort used chronically for six months appears to be the cause of severe hypotension following induction of anesthesia in an otherwise healthy patient. St. John's wort might cause adrenergic desensitization and decreased responsiveness to vasopressors, similar to the effects of antidepressants (8931).
BIPOLAR DISORDER: St. John's wort can induce hypomania or mania when used in patients with bipolar disorder or depressed patients with occult bipolar disorder (3555,3568). In some cases, mania occurred after two to eight weeks of treatment with St. John's wort and was effectively managed by decreasing the dose of St. John's wort and increasing the dose of mood stabilizers such as lithium (3568). Theoretically, like other antidepressants, St. John's wort may also induce rapid cycling between depression and mania in patients with bipolar disorder (3555).
DEPRESSION: St. John's wort can induce hypomania with typical doses in patients with major depression (325,3524,3568). In one case, hypomania occurred after four to eight weeks of treatment with St. John's wort and was effectively managed by decreasing the dose and initiating valproic acid (3568).
INFERTILITY: Preliminary evidence suggests that St. John's wort might inhibit oocyte fertilization and alter sperm DNA (4239,4240). This effect has not yet been demonstrated in humans, and animal studies suggest that St. John's wort doesn't adversely affect fertility or gestation (10846). However, until more is known, use with caution in couples attempting to conceive, and avoid use in couples having difficulty conceiving.
SCHIZOPHRENIA: St. John's wort might induce psychosis in patients with schizophrenia. There are two cases of relapse in non-medicated schizophrenia patients in remission who started taking St. John's wort. Psychotic symptoms resolved with readministration of antipsychotics and discontinuation of St. John's wort (6478).

Dosage and Administration

ORAL: For mild to moderate depression, most clinical trials have used St. John's wort extract standardized to 0.3% hypericin content. Doses are most commonly 300 mg three times daily (3548,3549). Doses of 1200 mg daily have also been used (5096). Some studies have also used a 0.2% hypericin extract dosed at 250 mg twice daily (4897,6434). A St. John's wort extract standardized to 5% hyperforin and dosed at 300 mg three times daily has also been used (761,4630). For children under 12 years of age with depression, St. John's wort extract standardized to 0.3% hypericin 300 mg daily has been used (4538). For obsessive-compulsive disorder (OCD), one study used an extended-release preparation of St. John's wort extract standardized to 0.3% hypericin content, dosed at 450 mg twice daily (5075). For premenstrual syndrome (PMS), one study used St. John's wort extract standardized to 0.3% hypericin dosed at 300 mg once daily (6429). For somatic symptoms associated with depression, 300 mg three times daily of the standardized hypericin extract has been used (376). Advise patients to avoid abrupt discontinuation of St. John's wort due to the risk

of adverse withdrawal effects (3569). For anxiety, 600 mg per day of the standardized extract Lichtwer LI 160, which contains 0.3% hypericin, has been used (9476).
TOPICAL: No typical dosage.

Comments

St. John's wort is native to Europe but is commonly found in the US and Canada in the dry ground of roadsides, meadows, and woods. Although not indigenous to Australia and long considered a weed, St. John's wort is now grown as a cash crop and produces 20 percent of the world's supply (6200).
The use of St. John's wort dates back to the ancient Greeks. Hippocrates documented the medical use of St. John's wort flowers. St. John's wort is so named because it blooms about June 24th, the birthday of John the Baptist. "Wort" is an old English word for plant (11804).
France has banned the use of St. John's wort products. The ban appears to be based on a report issued by the French Health Product Safety Agency warning of significant drug-herb interactions. Several other countries including Japan, the United Kingdom, and Canada are in the process of including drug-herb interaction cautionary language on St. John's wort products (4892).

STAR ANISE

Also Known As

Aniseed Stars, Anisi stellati fructus, Badiana, Chinese Anise, Chinese Star Anise, Eight-Horned Anise, Eight Horns, Illicium.
CAUTION: See separate listing for Anise.

Scientific Names

Illicium verum.
Family: Illiciaceae.

People Use This For

Orally, star anise is used for respiratory tract mucous membrane inflammation, peptic discomfort, flatulence, loss of appetite, infant colic, cough, and bronchitis. Star anise is also used orally for increasing milk secretion, promoting menstruation, facilitating childbirth, increasing libido, and treating symptoms of male climacteric.
As an inhalant, star anise is used for respiratory tract congestion.
In foods and beverages, star anise is considered a culinary spice; both the seed and oil are used as flavoring.
In manufacturing, the oil is used as a fragrance component in soaps, cosmetics, perfumes, and toothpaste, and to mask undesirable odors in drug products.

Safety

LIKELY SAFE ...when used orally in amounts commonly found in foods. Star anise has Generally Recognized As Safe (GRAS) status in the US (4912).
POSSIBLY SAFE ...when used orally and appropriately for medicinal purposes (12).
UNSAFE ...when consumed as a "tea" contaminated with Japanese star anise (Illicium anisatum). Japanese star anise is similar in appearance to Chinese star anise. However, Japanese star anise is toxic and should not be taken orally (10407).
There is insufficient reliable information available about the safety of star anise as an inhalant.
CHILDREN: UNSAFE ...when used orally in infants. Star anise has been associated with adverse neurological reactions, including irritability, vomiting, and seizures. The symptoms may be attributed to star anise alone or in combination with Japanese star anise (Illicium anisatum) (11384). There is insufficient reliable information available about the safety of star anise for older children.
PREGNANCY AND LACTATION: Insufficient reliable information available; avoid using.

Effectiveness

There is insufficient reliable information available about the effectiveness of star anise.

Mechanism of Action

The applicable part of star anise is the seed. Star anise seed contains a volatile oil, 75% of which is anethole (11384). Anethole has antiflatulent and expectorant effects. It also can have insecticidal and antifungal activity (11). At one time anethole was considered the active estrogenic agent in the essential oil. However, more recent information suggests the active estrogenic compounds are the anethole polymers, dianethole and photoanethole (11). Anethole might be mutagenic (11).

Adverse Reactions

Orally, star anise (Illicium verum) is usually well tolerated. However, some types of star anise have been contaminated with Japanese star anise (Illicium anisatum), which is toxic and should not be taken orally. Symptoms resulting from drinking tea made from contaminated star anise include seizures, vomiting, nervousness, rapid eye movements, and other serious neurological effects (10407).

In infants aged 2 weeks to 3 months, star anise tea can cause acute onset irritability, jitteriness, clonus or myoclonus, increased deep tendon reflexes, nystagmus, vomiting, and seizures. It is unclear whether this toxicity is caused by star anise alone or by contamination with Japanese star anise (11384).

Topically, use of the constituent anethole can cause dermatitis, including erythema, scaling, and vesiculation (11). Sensitization rarely occurs (18).

Interactions with Herbs & Other Dietary Supplements

None known.

Interactions with Drugs

None known.

Interactions with Foods

None known.

Interactions with Lab Tests

None known.

Interactions with Diseases or Conditions

HORMONE SENSITIVE CANCERS/CONDITIONS: Star anise might have estrogenic effects (11), women with hormone sensitive conditions should avoid star anise. Some of these conditions include breast cancer, uterine cancer, and ovarian cancer, endometriosis, and uterine fibroids.

Dosage and Administration

No typical dosage.

Comments

Star anise oil is the distilled oil of the seed (fruit) of star anise (Illicium verum). In the US, star anise oil (derived from Illicium verum) and anise oil (derived from Pimpinella anisum) are used interchangeably and both are recognized as "anise oil" in the USP (11). Avoid confusing star anise with Japanese star anise (Illicium anisatum), a highly poisonous species. Japanese star anise is similar in appearance to Chinese star anise. Some products described as "tea" have become contaminated with Japanese star anise, resulting in severe neurological toxicity. Until the safety of star anise tea can be determined, by chemical analysis, they should not be used (10407).

Star anise tea is used to treat infant colic, particularly in Caribbean and Hispanic cultures. Star anise should not be given to infants. It can cause severe neurologic toxicity (11384).

STAVESACRE

Also Known As

Lousewort.

Scientific Names

Delphinium staphisagria.

Family: Ranunculaceae.

People Use This For

Topically, stavesacre seeds are used to treat lice infestation and neuralgia.

Safety

LIKELY UNSAFE ...when used orally. The seeds are poisonous (18).

There is insufficient reliable information available about the safety of the topical use of stavesacre and the use of stavesacre extracts.

PREGNANCY AND LACTATION: LIKELY UNSAFE ...when used orally (18); avoid using.

Effectiveness

There is insufficient reliable information available about the effectiveness of stavesacre.

Mechanism of Action

Stavesacre contains diterpene alkaloids including delphinine, staphisine, and staphisagroine, which are reported to have effects similar to aconitine (18). Aconitine is a nor-diterpene alkaloid found in Monkshood, a highly toxic plant.

Adverse Reactions

Orally, stavesacre extract can cause inflammation of the alimentary tract (18,19), nausea, pruritus, urinary and stool urgency (18). Ingesting 2 teaspoons of seeds can cause weakened pulse, stomach pain, labored breathing, and collapse (18).
Topically, use of stavesacre can cause inflammation, eczema, and reddening of the skin (18).

Interactions with Herbs & Other Dietary Supplements

None known.

Interactions with Drugs

None known.

Interactions with Foods

None known.

Interactions with Lab Tests

None known.

Interactions with Diseases or Conditions

GASTROINTESTINAL IRRITATION: Can aggravate inflammation of the alimentary tract by irritating mucosal membranes (19).

Dosage and Administration

ORAL: No typical dosage.
TOPICAL: Washes and ointments are used to treat lice.

STEVIA

Also Known As

Azucacaa, Ca-A-Jhei, Ca-A-Yupi, Caa-He-É, Capim Doce, Eira-Caa, Erva Doce, Kaa Jhee, Paraguayan Sweet Herb, Stevioside, Sweetleaf, Sweet Herb of Paraguay, Sweet Leaf of Paraguay, Yerba Dulce.

Scientific Names

Stevia rebaudiana, synonym Eupatorium rebaudianum; Stevia eupatoria, synonyms Mustelia eupatoria, Stevia purpurea.
Family: Asteraceae/Compositae.

People Use This For

Orally, stevia is used as a weight loss aid, for treating diabetes, contraception, hypertension, heartburn, lowering uric acid levels, and as a cardiotonic and diuretic.
In foods, stevia is used as a non-caloric sweetener and flavor enhancer.

Safety

POSSIBLY SAFE ...when used orally in small amounts commonly found in foods and beverages as a sweetener. An acceptable daily dose is 25 mg per kg of body weight (11811). ...when stevioside, a constituent of stevia, is used orally. Doses up to 1500 mg per day for 2 years have been used (11809,11810).
There is insufficient reliable information about the safety of stevia used long-term. The FDA, regulatory agencies in Europe, and the World Health Organization have not approved stevia due to unanswered questions regarding chronic use and toxicity (5037).
PREGNANCY: POSSIBLY UNSAFE ...when used orally. There is preliminary evidence from animal studies that suggests a constituent of stevia called steviol might reduce birth weight of offspring (5036).
LACTATION: Insufficient reliable information available; avoid using.

Effectiveness

POSSIBLY EFFECTIVE

Hypertension. Taking stevioside, a constituent of stevia, orally seems to reduce blood pressure in people with hypertension. Doses of 750 or 1500 mg per day appear to reduce systolic blood pressure by 10-14 mmHg, and diastolic blood pressure by 6-14 mmHg. In patients with hypertension, the onset of decreased blood pressure begins within one week of initiation of treatment (11809,11811). Use of stevioside 1500 mg daily for 2 years might reduce the risk of left ventricular hypertrophy (11809).

INSUFFICIENT RELIABLE EVIDENCE to RATE

Diabetes. Preliminary clinical research suggests that stevioside, a constituent of stevia might reduce postprandial glucose levels by 18% in people with type 2 diabetes (11812). More evidence is needed to rate stevia for this use.

Mechanism of Action

The applicable part of stevia is the leaf. Stevia leaf contains the glycoside stevioside which is non-caloric, heat and acid stable, and 300 times sweeter than a 0.4% sucrose solution. Animal research suggests that stevioside is metabolized to steviol in the intestine, but significant amounts of steviol may not reach the blood stream (11809,11811). Stevia extract, and stevioside, seem to decrease blood pressure, according to human and animal studies (3745,3747). Stevia extract has vasodilating and diuretic activity in rats (3746,3747). Stevioside might also act as a calcium channel blocker (11809,11811).

Preliminary evidence suggests that the stevia constituents, stevioside and steviol, might stimulate insulin secretion via a direct action on beta cells (5032). Additional evidence suggests that steviol might inhibit GI glucose absorption (5035). Other research suggests that stevioside increases insulin sensitivity and improves skeletal muscle glucose transport (11813). Stevioside increases hepatic glycogen synthesis in animal experiments (3750). An aqueous stevia leaf extract increased glucose tolerance and reduced plasma glucose levels in a small group of healthy people (3301).

A fermented aqueous extract of stevia is bactericidal against many food-borne pathogenic bacteria in vitro, including E. coli 0157:H7, the enterohemorrhagic E. coli responsible for outbreaks of severe food poisoning in recent years (3300). Stevioside has shown no evidence of mutagenic, genotoxic, antifertility, or teratogenic effects (11811). However, the stevia constituent steviol, and metabolized steviol, are mutagenic in vitro (3748,3749). Some evidence suggests that stevia might adversely affect reproduction. An aqueous stevia extract reduced sperm production and testis weight in male rats (5033). Steviol fed to female hamsters reduced the number and birth weight of offspring (5036).

Adverse Reactions

Orally, stevioside, a constituent of stevia, can cause gastrointestinal adverse effects such as abdominal fullness and nausea. It can also cause headache, dizziness, myalgia, and numbness (11809,11810). Theoretically, stevia might cause allergic reactions in individuals sensitive to Asteraceae/Compositae family plants (11811). Members of this family include ragweed, chrysanthemums, marigolds, daisies, and many other herbs.

Interactions with Herbs & Other Dietary Supplements

HERBS AND SUPPLEMENTS WITH HYPOGLYCEMIC POTENTIAL: Stevioside, a stevia derivative, can lower blood glucose levels (3301,11802) and might have additive effects when used with other herbs and supplements that also lower glucose levels. This might increase the risk of hypoglycemia in some patients. Some herbs and supplements with hypoglycemic effects include alpha-lipoic acid, bitter melon, chromium, devil's claw, fenugreek, garlic, guar gum, horse chestnut, Panax ginseng, psyllium, Siberian ginseng, and others.

HERBS AND SUPPLEMENTS WITH HYPOTENSIVE EFFECTS: Stevioside, a stevia derivative, might have hypotensive effects (11809,11810). Theoretically, concurrent use of stevia with other herbs and supplements that decrease blood pressure might increase risk of hypotension. Some of these products include danshen, ginger, Panax ginseng, turmeric, valerian, and others.

Interactions with Drugs

ANTIDIABETES DRUGS: Theoretically, stevia might enhance blood glucose control requiring dosing adjustment of diabetes drug therapy in patients with type 2 diabetes (3301,5032,5035,11812).

ANTIHYPERTENSIVE DRUGS: Concomitant use with stevia might cause additive hypotensive effects; use with caution (11809,11810). Some medications for high blood pressure include captopril (Capoten), enalapril (Vasotec), losartan (Cozaar), valsartan (Diovan), amlodipine (Norvasc), hydrochlorothiazide (HydroDIURIL), furosemide (Lasix), and many others.

CALCIUM CHANNEL BLOCKERS: Stevioside, a constituent of stevia, might have calcium antagonist properties (11809,11811). Using stevia with calcium channel blockers such as verapamil (Calan, Covera-HS, Verelan), nifedipine (Procardia), diltiazem (Cardizem, Dilacor, Tiazac), and others might cause additive effects on blood pressure and the heart.

Interactions with Foods

None known.

Interactions with Lab Tests

BLOOD PRESSURE: Stevia might reduce blood pressure and blood pressure readings. Stevia extract and stevioside, contained in stevia, can lower blood pressure (3745,3747,5031,11809,11810).

GLUCOSE: Stevia might decrease blood glucose concentrations and test results (3301,5032,5035,11812).

Interactions with Diseases or Conditions

CROSS-ALLERGENICITY: Theoretically, stevia might cause allergic reactions in individuals sensitive to Asteraceae/Compositae family plants (11811). Members of this family include ragweed, chrysanthemums, marigolds, daisies, and many other herbs.
DIABETES: Stevia might reduce blood glucose and alter blood glucose control in patients with type 2 diabetes (3301,5032,5035,11812).
HYPOTENSION: Stevioside, a stevia derivative, has hypotensive effects (11809,11810). Theoretically, use in people with existing low blood pressure might exacerbate hypotension and possibly lead to syncope.
KIDNEY DISEASE: Theoretically, stevia might cause kidney damage. Preliminary evidence suggests that very large amounts of steviol, a metabolite of stevia, might cause acute renal damage (5034).

Dosage and Administration

Oral: For hypertension, stevioside, a constituent of stevia, 250 to 500 mg three times daily has been used (11809,11810).

Comments

The FDA classifies stevia as an "unsafe food additive." Stevia is considered "unsafe" because no one has ever provided FDA with adequate evidence that stevia is safe. Since stevia is not patentable, funding for safety studies seems unlikely (11808).
Dietary supplements are not regulated as food additives, so the FDA allows stevia to be imported "explicitly labeled as a dietary supplement or for use as a dietary ingredient of a dietary supplement" (11808). Canada and the European Community prohibit stevia as a food additive (5030). The FDA, regulatory agencies in Europe, and the World Health Organization have not approved stevia due to unanswered safety questions (5037). Stevia is approved for use in foods in Brazil, Japan, China and other countries in Asia and South America (11811).

STINGING NETTLE above ground parts

Also Known As

Common Nettle, Great Stinging Nettle, Nettle, Nettles, Ortie, Small Nettle, Urtica, Urticae herba et folium.
CAUTION: See separate listings for Stinging Nettle root and White Dead Nettle Flower.

Scientific Names

Urtica dioica; Urtica urens; and hybrid species.
Family: Urticaceae.

People Use This For

Orally, stinging nettle above ground parts are used for allergies, allergic rhinitis, and musculoskeletal aches and pains such as osteoarthritis. It is also used orally in conjunction with copious fluid intake in so-called "irrigation therapy" for urinary tract infections (UTI), and urinary tract inflammation, and kidney stones (nephrolithiasis). People also use stinging nettle for internal bleeding, including uterine bleeding, epistaxis, and melena; anemia; poor circulation; splenomegaly; diabetes and other endocrine disorders; gastric hyperacidity; biliary complaints; diarrhea and dysentery; asthma; pulmonary congestion; rash and eczema; cancer; prevention of signs of aging; blood purification; wound-healing; and as a general tonic.
Topically, stinging nettle above ground parts are used for musculoskeletal aches and pains, scalp seborrhea and oily hair, and hair loss (alopecia).
In foods, young stinging nettle is eaten as a cooked vegetable.
In manufacturing, stinging nettle extract is used as an ingredient in hair and skin products.

Safety

POSSIBLY SAFE ...when used orally and appropriately (1,2,12). There is insufficient reliable information available about the safety of the topical use of stinging nettle above ground parts.
PREGNANCY: LIKELY UNSAFE ...when used orally due to possible abortifacient and uterine-stimulant effects (4,6,19).
LACTATION: There is insufficient reliable information available about the safety of stinging nettle above ground parts during lactation; avoid using.

Effectiveness

POSSIBLY EFFECTIVE

Osteoarthritis. There is evidence that oral use of stinging nettle leaf extract might improve symptoms of pain in patients with osteoarthritis (1,6500). Some clinicians use stinging nettle leaf extract in combination with conventional nonsteroidal anti-inflammatory drugs (NSAIDs) or other analgesics. Evidence suggests that adding stinging nettle might allow for using lower analgesic doses in some patients (6500).

INSUFFICIENT RELIABLE EVIDENCE to RATE

Allergic rhinitis (hayfever). There is preliminary evidence that stinging nettle might improve symptoms of allergic rhinitis. Starting stinging nettle at the first sign of symptoms seems to provide subjective improvement (7035). More evidence is needed to rate stinging nettle above ground parts for this use.

Mechanism of Action

Stinging nettle leaf contains several nutrients and active constituents. The plant has traditionally been used as a food because of significant amounts of nutrients including carotene, vitamin C, vitamin K, potassium (2,8,11,18,19), and calcium (2,11). There is about as much vitamin C and carotene in stinging nettle as spinach and other greens (5). Stinging nettle is also a good source of chlorophyll. Stinging nettle contains the sterol beta-sitosterol and the flavonoids quercetin, rutin, kaempferol, and others. Stinging nettle seems to have a variety of pharmacological effects including analgesic (1,4), anti-inflammatory (19), local anesthetic (1), hemostatic (4), antibacterial (11), antiviral (6). For osteoarthritis and other musculoskeletal conditions, stinging nettle might work due to potential analgesic and anti-inflammatory effects. Some researchers think that stinging nettle might be beneficial for allergic rhinitis due to quercetin content. Quercetin is thought to have anti-inflammatory and mast-cell stabilizing effects. It decreases histamine release from basophils and mast cells (483). There is evidence that it might inhibit adrenergic stimulation, tumor necrosis factor (TNF), and platelet activation factor (PAF) (1). Stinging nettle seems to also act as a diuretic. The leaf juice can increase urine output and slightly decrease systolic blood pressure and body weight in people with venous insufficiency (1,11). Because of these effects, some people use stinging nettle for urinary tract disorders, including urinary tract infections (UTIs) and kidney stones. Stinging nettle also seems to lower body temperature and have CNS depressant (4,6,11) and anti-seizure activity (4). When given intravenously stinging nettle also seems to decrease blood pressure and heart rate (1,4). Stinging nettle leaf is well known to cause skin irritation when touched. The stinging nettle hairs of the leaf contain histamine, acetylcholine (1,4,5,8,11,18), and serotonin (1,4,8,11,18), that can cause local irritation.

Adverse Reactions

Orally, stinging nettle is typically well tolerated. The stinging nettle juice can sometimes cause diarrhea (1). Topically, fresh stinging nettle leaves applied or touched accidentally can cause local irritation (4,19).

Interactions with Herbs & Other Dietary Supplements

HERBS WITH CLOTTING POTENTIAL: Excessive use of herbs that contain vitamin K, an essential coagulation factor, can increase the risk of clotting in people using anticoagulants. These herbs include alfalfa, parsley, nettle, plantain, and others.

Interactions with Drugs

ANTIDIABETES DRUGS: There is some evidence that stinging nettle can decrease blood glucose levels. Theoretically, concomitant use of excessive amounts of stinging nettle might interfere with blood glucose control (4).

ANTIHYPERTENSIVE DRUGS: There is some evidence that stinging nettle might have blood pressure lowering effects. Theoretically, concomitant use of excessive amounts of stinging nettle might have additive effects with antihypertensive drugs on blood pressure (4).

CNS DEPRESSANTS: There is some evidence that stinging nettle preparations might have CNS depressant activity. Theoretically, concomitant use of excessive amounts of stinging nettle might have additive effects with CNS depressant drugs (4).

WARFARIN (Coumadin): There is some concern that stinging nettle might decrease the effects of anticoagulant drugs such as warfarin (Coumadin). Stinging nettle contains a significant amount of vitamin K (19); use cautiously. Dose adjustment of anticoagulants may be needed.

Interactions with Foods

None known.

Interactions with Lab Tests

None known.

Interactions with Diseases or Conditions

CONGESTIVE HEART FAILURE (CHF): Stinging nettle tea is often given as "irrigation therapy" and given in conjunction with large amounts of fluids. This should be avoided in patients with CHF. Large amounts of fluids might worsen symptoms of CHF (2,18).

DIABETES: There is some evidence stinging nettle can increase blood glucose levels (4). Theoretically, stinging nettle might worsen blood glucose control in patients with diabetes; use with caution.

HYPERTENSION: There is some evidence that stinging nettle above ground parts might have blood pressure lowering effects (4). Theoretically, stinging nettle might have additive effects with medications used to treat high blood pressure; use with caution.

RENAL INSUFFICIENCY: Stinging nettle tea is often used as "irrigation therapy" and given in conjunction with large amounts of fluids. This should be avoided in patients with kidney dysfunction. Large amounts of fluids might worsen this condition (2,18).

Dosage and Administration

ORAL: For osteoarthritis, people typically use crude stinging nettle leaf 9 grams daily (6500). For allergic rhinitis, people typically use stinging nettle extract 300 mg three times daily. However, in some cases, 300 mg up to seven times daily has been used (7035). Stinging nettle is often taken as a tea. One cup of tea is made by steeping 1.5-5 grams above ground parts in 150 mL boiling water for 10 minutes and then straining. Tea is typically taken in doses of one cup up to three times per day (1,2,4,8). Fresh juice from stinging nettle, 10-15 mL three times daily has been used (1). A dried extract of stinging nettle (7:1), 770 mg twice daily has also been used (1). Liquid extract of stinging nettle (1:1 in 25% alcohol), 3-4 mL three times daily has also been used (1,4).
TOPICAL: Tincture/spirit (1:10) has been used (18).

Comments

Stinging nettle leaf has a long history of use. It was used primarily as a diuretic and laxative as early as the times of the Greek physicians Dioscorides and Galen.

STINGING NETTLE root

Also Known As

Common Nettle, Great Stinging Nettle, Nettle, Nettles, Small Nettle, Urtica, Urticae Radix.
CAUTION: See separate listing for Stinging Nettle above ground parts and White Dead Nettle Flower.

Scientific Names

Urtica dioica; Urtica urens.
Family: Urticaceae.

People Use This For

Orally, stinging nettle root is used for urination disorders associated with benign prostatic hyperplasia (BPH), including nocturia, frequency, dysuria, urinary retention, and irritable bladder. Stinging nettle root is also used orally for joint ailments, as a diuretic, and an astringent.

Safety

POSSIBLY SAFE ...when used orally and appropriately. Stinging nettle root has been used safely for up to six months (5093,11230). The long term safety of stinging nettle root is unknown.
PREGNANCY AND LACTATION: Insufficient reliable information available; avoid using.

Effectiveness

POSSIBLY INEFFECTIVE

Benign prostatic hyperplasia (BPH). Taking an herbal blend containing stinging nettle root extract orally doesn't seem to be effective for treating symptoms of BPH. In a double-blind, placebo controlled trial, an herbal product containing stinging nettle root extract 80 mg, saw palmetto lipoidal extract 106 mg, pumpkin seed oil extract 160 mg, lemon bioflavonoid extract 33 mg, and vitamin A (100% as beta-carotene) 190 IU taken three times daily for six months failed to significantly improve symptoms in a group of men with BPH (5093).

There is insufficient reliable information available about the effectiveness of stinging nettle root for its other uses.

Mechanism of Action

Stinging nettle root contains polysaccharides with immunomodulating and weak anti-inflammatory effects (1,7). Stinging nettle seems to have an antiproliferative effect on prostatic epithelial and stromal cells (11227,11229). It may also lessen the effects of androgenic hormones by competitively blocking access to human sex hormone binding globulin (SHBG) (11228).

Adverse Reactions

Orally, stinging nettle root can cause gastrointestinal complaints, sweating, and allergic skin reactions (1,7). One case is reported of decreased ejaculatory volume associated with an herbal blend product containing nettle root extract, saw palmetto extract, pumpkin seed oil extract, lemon bioflavonoid extract, and beta-carotene (5093).

Interactions with Herbs & Other Dietary Supplements

None known.

Interactions with Drugs
None known.

Interactions with Foods
None known.

Interactions with Lab Tests
None known.

Interactions with Diseases or Conditions
None known.

Dosage and Administration
ORAL: For symptomatic treatment of benign prostatic hyperplasia (BPH), stinging nettle root extract 80 mg, in combination with saw palmetto lipoidal extract 106 mg, pumpkin seed oil extract 160 mg, lemon bioflavonoid extract 33 mg, and vitamin A (100% as beta-carotene) 190 IU taken three times daily has been used (5093).

Comments
Avoid confusing stinging nettle with white dead nettle. Stinging nettle root is used predominantly for urinary disorders, including BPH. White dead nettle herb is used for gastrointestinal complaints. White dead nettle flower is used for inflammation of the mucous membranes of the upper respiratory tract and vaginal discharge.

STONE ROOT

Also Known As
Citronella, Colinsonia, Hardback, Hardhack, Heal-all, Horse Balm, Horseweed, Knob Grass, Knob Root, Knobweed, Richleaf, Rich Weed.
CAUTION: See separate listings for Citronella Oil and Lemongrass.

Scientific Names
Collinsonia canadensis.
Family: Lamiaceae/Labiatae.

People Use This For
Orally stone root is used to treat bladder inflammation, edema, gastrointestinal disorders, headaches, hyperuricuria, indigestion, kidney stones, urea "bladder semolina", urinary calculus, water retention, and as a tonic.

Safety
POSSIBLY SAFE ...when used orally and appropriately. There are no reports of serious adverse effects (4,12,18).
PREGNANCY AND LACTATION: Insufficient reliable information available; avoid using (4).

Effectiveness
There is insufficient reliable information available about the effectiveness of stone root.

Mechanism of Action
The applicable parts of stone root are the rhizome and root. Stone root rhizome or root contains a volatile oil, caffeic acid derivatives including rosmaric acid (18), saponins, tannin, mucilage, and resin (4). Constituents of the volatile oil include caryophyllene, germacrene D, limonene, alpha- and beta-pinenes (18). Although no pharmacologic data are documented (4), stone root is said to have diuretic effects (4,6), stimulate stomach function (18), cause sweating (4), and reduce occurrence of urinary stones and help rid the body of stones (4).

Adverse Reactions
Orally, ingesting large amounts of stone root can cause intestinal tract irritation and colic-like pain, dizziness, nausea, and painful urination (18).

Interactions with Herbs & Other Dietary Supplements
HERBS WITH DIURETIC PROPERTIES: Theoretically, due to the diuretic effects of stone root (4,6), there may be additive effects and side effects with herbs having diuretic activity.

Interactions with Drugs
DIURETIC DRUGS: Theoretically, due to the diuretic effects of stone root (4,6), there may be additive effects and side effects with drugs having diuretic activity.

Interactions with Foods
None known.

Interactions with Lab Tests
None known.

Interactions with Diseases or Conditions
None known.

Dosage and Administration
ORAL: A typical dose of dried root is 1-4 grams or as tea three times daily (4). To make tea, simmer 1-4 grams root or rhizome in 150 mL of boiling water for 5-10 minutes, strain. As liquid extract: (1:1 in 25% alcohol) 1-4 mL three times daily (4). Tincture, (1:5 in 40% alcohol) 2-8 mL three times daily (4); tincture of Collinsonia, 2-8 mL (4).

Comments
This aromatic perennial herb has a strong, unpleasant smell that is reported to be numbing in large amounts (18).

STORAX

Also Known As
American Storax, Balsam Styracis, Balsamum Styrax Liquidus, Copalm, Estoraque Liquido, Gum Tree, Levant Storax, Liquid Amber, Liquid Storax, Opossum Tree, Red Gum, Styrax, Sweet Gum, White Gum.

Scientific Names
Liquidambar orientalis; Liquidambar styraciflua, synonym Liquidambar macrophylla.
Family: Hamamelidaceae or Altingiaceae.

People Use This For
Orally, storax is used for cancer, coughs, colds, diarrhea, epilepsy, sore throats, and parasitic infections.
Topically, storax is used to protect wounds, for ulcers, and scabies. Storax is an ingredient in Compound Benzoin Tincture.
As an inhalant, storax is placed in a vaporizer and used to treat coughs and bronchitis.
In foods, storax is used as a flavoring component or fixative.
In manufacturing, storax is used as a fragrance component or fixative in soaps and perfumes. Storax is also used as a fumigant and imbedding material in microscopy.

Safety
LIKELY SAFE ...when used orally in amounts commonly found in foods. Sorax has Generally Recognized As Safe (GRAS) status in the US (4912).
POSSIBLY SAFE ...when used orally. There are no published reports of toxicity from oral use (6). ...when used topically. Storax should not be used topically on large, open wounds (18).
POSSIBLY UNSAFE ...when large amounts are ingested. ...when applied to large open wounds. Systemic absorption can cause poisoning including kidney damage, e.g., albuminuria and hemorrhagic nephritis (18).
PREGNANCY AND LACTATION: Insufficient reliable information available; avoid using.

Effectiveness
There is insufficient reliable information available about the effectiveness of storax.

Mechanism of Action
The applicable part of storax is the balsam. American storax balsam and Levant storax balsam are very similar chemically. Both contain aromatic alcohols (18), cinnamic acid (18,271), cinnamic acid esters (6,18), storesins (13), styrene (6,18,271), a volatile oil (11,13), vanillin (6,11,18) and triterpenes (18). However, the amount of constituents varies between the species. In Levant storax, the volatile oil is usually less than 1%. In American storax, it ranges from 7 to over 20% (11). Storax has stimulant, antiseptic, and expectorant properties (11,13). It is also reported to have antimicrobial and anti-inflammatory properties (11).

Adverse Reactions

Orally, storax balsam can cause diarrhea (18).
Topically, storax balsam can cause skin sensitization and contact allergies (9,18). When applied to large, open wounds, systemic absorption can cause kidney damage (e.g., albuminuria and hemorrhagic nephritis) (18).

Interactions with Herbs & Other Dietary Supplements

None known.

Interactions with Drugs

None known.

Interactions with Foods

None known.

Interactions with Lab Tests

None known.

Interactions with Diseases or Conditions

None known.

Dosage and Administration

ORAL: No typical dosage.
TOPICAL/INHALATION: Storax is applied topically and administered by inhalation via a vaporizer (6,18). It is available commercially in combination products.

Comments

Storax is a medicinal balsam obtained from the tree trunks of Liquidambar orientalis (Levant storax) or Liquidambar styraciflua (American storax) (13,271). It is obtained by traumatizing the bark of the tree in early summer and stripping the bark later, perhaps as late as autumn. The bark is pressed in cold water, alternating with boiling water, and the crude liquid storax is collected (6). Storax is considered to be similar to Peru balsam in its effects (9).

STRAWBERRY

Also Known As

Alpine Strawberry, Fragariae folium, Mountain Strawberry, Strawberries, Virginian Strawberry, Wild Strawberry, Wood Strawberry.

Scientific Names

Fragaria vesca, synonyms Fragaria insularis Potentilla vesca; Fragaria virginiana, synonym Potentilla virginiana; Fragaria viridis, synonym Potentilla viridis, Fragaria collina.
Family: Rosaceae.

People Use This For

Orally, strawberry is used for GI tract mucous membrane inflammation, diarrhea, intestinal sluggishness, liver disease, jaundice, upper and lower respiratory tract mucous membrane inflammation, gout, arthritis, nervous tension, kidney ailments involving gravel and stones, diuretic, supportive for heart and circulatory ailments, fever, night sweats, blood purification, for stimulating metabolism, anemia, as a tonic, for inhibiting menstruation, and supporting "natural weight loss".
Topically, strawberry is used as a compress for rashes.

Safety

POSSIBLY SAFE ...when used orally and appropriately (12).
PREGNANCY AND LACTATION: Insufficient reliable information available; avoid using.

Effectiveness

There is insufficient reliable information available about the effectiveness of strawberry.

Mechanism of Action

The applicable part of strawberry is the leaf and fruit. Strawberry leaf contains ellagic acid tannins, oligomeric proanthocyanidins, and flavonoids including rutin and quercetin. People claim that strawberry leaf has astringent and diuretic activity (18); however, there are no data to support these claims (18). Strawberry leaves are rich in vitamin C (19). Preliminary research suggests that compounds contained in strawberry fruit might slow aging effects on the nervous system (1418,1419).

Adverse Reactions
Orally, allergic reactions may occur in people sensitive to strawberries (2).

Interactions with Herbs & Other Dietary Supplements
None known.

Interactions with Drugs
None known.

Interactions with Foods
None known.

Interactions with Lab Tests
None known.

Interactions with Diseases or Conditions
STRAWBERRY HYPERSENSITIVITY: Contraindicated (18).

Dosage and Administration
ORAL: Diarrhea, one cup tea (steep 1 gram dried leaf in 250 mL boiling water 5-10 minutes, strain); several cups daily (18).

STRONTIUM

Also Known As
Stable Strontium, Strontium Chloride, Strontium-89 Chloride, Strontium Citrate, Strontium Ranelate.

Scientific Names
Strontium; Sr; atomic number 38.

People Use This For
Orally, strontium is used for the prevention and treatment of osteoporosis. It is also used orally for metastatic cancer, bone pain, osteoarthritis, cough, seizures, sensitive teeth, and for preventing dental caries.
Intravenously, the strontium-89 isotope is used for skeletal metastases and prostate cancer.
Topically, strontium is used in toothpaste for sensitive teeth.

Safety
LIKELY SAFE ...when strontium-89 chloride is used intravenously, and appropriately. Strontium-89 chloride is an FDA-approved product (4948). ...when strontium chloride is used topically, and appropriately as a toothpaste.
Strontium chloride hexahydrate (Sensodyne-SC) is an FDA-approved product (9). The safety of strontium chloride when used orally is not known. Most dietary supplements with strontium contain the salt form of strontium chloride.
POSSIBLY SAFE ...when strontium ranelate is used orally and appropriately. Strontium ranelate seems to be safe when used for up to 3 years (11392,11393,11395).
There is insufficient reliable information about the safety of other strontium salts.
PREGNANCY AND LACTATION: LIKELY SAFE ...when strontium chloride is used topically and appropriately as a toothpaste (9). Strontium chloride hexahydrate (Sensodyne-SC) is an FDA approved product. Advise patients not to swallow the toothpaste.
Most dietary supplements with strontium contain the salt form of strontium chloride. The safety of using strontium chloride orally during pregnancy or lactation is not known; avoid using.

Effectiveness
EFFECTIVE

Dental hypersensitivity. Topical use of strontium chloride 10% in toothpaste relieves the pain of sensitive teeth (11745,11746). Best results are obtained with twice daily brushing (11756).

Painful bony metastases. Intravenous administration of strontium-89 chloride is effective for metastatic bone pain (11749,11750,11751,11752).

POSSIBLY EFFECTIVE

Osteoporosis. Taking strontium ranelate orally appears to reduce the risk of vertebral fractures by 40% in postmenopausal women with osteoporosis and a history of vertebral fracture. There is some evidence that it might actually increase bone mineral density (BMD) in these patients by 14% at the lumbar spine and 8% at the femoral neck (11392,11393,11395).

Prostate cancer. Intravenous administration of strontium-89 chloride seems to slow the progression of treatment-resistant prostate cancer and to relieve pain (11747,11748).

There is insufficient reliable information available about the effectiveness of strontium chloride, the form most commonly used in dietary supplements, when used orally for any condition.

Mechanism of Action

Strontium is an alkaline earth element, like calcium. It is physically and chemically similar to calcium.
Ninety-nine percent of strontium is found in bone (11396,11753). Strontium is a silvery metal found naturally as a non-radioactive element. It has four known stable forms and twelve known radioactive isotopes (11399).
Strontium has a beneficial effect on bone. It seems to enhance the replication of preosteoblastic cells. It also appears to increase bone formation by stimulating preosteoblast replication. It may also reduce bone resorption by inhibiting osteoclast activity (11396,11399,11753). Animal research suggests that strontium doesn't have adverse effects on bone mineral profile, bone mineral chemistry, or bone matrix mineralization (11754).
Bone strontium levels rapidly decrease with withdrawal of treatment. Plasma levels seem to correlate well with bone strontium levels after 4 weeks of treatment (11753). Strontium is excreted renally (11394,11400,11755).
Most of the research studies on strontiums effects on bone have used the strontium ranelate salt (11753). Strontium ranelate consists of two atoms of stable strontium and an organic moiety called ranelic acid (11399). There is interest in using strontium ranelate for osteoarthritis and bone pain due to metastatic cancer. Preliminary evidence suggests strontium ranelate may increase cartilage matrix formation, and remineralize bone lesions (11397,11402).
Strontium chloride is the most common salt form used in dietary supplements. But there isn't much research evaluating oral use of these formulations.
For cancer, radioactive strontium-89 is used. Strontium is preferentially taken up in areas of bone undergoing active bone turnover (11753,11755). This causes much greater concentrations of strontium-89 in tumorous bone than normal bone. Strontium-89 selectively irradiates metastatic bone with minimal effect on normal tissue (11755).
For dental hypersensitivity, strontium ions in toothpaste seem to relieve pain by blocking fluid flow in dentinal tubules, microscopic canals in the dentin (11756).
An inverse relationship also appears to exist between dental caries and content of stable strontium in drinking water (11402).

Adverse Reactions

Orally, strontium ranelate is usually well tolerated. However, strontium ranelate can cause epigastric pain and diarrhea (11392,11393,11395).
Intravenously, strontium-89 can cause a transient increase in bone pain. It can also cause bone marrow toxicity. In clinical studies, the nadir of platelet and white blood cell counts appears at approximately 4 to 8 weeks following injection, partially returning to baseline by 12 weeks (11752,11755). Patient should be given instructions about avoiding environmental radioactive contamination.

Interactions with Herbs & Other Dietary Supplements

None known.

Interactions with Drugs

None known.

Drug Influences on Nutrient Levels and Depletion

SOME DRUGS CAN AFFECT STRONTIUM LEVELS:
ANDROGENS: Androgens may decrease urinary excretion rates of strontium. Dosage adjustments may be necessary (11405).
CORTICOSTEROIDS: Corticosteroids may increase urinary excretion rates of strontium. Dosage adjustments may be necessary (11405).
ESTROGEN: Estrogens may decrease urinary excretion rates of strontium. Dosage adjustments may be necessary (11405).

Interactions with Foods

SODIUM: A sodium-poor diet increases the fecal elimination of calcium and may reduce the intestinal absorption of strontium (11403).

Interactions with Lab Tests

BLOOD CELL COUNTS: Strontium-89 depresses blood cell counts, particularly white cells and platelets. Monitor blood cell counts at least once every other week (11755).
CREATINE PHOSPHOKINASE: Strontium may cause a small rise in serum creatine phosphokinase. The clinical significance of this appears insignificant (11392,11395).

Interactions with Diseases or Conditions

BONE DISEASE: Delayed intestinal absorption of strontium may occur in patients with bone disease, such as postmenopausal osteoporosis or osteomalacia (11400,11404).
RENAL INSUFFICIENCY: Strontium is eliminated renally and, theoretically, might accumulate in patients with renal impairment (e.g., creatinine clearance less than 40 ml/minute) (11394,11400); use with caution.

Dosage and Administration

ORAL: For postmenopausal osteoporosis, strontium ranelate 2 grams daily has been used (11392,11395).
INTRAVENOUS: For treating bony metastases, 148MBq (MegaBequerel) strontium-89 chloride is given over 1 to 2 minutes. Or, a dose of 1.5 to 2.2 MBq per kilogram, 40 to 60 microCI (curie) per kilogram may be used (11755).

Comments

Strontium ranelate is being evaluated as a potential prescription treatment for osteoporosis. This is a different form than the strontium that is contained in most dietary supplements. Most supplements contain strontium chloride. But there isn't much scientific information about the oral use of strontium chloride in people. Advise patients against dietary supplements containing strontium chloride until more is known about long-term safety.

STROPHANTHUS

Also Known As

Kombe, Kombe-Strophanthus Seeds, Strophanthi Grati Semen, Strophanthi Kombe Semen, Strophanthus Seeds.

Scientific Names

Strophanthus gratus, synonym Roupellia grata; Strophanthus kombe.
Family: Apocynaceae.

People Use This For

Orally, strophanthus is used for arteriosclerosis, cardiac insufficiency, gastrocardiac symptoms, hypertension, and neurodystonia.

Safety

UNSAFE ...when used orally for self-medication (12,4077).
PREGNANCY: UNSAFE ...when used orally due to possible uterine stimulating effects (19); avoid using.
LACTATION: UNSAFE ...when used orally; avoid using (4077).

Effectiveness

There is insufficient reliable information available about the effectiveness of strophanthus.

Mechanism of Action

The applicable part of strophanthus is the seed. Strophanthus gratus contains a cardiac glycoside strophanthin-G (ouabain) which has digitalis-like effects, but milder. The cardiac glycoside in Strophanthus kombe, strophanthin-K (strophoside), has milder effects than strophanthin-G (18,4077).

Adverse Reactions

Orally, side effects include nausea, vomiting, headache, stupor, disturbance of color vision, and cardiac arrhythmias, particularly when strophanthin-G is administered parenterally and during overdose (18).

Interactions with Herbs & Other Dietary Supplements

ANTHRAQUINONE-CONTAINING HERBS AND LAXATIVE HERBS: Anthraquinone-containing herbs such as aloe, alder buckthorn, European buckthorn, cascara sagrada, frangula, rhubarb, and senna; laxative herbs such as castor bean can worsen strophanthus seed toxicity, particularly with long-term use, due to electrolyte loss (19).
CARDIAC GLYCOSIDE-CONTAINING HERBS: Contraindicated, and concomitant use can increase the risk of cardiac glycoside toxicity. Cardiac glycoside-containing herbs include black hellebore, Canadian hemp roots, digitalis leaf, hedge mustard, figwort, lily of the valley roots, motherwort, oleander leaf, pheasant's eye plant, pleurisy root, squill bulb leaf scales, and uzara (19).
CINCHONA and EPHEDRA: Use with strophanthus seed may increase risk of toxicity (19).
LICORICE: Can worsen effects of strophanthus seed due to hypokalemia (19).

Interactions with Drugs

CALCIUM SUPPLEMENTS: Calcium supplements may enhance the therapeutic effects of strophanthus (18).
CORTICOSTEROIDS: Use of corticosteroids may cause electrolyte depletion and increase the risk of

strophanthus toxicity (19).
DIGOXIN (Lanoxin): Contraindicated; therapeutic duplication increases risk of cardiac glycoside toxicity (2).
DIURETIC DRUGS: Theoretically, concomitant use of potassium-depleting diuretics and strophanthus can increase the risk of cardiac glycoside toxicity due to potassium depletion (19). Some diuretics that can deplete potassium include chlorothiazide (Diuril), chlorthalidone (Thalitone), furosemide (Lasix), hydrochlorothiazide (HCTZ, HydroDIURIL, Microzide), and others.
QUINIDINE: Contraindicated; cardiac medications, including quinidine, may increase the risk of cardiac glycoside toxicity; (18).
QUININE: Taking quinine with strophanthus may increase the risk of cardiac glycoside toxicity (18).
STIMULANT LAXATIVES: Overuse or misuse of laxatives may cause electrolyte depletion and increase risk of strophanthus toxicity (19).

Interactions with Foods
None known.

Interactions with Lab Tests
None known.

Interactions with Diseases or Conditions
CARDIAC CONDITIONS: CAUTION, strophanthus seed may cause arrhythmias (18).

Dosage and Administration
No typical dosage.

Comments
Strophanthus seeds can be confused with other African Strophanthus species (18). Strophanthus is used as an arrow poison in Africa (4077).

SULFORAPHANE

Also Known As
Sulphorafane, Sulforafane, SFN.

Scientific Names
1-isothiocyanate-4-methyl-sulfonyl butane.

People Use This For
Orally, sulforaphane is used for the prevention of prostate cancer and other types of cancer.

Safety
LIKELY SAFE ...when used orally in amounts found in foods (10264). There is insufficient reliable information available about the safety of sulforaphane in medicinal amounts.
CHILDREN: LIKELY SAFE ...when used orally in amounts found in foods (10264). There is insufficient reliable information available about the safety of sulforaphane in medicinal amounts.
PREGNANCY AND LACTATION: LIKELY SAFE ...when used orally in amounts found in foods (10264). There is insufficient reliable information available about the safety of sulforaphane in medicinal amounts.

Effectiveness
There is insufficient reliable information available about the effectiveness of sulforaphane.

Mechanism of Action
Sulforaphane, a sulfur-containing isothiocyanate, is a phytochemical found in cruciferous vegetables such as broccoli (particularly broccoli sprouts), cabbage, cauliflower, radish, and mustard (10264,10463,10681). After oral consumption, cruciferous vegetables containing glucosinolates are degraded to isothiocyanates. These isothiocyanates are conjugated to glutathione before excretion in the urine as an isothiocyanate mercapturic acid (10679). Cooking sulforaphane-containing vegetables seems to reduce the bioavailability of sulforaphane (10462).
Epidemiologic evidence suggests that consumption of cruciferous vegetables is inversely associated with various types of cancers, including leukemia and prostate and liver cancer (10264). Preliminary evidence suggests several theories of action, including the induction of carcinogen defense enzymes, inhibition of carcinogen-activating enzymes, induction of cell cycle arrest, and anti-inflammatory mechanisms (10265,10678,10681,10682). A combination of sulforaphane and selenium may also synergistically protect cells against oxidative damage. This synergy appears to occur at the levels of transcription and translation (10680). Sulforaphane increases the action of phase 2 enzymes,

which inactivate many carcinogens. Sulforaphane may also inhibit the activity of phase 1 enzymes, which increase the carcinogenic activity of some substances (10462,10463).

Adverse Reactions
None reported.

Interactions with Herbs & Other Dietary Supplements
None known.

Interactions with Drugs
None known.

Interactions with Foods
None known.

Interactions with Lab Tests
None known.

Interactions with Diseases or Conditions
None known.

Dosage and Administration
No typical dosage.

SUMA

Also Known As
Brazilian Ginseng, Pfaffia.

Scientific Names
Hebanthe eriantha, synonyms Pfaffia paniculata, Hebanthe paniculata, Gomphrena paniculata.
Family: Amaranthaceae.

People Use This For
Orally, suma is used as an immune enhancer or adaptogen to help the body adapt to all types of stress by enhancing or restoring the immune system. Suma is also used orally for cancer, diabetes, tumors, and as a tonic to restore body function.
Topically, suma is used for wounds and skin problems.

Safety
POSSIBLY SAFE ...when used orally short-term (12).
There is insufficient reliable information available about the safety of the topical use of suma.
PREGNANCY AND LACTATION: Insufficient reliable information available; avoid using.

Effectiveness
There is insufficient reliable information available about the effectiveness of suma.

Mechanism of Action
The applicable part of suma is the root. Cell culture data suggests that the isolated constituents pfaffic acid, a nortriterpene, and saponin derivatives pfaffosiges A through F may inhibit melanoma growth. An ethanolic extract has been shown to have mild anti-inflammatory and analgesic effect, but did not relieve noninflammatory pain (515). At present, we don't know how these components relate to the uses of suma.

Adverse Reactions
Powdered suma root can cause occupational asthma during industrial exposure to the root powder (515).

Interactions with Herbs & Other Dietary Supplements
None known.

Interactions with Drugs
None known.

Interactions with Foods
None known.

Interactions with Lab Tests
None known.

Interactions with Diseases or Conditions
None known.

Dosage and Administration
No typical dosage.

Comments
Suma is called Brazilian ginseng, presumably to present the herb in terms that consumers understand. It is unrelated to the ginsengs (American Ginseng, Panax Ginseng, etc.) or other plants which use ginseng as an alternate common name as well (Blue Cohosh, Canaigre, Codonopsis, Siberian Ginseng, Ashwagandha) (515).

SUMBUL

Also Known As
Ferrula, Musk Root.

Scientific Names
Ferula sumbul.
Family: Apiaceae/Umbelliferae

Comments
At the date of publication, this product was not a common ingredient used in brand name supplements marketed to consumers. Details about this product are available at the online version of *Natural Medicines Comprehensive Database*. See www.naturaldatabase.com.

SUMMER SAVORY

Also Known As
Bean Herb, Bohnenkraut, Savory.
CAUTION: See separate listing for Winter Savory.

Scientific Names
Satureja hortensis, synonym Calamintha hortensis.
Family: Lamiaceae/Labiatae.

People Use This For
Orally, summer savory is used as an appetite stimulant or expectorant, for coughs, flatulence, intestinal disorders including cramps, indigestion, diarrhea, nausea, and to relieve frequent thirst in people with diabetes. It is also used orally as a tea for sore throats, as a tonic, astringent, antiflatulent, and as an aphrodisiac.
Topically, summer savory is used for insect bites.
In foods, summer savory is used in cooking as a culinary spice. The oil is used as a flavoring agent.

Safety
LIKELY SAFE ...when used orally in amounts commonly found in foods. Summer savory has Generally Recognized As Safe (GRAS) status in the US (4912).
POSSIBLY SAFE ...when used orally and appropriately in medicinal amounts (5,6,18). ...when used topically as dilute oil (6,11), summer savory is nonirritating and nonsensitizing (11). Undiluted oil is a severe topical irritant (6).
PREGNANCY AND LACTATION: Insufficient reliable information available; avoid using amounts in excess of foods.

Effectiveness
There is insufficient reliable information available about the effectiveness of summer savory.

Mechanism of Action
The applicable parts of summer savory are the leaves and stem. Summer savory contains tannins (18), and a volatile oil (0.2-3.0 %) including thymol, carvacrol, p-cymene, limonene, and camphene (5,6,11,18). Other constituents also present include vitamin A, calcium, potassium, and proteins (11). Summer savory oil has antifungal, antibacterial, and spasmolytic properties (6,11). The mild antiseptic activity is due to cymene and carvacrol (5,18). A mild antidiarrheal effect is reportedly due to the astringent activity of the tannins (5,6,18).

Adverse Reactions
Topically, summer savory can cause skin eruptions (12). The concentrated oil of summer savory is strongly irritating (6).

Interactions with Herbs & Other Dietary Supplements
None known.

Interactions with Drugs
None known.

Interactions with Foods
None known.

Interactions with Lab Tests
None known.

Interactions with Diseases or Conditions
None known.

Dosage and Administration
ORAL: A typical dose is 3 teaspoons. In making the drink, do not boil, allow plant to soak (18).
TOPICAL: No typical dosage.

SUNDEW

Also Known As
Dew Plant, Drosera, Lustwort, Red Rot, Round-Leafed Sundew, Youthwort.

Scientific Names
Drosera intermedia; Drosera anglica, synonym Drosera longifolia; Drosera ramentacea; Drosera rotundifolia.
Family: Droseraeae.

People Use This For
Orally, sundew is used for bronchitis, asthma, pertussis, tracheitis, gastric ulceration, cancer, coughing fits, and dry cough.

Safety
POSSIBLY SAFE ...when used orally and appropriately (2,4).
PREGNANCY AND LACTATION: Insufficient reliable information available; avoid using.

Effectiveness
There is insufficient reliable information available about the effectiveness of sundew.

Mechanism of Action
Sundew seems to cause antispasmodic, demulcent, and expectorant effects (4). Researchers wonder if the antitussive effect demonstrated in animals is due to naphthoquinone constituents (4). Antimicrobial activity reported in vitro for naphthaquinone constituents (4).

Adverse Reactions
None reported.

Interactions with Herbs & Other Dietary Supplements
None known.

Interactions with Drugs
None known.

Interactions with Foods
None known.

Interactions with Lab Tests
None known.

Interactions with Diseases or Conditions
None known.

Dosage and Administration
ORAL: 1-2 grams dried plant three times daily, or one cup tea (made by steeping 1-2 grams dried plant in 150 mL boiling water 5-10 minutes, strain) three times daily (4); 3 grams dried plant is the average daily dose (2). Liquid extract (1:1 in 25% alcohol), 0.5-2 mL three times daily (4). Tincture (1:5 in 60% alcohol), 0.5-1 mL three times daily (4).

SUNFLOWER OIL

Also Known As
Corona Solis, Helianthi Annui Oleum, Marigold of Peru, Sunflower, Sunflower Oils, Sunflower Seed Oil.

Scientific Names
Helianthus annuus.
Family: Asteraceae/Compositae.

People Use This For
Orally, sunflower oil is used for constipation.
Topically, it is used for poorly healing wounds, skin lesions, psoriasis, arthritis, and as a massage oil.
In foods, sunflower oil is used as a cooking oil.

Safety
LIKELY SAFE ...when used orally and appropriately (9780).
There is insufficient reliable information available about the safety of topical medicinal uses for sunflower oil.
PREGNANCY AND LACTATION: Insufficient reliable information available; avoid using.

Effectiveness
INSUFFICIENT RELIABLE EVIDENCE to RATE

Hypercholesterolemia. There is evidence that using sunflower oil in the diet is more effective than olive oil for decreasing low density lipoprotein (LDL) cholesterol and apolipoprotein B (9780). More evidence is needed to rate sunflower oil for this use.

Mechanism of Action
Sunflower oil is cold pressed from the seeds of Helianthus annuus. Sunflower oil is high in linoleic acid and is used as a source of polyunsaturated fat in the diet (8132).

Adverse Reactions
Orally, sunflower oil seems to be well tolerated (8132). Sunflower oil can cause an allergic reaction in individuals sensitive to the Asteraceae/Compositae family. Members of this family include ragweed, chrysanthemums, marigolds, daisies, and many other herbs.

Interactions with Herbs & Other Dietary Supplements
None known.

Interactions with Drugs
None known.

Interactions with Foods
None known.

Interactions with Lab Tests

FASTING BLOOD GLUCOSE: A diet using sunflower oil as a fat source can cause increased fasting blood glucose levels in patients with type 2 diabetes (8132).
FASTING INSULIN: A diet using sunflower oil as a fat source can cause increased fasting insulin levels in patients with type 2 diabetes (8132).

Interactions with Diseases or Conditions

CROSS-ALLERGENICITY: Sunflower oil can cause an allergic reaction in individuals sensitive to the Asteraceae/Compositae family. Members of this family include ragweed, chrysanthemums, marigolds, daisies, and many other herbs.
DIABETES: A diet using sunflower oil as a fat source seems to increase fasting insulin and glucose levels. It also seems to increase postprandial lipids, which might increase the risk of atherosclerosis in patients with type 2 diabetes (8132).

Dosage and Administration

No typical dosage.

SUPEROXIDE DISMUTASE

Also Known As

Orgotein, S.O.D., SOD, Super-Oxide Dismutase, Super Dioxide Dismutase.

Scientific Names

Superoxide dismutase.

People Use This For

Orally, superoxide dismutase is used for removing wrinkles, regenerating tissue, and extending the length of life.
As an injection, superoxide dismutase is used for inflammatory diseases including osteoarthritis, sports injuries, rheumatoid arthritis, radiation-induced or interstitial cystitis, hyperuricemic syndromes, acute paraquat poisoning, for improving tolerance to radiation therapy, treating cancer, improving rejection rates in kidney transplantation, managing reperfusion injury in acute myocardial infarction, and treating respiratory distress syndrome.

Safety

POSSIBLY SAFE ...when used parenterally, short term. Intravenous, intramuscular, and local injections of superoxide dismutase (SOD) appear to be safe for short-term use (2230,2231,2232,2242,2233,2241,2243). However, since some SOD preparations are derived from animals, there is concern about contamination with diseased animal parts (1825). So far, there are no reports of disease transmission to humans due to use of contaminated SOD preparations.
PREGNANCY AND LACTATION: Insufficient reliable information available; avoid using.

Effectiveness

POSSIBLY EFFECTIVE

Bronchopulmonary dysplasia. Giving superoxide dismutase as an injection seems to reduce bronchopulmonary dysplasia in neonates with respiratory distress syndrome (2242).
Interstitial cystitis. Giving superoxide dismutase as an injection seems to be effective for treating interstitial cystitis (2233).
Osteoarthritis. Giving superoxide dismutase as an injection seems to be effective for treating osteoarthritis (2228,2229).
Rheumatoid arthritis (RA). Giving superoxide dismutase as an injection seems to be effective for treating RA (2230,2231,2232).

LIKELY INEFFECTIVE

Myocardial infarction (MI). Giving superoxide dismutase as an injection doesn't seem to be effective for managing reperfusion injury in acute MI (2241,2243).

Mechanism of Action

Superoxide dismutase (SOD) is an essential enzyme found in all living cells. Some cellular processes produce reactive oxygen species (ROS) such as superoxide radicals that can impair the function of cells and tissues. SOD catalyzes the conversion of superoxide to oxygen and hydrogen peroxide. SOD isoenzymes contain copper and zinc, and iron or manganese. Copper and zinc SOD is the most common. Researchers are interested in the role of SOD in variety of diseases including familial amyotrophic lateral sclerosis, Parkinson's disease, Alzheimer's disease, dengue fever, cancer, Down's syndrome, cataract, and neurological disorders such as Creutzfeldt-Jakob disease (11157).
SOD is found in yeast, spinach, chicken liver, and bovine blood (11157). Commercially, it is typically obtained from bovine liver (11008).

Adverse Reactions
As an injection, SOD can cause pain or allergic reactions at injection site (2235). It can also cause anaphylactic shock, which may be caused by product impurities (11008).
SOD may be prepared from bovine liver. Products made from contaminated or diseased organs might present a human health hazard. There is also concern that spleen extracts produced from cows in countries where bovine spongiform encephalitis (BSE) has been reported might be contaminated with diseased tissue. Countries where BSE has been reported include Great Britain, France, The Netherlands, Portugal, Luxembourg, Ireland, Switzerland, Oman, and Belgium (1825). There have been no reports of BSE transfer to humans from contaminated SOD products. Until more is known, tell patients to avoid these products unless country of origin can be determined. Patients should avoid products that are produced in countries where BSE has been found.

Interactions with Herbs & Other Dietary Supplements
None known.

Interactions with Drugs
None known.

Interactions with Foods
None known.

Interactions with Lab Tests
None known.

Interactions with Diseases or Conditions
None known.

Dosage and Administration
ORAL: No typical dosage.
INJECTION: For osteoarthritis, 16 mg as an intra-articular injection is used twice (2228,2229). For rheumatoid arthritis a typical dose is 4 mg as an intra-articular injection per week (2230,2232). A typical dose for interstitial or radiation-induced cystitis is 12 mg injected into the bladder wall, up to 6 times (2233). For radiation-induced cystitis, a typical dose is 8 mg injected intramuscularly per day (2234). For reducing rejection risk in kidney transplantation, a typical dose is 200 mg intravenously during surgery (2239). For reducing bronchopulmonary dysplasia in neonatal respiratory distress syndrome, 0.25 mg/kg subcutaneously twice daily until ventilator support is no longer required (2242).

Comments
Bovine or recombinant (rh-SOD) source parenteral SOD products are available (2238). There is no evidence that oral SOD products are absorbed.

SWAMP MILKWEED

Also Known As
Rose-Colored Silkweed, Swamp Silkweed.

Scientific Names
Asclepias incarnata.
Family: Asclepiadaceae or Apocynaceae.

People Use This For
Orally, swamp milkweed is used for digestive disorders.

Safety
LIKELY UNSAFE ...when used orally. It contains cardenolides, a type of cardioactive steroid. Digitalis-like poisonings are possible (18).
PREGNANCY AND LACTATION: LIKELY UNSAFE ...when used orally due to presence of cardioactive steroids (18); avoid using.

Effectiveness
There is insufficient reliable information available about the effectiveness of swamp milkweed.

Mechanism of Action

The applicable parts of swamp milkweed are the root and rhizome. Swamp milkweed contains cardioactive steroids known as cardenolides. In swamp milkweed, they have little therapeutic significance (18), but the concentration of the specific cardenolide present is not reported. In large amounts, swamp milkweed has an emetic effect (18).

Adverse Reactions

Orally, large amounts of swamp milkweed can cause vomiting (18).
Topically, the plant can cause local inflammation (19).

Interactions with Herbs & Other Dietary Supplements

CARDIAC GLYCOSIDE-CONTAINING HERBS: Contraindicated; concomitant use increases the risk of cardiac glycoside toxicity. Cardiac glycoside-containing herbs include black hellebore, Canadian hemp roots, digitalis leaf, hedge mustard, figwort, lily of the valley roots, motherwort, oleander leaf, pheasant's eye plant, pleurisy root, squill bulb leaf scales, and strophanthus seeds (19).
LICORICE/HORSETAIL: Theoretically, overuse/misuse of licorice rhizome or horsetail plant with cardiac glycoside-containing herbs increases the risk of cardiac toxicity due to potassium depletion (19).
OTHER CARDIOACTIVE HERBS: Avoid concomitant use with other cardioactive herbs due to unpredictability of effects and adverse effects. Other cardioactive herbs include calamus, cereus, cola, coltsfoot, devil's claw, European mistletoe, fenugreek, fumitory, ginger, Panax ginseng, hawthorn, white horehound, mate, parsley, quassia, scotch broom flower, shepherd's purse, and wild carrot (4).
STIMULANT LAXATIVE HERBS: Theoretically, overuse or misuse of stimulant laxatives with cardiac glycoside-containing herbs increases the risk of cardiac toxicity due to potassium depletion. Stimulant laxative herbs include aloe dried leaf sap, blue flag rhizome, alder buckthorn, European buckthorn, butternut bark, cascara bark, castor oil, colocynth fruit pulp, gamboge bark exudate, jalap root, black root, manna bark exudate, podophyllum root, rhubarb root, senna leaves and pods, wild cucumber fruit (Ecballium elaterium), and yellow dock root (19).

Interactions with Drugs

DIGOXIN (Lanoxin): Contraindicated; therapeutic duplication increases risk of cardiac glycoside toxicity (2).
DIURETIC DRUGS: Theoretically, concomitant use of potassium-depleting diuretics and swamp milkweed can increase the risk of cardiac glycoside toxicity due to potassium depletion (506). Some diuretics that can deplete potassium include chlorothiazide (Diuril), chlorthalidone (Thalitone), furosemide (Lasix), hydrochlorothiazide (HCTZ, HydroDIURIL, Microzide), and others.
MACROLIDE ANTIBIOTICS: Theoretically, concomitant use may increase risk of cardiac glycoside toxicity (17).
QUININE: Theoretically, concomitant use of swamp milkweed and quinine might increase risk of cardiac toxicity (506).
STIMULANT LAXATIVES: Theoretically, overuse or misuse of stimulant laxatives with swamp milkweed may increase risk of cardiac glycoside toxicity due to potassium depletion (19).
TETRACYCLINE ANTIBIOTICS: Theoretically, concomitant use may increase risk of cardiac glycoside toxicity (17).

Interactions with Foods

None known.

Interactions with Lab Tests

None known.

Interactions with Diseases or Conditions

HEART DISEASE: Contraindicated; theoretically the cardiac glycosides contained in swamp milkweed (18) might exacerbate the condition or interfere with existing drug therapy.

Dosage and Administration

No typical dosage.

SWEET ALMOND

Also Known As

Almond, Almonds, Almond Oil, Amygdala Dulcis, Expressed Almond Oil, Fixed Almond Oil, Sweet Almond Oil.
CAUTION: See separate listing for Bitter Almond.

Scientific Names

Prunus amygdalus dulcis. Family: Rosaceae.

People Use This For

Orally, sweet almond is used as a mild laxative, and as a remedy for cancer of the bladder, breast, mouth, spleen, and uterus.
Topically, sweet almond is used as an emollient for chapped skin, to soothe mucous membranes (as a demulcent), and as a weak antibacterial.
Parenterally, sweet almond is also used as a solvent for injectable drugs.
Sweet almonds, themselves, are a familiar food.
In manufacturing, sweet almond is used widely in cosmetics.

Safety

LIKELY SAFE ...when used orally (11). Unlike bitter almond oil, sweet almond oil contains no benzaldehyde and no (or only trace) poisonous hydrocyanic acid HCN (11,12). ...when used topically. Almond oil is nonirritating and nonsensitizing to skin (11).
PREGNANCY AND LACTATION: Insufficient reliable information available; avoid using.

Effectiveness

POSSIBLY EFFECTIVE

Constipation. Taking sweet almond orally seems to relieve constipation due to its laxative effects (11).
Skin irritation. Applying sweet almond topically may act as an emollient and demulcent (11).

Mechanism of Action

The applicable part of sweet almond is the fixed oil. Researchers believe the effects of sweet almond oil are due to the presence of many triglycerides (largely triolein and dioleolinolein) and fatty acids (oleic, linoleic, palmitic, stearic, lauric, myristic and palmitoleic acids) (11). A Japanese patent claims isolation of low molecular weight peptides with analgesic and anti-inflammatory properties (11).

Adverse Reactions

None reported.

Interactions with Herbs & Other Dietary Supplements

None known.

Interactions with Drugs

None known.

Interactions with Foods

None known.

Interactions with Lab Tests

None known.

Interactions with Diseases or Conditions

None known.

Dosage and Administration

ORAL: As a laxative typical doses used are up to 30 mL (11).

Comments

Avoid confusion between volatile almond oil and fixed almond oil. Fixed almond oil (sweet almond oil) is prepared by pressing the kernels of both sweet almond and bitter almond. It does not contain benzaldehyde or hydrocyanic acid (HCN). Sweet almond does not yield a volatile oil. Volatile almond oil (bitter almond oil) contains 95% benzaldehyde and 2-4% poisonous HCN. It is made by water maceration and steam distillation of partially defatted bitter almond (Prunus dulcis amara), apricot (Prunus armeniaca), peach (Prunus persica), and plum (Prunus domestica) kernels (11).

SWEET ANNIE

Also Known As
Annual Mugwort, Annual Wormwood, Artemisinin, Chinese Wormwood, Ching-hao, Qing Hao, Qinghao, Qinghaosu, Sweet Wormwood.

Scientific Names
Artemisia annua.
Family: Asteraceae/Compositae.

People Use This For
Orally, sweet Annie is used for malaria, dysentery, dyspepsia, fever (antipyretic), jaundice, scabies, tuberculosis, cryptosporidiosis in people with AIDS, preventing pneumocystis carinii infections in people with AIDS, psoriasis, systemic lupus erythematosus and other auto-immune disorders, bacterial and fungal infections, inflammatory conditions, anorexia, circulatory disorders, common cold, constipation, gallbladder disorders, gastritis, nematode infestation, painful menstruation, and rheumatism.
Topically, sweet Annie is used for bacterial and fungal infections, arthritis, rheumatism, bruises, neuralgia, and sprains.

Safety
POSSIBLY SAFE ...when used orally and appropriately (12).
There is insufficient reliable information available about the safety of sweet Annie when used topically.
PREGNANCY: LIKELY UNSAFE ...when used orally; avoid using (12,19).
LACTATION: Insufficient reliable information available; avoid using.

Effectiveness
There is insufficient reliable information available about the effectiveness of sweet Annie.

Mechanism of Action
The applicable parts of sweet Annie are the above ground parts (12). The constituent, artemisinin (qinghaosu), is a sesquiterpene lactone with antimalarial activity. Preliminary evidence suggests that artemisinin and quercetagetin 6,7,3',4'-tetramethyl ether might have cytotoxic effects against some types of tumor cells (3183). Extracts of sweet Annie are reported to have antipyretic, anti-inflammatory, and bacteriostatic properties (3184). Evidence suggests that sweet Annie promotes cell-mediated immunity and inhibits antibody responses (3177). Preliminary research suggests that capsules containing sweet Annie herb might have antimalarial activity (3185).

Adverse Reactions
The use of artemether, the semisynthetic derivative of artemisinin, which is a constituent of sweet Annie, has been associated with hypoglycemia, prolongation of the QT interval on the electrocardiogram, abdominal pain, and local injection site pain (3180). Artesunate has been associated with prolonged ataxic gait and slurred speech (450). Sweet Annie might cause an allergic reaction in people sensitive to the Asteraceae/Compositae family. Members of this family include ragweed, chrysanthemums, marigolds, daisies, and many other herbs.

Interactions with Herbs & Other Dietary Supplements
None known.

Interactions with Drugs
None known.

Interactions with Foods
None known.

Interactions with Lab Tests
None known.

Interactions with Diseases or Conditions
CROSS-ALLERGENICITY: Sweet Annie might cause an allergic reaction in people sensitive to the Asteraceae/Compositae family. Members of this family include ragweed, chrysanthemums, marigolds, daisies, and many other herbs.

Dosage and Administration
ORAL: Daily doses of 3-9 grams of sweet Annie above ground parts have been used (3176,3177).

Comments
The semisynthetic derivatives of artemisinin (a constituent of sweet Annie); artemether, arteether, and artesunate, are used as prescription antimalarial drugs in Asia, Africa, and Europe (3181,3182).

SWEET BAY

Also Known As
Bay, Bay Laurel, Bay Leaf, Bay Tree, Daphne, Grecian Laurel, Laurel, Mediterranean Bay, Noble Laurel, Roman Laurel, True Bay.

Scientific Names
Laurus nobilis.
Family: Lauraceae.

People Use This For
Orally, sweet bay is used to treat cancer, and as a bile and general stimulant, antiflatulent, diaphoretic, and herb for foods.
Topically, sweet bay is used as an anti-dandruff agent, as a counterirritant, and to treat rheumatic conditions.
In veterinary medicine, sweet bay is used as an udder ointment.
Historically, the fruit essential and fatty oils of sweet bay have been used for treating furuncles, a localized infection of hair follicles.
For food uses, sweet bay is used as a seasoning.
In food manufacturing, it is used as an herb and oil in processed foods.
In manufacturing, the oil is used in cosmetics, soaps, and detergents.

Safety
LIKELY SAFE ...when used orally in amounts found in foods (12). The highest levels of sweet bay used in food are 0.1% as a herb and 0.02% as an oil (11).
LIKELY UNSAFE ...when the whole, intact leaf is swallowed. The whole leaf is indigestible and can become lodged in the esophagus, hypopharynx (132,133,134,137), or perforate the intestinal lining (135,136).
PREGNANCY AND LACTATION: Insufficient reliable information available; avoid using in amounts exceeding those commonly found in foods.

Effectiveness
There is insufficient reliable information available about the effectiveness of sweet bay.

Mechanism of Action
The applicable part of sweet bay is the dried leaf. The sweet bay constituent, methyl eugenol, has sedative and narcotic properties in mice. The essential oil has bactericidal and fungicidal properties (11). The other constituents of sweet bay include proanthocyanidins, alkaloids, and plant acids (11).

Adverse Reactions
Sweet bay can cause allergic reactions, including contact dermatitis (11). The whole, intact leaf is indigestible and can become lodged in the esophagus and hypopharynx (132,133,134,137) and perforate the intestinal lining (135,136).

Interactions with Herbs & Other Dietary Supplements
None known.

Interactions with Drugs
CNS DEPRESSANTS: Because sweet bay theoretically can enhance the therapeutic and adverse effects of sedatives, concomitant use should be avoided.
NARCOTIC DRUGS: Theoretically, sweet bay can enhance the therapeutic and adverse effects of narcotics. Avoid concomitant use.

Interactions with Foods
None known.

Interactions with Lab Tests
None known.

Interactions with Diseases or Conditions
SWEET BAY ALLERGY: Because of contact dermatitis, sweet bay should be avoided in those having sensitivity to it.

Dosage and Administration
TOPICAL: An extract of sweet bay is typically used in baths and soaks (6002).
ORAL: No typical dosage.

Comments
The ancient Greeks and Romans crowned their victors with the leafy branches of sweet bay (11).

SWEET CICELY

Also Known As
British Myrrh, Shepherd's Needle, Sweet Bracken, Sweet Chervil, Sweet-Cus, Sweet-Fern, Sweet-Humlock, Sweets, The Roman Plant.

Scientific Names
Myrrhis odorata.
Family: Apiaceae/Umbelliferae.

Comments
At the date of publication, this product was not a common ingredient used in brand name supplements marketed to consumers. Details about this product are available at the online version of *Natural Medicines Comprehensive Database*. See www.naturaldatabase.com.

SWEET CLOVER

Also Known As
Common Melilot, Field Melilot, Hart's Tree, Hay Flower, King's Clover, Melilot, Meliloti herba, Melilotus, Sweet Lucerne, Sweet Melilot, Tall Melilot, Wild Laburnum, Yellow Melilot, Yellow Sweet Clover.
CAUTION: See separate listings for Red Clover.

Scientific Names
Melilotus altissimus, synonyms Melilotus macrorrhizus, Trifolium macrorrhizum; Melilotus officinalis, synonyms Melilotus arvensis, Melilotus vulgaris, Trifolium officinale.
Family: Fabaceae/Leguminosae.

People Use This For
Orally, sweet clover is used as a diuretic; and for symptoms of chronic venous insufficiency and varicose veins, including leg pain and heaviness, night cramps, pruritus and edema, supportive treatment of thrombophlebitis, hemorrhoids, post-thrombotic syndromes, and lymphatic congestion.
Topically, sweet clover is used for contusions and ecchymoses.

Safety
LIKELY SAFE ...when preparations of the flowering branch and leaf are used orally in moderate amounts (1,2,18).
LIKELY UNSAFE ...when excessive amounts are used orally because it can cause transient liver injury (18).
PREGNANCY: Insufficient reliable information available. A study of 30 second and third trimester pregnant women did not report any adverse effects (1).
LACTATION: Insufficient reliable information available; avoid using.

Effectiveness
POSSIBLY EFFECTIVE

Chronic venous insufficiency. Taking sweet clover orally seems to be effective for problems associated with chronic venous insufficiency such as varicose veins (1).

There is insufficient reliable information available about the effectiveness of sweet clover for its other uses.

Mechanism of Action
The applicable parts of sweet clover are the flowering branch and leaf. Fresh herb contains coumarinic acids (18), which are converted to free coumarins during drying (1,8,18). Dicoumarol, which has anticoagulant activity, can be

formed if the fresh herb is allowed to spoil (1). There is some evidence to suggest that sweet clover aids wound healing (2,8), and a locally perfused sweet clover extract might eliminate adrenaline-induced vasoconstriction. This would indicate peripheral vasodilation (1). Coumarin isolated from sweet clover reduces experimentally-induced paw inflammation in rats (1). Intravenous administration decreases pain, edema, and improves wound healing in people with phlebitis, and relieves symptoms of varicose veins (1). Sweet clover seems to increase venous reflux and improve lymphatic kinetics, and therefore reduces edema (2).

Adverse Reactions
Orally, headaches are rare (1,2,18), and large amounts can cause stupor and transient liver injury in susceptible individuals (18). There was one case report of bleeding diathesis following two months ingestion of large amounts of a multi-herb, "seasonal tonic" tea containing melilot, sweet woodruff, and tonka bean (all coumarin-containing herbs) (809).

Interactions with Herbs & Other Dietary Supplements
HERBS WITH ANTICOAGULANT/ANTIPLATELET POTENTIAL: Concomitant use of herbs that have constituents that might affect platelet aggregation could theoretically increase the risk of bleeding in some people. These herbs include angelica, clove, danshen, garlic, ginger, ginkgo, Panax ginseng, horse chestnut, red clover, turmeric, and others.

Interactions with Drugs
ANTICOAGULANT/ANTIPLATELET DRUGS: Theoretically, concomitant use might increase bleeding risk (19).
HEPATOTOXIC DRUGS: Theoretically, concomitant use might increase risk of hepatotoxicity.

Interactions with Foods
None known.

Interactions with Lab Tests
LIVER ENZYMES: Sweet clover might cause an increase in liver enzymes and test results, indicating liver damage; monitor (18).

Interactions with Diseases or Conditions
LIVER DISEASE: Theoretically, sweet clover might exacerbate liver disease (see Adverse Reactions) (18); avoid using.

Dosage and Administration
ORAL: Average amount, sweet clover preparations equivalent to 3-30 mg coumarin per day (1,2). Phlebitis or varicose veins, one cup (made by steeping 1-2 teaspoons finely chopped sweet clover in 150 mL boiling water 5-10 minutes, strain) two to three cups per day (8,18); 6 mL Melilotus/rutin preparation (600 mg Melilotus extract containing 3 mg coumarin and 150 mg rutin) per day reported in one clinical trial (1). CAUTION: Monitor liver enzymes with oral use (18), especially in people at risk for liver damage.
TOPICAL: Sweet clover extract in semi-solid preparations containing 3-5 mg/g coumarin (2,8,18). As a poultice for sores and hemorrhoids, wrap sweet clover in linen, thoroughly soak with hot water, place on the affected area (8).
INJECTION: Liquid forms for parenteral use corresponding to 1-7.5 mg coumarin per day (2,8).

Comments
Avoid confusion with red clover (Trifolium pratense) and hay flower, the sieved flower and fruit from cut hay grass (Poaceae family) plants.

SWEET GALE

Also Known As
Bayberry, Bog Myrtle, Dutch Myrtle.
CAUTION: See separate listing for Bayberry.

Scientific Names
Myrica gale.
Family: Myricaceae.

People Use This For
Orally, sweet gale is used for digestive disorders.
In Sweden, a strong brew of sweet gale dried bark is used as an anthelmintic and to cure itching.

Safety
There is insufficient reliable information available about the safety of sweet gale. The volatile oil of sweet gale is considered toxic (18).
Pregnancy and Lactation: Insufficient reliable information available; avoid using.

Effectiveness
There is insufficient reliable information available about the effectiveness of sweet gale.

Mechanism of Action
The applicable parts of sweet gale are the leaf, branch, and wax from catkin. Sweet gale contains 0.4-0.7% of a volatile oil that contains alpha-pinene, delta-cadinene, gamma-cadinene, limonene, beta-myrcene, beta-phellandrene, and 1,8 cineole. It also contains flavonoids including myricitrin (18). Sweet gale is thought to have astringent and aromatic properties (18).

Adverse Reactions
Orally, the volatile oil is considered toxic.

Interactions with Herbs & Other Dietary Supplements
None known.

Interactions with Drugs
None known.

Interactions with Foods
None known.

Interactions with Lab Tests
None known.

Interactions with Diseases or Conditions
None known.

Dosage and Administration
No typical dosage.

Comments
In the Middle ages, sweet gale was mixed with beer, and is said to have led to periods of extreme excitation (18).

SWEET ORANGE

Also Known As
Citri Sinensis, Jaffa Orange, Navel Orange, Orange, Pericarpium, Valencia Orange.
CAUTION: See separate listings for Bergamot Oil, Oswego Tea, and Bitter Orange.

Scientific Names
Citrus sinensis, synonyms Citrus aurantium var. sinensis, Citrus macracantha, Citrus aurantium var. dulcis.
Family: Rutaceae.

People Use This For
Orally, the peel of sweet orange is used as an appetite stimulant. Sweet orange peel is also used to reduce phlegm, treat coughs, colds, anorexia, and malignant breast sores. It is also used as a tonic, antiflatulent, and for dyspepsia. In conjunction with other fruits and vegetables, sweet orange juice is used orally for the prevention of hypertension and stroke, and for the improvement of blood lipid profiles.

Safety
LIKELY SAFE ...when sweet orange juice or fruit is used orally in amounts commonly found in foods (1310,3340).
CHILDREN: LIKELY SAFE ...when sweet orange juice or fruit is used orally in amounts commonly found in foods (1310,3340). LIKELY UNSAFE ...when the sweet orange peel is used orally in excessive amounts. There are reports of intestinal colic, convulsions, and death in children given large amounts of sweet orange peel (11).
PREGNANCY AND LACTATION: LIKELY SAFE ...when sweet orange juice or fruit is used orally in amounts commonly found in foods (1310,3340).

Effectiveness

POSSIBLY EFFECTIVE

Hypercholesterolemia. Consuming sweet orange juice seems to help improve blood lipid profiles. Large amounts of orange juice (750 mL daily for four weeks) seems to increase high-density lipoprotein (HDL) cholesterol by 21%, and reduce the ratio of low-density lipoprotein (LDL) to HDL cholesterol by 16% in hypercholesterolemic patients. Because consumption of this large amount of juice daily consists of approximately 20% of the daily energy requirement, consuming a combination of fruits, vegetables, and orange juice in equivalent amounts to the 750 mL of orange juice on a daily basis is probably a more practical approach. However, this combination was not specifically studied (3340).

Hypertension and stroke. Consuming sweet orange juice seems to help lower the risk of hypertension and stroke. Sweet orange juice products that provide at least 350 mg of potassium per serving and are low in sodium, saturated fat, and cholesterol are permitted by the FDA to make labeling claims that they might reduce the risk of developing high blood pressure and stroke (1310).

INSUFFICIENT RELIABLE EVIDENCE to RATE

Asthma. There is some evidence that consumption of vitamin C-rich citrus fruits, including sweet orange and others, might improve lung function in people with asthma. However, this is controversial. Some studies show that intake of citrus fruits 1-2 times per week produces significant benefit (6049,6055,6056). However, other studies have not found this benefit (6057,6058). More evidence is needed to rate sweet orange for this use.

Mechanism of Action

The applicable parts of sweet orange are the peel, juice and fruit. Orange peel contains essential oil and bitter principles. Limonene is the most abundant monoterpene in sweet orange (4946). The flavonoid constituents naringin and nobiletin might have anti-inflammatory activity (1281). Potential benefits of sweet orange fruit in asthma have been attributed to antioxidant properties of vitamin C or other fruit constituents (6049,6054,6055). For preventing high blood pressure and stroke, sweet orange juice is thought to be beneficial due to high concentrations of potassium. Potassium consumption seems to reduce the risk of developing hypertension and stroke (1310).

There is conflicting data about the effects of sweet orange juice on P-glycoprotein. In animal models, an ethyl acetate extract of orange juice seems to inhibit drug efflux by P-glycoprotein. Theoretically, this would increase absorption of certain drugs that are transported by P-glycoprotein (12116). But in humans, drinking large amounts of sweet orange juice seems to decrease absorption and blood levels of celiprolol. This suggests that orange juice affects P-glycoprotein by actually inducing drug efflux by P-glycoprotein (12115). Other researchers speculate that sweet orange juice might inhibit the drug transporter organic anion transporting polypeptide (OATP) (7046). More evidence is needed to determine sweet orange juice's effects on P-glycoprotein.

Sweet orange juice does not seem to affect cytochrome P450 3A4 (12116).

Adverse Reactions

There have been reports of intestinal colic, convulsions, and death in children following ingestion of large amounts of sweet orange peel (11).

Interactions with Herbs & Other Dietary Supplements

None known.

Interactions with Drugs

CELIPROLOL (Celicard): Sweet orange can decrease oral absorption and blood levels of celiprolol. Celiprolol levels, after a single dose of 100 mg, are decreased by about 80% to 90% in people who concurrently drink large amounts of sweet orange juice, 200 mL three times daily. It's not known if more moderate consumption of sweet orange juice affects celiprolol levels. Researchers theorize that this interaction might be due to sweet orange inhibiting the drug transporter in the gut, called organic anion transporting polypeptide (OATP), or inducing P-glycoprotein (12115).

FEXOFENADINE (Allegra): Sweet orange juice can significantly decrease oral absorption and blood levels of fexofenadine when used together. Sweet orange decreases bioavailability of fexofenadine by about 72%. Sweet orange juice seems to inhibit organic anion transporting polypeptide (OATP), which is a drug transporter in the gut, liver, and kidney (7046). It's not yet known how long sweet orange juice inhibits OATP. Separating administration times might not prevent this interaction. Tell patients it's best to take their medications with a plain glass of water.

IVERMECTIN: Taking ivermectin orally with sweet orange juice 750 mL over 4 hours seems to significantly reduce the bioavailability of ivermectin. This effect does not seem to be related to effects on p-glycoprotein. The effect on ivermectin is more pronounced in males compared to females (12154).

Interactions with Foods

None known.

Interactions with Lab Tests

None known.

Interactions with Diseases or Conditions
None known.

Dosage and Administration
ORAL: For improving lipid profiles, 750 mL sweet orange juice per day has been used (3340).
For appetite stimulation or as a digestive aid, 10-15 grams fresh or dry peel (free of white pulp layer) per day has been used (2). Peel may be used to prepare a tea (steep peel in boiling water 10-15 minutes, strain) or in other herbal preparations (2).

SWEET SUMACH

Also Known As
Aromatic Sumac, Fragrant Sumac, Polecatbush, Skunkbrush, Squawbush.

Scientific Names
Rhus aromatica, synonym Rhus canadensis.
Family: Anacardiaceae.

Comments
At the date of publication, there was very little scientific information about this product. Our staff is continually analyzing the available information on natural medicines and will add data to the online version of *Natural Medicines Comprehensive Database* as it becomes available. See www.naturaldatabase.com.

SWEET VERNAL GRASS

Also Known As
Grass, Spring Grass.

Scientific Names
Anthoxanthum odoratum.
Family: Poaceae/Gramineae.

People Use This For
Orally, sweet vernal grass is used for headache, nausea, sleeplessness, and conditions of the urinary tract.
In Russia, sweet vernal grass is used as an ingredient in certain brandies.
In foods, sweet vernal grass is used as a flavoring agent.

Safety
LIKELY UNSAFE ...when used orally. Sweet vernal grass contains the constituent, dicoumarol that has anticoagulant properties (6,18).
There is insufficient reliable information available about the safety of the topical use of sweet vernal grass.
PREGNANCY AND LACTATION: LIKELY UNSAFE ...when used orally (6,18): avoid using.

Effectiveness
There is insufficient reliable information available about the effectiveness of sweet vernal grass.

Mechanism of Action
Sweet vernal grass contains hydroxycinnamic acid glycosides that form dicoumarol (up to 1.5%) when the harvested plant is dehydrated (18). After an outbreak of hemorrhagic diathesis in cattle fed sweet vernal grass hay, veterinary experiments identified dicumarol, a known anticoagulant, in the hay (6).

Adverse Reactions
Orally, use of high levels of sweet vernal grass can cause headaches and dizziness (18). Cattle poisoned by sweet vernal hay showed characteristically rapid onset of symptoms including progressive weakness, mucosal pallor, stiff gait, tachypnea, tachycardia, and hematomata, quickly resulting in death (6).

Interactions with Herbs & Other Dietary Supplements

HERBS WITH ANTICOAGULANT/ANTIPLATELET POTENTIAL: Concomitant use with herbs that have constituents that might affect platelet aggregation could theoretically increase the risk of bleeding in some people. These herbs include angelica, clove, danshen, garlic, ginger, ginkgo, Panax ginseng, horse chestnut, red clover, turmeric, and others.

Interactions with Drugs

ANTICOAGULANT/ANTIPLATELET DRUGS: Theoretically, sweet vernal grass might cause additive effects and side effects with drugs having anticoagulant or antiplatelet properties (19).

Interactions with Foods

None known.

Interactions with Lab Tests

None known.

Interactions with Diseases or Conditions

None known.

Dosage and Administration

ORAL: No typical dosage.
TOPICAL: Sweet vernal grass is sometimes used as an extract (18).

Comments

This aromatic plant has been used as a flavoring agent due to its vanilla-like aroma (6).

SWEET VIOLET

Also Known As

Banafshah, Garden Violet, Neelapushpa, Neelapuspha, Sweet Violet Herb, Sweet Violet Root, Violae Odoratae Rhizoma, Herba, Violet.
CAUTION: See separate listing for Garden Violet.

Scientific Names

Viola odorata.
Family: Violaceae.

People Use This For

Orally, sweet violet is used for calming and relaxing nerves, physical and mental exhaustion, physical and psychological symptoms associated with menopause (hot flashes), metabolic imbalances, and to "detoxify blood". It is also used orally for depression, irritability, anxiety, GI complaints, abdominal pain, gallbladder complaints, mucous membrane inflammation of the stomach and intestines, enteritis, duodenitis, digestion problems caused by improper diet, flatulence, heartburn, and loss of appetite , respiratory tract conditions, particularly dry mucous membrane inflammation, rheumatism of the minor joints, fever, skin diseases, inflammation of the oral mucosa, nervous strain, headache, and insomnia, coughs, hoarseness, tuberculosis, throat inflammation, bronchitis accompanied by fixed mucous, nervous strain, insomnia, and hysteria.
Topically, sweet violet is used for skin impurities and disorders, and as a skin cleanser.
In herbal combinations, sweet violet is used for acute and chronic bronchitis, bronchial asthma, acute and chronic mucous inflammations of the upper and lower respiratory tract, cold symptoms of the upper respiratory tract, hoarseness, cough, mucous congestion, bronchial inflammation, and late "flu" symptoms. It is also used for chesty, spastic and whooping coughs, emphysema, "dust-damaged" lung, urinary incontinence due to senility, irritable bladder, enuresis nocturna or prostate condition, insomnia, and improving deep sleep.

Safety

POSSIBLY SAFE ...when used orally in appropriate amounts (2,18).
There is insufficient reliable information available about the safety of the topical use of sweet violet.
PREGNANCY AND LACTATION: Insufficient reliable information available; avoid using.

Effectiveness

There is insufficient reliable information available about the effectiveness of sweet violet.

Mechanism of Action
The applicable parts of sweet violet are the root and above ground parts. Sweet violet contains saponins (2), which have expectorant properties, and in high doses irritate mucous membranes (2).

Adverse Reactions
None reported.

Interactions with Herbs & Other Dietary Supplements
None known.

Interactions with Drugs
None known.

Interactions with Foods
None known.

Interactions with Lab Tests
None known.

Interactions with Diseases or Conditions
None known.

Dosage and Administration
ORAL: The typical dose of sweet violet as an herb is one cup tea (steep 2 teaspoons herb in 250 mL boiling water 10-15 minutes, strain) 2-3 times daily (18). As a root (5% w/v), take 1 tablespoon 5-6 times daily (simmer 20 grams in boiling water for 10-15 minutes, and strain) (18).
TOPICAL: No typical dosage.

SWEET WOODRUFF

Also Known As
Galii odorati herba, Master of the Wood, Waldmeister, Woodruff, Wordward.

Scientific Names
Galium odorata, synonym Asperula odorata.
Family: Rubiaceae.

People Use This For
Orally, sweet woodruff is used for preventing and treating respiratory tract, gastrointestinal tract, liver, gallbladder, and urinary tract disorders; for blood purification; venous complaints; weak veins; hemorrhoids; vasodilation; spasms; abdominal discomforts; strengthening the nervous system; agitation; hysteria; nervous menstrual disorders; restlessness; insomnia; neuralgia; strengthening heart function; cardiac irregularity; stomachache; migraine; and bladder stones. Sweet woodruff is also used orally for inducing sweating, as an antispasmodic, diuretic, or expectorant.
Topically, sweet woodruff is used for skin diseases, treating wounds, venous conditions, hemorrhoids, and for reducing inflammation.
In foods and beverages, sweet woodruff is used as a flavoring component.
In manufacturing, the extracts of sweet woodruff above ground parts are used as fragrance components in perfumes.

Safety
LIKELY SAFE ...when used orally in amounts commonly found in foods. Sweet woodruff has Generally Recognized As Safe (GRAS) status in the US (4912).
POSSIBLY SAFE ...when used orally and appropriately for medicinal uses on a short-term basis (12,18). There is insufficient reliable information available about the safety of the topical use of sweet woodruff.
PREGNANCY AND LACTATION: Insufficient reliable information available; avoid using.

Effectiveness
There is insufficient reliable information available about the effectiveness of sweet woodruff.

Mechanism of Action

The applicable parts of sweet woodruff are the above ground parts. Sweet woodruff leaves and the constituent asperuloside show evidence of anti-inflammatory activity (11). Sweet woodruff also demonstrates antibacterial activity (4009). The fresh plant contains up to 1% coumarin as a bound glycoside. Coumarin is supposedly enzymatically released during dehydration (11). Interestingly, one investigation failed to detect any coumarins in sweet woodruff (11). The coumarin constituent is thought to have anti-inflammatory, anti-edema, spasmolytic, and lymphokinetic effects, but the levels found in sweet woodruff are so low that therapeutic effects are doubtful (18). Other constituents present in sweet woodruff include monotopein, tannins, anthracene and naphthalene derivatives, plus traces of nicotinic acid, a fixed oil, and a bitter principle (11).

Adverse Reactions

Orally, sweet woodruff above ground parts can be associated with headache (12), and in larger amounts, stupor (18). Long-term use can cause liver damage (18).

Interactions with Herbs & Other Dietary Supplements

None known.

Interactions with Drugs

None known.

Interactions with Foods

None known.

Interactions with Lab Tests

None known.

Interactions with Diseases or Conditions

None known.

Dosage and Administration

ORAL: A typical dose is one cup tea. To make tea, use 2 teaspoons (1.8 grams) in a glass of water (18). The average single dose is 1 gram during the day or shortly before bedtime (18).
TOPICAL: No typical dosage.

Comments

Sweet woodruff root contains a red dye (6). Sweet woodruff is considered obsolete for medicinal use in many countries (18). Avoid confusing sweet woodruff, Galium odoratum, with Asperula odorata which is also referred to as woodruff.

TAGETES

Also Known As

African Marigold, Aztec Marigold, Big Marigold, Chinchilla Enana, Dwarf Marigold, French Marigold, Huacatay, Marigold, Mexican Marigold, Muster John Henry, Saffron Marigold, Stinking Roger.
CAUTION: See separate listing for Calendula.

Scientific Names

Tagetes erecta; Tagetes minuta, synonym Tagetes glandulifera; Tagetes patula.
Family: Asteraceae/Compositae.

People Use This For

Orally, tagetes is used as an anthelmintic, a menstrual flow stimulant, and for treating colic. Tagetes is also used orally for treating coughs, colds, mumps, mastitis, sore eyes, and dysentery.
Additionally, tagetes is used orally for improving digestion, inducing sweating, as an antiflatulent, sedative in gastric pain, bile flow and appetite stimulant, diuretic, and as an anti-abortifacient.
Topically, the leaves are used for treating sores and ulcers; and the flowers are used as a mosquito repellant. The juice of the leaves are used topically for eczema; and the oil is used for treating wound maggots.
In foods and beverages, tagetes is used as a flavor component.
In manufacturing, the oil is used as a fragrance in perfumes. The dried, ground flowers are used as chicken feed to enhance the characteristic yellow color of chicken skin and egg yolk.

Safety

LIKELY SAFE ...when used orally in amounts commonly found in foods. Tagetes has Generally Recognized As Safe (GRAS) status in the US (4912).

There is insufficient reliable information available about the safety of tagetes used in amounts greater than those found in foods.

PREGNANCY AND LACTATION: Insufficient reliable information available; avoid amounts greater than those commonly found in foods.

Effectiveness

There is insufficient reliable information available about the effectiveness of tagetes.

Mechanism of Action

The applicable parts of tagetes are the above ground parts. Some evidence suggests tagetes oil might have tranquilizing, hypotensive, bronchodilatory, spasmolytic, and anti-inflammatory properties (11). The constituent ocimenone demonstrates cidal activity against mosquito larvae (11). Alpha-terthienyl exhibits nematocidal and larvicidal activity (11). Patulin has demonstrated antispasmodic activity; and may reduce capillary permeability, and increase blood pressure (11).

Adverse Reactions

Topically, tagetes can cause contact dermatitis (11). Tagetes can also cause an allergic reaction in individuals sensitive to the Asteraceae/Compositae family. Members of this family include ragweed, chrysanthemums, marigolds, daisies, and many other herbs.

Interactions with Herbs & Other Dietary Supplements

None known.

Interactions with Drugs

None known.

Interactions with Foods

None known.

Interactions with Lab Tests

None known.

Interactions with Diseases or Conditions

CROSS-ALLERGENICITY: Tagetes can cause an allergic reaction in individuals sensitive to the Asteraceae/Compositae family. Members of this family include ragweed, chrysanthemums, marigolds, daisies, and many other herbs.

Dosage and Administration

No typical dosage.

Comments

Tagetes oil is distilled from the above ground parts of Tagetes erecta, minuta, and patula (11).

TAMARIND

Also Known As

Imlee, Tamarindo.

CAUTION: See separate listing for Garcinia.

Scientific Names

Tamarindus indica.

Family: Fabaceae/Leguminosae.

People Use This For

Orally, tamarind is used for chronic or acute constipation, liver and gallbladder disorders, to decrease fever, to treat pregnancy-related nausea, as an anthelmintic for children, for stomach disorders, and to treat colds. Topically, a thick paste of the seeds is used as a cast for broken bones. In foods and beverages, tamarind is used as a flavoring agent. It is also widely used in Asian cuisine for chutneys and curries.

Safety
LIKELY SAFE ...when used orally in amounts commonly found in foods. Tamarind has Generally Recognized As Safe (GRAS) status in the US (4912).
There is insufficient reliable information available about the safety of tamarind used in amounts greater than those found in food.
PREGNANCY AND LACTATION: Insufficient reliable information available; avoid using in amounts greater than those found in foods.

Effectiveness
There is insufficient reliable information available about the effectiveness of tamarind.

Mechanism of Action
The partially dried, fruit/pod of tamarind is used medicinally. It contains plant acids, largely d-tartaric acid, sugars, pectin, protein, vitamins, and minerals. The volatile oil contains over 60 compounds including methyl salicylate and safrole. The fruit pulp has mild laxative properties, but heat causes loss of this effect. Some evidence suggests an aqueous extract is highly toxic to the trematode Schistosoma mansoni, and the parasite-carrying snail Bulinus trucatus. Other evidence suggests that the tamarind constituent, tamarindienal might have antifungal activity against Aspergillus niger and Candida albicans, and antibacterial activity against Bacillus subtilis, Staphylococcus aureus, Escherichia coli, and Pseudomonas aeruginosa (11).

Adverse Reactions
None reported.

Interactions with Herbs & Other Dietary Supplements
None known.

Interactions with Drugs
IBUPROFEN: Taking tamarind fruit extract as a component of the food millet porridge concurrently with ibuprofen seems to increase ibuprofen absorption and blood levels (12093). Theoretically, this could increase the risk of ibuprofen side effects.

Interactions with Foods
None known.

Interactions with Lab Tests
None known.

Interactions with Diseases or Conditions
None known.

Dosage and Administration
ORAL: As a laxative, 10-50 grams of tamarind paste is used orally as fruit cubes (18). This is a paste prepared from the fermented fruit of Tamarindus indica (18).
TOPICAL: No typical dosage.

TANNIC ACID

Also Known As
None.

Scientific Names
Tannic acid.

People Use This For
Topically, tannic acid is used for cold sores and fever blisters, diaper rash and prickly heat, poison ivy, ingrown toenails, sore throat, inflamed tonsils, spongy or receding gums, acute dermatitis, and as a styptic. Tannic acid is used orally and topically for bleeding, chronic diarrhea, dysentery, bloody urine, painful joints, persistent coughs, and cancer. Vaginally, tannic acid is used as a douche for leukorrhea. In foods and beverages, tannic acid is used as a flavoring agent. In manufacturing, tannic acid is used in hemorrhoidal ointments and suppositories, for tanning hides and manufacturing ink, and to kill dust mites on furniture.

Safety

LIKELY SAFE ...when used orally in amounts commonly found in foods. Tannic acid has Generally Recognized As Safe (GRAS) status in the US (4912).
POSSIBLY UNSAFE ...when used topically to treat diaper rash and prickly heat (272), and minor burn or sunburn (272).
There is insufficient reliable information available about the safety of the topical use of tannic acid to treat cold sores and fever blisters. The FDA's concern about potential oral absorption and toxicity has prompted requests for further data (272).
PREGNANCY AND LACTATION: LIKELY UNSAFE ...when used topically on damaged skin or large areas of skin (2). There is insufficient reliable information available about the safety of the oral use of tannic acid during pregnancy and lactation; avoid using amounts greater than those found in foods.

Effectiveness

POSSIBLY INEFFECTIVE
Burns. Applying tannic acid doesn't seem to be effective for treating minor burn or sunburn (272).
Diaper rash. Applying tannic acid doesn't seem to be effective for treating diaper rash (272).
Herpes labialis (cold sores). Applying tannic acid doesn't seem to be effective for treating cold sores and fever blisters (272).
Prickly heat. Applying tannic acid doesn't seem to be effective for treating prickly heat (272).
There is insufficient reliable information available about the effectiveness of tannic acid for its other uses.

Mechanism of Action

Tannic acid is a mixture of glycosides of phenolics, mainly gallic acid (11). Pharmaceutical grade tannic acid is generally considered to be pentadigalloylglucose (11). Tannic acid has astringent effects (11,12). It dehydrates tissue, internally reducing secretions, and externally forming a protective layer of harder, constricted cells (12). Tannins show some evidence of antiviral, antimicrobial, CNS depressant, and cariostatic effects (11). Some evidence suggests that tannins might cause cancer, but other evidence shows tannins might prevent it (12). Regular consumption of herbs with high tannin concentrations correlates with increased incidence of esophageal or nasal cancer (12).

Adverse Reactions

Orally, large amounts of tannic acid can cause gastric irritation, nausea, and vomiting (11). Tannins have been associated with fatal liver damage from extensive use on burns or in enemas (11). However, the toxicity may be due to an impurity, digallic acid, rather than the tannins themselves (11).

Interactions with Herbs & Other Dietary Supplements

TANNIN-CONTAINING HERBS: Theoretically, herbs that contain high percentages of tannins (such as oak bark) might precipitate alkaloids and other alkaline constituents of herbs (19).

Interactions with Drugs

ORAL DRUGS: Theoretically, avoid concomitant administration due to potential of tannic acid to precipitate alkaloids and other basic drugs (19). Separate administration of oral drugs and tannic acid by the longest period of time practical (19).

Interactions with Foods

None known.

Interactions with Lab Tests

None known.

Interactions with Diseases or Conditions

KIDNEY DYSFUNCTION: Theoretically, oral use of tannic acid is contraindicated in individuals with kidney dysfunction. Tannic acid can cause kidney damage, potentially exacerbating a pre-existing condition (12).
LIVER DYSFUNCTION: Theoretically, oral use of tannic acid is contraindicated in individuals with liver dysfunction. Tannic acid can cause liver damage, potentially exacerbating a pre-existing condition (12).
PRE-EXISTING CONDITIONS: Theoretically, full baths are contraindicated in individuals with fever or infectious diseases, NYHA III and IV heart failure, or hypertonia stage IV (WHO) (2).
SKIN CONDITIONS: Full baths with tannic acid tea are contraindicated in individuals with weeping eczema and extensive skin damage (12).

Dosage and Administration

No typical dosage.

Comments

New York Heart Association (NYHA) stage I and II heart disease refers to people with heart disease without resulting limitations of physical activity and who are comfortable at rest and in whom ordinary physical activity results in fatigue, palpitation, trouble breathing, or anginal pain (2). Tannic acid is extracted from the nutgalls formed on twigs of certain oak trees by insects (Quercus infectoria and other Quercus species). The "universal antidote", formerly used for poisoning, contained tannic acid, activated charcoal, and magnesium oxide. These three ingredients in combination were believed to synergistically reduce the absorption of poisons. Unfortunately, tannic acid was instead adsorbed by activated charcoal, which diminished the benefit of the combination (272).

TANSY

Also Known As

Bitter Buttons, Buttons, Chrysanthemi vulgaris flos, Chrysanthemi vulgaris herba, Daisy, Hind Heal, Parsley Fern, Tansy Flower, Tansy Herb, Scented Fern, Stinking Willie.
CAUTION: See separate listing for Wood Sage.

Scientific Names

Tanacetum vulgare, synonyms Chrysanthemum vulgare, Tanacetum boreale.
Family: Asteraceae/Compositae.

People Use This For

Orally, tansy is used as an abortifacient, as an anthelmintic for roundworm or threadworm infestation in children, migraines, neuralgia, epilepsy, rheumatism, improving digestion and stimulating appetite, as an antispasmodic, for flatulence, bloating due to intestinal or peritoneal gas, stomach and duodenal ulcers, noninflammatory gallbladder conditions, palpitation, sciatica, stomachache, edema associated with weak heart, colds, fever, hysteria, calming nerves, gout, kidney problems, and tuberculosis. Tansy is also used as an antioxidant, antiseptic, bactericide, cordial, emmenagogue, diaphoretic, narcotic, pediculicide, tonic, and stimulant.
Topically, tansy is used for scabies, pruritus ani, bruises, sores, sprains, swelling, freckles, inflammation, leukorrhea, sunburn, swelling, toothache, tumors, and as an insect repellent.
In foods and manufacturing, tansy extracts are used in perfume, as a flavoring agent in foods and beverages, and a source of green dye.

Safety

POSSIBLY UNSAFE ...when used topically. Tansy can cause severe contact dermatitis (6,18,19).
LIKELY UNSAFE ...when varieties containing the toxic constituent thujone are used orally (2,6,515). Fatalities have been associated with ingestion of as little as 10 drops of tansy oil, although one individual recovered after ingesting 15 mL (6). Fatalities have also been reported from prepared teas or powdered forms (4,6). However, thujone concentration varies widely amongst tansy species (4,6,515).
PREGNANCY: LIKELY UNSAFE ...when used topically due to potential abortifacient, menstrual flow, and uterine stimulant effects (12,19).
LACTATION: POSSIBLY UNSAFE ...when used topically due to thujone content (2,6).

Effectiveness

There is insufficient reliable information available about the effectiveness of tansy.

Mechanism of Action

The applicable parts of tansy are the above ground parts. The activity and toxicity of the above ground parts of tansy vary greatly according to the subspecies (515). Thujone, a constituent with both activity and toxicity ranging from a concentration of 0-95% in the volatile oil (4,515). The thujone constituent causes an increase in salivation and an increase in blood flow to the mucous membranes and pelvic viscera (7). Researchers think thujone has a mind-altering effect similar to tetrahydrocannabinol (THC), the active principle in marijuana (515). Thujone also shows evidence of neurotoxicity (2), hepatotoxicity, and it might be harmful to individuals with defects in hepatic heme synthesis (4,12). Chronic thujone poisoning leads to seizures, delirium, and hallucinations (7). Tansy extracts have demonstrated effects in alleviating pain, stimulating bile, and increasing appetite in individuals with liver and gallbladder disorders (4). Some evidence suggests tansy extracts might also have antispasmodic activity (4). Other evidence suggests the constituent, caffeic acid, might have a role in the bile-stimulating effects (4). Tansy shows evidence that it might reduce serum lipid levels and has some hypoglycemic effects (4). Tansy demonstrates antifungal activity (4). Some evidence suggests tansy oil has antibacterial activity (6). In addition, tansy oil, ether extract, and the constituent beta-thujone show evidence of anthelmintic activity (4). Aqueous extracts of tansy can partially inactivate tick-borne encephalitis in vitro. They also induce resistance in experimental animals (6). Preliminary studies suggest tansy has some antitumor effects (4). The constituents believed to be responsible for allergic contact dermatitis are the sesquiterpene lactones (4,6,19).

Adverse Reactions

Orally, large amounts of thujone or using thujone-containing products long-term can cause restlessness, vomiting, vertigo, tremors, renal damage, and convulsions (12). Symptoms of toxicity include rapid, feeble pulse (4,6), severe gastroenteritis (2), severe spasms (4), convulsions (2,4), rapid breathing (2), vomiting, abdominal pain, facial flushing, loss of consciousness, irregular heartbeat, dilated pupils, pupillary rigidity, uterine bleeding, abortion, kidney damage, and liver damage (2,18). Death can occur 1-3.5 hours after ingestion (18).
Topically, tansy is associated with severe contact dermatitis (6,19) and local mucosal membrane irritation (19). It can cause an allergic reaction in individuals sensitive to the Asteraceae/Compositae family. Members of this family include ragweed, chrysanthemums, marigolds, daisies, and many other herbs.

Interactions with Herbs & Other Dietary Supplements

THUJONE-CONTAINING HERBS: Concomitant use of herbs containing thujone can increase the risk of thujone toxicity. Thujone-containing herbs include oak moss, oriental arborvitae, sage, wormwood, thuja (cedar), and tree moss (12); avoid using.

Interactions with Drugs

ALCOHOL (Ethanol): The constituent, thujone, heightens and alters the effect of alcohol (7).

Interactions with Foods

None known.

Interactions with Lab Tests

None known.

Interactions with Diseases or Conditions

CROSS-ALLERGENICITY: Tansy can cause an allergic reaction in individuals sensitive to the Asteraceae/Compositae family. Members of this family include ragweed, chrysanthemums, marigolds, daisies, and many other herbs.
PORPHYRIA: Theoretically, tansy can exacerbate porphyria in people with underlying defects in hepatic heme synthesis (12).

Dosage and Administration

No typical dosage.

Comments

The name tansy is derived from the Greek word, athanasia, for immortality. Tansy was thought to impart mortality and it was used for embalming (6). Avoid confusion with tansy ragwort (Senecio species) and other plants generically referred to as "tansy".

TANSY RAGWORT

Also Known As

Cankerwort, Common Ragwort, Dog Standard, European Ragwort, Ragweed, Ragwort, St. James' Wort, Staggerwort, Stammerwort, Stinking Nanny.
CAUTION: See separate listings for Golden Ragwort and Tansy.

Scientific Names

Senecio jacobaea.
Family: Asteraceae/Compositae.

People Use This For

Orally, tansy ragwort is used for cancer, colic, wound-healing, spasms, as a laxative, to induce sweating and menstruation, and for "cleansing and purification".

Safety

UNSAFE ...when used orally. Tansy ragwort contains hepatotoxic unsaturated pyrrolizidine alkaloids (UPAs) (12,19). Repeated exposure to low concentrations of UPAs linked to veno-occlusive disease, a serious condition (4,12). UPAs may also be carcinogenic and mutagenic (12). Topical use on abraded or broken skin might be unsafe due to potential for systemic absorption (12,19).

PREGNANCY: UNSAFE ...when used orally because of possible menstruation promoting and oxytocic activity, and teratogenic effects (19).
LACTATION: UNSAFE ...when used orally due to pyrrolizidine alkaloid (19).

Effectiveness

There is insufficient reliable information available about the effectiveness of tansy ragwort.

Mechanism of Action

The applicable parts of tansy ragwort are the above ground flowering parts. Some pyrrolizidine alkaloids have shown carcinogenic and mutagenic properties, and there are reports of renal toxicity. However, the primary concern is veno-occlusive disease (12). Unsaturated pyrrolizidine alkaloids are known to be hepatotoxic in animals and humans (4).

Adverse Reactions

Chronic exposure to plants containing UPA constituents has been associated with veno-occlusive disease (4021). Symptoms of acute veno-occlusive disease are characterized by a dull, dragging ache in the right upper abdomen and marked distention of the abdomen. These symptoms are sometimes accompanied by reduced urine output. Subacute veno-occlusive disease is associated with vague symptoms and persistent liver enlargement (4021). Tansy ragwort can cause an allergic reaction in individuals sensitive to the Asteraceae/Compositae family. Members of this family include ragweed, chrysanthemums, marigolds, daisies, and many other herbs.

Interactions with Herbs & Other Dietary Supplements

EUCALYPTUS: Theoretically, concomitant use might increase the risk of unsaturated pyrrolizidine alkaloid toxicity due to enzyme induction by eucalyptus (19).
PYRROLIZIDINE ALKALOID-CONTAINING HERBS: Concomitant use is contraindicated due to the risk of additive toxicity. Herbs containing unsaturated pyrrolizidine alkaloids include alkanna (12), borage (271), gravel root (4), hemp agrimony (271), hound's tongue (19), petasites (19), comfrey (271), coltsfoot, and the Senecio species plants; dusty miller (19), alpine ragwort (19), groundsel (271), golden ragwort (19), and tansy ragwort (271).

Interactions with Drugs

None known.

Interactions with Foods

None known.

Interactions with Lab Tests

None known.

Interactions with Diseases or Conditions

CROSS-ALLERGENICITY: Can cause an allergic reaction in individuals sensitive to the Asteraceae/Compositae family. Members of this family include ragweed, chrysanthemums, marigolds, daisies, and many other herbs.
LIVER DISEASE: Tansy ragwort is contraindicated in people with liver disease.

Dosage and Administration

No typical dosage.

Comments

Both tansy ragwort and golden ragwort are known as ragweed and can therefore be confused (see separate listing). American Herbal Products Association recommends labeling all botanical products that contain toxic pyrrolizidine alkaloids "For external use only. Do not apply to broken or abraded skin; do not use when nursing" (12).

TARRAGON

Also Known As

Estragon, Little Dragon, Mugwort.
CAUTION: See separate listing for Mugwort (Artemisia vulgaris).

Scientific Names

Artemisia dracunculus, synonym Artemisia glauca.
Family: Asteraceae/Compositae.

People Use This For

Orally, tarragon is used for digestive disorders, toothache, to promote menstruation, as a diuretic, appetite stimulant, and hypnotic.
In foods and beverages, tarragon is used as a culinary herb and a flavor component.
In manufacturing, tarragon is used as a fragrance component in soaps and cosmetics.

Safety

LIKELY SAFE ...when used orally in amounts commonly found in foods. Tarragon has Generally Recognized As Safe (GRAS) status in the US (4912).
POSSIBLY SAFE ...when used orally short-term in medicinal amounts (12).
POSSIBLY UNSAFE ...when used orally, long-term due to estragole, which can be carcinogenic (12).
PREGNANCY AND LACTATION: LIKELY UNSAFE ...when used in medicinal amounts due to possible menstrual promoting effects (11); avoid using.

Effectiveness

There is insufficient reliable information available about the effectiveness of tarragon.

Mechanism of Action

The applicable parts of tarragon are the above ground parts. Estragole is the main constituent of tarragon's essential oil (81%). The constituent estragole is a procarcinogen but the carcinogenic risk is minimal. It is not directly hepatotoxic or hepatocarcinogenic but requires activation by liver enzymes to reach full toxicity. In the liver other enzymes inactivate the carcinogenic metabolites, limiting possible damage to the liver (12). Tarragon shows evidence of antibacterial activity, but estragole does not appear to be responsible. Some information suggests undiluted tarragon oil can irritate the skin, but a concentration of 4% in petrolatum appears to be nonirritating and nonsensitizing (11).

Adverse Reactions

Tarragon can cause an allergic reaction in individuals sensitive to the Asteraceae/Compositae family. Members of this family include ragweed, chrysanthemums, marigolds, daisies, and many other herbs.

Interactions with Herbs & Other Dietary Supplements

None known.

Interactions with Drugs

None known.

Interactions with Foods

None known.

Interactions with Lab Tests

None known.

Interactions with Diseases or Conditions

CROSS-ALLERGENICITY: Can cause an allergic reaction in individuals sensitive to the Asteraceae/Compositae family. Members of this family include ragweed, chrysanthemums, marigolds, daisies, and many other herbs.

Dosage and Administration

No typical dosage.

Comments

Tarragon is also known as mugwort. Be careful not confuse it with mugwort (Artemisia vulgaris). Tarragon is a rich plant source of potassium (19). Adulteration of tarragon oil is common (11).

TAUMELLOOLCH

Also Known As

Bearded Darnel, Cheat, Darnel, Drake, Ray-Grass, Tare.

Scientific Names

Lolium temulentum.
Family: Poaceae/Gramineae.

People Use This For
Orally, taumelloolch is used for blood poisoning, cancer, cysts, dizziness, eczema, hemorrhage, idiocy, indurations, "knots", leprosy, gangrene, migraine, headache, nerve pain, nose bleeds, putrid flesh, sleeplessness, stomach cramps, involuntary dyskinetic movements, neuralgia, rheumatism, and sciatica, toothache, tumors, meningitis, urinary incontinence, and colic.
Topically, taumelloolch is used as a poultice for skin diseases, to draw out splinters, and for broken bones.

Safety
LIKELY UNSAFE ...when used orally. Symptoms of toxicity range from confusion and giddiness to weakness and death from respiratory failure (18,4502).
There is insufficient reliable information available about the safety of the topical use of taumelloolch.
PREGNANCY AND LACTATION: LIKELY UNSAFE ...when used orally (18,4502); avoid using.

Effectiveness
There is insufficient reliable information available about the effectiveness of taumelloolch.

Mechanism of Action
The applicable part of taumelloolch is the seed. The active agents of taumelloolch are temulentin, temultin acid, tannin, and glycoside (18). It has analgesic and narcotic properties, as well as toxicity (4502). Poisoning has been reported from ingestion of the grain, the berries mixed with grains, and the seed infected with a bacterial toxin (18,4502). To date, the toxic principle has not been identified (18,4502). No cases of poisonings have been reported in recent times, although the plant has become extremely rare through intensive seed-corn purification (18).

Adverse Reactions
Symptoms of taumelloolch toxicity include colic, confusion, giddiness, weakness, dizziness, dilated pupils, headache, confusion, staggering, somnolence, trembling, vision and speech disorders, vomiting, delirium, and death from respiratory failure (18,4502).

Interactions with Herbs & Other Dietary Supplements
None known.

Interactions with Drugs
None known.

Interactions with Foods
None known.

Interactions with Lab Tests
None known.

Interactions with Diseases or Conditions
None known.

Dosage and Administration
No typical dosage.

Comments
Taumelloolch is believed to be the tares of the biblical parable of the wheat and the tares (4502). Some information suggests that an ergot component extracted from the grass and seeds of taumelloolch is used by a mystic cult to induce religious ecstasy (4502).

TAURINE

Also Known As
Aminoethanesulfonate, L-Taurine.

Scientific Names
2-Aminoethane sulfonic acid.

People Use This For

Orally, taurine is used in the treatment of congestive heart failure (CHF), high blood pressure, hepatitis, high cholesterol (hypercholesterolemia), and cystic fibrosis. Other uses include seizure disorders (epilepsy), autism, attention deficit-hyperactivity disorder (ADHD), retinal degeneration, diabetes, and alcoholism. It is also used to improve mental performance and as an antioxidant.

Safety

POSSIBLY SAFE ...when used orally and appropriately. Taurine has been used safely in studies lasting up to one year (5248,5271,8217,8221).
CHILDREN: POSSIBLY SAFE ...when used orally and appropriately. Taurine has been given to children with apparent safety for up to 4 months (10455).
PREGNANCY AND LACTATION: Insufficient reliable information available; avoid using.

Effectiveness

POSSIBLY EFFECTIVE

Congestive heart failure (CHF). Taking taurine orally seems to improve left ventricular function (5248,5271,8221) and symptoms of heart failure (5271,5306,8221) in patients with New York Heart Association (NYHA) functional class II to IV. Some patients with severe heart failure rapidly improve from NYHA class IV to II after 4-8 weeks of treatment. Improvement seems to continue for as long as taurine treatment is continued, up to one year (5306,8217,8218,8221).

Hepatitis. Taking taurine orally might improve liver function in patients with acute hepatitis (10454).

INSUFFICIENT RELIABLE EVIDENCE to RATE

Cystic fibrosis. Taurine supplementation might be useful as adjunctive therapy to reduce steatorrhea in children with cystic fibrosis. However, it does not seem to improve growth, lung function, or other symptoms of cystic fibrosis (10455).

Mental performance. Preliminary clinical research suggests that taurine in combination with caffeine can produce minor improvements in mental performance. It might improve attention and verbal reasoning, but doesn't seem to have any effect on memory (9899).

More evidence is needed to rate taurine for these uses.

Mechanism of Action

Taurine is a conditionally essential amino sulfonic acid present in high amounts in meat and fish. The most abundant dietary source of taurine is human breast milk (3467). Large amounts of taurine are also found in the human brain, retina, heart, and platelets (8219,8220). Taurine is normally synthesized in the human body in adequate amounts from cysteine and hypotaurine (3467).

During prolonged times of insufficient intake, such as during parenteral nutrition, the body cannot maintain adequate levels of taurine and supplementation becomes necessary (3467). Supplementation is also necessary in non-breast-fed infants because their ability to synthesize taurine is undeveloped and cow's milk does not provide a sufficient amount (3467). Taurine is often added to human infant formulas, enteral products, and some parenteral nutritional solutions. Excess taurine is excreted by the kidneys (3467).

Taurine is involved in retinal photoreceptor activity, bile acid conjugation, white blood cell antioxidant activity, central nervous system neuromodulation, platelet aggregation, cardiac contractility, sperm motility, growth, insulin activity (8220), and osmoregulation (5280).

Taurine is thought to be beneficial in the treatment of congestive heart failure (CHF), although the exact mechanism of action remains unclear. The concentration of taurine increases in the left ventricle of patients with CHF; its function here is an area of active research (9900). Oral taurine alters intracellular calcium movement, increasing left ventricular function without any adverse changes in arterial pressure in patients with CHF (3467,5315,8222). Taurine might also improve heart failure because it seems to lower blood pressure and might normalize excessive sympathetic nervous system activity that often occurs in people with hypertension and CHF (3467,8219,8221,8222). Preliminary studies also suggest taurine might have natriuretic and diuretic activity. Taurine might also have a cholesterol-lowering effect. Taurine seems to stimulate bile acid synthesis. There is some evidence that taurine might also have antioxidant and free radical scavenging activity. Platelets normally have high levels of taurine, and can become more prone to aggregation during taurine depletion. However, it is unknown if taurine supplementation has any effect on platelet coagulation (3467).

Adverse Reactions

None reported.

Interactions with Herbs & Other Dietary Supplements

None known.

Interactions with Drugs

None known.

Interactions with Foods
None known.

Interactions with Lab Tests
None known.

Interactions with Diseases or Conditions
None known.

Dosage and Administration
ORAL: For the treatment of congestive heart failure, 2-6 grams per day in two or three divided doses has been used in clinical studies (3467,5248,5306,8217,8221). For the treatment of acute hepatitis, taurine 4 grams 3 times daily has been used for 6 weeks (10454). For treatment of steatorrhea in children with cystic fibrosis, taurine 30 mg/kg daily for 4 months in addition to pancreatic enzyme supplementation (10455).

TEA TREE OIL

Also Known As
Australian Tea Tree Oil, Melaleuca Oil, Oil of Melaleuca, Oleum Melaleucae.
CAUTION: See separate listings for Cajeput Oil and Niauli Oil.

Scientific Names
Melaleuca alternifolia.
Family: Myrtaceae.

People Use This For
Topically, tea tree oil is commonly used for skin and skin surface infections such as acne, onychomycosis, lice, scabies, athlete's foot, and ringworm. It is also used topically as a local antiseptic for cuts and abrasions, for burns, insect bites and stings, boils, vaginal infections, recurrent herpes labialis, toothache, infections of the mouth and nose, sore throat, and for ear infections such as otitis media and otitis externa.
It is also used as a bath additive to treat cough, bronchial congestion, and pulmonary inflammation.

Safety
POSSIBLY SAFE ...when used topically and appropriately (4028,4445,8573).
LIKELY UNSAFE ...when used orally. Like other essential oils, tea tree oil can cause significant toxicity if used orally (4028,10011).
CHILDREN: POSSIBLY SAFE ...when used topically and appropriately (8573). LIKELY UNSAFE ...when used orally. Ingestion of tea tree oil can be toxic (4030,10010,10013,11799).
PREGNANCY AND LACTATION: POSSIBLY SAFE ...when used topically and appropriately (512).
LIKELY UNSAFE ...when used orally. Ingestion of tea tree oil can be toxic (515).

Effectiveness
POSSIBLY EFFECTIVE

Acne. Applying a 5% tea tree oil gel appears to be as effective as 5% benzoyl peroxide (Oxy-5, Benzac AC, and others) for treating acne. Tea tree oil might work more slowly than benzoyl peroxide, but seems to be less irritating to facial skin (8573).

Onychomycosis. Topical application of 100% tea tree oil solution twice daily for 6 months can produce a mycological cure in about 18% of patients with toenail infections. It can also improve nail appearance and symptoms in about 56% of patients after three months and 60% of patients after six months of treatment. It seems to be comparable to twice daily application of clotrimazole 1% solution (Fungoid, Lotrimin, Lotrimin AF) (7031). Lower concentrations of tea tree oil do not seem to be as effective. For example, there is some evidence that a 5% tea tree oil cream applied three times daily for two months has no beneficial effect (7032).

Tinea pedis (athlete's foot). Topical application of a 10% tea tree oil cream seems comparable to tolnaftate 1% cream (Genaspor, Tinactin, Ting, and others) for relieving symptoms of athlete's foot, including scaling, inflammation, itching, and burning. Application of 25% or 50% tea tree oil solution appears to produce both clinical improvement and a mycological cure in 48%-50% of patients after 4 weeks of treatment (10033). However, application of 10% tea tree oil cream appears no more effective than placebo in producing a mycological cure for tinea pedis (4031).

POSSIBLY INEFFECTIVE

Herpes labialis (cold sores). Application of 6% tea tree oil gel 5 times daily does not significantly improve recurrent herpes labialis (2035).

INSUFFICIENT RELIABLE EVIDENCE to RATE

Bacterial vaginosis. Preliminary evidence suggests tea tree oil may be beneficial for anaerobic bacterial vaginosis (10017).

Oropharyngeal candidiasis. There is preliminary evidence that tea tree oil might be beneficial for oropharyngeal candidiasis in patients with HIV/AIDS refractory to fluconazole. Swishing and expelling tea tree oil solution for two to four weeks seems to improve oral candidiasis (4445).

More evidence is needed to rate tea tree oil for these uses.

Mechanism of Action

Tea tree oil is obtained by the distillation of the leaves of the tea tree. The oil contains more than 100 monoterpenoid, sesquiterpenoid, and alcohol compounds. Up to 90% is made up of terpinen-4-ol, 1,8-cineole, alpha-terpineol, terpinolene, and alpha- and gamma-terpinene (4027,7111). The primary constituent terpinen-4-ol is active against numerous pathogenic bacteria and fungi but seems to spare normal skin flora. The constituents, alpha-terpineol and linalool, may also contribute to its antimicrobial activity (10012,10026). Tea tree oil appears to disrupt the permeability barrier of microbial cell membrane structures, causing loss of chemiosmotic control (10028).

Tea tree oil has been found to inhibit growth of the yeast Candida albicans (4445,4446,10012). The oil has in vitro activity against Enterococcus faecium and Enterococcus faecalis, including vancomycin-resistant strains, Klebsiella pneumoniae, including gentamicin-resistant strains, and Stenotrophomonas maltophilia (4448,4451,7111,10012,10026). Tea tree oil also has in vitro activity against both methicillin-sensitive Staphylococcus aureus and methicillin-resistant Staphylococcus aureus (4448,4451,7111,10014,10027). The oil seems to have limited activity against Pseudomonas aeruginosa (7111,10012,10026). Oils produced with increased concentrations of terpinen-4-ol seem to have greater activity against these organisms (7111). Tea tree oil has also been found to inhibit in-vitro growth of the yeast species malassezia, commonly found on human skin (4450). It is also active against Propionibacterium acnes, Escherichia coli, Aspergillus flavus, Trichophyton mentagrophytes, and Trichophyton rubrum (8573). Additional evidence suggests tea tree oil may reduce histamine-induced skin inflammation caused by invading organisms. Tea tree oil applied to histamine-induced inflammation of the skin can decrease mean weal volume (10009). The constituents eucalyptol and limonene may be responsible for the adverse effect of contact eczema (10015,10029).

Adverse Reactions

Orally, tea tree oil and other essential oils can cause significant toxicity. Tea tree oil can cause confusion, inability to walk, disorientation, ataxia, systemic contact dermatitis (4028,10011,10016), and a eucalyptus-like odor on the breath (4028). There is at least one case of coma following ingestion of 120 mL of tea tree oil (4028). Ingestion of as little as 2.5 mL of tea tree oil can cause petechial body rash and neutrophil leukocytosis. It can take up to a week for symptoms to resolve (10011). In young children, ingestion of 10 mL or less of tea tree oil can cause significant ataxia, drowsiness, eucalyptus-like odor on the breath, respiratory failure, disorientation, and coma (4030,10010,11799). As a general rule never use undiluted volatile oils internally.

Topically, tea tree oil is usually well tolerated; however, it can cause local irritation and inflammation, allergic contact eczema, and allergic contact dermatitis in some patients (658,4027,4029,10015,10029,10030,10031,10032). Tea tree oil can cause skin dryness, and less frequently pruritus, stinging, burning, and redness in patients with acne (8573). It may also cause mild oral mucosal burning (4445). There is some concern that topical use of tea tree oil in the middle ear for treatment of ear infections might cause ototoxicity. There is preliminary evidence that preparations of 100% tea tree oil can cause ototoxicity and impaired hearing. However, so far there are no reports of ototoxicity in humans. Until more is known, tell patients to avoid such highly concentrated tea tree oil preparations. Lower concentrations of 2% tea tree oil seem less likely to have this effect (7025).

Interactions with Herbs & Other Dietary Supplements

None known.

Interactions with Drugs

None known.

Interactions with Foods

None known.

Interactions with Lab Tests

None known.

Interactions with Diseases or Conditions

None known.

Dosage and Administration

TOPICAL: For onychomycosis, 100% tea tree oil solution applied twice daily for six months has been used (7031). For tinea pedis (athlete's foot), 25% or 50% tea tree oil solution applied twice daily for one month has been used (10033). Tea tree oil 10% cream applied twice daily for one month has also been used (4031). For acne, 5% tea tree oil gel applied daily has been used (8573). For oropharyngeal candidiasis, 15 ml tea tree oil solution swished and expelled four times daily for two to four weeks has been used (4445). For anaerobic bacterial vaginosis, 200 mg tea tree oil pessaries inserted vaginally once daily for 5 days have been used (10017).

Comments
Tea tree oil has the aroma of nutmeg (515). The tea tree was named by eighteenth century sailors who made an aromatic tea from the leaves of the tree growing on the swampy southeast Australian coast (515). Do not confuse the tea tree with the unrelated common tea plant that is used to make black and green teas. Avoid confusion with cajeput oil and niauli oil.

TEAZLE

Also Known As
Barber's Brush, Brushes and Combs, Card Thistle, Church Broom, Teasel, Venus' Basin.

Scientific Names
Dipsacus fullonum, synonym Dipsacus sylvestris.
Family: Dipsacaceae.

Comments
At the date of publication, this product was not a common ingredient used in brand name supplements marketed to consumers. Details about this product are available at the online version of *Natural Medicines Comprehensive Database*. See www.naturaldatabase.com.

TERMINALIA

Also Known As
Arjuna, Axjun Argun, Bahera, Bahira, Bala Harade, Balera, Behada, Beleric Myrobalan, Bihara, Chebulic Myrobalan, Hara, Harada, Haritaki, He Zi, Hirala, Indian Almond, Kalidruma, Karshaphala, Myrobalan, Tropical Almond, Vibhitaki.

Scientific Names
Terminalia arjuna, synonyms Pentaptera arjuna, Pentaptera glabra; Terminalia bellirica, synonym Myrobalanus bellirica; Terminalia chebula.
Family: Combretaceae.

People Use This For
Orally, Terminalia arjuna is used for cardiovascular conditions, including ischemic heart disease and angina, hypertension, and hyperlipidemia. It is also used orally as a diuretic, for earaches, dysentery, venereal and urogenital diseases, and as an aphrodisiac.
Orally, Terminalia belerica and Terminalia chebula are used for hyperlipidemia and digestive disorders, including both diarrhea and constipation, and indigestion. They have also been used for HIV infection. Terminalia belerica is also used orally as a hepatoprotectant and for respiratory conditions, including respiratory tract infections, cough, and sore throat. Terminalia chebula is also used orally for dysentery.
Topically, Terminalia belerica and Terminalia chebula are used as a lotion for sore eyes. Terminalia chebula is also used topically as a mouthwash and gargle.
Intravaginally, Terminalia chebula is used as a douche for treating vaginitis.
In traditional Ayurvedic medicine, Terminalia belerica has been used as a "health-harmonizer" in combination with Terminalia chebula and Emblica officinalis. This combination is also used to lower cholesterol and to prevent necrosis of cardiac tissue. In traditional Ayurvedic medicine, Terminalia arjuna has been used to balance the three humors, kapha, pitta, and vata. It has also been used for asthma, bile duct disorders, scorpion stings, and for poisonings.

Safety
POSSIBLY SAFE ...when used orally and appropriately, short term. Several small studies have used the powdered bark of Terminalia arjuna safely in cardiac patients in trials lasting from 2 weeks to 3 months (2502,2503,2504); however, patients should avoid self-treatment with this product, due to the potentially significant cardiovascular effects. Further study is needed to determine the safety of Terminalia arjuna for long-term use.
There is insufficient reliable information available about the safety of Terminalia belerica and Terminalia chebula (6).
PREGNANCY: POSSIBLY UNSAFE ...when used orally. One source warns against using Terminalia belerica and

Terminalia chebula during pregnancy; however, the reason for this warning is not described (33); avoid using. There is insufficient reliable information available about the safety of Terminalia arjuna in pregnancy; avoid using. **LACTATION**: Insufficient reliable information available; avoid using.

Effectiveness

POSSIBLY EFFECTIVE

Angina. Taking terminalia orally seems to be effective as a short-term adjunct to conventional therapy for treating postmyocardial infarction angina. In one small clinical trial, postmyocardial infarction patients with angina taking Terminalia experienced significantly less angina, improved left ventricular ejection fractions, and decreased left ventricular mass compared to patients receiving the standard therapy alone (2502,2503).

Congestive heart failure (CHF). Taking Terminalia orally as a short-term adjunct to conventional therapy seems to be effective for treating severe congestive heart failure. In a small cross-over trial, patients with severe, refractory congestive heart failure had significant reductions in symptoms and improved left ventricular function after 2 weeks of treatment (2504).

Large-scale, long-term trials are necessary to clarify Terminalia's potential role in the treatment of cardiovascular conditions.

There is insufficient reliable information available about the effectiveness of Terminalia for its other uses.

Mechanism of Action

There are three species of terminalia of medicinal interest: Terminalia arjuna, Terminalia belerica and Terminalia chebula (6,33). The applicable part of Terminalia arjuna is the bark. The bark contains several active constituents, including Terminalia arjuna gallic acid, ethyl gallate, and the flavone luteolin. Luteolin may have anticancer properties (2506). The bark of Terminalia arjuna is reported to be beneficial in cardiovascular conditions; however, the exact mechanism is not known. Terminalia arjuna is reported to lower serum cholesterol and low-density lipoprotein (LDL) levels (2505,2517,2519). It is also thought to have an antihypertensive effect and act as a cardiac stimulant. However, studies have been conflicting; some indicating that it may actually increase blood pressure (33).

The applicable part of Terminalia belerica and Terminalia chebula is the fruit (6). These species also have been reported to improve lipid profiles, but to a lesser degree than Terminalia arjuna. Terminalia chebula is reported to have a greater effect on lipids than Terminalia belerica (2517,2519). The astringent properties of Terminalia belerica and Terminalia chebula are attributed to their beneficial effects in bowel irregularity and indigestion (33). Terminalia belerica also contains gallic acid, and is thought to have hepatoprotective properties (2507). An ethanolic extract of Terminalia chebula containing gallic acid and its ethyl ester may have activity against methicillin-resistant Staphylococcus aureus (2508). Terminalia chebula may also have activity against cytomegalovirus (CMV), herpes simplex I, Streptococcus mutans, Salmonella sp., Shigella, and retroviral reverse transcriptase (2509,2510,2511,2512,2513,2514). Both Terminalia belerica and Terminalia chebula may have activity against HIV (2518). The gallic acid and chebulagic acid in Terminalia chebula may have immunosuppressive effects against cytotoxic T lymphocytes (2515).

Adverse Reactions

None reported in humans. In animal studies, Terminalia chebula has caused hepatic and renal lesions (2516).

Interactions with Herbs & Other Dietary Supplements

None known.

Interactions with Drugs

None known.

Interactions with Foods

None known.

Interactions with Lab Tests

None known.

Interactions with Diseases or Conditions

None known.

Dosage and Administration

ORAL: For improving left ventricular function, treating postmyocardial infarction anginal pain as an adjunct to conventional therapy, and congestive failure, a dose of the powdered bark of Terminalia arjuna 500 mg every 8 hours has been used (2502,2503,2504).

Comments

The bark of Terminalia arjuna has been used in India for more than 3000 years, primarily as a heart remedy. An Indian physician named Vagbhata has been credited as the first to use this product for heart conditions in the seventh century A.D. Research on Terminalia has been going on since the 1930s, but pharmacological studies have provided mixed results. Its role in heart disease remains unclear.

THEANINE

Also Known As

Gamma-glutamylethylamide, L-theanine.
CAUTION: See separate listings for Green Tea and Threonine.

Scientific Names

5-N-ethylglutamine.

People Use This For

Orally, theanine is used for preventing dementia including Alzheimer's disease, treating hypertension, and enhancing the effects of chemotherapy drugs.

Safety

There is insufficient reliable information available about the safety of theanine.
Pregnancy and Lactation: Insufficient reliable information available.

Effectiveness

There is insufficient reliable information available about the effectiveness of theanine.

Mechanism of Action

Theanine is the major amino acid found in green tea. Green tea contains 1% to 3% theanine (7685,7690). There is interest in using theanine to prevent and treat dementia. Theanine is an analog of glutamate, which is an excitatory neurotransmitter. Levels of glutamate increase and cause neuronal death during periods of cerebral ischemia. Theanine demonstrates a protective effect by decreasing ischemic neuronal death in the forebrains of animal models (7685). The antagonistic effects of theanine on glutamate and N-methyl-D-aspartate (NMDA) receptors might provide neuroprotection (7685).

There is also interest in using theanine for hypertension. Theanine affects catecholamines that can cause vasoconstriction and lead to elevations in blood pressure. In animal models, theanine decreases norepinephrine levels (7686), decreases systolic and diastolic blood pressure (7687), and suppresses the stimulatory effects of caffeine (7685,8665). However, there is also some evidence theanine might induce an excitatory effect when used in very small doses, suggesting the effects of theanine are dose dependent (8665).

Green tea might prevent atherosclerosis by inhibiting the proliferation of smooth muscle cells in blood vessel walls, but theanine doesn't seem to affect smooth muscle (8666). Additionally, there is evidence that suggests theanine might prevent the development of atherosclerosis by inhibiting lipid peroxidation of low-density lipoproteins (LDL) (8667).

There is also interest in using theanine adjunctively for cancer. In studies involving doxorubicin, theanine increases the concentration of doxorubicin and adriamycin in tumors by blocking efflux of the drug from tumor cells (7688,7690,8668,8669). Theanine seems to enhance the effects of doxorubicin and adriamycin on drug sensitive and multi-drug resistant tumors (7688,8668,8669). Theanine may also enhance the suppressive action of doxorubicin on metastatic tumors (8312). Theanine also inhibits the efflux of idarubicin from leukemia cells in animal models (7689). Additionally, theanine seems to decrease the toxicity of idarubicin by reversing adverse effects on leukocytes and bone marrow cells (7689).

There is also some evidence that theanine might decrease serotonin and 5-hydroxyindole acetic acid (5HIAA) concentrations in the brain. Theanine might enhance the degradation of serotonin, and it might also directly inhibit the enzyme responsible for serotonin synthesis (8670).

Animal research suggests theanine may act synergistically with caffeine and other constituents in green tea to cause weight loss (11960).

Adverse Reactions

None reported.

Interactions with Herbs & Other Dietary Supplements

None known.

Interactions with Drugs

ANTIHYPERTENSIVE DRUGS: Theoretically, concomitant use of theanine might potentiate the activity of antihypertensive medications (7687).

STIMULANT DRUGS: Theoretically, concomitant use of theanine might decrease the effects of stimulant drugs such as caffeine (7685,7686).

Interactions with Foods
None known.

Interactions with Lab Tests
None known.

Interactions with Diseases or Conditions
None known.

Dosage and Administration
No typical dosage.

THIAMINE (VITAMIN B1)

Also Known As
Antiberiberi Factor, Antiberiberi Vitamin, Antineuritic Factor, Antineuritic Vitamin, Anurine, Aneurine Hydrochloride, B complex Vitamin, Thiamin Chloride, Thiamin Hydrochloride, Thiamine Chloride, Thiamine Hydrochloride, Thiaminium Chloride Hydrochloride.

Scientific Names
Thiamine; Thiamin; Vitamin B1; Vitamin B-1.

People Use This For
Orally, thiamine is used for thiamine deficiency syndromes, including beriberi, peripheral neuritis associated with pellagra, and neuritis of pregnancy. It is used for poor appetite, ulcerative colitis, chronic diarrhea, GI disorders, cerebellar syndrome, an insect repellent, diabetic neuropathy, AIDS, maintaining a positive mental attitude, enhancing learning abilities, heart disease, alcoholism, stress, improving athletic performance, and aging. Thiamine is also used orally for canker sores, immunodepression, memory loss including Alzheimer's disease, vision problems such as cataracts and glaucoma, motion sickness, and increasing energy.

By injection, thiamine is used for Wernicke's encephalopathy syndrome, other thiamine deficiency syndromes in critically ill people, acute alcohol withdrawal, and coma or hypothermia of unknown origin.

Safety
LIKELY SAFE ...when used orally and is generally considered nontoxic; although, rare hypersensitivity reactions have occurred (15). ...when used appropriately as the injectable FDA-approved prescription product.

PREGNANCY AND LACTATION: LIKELY SAFE ...when used orally at the recommended dietary allowance (RDA) of 1.4 mg per day (3094). There is insufficient reliable information available about the safety of using larger amounts during pregnancy or lactation.

Effectiveness
EFFECTIVE

Metabolic disorders. Taking thiamine orally helps to temporarily correct metabolic disorders associated with genetic diseases such as subacute necrotizing encephalopathy (SNE, Leigh's disease), maple syrup urine disease (branched-chain aminoacidopathy), and lactic acidosis associated with pyruvate carboxylase deficiency and hyperalaninemia (15).

Thiamine deficiency. Taking thiamine orally helps to prevent and treat thiamine deficiency syndromes including beriberi and peripheral neuritis associated with pellagra or neuritis of pregnancy. Thiamine deficiency can occur in people with malabsorption conditions such as alcoholism, cirrhosis, and gastrointestinal (GI) diseases; and in those with inadequate intake due to anorexia, nausea, and vomiting; and in those with increased requirements, including pregnancy, increased carbohydrate intake, increased physical activity, hyperthyroidism, infection, and hepatic disease; however, deficiency is rare with these conditions (15).

POSSIBLY EFFECTIVE

Cataracts. Taking thiamine orally seems to reduce the occurrence of cataracts. A large-scale population-based study found high dietary intake of thiamine was associated with a reduced risk of nuclear cataracts (6378).

INSUFFICIENT RELIABLE EVIDENCE to RATE

Athletic performance. Some clinical research suggests that thiamine (given as allithiamin), in combination with pantethine and pantothenic acid (vitamin B5) does not improve muscular strength or endurance in well-trained athletes (10432). More evidence is needed to rate thiamine for this use.

Mechanism of Action

Thiamine is required for carbohydrate metabolism. It combines with adenosine triphosphate (ATP) to form thiamine diphosphate, a coenzyme in carbohydrate metabolism, wherein the decarboxylation of pyruvic acid and alpha-ketoglutaric acid occurs. This coenzyme is also a part of transketolation reactions. Thiamine is also a coenzyme in the utilization of pentose in the hexose monophosphate shunt (15).

Thiamine deficiency leads to decreased transketolase activity in erythrocytes and increased pyruvic acid concentration in the blood (15). Pyruvic acid is converted to lactic acid. Therefore, lactic acidosis can also occur in patients with thiamine deficiency (15).

Thiamine might also be involved in neuromuscular transmission (10541).

Syndromes associated with thiamine deficiency are beriberi and Wernicke-Korsakoff syndrome (3041). Beriberi is characterized by anorexia; abdominal discomfort; constipation; peripheral neurologic changes; sleep disturbance; poor memory; and, sometimes, cardiovascular symptoms, including dyspnea, edema, palpitations, vasodilation, warm extremities, and high output cardiac failure. Wernicke-Korsakoff syndrome is characterized by confusion, aphonia, confabulation, nystagmus, ophthalmoplegia, and coma.

In Crohn's disease, decreased serum thiamine levels have been reported (6269). Preliminary animal data also suggests thiamine deficiency in diabetics may exacerbate the development of diabetic nephropathy (11467).

Adverse Reactions

Orally, thiamine is usually well tolerated, but in rare cases can cause dermatitis and other hypersensitivity reactions (15).

Injection of thiamine can cause feelings of warmth, tingling, pruritus, pain, urticaria, weakness, sweating, nausea, restlessness, tightness of the throat, angioedema, respiratory distress, cyanosis, pulmonary edema, GI bleeding, transient vasodilation and hypotension, vascular collapse, and death. Tenderness and induration can occur at IM injection sites (15).

Interactions with Herbs & Other Dietary Supplements

ARECA: Areca (betel) nuts reduce thiamine activity, probably by chemical inactivation (10538). Chronic, regular chewing of betel nuts may contribute to thiamine deficiency (10537,10538).

HORSETAIL: Horsetail (Equisetum) contains a thiaminase-like compound that can destroy thiamine in the stomach and theoretically cause symptomatic thiamine deficiency (10573). The Canadian Government requires that equisetum-containing products be certified free of thiaminase activity (10573). Avoid use of this herb in people at risk for thiamine deficiency.

Interactions with Drugs

None known.

Drug Influences on Nutrient Levels and Depletion

SOME DRUGS CAN AFFECT THIAMINE LEVELS:

ANTIBIOTICS: Interference with the normal gastrointestinal (GI) flora by antibiotics may reduce bacterial synthesis of thiamine. However, the majority of the daily thiamine requirement is obtained from the diet, rather than synthesis by the GI flora (9502). Therefore this isn't likely to be clinically significant, and thiamine supplements aren't necessary.

CONTRACEPTIVE DRUGS: Some studies have reported a small reduction in activity of the thiamine-dependent enzyme erythrocyte transketolase in women taking oral contraceptives, suggesting mild thiamine deficiency (10548,10555). However, other studies have found no effect (10527,10556). Routine use of thiamine supplements with oral contraceptives isn't necessary.

DIURETICS: Increased urinary thiamine excretion and biochemical evidence of thiamine deficiency may occur in some people treated with diuretics, especially in high doses (e.g., >80 mg furosemide per day) for several months (1283,1284,1286,10507,10508). Although most case reports involve furosemide (Lasix), animal data suggest that the effect is related to increased urinary flow and may occur with any diuretic (10509). Diuretic-induced thiamine deficiency appears to be rare in people less than 60 years of age (10506). Most reports involve elderly people who may have inadequate dietary vitamin intake (1283,10507). The potential for thiamine deficiency in people taking diuretics is a concern because it could worsen heart failure (1284,1285,1286,10507). Limited research suggests that supplementation with thiamine 200 mg/day may improve left ventricular ejection fraction and functional capacity in some thiamine-deficient people treated with high doses of furosemide for heart failure (1284,1286,10508). However, other studies have found no improvement (1285). It's too soon to recommend routine thiamine supplementation for people on prolonged, high-dose diuretic therapy. Monitor for thiamine deficiency.

FLUOROURACIL (5-fluorouracil, 5-FU, Adrucil): People receiving fluorouracil-containing chemotherapy regimens may be at risk for thiamine deficiency. Fluorouracil might interfere with activation of thiamine or increase its breakdown (10522). However, there isn't enough research to recommend routine thiamine supplements. Thiamine deficiency has been reported with other chemotherapy regimens, but this is likely due to reduced dietary intake associated with cancer and its treatment (10553,10554).

METFORMIN (Glucophage): Theoretically, metformin might reduce thiamine activity. Thiamine is involved in the entrance of glycolytic pyruvate into the mitochondrial Kreb's cycle. Reducing thiamine activity might lead to

increased amounts of pyruvate being converted to lactic acid. This effect might be responsible for some of the cases of lactic acidosis associated with Metformin. This theoretical effect is based on preclinical animal research with metformin's predecessor, phenformin (9536). This has not yet been substantiated in people taking metformin (11466).
PHENYTOIN (Dilantin): Some evidence suggests that chronic treatment with phenytoin might reduce levels of thiamine in plasma and cerebrospinal fluid, and reduce uptake of thiamine into nervous tissues (10510,10511,10512). Theoretically, this could contribute to side effects of phenytoin such as polyneuropathy and cerebellar ataxia (10510,10511). However, it isn't clear whether the patients affected also have other factors contributing to thiamine deficiency, such as dietary insufficiency. There isn't enough evidence to recommend routine thiamine supplementation for all patients taking phenytoin.

Interactions with Foods

COFFEE, TEA: Polyphenols, such as tannins, in coffee and tea can react with thiamine, converting it to an unabsorbable and inactive form (9535,10539,10540,10544). Biochemical evidence of thiamine deficiency has been found in a rural Thai population consuming large quantities of tea (> 1 liter per day) or chewing fermented tea leaves chronically (10537,10538). However, this effect hasn't been found Western populations, despite regular tea consumption (10539). The interaction isn't likely to be clinically significant, especially when the diet is adequate in thiamine and also ascorbic acid, which can prevent the reaction between thiamine and polyphenols (10538,10540).
SEAFOOD: Raw freshwater fish and shellfish contain thiaminase enzymes that destroy thiamine. Frequent ingestion of raw fish or shellfish can contribute to thiamine deficiency (9535,10537,10538). The enzymes are destroyed by cooking; therefore consumption of cooked seafood doesn't affect thiamine levels.

Interactions with Lab Tests

SERUM THEOPHYLLINE: Large amounts of thiamine can interfere with Schack and Waxler spectrophotometric determination of serum theophylline concentrations (15).
URIC ACID: Thiamine can cause false positive results in the phosphotungstate method for uric acid determination (15).
UROBILINOGEN: Thiamine can cause false positive results in the urine spot test with Ehrlich's reagent for urobilinogen (15).

Interactions with Diseases or Conditions

ALCOHOLISM, CIRRHOSIS, MALABSORPTION SYNDROMES: Thiamine absorption is decreased in these conditions (15).

Dosage and Administration

ORAL: As a dietary supplement in adults, 1-2 mg per day is commonly used. For mild thiamine deficiency syndromes in adults, the usual dose of thiamine is 5-30 mg daily in either a single dose or divided doses for one month (15). The typical dose for severe deficiency can be up to 300 mg per day (15). Parenteral thiamine is recommended for critically ill people (15). For genetic enzyme deficiency disorders, 10-20 mg daily is recommended, although 600-4000 mg daily in divided doses may be needed for Leigh's disease (15). A daily dietary intake of approximately 10 mg of thiamine has been associated with reducing the risk of nuclear cataracts (6378).
The daily recommended dietary allowances (RDAs) of thiamine are: Infants 0-6 months, 0.2 mg; Infants 7-12 months, 0.3 mg; Children 1-3 years, 0.5 mg; Children 4-8 years, 0.6 mg; Males 9-13 years, 0.9 mg; Males 14 years and older, 1.2 mg; Females 9-13 years, 0.9 mg; Women 14-18 years, 1 mg; Women over 18 years, 1.1 mg; Pregnant women, 1.4 mg; and Lactating women, 1.5 mg (3094).

Comments

Thiamine is frequently used in combination with other B vitamins in vitamin B complex formulations. Vitamin B complexes generally include vitamin B1 (thiamine), vitamin B2 (riboflavin), vitamin B3 (niacin/niacinamide), vitamin B5 (pantothenic acid), vitamin B6 (pyridoxine), vitamin B12 (cyanocobalamin), and folic acid. However, some products do not contain all of these ingredients and some may include others, such as biotin, para-aminobenzoic acid (PABA), choline bitartrate, and inositol.

THREONINE

Also Known As

None.
CAUTION: See separate listing for theanine.

Scientific Names

L-threonine.

People Use This For
Orally, threonine is used for spinal spasticity, multiple sclerosis, familiar spastic paraparesis, and amyotrophic lateral sclerosis (ALS, Lou Gehrig's disease).

Safety
POSSIBLY SAFE ...when used orally and appropriately. Taking threonine is doses of 2 grams to 4 grams daily for up to 12 months seems to be safe (681,12056,12057,12059).
PREGNANCY AND LACTATION: Insufficient reliable information; avoid using.

Effectiveness
POSSIBLY EFFECTIVE
Spinal spasticity. Taking threonine 6 grams/day orally seems to modestly decrease spasticity (12056).
POSSIBLY INEFFECTIVE
Amyotrophic lateral sclerosis (ALS, Lou Gehrig's disease). Taking threonine 2 grams to 4 grams daily for up to 12 months does not seem to slow the progression of ALS or reduce symptoms (681,12057). There is also concern that threonine might actually worsen pulmonary function in these patients. A significantly higher number of patients treated with threonine seem to have reduced pulmonary function compared to placebo (681).
INSUFFICIENT RELIABLE EVIDENCE to RATE
Familial spastic paraparesis (FSP). There is preliminary evidence that taking threonine 4.5 grams to 6 grams daily might improve some measures of motor impairment and spasticity. But the improvement does not seem to be clinically significant (12059).

Mechanism of Action
Threonine is a large neutral amino acid. Researchers are investigating threonine as a potential treatment for spasticity and amyotrophic lateral sclerosis (ALS) because it is a precursor to glycine. Glycine is the major inhibitory neurotransmitter in the spinal cord. But glycine itself poorly penetrates the central nervous system (CNS). Threonine has better penetration of the CNS. Threonine seems to boost glycine levels in the spinal cord (681,12056,12058). But it doesn't significantly increase glycine levels in the brain (12058).
In patients with spasticity, increasing glycine might reduce spasticity related to spinal cord injury (12056).
ALS is theorized to be cause by excess excitatory amino acids in the CNS such as glutamate. Increasing the inhibitory neurotransmitter, glycine, is thought to counter these excitatory amino acids (681,12057).
Following oral ingestion, plasma threonine levels rise rapidly. Fasting levels of threonine are approximately 113 mcgMol/L (681). After 2 weeks of taking 6 grams daily, plasma threonine levels rose to an average of 498 mcgMol/L (12056). Peak levels of threonine occur within 2 hours following administration (681).

Adverse Reactions
Orally, threonine seems to be well tolerated. Some patients can experience minor gastrointestinal upset including diarrhea (12056).
Other side effects reported in people have taken threonine including headache, rhinorrhea, flatus, constipation, and skin rash. One patient had a two-fold increase in serum ammonia levels following administration of threonine 4 grams daily (681).

Interactions with Herbs & Other Dietary Supplements
ALANINE: Threonine might compete with other amino acids to cross the blood brain barrier into the central nervous system (CNS). Theoretically, high plasma levels of amino acids such as alanine might decrease how much threonine enters the CNS and therefore decrease the effectiveness of threonine (12058).
BRANCHED-CHAIN AMINO ACIDS: Threonine competes with other amino acids to cross the blood brain barrier into the central nervous system (CNS). Theoretically, high plasma levels of other amino acids might decrease how much threonine enters the CNS and therefore decrease the effectiveness of threonine (12058). The branch-chained amino acids include leucine, isoleucine, and valine.
PHENYLALANINE: Threonine might compete with other amino acids to cross the blood brain barrier into the central nervous system (CNS). Theoretically, high plasma levels of amino acids such as phenylalanine might decrease how much threonine enters the CNS and therefore decrease the effectiveness of threonine (12058).
SERINE: Threonine might compete with other amino acids to cross the blood brain barrier into the central nervous system (CNS). Theoretically, high plasma levels of amino acids such as serine might decrease how much threonine enters the CNS and therefore decrease the effectiveness of threonine (12058).
TRYPTOPHAN: Threonine might compete with other amino acids to cross the blood brain barrier into the central nervous system (CNS). Theoretically, high plasma levels of amino acids such as tryptophan might decrease how much threonine enters the CNS and therefore decrease the effectiveness of threonine (12058).
TYROSINE: Threonine might compete with other amino acids to cross the blood brain barrier into the central nervous system (CNS). Theoretically, high plasma levels of amino acids such as tyrosine might decrease how much threonine enters the CNS and therefore decrease the effectiveness of threonine (12058).

Interactions with Drugs
NMDA ANTAGONISTS: Threonine increases central nervous system (CNS) glycine levels (12058). Glycine seems to bind a site on NMDA receptors and enhance the activity of the receptor (681,12057). Theoretically, this might decrease the effects of NMDA receptor antagonists such as memantine (Namenda).

Interactions with Foods
None known.

Interactions with Lab Tests
None known.

Interactions with Diseases or Conditions
AMYOTROPHIC LATERAL SCLEROSIS (ALS, Lou Gehrig's disease): There is some concern that threonine might decrease pulmonary function in patients with ALS. In one study, ALS patients taking threonine 4 grams/day had significantly reduced forced vital capacity (FVC) compared to patients on placebo (681). More evidence is needed to determine if threonine was actually the cause of this adverse outcome.

Dosage and Administration
ORAL: For spinal spasticity, threonine 6 grams/day has been used (12056). For familial spastic paraparesis (FSP), threonine 4.5 gram to 6 grams daily has been used (12059).

THUNDER GOD VINE

Also Known As
Huang-T'eng Ken, Lei Gong Teng, Lei-Kung T'eng, Taso-Ho-Hua, Threewingnut, Yellow Vine.

Scientific Names
Tripterygium wilfordii.
Family: Celastraceae.

People Use This For
Orally, thunder god vine is used for rheumatoid arthritis, excessive menstrual periods, multiple sclerosis, and as a male contraceptive. It is also used for abscesses, boils, fever, inflammation, systemic lupus erythematosus (SLE), psoriasis, and Behcet's disease.
Topically, thunder god vine is used for rheumatoid arthritis.
Thunder god vine has also been used non-medicinally as an insecticide against maggots or larvae, and as a rat and bird poison.

Safety
POSSIBLY SAFE ...when used orally and appropriately (4046,10231,10674,10675,10676). Thunder god vine has been used with apparent safety for up to 5 years (10231). ...when used topically (10233).
PREGNANCY: LIKELY UNSAFE ...when used orally. Thunder god vine is thought to be teratogenic (4047); avoid using.
LACTATION: Insufficient reliable information available; avoid using.

Effectiveness
POSSIBLY EFFECTIVE

Rheumatoid arthritis (RA). Taking thunder god vine orally appears to produce symptom relief in patients with RA, including improvements in pain, tender and swollen joints, and physical function (10674,10675,10676). Additive symptom relief with nonsteroidal anti-inflammatory drugs (NSAIDs) has also been observed (4046). Applying a tincture of thunder god vine topically over affected joints seems to decrease joint tenderness, stiffness, and swelling (10233).

INSUFFICIENT RELIABLE EVIDENCE to RATE

Contraception. Taking thunder god vine orally might be effective as a male contraceptive. Normalization of sperm function seems to return six weeks after discontinuation of treatment (4046,11133).
Nephrotic syndrome. Preliminary evidence suggests thunder god vine may be effective for nephrotic syndrome in children (10677).
Systemic lupus erythematosus (SLE). There is preliminary evidence that thunder god vine may be effective for nephritis associated with SLE (10232).
More evidence is needed to rate thunder god vine for these uses.

Mechanism of Action

The applicable parts of thunder god vine are the leaf and root. The active constituents of thunder god vine are triterpenoids. At least 21 types of triterpenoids have been identified including tripchlorolide, triptolidenol, triptolide, tripdiolide, and 16-hydroxytriptolide (840,10230). Thunder god vine leaf and root seems to have antifertility effects in males by inhibiting sperm transformation, maturation, and mobility. Triptolide, tripdiolide, and possibly other compounds seem to be responsible for the contraceptive effect (11130,11131). Male fertility appears to return to normal six weeks after discontinuation (4046,11133).

Thunder god vine also seems to have immunosuppressive, anti-inflammatory, and anti-proliferative effects. The immunosuppressive effects of thunder god vine are attributed to the constituent triptolide. Triptolide inhibits lymphocyte activation and T-cell expression of interleukin-2 (5305,11132). An alcoholic extract, known as T2, that contains triptolide and tripdiolide, inhibits T-cell and B-cell proliferation, as well as immunoglobulin production by B-cells (1442). T2 also inhibits the release of prostaglandin 2 (PGE 2) from mononuclear leukocytes (5305). A water extract of thunder god vine inhibits the activity of cellular adhesion molecules of leukocytes and endothelial cells, including integrins and selectins (1206,8409).

The Neotripterifordin, tripterifordin, and salaspermic acid constituents of thunder god vine exhibit potent anti-HIV replication activity in vitro (4048,4049).

Adverse Reactions

Orally, thunder god vine can cause gastrointestinal (GI) upset, diarrhea, headache, and hair loss (10675,10676). Infertility, lymphocyte suppression, menstrual changes, amenorrhea, and skin reactions may also occur (4046,10675,10676,11009). Decreased bone mineral content may occur in women taking thunder god vine for 5 or more years (10231). There is one report of a young male with some evidence of pre-existing heart damage who developed vomiting, diarrhea, leukopenia, renal failure, hypotension, and shock, and died three days after ingestion of thunder god vine (8658). There is also one report of an infant born with meningoencephalocele after the mother used thunder god vine for rheumatoid arthritis (RA) during pregnancy (4047). Thunder god vine extract may suppress immune function. However, this action only occurs at doses much higher than those typically used (10230).

Interactions with Herbs & Other Dietary Supplements

None known.

Interactions with Drugs

IMMUNOSUPPRESSANTS: Large doses of thunder god vine may suppress immune function (10230). Theoretically, concomitant use might enhance the effects of immunosuppressant drugs. Immunosuppressant drugs include azathioprine (Imuran), basiliximab (Simulect), cyclosporine (Neoral, Sandimmune), daclizumab (Zenapax), muromonab-CD3 (OKT3, Orthoclone OKT3), mycophenolate (CellCept), tacrolimus (FK506, Prograf), sirolimus (Rapamune), prednisone (Deltasone, Orasone), and other corticosteroids (glucocorticoids).

Interactions with Foods

None known.

Interactions with Lab Tests

None known.

Interactions with Diseases or Conditions

IMMUNE SYSTEM COMPROMISE: Large doses of thunder god vine may suppress immune function. Theoretically, thunder god vine might exacerbate these conditions (10230).

OSTEOPOROSIS: Thunder god vine can cause decreased bone mineral density. It should not be used by people with osteoporosis or people who are at risk for osteoporosis (10231).

Dosage and Administration

ORAL: For rheumatoid arthritis (RA), 180-570 mg thunder god vine extract per day has been used up to 20 weeks (10675,10676). For nephrotic syndrome in children, 1 mg per kg body weight daily has been used for up to 20 weeks (10677).

TOPICAL: For rheumatoid arthritis (RA), a tincture of thunder god vine applied over affected joints five to six times daily has been used (10232).

THYME flower, leaf

Also Known As

Common Thyme, French Thyme, Garden Thyme, Rubbed Thyme, Spanish Thyme, Thymi herba.
CAUTION: See separate listings for Thyme Oil and Wild Thyme.

Scientific Names

Thymus vulgaris; Thymus zygis.
Family: Lamiaceae/Labiatae.

People Use This For

Orally, thyme is used for bronchitis, pertussis, sore throat, colic, as an appetite stimulant, for dyspepsia, chronic gastritis, diarrhea in children, enuresis in children, as an antiflatulent, diuretic, urinary disinfectant, anthelmintic, and for rheumatic and skin disorders.
Topically, thyme is used for upper respiratory tract mucous membrane inflammation, laryngitis, tonsillitis, stomatitis, and halitosis.
In foods, thyme is used as a culinary herb.

Safety

LIKELY SAFE ...when used in the amounts commonly found in foods. Thyme has Generally Recognized As Safe (GRAS) status in the US (4912).
POSSIBLY SAFE ...when used orally and appropriately (1,12). ...when used topically and appropriately (18).
PREGNANCY: LIKELY UNSAFE ...when used in medicinal amounts because it might induce menstruation (4,19).
LACTATION: Insufficient reliable information.

Effectiveness

There is insufficient reliable information available about the effectiveness of thyme flower and leaf.

Mechanism of Action

Thyme contains thymol, carvacrol, and flavonoid constituents, which are responsible for the antispasmodic, antitussive, and expectorant effects (4). This explains why thyme is used as an antiflatulent, antispasmodic, antitussive, astringent, expectorant, antibacterial, anthelmintic, and to stimulate saliva (4,18). There may also be phenolic compounds of the volatile oil and flavonoids associated with antispasmodic activity. This mechanism may involve calcium channel blockade. However, some scientists question whether the phenolic components are involved (4). The antibacterial and antifungal activity is associated with the thymol and carvacrol (1). Thymol also demonstrates anthelmintic activity (4). The constituent, rosmarinic acid, reduces experimentally-induced edema, inhibits passive cutaneous anaphylaxis, and impairs experimental activation of macrophages in vivo (1). In animals, the thyme extract seems to have analgesic and antipyretic effects (4). The thymus vulgaris also has antithyrotropic activity (11). The fluid extracts show antispasmodic activity in smooth muscle, but the active constituents causing this activity have not been identified (11).

Adverse Reactions

Topically, thyme oil can lead to irritation (4). There is a low potential for sensitization (18).

Interactions with Herbs & Other Dietary Supplements

None known.

Interactions with Drugs

None known.

Interactions with Foods

None known.

Interactions with Lab Tests

None known.

Interactions with Diseases or Conditions

CROSS-ALLERGENICITY: CAUTION, cross-reactivity to oregano and other Labiatae species reported in an individual allergic to thyme (3808).
GASTROINTESTINAL (GI) IRRITATION (e.g., ulcers, etc.): CAUTION, use might exacerbate inflammation (19).

OTHER: When used as a bath, be cautious in cases of extensive skin injuries or disease, or in cases involving high fever or infectious disease, cardiac insufficiency or hypertonia (18).
URINARY TRACT INFLAMMATION: CAUTION, use might exacerbate inflammation (19).

Dosage and Administration

ORAL: 1-2 grams dried leaf/flower several times daily, or one cup tea (steep 1-2 grams dried leaf/flower in 150 mL boiling water for 10 minutes, strain) several times daily as needed (1,18); not to exceed 10 grams dried leaf with 0.03% phenol (calculated as thymol) per day (18). Fluid extract, 1-2 grams up to three times daily (2).
TOPICAL: Gargle (1) or compress (2,18), steep 5 grams dried leaf per 100 mL boiling water 10 minutes, strain (1,18).

Comments

Thyme is a plant rich in iron (19).

THYME OIL

Also Known As

Common Thyme, Red Thyme Oil, Spanish Thyme, Thyme Aetheroleum, Thyme Oil, White Thyme Oil.
CAUTION: See separate listings for Thyme, Spanish Origanum Oil, and Wild Thyme.

Scientific Names

Thymus vulgaris; Thymus zygis.
Family: Lamiaceae/Labiatae.

People Use This For

Orally, thyme oil is used for bedwetting in children, as an antispasmodic, for dyspraxia in children, and as an antiflatulent.
Topically, thyme oil is used as a counterirritant, an antiseptic in mouthwashes and liniments, and as a counterirritant in douche products. Thyme oil is also used for alopecia areata.
Otically, thyme oil is used as an antibacterial and antifungal ingredient.
In foods, thyme oil is used as a flavoring agent.
In manufacturing, red thyme oil is used in perfumes. It is also used in soaps, cosmetics, toothpastes.

Safety

LIKELY SAFE ...when used in amounts commonly found in foods. Thyme oil has Generally Recognized As Safe (GRAS) status in the US (4912).
POSSIBLY SAFE ...when used topically and appropriately (5177). Diluted thyme oil has been used safely for up to 7 months (5177).
LIKELY UNSAFE ...when used orally in medicinal amounts (4).
PREGNANCY: LIKELY UNSAFE ...when used orally in medicinal amounts; thyme oil might induce menstruation (4,12); avoid using.
LACTATION: There is insufficient reliable information available about the safety of thyme oil in medicinal amounts during breast-feeding; avoid using.

Effectiveness

POSSIBLY EFFECTIVE

Alopecia areata. Thyme oil applied topically in combination with the essential oils from rosemary, lavender, and cedarwood seem to improve hair growth by 44% after 7 months of treatment (5177).

Dyspraxia. Taking thyme oil in combination with evening primrose oil, fish oils, and vitamin E seems to improve movement disorders in children with dyspraxia (5708).

There is insufficient reliable information available about the effectiveness of thyme oil for its other uses.

Mechanism of Action

Thyme oil contains the volatile oils thymol and carvacrol. These constituents may have antispasmodic, antitussive, and expectorant effects (4). Thymol has fungicidal, antibacterial, anthelmintic (especially hookworms), and counterirritant properties (4,11). It's not clear how thyme oil works in alopecia areata (5177); however, it may be related to its effects as a counterirritant.

Adverse Reactions

Orally, thyme oil can cause nausea, vomiting, gastric pain, headache, dizziness, convulsions, coma, and cardiac and respiratory arrest (4).
Topically, it can cause skin or mucous membrane irritation, cheilitis, and glossitis (4).

Interactions with Herbs & Other Dietary Supplements
None known.

Interactions with Drugs
None known.

Interactions with Foods
None known.

Interactions with Lab Tests
None known.

Interactions with Diseases or Conditions
CARDIAC INSUFFICIENCY AND HYPERTONIA: Medical consultation needed before use in individuals with cardiac insufficiency or hypertonia (18).
INFECTION: Medical consultation needed before use in individuals with high fever or infectious disease.
SKIN INJURIES: Medical consultation needed before use in individuals with extensive skin injuries/disease (18).

Dosage and Administration
ORAL: A typical dose is 2 to 3 drops on a sugar cube, 2 or 3 times a day (5263).
TOPICAL: Must be diluted (4). Thyme oil is commonly applied as needed in 1% to 2% ointments (6002). For the treatment of alopecia areata, a combination of the essential oils including thyme 2 drops or 88 mg, rosemary 3 drops or 114 mg, lavender 3 drops or 108 mg, and cedarwood 2 drops or 94 mg, all mixed with 3 mL jojoba oil and 20 mL grapeseed oil has been used. Each night, the mixture is massaged into the scalp for 2 minutes with a warm towel placed around the head to increase absorption (5177).

Comments
Thyme oil is obtained by distillation of the leaves and flowering tops of thyme (Thymus vulgaris and/or Thymus zygis). White thyme oil (redistilled red thyme oil) is often adulterated (11).

THYMUS EXTRACT

Also Known As
Predigested Thymus Extract, Pure Thymic Extract, Thymomodulin, Thymosin, Thymostimulin, Thymus, Thymus Acid Lysate Derivative, Thymus Complex, Thymus Concentrate, Thymus-Derived Polypeptides, Thymus Factors, Thymus Polypeptides, Thymus Substance.

Scientific Names
None.

People Use This For
Orally, thymus extract is used for infectious diseases including recurrent respiratory infections, colds, flu, hepatitis B, hepatitis C, Epstein-Barr virus (EBV), mononucleosis, herpes and shingles, sinusitis, and AIDS/HIV. It is also used orally for asthma, hay fever, food allergies, cancer, rheumatoid arthritis, chronic fatigue syndrome (CFS), and systemic lupus erythematosus (SLE). It is also used orally for maintaining white cell production in cancer patients treated with radiation or chemotherapy, and preventing the effects of aging.

Safety
POSSIBLY SAFE ...when used orally and appropriately. No adverse effects have been reported in human studies with purified thymus extract (938,1010,1175,1176,1177,1178,6691,6694,6696,6697,6698,6699). Although some evidence suggests these products are safe, since they are derived from animals, there is concern about contamination with diseased animal parts (1825). However, so far there are no reports of disease transmission to humans due to use of contaminated thymus extract.
PREGNANCY AND LACTATION: Insufficient reliable information available; avoid using.

Effectiveness
POSSIBLY EFFECTIVE

Allergic rhinitis (hayfever). There is some evidence that treatment for 4 months with thymomodulin (calf thymus extract) might reduce the frequency of allergic episodes in patients with allergic rhinitis (1010).
Asthma. Taking thymus extract orally may reduce acute asthma attacks in children with asthma. Thymomodulin (calf thymus extract) seems to improve immune function and reduce the number of asthma attacks up to one year

after discontinuing intermittent treatment in children with asthma (6694).

Food allergies. Thymomodulin (calf thymus extract) plus an elimination diet might prevent allergic reactions to allergenic foods after completion of the elimination diet, compared to an elimination diet alone (1175,1176).

Respiratory infections. Taking thymus extract orally may be effective for treating adults and children with recurrent respiratory infections (938,6696,6697,6698,6699). Thymomodulin (calf thymus extract) treatment seems to reduce the number of infections or coughing attacks in patients with recurrent respiratory infections (6697,6698,6699). Thymomodulin (calf thymus extract) alone, or in combination with vaccine, seems to be more effective than vaccine alone or antibiotics in reducing the number and duration of infections in adults with recurrent respiratory infections (938).

There is insufficient reliable information available about the effectiveness of thymus extract for its other uses.

Mechanism of Action

Thymus extract is derived from bovine thymus glands (6614). Purified thymus extract induces immune response in spleen cells from athymic animals in vitro (6688). Preliminary human data suggests that a semipurified calf thymus extract might be useful for treating immunodeficiency conditions, bone marrow failure, auto-immune disorders, chronic skin diseases, recurrent viral and bacterial infections, and some cancers (6677).

Thymomodulin is a purified acid lysate derivative of calf thymus extract containing several polypeptides (6614,6689). It induces T-lymphocyte maturation, enhances the function of mature T-cells, and has indirect effects on B-cell and macrophage functions in vitro (6689). Thymomodulin improves immune function in patients with asthma, chronic bronchitis, recurrent respiratory infections, perennial allergic rhinitis, food allergies, chronic active hepatitis B, and HIV infection (938,1010,1175,1176,1178,6694,6696,6697,6698,6699). It reduces airway hyperresponsiveness to methacholine in atopic patients with asthma (6695). Limited human data suggest that thymomodulin might be useful for treating chronic active hepatitis B (1015,1177) and improving symptoms in patients with HIV infection (1178). Thymomodulin demonstrates activity when administered orally in elderly patients (6691).

Thymosin is a polypeptide extracted from fetal calf thymus glands that stimulates in vitro T-cell proliferation when incubated with T-lymphocytes from people with low T-cell counts (511,6687).

Thymostimulin is a polypeptide extracted from bovine thymus glands (6680). Preliminary human evidence suggests that parenteral thymostimulin might be useful for improving immune function in infants with inadequate B-lymphocyte or T-lymphocyte function (6682,6683), children with recurrent respiratory infections (6679,6684), and patients with primary immunodeficiencies (6685). Limited human evidence also suggests that parenteral thymostimulin might be useful for preventing recurrent herpes simplex labialis (HSL) episodes (6678), preventing exacerbations in patients with chronic obstructive pulmonary disease (COPD) (6681), and preventing cystitis, conjunctivitis, stomatomucositis, and myelotoxicity in women with breast cancer treated with chemotherapy (6680). Thymostimulin is not beneficial for treating patients with auto-immune chronic active hepatitis (6686).

Adverse Reactions

Adverse effects have not been reported. However, there is some concern about potential contamination. Thymus extract is derived from raw bovine thymus glands gathered from slaughterhouses, possibly from sick or diseased animals (6620). Products made from contaminated or diseased organs might present a human health hazard. There is also concern that thymus extract produced from cows in countries where bovine spongiform encephalitis (BSE) has been reported might be contaminated with diseased tissue. Countries where BSE has been reported include Great Britain, France, The Netherlands, Portugal, Luxembourg, Ireland, Switzerland, Oman, and Belgium (1825). However, there have been no reports of BSE transfer to humans from contaminated thymus extract products. Until more is known, tell patients to avoid these products unless country of origin can be determined. Patients should avoid products that are produced in countries where BSE has been found.

Interactions with Herbs & Other Dietary Supplements

None known.

Interactions with Drugs

IMMUNOSUPPRESSANTS: Patients using immunosuppressive drugs are cautioned to avoid thymus extract products, unless they are certified pathogen-free. Immunosuppressant drugs include azathioprine (Imuran), basiliximab (Simulect), cyclosporine (Neoral, Sandimmune), daclizumab (Zenapax), muromonab-CD3 (OKT3, Orthoclone OKT3), mycophenolate (CellCept), tacrolimus (FK506, Prograf), sirolimus (Rapamune), prednisone (Deltasone, Orasone), and other corticosteroids (glucocorticoids).

Interactions with Foods

None known.

Interactions with Lab Tests

None known.

Interactions with Diseases or Conditions

IMMUNE COMPROMISE, IMMUNOSUPPRESSION: Patients with compromised immune systems or using immunosuppressive drugs should be cautioned to avoid thymus extract products, unless they are certified pathogen-free, to reduce their risk of infection. This includes patients with HIV/AIDS and organ transplant recipients using immunosuppressive drugs.

Dosage and Administration

ORAL: A typical daily dose is 750 mg of crude thymus polypeptide fraction or 120 mg of pure thymus polypetides (thymomodulin) (6614).

Comments

The quality and potency of thymus extract products can vary greatly (6614).

TIRATRICOL

Also Known As

Triac, Triiodothyroacetic Acid.

Scientific Names

3,3',5-triiodothyroacetic acid.

People Use This For

Orally, tiratricol is used for treating pituitary resistance to thyroid hormone (PRTH), treating thyroid cancer (orphan drug designation), treating fetal hypothyroidism, increasing metabolic rate for weight loss, and reducing cellulite.

Safety

LIKELY SAFE ...when used orally under medical supervision for treating thyroid cancer (1616,1617,1618,1691). ...when used orally under medical supervision for treating pituitary resistance to thyroid hormone (PRTH) (1607,1608,1609,1610,1615).
POSSIBLY SAFE ...when used orally under medical supervision for treating fetal hypothyroidism (1613,1614).
POSSIBLY UNSAFE ...when used orally in the elderly, tiratricol might aggravate occult cardiac disease (15); avoid using.
LIKELY UNSAFE ...when used orally for increasing metabolic rate for weight loss or reducing cellulite (1620,1621,1622,1623,1624,1625). The FDA has issued a warning against tiratricol use for weight loss (1605).
PREGNANCY: POSSIBLY SAFE ...when used orally under medical supervision for treating fetal hypothyroidism (1613,1614). LIKELY UNSAFE ...when used orally for other purposes during pregnancy due to possible risk of fetal heart damage (1627,1628); avoid using.
LACTATION: Insufficient reliable information available; avoid using.

Effectiveness

LIKELY EFFECTIVE

Pituitary resistance to thyroid hormone (PRTH). Taking tiratricol orally is effective for treating pituitary resistance to thyroid hormone (PRTH) (1607,1608,1609,1610,1615).

POSSIBLY EFFECTIVE

Hypothyroidism. Taking tiratricol orally seems to be effective for treating fetal hypothyroidism (1613,1614).

Thyroid cancer. Taking tiratricol orally in combination with levo-thyroxine seems to be effective for treating thyroid cancer (1616,1617,1618). Tiratricol is an FDA designated orphan drug under study for use in combination with levo-thyroxine to suppress thyroid stimulating hormone (TSH) in patients with well-differentiated thyroid cancer who are intolerant to adequate doses of levo-thyroxine alone (1691).

LIKELY INEFFECTIVE

Weight loss. Taking tiratricol orally isn't effective for increasing metabolic rate for weight loss in people with normal thyroid function (1611,1612).

There is insufficient reliable information available about the effectiveness of tiratricol for its other uses.

Mechanism of Action

Tiratricol is a naturally occurring metabolite of T4 (thyroxine) and a structural analog of T3 (triiodothyronine) (1633,1634). Low concentrations of tiratricol are found in plasma, but tiratricol has no known role in thyroid physiology (1633). Tiratricol has a high affinity for T3 receptors and suppresses thyroid stimulating hormone (TSH) secretion at therapeutic doses without causing significant peripheral effects, such as increased basal metabolism rate and heart rate (1634). Tiratricol might lower total and LDL cholesterol, and stimulate bone formation (1632). About 67% of an oral dose of tiratricol is absorbed; the half-life is 6 hours (1631).

Adverse Reactions

Orally, tiratricol can cause severe diarrhea, fatigue, lethargy, and profound weight loss (1605). Heart attacks and strokes are possible, as well as symptoms of hyperthyroidism, including increased appetite, abdominal cramps, tremors, menstrual irregularities, nervousness, insomnia, sweating, intolerance to heat, fever, palpitations, tachycardia, increased pulse and blood pressure, chest pain, and cardiac arrhythmias (15,1605). Case reports have implicated tiratricol in centrally-mediated hypothyroidism, pseudohypothyroidism, internuclear ophthalmoplegia, and hepatotoxicity (1621,1623,1624,1625).

Interactions with Herbs & Other Dietary Supplements

HERBS AND SUPPLEMENTS WITH SYMPATHOMIMETIC ACTIVITY: Theoretically, large doses of tiratricol might enhance the effects and adverse effects of herbs and supplements that have sympathomimetic activity, including caffeine, guarana, and ephedra (15).
HERBS WITH THYROID ACTIVITY: Theoretically, tiratricol might enhance the effects and adverse effects of herbs that affect thyroid function, including bugleweed, balm leaf, and wild thyme.
VITAMIN K: Theoretically, tiratricol might antagonize the prothrombinemic effects of vitamin K by increasing catabolism of vitamin K-dependent clotting factors (15).

Interactions with Drugs

ANTICOAGULANT/ANTIPLATELET DRUGS: Theoretically, tiratricol might potentiate the hypoprothrombinemic effects of oral anticoagulants, including warfarin (Coumadin), by increasing catabolism of vitamin K-dependent clotting factors (15).
ANTIDIABETES DRUGS: Theoretically, tiratricol might interfere with blood glucose control requiring adjustment of diabetes drug therapy (15); monitor closely.
CHOLESTYRAMINE (Questran): Theoretically, cholestyramine might decrease tiratricol absorption (15).
STIMULANT DRUGS: Theoretically, large doses of tiratricol might enhance the effects and adverse effects of sympathomimetic drugs (15).
THYROID HORMONE: Concurrent use of tiratricol with thyroid hormones can have additive effects (1617); use only under medical supervision.

Interactions with Foods

None known.

Interactions with Lab Tests

PROTHROMBIN TIME (PT), INTERNATIONAL NORMALIZATION RATIO (INR): Theoretically, tiratricol might increase prothrombin time, increasing PT and INR test results, by increasing catabolism of vitamin K-dependent clotting factors (15).
THYROID FUNCTION TESTS: Abnormalities have been reported in people taking tiratricol (1691).
THYROID-STIMULATING HORMONE (TSH): Tiratricol reduces serum TSH levels, and test results (1631).
THYROTROPIN-RELEASING HORMONE (TRH) STIMULATION: Tiratricol reduces TSH secretion, serum levels and test results, to exogenous TRH stimulation (1609,1611,1617,1623,1633).

Interactions with Diseases or Conditions

ADRENAL INSUFFICIENCY, DIABETES, HYPOPITUITARISM: Theoretically, tiratricol might unmask symptoms of these conditions in patients with untreated hypothyroidism (15).
ANGINA, CARDIOVASCULAR DISEASE, HYPERTENSION: Theoretically, tiratricol might aggravate symptoms of these conditions (15); avoid using.
DIABETES: Theoretically, tiratricol might interfere with blood glucose control requiring adjustment of diabetes drug therapy (15), monitor closely.
LIVER DISEASE: Tiratricol is potentially hepatotoxic and might worsen liver disease (1624); avoid using.
MYXEDEMA: Patients with myxedema might be particularly sensitive to thyroid agents, including tiratricol (15).
PROLONGED CLOTTING TIME: Theoretically, tiratricol might increase the risk of bleeding in people with prolonged clotting time by increasing catabolism of vitamin K-dependent clotting factors (15).

Dosage and Administration

ORAL: The dose for TSH suppression tests used in clinical trials is 10-24 mcg twice daily initially, titrated to a TSH concentration of less than 0.1 mU/L (1632,1633).

Comments

Tiratricol is a thyroid supplement and should not be used by anyone with normal thyroid function (1605). The drug, which is available by prescription in France, has been studied since the fifties, mostly for thyroid disease (1629,1630). The FDA has determined that the product Triax (TRIAC, tiratricol) is not a dietary supplement but an unapproved new drug containing a potent thyroid hormone, which may cause serious health consequences. The State of Missouri embargoed the product at its distributor (Syntrax) and the Utah-based manufacturer (Pharmatech) has agreed to stop distributing any product containing the ingredient TRIAC. The FDA has issued recalls for other tiratricol-containing products, including Tricana Metabolic Hormone Analogue, Tria-Cutz Thyroid Stimulator Dietary Supplement Capsules, and Sci-Fi-Tri-Cuts Dietary Supplement Capsules (6675).

TOLU BALSAM

Also Known As

Balsam, Balsam of Tolu, Balsam Tolu, Balsamum Tolutanum, Myroxylan balsamum, Myroxylan toluiferum, Opobalsam, Resin Tolu, Resina Tolutana, Thomas Balsam, Tolu, Toluiferum Balsamum.
CAUTION: See separate listing for Peru Balsam.

Scientific Names

Myroxylon balsamum; Myroxylon balsamum var. balsamum, synonym Toluifera balsamum.
Family: Fabaceae/Leguminosae.

People Use This For

Orally, tolu balsam is used for cough, bronchitis, inflammation of respiratory tract mucous membranes, as an expectorant, and for cancer.
Topically, tolu balsam is used to treat of bedsores, cracked nipples, lips, and minor skin cuts.
As an inhalant, tolu balsam is used to treat laryngitis and croup.
In foods, tolu balsam is also used to flavor chewing gum, foods, and beverages.
In manufacturing, tolu balsam is used as a fixative, as fragrances in soaps and cosmetics, and as a flavoring in cough medicines.

Safety

LIKELY SAFE ...when the oleo resin and extract are used orally in amounts commonly found in foods. Tolu balsam has Generally Recognized As Safe (GRAS) status in the US (4912).
POSSIBLY SAFE ...when used orally and appropriately for medicinal purposes (2).
There is insufficient reliable information available about the safety of the topical use of tolu balsam.
PREGNANCY AND LACTATION: Insufficient reliable information available; avoid using.

Effectiveness

There is insufficient reliable information available about the effectiveness of tolu balsam.

Mechanism of Action

The applicable part of tolu balsam is the oleo resin. Tolu balsam has mild antiseptic action and expectorant properties (11).

Adverse Reactions

Orally, tolu balsam may cause kidney irritation (12).
Topically, it may cause allergic reactions (11).

Interactions with Herbs & Other Dietary Supplements

None known.

Interactions with Drugs

None known.

Interactions with Foods

None known.

Interactions with Lab Tests

None known.

Interactions with Diseases or Conditions

FEVER: Theoretically, tolu balsam is contraindicated in individuals with fever or inflammation (12,19).
KIDNEY DISEASE: Theoretically, tolu balsam might exacerbate kidney disease.
TOLU BALSAM ALLERGY: Avoid use of tolu balsam (11).

Dosage and Administration

ORAL: A typical dosage is 500-600 mg per day (2,18).
TOPICAL: No typical dosage.

Comments

Avoid confusion with Peru balsam. Tolu balsam is the oleo resin exuded from slits cut in the trunk of Myroxylon balsamum.

TOMATO

Also Known As

Love Apple.
CAUTION: See separate listing for Lycopene.

Scientific Names

Lycopersicon esculentum.
Family: Solanaceae.

People Use This For

Orally, tomato is used for reducing the risk of cancer, cardiovascular disease, and cataracts; and for treating arthritis, colds, chills, and digestive disorders.

Safety

LIKELY SAFE ...when the tomato fruit or its products are consumed in amounts found in foods (2406,9439,10418).
POSSIBLY UNSAFE ...when the leaf is used orally (18).
There is insufficient reliable information about the safety of the tomato vine.
PREGNANCY AND LACTATION: LIKELY SAFE ...when the tomato fruit or its products are consumed in typical food amounts. Avoid using amounts greater than those typically consumed in foods.

Effectiveness

POSSIBLY EFFECTIVE

Cardiovascular disease. Epidemiologic evidence suggests that increased consumption of tomato-based foods can decrease the risk myocardial infarction, stroke, and other cardiovascular events in women (10418).

Cataracts. Eating more than 3 servings of tomatoes each week may decrease the risk of developing cataracts (9439).

Prostate cancer. Consuming tomato fruit products seems to reduce the risk of prostate cancer. Epidemiological studies suggest that the risk of prostate cancer is decreased slightly in men who consume four or more weekly servings of tomato products, including tomatoes, tomato sauce, pizza, and tomato juice (2406,7895).

POSSIBLY INEFFECTIVE

Bladder cancer. Epidemiological studies have found no association between consuming tomatoes and tomato-based products, and the risk of bladder cancer (2407).

INSUFFICIENT RELIABLE EVIDENCE to RATE

Cancer. Epidemiological studies investigating consumption of tomatoes and tomato-based products, and the risk of breast cancer, cervical cancer, colon cancer, esophageal cancer, laryngeal cancer, lung cancer, oral cancer, ovarian cancer, pancreatic cancer, pleural cancer, rectal caner, and stomach cancer are inconclusive (1444,2404,2407). More evidence is needed to rate tomato for these uses.

Mechanism of Action

The applicable parts of tomato are the fruit, leaf, and vine. Tomatoes are the major dietary source of the carotenoid, lycopene. Lycopene is better absorbed from tomato products, such as tomato paste, than from fresh tomatoes (1497). Consumption of tomato juice can also significantly increase serum lycopene levels (1498,6607). One cup (240 mL) of tomato juice contains approximately 23 mg lycopene, depending on the brand (1499). Decreased serum or tissue lycopene concentrations are associated with an increased risk of prostate cancer (1447,1496,2405,2406,2407). Researchers have speculated that tomato products might stimulate immune function. However, there is evidence that long-term consumption of tomato juice has no effect on cell-mediated immune function (6607).

Adverse Reactions

Orally, symptoms of toxicity may include severe mucous membrane irritation, including vomiting, diarrhea, and colic. This is followed by dizziness, stupor, headache, bradycardia, respiratory disturbances, and mild spasms. In very severe cases, death by respiratory failure might occur (18). Signs of oral poisoning are not expected with ingestion of less than 100 grams of tomato leaves.

Interactions with Herbs & Other Dietary Supplements

None known.

Interactions with Drugs
None known.

Interactions with Foods
None known.

Interactions with Lab Tests
None known.

Interactions with Diseases or Conditions
None known.

Dosage and Administration
ORAL: For preventing prostate cancer, four or more servings of tomato products per week (equivalent to a dietary lycopene intake of greater than 6 mg daily) has been used (2406).

Comments
US Department of Agriculture (USDA) and Purdue University researchers are developing a tomato that contains more than twice as much lycopene and has a longer shelf life than currently available tomatoes (6671). The tomato, which is still in development, is modified with a yeast gene that slows the ripening process, allowing more time for lycopene to accumulate. Researchers think it will be several years before the tomato is commercially available.

TONKA BEAN

Also Known As
Coumarouna Odorata, Cumaru, Dutch Tonka, English Tonka, Legume, Tonka, Tonka Seed, Tonquin Bean, Torquin Bean.

Scientific Names
Dipteryx odorata, synonym Coumarouna odorata.
Family: Fabaceae/Leguminosae.

People Use This For
Orally, tonka bean is used as a tonic, an aphrodisiac, to treat cachexia, cramps, lymphedema, nausea, cough, schistosomiasis, spasms, and tuberculosis.
Topically, tonka bean is used for mouth ulcers, earache, and sore throat.
In manufacturing, coumarin, one of the active constituents of tonka bean is used as a flavoring and fragrance in various products in the food, liquor, tobacco, soap, and cosmetic industries.
In foods, the seeds are used to make a nutty-flavored beverage.

Safety
LIKELY UNSAFE ...when used orally. The FDA deems any food containing tonka bean or tonka bean extract to be impure (6). Rarely, coumarin, a constituent, has been associated with hepatotoxicity ranging from elevated liver enzymes to severe hepatic damage (6,297).
There is insufficient reliable information available about the safety of the topical use of tonka bean.
PREGNANCY AND LACTATION: LIKELY UNSAFE ...when used orally (6,297); avoid using.

Effectiveness
There is insufficient reliable information available about the effectiveness of tonka bean.

Mechanism of Action
The applicable parts of tonka bean are the fruit and seed. Tonka bean seeds usually contain 1-3% coumarin but may contain up to 10% (6,4502). Tonka bean seeds also contain coumaric-acid-beta-glucoside, o-coumaric acid, linoleic acid, oleic-acid, sitosterol, stearic acid, stigmasterol, and umbelliferone (296). The fruit contains melilotoside-1-p-coumaryl-beta-d-glucose (296). There is some evidence that coumarin can reduce edema and inflammation by increasing venous and lymphatic return (295). Other information suggests tonka bean might have narcotic and spasmolytic properties (4502,18).

Adverse Reactions
Orally, coumarin can be associated with nausea, vomiting (286), diarrhea, dizziness, insomnia (287), asymptomatic SGOT elevations (286), and rarely, liver toxicity (6,297). Large doses of the extract can paralyze the heart (4502).

Interactions with Herbs & Other Dietary Supplements
None known.

Interactions with Drugs
None known.

Interactions with Foods
None known.

Interactions with Lab Tests
None known.

Interactions with Diseases or Conditions
LIVER DISEASE: Although it is rare, the tonka bean constituent, coumarin, can cause liver toxicity (298).

Dosage and Administration
ORAL: Some people use an amount of tonka bean based on its coumarin content, and the typical dose of coumarin used is 60 mg daily (6002).
TOPICAL: No typical dosage.

Comments
The term coumarin is derived from Coumarou, the Caribbean name for the tonka tree (13). In plants, more than 700 different coumarins have been identified. Coumarin, itself, is widely distributed and has the characteristic odor of new-mown hay (13). Do not confuse coumarin with the potent anticoagulants bishydroxycoumarin, dicumarol, (13,295) or warfarin (a derivative of 4-hydroxycoumarin) (16).

TORMENTIL

Also Known As
Biscuits, Bloodroot, Cinquefoil, Earthbank, English Sarsaparilla, Ewe Daisy, Flesh And Blood, Potentilla, Septfoil, Shepherd's Knapperty, Shepherd's Knot, Thormantle, Tormentilla, Tormentillae rhizoma.
CAUTION: See separate listings for German Sarsaparilla, Potentilla, and Sarsaparilla.

Scientific Names
Potentilla erecta, Potentilla tormentilla.
Family: Rosaceae.

People Use This For
Orally, tormentil is used to treat diarrhea, acute and subacute gastroenteritis, and fever.
Topically, tormentil is used for reducing superficial bleeding and treating mild inflammation of the oral and pharyngeal mucous membranes.

Safety
POSSIBLY SAFE ...when used orally and appropriately (12). ...when used topically and appropriately (12).
CHILDREN: POSSIBLY SAFE ...when used orally and appropriately up to 5 days (10667).
PREGNANCY AND LACTATION: Insufficient reliable information available; avoid using.

Effectiveness
There is insufficient reliable information available about the effectiveness of tormentil.

Mechanism of Action
The applicable part of tormentil is the root. It contains 17-22% tannins, proanthocyanidins, flavonoids, and triterpenes (18). The astringent effect of tannins relieves diarrhea and soothes mucus membrane inflammation. Tannins reduce superficial bleeding by causing skin and superficial capillary contraction. Tannins also show some evidence of antiviral, antimicrobial, CNS depressant, and cariostatic effects (11). Some evidence suggests that tannins might cause cancer but other evidence shows tannins might prevent it (12). Regular consumption of herbs with high tannin concentrations correlates with increased incidence of esophageal or nasal cancer (12).

Adverse Reactions
Orally, tormentil can cause nausea, vomiting (7,12,18), and stomach complaints (2). Tormentil contains 17-22% tannins and theoretically has the potential to cause kidney damage and necrotic conditions of the liver (12).

Interactions with Herbs & Other Dietary Supplements
None known.

Interactions with Drugs
None known.

Interactions with Foods
MILK: When added to tormentil tea, milk can bind to the tannins and decrease their astringent and adverse effects (12).

Interactions with Lab Tests
None known.

Interactions with Diseases or Conditions
None known.

Dosage and Administration
ORAL: For diarrhea, a typical dose is one cup of the tea 2-4 times daily between meals, up to 4-6 grams of root per day. The tea is prepared by steeping 2-3 grams of the finely cut or powdered root in 150 mL boiling water for 10-15 minutes and then straining (18). In children with rotavirus diarrhea, tormentil root 1:10 extract in a dose of 3 drops per year of life has been used three times daily for up to 5 days (10667).
TOPICAL: The usual daily dose of the tincture, 1:10, is 10-20 drops in one glass of water used as a mouth or throat rinse (18).

Comments
Avoid confusion with potentilla (Potentilla anserina).

TRAGACANTH

Also Known As
Goat's Thorn, Green Dragon, Gum Dragon, Gum Tragacanth, Gummi Tragacanthae, Hog Gum, Syrian Tragacanth, Tragacanth Gum.
CAUTION: See separate listing for Astragalus.

Scientific Names
Astragalus gummifer.
Family: Fabaceae/Leguminosae.

People Use This For
Orally, tragacanth is used both for diarrhea and as a laxative.
Topically, tragacanth is an ingredient in toothpastes, hand lotions, and vaginal creams and jellies.
In foods, tragacanth is important for stabilizing, thickening, and suspending ingredients in salad dressings, foods, and beverages.
In pharmaceutical preparations, tragacanth is used as an emulsifier, binding agent, and demulcent. It is also a component of denture adhesives.

Safety
LIKELY SAFE ...when used orally in amounts commonly found in foods. Tragacanth has Generally Recognized As Safe (GRAS) status in the US (4912). ...when used topically, in the amounts found in cosmetics. Tragacanth is not considered to be irritating, sensitizing, or phototoxic (4072).
POSSIBLY SAFE ...when used orally in medicinal amounts (4068). However, insufficient fluid intake with tragacanth might lead to esophageal closure or obstruction ileus (18).
PREGNANCY AND LACTATION: Insufficient reliable information available; avoid using amounts greater than those found in foods.

Effectiveness
There is insufficient reliable information available about the effectiveness of tragacanth.

Mechanism of Action
Tragacanth contains water-soluble tragacanthin and water-insoluble bassorin (11). When added to water, tragacanthin dissolves to form a viscous colloidal solution; bassorin swells to form a thick gel (11). Among plant gums, tragacanth

produces the most viscous solution (11). When ingested, the bulk of tragacanth stretches the intestinal wall, increasing peristalsis (18). Although tragacanth increases stool weight and decreases GI transit time, it does not appear to affect cholesterol, triglyceride, or phospholipid levels as do other soluble fibers (6). Some preliminary data indicate that people with diabetes who ingest tragacanth along with a high sugar load have lower peak serum glucose and insulin levels (4069). However, this effect has not been consistent (6). The mucilaginous, adhesive properties of tragacanth justify its use as a component in denture adhesives (6). Tragacanth appears to inhibit growth of cancer cells (11). Preliminary evidence suggests tragacanthin polysaccharides might offer some protection from hantavirus infections (4070). Tragacanth is highly susceptible to bacterial digestion, even in the presence of preservatives (11).

Adverse Reactions
Orally, use of tragacanth requires ample fluid intake. Insufficient fluid intake can lead to obstruction ileus and esophageal closure (18). Tragacanth can cause asthma symptoms in people who are sensitive to quillaia bark (6).

Interactions with Herbs & Other Dietary Supplements
HERBS AND SUPPLEMENTS: Theoretically, concomitant administration might reduce absorption of supplements and/or herbs due to hydrocolloidal fiber content of tragacanth (19).

Interactions with Drugs
ORAL DRUGS: Theoretically, concomitant administration of oral drugs might reduce drug absorption due to hydrocolloidal fiber content of tragacanth (19).

Interactions with Foods
NUTRIENTS: Theoretically, concomitant administration might impair nutrient absorption from foods due to hydrocolloidal fiber content of tragacanth (19).

Interactions with Lab Tests
None known.

Interactions with Diseases or Conditions
QUILLAIA ALLERGY: Tragacanth can cause asthma symptoms in individuals sensitive to quillaia bark (19).

Dosage and Administration
No typical dosage.

Comments
Karaya gum is a common adulterant in tragacanth (16). It is important to use any amount with adequate fluid intake to prevent esophageal closure or obstruction of the ileus (18).

TRAILING ARBUTUS

Also Known As
Gravel Plant, Ground Laurel, Mountain Pink, Water Pink, Winter Pink.

Scientific Names
Epigaea repens.
Family: Ericaceae.

People Use This For
Orally, trailing arbutus is used for urinary tract conditions, as an astringent, and a diuretic.

Safety
POSSIBLY SAFE ...when the leaves are used orally short-term (12).
UNSAFE ...when the fresh or dried leaves are used orally long-term because they could cause hydroquinone toxicity (18).
PREGNANCY AND LACTATION: Insufficient reliable information available; avoid using.

Effectiveness
There is insufficient reliable information available about the effectiveness of trailing arbutus.

Mechanism of Action
The applicable parts of trailing arbutus are the above ground parts. Trailing arbutus is not suitable for long term use due to its hydroquinone glycoside content (18). Arbutin may have urinary antiseptic properties due to hydrolysis to its hydroquinone by the intestinal flora (7,11). As a result, long term use is stated to lead to hydroquinone toxicity (18).

Adverse Reactions
Orally, chronic use of trailing arbutus may lead to hydroquinone toxicity. Symptoms of toxicity include tinnitus, vomiting, delirium, convulsions, and collapse (11). Liver damage, cachexia, hemolytic anemia, and hair depigmentation may also occur with long term use (18). Overdosage could lead to inflammation of the mucous membranes of the bladder and urinary tract, and may be accompanied by bloody urine, difficulty with urination, and painful urination (18).

Interactions with Herbs & Other Dietary Supplements
None known.

Interactions with Drugs
None known.

Interactions with Foods
None known.

Interactions with Lab Tests
None known.

Interactions with Diseases or Conditions
None known.

Dosage and Administration
ORAL: Trailing arbutus is taken as a tea or extract (18).

Comments
Trailing arbutus's alternate name of gravel plant is similar to that of gravel root. Be careful not to confuse the two.

TRANSFER FACTOR

Also Known As
Bovine Dialyzable Leukocyte Extract, Bovine Dialyzable Transfer Factor, Bovine Transfer Factor, Dialyzable Leukocyte Extract, Dialyzable Transfer Factor, DLE, Human Dialyzable Leukocyte Extract, Human Transfer Factor, TF, TFd.
CAUTION: See separate listing for Bovine Colostrum.

Scientific Names
Transfer Factor

People Use This For
Orally and parenterally, transfer factor is used for infectious diseases in both immunocompetent and immunosuppressed patients, including cryptosporidiosis, septicemia, sinusitis and bronchitis, influenza, the common cold, herpes, varicella, hepatitis B, cytomegalovirus (CMV), Epstein-Barr virus, Pneumocystis carinii, Mycobacterium tuberculosis, Mycobacterium fortuitum, Mycobacterium avium, coccidioidomycosis, candidiasis, leishmaniasis, Cryptococcus, and lepromatous leprosy. Transfer factor is also used for diabetes, autism, infertility, systemic lupus erythematosus (SLE), fibromyalgia, chronic fatigue syndrome (CFS), Bechcet's syndrome, pemphigus vegetans, psoriasis, Wiskott-Aldrich syndrome, alopecia totalis, and Alzheimer's disease. It is also used for retinitis pigmentosa, chorioretinitis, amyotrophic lateral sclerosis (ALS, Lou Gehrig's disease), multiple sclerosis, osteosarcoma, bone metastasis, lung cancer, melanoma, epidermal dysplasia, food and chemical hypersensitivity, myasthenia gravis, subacute sclerosis panencephalitis, atopic dermatitis, and bronchial asthma.

Safety
POSSIBLY SAFE ...when used orally or parenterally and appropriately. Human-derived transfer factor has been used safely in studies lasting up to 2 years (3062,7562,7797,7798) and bovine-derived transfer factor has been safely used in small studies lasting up to 3 months (1445,1507). Some evidence suggests these products are safe; however, some preparations are derived from animals and there is concern about contamination with diseased animal parts (see

Adverse Reactions) (1825). There are no reports of disease transmission to humans due to use of contaminated bovine transfer factor.

CHILDREN: POSSIBLY SAFE ...when used orally or parenterally and appropriately. Human-derived transfer factor administered subcutaneously has been used safely for up to 6 years (7794). Oral bovine transfer factor has been used safely for up to 6 months (350).

PREGNANCY AND LACTATION: Insufficient reliable information available; avoid using.

Effectiveness

POSSIBLY EFFECTIVE

Herpes zoster (shingles). Administering transfer factor subcutaneously seems to prevent varicella-zoster in children with leukemia. Human-derived transfer factor prepared from donors with varicella-zoster antibodies seems to protect nonimmune children with acute lymphocytic leukemia (384). However, administering human-derived transfer factor subcutaneously doesn't seem to prevent recurrent varicella-zoster infection or restore immunity in people receiving bone marrow transplant for leukemia (3278).

POSSIBLY INEFFECTIVE

Amyotrophic lateral sclerosis (ALS, Lou Gehrig's disease). Human-derived transfer factor from healthy donors doesn't seem to affect the course of ALS (7795).

Chronic fatigue syndrome (CFS). Administering transfer factor intramuscularly doesn't seem to improve CFS. Transfer factor, obtained from relatives or other human donors, doesn't seem to improve CFS symptoms when administered biweekly, either alone or in combination with cognitive behavioral therapy (7562).

Lung cancer. Administering human-derived transfer factor intramuscularly, in combination with lung resection and chemotherapy, doesn't seem to significantly affect survival (5447,7800).

Malignant melanoma. Administering human-derived transfer factor intramuscularly or subcutaneously, as adjuvant therapy, doesn't seem to affect disease progression or prolong survival when used for up to two years following surgery for Stage I and Stage II melanoma (3062,3063).

INSUFFICIENT RELIABLE EVIDENCE to RATE

AIDS-related cryptosporidiosis. There's some preliminary evidence that oral transfer factor might be beneficial for people with cryptosporidiosis related to AIDS. Transfer factor from bovine sources seems to improve stool frequency and help eradicate oocysts in some patients (1445,1480).

Hepatitis B. Transfer factor derived from patients with acute hepatitis B might be useful for treating chronic active hepatitis B infection (7797).

Leishmania lesions. There's some evidence that transfer factor obtained from patients with antibodies to leishmania can heal persistent cutaneous leishmania lesions (3930,8105).

Multiple sclerosis (MS). There's conflicting research about the use of human-derived transfer factor for MS. It might slow disease progression in people with mild to moderate symptoms. A positive effect is seen only after 18 months to 2 years of therapy (7798,7799).

Woskott-Aldrich syndrome. Some research suggests that human-derived transfer factor might prolong survival in people with Wiskott-Aldrich syndrome, an x-linked recessive genetic disorder (7794).

More evidence is needed to rate transfer factor for these uses.

Mechanism of Action

Transfer factor refers to a variety of dialyzable polypeptide molecules extracted from leukocytes of humans and animals, such as cows and mice (1493,1494). Bovine transfer factor is structurally similar to human-derived transfer factor (7788). Transfer factor contains more than 200 different substances (7790).

Transfer factors are products of T-lymphocytes that transfer the ability to express delayed-type hypersensitivity and cell-mediated immunity from sensitized donors to non-immune recipients (7793). Transfer factors are derived from sources that have developed immunity to certain infectious diseases. For example, bovine transfer factor for cryptosporidiosis is prepared by first inoculating calves with cryptosporidium and then harvesting of lymph nodes (1410,1420,1445,1480,7791). Human-derived transfer factor is prepared from blood of donors with antigen-specific immune responses (1476,1507). The theory is that use of transfer factor from sensitized donors, human or animal, can cause deficient recipients to express cell-mediated immunity (1493). This effect is antigen-specific and results in expression of delayed type hypersensitivity and production of lymphokines (1493,1495,1507,7788).

Animal studies indicate that transfer factor prepared from bovine lymphocytes or bovine colostrum confers cell-mediated immunity to specific antigens on recipients of different species (1475,1477,1478,7791,7792). The exact mechanism of action of transfer factors is unknown; however, a specific amino acid sequence in transfer factor has been identified, and antigen specificity is well-established (1475,1477,1478,7793). Although the recipient of transfer factor acquires the ability to express the cell-mediated immune responses of the donor, the serum of the recipient will not cause a similar response if used to inoculate an unsensitized individual. The production of transfer factor appears to be regulated by immune response genes, but the immunologic activities of transfer factor are not (7789). It is possible that transfer factors might cause an immune response by different mechanisms than active immunization (7793). Research suggests that transfer factors specific to a variety of bacteria, viruses, protozoa, and other parasites might be useful for microbial diseases (7790). However, there is no evidence that non-specific transfer factor products, such as those marketed on the Internet, are effective for any indication.

Adverse Reactions
Orally or parenterally, transfer factor might cause fever in some patients (1507).
Parenterally, transfer factor is usually well tolerated (3062,3063,7562,7799). It can cause tenderness, pain, and swelling at the injection site (3062,7562,7799).
There is also some concern that bovine-derived transfer factor that is produced from cows in countries where bovine spongiform encephalitis (BSE) has been reported might be contaminated with diseased tissue. Countries where BSE has been reported include Great Britain, France, the Netherlands, Portugal, Luxembourg, Ireland, Switzerland, Oman, and Belgium (1825). However, there have been no reports of BSE transfer to humans from contaminated transfer factor products. Until more is known, tell patients to avoid these products unless country of origin can be determined. Patients should avoid products that are produced in countries where BSE has been found.

Interactions with Herbs & Other Dietary Supplements
None known.

Interactions with Drugs
None known.

Interactions with Foods
None known.

Interactions with Lab Tests
None known.

Interactions with Diseases or Conditions
None known.

Dosage and Administration
ORAL: For cryptosporidiosis, clinical studies used bovine transfer factor 1 unit (5 x 108 lymph node cell equivalents) weekly for 1-1/2 to 3 months (1420,1445).
SUBCUTANEOUS: For preventing varicella-zoster in nonimmune children with leukemia, a single dose of human-derived transfer factor, specific for varicella, of 100 million lymphocyte equivalents per 7 kg of body weight has been used (384).

Comments
Transfer factors thus far have been produced only in laboratories for experimental use. There's some evidence that they can be stored for 12 months and retain potency (7790).

TRAVELER'S JOY

Also Known As
Old Man's Beard, Travelers Joy.
CAUTION: See separate listings for Clematis, Fringetree, Usnea, and Woodbine.

Scientific Names
Clematis vitalba.
Family: Ranunculaceae.

People Use This For
Orally, traveler's joy is used for diseases of the male genitals and migraine headaches.
Topically, traveler's joy is used for poorly healing wounds and migraine headaches.

Safety
LIKELY UNSAFE ...when used orally or topically due to the constituent protoanemonin, which is a severe local irritant (18).
PREGNANCY AND LACTATION: LIKELY UNSAFE ...when used orally or topically (18).

Effectiveness
There is insufficient reliable information available about the effectiveness of traveler's joy.

Mechanism of Action
The applicable part of traveler's joy is the fresh leaf. When the fresh plant is crushed or cut into small pieces, the glycoside ranunculin is enzymatically changed into a severely irritating protoanemonin, which, in turn, rapidly degrades into the less toxic anemonin (18). Both protoanemonin and ranunculin are destroyed to an unknown extent during the drying process (2).

Adverse Reactions
Orally, traveler's joy can cause severe irritation of the gastrointestinal tract, including colic and diarrhea. Irritation of the urinary tract can also occur.
Topically, skin contact can cause blisters and burns that are difficult to heal (18).

Interactions with Herbs & Other Dietary Supplements
None known.

Interactions with Drugs
None known.

Interactions with Foods
None known.

Interactions with Lab Tests
None known.

Interactions with Diseases or Conditions
None known.

Dosage and Administration
No typical dosage.

TREE OF HEAVEN

Also Known As
A-Lan-Thus, Ailanthus Glandulosa, Ailanto, Chinese Sumach, Copal Tree, Heaven Tree, Paradise Tree, Stinktree, Varnish Tree, Vernis de Japon.

Scientific Names
Ailanthus altissima, Ailanthus cacodendron, Ailanthus giraldii, Ailanthus glandulosa, Ailanthus vilmoriniana, Rhus cacodendron, Toxicodendron altissimum.
Family: Simaroubaceae.

People Use This For
Orally, tree of heaven is used for pathological leukorrhea, diarrhea, chronic diarrhea, chronic dysentery, dysmenorrhea, and asthma, cramps, epilepsy, fast heart rate, gonorrhea, malaria, and tapeworms. It has also been used as a bitter and a tonic.
In foods, the young leaves of the tree of heaven are eaten.
In manufacturing, tree of heaven is used as insecticide.

Safety
There is insufficient reliable information available about the safety of tree of heaven. However, fatal poisonings have been reported in animal experiments (18).
Pregnancy and Lactation: Insufficient reliable information available; avoid using.

Effectiveness
There is insufficient reliable information available about the effectiveness of tree of heaven.

Mechanism of Action
The applicable parts of tree of heaven are the dried trunk and root bark. The bark of the tree of heaven is said to have astringent, antipyretic, and antispasmodic properties (18). Some evidence suggests the quassionoid constituents, including ailanthone and quassin, have antiprotozoan, anthelmintic, antileukemic, and cytotoxic properties (18). The bark also contains tannins and indole alkaloids of the beta-carbolic type (18).

Adverse Reactions
Orally, large amounts of the tree of heaven bark can cause queasiness, dizziness, headache, limb tingling, and diarrhea (18).

Interactions with Herbs & Other Dietary Supplements
None known.

Interactions with Drugs
None known.

Interactions with Foods
None known.

Interactions with Lab Tests
None known.

Interactions with Diseases or Conditions
None known.

Dosage and Administration
ORAL: A typical dose is 6-9 grams (18).

Comments
Until recently, tree of heaven was used only in folk medicine. Currently, it is being investigated as a potential drug (18).

TRYPSIN

Also Known As
Proteinase, Proteolytic Enzyme, Tripsin.

Scientific Names
Trypsin.

People Use This For
Orally, trypsin is used for digestive enzyme supplementation in conjunction with lipase, amylase, and other proteases.
In combination with bromelain and rutin, trypsin is used for osteoarthritis.
Topically, trypsin is used for wound and ulcer cleansing to remove necrotic tissue and debris. Also, the prescription aerosol products containing trypsin, Peru balsam, and castor oil are applied topically for enzymatic debridement, promotion of normal wound healing, and promoting the healing of necrotic oral mucosa ulcers.

Safety
POSSIBLY SAFE ...when used topically by health care professionals trained in wound debridement (506). The topical combination containing trypsin, Peru balsam, and castor oil is an FDA-approved prescription aerosol product. There is insufficient reliable information available about the safety of trypsin for its other uses.
PREGNANCY AND LACTATION: Insufficient reliable information available; avoid using.

Effectiveness
POSSIBLY EFFECTIVE

Osteoarthritis. In a double-blind trial, 73 patients with painful osteoarthritis of the knee were randomly assigned the combination enzyme product (Phlogenzym) or diclofenac (Voltaren) 50 mg three times daily during the first week and then twice daily in weeks 2 and 3. The enzyme product was similar to diclofenac in relieving pain and improving knee function (6252).

Wound healing. Applying trypsin topically seems to be helpful for cleansing wounds of necrotic material and enhancing wound healing (715,716).

There is insufficient reliable information available about the effectiveness of trypsin for its other uses.

Mechanism of Action
Trypsin is a proteolytic enzyme formed in the small intestines by the action of enteropeptidase on trypsinogen (511). Trypsin supplements are derived from fungi or bacterial sources, pancreas of livestock, or from plant sources. It is

used to remove dead tissue that remains after trauma, infections such as decubitus ulcers, and surgical procedures. The removal of dead cells allows the growth of healthy tissues (13). Some topical preparations that are available contain balsam of Peru and castor oil to protect the skin and prevent premature epithelial destruction (13). Evidence from in vitro studies of necroses and purulent exudates (2648) and a human study (2649) shows streptokinase-streptodornase can have better proteolytic activity than trypsin alone.

Adverse Reactions

Topically, trypsin can cause localized pain and transient burning (506).

Interactions with Herbs & Other Dietary Supplements

None known.

Interactions with Drugs

None known.

Interactions with Foods

None known.

Interactions with Lab Tests

None known.

Interactions with Diseases or Conditions

None known.

Dosage and Administration

ORAL: For osteoarthritis, a combination enzyme product (Phlogenzym), which contains rutin 100 mg, trypsin 48 mg, and bromelain 90 mg, has been given 2 tablets three times daily (6252).
TOPICAL: Wound debridement products (Dermuspray, Granulderm, Granulex, and GranuMed) containing trypsin, Peru balsam, and castor oil (506) are FDA-approved prescription products.

Comments

Commercial trypsin is prepared from animal sources, such as ox pancreas (13).

TUNG SEED

Also Known As

Balucanat, Candleberry, Candleberry Tree, Candlenut, China-Wood Oil, Country Walnut, Indian Walnut, Kukui, Otaheite Walnut, Tung, Varnish Tree.
CAUTION: See separate listing for Bayberry.

Scientific Names

Aleurites moluccanus, synonyms Aleurites javanicus, Aleurites pentaphyllus, Aleurites remyi, Aleurites trilobus, Jatropha moluccana; Vernicia cordata, synonym Aleurites cordatus.
Family: Euphorbiaceae.

People Use This For

Orally, tung seed is used for asthma, bloody diarrhea, dysentery, sprue, and as a bowel stimulant.
Topically, tung seed is used to stimulate hair growth and for constipation.
In manufacturing, the oil of tung seed is used in soaps, rubber substitutes, linoleum, and insulation. The seed cake of tung seed is used as a fertilizer. The seed is also the source of the oil that is widely used as a wood preservative and varnish.

Safety

LIKELY UNSAFE ...when used orally (6). Tung seed is believed to contain toxalbumin and hydrogen cyanide (6). Toxicity ranges from severe gastrointestinal irritation to death (6,4502). Even a single seed might cause severe poisoning (4502).
There is insufficient reliable information available about the safety of the topical use of tung seed.
PREGNANCY AND LACTATION: LIKELY UNSAFE ...when used orally (6,); avoid using.

Effectiveness

There is insufficient reliable information available about the effectiveness of tung seed.

Mechanism of Action
Tung seed contains an oil that consists of eleostearic acid, linolenic, linoleic, and oleic acid. It is also thought to contain a toxalbumin and hydrogen cyanide (6). Internally, tung seed has cathartic effects (6,4502). The kernels have laxative and stimulant effects. They also promote sweating (4502).

Adverse Reactions
Orally, tung seed can cause severe stomach pain, violent vomiting, debility, diarrhea, slowed reflexes, slowed breathing, and possibly death (6,4502). Skin contact with tung seed can cause acute dermatitis (4502).

Interactions with Herbs & Other Dietary Supplements
None known.

Interactions with Drugs
None known.

Interactions with Foods
None known.

Interactions with Lab Tests
None known.

Interactions with Diseases or Conditions
None known.

Dosage and Administration
No typical dosage.

Comments
The seeds of the fruit from this plant resemble a walnut, and the term walnut is applied to this species. Tung seed should never be confused with the common walnut. Unlike the walnut, if tung seeds are eaten raw they are toxic. When roasted, the kernels are reported to be edible (6). It is said that fishermen throw tung seeds into the water to stupefy the fish (6,4502).

TURKEY CORN

Also Known As
Bleeding Heart, Dutchman's Breeches, Squirrel Corn, Staggerweed.

Scientific Names
Dicentra cucullaria.
Family: Fumariaceae.

People Use This For
Orally, turkey corn is used for digestive and menstrual disorders, urinary tract diseases, and skin rashes.

Safety
POSSIBLY UNSAFE ...when used orally. Theoretically, the constituent bicuculline, an antagonist of gamma-aminobutyric acid (GABA), could cause poisoning (18).
PREGNANCY AND LACTATION: POSSIBLY UNSAFE ...when used orally (18); avoid using.

Effectiveness
There is insufficient reliable information available about the effectiveness of turkey corn.

Mechanism of Action
The applicable part of turkey corn is the dried tuber. Turkey corn is thought to have diuretic and tonic properties (18). It contains various isoquinoline alkaloids, including bicuculline, corlumine, protopine, cryptopine, and cularine. Bicuculline is a centrally-acting, spasmogenic antagonist of GABA (18).

Adverse Reactions
None reported.

Interactions with Herbs & Other Dietary Supplements
None known.

Interactions with Drugs
None known.

Interactions with Foods
None known.

Interactions with Lab Tests
None known.

Interactions with Diseases or Conditions
None known.

Dosage and Administration
ORAL: Turkey corn is used as a liquid extract (18).

TURMERIC

Also Known As
Curcuma, Curcumae Longae Rhizoma, Curcumin, Haridra, Indian Saffron, Nisha, Rajani, Tumeric, Turmeric Root.
CAUTION: See separate listings for Javanese Turmeric, Zedoary, and Goldenseal.

Scientific Names
Curcuma longa, synonym Curcuma domestica; Curcuma aromatica.
Family: Zingiberaceae.

People Use This For
Orally, turmeric is used for dyspepsia, abdominal pain, hemorrhage, diarrhea, flatulence, abdominal bloating, loss of appetite, jaundice, hepatitis, and liver and gallbladder complaints. It is also used for headaches, bronchitis, colds, chest infections, leprosy, fever, amenorrhea, and cancer. Other uses include depression, edema, worms, kidney inflammation, and cystitis.
Topically, turmeric is used for analgesia, ringworm, bruising, leech bites, eye infections, inflammatory skin conditions, inflammation of the oral mucosa, and infected wounds.
In food and manufacturing, the essential oil is used in perfumes, and turmeric and its resin are used as a flavor and color component in foods. Turmeric is also a culinary spice and a major ingredient in curry powder.

Safety
LIKELY SAFE ...when used in amounts commonly found in foods. Turmeric has Generally Recognized As Safe (GRAS) status in the US (4912).
POSSIBLY SAFE ...when used orally or topically in medicinal amounts (10453,11144,11148,11149,11150).
PREGNANCY: LIKELY UNSAFE ...when used orally in medicinal amounts; turmeric might stimulate menstrual flow and the uterus (12).
LACTATION: There is insufficient reliable information available about the safety of turmeric in medicinal amounts during lactation.

Effectiveness
POSSIBLY EFFECTIVE

Dyspepsia. Taking turmeric orally seems to relieve dyspeptic symptoms (11144).

INSUFFICIENT RELIABLE EVIDENCE to RATE

Anterior uveitis. Clinical research suggests curcumin given orally might be useful for treating chronic anterior uveitis (11150).

Colorectal cancer. Preliminary clinical research suggests an extract of turmeric might stabilize colorectal cancer refractory to other treatments in some patients (10453).

Rheumatoid arthritis (RA). Curcumin, a constituent of turmeric, might relieve some symptoms of rheumatoid arthritis (RA) (11149).

Skin cancer. Other preliminary clinical research suggests that an ethanol extract of turmeric in combination with turmeric ointment might relieve odor and itching associated with skin cancers (11148).

More evidence is needed to rate turmeric for these uses.

Mechanism of Action
The applicable part of turmeric is the rhizome. Turmeric's major active constituents are curcuminoids including curcumin (diferuloylmethane), a yellow pigment. It seems to have anti-inflammatory activity, possibly by inhibiting cyclooxygenase-2 (COX-2), prostaglandins, and leukotrienes (11138,11139,11140).
Turmeric also exhibits chemopreventive and growth inhibitory activity against several tumor cell lines. It seems to induce apoptosis in cancer cells and may inhibit angiogenesis (11141,11142).
Curcumin might have antithrombotic effects. Preliminary research suggests it might inhibit platelet-activating factor and arachidonic acid platelet aggregation, possibly by interfering with thromboxane synthesis (11143).
Other preliminary research suggests that turmeric might also have antioxidant and immunostimulatory effects (11140,11147). It also seems to have activity against some bacteria, human immunodeficiency virus (HIV), and the protozoan Leishmania amazonensis (11140).
The bioavailability of curcumin is very low after oral administration (10453). Bromelain is sometimes recommended to enhance curcumin absorption, but there's no reliable evidence to support this.

Adverse Reactions
Orally, turmeric is generally well tolerated (10453,11144,11148,11149,11150). It can cause gastrointestinal (GI) adverse effects such as nausea and diarrhea (10453).
Topically, turmeric can cause allergic dermatitis (11146).

Interactions with Herbs & Other Dietary Supplements
HERBS WITH ANTICOAGULANT/ANTIPLATELET POTENTIAL: Concomitant use of turmeric with herbs might affect platelet aggregation could theoretically increase the risk of bleeding in some people (11143). These herbs include angelica, clove, danshen, garlic, ginger, ginkgo, Panax ginseng, red clover, willow, and others.

Interactions with Drugs
ANTICOAGULANT/ANTIPLATELET DRUGS: Concomitant use of turmeric with these drugs might increase the risk of bleeding due to decreased platelet aggregation. Turmeric has been reported to have antiplatelet effects (11143); avoid concomitant use. Some of these drugs include aspirin, clopidogrel (Plavix), dalteparin (Fragmin), enoxaparin (Lovenox), heparin, ticlopidine (Ticlid), warfarin (Coumadin), and others.

Interactions with Foods
None known.

Interactions with Lab Tests
None known.

Interactions with Diseases or Conditions
BILE DUCT OBSTRUCTION AND GALLSTONES: Turmeric can cause gallbladder contractions (11145). Use with caution in patients with gallstones or gallbladder disease.

Dosage and Administration
ORAL: For dyspepsia, 500 mg of turmeric four times daily has been used (11144). For colorectal cancer, curcuma extract 440 to 2200 mg, containing curcumin 36 to 180 mg, has been given daily for up to 4 months (10453).
TOPICAL: No typical dosage.

Comments
Turmeric has a warm, bitter taste and is frequently used to flavor or color curry powders, mustards, butters, and cheeses (6002). Avoid confusion with Javanese turmeric root (Curcuma zedoaria).

TURPENTINE OIL

Also Known As
Purified Turpentine Oil, Spirits Of Turpentine, Terebinthinae aetheroleum, Turpentine.

Scientific Names
Pinus palustris, synonym Pinus australis; Pinus pinaster; other Pinus species.
Family: Pinaceae.

People Use This For
Topically, turpentine oil is used for rheumatic and neuralgic ailments, muscle pain, toothaches, and disseminated sclerosis.

By inhalation, the vapors of turpentine oil are used to reduce the thickened secretions associated with chronic diseases of the bronchi.
In foods and beverages, distilled turpentine oil is used as a flavoring ingredient.
In manufacturing, turpentine oil is used as an ingredient in soap and cosmetics. Turpentine oil is also used as a paint solvent.

Safety

POSSIBLY SAFE ...when used topically and appropriately (2). ...when the vapors are inhaled appropriately (2).
POSSIBLY UNSAFE ...when applied topically to large areas (2).
LIKELY UNSAFE ...when used orally for medicinal purposes. 2 mL/kg of turpentine oil is considered toxic (17). 120-180 mL is potentially lethal in adults (17). Pulmonary aspiration can cause hemorrhagic pulmonary edema (17).
CHILDREN: LIKELY UNSAFE ...when used orally, 15 mL is potentially lethal (17). There is insufficient reliable information available about the safety of turpentine oil applied topically or inhaled as vapors in children.
PREGNANCY AND LACTATION: LIKELY UNSAFE ...when used orally. It might be an abortifacient (19). There is insufficient reliable information available about the safety of turpentine oil applied topically or inhaled as vapors during pregnancy and lactation.

Effectiveness

There is insufficient reliable information available about the effectiveness of turpentine oil.

Mechanism of Action

Turpentine oil is a central nervous system depressant and a pulmonary aspiration hazard. When applied topically, turpentine oil is irritating and exhibits rubefacient and counterirritant effects (6,11). When inhaled, turpentine oil can have a decongestant effect, possibly by stimulating the cold receptors, which results in reflex vasoconstriction (7).

Adverse Reactions

Orally, turpentine oil can cause headache, insomnia, coughing, vomiting, hematuria, albuminuria (6), urinary tract inflammation (17), coma (6), and death (17). Pulmonary aspiration produces hemorrhagic pulmonary edema (17). As inhalation therapy, it can cause mild respiratory tract inflammation (17). Turpentine oil can exacerbate bronchial spasms in people with asthma and whooping cough (7).
Topically, it can cause skin irritation, contact allergies, and hypersensitivity (6). Symptoms of poisoning can occur when turpentine oil is applied extensively, including kidney and central nervous system damage (2).

Interactions with Herbs & Other Dietary Supplements

None known.

Interactions with Drugs

None known.

Interactions with Foods

None known.

Interactions with Lab Tests

None known.

Interactions with Diseases or Conditions

ACUTE RESPIRATORY TRACT INFLAMMATION: Inhalation of turpentine is contraindicated (2).
ASTHMA, WHOOPING COUGH: Turpentine can exacerbate bronchial spasms (7).
HYPERSENSITIVITY: Contraindicated (2).

Dosage and Administration

TOPICAL: Several drops of the oil are typically rubbed onto the affected area. The liquid and semi-solid preparations are commonly made in concentrations of 10-50% (2). Application of turpentine should not exceed three to four times per day (3).
INHALATION: The vapors of turpentine are often inhaled as several drops of the oil in hot water (2).

Comments

Turpentine oil is obtained by the distillation of the oleoresin (gum turpentine) of longleaf pine (Pinus palustris) and other Pinus species. Terpin hydrate is a semi-synthetic derivative of turpentine (6). Turpentine oil has been used to adulterate juniper berry oil (512). Avoid confusion with gum turpentine, which is the oleoresin (6).

TURTLE HEAD

Also Known As
Balmony, Bitter Herb, Chelone, Hummingbird Tree, Salt-rheum Weed, Shellflower, Snakehead, Turtlebloom.

Scientific Names
Chelone glabra.
Family: Scrophulariaceae.

People Use This For
Orally, turtle head is used as a cathartic tonic.

Safety
POSSIBLY SAFE ...when used orally (12,18).
PREGNANCY AND LACTATION: Insufficient reliable information available; avoid using.

Effectiveness
There is insufficient reliable information available about the effectiveness of turtle head.

Mechanism of Action
The applicable parts of turtle head are the above ground parts and root. Turtle head contains iridoide monoterpenes including catalpol and a bitter-tasting resin (18).

Adverse Reactions
None reported.

Interactions with Herbs & Other Dietary Supplements
None known.

Interactions with Drugs
None known.

Interactions with Foods
None known.

Interactions with Lab Tests
None known.

Interactions with Diseases or Conditions
None known.

Dosage and Administration
No typical dosage.

Comments
Avoid confusion with Chelone obliqua which is commonly known as red turtle head (4500).

TYROSINE

Also Known As
L-tyrosine, Tyr, Tyrosinum.

Scientific Names
2-amino-3-(4-hydroxyphenyl)propionic acid.

People Use This For
Orally, tyrosine is used for depression, attention deficit disorder (ADD), attention deficit-hyperactivity disorder (ADHD), phenylketonuria (PKU), improving alertness following sleep depravation. It is also used for stress, premenstrual syndrome (PMS), Parkinson's disease, chronic fatigue syndrome (CFS), narcolepsy, alcohol and cocaine withdrawal, Alzheimer's disease, cardiovascular disease, impotence, loss of libido,

schizophrenia, and as a suntan agent and appetite suppressant.
Topically, tyrosine is used for signs of aging skin such as wrinkles.

Safety

LIKELY SAFE ...when used orally in amounts commonly found in foods. Tyrosine has Generally Recognized As Safe (GRAS) status in the US (4912).
POSSIBLY SAFE ...when used orally and appropriately, short-term. Tyrosine seems to be safe when used in doses up to 150 mg/kg per day for up to 3 months (7210,7211,7215). ...when used topically and appropriately (6155).
PREGNANCY AND LACTATION: There is insufficient reliable information available about the safety of tyrosine during pregnancy and lactation when used in medicinal amounts.

Effectiveness

EFFECTIVE

Phenylketonuria (PKU). Tyrosine is used as a component of protein supplements for people with phenylketonuria (PKU), a genetic disorder in which there is an inability to metabolize phenylalanine, a precursor of tyrosine (7212,7213,7232). The current recommendation for people with PKU is the incorporation of 6 grams of tyrosine per 100 grams of protein. However, additional separate supplementation with free tyrosine is not recommended because it can produce wide variations in tyrosine plasma concentrations and side effects (7212).

POSSIBLY EFFECTIVE

Sleep deprivation. Taking tyrosine orally seems to improve alertness following sleep deprivation (7215). Tyrosine 150 mg/kg seems to delay performance decline in psychomotor tests by about 3 hours after loss of a night's sleep (7215).

POSSIBLY INEFFECTIVE

Attention deficit disorder (ADD). Taking tyrosine orally doesn't seem to improve symptoms of adult ADD. Some patients might have transient improvement in symptoms after starting tyrosine, but adult patients quickly acquire tolerance (7210,7211).

Attention deficit-hyperactivity disorder (ADHD). Taking tyrosine orally doesn't seem to improve symptoms of childhood ADHD (7209).

Depression. Taking tyrosine orally doesn't seem to improve symptoms of moderate depression (7208).

INSUFFICIENT RELIABLE EVIDENCE to RATE

Wrinkled skin. A topical preparation containing 10% vitamin C as L-ascorbic acid, acetyl tyrosine, zinc sulfate, sodium hyaluronate, and bioflavonoids (Cellex-C High Potency Serum) applied for 3 months to photo-aged facial skin seems to improve fine and coarse wrinkling, yellowing and sallowness, roughness, and skin tone compared to placebo (6155). More evidence is needed to rate the effectiveness of tyrosine for this use.

Mechanism of Action

Tyrosine is a nonessential amino acid that the body synthesizes from phenylalanine. For people with phenylketonuria (PKU) who cannot synthesize tyrosine from phenylalanine, tyrosine is an essential amino acid (7212). Tyrosine can also be obtained from dietary proteins in dairy products, meats, fish, eggs, nuts, beans, oats, and wheat. When dietary intake of tyrosine is inadequate, phenylalanine is converted to tyrosine (7217). Dietary needs of tyrosine are dependent on phenylalanine intake. When phenylalanine intake is adequate (about 9 mg/kg/day), dietary tyrosine intake should be about 7 mg/kg/day (7214). Inadequate tyrosine intake is rare in developed nations. Tyrosine is incorporated into all proteins. Tyrosine is a precursor of thyroxine and melanin (7212); it is also a precursor for the synthesis of catecholamines, norepinephrine, epinephrine, and dopamine (7215,7217). Tyrosine is classified as a large neutral amino acid (LNAA) and is transported across the blood brain barrier by the LNAA transporter. Tyrosine competes with other LNAAs, such as tryptophan, to get into the brain (7217). There is interest in tyrosine for preventing the negative effects related to stress. Some scientists think that the brain may not be able to synthesize enough tyrosine from phenylalanine under stressful conditions (7217). Catecholamines like epinephrine, norepinephrine, and dopamine that are synthesized from tyrosine can become depleted during stress. There is speculation that increasing the availability of tyrosine to the brain allows increased catecholamine synthesis, and avoidance of the negative effects of stress. There is some evidence in animals and humans that supplemental tyrosine might improve performance, memory, and learning, under extreme environmental conditions, intense exercise, or psychological stress (7215,7217).

Adverse Reactions

Orally, tyrosine can cause nausea, headache, fatigue, heartburn, and arthralgia (7211).

Interactions with Herbs & Other Dietary Supplements

None known.

Interactions with Drugs

LEVODOPA: There is some concern that tyrosine might decrease the effectiveness of L-dopa. Tyrosine and levodopa compete for absorption in the proximal duodenum by the large neutral amino acid (LNAA) transport system (2719). Advise patients to separate doses of tyrosine and L-dopa by at least 2 hours.
THYROID HORMONE: There is some concern that tyrosine might have additive effects with thyroid hormone

medications. Tyrosine is a precursor to thyroid hormone and might boost levels (7212). These drugs include levothyroxine (Synthroid, Levoxyl) and liothyronine (Cytomel).

Interactions with Foods

None known.

Interactions with Lab Tests

THYROID STIMULATING HORMONE (TSH): Theoretically, tyrosine might decrease TSH levels. Tyrosine is a precursor of thyroxine and might boost thyroid hormone levels, which can decrease TSH results (7212).

Interactions with Diseases or Conditions

HYPERTHYROIDISM, GRAVES' DISEASE: Theoretically, tyrosine might exacerbate hyperthyroidism and Graves' disease. Tyrosine is a precursor of thyroxine and might boost thyroid hormone levels (7212). Tell patients with hyperthyroidism or Grave's disease not to take tyrosine supplements.

Dosage and Administration

ORAL: For improving alertness after sleep depravation, 150 mg/kg/day of tyrosine has been used (7215).

USNEA

Also Known As

Beard Moss, Old Man's Beard, Sodium Usniate, Tree Moss, Tree's Dandruff, Usnea Lichen, Usnic Acid, Woman's Long Hair.
CAUTION: See separate listing for Oak Moss.

Scientific Names

Usnea barbata; Usnea florida; Usnea hirta; Usnea plicata.
Family: Usneaceae.

People Use This For

Orally, usnea is used for weight loss, pain relief, fever control, wound healing, and as an expectorant.
Topically, usnea is used for mild inflammation of the mouth and pharynx.

Safety

POSSIBLY SAFE ...when used topically and appropriately (12). There is insufficient reliable information available about the safety of usnea taken orally.
PREGNANCY AND LACTATION: Insufficient reliable information available; avoid using.

Effectiveness

There is insufficient reliable information available about the effectiveness of usnea.

Mechanism of Action

The applicable part of usnea is the plant body. Usnea contains a variety of lichen acids including usnic acid, thamnolic acid, lobaric acid, stictinic acid, evernic acid, barbatic acid, diffractaic acid, and protocetraric acid. However, the exact composition varies significantly among species (11720). The hydroalcoholic extracts of Usnea barbata and Usnea hirta have anti-inflammatory, analgesic, and antipyretic activity (852). The usnic acid constituent of usnea has antibacterial, antifungal, antiviral, and antiprotozoal activity. It also seems to have antipyretic, anti-inflammatory, and analgesic effects that may result from inhibition of prostaglandin synthesis. Preliminary research on leukemia cells suggests that usnic acid might also have antiproliferative activity (11720).

Adverse Reactions

Orally, usnic acid as an ingredient in the product LipoKinetix has been associated with hepatoxicity (7091).
Topically, usnea can cause local irritation, contact dermatitis, and conjunctivitis (11720).

Interactions with Herbs & Other Dietary Supplements

None known.

Interactions with Drugs

None known.

Interactions with Foods

None known.

Interactions with Lab Tests
None known.

Interactions with Diseases or Conditions
None known.

Dosage and Administration
No typical dosage.

Comments
Sodium usniate (usnic acid) is a constituent of Usnea. Sodium usniate is also an ingredient of the brand named product LipoKinetix. There are serious concerns about the safety of LipoKinetix, which is marketed for weight loss. From July to December 2000 there were at least seven cases of acute hepatotoxicity in patients taking LipoKinetix. Symptoms including nausea, weakness and fatigue, abdominal pain, and yellowing of the skin usually develop from 2 weeks to 3 months after starting LipoKinetix. Symptoms resolve when it is discontinued (7091). It is unclear if the sodium usniate ingredient is the cause of these adverse events. Tell patients not to use this product.
Usnea species are whitish, reddish, or black lichens that grow on a variety of trees. Avoid confusion with oak moss (Evernia prunastri), also referred to as tree moss.

UVA URSI

Also Known As
Arberry, Arcostaphylos, Bear's Grape, Bearberry, Beargrape, Bearsgrape, Common Bearberry, Hogberry, Kinnikinnik, Manzanita, Mountain Box, Mountain Cranberry, Ptarmigan Berry, Raisin D'Ours, Red Bearberry, Redberry, Rockberry, Sagackhomi, Sandberry, Uva-Ursi, Uvae ursi folium.
CAUTION: See separate listings for Alpine Cranberry, Cramp Bark, and Cranberry.

Scientific Names
Arctostaphylos uva-ursi, synonym Arbutus uva-ursi.
Family: Ericacea.

People Use This For
Orally, uva ursi is used for urinary tract infections (UTIs), inflammatory conditions of the efferent urinary tract, cystitis, urethritis, diuresis, constipation, lithuria, dysuria, acidic urine, pyelonephritis, and bronchitis.
In combination, an herbal preparation containing uva ursi, hops, and peppermint is used to treat people with compulsive, strangury enuresis and painful urination.

Safety
POSSIBLY SAFE ...when used orally and appropriately, short-term (2,4,12).
POSSIBLY UNSAFE ...when used orally for extended periods. There is some concern about the safety of long-term use because of the hydroquinone constituent of uva ursi. Hydroquinone can have mutagenic and carcinogenic effects, and long-term use might result in significant adverse effects. Tell patients to avoid using uva ursi for more than one week or more than five times per year (2,7,18).
CHILDREN: LIKELY UNSAFE ...when used orally due to the risk of hepatotoxicity in children less than 12 years old (2,7,18).
PREGNANCY: LIKELY UNSAFE ...when used orally (2,4,6,7,12,18). Uva ursi can have oxytocic effects (19); avoid using.
LACTATION: Insufficient reliable information available; avoid using.

Effectiveness
POSSIBLY EFFECTIVE
Urinary tract infections (UTIs). Taking a combination product containing both uva ursi and dandelion orally seems to significantly reduce the recurrence rate of UTIs in women (1932). However, since it isn't clear if this kind of extended use is safe, tell patients not to use uva ursi for long term prevention of UTIs.
There is insufficient reliable information available about the effectiveness of uva ursi for its other uses.

Mechanism of Action
The applicable part of uva ursi is the leaf. Uva ursi can have urinary antiseptic and astringent effects (4). Some references report diuretic activity, but others disagree (6,8). Its constituents include arbutin (a phenol), tannins, and hydroquinone (4,6,7). The tannins can be responsible for adverse gastrointestinal tract effects (5) and limit the duration of use (4). Uva ursi and the constituent, arbutin, exhibit antimicrobial activity in vitro (2,4). Arbutin is absorbed from

the gastrointestinal tract unchanged and is hydrolyzed to hydroquinone in alkaline urine. There it can exert antiseptic and astringent effects (4,5,7). For this reason, urinary acidifying agents may decrease the effectiveness of uva ursi, and urinary alkalinizing agents may increase its effectiveness (19).
Hydroquinone is cytotoxic in vitro (4). Crude uva ursi extract can be more effective than the constituent arbutin as an astringent and antiseptic (4). In rats, uva ursi shows anti-inflammatory activity against experimentally-induced inflammation (4). Large amounts of uva ursi are reported to be oxytocic, although in vitro studies show no utero activity (4).

Adverse Reactions

Orally, uva ursi can cause nausea, vomiting (2), gastrointestinal discomfort, and a greenish-brown discoloration of the urine (4). Large amounts can be oxytocic, increasing the rapidity of labor (4). One gram of hydroquinone, equivalent to 6-20 grams of uva ursi, can cause tinnitus, nausea, vomiting, shortness of breath, cyanosis, convulsions, delirium, and collapse (4). Five grams of hydroquinone, equivalent to 30-100 grams of uva ursi, can cause death (4). Other adverse effects due to uva ursi include hepatotoxicity and irritation and inflammation of the urinary tract mucous membranes (18). Chronic use, especially in children (18), can cause liver impairment due to its tannin content (4).

Interactions with Herbs & Other Dietary Supplements

None known.

Interactions with Drugs

None known.

Interactions with Foods

None known.

Interactions with Lab Tests

COLORIMETRIC URINE TESTS: Theoretically, uva ursi can interfere with colorimetric urine tests and can turn urine greenish-brown (4).

Interactions with Diseases or Conditions

GI IRRITATION: Because excessive use of uva ursi can lead to stomach distress due to its tannin content, its use is contraindicated in patients with GI irritation (12,19).
KIDNEY DISORDERS: Contraindicated (12,19).

Dosage and Administration

ORAL: The typical dose of dried herb is 1.5-4 grams daily (4). It's also commonly used as a tea. The tea is prepared by steeping 3 grams of the dried leaf in 150 mL cold water for 12-24 hours and then straining. One cup of tea is usually taken up to 4 times daily (2,7,515). Uva ursi leaf teas should be prepared with cold water to minimize the tannin content (515). The hydroquinone derivative, calculated as water-free arbutin, is commonly dosed as 100-210 mg up to 4 times daily (2,7,515). The fluid extract (1:1 in 25% alcohol) is given 1.5-4 mL three times daily (4). Medical consultation is needed for urinary tract symptoms persisting longer than 48 hours (4). Uva ursi should not be used longer than one week without monitoring due to its potential risks (7). Limit its use to less than five times per year (7).

Comments

Bears are particularly fond of the fruit, which is implied in the Latin name "uva ursi", which means "bear's grape". Most authorities refer to Arctostaphylos uva-ursi as uva ursi. However, the related plants, Arctostaphylos adentricha and Arctostaphylos coactylis, have also been termed uva ursi by some authors (6).

UZARA

Also Known As

Uzara, Uzarae radix.

Scientific Names

Xysmalobium undulatum.
Family: Asclepiadaceae.

People Use This For

Orally, uzara is used for diarrhea.

Safety

POSSIBLY SAFE ...when used orally for short-term use (2). Medical consultation is needed for diarrhea persisting more than three to four days (2).
LIKELY UNSAFE ...when used parenterally. Deaths have occurred after administration of uzara products (18).
PREGNANCY AND LACTATION: Insufficient reliable information available; avoid using.

Effectiveness

There is insufficient reliable information available about the effectiveness of uzara.

Mechanism of Action

The applicable part of uzara is the root. It inhibits intestinal motility (2), and in larger amounts, it can have digitalis-like effects on the heart (2). Uzara contains a cardiac glycoside mixture of cardenolides, which include uzarone, xysmalobin, and uzarin. The glycosides can be poorly absorbed (18).

Adverse Reactions

Orally, there have been no reports of adverse reactions associated with white uzara, but it is theoretically possible due to the cardiac glycoside content (18).
Parenterally, deaths have occurred after administration of uzara products (18).

Interactions with Herbs & Other Dietary Supplements

CARDIAC GLYCOSIDE-CONTAINING HERBS: Uzara is contraindicated with these herbs, and concomitant use can increase the risk of cardiac glycoside toxicity. Cardiac glycoside containing herbs include black hellebore, Canadian hemp roots, digitalis leaf, hedge mustard, figwort, lily of the valley roots, motherwort, oleander leaf, pheasant's eye plant, pleurisy root, squill bulb leaf scales, and strophanthus seeds (19).
LICORICE/HORSETAIL: Theoretically, overuse or misuse of the licorice rhizome or horsetail plant with cardiac glycoside-containing herbs, like uzara, increases the risk of cardiac toxicity due to potassium depletion (19).
OTHER CARDIOACTIVE HERBS: Avoid concomitant use of uzara with other cardioactive herbs due to the unpredictability of therapeutic and adverse effects. Other cardioactive herbs include calamus, cereus, cola, coltsfoot, devil's claw, European mistletoe, fenugreek, fumitory, ginger, panax ginseng, hawthorn, white horehound, mate, parsley, quassia, scotch broom flower, shepherd's purse, and wild carrot (4).
STIMULANT LAXATIVE HERBS: Theoretically, overuse or misuse of stimulant laxatives with cardiac glycoside-containing herbs, like uzara, increases the risk of cardiac toxicity due to potassium depletion. Stimulant laxative herbs include the dried leaf sap of aloe, blue flag rhizome, alder buckthorn, European buckthorn, butternut bark, cascara bark, castor oil, colocynth fruit pulp, gamboge bark exudate, jalap root, black root, manna bark exudate, podophyllum root, rhubarb root, senna leaves and pods, wild cucumber fruit (Ecballium elaterium), and yellow dock root (19).

Interactions with Drugs

DIGOXIN (Lanoxin): Using uzara with digoxin is contraindicated due to therapeutic duplication and an increased risk of cardiac glycoside toxicity (2).
DIURETIC DRUGS: Theoretically, concomitant use of potassium-depleting diuretics and uzara can increase the risk of cardiac glycoside toxicity due to potassium depletion (506). Some diuretics that can deplete potassium include chlorothiazide (Diuril), chlorthalidone (Thalitone), furosemide (Lasix), hydrochlorothiazide (HCTZ, HydroDIURIL, Microzide), and others.
MACROLIDE ANTIBIOTICS: Theoretically, concomitant use may increase risk of cardiac glycoside toxicity (17).
QUININE: Theoretically, concomitant use of quinine and uzara can increase the risk of cardiac toxicity (506).
STIMULANT LAXATIVES: Theoretically, overuse or misuse of stimulant laxatives can increase the risk of cardiac glycoside toxicity due to potassium depletion (2).
TETRACYCLINE ANTIBIOTICS: Theoretically, concomitant use may increase risk of cardiac glycoside toxicity (17).

Interactions with Foods

None known.

Interactions with Lab Tests

None known.

Interactions with Diseases or Conditions

HEART DISEASE: Uzara is contraindicated in individuals with heart disease (18). Theoretically, the cardiac glycosides contained in uzara can exacerbate this condition or interfere with existing drug therapy.
HYPOKALEMIA: Theoretically, the use of uzara can increase the risk of cardiac toxicity in hypokalemic patients.

Dosage and Administration

ORAL: Uzara is commonly taken as liquid ethanol-water extracts or dry extracts obtained from methanol-water extractions (2). The initial dose is 75 mg of the total glycosides calculated as uzarin or the equivalent to 1 gram of the dried root (2). Then the dose is 45-90 mg per day of the total glycosides calculated as uzarin (2). Seek medical consultation for diarrhea persisting more than three to four days (2).

VALERIAN

Also Known As

Amantilla, All-Heal, Baldrian, Baldrianwurzel, Belgium Valerian, Common Valerian, Fragrant Valerian, Garden Heliotrope, Garden Valerian, Indian Valerian, Mexican Valerian, Pacific Valerian, Tagara, Valeriana, Valeriana officinalis, Valeriana rhizome, Valerianae radix, Valeriane.

Scientific Names

Valeriana officinalis; Valeriana edulis; Valeriana jatamansii, synonym Valeriana wallichii; Valeriana sitchensis.
Family: Valerianaceae.

People Use This For

Orally, valerian is used as a sedative-hypnotic for insomnia and as an anxiolytic for restlessness and sleeping disorders associated with anxiety. It has also been used for mood disorders such as depression, infantile convulsions, mild tremors, epilepsy, and attention deficit-hyperactivity disorder (ADHD). It is also used orally for muscle and joint pain, and conditions associated with anxiety and psychological stress including nervous asthma, hysterical states, excitability, hypochondria, headaches, migraine, and stomach upset. Valerian is also used for menstrual cramps and symptoms associated with menopause, including hot flashes and anxiety.
Topically, valerian is used as a bath additive for restlessness and sleep disorders.
In manufacturing, the extracts and essential oil are used as flavoring in foods and beverages.

Safety

LIKELY SAFE ...when used in amounts commonly found in foods. Valerian has Generally Recognized As Safe (GRAS) status in the US (4912).
POSSIBLY SAFE ...when used orally and appropriately, short-term. Clinical studies have reported safe use of valerian for medicinal purposes in over 12,000 patients in trials lasting up to 28 days (2074,3484,3485,4032,6480). The safety of long-term use is unknown.
There is insufficient reliable information available about the safety of valerian when used topically.
CHILDREN: POSSIBLY SAFE ...when used orally and appropriately for up to 8 weeks (10207).
PREGNANCY AND LACTATION: Insufficient reliable information available; avoid using.

Effectiveness

POSSIBLY EFFECTIVE

Anxiety. Taking valerian orally seems to reduce self-reported stress in social anxiety and anxiety disorder (9893,9895,9896).

Insomnia. Taking valerian orally seems to reduce the time to sleep onset (sleep latency), and improve subjective sleep quality. The greatest benefit is usually seen in patients using 400-900 mg valerian extract up to two hours before bedtime (6248,6249,8250,8296). Valerian seems to improve the sleep quality of insomniacs who have recently withdrawn from benzodiazepines. After tapering the benzodiazepine over two weeks, 300 mg valerian extract in three divided daily doses might subjectively improve sleep quality (8006). Valerian does not always relieve insomnia as fast as benzodiazepines (6480). Continuous nightly use for several days to four weeks is required for significant effect (6249,10209). Some research suggests that valerian is inferior to temazepam (Restoril) and diphenhydramine (Benadryl) for causing sedation in elderly people (10424). A combination of valerian with lemon balm might improve the quality and quantity of sleep in healthy people (10423). There is also preliminary clinical research that suggests valerian might help improve sleep in intellectually impaired children (10207).

There is insufficient reliable information available about the effectiveness of valerian for its other uses.

Mechanism of Action

The applicable part of valerian is the root. Valerian is reported to have sedative-hypnotic, anxiolytic, antidepressant, anticonvulsant, and antispasmodic effects (3484,3485). Valerian might also have hypotensive properties (9893). The pharmacological effects of valerian have primarily been attributed to valepotriates (iridoid esters), volatile oils, monoterpenes, and sesquiterpenes constituents. The primary monoterpene is berneol and the primary sesquiterpenes are valerenic acid, valerenone, and kessyl glycol (3484,3486). However, because valerian extracts without some of these constituents have similar effects, it is likely that multiple constituents are responsible for its pharmacological effects. Valepotriate constituents are known to have sedative-hypnotic and spasmolytic effects. Valepotriates have also been shown to decrease benzodiazepine withdrawal in an animal model and to bind dopamine

receptors (3484,3486). The valepotriates might act as prodrugs. They are thought to rapidly decompose to homobaldrinal in the intestine after ingestion (3486). Valepotriates are highly unstable and rapidly decompose in acid or alkaline environments and at high temperatures. Although there are published reports of toxicity due to the valepotriate constituents, these constituents are poorly absorbed and quickly degraded to less toxic metabolites and are not likely to cause acute adverse reactions (3486). The presence of an epoxide group on the valepotriates has raised concern about possible cytotoxicity and carcinogenicity (3485,3486); however, in vivo studies to date have failed to show any carcinogenic effects (3486). The sesquiterpenes, valerenic acid and kessyl glycol, have been shown to cause sedation in animals (3486). Valerenic acid also appears to inhibit the enzyme system responsible for the central catabolism of GABA, increasing GABA concentrations and decreasing central nervous system (CNS) activity (3486). There is some evidence that valerian might also contain other constituents such as lignans and GABA which may also be responsible for the sedative effects of valerian (3486).
Valerian doesn't seem to have a negative impact on reaction time, alertness, and concentration the morning after intake (2074). In healthy elderly people, valerian doesn't seem to affect psychomotor performance (10424).

Adverse Reactions

Orally, valerian can cause headache, excitability, uneasiness, cardiac disturbances, and insomnia (3484). Occasionally, valerian may cause gastric discomfort, dry mouth, vivid dreams (4032), and morning drowsiness (2074). Although residual morning effects on alertness and concentration appear uncommon, impaired alertness and information processing may sometimes occur (2074). Impairment is dose-dependent and peaks within the first few hours after an oral valerian dose (2074). Warn patients against driving or operating dangerous machinery after taking valerian.
There is little information regarding valerian overdose. In one individual, 20 times the normal dose caused fatigue, tight chest, abdominal cramping, and tremor of the hand and foot (659). Benzodiazepine-like withdrawal symptoms have been reported when treatment is discontinued (3487). Patients should taper doses slowly after extended use.
There have been several case reports of hepatotoxicity associated with the use of multi-ingredient preparations containing valerian. It is possible, however, that these preparations may have been adulterated with hepatotoxic agents (8243). Hepatotoxicity involving long-term use of single-ingredient valerian preparations has also been reported (3484). Because a variety of doses were used in these cases, and many people have used higher doses safely, these hepatotoxic reactions might have been idiosyncratic. Tell patients the long-term effect of valerian on liver function is unknown.

Interactions with Herbs & Other Dietary Supplements

HERBS AND SUPPLEMENTS WITH SEDATIVE PROPERTIES: Use of valerian with other herbs and supplements that have sedative properties might enhance therapeutic and possibly adverse effects (3496). Some of these products include calamus, California poppy, catnip, hops, Jamaican dogwood, kava, L-tryptophan, melatonin, sage, SAMe, St. John's wort, sassafras, scullcap, and others.

Interactions with Drugs

ALCOHOL (Ethanol): Theoretically, valerian might have an additive sedative effect with alcohol (9894).
BENZODIAZEPINES: Theoretically, concomitant use with benzodiazepines may cause additive therapeutic and adverse effects (3486).
CNS DEPRESSANTS: Theoretically, concomitant use of valerian and drugs with sedative properties may cause additive therapeutic and adverse effects (3486).
CYTOCHROME P450 3A4 (CYP3A4) SUBSTRATES: There is preliminary evidence that valerian may inhibit the cytochrome P450 3A4 (CYP3A4) enzyme (6450). Theoretically, valerian might increase levels of drugs metabolized by CYP3A4. However, so far, this interaction has not been reported in humans. Some drugs metabolized by CYP3A4 include lovastatin (Mevacor), ketoconazole (Nizoral), itraconazole (Sporanox), fexofenadine (Allegra), triazolam (Halcion), chemotherapeutic agents (etoposide, paclitaxel, vinblastine, vincristine, vindesine), and numerous others. Use valerian cautiously or avoid in patients taking these drugs.

Interactions with Foods

ALCOHOL: Theoretically, valerian might have an additive sedative effect with alcohol (9894).

Interactions with Lab Tests

None known.

Interactions with Diseases or Conditions

None known.

Dosage and Administration

ORAL: For decreasing sleep latency and improving sleep quality, most studies have used 400-900 mg valerian extract up to two hours before bedtime for as long as 28 days (2074,3484,6480,8006,8250,8296,10424). Other studies have used valerian extract 300-450 mg given in three divided doses (3484,8006). Valerian extract 120 mg, with lemon balm extract 80 mg, has been used 3 times daily for up to 30 days (10423). Valerian should be given 30 minutes to 2 hours before bedtime (9894).

VANADIUM

Also Known As
Metavanadate, Orthovanadate, Vanadate, Vanadium Pentoxide, Vanadyl, Vanadyl Sulfate.

Scientific Names
Vanadium; V; atomic number 23.

People Use This For
Orally, vanadium is used for diabetes, hypoglycemia, hyperlipidemia, heart disease, edema, improving athletic performance in weight training, and preventing cancer. Vanadium is also used for treating tuberculosis, diabetes, syphilis, and a form of microcytic anemia (chlorosis).

Safety
LIKELY SAFE ...when used orally and appropriately. Vanadium is safe when taken in amounts below the tolerable upper intake level (UL) of 1.8 mg per day (7135).
POSSIBLY UNSAFE ...when used orally in high doses. Taking more than the tolerable upper intake level (UL) of 1.8 mg per day can increase the risk of gastrointestinal side effects and theoretically, renal toxicity (7135). In some cases, patients with diabetes have used very high doses (100 mg per day) safely for up to 4 weeks (3055,3056,3057). However, there is concern that prolonged use of high doses might cause serious side effects including kidney damage (7135). Tell patients to avoid exceeding the UL.
CHILDREN: LIKELY SAFE ...when used orally in amounts found in foods (7135). There is insufficient reliable information available about the safety of vanadium when used in children in amounts greater than those typically found in foods.
PREGNANCY AND LACTATION: LIKELY SAFE ...when used orally in amounts found in foods (7135). There is insufficient reliable information available about the safety of vanadium when used in pregnant or breast-feeding women in amounts greater than those typically found in foods.

Effectiveness
POSSIBLY EFFECTIVE

Diabetes. There is some evidence that high oral doses of vanadyl sulfate (100 mg daily, 31 mg elemental vanadium), can improve hepatic and peripheral insulin sensitivity in patients with type 2 diabetes and possibly reduce blood glucose levels (3055,3056,3057); however, prolonged use of these high doses might not be safe (7135). It's not known if lower doses have the same benefit. Until more is known, tell patients not to use vanadium for treating type 2 diabetes.

There is insufficient reliable information available about the effectiveness of vanadium for its other uses.

Mechanism of Action
Vanadium is a trace mineral. Good sources of dietary vanadium include mushrooms; shellfish; black pepper; parsley; dillseed; grains and grain products; and beverages such as beer, wine, and artificially sweetened drinks (7135). Drinking water can also contain trace amounts of vanadium (3011). Vanadyl sulfate contains 31% elemental vanadium. Sodium metavanadate contains 42% elemental vanadium. Sodium orthovanadate contains 28% elemental vanadium (16). The vanadium pentoxide form, which is considered toxic, is not found in foods or supplements. An average diet provides 6 to 18 mcg vanadium per day. Only about 5% of ingested vanadium is absorbed. In vivo, vanadium is converted to the vanadyl cation, which can form complexes with ferritin and transferrin. Highest concentrations are found in the liver, kidney, and bone (7135).
Vanadium appears to be important in normal bone growth and as a cofactor for various enzyme reactions. Vanadium inhibits ATPases, phosphatases, and phosphoryl-transfer enzymes (7135).
Vanadium also seems to have cardiovascular effects. There is some evidence that prolonged administration might be associated with dose-dependent increases in blood pressure (3012). Vanadium also inhibits cholesterol synthesis from mevalonic acid (3012).
Some evidence suggests that vanadium can mimic the actions of insulin, possibly by causing phosphorylation of insulin receptor proteins. Vanadium activates the receptor; stimulates glucose oxidation and transport; inhibits lipolysis in adipose tissue; stimulates glycogen synthesis in the liver; inhibits hepatic gluconeogenesis; inhibits intestinal glucose transport; and increases glucose uptake, utilization, and glycogen synthesis in skeletal muscle (3012,3013). It appears to augment the effects of insulin in insulin-resistant type 2 diabetes, but might not have an effect in type 1 diabetes (482). Preliminary evidence suggests that L-glutamic acid gamma-monohydroxamate might activate endogenous vanadium, facilitating glucose metabolism through conversion of intracellular vanadium into an active insulinomimetic compound (388).
There is also some evidence that vanadium might protect against dental caries (3012). A few preliminary studies suggest vanadium might offer protection against hematological toxicity and the development of hepatic carcinoma (3014,3016), but others suggest that vanadium is potentially mutagenic, carcinogenic (3019), and might interfere with mitosis and chromosome distribution (3051).

Adverse Reactions

Orally, vanadium most commonly causes mild gastrointestinal upset (7135). There is concern that taking doses exceeding the tolerable upper intake level (UL) of 1.8 mg per day can increase the risk of gastrointestinal side effects and possibly lead to more severe toxicity. In some cases, patients with diabetes have used very high doses (100 mg per day) safely for up to 4 weeks (3055,3056,3057). However, there is concern that prolonged use of high doses might cause serious side effects including kidney damage (7135). Doses of 22.5 mg daily for five months can cause cramps and diarrhea (3012). Vanadium has also been associated with green discoloration of tongue, fatigue, lethargy, and focal neurological lesions, which were unrelated to dose (7135).

Significant toxic effects have been observed in animal studies of vanadium including decreased weight gain, deterioration in health, pro-oxidant effects, alteration in renal function, increased serum urea and creatinine levels, tissue vanadium accumulation, and some deaths (3017,3018,3021). High body levels of vanadium have been associated with an increased incidence of renal stone disease, distal renal tubular acidosis, hypokalemic periodic paralysis, sudden unexplained nocturnal death, and malnutrition-related diabetes mellitus (3020).

Ingestion of vanadium pentoxide form of vanadium can cause significant toxicity. It has been associated with gastrointestinal disturbances, abnormalities of renal function tests, and nervous system effects (3011). Severe and chronic respiratory tract disorders have been reported from occupational exposure to vanadium dusts (17). This form of vanadium is not found in foods or vanadium supplements.

Interactions with Herbs & Other Dietary Supplements

None known.

Interactions with Drugs

ANTICOAGULANT/ANTIPLATELET DRUGS: Theoretically, the sodium orthovanadate form of vanadium might potentiate anticoagulant therapeutic and adverse effects (3054).

ANTIDIABETES DRUGS: The vanadyl sulfate form of vanadium might have additive effects with diabetes drug therapy. The vanadyl sulfate form of vanadium increases insulin sensitivity (3055,3056,3057) and might lower blood glucose (3057) in individuals with type 2 diabetes. Monitor carefully.

Interactions with Foods

None known.

Interactions with Lab Tests

BLOOD GLUCOSE: The vanadyl sulfate form of vanadium might lower blood glucose levels and test results in people with type 2 diabetes (3057).

SERUM CREATININE: There is preliminary evidence that vanadium might adversely affect renal function (7135). Theoretically, renal function tests might be altered in people taking high doses of vanadium for extended periods.

Interactions with Diseases or Conditions

DIABETES: The vanadyl sulfate form of vanadium might alter blood glucose control in patients with type 2 diabetes. The vanadyl sulfate form of vanadium increases insulin sensitivity (3055,3056,3057) and might lower blood glucose (3057) in individuals with type 2 diabetes. Monitor carefully.

RENAL DYSFUNCTION: There is preliminary evidence that vanadium might cause nephrotoxicity (7135). People with renal dysfunction should avoid vanadium supplements.

Dosage and Administration

ORAL: For type 2 diabetes, the vanadyl sulfate form of vanadium 50 mg twice daily has been used (3055,3056,3057). The National Institute of Medicine has set the tolerable upper intake level (UL) of vanadium at 1.8 mg per day of elemental vanadium for adults (7135). No UL has been set for infants, children, and pregnant or lactating women (7135). Vanadium intake should be limited to food or infant formula in these groups (7135). An average diet provides 6 to 18 mcg vanadium per day (7135). Vanadyl sulfate contains 31% elemental vanadium. Sodium metavanadate contains 42% elemental vanadium. Sodium orthovanadate contains 28% elemental vanadium (16).

Comments

Vanadium was named for the Norse goddess of beauty, Vanadis, because of its beautiful multicolored compounds.

VANILLA

Also Known As
Bourbon Vanilla, Common Vanilla, Madagascar Vanilla, Mexican Vanilla, Réunion Vanilla, Tahiti Vanilla, Tahitian Vanilla, Vanillin.

Scientific Names
Vanilla planifolia, synonyms Vanilla fragrans, Myrobroma fragrans; Vanilla tahitensis.
Family: Orchidaceae.

People Use This For
Orally, vanilla is used as an aphrodisiac, antiflatulent, antipyretic, and stimulant.
In foods and beverages, vanilla is used as a flavoring agent. It is added to foods to reduce the amount of sugar needed for sweetening and inhibit the development of dental caries.
In manufacturing, vanilla is used as a flavoring agent in syrups for pharmaceutical use. It is also used as a fragrance in perfumes.

Safety
LIKELY SAFE ...when used orally in amounts commonly found in foods. Vanilla has Generally Recognized As Safe (GRAS) status in the US (4912).
PREGNANCY AND LACTATION: Insufficient reliable information available; avoid amounts in excess of those found in foods.

Effectiveness
There is insufficient reliable information available about the effectiveness of vanilla.

Mechanism of Action
The applicable part of vanilla is the fruit. Although the constituent vanillin is primarily responsible for the flavor of vanilla (11), over 150 aromatic compounds contribute to its fragrance (11,6). The catechin content of vanilla shows evidence of an anti-caries effect (6). In controlled studies, meals flavored with vanilla provided a higher degree of satisfaction than identical meals without vanilla flavoring (6). Contact dermatitis associated with the vanilla plant is thought to be due to the calcium oxalate crystals in the plant (6).

Adverse Reactions
Orally and topically, vanilla has been associated with allergic responses including contact dermatitis (6,11). Workers preparing vanilla have reported headache, dermatitis, and insomnia, characterized as "vanillism."

Interactions with Herbs & Other Dietary Supplements
None known.

Interactions with Drugs
None known.

Interactions with Foods
None known.

Interactions with Lab Tests
None known.

Interactions with Diseases or Conditions
None known.

Dosage and Administration
No typical dosage.

Comments
Synthetically-produced vanillin is often used as a substitute for vanilla (6), even though the fragrance, rather than the vanillin content, determines the value of vanilla (11). Vanilla extracts have been extensively adulterated (11). Extracts of Mexican origin have been adulterated with coumarin, often due to tonka beans (6). Since 1954, the FDA has prohibited the use of coumarin in food (6).

VERBENA

Also Known As

Blue Vervain, Common Verbena, Common Vervain, Eisenkraut, Enchanter's Plant, European Vervain, Herb of Grace, Herb of the Cross, Holywort, Juno's Tears, Ma Bian Cao, Pigeon's Grass, Pigeonweed, Simpler's Joy, Turkey Grass, Verbenae herba, Vervain.
CAUTION: See separate listing for Lemon Verbena.

Scientific Names

Verbena officinalis.
Family: Verbenaceae.

People Use This For

Orally, verbena is used for sore throats and other oral and pharyngeal inflammation, respiratory tract diseases such as asthma and whooping cough, and angina. Verbena is also used orally for depression, melancholia, hysteria, generalized seizure, gallbladder pain, fever, debility of convalescence after fevers, pains, spasms, exhaustion, angina, nervous conditions, digestive disorders, liver and gallbladder diseases, jaundice, kidney and lower urinary tract ailments and diseases, menopausal complaints, irregular menstruation, for lactation during nursing, arthritic conditions, gout, metabolic disorders, anemia, and edema associated with weak heart.
Topically, verbena is used for poorly healing wounds, abscesses and burns, as a gargle for cold symptoms and oral/pharyngeal cavity diseases, arthritis, rheumatism, dislocations, contusions, itching, and minor burns.
In combination with gentian root, European elder flower, cowslip flower, and sorrel, verbena is used orally for maintaining healthy sinuses and treating sinusitis.
In manufacturing, verbena flowers are used as a flavoring agent in alcoholic beverages.

Safety

LIKELY SAFE ...when used orally in amounts commonly found in foods. Verbena has Generally Recognized As Safe (GRAS) status in the US (4912).
POSSIBLY SAFE ...when used orally and appropriately in medicinal amounts (12). ...when verbena is used orally in a combination with gentian root, European elder flower, cowslip flower, and sorrel (Quanterra Sinus Defense, Sinupret) (7,374,379).
LIKELY UNSAFE ...when used orally in excessive amounts because the constituent, verbenalin, can cause stupor and convulsions (4).
There is insufficient reliable information available about the safety of the topical use of verbena.
PREGNANCY: LIKELY UNSAFE ...when used orally; verbena is believed to be an abortifacient and oxytoxic agent (4). There is insufficient reliable information available about the safety of the topical use of verbena during pregnancy.
LACTATION: Insufficient reliable information available; avoid using.

Effectiveness

POSSIBLY EFFECTIVE

Sinusitis. Taking verbena orally in combination with gentian root, European elder flower, cowslip flower, and sorrel (Quanterra Sinus Defense, Sinupret) seems to be effective for treating acute or chronic sinusitis (7,374,379).

There is insufficient reliable information available about the effectiveness of verbena for its other uses.

Mechanism of Action

The applicable parts of verbena are the above ground parts. They contain the iridoid glycosides verbascoside (acetoside), verbenalin, and verbenin (aucubin) (4). Verbena possesses weak parasympathetic properties and can cause a slight contraction of the uterus. The herb shows evidence of luteinizing activity, perhaps by inhibiting the gonadotrophic activity of the posterior pituitary (4). Some evidence indicates the iridoid glycosides have a mild laxative effect. Small amounts of the constituent, verbenin, appear to stimulate sympathetic activity. Larger amounts of verbenin inhibit sympathetic activity (4). Preliminary evidence suggests verbenin might also stimulate milk secretion (4). The constituent, verbenalin, shows evidence of uterine stimulant activity (4). The constituent verbascoside shows evidence of analgesic and antihypertensive activity. Verbascoside also appears to enhance the antitremor action of levodopa (4).

Adverse Reactions

Orally, excessive amounts of the constituent, verbenalin, can cause CNS paralysis, stupor, and convulsions (4).

Interactions with Herbs & Other Dietary Supplements

None known.

Interactions with Drugs
ANTIHYPERTENSIVE DRUGS: Theoretically, excessive amounts of verbena can interfere with drug therapy for hypertension due to the antihypertensive effects of the constituent verbascoside (4).

Interactions with Foods
None known.

Interactions with Lab Tests
None known.

Interactions with Diseases or Conditions
HYPERTENSION: Theoretically, excessive amounts of verbena might reduce blood pressure (4).
HYPOTENSION: Theoretically, excessive amounts of verbena might exacerbate this condition (4).

Dosage and Administration
ORAL: A typical dose is one cup tea three times daily (4). To make tea, steep 2-4 grams dried above ground parts in 150 mL boiling water for 5 10 minutes and strain (4). 2-4 mL of the liquid extract, 1:1 in 25% ethanol, has been used three times daily (4). 5-10 mL of the tincture, 1:1 in 40% ethanol, has been used three times daily (4).
For acute or chronic sinusitis, two Sinupret tablets three times daily for up to two weeks has been used in clinical trials (7,374,379), equivalent to gentian root 12 mg, European elder flower 36 mg, verbena 36 mg, cowslip flower 36 mg, and sorrel 36 mg three times daily.
TOPICAL: No typical dosage.

VERONICA

Also Known As
Ehrenpreiskraut, Gypsy Weed, Speedwell, Veronica Herb, Veronicae herba.
CAUTION: See separate listings for Bugleweed, and for Black Root (Leptandra virginica) and Brooklime (Veronica beccabungo) which are both known also as Speedwell.

Scientific Names
Veronica officinalis.
Family: Scrophulariaceae.

People Use This For
Orally, veronica is used for diseases and discomforts of the respiratory tract, gastrointestinal tract, liver, kidney, and lower urinary tract. Veronica is also used orally for gout, arthritis, rheumatic complaints, diseases of the spleen, scrofulosis, as an appetite stimulant and tonic, to induce sweating, for nervous irritation, "blood purification," and promotion of metabolism.
Topically, veronica is used as a gargle for inflammation of the oral and pharyngeal mucosa, for perspiration of the feet, stimulation of wound healing, chronic skin conditions, and itching.

Safety
LIKELY SAFE ...when consumed in amounts commonly found in foods. Veronica has Generally Recognized As Safe (GRAS) status in the US (4912).
POSSIBLY SAFE ...when used orally and appropriately in medicinal amounts (12).
There is insufficient reliable information available about the safety of the topical use of veronica.
PREGNANCY AND LACTATION: Insufficient reliable information available; avoid using.

Effectiveness
There is insufficient reliable information available about the effectiveness of veronica.

Mechanism of Action
The applicable parts of veronica are the above ground parts. Extracts of veronica may protect against ulcers induced by nonsteroidal anti-inflammatory drugs (NSAIDs). Veronica may enhance gastric mucosa regeneration (4010).

Adverse Reactions
None reported.

Interactions with Herbs & Other Dietary Supplements
None known.

Interactions with Drugs
None known.

Interactions with Foods
None known.

Interactions with Lab Tests
None known.

Interactions with Diseases or Conditions
GASTRIC ULCERS: Theoretically, veronica may enhance ulcer healing (4010).

Dosage and Administration
ORAL: As an expectorant, 1 cup tea (steep 1.5 grams finely cut above ground parts in 150 mL boiling water 10 minutes, strain) 2-3 times daily is commonly used (18).
TOPICAL: For lavages and compresses for eczema, ulcers, and wounds, boil 1 handful above ground parts in 1 L water for 10 minutes (18).

Comments
Avoid confusion with other Veronica species, including Veronica allionii and Veronica chamaedrys (18).

VETIVER

Also Known As
Chiendent Odorant, Cuscus, Cuscus Grass, Khas-khas, Khus Khus, Khus-khus Grass, Reshira, Sugandhimula, Ushira, Vétiver, Vetivergras, Zacate Violeta.

Scientific Names
Chrysopogon zizanioides, synonyms Vetiveria zizanioides, Anatherum zizanioides, Andropogon odoratus, Phalaris zizanioides.
Family: Poaceae/Gramineae.

People Use This For
Orally, vetiver is used as a uterine stimulant to promote menses and to cause abortion. It is also used orally for nervous and circulatory problems.
Topically, vetiver is used for stress relief, recovery from emotional traumas and shocks, treatment of lice, and as an insect repellent.
As an inhalant, vetiver is used for "aroma therapy" for nervousness, insomnia, rheumatism, and muscle relaxation.
In manufacturing, vetiver is used as a flavoring in alcoholic beverages.

Safety
LIKELY SAFE ...when used in amounts commonly found in foods. Vetiver has Generally Recognized As Safe (GRAS) status in the US (4912).
POSSIBLY SAFE ...when used orally (12).
PREGNANCY: LIKELY UNSAFE ...when used orally because it is a potential abortifacient and it has menstrual and uterine stimulant effects (12).
LACTATION: Insufficient reliable information available: avoid using.

Effectiveness
There is insufficient reliable information available about the effectiveness of vetiver.

Mechanism of Action
The applicable part of vetiver is the root. Vetiver root contains numerous constituents including limonene, p-cymene, palmitic acid, benzoic acid, delta-3-carene (513). Vetiver may contain a volatile oil which accounts for its use as a repellent to flies, cockroaches, bedbugs, and clothes moths (5279).

Adverse Reactions
None reported.

Interactions with Herbs & Other Dietary Supplements
None known.

Interactions with Drugs
None known.

Interactions with Foods
None known.

Interactions with Lab Tests
None known.

Interactions with Diseases or Conditions
None known.

Dosage and Administration
No typical dosage.

VINPOCETINE

Also Known As
AY-27255, Cavinton, Ethyl Apovincaminate, Ethylapovincaminoate, RGH-4405, TCV-3b, Vinpocetin.

Scientific Names
Eburnamenine-14-carboxylic acid, Ethyl Ester.

People Use This For
Orally, vinpocetine is used for enhancing memory, improving cerebral blood flow, improving cerebral oxygen and glucose utilization, protecting against age-related cognitive decline and Alzheimer's disease, treating cerebrovascular disease, preventing post-stroke morbidity and mortality, treating organic psychosyndromes, treating intractable tumoral calcinosis in people undergoing hemodialysis, decreasing stroke risk, treating menopausal symptoms, seizure disorders, and preventing motion sickness.
Intravenously, vinpocetine is injected for treating seizure disorders and stroke.

Safety
POSSIBLY SAFE ...when used orally and appropriately (1784). No significant adverse effects were reported in a study of people with Alzheimer's disease treated with large doses of vinpocetine (60 mg per day) for one year (1784).
PREGNANCY AND LACTATION: Insufficient reliable information available; avoid using.

Effectiveness
POSSIBLY EFFECTIVE

Dementia. Vinpocetine is used to treat cognitive impairment due to vascular disease, Alzheimer's disease, and other kinds of dementias. It might have a modest effect on cognitive impairment from various causes, but most studies have lasted 6 months or less (1784,1787,1789). Most of the studies were published prior to 1990 and used a variety of terms and criteria for cognitive decline and dementia (10221,10827).

INSUFFICIENT RELIABLE EVIDENCE to RATE

Memory. Preliminary clinical research suggests vinpocetine might enhance memory in normal volunteers (1796,1797).

Stroke. Preliminary clinical research suggests vinpocetine might modestly reduce the residual effects of acute ischemic stroke (1785). There have been few clinical studies investigating the use of vinpocetine for stroke, and most have been published in languages other than English. Two meta-analyses of these studies found insufficient conclusive information to determine the effectiveness of vinpocetine for acute ischemic stroke (10222,10828).

More evidence is needed to rate vinpocetine for these uses.

Mechanism of Action
Vinpocetine is a synthetic derivative of apovincamine, a compound found in the periwinkle plant, Vinca minor. Vinpocetine appears to have many varied pharmacologic effects; but mechanisms of action are unclear and well-designed clinical studies to substantiate activity have not been published (10827). Some studies indicate that vinpocetine might enhance cerebral blood flow without affecting peripheral blood flow (1786,1793). Preliminary evidence indicates that vinpocetine stimulates cerebral metabolism and increases glucose and oxygen consumption by the brain (10827). Potential mechanisms for the nootropic-like effects of vinpocetine include indirect or direct cholinergic activity, augmented norepinephrine effects on cortical cyclic adenosine monophosphate (AMP), and increased turnover of brain catecholamines (1800). It might also improve microcirculation in the brain and increase cerebral blood flow by improving red blood cell deformability, reducing cerebral vascular resistance, and inhibiting

platelet aggregation (10827). Vinpocetine inhibits drug-induced platelet aggregation (1801). Pharmacological effects that might be useful in treating stroke include a possible neuroprotective and anticonvulsant effect by blocking voltage-gated sodium channels. It also might protect neurons by enhancing the effect of adenosine in preventing hypoxia. Animal studies suggest that vinpocetine decreases neuronal death in ischemia and decreases the size of cerebral infarction in experimental strokes (10728). The bioavailability of vinpocetine varies from 7-57%; food significantly enhances absorption (1802).

Adverse Reactions

Orally, adverse effects include gastric discomfort, vertigo, anxiety, nausea, facial flushing, sleep disturbances, and headache (10221).

Interactions with Herbs & Other Dietary Supplements

HERBS WITH ANTICOAGULANT/ANTIPLATELET POTENTIAL: Theoretically, concomitant use with herbs that might affect platelet aggregation might increase the risk of bleeding in some people (1821). These herbs include angelica, clove, danshen, fenugreek, feverfew, garlic, ginger, ginkgo, Panax ginseng, poplar, red clover, turmeric, and others.

Interactions with Drugs

ANTICOAGULANT/ANTIPLATELET DRUGS: Vinpocetine seems to have antiplatelet effects (1801). Theoretically, taking vinpocetine with antiplatelet or anticoagulant drugs might increase the risk of bruising and bleeding. Some of these drugs include aspirin, clopidogrel (Plavix), nonsteroidal anti-inflammatory drugs (NSAIDs) such as diclofenac (Voltaren, Cataflam, others), ibuprofen (Advil, Motrin, others), naproxen (Anaprox, Naprosyn, others), dalteparin (Fragmin), enoxaparin (Lovenox), heparin, warfarin (Coumadin), and others.
WARFARIN (Coumadin): The combination of warfarin and vinpocetine leads to slight increases in the area under the concentration curve and prothrombin time. In most patients, this interaction is likely to be clinically insignificant (10829).

Interactions with Foods

FOODS: Administration of oral vinpocetine with food enhances its absorption (1802).

Interactions with Lab Tests

PROTHROMBIN TIME (PT)/ INTERNATIONAL NORMALIZATION RATIO (INR): Vinpocetine might increase PT and INR. It has been reported to modestly increase warfarin AUC, PT, and factor VII clotting time (10829).

Interactions with Diseases or Conditions

COAGULOPATHIES: Vinpocetine should not be used by people with blood-clotting disorders because it might increase the risk of bleeding (1801).

Dosage and Administration

ORAL: For treating cognitive impairment due to vascular disease, Alzheimer's disease, and other kinds of dementias, 5-10 mg three times daily has been used (1784,1787,1789).

Comments

Vinpocetine is a synthetic derivative of apovincamine which is found in periwinkle, Vinca minor (10827). Vinpocetine synthesis requires considerable laboratory manipulation, stretching the Dietary Supplement Health and Education Act (DSHEA) definition of a dietary supplement. Vinpocetine is sold by prescription in Germany under the brand name, Cavinton. It has also been referred to generically as cavinton. Although website advertising claims that "more than a hundred" safety and effectiveness studies have been funded by the Hungarian manufacturer Gedeon Richter, few double-blind controlled clinical studies have been published (1785).

VITAMIN A

Also Known As

3-Dehydroretinol, Antixerophthalmic Vitamin, Axerophtholum, Dehydroretinol, Oleovitamin A, Retinoids, Retinol, Retinol Acetate, Retinol Palmitate, Retinyl Acetate, Retinyl Palmitate, Vitamin A1, Vitamin A2, Vitaminum A. CAUTION: See separate listings for Beta-Carotene and Lutein.

Scientific Names

Vitamin A.

People Use This For

Orally, vitamin A is used to prevent and treat the symptoms of vitamin A deficiency, promote good vision, prevent glaucoma and cataracts, prevent and speed recovery from infections, and improve immune function. It is also used for skin conditions including acne, eczema, psoriasis, cold sores, wounds and burns, sunburn, keratosis follicularis (Darier's disease), ichthyosis (noninflammatory skin scaling), lichen planus pigmentosus, and pityriasis rubra pilaris. Vitamin A is also used orally to prevent and treat vitamin A deficiency due to abnormal storage and transport of vitamin A in people with abetalipoproteinemia, protein deficiency, diabetes mellitus, hyperthyroidism, fever, liver disease, or cystic fibrosis with liver involvement. It is also used orally for heavy menses, premenstrual syndrome, atrophic vaginitis, candidiasis, fibrocystic breast disease, reduced sperm count, gastrointestinal ulcers, Crohn's disease, periodontal disease, diabetes, Hurler syndrome (mucopolysaccharidosis), sinusitis, allergic rhinitis, and urinary tract infections. It is also used for reducing complications of measles, with antibiotics for hastening clinical shigellosis cure, atrophic rhinitis, loss of sense of smell, asthma, persistent headaches, kidney stones, hyperthyroidism, anemia, deafness, tinnitus, and leukoplakia. Other uses include preventing and treating cancer, degenerative diseases of the nervous system, protecting the heart and cardiovascular system (antioxidant effects), and slowing the aging process. Vitamin A is used orally to decrease morbidity associated with malaria in children, and to reduce morbidity and mortality from pneumonia and HIV in children with vitamin A deficiency. Vitamin A is also used orally to decrease the risk of HIV transmission to the fetus during pregnancy and transmission to the newborn during childbirth and early breast-feeding periods.

Topically, vitamin A is used to improve wound healing, reduce wrinkles, and to protect the skin against UV radiation.

Intramuscularly, vitamin A is used for preventing and treating the symptoms of vitamin A deficiency, including xerophthalmia and night blindness; preventing vitamin A deficiency in people with malabsorption; preventing bronchopulmonary dysplasia in premature infants; and preventing stress ulcers in severely ill hospitalized patients.

Safety

LIKELY SAFE ...when used orally or intramuscularly and appropriately. Vitamin A is safe in adults when used in doses less than 10,000 units per day (7135).

POSSIBLY SAFE ...when used intravaginally and appropriately. All-trans-retinoic acid in concentrations up to 0.372% appears to be safe when used topically on the cervix (9199).

POSSIBLY UNSAFE ...when used orally in excessive doses. Prolonged use of excessive doses can cause significant side effects such as hypervitaminosis A. The risk for developing hypervitaminosis A is related to total cumulative dose of vitamin A rather than a specific daily dose (1467,1469). Tell patients to avoid extended use of doses greater than 10,000 units per day (7135).

CHILDREN: LIKELY SAFE ...when used orally or intramuscularly and appropriately. The amount of vitamin A that is safe depends on age. For children up to 3 years of age, doses less than 2000 units per day seem to be safe. For children ages 4 to 8, doses less than 3000 units per day seem to be safe. For children ages 9 to 13, doses less than 5700 units per day seem to be safe. For children 14 to 18, doses of 9300 units per day seem to be safe (7135).
POSSIBLY UNSAFE ...when used orally in excessive doses. For children up to 3 years of age, avoid doses greater than 2000 units per day. For children ages 4 to 8, avoid doses greater than 3000 units per day. For children ages 9 to 13, avoid doses greater than 5700 units per day. For children 14 to 18, avoid doses greater than 9300 units per day (7135). Higher doses of vitamin A supplementation have been associated with increased risk of side effects such as pneumonia and diarrhea (319). Long-term supplementation with low to moderate doses on a regular basis can cause severe, but usually reversible, liver damage (11978).

PREGNANCY AND LACTATION: LIKELY SAFE ...when used orally or intramuscularly and appropriately. Vitamin A is safe during pregnancy and lactation when used in doses less than 10,000 units per day (7135).
POSSIBLY UNSAFE ...when used orally or intramuscularly in excessive doses. Daily intake of greater than 10,000 units can cause fetal malformations (3066,7135). Excessive dietary intake of vitamin A has also been associated with teratogenicity (11978). The first trimester of pregnancy seems to be the critical period for susceptibility to vitamin A-associated birth defects such as craniofacial abnormalities and abnormalities of the central nervous system (7135). Pregnant women should monitor vitamin A intake from all sources. Forms of vitamin A are found in several foods including animal products, primarily liver, some fortified breakfast cereals, and dietary supplements (3066).

Effectiveness

EFFECTIVE

Vitamin A deficiency. Taking vitamin A orally is effective for preventing and improving symptoms of vitamin A deficiency, including xerophthalmia and night blindness. Vitamin A deficiency can occur due to abnormal storage and transport of vitamin A in people with abetalipoproteinemia, protein deficiency, diabetes mellitus, hyperthyroidism, fever, liver disease, and cystic fibrosis (7135).

POSSIBLY EFFECTIVE

Breast cancer. Epidemiological evidence shows an association between high dietary intake of vitamin A and a reduced risk of breast cancer among premenopausal women with a positive family history of breast cancer (1444). However, it's not known if supplemental vitamin A has a similar benefit.

Cataracts. A large-scale population-based study found high dietary intake of vitamin A was associated with a reduced risk of nuclear cataracts (6378).

HIV-related diarrhea. Taking vitamin A in combination with conventional medicines seems to decrease mortality rate from diarrhea in HIV-infected children with vitamin A deficiency (1465).
Malaria. Taking vitamin A orally seems to help decrease symptoms of malaria in children less than 3 years of age living in endemic malaria areas (1464).
Measles. Taking vitamin A orally seems to reduce the complications of measles in children with vitamin A deficiency (7135).
Photoreactive keratectomy. Taking vitamin A orally in combination with vitamin E seems to improve healing after photoreactive keratectomy. High dose (50,000 to 75,000 units) vitamin A in the form of retinol palmitate taken daily with 230 mg vitamin E (alpha-tocopheryl nicotinate) seems to accelerate re-epithelialization, reduce haze formation, and improve visual acuity in patients undergoing laser surgery for myopia (348).
Post-partum complications. Taking vitamin A orally seems to reduce the occurrence of post-partum diarrhea and fever in malnourished women. Retinyl acetate taken weekly before, during, and after pregnancy reduces, but does not eliminate, the occurrence of post partum diarrhea and fever (2581).
Pregnancy-related complications. Taking vitamin A orally seems to reduce pregnancy-related maternal mortality and night blindness in malnourished women. Retinyl acetate taken weekly before, during, and after pregnancy seems to reduce pregnancy-related mortality and night blindness (6153,6154). In one trial, 23,300 IU retinyl acetate reduced pregnancy-related mortality by 40% (6153). Some evidence suggests zinc supplements might potentiate the effects of vitamin A in restoring sight in zinc-deficient pregnant women affected by night-blindness (8630).
Weight loss. Vitamin A 5000 IU per day in combination with calcium 1000 mg per day for two years seems to cause a modest weight reduction (1.04 kg) and body fat reduction (2.10 kg) in women 18 to 31 years of age (8830).

POSSIBLY INEFFECTIVE

Anemia. In developing nations with a high prevalence of anemia, taking 3,000 mcg retinol equivalent of vitamin A in combination with iron and folate orally doesn't seem to improve hemoglobin and erythropoietin concentrations any better than iron and folate alone (9188).
Chemotherapy-induced gastrointestinal (GI) adverse effects. Taking vitamin A orally by children receiving chemotherapy doesn't seem to prevent GI adverse effects. Vitamin A supplements don't seem to have any effect on the incidence or severity of symptoms such as diarrhea and mouth pain (9802).
Fetal and early infant mortality. Taking oral retinyl acetate 23,300 IU weekly before, during, and after pregnancy by malnourished women doesn't seem to reduce fetal and early infant mortality (6152).
HIV transmission. Taking vitamin A orally doesn't seem to decrease the risk of HIV transmission to the fetus during pregnancy, to newborns during delivery, or during the early breast-feeding periods (6376). Preliminary clinical research suggests vitamin A supplementation of pregnant women with HIV infection might increase the risk of HIV transmission to their babies through breast milk (9801).

LIKELY INEFFECTIVE

Head and neck cancer. Taking vitamin A orally doesn't reduce the risk of second primary tumors and tumor reoccurrence in patients with head and neck cancer. Vitamin A does not improve survival or event-free survival (1710).
Pneumonia. Taking vitamin A orally doesn't decrease the severity of pneumonia in children living in developing countries (1466).

INSUFFICIENT RELIABLE EVIDENCE to RATE

Cervical dysplasia. Preliminary clinical research suggests that a specific form of vitamin A, 13-cis-retinoic acid, taken orally might improve cervical dysplasia in women with human papillomavirus (HPV) infection (9198).
Cervical neoplasia. Research suggests that all-trans-retinoic acid, delivered topically with a collagen sponge or cervical cap can reduce mild to moderate cervical neoplasia (9199).
Lung cancer. There is preliminary evidence that taking vitamin A orally might improve survival and reduce the reoccurrence of tumors in people with lung cancer (7875).
Ovarian cancer. Population research suggests that vitamin A consumption doesn't effect the risk of developing ovarian cancer (9193).
More evidence is needed to rate vitamin A for these uses.

Mechanism of Action

Vitamin A is a fat-soluble vitamin. Vitamin A includes a family of molecules containing a 20-carbon structure with various chemical groups at the 15 carbon position. Variations at the 15 carbon position yield different vitamin A forms, including retinol, retinal, retinoic acid, and retinyl ester. These different forms of vitamin A are often collectively referred to as "retinoids." The most potent form of vitamin A, all-trans retinol, is the form of retinol in the diet. It reverses signs and symptoms of vitamin A deficiency and is the standard for vitamin A activity (9191). The vitamin A family also includes provitamin A carotenoids, which are dietary precursors to retinol.
Vitamin A is found in foods in several forms. Retinol, also called preformed vitamin A, is present in esterified form in animal-derived products including eggs, whole milk, butter, fortified margarine, meat, and oily salt-water fish (7135). Animal liver contains the highest amount of dietary retinol. About two-thirds of vitamin A intake comes from dietary retinol (9189). Fresh water fish contain a form of vitamin A called 3-dehydroretinol, but have only 30% to 40% of the biologic activity of retinol (15). About a third of dietary vitamin A comes from plants, which synthesize carotenoids that are converted to vitamin A in the body (7135). Carotenoid pigments (including alpha-, beta-, and

gamma-carotene and cryptoxanthin) are present in grains, oils, green and yellow vegetables, and especially in carrots and fruits (8044). The amount of carotenoids absorbed and converted to vitamin A depends upon the amount of carotenoids ingested, the individual's vitamin A status, and carotenoid body stores. Carotenoids provide approximately 50% of the vitamin A needed in the American diet (8044).

The liver seems to maintain vitamin A concentrations within a relatively narrow range by storage and release of vitamin A (9595). Dietary retinyl esters are hydrolyzed by pancreatic and intestinal enzymes. Unesterified retinol is directly absorbed intestinal cells, mostly by active transport at lower concentrations and by diffusion at higher concentrations (9186,9187). There seem to be differences in the absorption of various forms of vitamin A, but more research is needed to determine the clinical significance (9187). Ingested vitamin A is stored in the body as retinol, predominantly in the liver, but also in the retina, kidneys, lungs, adrenal glands, and intraperitoneal fat (1467). Retinol-binding protein (RBP) is required to transport retinol from the liver and accumulates in the liver during periods of vitamin A deficiency (6377). When vitamin A as retinol is available, it binds to accumulated RBP and is promptly released into the blood when needed (6377). A serum retinol level of 1.05 micromoles/liter or less is considered normal. Serum retinol levels increase with age (9197).

Transport protein levels can be reduced in people with protein malnutrition, causing signs of vitamin A deficiency. In alcoholism, vitamin A deficiency is common since alcohol accelerates the breakdown of retinol through induction of cytochrome isoenzymes and interferes with the conversion of beta-carotene to retinol (1488,7139). Serum retinol levels decrease transiently in acute response to infection, but overall vitamin A stores are not affected (9197).

The majority of vitamin A is excreted in the urine. Lesser amounts are lost through the breath and feces, as inactive metabolites (7135). In vitamin A excess, biliary excretion increases (7135).

Vitamin A is required for vision, growth and bone development, reproduction, cell proliferation and differentiation, immune function, and the integrity of mucosal and epithelial surfaces. All-trans retinol is converted in the body to all-trans retinoic acid by an unknown mechanism. All-trans retinoic acid is the active form of vitamin A in almost all biological processes. Retinoic acid regulates the expression of various genes that encode for structural proteins, such as keratins in the skin; enzymes, such as alcohol dehydrogenase; extracellular matrix proteins, such as the basement membrane protein laminin; and retinol binding proteins and receptors (7135,9189). Vitamin A acts as a cofactor in mucopolysaccharide synthesis, cholesterol synthesis, hydroxysteroid metabolism, and glycoprotein glycosylation (15). Vitamin A seems to have the opposite effect of steroids on wound healing. It stimulates the expression of transforming growth factor-beta (TGF-beta) and insulin-like growth factor (IGF), and increases collagen production, resulting in improved wound healing (320). Vitamin A is also important for immune function. Retinoic acid is required in maintaining sufficient levels of natural killer cells, and preliminary evidence suggests that retinoic acid might increase the production of cytokines, such as interleukin 1 (IL-1). Additionally, B lymphocyte growth, differentiation, and activation are dependent on retinol (7135). Retinol also seems to affect pulmonary function. Higher retinol levels have been associated with higher forced expiratory volume (FEV) and forced vital capacity (FVC) (9195).

Vitamin A is important for the normal utilization of iron and prevention of anemia. Deficiency of vitamin A impairs maturation of hematopoietic cells in the bone marrow. Vitamin A may facilitate mobilization of body stores of iron. Preliminary evidence also indicates that vitamin A and beta-carotene enhance non-heme iron absorption from iron-fortified wheat and corn flour, and rice. It's suggested that these vitamins bind to iron in the gut, improving its solubility and preventing binding by dietary polyphenols and phytate, which reduce iron absorption. In addition, vitamin A appears to be involved with production of erythropoietin by the liver and kidney (9518,9569,9586,).

In embryonic development, vitamin A plays an important role in neural development, and is also involved in the development of the limbs, lung, heart, eyes, and ears (7135,11978). Vitamin A deficiency seems to adversely affect fetal immune status. Maternal-fetal transmission of HIV is higher in the presence of low vitamin A status. However, excessive vitamin A is teratogenic, causing central nervous system, craniofacial, cardiovascular, and thymus malformations (11978).

In the retina, retinol is converted to cis-retinal, which combines with opsin to form rhodopsin, the visual pigment. Retinal is required by the eye for the transduction of light into the neural signals that produce vision. The most specific indicator of vitamin A deficiency is xerophthalmia, which is initially manifested by night blindness that progresses to complete visual loss if untreated. Vitamin A deficiency is also associated with follicular hyperkeratosis and increased risk of infectious morbidity and mortality (7135). Some research has linked retinol deficiency to development of cervical neoplasms in women with human immunodeficiency virus (HIV) infection (9800).

In vitro studies suggest retinoids might help prevent cancer by inducing tumor suppressor genes known as retinoic acid receptors (RAR). Tumor suppressor gene RAR-beta2 is absent in many malignant tumor cells, possibly due to methylation of the gene. When demethylated, the RAR-beta2 gene can be induced by retinoic acid to function and suppress growth of cancer cells (6380,6381). However, there is evidence that some forms of retinoic acid, such as all-trans-retinoic acid, do not use the RAR receptor to inhibit cancer growth and may use other mechanisms and pathways to inhibit growth (8045). There is also evidence that the inhibitory effect on cancer cell growth by certain statin drugs with a closed ring structure, such as mevastatin and lovastatin (Mevacor), may be enhanced when used with 13-cis retinoic acid (8046). Ethanol may compete with retinol for alcohol dehydrogenase and inhibit retinoic acid synthesis, interfering with normal retinoid signaling of RAR genes and cause malignant transformation of hepatic cells (6377). Preliminary evidence suggests that all-trans-retinoic acid applied topically might help protect the skin against UV radiation damage. UV radiation seems to cause a functional vitamin A deficiency in the skin (1468).

Based on cell culture and animal studies, it's been suggested that vitamin E affects the activity of vitamin A. These include preventing oxidation in the gut and increasing absorption, enhancing utilization, promoting liver storage, protecting against cell damage caused by high vitamin A levels, and reducing some of the symptoms of hypervitaminosis A (10545,10557,10558,10560). Supportive data in humans is very limited. There is some preliminary evidence that vitamin E increases the effects of vitamin A in the treatment of some skin conditions (10562). Small studies have reported increased vitamin A absorption and excretion, and both increases and decreases in vitamin A levels when vitamin E is taken concurrently (10559,10561,10563,10564). Despite the lack of good evidence of efficacy or necessity, vitamin E has been added to the intermittent, high doses of vitamin A sometimes used to treat deficiency in developing countries (10558,10560). Further research is needed to determine whether vitamin E affects the activity of vitamin A in humans.

Vitamin A toxicity can occur when vitamin A intake exceeds the storage capacity of the liver or when liver function is compromised. Vitamin A is released into the circulation as retinyl esters rather than bound to retinol-binding protein (RBP). The retinyl esters expose target tissues to free retinol, resulting in the damaging effects of hypervitaminosis A (9196).

Both human and animal studies suggest excessive vitamin A intake can have a negative effect on bone. It seems to suppress osteoblast activity, stimulate osteoclast formation, and antagonize the ability of vitamin D to maintain normal serum calcium levels (7712,9190,9191,9192). Some evidence suggests that older people can't metabolize vitamin A as well younger people, which could increase the risk of osteoporosis (9191).

Adverse Reactions

Orally, vitamin A is generally well tolerated at doses below the Tolerable Upper Intake Level (UL). For adults, the UL is 3,000 mcg per day (10,000 units). Acute toxicity following doses of 15,000 mcg (50,000 units) are characterized by nausea, vomiting, headache, increased cerebrospinal fluid pressure, vertigo, blurred vision, muscular incoordination, and bulging fontanelle in infants. These are usually transient effects involving single or short-term large doses (7135). Toxicity from a single ingestion of a large dose of vitamin A is more common in young children than adults (15). In children, approximately 25,000 units/kg can cause irritability, drowsiness, dizziness, delirium, coma, vomiting, diarrhea, increased intracranial pressure with bulging fontanelles in infants, headache, swelling of the optic disk, bulging eyeballs, and visual disturbances. Skin redness and generalized peeling of the skin occur a few days later and may last for several weeks (15).

Chronic toxicity is usually associated with ingestion of large doses greater than or equal to 30,000 mcg (100,000 units) for months or years. The liver is the main storage site and the primary target of vitamin A toxicity. Hepatotoxicity ranges from reversibly elevated liver enzymes, alanine aminotransferase (ALT, formerly SGPT) and aspartate aminotransferase (AST, formerly SGOT), to widespread fibrosis and cirrhosis and death (6377,7135). Chronic use of large amounts of vitamin A causes symptoms of vitamin A toxicity including fatigue, malaise, lethargy, irritability, psychiatric changes mimicking severe depression or schizophrenic disorder, anorexia, abdominal discomfort, nausea and vomiting, mild fever, and excessive sweating (7135). Other symptoms include dry skin and lips; cracking, scaling, and itchy skin; skin redness; hyperpigmentation; and massive skin peeling. Hypervitaminosis A can cause brittle nails, cheilitis, gingivitis, hair loss, reduced menstrual flow, spider angiomas, anemia, leukopenia, leukocytosis, and thrombocytopenia (15). Slow growth, premature epiphyseal closure, painful hyperostosis of the long bones, osteosclerosis, joint pain, muscle pain, hypercalcemia, and hypercalciuria have also been reported (15). Sometimes children fail to gain weight normally. Adults may lose weight (15). There is also some evidence that vitamin A supplementation might increase the risk of pneumonia and diarrhea in children. Although vitamin A can prevent diarrhea and reduce mortality in malnourished children, doses as low as 10,000 units weekly for 40 weeks have been associated with diarrhea and pneumonia in well-nourished children (319). Discourage vitamin A supplementation in healthy, well-nourished children.

Vitamin A can increase the risk for osteoporosis. Chronic, high intake of vitamin A 10,000 IU or more per day seems to increase the risk of osteoporosis and hip fracture in postmenopausal women (7712,7713) and overall risk of fracture in middle-aged men (9190). High serum retinol levels also increase the risk of fracture in men. Men with high serum retinol levels are seven times more likely to fracture a hip than men with lower serum retinol levels (9190). Vitamin A damage to bone can occur subclinically, without signs or symptoms of hypervitaminosis A. Some researchers are concerned that consumption of vitamin A fortified foods such as margarine and low-fat dairy products in addition to in addition to vitamin A or multivitamin supplements might cause excessive serum retinol levels. Older people have higher levels of vitamin A and might be at increased risk for vitamin A induced osteoporosis. Recommendations for vitamin A intake are likely to be reassessed. For now, tell patients who eat a lot of low-fat dairy products, fruits, and vegetables that they don't need a vitamin A supplement (7712,9189,9190,9191,9192). Population research suggests high vitamin A intake might increase the risk of gastric carcinoma (9194).

Intravaginally, all-trans retinoic acid can cause vaginal discharge, itching, irritation, and burning (9199).

Interactions with Herbs & Other Dietary Supplements

IRON: Vitamin A may improve hemoglobin levels in people with anemia and low serum retinol levels. It's unlikely that vitamin A supplements would have significant effects on iron status in people without vitamin A deficiency (9518,9569,9586).

Interactions with Drugs

HEPATOTOXIC DRUGS: Excessive doses of vitamin A can cause hepatotoxicity ranging from elevated liver enzymes to liver failure (7135). Taking high doses of vitamin A in combination with other potentially hepatotoxic drugs might increase the risk of liver disease. Advise patients against combining high doses of vitamin A with other hepatotoxic drugs. Some drugs that can adversely affect the liver include acetaminophen (Tylenol), amiodarone (Cordarone), carbamazepine (Tegretol), isoniazid (INH), methotrexate (Rheumatrex), methyldopa (Aldomet), and many others.
RETINOIDS: These vitamin A derivatives could have additive toxic effects with vitamin A supplements (3046). Advise patients taking retinoids to avoid vitamin A supplements. Some of these retinoids include acitretin (Soriatane), bexarotene (Targretin), etretinate (Tegison), and isotretinoin (Accutane), tretinoin (Retin-A, Renova), and tazarotene (Avage).
TETRACYCLINE ANTIBIOTICS: Benign intracranial hypertension (pseudotumor cerebri) can occur with tetracyclines and with vitamin A intoxication (either an acute overdose, or chronic accumulation from doses of 40,000 units/day or more). Case reports suggest that taking tetracyclines and vitamin A concurrently can increase the risk of this condition (10545,10546,10547). Avoid high doses of vitamin A in people taking tetracyclines chronically. Tetracyclines include demeclocycline (Declomycin), minocycline (Minocin), and tetracycline (Achromycin).
WARFARIN (Coumadin): Vitamin A toxicity is associated with hemorrhage and hypoprothrombinemia, possibly due to vitamin K antagonism (505). High doses of vitamin A could increase the risk of bleeding with warfarin. Advise patients taking warfarin to avoid doses of vitamin A above the Tolerable Upper Intake Level of 10,000 units/day for adults.

Drug Influences on Nutrient Levels and Depletion

SOME DRUGS CAN AFFECT VITAMIN A LEVELS:
BILE ACID SEQUESTRANTS: By reducing absorption of dietary fats, cholestyramine (Questran) and colestipol (Colestid) may also reduce absorption of fat-soluble vitamins such as vitamin A. Some studies have reported a fall in serum vitamin A levels, but they rarely fall below the normal range with therapy of up to 2 years' duration (4455,4457,4460). Since some of the vitamin A in plasma is carried on lipids, part of this fall in plasma vitamin A levels may be due to decreased plasma lipid levels (4457,4460). Other studies have reported no change in plasma vitamin A levels with colestipol, up to 30 grams/day for 6 months, or cholestyramine 12 to 24 grams/day for up to 10 years (4461,10566,10567,10568,10569). Routine vitamin A supplements aren't necessary in people taking bile acid sequestrants, but check vitamin A levels in people taking high doses for more than 2 years.
ESTROGENS, ORAL CONTRACEPTIVES: Women taking oral contraceptives have higher plasma levels of vitamin A than non-users, but may have reduced liver stores of the vitamin. It's thought that estrogens stimulate production of retinol binding protein which carries vitamin A in the blood, and may pull more vitamin A out of storage sites such as the liver (9373,9505,10523,10548). Supplementation with up to 5000 IU/day in women taking oral contraceptives doesn't significantly affect plasma vitamin A levels, but might maintain liver stores (9373,9505,10548). There isn't enough data to recommend routine use of vitamin A supplements.
MINERAL OIL: Mineral oil has been reported to reduce absorption of all fat-soluble vitamins (4454,4495). However, there was no change in serum vitamin A levels in children who used mineral oil for up to four months (4496). Mineral oil should not be used on a regular basis due to its side effects. Its effect on vitamin A levels with occasional use is unlikely to be clinically significant.
NEOMYCIN: Neomycin (Mycifradin, Neo-Fradin) can bind and precipitate fatty acids and bile acids in the gut, reducing fat absorption. There is limited evidence that this can affect fat-soluble vitamin absorption. Single doses of neomycin reduced absorption of large doses (300,000 units) of vitamin A given concurrently (10565). However, there was no change in serum vitamin A levels in adults who took neomycin 1 to 2 grams/day for 18 weeks for treatment of hyperlipoproteinemia (10566). It's unlikely that neomycin, or the other oral aminoglycosides such as kanamycin (Kantrex), and paromomycin (Humatin), will cause clinically significant vitamin A depletion.
ORLISTAT (Xenical): Orlistat can decrease absorption of fat soluble vitamins including vitamin A, leading to low plasma levels in some patients (1730). Several studies suggest that vitamin A is not affected as much by orlistat as some other fat-soluble vitamins (1727,9595,10570,10571). However, the manufacturer of orlistat recommends that all patients take a multivitamin supplement containing all the fat soluble vitamins, separating the dosing time by at least 2 hours from orlistat (1730).

Interactions with Foods

FAT: Dietary fat increases vitamin A absorption (7135).

Interactions with Lab Tests

BILIRUBIN: Vitamin A can cause false increase in bilirubin test results using Ehrlich's reagent (15).
CHOLESTEROL: There are unsubstantiated reports that vitamin A can produce false increases in serum cholesterol test results measured by the Zlatkis-Zak reaction (15).

Interactions with Diseases or Conditions

ALCOHOLISM: Chronic alcohol ingestion might potentiate the adverse effects of vitamin A, particularly hepatotoxicity (7135,7139). There is some evidence that chronic and excessive ethanol intake induces cytochrome P450

2E1 (CYP2E1) metabolism of vitamin A, which can increase production of hepatotoxic and carcinogenic vitamin A metabolites (1488,7135,7139).
ANEMIA: Anemia may not be adequately treated by iron supplements alone in patients with vitamin A deficiency. Vitamin A deficiency impairs iron mobilization from body stores. Combining vitamin A with iron supplementation in anemic patients with concurrent vitamin A deficiency seems to improve hemoglobin concentrations better than iron alone (7135).
FAT MALABSORPTION DISORDERS: Oral vitamin A absorption is decreased in conditions where fat absorption is reduced, such as celiac disease, short gut syndrome, obstructive jaundice, cystic fibrosis, pancreatic disease, and cirrhosis of the liver (7135). Water-miscible oral vitamin A preparations should be used in patients with fat malabsorption disorders.
HYPERLIPIDEMIA: Type V hyperlipoproteinemia increases risk of vitamin A hypervitaminosis (7135).
INTESTINAL INFECTIONS AND INFESTATIONS: Ascariasis, giardiasis, hookworm, salmonellosis, schistosomiasis, and other intestinal infections and infestations can reduce oral vitamin A absorption (7135).
LIVER DISEASE: Patients with liver disease can have an increased risk of hypervitaminosis and hepatotoxicity, especially if they take excessive doses of vitamin A (7135).
MALNUTRITION: In severe protein energy malnutrition (marasmus and kwashiorkor), there is reduced release of retinol from the liver. Until nutrition status is normalized, there is increased risk of vitamin A hypervitaminosis (7135).
ZINC DEFICIENCY: Zinc is required in hepatic synthesis of retinol binding protein. Without adequate zinc, symptoms of vitamin A deficiency can appear, despite vitamin A supplementation (8630). Zinc in combination with vitamin A seems to improve measures of vitamin A adequacy in undernourished children better than vitamin A or zinc alone (8636).

Dosage and Administration

ORAL: Treatment of deficiency in adults without corneal changes is 10,000 to 25,000 units daily until clinical improvement occurs, usually 1-2 weeks. Individuals with fat malabsorption, low protein intake, or hepatic or pancreatic disease might benefit from water-miscible oral preparations. If oral absorption is still insufficient, parenteral administration may be necessary. For prevention of nuclear cataracts, 10,000 units per day has been used (6378). For accelerating re-epithelialization following photoreactive keratectomy, vitamin A (retinol palmitate) 25,000 units and 230 mg vitamin E (alpha-tocopheryl nicotinate) have been used 3 times daily for 30 days, followed by twice daily for 2 months (348). Adequate Intake (AI) levels of vitamin A for infants have been established: birth to 6 months, 400 mcg/day (1300 units); 7 to 12 months, 500 mcg/day (1700 units). Recommended Dietary Allowance (RDA) levels for children and adults have been established: children 1 to 3 years, 300 mcg/day (1000 units); 4 to 8 years, 400 mcg/day (1300 units); 9 to 13 years, 600 mcg/day (2000 units); men 14 years and older, 900 mcg/day (3000 units); women 14 years and older, 700 mcg/day (2300 units); pregnancy 14 to 18 years, 750 mcg/day (2500 units); 19 years and older, 770 mcg/day (2600 units); lactation 14 to 18 years, 1200 mcg/day (4000 units); 19 years and older 1300 mcg/day (4300 units) (7135). Tolerable Upper Intake Levels (UL) for vitamin A have also been established. The UL is the highest level of intake that is likely to pose no risk of adverse effects. The ULs for vitamin A are for preformed vitamin A (retinol) and do not include provitamin A carotenoids: infants and children from birth to 3 years, 600 mcg/day (2000 units); children 4 to 8 years, 900 mcg/day (3000 units); 9 to 13 years 1700 mcg/day (6000 units); 14 to 18 years (including pregnancy and lactation) 2800 mcg/day (9000 units); adults age 19 and older (including pregnancy and lactation) 3000 mcg/day (10,000 units). Vitamin A dosage is most commonly expressed in units, but dosage in micrograms is sometimes used. One mcg of vitamin A equals 3.33 units of vitamin A. Vitamin A recommendations are for retinol, or preformed vitamin A. Formerly, vitamin A RDA recommendations were expressed as retinol equivalents (RE) to account for the differences in bioconversion of the various vitamin A forms to retinol. Retinol activity equivalents (RAE) are now used: 1 mcg of retinol equals 1 RAE which equals 2 mcg supplemental beta-carotene, 12 mcg of dietary beta-carotene, and 24 mcg dietary alpha-carotene or beta-cryptoxanthin. Either preformed vitamin A from animal products (retinol) or provitamin A carotenoids from plant products is an acceptable vitamin A source, although provitamin A carotenoids must be consumed in larger quantities (7135). Consumption of 5 servings of fruits and vegetables per day supplies 5 to 6 mg per day of provitamin A carotenoids, which provides about 50-65% of the adult RDA for vitamin A (7135).

VITAMIN B12

Also Known As

B-12, B Complex, B Complex Vitamin, Bedumil, Cobalamin, Cobalamins, Cobamin, Cyanocobalamin, Cyanocobalaminum, Cycobemin, Hydroxocobalamin, Hydroxocobalaminum, Hydroxocobemine, Idrossocobalamina, Methylcobalamin, Vitadurin, Vitamin B-12.
CAUTION: See separate listing for Dibencozide.

Scientific Names

Vitamin B12; Cyanocobalamin; Hydroxocobalamin; Methylcobalamin.

People Use This For

Orally, vitamin B12 is used for treating pernicious anemia and preventing and treating vitamin B12 deficiency. It is also used orally for treating primary hyperhomocysteinemia, heart disease, male infertility, diabetes, memory loss, circadian rhythm sleep disorders, Alzheimer's disease, depression, psychiatric disorders, osteoporosis, tendonitis, immunosuppression, AIDS, inflammatory bowel disease, asthma, allergies, vitiligo, and seborrheic dermatitis. It is also used orally for thyrotoxicosis, amyotrophic lateral sclerosis (Lou Gehrig's disease), multiple sclerosis, periodontal disease, tinnitus, hemorrhage, malignancy, and liver and kidney disease. Vitamin B12 is also used orally for aging, improving concentration, mood elevation, boosting energy, maintaining fertility, and protection against the toxins and allergens from tobacco smoke.

Topically, a vitamin B12 nasal gel is applied for pernicious anemia and preventing and treating vitamin B12 deficiency.

Parenterally, vitamin B12 is used for pernicious anemia and preventing and treating vitamin B12 deficiency. It is also used parenterally for tremor associated with shaky-leg syndrome or orthostatic tremor. Vitamin B12 is also used parenterally to treat tiredness or fatigue, chronic fatigue syndrome, thyrotoxicosis, hemorrhage, malignancy, and liver and kidney disease.

Safety

LIKELY SAFE ...when used orally, intravenously, or intranasally and appropriately. Vitamin B12 is generally considered safe, even in large doses (15).

PREGNANCY: LIKELY SAFE ...when used orally in amounts that do not exceed the recommended dietary allowance (RDA). The RDA for vitamin B12 in pregnant women is 2.6 mcg per day (6243). There is insufficient reliable information available about the safety of larger amounts of vitamin B12 during pregnancy.

LACTATION: LIKELY SAFE ...when used orally in amounts that do not exceed the recommended dietary allowance (RDA). The RDA of vitamin B12 during lactation is 2.8 mcg per day (6243). There is insufficient reliable information available about the safety of larger amounts of vitamin B12 while nursing.

Effectiveness

EFFECTIVE

Imerslund-Grasbeck disease. Administering vitamin B12 intramuscularly is effective for treating familial selective vitamin B12 malabsorption (Imerslund-Grasbeck disease) (15).

Pernicious anemia. Administering vitamin B12 intramuscularly, intranasally, or orally is effective for treating pernicious anemia. Both the cyanocobalamin and hydroxocobalamin forms of vitamin B12 are used intramuscularly. Cyanocobalamin is used for intranasal administration (15). Oral vitamin B12 is as effective as intramuscular administration (2900,2902,2909,2910,3024). However, oral preparations should not be used in patients with diarrhea or vomiting, severe neurologic involvement, nor in patients likely to be nonadherent (2900).

Vitamin B12 deficiency. Administering vitamin B12 orally, intramuscularly, or intranasally is effective for preventing and treating dietary vitamin B12 deficiency. People at risk for vitamin B12 deficiency include strict vegetarians and people with increased vitamin B12 requirements associated with pregnancy, thyrotoxicosis, hemolytic anemia, hemorrhage, malignancy, and hepatic and renal disease. Moderate consumption of animal products may not be sufficient to restore and maintain vitamin B12 levels in adolescents (age 9-15 years) who have eaten a strict vegetarian diet with inadequate intake of vitamin B12 from infancy to six years of age. A higher dietary intake of vitamin B12 or supplements is usually needed in order to restore and maintain optimal vitamin B12 levels in these adolescents (10125). Vitamin B12 is used intramuscularly for vitamin B12 deficiency with hyperhomocysteinemia in adult vegetarians. There is some evidence a single injection of intramuscular cyanocobalamin (1000 mcg) can decrease homocysteine levels up to 36% and normalize serum vitamin B12 levels in adult vegetarians (9512). Vitamin B12 deficiency is especially common in older adults (2915,2919,9335). Vitamin B12 in foods such as milk and fortified bread is approximately 55-60% absorbed by people over 60 years of age (10124). Older adults who take oral vitamin B12 supplements in doses of 25 to 37.5 mcg/day are more likely to have normal vitamin B12 levels than those who don't take supplements (9335). However, some older adults with vitamin B12 deficiency might require daily supplementation of vitamin B12 in doses of 50-100 mcg/day in order to restore levels to normal (10126). Oral therapy is as effective as intramuscular administration, even in patients with malabsorption disorders (2900,2901,2911,2915,9335). However, oral preparations should not be used in patients with diarrhea, vomiting, severe neurologic involvement, nor in patients likely to be nonadherent (2900).

LIKELY EFFECTIVE

Hyperhomocysteinemia. Taking vitamin B12 orally in combination with folic acid, and sometimes with pyridoxine (vitamin B6), can reduce serum concentrations of homocysteine. Folic acid 0.5 to 5 mg/day lowers fasting homocysteine levels by an average of 25% (9400,9405,9408,9409,9410). Adding vitamin B12 (mean dose, 0.5 mg/day) produces an additional decrease in homocysteine levels of about 7% on average (6883,9400,9401,9405,9409), but probably only in people with vitamin B12 deficiency (2147,3047). Vitamin B12 in combination with folic acid and other vitamins also seems to significantly reduce homocysteine levels in patients with end-stage renal disease (ESRD) (1489,6883,6884,7289,7881,9414,9415,9416). A supplement containing vitamin B12 500 mcg with folic acid 2.5 mg and pyridoxine 25 mg, taken daily, may reduce the increase in homocysteine concentrations associated with nitrous oxide general anesthesia (9481). Some researchers recommend routine use of vitamin B12 in homocysteine-lowering regimens to avoid the risk of neuropathy in people with undetected vitamin B12 deficiency (9405). There is also preliminary evidence that that daily intake of 4.2-6.0 mcg of vitamin B12 in combination with 700 mcg of folic acid and 4.2-6.0 mg of pyridoxine (vitamin B6) might lower homocysteine levels in patients with sickle cell disease (SCD), but it is unknown if this effect will reduce endothelial damage in these patients (9324). Using vitamin B12 alone has a limited effect on homocysteine levels, and probably only in those people with vitamin B12 deficiency (2149,9410,9512). Hyperhomocysteinemia is a risk factor for coronary, cerebral, and peripheral atherosclerosis; recurrent thromboembolism; deep vein thrombosis; myocardial infarction; and ischemic stroke (1899,2147,3047,3323,9402,9405,9408,9409). But elevated homocysteine levels may be a marker instead of a cause of vascular disease (11387,11388). A 5 micromole increase in plasma homocysteine increases the risk of cerebrovascular disease by 50%, and the risk of coronary heart disease by 60% in men and 80% in women (9407,9411). However, it's not clear if lowering homocysteine levels results in reduced cardiovascular morbidity and mortality (1489,6883,6884,7229,9308,9400,9405,9409). Folic acid, pyridoxine (vitamin B6), and vitamin B12 supplementation can reduce total homocysteine from 13.4 to 11.0 micromoles per liter. However, this reduction doesn't seem to help with secondary prevention of death or cardiovascular events such as stroke or myocardial infarction in people with prior stroke (11387). More evidence is needed to fully explain the association of total homocysteine levels with vascular risk. Until definitive data are available, the current recommendation is screening of 40-year-old men and 50-year-old women for hyperhomocysteinemia. For patients with homocysteine levels greater than 11 micromoles/L, supplement with folic acid and vitamin B12 (9308).

POSSIBLY INEFFECTIVE

Circadian rhythm sleep disorders. Taking vitamin B12 orally, in methylcobalamin form, doesn't seem to be effective for treating delayed sleep phase syndrome. Methylcobalamin 0.5 to 1 mg three times daily, with or without bright light therapy, doesn't seem to help people with primary circadian rhythm sleep disorders (1344,1345,1346,1347,1348).

Stroke. Taking vitamin B12 orally doesn't seem to be useful for preventing stroke recurrence. In people with a history of stroke, neither high dose vitamin B12 combinations containing 25 mg of pyridoxine, 0.4 mg of vitamin B12, and 2.5 mg of folic acid nor low dose combinations containing 200 mcg of pyridoxine, 6 mcg of vitamin B12, and 20 mcg of folic acid seem to affect risk of recurring stroke (11387).

INSUFFICIENT RELIABLE EVIDENCE to RATE

Angioplasty. There are conflicting findings about the benefits of taking folic acid plus vitamin B6 and vitamin B12 following angioplasty. Some evidence suggests that folic acid 1 mg plus vitamin B12 400 mcg and pyridoxine 10 mg daily can decrease the rate of restenosis in patients treated with balloon angioplasty (8009,9412). But this combination does not seem to be as effective for reducing restenosis in patients after coronary stenting (8009). An intravenous loading dose of folic acid, vitamin B6, and vitamin B12 followed by oral administration of folic acid 1.2 m plus vitamin B6 48 mg and vitamin B12 60 mcg taken daily after coronary stenting also does not seem to reduce restenosis and might actually increase restenosis (12150,12151). Due to the lack of evidence of benefit and potential for harm, this combination of vitamins should not be recommended for patients receiving coronary stents (12151).

Breast cancer. Higher dietary folate intake is associated with a reduced risk of breast cancer. The risk may even be further reduced in women who also consume high amounts of dietary vitamin B12 in combination with dietary pyridoxine and methionine. However, there is no evidence that dietary vitamin B12 alone reduces the risk of breast cancer (9328).

Fatigue. There is some evidence intramuscular injections of vitamin B12 5 mg given twice per week might improve the general well being and happiness of patients complaining of tiredness or fatigue (10127).

Hypertriglyceridemia. Some evidence suggests that 7.5 mcg of vitamin B12 in combination with 5 grams of fish oil might be superior to fish oil alone when used daily to reduce total serum cholesterol and triglycerides. This suggests vitamin B12 might have an independent effect in lowering serum cholesterol and triglycerides, but further investigation is needed to confirm this effect (8694).

Lung cancer. Preliminary evidence suggests that there is no relationship between vitamin B12 status and lung cancer (9454).

Shaky leg syndrome. There are some preliminary clinical reports that the cyanocobalamin form of vitamin B12 can help relieve tremor associated with shaky-leg syndrome (6358).

More evidence is needed to rate vitamin B12 for these uses.

Mechanism of Action

Vitamin B12 is a naturally occurring B complex vitamin that is formed by microorganisms. It is also found in some foods from animal origin (e.g., meat, fish, shellfish, liver) in coenzyme form, mainly adenosylcobalamin and methylcobalamin. Cyanocobalamin and hydroxocobalamin are synthetic forms of vitamin B12.

Vitamin B12 is required for nucleoprotein and myelin synthesis, cell reproduction, normal growth, and normal erythropoiesis. Synthetic vitamin B12 can be converted to coenzyme B12, which is essential for the conversion of methylmalonate to succinate, and the synthesis of methionine from homocysteine (15,9320). Vitamin B12 is involved in maintaining sulfhydryl groups in the reduced form required by enzymes involved in fat and carbohydrate metabolism and protein synthesis. Vitamin B12 is essential for folate utilization, and its absence results in a functional folate deficiency (15).

Vitamin B12 deficiency can take months to years to become symptomatic due to large body stores. Normal serum vitamin B12 levels range between 200-900 pg/mL. Serum concentrations less than 200 pg/mL indicate deficiency, and concentrations less than 100 pg/mL usually result in megaloblastic anemia or neurologic damage (15). Vitamin B12 deficiency results in megaloblastic anemia, gastrointestinal lesions, and neurologic damage, beginning with an inability to produce myelin and progressing to degeneration of the axon and nerve head (15). Neurologic symptoms caused by vitamin B12 deficiency can include neuropsychiatric disorders such as depression (6357), paresthesias, ataxia, memory loss, weakness, and personality and mood changes without anemia (1484,1485,3235,5646). Some neurologic symptoms and elevated homocysteine levels can occur without any signs of B12 deficiency anemia (1484,1485,3235). Vitamin B12 deficiency is associated with impaired cognitive performance in adolescents (aged 10-16 years) who have been fed a strict vegetarian diet from infancy to 6 years of age. Consequences of low vitamin B12 intake during childhood and its effect on cognitive functioning in adulthood are unknown (10125). Elevated methylmalonate or methylmalonic acid (MMA) levels occur early in vitamin B12 deficiency, and may precede other symptoms (1484,1485,5646). In combination with homocysteine levels, MMA levels can be used to diagnose vitamin B12 deficiency (5646).

Vitamin B12 is absorbed via an active transport mechanism in the terminal ileum. This requires the glycoprotein, intrinsic factor, which is produced by the stomach. At normal gastric pH, vitamin B12 is cleaved from proteins in food. It then binds to intrinsic factor and is absorbed by ileal transport. Absorption can be reduced by increased gastric pH such as in atrophic gastritis, use of acid-suppressing drugs, or partial gastrectomy. Reduced absorption also occurs with loss of intrinsic factor in conditions such as pernicious anemia (an autoimmune disorder in which the ability to produce intrinsic factor is lost) and total gastrectomy. Intramuscular administration is often used to avoid these absorption problems. However, there is also a lesser-known transport system for vitamin B12 that does not rely on either intrinsic factor or the terminal ileum. Absorption is more efficient by the intrinsic factor route (about 60%), but 1% of an oral dose of vitamin B12 can be absorbed without intrinsic factor or stomach acid. Large oral doses (300 to 1000 mcg) can be sufficiently absorbed to treat pernicious anemia and malabsorption from food (2900,2901,2909,9518). The risk for vitamin B12 deficiency is higher with increased age, male gender, and in people of Caucasian and Latin American descent. Deficiency in vitamin B12 results from insufficient intake, malabsorption from food, and other medical conditions (1484,1485). However, body stores of vitamin B12 are large, and it is widely available in food. Vitamin B12 deficiency is almost always caused by a disorder of absorption (9518).

Deficiency of vitamin B12 can be masked by folic acid, particularly in large doses. Folate will improve vitamin B12 associated anemia, but it will allow the neurologic abnormalities to progress. There is some concern that food fortified with folic acid can cause under-recognition of vitamin B12 deficiency, particularly in the elderly (5646).

Vitamin B12 is required in one of the pathways for homocysteine metabolism. Remethylation of homocysteine to methionine requires folate and the methylcobalamin form of vitamin B12 as a cofactor (3047,9407,9409). Some evidence suggests elevated homocysteine levels might cause vascular endothelial cell damage, impaired endothelium-dependent vasodilation due to reduced nitric oxide activity, increased oxidation and arterial deposition of low-density lipoproteins (LDL), increased platelet adhesiveness, and activation of the clotting cascade (2147,3047,9403,9408). Vitamin B12 supplements have a small additive effect to folic acid in lowering fasting homocysteine levels, but probably only in people with vitamin B12 deficiency (2147,3047). Elevated homocysteine concentrations are possibly associated with other conditions such as decreased cognitive function, impaired memory, Alzheimer's disease, and vascular dementia (5646,9330,9331).

Low vitamin B12 levels are also associated with other conditions such as hearing loss in elderly women (1482) and possibly chronic fatigue syndrome (6082). Some researchers think that vitamin B12 supplements could help symptoms of chronic fatigue syndrome by correcting red blood cell abnormalities and improving oxygen delivery to tissues (6082). The methylcobalamin form of vitamin B12 might also influence melatonin levels. Methylcobalamin seems to improve alertness and reduce sleep time in humans with normal sleep patterns, possibly due to affects on melatonin (1349).

Adverse Reactions

Orally and intramuscularly, vitamin B12 does not usually cause adverse effects, even in large doses (6243). In some people, vitamin B12 can cause diarrhea, peripheral vascular thrombosis, itching, transitory exanthema, urticaria, feelings of swelling of the entire body, and anaphylaxis, possibly due to impurities in vitamin B12 preparations. Treatment of vitamin B12 deficiency can unmask polycythemia vera, which is an increase in blood volume and the number of red blood cells (15).

Vitamin B12 (20 micrograms/day) and pyridoxine (80 mg/day) may cause rosacea fulminans, characterized by intense erythema with nodules, papules, and pustules. Symptoms may persist for up to 4 months after the supplement is stopped, and may require treatment with systemic corticosteroids and topical therapy (10998).

Interactions with Herbs & Other Dietary Supplements

FOLIC ACID: Folic acid, particularly in large doses, can mask vitamin B12 deficiency (5646). In vitamin B12 deficiency, folic acid can produce hematologic improvement in megaloblastic anemia, while allowing potentially irreversible neurological damage to progress. Vitamin B12 status should be determined before folic acid is given as monotherapy (2677,3092,5646).

POTASSIUM: Potassium supplements can reduce absorption of vitamin B12 in some people (4511,4512). This might be due to acidification of the ileal contents, which reduces the activity of intrinsic factor (4512). This effect has been reported with potassium chloride and, to a lesser extent, with potassium citrate (10501). Potassium might contribute to vitamin B12 deficiency in some people with other risk factors, but routine supplements aren't necessary.

VITAMIN C: Preliminary evidence suggests that vitamin C supplements can destroy dietary vitamin B12. However, other components of food, such as iron and nitrates, might counteract this effect (9511). It isn't clear whether this interaction is clinically significant, and it can likely be avoided if vitamin C supplements are taken at least 2 hours after meals.

Interactions with Drugs

CHLORAMPHENICOL: Limited case reports suggest that chloramphenicol can delay or interrupt the reticulocyte response to supplemental vitamin B12 in some patients (3072). Monitor blood counts closely if this combination can't be avoided.

Drug Influences on Nutrient Levels and Depletion

SOME DRUGS CAN AFFECT VITAMIN B12 LEVELS:

AMINOSALICYLIC ACID (para-aminosalicylic acid, PAS, Paser): Aminosalicylic acid can reduce oral vitamin B12 absorption, possibly by as much as 55%, as part of a general malabsorption syndrome (9574). Megaloblastic changes, and occasional cases of symptomatic anemia have occurred, usually after doses of 8 to 12 grams/day for several months (4558,9395,9397). Monitor vitamin B12 levels in people taking aminosalicylic acid for more than one month.

ANTIBIOTICS: Disruption of the normal gastrointestinal (GI) flora may interrupt enterohepatic recirculation of vitamin B12 and increase fecal excretion (4436). Vitamin B12 is also synthesized by the GI flora, but mainly in the colon where absorption is poor. The majority of bacterially synthesized vitamin B12 is therefore excreted in the feces and does not significantly contribute to the body's store of vitamin B12 (4437,9502). The effects of antibiotics on gastrointestinal bacteria are unlikely to have clinically significant effects on vitamin B12 levels. In people with bacterial overgrowth of the small bowel, antibiotics such as metronidazole (Flagyl) can actually improve vitamin B12 status. An increased bacterial load can bind significant amounts of vitamin B12 in the gut, preventing its absorption (4437,9502).

COBALT IRRADIATION: Cobalt irradiation of the small bowel can decrease gastrointestinal (GI) absorption of vitamin B12 (15).

COLCHICINE: Colchicine in doses of 1.9 to 3.9 mg/day can disrupt normal intestinal mucosal function, leading to malabsorption of several nutrients, including vitamin B12 (4543,4544,4545). Lower doses don't seem to have a significant effect on vitamin B12 absorption after 3 years of colchicine therapy (5921). The significance of this interaction isn't clear. Monitor vitamin B12 levels in people taking large doses of colchicine for prolonged periods.

COLESTIPOL (Colestid), CHOLESTYRAMINE (Questran): These resins can decrease gastrointestinal (GI) absorption of vitamin B12 by binding intrinsic factor and vitamin B12-intrinsic factor complexes (10542,10543). However, absorption isn't completely prevented (10542). It's unlikely that this interaction will deplete body stores of vitamin B12 unless there are other factors contributing to deficiency. In a group of children treated with cholestyramine for up to 2.5 years there wasn't any change in serum vitamin B12 levels (4455). Routine supplements aren't necessary.

H2-BLOCKERS: Reduced secretion of gastric acid and pepsin produced by H2-blockers can reduce absorption of protein-bound (dietary) vitamin B12, but not supplemental vitamin B12 (4539,4540,4541,9513,9514,9528). Gastric acid is needed to release vitamin B12 from protein for absorption (4541,9513,9514,9528). Clinically significant vitamin B12 deficiency and megaloblastic anemia are unlikely, unless H2-blocker therapy is prolonged (2 years or more), or the person's diet is poor (4539,9513,9514). It is also more likely if the person is rendered achlorhydric (4483), which occurs more frequently with proton pump inhibitors than H2-blockers. Monitor vitamin B12 levels in people taking high doses of H2 blockers for prolonged periods. The H2-blockers include cimetidine (Tagamet), ranitidine (Zantac), nizatidine (Axid), and famotidine (Pepcid).

METFORMIN (Glucophage): Metformin may reduce serum folic acid and vitamin B12 levels (32,4490,8834). These changes can lead to hyperhomocysteinemia, adding to the risk of cardiovascular disease in people with diabetes (32,4490,7839). There are also rare reports of megaloblastic anemia in people who have taken metformin for 5 years or more (9520,9521,9522). Possible mechanisms for lowered vitamin B12 levels are decreased intrinsic factor secretion, reduced uptake of vitamin B12-intrinsic factor complexes, altered bowel motility, and bacterial overgrowth (32,9521). Reduced absorption of vitamin B12 can be measured with the Schilling test after a few weeks of metformin therapy (7841). Reduced serum levels of vitamin B12 occur in up to 30% of people taking metformin chronically (4490,9520,9521,9523). However, clinically significant deficiency isn't likely to develop if dietary intake of vitamin B12 is adequate (9521). Deficiency can be corrected with vitamin B12 supplements even if metformin is continued (9520,9522). The metformin-induced malabsorption of vitamin B12 is reversible by oral calcium supplementation (8834,9523). A multivitamin preparation may also be valuable for some patients. Monitor for signs and symptoms of vitamin B12 and folic acid deficiency. Advise people taking metformin chronically to include adequate amounts of vitamin B12 in their diet, and have their serum vitamin B12 and homocysteine levels checked annually.

NEOMYCIN: Absorption of vitamin B12 can be reduced by neomycin, but prolonged use of large doses is needed to induce pernicious anemia (3046,8434). Supplements aren't needed with normal doses.

NITROUS OXIDE: Nitrous oxide inactivates the cobalamin form of vitamin B12 by oxidation. Symptoms of vitamin B12 deficiency, including sensory neuropathy, myelopathy, and encephalopathy, can occur within days or weeks of exposure to nitrous oxide anesthesia in people with subclinical vitamin B12 deficiency. Symptoms are treated with high doses of vitamin B12, but recovery can be slow and incomplete. People with normal vitamin B12

levels have sufficient vitamin B12 stores to make the effects of nitrous oxide insignificant, unless exposure is repeated and prolonged (nitrous oxide abuse) (9527,9532). In people with risk factors for vitamin B12 deficiency, check vitamin B12 levels prior to using nitrous oxide anesthesia.
ORAL CONTRACEPTIVES: The data regarding the effects of oral contraceptives on vitamin B12 serum levels are conflicting. Some studies have found reduced serum levels in oral contraceptive users (4547,9371,9373,9505), but others have found no effect despite use of oral contraceptives for up to 6 months (4498,7843,9372). When reduced serum levels are detected, vitamin B12 absorption, urinary excretion, tissue and erythrocyte levels, methylmalonic acid levels, and homocysteine are normal (9371,9373,9505,10123). When oral contraceptive use is stopped, normalization of vitamin B12 levels usually occurs (10123). It's suggested that oral contraceptives reduce production of transcobalamin I, the protein which transports vitamin B12 in the blood (4547,9373,9505). Thus more of the vitamin is available for tissue uptake and serum levels may be reduced. Vitamin B12 supplements don't seem to increase serum levels of vitamin B12 (9373). Lower vitamin B12 serum levels seen with oral contraceptives probably aren't clinically significant.
PHENYTOIN (Dilantin), PHENOBARBITAL, PRIMIDONE (Mysoline): These anticonvulsants have been associated with reduced vitamin B12 absorption, and reduced serum and cerebrospinal fluid levels in some patients. This may contribute to the megaloblastic anemia, primarily caused by folate deficiency, associated with these drugs (7843,10502,10503,10504). It's also suggested that reduced vitamin B12 levels may contribute to the neuropsychiatric side effects of these drugs (10504,10505). Encourage patients to maintain adequate dietary vitamin B12 intake, and check folate and vitamin B12 status if symptoms of anemia develop.
PROTON PUMP INHIBITORS (PPIs): The reduced secretion of gastric acid and pepsin produced by PPIs can reduce absorption of protein-bound (dietary) vitamin B12, but not supplemental vitamin B12 (4483,4484,4485,4486,9513,9528). Gastric acid is needed to release vitamin B12 from protein for absorption (4484,4486,9513,9528). Reduced vitamin B12 levels may be more common with PPIs than with H2-blockers, because they are more likely to produce achlorhydria (complete absence of gastric acid secretion) (4483,4486). However, clinically significant vitamin B12 deficiency is unlikely, unless PPI therapy is prolonged (2 years or more) or dietary vitamin intake is low (4483,4484,9513). Monitor vitamin B12 levels in people taking high doses of PPIs for prolonged periods. The PPIs include omeprazole (Prilosec, Losec), lansoprazole (Prevacid), rabeprazole (Aciphex), pantoprazole (Protonix, Pantoloc), and esomeprazole (Nexium).
ZIDOVUDINE (AZT, Combivir, Retrovir): Reduced serum vitamin B12 levels may occur when zidovudine therapy is started (30,10531). This adds to other factors that cause low vitamin B12 levels in people with HIV, and might contribute to the hematological toxicity associated with zidovudine (10531,10532). However, data suggest vitamin B12 supplements aren't helpful for people taking zidovudine (10532,10533).

Interactions with Foods

ALCOHOL (Ethanol): Excessive alcohol intake lasting longer than two weeks can decrease vitamin B12 absorption from the gastrointestinal tract (15).

Interactions with Lab Tests

INTRINSIC FACTOR: Vitamin B12 can cause a false-positive test result for intrinsic factor antibodies (15).

Interactions with Diseases or Conditions

ANGIOPLASTY: An intravenous loading dose of folic acid, vitamin B6, and vitamin B12 followed by oral administration of folic acid 1.2 m plus vitamin B6 48 mg and vitamin B12 60 mcg taken daily after coronary stenting might actually restenosis rates (12150). Due to the potential for harm this combination of vitamins should not be recommended for patients receiving coronary stents (12151).
COBALAMIN OR COBALT HYPERSENSITIVITY: Contraindicated (15).
LEBER'S DISEASE: Vitamin B12 is contraindicated in early Leber's disease, which is hereditary optic nerve atrophy. Vitamin B12 can cause severe and swift optic atrophy (15).
MEGALOBLASTIC ANEMIA: The correction of megaloblastic anemia with vitamin B12 can result in fatal hypokalemia and gout in susceptible individuals, and it can obscure folate deficiency in megaloblastic anemia (15); use with caution.
POLYCYTHEMIA VERA: The treatment of vitamin B12 deficiency can unmask the symptoms of polycythemia vera (15).

Dosage and Administration

ORAL: For malabsorption of vitamin B12 from food or pernicious anemia, cyanocobalamin doses of 300 to 2000 mcg daily have been used (2900,2901,2909). For hyperhomocysteinemia, vitamin B12 in a dose of 500 mcg in combination with 0.5 to 5 mg folic acid and 16.5 mg pyridoxine has been used (9400,9405). To decrease the rate of restenosis after coronary angioplasty, a combination of vitamin B12 400 mcg plus pyridoxine (vitamin B6) 10 mg and folic acid 1 mg taken daily has been used (8008). For reducing increased homocysteine concentrations associated with nitrous oxide general anesthesia, a supplement containing vitamin B12 500 mcg with pyridoxine (vitamin B6) 25 mg and folic acid 2.5 mg taken daily for one week before surgery has been used (9481). The typical general supplemental dose of vitamin B12 is 1-25 mcg per day (15). The recommended dietary allowances (RDAs) of vitamin B12 are: Infants 0-6 months, 0.4 mcg; Infants 7-12 months, 0.5 mcg; Children 1-3 years, 0.9 mcg;

Children 4-8 years, 1.2 mcg; Children 9-13 years, 1.8 mcg; Older children and adults, 2.4 mcg; Pregnant women 2.6 mcg; and Lactating women, 2.8 mcg (3094). Because 10-30% of older people do not absorb food-bound vitamin B12 efficiently, those over 50 years should meet the RDA by eating foods fortified with B12 or by taking a vitamin B12 supplement (6243). Supplementation of 25-100 mcg per day has been used to maintain vitamin B12 levels in older people (2911,9335,10126).
INTRAMUSCULAR (IM): For treatment of vitamin B12 deficiency, the usual dose is 30 mcg daily for 5-10 days. For maintenance therapy, 100-200 mcg once monthly is commonly used. Both cyanocobalamin and hydroxocobalamin forms are used (15). For familial selective vitamin B12 malabsorption, cyanocobalamin 1000 mcg weekly for 3 weeks, followed by 250 mcg monthly is commonly used (15). For relief of tremor associated with shaky-leg syndrome, injections of 1000 mcg of the cyanocobalamin form of vitamin B12 daily for two weeks, then weekly for two months, and once a month thereafter has been used (6358). For decreasing homocysteine levels and normalizing B12 levels in adult vegetarians, cyanocobalamin 1000 mcg has been used (9512).

Comments
Vitamin B12 is frequently used in combination with other B vitamins in vitamin B complex formulations. Vitamin B complex generally includes vitamin B1 (Thiamine), vitamin B2 (Riboflavin), vitamin B3 (Niacin/Niacinamide), vitamin B5 (Pantothenic Acid), vitamin B6 (Pyridoxine), vitamin B12 (Cyanocobalamin), and folic acid. However, some products do not contain all of these ingredients and some may include others, such as biotin, para-aminobenzoic acid (PABA), choline bitartrate, and inositol (3022).

VITAMIN C (ASCORBIC ACID)

Also Known As
Antiscorbutic Vitamin, Ascorbate, Ascorbyl Palmitate, Calcium Ascorbate, Cevitamic Acid, Iso-Ascorbic Acid, L-Ascorbic Acid, Sodium Ascorbate.
CAUTION: See separate listings for Acerola, Cherokee Rosehip, and Rose Hip.

Scientific Names
Ascorbic acid.

People Use This For
Orally, vitamin C is used for preventing and treating scurvy; preventing deficiency in people with gastrointestinal diseases and those on chronic total parenteral nutrition or chronic hemodialysis; increasing iron absorption from the gastrointestinal tract; and increasing the healing rate of wounds, burns, fractures, ulcers, and pressure sores. It is used for urine acidification, treating idiopathic methemoglobinemia, correcting tyrosinemia in premature infants on high-protein diets, increasing iron excretion (in combination with deferoxamine), preventing and treating the common cold and other viral infections, bronchitis, human immunodeficiency virus (HIV) disease, Helicobacter pylori infection, tuberculosis, dysentery, furunculosis, hematuria, retinal hemorrhages, hemorrhagic states, and anemia. Vitamin C is also used orally for atherosclerosis, preventing vascular thrombosis, myocardial infarction, stroke, hypertension, lowering cholesterol, glaucoma, preventing cataracts, preventing gallbladder disease, dental caries, pyorrhea, gum infections, constipation, peptic ulcer, acne, dermatitis, improving immune function, hay fever, asthma, bronchitis, cystic fibrosis, cystitis, prostatitis, infertility, and diabetes. It is also used orally for mental depression, cognitive impairment, dementia, Alzheimer's disease, physical and mental stress, fatigue, attention deficit-hyperactivity disorder (ADHD), autism, collagen disorders, arthritis and bursitis, back pain and disc inflammation, cancer, osteogenesis imperfecta, and osteoporosis. Other uses include improving physical endurance, reducing aging, heat prostration, for counteracting the side effects of cortisone and related drugs, aiding drug withdrawal in addiction, and in the treatment of levodopa, succinylcholine, interferon, aspirin, and arsenic toxicity. Other uses include use as an adjunct to radiation therapy and treating chronic radiation proctitis. It is also used to prevent human immunodeficiency virus (HIV) transmission to breast-fed babies.
Topically, vitamin C is used for improving skin conditions, protecting against free radicals and pollutants, and for improving photo-aged skin. It is also applied topically for ulcerative mucositis associated with radiation therapy.
Parenterally, vitamin C is used for preventing and treating vitamin C deficiency and correcting tyrosinemia in premature infants on high-protein diets.

Safety
LIKELY SAFE ...when used orally, topically, intramuscularly, or intravenously and appropriately. Vitamin C is safe when taken orally in doses below the tolerable upper intake level (UL). Tell patients not to exceed the UL of 2000 mg per day (1959,4713,4714,4844). ...when used intravenously or intramuscularly and appropriately. Injectable vitamin C is an FDA-approved prescription product (15).
POSSIBLY UNSAFE ...when used orally in excessive doses. Doses greater than the tolerable upper intake level (UL) of 2000 mg per day can significantly increase the risk of adverse effects such as osmotic diarrhea and gastrointestinal upset (4844).

CHILDREN: LIKELY SAFE ...when used orally and appropriately (4844,10352). POSSIBLY UNSAFE ...when used orally in excessive amounts. Tell patients not to use doses above the tolerable upper intake level (UL) of 400 mg per day for children ages 1 to 3 years, 650 mg per day for children 4 to 8 years, 1200 mg per day for children 9 to 13 years, and 1800 mg per day for adolescents 14 to 18 years. Higher doses can cause osmotic diarrhea and gastrointestinal upset (4844).

PREGNANCY AND LACTATION: LIKELY SAFE ...when used orally and appropriately (4844). POSSIBLY UNSAFE ...when used orally in excessive doses. Tell patients not to use doses exceeding the UL of 2000 mg per day for pregnant or breast-feeding women over age 19; and 1800 mg per day for pregnant and breast-feeding women 14 to 18 years. Higher doses can cause osmotic diarrhea and gastrointestinal upset. Large doses of vitamin C during pregnancy can also cause newborn scurvy (4844); avoid using.

Effectiveness

EFFECTIVE

Vitamin C deficiency. Administering vitamin C orally or intramuscularly prevents and treats vitamin C deficiency, including scurvy. Vitamin C administration can reverse complications of scurvy within two days to three weeks (4844).

LIKELY EFFECTIVE

Iron absorption. Concurrent administration of at least 200 mg vitamin C per 30 mg iron increases iron absorption (3042,9518).

Tyrosinemia. Administering vitamin C orally or intramuscularly improves tyrosinemia in premature infants on high protein diets (15).

POSSIBLY EFFECTIVE

Age-related macular degeneration (AMD). Taking vitamin C 500 mg orally, in combination with elemental zinc 80 mg, vitamin E 400 IU, and beta-carotene 15 mg daily seems to provide a risk reduction of 27% for visual acuity loss and a risk reduction of 25% for progression of AMD in patients with advanced AMD (7303). Patients with monocular or binocular intermediate AMD or monocular advanced AMD are at high risk for advanced AMD. Theoretically, these patients may also benefit from vitamin C and antioxidant-zinc supplementation (11326). There isn't enough evidence to know if this combination is beneficial for people with less advanced macular disease or for preventing AMD. Vitamin C with other antioxidants, but without zinc, doesn't seem to have any effect on AMD (7303,7304). Epidemiological evidence suggests that increased vitamin C dietary intake and supplements might actually increase the risk of age-related maculopathy (9823).

Albuminuria. Taking vitamin C plus vitamin E can reduce the excretion of albumin by about 19% when given for 4 weeks in patients with type 2 diabetes. This might also reduce the risk of end-stage renal disease in patients with type 2 diabetes (10434).

Atherosclerosis and peripheral arterial disease. Taking vitamin C orally seems to decrease the risk of atherosclerosis and peripheral arterial disease. Patients with peripheral arterial disease, appear to have lower levels of vitamin C and higher levels of C-reactive protein, a marker of inflammation (9813). In women, there is some epidemiological evidence suggesting that dietary vitamin C can decrease the risk of peripheral arterial disease. However, it does not seem to have this effect in men (10130). However, other research suggests that slow release vitamin C 250 mg in combination with vitamin E 136 IU twice daily might slow the progression of atherosclerosis of the carotid artery. This combination appears to benefit both smoking and nonsmoking men, but has a marginal effect in postmenopausal women (1918,10473). Epidemiological evidence also suggests that dietary intake of vitamin C doesn't affect atherosclerotic markers such as carotid artery wall thickness or carotid artery plaque (9814). In children with familial hypercholesterolemia, vitamin C and vitamin E may increase flow mediated dilation, when used with a National Cholesterol Education Program Step II (NCEP-II) diet (10352). There's also some evidence that the combination of vitamin C and vitamin E might help prevent cardiac transplant-associated arteriosclerosis (5197). Overall, vitamin C appears to slow progression of atherosclerosis. The effects of dietary and supplemental vitamin C on atherosclerosis requires further study to determine if it is generally beneficial or more useful in specific patient populations (9815).

Cancer. Dietary vitamin C might decrease the risk of developing mouth cancer, esophageal cancer, and stomach cancer (10819,10821,10822). Some evidence suggests that a diet low in vitamin C might increase the risk of mortality due to cancer in men, but not in women (3910,5878). Research on the protective effects of vitamin C against developing breast cancer is mixed. Some research suggests that dietary vitamin C reduces breast cancer risk (1444,10823,10824); other research suggests no association between vitamin C intake and breast cancer risk (10825,10826). There is currently no evidence that vitamin C from supplements has any effect on breast cancer risk. Some researchers project that plasma ascorbic acid increases to theoretically protective levels against cancer with an increase of one serving of fruits and vegetables per day (3910). The use of high-dose vitamin C, as adjunctive therapy, in combination with other antioxidants to treat cancer is controversial. Some experts think these supplements might increase the sensitivity of tumor cells to radiation and reduce toxicity in normal cells. Other experts worry that antioxidants might protect cancer cells from the effects of radiation (9826). High dose oral vitamin C, 10 grams daily in patients with advanced cancer regardless of prior chemotherapy, does not seem to improve survival or decrease disease progression (4842,4843). Preliminary clinical evidence suggests high doses of vitamin C given intravenously might have a beneficial effect on survival rate in patients with terminal cancer. Thus far, this has not been tested in well-designed clinical trials (9809). Some observational research in children with lymphoblastic leukemia suggests that greater dietary vitamin C intake is associated with fewer delays in chemotherapy, less toxicity, and fewer hospitalization days (11997).

Common cold. There is a lot of controversy about the effectiveness of vitamin C for treating the common cold (1969,1989,7100,9835,9836). However, the majority of evidence shows that taking high doses of vitamin C orally might decrease the duration of cold symptoms by 1-1.5 days in some patients (1966,1967,1968,1987,6458,7102,9832). Other studies have found no effect with doses up to 3 grams daily (9833). Some research suggests vitamin C may be more effective for treating cold symptoms in children than in adults. There may also be a dose-dependent response, doses of at least 2 grams per day seems to work better than 1 gram doses (9834). Tell patients that the high doses used for treating the common cold, 1-3 grams daily, can increase the risk of side effects. Some patients might not think the modest benefit is worth the risk. Explain to patients that taking vitamin C supplements prophylactically does not decrease the risk of catching a cold (1966,1967,1968,1987,3042,6458,7101,9832). Dietary intake of vitamin C also doesn't seem to affect the risk of getting a cold (10780).

Erythema. There is some evidence that an aqueous formulation of topical vitamin C can decrease the degree and duration of erythema following cutaneous carbon dioxide laser resurfacing for scar and wrinkle removal (1959).

Exercise-induced respiratory infections. Some evidence suggests that prophylactic use of vitamin C in doses of 600 mg to 1 gram per day before heavy physical exercise, such as a marathon, might prevent upper respiratory infections that sometimes follow heavy exercise (9831).

Gallbladder disease. There is some evidence that vitamin C supplementation and increased vitamin C serum levels decreases the risk of developing gallbladder disease in women; however, it doesn't seem to have this effect in men (5877).

Gastric cancer. Taking vitamin C orally seems to promote regression of premalignant gastric lesions in people at high risk for gastric cancer. Vitamin C 1 gram twice daily seems to cause regression of intestinal metaplasia and multifocal nonmetaplastic atrophy (2579).There is conflicting epidemiological evidence regarding the effects of dietary and supplemental vitamin C on preventing gastric cancer (9194,9838). More evidence is needed.

Helicobacter pylori (H pylori) infection. Taking vitamin C orally seems to decrease gastritis associated with acid suppressive therapy in patients with H. pylori infection (10359). After H. pylori is eradicated, vitamin C appears to decrease the incidence of precancerous changes in stomach tissue (10360).

HIV transmission. Taking vitamin C orally during pregnancy and breast-feeding seems to reduce HIV transmission. Supplementation of mothers with HIV disease with vitamin B, vitamin C, and vitamin E seems to reduce child mortality and HIV transmission through breast milk (9801).

Hypertension. Taking vitamin C orally, added to a conventional antihypertensive medication regimen, appears to decrease both systolic and mean blood pressure, but does not seem to decrease diastolic pressure (2044). In patients with type 2 diabetes, vitamin C 500 mg taken daily for 4 weeks, in addition to antihypertensives, seems to reduce arterial blood pressure and improve arterial stiffness (9822). But supplemental vitamin C 500 mg per day taken without antihypertensives doesn't seem to reduce systolic or diastolic blood pressure (9821). Dietary restriction of vitamin C is associated with increases in both diastolic and systolic blood pressure (10354).

Lead toxicity. Consuming vitamin C from dietary sources seems to lower blood concentrations of lead (3097,3098,3099).

Nitrate tolerance. Taking vitamin C orally seems to prevent the development of nitrate tolerance in patients taking sublingual nitroglycerin. There is some evidence that short-term vitamin C supplementation can prevent attenuation of tolerance to the vasodilatory effects of nitrates (1441,1961).

Osteoarthritis. Consuming vitamin C from dietary sources seems to reduce the risk of cartilage loss and disease progression in people with osteoarthritis (5881).

Pre-eclampsia. Taking vitamin C orally with vitamin E seems to prevent pre-eclampsia in high-risk pregnancies (3236).

Reflex sympathetic dystrophy (RSD). Patients given vitamin C supplements for 50 days after a wrist fracture seem to be significantly less likely to develop RSD (2045).

Sunburn. Taking vitamin C orally in combination with vitamin E seems to prevent ultraviolet (UV) radiation-induced erythema (sunburn) (4715,4716). Vitamin C in combination with high dose oral RRR-alpha-tocopherol (natural vitamin E) seems to protect against skin inflammation after exposure to ultraviolet (UV) radiation (1416,4715). This effect is not found when vitamin C is used without vitamin E (1417). Applying vitamin C topically, in combination with vitamin E and melatonin, also seems to prevent ultraviolet (UV) radiation-induced erythema (sunburn). Topical vitamin C in combination with topical vitamin E and melatonin seems to provide modest photo-protective effects when used prior to UV exposure. However, it has no effect when used during or after UV exposure (4713,4714).

Wrinkled skin. Topical preparations containing 5-10% vitamin C seem to improve the appearance of wrinkled skin. In one trial, a topical preparation containing 10% vitamin C as L-ascorbic acid and acetyl tyrosine, zinc sulfate, sodium hyaluronate, and bioflavonoids (Cellex-C High Potency Serum) used for 3 months and applied to photo-aged facial skin improved fine and coarse wrinkling, yellowing and sallowness, roughness, and skin tone compared to placebo (6155).

POSSIBLY INEFFECTIVE

Acute bronchitis. Taking vitamin C orally 500 mg on day 1, then 250 mg on days 2 through 5 (similar to an azithromycin regimen) doesn't seem to have any effect on acute bronchitis duration or symptoms (9827).

Alzheimer's disease or vascular dementia. Consuming vitamin C from dietary sources, as a supplement alone, or in combination with vitamin E, doesn't seem to affect the risk of developing Alzheimer's disease or vascular dementia (4636,9824,10131). However, some epidemiological research suggests that long-term use of vitamin C and vitamin E supplements in combination, and in higher doses than typically found in multivitamins, is associated with a reduced prevalence and incidence of Alzheimer's disease (11390).

Attention deficit-hyperactivity disorder (ADHD). Taking megadose vitamins including vitamin C orally doesn't seem to help ADHD symptoms (9957,9958,9959).

Interferon-related retinopathy. Taking vitamin C 600 mg per day orally doesn't seem to reduce the risk of retinopathy associated with interferon therapy in patients with chronic hepatitis C (10355).

Radiation dermatitis. Applying a 10% vitamin C solution does not appear to have a protective effect when applied to the scalps of patients treated with radiation for intracranial tumors (789).

Stroke. Most population studies show that taking vitamin C orally doesn't seem to affect the risk of ischemic or hemorrhagic stroke (1449,1958,7390,7716). Lower plasma levels of vitamin C have been associated with increased stroke risk (1957,7714). Higher consumption of fruits and vegetables has been associated with reduced ischemic stroke risk (7394). Suggest a diet high in fruits and vegetables rather than vitamin C supplements to reduce stroke risk.

INSUFFICIENT RELIABLE EVIDENCE to RATE

Aspirin-associated gastric damage. Some clinical evidence suggests that vitamin C might prevent gastric damage associated with aspirin therapy by decreasing blood loss and preventing decreased gastric blood flow (10357).

Asthma. There is some evidence that low levels of vitamin C are associated with certain conditions. Vitamin C levels might be decreased in some asthmatics (5873). Some clinical evidence also suggests that oral vitamin C might decrease exercise-induced asthma (1443).

Bladder cancer. Epidemiological research suggests that supplemental vitamin C use does not affect mortality rate associated with bladder cancer (9839).

Cardiovascular disease. Using antioxidants such as vitamin C for preventing heart disease and cardiovascular events such as myocardial infarction (MI) is controversial. There have been lots of studies, but results have been mixed (11001). In populations with relatively low or deficient vitamin C intake, vitamin C seems to lower the risk of death from coronary heart disease, although not all studies have shown benefit (1958,7714,7715,10815,11001). Some large population studies have shown a reduction in mortality from coronary heart disease either from dietary sources or supplements (3910,7394,10358,10814,10816,10817,11003), but similar studies have shown no effect on mortality risk with increased vitamin C intake (1958,3933,3934,3938,7724). Interestingly, two of the positive studies found a 25-28% reduction of cardiovascular disease and cardiovascular disease mortality in women only who took vitamin C supplements (10358,11002). Some population studies that found benefit have been criticized for not considering concurrent vitamin E intake (7715,11002). Some research suggests that a combination of vitamin C and vitamin E might offer additional benefit for preventing coronary heart disease (3938). In people with coronary heart disease, the few studies that have been done haven't shown vitamin C to be beneficial (10817,10818,11000). Vitamin C in combination with selenium, beta-carotene, vitamin E also doesn't seem to protect against cardiovascular disease progression and related events such as MI (7388). Studies investigating serum vitamin C concentrations and cardiovascular mortality risk are inconclusive. One study found decreased mortality with increasing concentrations (3910); the other found no effect (5878). Tell patients more research is needed before supplemental vitamin C can be recommended for preventing coronary heart disease. Increasing fruit and vegetable intake by one serving per day in the average person could boost plasma ascorbic acid to theoretically protective levels (3910). A Science Advisory from the American Heart Association also states that the evidence does not justify use of antioxidants such as vitamin C for reducing the risk of cardiovascular disease (12142). Tell patients more research is needed before supplemental vitamin C can be recommended for preventing coronary heart disease. Increasing fruit and vegetable intake by one serving per day in the average person could boost plasma ascorbic acid to theoretically protective levels (3910).

Cataracts. There is conflicting information about the use of vitamin C to prevent cataracts. Vitamin C plus vitamin E and beta-carotene doesn't seem to have any significant effect on age-related loss of vision due to cataracts in well-nourished people who took the supplement for an average of 6.3 years (7304). However, population research suggests that vitamin C use in multivitamins or any supplement containing vitamin C for 10 years appears to reduce the incidence of nuclear and cortical cataracts by 60%. Use of supplements for shorter periods doesn't appear to reduce the risk for cataract development (4208).

Chronic radiation proctitis. Preliminary clinical research suggests that vitamin C 500 mg plus vitamin E 400 IU three times daily might improve symptoms of chronic radiation proctitis (9825).

HIV/AIDS. Taking vitamin C 250 mg daily in combination with vitamin A, beta-carotene, vitamin E, selenium, and coenzyme Q-10 seems to improve markers of oxidative defense and oxidative stress in men with human immunodeficiency virus (HIV) disease. However, higher doses of vitamin C, 1000 mg, and the other antioxidants don't seem to provide any additional effect. Neither high-dose nor low-dose antioxidants affect viral load (9830).

Infertility. There is preliminary evidence that women with infertility, due to luteal phase defect, might increase their progesterone levels by taking vitamin C 750 mg daily (12010). It's not currently known if vitamin C can significantly increase pregnancy rates.

Leukemia. There is some evidence that vitamin C might have a synergistic effect with arsenic trioxide (Trisenox) on myeloid leukemia cells. Preclinical evidence suggests that vitamin C might enhance the apoptotic effect of

arsenic trioxide in patients with acute myeloid leukemia (9837).
Mental stress. Preliminary evidence suggests that vitamin C might reduce blood pressure and subjective symptoms during psychological or mental stress (10353).
Osteoporosis. Some evidence suggests that vitamin C intake might be related to bone mineral density in premenopausal women and men. In postmenopausal women who use estrogen and smoke, higher vitamin C levels might reduce fracture risk. However, in postmenopausal women without a history of smoking or estrogen use, higher serum vitamin C levels have been associated with lower bone mineral density. At present, there is not enough information to make recommendations about vitamin C and bone density (9828).
Ovarian cancer. Epidemiological research suggests that dietary vitamin C does not affect risk of developing ovarian cancer (9193).
Overall mortality. Some research suggests that plasma vitamin C levels are positively associated with a reduced risk of mortality from all causes (3910). However, in high-risk patients, vitamin C 250 mg in combination with vitamin E 600 mg and beta-carotene 20 mg daily doesn't seem to affect overall mortality risk. Additionally this combination doesn't seem to reduce mortality rate or illness from vascular disease in people with diabetes, coronary disease, or occlusive arterial disease. This vitamin combination also doesn't seem to reduce the risk of cancer or hospitalization for any other nonvascular cause (9817).
Sickle cell disease. Vitamin C, in combination with aged garlic extract and vitamin E might be useful for sickle cell disease (5056).
More evidence is needed to rate the effectiveness of vitamin C for these uses.

Mechanism of Action

Vitamin C is a commonly used water-soluble vitamin. Although many mammals can produce vitamin C, humans must obtain vitamin C from foods and other sources (1964). It's contained in the high concentration in fresh fruits and vegetables, especially the citrus fruits. Vitamin C is labile, and the amount in foods can decrease significantly with cooking and storage (3042). Vitamin C has a role in several physiological functions. It is involved in tyrosine metabolism and is a cofactor in the synthesis of carnitine, thyroxin, norepinephrine, dopamine, and tryptophan (3042). Vitamin C is also involved in a variety of metabolic processes including oxidation-reduction reactions and cellular respiration, carbohydrate metabolism, synthesis of lipids and proteins, catabolism of cholesterol to bile acids, conversion of folic acid to folinic acid, and iron metabolism (5877). Vitamin C is probably best known for its effects as an antioxidant and its role in maintaining proper immune function (15). Normal plasma vitamin C levels typically exceed 0.3 mg/dL. When plasma levels exceed 1.4 mg/dL, excretion of vitamin C greatly increases (1965,1969). Concentrations below 0.2 mg/dL indicate significant deficiency (1964).
Vitamin C deficiency can cause fatigue, personality changes, and decline in psychomotor performance and motivation within 84 to 97 days. Some evidence suggests that subclinical vitamin C deficiency is more common in healthy people than generally recognized (9810). Since the nonspecific symptom of fatigue is often the first symptom of deficiency, vitamin C depletion may go undiagnosed (9809). Sustained vitamin C deficiency over 3 to 5 months results in symptomatic scurvy characterized by gingival swelling and bleeding, loosening of the teeth, hyperkeratosis, perifollicular hemorrhages, petechial hemorrhages in the viscera, and hemorrhages into the muscles of the arms, legs, and joints (1964). Severe scurvy may progress to neuritis, jaundice, fever, dyspnea, and death. In infants, vitamin C deficiency is initially manifested by listlessness, anorexia, irritability, and failure to thrive. Later symptoms result from hemorrhage and collagen deficiency, with seizures, shock, and death if left untreated (1965).
Because of vitamin C's role in maintaining normal immune function, a lot of people use it for treating and preventing infectious conditions such as the common cold. T-lymphocyte activity, phagocyte function, leukocyte mobility, and possibly antibody and interferon production seem to be increased by vitamin C (1963,1965). Vitamin C levels in phagocytes and lymphocytes are up to 100 times greater than in plasma (7101). Some researchers think that vitamin C levels in white blood cells decrease at the onset of a cold and that boosting vitamin C intake might be beneficial. There is some evidence vitamin C might have other effects in patients with the common cold. Vitamin C might protect normal tissues against reactive oxygen species that are produced by phagocytes during a viral infection. It might also enhance the proliferative responses of T-lymphocytes (1988). There is some evidence that vitamin C might also have weak antihistamine properties (1969). There is preliminary evidence vitamin C excretion might actually decrease during a cold, indicating that patients may retain vitamin C. However, absorption of vitamin C is unchanged during a cold (1986).
Other potentially beneficial effects of vitamin C are attributed primarily to its role as an antioxidant and free radical scavenging effects. Vitamin C readily undergoes reversible oxidation and reduction in the body (1963). Vitamin C decreases oxidants in gastric juice, lipid peroxidation, and oxidative DNA and protein damage (3042). Damage by reactive oxygen species are thought to be a contributing factor to a number of diseases, including dementia, asthma, hypertension, osteoarthritis, and cancer. Researchers theorized that antioxidants such as vitamin C might protect against some diseases associated with oxidative damage. For example, in hypertension, endothelium-derived nitric oxide (NO), which causes vasodilation, might be inhibited by superoxide anions. Vitamin C can scavenge the superoxide anions and theoretically might help patients with hypertension. However, in this case there is some evidence that oral doses might not reach concentrations high enough for this effect (5879). In people with chronic heart failure, intra-arterial vitamin C seems to improve endothelial dysfunction and flow-dependent dilation of the arteries. Vitamin C appears to prevent inactivation of NO-mediated vasodilation. Four weeks of oral vitamin C 1 gram twice daily appears to produce a similar effect (2434). There's also some evidence that vitamin C might

suppress the apoptosis (death) of endothelial cells of patients with congestive heart failure, but the clinical relevance of this isn't known (9816). Intracoronary infusion of vitamin C has been shown to enhance the inotropic response to dobutamine (Dobutrex), possibly by reducing oxidative stress caused by beta-adrenergic stimulation of the ventricle (2432). Some researchers think vitamin C might prevent or slow atherosclerosis by inhibiting low-density lipoprotein (LDL) cholesterol; by impairing the products of reactive oxygen species from vascular cells; and by limiting the cellular responses to oxidized LDL, such as production of endothelium-derived NO (9812). In patients with coronary spastic angina, vitamin C seems to improve endothelial function when given by intravenous infusion as a single 2 gram dose (9819). Some research suggests that endothelial function may relate to insulin resistance in patients with hypertension. Single-dose intravenous vitamin C seems to improve endothelial function and restore insulin-mediated vasodilatation, but doesn't seem to improve glucose uptake (9820). Oral vitamin C seems to improve endothelial function in healthy young smokers, short term; the improvements in endothelial function diminish within 8 weeks, even though vitamin C levels remain elevated (9818).

In smokers, a single 3 gram dose given by intravenous infusion appears to restore coronary microcirculatory responsiveness and impaired coronary flow reserve induced by the oxidant effects of smoking. Vitamin C might reduce oxidative stress caused by the large number of oxidants in cigarette smoke (1956). Whether these effects are sustained when vitamin C is taken chronically is unknown. Pulmonary function is also positively related to dietary vitamin C intake in smokers and nonsmokers (2400). For radiation-induced oral mucositis, the reduced form of vitamin C might be beneficial due to its antioxidant effect and role in maintaining connective tissue integrity (6103). Vitamin C may also reduce toxicity of reactive oxygen during radio-immunotherapy due to its antioxidant effects (5878).

Research in marathon runners suggests vitamin C might help post-race immune suppression. Vitamin C 1500 mg taken daily for 7 days before running seems to reduce post exercise serum cortisol and cytokines (11961).

Free radicals are also generated in the skin by exposure to ultraviolet light and cause photo-aging. Vitamin C in the skin is believed to play a key role in neutralizing these free radicals and reducing UV skin damage. Topical application of vitamin C is thought to prevent skin damage when applied prior to UV exposure due to vitamin C's antioxidant effects (6062,6155). Topical preparations are thought to help treat photo-aged and wrinkled skin due to vitamin C's antioxidant properties and by possibly by increasing collagen production and improving collagen organization (6155). Topical preparations containing 10% vitamin C might be most effective for increasing vitamin C concentrations in the skin. Because vitamin C is water soluble, oral supplementation of vitamin C might not produce high enough concentrations in the skin to treat photo-aged skin (6064,6155).

Vitamin C is well absorbed orally at lower does, but absorption decreases as the dose increases. Approximately 87% of a 30 mg oral dose is absorbed, 80% of a 100 mg dose is absorbed, 63 % of a 500 mg dose is absorbed, and less than 50% of a 1250 mg does is absorbed. Most of what is absorbed is excreted in the urine. Decreased bioavailability with increasing dosages and increased renal excretion limits the plasma levels attainable with oral vitamin C supplementation (9809).

Adverse Reactions

Orally, the adverse effects of vitamin C are dose-related (3042) and include nausea, vomiting, esophagitis, heartburn, abdominal cramps, gastrointestinal obstruction, fatigue, flushing, headache, insomnia, sleepiness, and diarrhea. Doses greater than the tolerable upper intake level (UL) of 2000 mg per day can increase the risk of significant adverse effects such as osmotic diarrhea and gastrointestinal upset (4844).

Vitamin C may also cause precipitation of urate, oxalate, or cysteine stones or drugs in the urinary tract (10356). Hyperoxaluria, hyperuricosuria, hematuria, and crystalluria have occurred in people taking 1 gram or more per day (3042). Large amounts of vitamin C are associated with deep vein thrombosis. Prolonged use of large amounts of vitamin C can also result in increased metabolism of vitamin C, and scurvy can occur when vitamin C intake is reduced (15).

Oral supplementation with vitamin C has also been associated with an increased rate of carotid inner wall thickening in men. There is preliminary evidence that supplemental intake of vitamin C 500 mg daily for 18 months can cause a 2.5-fold increased rate of carotid inner wall thickening in non-smoking men and a 5-fold increased rate in men who smoked. The men in this study were 40-60 years old. This effect was not associated with vitamin C from dietary sources (1355). There is also some concern that supplements of vitamin C 200 mg might increase production reactive oxygen molecules capable of damaging DNA. This is based on very preliminary in vitro evidence that vitamin C can induce decomposition of lipid hydroperoxides to reactive molecules. More evidence is needed to determine if this is clinically relevant in humans taking vitamin C supplements (7088).

Topically, vitamin C might cause tingling or irritation at the site of application (6166).

Interactions with Herbs & Other Dietary Supplements

IRON: Concomitant use of 200 mg of vitamin C per 30 mg of elemental iron increases oral iron absorption, especially ferric iron (3042,9518). Ascorbic acid reduces elemental iron to its ferrous form, the most absorbable form (1960).

VITAMIN E: Vitamin E can increase the serum concentration of vitamin C, and reciprocally, vitamin C can increase the serum concentration of vitamin E. The mechanism for the vitamin E-induced increase in vitamin C concentrations is unknown but might result from increased absorption or decreased plasma clearance of ascorbic acid (10472). In patients taking vitamin C and vitamin E doses below tolerable upper intake levels (UL), this interaction appears unlikely to cause toxicity.

Interactions with Drugs

ACETAMINOPHEN (Tylenol, Others): High doses of vitamin C, 3 grams or more, can decrease the elimination rate of acetaminophen by approximately 75% and might increase the risk of acetaminophen side effects. Vitamin C seems to competitively inhibit sulfate conjugation of acetaminophen (6451).

ALUMINUM: Concomitant use might increase aluminum absorption. The clinical significance of this is unknown (3046). Administer vitamin C two hours before, or four hours after, taking an antacid (3046).

ASPIRIN: Concomitant use can increase urinary excretion of vitamin C and decrease excretion of salicylates. However, it might not have a clinically significant effect on salicylate plasma levels (3046).

CHEMOTHERAPY: Theoretically, concomitant use might decrease the effectiveness of chemotherapy. Preliminary evidence from an unpublished study suggests that antioxidants such as vitamin E, vitamin C, and vitamin A might decrease the effectiveness of chemotherapy (391).

CHOLINE MAGNESIUM TRISALICYLATE (Trilisate): Concomitant use can increase urinary excretion of vitamin C and decrease excretion of salicylates. However, it might not have a clinically significant effect on salicylate plasma levels (3046).

ESTRADIOL: Vitamin C might interfere with the metabolism of estradiol, resulting in higher blood levels, particularly in women with low estradiol levels (129,11161). However, this effect appears to be less pronounced in women with higher initial ascorbic acid levels (3712,11161).

FLUPHENAZINE (Prolixin): Concomitant use of fluphenazine and vitamin C might decrease fluphenazine blood levels (11017). Advise patients not to take large amounts of vitamin C while taking fluphenazine.

HEPARIN: There is some evidence that high dose vitamin C might decrease the effectiveness of heparin (1962,6452). However, vitamin C in combination with B vitamin infusion appears to have no effect on the anticoagulant effects of heparin when mixed together in the same IV bag (1962).

HMG-CoA REDUCTASE INHIBITORS ("Statins"): Concomitant use of vitamin C in combination with beta-carotene, selenium, and vitamin E appears to decrease the effectiveness of simvastatin (Zocor) plus niacin (7388). This combination of antioxidants can lower high-density lipoprotein-2 (HDL-2) levels by 15%, and reduce the HDL-2 raising effects of HMG-CoA reductase inhibitors and niacin by more than 50%, in people with heart disease (7388).

NIACIN: Concomitant use of vitamin C with beta-carotene, selenium, and vitamin E appears to decrease the effectiveness simvastatin (Zocor) plus niacin (7388). This combination can lower high-density lipoprotein-2 (HDL-2) levels by 15%, and reduce the HDL-2 raising effects of HMG-CoA reductase inhibitors and niacin by more than 50%, in people with heart disease (7388).

PROTEASE INHIBITORS (PIs): Vitamin C seems to modestly reduce indinavir (Crixivan) levels. Vitamin C 1 gram daily for 7 days given with indinavir reduces the area under the concentration curve by 14%. The mechanism for this interaction is unknown. This is unlikely to be clinically significant in most patients. However, the effect of higher doses of vitamin C is unknown (11300). Protease inhibitors include amprenavir (Agenerase), nelfinavir (Viracept), ritonavir (Norvir), and saquinavir (Fortovase, Invirase).

SALSALATE (Disalcid): Concomitant use can increase urinary excretion of vitamin C and decrease excretion of salicylates. However, it might not have a clinically significant effect on salicylate plasma levels (3046).

WARFARIN (Coumadin): Theoretically, concomitant use with large amounts of vitamin C might impair response to warfarin (3046,9804,9806). Doses of vitamin C up to 10 grams per day don't seem to affect coagulation time in patients taking warfarin (3046,9805,9807). Higher doses of vitamin C might affect warfarin absorption or antagonize the anticoagulant effect of warfarin by an unknown mechanism (3046,9807).

Drug Influences on Nutrient Levels and Depletion

SOME DRUGS CAN AFFECT VITAMIN C LEVELS:

ASPIRIN and OTHER SALICYLATES: Concomitant use can increase urinary excretion of vitamin C. However, there is no evidence of vitamin C deficiency associated with use of aspirin and other salicylates. Consider supplementation only in patients on long-term salicylate therapy with signs of vitamin C deficiency (3046).

DIHYDROPYRIDINE CALCIUM CHANNEL BLOCKERS (DCCBs): Dihydropyridine calcium channel blockers, amlodipine (Norvasc), felodipine (Plendil), isradipine (DynaCirc), nicardipine (Cardene), nifedipine (Adalat, Procardia), and nisoldipine (Sular), might reduce plasma ascorbic acid levels. DCCBs seem to inhibit vitamin C accumulation in intestinal cells and increase vitamin C's elimination (9808). Consider supplementation if clinical judgment warrants it.

ESTROGENS and ESTROGEN-CONTAINING ORAL CONTRACEPTIVES: Estrogens can increase elimination of vitamin C (11875,11876). Consider supplementation if clinical judgment warrants it.

NICOTINE and SMOKING: Nicotine can increase elimination of vitamin C. Smokers have been reported to have lower plasma levels of vitamin C than nonsmokers with similar diets. These low levels can be corrected with moderate supplementation or by an increasing fruit and vegetable intake to recommended dietary levels (5875). Consider supplementation only if clinical judgment warrants it.

Interactions with Foods

None known.

Interactions with Lab Tests

ACETAMINOPHEN: Vitamin C can cause false-negative urine results with methods based on hydrolysis and formation of an indophenol blue chromogen (275).
ASPARTATE AMINOTRANSFERASE (AST, SGOT): Large amounts of ascorbic acid can cause a false increase in results of serum tests relying on color reactions (Redox reactions) and Technicon SMA 12/60 (275).
BILIRUBIN: Large amounts of vitamin C can cause a false increase in serum test results measured by Technicon SMA 12/60 or colorimetric methods (275).
CALCIUM/SODIUM: Daily vitamin C 3-6 grams can cause an increase in urinary calcium and test results, and a decrease in urinary sodium and test results (15).
CARBAMAZEPINE (Tegretol): Large doses of vitamin C can cause falsely increased serum assay results measured by Ames ARIS method (275).
CREATININE: Vitamin C can cause a false increase in serum creatinine or urine test results (275).
GLUCOSE: Large amounts of vitamin C can cause false increases in urine test results measured by copper reduction methods (e.g., Clinitest), and false decreases in results measured by glucose oxidase methods (e.g., Clinistix, Tes-Tape) (15).
HIGH-DENSITY LIPOPROTEIN-2 (HDL-2): Vitamin C in combination with beta-carotene, selenium, and vitamin E seems to lower HDL-2 levels. This combination can lower HDL-2 levels by 15% in people with heart disease (7388).
IRON: Vitamin C can increase the absorption of iron and measures of iron status, such as serum iron and ferritin (9518).
LACTIC DEHYDROGENASE (LDH): Vitamin C can cause a false decrease in test results measured by Technicon SMA 12/60 and Abbott 100 methods (275).
OCCULT BLOOD: False-negative guaiac results occur with 250 mg or more of vitamin C per day (3042).
THEOPHYLLINE: Large amounts of vitamin C can cause a false decrease in serum assay results when measured by the ARIS system or Ames Seralyzer photometer (275).
URIC ACID: Large amounts of vitamin C can cause a decrease in serum uric acid concentrations and test results measured by enzymatic method assays (15).
VITAMIN B12: Large amounts of vitamin C can interfere with vitamin B12 assay, resulting in false decrease in vitamin B12 levels (1965).

Interactions with Diseases or Conditions

ANGIOPLASTY: There is some concern that when antioxidant vitamins, including vitamin C, are used in combination they might have harmful effects in patients after angioplasty. A combination of beta-carotene 30,000 IU, vitamin C 500 mg, and vitamin E 700 IU daily started 30 days before angioplasty, and continued for 6 months thereafter, seems to prevent beneficial vascular remodeling in patients by promoting fibrosis at the site of angioplastic intervention (11000). Tell patients to avoid taking supplements containing these vitamins immediately before and following angioplasty without the supervision of a health care professional.
CANCER: Cancerous cells accumulate high concentrations of vitamin C. Cancer cells uptake the oxidized form of vitamin C, dehydroascorbic acid, then convert it back to vitamin C (4838,4839,4840,4841). However, it is not yet known if this benefits growth of cancer cells or has any detrimental effect of cancer treatments. Until more is known, patients with cancer should only use high doses of vitamin C under the direction of their oncologist.
DIABETES: Vitamin C can affect glycogenolysis and increase blood sugar, but this effect remains controversial (15).
GLUCOSE-6-PHOSPHATE DEHYDROGENASE DEFICIENCY: Large amounts of vitamin C can cause hemolysis in individuals with glucose-6-phosphate dehydrogenase deficiency (15).
INCREASED NEEDS: Vitamin C requirements are increased in pregnancy, lactation, hyperthyroidism, stress, fever, infection, trauma, burns, smoking, and cold exposure (7722).
IRON OVERLOAD, HEMOCHROMATOSIS, THALASSEMIA, SIDEROBLASTIC ANEMIA: Use vitamin C with caution, vitamin C can increase iron absorption, which could worsen these conditions (1960).
KIDNEY STONES: Large amounts of vitamin C can increase the risk of oxalate stone formation. Vitamin C is metabolized to oxalic acid, so increased consumption increases the urinary concentration of oxalic acid (10356). Tell patients prone to kidney stone formation to avoid high doses of vitamin C.
MYOCARDIAL INFARCTION (MI): Vitamin C levels are significantly reduced during the acute phase after a MI. However, low plasma levels of vitamin C have not been associated with an increased risk of MI (5876).
SICKLE CELL DISEASE: Vitamin C can decrease blood pH, which can rarely precipitate sickle cell crisis (15).

Dosage and Administration

ORAL: For scurvy, 100-250 mg once or twice daily for several days is commonly used (15). For treating the common cold, 1-3 grams daily has been used (6458). For preventing the common cold, in people under physical stress, vitamin C 600-1000 mg daily has been used (9831). During acute stress, vitamin C 1 gram 3 times daily, as a sustained release preparation, has been used for up to 14 days (10353). For chronic hemodialysis in adults, 100-200 mg per day is recommended (15). For preventing nitrate tolerance, 3-6 grams of vitamin C daily has been used (1961). For preventing sunburn, 2 grams of vitamin C in combination with RRR-alpha-tocopherol (natural vitamin E) 1000 IU has been used (4716). For treatment of premalignant gastric lesions, vitamin C 1 gram twice daily has been used (2579). For slowing progression of atherosclerosis, slow release vitamin C 250 mg in combination with 91 mg (136 IU) of vitamin E has been given twice daily for up to 6 years (1918,10473). For treatment of familial hypercholesterolemia in children, vitamin C 500 mg daily and vitamin E 400 IU daily have been used for up to 6 months with a National Cholesterol Education Program Step II (NCEP-II) diet (10352). For tyrosinemia in premature infants on high protein diets, 100 mg of vitamin C has been used (15). For reducing albinuria in patients with type 2 diabetes, vitamin C 1250 mg with vitamin E 680 IU daily has been used for 4 weeks (10434). For infertility associated with luteal phase defect, 750 mg per day has been used (12010).

The daily recommended dietary allowances (RDAs) are: Infants 0 to 12 months, human milk content (older recommendations specified 30-35 mg); Children 1 to 3 years, 15 mg; Children 4 to 8 years, 25 mg; Children 9 to 13 years, 45 mg; Adolescents 14 to 18 years, 75 mg for boys and 65 mg for girls; Adults age 19 and greater, 90 mg for men and 75 mg for women; Pregnancy and Lactation: age 18 or younger, 115 mg; ages 19 to 50 years 120 mg. People who use tobacco should take an additional 35 mg per day (4844).

The tolerable upper intake levels (UL) for vitamin C are 400 mg per day for children ages 1 to 3 years, 650 mg per day for children 4 to 8 years, 1200 mg per day for children 9 to 13 years, and 1800 mg per day for adolescents and pregnant and lactating women 14 to 18 years, and 2000 mg per day for adults and pregnant and lactating women (4844).

TOPICAL: Most topical preparations used for aged or wrinkled skin are applied daily. Studies have used creams containing 5% to 10% vitamin C (6155). In one study a specific vitamin C formulation (Cellex-C High Potency Serum) used 3 drops applied daily to areas of facial skin (6155). Avoid application to eye area or eyelids. Also avoid contact with hair or clothes. It can cause discoloration (6166).

Comments

Most experts recommend getting antioxidants, including vitamin C, from a diet high in fruits, vegetables, and whole grains rather than taking supplements (1440,3042). Ready-to-drink orange juice contains 25% less active vitamin C than frozen orange juice. Oxidized vitamin C is not readily absorbed across the intestinal mucosa. Much, 51-76%, of the vitamin C in ready-to-drink orange juice is oxidized, compared with only 20% of vitamin C in frozen orange juice. Frozen orange juice consumed within one week of reconstitution is the most reliable source of vitamin C. Tell patients who prefer ready-to-drink orange juice that these products should be purchased 3 to 4 weeks before the expiration date and consumed within one week of opening (9811).

VITAMIN D

Also Known As

Alfacalcidol: 1-alpha-hydroxycholecalciferol, 1 alpha (OH)D3.
Calcifediol: 25-HCC, 25-hydroxycholecalciferol, 25-hydroxyvitamin D3, 25-OHCC, 25-OHD3.
Calcipotriene: Calcipotriol.
Calcitriol: 1,25-DHCC, 1,25-dihydroxycholecalciferol, 1,25-dihydroxyvitamin D3, 1,25-diOHC, 1,25(0H)2D3.
Cholecalciferol: Activated 7-dehydrocholesterol, colecalciferol, Vitamin D3.
Dihydrotachysterol: DHT, dihydrotachysterol 2, dichysterol.
Ergocalciferol: Activated ergosterol, Calciferol, Ergocalciferolum, Irradiated ergosterol, Viosterol, Vitamin D2.
Paricalcitol: 19-nor-1,25-dihydroxyvitamin D2, Paracalcin.

Scientific Names

1,25-dihydroxycholecalciferol; 25-hydroxycholecalciferol; Alfacalcidol; Calcifediol; Calcipotriene; Calcitriol; Cholecalciferol; Dihydrotachysterol; Ergocalciferol; Paricalcitol.

People Use This For

Orally, vitamin D is used for building bone mass and preventing bone loss, protecting against muscle weakness, promoting strong teeth, enhancing immune function, preventing auto-immune diseases, reducing risk of multiple sclerosis, rheumatoid arthritis, treating cancer, and reducing risk of colon, breast, and prostate cancer. It is also used orally for preventing and treating rickets, postmenopausal osteoporosis, to prevent falls and fractures in people at risk for osteoporosis, corticosteroid-induced osteoporosis, osteomalacia, anticonvulsant-induced osteomalacia, renal osteodystrophy, osteitis fibrosa in people on dialysis, hepatic osteodystrophy, and osteogenesis imperfecta. Vitamin D is also used for preventing and treating hypocalcemia and tetany in premature infants, hypocalcemic tetany, bone disorders in people with familial hypophosphatemia, hypophosphatemia associated with Fanconi syndrome, and hypocalcemia associated with postoperative or idiopathic hypoparathyroidism or pseudohypoparathyroidism. Other uses include plaque-type psoriasis, actinic keratoses, lupus vulgaris, squamous cell carcinomas, vitiligo, scleroderma, myelodysplastic syndrome, and preventing type 1 diabetes. Vitamin D is also used orally to treat severe proximal myopathy associated with vitamin D deficiency and to maintain bone density in prostatic cancer patients at risk for osteoporosis when treated with luteinizing hormone-releasing hormone analogue (LHRH-a).

Topically, vitamin D is used as calcitriol or calcipotriene for plaque-type psoriasis.

Intravenously, vitamin D, administered as calcitriol, is used for hypocalcemic tetany in premature infants, hypocalcemia and hyperparathyroidism in renal dialysis patients, and osteitis fibrosa.

Intramuscularly, vitamin D is administered as ergocalciferol for hepatic osteodystrophy, as an injectable source of vitamin D, and to treat severe proximal myopathy associated with vitamin D deficiency.

Safety

LIKELY SAFE ...when used orally and appropriately (7555). Vitamin D is safe when used in doses below the tolerable upper intake level (UL). Tell patients not to exceed the UL 50 mcg (2000 units) per day (7555).
POSSIBLY UNSAFE ...when used orally in excessive doses. Doses greater than the tolerable upper intake level (UL) of 50 mcg (2000 units) per day can increase the risk of hypercalcemia (7555).
CHILDREN: LIKELY SAFE ...when used orally and appropriately. Vitamin D is safe when used in doses below the tolerable upper intake level (UL). Children older than one year should not exceed the UL 50 mcg (2000 units) per day; children younger than one year should not exceed the UL 25 mcg (1000 units) per day (7555).
POSSIBLY UNSAFE ...when used orally in excessive amounts. Tell patients not to use doses above the tolerable upper intake level (UL) of 50 mcg (2000 units) per day for children older than one year; children younger than one year should not exceed the UL 25 mcg (1000 units) per day. Higher doses can cause hypercalcemia (7555).
PREGNANCY: LIKELY SAFE ...when used orally and appropriately. Vitamin D is safe when used in doses below the tolerable upper intake level (UL) of 50 mcg (2000 units) per day (7555). POSSIBLY UNSAFE ...when used orally in excessive amounts. Tell patients not to use doses above the tolerable upper intake level (UL) of 50 mcg (2000 units) per day. Hypercalcemia during pregnancy due to excessive vitamin D intake can lead to suppression of parathyroid hormone, hypocalcemia, tetany, seizures, aortic valve stenosis, retinopathy, and mental and/or physical retardation in the infant (7555).
LACTATION: LIKELY SAFE ...when used orally and appropriately. Vitamin D is safe when used in doses below the tolerable upper intake level (UL) of 50 mcg (2000 units) per day (7555). POSSIBLY UNSAFE ...when used orally in excessive amounts. Tell patients not to use doses above the tolerable upper intake level (UL) of 50 mcg (2000 units) per day.

Effectiveness

EFFECTIVE

Familial hypophosphatemia. Taking calcitriol or dihydrotachysterol orally in conjunction with phosphate supplements is effective for treating bone disorders in people with familial hypophosphatemia (11818).
Fanconi syndrome. Taking ergocalciferol orally is effective for treating hypophosphatemia associated with Fanconi syndrome (11819).
Hypoparathyroidism. Taking dihydrotachysterol or calcitriol orally is effective for increasing serum calcium concentrations in people with hypoparathyroidism or pseudohypoparathyroidism. Ergocalciferol is effective in high doses for increasing serum calcium concentrations in people with hypoparathyroidism or pseudohypoparathyroidism (11820).
Osteomalacia. Taking cholecalciferol is effective for treating osteomalacia. Calcifediol orally is effective for treating osteomalacia secondary to liver disease (hepatic osteodystrophy), and anticonvulsant-induced osteomalacia. Ergocalciferol is effective for osteomalacia due to malabsorption syndromes and corticosteroid-induced osteomalacia (11821).
Psoriasis. Applying calcipotriene topically effectively treats plaque-type psoriasis in some patients (11822).
Renal osteodystrophy. Taking calcifediol orally manages hypocalcemia and prevents renal osteodystrophy in people with chronic renal failure undergoing dialysis (11823).
Rickets. Ergocalciferol is effective for treating rickets. Calcitriol should be used in patients with renal failure (11824).

LIKELY EFFECTIVE

Corticosteroid-induced osteoporosis. Taking calcifediol or cholecalciferol orally prevents corticosteroid-induced osteopenia and osteoporosis (7555).
Fall prevention. Vitamin D seems to reduce falls by 22% in older adults. To prevent one fall, 15 older adults would need to be given supplemental vitamin D. This risk reduction appears to be independent of calcium supplementation, but some experts think a combination of calcium and vitamin D may be important (11916). Vitamin D, in combination with calcium, but not calcium alone, may prevent falls by decreasing body sway and systolic blood pressure instead of increasing bone mass strength (6362,11939). Vitamin D deficiency is linked to increased risk of falls (11917,11918).
Osteoporosis. Taking vitamin D orally in conjunction with calcium supplements seems to help treat postmenopausal osteoporosis (7555,11827). Vitamin D with calcium taken orally also seems to decrease the risk of non-vertebral fractures in elderly women (6362). Taking alfacalcidol orally seems to maintain bone density in prostatic carcinoma patients at risk for osteoporosis when treated with luteinizing hormone-releasing hormone analogue (LHRH-a). Alfacalcidol maintains but does not increase bone mineral density (6360). Taking cholecalciferol alone does not seem to prevent fractures in frail elderly people. Daily supplementation for 2 years with 10 mcg vitamin D3 contained in 5 mL of cod liver oil does not prevent hip fracture or other osteoporotic fractures in institutionalized elderly people (10140). However, giving cholecalciferol orally to breast-fed infants also seems to help increase bone mineral density. In a retrospective study, prepubertal girls who received cholecalciferol in infancy had significantly greater bone mineral density at some skeletal sites compared to girls that did not receive vitamin D during infancy (3464).

POSSIBLY EFFECTIVE

Diabetes. Administering calcitriol orally to infants might help prevent the development of type 1 diabetes. Daily vitamin D supplementation in infants during the first year of life is associated with a reduced incidence of type 1 diabetes development later in life (10139).

Hyperparathyroidism-related bone loss. Taking cholecalciferol orally seems to help decrease secondary hyperparathyroidism and bone turnover in women. In one study, supplementation with cholecalciferol resulted in increased serum levels of 25-hydroxyvitamin D, reduced levels of parathyroid hormone, and decreased production of markers of bone turnover (3463).

Multiple sclerosis (MS). Population research suggests that long-term vitamin D supplementation decreases the risk of MS in women by up to 40%. The effect seems to be dose-dependent. Consumption of at least 400 IU per day, mainly in the form of a multivitamin supplement, appears to have the greatest protective effect (11356).

Osteogenesis imperfecta. Taking vitamin D orally seems to help treat osteogenesis imperfecta (11826).

POSSIBLY INEFFECTIVE

Muscle strength. Oral cholecalciferol 1000 IU per day doesn't seem to increase muscle strength or improve physical performance in healthy older men who are not vitamin D deficient (11814).

Renal transplant-related bone loss. Calcitriol 0.25 mcg per day in combination with calcium carbonate 500 mg per day doesn't significantly decrease bone loss associated with long-term renal transplantation; however, calcitriol might reduce osteoclast suppression, help maintain trabecular bone volume and wall thickness, and improve axial bone mineral density (4823).

INSUFFICIENT RELIABLE EVIDENCE to RATE

Myelodysplastic syndrome. Taking calcitriol or calcifediol orally seems to help myelodysplastic syndrome (11825).

Proximal myopathy. Administering ergocalciferol intramuscularly or taking ergocalciferol orally seems to help treat severe proximal myopathy associated with severe vitamin D deficiency. Several case reports suggest vitamin D therapy can provide prompt relief of muscle weakness and restore mobility (6359).

Mechanism of Action

Vitamin D is a fat-soluble vitamin. The term vitamin D refers to several forms of vitamin D. There are 2 forms that are physiologically important, ergocalciferol (vitamin D2) and cholecalciferol (vitamin D3). Ergocalciferol comes from ergosterol, a plant sterol, and yeast. Cholecalciferol is synthesized in the skin via 7-dehydrocholesterol, a cholesterol precursor. Both ergocalciferol and cholecalciferol are biologically inert and require hydroxylation in the body to form the active metabolite, calcitriol (7555). Some research suggests that vitamin cholecalciferol may be more efficient in raising 25-hydroxyvitamin D serum levels, the best measure of vitamin D status (11937,11938).

Very few foods naturally contain vitamin D. Dietary sources include eggs from hens that have been fed vitamin D and fatty fish such as herrings, mackerel, sardines, and tuna. In the US, Canada, and many other countries the main source of dietary vitamin D is fortified milk and other foods. But these are relatively minor sources of vitamin D (7555).

Brief exposure to sunlight (about 25% of the amount of time it would take to cause light pinkness to the skin) is the most efficient way to get vitamin D (11935). Skin exposure to the sun provides as much as 80% to 90% of the body's vitamin D stores (7133). Full-body sun exposure can lead to the synthesis of as much as 10,000 units of vitamin D per day (6855). Vitamin D is stored in body fat for use during periods without sun exposure. Conversely, excessive sun exposure causes photodegradation of vitamin D produced in the skin, limiting the risk of vitamin D toxicity from such exposure (11936). Use of sunscreens can reduce vitamin D synthesis in the body, although this is unlikely to lead to deficiencies, since exposure of the face and arms to the sun for 5-10 minutes, 2-3 times per week ensures adequate synthesis (6855). However, vitamin D supplements may be needed by elderly people with limited sun exposure, people living in northern latitudes, dark-skinned African Americans, Asian Indians living in the western hemisphere, as well as people with gastrointestinal diseases leading to malabsorption of vitamin D from the diet (6855,7133).

The elderly, who generally have less sun exposure and less dietary vitamin D intake, may be at the greatest risk for insufficient vitamin D. Factors such as lack of exposure to sunlight, reduced skin synthesis of vitamin D, lower dietary intake, impaired intestinal absorption, and reduced metabolism to active forms of vitamin D by the kidneys increase with aging (11919). Also, vitamin D receptors seem to decrease with age (11921).

Dark-skinned people need increased exposure to sunlight to produce the same amount of vitamin D as fair-skinned people, because the skin pigment melanin competes with vitamin D precursors in the skin for photons from UV-B light (6857). This also affects vitamin D in breast milk. For example, breast milk from African Americans is generally lower in vitamin D content than that from Caucasian women (35 units/L compared with 68 units/L, respectively) (6857). African American infants who are exclusively breast-fed are therefore at risk for vitamin D deficiency and rickets, even if they live in sunny climates such as the southern US (6857).

Obese people (body mass index >30kg/m2) may have reduced serum vitamin D levels and reduced bioavailability of vitamin D from both cutaneous synthesis and gastrointestinal absorption. In response to similar UV-B exposures, the increase in serum vitamin D levels can be 57% less in obese people than in those who were slim. The content of vitamin D precursors in the skin are similar in both groups, suggesting that vitamin D synthesis is not affected in obese people, but that vitamin D is sequestered into body fat, reducing its availability (6856).

The main function of vitamin D is to regulate serum calcium and phosphorus concentrations. Vitamin D enhances the efficiency of the intestinal absorption of calcium, primarily in the duodenum and jejunum, and phosphorus, particularly in the jejunum and ilium. Vitamin D can increase serum calcium levels, but this effect is modest in healthy people in doses less than 1200 IU per day. If dietary intake of calcium is inadequate, calcitriol in combination with parathyroid hormone mobilizes calcium stores from bone. Calcitrol also appears to have effects in the brain, heart, pancreas, mononuclear cells, activated lymphocytes, and skin, but its exact physiologic role is unclear (7555).

The hydroxylation of vitamin D to calcitriol occurs in the kidneys. People with chronic renal failure may require forms of vitamin D such as calcitriol, dihydrotachysterol, or calcifediol that don't require renal hydroxylation (7555).

In people with granulomatous disorders such as tuberculosis, sarcoidosis, and histoplasmosis, vitamin D metabolism is disturbed. Vitamin D is converted to calcitriol by activated macrophages trapped in the pulmonary alveoli and granulomatous inflammation, in addition to the kidneys. This may increase the risk of hypercalcemia (7555,11881).

Since vitamin D is important for calcium homeostasis and for bone health, it is used to help prevent osteoporosis. Some researchers suggest that postmenopausal women need serum levels of 25-hydroxy-vitamin D (calcifediol) of at least 40 mmol/L for optimal bone health (6854). When intake of calcium is low in healthy elderly women, 25-hydroxy-vitamin D (calcifediol) seems to be more biologically active and a more important determinant of gut calcium absorption than calcitriol (10141). Osteopenia in elderly men also seems to correlate with circulating levels of vitamin D and vitamin K (7132). Vitamin D deficiency causes muscle pain and proximal muscle weakness with symptoms such as sensation of heaviness in the legs, rapid fatigue, and problems with climbing stairs and getting up from a chair. Vitamin D deficiency also increases postural sway and affects psychomotor function (11922,11923,11924,11925).

Vitamin D may prevent falls by increasing muscle strength and neuromuscular function in addition to strengthening bone. It seems to increase muscle protein synthesis, possibly by activating second messengers and phosphorylation (11919,11922). The standard dose of 400 units that is found in most multivitamin tablets appears to be too low to prevent falls or reduce fracture risk, but the optimal dose is unknown (11926,11927,11928). Fractures were reduced in clinical trials using 700 to 800 units of vitamin D daily (980,11930,11931). Some research suggests that sufficient calcium intake along with vitamin D is necessary to prevent falls (11932).

There is some epidemiological evidence that people with vitamin D deficiency might be at an increased risk of colon, breast, and prostate cancer, but more research is needed to know if vitamin D affects cancer risk (7555). Some researchers think vitamin D might have antiproliferative effects in these cancers (6855).

Some evidence suggests vitamin D supplementation during infancy might prevent the development of type 1 diabetes later on in life. Type 1 diabetes is believed to be an autoimmune disease. Vitamin D supplementation might inhibit an autoimmune reaction that targets the beta cells of the pancreas (10139).

Adverse Reactions

Orally, vitamin D is well tolerated. Vitamin D intoxication can occur when vitamin D supplements are taken in excessive doses. Symptoms of vitamin D toxicity include hypercalcemia, azotemia, and anemia. Symptoms of hypercalcemia include weakness, fatigue, sleepiness, headache, loss of appetite, dry mouth, metallic taste, nausea, vomiting, abdominal cramps, constipation, diarrhea, dizziness, ringing in the ears, trouble walking, skin eruptions, hypotonia in infants, muscle pain, bone pain, and irritability. Advanced symptoms may include runny nose, itching, decreased libido, and kidney insufficiency due to precipitation of calcium phosphate in the tubules. Symptoms of renal impairment include frequency, nighttime awakening to urinate, thirst, inability to concentrate urine, and proteinuria. Renal impairment is usually reversible with discontinuation of vitamin D supplements (10142). Other symptoms of vitamin D toxicity include osteoporosis in adults, decreased growth in children, weight loss, anemia, calcific conjunctivitis, photophobia, metastatic calcification, pancreatitis, generalized vascular calcification, and seizures. Rarely, people develop hypertension and psychosis. Lab values of urinary calcium, phosphate, albumin, blood urea nitrogen, serum cholesterol, aspartate aminotransferase, and alanine aminotransferase concentrations might increase (10142). Serum alkaline phosphatase concentrations usually decrease in vitamin D deficiency (7555).

Interactions with Herbs & Other Dietary Supplements

None known.

Interactions with Drugs

PHENYTOIN (Dilantin): Concomitant use might reduce plasma concentrations of the active 25-hydroxylated vitamin D analogs and increase metabolism to inactive metabolites. Vitamin D analogs that require 25-hydroxylation in the body for activity might be ineffective when used with phenytoin (7555).

PHENOBARBITAL (Luminal): Concomitant use might reduce plasma concentrations of the active 25-hydroxylated vitamin D analogs and increase metabolism to inactive metabolites. Vitamin D analogs that require 25-hydroxylation in the body for activity might be ineffective when used with phenobarbital (7555).

THIAZIDE DIURETICS: Concomitant use of thiazides and pharmacologic amounts of vitamin D in people with hyperparathyroidism might result in hypercalcemia (7555).

Drug Influences on Nutrient Levels and Depletion

SOME DRUGS CAN AFFECT VITAMIN D LEVELS:

CARBAMAZEPINE (Tegretol): Carbamazepine increases vitamin D metabolism and reduces vitamin D serum levels. The necessity for supplementation with vitamin D has not been adequately studied (4430,4431).

CHOLESTYRAMINE (Questran, LoCholest, Prevalite): Concomitant use can decrease vitamin D absorption in the gastrointestinal tract. However, there is no clinical evidence that supplementation is necessary (4454,4455,4456,4457,4458,4459).
COLESTIPOL (Colestid): Concomitant use can decrease vitamin D absorption in the gastrointestinal tract. In some cases, supplementation may be appropriate (4460,4461).
CORTICOSTEROIDS: Use of corticosteroids can cause osteoporosis and calcium depletion with long-term administration. This calcium depletion creates a greater need for both supplemental calcium and vitamin D, which is necessary for calcium absorption. It might be prudent to supplement calcium and vitamin D (calcitriol) before, during, and after long-term and/or high-dose corticosteroid therapy (4462,4463,4464,4465,4466,4467).
MINERAL OIL: Mineral oil can reduce dietary vitamin D absorption. Avoid long-term use of mineral oil (4495).
ORLISTAT (Xenical): Orlistat can reduce vitamin D levels (1725,1726,1727,1730). Consider a multivitamin with fat-soluble vitamins, taken at least 2 hours before or after orlistat, or at bedtime.
PHENOBARBITAL (Luminal): Phenobarbital can cause vitamin D deficiency when used long-term. Some authors recommended that patients receiving long-term phenobarbital therapy take 400-800 IU/day of vitamin D and maintain a diet rich in calcium. Other authors suggest that vitamin D should be supplemented only if deficiencies are noted (4531).
PHENYTOIN (Dilantin) and FOSPHENYTOIN (Cerebyx): Use of phenytoin and fosphenytoin can cause vitamin D deficiency when used long-term. Some authors suggest that patients receiving long-term phenytoin therapy should receive 400-800 IU/day of vitamin D and maintain a diet rich in calcium (4475).
RIFAMPIN (Rimactane): Rifampin increases vitamin D metabolism and reduces vitamin D serum levels. The need for vitamin D supplementation has not been adequately studied (4514).
STIMULANT LAXATIVES: Stimulant laxatives can reduce dietary vitamin D absorption. Limit stimulant laxatives to short-term use (4425). Some stimulant laxatives include cascara (CitraMax Plus), senna (Senokot), bisacodyl (Dulcolax), and others.

Interactions with Foods

None known.

Interactions with Lab Tests

None known.

Interactions with Diseases or Conditions

ARTERIOSCLEROSIS: Hypercalcemia can contribute to arteriosclerosis, particularly in patients with kidney disease. Use supplemental vitamin D cautiously (11815,11816).
HISTOPLASMOSIS: Vitamin D may increase calcium levels in people with histoplasmosis. The metabolism to calcitriol is increased in people with histoplasmosis, which may cause hypercalcemia and complications such as kidney stones and calcified tissue. Use supplemental vitamin D cautiously (11881).
HYPERCALCEMIA: Vitamin D supplements may worsen hypercalcemia (11815).
HYPERPARATHYROIDISM: Vitamin D may increase calcium levels in people with hyperparathyroidism. Use supplemental vitamin D cautiously (11815).
LYMPHOMA: Vitamin D may increase calcium levels in people with lymphoma. In some kinds of lymphoma, vitamin D is more readily converted to calcitriol and may result in hypercalcemia and complications such as kidney stones and calcified tissue. Use supplemental vitamin D cautiously (11815,11881).
RENAL DISEASE: Vitamin D may increase calcium levels and increase the risk of arteriosclerosis in renal failure. This must be balanced with the need to prevent renal osteodystrophy. Monitor calcium levels carefully (11816).
SARCOIDOSIS: Vitamin D may increase calcium levels in people with sarcoidosis. The metabolism to calcitriol is increased in people with sarcoidosis, which may cause hypercalcemia and complications such as kidney stones and calcified tissue. Use supplemental vitamin D cautiously (11881).
TUBERCULOSIS: Vitamin D may increase calcium levels in people with tuberculosis. The metabolism to calcitriol is increased in people with tuberculosis, which may cause hypercalcemia and complications such as kidney stones and calcified tissue. Use supplemental vitamin D cautiously (11881).

Dosage and Administration

ORAL: Most vitamin supplements contain the equivalent of 10 mcg (400 units) vitamin D as calcifediol, calcitriol, cholecalciferol, and ergocalciferol. The National Academy of Sciences publishes an Adequate Intake (AI) recommendation which is an estimate of the amount of vitamin D that appears to sustain normal functioning. The current daily AI of vitamin D used as cholecalciferol or ergocalciferol to prevent rickets in healthy children and osteomalacia in adults is based on age. Birth through 50 years of age, 5 mcg (200 units); Adults (ages 51 to 70), 10 mcg (400 units); Adults (greater than 70 years of age), 15 mcg (600 units) daily (7555). Some authorities recommend 1000 units per day for older adults who are not exposed to sunlight (11933).
The upper intake levels (UL) for vitamin D are 25 mcg for infants 0-12 months and 50 mcg for everyone over one year of age (7555).
For preventing multiple sclerosis (MS), long-term consumption of at least 400 IU per day, mainly in the form of a multivitamin supplement, has been used (11356).

For preventing falls, 800 IU per day has been used in combination with calcium 1200 mg per day (11939). Other vitamin D analogs and vitamin D products for other routes of administration are available as FDA-approved prescription drugs.

Comments

One unit of vitamin D equals the biologic activity of 25 nanograms of ergocalciferol or cholecalciferol (7555). Canada recognizes the importance of vitamin D in the prevention of osteoporosis in its health claim for foods that contain calcium: "A healthy diet with adequate calcium and vitamin D, and regular physical activity, help to achieve strong bones and may reduce the risk of osteoporosis" (11940). The US version of this osteoporosis health claim does not yet include vitamin D.

VITAMIN E

Also Known As

All Rac-Alpha-Tocopherol, Alpha-Tocopherol, Alpha Tocopherol Acetate, Alpha Tocopheryl Acetate, d-Alpha-Tocopherol, d-Alpha-Tocopheryl, d-Alpha-Tocopheryl Acetate, d-Alpha-Tocopheryl Succinate, dl-Alpha-Tocopherol, dl-Alpha-Tocopheryl, dl-Alpha-Tocopheryl Acetate, d-Tocopherol, d-Tocopheryl Acetate, dl-Tocopherol, d-Beta-Tocopherol, d-Delta-Tocopherol, d-Gamma-Tocopherol, Mixed Tocopherols, RRR-Alpha-Tocopherol, Tocopherol, Tocopheryl Acetate, Tocopheryl Acid Succinate, Tocopheryl Succinate, Tocotrienol, Tocotrienol Concentrate.

Scientific Names

Alpha-tocopherol; alpha tocotrienol; beta-tocopherol; beta tocotrienol; delta-tocopherol; delta tocotrienol; gamma-tocopherol; gamma tocotrienol.

People Use This For

Orally, vitamin E is used for replacement therapy in vitamin E deficiency, treating and preventing cardiovascular disease, including slowing atherogenesis and preventing heart attacks. It is used orally for angina, thrombophlebitis, intermittent claudication, hypertension, and preventing ischemia-reperfusion injury after coronary artery bypass surgery. Vitamin E is also used orally for treating diabetes and its complications. Vitamin E is used orally for preventing cancer, particularly lung and oral cancer in smokers; colorectal cancer and polyps; and gastric, prostate, and pancreatic cancer. Vitamin E is used orally for Alzheimer's disease and other dementias, Parkinson's disease, night cramps, restless leg syndrome, and as an adjunct in the treatment of epilepsy. Vitamin E is also used orally for preventing pre-eclampsia in high-risk women, for improving physical endurance, increasing energy, preventing allergies, for asthma and respiratory infections, for protecting against negative effects of air pollution, preventing aging, preventing cataracts, and improving healing after photoreactive keratectomy. It is also used orally for inflammatory skin disorders, aging skin, sunburns, cystic fibrosis, oral leukoplakia, premenstrual syndrome (PMS), dysmenorrhea, habitual abortion, menopausal syndrome, hot flashes associated with breast cancer, infertility, impotence, chronic cystic mastitis, mammary dysplasia, peptic ulcers, porphyria, tardive dyskinesia, neuromuscular disorders, Huntington's disease, chronic progressive hereditary chorea, and myotonic dystrophy. Additionally, vitamin E is used orally for preventing vitamin E deficiency in people with malabsorption syndromes or abetalipoproteinemia, treating hemolytic anemia caused by vitamin E deficiency in premature neonates, preventing retinopathy of prematurity, preventing bronchopulmonary dysplasia secondary to oxygen therapy in neonates, and preventing intraventricular hemorrhage in premature neonates. Vitamin E is used orally for correcting erythrocyte membrane abnormalities in people with beta-thalassemia, for hereditary spherocytosis, glucose-6-phosphate dehydrogenase deficiency or sickle-cell anemia, treating anemia in conjunction with erythropoietin in people on dialysis, reducing doxorubicin-induced hair loss, reducing amiodarone-induced pulmonary toxicity, and for radiation-induced fibrosis. Vitamin E is also used orally to treat retinitis pigmentosa, osteoarthritis, nonalcoholic steatohepatitis in children, reduce muscle damage after exercise, and improve muscle strength.

Topically, vitamin E is used for dermatitis, aging skin, granuloma annulare, and protecting against skin ulceration caused by extravasation of chemotherapy drugs.

Safety

LIKELY SAFE ...when used orally or topically and appropriately. Vitamin E is generally considered non-toxic, even at doses exceeding the recommended dietary allowance (RDA); however, adverse effects are more likely to occur with higher doses. The tolerable upper intake level (UL) for vitamin E is 1000 mg per day, equivalent to 1100 IU of synthetic vitamin E and 1500 IU of natural vitamin E (4668,4681,4713,4714,4844).

POSSIBLY UNSAFE ...when used orally in excessive amounts. Repeated administration of doses exceeding the tolerable upper intake level (UL) of 1000 mg per day has been associated with significant side effects (4844). Mega-dosing should be avoided. ...when used intravenously in large doses. Large repeated intravenous doses of all-rac-alpha-tocopherol (synthetic vitamin E) were associated with decreased activity of clotting factors and bleeding in one report (3074).

PREGNANCY: LIKELY SAFE ...when used orally in amounts that do not exceed the recommended dietary allowance (RDA); however, maternal supplementation is not generally recommended unless dietary vitamin E falls below the RDA (4260). POSSIBLY SAFE ...when used orally and appropriately in amounts exceeding the recommended dietary allowance (RDA). No adverse effects were reported with oral intake of 400 IU per day starting at weeks 18-22 of pregnancy in women at high risk for pre-eclampsia (3236), or with 600-900 IU daily during the last two months of pregnancy (4260). There is insufficient reliable information available about the safety of the topical use of vitamin E during pregnancy.

LACTATION: LIKELY SAFE ...when used orally in amounts that do not exceed the recommended dietary allowance (RDA) (4844). There is insufficient reliable information about the safety of vitamin E supplementation in amounts greater than the RDA while nursing.

Effectiveness

EFFECTIVE

Vitamin E deficiency. Taking vitamin E orally is effective for preventing and treating vitamin E deficiency (4844). However, vitamin E deficiency is rare in humans. It most commonly occurs in people with malabsorption disorders such as abetalipoproteinemia; cystic fibrosis; gastrectomy; hepatitic-biliary tract disease including chronic cholestasis, hepatic cirrhosis, biliary atresia, and obstructive jaundice; in infants receiving formula with insufficient vitamin E; intestinal diseases including celiac and tropical sprue; and regional enteritis (4844).

POSSIBLY EFFECTIVE

Age-related macular degeneration (AMD). Taking vitamin E 400 IU orally, plus elemental zinc 80 mg, vitamin C 500 mg, and beta-carotene 15 mg daily seems to provide a risk reduction of 27% for visual acuity loss and a risk reduction of 25% for progression of AMD in patients with advanced AMD (7303). Patients with monocular or binocular intermediate AMD or monocular advanced AMD are at high risk for advanced AMD. Theoretically, these patients may also benefit from vitamin E and antioxidant-zinc supplementation (11326). There isn't enough evidence to know if this combination is beneficial for people with less advanced macular disease or for preventing AMD. Vitamin E with antioxidants, but without zinc, doesn't seem to have any effect on AMD (7303,7304). Vitamin E alone doesn't seem to prevent age-related maculopathy in men who smoke (4667).

Alzheimer's disease. There's some evidence that all-rac-alpha-tocopherol (synthetic vitamin E) 2000 IU per day is similar to selegiline (Eldepryl), and superior to placebo, for slowing cognitive function decline in patients with moderately severe Alzheimer's disease. But there doesn't appear to be an additive effect when vitamin E is used in combination with selegiline (Eldepryl) (4635). Retrospective data suggests that long-term combination therapy with donepezil (Aricept) 5 mg and vitamin E 1000 IU per day may help slow cognitive decline in patients with Alzheimer's disease (11472).

There's conflicting evidence about whether or not vitamin E can decrease the risk of Alzheimer's disease. There's some evidence that long-term use of either vitamin E or vitamin C supplements, or the combination, in doses higher than those typically found in multivitamins, reduces risk of Alzheimer's disease (11390). But other research suggests that vitamin E from dietary sources or supplements does not affect the risk of developing Alzheimer's disease or vascular dementia (4636,9824,10131).

Anemia. Two small studies in adults and children on chronic hemodialysis have shown improved response to erythropoietin with vitamin E supplementation (4640,4647). In one study, children given vitamin E 15 mg/kg in combination with erythropoietin had significantly increased hemoglobin (Hgb) and hematocrit (Hct) levels after two weeks of combination treatment compared to eight and five weeks in patients without combination treatment (4640). In the other study of adults, concurrent supplementation with vitamin E 500 mg daily allowed dose reductions of erythropoietin from an average of 93 U/kg/week to 74 U/kg/week with the same results on Hgb levels (4647). However, vitamin E 50 IU daily does not appear does not increase the response of preterm infants to erythropoietin and iron in anemia of prematurity (10362).

Beta-thalassemia. Taking vitamin E orally seems to be effective for correcting erythrocyte membrane abnormalities in children with beta-thalassemia and low vitamin E plasma concentrations (4642).

Bladder cancer. Taking vitamin E 200 IU orally for greater than 10 years seems to be associated with a reduced risk of bladder cancer mortality (9839).

Chemotherapy extravasation. Applying vitamin E topically, in combination with dimethylsulfoxide (DMSO), seems to be effective for treating chemotherapy extravasation (4668).

Cisplatin-induced neurotoxicity. Alpha-tocopherol administered before chemotherapy, and continued for 3 months after the completion of treatment, seems to reduce the incidence of peripheral neurotoxicity by 55% without affecting cisplatin efficacy (10366).

Colorectal cancer. Taking vitamin E orally, in combination with vitamin A and vitamin C or a multivitamin, seems to have a protective effect in patients with previous colorectal adenomas (3954,3956). A retrospective study has also associated oral vitamin E and multivitamin use with a lower incidence of colorectal cancer (3958); however, vitamin E alone has not been shown to be beneficial (3953,3955,3957).

Dementia. A longitudinal cohort study of 3,385 elderly men aged 71 to 93 years found that men who consumed supplemental vitamin E and vitamin C had a decreased risk of developing vascular and mixed or other dementias; however, there was no protective effect for Alzheimer's dementia. This study did not distinguish between different forms of vitamin E (4636).

Dyspraxia. Taking vitamin E orally, in combination with evening primrose oil, thyme oil, and fish oils seems to improve movement disorders in children with dyspraxia (5708).

Gastroesophageal cancer. In a large-scale study of 29,584 people in China, the combination of oral vitamin E, beta-carotene, and selenium over 5.25 years significantly reduced total mortality, total cancer mortality, and stomach cancer mortality. However, this population has a high risk of gastric cancer, which is thought to be related to poor vitamin and mineral intake (4679). It is unknown if supplementation with these vitamins and minerals would be beneficial in people with adequate nutrition. Although there has been some conflicting evidence (4677), vitamin E alone does not seem to offer this benefit (3960,4676). However, there is preliminary evidence that increasing dietary consumption of vitamin E can slow progression of gastric carcinoma (3360).

Glomerulosclerosis. There is some evidence that vitamin E taken orally might reduce proteinuria in children with focal segmental glomerulosclerosis who are refractory to standard medical management (4675).

Glucose-6-phosphate dehydrogenase (G6PD) deficiency. There is renewed interest in vitamin E taken orally for G6PD deficiency (4685). In two open studies, vitamin E 800 IU alone or in combination with selenium reduced hemolysis and reticulocytosis and increased red blood cell (RBC) half-life and vitamin E levels in patients with G6PD deficiency (4682,4683). In one study, vitamin E plus selenium 25 mcg daily offered significantly more improvement compared to vitamin E alone (4683). These findings are contrary to an earlier study that found no effect with vitamin E at 2000 to 2400 IU per day (4684).

Granuloma annulare. Topical vitamin E seems to clear granuloma annulare lesions within one to three weeks (4681).

Huntington's disease. RRR-alpha-tocopherol (natural vitamin E) can significantly improve symptoms in patients with early Huntington's disease, but this benefit is not seen in patients with more advanced disease (4686).

Infertility. In one study, males with asthenospermia or oligoasthenospermia, receiving oral vitamin E supplementation, achieved impregnation at a rate of 21% compared to none for similar patients receiving placebo (4695). In another study, males enrolled in an in vitro fertilization program who had previously had low fertilization rates were treated with oral vitamin E for three months. Fertilization rates increased significantly from 19% to 29% after one month of treatment (3583). In a crossover trial, males found to have elevated reactive oxygen species in their semen, which might be associated with infertility, were treated with oral vitamin E. After treatment, in vitro sperm binding to the zona pellucida was significantly increased (4693). Interestingly, high-dose vitamin E in combination with vitamin C does not seem to offer any benefit to sperm functionality (4696). Vitamin E plus selenium seems to improve sperm functionality, but doesn't improve fertilization rates (3585). Although vitamin E preparations used alone appear to offer some benefit in men with asthenospermia or oxidative damage to sperm, combining vitamin E with vitamin C or selenium does not appear to be beneficial. Studies did not differentiate between different forms of vitamin E.

Intracranial hemorrhage. Taking vitamin E orally seems to be effective for treating intracranial hemorrhage in premature neonates (4655).

Intraventricular hemorrhage. Taking vitamin E orally seems to be effective for treating intraventricular hemorrhage in premature neonates (4656).

Ischemic reperfusion injury. Taking vitamin E orally with vitamin C and allopurinol two days prior to coronary bypass surgery and one day postoperatively, patients had fewer perioperative infarctions and less creatine kinase-MB release (4699); however, this benefit was not found when using vitamin E alone or in combination with vitamin C without allopurinol (4697,4698).

Nitrate tolerance. In a small placebo-controlled study, patients with ischemic heart disease and healthy volunteers receiving vitamin E had a decreased attenuation of response to nitroglycerin compared to placebo (4705).

Osteoarthritis. Taking vitamin E orally might slow progression of osteoarthritis but does not seem to improve symptoms of pain or stiffness (5264,5881). Vitamin E also does not seem to help prevent osteoarthritis from developing (5881).

Parkinson's disease. Preliminary evidence suggests that dietary vitamin E intake might be associated with a decreased occurrence of Parkinson's disease (4712). But taking all rac-alpha-tocopherol (synthetic vitamin E) 2000 IU supplements daily does not seem to have any benefit for patients who have Parkinson's disease (4709,4710,4711).

Photoreactive keratectomy. High dose (50,000 to 75,000 units) vitamin A in the form of retinol palmitate taken orally with 230 mg vitamin E (alpha-tocopheryl nicotinate) daily seems to accelerate re-epithelialization, reduce haze formation, and improve visual acuity in patients undergoing laser surgery for myopia (348).

Pre-eclampsia. Taking a combination of vitamin E 400 IU and vitamin C 1000 mg daily significantly reduced the risk of proteinuric hypertension in high-risk women when started in weeks 16 to 22 of pregnancy (3236). Other researchers using vitamin E in combination with vitamin C and allopurinol beginning at 24 to 32 weeks gestation found the combination similar to placebo (4718).

Premenstrual syndrome (PMS). Taking vitamin E orally seems to reduce symptoms of anxiety, craving, and depression in patients with PMS (4719,4720).

Prostate cancer. In one study, 29,133 smokers taking 50 mg per day of all-rac-alpha-tocopherol (synthetic vitamin E), either alone or in combination with beta-carotene, had a significantly lower incidence of prostate cancer and mortality associated with prostate cancer (3959,11303). Epidemiological studies also support an inverse relationship between vitamin E consumption and the risk of prostate cancer. These epidemiological studies did not distinguish between different forms of vitamin E (4644,4645,4646).

Radiation-induced fibrosis. Taking vitamin E 1000 IU orally with pentoxifylline 800 mg daily seems to reverse radiation-induced fibrosis (4672,4673). Regression of radiation-induced fibrosis becomes significant after three months of treatment and continues to improve thereafter. After 12 months of treatment, mean surface area of fibrosis can decrease by 66% (4672). However, vitamin E alone doesn't seem to be effective (10363).

Retrolental fibroplasia. Taking vitamin E orally seems to be effective for treating retrolental fibroplasia in premature neonates (10).

Rheumatoid arthritis (RA). Vitamin E taken orally in conjunction with standard therapy is superior to standard therapy alone for reducing pain, but not inflammation in patients with RA (4723).

Sunburn. High dose oral RRR-alpha-tocopherol (natural vitamin E) in combination with vitamin C protected against skin inflammation after exposure to ultraviolet (UV) radiation in two small, double-blind, placebo-controlled studies (4715,4716). Alpha-tocopherol acetate 400 IU alone does not seem to offer this benefit (4715). In one study, topically applied vitamin E in combination with topical vitamin C and melatonin provided modest photoprotective effect when used prior to UV exposure, but had no effect when used during or after UV exposure (4713,4714).

Tardive dyskinesia. Taking vitamin E orally seems to significantly improve Abnormal Involuntary Movement Scale (AIMS) scores in people with tardive dyskinesia. It seems to be more effective in higher doses and in people who have had tardive dyskinesia for less than five years (3942,3943,3944,3945,3946,3948). In the largest study to date, conflicting findings have been reported; however, this study has not yet been published, preventing further evaluation of its findings (3947). Both RRR-alpha-tocopherol (natural vitamin E) and unspecified forms were used in clinical trials.

Uveitis. Taking vitamin E orally with vitamin C seems to improve visual acuity in patients with acute anterior uveitis, but does not seem to decrease inflammation measured by laser flare (4730).

POSSIBLY INEFFECTIVE

Angina. Taking vitamin E orally may have some effect on endothelial dysfunction, but doesn't seem to help nonsmokers or smokers with angina (3896,4634,4649,4650,4651,4652).

Atherosclerosis. Taking RRR-alpha-tocopherol (natural vitamin E) orally doesn't appear to have any effect on atherosclerosis progression or mortality in patients with atherosclerosis (3899,3936). However, there is preliminary evidence that a combination of vitamin E and vitamin C, might help prevent the progression of atherosclerosis in men, particularly smokers and cardiac transplant patients (1918).

Breast cancer-related hot flashes. Taking vitamin E orally does not seem to significantly reduce hot flashes in women who have had breast cancer (454). There have been no clinical trials using vitamin E supplementation for postmenopausal symptoms.

Bronchopulmonary dysplasia. In one study, taking vitamin E orally had no benefit for treating bronchopulmonary dysplasia in premature infants weighing less than 1500 grams at birth (4657).

Congestive heart failure (CHF). Taking vitamin E orally for 12 weeks doesn't seem to improve prognostic or functional indices of CHF or improve quality-of-life measurements (3906).

Duchenne muscular dystrophy. A double-blind study in 106 boys for 18 months found no difference between placebo and combination oral vitamin E and penicillamine for slowing disease progression (4703). Hemolytic anemia. Vitamin E 25 IU per day given to premature infants for six weeks seems to have no beneficial effects on hemolytic anemia (4648).

Hypertension. Taking vitamin E orally for 3 to 4 years doesn't seem to lower blood pressure in patients already on hypertension treatment (5210).

Intermittent claudication. Taking all rac-alpha-tocopherol (synthetic vitamin E) orally doesn't appear to have any effect when used alone or in combination with beta-carotene for treating symptoms or disease progression in male smokers (4732).

Lung cancer. Taking all rac-alpha-tocopherol (synthetic vitamin E) 50 mg per day for 5 to 8 years is not associated with a lower risk of developing lung cancer for male smokers (3949).

Myotonic dystrophy. A small study comparing placebo to combination vitamin E and selenium taken orally showed no difference in functional deterioration over two years (4704).

Oral mucosal lesions. Although there is some conflicting evidence (3951,4708), the largest and most significant controlled trial indicates that supplementation with all rac-alpha-tocopherol (synthetic vitamin E) 50 mg daily for five to seven years has no effect on the incidence of oral lesions in male cigarette smokers (3951).

Pancreatic cancer. Taking all rac-alpha-tocopherol (synthetic vitamin E) 50 mg daily supplements for 5 to 8 years by male smokers does not reduce the incidence or mortality of carcinoma of the pancreas (3961).

Respiratory infections. Taking oral vitamin E 200 mg daily, alone or in supplemental multivitamin form, does not appear to decrease the incidence, duration, or severity of upper or lower respiratory infections in elderly persons (10788,12094). But some evidence suggests that vitamin E might reduce the incidence of the common cold in elderly long-term care patients (12094). More evidence is needed to determine how effective vitamin E might be for reducing the incidence of the common cold.

Retinitis pigmentosa. Taking all rac-alpha-tocopherol (synthetic vitamin E) orally does not appear to slow visual decline is people with retinitis pigmentosa and has been associated with more rapid loss of visual acuity, although the validity of the study with these findings has been questioned (83,84,85,86,87,88).

Scarring. Applying vitamin E topically doesn't seem to reduce surgical wound scarring (4721,4722).

LIKELY INEFFECTIVE

Breast cancer. Neither dietary nor supplemental vitamin E intake has shown any protective effect for breast cancer or mammary dysplasia (4658,4659,4660,4661,4662). However, there is some evidence that an inverse association might exist between serum vitamin E levels and the risk of developing breast cancer (10132).

Cardiovascular disease. Taking vitamin E supplements orally is not effective for preventing heart disease and cardiovascular events such as myocardial infarction (MI). Observational studies have associated vitamin E with reductions in cardiovascular events (3898,3933,3934). Some evidence also suggests dietary vitamin E can decrease the risk of peripheral arterial disease in men, but not in women (10130). However, clinical trials using vitamin E supplements do not support the epidemiological evidence (10365). With few exceptions (3357,3936), large-scale controlled clinical trials show that vitamin E supplements offer no benefit for primary prevention in high risk patients (3907,3935,3937), or secondary prevention of heart disease and cardiovascular events such as MI, stroke, and death (3896,3899). Based on these findings, the FDA has refused to allow labeling claims for vitamin E supplements for prevention of cardiovascular disease (3939). Tell patients not to rely on vitamin E supplements for preventing heart disease. Recommend increasing dietary vitamin E consumption instead. A Science Advisory from the American Heart Association also states that the evidence does not justify use of antioxidants such as vitamin E for reducing the risk of cardiovascular disease (12142). Tell patients not to rely on vitamin E supplements for preventing heart disease. Recommend increasing dietary vitamin E consumption instead.

INSUFFICIENT RELIABLE EVIDENCE to RATE

Cataracts. There is conflicting information about the use of vitamin E to prevent cataracts. Vitamin E alone or in combination with other vitamins does not seem to prevent the development and progression of age-related cataracts and vision loss (4666,7304). Vitamin E plus vitamin C and beta-carotene with zinc doesn't seem to have any significant effect on age-related loss of vision due to cataracts in well-nourished people when taken for an average of 6.3 years (7304), but most population research suggests a beneficial effect of vitamin E (2395,4208,4663,4664,4665,4759). Vitamin E use in multivitamins or any supplement containing vitamin E for ten years appears to reduce the incidence of nuclear and cortical cataracts by 60%, according to epidemiological research. Use of supplements for shorter periods doesn't appear to reduce the risk for cataract development (4208).

Chemotherapy-related infection. Observational research suggests that greater dietary intake of vitamin E may lower the incidence of infection in children undergoing chemotherapy for lymphoblastic leukemia (11997).

Common cold. Preliminary evidence suggests that elderly patients in long-term care facilities, who take vitamin E 200 IU daily, have a lower incidence of the common cold (12094).

Diabetes. Vitamin E might be beneficial in diabetes and diabetic neuropathy, retinopathy, and nephropathy. Some evidence suggests it improves glucose disposal in type 2 diabetics (4726,4727), improves monocyte function, which lessens atherogenesis (95), improves nerve conduction in diabetic neuropathy (4724), improves retinal blood flow, and decreases creatinine clearance (4725).

In type 1 diabetes, clinical research indicates that vitamin E might have a role in the management of early vascular disease by improving endothelial vasodilator function (94). One study has shown that 750 IU (503 mg) RRR-alpha-tocopherol daily for one year decreased lipoprotein susceptibility to copper oxidization in type 1 diabetics (3358).

Dysmenorrhea. Preliminary clinical research suggests vitamin E supplementation might reduce menstrual pain in teenaged girls with primary dysmenorrhea (10361).

Epilepsy. There is preliminary evidence that vitamin E might reduce seizure frequency in refractory epilepsy; however, trials have been few and contradictory (4670,4671,6066).

Hyperlipidemia. Some preliminary clinical research suggests that vitamin E in combination with vitamin C might restore endothelial function in hyperlipidemic children, which might slow progression of atherosclerosis (10352).

Ischemic stroke. There is some evidence that all rac-alpha-tocopherol (synthetic vitamin E) might reduce the risk of ischemic stroke in male smokers with hypertension and diabetes (3359).

Liver transplant. A water soluble form of vitamin E, tocopheryl succinate polyethylene glycol 10,000 (TPGS), may improve absorption of cyclosporine after liver transplant (10368).

Nocturnal leg cramps. Limited evidence suggests vitamin E might offer some benefit for nocturnal leg cramps (4700,4701), but there is conflicting evidence (4702).

Sickle cell disease. Taking vitamin E orally with aged garlic extract and vitamin C might be useful for sickle cell anemia (5056).

Steatohepatitis. Preliminary clinical evidence indicates that vitamin E may be helpful in nonalcoholic steatohepatitis in children; however, long-term studies have not been performed (89).

More evidence is needed to rate vitamin E for these uses.

Mechanism of Action

Vitamin E is a fat-soluble vitamin present in many foods including vegetable oils, cereal grains, animal fats, meat, poultry, eggs, fruits, and vegetables (96). Wheat germ oil is a particularly rich source of vitamin E. Maximum vitamin E intake from diet alone typically reaches about 60 IU per day (97). Vitamin E deficiency is rare and most typically seen in genetic abnormalities that prevent maintenance of normal blood concentrations of vitamin E or conditions that prevent absorption. Vitamin E deficiency does not cause specific disease in adults, although creatinuria, ceroid deposition, muscle weakness, and decreased erythrocyte survival are associated with low serum vitamin E concentrations. In adults, total body stores of vitamin E, found in adipose tissue, have been estimated to be 3-8 grams and are sufficient to meet the body's requirements for four or more years of a deficient diet. In premature infants,

vitamin E deficiency can cause irritability, edema, thrombosis, and hemolytic anemia (15).
Unlike most nutrients, vitamin E does not appear to have a specific role in a required metabolic process. The major function of vitamin E is probably that of a chain-breaking antioxidant that prevents the formation of free radicals. Vitamin E's therapeutic benefits have primarily been attributed to its antioxidant effects. Vitamin E exists in eight forms, including alpha-, beta-, gamma-, and delta-tocopherols and four tocotrienols. Although vitamin E exists in numerous forms, supplemental vitamin E usually refers to alpha-tocopherol. For biological activity, vitamin E is dependent on hepatic alpha-tocopherol transfer protein (alpha-TTP) for distribution. Although the typical diet contains other forms of vitamin E (beta-, gamma-, and delta-tocopherols), these have very limited systemic bioavailability because they do not bind with alpha-TTP. Supplemental beta-, gamma-, and delta-tocopherols, and tocotrienols appear to have little in vivo activity in humans and do not contribute toward meeting established vitamin E requirements (4844). Only the alpha-tocopherol form of vitamin E is maintained in plasma and thought to be therapeutically useful. Alpha-tocopherol exists as eight stereoisomers. The RRR-alpha-tocopherol isomer, formerly called d-alpha-tocopherol, has the greatest affinity for alpha-TTP and the most biologic activity (4844). RRR-alpha-tocopherol is sometimes called natural vitamin E and occurs naturally in foods (3940,4844). The racemic mixture of all eight alpha-tocopherol isomers, or all rac-alpha-tocopherol, was formerly known as dl-alpha-tocopherol (4844). All rac-alpha-tocopherol, sometimes called synthetic vitamin E, is found in vitamin E-fortified foods. Both forms of vitamin E, natural and synthetic, can be found in vitamin E supplements. All rac-alpha-tocopherol has lower affinity for alpha-TTP and thus has less biologic activity than RRR-alpha-tocopherol (4627,4844). Based on weight, 15 mg of RRR-alpha tocopherol is approximately equivalent in potency to 30 mg of all rac-alpha-tocopherol (99,200,218,4844). Although higher bioavailability for the natural form is well-known, the relative potency of natural and synthetic vitamin E is controversial. Some researchers cite the potency of the natural to synthetic form as 1.36, rather than 2.0 (100,202,247,248). Therapeutic benefits of vitamin E have largely been attributed to its role as an antioxidant. Oxidative damage has been attributed to many conditions for which vitamin E is used, including lipid peroxidation in heart disease (6204). Some preliminary research suggests that vitamin E might inhibit the local inflammatory process and oxidation of low-density lipoprotein (LDL) cholesterol that is associated with atherosclerosis (97,249), but when this theory was tested in healthy adults without heart disease, RRR-alpha-tocopherol, even at 2000 IU per day, did not produce markers that indicate a reduction in lipid oxidation (3370). This appears to be another case where promising laboratory data turns out to be clinically irrelevant. Vitamin E also doesn't appear to improve endothelium-dependent vasodilation in older adults with hypercholesterolemia (11286).
Some researchers think the antioxidant activity of vitamin E may slow progression of renal disease. Oxidative metabolites may accumulate in renal dysfunction. Vitamin E could theoretically slow the rate of decline in chronic inflammatory kidney diseases such as IgA nephropathy, diabetic nephropathy, and glomerulosclerosis; and poisoning by nephrotoxic drugs and other compounds (10369).
In tardive dyskinesia, it is thought that some patients may have increased dopamine turnover resulting in increased production of free radicals and structural damage. Additionally, people with tardive dyskinesia may have decreased levels of vitamin E and vitamin C (3598). Oxidative damage has also been associated with diabetes and related complications.
Oxidative damage has also long been associated with the development of cancers. Vitamin E and other antioxidants are theorized to minimize this damage (5882). Several mechanisms have been theorized for reducing bladder carcinogenesis, including the neutralization of reactive oxygen species, the inhibition of the formation of nitrosamines, and an enhancement of immune function (9839). Preliminary evidence also suggests vitamin E and other antioxidants can decrease oxidative damage associated with tumor-directed radio-immunotherapy (5882). Vitamin E is used for photo-aged skin and to prevent oxidative skin damage related to ultraviolet (UV) radiation (e.g., sunburn) due to its antioxidant effects. However, some researchers think that this benefit requires concomitant use with other antioxidants such as vitamin C to prevent degradation of vitamin E (6062,6064). Chemotherapy and radiation therapy also adversely affect vitamin E status (98).
Vitamin E status may also decline with standard parenteral nutrition formulas. Lipid emulsions and amino acid solutions appear to be susceptible to oxidative degradation with storage (98).
Vitamin E appears to slow the progression of Alzheimer's disease, possibly due to an interaction with free radicals and a disruption of cellular damage (11472). Preliminary data suggests vitamin E might improve cognitive function by decreasing beta-amyloid damage (4637,4638,4639).
Some evidence links asthma to increased oxidative stress and vitamin E deficiency (315,401,409,422,6058). Epidemiological and case-control studies have associated asthma with lower vitamin E intake, lower vitamin E serum levels, and lower vitamin levels in lung lining fluid, but clinical studies using vitamin E supplementation for asthma have not been performed (315,401,409,422,6058).
Lower vitamin E serum levels have also been associated with higher IgE levels and positive allergen skin tests (5275).
In addition to its antioxidant function, vitamin E inhibits protein kinase C activity, which is involved in cell proliferation and differentiation in several cell types, including smooth muscle, platelets, and monocytes (4844).
Preliminary research suggests that vitamin E might have an antiproliferative effect on benign hyperplastic prostate cells (11235).
Large amounts of vitamin E interfere with vitamin K-dependent clotting factor production, producing hypoprothrombinemic effects, especially in people with vitamin K deficiency or those who are taking oral anticoagulants (3073,3074). Mixed tocopherols seem to have a greater effect on platelet aggregation than alpha-tocopherol alone, which might explain the discrepancy between the effects of dietary vitamin E intake and

supplemental vitamin E (alpha-tocopherol) in cardiovascular disease. Mixed tocopherols seem to increase nitric oxide (NO) release and superoxide dismutase (SOD) protein content in platelets, which may contribute to the effect on platelet aggregation (10364).

For immune function in the elderly, vitamin E supplementation might replenish an inapparent deficiency. Deficiency of vitamin E and other micronutrients are common in apparently well-nourished people over age 90 and might affect the number and function of natural killer cells in old age (4688). Most research suggests that vitamin E supplementation in healthy elderly people improves response to delayed-type hypersensitivity skin testing (DTH), an indicator of immune function, and antibody response to hepatitis B, tetanus and diphtheria, and pneumococcal vaccines (4676,4689,4690,4691). But whether vitamin E supplementation results in better health in elderly people is unknown.

In the treatment of epilepsy, vitamin E is primarily used because some patients taking anti-epileptic drugs have decreased blood levels of vitamin E. Vitamin E might also act as a membrane stabilizer and enzyme repressor in these patients (3356,6066).

Although biological activity of other forms is significantly less and current guidelines do not include forms of vitamin E other than alpha-tocopherol for meeting dietary requirements (4844), the other forms, such as gamma-tocopherol and the tocotrienols, have been associated with some pharmacological activity. For example, gamma-tocopherol appears to decrease the programmed death of human coronary artery endothelial cells, possibly by decreasing LDL oxidation (4092). Gamma-tocopherol inhibits prostate cancer cell growth in vitro (4089). Gamma-tocopherol also appears to prolong prothrombin and partial thromboplastin times and has caused hemorrhage in experimental animals (4098). Beta- and delta-tocopherol have also been shown to prolong prothrombin and partial thromboplastin times in laboratory animals (4098). RRR-alpha-tocopheryl succinate, known as vitamin E succinate (VES), is currently being researched for its chemotherapeutic and chemopreventive potential. VES has been shown to inhibit tumor cell growth, primarily by triggering apoptosis in human prostate carcinoma (3361). There is some evidence that the inhibitory effect on cancer cell growth by statin drugs with a closed ring structure, such as mevastatin and lovastatin (Mevacor), may be enhanced when used with alpha tocopheryl succinate (8046). The tocotrienols from rice and barley bran might lower total cholesterol and LDL, possibly by decreasing activity of HMG CoA reductase, but in a different way than "statin" drugs (3237,3238,3239,3240,3241). Tocotrienols might also be capable of decreasing carotid artery plaque size in some people, possibly by decreasing platelet aggregation (3239).

Some people think that taking vitamin E with a high fat meal is necessary to increase absorption. However, vitamin E (d-alpha-tocopherol) is similarly absorbed when taken with high-fat (36 grams) or low-fat (3 grams) meals (6133).

In conditions with severe fat malabsorption such as short bowel syndrome, lipid soluble forms of vitamin E, such as those in food, may not be absorbed. A water soluble form of vitamin E such as tocopheryl succinate polyethylene glycol 10,000 (TPGS), may improve vitamin E status in these people (10367).

Adverse Reactions

Orally, vitamin E seldom causes adverse effects. In uncommon cases, vitamin E can cause nausea, diarrhea, intestinal cramps, fatigue, weakness, headache, blurred vision, rash, gonadal dysfunction, and creatinuria. It is unclear if vitamin E contributes to increased risk of hemorrhagic stroke. One study suggested a higher incidence of hemorrhagic stroke in male smokers taking all rac-alpha-tocopherol (synthetic vitamin E), but several other studies lasting from 1.4 years to 4.5 years with study participants taking either all rac-alpha-tocopherol (synthetic vitamin E) or RRR-alpha-tocopherol (natural vitamin E) showed no increased risk for stroke (2307,3896,3936,3949,4635). High doses of vitamin E might increase the risk of bleeding due to antagonism of vitamin K-dependent clotting factors and platelet aggregation. Patients with vitamin K deficiencies or taking anticoagulant or antiplatelet drugs are at a greater risk for bleeding (4844,11999).

There is some evidence that vitamin E in combination with simvastatin (Zocor), niacin, selenium, vitamin C, and beta-carotene might lower high density lipoprotein-2 (HDL-2) by 15%, HDL-2 is considered to be the most cardioprotective component of HDL (7388). However, vitamin E and a statin alone don't seem to negatively affect HDL (11286,11287).

Although only certain isomers of vitamin E are included for determination of dietary requirements, all isomers are considered for determining safe intake levels. All the isomers are thought to potentially contribute to toxicity.

Topically, vitamin E has been associated with contact dermatitis, inflammatory reactions, and eczematous lesions (11998).

Interactions with Herbs & Other Dietary Supplements

HERBS WITH ANTICOAGULANT/ANTIPLATELET POTENTIAL: Vitamin E inhibits platelet aggregation and adhesion (4844). Concomitant use with herbs that also affect platelet aggregation could theoretically increase the risk of bleeding in some people. These herbs include angelica, asafoetida, clove, danshen, garlic, ginger, ginkgo, Panax ginseng, horse chestnut, meadowsweet, poplar, quassia, red clover, willow, and others.

IRON: Concomitant use of vitamin E in amounts greater than 10 units/kg per day can delay the response to iron therapy in children with iron-deficiency anemia (15).

NIACIN, NIACINAMIDE (VITAMIN B3): There is some evidence that niacin, simvastatin (Zocor), and vitamin E in combination with selenium, vitamin C, and beta-carotene might lower high density lipoprotein-2 (HDL-2) by 15%, HDL-2 is considered to be the most cardioprotective component of HDL (7388).

OMEGA-6 FATTY ACIDS: Increased intake of omega-6 fatty acids may increase vitamin E requirements,

particularly at higher doses (4844).
VITAMIN A: Based on cell culture and animal studies, it's been suggested that vitamin E affects the activity of vitamin A. These include preventing oxidation in the gut and increasing absorption, enhancing utilization, promoting liver storage, protecting against cell damage caused by high vitamin A levels, and reducing some of the symptoms of hypervitaminosis A (10545,10557,10558,10560).

Interactions with Drugs

ANTICOAGULANT/ANTIPLATELET DRUGS: Concomitant use of vitamin E and anticoagulant or antiplatelet agents might increase the risk of bleeding, possibly through inhibition of platelet aggregation and antagonism of vitamin K-dependent clotting factors (4733,4844). Mixed tocopherols, such as those found in food, seem to have a greater antiplatelet effect than alpha-tocopherol (10364). RRR alpha-tocopherol 1000 IU per day antagonizes vitamin K dependent clotting factors (11999). Anticoagulant and antiplatelet drugs that might interact with vitamin E include aspirin, clopidogrel (Plavix), dalteparin (Fragmin), enoxaparin (Lovenox), heparin, ticlopidine (Ticlid), warfarin (Coumadin), and others.
CHEMOTHERAPY: Preliminary evidence suggests antioxidants such as vitamin E and vitamin A might reduce the effectiveness of cancer chemotherapy (391). Patients undergoing chemotherapy should not use vitamin E and other antioxidants without the supervision of a healthcare provider.
HMG-CoA REDUCTASE INHIBITORS ("Statins"): There is some evidence that simvastatin, niacin, and vitamin E in combination with selenium, vitamin C, and beta-carotene might lower high density lipoprotein-2 (HDL-2) by 15%, HDL-2 is considered to be the most cardioprotective component of HDL (7388). However, vitamin E and a statin alone don't seem to negatively affect HDL (11286,11287). HMG-CoA reductase inhibitors include atorvastatin (Lipitor), cerivastatin (Baycol), fluvastatin (Lescol), lovastatin (Mevacor), pravastatin (Pravachol), and simvastatin (Zocor).
NIACIN: There is some evidence that niacin, simvastatin (Zocor), and vitamin E in combination with selenium, vitamin C, and beta-carotene might lower high density lipoprotein-2 (HDL-2) by 15%, HDL-2 is considered to be the most cardioprotective component of HDL (7388).
WARFARIN (Coumadin): Use of more than 400 IU of vitamin E per day with warfarin might prolong prothrombin time (PT), INR, and increase the risk of bleeding, due to interference with production of vitamin K-dependent clotting factors (91,92,93). At a dose of 1000 IU per day, vitamin E can antagonize vitamin K dependent clotting factors even in people not taking warfarin (11999). The risk for vitamin E interaction with warfarin is greater in people who are already deficient in vitamin K (91,92,93). Limited clinical evidence suggests that doses up to 1200 IU daily may be used safely by patients taking warfarin, but this may not be applicable in all patient populations (90). Monitor INR closely in patients taking warfarin who start vitamin E in doses of 400 IU or more.

Drug Influences on Nutrient Levels and Depletion

SOME DRUGS CAN AFFECT VITAMIN E LEVELS:
CHOLESTYRAMINE (Questran): Cholestyramine can reduce dietary vitamin E absorption and serum levels (4455,4456).
COLESTIPOL (Colestid): Colestipol can reduce dietary vitamin E absorption and serum levels (4460,4461).
ETHANOL: Theoretically, ethanol might decrease serum levels of alpha- and gamma-tocopherol, contributing to liver injury (4097).
FISH OILS: Dietary fish oils can reduce vitamin E levels. The mechanism is unknown, but might result from reduced vitamin E absorption or increased vitamin E utilization by tissues to reduce free radicals and prevent peroxidative damage (7384).
GEMFIBROZIL (Lopid): Gemfibrozil can decrease serum levels of both alpha- and gamma-tocopherol, but the clinical significance of this is not known (4096).
MINERAL OIL: Mineral oil can reduce dietary vitamin E absorption and serum levels. Avoid long-term use of mineral oil (4495,4496).
ORLISTAT (Xenical): Orlistat can reduce the absorption of beta-carotene and some fat-soluble vitamins (1725,1726,1727). Consider a multivitamin with fat-soluble vitamins, taken at least 2 hours before or after orlistat, or at bedtime.

Interactions with Foods

FOODS HIGH IN FAT: High-fat meals might increase vitamin E absorption; however, the amount of fat required to facilitate vitamin E absorption has not been established (4844).

Interactions with Lab Tests

PROTHROMBIN TIME (PT)/INTERNATIONAL NORMALIZED RATIO (INR): High dose vitamin E might increase PT and INR in patients concurrently taking warfarin or other anticoagulant agents (4844). People with vitamin K deficiency are at greater risk for vitamin E interference with clotting and increased PT and INR (91,92,93).

Interactions with Diseases or Conditions

ANGIOPLASTY: There is some concern that when antioxidant vitamins, including vitamin E, are used together they might have harmful effects in patients after angioplasty. A combination of beta-carotene 30,000 IU, vitamin C

500 mg, and vitamin E 700 IU daily started 30 days before angioplasty, and continued for 6 months thereafter, seems to prevent beneficial vascular remodeling in patients after angioplasty by promoting fibrosis at the site of angioplastic intervention (11000). Tell patients to avoid taking supplements of these vitamins immediately before and following angioplasty without the supervision of a healthcare professional.
BLEEDING DISORDERS: Vitamin E in doses of 1000 IU per day can decrease vitamin K dependent clotting factors and may exacerbate bleeding disorders (11999); use with caution.
PRE-ECLAMPSIA: Vitamin E with vitamin C helps prevent pre-eclampsia in high-risk women (3236).
RETINITIS PIGMENTOSA: All rac-alpha-tocopherol (synthetic vitamin E) 400 IU has been associated with accelerated visual decline in people with retinitis pigmentosa. However, much lower doses (3 IU) does not seem to produce this effect (83).
VITAMIN K DEFICIENCY: Vitamin E might worsen coagulation defects in people with vitamin K deficiency (11999); use cautiously.

Dosage and Administration

ORAL: A typical dose for vitamin E deficiency in adults is RRR-alpha tocopherol (natural vitamin E) 60-75 IU per day (15). For tardive dyskinesia, most studies used RRR-alpha-tocopherol (natural vitamin E) 1600 IU daily (3942,3943,3944). For improving male fertility, vitamin E (type unspecified) 200 to 600 IU daily has been used (4693). For Alzheimer's disease, a typical dose is up to 2000 IU daily (4635). Combination therapy of donepezil (Aricept) 5 mg and vitamin E 1000 IU per day has been used for slowing cognitive decline in patients with Alzheimer's disease (11472). For early Huntington's chorea, one study used RRR-alpha-tocopherol (natural vitamin E) 3000 IU (4686). Rheumatoid arthritis pain has been treated with vitamin E (type unspecified) 600 IU twice daily (4723). For diabetic neuropathy, vitamin E (type unspecified) 900 mg daily has been used (4724). For preventing neurotoxicity caused by cisplatin, vitamin E (alpha-tocopherol) 300 mg daily has been used with each chemotherapy treatment and for up to 3 months after stopping cisplatin therapy (10366). For improving retinal blood flow and creatinine clearance in type 1 diabetes, vitamin E (type unspecified) 1800 IU has been used (4725). For enhancing immune function in elderly people, vitamin E (type unspecified) 100 to 200 mg daily has been used (4687,4689,4690). For preventing nitrate tolerance, vitamin E (type unspecified) 200 mg three times daily has been used (4705). For improving response to erythropoietin in people on dialysis, adults have received vitamin E (type unspecified) 300 to 500 mg daily, and children have received 15 mg per kg per day (4640,4641,4647). For children with focal segmental glomerulosclerosis, vitamin E (type unspecified) 200 IU has been used to reduce proteinuria (4675). For G6PD deficiency, vitamin E (type unspecified) 800 IU daily has been used (4682,4683). For children with familial hypercholesterolemia, vitamin E 200 IU, with vitamin C 250 mg, 2 times daily has been used for up to 6 months, with a National Cholesterol Education Program Step II (NCEP-II) diet (10352). For premenstrual syndrome (PMS), RRR-alpha-tocopherol (natural vitamin E) 400 IU daily has been used (4719). For treatment of dysmenorrhea, vitamin E 500 IU daily has been used starting 2 days before the menstrual period began and continuing through the first 3 days of bleeding (10361). For accelerating re-epithelialization following photoreactive keratectomy, 230 mg vitamin E (alpha-tocopheryl nicotinate) and vitamin A (retinol palmitate) 25,000 units have been used 3 times daily for 30 days, followed by twice daily for 2 months (348). In premature neonates, oral vitamin E (type unspecified) 15 to 30 IU per kg per day has been used to prevent retinopathy and bronchopulmonary dysplasia (15). For nocturnal leg cramps, vitamin E (type unspecified) 400 IU at bedtime has been used (4701). Radiation-induced fibrosis has been treated with vitamin E (type unspecified) 1000 IU daily in combination with pentoxifylline 800 mg (4672,4673). For beta-thalassemia, vitamin E 750 IU daily has been used (15). For preventing sunburn, RRR-alpha-tocopherol 1000 IU in combination with 2 grams of ascorbic acid has been used (4716). For preventing prostate cancer, vitamin E (type unspecified) 50 to 100 IU daily has been used (3959,4646,11303). For sickle cell anemia, 450 IU daily has been used (15). For preventing pre-eclampsia in high risk women, vitamin E 400 IU with vitamin C 1000 mg daily has been used (3236). The oral dose of palm oil tocotrienols (Palmvitee) used to reduce lipids is 200-260 mg per day (3238,3239,3240). For restless leg syndrome, 400 IU twice daily has been used (6670). For treatment of anemia of prematurity, 50 IU daily has been used for up to 6 weeks (10362).
The recommended daily intake of vitamin E for adults was recently increased. Both women and men should consume 15 mg of vitamin E from food (4844). This is equivalent to 22 IU of the RRR-alpha-tocopherol (natural vitamin E) or 33 IU of the all rac-alpha-tocopherol (synthetic vitamin E) (4844). For Infants 7-12 months, 6 mg; Children 1-3 years, 7 mg; Children 4 -8 years, 11 mg; Older children and adults, 15 mg; Pregnant women, 15 mg; Lactating women, 19 mg (4844). The recommended upper dosage limit for all forms of supplemental alpha-tocopherol is 1000 mg (4844). Dosing for vitamin E can be confusing. Some sources and clinical studies choose to express vitamin E dosing based on mg or International Units (IU). Current guidelines have expressed recommended dietary allowance (RDA) and upper tolerable limits for vitamin E in milligrams. However, most products are still labeled in IUs. It becomes important to understand how to convert between IUs and milligrams of vitamin E. The appropriate method for doing this depends of the formulation of vitamin E being considered and whether or not you are determining RDA or tolerable upper limit. For conversions related to RDA and to convert IUs of RRR-alpha-tocopherol (natural vitamin E) to milligrams of alpha-tocopherol, multiply by a factor of 0.67. For example, 30 IU of RRR-alpha-tocopherol is 20 mg RRR-alpha-tocopherol (natural vitamin E). To convert IUs of all-rac-tocopherol (synthetic vitamin E) to milligrams of alpha-tocopherol, multiply by a factor of 0.45. For example, 30 IU all rac-tocopherol equals 13.5 mg of all rac-alpha-tocopherol (synthetic vitamin E). The tolerable upper limit conversion factor for racemic and RRR-alpha tocopherol assumes that all isomers of vitamin E might contribute to toxicity so

the conversion factor for all rac-alpha tocopherol (synthetic vitamin E) is different. For conversions related to upper limit and to convert IUs all rac-alpha tocopherol (synthetic vitamin E), multiply by a factor of 0.91. For example, 2000 IUs all rac-alpha tocopherol (synthetic vitamin E) is equivalent to 1820 mg. The conversion factor of 0.67 is the same for calculating upper limit for RRR-alpha tocopherol (natural vitamin E). The same factors are used for either acetate or succinate salts because the content has been adjusted for the molecular weights of the salts (4844). Natural vitamin E (d-alpha-tocopherol) is similarly absorbed when taken with high-fat (36 grams) or low-fat (3 grams fat) meals (6133). Synthetic vitamin E (all rac-alpha-tocopherol) should be taken with food for best absorption (6405).
TOPICAL: For treating chemotherapy extravasation, 10% vitamin E (type unspecified) has been used topically in combination with 90% dimethyl sulfoxide (DMSO) (4713).

Comments

The American Heart Association recommends obtaining antioxidants, including vitamin E, by eating a well-balanced diet high in fruits, vegetables, and whole grains rather than from supplements until more is known about the risks and benefits of supplementation (1440).

VITAMIN K

Also Known As

Vitamin K1: Methylphytyl Naphthoquinone, Phylloquinone, Phytomenadione, Phytonadione, 2-Methyl-3-Phytyl-1,4-Naphthoquinone.
Vitamin K2: Menaquinone, Menatetrenone, MK-1, MK-2, MK-4, MK-5, MK-6, MK-7, MK-8, MK-9, MK-10, MK-11, MK-12, MK-13.
Vitamin K3: Menadione, Menadione Sodium Bisulfite, 2-Methyl-1,4-Naphthoquinone.
Vitamin K4: Menadiol Diacetate, Menadiol Sodium Diphosphate, Menadiol Sodium Phosphate, Menadiolum Solubile Methylnaphthohydroquinone.
Vitamin K5: 4-Amino-2-Methyl-1-Naphthol.

Scientific Names

Phytonadione (K1); menaquinone (K2); menadione (K3); menadiol acetate (K4); 4-amino-2-methyl-1-naphthol (K5).

People Use This For

Orally, vitamin K1 (phytonadione) is used for preventing and treating hypoprothrombinemia caused by vitamin K deficiency; to counteract excessive doses of oral anticoagulants; to prevent hemorrhagic disease of the newborn; to treat hypoprothrombinemia induced by salicylates, sulfonamides, quinine, quinidine, or broad-spectrum antibiotic therapy; to prevent and treat osteoporosis; and relieve itching associated with primary biliary cirrhosis. Vitamin K2 (menaquinone) is used orally to treat osteoporosis and steroid-induced bone loss, and to lower total cholesterol in dialysis patients. Vitamin K3 (menadiol acetate) is used orally in combination with vitamin C for treating prostate and breast cancers. Vitamin K4 (menadiol sodium diphosphate) is used orally for treating hypoprothrombinemia resulting from impaired absorption or synthesis of vitamin K.
Topically, vitamin K1 (phytonadione) is used for eliminating spider veins, bruises, scars, stretch marks and burns, treating rosacea, speeding healing, and reducing postoperative bruising and swelling.
Parenterally, vitamin K1 (phytonadione) is used to prevent and treat hypoprothrombinemia caused by vitamin K deficiency, especially that associated with malabsorption syndromes or prolonged parenteral nutrition; to counteract excessive doses of oral anticoagulants; to prevent and treat hemorrhagic disease of the newborn; and to treat hypoprothrombinemia induced by salicylates, sulfonamides, quinine, quinidine, or broad-spectrum antibiotic therapy. Vitamin K4 (menadiol sodium diphosphate) is injected for treating hypoprothrombinemia resulting from impaired absorption or synthesis of vitamin K.

Safety

LIKELY SAFE ...when vitamin K1 is used orally or parenterally, and appropriately. Vitamin K1 (phytonadione) in oral and injectable form is an FDA-approved drug (15). A tolerable upper intake level for vitamin K has not been set (7135).
CHILDREN: LIKELY SAFE ...when vitamin K1 is used orally or parenterally and appropriately. Vitamin K1 (phytonadione) in oral and injectable form is FDA approved for use in children (15). A tolerable upper intake level for vitamin K in children has not been set (7135).
PREGNANCY AND LACTATION: LIKELY SAFE ...when used orally in amounts that do not exceed the recommended dietary allowance (RDA) (15). A tolerable upper intake level for vitamin K in pregnancy and lactation has not been set (7135).

Effectiveness

EFFECTIVE

Hemorrhagic disease. Vitamin K1 (phytonadione) administered orally can prevent hemorrhagic disease of newborns (15).

Hypoprothrombinemia. Vitamin K1 (phytonadione) used orally or parenterally can prevent and treat hypoprothrombinemia caused by vitamin K deficiency or induced by salicylates, sulfonamides, quinine, quinidine, or broad-spectrum antibiotic therapy (15).

Warfarin anticoagulation. Taking vitamin K1 (phytonadione) orally or parenterally will counteract excessive oral warfarin anticoagulation (15).

INSUFFICIENT RELIABLE EVIDENCE to RATE

Hypercholesterolemia. There is preliminary clinical evidence that vitamin K2 (menaquinone) might reduce serum cholesterol in patients on continuous ambulatory peritoneal dialysis with elevated cholesterol levels (59).

Osteoporosis. There is some preliminary clinical evidence that vitamin K2 (menaquinone) might help to treat osteoporosis by slowing bone loss and possibly decreasing fractures (54,55), but vitamin K2 (menaquinone) seems to be ineffective for preventing osteoporosis in postmenopausal women (58). Vitamin K2 (menaquinone) might also decrease steroid-induced osteoporosis (6799).

More evidence is needed to rate vitamin K for these uses.

Mechanism of Action

Vitamin K is a generic term for a group of related compounds. Vitamin K compounds have a common central ring structure, which results in similar activity. Varying side chains differentiate the compounds in terms of intestinal absorption, transport, tissue distribution, and bioavailability (57). Only small amounts of vitamin K are stored in body tissues (64). Vitamin K1 (phytonadione) is obtained from dietary sources, such as leafy green vegetables, broccoli, Brussels sprouts, plant oils, and margarine (57,7135). Vitamin K2 (menaquinone) is obtained from meat and cheeses and synthesis by bacteria in the colon (64). Vitamin K4 (menadiol sodium diphosphate) is a synthetic, water-soluble salt of vitamin K3 (menadione) and is converted to vitamin K3 in the liver. Bile salts are required for oral absorption of vitamin K1 (phytonadione) and vitamin K2 (menaquinone), but not vitamin K4 (menadiol sodium diphosphate) (15). Vitamin K is a coenzyme for the hepatic synthesis of blood coagulation factors II (prothrombin), VII (proconvertin), IX (Christmas factor or plasma thromboplastin component), and X (Stuart-Prower factor), and proteins C and S in the liver (57,7131,7135). Vitamin K is also involved in carboxylation of gamma-carboxyglutamate (Gla) proteins that facilitate binding of coagulation factors to platelets (57). In adequate doses, vitamin K reverses the inhibitory effects of coumarin and warfarin derivatives on the synthesis of clotting factors (15). Besides its classic role in blood coagulation, vitamin K is involved in other physiologic processes. People try supplementing vitamin K for osteoporosis because there is evidence that low vitamin K intake or serum levels are associated with reduced bone mineral density and fractures in people with osteoporosis (55,60,61,62,837,6193,7131). Osteopenia in elderly men seems to correlate with circulating levels of vitamins K and D (7132). Whether people taking vitamin K antagonists or oral anticoagulants are at increased risk of fracture is controversial (51,52,63,7134). Oral anticoagulants might have some effect on the bone mineral density of the radius of the arm, but no effect on the bones of the hip and back (7135). The most pronounced effects of vitamin K antagonists appear to be on rapidly growing bone (7133). Endogenous vitamin K is responsible for activation of osteocalcin (bone Gla protein) that provides calcium-attracting properties to bone (6797,7130). Supplementing vitamin K increases osteocalcin levels in postmenopausal women (56,6797,6798). Vitamin K is known to act as a cofactor for carboxylation of osteocalcin, leading to the suggestion that undercarboxylated osteocalcin (ucOC) levels could be used as an indicator of vitamin K nutritional status (7130,7131,7135). However, variations in testing methodology and inconsistent clinical findings indicate that the usefulness of ucOC levels is undecided (7135). Higher ucOC levels are seen in elderly women with hip fracture, and supplemental vitamin K1 normalizes ucOC levels and increases bone mass (7130). Preliminary evidence suggests that vitamin K may affect calcium balance, urinary calcium excretion, and the production of prostaglandin E2 and interleukin 6 (7131). Vitamin K might also play a role in prevention of atherosclerosis (53,57). Atherosclerosis has been linked to low serum vitamin K levels (53). Laboratory evidence suggests vitamin K supplementation might protect against atherosclerosis (65).

Adverse Reactions

Orally, oral vitamin K causes few adverse effects.

Intravenously, vitamin K can cause reactions that resemble hypersensitivity or anaphylaxis. These reactions are rare. It is unclear whether the adverse effect is caused by the drug or a component of the solution. There have been very rare cases of hyperbilirubinemia, particularly premature neonates, following large doses of vitamin K (15).

Interactions with Herbs & Other Dietary Supplements

COENZYME Q10: Coenzyme Q10 is chemically similar to vitamin K2 (menaquinone) and can have vitamin K-like effects, including antagonism of warfarin (2128,6048). Concomitant use of coenzyme Q10 and vitamin K might cause additive effects and increase the risk of clotting in people taking anticoagulants.

HERBS WITH CLOTTING POTENTIAL: Concomitant use of vitamin K with herbs that contain vitamin K can have additive effects and increase the risk of clotting in people using anticoagulants (57,7131,7135). Some of these herbs include alfalfa, cabbage, parsley, nettle, plantain, and others.

TIRATRICOL: Theoretically, tiratricol might antagonize the prothrombinemic effects of vitamin K by increasing catabolism of vitamin K-dependent clotting factors (15).
VITAMIN A: High doses of vitamin A antagonize effects of vitamin K in animals. However, it isn't known if this can occur in humans (7135,10560).
VITAMIN E: High doses of vitamin E (e.g., >800 units/day) can antagonize the effects of vitamin K, increasing the risk of bleeding in people who are taking warfarin or have low vitamin K intakes (93,7135). Vitamin E appears to reduce the absorption of vitamin K and to bind to vitamin K dependent enzymes, preventing their activity (7135,11512).

Interactions with Drugs

WARFARIN (Coumadin): Vitamin K antagonizes the effects of oral anticoagulants such as warfarin (Coumadin) (15). Excessive vitamin K intake, either from supplements or from changes in the diet, can reduce the anticoagulant effect (15).

Drug Influences on Nutrient Levels and Depletion

SOME DRUGS CAN AFFECT VITAMIN K LEVELS:
ANTIBIOTICS: Vitamin K produced by intestinal bacteria is absorbed from the ileum and taken up by the liver (4437,4439,9502). The contribution of this source to overall vitamin K status in humans is unclear, and likely varies (4439,7135). Destruction of vitamin K-producing bacteria by antibiotics can sometimes lead to vitamin K deficiency, prolonged clotting times, and bleeding (3092,4439,9502,11513,11514,11515,11516). It's suggested that antibiotics such as cefamandole (Mandol) that are secreted into the bile in large amounts have a greater effect on vitamin K-producing bacteria (11514). Also, some cephalosporins have a methylthiotetrazole side chain that may interfere with vitamin K activity, directly inhibiting clotting factor production in the liver (4439,11516). These cephalosporins include cefamandole (Mandol), cefoperazone (Cefobid), cefmetazole (Zefazone), and cefotetan (Cefotan). Problems due to interference of antibiotics with vitamin K are most likely to occur with prolonged antibiotic therapy (10 days or more) in people with poor dietary vitamin K intake (e.g., hospitalized patients with limited nutrient intake, or infants who have not built up stores of vitamin K) (11514,11515,11516). Vitamin K supplements aren't necessary for otherwise healthy people taking short courses of antibiotics.
ANTICONVULSANTS: When taken during pregnancy, anticonvulsants that induce hepatic enzymes (e.g., phenobarbital, phenytoin, carbamazepine) can reduce vitamin K levels in the fetus and increase the risk of intracranial hemorrhage soon after birth (11521,11522,11523,11524,11525). It's thought that liver enzyme induction by these drugs increases vitamin K metabolism (11521,11522,11523,11525). This has a significant effect on vitamin K levels in infants, who haven't built up stores of the vitamin (11525). It's recommended that women who need these anticonvulsants during pregnancy take vitamin K 10 to 20 mg/day orally for the last month of pregnancy, and the baby should receive vitamin K immediately after delivery (11522,11525). There's limited evidence that chronic carbamazepine or phenytoin therapy can cause subclinical reductions in vitamin K activity in adults. There are rare reports of prolonged clotting times and bleeding in people with additional risk factors for vitamin K deficiency, such as poor nutritional intake (10582,11533,11534). These anticonvulsants don't significantly affect vitamin K and clotting parameters in most children and adults.
BILE ACID SEQUESTRANTS: By reducing absorption of dietary fats, cholestyramine (Questran) and colestipol (Colestid) may also reduce absorption of fat-soluble vitamins such as vitamin K. Some studies have found no changes in vitamin K levels or prothrombin times with up to 2 years of cholestyramine or colestipol therapy (4455,4460,10566). However, there are a few case reports of hypoprothrombinemia and bleeding, usually in people with other risk factors (4458,11519). Monitor patients closely.
MINERAL OIL: Mineral oil can reduce absorption of fat soluble vitamins including vitamin K. Chronic use, both daily and intermittently, has been associated with prolonged clotting times (4495). Advise patients against regular or long-term use of mineral oil.
ORLISTAT (Xenical): Orlistat can reduce the absorption of some fat-soluble vitamins, although the extent of its effect on food-derived vitamin K hasn't been determined (1730). In healthy people, small decreases in plasma vitamin K levels can occur, but usually without any change in clotting times (9595,10570). However, prolonged clotting times might occur when orlistat is added to warfarin therapy. This may be due to both direct effects of orlistat on vitamin K absorption, and reduced intake of vitamin K-rich fatty foods that cause unpleasant side effects with orlistat (11520). The manufacturer of orlistat recommends that all patients take a multivitamin supplement containing all the fat soluble vitamins, separating the dosing time by at least 2 hours from orlistat (1730).
RIFAMPIN (Rifadin, Rimactane): There are occasional reports of vitamin K deficiency associated with rifampin therapy, leading to prolonged clotting times and, in one case, a cerebral bleed (11517,11518). Suggested mechanisms are reduced intestinal absorption of vitamin K, destruction of vitamin K-producing intestinal bacteria, and interference with the enzyme which regenerates vitamin K from an inactive metabolite. Symptomatic vitamin K deficiency is most likely to occur in people with poor dietary intake or other contributory factors (11517,11518). Monitor patients closely.

Interactions with Foods

None known.

Interactions with Lab Tests

17-HYDROXYCORTICOSTEROIDS: Might cause false increase in urine test results due to in vitro interference with Reddy method (275).
BILIRUBIN: Large amounts of vitamin K can increase serum bilirubin and test results in neonates or people with G-6-PD deficiency (275).
CALCIUM: Can reduce urinary calcium excretion and test results (275).
ERYTHROCYTES: Can decrease blood erythrocyte levels and test results (275).
HEMATOCRIT: Vitamin K3 and vitamin K4 might decrease hematocrit and test results, especially in people with G-6-PD deficiency (275).
HEMOGLOBIN: Vitamin K3 and vitamin K4 might decrease blood hemoglobin level and test results, especially in people with G-6-PD deficiency (275). Vitamin K can increase urine hemoglobin levels and test results (275).
HYDROXYPROLINE: Can decrease urine levels and test results (275).
LEUKOCYTES, PLATELETS: Vitamin K3 and vitamin K4 can decrease blood levels and test results due to pancytopenia (275).
OSTEOCALCIN: Can increase serum levels and test results in postmenopausal women (275).
PORPHYRINS: Can increase urine levels and test results (275).
PROTEIN: Can increase urine levels and test results (275).
PROTHROMBIN TIME (PT): Can decrease PT due to procoagulation effects of vitamin K (275).
UROBILINOGEN: May increase urine levels and test results due to hemolytic anemia in G-6-PD deficiency (275).

Interactions with Diseases or Conditions

HEMODIALYSIS: Excessive vitamin K intake has been associated with soft tissue calcification in patients receiving hemodialysis (11744).
LIVER DISEASE: Vitamin K is not effective for treating hypoprothrombinemia caused by severe liver disease. High doses may worsen coagulation defects (15).
REDUCED BILE SECRETION: People with decreased bile secretion may require co-administration of supplemental bile salts to ensure adequate vitamin K absorption (15).

Dosage and Administration

ORAL: There is no typical dose for vitamin K. Doses should be individualized and medically supervised (15). People with decreased bile secretion might require co-administration of supplemental bile salts to ensure adequate vitamin K absorption (15). Efficient absorption of vitamin K from the intestine requires dietary fat, although the amount needed for optimal absorption has not been determined (7135). For osteoporosis, clinical studies used vitamin K2 (menaquinone) 45 mg per day (54,55,59). Vitamin K2 (menaquinone) is not currently available in the US. There is insufficient information to determine recommended dietary allowances (RDAs) for vitamin K, so daily adequate intake (AI) recommendations have been formed: Infants 0-6 months, 2 mcg; Infants 6-12 months, 2.5 mcg; Children 1-3 years, 30 mcg; Children 4-8 years, 55 mcg; Children 9-13 years, 60 mcg; Adolescents 14-18 years (including those pregnant or lactating), 75 mcg; Men over 19 years, 120 mcg; Women over 19 years (including those pregnant and lactating), 90 mcg (7135).
PARENTERAL: Injectable vitamin K is an FDA-approved prescription product.

Comments

The name vitamin K comes from the German word Koagulationsvitamin (57). Vitamin K1 (phytonadione) is the only form of vitamin K available in the US. Vitamin K1 (phytonadione) is generally the preferred form of vitamin K, due to lower toxicity, rapid effects, greater potency, and superior efficacy in some indications, such as oral anticoagulant-induced hypoprothrombinemia (15,17). Vitamin K3 (menadione) is no longer used therapeutically because it has been linked to hepatic toxicity (7135). Vitamin K4 (menadiol), which was marketed as Synkayvite tablets and injection, is no longer available in the US. A specific form of vitamin K2 (menaquinone), MK-4, is an accepted treatment for osteoporotic osteopenia in Japan (57,58). An increased understanding of the physiologic role of vitamin K beyond blood coagulation has led some researchers to suggest that the guidelines for nutritional intake of vitamin K should be increased (57). The 2001 National Institute of Medicine Food and Nutrition Board slightly increased recommendations for adequate intake, but cited insufficient conclusive evidence for substantial increases (7135).

VITAMIN O

Also Known As

Liquid Oxygen, Stabilized Liquid Oxygen, Stabilized Oxygen.

Scientific Names

None.

People Use This For

Orally, vitamin O is used for increasing energy; improving immune function; eliminating bacteria, viruses, fungi and parasites; treating yeast infections; eliminating toxins and poisons from the body; and healing mouth sores. Vitamin O is also used for improving concentration, memory and alertness; calming the nervous system; easing depression, irritability, unexplained hostility and dizziness; relieving arthritis, muscle aches and pains, asthma, bronchial problems, emphysema and lung disease, sinus infection, diabetes, body weakness, chronic fatigue, and heart and circulation problems. Vitamin O has been used for obesity; constipation; gas and bloating; loss of appetite; poor digestion; stomach acid; premenstrual syndrome (PMS); menopause; sexual dysfunction; headaches; migraines; premature aging; rashes; skin problems; itchy ears, nose and anus; and tumors and deposit buildup.
Topically, it is used as an antiseptic.

Safety

There is insufficient reliable information available about the safety of vitamin O.
Pregnancy and Lactation: Insufficient reliable information available; avoid using.

Effectiveness

There is insufficient reliable information available about the effectiveness of vitamin O.

Mechanism of Action

The chemical formula of the oxygen compound in vitamin O is not disclosed in promotional information. One supplier describes its product as a mildly buffered solution of deionized water and sodium chloride with a pH of 7.2 (5318). Another supplier lists magnesium peroxide as the active ingredient (5320). Still another claims the ingredients are secret (5321).

Adverse Reactions

None reported.

Interactions with Herbs & Other Dietary Supplements

None known.

Interactions with Drugs

None known.

Interactions with Foods

None known.

Interactions with Lab Tests

None known.

Interactions with Diseases or Conditions

None known.

Dosage and Administration

ORAL: In capsule form of unspecified strength, the dose is typically two capsules three times per day with water (5320). Various quantities, usually measured in drops, of solutions are recommended (e.g., 6 drops in 8 ounces of water, juice, milk, etc; 20 drops 3 times a day in a glass of water; 20 drops per gallon of water) (5321).

Comments

Although vitamin O is called liquid oxygen, remember that oxygen only exists in a liquid form at temperatures below -183 degrees C and that water, by weight, is about 88% oxygen (16). The FTC states that Vitamin O appears to be nothing more than saltwater (311).
In May 2000, Rose Creek Health Products agreed to pay $375,000 to settle Federal Trade Commission charges that they made false and unsubstantiated health claims in their advertising for "Vitamin O". The settlement prohibits the company from making unsupported representations that "Vitamin O" is an effective treatment for any life-threatening diseases, or that the effectiveness of "Vitamin O" is established by medical or scientific research or studies (5076).

WAFER ASH

Also Known As

Pickaway Anise, Prairie Grub, Scubby Trefoil, Stinking Prairie Bush, Swamp Dogwood, Three-Leaved Hop Tree, Wingseed.

Scientific Names

Ptelea trifoliata.
Family: Rutaceae.

Comments

At the date of publication, this product was not a common ingredient used in brand name supplements marketed to consumers. Details about this product are available at the online version of *Natural Medicines Comprehensive Database*. See www.naturaldatabase.com.

WAHOO

Also Known As

Arrowwood, Bitter Ash, Bleeding Heart, Burning Bush, Bursting Heart, Eastern Burning Bush, Fish Wood, Fusanum, Fusoria, Gadrose, Gatten, Gatter, Indian Arrowroot, Indian Arrowwood, Pegwood, Pigwood, Prickwood, Skewerwood, Spindle Tree, Strawberry Bush, Strawberry Tree.
CAUTION: See separate listing for Burning Bush.

Scientific Names

Euonymus atropurpureus.
Family: Celastraceae.

People Use This For

Orally, wahoo root bark is used orally for indigestion, to stimulate bile production, and as a laxative, diuretic, or tonic.

Safety

LIKELY UNSAFE ...when the bark, seeds or berries are used orally. Ingesting 36 berries can be fatal (18). The poisonous principle has not been identified (17).
PREGNANCY AND LACTATION: LIKELY UNSAFE ...when used orally (18).

Effectiveness

There is insufficient reliable information available about the effectiveness of wahoo.

Mechanism of Action

The applicable parts of wahoo are the trunk, root bark, and fruit. The seeds contain cardioactive steroids known as cardenolides. The trunk, root bark, and fruit also contain varied alkaloids, caffeine, and theobromine (18). Wahoo is thought to stimulate bile flow and have laxative effects. In larger amounts, it can affect the heart (18).

Adverse Reactions

Wahoo is considered poisonous (17). Several hours after ingesting wahoo seeds, people experience severe upset stomach, sometimes with bloody diarrhea, fever, shortness of breath, circulatory problems, signs of collapse, stupor increasing to unconsciousness, alternating with motor restlessness, severe tonic-clonic spasms with locked jaw muscles and coma.

Interactions with Herbs & Other Dietary Supplements

CARDIAC GLYCOSIDE-CONTAINING HERBS: Contraindicated; concomitant use increases the risk of cardiac glycoside toxicity. Cardiac glycoside-containing herbs include black hellebore, Canadian hemp roots, digitalis leaf, hedge mustard, figwort, lily of the valley roots, motherwort, oleander leaf, pheasant's eye plant, pleurisy root, squill bulb leaf scales, and strophanthus seeds (19).
LICORICE/HORSETAIL: Theoretically, overuse/misuse of licorice rhizome or horsetail plant with wahoo increases the risk of cardiac toxicity due to potassium depletion (19).
OTHER CARDIOACTIVE HERBS: Avoid concomitant use with other cardioactive herbs due to unpredictability of effects and adverse effects. Other cardioactive herbs include calamus, cereus, cola, coltsfoot, devil's claw, European mistletoe, fenugreek, fumitory, ginger, Panax ginseng, hawthorn, white horehound, mate, parsley, quassia, scotch broom flower, shepherd's purse, and wild carrot (4).

STIMULANT LAXATIVE HERBS: Theoretically, use of stimulant laxatives can have additive effects and adverse effects. Use also increases the risk of cardiac toxicity due to potassium depletion. Stimulant laxative herbs include aloe dried leaf sap, blue flag rhizome, alder buckthorn, European buckthorn, butternut bark, cascara bark, castor oil, colocynth fruit pulp, gamboge bark exudate, jalap root, black root, manna bark exudate, podophyllum root, rhubarb root, senna leaves and pods, wild cucumber fruit (Ecballium elaterium), and yellow dock root (19).

Interactions with Drugs

DIGOXIN (Lanoxin): Contraindicated; using wahoo with digoxin increases risk of cardiac glycoside toxicity due to therapeutic duplication (2).
DIURETIC DRUGS: Theoretically, concomitant use of potassium-depleting diuretics with wahoo can increase the risk of cardiac glycoside toxicity due to potassium depletion (506). Some diuretics that can deplete potassium include chlorothiazide (Diuril), chlorthalidone (Thalitone), furosemide (Lasix), hydrochlorothiazide (HCTZ, HydroDIURIL, Microzide), and others.
MACROLIDE ANTIBIOTICS: Theoretically, concomitant use may increase risk of cardiac glycoside toxicity (17).
QUININE: Theoretically, concomitant use of quinine and wahoo might increase risk of cardiac toxicity (506).
STIMULANT LAXATIVES: Theoretically, use of stimulant laxatives with wahoo might have additive laxative effects, and can increase the risk of cardiac glycoside toxicity due to potassium depletion (2).
TETRACYCLINE ANTIBIOTICS: Theoretically, concomitant use may increase risk of cardiac glycoside toxicity (17).

Interactions with Foods

None known.

Interactions with Lab Tests

None known.

Interactions with Diseases or Conditions

GASTROINTESTINAL (GI) CONDITIONS: Theoretically, wahoo can increase gastric secretions and stimulate peristalsis. These effects might exacerbate GI irritation or inflammation (18).

Dosage and Administration

No typical dosage.

Comments

Avoid confusion with Euonymus europaeus (18).

WALLFLOWER

Also Known As

Beeflower, Gillyflower, Giroflier, Handflower, Keiri, Wallstock-Gillofer.

Scientific Names

Erysimum cheiri, synonym Cheiranthus cheiri.
Family: Brassicaceae/Cruciferae.

People Use This For

Orally, wallflower is used for cardiac insufficiency, to encourage menstruation, and as a laxative. It is also used orally for liver and gallbladder diseases because of its bitter taste.

Safety

POSSIBLY UNSAFE ...when used orally (18).
PREGNANCY AND LACTATION: POSSIBLY UNSAFE ...when used orally due to its possible toxic effects (18); avoid using.

Effectiveness

There is insufficient reliable information available about the effectiveness of wallflower.

Mechanism of Action

The applicable parts of wallflower are the above ground parts. It does contain cardiac glycosides, but they may be poorly absorbed when wallflower is taken orally (18).

Adverse Reactions
Poisoning may occur with parenteral administration, but is expected to be low with oral administration due to poor absorption of the cardiac glycosides (18).

Interactions with Herbs & Other Dietary Supplements
CARDIAC GLYCOSIDE-CONTAINING HERBS: Contraindicated, concomitant use may increase the risk of cardiac glycoside toxicity. Cardiac glycoside-containing herbs include black hellebore, Canadian hemp roots, digitalis leaf, hedge mustard, figwort, lily-of-the-valley roots, motherwort, oleander leaf, pheasant's eye plant, pleurisy root, squill bulb leaf scales, and strophanthus seeds (19).
CINCHONA and EPHEDRA: Use with wallflower seed may increase risk of toxicity (19).
LICORICE/HORSETAIL: Theoretically, overuse/misuse of licorice rhizome or horsetail plant with cardiac glycoside-containing herbs increases the risk of cardiac toxicity due to potassium depletion (19).
OTHER CARDIOACTIVE HERBS: Avoid concomitant use with other cardioactive herbs due to unpredictability of effects and adverse effects. Other cardioactive herbs include calamus, cereus, cola, coltsfoot, devil's claw, European mistletoe, fenugreek, fumitory, ginger, Panax ginseng, hawthorn, white horehound, mate, parsley, quassia, scotch broom flower, shepherd's purse, and wild carrot (4).
STIMULANT LAXATIVE HERBS: Theoretically, overuse or misuse of stimulant laxatives with cardiac glycoside-containing herbs increases the risk of cardiac toxicity due to potassium depletion. Stimulant laxative herbs include aloe dried leaf sap, blue flag rhizome, alder buckthorn, European buckthorn, butternut bark, cascara bark, castor oil, colocynth fruit pulp, gamboge bark exudate, jalap root, black root, manna bark exudate, podophyllum root, rhubarb root, senna leaves and pods, wild cucumber fruit (Ecballium elaterium), and yellow dock root (19).

Interactions with Drugs
CALCIUM SUPPLEMENTS: Calcium supplements may enhance the therapeutic effects of wallflower (18).
CORTICOSTEROIDS: Use of corticosteroids may cause electrolyte depletion and increase risk of cardiac glycoside toxicity (19).
DIGOXIN (Lanoxin): Contraindicated; therapeutic duplication increases risk of cardiac glycoside toxicity (2).
DIURETIC DRUGS: Theoretically, concomitant use of potassium-depleting diuretics and wallflower can increase the risk of cardiac glycoside toxicity due to potassium depletion (506). Some diuretics that can deplete potassium include chlorothiazide (Diuril), chlorthalidone (Thalitone), furosemide (Lasix), hydrochlorothiazide (HCTZ, HydroDIURIL, Microzide), and others.
STIMULANT LAXATIVES: Overuse or misuse of stimulant laxatives may cause electrolyte depletion and increase the risk of cardiac glycoside toxicity (19).
QUINIDINE: Cardiac medications, including quinidine may increase the risk of cardiac glycoside toxicity; contraindicated (18).
QUININE: Taking quinine with wallflower may increase the risk of cardiac glycoside toxicity (18).

Interactions with Foods
None known.

Interactions with Lab Tests
None known.

Interactions with Diseases or Conditions
CARDIAC CONDITIONS: Wallflower may cause arrhythmias (18); use with caution.

Dosage and Administration
No typical dosage.

Comments
Canadian hemp is also known as wallflower (Cheiranthus cheiri). Wallflower is considered obsolete as a medicinal herb (18).

WATER AVENS

Also Known As
Chocolate Root, Cure All, Indian Chocolate, Throat Root, Water Chisch, Water Flower.

Scientific Names
Geum rivale.
Family: Rosaceae.

Comments
At the date of publication, this product was not a common ingredient used in brand name supplements marketed to consumers. Details about this product are available at the online version of *Natural Medicines Comprehensive Database*. See www.naturaldatabase.com.

WATER DOCK

Also Known As
None.

Scientific Names
Rumex aquaticus.
Family: Polygonaceae.

People Use This For
Orally, water dock is used for "blood purification" and constipation.
Topically, water dock is used for mouth ulcers, skin sores, scorbutic conditions, and for cleaning the teeth.
In foods, water dock leaves are used in salads.

Safety
There is insufficient reliable information available about the safety of water dock.
Pregnancy and Lactation: Insufficient reliable information is available; avoid using.

Effectiveness
There is insufficient reliable information available about the effectiveness of water dock.

Mechanism of Action
The applicable part of water dock is the dried root. Water dock contains anthracene derivatives, oxalic acid and calcium oxalate, and tannins (18), an essential oil, fat, protein, quercitrin, starch, and tannin. Water dock is considered to have digestive properties (18).

Adverse Reactions
None reported.

Interactions with Herbs & Other Dietary Supplements
CALCIUM, IRON, ZINC: Concurrent use might decrease mineral absorption. Water dock contains oxalate (7,12), which can bind multivalent metal ions in the gastrointestinal tract and decrease mineral absorption.

Interactions with Drugs
None known.

Interactions with Foods
CALCIUM, IRON, ZINC: Concurrent use might decrease mineral absorption from foods. Water dock contains oxalate (7,12), which can bind multivalent metal ions in the gastrointestinal tract and decrease mineral absorption.

Interactions with Lab Tests
None known.

Interactions with Diseases or Conditions
COAGULATION DISORDERS: Oxalate constituents can alter serum calcium concentrations, possibly decreasing coagulation time (12).
KIDNEY DISEASE: Use with caution in individuals with a history of kidney stones. Insoluble oxalate crystals may form in the kidneys, causing further damage (12).

Dosage and Administration
ORAL: Water dock is used orally or topically as a liquid extract or as a powder.

WATER FENNEL

Also Known As
Horsebane, Water Dropwort.

Scientific Names
Oenanthe aquatica.

Interactions with Diseases or Conditions
None known.

Comments
At the date of publication, this product was not a common ingredient used in brand name supplements marketed to consumers. Details about this product are available at the online version of *Natural Medicines Comprehensive Database*. See www.naturaldatabase.com.

WATER GERMANDER

Also Known As
None.

Scientific Names
Teucrium scordium.
Family: Lamiaceae/Labiatae.

Comments
At the date of publication, this product was not a common ingredient used in brand name supplements marketed to consumers. Details about this product are available at the online version of *Natural Medicines Comprehensive Database*. See www.naturaldatabase.com.

WATER HEMLOCK

Also Known As
Beaver Poison, Brook-Tongue, Carotte a Moreau, Children's Bane, Cique Vireuse, Cowbane, Death-of-Man, European Water Hemlock, False Parsley, Fever Root, Mockeel Root, Muskrat Weed, Musquash Root, Poison Parsnip, Snake Weed, Snakeroot, Spotted Cowbane, Spotted Hemlock, Spotted Parsley, Wasser-Schierling, Wild Carrot, Wild Dill, Wild Parsnip.
CAUTION: See separate listings for Hemlock and Hemlock Water Dropwort.

Scientific Names
Cicuta virosa, synonym Cicuta mackenzieana; Cicuta maculata; Cicuta douglasii, synonyms Cicuta californica, Cicuta vagans, Sium douglasii; Cicuta occidentalis; Cicuta bulbifera.
Family: Apiaceae/Umbelliferae.

People Use This For
Orally, water hemlock is used for migraine headaches, painful menstruation, and worm infestations.
Topically, water hemlock is used for inflammation of the skin.

Safety
UNSAFE ...when used orally. Water hemlock is considered to be the most poisonous plant growing in North America (6349). Intoxication can result from chewing or ingestion any part of the plant (6348). The usual lethal adult dose is one rhizome (6347) or a 2-3 cm portion of root (6349). ...when used topically (6348). Death can result when hemlock is applied topically (6348,6349).
CHILDREN: UNSAFE ...when used orally or topically (6347,6351,6355). Fatalities have resulted when hollow stems of water hemlock are used as whistles (6347), when hemlock is ingested (6355), or when hemlock has been applied topically (6351).
PREGNANCY AND LACTATION: UNSAFE ...when used orally or topically. Water hemlock is toxic; avoid using (6349,6348).

Effectiveness

There is insufficient reliable information available about the effectiveness of water hemlock.

Mechanism of Action

All parts of water hemlock at all stages of growth, including leaves and stems, are considered poisonous and can be lethal if ingested (6346,6349). The freshly harvested root is considered most toxic in early spring (6346). All plant parts contain the toxin cicutoxin, but it is especially concentrated in the root (6350). Cicutoxin is a highly unsaturated aliphatic alcohol (6346,6347,6348) that is found in a yellow oily liquid of roots and stems (6354). Water hemlock poisoning consists of cholinergic effects such as salivation, perspiration, diaphoresis, abdominal discomfort, and nausea (6350); and occurs almost immediately after ingestion (6346). Convulsions, seizures, and spastic-tonic movements follow (6346,6350,6353) which are believed to be due to cholinergic stimulation of the brain stem (reticular formation) or the basal ganglia (6346,6350). Narrow pupils, most likely due to the cholinergic effects of the toxin, and dilated pupils, due to brain hypoxia or ischemia, have been reported (6346). Increases in creatine phosphokinase occur indicating the severity of muscle rigors, rigidity and convulsions, and increases in serum lactic dehydrogenase also may occur that indicate possible liver or skeletal muscle damage (6347). Cicutoxin can also be absorbed through the skin (6349). Death usually results from cyanosis, exhaustion, and respiratory paralysis (6347,6348,6350).

Adverse Reactions

Orally, toxic effects occur immediately (6350). Prompt medical attention is advised after ingestion of water hemlock (6346). Death can result 15 minutes to 8 hours after ingestion (6351,6353). The usual lethal adult dose is one rhizome (6347) or a 2-3 cm portion of root (6349). The first symptoms of water hemlock poisoning are nausea, vomiting, wheezing, salivation, sweating, dizziness, abdominal pain, flushing, lethargy, delirium, and defecation (6346,6347,6349,6350,6351). These symptoms are followed by respiratory distress, muscle spasms, restless movements, bronchial secretions, convulsions, mydriasis, miosis, eyeball protrusion, glycosuria, proteinuria, abnormal EEG, metabolic acidosis, hypertension, supraventricular tachycardia, hypotension, bradycardia, muscle rigidity, tremors, grinding of teeth, tonic-clonic movements, grand-mal seizures, rhabdomyolysis, acute renal failure, cerebral edema, unconsciousness, and coma (6346,6347,6348,6349,6350,6351,6353). Elevated serum CPK, LDH, AST and alkaline phosphatase levels also occur (6346). Death can occur during convulsions and from respiratory paralysis, exhaustion, or heart failure (6347,6348,6350).

Interactions with Herbs & Other Dietary Supplements

None known.

Interactions with Drugs

None known.

Interactions with Foods

None known.

Interactions with Lab Tests

SERUM LIVER ENZYMES: Ingestion of water hemlock can cause elevations in serum liver enzymes such as lactic dehydrogenase (LDH), aspartate aminotransferase (AST), and alkaline phosphatase (6346,6347).
SERUM MUSCLE ENZYMES: Ingestion of water hemlock can cause elevations in serum muscle enzymes such as creatine phosphokinase (CPK) and lactic dehydrogenase (LDH isoenzyme fraction 5) levels (6346,6347).

Interactions with Diseases or Conditions

None known.

Dosage and Administration

No typical dosage.

Comments

Water hemlock is found in marshy, swampy areas of meadows, along banks of streams, pools, and rivers. Accidental ingestion usually occurs when water hemlock is mistaken for edible plants such as artichokes, celery, sweet potatoes, sweet anise, and wild parsnip (6346). There are approximately 20 species of water hemlock (Cicuta) and most are found in North America (6339). The most commonly encountered are Cicuta maculata in southern Missouri and the eastern US, Cicuta vagans in the Pacific Northwest, Cicuta bulbifera in the Middle Northwest, Cicuta occidentalis in the Rocky Mountain region (6351) and Cicuta virosa which is found throughout the US and is known as the common European water hemlock (6346,6347,6348). All species of water hemlock are considered poisonous (6351). The rhizome has an extremely unpleasant smell and is the most toxic portion of the plant.

WATER PLANTAIN

Also Known As
Alisma, Mad-Dog Weed.
CAUTION: See separate listings for Great Plantain, Buckhorn Plantain, Blond Psyllium, Black Psyllium.

Scientific Names
Alisma plantago-aquatica; Alisma plantago-aquatica subsp. orientale, synonyms Alisma orientale, Alisma plantago-aquatica var. orientale .
Family: Alismataceae.

People Use This For
Orally, water plantain is used for bladder and urinary tract diseases.

Safety
POSSIBLY UNSAFE ...when used orally (18).
PREGNANCY AND LACTATION: POSSIBLY UNSAFE ...when used orally due to its toxic potential (18); avoid using.

Effectiveness
There is insufficient reliable information available about the effectiveness of water plantain.

Mechanism of Action
The applicable part of water plantain is the root/rhizome. The fresh rootstock is thought to be poisonous. It contains the cyanogenic chlorogenic acid sulfate (18).

Adverse Reactions
None reported.

Interactions with Herbs & Other Dietary Supplements
None known.

Interactions with Drugs
None known.

Interactions with Foods
None known.

Interactions with Lab Tests
None known.

Interactions with Diseases or Conditions
None known.

Dosage and Administration
No typical dosage.

Comments
Water plantain rootstock is said to be bitter in taste (18). It sounds similar to the common and species names of great plantain, and buckhorn plantain. Be careful not to confuse them.

WATERCRESS

Also Known As

Agrião, Berro, Berro Di Agua, Brunnenkresse, Crescione Di Fonte, Cresson au Poulet, Cresson D'eau, Cresson De Fontaine, Indian Cress, Mizu-Garashi, Nasilord, Nasturtii herba, Oranda-Garashi, Scurvy Grass, Selada-Air, Tall Nasturtium, Wasserkresse, Waterkres.
CAUTION: See separate listings for Nasturtium and Scurvy Grass.

Scientific Names

Nasturtium officinale, synonyms Radicula nasturtium, Rorippa nasturtium, Sisymbrium nasturtium.
Family: Brassicaceae/Cruciferae.

People Use This For

Orally, watercress is used for respiratory tract mucous membrane inflammation, coughs, bronchitis, as a spring tonic, an appetite stimulant, improving digestion, alopecia, cancer, flu, goiter, polyps, scurvy, tuberculosis, gland tumors, as an abortifacient, aphrodisiac, bactericide, laxative, restorative, stimulant, and anthelmintic.
Topically, watercress is used for arthritis, rheumatoid arthritis, earache, eczema, scabies, and warts.
In foods, watercress is widely used in leaf salads and as a culinary spice.

Safety

LIKELY SAFE ...when consumed in amounts commonly found in foods.
POSSIBLY SAFE ...when used orally in medicinal amounts, short-term (2,8,12).
POSSIBLY UNSAFE ...when used orally in excessive amounts (8,12,19). ...when used orally long term (8,12,19). Watercress can cause gastric mucosal irritation (8,12) or damage (19).
There is insufficient reliable information available about the safety of watercress for its other uses.
CHILDREN: LIKELY UNSAFE ...when used orally in medicinal amounts; avoid using in children younger than 4 years old (12,19).
PREGNANCY: LIKELY UNSAFE ...when used in medicinal amounts. Watercress might stimulate menstruation or have abortifacient effects (19).
LACTATION: Insufficient reliable information available; avoid using.

Effectiveness

There is insufficient reliable information available about the effectiveness of watercress.

Mechanism of Action

The applicable parts of watercress are the above ground parts. Watercress is thought to have antibiotic and diuretic activity (18). The above ground parts contain mustard oil (18), vitamin C, and beta-carotene, and vitamin K (19). Mustard oil is believed responsible for diuretic effects and gastrointestinal irritation after consumption of large amounts of watercress (18). The constituent, phenethyl isothiocyanate, released by chewing watercress, might inhibit metabolic activation of a lung carcinogens (4019).

Adverse Reactions

Orally, large amounts of watercress can cause gastrointestinal irritation (18). Theoretically, excessive or prolonged use might cause kidney damage (19).

Interactions with Herbs & Other Dietary Supplements

None known.

Interactions with Drugs

CHLORZOXAZONE (Parafon Forte, Paraflex): Concomitant use with watercress may potentiate the effects of chlorzoxazone due to reduced metabolism and elimination (4018).
WARFARIN (Coumadin): Theoretically, consuming large amounts of watercress with high vitamin K content might antagonize the anticoagulant effects of warfarin (11285).

Interactions with Foods

None known.

Interactions with Lab Tests

INTERNATIONAL NORMALIZED RATIO (INR)/PROTHROMBIN TIME (PT): Theoretically, watercress might decrease coagulation test results due to high vitamin K content (11285).

Interactions with Diseases or Conditions

GASTRIC OR DUODENAL ULCERS: Watercress is contraindicated in people with gastric or duodenal ulcers (12,19).
INFLAMMATORY KIDNEY DISEASES: Watercress is contraindicated in people with inflammatory kidney disease (12,19).

Dosage and Administration

No typical dosage.

Comments

Avoid confusing watercress with nasturtium (Tropaeolum majus).

WHEAT BRAN

Also Known As

Bran, Cereal Fiber, Dietary Fiber.
CAUTION: See separate listings for Oat Bran and Rice Bran.

Scientific Names

Triticum aestivum.
Family: Poaceae/Gramineae.

People Use This For

Orally, wheat bran is used as a supplemental source of dietary fiber for preventing colon diseases (including cancer), preventing gastric cancer, treating irritable bowel syndrome (IBS), reducing the risk of hemorrhoids and hiatal hernia, hypercholesterolemia, hypertension, reducing the risk of breast cancer and gallbladder disease, and type 2 diabetes.

Safety

LIKELY SAFE ...when used orally and appropriately (10326,10328).
PREGNANCY AND LACTATION: LIKELY SAFE ...when used orally (5).

Effectiveness

POSSIBLY EFFECTIVE

Constipation. Taking wheat bran orally seems to be effective for treating mild constipation and restoring normal bowel function. Wheat bran seems to increase stool output and improve colonic transit, but does not soften normal-viscosity stool (6265,11004,11116,11117).

Gastric cancer. Epidemiologic evidence suggests that dietary cereal fiber can reduce the risk of gastric cancer (10435).

Hemorrhoids. Taking wheat bran orally seems to be effective for reducing the risk of hemorrhoids (11118,11119).

Hypertension. Taking wheat bran orally seems to produce modest, but significant reductions in systolic, diastolic, and mean arterial blood pressures (4963,11463).

Irritable bowel syndrome (IBS). Taking wheat bran orally may reduce abdominal pain and improve bowel function in patients with mild to moderate IBS. However, it may not be as effective as guar gum (10326).

POSSIBLY INEFFECTIVE

Colorectal cancer. Several large well-designed studies showed that fiber, including wheat-bran fiber, does not prevent the recurrence of colorectal adenomas, despite earlier evidence that suggested a beneficial effect (160,4819,4820,4821).

Diabetes. Taking wheat bran orally does not seem to consistently improve indices of blood sugar control. It does not improve blood pressure, lipids, clotting factors, homocysteine, C-reactive protein, or other factors associated with cardiovascular disease in patients with type 2 diabetes (6266,10328).

There is insufficient reliable information available about the effectiveness of wheat bran for its other uses.

Mechanism of Action

The applicable part of wheat bran is the outer hull of the grain, which is largely composed of insoluble fiber (4963). The laxative effect of wheat bran is dependent on particle size; larger particles have a greater laxative effect than smaller particles (6265). Wheat bran has negligible water-holding capacity and no stool softening effect in people with normal stools (6265). Wheat bran increases colonic transit time, stool output, and bowel movement frequency (6265,11463). Preliminary evidence suggests consumption of wheat bran might move the digestion site of foods from the proximal to distal portion of the colon (375). In the distal colon, butyrate produced from digestion of grains and starches reduces ammonia produced by fermentation of foods high in fat and sugar, possibly preventing cell damage and reducing the risk of colon cancer (375).

Adverse Reactions

Orally, wheat bran may cause flatulence and GI discomfort, especially with initial use. One carefully controlled study designed to look at side effects noted no increase in GI symptoms in subjects taking 20 to 40 grams of wheat bran per day (6265).

Interactions with Herbs & Other Dietary Supplements

None known.

Interactions with Drugs

DIGOXIN (Lanoxin): Theoretically, wheat bran may interfere with absorption (156).

Interactions with Foods

IRON: Wheat bran inhibits dietary iron absorption (156).

Interactions with Lab Tests

BLOOD PRESSURE: Wheat bran might lower blood pressure and blood pressure readings in individuals with hypertension (4963).

Interactions with Diseases or Conditions

None known.

Dosage and Administration

ORAL: For laxative effects, 20 to 25 grams per day has been used (6265,11004,11116,11117). It appears that 40 grams per day is no more effective than 20 grams per day (6265). For the treatment of irritable bowel syndrome (IBS), wheat bran 30 grams per day has been used for up to 12 weeks (10326). For hypertension, 3-6 grams whole-wheat flour, wheat flakes, and brown rice, combined with a National Cholesterol Education Program (NCEP) step 1 diet has been used (11463).

Adequate intake (AI) levels for dietary fiber intake per day have been set. For children 1 to 3 years, the AI is 19 grams and 4 to 8 years, 25 grams. For boys 9 to 13 years, the AI is 31 grams, and 38 grams for boys 14 to 18 years. For girls 9 to 18 years, the AI is 26 grams. For men 19 to 50 years, the AI is 38 grams, and 30 grams for men older than 51 years. For women 19 to 50 years, the AI is 25 grams, and 21 grams for women older than 51 years. For pregnant women, the AI is 28 grams, and 29 grams for lactating women (11120). AI for children less than one year has not been set. A tolerable upper intake levels (UL) for fiber has not been set (11120).

Comments

Wheat bran is the outer grain hull of wheat (Triticum aestrivum).

WHEATGRASS

Also Known As

Agropyron, Couchgrass, Cutch, Dog Grass, Durfa Grass, Graminis rhizoma, Quack Grass, Quitch Grass, Scotch Quelch, Triticum, Twitchgrass, Witch Grass.

Scientific Names

Elytrigia repens, synonyms Agropyron repens, Agropyron firmum, Elymus repens, Triticum firmum, Triticum repens.

Family: Poaceae/Gramineae.

People Use This For

Orally, wheatgrass is primarily used as a concentrated source of nutrients. It is used therapeutically for increasing hemoglobin production, improving blood sugar disorders such as diabetes, preventing tooth decay, improving wound healing, and preventing bacterial infections. It is also used orally for removing deposits of drugs, heavy metals, and carcinogens from the body and neutralizing toxins, removing toxins from the liver and removing toxins from the blood stream. Additionally, wheatgrass is used orally for preventing gray hair, reducing high blood pressure, improving digestion, and blocking intestinal cholesterol absorption. It is used orally to treat cystitis, urethritis, prostatitis, benign prostatic hypertrophy (BPH), renal calculus (kidney stones), and in "irrigation therapy" (use of a mild diuretic and copious fluid intake to increase urine flow). It is also used orally for common cold, cough and bronchitis, fever and colds, inflammation of mouth and pharynx, tendency to infection, gout, liver disorders, ulcerative colitis, cancer, rheumatic pain, and chronic skin problems.

Wheatgrass is used for cancer and arthritis in alternative treatment programs.

In foods and beverages, wheatgrass extracts are used as a flavoring component.

Safety

LIKELY SAFE ...when consumed in amounts commonly found in foods (5286).
POSSIBLY SAFE ...when wheatgrass juice is taken orally, and appropriately, in medicinal amounts. Wheatgrass has been used safely for up to one month (11165).
There is insufficient reliable information available about the long-term safety of wheatgrass when used medicinally.
PREGNANCY AND LACTATION: Insufficient reliable information available; avoid using.

Effectiveness

INSUFFICIENT RELIABLE EVIDENCE to RATE

Ulcerative colitis. There is some evidence that wheatgrass juice taken orally might help active distal ulcerative colitis. Freshly extracted wheatgrass juice might reduce overall disease activity, and the severity of rectal bleeding (11165). More evidence is needed to rate wheatgrass for this use.

Mechanism of Action

The applicable parts of wheatgrass are the above ground parts, root, and rhizome. A constituent of wheatgrass, agropyrene, seems to have antibiotic activity (7162). The constituent, apigenin, may have antioxidant and anti-inflammatory activity, which might explain its use for ulcerative colitis (11165). Wheatgrass contains large amounts of chlorophyll. High-chlorophyll beverages are sometimes included in diets purported to treat diseases such as cancer and rheumatoid arthritis (5286,6982). It also contains vitamin A, vitamin C, and vitamin E, iron, calcium, magnesium and amino acids.
Wheatgrass juice is a popular health drink. It is thought to possess therapeutic qualities only when fresh and consumed on an empty stomach immediately after extraction. But there is no research to determine the effect of freshness on effectiveness or bioavailability of its constituents (11165).

Adverse Reactions

Orally, wheatgrass can cause nausea, anorexia, and constipation (11165).

Interactions with Herbs & Other Dietary Supplements

None known.

Interactions with Drugs

None known.

Interactions with Foods

None known.

Interactions with Lab Tests

None known.

Interactions with Diseases or Conditions

None known.

Dosage and Administration

For treating ulcerative colitis, 100 ml of wheatgrass juice daily for 1 month has been used (11165).

WHEY PROTEIN

Also Known As

Bovine Whey Protein Concentrate.
CAUTION: See separate listing for Branched Chain Amino Acids.

Scientific Names

None.

People Use This For

Orally, whey protein is used as a food supplement, as an alternative to milk for people with lactose intolerance, for protein allergy, asthma, hyperlipidemia, obesity and weight loss, replacing or supplementing milk-based infant formulas, atopic disease in infants, treating metastatic carcinoma, colon cancer, and reversing weight loss and increasing glutathione (GSH) in people with HIV disease.

Safety

LIKELY SAFE ...when quality products are used orally and appropriately. There are no reports of toxicity in clinical trials (4926,4927,4929,4930,4932,4935,4936,4941).
PREGNANCY AND LACTATION: LIKELY SAFE ...when quality products are used orally and appropriately (4929).

Effectiveness

POSSIBLY EFFECTIVE

Atopic disease. Taking whey protein orally seems to decrease the risk of developing atopic disease in infants genetically predisposed to allergy (4927,4929).

HIV/AIDS-related weight loss. Taking whey protein orally seems to help reverse weight loss in patients with HIV (4926,4932,4935,4936).

INSUFFICIENT RELIABLE EVIDENCE to RATE

Cancer. There is preliminary evidence that taking whey protein orally might help produce tumor regression in some patients with metastatic carcinoma (4930). More evidence is needed to rate whey protein for this use.

Mechanism of Action

Whey is a by-product of cheese manufacturing which contains carbohydrates including lactose; minerals including calcium, sodium, phosphorus, and potassium (2640); proteins including alpha-lactalbumin, beta-lactoglobulin, lactoferrin, serum albumin, lysozyme, and immunoglobulins A, G, and M (2640); and cysteine (4937).

Whey protein may vary in the amount and activity of immunoglobulins and other proteins present, depending on the production methods used (2640). Whey protein typically contains 24% branched chain amino acids which are readily oxidized as an energy source during stress. Whey protein is also a source of gamma-glutamylcysteine, a precursor of glutathione (GSH), which acts as an intracellular antioxidant (2640). GSH is depleted by oxidative stress, which occurs during infections, trauma, or major surgery (2640). Low levels of GSH in patients with HIV have been associated with impaired T-cell function (2640). A specific whey protein formulation (Immunocal) might enhance the reduced-to-oxidized glutathione ratio (GSH/GSSG) in lymphocytes, a marker of oxidative stress in reactive oxygen species (ROS)-mediated diseases, including AIDS-related wasting (1382). Whey products also has anti-HIV and anti-apoptotic effects in vitro (4937).

In patients with HIV infection, whey protein increases body weight (4926,4935,4936), elevates GSH in mononuclear cells (4926), increases albumin, increases CD4 and CD8 counts (4935), and reduces diarrhea (4932,4936).

Whey protein also has immunomodulating activity (4939,4940). It's thought that immunoglobulins in whey protein may bind antigens in the gut and prevent their absorption (2640). Whey protein formulations can be produced that are high in specific immunoglobulins. For example, whey proteins derived from the milk of cows infected with Cryptosporidium may be a rich source of antibodies against Cryptosporidium (2640). These types of whey protein formulations can reduce gastrointestinal Cryptosporidium parvum infection in animal models (4934).

Some researchers are interested in using whey protein to prevent cancer. It's thought that whey protein might prevent cancer by providing GSH substrates and increasing tissue GSH levels (4943). Whey protein might exert antitumor effects by depleting tumor cells of GSH, making them more vulnerable to chemotherapy (2640,4930). Animal models of cancer indicated that whey protein diets might protect against certain cancers (3976,4928,4933).

Researchers are also interested in whey protein for cardiovascular conditions. There is preliminary evidence that a unique combination of hydrolyzed whey protein isolates inhibits angiotensin converting enzyme (ACE) (6171).

There is also interest in whey protein as a protein source in high-protein diets used for weight loss. In animal models, a whey protein diet seems to reduce weight and improve insulin sensitivity compared to red meat (12111).

Adverse Reactions

Orally, whey protein is usually well tolerated. High doses from 2.3 to 6.5 g/kg/day can cause increased stool frequency, nausea, thirst, bloating, cramps, reduced appetite, fatigue, and headache. Whey protein can also increase blood urea nitrogen (BUN) levels twofold (2640).

Interactions with Herbs & Other Dietary Supplements

None known.

Interactions with Drugs

ALENDRONATE (Fosamax): Theoretically, use of whey protein with alendronate might decrease absorption. Whey protein contains minerals that might bind alendronate in the gut (9).
LEVODOPA: Theoretically, concomitant use might decrease levodopa (Larodopa) absorption (4944).
QUINOLONE ANTIBIOTICS: Theoretically, use of whey protein with quinolones might decrease absorption. Whey protein contains minerals that might bind quinolones in the gut (9).
TETRACYCLINE ANTIBIOTICS: Theoretically, use of whey protein with tetracyclines might decrease absorption. Whey protein contains minerals that might bind tetracyclines in the gut (9).

Interactions with Foods
None known.

Interactions with Lab Tests
BLOOD UREA NITROGEN (BUN): Whey protein in amounts of 2.3 g/kg/day or more, in addition to a normal diet, can produce twofold increases in BUN concentrations (2640). However, whey protein does not change serum creatinine, indicating that the effect is due to protein loading, rather than reduced renal function (2640).

Interactions with Diseases or Conditions
MILK ALLERGY: Individuals allergic to bovine milk products should avoid using whey protein (4942).

Dosage and Administration
ORAL: A typical dose as a dietary supplement in people with HIV disease is 8.4-84 grams per day (4926,4935), or 2.4 g/kg per day in a calorie-enriched formula (4941), or 42-84 grams per day in a glutamine enriched formula (4935). A dose for treating metastatic carcinoma is 30 grams per day (4930).

Comments
Whey protein is the soluble protein contained in whey, the watery portion of milk that separates from the curds in the process of cheese making.

WHITE COHOSH

Also Known As
Baneberry, Coralberry, Doll's Eye, Red BaneBerry, Snakeberry, White Baneberry.
CAUTION: See separate listings for Black Cohosh, Blue Cohosh, and European Baneberry.

Scientific Names
Actaea pachypoda, synonym Actaea alba; Actaea rubra.
Family: Ranunculaceae.

People Use This For
Orally, white cohosh has been used to stimulate menstruation and to treat other female disorders. White cohosh is also used orally for colds and cough, urogenital disorders, stomach disorders, reviving those near death, as a purgative, in childbirth, and for curing itching.

Safety
LIKELY UNSAFE ...when used orally. The entire plant is toxic (6).
PREGNANCY AND LACTATION: LIKELY UNSAFE ...when used orally due to toxicity (6); avoid using.

Effectiveness
There is insufficient reliable information available about the effectiveness of white cohosh.

Mechanism of Action
The constituent protoanemonin is believed to cause irritant effects (6). The fruit and berries are especially toxic. They contain toxic glycosides and an essential oil (6).

Adverse Reactions
Orally, white cohosh can cause gastrointestinal (GI) irritation (19), acute stomach cramping, headache, tachycardia, vomiting, delirium, and circulatory failure (6).
Topically, the application of white cohosh can lead to inflammation and skin blistering (6).

Interactions with Herbs & Other Dietary Supplements
None known.

Interactions with Drugs
None known.

Interactions with Foods
None known.

Interactions with Lab Tests
None known.

Interactions with Diseases or Conditions
GASTROINTESTINAL (GI) CONDITIONS: White cohosh can irritate the GI tract. Avoid using in individuals with infectious or inflammatory GI conditions (19).

Dosage and Administration
No typical dosage.

Comments
White cohosh appears to be a substance with no reliable evidence to support its use, yet with documented toxicity. It should not be confused with black cohosh, used for symptoms of menopause, nor with blue cohosh, a substance used as a uterine stimulant and antispasmodic (6). White cohosh is also known as baneberry but it should not be confused with European baneberry.

WHITE DEAD NETTLE FLOWER

Also Known As
Archangel, Bee Nettle, Blind Nettle, Deaf Nettle, Dumb Nettle, Lamii Albi Flos, Stingless Nettle, White Archangel.
CAUTION: See separate listings for Stinging Nettle above ground parts and Stinging Nettle root.

Scientific Names
Lamium album.
Family: Lamiaceae/Labiatae.

People Use This For
Orally, white dead nettle flower is used for mild inflammation of mucous membranes in the upper respiratory tract, and as a sedative.
Topically, white dead nettle flower is used for mild inflammation of the mouth, throat, and skin, and for non-specific vaginal discharge.

Safety
LIKELY SAFE ...when used orally and appropriately (2,18).
There is insufficient reliable information available about the safety of white dead nettle flower for its other uses.
PREGNANCY AND LACTATION: Insufficient reliable information available; avoid using.

Effectiveness
There is insufficient reliable information available about the effectiveness of white dead nettle flower.

Mechanism of Action
White dead nettle flowers contain tannin, mucilage, and saponins (2). These give nettle expectorant and astringent effects.

Adverse Reactions
None reported.

Interactions with Herbs & Other Dietary Supplements
None known.

Interactions with Drugs
None known.

Interactions with Foods
None known.

Interactions with Lab Tests
None known.

Interactions with Diseases or Conditions
None known.

Dosage and Administration
ORAL: The average daily dose is 3 grams (2).
TOPICAL: The typical dosage is 5 grams of the white dead nettle flower is commonly added to a sitz bath (2).

Comments
Avoid confusion with stinging nettle herb and stinging nettle root.

WHITE HELLEBORE

Also Known As
European Hellebore, European White Hellebore, Langwort.
CAUTION: See separate listings for Black Hellebore, American Hellebore, and Pheasant's Eye (false hellebore).

Scientific Names
Veratrum album, synonym Veratrum lobelianum.
Family: Melanthiaceae or Liliaceae.

People Use This For
Orally, white hellebore is used to treat cholera, gout, and hypertension.
Topically, white hellebore is used for herpetic lesions.
In manufacturing, white hellebore is used as an insecticide against flies and mosquitoes.

Safety
LIKELY UNSAFE ...when used orally. All plant parts are considered toxic (6). Between 10-20 mg of alkaloids (1-2 grams of rhizome/root) are lethal (6,18). ...when used topically. Toxic alkaloids can be absorbed through intact skin (6,18).
PREGNANCY: LIKELY UNSAFE ...when used orally or topically because it could be teratogenic (6); avoid using.
LACTATION: LIKELY UNSAFE ...when used orally or topically (6); avoid using.

Effectiveness
There is insufficient reliable information available about the effectiveness of white hellebore.

Mechanism of Action
The applicable parts of white hellebore are the rhizome and root. White hellebore contains the toxic ester-alkaloids protoveratrine A and B (13), which are sensory nerve irritants (18). These alkaloids inhibit the inactivation of the sodium ion channels and thus have a paralyzing effect on many excitable cells, including those of the heart (18).

Adverse Reactions
Orally, white hellebore can cause mucous membrane irritation (18), a burning sensation in upper abdomen, salivation, vomiting, gastric erosion, severe hypotension, bradycardia, and shock (6,553). Large doses may cause central respiratory depression, blindness, paralysis, convulsions, cardiac arrhythmias, and death (6).
Topically, it can cause skin irritation (18) and the toxic alkaloids could be absorbed.
By inhalation, the powdered root induces violent sneezing and runny nose (6).

Interactions with Herbs & Other Dietary Supplements
None known.

Interactions with Drugs
None known.

Interactions with Foods
None known.

Interactions with Lab Tests
None known.

Interactions with Diseases or Conditions
None known.

Dosage and Administration
No typical dosage.

Comments
Crude white hellebore is not used therapeutically (13), though it is sometimes used in homeopathic dilutions (18). In Roman times, white hellebore was used as a poison. An extract has been used as an arrow tip poison.

WHITE HOREHOUND

Also Known As
Common Hoarhound, Hoarhound, Horehound, Houndsbane, Marrubii herba, Marrubium, Mastranzo.
CAUTION: See separate listing for Black Horehound.

Scientific Names
Marrubium vulgare.
Family: Lamiaceae/Labiatae.

People Use This For
Orally, white horehound is used for loss of appetite, cough, bronchitis, respiratory tract mucous membrane inflammation, whooping cough, asthma, tuberculosis, indigestion, bloating and flatulence, diarrhea, jaundice, debility, liver and gallbladder complaints, and for painful menstruation. It is also used orally as a laxative, an anthelmintic, as a diuretic, and to induce sweating.
Topically, white horehound is used for skin damage, ulcers, and wounds.
In manufacturing, the extracts of white horehound are used as flavoring in foods and beverages, and as an expectorant in cough syrups and lozenges.

Safety
LIKELY SAFE ...when used orally in amounts commonly found in foods. White horehound has Generally Recognized As Safe (GRAS) status in the US (4912).
POSSIBLY SAFE ...when used orally and appropriately (2,12).
POSSIBLY UNSAFE ...when used orally in excessive amounts; white horehound may have a purgative effects (4,12).
There is insufficient reliable information available about the safety of the topical use of white horehound.
PREGNANCY: LIKELY UNSAFE ...when used orally; white horehound might have abortifacient effect (19), or stimulate menstrual flow and the uterus (12). There is insufficient reliable information available about the safety of topical use during pregnancy; avoid using.
LACTATION: There is insufficient reliable information available about the safety of oral use during lactation; avoid amounts greater than those commonly found in foods. There is insufficient reliable information available about the safety of topical use during lactation; avoid using.

Effectiveness
There is insufficient reliable information available about the effectiveness of white horehound.

Mechanism of Action
The applicable parts of white horehound are the above ground parts. White horehound contains marrubiin, bitter ingredients, volatile oil, and tannins (515). The constituent, marrubiin does not exist in the fresh plant; it is formed from premarrubiin during processing (515). The volatile oil of white horehound exhibits vasodilation, expectorant (11), and antischistosomal activity (4). Preliminary evidence suggests the hydroxycinnamic derivatives might have weak antioxidant activity (11). Other evidence suggests marrubinic acid may stimulate bile secretion (515). Marrubiin's expectorant effects may result from direct stimulation of bronchial mucosal secretions (512). Marrubiin may act to normalize extrasystolic arrhythmias (4,11), but large amounts might cause arrhythmias (4). An alcoholic extract reduces spasms of gastrointestinal (GI) tract (515). An aqueous extract demonstrates evidence that it can antagonize serotonin (11) and exerts anti-inflammatory activity (4,11).

Adverse Reactions
Orally, large amounts of white horehound can cause purgative effects (4,12).
Topically, skin contact with the plant juice may cause contact dermatitis (4).

Interactions with Herbs & Other Dietary Supplements
None known.

Interactions with Drugs
None known.

Interactions with Foods
None known.

Interactions with Lab Tests
None known.

Interactions with Diseases or Conditions
HEART CONDITIONS: Theoretically, large amounts of white horehound might cause arrhythmias (4).

Dosage and Administration
ORAL: A typical dose is 1-2 grams dried above ground parts or one cup of tea of three times daily before meals to stimulate bile secretion or during the day as an expectorant (8). To make tea, steep 1-2 grams dried above ground parts in 150 mL boiling water 5-10 minutes, and strain (4,8). Up to 4.5 grams dried above ground parts or 2-6 tablespoons of pressed juice (or equivalent preparations) are used per day (2). A typical dose of pressed juice is 30-60 mL daily (18). 1-3 mL of the liquid extract, 1:1 in 25% ethanol, has been used three times daily (4). 1-2 mL of the tincture, 1:10 in 45% alcohol, has been used three times daily (4).
TOPICAL: No typical dosage.

Comments
White horehound derives its name from ancient Greece where it was used for treating mad-dog bites (515).

WHITE LILY

Also Known As
Baurenlilien, Farmer's Lily, Madonna Lily, Meadow Lily, White Pond Lily.

Scientific Names
Lilium candidum.
Family: Liliaceae.

Comments
At the date of publication, there was very little scientific information about this product. Our staff is continually analyzing the available information on natural medicines and will add data to the online version of *Natural Medicines Comprehensive Database* as it becomes available. See www.naturaldatabase.com.

WHITE MUSTARD

Also Known As
Sinapis albae semen, Weibe Senfsamen.
CAUTION: See separate listings for Black Mustard, Black Mustard Oil, and Hedge Mustard.

Scientific Names
Sinapis alba, synonym Brassica alba.
Family: Brassicaceae/Cruciferae.

People Use This For
Orally, white mustard is used "to brighten and clear" the voice, for those with a tendency for infection, as an emetic, diuretic, and as an appetite stimulant.
Topically, white mustard is used for cough and colds, pulmonary congestion, bronchitis, joint and soft tissue inflammation, rheumatism, arthritis, lumbago, inflammation of the mouth and pharynx, hyperemization of the skin, a counterirritant, and a bath to treat paralytic symptoms.
In foods and condiments, white mustard is a common flavoring agent, and is considered a culinary spice.

Safety
LIKELY SAFE ...when used orally in the amounts commonly found in foods. White mustard has Generally Recognized As Safe (GRAS) status in the US (4912).
POSSIBLY SAFE ...when used orally and appropriately for medicinal purposes (12). ...when used topically and appropriately (12,19).
LIKELY UNSAFE ...when used orally as an emetic because mustard is an irritant. Used as an emetic, the esophageal tissue is twice exposed to the corrosive effects of white mustard (19). Ingestion of a large quantity can

cause irritant poisoning (12,19). ...when used topically for more than 15-30 minutes because severe burns can occur (12,19). ...when used topically on a regular basis for more than 2 weeks (2,12,19).
CHILDREN: LIKELY UNSAFE ...when used orally in medicinal amounts. ...when used topically in children under 6 years of age (2,12,19).
PREGNANCY: LIKELY UNSAFE ...when used orally in medicinal amounts; white mustard can have abortifacient and menstrual-stimulant properties (19).
LACTATION: Insufficient reliable information available; avoid using.

Effectiveness
There is insufficient reliable information available about the effectiveness of white mustard.

Mechanism of Action
The applicable part of white mustard is the seed. White mustard seeds contain mustard oil glycosides and mustard oils (2). White mustard contains the glucosinolate sinalbin, which on hydrolysis yields p-hydroxybenzyl isothiocyanate, p-hydroxybenzylamine, and other constituents, such as proteins, fatty oil, and sinapine (11,18). These products of hydrolysis possess irritant and bacteriostatic properties (18). White mustard's pungent taste comes from p-hydroxybenzyl isothiocyanate (11). Some evidence suggests the glucosinolate products can have protective effects against carcinogens (11).

Adverse Reactions
Orally, long-term use of white mustard can increase the risk of nerve damage (2,18). Isothiocyanates, such as those in mustard, can cause endemic goiters (6,11).
Topically, white mustard can cause blistering and skin ulceration, as well as nerve damage (2,12,18,19).

Interactions with Herbs & Other Dietary Supplements
None known.

Interactions with Drugs
None known.

Interactions with Foods
None known.

Interactions with Lab Tests
None known.

Interactions with Diseases or Conditions
KIDNEY DISEASE: Irritant poisoning from white mustard can occur in people with kidney disorders (12,19).

Dosage and Administration
ORAL: The average amount of white mustard is 60-150 grams daily (18). To "brighten and clear" the voice, mustard flour, or powdered mustard, is stirred with honey to form balls (18). One or two of these honey balls are taken on an empty stomach (18).
TOPICAL: As a foot bath, 20 to 30 grams of mustard flour is typically mixed in 1 liter of water (18). For a mustard bath, 150 grams of mustard flour in a pouch is commonly placed in the bath (18). For local application, 4 tablespoons (50-70 grams) of the powdered seeds are usually mixed with warm water to form a soft material, which is applied for 10-15 minutes for adults and 5-10 minutes for children older than 6 years of age (2,18). Decrease the application time in individuals with sensitive skin (2). Treatment should not exceed two weeks (2,12,18,19).

Comments
Avoid confusion black mustard (Brassica nigra) and hedge mustard (Sisymbrium officinale).

WHITE SANDALWOOD OIL

Also Known As
Chandana Oil, East Indian Sandalwood Oil, Sanderswood, Santal Oil, White Saunders Oil, Yellow Sandalwood Oil, Yellow Saunders Oil.
CAUTION: See separate listings for Red Sandalwood and White Sandalwood wood.

Scientific Names
Santalum album.
Family: Santalaceae.

People Use This For
Orally, white sandalwood oil is used as an adjuvant therapy for lower urinary tract infection, common cold, cough/bronchitis, fevers, urinary tract inflammatory conditions, mouth and pharynx inflammation, liver and gallbladder complaints, infection, stomachache, vomiting, gonorrhea, pains, "strengthening the heart", headache, urogenital disorders, to reduce libido, for heatstroke, sunstroke, and resulting fever.
In food and beverages, it is used as a flavor component.
In manufacturing, white sandalwood oil is used as a fragrance ingredient in soaps, cosmetics, and perfumes.

Safety
LIKELY SAFE ...when used orally in amounts commonly found in foods. White sandalwood oil has Generally Recognized As Safe (GRAS) status in the US (4912). ...when used topically (11).
POSSIBLY SAFE ...when used orally for short-term medicinal use as enteric-coated products (2).
POSSIBLY UNSAFE ...when used orally for longer than 6 weeks, condition should be medically evaluated (2,19). There is insufficient reliable information available about the safety of the topical use of white sandalwood oil in amounts greater than those found in cosmetics.
PREGNANCY: LIKELY UNSAFE ...when used orally in medicinal amounts because it might have an abortifacient effect (19); avoid using. There is insufficient reliable information available about the safety of topical use during pregnancy.
LACTATION: Insufficient reliable information available; avoid using amounts greater than those found in foods.

Effectiveness
There is insufficient reliable information available about the effectiveness of white sandalwood oil.

Mechanism of Action
White sandalwood oil is reported to have antifungal, antiseptic, diuretic (11), antibacterial, and spasmolytic activity (2). It is considered to be a kidney irritant (19). Although some evidence suggests it is not irritating, sensitizing, or phototoxic when applied to the skin, the constituent, santalol, can cause contact dermatitis (11).

Adverse Reactions
Orally, use of white sandalwood oil can cause itching, nausea, gastrointestinal complaints, and blood in the urine (18). Topically, use can cause contact dermatitis in sensitive individuals (11).

Interactions with Herbs & Other Dietary Supplements
None known.

Interactions with Drugs
None known.

Interactions with Foods
None known.

Interactions with Lab Tests
None known.

Interactions with Diseases or Conditions
KIDNEY DISEASE: Contraindicated in kidney disease, particularly in individuals with diseases of the kidney parenchyma (2,19).

Dosage and Administration
ORAL: A typical oral dose is 1-1.5 grams of oil per day in an enteric-coated form; maximum use 6 weeks without medical evaluation (2).

WHITE SANDALWOOD wood

Also Known As
Chandana, East Indian Sandalwood, Sandalwood, Santali Lignum Albi, Tan Xiang, White Saunders, Yellow Sandalwood, Yellow Saunders.
CAUTION: See separate listings for Red Sandalwood and White Sandalwood Oil.

Scientific Names
Santalum album. Family: Santalaceae.

People Use This For

Orally, white sandalwood wood is used as an adjunct therapy for lower urinary tract infections, treating colds, cough, bronchitis, fevers, inflammatory conditions of the mouth, pharynx, or efferent urinary tract, for liver and gallbladder complaints, heat stroke, sun stroke and associated fever, gonorrhea, and as an anti-aphrodisiac.

Safety

POSSIBLY SAFE ...when the wood is used orally and appropriately short-term, for less than 6 weeks (2,12).
POSSIBLY UNSAFE ...when used orally longer than 6 weeks (2,12,18).
PREGNANCY: LIKELY UNSAFE ...when used orally because it is believed to have abortifacient effects (19); avoid using.
LACTATION: Insufficient reliable information available; avoid using.

Effectiveness

There is insufficient reliable information available about the effectiveness of white sandalwood wood.

Mechanism of Action

White sandalwood wood has antibacterial, spasmolytic, and urinary disinfectant activities (2,18).

Adverse Reactions

Orally, white sandalwood wood can cause nausea, gastrointestinal complaints, itching, and hematuria (blood in the urine) (2,18). High doses or use longer than six weeks can cause kidney toxicity (2,12,18). White sandalwood has minimal potential for sensitization (18).

Interactions with Herbs & Other Dietary Supplements

None known.

Interactions with Drugs

None known.

Interactions with Foods

None known.

Interactions with Lab Tests

None known.

Interactions with Diseases or Conditions

KIDNEY DISEASE: White sandalwood wood is contraindicated in diseases of kidney parenchyma (2,12,18).

Dosage and Administration

ORAL: The typical dose is 10-20 grams of the wood per day, brewed as a tea or other preparations (2). White sandalwood wood should not be used for more than a six-week duration (2,12).

Comments

Sandalwood has a very dense composition and is valued as a wood for carving (6). Avoid confusion with red sandalwood (Pterocarpus santalinus) and white sandalwood oil.

WHITE SOAPWORT

Also Known As

Gypsophilae radix, Soapwort.
CAUTION: See separate listing for Red Soapwort.

Scientific Names

Gypsophila paniculata.
Family: Caryophyllaceae.

People Use This For

Orally, white soapwort is used for cough, bronchitis, and inflammation of the mucous membranes in the upper and lower respiratory tract.
Topically, white soapwort is used for chronic skin disorders and eczema.

Safety

POSSIBLY SAFE ...when used orally and appropriately (2).
PREGNANCY AND LACTATION: Insufficient reliable information; avoid using.

Effectiveness

There is insufficient reliable information available about the effectiveness of white soapwort.

Mechanism of Action

The applicable part of white soapwort is the root. White soapwort has expectorant, emetic, antibiotic, and insecticidal effects (18). In large amounts, it is cytotoxic (2). The saponin constituents exhibit expectorant effects (2), and they irritate the gastric mucosa to stimulate the bronchial mucous glands via parasympathetic sensory pathways (7). Saponins can cause stomach upset, nausea, and vomiting (7).

Adverse Reactions

Orally, white soapwort can cause stomach irritation (2), nausea, and vomiting (7).

Interactions with Herbs & Other Dietary Supplements

None known.

Interactions with Drugs

None known.

Interactions with Foods

None known.

Interactions with Lab Tests

None known.

Interactions with Diseases or Conditions

GI IRRITATION: Theoretically, the saponin content of white soapwort can exacerbate existing gastrointestinal mucosal irritation (6).

Dosage and Administration

ORAL: The typical dose of white soapwort is 30-150 mg per day of the dried root or 3-15 mg per day of the gypsophila saponin or equivalent preparations (2).

Comments

In the Middle Ages, Franciscan and Dominican monks viewed soapwort as a divine gift that was meant to keep them clean (6). Avoid confusion with the red soapwort root.

WILD CARROT

Also Known As

Beesnest Plant, Bird's Nest Root, Daucus, Garijara, Queen Anne's Lace, Shikha-Mula.
CAUTION: See separate listings for Hemlock and Water Hemlock.

Scientific Names

Daucus carota subsp. carota.
Family: Apiaceae/Umbelliferae.

People Use This For

Orally, wild carrot is used for urinary calculus or stones, and high uric acid in urine, cystitis, and gout. The seed oil is used for dysentery, indigestion, uterine pain, heart disease, cancer, kidney problems, as a nerve tonic, a diuretic, an antiflatulent, an aphrodisiac, to induce menstruation, and as an anthelmintic.
In foods wild carrot oil is used as a flavoring agent in alcoholic and non-alcoholic beverages, frozen dairy desserts, candy, baked goods, gelatins, puddings, meat and meat products, condiments relishes, and soups.
In manufacturing, wild carrot seed oil is used as a fragrance in soaps, detergents, creams, lotions, and perfumes.

Safety

LIKELY SAFE ...when used orally in amounts commonly found in foods. Wild carrot oil has Generally Recognized As Safe (GRAS) status in the US (4912).

POSSIBLY SAFE ...when wild carrot seed oil is used orally and appropriately in medicinal amounts (4,11).
LIKELY UNSAFE ...when an excessive amount of wild carrot seed oil is used orally, it can cause renal irritation (4). Theoretically, high doses of oil could cause neurological effects (6) because the seed contains the psychoactive agent myristicin.
There is insufficient reliable information available about the safety of the oral use of the above ground parts of wild carrot.
PREGNANCY: LIKELY UNSAFE ...when used orally. The seeds, oil, and above ground parts can cause uterine stimulant, abortifacient, and menstrual stimulant effects (19).
LACTATION: POSSIBLY UNSAFE ...when the seed oil is used orally. Wild carrot seed oil has mild estrogenic activity and irritant effects (4). There is insufficient reliable information available about the safety of the oral use of the seeds or above ground parts during lactation.

Effectiveness

There is insufficient reliable information available about the effectiveness of wild carrot.

Mechanism of Action

The applicable parts of wild carrot are the fruit and seed. Wild carrot fruit/seed contains flavones including apigenin, chrysin, luteolin; flavonols including kaempferol and quercetin and various glycosides. The amount and composition of the volatile oil contained in the fruit/seed varies between different cultivars. The furanocoumarins, 8-methoxypsoralen and 5 methoxypsoralen are found in the plant (4). Some evidence suggests that wild carrot might have significant antifertility activity (4,3858). Other evidence suggests that wild carrot has cholinergic-type actions, perhaps due to the choline constituents (4). Wild carrot seed oil shows some evidence of vasodilation, cardiac depressant, and smooth muscle relaxation effects (11). Terpinen-4-ol, a component of the seed oil, is a renal irritant and believed to cause a diuretic effect (4). A tertiary base isolated from wild carrot seed appears to have papaverine-like antispasmodic activity.

Adverse Reactions

Orally, ingesting excessive doses can cause renal irritation or neurological effects. Hypersensitivity reactions and increased sensitivity to UV light and sunburn might occur (19,4).
Topically, contact with the plant can cause dermatitis (4).

Interactions with Herbs & Other Dietary Supplements

HERBS WITH SEDATIVE PROPERTIES: Theoretically, concomitant use with herbs that have sedative properties might enhance therapeutic and adverse effects. These include California poppy, catnip, German chamomile, hops, Jamaican dogwood, kava, lemon balm, scullcap, valerian, and others.

Interactions with Drugs

ANTIHYPERTENSIVE DRUGS: Theoretically, excessive doses of wild carrot seed oil might interfere with antihypertensive therapy due to cardiotonic effects (4).
ESTROGENS: Theoretically, excessive use of the above ground parts of wild carrot might interfere with hormonal therapy due to estrogenic effects of wild carrot (4).
PHOTOSENSITIZING DRUGS: Theoretically, concomitant use might result in increased photosensitivity (19). Some drugs that cause photosensitivity include amitriptyline (Elavil), quinolones (Ciprofloxacin, others), sulfa drugs (Septra, Bactrim, others), and tetracycline.

Interactions with Foods

None known.

Interactions with Lab Tests

None known.

Interactions with Diseases or Conditions

RENAL INFLAMMATION/IRRITATION: Contraindicated due to renal irritant properties (4,19).
UV LIGHT THERAPY: Contraindicated due to photosensitizing effect; avoid excessive periods in the sun (19).

Dosage and Administration

ORAL: No typical dosage. But, the dried above ground parts is 2-4 grams or as tea has been used three times daily. To make tea, steep 2-4 grams of above ground parts in boiling water for 5-10 minutes, strain (4). A liquid extract (1:1 in 25% alcohol) 2-4 mL three times daily has been used (4).

Comments

Carrot seed oil is steam-distilled from the dried root of both the familiar vegetable known as carrot, and the wild carrot. Avoid confusing wild carrot (which has an inedible white tap root) with the common carrot (Daucus carota subspecies sativus) (4).

WILD CHERRY

Also Known As
Black Cherry, Black Choke, Choke Cherry, Rum Cherry Bark, Virginian Prune, Wild Black Cherry.
CAUTION: See separate listing for Cherry Laurel Water.

Scientific Names
Prunus serotina; Prunus virginiana.
Family: Rosaceae.

People Use This For
Orally, wild cherry is used for colds, whooping cough, bronchitis and other lung problems, diarrhea, gout, digestive disorders, pain, and cancer. It is also used in cough syrups because of its sedative, expectorant, astringent, and antitussive effects.
In foods and beverages, wild cherry is used as a flavoring agent.

Safety
LIKELY SAFE ...when used orally in amounts commonly found in foods and beverages. Wild cherry has Generally Recognized As Safe (GRAS) status in the US (4912).
POSSIBLY SAFE ...when used orally and appropriately short-term, in limited amounts (12).
POSSIBLY UNSAFE ...when used orally and long-term or in excessive amounts (12,19). The constituent, prunasin, hydrolyzes to hydrocyanic acid (HCN) (11,12,13,18).
PREGNANCY: LIKELY UNSAFE ...when used orally because prunasin is potentially teratogenic (19).
LACTATION: Insufficient reliable information available; avoid using.

Effectiveness
There is insufficient reliable information available about the effectiveness of wild cherry.

Mechanism of Action
The applicable part of wild cherry is the stem bark. Wild cherry bark has astringent, antitussive, and sedative effects (18). It contains prunasin, a cyanogenic glycoside that is hydrolyzed to toxic hydrocyanic acid (HCN) and benzaldehyde (11). Bark collected in the fall has a higher HCN yield (approximately 0.15%) than bark collected in the spring (approximately 0.05%). Leaves collected in the spring have the highest HCN yield (approximately 0.25%) (11).

Adverse Reactions
Orally, large amounts of wild cherry can lead to fatal poisonings (18).

Interactions with Herbs & Other Dietary Supplements
None known.

Interactions with Drugs
CYTOCHROME P450 3A4 (CYP3A4) SUBSTRATES: There's preliminary evidence that wild cherry can inhibit CYP3A4 enzymes (6450). Theoretically, wild cherry might increase levels of drugs metabolized by CYP3A4. However, so far, this interaction has not been reported in humans. Some drugs metabolized by CYP3A4 include lovastatin (Mevacor), ketoconazole (Nizoral), itraconazole (Sporanox), fexofenadine (Allegra), triazolam (Halcion), and numerous others. Use wild cherry cautiously or avoid in patients taking these drugs.

Interactions with Foods
None known.

Interactions with Lab Tests
None known.

Interactions with Diseases or Conditions
None known.

Dosage and Administration
ORAL: People use 5 to 12 drops of the liquid extract containing wild cherry bark (12-14% by volume) in water two to three times daily (5023).

Comments
Avoid confusion with cherry laurel water. In Chinese medicine, the stem and bark of related species (Prunus armeniaca) may be effective as an antidote for apricot kernel poisoning (18).

WILD DAISY

Also Known As
Bruisewort.

Scientific Names
Bellis perennis.
Family: Asteraceae/Compositae.

Comments
At the date of publication, there was very little scientific information about this product. Our staff is continually analyzing the available information on natural medicines and will add data to the online version of *Natural Medicines Comprehensive Database* as it becomes available. See www.naturaldatabase.com.

WILD INDIGO

Also Known As
American Indigo, Baptista, False Indigo, Horsefly Weed, Indigo Broom, Rattlebush, Yellow Broom, Yellow Indigo.

Scientific Names
Baptisia tinctoria.
Family: Fabaceae/Leguminosae.

People Use This For
Orally, wild indigo is used for diphtheria, influenza, malaria, septic angina, and typhoid fever with prostration. It is also used orally for upper respiratory tract infections, common head cold, tonsillitis, stomatitis, inflammation of the mouth and throat mucous membranes, fever, lymphadenitis, furunculosis, Crohn's disease, scarlet fever, typhoid, and pharyngitis.
Topically, wild indigo is used for painless ulcers, inflamed nipples, as a douche for leukorrhea, and for cleaning open and inflamed wounds.

Safety
UNSAFE ...when used orally or topically, long-term; contraindicated due to potential toxicity (12,19).
PREGNANCY AND LACTATION: UNSAFE ...when used orally or topically due to its toxic potential (12,19).

Effectiveness
There is insufficient reliable information available about the effectiveness of wild indigo.

Mechanism of Action
The applicable part of wild indigo is the root. Preliminary evidence suggests that glycoprotein constituents might have lymphocyte stimulating activity (393). Quinolizidine alkaloids cause gastrointestinal symptoms with high doses (18).

Adverse Reactions
Orally, large doses of wild indigo can cause vomiting, diarrhea, gastrointestinal complaints, and spasms (12).

Interactions with Herbs & Other Dietary Supplements
None known.

Interactions with Drugs
None known.

Interactions with Foods
None known.

Interactions with Lab Tests
None known.

Interactions with Diseases or Conditions
GASTRIC DISORDERS: Use of wild indigo is contraindicated in patients with inflammatory gastrointestinal conditions, particularly with accompanying capillary congestion (19).

Dosage and Administration
ORAL: One cup of tea is typically taken orally 3 times daily. The tea is prepared by simmering 0.5-1 grams dried root in 150 mL of boiling water for 10-15 minutes and straining (18).
TOPICAL: An ointment is prepared using one part of liquid extract to 8 parts of ointment base and applied to the affected area (18).

WILD LETTUCE

Also Known As
Acrid Lettuce, Bitter Lettuce, German Lactucarium, Green Endive, Lactucarium, Lettuce Opium, Poison Lettuce, Strong-Scented Lettuce.

Scientific Names
Lactuca virosa.
Family: Asteraceae/Compositae.

People Use This For
Orally, wild lettuce is used for whooping cough, mucous inflammations of the bronchial tract, asthma, urinary tract diseases, irritable cough, insomnia, restlessness, excitability in children, priapism, painful menses, nymphomania, muscular or joint pains, for aiding circulation, swollen genitals, and as an opium substitute in cough preparations.
The seed oil is used orally for arteriosclerosis and as a substitute for wheat germ oil.
Topically, wild lettuce latex is used as an antiseptic.
By inhalation, wild lettuce is used for a recreational "high" or hallucinogenic effect.

Safety
POSSIBLY SAFE ...when used orally and appropriately (12,4).
LIKELY UNSAFE ...when used orally in large doses because they can cause stupor, depressed respiration, and death (4).
PREGNANCY AND LACTATION: Insufficient reliable information available; avoid using.

Effectiveness
There is insufficient reliable information available about the effectiveness of wild lettuce.

Mechanism of Action
The applicable parts of wild lettuce are the latex and leaf. Wild lettuce is thought to have mild sedative, analgesic, and hypnotic or tranquilizing effects (4,18). Wild lettuce contains lactucin and lactupicrin (4). The milky latex, known as lactucarium, can cause mydriasis (4). This effect is theorized to be due to the presence of hyoscyamine (4); however, the dried sap contains no hyoscyamine (4). Wild lettuce has sedative activity (4). Lactucin, lactupicrin, and hyoscyamine have all been proposed responsible for this activity, but the active constituent(s) has not been identified (4). Low concentrations (nanogram amounts) of morphine have been found in Lactuca species and are considered too low to have a pharmacological effect (4).

Adverse Reactions
Orally, large amounts can cause sweating, increased respiration, tachycardia, pupil dilation, dizziness, ringing in the ears, vision disorders, pressure in the head, somnolence, excitatory states (18), respiratory depression, coma, and death (4).
Topically, wild lettuce can cause contact dermatitis (4). It can cause an allergic reaction in individuals sensitive to the Asteraceae/Compositae family. Members of this family include ragweed, chrysanthemums, marigolds, daisies, and many other herbs.

Interactions with Herbs & Other Dietary Supplements
HERBS WITH ANTICOAGULANT/ANTIPLATELET POTENTIAL: Concomitant use of herbs that have antiplatelet/anticoagulant effects could theoretically increase the risk of bleeding in some people. These herbs include clove, danshen, garlic, ginger, ginkgo, ginseng, meadowsweet, poplar, red clover, and others.

HERBS WITH SEDATIVE PROPERTIES: Theoretically, concomitant use with herbs that have sedative properties might enhance therapeutic and adverse effects. These include calamus, California poppy plant, catnip leaves, hops, Jamaican dogwood bark, kava root, passionflower, sage, St. John's wort, sassafras bark, scullcap plant, valerian, and others.

Interactions with Drugs

CNS DEPRESSANTS: Theoretically, concomitant use with drugs with sedative effects might cause additive therapeutic effects and adverse effects (19).

Interactions with Foods

None known.

Interactions with Lab Tests

None known.

Interactions with Diseases or Conditions

BENIGN PROSTATIC HYPERPLASIA (BPH): Contraindicated in prostate enlargement (12). Wild lettuce might contain hyoscyamine (4) which is contraindicated in conditions involving urinary retention, including BPH (15).
CROSS-ALLERGENICITY: Wild lettuce can cause an allergic reaction in individuals sensitive to members of the Asteraceae/Compositae plant family. Members of this family include ragweed, chrysanthemums, marigolds, daisies, and many other herbs.
NARROW-ANGLE GLAUCOMA: Contraindicated (12). Wild lettuce might contain hyoscyamine (4) which can exacerbate narrow-angle (closed-angle) glaucoma (15).

Dosage and Administration

ORAL: A typical dose is 0.5-3 grams dried leaves or as tea three times daily. To make tea, steep 0.5 - 3 grams dried leaves in 150 mL of boiling water, strain (4). As the liquid extract (1:1 in 25% alcohol), 0.5 - 3 mL three times daily (4). For the dried latex extract, lactucarium, 0.3 -1 grams three times daily (4). Also available as a soft extract, with the usual dose of 0.3 - 1 grams three times daily (4).

WILD MINT

Also Known As

Hairy Mint, Marsh Mint, Water Mint.

Scientific Names

Mentha aquatica, synonym Mentha palustris.
Family: Lamiaceae/Labiatae.

Comments

At the date of publication, this product was not a common ingredient used in brand name supplements marketed to consumers. Details about this product are available at the online version of *Natural Medicines Comprehensive Database*. See www.naturaldatabase.com.

WILD RADISH

Also Known As

Joint-Podded Charlock.

Scientific Names

Raphanus raphanistrum.
Family: Brassicaceae/Cruciferae.

Comments

At the date of publication, this product was not a common ingredient used in brand name supplements marketed to consumers. Details about this product are available at the online version of *Natural Medicines Comprehensive Database*. See www.naturaldatabase.com.

WILD THYME

Also Known As
Mother of Thyme, Serpyllum, Shepherd's Thyme.
CAUTION: See separate listings for Thyme, Spanish Origanum Oil, and Thyme Oil.

Scientific Names
Thymus serpyllum.
Family: Lamiaceae/Labiatae.

People Use This For
Orally, wild thyme is used for cough, bronchitis, inflammation of the respiratory tract, kidney and bladder disorders, to relieve flatulence and colic, as a digestive aid, expectorant, aromatic, and antimicrobial.
Topically, wild thyme is used for arthritis and sprains.

Safety
LIKELY SAFE ...when used in amounts commonly found in foods. Wild thyme has Generally Recognized As Safe (GRAS) status in the US (4912).
POSSIBLY SAFE ...when preparations of the above ground flowering parts are used orally and appropriately (12).
PREGNANCY AND LACTATION: Insufficient reliable information; avoid using in medicinal amounts.

Effectiveness
There is insufficient reliable information available about the effectiveness of wild thyme.

Mechanism of Action
The applicable parts of wild thyme are the above ground, flowering parts. There is insufficient reliable information available about the possible mechanism of action and active ingredients.

Adverse Reactions
None reported.

Interactions with Herbs & Other Dietary Supplements
None known.

Interactions with Drugs
None known.

Interactions with Foods
None known.

Interactions with Lab Tests
None known.

Interactions with Diseases or Conditions
THYROID DISORDERS: Can suppress thyroid function by decreasing hormone production and/or release (19).

Dosage and Administration
ORAL: One cup of tea taken orally before meals. The tea is prepared by steeping 1.5-2 grams dried plant in 150 mL of boiling water for 10 minutes and straining. The daily dose is equivalent to 4-6 grams dried herb (18).

WILD YAM

Also Known As
Atlantic Yam, Barbasco, China Root, Colic Root, Devil's Bones, Dioscorea, Dioscoreae, Mexican Yam, Natural DHEA, Phytoestrogen, Rheumatism Root, Rhizoma Dioscoreae, Wild Mexican Yam, Yam, Yuma.
CAUTION: See separate listings for Pregnenolone and Progesterone.

Scientific Names
Dioscorea composita, synonym Dioscorea tepinapensis; Dioscorea floribunda; Dioscorea mexicana, synonym Dioscorea macrostachya; Discorea villosa, synonym Dioscorea hirticaulis. Family: Dioscoreaceae.

People Use This For

Orally, wild yam is used as a "natural alternative" for estrogen replacement therapy, postmenopausal vaginal dryness, premenstrual syndrome, osteoporosis, increasing energy and libido in men and women, and for breast enlargement. Wild yam is also used orally for treating diverticulosis, gallbladder colic, painful menstruation, cramp, rheumatoid arthritis, and for increasing energy.

Topically, wild yam is used for menopausal vasomotor symptoms such as hot flashes.

In manufacturing, the constituent of wild yam root, diosgenin, is used as a precursor for commercial chemical synthesis of human steroidal hormones.

Safety

POSSIBLY SAFE ...when used orally (12). ...when used topically (10989).

PREGNANCY AND LACTATION: Insufficient reliable information available; avoid using.

Effectiveness

POSSIBLY INEFFECTIVE

Menopausal symptoms. Wild yam applied topically appears to be no better than placebo for relieving vasomotor symptoms such as hot flashes and night sweats in menopausal women using wild yam cream for 3 months. It doesn't appear to cause changes in serum follicle stimulating hormone (FSH), estradiol, or progesterone (10989).

There is insufficient reliable information available about the effectiveness of wild yam for its other uses.

Mechanism of Action

The applicable parts of wild yam are the root and rhizome. The tubers of Dioscorea species contain the glycoside diosgenin, a steroid precursor that was used in the first commercial production of oral contraceptives, topical hormones, systemic corticosteroids, androgens, estrogens, progestogens, and other sex hormones (515). Dioscorea continues to be used as the precursor for manufacturing progesterone contained in some "natural progesterone" cosmetic products. The chemical transformation of diosgenin to estrogen, progesterone, or any other steroidal compound does not occur in the human body (515). Diosgenin prevents estrogen-induced bile flow suppression (5129). It shows some evidence that it might stimulate growth of mammary tissue (5130), and attenuate indomethacin-induced intestinal inflammation (5131). A wild yam extract enhances estradiol binding to estrogen receptors and induces transcription activity in estrogen-responsive cells (6180). Topically applied wild yam doesn't appear to cause changes in serum follicle stimulating hormone (FSH), estradiol, or progesterone (10989).

Adverse Reactions

Orally, ingestion of large amounts of wild yam tincture has caused emesis (12).

Interactions with Herbs & Other Dietary Supplements

None known.

Interactions with Drugs

None known.

Interactions with Foods

None known.

Interactions with Lab Tests

None known.

Interactions with Diseases or Conditions

HORMONE SENSITIVE CANCERS/CONDITIONS: Wild yam has in vitro estrogenic effects, but doesn't appear to affect hormone levels when used topically (6180,10989). Women with hormone sensitive conditions should avoid wild yam until more is known. Some hormone sensitive conditions include breast cancer, uterine cancer, ovarian cancer, endometriosis, and uterine fibroids.

Dosage and Administration

No typical dosage.

Comments

Diosgenin, a component of wild yam, is promoted as a natural precursor to dehydroepiandrosterone (DHEA). Some wild yam products are promoted as "natural DHEA". Although diosgenin can be converted to steroidal compounds, including DHEA, in the laboratory, this chemical synthesis does not occur in the human body. So taking wild yam extract will not increase DHEA levels in humans (515,2112). People interested in taking DHEA should avoid wild yam products labeled as "natural DHEA."

WILLARD WATER

Also Known As
Biowater, Carbonaceous Activated Water, Catalyst Altered Water, Williard's Water.

Scientific Names
None.

People Use This For
Orally, Willard water is used for arthritis, acne, anxiety, nervous stomach, hypertension, ulcers, and hair growth. In manufacturing, Willard water is used as a food preserver, laundry aid, and a treatment for bovine and feline leukemia.

Safety
There is insufficient reliable information available about the safety of Willard water.
Pregnancy and Lactation: Insufficient reliable information available; avoid using.

Effectiveness
There is insufficient reliable information available about the effectiveness of Willard water.

Mechanism of Action
The formula for Willard water has changed over time. Some of the ingredients found in products analyzed by the FDA included rock salt in various combinations, lignite, sodium metasilicate, sulfated castor oil, calcium chloride, and magnesium sulfate (18).

Adverse Reactions
None reported.

Interactions with Herbs & Other Dietary Supplements
None known.

Interactions with Drugs
None known.

Interactions with Foods
None known.

Interactions with Lab Tests
None known.

Interactions with Diseases or Conditions
None known.

Dosage and Administration
No typical dosage.

Comments
Willard water was developed in the early twentieth century at the South Dakota School of Mines by a chemistry professor named John Wesley Willard, Ph.D. It was developed and patented as an industrial cleanser to clean and degrease train parts. However, it became legendary among townsfolk who used Willard water to treat almost every disease known to humans and animals, and as a plant fertilizer. It is not recognized as safe or effective by the FDA (6).

WILLOW BARK

Also Known As
Basket Willow, Bay Willow, Brittle Willow, Crack Willow, Daphne Willow, Knackweide, Laurel Willow, Lorbeerweide, Osier Rouge, Pupurweide, Purple Osier, Purple Osier Willow, Reifweide, Salicis cortex, Silberweide, Violet Willow, Weidenrinde, White Willow, White Willow Bark.

Scientific Names
Salix alba; Salix daphnoides; Salix fragilis; Salix pentandra; Salix purpurea; other Salix species.
Family: Salicaceae.

People Use This For
Orally, willow bark is used for mild feverish colds and infections, headaches, pain caused by inflammation, muscle and joint aches, influenza, respiratory tract mucous membrane inflammation, gouty arthritis, ankylosing spondylitis, rheumatoid arthritis (RA), systemic connective tissue disorders characterized by inflammatory changes, diseases accompanied by fever, rheumatic ailments, gout, and inflammatory joint disease.

Safety
POSSIBLY SAFE ...when used orally and appropriately, short-term (6456). Willow bark has been used safely up to 4 weeks in one study (6456).
CHILDREN: POSSIBLY UNSAFE ...when used orally for viral infections. Although Reye's syndrome has not been reported (12), the salicin constituent in willow bark is similar to aspirin and might pose the same risk (15).
PREGNANCY: Insufficient reliable information available; avoid using.
LACTATION: POSSIBLY UNSAFE ...when used orally. Willow bark contains salicylates which are excreted in breast milk and have been linked to macular rashes in breast-fed infants (4).

Effectiveness
POSSIBLY EFFECTIVE

Back pain. There's some evidence that a willow bark extract providing 120-240 mg of the salicin constituent daily can reduce low back pain in some patients. The higher concentration of 240 mg salicin is more effective. However, it can take up to 1 week for significant relief (6456).

There is insufficient reliable information available about the effectiveness of willow bark for its other uses.

Mechanism of Action
Willow bark constituents include flavonoids, tannins, and salicylates. Most of the information about willow bark is based on documented pharmacology for salicylates. These actions include anti-inflammatory, antipyretic, dose-dependent hyperglycemic/hypoglycemic, uricosuric/antiuricosuric activities, and increases in blood clotting time and plasma-albumin binding (4). These phenolic glycosides are heat labile and they convert to salicin if willow bark is dried (512). Salicin is a prodrug that is metabolized to saligenin in the gastrointestinal tract and to salicylic acid after absorption (4). Because time is required for the prodrugs to convert to salicylic acid, the properties of willow bark have a slower onset and a longer effectiveness than salicylate itself (3). In vitro tests show that salicin and salicortin inhibit cyclooxygenase. This means irreversible inhibition of thrombocytes is unlikely and there should be no increased interaction with blood coagulants (8). The tannin constituents have astringent properties (4). Tannins also show some evidence of antiviral, antimicrobial, non-specific CNS depressant and cariostatic effects (11). Tannins exert an astringent effect on mucosal tissue. This effect dehydrates the tissue, internally reducing secretions, and externally forming a protective layer of harder, constricted cells (12). Plants with at least 10% tannins can cause gastrointestinal disturbances, kidney damage, and necrotic conditions of the liver (12). Some evidence suggests that tannins might cause cancer, while other evidence shows they may prevent it (12). Regular consumption of herbs with high tannin concentrations correlates with increased incidence of esophageal or nasal cancer (12).

Adverse Reactions
Orally, gastrointestinal disturbances, kidney damage, and necrotic conditions of the liver are possible due to the tannin content in willow bark. Adverse reactions associated with salicylates are possible including gastric and renal irritation, hypersensitivity, blood in stool, tinnitus, nausea, and vomiting (12). Willow bark may cause serious allergic reactions, including anaphylaxis, in people who are allergic to aspirin (10392).
Topically, salicin has been associated with skin rashes (4).

Interactions with Herbs & Other Dietary Supplements
HERBS WITH ANTICOAGULANT/ANTIPLATELET POTENTIAL: Concomitant use of herbs that have antiplatelet/anticoagulant effects could theoretically increase the risk of bleeding in some people. These herbs include clove, danshen, garlic, ginger, ginkgo, ginseng, meadowsweet, red clover, and others.
SALICYLATE-CONTAINING HERBS: Theoretically, concomitant use may potentiate salicylate effects and adverse effects. Salicylate-containing herbs include aspen bark, poplar, sweet birch.

TANNIN-CONTAINING HERBS: Theoretically, herbs such as willow bark that contain a high percentage of tannins might precipitate alkaloids of other herbs.

Interactions with Drugs

ANTICOAGULANT/ANTIPLATELET DRUGS: Irreversible inhibition of thrombocytes is unlikely with plant salicylates and there should not be an interaction with blood coagulants (8).
ASPIRIN: Willow bark contains salicin, a plant salicylate. Theoretically, willow bark might have an additive effect with other salicylate-containing drugs such as aspirin. Salicin doesn't seem to have the antiplatelet effects of aspirin (12).
CHOLINE MAGNESIUM TRISALICYLATE (Trilisate): Willow bark contains salicin, a plant salicylate. Theoretically, willow bark might have an additive effect with other salicylate-containing drugs such as choline magnesium trisalicylate (12).
ORAL DRUGS: Theoretically, concomitant oral administration might cause precipitation of some drugs due to the high tannin content of willow bark (19). Separate administration of oral drugs and tannin-containing herbs by the longest period of time practical (19).
SALSALATE (Disalcid): Willow bark contains salicin, a plant salicylate. Theoretically, willow bark might have an additive effect with other salicylate-containing drugs such as salsalate (12).

Interactions with Foods

None known.

Interactions with Lab Tests

None known.

Interactions with Diseases or Conditions

KIDNEY OR LIVER DYSFUNCTION: Theoretically, oral use of willow bark is contraindicated in people with kidney or liver dysfunction because it might exacerbate these conditions. Plants with at least 10% tannins are reported to have the potential to cause kidney damage and liver necrosis (12).
SALICYLATE PRECAUTIONS: Avoid or use cautiously in individuals with aspirin hypersensitivity, asthma, active peptic ulcer disease, diabetes, gout, hemophilia, hypoprothrombinemia, kidney or liver disease (4). Willow bark may cause serious allergic reactions, including anaphylaxis, in people who are allergic to aspirin (10392).

Dosage and Administration

ORAL: For back pain, willow bark extract providing 120-240 mg salicin has been used in a clinical study. The higher 240 mg dose might be more effective (6456). A typical dose for other uses is 1-3 grams dried bark 3-4 times daily, or one cup tea. To make tea, steep 1-3 grams bark in 150 mL of boiling water for 5 minutes, and strain (8). Liquid extract (1:1 in 25% alcohol), 1-3 mL three times daily has been used (4).

Comments

Salicylate concentrations vary greatly among Salix species (512). Salix alba bark is reported to contain 0.49-0.98% salicin (4); Salix purpurea bark contains 3-9%; Salix daphnoides 4.9-5.6%; Salix fragilis 3.9-10.2% (8).

WINE

Also Known As

Alcohol, Ethanol.
CAUTION: See separate listing for Resveratrol.

Scientific Names

Vitis vinifera.
Family: Vitaceae.

People Use This For

Orally, wine is used for reducing the risk of cardiovascular disease, including coronary heart disease (CHD), atherosclerosis, and myocardial infarction (MI); and for reducing the risk of ischemic stroke and type 2 diabetes. It is also used orally to prevent cognitive decline in later life and to prevent Alzheimer's disease. Wine is also used orally for anxiety, achlorhydria, malabsorption syndromes, and as an appetite stimulant.
Topically, wine is used to stimulate wound healing and improve rheumatoid skin ulcerations.

Safety

LIKELY SAFE ...when used orally, responsibly, and in moderation (11880).
POSSIBLY UNSAFE ...when used orally in excess of 1 to 2 five-ounce glasses of wine per day. Larger amounts

can cause minimal to significant adverse effects (11880).
PREGNANCY: LIKELY UNSAFE ...when used orally; alcohol is a teratogen. Use during pregnancy, especially during the first two months after conception, is associated with significant risk of spontaneous abortion, fetal alcohol syndrome, and developmental and behavioral dysfunction in infants and children exposed to alcohol in utero (8100); avoid using.
LACTATION: LIKELY UNSAFE ...when used orally. Alcohol is secreted in breast milk. Chronic use can cause abnormal psychomotor development, and disrupt the infant's sleep wake pattern. Alcohol also seems to reduce milk production (11878); avoid using.

Effectiveness

LIKELY EFFECTIVE

Cardiovascular disease. Consumption of alcoholic drinks, including wine, by otherwise healthy people seems to reduce the risk of developing cardiovascular disease. Moderate alcohol use (one to two drinks per day) reduces the risk of coronary heart disease, atherosclerosis, and myocardial infarction (MI), by approximately 30% to 50% when compared with nondrinkers (2267,2268,2271,6888,6892,8648,8649,10128,11879). Light to moderate alcohol consumption reduces ischemic stroke risk, but there is evidence that consuming any amount of alcohol can increase the risk of hemorrhagic stroke (841,2271,2279,6834,6842,6893). There is some evidence that light to moderate consumption of alcoholic drinks (one to two drinks per day) including wine, can reduce the risk of all-cause mortality in people who are middle-aged or older (2058,6823,6837,6843). Light to moderate consumption of alcohol might also reduce the risk of cardiovascular mortality in otherwise healthy people (2058,2270,6835,6837). Light to moderate alcohol consumption in the year prior to first acute MI is associated with a reduced cardiovascular- and all-cause mortality risk compared with non-drinkers (8650). Consumption of one alcoholic beverage per day or consuming alcohol on at least 3 to 4 days per week is a good rule of thumb for people who drink alcohol. Tell patients not to exceed two drinks per day. More than two drinks daily can increase the risk of cardiovascular and overall mortality (841,2060,2261,6173,6890,8648,11879). In men with established coronary heart disease (CHD), consumption of 1-14 alcoholic drinks per week, including wine, doesn't seem to have any effect on cardiovascular disease or all-cause mortality compared with men who drink less than one drink per week. Consuming three or more drinks per day is associated with increased mortality in men with a history of heart attacks (6173).

POSSIBLY EFFECTIVE

Cognitive function. Elderly men who have a history of consuming up to one alcoholic drink per day seem to maintain better general cognitive function during their late 70's and 80's compared to non-drinkers (6824,6829). However, consumption of more than four drinks per day during middle age seems to be associated with significantly poorer cognitive function in later life (6824).

Diabetes. Light to moderate alcohol consumption from wine and other sources, is associated with a reduced risk of type 2 diabetes in healthy men (6172,6891). Light to moderate alcohol consumption is also associated with a reduced risk of coronary heart disease (CHD) in men and women with type 2 diabetes compared with non-drinkers with type 2 diabetes. The risk reduction of CHD associated with light to moderate alcohol consumption in people with type 2 diabetes is similar to that found in people without diabetes who consume light to moderate amounts of alcohol (8653,8654).

Heart failure. Consuming one to four alcoholic drinks per day is associated with a reduced risk of heart failure in persons aged 65 years or older (8104). Consumption of 1-14 alcoholic drinks per week is associated with reduced all-cause mortality in people with ischemic left ventricular (LV) dysfunction compared with non-drinkers with ischemic LV dysfunction. However, this benefit does not seem to occur for those patients with non-ischemic LV dysfunction (6827).

Helicobacter pylori (H pylori). There is some evidence that moderate to high (more than 75 grams) consumption of alcohol per week from beverages such as beer and wine can reduce the risk of H. pylori infection (8034).

INSUFFICIENT RELIABLE EVIDENCE to RATE

Alzheimer's disease. There is some evidence that 1 to 2 drinks per day can reduce the risk of developing Alzheimer's disease in both men and women compared with non-drinkers (6603).

Anxiety. The effect of alcohol on anxiety is complex, and may be affected by the psychological state of the user. It sometimes reduces anxiety, sometimes increases it, and sometimes has no effect (2266).

Cancer. There is some preliminary evidence that intake of up to 21 alcoholic drinks per week, including wine, might slightly reduce the risk of cancer-related mortality (6823).

Post-menopausal osteoporosis. There is preliminary evidence that moderate alcohol consumption in postmenopausal women is associated with increased bone mineral density in the trochanter, femoral neck, mid-radius, and lumbar spine (6825,6836,8655). Alcohol intake of one-half to one drink per day seems to have the greatest effect on bone mineral density compared with non-drinkers and heavy drinkers of alcohol (8655).

More evidence is needed to rate wine for these uses.

Mechanism of Action

Wine is the natural yeast fermentation product of the juice of sun-ripened grapes, the fruit of Vitis vinifera. Wine normally contains 10% to 14% alcohol, predominantly as ethanol, which is a central nervous system (CNS) depressant (2263).
Several mechanisms have been proposed for the protective effects of alcohol against coronary heart

disease (CHD) (2060,2268,2270,6839,6840). One to two alcoholic drinks per day increases high-density lipoprotein (HDL) cholesterol by about 12% (6892) and apolipoprotein A-I by about 2.2% (8649). This increase in HDL cholesterol levels may account for about 50% of the cardioprotective effect of moderate alcohol consumption (2261,6838,6841). Moderate alcohol consumption also decreases low-density lipoprotein (LDL) cholesterol by 5% to 17% (6841,8649), triglycerides by 5% to 10%, and apolipoprotein B levels by 3.7% (8649). There is concern that moderate alcohol consumption can increase systolic blood pressure (6841). However, there is evidence that light to moderate alcohol consumption does not increase the risk of hypertension and may actually decrease the risk (8102). Effects of alcohol on blood clotting include a reduction in clotting potential and enhancement of clot breakdown (2261). Alcohol consumption decreases platelet aggregation, possibly via inhibition of prostaglandin synthesis (6892). Moderate alcohol consumption is also associated with an increase in plasma levels of tissue-type plasminogen activator, an indicator of fibrinolytic capacity (6894). Alcohol also seems to lower fibrinogen and interleukin-1 alpha concentrations (11943). Light to moderate alcohol consumption also seems to produce a reduction in coronary narrowing due to atherosclerosis (2261,6840,8652). Wine may also have anti-inflammatory effects. It reduces high sensitivity C-reactive protein (hs-CRP) and expression of adhesion molecules, markers of inflammation that seem to be related to early atherosclerosis (11943). There is also evidence that an increased intake of dietary folate or the use of supplemental folate (400 mcg/day) in moderate alcohol users can lower homocysteine levels compared with nonusers of alcohol (8101). High levels of homocysteine are a risk factor for cardiovascular disease. Homocysteine breakdown and removal requires folate, and alcohol is an antagonist of folate metabolism (8101). The protective effect of alcohol against cardiovascular disease is lost at higher intakes of alcohol (greater than one to two drinks per day). High alcohol consumption can cause increased homocysteine levels, hypertension, hemorrhagic stroke, fatal arrhythmias, and direct damage to heart muscle (alcoholic cardiomyopathy) (2060,2261,2267,2270,8101,8102,8103).

Some alcoholic beverages, in particular red wine, have constituents that may be more protective than others against coronary heart disease, but there is no conclusive evidence of this from clinical studies (2267,2268,6892). Red wine has higher concentrations of polyphenolic compounds than other alcoholic drinks. The antioxidant properties of these polyphenols may contribute to protection against coronary heart disease by reducing oxidation of LDL cholesterol (2268). The polyphenolic compounds in red wine include trans-resveratrol; proanthocyanidins; anthocyanins; and flavonoids such as quercetin, kaempferol, and catechins (1262,2057,8976). However, the polyphenol content of wine is highly dependent on grape type, climate, and practices used to make the wine (2057). Unlike red wines, white wines have very low polyphenol concentrations (2030). The antioxidant potential of plasma and erythrocytes is increased for up to 4.5 hours after red wine consumption (6828). However, there is some evidence that the increase of polyphenols in plasma after red wine consumption is not sufficient to acutely influence lipoprotein oxidation (1262,6826,8976). There is evidence that other foods such as onions and black tea may be better sources of polyphenols than red wine (8976). Additionally, a difference in lifestyle among wine, beer, and other alcohol beverage drinkers, including diet and social class, might also explain why some alcoholic beverages appear to offer more protection than others against CHD (10129).

Several red wine components also have in vitro antiplatelet effects, including trans-resveratrol, quercetin, and catechins (2057). Red wine and white wine seem to have similar activity on platelets (2057,2949). Human data also suggest rebound hypercoagulability can normally occur when acute or chronic alcohol consumption stops, but that red wine attenuates this effect (2060,2061). Red wine might also reduce mutagenic DNA damage and improve endothelial function when added to a high fat diet. Red wine also might have additive vasorelaxing benefits with a low-fat, high plant material diet (2059).

Possible mechanisms by which alcohol could have a protective effect against ischemic stroke include increasing HDL and prostacyclin, decreasing fibrinogen, and inhibiting platelet aggregation (6842). There is evidence that moderate alcohol increases cerebral blood flow (8651). Moderate alcohol consumption is associated with a lower prevalence of white matter changes and brain infarcts on magnetic resonance imaging in adults 65 years of age or older compared to non-drinkers and heavy drinkers (8651).

Moderate alcohol intake may be protective against the development of type 2 diabetes due to an increase in insulin sensitivity (6891). Wine stimulates gastric acid secretion and gastrin release. This may explain why moderate to high alcohol consumption from beverages such as wine seems to prevent Helicobacter pylori infection (8034). Moderate alcohol consumption may be protective against postmenopausal bone loss due to an increase in estrogen levels, increased calcitonin secretion, and reduced parathyroid hormone secretion (6825,6836,8655). However, heavy and chronic alcohol consumption reduces bone mineral density, possibly due to increased calcium and magnesium excretion, increased cortisol secretion, and reduced osteoblast activity (6836,8656). Chronic alcoholics also often have other risk factors for osteoporosis, including poor nutrition, smoking, sedentary lifestyle, and lower body weight (6825,6836).

Adverse Reactions

Orally, wine can cause a variety of side effects due to the alcohol content. The side effects depend on the amount ingested and can vary among individuals. Some common side effects include flushing, confusion, emotional lability, perceptual and sensational disturbances, blackouts, lack of coordination and trouble walking, central nervous system (CNS) depression, drowsiness, respiratory depression, hypothermia, hypoglycemia, nausea, vomiting, diarrhea, abdominal pain, and others. Chronic heavy ethanol ingestion (three or more alcoholic drinks per day) can lead to physical dependence, malnutrition, amnesia, dementia, somnolence, cardiac myopathy, hepatotoxicity, and cirrhosis. Other effects of chronic abuse are pancreatitis, hypomagnesemia, skeletal myopathies, Wernicke's encephalopathy,

Korsakoff's psychosis, chronic cerebellar syndrome, mouth cancer, esophageal cancer, pharyngeal cancer, laryngeal cancer, and liver cancer (6843,8972,9004). There is evidence that heavy alcohol consumption is associated with the mutation of the p53 gene in individuals with esophageal carcinoma (9005). There is also some evidence heavy consumption of wine is associated with the highest risk of esophageal cancer compared to heavy consumption of beer and spirits (8972). Chronic intake of three or more drinks per day is associated with an increased risk of all-cause mortality, ischemic stroke, and hypertension (2261,6892,8102). Heavy alcohol consumption (fifteen or more drinks per week) is also associated with a higher percentage of white matter changes and larger ventricular and sulcal size on magnetic resonance imaging of the brain, suggesting heavy alcohol consumption decreases cerebral blood flow and may contribute to brain atrophy (8651). Consumption of any amount of alcohol can increase the risk of hemorrhagic stroke (841,2271).

Daily consumption one or more alcoholic drinks in women might increase the risk of breast cancer by 2% to 15% and increase mortality from breast cancer by as much as 30% (6843,8100,8974). There is also evidence in women who consume alcohol daily that the risk for breast cancer increases when the daily intake of folate is 300 mcg or less (8974).

Some research suggests an association between alcohol consumption and an increased risk for pancreatic cancer, but other studies do not support this association (8038).

Wine is associated with triggering asthmatic reactions in people with a history of asthma, possibly due to salicylates and/or added sulfites contained in wines (6174). People who are allergic to sulfites and/or yeast might react to wine.

There is some evidence consumption of more than six beers per week is associated with a larger waist-to-hip ratio than those consuming an equivalent amount of hard liquor or wine. However, an association between moderate alcohol intake equivalent to approximately three beers per week or less and waist-to-hip ratio does not seem to exist (10164,10165). It is also unclear whether waist-to-hip ratios associated with the intake of wine, beer, or other alcoholic beverages have any clinical significance (9007).

Interactions with Herbs & Other Dietary Supplements

HERBS/SUPPLEMENTS WITH SEDATIVE PROPERTIES: Theoretically, concomitant use of wine with herbs that have sedative properties might enhance adverse effects (2262). Some of these supplements include 5-HTP, calamus, California poppy, catnip, hops, Jamaican dogwood, kava, St. John's wort, scullcap, valerian, yerba mansa, and others.

Interactions with Drugs

ASPIRIN: Concomitant use of aspirin with alcohol may increase the risk of gastrointestinal (GI) bleeding (2262).

BARBITURATES: Concomitant consumption of large amounts of alcohol may decrease metabolism of barbiturates (2262). Some of these sedative medications include pentobarbital (Nembutal), phenobarbital (Luminal), secobarbital (Seconal), and others.

BENZODIAZEPINES: Concomitant consumption of large amounts of alcohol may decrease metabolism of benzodiazepines (2262).

CEFAMANDOLE (Mandol): Cefamandole antibiotics can cause a disulfiram-like reaction when taken with alcohol (2262).

CEFOPERAZONE (Cefobid): Cefoperazone can cause a disulfiram-like reaction when taken with alcohol (2262).

CHLORPROPAMIDE (Diabinese): Chlorpropamide can cause a disulfiram-like reaction when taken with alcohol (506).

CISAPRIDE (Propulsid): Concomitant use of cisapride might increase blood alcohol levels and effects, due to the alcohol in wine (2262). Red wine increases plasma cisapride concentrations, possibly by reducing metabolism (1383).

CNS DEPRESSANTS: Concomitant use of antihistamines, barbiturates, benzodiazepines, and tricyclic antidepressants with alcohol may increase sedative and other adverse effects (2262).

CYCLOSPORINE (Neoral, Sandimmune): Red wine reduces plasma cyclosporine concentrations, possibly by reducing cyclosporine absorption. There is evidence the reduction in cyclosporine AUC by red wine is less in Asians (8% to 14%) than Caucasians (35% to 36%) (1384,1387,8977).

DISULFIRAM (Antabuse): The alcohol content of wine can cause a disulfiram reaction when taken within 12 hours of disulfiram (2262). Patients taking disulfiram should not drink any alcoholic beverages including wine.

ERYTHROMYCIN: Concomitant use of erythromycin with alcohol may increase blood alcohol levels and effect (2262).

FELODIPINE (Plendil): Red wine can cause "dose dumping" of extended release felodipine. Red wine taken on an empty stomach with felodipine can alter the pharmacokinetics of extended release felodipine, possibly by changing absorption or metabolism. Red wine can delay the appearance of felodipine in plasma until 4 hours after dosing and can rapidly increase its plasma concentration, producing peak serum levels 3 to 4 times higher than when felodipine is given with water. This can cause an increase in adverse effects 5 hours after dosing (11976).

GRISEOFULVIN (Fulvicin): Griseofulvin can cause a disulfiram-like reaction when taken with alcohol (2262).

H2-BLOCKERS: Concomitant use of cimetidine (Tagamet) and ranitidine (Zantac) with alcohol may increase blood alcohol levels and adverse effects (2262).

HEPATOTOXIC DRUGS: Concomitant use with acetaminophen, isoniazid, and phenylbutazone may increase the risk of hepatotoxicity (2262).

METFORMIN (Glucophage): Concomitant consumption of large amounts of alcohol may increase the risk of

lactic acidosis with metformin (2262).
METRONIDAZOLE (Flagyl): Metronidazole can cause a disulfiram-like reaction when taken with alcohol (2262).
MONOAMINE OXIDASE INHIBITORS (MAOIs): Concomitant use of MAOIs with red wine may cause hypertensive crisis due to the tyramine content of wines (506).
NARCOTIC DRUGS: Concomitant consumption of large amounts of alcohol may decrease metabolism of narcotics (2262).
NONSTEROIDAL ANTI-INFLAMMATORY DRUGS (NSAIDs): Concomitant use of nonsteroidal anti-inflammatory drugs with alcohol may increase the risk of gastrointestinal (GI) bleeding (2262).
PHENYTOIN (Dilantin): Concomitant consumption of large amounts of alcohol may induce metabolism, reducing therapeutic effectiveness of phenytoin (2262).
SULFONAMIDE ANTIBIOTICS: Sulfonamide antibiotics can cause a disulfiram-like reaction when taken with alcohol (2262).
TOLBUTAMIDE (Orinase): Tolbutamide can cause a disulfiram-like reaction when taken with alcohol (2262).
WARFARIN (Coumadin): Acute alcohol intoxication can decrease metabolism and increase effects of warfarin (2262). In contrast, chronic intoxication can induce metabolism of warfarin, reducing therapeutic effectiveness (2262).

Drug Influences on Nutrient Levels and Depletion

B VITAMINS: Concomitant chronic use with alcohol might interfere with absorption of B vitamins and other nutrients (2263).

Interactions with Foods

None known.

Interactions with Lab Tests

LIVER FUNCTION TESTS: Chronic alcohol ingestion may increase alkaline phosphatase (Alk phos), alanine aminotransferase (ALT), aspartate aminotransferase (AST), gamma-glutamyltransferase (GGT), and bilirubin test results (2263).
MEAN CORPUSCULAR VOLUME (MCV): Chronic alcohol ingestion may increase MCV (2263).
TRIGLYCERIDES: Chronic alcohol ingestion may increase triglycerides (2263).

Interactions with Diseases or Conditions

ASTHMA: Wine is associated with triggering asthma reactions, possibly due to salicylates and/or added sulfites contained in wines (6174).
GOUT: Alcohol use may exacerbate gout (2263).
HEART CONDITIONS: Alcohol use may exacerbate congestive heart failure (2261,2263,6889) and idiopathic cardiomyopathy (6889).
HIGH BLOOD PRESSURE: Consuming three or more alcoholic drinks a day may increase blood pressure and exacerbate hypertension (2261).
HYPERTRIGLYCERIDEMIA: Alcohol use may exacerbate hypertriglyceridemia (2261,2263,6892).
INSOMNIA: Alcohol use may exacerbate insomnia (2263).
LIVER DISEASE: Alcohol use may exacerbate liver disease (2261).
NEUROLOGICAL CONDITIONS: Alcohol use may exacerbate degenerative neurological conditions (6889).
PANCREATITIS: Alcohol use may exacerbate pancreatitis (2261).
PEPTIC ULCER DISEASE (PUD)/GASTROESOPHAGEAL REFLUX DISEASE (GERD): Alcohol use may exacerbate PUD and GERD (2261,2263).
PORPHYRIA: Alcohol use may exacerbate porphyria (2261).
PSYCHIATRIC DISORDERS: Consuming three or more drinks of alcohol a day may exacerbate psychiatric disorders and increase cognitive impairment (2261).

Dosage and Administration

ORAL: For reducing the risk of cardiovascular disease, ischemic stroke, and all-cause mortality, 1-2 glasses (120-240 mL) per day has been used (2261,2271,6835,6837,6840,6841,6842,6888) (6892,6893,8648,8649,8650,10128). Up to four glasses per day has been used to reduce the risk for heart failure (8104). Up to one drink per day has been used to lessen cognitive decline in older men (6824,6829). Between two drinks per week and three or four drinks per day has been used to reduce risk of type 2 diabetes in healthy men (6172,6891). Up to seven drinks per week has been used to reduce the risk of coronary heart disease (CHD) in people with type 2 diabetes (8653,8654). Consumption of more than 75 grams of alcohol from beverages such as wine has been used to reduce the risk of Helicobacter pylori infection (8034).
TOPICAL: No typical dosage.

Comments

One report disputes the "French paradox" and suggests that reduced risk of heart disease in the French population is not due to red wine consumption, but due to the traditional French diet, which is low in animal fat (835).

WINTER CHERRY

Also Known As
Cape Gooseberry, Chinese Latern, Coqueret, Japanaese Latern, Strawberry Tomato.
CAUTION: See separate listing for Ashwagandha.

Scientific Names
Physalis alkekengi.
Family: Solanaceae.

Comments
At the date of publication, there was very little scientific information about this product. Our staff is continually analyzing the available information on natural medicines and will add data to the online version of *Natural Medicines Comprehensive Database* as it becomes available. See www.naturaldatabase.com.

WINTER SAVORY

Also Known As
Mountain Savory Oil, Savory.
CAUTION: See separate listing for Summer Savory.

Scientific Names
Satureja montana; Satureja obovata, synonym Calamintha montana.
Family: Lamiaceae/Labiatae.

People Use This For
Orally, winter savory is used for intestinal disorders including cramps, indigestion, diarrhea, nausea, flatulence, sore throat, as a tonic, expectorant, and to decrease libido.
In manufacturing, the oleoresin of winter savory oil is used as a flavoring agent.

Safety
LIKELY SAFE ...when used orally in amounts commonly found in foods. Summer savory has Generally Recognized As Safe (GRAS) status in the US (4912).
There is insufficient reliable information available about the safety of the medicinal use of winter savory.
PREGNANCY AND LACTATION: Insufficient reliable information available; avoid using.

Effectiveness
There is insufficient reliable information available about the effectiveness of winter savory.

Mechanism of Action
The applicable parts of winter savory are the leaf and stem. Winter savory contains flavonoids (11), ursolic and oleanolic acids, and 1.6% volatile oil. Constituents of the volatile oil include carvacrol, p-cymene, and thymol (6,11). Some evidence suggests the flavonoid, eriodictyol, might have a vasodilator effect (4124). Other information indicates carvacrol, found in both savories, might have diuretic effects (6,11).

Adverse Reactions
None reported.

Interactions with Herbs & Other Dietary Supplements
None known.

Interactions with Drugs
None known.

Interactions with Foods
None known.

Interactions with Lab Tests
None known.

Interactions with Diseases or Conditions
None known.

Dosage and Administration
No typical dosage.

Comments
Although summer savory and winter savory are both used as spices, in the United States summer savory is the most common (6).

WINTER'S BARK

Also Known As
Pepper Bark, Wintera, Wintera Aromatica, Winters Bark, Winter's Cinnamon, Winters Cinnamon.

Scientific Names
Drimys winteri, synonym Drimys chilensis.
Family: Winteraceae.

Comments
At the date of publication, this product was not a common ingredient used in brand name supplements marketed to consumers. Details about this product are available at the online version of *Natural Medicines Comprehensive Database*. See www.naturaldatabase.com.

WINTERGREEN leaf

Also Known As
Boxberry, Canada Tea, Checkerberry, Deerberry, Ground Berry, Hilberry, Mountain Tea, Partridge Berry, Spiceberry, Teaberry, Wax Cluster.
CAUTION: See separate listing for Wintergreen Oil.

Scientific Names
Gaultheria procumbens.
Family: Ericaceae.

People Use This For
Orally, wintergreen leaf is used for headache, stomachache, flatulence, fever, kidney disorders, asthma, neuralgia (particularly sciatica), pleurisy (and pain associated with pleurisy), ovarian pain, inflammation of the testis or epididymis, inflammation of the diaphragm, gouty arthritis, and dysmenorrhea.
Topically, wintergreen leaf is used as a wash for rheumatism, sore muscles, and lumbago.
In manufacturing, wintergreen leaf is used as a flavoring agent in food, candies, teas and pharmaceutical products.

Safety
LIKELY SAFE ...when used orally and appropriately in medicinal amounts (12). ...when consumed as a flavoring agent in amounts found in foods (12).
CHILDREN: POSSIBLY UNSAFE ...when used orally; potentially toxic to small children (19).
PREGNANCY: Insufficient reliable information; avoid using in amounts greater than those found in foods.
LACTATION: POSSIBLY UNSAFE ...when used orally or topically; potentially toxic to infants (19).

Effectiveness
There is insufficient reliable information available about the effectiveness of wintergreen leaf.

Mechanism of Action
When freshly harvested, the plant contains galutherin that changes into methyl salicylate as the plant is dried (18). The leaves contain 0.5-0.8% wintergreen oil (6).

Adverse Reactions
Topically, use of wintergreen leaf can cause contact dermatitis due to the essential oils (18). Symptoms of toxicity (salicylism) include tinnitus, nausea, vomiting (6), diarrhea, headache, stomach pain, and confusion (3805).

Interactions with Herbs & Other Dietary Supplements
None known.

Interactions with Drugs
None known.

Interactions with Foods
None known.

Interactions with Lab Tests
None known.

Interactions with Diseases or Conditions
GI CONDITIONS: Contraindicated; may aggravate gastrointestinal irritation or inflammation (19).

Dosage and Administration
ORAL: People typically prepare wintergreen leaf as a tea with 1 teaspoon of the dried leaves added to 1 cup boiling water. The tea is taken cold, 1 cup per day (5253,5254).
TOPICAL: No typical dosage.

WINTERGREEN OIL

Also Known As
Boxberry, Canada Tea, Checkerberry, Deerberry, Gaultheria Oil, Ground Berry, Hilberry, Mountain Tea, Partridge Berry, Spiceberry, Teaberry, Wax Cluster.
CAUTION: See separate listing for Wintergreen leaf.

Scientific Names
Gaultheria procumbens.
Family: Ericaceae.

People Use This For
Orally, small doses of wintergreen oil have been used to stimulate gastric secretion and aid digestion.
Topically, wintergreen oil is used as a counterirritant, for musculoskeletal pain, and as an antiseptic.
In manufacturing, the oil is used as a flavoring agent in food, candies, teas, and in pharmaceutical products.

Safety
LIKELY SAFE ...when used in amounts commonly found in foods. Wintergreen oil has Generally Recognized As Safe (GRAS) status in the US (4912). ...when used topically and appropriately (272).
LIKELY UNSAFE ...when used orally for medicinal purposes, unless the methyl salicylate content is highly diluted (6,272).
CHILDREN: LIKELY UNSAFE ...when used orally; 4-10 mL can be lethal (159). ...when used topically in children less than 2 years old (272). Children can be poisoned by ingesting topical liniment. One teaspoon of topical liniment contains 7 grams salicylates or approximately 22 adult aspirin tablets (159). Child-resistant containers are required for topical liquid preparations containing more than 5% methyl salicylate (6,272).
PREGNANCY: There is insufficient reliable information available about the safety of the oral use wintergreen oil in medicinal amounts; avoid using.
LACTATION: LIKELY UNSAFE ...when used orally. It might be toxic to nursing infants (19).

Effectiveness
There is insufficient reliable information available about the effectiveness of wintergreen oil.

Mechanism of Action
Wintergreen oil contains 98% methyl salicylate (6). It has antipyretic, anti-inflammatory, and analgesic properties (11), possibly due to its counterirritant effect (6).

Adverse Reactions
Topically, contact dermatitis can occur due to the essential oils (18). Other symptoms of toxicity (salicylism) include tinnitus, nausea, vomiting (6), diarrhea, headache, stomach pain, and confusion (3805). When applied topically and covered with an occlusive dressing, 12-20% of methyl salicylate was absorbed systemically over ten hours (272).

Interactions with Herbs & Other Dietary Supplements
None known.

Interactions with Drugs
ASPIRIN: Topical use of wintergreen oil in large amounts, with occlusive dressings, or for prolonged periods of time, can cause additive salicylate toxicity (159,272).
WARFARIN (Coumadin): Concomitant use of topical wintergreen oil-containing products and warfarin can increase INR and bleeding risk due to systemic absorption of the methyl salicylate contained in wintergreen oil (3811,6181). Topical analgesic gels, lotions, creams, ointments, liniments, and sprays can contain up to 55% methyl salicylate (6181).

Interactions with Foods
None known.

Interactions with Lab Tests
None known.

Interactions with Diseases or Conditions
GASTROINTESTINAL INFLAMMATION: Oral use is contraindicated because it can aggravate inflammation (19).
SALICYLATE ALLERGY/ASTHMA: Individuals with salicylate allergy, asthma, or nasal polyps should use cautiously due to its potential for allergic reaction (272).

Dosage and Administration
TOPICAL: Apply as gels, lotion, ointments, or liniments (containing 10-60% methyl salicylate) 3-4 times daily (3). Heat can increase skin absorption; do not apply after strenuous exercise or use a heating pad after application (3).

Comments
Wintergreen oil is obtained by steam distillation of warmed, water-macerated leaves.

WITCH HAZEL

Also Known As
Hamamelis, Hazel, Snapping Tobacco Wood, Spotted Elder, Winter Bloom, Witchazel.

Scientific Names
Hamamelis virginiana.
Family: Hamamelidaceae.

People Use This For
Orally, witch hazel is used for diarrhea, mucus colitis, vomiting blood, coughing up blood, tuberculosis, colds, fevers, tumors and cancer.
Topically, witch hazel is used for itching, skin inflammation, eye inflammation, skin injury, mucous membrane inflammation, varicose veins, hemorrhoids, bruises, insect bites, minor burns, and other skin irritations.
In manufacturing, witch hazel leaf extract, bark extract, and witch hazel water are used as astringents and hemostatics in preparations for insect bites, stings, teething, hemorrhoids, itching, irritations, and minor pain.

Safety
LIKELY SAFE ...when witch hazel water is used topically and appropriately (272).
POSSIBLY SAFE ...when used orally and appropriately (12). In high doses, tannins in witch hazel bark can cause liver damage (8). The volatile oil contains safrole, a known carcinogen, but in amounts too small for concern (4).
PREGNANCY AND LACTATION: Insufficient reliable information available; avoid using.

Effectiveness
POSSIBLY EFFECTIVE

Hemorrhoids. Applying witch hazel water topically may help to temporarily relieve itching, discomfort, irritation, and burning associated with anorectal disorders (272).
Minor bleeding. Applying witch hazel bark, leaf, or water as a styptic seems to reduce minor bleeding (7,8).
Skin irritation. Applying witch hazel cream topically relieve mild skin irritation, but less so than hydrocortisone (11151).

There is insufficient reliable information available about the effectiveness of witch hazel for its other uses.

Mechanism of Action

The applicable parts of witch hazel are the leaf and bark. The active constituents include gallotannins, gallic acid, myricetin, quercetin, kaempferol, and catechol derivatives. Witch hazel leaf and bark possess astringent, styptic, and anti-inflammatory properties (10377). The leaf contains 8-10% tannins (512). The bark contains up to 12% tannins (10377).

Tannins, applied topically to broken skin or mucous membranes induce protein precipitation. They tighten up superficial cell layers and shrink colloidal structures thereby causing capillaries to constrict. The decrease in vascular permeability approximates an anti-inflammatory effect. The astringent activity of tannins also causes an indirect antibacterial effect (7).

Steam distillation used for producing Hamamelis water removes the tannins (13). Thus, the astringent properties of Hamamelis water result from its 14-15% alcohol content (13).

Adverse Reactions

Orally, plants with at least 10% tannins can cause gastrointestinal disturbances, kidney damage, and necrotic conditions of the liver (12). Some evidence suggests that tannins might cause cancer; other evidence shows tannins may prevent it (12). Regular consumption of herbs with high tannin concentrations correlates with increased incidence of esophageal or nasal cancer (12).

Topically, witch hazel can cause contact dermatitis (6).

Interactions with Herbs & Other Dietary Supplements

None known.

Interactions with Drugs

None known.

Interactions with Foods

None known.

Interactions with Lab Tests

None known.

Interactions with Diseases or Conditions

None known.

Dosage and Administration

ORAL: A typical dose is 2 grams of dried leaves three times daily or as tea. To make tea, steep 2 grams in 150 mL of boiling water for 5-10 minutes, and strain (4). Hamamelis Liquid Extract (1:1 in 45% alcohol), 2-4 mL three times daily, has also been used (4).

TOPICAL: For compresses and irrigations, simmer 5-10 grams leaf and bark per 250 mL of water (2). For poultice, use witch hazel water (Hamamelis water) undiluted or diluted 1:3 with water. Semi-solid preparations 20-30% (2). Extracts, semi solid and liquid preparations corresponding to 5-10% leaf and bark (2).

RECTAL: Suppositories, corresponding to 0.1-1 grams leaf and bark applied 1-3 times daily (2). Anorectal disorders, Hamamelis water applied externally up to six times a day or after each bowel movement (272).

Comments

Witch hazel water (Hamamelis water, distilled witch hazel extract) is distilled from dried leaves, bark, and partially dormant twigs of Hamamelis virginiana (11).

WOOD ANEMONE

Also Known As

Crowfoot, Smell Fox, Wind Flower.

Scientific Names

Anemone nemorosa.
Family: Ranunculaceae.

People Use This For

Orally, wood anemone is used orally for stomach pains, delayed menstruation, gout, whooping cough, and asthma.

Safety
LIKELY UNSAFE ...when the fresh plant is used orally. Freshly harvested wood anemone can cause severe irritation to the gastrointestinal tract. Ingesting 30 freshly harvested plants is believed to be fatal (18).
There is insufficient reliable information available about the safety of the dried, cut above ground parts.
PREGNANCY AND LACTATION: LIKELY UNSAFE ...when the fresh plant is used orally or topically (18).
There is insufficient reliable information available about the safety of the oral or topical use of the dried, cut plant during pregnancy and lactation; avoid using.

Effectiveness
There is insufficient reliable information available about the effectiveness of wood anemone.

Mechanism of Action
The applicable parts of wood anemone are the above ground parts. When the fresh plant is crushed or cut into small pieces, the glycoside ranunculin is enzymatically changed into a severely irritating protoanemonin, which, in turn, rapidly degrades into the less toxic anemonin (18). Both protoanemonin and ranunculin are destroyed to an unknown extent during the drying process (2).

Adverse Reactions
Orally, the ingestion of freshly harvested wood anemone can cause colic, diarrhea, and severe irritation to the gastrointestinal tract and the urinary drainage passages (18).
Topically, wood anemone can cause slow-healing blisters and burns after prolonged skin contact (18).

Interactions with Herbs & Other Dietary Supplements
None known.

Interactions with Drugs
None known.

Interactions with Foods
None known.

Interactions with Lab Tests
None known.

Interactions with Diseases or Conditions
None known.

Dosage and Administration
No typical dosage.

Comments
Avoid confusion with the poisonous plant, pasque flower (Pulsatilla pratensis). Although the two plants are from the same botanical family and have similar pharmacological compounds, they are not synonymous (2,18). Wood anemone was traditionally used in Russian folk medicine.

WOOD SAGE

Also Known As
Ambroise, Garlic Sage, Hind Heal, Large-Leaved Germander.
CAUTION: See separate listings for Sage and Tansy.

Scientific Names
Teucrium scorodonia.
Family: Lamiaceae/Labiatae.

People Use This For
Orally, wood sage is used for gastrointestinal tract disorders, tuberculosis, mucous membrane inflammation of the bronchi and nose, throat spasms, hypertension, healing wounds, and liver disorders.

Safety
There is insufficient reliable information available about the safety of wood sage.
Pregnancy and Lactation: Insufficient reliable information is available; avoid using.

Effectiveness
There is insufficient reliable information available about the effectiveness of wood sage.

Mechanism of Action
The applicable parts of wood sage are the above ground parts. Wood sage is thought to have spasmolytic and expectorant properties (18). It contains flavonoids, a volatile oil, diterpenes, and iridoide monoterpenes (18).

Adverse Reactions
None reported.

Interactions with Herbs & Other Dietary Supplements
None known.

Interactions with Drugs
None known.

Interactions with Foods
None known.

Interactions with Lab Tests
None known.

Interactions with Diseases or Conditions
None known.

Dosage and Administration
ORAL: A typical dose for bronchitis is one cup of tea. To make tea, steep 2 teaspoons of dried herb in 150 mL water for 10-15 minutes, and strain.

Comments
Wood sage smells faintly of leeks when being dried. In most countries, wood sage is obsolete as a drug (18).

WOOD SORREL

Also Known As
Common Sorrel, Cuckoo Bread, Cuckowes Meat, Fairy Bells, Green Sauce, Hallelujah, Mountain Sorrel, Shamrock, Sour Trefoil, Stickwort, Stubwort, Surelle, Three-Leaved Grass, White Sorrel, Wood Sour.

Scientific Names
Oxalis acetosella, synonym Oxalis montana.
Family: Oxalidaceae.

People Use This For
Orally, wood sorrel is used for liver and digestive disorders, scurvy, wounds, and inflammation of the gums.

Safety
POSSIBLY UNSAFE ...when used orally, particularly in large amounts (6,17).
CHILDREN: POSSIBLY UNSAFE ...when used orally. One four-year old child died after consuming rhubarb leaves, which is also a source of oxalic acid (17).
PREGNANCY: LIKELY UNSAFE ...when used orally because it might stimulate menses (19): avoid using.
LACTATION: POSSIBLY UNSAFE ...when used orally (6,17); avoid using.

Effectiveness
There is insufficient reliable information available about the effectiveness of wood sorrel.

Mechanism of Action

The applicable part of wood sorrel is the whole flowering plant. It contains 0.3-1.25% oxalic acid (18). Oxalate content is high in fresh leaves and roots (17,19). Once absorbed, the oxalic acid reacts with calcium in plasma and resulting insoluble calcium oxalate may precipitate in the kidneys, blood vessels, heart, lungs, and liver. This may also cause hypocalcemia (12,17). Oxalate crystals damage mucosal tissue, resulting in severe irritation and possible damage. The systemic absorption of oxalates may result in kidney damage, both in people with pre-existing kidney disease and in healthy kidneys (19).

Adverse Reactions

Orally, consuming excessive amounts of wood sorrel can cause diarrhea, nausea, polyuria (6), dermatitis (4) and gastrointestinal symptoms due to its oxalic acid content. Oxalic acid poisoning affects skin, eyes, respiratory system and kidneys. Oral symptoms of oxalate irritation include swelling of the mouth, tongue and throat, with difficulty in speaking and suffocation. It has a corrosive effect on the digestive tract. It can lead to oxalic acid crystals in the kidneys, blood vessels, heart, lungs, liver, and/or hypocalcemia (17).

Interactions with Herbs & Other Dietary Supplements

CALCIUM, IRON, ZINC: Concurrent use might decrease mineral absorption. Wood sorrel contains oxalate (7,12), which can bind multivalent metal ions in the gastrointestinal tract and decrease mineral absorption.

Interactions with Drugs

None known.

Interactions with Foods

CALCIUM, IRON, ZINC: Concurrent use might decrease mineral absorption from foods. Wood sorrel contains oxalate (7,12), which can bind multivalent metal ions in the gastrointestinal tract and decrease mineral absorption.

Interactions with Lab Tests

None known.

Interactions with Diseases or Conditions

COAGULATION DISORDERS: Oxalate constituents can alter the calcium concentrations and decrease coagulation time (4,12).
GI CONDITIONS: Theoretically can exacerbate stomach and intestinal ulcers due to mucosal irritant effect (19).
KIDNEY DISEASE: Can damage kidneys with formation of insoluble oxalate; use with caution or avoid in individuals with history of kidney stones (12,19).

Dosage and Administration

No typical dosage.

Comments

Wood sorrel is also called common sorrel, and could be confused with sorrel.

WOODBINE

Also Known As

Clematis, Devil's Darning Needle, Old Man's Beard, Traveler's Joy, Vine Bower, Virgin's Bower.
CAUTION: See separate listings for Clematis, Fringetree, Traveler's Joy, and Usnea.

Scientific Names

Clematis virginiana.
Family: Rananculaceae.

People Use This For

Orally, woodbine is used for skin sores, cuts, itching, venereal disorders, cancer, tumors, itching, fever, nephrosis, ulcers, diuretic, purgative, tuberculosis, and cervical lymphadenitis.

Safety

LIKELY UNSAFE ...when used orally or topically because it is a powerful irritant (6).
PREGNANCY AND LACTATION: LIKELY UNSAFE ...when used orally or topically (6); avoid using.

Effectiveness
There is insufficient reliable information available about the effectiveness of woodbine.

Mechanism of Action
The applicable part of woodbine is the leaf. There is insufficient reliable information available about the possible mechanism of action and active ingredients.

Adverse Reactions
Orally, the juice derived from the woodbine leaf is said to be a powerful local irritant (6).

Interactions with Herbs & Other Dietary Supplements
None known.

Interactions with Drugs
None known.

Interactions with Foods
None known.

Interactions with Lab Tests
None known.

Interactions with Diseases or Conditions
None known.

Dosage and Administration
ORAL: People typically make a liquid preparation of woodbine, combining one heaping teaspoon of leaves and flowers with one cup of water and allowing the mixture to stand for 30 minutes. The dose is one tablespoon 4 to 6 times daily (5263).

Comments
Avoid confusion with American ivy, gelsemium or honeysuckle, which are also known as woodbine.

WORMSEED

Also Known As
Levant, Santonica, Sea Wormwood, Worm Seed.
CAUTION: See separate listings for Chenopodium Oil, Levant Berry, Mugwort. Wormwood, and Wormwood Oil.

Scientific Names
Artemisia cina, synonym Seriphidium cinum.
Family: Asteraceae/Compositae.

People Use This For
Orally, wormseed is used for ascaris and oxyuris infestations.

Safety
UNSAFE ...when used orally due to its highly toxic adverse effects (18).
PREGNANCY AND LACTATION: UNSAFE ...when used orally due to potential for toxicity (18); avoid using.

Effectiveness
There is insufficient reliable information available about the effectiveness of wormseed.

Mechanism of Action
The anthelmintic activity is attributed to the sesquiterpene lactone beta-santonin. When wormseed is used with a laxative, it appears to paralyze the muscles of ascarids and facilitate their elimination from the body. Some data suggest wormseed lowers body temperature when a fever is present (18).

Adverse Reactions
Orally, death has been reported with less than 10 grams of herb. Symptoms of poisoning are possible in amounts used to treat parasitic infestations. Symptoms may include kidney irritation, gastroenteritis, stupor, visual disorders,

muscle twitching, and epileptiform spasms (18). It can cause an allergic reaction in individuals sensitive to the Asteraceae/Compositae family. Members of this family include ragweed, chrysanthemums, marigolds, daisies, and many other herbs.

Interactions with Herbs & Other Dietary Supplements
None known.

Interactions with Drugs
None known.

Interactions with Foods
None known.

Interactions with Lab Tests
None known.

Interactions with Diseases or Conditions
CROSS-ALLERGENICITY: Can cause an allergic reaction in individuals sensitive to the Asteraceae/Compositae family. Members of this family include ragweed, chrysanthemums, marigolds, daisies, and many other herbs.

Dosage and Administration
No typical dosage.

Comments
Avoid confusing wormseed with chenopodium oil (or wormseed oil), wormwood oil, or wormwood. Avoid confusing wormseed, also referred to as levant, with levant berry.

WORMWOOD above ground parts

Also Known As
Absinth, Absinthe, Absinthii Herba, Absinthites, Absinthium, Ajenjo, Armoise, Artesian Absinthium, Artemisia, Common Wormwood, Green Ginger, Herbe d'Absinthe, Indhana, Wermut, Wermutkraut, Wurmkraut.
CAUTION: See separate listings for Wormwood Oil and Mugwort.

Scientific Names
Artemisia absinthium.
Family: Asteraceae/Compositae.

People Use This For
Orally, wormwood above ground parts are used for loss of appetite, indigestion, biliary dyskinesia, and gastrointestinal complaints such as low acidity gastritis.
Topically, wormwood above ground parts are used for healing wounds and insect bites.
In combination with other herbs, wormwood above ground parts are used for indigestion, particularly functional disorders of the gallbladder drainage system, loss of appetite, and discomfort due to fullness and flatulence.
Historically, wormwood above ground parts were used as an anthelmintic, aphrodisiac, tonic, antispasmodic, and to stimulate sweating.
In manufacturing, wormwood above ground parts are used for flavoring alcoholic bitters and vermouth.

Safety
LIKELY SAFE ...when used orally in the amounts commonly found foods including bitters and vermouth. Wormwood products that are thujone-free have Generally Recognized As Safe (GRAS) status in US (4912).
POSSIBLY SAFE ...when used orally and appropriately short-term (12). Although aqueous extracts or brewed teas are reported to contain the toxic constituent thujone, the amount is low (12).
LIKELY UNSAFE ...when used orally long-term or in excessive amounts.
There is insufficient reliable information available about the safety of the topical use of wormwood above ground parts.
PREGNANCY: UNSAFE ...when used orally. Thujone has potential uterine and menstrual stimulant effects (12). There is insufficient reliable information available about the safety of the topical use of wormwood above ground parts during pregnancy.
LACTATION: Insufficient reliable information available; avoid using.

Effectiveness

There is insufficient reliable information available about the effectiveness of wormwood above ground parts.

Mechanism of Action

Wormwood contains bitter principles (absinthin and anabsinthin) and a volatile oil composed of up to 70% thujone (7). In small doses, wormwood acts as an aromatic bitter (7). As the amount ingested increases, the toxic effects of thujone become more pronounced leading to increased salivation and increased blood flow to mucous membranes and pelvic viscera (7). Thujone heightens and alters the effect of alcohol (7). Chronic thujone poisoning leads to seizures, delirium, and hallucinations (7). Researchers think thujone has a mind-altering effect similar to tetrahydrocannabinol, the active principle in marijuana (515). Some evidence suggests that thujone exposure might be harmful to individuals with underlying defects in hepatic heme synthesis (12). Thujone also induces synthesis of a rate-controlling enzyme for the 5-aminolevulinic acid synthase pathway. This effect is similar to that of phenobarbital and glutethimide, drugs with known porphyrinogenic activity (12). Thujone shows evidence of antioxidant, antimicrobial and antifungal activity (12).

Adverse Reactions

Orally, habitual use of large amounts of wormwood can cause restlessness, insomnia, nightmares, vomiting, stomach and intestinal cramps (8), dizziness, tremors (11,12), urine retention (8), renal damage, and convulsions (11,12). Absinthism, a group of neurological symptoms, is characterized by digestive disorders, thirst, restlessness, vertigo, tremor, numbness of extremities, diminished intellect, delirium, paralysis, and death (17).

Topically, skin contact with fresh wormwood can cause contact dermatitis (19). Wormwood can also cause an allergic reaction in people sensitive to the Asteraceae/Compositae family. Members of this family include ragweed, chrysanthemums, marigolds, daisies, and many other herbs.

Interactions with Herbs & Other Dietary Supplements

THUJONE-CONTAINING HERBS: Concomitant use with other herbs that contain thujone might increase risk of thujone toxicity. Thujone-containing herbs include oak moss, oriental arborvitae, sage, tansy, thuja (cedar), and tree moss (12).

Interactions with Drugs

ANTACIDS: Theoretically, due to reports that wormwood increases stomach acid, wormwood might decrease the effectiveness of antacids (19).

ANTICONVULSANTS: Theoretically, concomitant use might interfere with the effectiveness of anticonvulsant drugs due to wormwood's potential to cause seizures (8,11,12).

H2-BLOCKERS: Theoretically, due to reports that wormwood increases stomach acid, wormwood might decrease the effectiveness of H2-blockers (19). The H2 blockers include cimetidine (Tagamet), ranitidine (Zantac), nizatidine (Axid), and famotidine (Pepcid).

PROTON PUMP INHIBITORS (PPIs): Theoretically, due to reports that wormwood increases stomach acid, wormwood might decrease the effectiveness of PPIs (19). PPIs include omeprazole (Prilosec), lansoprazole (Prevacid), rabeprazole (Aciphex), pantoprazole (Protonix), and esomeprazole (Nexium).

Interactions with Foods

None known.

Interactions with Lab Tests

None known.

Interactions with Diseases or Conditions

CROSS-ALLERGENICITY: Wormwood above ground parts can cause an allergic reaction in people sensitive to the Asteraceae/Compositae family. Members of this family include ragweed, chrysanthemums, marigolds, daisies, and many other herbs (4).

ULCERS: Contraindicated in individuals with gastric or duodenal ulcers due to potential for stomach irritation and intestinal tract stimulation (8,19).

Dosage and Administration

ORAL: A typical dose is one cup tea before eating as an appetite stimulant or after meals as a bile flow stimulant (8). To make tea, steep 1-1.5 grams (1 teaspoon) finely chopped above ground parts in 150 mL boiling water 10 minutes, and strain. Total daily dose is up to 3 grams per day (2). Do not exceed 1.5 grams above ground parts per dose (8).

Comments

Wormwood is the principal flavor ingredient in absinthe, a 136-proof alcoholic beverage popular at the turn of the century (515). Absinthe is historically associated with addiction, acts of violence (515), damage to the nervous system, and mental deterioration (17). Vincent van Gogh's self-amputation of his left ear is attributed to his absinthe addiction (11,515). Absinthe was banned in many countries by 1915, including the US (11).

WORMWOOD OIL

Also Known As

Artemisia.
CAUTION: See separate listing for Wormwood above ground parts.

Scientific Names

Artemisia absinthium.
Family: Asteraceae/Compositae.

People Use This For

Topically, wormwood oil is used as a counterirritant.
In foods, wormwood oil is used as a flavoring agent.
In manufacturing, wormwood oil is used as a fragrance component in soaps, cosmetics, and perfumes.

Safety

POSSIBLY SAFE ...when used orally in amounts commonly found in foods. Thujone-free wormwood oil has Generally Recognized As Safe (GRAS) status in the US (4912).
LIKELY UNSAFE ...when thujone-containing wormwood oil is used orally. One-half ounce of thujone-containing volatile oil can cause convulsions and unconsciousness (17,515).
There is insufficient reliable information available about the safety of wormwood oil when used topically in amounts greater than those found in cosmetics.
PREGNANCY: LIKELY UNSAFE ...when used topically; avoid using. Wormwood oil might have uterine and menstrual stimulant effects (12,19) and thujone could be toxic.
LACTATION: LIKELY UNSAFE ...when used topically; avoid using. There is concern about the toxic potential of thujone (11).

Effectiveness

There is insufficient reliable information available about the effectiveness of wormwood oil.

Mechanism of Action

The volatile oil of wormwood is considered an active narcotic poison (17). The major constituents of the oil are azulenes (11,515), but it also contains 3-12% thujone (11,515). The azulene constituents have anti-inflammatory and antipyretic activity (11). They also have antibacterial effects against Staphylococcus aureus, the penicillin-resistant strain S. aureus, Klebsiella pneumoniae, and Pseudomonas aeruginosa (11). The constituent, thujone is chemically related to camphor (12). As the amount of thujone ingested is increased, the toxic effect becomes pronounced, leading to increased salivation and erythema of the mucous membranes and pelvic viscera. Thujone heightens and alters the effect of alcohol. Researchers think thujone has a mind-altering effect similar to tetrahydrocannabinol, the active constituent marijuana (4). Chronic thujone poisoning leads to epileptic seizures, delirium, and hallucinations (7). Some evidence suggests thujone might be harmful to individuals with underlying defects in hepatic heme synthesis. Other evidence suggests thujone induces synthesis of a rate-controlling enzyme for the 5-aminolevulinic acid synthase pathway. Phenobarbital and glutethimide have similar effects, suggesting thujone might have porphyrinogenic activity (12).

Adverse Reactions

Orally, wormwood oil can cause nausea, vomiting, diffuse muscle aches, acute renal toxicity, seizures, rhabdomyolysis, and acute renal failure (661,662). Wormwood oil can cause an allergic reaction in people sensitive to the Asteraceae/Compositae family. Members of this family include ragweed, chrysanthemums, marigolds, daisies, and many other herbs.

Interactions with Herbs & Other Dietary Supplements

THUJONE-CONTAINING HERBS: Concomitant use might increase the risk of thujone toxicity. Thujone-containing herbs include oak moss, oriental arborvitae, sage, tansy, thuja (cedar), and tree moss (12); avoid using.

Interactions with Drugs
None known.

Interactions with Foods
None known.

Interactions with Lab Tests
None known.

Interactions with Diseases or Conditions
CROSS-ALLERGENICITY: Wormwood oil can cause an allergic reaction in individuals sensitive to the Asteraceae/Compositae family. Members of this family include ragweed, chrysanthemums, marigolds, daisies, and many other herbs.

Dosage and Administration
No typical dosage.

Comments
Wormwood oil is distilled from leaves and flowers of Artemisia absinthium just before or during flowering. Thujone-containing wormwood oil is highly toxic.

XANTHAN GUM

Also Known As
Bacterial Polysaccharide, Corn Sugar Gum, Xanthan.

Scientific Names
Xanthomonas campestris (Bacterium).

People Use This For
Orally, xanthan gum is used for lowering blood glucose and total plasma cholesterol in people with diabetes. It is also used orally as a laxative.
Topically, xanthan gum is used as a saliva substitute in people with Sjogren's syndrome.
In manufacturing, xanthan gum is used as a thickening, suspending, emulsifying, and stabilizing agent in foods, toothpastes, and pharmaceutical products.

Safety
LIKELY SAFE ...when consumed in amounts found in foods, up to 10 mg/kg per day (4914). It has Generally Recognized As Safe (GRAS) status in the US (4912). ...when used orally for medicinal use in amounts up to 15 grams per day (4914,4916,4917,4918). ...when used topically and appropriately (4914).
PREGNANCY AND LACTATION: Insufficient reliable information is available; avoid using in amounts greater than those found in foods.

Effectiveness
POSSIBLY EFFECTIVE

Constipation. Taking xanthan gum orally as a bulk-forming laxative seems to decrease constipation (4917,4918).
Diabetes. Taking xanthan gum orally seems to lower blood glucose and cholesterol in people with diabetes (4916).
Sjogren's syndrome. Applying xanthan gum topically seems to help as a saliva substitute in people with Sjogren's syndrome (4915).

Mechanism of Action
Xanthan gum is a polysaccharide produced by fermenting carbohydrate with the bacterium Xanthomonas campestris. It is a bulk-forming laxative. In the body it forms an emollient gel that stimulates peristalsis and passage of intestinal contents (4917). Xanthan gum slows gastric emptying and intestinal absorption of glucose (4916). It mimics saliva as a lubricating and wetting agent in humans (4915), and shows evidence that it might reduce demineralization of tooth enamel (4920).

Adverse Reactions
Orally, xanthan gum can cause flatulence and abdominal distention (4916,4918). Occupational exposure in workers handling xanthan gum powder can cause flu-like symptoms, and nose and throat irritation without acute or chronic loss of pulmonary function (4913).

Interactions with Herbs & Other Dietary Supplements

BULK-FORMING LAXATIVE HERBS AND SUPPLEMENTS: Theoretically, concomitant use may increase likelihood of flatulence and abdominal distention.
HERBS WITH HYPOGLYCEMIC POTENTIAL: Theoretically, concomitant use with pharmacologically active amounts of xanthan gum could result in excessive lowering of blood glucose.

Interactions with Drugs

ANTIDIABETES DRUGS: Xanthan gum seems to lower blood glucose in people with diabetes (4916). Concomitant use of xanthan gum with antidiabetes medication might have additive effects. Monitor blood glucose levels closely. Some antidiabetes drugs include glimepiride (Amaryl), glyburide (DiaBeta, Glynase PresTab, Micronase), insulin, pioglitazone (Actos), rosiglitazone (Avandia), and others.

Interactions with Foods

None known.

Interactions with Lab Tests

BLOOD GLUCOSE: Might lower blood glucose and test results (4916).
CHOLESTEROL: Might lower serum cholesterol and test results (4916).

Interactions with Diseases or Conditions

CONTRAINDICATIONS: Bulk forming laxative are contraindicated in individuals with nausea, vomiting, appendicitis, fecal impaction, intestinal obstruction, or undiagnosed abdominal pain.

Dosage and Administration

ORAL: The World Health Organization (WHO) has set the maximum acceptable intake for xanthan gum as a food additive at 10 mg/kg per day (4914), and as a laxative at 15 grams per day (4918). For safety and effectiveness, bulk laxatives require adequate fluid intake (272). For diabetes a typical dose is 12 grams per day as an ingredient in muffins (4916).
TOPICAL: Saliva substitutes, 0.018% or 0.092% aqueous solutions with added electrolytes and peppermint flavoring (4915).

Comments

Xanthan gum is an ingredient in some sustained release matrix tablets (4914).

XYLITOL

Also Known As

Birch Sugar, E967, Meso-Xylitol, Xylit, Xylite.

Scientific Names

Xylitol; xylo-pentane-1,2,3,4,5-pentol.

People Use This For

Orally, xylitol is used to prevent acute otitis media in young children, and as a sugar substitute for people with diabetes.
Topically, xylitol is used in chewing gums and other oral care products to prevent dental caries and dry mouth.
Intravenously, xylitol is used as an energy source in parenteral nutrition.
In foods, xylitol is used as a sweetener, including sugar-free preparations.

Safety

LIKELY SAFE ...when used orally in amounts commonly found in foods. Xylitol has Generally Recognized As Safe (GRAS) status in the US (4912).
POSSIBLY SAFE ...when used orally and topically, and appropriately in medicinal amounts. Xylitol has been used safely in doses from 20-53 grams per day for up to three years (6815,6819,6821).
POSSIBLY UNSAFE ...when used orally in very high doses, long-term. There is some concern that very high doses for extended periods of use can induce tumor growth (6815,6820). However, this effect has not yet been demonstrated in humans.
CHILDREN: POSSIBLY SAFE ...when used orally and topically, and appropriately in medicinal amounts. Xylitol has been used safely in children in doses up to 20 grams per day for up to three years (6815,6819).
PREGNANCY AND LACTATION: There insufficient reliable information available about the use of xylitol in medicinal amounts during pregnancy and lactation; avoid using.

Effectiveness

LIKELY EFFECTIVE

Dental caries. Use of xylitol-containing products such as foods, chewing gum, candies, soluble dragees, and toothpaste that provide 1-20 grams of xylitol per day can significantly reduce the rate of cavity formation in both adults and children (6815,6819,6822). Xylitol products appear to be more effective than products containing sorbitol for preventing cavity formation (6822).

POSSIBLY EFFECTIVE

Otitis media. Xylitol 8.4-10 grams per day given orally as a chewing gum, lozenge, or syrup five times a day after meals to preschool children, seems to significantly reduce the number of episodes of acute otitis media and the usage of antibiotics (6816,6817). However, xylitol gum, lozenges, or liquid 8.4-10 grams per day administered at the onset of symptoms of an acute respiratory infection does not seem to prevent acute otitis media (3846).

Mechanism of Action

Xylitol is a polyhydric alcohol (polyol) related to the pentose sugar, xylose (9). Xylitol is found in almost all plant material, including fruits such as raspberries, strawberries, and plums; vegetables; and mushrooms. Commercial preparations are extracted from birch wood (268). In the body, it is produced during metabolism of glucose in the liver (268). Xylitol has several properties that might provide a locally protective effect against dental caries. Xylitol is not fermented by plaque flora to the low pH associated with caries. Xylitol lowers plaque and salivary levels of Streptococcus mutans and lactobacilli, which cause caries. Most children acquire Streptococcus mutans from their mothers after birth. Habitual chewing of xylitol gum by mothers with high bacterial levels beginning three months after delivery appears to significantly reduce transmission of Streptococcus mutans to their children (6818). Xylitol also reduces bacterial adhesiveness. Xylitol increases salivary flow rates and calcium and phosphate concentrations in saliva, which promote buffering and remineralization of tooth surfaces. Xylitol also stimulates activity of the antimicrobial enzyme lactoperoxidase in saliva (6815,6819).

Due to its five-carbon structure, xylitol is not a substrate for growth of most bacteria, and it may inhibit some bacterial enzymes and interfere with their metabolism of six carbon sugars (6819). In the prevention of acute otitis media, xylitol may work by inhibiting growth of bacteria including Streptococcus pneumoniae, and preventing adhesion of pneumococci and Haemophilus influenzae to nasopharyngeal cells (3846,6819). There is also some preliminary evidence from animal models that suggests xylitol might increase the calcium and phosphorus content of bone and protect against osteoporosis (6819).

Adverse Reactions

Orally, acute administration of large amounts of xylitol (30 to 40 grams) can cause osmotic diarrhea and flatulence. However, if the dose is increased gradually, tolerance to this effect can occur and prevent development of diarrhea and flatulence (9). Intravenous infusion of high doses has been associated with hyperuricemia, changes in liver function tests, and acidosis, including lactic acidosis (6815).

Interactions with Herbs & Other Dietary Supplements

None known.

Interactions with Drugs

None known.

Interactions with Foods

None known.

Interactions with Lab Tests

None known.

Interactions with Diseases or Conditions

None known.

Dosage and Administration

ORAL: For acute otitis media, total daily doses of 8.4 to 10 grams have been used in chewing gum, lozenges, or syrup given in five divided doses, after meals for prevention (3846,6816,6817).

TOPICAL: For prevention of dental caries in adults and children, a wide range of doses has been used. Typically, doses are from 7 to 20 grams per day divided into three to five doses, usually given as candies or chewing gum (6815,6819).

INTRAVENOUS: No typical dosage.

Comments

Xylitol is widely used in other countries as a sugar substitute and in chewing gums, mints, and other candies. Its use in the United States is relatively limited. Sorbitol is the most commonly used sweetener in sugarless gums because it is less expensive than xylitol and easier to formulate into commercial products (8329). Some national brands of chewing gum contain milligram amounts of xylitol, far from the gram doses that seem to prevent tooth decay.

YARROW

Also Known As

Achilee, Achillea, Acuilee, Band Man's Plaything, Bauchweh, Birangasifa, Birangasipha, Biranjasipha, Bloodwort, Carpenter's Weed, Civan Percemi, Common Yarrow, Devil's Nettle, Devil's Plaything, Erba Da Cartentieri, Erba Da Falegname, Gandana, Gemeine Schafgarbe, Green Arrow, Herbe Aux Charpentiers, Katzenkrat, Milefolio, Milfoil, Millefeuille, Millefolii flos, Millefolii herba, Millefolium, Millegoglie, Noble Yarrow, Nosebleed, Old Man's Pepper, Roga Mari, Sanguinary, Soldier's Wound Wort, Staunchweed, Tausendaugbram, Thousand-Leaf, Wound Wort.
CAUTION: See separate listing for Bloodroot.

Scientific Names

Achillea millefolium, synonyms Achillea borealis, Achillea lanulosa, Achillea magna.
Family: Asteraceae/Compositae.

People Use This For

Orally, yarrow is used for fever, common cold, allergic rhinitis, amenorrhea, dysentery, diarrhea, loss of appetite, mild or spastic gastrointestinal (GI) tract discomfort, and to induce sweating. Specifically, yarrow is used orally for thrombotic conditions with hypertension, including cerebral and coronary thromboses.
Orally, the fresh leaves of yarrow are chewed to relieve toothache.
Topically, yarrow is used as a styptic; for bleeding hemorrhoids; for wounds; and as a sitz bath for painful, lower pelvic, cramp-like conditions of psychosomatic origin in women.
In combination with other herbs, yarrow is used for bloating, flatulence, mild gastrointestinal (GI) cramping, and nervous gastrointestinal complaints.
In foods, the young leaves and flowers of yarrow are used in salads.
In manufacturing, yarrow is also used as a cosmetic cleanser and in snuff. Yarrow oil is used in shampoos.

Safety

LIKELY SAFE ...when used orally in amounts commonly found in foods. Yarrow has Generally Recognized As Safe (GRAS) status in the US (4912).
POSSIBLY SAFE ...when used orally and appropriately for medicinal purposes (2,12).
PREGNANCY: LIKELY UNSAFE ...when used orally; yarrow is believed to be an abortifacient and affect the menstrual cycle (12).
LACTATION: Insufficient reliable information available; avoid excessive amounts during lactation (4).

Effectiveness

There is insufficient reliable information available about the effectiveness of yarrow.

Mechanism of Action

The applicable parts of yarrow are the above ground parts. Yarrow has diaphoretic, antipyretic, hypotensive, astringent, diuretic, urinary antiseptic, spasmolytic, and antiflatulent effects (4). Yarrow contains amino acids, fatty acids, ascorbic acid, caffeic acid, folic acid, salicylic acid, succinic acid, alkaloids, flavonoids including rutin, tannins, volatile oil, an unknown cyanogenetic compound, and sugars (4). The volatile oil contains chamazulene, other azulenes (11), and trace amounts of thujone (4,11) The volatile oil content, and especially the azulene content, varies considerably depending on the source (11). Some evidence suggests that achilleine, an alkaloid constituent, might decrease clotting time (4). The alkaloid fraction has shown evidence of antipyretic and hypotensive effects (4). An aqueous extract shows some evidence of anti-inflammatory and diuretic activity (4). Anti-inflammatory and anti-allergy activities may be associated with the constituent chamazulene (6). Not all species contain azulene constituents (6). An ethanolic extract shows moderate antibacterial activity against Staphylococcus aureus, Bacillus subtilis, Mycobacterium smegmatis, Escherichia coli, Shigella sonnei, and Shigella flexneri (4). Some evidence suggests that the volatile oil of yarrow might have CNS depressant activity (4).

Adverse Reactions

Orally, large amounts of yarrow might cause sedative and diuretic effects (4,5).
Topically, yarrow can cause dermatitis (4).
Yarrow may cause an allergic reaction in individuals sensitive to the Asteraceae/Compositae family. Members of this family include ragweed, chrysanthemums, marigolds, daisies, and many other herbs.

Interactions with Herbs & Other Dietary Supplements

THUJONE CONTAINING HERBS: Concomitant use can increase the risk of thujone toxicity. Thujone-containing herbs include oak moss, oriental arborvitae, sage, tansy, thuja (cedar), tree moss, and wormwood (2,4,11,12); avoid using.

Interactions with Drugs

ANTACIDS: Theoretically, due to reports that yarrow increases stomach acid, yarrow might decrease the effectiveness of antacids (19).
ANTICOAGULANT/ANTIPLATELET DRUGS: Theoretically, concomitant use might cause increased effects and adverse effects (4).
BARBITURATES: Theoretically, concomitant use might prolong barbiturate-induced sleep time (4). Some of these sedative medications include pentobarbital (Nembutal), phenobarbital (Luminal), secobarbital (Seconal), and others.
H2-BLOCKERS: Theoretically, due to reports that yarrow increases stomach acid, yarrow might decrease the effectiveness of H2-blockers (19). The H2 blockers include cimetidine (Tagamet), ranitidine (Zantac), nizatidine (Axid), and famotidine (Pepcid).
PROTON PUMP INHIBITORS (PPIs): Theoretically, due to reports that yarrow increases stomach acid, yarrow might decrease the effectiveness of PPIs (19). PPIs include omeprazole (Prilosec), lansoprazole (Prevacid), rabeprazole (Aciphex), pantoprazole (Protonix), and esomeprazole (Nexium).

Interactions with Foods

None known.

Interactions with Lab Tests

None known.

Interactions with Diseases or Conditions

CROSS-ALLERGENICITY: Yarrow may cause an allergic reaction in individuals sensitive to the Asteraceae/Compositae family. Members of this family include ragweed, chrysanthemums, marigolds, daisies, and many other herbs.

Dosage and Administration

ORAL: No typical dosage.
But, traditionally an oral dose of 2-4 grams of the dried flowerheads or one cup tea three times daily has been used. To make tea, steep 2-4 grams dried flowerhead or 2 grams finely cut above ground parts in 150 mL of boiling water for 10-15 minutes, and strain (4). A daily dose is up to 4.5 grams above ground parts, 3 grams flowerheads, 3 teaspoons pressed juice from fresh plants, or equivalent preparations per day. The liquid extract, 1:1 in 25% alcohol, is typically dosed at 2-4 mL three times daily (4). The tincture, 1:5 in 45% alcohol, is typically dosed at 2-4 mL three times daily (4).
TOPICAL: No typical dosage.
But, traditionally as a sitz bath, 100 grams above ground parts per 20 L of water has been used (2).

YELLOW DOCK

Also Known As

Broad-Leaved Dock, Curled Dock, Curly Dock, Field Sorrel, Narrow Dock, Rumex, Sheep Sorrel, Sorrel, Sour Dock, Yellowdock.

Scientific Names

Rumex crispus; Rumex obtusifolius.
Family: Polygonaceae.

People Use This For

Orally, yellow dock is used for acute and chronic inflammation of nasal passages and the respiratory tract, as an adjunct to antibacterial therapy, a laxative, tonic, and for treating venereal diseases.
Topically, yellow dock is used as a dentifrice.
Historically, yellow dock has been used for chronic skin diseases, dermatitis, rashes, scurvy, obstructive jaundice, and psoriasis with constipation.
For food uses, yellow dock is used in salads.

Safety

POSSIBLY SAFE ...when consumed in amounts commonly found in foods. Young leaves must be boiled to remove the oxalate content; death has occurred after consuming uncooked leaves (6,18). ...when used orally and appropriately for medicinal purposes.
PREGNANCY: POSSIBLY UNSAFE ...when used orally; avoid using. Contains anthraquinone glycosides, and unstandardized laxatives are not desirable during pregnancy (4)
LACTATION: POSSIBLY UNSAFE ...when used orally; avoid using. Anthraquinones are secreted into breast milk (4,5).

Effectiveness

There is insufficient reliable information available about the effectiveness of yellow dock.

Mechanism of Action

The applicable parts of yellow dock are the root and rhizome. Yellow dock contains anthraquinone glycosides (chrysophanic acid, emodin, physcion), oxalates (oxalic acid and calcium oxalate), and tannins (4,5,6,12). Oxalate content is high in the leaves and low in the stalks (17). The anthroquinones (2-4%) have a mild stimulant laxative effect (4,6,12). Anthroid laxative use is not associated with an increased risk of developing colorectal adenoma or carcinoma (6138). The tannins (12-20%) (12,19) are responsible for the astringent effect (5). Yellow dock is reported to stimulate bile production (4). The leaves of yellow dock contain provitamin A (beta-carotene) and iron (19).

Adverse Reactions

Orally, vomiting may occur after ingestion of fresh rhizome (18). Consuming excessive amounts can cause diarrhea, nausea, polyuria (6), or dermatitis (4). Excessive oral use can also cause abdominal cramps, hypokalemia, and intestinal atrophy (4). There is one report of a death, preceded by vomiting, diarrhea, coma, respiratory depression, liver and kidney failure, severe metabolic acidosis, and ventricular fibrillation, after ingestion of 500 grams of yellow dock (17). Oxalic acid reacts with calcium in plasma, forming insoluble calcium oxalate, which can cause hypocalcemia; the crystals may precipitate in the kidneys, blood vessels, heart, lungs, and liver. Individuals with a history of kidney stones should use yellow dock cautiously (12).
Topically, contact with the plant may cause dermatitis in people sensitive to yellow dock (6). Older or uncooked leaves should be avoided (6). Yellow dock can cause allergic reaction in individuals allergic to ragweed (4117).

Interactions with Herbs & Other Dietary Supplements

CALCIUM, IRON, ZINC: Concurrent use might decrease mineral absorption. Yellow dock contains oxalate (7,12), which can bind multivalent metal ions in the gastrointestinal tract and decrease mineral absorption.
CARDIAC-GLYCOSIDE-CONTAINING HERBS: Theoretically, concomitant use may increase the risk of cardiac glycoside toxicity because of the presence of stimulant laxatives in yellow dock, which can decrease serum potassium (19).
STIMULANT LAXATIVE HERBS: Theoretically, concomitant use of yellow dock with other stimulant laxative herbs can increase the risk of potassium depletion. Stimulant laxative herbs include aloe dried leaf sap, blue flag rhizome, alder buckthorn, European buckthorn, butternut bark, cascara bark, castor oil, colocynth fruit pulp, gamboge bark exudate, jalap root, black root, manna bark exudate, podophyllum root, rhubarb root, senna leaves and pods, and wild cucumber fruit (19).

Interactions with Drugs

DIGOXIN (Lanoxin): Toxic effects due to hypokalemia are possible when yellow dock is used chronically or in large amounts (4,19).
DIURETIC DRUGS: Overuse of yellow dock might compound diuretic-induced potassium loss (19). There is some concern that people taking yellow dock along with potassium-depleting diuretics might have an increased risk for hypokalemia. Initiation of potassium supplementation or an increase in potassium supplement dose may be necessary for some patients. Some diuretics that can deplete potassium include chlorothiazide (Diuril), chlorthalidone (Thalitone), furosemide (Lasix), hydrochlorothiazide (HCTZ, HydroDIURIL, Microzide), and others.

Interactions with Foods

CALCIUM, IRON, ZINC: Concurrent use might decrease mineral absorption from foods. Yellow dock contains oxalate (7,12), which can bind multivalent metal ions in the gastrointestinal tract and decrease mineral absorption.

Interactions with Lab Tests

COLORIMETRIC TESTS: Yellow dock might discolor urine (pink, red, purple, orange, rust), interfering with diagnostic tests that depend on a color change, due to its anthraquinone content (12,275).
SERUM POTASSIUM: Excessive use of yellow dock might cause potassium depletion, reducing serum potassium concentrations and test results (4,19).

Interactions with Diseases or Conditions

COAGULATION DISORDERS: Oxalate constituents of yellow dock can alter calcium concentrations and decrease coagulation time (4,12).
GI CONDITIONS: Avoid use in individuals with intestinal obstruction (4). Theoretically, yellow dock can exacerbate stomach and intestinal ulcers due to its mucosal irritant effect (19).
KIDNEY DISEASE: Yellow dock can damage kidneys with formation of insoluble oxalate; use with caution or avoid in individuals with a history of kidney stones (12,19). Yellow dock contains oxalates, and thus should be avoided in individuals with kidney disease (12).

Dosage and Administration

ORAL: Typical dose of the dried root is 2-4 grams or as a tea (Simmer 2-4 grams root in 150 mL of boiling water for 5-10 minutes, strain) 3 times daily (4). The liquid extract 2-4 mL (1:1 in 25% alcohol) 3 times daily (4) and a tincture 1-2 mL (1:5 in 45% alcohol) have also been used (4).

YELLOW LUPIN

Also Known As

Hasenklee, Lupin Jaune.

Scientific Names

Lupinus luteus.
Family: Fabaceae/Leguminosae.

People Use This For

Orally, yellow lupin is used for urinary tract disorders, as an anthelmintic for worm infestations, and as a diuretic. Topically, yellow lupin is used for ulcers.

Safety

POSSIBLY UNSAFE ...when the seeds or above ground parts are used orally (18).
There is insufficient reliable information available about the topical safety of yellow lupin.
PREGNANCY AND LACTATION: POSSIBLY UNSAFE ...when used orally (18); avoid using.

Effectiveness

There is insufficient reliable information available about the effectiveness of yellow lupin.

Mechanism of Action

Yellow lupin contains 0.6% to 1.6% quinolizidine alkaloids in the above ground plant parts, including sparteine, 13-hydroxylupanine, lupinines and p-cumaroyllupinine. The seed contain 0.4% to 3.3% quinolizidine alkaloids, including lupinines, sparteine, and in some cultivated strains, gramine. At present, we don't know how these components relate to the uses of lupin. Poisoning has been seen in animals, and is known as "lupinosis". It is due to the presence of mycotoxins that are produced by the fungus Phomopsis leptostromiformis, which sometimes lives in lupins (18).

Adverse Reactions

Orally, the symptoms of poisoning following ingestion include salivation, vomiting, dysphagia, cardiac arrhythmias, ascending paralysis and possibly death due to respiratory failure (18).

Interactions with Herbs & Other Dietary Supplements

None known.

Interactions with Drugs

None known.

Interactions with Foods

None known.

Interactions with Lab Tests

None known.

Interactions with Diseases or Conditions

None known.

Dosage and Administration
No typical dosage.

YELLOW TOADFLAX

Also Known As
Brideweed, Butter and Eggs, Buttered Hayhocks, Calves' Snout, Churnstaff, Devil's Head, Devil's Ribbon, Doggies, Dragon-Bushes, Eggs and Bacon, Eggs and Collops, Flaxweed, Fluelli, Gallwort, Larkspur Lion's Mouth, Monkey Flower, Pattens and Clogs, Pedlar's Basket, Pennywort, Rabbits, Ramsted, Snapdragon, Toadpipe, Yellow Rod.

Scientific Names
Linaria vulgaris.
Family: Scrophulariaceae.

Comments
At the date of publication, this product was not a common ingredient used in brand name supplements marketed to consumers. Details about this product are available at the online version of *Natural Medicines Comprehensive Database*. See www.naturaldatabase.com.

YERBA MANSA

Also Known As
Lizard's Tail, Swamp Root, Yerba Manza.

Scientific Names
Anemopsis californica, synonym Anemia californica.
Family: Saururaceae.

People Use This For
Orally, yerba mansa is used for cancer; catarrh; common cold; cough; gastrointestinal disturbances; orthopedic, skin, and throat ailments; tuberculosis; venereal diseases; and women's ailments. It is also used orally as an analgesic, disinfectant, emetic, laxative, tonic, and to induce sweating.

Safety
There is insufficient reliable information available about the safety of yerba mansa.
Pregnancy and Lactation: Insufficient reliable information is available; avoid using.

Effectiveness
There is insufficient reliable information available about the effectiveness of yerba mansa.

Mechanism of Action
The applicable parts of yerba mansa are the root and rhizome. Yerba mansa is believed to have sedative effects. It is also a urinary irritant (19). In animals, methyleugenol, a constituent of the volatile oil, prolongs the hypnotic effect of barbiturates and CNS depressant effects of chlorpromazine (19).

Adverse Reactions
None reported.

Interactions with Herbs & Other Dietary Supplements
HERBS WITH SEDATIVE PROPERTIES: Theoretically, concomitant use with herbs that have sedative properties might enhance therapeutic and adverse effects. Some of these supplements include 5-HTP, calamus, California poppy, catnip, hops, Jamaican dogwood, kava, St. John's wort, scullcap, valerian, yerba mansa, and others.

Interactions with Drugs
CNS DEPRESSANTS: Theoretically, concomitant use might cause additive or prolonged sedative effects (19).

Interactions with Foods
None known.

Interactions with Lab Tests
None known.

Interactions with Diseases or Conditions
URINARY TRACT INFLAMMATION: Contraindicated due to urinary irritant effects (19).

Dosage and Administration
No typical dosage.

Comments
There is very little scientific information about this product. Our staff is continually analyzing the available information on natural medicines and will add data here as it becomes available.

YERBA SANTA

Also Known As
Bear's Weed, Consumptive's Weed, Eriodictyon, Gum Bush, Gum Plant, Hierba Santa, Holy Herb, Holy Weed, Mountain Balm, Sacred Herb, Tarweed.

Scientific Names
Eriodictyon californicum; Eriodictyon glutinosum; Wigandia californicum.
Family: Hydrophyllaceae.

People Use This For
Orally, yerba santa is used for coughs, colds, tuberculosis, asthma, chronic bronchitis, xerostomia, as an antispasmodic, tonic, an antipyretic, and as an expectorant.
Topically, yerba santa is used as a poultice to treat bruises, sprains, wounds, insect bites, and to relieve rheumatism.
In foods and beverages, a fluid extract of yerba santa is used as a flavoring component.
In manufacturing, yerba santa is used as a pharmaceutical flavoring agent to mask the bitter taste of other drugs.

Safety
LIKELY SAFE ...when consumed in food amounts (11). ...when used orally as a medicinal (6,12).
There is insufficient reliable information about the safety of the topical use of yerba santa.
PREGNANCY AND LACTATION: Insufficient reliable information available.

Effectiveness
There is insufficient reliable information available about the effectiveness of yerba santa.

Mechanism of Action
The applicable part of yerba santa is the leaf. Yerba santa contains several flavonoids including eriodictyonine (6%), eriodictyol (0.5%) (6,11), chrysoeriol, and cirsimaritin (4118); tannins (11); and a trace amount of volatile oil (6,11). Yerba santa may have a mild diuretic effect (18). Eriodictyol is reported to exert an expectorant effect (6,11).

Adverse Reactions
None reported.

Interactions with Herbs & Other Dietary Supplements
None known.

Interactions with Drugs
None known.

Interactions with Foods
None known.

Interactions with Lab Tests
None known.

Interactions with Diseases or Conditions
None known.

Dosage and Administration

ORAL: People typically prepare yerba santa using 1 teaspoon of the leaves added to 1 cup boiling water. The liquid is taken warm, 30 minutes before bedtime or a mouthful taken 3 times a day (5254).

YEW

Also Known As

Chinwood, Common Yew, English Yew, Pacific Yew, Western Yew.

Scientific Names

Taxus brevifolia; Taxus baccata; and other Taxus species.
Family: Taxaceae.

People Use This For

Orally, yew is used for promoting menstruation, inducing abortion, treating diphtheria, tapeworm infestation, tonsillitis, epilepsy, rheumatism, urinary tract conditions, and liver conditions.
Yew is FDA-approved for the treatment of breast and ovarian cancer.

Safety

LIKELY UNSAFE ...when used orally (6,18). All parts of the yew plant are considered poisonous (5604). Ingestion of 50-100 grams of yew needles can cause death (18,5604). Yew can cause severe gastrointestinal irritation and can cause heart rate to slow dangerously (17,159). Many of the reported fatalities have occurred after ingestion of large amounts of plant material, especially yew needles (5603,5604,5605).
CHILDREN: UNSAFE ...when the berries are used orally. One chewed berry is potentially lethal (159).
PREGNANCY AND LACTATION: UNSAFE ...when the needles are used orally. Yew needles have been used as an abortifacient (16,18).

Effectiveness

There is insufficient reliable information available about the effectiveness of yew.

Mechanism of Action

The applicable parts of yew are the bark, branch tip, and needle. The yew bark is reported to have antispasmodic, nerve toxicant, and cardiac metabolism effects (6,18). It contains many alkaloids of which taxine A and B are considered to be cardiotoxic (5603,5604). Taxine B affects myocardial cells of the heart by inhibiting both calcium and sodium transport across cell membranes (5604). Yew also contains flavonoids (18). Old growth Pacific yew bark contains 0.01% paclitaxel (13,512). Initially, the small yield from the bark limited the amount of drug that could be produced. Efforts to increase the drug without decimating the supply of the Pacific yew resulted in a semi-synthetic process that produces larger yields (512). English yew needles can be used to isolate 10 desacetylbaccatin III which is converted to paclitaxel (13,512). Paclitaxel is available as the prescription drug, Taxol, for treating advanced ovarian cancer, non-small cell lung cancer, metastatic breast cancer, esophageal cancer, bladder cancer, head and neck cancer, and AIDS-related Kaposi's sarcoma (15).

Adverse Reactions

Orally, death has occurred with ingestion of 50-100 grams of yew needles (18,5604). Symptoms of poisoning include queasiness, dry mouth, (18) vomiting, vertigo, severe abdominal pain, weakness (5604), nervousness, trembling, dyspnea, incoordination (5603), tachycardia, bradycardia, arrhythmias, hypotension, unconsciousness, coma (5604), mydriasis, reddening of the lips, pale and cyanotic skin (6,18), and death secondary to cardiac arrest (5604).

Interactions with Herbs & Other Dietary Supplements

None known.

Interactions with Drugs

None known.

Interactions with Foods

None known.

Interactions with Lab Tests

None known.

Interactions with Diseases or Conditions
None known.

Dosage and Administration
No typical dosage.

YIN CHEN

Also Known As
Armoise Capillaire, Capillary Wormwood, Chiu, In Chen, Inchin-Ko-To, Inchinko, Kawara-Yomogi, Kyunchinho, Rumput Roman, Shih Yin Ch'en, Yin Ch'en, Yin Ch'en Hao, Yin Chen Hao.

Scientific Names
Artemisia capillaris; Artemisia scoparia.
Family: Asteraceae/Compositae.

People Use This For
Orally, yin chen is used to treat hepatitis, infectious cholecystitis, and hyperlipidemia. Yin chen is also used to stimulate the bile flow, liver, and gallbladder. It is used orally for newborn kernicterus, for symptoms of intermittent fever and chills, bitter taste in the mouth, chest constriction, flank pain, dizziness, nausea, and loss of appetite. In addition, it is used for headache, constipation, painful urination, fever, itching, tumors, catarrh, rheumatism, painful menses, malaria, and spasms.
In Chinese and Japanese herbal combinations, yin chen is used orally for jaundice with fever, urinary dysfunction, constipation, and abdominal distention.
Yin chen is contained in inchin-ko-to, a Kampo (Chinese/Japanese) medicine used to treat hepatitis C.

Safety
POSSIBLY SAFE ...when the above ground parts are used orally and appropriately (12,4342). However, serious conditions such as hepatitis require medical management by a physician and should not be self-treated.
CHILDREN: POSSIBLY UNSAFE ...when used orally. Children under the age of 12 years should not use except under care of physician (4344).
PREGNANCY AND LACTATION: LIKELY UNSAFE ...when used orally (12); avoid using.

Effectiveness
There is insufficient reliable information available about the effectiveness of yin chen.

Mechanism of Action
The applicable parts of yin chen are the above ground parts which contain varied constituents. Scoparone, chlorogenic acid, and caffeic acid have demonstrated effects in stimulating bile secretion and protecting the liver against carbon tetrachloride injury (4343). The essential oils cause yin chen to have antipyretic (4343) and antifungal properties (4344). Yin chen is also believed to have bactericide, anti-inflammatory, and diuretic properties (4342,4343,4344). Some evidence suggests yin chen can reduce blood pressure, cholesterol levels, and act as an antiasthmatic agent (4342,4343). Inchin-ko-to, a medicine that contains yin chen, shows evidence that it can prevent apoptosis that is believed to be the mechanism of cell death in viral and fulminant hepatitis (4345). Genepin, a metabolite of inchin-ko-to, appears to be responsible for therapeutic effects (4346).

Adverse Reactions
Orally, use of yin chen is associated with nausea, abdominal distention, and dizziness (4343). One study using yin chen and da zao (Fructus Zizyphi Jujubae) orally to treat infectious hepatitis reported 2 women developed Adams-Stokes syndrome. This syndrome is usually associated with heart block (4342). Yin chen can cause an allergic reaction in individuals sensitive to the Asteraceae/Compositae family. Members of this family include ragweed, chrysanthemums, marigolds, daisies, and many other herbs.

Interactions with Herbs & Other Dietary Supplements
None known.

Interactions with Drugs
None known.

Interactions with Foods
None known.

Interactions with Lab Tests
None known.

Interactions with Diseases or Conditions
None known.

Dosage and Administration
ORAL: A typical dose of yin chen is 9-15 grams. In very serious conditions up to 30 grams might be used three times daily (4342). Yin chen is most often used in herbal combinations.

Comments
Traditional Chinese medicine nearly always uses herbal combinations. A well accepted motto in herbal medicine translates as "One ruler, two ministers, three aides, and four guides." In this expression, the active principle is the ruler and the other nine are helpers with different degrees of strength (4343).

YLANG YLANG OIL

Also Known As
Ylang Ylang.
CAUTION: See separate listing for Cananga Oil (Cananga odorata macrophylla).

Scientific Names
Cananga odorata forma. genuina, synonym Canangium odoratum forma. genuina.
Family: Annonaceae.

People Use This For
Topically, ylang ylang oil is used as a sedative, antiseptic, hypotensive, and aphrodisiac.
In foods and beverages, ylang ylang oil is used as a flavoring agent.
In manufacturing, it is used as a fragrance for cosmetics (maximum levels 1% in perfumes) and soaps.

Safety
LIKELY SAFE ...when used in amounts commonly found in foods. Ylang ylang has Generally Recognized As Safe (GRAS) status in the US (4912). ...when applied topically in amounts found in cosmetics and soaps (11) it is nonirritating and nonsensitizing to skin, and no phototoxicity is reported (11).
PREGNANCY AND LACTATION: Insufficient reliable information available; avoid using.

Effectiveness
There is insufficient reliable information available about the effectiveness of ylang ylang oil.

Mechanism of Action
There is insufficient reliable information available about the possible mechanism of action and active ingredients.

Adverse Reactions
None reported.

Interactions with Herbs & Other Dietary Supplements
None known.

Interactions with Drugs
None known.

Interactions with Foods
None known.

Interactions with Lab Tests
None known.

Interactions with Diseases or Conditions
None known.

Dosage and Administration
No typical dosage.

Comments
Ylang ylang oil is the distilled oil from freshly harvested Cangana odorata genuina flower.

YOGURT

Also Known As
Acidophilus Milk, Bulgarian Yogurt, Live Culture Yogurt, Probiotics, Yoghurt, Yougurt.
CAUTION: See separate listings for Bifidobacteria, Lactobacillus, and Saccharomyces boulardii.

Scientific Names
None.

People Use This For
Orally, yogurt is used for restoring gastrointestinal normal flora after antibiotic therapy, reducing antibiotic-associated diarrhea, acute diarrhea in children, treating and preventing vaginal candidiasis, bacterial vaginosis, and preventing urinary tract infections. Yogurt is also used orally for lactose intolerance, reducing the risk of colorectal cancer, treating hyperlipidemia, eradicating Helicobacter pylori infection in peptic ulcer disease, and preventing sunburns.
Intravaginally, yogurt is used for treating vaginal candidiasis and bacterial vaginosis in pregnancy.
Yogurt is also eaten as a food and used as an alternative to milk in lactose-intolerant individuals.

Safety
LIKELY SAFE ...when consumed in food amounts.
...when used orally for medicinal purposes (1240,1241,1242,1246,1253,1256,3590,8526).
POSSIBLY SAFE ...when used intravaginally. There are no adverse reactions reported in a small clinical study (1248).
PREGNANCY: LIKELY SAFE ...when consumed in food amounts. POSSIBLY SAFE ...when used intravaginally. There are no adverse reactions reported in a small clinical study in pregnant women (1248).
LACTATION: LIKELY SAFE ...when consumed in amounts commonly found in foods. There is insufficient reliable information available about the safety of the intravaginal use of yogurt during breast-feeding.

Effectiveness
POSSIBLY EFFECTIVE

Antibiotic-associated diarrhea. There is some clinical evidence that consuming a specific yogurt product fermented with Lactobacillus rhamnosus GG can significantly decrease symptoms of diarrhea, abdominal distress, stomach pain, and flatulence in people taking erythromycin (1255,3589). It's not known if other yogurt products offer the same benefits.

Bacterial vaginosis. Taking yogurt orally seems to help treat bacterial vaginosis (1245,1248).

Diarrhea. Yogurt formula given as a replacement for milk formula in infants and young children seems to relieve persistent diarrhea (1250,1254).

Helicobacter pylori (H pylori). Supplementation with Lactobacillus- and Bifidobacterium-containing yogurt can improve eradication rates of H. pylori by increasing compliance in patients treated for peptic ulcer with standard triple-drug therapy, including lansoprazole (Prevacid), amoxicillin (Amoxil, others), and clarithromycin (Biaxin). It can also restore Bifidobacterium in stools after depletion by triple therapy (8525). However, consuming yogurt without standard triple-drug therapy does not appear to effectively eradicate H. pylori (10053).

Hyperlipidemia. Taking yogurt orally seems to decrease cholesterol in patients with borderline to moderate hyperlipidemia (1240,1241,3590). Fermented milk or yogurt products fermented with specific organisms including Lactobacillus acidophilus and a combination of Enterococcus faecium and Streptococcus thermophilus have been shown to produce mild to moderate reductions in serum cholesterol (1240,1241,3590). In one crossover study, four weeks of treatment with a human strain of Lactobacillus acidophilus resulted in a significant reduction in total serum cholesterol (3.2%) (1240). In another small crossover study, a milk preparation fermented with Lactobacillus acidophilus plus added fructo-oligosaccharides was tested in men. After three weeks of treatment, there was a significant decrease in total cholesterol (4.4%), low-density lipoprotein (LDL) levels (5.4%), and the LDL/high-density lipoprotein (HDL) ratio (5.3%). There were not significant changes in triglyceride or HDL levels (1241). In a larger study, borderline hyperlipidemic men and women taking a specific yogurt fermented with a strain of Enterococcus faecium and two strains of Streptococcus thermophilus (CAUSIDO culture), for an eight week period, had a significant average LDL reduction of 8.4% after adjusting for changes in body mass. Yogurts in this study fermented with a Streptococcus thermophilus/Lactobacillus acidophilus combination and a Streptococcus thermophilus/Lactobacillus rhamnosus combination did not significantly reduce LDL cholesterol (3590).

Lactose intolerance. Continuous consumption of yogurt with live bacterial cultures seems to improve lactose tolerance in children and adults with lactose malabsorption. The presence of actively growing bacteria cultures or the fat content does not seem to influence tolerability (1246,1256,8526,8943,9220).

Vaginal candidiasis. Taking yogurt orally seems to help prevent vaginal candidiasis (1245,1249).

POSSIBLY INEFFECTIVE

Asthma. Taking yogurt orally as an adjunctive treatment doesn't seem to improve asthma (1244,3589).

Malnourishment-related diarrhea. Yogurt formula given as a replacement for milk formula doesn't seem to help acute, noninfectious diarrhea in malnourished infants and children (1242).

INSUFFICIENT RELIABLE EVIDENCE to RATE

Urinary tract infections (UTIs). Preliminary research indicates that consuming a yogurt drink containing Lactobacillus does not seem to prevent recurrent UTIs when used up to 6 months in women with a history of UTIs (8253). More evidence is needed to rate yogurt for this use.

Mechanism of Action

Yogurt is a dairy preparation produced by fermenting milk using one or more of a variety of specific organisms such as Lactobacillus acidophilus, Lactobacillus rhamnosus, Lactobacillus bulgaricus, Enterococcus faecium, Streptococcus thermophilus, and others (1240,1241,3589,3590). The bacteria in yogurt provides the active constituents, peptidoglycans, polysaccharide, and techoic acid, which modulates the immune system, and beta-galactosidase, which improves lactose tolerance (3589,8517). The partial digestion of milk products results in production of solubilized forms of calcium, which are easily absorbed (3589).

The medicinal benefit of yogurt is primarily attributed to the live cultures it contains as a source of probiotics. Probiotics are symbiotic micro-organisms similar to the human gastrointestinal normal flora that, when ingested, can pass through the stomach and potentially colonize the lower gastrointestinal tract. It is thought that this colonization might restore the normal flora after antibiotic therapy and maintain the balance of flora to prevent or minimize antibiotic-associated diarrhea (3589). Probiotics contained in yogurt are also thought to help restore normal flora and normal bowel function in other causes of diarrhea. The lactic acid bacteria found in yogurt seem to suppress growth of pathogenic bacteria such as Salmonella typhimurium (3589). The lactobacillus species in yogurt can also stimulate the production of mucin by intestinal goblet cells, which improves the intestinal environment (8513).

There is preliminary evidence that yogurt might stimulate the immune system (3589). In vitro studies have produced an increase of immune related substances after yogurt consumption or exposure to lactic acid bacteria (3589). Other components of yogurt, such as whey protein, short peptides, and conjugated linoleic acid, may contribute to its proposed immune effects (3589). Yogurt may have an effect on IgE-mediated diseases such as asthma by decreasing IgE production, but human studies have produced conflicting results (3589).

Yogurt may reduce nitrite concentrations in the gastrointestinal tract (3589). Preliminary evidence indicates that nitrites lead to the formation of carcinogenic compounds.

In healthy infants, milk fermented with Lactobacillus casei increases fecal lactobacilli and decreases potentially harmful beta-glucosidase enzyme activity. Beta-glucosidase is a bacterial enzyme that has been associated with enterohepatic circulation of toxins and carcinogens. Beta-glucosidase has been shown to be elevated in diets high in meat (1243).

Lactobacillus is part of the normal vaginal flora. Probiotics, particularly Lactobacillus acidophilus strains, are thought to be beneficial for candidal vaginal infections by helping to restore the normal flora of the vagina. Lactobacillus acidophilus has also been found to inhibit growth of Candida albicans. Presence of lactobacillus species in the rectum has been associated with lactobacillus colonization in the vagina (1245,1249).

For lowering cholesterol in hyperlipidemia, it is thought that certain culture strains found in yogurt might deconjugate bile salts. This action reduces the serum concentrations of low-density lipoprotein (LDL) cholesterol (3590). Other evidence suggests yogurt with live bacterial cultures can increase short-chain fatty acid production, which might improve lipid and glucose metabolism with chronic yogurt consumption (8943).

People with lactase deficiency seem to tolerate and digest pasteurized yogurt or yogurt with live bacterial cultures better than milk. However, lactose absorption seems to be greater with live culture yogurt than pasteurized yogurt. Yogurt seems to have an immediate beneficial effect on lactose digestion and a delayed effect as the intestinal flora adapts to chronic yogurt ingestion (8943). Some evidence suggests yogurt might induce production of endogenous lactase in the intestine, or active bacteria cultures might produce beta-galactosidase and partially replace deficient lactase (1256,8517,8526,8943).

Yogurt, like milk, is rich in B vitamins. However, yogurt might not be a good source of B vitamins because the bioavailability of B vitamins in yogurt is low. It is likely that bacteria in yogurt consume B vitamins, especially thiamine (vitamin B1), riboflavin (vitamin B2), and pyridoxine (vitamin B6), making them less available for intestinal absorption (10464).

Adverse Reactions

Orally, yogurt is usually well tolerated (8561). Fatal Lactobacillus rhamnosus septicemia has been reported in an immunocompromised patient consuming yogurt and taking prolonged courses of multiple broad spectrum antibiotics (8561).

Interactions with Herbs & Other Dietary Supplements
None known.

Interactions with Drugs
CIPROFLOXACIN (Cipro): Concomitant administration can significantly reduce absorption of ciprofloxacin (Cipro) (1252).
IMMUNOSUPPRESSANTS: Theoretically, yogurt could cause infection in patients taking medications that suppress the immune system. These include cyclosporine (Neoral, Sandimmune), tacrolimus (Prograf), azathioprine (Imuran), and cancer chemotherapeutic agents like cyclophosphamide (Cytoxan) and cisplatin (Platinol) (4380,4391,4393,4398).
TETRACYCLINE ANTIBIOTICS: Concomitant administration can reduce the absorption of tetracyclines (15).

Interactions with Foods
None known.

Interactions with Lab Tests
None known.

Interactions with Diseases or Conditions
IMMUNODEFICIENCY: There is some concern that yogurt might cause pathogenic colonization, especially in patients who are immunocompromised. Yogurt and probiotics have caused bacteremia and fungemia in seriously ill, immunocompromised patients, but very rarely. Pathogenic colonization is more likely to occur in severely immunocompromised patients (8561).

Dosage and Administration
ORAL: Yogurt should be labeled with a "Live and Active Cultures" seal from the National Yogurt Association, indicating the product reliably contains at least 100 million active cultures per gram of yogurt (e.g., Dannon, Yoplait). For preventing antibiotic-induced diarrhea, 125 mL (approximately 4 ounces) of yogurt containing Lactobacillus GG taken twice daily throughout the antibiotic treatment course has been used (1255). Some researchers recommend taking 240 mL (8 ounces) of other yogurt preparations twice daily (1736). Separate antibiotic administration and yogurt by at least two hours. For acute diarrhea, 125 grams of yogurt containing Lactobacillus casei twice daily has been used (1253). For reducing cholesterol, several different doses have been tried depending on the preparation. A typical dose of 200 mL of yogurt containing Lactobacillus acidophilus per day has been used (1240). A combination product of 125 mL Lactobacillus acidophilus yogurt with 2.5% fructo-oligosaccharides three times daily has also been used (1241). A dose of 450 mL daily of yogurt containing the CAUSIDO culture has also been used (3590). For preventing vaginal candidiasis and bacterial vaginosis, a typical dose is 150 mL Lactobacillus acidophilus yogurt per day (1245).
INTRAVAGINAL: No typical dosage.

YOHIMBE

Also Known As
Johimbi, Yohimbehe, Yohimbehe cortex, Yohimbine.

Scientific Names
Pausinystalia yohimbe, synonyms Pausinystalia johimbe, Corynanthe johimbi, Corynanthe yohimbi.
Family: Rubiaceae.

People Use This For
Orally, yohimbe is used as an aphrodisiac, for impotence, exhaustion, angina, hypertension, diabetic neuropathy, and postural hypotension. Yohimbe is also used for general sexual dysfunction in men and women, sexual dysfunction caused by selective-serotonin reuptake inhibitors (SSRI), and as an adjunct to conventional antidepressants for refractory depression.
Yohimbe bark is also smoked or snuffed for its hallucinogenic effects.

Safety
POSSIBLY SAFE ...when used orally and appropriately with medical supervision. The primary active constituent, yohimbine has been shown to be safe in several clinical trials lasting up to 10 weeks (3305,3307,3311,3313). However, yohimbe is not appropriate for self-treatment.
LIKELY UNSAFE ...when used orally in excessive doses or without medical supervision. The primary active ingredient, yohimbine, is considered unsafe for unmonitored nonprescription use (515). Large doses can cause

significant toxicity including severe hypotension, heart conduction disorders, and death (18).
There is insufficient reliable information available about the safety of inhaling yohimbe bark.
CHILDREN: LIKELY UNSAFE ...when used orally. Children can be extra sensitive to the adverse effects of yohimbe (19).
PREGNANCY AND LACTATION: LIKELY UNSAFE ...when used orally. Yohimbe might have uterine relaxant effects and also cause fetal toxicity (19).

Effectiveness

POSSIBLY EFFECTIVE

Erectile dysfunction (ED). There is evidence suggesting that the primary constituent, yohimbine, can be helpful for impotence. Yohimbine seems to help men with organic, psychogenic, mixed, and unknown vascular erectile dysfunction (3305,3307,3311,3313,10629). Some herbalists suggest that the yohimbe bark actually works better than the isolated yohimbine constituent; however, yohimbe bark has not been evaluated in studies.

Sexual dysfunction. There is evidence from multiple clinical trials that the primary constituent, yohimbine, can improve sexual dysfunction associated with selective-serotonin reuptake inhibitors (SSRIs) (3305,3306,3307,3311,3313,3970,3971,3972,3973). However, this benefit has not been described specifically for the yohimbe bark.

There is insufficient reliable information available about the effectiveness of yohimbe for its other uses.

Mechanism of Action

The applicable part of yohimbe is the bark. The constituent thought to be responsible for yohimbe's effects is the alkaloid yohimbine (10629). Yohimbe bark contains approximately 6% yohimbine. Aphrodisiac activity of yohimbe has been attributed to genital blood vessel dilation, nerve impulse transmission to genital tissue, and increased reflex excitability in the sacral region of the spinal cord (11). The yohimbine constituent readily penetrates the central nervous system (CNS) and works primarily through alpha 2-adrenergic receptor blockade (3305). It also has monoamine oxidase (MOA) inhibiting, calcium channel blocking, and peripheral serotonin receptor blocking effects (11). Yohimbine likely works several ways to affect impotence since it has been effective in men with organic, psychogenic, mixed, and unknown vascular erectile dysfunction (3305,3310,3311,10629). Yohimbine's effect on impotence might be mediated through both increased penile blood flow and increased central sympathetic excitatory impulses to the genital tissue (3305,3309). In women, a nitric oxide-enhanced form of yohimbine (NMI-870) is theorized to improve sexual arousal by increasing vaginal blood flow by dilating vaginal blood vessels (6198).

Adverse Reactions

Orally, yohimbe and the constituent yohimbine in typical doses can cause excitation, tremor, insomnia, anxiety, hypertension, tachycardia, dizziness, gastric intolerance, salivation, sinusitis, irritability, headache, urinary frequency, fluid retention, rash, nausea, and vomiting (3303,3304,3305,3309,3311,3313,10629). Although low doses can stimulate respiration, high doses can cause respiratory depression (11). High doses can also cause other severe toxicities including paralysis, severe hypotension, cardiac conduction disorders, cardiac failure, and death (18). There is also one report of a hypersensitivity reaction including fever; chills; malaise; itchy, scaly skin; progressive renal failure; and lupus-like syndrome associated with ingestion of a one-day dose of yohimbine (6169).

Interactions with Herbs & Other Dietary Supplements

CAFFEINE-CONTAINING HERBS: Theoretically, concomitant use of yohimbe with large amounts of caffeine-containing herbs or products can increase the risk of hypertensive crisis (12). Caffeine-containing herbs include coffee, cola, guarana, mate, and tea.
EPHEDRA: Theoretically, concomitant use of large amounts of ephedra can increase the risk of hypertensive crisis due to ephedrine content (12).
HERBS WITH MONOAMINE OXIDASE INHIBITING (MAOI) ACTIVITY: Theoretically, concomitant use of these herbs with yohimbe can have additive therapeutic and adverse effects (12). Herbs with MAOI activity include California poppy, ginkgo, mace, and St. John's wort (12).

Interactions with Drugs

ANTIHYPERTENSIVE DRUGS: Concomitant use of yohimbe can interfere with blood pressure control and should be used with caution (11).
CLONIDINE (Catapres): Avoid concomitant use; yohimbine antagonizes the effect of clonidine (11,19).
GUANABENZ (Wytensin): Avoid concomitant use; yohimbine antagonizes the effect of guanabenz (11,19).
MONOAMINE OXIDASE INHIBITORS (MAOIs): Concomitant use with yohimbe can result in additive effects (11,12).
NALOXONE (Narcan): Concomitant use can have additive therapeutic and adverse effects (19).
PHENOTHIAZINES: Yohimbe is contraindicated with phenothiazines due to the risk of increased alpha 2-adrenergic antagonism (19).
STIMULANT DRUGS: Yohimbe is contraindicated because concomitant use increases the risk of hypertensive crisis due to yohimbe monoamine oxidase inhibitor MAOI activity (11,12).

TRICYCLIC ANTIDEPRESSANTS (TCAs): Yohimbe is contraindicated due to its potential to increase or decrease blood pressure (19).

Interactions with Foods

TYRAMINE-CONTAINING FOODS: Avoid concomitant consumption of large amounts of tyramine-containing foods, due to the risk of hypertensive crisis (11). Tyramine-containing foods include aged cheeses, fermented meats, red wines, and others (506).
VASOPRESSOR-CONTAINING FOODS: Avoid concomitant consumption of large amounts of vasopressor-containing foods due to the risk of hypertensive crisis (11). Vasopressor-containing foods include overripe fava beans, coffee, tea, colas, and chocolate (506).

Interactions with Lab Tests

None known.

Interactions with Diseases or Conditions

ANGINA, HEART DISEASE: Contraindicated, due to the cardiovascular effects of the yohimbe constituent, yohimbine (515).
ANXIETY: Contraindicated; the yohimbe constituent, yohimbine, might cause anxiety (515).
BENIGN PROSTATIC HYPERPLASIA (BPH): Theoretically, yohimbe might exacerbate symptoms of BPH due to antagonism of alpha-2 receptors and decreased circulation (19).
DEPRESSION: Contraindicated. The constituent yohimbine might elicit manic-like symptoms in individuals with bipolar depression or suicidal tendencies in individuals with endogenous depression (19).
DIABETES: Avoid, due to the monoamine oxidase inhibiting (MAOI) activity of yohimbe (515). Use of MAO inhibitors in patients receiving insulin or oral antidiabetes drugs has been associated with hypoglycemic episodes (15).
HYPERTENSION: Avoid; small amounts of yohimbine can increase blood pressure (19).
HYPOTENSION: Contraindicated; large amounts of yohimbine can cause hypotension (515).
KIDNEY DISEASE: Contraindicated. Theoretically, yohimbine might have antidiuretic effects (19).
LIVER DISEASE: Contraindicated. Theoretically, liver disease might alter metabolism of the constituent yohimbine (19).
POST-TRAUMATIC STRESS DISORDER (PTSD): Avoid; the constituent yohimbine has been associated with triggering acute symptoms in four individuals with PTSD (1294).
SCHIZOPHRENIA: Use with caution; the constituent yohimbine might activate psychoses in patients with schizophrenia (19,515).
YOHIMBE HYPERSENSITIVITY: Contraindicated (19).

Dosage and Administration

ORAL: For sexual dysfunction, including impotence, a typical dose of the constituent yohimbine is 15-30 mg daily (3303,3305,3307,3313,10629). Doses of yohimbine up to 100 mg daily have been used. However, significantly more severe adverse effects would be expected with such a high dose (3312).

Comments

Yohimbe is the name of an evergreen tree that is native to Zaire, Cameroon, and Gabon. The bark of the yohimbe tree contains the alkaloid yohimbine (4201).

YUCCA

Also Known As

Adam's Needle (Yucca filamentosa), Aloe Yucca (Yucca aloifolia), Bear Grass (Yucca filamentosa), Dagger Plant (Yucca aloifolia), Joshua Tree (Yucca brevifolia), Mohave Yucca (Yucca schidigera), Our-Lord's-Candle (Yucca whipplei), Soapweed (Yucca glauca), Spanish Bayonet (Yucca aloifolia).

Scientific Names

Yucca aloifolia; Yucca brevifolia, synonym Yucca arborescens; Yucca filamentosa; Yucca glauca, synonym Yucca angustifolia; Yucca schidigera, synonym Yucca mohavensis; Yucca whipplei; other Yucca species.
Family: Agavaceae.

People Use This For

Orally, yucca is used for osteoarthritis, hypertension, migraine headaches, colitis, hypercholesterolemia, stomach disorders, diabetes, poor circulation, and liver and gallbladder disorders.
Topically, yucca is used for sores, skin diseases, inflammation, bleeding, sprains, broken limbs, joint pain, baldness and dandruff.
In foods, yucca is fried like potatoes.

In manufacturing, yucca extract is used as a foaming and flavoring agent in carbonated beverages. Many compounds from yucca have been used in the synthesis of new drugs.

Safety

LIKELY SAFE ...when used orally in amounts commonly found in foods. Mojave yucca and Joshua tree have Generally Recognized As Safe (GRAS) status in the US (4912).
POSSIBLY SAFE ...when used orally and appropriately, short-term (12).
There is insufficient reliable information available about the safety of yucca used long-term or applied topically.
PREGNANCY AND LACTATION: There is insufficient reliable information about the safety of yucca in medicinal amounts during pregnancy and breast-feeding; avoid using.

Effectiveness

INSUFFICIENT RELIABLE EVIDENCE to RATE

Hypercholesterolemia. Taking yucca orally, in combination with diet and exercise, seems to help lower triglycerides and cholesterol levels (4,6).
Hypertension. Taking yucca orally, in combination with diet and exercise, might help lower blood pressure (4,6).
Osteoarthritis. There is preliminary evidence that a yucca extract might reduce symptoms of osteoarthritis such as pain, swelling, and stiffness (4,6).
More evidence is needed to rate yucca for these uses.

Mechanism of Action

The applicable part of yucca is the root of the non-flowering plant. Yucca contains saponins that are believed responsible for the pharmacologic activity of the plant (4,6,11). However, the mechanism for these effects is unclear because yucca saponins don't seem to be absorbed in the gastrointestinal tract (4). The saponins in yucca are often irritating to mucous membranes and might cause GI irritation (4077). In vitro, saponins have hemolytic activity (11). There is preliminary evidence that yucca has anti-inflammatory, antitumor, and antiviral activity (4,6,11).

Adverse Reactions

Orally, yucca can cause stomach upset, mucous membrane irritation, bitter taste, nausea, and vomiting (7).
Intravenously, yucca administration may result in hemolysis (11).

Interactions with Herbs & Other Dietary Supplements

None known.

Interactions with Drugs

None known.

Interactions with Foods

None known.

Interactions with Lab Tests

None known.

Interactions with Diseases or Conditions

None known.

Dosage and Administration

ORAL: No typical dosage. However, traditionally 380 to 490 mg of the powdered yucca stalk or root has been used two to three times daily. Yucca can be prepared as a decoction by boiling one-fourth ounce of the root in 16 ounces of water for 15 minutes. People have taken 3 to 5 cups of this liquid per day (6006).
TOPICAL: No typical dosage.

ZEDOARY

Also Known As

Cedoaria, Cetoal, E Zhu, E-Zhu, Indian Arrowroot, Kua, Sati, Shati, Temu Kuning, Temu Putih, Turmeric, Zedoaire, Zedoária, Zedoarie rhizoma, Zitwer, Zitwerwirtzelstock.
CAUTION: See separate listings for Turmeric, Goldenseal, and Javanese Turmeric.

Scientific Names

Curcuma zedoaria, synonym Amomum zedoaria.
Family: Zingiberaceae.

People Use This For

Orally, zedoary is used for colic, spasms, stimulating appetite, improving digestion, stimulating bile flow, nervous diseases, and as an anti-inflammatory.
In combination herbal products, zedoary extracts are used for gastrointestinal complaints and stimulating bile flow.

Safety

POSSIBLY SAFE ...when used orally and appropriately (12).
PREGNANCY: LIKELY UNSAFE ...when used orally; avoid using (12) due to potential abortifacient effects (19).
LACTATION: Insufficient reliable information available; avoid using.

Effectiveness

There is insufficient reliable information available about the effectiveness of zedoary.

Mechanism of Action

The applicable part of zedoary is the rhizome. Zedoary contains a volatile oil and curcuminoids (18). Zedoary is thought to stimulate bile production and gallbladder emptying (512). The volatile oil contains sesquiterpene ketones known as turmerones that are believed responsible for increasing bile production (512). The curcuminoid constituents are believed to be responsible for gallbladder emptying effects (512). The isolated sesquiterpene constituent dehydrocurdione shows some evidence of anti-inflammatory activity (4011). Experimental evidence suggests other sesquiterpenes isolated from zedoary might be hepatoprotective (4012). Compounds isolated from zedoary demonstrate some evidence of antifungal (4013) and cytotoxic (4014) activity.

Adverse Reactions

None reported.

Interactions with Herbs & Other Dietary Supplements

None known.

Interactions with Drugs

None known.

Interactions with Foods

None known.

Interactions with Lab Tests

None known.

Interactions with Diseases or Conditions

MENORRHAGIA: Some experts suggest that zedoary should not be used by women who have heavy menstrual periods (12).

Dosage and Administration

ORAL: One cup of tea is typically taken three times daily at meals. To make tea, steep 1-1.5 grams powdered dried rhizome in 150 mL boiling water, 5-10 minutes, and strain (18).

Comments

Traditional methods for preparing zedoary involve prolonged washing with water to remove most of the protein, water-soluble nutrients, and presumably, an unidentified toxic constituent (4015).

ZINC

Also Known As

Zinc Acetate, Zinc Acexamate, Zinc Aspartate, Zinc Citrate, Zinc Gluconate, Zinc Methionine, Zinc Monomethionine, Zinc Oxide, Zinc Picolinate, Zinc Pyrithione, Zinc Sulfate.

Scientific Names

Zinc; Zn; atomic number 30.

People Use This For

Orally, zinc is used for treatment and prevention of zinc deficiency. It is also used orally for treating the common cold, recurrent ear infections, and preventing acute lower respiratory infections. Other oral uses include macular degeneration, night blindness, cataracts, diabetes, hypertension, acquired immunodeficiency syndrome (AIDS), psoriasis, eczema, and acne. It is also used orally for anorexia nervosa, acute diarrhea in children with zinc deficiency, attention deficit-hyperactivity disorder (ADHD), blunted sense of taste (hypogeusia), aphthous ulcers, Crohn's disease, ulcerative colitis, and peptic ulcers. Other oral uses include benign prostatic hyperplasia (BPH); male infertility, male impotence; osteoporosis, rheumatoid arthritis, and muscle cramps in patients with cirrhosis. It is also used orally for sickle cell disease, thalassemia, Alzheimer's disease, Down syndrome, Wilson's disease, Hansen's disease, acrodermatitis enteropathica, necrolytic acral erythema, and delayed wound healing associated with zinc deficiency. Zinc is also used orally for improving athletic performance and strength, improving immune function, improving growth and health in zinc-deficient stunted children, tinnitus, and severe head injuries. It is also used orally and locally for parasitic infections, including prevention and treatment of malaria.

Topically, zinc is used for treating acne, aging skin, herpes simplex infections, resistant trichomonas infection, and speeding wound healing. Zinc citrate is used in toothpaste and mouthwash to prevent dental plaque formation and gingivitis.

Intranasally, zinc is used for treating the common cold.

Ophthalmically, zinc sulfate is used in products for eye irritation.

Intravenously, zinc is used as a component of total parenteral nutrition and for improving outcomes in burn patients.

Safety

LIKELY SAFE ...when used orally or topically and appropriately. Zinc is safe in amounts that do not exceed the tolerable upper intake level (UL) of 40 mg per day (7135).

POSSIBLY SAFE ...when used orally and appropriately in doses higher than the tolerable upper intake level (UL). There is some concern that doses higher than the UL of 40 mg per day might decrease copper absorption and result in anemia. However, there is some evidence doses of elemental zinc as high as 80 mg daily in combination with copper 2 mg can be used safely for approximately six years without significant adverse effects (7303,8622).

POSSIBLY UNSAFE ...when used intranasally. Case reports and animal research suggest that intranasal zinc might cause permanent anosmia (loss of sense of smell) (11155,11156,11703,11704,11705,11706,11707). Until more is known, use intranasal zinc with caution.

LIKELY UNSAFE ...when taken orally in excessive amounts. Chronic intake of 450-1600 mg daily can cause sideroblastic anemia. Ingestion of 10-30 grams of zinc sulfate can be lethal in adults (7135).

CHILDREN: LIKELY SAFE ...when used orally and appropriately (7135). Zinc is safe in amounts that do not exceed the tolerable upper intake level (UL). The UL for children is based on age; 4 mg per day for infants birth to 6 months, 5 mg per day for infants 7 to 12 months, 7 mg per day for children 1 to 3 years, 12 mg per day for children 4 to 8 years, 23 mg per day for children 9 to 13 years, and 34 mg per day for adolescents ages 14 to 18 years (7135). POSSIBLY UNSAFE ...when used orally in high doses. Taking amounts greater than the tolerable upper intake level (UL) can cause sideroblastic anemia and copper deficiency (7135).

PREGNANCY: LIKELY SAFE ...when used orally and appropriately. Zinc is safe in amounts that do not exceed the tolerable upper intake level (UL) of 34 mg per day for pregnant women 14 to 18 years, and 40 mg per day for pregnant women age 19-50 (7135). LIKELY UNSAFE ...when used orally in high doses. Tell pregnant patients not to exceed the tolerable upper intake level (UL) (7135). Taking higher doses during the third trimester can cause premature births and stillbirths (332).

LACTATION: LIKELY SAFE ...when used orally and appropriately. Zinc is safe in amounts that do not exceed the tolerable upper intake level (UL) of 34 mg per day for lactating women age 14 to 18 years, and 40 mg per day for pregnant women age 19-50 (7135). POSSIBLY UNSAFE ...when used orally in high doses. Tell breast-feeding patients not to exceed the tolerable upper intake level (UL). Higher doses can cause zinc-induced copper deficiency in nursing infants (7135).

Effectiveness

EFFECTIVE

Wilson's disease. Taking zinc orally improves symptoms of Wilson's disease (822,823,2693). Zinc blocks copper absorption and increases copper elimination in the stool of people with Wilson's disease (2692).

Zinc deficiency. Taking zinc orally or intravenously prevents and treats zinc deficiency (2619). However, routine zinc supplementation is not recommended (403). Zinc deficiency requiring supplementation may occur in severe diarrhea, malabsorption syndromes, liver cirrhosis and alcoholism, after major surgery, and during long-term administration of total parenteral nutrition (TPN) (3900). Zinc supplementation (136 mg elemental zinc per day) in patients with cirrhosis and zinc deficiency seems to improve liver function and glucose tolerance, possibly by increasing insulin-like growth factor (8624).

LIKELY EFFECTIVE

Diarrhea. Taking zinc orally reduces the duration and severity of acute and persistent diarrhea in malnourished or zinc-deficient children (825,826,827,3455,3456,8633,8638). Zinc supplements lower the probability of continuing diarrhea by approximately 24% in acute diarrhea and lower the rate of treatment failure or mortality by approximately 42% in persistent diarrhea (8633,10248). Zinc also seems to reduce hospital admissions due to acute diarrhea by approximately 23% (10248). Severe zinc deficiency in children is common in developing countries.

POSSIBLY EFFECTIVE

Acne. Taking zinc orally might help treat acne. Research suggests that people with acne might have lower serum and skin zinc levels (2686,6507,6508,6509). Clinical trials have been small, but most suggest that zinc can improve acne (6297,6298,6299,6501,6502,6503,6504). So far, it is not clear how zinc compares to other treatments. Comparative trials with tetracycline have yielded conflicting results (6505,6506). Topically, in combination with erythromycin, zinc also seems to help treat acne (819,820,2687,2688).

Acrodermatitis enteropathica. Taking zinc orally seems to help improve acrodermatitis enteropathica (821,2689,2690,2691). There is one case report of oral zinc sulfate 225 mg twice daily plus interferon alfa-2b for six months resolving all lesions in a woman with necrolytic acral erythema and hepatitis C. Necrolytic acral erythema is categorized in the family of necrolytic erythemas which includes acrodermatitis enteropathica (6192).

Age-related macular degeneration (AMD). Taking zinc orally in combination with antioxidant vitamins might slow the progression of advanced age-related macular degeneration (AMD). Elemental zinc 80 mg plus vitamin C 500 mg, vitamin E 400 IU, and beta-carotene 15 mg daily seems to provide a risk reduction of 27% for visual acuity loss and a risk reduction of 24% for progression of AMD in patients with advanced AMD (7303). Patients with monocular or binocular intermediate AMD or monocular advanced AMD are at high risk for advanced AMD. Theoretically, these patients may also benefit from zinc and antioxidant supplementation (11326). There isn't enough information to determine if zinc plus antioxidants is beneficial for people with less advanced macular disease or for preventing AMD (6583,6584,7303). However, dietary zinc or zinc supplementation alone does not seem to reduce the risk of developing of AMD (6579,6580,6581).

Anorexia nervosa. Taking zinc supplements orally might help increase weight gain and improve depressive symptoms in patients with anorexia nervosa (6905,6906).

Attention deficit-hyperactivity disorder (ADHD). Taking zinc orally in combination with conventional treatment might modestly improve symptoms of hyperactivity, impulsivity, and impaired socialization in some children with ADHD (11350,12060). But zinc might not improve attention deficit (11350). There is some evidence that zinc could be most helpful in children with a high body mass index (BMI), low zinc levels, and low free fatty acid levels (11350). Some research suggests that children with ADHD have lower serum zinc levels than children without ADHD (9965,9966). Other research suggests ADHD patients with lower zinc levels might not respond adequately to stimulant therapy (9967). Studies using zinc for ADHD have taken place in the Middle East where zinc deficiency is relatively common compared to Western countries. It's not known if zinc would have the same potential benefits when used for ADHD in patient populations from Western countries.

Burns. Administering zinc intravenously in combination with other minerals seems to improve the outcomes of burn patients (6520). Supplementation with zinc, copper, and selenium significantly reduced pulmonary infections and shortened intensive care unit stay in patients with serious burns (6520).

Common cold. Using zinc oral lozenges seems to help decrease the duration of the common cold in adults. The majority of studies show a significant decrease in the duration of symptoms of the common cold when adults take zinc gluconate or acetate lozenges providing 9-24 mg elemental zinc per dose. Lozenges should be taken every 2 hours while awake starting within 48 hours of symptom onset (333,334,335,337,6703,6705). However, not all studies have been positive (333,338,339,6521,6522,6700). The reasons for these different findings are not clear, but might be due to differences in zinc formulations and study methodologies. In some cases, flavoring agents such as citric acid, mannitol, and sorbitol might chelate zinc and decrease zinc ionization. Since zinc ionization is thought to be an important step involved in the effectiveness of zinc, a decrease in zinc ionization could decrease effectiveness (300,340,6522). Some of the positive studies have also been criticized for inadequately blinding the unpleasant, distinctive taste of zinc (6522,6706). Overall, zinc products seem to be beneficial for reducing the duration of symptoms of the common cold in adults. Zinc from supplements taken prophylactically does not seem to prevent the common cold (10780,10784). Research on zinc lozenges in children is conflicting (341,10803).

The role of intranasal zinc to prevent or treat the common cold is controversial. Zinc nasal spray (as a sulfate, gluconate emulsion, or gluconium gel) reduces the severity and duration of cold symptoms according to some research, while other research has found no effect (6471,8628,8629,10247). Zinc nasal spray doesn't seem to prevent experimentally induced colds (8628).

Gingivitis. Using zinc toothpaste or mouthwash alone or in combination with triclosan seems to prevent plaque accumulation, gingivitis, or formation of calculus (6523,6524,6525,6526,6527,6528,6529). Most studies used zinc citrate in combination with triclosan, which is not available in the US (6523).

Herpes simplex virus (HSV). Applying zinc topically seems to help treat herpes simplex infection (6538,6539,6540). Zinc sulfate seems to reduce the severity and duration of symptoms in both orolabial and genital herpes (6538,6539,6540,8623). Zinc oxide (0.3%) in combination with glycine cream applied topically every 2 hours to facial and circumoral herpes seems to reduce symptoms such as blistering, soreness, itching, and tingling. It can also reduce the duration of lesions from 6.5 days to 5 days when treatment is begun within 24 hours of onset of symptoms (8623).

Hypogeusia. Taking zinc orally might be effective for taste dysfunction in some patients with zinc depletion (6542,6546). Zinc also seems to improve hypogeusia conditions unrelated to zinc deficiency, such as gustin/carbonic anhydrase VI deficiency, captopril-induced taste disturbances, hypogeusia secondary to head and neck radiation, and post-traumatic olfactory disorder (6543,6544,6545,6547). In uremic adults, zinc supplementation, orally or via dialysate, might improve taste acuity; but it appears to be ineffective for pediatric dialysis patients (6548,6549,6550).

Leprosy. Taking zinc orally in combination with anti-leprosy drugs seems to help treat leprosy (6534,6535,6536,6537). Zinc levels appear to be reduced in people with leprosy. Early clinical evidence suggests that the addition of zinc to the anti-leprosy drug regimen might allow for lowering or eliminating steroid doses in a severe form of leprosy, erythema nodosum leprosum (6534,6535,6536).

Muscle cramps. Taking zinc orally by people with cirrhosis seems to help treat muscle cramps in zinc-deficient patients (1352).

Peptic ulcers. Taking zinc orally seems to help treat and prevent peptic ulcers (6588,6589,6590,6591). Zinc acexamate (not available in the US) seems to improve peptic ulcers when compared to placebo or H2 receptor antagonist drugs (6589). It is not known if other zinc salts are effective.

Pneumonia. Zinc supplementation seems to reduce the incidence of pneumonia in undernourished children aged six months to three years in developing countries by 25% (8637). However, zinc supplementation does not show any additional benefit, compared with antibiotics and vitamin A alone, when used to reduce the severity of illness in children with both measles and pneumonia (9589). Taking 10 mg of zinc daily for six months seems to help reduce the incidence of acute lower respiratory infection in 45% of children ages 6 to 35 months living in developing countries (8920).

Sickle cell disease. Taking zinc orally seems to help treat sickle cell disease in people with zinc deficiency (6594,6595,6596,8626), and decrease the incidence of sickle-cell crisis and infections (6594,6596). Although zinc might reduce the number of hospitalizations for sickle cell crisis, the severity of a crisis does not appear to be reduced, based on length of hospital stay (6594,6596). In prepubertal children with homozygous sickle cell disease, supplementation with elemental zinc 10 mg per day seems to improve growth, height, and weight gain (8626).

Venous leg ulcers. Taking zinc orally might help treat arterial and venous leg ulcers in people with low zinc levels (6903), and recurrent aphthous ulcers in people with low zinc levels (6593). However, it's not helpful for recurring aphthous ulcers (6592,6593) or arterial and venous leg ulcers (6902) in people with adequate zinc levels. Topical zinc also seems to help treat leg ulcers (2694,6901).

Vitamin A deficiency. Taking zinc orally in combination with vitamin A seems to improve measures of vitamin A adequacy in undernourished children better than vitamin A or zinc alone (8636).

POSSIBLY INEFFECTIVE

AIDS diarrhea-wasting syndrome. Taking zinc orally in combination with vitamins doesn't seem to help treat AIDS diarrhea-wasting syndrome (6564).

Alopecia areata. Although there is preliminary evidence that suggests zinc in combination with biotin might be helpful for alopecia areata (6932), most studies indicate that zinc is not effective for alopecia areata, alopecia totalis, or alopecia universalis (6931,6932).

Atopic dermatitis (eczema). Taking zinc orally doesn't appear to improve the surface area affected and degree of erythema, symptom scores of itch and sleep disturbance, or topical steroid use in children with eczema. Zinc levels appear to be normal in children with eczema (6911).

Cataracts. Taking zinc orally in combination with antioxidant vitamins doesn't seem to help treat or prevent cataracts. Taking elemental zinc 80 mg plus vitamin C 500 mg, vitamin E 400 IU, and beta-carotene 15 mg daily does not seem to have any effect on the development or progression of age-related lens opacities (cataracts) or the need for cataract surgery in well-nourished people 55-80 years of age. However, it is unknown whether earlier intervention and/or a longer period of treatment with supplements would have any effect on cataracts (7304).

Inflammatory bowel disease (IBD). Taking zinc orally doesn't seem to help treat IBD (6913,6915,6916).

Influenza. Supplemental zinc seems to improve cell-mediated immune response in elderly people (824), but it doesn't seem to have a significant effect on antibody response and incidence of flu infection after flu vaccine (6553,6563). Additionally, zinc supplementation in patients on hemodialysis, who have a high risk of zinc deficiency, doesn't seem to improve response to influenza vaccine (10809). Taking zinc supplements orally is unlikely to improve immune function in people without risk factors for zinc deficiency (10789). However, there is preliminary evidence that suggests zinc along with selenium might reduce the incidence of infections in institutionalized older patients (8921).

Malaria. Taking zinc orally doesn't seems to help prevent or treat malaria in undernourished children in developing countries. Zinc supplements don't seem to protect against infection by Plasmodium falciparum (8638). In acute malaria, zinc supplements do not affect fever, parasitemia, or hemoglobin in zinc-deficient children (10246).

Pregnancy-related iron deficiency. Taking zinc orally doesn't seem to help improve iron status in pregnant women taking supplemental iron and folic acid (6104).

Psoriasis. Taking zinc orally doesn't seem to help treat psoriasis (6513,6514,6912). Zinc epidermal levels are reportedly lower in people with psoriasis (6509). However, zinc has no effect on the psoriasis area and severity index (6513,6514).

Psoriatic arthritis. Taking zinc orally, alone or in combination with nonsteroidal anti-inflammatory drugs (NSAIDs), has no effect on the course of psoriatic arthritis (6514,6515).

Rheumatoid arthritis (RA). Taking zinc orally doesn't seem to help treat RA (2823,6516,6517,6518,6519).

Tinnitus. Taking zinc orally doesn't seem to help treat tinnitus (6914,6917,6921).

INSUFFICIENT RELIABLE EVIDENCE to RATE

AIDS-related opportunistic infections. There is some preliminary clinical evidence that taking zinc supplements orally in combination with zidovudine (AZT, Retrovir, a component of Combivir) might reduce opportunistic infections of Pneumocystis carinii and Candida in patients with AIDS (6566). However, zinc supplementation might also adversely affect the overall survival in people with AIDS (6565).

Alzheimer's disease. Preliminary clinical evidence has shown a modest slowing of cognitive decline in patients with Alzheimer's disease who take zinc supplements (2824).

Impotence. Taking zinc orally to treat male impotence secondary to disease or medical treatment has produced varying results (6568,6569,6570,6571,6572,6708).

Neurological trauma. Administering zinc parenterally immediately following post-head trauma seems to improve the rate of neurological recovery (2696).

Wrinkled skin. A topical preparation containing 10% vitamin C as L-ascorbic acid and acetyl tyrosine, zinc sulfate, sodium hyaluronate, and bioflavonoids (Cellex-C High Potency Serum) applied to photo-aged facial skin for 3 months seems to improve fine and coarse wrinkling, yellowing and sallowness, roughness, and skin tone compared to placebo (6155).

More evidence is needed to rate zinc for these uses.

Mechanism of Action

Zinc is a biologically essential trace element and is the second most abundant trace element in the body. The total body content is about 2 grams (8621). It is a cofactor in many biological processes including DNA, RNA, and protein synthesis. About 30% of cellular zinc is found within the nucleus. A large number of proteins that play a role in the regulation of gene expression are thought to contain zinc (8619). Zinc also plays a role in immune function, wound healing, reproduction, growth and development, behavior and learning, taste and smell, blood clotting, thyroid hormone function, and insulin action (331). Zinc is found in more than 300 enzymes (8619). Nearly 100 enzymes depend on zinc as a catalyst (7135). Zinc is also required in hepatic synthesis of retinol binding protein, the transport protein of vitamin A (8630). Without adequate zinc, symptoms of vitamin A deficiency can appear, despite vitamin A supplementation (8630). Meat, seafood, dairy products, nuts, legumes, and whole grains contain relatively high concentrations of zinc (331). Many breakfast cereals are fortified with zinc (7135). Zinc oxide and zinc sulfate are typically used to fortify wheat products (10668). 15-40% of the zinc in foods is absorbed. Bioavailability is influenced by zinc ionic status. Zinc is mostly absorbed in the small intestine, particularly the jejunum. Zinc absorption is increased during states of zinc deficiency (7135). During lactation, zinc excretion increases via breast milk. The body seems to compensate for this increased demand by increasing zinc absorption and conserving endogenous zinc (8631). More than 85% of the total zinc in the body is in skeletal muscle and bone; plasma zinc is tightly regulated at approximately 10 to 15 micromol/L (7135). Zinc deficiency is characterized by growth retardation, low insulin levels, reduced levels of insulin-like growth factor (IGF) -1, anorexia, mental lethargy, irritability, low sperm count, generalized hair loss, rough and dry skin, skin lesions, slow wound healing, decreased thyroid function, delayed onset of puberty, poor sense of smell and taste, diarrhea, and nausea (8619). Although zinc deficiency and tri-iodothyronine (T3) have complementary roles in growth and development, growth failure in zinc deficiency does not seem to be the result of impaired T3 function (8619).

Zinc deficiency is not uncommon world-wide, but deficiency is rare in the United States; most diets provide more than the recommended dietary allowance (RDA) (8632). Moderate zinc deficiency is associated with malabsorption syndromes, alcoholism, chronic renal disease, and chronic debilitating diseases (8621). There is no reliable test in clinical use to determine zinc deficiency. Serum or plasma zinc on its own is neither sensitive nor specific. It seems to be useful to measure zinc status on a population basis, but is an inaccurate measure in individuals, particularly in people with chronic infections or inflammatory conditions (8625). The most reliable method for diagnosing marginal zinc deficiency is a positive response to zinc supplementation and improvement in subtle symptoms such as growth retardation or altered ability to taste or smell (8621). Zinc plays a key role in the maintenance of vision. It is present in high concentrations in the eye, particularly in the retina and choroid. Zinc deficiency can alter vision, and severe deficiency causes changes in the retina and retinal pigment epithelium (RPE). Zinc interacts with taurine and vitamin A in the retina, modifies plasma membranes in the photoreceptors, regulates the light-rhodopsin reaction within the photoreceptor, modulates synaptic transmission, and serves as an antioxidant in both the RPE and retina. It seems to slow the progression of some degenerative retinal diseases (8621). Topically, zinc sulfate ophthalmic solution acts as a mild astringent, precipitating protein and clearing mucus from the outer surface of the eye (15).

Zinc is responsible for neutrophil, natural killer cell, and T-lymphocyte function (6551). Even mild zinc deficiency might adversely affect T-cell functions (6552). Interestingly, high-dose zinc supplementation, 20 times the RDA, can have a negative effect similar to deficiency on immune function (8625).

For the common cold, zinc doesn't have any effect on interleukin-8 in nasal secretions, suggesting that zinc doesn't affect immune response to colds (10783,10784).

The amount of available ionized zinc might influence the effectiveness of zinc (336). The extent of zinc ionization varies with different lozenge formulations (340). The addition of flavoring agents such as citric acid, mannitol, or sorbitol to zinc gluconate lozenge preparations decreases the extent of zinc ionization, while the addition of glycine to zinc gluconate lozenges does not (300). Some researchers question the clinical relevance of oral zinc levels since the rhinovirus replicates in the nasal mucosa (8628,8629). Also, zinc inhibits rhinovirus replication in vitro, but there's no evidence this happens in vivo (10783,10784).

Zinc ions might also have effects against other viruses. There's some evidence that zinc ions also have antiviral activity against the herpes virus (6538,6539,6541). Plasma zinc levels are low in people with HIV infection, but this appears to be a marker of disease progression rather than an indication that zinc deficiency. Some evidence suggests that zinc supplementation might increase disease progression and mortality in HIV infected patients, but other evidence suggests that avoiding zinc deficiency might allow normal or improved immune function, particularly T-lymphocyte mediated cellular immunity. It also might inhibit susceptibility of T-lymphocytes to apoptosis (8625).

More research is needed to tell if zinc should be avoided or prescribed for zinc deficiency in HIV disease.
People with sickle cell disease (SCD) are commonly zinc deficient. Zinc deficiency in SCD might cause a cell-mediated immune disorder, and increase the risk of infection in SCD. Some researchers think zinc deficiency leads to increased production of tumor necrosis factor (TNF)-alpha and interleukin-1 (IL-1) which might result in vaso-occlusive pain. This may explain the benefit of zinc supplementation in some patients with SCD (8627).
Topical zinc might be effective for treating acne (819,820,2687,2688) due to anti-inflammatory activity resulting from inhibition of polymorphonuclear leukocyte chemotaxis induced by decreased granulocyte zinc levels (2686). Male fertility appears to be influenced by zinc (6573,6574,6575,6576). Infertile males have lower seminal plasma zinc, with normal or reduced blood zinc (6575,6577). Clinical research suggests that short-term dietary zinc depletion results in reduced serum testosterone concentrations, seminal volume, and total seminal zinc loss per ejaculate (6576). Supplementation with zinc improves sperm parameters in men with reduced sperm mobility (6578); excess zinc might reduce sperm motility (6573). Zinc levels appear to decrease in the prostate tissue and prostatic fluid in men with prostatic carcinoma (6909,6910).
Zinc blocks copper absorption and increases copper elimination in the stool of people with Wilson's disease (2692). In acrodermatitis enteropathica, zinc seems to regulate linoleic acid and serum lipoprotein metabolism (2689). In children with thalassemia major, zinc deficiency is common (6597,6598,6599). The role of zinc in Alzheimer's disease might be both protective and causative. Laboratory studies suggest that zinc might contribute to aggregation of amyloid beta peptide, but protect against subsequent neurotoxicity as an antioxidant (6510,6511,6512). Zinc levels appear to be reduced in some people with major depression (6562).
Preliminary research suggests some people with type 2 diabetes might be zinc deficient, possibly as a result of altered zinc metabolism (6531,6532). There's some evidence that zinc can increase glucose transport into cells and potentiate insulin-induced glucose transport, possibly by affecting the insulin intracellular signaling pathway (second messenger system) (8620). In patients with cirrhosis and impaired glucose tolerance, zinc can increase serum levels of insulin-like growth factor (IGF) -1 by 30% and improve glucose tolerance (8624). Whether zinc deficiency is involved in the development of insulin resistance is unknown. In type 1 diabetes with zinc deficiency, zinc supplementation might reduce lipid peroxidation (6533). In people with osteoporosis, urinary zinc excretion is increased, possibly as a result of bone resorption (6918). Serum zinc levels have been variably reported as normal or decreased in people with osteoporosis (6918,6920). Early clinical evidence suggests that zinc in combination with copper, manganese, and calcium might slow bone loss (1994).
For aiding in wound healing, topical zinc might enhance re-epithelialization, decrease inflammation, and inhibit bacterial growth (2699). Zinc oxide absorption is best in an acidic environment (2809). Zinc acetate is absorbed over a wide pH range and might be a better choice in people with reduced stomach acid (2809). An enteric-coated zinc aspartate preparation (Taurizine) showed no absorption (2740). Zinc uptake in human intestinal epithelial cells is similar for zinc chloride, zinc methionine, and zinc propionate (2739). Most zinc is excreted in the feces, with a small amount eliminated in the urine (7135).

Adverse Reactions

Orally, zinc can cause nausea, vomiting, and a metallic taste in the mouth (2619,11350). There is concern that high daily doses above the tolerable upper intake level (UL) of 40 mg per day might increase the risk of copper deficiency (7135). To prevent copper deficiency, some clinicians give a small dose of copper when zinc is used in high doses, long-term (7303). In overdose, zinc can cause watery diarrhea, irritation and corrosion of the gastrointestinal (GI) tract, acute renal tubular necrosis, and interstitial nephritis (331,1352). Other symptoms of toxicity include flu-like and central nervous system (CNS) symptoms including fever, coughing, nausea, vomiting, diarrhea, epigastric pain, lethargy, fatigue and neuropathy, dehydration, severe vomiting (2663,2681); and zinc-induced copper deficiency with symptoms including sideroblastic anemia, neutropenia, impaired immune function, and an increase in the ratio of low-density-lipoprotein to high-density-lipoprotein (LDL/HDL) cholesterol (2619,2681). However, daily doses of 80 mg elemental zinc in combination with copper 2 mg for five years doesn't seem to cause changes in serum cholesterol or hematocrit (8622). Daily doses of 300 mg of supplemental zinc for six weeks appear to impair immune response (7135). There is preliminary evidence that higher dietary zinc intake might increase the risk for benign prostatic hyperplasia (BPH) (6908). Epidemiological evidence suggests that taking more than 100 mg of supplemental zinc daily or taking supplemental zinc for 10 or more years doubles the risk of developing prostate cancer (10306).
Topically, zinc can cause burning, stinging, itching, and tingling when applied to inflamed tissue (8623). Zinc oxide can be deposited in the submucosal tissue and cause dark discoloration of the skin. This can occur with prolonged topical application to intact skin, application to eroded or ulcerated skin, or penetrating traumatic exposure, and also parenteral administration (8618).
Intranasally, zinc can cause nasal irritation, headache, bad taste, bloody nose, dry nose, loss of sense of smell, dry mouth, and burning and irritation of the throat (8628,8629,11306,11155). There are case reports of complete loss of sense of smell (anosmia) that may be permanent with use of zinc gluconate nasal gel (Zicam). Loss of sense of smell appears to be dose related but has been reported following a single application (11306,11155,11707). Zinc sulfate nasal spray was used unsuccessfully for polio prophylaxis before the polio vaccine was developed. It caused loss of smell and/or taste, which was sometimes permanent (11713). Animal studies suggest that zinc sulfate negatively affects smell, possibly by damaging the olfactory epithelium and neurons (11156,11703,11704,11705,11706). Zinc gluconate nasal spray has not been tested for safety in animals or humans. The clinical studies of intranasal zinc have not described anosmia as an adverse effect, but testing was not done to see if zinc use adversely affected sense of

smell (6471,8628,8629,10247).
Occupational inhalation of zinc oxide fumes can cause metal fume fever with symptoms including fatigue, chills, fever, myalgias, cough, dyspnea, leukocytosis, thirst, metallic taste, and salivation (331).

Interactions with Herbs & Other Dietary Supplements

COPPER: Concomitant use with zinc may impair copper absorption (2693).
IP-6 (Phytic Acid): IP-6 in foods can decrease zinc absorption (7135). Theoretically, IP-6 supplements could also interfere with zinc absorption. IP-6 chelates multivalent metal ions in the gastrointestinal tract, preventing absorption (1858).
IRON: Non-heme iron might decrease zinc absorption. Non-heme iron and zinc compete for a common absorption pathway in the gut. However, when iron and zinc are taken concomitantly with food, this interaction is not likely to occur. When taken with food, zinc absorption is facilitated by proteins in food through an alternate pathway that does not compete with iron (7357). Protein-bound heme iron (found in red meats) does not affect zinc absorption (7135).

Interactions with Drugs

CISPLATIN (Platinol-AQ): Concomitant use with zinc might increase the cytotoxicity of cisplatin when in the presence of the chelate ethylenediaminetetraacetic acid (EDTA), as compared to cisplatin treatment alone (2668).
PENICILLAMINE: Penicillamine chelates zinc and can reduce the effects of supplemental zinc (2678). Separate dose times by at least 2 hours.
POTASSIUM-SPARING DIURETICS: Concomitant use with zinc can lead to zinc accumulation and increase risk of adverse effects (830).
QUINOLONE ANTIBIOTICS: Concomitant use with zinc reduces drug absorption and serum levels of quinolones due to zinc binding (828,2682). Concomitant use can also reduce the effects of zinc supplementation due to reduced zinc absorption.
TETRACYCLINE ANTIBIOTICS: Concomitant use with zinc decreases absorption and serum levels of demeclocycline (Declomycin), minocycline (Minocin), and tetracycline (Achromycin) due to zinc binding. Concomitant use can also reduce the effects of zinc supplementation due to reduced zinc absorption. Doxycycline (Vibramycin) does not interact with zinc (4945).
THIAZIDE DIURETICS: Concomitant use with zinc can interfere with zinc supplementation by increasing urinary zinc elimination (830,831).

Drug Influences on Nutrient Levels and Depletion

SOME DRUGS CAN AFFECT ZINC LEVELS:
AMILORIDE (Midamor): Amiloride reduces urinary zinc excretion and can increase zinc levels (830).
CAPTOPRIL (Capoten): Captopril might increase urinary zinc excretion in patients with hypertension. There is no data on other ACE-inhibitors (ACEIs). The clinical consequence of urinary zinc loss in hypertensive patients is unknown (25,26). Patients receiving high doses, greater than 200 mg daily, long-term have developed taste disturbances which resolved in some patients with zinc supplementation (6543).
DEFEROXAMINE (Desferal): Deferoxamine increases urinary zinc elimination (6597,6598).
DIURETICS: Use of loop diuretics and thiazide diuretics can increase urinary zinc loss and reduce serum levels. This is more likely with higher doses or when used in combination with diuretics of another class (4412,4425).
PENICILLAMINE (Cuprimine): Penicillamine can reduce serum zinc levels and might cause zinc depletion in some patients (4453,4531,4534,9630).
QUINOLONES: Treatment with fluoroquinolones can reduce dietary zinc absorption. The clinical significance is yet to be determined, and the need for supplementation has not been adequately studied. Consider zinc supplementation in patients on long-term fluoroquinolone therapy (828,2682).
TETRACYCLINES: Tetracyclines, except doxycycline (Vibramycin), can reduce dietary zinc absorption and serum levels due to zinc binding. The clinical significance is yet to be determined, and the need for supplementation has not been adequately studied. Consider zinc supplementation in patients on long-term tetracycline therapy (4945).

Interactions with Foods

FOODS: Concomitant administration with foods containing bran, phytates, calcium, or phosphorus may decrease supplemental zinc absorption (506).
VEGETARIANISM: Absorption of zinc from vegetarian diets is lower than from non-vegetarian diets most likely due to the higher amount of phytate, calcium, and other inhibitors of zinc absorption (7135). Dietary zinc requirements, particularly in strict vegetarians, may be 50% greater when the major food sources are grains and legumes (7135).

Interactions with Lab Tests

BLOOD ZINC ASSAYS: Avoid using powdered gloves when drawing blood for zinc assays, due to potential for sample contamination (2663).
HEMOGLOBIN A1C (HgbA1c): Supplementation with elemental zinc 50 mg per day has increased HgbA1c in type 1 diabetics (6530).
LIPID PROFILES: Zinc supplementation might reduce high-density lipoprotein (HDL) cholesterol levels and test

results (2681). Zinc supplementation might increase the ratio of low-density-lipoprotein to high-density-lipoprotein (LDL/HDL) cholesterol and test results (2681).

Interactions with Diseases or Conditions

ALCOHOLISM: Long-term excessive alcohol consumption is associated with impaired zinc absorption and increased excretion of zinc in the urine (7135).

HUMAN IMMUNODEFICIENCY VIRUS (HIV): Use zinc with caution in people with HIV infection. Some evidence suggests an association between higher intakes of zinc and reduced survival time (6565). However, other researchers have reported no association. Some research suggests that avoiding zinc deficiency in patients with HIV disease might allow normal or improved immune function (8625).

MALABSORPTION SYNDROMES (Sprue, Crohn's Disease, Short Bowel Syndrome, etc.): People with malabsorption syndromes may be zinc deficient due to decreased zinc absorption and increased urinary zinc losses (7135).

RHEUMATOID ARTHRITIS (RA): Zinc absorption is reduced in people with rheumatoid arthritis (2823).

Dosage and Administration

ORAL: The typical dose for treating the common cold is one zinc gluconate or acetate lozenge, providing 9-24 mg elemental zinc, dissolved in the mouth every two hours while awake when cold symptoms are present (333,335,336).

For acute diarrhea in malnourished or zinc-deficient children, 10-40 mg elemental zinc is given daily (825,826,827,3455,3456,10248).

For preventing pneumonia in babies and children in developing countries, 10 mg per day has been used (8920).

For hypogeusia, 25-100 mg oral zinc has been used in clinical trials (6542). Anorexia nervosa has been treated with 100 mg of zinc gluconate daily (6905).

For treating gastric ulcers, zinc sulfate 200 mg three times daily has been used (6591).

For muscle cramps in zinc deficient patients with cirrhosis, zinc sulfate 220 mg twice daily has been used (1352).

Sickle cell disease has been treated with zinc sulfate 220 mg three times daily (6594).

To increase growth and weight gain in prepubertal children with sickle cell disease, 10 mg elemental zinc per day has been used (8626).

For treating attention deficit-hyperactivity disorder (ADHD) in children, doses of zinc sulfate 55 mg (15 mg elemental zinc) to 150 mg (40 mg elemental zinc) daily has been used (11350,12060).

For treating acne, clinical trials have used 30 to 135 mg elemental zinc daily (6297,6298,6299,6501,6502).

For treating age-related macular degeneration (AMD), elemental zinc 80 mg plus vitamin C 500 mg, vitamin E 400 IU, and beta-carotene 15 mg has been given daily (7303).

For treating advanced cirrhosis, zinc sulfate 200 mg three times daily has been used (8624).

The National Institute of Medicine has established Adequate Intake (AI) levels of zinc for infants birth to 6 months is 2 mg/day (7135). For older infants, children, and adults, Recommended Dietary Allowance (RDA) quantities of zinc have been established: infants and children 7 months to 3 years, 3 mg/day; 4 to 8 years, 5 mg/day; 9 to 13 years, 8 mg/day; girls 14 to 18 years, 9 mg/day; boys and men age 14 and older, 11 mg/day; women 19 and older, 8 mg/day; pregnant women 14 to 18, 13 mg/day; pregnant women 19 and older, 11 mg/day; lactating women 14 to 18, 14 mg/day; lactating women 19 and older, 12 mg/day (7135).

The typical North American male consumes about 13 mg/day of dietary zinc; women consume approximately 9 mg/day (7135).

The Tolerable Upper Intake Levels (UL) of zinc for people who are not receiving zinc under medical supervision: Infants birth to 6 months, 4 mg/day; 7 to 12 months, 5 mg/day; children 1 to 3 years, 7 mg/day; 4 to 8 years, 12 mg/day; 9 to 13 years, 23 mg/day; 14 to 18 years (including pregnancy and lactation), 34 mg/day; adults 19 years and older (including pregnancy and lactation), 40 mg/day (7135).

Different salt forms provide different amounts of elemental zinc. Zinc sulfate contains 23% elemental zinc; 220 mg zinc sulfate contains 50 mg zinc. Zinc gluconate contains 14.3% elemental zinc; 10 mg zinc gluconate contains 1.43 mg zinc (506).

INTRANASAL: For treating or preventing the common cold 2.1 mg of elemental zinc per day has been used (10247).

TOPICAL: For acne vulgaris, zinc acetate 1.2% with erythromycin 4% as a lotion has been applied twice daily (819).

For herpes simplex infections, zinc sulfate 0.25% applied 8 to 10 times daily or zinc oxide, 0.3%, with glycine applied every 2 hours while awake has been used (8623). Lower concentrations have shown variable efficacy (6538).

Comments

Zinc acetate (Galzin) is an FDA-approved orphan drug for treating Wilson's disease. Zinc and cadmium are chemically similar and often occur together in nature. Cadmium is not an essential element, and excessive long-term exposure can lead to kidney dysfunction. The concentration of cadmium in zinc-containing supplements can vary as much as 37-fold. Zinc gluconate consistently contains the lowest cadmium concentration (10669).

1 Monographs on the medicinal uses of plant drugs. Exeter, UK: European Scientific Co-op Phytother., 1997.

2 Blumenthal M, ed. The Complete German Commission E Monographs: Therapeutic Guide to Herbal Medicines. S. Klein, transl. Boston, MA: American Botanical Council, 1998.

3 Tyler VE. Herbs of Choice. Binghamton, NY: Pharmaceutical Products Press, 1994.

4 Newall CA, Anderson LA, Philpson JD. Herbal Medicine: A Guide for Healthcare Professionals. London, UK: The Pharmaceutical Press, 1996.

5 Foster S, Tyler VE. Tyler's Honest Herbal: A Sensible Guide to the Use of Herbs and Related Remedies. 3rd ed., Binghamton, NY: Haworth Herbal Press, 1993.

6 The Review of Natural Products by Facts and Comparisons. St. Louis, MO: Wolters Kluwer Co., 1999.

7 Schulz V, Hansel R, Tyler VE. Rational Phytotherapy: A Physician's Guide to Herbal Medicine. Terry C. Telger, transl. 3rd ed. Berlin, GER: Springer, 1998.

8 Wichtl MW. Herbal Drugs and Phytopharmaceuticals. Ed. N.M. Bisset. Stuttgart: Medpharm GmbH Scientific Publishers, 1994.

9 Martindale W. Martindale: The Extra Pharmacopoeia. Pharmaceutical Press, 1999.

10 United States Pharmacopeial Convention, Inc., ed. Drug Information for the Health Care Professional. 19th ed., Englewood, CO: Micromedex Inc., 1999.

11 Leung AY, Foster S. Encyclopedia of Common Natural Ingredients Used in Food, Drugs and Cosmetics. 2nd ed., New York, NY: John Wiley & Sons, 1996.

12 McGuffin M, Hobbs C, Upton R, Goldberg A, eds. American Herbal Products Association's Botanical Safety Handbook. Boca Raton, FL: CRC Press, 1997.

13 Robbers JE, Speedie MK, Tyler VE. Pharmacognosy and Pharmacobiotechnology. Baltimore, MD: Williams & Wilkins, 1996.

15 McKevoy GK, ed. AHFS Drug Information. Bethesda, MD: American Society of Health-System Pharmacists, 1998.

16 Gennaro A. Remington: The Science and Practice of Pharmacy. 19th ed., Lippincott: Williams & Wilkins, 1996.

17 Ellenhorn MJ, et al. Ellenhorn's Medical Toxicology: Diagnoses and Treatment of Human Poisoning. 2nd ed. Baltimore, MD: Williams & Wilkins, 1997.

18 Gruenwald J, Brendler T, Jaenicke C. PDR for Herbal Medicines. 1st ed. Montvale, NJ: Medical Economics Company, Inc., 1998.

19 Brinker F. Herb Contraindications and Drug Interactions. 2nd ed. Sandy, OR: Eclectic Medical Publications, 1998.

21 Miller LG. Herbal medicinals: selected clinical considerations focusing on known or potential drug-herb interactions. *Arch Intern Med* 1998;158:2200-11.

22 Adams ME. Hype about glucosamine. *Lancet* 1999;354:353.

23 O'Mara NB. PremesisRx. *Pharmacist's Letter/Prescriber's Letter* 1999:15;151206.

25 Golik A, Zaidensttein R, Dishi V, et al. Effects of captopril and enalapril on zinc metabolism in hypertensive patients. *J Am Coll Nutr* 1998;17:75-8.

26 Golik A, Modai D, Averbukh Z, et al. Zinc metabolism in patients treated with captopril versus enalapril. *Metabolism* 1990;39:665-7.

27 Kung AWC, Pun KK. Bone mineral density in premenopausal women receiving long-term physiological doses of levothyroxine. *JAMA* 1991;265:2688-91.

28 Schneider DL, Barrett-Connor EL, Morton DJ. Thyroid hormone use and bone mineral density in elderly men. *Arch Intern Med* 1995;155:2005-7.

29 Franklyn AJ, Bettenridge J, Daykin J, et al. Long-term thyroxine treatment and bone mineral density. *Lancet* 1992;340:9-13.

30 Paltiel O, Falutz J, Veilleux M, et al. Clinical correlates of subnormal vitamin B12 levels in patients infected with the human immunodeficiency virus. *Am J Hematol* 1995;49:318-22.

31 Tang G, Serfaty-Lacrosniere C, Camilo ME, et al. Gastric acidity influences the blood response to a beta-carotene dose in humans. *Am J Clin Nutr* 1996;64:622-6.

32 Carlsen SM, Folling I, Grill V, et al. Metformin increases total homocysteine levels in non-diabetic male patients with coronary heart disease. *Scand J Clin Lab Invest* 1997;57:521-7.

33 Chevallier A. Encyclopedia of Medicinal Plants. New York, NY: DK Publishing, 1996.

34 Leatherdale B, et al. Improvement in glucose tolerance due to Momordica charantia. *Br Med J* (Clin Res Ed) 1981;282:1823-4.

35 Welihinda J, et al. Effect of Momordica charantia on the glucose tolerance in maturity onset diabetes. *J Ethnopharmacol* 1986;17:277-82.

36 Srivastava Y, Venkatakrishna-Bhatt H, Verma Y, et al. Antidiabetic and adaptogenic properties of Momordica charantia extract: An experimental and clinical evaluation. *Phytother Res* 1993;7:285-9.

37 Raman A, et al. Anti-diabetic properties and phytochemistry of Momordica charantia L. (Cucurbitaceae). *Phytomedicine* 1996;294.

38 Baldwa VS, Bhandari CM, Pangaria A, Goyal RK. Clinical trial in patients with diabetes mellitus of an insulin-like compound obtained from plant sources. *Upsala J Med Sci* 1977;82:39-41.

39 Perossini M, Guidi G, Chiellini S, Siravo D. [Diabetic and hypertensive retinopathy therapy with Vaccinium myrtillus anthocyanosides (Tegens). Double blind, placebo-controlled clinical trial]. [Article in Italian]. *Ann Ottalmol Clin Ocul* 1987;113:1173-7.

40 Scharrer A, Ober M. Anthocyanosides in the treatment of retinopathies. *Kiln Monastbl Augenheilkd* 1981;178:386-9.

41 Coleman M, Steinberg G, Tippett J, et al. A preliminary study of the effect of pyridoxine administration in a subgroup of hyperkinetic children: A double-blind crossover comparison with methylphenidate. *Biol Psych* 1979;14:741-51.

42 Cucinotta D, Passeri M, Ventura S, et al. Multicenter clinical placebo-controlled study with acetyl-L-carnitine (ALC) in the treatment of mildly demented elderly patients. *Drug Development Res* 1988;14:213-6.

43 Kidd PM. A review of nutrients and botanicals in the integrative management of cognitive dysfunction. *Alternative Medicine Review* 1999;4:144-61.

44 Mayeux R, Sano M. Treatment of Alzheimer's Disease. *N Engl J Med* 1999;341:1670-9.

45 Shanmugasundaram ER, Rajeswari G, Baskaran K, et al. Use of Gymnema sylvestre leaf extract in the control of blood glucose in insulin-dependent diabetes mellitus. *J Ethnopharmacol* 1990;30:281-94.

46 Baskaran K, Kizar-Ahamath B, Shanmugasundaram MR, Shanmugasundaram ERB. Antidiabetic effect of leaf extract from Gymnema sylvestre in non-insulin-dependent diabetes mellitus patients. *J Ethnopharmacol* 1990;30:295-300.

47 Head KA. Type 1 diabetes: prevention of the disease and its complications. *Townsend Letter for Doctors & Patients* 1998;180:72-84.

48 Sinsheimer JE, Subba-Rao G, McIlhenny HM. Constitents from G sylvestre leaves: isolation and preliminary characterization of the gymnemic acids. *J Pharmacol Sci* 1970;59:622-8.

49 Awang DV. Parthenocide: demise of a facile theory of feverfew activity. *J Herbs Spices Med Plants* 1998;5:95-8.

50 Murch SJ, Simmons CB, Saxena PK. Melatonin in feverfew and other medicinal plants. *Lancet* 1997;350:1598-9.

51 Matsunaga S, Ito H, Sakou T. The effect of vitamin K and D supplementation on ovariectomy-induced bone loss. *Calcif Tissue Int* 1999;65:285-9.

52 Caraballo PJ, Heit JA, Atkinson EJ, et al. Long-term use of oral anticoagulants and the risk of fracture. *Arch Intern Med* 1999;159:1750-6.

53 Jie KG, Bots ML, Vermeer C, et al. Vitamin K status and bone mass in women with and without aortic atherosclerosis: a population-based study. *Calcif Tissue Int* 1996;59:352-6.

54 Shiraki M, Shiraki Y, Aoki C, Miura M. Vitamin K2 (menatetrenone) effectively prevents fractures and sustains lumbar bone mineral density in osteoporosis. *J Bone Miner Res* 2000;15:515-21.

55 Olson RE. Osteoporosis and vitamin K intake. *Am J Clin Nutr* 2000;71:1031-2.

56 Vermeer C, Gijsbers BL, Craciun AM, et al. Effects of vitamin K on bone mass and bone metabolism. *J Nutr* 1996;126:1187S-91S.

57 Vermeer C, Schurgers LJ. A comprehensive review of vitamin K and vitamin K antagonists. *Hematol Oncol Clin North Am* 2000;14:339-53.

58 Iwamoto I, Kosha S, Noguchi S, et al. A longitudinal study of the effect of vitamin K2 on bone mineral density in postmenopausal women a comparative study with vitamin D3 and estrogen-progestin therapy. *Maturitas* 1999;31:161-4.

59 Nagasawa Y, Fujii M, Kajimoto Y, et al. Vitamin K2 and serum cholesterol in patients on continuous ambulatory peritoneal dialysis. *Lancet* 1998;351:724.

60 Bitensky L, Hart JP, Catterall A, et al. Circulating vitamin K levels in patients with fractures. *J Bone Joint Surg Br* 1988;70:663-4.

61 Hart JP, Shearer MJ, Klenerman L, et al. Electrochemical detection of depressed circulating levels of vitamin K1 in osteoporosis. *J Clin Endocrinol Metab* 1985;60:1268-9.

62 Hodges SJ, Akesson K, Vergnaud P, et al. Circulating levels of vitamins K1 and K2 decreased in elderly women with hip fracture. *J Bone Miner Res* 1993;8:1241-5.

63 Kanai T, Takagi T, Masuhiro K, et al. Serum vitamin K level and bone mineral density in post-menopausal women. *Int J Gynaecol Obstet* 1997;56:25-30.

64 Shearer MJ, Bach A, Kohlmeier M. Chemistry, nutritional sources, tissue distribution and metabolism of vitamin K with special reference to bone health. *J Nutr* 1996;126:1181S-6S.

65 Kawashima H, Nakajima Y, Matubara Y, et al. Effects of vitamin K2 (menatetrenone) on atherosclerosis and blood coagulation in hypercholesterolemic rabbits. *Jpn J Pharmacol* 1997;75:135-43.

66 Rosen HM, Yoshimura N, Hodgman JM, Fischer JE. Plasma amino acid patterns in hepatic encephalopathy of differing etiology. *Gastroenterology* 1977;72:483-7.

68 O'Keefe SJ, Ogden J, Dicker J. Enteral and parenteral branched chain amino acid-supplemented nutritional support in patients with encephalopathy due to alcoholic liver disease. *JPEN J Parenter Enteral Nutr* 1987;11:447-53.

69 Marchesini G, Bianchi G, Rossi B, et al. Nutritional treatment with branched-chain amino acids in advanced liver cirrhosis. *J Gastroenterol* 2000;35:7-12.

70 Vorgerd M, Grehl T, Jager M, et al. Creatine therapy in myophosphorylase deficiency (McArdle disease): a placebo-controlled crossover trial. *Arch Neurol* 2000;57:956-63.

71 Cangiano C, Laviano A, Meguid MM, et al. Effects of administration of oral branched-chain amino acids on anorexia and caloric intake in cancer patients. *J Natl Cancer Inst* 1996;88:550-2.

72 Richardson MA, Bevans ML, Weber JB, et al. Branched chain amino acids decrease tardive dyskinesia symptoms. *Psychopharmacology* (Berl) 1999;143:358-64.

73 Mori N, Adachi Y, Takeshima T, et al. Branched-chain amino acid therapy for spinocerebellar degeneration: a pilot clinical crossover trial. *Intern Med* 1999;38:401-6.

74 Stein TP, Schluter MD, Leskiw MJ, Boden G. Attenuation of the protein wasting associated with bed rest by branched-chain amino acids. *Nutrition* 1999;15:656-60.

75 Institute of Medicine. The role of protein and amino acids in sustaining and enhancing performance. Washington, DC: National Academy Press, 1999. Available at: http://books.nap.edu/books/0309063469/html/309.html#pagetop

77 Blomstrand E, Ek S, Newsholme EA. Influence of ingesting a solution of branched-chain amino acids on plasma and muscle concentrations of amino acids during prolonged submaximal exercise. *Nutrition* 1996;12:485-90.

78 Suryawan A, Hawes JW, Harris RA, et al. A molecular model of human branched-chain amino acid metabolism. *Am J Clin Nutr* 1998;68:72-81.

79 Branchey L, Branchey M, Shaw S, Lieber CS. Relationship between changes in plasma amino acids and depression in alcoholic patients. *Am J Psychiatry* 1984;141:1212-5.

80 Majumdar SK, Shaw GK, Thomson AD, et al. Changes in plasma amino acid patterns in chronic alcoholic patients during ethanol withdrawal syndrome: their clinical implications. *Med Hypotheses* 1983;12:239-51.

81 Naylor CD, O'Rourke K, Detsky AS, Baker JP. Parenteral nutrition with branched-chain amino acids in hepatic encephalopathy. A meta-analysis. *Gastroenterology* 1989;97:1033-42.

82 Fabbri A, Magrini N, Bianchi G, et al. Overview of randomized clinical trials of oral branched-chain amino acid treatment in chronic hepatic encephalopathy. *JPEN J Parenter Enteral Nutr* 1996;20:159-64.

83 Berson EL, Rosner B, Sandberg MA, et al. A randomized trial of vitamin A and vitamin E supplementation for retinitis pigmentosa. *Arch Ophthalmol* 1993;111:761-72.

84 Gamel JW, Barr CC. A randomized trial of vitamin A and vitamin E supplementation for retinitis pigmentosa. *Arch Ophthalmol* 1993;111:1462-3.

85 Fielder AR. A randomized trial of vitamin A and vitamin E supplementation for retinitis pigmentosa. *Arch Ophthalmol* 1993;111:1463;discussion 1463-6.

86 Clowes DD. A randomized trial of vitamin A and vitamin E supplementation for retinitis pigmentosa. *Arch Ophthalmol* 1993;111:1461-2.

87 Norton EW. A randomized trial of vitamin A and vitamin E supplementation for retinitis pigmentosa. *Arch Ophthalmol* 1993;111:1460.

88 Marmor MF. A randomized trial of vitamin A and vitamin E supplementation for retinitis pigmentosa. *Arch Ophthalmol* 1993;111:1460-1.

89 Lavine JE. Vitamin E treatment of nonalcoholic steatohepatitis in children: a pilot study. *J Pediatr* 2000;136:734-8.

90 Kim JM, White RH. Effect of vitamin E on the anticoagulant response to warfarin. *Am J Cardiol* 1996;77:545-6.

91 Corrigan JJ Jr. The effect of vitamin E on warfarin-induced vitamin K deficiency. *Ann N Y Acad Sci* 1982;393:361-8.

92 Corrigan JJ Jr. Coagulation problems relating to vitamin E. *Am J Pediatr Hematol Oncol* 1979;1:169-73.

93 Corrigan JJ Jr, Marcus FI. Coagulopathy associated with vitamin E ingestion. *JAMA* 1974;230:1300-1.

94 Skyrme-Jones RA, O'Brien RC, Berry KL, Meredith IT. Vitamin E supplementation improves endothelial function in type I diabetes mellitus: a randomized, placebo-controlled study. *J Am Coll Cardiol* 2000;36:94-102.

95 Devaraj S, Jialal I. Low-density lipoprotein postsecretory modification, monocyte function, and circulating adhesion molecules in type 2 diabetic patients with and without macrovascular complications: the effect of alpha-tocopherol supplementation. *Circulation* 2000;102:191-6.

96 Surai PF, MacPherson A, Speake BK, Sparks NH. Designer egg evaluation in a controlled trial. *Eur J Clin Nutr* 2000;54:298-305.

97 Meydani M. Effect of functional food ingredients: vitamin E modulation of cardiovascular diseases and immune status in the elderly. *Am J Clin Nutr* 2000;71:1665S-8S.

98 Jonas CR, Puckett AB, Jones DP, et al. Plasma antioxidant status after high-dose chemotherapy: a randomized trial of parenteral nutrition in bone marrow transplantation patients. *Am J Clin Nutr* 2000;72:181-9.

99 Burton GW, Traber MG, Acuff RV, et al. Human plasma and tissue alpha-tocopherol concentrations in response to supplementation with deuterated natural and synthetic vitamin E. *Am J Clin Nutr* 1998;67:669-84.

100 Vatassery GT, Bauer T, Dysken M. On the biological activity of vitamin E. *Am J Clin Nutr* 2000;72:202-3.

101 Klein AD, Penneys NS. Aloe vera. *J Am Acad Dermatol* 1988;18:714-20.

102 Lyss G, Schmidt TJ, Merfort I, Pahl HL, et al. Helenalin, an antiinflammatory sesquiterpene lactone from Arnica, selectively inhibits transcription factor NF-kappa B. *Biol Chem* 1997;378:951-61.

103 Baillargeon L, Drouin J, Desjardins L, et al. [The effects of Arnica montana on blood coagulation. Radomized controlled trial]. [Article in French]. *Can Fam Physician* 1993;39:2362-7.

104 Schroder H, Losche W, Strobach H, et al. Helenalin and 11 alpha, 13-dihydrohelenalin, two constituents from Arnica montana L., inhibit human platelet function via thiol-dependent pathways. *Thromb Res* 1990;57:839-45.

105 Sabeel AI, Kurkus J, Lindholm T. Intensive Hemodialysis and Hemoperfusion Treatment of Amanita Mushroom Poisoning. *Mycopathologia* 1995;131:107-14.

106 Bustamante J, Lodge JK, Marcocci L, et al. Alpha-lipoic acid in liver metabolism and disease. *Free Radic Biol Med* 1998;24:1023-39.

107 Ehren I, Lundberg JO, Adolfsson J, Wiklund NP. Effects of L-arginine treatment on symptoms and bladder nitric oxide levels in patients with interstitial cystitis. *Urology* 1998;52:1026-9.

108 Bode-Boger SM, Boger RH, Galland A, et al. L-arginine-induced vasodilation in healthy humans: pharmacokinetic-pharmacodynamic relationship. *Br J Clin Pharmacol* 1998;46:489-97.

109 Sandrini G, Franchini S, Lanfranchi S, et al. Effectiveness of ibuprofen-arginine in the treatment of acute migraine attacks. *Int J Clin Pharmacol Res* 1998;18:145-50.

110 Lerman A, Burnett JC Jr, Higano ST, et al. Long-term L-arginine improves small-vessel coronary endothelial function in humans. *Circulation* 1998;97:2123-8.

111 Chuntrasakul C, Siltharm S, Sarasombath S, et al. Metabolic and immune effects of dietary arginine, glutamine, and omega-3 fatty acids supplementation in immunocompromised patients. *J Med Assoc Thai* 1998;81:334-43.

112 Andres A, Morales JM, Praga M, et al. L-arginine reverses the antinatriuretic effect of cyclosporin in renal transplant patients. *Nephrol Dial Transplant* 1997;12:1437-40.

113 Pichard C, Sudre P, Karsegard V, et al. A randomized double-blind controlled study of 6 months of oral nutritional supplementation with arginine and omega-3 fatty acids in HIV-infected patients. Swiss HIV Cohort Study. *AIDS* 1998;12:53-63.

114 Wheeler MA, Smith SD, Saito N, et al. Effect of long-term oral L-arginine on the nitric oxide synthase pathway in the urine from patients with interstitial cystitis. *J Urol* 1997;158:2045-50.

115 Saffle JR, Wiebke G, Jennings K, et al. Randomized trial of immune-enhancing enteral nutrition in burn patients. *J Trauma* 1997;42:793-800, discussion 800-2.

116 Adams MR, McCredie R, Jessup W, et al. Oral L-arginine improves endothelium-dependent dilatation and reduces monocyte adhesion to endothelial cells in young men with coronary artery disease. *Atherosclerosis* 1997;129:261-9.

117 Takano H, Lim HB, Miyabara Y, et al. Oral administration of L-arginine potentiates allergen-induced airway inflammation and expression of interleukin-5 in mice. *J Pharmacol Exp Ther* 1998;286:767-71.

118 Hibbard MK, Sandri-Goldin, RM. Arginine-rich regions succeeding the nuclear localization region of the herpes simplex virus type 1 regulatory protein ICP27 are required for efficient nuclear localization and late gene expression. *J Virol* 1995;69:4656-7.

119 Griffith RS, DeLong DC, Nelson JD. Relation of arginine-lysine antagonism to herpes simplex growth in tissue culture. *Chemotherapy* 1981;27:209-13.

120 McCaffrey MJ, Bose CL, Reiter PD, Stiles AD. Effect of L-arginine infusion on infants with persistent pulmonary hypertension of the newborn. *Biol Neonate* 1995;67:240-3.

121 Sapienza MA, Kharitonov SA, Horvath I, et al. Effect of inhaled L-arginine on exhaled nitric oxide in normal and asthmatic subjects. *Thorax* 1998;53:172-5.

122 Saijyo T, Nomura M, Nakaya Y, Saito K, et al. Autonomic nervous system activity during infusion of L-arginine in patients with liver cirrhosis. *Liver* 1998;18:27-31.

123 Newcomer AD, Park HS, O'Brien PC, McGill DB. Response of patients with irritable bowel syndrome and lactase deficiency using unfermented acidophilus milk. *Am J Clin Nutr* 1983;38:257-63.

124 Gotz V, Romankiewicz JA, Moss J, Murray HW. Prophylaxis against ampicillin-associated diarrhea with a lactobacillus preparation. *Am J Hosp Pharm* 1979;36:754-7.

125 Contardi I. [Oral bacterial therapy in prevention of antibiotic-induced diarrhea in childhood]. [Article in Italian]. *Clin Ter* 1991;136:409-13.

126 Kaaja RJ, Kontula KK, Raiha A, Laatikainen T. Treatment of cholestasis of pregnancy with peroral activated charcoal. A preliminary study. *Scand J Gastroenterol* 1994;29:178-81.

127 Bowry VW, Ingold KU, Stocker R. Vitamin E in human density lipoprotein. When and how this antioxidant becomes a pro-oxidant. *Biochem J* 1992;288(Pt 2):341-4.

128 Kagan VE, Serbinova EA, Forte T, et al. Recycling of vitamin E in human low density lipoproteins. *J Lipid Res* 1992;33:385-97.

129 Back DJ, Breckenridge AM, MacIver M, et al. Interaction of ethinyloestradiol with ascorbic acid in man. *Br Med J* (Clin Res Ed) 1981;282:1516.

130 Morris JC, Beeley L, Ballantine N. Interaction of ethinyloestradiol with ascorbic acid in man. [letter] *Br Med J* (Clin Res Ed) 1981;283:503.

131 Levine M, Conry-Cantilena C, Wang Y, et al. Vitamin C pharmacokinetics in healthy volunteers: evidence for recommended dietary allowance. *Proc Natl Acad Sci U S A* 1996;93:3704-9.

132 Buto SK, Tsang TK, Sielaff GW, et al. Bay leaf impaction in the esophagus and hypopharynx. *Ann Intern Med* 1990;113:82-3.

133 Johns AN. Beware of the bay leaf. *Br Med J* 1980;281:1682.

134 Belitsos NJ. Bay leaf impaction. *Ann Intern Med* 1990;113:483-4.

135 Bell CD, Mustar, RA. Bay leaf perforation of Meckel's diverticulum. *JCC* 1997;40:146.

136 Palin WE, Richardson JD. Complications from bay leaf ingestions. *JAMA* 1983;289:729-30.

137 Brokaw SA. Complications of bay leaf ingestion [letter]. *JAMA* 1983;250:729.

138 Price JF. Antioxidant vitamins in the prevention of cardiovascular disease. The epidemiological evidence. *Eur Heart J* 1997;18:719-27.

139 Omenn GS. Chemoprevention of lung cancer: the rise and demise of beta-carotene. *Annu Rev Public Health* 1998;19:73-99.

140 Giuliano AR, Gapstur S. Can cervical dysplasia and cancer be prevented with nutrients? *Nutr Rev* 1998;56:9-16.

141 Lieberman S. A Review of the effectiveness of cimicifuga racemosa (Black Cohosh) for the symptoms of menopause. *J Womens Health* 1998;7:525-9.

142 Jarboe CH, Schmidt CM, Nicholson JA, Zirvi KA. Uterine relaxant properties of Viburnum. *Nature* 1966;212:837.

143 Soderling E, Le Bell A, Kirstila V, Tenovuo J. Betaine-containing toothpaste relieves subjective symptoms of dry mouth. *Acta Odontol Scand* 1998;56:65-9.

144 Barak AJ, Beckenhauer HC, Tuma DJ. Betaine, ethanol, and the liver, a review. *Alcohol* 1996;13:395-8.

145 Wilcken DE, Wilcken B, Dudman NP, Tyrrell PA. Homocystinuria - the effects of betaine in the treatment of patients not responsive to pyridoxine. *N Engl J Med* 1983;309:448-53.

146 Duell PG, Malinow MR. Homocysteine: An important risk factor for atherosclerotic vascular disease. *Curr Opin Lipidol* 1997;8:28-34.

147 Bakker RC, Brandjes DP. Hyperhomocysteinaemia and associated disease. *Pharm World Sci* 1997;19:126-32.

148 Daviglus ML, Dyer AR, Persky V, et al. Dietary beta-carotene, vitamin C, and risk of prostate cancer: results from the Western Electric Study. *Epidemiology* 1996;7:472-7.

149 Simopoulos AP, Leaf A, Salem N. Workshop statement on the essentiality of and recommended dietary intakes for Omega-6 and Omega-3 fatty acids. *Prostaglandins Leukot Essent Fatty Acids* 2000;63:119-21.

150 Johnson JA, Lalonde RL. Congestive Heart Failure. Eds. DiPiro JT, et al. Pharmacotherapy, third ed. Stamford: Appleton and Lange, 1997.

151 Sklar S, et al. Drug therapy screening system. Indianapolis, IN: First Data Bank 99.1-99. 2 eds.

152 Bourgoin BP, Evans DR, Cornett JR, et al. Lead content in 70 brands of dietary calcium supplements. *Am J Public Health* 1993;83:1155-60.

153 Elmer GW, Surawicz CM, McFarland LV. Biotherapeutic Agents, A neglected modality for the treatment and prevention of selected intestinal and vaginal infections. *JAMA* 1996;275:870-5.

155 Scarpignato C, Rampal P. Prevention and treatment of traveler's diarrhea: A clinical pharmacological approach. *Chemotherapy* 1995;41:48-81.

156 Chiesara E, Borghini R, Marabini. Dietary fibre and drug interactions. *Eur J Clin Nutr* 1995;49:S123-8.

157 Drug Facts and Comparisons. Olin BR, ed. St. Louis, MO: Facts and Comparisons. (updated monthly).

158 Pandya DP. Nutrition and coronary heart disease. *Comp Ther* 1998;24:198-204.

159 Gossel TA, Bricker JD. Principles of Clinical Toxicology. New York, NY:Raven Press, 1994.

160 ECP consensus panel on cereals and cancer. *Eur J Cancer Prev* 1998;7S1-S2.

161 Saavedra JM, et al. Feeding of bifidobacterium bifidum and streptococcus thermophilus to infants in hospital for prevention of diarrhea and shedding of rotavirus. *Lancet* 1994;344:1046-9.

162 Bouhnik Y, Pochart P, Marteau P, et al. Fecal recovery in humans of viable bifidobacterium ingested in fermented milk. *Gastroenterology* 1992;102:875-8.

163 Sauvaire Y, et al. 4-hydroxyisoleucine. A novel amino acid potentiator of insulin secretion. *Diabetes* 1998;47:206-10.

164 Madar Z, Thorne R. Dietary fiber. *Prog Food Nutr Sci* 1987;11:153-74.

165 Ultee A, Kets EP, Smid EJ. Mechanisms of action of carvacrol on the food-borne pathogen Bacillus cereus. *Appl Environ Microbiol* 1999;65:4606-10.

166 Miller LG. Herbal Medicinals. Selected clinical considerations focusing on known or potential drug-herb interactions. *Arch Intern Med* 1998;158:2200-11.

167 Bennett DA Jr, Phun L, Polk JF, et al. Neuropharmacology of St. John's Wort (Hypericum). *Ann Pharmacother* 1998;32:1201-8.

168 Hippius H. St. John's Wort (Hypericum perforatum) an herbal antidepressant. *Curr Med Res Opin* 1998;14:171-84.

169 Wagner J, Wagner ML, Hening WA. Beyond benzodiazepines: alternative pharmacologic agents for the treatment of insomnia. *Ann Pharmacother* 1998;32:680-91.

170 Henry JG, Sobki S, Afafat N. Interference by biotin therapy on measurement of TSH and FT4 by enzyme immunoassay on Boehringer Mannheim ES 700 analyzer. *Ann Clin Biochem* 1996;33:162-3.

171 Hochman LG, Scher RK, Meyerson MS. Brittle nails: response to daily biotin supplementation. *Cutis* 1993;51:303-5.

172 Said HM, Redha R, Nylander W. Biotin transport in the human intestine: inhibition by anticonvulsant drugs. *Am J Clin Nutr* 1989;49:127-31.

173 Bonjour JP. Biotin in human nutrition. *Ann N Y Acad Sci* 1985;447:97-104.

174 Nyhan WL. Clinical problems relating to biotin. *Ann N Y Acad Sci* 1985;447:222-4.

175 Krause KH, et al. Biotin Status of Epileptics. *Ann N Y Acad Sci* 1985;447:297-313.

176 Mock DM, et al. Disturbances in biotin metabolism in children undergoing long-term anticonvulsant therapy. *J Pediatr Gastroentereol Nutr* 1998;26(3):245-50.

177 Coggeshall JC, et al. Biotin status and plasma glucose in diabetics. *Annals New York Academy of Sciences* 1985;447:389-92.

178 Arvill A, Bodin L. Effect of short-term ingestion of konjac glucomannan on serum cholesterol in healthy men. *Am J Clin Nutr* 1995;61:585-9.

179 Vido L, Facchin P, Antonello I, et al. Childhood obesity treatment: double blinded trial on dietary fibres (glucomannan) versus placebo. *Padiatr Padol* 1993;28:133-6.

180 Livieri C, Novazi F, Lorini R. [The use of highly purified glucomannan-based fibers in childhood obesity]. [Article in Italian]. *Pediatr Med Chir* 1992;14:195-8.

181 Vita PM, Restelli A, Caspani P, et al. [Chronic use of glucomannan in the dietary treatment of severe obesity]. [Article in Italian]. *Minerva Med* 1992;83:135-9.

182 Walsh DE, Yaghoubian V, Behforooz A. Effect of glucomannan on obese patients: a clinical s tudy. *Int J Obes* 1984;8:289-93.

183 Cairella M, Marchini GAD. [Evaluation of the action of glucomannan on metabolic parameters and on the sensation

REFERENCES

of satiation in overweight and obese patients]. [Article in Italian]. *Clin Ter* 1995;146:269-74.

184 Koshy KM, Griswold E, Schneeberger EE. Interstitial nephritis in a patient taking creatine. *N Engl J Med* 1999;340:814-5.

185 Kubota K, Sakurai T, Nakazato K, et al. [Effect of green tea on iron absorption in elderly patients with iron deficiency anemia]. [Article in Japanese]. *Nippon Ronen Igakkai Zasshi* 1990;27:555-8.

186 Barker G, Loftus L, Cuddy P, Barker B. The effects of sucralfate suspension and diphenhydramine syrup plus kaolin-pectin on radiotherapy-induced mucositis. *Oral Surg Oral Med Oral Pathol* 1991;71:288-93.

187 Carnel SB, Blakeslee DB, Oswald SG, Barnes M. Treatment of radiation- and chemotherapy-induced stomatitis. *Otolaryngol Head Neck Surg* 1990;102:326-30.

188 Epstein WL. Topical prevention of poison ivy/oak dermatitis. *Arch Dermatol* 1989;125:499-501.

189 Juch RD, et al. Pharmazeutische Praparate, Egerkingen, Schweiz. Pastes: what do they contain? How do they work? *Dermatology* 1994;189(4):373-7.

190 Tart RP, Li KC, Storm BL, et al. Enteric MRI contrast agents: comparative study of five potential agents in humans. *Magn Reson Imaging* 1991;9:559-68.

191 Mitchell DG, Vinitski S, Mohamed FB, et al. Comparison of Kaopectate with barium for negative and positive enteric contrast at MR imaging. *Radiology* 1991;181:475-80.

192 Despotis GJ, Alsoufiev AL, Spitznagel E, et al. DG Response of kaolin ACT to heparin: evaluation with an automated assay and higher heparin doses. *Ann Thorac Surg* 1996;61:795-9.

193 Paquet C. Assessment of kaolin agglutination test. *Tuber Lung Dis* 1994;75:397.

194 Sarnaik RM, Sharma M, Kate SK, Jindal SK. Serodiagnosis of tuberculosis: assessment of kaolin agglutination test. *Tuber Lung Dis* 1993;74:405-6.

195 Levin JL, Frank AL, Williams MG, et al. Kaolinosis in a cotton mill worker. *Am J Ind Med* 1996;29:215-21.

196 Chaudhary BA, Kanes GJ, Pool WH. Pleural thickening in mild kaolinosis. *South Med J* 1997;90:1106-9.

197 Altekruse EB, Chaudhary BA, Pearson MG, Morgan WK. Kaolin dust concentrations and pneumoconiosis at a kaolin mine. *Thorax* 1984;39:436-41.

198 Rodin SM, Johnson BF. Pharmacokinetic interactions with digoxin. *Clin Pharmacokinet* 1988;15:227-44.

199 Babhair SA, Tariq M. Effect of magnesium trisilicate and kaolin-pectin on the bioavailability of trimethoprim. *Res Commun Chem Pathol Pharmacol* 1983;40:165-8.

200 Kayden HJ, Wisniewski T. On the biological activity of vitamin E. *Am J Clin Nutr* 2000;72:201-3.

202 Cohn W. Evaluation of vitamin E potency. *Am J Clin Nutr* 1999;69:156-8.

203 Vorbach EU, Arnoldt KH, Hubner WD. Efficacy and tolerability of St. John's wort extract LI 160 versus imipramine in patients with severe depressive episodes according to ICD- 10. *Pharmacopsychiatry* 1997;30:81-5.

204 Wheatley D. LI 160, an extract of St. John's wort, versus amitriptyline in mildly to moderately depressed outpatients - a controlled 6-week clinical trial. *Pharmacopsychiatry* 1997;30 Suppl 2:77-80.

205 Volz HP. Controlled clinical trials of hypericum extracts in depressed patients - an overview. *Pharmacopsychiatry* 1997;30 Suppl 2:72-6.

206 Gulick RM, McAuliffe V, Holden-Wiltse J, et al. Phase I studies of hypericin, the active compound in St. John's Wort, as an antiretroviral agent in HIV-infected adults. AIDS Clinical Trials Group Protocols 150 and 258. *Ann Intern Med* 1999;130:510-4.

207 Ashton AK, Ahrens K, Gupta S, Masand PS. Antidepressant-induced sexual dysfunction and Ginkgo biloba. *Am J Psychiatry* 2000;157:836-7.

208 Davydov L, Stirling AL. Stevens-Johnson syndrome with Ginkgo biloba. *J Herb Pharmacother* 2001;1:65-69.

209 Kostyuk VA, Potapovich AI. Antiradical and chelating effects in flavonoid protection against silica-induced cell injury. *Arch Biochem Biophys* 1998;355:43-8.

211 Drewa G, Schachtschabel DO, Palgan K, et al. The influence of rutin on the weight, metastasis and melanin content of B16 melanotic melanoma in C57BL/6 mice. *Neoplasma* 1998;45(4):266-71.

212 Kehoe WA. Ginkgo biloba for SSRI-induced sexual dysfunction. *Pharmacist's Letter/Prescriber's Letter* 1997;13:130916.

213 Paick J, Lee J. An experimental study of the effect of ginkgo biloba extract on the human and rabbit corpus cavernosum tissue. *J Urol* 1996;156:1876-80.

215 Osol and Farar. The Dispensatory of the United States of America. 25th ed. JB Lippincott Co., 1955.

216 Dorland's Illustrated Medical Dictionary, 25th ed. WB Saunders Company, 1974.

218 Horwitt MK, Elliott WH, Kanjananggulpan P, Fitch CD. Serum concentrations of alpha-tocopherol after ingestion of various vitamin E preparations. *Am J Clin Nutr* 1984;40:240-5.

219 Pratt S. Dietary prevention of age-related macular degeneration. *J Am Optom Assoc* 1999;70:39-47.

220 Hertog MGL, Sweetnam PM, Fehily AM, et al. Antioxidant flavonols and ischemic heart disease in a Welsh population of men: the Caerphilly Study. *Am J Clin Nutr* 1997;65:1489-94.

221 Drew S, Davies E. Effectiveness of Ginkgo biloba in treating tinnitus: double blind, placebo controlled trial. *BMJ* 2001;322:73.

222 Chen J, Wollman Y, Chernichovsky T, et al. Effect of oral administration of high-dose nitric oxide donor L-arginine in men with organic erectile dysfunction: results of a double-blind, randomized, placebo-controlled study. *BJU Int* 1999;83:269-73.

223 Williamson EM, Evans FJ, eds. Potter's new cyclopaedia of botanical drugs and preparations. Essex, England: CW Daniel Company Ltd., 1998.

224 Leonetti HB, Longo S, Anasti JN. Transdermal progesterone cream for vasomotor symptoms and postmenopausal bone loss. *Obstet Gynecol* 1999;94:225-8.

225 Bracco GL, Carli P, Sonni L, et al. Clinical and histologic effects of topical treatments of vulval lichen sclerosus. A critical evaluation. *J Reprod Med* 1993;38:37-40.

226 Langer RD. Micronized progesterone: a new therapeutic option. *Int J Fertil Womens Med* 1999;44:67-73.

227 Licciardi FL, Kwiatkoski A, Noyes NL, et al. Oral versus intramuscular progesterone for in vitro fertilization: a prospective randomized study. *Fertil Steril* 1999;71:614-8.

228 Greendale GA, Reboussin BA, Hogan P, et al. Symptom relief and side effects of postmenopausal hormones: results from the Postmenopausal Interventions Trial. *Obstet Gynecol* 1998;92:982-8.

230 Sloane P. Advances in the treatment of Alzheimer's disease. *Am Fam Physician* 1998;58:1577-86, 1589-90.

231 Morris M, Beckett L, Scherr P, et al. Vitamin E and vitamin C supplement use and risk of incident Alzheimer's disease. *Alzheimer Dis Assoc Disord* 1998;12:121-6.

232 Sano M, Ernesto C, Thomas R, et al. A controlled trial of selegiline, alpha-tocopherol, or both as treatment for Alzheimer's disease. The Alzheimer's Disease Cooperative Study. *N Engl J Med* 1997;336:1216-22.

233 Chakravarty N. Inhibition of histamine release from mast cells by nigellone. *Ann Allergy* 1993;70(3):237-42.

234 Haq A, Abdullatif M, Lobo PI, et al. Black seed: effect on human lymphocytes and polymorphonuclear leukocyte phagocytic activity. *Immunopharmacology* 1995;30(2):147-55.

235 Houghton PJ, Zarka R, de las Heras B, Hoult JR. Fixed oil of Black seed and derived thymoquinone inhibit eicosanoid generation in leukocytes and membrane lipid peroxidation. *Planta Med* 1995;61(1):33-6.

236 Salomi NJ, Nair SC, Jayawardhanan KK, et al. Antitumour principles from Black seed seeds. *Cancer Lett* 1992;63(1):41-6.

237 Daba MH, Abdel-Rahman MS. Hepatoprotective activity of thymoquinone in isolated rat hepatocytes. *Toxicol Lett* 1998;95(1):23-9.

238 Worthen DR, Ghosheh OA, Crooks PA. The in vitro anti-tumor activity of some crude and purified components of blackseed, Black seed L. *Anticancer Res* 1998;18(3A):1527-32.

239 Badary OA, Al-Shabanah OA, Nagi MN, et al. Inhibition of benzo(a)pyrene-induced forestomach carcinogenesis in mice by thymoquinone . *Eur J Cancer Prev* 1999;8:435-40.

240 Nagi MN, Alam K, Badary OA, et al. Thymoquinone protects against carbon tetrachloride hepatotoxicity in mice via an antioxidant mechanism. *Biochem Mol Biol Int* 1999;47(1):153-9.

241 Aqel M, Shaheen R. Effects of the volatile oil of Black seed seeds on the uterine smooth muscle of rat and guinea pig. *J Ethnopharmacol* 1996;52:23-6.

242 Keshri G, Singh MM, Lakshmi V, Kamboj VP. Post-coital contraceptive efficacy of the seeds of Black seed in rats. *Indian J Physiol Pharmacol* 1995;39:59-62.

243 Hanafy MS, Hatem ME. Studies on the antimicrobial activity of Black seed seed (black cumin). *J Ethnopharmacol* 1991;34:275-8.

244 Benjamin J, Muir T, Briggs K, Pentland B. A case of cerebral haemorrhage-can Ginkgo biloba be implicated? *Postgrad Med J* 2001;77:112-3.

245 Tennekoon KH, Jeevathayaparan S, Kurukulasooriya AP, Karunanayake EH. Possible hepatotoxicity of Nigella sativa seeds and Dregea volubilis leaves. *J Ethnopharmacol* 1991;31(3):283-9.

246 Medenica RD. Use of Black seed to increase immune function. U.S. Patent 5,482,711, issued January 9, 1996. Obtained from US Patent and Trademark Ofc on April 12, 2000. www.uspto.gov/patft/index.htm.

247 Kiyose C, Muramatsu R, Kameyama Y, et al. Biodiscrimination of alpha-tocopherol stereoisomers in humans after oral administration. *Am J Clin Nutr* 1997;65:785-9.

248 Baker H, Handelman GJ, Short S, et al. Comparison of plasma alpha and gamma tocopherol levels following chronic oral administration of either all-rac-alpha-tocopheryl acetate or RRR-alpha-tocopheryl acetate in normal adult male subjects. *Am J Clin Nutr* 1986;43:382-7.

249 van Tits LJ, Demacker PN, de Graaf J, et al. Alpha-tocopherol supplementation decreases production of superoxide and cytokines by leukocytes ex vivo in both normolipidemic and hypertriglyceridemic individuals. *Am J Clin Nutr* 2000;71:458-64.

250 Bucci AJ, Myre SA, Tan HS, Shenouda LS. In vitro interaction of quinidine with kaolin and pectin. *J Pharm Sci* 1981;70:999-1002.

251 Allen MD, Greenblatt DJ, Harmatz JS, Smith TW. Effect of magnesium-aluminum hydroxide and kaolin-pectin on absorption of digoxin from tablets and capsules. *J Clin Pharmacol* 1981;21:26-30.

252 Albert KS, Ayres JW, DiSanto AR, et al. Influence of kaolin-pectin suspension on digoxin bioavailability. *J Pharm Sci* 1978;67:1582-6.

253 Albert KS, et al. Pharmacokinetic evaluation of a drug interaction between kaolin-pectin and clindamycin. *J Pharm Sci* 1978 67:1579-82.

254 Huyzen RJ, Harder MP, Huet RC, et al. Alternative perioperative anticoagulation monitoring during cardiopulmonary bypass in aprotinin-treated patients. *J Cardiothorac Vasc Anesth* 1994;8:153-6.

255 Grim W, Muller H. A randomized controlled trial of the effect of fluid extract of Echinacea purpurea on the incidence and severity of colds and respiratory infections. *Am J Med* 106:138-43.

256 He K, Zhao GX, Shi G, et al. Additional bioactive annonaceous acetogenins from Asminia triloba (Annonaceae). *Bioorg Med Chem* 1997;5:501-6.

257 Ratnayake S, Rupprecht JK, Potter WM, McLaughlin JL. Evaluation of various parts of the paw paw tree, Asmina triloba (Annonaceae), as commercial sources for the pesticidal annonaceous acetogenins. *J Econ Entomol* 1992;85:2353-6.

258 Zhao GX, Miesbauer LR, Smith DL, et al. Asimin, asiminacin, and asiminecin: novel highly cytotoxic asimicin isomers from Asiminia triloba. *J Med Chem* 1994;37:1971-6.

259 Salonen JT, Seppanen K, Nyyssonen K, et al. Intake of mercury from fish, lipid peroxidation, and the risk of myocardial infarction and coronary, cardiovascular, and any death in eastern Finnish men. *Circulation* 1995;91:645-55.

260 Cone EH, Lange R, Darwin WD. In vivo adulteration: excess fluid ingestion causes false-negative marijuana and cocaine urine test results. *J Anal Toxicol* 1998;22:460-73.

261 Wu AH, Forte E, Casella G, et al. CEDIA for screening drugs of abuse in urine and the effect of adulterants. *J Forensic Sci* 1995;40:614-8.

262 Rabbani GH, et al. Randomized controlled trial of berberine sulfate therapy for diarrhea due to enterotoxigenic Escherichia coli and Vibrio cholerae. *J Infect Dis* 1987;155(5):979-84.

263 Sheng WD, Jiddawi MS, Hong XQ, Abdulla SM. Treatment of chloroquine-resistant malaria using pyrimethamine in combination with berberine, tetracycline, or cotrimoxazole. *East Afr Med J* 1997;74:283-4.

264 Khosla PG, et al. Berberine, a potential drug for trachoma. *Rev Int Trach Pathol Ocul Trop Subtrop Sante Publique* 1992;69:147-65.

265 Tamminga C, Smith RC, Chang S, et al. Depression associated with oral choline. [letter] *Lancet* 1976;2:905.

266 Facts and Comparisons staff. Drug Facts and Comparisons. St Louis: Wolters Kluwer Company (updated monthly).

267 Anon. Chaparral-containing Herp-Eeze on the market. *Pharmacist's Letter/Prescriber's Letter* 1999;15:150215.

268 Merck Index, 12th ed. Whitehouse Station: Merck Research Laboratories, 1996.

269 Neal H. Dictionary of Chemical Names and Synonyms. Chelsea: Lewis Publishers, 1992.

270 Parker SP. ed. McGaw Hill Dictionary of Chemistry. New York: McGraw-Hill Book Company 1984.

271 Bruneton J. Pharmacognosy, Phytochemistry, Medicinal Plants. Paris: Lavoisier Publishing, 1995.

272 Covington TR, et al. Handbook of Nonprescription Drugs. 11th ed. Washington, DC: Am Pharmaceutical Assn, 1996.

274 Chenoy R, Hussain S, Tayob Y, et al. Effect of oral gamolenic acid from evening primrose oil on menopausal flushing. *BMJ* 1994;308:501-3.

275 Young DS. Effects of Drugs on Clinical Laboratory Tests 4th ed. Washington: AACC Press, 1995.

276 Balch JF, Balch PA. Prescription for Nutritional Healing. Garden City Park: Avery Publishing Group, 1997.

277 Silagy CA, Neil HA. A meta-analysis of the effect of garlic on blood pressure. *J Hypertension* 1994;12:463-8.

REFERENCES

278 McMahon FG, Vargas R. Can garlic lower blood pressure? A pilot study. *Pharmacotherapy* 1993;13:406-7.

279 Auer W, Eiber A, Hertkorn E, et al. Hypertension and hyperlipidaemia: garlic helps in mild cases. *Br J Clin Pract Symp Suppl* 1990;69:3-6.

280 Hentschel C, Dressler S, Hahn EG. Fumaria officinalis (fumitory)-clinical applications. *Fortschr Med* 1995;113:291-2.

281 Pittler MH, Ernst E. Horse-chestnut seed extract for chronic venous insufficiency. A criteria-based systematic review. *Arch Dermatol* 1998;134:1356-60.

282 Greeske K, Pohlmann BK. Horse chestnut seed extract-an effective therapy principle in general practice. Drug therapy of chronic venous insufficiency. *Fortschr Med* 1996;114:196-200.

283 Diehm C, Trampisch HJ, Lange S, Schmidt C. Comparison of leg compression stocking and oral horse-chestnut seed extract in patients with chronic venous insufficiency. *Lancet* 1996;347:292-4.

284 Diehm C, Vollbrecht D, Amendt K, Comberg HU. Medical edema protection-clinical benefit in patients with chronic deep vein incompetence. *Vasa* 1992;21:188-92.

285 Bisler H, Pfeifer R, Kluken N, Pauschinger P. [Effects of horse-chestnut seed on transcapillary filtration in chronic venous insufficiency]. [Article in German]. *Dtsch Med Wochenschr* 1986;111:1321-9.

286 Mohler JL, Gomella LG, Crawford ED, et al. Phase II evaluation of coumarin (1,2-benzopyrone) in metastatic prostatic carcinoma. *Prostate* 1992;20:123-31.

287 Marshall ME, Butler K, Fried A. Phase I evaluation of coumarin (1,2 benzopyrone) and cimetidine in patients with advanced malignancies. *Mol Biother* 1991;3:170-8.

288 Howanitz JH, Howanitz PJ, eds. Renal Function by D.O. Rogerson Laboratory Medicine Test Selection and Interpretation. New York: Churchill Livingstone, 1991.

289 van Joost T, Smitt JH, van Ketel WG. Sensitization to olive oil (olea europeae). *Contact Dermatitis* 1981;7:309-10.

291 Bakerink JA, Gospe SM Jr, Dimand RJ, Eldridge MW. Multiple organ failure after ingestion of pennyroyal oil from herbal tea in two infants. *Pediatrics* 1996;98(5):944-7.

292 Sudekum M, Poppenga RH, Raju N, Braselton WE Jr. Pennyroyal oil toxicosis in a dog. *J Am Vet Med Assoc* 1992;200:817-8.

295 Ritschel WA, Brady ME, Tan HIS, et al. Pharmacokinetics of Coumarin and its 7-hyroxy-metabolites upon intravenous and peroral administration of coumarin in man. *Eur J Clin Pharmacol* 1997;12:457-61.

296 Agriculture Res Svc. Dr. Duke's phytochemical and ethnobotanical databases. www.ars-grin.gov/duke/ (Accessed 7 July 1999).

297 Cox D, O'Kennedy R, Thornes RD. The rarity of toxicity in patients treated with coumarin (1,2-benzopyrone). *Hum Toxicol* 1989;8:501-6.

298 Mann J, Truswell AS, eds. Essentials of Human Nutrition. Oxford: Oxford Univ Press 1998.

299 Rozanova IA, et al. Effect of antiatherosclerotic diet, containing polyunsaturated fatty acids of the omega-3 family from flax oil, on fatty acid composition of cell membranes of patients with ischemic heart disease. Hypertensive disease and hyperlipoproteinemia. *Vopr Pitan* 1997;(5):15-7.

300 Zarembo JE, Godfrey JC, Godfrey NJ. Zinc(II) in saliva: determination of concentrations produced by different formulations of zinc gluconate lozenges containing common excipients. *J Pharm Sci* 1992;81:128-30.

301 Goldenberg RL, Tamura T, Neggers Y, et al. The effect of zinc supplementation on pregnancy outcome. *JAMA* 1995;274:463-8.

303 Upton R, ed. Astragalus Root: Analytical, quality control, and therapeutic monograph. Santa Cruz, CA: American Herbal Pharmacopoeia. 1999:1-25.

304 Upton R, ed. Valerian Root: Analytical, quality control, and therapeutic monograph. Santa Cruz, CA: American Herbal Pharmacopoeia 1999:1-25.

310 Penzak SR, Gubbins PO, Gurley BJ, et al. Grapefruit juice decreases the systemic availability of itraconazole capsules in healthy volunteers. *Ther Drug Monit* 1999;21:304-9.

311 FTC. FTC charges marketer of vitamin O of making false claims. Fed Trade Comm. 1999. Available at: www.ftc.gov/opa/1999/03/rosecreek.htm

313 Mehta DK (Ex Ed). British National Formulary, Number 37. British Medical Association and Royal Pharmaceutical Society of Great Britain: London, England, March 1999.

314 Horton TJ, Geissler CA. Aspirin potentiates the effect of ephedrine on the thermogenic response to a meal in obese but not lean women. *Int J Obes* 1991;15:359-66.

315 Baker JC, Tunnicliffe WS, Duncanson RC, Ayres JG. Dietary antioxidants and magnesium in type 1 brittle asthma: a case control study. *Thorax* 1999;54:115-8.

316 Hammer KA, Carson CF, Riley TV. Antimicrobial activity of essential oils and other plant extracts. *J Appl Microbiol* 1999;86:985-90.

317 Fernandez-Anaya S, Crespo JF, Rodriguez JR, et al. Beer anaphylaxis. *J Allergy Clin Immunol* 1999;103:959-60.

318 Katz DL. Acute nutrient effects in endothelial function: a randomized, single-blind, crossover trial in healthy adults. Am Coll of Nutr 40th Ann Meeting. Oct 1999, Wash, DC.

319 Griffiths JK. The vitamin A paradox. *J Pediatr* 2000;137:604-7.

320 Wicke C, Halliday B, Allen D, et al. Effects of steroids and retinoids on wound healing. *Arch Surg* 2000;135:1265-70.

322 Morreale P, Manopulo R, Galati M, et al. Comparison of the anti-inflammatory efficacy of chondroitin sulfate and diclofenac sodium in patients with knee osteoarthritis. *J Rheumatol* 1996;23:1385-91.

323 Conrozier T. [Anti-arthrosis treatments: efficacy and tolerance of chondroitin sulfates]. [Article in French]. *Presse Med* 1998;27:1862-5.

324 Mazieres B, Loyau G, Menkes CJ, et al. [Chondroitin sulfate in the treatment of gonarthrosis and coxarthrosis. 5-months result of a multicenter double-blind controlled prospective study using placebo]. [Article in French]. *Rev Rhum Mal Osteoartic* 1992;59:466-72.

325 O'Breasail AM, Argouarch S. Hypomania and St John's wort. *Can J Psychiatry* 1998;43:746-7.

326 Trivedy C, Warnakulasuriya S, Peters TJ. Areca nuts can have deleterious effects. *BMJ* 1999;318:1287.

327 Cox SC, Walker DM. Oral submucous fibrosis. A review. *Aust Dent J* 1996;41:294-9.

328 Gupta PC, Sinor PN, Bhonsle RB, et al. Oral submucous fibrosis in India: a new epidemic? *Natl Med J India* 1998;11:113-6.

329 VanWyk CW. Oral submucous fibrosis. The South African experience. *Indian J Dent Res* 1997;8:39-45.

330 Wiid I, Hoal-van Helden E, Hon D, et al. Potentiation of isoniazid activity against Mycobacterium tuberculosis by melatonin. *Antimicrob Agents Chemother* 1999;43:975-7.

331 Barceloux DG. Zinc. *J Toxicol Clin Toxicol* 1999;37:279-92.

332 Anon. Zinc for the common cold. *Med Lett Drugs Ther* 1997;39:9-10.

333 Mossad SB, Macknin ML, Medendorp SV, Mason P. Zinc gluconate lozenges for treating the common cold. A randomized, double-blind, placebo-controlled study. *Ann Intern Med* 1996;125:81-8.

334 Godfrey JC, Conant Sloane B, Smith DS, et al. Zinc gluconate and the common cold: a controlled clinical study. *J Int Med Res* 1992;20:234-6.

335 Al-Nakib W, Higgins PG, Barrow I, et al. Prophylaxis and treatment of rhinovirus colds with zinc gluconate lozenges. *J Antimicrob Chemother* 1987;20:893-901.

336 Eby GA, Davis DR, Halcomb WW. Reduction in duration of common colds by zinc gluconate lozenges in a double-blind study. *Antimicrob Agents Chemother* 1984;25:20-4.

337 Farr BM, Conner EM, Betts RF, et al. Two randomized controlled trials of zinc gluconate lozenge therapy of experimentally induced rhinovirus colds. *Antimicrob Agents Chemother* 1987;31:1183-7.

338 Smith DS, Helzner EC, Nuttall CE Jr, et al. Failure of zinc gluconate in treatment of acute upper respiratory tract infections. *Antimicrob Agents Chemother* 1989;33:646-8.

339 Weismann K, Jakobsen JP, Weismann JE, et al. Zinc gluconate lozenges for common cold. A double-blind clinical trial. *Dan Med Bull* 1990;37:279-81.

340 Eby GA. Zinc ion availability--the determinant of efficacy in zinc lozenge treatment of common colds. *J Antimicrob Chemother* 1997;40:483-93.

341 Macknin ML, Piedmonte M, Calendine C, et al. Zinc gluconate lozenges for treating the common cold in children: a randomized, controlled trial. *JAMA* 1998;279:1962-7.

345 Carta A, Calvani M, Bravi D, Bhuachalla SN. Acetyl-L-carnitine and Alzheimer's disease: pharmacological considerations beyond the cholinergic sphere. *Ann N Y Acad Sci* 1993;695:324-6.

347 SAMe for depression. *Medical Letter* 1999;41:107-8.

348 Vetrugno M, Maino A, Cardia G, et al. A randomised, double masked, clinical trial of high dose vitamin A and vitamin E supplementation after photorefractive keratectomy. *Br J Ophthalmol* 2001;85:537-9.

349 Garfinkel D, Zisapel N, Wainstein J, Laudon M. Facilitation of benzodiazepine discontinuation by melatonin, a new clinical approach. *Arch Intern Med* 1999;159:2456-60.

350 Jones JF, Minnich LL, Jeter WS, et al. Treatment of childhood combined Epstein-Barr virus/cytomegalovirus infection with oral bovine transfer factor. *Lancet* 1981;2:122-4.

354 Kobashi Y, Nakajima M, Niki Y, Matsushima T. [A case of acute eosinophilic pneumonia due to Sho-saiko-to]. [Article in Japanese]. *Nippon Kyobu Shikkan Gakkai Zasshi* 1997;35:1372-7.

355 Wada Y, Kubo M. [Acute lymphoblastic leukemia complicated by type C hepatitis during treatment and further by acute interstitial pneumonia due to sho-saiko-to in 7-year-old]. [Article in Japanese]. *Arerugi* 1997;46(11):1148-55.

356 Sato A, Toyoshima M, Kondo A, et al. [Pneumonitis induced by the herbal medicine Sho-saiko-to in Japan]. [Article in Japanese]. *Nippon Kyobu Shikkan Gakkai Zasshi* 1997;35:391-5.

357 Daibo A, Yoshida Y, Kitazawa S, et al. [A case of pneumonitis and hepatic injury caused by a herbal drug (sho-saiko-to)]. [Article in Japanese]. *Nippon Kyobu Shikkan Gakkai Zasshi* 1992;30(8):1583-8.

358 Sugiyama H, Nagai M, Kotajima F, et al. [A case of interstitial pneumonia with chronic hepatitis C following interferon-alfa and sho-saiko-to therapy]. [Article in Japanese]. *Arerugi* 1995;44:711-4.

359 Ishizaki T, Sasaki F, Ameshima S, et al. Pneumonitis during interferon and/or herbal drug therapy in patients with chronic active hepatitis. *Eur Respir J* 1996;9(12):2691-6.

360 Nakagawa A, Yamaguchi T, Takao T, Amano H. [Five cases of drug induced pneumonitis due to Sho-saiko-to or interferon-alpha or both]. [Article in Japanese]. *Nippon Kyobu Shikkan Gakkai Zasshi* 1995;33:1361-6.

361 Miyazaki E, Ando M, Ih K, et al. [Pulmonary edema associated with the Chinese medicine shosaikoto]. [Article in Japanese]. *Nihon Kokyuki Gakkai Zasshi* 1998;36:776-80.

362 Piras G, Makino M, Baba M. Sho-saiko-to, a traditional Kampo medicine, enhances the anti-HIV-1 activity of lamivudine (3TC) in vitro. *Microbiol Immunol* 1997;41:835-9.

363 Benninger J, Schneider HT, Schuppan D, et al. Acute hepatitis induced by greater celandine (Chelidonium majus). *Gastroenterol* 1999;117:1234-7.

365 FDA. Guide to Inspections of Cosmetic Product Manufacturers: products containing estrogenic hormones, placental extract or vitamins. 2001. Available at: http://www.fda.gov/ora/inspect_ref/igs/cosmet.html

366 Nityanand S, Srivastava JS, Asthana OP. Clinical trials with gugulipid. A new hypolipidaemic agent. *J Assoc Phys India* 1989;37:323-8.

367 Arandjelovic C. Canadian health officials pull Chinese herbal drugs. (Reprinted from Reuters). *Richters HerbLetter* November 23, 1999.

368 Skopnik H, Heimann G. [Manifestation of intolerance to cow's milk protein in mucoviscidosis with the symptom triad of hypoproteinemia, edema and anemia]. [Article in German]. *Klin Padiatr* 1987;199:453-6.

370 Benowitz LI, Goldberg DE, Madsen JR, et al. Inosine stimulates extensive axon collateral growth in the rat corticospinal tract after injury. *Proc Natl Acad Sci U S A* 1999;96:13486-90.

371 Balkan B, Dunning BE. Glucosamine inhibits glucokinase in vitro and produces a glucose-specific impairment of in vivo insulin secretion in rats. *Diabetes* 1994;43:1173-9.

372 Giaccari A, Morviducci L, Zorretta D, et al. In vivo effects of glucosamine on insulin secretion and insulin sensitivity in the rat: possible relevance to the maladaptive responses to chronic hyperglycaemia. *Diabetologia* 1995;38:518-24.

374 Neubauer N, Marz RW. Placebo-controlled, randomized, double-blind, clincal trial with Sinupret sugar coated tablets on the basis of a therapy with antibiotics and decongestant nasal drops in acute sinusitis. *Phytomedicine* 1994;1:177-81.

375 Govers MJ, Gannon NJ, Dunshea FR, et al. Wheat bran affects the site of fermentation of resistant starch and luminal indexes related to colon cancer risk: a study in pigs. *Gut* 1999;45:840-7.

376 Hubner WD, Lande S, Podzuweit H. Hypericum treatment of mild depressions with somatic symptoms. *J Geriatr Psychiatry Neurol* 1994;7 Suppl 1:S12-4.

377 Stevinson C, Dixon M, Ernst E. Hypericum for fatigue. *Phytomedicine* 1998;5:443-7.

379 Marz RW, Ismail C, Popp MA. Action profile and efficacy of a herbal combination preparation for the treatment of sinusitis. *Wien Med Wochenschr* 1999;149:202-8.

380 Dupuis C. Poison ivy. *Pharmacy Practice* 1995;11:51-2,54-5.

381 Malinow MR, Bardana EJ Jr, Goodnight SH Jr. Pancytopenia during ingestion of alfalfa seeds. *Lancet* 1981 March;14(8220 Pt1):615.

382 Johne A, Brockmoller J, Bauer S, et al. Pharmacokinetic interaction of digoxin with an herbal extract from St John's wort (Hypericum perforatum). *Clin Pharmacol Ther* 1999;66:338-45.

383 Dalvi SS, Nayak VK, Pohujani SM, et al. Effect of gugulipid on bioavailability of diltiazem and propranolol. *J Assoc Phys India* 1994;42:454-5.

384 Steele RW, Myers MG, Vincent MM. Transfer factor for the prevention of varicella-zoster infection in childhood leukemia. *N Engl J Med* 1980;303:355-9.

387 FDA Talk Paper. FDA takes action against firm marketing unapproved drugs. 1999. Available at: www.fda.gov/bbs/topics/ANSWERS/ANS00988.html

388 Goldwaser I, Li J, Gershonov E, et al. L-Glutamic acid gamma-monohydroxamate. A potentiator of vanadium-evoked glucose metabolism in vitro and in vivo. *J Biol Chem* 1999;274(37):26617-24.

389 Duda RB, Zhong Y, Navas V, et al. American ginseng and breast cancer therapeutic agents synergistically inhibit MCF-7 breast cancer cell growth. *J Surg Oncol* 1999;72:230-9.

390 Strahl S, Ehret V, Dahm HH, Maier KP. [Necrotizing hepatitis after taking herbal medication]. [Article in German]. *Dtsch Med Wochenschr* 1998;123:1410-4.

391 Labriola D, Livingston R. Possible interactions between dietary antioxidants and chemotherapy. *Oncology* 1999;13:1003-8.

393 Beuscher N, Scheit KH, Bodinet C, Kopanski L. [Immunologically active glycoproteins of Baptisia tinctoria]. [Article in German]. *Planta Med* 1989;55:358-63.

394 Anon. A better treatment for depression? *UC Berkeley Wellness Letter* 1997;13:1-2.

395 Subrahmanyam M. A prospective randomized, clinical and histological study of superficial burn wound healing with honey and silver sulfadiazine. *Burns* 1998;24(2):157-61.

396 Subrahmanyam M. Honey dressing vs boiled potato peel in the treatment of burns: a prospective randomized study. *Burns* 1996;22(6):491-3.

397 Subrahmanyam M. Honey impregnated gauze vs amniotic membrane in the treatment of burns. *Burns* 1994;20(4):331-3.

398 Subrahmanyam M. Honey impregnated gauze versus polyurethane film (OpSite) in the treatment of burns- a prospective randomized study. *Br J Plast Surg* 1993;46(4):322-3.

399 Subrahmanyam M. Topical application of honey in treatment of burns. *Br J Surg* 1991;78(4):497-8.

401 Kelly FJ, Mudway I, Blomberg A, et al. Altered lung antioxidant status in patients with mild asthma. *Lancet* 1999;354:482-3.

403 Whitney E, Cataldo CB, Rolfes SR, eds. Understanding Normal and Clinical Nutrition. Belmont, CA: Wadsworth, 1998.

404 Kehoe WA. Grapefruit juice and lovastatin: Is this an important interaction? *Pharmacist's Letter*, Dec. 1998:Detail Document #141204.

405 Cook IJ, et al. Effect of dietary fiber on rectosigmoid motility in patients with irritable bowel syndrome: A controlled, crossover study. *Gastroenterol* 1990;98:66-72.

406 Upton R, ed. Hawthorn Leaf with Flower: Analytical, quality control, and therapeutic monograph. Santa Cruz, CA: American Herbal Pharmacopoeia 1999:1-29.

409 Powell CV, Nash AA, Powers HJ, Primhak RA. Antioxidant status in asthma. *Pediatr Pulmonol* 1994;18:34-8.

410 A Modern Herbal (Mrs.M.Grieve) website. Available at: http://botanical.com/botanical/mgmh/s/squawv85.html (Accessed 25 November 1999).

412 Woo KS, Chook P, Lolin YI, et al. Folic acid improves arterial endothelial function in adults with hyperhomocysteinemia. *J Am Coll Cardiol* 1999;34:2002-6.

416 Pajaron MJ, Vila L, Prieto I, et al. Cross-reactivity of Olea europaea with other Oleaceae species in allergic rhinitis and bronchial asthma. *Allergy* 1997;52(8):829-35.

417 Batanero E, Gonzalez De La Pena MA, Villalba M, et al. Isolation, cDNA cloning and expression of Lig v 1, the major allergen from privet pollen. *Clin Exp Allergy* 1996;26(12):1401-10.

418 Khoo KS, Ang PT. Extract of astragalus membranaceus and ligustrum lucidum does not prevent cyclophosphamide-induced myelosuppression. *Singapore Med J* 1995;36(4):387-90.

419 Lau BH, Ruckle HC, Botolazzo T, Lui PD. Chinese medicinal herbs inhibit growth of murine renal cell carcinoma. *Cancer Biother* 1994;9(2):153-61.

420 Niikawa M, Hayashi H, Sato T, et al. Isolation of substances from glossy privet (Ligustrum lucidum Ait.) inhibiting the mutagenicity of benzo[a]pyrene in bacteria. *Mutat Res* 1993;319(1):1-9.

421 Rittenhouse JR, Lui PD, Lau BH. Chinese medicinal herbs reverse macrophage suppression induced by urological tumors. *J Urol* 1991;146(2):486-90.

422 Kalayci O, Besler T, Kilinc K, et al. Serum levels of antioxidant vitamins (alpha tocopherol, beta carotene, and ascorbic acid) in children with bronchial asthma. *Turk J Pediatr* 2000;42:17-21.

423 Sun Y, Hersh EM, Talpaz M, et al. Immune restoration and/or augmentation of local graft versus host reaction by traditional Chinese medicinal herbs. *Cancer* 1983;52:70-3.

424 Lucas A, Stafford M, Morley R, et al. Efficacy and safety of long-chain polyunsaturated fatty acid supplementation of infant-formula milk: a randomized trial. *Lancet* 1999;354:1948-54.

425 Gibson RA. Long-chain polyunsaturated fatty acids and infant development (editorial). *Lancet* 1999;354:1919.

426 Arjmandi BH, Birnbaum RS, Juma S, et al. The synthetic phytoestrogen, ipriflavone, and estrogen prevent bone loss by different mechanisms. *Calcif Tissue Int* 2000;66(1):61-5.

427 Melis GB, Paoletti AM, Bartolini R, et al. Ipriflavone and low doses of estrogens in the prevention of bone mineral loss in climacterium. *Bone Miner* 1992;19,Suppl 1:S49-56.

428 Agnusdei D, Adami S, Cervetti R, et al. Effects of ipriflavone on bone mass and calcium metabolism in postmenopausal osteoporosis. *Bone Miner* 1992;19,Suppl 1:S43-8.

429 Sato Y, Kuno H, Kaji M, et al. Effect of ipriflavone on bone in elderly hemiplegic stroke patients with hypovitaminosis D. *Am J Phys Med Rehabil* 1999;78(5):457-63.

430 Ohta H, Komukai S, Makita K, et al. Effects of 1-year ipriflavone treatment on lumbar bone mineral density and bone metabolic markers in postmenopausal women with low bone mass. *Horm Res* 1999;51(4):178-83.

431 Head KA. Ipriflavone: an important bone-building isoflavone. *Altern Med Rev* 1999;4(1):10-22.

432 Agnusdei D, Bufalino L. Efficacy of ipriflavone in established osteoporosis and long-term safety. *Calcif Tissue Int* 1997;61,Suppl 1:S23-7.

433 Gennari C, Adami S, Agnusdei D, et al. Effect of chronic treatment with ipriflavone in postmenopausal women with low bone mass. *Calcif Tissue Int* 1997;61,Suppl 1:S19-22.

434 Petilli M, Fiorelli G, Benvenuti S, et al. Interactions between ipriflavone and the estrogen receptor. *Calcif Tissue Int* 1995;56(2):160-5.

441 Hirazumi A, Furusawa E. An immunomodulatory polysaccharide-rich substance from the fruit juice of Morinda citrifolia (noni) with antitumour activity. *Phytother Res* 1999;13:380-7.

442 Hiwasa T, Arase Y, Chen Z, et al. Stimulation of ultraviolet-induced apoptosis of human fibroblast UVr-1 cells by tyrosine kinase inhibitors. *FEBS Lett* 1999;444:173-6.

443 Hiramatsu T, Imoto M, Koyano T, Umezawa K. Induction of normal phenotypes in ras-transformed cells by

damnacanthal from Morinda citrifolia. *Cancer Lett* 1993;73:161-6.

444 Younos C, Rolland A, Fleurentin J, et al. Analgesic and behavioural effects of Morinda citrifolia. *Planta Med* 1990;56:430-4.

448 Yoshikawa M, Yamaguchi S, Nishisaka H, et al. Chemical constituents of Chinese natural medicine, morindae radix, the dried roots of morinda officinalis how: structures of morindolide and morofficinaloside. *Chem Pharm Bull* (Tokyo) 1995;43(9):1462-5.

449 Cui C, Yang M, Yao Z, et al. [Antidepressant active constituents in the roots of Morinda officinalis how]. [Article in Chinese]. *Chung Kuo Chung Yao Tsa Chih* 1995;20:36-9, 62-3.

450 Miller LG, Panosian CB. Ataxia and slurred speech after artesunate treatment for falciparum malaria [letter]. *N Engl J Med* 1997;336:1328.

451 Yang YJ, Shu HY, Min ZD. [Anthraquinones isolated from Morinda officinalis and Damnacanthus indicus]. [Article in Chinese]. *Yao Hsueh Hsueh Pao* 1992;27:358-64.

452 Li S, Ouyang Q, Tan X, et al. [Chemical constituents of Morinda officinalis how]. [Article in Chinese]. *Chung Kuo Chung Yao Tsa Chih* 1991;16:675-6, 703.

453 Qiao ZS, Wu H, Su ZW. [Comparison with the pharmacological actions of Morinda officinalis, Damnacanthus officinarum and Schisandra propinqua]. [Article in Chinese]. *Chung Hsi I Chieh Ho Tsa Chih* 1991;11:390,415-7.

454 Barton DL, Loprinzi CL, Quella SK, et al. Prospective evaluation of vitamin E for hot flashes in breast cancer survivors. *J Clin Oncol* 1998;16:495-500.

455 Nagao T, Ibayashi S, Fujii K, et al. Treatment of warfarin-induced hair loss with ubidecarenone. *Lancet* 1995;346:1104-5.

456 Henriksen JE, Andersen CB, Hother-Nielsen O, et al. Impact of ubiquinone (coenzyme Q10) treatment on glycaemic control, insulin requirement and well-being in patients with Type 1 diabetes mellitus. *Diabet Med* 1999;16:312-8.

457 Weis M, Mortensen SA, Rassing MR, et al. Bioavailability of four oral coenzyme Q10 formulations in healthy volunteers. *Mol Aspects Med* 1994;15:s273-80.

461 KeDi High-Tech Ind Co (Xiamen Office). www.eckorea.net/co/kedi/3.asp (Accessed 10 January 2000).

462 Seabuckthorn seed oil. RichNature Inc. www.richnature.com/products/herbal/seaseed.htm (Accessed 10 January 2000).

463 Seabuckthorn berry oil. RichNature Inc. www.richnature.com/products/herbal/seaberry.htm (Accessed 10 January 2000).

466 Amosova EN, Zueva EP, Razina TG, et al. [The search for new anti-ulcer agents from plants in Siberia and the Far East]. [Article in Russian]. *Eksp Klin Farmakol* 1998;61:31-5.

467 Ianev E, Radev S, Balutsov M, et al. [The effect of an extract of sea buckthorn (Hippophae rhamnoides L.) on the healing of experimental skin wounds in rats]. [Article in Bulgarian]. *Khirurgiia* (Sofiia) 1995;48:30-3.

468 Li Y, Liu H. Prevention of tumour production in rats fed aminopyrine plus nitrite by sea buckthorn juice. *IARC Sci Publ* 1991;105:568-70.

469 Cheng TJ, Pu JK, Wu LW, et al. [A preliminary study on hepato-protective action of seed oil of Hippophae rhamnoides L. (HR) and mechanism of the action]. [Article in Chinese]. *Chung Kuo Chung Yao Tsa Chih* 1994;19:367-70, 384.

470 Cheng TJ. [Protective action of seed oil of Hippophae rhamnoides L. (HR) against experimental liver injury in mice]. [Article in Chinese]. *Chung Hua Yu Fang I Hsueh Tsa Chih* 1992;26:227-9.

471 Wang Y, Lu Y, Liu X, et al. [The protective effect of Hippophae rhamnoides L. on hyperlipidemic serum cultured smooth muscle cells in vitro]. [Article in Chinese]. *Chung Kuo Chung Yao Tsa Chih* 1992;17:601, 624-6 (inside back cover).

472 Xiao M, Yang Z, Jiu M, et al. [The antigastroulcerative activity of beta-sitosterol-beta-D-glucoside and its aglycone in rats]. [Article in Chinese]. *Hua Hsi I Ko Ta Hsueh Hsueh Pao* 1992;23:98-101.

473 Satietrol press releases. PacificHealth Labs, Inc., Woodbridge, NJ. www.satietrol.com/press.htm and www.satietrol.com/press1.htm (Accessed 10 January 2000).

474 Klement P, Liao P, Bajzar L. A novel approach to arterial thrombolysis. *Blood* 1999;94(8):2735-43.

475 Redlitz A, Nicolini FA, Malycky JL, et al. Inducible carboxypeptidase activity. A role in clot lysis in vivo. *Circulation* 1996;93(7):1328-30.

476 Kopin AS, Mathes WF, McBride EW, et al. The cholecystokinin-A receptor mediates inhibition of food intake yet is not essential for the maintenance of body weight. *J Clin Invest* 1999;103:383-91.

477 Lam WF, Gielkens HA, de Boer SY, et al. Influence of hyperglycemia on the satiating effect of CCK in humans. *Physiol Behav* 1998;65(3):505-11.

478 Zhongrui L, Shuzhen T. [Clinical observation on curative effect of oral seabuckthorn seed oil on cancers under chemotherapy]. [Article in Chinese]. *Hippophae* 1993;6:39-41.

479 Changshun L, Xinming C, Fenrong W, et al. [Clinical observation on reflux esophagitis treated with seabuckthorn seed oil]. [Article in Chinese]. *Hippophae* 1996;9:40-1.

480 Gengquan Q, Xiang Q. [A clinical report on the therapeutics of seabuckthorn oil softgels on peptic ulcer in 30 cases]. [Article in Chinese]. *Hippophae* 1997;10:39-41.

481 Shoskes DA, Zeitlin SI, Shahed A, Rajfer J. Quercetin in men with category III chronic prostatitis: A preliminary prospective, double-blind, placebo-controlled trial. *Urol* 1999;54:960-3.

482 Aharon Y, Mevorach M, Shamoon H. Vanadyl sulfate does not enhance insulin action in patients with type 1 diabetes. *Diabetes Care* 1998;21:2194-5.

483 Anon. Quercetin. *Alt Med Rev* 1998;3(2):140-3.

484 Miodini P, Fioravanti L, Di Fronzo G, Cappelletti V. The two phyto-oestrogens genistein and quercetin exert different effects on oestrogen receptor function. *Br J Cancer* 1999;80:1150-5.

485 El Attar TM, Virji AS. Modulating effect of resveratrol and quercetin on oral cancer cell growth and proliferation. *Anticancer Drugs* 1999;10:187-93.

486 Wiseman H. The bioavailability of non-nutrient plant factors: dietary flavonoids and phyto-oestrogens. *Proc Nutr Soc* 1999;58(1):139-46.

487 McAnlis GT, McEneny J, Pearce J, Young IS. Absorption and antioxidant effects of quercetin from onions, in man. *Eur J Clin Nutr* 1999;53(2):92-6.

488 Hansten PD, Horn JR. Hansten and Horn's Drug Interactions Analysis and Management. Vancouver, CAN:Appl Therapeut, 1999.

489 Huang Z, Fasco MJ, Kaminsky LS. Inhibition of estrone sulfatase in human liver microsomes by quercetin and other flavonoids. *J Steroid Biochem Mol Biol* 1997;63(1-3):9-15.

490 Garg R, Malinow MR, Pettinger M, et al. Niacin treatment increases plasma homocysteine levels. *Am Heart J* 1999;138:1082-7.

492 Eriksson JG, Forsen TJ, Mortensen SA, Rohde M. The effect of coenzyme Q10 administration on metabolic control in

REFERENCES

patients with type 2 diabetes mellitus. *Biofactors* 1999;9:315-8.

496 Anon. Inositol hexaniacinate. *Altern Med Rev* 1998;3(3):222-3.

497 Mehta DK (Executive Editor). British National Formulary 38. British Medical Association and Royal Pharmaceutical Society of Great Britain, London, UK, 1999. pg 104.

498 Sunderland GT, Belch JJ, Sturrock RD, et al. A double-blind, randomized, placebo-controlled trial of hexopal in primary Raynaud's disease. *Clin Rheumatol* 1988;7:46-9.

499 Hutt V, Wechsler JG, Klor HU, Ditschuneit H. [Effect of a clofibrate-inositol nicotinate combination on lipids and lipoproteins in primary hyperlipoproteinemia of types IIa, IV and V]. [Article in German]. *Arzneimittelforschung* 1983;33(5):776-9.

500 Brinker F. Herb Contraindications and Drug Interactions. Sandy, OR: Eclectic Medical Publ, 1997.

501 De Smet PAGM, Keller K, Hansel R, Chandler RF, Eds. Adverse Effects of Herbal Drugs 1. Verlag, Berlin: Springer, 1992.

502 De Smet PAGM, Keller K, Hansel R, Chandler RF, Eds. Adverse Effects of Herbal Drugs 2. Verlag, Berlin: Springer, 1993.

503 Duke, JA. The Green Pharmacy. Emmaus, PA: Rodale Press, 1997.

504 Holt GA. Food & Possible Interactions with Drugs: Revised and Expanded Ed. Chicago, IL: Precept Press, 1998.

505 Hardman JG, Limbird LL, Molinoff PB, eds. Goodman and Gillman's The Pharmacological Basis of Therapeutics, 9th ed. New York, NY: McGraw-Hill, 1996.

506 Burnham TH, ed. Drug Facts and Comparisons, Updated Monthly. Facts and Comparisons, St. Louis, MO.

507 Pheatt N, ed. Nonherbal Dietary Supplements Continuing Education Booklet. Stockton, CA: Therapeutic Research Center, 1998. pgs. 1-51.

508 Lieberman S. The Real Vitamin and Mineral Book. Honesdale, PA: Paragon Press, 1997.

509 Dukes, MNG. Meyler's Side Effects of Drugs. 13th ed. Elsevier: Amsterdam, 1997.

510 Meuss AR, transl. Phytotherapy in Paediatrics - Handbook for Physicians and Pharmacists by H Schilcher. 2nd edition. Stuttgart, Germany: Medpharm GmbH Scientific Publishers, 1997.

511 Spraycar M, ed. Stedman's Medical Dictionary. 26th ed. Baltimore, MD: Williams & Wilkins, 1995.

512 Robbers JE, Tyler VE. Tyler's Herbs of Choice: The Therapeutic Use of Phytomedicinals. New York, NY: The Haworth Herbal Press, 1999.

513 Agri Res Svc: Dr. Duke's phytochemical and ethnobotanical databases. www.ars-grin.gov/duke (Accessed 3 November 1999).

515 Foster S, Tyler VE. Tyler's Honest Herbal, 4th ed., Binghamton, NY: Haworth Herbal Press, 1999.

516 Morrix W, ed. The American Heritage Dictionary of the English Language. New York, NY: Am Heritage Publ, 1969.

517 Duke JA, Vasquez R. Amazonian Ethnobotanical Dictionary. Boca Raton, FL: CRC Press, 1994.

518 Schultes RE, Raffauf RF. The Healing Forest, Medicinal and Toxic Plants of the Northwest Amazonia. Portland, OR: Dioscorides Press, 1990.

519 Foster S, Duke JA. Eastern/Central Medicinal Plants. New York, NY: Houghton Mifflin Co., 1990.

520 Richter W, et al. Interaction between fibre and lovastatin. *Lancet* 1991;338:706.

522 Ioannides-Demos LL, Christophidis N, et al. Dosing implications of a clinical interaction between grapefruit juice and cyclosporine and metabolite concentrations in patients with autoimmune diseases. *J Rheumatol* 1997;24:49-54.

523 Josefsson M, Zackrisson AL, Ahlner J. Effect of grapefruit juice on the pharmacokinetics of amlodipine in healthy volunteers. *Eur J Clin Pharmacol* 1996;51:189-93.

524 Garg SK, Kumar N, Bhargava VK, Prabhakar SK. Effect of grapefruit juice on carbamazepine bioavailability in patients with epilepsy. *Clin Pharmacol Ther* 1998;64:286-8.

525 Weber A, Jager R, Borner A, et al. Can grapefruit juice influence ethinylestradiol bioavailability? *Contraception* 1996;53:41-7.

526 Schubert W, Cullberg G, Edgar B, Hedner T. Inhibition of 17 beta-estradiol metabolism by grapefruit juice in ovariectomized women. *Maturitas* 1994;20:155-63.

527 Kantola T, Kivisto KT, Neuvonen PJ, et al. Grapefruit juice greatly increases serum concentrations of lovastatin and lovastatin acid. *Clin Pharmacol Ther* 1998 63:397-402.

528 Bailey DG, Spence JD, Munoz C, Arnold JM. Interaction of citrus juices with felodipine and nifedipine. *Lancet* 1991;337:268-9.

529 Bailey DG, Arnold JM, Strong HA, et al. Effect of grapefruit juice and naringin on nisoldipine pharmacokinetics. *Clin Pharmacol Ther* 1993;54:589-94.

530 Rau SE, Bend JR, Arnold MO, et al. Grapefruit juice-terfenadine single-dose interaction: magnitude, mechanism, and relevance. *Clin Pharmacol Ther* 1997 61:401-9.

531 Robbins RC, Martin FG, Roe JM. Ingestion of grapefruit lowers elevated hematocrits in human subjects. *Int J Vitam Nutr Res* 1988;58:414-7.

532 Gin H, et al. The influence of Guar gum on absorption of metformin from the gut in healthy volunteers. *Horm Metab Res* 1989;21:81-3.

533 Huupponen R, et al. Effect of guar gum, a fibre preparation, on digoxin and penicillin absorption in man. *Eur J Clin Pharmacol* 1984;26:279-81.

534 Spillane PK, et al. Neurological manifestations of kava intoxication. *Med J Aust* 1997;167:172-3.

535 Swensen JN. Man convicted of driving under the influence of kava. Salt Lake City, UT: Deseret News, 1996.

536 Almeida JC, Grimsley EW. Coma from the health food store: interaction between kava and alprazolam. *Ann Intern Med* 1996;125:940-1.

537 Bano G, Amla V, Raina RK, et al. The effect of piperine on pharmacokinetics of phenytoin in healthy volunteers. *Planta Med* 1987;53:568-9.

538 Bano G, et al. Effect of piperine on bioavailability and pharmacokinetics of propranolol and theophylline in healthy volunteers. *Eur J Clin Pharmacol* 1991;41;615-7.

539 Etman M. Effect of a bulk forming laxative on the bioavailablility of caramazepine in man. *Drug Dev Ind Pharm* 1995;21:1901-6.

540 Perlman BB. Interaction between lithium salts and ispaghula husk. *Lancet* 1990;35:416.

541 Amabeoku, GJ, et al. Pharmacokinetic interaction of single doses of quinine and carbamazepine, phenobarbitone and phenytoin in healthy volunteers. *East Afr Med J* 1993;70:90-3.

542 Gordon JB. SSRIs and St. John's Wort: possible toxicity? *Am Fam Physician* 1998;57:950,953.

543 McRae S. Elevated serum digoxin levels in a patient taking digoxin and Siberian ginseng. *CMAJ* 1996;155:293-5.

544 Tatro D, Ed. Anticoagulants-Vitamin E: in Drug Interaction Facts, Facts and Comparisons. St. Louis, MO, January 1997.

545 Dunbain DW, et al. Lead poisoning from Indian herbal medicine (Ayurveda). *Med J Aust* 1992;157:835-6.

546 Sheerin NS, et al. Simultaneous exposure to lead, arsenic and mercury from Indian ethnic remedies. *Br J Clin Pract* 1994;48:332-3.

547 Markowitz SB, Nunez CM, Klitzman S, et al. Lead poisoning due to Hai Ge Fan, the porphyrin content of individual erythrocytes. *JAMA* 1994;271:932-4.

548 Tay CH, Seah CS. Arsenic poisoning from anti-asthmatic herbal preparations. *Med J Aust* 1975;2:424-8.

549 Colgrove ML, Atkinson JM, Collins T, et al. Lead poisoning-associated death from Asian Indian folk remedies, Florida. *MMWR Morb Mortal Wkly Rep* 1984;33:642-5.

550 Schaumburg HH, Berger A. Alopecia and sensory polyneuropathy from thallium in a Chinese herbal medication. *JAMA* 1992;268:3430-1.

551 Espinoza EO, Mann MJ, Bleasdell B, et al. Toxic metals in selected traditional Chinese medicinals. *J Forensic Sci* 1996;41:453-6.

552 Takegoshi K, Tohyama T, Okuda K, et al. A case of Venoplant-induced hepatic injury. *Gastroenterol Jpn* 1986;21:62-5.

553 Jaspersen-Schib R, Theus L, Guirguis-Oeschger M, et al. [Serious plant poisonings in Switzerland 1966-1994. Case analysis from the Swiss Toxicology Information Center]. [Article in German]. *Schweiz Med Wochenschr* 1996;126:1085-98.

554 Cerulli J, Grabe DW, Gauthier I, et al. Chromium picolinate toxicity. *Ann Pharmacother* 1998;32:428-31.

555 Lin JL, et al. Flavonoid-induced acute nephropathy. *Am J Kidney Dis* 1994;23:433-40.

556 Becker BN. Ginseng-induced diuretic resistance. *JAMA* 1996 276:606-7.

557 Tao SH, Bolger, PM. Hazard assessment of germanium supplements. *Regul Toxicol Pharmacol* 1997;25:211-9.

558 Tai YT. Adverse effects from traditional Chinese medicine. *Lancet* 1993;341:892.

559 Tai YT, et al. Cardiotoxicity after accidental herb-induced aconite poisoning. *Lancet* 1992;340:1254-6.

560 Osher HL, Katz KH, Wagner DJ. Khellin in the treatment of angina pectoris. *N Engl J Med* 1951;244:315-21.

561 Fatovich DM. Aconite: a lethal Chinese herb. *Ann Emerg Med* 1992;21:309-11.

562 Tomlinson B, Chan TY, Chan JC, Critchley JA. Herb-induced aconite poisoning. *Lancet* 1993;341:370-1.

563 Chan TY, Tomlinson B, Critchley JA. Aconitine poisoning following the ingestion of Chinese herbal medicines: a report of eight cases. *Aust N Z J Med* 1993;23:268-71.

564 van Ypersele de Strihou C, Vanherweghem JL. The tragic paradigm of Chinese herbs nephropathy. *Nephrol Dial Transplant* 1995;10:157-60.

565 Blumenthal HJ, Vance DA. Chewing gum headaches. *Headache* 1997;37:665-6.

566 Jones TK, Lawson BM. Profound neonatal congestive heart failure caused by maternal consumption of blue cohosh herbal medication. *J Pediatr* 1998;132:550-2.

567 Subiza J, Subiza JL, Hinojosa M, et al. Anaphylactic reaction after the ingestion of chamomile tea; a study of cross-reactivity with other composite pollens. *J Allergy Clin Immunol* 1989;84:353-8.

568 Smith BC, Desmond PV. Acute hepatitis induced by ingestion of the herbal medication chaparral. *Aust N Z J Med* 1993;23:526.

569 Gordon DW, Rosenthal G, Hart J, et al. Chaparral ingestion: the broadening spectrum of liver injury caused by herbal medications. *JAMA* 1995;273:489-90.

570 Batchelor WB, Heathcote J, Wanless IR. Chaparral-induced hepatic injury. *Am J Gastroenterol* 1995;90:831-3.

571 Katz M, Saibil F. Herbal hepatitis: subacute hepatic necrosis secondary to chaparral leaf. *J Clin Gastroenterol* 1990;12:203-6.

572 Ko RJ, Greenwald MS, Loscutoff SM, et al. Lethal ingestion of Chinese herbal tea containing ch'an su. *West J Med* 1996;164:71-5.

573 Chan JC, Chan TY, Chan KL, et al. Anticholinergic poisoning from Chinese herbal medciines. *Aust N Z J Med* 1994;24:317-8.

574 Sperl W, Stuppner H, Gassner I, et al. Reversible hepatic veno-occlusive disease in an infant after consumption of pyrrolizidine-containing herbal tea. *Eur J Pediatr* 1995;154:112-6.

575 Roulet M, Laurini R, Rivier L, Calame A. Hepatic veno-occlusive disease in newborn infant of a woman drinking herbal tea. *J Pediatr* 1988;112:433-6.

576 Matthews, MK. Association of Ginkgo biloba with intracerebral hemorrhage. *Neurology* 1998;50:1934.

577 Gilbert GJ. Ginkgo biloba. *Neurology* 1997;48:1137.

578 Rowin J, Lewis SL. Spontaneous bilateral subdural hemotomas with chronic Gingko biloba ingestion. *Neurology* 1996;46:1775-6.

579 Rosenblatt M, Mindel T. Spontaneous hyphema associated with ingestion of Gingko biloba extract. *N Engl J Med* 1997;336:1108.

580 Jaakkola MS, et al. Asthma caused by occupational exposure to pectin. *J Allergy Clin Immunol* 1997;100:575-6.

581 Westphal W, et al. [Exogenous allergic asthma following pectin exposure-a new occupational allergen].[Article in German]. *Pneumologie* 1990;44(Suppl 1):337-8.

582 Baldwin JL, et al. Pectin-induced occupational asthma. *Chest* 1993;104:1936-7.

583 Cohen AJ, et al. Occupational asthma caused by pectin inhalation during the manufacture of jam. *Chest* 1993;103:309-11.

584 Kraut A, et al. Christmas candy maker's asthma. IgG4-mediated pectin allergy. *Chest* 1992;102:1605-7.

585 Garty BZ. Garlic burns. *Pediatrics* 1993;91:658-9.

586 Rose KD, et al. Spontaneous spinal epidural hematoma with associated platelet dysfunction from excessive garlic ingestion: a case report. *Neurosurg* 1990;26:880-2.

587 Burnham BE. Garlic as a possible risk for postoperative bleeding. *Plast Reconstr Surg* 1995;95:213.

588 Shuster J. Black cohosh root? Chasteberry Tree? Seizures! *Hosp Pharm* 1996;31:1553-4.

589 Scaglione F, Cattaneo G, Alessandria M, Cogo R. Efficacy and safety of the standardized Ginseng extract G115 for potentiating vaccination against the influenza syndrome and protection against the common cold. *Drugs Exp Clin Res* 1996;22:65-72.

590 Palmer BV, Montgomery AC, Monteiro JC, et al. Gin Seng and mastalgia [letter]. *BMJ* 1978;1:1284.

591 Hopkins MP, Androff L, Benninghoff AS. Ginseng face cream and unexplained vaginal bleeding. *Am J Obstet Gynecol* 1988;159:1121-2.

592 Greenspan EM. Ginseng and vaginal bleeding [letter]. *JAMA* 1983;249:2018.

593 Koren G, Randor S, Martin S, Danneman D. Maternal ginseng use associated with neonatal androgenization. *JAMA* 1990;264:2866.

594 Gonzalez-Seijo JC, Ramos YM, Lastra I. Manic episode and ginseng: Report of a possible case. *J Clin Psychopharmacol* 1995;15:447-8.

595 Ryu S, Chien Y. Ginseng-associated cerebral arteritis. *Neurology* 1995;45:829-30.

596 Dega H, Laporte JL, Frances C, et al. Ginseng as a cause of Stevens-Johnson syndrome. *Lancet* 1996;313:756.

597 Brown R. Potential interactions of herbal medicines with antipsychotics, antidepressants and hypnotics. *Eur J Herbal Med* 1997;3:25-8.

REFERENCES

598 Hamid S, Rojter S, Vierling J. Protracted cholestatic hepatitis after the use of Prostata. *Ann Intern Med* 1997;127:169-70.

600 Malo JL, Cartier A, L'Archeveque J, et al. Prevalence of occupational asthma and immunologic sensitization to guar gum among employees at a carpet-manufacturing plant. *J Allergy Clin Immunol* 1990;86:562-9.

601 Lagier F, Cartier A, Somer J, et al. Occupational asthma caused by guar gum. *J Allergy Clin Immunol* 1990;85:785-90.

602 Lewis JH. Esophageal and small bowel obstruction from guar gum-containing diet pills: analysis of 26 cases reported to the FDA. *Am J Gastroenterol* 1992;87:1424-8.

603 Norton SA, et al. Kava dermopathy. *J Am Acad Dermatol* 1994;31(1):89-97.

604 Agha FP, et al. Giant colonic bezoar: a medication bezoar due to psyllium seed husks. *Am J Gastroenterol* 1984;79:319-21.

605 Brown R. Potential interactions of herbal medicines with antipsychotics, antidepressants and hypnotics. *Eur J Herbal Med* 1997;3:25-8.

606 Harder S, Fuhr U, Staib AH, Wolff T. Ciprofloxacin-caffeine: a drug interaction established using in vivo and in vitro investigations. *Am J Med* 1989;87:89S-91S.

607 Carbo M, Segura J, De la Torre R, et al. Effect of quinolones on caffeine disposition. *Clin Pharmacol Ther* 1989;45:234-40.

608 Healy DP, Polk RE, Kanawati L, et al. Interaction between oral ciprofloxacin and caffeine in normal volunteers. *Antimicrob Agents Chemother* 1989;33:474-8.

609 Mester R, Toren P, Mizrachi I, et al. Caffeine withdrawal increases lithium blood levels. *Biol Psychiatry* 1995;37:348-50.

610 Jefferson JW. Lithium tremor and caffeine intake: two cases of drinking less and shaking more. *J Clin Psychiatry* 1988;49:72-3.

611 Yu CM, et al. Chinese herbs and warfarin potentiation by Danshen. *J Intern Med* 1997;241:337-9.

612 Tam LS, et al. Warfarin interacions with Chinese traditional medicines: danshen and methyl salicylate medicated oil. *Aust N Z J Med* 1995;25:258.

613 Shaw D, Leon C, Kolev S, Murray V. Traditional remedies and food supplements: a 5-year toxicological study (1991-1995). *Drug Saf* 1997;17:342-56.

615 Richter WO, Jacob BG, Schwandt P. Interaction between fibre and lovastatin. *Lancet* 1991;338:706.

616 Sunter WH. Warfarin and garlic. *Pharm J* 1991;246:722.

617 Shader RI, Greenblatt DJ. Phenylzine and the dream machine-ramblings and reflections. *J Clin Psychopharmacol* 1985;5:65.

618 Jones BD, Runikis AM. Interaction of ginseng with phenelzine. *J Clin Psychopharmacol* 1987;7:201-2.

619 Janetzky K, Morreale AP. Probable interaction between warfarin and ginseng. *Am J Health Syst Pharm* 1997;54:692-3.

620 Golsch S, Vocks E, Rakoski J, et al. [Reversible increase in photosensitivity to UV-B caused by St. John's wort extract]. [Article in German]. *Hautarzt* 1997;48:249-52.

621 Bove GM. Acute neuropathy after exposure to sun in a patient treated with St. John's Wort. *Lancet* 1998;352:1121-2.

622 Sharma RD, Raghuram TC, Rao NS. Effect of fenugreek seeds on blood glucose and serum lipids in type I diabetes. *Eur J Clin Nutr* 1990;44:301-6.

623 Thys-Jacobs S, Starkey P, Bernstein D, Tian J. Calcium carbonate and the premenstrual syndrome: Effects on premenstrual and menstrual symptoms. *Am J Obstet Gynecol* 1998;179:444-52.

624 Chang T, Benet LZ, Hebert MF. The effect of water-soluble vitamin E on cyclosporine pharmacokinetics in healthy volunteers. *Clin Pharmacol Ther* 1996;59:297-303.

625 Pan SH, Lopez RR Jr, Sher LS, et al. Enhanced oral cyclosporine absorption with water-soluble vitamin E early after liver transplantation. *Pharmacother* 1996;16:59-65.

626 Lasswell WL Jr, Weber SS, Wilkins JM. In vitro interaction of neuroleptics and tricylic antidepressants with coffee, tea, and gallotannic acid. *J Pharm Sci* 1984;73:1056-8.

627 Kulhanek F, Linde OK, Meisenberg G. Precipitation of Antipsychotic drugs in interaction with coffee or tea. *Lancet* 1979;2:1130.

628 Brockmoller J, Reum T, Bauer S, et al. Hypericin and pseudohypericin: pharmacokinetics and effects on photosensitivity in humans. *Pharmacopsychiatry* 1997;30:94-101.

629 Kang-Yum E, Oransky SH. Chinese patent medicine as a potential source of mercury poisoning. *Vet Hum Toxicol* 1992;34:235-8.

630 Prussick R, Ali MA, Rosenthal D, Guyatt G. The protective effect of vitamin E on the hemolysis associated with Dapsone treatment in patients with dermatitis herpetiformis. *Arch Dermatol* 1992;128:210-3.

631 Merhav H, Amitai Y, Palti H, Godfrey S. Tea drinking and microcytic anemia in infants. *Am J Clin Nutr* 1985;41:1210-3.

632 Ridker PM, McDermott WV. Comfrey herb tea and hepatic veno-occlusive disease. *Lancet* 1989;2:657-8.

633 Weston CF, Cooper BT, Davies JD, Levine DF. Veno-occlusive disease of the liver secondary to ingestion of comfrey. *BMJ* 1987;295:183.

634 Bach N, Thung SN, Schaffner F. Comfrey herb tea-induced heapatic veno-occlusive disesae. *Am J Med* 1989;87:97-9.

635 Yeong ML, Swinburn B, Kennedy M, Nicholson G. Hepatic veno-occlusive disease associated with comfrey ingestion. *J Gastroenterol Hepatol* 1990;5:211-4.

636 Hassell LH, MacMillan MW. Acute anticholinergic syndrome following ingestion of Angel's trumpet tea. *Hawaii Med J* 1995;54:669-70.

637 Kamiyama T, Nouchi T, Kojima S, et al. Autoimmune hepatitis triggered by administration of an herbal medicine. *Am J Gastroenterol* 1997;92:703-4.

638 Mullins RJ. Echinacea-associated anaphylaxis. *Med J Aust* 1998;168:170-1.

639 Doyle H, Kargin M. Herbal stimulant containing ephedrine has also caused psychosis. *BMJ* 1996;313:756.

640 Castot A, et al. [Pharmacovigilance off the beaten track: herbal surveillance or pharmacovigilance of medicinal plants]. [Article in French]. *Therapie* 1997;52:97-103.

641 Mostefa-Kara N, et al. Fatal hepatitis after herbal tea. *Lancet* 1992;340:674.

642 Larrey D, et al. Hepatitis after germander (Teucrium chamaedrys) administration: another instance of herbal medicine hepatotoxicity. *Ann Intern Med* 1992;117:129-32.

643 Woolf, GM. Jin Bu Huan toxicity in adults- Los Angeles, 1993. *MMWR Morb Mortal Wkly Rep* 1993;42:920-2.

644 Horowitz RS, et al. Jin Bu Huan toxicity in children-Colorado, 1993. *MMWR Morb Mortal Wkly Rep* 1993;42:633-5.

645 Pye KG, Kelsey SM, House IM, et al. Severe dyserythropoeisis and autoimmune thrombocytopenia associated with ingestion of kelp supplement. *Lancet* 1992;339:1540.

646 Spiller HA, et al. Retrospective study of misletoe ingestion. *J Toxicol Clin Toxicol* 1996;34:405-8.

647 Harvey J, et al. Mistletoe hepatitis. *Br Med J* (Clin Res Ed) 1981;282:186-7.

648 Krenzelok EP, et al. American mistletoe exposures. *Am J Emerg Med* 1997;15:516-20.

649 Solbakken AM, Rorbakken G, Gundersen T. [Nature medicine as intoxicant]. [Article in Norwegian]. *Tidsskr Nor Laegeforen* 1997;117:1140-1.

650 Anderson IB, et al. Pennyroyal toxicity: measurement of toxic metabolite levels in two cases and review of the literature. *Ann Intern Med* 1996;124:726-34.

651 Takahashi M, et al. Contact dermatitis due to honeybee royal jelly. *Contact Dermatitis* 1983;9:452-5.

652 Bullock RJ, et al. Fatal royal jelly-induced asthma. *Med J Aust* 1994;160:44.

653 Thien FCK, et al. Royal jelly-induced asthma. *Med J Aust* 1993;159:639.

654 Beuers U. Hepatitis after chronic abuse of senna. *Lancet* 1991;337:372-3.

655 Ortiz Cansado A, et al. [Veno-occlusive liver disease due to intake of Senecio vulgaris tea]. [Article in Spanish]. *Gastroenterol Hepatol* 1995;18:413-6.

656 Tomioka M, et al. [Hepatic veno-occlusive disease associated with ingestion of Senecio tephrosioides]. [Article in Spanish]. *Rev Gastroenterol Peru* 1995;15:299-302.

658 De Groot AC. Airborn allergic contact dermatitis from tea tree oil. *Contact Dermatitis* 1996;35:304-5.

659 Willey LB, et al. Valerian overdose: a case report. *Vet Hum Toxicol* 1995;37:364-5.

660 Cahill DJ, et al. Multiple follicular development associated with herbal medicine. *Hum Reprod* 1994;9:1469-70.

661 Berlin R, et al. Wormwood: Oregon Poison Ctr. Portland, OR: Oregon Health Sci Univ 1996.

662 Weisbord SD, Soule JB, Kimmel PL. Poison on line-acute renal failure caused by oil of wormwood purchased through the internet. *N Engl J Med* 1997;337:825-7.

663 Graedon J, Graedon T. The People's Guide to Deadly Possible Interactions with Drugs. New York, NY: St. Martin's Press, 1995.

664 Blumenthal M. Herb and Conventional Possible Interactions with Drugs. Austin, TX: Am Botanical Council, 1997.

665 LoVecchio F, Curry SC, Bagnasco T. Butyrolactone-induced central nervous system depression after ingestion of RenewTrient, a dietary supplement. *N Engl J Med* 1998;339:847-8.

667 Blickstein D, et al. Warfarin antagonism by avocado. *Lancet* 1991;337:914-5.

668 Colquhoun DM, et al. Comparison of the effects on lipoproteins and apolipoproteins of a diet high in monounsaturated fatty acids, enriched with avocado, and a high-carbohydrate diet. *Am J Clin Nutr* 1992;56(4):671-77.

669 Lopez Ledesma R, et al. Monounsaturated fatty acid (avocado) rich diet for mild hypercholesterolemia. *Arch Med Res* 1996;27(4):519-23.

670 Carranza J, et al. [Effects of avocado on the level of blood lipids in patients with phenotype II and IV dyslipidemias].[Article in Spanish]. *Arch Inst Cardiol Mex* 1995;65(4):342-8.

671 Lerman-Garber I, et al. Effect of a high-monounsaturated fat diet enriched with avocado in NIDDM patients. *Diabetes Care* 1994;17(4):311-5.

672 van Weerden WM, et al. Effects of adrenal androgens on the transplantable human prostate tumor PC-82. *Endocrinol* 1992;131:2909-13.

673 Mecenas CA, Giussani DA, Owiny JR, et al. Production of premature delivery in pregnant rhesus monkeys by androstenedione infusion. *Nat Med* 1996;2:443-8.

674 Anon. Creatine and androstenedione, two dietary supplements. *Med Lett Drugs Ther* 1998;40:105-6.

675 Alvizouri-Munoz M, Carranza-Madrigal J, Herrera-Abarca JE, et al. Effects of avocado as a source of monounsaturated fatty acids on plasma lipid levels. *Arch Med Res* 1992;23:163-7.

676 Chen Z, Posch A, Cremer R, et al. Identification of hevein (Hev b 6.02) in Hevea latex as a major cross- reacting allergen with avocado fruit in patients with latex allergy. *J Allergy Clin Immunol* 1998;102:476-81.

677 Diehl HW, May EL. Cetyl myristoleate isolated from Swiss albino mice: an apparent protective agent against adjuvant arthritis in rats. *J Pharm Sci* 1994;83:296-9.

678 Plaitakis A, Smith J, Mandeli J, Yahr MD. Pilot trial of branched-chain aminoacids in amyotrophic lateral sclerosis. *Lancet* 1988;1:1015-8.

679 Anon. Branched-chain amino acids and amyotrophic lateral sclerosis: a treatment failure? The Italian ALS Study Group. *Neurology* 1993;43:2466-70.

680 Testa D, Caraceni T, Fetoni V. Branched-chain amino acids in the treatment of amyotrophic lateral sclerosis. *J Neurol* 1989;236:445-7.

681 Tandan R, Bromberg MB, Forshew D, et al. A controlled trial of amino acid therapy in amyotrophic lateral sclerosis: I. Clinical, functional, and maximum isometric torque data. *Neurology* 1996;47:1220-6.

682 FDA. FDA warns about products containing gamma butyrolactone or GBL and asks companies to issue a recall. Talk Paper, 21 January 1999.

684 Plauth M, Egberts EH, Hamster W, et al. Long-term treatment of latent portosystemic encephalopathy with branched-chain amino acids. A double-blind placebo-controlled crossover study. *J Hepatol* 1993;17:308-14.

685 Egberts EH, Schomerus H, Hamster W, Jurgens P. Branched chain amino acids in the treatment of latent portosystemic encephalopathy. A double-blind, placebo-controlled, crossover study. *Gastroenterol* 1985;88:887-95.

686 Rossi Fanelli F, Cangiano C, Capocaccia L, et al. Use of branched chain amino acids for treating hepatic encephalopathy: clinical experiences. *Gut* 1986;27:111-5.

687 Wahren J, Denis J, Desurmont P, Eriksson LS, et al. Is intravenous administration of branched chain amino acids effective in the treatment of hepatic encephalopathy? A multicenter study. *Hepatol* 1983;3:475-80.

688 Michel H, Bories P, Aubin JP, et al. Treatment of acute hepatic encephalopathy in cirrhotics with a branched-chain amino acids enriched versus a conventional amino acids mixture. A controlled study of 70 patients. *Liver* 1985;5:282-9.

689 Vilstrup H, Gluud C, Hardt F, et al. Branched chain enriched amino acid versus glucose treatment of hepatic encephalopathy. A double-blind study of 65 patients with cirrhosis. *J Hepatol* 1990;10:291-6.

690 Marchesini G, Dioguardi FS, Bianchi GP, et al. Long-term oral branched-chain amino acid treatment in chronic hepatic encephalopathy. A randomized double-blind casein-controlled trial. The Italian Multicenter Study Group. *J Hepatol* 1990;11:92-101.

691 Chuah SY, Ellis BJ, Mayberry JF. Exacerbation of hepatic encephalopathy by branched-chain amino acids-a case report. *J Hum Nutr Diet* 1992;5:53-6.

692 Blomstrand E, Hassmen P, Ek S, et al. Influence of ingesting a solution of branched-chain amino acids on perceived exertion during exercise. *Acta Physiol Scand* 1997;159:41-9.

693 MacLean DA, Graham TE. Branched-chain amino acid supplementation augments plasma ammonia responses during exercise in humans. *J Appl Physiol* 1993;74:2711-7.

694 MacLean DA, Graham TE, Saltin B. Branched-chain amino acids augment ammonia metabolism while attenuating protein breakdown during exercise. *Am J Physiol* 1994;267:E1010-22.

695 Breum L, Pedersen JK, Ahlstrom F, et al. Comparison of an ephedrine/caffeine combination and dexfenfluramine in the treatment of obesity. A double-blind multi-centre trial in

REFERENCES

general practice. *Int J Obes Relat Metab Disord* 1994;18:99-103.

696 Toubro S, Astrup AV, Breum L, Quaade F. The acute and chronic effects of ephedrine/caffeine mixtures on energy expenditure and glucose metabolism in humans. *Int J Obes Relat Metab Disord* 1993;17:S73-7.

697 Toubro S, Astrup AV, Breum L, Quaade F. Safety and efficacy of long-term treatment with ephedrine, caffeine and an ephedrine/caffeine mixture. *Int J Obes Relat Metab Disord* 1993;17:S69-72.

698 Cystadane (betaine anhydrous for oral solution) Package insert. Orphan Med. October 1996.

699 Feldman J, Menkes CJ, Pallardy G, et al. [Double-blind study of the treatment of disc lumbosciatica by chemonucleolysis]. [Article in French]. *Rev Rhum Mal Osteoartic* 1986;53:147-52.

700 Nordby EJ. A comparison of discectomy and chemonucleolysis. *Clin Orthop* 1985;:279-83.

701 Javid MJ. Chemonucleolysis versus laminectomy. A cohort comparison of effectiveness and charges. *Spine* 1995;20:2016-22.

703 Clarkson PM, Haymes EM. Trace mineral requirements for athletes. *Int J Sport Nutr* 1994;4:104-19.

704 Clarkson PM. Minerals: exercise performance and supplementation in athletes. *J Sports Sci* 1991;9:91-116.

705 Campbell WW, Anderson RA. Effects of aerobic exercise and training on the trace minerals chromium, zinc and copper. *Sports Med* 1987 4:9-18.

706 Broun ER, Greist A, Tricot G, Hoffman R. Excessive zinc ingestion. A reversible cause of sideroblastic anemia and bone marrow depression. *JAMA* 1990;264:1441-3.

707 Sandstead HH. Requirements and toxicity of essential trace elements, illustrated by zinc and copper. *Am J Clin Nutr* 1995;61:621S-4S.

708 Brewer GJ, Dick RD, Johnson VD, et al. Treatment of Wilson's disease with zinc: XV long-term follow-up studies. *J Lab Clin Med* 1998;132:264-78.

709 Weight LM, Noakes TD, Labadarios D, et al. Vitamin and mineral status of trained athletes including the effects of supplementation. *Am J Clin Nutr* 1988;47:186-91.

710 Finley EB, Cerklewski FL. Influence of ascorbic acid supplementation on copper status in young adult men. *Am J Clin Nutr* 1983;37:553-6.

711 Scharf MB, Hauck M, Stover R, et al. Effect of gamma-hydroxybutyrate on pain, fatigue, and the alpha sleep anomaly in patients with fibromyalgia. Preliminary report. *J Rheumatol* 1998;25:1986-90.

712 Chin RL, Sporer KA, Cullison B, et al. Clinical course of gamma-hydroxybutyrate overdose. *Ann Emerg Med* 1998;31:716-22.

713 Tunnicliff, G. Sites of action of gamma-hydroxybutyrate (GHB)-a neuroactive drug with abuse potential. *J Toxicol Clin Toxicol* 1997;35:581-90.

714 FDA Talk Paper. FDA re-issues warning on GHB. February 18, 1997.

715 Latha B, Ramakrishnan M, Jayaraman V, Babu M. The efficacy of trypsin: chymotrypsin preparation in the reduction of oxidative damage during burn injury. *Burns* 1998;24:532-8.

716 Latha B, Ramakrishnan M, Jayaraman V, Babu M. Serum enzymatic changes modulated using trypsin: chymotrypsin preparation during burn wounds in humans. *Burns* 1997;23:560-4.

717 Shaw PC. The use of a trypsin-chymotrypsin formulation in fractures of the hand. *Br J Clin Pract* 1969;23:25-6.

718 McCue FC, Webster TM, Gieck J. Clinical effects of proteolytic enzymes after reconstructive hand surgery. *Int Surg* 1972;57:479-82.

719 Patil SP, Niphadkar PV, Bapat MM. Allergy to fenugreek (Trigonella foenum graecum). *Ann Allergy Asthma Immunol* 1997;78:297-300.

720 Ahsan SK, Tariq M, Ageel AM, et al. Effect of Trigonella foenum-graecum and Ammi majus on calcium oxalate urolithiasis in rats. *J Ethnopharmacol* 1989;26:249-54.

721 Fischer-Rasmussen W, Kjaer SK, Dahl C, Asping U. Ginger treatment of hyperemesis gravidarum. *Eur J Obstet Gynecol Reprod Biol* 1991;38:19-24.

722 Phillips S, Ruggier R, Hutchinson SE. Zingiber officinale (ginger)-an antiemetic for day case surgery. *Anaesthesia* 1993;48:715-7.

723 Bone ME, Wilkinson DJ, Young JR, et al. Ginger root-a new antiemetic. The effect of ginger root on postoperative nausea and vomiting after major gynaecological surgery. *Anaesthesia* 1990;45:669-71.

724 Foster S. Feverfew, Tanacetum parthenium, botanical series #310. Austin, TX: Am Botanical Council, 1996.

725 Awang, DVC. Feverfew effective in Migraine prevention. *HerbalGram* 1998;42:18.

726 Awang, DVC. Feverfew trials: the promise of- and the problem with standardized extracts. *HerbalGram* 1997;41:16-7.

727 Kuritzky A, Elhacham Y, Yerushalmi Z, et al. Feverfew in the treatment of migraine: its effect on serotonin uptake and platelet activity. *Neurology* 1994;44(Suppl 2):A201. (Abstract 293P)

728 Heymsfield SB, Allison DB, Vasselli JR, et al. Garcinia cambogia (hydroxycitric acid) as a potential antiobesity agent: a randomized controlled trial. *JAMA* 1998;280:1596-600.

729 Dulloo AG, Miller DS. Aspirin as a promoter of ephedrine-induced thermogenesis: potential use in the treatment of obesity. *Am J Clin Nutr* 1987;45:564-9.

730 Williams M. Immuno-protection against herpes simplex type II infection by eleutherococcus root extract. *Int J Altern Complem Med* 1995;13:9-12.

731 Isaacsohn JL, Moser M, Stein EA, et al. Garlic powder and plasma lipids and lipoproteins, a multicenter, randomized, placebo-controlled trial. *Arch Intern Med* 1998;158:1189-94.

732 Berthold HK, Sudhop T, von Bergmann K. Effect of a garlic oil preparation on serum lipoproteins and cholesterol metabolism. *JAMA* 1998;279:1900-2.

733 Mitscher LA, Mitscher LA, Jung M, Shankel D, et al. Chemoprotection: a review of the potential therapeutic antioxidant properties of green tea (Camellia sinensis) and certain of its constituents. *Med Res Rev* 1997;17:327-65.

734 Kono S, Shinchi K, Ikeda N, et al. Green tea consumption and serum lipid profiles: a cross-sectional study in northern Kyushu, Japan. *Prev Med* 1992;21:526-31.

735 Kingsbury JM. Poison ivy, poison sumac, and other rash-producing plants. York State Coll of Agri, Life Sci, Info Bull. #105;1976.

736 Liu JH, Xu SX, Yao XS, Kobayashi H. Angelol-type coumarins from Angelica pubescence F. biserrata and their inhibitory effect on platelet aggregation. *Phytochem* 1995;39:1099-101.

737 Lo AC, Chan K, Yeung JH, Woo KS. Danggui (Angelica sinensis) affects the pharmacodynamics but not the pharmacokinetics of warfarin in rabbits. *Eur J Drug Metab Pharmacokinet* 1995;20:55-60.

738 Hirata JD, Swiersz LM, Zell B, et al. Does dong quai have estrogenic effects in postmenopausal women? A double-blind, placebo-controlled trial. *Fertil Steril* 1997;68:981-6.

739 Cooper RL, Cooper MM. Red pepper-induced dermatitis in breast-fed infants. *Dermatol* 1996;93:61-2.

740 Stone-Dorshow T, Levitt MD. Gaseous response to ingestion of a poorly absorbed fructo-oligosaccharide sweetener. *Am J Clin Nutr* 1987;46:61-5.

741 Bornet FR. Undigestible sugars in food products. *Am J Clin Nutr* 1994;59:763S-9S.

743 Schaafsma G, Meuling WJ, van Dokkum W, Bouley C. Effects of a milk product, fermented by Lactobacillus acidophilus and with fructo-oligosaccharides added, on blood lipids in male volunteers. *Eur J Clin Nutr* 1998;52:436-40.

744 Roberfroid M. Dietary fiber, inulin, and oligofructose: a review comparing their physiological effects. *Crit Rev Food Sci Nutr* 1993;33:103-48.

745 Briet F, et al. Symptomatic response to varying levels of fructo-oligosaccharides consumed occasionally or regularly. *Eur J Clin Nutr* 1995;49:501-7.

746 Mitsouka T, Hidaka H, Eida T. Effect of fructo-oligosaccharides on intestinal microflora. *Nahrung* 1987;31:427-36.

747 Alles MS, et al. Fate of fructo-oligosaccharides in the human intestine. *Br J Nutr* 1996;76:211-21.

748 Pierre F, et al. Short-chain fructo-oligosaccharides reduced the occurrence of colon tumors and develop gut-associated lymphoid tissue in Min mice. *Cancer Res* 1997;57:225-8.

749 Gibson GR. Dietary modulation of the human gut microflora using prebiotics. *Br J Nutr* 1998;80:S209-12.

750 Bouhnik Y, et al. Short-chain fructo-oligosaccharide administration dose-dependently increases fecal bifidobacteria in healthy humans. *J Nutr* 1999;129:113-6.

751 Fry AC, et al. The effects of gamma-oryzanol supplementation during resistance exercise training. *Int J Sport Nutr* 1997;7:318-29.

752 Sasaki J, et al. Effects of gamma-oryzanol on serum lipids and apolipoproteins in dyslipidemic schizophrenics receiving major tranquilizers. *Clin Ther* 1990;12:263-8.

753 Shimomura Y, et al. Effect of gamma-oryzanol on serum TSH concentrations in primary hypothyroidism. *Endocrinol Jpn* 1980;27:83-6.

754 Sugano M, Tsuji E. Rice bran oil and human health. *Biomed Environ Sci* 1996;9:242-6.

755 Wheeler KB, Garleb KA. Gamma oryzanol-plant sterol supplementation: metabolic, endocrine, and physiologic effects. *Int J Sport Nutr* 1991;1:170-7.

756 Seetharamaiah GS, Chandrasekhara N. Effect of oryzanol on cholesterol absorption and biliary and fecal bile acids in rats. *Indian J Med Res* 1990;92:471-5.

757 Ishihara M, et al. [Clinical effect of gamma-oryzanol on climacteric disturbance- on serum lipid peroxides]. [Article in Japanese]. *Nippon Sanka Fujinka Gakkai Zasshi* 1982;34:243-51.

758 Upton R, ed. St. John's wort, Hypericum perforatum: Quality control, analytical and therapeutic monograph. Santa Cruz, CA: American Herbal Pharmacopoeia 1997;1-32.

759 Chavez ML,Chavez PI. Saint John's wort. *Hosp Pharm* 1997;32:1621-32.

760 Chavez ML. Glucosamine sulfate and chondroitin sulfates. *Hosp Pharm* 1997;32:1275-85.

761 Laakmann G, Schule C, Baghai T, Kieser M. St. John's wort in mild to moderate depression: the relevance of hyperforin for the clinical efficacy. *Pharmacopsych* 1998;31:54-9.

762 Chatterjee SS, Noldner M, Koch E, Erdelmeier C. Antidepressant activity of hypericum perforatum and hyperforin: the neglected possibility. *Pharmacopsych* 1998;31:7-15.

763 Muller WE, Singer A, Wonnemann M, et al. Hyperforin represents the neurotransmitter reuptake inhibiting constituent of hypericum extract. *Pharmacopsychiatry* 1998;31:16-21.

764 Gerber GS, Zagaja GP, Bales GT, et al. Saw palmetto (Serenoa repens) in men with lower urinary tract symptoms: effects on urodynamic parameters and voiding symptoms. *Urol* 1998;51:1003-7.

767 Shiroky JB, Neville C, Esdaile JM, et al. Low-dose methotrexate with leucovorin (folinic acid) in the management of rheumatoid arthritis. Results of a multicenter randomized, double-blind, placebo-controlled trial. *Arthritis Rheum* 1993;36:795-803.

768 Duhra P. Treatment of gastrointestinal symptoms associated with methotrexate therapy for psoriasis. *J Am Acad Dermatol* 1993;28:466-9.

769 Voordouw BC, Euser R, Verdonk RE, et al. Melatonin and melatonin-progestin combinations alter pituitary-ovarian function in women and can inhibit ovulation. *J Clin Endocrinol Metab* 1992;74:108-17.

770 Becker BN. Ginseng-induced diuretic resistance. *JAMA* 1996;276:606-7.

771 Walaszek Z. Potential use of D-glucarate derivatives in cancer prevention. *Cancer Lett* 1990;54:1-8.

772 Dwivedi C, et al. Effect of calcium glucarate on B-glucuronidase activity and glucarate content on certain vegetables and fruits. *Biochem Med Metab Bio* 1990;43:83-92.

773 Heerdt AS, Young CW, Borgen PI. Calcium glucarate as a chemopreventive agent in breast cancer. *Isr J Med Sci* 1995;31:101-5.

774 Walaszek Z, et al. Metabolism, uptake and excretion of D-glucaric acid salt and its potential use in cancer prevention. *Cancer Detect Prev* 1997;21(2):178-90.

775 Walaszek Z, Hanausek-Walaszek M, Minton JP, Webb TE. Dietary glucarate as anti-promter of 7,12-dimethylbenz(a)anthracene-induced mammary tumorigenesis. *Carcinogenesis* 1986;7:1463-6.

776 Curley RW Jr., et al. Activity of D-glucarate analogues: synergistic antiproliferative effects with retinoid in cultured human mammary tumor cells appear to specifically require the D-glucarate structure. *Life Sci* 1994;54(18):1299-303.

777 Furuno K, et al. Preventive effect of D-glucarate against renal damage induced by kanamycin. *J Antibiot* (Tokyo) 1976;29(9):950-3.

778 Kampf D, Roots I, Hildenbrandt AG. Urinary excretion of D-glucarate, an indicator of drug metabolizing enzyme activity, in patients with impaired renal function. *Eur J Clin Pharmacol* 1980;18(3):255-61.

779 Mezey E. Increased urinary excretion of D-glucarate acid in alcoholism. *Res Commun Chem Pathol Pharmacol* 1976;15(4);735-42.

780 Pointel JP, et al. Titrated extract of Centella asiatica (TECA) in the treatment of venous insufficiency of the lower limbs. *Angiol* 1987;38(1 Pt 1):46-50.

781 Farese RV Jr, Biglieri EG, Shackleton CH, et al. Licorice-induced hypermineralocorticoidism. *N Engl J Med* 1991;325:1223-7.

782 Singh YN, Blumenthal M. Kava an overview. *HerbalGram* 1997;39:33-44, 46-55.

783 Cartier LC, Lehrer A, Malo JL. Occupational asthma caused by aromatic herbs. *Allergy* 1996;51:647-9.

784 Joy JE, Watson SJ Jr, Benson JA Jr, et al. Marijuana and medicine: assessing the science base. A summary of the 1999 Inst of Med report. *Arch Gen Psychiatr* 2000 Jun;57:547-52.

785 Hsu CK, Leo P, Shastry D, et al. Anticholinergic poisoning associated with herbal tea. *Arch Intern Med* 1995;155:2245-8.

787 Foster S. Peppermint, Menta x piperita, botanical series #306. Austin, TX: Am Botanical Council, 1990.

788 Kapil A, Moza N. Anticomplementary activity of boswellic acids-an inhibitor of C3-convertase of the classical

complement pathway. *Int J Immunopharmacol* 1992;14(7):1139-43.

789 Halperin EC, Gaspar L, George S, et al. A double-blind, randomized, prospective trial to evaluate topical vitamin C solution for the prevention of radiation dermatitis. *Int J Radiat Oncol Biol Phys* 1993;26:413-6.

790 Wslbling RH, Leonhardt K. Local therapy of herpes simplex with dried extract from Melissa officinalis. *Phytomedicine* 1994;1:25-31.

791 Takahashi M, Matsuo I, Ohkido M. Contact dermatitis due to honeybee royal jelly. *Contact Dermatitis* 1983;9:452-5.

792 Bullock RJ, et al. Fatal royal jelly-induced asthma. *Med J Aust* 1994;160:44.

793 Reiter WJ, Pycha A, Schatzl G, et al. Dehydroepiandosterone in the treatment of erectile dysfunction: A prospective, double-blind, randomized, placebo-controlled study. *Urol* 1999;53:590-5.

795 Foster S. Milk Thistle, Silybum marianum, botanical series #305. Austin, TX: Am Botanical Council, 1996.

797 Awang DVC. Siberian ginseng toxicity may be case of mistaken identity. [Letter]. *CMAJ* 1996;155:1237.

798 Moretti S. Effect of L-carnitine on human immunodeficiency virus-1 infection-associated apoptosis: a pilot study. *Blood* 1998;91:3817-24.

799 Magro-Filho O, de Carvalho AC. Topical effect of propolis in the repair of sulcoplasties by the modified Kazanjian technique. Cytological and clinical evaluation. *J Nihon Univ Sch Dent* 1994;36:102-11.

800 Magro-Filho O, de Carvalho AC. Application of propolis to dental sockets and skin wounds. *J Nihon Univ Sch Dent* 1990;32(1):4-13.

806 Stanko RT, Mullick P, Clarke MR, et al. Pyruvate inhibits growth of mammary adenocarcinoma 13762 in rats. *Cancer Res* 1994;54:1004-7.

807 Stanko RT, Robertson RJ, Galbreath RW, et al. Enhanced leg exercise endurance with a high-carbohydrate diet and dihydroxyacetone and pyruvate. *J Appl Physiol* 1990;69:1651-6.

808 Stanko RT, Robertson RJ, Spina RJ, et al. Enhancement of arm exercise endurance capacity with dihydroxyacetone and pyruvate. *J Appl Physiol* 1990;68:119-24.

809 Hogan RP III. Hemorrhagic diathesis caused by drinking an herbal tea. *JAMA* 1983;249:2679-80.

810 Gonzalez M, Zarzuelo A, Gamez MJ, et al. Hypoglycemic activity of olive leaf. *Planta Med* 1992;58(6):513-5.

811 Heimann SW. Pycnogenol for ADHD? *J Am Acad Child Adolesc Psychiatr* 1999;38:357-8.

812 Mash DC, Kovera CA, Buck BE, et al. Medication development of ibogaine as a pharmacotherapy for drug dependence. *Ann N Y Acad Sci* 1998;844:274-92.

813 Glick SD, Maisonneuve IS. Mechanisms of antiaddictive actions of ibogaine. *Ann N Y Acad Sci* 1998;844:214-26.

815 Royal Botanical Gardens Kew online databases. www.rbgkew.org.uk/web.dbs/webdbsintro.html.

816 Germplasm Resources Info. www.ars-grin.gov/npgs (Accessed 3 November 1999).

817 Harrington C. Plant dubbed nature's Viagra. Calgary, CAN: Canadian Press; 15 Nov. 1998.

818 Dudley JP. Bilateral pneumothorax resulting from the bronchoscopic removal of a puncture vine fruit. *Ann Otol Rhinol Laryngol* 1983;92(4 Pt 1):396-7.

819 Pierard-Franchimont C, Goffin V, Visser JN, et al. A double-blind controlled evaluation of the sebosuppressive activity of topical erythromycin-zinc complex. *Eur J Clin Pharmacol* 1995;49:57-60.

820 Feucht CL, Allen BS, Chalker DK, et al. Topical erythromycin with zinc in acne. A double-blind controlled study. *J Am Acad Dermatol* 1980;3:483-91.

821 Mostafa WZ, al-Zayer AA. Acrodermatitis enteropathica in Saudi Arabia. *Int J Dermatol* 1990;29:134-8.

822 Hoogenraad TU, Van Hattum J, Van den Hamer CJ. Management of Wilson's disease with zinc sulphate. Experience in a series of 27 patients. *J Neurol Sci* 1987;77:137-46.

823 Anderson LA, Hakojarvi SL, Boudreaux SK. Zinc acetate treatment in Wilson's disease. *Ann Pharmacother* 1998;32:78-87.

824 Fortes C, Forastiere F, Agabiti N, et al. The effect of zinc and vitamin A supplementation on immune response in an older population. *J Am Geriatr Soc* 1998;46:19-26.

825 Faruque AS, Mahalanabis D, Haque SS, et al. Double-blind, randomized, controlled trial of zinc or vitamin A supplementation in young children with acute diarrhea. *Acta Paediatr* 1999;88:154-60.

826 Roy SK, Tomkins AM, Akramuzzaman SM, et al. Randomized, controlled trial of zinc supplementation in malnourished Bangladeshi children with acute diarrhea. *Arch Dis Child* 1997;77:196-200.

827 Sazawal S, Black RE, Bhan MK, et al. Zinc supplementation in young children with acute diarrhea in India. *N Engl J Med* 1995;333:839-44.

828 Blondeau JM. Expanded activity and utility of the new fluoroquinolones: a review. *Clin Ther* 1999;21:3-40.

829 Mountokalakis T, Dourakis S, Karatzas N, et al. Zinc deficiency in mild hypertensive patients treated with diuretics. *J Hypertens Suppl* 1984;2(3):S571-2.

830 Reyes AJ, Olhaberry JV, Leary WP, et al. Urinary zinc excretion, diuretics, zinc deficiency and some side-effects of diuretics. *S Afr Med J* 1983;64:936-41.

831 Cohanim M, Yendt ER. The effects of thiazides on serum and urinary zinc in patients with renal calculi. *Johns Hopkins Med J* 1975;136:137-44.

832 Ghio S, de Servi S, Perotti R, et al. Different susceptibility to the development of nitroglycerin tolerance in the arterial and venous circulation in humans- effects of N-acetylcysteine administration. *Circulation* 1992;86:798-802.

833 Blueberry. Eat 5 a day for better health. www.5aday.com/ (Accessed 12 October 2000).

834 Calabrese C, Myer S, Munson S, et al. A cross-over study of the effect of a single oral feeding of medium chain triglyceride oil vs canola oil on post-ingestion plasma triglyceride levels in healthy men. *Altern Med Rev* 1999;4:23-8.

835 Law M, Wald N. Why heart disease mortality is low in France: the time lag explanation. *BMJ* 1999;318:1471-80.

836 Nestel PJ, Pomeroy S, Kay S, et al. Isoflavones from red clover improve systemic arterial compliance but not plasma lipids in menopausal women. *J Clin Endocrinol Metab* 1999;84:895-8.

837 Feskanich D, Weber P, Willett WC, et al. Vitamin K intake and hip fractures in women: a prospective study. *Am J Clin Nutr* 1999;69:74-9.

838 Zheng GQ, Kenney PM, Lam LK. Sesquiterpenes from clove (Eugenia caryophyllata) as potential anticarcinogenic agents. *J Nat Prod* 1992;55:999-1003.

839 Anon. The wellness guide to dietary supplements. *UC Berkeley Wellness Letter* 1998;14:WNL SUPP.

840 Duan H, Takaishi Y, Momota H, et al. Triterpenoids from Tripterygium wilfordii. *Phytochemistry* 2000;53:805-10.

841 Hart CL, Smith GD, Hole DJ, Hawthorne VM. Alcohol consumption and mortality from all causes, coronary heart disease, and stroke: results from a prospective cohort study of Scottish men with 21 years of follow up. *BMJ* 1999;318:1725-9.

842 Potter SM, Baum JA, Teng H, et al. Soy protein and isoflavones: their effects on blood lipids and bone density in

postmenopausal women. *Am J Clin Nutr* 1998;68:1375S-9S.

845 Allman MA, Pena MM, Pang D. Supplementation with flaxseed oil versus sunflower seed oil in healthy young men consuming a low fat diet: effects on platelet composition and function. *Eur J Clin Nutr* 1995;49(3):169-78.

849 Tritrungtasna O, Jerasutus S, Suvanprakorn P. Treatment of alopecia areata with khellin and UVA. *Int J Dermatol* 1993;32:690.

850 Waller DP, Martin AM, Farnsworth NR, Awang DV. Lack of androgenicity of Siberian ginseng. *JAMA* 1992;267:2329.

851 Nestel PJ, Yamashita T, Sasahara T, et al. Soy isoflavones improve systemic arterial compliance but not plasma lipids in menopausal and perimenopausal women. *Arterioscler Thromb Vasc Biol* 1997;17:3392-8.

852 Dobrescu D, Tanasescu M, Mezdrea A, et al. Contributions to the complex study of some lichens-Usnea genus. Pharmacological studies on Usnea barbata and Usnea hirta species. *Rom J Physiol* 1993;30:101-7.

854 Wiesenauer M, Lydtke R. Mahonia aquifolium in patients with Psoriasis vulgaris; an intraindividual study. *Phytomedicine* 1996;3:231-5.

856 Natural Health Remedies. Health Canada. URL: hc-sc.gc.ca/english/archives/96-97/herbnae.html (Accessed 16 July 1999).

857 Gieler U, von der Weth A, Heger M. Mahonia aquifolium- a new type of topical treatment for psoriasis. *J Dermatol Treatment* 1995;6:31-4.

858 Hiermann A, Bucar F. Studies of Epilobium angustifolium extracts on growth of accessory sexual organs in rats. *J Ethnopharmacol* 1997;55(3):179-83.

859 Hiermann A, Reidlinger M, Juan H, Sametz W. [Isolation of the antiphlogistic principle from Epilobium angustifolium]. [Article in German]. *Planta Med* 1991;57(4):357-60.

860 Hiermann A, Juan H, Sametz W. Influence of Epilobium extracts on prostaglandin biosynthesis and carrageenin induced edema of the rat paw. *J Ethnopharmacol* 1986;17(2):161-9.

864 USDA nutrient database for standard reference, release 12 (March 1998), crude rice bran. www.nal.usda.gov/fnic/cgi-bin/list_nut.pl (Accessed 20 July 1999).

865 Gerhardt AL, Gallo NB. Full-fat rice bran and oat bran similarly reduce hypercholesterolemia in humans. *J Nutr* 1998;128:865-9.

866 Ghoneum M. Anti-HIV activity in vitro of MGN-3, an activated arabinoxylane from rice bran. *Biochem Biophys Res Commun* 1998;243:25-9.

867 Iida T, Nakagawa R, Hirakawa H, et al. Clinical trial of a combination of rice bran fiber and cholestyramine for promotion of fecal excretion of retained polychlorinated dibenzofuran and polychlorinated biphenyl in Yu-Cheng patients. *Fukuoka Igaku Zasshi* 1995;86:226-33.

868 Abdel-Fattah A, Aboul-Enein MN, Wassel GM, El-Menshawi BS. An approach to the treatment of vitiligo by khellin. *Dermatologica* 1982;165:136-40.

869 Duarte J, Torres AI, Zarzuelo A. Cardiovascular effects of visnagin on rats. *Planta Med* 2000;66:35-9.

870 Iida T, Hirakawa H, Matsueda T, et al. [Therapeutic trials for promotion of faecal excretion of PCDFs by the administration of rice bran fiber and cholestyramine in Yusho patients]. [Article in Japanese]. *Fukuoka Igaku Zasshi* 1993;84:257-62.

871 Weisburger JH, Reddy BS, Rose DP, et al. Protective mechanisms of dietary fibers in nutritional carcinogenesis. *Basic Life Sci* 1993;61:45-63.

872 Fujiwaki T, Furusho K. The effects of rice bran, broth bathing in patients with atopic dermatitis. *Acta Paediatr Jpn* 1992;34:505-10.

873 Sanders TA, Reddy S. The influence of rice bran on plasma lipids and lipoproteins in human volunteers. *Eur J Clin Nutr* 1992;46(3):167-72.

874 Jahnen A, Heynck H, Gertz B, et al. Dietary fibre: the effectiveness of a high bran intake in reducing renal calcium excretion. *Urol Res* 1992;20:3-6.

875 Cara L, Dubois C, Borel P, et al. Effects of oat bran, rice bran, wheat fiber, and wheat germ on postprandial lipemia in healthy adults. *Am J Clin Nutr* 1992;55:81-8.

876 Ebisuno S, Morimoto S, Yasukawa S, Ohkawa T. Results of long-term rice bran treatment on stone recurrence in hypercalciuric patients. *Br J Urol* 1991;67:237-40.

877 Kestin M, Moss R, Clifton PM, Nestel PJ. Comparative effects of three cereal brans on plasma lipids, blood pressure, and glucose metabolism in mildly hypercholesterolemic men. *Am J Clin Nutr* 1990;52:661-6.

878 Noronha IL, Andriolo A, Lucon AM, et al. [Rice bran in the treatment of idiopathic hypercalciuria in patients with urinary calculosis]. [Article in Portugese]. *Rev Paul Med* 1989;107:19-24.

879 Tomlin J, Read NW. Comparison of the effects on colonic function caused by feeding rice bran and wheat bran. *Eur J Clin Nutr* 1988;42:857-61.

880 Ebisuno S, Morimoto S, Yoshida T, et al. Rice-bran treatment for calcium stone formers with idiopathic hypercalciuria. *Br J Urol* 1986;58:592-5.

881 Ohkawa T, Ebisuno S, Kitagawa M, et al. Rice bran treatment for patients with hypercalciuric stones: experimental and clinical studies. *J Urol* 1984;132:1140-5.

882 Ohkawa T, Ebisuno S, Kitagawa M, et al. Rice bran treatment for hypercalciuric patients with urinary calculous disease. *J Urol* 1983;129:1009-11.

883 Tsuda M. Purification and characterization of a lectin from rice bran. *J Biochem* (Tokyo) 1979;86:1451-61.

884 Kumar B, Chaudhuri DK. Isolation, partial characterization of antithiamine factor present in rice-bran and its effect on TPP-transketolase system and Staphylococcus aureus. *Int J Vitam Nutr Res* 1976;46:154-9.

885 Guerra MJ, Jaffe WG [Nutritional studies with rice bran]. [Article in Spanish]. *Arch Latinoam Nutr* 1975;25:401-17.

887 Fessenden JM, Wittenborn W, Clarke L. Gingko biloba: a case report of herbal medicine and bleeding postoperatively from a laparoscopic cholecystectomy. *Am Surg* 2001;67:33-5.

888 Bomser J, Madhavi DL, Singletary K, Smith MA. In vitro anticancer activity of fruit extracts from Vaccinium species. *Planta Med* 1996;62:212-6.

889 Joseph JA, Shukitt-Hale B, Denisova NA, et al. Reversals of age-related declines in neuronal signal transduction, cognitive, and motor behavioral deficits with blueberry, spinach, or strawberry dietary supplementation. *J Neurosci* 1999;19:8114-21.

900 Youdim KA, Shukitt-Hale B, MacKinnon S, et al. Polyphenolics enhance red blood cell resistance to oxidative stress: in vitro and in vivo (1). *Biochim Biophys Acta* 2000;1519:117-22.

901 Birdsall TC. 5-Hydroxytryptophan: A Clinically-Effective Serotonin Precursor. *Altern Med Rev* 1998;3:271-80.

902 Michelson D, Page SW, Casey R, et al. An eosinophilia-myalgia syndrome related disorder associated with exposure to L-5-hydroxytryptophan. *J Rheumatol* 1994;21:2261-5.

903 Nakajima T, Kudo Y, Kaneko Z. Clinical evaluation of 5-hydroxy-L-tryptophan as an antidepressant drug. *Folia Psychiatr Neurol Jpn* 1978;32:223-30.

904 Coppen A, Whybrow PC, Noguera R, et al. The comparative antidepressant value of L-tryptophan and imipramine with and without attempted potentiation by liothyronine. *Arch Gen Psychiatr* 1972;26:234-41.

REFERENCES

906 Rao B, Broadhurst AD. Tryptophan and depression [letter]. *Br Med J* 1976;1:460.

907 Cao G, Shukitt-Hale B, Bickford PC, et al. Hyperoxia-induced changes in antioxidant capacity and the effect of dietary antioxidants. *J Appl Physiol* 1999;86:1817-22.

908 Bickford PC, Gould T, Briederick L, et al. Antioxidant-rich diets improve cerebellar physiology and motor learning in aged rats. *Brain Res* 2000;866:211-7.

909 Cignarella A, Nastasi M, Cavalli E, Puglisi L. Novel lipid-lowering properties of Vaccinium myrtillus L. leaves, a traditional antidiabetic treatment, in several models of rat dyslipidaemia: a comparison with ciprofibrate. *Thromb Res* 1996;84:311-22.

910 Vorberg G. Ginkgo biloba extract (GBE): A long-term study of chronic cerebral insufficiency in geriatric patients. *Clin Trials J* 1985;22:149-57.

911 Zheng GQ, Kenney PM, Lam LK. Anethofuran, carvone, and limonene: potential cancer chemopreventive agents from dill weed oil and caraway oil. *Planta Med* 1992;58:338-41.

912 Van Hiele LJ. L-5-hydroxytryptophan in depression: the first substitution therapy in psychiatry: the treatment of 99 out-patients with therapy-resistant depressions. *Neuropsychobiol* 1980;6:230-40.

913 Puttini PS, Caruso I. Primary fibromyalgia syndrome and 5-hydroxy-L-tryptophan: a 90-day open study. *J Int Med Res* 1992;20:182-9.

914 Cangiano C, Ceci F, Cancino A, et al. Eating behavior and adherence to dietary prescriptions in obese adult subjects treated with 5-hydroxytryptophan. *Am J Clin Nutr* 1992;56:863-7.

915 Kahn RS, Westenberg HGM. L-5-hydroxytryptophan in the treatment of anxiety disorders. *J Affect Disord* 1985;8:197-200.

916 Trouillas P, Brudon F, Adeleine P. Improvement of cerebellar ataxia with levorotatory form of 5-hydroxytryptophan: a double-blind study with quantified data processing. *Arch Neurol* 1988;45:1217-22.

917 Williams A, Goodenberger D, Caline DB, et al. Palatal myclonus following herpes zoster amellorated by 5-hydroxytryptophan and carbidopa. *Neurology* 1978;28:358-9.

918 Meyer JS, Welch KM, Deshmukh VD, et al. Neurotransmitter precursor amino acids in the treatment of multi-infarct dementia and Alzheimer's disease. *J Amer Geriat Soc* 1977;25:289-98.

919 FDA Talk Paper. Impurities confirmed in dietary supplement 5-hydroxy-L-tryptophan. August 31, 1998. Available at: http://vm.cfsan.fda.gov/~lrd/tp5htp.html

920 Kaplan PW, Tusa RJ, Shankroff J, et al. Visual evoked potentials in adrenoleukodystrophy: a trial with glycerol trioleate and Lorenzo oil. *Ann Neurol* 1993;34:169-74.

921 Poulos A, Gibson R, Sharp P, et al. Very long chain fatty acids in X-linked adrenoleukodystrophy brain after treatment with Lorenzo's oil. *Ann Neurol* 1994;36:741-6.

922 Duchesne N, Dufour M, Bouchard G, et al. Adrenoleukodystrophy: magnetic resonance follow-up after Lorenzo's oil therapy. *Can Assoc Radiol J* 1995;46:386-91.

923 Moser HW. Clinical and therapeutic aspects of adrenoleukodystrophy and adrenomyeloneuropathy. *J Neuropathol Exp Neurol* 1995;54:740-5.

924 Aubourg P, Adamsbaum C, Lavallard-Rousseau MC, et al. A two-year trial of oleic and erucic acids (Lorenzo's oil) as treatment for adrenomyeloneuropathy. *N Engl J Med* 1993;329:745-52.

925 Kickler TS, Zinkham WH, Moser A, et al. Effect of erucic acid on platelets in patients with adrenoleukodystrophy. *Biochem Mol Med* 1996;57:125-33.

926 Chai BC, Etches WS, Stewart MW, Siminoski K. Bleeding in a patient taking Lorenzo's oil: evidence for a vascular defect. *Postgrad Med J* 1996;72:113-4.

927 Revell P, Green A, Green S. Platelets in treated adrenoleukodystrophy: a brief report. *J Inherit Metab Dis* 1995;18:635-7.

928 Moser HW. Komrower Lecture. Adrenoleukodystrophy: natural history, treatment and outcome. *J Inherit Metab Dis* 1995;18:435-47.

929 Maeda K, Suzuki Y, Yajima S, et al. Improvement of clinical and MRI findings in a boy with adrenoleukodystrophy by dietary erucic acid therapy. *Brain Dev* 1992;14:409-12.

930 Wong V. Adrenoleukodystrophy in a Chinese boy. *Brain Dev* 1992;14:276-7.

931 Rasmussen M, Moser AB, Borel J, et al. Brain, liver, and adipose tissue erucic and very long chain fatty acid levels in adrenoleukodystrophy patients treated with glyceryl trierucate and trioleate oils (Lorenzo's oil). *Neurochem Res* 1994;19:1073-82.

932 Miller TE, Dodd J, Ormrod DJ, Geddes R. Anti-inflammatory activity of glycogen extracted from Perna canaliculus (NZ green-lipped mussel). *Agents Actions* 1993;38 Spec No:C139-42.

933 Couch RA, Ormrod DJ, Miller TE, Watkins WB. Anti-inflammatory activity in fractionated extracts of the green-lipped mussel. *N Z Med J* 1982;95:803-6.

934 Miller TE, Ormrod D. The anti-inflammatory activity of Perna canaliculus (NZ green lipped mussel). *N Z Med J* 1980;92:187-93.

935 Larkin JG, Capell HA, Sturrock RD. Seatone in rheumatoid arthritis: a six-month placebo-controlled study. *Ann Rheum Dis* 1985;44:199-201.

936 Miller T, Wu H. In vivo evidence for prostaglandin inhibitory activity in New Zealand green-lipped mussel extract. *N Z Med J* 1984;97:355-7.

937 Naghii MR, Samman S. The effect of boron supplementation on its urinary excretion and selected cardiovascular risk factors in healthy male subjects. *Biol Trace Elem Res* 1997;56:273-86.

938 Vettori G, Lazzaro A, Mazzanti P, Cazzola P. [Prevention of recurrent respiratory infections in adults]. [Article in Italian]. *Minerva Med* 1987;78:1281-9.

939 Usuda K, Kono K, Iguchi K, et al. Hemodialysis effect on serum boron level in the patients with long term hemodialysis. *Sci Total Environ* 1996;191:283-90.

940 Meacham SL, Taper LJ, Volpe SL. Effect of boron supplementation on blood and urinary calcium, magnesium, and phosphorus, and urinary boron in athletic and sedentary women. *Am J Clin Nutr* 1995;61:341-5.

941 Newnham RE. Essentiality of boron for healthy bones and joints. *Environ Health Perspect* 1994;102:83-5.

942 Meacham SL, Taper LJ, Volpe SL. Effects of boron supplementation on bone mineral density and dietary, blood, and urinary calcium, phosphorus, magnesium, and boron in female athletes. *Environ Health Perspect* 1994;102(Suppl 7):79-82.

943 Penland JG. Dietary boron, brain function, and cognitive performance. *Environ Health Perspect* 1994;102:65-72.

944 Green NR, Ferrando AA. Plasma boron and the effects of boron supplementation in males. *Environ Health Perspect* 1994;102:73-7.

945 Shils M, Olson A, Shike M. Modern Nutrition in Health and Disease. 8th ed. Philadelphia, PA: Lea and Febiger, 1994.

946 Wyatt RJ, Engelman K, Kupfer DJ, et al. Effects of L-tryptophan (a natural sedative) on human sleep. *Lancet* 1970;2(7678):842-6.

947 Hunt MJ, Barnetson R. A comparative study of gluconolactone versus benzoyl peroxide in the treatment of acne. *Australas J Dermatol* 1992;33:131-4.

948 Thueson DO, Chan EK, Oechsli LM, Hahn GS. The roles of pH and concentration in lactic acid-induced stimulation of epidermal turnover. *Dermatol Surg* Jun 1998;24(6):641-5.

949 Kempers S, Katz HI, Wildnauer R, Green B. An evaluation of the effect of an alpha hydroxy acid-blend skin cream in the cosmetic improvement of symptoms of moderate to severe xerosis, epidermolytic hyperkeratosis, and ichthyosis. *Cutis* 1998;61:347-50.

950 Berardesca E, Distante F, Vignoli GP, et al. Alpha hydroxyacids modulate stratum corneum barrier function. *Br J Dermatol* 1997;137:934-8.

951 Rawlings AV, Davies A, Carlomusto M, et al. Effect of lactic acid isomers on keratinocyte ceramide synthesis, stratum corneum lipid levels and stratum corneum barrier function. *Arch Dermatol Res* 1996;288:383-90.

952 Stiller MJ, Bartolone J, Stern R, et al. Topical 8% glycolic acid and 8% L-lactic acid creams for the treatment of photodamaged skin. A double-blind, vehicle-controlled clinical trial. *Arch Dermatol* 1996;132:631-6.

953 Piacquadio D, Dobry M, Hunt S, et al. Short contact 70% glycolic acid peels as a treatment for photodamaged skin. A pilot study. *Dermatol Surg* 1996;22:449-52.

954 Ditre CM, Griffin TD, Murphy GF, et al. Effects of alpha-hydroxy acids on photoaged skin: a pilot clinical, histologic, and ultrastructural study [see comments]. *J Am Acad Dermatol* 1996;34:187-95.

955 Wehr R, Krochmal L, Bagatell F, Ragsdale W. A controlled two-center study of lactate 12 percent lotion and a petrolatum-based creme in patients with xerosis. *Cutis* 1986;37:205-7, 209.

956 Barnes S. Phytoestrogens and breast cancer. *Baillieres Clin Endocrinol Metab* 1998;12:559-79.

957 Hotz G, Frank T, Zoller J, Wiebelt H. [Antiphlogistic effect of bromelaine following third molar removal]. [Article in German]. *Dtsch Zahnarztl Z* 1989;44:830-2.

958 Valueva TA, Revina TA, Mosolov VV. Potato tuber protein proteinase inhibitors belonging to the Kunitz soybean inhibitor family. *Biochemistry* (Mosc) 1997;62:1367-74.

959 Tanabe S, Tesaki S, Watanabe M, Yanagihara Y. [Cross-reactivity between bromelain and soluble fraction from wheat flour]. [Article in Japanese]. *Arerugi* 1997;46:1170-3.

960 Masson M. [Bromelain in blunt injuries of the locomotor system. A study of observed applications in general practice]. [Article in German]. *Fortschr Med* 1995;113:303-6.

961 Zimacheva AV, Mosolov VV. [Cysteine proteinase inhibitors from soy seeds]. [Article in Russian]. *Biokhimiia* 1995;60:118-23.

962 Zavadova E, Desser L, Mohr T. Stimulation of reactive oxygen species production and cytotoxicity in human neutrophils in vitro and after oral administration of a polyenzyme preparation. *Cancer Biother* 1995;10:147-52.

963 Diez-Gomez ML, Quirce S, Aragoneses E, Cuevas M. Asthma caused by Ficus benjamina latex: evidence of cross-reactivity with fig fruit and papain. *Ann Allergy Asthma Immunol* 1998;80:24-30.

964 Raus I. [Clinical studies on Frubienzyme in a controlled double-blind trial]. [Article in German]. *Fortschr Med* 1976;94:1579-82.

965 Billigmann P. [Enzyme therapy-an alternative in treatment of herpes zoster. A controlled study of 192 patients]. [Article in German]. *Fortschr Med* 1995;113:43-8.

966 Shuttleworth D, Hill S, Marks R, Connelly DM. Relief of experimentally induced pruritus with a novel eutectic mixture of local anaesthetic agents. *Br J Dermatol* 1988;119:535-40.

967 Mansfield LE, Ting S, Haverly RW, Yoo TJ. The incidence and clinical implications of hypersensitivity to papain in an allergic population, confirmed by blinded oral challenge. *Ann Allergy* 1985;55:541-3.

968 Bienen H, Raus I. [Therapeutic comparison of throat lozenges; (author's transl)]. [Article in German]. *MMW Munch Med Wochenschr* 1981;123:745-7.

969 Reinecke M. [Treatment of inflammatory diseases of the mouth and throat with Larypront in ENT practice; (author's transl)]. [Article in German]. *MMW Munch Med Wochenschr* 1976;118:1253-4.

970 Baron JA, Beach M, Mandel JS, et al. Calcium supplements for the prevention of colorectal adenomas. Calcium Polyp Prev Study Group. *N Engl J Med* 1999;340:101-7.

971 Levine RJ, Hauth JC, Curet LB, et al. Trial of calcium to prevent preeclampsia. *N Engl J Med* 1997;337:69-76.

972 Whelton PK, Kumanyika SK, Cook NR, et al. Efficacy of nonpharmacologic interventions in adults with high-normal blood pressure: results from phase 1 of the trials of hypertension prevention (TOHP). Trials of Hypertension Prev (TOHP) Collab Res Group. *Am J Clin Nutr* 1997;65:652S-60S.

973 Purwar M, Kulkarni H, Motghare V, Dhole S. Calcium supplementation and prevention of pregnancy induced hypertension. *J Obstet Gynaecol Res* 1996;22:425-30.

974 Yamamoto ME, Applegate WB. Klag MJ, et al. Lack of blood pressure effect with calcium and magnesium supplementation in adults with high-normal blood pressure. Results from phase I of the trials of hypertension prevention (TOHP). Trials of Hypertension Prev (TOHP) Collab Res Group. *Ann Epidemiol* 1995;5:96-107.

975 Petersen LJ, Rudnicki M, Hojsted J. Long-term oral calcium supplementation reduces diastolic blood pressure in end stage renal disease. A randomized, double-blind, placebo-controlled study. *Int J Artif Organs* 1994;17:37-40.

976 Weinberger MH, Wagner UL, Fineberg NS. The blood pressure effects of calcium supplementation in humans of known sodium responsiveness. *Am J Hypertens* 1993;6:799-805.

977 Storm D, Eslin R, Porter ES, et al. Calcium supplementation prevents seasonal bone loss and changes in biochemical markers of bone turnover in elderly New England women: a randomized, placebo-controlled trial. *J Clin Endocrinol Metab* 1998;83:3817-25.

978 Baeksgaard L, Andersen KP, Hyldstrup L. Calcium and vitamin D supplementation increases spinal BMD in healthy, postmenopausal women. *Osteoporos Int* 1998;8:255-60.

979 Riggs BL, O'Fallon WM, Muhs J, et al. Long-term effects of calcium supplementation on serum parathyroid hormone level, bone turnover, and bone loss in elderly women. *J Bone Miner Res* 1998;13:168-74.

980 Dawson-Hughes B, Harris SS, Krall EA, Dallal GE. Effect of calcium and vitamin D supplementation on bone density in men and women 65 years of age or older. *N Engl J Med* 1997;337:670-6.

981 Devine A, Dick IM, Heal SJ, et al. A 4-year follow-up study of the effects of calcium supplementation on bone density in elderly postmenopausal women. *Osteoporos Int* 1997;7:23-8.

982 Bernstein CN, Seeger LL, Anton PA, et al. A randomized, placebo-controlled trial of calcium supplementation for decreased bone density in corticosteroid-using patients with inflammatory bowel disease: a pilot study. *Aliment Pharmacol Ther* 1996;10:777-86.

983 Ilich-Ernst JZ, McKenna AA, Badenhop NE, et al. Iron status, menarche, and calcium supplementation in adolescent girls. *Am J Clin Nutr* 1998;68:880-7.

984 Dwyer JH, Dwyer KM, Scribner RA, et al. Dietary calcium, calcium supplementation, and blood pressure in

African American adolescents. *Am J Clin Nutr* 1998;68:648-55.

985 Thys-Jacobs S, Starkey P, Bernstein D, Tian J. Calcium carbonate and the premenstrual syndrome: effects on premenstrual and menstrual symptoms. Premenstrual Syndrome Study Group. *Am J Obstet Gynecol* 1998;179:444-52.

986 Reid IR. The roles of calcium and vitamin D in the prevention of osteoporosis. *Endocrinol Metab Clin North Am* 1998;27:389-98.

987 Ricci TA, Chowdhury HA, Heymsfield SB, et al. Calcium supplementation suppresses bone turnover during weight reduction in postmenopausal women. *J Bone Miner Res* 1998;13:1045-50.

988 Kalkwarf HJ, Specker BL, Bianchi DC, et al. The effect of calcium supplementation on bone density during lactation and after weaning. *N Engl J Med* 1997;337:523-8.

989 McKenna AA, Ilich JZ, Andon MB, et al. Zinc balance in adolescent females. *Am J Clin Nutr* 1997;65:1460-4.

990 Gupta SK, Gupta RC, Seth AK, Gupta A. Reversal of fluorosis in children. *Acta Paediatr Jpn* 1996;38:513-9.

991 Steinbach G, Lupton J, Reddy BS. Calcium carbonate treatment of diarrhea in intestinal bypass patients. *Eur J Gastroenterol Hepatol* 1996;8:559-62.

992 Lupton JR, Steinbach G, Chang WC, et al. Calcium supplementation modifies the relative amounts of bile acids in bile and affects key aspects of human colon physiology. *J Nutr* 1996;126:1421-8.

993 Alberts DS, Ritenbaugh C, Story JA, et al. Randomized, double-blind, placebo-controlled study of effect of wheat bran fiber and calcium on fecal bile acids in patients with resected adenomatous colon polyps. *J Natl Cancer Inst* 1996;88:81-92.

994 Baron JA, Tosteson TD, Wargovich MJ, et al. Calcium supplementation and rectal mucosal proliferation: a randomized controlled trial. *J Natl Cancer Inst* 1995;87:1303-7.

995 Gallagher JC, Riggs BL, DeLuca. Effect of estrogen on calcium absorption and serum vitamin D metabolites in postmenopausal osteoporosis. *J Clin Endocrinol Metab* 1980;51:1359-64.

996 Whiting SJ. Safety of some calcium supplements questioned. *Nutr Rev* 1994;52:95-7.

997 Roberts HJ. Potential toxicity due to dolomite and bonemeal. *South Med J* 1983;76:556-9.

999 Akedo I, Ishikawa H, Nakamura T, et al. Three cases with familial adenomatous polyposis diagnosed as having malignant lesions in the course of a long-term trial using docosahexanoic acid (DHA)-concentrated fish oil capsules. *Jpn J Clin Oncol* 1998;28:762-5.

1000 Danno K, Sugie N. Combination therapy with low-dose etretinate and eicosapentaenoic acid for psoriasis vulgaris. *J Dermatol* 1998;25:703-5.

1001 Prisco D, Paniccia R, Bandinelli B, et al. Effect of medium-term supplementation with a moderate dose of n-3 polyunsaturated fatty acids on blood pressure in mild hypertensive patients. *Thromb Res* 1998;1:105-12.

1002 Gans RO, Bilo HJ, Weersink EG, et al. Fish oil supplementation in patients with stable claudication. *Am J Surg* 1990;160:490-5.

1003 Vognild E, Elvevoll EO, Brox J, et al. Effects of dietary marine oils and olive oil on fatty acid composition, platelet membrane fluidity, platelet responses, and serum lipids in healthy humans. *Lipids* 1998;33:427-36.

1004 Mayser P, Mrowietz U, Arenberger P, et al. Omega-3 fatty acid-based lipid infusion in patients with chronic plaque psoriasis: results of a double-blind, randomized, placebo-controlled, multicenter trial. *J Am Acad Dermatol* 1998;38:539-47.

1005 Campan P, Planchand PO, Duran D. Pilot study on n-3 polyunsaturated fatty acids in the treatment of human experimental gingivitis. *J Clin Periodontol* 1997;24:907-13.

1006 Thies N. The effect of 12 months' treatment with eicosapentaenoic acid in five children with cystic fibrosis. *J Paediatr Child Health* 1997;33:349-51.

1007 Singh RB, Niaz MA, Sharma JP, et al. Randomized, double-blind, placebo-controlled trial of fish oil and mustard oil in patients with suspected acute myocardial infarction: the Indian experiment of infarct survival-4. *Cardiovasc Drugs Ther* 1997;11:485-91.

1008 Sagar PS, Das UN, Koratkar R, et al. Cytotoxic action of cis-unsaturated fatty acids on human cervical carcinoma (HeLa) cells: relationship to free radicals and lipid peroxidation and its modulation by calmodulin antagonists. *Cancer Lett* 1992;63:189-98.

1009 Grimsgaard S, Bonaa KH, Hansen JB, Nordoy A. Highly purified eicosapentaenoic acid and docosahexaenoic acid in humans have similar triacylglycerol-lowering effects but divergent effects on serum fatty acids. *Am J Clin Nutr* 1997;66:649-59.

1010 Marzari R, Mazzanti P, Cazzola P, Pirodda E. [Perennial allergic rhinitis. Prophylaxis of acute episodes using thymomodulin]. [Article in Italian]. *Minerva Med* 1987;78(22):1675-81.

1011 Allard JP, Kurian R, Aghdassi E, et al. Lipid peroxidation during n-3 fatty acid and vitamin E supplementation in humans. *Lipids* 1997;32:535-41.

1012 Andreassen AK, Hartmann A, Offstad J, et al. Hypertension prophylaxis with omega-3 fatty acids in heart transplant recipients. *J Am Coll Cardiol* 1997;29:1324-31.

1013 Badalamenti S, Salerno F, Salmeron JM, et al. Lack of renal effects of fish oil administration in patients with advanced cirrhosis and impaired glomerular filtration. *Hepatol* 1997;25:313-6.

1014 Agren JJ, Hanninen O, Julkunen A, et al. Fish diet, fish oil and docosahexaenoic acid rich oil lower fasting and postprandial plasma lipid levels. *Eur J Clin Nutr* 1996;50:765-71.

1015 Zeman K, Dworniak D, Tchorzewski H, et al. Effect of thymic extract on allogeneic MLR and mitogen-induced responses in patients with chronic active hepatitis B. *Immunol Invest* 1991;20(7):545-55.

1016 Saynor R, Gillott T. Changes in blood lipids and fibrinogen with a note on safety in a long term study on the effects of n-3 fatty acids in subjects receiving fish oil supplements and followed for seven years. *Lipids* 1992;27:533-8.

1017 van der Tempel H, Tulleken JE, Limburg PC, et al. Effects of fish oil supplementation in rheumatoid arthritis. *Ann Rheum Dis* 1990;49:76-80.

1018 Vuksan V, Sievenpiper JL, Koo VY, et al. American ginseng (Panax quinquefolius L) reduces postprandial glycemia in nondiabetic subjects and subjects with type 2 diabetes mellitus. *Arch Intern Med* 2000;160:1009-13.

1020 Toft I, Bonaa KH, Ingebretsen OC, et al. Effects of n-3 polyunsaturated fatty acids on glucose homeostasis and blood pressure in essential hypertension. A randomized, controlled trial. *Ann Intern Med* 1995;123:911-8.

1021 Badalamenti S, Salerno F, Lorenzano E, et al. Renal effects of dietary supplementation with fish oil in cyclosporine-treated liver transplant recipients. *Hepatol* 1995;22:1695-71.

1022 Sacks FM, Stone PH, Gibson CM, et al. Controlled trial of fish oil for regression of human coronary atherosclerosis. HARP Res Group. *J Am Coll Cardiol* 1995;25:1492-8.

1023 Sakakibara H, Hirose K, Matsushita K, et al. Effect of supplementation with eicosapentaenoic acid ethylster MND-21, on generation of leukotrienes by calcium ionophore-activated leukocytes in bronchial asthma. *Nihon Kyobu Shikkan Gakkai Zasshi* 1995;33:395-402.

1024 Eritsland J, Arnesen H, Seljeflot I, Hostmark AT. Long-term metabolic effects of n-3 polyunsaturated fatty acids in patients with coronary artery disease. *Am J Clin Nutr* 1995;61:831-6.

1025 Shimizu H, Ohtani K, Tanaka Y, et al. Long-term effect of eicosapentaenoic acid ethyl (EPA-E) on albuminuria of non-insulin dependent diabetic patients. *Diabetes Res Clin Pract* 1995;28:35-40.

1026 Onwude JL, Lilford RJ, Hjartardottir H, et al. A randomised double blind placebo controlled trial of fish oil in high risk pregnancy. *Br J Obstet Gynaecol* 1995;102:95-100.

1027 Bulstra-Ramakers MT, Huisjes HJ, Visser GH. The effects of 3g eicosapentaenoic acid daily on recurrence of intrauterine growth retardation and pregnancy induced hypertension. *Br J Obstet Gynaecol* 1995;102:123-6.

1028 Leaf A, Jorgensen MB, Jacobs AK, et al. Do fish oils prevent restenosis after coronary angioplasty? *Circulation* 1994;90:2248-57.

1029 McVeigh GE, Brennan GM, Cohn JN, et al. Fish oil improves arterial compliance in non-insulin-dependent diabetes mellitus. *Arterioscler Thromb* 1994;14:1425-9.

1030 Sacks FM, Hebert P, Appel LJ, et al. Short report: the effect of fish oil on blood pressure and high-density lipoprotein-cholesterol levels in phase I of the trials of hypertension prevention. *J Hypertens* 1994;12:209-13.

1031 Lau CS, Morley KD, Belch JJ. Effects of fish oil supplementation on non-steroidal anti-inflammatory drug requirement in patients with mild rheumatoid arthritis- a double-blind, placebo-controlled study. *Br J Rheumatol* 1993;32:982-9.

1032 Rossi E, Costa M. Fish oil derivatives as a prophylaxis of recurrent miscarriage associated with antiphospholipid antibodies (APL): a pilot study. *Lupus* 1993;2:319-23.

1033 Vandongen R, Mori TA, Burke V, et al. Effects on blood pressure of omega 3 fats in subjects at increased risk of cardiovascular disease. *Hypertension* 1993;22:371-9.

1034 Grimminger F, Mayser P, Papavassilis C, et al. A double-blind, randomized, placebo-controlled trial of n-3 fatty acid based lipid infusion in acute, extended guttate psoriasis. Rapid improvement of clinical manifestations and changes in neutrophil leukotriene profile. *Clin Invest* 1993;71:634-43.

1035 Soyland E, Funk J, Rajka G, et al. Effect of dietary supplementation with very-long-chain n-3 fatty acids in patients with psoriasis. *N Engl J Med* 1993;328:1812-6.

1036 Thien FC, Mencia-Huerta J, Lee TH. Dietary fish oil effects on seasonal hay fever and asthma in pollen- sensitive subjects. *Am Rev Respir Dis* 1993;147:1138-43.

1037 Greenfield SM, Green AT, Teare JP, et al. A randomized controlled study of evening primrose oil and fish oil in ulcerative colitis. *Aliment Pharmacol Ther* 1993;7:159-66.

1038 Bellamy CM, Schofield PM, Faragher EB, et al. Can supplementation of diet with omega-3 polyunsaturated fatty acids reduce coronary angioplasty restenosis. *Eur Heart J* 1992;13:1626-31.

1039 Kjeldsen-Kragh J, Lund JA, Riise T, et al. Dietary omega-3 fatty acid supplementation and naproxen treatment in patients with rheumatoid arthritis. *J Rheumatol* 1992;19:1531-6.

1040 Hawthorne AB, Daneshmend TK, Hawkey CJ, et al. Treatment of ulcerative colitis with fish oil supplementation: a prospective 12 month randomised controlled trial. *Gut* 1992;33:922-8.

1041 Astorga G, Cubillos A, Masson L, Silva JJ. Active rheumatoid arthritis: effect of dietary supplementation with omega-3 oils. A controlled double-blind trial. *Rev Med Chil* 1991;119:267-72.

1042 D'Almeida A, Carter JP, Anatol A, Prost C. Effects of a combination of evening primrose oil (gamma linolenic acid) and fish oil (eicosapentaenoic + docahexaenoic acid) versus magnesium, and versus placebo in preventing pre-eclampsia. *Women Health* 1992;19:117-31.

1043 Hamazaki T, Sawazaki S, Itomura M, et al. The effect of docosahexaenoic acid on aggression in young adults. A placebo-controlled double-blind study. *J Clin Invest* 1996;97:1129-33.

1044 Conquer JA, Holub BJ. Supplementation with an algae source of docosahexaenoic acid increases (n-3) fatty acid status and alters selected risk factors for heart disease in vegetarian subjects. *J Nutr* 1996;126:3032-9.

1045 Carlson SE, Werkman SH. A randomized trial of visual attention of preterm infants fed docosahexaenoic acid until two months. *Lipids* 1996;31:85-90.

1046 Buckley LM, Leib ES, Cartularo KS, et al. Calcium and vitamin D3 supplementation prevents bone loss in the spine secondary to low-dose corticosteroids in patients with rheumatoid arthritis. A randomized double-blind, placebo-controll ed trial. *Ann Intern Med* 1996;125:961-8.

1047 White E, Shannon JS, Patterson RE. Relationship between vitamin and calcium supplement use and colon cancer. *Cancer Epidemiol Biomarkers Prev* 1997;6:769-74.

1048 Mindell E. Earl Mindell's Supplement Bible. New York, NY: Simon and Schuster, 1998.

1049 Suhner A, Schlagenhauf P, Johnson R, et al. Comparative study to determine the optimal melatonin dosage form for the alleviation of jet lag. *Chronobiol Int* 1998;15:655-6.

1052 Wright SW, Lawrence LM, Wrenn KD, et al. Randomized clinical trial of melatonin after night-shift work: efficacy and neuropsychologic effects. *Ann Emerg Med* 1998 32(3 Pt 1):334-40.

1053 Dolberg OT, Hirschmann S, Grunhaus L. Melatonin for the treatment of sleep disturbances in major depressive disorder. *Am J Psychiatr* 1998;155:1119-21.

1054 James M, Tremea MO, Jones JS, Krohmer JR. Can melatonin improve adaptation to night shift? *Am J Emerg Med* 1998;16:367-70.

1055 Arunachalam K, Gill HS, Chandra RK. Enhancement of natural immune function by dietary consumption of Bifidobacterium lactis (HN019). *Eur J Clin Nutr* 2000;54:263-7.

1056 McArthur AJ, Budden S. Sleep dysfunction in Rett syndrome: a trial of exogenous melatonin treatment. *Dev Med Child Neurol* 1998;40:186-92.

1057 Lorenz RT, Cysewski GR. Commercial potential for Haematococcus microalgae as a natural source of astaxanthin. *Trends Biotechnol* 2000;18:160-7 .

1058 Benes L, Claustrat B, Horriere F, et al. Transmucosal, oral controlled-release, and transdermal drug administration in human subjects: a crossover study with melatonin. *J Pharm Sci* 1997;86:1115-9.

1059 Leibenluft E, Feldman-Naim S, Turner EH, et al. Effects of exogenous melatonin administration and withdrawal in five patients with rapid-cycling bipolar disorder. *J Clin Psychiatr* 1997;58:383-8.

1060 Lievin V, Peiffer I, Hudault S, et al. Bifidobacterium strains from resident infant human gastrointestinal microflora exert antimicrobial activity. *Gut* 2000;47:646-52.

1061 Worobec S, LaChine A. Dangers of orally administered para-aminobenzoic acid. *JAMA* 1984;251:2348.

1062 Van Den Heuvel CJ, Reid KJ, Dawson D. Effect of atenolol on nocturnal sleep and temperature in young men: reversal by pharmacological doses of melatonin. *Physiol Behav* 1997;61:795-802.

1063 Wikner J, Wetterberg L, Rojdmark S. Does hypercalcaemia or calcium antagonism affect human melatonin secretion or renal excretion? *Eur J Clin Invest* 1997;27:374-9.

1064 Lissoni P, Brivio O, Brivio F, et al. Adjuvant therapy with the pineal hormone melatonin in patients with lymph node relapse due to malignant melanoma. *J Pineal Res* 1996;21:239-42.

1065 Zarafonetis CJ, Dabich L, DeVol EB, et al. Potassium para-aminobenzoate and liver function test findings. *J Am Acad Dermatol* 1986;15:144-9.

1066 Bangha E, Elsner P, Kistler GS. Suppression of UV-induced erythema by topical treatment with melatonin (N-acetyl-5-methoxytryptamine). A dose response study. *Arch Dermatol Res* 1996;288:522-6.

1067 Carson CC. Potassium para-aminobenzoate for the treatment of Peyronie's disease: is it effective? *Tech Urol* 1997;3:135-9.

1068 Attenburrow ME, Cowen PJ, Sharpley AL. Low dose melatonin improves sleep in healthy middle-aged subjects. *Psychopharmacol* (Berl) 1996;126:179-81.

1069 Lissoni P, Pittalis S, Ardizzoia A, et al. Prevention of cytokine-induced hypotension in cancer patients by the pineal hormone melatonin. *Support Care Cancer* 1996;4:313-6.

1070 Ellis CM, Lemmens G, Parkes JD. Melatonin and insomnia. *J Sleep Res* 1996;5:61-5.

1071 Zarafonetis CJ, Dabich L, Skovronski JJ, et al. Retrospective studies in scleroderma: skin response to potassium para-aminobenzoate therapy. *Clin Exp Rheumatol* 1988;6:261-8.

1072 Garfinkel D, et al. Improvement of sleep quality in elderly people by controlled-release melatonin. *Lancet* 1995;346:541-44.

1073 Zarafonetis CJ, Dabich L, Negri D, et al. Retrospective studies in scleroderma: effect of potassium para-aminobenzoate on survival. *J Clin Epidemiol* 1988;41:193-205.

1074 Clegg DO, Reading JC, Mayes MD, et al. Comparison of aminobenzoate potassium and placebo in the treatment of scleroderma. *J Rheumatol* 1994;21:105-10.

1075 Zarafonetis CJ, Dabich L, Devol EB, et al. Retrospective studies in scleroderma: pulmonary findings and effect of potassium p-aminobenzoate on vital capacity. *Respiration* 1989;56:22-33.

1076 Valcavi R, Zini M, Maestroni GJ, et al. Melatonin stimulates growth hormone secretion through pathways other than the growth hormone-releasing hormone. *Clin Endocrinol* (Oxf) 1993;39:193-9.

1077 Petrie K, Dawson AG, Thompson L, Brook R. A double-blind trial of melatonin as a treatment for jet lag in international cabin crew. *Biol Psychiatr* 1993;33:526-30.

1078 Dollins AB, Lynch HJ, Wurtman RJ, et al. Effect of pharmacological daytime doses of melatonin on human mood and performance. *Psychopharmacol* (Berl) 1993;112:490-6.

1079 Claustrat B, Brun J, David M, et al. Melatonin and jet lag: confirmatory result using a simplified protocol. *Biol Psychiatr* 1992;32:705-11.

1080 Lissoni P, Barni S, Ardizzoia A, et al. Randomized study with the pineal hormone melatonin versus supportive care alone in advanced nonsmall cell lung cancer resistant to a first-line chemotherapy containing cisplatin. *Oncol* 1992;49:336-9.

1081 Dahlitz M, Alvarez B, Vignau J, et al. Delayed sleep phase syndrome response to melatonin. *Lancet* 1991;337:1121-4.

1082 Sack RL, Lewy AJ, Blood ML, et al. Melatonin administration to blind people: phase advances and entrainment. *J Biol Rhythms* 1991;6:249-61.

1083 James SP, Sack DA, Rosenthal NE, Mendelson WB. Melatonin administration in insomnia. *Neuropsychopharmacol* 1990;3:19-23.

1084 Ludwig G. Evaluation of conservative therapeutic approaches to Peyronie's disease (fibrotic induration of the penis). *Urol Int* 1991;47:236-9.

1085 Petrie K, Conaglen JV, Thompson L, Chamberlain K. Effect of melatonin on jet lag after long haul flights. *BMJ* 1989;298:705-7.

1086 Hughes CG. Oral PABA and vitiligo. *J Am Acad Dermatol* 1983;9:770.

1087 Carnielli VP, Da Riol R, Montini G. Iron supplementation enhances response to high doses of recombinant human erythropoietin in preterm infants. *Arch Dis Child Fetal Neonatal Ed* 1998;79:F44-8.

1088 Silva J, Andrade S, Ventura H, et al. Iron supplementation in haemodialysis-practical clinical guidelines. *Nephrol Dial Transplant* 1998;13:2572-7.

1089 Brolin RE, Gorman JH, Gorman RC, et al. Prophylactic iron supplementation after Roux-en-Y gastric bypass: a prospective, double-blind, randomized study. *Arch Surg* 1998;133:740-4.

1090 Fudin R, Jaichenko J, Shostak A, et al. Correction of uremic iron deficiency anemia in hemodialyzed patients: a prospective study. *Nephron* 1998;79:299-305.

1091 Sowade O, Messinger D, Franke W, et al. The estimation of efficacy of oral iron supplementation during treatment with epoetin beta (recombinant human erythropoietin) in patients undergoing cardiac surgery. *Eur J Haematol* 1998;60:252-9.

1093 Sever Y, Ashkenazi A, Tyano S, Weizman A. Iron treatment in children with attention deficit hyperactivity disorder. A preliminary report. *Neuropsychobiology* 1997;35:178-80.

1094 Kantor GR, Ratz JL. Liver toxicity from potassium para-aminobenzoate. *J Am Acad Dermatol* 1985;13:671-2.

1095 Bruner AB, Joffe A, Duggan AK, et al. Randomized study of cognitive effects of iron supplementation in non- anaemic iron-deficient adolescent girls. *Lancet* 1996;348:992-6.

1096 Bamford DS, Percival RC, Tothill AU. Raspberry leaf tea: a new aspect to an old problem. *Br J Pharmacol* 1970;40:161P+.

1097 Corti MC, Guralnik JM, Salive ME, et al. Serum iron level, coronary artery disease, and all-cause mortality in older men and women. *Am J Cardiol* 1997;79:120-7.

1098 Ullen H, Augustsson K, Gustavsson C, Steineck G. Supplementary iron intake and risk of cancer: reversed causality? *Cancer Lett* 1997;114:215-6.

1099 Reunanen A, Takkunen H, Knekt P, et al. Body iron stores, dietary iron intake and coronary heart disease mortality. *J Intern Med* 1995;238:223-30.

1100 Lund EK, Wharf SG, Fairweather-Tait SJ, Johnson IT. Oral ferrous sulfate supplements increase the free radical-generating capacity of feces from healthy volunteers. *Am J Clin Nutr* 1999;69:250-5.

1101 Schumann K, Elsenhans B, Maurer A. Iron supplementation. *J Trace Elem Med Biol* 1998;12:129-40.

1102 Rehman A, Collis CS, Yang M, et al. The effects of iron and vitamin C co-supplementation on oxidative damage to DNA in healthy volunteers. *Biochem Biophys Res Comm* 1998;246:293-8.

1103 Recommended Dietary Allowances. Inst Med of Natl Acad Sci, 1989.

1104 Soewondo S. The effect of iron deficiency and mental stimulation on Indonesian children's cognitive performance and development. *Kobe J Med Sci* 1995;41:1-17.

1105 Budeiri D, Li Wan Po A, Dornan JC. Is evening primrose oil of value in the treatment of premenstrual syndrome? *Control Clin Trials* 1996;17:60-8.

1106 Khoo SK, Munro C, Battistutta D. Evening primrose oil and treatment of premenstrual syndrome. *Med J Aust* 1990;153:189-92.

1107 Gordon M, et al. A phase II controlled study of a combination of the immune modulator, lentinan, with didanosine (ddI) in HIV patients with CD4 cells of 200-500/mm3. *J Med* 1995;26(5-6):193-207.
1108 Yoshiyuki T, et al. Treatment for peritoneal dissemination of gastric cancer by intraperitoneal administration of CDDP through Infuse-a-Port. *Gan To Kagaku Ryoho* 1994;21(13):2323-5.
1109 Tari K, et al. [Effect of lentinan for advanced prostate carcinoma]. [Article in Japanese]. *Hinyokika Kiyo* 1994;40:119-23.
1110 Nishihira T, Akimoto M, Mori S. Anti-cancer effects of BRMs associated with nutrition in cancer patients. *Gan To Kagaku Ryoho*1988;15(4 Pt 2-3):1615-20.
1111 Wada T, et al. A comparative clinical trial with tegafur plus lentinan treatment at two different doses in advanced cancer. *Gan To Kagaku Ryoho* 1987;14(8):2509-11.
1112 Kosaka A, et al. Synergistic action of lentinan (LNT) with endocrine therapy of breast cancer in rats and humans. *Gan To Kagaku Ryoho* 1987;14(2):516-22.
1113 Taguchi T. Clinical efficacy of lentinan on patients with stomach cancer: end point results of a four-year follow-up survey. *Cancer Detect Prev Suppl* 1987;1:333-49.
1114 Thein DJ, Hurt WC. Lysine as a prophylactic agent in the treatment of recurrent herpes simplex labialis. *Oral Surg Oral Med Oral Pathol* 1984;58(6):659-66.
1115 McCune MA, et al. Treatment of recurrent herpes simplex infections with L-lysine monohydrochloride. *Cutis* 1984;34(4):366-73.
1116 DiGiovanna JJ, Blank H. Failure of lysine in frequently recurrent herpes simplex infection. Treatment and prophylaxis. *Arch Dermatol* 1984;120(1):48-51.
1117 Chiang BL, Sheih YH, Wang LH, et al. Enhancing immunity by dietary consumption of a probiotic lactic acid bacterium (Bifidobacterium lactis HN019): optimization and definition of cellular immune responses. *Eur J Clin Nutr* 2000;54:849-55.
1118 Milman N, Scheibel J, Jessen O. Lysine prophylaxis in recurrent herpes simplex labialis: a double-blind, controlled crossover study. *Acta Derm Venereol* 1980;60(1):85-7.
1119 Griffith RS, Norins A, Kagan C. A multicentered study of lysine therapy in Herpes simplex infection. *Dermatologica* 1978;156(5):257-67.
1120 Griffith RS, et al. Success of L-lysine therapy in frequently recurrent herpes simplex infection. Treatment and prophylaxis. *Dermatologica* 1987;175(4):183-90.
1121 Lo JC, et al. Fanconi's syndrome and tubulointerstitial nephritis in association with L-lysine ingestion. *Am J Kidney Dis* 1996;28(4):614-7.
1122 McFarlin BL, Gibson MH, O'Rear J, Harman P. A national survey of herbal preparation use by nurse-midwives for labor stimulation. Review of the literature and recommendations for practice. *J Nurse Midwifery* 1999;44:205-16.
1123 Nurnberger JI Jr, Adkins S, Lahiri DK, et al. Melatonin suppression by light in euthymic bipolar and unipolar patients. *Arch Gen Psychiatr* 2000;57:572-9.
1124 Flodin NW. The metabolic roles, pharmacology, and toxicology of lysine. *J Am Coll Nutr* 1997;16(1):7-12.
1125 Naguib M, Samarkandi AH. The comparative dose-response effects of melatonin and midazolam for premedication of adult patients: a double-blinded, placebo-controlled study. *Anesth Analg* 2000;91:473-9.
1126 DeMuro RL, Nafziger AN, Blask DE, et al. The absolute bioavailability of oral melatonin. *J Clin Pharmacol* 2000;40:781-4.
1127 Leone M, D'Amico D, Moschiano F, et al. Melatonin versus placebo in the prophylaxis of cluster headache: a double-blind pilot study with parallel groups. *Cephalalgia* 1996;16:494-6.
1128 Peres MF, Seabra ML, Zukerman E, Tufik S. Cluster headache and melatonin. *Lancet* 2000;355:147.
1129 Blau JN, Engel HO. A new cluster headache precipitant: increased body heat. *Lancet* 1999;354:1001-2.
1130 Hall SL, Greendale GA. The relation of dietary vitamin C intake to bone mineral density: results from the PEPI study. *Calcif Tissue Int* 1998;63(3):183-9.
1131 Civitelli R, et al. Dietary L-lysine and calcium metabolism in humans. *Nutr* 1992;8(6):400-5.
1132 Cagnacci A, Krauchi K, Wirz-Justice A, Volpe A. Homeostatic versus circadian effects of melatonin on core body temperature in humans. *J Biol Rhythms* 1997;12:509-17.
1133 Smith KA, Fairburn CG, Cowen PJ. Symptomatic relapse in bulimia nervosa following acute tryptophan depletion. *Arch Gen Psychiatr* 1999;56:171-6.
1134 Sharma RP, Shapiro LE, Kamath SK. Acute dietary tryptophan depletion: effects on schizophrenic positive and negative symptoms. *Neuropsychobiol* 1997;35:5-10.
1135 van Hall G, Raaymakers JS, Saris WH. Ingestion of branched-chain amino acids and tryptophan during sustained exercise in man: failure to affect performance. *J Physiol* (Lond) 1995;486:789-94.
1136 Delgado PL, Price LH, Miller HL. Serotonin and the neurobiology of depression. Effects of tryptophan depletion in drug-free depressed patients. *Arch Gen Psychiatr* 1994;51:865-74.
1137 Macfarlane GT, Cummings JH. Probiotics and prebiotics: can regulating the activities of intestinal bacteria benefit health? *BMJ* 1999;318:999-1003.
1138 Bowen DJ, Spring B, Fox E. Tryptophan and high-carbohydrate diets as adjuncts to smoking cessation therapy. *J Behav Med* 1991;14:97-110.
1139 Etzel KR, Stockstill JW, Rugh JD. Tryptophan supplementation for nocturnal bruxism: report of negative results. *Rugh JDJ Craniomandib Disord* 1991;5:115-20.
1140 Stockstill JW, McCall D Jr., Gross AJ. The effect of L-tryptophan supplementation and dietary instruction on chronic myofascial pain. *J Am Dent Assoc* 1989;118:457-60.
1141 Messiha FS. Fluoxetine: adverse effects and drug-drug interactions. *J Toxicol Clin Toxicol* 1993;31:603-30.
1142 Devoe LD, Castillo RA, Searle NS. Maternal dietary substrates and human fetal biophysical activity. The effects of tryptophan and glucose on fetal breathing movements. *Am J Obstet Gynecol* 1986;155:135-9.
1143 Lieberman HR, Corkin S, Spring BJ. The effects of dietary neurotransmitter precursors on human behavior. *Am J Clin Nutr* 1985;42:366-70.
1144 Schmidt HS. L-tryptophan in the treatment of impaired respiration in sleep. *Bull Eur Physiopathol Respir* 1983;19:625-9.
1145 Seltzer S, Dewart D, Pollack R. The effects of dietary tryptophan on chronic maxillofacial pain and experimental pain tolerance. *J Psychiatr Res* 1982-83;17:181-6.
1146 Hartmann E, Spinweber CL. Sleep induced by L-tryptophan. Effect of dosages within the normal dietary intake. *J Nerv Ment Dis* 1979;167:497-9.
1147 Hitosugi M, Kitamura O, Takatsu A, Yoshino Y. Autopsy case of duodenal obstruction from impacted mushroom. *J Gastroenterol* 1998;33:562-5.
1148 Hanada K, Hashimoto I. Flagellate mushroom (Shiitake) dermatitis and photosensitivity. *Dermatol* 1998;197:255-7.
1149 Levy AM, Kita H, Phillips SF, et al. Eosinophilia and gastrointestinal symptoms after ingestion of shiitake mushrooms. *J Allergy Clin Immunol* 1998;101:613-20.

1150 Murakami M, Kawabe K, Hosoi Y, et al. Decreased pulmonary perfusion in hypersensitivity pneumonitis caused by Shiitake mushroom spores. *J Intern Med* 1997;241:85-8.

1151 Matsui S, Nakazawa T, Umegae Y, Mori M. Hypersensitivity pneumonitis induced by Shiitake mushroom spores. *Intern Med* 1992;31:1204-6.

1152 Nakamura T. Shiitake (Lentinus edodes) dermatitis. *Contact Dermatitis* 1992;27:65-70.

1153 Ueda A, Obama K, Aoyama K, et al. Allergic contact dermatitis in shiitake (Lentinus edodes (Berk) Sing) growers. *Contact Dermatitis* 1992;26:228-33.

1154 Hirayama K, Rafter J. The role of probiotic bacteria in cancer prevention. *Microbes Infect* 2000;2:681-6.

1155 Otsuka M, Shinozuka K, Hirata G, Kunitomo M. [Influences of a shiitake (Lentinus edodes)-fructo-oligosaccharide mixture (SK-204) on experimental pulmonary thrombosis in rats]. [Article in Japanese]. *Yakugaku Zasshi* 1996;116:169-73.

1157 Colloidal minerals in brief. www.colloidal.com.au/ (Accessed 23 July 1999).

1158 Wallach J. Dr. Joel Wallach's colloidal minerals. www.elementsofhealth.com/b1.html (Accessed 23 July 1999).

1159 Schauss A. Colloidal minerals: Clinical implications of clay suspension products sold as dietary supplements. *Amer J of Nat Med* 1997;4:5-10.

1160 Sposito G, Skipper NT, Sutton R, et al. Surface geochemistry of the clay minerals. *Proc Natl Acad Sci U S A* 1999;96(7):3358-64.

1161 Schrauzer G. An overview of liquid mineral supplements. *Int J of Integrative Med* 1999;1:18-22.

1162 Branton SL, Lott BD, Maslin WR, et al. Fatty liver-hemorrhagic syndrome observed in commercial layers fed diets containing chelated minerals. *Avian Dis* 1995;39:631-5.

1167 Durlach J, Bac P, Durlach V, et al. Magnesium status and ageing: an update. *Magnes Res* 1998;11:25-42.

1168 Scheen AJ. Perspective in the treatment of insulin resistance. *Hum Reprod* 1997;12:63-71.

1169 Ziment I. Alternative therapies for asthma. *Curr Opin Pulm Med* 1997;3:61-7.

1170 Preuss HG, Gondal JA, Lieberman S. Association of macronutrients and energy intake with hypertension. *J Am Coll Nutr* 1996;15:21-35.

1171 de Valk HW, Verkaaik R, van Rijn HJ, et al. Oral magnesium supplementation in insulin-requiring Type 2 diabetic patients. *Diabet Med* 1998;15:503-7.

1172 Lima M, Cruz T, Pousada JC, et al. The effect of magnesium supplementation in increasing doses on the control of type 2 diabetes. *Diabetes Care* 1998;21:682-6.

1173 Hill J, Micklewright A, Lewis S, et al. Investigation of the effect of short-term change in dietary magnesium intake in asthma. *Eur Respir J* 1997;10:2225-9.

1174 Zehender M, Meinertz T, Faber T, et al. Antiarrhythmic effects of increasing the daily intake of magnesium and potassium in patients with frequent ventricular arrhythmias. Magnesium in Cardiac Arrhythmias (MAGICA)Investigators. *J Am Coll Cardiol* 1997;29:1028-34.

1175 Cavagni G, Piscopo E, Rigoli E, et al. Food allergy in children: an attempt to improve the effects of the elimination diet with an immunomodulating agent (thymomodulin). A double-blind clinical trial. *Immunopharmacol Immunotoxicol* 1989;11:131-42.

1176 Genova R, Guerra A. Thymomodulin in management of food allergy in children. *Int J Tissue React* 1986;8(3):239-42.

1177 Galli M, Crocchiolo P, Negri C, et al. Attempt to treat acute type B hepatitis with an orally administered thymic extract (thymomodulin): preliminary results. *Drugs Exp Clin Res* 1985;11(9):665-9.

1178 Valesini G, Barnaba V, Benvenuto R, et al. A calf thymus acid lysate improves clinical symptoms and T-cell defects in the early stages of HIV infection: second report. *Eur J Cancer Clin Oncol* 1987;23(12):1915-9.

1179 Withanachchi J, Al-Faleh H, Griffiths J, Senaratne MP. Dichotomous and modest response to folic acid and lack of additional effect of vitamin B-12 in hyperhomocystinemia. *Clin Invest Med* 2000;23:S5.

1180 Witteman JC, Grobbee DE, Derkx FH, et al. Reduction of blood pressure with oral magnesium supplementation in women with mild to moderate hypertension. *Am J Clin Nutr* 1994;60:129-35.

1181 Lasserre B, Spoerri M, Moullet V, et al. Should magnesium therapy be considered for the treatment of coronary heart disease? II. Epidemiological evidence in outpatients with and without coronary heart disease. *Magnes Res* 1994;7:145-53.

1182 Yamori Y, Nara Y, Mizushima S, et al. Nutritional factors for stroke and major cardiovascular diseases: international epidemiological comparison of dietary prevention. *Health Rep* 1994;6:22-7.

1183 Mauskop A, Altura BT, Cracco RQ, et al. Deficiency in serum ionized magnesium but not total magnesium in patients with migraines. Possible role of ICa2+/IMg2+ ratio. *Headache* 1993;33:135-8.

1184 Mauskop A, Altura BT, Cracco RQ, et al. Intravenous magnesium sulfate relieves cluster headaches in patients with low serum ionized magnesium levels. *Headache* 1995;35:597-600.

1185 Mauskop A, Altura BT, Cracco RQ, Altura BM. Intravenous magnesium sulphate relieves migraine attacks in patients with low serum ionized magnesium levels: a pilot study. *Clin Sci* (Colch) 1995;89:633-6.

1186 Facchinetti F, Sances G, Borella P, et al. Magnesium prophylaxis of menstrual migraine: effects on intracellular magnesium. *Headache* 1991;31:298-301.

1187 Facchinetti F, Borella P, Sances G, et al. Oral magnesium successfully relieves premenstrual mood changes. *Obstet Gynecol* 1991;78:177-81.

1188 Walker AF, De Souza MC, Vickers MF, et al. Magnesium supplementation alleviates premenstrual symptoms of fluid retention. *J Womens Health* 1998;7:1157-65.

1189 Starobrat-Hermelin B, Kozielec T. The effects of magnesium physiological supplementation on hyperactivity in children with attention deficit hyperactivity disorder (ADHD). Positive response to magnesium oral loading test. *Magnes Res* 1997;10:149-56.

1190 Thel MC, Armstrong AL, McNulty SE, et al. Randomised trial of magnesium in in-hospital cardiac arrest. Duke Internal Medicine Housestaff. *Lancet* 1997;350:1272-6.

1191 Lichodziejewska B, Klos J, Rezler J, et al. Clinical symptoms of mitral valve prolapse are related to hypomagnesemia and attenuated by magnesium supplementation. *Am J Cardiol* 1997;79(6):768-72.

1192 Sanjuliani AF, de Abreu Fagundes VG, Francischetti EA. Effects of magnesium on blood pressure and intracellular ion levels of Brazilian hypertensive patients. *Int J Cardiol* 1996;56:177-83.

1193 Hoogerbrugge N, Cobbaert C, de Heide L, et al. Oral physiological magnesium supplementation for 6 weeks with 1 g/d magnesium oxide does not affect increased Lp(a) levels in hypercholesterolaemic subjects. *Magnes Res* 1996;9:129-32.

1194 Dahle LO, Berg G, Hammar M, et al. The effect of oral magnesium substitution on pregnancy-induced leg cramps. *Am J Obstet Gynecol* 1995;173:175-80.

1195 Plum-Wirell M, Stegmayr BG, Wester PO. Nutritional magnesium supplementation does not change blood pressure nor serum or muscle potassium and magnesium in untreated hypertension. A double-blind crossover study. *Magnes Res* 1994;7:277-83.

1196 Alexandersen P, Toussaint A, Christiansen C, et al. Ipriflavone in the treatment of postmenopausal osteoporosis: A randomized comtrolled trial. *JAMA* 2001;285:1482-8.

1197 Purvis JR, Cummings DM, Landsman P, et al. Effect of oral magnesium supplementation on selected cardiovascular risk factors in non-insulin-dependent diabetics. *Arch Fam Med* 1994;3:503-8.

1198 Galloe AM, Rasmussen HS, Jorgensen LN, et al. Influence of oral magnesium supplementation on cardiac events among survivors of an acute myocardial infarction. *BMJ* 1993;307:585-7.

1199 Widman L, Wester PO, Stegmayr BK, et al. The dose-dependent reduction in blood pressure through administration of magnesium. A double blind placebo controlled cross-over study. *Am J Hypertens* 1993;6:41-5.

1201 Rattan V, Sidhu H, Vaidyanathan S. Effect of combined supplementation of magnesium oxide and pyridoxine in calcium-oxalate stone formers. *Urol Res* 1994;22:161-5.

1202 Brodsky MA, Orlov MV, Capparelli EV, et al. Magnesium therapy in new-onset atrial fibrillation. *Am J Cardiol* 1994;73:1227-9.

1203 Holmang A, Nilsson C, Niklasson M, et al. Induction of insulin resistance by glucosamine reduces blood flow but not interstitial levels of either glucose or insulin. *Diabetes* 1999;48:106-11.

1204 Kim YB, Zhu JS, Zierath JR, et al. Glucosamine infusion in rats rapidly impairs insulin stimulation of phosphoinositide 3-kinase but does not alter activation of Akt/protein kinase B in skeletal muscle. *Diabetes* 1999;48:310-20.

1205 Attias J, Weisz G, Almog S, et al. Oral magnesium intake reduces permanent hearing loss induced by noise exposure. *Am J Otolaryngol* 1994;15:26-32.

1206 Chang DM, Kuo SY, Lai JH, Chang ML. Effects of anti-rheumatic herbal medicines on cellular adhesion molecules. *Ann Rheum Dis* 1999;58:366-71.

1207 Wright IM. Neonatal effects of maternal consumption of blue cohosh. *J Pediatr* 1999;134:384-5.

1208 Skorodin MS, Tenholder MF, Yetter B, et al. Magnesium sulfate in exacerbations of chronic obstructive pulmonary disease. *Arch Intern Med* 1995;155:496-500.

1211 Kubo K, Nanba H. The effect of maitake mushrooms on liver and serum lipids. *Alt Ther Health Med* 1996;2:62-6.

1212 Kubo K, Aoki H, Nanba H. Anti-diabetic activity present in the fruit body of Grifola frondosa (Maitake). I. *Biol Pharm Bull* 1994;17:1106-10.

1213 Kabir Y, Kimura S. Dietary mushrooms reduce blood pressure in spontaneously hypertensive rats (SHR). *J Nutr Sci Vitaminol* (Tokyo) 1989;35:91-4.

1214 Kabir Y, Yamaguchi M, Kimura S. Effect of shiitake (Lentinus edodes) and maitake (Grifola frondosa) mushrooms on blood pressure and plasma lipids of spontaneously hypertensive rats. *J Nutr Sci Vitaminol* (Tokyo) 1987;33:341-6.

1215 Espeland MA, Hogan PE, Fineberg SE, et al. Effect of postmenopausal hormone therapy on glucose and insulin concentrations. PEPI Investigators. Postmenopausal Estrogen/Progestin Interventions. *Diabetes Care* 1998;21:1589-95.

1216 Chen FP, Lee N, Soong YK. Changes in the lipoprotein profile in postmenopausal women receiving hormone replacement therapy. Effects of natural and synthetic progesterone. *J Reprod Med* 1998;43:568-74.

1217 Espeland MA, Marcovina SM, Miller V, et al. Effect of postmenopausal hormone therapy on lipoprotein(a) concentration. Postmenopausal Estrogen/Progestin Interventions (PEPI) Investigators. *Circulation* 1998;97:979-86.

1218 Perino M, Brigandi FG, Abate FG, et al. Intramuscular versus vaginal progesterone in assisted reproduction: a comparative study. *Clin Exp Obstet Gynecol* 1997;24:228-31.

1219 Steingrub JS, Lopez T, Teres D, et al. Amniotic fluid embolism associated with castor oil ingestion. *Crit Care Med* 1988;16:642-3.

1220 Freeman EW, Rickels K, Sondheimer SJ, et al. A double-blind trial of oral progesterone, alprazolam, and placebo in treatment of severe premenstrual syndrome. *JAMA* 1995;274:51-7.

1221 Schweizer E, Case WG, Garcia-Espana F, et al. Progesterone co-administration in patients discontinuing long-term benzodiazepine therapy: effects on withdrawal severity and taper outcome. *Psychopharmacol* (Berl) 1995;117:424-9.

1222 Simon JA, Robinson DE, Andrews MC, et al. The absorption of oral micronized progesterone: the effect of food, dose proportionality, and comparison with intramuscular progesterone. *Fertil Steril* 1993;60:26-33.

1223 Nappi C, Affinito P, Di Carlo C, et al. Double-blind controlled trial of progesterone vaginal cream treatment for cyclical mastodynia in women with benign breast disease. *J Endocrinol Invest* 1992;15:801-6.

1224 Freeman EW, Weinstock L, Rickels K, et al. A placebo-controlled study of effects of oral progesterone on performance and mood. *Br J Clin Pharmacol* 1992;33:293-8.

1225 Smitz J, Devroey P, Faguer B, et al. A prospective randomized comparison of intramuscular or intravaginal natural progesterone as a luteal phase and early pregnancy supplement. *Hum Reprod* 1992;7:168-75.

1226 Darj E, Nilsson S, Axelsson O, et al. Clinical and endometrial effects of oestradiol and progesterone in post-menopausal women. *Maturitas* 1991;13(2):109-15.

1227 Bassetti S, Frei R, Zimmerli W. Fungemia with Saccharomyces cerevisiae after treatment with Saccharomyces boulardii. *Am J Med* 1998;105:71-2.

1228 Cooper A, Spencer C, Whitehead MI, et al. Systemic absorption of progesterone cream from Progest cream in postmenopausal women. *Lancet* 1998;351:1255-6.

1229 Burry KA, Paton PE, Hermsmeyer K. Percutaneous absorption of progesterone in postmenopausal women treated with transdermal estrogen. *Am J Obstet Gynecol* 1999;180:1504-11.

1230 FDA. www.verity.fda.gov/default.html.

1231 Cooper AJ, Whitehead MI. Correspondence. *Lancet* 1998;352:906.

1233 Colombel JF, Cortot A, Neut C, Romond C. Yoghurt with Bifidobacterium longum reduces erythromycin-induced gastrointestinal effects. *Lancet* 1987;2:43.

1234 Abul-Ezz SR, Barone GW, Gurley BJ, et al. Effect of herbal supplements on cyclosporine blood levels and associated acute rejection. Am Soc of Nephrol Ann Mtg, Toronto, CAN 2000;Oct. 11-16:abstract A3754.

1236 Ha GY, Yang CH, Kim H, Chong Y. Case of sepsis caused by Bifidobacterium longum. *J Clin Microbiol* 1999;37:1227-8.

1238 Ascherio A, Zhang SM, Hernan MA, et al. Prospective study of caffeine intake and risk of Parkinson's disease in men and women. Proceedings 125th Ann Mtg Am Neurological Assn. Boston, MA: 2000;Oct 15-18:42 (abstract 53).

1239 Wasowicz W, Gromadzinska J, Szram K, et al. Selenium, zinc, and copper concentrations in the blood and milk of lactating women. *Biol Trace Elem Res* 2001;79:221-33.

REFERENCES

1240 Anderson JW, Gilliland SE. Effect of fermented milk (yogurt) containing Lactobacillus acidophilus L1 on serum cholesterol in hypercholesterolemic humans. *J Am Coll Nutr* 1999;18:43-50.

1241 Schaafsma G, Meuling WJ, van Dokkum W, Bouley C. Effects of a milk product, fermented by Lactobacillus acidophilus and with fructo-oligosaccharides added, on blood lipids in male volunteers. *Eur J Clin Nutr* 1998;52:436-40.

1242 Bhatnagar S, Singh KD, Sazawal S, et al. Efficacy of milk versus yogurt offered as part of a mixed diet in acute noncholera diarrhea among malnourished children. *J Pediatr* 1998;132:999-1003.

1243 Guerin-Danan C, Chabanet C, Pedone C, et al. Milk fermented with yogurt cultures and Lactobacillus casei compared with yogurt and gelled milk: influence on intestinal microflora in healthy infants. *Am J Clin Nutr* 1998;67:111-7.

1244 Wheeler JG, Shema SJ, Bogle ML, et al. Immune and clinical impact of Lactobacillus acidophilus on asthma. *Ann Allergy Asthma Immunol* 1997;79:229-33.

1245 Shalev E, Battino S, Weiner E, et al. Ingestion of yogurt containing Lactobacillus acidophilus compared with pasteurized yogurt as prophylaxis for recurrent candidal vaginitis and bacterial vaginosis. *Arch Fam Med* 1996;5:593-6.

1246 Nizami SQ, Bhutta ZA, Molla AM. Efficacy of traditional rice-lentil-yogurt diet, lactose free milk protein-based formula and soy protein formula in management of secondary lactose intolerance with acute childhood diarrhea. *J Trop Pediatr* 1996;42:133-7.

1247 Niault M, Thomas F, Prost J, et al. Fungemia due to Saccharomyces species in a patient treated with enteral Saccharomyces boulardii. *Clin Infect Dis* 1999;28:930.

1248 Neri A, Sabah G, Samra Z. Bacterial vaginosis in pregnancy treated with yogurt. *Acta Obstet Gynecol Scand* 1993;72:17-9.

1249 Hilton E, Isenberg HD, Alperstein P, et al. Ingestion of yogurt containing Lactobacillus acidophilus as prophylaxis for candidal vaginitis. *Ann Intern Med* 1992;116:353-7.

1250 Touhami M, Boudraa G, Mary JY, et al. Clinical consequences of replacing milk with yogurt in persistent infantile diarrhea. *Ann Pediatr* (Paris) 1992;39:79-86.

1251 McCullough MJ, Clemons KV, McCusker JH, Stevens DA. Species identification and virulence attributes of Saccharomyces boulardii (nom. inval.). *J Clin Microbiol* 1998;36:2613-7.

1252 Neuvonen PJ, Kivisto KT, Lehto P. Interference of dairy products with the absorption of ciprofloxacin. *Clin Pharmacol Ther* 1991;50:498-502.

1253 Isolauri E, Juntunen M, Rautanen T, et al. A human Lactobacillus strain (Lactobacillus casei sp strain GG) promotes recovery from acute diarrhea in children. *Pediatrics* 1991;8:90-7.

1254 Boudraa G, Touhami M, Pochart P, et al. Effect of feeding yogurt versus milk in children with persistent diarrhea. *J Pediatr Gastroenterol Nutr* 1990;11:509-12.

1255 Siitonen S, Vapaatalo H, Salminen S, et al. Effect of Lactobacillus GG yogurt in prevention of antibiotic associated diarrhea. *Ann Med* 1990;22:57-9.

1256 Lerebours E, N'Djitoyap NC, Lavoine A, et al. Yogurt and fermented-then-pasteurized milk: effects of short-term and long-term ingestion on lactose absorption and mucosal lactase activity in lactase-deficient subjects. *Am J Clin Nutr* 1989;49:823-7.

1258 Alexandrakis G, Tse DT, Rosa RH Jr, Johnson TE. Nasolacrimal duct obstruction and orbital cellulitis associated with chronic intranasal cocaine abuse. *Arch Ophthalmol* 1999;117(12):1617-22.

1259 Ros JJ, Pelders MG, De Smet PA. A case of positive doping associated with a botanical food supplement. *Pharm World Sci* 1999;21:44-6.

1260 Joeres R, Klinker H, Heusler H, et al. Influence of mexiletine on caffeine elimination. *Pharmacol Ther* 1987;33:163-9.

1261 Cooper RA, Molan PC, Harding KG. Antibacterial activity of honey against strains of Staphylococcus aureus from infected wounds. *J R Soc Med* 1999;92(6):283-5.

1262 Caccetta RA, Croft KD, Beilin LJ, Puddey IB. Ingestion of red wine significantly increases plasma phenolic acid concentrations but does not acutely affect ex vivo lipoprotein oxidizability. *Am J Clin Nutr* 2000;71:67-74.

1263 Jurkiewicz E, Panse P, Jentsch KD, et al. In vitro anti-HIV-1 activity of chondroitin polysulphate. *AIDS* 1989;3:423-7.

1264 Cignarella A, Nastasi M, Cavalli E, Puglisi L. Novel lipid-lowering properties of Vaccinium myrtillus L. leaves, a traditional antidiabetic treatment, in several models of rat dyslipidaemia: a comparison with ciprofibrate. *Thromb Res* 1996;84(5):311-22.

1265 Fraisse D, Carnat A, Lamaison JL. [Polyphenolic composition of the leaf of bilberry]. [Article in French]. *Ann Pharm Fr* 1996;54(6):280-3.

1266 Kunsman GW, Levine B, Smith ML. Vitamin B2 interference with TDx drugs-of-abuse assays. *J Forensic Sci* 1998;43:1225-7.

1268 Merritt JC, Crawford WJ, Alexander PC, et al. Effect of marihuana on intraocular and blood pressure in glaucoma. *Ophthalmol* 1980;87:222-8.

1269 Magainin Pharmaceuticals announces new research program for anti-angiogenesis agent - Squalamine - at Georgetown Univ Med Ctr. PRNewswire. www.prnewswire.com (Accessed 22 January 2000).

1270 Okada S, Rohan PJ, Miller FW, et al. Myopathies following ingestion of special nutritional products. *Arthritis Rheum* 1996;39:349.

1271 Zaacks SM, Klein L, Tan CD, et al. Hypersensitivity myocarditis associated with ephedra use. *J Toxicol Clin Toxicol* 1999;37:485-9.

1272 Powell T, Hsu FF, Turk J, Hruska K. Ma-huang strikes again: ephedrine nephrolithiasis. *Am J Kidney Dis* 1998;32:153-9.

1273 Nadir A, Agrawal S, King PD, Marshall JB. Acute hepatitis associated with the use of a Chinese herbal product, ma-huang. *Am J Gastroenterol* 1996;91:1436-8.

1274 Theoharides TC. Sudden death of a healthy college student related to ephedrine toxicity from a ma-huang containing drink. *J Clin Psychopharmacol* 1997;17:437-9.

1275 Vahedi K, Domingo V, Amarenco P, Bousser MG. Ischemic stroke in a sportsman who consumed MaHuang extract and creatine monohydrate for bodybuilding. *J Neurol Neurosurg Psychiatr* 2000;68:112-3.

1276 Doyle H, Kargin M. Herbal stimulant containing ephedrine has also caused psychosis. *BMJ* 1996;313:756.

1278 Tapiainen T, Luotonen L, Kontiokari T, et al. Xylitol administered only during respiratory infections failed to prevent acute otitis media. *Pediatrics* 2002 Feb;109(2):E19.

1279 Hussain MD, Teixeira MG. Saint John's wort and analgesia: effect of Saint John's wort on morphine induced analgesia. AAPS Ann Mtg & Expo Indianapolis, IN:2000;Oct 29- Nov 2:presentation #3453.

1280 Baur A, Harrer T, Peukert M, et al. Alpha-lipoic acid is an effective inhibitor of human immuno-deficiency virus (HIV-1) replication. *Klin Wochenschr* 1991;69:722-4.

1281 Ishiwa J, Sato T, Mimaki Y, et al. A citrus flavonoid, nobiletin, suppresses production and gene expression of matrix metalloproteinase 9/gelatinase B in rabbit synovial fibroblasts. *J Rheumatol* 2000;27:20-5.

1282 McFarland LV. Saccharomyces boulardii is not Saccharomyces cerevisiae. *Clin Infect Dis* 1996;22:200-1.

1283 Brady JA, Rock CL, Horneffer MR. Thiamin status, diuretic medications, and the management of congestive heart failure. *J Am Diet Assoc* 1995;95:541-4.

1284 Shimon I, Almog S, Vered Z, et al. Improved left ventricular function after thiamine supplementation in patients with congestive heart failure receiving long-term furosemide therapy. *Am J Med* 1995;98:485-90.

1285 Pfitzenmeyer P, Guilland JC, d'Athis P, et al. Thiamine status of elderly patients with cardiac failure including the effects of supplementattion. *Int J Vitam Nutr Res* 1994;64:113-8.

1286 Seligmann H, Halkin H, Rauchfleisch S, et al. Thiamine deficiency in patients with congestive heart failure receiving long-term furosemide therapy: a pilot study. *Am J Med* 1991;91:151-5.

1287 Schubert SY, Lansky EP, Neeman I. Antioxidant and eicosanoid enzyme inhibition properties of pomegranate seed oil and fermented juice flavonoids. *J Ethnopharmacol* 1999;66:11-7.

1288 Cheng TO. Ginseng-warfarin interaction. ACC Current Journal Review 2000;9:84.

1290 Piscitelli SC, Burstein AH, Chaitt D, et al. Indinavir concentrations and St. John's wort. *Lancet* 2000;355:547-8.

1292 Yue QY, Bergquist C, Gerden B. Safety of St John's wort (Hypericum perforatum). *Lancet* 2000;355:576-7.

1293 Ruschitzka F, Meier PJ, Turina M, et al. Acute heart transplant rejection due to Saint John's wort. *Lancet* 2000;355:548-9.

1294 Southwick SM, Morgan CA III, Charney DS, High JR. Yohimbine use in a natural setting: effects on post-traumatic stress disorder. *Biol Psychiatr* 1999;46:442-4.

1296 Roberts JE, Wang RH, Tan IP, et al. Hypericin (active ingredient in St. John's wort) photo-oxidation of lens proteins. *Photochem Photobiol* 1999;69:42S.

1297 Frieling UM, Schaumberg DA, Kupper TS, et al. A randomized, 12-year primary-prevention trial of beta carotene supplementation for nonmelanoma skin cancer in the physicians' health study. *Arch Dermatol* 2000;136:179-84.

1298 Mueller BA, Scott MK, Sowinski KM, Prag KA. Noni juice (Morinda citrifolia): hidden potential for hyperkalemia? *Am J Kidney Dis* 2000;35:310-2.

1299 Speetjens JK, Collins RA, Vincent JB, Woski SA. The nutritional supplement chromium(III) tris(picolinate) cleaves DNA. *Chem Res Toxicol* 1999;12:483-7.

1300 Weiss W, Huber G, Engel KH, et al. Identification and characterization of wheat grain albumin/globulin allergens. *Electrophoresis* 1997;18:826-33.

1301 Gurley BJ, Barone GW. Herb-drug interaction involving St. John's wort and cyclosporine. AAPS Ann Mtg & Expo Indianapolis, IN:2000;Oct29- Nov2: presentation #3443.

1302 Singh AK, Granley K, Misrha U, et al. Screening and confirmation of drugs in urine: interference of hordenine with the immunoassays and thin layer chromatography methods. *Forensic Sci Int* 1992;54:9-22.

1303 Gurley BJ, Gardner SF, Hubbard MA. Clinical assessment of potential cytochrome P450-mediated herb-drug interactions. AAPS Ann Mtg & Expo Indianapolis, IN: 2000; Oct 29 - Nov 2:presentation #3460.

1304 Millet Y, Jouglard J, Steinmetz MD, et al. Toxicity of some essential plant oils. Clinical and experimental study. *Clin Toxicol* 1981;18:1485-98.

1305 Gohla SH, Haubeck HD, Neth RD. Mitogenic activity of high molecular polysaccharide fractions isolated from the Cupressaceae Thuja occidentale L. I. Macrophage-dependent injuction of CD-4-positive T-helper (Th+) lymphocytes. *Leukemia* 1988;2(8):528-33.

1306 Offergeld R, Reinecker C, Gumz E, et al. Mitogenic activity of high molecular polysaccharide fractions isolated from the cuppressaceae Thuja occidentalis L. enhanced cytokine-production by thyapolysaccharide, g-fraction (TPSg). *Leukemia* 1992;6(Suppl 3):189S-91S.

1307 Wu ZL, Chen JK, Ong T, et al. Antitransforming activity of chlorophyllin against selected carcinogens and complex mixtures. *Teratog Carcinog Mutagen* 1994;14:75-81.

1309 Dashwood RH, Breinholt V, Bailey GS. Chemopreventive properties of chlorophyllin: Inhibition of aflatoxin B1 (AFB1)-DNA binding in vivo and anti-mutagenic activity against AFB1 and two heterocyclic amines in the Salmonella mutagenicity assay. *Carcinogenesis* 1991;12(5):939-42.

1310 FDA, CFSAN. FDA approved potassium health claim notification for potassium containing foods. 2000. Available at: www.cfsan.fda.gov/~dms/hclm-k.html

1311 Sarkar D, Sharma A, Talukder G. Clastogenic activity of pure chlorophyll and anticlastogenic effects of equivalent amounts of crude extract of Indian spinach leaf and chlorophyllin following dietary supplementation to mice. *Environ Mol Mutagen* 1996;28:121-6.

1312 Amara-Mokrane YA, Lehucher-Michel MP, Balansard G, et al. Protective effects of alpha-hederin, chlorophyllin and ascorbic acid towards the induction of micronuclei by doxorubicin in cultured human lymphocytes. *Mutagenesis* 1996;11:161-7.

1313 US Food and Drug Administration. Center for Food Safety and Applied Nutrition. Letter regarding dietary supplement health claim for omega-3 fatty acids and coronary heart disease. Available at: http://vm.cfsan.fda.gov/~dms/ds-ltr11.html.

1314 Dai R, Shoemaker R, Farrens D, et al. Characterization of silkworm chlorophyll metabolites as an active photosensitizer for photodynamic therapy. *J Nat Prod* 1992;55(9):1241-51.

1315 Lee WY, Park JH, Kim BS, et al. Chlorophyll derivatives (CpD) extracted from silk worm excreta are specifically cytotoxic to tumor cells in vitro. *Yonsei Med J* 1990;31:225-33.

1316 Foerster KK, Schmid K, Rovati LC. Efficacy of glucosamine sulfate in osteoarthritis of the lumbar spine: a placebo-controlled, randomized, double-blind study. Am Coll Rheumatol 64th Ann Scientific Mtg, Philadelphia, PA: 2000;Oct 29- Nov 2:abstract 1613.

1317 Anon. High-dose multivitamins adversely affect coronary plaque composition. Reuters Health. www.medscape.com/reuters/prof/2000/11/11.02/20001101clin013.html (Accessed 2 November 2000).

1318 Smith SW, Zvosec DL. Death and central nervous system depression after ingestion of 1.4-butanediol, a gamma-hydroxybutyrate-related dietary supplement. *Ann Emerg Med* 2000;36:S85.

1319 ORCHIC PMG (Protomorphogen). Natural Health Cod. www.nbizz.com/naturalhealthdoc/listings/184.html (Accessed 9 November 2000).

1320 Gambos J. Fooling the bladder cops: the complete drug testing guide. www.csun.edu/~hbcsc096/dt/ftbc.txt (Accessed 9 November 2000).

1321 Young RW, Beregi JS Jr. Use of chlorophyllin in the care of geriatric patients. *J Am Geriatr Soc*, 1980; 28(1):46-7.

1322 Christiansen SB, Byel SR, Stromsted H, et al. [Can chlorophyll reduce fecal odor in colostomy patients]?[Article in Danish]. *Ugeskr Laeger*, 1989; 151(27):1753-4.

1323 Nahata MC, Slencsak CA, Kamp J. Effect of chlorophyllin on urinary odor in incontinent geriatric patients. *Drug Intell Clin Pharm* 1983; 17(10):732-4.

REFERENCES

1324 Yoshida A, Yokono O, Oda T. Therapeutic effect of chlorophyll-a in the treatment of patients with chronic pancreatitis. *Gastroenterol Jpn* 1980; 15(1):49-61.

1326 Mathews-Roth MM. Carotenoids in erythropoietic protoporphyria and other photosensitivity diseases. *Ann N Y Acad Sci* 1993; 691:127-38.

1329 Cardiovascular Benefits Claimed For Cocoa Flavonoids. www.medscape.com/reuters/prof/2000/02/02.21/dd02210b.html (Accessed 21 February 2000).

1330 Rindone JP, Hiller D, Collacott E, et al. Randomized, controlled trial of glucosamine for treating osteoarthritis of the knee. *West J Med* 2000;172:91-4.

1331 Duker EM, Kopanski L, Jarry H, Wuttke W. Effects of extracts from Cimicifuga racemosa on gonadotropin release in menopausal women and ovariectomized rats. *Planta Med* 1991;57:420-4.

1332 Hamerski D, Schmitt D, Matern U. Induction of two prenyltransferases for the accumulation of coumarin phytoalexins in elicitor-treated Ammi majus cell suspension cultures. *Phytochemistry* 1990;29:1131-5.

1333 Bourinbaiar AS, Tan X, Nagorny R. Inhibitory effect of coumarins on HIV-1 replication and cell-mediated or cell-free viral transmission. Acta Virol 1993;37:241-50.

1334 Harvei S, Bjerve KS, Tretli S, et al. Prediagnostic level of fatty acids in serum phospholipids: omega-3 and omega-6 fatty acids and the risk of prostate cancer. *Int J Cancer* 1997;71:545-51.

1335 Bagasra O, Whittle P, Heins B, Pomerantz RJ. Anti-human immunodeficiency virus type 1 activity of sulfated monosaccharides: comparison with sulfated polysaccharides and other polyions. *J Infect Dis* 1991;164:1082-90.

1336 Gann PH, Hennekens CH, Sacks FM, et al. Prospective study of plasma fatty acids and risk of prostate cancer. *J Natl Cancer Inst* 1994;86:281-6.

1337 Kolonel LN, Nomura AM, Cooney RV. Dietary fat and prostate cancer: current status. *J Natl Cancer Inst* 1999;91:414-28.

1338 Okamoto M, Mitsunobu F, Ashida K, et al. Effects of perilla seed oil supplementation on leukotriene generation by leucocytes in patients with asthma associated with lipometabolism. *Int Arch Allergy Immunol* 2000;122:137-42.

1339 Burstein AH, Horton RL, Dunn T, et al. Lack of effect of St John's Wort on carbamazepine pharmacokinetics in healthy volunteers. *Clin Pharmacol Ther* 2000;68:605-12.

1340 Durr D, Stieger B, Kullak-Ublick GA, et al. St. John's Wort induces intestinal P-glycoprotein/MDR1 and intestinal and hepatic CYP3A4. *Clin Pharmacol Ther* 2000;68:598-604.

1341 Jepsen S, Hansen AB. The influence of N-acetylcysteine on the measurement of prothrombin time and activated partial thromboplastin time in healthy subjects. *Scand J Clin Lab Invest* 1994;54:543-7.

1342 Leeb BF, Schweitzer H, Montag K, Smolen JS. A meta-analysis of chondroitin sulfate in the treatment of osteoarthritis. *J Rheumatol* 2000;27:205-11.

1343 Mosbech H, Muller U. Side-effects of insect venom immunotherapy: results from an EAACI multicenter study. *Allergy* 2000;55:1005-10.

1344 Yamadera W, Sasaki M, Itoh H, et al. Clinical features of circadian rhythm sleep disorders in outpatients. *Psychiatry Clin Neurosci* 1998;52:311-6.

1345 Okawa M, Uchiyama M, Ozaki S, et al. Circadian rhythm sleep disorders in adolescents: clinical trials of combined treatments based on chronobiology. *Psychiatry Clin Neurosci* 1998;52:483-90.

1346 Okawa M, Takahashi K, Egashira K, et al. Vitamin B12 treatment for delayed sleep phase syndrome: a multi-center double-blind study. *Psychiatry Clin Neurosci* 1997;51:275-9.

1347 Yamadera H, Takahashi K, Okawa M. A multicenter study of sleep-wake rhythm disorders: therapeutic effects of vitamin B12, bright light therapy, chronotherapy and hypnotics. *Psychiatry Clin Neurosci* 1996;50:203-9.

1348 Ohta T, Ando K, Iwata T, et al. Treatment of persistent sleep-wake schedule disorders in adolescents with methylcobalamin (vitamin B12). *Sleep* 1991;14:414-8.

1349 Mayer G, Kroger M, Meier-Ewert K. Effects of vitamin B12 on performance and circadian rhythm in normal subjects. *Neuropsychopharmacology* 1996;15:456-64.

1350 Reimund E. Sleep deprivation-induced dermatitis: further support of nicotinic acid depletion in sleep deprivation. *Med Hypotheses* 1991;36:371-3.

1351 Shad JA, Chinn CG, Brann OS. Acute hepatitis after ingestion of herbs. *South Med J* 1999;92:1095-7.

1352 Kugelmas M. Preliminary observation: oral zinc sulfate replacement is effective in treating muscle cramps in cirrhotic patients. *J Am Coll Nutr* 2000;19:13-5.

1353 Grubben MJ, Boers GH, Blom HJ, et al. Unfiltered coffee increases plasma homocysteine concentrations in healthy volunteers: a randomized trial. *Am J Clin Nutr* 2000;71:480-4.

1354 Watkins TR, Geller M, Kooyenga DK, Bierenbaum ML. Hypocholesterolemic and antioxidant effect of rice bran oil non-saponifiables in hypercholesterolemic subjects. *Environmental & Nutritional Interactions* 1999;3:115-22.

1355 Dwyer JH, Merz NB, Shirocre AM, et al. Progression of early atherosclerosis and intake of vitamin C and vitamin E from supplements and food. The Los Angeles Atherosclerosis Study. 41st Annual Conference on Cardiovascular Disease Epidemiology and Prevention - Abstract P77. *Circulation* 2001;103:1365d.

1356 Marijuana Use by Middle-Aged Adults Linked to Increased Risk of MI. www.medscape.com/reuters/prof/2000/03/03.03/ep03030b.html (Accessed 3 March 2000).

1357 Feigin A, Kieburtz K, Como P, et al. Assessment of coenzyme Q10 tolerability in Huntington's disease. *Mov Disord* 1996;11:321-3.

1358 Mullins RJ. Allergic reactions to Echinacea. *J Allergy Clin Immunol* 2000;104:S340-341 (Abstract 1003).

1359 Elmets CA, Singh D, Tubesing K, et al. Cutaneous photoprotection from ultraviolet injury by green tea polyphenols. *J Am Acad Dermatol* 2001;44:425-32.

1360 McGuire JK, Kulkarni MS, Baden HP. Fatal hypermagnesemia in a child treated with megavitamin/megamineral therapy. *Pediatrics* 2000;105:e18.

1361 Blum A, Hathaway L, Mincemoyer R, et al. Effects of oral L-arginine on endothelium-dependent vasodilation and markers of inflammation in healthy postmenopausal women. *J Am Coll Cardiol* 2000;35(2):271-6.

1362 Creager MA, Gallagher SJ, Girerd XJ, et al. L-arginine improves endothelium-dependent vasodilation in hypercholesterolemic humans. *J Clin Invest* 1992;90:1248-53.

1363 Clarkson P, Adams MR, Powe AJ, et al. Oral L-arginine improves endothelium-dependent dilation in hypercholesterolemic young adults. *J Clin Invest* 1996;97:1989-94.

1364 Desser L, Rehberger A, Paukovits W. Proteolytic enzymes and amylase induce cytokine production in human peripheral blood mononuclear cells in vitro. *Cancer Biother* 1994;9:253-63.

1365 Wallace MB, Lim J, Cutler A, Bucci L. Effects of dehydroepiandrosterone vs androstenedione supplementation in men. *Med Sci Sports Exerc* 1999;31:1788-92.

1366 Phan TG, Estell J, Duggin G, et al. Lead poisoning from drinking Kombucha tea brewed in a ceramic pot. *Med J Aust* 1998;169(11-12):644-6.

1367 Schilling BK, Stone MH, Utter A, et al. Creatine supplementation and health variables: a retrospective study. *Med Sci Sports Exerc* 2001;33:183-8.

1368 Greenhaff P. Renal dysfunction accompanying oral creatine supplements. *Lancet* 1998;352:233-4.

1369 Ferraro S, Codella C, Palumbo F, et al. Hemodynamic effects of creatine phosphate in patients with congestive heart failure: a double-blind comparison trial versus placebo. *Clin Cardiol* 1996;19:699-703.

1370 Lyon MJ, Shaw JC. Allergic contact dermatitis reaction to henna. *Arch Dermatol* 2000;136:124-5.

1371 Leppala JM, Virtamo J, Fogelholm R, et al. Controlled trial of alpha-tocopherol and beta-carotene supplements on stroke incidence and mortality in male smokers. *Arterioscler Thromb Vasc Biol* 2000;20:230-5.

1372 Sigurjonsdottir HA, Ragnarsson J, Franzson L, Sigurdsson G. Is blood pressure commonly raised by moderate consumption of liquorice? *J Hum Hypertens* 1995;9:345-8.

1373 Baron AM, Donnerstein RL, Samson RA, et al. Hemodynamic and electrophysiologic effects of acute chocolate ingestion in young adults. *Am J Cardiol* 1999;84:370-3.

1374 Friedman G. Diet and the irritable bowel syndrome. *Gastroenterol Clin North Am* 1991;20:313-24.

1375 Blue-Green Algae Protein Is a Promising Anti-HIV Microbicide Candidate. www.medscape.com/reuters/prof/2000/03/03.16/dd03160g.html (Accessed 16 March 2000).

1376 Anderson JW, Allgood LD, Lawrence A, et al. Cholesterol-lowering effects of psyllium intake adjunctive to diet therapy in men and women with hypercholesterolemia: meta-analysis of 8 controlled trials. *Am J Clin Nutr* 2000;71:472-9.

1377 Lee A, Minhas R, Ito S, et al. Safety of St. John's wort during breastfeeding. *Clin Pharmacol Ther* 2000;67:130, abstract PII-64.

1378 Roots I, Johne A, Schmider J, Brockmoller J, et al. Interaction of a herbal extract from St. John's wort with amitriptyline and its metabolites. *Clin Pharmacol Ther* 2000;67:159, abstract PIII-69.

1379 Carson SW, Hill-Zabala CE, Roberts SH, Hawke RL. Inhibitory effect of methanolic solution of St. John's wort (hypericum perforatum) on cytochrome p450 3A4 activity in human liver microsomes. *Clin Pharmacol Ther* 2000;67(2):99 (abstract PI-39).

1380 For Dieter, Nearly the Ultimate Loss. www.washingtonpost.com/wp-dyn/articles/A33421-2000Mar17.html (Accessed 19 March 2000).

1381 FDA Takes Aim at Ephedra. www.washingtonpost.com/wp-dyn/articles/A33439-2000Mar17.html (Accessed 19 March 2000).

1382 Dallas S, Stempak D, Koren G, et al. Whey protein concentrate (WPC) modulation of lymphocyte glutathione levels in vitro. *Clin Pharmacol Ther* 2000;67:156 (abstract PIII-56).

1383 Offman EM, Freeman DJ, Dresser GK, et al. Cisapride interaction with grapefruit juice and red wine. *Clin Pharmacol Ther* 2000;67:110 (abstract PI-83).

1384 Tsunoda SM, Christians U, Velez RL, et al. Red wine (RW) effects on cyclosporine (CyA) metabolites. *Clin Pharmacol Ther* 2000;67:150 (abstract PIII-35).

1385 Bertino JS, Demuro RL, Blask DE, et al. Absolute bioavailability (F) of oral melatonin (M). *Clin Pharmacol Ther* 2000;67:106 (abstract PI-72).

1386 Veronese M, Burke J, Dorval E, et al. Grapefruit juice (GFJ) inhibits hepatic and intestinal CYP3A4 dose-dependently. *Clin Pharmacol Ther* 2000;67:151 (abstract PIII-37).

1387 Tsunoda SM, Harris RZ, Velez RL, et al. Red wine (RW) effects on cyclosporine (CyA) Pharmacokinetics. *Clin Pharmacol Ther* 1998;65:159 (abstract PII-51).

1388 Bailey DG, Dresser GK, Kreeft JH, et al. Grapefruit juice-felodipine interaction: Effect of segments and an extract from unprocessed fruit. *Clin Pharmacol Ther* 2000;67:107 (abstract PI-71).

1389 Frye RF, Kroboth PD, Folan MM, et al. Effect of DHEA on CYP3A-mediated metabolism of triazolam. *Clin Pharmacol Ther* 2000;67:109 (abstract PI-82).

1390 Soldner A, Christians U, Susanto M, et al. Grapefruit juice activates P-glycoprotein-mediated drug transport. *Pharm Res* 1999;16:478-85.

1391 Zaidenstein R, Avni B, Dishi V, et al. Effect of grapefruit juice on the pharmacokinetics of losartan in healthy volunteers. *Clin Pharmacol Ther* 1998;65:(abstract PI-60).

1392 Dresser GK, Bailey DG, Carruthers SG. Grapefruit juice-felodipine interaction in healthy seniors. *Clin Pharmacol Ther* 1998;65:(abstract PIII-63).

1393 Martin KJ, Chen SF, Clark GM, et al. Evaluation of creatine analogues as a new class of anticancer agents using freshly explanted human tumor cells. *J Natl Cancer Inst* 1994;86:608-13.

1394 John Mendelson J, Tolliver B, Delucchi K, Berger P. Capsaicin increases the lethality of cocaine. *Clin Pharmacol Ther* 1998;65:(abstract PII-27).

1395 Johnson MA, Robin P, Smith RP, et al. Large lung bullae in marijuana smokers. *Thorax* 2000;55:340-2.

1396 Sandor PS, Afra J, Ambrosini A, Schoenen J. Prophylactic treatment of migraine with beta-blockers and riboflavin: differential effects on the intensity dependence of auditory evoked cortical potentials. *Headache* 2000;40:30-5.

1397 Schoenen J, Lenaerts M, Bastings E. High-dose riboflavin as a prophylactic treatment of migraine: results of an open pilot study. *Cephalalgia* 1994;14:328-9.

1398 Schoenen J, Jacquy J, Lenaerts M. Effectiveness of high-dose riboflavin in migraine prophylaxis. A randomized controlled trial. *Neurology* 1998;50:466-70.

1401 Jardim LB, Palma-Dias R, Silva LC, et al. Maternal hyperphenylalaninaemia as a cause of microcephaly and mental retardation. *Acta Paediatr* 1996;85:943-6.

1402 Rouse B, Azen C, Koch R, et al. Maternal phenylketonuria collaborative Study (MPKUCS) offspring: facial anomalies, malformations, and early neurological sequelae. *Am J Med Genet* 1997;69:89-95.

1403 Sternberg EM, Van Woert MH, Young SN, et al. Development of a scleroderma-like illness during therapy with L-5-hydroxytryptophan and carbidopa. *N Engl J Med* 1980;303:782-7.

1404 Joly P, Lampert A, Thomine E, et al. Development of pseudobullous morphea and scleroderma-like illness during therapy with L-5-hydroxytryptophan and carbidopa. *J Am Acad Dermatol* 1991;25:332-3.

1405 Anderson JW, Allgood LD, Turner J, et al. Effects of psyllium on glucose and serum lipid responses in men with type 2 diabetes and hypercholesterolemia. *Am J Clin Nutr* 1999;70:466-73.

1406 Miller EE, Evans AE, Cohn M. Inhibition of rate of tumor growth by creatine and cyclocreatine. *Proc Natl Acad Sci U S A* 1993;90:3304-8.

1407 O'Brien PM, Pipkin FB. The effect of essential fatty acid and specific vitamin supplements on vascular sensitivity in the mid trimester of human pregnancy. *Clin Exp Hypertens B* 1983;2:247-54.

1408 O'Brien PM, Morrison R, Pipken FB. Effect of dietary supplementation with linoleic and gammalinolenic acids on the pressor response to angiotensin II--possible role in pregnancy induced hypertension? *Br J Clin Pharmacol* 1985;19:335-42.

1409 Laivuori H, Hovatta O, Viinikka L, et al. Dietary supplementation with primrose oil or fish oil does not change urinary excretion of prostacyclin and thromboxane metabolites in pre-eclamptic women. *Prostaglandins Leukot Essent Fatty Acids* 1993;49:691-4.

1410 Ritchie DJ, Becker ES. Update on the management of intestinal cryptosporidiosis in AIDS. *Ann Pharmacother* 1994;28:767-78.

1411 Dove D, Johnson P. Oral evening primrose oil: its effect on length of pregnancy and selected intrapartum outcomes in low-risk nulliparous women. *J Nurse Midwifery* 1999;44:320-4.

1412 Brinkeborn RM, Shah DV, Degenring FH. Echinaforce and other Echinacea fresh plant preparations in the treatment of the common cold. A randomized, placebo controlled, double-blind clinical trial. *Phytomedicine* 1999;6:1-6.

1413 Mengs U, Clare CB, Poiley JA. Toxicity of Echinacea purpurea. Acute, subacute and genotoxicity studies. *Arzneimittelforschung* 1991;41:1076-81.

1414 Awang DVC, Kindack DG. Echinacea. *Can Pharm J* November 1999:512-6.

1415 D'Avanzo B, La Vecchia C, Franceschi S, et al. Coffee consumption and bladder cancer risk. *Eur J Cancer* 1992;28A(8-9):1480-4.

1416 Pannelli F, La Rosa F, Saltalamacchia G, et al. Tobacco smoking, coffee, cocoa and tea consumption in relation to mortality from urinary bladder cancer in Italy. *Eur J Epidemiol* 1989;5:392-7.

1417 Slattery ML, West DW, Robison LM. Fluid intake and bladder cancer in Utah. *Int J Cancer* 1988;42:17-22.

1418 Joseph JA, Shukitt-Hale B, Denisova NA, et al. Long-term dietary strawberry, spinach, or vitamin E supplementation retards the onset of age-related neuronal signal-transduction and cognitive behavioral deficits. *J Neurosci* 1998;18:8047-55.

1419 Joseph JA, Shukitt-Hale B, Denisova NA, et al. Reversals of age-related declines in neuronal signal transduction, cognitive, and motor behavioral deficits with blueberry, spinach, or strawberry dietary supplementation. *J Neurosci* 1999;19:8114-21.

1420 Chng HH, Shaw D, Klesius P, Saxon A. Inability of oral bovine transfer factor to eradicate cryptosporidial infection in a patient with congenital dysgammaglobulinemia. *Clin Immunol Immunopathol* 1989;50:402-6.

1421 Gebhardt R. Hepatoprotection with artichoke extract. *Pharm Ztg* 1995;140:34-7.

1422 Gebhardt R. Antioxidative and protective properties of extracts from leaves of the artichoke (Cynara scolymus L.) against hydroperoxide-induced oxidative stress in cultured rat hepatocytes. *Toxicol Appl Pharmacol* 1997;144:279-86.

1423 Hammerl WH, Kindler K, Kranzl C, et al. Effect of cynarin (cynarine) on hyperlipidemia, especially on hypercholesterolemia. *Wien Med Wochenschr* 1973;123:601-5.

1424 Heckers H, Dittmar K, Schmahl FW, et al. Inefficiency of cynarin as therapeutic regimen in familial type II hyperlipoproteinaemia. *Atherosclerosis* 1977;26:249-53.

1425 Gebhardt R. Inhibition of cholesterol biosynthesis in primary cultured rat hepatocytes by artichoke (Cynara scolymus L.) extracts. *J Pharmacol Exp Therap* 1998;386:1122-8.

1426 Brown JE, Rice-Evans CA. Luteolin-rich artichoke extract protects low density lipoprotein from oxidation in vitro. *Free Radic Res* 1998;29:247-55.

1427 Vogler BK, Pittler MH, Ernst E. The efficacy of ginseng. A systemic review of randomized clinical trials. *Eur J Clin Pharmacol* 1999;55:567-75.

1428 Osato MS, Reddy SG, Graham DY. Osmotic effect of honey on growth and viability of Helicobacter pylori. *Dig Dis Sci* 1999;44(3):462-4.

1430 Anon. Adverse events associated with ingestion of gamma-butyrolactone--Minnesota, New Mexico, and Texas, 1998-1999. *MMWR Morb Mortal Wkly Rep* 1999;48:137-40.

1431 Harrington RD, Woodward JA, Hooton TM, et al. Life-threatening interactions between HIV-1 protease inhibitors and the illicit drugs MDMA and gamma-hydroxybutyrate. *Arch Intern Med* 1999;159:2221-4.

1432 Bergnes G, Yuan W, Khandekar VS, et al. Creatine and phosphocreatine analogs: anticancer activity and enzymatic analysis. *Oncol Res* 1996;8:121-30.

1433 Ellaway CM, Williams K, Leonard H, et al. Rett syndrome: randomized controlled trial of L-carnitine. *J Child Neurol* 1999;14:162-7.

1434 Brevetti G, Diehm C, Lambert D, et al. European multicenter study on propionyl-L-carnitine in intermittent claudication. *J Am Coll Cardiol* 1999;34:1618-24.

1435 Brevetti G, Perna S, Sabba C, et al. Propionyl-L-carnitine in intermittent claudication: double-blind, placebo-controlled, dose titration, multicenter study. *J Am Coll Cardiol* 1995;26:1411-6.

1436 Brevetti G, Perna S, Sabba C, et al. Effect of propionyl-L-carnitine on quality of life in intermittent claudication. *Am J Cardiol* 1997;79:777-80.

1437 Brevetti G, Perna S, Sabba C, et al. Superiority of L-propionylcarnitine vs L-carnitine in improving walking capacity in patients with peripheral vascular disease: an acute, intravenous, double-blind, cross-over study. *Eur Heart J* 1992;13:251-5.

1438 Ishikura H, Matsuo N, Matsubara M, et al. Valproic acid overdose and L-carnitine therapy. *J Anal Toxicol* 1996;20:55-8.

1439 Siliprandi N, Di Lisa F, Menabo R. Propionyl-L-carnitine: biochemical significance and possible role in cardiac metabolism. *Cardiovasc Drugs Ther* 1991;5 Suppl 1:11-5.

1440 Tribble DL. AHA Science Advisory. Antioxidant consumption and risk of coronary heart disease: emphasis on vitamin C, vitamin E, and beta-carotene: A statement for healthcare professionals from the American Heart Association. *Circulation* 1999;99:591-5.

1441 Watanabe H, Masaaki K, Ohtsuka S, et al. Randomized, double-blind, placebo-controlled study of the preventative effect of supplemental oral vitamin C on attenuation of development of nitrate tolerance. *J Am Coll Cardiol* 1998;31:1323-9.

1442 Tao X, Davis LS, Lipsky PE. Effect of an extract of the Chinese herbal remedy Tripterygium wilfordii Hook F on human immune responsiveness. *Arthritis Rheum* 1991;34:1274-81.

1443 Cohen HA, Neuman I, Nahum H. Blocking effect of vitamin C in exercise-induced asthma. *Arch Pediatr Adolesc Med* 1997;151:103-9.

1444 Zhang S, Hunter DJ, Forman MR, et al. Dietary carotenoids and vitamins A, C, and E and risk of breast cancer. *J Natl Cancer Inst* 1999;91:547-56.

1445 Louie E, Borkowsky W, Klesius PH, et al. Treatment of cryptosporidiosis with oral bovine transfer factor. *Clin Immunol Immunopathol* 1987;44:329-34.

1446 Klipstein-Grobusch K, Launer LJ, Geleijnse JM, et al. Serum carotenoids and atherosclerosis. The Rotterdam Study. *Atherosclerosis* 2000;148:49-56.

1447 Gann PH, Ma J, Giovannucci E, et al. Lower prostate cancer risk in men with elevated plasma lycopene levels: results of a prospective analysis. *Cancer Res* 1999;59:1225-30.

1448 Lee IM, Cook NR, Manson JE, et al. Beta-carotene supplementation and incidence of cancer and cardiovascular disease: the Women's Health Study. *J Natl Cancer Inst* 1999;91:2102-6.

1449 Ascherio A, Rimm EB, Hernan MA, et al. Relation of consumption of vitamin E, vitamin C, and carotenoids to risk for stroke among men in the United States. *Ann Intern Med* 1999;130:963-70.

1451 Wakabayashi K, Kono S, Shinchi K, et al. Habitual coffee consumption and blood pressure: A study of self-defense officials in Japan. *Eur J Epidemiol* 1998;14:669-73.

1452 Hodgson JM, Puddey IB, Burke V, et al. Effects on blood pressure of drinking green and black tea. *J Hypertens* 1999;17:457-63.

1453 Dulloo AG, Duret C, Rohrer D, et al. Efficacy of a green tea extract rich in catechin polyphenols and caffeine in increasing 24-h energy expenditure and fat oxidation in humans. *Am J Clin Nutr* 1999;70:1040-5.

1454 Garbisa S, Biggin S, Cavallarin N, et al. Tumor invasion: molecular shears blunted by green tea. *Nat Med* 1999;5:1216.

1455 Cao Y, Cao R. Angiogenesis inhibited by drinking tea. *Nature* 1999;398:381.

1456 L'Allemain G. [Multiple actions of EGCG, the main component of green tea]. [Article in French]. *Bull Cancer* 1999;86:721-4.

1457 Bushman JL. Green tea and cancer in humans: a review of the literature. *Nutr Cancer* 1998;31:151-9.

1458 Wakai K, Ohno Y, Obata K. Prognostic significance of selected lifestyle factors in urinary bladder cancer. *Jpn J Cancer Res* 1993;84:1223-9.

1459 Ohno Y, Aoki K, Obata K, et al. Case-control study of urinary bladder cancer in metropolitan Nagoya. *Natl Cancer Inst Monogr* 1985;69:229-34.

1460 Booth SL, Madabushi HT, Davidson KW, et al. Tea and coffee brews are not dietary sources of vitamin K-1 (phylloquinone). *J Am Diet Assoc* 1995;95:82-3.

1461 Lou FQ, Zhang MF, Zhang XG, et al. A study on tea-pigment in prevention of atherosclerosis. *Chin Med J* (Engl) 1989;102:579-83.

1463 Graham HN. Green tea composition, consumption, and polyphenol chemistry. *Prev Med* 1992;21:334-50.

1464 Shankar AH, Genton B, Semba RD, et al. Effect of vitamin A supplementation on morbidity due to Plasmodium falciparum in young children in Papua New Guinea: a randomised trial. *Lancet* 1999;354:203-9.

1465 Fawzi WW, Mbise RL, Hertzmark E, et al. A randomized trial of vitamin A supplements in relation to mortality among human immunodeficiency virus-infected and uninfected children in Tanzania. *Pediatr Infect Dis J* 1999;18:127-33.

1466 Fawzi WW, Mbise RL, Fataki MR, et al. Vitamin A supplementation and severity of pneumonia in children admitted to the hospital in Dar es Salaam, Tanzania. *Am J Clin Nutr* 1998;68:187-92.

1467 Kowalski TE, Falestiny M, Furth E, Malet PF. Vitamin A hepatotoxicity: a cautionary note regarding 25,000 IU supplements. *Am J Med* 1994;97(6):523-8.

1468 Wang Z, Boudjelal M, Kang S, et al. Ultraviolet irradiation of human skin causes functional vitamin A deficiency, preventable by all-trans retinoic acid pre-treatment. *Nat Med* 1999;5:418-22.

1469 Meyers DG, Maloley PA, Weeks D. Safety of antioxidant vitamins. *Arch Intern Med* 1996;156(9):925-35.

1470 Cooper DA, Eldridge AL, Peters JC. Dietary carotenoids and certain cancers, heart disease, and age-related macular degeneration: a review of recent research. *Nutr Rev* 1999;57:201-14.

1471 Cooper DA, Eldridge AL, Peters JC. Dietary carotenoids and lung cancer: a review of recent research. *Nutr Rev* 1999;57:133-45.

1472 Garewal HS, Katz RV, Meyskens F, et al. Beta-carotene produces sustained remissions in patients with oral leukoplakia: results of a multicenter prospective trial. *Arch Otolaryngol Head Neck Surg* 1999;125:1305-10.

1473 Cook NR, Stampfer MJ, Ma J, et al. Beta-carotene supplementation for patients with low baseline levels and decreased risks of total and prostate carcinoma. *Cancer* 1999;86:1783-92.

1474 Neuman I, Nahum H, Ben-Amotz A. Prevention of exercise-induced asthma by a natural isomer mixture of beta-carotene. *Ann Allergy Asthma Immunol* 1999;82:549-53.

1475 Radosevich JK, Scott GH, Olson GB. Delayed-type hypersensitivity responses induced by bovine colostral components. *Am J Vet Res* 1985;46:875-8.

1476 Sharma MK, Foroozanfar N, Ala FA. Progressive BCG infection in an immunodeficient child treated with transfer factor. *Clin Immunol Immunopathol* 1978;10:369-80.

1477 Klesius PH, Fudenberg HH. Bovine transfer factor: in vivo transfer of cell-mediated immunity to cattle with alcohol precipitates. *Clin Immunol Immunopathol* 1977;8:238-46.

1478 Klesius PH, Qualls DF, Elston AL, Fudenberg HH. Effects of bovine transfer factor (TFd) in mouse coccidiosis (Eimeria ferrisi). *Clin Immunol Immunopathol* 1978;10:214-21.

1479 Devaraj S, Jialal I. Alpha-tocopherol decreases interleukin-1 beta release from activated human monocytes by inhibition of 5-lipoxygenase. *Arterioscler Thromb Vasc Biol* 1999;19(4):1125-33.

1480 McMeeking A, Borkowsky W, Klesius PH, et al. A controlled trial of bovine dialyzable leukocyte extract for cryptosporidiosis in patients with AIDS. *J Infect Dis* 1990;161:108-12.

1481 Lillie JW, O'Keefe M, Valinski H, et al. Cyclocreatine (1-carboxymethyl-2-iminoimidazolidine) inhibits growth of a broad spectrum of cancer cells derived from solid tumors. *Cancer Res* 1993;53:3172-3178.

1482 Houston DK, Johnson MA, Nozza RJ, et al. Age-related hearing loss, vitamin B-12, and folate in elderly women. *Am J Clin Nutr* 1999;69:564-71.

1483 Selhub J, Jacques PF, Wilson PW, et al. Vitamin status and intake as primary determinants of homocysteinemia in an elderly population. *JAMA* 1993;270:2693-8.

1484 Carmel R, Green R, Jacobsen DW, et al. Serum cobalamin, homocysteine, and methylmalonic acid concentrations in a multiethnic elderly population: ethnic and sex differences in cobalamin and metabolite abnormalities. *Am J Clin Nutr* 1999;70:904-10.

1485 Stabler SP, Allen RH, Fried LP, et al. Racial differences in prevalence of cobalamin and folate deficiencies in disabled elderly women. *Am J Clin Nutr* 1999;70:911-9.

1486 Laser Reutersward A, Skog K, Jagerstad M. Mutagenicity of pan-fried bovine tissues in relation to their content of creatine, creatinine, monosaccharides and free amino acids. *Food Chem Toxicol* 1987;25:755-62.

1487 Manabe S, Kurihara N, Wada O, et al. Formation of PhIP in a mixture of creatinine, phenylalanine and sugar or aldehyde by aqueous heating. *Carcinogenesis* 1992;13:827-830.

1488 Liu C, Russell RM, Seitz HK, et al. Ethanol enhances retinoic acid metabolism into polar metabolites in rat liver via induction of cytochrome P4502E1. *Gastroenterol* 2001;120:179-89.

1489 Bostom AG, Gohh RY, Beaulieu AJ, et al. Treatment of hyperhomocysteinemia in renal transplant recipients. A randomized, placebo-controlled trial. *Ann Intern Med* 1997;127:1089-92.

1492 Klipstein-Grobusch K, Grobbee DE, den Breeijen JH, et al. Dietary iron and risk of myocardial infarction in the Rotterdam Study. *Am J Epidemiol* 1999;149:421-8.

1493 Kirkpatrick CH. Structural nature and functions of transfer factors. *Ann N Y Acad Sci* 1993;685:362-8.

1494 Kirkpatrick CH. Biological response modifiers. Interferons, interleukins, and transfer factor. *Ann Allergy* 1989;62:170-6.

1495 Hassner A, Adelman DC. Biologic response modifiers in primary immunodeficiency disorders. *Ann Intern Med* 1991;115:294-307.

1496 Clinton SK, Emenhiser C, Schwartz SJ, et al. Cis-trans lycopene isomers, carotenoids, and retinol in the human prostate. *Cancer Epidemiol Biomarkers Prev* 1996;5:823-33.

1497 Gartner C, Stahl W, Sies H. Lycopene is more bioavaiable from tomato paste than from fresh tomatoes. *Am J Clin Nutr* 1997;66:116-22.

1498 Paetau I, Khachik F, Brown ED, et al. Chronic ingestion of lycopene-rich tomato juice or lycopene supplements significantly increases plasma concentrations of lycopene and related tomato carotenoids in humans. *Am J Clin Nutr* 1998;68:1187-95.

1499 USDA. NCC Carotenoid Database for U.S. Foods. 1998. Available at: http://www.nal.usda.gov/fnic/foodcomp/Data/car98/car98.html

1500 Rueff F, Schoepf P, Pfuetzner W, Przybilla B. Sensitization to condurango bark is frequent in patients with allergy to natural rubber latex. *J Allergy Clin Immunol* 1998;101:S207.

1501 Pfutzner W, Thomas P, Rueff F, Przybilla B. Anaphylactic reaction elicited by condurango bark in a patient allergic to natural rubber latex. *J Allergy Clin Immunol* 1998;101:281-2.

1502 Medicinal Plants. Springer Verlag: Lavoisier, NY, 1995.

1503 Reichert R. Sedative Effects of California Poppy and Corydalis. Quarterly Review of Natural Medicine, Winter 1996:256.

1505 Trivedi CP, Modi NT, Sarin RK, Rao SS. Bronchodilator and anti-inflammatory effect of glycosidal fraction of Acacia farnesiana. *Indian J Physiol Pharmacol* 1986;30:267-8.

1507 Fudenberg HH. Transfer factor: past, present and future. *Annu Rev Pharmacol Toxicol* 1989;29:475-516.

1512 Anon. In vitro screening of traditional medicines for anti-HIV activity: memorandum from a WHO meeting. *Bull World Health Organ* 1989;67:613-8.

1514 Le Bars PL, Katz MM, Berman N, et al. A placebo-controlled, double-blind, randomized trial of an extract of Ginkgo biloba for dementia. North American EGb Study Group. *JAMA* 1997;278:1327-32.

1515 Oken BS, Storzbach DM, Kaye JA. The efficacy of Ginkgo biloba on cognitive function in Alzheimer disease. *Arch Neurol* 1998;55:1409-15.

1516 Akhtar MS, et al. Field trial of Saussurea lappa roots against nematodes and Nigella sativa seeds against cestodes in children. *JPMA J Pak Med Assoc* 1991 Aug;41(8)185-7.

1519 Tona L, et al. Antiamoebic and phytochemical screening of some Congolese medicinal plants. *J Ethnopharmacol* 1998 May, 61(1):57-65.

1520 Houpt JB, McMillan R, Wein C, Paget-Dellio SD. Effect of glucosamine hydrochloride in the treatment of pain of osteoarthritis of the knee. *J Rheumatol* 1999;26:2423-30.

1522 Park HJ, Lee JH, Song YB, Park KH. Effects of dietary supplementation of lipophilic fraction from Panax ginseng on cGMP and cAMP in rat platelets and on blood coagulation. *Biol Pharm Bull* 1996;19:1434-9.

1523 Lin RC, Li TK. Effects of isoflavones on alcohol pharmacokinetics and alcohol-drinking behavior in rats. *Am J Clin Nutr* 1998;68:1512S-5S.

1524 Xie CI, Lin RC, Antony V, et al. Daidzin, an antioxidant isoflavonoid, decreases blood alcohol levels and shortens sleep time induced by ethanol intoxication. *Alcohol Clin Exp Res* 1994;18:1443-7.

1525 Avalos J, Rupprecht JK, McLaughlin JL, et al. Guinea pig maximization test of the bark extract from pawpaw, Asimina triloba (Annonaceae). *Contact Dermatitis* 1993;29:33-5.

1526 Tomoda M, Gonda R, Shimizu N, Yamada H. Plant mucilages. XLII. An anti-complementary mucilage from the leaves of Malva sylvestris var. mauritiana. *Chem Pharm Bull* 1989;37:3029-32.

1527 Stefanova Z, Neychev H, Ivanovska N, Kostova I. Effect of a total extract from Fraxinus ornus stem bark and esculin on zymosan- and carrageenan-induced paw oedema in mice. *J Ethnopharmacol* 1995;46:101-6.

1528 Pintos J, Franco EL, Oliveira BV, et al. Mate, coffee, and tea consumption and risk of cancers of the upper aerodigestive tract in southern Brazil. *Epidemiology* 1994;5:583-90.

1529 De Stefani E, Fierro L, Mendilaharsu M, et al. Meat intake, 'mate' drinking and renal cell cancer in Uruguay: a case-control study. *Br J Cancer* 1998;78:1239-43.

1530 De Stefani E, Correa P, Fierro L, et al. Black tobacco, mate, and bladder cancer. A case-control study from Uruguay. *Cancer* 1991;67:536-40.

1531 De Stefani E, Fierro L, Correa P, et al. Mate drinking and risk of lung cancer in males: a case-control study from Uruguay. *Cancer Epidemiol Biomarkers Prev* 1996;5:515-9.

1532 Kong YC, Yeung HW, Cheung YM, et al. Isolation of the uterotonic principle from Leonurus artemisia, the Chinese motherwort. *Am J Chin Med* 1976;4:373-82.

1533 Zou QZ, Bi RG, Li JM, et al. Effect of motherwort on blood hyperviscosity. *Am J Chin Med* 1989;17:65-70.

1534 Zgorniak-Nowosielska I, Grzybek J, Manolova N, et al. Antiviral activity of Flos verbasci infusion against influenza and Herpes simplex viruses. *Arch Immunol Ther Exp* 1991;39:103-8.

1535 al-Harbi MM, Qureshi S, Raza M, et al. Gastric antiulcer and cytoprotective effect of Commiphora molmol in rats. *J Ethnopharmacol* 1997;55:141-50.

1536 al-Harbi MM, Qureshi S, Raza M, et al. Anticarcinogenic effect of Commiphora molmol on solid tumors induced by Ehrlich carcinoma cells in mice. *Chemotherapy* 1994:40:337-47.

1537 Pintao AM, Pais MS, Coley H, et al. In vitro and in vivo antitumor activity of benzyl isothiocyanate: a natural product from Tropaeolum majus. *Planta Med* 1995;61:233-6.

1538 Buck DS, Nidorf DM, Addino JG. Comparison of two topical preparations for the treatment of onychomycosis: Melaleuca alternifolia (tea tree) oil and clotimazole. *J Fam Pract* 1994;38:601-5.

1539 De Rosa SC, Zaretsky MD, Dubs JG, et al. N-acetylcysteine replenishes glutathione in HIV infection. *Eur J Clin Invest* 2000;30:915-29.

1540 Cherif S, Rahal N, Haouala M, et al. [A clinical trial of a titrated Olea extract in the treatment of essential arterial hypertension]. *J Pharm Belg* 1996;51:69-71.

1541 Aziz NH, Farag SE, Mousa LA, et al. Comparative antibacterial and antifungal effects of some phenolic compounds. *Microbios* 1998;93:43-54.

1542 Pieroni A, Heimler D, Pieters L, et al. In vitro anti-complementary activity of flavonoids from olive (Olea europaea L.) leaves. *Pharmazie* 1996;51:765-8.

1543 Liccardi G, D'Amato M, D'Amato G. Oleaceae pollinosis: a review. *Int Arch Allergy Immunol* 1996;111:210-7.

1544 Holti G. An experimentally controlled evaluation of the effect of inositol nicotinate upon the digital blood flow in

patients with Raynaud's phenomenon. *J Int Med Res* 1979;7:473-83.
1545 Ring EF, Bacon PA. Quantitative thermographic assessment of inositol nicotinate therapy in Raynaud's phenomena. *J Int Med Res* 1977;5:217-22.
1546 Wilke H, Frahm H. [Treatment of hyperlipoproteinaemia types IIa, IIb, IV and V with a combination of clofibrate and inositol nicotinate]. [Article in German]. *Dtsch Med Wochenschr* 1976;101:401-5.
1547 Anon. Alpha-lipoic acid. *Altern Med Rev* 1998;3:308-10.
1548 Berkson BM. Thioctic acid in treatment of hepatotoxic mushroom (Phalloides) poisoning (letter). *N Engl J Med* 1979;300:371.
1549 Roldan EJ, Perez Lloret A. Thioctic acid in Amanita poisoning (letter). *Crit Care Med* 1986;14:753-4.
1550 Biewenga GP, Haenen GR, Bast A. The pharmacology of the antioxidant lipoic acid. *Gen Pharmacol* 1997;29:315-31.
1554 Matalon R, Stumpf DA, Michals K, et al. Lipoamide dehydrogenase deficiency with primary lactic acidosis: favorable response to treatment with oral lipoic acid. *J Pediatr* 1984;104:65-9.
1555 Yoshida I, Sweetman L, Kulovich S, et al. Effect of lipoic acid in patient with defective activity of pyruvate dehydrogenase, 2-oxoglutarate dehydrogenase, and branched-chain keto acid dehydrogenase. *Pediatr Res* 1990;27:75-9.
1556 Dana Consortium on the therapy of HIV dementia and related cognitive disorders. A randomized, double-blind, placebo-controlled trial of deprenyl and thioctic acid in human immunodeficiency virus-associated cognitive impairment. *Neurology* 1998;50:645-51.
1557 Maesaka H, Komiya K, Misugi K, Tada K. Hyperalaninemia hyperpyruvicemia and lactic acidosis due to pyruvate carboxylase deficiency of the liver; treatment with thiamine and lipoic acid. *Eur J Pediatr* 1976;122:159-68.
1561 Packer L, Tritschler HJ, Wessel K. Neuroprotection by the metabolic antioxidant alpha-lipoic acid. *Free Radic Biol Med* 1997;22:359-78.
1562 Merin JP, Matsuyama M, Kira T, et al. Alpha-lipoic acid blocks HIV-1 LTR-dependent expression of hygromycin resistance in THP-1 stable transformants. *FEBS Lett* 1996;394:9-13.
1563 Suzuki YJ, Aggarwal BB, Packer L. Alpha-lipoic acid is a potent inhibitor of NF-kappa B activation in human T cells. *Biochem Biophys Res Commun* 1992;189:1709-15.
1571 Chiddo A, Gaglione A, Musci S, et al. Hemodynamic study of intravenous propionyl-L-carnitine in patients with ischemic heart disease and normal left ventricular function. *Cardiovasc Drugs Ther* 1991;5 Suppl 1:107-11.
1572 Bartels GL, Remme WJ, Pillay M, et al. Acute improvement of cardiac function with intravenous L-propionylcarnitine in humans. *J Cardiovasc Pharmacol* 1992;20:157-64.
1573 Bartels GL, Remme WJ, Pillay M, et al. Effects of L-propionylcarnitine on ischemia-induced myocardial dysfunction in men with angina pectoris. *Am J Cardiol* 1994;74:125-30.
1574 Persico G, Amato B, Aprea G, et al. The early effects of intravenous L-propionyl carnitine on ulcerative trophic lesions of the lower limbs in arteriopathic patients: a controlled randomized study. *Drugs Exp Clin Res* 1995;21:187-98.
1575 Anand I, Chandrashekhan Y, De Giuli F, et al. Acute and chronic effects of propionyl-L-carnitine on the hemodynamics, exercise capacity, and hormones in patients with congestive heart failure. *Cardiovasc Drugs Ther* 1998;12:291-9.
1576 Dal Lago A, De Martini D, Flore R, et al. Effects of propionyl-L-carnitine on peripheral arterial obliterative disease of the lower limbs: a double-blind clinical trial. *Drugs Exp Clin Res* 1999;25:29-36.
1577 Ferrari R, De Giuli F. The propionyl-L-carnitine hypothesis: an alternative approach to treating heart failure. *J Card Fail* 1997;3:217-24.
1578 Wiseman LR, Brogden RN. Propionyl-L-carnitine. *Drugs Aging* 1998;12:243-8; discussion 249-50.
1579 Cherchi A, Lai C, Onnis E, et al. Propionyl carnitine in stable effort angina. *Cardiovasc Drugs Ther* 1990;4:481-6.
1580 Bartels GL, Remme WJ, den Hartog FR, et al. Additional anti-ischemic effects of long-term L-propionylcarnitine in anginal patients treated with conventional antianginal therapy. *Cardiovasc Drugs Ther* 1995;9:749-53.
1581 Bartels GL, Remme WJ, Holwerda KJ, Kruijssen DA. Anti-ischaemic efficacy of L-propionylcarnitine - a promising novel metabolic approach to ischaemia? *Eur Heart J* 1996;17:414-20.
1582 Caponnetto S, Canale C, Masperone MA, et al. Efficacy of L-propionylcarnitine treatment in patients with left ventricular dysfunction. *Eur Heart J* 1994;15:1267-73.
1583 Mancini M, Rengo F, Lingetti M, et al. Controlled study on the therapeutic efficacy of propionyl-L-carnitine in patients with congestive heart failure. *Arzneimittelforschung* 1992;42:1101-4.
1584 Stoy DB, LaRosa JC, Brewer BK, et al. Cholesterol-lowering effects of ready-to-eat cereal containing psyllium. *J Am Diet Assoc* 1993;93:910-2.
1586 Hernandez-Avila M, Gonzalez-Cossio T, Hernandez-Avila JE, et al. Dietary calcium supplements to lower blood lead levels in lactating women: a randomized placebo-controlled trial. *Epidemiology* 2003;14:206-12.
1588 De Falco FA, D'Angelo E, Grimaldi G, et al. [Effect of the chronic treatment with L-acetylcarnitine in Down's syndrome]. [Article in Italian]. *Clin Ter* 1994;144:123-7.
1589 Tempesta E, Troncon R, Janiri L, et al. Role of acetyl-L-carnitine in the treatment of cognitive deficit in chronic alcoholism. *Int J Clin Pharmacol Res* 1990;10:101-7.
1590 Mezzina C, De Grandis D, Calvani M, et al. Idiopathic facial paralysis: new therapeutic prospects with acetyl-L-carnitine. *Int J Clin Pharmacol Res* 1992;12:299-304.
1591 Postiglione A, Soricelli A, Cicerano U, et al. Effect of acute administration of L-acetyl carnitine on cerebral blood flow in patients with chronic cerebral infarct. *Pharmacol Res* 1991;23:241-6.
1592 Rosadini G, Marenco S, Nobili F, et al. Acute effects of acetyl-L-carnitine on regional cerebral blood flow in patients with brain ischaemia. *Int J Clin Pharmacol Res* 1990;10:123-8.
1593 Onofrj M, Fulgente T, Melchionda D, et al. L-acetylcarnitine as a new therapeutic approach for peripheral neuropathies with pain. *Int J Clin Pharmacol Res* 1995;15:9-15.
1594 Thal LJ, Carta A, Clarke WR, et al. A 1-year multicenter placebo-controlled study of acetyl-L-carnitine in patients with Alzheimer's Disease. *Neurology* 1996;47:705-11.
1595 Sano M, Bell K, Cote L, et al. Double-blind parallel design pilot study of acetyl levocarnitine in patients with Alzheimer's Disease. *Arch Neurol* 1992;49:1137-41.
1596 Spagnoli A, Lucca U, Menasce G, et al. Long-term acetyl-L-carnitine treatment in Alzheimer's Disease. *Neurology* 1991;41:1726-32.
1597 Brooks JO 3rd, Yesavage JA, Carta A, Bravi D. Acetyl L-carnitine slows decline in younger patients with Alzheimer's disease: a reanalysis of a double-blind, placebo-controlled study using the trilinear approach. *Int Psychoger* 1998;10:193-203.

1598 Pettegrew JW, Klunk WE, Panchalingam K, et al. Clinical and neurochemical effects of acetyl-L-carnitine in Alzheimer's disease. *Neurobiol Aging* 1995;16:1-4.

1599 Rai G, Wright G, Scott L, et al. Double-blind, placebo controlled study of acetyl-l-carnitine in patients with Alzheimer's dementia. *Curr Med Res Opin* 1990;11:638-47.

1600 Dong Y, Yang MM, Kwan CY. In vitro inhibition of proliferation of HL-60 cells by tetrandrine and coriolus versicolor peptide derived from Chinese medicinal herbs. *Life Sci* 1997;60:PL135-40.

1605 FDA. FDA warns against consuming triax metabolic accelerator. Available at: www.fda.gov/bbs/topics/ANSWERS/ANS00984.html

1607 McDermott MT, Ridgway EC. Central hyperthyroidism. *Endocrinol Metab Clin North Am* 1998;27(1):187-203.

1608 Takeda T, Suzuki S, Liu RT, et al. Triiodothyroacetic acid has unique potential for therapy of resistance to thyroid hormone. *J Clin Endocrinol Metab* 1995;80:2033-40.

1609 Kunitake JM, Hartman N, Henson LC, et al. 3,5,3'-triiodothyroacetic acid therapy for thyroid hormone resistance. *J Clin Endocrinol Metab* 1989;69:461-6.

1610 Dulgeroff AJ, Geffner ME, Koyal SN, et al. Bromocriptine and Triac therapy for hyperthyroidism due to pituitary resistance to thyroid hormone. *J Clin Endocrinol Metab* 1992;75(4):1071-5.

1611 Beck-Peccoz P, Sartorio A, De Medici C, et al. Dissociated thyromimetic effects of 3, 5, 3'-triiodothyroacetic acid (TRIAC) at the pituitary and peripheral tissue levels. *J Endocrinol Invest* 1988;11(2):113-8.

1612 Lind P, Langsteger W, Koltringer P, et al. 3,5,3'-Triiodothyroacetic acid (TRIAC) effects on pituitary thyroid regulation and on peripheral tissue parameters. *Nuklearmedizin* 1989;28(6):217-20.

1613 Nicolini U, Venegoni E, Acaia B, et al. Prenatal treatment of fetal hypothyroidism: is there more than one option? *Prenat Diagn* 1996;16(5):443-8.

1614 Asteria C, Rajanayagam O, Collingwood TN, et al. Prenatal diagnosis of thyroid hormone resistance. *J Clin Endocrinol Metab* 1999;84(2):405-10.

1615 Radetti G, Persani L, Molinaro G, et al. Clinical and hormonal outcome after two years of triiodothyroacetic acid treatment in a child with thyroid hormone resistance. *Thyroid* 1997;7(5):775-8.

1616 Jaffiol C, Daures JP, Nsakala N, et al. [Long term follow up of medical treatment of differentiated thyroid cancer]. [Article in French]. *Ann Endocrinol* (Paris) 1995;56:119-26.

1617 Mueller-Gaertner HW, Schneider C. 3,5,3'-Triiodothyroacetic acid minimizes the pituitary thyrotrophin secretion in patients on levo-thyroxine therapy after ablative therapy for differentiated thyroid carcinoma. *Clin Endocrinol* (Oxf) 1988;28(4):345-51.

1618 Mechelany C, Schlumberger M, Challeton C, et al. TRIAC (3,5,3'-triiodothyroacetic acid) has parallel effects at the pituitary and peripheral tissue levels in thyroid cancer patients treated with L-thyroxine. *Clin Endocrinol* (Oxf) 1991;35(2):123-8.

1620 Chow WS, Lam KS. An overweight woman with galactorrhoea. *Postgrad Med J* 1998;74:121-2.

1621 Lledo Carreres M, Lajo Garrido JL, Gonzalez Rico M, et al. Toxic internuclear ophthalmoplegia related to antiobesity treatment. *Ann Pharmacother* 1992;26:1457-8.

1622 Ferner RE, Burnett A, Rawlins MD. Triiodothyroacetic acid abuse in a female body builder. *Lancet* 1986;1:383.

1623 Heim J. [Hypothyroidism of central origin corrected by the cessation of Triac therapy]. [Article in French]. *Ann Med Interne* (Paris) 1982;133:588-9.

1624 Jean-Pastor MJ, Jean P, Biour M, et al. [Hepatopathies from treatment with a specialty drug combination of tiratricol-cyclovalone-retinol]. [Article in French]. *J Toxicol Clin Exp* 1986;6:115-21.

1625 Bentin J, Desir D, Mockel J. Triac (3,5,3'-triiodo-thyroacetic acid) induced "pseudohypothyroidism". *Acta Clin Belg* 1984;39:285-9.

1627 Hawkey CM, Olsen EG, Symons C. Production of cardiac muscle abnormalities in offspring of rats receiving triiodothyroacetic acid (triac) and the effect of beta adrenergic blockade. *Cardiovasc Res* 1981;15:196-205.

1628 Olsen EG, Symons C, Hawkey C. Effect of triac on the developing heart. *Lancet* 1977;2:221-3.

1629 Pitt-Rivers R. Physiological activity of the acetic acid analogues of some iodinated thyronines. *Lancet* 1953;2:234.

1630 Lerman JL, Pitt-rivers R. Physiological activity of triiodo and tetraiodothyroacetic acid on blood-cholesterol levels. *Lancet* 1956;1:885-9.

1631 Menegay C, Juge C, Burger AG. Pharmacokinetics of 3,5,3'-triiodothyroacetic acid and its effects on serum TSH levels. *Acta Endocrinol* (Copenh) 1989;121(5):651-8.

1632 Sherman SI, Ringel MD, Smith MJ, et al. Augmented hepatic and skeletal thyromimetic effects of tiratricol in comparison with levothyroxine. *J Clin Endocrinol Metab* 1997;82:2153-8.

1633 Sherman SI, Ladenson PW. Organ-specific effects of tiratricol: a thyroid hormone analog with hepatic, not pituitary, superagonist effects. *J Clin Endocrinol Metab* 1992;75(3):901-5.

1634 Bracco D, Morin O, Schutz Y, et al. Comparison of the metabolic and endocrine effects of 3,5,3'-triiodothyroacetic acid and thyroxine. *J Clin Endocrinol Metab* 1993;77:221-8.

1635 Ng TB. A review of research on the protein-bound polysaccharide (polysaccharopeptide, PSP) from the mushroom Coriolus versicolor (Basidiomycetes: Polyporaceae). *Gen Pharmacol* 1998;30:1-4.

1636 Mizutani Y, Yoshida O. Activation by the protein-bound polysaccharide PSK (krestin) of cytotoxic lymphocytes that act on fresh autologous tumor cells and T24 human urinary bladder transitional carcinoma cell line in patients with urinary bladder cancer. *J Urol* 1991;145:1082-7.

1637 Kobayashi H, Matsunaga K, Oguchi Y. Antimetastatic effects of PSK (Krestin), a protein-bound polysaccharide obtained from basidiomycetes: an overview. *Cancer Epidemiol Biomarkers Prev* 1995;4:275-81.

1638 Dong Y, Kwan CY, Chen ZN, et al. Antitumor effects of a refined polysaccharide peptide fraction isolated from Coriolus versicolor: in vitro and in vivo studies. *Res Commun Mol Pathol Pharmacol* 1996;92:140-8.

1639 Kanoh T, Saito K, Matsunaga K, et al. Enhancement of the antitumor effect by the concurrent use of a monoclonal antibody and the protein bound polysaccharide PSK in mice bearing a human cancer cell line. *In Vivo* 1994;8:241-5.

1640 Maehara Y, Inutsuka S, Takeuchi H, et al. Postoperative PSK and OK-432 immunochemotherapy for patients with gastric cancer. *Cancer Chemother Pharmacol* 1993;33:171-5.

1641 Harada M, Matsunaga K, Oguchi Y, et al. Oral administration of PSK can improve the impaired anti-tumor CD4+ T-cell response in gut associated lymphoid tissue (GALT) of specific-pathogen-free mice. *Int J Cancer* 1997;70:362-72.

1642 Tsukagoshi S, Hashimoto Y, Fujii G, et al. Krestin (PSK). *Cancer Treat Rev* 1984;11:131-55.

1643 Collins RA, Ng TB. Polysaccharopeptide from Coriolus versicolor has potential for use against human

immunodeficiency virus type 1 infection. *Life Sci* 1997;60:PL383-7.
1644 Tochikura TS, Nakashima H, Hirose K, et al. A biological response modifier, PSK, inhibits human immunodeficiency virus infection in vitro. *Biochem Biophys Res Commun* 1987;148:726-33.
1645 Gong S, Zhang HQ, Yin WP, et al. Involvement of interleukin-2 in analgesia produced by Coriolus versicolor polysaccharide peptides. *Chung Kuo Yao Li Hsueh Pao* 1998;19:67-70.
1646 Ng TB, Chan WY. Polysaccharopeptide from the mushroom Coriolus versicolor possesses analgesic activity but does not produce adverse effects on female reproductive or embryonic development in mice. *Gen Pharmacol* 1997;29:269-73.
1647 Yeung JH, Chiu LC, Ooi VE. Effect of polysaccharide peptide (PSP) on glutathione and protection against paracetamol-induced hepatotoxicity in the rat. *Methods Find Exp Clin Pharmacol* 1994;16:723-9.
1648 Iino Y, Yokoe T, Maemura M, et al. Immunochemotherapies versus chemotherapy as adjuvant treatment after curative resection of operable breast cancer. *Anticancer Res* 1995;15:2907-11.
1649 Ogoshi K, Satou H, Isono K, et al. Immunotherapy for esophageal cancer. A randomized trial in combination with radiotherapy and radiochemotherapy. Cooperative Study Group for Esophageal Cancer in Japan. *Am J Clin Oncol* 1995;18:216-22.
1650 Yokoe T, Iino Y, Takei H, et al. HLA antigen as predictive index for the outcome of breast cancer patients with adjuvant immunochemotherapy with PSK. *Anticancer Res* 1997;17:2815-8.
1651 Nakazato H, Koike A, Saji S, et al. Efficacy of immunochemotherapy as adjuvant treatment after curative resection of gastric cancer. Study Group of Immunochemotherapy with PSK for Gastric Cancer. *Lancet* 1994;343:1122-6.
1652 Sugimachi K, Maehara Y, Ogawa M, et al. Dose intensity of uracil and tegafur in postoperative chemotherapy for patients with poorly differentiated gastric cancer. *Cancer Chemother Pharmacol* 1997;40:233-8.
1653 Hayakawa K, Mitsuhashi N, Saito Y, et al. Effect of Krestin as adjuvant treatment following radical radiotherapy in non-small cell lung cancer patients. *Cancer Detect Prev* 1997;21:71-7.
1654 Morimoto T, Ogawa M, Orita K, et al. Postoperative adjuvant randomised trial comparing chemoendocrine therapy, chemotherapy and immunotherapy for patients with stage II breast cancer: 5-year results from the Nishinihon Cooperative Study Group of Adjuvant Chemoendocrine Therapy for Breast Cancer (ACETBC) of Japan. *Eur J Cancer* 1996;32A:235-42.
1655 Suto T, Fukuda S, Moriya N, et al. Clinical study of biological response modifiers as maintenance therapy for hepatocellular carcinoma. *Cancer Chemother Pharmacol* 1994;33 Suppl:S145-8.
1656 Toi M, Hattori T, Akagi M, et al. Randomized adjuvant trial to evaluate the addition of tamoxifen and PSK to chemotherapy in patients with primary breast cancer. 5-Year results from the Nishi-Nippon Group of the Adjuvant Chemoendocrine Therapy for Breast Cancer Organization. *Cancer* 1992;70:2475-83.
1657 Mitomi T, Tsuchiya S, Iijima N, et al. Randomized, controlled study on adjuvant immunochemotherapy with PSK in curatively resected colorectal cancer. The Cooperative Study Group of Surgical Adjuvant Immunochemotherapy for Cancer of Colon and Rectum (Kanagawa). *Dis Colon Rectum* 1992;35:123-30.
1658 Nio Y, Tsubono M, Tseng CC, et al. Immunomodulation by orally administered protein-bound polysaccharide PSK in patients with gastrointestinal cancer. *Biotherapy* 1992;4:117-28.
1659 Kondo T, Sakamoto J, Nakazato H. Alternating immunochemotherapy of advanced gastric carcinoma: a randomized comparison of carbazilquinone and PSK to carbazilquinone in patients with curative gastric resection. *Biotherapy* 1991;3:287-95.
1660 Torisu M, Hayashi Y, Ishimitsu T, et al. Significant prolongation of disease-free period gained by oral polysaccharide K (PSK) administration after curative surgical operation of colorectal cancer. *Cancer Immunol Immunother* 1990;31:261-8.
1661 Go P, Chung CH. Adjuvant PSK immunotherapy in patients with carcinoma of the nasopharynx. *J Int Med Res* 1989;17:141-9.
1662 Fukushima M. Adjuvant therapy of gastric cancer: the Japanese experience. *Semin Oncol* 1996;23:369-78.
1664 Arnaud J, Malvy D, Richard MJ, et al. Selenium status in an iodine deficient population of the West Ivory Coast. *J Physiol Anthropol Appl Human Sci* 2001;20:81-4.
1665 Neve J. New approaches to assess selenium status and requirement. *Nutr Rev* 2000;58:363-9.
1668 Davies C, Maidment S, Hanley P, et al. Dimethylaminoethanol (DMAE). HSE. Risk assessment document; EH72/2;1997. (TOXLINE).
1669 Re O. 2-Dimethylaminoethanol (deanol): a brief review of its clinical efficacy and postulated mechanism of action. *Curr Ther Res Clin Exp* 1974;16:1238-42.
1671 Pieralisi G, Ripari P, Vecchiet L. Effects of a standardized ginseng extract combined with dimethylaminoethanol bitartrate, vitamins, minerals, and trace elements on physical performance during exercise. *Clin Ther* 1991;13:373-82.
1672 George J, Pridmore S, Aldous D. Double blind controlled trial of deanol in tardive dyskinesia. *Aust N Z J Psychiatry* 1981;15:68-71.
1673 Penovich P, Morgan JP, Kerzner B, et al. Double-blind evaluation of deanol in tardive dyskinesia. *JAMA* 1978;239:1997-8.
1674 de Montigny C, Chouinard G, Annable L. Ineffectiveness of deanol in tardive dyskinesia: a placebo controlled study. *Psychopharmacology* (Berl) 1979;65:219-23.
1675 Lindeboom SF, Lakke JP. Deanol and physostigmine in the treatment of L-dopa-induced dyskinesias. *Acta Neurol Scand* 1978;58:134-8.
1676 Jus A, Villeneuve A, Gautier J, et al. Deanol, lithium and placebo in the treatment of tardive dyskinesia. A double-blind crossover study. *Neuropsychobiology* 1978;4:140-9.
1677 Oettinger L Jr. Pediatric psychopharmacology. A review with special reference to deanol. *Dis Nerv Syst* 1977;38:25-31.
1679 Lewis JA, Young R. Deanol and methylphenidate in minimal brain dysfunction. *Clin Pharmacol Ther* 1975;17:534-40.
1680 Fisman M, Mersky H, Helmes E. Double-blind trial of 2-dimethylaminoethanol in Alzheimer's disease. *Am J Psychiatry* 1981;138:970-2.
1681 Ferris SH, Sathananthan G, Gershon S, et al. Senile dementia: treatment with deanol. *J Am Geriatr Soc* 1977;25:241-4.
1682 Cherkin A, Exkardt MJ. Effects of dimethylaminoethanol upon life-span and behavior of aged Japanese quail. *J Gerontol* 1977;32:38-45.
1683 Stenback F, Weisburger JH, Williams GM. Effect of lifetime administration of dimethylaminoethanol on longevity, aging changes, and cryptogenic neoplasms in C3H mice. *Mech Ageing Dev* 1988;42:129-38.

REFERENCES

1684 Haug BA, Holzgraefe M. Orofacial and respiratory tardive dyskinesia: potential side effects of 2-dimethylaminoethanol (deanol)? *Eur Neurol* 1991;31:423-5.

1685 Casey DE. Mood alterations during deanol therapy. *Psychopharmacology* (Berl) 1979;62:187-91.

1686 Sergio W. Use of DMAE (2-dimethylaminoethanol) in the induction of lucid dreams. *Med Hypotheses* 1988;26:255-7.

1688 Lissoni P, Barni S, Cattaneo G, et al. Clinical results with the pineal hormone melatonin in advanced cancer resistant to standard antitumor therapies. *Oncology* 1991;48:448-50.

1689 Claustrat B, Brun J, Geoffriau M, et al. Nocturnal plasma melatonin profile and melatonin kinetics during infusion in status migrainosus. *Cephalalgia* 1997;17:511-7;487.

1690 Mallo C, Zaidan R, Galy G, et al. Pharmacokinetics of melatonin in man after intravenous infusion and bolus injection. *Eur J Clin Pharmacol* 1990;38:297-301.

1691 FDA. List of orphan designations and approvals. Office of Orphan Products Development. Available at: www.fda.gov/orphan/designat/list.htm.

1692 Lissoni P, Tisi E, Barni S, et al. Biological and clinical results of a neuroimmunotherapy with interleukin-2 and the pineal hormone melatonin as a first line treatment in advanced non-small cell lung cancer. *Br J Cancer* 1992;66:155-8.

1693 Lissoni P, Barni S, Ardizzoia A, et al. A randomized study with the pineal hormone melatonin versus supportive care alone in patients with brain metastases due to solid neoplasms. *Cancer* 1994;73:699-701.

1694 Lissoni P, Tancini G, Paolorossi F, et al. Chemoneuroendocrine therapy of metastatic breast cancer with persistent thrombocytopenia with weekly low-dose epirubicin plus melatonin: a phase II study. *J Pineal Res* 1999;26:169-73.

1695 Lissoni P, Tancini G, Barni S, et al. The pineal hormone melatonin in hematology and its potential efficacy in the treatment of thrombocytopenia. *Recenti Prog Med* 1996;87:582-5.

1696 Lissoni P, Barni S, Brivio F, et al. A biological study on the efficacy of low-dose subcutaneous interleukin-2 plus melatonin in the treatment of cancer-related thrombocytopenia. *Oncology* 1995;52:360-2.

1697 Bregani ER, Lissoni P, Rossini F, et al. Prevention of interleukin-2-induced thrombocytopenia during the immunotherapy of cancer by a concomitant administration of the pineal hormone melatonin. *Recenti Prog Med* 1995;86:231-3.

1698 Perna AF, Castaldo P, Ingrosso D, et al. Homocysteine, a new cardiovascular risk factor, is also a powerful uremic toxin. *J Nephrol* 1999;12:230-40.

1699 Fauteck J, Schmidt H, Lerchl A, et al. Melatonin in epilepsy: first results of replacement therapy and first clinical results. *Biol Signals Recept* 1999;8:105-10.

1700 Brendler T. Herbal Remedies Disk. 1st ed. Berlin:1996.

1701 Wallach J. Interpretation of Diagnostic Tests. A synopsis of Laboratory Medicine. Fifth ed; Boston, MA: Little Brown, 1992.

1704 Toubro S, Astrup A. Randomised comparison of diets for maintaining obese subjects' weight after major weight loss: ad lib, low fat, high carbohydrate diet v fixed energy intake. *BMJ* 1997;314:29-34.

1705 van Zandwijk N. N-acetylcysteine for lung cancer prevention. *Chest* 1995;107:1437-41.

1706 Ammon HP, Safayhi H, Mack T, Sabieraj J. Mechanism of antiinflammatory actions of curcumine and boswellic acids. *J Ethnopharmacol* 1993;38:1139.

1707 De Smet PAGM, Keller K, Hansel R, Chandler RF. Adverse Effects of Herbal Drugs Vol. 3, Springer-Verlag, Berlin, 1997.

1708 Gupta I, Gupta V, Parihar A, et al. Effects of Boswellia serrata gum resin in patients with bronchial asthma: results of a double-blind, placebo-controlled, 6-week clinical study. *Eur J Med Res* 1998;3:511-4.

1709 Gupta I, Parihar A, Malhotra P, et al. Effects of Boswellia serrata gum resin in patients with ulcerative colitis. *Eur J Med Res* 1997;2:37-43.

1710 van Zandwijk N, Dalesio O, Pastorino U, et al. EUROSCAN, a randomized trial of vitamin A and N-acetylcysteine in patients with head and neck cancer or lung cancer. For the European Organization for Research and Treatment of Cancer Head and Neck and Lung Cancer Cooperative Groups. *J Natl Cancer Inst* 2000;92:977-86.

1711 Horowitz RS, Dart RC, Jarvie DR, et al. Placental transfer of N-acetylcysteine following human maternal acetaminophen toxicity. *J Toxicol Clin Toxicol* 1997;35:447-51.

1712 Mato JM, Camara J, Fernandez de Paz J, et al. S-adenosylmethionine in alcoholic liver cirrhosis: a randomized, placebo-controlled, double-blind, multicenter clinical trial. *J Hepatol* 1999;30:1081-9.

1713 Loehrer FM, Schwab R, Angst CP, et al. Influence of oral S-adenosylmethionine on plasma 5-methyltetrahydrofolate, S-adenosylhomocysteine, homocysteine and methionine in healthy humans. *J Pharmacol Exp Ther* 1997;22:845-50.

1714 Loehrer FM, Angst CP, Haefeli WE, et al. Low whole-blood S-adenosylmethionine and correlation between 5-methyltetrahydrofolate and homocysteine in coronary artery disease. *Arterioscler Thromb Vasc Biol* 1996;16:727-33.

1715 Louis E. Tremor disorders: identification and treatment. *Medical Update for Psychiatrists* 1997;2:172-6.

1716 Bailey B, McGuigan MA. Management of anaphylactoid reactions to intravenous N-acetylcysteine. *Ann Emerg Med* 1998;31:710-5.

1719 American College of Rheumatology ad hoc committee on clinical guidelines. Guidelines for monitoring drug therapy in rheumatoid arthritis. *Arthritis Rheum* 1996;39:723-31.

1721 Jorgensen KM, Witting MD. Does exogenous melatonin improve day sleep or night alertness in emergency physicians working night shifts? *Ann Emerg Med* 1998;31:699-704.

1722 Sanders DC, Chaturvedi AK, Hordinsky JR. Melatonin: aeromedical, toxicopharmacological, and analytical aspects. *J Anal Toxicol* 1999;23:159-67.

1724 Arangino S, Cagnacci A, Angiolucci M, et al. Effects of melatonin on vascular reactivity, catecholamine levels, and blood pressure in healthy men. *Am J Cardiol* 1999;83:1417-9.

1725 Zhi J, Jelia AT, Koss-Twardy SG, et al. The effect of orlistat, an inhibitor of dietary fat absorption, on the pharmacokinetics of beta-carotene in healthy volunteers. *J Clin Pharmacol* 1996;36:152-9.

1726 James WP, Avenell A, Broom J, et al. A one-year trial to assess the value of orlistat in the management of obesity. *Int J Obes Relat Metab Disord* 1997;21:S24-S30.

1727 Melia AT, Koss-Twardy SG, Zhi J. The effect of orlistat, an inhibitor of dietary fat absorption, on the absorption of vitamins A and E in healthy volunteers. *J Clin Pharmacol* 1996;36:647-53.

1728 Brusco LI, Marquez M, Cardinali DP. Monozygotic twins with Alzheimer's disease treated with melatonin: Case report. *J Pineal Res* 1998;25:260-3.

1729 Brusco LI, Fainstein I, Marquez M, et al. Effect of melatonin in selected populations of sleep-disturbed patients. *Biol Signals Recept* 1999;8:126-31.

1730 Roche, Inc. Xenical package insert. Nutley, NJ. May 1999.

1731 Chen RM, Wu JJ, Lee SC, et al. Increase of intestinal Bifidobacterium and suppression of coliform bacteria with short-term yogurt ingestion. *J Dairy Sci* 1999:82:2308-14.

1733 Garg R, Malinow M, Pettinger M. Niacin treatment increases plasma homocyst(e)ine levels. *Am Heart J* 1999;138:1082-7.

1735 Dawson D, Rogers NL, van den Heuvel CJ, et al. Effect of sustained nocturnal transbuccal melatonin administration on sleep and temperature in elderly insomniacs. *J Biol Rhythms* 1998;13:532-8.

1736 Anon. Yogurt cuts down diarrhea. HealthNews, November 1999.

1738 Haimov I, Lavie P, Laudon M, et al. Melatonin replacement therapy of elderly insomniacs. *Sleep* 1995;18:598-603.

1739 Luboshitzky R, Wagner O, Lavi S, et al. Abnormal melatonin secretion in hypogonadal men: the effect of testosterone treatment. *Clin Endocrinol* (Oxf) 1997;47:463-9.

1740 Pierce A. The American Pharmaceutical Association Practical Guide to Natural Medicines. New York: The Stonesong Press, 1999:19.

1741 Nordlund JJ, Lerner AB. The effects of oral melatonin on skin color and on the release of pituitary hormones. *J Clin Endocrinol Metab* 1977;45:768-74.

1742 Cavallo A, Ritschel WA. Pharmacokinetics of melatonin in human sexual maturation. *J Clin Endocrinol Metab* 1996;81:1882-6.

1743 Commentz JC, Uhlig H, Henke A, et al. Melatonin and 6-hydroxymelatonin sulfate excretion is inversely correlated with gonadal development in children. *Horm Res* 1997;47:97-101.

1744 Palm L, Blennow G, Wetterberg L. Long-term melatonin treatment in blind children and young adults with circadian sleep-wake disturbances. *Dev Med Child Neurol* 1997;39:319-25.

1745 Lancioni GE, O'Reilly MF, Basili G. Review of strategies for treating sleep problems in persons with severe or profound mental retardation or multiple handicaps. *Am J Ment Retard* 1999;104:170-86.

1746 Jan JE, O'Donnell ME. Use of melatonin in the treatment of paediatric sleep disorders. *J Pineal Res* 1996;21:193-9.

1747 O'Callaghan FJ, Clarke AA, Hancock E, et al. Use of melatonin to treat sleep disorders in tuberous sclerosis. *Dev Med Child Neurol* 1999;41:123-6.

1749 Skene DJ, Lockley SW, Arendt J. Melatonin in circadian sleep disorders in the blind. *Biol Signals Recept* 1999;8:90-5.

1751 Dagan Y, Zisapel N, Nof D, et al. Rapid reversal of tolerance to benzodiazepine hypnotics by treatment with oral melatonin: a case report. *Eur Neuropsychopharmacol* 1997;7:157-60.

1752 Holt S, Goodier D, Marley R, et al. Improvement in renal function in hepatorenal syndrome with N-acetylcysteine. *Lancet* 1999;353:294-5.

1753 Waldhauser F, Saletu B, Trinchard-Lugan I. Sleep laboratory investigations on hypnotic properties of melatonin. *Psychopharmacology* (Berl) 1990;100:222-6.

1754 Garfinkel D, Laudon M, Nof D, et al. Improvement of sleep quality in elderly people by controlled-release melatonin. *Lancet* 1995;346:541-4.

1755 Spiller HA, Krenzelok EP, Grande GA, et al. A prospective evaluation of the effect of activated charcoal before oral N-acetylcysteine in acetaminophen overdose. *Ann Emerg Med* 1994;23:519-23.

1756 Dollins AB, Zhdanova IV, Wurtman RJ, et al. Effect of inducing nocturnal serum melatonin concentrations in daytime on sleep, mood, body temperature, and performance. *Proc Natl Acad Sci U S A* 1994;91:1824-8.

1757 Zhdanova IV, Wurtman RJ, Lynch HJ, et al. Sleep-inducing effects of low doses of melatonin ingested in the evening. *Clin Pharmacol Ther* 1995;57:552-8.

1758 Nave R, Peled R, Lavie P. Melatonin improves evening napping. *Eur J Pharmacol* 1995;275:213-6.

1759 Zhdanova IV, Wurtman RJ, Morabito C, et al. Effects of low oral doses of melatonin, given 2-4 hours before habitual bedtime, on sleep in normal young humans. *Sleep* 1996;19(5):423-31.

1761 Kelly GS. Clinical applications of N-acetylcysteine. *Altern Med Rev* 1998;3:114-27.

1762 Chyka PA, Butler AY, Holliman BJ, Herman MI. Utility of acetylcysteine in treating poisonings and adverse drug reactions. *Drug Saf* 2000;22:123-48.

1763 Gillissen A, Nowak D. Characterization of N-acetylcysteine and ambroxol in anti-oxidant therapy. *Respir Med* 1998;92:609-23.

1764 Carman JS, Post RM, Buswell R, et al. Negative effects of melatonin on depression. *Am J Psychiatry* 1976;133:1181-1186.

1765 Marchetti G, Lodola E, Licciardello L, Colombo A. Use of N-acetylcysteine in the management of coronary artery diseases. *Cardiologia* 1999;44:633-7.

1766 Leibenluft E, Feldman-Naim S, Turner EH, et al. Effects of exogenous melatonin administration and withdrawal in five patients with rapid-cycling bipolar disorder. *J Clin Psychiatry* 1997;58:383-8.

1767 Morini M, Cai T, Aluigi MG, et al. The role of the thiol N-acetylcysteine in the prevention of tumor invasion and angiogenesis. *Int J Biol Markers* 1999;14:268-71.

1768 Bangha E, Elsner P, Kistler GS. Suppression of UV-induced erythema by topical treatment with melatonin (N-acetyl-5-methoxytryptamine). Influence of the application time point. *Dermatology* 1997;195:248-52.

1769 Fischer T, Bangha E, Elsner P, et al. Suppression of UV-induced erythema by topical treatment with melatonin. Influence of the application time point. *Biol Signals Recept* 1999;8:132-5.

1770 Naguib M, Samarkandi AH. Premedication with melatonin: a double-blind, placebo-controlled comparison with midazolam. *Br J Anaesth* 1999;82:875-80.

1771 Jan JE, Freeman RD, Fast DK. Melatonin treatment of sleep-wake cycle disorders in children and adolescents. *Dev Med Child Neurol* 1999;41:491-500.

1772 Avery D, Lenz M, Landis C. Guidelines for prescribing melatonin. *Ann Med* 1998;30:122-30.

1773 Brzezinski A. Melatonin in humans. *N Engl J Med* 1997;336:186-95.

1774 Arendt J. Melatonin. *BMJ* 1996;312:1242-3.

1775 Nathan PJ, Burrows GD, Norman TR. The effect of age and pre-light melatonin concentration on the melatonin sensitivity to dim light. *Int Clin Psychopharmacol* 1999;14:189-92.

1776 Fraschini F, Cesarani A, Alpini D, et al. Melatonin influences human balance. *Biol Signals Recept* 1999;8:111-9.

1777 Meeking DR, Wallace JD, Cuneo RC, et al. Exercise-induced GH secretion is enhanced by the oral ingestion of melatonin in healthy adult male subjects. *Eur J Endocrinol* 1999;141:22-6.

1778 Ebadi M, Govitrapong P, Phansuwan-Pujito P, et al. Pineal opioid receptors and analgesic action of melatonin. *J Pineal Res* 1998;24:193-200.

1779 Forsling ML, Wheeler MJ, Williams AJ. The effect of melatonin administration on pituitary hormone secretion in man. *Clin Endocrinol* (Oxf) 1999;51:637-42.

1780 Stoschitzky K, Sakotnik A, Lercher P, et al. Influence of beta-blockers on melatonin release. *Eur J Clin Pharmacol* 1999;55:111-5.

1781 Zeitzer JM, Daniels JE, Duffy JF, et al. Do plasma melatonin concentrations decline with age? *Am J Med* 1999;107:432-6.

REFERENCES

1784 Thal LJ, Salmon DP, Lasker B, et al. The safety and lack of efficacy of vinpocetine in Alzheimer's disease. *J Am Geriatr Soc* 1989;37:515-20.

1785 Bereczki D, Fekete I. A systematic review of vinpocetine therapy in acute ischaemic stroke. *Eur J Clin Pharmacol* 1999;55:349-52.

1786 Szakall S, Boros I, Balkay L, et al. Cerebral effects of a single dose of intravenous vinpocetine in chronic stroke patients: a PET study. *J Neuroimaging* 1998;8:197-204.

1787 Hindmarch I, Fuchs HH, Erzigkeit H. Efficacy and tolerance of vinpocetine in ambulant patients suffering from mild to moderate organic psychosyndromes. *Int Clin Psychopharmacol* 1991;6:31-43.

1788 Ueyoshi A, Ota K. Clinical appraisal of vinpocetine for the removal of intractable tumoral calcinosis in haemodialysis patients with renal failure. *J Int Med Res* 1992;20(5):435-43.

1789 Balestreri R, Fontana L, Astengo F. A double-blind placebo controlled evaluation of the safety and efficacy of vinpocetine in the treatment of patients with chronic vascular senile cerebral dysfunction. *J Am Geriatr Soc* 1987;35:425-30.

1790 Hayakawa M. Effect of vinpocetine on red blood cell deformability in stroke patients. *Arzneimittelforschung* 1992;42(4):425-7.

1791 Hayakawa M. Comparative efficacy of vinpocetine, pentoxifylline and nicergoline on red blood cell deformability. *Arzneimittelforschung* 1992;42(2):108-10.

1792 Kiss E. Adjuvant effect of cavinton in the treatment of climacteric symptoms. *Ther Hung* 1990;38(4):170-3.

1793 Miyazaki M. The effect of a cerebral vasodilator, vinpocetine, on cerebral vascular resistance evaluated by the Doppler ultrasonic technique in patients with cerebrovascular diseases. *Angiology* 1995;46:53-8.

1794 Dutov AA, Gal'tvanitsa GA, Volkova VA, et al. [Cavinton in the prevention of the convulsive syndrome in children after birth injury]. [Article in Russian]. *Zh Nevropatol Psikhiatr Im S S Korsakova* 1991;91:21-2.

1795 Dutov AA, Tolpyshev BA, Petrov AP, et al. [Use of cavinton in epilepsy]. [Article in Russian]. *Zh Nevropatol Psikhiatr Im S S Korsakova* 1986;86:850-5.

1796 Bhatti JZ, Hindmarch I. Vinpocetine effects on cognitive impairments produced by flunitrazepam. *Int Clin Psychopharmacol* 1987;2:325-31.

1797 Subhan Z, Hindmarch I. Psychopharmacological effects of vinpocetine in normal healthy volunteers. *Eur J Clin Pharmacol* 1985;28:567-71.

1798 Bodo D, Kotovskaia AR, Galle RR, et al. [Effectiveness of the preparation Gavinton in preventing motion sickness]. [Article in Russian]. *Kosm Biol Aviakosm Med* 1982;16(3):49-51.

1799 The Natural Pharmacist. Vinpocetine. www.tnp.com/substance.asp?ID=573. (Accessed 16 December 1999).

1800 Nicholson CD. Pharmacology of nootropics and metabolically active compounds in relation to their use in dementia. *Psychopharmacology* (Berl) 1990;101:147-59.

1801 Akopov SE, Gabrielian ES. Effects of aspirin, dipyridamole, nifedipine and cavinton which act on platelet aggregation induced by different aggregating agents alone and in combination. *Eur J Clin Pharmacol* 1992;42:257-9.

1802 Lohmann A, Dingler E, Sommer W, et al. Bioavailability of vinpocetine and interference of the time of application with food intake. *Arzneimittelforschung* 1992;42:914-7.

1803 McGrath JJ, Soares KVS. Cholinergic medication for neuroleptic-induced tardive dyskinesia. *Cochrane Database Syst Rev* 2000;2:CD000207.

1804 Soares KV, McGrath JJ. The treatment of tardive dyskinesia- a systematic review and meta-analysis. *Schizophr Res* 1999;39:1-16; discussion 17-18.

1805 Krizek M, Senft V, Motan J. Influence of hemodialysis on selenium blood levels. *Sb Lek* 2000;101:241-8.

1816 Allen LV. Nutritional Products. In: Covington TR, Ed. Handbook of Nonprescription Drugs. Washington, DC: American Pharmaceutical Association;1996:361-92.

1817 Valimaki MJ, Kinnunen K, Volin L, et al. A prospective study of bone loss and turnover after allogeneic bone marrow transplantation: effect of calcium supplementation with or without calcitonin. *Bone Marrow Transplant* 1999;23:355-61.

1818 Allender PS, Cutler JA, Follmann D, et al. Dietary calcium and blood pressure: a meta-analysis of randomized clinical trials. *Ann Intern Med* 1996;124:825-31.

1819 Bucher HC, Cook RJ, Guyatt GH, et al. Effects of dietary calcium supplementation on blood pressure. A meta-analysis of randomized controlled trials. *JAMA* 1996;275:1016-22.

1820 Kawano Y, Yoshimi H, Matsuoka H, et al. Calcium supplementation in patients with essential hypertension: assessment by office, home and ambulatory blood pressure. *J Hypertens* 1998;16:1693-9.

1821 Griffith LE, Guyatt GH, Cook RJ, et al. The influence of dietary and nondietary calcium supplementation on blood pressure: an updated meta-analysis of randomized controlled trials. *Am J Hypertens* 1999;12:84-92.

1822 Thys-Jacobs S, Starkey P, Bernstein D, Tian J. Calcium carbonate and the premenstrual syndrome: effects on premenstrual and menstrual symptoms. Premenstrual Syndrome Study Group. *Am J Obstet Gynecol*, 1998;179:444-52.

1823 Alvir JM, Thys-Jacobs S. Premenstrual and menstrual symptom clusters and response to calcium treatment. *Psychopharmacol Bull* 1991;27:145-8.

1824 Thys-Jacobs S, Ceccarelli S, Bierman A, et al. Calcium supplementation in premenstrual syndrome: a randomized crossover trial. *J Gen Intern Med* 1989;4:183-9.

1825 Lewis CJ. Letter to reiterate certain public health and safety concerns to firms manufacturing or importing dietary supplements that contain specific bovine tissues. FDA. Available at: www.cfsan.fda.gov/~dms/dspltr05.html.

1826 Steinbach G, Lupton J, Reddy BS, et al. Effect of calcium supplementation on rectal epithelial hyperproliferation in intestinal bypass subjects. *Gastroenterology* 1994;106:1162-7.

1827 Barsotti G, Cupisti A, Morelli E, et al. Secondary hyperparathyroidism in severe chronic renal failure is corrected by very-low dietary phosphate intake and calcium carbonate supplementation. *Nephron* 1998;79:137-41.

1828 Tsukamoto Y, Moriya R, Nagaba Y, et al. Effect of administering calcium carbonate to treat secondary hyperparathyroidism in nondialyzed patients with chronic renal failure. *Am J Kidney Dis* 1995;25:879-86.

1829 Rudnicki M, Hojsted J, Petersen LJ, et al. Oral calcium effectively reduces parathyroid hormone levels in hemodialysis patients: a randomized double-blind placebo-controlled study. *Nephron* 1993;65:369-74.

1830 Adachi JD, Ioannidis G. Calcium and vitamin D therapy in corticosteroid-induced bone loss: what is the evidence? *Calcif Tissue Int* 1999;65:332-6.

1831 Adachi JD, Bensen WG, Bianchi F, et al. Vitamin D and calcium in the prevention of corticosteroid induced osteoporosis: a 3 year followup. *J Rheumatol* 1996;23:995-1000.

1832 Recommendations for the prevention and treatment of glucocorticoid-induced osteoporosis. American College of Rheumatology Task Force on Osteoporosis Guidelines. *Arthritis Rheum* 1996;39:1791-801.

1833 Crowther CA, Hiller JE, Pridmore B, et al. Calcium supplementation in nulliparous women for the prevention of pregnancy-induced hypertension, preeclampsia and preterm birth: an Australian randomized trial. FRACOG and the ACT Study Group. *Aust N Z J Obstet Gynaecol* 1999;39:12-8.

1834 Power ML, Heaney RP, Kalkwarf HJ, et al. The role of calcium in health and disease. *Am J Obstet Gynecol* 1999;181:1560-9.

1835 Dawson-Hughes B, Harris SS, Krall EA, Dallal GE. Effect of calcium and vitamin D supplementation on bone density in men and women 65 years of age or older. *N Engl J Med* 1997;337:670-6.

1836 Chapuy MC, Arlot ME, Duboeuf F, et al. Vitamin D3 and calcium to prevent hip fractures in the elderly women. *N Engl J Med* 1992;327:1637-42.

1837 Celotti F, Bignamini A. Dietary calcium and mineral/ vitamin supplementation: a controversial problem. *J Int Med Res* 1999;27:1-14.

1838 Heller HJ, Stewart A, Haynes S, Pak CY. Pharmacokinetics of calcium absorption from two commercial calcium supplements. *J Clin Pharmacol* 1999;39:1151-4.

1839 Fujita T, Ohue T, Fujii Y, et al. Heated oyster shell-seaweed calcium (AAA Ca) on osteoporosis. *Calcif Tissue Int* 1996;58:226-30.

1840 Fujita T, Ohue T, Fujii Y, et al. Effect of calcium supplementation on bone density and parathyroid function in elderly subjects. *Miner Electrolyte Metab* 1995;21:229-31.

1841 Talbot JR, Guardo P, Seccia S, etal. Calcium bioavailability and parathyroid hormone acute changes after oral intake of dairy and nondairy products in healthy volunteers. *Osteoporos Int* 1999;10:137-42.

1842 Heaney RP, Dowell MS, Barger-Lux MJ. Absorption of calcium as the carbonate and citrate salts, with some observations on method. *Osteoporos Int* 1999;9:19-23.

1843 Maton PN, Burton ME. Antacids revisited: a review of their clinical pharmacology and recommended therapeutic use. *Drugs* 1999;57:855-70.

1844 Clemens JD, Feinstein AR. Calcium carbonate and constipation: a historical review of medical mythopoeia. *Gastroenterology* 1977;72:957-61.

1845 Saunders D, Sillery J, Chapman R. Effect of calcium carbonate and aluminum hydroxide on human intestinal function. *Dig Dis Sci* 1988;33:409-13.

1846 Krall EA, Dawson-Hughes B. Smoking increases bone loss and decreases intestinal calcium absorption. *J Bone Miner Res* 1999;14:215-20.

1847 Praet JP, Peretz A, Mets T, Rozenberg S. Comparative study of the intestinal absorption of three salts of calcium in young and elderly women. *J Endocrinol Invest* 1998;21:263-7.

1848 Minihane AM, Fairweather-Tait SJ. Effect of calcium supplementation on daily nonheme-iron absorption and long-term iron status. *Am J Clin Nutr* 1998;68:96-102.

1849 Sokoll LJ, Dawson-Hughes B. Calcium supplementation and plasma ferritin concentrations in premenopausal women. *Am J Clin Nutr* 1992;56:1045-8.

1850 Kalkwarf HJ, Harrast SD. Effects of calcium supplementation and lactation on iron status. *Am J Clin Nutr* 1998;67:1244-9.

1854 Steinmetz KA, Potter JD. Vegetables, fruit, and cancer prevention: a review. *J Am Diet Assoc* 1996;96:1027-39.

1855 Graf E, Eaton JW. Antioxidant functions of phytic acid. *Free Radic Biol Med* 1990;8:61-69.

1857 Shamsuddin AM, Vucenik I, Cole KE. IP6: a novel anti-cancer agent. *Life Sci* 1997;61:343-54.

1858 Zhou JR, Erdman JW Jr. Phytic acid in health and disease. *Crit Rev Food Sci Nutr* 1995;35:495-508.

1859 Shamsuddin AM. Metabolism and cellular functions of IP6: a review. *Anticancer Res* 1999;19:3733-6.

1860 Shamsuddin AM, Vucenik I. Mammary tumor inhibition by IP6: a review. *Anticancer Res* 1999;19:3671-4.

1861 Challa A, Rao DR, Reddy BS. Interactive suppression of aberrant crypt foci induced by azoxymethane in rat colon by phytic acid and green tea. *Carcinogenesis* 1997;18:2023-6.

1862 Saied IT, Shamsuddin AM. Up-regulation of the tumor suppressor gene p53 and WAF1 gene expression by IP6 in HT-29 human colon carcinoma cell line. *Anticancer Res* 1998;18:1479-84.

1863 Thompson LU, Zhang L. Phytic acid and minerals: effect on early markers of risk for mammary and colon carcinogenesis. *Carcinogenesis* 1991;12:2041-5.

1864 Vucenik I, Zhang ZS, Shamsuddin AM. IP6 in treatment of liver cancer. II. Intra-tumoral injection of IP6 regresses pre-existing human liver cancer xenotransplanted in nude mice. *Anticancer Res* 1998;18:4091-6.

1865 Shamsuddin AM, Yang GY. Inositol hexaphosphate inhibits growth and induces differentiation of PC-3 human prostate cancer cells. *Carcinogenesis* 1995;16:1975-9.

1866 Shamsuddin AM, Elsayed AM, Ullah A. Suppression of large intestinal cancer in F344 rats by inositol hexaphosphate. *Carcinogenesis* 1988;9:577-80.

1867 Vucenik I, Podczasy JJ, Shamsuddin AM. Antiplatelet activity of inositol hexaphosphate. *Anticancer Res* 1999;19:3689-93.

1868 Jariwalla RJ. Inositol hexaphosphate (IP6) as an anti-neoplastic and lipid-lowering agent. *Anticancer Res* 1999;19:3699-3702.

1869 Sandberg AS, Brune M, Carlsson NG, et al. Inositol phosphates with different numbers of phosphate groups influence iron absorption in humans. *Am J Clin Nutr* 1999;70:240-6.

1870 Sandstrom B, Sandberg AS. Inhibitory effects of isolated inositol phosphates on zinc absorption in humans. *J Trace Elem Electrolytes Health Dis* 1992;6:99-103.

1871 Ide N, Lau BH. Garlic compounds protect vascular endothelial cells from oxidized low density lipoprotein-induced injury. *J Pharm Pharmacol* 1997;49:908-11.

1873 Steiner M, Khan AH, Holbert D, Lin RI. A double-blind crossover study in moderately hypercholesterolemic men that compared the effect of aged garlic extract and placebo administration on blood lipids. *Am J Clin Nutr* 1996;64:866-70.

1874 Steiner M, Lin RS. Changes in platelet function and susceptibility of lipoproteins to oxidation associated with administration of aged garlic extract. *J Cardiovasc Pharmacol* 1998;31:904-8

1875 Lau BS, Lam F, Wang-Cheng R. Effect of an odor-modified garlic preparation on blood lipids. *Nutrition Research* 1987;7:139-49.

1876 Munday JS, James KA, Fray LM, et al. Daily supplementation with aged garlic extract, but not raw garlic, protects low density lipoprotein against in vitro oxidation. *Atherosclerosis* 1999;143:399-404.

1877 Imai J, Ide N, Nagae S, et al. Antioxidant and radical scavenging effects of aged garlic extract and its constituents. *Planta Med* 1994;60:417-20.

1878 Moriguchi T, Saito H, Nishiyama N. Aged garlic extract prolongs longevity and improves spatial memory deficit in senescence-accelerated mouse. *Biol Pharm Bull* 1996;19:305-7.

1879 Efendy JL, Simmons DL, Campbell GR, Campbell JH. The effect of the aged garlic extract, 'Kyolic', on the development of experimental atherosclerosis. *Atherosclerosis* 1997;132:37-42.

1880 Ide N, Lau BH. Aged garlic extract attenuates intracellular oxidative stress. *Phytomedicine* 1999;6:125-31.

1881 Sigounas G, Hooker J, Anagnostou A, Steiner M. S-allylmercaptocysteine inhibits cell proliferation and reduces

REFERENCES

the viability of erythroleukemia, breast, and prostate cancer cell lines. *Nutr Cancer* 1997;27:186-91.

1882 Zhang Y, Moriguchi T, Saito H, Nishiyama N. Functional relationship between age-related immunodeficiency and learning deterioration. *N Eur J Neurosci* 1998;10:3869-75.

1883 Wang BH, Zuzel KA, Rahman K, Billington D. Treatment with aged garlic extract protects against bromobenzene toxicity to precision cut rat liver slices. *Toxicology* 1999;132:215-25.

1884 Gwilt PR, Lear CL, Tempero MA, et al. The effect of garlic extract on human metabolism of acetaminophen. *Cancer Epidemiol Biomarkers Prev* 1994;3:155-60.

1885 Horie T, Matsumoto H, Kasagi M, et al. Protective effect of aged garlic extract on the small intestinal damage of rats induced by methotrexate administration. *Planta Med* 1999;65:545-8.

1886 Nguyen TT, Dale LC, von Bergmann K, Croghan IT. Cholesterol-lowering effect of stanol ester in a US population of mildly hypercholesterolemic men and women: a randomized controlled trial. *Mayo Clin Proc* 1999;74:1198-206.

1888 Ostlund RE Jr, Spilburg CA, Stenson WF. Sitostanol administered in lecithin micelles potently reduces cholesterol absorption in humans. *Am J Clin Nutr* 1999;70:826-31.

1889 Mook-Jung I, Shin JE, Yun SH, et al. Protective effects of asiaticoside derivatives against beta-amyloid neurotoxicity. *J Neurosci Res* 1999;58:417-25.

1890 Maquart FX, Chastang F, Simeon A, et al. Triterpenes from Centella asiatica stimulate extracellular matrix accumulation in rat experimental wounds. *Eur J Dermatol* 1999;9:289-96.

1891 Refsum H, Ueland PM, Nygard O, Vollset SE. Homocysteine and cardiovascular disease. *Annu Rev Med* 1998;49:31-62.

1892 Malinow MR, Bostom AG, Krauss RM. Homocyst(e)ine, diet, and cardiovascular diseases: a statement for healthcare professionals from the Nutrition Committee, American Heart Association. *Circulation* 1999;99:178-82.

1896 Investigator's Brochure: Ademetionine 1,4-butanedisulfonate. Knoll Pharmaceuticals.

1897 Stramentinoli G, Gualano M, Galli-Kienle M. Intestinal absorption of S-adenosyl-L-methionine. *J Pharmacol Exp Ther* 1979;209:323-6.

1898 Morrow LE, Grimsley EW. Long-term diuretic therapy in hypertensive patients: effects on serum homocysteine, vitamin B6, vitamin B12, and red blood cell folate concentrations. *South Med J* 1999;92:866-70.

1899 Christensen B, Landaas S, Stensvold I, et al. Whole blood folate, homocysteine in serum, and risk of first acute myocardial infarction. *Atherosclerosis* 1999;147:317-26.

1900 Lininger SW. The Natural Pharmacy. 1st ed. Rocklin, CA: Prima Publishing; 1998.

1901 Brewster MA, Schedewie H. Trimethylaminuria. *Ann Clin Lab Sci* Jan.-Feb. 1983; 13(1):20-4.

1902 Friedman PA, Bushinsky DA. Diuretic effects on calcium metabolism. *Semin Nephrol* 1999;19:551-6.

1903 Wesnes KA, Ward T, McGinty A, Petrini O. The memory enhancing effects of a Ginkgo biloba/Panax ginseng combination in healthy middle-aged volunteers. *Psychopharmacology* 2000;152:353-361.

1905 Broeder CE, Quindry J, Brittingham K, et al. The Andro Project: physiological and hormonal influences of androstenedione supplementation in men 35 to 65 years old participating in a high-intensity resistance training program. *Arch Intern Med* 2000;160:3093-104.

1906 Catlin DH, Leder BZ, Ahrens B, et al. Trace contamination of over-the-counter androstenedione and positive urine test results for a nandrolone metabolite. *JAMA* 2000;284:2618-21.

1907 Hudsin J, Towers GHN. Phytomedicines as antivirals. *Drugs Fut* 1999;24:295-320.

1908 Abdel-Fattah A, Aboul-Enein MN, Wassel G, El-Menshawi B. Preliminary report on the therapeutic effect of khellin in psoriasis. *Dermatologica* 1983;167:109-10.

1909 Clark RH, Feleke G, Din M, et al. Nutritional treatment for acquired immunodeficiency virus-associated wasting using beta-hydroxy beta-methylbutyrate, glutamine, and arginine: a randomized, double-blind, placebo-controlled study. *JPEN J Parenter Enteral Nutr* 2000;24:133-9.

1910 Thom H, Carter PE, Cole GF, et al. Ammonia and carnitine concentrations in children treated with sodium valproate compared with other anticonvulsant drugs. *Dev Med Child Neurol* 1991;33:795-802.

1911 Hug G, McGraw CA, Bates SR, et al. Reduction of serum carnitine concentrations during anticonvulsant therapy with phenobarbital, valproic acid, phenytoin, and carbamazepine in children. *J Pediatr* 1991;119:799-802.

1912 Riva R, Albani F, Gobbi G, et al. Carnitine disposition before and during valproate therapy in patients with epilepsy. *Epilepsia* 1993;34:184-7.

1913 Zelnik N, Fridkis I, Gruener N. Reduced carnitine and antiepileptic drugs: cause relationship or co-existence? *Acta Paediatr* 1995;84:93-5.

1914 Bohles H, Sewell AC, Wenzel D. The effect of carnitine supplementation in valproate-induced hyperammonaemia. *Acta Paediatr* 1996;85:446-9.

1915 Altunbasak S, Baytok V, Tasouji M, et al. Asymptomatic hyperammonemia in children treated with valproic acid. *J Child Neurol* 1997;12:461-3.

1916 Coulter DL. Prevention of hepatotoxicity recurrence with valproate monotherapy and carnitine. *Ann Neurol* 1988;24:301.

1917 Vance CK, Vance H, Winter SC, et al. Control of valproate-induced hepatotoxicity with carnitine. *Ann Neurol* 1989;26:456.

1918 Salonen JT, Nyyssonen K, Salonen R, et al. Antioxidant Supplementation in Atherosclerosis Prevention (ASAP) study: a randomized trial of the effect of vitamins E and C on 3-year progression of carotid atherosclerosis. *J Intern Med* 2000;248:377-86.

1919 Ernst E, Pittler MH. Efficacy of ginger for nausea and vomiting: a systematic review of randomized clinical trials. *Br J Anaesth* 2000;84:367-71.

1920 Anon. Case problem: presenting conventional and complementary approaches for relieving nausea in a breast cancer patient undergoing chemotherapy. *J Am Diet Assoc* 2000;100:257-9.

1921 Wilkinson JM. What do we know about herbal morning sickness treatments? A literature survey. *Midwifery* 2000;16:224-8.

1922 Jewell D, Young G. Interventions for nausea and vomiting in early pregnancy. *Cochrane Database Syst Rev* 2000;2:CD000145.

1923 Micklefield GH, Redeker Y, Meister V, et al. Effects of ginger on gastroduodenal motility. *Int J Clin Pharmacol Ther* 1999;37:341-6.

1924 Lumb AB. Mechanism of antiemetic effect of ginger. *Anaesthesia* 1993;48:1118.

1926 Vynograd N, Vynograd I, Sosnowski Z. A comparative multi-centre study of the efficacy of propolis, acyclovir and placebo in the treatment of genital herpes (HSV). *Phytomedicine* 2000;7(1):1-6.

1927 Spasov AA, Wikman GK, Mandrikov VB, et al. A double-blind, placebo-controlled pilot study of the stimulating and adaptogenic effect of Rhodiola rosea SHR-5 extract on the fatigue of students caused by stress during an examination

period with a repeated low-dose regimen. *Phytomedicine* 2000;7:85-89.
1928 Rao AV, Agarwal S. Role of antioxidant lycopene in cancer and heart disease. *J Am Coll Nutr* 2000;19:563-9.
1929 Panton LB, Rathmacher JA, Baier S, et al. Nutritional supplementation of the leucine metabolite beta-hydroxy-beta-methylbutyrate (hmb) during resistance training. *Nutrition* 2000;16:734-9.
1930 Kelly GS. L-carnitine: therapeutic applications of a conditionally-essential amino acid. *Altern Med Rev* 1998;3(5):345-60.
1931 Krahenbuhl S. Carnitine metabolism in chronic liver disease. *Life Sci* 1996;59:1579-99.
1932 Larsson B, Jonasson A, Fianu S. Prophylactic effect of UVA-E in women with recurrent cystitis: a preliminary report. *Curr Ther Res* 1993;53:441-3.
1933 Brass E. Pharmacokinetic considerations for the therapeutic use of carnitine in hemodialysis patients. *Clin Ther* 1995;17:176-85.
1934 Lee NA, Reasner CA. Beneficial effect of chromium supplementation on serum triglyceride levels in NIDDM. *Diabetes Care* 1994;17:1449-52.
1935 Fox GN, Sabovic Z. Chromium picolinate supplementation for diabetes mellitus. *J Fam Pract* 1998;46:83-6.
1936 Reading SA. Chromium picolinate. *J Fla Med Assoc* 1996 Jan;83:29-31.
1937 Urberg M, Zemel MB. Evidence for synergism between chromium and nicotinic acid in the control of glucose tolerance in elderly humans. *Metabolism* 1987;36:896-9.
1938 Mohamedshah FY, Moser-Veillon PB, Yamini S, et al. Distribution of a stable isotope of chromium (53Cr) in serum, urine, and breast milk in lactating women. *Am J Clin Nutr* 1998;67:1250-5.
1939 Grant KE, Chandler RM, Castle AL, Ivy JL. Chromium and exercise training: effect on obese women. *Med Sci Sports Exerc* 1997;29:992-8.
1942 Jing SB, Li L, Ji D, et al. Effect of chitosan on renal function in patients with chronic renal failure. *J Pharm Pharmacol* 1997;49:721-3.
1943 Rao SB, Sharma CP. Use of chitosan as a biomaterial: studies on its safety and hemostatic potential. *J Biomed Mater Res* 1997;34:21-28.
1944 Biagini G, Bertani A, Muzzarelli R, et al. Wound management with N-carboxybutyl chitosan. *Biomaterials* 1991;12:281-6.
1945 Muzzarelli R, Biagini G, Pugnaloni A, et al. Reconstruction of parodontal tissue with chitosan. *Biomaterials* 1989;10:598-603.
1946 Tsoko M, Beauseigneur F, Gresti J, et al. Enhancement of activities relative to fatty acid oxidation in the liver of rats depleted of L-carnitine by D-carnitine and a gamma-butyrobetaine hydroxylase inhibitor. *Biochem Pharmacol* 1995;49:1403-10.
1947 Colombani P, Wenk C, Kunz I, et al. Effects of L-carnitine supplementation on physical performance and energy metabolism of endurance-trained athletes: a double-blind crossover field study. *Eur J Appl Physiol* 1996;73:434-9.
1948 Krahenbuhl S, Reichen J. Carnitine metabolism in patients with chronic liver disease. *Hepatology* 1997;25:148-53.
1949 Zeisel SH. Choline: needed for normal development of memory. *J Am Coll Nutr* 2000;19:528S-31S.
1950 Hahn CJ, Evans GW. Absorption of trace metals in the zinc-deficient rat. *Am J Physiol* 1975;228:1020-3.
1951 Wasser WG, Feldman NS, D'Agati VD. Chronic renal failure after ingestion of over-the-counter chromium picolinate. [letter] *Ann Intern Med* 1997;126:410.
1952 Mertz W. Interaction of chromium with insulin: a progress report. *Nutr Rev* 1998;56:174-7.
1953 Anderson RA. Chromium, glucose intolerance and diabetes. *J Am Coll Nutr* 1998;17:548-55.
1954 Davydov M, Krikorian AD. Eleutherococcus senticosus (Rupr. & Maxim.) Maxim. (Araliaceae) as an adaptogen: a closer look. *J Ethnopharmacol* 2000;72:345-93.
1955 Morrison LM, Enrick N. Coronary heart disease: reduction of death rate by chondroitin sulfate A. *Angiology* 1973;24:269-87.
1956 Kaufmann PA, Gnecchi-Ruscone T, di Terlizzi M, et al. Coronary heart disease in smokers: vitamin C restores coronary microcirculatory function. *Circulation* 2000;102:1233-8.
1957 Yokoyama T, Date C, Kokubo Y, et al. Serum vitamin C concentration was inversely associated with subsequent 20-year incidence of stroke in a Japanese rural community : the shibata study. *Stroke* 2000;31:2287-94.
1958 Gale CR, Martyn CN, Winter PD, Cooper C. Vitamin C and risk of death from stroke and coronary heart disease in cohort of elderly people. *BMJ* 1995;310:1563-6.
1959 Alster TS, West TB. Effect of topical vitamin C on postoperative carbon dioxide laser resurfacing erythema. *Dermatol Surg* 1998;24:331-4.
1960 Slivka A, Kang JO, Cohen G. Ascorbic acid. *N Engl J Med* 1986;315:708-9.
1961 Daniel TA, Nawarskas JJ. Vitamin C in the prevention of nitrate tolerance. *Ann Pharmacother* 2000;34:1193-7.
1962 Hodby ED, Hirsh J, Adeniyi-Jones C. The influence of drugs upon the anticoagulant activity of heparin. *Can Med Assoc J* 1972;106:562-4.
1963 Leibovitz B, Siegel BV. Ascorbic acid and the immune response. *Adv Exp Med Biol* 1981;135:1-25.
1964 Kasa RM. Vitamin C: from scurvy to the common cold. *Am J Med Technol* 1983;49:23-6.
1965 Vilter RW. Nutritional aspects of ascorbic acid: uses and abuses. *West J Med* 1980;133:485-92.
1966 Martin NG, Carr AB, Oakeshott JG, Clark P. Co-twin control studies: vitamin C and the common cold. *Prog Clin Biol Res* 1982;103:365-73.
1967 Pitt HA, Costrini AM. Vitamin C prophylaxis in marine recruits. *JAMA* 1979;241:908-11.
1968 Anderson TW. Vitamin C and the common cold. *J Med Soc N J* 1979;76:765-6.
1969 Coulehan JL. Ascorbic acid and the common cold: reviewing the evidence. *Postgrad Med* 1979;66:153-60.
1970 Uebelhart D, Thonar EJ, Delmas PD, et al. Effects of oral chondroitin sulfate on the progression of knee osteoarthritis: a pilot study. *Osteoarthritis Cartilage* 1998;6:39-46.
1971 Bourgeois P, Chales G, Dehais J, et al. Efficacy and tolerability of chondroitin sulfate 1200 mg/day vs chondroitin sulfate 3 x 400 mg/day vs placebo. *Osteoarthritis Cartilage* 1998;6:25-30.
1972 Bucsi L, Poor G. Efficacy and tolerability of oral chondroitin sulfate as a symptomatic slow-acting drug for osteoarthritis (SYSADOA) in the treatment of knee osteoarthritis. *Osteoarthritis Cartilage* 1998;6 Suppl A:31-6.
1973 Kelly GS. The role of glucosamine sulfate and chondroitin sulfates in the treatment of degenerative joint disease. *Altern Med Rev* 1998;3:27-39.
1974 Limberg MB, McCaa C, Kissling GE, Kaufman HE. Topical application of hyaluronic acid and chondroitin sulfate in the treatment of dry eyes. *Am J Ophthalmol* 1987;103:194-7.
1975 Fan YY, Chapkin RS. Importance of dietary gamma-linolenic acid in human health and nutrition. *J Nutr* 1998;128:1411-4.
1976 Johnson MM, Swan DD, Surette ME. Dietary supplementation with gamma-linolenic acid alters fatty acid content and eicosanoid production in healthy humans. *J Nutr* 1997;127:1435-44.

1977 Stainforth JM, Layton AM, Goodfield MJ. Clinical aspects of the use of gamma linolenic acid in systemic sclerosis. *Acta Derm Venereol* 1996;76:144-6.

1978 McCaul JA, Lamey PJ. Multiple oral mucoceles treated with gamma-linolenic acid: report of a case. *Br J Oral Maxillofac Surg* 1994;32:392-3.

1979 Guivernau M, Meza N, Barja P, Roman O. Clinical and experimental study on the long-term effect of dietary gamma-linolenic acid on plasma lipids, platelet aggregation, thromboxane formation, and prostacyclin production. *Prostaglandins Leukot Essent Fatty Acids* 1994;51:311-6.

1980 Jamal GA. The use of gamma linolenic acid in the prevention and treatment of diabetic neuropathy. *Diabet Med* 1994;11:145-9.

1981 Horrobin DF. The use of gamma-linolenic acid in diabetic neuropathy. *Agents Actions Suppl* 1992;37:120-44.

1982 Cant A, Shay J, Horrobin DF. The effect of maternal supplementation with linoleic and gamma- linolenic acids on the fat composition and content of human milk: a placebo-controlled trial. *J Nutr Sci Vitaminol* (Tokyo) 1991;37:573-9.

1983 van der Merwe CF, Booyens J, Joubert HF, van der Merwe CA. The effect of gamma-linolenic acid, an in vitro cytostatic substance contained in evening primrose oil, on primary liver cancer. A double- blind placebo controlled trial. *Prostaglandins Leukot Essent Fatty Acids* 1990;40:199-202.

1984 Jamal GA, Carmichael H. The effect of gamma-linolenic acid on human diabetic peripheral neuropathy: a double-blind placebo-controlled trial. *Diabet Med* 1990;7:319-23.

1985 Pullman-Mooar S, Laposata M, Lem D. Alteration of the cellular fatty acid profile and the production of eicosanoids in human monocytes by gamma-linolenic acid. *Arthritis Rheum* 1990;33:1526-33.

1986 Davies JE, Hughes RE, Jones E, et al. Metabolism of ascorbic acid (vitamin C) in subjects infected with common cold viruses. *Biochem Med* 1979;21:78-85.

1987 Hemila H. Does vitamin C alleviate the symptoms of the common cold?- a review of current evidence. *Scand J Infect Dis* 1994;26:1-6.

1988 Hemila H, Herman ZS. Vitamin C and the common cold: a retrospective analysis of Chalmers' review. *J Am Coll Nutr* 1995;14:116-23.

1989 Hemila H. Vitamin C, the placebo effect, and the common cold: a case study of how preconceptions influence the analysis of results. *J Clin Epidemiol* 1996;49:1079-84.

1990 Barrington WW, Angle CR, Willcockson NK, et al. Autonomic function in manganese alloy workers. *Environ Res* 1998;78:50-8.

1991 Greger JL. Dietary standards for manganese: overlap between nutritional and toxicological studies. *J Nutr* 1998;128:368S-71S.

1992 Hauser RA, Zesiewicz TA, Martinez C, et al. Blood manganese correlates with brain magnetic resonance imaging changes in patients with liver disease. *Can J Neurol Sci* 1996;23:95-8.

1993 Okano T. Effects of essential trace elements on bone turnover-in relation to the osteoporosis. *Nippon Rinsho* 1996;54:148-54.

1994 Strause L, Saltman P, Smith KT, et al. Spinal bone loss in postmenopausal women supplemented with calcium and trace minerals. *J Nutr* 1994;124:1060-4.

1995 Lean ME, Noroozi M, Kelly I. Dietary flavonols protect diabetic human lymphocytes against oxidative damage to DNA. *Diabetes* 1999 Jan;48(1):176-81.

1996 Rachkauskas GS. The efficacy of enterosorption and a combination of antioxidants in schizophrenics. *Lik Sprava* 1998 Jun;(4):122-4.

1997 Kuo SM, Leavitt PS, Lin CP. Dietary flavonoids interact with trace metals and affect metallothionein level in human intestinal cells. *Biol Trace Elem Res* 1998;62:135-53.

1998 Conquer JA, Maiani G, Azzini E, et al. Supplementation with quercetin markedly increases plasma quercetin concentration without effect on selected risk factors for heart disease in healthy subjects. *J Nutr* 1998;128:593-7.

1999 Janssen K, Mensink RP, Cox FJ, et al. Effects of the flavonoids quercetin and apigenin on hemostasis in healthy volunteers: results from an in vitro and a dietary supplement study. *Am J Clin Nutr* 1998 Feb;67(2):255-62.

2000 Freeland-Graves JH, Lin PH. Plasma uptake of manganese as affected by oral loads of manganese, calcium, milk, phosphorus, copper, and zinc. *J Am Coll Nutr* 1991;10:38-43.

2001 Krieger D, Krieger S, Jansen O, et al. Manganese and chronic hepatic encephalopathy. *Lancet* 1995;346:270-4.

2002 O'Dell BL. Mineral interactions relevant to nutrient requirements. *J Nutr* 1989;119:1832-8.

2003 Moghissi KS. Risks and benefits of nutritional supplements during pregnancy. *Obstet Gynecol* 1981;58:68S-78S.

2004 Penland JG, Johnson PE. Dietary calcium and manganese effects on menstrual cycle symptoms. *Am J Obstet Gynecol* 1993;168:1417-23.

2005 Freeland-Graves JH, Turnlund JR. Deliberations and evaluations of the approaches, endpoints and paradigms for manganese and molybdenum dietary recommendations. *J Nutr* 1996;126:2435S-40S.

2006 Li MK, Blacklock NJ, Garside J. Effects of magnesium on calcium oxalate crystallization. *J Urol* 1985;133:23.

2007 Johansson G, Backman U, Danielson BG, et al. Biochemical and clinical effects of the prophylactic treatment of renal calcium stones with magnesium hydroxide. *J Urol* 1980;124:770–4.

2008 Freeland-Graves JH. Manganese: an essential nutrient for humans. *Nutr Today* 1988;23:13-9.

2009 Prudden JF, Balassa LL. The biological activity of bovine cartilage preparations. Clinical demonstration of their potent anti-inflammatory capacity with supplementary notes on certain relevant fundamental supportive studies. *Semin Arthritis Rheum* 1974;3:287-321.

2010 Prudden JF. The treatment of human cancer with agents prepared from bovine cartilage. *J Biol Response Mod* 1985 Dec;4(6):551-84.

2011 Durk H, Haase K, Saal J, et al. Nephrotic syndrome after injections of bovine cartilage and marrow extract. [letter] *Lancet* 1989;1:614.

2012 Ashar B, Vargo E. Shark cartilage-induced hepatitis [let er]. *Ann Intern Med* 1996;125:780-1.

2013 Hunt TJ, Connelly JF. Shark cartilage for cancer treatment. *Am J Health Syst Pharm* 1995;52:1756-60.

2014 Lane IW, Comac L. Sharks don't get cancer. Garden City, NY: Avery Publishing Group; 1992.

2015 Miller DR, Anderson GT, Stark JJ, et al. Phase I/II trial of the safety and efficacy of shark cartilage in the treatment of advanced cancer. *J Clin Oncol* 1998;16:3649-55.

2020 Sturtevant FM. Use of aspartame in pregnancy. *Int J Fertil* 1985;30(1):85-7.

2021 Silkaitis RP, Mosnaim AD. Pathways linking L-phenylalanine and 2-phenylethylamine with p-tyramine in rabbit brain. *Brain Res* 1976;114:105-15.

2023 PKU - Dietary Treatment of the Untreated Adult PKU. National Society for Phenylketonuria (NSPKU). 1996-2001. Available at: web.ukonline.co.uk/nspku/untreatd.htm

2024 Fouty B, Frerman F, Reves R. Riboflavin to treat nucleoside analogue-induced lactic acidosis. *Lancet* 1998;352:291-2.

2025 Levine J, Mishori A, Susnosky M, et al. Combination of inositol and serotonin reuptake inhibitors in the treatment of depression. *Biol Psychiatry* 1999;45:270-3.

2026 Levine J, Barak Y, Kofman O, Belmaker RH. Follow-up and relapse analysis of an inositol study of depression. *Isr J Psychiatry Relat Sci* 1995;32:14-21.

2027 Souza FG, Mander AJ, Foggo M, et al. The effects of lithium discontinuation and the non-effect of oral inositol upon thyroid hormones and cortisol in patients with bipolar affective disorder. *J Affect Disord* 1991;22:165-70.

2028 Nestler JE, Jakubowicz DJ, Reamer P, et al. Ovulatory and metabolic effects of D-chiro-inositol in the polycystic ovary syndrome. *N Engl J Med* 1999;340:1314-20.

2030 Soleas GJ, Diamandis EP, Goldberg DM. Resveratrol: a molecule whose time has come? And gone? *Clin Biochem* 1997;30:91-113.

2031 Ross D, Cooper AJ, Pryse-Davies J, et al. Randomized, double-blind, dose-ranging study of the endometrial effects of a vaginal progesterone gel in estrogen-treated postmenopausal women. *Am J Obstet Gynecol* 1997;177:937-41.

2032 Pouly JL, Bassil S, Frydman R, et al. Luteal support after in-vitro fertilization: Crinone 8%, a sustained release vaginal progesterone gel, versus Utrogestan, an oral micronized progesterone. *Hum Reprod* 1996;11:2085-9.

2033 Affinito P, Di Carlo C, Di Mauro P, et al. Endometrial hyperplasia: efficacy of a new treatment with a vaginal cream containing natural micronized progesterone. *Maturitas* 1994;20:191-8.

2034 Miles RA, Paulson RJ, Lobo RA, et al. Pharmacokinetics and endometrial tissue levels of progesterone after administration by intramuscular and vaginal routes: a comparative study. *Fertil Steril* 1994;62:485-90.

2035 Carson CR, Ashton L, Dry L, et al. Melaleuca alternifolia (tea tree) oil gel (6%) for the treatment of recurrent herpes labialis. *J Antimicrob Chemother* 2001;48:450-1.

2036 Zorgniotti AW, Lizza EF. Effect of large doses of the nitric oxide precursor, L-arginine, on erectile dysfunction. *Int J Impot Res* 1994;6:33-5.

2038 Klotz T, Mathers MJ, Braun M, et al. Effectiveness of oral L-arginine in first-line treatment of erectile dysfunction in a controlled crossover study. *Urol Int* 1999;63:220-3.

2039 Morse PF, Horrobin DF, Manku MS, et al. Meta-analysis of placebo-controlled studies of the efficacy of Epogam in the treatment of atopic eczema. Relationship between plasma essential fatty acid changes and clinical response. *Br J Dermatol* 1989;121:75-90.

2040 Penzak SR, Jann MW, Cold JA, et al. Seville (sour) orange juice: synephrine content and cardiovascular effects in normotensive adults. *J Clin Pharmacol* 2001;41:1059-63.

2041 Warren MP, Biller BMK, Shangold MM. A new clinical option for hormone replacement therapy in women with secondary amenorrhea: effects of cyclic administration of progesterone from the sustained-release vaginal gel Crinone (4% and 8%) on endometrial morphologic features and withdrawal bleeding. *Am J Obstet Gynecol* 1999;180:42-8.

2042 van den Berg H. Carotenoid interactions. *Nutr Rev* 1999;57:1-10.

2043 Mazzotta G, Sarchielli P, Alberti A, Gallai V. Intracellular Mg++ concentration and electromyographical ischemic test in juvenile headache. *Cephalalgia* 1999;19(9):802-9.

2044 Duffy SJ, Gokce N, Holbrook M, et al. Treatment of hypertension with ascorbic acid. *Lancet* 1999;354:2048-9.

2045 Zollinger PE, Tuinebreijer WE, Kreis RW, Breederveld RS. Effect of vitamin C on frequency of reflex sympathetic dystrophy in wrist fractures: a randomized trial. *Lancet* 1999;354:2025-8.

2047 Colodny L, Hoffman RL. Inositol--clinical applications for exogenous use. *Altern Med Rev* 1998;3:432-47.

2048 Nomenclature of Cyclitols. IUPAC Commission on the Nomenclature of Organic Chemistry (CNOC) and IUPAC-IUB Commission on Biochemical Nomenclature (CBN). Available at: http://www.chem.qmw.ac.uk/iupac/cyclitol/ (Accessed 23 January 2004).

2049 Mori TA, Bao DQ, Burke V, et al. Dietary fish as a major component of a weight-loss diet: effect on serum lipids, glucose, and insulin metabolism in overweight hypertensive subjects. *Am J Clin Nutr* 1999;70:817-25.

2050 Stryer L. Biochemistry, third edition. W.H. Freeman and Co., New York, 1988.

2052 Lehmann WD, Theobald N, Fischer R, Heinrich HC. Stereospecificity of phenylalanine plasma kinetics and hydroxylation in man following oral application of a stable isotope-labelled pseudo-racemic mixture of L- and D-phenylalanine. *Clin Chim Acta* 1983;128:181-98.

2056 Kraft K. Artichoke leaf extract- recent findings reflecting effects on lipid metabolism, liver and gastrointestinal tracts. *Phytomedicine* 1997;4:369-78.

2057 Soleas GJ, Diamandis EP, Goldberg DM. Wine as a biological fluid: history, production, and role in disease prevention. *J Clin Lab Anal* 1997;11:287-313.

2058 Renaud SC, Gueguen R, Siest G, Salamon R. Wine, beer, and mortality in middle-aged men from eastern France. *Arch Intern Med* 1999;159:1865-70.

2059 Leighton F, Cuevas A, Guasch V, et al. Plasma polyphenols and antioxidants, oxidative DNA damage and endothelial function in a diet and wine intervention study in humans. *Drugs Exp Clin Res* 1999;25:133-41.

2060 Criqui MH. Alcohol and coronary heart disease: consistent relationship and public health implications. *Clin Chim Acta* 1996;246:51-7.

2061 Renaud SC, Ruf JC. Effects of alcohol on platelet functions. *Clin Chim Acta* 1996;246:77-89.

2063 Yun TK, Choi SY. Non-organ specific cancer prevention of ginseng: a prospective study in Korea. *Int J Epidemiol* 1998;27:359-64.

2064 Sorensen H, Sonne J. A double-masked study of the effects of ginseng on cognitive functions. *Curr Ther Res* 1996;57:959-68.

2065 Bitzan MM, Gold BD, Philpott DJ, et al. Inhibition of Helicobacter pylori and Helicobacter mustelae binding to lipid receptors by bovine colostrum. *J Infect Dis* 1998;177:955-61.

2067 Huppertz HI, Rutkowski S, Busch DH, et al. Bovine colostrum ameliorates diarrhea in infection with diarrheogenic Escherichia coli, shiga toxin-producing E. Coli, and E. coli expressing intimin and hemolysin. *J Pediatr Gastroenterol Nutr* 1999;29:452-6.

2068 Freedman DJ, Tacket CO, Delehanty A, et al. Milk immunoglobulin with specific activity against purified colonization factor antigens can protect against oral challenge with enterotoxigenic Escherichia coli. *J Infect Dis* 1998;177:662-7.

2069 Tacket CO, Losonsky G, Link H, et al. Protection by milk immunoglobulin concentrate against oral challenge with enterotoxigenic Escherichia coli. *N Engl J Med* 1988;318:1240-3.

2070 Tacket CO, Binion SB, Bostwick E, et al. Efficacy of bovine milk immunoglobulin concentrate in preventing illness after Shigella flexneri challenge. *Am J Trop Med Hyg* 1992;47:276-83.

2071 Tacket CO, Losonsky G, Livio S, et al. Lack of prophylactic efficacy of an enteric-coated bovine hyperimmune milk product against enterotoxigenic Escherichia coli challenge administered during a standard meal. *J Infect Dis* 1999;180:2056-9.

2072 Petschow BW, Talbott RD. Reduction in virus-neutralizing activity of a bovine colostrum immunoglobulin concentrate by gastric acid and digestive enzymes. *J Pediatr Gastroenterol Nutr* 1994;19:228-35.

2074 Kuhlmann J, Berger W, Podzuweit H, Schmidt U. The influence of valerian treatment on "reaction time, alertness and concentration" in volunteers. *Pharmacopsychiatry* 1999;32:235-41.

2075 Dev S. Ancient-modern concordance in Ayurvedic plants: some examples. *Environ Health Perspect* 1999;107:783-9.

2076 GRIN Taxonomy search page http://www.ars-grin.gov/cgi-bin/npgs/html/tax_search.pl? (Accessed 27 February 2000).

2077 Jacob A, Pandey M, Kapoor S, Saroja R. Effect of the Indian gooseberry (amla) on serum cholesterol levels in men aged 35-55 years. *Eur J Clin Nutr* 1988;42:939-44.

2078 Asmawi MZ, Kankaanranta H, Moilanen E, Vapaatalo H. Anti-inflammatory activities of Emblica officinalis Gaertn leaf extracts. *J Pharm Pharmacol* 1993;45:581-4.

2079 Ihantola-Vormisto A, Summanen J, Kankaanranta H, et al. Anti-inflammatory activity of extracts from leaves of Phyllanthus emblica. *Planta Med* 1997;63:518-24.

2080 Hu JF. [Inhibitory effects of Phyllanthus emblica juice on formation of N-nitrosomorpholine in vitro and N-nitrosoproline in rat and human]. [Article in Chinese]. *Chung Hua Yu Fang I Hsueh Tsa Chih* 1990;24:132-5.

2081 Bhattacharya A, Chatterjee A, Ghosal S, Bhattacharya SK. Antioxidant activity of active tannoid principles of Emblica officinalis (amla). *Indian J Exp Biol* 1999;37:676-80.

2082 Janicak PG, Lipinski J, Davis JM, et al. S-adenosylmethionine in depression. A literature review and preliminary report. *Ala J Med Sci* 1988;25:306-13.

2083 De Vanna M, Rigamonti R. Oral S-adenosyl-L-methionine in depression. *Curr Ther Res* 1992;52:478-85.

2084 Zhao G. [Inherited metabolic aberration of phenylalanine in the family members of patients with essential hypertension and stroke]. [Article in Chinese]. *Chung Hua I Hsueh Tsa Chih* (Taipei) 1991;71:28, 388-90.

2086 Damario MA, Goudas VT, Session DR, et al. Crinone 8% vaginal progesterone gel results in lower embryonic implantation efficiency after in vitro fertilization-embryo transfer. *Fertil Steril* 1999;72:830-6.

2089 Gibbons WE, Toner JP, Hamacher P, Kolm P. Experience with a novel vaginal progesterone preparation in a donor oocyte program. *Fertil Steril* 1998;69:96-101.

2091 FDA MedWatch. Summary of safety-related drug labeling changes approved by FDA May 1998. Crinone (progesterone) Gel. May 11, 1998. Available at: http://www.fda.gov/medwatch/safety/1998/may98.htm#crinon

2092 Woelk H, Kapoula O, Lehrl S, et al. [Comparison of kava special extract WS 1490 and benzodiazepines in patients with anxiety]. [Article in German]. *Z Allg Med* 1993;69:271–7.

2093 Pittler MH, Ernst E. Efficacy of kava extract for treating anxiety: systematic review and meta-analysis. *J Clin Psychopharmacol* 2000;20:84-9.

2094 Volz HP, Kieser M. Kava-kava extract WS 1490 versus placebo in anxiety disorders--a randomized placebo-controlled 25-week outpatient trial. *Pharmacopsychiatry* 1997;30:1-5.

2095 Lehmann E, Kinzler E, Friedemann J. Efficacy of a special Kava extract (Piper methysticum) in patients with states of anxiety, tension and excitedness of non-mental origin- a double-blind placebo-controlled study of four weeks treatment. *Phytomedicine* 1996;3:113-9.

2096 Warnecke G. [Psychosomatic dysfunctions in the female climacteric. Clinical effectiveness and tolerance of Kava extract WS 1490]. [Article in German]. *Fortschr Med* 1991;109:119-22.

2097 Heinze HJ, Munthe TF, Steitz J, Matzke M. Pharmacopsychological effects of oxazepam and kava-extract in a visual search paradigm assessed with event-related potentials. *Pharmacopsychiatry* 1994;27:224-30.

2098 Munte TF, Heinze HJ, Matzke M, Steitz J. Effects of oxazepam and an extract of kava roots (Piper methysticum) on event-related potentials in a word recognition task. *Neuropsychobiology* 1993;27:46-53.

2100 Kreider RB, Ferreira M, Wilson M, et al. Effects of creatine supplementation on body composition, strength, and sprint performance. *Med Sci Sports Exerc* 1998;30:73-82.

2101 Vandenberghe K, Goris M, Van Hecke P, et al. Long-term creatine intake is beneficial to muscle performance during resistance training. *J Appl Physiol* 1997;83:2055-63.

2102 Earnest CP, Snell PG, Rodriguez R, et al. The effect of creatine monohydrate ingestion on anerobic power indices, muscular strength and body composition. *Acta Physiol Scand* 1995;153:207-9.

2103 Balsom PD, Soderland K, Ekblom B. Creatine in humans with special reference to creatine supplementation. *Sports Med* 1994;18:268-80.

2104 Hultman E, Soderlund K, Timmons JA, et al. Muscle creatine loading in men. *J Appl Physiol* 1996;81:232-7.

2105 Burke LM, Pyne DB, Telford RD. Oral creatine supplementation does not improve sprint performance in elite swimmers. *Med Sci Sports Exerc* 1995;27:S146.

2106 Mujika I, Chatard J, Lacoste L, et al. Creatine supplementation does not improve sprint performance in competitive swimmers. *Med Sci Sports Exerc* 1996;28:1435-41.

2107 Hanioka T, Tanaka M, Ojima M, et al. Effect of topical application of coenzyme Q10 on adult periodontitis. *Molec Aspects Med* 1994;15:S241-8.

2108 Watts TLP. Coenzyme Q10 and periodontal treatment: is there any beneficial effect? *Br Dent J* 1995;178:209-13.

2109 Malm C, Svensson M, Ekblom B, et al. Effects of ubiquinone-10 supplementation and high intensity training on physical performance in humans. *Acta Physiol Scand* 1997;161:379-84.

2110 Weston SB, Zhou S, Weatherby RP, et al. Does exogenous coenzyme Q10 affect aerobic capacity in endurance athletes? *Int J Sport Nutr* 1997;7:197-206.

2111 Kuritzky L. DHEA: Science or Wishful Thinking? *Hosp Pract* 1998;33:85-6.

2112 Skolnick AA. Scientific verdict still out on DHEA. *JAMA* 1996;276:1365-7.

2113 Van Vollenhoven RF, Morabito LM, Engleman EG, et al. Treatment of Systemic Lupus Erythematosus with Dehydroepiandrosterone: 50 Patients Treated up to 12 Months. *J Rheumatol* 1998;25:285-9.

2114 Van Vollenhoven RF, Engleman EG, McGurie JL. Dehydroepiandrosterone in Systemic Lupus Erythematosus. *Arth Rheum* 1995;38:1826-31.

2115 Ebeling P, Koivisto VA. Physiological Importance of dehydroepiandrosterone. *Lancet* 1994;343:1479-81.

2116 Dehydroepiandrosterone (DHEA). *Med Lett Drugs Ther* 1996;38:91-2.

2117 Vandeberghe K, Gillis N, Van Leemputte M, et al. Caffeine counteracts the ergogenic action of muscle creatine loading. *J Appl Physiol* 1996;80:452-7.

2118 Pritchard NR, Kalra PA. Renal dysfunction accompanying oral creatine supplements. *Lancet* 1998;351:1252-3.

2119 Braverman Y, Chizov-Ginzburg A. Repellency of synthetic and plant-derived preparations for Culicoides imicola. *Med Vet Entomol* 1997;11:355-60.

2120 Poortmans JR, Auquier H, Renaut V, et al. Effect of short-term creatine supplementation on renal responses in men. *Eur J Appl Physiol* 1997;76:566-7.

2121 Kamikawa T, Kobayashi A, Yamashita T, et al. Effects of coenzyme Q10 on exercise tolerance in chronic stable angina pectoris. *Am J Cardiol* 1985;56:247-51.

2122 Langsjoen P, Willis R, Folkers K. Treatment of essential hypertension with coenzyme Q10. *Mol Aspects Med* 1994;S265-72.

2123 Folkers K, Hanioka T, Xia LJ, et al. Coenzyme Q10 increases T4/T8 ratios of lymphocytes in ordinary subjects and relevance to patients having the AIDS related complex. *Biochem Biophys Res Commun* 1991;176:786-91.

2124 Folkers K, Langsjoen P, Nara Y, et al. Biochemical deficiencies of coenzyme Q10 in HIV-infection and exploratory treatment. *Biochem Biophys Res Commun* 1988;153:888-96.

2125 Suzuki S, Hinokio Y, Ohtomo M, et al. The effects of coenzyme Q10 treatment on maternally inherited diabetes mellitus and deafness, and mitochondrial DNA 3243 (A to G) mutation. *Diabetologia* 1998;41:584-8.

2126 Andersen CB, Henriksen JE, Hother-Nielsen O, et al. The effect of coenzyme Q10 on blood glucose and insulin requirement in patients with insulin dependent diabetes mellitus. *Mol Aspects Med* 1997;18 Suppl:S307-9.

2127 Folkers K, Simonsen R. Two successful double-blind trials with coenzyme Q10 (vitamin Q10) on muscular dystrophies and neurogenic atrophies. *Biochem Biophys Acta* 1995;1271:281-6.

2128 Spigset O. Reduced effect of warfarin caused by ubidecarenone. *Lancet* 1994;334:1372-3.

2129 Daferera DJ, Ziogas BN, Polissiou MG. GC-MS analysis of essential oils from some Greek aromatic plants and their fungitoxicity on Penicillium digitatum. *J Agric Food Chem* 2000;48:2576-81.

2130 Dorman HJ, Deans SG. Antimicrobial agents from plants: antibacterial activity of plant volatile oils. *J Appl Microbiol* 2000;88:308-16.

2131 Buckle J. Use of aromatherapy as a complementary treatment for chronic pain. *Altern Ther Health Med* 1999;5:42-51.

2132 Degelau J, Guay D, Hallgren H. The effect of DHEAS on influenza vaccination in aging adults. *J Am Geriatr Soc* 1997;45(6):747-51.

2133 Yen SS, Morales AJ, Khorram O. Replacement of DHEA in aging men and women. Potential remedial effects. *Ann N Y Acad Sci* 1995;774:128-42.

2134 Greenberg S, Fishman WH. Coenzyme Q10: A New Drug for Cardiovascular Disease. *J Clin Pharmacol* 1990;30:596-608.

2135 Lewin A, Lavon H. The effect of coenzyme Q10 on sperm motility and function. *Mol Aspects Med* 1997;18 Suppl:S213-9.

2136 van Vollenhoven RF, Engleman EG, McGuire JL. Dehydroepiandrosterone in Systemic Lupus Erythematosus. *Arthritis Rheum* 1994;37:1305-10.

2138 Goodman GA, Rall TW, Nies AS, Taylor P. The Pharmacological Basis of Therapeutics, 9th ed.

2139 Ma J, Stampfer MJ, Giovannucci E, et al. Methylenetetrahydrofolate reductase polymorphism, dietary interactions, and risk of colorectal cancer. *Cancer Res* 1997;57:1098-102.

2140 Lashner BA, Provencher KS, Seidner DL, et al. The effect of folic acid supplementation on the risk for cancer or dysplasia in ulcerative colitis. *Gastroenterol* 1997;112:29-32.

2141 La Vecchia C, Braga C, Negri E et al. Intake of selected micronutrients and risk of colorectal cancer. *Int J Cancer* 1997;73:525-30.

2142 Tseng M, Murray SC, Kupper LL, Sandler RS. Micronutrients and the risk of colorectal adenomas. *Am J Epidemiol* 1996;144:1005-14.

2143 Baron JA, Sandler RS, Haile RW, et al. Folate intake, alcohol consumption, cigarette smoking, and risk of colorectal adenomas. *J Natl Cancer Inst* 1998;90:57-62.

2144 Slattery ML, Schaffer D, Edwards SL, et al. Are dietary factors involved in DNA methylation associated with colon cancer? *Nutr Cancer* 1997;28:52-62.

2145 Freudenheim JL, Graham S, Marshall JR, et al. Folate intake and carcinogenesis of the colon and rectum. *Int J Epidemiol* 1991;20:368-74.

2146 Brouwer IA, van Dusseldorp M, Thomas CM, et al. Low-dose folic acid supplementation decreases plasma homocysteine concentrations: a randomized trial. *Am J Clin Nutr* 1999;69:99-104.

2147 Landgren F, Israelsson B, Lindgren A, et al. Plasma homocysteine in acute myocardial infarction: homocysteine-lowering effect of folic acid. *J Intern Med* 1995;237:381-8.

2148 Woodside JV, Yarnell JW, McMaster D, et al. Effect of B-group vitamins and antioxidant vitamins on hyperhomocysteinemia: a double-blind, randomized, factorial-design, controlled trial. *Am J Clin Nutr* 1998;67:858-66.

2149 Brattstrom LE, Israelsson B, Jeppsson JO, et al. Folic acid-an innocuous means to reduce plasma homocysteine. *Scand J Clin Lab Invest* 1988;48:215-21.

2150 Brown RS, Di Stanislao PT, Beaver WT, et al. The administration of folic acid to institutionalized epileptic adults with phenytoin-induced gingival hyperplasia. A double-blind, randomized, placebo-controlled, parallel study. *Oral Surg Oral Med Oral Pathol* 1991;70:565-8.

2151 Drew HJ, Vogel RI, Molofsky W, et al. Effect of folate on phenytoin hyperplasia. *J Clin Periodontol* 1987;14:350-6.

2152 Pack AR, Thomson ME. Effects of topical and systemic folic acid supplementation on gingivitis in pregnancy. *J Clin Periodontol* 1980;7:402-14.

2153 Juhlin L, Olsson MJ. Improvement of vitiligo after oral treatment with vitamin B12 and folic acid and the importance of sun exposure. *Acta Derm Venereol* 1997;77:460-2.

2154 Montes LF, Diaz ML, Lajous J, et al. Folic acid and vitamin B12 in vitiligo: a nutritional approach. *Cutis* 1992;50:39-42.

2155 Strom CM, Brusca RM, Pizzi WJ. Double-blind, placebo-controlled crossover study of folinic acid Leucovorin for the treatment of fragile X syndrome. *Am J Med Genet* 1992;44:676-82.

2156 Fisch GS, Cohen IL, Gross AC, et al. Folic acid treatment of fragile X males: a further study. *Am J Med Genet* 1988;30:393-9.

2157 Gillberg C, Wahlstrom J, Johansson R, et al. Folic acid as an adjunct in the treatment of children with the autism fragile-X syndrome (AFRAX). *Dev Med Child Neurol* 1986;28:624-7.

2158 Rosenblatt DS, Duschenes EA, Hellstrom FV, et al. Folic acid blinded trial in identical twins with fragile X syndrome. *Am J Hum Genet* 1985;37:543-52.

2159 Hagerman RJ, Jackson AW, Levitas A, et al. Oral folic acid versus placebo in the treatment of males with the fragile X syndrome. *Am J Med Genet* 1986;23:241-62.

2160 Brown WT, Cohen IL, Fisch GS, et al. High dose folic acid treatment of fragile (X) males. *Am J Med Genet* 1986;23:263-71.

2161 Muggia FM, Synold TW, Newman EM, et al. Failure of pretreatment with intravenous folic acid to alter the cumulative hematologic toxicity of lometrexol. *J Natl Cancer Inst* 1996;88:1495-6.

2162 Morgan SL, Baggott JE, Vaughn WH, et al. Supplementation with folic acid during methotrexate therapy for rheumatoid arthritis. A double-blind, placebo-controlled tri al. *Ann Intern Med* 1994;121:833-41.

2163 Morgan SL, Baggott JE, Vaughn WH, et al. The effect of folic acid supplementation on the toxicity of low-dose

REFERENCES

methotrexate in patients with rheumatoid arthritis. *Arthritis Rheum* 1990;33:9-18.

2164 Ortiz Z, Shea B, Suarez-Almazor ME, et al. The efficacy of folic acid and folinic acid in reducing methotrexate gastrointestinal toxicity in rheumatoid arthritis. A metaanalysis of randomized controlled trials. *J Rheumatol* 1998;25:36-43.

2165 Kelly GS. Folates: supplemental forms and therapeutic applications. *Altern Med Rev* 1998;3(3):208-20.

2166 Pack AR. Effects of folate mouthwash on experimental gingivitis in man. *J Clin Periodontol* 1986;13(7):671-6.

2167 Slater G, Jenkins D, Logan P, et al. Beta-hydroxy-beta-methylbutyrate (HMB) supplementation does not affect changes in strength or body composition during resistance training in trained men. *Int J Sport Nutr Exerc Metab* 2001;11:384-96.

2168 Nissen S, Sharp R, Ray M, et al. Effect of leucine metabolite beta-hydroxy-beta-methylbutyrate on muscle metabolism during resistance-exercise training. *J Appl Physiol* 1996;81:2095-104.

2169 Gennari C, Agnusdei D, Crepaldi G, et al. Effect of ipriflavone-a synthetic derivative of natural isoflavones-on bone mass loss in the early years after menopause. *Menopause* 1998;5(1):9-15.

2170 Agnusdei D, Crepaldi G, Isaia G, et al. A double blind, placebo-controlled trial of ipriflavone for prevention of postmenopausal spinal bone loss. *Calcif Tissue Int* 1997;61:142-7.

2171 Gambacciani M, Ciaponi M, Cappagli B, et al. Effects of combined low dose of the isoflavone derivative ipriflavone and estrogen replacement on bone mineral density and metabolism in postmenopausal women. *Maturitas* 1997;28(1):75-81.

2172 Agnusdei D, Gennari C, Bufalino L. Prevention of early postmenopausal bone loss using low doses of conjugated estrogens and the non-hormonal, bone-active drug ipriflavone. *Osteoporos Int* 1995;5(6):462-6.

2173 Valente M, Bufalino L, Castiglione GN, et al. Effects of 1-year treatment with ipriflavone on bone in postmenopausal women with low bone mass. *Calcif Tissue Int* 1994;54(5):377-80.

2174 Ushiroyama T, Okamura S, Ikeda A, et al. Efficacy of ipriflavone and 1 alpha vitamin D therapy for the cessation of vertebral bone loss. *Int J Gynaecol Obstet* 1995;48(3):283-8.

2175 Agnusdei D, Zacchei F, Bigazzi S, et al. Metabolic and clinical effects of ipriflavone in established post-menopausal osteoporosis. *Drugs Exp Clin Res* 1989;15(2):97-104.

2176 Agnusdei D, Camporeale A, Gonnelli S, et al. Short-term treatment of Paget's disease of bone with ipriflavone. *Bone Miner* 1992;19 Suppl 1:S35-42.

2177 Hyodo T, Ono K, Koumi T, et al. A study of the effects of ipriflavone administration on hemodialysis patients with renal osteodystrophy: preliminary report. *Nephron* 1991;58(1):114-5.

2178 Monostory K, Vereczkey L, Levai F, et al. Ipriflavone as an inhibitor of human cytochrome P450 enzymes. *Br J Pharmacol* 1998;123(4):605-10.

2179 Melis GB, Paoletti AM, Cagnacci A, et al. Lack of any estrogenic effect of ipriflavone in postmenopausal women. *J Endocrinol Invest* 1992;15(10):755-61.

2184 Benjamin J, Levine J, Fux M, et al. Double-blind, placebo-controlled, crossover trial of inositol treatment for panic disorder. *Am J Psychiatry* 1995;152:1084-6.

2185 Levine J, Barak Y, Gonzalves M, et al. Double-blind, controlled trial of inositol treatment of depression. *Am J Psychiatry* 1995;152:792-4.

2186 Fux M, Levine J, Aviv A, Belmaker RH. Inositol treatment of obsessive-compulsive disorder. *Am J Psychiatry* 1996;153:1219-21.

2187 Levine J. Controlled trials of inositol in psychiatry. *Eur Neuropsychopharmacol* 1997;7:147-55.

2188 Levine J, Goldberger I, Rapaport A, et al. CSF inositol in schizophrenia and high-dose inositol treatment of schizophrenia. *Eur Neuropsychopharmacol* 1994;4:487-90.

2189 Barak Y, Levine J, Glasman A, et al. Inositol treatment of Alzheimer's disease: a double blind, cross-over placebo controlled trial. *Prog Neuropsychopharmacol Biol Psychiatry* 1996;20:729-35.

2190 Levine J, Aviram A, Holan A, et al. Inositol treatment of autism. *J Neural Transm* 1997;104:307-10.

2191 Hallman M, et al. Inositol supplementation in premature infants with respiratory distress syndrome. *N Engl J Med* 1992;326:1233-9.

2192 Hallman M, Pohjavuori M, Bry K. Inositol supplementation in respiratory distress syndrome. *Lung* 1990;168:877-82.

2193 Gregersen G, Bertelsen B, Harbo H, et al. Oral supplementation of myoinositol: effects on peripheral nerve function in human diabetics and on the concentration in plasma, erythrocytes, urine and muscle tissue in human diabetics and normals. *Acta Neurol Scand* 1983;67:164-72.

2194 Salway JG, Whitehead L, Finnegan JA. Effect of myo-inositol on peripheral-nerve function in diabetes. *Lancet* 1978;2:1282-4.

2195 Gregersen G, Borsting H, Theil P, Servo C. Myoinositol and function of peripheral nerves in human diabetics. A controlled clinical trial. *Acta Neurol Scand* 1978;58:241-8.

2197 Ghent WR, Eskin BA, Low DA, Hill LP. Iodine replacement in fibrocystic disease of the breast. *Can J Surg* 1993;36:453-60.

2198 Adamietz IA, Rahn R, Bottcher HD, et al. Prophylaxis with povidone-iodine against induction of oral mucositis by radiochemotherapy. *Support Care Cancer* 1998;6:373-7.

2199 Rahn R, Adamietz IA, Boettcher HD, et al. Povidone-iodine to prevent mucositis in patients during antineoplastic radiochemotherapy. *Dermatology* 1997;195(Suppl 2):57-61.

2200 Apelqvist J, Ragnarson Tennvall G. Cavity foot ulcers in diabetic patients: a comparative study of cadexomer iodine ointment and standard treatment. An economic analysis alongside a clinical trial. *Acta Derm Venereol* 1996; 76(3):231-5.

2203 Poldinger W, Calanchini B, Schwarz W. A functional-dimensional approach to depression: serotonin deficiency as a target syndrome in a comparison of 5-hydroxytryptophan and fluvoxamine. *Psychopathology* 1991;24:53-81.

2204 Ribeiro CA. L-5-Hydroxytryptophan in the prophylaxis of chronic tension-type headache: a double-blind, randomized, placebo-controlled study. *Headache* 2000;40:451-6.

2205 Facts and Comparisons. Drug Facts and Comparisons. St. Louis: Wolters Kluwer Co., 1998.

2207 Ovrum E, Tangen G, Holen EA, et al. Conversion of postischemic ventricular fibrillation with intraaortic infusion of potassium chloride. *Ann Thorac Surg* 1995;60:156-9.

2208 Breslau NA, Heller HJ, Reza-Albarran AA, Pak CY. Physiological effects of slow release potassium phosphate for absorptive hypercalciuria: a randomized double-blind trial. *J Urol* 1998;160:664-8.

2209 Heller HJ, et al. Sustained reduction in urinary calcium during long-term treatment with slow release neutral potassium phosphate in absorptive hypercalciuria. *Urol* 1998;159:1451-5;discussion 1455-6.

2210 Singh RB, Singh NK, Niaz MA, Sharma JP. Effect of treatment with magnesium and potassium on mortality and reinfarction rate of patients with suspected acute myocardial infarction. *Int J Clin Pharmacol Ther* 1996;34:219-25.

2212 Albert KS, Ayres JW, DiSanto AR, et al. Influence of kaolin-pectin suspension on digoxin bioavailability. *J Pharm Sci* 1978;67:1582-6.

2213 Albert KS, Welch RD, DeSante KA, et al. Decreased tetracycline bioavailability caused by a bismuth subsalicylate antidiarrheal mixture. *J Pharm Sci* 1979;68:586-8.

2214 Veldman FJ, Nair CH, Vorster HH, et al. Dietary pectin influences fibrin network structure in hypercholesterolaemic subjects. *Thromb Res* 1997;86:183-96.

2215 Davidson MH, Dugan LD, Stocki J, et al. A low-viscosity soluble-fiber fruit juice supplement fails to lower cholesterol in hypercholesterolemic men and women. *J Nutr* 1998;128:1927-32.

2216 Cerda JJ, Robbins FL, Burgin CW, et al. The effects of grapefruit pectin on patients at risk for coronary heart disease without altering diet or lifestyle. *Clin Cardiol* 1988;11:589-94.

2217 Hillman LC, Peters SG, Fisher CA, et al. The effects of the fiber components pectin, cellulose and lignin on serum cholesterol levels. *Am J Clin Nutr* 1985;42:207-13.

2218 Marti J. The Alternative Health & Medicine Encyclopedia. 2nd ed. Detroit, MI: Gale Research International Limited; 1998.

2219 Trevisan M, Krogh V, Freudenheim J, et al. Consumption of olive oil, butter, and vegetable oils and coronary heart disease risk factors. The Research Group ATS-RF2 of the Italian National Research Council. *JAMA* 1990;263:688-92.

2220 Keys A, Menotti A, Karvonen MJ , et al. The diet and 15-year death rate in the seven countries study. *Am J Epidemiol* 1986;124:903-15.

2221 Martin-Moreno JM, Willett WC, Gorgojo L, et al. Dietary fat, olive oil intake and breast cancer risk. *Int J Cancer* 1994;58:774-80.

2222 la Vecchia C, Negri E, Franceschi S, et al. Olive oil, other dietary fats, and the risk of breast cancer (Italy). *Cancer Causes Control* 1995;6:545-50.

2223 Trichopoulou A, Katsouyanni K, Stuver S, et al. Consumption of olive oil and specific food groups in relation to breast cancer risk in Greece. *J Natl Cancer Inst* 1995;87:110-6.

2224 Katan MB, Zock PL, Mensink RP. Dietary oils, serum lipoproteins, and coronary heart disease. *Am J Clin Nutr* 1995;61:1368S-73S.

2225 Rock CL, Swendseid ME. Plasma beta-carotene response in humans after meals supplemented with dietary pectin. *Am J Clin Nutr* 1992;55:96-9.

2228 McIlwain H, Silverfield JC, Cheatum DE, et al. Intra-articular orgotein in osteoarthritis of the knee: a placebo-controlled efficacy, safety, and dosage comparison. *Am J Med* 1989;87:295-300.

2229 Gammer W, Broback LG. Clinical comparison of orgotein and methylprednisolone acetate in the treatment of osteoarthrosis of the knee joint. *Scand J Rheumatol* 1984;13(2):108-12.

2230 Goebel KM, Storck U, Neurath F. Intrasynovial orgotein therapy in rheumatoid arthritis. *Lancet* 1981;1:1015-7.

2231 Walravens M, Dequeker J. Comparison of gold and orgotein treatment in rheumatoid arthritis. *Curr Ther Res Clin Exp* 1976;20:62-9.

2232 Goebel KM, Storck U. Effect of intra-articular orgotein versus a corticosteroid on rheumatoid arthritis of the knees. *Am J Med* 1983;74:124-8.

2233 Kadrnka F. Results of a multicenter orgotein study in radiation induced and interstitial cystitis. [Article in German]. *Eur J Rheumatol Inflamm* 1981;4(2):237-43.

2234 Sanchiz F, Milla A, Artola N, et al. Prevention of radioinduced cystitis by orgotein: a randomized study. *Anticancer Res,* 1996;16(4A):2025-8.

2235 Nielsen OS, Overgaard J, Overgaard M, et al. Orgotein in radiation treatment of bladder cancer. A report on allergic reactions and lack of radioprotective effect. *Acta Oncol* 1987;26(2):101-4.

2236 Marberger H, Bartsch G, Huber W, et al. Orgotein: a new drug for the treatment of radiation cystitis. *Curr Ther Res Clin Exp,* 1975;18(3):466-75.

2237 Chan TY. Interaction between warfarin and danshen (Salvia miltiorrhiza). *Ann Pharmacother* 2001;35:501-4.

2238 Pollak R, Andrisevic JH, Maddux MS, et al. A randomized double-blind trial of the use of human recombinant superoxide dismutase in renal transplantation. *Transplantation* 1993 Jan;55(1):57-60.

2239 Land W, Schneeberger H, Schleibner S, et al. The beneficial effect of human recombinant superoxide dismutase on acute and chronic rejection events in recipients of cadaveric renal transplants. *Transplantation* 1994;57(2):211-7.

2240 Schneeberger H, Schleibner S, Illner WD, et al. The impact of free radical-mediated reperfusion injury on acute and chronic rejection events following cadaveric renal transplantation. *Clin Transpl* 1993;:219-32.

2241 Flaherty JT, Pitt B, Gruber JW, et al. Recombinant human superoxide dismutase (h-SOD) fails to improve recovery of ventricular function in patients undergoing coronary angioplasty for acute myocardial infarction. *Circulation* 1994;89:1982-91.

2242 Rosenfeld W, Evans H, Concepcion L, et al. Prevention of bronchopulmonary dysplasia by administration of bovine superoxide dismutase in preterm infants with respiratory distress syndrome. *J Pediatr* 1984;105(5):781-5.

2243 Murohara Y, Yui Y, Hattori R, et al. Effects of superoxide dismutase on reperfusion arrhythmias and left ventricular function in patients undergoing thrombolysis for anterior wall acute myocardial infarction. *Am J Cardiol* 1991;67:765-7.

2245 Ardissino D, Merlini PA, Savonitto S, et al. Effect of transdermal nitroglycerin or N-acetylcysteine, or both, in the long-term treatment of unstable angina pectoris. *J Am Coll Cardiol* 1997;29:941-7.

2246 Horowitz JD, Henry CA, Syrjanen ML, et al. Nitroglycerine/N-acetylcysteine in the management of unstable angina pectoris. *Eur Heart J* 1988;9:95-100.

2247 Brown DM. Bile plug syndrome: successful management with a mucolytic agent. *Pediatr Surg* 1990;25:351-2.

2248 Evans JS, George DE, Mollit D. Biliary infusion therapy in the inspissated bile syndrome of cystic fibrosis. *J Pediatr Gastroenterol Nutr* 1991;12(1):131-5.

2249 Mulvaney WP, Quilter T, Mortera A. Experiences with acetylcysteine in cystinuric patients. *J Urol* 1975;114(1):107-8.

2250 Giovannucci E, Stampfer MJ, Colditz GA, et al. Multivitamin use, folate, and colon cancer in women in the Nurses' Health Study. *Ann Intern Med* 1998;129:517-24.

2251 Drew HJ, Vogel RI, Molofsky W, et al. Effect of folate on phenytoin hyperplasia. *J Clin Periodontol* 1987;14(6):350-6.

2252 Unverferth DV, Jagadeesh JM, Unverferth BJ, et al. Attempt to prevent doxorubicin-induced acute human myocardial morphologic damage with acetylcysteine. *J Natl Cancer Inst* 1983;71:917-20.

2253 Dresdale AR, Barr LH, Bonow RO, et al. Prospective randomized study of the role of N-acetyl cysteine in reversing doxorubicin-induced cardiomyopathy. *Am J Clin Oncol* 1982;5:657-63.

2254 Louwerse ES, Weverling GJ, Bossuyt PM, et al. Randomized, double-blind, controlled trial of acetylcysteine in amyotrophic lateral sclerosis. *Arch Neurol* 1995;52:559-64.

REFERENCES

2255 Heiss WD, Kessler J, Mielke R, et al. Long-term effects of phosphatidylserine, pyritinol, and cognitive training in Alzheimer's disease. A neuropsychological, EEG, and PET investigation. *Dementia* 1994;5:88-98.

2256 Wiklund O, Fager G, Andersson A, et al. N-acetylcysteine treatment lowers plasma homocysteine but not serum lipoprotein(a) levels. *Atherosclerosis* 1996;119:99-106.

2257 Kroon AA, Demacker PN, Stalenhoef AF. N-acetylcysteine and serum concentrations of lipoprotein(a). *J Intern Med* 1991;230:519-26.

2258 Bostom AG, Shemin D, Yoburn D, et al. Lack of effect of oral N-acetylcysteine on the acute dialysis-related lowering of total plasma homocysteine in hemodialysis patients. *Atherosclerosis* 1996;120:241-4.

2259 Hurd RW, Wilder BJ, Helveston WR, et al. Treatment of four siblings with progressive myoclonus epilepsy of the Unverricht-Lundborg type with N-acetylcysteine. *Neurology* 1996;47:1264-8.

2260 De Flora S, Grassi C, Carati L. Attenuation of influenza-like symptomatology and improvement of cell-mediated immunity with long-term N-acetylcysteine treatment. *Eur Respir J* 1997;10:1535-41.

2261 Pearson TA. Alcohol and heart disease. *Circulation* 1996;94:3023-5.

2262 Fraser AG. Pharmacokinetic interactions between alcohol and other drugs. *Clin Pharmacokinet* 1997;33:79-90.

2263 Isselbacher KJ, Braunwald E, Wilson JD, et al. Harrison's Principles of Internal Medicine. 13th Ed. New York, NY: McGraw-Hill, 1994.

2264 Fahey TD, Pearl MS. The hormonal and perceptive effects of phosphatidylserine administration during two weeks of resistive exercise-induced overtraining. *Biol Sport* 1998;15:135-44.

2265 Kushner MG, Mackenzie TB, Fiszdon J, et al. The effects of alcohol consumption on laboratory-induced panic and state anxiety. *Arch Gen Psychiatry* 1996;53(3):264-70.

2266 de Boer MC, Schippers GM, van der Staak CP. Alcohol and social anxiety in women and men: pharmacological and expectancy effects. *Addict Behav* 1993;18:117-26.

2267 Kiechl S, Willeit J, Rungger G, et al. Alcohol consumption and atherosclerosis: what is the relation? Prospective results from the Bruneck Study. *Stroke* 1998;29:900-7.

2268 Klatsky AL, Armstrong MA, Friedman GD. Red wine, white wine, liquor, beer, and risk for coronary artery disease hospitalization. *Am J Cardiol* 1997;80:416-20.

2269 Siscovick DS, Weiss NS, Fox N. Moderate alcohol consumption and primary cardiac arrest. *Am J Epidemiol* 1986;123:499-503.

2270 Hennekens CH, Willett W, Rosner B, et al. Effects of beer, wine, and liquor in coronary deaths. *JAMA* 1979;242:1973-4.

2271 Stampfer MJ, Colditz GA, Willett WC, et al. A prospective study of moderate alcohol consumption and the risk of coronary disease and stroke in women. *N Engl J Med* 1988;319:267-73.

2273 Sills MA, Forsythe WI, Haidukewych D, et al. The medium chain triglyceride diet and intractable epilepsy. *Arch Dis Child* 1986;61:1168-72.

2274 Trauner DA. Medium-chain triglyceride (MCT) diet in intractable seizure disorders. *Neurology* 1985;35:237-8.

2275 Nijveldt RJ, Tan AM, Prins HA, et al. Use of a mixture of medium-chain triglycerides and longchain triglycerides versus long-chain triglycerides in critically ill surgical patients: a randomized prospective double-blind study. *Clin Nutr* 1998;17:23-9.

2276 Ball MJ. Parenteral nutrition in the critically ill: use of a medium chain triglyceride emulsion. *Intensive Care Med* 1993;19:89-95.

2277 Jiang ZM, Zhang SY, Wang XR, et al. A comparison of medium-chain and long-chain triglycerides in surgical patients. *Ann Surg* 1993;217:175-84.

2278 Clarke PJ, Ball MJ, Hands LJ, et al. Use of a lipid containing medium chain triglycerides in patients receiving TPN: a randomized prospective trial. *Br J Surg* 1987;74:701-4.

2279 Truelsen T, Gronbaek M, Schnohr P, et al. Intake of beer, wine, and spirits and risk of stroke: the copenhagen city heart study. *Stroke* 1998;29:2467-72.

2280 Iversen HK. N-acetylcysteine enhances nitroglycerin-induced headache and cranial arterial responses. *Clin Pharmacol Ther* 1992;52:125-33.

2281 Hogan JC, Lewis MJ, Henderson AH. N-acetylcysteine fails to attenuate haemodynamic tolerance to glyceryl trinitrate in healthy volunteers. *Br J Clin Pharmacol* 1989;28:421-6.

2282 Hogan JC, Lewis MJ, Henderson AH. Chronic administration of N-acetylcysteine fails to prevent nitrate tolerance in patients with stable angina pectoris. *Br J Clin Pharmacol* 1990;30:573-7.

2283 American Pharmaceutical Association. Handbook of Nonprescription Drugs. 11th Ed. Washington, DC: American Pharmaceutical Association; 1996.

2284 Uenotsuchi T, Satoh E, Kiryu H, Yano Y. Pyemotes dermatitis caused by indirect contact with husk rice. *Br J Dermatol* 2000;143:680-2.

2286 Soroka N, Silverberg DS, Greemland M, et al. Comparison of a vegetable-based (soya) and an animal-based low-protein diet in predialysis chronic renal failure patients. *Nephron* 1998;79:173-80.

2287 Gentile MG, Fellin G, Cofano F, et al. Treatment of proteinuric patients with a vegetarian soy diet and fish oil. *Clin Nephrol* 1993;40:315-20.

2288 D'Amico G, Gentile MG. Effect of dietary manipulation on the lipid abnormalities and urinary protein loss in nephrotic patients. *Miner Electrolyte Metab* 1992;18:203-6.

2290 Franke AA, Custer LJ, Tanaka Y. Isoflavones in human breast milk and other biological fluids. *Am J Clin Nutr* 1998;68:1466-73.

2291 Brown KH, Perez F, Peerson JM, et al. Effect of dietary fiber (soy polysaccharide) on the severity, duration, and nutritional outcome of acute, watery diarrhea in children. *Pediatrics* 1993;92:241-7.

2292 Vanderhoof JA, Murray ND, Paule CL, et al. Use of soy fiber in acute diarrhea in infants and toddlers. *Clin Pediatr* (Phila) 1997;36:135-9.

2293 Wong WW, Smith EO, Stuff JE, et al. Cholesterol-lowering effect of soy protein in normocholesterolemic and hypercholesterolemic men. *Am J Clin Nutr* 1998;68:1385S-9.

2294 Nilausen K, Meinertz H. Variable lipemic response to dietary soy protein in healthy, normolipemic men. *Am J Clin Nutr* 1998;68:1380S-4.

2295 Bakhit RM, Klein BP, Essex-Sorlie D, et al. Intake of 25 g of soybean protein with or without soybean fiber alters plasma lipids in men with elevated cholesterol concentrations. *J Nutr* 1994;124:213-22.

2296 Washburn S, Burke GL, Morgan T, et al. Effect of soy protein supplementation on serum lipoproteins, blood pressure, and menopausal symptoms in perimenopausal women. *Menopause* 1999;6:7-13.

2297 Albertazzi P, Pansini F, Bonaccorsi G, et al. The effect of dietary soy supplementation on hot flushes. *Obstet Gynecol* 1998;91:6-11.

2298 Jacobsen BK, Knutsen SF, Fraser GE. Does high soy milk intake reduce prostate cancer incidence? The Adventist Health Study. *Cancer Causes Control* 1998;9:553-7.

2299 Montori VM, Farmer A, Wollan PC, Dinneen SF. Fish oil supplementation in type 2 diabetes: a quantitative systemic review. *Diabetes Care* 2000;23:1407-15.

2300 Patti L, Maffettone A, Iovine C, et al. Long-term effects of fish oil on lipoprotein subfractions and low density lipoprotein size in non-insulin- dependent diabetic patients with hypertriglyceridemia. *Atherosclerosis* 1999;146:361-7.

2301 Yosefy C, Viskoper JR, Laszt A, et al. The effect of fish oil on hypertension, plasma lipids and hemostasis in hypertensive, obese, dyslipidemic patients with and without diabetes mellitus. *Prostaglandins Leukot Essent Fatty Acids* 1999;61:83-7.

2302 Eritsland J, Seljeflot I, Abdelnoor M, et al. Long-term effects of n-3 fatty acids on serum lipids and glycaemic control. *Scand J Clin Lab Invest* 1994;54:273-80.

2303 Akhondzadeh S, Kashani L, Mobaseri M, et al. Passionflower in the treatment of opiates withdrawal: a double-blind randomized controlled trial. *J Clin Pharm Ther* 2001;25:369-73.

2304 Daviglus ML, Stamler J, Orencia AJ, et al. Fish consumption and the 30-year risk of fatal myocardial infarction. *N Engl J Med* 1997;336:1046-53.

2305 Guallar E, Hennekens CH, Sacks FM, et al. A prospective study of plasma fish oil levels and incidence of myocardial infarction in U.S. male physicians. *J Am Coll Cardiol* 1995;25(2):387-94.

2306 Guallar E, Aro A, Jimenez FJ, et al. Omega-3 fatty acids in adipose tissue and risk of myocardial infarction: the EURAMIC study. *Arterioscler Thromb Vasc Biol* 1999;19(4):1111-8.

2307 Anon. Dietary supplementation with n-3 polyunsaturated fatty acids and vitamin E after myocardial infarction: results of the GISSI-Prevenzione trial. Gruppo Italiano per lo Studio della Soprawivenza nell'Infarto miocardico. *Lancet* 1999;354:447-55.

2308 Burr ML, Sweetham PM, Fehily AM. Diet and reinfarction. *Eur Heart J* 1994;15:1152-3.

2309 Ascherio A, Rimm EB, Stampfer MJ, et al. Dietary intake of marine n-3 fatty acids, fish intake, and the risk of coronary disease among men. *N Engl J Med* 1995;332:977-82.

2310 Pietinen P, Ascherio A, Korhonen P, et al. Intake of fatty acids and risk of coronary heart disease in a cohort of Finnish men. The Alpha-Tocopherol, Beta-Carotene Cancer Prevention Study. *Am J Epidemiol* 145:876-87.

2311 von Schacky C, Angerer P, Kothny W, et al. The effect of dietary omega-3 fatty acids on coronary atherosclerosis. A randomized, double-blind, placebo-controlled tr ial. *Ann Intern Med* 1999;130:554-62.

2312 Siscovick DS, Raghunathan TE, King I, et al. Dietary intake and cell membrane levels of long-chain n-3 polyunsaturated fatty acids and the risk of primary cardiac arrest. *JAMA* 1995;274:1363-7.

2313 Albert CM, Hennekens CH, O'Donnell CJ, et al. Fish consumption and risk of sudden cardiac death. *JAMA* 1998;279:23-8.

2314 Eritsland J, Amesen H, Gronseth K, et al. Effect of dietary supplementation with n-3 fatty acids on coronary artery bypass graft patency. *Am J Cardiol* 1996;77:31-6.

2315 Marckmann P, Bladbjerg EM, Jespersen J. Dietary fish oil (4 g daily) and cardiovascular risk markers in healthy men. *Arterioscler Thromb Vasc Biol* 1997;17:3384-91.

2316 Jalihal A, Kurian G. Ispaghula therapy in irritable bowel syndrome: Improvement in overall well-being is related to reduction bowel dissatisfaction. *J Gastroenterol Hepatol* 1990;5:507-13.

2317 Layne KS, Goh YK, Jumpsen JA, et al. Normal subjects consuming physiological levels of 18:3(n-3) and 20:5(n-3 from flaxseed or fish oils have characteristic differences in plasma lipid and lipoprotein fatty acid levels. *J Nutr* 1996;126:2130-40.

2318 Adler A, Holub BJ. Effect of garlic and fish-oil supplementation on serum lipid and lipoprotein concentrations in hypercholesterolemic men. *Am J Clin Nutr* 1997;65:445-50.

2319 Morcos NC. Modulation of lipid profile by fish oil and garlic combination. *J Natl Med Assoc* 1997;89:673-8.

2320 Cairns JA, Gill J, Morton B, et al. Fish oils and low-molecular-weight heparin for the reduction of restenosis after percutaneous transluminal coronary angioplasty. The EMPAR Study. *Circulation* 1996;94:1553-60.

2321 Chan EK, Schroeder DJ. Psyllium in hypercholesterolemia. *Ann Pharmacother* 1995;29:625-7.

2322 de Deckere EAM, Korver O, Verschuren PM, Katan MB. Health aspects of fish n-3 polyunsaturated fatty acids from plant and marine origin. *Eur J Clin Nutr* 1998;52:749-53.

2323 Higdon JV, Liu J, Du S, et al. Supplementation of postmenopausal women with fish oil rich in eicosapentaenoic acid and docosahexaenoic acid is not associated with greater in vivo lipid peroxidation compared with oils rich in oleate and linoleate as assessed by plasma malondialdehyde and F(2)- isoprostanes. *Am J Clin Nutr* 2000;72:714-22.

2324 Sprecher DL, Harris BV, Goldberg AC. Efficacy of psyllium in reducing serum cholesterol levels in hypercholesterolemic patients on high- or low-fat diets. *Ann Intern Med* 1993;119:545-54.

2326 Schectman G, Hiatt J, Hartz A. Evaluation of the effectiveness of lipid-lowering therapy (bile acid sepquestrants, niacin, psyllium and lovastatin) for treating hypercholesterolemia in veterans. *Am J Cardiol* 1993;71:759-65.

2327 Erratum. *Am J Clin Nutr* 1998;67:1286.

2328 Suhonen R, Kantola I, Bjorksten F. Anaphylactic shock due to ingestion of psyllium laxative. *Allergy* 1983;38:363-5.

2329 Vaswani SK, Hamilton RG, Valentine MD, Adkinson NF. Psyllium laxative-induced anaphylaxis, asthma, and rhinitis. *Allergy* 1996;51:266-8.

2330 Freeman GL. Psyllium hypersensitivity. *Ann Allergy* 1994;73:490-2.

2331 Burton Goldberg Group. Alternative Medicine: The Definitive Guide. Puyallup, WA: Burton Goldberg Group, 1994.

2333 Balch JF, Balch PA. Prescription for Nutritional Healing. 2nd ed., Garden City Park, NY: Avery Publishing Group, 1997.

2334 Scolapio JS, Camilleri M, Fleming CR, et al. Effect of growth hormone, glutamine, and diet on adaptation in short-bowel syndrome: a randomized, controlled study. *Gastroenterology* 1997;113:1074-81.

2335 Eschbach LF, Webster MJ, Boyd JC, et al. The effect of siberian ginseng (Eleutherococcus senticosus) on substrate utilization and performance. *Int J Sport Nutr Exerc Metab* 2000;10:444-51.

2336 Anderson PM, Schroeder G, Skubitz KM. Oral glutamine reduces the duration and severity of stomatitis after cytotoxic cancer chemotherapy. *Cancer* 1998;83:1433-9.

2337 Noyer CM, Simon D, Borczuk A, et al. A double-blind placebo-controlled pilot study of glutamine therapy for abnormal intestinal permeability in patients with AIDS. *Am J Gastroenterol* 1998;93:972-5.

2338 Den Hond E, Hiele M, Peeters M, et al. Effect of long-term oral glutamine supplements on small intestinal permeability in patients with Crohn's disease. *J Parenter Enteral Nutr* 1999;23:7-11.

2339 Van Den Berg CJ, Jones JD, Wilson DM, et al. Glutamine therapy of cystinuria. *Invest Urol* 1980;18:155-7.

REFERENCES

2340 Fernandez R, Phillips SF. Components of fiber impair iron absorption in the dog. *Am J Clin Nutr* 1982;35:107-12.

2341 Haub MD, Potteiger JA, Nau KL, et al. Acute L-glutamine ingestion does not improve maximal effort exercise. *J Sports Med Phys Fitness* 1998;38:240-4.

2342 Castell LM, Newsholme EA. The effects of oral glutamine supplementation on athletes after prolonged, exhaustive exercise. *Nutrition* 1997;13:738-42.

2343 Shils ME, Young VR, eds. Modern Nutrition in Health and Disease. 7th ed., Philadelphia: Lea and Febiger, 1988.

2347 Gerber DA, Tanenbaum L, Ahrens M. Free serum histidine levels in patients with rheumatoid arthritis and control subjects following an oral load of free L-histidine. *Metabolism* 1976; 25(6):655-7.

2348 Discontinued citation (see Ref 2352).

2349 Dixon JS, et al. The effect of drugs on serum histidine levels in rheumatoid arthritis. *Rheumatol Int* 1983; 3(4):145-9.

2350 Pinals RS, et al. Treatment of rheumatoid arthritis with L-histidine: a randomized, placebo-controlled, double-blind trial. *J Rheumatol* 1977; 4(4):414-9.

2351 Gerber DA, Tanenbaum L, Ahrens M. Free serum histidine levels in patients with rheumatoid arthritis and control subjects following an oral load of free L-histidine. *Metabolism* 1976; 25(6):655-7.

2352 Blumenkrantz MJ, et al. Histidine supplementation for treatment of anaemia of uraemia. *Br Med J* 1975;2(5970):530-3.

2353 Reeves RD, Barbour GL, Robertson CS, Crumb CK. Failure of histidine supplementation to improve anemia in chronic dialysis patients. *Am J Clin Nutr* 1977;30:579-81.

2354 Bigwood EJ, ed. Protein and amino acid functions. Oxford, NY: Pergamon Press, 1972.

2355 Sacher RA, McPherson RA, eds. Widdmann's Clinical Interpretation of Laboratory Tests. 10th ed., Philadelphia: FA Davis Company, 1991.

2360 Tao SH, Bolger PM. Hazard assessment of germanium supplements. *Regul Toxicol Pharmacol* 1997;25:211-9.

2361 Byrne TA, Persinger RL, Young LS, et al. A new treatment for patients with short-bowel syndrome. Growth hormone, glutamine, and a modified diet. *Ann Surg* 1995;222:243-54.

2362 Byrne TA, Morrissey TB, Nattakom TV, et al. Growth hormone, glutamine, and a modified diet enhance nutrient absorption in patients with severe short bowel syndrome. *JPEN J Parenter Enteral Nutr* 1995;19:296-302.

2363 Morlion BJ, Stehle P, Wachtler P, et al. Total parenteral nutrition with glutamine dipeptide after major abdominal surgery: a randomized, double-blind, controlled study. *Ann Surg* 1998;227:302-8.

2364 Skubitz KM, Anderson PM. Oral glutamine to prevent chemotherapy induced stomatitis: a pilot study. *J Lab Clin Med* 1996;127:223-8.

2365 Jebb SA, Osborne RJ, Maughan TS, et al. 5-fluorouracil and folinic acid-induced mucositis: no effect of oral glutamine supplementation. *Br J Cancer* 1994;70:732-5.

2366 Ziegler TR, Young LS, Benfell K, et al. Clinical and metabolic efficacy of glutamine-supplemented parenteral nutrition after bone marrow transplantation. A randomized, double-blind, controlled study. *Ann Intern Med* 1992;116:821-8.

2367 Fernandez R, Phillips SF. Components of fiber bind iron in vitro. *Am J Clin Nutr* 1982;35:100-6.

2368 Anderson PM, Ramsay NK, Shu XO, et al. Effect of low-dose oral glutamine on painful stomatitis during bone marrow transplantation. *Bone Marrow Transplant* 1998;22:339-44.

2369 Starling RD, Trappe TA, Short KR, et al. Effect of inosine supplementation on aerobic and anaerobic cycling performance. *Med Sci Sports Exerc* 1996;28:1193-8.

2370 Williams MH, Kreider RB, Hunter DW, et al. Effect of inosine supplementation on 3-mile treadmill run performance and VO2 peak. *Med Sci Sports Exerc* 1990;22:517-22.

2371 Ramirez FC, Lee K, Graham DY. All lactase preparations are not the same: results of a prospective, randomized, placebo-controlled trial. *Am J Gastroenterol* 1994;89:566-70.

2372 Sanders SW, Tolman KG, Reitberg DP. Effect of a single dose of lactase on symptoms and expired hydrogen after lactose challenge in lactose-intolerant subjects. *Clin Pharm* 1992;11:533-8.

2373 Lin MY, Dipalma JA, Martini MC, et al. Comparative effects of exogenous lactase (beta-galactosidase) preparations on in vivo lactose digestion. *Dig Dis Sci* 1993;38:2022-7.

2374 DairyEase product information. McNeil-PPC Inc. Fort Washington, PA 19034.

2375 Lami F, et al. Efficacy of addition of exogenous lactase to milk in adult lactase deficiency. *Am J Gastroenterol* 1988;83(10):1145-9.

2376 Horowitz M, Wishart J, Mundy L, Nordin BE. Lactose and calcium absorption in postmenopausal osteoporosis. *Arch Intern Med* 1987;147:534-6.

2377 Newcomer AD, et al. Lactase deficiency: prevalence in osteoporosis. *Ann Intern Med* 1978;89:218-20.

2379 Lloyd-Still JD. Cystic fibrosis and colonic strictures. A new "iatrogenic" disease. *J Clin Gastroenterol* 1995; 21(1):2-5.

2380 Croft NM, Marshall TG, Ferguson A. Gut inflammation in children with cystic fibrosis on high-dose enzyme supplements. *Lancet* 1995;346:1265-7.

2381 Smyth RL, et al. Fibrosing colonopathy in cystic fibrosis: results of a case-control study. *Lancet* 1995;346:1247-51.

2382 Smyth RL, et al. Strictures of ascending colon in cystic fibrosis and high-strength pancreatic enzymes. *Lancet* 1994;343:85-6.

2383 Tursi JM, Phair PG, Barnes GL. Plant sources of acid stable lipases: potential therapy for cystic fibrosis. *J Paediatr Child Health* 1994; 30(6):539-43.

2384 Malesci A. New enteric-coated high-lipase pancreatic extract in the treatment of pancreatic steatorrhea. *J Clin Gastroenterol* 1994; 18(1):32-5.

2385 Fernandez-Banares F, Hinojosa J, Sanchez-Lombrana JL, et al. Randomized clinical trial of Plantago ovata seeds (dietary fiber) as compared with mesalamine in maintaining remission in ulcerative colits (GETECCU). *Am J Gastroenterol* 1999;94:427-33.

2387 Schwesinger WH, Kurtin WE, Page CP, et al. Soluble dietary fiber protects against cholesterol gallstone formation. *Am J Surg* 1999;177:307-10.

2388 Snodderly DM. Evidence for protection against age-related macular degeneration by carotenoids and antioxidant vitamins. *Am J Clin Nutr* 1995;62:1448S-61S.

2389 Landrum JT, Bone RA, Joa H, et al. A one year study of the macular pigment: the effect of 140 days of a lutein supplement. *Exp Eye Res* 1997;65:57-62.

2390 van den Berg H, van Vliet T. Effect of simultaneous, single oral doses of beta-carotene with lutein or lycopene on the beta-carotene and retinyl ester responses in the triacylglycerol-rich lipoprotein fraction of men. *Am J Clin Nutr* 1998;68:82-9.

2391 Kostic D, White WS, Olson JA. Intestinal absorption, serum clearance, and interactions between lutein and beta-carotene when administered to human adults in separate or combined oral doses. *Am J Clin Nutr* 1995;62:604-10.

2392 Koonsvitsky BP, Berry DA, et al. Olestra affects serum concentrations of alpha-tocopherol and carotenoids but not vitamin D or vitamin K status in free-living subjects. *J Nutr* 1997;127:1636S-45S.

2393 Wolever TM, Robb PA. Effect of guar, pectin, psyllium, soy polysaccharide, and cellulose on breath hydrogen and methane in healthy subjects. *Am J Gastroenterol* 1992:87:305-10.

2394 Seddon JM, Ajani UA, Sperduto RD, et al. Dietary carotenoids, vitamins A, C, and E, and advanced age-related macular degeneration. Eye Disease Case-Control Study Group. *JAMA* 1994;272:1413-20.

2395 Hankinson SE, Stampfer MJ, Seddon JM, et al. Nutrient intake and cataract extraction in women: a prospective study. *BMJ* 1992;305:335-9.

2398 Lyle BJ, Mares-Perlman JA, Klein BE, et al. Antioxidant intake and risk of incident age-related nuclear cataracts in the Beaver Dam Eye Study. *Am J Epidemiol* 1999;149:801-9.

2400 Chen R, Tunstall-Pedoe H, Bolton-Smith C, et al. Association of dietary antioxidants and waist circumference with pulmonary function and airway obstruction. *Am J Epidemiol* 2001:153:157-63.

2401 Rao AV, Agarwal S. Bioavailability and in vivo antioxidant properties of lycopene from tomato products and their possible role in the prevention of cancer. *Nutr Cancer* 1998;31:199-203.

2403 Johnson EJ, Qin J, Krinsky NI, Russell RM. Ingestion by men of a combined dose of beta-carotene and lycopene does not affect the absorption of beta-carotene but improves that of lycopene. *J Nutr* 1997;127:1833-7.

2404 La Vecchia C. Mediterranean epidemiological evidence on tomatoes and the prevention of digestive-tract cancers. *Proc Soc Exp Biol Med* 1998;218(2):125-8.

2405 Tzonou A, Signorello LB, Lagiou P, et al. Diet and cancer of the prostate: a case-control study in Greece. *Int J Cancer* 1999;80:704-8.

2406 Giovannucci E, Ascherio A, Rimm EB, et al. Intake of carotenoids and retinol in relation to risk of prostate cancer. *J Natl Cancer Inst* 1995;87:1767-76.

2407 Giovannucci E. Tomatoes, tomato-based products, lycopene, and cancer: review of the epidemiologic literature. *J Natl Cancer Inst* 1999;91:317-31.

2409 La Vecchia C, Negri E, Franceschi S, Decarli A. Case-control study on influence of methionine, nitrite, and salt on gastric carcinogenesis in northern Italy. *Nutr Cancer* 1997;27:65-8.

2410 Bellamy MF, McDowell IF, Ramsey MW, et al. Hyperhomocysteinemia after an oral methionine load acutely impairs endothelial function in healthy adults. *Circulation* 1998;98:1848-52.

2411 Hladovec J, Sommerova Z, Pisarikova A. Homocysteinemia and endothelial damage after methionine load. *Thromb Res* 1997;88:361-4.

2412 Bellone J, Farello G, Bartolotta E, et al. Methionine potentiates both basal and GHRH-induced GH secretion in children. *Clin Endocrinol* (Oxf) 1997;47:61-4.

2413 Vale JA, Meredith TJ, Goulding R. Treatment of acetaminophen poisoning. The use of oral methionine. *Arch Intern Med* 1981;141:394-6.

2414 Christensen B, Guttormsen AB, Schneede J, et al. Preoperative methionine loading enhances restoration of the cobalamin-dependent enzyme methionine synthase after nitrous oxide anesthesia. *Anesthesiology* 1994;80:1046-56.

2415 Meakins TS, Persaud C, Jackson AA. Dietary supplementation with L-methionine impairs the utilization of urea-nitrogen and increases 5-L-oxoprolinuria in normal women consuming a low protein diet. *J Nutr* 1998;128:720-7.

2417 Bucci LR, Hickson JF Jr, Wolinsky I, Pivarnik JM. Ornithine supplementation and insulin release in bodybuilders. *Int J Sport Nutr* 1992;2:287-91.

2418 Fogelholm GM, Naveri HK, Kiilavuori KT, Harkonen MH. Low-dose amino acid supplementation: no effects on serum human growth hormone and insulin in male weightlifters. *Int J Sport Nutr* 1993;3:290-7.

2424 Zhdanova IV, Piotrovskaya VR. Melatonin treatment attenuates symptoms of acute nicotine withdrawal in humans. *Pharmacol Biochem Behavior* 2000;67:131-5.

2425 Bellipanni G, Bianchi P, Pierpaoli W, et al. Effects of melatonin in perimenopausal and menopausal women: a randomized and placebo controlled study. *Exp Gerontol* 2001;36:297-310.

2426 Erdman JW. AHA Science Advisory: Soy protein and cardiovascular disease. A statement for healthcare professionals from the Nutrition Committee of the AHA. *Circulation* 2000;102:2555-9.

2427 Domino EF, et al. Lack of clinically significant improvement of patients with tardive dyskinesia following phosphatidylcholine therapy. *Biol Psychiatry* 1985; 20(11): 1189-96.

2428 McFadyen IJ, Chetty U, Setchell KDR, et al. A randomized double blind, cross over trial of soya protein for the treatment of cyclical breast pain. *Breast* 2000;9:271-6.

2429 Lu LJ, Anderson KE, Grady JJ, et al. Decreased ovarian hormones during a soya diet: implications for breast cancer prevention. *Cancer Res* 2000;60:4112-21.

2430 Xu X, Duncan AM, Wangen KE, Kurzer MS. Soy consumption alters endogenous estrogen metabolism in postmenopausal women. *Cancer Epidemiol Biomarkers Prev* 2000;9:781-6.

2431 Grosse Duweler K, Rohdewald P. Urinary metabolites of French maritime pine bark extract in humans. *Pharmazie* 2000;55:364-8.

2432 Mak S, Newton GE. Vitamin C augments the inotropic response to dobutamine in humans with normal left ventricular function. *Circulation* 2001;103:826-30.

2433 Packer L, Midori H, Toshikazu Y, eds. Antioxidant Food Supplements in Human Health. San Diego: Academic Press, 1999.

2434 Hornig B, Arakawa N, Kohler C, Drexler H. Vitamin C improves endothelial function of conduit arteries in patients with chronic heart failure. *Circulation* 1998;97:363-8.

2435 Rice-Evans CA, Packer L, eds. Flavonoids in Health and Disease. Manhattan, NY: Marcel Dekker, Inc., 1998.

2437 Crook T, Petrie W, Wells C, Massari DC. Effects of phosphatidylserine in Alzheimer's disease. *Psychopharmacol Bull* 1992;28:61-6.

2438 Delwaide PJ, Gyselynck-Mambourg AM, Hurlet A, Ylieff M. Double-blind, randomized, controlled study of phosphatidylserine in senile demented patients. *Acta Neurol Scand* 1986;73:136-40.

2439 Engel RR, Satzger W, Gunther W, et al. Double-blind cross-over study of phosphatidylserine vs. placebo in patients with early dementia of the Alzheimer type. *Eur Neuropsychopharmacol* 1992;2:149-55.

2440 Cenacchi T, Bertoldin T, Farina C, et al. Cognitive decline in the elderly: a double-blind, placebo-controlled multicenter study on efficacy of phosphatidylserine administration. *Aging* (Milano) 1993;5:123-33.

2441 Crook TH, Tinklenberg J, Yesavage J, et al. Effects of phosphatidylserine in age-associated memory impairment. *Neurology* 1991;41:644-9.

2443 De Bandt JP, et al. A randomized controlled trial of the influence of the mode of enteral ornithine alpha-ketoglutarate administration in burn patients. *J Nutr* 1998;128(3):563-9.

2444 Moukarzel AA, et al. Growth retardation in children receiving long-term total parenteral nutrition: effects of ornithine alpha-ketoglutarate. *Am J Clin Nutr* 1994;60(3):408-13.

2445 Wernerman J, et al. Glutamine and ornithine-alpha-ketoglutarate but not branched-chain amino acids reduce the loss of muscle glutamine after surgical trauma. *Metabolism* 1989;38(8 Suppl 1):63-6.

2446 Wernerman J, et al. Ornithine-alpha-ketoglutarate improves skeletal muscle protein synthesis as assessed by ribosome analysis and nitrogen use after surgery. *Ann Surg* 1987;206(5):674-8.

2447 Woollard ML, Pearson RM, Dorf G, et al. Controlled trial of ornithine alpha ketoglutarate (OAKG) in patients with stroke. *Stroke* 1978;9:218-22.

2448 Blomqvist BI, et al. Glutamine and alpha-ketoglutarate prevent the decrease in muscle free glutamine concentration and influence protein synthesis after total hip replacement. *Metabolism* 1995;44(9):1215-22.

2449 Chainuvati T, Plengvanit U, Viranuvatti V. Ornicetil on encephalopathy. Effect of ornicetil (ornithine alpha-ketoglutarate) on encephalopathy in patients with acute and chronic liver disease. *Acta Hepatogastroenterol* (Stuttg) 1977;24(6):434-9.

2450 Gay G, et al. Effects of ornithine alphaketoglutarate on blood insulin, glucagon and aminoacids in alcoholic cirrhosis. *Biomedicine* 1979;30(3):173-7.

2451 Arcangeli P. Pycnogenol in chronic venous insufficiency. *Fitoterapia* 2000;71:236-44.

2452 Marconi C, Sassi G, Cerretelli P. The effect of an alpha-ketoglutarate-pyridoxine complex on human maximal aerobic and anaerobic performance. *Eur J Appl Physiol* 1982;49(3):307-17.

2454 Cotzias GC, Van Woert MH, Schiffer LM. Aromatic amino acids and modification of parkinsonism. *N Engl J Med,* 1967;276:374-9.

2455 Heller B, Fischer BE, Martin R. Therapeutic action of D-phenylalanine in Parkinson's disease. *Arzneimittelforschung* 1976;26:577-9.

2456 Kitade T, Odahara Y, Shinohara S, et al. Studies on the enhanced effect of acupuncture analgesia and acupuncture anesthesia by D-phenylalanine (2nd report)- schedule of administration and clinical effects in low back pain and tooth extraction. *Acupunct Electrother Res* 1990;15:121-35.

2457 Mosnik DM, Spring B, Rogers K, Baruah S. Tardive dyskinesia exacerbated after ingestion of phenylalanine by schizophrenic patients. *Neuropsychopharmacology* 1997;16:136-46.

2458 Gardos G, Cole JO, Matthews JD, et al. The acute effects of a loading dose of phenylalanine in unipolar depressed patients with and without tardive dyskinesia. *Neuropsychopharmacology* 1992;6:241-7.

2459 Walsh NE, Ramamurthy S, Schoenfeld L, Hoffman J. Analgesic effectiveness of D-phenylalanine in chronic pain patients. *Arch Phys Med Rehabil* 1986;67:436-9.

2460 Mitchell MJ, Daines GE, Thomas BL. Effect of L-tryptophan and phenylalanine on burning pain threshold. *Phys Ther* 1987;67:203-5.

2461 Antoniou C, Schulpis H, Michas T, et al. Vitiligo therapy with oral and topical phenylalanine with UVA exposure. *Int J Dermatol* 1989;28:545-7.

2462 Petrassi C, Mastromarino A, Spartera C. Pycnogenol in chronic venous insufficiency. *Phytomedicine* 2000;7:383-8.

2463 Siddiqui AH, Stolk LM, Bhaggoe R, et al. L-phenylalanine and UVA irradiation in the treatment of vitiligo. *Dermatology* 1994;88:215-8.

2464 Thiele B, Steigleder GK. [Repigmentation treatment of vitiligo with L-phenylalanine and UVA irradiation]. [Article in German]. *Z Hautkr* 1987;62:519-23.

2465 Cormane RH, Siddiqui AH, Westerhof W, Schutgens RB. Phenylalanine and UVA light for the treatment of vitiligo. *Arch Dermatol Res* 1985;277:126-30.

2466 Kuiters GR, et al. Oral phenylalanine loading and sunlight as source of UVA irradiation in vitiligo on the Caribbean island of Curacao NA. *J Trop Med Hyg* 1986;89:149-55.

2467 Schulpis CH, Antoniou C, Michas T, Strarigos J. Phenylalanine plus ultraviolet light: preliminary report of a promising treatment for childhood vitiligo. *Pediatr Dermatol* 1989;6: 332-5.

2468 Beckmann H, Athen D, Olteanu M, Zimmer R. DL-phenylalanine versus imipramine: a double-blind controlled study. *Arch Psychiatr Nervenkr* 1979;227:49-58.

2469 Birkmayer W, Riederer P, Linauer W, Knoll J. L-deprenyl plus L-phenylalanine in the treatment of depression. *J Neural Transm* 1984;59:81-7.

2470 Henry JB, ed. Clinical Diagnosis and Management by Laboratory Methods. 19th ed. Philadelphia,PA: W.B. Saunders, 1996.

2472 Stanko RT, Tietze DL, Arch JE. Body composition, energy utilization, and nitrogen metabolism with a 4.25-MJ/d low-energy diet supplemented with pyruvate. *Am J Clin Nutr* 1992;56:630-5.

2473 Matthys D, Van Coster R, Verhaaren H. Fatal outcome of pyruvate loading test in child with restrictive cardiomyopathy. *Lancet* 1991;338:1020-1.

2474 Stanko RT, Reynolds HR, Hoyson R, et al. Pyruvate supplementation of a low-cholesterol, low-fat diet: effects on plasma lipid concentrations and body composition in hyperlipidemic patients. *Am J Clin Nutr* 1994;59:423-7.

2475 Wagner DR. Hyperhydrating with glycerol: implications for athletic performance. *J Am Diet Assoc* 1999;99:207-12.

2476 Murray R, Eddy DE, Paul GL, et al. Physiological responses to glycerol ingestion during exercise. *J Appl Physiol* 1991;71:144-9.

2477 Robergs RA, Griffin SE. Glycerol. Biochemistry, pharmacokinetics and clinical and practical applications. *Sports Med* 1998;26:145-67.

2478 Arnall DA, Goforth HW. Failure to reduce body water loss in cold-water immersion by glycerol ingestion. *Undersea Hyperb Med* 1993;20:309-20.

2479 Montner P, Stark DM, Riedesel ML, et al. Pre-exercise glycerol hydration improves cycling endurance time. *Int J Sports Med* 1996;17:27-33.

2480 Yu YL, Kumana CR, Lauder IJ, et al. Treatment of acute cortical infarct with intravenous glycerol. A double-blind, placebo-controlled randomized trial. *Stroke* 1993;24:1119-24.

2481 Yu YL, Kumana CR, Lauder IJ, et al. Treatment of acute cerebral hemorrhage with intravenous glycerol. A double-blind, placebo-controlled, randomized trial. *Stroke* 1992;23:967-71.

2482 Frei A, Cottier C, Wunderlich P, Ludin E. Glycerol and dextran combined in the therapy of acute stroke. A placebo-controlled, double-blind trial with a planned interim analysis. *Stroke* 1987;18:373-9.

2483 Bayer AJ, Pathy MS, Newcombe R. Double-blind randomised trial of intravenous glycerol in acute stroke. *Lancet* 1987;:405-8.

2484 Friedli W, Imbach P, Ghisleni-Steinegger S, et al. [Treatment with 10% glycerin in acute ischemic cerebral infarct. Doubleblind study]. [Article in German]. *Schweiz Med Wochenschr* 1979;109:737-42.

2485 Bjorvell H, Hylander B, Rossner S. Effects of glycerol addition to diet in weight-reducing clubs. *Int J Obes* 1984;8:129-33.

2486 Fawer R, Justafre JC, Berger JP, Schelling JL. Intravenous glycerol in cerebral infarction: a controlled 4-month trial. *Stroke* 1978;9:484-6.

2487 Ivy JL, Cortez MY, Chandler RM, et al. Effects of pyruvate on the metabolism and insulin resistance of obese Zucker rats. *Am J Clin Nutr* 1994;59:331-7.

2488 DeBoer LW, Bekx PA, Han L, Steinke L. Pyruvate enhances recovery of rat hearts after ischemia and reperfusion by preventing free radical generation. *Am J Physiol* 1993;265:H1571-6.

2490 Yamauchi K, Wakabayashi H, Hashimoto S, et al. Effects of orally administered bovine lactoferrin on the immune system of healthy volunteers. *Adv Exp Med Biol* 1998;443:261-5.

2491 Bellamy W, Takase M, Wakabayashi H, et al. Antibacterial spectrum of lactoferricin B, a potent bactericidal peptide derived from the N-terminal region of bovine lactoferrin. *J Appl Bacteriol* 1992;73:472-9.

2492 Inder WJ, Swanney MP, Donald RA, et al. The effect of glycerol and desmopressin on exercise performance and hydration in triathletes. *Med Sci Sports Exerc* 1998;30:1263-9.

2493 Schmidtke I, Schoop W. Pycnogenol: stasis oedema and its medical treatment. *Schweizerische Zeitschrift fur GanzheitsMedizin* 1995;3:114-5.

2494 Hill AG, et al. Cellular potassium depletion predisposes to hypokalaemia after oral sodium phosphate. *Aust N Z J Surg* 1998;68(12):856-8.

2495 Clarkston WK, Tsen TN, Dies DF, et al. Oral sodium phosphate versus sulfate-free polyethylene glycol electrolyte lavage solution in outpatient preparation for colonoscopy: a prospective comparison. *Gastrointest Endosc* 1996;43:42-8.

2496 Fine A, Patterson J. Severe hyperphosphatemia following phosphate administration for bowel preparation in patients with renal failure: two cases and a review of the literature. *Am J Kidney Dis* 1997;29:103-5.

2497 DiPalma JA, Buckley SE, Warner BA, et al. Biochemical effects of oral sodium phosphate. *Dig Dis Sci* 1996;41:749-53.

2498 Helikson MA, Parham WA, Tobias JD. Hypocalcemia and hyperphosphatemia after phosphate enema use in a child. *J Pediatr Surg* 1997;32:1244-6.

2499 Galloway SD, Tremblay MS, Sexsmith JR, Roberts CJ. The effects of acute phosphate supplementation in subjects of different aerobic fitness levels. *Eur J Appl Physiol* 1996;72:224-30.

2500 Uebelhack R, Franke L, Schewe HJ. Inhibition of platelet MAO-B by kava pyrone-enriched extract from Piper methysticum Forster (kava-kava). *Pharmacopsychiatry* 1998;31:187-92.

2501 Gleitz J, Beile A, Wilkens P, et al. Antithrombotic action of the kava pyrone (+)-kavain prepared from Piper methysticum on human platelets. *Planta Med* 1997;63:27-30.

2502 Dwivedi S, Jauhari R. Beneficial effects of Terminalia arjuna in coronary artery disease. *Indian Heart J* 1997;49:507-10.

2503 Dwivedi S, Agarwal MP. Antianginal and cardioprotective effects of Terminalia arjuna, an indigenous drug, in coronary artery disease. *J Assoc Physicians India* 1994;42:287-9.

2504 Bharani A, Ganguly A, Bhargava KD. Salutary effect of Terminalia Arjuna in patients with severe refractory heart failure. *Int J Cardiol* 1995;49(3):191-9.

2505 Ram A, Lauria P, Gupta R, et al. Hypocholesterolaemic effects of Terminalia arjuna tree bark. *J Ethnopharmacol* 1997;55(3):165-9.

2506 Pettit GR, Hoard MS, Doubek DL, et al. Antineoplastic agents 338. The cancer cell growth inhibitory. Constituents of Terminalia arjuna (Combretaceae). *J Ethnopharmacol* 1996;53(2):57-63.

2507 Anand KK, Singh B, Saxena AK, et al. 3,4,5-Trihydroxy benzoic acid (gallic acid), the hepatoprotective principle in the fruits of Terminalia belerica-bioassay guided activity. *Pharmacol Res* 1997;36:315-21.

2508 Sato Y, Oketani H, Singyouchi K, et al. Extraction and purification of effective antimicrobial constituents of Terminalia chebula RETS. against methicillin-resistant Staphylococcus aureus. *Biol Pharm Bull* 1997 Apr;20(4):401-4.

2509 Yukawa TA, Kurokawa M, Sato H, et al. Prophylactic treatment of cytomegalovirus infection with traditional herbs. *Antiviral Res* 1996;32(2):63-70.

2510 Shiraki K, Yukawa T, Kurokawa M, Kageyama S. [Cytomegalovirus infection and its possible treatment with herbal medicines]. [Article in Japanese]. *Nippon Rinsho* 1998;56(1):156-60.

2511 Suthienkul O, Miyazaki O, Chulasiri M, et al. Retroviral reverse transcriptase inhibitory activity in Thai herbs and spices: screening with Moloney murine leukemia viral enzyme. *Southeast Asian J Trop Med Public Health* 1993;24(4):751-5.

2512 Kurokawa M, Nagasaka K, Hirabayashi T, et al. Efficacy of traditional herbal medicines in combination with acyclovir against herpes simplex virus type 1 infection in vitro and in vivo. *Antiviral Res* 1995;27(1-2):19-37.

2513 Jagtap AG, Karkera SG. Potential of the aqueous extract of Terminalia chebula as an anticaries agent. *J Ethnopharmacol* 1999 Dec 15;68(1-3):299-306.

2514 Phadke SA, Kulkarni SD. Screening of in vitro antibacterial activity of Terminalia chebula, Eclapta alba and Ocimum sanctum. *Indian J Med Sci* 1989;43(5):113-7.

2515 Hamada S, Kataoka T, Woo JT, et al. Immunosuppressive effects of gallic acid and chebulagic acid on CTL-mediated cytotoxicity. *Biol Pharm Bull* 1997;20:1017-9.

2516 Arseculeratne SN, Gunatilaka AA, Panabokke RG. Studies of medicinal plants of Sri Lanka. Part 14: Toxicity of some traditional medicinal herbs. *J Ethnopharmacol* 1985;13(3):323-35.

2517 Shaila HP, Udupa SL, Udupa AL. Hypolipidemic activity of three indigenous drugs in experimentally induced atherosclerosis. *Int J Cardiol* 1998;67(2):119-214.

2518 el-Mekkawy S, Meselhy MR, Kusumoto IT, et al. Inhibitory effects of Egyptian folk medicines on human immunodeficiency virus (HIV) reverse transcriptase. *Chem Pharm Bull* (Tokyo) 1995;43(4):641-8.

2519 Thakur CP, Thakur B, Singh S, et al. The Ayurvedic medicines Haritaki, Amala and Bahira reduce cholesterol-induced atherosclerosis in rabbits. *Int J Cardiol* 1988;21(2):167-75.

2520 Kiistala R, Makinen-Kiljunen S, Heikkinen K, et al. Occupational allergic rhinitis and contact urticaria caused by bishop's weed (Ammi majus). *Allergy* 1999;54(6):635-9.

2521 Ossenkoppele PM, van der Sluis WG, van Vloten WA. [Phototoxic dermatitis following the use of Ammi majus fruit for vitiligo]. [Article in Dutch]. *Ned Tijdschr Geneeskd* 1991;135(11):478-80.

2522 Harvengt C, Desager JP. HDL-cholesterol increase in normolipaemic subjects on khellin: a pilot study. *Int J Clin Pharmacol Res* 1983;3(5):363-6.

2523 Durate J, Vallejo I, Perez-Vizcaino F, et al. Effects of visnadine on rat isolated vascular smooth muscles. *Planta Med* 1997;63(3):233-6.

2524 Duarte J, Perez-Vizcaino F, Torres AI, et al. Vasodilator effects of visnagin in isolated rat vascular smooth muscle. *Eur J Pharmacol* 1995;286(2):115-22.

2525 Rauwald HW, Brehm O, Odenthal KP. The involvement of a Ca2+ channel blocking mode of action in the pharmacology of Ammi visnaga fruits. *Planta Med* 1994;60(2):101-5.

2526 Ahsan SK, Tariq M, Ageel AM, et al. Effect of Trigonella foenum-graecum and Ammi majus on calcium oxalate urolithiasis in rats. *J Ethnopharmacol* 1989;26:249-54.

2527 Shlosberg A, Egyed MN. Examples of poisonous plants in Israel of importance to animals and man. *Arch Toxicol Suppl* 1983;6:194-6.

2528 Bethea D, Fullmer B, Syed S, et al. Psoralen photobiology and photochemotherapy: 50 years of science and medicine. *J Dermatol Sci* 1999;19(2):78-88.

2529 McKevoy GK, ed. AHFS Drug Information. Bethesda, MD: American Society of Health-System Pharmacists, 2000.

2530 Rehman J, Dillow JM, Carter SM, et al. Increased production of antigen-specific immunoglobulins G and M following in vivo treatment with the medicinal plants Echinacea angustifolia and Hydrastis canadensis. *Immunol Lett* 1999;68:391-5.

2531 Zhu M, Chan KW, Ng LS, et al. Possible influences of ginseng on the pharmacodynamics of warfarin in rats. *J Pharm Pharmacol* 1999;51:175-80.

2532 Eddleston M, Rajapakse S, Rajakanthan K, et al. Anti-digoxin Fab fragments in cardiotoxicity induced by ingestion of yellow oleander: a randomized controlled trial. *Lancet* 2000;355(9208):967-72.

2533 McAlindon TE, LaValley MP, Gulin JP, Felson DT. Glucosamine and Chondroitin for Treatment of Osteoarthritis A Systematic Quality Assessment and Meta-analysis. *JAMA* 2000;283:1469-75.

2534 Jensen GS, Ginsberg DJ, Huerta P, et al. Consumption of Aphanizomenon flos-aquae has rapid effects on the circulation and function of immune cells in humans. A novel approach to nutritional mobilization of the immune system. *JANA* 2000;2:50;50-6.

2535 Kushak RI, Drapeau C, Van Cott EM, Winter HH. Favorable effects of blue-green algae Aphanizomenon flos-aquae on rat plasma lipids. *JANA* 2000;2:50;59-65.

2536 Spadea L, Balestrazzi E. Treatment of vascular retinopathies with pycnogenol. *Phytother Res* 2001;15:219-23.

2537 Choi HK, Jung GW, Moon KH, et al. Clinical study of SS-Cream in patients with lifelong premature ejaculation. *Urology* 2000;55:257-61.

2538 Kiesewetter H, Koscielny J, Kalus U, et al. Efficacy of orally administered extract of red vine leaf AS 195 (folia vitis viniferae) in chronic venous insufficiency (stages I-II). A randomized, double-blind, placebo-controlled trial. *Arzneimittelforschung* 2000;50:109-17.

2539 Xiao Dong S, Zhi Ping Z, Zhong Xiao W, et al. Possible enhancement of the first-pass metabolism of phenacetin by ingestion of grape juice in Chinese subjects. *Br J Clin Pharmacol* 1999;48:638-40.

2540 Ozturk HS, Kacmaz M, Cimen MY, Durak I. Red wine and black grape strengthen blood antioxidant potential. *Nutrition* 1999;15:954-5.

2541 Bombardelli E, Morazzoni P. Vitis vinifera L. *Fitoterapia* 1995;LXVI:291-317.

2542 Watson RR. Reduction of cardiovascular disease risk factors by French maritime pine bark extract. *CVR&R* 1999;June:326-9.

2543 Rohdewald P. Bioavailability and metabolism of pycnogenol. *Eur Bull Drug Res* 1999;7:5-7.

2544 Gulati OP. Pycnogenol in venous disorders: a review. *Eur Bull Drug Res* 1999;7:8-13.

2545 Rohdewald P. Reducing the risk for stroke and heart infarction with pycnogenol. *Eur Bull Drug Res* 1999;7:14-18.

2546 Lee JY, Lee KS, Kim TS, et al. Squalene-induced extrinsic lipoid pneumonia: serial radiologic findings in nine patients. *J Comput Assist Tomogr* 1999;23:730-5.

2547 Lee JS, Im JG, Song KS, et al. Exogenous lipoid pneumonia: high-resolution CT findings. *Eur Radiol* 1999;9(2):287-91.

2548 Asnis DS, Saltzman HP, Melchert A. Shark oil pneumonia. An overlooked entity. *Chest* 1993,103(3):976-7.

2549 Skopinska-Rozewska E, Krotkiewski M, Sommer E, et al. Inhibitory effect of shark liver oil on cutaneous angiogenesis induced in Balb/c mice by syngeneic sarcoma L-1, human urinary bladder and human kidney tumour cells. *Oncol Rep* 1999;6(6):1341-4.

2550 Hichami A, Duroudier V, Leblais V, et al. Modulation of platelet-activating-factor production by incorporation of naturally occurring 1-O-alkylglycerols in phospholipids of human leukemic monocyte-like THP-1 cells. *Eur J Biochem* 1997;250:242-8.

2551 Loftsson T, Petersen DS, Le Goffic F, Olafsson JH. Unsaturated glycerol monoethers as novel skin penetration enhancers. *Pharmazie* 1997;52:463-5.

2552 Hasle H, Rose C. [Shark liver oil (alkoxyglycerol) and cancer treatment]. [Article in Danish]. *Ugeskr Laeger* 1991;153:343-6.

2553 Wang S, Tan D, Zhao Y, et al. The effect of pycnogenol on the microcirculation, platelet function and ischemic myocardium in patients with coronary artery diseases. *Eur Bull Drug Res* 1999;7:19-25.

2554 Pavlovic P. Improved endurance by use of antioxidants. *Eur Bull Drug Res* 1999;7:26-9.

2555 Kohama T, Suzuki N. The treatment of gynecological disorders with pycnogenol. *Eur Bull Drug Res* 1999;7:30-2.

2556 Roseff SJ, Gulati R. Improvement of sperm quality by pycnogenol. *Eur Bull Drug Res* 1999;7:33-6.

2557 Bell L, Halstenson CE, Halstenson CJ, et al. Cholesterol-lowering effects of calcium carbonate in patients with mild to moderate hypercholesterolemia. *Arch Intern Med* 1992;152:2441-4.

2558 Ramon JM, Bou R, Romea S, et al. Dietary fat intake and prostate cancer risk: a case-control study in Spain. *Cancer Causes Control* 2000;11:679-85.

2559 Colditz GA. Changing dietary patterns and cancer prevention: alpha-linolenic acid health risks and benefits. *Cancer Causes Control* 2000;11:677-8.

2560 Costa RL, Summa MA. Soy protein in the management of hyperlipidemia. *Ann Pharmacother* 2000;34:931-5.

2561 Ezaki O, Takahashi M, Shigematsu T, et al. Long-term effects of dietary alpha-linolenic acid from perilla oil on serum fatty acids composition and on the risk factors of coronary heart disease in Japanese elderly subjects. *J Nutr Sci Vitaminol* 1999;45:759-72.

2562 Walker AF, Middleton RW, Petrowicz O. Artichoke leaf extract reduces symptoms of irritable bowel syndrome in a post-marketing surveillance study. *Phytother Res* 2001;15:58-61.

2563 Sangalli BC, Chiang W. Toxicology of nutmeg abuse. *Clin Toxicol* 2000;38:671-8.

2564 Lissoni P, Tancini G, Barni S, et al. Treatment of cancer chemotherapy-induced toxicity with the pineal hormone melatonin. *Support Care Cancer* 1997;5:126-9.

2565 Lissoni P, Bucovec R, Bonfanti A, et al. Thrombopoietic properties of 5-methoxytryptamine plus melatonin versus melatonin alone in the treatment of cancer-related thrombocytopenia. *J Pineal Res* 2001;30:123-6.

2566 Lissoni P, Giani L, Zerbini S, et al. Biotherapy with the pineal immunomodulating hormone melatonin versus melatonin plus Aloe vera in untreatable advanced solid neoplasms. *Nat Immun* 1998;16:27-33.

2567 Hammar M, Larsson L, Tegler L. Calcium treatment of leg cramps in pregnancy. Effect on clinical symptoms and total serum and ionized serum calcium concentrations. *Acta Obstet Gynecol Scand* 1981;60:345-7.

2568 Lissoni P. Modulation of anticancer cytokines IL-2 and IL-12 by melatonin and the other pineal indoles 5-methoxytryptamine and 5-methoxytryptophol in the treatment of human neoplasms. *Ann N Y Acad Sci* 2000;917:560-7.

2569 Heaney RP. Calcium, dairy products and osteoporosis. *J Am Coll Nutr* 2000;19:83S-99S.

2570 Chiu KM. Efficacy of calcium supplements on bone mass in postmenopausal women. *J Gerontol A Biol Sci Med Sci* 1999;54:M275-80.

2571 McGarry KA, Kiel DP. Postmenopausal osteoporosis. Strategies for preventing bone loss, avoiding fracture. *Postgrad Med* 2000;108:79-82,85-88, 91.

2572 Nieves JW, Komar L, Cosman F, Lindsay R. Calcium potentiates the effect of estrogen and calcitonin on bone mass: review and analysis. *Am J Clin Nutr* 1998;67:18-24.

2574 Winther K, Ranlov C, Rein E, et al. Russian root (Siberian ginseng) improves cognitive functions in middle-aged people, whereas Ginkgo biloba seems effective only in the elderly. *J Neurological Sci* 1997;150:S90.

2575 Deal C. Can calcium and vitamin D supplementation adequately treat most patients with osteoporosis? *Cleve Clin J Med* 2000;67:696-8.

2576 Kanis JA. The use of calcium in the management of osteoporosis. *Bone* 1999;24:279-90.

2577 Mackerras D, Lumley T. First- and second-year effects in trials of calcium supplementation on the loss of bone density in postmenopausal women. *Bone* 1997;21:527-33.

2578 Bryant RJ, Cadogan J, Weaver CM. The new dietary reference intakes for calcium: implications for osteoporosis. *J Am Coll Nutr* 1999;18:406S-412S.

2579 Correa P, Fontham ETH, Bravo JC, et al. Chemoprevention of gastric dysplasia: randomized trial of antioxidant supplements and anti-Helicobacter pylori therapy. *J Natl Cancer Inst* 2000;92:1881-8.

2580 Rautalahti M, Virtamo J, Haukka J, et al. The effect of alpha-tocopherol and beta-carotene supplementation on COPD symptoms. *Am J Respir Crit Care Med* 1997;156:1447-52.

2581 Christian P, West KP, Khatry SK, et al. Vitamin A or beta-carotene supplementation reduces symptoms of illness in pregnant and lactating Nepali women. *J Nutr* 2000;130:2675-82.

2582 Albanes D, Heinonen OP, Taylor PR, et al. Alpha-tocopherol and beta-carotene supplements and lung cancer incidence in the alpha-tocopherol, beta-carotene cancer prevention study: effects of baseline characteristics and study compliance. *J Natl Cancer Inst* 1996;88:1560-70.

2583 Sun D, Abraham SN, Beachey EH. Influence of berberine sulfate on synthesis and expression of Pap fimbrial adhesin in uropathogenic Escherichia coli. *Antimicrob Agents Chemother* 1988;32:1274-7.

2584 Sun D, Courtney HS, Beachey EH. Berberine sulfate blocks adherence of Streptococcus pyogenes to epithelial cells, fibronectin, and hexadecane. *Antimicrob Agents Chemother* 1988;32(9):1370-4.

2585 Takatsuka N, Nagata C, Kurisu Y, et al. Hypocholesterolemic effect of soymilk supplementation with usual diet in premenopausal normolipidemic Japanese women. *Prev Med* 2000;31:308-14.

2586 Wiseman H, O'Reilly JD, Adlercreutz H, et al. Isoflavone phytoestrogens consumed in soy decrease F2-isoprostane concentrations and increase resistance of low-density lipoprotein to oxidation in humans. *Am J Clin Nutr* 2000;72:395-400.

2587 Kaneda Y, Torii M, Tanaka T, Aikawa M. In vitro effects of berberine sulphate on the growth and structure of Entamoeba histolytica, Giardia lamblia and Trichomonas vaginalis. *Ann Trop Med Parasitol* 1991;85:417-25.

2588 Gupte S. Use of berberine in treatment of giardiasis. *Am J Dis Child* 1975; 129:866.

2589 Chan E. Displacement of bilirubin from albumin by berberine. *Biol Neonate* 1993;63:201-8.

2590 Winek CL, Elzein EO, Wahba WW, Feldman JA. Interference of herbal drinks with urinalysis for drugs of abuse. *J Anal Toxicol* 1993;17:246-7.

2591 Bhide MB, Shaven SR, Dutta NK. Absorption, distribution, and excretion of berberine. *Indian J Med Res* 1969;57:2128-31.

2592 van der Vliet A. Cigarettes, cancer and the carotenoids: a continuing, unresolved antioxidant paradox. *Am J Clin Nutr* 2000;72:1421-3.

2593 Alberg AJ, Chen JC, Zhao H, et al. Household exposure to passive cigarette smoking and serum micronutrient concentrations. *Am J Clin Nutr* 2000;72:1576-82.

2594 Normen L, Dutta P, Lia A, et al. Soy sterol esters and B-sitostanol ester as inhibitors of cholesterol absorption in human small bowel. *Am J Clin Nutr* 2000;71:908-13.

2595 Michaud DS, Feskanich D, Rimm EB, et al. Intake of specific carotenoids and risk of lung cancer in 2 prospective US cohorts. *Am J Clin Nutr* 2000;72:990-7.

2596 Osterhoudt KC, Lee SK, Callahan JM, Henretig FM. Catnip and the alteration of human consciousness. *Vet Hum Toxicol* 1997 Dec;39(6):373-5.

2597 Just MJ, Recio MC, Giner RM, et al. Anti-inflammatory activity of unusual lupane saponins from Bupleurum fruticescens. *Planta Med* 1998;64(5):404-7.

2598 Matsumoto T, Yamada H. Regulation of immune complexes binding of macrophages by pectic polysaccharide from Bupleurum falcatum L.: pharmacological evidence for the requirement of intracellular calcium/calmodulin on Fc receptor up-regulation by bupleuran 2IIb. *J Pharm Pharmacol* 1995;47:152-6.

2599 Green A, Williams G, Neale R, et al. Daily sunscreen applications and beta-carotene supplementation in prevention of basal-cell and squamous-cell carcinomas of the skin: a randomized controlled trial. *Lancet* 1999;354:723-9.

2600 Drovanti A, Bignamini AA, Rovati AA. Therapeutic activity of oral glucosamine sulfate in osteoarthrosis: a placebo-controlled, double-blind investigation. *Clin Ther* 1980;3:260-72.

2601 da Camara CC, Dowless GV. Glucosamine sulfate for osteoarthritis. *Ann Pharmacother* 1998;32:580-7.

2602 Lopes Vaz AL. Double-blind, clinical evaluation of the relative efficacy of ibuprofen and glucosamine sulphate in the management of osteoarthrosis of the knee in out-patients. *Curr Med Res Opin* 1982;8:145-9.

2603 Pujalte JM, Llavore EP, Ylescupidez FR. Double-blind clinical evaluation of oral glucosamine sulphate in the basic treatment of osteoarthrosis. *Curr Med Res Opin* 1980;7:110-4.

2604 Qiu GX, Gao SN, Giacovelli G, et al. Efficacy and safety of glucosamine sulfate versus ibuprofen in patients with knee osteoarthritis. *Arzneimittelforschung* 1998;48:469-74.

2605 Reichelt A. Efficacy and safety of intramuscular glucosamine sulfate in osteoarthritis of the knee. A randomised, placebo-controlled, double-blind study. *Arzneimittelforschung* 1994;44:75-80.

2606 Forster K, Schmid K, Rovati L, et al. Longer-term treatment of mild-to-moderate osteoarthritis of the knee with glucosamine sulfate- a randomized controlled, double-blind clinical study. *Euro J Clin Pharmacol* 1996;50:542.

2607 Setnikar I, Palumbo R, Canali S, et al. Pharmacokinetics of glucosamine in man. *Arzneimittelforschung* 1993;43:1109-13.

2608 Barclay TS, Tsourounis C, McCart GM. Glucosamine. *Ann Pharmacother* 1998;32:574-9.

REFERENCES

2609 Burton AF, Anderson FH. Decreased incorporation of 14C-glucosamine relative to 3H-N-acetyl glucosamine in the intestinal mucosa of patients with inflammatory bowel disease. *Am J Gastroenterol* 1983;78:19-22.

2610 Goodman MJ, Kent PW, Truelove SC. Glucosamine synthetase activity of the colonic mucosa in ulcerative colitis and Crohn's disease. *Gut* 1977;18:219-28.

2612 Leite JR, Seabra Mde L, Maluf E, et al. Pharmacology of lemongrass (Cymbopogon citratus Stapf). III. Assessment of eventual toxic, hypnotic and anxiolytic effects on humans. *J Ethnopharmacol* 1986;17:75-83.

2613 Feher J, Deak G, Muzes G, et al. [Liver-protective action of silymarin therapy in chronic alcoholic liver diseases]. [Article in Hungarian]. *Orv Hetil* 1989;130:2723-7.

2614 Szilard S, Szentgyorgyi D, Demeter I. Protective effect of Legalon in workers exposed to organic solvents. *Acta Med Hung* 1988;45:249-56.

2615 Hruby K, Csomos G, Fuhrmann M, Thaler H. Chemotherapy of Amanita phalloides poisoning with intravenous silibinin. *Hum Toxicol* 1983;2:183-95.

2616 Ferenci P, Dragosics B, Dittrich H, et al. Randomized controlled trial of silymarin treatment in patients with cirrhosis of the liver. *J Hepatol* 1989;9:105-13.

2617 Velussi M, Cernigoi AM, De Monte A, et al. Long-term (12 months) treatment with an anti-oxidant drug (silymarin) is effective on hyperinsulinemia, exogenous insulin need and malondialdehyde levels in cirrhotic diabetic patients. *J Hepatol* 1997;26:871-9.

2618 Salmi HA, Sarna S. Effect of silymarin on chemical, functional, and morphological alterations of the liver. A double-blind, controlled study. *Scand J Gastroenterol* 1982;17:517-21.

2619 Hebel SK, ed. Drug Facts and Comparisons. 52nd ed. St. Louis: Facts and Comparisons, 1998.

2620 Tyrey L. Delta 9-Tetrahydrocannabinol: a potent inhibitor of episodic luteinizing hormone secretion. *J Pharmacol Exp Ther* 1980;213:306-8.

2621 Sallan SE, Zinberg NE, Frei E III. Antiemetic effect of delta-9-tetrahydrocannabinol in patients receiving cancer chemotherapy. *N Engl J Med* 1975;293:795-7.

2622 Schwartz RH, Beveridge RA. Marijuana as an antiemetic drug: how useful is it today? Opinions from clinical oncologists. *J Addict Dis* 1994;13:53-65.

2623 FDA Office of Regulatory Affairs. Sec. 457.100 Pangamic Acid and Pangamic Acid Products Unsafe for Food and Drug Use. (CPG 7121.01). 1995. Available at: www.fda.gov/ora/compliance_ref/cpg/cpgdrg/cpg457-100.html (Accessed 16 July 1999).

2624 Heber D, Yip I, Ashley JM, et al. Cholesterol-lowering effects of a proprietary Chinese red-yeast-rice dietary supplement. *Am J Clin Nutr* 1999;69:231-6.

2625 FDA Talk Paper. FDA determines Cholestin to be unapproved drug. May 20, 1998. Available at: www.fda.gov/bbs/topics/ANSWERS/ANS00871.html

2627 Puente S, et al. Eosinophilic gastroenteritis caused by bee pollen sensitization. Med Clin (Barc) 10 May 1997;108(18):698-700.

2628 Patrick L. Beta-carotene: the controversy continues. *Alt Med Rev* 2000;5:530-45.

2629 Lee SK, et al. Modulation of in vitro biomarkers of the carcinogenic process by chemopreventive agents. *Anticancer Res* 1999;19(1A):35-44.

2630 Mirzoeva OK, Calder PC. The effect of propolis and its components on eicosanoid production during the inflammatory response. *Prostaglandins Leukot Essent Fatty Acids* 1996;55:441-9.

2631 Park YK, et al. Antimicrobial activity of propolis on oral microorganisms. *Curr Microbiol* 1998;36:24-8.

2632 Hay KD, Greig DE. Propolis allergy: a cause of oral mucositis with ulceration. *Oral Surg Oral Med Oral Pathol* 1990;70:584-6.

2633 Hashimoto T, et al. Synthesis of two allergenic constituents of propolis and poplar bud excretion. *Z Naturforsch* [C] 1988;43:470-2.

2634 Yeih DF, Chiang FT, Huang SKS. Successful treatment of aconitine induced life threatening ventricular tachyarrhythmia with amiodarone. *Heart* 2000;84(4):E8.

2635 Tixier JM, et al. Evidence by in vivo and in vitro studies that binding of pycnogenols to elastin affects its rate of degradation by elastases. *Biochem Pharmacol* 1984;33:3933-9.

2636 Liu FJ, Zhang YX, Lau BH. Pycnogenol enhances immune and haemopoietic functions in senescence-accelerated mice. *Cell Mol Life Sci* 1998;54:1168-72.

2637 Fitzpatrick DF, Bing, Rohdewald P. Endothelium-dependent vascular effects of Pycnogenol. *J Cardiovasc Pharmacol* 1998;32:509-15.

2639 Thys-Jacobs S. Micronutrients and the premenstrual syndrome: The case for calcium. *J Am Coll Nutr* 2000;19:220-7.

2640 Bell SJ. Whey protein concentrates with and without immunoglobulins: a review. *J Med Food* 2000;3:1-13.

2641 Dauer A, Metzner P, Schimmer O. Proanthocyanidins from the bark of Hamamelis virginiana exhibit antimutagenic properties against nitroaromatic compounds. *Planta Med* 1998;64:324-7.

2642 Omenn GS, Goodman GE, Thornquist MD, et al. Effects of a combination of beta-carotene and vitamin A on lung cancer and cardiovascular disease. *N Engl J Med* 1996;334:1150-5.

2644 Tveskov C, Djurhuus MS, Klitgaard NAH, Egstrup K. Potassium and magnesium distribution, ECG changes, and ventricular ectopic beats during beta-2-adrenergic stimulation with terbutaline in healthy subjects. *Chest* 1994;106:1654-9.

2645 Gray ME, Titlow LW. The effect of pangamic acid on maximal treadmill performance. *Med Sci Sports Exerc* 1982;14:424-7.

2646 Hennekens CH, Buring JE, Manson JE, et al. Lack of effect of long-term supplementation with beta-carotene on the incidence of malignant neoplasms and cardiovascular disease. *N Engl J Med* 1996;334:1145-9.

2648 Hellgren L, Vincent J. Degradation and liquefication effect of streptokinase-streptodornase and stabilised trypsin on tissue necroses, crusts of fibrinoid, purulent exudate and clotted blood from leg ulcers. *J Int Med Res* 1977;5:334-7.

2649 Suomalainen O. Evaluation of two enzyme preparations-Trypure and Varidase in traumatic ulcers. *Ann Chir Gynaecol* 1983;72:62-5.

2650 FDA Talk Paper. FDA Cautions Consumers on "Kombucha Mushroom Tea." Available at: www.vm.cfsan.fda.gov/~lrd/TPMUSHRM.html

2651 Sadjadi J. Anthrax associated with the Kombucha mushroom in Iran. *JAMA* 1998;280:1567-8.

2652 Kombucha-toxicity alert. *Crit Path AIDS Proj* 1994;30:31-32 1994-5.

2653 Gamundi R, Valdivia M. The Kombucha mushroom: two different opinions. *Sidahora* 1995;90:34-5.

2654 Majchrowicz M. Kombucha: a dubious "cure". *GMHC Treat Issues* 1995;9:10.

2655 CDC. Unexplained severe illness possibly associated with consumption of Kombucha tea-Iowa, 1995. *MMWR Morb Mortal Wkly Rep* 1995;44:892-3,899-900.

2656 Srinivasan R, Smolinske S, Greenbaum DJ. Probable gastrointestinal toxicity of Kombucha tea: is this beverage healthy or harmful? *Gen Intern Med* 1997;12:643-4.

2657 Greenberg ER, Baron JA, Karagas MR, et al. Mortality associated with low plasma concentration of beta carotene and the effect of oral supplementation. *JAMA* 1996;275:699-703.

2658 Blot WJ, Li JY, Taylor PR. Nutritional intervention trials in Linxian, China: supplementation with specific vitamin/mineral combinations, cancer incidence, and disease-specific mortality in the general population. *J Natl Cancer Inst* 1993;85:1483-92.

2659 McLeod MN, Gaynes BN, Golden RN. Chromium potentiation of antidepressant pharmacotherapy for dysthymic disorder in 5 patients. *J Clin Psych* 1999;60:237-40.

2660 Logani S, Chen MC, Tran T, et al. Actions of Ginkgo Biloba related to potential utility for the treatment of conditions involving cerebral hypoxia. *Life Sciences* 2000;67:1389-96.

2661 May SW, Pollock SH. Selenium-based antihypertensives. Rationale and potential. *Drugs* 1998;56(6):959-64.

2662 Aaseth J, Haugen M, Forre O. Rheumatoid arthritis and metal compounds-perspectives on the role of oxygen radical detoxification. *Analyst* 1998;123:3-6.

2663 Chan S, Gerson B, Subramaniam S. The role of copper, molybdenum, selenium, and zinc in nutrition and health. *Clin Lab Med* 1998;18:673-85.

2664 Clark LC, Combs GF Jr, Turnbull BW, et al. Effects of selenium supplementation for cancer prevention in patients with carcinoma of the skin. A randomized controlled trial. *JAMA* 1996;276:1957-63.

2665 Wesnes K, Simmons D, Rook M, Simpson P. A double-blind placebo-controlled trial of Tanakan in the treatment of idiopathic cognitive impairment in the elderly. *Human Psychopharmacol* 1987;2:159-69.

2666 Hofferberth B. The efficacy of Egb 761 in patients with senile dementia of the Alzheimer type, A double-blind, palcebo-controlled study on different levels of investigation. *Human Psychopharmacol* 1994;9:215-22.

2667 Clark LC, Dalkin B, Krongrad A, et al. Decreased incidence of prostate cancer with selenium supplementation: results of a double-blind cancer prevention trial. *Br J Urol* 1998;81:730-4.

2668 Maier RH, Purser SM, Nicholson DL, Pories WJ. The cytotoxic interaction of inorganic trace elements with EDTA and cisplatin in sensitive and resistant human ovarian cancer cells. *In Vitro Cell Dev Biol Anim* 1997;33:218-21.

2669 Rapuri PB, Gallagher JC, Kinyamu HK, Ryschon KL. Caffeine intake increases the rate of bone loss in elderly women and interacts with vitamin D receptor genotypes. *Am J Clin Nutr* 2001;74:694-700.

2670 Heaney RP, Rafferty K. Carbonated beverages and urinary calcium excretion. *Am J Clin Nutr* 2001;74:343-7.

2671 Koller LD, Exon JH. The two faces of selenium-deficiency and toxicity--are similar in animals and man. *Can J Vet Res* 1986;50:297-306.

2672 Hoogwerf BJ, Hibbard DM, Hunninghake DB. Effects of long-term cholestyramine administration on vitamin D and parathormone levels in middle-aged men with hypercholesterolaemia. *J Lab Clin Med* 1992;119:407-11.

2673 Mark SD, Wang W, Fraumeni JF Jr, et al. Do nutritional supplements lower the risk of stroke or hypertension? *Epidemiology* 1998;9:9-15.

2674 Knoben JE, Anderson PO. Handbook of Clinical Drug Data. 7th ed. Hamilton, IL: Drug Intelligence Publications, Inc., 1993.

2675 Gough H, Goggin T, Bissessar A, et al. A comparative study of the relative influence of different anticonvulsant drugs, UV exposure and diet on vitamin D and calcium metabolism in out-patients with epilepsy. *Quart J Med* 1986;59:569-77.

2676 Neve J. Selenium as a risk factor for cardiovascular diseases. *J Cardiovasc Risk* 1996;3:42-7.

2677 Shils ME, Olson JA, Shike M, Ross AC, eds. Modern Nutrition in Health and Disease. 9th ed. Baltimore, MD: Williams & Wilkins, 1999.

2678 Brewer GJ, Yuzbasiyan-Gurkan V, Johnson V, et al. Treatment of Wilson's disease with zinc: XI. Interaction with other anticopper agents. *J Am Coll Nutr* 1993;12:26-30.

2679 Brewer GJ, Johnson V, Kaplan J. Treatment of Wilson's disease with zinc: XIV. Studies of the effect of zinc on lymphocyte function. *J Lab Clin Med* 1997;129(6):649-52.

2680 Fuchs GJ. Possibilities for zinc in the treatment of acute diarrhea. *Am J Clin Nutr* 1998;68(2 Suppl):480S-3.

2681 Fosmire GJ. Zinc toxicity. *Am J Clin Nutr* 1990;51:225-7.

2682 Lomaestro BM, Bailie GR. Absorption interactions with fluoroquinolones. 1995 update. *Drug Saf* 1995;12:314-33.

2684 Perry HM. Thyroid replacement and osteoporosis (editorial). *Arch Intern Med* 1986;146:41-2.

2685 Coindre JM, David JP, Riviere L, et al. Bone loss in hypothyroidism with hormone replacement: A histomorphometric study. *Arch Intern Med* 1986;146:48-53.

2686 Dreno B, Trossaert M, Boiteau HL, Litoux P. Zinc salts effects on granulocyte zinc concentration and chemotaxis in acne patients. *Acta Derm Venereol* 1992;72:250-2.

2687 Schachner L, Eaglstein W, Kittles C, Mertz P. Topical erythromycin and zinc therapy for acne. *J Am Acad Dermatol* 1990;22:253-60.

2688 Habbema L, Koopmans B, Menke HE, et al. A 4% erythromycin and zinc combination (Zineryt) versus 2% erythromycin (Eryderm) in acne vulgaris: a randomized, double-blind comparative study. *Br J Dermatol* 1989;121:497-502.

2689 Walldius G, Michaelsson G, Hardell LI, Aberg H. The effects of diet and zinc treatment on the fatty acid composition of serum lipids and adipose tissue and on serum lipoproteins in two adolescent patients with acrodermatitis enteropathica. *Am J Clin Nutr* 1983;38:512-22.

2690 Koletzko B, Bretschneider A, Bremer HJ. Fatty acid composition of plasma lipids in acrodermatitis enteropathica before and after zinc supplementation. *Eur J Pediatr* 1985;143:310-4.

2691 Borroni G, Brazzelli V, Vignati G, et al. Bullous lesions in acrodermatitis enteropathica. Histopathologic findings regarding two patients. *Am J Dermatopathol* 1992;14:304-9.

2692 Sturniolo GC, Mestriner C, Irato P, et al. Zinc therapy increases duodenal concentrations of metallothionein and iron in Wilson's disease patients. *Am J Gastroenterol* 1999;94:334-8.

2693 Brewer GJ, Dick RD, Johnson VD, et al. Treatment of Wilson's disease with zinc: XV long-term follow-up studies. *J Lab Clin Med* 1998;132:264-78.

2694 Rittenhouse T. The management of lower-extremity ulcers with zinc-saline wet dressings versus normal saline wet dressings. *Adv Ther* 1996;13:88-94.

2695 Paul TL, Kerrigan J, Kelly AM, et al. Long-term L-thyroxine therapy is associated with decreased hip bone density in premenopausal women. *JAMA* 1988;259:3137-41.

2696 Young B, Ott L, Kasarskis E, et al. Zinc supplementation is associated with improved neurologic recovery rate and visceral protein levels of patients with severe closed head injury. *J Neurotrauma* 1996;13:25-34.

2697 Stall GM, Harris S, Sokoll LJ, Dawson-Hughes B. Accelerated bone loss in hypothyroid patients overtreated with L-thyroxine. *Ann Intern Med* 1990;113:265-9.

2698 Greenspan SL, Greenspan FS, Resnick NM, et al. Skeletal integrity in premenopausal and postmenopausal women receiving long-term L-thyroxine therapy. *Am J Med* 1991;91:5-14.

2699 Agren MS. Studies on zinc in wound healing. *Acta Derm Venereol Suppl* (Stockh) 1990;154:1-36.

2700 Shukla A, Rasik AM, Jain GK, et al. In vitro and in vivo wound healing activity of asiaticoside isolated from Centella asiatica. *J Ethnopharmacol* 1999;65:1-11.

2702 Shabert JK, Winslow C, Lacey JM, Wilmore DW. Glutamine-antioxidant supplementation increases body cell mass in AIDS patients with weight loss: a randomized, double-blind controlled trial. *Nutrition* 1999;15:860-4.

2703 Scolapio JS. Effect of growth hormone, glutamine, and diet on body composition in short bowel syndrome: a randomized, controlled study. *JPEN J Parenter Enteral Nutr* 1999;23:309-12.

2704 Rubio IT, Cao Y, Hutchins LF, et al. Effect of glutamine on methotrexate efficacy and toxicity. *Ann Surg* 1998;227:772-8.

2705 Yoshida S, Matsui M, Shirouzu Y, et al. Effects of glutamine supplements and radiochemotherapy on systemic immune and gut barrier function in patients with advanced esophageal cancer. *Ann Surg* 1998;227:485-91.

2706 Osol A, Hoover JE, eds. Remington's Pharmaceutical Science, 15th ed. Easton, PA: Mack Publishing Company, 1975.

2708 The National Toxicology Program (NTP). Caffeine. Center for the Evaluation of Risks to Human Reproduction (CERHR). Available at: http://cerhr.niehs.nih.gov/genpub/topics/caffeine-ccae.html.

2709 Klebanoff MA, Levine RJ, DerSimonian R, et al. Maternal serum paraxanthine, a caffeine metabolite, and the risk of spontaneous abortion. *N Engl J Med* 1999;341:1639-44.

2710 Eskenazi B. Caffeine—filtering the facts. *N Engl J Med* 1999;341:1688-9.

2711 Fernandes O, Sabharwal M, Smiley T, et al. Moderate to heavy caffeine consumption during pregnancy and relationship to spontaneous abortion and abnormal fetal growth: a meta-analysis. *Reprod Toxicol* 1998;12:435-44.

2712 Stookey JD. The diuretic effects of alcohol and caffeine and total water intake misclassification. *Eur J Epidemiol* 1999;15:181-8.

2713 Wemple RD, Lamb DR, McKeever KH. Caffeine vs caffeine-free sports drinks: effects on urine production at rest and during prolonged exercise. *Int J Sports Med* 1997;18:40-6.

2714 Pollock BG, Wylie M, Stack JA, et al. Inhibition of caffeine metabolism by estrogen replacement therapy in postmenopausal women. *J Clin Pharmacol* 1999;39:936-40.

2715 Goldstein J, Hoffman HD, Armellino JJ, et al. Treatment of severe, disabling migraine attacks in an over-the-counter population of migraine sufferers: results from three randomized, placebo-controlled studies of the combination of acetaminophen, aspirin, and caffeine. *Cephalalgia* 1999;19:684-91.

2716 Lipton RB, Stewart WF, Ryan RE Jr, et al. Efficacy and safety of acetaminophen, aspirin, and caffeine in alleviating migraine headache pain: three double-blind, randomized, placebo-controlled trials. *Arch Neurol* 1998;55:210-7.

2717 Silberstein SD, Armellino JJ, Hoffman HD, et al. Treatment of menstruation-associated migraine with the nonprescription combination of acetaminophen, aspirin, and caffeine: results from three randomized, placebo-controlled studies. *Clin Ther* 1999;21:475-91.

2718 Migliardi JR, Armellino JJ, Friedman M, et al. Caffeine as an analgesic adjuvant in tension headache. *Clin Pharmacol Ther* 1994;56:576-86.

2719 DiPiro JT, Talbert RL, Yee GC, et al; eds. Pharmacotherapy: A pathophysiologic approach. 4th ed. Stamford, CT: Appleton & Lange, 1999.

2720 Rees K, Allen D, Lader M. The influences of age and caffeine on psychomotor and cognitive function. *Psychopharmacology* (Berl) 1999;145:181-8.

2721 Ross DS. Monitoring L-thyroxine therapy: lessons from the effects of L-thyroxine on bone density (editorial). *Am J Med* 1991;91:1-4.

2722 Nurminen ML, Niittynen L, Korpela R, Vapaatalo H. Coffee, caffeine and blood pressure: a critical review. *Eur J Clin Nutr* 1999;53:831-9.

2723 Dews PB, Curtis GL, Hanford KJ, O'Brien CP. The frequency of caffeine withdrawal in a population-based survey and in a controlled, blinded pilot experiment. *J Clin Pharmacol* 1999;39:1221-32.

2724 Akhtar S, Wood G, Rubin JS, et al. Effect of caffeine on the vocal folds: a pilot study. *J Laryngol Otol* 1999;113:341-5.

2725 Weber JG, Klindworth JT, Arnold JJ, et al. Prophylactic intravenous administration of caffeine and recovery after ambulatory surgical procedures. *Mayo Clin Proc* 1997;72:621-6.

2726 Hampl KF, Schneider MC, Ruttimann U, et al. Perioperative administration of caffeine tablets for prevention of postoperative headaches. *Can J Anaesth* 1995;42:789-92.

2727 Yucel A, Ozyalcin S, Talu GK, et al. Intravenous administration of caffeine sodium benzoate for postdural puncture headache. *Reg Anesth Pain Med* 1999;24:51-4.

2728 Camann WR, Murray RS, Mushlin PS, Lambert DH. Effects of oral caffeine on postdural puncture headache. A double-blind, placebo-controlled trial. *Anesth Analg* 1990;70:181-4.

2729 FDA. Proposed rule: dietary supplements containing ephedrine alkaloids. Available at: www.verity.fda.gov (Accessed 25 January 2000).

2730 Rasmussen HS, Cintin C, Aurup P, et al. The effect of intravenous magnesium therapy on serum and urine levels of potassium, calcium and sodium in patients with ischemic heart disease, with and without acute myocardial infarction. *Arch Intern Med* 1988;148:1801-5.

2731 Cholst IN, Steinberg SF, Tropper PJ, et al. The influence of hypermagnesemia on serum calcium and parathyroid hormone levels in human subjects. *N Engl J Med* 1984;310:1221-5.

2732 Wilt TJ, Ishani A, Stark G, et al. Saw palmetto extracts for treatment of benign prostatic hyperplasia: a systematic review. *JAMA* 1998;280:1604-9.

2733 Gerber GS, Zagaja GP, Bales GT, et al. Saw palmetto (Serenoa repens) in men with lower urinary tract symptoms: effects on urodynamic parameters and voiding symptoms. *Urology* 1998;51:1003-7.

2734 Lowe FC, Fagelman E. Phytotherapy in the treatment of benign prostatic hyperplasia: an update. *Urology* 1999;53:671-8.

2735 Marks LS, Tyler VE. Saw palmetto extract: newest (and oldest) treatment alternative for men with symptomatic benign prostatic hyperplasia. *Urology* 1999;53:457-61.

2736 USRF Research. Clinical effects of saw palmetto extract in men with symptomatic BPH webpage: www.usrf.org/spepapers.html (Accessed 23 June 2004).

2737 Ludwig DS, Pereira MA, Kroenke CH, et al. Dietary fiber, weight gain, and cardiovascular disease risk factors in young adults. *JAMA* 1999;282:1539-46.

2738 Sherwood JK, Ackroyd FW, Garcia M. Effect of cimetidine on circulating parathyroid hormone in primary hyperparathyroidism. *Lancet* 1980;1:616-20.

2739 Beutler KT, Pankewycz O, Brautigan DL. Equivalent uptake of organic and inorganic zinc by monkey kidney fibroblasts, human intestinal epithelial cells, or perfused mouse intestine. *Biol Trace Elem Res* 1998;61:19-31.

2740 Duisterwinkel FJ, Wolthers BG, Koopman BJ, et al. Bioavailability of orally administered zinc, using Taurizine. *Pharm Weekbl Sci* 1986;8:85-8.

2743 Dr. Duke's Phytochemical and Ethnobotanical Databases. Ethnobotanical uses: Andrographis paniculata. www.ars-grin.gov/cgi-bin/duke/ethnobot.pl?andrographis%20pnaiculata (Accessed 27 January 2000).

2744 Caceres DD, Hancke JL, Burgos RA, et al. Use of visual analogue scale measurements (VAS) to assess the effectiveness of standardized Andrographis paniculata extract SHA-10 in reducing the symptoms of common cold. A randomized, double-blind, placebo study. *Phytomedicine* 1999;6:217-23.

2746 Indian Herbs. Andrographis paniculata. www.indianherbs.com (Accessed 23 June 2004).

2748 Thamlikitkul V, Dechatiwongse T, Theerapong S, et al. Efficacy of Andrographis paniculata, Nees for pharyngotonsillitis in adults. *J Med Assoc Thai* 1991;74:437-42.

2750 Madav S, Tripathi HC, Tandan SK, et al. Antiallergic activity of andrographolide. *Indian J Pharm Sci* 1998;60:176-8.

2751 Gupta PP, Tandon JS, Patnaik GK. Antiallergic activity of andrographolides isolated from Andrographis paniculata (Burm. F) Wall. *Pharm Biol* 1998;36:72-4.

2752 Kumar S, Gopal K. Screening of plant species for inhibition of bacterial population of raw water. *Journal of Environmental Science And Health Part A Toxic-Hazardous Engineering* 1999;34:975-87.

2753 Madav S, Tripathi HC, Tandan Mishra SK. Analgesic, antipyretic and antiulcerogenic effects of andrographolide. *Indian J Pharm Sci* 1995;57:121-5.

2754 Vedavathy S, Rao KN. Antipyretic activity of six indigenous medicinal plants of Tirumala Hills, Andhra Pradesh, India. *J Ethnopharmacol* 1991;33:193-6.

2755 Zhang CY, Tan BK. Mechanisms of cardiovascular activity of Andrographis paniculata in the anaesthetized rat. *J Ethnopharmacol* 1997;56:97-101.

2756 Guo ZL, Zhao HY, Zheng XH. The effect of andrographis paniculata nees (APN) in alleviating the myocardial ischemic reperfusion injury. *J Tongji Med Univ* 1994;14:49-51.

2757 Guo Z, Zhao H, Fu L. Protective effects of API0134 on myocardial ischemia and reperfusion injury. *J Tongji Med Univ* 1996;16:193-7.

2758 Zhao HY, Fang WY. Antithrombotic effects of Andrographis paniculata nees in preventing myocardial infarction. *Chin Med J* (Engl) 1991;104:770-5.

2759 Amroyan E, Gabrielian E, Panossian A, et al. Inhibitory effect of andrographolide from Andrographis paniculata on PAF-induced platelet aggregation. *Phytomedicine* 1999;6:27-31.

2760 Zhang C, Kuroyangi M, Tan BK. Cardiovascular activity of 14-deoxy-11,12-didehydroandrographolide in the anaesthetised rat and isolated right atria. *Pharmacol Res* 1998;38:413-7.

2761 Shukla B, Visen PK, Patnaik GK, Dhawan BN. Choleretic effect of andrographolide in rats and guinea pigs. *Planta Med* 1992;58:146-9.

2762 Visen PK, Shukla B, Patnaik GK, Dhawan BN. Andrographolide protects rat hepatocytes against paracetamol-induced damage. *J Ethnopharmacol* 1993;40:131-6.

2763 Rana AC, Avadhoot Y. Hepatoprotective effects of Andrographis paniculata against carbon tetrachloride-induced liver damage. *Arch Pharm Res* 1991;14:93-5.

2764 Leelarasamee A, Trakulsomboon S, Sittisomwong N. Undetectable anti-bacterial activity of Andrographis paniculata (Burma) wall. ex ness. *J Med Assoc Thai* 1990;73:299-304.

2765 Chang RS, Ding L, Chen GQ, et al. Dehydroandrographolide succinic acid monoester as an inhibitor against the human immunodeficiency virus. *Proc Soc Exp Biol Med* 1991;197:59-66.

2766 Puri A, Saxena R, Saxena RP, et al. Immunostimulant agents from Andrographis paniculata. *J Nat Prod* 1993;56:995-9.

2767 Raj RK. Screening of indigenous plants for anthelmintic action against human Ascaris lumbricoides:Part II. *Ind J Physiol Pharmacol* 1975;19(1);47-9.

2768 Matsuda T, Kuroyanagi M, Sugiyama S, et al. Cell differentiation-inducing diterpenes from Andrographis paniculata Nees. *Chem Pharm Bull* (Tokyo) 1994;42:1216-25.

2769 Akbarsha MA, Manivannan B, Hamid KS, Vijayan B. Antifertility effect of Andrographis paniculata (Nees) in male albino rat. *Indian J Exp Biol* 1990;28:421-6.

2770 Burgos RA, Caballero EE, Sanchez NS, et al. Testicular toxicity assessment of Andrographis paniculata dried extract in rats. *J Ethnopharmacol* 1997;58:219-24.

2771 Panossian A, Kochikian A, Gabrielian E, et al. Effect of Andrographis paniculata extract on progesterone in blood plasma of pregnant rats. *Phytomedicine* 1999;6:157-61.

2772 Caceres DD, Hancke JL, Burgos RA, Wikman GK. Prevention of common colds with Andrographis Paniculata dried extract: a pilot, double-blind trial. *Phytomedicine* 1997;4:101-4.

2773 Melchior J, Palm S, Wikman G. Controlled clinical study of standardized Andrographis paniculata in common cold- a pilot trial. *Phytomedicine* 1996;97;3:315-8.

2774 Hancke J, Burgos R, Caceres D, Wikman G. A double-blind study with a new monodrug Kan Jang: decrease of symptoms and improvement in the recovery from common colds. *Phytotherapy Res* 1995;9:559-62.

2775 GRIN/NPGS Taxonomy Info. Taxon: Andrographis paniculata (Burm. f.) www.ars-grin.gov/cgi-bin/npgs/html/taxon.pl?414228 (Accessed 27 January 2000).

2776 Zoha MS, Hussain AH, Choudhury SA. Antifertility effect of andrographis paniculata in mice. *Bangladesh Med Res Counc Bull* 1989;15:34-7.

2777 Gozalbes R, Galvez J, Garcia-Domenech R, Derouin F. Molecular search of new active drugs against Toxoplasma gondii. *SAR QSAR Environ Res* 1999;10:47-60.

2778 Kapil A, Koul IB, Banerjee SK, Gupta BD. Antihepatotoxic effects of major diterpenoid constituents of Andrographis paniculata. *Biochem Pharmacol* 1993;46:182-5.

2779 Gupta S, Yadava JN, Tandon JS. Antisecretory (antidiarrheal) activity of Indian medicinal plants against Escherchia coli enterotoxin-induced secretion in rabbit and guinea pig ileal loop models. *Int J Pharmacogn* 1993;31:198-204.

2780 Najib NA, Rahman N, Furuta T, et al. Antimalarial activity of extracts of Malaysian medicinal plants. *J Ethnopharmacol* 1999;64:249-54.

2781 Misra P, Pal NL, Guru PY, et al. Antimalarial activity of Andrographis paniculata (Kalmegh) against Plasmodium berghei NK 65 in Mastomys natalensis. *Int J Pharmacogn* 1992;30:263-74.

2782 Wang DW, Zhao HY. Prevention of atherosclerotic arterial stenosis and restenosis after angioplasty with Andrographis paniculata nees and fish oil. Experimental studies of effects and mechanisms. *Chin Med J* (Engl) 1994;107:464-70.

2783 Wang DW, Zhao HY. Experimental studies on prevention of atherosclerotic arterial stenosis and restenosis after

REFERENCES

angioplasty with Andrographis Paniculata Nees and fish oil. *J Tongji Med Univ* 1993;13:193-8.
2784 Holodniy M, Koch J, Mistal M, et al. A double blind, randomized, placebo-controlled phase II study to assess the safety and efficacy of orally administered SP-303 for the symptomatic treatment of diarrhea in patients with AIDS. *Am J Gastroenterol* 1999;94:3267-73.
2786 Gabriel SE, Davenport SE, Steagall RJ, et al. A novel plant-derived inhibitor of cAMP-mediated fluid and chloride secretion. *Am J Physiol* 1999;276:G58-G63.
2787 Safrin S, McKinley G, McKeough M, et al. Treatment of acyclovir-unresponsive cutaneous herpes simplex virus infection with topically applied SP-303. *Antiviral Res* 1994;25:185-92.
2788 Orozco-Topete R, Sierra-Madero J, Cano-Dominguez C, et al. Safety and efficacy of Virend for topical treatment of genital and anal herpes simplex lesions in patients with AIDS. *Antiviral Res* 1997;35:91-103.
2789 King SR, Tempesta MS. From shaman to human clinical trials: the role of industry in ethnobotany, conservation and community reciprocity. *Ciba Found Symp* 1994;185:197-206.
2790 Barnard DL, Smee DF, Huffman JH, et al. Antiherpesvirus activity and mode of action of SP-303, a novel plant flavonoid. *Chemotherapy* 1993;39:203-11.
2791 Wyde PR, Ambrose MW, Meyerson LR, Gilbert BE. The antiviral activity of SP-303, a natural polyphenolic polymer, against respiratory syncytial and parainfluenza type 3 viruses in cotton rats. *Antiviral Res* 1993;20:145-54.
2792 Barnard DL, Huffman JH, Meyerson LR, Sidwell RW. Mode of inhibition of respiratory syncytial virus by a plant flavonoid, SP-303. *Chemotherapy* 1993;39:212-7.
2793 Sidwell RW, Huffman JH, Moscon BJ, Warren RP. Influenza virus-inhibitory effects of intraperitoneally and aerosol-administered SP-303, a plant flavonoid. *Chemotherapy* 1994;40:42-50.
2794 Gilbert BE, Wyde PR, Wilson SZ, Meyerson LR. SP-303 small-particle aerosol treatment of influenza A virus infection in mice and respiratory syncytial virus infection in cotton rats. *Antiviral Res* 1993;21:37-45.
2795 Perdue GP, Blomster RN, Blake DA, Farnsworth NR. South American plants II: taspine isolation and anti-inflammatory activity. *J Pharm Sci* 1979;68:124-6.
2796 Vaisberg AJ, Milla M, Planas MC, et al. Taspine is the cicatrizant principle in Sangre de Grado extracted from Croton lechleri. *Planta Med* 1989;55:140-3.
2797 Pieters L, de Bruyne T, Claeys M, et al. Isolation of a dihydrobenzofuran lignan from South American dragon's blood (Croton spp.) as an inhibitor of cell proliferation. *J Nat Prod* 1993;56:899-906.
2798 Chen ZP, Cai Y, Phillipson JD. Studies on the anti-tumour, anti-bacterial, and wound-healing properties of dragon's blood. *Planta Med* 1994;60:541-5.
2799 Desmarchelier C, Witting Schaus F, Coussio J, Cicca G. Effects of Sangre de Drago from Croton lechleri Muell.-Arg. on the production of active oxygen radicals. *J Ethnopharmacol* 1997;58:103-8.
2804 Raintree Nutrition. Sangre de Grado website: www.rain-tree.com/sangre.htm (Accessed 31 January 2000).
2805 USDA, ARS, National Genetic Resources Program. Germplasm Resources Information Network - (GRIN). Taxon: Croton lechleri mull. Arg website: www.ars-grin.gov/cgi-bin/npgs/html/tax_search.pl?croton+lechleri (Accessed 31 January 2000).
2806 Dicesare D, Dupont HL, Mathewson JJ, et al. A double-blind randomized, placebo-controlled study of SP-303 (Provir) in the symptomatic treatment of acute diarrhea among travelers to Mexico and Jamaica. Infectious Diseases Society of America Annual Meeting, 1998 (abstract).
2807 BioWorld Today. Shaman will sidestep FDA by selling product over internet website: http://www.bioworld.com(Accessed 6 January 2000).
2809 Henderson LM, Brewer GJ, Dressman JB, et al. Effect of intragastric pH on the absorption of oral zinc acetate and zinc oxide in young healthy volunteers. *JPEN J Parenter Enteral Nutr* 1995;19:393-7.
2810 Kelley DS, Simon VA, Taylor PC, et al. Dietary supplementation with conjugated linoleic acid increased its concentration in human peripheral blood mononuclear cells, but did not alter their function. *Lipids* 2001;36:669-74.
2811 Schlager TA, Anderson S, Trudell J, Hendley JO. Effect of cranberry juice on bacteriuria in children with neurogenic bladder receiving intermittent catheterization. *J Pediatr* 1999;135:698-702.
2812 Sobota AE. Inhibition of bacterial adherence by cranberry juice: potential use for the treatment of urinary tract infections. *J Urol* 1984;131:1013-6.
2813 Howell AB, Vorsa N, Foo LY, et al. Inhibition of the Adherence of P-Fimbriated Escherichia coli to Uroepithelial-Cell Surfaces by Proanthocyanidin Extracts from Cranberries (letter). *N Engl J Med* 1998;339:1085-6.
2814 Ahuja S, Kaack B, Roberts J. Loss of fimbrial adhesion with the addition of Vaccinum macrocarpon to the growth medium of P-fimbriated Escherichia coli. *J Urol* 1998;159:559-62.
2815 Habash MB, Van der Mei HC, Busscher HJ, Reid G. The effect of water, ascorbic acid, and cranberry derived supplementation on human urine and uropathogen adhesion to silicone rubber. *Can J Microbiol* 1999;45:691-4.
2816 Weiss EI, Lev-Dor R, Kashamn Y, et al. Inhibiting interspecies coaggregation of plaque bacteria with a cranberry juice constituent. *J Am Dent Assoc* 1998;129:1719-23.
2819 Smedman A, Vessby B. Conjugated linoleic acid supplementation in humans--metabolic effects. *Lipids* 2001;36:773-81.
2820 Ens JG, Ma DW, Cole KS, et al. An assessment of c9,t11 linoleic acid intake in a small group of young Canadians. *Nutr Res* 2001;21:955-60.
2821 Riserus U, Arner P, Brismar K, Vessby B. Treatment with dietary trans10cis12 conjugated linoleic acid causes isomer-specific insulin resistance in obese men with the metabolic syndrome. *Diabetes Care* 2002;25:1516-21.
2822 www.healthlink.com.au/nat_lib/htm-data/htm-herb/bhp770.htm (Accessed 8 February 2000).
2823 Naveh Y, Schapira D, Ravel Y, et al. Zinc metabolism in rheumatoid arthritis: plasma and urinary zinc and relationship to disease activity. *J Rheumatol* 1997;24:643-6.
2824 Potocnik FC, van Rensburg SJ, Park C, et al. Zinc and platelet membrane microviscosity in Alzheimer's disease. The in vivo effect of zinc on platelet membranes and cognition. *S Afr Med J* 1997;87:1116-9.
2825 de Haan A, van Doorn JE, Westra HG. Effects of potassium plus magnesium aspartate on muscle metabolism and force development during short intensive static exercise. *Int J Sports Med* 1985;6:44-9.
2826 Golf SW, Bender S, Gruttner J. On the significance of magnesium in extreme physical stress. *Cardiovasc Drugs Ther* 1998;12:197-202.
2827 Golf SW, Happel O, Graef V, Seim KE. Plasma aldosterone, cortisol and electrolyte concentrations in physical exercise after magnesium supplementation. *J Clin Chem Clin Biochem* 1984;22:717-21.
2828 Hagan RD, Upton SJ, Duncan JJ, et al. Absence of effect of potassium-magnesium aspartate on physiologic responses to

prolonged work in aerobically trained men. *Int J Sports Med* 1982;3:177-81.

2829 Maughan RJ, Sadler DJ. The effects of oral administration of salts of aspartic acid on the metabolic response to prolonged exhausting exercise in man. *Int J Sports Med* 1983;4:119-23.

2830 Weller E, Bachert P, Meinck HM, et al. Lack of effect of oral Mg-supplementation on Mg in serum, blood cells, and calf muscle. *Med Sci Sports Exerc* 1998;30:1584-91.

2900 Kuzminski AM, Del Giacco EJ, et al. Effective treatment of cobalamin deficiency with oral cobalamin. *Blood* 1998;92:1191-1198.

2901 Andres E, Kurtz JE, Perrin AE, et al. Oral cobalamin therapy for the treatment of patients with food-cobalamin malabsorption. *Am J Med* 2001;111:126-9.

2902 Lederle FA. Oral cobalamin for pernicious anemia. Medicine's best kept secret? *JAMA* 1991;265:94-95.

2903 Gunnes P, Rasmussen K. Haemodynamic effects of pharmacological doses of secretin in patients with impaired left ventricular function. *Eur Heart J* 1986; 7(2): 146-9.

2904 Gunnes P, et al. Cardiovascular effects of secretin infusion in man. *Scand J Clin Lab Invest* 1983;43(7):637-42.

2905 Tulassay Z, et al. [Secretin versus cimetidine in the therapy of active bleeding from peptic gastroduodenal lesions. A prospective, randomized, double-blind, multicentric study]. [Article in German]. *Wien Med Wochenschr* 1990;140(13):361-4.

2906 Wagner PK, Rothmund M. [Effect of cimetidine and synthetic secretin as treatment of acute upper gastrointestinal bleeding-a prospective alternate trial]. [Article in German]. *Z Gastroenterol* 1980;18(6):337-41.

2908 Rothmund M, Wagner PK. [Effect of cimetidine and secretin on acute bleedings from gastroduodenal ulcers and erosions: a prospective study]. [Article in German]. *Dtsch Med Wochenschr* 1982;107(7):245-8.

2909 Elia M. Oral or parenteral therapy for B12 deficiency. *Lancet* 1998;352:1721-1722.

2910 Andres E, Goichot B, Schlienger JL. Food cobalamin malabsorption: a usual cause of vitamin B12 deficiency. *Arch Intern Med* 2000;160:2061-2.

2911 Verhaeverbeke I, Mets T, Mulkens K, Vandewoude M. Normalization of low vitamin B12 serum levels in older people by oral treatment. *J Am Geriatr Soc* 1997;45:124-125.

2912 Spilker G, et al. [Long-acting secretin for the prevention of stress ulcers in surgery]. [Article in French]. *Nouv Presse Med* 1982; 11(4): 267-9.

2913 Theisinger W, Spilker G, Bader M . [Prevention of stress ulcers with synthetic depot secretin]. [Article in German]. *Med Klin* 1981;76(10):291-3.

2915 Allen LH, Casterline J. Vitamin B-12 deficiency in elderly individuals: diagnosis and requirements. *Am J Clin Nutr* 1994;60:12-14

2916 Product information. Secretin. Ferring Pharmaceuticals, Tarrytown, NY; 6/88.

2917 Horvath K, Stefatos G, Sokolski KN. Improved social and language skills after secretin administration. *J Assoc Acad Minor Phys* 1998;9(1):9-15.

2918 Tympner F, Rosch W. The treatment of chronic recurrent pancreatitis with depot secretin-a preliminary report. *Hepatogastroenterology* 1986;33:159-62.

2919 Lindenbaum J, Rosenberg IH, Wilson PW, et al. Prevalence of cobalamin deficiency in the Framingham elderly population. *Am J Clin Nutr* 1994;60:2-11.

2920 Snider SR. Octacosanol in parkinsonism. *Ann Neurol* 1984;16:723.

2921 Norris FH, Denys EH, Fallat RJ. Trial of octacosanol in amyotrophic lateral sclerosis. *Neurology* 1986;36:1263-4.

2924 Kato S, Karino K, Hasegawa S, et al. Octacosanol affects lipid metabolism in rats fed on a high-fat diet. *Br J Nutr* 1995;73:433-41.

2925 Kabir Y, Kimura S. Distribution of radioactive octacosanol in response to exercise in rats. *Nahrung* 1994;38:373-7.

2926 Beltz SD, Doering PL. Efficacy of nutritional supplements used by athletes. *Clin Pharm* 1993;12(12):900-8.

2927 Canetti M, Moreira M, Mas R, et al. A two-year study on the efficacy and tolerability of policosanol in patients with type II hyperlipoproteinaemia. *Int J Clin Pharmacol Res* 1995;15:159-65.

2928 Pons P, Rodriguez M, Robaina C, et al. Effects of successive dose increases of policosanol on the lipid profile of patients with type II hypercholesterolaemia and tolerability to treatment. *Int J Clin Pharmacol Res* 1994;14:27-33.

2929 Torres O, Agramonte AJ, Illnait J, et al. Treatment of hypercholesterolemia in NIDDM with policosanol. *Diabetes Care* 1995;18:393-7.

2930 Batista J, Stusser R, Saez F, Perez B. Effect of policosanol on hyperlipidemia and coronary heart disease in middle-aged patients. A 14-month pilot study. *Int J Clin Pharmacol Ther* 1996;34:134-7.

2931 Castano G, Mas R, Roca J, et al. A double-blind, placebo-controlled study of the effects of policosanol in patients with intermittent claudication. *Angiology* 1999;50:123-30.

2933 Arruzazabala ML, Mas R, Molina V, et al. Effect of policosanol on platelet aggregation in type II hypercholesterolemic patients. *Int J Tissue React* 1998;20:119-24.

2934 Menendez R, Arruzazabala L, Mas R, et al. Cholesterol-lowering effect of policosanol on rabbits with hypercholesterolaemia induced by a wheat starch-casein diet. *Br J Nutr* 1997;77:923-32.

2935 Arruzazabala ML, Valdes S, Mas R, et al. Effect of policosanol successive dose increases on platelet aggregation in healthy volunteers. *Pharmacol Res* 1996;34:181-5.

2936 Carbajal D, Arruzazabala ML, Valdes S, Mas R. Effect of policosanol on platelet aggregation and serum levels of arachidonic acid metabolites in healthy volunteers. *Prostaglandins Leukot Essent Fatty Acids* 1998;58:61-4.

2937 Arruzazabala ML, Valdes S, Mas R, et al. Comparative study of policosanol, aspirin and the combination therapy policosanol-aspirin on platelet aggregation in healthy volunteers. *Pharmacol Res* 1997;36:293-7.

2938 Valdes S, Arruzazabala ML, Fernandez L. Effect of policosanol on platelet aggregation in healthy volunteers. *Int J Clin Pharmacol Res* 1996;16:67-72.

2939 Menendez R, Fernandez SI, Del Rio A, et al. Policosanol inhibits cholesterol biosynthesis and enhances low density lipoprotein processing in cultured human fibroblasts. *Biol Res* 1994;27:199-203.

2941 Stusser R, Batista J, Padron R, et al. Long-term therapy with policosanol improves treadmill exercise-ECG testing performance of coronary heart disease patients. *Int J Clin Pharmacol Ther* 1998;36:469-73.

2943 Castano G, Canetti M, Moreira M, et al. Efficacy and tolerability of policosanol in elderly patients with type II hypercholesterolemia: A 12-month study. *Curr Ther Res* 1995;56:819-23.

2944 Castano G, Tula L, Canetti M, et al. Effects of policosanol in hypertensive patients with type II hypercholesterolemia. *Curr Ther Res* 1996;57:691-5.

2948 Jang M, Cai L, Udeani GO, et al. Cancer chemopreventive activity of resveratrol, a natural product derived from grapes. *Science* 1997;275:218-20.

2949 Pace-Asciak CR, Rounova O, Hahn SE, et al. Wines and grape juices as modulators of platelet aggregation in healthy human subjects. *Clin Chim Acta* 1996;246:163-82.

2950 Bertelli AA, Giovannini L, Bernini W, et al. Antiplatelet activity of cis-resveratrol. *Drugs Exp Clin Res* 1996;22:61-3.

2951 Pace-Asciak CR, et al. The red wine phenolics trans-resveratrol and quercetin block human platelet aggregation and eicosanoid synthesis: implications for protection against coronary heart disease. *Clin Chim Acta* 1995; 235(2): 207-19.

2952 Bertelli A, et al. Plasma and tissue resveratrol concentrations and pharmacological activity. *Drugs Exp Clin Res* 1998; 24(3): 133-8.

2954 Chen CK, Pace-Asciak CR. Vasorelaxing activity of resveratrol and quercetin in isolated rat aorta. *Gen Pharmacol* 1996;27:363-6.

2956 Davy BM, Melby CL, Beske SD, et al. Oat consumption does not affect resting casual and ambulatory 24-h arterial blood pressure in men with high-normal blood pressure to stage I hypertension. *J Nutr* 2002;132:394-8.

2958 Huang C, et al. Resveratrol suppresses cell transformation and induces apoptosis through a p53-dependent pathway. *Carcinogenesis* 1999; 20(2): 237-42.

2959 Carbo N, et al. Resveratrol, a natural product present in wine, decreases tumour growth in a rat tumour model. *Biochem Biophys Res Commun*, 1999;254(3):739-43.

2960 Gehm BD, et al. Resveratrol, a polyphenolic compound found in grapes and wine, is an agonist for the estrogen receptor. *Proc Natl Acad Sci U S A* 1997; 94(25): 14138-43.

2961 Bertelli AA, et al. Antiplatelet activity of synthetic and natural resveratrol in red wine. *Int J Tissue React* 1995; 17(1): 1-3.

2971 Concannon MJ, Puckett CL. Microsurgical replantation of an ear in a child without venous repair. *Plast Reconstr Surg* 1998;102:2088-93; discussion 2094-6.

3001 Johnson, LW. Conjugated linoleic acids for body fat mass reduction. *Integrative Medicine Consult* 2001;3:17,21.

3005 George MS, Guidotti A, Rubinow D, et al. CSF neuroactive steroids in affective disorders: pregnenolone, progesterone, and DBI. *Biol Psych* 1994;35:775-80.

3006 Wang M, Seippel L, Purdy RH, Backstrom T. Relationship between symptom severity and steroid variation in women with premenstrual syndrome: study on serum pregnenolone, pregnenolone sulfate, 5 alpha-pregnane-3,20-dione and 3 alpha-hydroxy-5 alpha-pregnan-20-one. *J Clin Endocrinol Metab* 1996;81:1076-82.

3007 Steiger A, et al. Neurosteroid pregnenolone induces sleep-EEG changes in man compatible with inverse agonistic GABAA-receptor modulation. *Brain Res* 1993; 615(2): 267-74.

3008 Devlin TM, ed. Textbook of Biochemistry With Clinical Correlations. third ed. New York: Wiley-Liss Inc., 1992.

3011 Klaassen CD, ed. Casarett and Doull's Toxicology: The Basic Science of Poisons. fifth ed. New York: McGraw-Hill, 1996.

3012 Harland BF, Harden-Williams BA. Is vanadium of human nutritional importance yet? *J Am Diet Assoc* 1994;94:891-4.

3013 Malabu UH, Dryden S, McCarthy HD, et al. Effects of chronic vanadate administration in the STZ-induced diabetic rat. *Diabetes* 1994;43:9-15.

3014 Bishayee A, Karmakar R, Mandal A, et al. Vanadium mediated chemoprotection against chemical hepatocarcinogenesis in rats: haematological and histological characteris tics. *Eur J Cancer Prev* 1997;6:58-70.

3016 Chakraborty A, Chatterjee M. Enhanced erythropoietin and suppression of gamma-glutamyl-transpeptidase (GGT) activity in murine lymphoma following administration of vanadium. *Neoplasma* 1994;41:291-6.

3017 Domingo JL, Sanchez DJ, Gomez M, et al. Oral vanadate and Tiron in treatment of diabetes mellitus in rats: improvement of glucose homeostasis and negative side effects. *Vet Human Toxicol* 1993;35:495-500.

3018 Oster MH, Llobet JM, Domingo JL, et al. Vanadium treatment of diabetic Sprague-Dawley rats results in tissue vanadium accumulation and pro-oxidant effects. *Toxicology* 1993;83:115-30.

3019 Stern A, Yin X, Tsang SS, et al. Vanadium as a modulator of cellular regulatory cascades and oncogene expression. *Biochem Cell Biol* 1993;71:103-12.

3020 Sitprija V, Tungsanga K, Tosukhowong P, et al. Metabolic problems in northeastern Thailand: possible role of vanadium. *Mineral Electrolyte Metab* 1998;19:51-6.

3021 Domingo JL, Gomez M, Llobet JM, et al. Oral vanadium administration to streptozocin-diabetic rats has marked negative side-effects which are independent of the form of vanadium used. *Toxicology* 1991;66:279-87.

3022 Kastrup EK. Drug Facts and Comparisons. 1998 ed. St. Louis, MO: Facts and Comparisons, 1998.

3023 Lacy C, et al. Drug Information Handbook. fifth ed. Hudson, OH: Lexi-Comp Inc., 1997.

3024 Hathcock JN, Troendle GJ. Oral cobalamin for treatment of pernicious anemia? *JAMA* 1991;265:96-97.

3025 Arai Y, Watanabe S, Kimira M, et al. Dietary intake of flavonols, flavones and isoflavones by Japanese women and the inverse correlation between quercetin intake and plasma LDL cholesterol concentration. *J Nutr* 2000;130:2243-50.

3026 Margolin KA, Green MR. Polymicrobial enteric septicemia from coffee enemas. *West J Med* 1984;140:460.

3041 Beers MH, Berkow R. The Merck Manual of Diagnosis and Therapy. 17th ed. West Point, PA: Merck and Co., Inc., 1999.

3042 Levine M, Rumsey SC, Daruwala R, et al. Criteria and recommendations for vitamin C intake. *JAMA* 1999;281:1415-23.

3046 Hansten PD, Horn JR. Drug Interactions Analysis and Management. Vancouver, WA: Applied Therapeutics Inc., 1997 and updates.

3047 Mayer EL, Jacobsen DW, Robinson K. Homocysteine and coronary atherosclerosis. *J Am Coll Cardiol* 1996;27:517-27.

3048 Robinson K, Arheart K, Refsum H, et al. Low circulating folate and vitamin B6 concentrations: Risk factors for stroke, peripheral vascular disease, and coronary artery disease. *Circulation* 1998;97:437-43.

3049 Omenn GS, Beresford SAA, Motulsky AG. Preventing coronary heart disease: B vitamins and homocysteine. *Circulation* 1998;97:421-4.

3050 Rimm EB, Willett WC, Hu FB, et al. Folate and vitamin B6 from diet and supplements in relation to risk of coronary heart disease among women. *JAMA* 1998;279:359-64.

3051 Leonard A, Gerber GB. Mutagenicity, carcinogenicity and teratogenicity of vanadium Compounds. *Mutat Res* 1994;317:81-8.

3052 Fawcett JP, Farquhar SJ, Thou T, Shand BI. Oral vanadyl sulphate does not affect blood cells, viscosity or biochemistry in humans. *Pharmacol Toxicol* 1997;80:202-6.

3053 Fawcett JP, Farquhar SJ, Walker RJ, et al. The effect of oral vanadyl sulfate on body composition and performance in weight-training athletes. *Int J Sport Nutr* 1996;6:382-90.

3054 Funakoshi T, Shimada H, Kojima S, et al. Anticoagulant action of vanadate. *Chem Pharmaceut Bull* 1992;40:174-6.

3055 Halberstam M, Cohen N, Shlimovich P, et al. Oral vanadyl sulfate improves insulin sensitivity in NIDDM but not in obese nondiabetic subjects. *Diabetes* 1996;45:659-66.

3056 Cohen N, Halberstam M, Shlimovich P, et al. Oral vanadyl sulfate improves hepatic and peripheral insulin sensitivity in patients with non-insulin-dependent diabetes mellitus. *J Clin Invest* 1995;95:2501-9.

3057 Boden G, Chen X, Ruiz J, et al. Effects of vanadyl sulfate on carbohydrate and lipid metabolism in patients with non-insulin-dependent diabetes mellitus. *Metabolism* 1996;45:1130-5.

3062 Miller LL, Spitler LE, Allen RE, Minor DR. A randomized, double-blind, placebo-controlled trial of transfer factor as adjuvant therapy for malignant melanoma. *Cancer* 1988;61:1543-9.

3063 Bukowski RM, Deodhar S, Hewlett JS, Greenstreet R. Randomized controlled trial of transfer factor in Stage II malignant melanoma. *Cancer* 1983;51:269-72.

3066 FDA Talk Paper. Vitamin A and birth defects (T95-56). Food and Drug Administration, U.S.Department of Health and Human Services, Rockville, MD. October 6, 1995.

3070 Miner JL, Cederberg CA, Nielsen MK, et al. Conjugated linoleic acid (CLA), body fat, and apoptosis. *Obes Res* 2001;9:129-34.

3072 Tatro DS, ed. Drug Interactions Facts. Facts and Comparisons Inc., St. Louis, MO. 1999.

3073 Frank J, Weiser H, Biesalski HK. Interaction of vitamins E and K: effect of high dietary vitamin E on phylloquinone activity in chicks. *Int J Vit Nutr Res* 1997;67:242-7.

3074 Helson L. The effect of intravenous vitamin E and menadiol sodium diphosphate on vitamin K dependent clotting factors. *Thromb Res* 1984;35:11-8.

3082 Budavari S, ed. The Merck Index. 12th ed. Whitehouse Station, NJ: Merck & Co., Inc., 1996.

3083 Bushehri N, Jarrell ST, Lieberman S, et al. Oral reduced B-nicotinamide adenine dinucleotide (NADH) affects blood pressure, lipid peroxidation, and lipid profile in hypertensive rats (SHR). *Geriatr Nephrol Urol* 1998;8:95-100.

3085 Swerdlow RH. Is NADH effective in the treatment of Parkinson's disease?. *Drugs Aging* 1998; 13(4):263-8.

3086 Kuhn W, Muller T, Winkel R, et al. Parenteral application of NADH in Parkinson's disease: clinical improvement partially due to stimulation of endogenous levodopa biosynthesis. *J Neural Transmiss* (Budapest), 1996; 103(10):1187-93.

3087 Birkmayer JG. Coenzyme nicotinamide adenine dinucleotide: new therapeutic approach for improving dementia of the Alzheimer type. *Ann Clin Lab Sci* 1996; 26(1):1-9.

3088 Vrecko K, Birkmayer JG, Krainz J. Stimulation of dopamine biosynthesis in cultured PC 12 phaeochromocytoma cells by the coenzyme nicotinamide adeninedinucleotide (NADH). *J Neural Transmiss* (Parkinsons Disease & Dementia Section), 1993; 5(2):147-56.

3089 Birkmayer JG, Vrecko C, Volc D, Birkmayer W. Nicotinamide adenine dinucleotide (NADH) - a new therapeutic approach to Parkinson's disease. Comparison of oral and parenteral application. *Acta Neurol Scand Suppl* 1993; 146:32-5.

3090 Dizdar N, Kagedal B, Lindvall B. Treatment of Parkinson's disease with NADH. *Acta Neurol Scand* 1994; 90(5):345-7.

3091 Vrecko K, Storga D, Birkmayer JG, et al. NADH stimulates endogenous dopamine biosynthesis by enhancing the recycling of tetrahydrobiopterin in rat phaeochromocytoma cells. *Biochim Biophys Acta* 1997;1361:59-65.

3092 Fauci AS, Braunwald E, Isselbacher KJ, et al. Harrison's Principles of Internal Medicine, 14th ed. New York, NY: McGraw-Hill, 1998.

3093 Wyatt KM, Dimmock PW, Jones PW, O'Brien PM. Efficacy of vitamin B6 in the treatment of premenstrual syndrome. *BMJ* 1999;318:1375-81.

3094 Yates AA, Schlicker SA, Suitor CW. Dietary reference intakes: The new basis for recommendations for calcium and related nutrients, B vitamins, and choline. *J Am Diet Assoc* 1998;98:699-706.

3095 Song Z, Johansen HK, Faber V, et al. Ginseng treatment reduces bacterial load and lung pathology in chronic Pseudomonas aeruginosa pneumonia in rats. *Antimicrob Agents Chemother* 1997;41:961-4.

3096 Song Z, Kharazmi A, Wu H, et al. Effects of Ginseng treatment on neutrophil chemiluminescence and immunoglobulin G subclasses in a rat model of chronic Pseudomonas aeruginosa pneumonia. *Clin Diagn Lab Immunol* 1998;5:882-7.

3097 Simon JA, Hudes ES. Relationship of ascorbic acid to blood lead levels. *JAMA* 1999;281:2289-93.

3098 Dawson EB, Evans DR, Harris WA, et al. The effect of ascorbic acid supplementation on the blood lead levels of smokers. *J Am Coll Nutr* 1999;18:166-70.

3099 Cheng Y, Willett WC, Schwartz J, et al. Relation of nutrition to bone lead and blood lead levels in middle-aged to elderly men. The Normative Aging Study. *Am J Epidemiol* 1998;147:1162-74.

3100 Escarpa A, Gonzalez MC. High-performance liquid chromatography with diode-array detection for the determination of phenolic compounds in peel and pulp from different apple varieties. *J Chromatogr A* 1998;823:331-7.

3101 Cruz T, Galvez J, Ocete MA, et al. Oral administration of rutoside can ameliorate inflammatory bowel disease in rats. *Life Sci* 1998;62:687-95.

3102 Galvez J, Cruz T, Crespo E, et al. Rutoside as mucosal protective in acetic acid-induced rat colitis. *Planta Med* 1997;63:409-14.

3103 Kostyuk VA, Potapovich AI, Speransky SD, Maslova GT. Protective effect of natural flavonoids on rat peritoneal macrophages injury caused by asbestos fibers. *Free Radical Biol Med* 1996;21:487-93.

3104 Webster RP, Gawde MD, Bhattacharya RK. Protective effect of rutin, a flavonol glycoside, on the carcinogen-induced DNA damage and repair enzymes in rats. *Cancer Lett* 1996;109:185-91.

3105 Schmitt A, Salvayre R, Delchambre J, Negre-Salvayre A. Prevention by alpha-tocopherol and rutin of glutathione and ATP depletion induced by oxidized LDL in cultured endothelial cells. *Br J Pharmacol* 1995;116:1985-90.

3106 Rueff J, Gaspar J, Laires A. Structural requirements for mutagenicity of flavonoids upon nitrosation. A structure-activity study. *Mutagenesis* 1995;10:325-8.

3107 Perez Guerrero C, Martin MJ, Marhuenda E. Prevention by rutin of gastric lesions induced by ethanol in rats: role of endogenous prostaglandins. *Gen Pharmacol* 1994;25:575-80.

3108 Deschner EE, Ruperto J, Wong G, Newmark HL. Quercetin and rutin as inhibitors of azoxymethanol-induced colonic neoplasia. *Carcinogenesis* 1991;12:1193-6.

3109 Lewis R, Wake G, Court G, et al. Non-ginsenoside nicotinic activity in ginseng species. *Phytother Res* 1999;13;59-64.

3111 Barnett ML, Kremer JM, St.Clair W, et al. Treatment of rheumatoid arthritis with oral type II collagen. *Arthritis Rheum* 1998;41:290-7.

3112 Barnett ML, Combitchi D, Trentham DE. A pilot trial of oral type II collagen in the treatment of juvenile rheumatoid arthritis. *Arthritis Rheum* 1996;39:623-8.

3113 Ghoneum M. Anti-HIV activity in vitro of MGN-3, an activated arabinoxylane from rice bran. *Biochem Biophys Res Commun* 1998;243:25-9.

3116 Ghoneum M, Namatalla G, Kim C. Effect of MGN-3 on human natural killer cell activity and interferon-gamma synthesis in vitro [abstract]. *Federation of American Societies for Experimental Biology Journal* 1996;10:26-32.

REFERENCES

REFERENCES

3117 Ghoneum M, Jewett A. Synergistic effect of modified arabinoxylane (MGN-3) and low dose of recombinant IL-2 on human NK cell activity and TNF production [abstract]. American Acadamy of Anti-Aging Medicine Educational Conference, August 15-6, 1998.

3118 Ghoneum M. Enhancement of human natural killer cell activity by modified arabinoxylane from rice bran (MGN-3). *Int J Immunotherapy* 1998;14:89-99.

3119 Ghoneum M, Namatalla G. NK immunomodulatory function in 27 cancer patients by MGN-3, a modified arabinoxylane from rice bran [abstract]. 87th Annual Meeting of the American Association for Cancer Research. April 20-4, 1996.

3120 Ghoneum M. Immunomodulatory and anti-cancer properties of MGN-3, a modified xylose from rice bran, in 5 patients with breast cancer [abstract]. American Association for Cancer Research Special Conference. November 5-8, 1995.

3121 Belogortseva NI, Yoon JY, Kim KH. Inhibition of Helicobacter pylori hemagglutination by polysaccharide fractions from roots of Panax ginseng. *Planta Med* 2000;66:217-20.

3122 Shin HR, Kim JY, Yun TK, et al. The cancer-preventive potential of Panax ginseng: a review of human and experimental evidence. *Cancer Causes Control* 2000;11:565-76.

3123 Varis T, Kivisto KT, Neuvonen PJ. Grapefruit juice can increase the plasma concentration of methylprednisolone. *Eur J Clin Pharmacol* 2000;56:489-93.

3125 Kalden JR, Sieper J. Oral collagen in the treatment of rheumatoid arthritis [editorial]. *Arthritis Rheum* 1998;41:191-4.

3126 Trentham DE. Oral tolerization as a treatment of rheumatoid arthritis. *Rheum Dis Clin North Am* 1998;24:525-36.

3127 Mullins RJ, Richards C, Walker T. Allergic reactions to oral, surgical and topical bovine collagen. Anaphylactic risk for surgeons. *Aust N Z J Ophthalmol* 1996;24:257-60.

3128 AutoImmune Inc. announces phase III trial results for Colloral. URL http://www.autoimmune.com/clinic/coll.html (Accessed 24 October 1999).

3129 Wang XD, Zhang JM, Yang HH, Hu GY. Modulation of NMDA receptor by huperzine A in rat cerebral cortex. *Chung Kuo Yao Li Hsueh Pao* 1999;20:31-5.

3131 Skolnick AA. Old Chinese herbal medicine used for fever yields possible new Alzheimer Disease therapy. *JAMA* 1997;277:776.

3132 Wang H, Tang XC. Anticholinesterase effects of huperzine A, E2020, and tacrine in rats. *Chung Kuo Yao Li Hsueh Pao* 1998;19:27-30.

3133 Xiong ZQ, Cheng DH, Tang XC. Effects of huperzine A on nucleus basalis magnocellularis lesion-induced spatial working memory deficit. *Chung Kuo Yao Li Hsueh Pao* 1998;19:128-32.

3134 Ye JW, Cai JX, Wang LM, Tang XC. Improving effects of huperzine A on spatial working memory in aged monkeys and young adult monkeys with experimental cognitive impairment. *J Pharmacol Exp Ther* 1999;288:814-9.

3135 Wang T, Tang XC. Reversal of scopolamine-induced deficits in radial maze performance by (-)-huperzine A: comparison with E2020 and tacrine. *Eur J Pharmacol* 1998;349:137-42.

3136 Cheng DH, Tang XC. Comparative studies of huperzine A, E2020, and tacrine on behavior and cholinesterase activities. *Pharmacol Biochem Behav* 1998;60:377-86.

3137 Lallement G, Veyret J, Masqueliez C, et al. Efficacy of huperzine in preventing soman-induced seizures, neuropathological changes and lethality. *Fundam Clin Pharmacol* 1997;11:387-94.

3138 Xu SS, Gao ZX, Weng Z, et al. Efficacy of tablet huperzine-A on memory, cognition, and behavior in Alzheimer's disease. *Zhongguo Yao Li Xue Bao* 1995;16:391-5.

3139 Grunwald J, Raveh L, Doctor BP, Ashani Y. Huperzine A as a pretreatment candidate drug against nerve agent toxicity. *Life Sci* 1994;54:991-7.

3140 Zhang RW, Tang XC, Han YY, et al. [Drug evaluation of huperzine A in the treatment of senile memory disorders]. [Article in Chinese]. *Chung Kuo Yao Li Hsueh Pao* 1991;12:250-2.

3141 Tang XC, De Sarno P, Sugaya K, Giacobini E. Effect of huperzine A, a new cholinesterase inhibitor, on the central cholinergic system of the rat. *J Neurosci Res* 1989;24:276-85.

3142 Safety Briefs, ISMP Medication Safety Alert, vol.4, #4. Institute for Safe Medication Practices, Warminster, PA. February 24, 1999.

3148 Bupleurum falcatum Bitter & cool. The Australian Naturopath Network web site. Available at: www.comcen.com.au/~sburgess/herbs/Monographs/bupleuru.htm.

3151 Jing H, Jiang Y, Luo S. [Chemical constituents of the roots of Bupleurum longicaule Wall. ex DC. var. franchetii de Boiss and B. chaishoui Shan et Sheh]. [Article in Chinese]. *Chung Kuo Chung Yao Tsa Chih* 1996;21:739-41,762.

3152 Yen MH, Lin CC, Chuang CH, Liu SY. Evaluation of root quality of Bupleurum species by TLC scanner and the liver protective effects of xiao-chai-hu-tang prepared using three different Bupleurum species. *J Ethnopharmacol* 1991;34:155-65.

3153 Blankson H, Stakkestad JA, Fagertun H, et al. Conjugated linoleic acid reduces body fat mass in overweight and obese humans. *J Nutr* 2000;130:2943-8.

3154 Yamada H. [Structure and pharmacological activity of pectic polysaccharides from the roots of Bupleurum falcatum L]. [Article in Japanese]. *Nippon Yakurigaku Zasshi* 1995;106:229-37.

3155 Matsumoto T, Moriguchi R, Yamada H. Role of polymorphonuclear leucocytes and oxygen-derived free radicals in the formation of gastric lesions induced by HCl/ethanol, and a possible mechanism of protection by anti-ulcer polysaccharide. *J Pharm Pharmacol* 1993;45:535-9.

3156 Hattori T, Ito M, Suzuki Y. [Studies on antinephritic effects of plant components in rats (1). Effects of saikosaponins original-type anti-GBM nephritis in rats and its mechanisms]. [Article in Japanese]. *Nippon Yakurigaku Zasshi* 1991;97:13-21.

3157 Ahn BZ, Yoon YD, Lee YH, et al. Inhibitory effect of bupleuri radix saponins on adhesion of some solid tumor cells and relation to hemolytic action: screening of 232 herbal drugs for anti-cell adhesion. *Planta Med* 1998;64:220-4.

3158 Elias SL, Innis SM. Infant plasma trans, n-6, and n-3 fatty acids and conjugated linoleic acids are related to maternal plasma fatty acids, length of gestation, and birth weight and length. *Am J Clin Nutr* 2001;73:807-814.

3159 Chang WC, Hsu FL. Inhibition of platelet activation and endothelial cell injury by flavan-3-ol and saikosaponin compounds. *Prostaglandins Leukot Essent Fatty Acids* 1991;44:51-6.

3160 Kato M, Pu MY, Isobe K, et al. Characterization of the immunoregulatory action of saikosaponin-d. Cell Immunol, 1994;159(1):15-25.

3161 Ushio Y, Oda Y, Abe H. Effect of saikosaponin on the immune responses in mice. *Int J Immunopharmacol* 1991;13:501-8.

3162 Hoyos AB. Reduced incidence of necrotizing enterocolitis associated with enteral administration of Lactobacillus acidophilus and Bifidobacterium infantis to neonates in an intensive care unit. *Int J Infect Dis* 1999;3:197-202.

3163 Chiu HF, Lin CC, Yen MH, et al. Pharmacological and pathological studies on hepatic protective crude drugs from

Taiwan (V): The effects of Bombax malabarica and Scutellaria rivularis. *Am J Chin Med* 1992;20:257-64.

3164 Izumi S, Ohno N, Kawakita T, et al. Wide range of molecular weight distribution of mitogenic substance(s) in the hot water extract of a Chinese herbal medicine, Bupleurum chinense. *Biol Pharm Bull* 1997;20:759-64.

3165 Guinea MC, Parellada J, Lacaille-Dubois MA, Wagner H. Biologically active triterpene saponins from Bupleurum fruticosum. *Planta Med* 1994;60:163-7.

3166 Martin S, Padilla E, Ocete MA, et al. Anti-inflammatory activity of the essential oil of Bupleurum fruticescens. *Planta Med* 1993;59(6):533-6.

3167 Lorente I, Ocete MA, Zarzuelo A, et al. Bioactivity of the essential oil of Bupleurum fruticosum. *J Nat Prod* 1989;52:267-72.

3168 Bermejo Benito P, Abad Martinez MJ, Silvan Sen AM, et al. In vivo and in vitro antiinflammatory activity of saikosaponins. *Life Sci* 1998;63:1147-56.

3169 Phuapradit P, Varavithya W, Vathanophas K, et al. Reduction of rotavirus infection in children receiving bifidobacteria-supplemented formula. *J Med Assoc Thai* 1999;82:S43-S48.

3170 Estevez-Braun A, Estevez-Reyes R, Moujir LM, et al. Antibiotic activity and absolute configuation of 8S-heptadeca-2(Z),9(Z)-diene-4,6-diyne-1,8-diol from Bupleurum salicifolium. *J Nat Prod* 1994;57:1178-82.

3171 Zhang SL. [Therapeutic effects of huperzine A on the aged with memory impairment]. [Article in Chinese]. *New Drugs and Clinical Remedies* 1986;5:260-2.

3172 Cheng YS, Lu CZ, Ying ZL, et al. [128 cases of myasthenia gravis treated with huperzine A]. [Article in Chinese]. *New Drugs and Clinical Remedies* 1986;5:197-9.

3176 HolisticOnLine website. URL: holisticonline.com/Herbal-Med/_scripts/getHerb_Dir.idc?Herb_Names=365 (Accessed 25 November 1999).

3177 Dharmananda S. PCP prophylaxis with drugs and herbs. Institute for Traditional Medicine Online. URL: www.rdi.gpo.or.th/NetZine/V3N42/pcp.htm (Accessed 25 November 1999).

3180 Pittler MH, Ernst E. Artemether for severe malaria: a meta-analysis of randomized clinical trials. *Clin Infect Dis* 1999;28:597-601.

3181 van Agtmael MA, Eggelte TA, van Boxtel CJ. Artemisinin drugs in the treatment of malaria: from medicinal herb to registered medication. *Trends Pharmacol Sci* 1999;20:199-205.

3182 Moneton P, Ducret JP. Positioning, labeling and control of medical information: artesunate strategy and Arsumax development story. *Med Trop* (Mars) 1998;58:70-2.

3183 Zheng GQ. Cytotoxic terpenoids and flavonoids from Artemisia annua. *Planta Med* 1994;60:54-7.

3184 Huang L, Liu JF, Liu LX, et al. [Antipyretic and anti-inflammatory effects of Artemisia annua L]. [Article in Chinese]. *Chung Kuo Chung Yao Tsa Chih* 1993;18:44-48,63-4.

3185 Wan YD, Zang QZ, Wang JS. [Studies on the antimalarial action of gelatin capsule of Artemisia annua]. [Article in Chinese]. *Chung Kuo Chi Sheng Chung Hsueh Yu Chi Sheng Chung Ping Tsa Chih* 1992;10:290-4.

3187 PlanetHerbs Online website. URL http://www.planetherbs.com/articles/rhodiola%20rosea.htm (Accessed 22 November 1999).

3188 Mother Nature's General Store, Inc. website. URL http://www.herbalphen.com/rhod.htm (Accessed 22 November 1999).

3189 Nutri-Mart Cyberstore. URL http://www.nutrimart.com/Bulk/Description/rhodiola_rosea.htm (Accessed 22 November 1999).

3190 Salikhova RA, Aleksandrova IV, Mazurik VK, et al. [Effect of Rhodiola rosea on the yield of mutation alterations and DNA repair in bone marrow cells]. [Article in Russian]. *Patol Fiziol Eksp Ter* 1997;(4):22-4.

3191 Lishmanov IB, Naumova AV, Afanas'ev SA, Maslov LN. [Contribution of the opioid system to realization of inotropic effects of Rhodiola rosea extracts in ischemic and reperfusion heart damage in vitro]. [Article in Russian]. *Eksp Klin Farmakol* 1997;60(3):34-6.

3192 Maimeskulova LA, Maslov LN, Lishmanov IB, Krasnov EA. [The participation of the mu-, delta- and kappa-opioid receptors in the realization of the anti-arrhythmia effect of Rhodiola rosea]. [Article in Russian]. *Eksp Klin Farmakol* 1997;60(1):38-9.

3193 Maslova LV, Kondrat'ev BI, Maslov LN, Lishmanov IB. [The cardioprotective and antiadrenergic activity of an extract of Rhodiola rosea in stress]. [Article in Russian]. *Eksp Klin Farmakol* 1994;57(6):61-3.

3194 Bocharova OA, Matveev BP, Baryshnikov AI, et al. [The effect of a Rhodiola rosea extract on the incidence of recurrences of a superficial bladder cancer]. [Article in Russian]. *Urol Nefrol* (Mosk) 1995;(2):46-7.

3195 Lishmanov IB, Maslova LV, Maslov LN, Dan'shina EN. [The anti-arrhythmia effect of Rhodiola rosea and its possible mechanism]. [Article in Russian]. *Bull Eksp Biol Med* 1993;116(8):175-6.

3196 Udintsev SN, Krylova SG, Fomina TI. [The enhancement of the efficacy of adriamycin by using hepatoprotectors of plant origin in metastases of Ehrlich's adenocarcinoma to the liver in mice]. [Article in Russian]. *Vopr Onkol* 1992;38(10):1217-22.

3197 Udintsev SN, Shakhov VP. [Changes in clonogenic properties of bone marrow and transplantable mice tumor cells during combined use of cyclophosphane and biological response modifiers of adaptogenic origin]. [Article in Russian]. *Eksp Onko* 1990;12(6):55-6.

3198 Petkov VD, Yonkov D, Mosharoff A, et al. Effects of alcohol aqueous extract from Rhodiola rosea L. roots on learning and memory. *Acta Physiol Pharmacol Bulg* 1986;12(1):3-16.

3219 Brown L, Rimm EB, Seddon JM, et al. A prospective study of carotenoid intake and risk of cataract extraction in US men. *Am J Clin Nutr* 1999;70:517-24.

3220 Chasan-Taber L, Willett WC, Seddon JM, et al. A prospective study of carotenoid and vitamin A intakes and risk of cataract extraction in US women. *Am J Clin Nutr* 1999;70:509-16.

3221 Lyle BJ, Mares-Perlman JA, Klein BE, et al. Antioxidant intake and risk of incident age-related nuclear cataracts in the Beaver Dam Eye Study. *Am J Epidemiol* 1999;149:801-9.

3222 Teikari JM, Rautalahti M, Haukka J, et al. Incidence of cataract operations in Finnish male smokers unaffected by alpha tocopherol or beta carotene supplements. *J Epidemiol Community Health* 1998;52:468-72.

3223 Teikari JM, Virtamo J, Rautalahti M, et al. Long-term supplementation with alpha-tocopherol and beta-carotene and age-related cataract. *Acta Ophthalmol Scand* 1997;75:634-40.

3224 Sommerburg O, Keunen JE, Bird AC, van Kuijk FJ. Fruits and vegetables that are sources for lutein and zeaxanthin: the macular pigment in human eyes. *Br J Ophthalmol* 1998;82:907-10.

3225 Hammond BR Jr, Wooten BR, Snodderly DM, et al. Density of the human crystalline lens is related to the macular pigment carotenoids, lutein and zeaxanthin. *Optom Vis Sci* 1997;74:499-504.

3226 Gross AS, Goh YD, Addison RS, et al. Influence of grapefruit juice on cisapride pharmacokinetics. *Clin Pharmacol Ther* 1999;65:395-401.

3227 Lilja JJ, Kivisto KT, Neuvonen PJ. Grapefruit juice increases serum concentrations of atorvastatin and has no effect on pravastatin. *Clin Pharmacol Ther* 1999;66:118-27.

3228 Ozdemir M, Aktan Y, Boydag BS. Interaction between grapefruit juice and diazepam in humans. *Eur J Drug Metab Pharmacokinet* 1998;23:55-9.

3229 Grapefruit-drug interactions. URL: powernetdesign.com/grapefruit (Accessed 26 September 1999).

3230 Zaidenstein R, Dishi V, Gips M, et al. The effect of grapefruit juice on the pharmacokinetics of orally administered verapamil. *Eur J Clin Pharmacol* 1998;54:337-40.

3231 Arlt W, Callies F, van Vlijmen JC, et al. Dehydroepiandosterone replacement in women with adrenal insufficiency. *N Engl J Med* 1999;341:1013-20.

3232 Oelkers W. Dehydroepiandosterone for adrenal insufficiency (editorial). *N Engl J Med* 1999;341:1073-4.

3233 Selhub J, Jacques PF, Rosenberg IH, et al. Serum total homocysteine concentrations in the Third National Health and Nutrition Examination Survey (1991-4): population reference ranges and contribution of vitamin status to high serum concentrations. *Ann Intern Med* 1999;131:331-9.

3234 Rahman K, Billington D. Dietary supplementation with aged garlic extract inhibits ADP-induced platelet aggregation in humans. *J Nutr* 2000;130:2662-5.

3235 Lindenbaum J, Healton EB, Savage DG, et al. Neuropsychiatric disorders caused by cobalamin deficiency in the absence of anemia or macrocytosis. *N Engl J Med* 1988;318:1720-8.

3236 Chappell LC, Seed PT, Briley AL, et al. Effect of antioxidants on the occurrence of pre-eclampsia in women at increased risk: a randomized trial. *Lancet* 1999;354:810-6.

3237 Mensink RP, van Houwelingen AC, Kromhout D, Hornstra G. A vitamin E concentrate rich in tocotrienols had no effect on serum lipids, lipoproteins, or platelet function in men with mildly elevated serum lipid concentrations. *Am J Clin Nutr* 1999;69:213-9.

3238 Qureshi AA, Qureshi N, Wright JJ, et al. Lowering of serum cholesterol in hypercholesterolemic humans by tocotrienols (palmvitee). *Am J Clin Nutr* 1991;53:1021S-6S.

3239 Tomeo AC, Geller M, Watkins TR, et al. Antioxidant effects of tocotrienols in patients with hyperlipidemia and carotid stenosis. *Lipids* 1995;30:1179-83.

3240 Qureshi AA, Bradlow BA, Brace L, et al. Response of hypercholesterolemic subjects to administration of tocotrienols. *Lipids* 1995;30:1171-7.

3241 Qureshi AA, Bradlow BA, Slaser WA, et al. Novel tocotrienols of rice bran modulate cardiovascular disease risk parameters of hypercholesterolemic humans. *Nutr Biochem* 1997;8:290-8.

3242 Conte A, de Bernardi M, Palmieri L, et al. Metabolic fate of exogenous chondroitin sulfate in man. *Arzneimittelforschung* 1991; 41:768-72.

3243 Pittler MH, Abbot NC, Harkness EF, Ernst E. Randomized, double-blind trial of chitosan for body weight reduction. *Eur J Clin Nutr* 1999;53:379-81.

3244 Wuolijoki E, Hirvela T, Ylitalo P. Decrease in serum LDL cholesterol with microcrystalline chitosan. *Methods Find Exp Clin Pharmacol* 1999;21:357-61.

3245 Takahashi K, Yoshino K, Shirai T, et al. Effect of a traditional herbal medicine (shakuyaku-kanzo-to) on testosterone secretion in patients with polycystic ovary syndrome detected by ultrasound. *Nippon Sanka Fujinka Gakkai Zasshi* 1988;40:789-92.

3246 Armanini D, Bonanni G, Palermo M, et al. Reduction of serum testosterone in men by licorice. *N Engl J Med* 1999;341:1158.

3247 Abe Y, Ueda T, Kato T, Kohli Y. [Effectiveness of interferon, glycyrrhizin combination therapy in patients with chronic hepatitis C]. *Nippon Rinsho* 1994;52:1817-22.

3248 Takahara T, Watanabe A, Shiraki K. Effects of glycyrrhizin on hepatitis B surface antigen: a biochemical and morphological study. *J Hepatol* 1994;21:601-9.

3249 Sato H, Goto W, Yamamura J, et al. Therapeutic basis of glycyrrhizin on chronic hepatitis B. *Antiviral Res* 1996;30:171-7.

3250 Acharya SK, Dasarathy S, Tandon A, Joshi YK, Tandon BN. A preliminary open trial on interferon stimulator (SNMC) derived from Glycyrrhiza glabra in the treatment of subacute hepatic failure. *Indian J Med Res* 1993;98:69-74.

3251 Zhang XH, Lowe D, Giles P, et al. Gender may affect the action of garlic oil on plasma cholesterol and glucose levels of normal subjects. *J Nutr* 2001;131:1471-8.

3252 Armanini D, Lewicka S, Pratesi C, et al. Further studies on the mechanism of the mineralocorticoid action of licorice in humans. *J Endocrinol Invest* 1996;19:624-9.

3253 Krahenbuhl S, Hasler F, Frey BM, et al. Kinetics and dynamics of orally administered 18 beta-glycyrrhetinic acid in humans. *J Clin Endocrinol Metab* 1994;78:581-5.

3254 Lee YS, Lorenzo BJ, Koufis T, et al. Grapefruit juice and its flavonoids inhibit 11 beta-hydroxysteroid dehydrogenase. *Clin Pharmacol Ther* 1996;59:62-71.

3255 Zhang YD, Lorenzo B, Reidenberg MM. Inhibition of 11 beta hydroxysteroid dehydrogenase obtained from guinea pig kidney by furosemide, naringenin and some other compounds. *J Steroid Biochem Mol Biol* 1994;49:81-5.

3256 Hiai S, Yokoyama H, Oura H, et al. Stimulation of pituitary-adrenocortical system by ginseng saponin. *Endocrinol Jpn* 1979;26:661-5.

3257 Kase Y, Saitoh K, Ishige A, et al. Mechanisms by which Hange-shashin-to reduces prostaglandin E2 levels. *Biol Pharm Bull* 1998;21:1277-81.

3259 Peters H, Noble NA. Dietary L-arginine in renal disease. *Semin Nephrol* 1996;16:567-75.

3260 Wang R, Ghahary A, Shen YJ, et al. Human dermal fibroblasts produce nitric oxide and express both constitutive and inducible nitric oxide synthase isoforms. *J Invest Dermatol* 1996;106:419-27.

3261 Venturi A, Gionchetti P, Rizzello F, et al. Impact on the composition of the faecal flora by a new probiotic preparation: preliminary data on maintenance treatment of patients with ulcerative colitis. *Aliment Pharmacol Ther* 1999;13:1103-8.

3262 Russell IJ, Michalek JE, Flechas JD, et al. Treatment of fibromyalgia syndrome with Super Malic: a randomized, double blind, placebo controlled, crossover pilot study. *J Rheumatol* 1995;22:953-8.

3263 Koo WK, Walters JC, Esterlitz J, et al. Maternal calcium supplementation and fetal bone mineralization. *Obstet Gynecol* 1999;94:577-82.

3264 Raman L, Rajalakshmi K, Krishnamachari KAVR, et al. Effect of calcium supplementation to undernourished mothers during pregnancy on the bone density of the neonates. *Am J Clin Nutr* 1978; 31:466-9.

3265 Roth JA, Kim B-G, Lin W-L, et al. Melatonin promotes osteoblast differentiation and bone formation. *J Biol Chem* 1999;274:22041-7.

3267 Singh RB, Niaz MA, Ghosh S. Hypolipidemic and antioxidant effects of Commiphora mukul as an adjunct to dietary therapy in patients with hypercholesterolemia. *Cardiovasc Drugs Ther* 1994;8:659-64.

3268 Thappa DM, Dogra J. Nodulocystic acne: oral gugulipid versus tetracycline. *J Dermatol* 1994;21:729-31.

3269 Adzet T, Camarasa J, Laguna JC. Hepatoprotective activity of polyphenolic compounds from Cynara scolymus against CCl4 toxicity in isolated rat hepatocytes. *J Nat Prod* 1987;50:612-7.

3270 Wolkowitz OM, Reus VI, Keebler A, et al. Double-blind treatment of major depression with dehydroepiandosterone. *Am J Psychiatry* 1999;156:646-9.

3273 The IOOC's Trade Standard Applying to Olive Oil and Olive Pomace Oil. Available at: sovrana.com/ioocdef.htm (Accessed 23 June 2004).

3274 Kamien M. Practice tip. Which cerumenolytic? *Aust Fam Physician* 1999;28:817,828.

3275 Isaksson M, Bruze M. Occupational allergic contact dermatitis from olive oil in a masseur. *J Am Acad Dermatol* 1999;41:312-5.

3276 Hoberman A, Paradise JL, Reynolds EA, et al. Efficacy of Auralgan for treating ear pain in children with acute otitis media. *Arch Pediatr Adolesc Med* 1997;151:675-8.

3278 Bowden RA, Siegel MS, Steele RW, et al. Immunologic and clinical responses to varicella-zoster virus-specific transfer factor following marrow ransplantation. *J Infect Dis* 1985;152:1324-7.

3279 Chavez ML, Chavez PI. Echinacea. *Hosp Pharm* 1998;33:180-8.

3280 Gunning K. Echinacea in the treatment and prevention of upper respiratory tract infections. *West J Med* 1999;171:198-200.

3281 Barrett B, Vohmann M, Calabrese C. Echinacea for upper respiratory infection. *J Fam Pract* 1999;48:628-35.

3282 Grimm W, Muller HH. A randomized controlled trial of the effect of fluid extract of Echinacea purpurea on the incidence and severity of colds and respiratory infections. *Am J Med* 1999;106:138-43.

3283 Putter M, Grotemeyer KH, Wurthwein G, et al. Inhibition of smoking-induced platelet aggregation by aspirin and pycnogenol. *Thromb Res* 1999;95:155-61.

3284 Bisignano G, Tomaino A, Lo Cascio R, et al. On the in-vitro antimicrobial activity of oleuropein and hydroxytyrosol. *J Pharm Pharmacol* 1999;51:971-4.

3285 Mensink RP, Katan MB. An epidemiological and an experimental study on the effect of olive oil on total serum and HDL cholesterol in healthy volunteers. *Eur J Clin Nutr* 1989;43 Suppl 2:43-8.

3286 Mata P, Alvarez-Sala LA, Rubio MJ, et al. Effects of long-term monounsaturated- vs polyunsaturated-enriched diets on lipoproteins in healthy men and women. *Am J Clin Nutr* 1992;55:846-50.

3287 Lichtenstein AH, Ausman LM, Carrasco W, et al. Effects of canola, corn, and olive oils on fasting and postprandial plasma lipoproteins in humans as part of a National Cholesterol Education Program Step 2 diet. *Arterioscler Thromb* 1993;13:1533-42.

3288 Zambon A, Sartore G, Passera D, et al. Effects of hypocaloric dietary treatment enriched in oleic acid on LDL and HDL subclass distribution in mildly obese women. *J Intern Med* 1999;246:191-201.

3289 Ruiz-Gutierrez V, Muriana FJ, Guerrero A, et al. Plasma lipids, erythrocyte membrane lipids and blood pressure of hypertensive women after ingestion of dietary oleic acid from two different sources. *J Hypertens* 1996;14:1483-90.

3290 Tsimikas S, Philis-Tsimikas A, Alexopoulos S, et al. LDL isolated from Greek subjects on a typical diet or from American subjects on an oleate-supplemented diet induces less monocyte chemotaxis and adhesion when exposed to oxidative stress. *Arterioscler Thromb Vasc Biol* 1999;19:122-30.

3291 Nutt JG, Woodward WR, Hammerstad JP, et al. The "on-off" phenomenon in Parkinson's disease. Relation to levodopa absorption and transport. *N Engl J Med* 1984;310:483-8.

3292 Baruzzi A, Contin M, Riva R, et al. Influence of meal ingestion time on pharmacokinetics of orally administered levodopa in parkinsonian patients. *Clin Neuropharmacol* 1987;10:527-37.

3293 Juncos JL, Fabbrini G, Mouradian MM, et al. Dietary influences on the antiparkinsonian response to levodopa. *Arch Neurol* 1987;44:1003-5.

3294 Eriksson T, Granerus AK, Linde A, et al. "On-off" phenomenon in Parkinson's disease: relationship between dopa and other large neutral amino acids in plasma. *Neurology* 1988;38:1245-8.

3300 Tomita T, Sato N, Arai T, et al. Bactericidal activity of a fermented hot-water extract from Stevia rebaudiana Bertoni towards enterohemorrhagic Escherichia coli O157:H7 and other food-borne pathogenic bacteria. *Microbiol Immunol* 1997;41:1005-9.

3301 Curi R, Alvarez M, Bazotte RB, et al. Effect of Stevia rebaudiana on glucose tolerance in normal adult humans. *Braz J Med Biol Res* 1986;19:771-4.

3302 Evans DA, Raj RK. Larvicidal efficacy of Quassin against Culex quinquefasciatus. *Indian J Med Res* 1991;93:324-7.

3303 Owen JA, Nakatsu SL, Fenemore J, et al. The pharmacokinetics of yohimbine in man. *Eur J Clin Pharmacol* 1987;3:877-82.

3304 Cappiello A, McDougle CJ, Malison RT, et al. Yohimbine augmentation of Fluvoxamine in refactory depression: a single blind study. *Biol Psychiatry* 1995;38:765-7.

3305 Montorsi F, Strambi LF, Guazzoni G, et al. Effect of yohimbine-trazodone on psychogenic impotence: a randomized, double-blind, placebo-controlled study. *Urology* 1994;44:732-6.

3306 Balon R. Fluoxetine-induced sexual dysfunction and yohimbine. *J Clin Psychiatry* 1993;54:161-2.

3307 Carey MP, Johnson BT. Effectiveness of yohimbine in the treatment of erectile disorder: four meta-analytic integrations. *Arch Sexual Behavior* 1996;25:341-60.

3309 Kunellius P, Hakkinen J, Lukkarinen O. Is high-dose yohimbine hydrochloride effective in the treatment of mixed-type impotence? A prospective, randomized, controlled, double-blind crossover study. *Urol* 1997;49:441-4.

3310 Wagner G, Saenz de Tejada IS. Update on male erectile dysfunction. *BMJ* 1998;316:678-82.

3311 Witt DK. Yohimbine for erectile dysfuntion. *J Fam Pract* 1998;46:282-3.

3312 Teloken C, Rhoden EL, Sogari P, et al. Therapeutic effects of high dose yohimbine hydrochloride on organic erectile dysfunction. *J Urol* 1998;159:122-4.

3313 Ashton AK. Yohimbine in the treatment of male erectile dysfunction. *Am J Psychiatr* 1994;151:1397.

3314 Anderson PO, Knoben JE, Troutman WG. Handbook of Clinical Drug Data. 9th ed. Stamford, CT: Appleton & Lange, 1999.

3315 Siegel G, Klubendorf D. The anti-atherosclerotic effect of Allium sativum: Statistics re-evaluated. *Atherosclerosis* 2000;150:437-8.

3316 Aydin A, Ersoz G, Tekesin O, et al. Garlic Oil and Helicobacter pylori Infection. *Am J Gastroenterol* 2000;95:563-4.

3317 Fernandez-Vozmediano JM, Armario-Hita JC, Manrique-Plaza A. Allergic contact dermatitis from diallyl disulfide. *Contact Dermatitis* 2000;42:108-9.

3318 Stjernberg L, Berglund J. Garlic as an Insect Repellant. *JAMA* 2000;284:831.

3319 Bloch AS. Pushing the Envelope of Nutrition Support: Complementary Therapies. *Nutrition* 2000;16:236-9.

3320 Fleischauer AT, Poole C, Arab L. Garlic consumption and cancer prevention: meta-analyses of colorectal and stomach cancers. *Am J Clin Nutr* 2000;72:1047-52.

R E F E R E N C E S

3321 Sato T, Miyata G. The Nutraceutical Benefit, Part IV: Garlic. *Nutrition* 2000;16:787-8.

3322 O'Gara EA, Hill DJ, Maslin DJ. Activities of Garlic Oil, Garlic Powder, and Their Diallyl Constituents against Helicobacter pylori. *Appl Environ Microbiol* 2000;66:2269-73.

3323 Voutilainen S, Lakka TA, Porkkala-Sarataho E, et al. Low serum folate concentrations are associated with an excess incidence of acute coronary events: the Kuopio Ischaemic Heart Disease Risk Factor Study. *Eur J Clin Nutr* 2000;54:424-8.

3324 Bostom AG, Shemin D, Bagley P, et al. Controlled Comparison of L-5-Methyltetrahydrofolate Versus Folic Acid for the Treatment of Hyperhomocysteinemia in the Hemodialysis Patients. *Circulation* 2000;101:2829-32.

3325 US Food and Drug Administration, Center for Food Safety, and Applied Nutrition, Office of Nutritional Products, Labeling, and Dietary Supplements. Letter regarding dietary supplement health claim for folic acid with respect to neural tube defects. 2000. Available at: http://vm.cfsan.fda.gov/~dms/ds-ltr7.html.

3330 Tenebaum A, Fisman EZ, Motro M. L-arginine: Rediscovery in progress. *Cardiology* 1998;90:153-5.

3331 Brittenden J, Park KGM, Heys SD, et al. L-Arginine stimulates host defenses in patients with breast cancer. *Surgery* 1994;115:205-12.

3332 Oomen CM, van Erk MJ, Feskens E, et al. Arginine intake and risk of coronary heart disease mortality in elderly men. *Arterioscler Thromb Vasc Biol* 2000;20:2134-9.

3333 Harkins K. What's the use of cranberry juice? *Age Ageing* 2000;29:9-12.

3334 Jackson B, Hicks LE. Effect of cranberry juice on urinary pH in older adults. *Home Healthc Nurse* 1997;15:199-202.

3335 Avorn J. The effect Of Cranberry Juice on the presence of bacteria and white blood cells in the urine of elderly women. What is the role of bacterial adhesion? *Adv Exp Med Biol* 1996;408:185-6.

3336 Kuzminski LN. Cranberry juice and urinary tract infections: Is there a beneficial relationship? *Nutr Rev* 1996;54:S87-S90.

3337 Fleet JC. New support for a folk remedy: Cranberry juice reduces bacteriuria and pyuria in elderly women. *Nutr Rev* 1994;52:168-70.

3338 Schmidt DR, Sobota AE. An examination of the anti-adherence activity of cranberry juice on urinary and nonurinary bacterial isolates. *Microbios* 1988;55:173-81.

3339 Kinney AB, Blount M. Effect of cranberry juice on urinary pH. *Nurs Res* 1979;28:287-90.

3340 Kurowska EM, Spence JD, Jordan J, et al. HDL-cholesterol-raising effect of orange juice in subjects with hypercholesterolemia. *Am J Clin Nutr* 2000;72:1095-100.

3341 Rayman MP. The importance of selenium to human health. *Lancet* 2000;356:233-41.

3342 Mark SD, Qiao YL, Dawsey SM, et al. Prospective study of serum selenium levels and incident esophageal and gastric cancers. *J Natl Cancer Inst* 2000;92:1753-63.

3343 Vinceti M, Rothman KJ, Bergomi KJ, et al. Excess melanoma incidence in a cohort exposed to high levels of environmental selenium. *Cancer Epidemiol Biomarkers Prev* 1998;7:853-6.

3344 Urgert R, Vliet TV, Zock PL, et al. Heavy coffee consumption and plasma homocysteine: a randomized controlled trial in healthy volunteers. *Am J Clin Nutr* 2000;72:1107-10.

3345 Leitzmann MF, Willett WC, Rimm EB, et al. A Prospective study of coffee consumption and the risk of symptomatic gallstone disease in men. *JAMA* 1999;281:2106-12.

3346 Ernst E. Colonic irrigation and the theory of autointoxication: A triumph of ignorance over science. *J Clin Gastroenterol* 1997;24:196-8.

3347 Green S. A critique of the rationale for cancer treatment with coffee enemas and diet. *JAMA* 1992;268:3224-7.

3348 Reed A, James N, Sikora K. Juices, coffee enemas, and cancer. *Lancet* 1990;336:677-8.

3349 Shils ME, Herman MG. Unproved dietary claims in the treatment of patients with cancer. *Bull N Y Acad Med* 1982;58:323-39.

3350 Geerling BJ, Dagnelie PC, Badart-Smook A, et al. Diet as a risk factor for the development of ulcerative colitis. *Am J Gastroenterol* 2000;95:1008-13.

3351 Brenner A. The effects of megadoses of selected B complex vitamins on children with hyperkinesis: controlled studies with long-term follow-up. *J Learn Disabil* 1982;15:258-64.

3353 Siegel RK. Ginseng Abuse Syndrome. *JAMA* 1979;241:1614-5.

3354 Palop-Larrea V, Gonzalvez-Perales JL, Catalan-Oliver C, et al. Metrorrhagia and ginseng. *Ann Pharmacother* 2000;34:1347-8.

3355 Fuller CJ, May MA, Martin KJ. The effect of Vitamin E and Vitamin C supplementation on LDL oxidizability and neutrophil respiratory burst in young smokers. *J Am Coll Nutr* 2000;19:361-9.

3356 Sullivan C, Capaldi N, Mack G, et al. Seizures and natural Vitamin E. *Med J Aust* 1990;152:613-4.

3357 Boaz M, Smetana S, Weinstein T, et al. Secondary prevention with antioxidants of cardiovascular disease in endstage renal disease: randomised placebo-controlled trial. *Lancet* 2000;356:1213-8.

3358 Engelen W, Keenoy BM, Vertommen J, Leeuw ID. Effects of long-term supplementation with moderate pharmacologic doses of vitamin E are saturable and reversible in patients with type 1 diabetes. *Am J Clin Nutr* 2000;72:1142-9.

3359 Leppala JM, Virtamo J, Fogelholm R, et al. Vitamin E and Beta Carotene supplementation in high risk for stroke: a subgroup analysis of the alpha-tocopherol, beta-carotene cancer prevention study. *Arch Neurol* 2000;57:1503-9.

3360 Palli D, Russo A, Saieva C, et al. Dietary and familial determinants of 10-year survival among patients with gastric carcinoma. *Cancer* 2000;89:1205-13.

3361 Israel K, Yu W, Sanders BG, Kline K. Vitamin E succinate induces apoptosis in human prostate cancer cells: role for Fas in vitamin E succinate-triggered apoptosis. *Nutr Cancer* 2000;36:90-100.

3362 Stoneham M, Goldacre M, Seagroatt V, Gill L. Olive oil, diet and colorectal cancer: an ecological study and a hypothesis. *J Epidemiol Community Health* 2000;54:756-60.

3363 Bartoli R, Fernandez-Bariares F, Navarro E, et al. Effect of olive oil on early and late events of colon carcinogenesis in rats: modulation of arachidonic acid metabolism and local prostaglandin E2 synthesis. *Gut* 2000;46:191-9.

3364 Hipkiss AR, Chana H. Carnosine protects proteins against methylglyoxal-mediated modifications. *Biochem Biophys Res Commun* 1998;248:28-32.

3365 Singh RB, Niaz MA, Rastogi SS, et al. Effect of hydrosoluble coenzyme Q10 on blood pressures and insulin resistance in hypertensive patients with coronary artery disease. *J Hum Hypertens* 1999;13:203-8.

3366 Rotig A, Appelkvist EL, Geromel V, et al. Quinone-responsive multiple respiratory-chain dysfunction due to widespread coenzyme Q10 deficiency. *Lancet* 2000;356:391-5.

3367 Laaksonen R, Jokelainen K, Sahi T, et al. Decreases in serum ubiquinone concentrations do not result in reduced levels in muscle tissue during short-term simvastatin treatment in humans. *Clin Pharmacol Ther* 1995;57:62-6.

3368 Kishi T, Watanabe T, Folkers K. Bioenergetics in clinical medicine. XV. Inhibition of coenzyme Q10 enzymes by clinically used adrenergic blockers of B-receptors. *Res Commun Chem Pathol Pharmacol* 1977;17:157-64.

3369 Kishi H, Kishi T, Folkers K. Bioenergetics in clinical medicine. III. Inhibition of coenzyme Q10 enzymes by clinically used anti-hypertensive drugs. *Res Commun Chem Pathol Pharmacol* 1975;12:533-40.

3370 Fuke C, Krikorian SA, Couris RR. Coenzyme Q10: A Review of essential functions and clinical trials. *US Pharmacist* 2000;28-41.

3371 Harmelin DL, Martin FR, Wark JD. Antacid-induced phosphate depletion syndrome presenting as nephrolithiasis. *Aust N Z J Med* 1990;20:803-5.

3372 Roberts DH, Knox FG. Renal phosphate handling and calcium nephrolithiasis: role of dietary phosphate and phosphate leak. *Semin Nephrol* 1990;10:24-30.

3373 Pino AM, Valladares LE, Palma MA, et al. Dietary isoflavones affect sex hormone-binding globulin levels in postmenopausal women. *J Clin Endocrinol Metab* 2000;85:2797-800.

3374 Nissen S, Sharp RL, Panton L, et al. B-Hydroxy-B-Methylbutyrate (HMB) supplementation in humans is safe and may decrease cardiovascular risk factors. *J Nutr* 2000;130:1937-45.

3375 Howes JB, Sullivan D, Lai N, et al. The effects of dietary supplementation with isoflavones from red clover on the lipoprotein profiles of postmenopausal women with mild to moderate hypercholesterolemia. *Atherosclerosis* 2000;152:143-7.

3376 Umland EM, Cauffield JS, Kirk JK, et al. Phytoestrogens as therapeutic alternatives to traditional hormone replacement in postmenopausal women. *Pharmacother* 2000;20:981-90.

3378 Nakagawa H, Yamamoto D, Kiyozuka Y, et al. Effects of genistein and synergistic action in combination with eicosapentaenoic acid on the growth of breast cancer cell lines. *J Cancer Res Clin Oncol* 2000;126:448-54.

3380 Lu LJ, Lin SN, Grady JJ, et al. Altered kinetics and extent of urinary daidzein and genistein excretion in women during chronic soya exposure. *Nutr Cancer* 1996;26:289-302.

3381 Kantha SS, Wada S, Tanaka H, et al. Carnosine sustains the retention of cell morphology in continuous fibroblast culture subjected to nutritional insult. *Biochem Biophys Res Commun* 1996;223:278-82.

3382 Anon. Black cohosh: was Lydia E. Pinkham on to something? *UC Berkeley Wellness Letter* 2001;17:5.

3383 Edmunds J. Blue cohosh and newborn myocardial infarction? *Midwifery Today Int Midwife* 1999;52:34-5.

3384 Davis BR, Oberman A, Blaufox MD, et al. Lack of effectiveness of a low-sodium/high-potassium diet in reducing antihypertensive medication requirements in overweight persons with mild hypertension. *Am J Hypertens* 1994;7:926-32.

3385 Whelton PK, He J, Cutler JA, et al. Effects of oral potassium on blood pressure. Meta-analysis of randomized controlled clinical trials. *JAMA* 1997;277:1624-32.

3386 Whelton PK, Buring J, Borhani NO, et al. The effect of potassium supplementation in persons with a high-normal blood pressure. Results from phase 1 of the trials of hypertension prevention (TOHP). *Ann Epidemiol* 1995;5:85-95.

3387 Zand RS, Jenkins DJ, Diamandis EP. Steroid hormone activity of flavonoids and related compounds. *Breast Cancer Res Treat* 2000;62:35-49.

3390 Zaloga GP, Roberts PR, Black KW, et al. Carnosine is a novel peptide modulator of intracellular calcium and contractility in cardiac cells. *Am J Physiol* 1997;272:H462-8.

3391 Maynard LM, Boissonneault GA, Chow CK, Bruckner GG. High levels of dietary carnosine are associated with increased concentrations of carnosine and histidine in rat soleus muscle. *J Nutr* 2001;131:287-90.

3392 Terkelsen LH, Eskild-Jensen A, Kjeldsen H, et al. Topical application of cod liver oil ointment accelerates wound healing: an experimental study in wounds in the ears of hairless mice. *Scand J Plast Reconstr Surg Hand Surg* 2000;34:15-20.

3393 Borchers AT, Stern JS, Hackman RM, et al. Mushrooms, tumors, and immunity. *Proc Soc Exp Biol Med* 1999;221:281-293.

3394 Ooi VE, Liu F. Immunomodulation and anti-cancer activity of polysaccharide-protein complexes. *Curr Med Chem* 2000;7:715-29.

3395 Veierod MB, Thelle DS, Laake P. Diet and risk of cutaneous malignant melanoma: a prospective study of 50,757 Norwegian men and women. *Int J Cancer* 1997;71:600-4.

3396 Dawson JK, Abernethy VE, Graham DR, Lynch MP. A woman who took cod-liver oil and smoked. *Lancet* 1996;347:1804.

3397 Lombardo YB, Chicco A, D'Alessandro ME, et al. Dietary fish oil normalize dyslipidemia and glucose intolerance with unchanged insulin levels in rats fed a high sucrose diet. *Biochim Biophys Acta* 1996;1299:175-82.

3398 Stammers T, Sibbald B, Freeling P. Efficacy of cod liver oil as an adjunct to non-steroidal anti-inflammatory drug treatment in the management of osteoarthritis in general practice. *Ann Rheum Dis* 1992;51:128-9.

3399 Jensen T, Stender S, Goldstein K, et al. Partial normalization by dietary cod-liver oil of increased microvascular albumin leakage in patients with insulin-dependent diabetes and albuminuria. *N Engl J Med* 1989;321:1572-7.

3400 Committee on Nutrition, American Academy of Pediatrics. Soy protein-based formulas: recommendations for use in infant feeding. *Pediatrics* 1998;101:148-53.

3401 Anderson JW, Johnstone BM, Cook-Newell ME. Meta-analysis of the effects of soy protein intake on serum lipids. *N Engl J Med* 1995;333:276-82.

3402 Crouse JR III, Morgan T, Terry JG, et al. A randomized trial comparing the effect of casein with that of soy protein containing varying amounts of isoflavones on plasma concentrations of lipids and lipoproteins. *Arch Intern Med* 1999;159:2070-6.

3403 Zhu JS, Halpern GM, Jones K. The scientific rediscovery of an ancient Chinese herbal medicine: Cordyceps sinensis: part I. *J Altern Complement Med* 1998;4:289-303.

3404 Zhu JS, Halpern GM, Jones K. The scientific rediscovery of a precious ancient Chinese herbal regimen: Cordyceps sinensis: part II. *J Altern Complement Med* 1998;4:429-57.

3405 Rossetti L, Hawkins M, Chen W, et al. In vivo glucosamine infusion induces insulin resistance in normoglycemic but not in hyperglycemic conscious rats. *J Clin Invest* 1995;96:132-40.

3406 Shankar RR, Zhu JS, Baron AD. Glucosamine infusion in rats mimics the beta-cell dysfunction of non-insulin-dependent diabetes mellitus. *Metabolism* 1998;47:573-7.

3407 Nakamura K, Yamaguchi Y, Kagota S, et al. Inhibitory effect of Cordyceps sinensis on spontaneous liver metastasis of Lewis lung carcinoma and B16 melanoma cells in syngeneic mice. *Jpn J Pharmacol* 1999;79:335-41.

3409 Chiu JH, Ju CH, Wu LH, et al. Cordyceps sinensis increases the expression of major histocompatibility complex class II antigens on human hepatoma cell line HA22T/VGH cells. *Am J Chin Med* 1998;26:159-70.

3410 Bok JW, Lermer L, Chilton J, et al. Antitumor sterols from the mycelia of Cordyceps sinensis. *Phytochemistry* 1999;51:891-8.

3411 Li LS, Zheng F, Liu ZH. [Experimental study on effect of Cordyceps sinensis in ameliorating aminoglycoside induced nephrotoxicity]. [Article in Chinese]. *Chung Kuo Chung Hsi I Chieh Ho Tsa Chih* 1996;16:733-7.

3412 Wang SM, Lee LJ, Lin WW, Chang CM. Effects of a water-soluble extract of Cordyceps sinensis on steroidogenesis and capsular morphology of lipid droplets in cultured rat adrenocortical cells. *J Cell Biochem* 1998;69:483-9.

3414 Chen YJ, Shiao MS, Lee SS, Wang SY. Effect of Cordyceps sinensis on the proliferation and differentiation of human leukemic U937 cells. *Life Sci* 1997;60:2349-59.

3415 Kiho T, Yamane A, Hui J, et al. Polysaccharides in fungi. XXXVI. Hypoglycemic activity of a polysaccharide (CS-F30) from the cultural mycelium of Cordyceps sinensis and its effect on glucose metabolism in mouse liver. *Biol Pharm Bull* 1996;19:294-6.

3416 Kuo YC, Tsai WJ, Shiao MS, et al. Cordyceps sinensis as an immunomodulatory agent. *Am J Chin Med* 1996;24:111-25.

3417 Zhou DH, Lin LZ. [Effect of Jinshuibao capsule on the immunological function of 36 patients with advanced cancer]. [Article in Chinese]. *Chung Kuo Chung Hsi I Chieh Ho Tsa Chih* 1995;15:476-8.

3418 Xu F, Huang JB, Jiang L, et al. Amelioration of cyclosporin nephrotoxicity by Cordyceps sinensis in kidney-transplanted recipients. *Nephrol Dial Transplant* 1995;10:142-3.

3419 Bao ZD, Wu ZG, Zheng F. [Amelioration of aminoglycoside nephrotoxicity by Cordyceps sinensis in old patients]. [Article in Chinese]. *Chung Kuo Chung Hsi I Chieh Ho Tsa Chih* 1994;14:271-3, 259.

3420 Kuo YC, Lin CY, Tsai WJ, et al. Growth inhibitors against tumor cells in Cordyceps sinensis other than cordycepin and polysaccharides. *Cancer Invest* 1994;12:611-5.

3421 Kiho T, Hui J, Yamane A, Ukai S. Polysaccharides in fungi. XXXII. Hypoglycemic activity and chemical properties of a polysaccharide from the cultural mycelium of Cordyceps sinensis. *Biol Pharm Bull* 1993;16:1291-3.

3424 Chen JR, Yen JH, Lin CC, et al. The effects of Chinese herbs on improving survival and inhibiting anti-ds DNA antibody production in lupus mice. *Am J Chin Med* 1993;21:257-62.

3425 Liu C, Lu S, Ji MR. [Effects of Cordyceps sinensis (CS) on in vitro natural killer cells]. [Article in Chinese]. *Chung Kuo Chung Hsi I Chieh Ho Tsa Chih* 1992;12:267-9, 259.

3427 Xu RH, Peng XE, Chen GZ, Chen GL. Effects of cordyceps sinensis on natural killer activity and colony formation of B16 melanoma. *Chin Med J* (English) 1992;105:97-101.

3428 Cheng Q. [Effect of cordyceps sinensis on cellular immunity in rats with chronic renal insufficiency]. [Article in Chinese]. *Chung Hua I Hsueh Tsa Chih* (Taipei) 1992;72:27-9, 63.

3429 Zhao Y. [Inhibitory effects of alcoholic extract of Cordyceps sinensis on abdominal aortic thrombus formation in rabbits]. [Article in Chinese]. *Chung Hua I Hsueh Tsa Chih* (Taipei) 1991;71:612-5, 42.

3431 Chen GZ, Chen GL, Sun T, et al. Effects of Cordyceps sinensis on murine T lymphocyte subsets. *Chin Med J* (English) 1991;104:4-8.

3432 Zhu XY, Yu HY. [Immunosuppressive effect of cultured Cordyceps sinensis on cellular immune response]. [Article in Chinese]. *Chung Hsi I Chieh Ho Tsa Chih* 1990;10:485-7, 454.

3434 Yamaguchi N, Yoshida J, Ren LJ, et al. Augmentation of various immune reactivities of tumor-bearing hosts with an extract of Cordyceps sinensis. *Biotherapy* 1990;2:199-205.

3435 Zhou L, Yang W, Xu Y, et al. [Short-term curative effect of cultured Cordyceps sinensis (Berk.) Sacc. Mycelia in chronic hepatitis B]. [Article in Chinese]. *Chung Kuo Chung Yao Tsa Chih* 1990;15:53-5, 65.

3436 Mei QB, Tao JY, Gao SB, et al. [Antiarrhythmic effects of Cordyceps sinensis (Berk.) Sacc]. [Article in Chinese]. *Chung Kuo Chung Yao Tsa Chih* 1989;14:616-8, 640.

3437 Yoshida J, Takamura S, Yamaguchi N, et al. Antitumor activity of an extract of Cordyceps sinensis (Berk.) Sacc. against murine tumor cell lines. *Jpn J Exp Med* 1989;59:157-61.

3450 Geleijnse JM, Launer LJ, Hofman A, et al. Tea flavonoids may protect against atherosclerosis: the Rotterdam Study. *Arch Intern Med* 1999;159:2170-4.

3451 Schechter JO. Treatment of disequilibrium and nausea in the SRI discontinuation syndrome. *J Clin Psychiatry* 1998;59:431-2.

3452 Arfeen Z, Owen H, Plummer JL, et al. A double-blind randomized controlled trial of ginger for the prevention of postoperative nausea and vomiting. *Anaesth Intensive Care* 1995;23:449-52.

3453 Visalyaputra S, Petchpaisit N, Somcharoen K, Choavaratana R. The efficacy of ginger root in the prevention of postoperative nausea and vomiting after outpatient gynaecological laparoscopy. *Anaesthesia* 1998;53:506-10.

3454 Linos A, Kaklamani VG, Kaklamani E, et al. Dietary factors in relation to rheumatoid arthritis: a role for olive oil and cooked vegetables? *Am J Clin Nutr* 1999;70:1077-82.

3455 Penny ME, Peerson JM, Marin RM, et al. Randomized, community-based trial of the effect of zinc supplementation, with and without other micronutrients, on the duration of persistent childhood diarrhea in Lima, Peru. *J Pediatr* 1999;135:208-17.

3456 Bhutta ZA, Black RE, Brown KH, et al. Prevention of diarrhea and pneumonia by zinc supplementation in children in developing countries: pooled analysis of randomized controlled trials. *J Pediatr* 1999;135:689-97.

3457 Korschunov VM, Smeyanov VV, Efimov BA, et al. Therapeutic use of an antibiotic-resistant Bifidobacterium preparation in men exposed to high-dose gamma-irradiation. *J Med Microbiol* 1996;44:70-4.

3458 Isolauri E, Arvola T, Sutas Y, et al. Probiotics in the management of atopic eczema. *Clin Exp Allergy* 2000;30:1604-10.

3460 Korting GE, Smith SD, Wheeler MA, et al. A randomized double-blind trial of oral L-arginine for treatment of interstitial cystitis. *J Urol* 1999;161:558-65.

3461 Schweizer J, Hautmann C. Comparison of two dosages of Ginkgo biloba extract Egb 761 in patients with peripheral arterial occlusive disease Fontain's stage llb / a randomised, double-blind, multicentric clinical trial. *Arzneimittelforschung* 1999;49:900-4.

3462 Hawkins EB. NADH: Advanced supplementation for more energy and slower aging. *Natural Pharmacy* 1998;2:10.

3463 Kyriakidou-Himonas M, Aloia JF, Yeh JK. Vitamin D supplementation in postmenopausal black women. *J Clin Endocrinol Metab* 1999;84:3988-90.

3464 Zamora SA, Rizzoli R, Belli DC, et al. Vitamin D supplementation during infancy is associated with higher bone mineral mass in prepubertal girls. *J Clin Endocrinol Metab* 1999;84:4541-4.

3465 Boger RH, Bode-Boger SM, Thiele W, et al. Restoring vascular nitric oxide formation by L-arginine improves the symptoms of intermittent claudication in patients with peripheral arterial occlusive disease. *J Am Coll Cardiol* 1998;32:1336-44.

3466 Boger RH, Bode-Boger SM, Thiele W, et al. Biochemical evidence for impaired nitric oxide synthesis in patients with peripheral arterial occlusive disease. *Circulation* 1997;95:2068-74.

3467 Niittynen L, Nurminen ML, Korpela R, et al. Role of arginine, taurine, and homocysteine in cardiovascular diseases. *Ann Med* 1999;31:318-26.

3469 Butland BK, Fehily AM, Elwood PC. Diet and lung function decline in a cohort of 2512 middle aged men. *Thorax* 2000;55(2):102-8.

3470 Le Marchand L, Murphy SP, Hankin JH, et al. Intake of flavonoids and lung cancer. *J Natl Cancer Inst* 2000;92(2):154-60.

3471 Gulyas A, Repges R, Dethlefsen U. Therapy of chronic obstructive pulmonary diseases in children. *Atemwegs und Lungenkrankheiten* 1997;23:291-4.

3472 Dekkers R. Apple juice and the chemical-contact softening of gallstones. *Lancet* 1999;354(9196):2171.

3473 Sinniah D, Baskaran G. Margosa oil poisoning as a cause of Reye's syndrome. *Lancet* 1981;1(8218):487-9.

3474 Sinniah D, Baskaran G, Looi LM, Leong KL. Reye-like syndrome due to margosa oil poisoning: report of a case with postmortem findings. *Am J Gastroenterol* 1982;77(3):158-61.

3475 Sinniah R, Sinniah D, Chia LS, Baskaran G. Animal model of margosa oil ingestion with Reye-like syndrome. Pathogenesis of microvesicular fatty liver. *J Pathol* 1989;159(3):255-64.

3476 Lai SM, Lim KW, Cheng HK. Margosa oil poisoning as a cause of toxic encephalopathy. *Singapore Med J* 1990;31:463-5.

3477 Furbee B, Wermuth M. Life-threatening plant poisoning. *Crit Care Clin* 1997;13(4):849-88.

3478 Lewis WH, Smith PR. Poke root herbal tea poisoning. *JAMA* 1979;242:2759-60.

3479 Roberge R, Brader E, Martin ML, et al. The root of evil-pokeweed intoxication. *Ann Emerg Med* 1986;15:470-3.

3480 Jaeckle KA, Freemon FR. Pokeweed poisoning. *South Med J* 1981;74(5):639-40.

3481 Barker BE, Farnes P, LaMarche PH. Haematological effects of pokeweed. *Lancet* 1967;1:437.

3482 Kell SO, Rosenberg SA, Conlon TJ, Spyker DA. A peek at poke: mitogenicity and epidemiology. *Vet Hum Toxicol* 1982;24:36.

3483 Anon. Toxic reactions to plant products sold in health food stores. *Med Lett Drugs Ther* 1979;21:29-32.

3484 Klepser TB, Klepser ME. Unsafe and potentially safe herbal therapies. *Am J Health Syst Pharm* 1999;56:125-38.

3485 Plushner SL. Valerian: Valerian officinalis. *Am J Health Syst Pharm* 2000;57:328,333,335.

3486 Houghton PJ. The scientific basis for the reputed activity of Valerian. *J Pharm Pharmacol* 1999;51(5):505-12.

3487 Garges HP, Varia I, Doraiswamy PM. Cardiac complications and delirium associated with Valerian root withdrawal. [Letter to the Editor] *JAMA* 1998;280:1566-7.

3488 Tuncok Y, Kozan O, Cavdar C, et al. Urginea maritima (squill) toxicity. *J Toxicol Clin Toxicol* 1995;33(1):83-6.

3489 Wax PM. Squill through the ages. *J Toxicol Clin Toxicol* 1995;33(1):86.

3490 But PP, Tai YT, Young K. Three fatal cases of herbal aconite poisoning. *Vet Hum Toxicol* 1994;36(3):212-5.

3491 Feldkamp A, Koster B, Weber HP. [Fatal poisoning caused by aconite monk's hood]. [Article in German]. *Monatsschr Kinderheilkd* 1991;139(6):366-7.

3492 Hallstrom H, Thuvander A. Toxicological evaluation of myristicin. *Nat Toxins* 1997;5(5):186-92.

3493 Jeong HG, Yun CH. Induction of rat hepatic cytochrome P450 enzymes by myristicin. *Biochem Biophys Res Commun* 1995;217:966-71.

3494 Dinakar HS. Acute psychosis associated with nutmeg toxicity. *Med Times* 1977;105:63-4.

3495 Haynes BE, Bessen HA, Wightman WD. Oleander tea: herbal draught of death. *Ann Emerg Med* 1985;14(4):350-3.

3496 Biberoglu S, Biberoglu K, Komsuoglu B. Mad honey. [Letter to the Editor] *JAMA* 1988;259:1943.

3497 Sheikh NM, Philen RM, Love LA. Chaparral-associated hepatotoxicity. *Arch Intern Med* 1997;157:913-9.

3499 Davies JH. Abrus precatorius (rosary pea). The most common lethal plant poison. *J Fla Med Assoc* 1978;65:188-91.

3500 Herschler R. Methylsulfonylmethane in dietary products. US patent no. 4,616,039; 1986.

3501 Richmond VL. Incorporation of methylsulfonylmethane sulfur into guinea pig serum proteins. *Life Sci* 1986;39:263-8.

3502 O'Dwyer PJ, et al. Use of polar solvents in chemoprevention of 1,2-dimethylhydrazine-induced colon cancer. *Cancer* 1988;62:944-8.

3503 McCabe D, et al. Polar solvents in the chemoprevention of dimethylbenzanthracene-induced rat mammary cancer. *Arch Surg* 1986;62:1455-9.

3504 Klandorf H, et al. Dimethyl sulfoxide modulation of diabetes onset in NOD mice. *Diabetes* 1998;62:194-7.

3508 Godley PA. Essential fatty acid consumption and risk of breast cancer. *Breast Cancer Res Treat* 1995;35:91-5.

3509 Malloy MJ, Kane JP. Agents used in hyperlipidemia. In: B. Katzung, ed. Basic and Clinical Pharmacology. 4th ed. Norwald, CT: Appleton and Lange, 1989.

3510 Rose DP. The mechanistic rationale in support of dietary cancer prevention. *Prev Med* 1996;25:34-7.

3511 Noguchi M, Rose DP, Earashi M, et al. The role of fatty acids and eicosanoid synthesis inhibitors in breast carcinoma. *Oncology* 1995;52:265-71.

3512 Balch JF, Balch PA. Prescription for Nutritional Healing. Garden City Park, NY: Avery Publ Group.

3513 Thien FC, Leung R, Baldo BA, et al. Asthma and anaphylaxis induced by royal jelly. *Clin Exp Allergy* 1996;26:216-22.

3514 Roger A, Rubira N, Nogueiras C, et al. [Anaphylaxis caused by royal jelly]. [Article in Spanish]. *Allergol Immunopathol* (Madr) 1995;23:133-5.

3515 Vittek J. Effect of royal jelly on serum lipids in experimental animals and humans with atherosclerosis. *Experientia* 1995;51:927-35.

3516 Yonei Y, Shibagaki K, Tsukada N, et al. Case report: haemorrhagic colitis associated with royal jelly intake. *J Gastroenterol Hepatol* 1997;12:495-9.

3521 Iruela LM, Minguez L, Merino J, Monedero G. Toxic interaction of S-adenosylmethionine and clomipramine. *Am J Psych* 1993;150:522.

3523 Carney MW, Chary TK, Bottiglieri T, et al. The switch mechanism and the bipolar/unipolar dichotomy. *Br J Psychiatry* 1989;154:48-51.

3524 Schneck C. St. John's wort and hypomania. *J Clin Psychiatry* 1998;59:689.

3525 Adverse Drug Reactions Advisory Committee. An adverse reaction to the herbal medication milk thistle (Silybum marianum). *Med J Aust* 1999;170:218-9.

3526 Page RL II, Lawrence JD. Potentiation of warfarin by dong quai. *Pharmacotherapy* 1999;19:870-6.

3529 D'Adamo P. Larch arabinogalactan. *J Naturopath Med* 1996;6:33-7.

3530 Kelly GS. Larch arabinogalactan: Clinical relevance of a novel immune-enhancing polysaccharide. *Alt Med Rev* 1999;4:96-103.

3531 Anon. Best herb for fighting off colds. *Bottom Line* 1999;20:1.

3535 Anon. Toxic algae in lake Sammamish. King County, WA. October 28, 1998; Available at: splash.metrokc.gov/wlr/waterres/lakes/bloom.htm (Accessed 5 December 1999).

3536 Anon. Health Canada announces results of blue-green algal products testing – only Spirulina found Microcystin-free. Health Canada, September 27, 1999; Available at: www.hc-

REFERENCES

sc.gc.ca/english/archives/releases/99_114e.htm (Accessed 27 October 1999).

3540 Ziegler D, Hanefeld M, Ruhnau K, et al. Treatment of symptomatic diabetic polyneuropathy with the antioxidant alpha-lipoic acid: A 7-month, multicenter, randomized, controlled trial (ALADIN III Study). *Diabetes Care* 1999;22:1296-301.

3541 Reljanovic M, Reichel G, Rett K, et al. Treatment of diabetic polyneuropathy with the antioxidant thioctic acid (alpha-lipoic acid): A 2-year, multicenter, randomized, double-blind, placebo-controlled trial (ALADIN II). Alpha Lipoic Acid in Diabetic Neuropathy. *Free Radic Res* 1999;31:171-7.

3542 Ziegler D, Schatz H, Conrad F, et al. Effects of treatment with the antioxidant alpha-lipoic acid on cardiac autonomic neuropathy in NIDDM patients. *Diabetes Care* 1997;20:369-73.

3544 Streeper RS, Henriksen EJ, Jacob S, et al. Differential effects of lipoic acid stereoisomers on glucose metabolism in insulin-resistant skeletal muscle. *Am J Physiol* 1997;273:E185-91.

3545 Konrad T, Vicini P, Kusterer K, et al. Alpha-lipoic acid treatment decreases serum lactate and pyruvate concentrations and improves glucose effectiveness in lean and obese patients with Type 2 diabetes. *Diabetes Care* 1999;22:280-7.

3546 Packer L. Antioxidant properties of lipoic acid and its therapeutic effects in prevention of diabetes complications and cataracts. *Ann N Y Acad Sci* 1994;738:257-64.

3547 Schempp CM, Winghofer B, Langheinrich M, et al. Hypericin levels in human serum and interstitial skin blister fluid after oral single-dose and steady state administration of Hypericum perforatum extract (St. John's Wort). *Skin Pharmacol Appl Skin Physiol* 1999;12:299-304.

3548 Kim HL, Streltzer J, Goebert D. St. John's wort for depression: A meta analysis of well-defined clinical trials. *J Nerv Ment Dis* 1999;187:532-9.

3549 Linde K, Ramirez G, Mulrow CD, et al. St. John's wort for depression: an overview and meta-analysis of randomized clinical trials. *BMJ* 1996;313:253-8.

3550 Harrer G, Schmidt U, Kuhn U, Biller A. Comparison of equivalence between the St. John's wort extract LoHyp-57 and fluoxetine. *Arzneimittelforschung* 1999;49:289-96.

3551 Philipp M, Kohnen R, Hiller KO. Hypericum extract versus imipramine or placebo in patients with moderate depression: randomized mulicentre study of treatment for eight weeks. *BMJ* 1999;319:1534-9.

3552 Gaster B, Holroyd J. St John's wort for depression. *Arch Intern Med* 2000;160:152-6.

3553 Singer A, Wonnemann M, Muller WE. Hyperforin, a major antidepressant constituent of St. John's wort, inhibits serotonin uptake by elevating free intracellular Na+11. *J Pharmacol Exp Ther* 1999;290:1363-8.

3554 Schempp C, Pelz K, Wittmer A, et al. Antibacterial activity of hyperforin from St. John's wort, against multiresistant Stapylococcus aureus and gram-positive bacteria. *Lancet* 1999;353:2129.

3555 Nierenberg AA, Burt T, Matthews J, et al. Mania associated with St. John's wort. *Biol Psychiatry* 1999;46:1707-8.

3556 Nebel A, Schneider BJ, Baker RA, et al. Potential metabolic interaction between St. John's wort and theophylline. *Ann Pharmacother* 1999;33:502.

3557 Ziegler D, Hanefeld M, Ruhnau KJ, et al. Treatment of symptomatic diabetic peripheral neuropathy with the antioxidant alpha-lipoic acid: A 3-week, multicenter, randomized, controlled trial (ALADIN Study). *Diabetologia* 1995;38:1425-33.

3558 Huang KC. The Pharmacology of Chinese Herbs. 2nd ed. Boca Raton, FL: CRC Press, 1999:267.

3559 Upton R, ed. Schisandra Berry: Analytical, quality control, and therapeutic monograph. Santa Cruz, CA: American Herbal Pharmacopoeia 1999;1-25.

3561 Pepping J. Huperzine A. *Am J Health Syst Pharm* 2000;57:530-4.

3562 Gaster B. S-adenosylmethionine (SAMe) for treatment of depression. *Alternative Medicine Alert* 1999;12:133-5.

3563 Chevallier A. Encyclopedia of Medicinal Plants. New York, NY: DK Publishing, 1996;202.

3564 Anon. Lapacho. The Natural Pharmacist 2000. Available at: http://www.tnp.com/substance.asp?ID=67 (Accessed 7 April 2000).

3567 Anon. Colostrum. The Natural Pharmacist. Prima Communications, Inc., 2000. Available at: http://www.tnp.com/substance.asp?ID=121 (Accessed 5 May 2000).

3568 Moses EL, Mallinger AG. St. John's wort: Three cases of possible mania induction. *J Clin Psychopharmacol* 2000;20:115-7.

3569 Beckman SE, Sommi RW, Switzer J. Consumer use of St. John's wort: A survey of effectiveness, safety, and tolerability. *Pharmacotherapy* 2000;20:568-74.

3570 Ereshefsky B, Gewertz N, Lam YMF, et al. Determination of SJW differential metabolism at CYP2D6 and CYP3A4, using dextromethorphan probe methodology. Abstract Poster Presentations, 39th NCDEU Annual Meeting, 1999:Poster 130 128.

3571 Gewertz N, Ereshefsky B, Lam YWF, et al. Determination of the differential effects of St. John's wort on the CYP1A2 and NAT2 metabolic pathways using caffeine probe methodology. Abstract Poster Presentations, 39th NCDEU Annual Meeting, 1999:Poster 131.

3573 Towheed TE, Anastassiades TP. Glucosamine and Chondriotin for treating symptoms of osteoarthritis. Evidence is widely touted but incomplete. *JAMA* 2000;238:1483-4.

3574 Anon. Bee Propolis. MotherNature.com 1999. Available at: http://www.mothernature.com/library/books/natmed/bee_propolis.asp (Accessed 28 May 2000).

3577 Anon. PC-SPES. UCSF Cancer Center Communications 2000. Available at: http://cc.ucsf.edu/clinical/uro_pc-spes.html (Accessed 2 June 2000).

3579 Meyer AS, Yi OS, Pearson DA, et al. Inhibition of human low-density lipoprotein oxidation in relation to composition of phenolic antioxidants in grapes (Vitis vinifera). *J Agric Food Chem* 1997;45:1638-43.

3580 Anon. OPCs (Oligomeric Proanthocyanidins). The Natural Pharmacist 2000. Available at: http://www.tnp.com/substance.asp?ID=181. (Accessed 3 June 2000).

3581 Murray MT. Natural Alternatives to Over-the-Counter and Prescription Drugs. New York, NY: Quill, 1994.

3582 Pizzorno JE, Murray MT, eds. Textbook of Natural Medicine. 2nd ed. New York, NY: Chuchill Livingstone, 1999.

3583 Geva E, Bartoov B, Zabludovsky N, et al. The effect of antioxidant treatment on human spermatozoa and fertilization rate in an in vitro fertilization program. *Fertil Steril* 1996;66:430-4.

3585 Vezina D, Mauffette F, Roberts KD, et al. Selenium-vitamin E supplementation in infertile men. Effects on semen parameters and micronutrient levels and distribution. *Biol Trace Elem Res* 1996;53:65-83.

3586 Cowart CL, London SN, Vernon MW, Pedigo NG. The effects of cyclic adenosine monophosphate, forskolin, and theophylline on motility parameters in gossypol-treated human sperm. *Fertil Steril* 1994;61:929-34.

3587 Gregory PJ. Probiotics for antibiotic-associated diarrhea. *Pharmacist's Letter/Prescriber's Letter* 2000;16:160103.

3588 Pizzorno JE, Murray MT, eds. Textbook of Natural Medicine. 2nd ed. Edinburgh: Churchill Livingstone, 1999.

3589 Meydani SN, Ha WK. Immunologic effects of yogurt. *Am J Clin Nutr* 2000;71:861-72.

3590 Agerholm-Larsen L, Raben A, Haulrik N, et al. Effect of 8 week intake of probiotic milk products on risk factors for cardiovascular diseases. *Eur J Clin Nutr* 2000;54:288-97.

3591 Anon. Female Viagra equivalent now available – Topical Natural Sensation from Strategic Science and Technologies, Inc. PRNewswire May 25, 2000.

3593 Blum A, Porat R, Rosenschein U, et al. Clinical and inflammatory effects of dietary L-arginine in patients with intractable angina pectoris. *Am J Cardiol* 1999;15:1488-90.

3594 Tentolouris C, Tousoulis D, Toutouzas P, et al. Effects of acute L-arginine administration in coronary atherosclerosis [letter]. *Circulation* 1999;99:1648.

3595 Rector TS, Bank AJ, Mullen KA, et al. Randomized, double-blind, placebo-controlled study of supplemental oral L-arginine in patients with heart failue. *Circulation* 1996;93:2135-41.

3596 Watanabe G, Tomiyama H, Doba N. Effects of oral administration of L-arginine on renal function in patients with heart failure. *J Hypertens* 2000;18:229-34.

3598 Kehoe WA. Vitamin E for neuroleptic-induced tardive dyskinesia. *Pharmacist's Letter/Prescriber's Letter* 1999;15:150105.

3599 Markowitz JS, DeVane CL, Boulton DW, et al. Effect of St. John's wort (Hypericum perforatum) on cytochrome P-450 2D6 and 3A4 activity in healthy volunteers. *Life Sci* 2000;66:PL133-9.

3600 Salvioli G, Neri M. L-acetylcarnitine treatment of mental decline in the elderly. *Drugs Exp Clin Res* 1994;20:169-76.

3601 Passeri M, Cucinotta D, Bonati PA, et al. Acetyl-L-carnitine in the treatment of mildly demented elderly patients. *Int J Clin Pharmacol Res* 1990;10:75-9.

3602 Bella R, Biondi R, Raffaele R, Pennisi G. Effect of acetyl-L-carnitine on geriatric patients suffering from dysthymic disorders. *Int J Clin Pharmacol Res* 1990;10:355-60.

3603 Garzya G, Corallo D, Fiore A, et al. Evaluation of the effects of L-acetylcarnitine on senile patients suffering from depression. *Drugs Exp Clin Res* 1990;16:101-6.

3604 Tempesta E, Casella L, Pirrongelli C, et al. L-acetylcarnitine in depressed elderly subjects. A cross-over study vs placebo. *Drugs Exp Clin Res* 1987;13:417-23.

3605 Di Marzio L, Moretti S, D'Alo S, et al. Acetyl-L-carnitine administration increases insulin-like growth factor 1 levels in asymptomatic HIV-1-infected subjects: correlation with its suppressive effect on lymphocyte apoptosis and ceramide generation. *Clin Immunol* 1999;92:103-10.

3606 Famularo G, Moretti S, Marcellini S, et al. Acetyl-carnitine deficiency in AIDS patients with neurotoxicity on treatment with antiretroviral nucleoside analogues. *AIDS* 1997;11:185-90.

3607 Moncada ML, Vicari E, Cimino C, et al. Effect of acetylcarnitine treatment in oligoasthenospermic patients. *Acta Europ Fertil* 1992;23:221-4.

3608 Jeulin C, Lewin LM. Role of free L-carnitine and acetyl-L-carnitine in post-gonadal maturation of mammalian spermatozoa. *Hum Reprod Update* 1996;2:87-102.

3609 Jeulin C, Soufir JC, Marson J, et al. [Acetylcarnitine and spermatozoa: relationship with epididymal maturation and motility in the boar and man]. [Article in French]. *Reprod Nutr Develop* 1988;28:1317-27.

3610 Golan R, Weissenberg R, Lewin LM. Carnitine and acetylcarnitine in motile and immotile human spermatozoa. *Int J Androl* 1984;7:484-94.

3611 Kohengkul S, Tanphaichitr V, Muangmun V, Tanphaichitr N. Levels of L-carnitine and L-O-acetylcarnitine in normal and infertile human semen: a lower level of L-O-acetycarnitine in infertile semen. *Fertil Steril* 1977;28:1333-6.

3612 Tanphaichitr N. In vitro stimulation of human sperm motility by acetylcarnitine. *Int J Fertil* 1977;22:85-91.

3616 Anon. *Carnitor* (levocarnitine) package insert. Sigma-Tau Pharmaceuticals Inc, Gaithersburg, MD. December 1999.

3617 Mintz M. Carnitine in human immunodeficiency virus type 1 infection/acquired immune deficiency syndrome. *J Child Neurol* 1995;10:S40-4.

3618 Dalakas MC, Leon-Monzon ME, Bernardini I, et al. Zidovudine-induced mitochondrial myopathy is associated with muscle carnitine deficiency and lipid storage. *Ann Neurol* 1994;35:482-7.

3619 Georgala S, Schulpis KH, Georgala C, Michas T. L-carnitine supplementation in patients with cystic acne on isotretinoin therapy. *J Eur Acad Dermatol Venereol* 1999;13:205-9.

3620 Ramos AC, Barrucand L, Elias PR, et al. Carnitine supplementation in diphtheria. *Indian Pediatr* 1992;29:1501-5.

3621 Ramos AC, Elias PR, Barrucand L, Da Silva JA. The protective effect of carnitine in human diphtheric myocarditis. *Pediatr Res* 1984;18:815-9.

3622 Plioplys AV, Kasnicka I. L-carnitine as a treatment for Rett syndrome. *South Med J* 1993;86:1411-2.

3623 Cacciatore L, Cerio R, Ciarimboli M, et al. The therapeutic effect of L-carnitine in patients with exercise-induced stable angina: a controlled study. *Drugs Exp Clin Res* 1991;17:225-35.

3624 Cherchi A, Lai C, Angelino F, et al. Effects of L-carnitine on exercise tolerance in chronic stable angina: a multicenter, double-blind, randomized, placebo-controlled, crossover study. *Int J Clin Pharmacol Ther Toxicol* 1985;23:569-72.

3625 Rizos I. Three-year survival of patients with heart failure caused by dilated cardiomyopathy and L-carnitine administration. *Am Heart J* 2000;139:S120-3.

3626 Ghidini O, Azzurro M, Vita G, Sartori G. Evaluation of the therapeutic efficacy of L-carnitine in congestive heart failure. *Int J Clin Pharmacol Ther Toxicol* 1988;26:217-20.

3627 Singh RB, Niaz MA, Agarwal P, et al. A randomized, double-blind, placebo-controlled trial of L-carnitine in suspected acute myocardial infarction. *Postgrad Med J* 1996;72:45-50.

3628 Iliceto S, Scrutinio D, Bruzzi P, et al. Effects of L-carnitine administration on left ventricular remodeling after acute anterior myocardial infarction: the L-Carnitine Ecocardiografia Digitalizzata Infarto Miocardico (CEDIM) Trial. *J Am Coll Cardiol* 1995;26:380-7.

3629 Davini P, Bigalli A, Lamanna F, Boem A. Controlled study on L-carnitine therapeutic efficacy in post-infarction. *Drugs Exp Clin Res* 1992;18:355-65.

3630 Plioplys AV, Plioplys S. Amantadine and L-carnitine treatment of Chronic Fatigue Syndrome. *Neuropsychobiology* 1997;35:16-23.

3631 Brevetti G, Chiariello M, Ferulano G, et al. Increases in walking distance in patients with peripheral vascular disease treated with L-carnitine: a double-blind, cross-over study. *Circulation* 1988;77:767-73.

3632 Cifone MG, Alesse E, Di Marzio L, et al. Effect of L-carnitine treatment in vivo on apoptosis and ceramide generation in peripheral blood lymphocytes from AIDS patients. *Proc Assoc Am Physicians* 1997;109:146-53.

3633 Scaglia F, Longo N. Primary and secondary alterations of neonatal carnitine metabolism. *Semin Perinatol* 1999;23:152-61.

3634 Bonner CM, DeBrie KL, Hug G, et al. Effects of parenteral L-carnitine supplementation on fat metabolism and nutrition in premature neonates. *J Pediatr* 1995;126:287-92.

3635 Schmidt-Sommerfeld E, Penn D. Carnitine and total parenteral nutrition of the neonate. *Biol Neonate* 1990;58:81-8.

3636 Melegh B, Kerner J, Sandor A, et al. Oral L-carnitine supplementation in low-birth-weight newborns: a study on neonates requiring combined parenteral and enteral nutrition. *Acta Paediatr Hung* 1986;27:253-8.

3637 Schmidt-Sommerfeld E, Penn D, Wolf H. Carnitine deficiency in premature infants receiving total parenteral nutrition: effect of L-carnitine supplementation. *J Pediatr* 1983;102:931-5.

3639 Heinonen OJ. Carnitine and physical exercise. *Sports Med* 1996;22:109-32.

3640 Berthillier G, Eichenberger D, Carrier HN, et al. Carnitine metabolism in early stages of Duchenne muscular dystrophy. *Clin Chim Acta* 1982;122:369-75.

3641 Marthaler NP, Visarius T, Kupfer A, Lauterburg BH. Increased urinary losses of carnitine during ifosfamide chemotherapy. *Cancer Chemother Pharmacol* 1999;44:170-2.

3642 Heuberger W, Berardi S, Jacky E, et al. Increased urinary excretion of carnitine in patients treated with cisplatin. *Eur J Clin Pharmacol* 1998;54:503-8.

3643 Schoderbeck M, Auer B, Legenstein E, et al. Pregnancy-related changes of carnitine and acylcarnitine concentrations of plasma and erythrocytes. *J Perinat Med* 1995;23:477-85.

3644 Novak M. Carnitine supplementation in soy-based formula-fed infants. *Biol Neonate* 1990;58:89-92.

3645 Goral S. Levocarnitine and muscle metabolism in patients with end-stage renal disease. *J Ren Nutr* 1998;8:118-21.

3646 Kletzmayr J, Mayer G, Legenstein E, et al. Anemia and carnitine supplementation in hemodialyzed patients. *Kidney Int* 1999;69:93-106.

3647 Ahmad S, Robertson HT, Golper TA, et al. Multicenter trial of L-carnitine in maintenance hemodialysis patients. II. Clinical and biochemical effects. *Kidney Int* 1990;38:912-8.

3648 Nuesch R, Rossetto M, Martina B. Plasma and urine carnitine concentrations in well-trained athletes at rest and after exercise. Influence of L-carnitine intake. *Drugs Exp Clin Res* 1999;25:167-71.

3649 Vecchiet L, Di Lisa F, Pieralisi G, et al. Influence of L-carnitine administration on maximal physical exercise. *Eur J Appl Physiol* 1990;61:486-90.

3650 Marconi C, Sassi G, Carpinelli A, Cerretelli P. Effects of L-carnitine loading on the aerobic and anaerobic performance of endurance athletes. *Eur J Appl Physiol* 1985;54:131-5.

3651 Mingrone G, Greco AV, Capristo E, et al. L-carnitine improves glucose disposal in type 2 diabetic patients. *J Am Coll Nutr* 1999;18:77-82.

3652 Capaldo B, Napoli R, Di Bonito P, et al. Carnitine improves peripheral glucose disposal in non-insulin-dependent diabetic patients. *Diabetes Res Clin Pract* 1991;14:191-5.

3653 Bertelli A, Ronca G. Carnitine and coenzyme Q10: biochemical properties and functions, synergism and complementary action. *Int J Tissue React* 1990;12:183-6.

3657 Coppen A, Bailey J. Enhancement of the antidepressant action of fluoxetine by folic acid: a randomised, placebo controlled trial. *J Affect Dis* 2000;60:121-31.

3658 Anon. W&B Associates Inc. website. URL http://www.wandb.com/cholesterol.6.htm (Accessed 30 March 2000).

3661 Patel SB, Honda A, Salen G. Sitosterolemia: exclusion of genes involved in reduced cholesterol biosynthesis. *J Lipid Res* 1998;39:1055-61.

3662 Salen G, Shore V, Tint GS, et al. Increased sitosterol absorption, decreased removal, and expanded body pools compensate for reduced cholesterol synthesis in sitosterolemia with xanthomatosis. *J Lipid Res* 1989;30:1319-30.

3663 Nguyen LB, Shefer S, Salen G, et al. Competitive inhibition of hepatic sterol 27-hydroxylase by sitosterol: decreased activity in sitosterolemia. *Proc Assoc Am Physicians* 1998;110:32-9.

3665 Jones PJ, MacDougall DE, Ntanios F, Vanstone CA. Dietary phytosterols as cholesterol-lowering agents in humans. *Can J Physiol Pharmacol* 1997;75(3):217-27.

3666 Heinemann T, Kullak-Ublick GA, Pietruck B, von Bergmann K. Mechanisms of action of plant sterols on inhibition of cholesterol absorption. Comparison of sitosterol and sitostanol. *Eur J Clin Pharmacol* 1991;40 Suppl 1:S59-63.

3667 Awad AB, von Holtz RL, Cone JP, et al. Beta-sitosterol inhibits growth of HT-29 human colon cancer cells by activating the sphingomyelin cycle. *Anticancer Res* 1998;18:471-3.

3668 Awad AB, Chen YC, Fink CS, Hennessey T. Beta-sitosterol inhibits HT-29 human colon cancer cell growth and alters membrane lipids. *Anticancer Res* 1996;16:2797-804.

3669 Bouic PJ, Etsebeth S, Liebenberg RW, et al. Beta-sitosterol and beta-sitosterol glucoside stimulate human peripheral blood lymphocyte proliferation: implications for their use as an immunomodulatory vitamin combination. *Int J Immunopharmacol* 1996;18:693-700.

3672 Hidaka H, Kojima H, Kawabata T, et al. Effects of an HMG-CoA reductase inhibitor, pravastatin, and bile sequestering resin, cholestyramine, on plasma plant sterol levels in hypercholesterolemic subjects. *J Atheroscler Thromb* 1995;2:60-5.

3673 Ntanios FY, Jones PJ, Frohlich JJ. Effect of 3-hydroxy-3-methylglutaryl coenzyme A reductase inhibitor on sterol absorption in hypercholesterolemic subjects. *Metabolism* 1999;48:68-73.

3678 Anon. FDA alert on misuse of consumer products containing GHB, GBL and BD. Food and Drug Administration, Rockville, MD. June 15, 1999. Available at: http://www.fda.gov/cder/graphics/ghb.gif.

3679 Anon. Important message for health professionals: Report serious adverse events associated with dietary supplements containing GBL, GHB or BD. Food and Drug Administration, Rockville, MD. August 25, 1999. Available at: http://vm.cfsan.fda.gov/~dms/mwgblghb.html.

3680 Otto A. Acquaintance rape drug may one day help instead of hurt (news). *Pharmacy Today*. American Pharmaceutical Association, Washington, DC. April 2000:17.

3681 Hillory J. Farias and Samantha Reid date-rape drug prohibition act of 2000. 106th Congress of the United States of America. HR 2130.

3682 Anon. Multistate outbreak of poisonings associated with illicit use of gamma hydroxy butyrate. *JAMA* 1991;265:447-8.

3683 Kalra MA, Hart LL. Gammahydroxybutyrate in narcolepsy. *Ann Pharmacother* 1992;26:647-8.

3684 Addolorato G, Cibin M, Caprista E, et al. Maintaining abstinence from alcohol with gamma hydroxybutyric acid. [Letter] *Lancet* 1998;351:38.

3685 Strong AJ. Gamma hydroxybutyric acid and intracranial pressure. [Letter] *Lancet* 1984;1(8389):1304.

3686 Gallimberti L, Canton G, Gentile N, et al. Gamma-hydroxybutyric acid for treatment of alcohol withdrawal syndrome. *Lancet* 1989;2:787-9.

3687 Smith KM. Drugs used in acquaintance rape. *J Am Pharm Assoc* 1999;39:519-25.

3688 Dyer JE. Gamma-Hydroxybutyrate: a health-food product producing coma and seizure-like activity. *Am J Emerg Med* 1991;9:321-4.

3689 Scrima L, Hartman PG, Johnson FH Jr, et al. The effects of gamma-hydroxybutyrate on the sleep of narcolepsy patients: a double-blind study. *Sleep* 1990;13:479-90.

3690 Scrima L, Hartman PG, Johnson FH Jr, Hiller FC. Efficacy of gamma-hydroxybutyrate versus placebo in treating narcolepsy-cataplexy: double-blind subjective measures. *Biol Psychiatry* 1989;26:331-43.

3691 Scharf MB, Brown D, Woods M, et al. The effects and effectiveness of gamma-hydroxybutyrate in patients with narcolepsy. *J Clin Psychiatry* 1985;46:222-5.

3692 Broughton R, Mamelak M. The treatment of narcolepsy-cataplexy with nocturnal gamma-hydroxybutyrate. *Can J Neurol Sci* 1979;6:1-6.

3693 Hoes MJ, Vree TB, Guelen PJ. Gamma-hydroxybutyric acid as hypnotic. Clinical and pharmacokinetic evaluation of gamma-hydroxybutyric acid as hypnotic in man. *Encephale* 1980;6:93-9.

3694 Gallimberti L, Schifano F, Forza G, et al. Clinical efficacy of gamma-hydroxybutyric acid in treatment of opiate withdrawal. *Eur Arch Psychiatry Clin Neurosci* 1994;244:113-4.

3695 Gallimberti L, Cibin M, Pagnin P, et al. Gamma-hydroxybutyric acid for treatment of opiate withdrawal syndrome. *Neuropsychopharmacology* 1993;9:77-81.

3696 Gallimberti L, Ferri M, Ferrara SD, et al. Gamma-Hydroxybutyric acid in the treatment of alcohol dependence: a double-blind study. *Alcohol Clin Exp Res* 1992;16:673-6.

3697 Kleinschmidt S, Schellhase C, Mertzlufft F. Continuous sedation during spinal anaesthesia: gamma-hydroxybutyrate vs. propofol. *Eur J Anaesthesiol* 1999;16:23-30.

3698 Kleinschmidt S, Grundmann U, Knocke T, et al. Total intravenous anaesthesia with gamma-hydroxybutyrate (GHB) and sufentanil in patients undergoing coronary artery bypass graft surgery: a comparison in patients with unimpaired and impaired left ventricular function. *Eur J Anaesthesiol* 1998;15:559-64.

3699 Tunnicliff G. Significance of gamma-hydroxybutyric acid in the brain. *Gen Pharmacol* 1992;23:1027-34.

3700 Goodman LS, Gilman A. The Pharmacological Basis of Therapeutics. 5th ed. New York, NY: Macmillan Publ. Co., Inc., 1975.

3701 Zava DT, Dollbaum CM, Blen M. Estrogen and progestin bioactivity of foods, herbs, and spices. *Proc Soc Exp Biol Med* 1998;217(3):369-78.

3702 Rodriguez M, Alvarez M, Zayas M. [Microbiological quality of spices consumed in Cuba]. [Article in Spanish]. *Rev Latinoam Microbiol* 1991;33(2-3):149-51.

3703 Kivanc M, Akgul A, Dogan A. Inhibitory and stimulatory effects of cumin, oregano and their essential oils on growth and acid production of Lactobacillus plantarum and Leuconostoc mesenteroides. *Int J Food Microbiol* 1991;13(1):81-5.

3704 Akgul A, Kivanc M. Inhibitory effects of selected Turkish spices and oregano components on some foodborne fungi. *Int J Food Microbiol* 1988;6(3):263-8.

3705 Benito M, Jorro G, Morales C, et al. Labiatae allergy: systemic reactions due to ingestion of oregano and thyme. *Ann Allergy Asthma Immunol* 1996;76(5): 416-8.

3706 Krenzelok EP, Jacobsen TD, Aronis J. American mistletoe exposures. *Am J Emerg Med* 1997;15:516-20.

3707 Friess H, Beger HG, Kunz J, et al. Treatment of advanced pancreatic cancer with mistletoe: results of a pilot trial. *Anticancer Res* 1996 Mar-Apr;16:915-20.

3709 Kuttan G, Menon LG, Antony S, et al. Anticarcinogenic and antimetastatic activity of Iscador. *Anticancer Drugs* 1997 Apr;8 Suppl 1:S15-6.

3710 Upton R, ed. Ashwagandha Root (Withania somnifera): Analytical, quality control, and therapeutic monograph. Santa Cruz, CA: American Herbal Pharmacopoeia 2000:1-25.

3711 Davis L, Kuttan G. Effect of Withania somnifera on cyclophosphamide-induced urotoxicity. *Cancer Lett* 2000;148:9-17.

3712 Zamah NM, Humpel M, Kuhnz W, et al. Absence of an effect of high vitamin C dosage on the systemic availability of ethinyl estradiol in women using a combination oral contraceptive. *Contraception* 1993;48:377-91.

3713 Chu DT, Wong WL, Mavligit GM. Immunotherapy with Chinese medicinal herbs. II. Reversal of cyclophosphamide-induced immune suppression by administration of fractionated Astragalus membranaceus in vivo. *J Clin Lab Immunol* 1988;25:125-9.

3714 Thie NM, Prasad NG, Major PW. Evaluation of glucosamine sulfate compared to ibuprofen for the treatment of temporomandibular joint osteoarthritis: a randomized double blind controlled 3 month clinical trial. *J Rheumatol* 2001;28:1347-55.

3715 Vehmeyer K, Hajto T, Hostanska K, et al. Lectin-induced increase in clonogenic growth of haematopoietic progenitor cells. *Eur J Haematol* 1998 Jan;60(1):16-20.

3716 Ortega N, Quiralte J, Blanco C, et al. Tobacco allergy: demonstration of cross-reactivity with other members of Solanaceae family and mugwort pollen. *Ann Allergy Asthma Immunol* 1999 Feb;82(2): 194-7.

3717 Lombardi C, Senna GE, Gatti B, et al. Allergic reactions to honey and royal jelly and their relationship with sensitization to compositae. *Allergol Immunopathol* (Madr) 1998;26(6):288-90.

3718 Westendorf J, Pfau W, Schulte A. Carcinogenicity and DNA adduct formation observed in ACI rats after long-term treatment with madder root, Rubia tinctorum L. *Carcinogenesis* 1998;19(12): 2163-8.

3719 Boozer CN, Nasser JA, Heymsfield SB, et al. An herbal supplement containing Ma Huang-Guarana for weight loss: a randomized, double-blind trial. *Int J Obes Relat Metab Disord* 2001;25:316-24.

3720 Bourinbaiar AS, Lee-Huang S. Potentiation of anti-HIV activity of anti-inflammatory drugs, dexamethasone and indomethacin, by MAP30, the antiviral agent from bitter melon. *Biochem Biophys Res Commun* 1995;208(2):779-85.

3721 Lee-Huang S, Huang PL, Chen HC, et al. Anti-HIV and anti-tumor activities of recombinant MAP30 from bitter melon. *Gene* 1995;161:151-6.

3722 Cunnick JE, Sakamoto K, Chapes SK, et al. Induction of tumor cytotoxic immune cells using a protein from the bitter melon (Momordica charantia). *Cell Immunol* 1990;126:278-89.

3723 Jilka C, Strifler B, Fortner GW, et al. In vivo antitumor activity of the bitter melon (Momordica charantia). *Cancer Res* 1983;43(11):5151-5.

3724 Leung SO, Yeung HW, Leung KN. The immunosuppressive activities of two abortifacient proteins isolated from the seeds of bitter melon (Momordica charantia). *Immunopharmacol* 1987;13(3):159-71.

3726 Tseng J, Chang JG. Suppression of tumor necrosis factor-alpha, interleukin-1 beta, interleukin-6 and granulocyte-monocyte colony stimulating factor secretion from human monocytes by an extract of Poria cocos. *Zhonghua Min Guo Wei Sheng Wu Ji Mian Yi Xue Za Zhi* 1992;25(1):1-11.

3727 Hattori T, Hayashi K, Nagao T, et al. Studies on antinephritic effects of plant components (3): Effect of pachyman, a main component of Poria cocos Wolf on original-type anti-GBM nephritis in rats and its mechanisms. *Jpn J Pharmacol* 1992;59(1):89-96.

3728 Cuellar MJ, Giner RM, Recio MC, et al. Effect of the basidiomycete Poria cocos on experimental dermatitis and

REFERENCES

other inflammatory conditions. *Chem Pharm Bull* (Tokyo) 1997;45(3):492-4.

3729 Kaminaga T, Yasukawa K, Kanno H, et al. Inhibitory effects of lanostane-type triterpene acids, the components of Poria cocos, on tumor promotion by 12-O tetradecanoylphorbol-13-acetate in two-stage carcinogenesis in mouse skin. *Oncology* 1996;53(5):382-5.

3730 Tai T, Akita Y, Kinoshita K, et al. Anti-emetic principles of Poria cocos. *Planta Med* 1995;61:527-30.

3731 Wang SS, Yang S, Ma Y. [Efficacy of poria-polyporus anti-diarrhea oral liquor in treating infantile rotavirus diarrhea: a controlled study with smicta]. [Article in Chinese]. *Chung Kuo Chung Hsi I Chieh Ho Tsa Chih* 1995;15:284-6.

3732 Li YL. [Clinical and experimental study on the treatment of children diarrhea by granule of children-diarrhea fast-stopping]. [Article in Chinese]. *Chung Hsi I Chieh Ho Tsa Chih* 1991;11:79-82, 67.

3733 Wang SQ, Du XR, Lu HW, et al. Experimental and clinical studies of Shen Yan Ling in treatment of chronic glomerulonephritis. *J Tradit Chin Med* 1989;9:132-4.

3734 Yang DJ. [Tinnitus treated with combined traditional Chinese medicine and Western medicine]. [Article in Chinese]. *Zhong Xi Yi Jie He Za Zhi* 1989;9:270-1, 259-60.

3735 Gong QM, Wang SL, Gan C. [A clinical study on the treatment of acute upper digestive tract hemorrhage with wen-she decoction]. [Article in Chinese]. *Chung Hsi I Chieh Ho Tsa Chih* 1989;9:272-3, 260.

3736 Yasukawa K, Kaminaga T, Kitanaka S, et al. 3 beta-p-hydroxybenzoyldehydrotumulosic acid from Poria cocos, and its anti-inflammatory effect. *Phytochemistry* 1998;48:1357-60.

3737 Nukaya H, Yamashiro H, Fukazawa H, et al. Isolation of inhibitors of TPA-induced mouse ear edema from Hoelen, Poria cocos. *Chem Pharm Bull* (Tokyo) 1996;44:847-9.

3740 Kouzi SA, McMurtry RJ, Nelson SD. Hepatotoxicity of germander (Teucrium chamaedrys L.) and one of its constituent neoclerodane diterpenes teucrin A in the mouse. *Chem Res Toxicol* 1994;7(6):850-6.

3741 Larrey D, Vial T, Pauwels A, et al. Hepatitis after germander (Teucrium chamaedrys) administration: another instance of herbal medicine hepatotoxicity. *Ann Intern Med* 1992;117(2):129-32.

3742 Pauwels A, Thierman-Duffaud D, Azanowsky JM, et al. [Acute hepatitis caused by wild germander. Hepatotoxicity of herbal remedies. Two cases]. [Article in French]. *Gastroenterol Clin Biol* 1992;16(1):92-5.

3743 Castot A, Djezzar S, Deleau N, et al. [Pharmacovigilance off the beaten track: herbal surveillance or pharmacovigilance of medicinal plants]. [Article in French]. *Therapie* 1997;52(2):97-103.

3744 Mostefa-Kara N, Pauwels A, Pines E, et al. Fatal hepatitis after herbal tea. *Lancet* 1992;340(8820):674.

3745 Chan P, Xu DY, Liu JC, et al. The effect of stevioside on blood pressure and plasma catecholamines in spontaneously hypertensive rats. *Life Sci* 1998;63:1679-84.

3746 Melis MS. A crude extract of Stevia rebaudiana increases the renal plasma flow of normal and hypertensive rats. *Braz J Med Biol Res* 1996;29:669-75.

3747 Melis MS. Chronic administration of aqueous extract of Stevia rebaudiana in rats: renal effects. *J Ethnopharmacol* 1995;47:129-34.

3748 Matsui M, Matsui K, Kawasaki Y, et al. Evaluation of the genotoxicity of stevioside and steviol using six in vitro and one in vivo mutagenicity assays. *Mutagenesis* 1996;11:573-9.

3749 Pezzuto JM, Compadre CM, Swanson SM, et al. Metabolically activated steviol, the aglycone of stevioside, is mutagenic. *Proc Natl Acad Sci U S A* 1985;82:2478-82.

3750 Hubler MO, Bracht A, Kelmer-Bracht AM. Influence of stevioside on hepatic glycogen levels in fasted rats. *Res Commun Chem Pathol Pharmacol* 1994;84:111-8.

3751 Fang HJ, Su XL, Liu HY, et al. [Studies on the chemical components and anti-tumor action of the volatile oils from Pelargonium graveoleus]. [Article in Chinese]. *Yao Hsueh Hsueh Pao* 1989;24:366-71.

3752 Lis-Balchin M, Buchbauer G, Hirtenlehner T, Resch M. Antimicrobial activity of Pelargonium essential oils added to a quiche filling as a model food system. *Lett Appl Microbiol* 1998;27:207-10.

3753 Pattnaik S, Subramanyam VR, Kole C. Antibacterial and antifungal activity of ten essential oils in vitro. *Microbios* 1996;86:237-46.

3754 Agarwal AK, Singh M, Gupta N, et al. Management of giardiasis by an immuno-modulatory herbal drug Pippali rasayana. *J Ethnopharmacol* 1994;44:143-6.

3755 Agarwal AK, Tripathi DM, Sahai R, et al. Management of giardiasis by a herbal drug Pippali Rasayana: a clinical study. *J Ethnopharmacol* 1997;56:233-6.

3756 Shah AH, Al-Shareef AH, Ageel AM, Qureshi S. Toxicity studies in mice of common spices, Cinnamomum zeylanicum bark and Piper longum fruits. *Plant Foods Hum Nutr* 1998;52:231-9.

3757 Khajuria A, Zutshi U, Bedi KL. Permeability characteristics of piperine on oral absorption-an active alkaloid from peppers and a bioavailability enhancer. *Indian J Exp Biol* 1998;36:46-50.

3758 Ghoshal S, Prasad BN, Lakshmi V. Antiamoebic activity of Piper longum fruits against Entamoeba histolytica in vitro and in vivo. *J Ethnopharmacol* 1996;50:167-70.

3759 el-Mofty MM, Khudoley VV, Shwaireb MH. Carcinogenic effect of force-feeding an extract of black pepper (Piper nigrum) in Egyptian toads (Bufo regularis). *Oncology* 1991;48:347-50.

3760 Singh A, Rao AR. Evaluation of the modulatory influence of black pepper (Piper nigrum, L.) on the hepatic detoxication system. *Cancer Lett* 1993;72:5-9.

3761 Nalini N, Sabitha K, Viswanathan P, Menon VP. Influence of spices on the bacterial (enzyme) activity in experimental colon cancer. *J Ethnopharmacol* 1998;62:15-24.

3762 Day C, Cartwright T, Provost J, Bailey CJ. Hypoglycaemic effect of Momordica charantia extracts. *Planta Med* 1990;56:426-9.

3763 Ali L, Khan AK, Mamun MI, et al. Studies on hypoglycemic effects of fruit pulp, seed, and whole plant of Momordica charantia on normal and diabetic model rats. *Planta Med* 1993;59:408-12.

3764 Cakici I, Hurmoglu C, Tunctan B, et al. Hypoglycaemic effect of Momordica charantia extracts in normoglycaemic or cyproheptadine-induced hyperglycaemic mice. *J Ethnopharmacol* 1994;44:117-21.

3765 Sarkar S, Pranava M, Marita R. Demonstration of the hypoglycemic action of Momordica charantia in a validated animal model of diabetes. *Pharmacol Res* 1996;33:1-4.

3766 Hansson A, Veliz G, Naquira C, et al. Preclinical and clinical studies with latex from Ficus glabrata HBK, a traditional intestinal anthelminthic in the Amazonian area. *J Ethnopharmacol* 1986;17:105-38.

3767 Lee IS, Jung KY, Oh SR, et al. Structure-activity relationships of lignans from Schisandra chinensis as platelet activating antagonists. *Biol Pharm Bull* 1999;22:265-7.

3768 Sun HD, Qiu SX, Lin LZ, et al. Nigranoic acid, a triterpenoid from Schisandra sphaerandra that inhibits HIV-1 reverse transcriptase. *J Nat Prod* 1996;59:525-7.

3769 Fukuda K, Ohta T, Oshima Y, et al. Specific CYP3A4 inhibitors in grapefruit juice: furocoumarin dimers as components of drug interaction. *Pharmacogenetics* 1997;7:391-6.

3770 Meagher EA, Barry OP, Lawson JA, et al. Effects of vitamin E on lipid peroxidation in healthy persons. *JAMA* 2001;285:1178-82.

3771 Lilja JJ, Kivisto KT, Backman JT, et al. Grapefruit juice substantially increases plasma concentrations of buspirone. *Clin Pharmacol Ther* 1998;64:655-60.

3773 Kupferschmidt HH, Fattinger KE, Ha HR, et al. Grapefruit juice enhances the bioavailability of the HIV protease inhibitor saquinavir in man. *Br J Clin Pharmacol* 1998;45:355-9.

3774 Lilja JJ, Kivisto KT, Neuvonen PJ. Grapefruit juice-simvastatin interaction: effect on serum concentrations of simvastatin, simvastatin acid, and HMG-CoA reductase inhibitors. *Clin Pharmacol Ther* 1998;64:477-83.

3775 Ameer B, Weintraub RA. Drug interactions with grapefruit juice. *Clin Pharmacokinet* 1997;33:103-21.

3800 Tyler VE, Brady LR, Robbers JE. Pharmacognosy. 7th ed. Philadelphia, PA: Lea & Febiger, 1976.

3801 Gobel H, Schmidt G, Soyka D. Effect of peppermint and eucalyptus oil preparations on neurophysiological and experimental algesimetric headache parameters. *Cephalalgia* 1994;14:228-34;discussion 182.

3802 Liu JH, Chen GH, Yeh HZ, et al. Enteric-coated peppermint-oil capsules in the treatment of irritable bowel syndrome: a prospective, randomized trial. *J Gastroenterol* 1997;32:765-8.

3803 Pittler MH, Ernst E. Peppermint oil for irritable bowel syndrome: a critical review and metaanalysis. *Am J Gastroenterol* 1998;93:1131-5.

3804 Tate S. Peppermint oil: a treatment for postoperative nausea. *J Adv Nurs* 1997;26:543-9.

3805 United States Pharmacopeial Convention I, editor. Drug Information for the Health Care Professional. 19th ed. Micromedex, 1999.

3807 Correa CM, Tibana A, Gontijo-Filho PP. Vegetables as a source of infection with Pseudomonas aeruginosa in a University and Oncology Hospital of Rio de Janeiro. *J Hosp Infect* 1991;18(4):301-6.

3808 Benito M, Jorro G, Morales C, et al. Labiatae allergy: systemic reactions due to ingestion of oregano and thyme. *Ann Allergy Asthma Immunol* 1996; 76(5):416-8.

3811 Chan TY. Potential dangers from topical preparations containing methyl salicylate. *Hum Exp Toxicol* 1996;15(9):747-50.

3818 Tsuda T, Sugaya A, Ohguchi H, et al. Protective effects of peony root extract and its components on neuron damage in the hippocampus induced by the cobalt focus epilepsy model. *Exp Neurol* 1997;146:518-25.

3822 Mossa JS, Tariq M, Mohsin A, et al. Pharmacological studies on aerial parts of Calotropis procera. *Am J Chin Med* 1991;19:223-31.

3823 Kumar VL, Basu N. Anti-inflammatory activity of the latex of Calotropis procera. *J Ethnopharmacol* 1994;44:123-5.

3824 Mascolo N, Sharma R, Jain SC, et al. Ethnopharmacology of Calotropis procera flowers. *J Ethnopharmacol* 1988;22:211-21.

3825 Sen T, Basu A, Chaudhuri AK. Studies on the possible mechanism of the gastric mucosal protection by Calotropis procera - involvement of 5-lipoxygenase pathway. *Fund Clin Pharmacol* 1998;12:82-7.

3826 Levy L. The activity of chaulmoogra acids against Mycobacterium leprae. *Am Rev Respir Dis* 1975;111:703-5.

3828 Mascolo N, Autore G, Capasso F. Local anti-inflammatory activity of Tamus communis. *J Ethnopharmacol* 1987;19:81-4.

3829 Schmidt RJ, Moult SP. The dermatitic properties of black bryony (Tamus communis L.). *Contact Dermatitis* 1983;9:390-6.

3830 Carotenuto A, De Feo V, Fattorusso E, et al. The flavonoids of Allium ursinum. *Phytochem* 1996;41:531-6.

3831 Rietz B, Isensee H, Strobach H, et al. Cardioprotective actions of wild garlic (allium ursinum) in ischemia and reperfusion. *Mol Cell Biochem* 1993;119:143-50.

3832 Rana BK, Singh UP, Taneja V. Antifungal activity and kinetics of inhibition by essential oil isolated from leaves of Aegle marmelos. *J Ethnopharmacol* 1997;57:29-34.

3833 Prakash D, Joshi BD, Pal M. Vitamin C in leaves and seed oil composition of the Amaranthus species. *Int J Food Sci Nutr* 1995;46:47-51.

3834 Sharma SR, Dwivedi SK, Swarup D. Hypoglycaemic, antihyperglycaemic and hypolipidemic activities of Caesalpinia bonducella seeds in rats. *J Ethnopharmacol* 1997;58:39-44.

3835 Ippen H. [Phytophotodermatitis caused by plant trimming (edger's rash)]. [Article in German]. *Derm Beruf Umwelt* 1990;38(6):190-2.

3836 Misra SB, Dixit SN. Antifungal properties of leaf extract of Ranunculus sceleratus L. *Experientia* 1978;34(11):1442-3.

3837 Goerz G, Wirth G, Maas B, et al. [Allergic contact dermatitis due to Asteraceae (Compositae). Cross reaction with Liatris spicata]. [Article in German]. *Derm Beruf Umwelt* 1985;33(3):95-8.

3838 Krenzelok EP, Jacobsen TD, Aronis JM. Poinsettia exposures have good outcomes...just as we thought. *Am J Emerg Med* 1996;14(7):671-4.

3839 Cohen LM, Cohen JL. Erythema multiforme associated with contact dermatitis to poison ivy: three cases and a review of the literature. *Cutis* 1998;62:139-42.

3841 Kuo SC, Chen SC, Chen LH, et al. Potent antiplatelet, anti-inflammatory and antiallergic isoflavanquinones from the roots of Abrus precatorius. *Planta Med* 1995;61:307-12.

3842 Wang JP, Hsu MF, Chang LC, et al. Inhibition of plasma extravasation by abruquinone A, a natural isoflavanquinone isolated from Abrus precatorius. *Eur J Pharmacol* 1995;273:73-81.

3846 Tapiainen T, Luotonen L, Kontiokari T, et al. Xylitol administered only during respiratory infections failed to prevent acute otitis media. *Pediatrics* 2002;109(2):E19.

3847 Respiratory illness associated with inhalation of mushroom spores - Wisconsin 1994. *MMWR Morb Mortal Wkly Rep* 1994;43(29):525-6.

3850 Sidhu GS, Oakenfull DG. A mechanism for the hypocholesterolaemic activity of saponins. *Br J Nutr* 1986;55(3):643-9.

3851 Wu JY, Gardner BH, Murphy CI, et al. Saponin adjuvant enhancement of antigen-specific immune responses to an experimental HIV-1 vaccine. *J Immunol* 1992;148(5):1519-25.

3852 Pillion DJ, Amsden JA, Kensil CR, et al. Structure-function relationship among Quillaja saponins serving as excipients for nasal and ocular delivery of insulin. *J Pharm Sci* 1996;85(5):518-24.

3853 Recchia J, Lurantos MH, Amsden JA, et al. A semisynthetic Quillajasaponin as a drug delivery agent for aminoglycoside antibiotics. *Pharm Res* 1995;12(12):1917-23.

3854 Mitscher LA, Bathala MS, Clark GW, et al. Antimicrobial agents from higher plants. The quaternary alkaloids of Ptelea trifoliata. *Lloydia* 1975;38:109-16.

3858 Majumder PK, Dasgupta S, Mukhopadhaya RK, et al. Anti-steroidogenic activity of the petroleum ether extract and fraction 5 (fatty acids) of carrot (Daucus carota L.) seeds in mouse ovary. *J Ethnopharmacol* 1997;57(3):209-12.

3859 Maher TJ. Chromium and other minerals in diabetes mellitus. *US Pharm* 1999;24:66-76.

3860 Nisley N, Klepser T. Phytoestrogens for the prevention and treatment of osteoporosis. *Alt Med Alert* 1999 Dec;138-42.

3861 Leder BZ, Longcope C, Catlin DH, et al. Oral androstenedione administration and serum testosterone concentrations in young men. *JAMA* 2000;283:779-82.

3862 Rasmussen BB, Volpi E, Gore DC, Wolfe RR. Androstenedione does not stimulate muscle anabolism in young healthy men. *J Clin Endocrinol Metab* 2000;85(1):55-9.

3863 Tode T, Kikuchi Y, Hirata J, et al. Effect of Korean red ginseng on psychological functions in patients with severe climacteric syndromes. *Int J Gynaecol Obstet* 1999;67:169-74.

3864 Rabkin JG, Ferrando SJ, Wagner GJ, Rabkin R. DHEA treatment for HIV positive patients: effects on mood, androgenic and anabolic parameters. *Psychoneuroendocrinol* 2000;25:53-68.

3865 Dyner TS, Lang W, Geaga J, et al. An open-label, dose-escalation trial of oral dehydroepiandrosterone tolerance and pharmacokinetics in patients with HIV disease. *J Acq Immun Def Synd* 1993;6:459-65.

3866 Henderson E, Yang JY, Schwartz A. Dehydroepiandrosterone (DHEA) and synthetic DHEA analogs are modest inhibitors of HIV-1 IIIB replication. *AIDS Res Hum Retroviruses* 1992;8:625-31.

3867 Christeff N, Gherbi N, Mammes O, et al. Serum cortisol and DHEA concentrations during HIV infection. *Psychoneuroendocrinol* 1997;22:S11-8.

3868 Ruhnau KJ, Meissner HP, Finn JR, et al. Effects of 3-week oral treatment with the antioxidant thioctic acid (alpha-lipoic acid) in symptomatic diabetic polyneuropathy. *Diabet Med* 1999;16:1040-3.

3869 Sachse G, Willms B. Efficacy of thioctic acid in the therapy of peripheral diabetic neuropathy. *Hormone Metab Res Suppl* 1980;9:105-7.

3870 Gleiter CH, Schreeb KH, Freudenthaler S, et al. Lack of interaction between thioctic acid, glibenclamide and acarbose. *Br J Clin Pharmacol* 1999;48:819-25.

3871 Packer L, Witt EH, Tritschler HJ. Alpha-Lipoic acid as a biological antioxidant. *Free Rad Biol Med* 1995;19:227-50.

3872 Teichert J, Kern J, Tritschler HJ. Investigations on the pharmacokinetics of alpha-lipoic acid in healthy volunteers. *Int J Clin Pharmacol Ther* 1998;36:625-8.

3873 Nagamatsu M, Nickander KK, Schmelzer JD, et al. Lipoic acid improves nerve blood flow, reduces oxidative stress, and improves distal nerve conduction in experimental diabetic neuropathy. *Diabetes Care* 1995;18:1160-7.

3874 Jacob S, Henriksen EJ, Tritschler HJ, et al. Improvement of insulin-stimulated glucose-disposal in type 2 diabetes after repeated parenteral administration of thioctic acid. *Exp Clin Endocrinol Diabetes* 1996;104:284-8.

3875 Jacob S, Henriksen EJ, Schiemann AL, et al. Enhancement of glucose disposal in patients with type 2 diabetes by alpha-lipoic acid. *Arzneimittelforschung* 1995;45:872-4.

3876 Jacob S, Ruus P, Hermann R, et al. Oral administration of RAC-alpha-lipoic acid modulates insulin sensitivity in patients with type-2 diabetes mellitus: a placebo-controlled, pilot trial. *Free Rad Biol Med* 1999;27:309-14.

3877 Haramaki N, Assadnazari H, Zimmer G, et al. The influence of vitamin E and dihydrolipoic acid on cardiac energy and glutathione status under hypoxia-reoxygenation. *Biochem Mol Biol Int* 1995;37:591-7.

3878 Kishi Y, Schmelzer JD, Yao JK, et al. Alpha-lipoic acid: effect on glucose uptake, sorbitol pathway, and energy metabolism in experimental diabetic neuropathy. *Diabetes* 1999;48:2045-51.

3879 Bustamante J, Lodge JK, Marcocci L, et al. Alpha-lipoic acid in liver metabolism and disease. *Free Rad Biol Med* 1998;24:1023-39.

3880 Marshall AW, Graul RS, Morgan MY, Sherlock S. Treatment of alcohol-related liver disease with thioctic acid: a six-month, randomized, double-blind trial. *Gut* 1982;23:1088-93.

3881 Conlon BJ, Aran JM, Erre JP, Smith DW. Attenuation of aminoglycoside-induced cochlear damage with the metabolic antioxidant alpha-lipoic acid. *Hear Res* 1999;128:40-4.

3882 Vilas GL, Aldonatti C, San Martin de Viale LC, Rios de Molina MC. Effect of Alpha-lipoic acid amide on hexachlorobenzene porphyria. *Biochem Mol Biol Int* 1999;47:815-23.

3883 Gurer H, Ozgunes H, Oztezcan S, Ercal N. Antioxidant role of alpha-lipoic acid in lead toxicity. *Free Rad Biol Med* 1999;27:75-81.

3884 Altenkirch H, Stoltenburg-Didinger G, Wagner HM, et al. Effects of lipoic acid in hexacarbon-induced neuropathy. *Neurotoxicol Teratol* 1990;12:619-22.

3885 Fuchs J, Schofer H, Milbradt R, et al. Studies on lipoate effects on blood redox state in human immunodeficiency virus infected patients. *Arzneimittelforschung* 1993;43:1359-62.

3886 Vermeulen EG, Stehouwer CD, Twisk JW, et al. Effect of homocysteine-lowering treatment with folic acid plus vitamin B6 on progression of subclinical atherosclerosis: a randomised, placebo-controlled trial. *Lancet* 2000;355:517-22.

3887 Bostom AG, Garber C. Endpoints for homocysteine-lowering trials. *Lancet* 2000;355:511-2.

3888 Vuorio AF, Gylling H, Turtola H, et al. Stanol ester margarine alone and with simvastatin lowers serum cholesterol in families with familial hypercholesterolemia caused by the FH-north karelia mutation. *Arterioscler Thromb Vasc Biol* 2000;20:500-6.

3889 Becker M, Staab D, Von Bergmann K. Treatment of severe familial hypercholesterolemia in childhood with sitosterol and sitostanol. *J Pediatr* 1993;122:292-6.

3891 Paice JA, Ferrans CE, Lashley FR, et al. Topical capsaicin in the management of HIV-associated peripheral neuropathy. *J Pain Symptom Manage* 2000;19:45-52.

3892 Bloch M, Schmidt PJ, Danaceau MA, et al. Dehydroepiandrosterone treatment of midlife dysthymia. *Biol Psychiatry* 1999;45:1533-41.

3893 Wolf OT, Neumann O, Hellhammer DH, et al. Effects of a two-week physiological dehydroepiandrosterone substitution on cognitive performance and well-being in healthy elderly women and men. *J Clin Endocrinol Metab* 1997;82:2363-7.

3894 Environmental Protection Agency. Cesium. 2002. Available at: www.epa.gov/radiation/radionuclides/cesium.htm

3896 Yusuf S, Dagenais G, Pogue J, et al. Vitamin E supplementation and cardiovascular events in high-risk patients. The heart outcomes prevention evaluation study investigators. *N Engl J Med* 2000;342:154-60.

3898 Stampfer MJ, Hennekens CH, Manson JE, et al. Vitamin E consumption and the risk of coronary disease in women. *N Engl J Med* 1993;328:1444-9.

3899 Lonn E, Yusuf S, Dzavik V, et al. Effects of ramipril and vitamin E on atherosclerosis: the study to evaluate carotid ultrasound changes in patients treated with ramipril and vitamin E (SECURE). *Circulation* 2001;103:919-25.

3900 Peirce A. The American Pharmaceutical Association Practical Guide to Natural Medicines. New York, NY: William Morrow and Co., 1999.

3901 Tyler VE, Brady LR, Robbers JB. Pharmacognosy. 8th ed. Philadelphia, PA: Lea and Fibiger, 1981.

3902 Barlet A, Albrecht J, Aubert A, et al. [Efficacy of Pygeum africanum extract in the medical therapy of urination disorders due to benign prostatic hyperplasia: evaluation of objective and subjective parameters. A placebo-controlled, double-blind, multicenter study]. [Article in German]. *Wien Klin Wochenschr* 1990;102:667-73.

3903 Breza J, Dzurny O, Borowka A, et al. Efficacy and acceptability of tadenan (Pygeum africanum extract) in the treatment of benign prostatic hyperplasia (BPH): a multicentre trial in central Europe. *Curr Med Res Opin* 1998;14:127-39.

3904 Dufour B, Choquenet C, Revol M, et al. Controlled study of the effects of Pygeum africanum extract on the functional symptoms of prostatic adenoma. *Ann Urol* (Paris) 1984;18:193-5.

3905 Whitmore A. FDA warns consumers against dietary supplement products that may contain Digitalis mislabeled as Plantain. Food and Drug Administration, U.S. Department of the Interior, Washington DC, 1997.

3906 Keith ME, Jeejeebhoy KN, Langer A, et al. A controlled clinical trial of vitamin E supplementation in patients with congestive heart failure. *Am J Clin Nutr* 2001;73:219-24.

3907 Collaborative Group of the Primary Prevention Project. Low-dose aspirin and vitamin E in people at cardiovascular risk: a randomised trial in general practice. *Lancet* 2001;357:89-95.

3908 Kleijnen J. Evening primrose oil. *BMJ* 1994;309:824-825.

3909 Head RJ, McLennan PL, Raederstorff D, et al. Prevention of nerve conduction deficit in diabetic rats by polyunsaturated fatty acids. *Am J Clin Nutr* 2000;71:386S-392S.

3910 Khaw KT, Bingham S, Welch A, et al. Relation between plasma ascorbic acid and mortality in men and women in EPIC-Norfolk prospective study: a prospective population study. European Prospective Investigation into Cancer and Nutrition. *Lancet* 2001;357:657-63.

3911 Singer P, Wirth M, Berger I. A possible contribution of decrease in free fatty acids to low serum triglyceride levels after diets supplemented with n-6 and n-3 polyunsaturated fatty acids. *Atherosclerosis* 1990; 83(2-3):167-75.

3912 Fischer S, Honigmann G, Hora C, et al. [Results of linseed oil and olive oil therapy in hyperlipoproteinemia patients]. [Article in German]. *Dtsch Z Verdau Stoffwechselkr* 1984;44(5):245-51.

3914 Debourdeau PM, Djezzar S, Estival JL, et al. Life-threatening eosinophilic pleuropericardial effusion related to vitamins B5 and H. *Ann Pharmacother* 2001;35(4):424-6.

3916 Manabe H, et al. Effects of Catuaba extracts on microbial and HIV infection. *In Vivo* 1992; 6(2):161-5.

3919 Agricultural Research Service. Dr. Duke's Phytochemical and Ethnobotanical Databases. Available at: www.ars-grin.gov/duke/.

3920 Burkill JD. A Dictionary of the Economic Products of the Malay Peninsula. Kuala Lumpur: Art Printing Works, 1966.

3921 Calixto JB. Antispasmodic effects of an alkaloid extracted from Phyllanthus sellowianus: A comparative study with papaverine. *Braz J Med Biol Res* 1984; 17:313-21. [primary reference in Taylor].

3922 Kao YH, Hiipakka RA, Liao S. Modulation of endocrine systems and food intake by green tea epigallocatechin gallate. *Endocrinology* 2000;141:980-7.

3924 Milne A, Hopkirk N, Lucas CR, et al. Failure of New Zealand hepatitis B carriers to respond to Phyllanthus amarus. *N Z Med J* 1994;107:243.

3925 Wang M, Cheng H, Li Y, et al. Herbs of the genus Phyllanthus in the treatment of chronic hepatitis B: observations with three preparations from different geographic sites. *J Lab Clin Med* 1995; 126:350-2.

3926 Inoue M, Tajima K, Mizutani M, et al. Regular consumption of green tea and the risk of breast cancer recurrence: follow-up study from the Hospital-based Epidemiologic Research Program at Aichi Cancer Center (HERPACC), Japan. *Cancer Lett* 2001;167:175-82.

3927 Qian-Cutrone J, et al. Niruriside, a new HIV REV/RRE binding inhibitor from Phyllanthus niruri. *J Nat Prod* 1996; 59(2):196-9.

3928 Srividya N, Periwal S. Diuretic, hypotensive and hypoglycaemic effect of Phyllanthus amarus. *Indian J Exp Biol* 1995; 33:861-4.

3929 Wilkins AL, et al. Photosensitivity in South Africa. IX. Structure elucidation of a beta-glucosidase-treated saponin from Tribulus terrestis, and the identification of saponin chemotypes of South African T. terrestis. *Onderstepoort Journal Veterinary Res* 1996; 63:327-34.

3930 Sharma MK, Anaraki F, Ala F. Preliminary results of transfer factor therapy of persistant cutaneous leishmania infection. *Clin Immunol Immunopathol* 1979;12:183-90.

3931 Wang B, Ma L, Liu T. 406 cases of angina pectoris in coronary heart disease treated with saponin of Tribulus terrestris. *Chung Hsi I Chieh Ho Tsa Chih* 1990; 10(2):85-7, 68.

3932 Harvey J, Colin-Jones DG. Mistletoe hepatitis. *Br Med J* (Clin Res Ed) 1981; 282:186-7.

3933 Rimm EB, Stampfer MJ, Ascherio A, et al. Vitamin E consumption and the risk of coronary heart disease in men. *N Engl J Med* 1993;328:1450-6.

3934 Kushi LH, Folsom AR, Prineas RJ, et al. Dietary antioxidant vitamins and death from coronary heart disease in postmenopausal women. *N Engl J Med* 1996;334:1156-62.

3935 Virtamo J, Rapola JM, Ripatti S, et al. Effect of vitamin E and beta carotene on the incidence of primary nonfatal myocardial infarction and fatal coronary heart disease. *Arch Intern Med* 1998;158:668-75.

3936 Stephens NG, Parsons A, Schofield PM, et al. Randomised controlled trial of vitamin E in patients with coronary disease: Cambridge Heart Antioxidant Study. *Lancet* 1996;347:781-6.

3937 Rapola JM, Virtamo J, Ripatti S, et al. Randomised trial of alpha-tocopherol and beta-carotene supplements on incidence of major coronary events in men with previous myocardial infarction. *Lancet* 1997;349:1715-20.

3938 Losonczy KG, Harris TB, Havlik RJ. Vitamin E and vitamin C supplement use and risk of all-cause and coronary heart disease mortality in older persons:epidemiologic studies of the elderly. *Am J Clin Nutr* 1996;64:190-6.

3939 Anon. Vitamin E health claim falls short of significant scientific agreement - FDA. *FDC Reports: The Tan Sheet.* January 24, 2000;10.

3940 Stammler G, Volm M. Green tea catechins (EGCG and EGC) have modulating effects on the activity of doxorubicin in drug-resistant cell lines. *Anticancer Drugs* 1997;8:265-8.

3941 Weisburger JH. Tea and health: the underlying mechanisms. *Proc Soc Exp Biol Med* 1999;220:271-5.

3942 Adler LA, Edson R, Lavori P, et al. Long-term treatment effects of vitamin E for tardive dyskinesia. *Biol Psychiatry* 1998;43:868-72.

3943 Sajjad SH. Vitamin E in the treatment of tardive dyskinesia: a preliminary study over 7 months at different doses. *Int Clin Psychopharmacol* 1998;13:147-55.

3944 Lohr JB, Caligiuri MP. A double-blind, placebo-controlled study of vitamin E treatment of tardive dyskinesia. *J Clin Psychiatry* 1996;57:167-73.

3945 Shriqui CL, Bradwejn J, Annable L, Jones BD. Vitamin E in the treatment of tardive dyskinesia: a double-blind, placebo-controlled study. *Am J Psychiatry* 1992;149:391-3.

3946 Dorfman-Etrog P, Hermesh H, Prilipko L, et al. The effect of vitamin E addition to acute neuroleptic treatment on the emergence of extrapyramidal side effects in schizophrenic patients: an open label study. *Eur Neuropsychopharmacol* 1999;9:475-7.

REFERENCES

3947 Boomershine KH, Shelton PS, Boomershine JE. Vitamin E in the treatment of tardive dyskinesia. *Ann Pharmacother* 1999;33:1195-202.

3948 Dabiri LM, Pasta D, Darby JK, Mosbacher D. Effectiveness of vitamin E for treatment of long-term tardive dyskinesia. *Am J Psychiatry* 1994;151:925-6.

3949 The Alpha-Tocopherol, Beta Carotene Cancer Prevention Study Group. The effect of vitamin E and beta carotene on the incidence of lung cancer and other cancers in male smokers. *N Engl J Med* 1994;330:1029-35.

3951 Liede K, Hietanen J, Saxen L, et al. Long-term supplementation with alpha-tocopherol and beta-carotene and prevalence of oral mucosal lesions in smokers. *Oral Dis* 1998;4:78-83.

3952 Pantuck EJ, Pantuck CB, Anderson KE, et al. Effect of brussels sprouts and cabbage on drug conjugation. *Clin Pharmacol Ther* 1984;35:161-169.

3953 Malila N, Virtamo J, Virtanen M, et al. The effect of alpha-tocopherol and beta-carotene supplementation on colorectal adenomas in middle-aged male smokers. *Cancer Epidemiol Biomarkers Prev* 1999;8:489-93.

3954 Roncucci L, Di Donato P, Carati L, et al. Antioxidant vitamins or lactulose for the prevention of the recurrence of colorectal adenomas. Colorectal Cancer Study Group of the Univ of Modena and the Health Care Dist 16. *Dis Colon Rectum* 1993;36:227-34.

3955 Greenberg ER, Baron JA, Tosteson TD, et al. A clinical trial of antioxidant vitamins to prevent colorectal adenoma. Polyp Prevention Study Group. *N Engl J Med* 1994;331:141-7.

3956 Paganelli GM, Biasco G, Brandi G, et al. Effect of vitamin A, C, and E supplementation on rectal cell proliferation in patients with colorectal adenomas. *J Natl Cancer Inst* 1992;84:47-51.

3957 McKeown-Eyssen G, Holloway C, Jazmaji V, et al. A randomized trial of vitamins C and E in the prevention of recurrence of colorectal polyps. *Cancer Res* 1988;48:4701-5.

3958 White E, Shannon JS, Patterson RE. Relationship between vitamin and calcium supplement use and colon cancer. *Cancer Epidemiol Biomarkers Prev* 1997;6:769-74.

3959 Heinonen OP, Albanes D, Virtamo J, et al. Prostate cancer and supplementation with alpha-tocopherol and beta-carotene: incidence and mortality in a controlled trial. *J Natl Cancer Inst* 1998;90:440-6.

3960 Varis K, Taylor PR, Sipponen P, et al. Gastric cancer and premalignant lesions in atrophic gastritis: a controlled trial on the effect of supplementation with alpha-tocopherol and beta-carotene. The Helsinki Gastritis Study Group. *Scand J Gastroenterol* 1998;33:294-300.

3961 Rautalahti MT, Virtamo JR, Taylor PR, et al. The effects of supplementation with alpha-tocopherol and beta-carotene on the incidence and mortality of carcinoma of the pancreas in a randomized, controlled trial. *Cancer* 1999;86:37-42.

3962 Slattery ML, Benson J, Curtin K, et al. Carotenoids and colon cancer. *Am J Clin Nutr* 2000;71:575-82.

3963 Steinmetz KA, Potter JD. Vegetables, fruit, and cancer. I. Epidemiology. *Cancer Causes Control* 1991;2:325-57.

3964 Slattery ML, Potter JD, Coates A, et al. Plant foods and colon cancer: an assessment of specific foods and their related nutrients (United States). *Cancer Causes Control* 1997;8:575-90.

3965 Cohen AJ, Bartlik B. Ginkgo biloba for antidepressant-induced sexual dysfunction. *J Sex Marital Ther* 1998;24:139-43.

3966 Balon R. Ginkgo biloba for antidepressant-induced sexual dysfunction? *J Sex Marital Ther* 1999;25:1-2.

3967 Ellison JM, DeLuca P. Fluoxetine-induced genital anesthesia relieved by Ginkgo biloba extract. *J Clin Psychiatry* 1998;59:199-200.

3968 Balon R. The effects of antidepressants on human sexuality: diagnosis and management update 1999. *Primary Psychiatry* 1999;6:40-54.

3969 Levine SB. Caution recommended. *J Sex Marital Ther* 1999;25:2-5.

3970 Jacobsen FM. Fluoxetine-induced sexual dysfunction and an open trial of yohimbine. *J Clin Psychiatry* 1992;53:119-22.

3971 Hollander E, McCarley A. Yohimbine treatment of sexual side effects induced by serotonin reuptake blockers. *J Clin Psychiatry* 1992;53:207-9.

3972 Harvey KV, Balon R. Clinical implications of antidepressant drug effects on sexual function. *Ann Clin Psychiatry* 1995;7:189-201.

3973 Balon R. The effects of anitdepressants on human sexuality: diagnosis and management update 1999. *Primary Psychiatry* 1999;6:40-54.

3974 Redondo P, Bauza A. Topical N-acetylcysteine for lamellar ichthyosis. *Lancet* 1999;354:1880.

3975 Sekharam M, Trotti A, Cunnick JM, Wu J. Suppression of fibroblast cell cycle progression in G1 phase by N-acetylcysteine. *Toxicol Appl Pharmacol* 1998;149:210-6.

3976 Hakkak R, Korourian S, Shelnutt SR, et al. Diets containing whey proteins or soy protein isolate protect against 7,12-dimethylbenz(a)anthracene-induced mammary tumors in female rats. *Cancer Epidemiol Biomarkers Prev* 2000;9:113-7.

3977 Henkel. FDA. Soy: Health Claims for Soy Protein, Questions About Other Components. May-June 2000. Available at: http://vm.cfsan.fda.gov/~dms/fdsoypr.html#health.

3978 Tham DM, Gardner CD, Haskell WL. Clinical review 97: Potential health benefits of dietary phytoestrogens: a review of the clinical, epidemiological, and mechanistic evidence. *J Clin Endocrinol Metab* 1998;83:2223-35.

3979 Setchell KD. Phytoestrogens: the biochemistry, physiology, and implications for human health of soy isoflavones. *Am J Clin Nutr* 1998;68:1333S-46S.

3980 McMichael-Phillips DF, Harding C, Morton M, et al. Effects of soy-protein supplementation on epithelial proliferation in the histologically normal human breast. *Am J Clin Nutr* 1998;68:1431S-5S.

3981 Petrakis NL, Barnes S, King EB, et al. Stimulatory influence of soy protein isolate on breast secretion in pre- and postmenopausal women. *Cancer Epidemiol Biomarkers Prev* 1996;5:785-94.

3982 Setchell KD. Absorption and metabolism of soy isoflavones-from food to dietary supplements and adults to infants. *J Nutr* 2000;130:654S-5S.

3983 Barnes S, Kim H, Darley-Usmar V, et al. Beyond ERalpha and ERbeta: Estrogen receptor binding is only part of the isoflavone story. *J Nutr* 2000;130:656S-7S.

3984 Evans BA, Griffiths K, Morton MS. Inhibition of 5 alpha-reductase in genital skin fibroblasts and prostate tissue by dietary lignans and isoflavonoids. *J Endocrinol* 1995;147:295-302.

3985 Adlercreutz H, Mazur W, Bartels P, et al. Phytoestrogens and prostate disease. *J Nutr* 2000;130:658S-9S.

3986 Brzezinski A, Adlercreutz H, Sheoul R, et al. Short-term effects of phytoestrogen-rich diet on postmenopausal women. *Menopause* 1997;4:89-94.

3987 Kurzer M. Hormonal effects of soy isoflavones: Studies in premenopausal and postmenopausal women. *J Nutr* 2000;130:660-1.

3988 Baird DD, Umbach DM, Lansdell L, et al. Dietary intervention study to assess estrogenicity of dietary soy among postmenopausal women. *J Clin Endocrinol Metab* 1995;80:1685-90.

3989 Duncan AM, Underhill KE, Xu X, et al. Modest hormonal effects of soy isoflavones in postmenopausal women. *J Clin Endocrinol Metab* 1999;84:3479-84.

3990 Ginsburg J, Prelevic GM. Lack of significant hormonal effects and controlled trials of phyto-oestrogens. *Lancet* 2000;355:163-4.

3991 Quella SK, Loprinzi CL, Barton DL, et al. Evaluation of soy phytoestrogens for the treatment of hot flashes in breast cancer survivors: a North Central Cancer Treatment Group trial. *J Clin Oncol* 2000;18:1068-74.

3992 Anthony MS. Soy and cardiovascular disease: Cholesterol lowering and beyond. *J Nutr* 2000;130:662S-3S.

3993 Lockwood K, Moesgaard S, Yamamoto T, Folkers K. Progress on therapy of breast cancer with vitamin Q10 and the regression of metastases. *Biochem Biophys Res Commun* 1995;212:172-7.

3994 Hargreaves DF, Potten CS, Harding C, et al. Two-week dietary soy supplementation has an estrogenic effect on normal premenopausal breast. *J Clin Endocrinol Metab* 1999;84:4017-24.

3995 Lockwood K, Moesgaard S, Folkers K. Partial and complete regression of breast cancer in patients in relation to dosage of coenzyme Q10. *Biochem Biophys Res Commun* 1994;199:1504-8.

3996 Poortmans JR, Francaux M. Long-term oral creatine supplementation does not impair renal function in healthy athletes. *Med Sci Sports Exerc* 1999;31:1108-10.

3997 Juhn MS, Tarnopolsky M. Potential side effects of oral creatine supplementation: a critical review. *Clin J Sport Med* 1998;8:298-304.

3998 Graham AS, Hatton RC. Creatine: a review of efficacy and safety. *J Am Pharm Assoc* (Wash) 1999;39:803-10.

3999 Pepping J. Creatine. *Am J Health Syst Pharm* 1999;56:1608-10.

4000 Medina JH, Viola H, Wolfman C, et al. Overview-flavonoids: a new family of benzodiazepine receptor ligands. *Neurochem Res* 1997;22:419-25.

4001 Salgueiro JB, Ardenghi P, Dias M, et al. Anxiolytic natural and synthetic flavonoid ligands of the central benzodiazepine receptor have no effect on memory tasks in rats. *Pharmacol Biochem Behav* 1997;58:887-91.

4002 Rommelspacher H, May T, Salewski B. (1-methyl-beta-carboline) is a natural inhibitor of monoamine oxidase type A in rats. *Eur J Pharmacol* 1994;252:51-9.

4003 Anon. Licensed fish-oil concentrate versus cod-liver oil. *Lancet* 1987;2:453.

4004 Henderson MJ, Jones RG. Cod liver oil or bust. *Lancet* 1987;2:274-5.

4005 Landymore RW, MacAulay M, Sheridan B, Cameron C. Comparison of cod-liver oil and aspirin-dipyridamole for the prevention of intimal hyperplasia in autologous vein grafts. *Ann Thorac Surg* 1986;41:54-7.

4006 Neef H, Augustijns P, Declercq P, et al. Inhibitory effects of Galega officinalis on glucose transport across monolayers of human intestinal epithelial cells (Caco-2). *Pharm Pharmacol Lett* 1996;6:86-9.

4007 Atanasov AT. Effect of Galega officinalis L. extract on platelet aggregation in rats. *J Herbs Spices Med Plants* 1995;3:71-6.

4008 Huxtable CR, Dorling RR, Colegate SM. Identification of galegine, an isoprenyl guanidine, as the toxic principle of Schoenus asperocarpus (poison sedge). *Aust Vet J* 1993;70:169-71.

4009 Duke JA. CRC Handbook of Medicinal Herbs. 1st ed. Boca Raton, FL: CRC Press, Inc., 1985.

4010 Scarlat M, Sandor V, Tamas M, Cuparencu B. Experimental anti-ulcer activity of Veronica officinalis L. extracts. *J Ethnopharmacol* 1985;13:157-63.

4011 Yoshioka T, Fujii E, Endo M, et al. Antiinflammatory potency of dehydrocurdione, a zedoary-derived sesquiterpene. *Inflamm Res* 1998;47(12):476-81.

4012 Matsuda H, Ninomiya K, Morikawa T, et al. Inhibitory effect and action mechanism of sesquiterpenes from Zedoariae Rhizoma on D-galactosamine/lipopolysaccharide-induced liver injury. *Bioorg Med Chem Lett* 1998;8:339-44.

4013 Gupta SK, Banerjee AB, Achari B. Isolation of Ethyl p-methoxycinnamate, the major antifungal principle of Curcumba zedoaria. *Lloydia* 1976;39:218-22.

4014 Syu WJ, Shen CC, Don MJ, et al. Cytotoxicity of curcuminoids and some novel compounds from Curcuma zedoaria. *J Nat Prod* 1998;61:1531-4.

4015 Latif MA, Morris TR, Miah AH, et al. Toxicity of shoti (Indian arrowroot: Curcuma zedoaria) for rats and chicks. *Br J Nutr* 1979;41:57-63.

4016 Wu D, Meydani M, Leka LS, et al. Effect of dietary supplementation with black currant seed oil on the immune response of healthy elderly subjects. *Am J Clin Nutr* 1999;70:536-43.

4018 Leclercq I, Desager JP, Horsmans Y. Inhibition of chlorzoxazone metabolism, a clinical probe for CYP2E1, by a single ingestion of watercress. *Clin Pharmacol Ther* 1998;64:144-9.

4019 Hecht SS, Chung FL, Richie JP Jr., et al. Effects of watercress consumption on metabolism of a tobacco-specific lung carcinogen in smokers. *Cancer Epidemiol Biomarkers Prev* 1995;4:877-84.

4020 Habtemariam S. Cistifolin, an integrin-dependent cell adhesion blocker from the anti- rheumatic herbal drug, gravel root (rhizome of Eupatorium purpureum). *Planta Med* 1998;64:683-5.

4021 WHO working group. Pyrrolizidine alkaloids. Environmental Health Criteria, 80. WHO: Geneva, 1988.

4022 Landymore RW, Kinley CE, Cooper JH, et al. Cod-liver oil in the prevention of intimal hyperplasia in autogenous vein grafts used for arterial bypass. *J Thorac Cardiovasc Surg* 1985;89:351-7.

4023 Dahlquist I, Fregert S. Contact allergy to atranorin in lichens and perfumes. *Contact Dermatitis* 1980;6:111-9.

4024 Lauterwein M, Oethinger M, Belsner K, et al. In vitro activities of the lichen secondary metabolites vulpinic acid, (+)-usnic acid, and (-)-usnic acid against aerobic and anaerobic microorganisms. *Antimicrob Agents Chemother* 1995;39:2541-3.

4025 Brox JH, Killie JE, Gunnes S, Nordoy A. The effect of cod liver oil and corn oil on platelets and vessel wall in man. *Thromb Haemost* 1981;46:604-11.

4026 Sanders TA, Vickers M, Haines AP. Effect on blood lipids and haemostasis of a supplement of cod-liver oil, rich in eicosapentainoic and docosahexaenoic acids, in healthy young men. *Clin Sci* (Colch) 1981;61:317-24.

4027 Rubel DM, Freeman S, Southwell IA. Tea tree oil allergy: what is the offending agent? Report of three cases of tea tree oil allergy and review of the literature. *Australas J Dermatol* 1998;39:244-7.

4028 Carson CF, Riley TV, Cookson BD. Efficacy and safety of tea tree oil as a topical antimicrobial agent. *J Hosp Infect* 1998;40:175-8.

4029 Bhushan M, Beck MH. Allergic contact dermatitis from tea tree oil in a wart paint. *Contact Dermatitis* 1997;36:117-8.

4030 Del Beccaro MA. Melaleuca oil poisoning in a 17-month old. *Vet Hum Toxicol* 1995;37:557-8.

REFERENCES

4031 Tong MM, Altman PM, Barnetson RS. Tea tree oil in the treatment of tinea pedis. *Australas J Dermatol* 1992;33:145-9.

4032 Wheatley D. Stress-induced insomnia treated with kava and valerian: singly and in combination. *Hum Psychopharmacol Clin Exp* 2001;16:353-6.

4033 Goncalo S. Contact sensitivity to lichens and compositae in Frullania dermatitis. *Contact Dermatitis* 1987;16:84-6.

4034 Goncalo S, Cabral F, Goncalo M. Contact sensitivity to oak moss. *Contact Dermatitis* 1988;19:355-7.

4037 Jussofie A, Schmiz A, Hiemke C. Kavapyrone enriched extract from Piper methysticum as modulator of the GABA binding site in different regions of rat brain. *Psychopharmacology* 1994;116:469-74.

4038 Davies LP, Drew CA, Duffield P, et al. Kava Pyrones and Resin: Studies on GABA-A, GABA-B, and Benzodiazepine Binding Sites in Rodent Brain. *Pharmacol Toxicol* 1992;71:120-6.

4039 Thune P, Solberg Y, McFadden N, et al. Perfume allergy due to oak moss and other lichens. *Contact Dermatitis* 1982;8:396-400.

4040 al-Bekairi AM, Qureshi S, Chaudhry MA, et al. Mitodepressive, clastogenic and biochemical effects of (+)-usnic acid in mice. *J Ethnopharmacol* 1991;33:217-20.

4041 Chen CP, Lin CC, Namba T. Screening of Taiwanese crude drugs for antibacterial activity against Streptococcus mutans. *J Ethnopharmacol* 1989;27:285-95.

4042 Akihisa T, Yasukawa K, Kimura Y, et al. Five D:C-friedo-oleanane triterpenes from the seeds of Trichosanthes kirilowii Maxim. and their anti-inflammatory effects. *Chem Pharm Bull* (Tokyo) 1994;42:1101-5.

4043 Ozaki Y, Xing L, Satake M. Anti-inflammatory effect of Trichosanthes kirilowii Maxim, and its effective parts. *Biol Pharm Bull* 1996;19:1046-8.

4044 Takano F, Yoshizaki F, Suzuki K, et al. Anti-ulcer effects of Trichosanthes fruits. *Chem Pharm Bull* (Tokyo) 1990;38:1313-6.

4045 Hikino H, Yoshizawa M, Suzuki Y, et al. Isolation and hypoglycemic activity of trichosans A, B, C, D, and E: glycans of Trichosanthes kirilowii roots. *Planta Med* 1989;55:349-50.

4046 Tao XL, Sun Y, Dong Y, et al. A prospective, controlled, double-blind, cross-over study of tripterygium wilfodii hook F in treatment of rheumatoid arthritis. *Chin Med J* 1989;102:327-32.

4047 Takei A, Nagashima G, Suzuki R, et al. Meningoencephalocele associated with Tripterygium wilfordii treatment. *Pediatr Neurosurg* 1997;27:45-8.

4048 Chen K, Shi QA, Fujioka T, et al. Anti-AIDS agents, 4. Tripterifordin, a novel anti-HIV principle from Tripterygium wilfordii: isolation and structural elucidation. *J Nat Prod* 1992;55:88-92.

4049 Chen K, Shi Q, Kashiwada Y, et al. Anti-aids agents, 6. Salaspermic acid, an anti-HIV principle from Tripterygium wilfordii, and the structure-activity correlation with its related compounds. *J Nat Prod* 1992;55:340-6.

4050 Attaguile G, Caruso A, Pennisi G, et al. Gastroprotective effect of aqueous extract of Cistus incanus L. in rats. *Pharmacol Res* 1995;3:29-32.

4051 Liu FJ, Sun DM. Studies on the active constituents lowering blood lipid in beeswax. *J Chin Mater Med* (Zhongguo Zhongyao Zazhi) 1996;21:553-4.

4052 Carbajal D, Molina V, Valdes S, et al. Anti-inflammatory activity of D-002: an active product isolated from beeswax. *Prostaglandins Leukot Essent Fatty Acids* 1998;59:235-8.

4053 Carbajal D, Molina V, Valdes S, et al. Possible cytoprotective mechanism in rats of D-002, an anti-ulcerogenic product isolated from beeswax. *J Pharm Pharmacol* 1996;48:858-60.

4054 Carbajal D, Molina V, Valdes S, et al. Anti-ulcer activity of higher primary alcohols of beeswax. *J Pharm Pharmacol* 1995;47:731-3.

4055 Schelosky L, Raffaup C, Jendroska K, Poewe W. Kava and dopamine antagonism. *J Neurol Neurosurg Psychiatry* 1995;58:639-40.

4056 White CM, Fan C, Chow M. An evaluation of the hemostatic effect of externally applied notoginseng and notoginseng total saponins. *J Clin Pharmacol* 2000; 40:1150-3.

4058 Roesyanto-Mahadi ID, Geursen-Reitsma AM, van Joost T, et al. Sensitization to fragrance materials in Indonesian cosmetics. *Contact Dermatitis* 1990;22:212-7.

4059 Arras G, Grella GE. Wild thyme, Thymus capitatus, essential oil seasonal changes and antimycotic activity. *J Hortic Sci* 1992;67:197-202.

4060 Thompson DP. Effect of phenolic compounds on mycelial growth of Fusarium and Penicillium species. *J Food Protection* 1997;60:1262-4.

4062 Stiles JC, Sparks W, Ronzio RA. The inhibition of Candida albicans by Oregano. *J Appl Nutrition* 1995;47:96-102.

4063 Viollon C, Chaumont JP. Antifungal properties of essential oils and their main components upon Cryptococcus neoformans. *Mycopathologia* 1994;128:151-3.

4064 Osawa K, Matsumoto T, Maruyama T, et al. Studies of the antibacterial activity of plant extracts and their constituents against periodontopathic bacteria. *Bull Tokyo Dent Coll* 1990;31:17-21.

4065 Ultee A, Gorris LG, Smid EJ. Bactericidal activity of carvacrol towards the food-borne pathogen Bacillus cereus. *J Appl Microbiol* 1998;85:211-8.

4066 Helander IM, Alakomi H-L, Latva-Kala K, et al. Characterization of the action of selected essential oil components on gram-negative bacteria. *J Agric Food Chem* 1998;46:3590-5.

4067 Aeschbach R, Loliger J, Scott BC. Antioxidant actions of thymol, carvacrol, 6-gingerol, zingerone and hydroxytyrosol. *Food Chem Toxicol* 1994;32:31-6.

4068 Eastwood MA, Brydon WG, Anderson DM, et al. The effects of dietary gum tragacanth in man. *Toxicol Lett* 1984;21:73-81.

4069 Jenkins DJ, Wolever TM, Leeds AR, et al. Dietary fibres, fibre analogues, and glucose tolerance: importance of viscosity. *Br Med J* 1978;1:1392-4.

4070 Smee DF, Sidwell RW, Huffman JH, et al. Antiviral activities of tragacanthin polysaccharides on Punta Toro virus infections in mice. *Chemotherapy* 1996;42:286-93.

4071 FAO and WHO working groups. Tragacanth gum. *WHO Food Additives Series* 1985;20:253-62.

4072 Anon. Final report on the safety assessment of Tragacanth Gum. *J Am Coll Toxicol* 1987;6:1-22.

4073 Vaswani SK, Hamilton RG, Carey RN, et al. Anaphylaxis recurrent urticaria and angioedema from grape hypersensitivity. *J All Clin Immunol* 1998;101:S31.

4074 BIBRA working group. Anthocyanins. Toxicity profile. *BIBRA Toxicol Int* 1991;6.

4075 Garcia Ortiz JC, Cosmes Martin P, Lopez-Asunsolo A. Melon sensitivity shares allergens with Plantago and grass pollens. *Allergy* 1995;50:269-73.

4076 Hollis S. The Country Diary Herbal. New York, NY: Henry Holt and Co., 1990.

4077 Tyler VE, Brady LR, Robbers JE. Pharmacognosy 9th ed. Philadelphia, PA: Lea & Febiger, 1988.

4078 Foster S, Duke JA. The Peterson Field Guide to Medicinal Plants: Eastern and Central North America. Boston, MA: Houghton Mifflin Co., 1990.

4079 Eigenmann PA, Burks AW, Bannon GA, et al. Identification of unique peanut and soy allergens in sera adsorbed with cross-reacting antibodies. *J Allergy Clin Immunol* 1996;98:969-78.

4080 Bardare M, Magnolfi C, Zani G. Soy sensitivity: personal observation on 71 children with food intolerance. *Allerg Immunol* (Paris) 1988;20:63-6.

4081 Van Hevelingen A. The orris iris. *The Herb Companion* 1992;4:32-5.

4082 Schmidt GD, Roberts LS. Foundations of Parasitology. St Louis, MO: Times Mirror/Mosby College Publ., 1985.

4084 Drugs in Pregnancy and Lactation. 4th ed. Baltimore, MD: Williams & Wilkens, 1994.

4085 Lichtenstein AH, Ausman LM, Jalbert SM, et al. Effects of different forms of dietary hydrogenated fats on serum lipoprotein cholesterol levels. *N Engl J Med* 1999;340:1933-40.

4087 FDA. Center for Science in the Public Interest. A Food Labeling Guide. Available at: http://www.cfsan.fda.gov/~dms/flg-6c html.

4089 Moyad MA, Brumfield SK, Pienta KJ. Vitamin E, alpha- and gamma-tocopherol, and prostate cancer. *Semin Urol Oncol* 1999;17:85-90.

4092 Li D, Saldeen T, Mehta JL. Gamma-tocopherol decreases ox-LDL-mediated activation of nuclear factor- kappaB and apoptosis in human coronary artery endothelial cells. *Biochem Biophys Res Commun* 1999;259:157-61.

4096 Aberg F, Appelkvist EL, Broijersen A, et al. Gemfibrozil-induced decrease in serum ubiquinone and alpha- and gamma- tocopherol levels in men with combined hyperlipidaemia. *Eur J Clin Invest* 1998;28:235-42.

4097 Sadrzadeh SM, Nanji AA, Meydani M. Effect of chronic ethanol feeding on plasma and liver alpha- and gamma-tocopherol levels in normal and vitamin E-deficient rats. Relationship to lipid peroxidation. *Biochem Pharmacol* 1994;47:2005-10.

4098 Takahashi O. Haemorrhagic toxicity of a large dose of alpha-, beta-, gamma- and delta-tocopherols, ubiquinone, beta-carotene retinol acetate and L-ascorbic acid in the rat. *Food Chem Toxicol* 1995;33:121-8.

4100 Scholz E, Rimpler R. Proanthocyanidins from Krameria triandra root. *Planta Med* 1989;55(4):379-84.

4101 The Bantam Medical Dictionary. rev ed. New York, NY: Bantam Books, 1990.

4104 Abdullaev FI, Gonzalez de Mejia E. Antitumor activity of natural substances: lectins and saffron. *Arch Latinoam Nutr* 1997;47:195-202.

4105 Nair SC, Pannikar B, Panikkar KR. Antitumor activity of Saffron (Crocus sativus). *Cancer Lett* 1991;57:109-14.

4106 Feo F, Martinez J, Martinez A, et al. Occupational allergy in saffron workers. *Allergy* 1997;52:633-41.

4107 Wuthrich B, Schmid-Grendelmeyer P, Lundberg M. Anaphylaxis to saffron. *Allergy* 1997;52:476-7.

4109 Miller TL, Willett SL, Moss ME, et al. Binding of crocetin to plasma albumin. *J Pharm Sci* 1982;71:173-7.

4110 Grainer JL, Jones JR. The Use of Crocetin in Experimental Atherosclerosis. *Experientia* 1975;31:548-9.

4111 Vandenplas O Depelchin S, Toussaint G, et al. Occupational asthma caused by sarsaparilla root dust. *J Allergy Clin Immunol* 1996;97:1416-8.

4112 Ahn YO. Diet and stomach cancer in Korea. *Int J Cancer* 1997;Suppl 10:7-9.

4113 Archana R, Namasivayam A. Antistressor effect of Withania somnifera. *J Ethnopharmacol* 1999;64:91-3.

4114 Davis L, Kuttan G. Suppressive effect of cyclophosphamide-induced toxicity by Withania somnifera extract in mice. *J Ethnopharmacol* 1998;62:209-14.

4116 Bhattacharya SK, Satyan KS, Ghosal S. Antioxidant activity of glycowithanolides from Withania somnifera. *Indian J Exp Biol* 1997 35:236-9.

4117 Shen HD, Chang LY, Gong YJ, et al. A monoclonal antibody against ragweed pollen cross-reacting with yellow dock pollen. *Chung Hua Min Kuo Wei Sheng Wu Chi Mien I Hsueh Tsa Chih* 1985;18:232-9.

4118 Liu YL, Ho DK, Cassady JM, et al. Isolation of potential cancer chemopreventive agents from Eriodictyon californicum. *J Nat Prod* 1992;55(3):357-63.

4119 Younos C, Rolland A, Fleurentin J, et al. Analgesic and behavioural effects of Morinda citrifolia. *Planta Med* 1990;56:430-4.

4120 Nakano M, Nakashima H, Itoh Y. Anti-human immunodeficiency virus activity of oligosaccharides from rooibos tea (Aspalathus linearis) extracts in vitro. *Leukemia* 1997;11:128-30.

4121 Nakano M, Itoh Y, Mizuno T, Nakashima H. Polysaccharide from Aspalathus linearis with strong anti-HIV activity. *Biosci Biotechnol Biochem* 1997;61:267-71.

4122 Shimoi K, Masuda S, Shen B, et al. Radioprotective effects of antioxidative plant flavonoids in mice. *Mutat Res* 1996;350:153-61.

4123 Inanami O, Asanuma T, Inukai N, et al. The suppression of age-related accumulation of lipid peroxides in rat brain by administration of Rooibos tea (Aspalathus linearis). *Neurosci Lett* 1995;196:85-8.

4124 Sanchez de Rojas VR, Somoza B, Ortega T, et al. Vasodilatory effect in rat aorta of eriodictyol obtained from Satureja obovata. *Planta Med* 1999;65:234-8.

4125 Lacy CF, Armstrong LL, Ingrim NB, Lance LL. Drug Information Handbook. Hudson, OH: Lexi Comp Inc; 1998-9.

4137 Sills AK Jr, Williams JI, Tyler BM, et al. Squalamine inhibits angiogenesis and solid tumor growth in vivo and perturbs embryonic vasculature. *Cancer Res* 1998;58:2784-92.

4138 Kikuchi K, Bernard EM, Sadownik A, et al. Antimicrobial activities of squalamine mimics. *Antimicrob Agents Chemother* 1997;41:1433-8.

4139 Moore KS, Wehrli S, Roder H, et al. Squalamine: an aminosterol antibiotic from the shark. *Proc Natl Acad Sci U S A* 1993;90:1354-8.

4140 Keynan N, Tamir R, Waisel Y, et al. Allergenicity of the pollen of Pistacia. *Allergy* 1997;52(3):323-30.

4141 Iauk L, Ragusa S, Rapisarda A, et al. In vitro antimicrobial activity of Pistacia lentiscus L. extracts: preliminary report. *J Chemother* 1996;8(3):207-9.

4142 Al-Said MS, Ageel AM, Parmar NS, Tariq M. Evaluation of mastic, a crude drug obtained from Pistacia lentiscus for gastric and duodenal anti-ulcer activity. *J Ethnopharmacol* 1986;15(3):271-8.

4143 Vallverdu A, Garcia-Ortega P, Martinez J, et al. Mercurialis annua: characterization of main allergens and cross-reactivity with other species. *Int Arch Allergy Immunol* 1997;112:356-64.

4144 Garcia-Ortega P, Martinez J, Martinez A, et al. Mercurialis annua pollen: a new source of allergic sensitization and respiratory disease. *J Allergy Clin Immunol* 1992;89:987-93.

4145 Mancini SD, Edwards JM. Cytotoxic principles from the sap of Kalmia latifolia. *J Nat Prod* 1979;42(5):483-8.

4146 Garcia Ortiz JC, Terron M, Bellido J. Contact allergy to henna. *Int Arch Allergy Immunol* 1997;114:298-9.

4147 Kandil HH, al-Ghanem MM, Sarwat MA, al-Thallab FS. Henna (Lawsonia inermis Linn.) inducing haemolysis among G6PD-deficient newborns. A new clinical observation. *Ann Trop Paediatr* 1996;16:287-91.

4148 Majoie IM, Bruynzeel DP. Occupational immediate-type hypersensitivity to henna in a hairdresser. *Am J Contact Dermat* 1996;7:38-40.

4149 Clarke DT, Jones GR, Martin MM. The anti-sickling drug lawsone (2-OH-1,4-naphthoquinone) protects sickled cells against membrane damage. *Biochem Biophys Res Commun* 1986;139:780-6.

4150 Sharma VK. Tuberculostatic activity of henna (Lawsonia inermis Linn.). *Tubercle* 1990;71:293-5.

4151 Van Damme EJ, Roy S, Barre A, et al. The major elderberry (Sambucus nigra) fruit protein is a lectin derived from a truncated type 2 ribosome-inactivating protein. *Plant J* 1997;12:1251-60.

4152 Todorov S, Philianos S, Petkov V, et al. Experimental pharmacological study of three species from genus Salvia. *Acta Physiol Pharmacol Bulg* 1984;10(2):13-20.

4200 Bak AA, Grobbee DE. The effect of serum cholesterol levels of coffee brewed by filtering or boiling. *N Engl J Med* 1989;321:1432-7.

4201 Chevallier A. The Encyclopedia of Medicinal Plants. London, UK: Dorling Kindersley, Ltd., 1996.

4202 Andermann G, Dietz M. The influence of the route of administration on the bioavailability of an endogenous macromolecule: chondroitin sulphate (CSA). *Eur J Drug Metab Pharmacokinet* 1982;7:11-6.

4203 Ronca F, Palmieri L, Panicucci P, et al. Anti-inflammatory activity of chondroitin sulfate. *Osteoarthritis Cartilage* 1998;6 Suppl A:14-21.

4204 Conte A, Volpi N, Palmieri L, et al. Biochemical and pharmacokinetic aspects of oral treatment with chondroitin sulfate. *Arzneimittelforschung* 1995;45:918-25.

4205 Silvestro L, Lanzarotti E, Marchi E, et al. Human pharmacokinetics of glycosaminoglycans using deuterium-labeled and unlabeled substances: evidence for oral absorption. *Semin Thromb Hemost* 1994;20:281-92.

4207 Vale S. Subarachnoid haemorrhage associated with Ginkgo biloba. *Lancet* 1998;352(9121):36.

4208 Mares-Perlman JA, Lyle BJ, Klein R, et al. Vitamin supplement use and incident cataracts in a population-based study. *Arch Ophthalmol* 2000;118:1556-63.

4209 Alic M. Green Tea for remission maintenance in Crohn's disease. *Am J Gastroenterol* 1999;94:1710-1.

4210 Gupta S, Ahmad N, Mukhtar H. Prostate chemoprevention by green tea. *Semin Urol Oncol* 1999; 17(2):70-6.

4211 Taylor JR, Wilt VM. Probable antagonism of warfarin by green tea. *Ann Pharmacother* 1999;33:426-8.

4212 Klaunig JE, Xu Y, Han C, et al. The effect of tea consumption on oxidative stress in smokers and nonsmokers. *Proc Soc Exp Biol Med* 1999;220:249-54.

4213 Li N, Sun Z, Han C, Chen J. The chemopreventive effects of tea on human oral precancerous mucosa lesions. *Proc Soc Exp Biol Med* 1999;220:218-24.

4215 Viereck EG. Alaska's Wilderness Medicines Healthful Plants of the Far North. Anchorage, AK: Alaska Northwest Books, 1998.

4216 Curhan GC, Willett WC, Speizer FE, Stamfer MJ. Beverage use and risk of kidney stones in women. *Ann Intern Med* 1998;128:534-40.

4217 Lee IP, Kim YH, Kang MH, et al. Chemopreventive effect of green tea (Camellia sinensis) against cigarette smoke induced mutations in humans. *J Cell Biochem Suppl* 1997;27:68-75.

4218 Kaegi E. Unconventional therapies for cancer: 2. Green tea. The Task Force on Alternative Therapies of the Canadian Breast Cancer Research Initiative. *CMAJ* 1998;158:1033-5.

4219 Hollman PC, Feskens EJ, Katan MB. Tea flavonols in cardiovascular disease and cancer epidemiology. *Proc Soc Exp Biol Med* 1999;220(4):198-202.

4221 Durlach PJ. The effects of a low dose of caffeine on cognitive performance. *Psychopharmacol* 1998;140:116-9.

4222 Sesso HD, Gaziano JM, Buring JE, et al. Coffee and tea intake and the risk of myocardial infarction. *Am J Epidemiol* 1999;149:162-7.

4224 Hindmarch I, Quinlan PT, Moore KL, Parkin C. The effects of black tea and other beverages on aspects of cognition and psychomotor performance. *Psychopharmacol* 1998;139:230-8.

4225 Sotaniemi EA, Haapakoski E, Rautio A. Ginseng therapy in non-insulin dependent diabetic patients. *Diabetes Care* 1995;18:1373-5.

4227 Lee BM, Lee SK, Kim HS. Inhibition of oxidative DNA damage, 8-OHdG, and carbonyl contents in smokers treated with antioxidants (vitamin E, vitamin C, beta-carotene and red ginseng.) *Cancer Lett* 1998;132:219-27.

4228 Oh M, Choi YH, Choi S, et al. Anti-proliferating effects of ginsenoside Rh2 on MCF-7 human breast cancer cells. *Int J Oncol* 1999;14(5):869-75.

4230 Allen JD, McLung J, Nelson AG, Welsch M. Ginseng supplementation does not enhance healthy young adult's peak aerobic exercise performance. *J Am Coll Nutr* 1998;17:462-6.

4231 Engels HJ, Wirth JC. No ergogenic effects of ginseng (Panax ginseng C.A. Meyer) during grades maximal aerobic exercise. *J Am Diet Assoc* 1997;97:1110-5.

4233 Wolkowitz OM, Reus VI, Manfredi F, et al. Dehydroepiandrosterone (DHEA) treatment of depression. *Biol Psychiatry* 1997;41:311-8.

4234 Salvati G, Genovesi G, Marcellini L, et al. Effects of Panax ginseng C.A. Meyer saponins on male fertility. *Panminerva Med* 1996;38:249-54.

4235 Yun TK. Experimental and epidemiological evidence of the cancer-preventive effects of Panax ginseng C.A. Meyer. *Nutr Rev* 1996;54:71-81.

4236 Morris AC, Jacobs I, McLellan TM, et al. No ergogenic effect of ginseng ingestion. *Int J Sport Nutr* 1996;6:263-71.

4237 Leffler CT, Philippi AF, Leffler SG, et al. Glucosamine, chondroitin, and manganese ascorbate for degenerative joint disease of the knee or low back: a randomized, double-blind, placebo-controlled pilot study. *Mil Med* 1999;164:85-91.

4239 Ondrizek RR, Chan PJ, Patton WC, King A. Inhibition of human sperm motility by specific herbs used in alternative medicine. *J Assist Reprod Genet* 1999;16:87-91.

4240 Ondrizek RR, Chan PJ, Patton WC, King A. An alternative medicine study of herbal effects on the penetration of zona-free hamster oocytes and the integrity of sperm deoxyribonucleic acid. *Fertil Steril* 1999;71:517-22.

4242 Labrie F, Diamond P, Cusan L, et al. Effect of 12 month dehydroepiandrosterone replacement therapy on bone, vagina, and endometrium in postmenopausal women. *J Clin Endocrinol Metab* 1997;82:3498-505.

4243 Ding DZ, Shen TK, Cui YZ. Effects of red ginseng on the congestive heart failure and its mechanism. *Chung Kuo Chung His I Chieh Ho Tsa Chih* 1995;15:325-7.

4244 Bahrke MS, Morgan WP. Evaluation of the ergogenic properties of ginseng. *Sports Med* 1994;18:229-48.

4245 Tyler, V. Herb News. *Prevention* 1999;9:105.

4248 Kroboth PD, Salek FS, Pittenger AL, et al. DHEA and DHEA-S: A review. *J Clin Pharmacol* 1999;39:327-48.

4249 Casson PR, Faquin LC, Stentz FB. Replacement of dehydroepiandrosterone enhances T-lymphocyte insulin binding in postmenopausal women. *Fertil Steril* 1995;63:1027-31.

4250 Bates GW, Egerman RS, Umstot ES, et al. Dehydroepiandrosterone attenuates study-induced declines in insulin sensitivity in postmenopausal women. *Ann N Y Acad Sci* 1995;774:291-3.

4251 Morales AJ, Haubrich RH, Hwang JY, et al. The effect of six months treatment with 100 mg daily dose of dehydroepiandrosterone (DHEA) on circulating sex steroids, body composition and muscle strength in age-advanced men and women. *Clin Endocrinol* 1998;49:421-32.

4252 Casson PR, Andersen RN, Herrod HG, et al. Oral dehyroepiandosterone in physiologic doses modulates immune function in postmenopausal women. *Am J Obstet Gynecol* 1995;1536-9.

4253 Arlt W, Justl H, Callies F, et al. Oral dehydroepiandrosterone for adrenal androgen replacement: pharmacokinetics and peripheral conversion to androgens and estrogens in young healthy females after dexamethasone suppression. *J Clin Endocrinol Metab* 1998;83:1928-34.

4254 Kudielka BM, Hellhammer J, Hellhammer D, et al. Sex differences in endocrine and psychological responses to psychosocial stress in healthy elderly subjects and the impact of a 2 week dehydroepiandrosterone treatment. *J Clin Endocrinol Metab* 1998;83:1756-61.

4255 Flynn MA, Weaver-Osterholtz D, Sharpe-Timms KL, et al. Dehydroepiandrosterone replacement in aging humans. *J Clin Endocrinol Metab* 1999;84:1527-33.

4258 Young LY, Koda-Kimble MA. Applied Therapeutics: The Clinical Use of Drugs. 6th ed. Vancouver, CAN: Applied Thera, Inc. 1995.

4259 FDA Talk Paper. FDA Warns About GBL-Related Products. 1999. Available at: vm.cfsan.fda.gov/~lrd/tpgbl2.html

4260 Briggs GB, Freeman RK, Yaffe SJ. Drugs in Pregnancy and Lactation. 5th ed. Philadelphia: Lippincott Williams & Wilkins; 1998.

4261 FDA Talk Paper. FDA Approves Xyrem for Cataplexy Attacks in Patients with Narcolepsy. Issued July 17, 2002. Availbale at: http://www.fda.gov/bbs/topics/ANSWERS/2002/ANS01157.html

4263 Sobolev VS, Cole RJ, Dorner JW, et al. Isolation, Purification, and Liquid Chromatographic Determination of Stilbene Phytoalexins in Peanuts. *J AOAC Intl* 1995;78:1177-82.

4264 Stampfer J, Manson JE, Rimm EB, et al. Frequent nut consumption and risk of coronary heart disease study. *BMJ* 1998; 17:1341-5.

4265 Kritchevsky D, Tepper SA, Klurfeld DM. Lectin may contribute to the atherogenicity of peanut oil. *Lipids* 1998;33:821-3.

4266 Kritchevsky D. Cholesterol vehicle in experimental atherosclerosis. A brief review with special reference to peanut oil. *Arch Pathol Lab Med* 1988;112:1041-4.

4267 la Vecchia C, Negri E, Franceschi S, et al. Olive oil, other dietary fats, and the risk of breast cancer. (Italy) *Cancer Causes Control* 1995;6(6):545-50.

4269 Muzzarelli RA, Biagini G, Bellardini, et al. Osteoconduction exerted by methylpyrrolidinone chitosan used in dental surgery. *Biomaterials* 1993;14:39-43.

4270 Muzzarelli R, Tarsi R, Fillippini O, et al. Antimicrobial properties of N-carboxybutyl chitosan. *Antimicrob Agents Chemother* 1990;34:2019-23.

4274 Riordan SM, Williams R. Treatment of Hepatic Encephalopathy. *N Engl J Med* 1997;337:473-9.

4275 Shipochliev T. Uterotonic action of extracts from a group of medicinal plants. *Vet Med Nauki* 1981;18(4):94-8.

4278 Olsen A, Siboska GE, Clark BF, Rattan SI. N(6)-Furfuryladenine, kinetin, protects against Fenton reaction-mediated oxidative damage to DNA. *Biochem Biophys Res Commun* 1999;265:499-502.

4282 National Genetics Resources Program. The Germplasm Resources Information Network. Available at: http://www.ars-grin.gov (Accessed 24 February 2000).

4283 Wang H, Nair MG, Strasburg GM, et al. Novel antioxidant compounds from tart cherries (Prunus cerasus). *J Nat Prod* 1999;62:86-8.

4284 Bruneton J. Pharmacognosy Phytochemistry Medicinal Plants. 2nd ed. Paris, FR: Lavoisier, 1999:142.

4289 Protocol Title: A Phase 1B Dose-Range Study to Evaluate the Safety, Pharmacokinetics, and Effects of (+)-calaonlide A on surrogate markers in HIV-positive patients with no previous antiretroviral therapy. Protocol ID numbers: FDA 297A.

4290 Reuters Health. Anti-HIV herbal product shows therapeutic potential in phase I trial. November 1, 1999.

4291 Newman RA, Chen W, Madden TL. Pharmaceutical properties of related calanolide compounds with activity against human immunodeficiency virus. *J Pharm Sci* 1998;87:1077-80.

4292 Buckheit RW, White EL, Fliakas-Boltz V, et al. Unique anti-human immunodeficiency virus activities of the nonnucleoside reverse transcriptase inhibitors calanolide A, costatolide, and dihydrocostatolide. *Antimicrob Agents Chemother* 1999;43(8):1827-34.

4293 Boyer PL, Currens MH, McMahon JB. Analysis of nonnucleoside drug-resistant variants of human immunodeficiency virus type 1 reverse transcriptase. *J Virol* 1993;67(4):2412-20.

4294 Currens MJ, Nariner JM, McMahon JB, Boyd MR. Kinetic analysis of inhibition of human immunodeficiency virus type-a reverse transcriptase by calanolide A. *J Pharmacol Exp Ther* 1996;279(2):652-61.

4295 Currens MJ, Gulakowski RJ, Mariner JM, et al. Antiviral activity and mechanism of action of calanolide A against the human immunodeficiency virus type-1. *J Pharmacol Exp Ther* 1996;279(2):645-51.

4299 Kanth VR, Diwan PV. Analgesic, anti-inflammatory and hypoglycaemic activities of Sida cordifolia. *Phytother Res* 1999;13(1):75-7.

4300 Fuhr U. Drug Interactions with Grapefruit Juice. *Drug Saf* 1998;18:251-72.

4301 Yablonsky F, Nicolas V, Riffaud JP, Bellamy F. Antiproliferative effect of Pygeum africanum extract on rat prostatic fibroblasts. *J Urol* 1997;157:2881-7.

4302 Andro MC, Riffaud JP. Pygeum africanum extract for the treatment of patients with benign prostatic hyperplasia. A review of 25 years of published experience. *Curr Ther Res* 1995;56:796-817.

4303 Homer KA, Manji F, Beighton D. Inhibition of peptidase and glycosidase activities of Porphyromonas gingivalis, Bacteroides intermedius and Treponema denticola by plant extracts. *J Clin Periodontol* 1992;19(5):305-10.

4304 Anon. Sida Cordifolia. Metro Marketing, Inc. Available at: http://metromkt.net/viable/1sidacor.shtml. (Accessed 9 March 2000).

4310 Anon. Sida Cordifolia Linn. Available at: http://www.modern-natural.com/sida_cordifolia.htm. (Accessed 9 March 2000).

4314 Anon. Strictly Medicinal Herb Seeds. Available at: http://www.chatlink.com/~herbseed/sida.html. (Accessed 9 March 2000).

4321 Maharishi Ayur-Ved Products Inc. 1998; Ayurvedic Herbs: Bala. Available at: http://www.mapi.com/cgi-local/shop.pl/page=herbbala.html/SID=1877132249. (Accessed 9 March 2000).

4322 Caron MF, Hotsko AL, Robertson S, et al. Electrocardiographic and hemodynamic effects of Panax ginseng. *Ann Pharmacother* 2002;36:758-63.

4326 Goodwin TW. Metabolism, nutrition, and function of carotenoids. *Annu Rev Nutr* 1986;6:273-97.

4330 Pettengell KE, Grayson MJ. Cimetidine and hyperparathyroidism. *Lancet* 1980;1:1134.

4331 Graziani G, Aroldi A, Colussi G, et al. Cimetidine and hyperparathyroidism. *Lancet* 1980;1:1134.

4332 Kobayashi M, Kakizono T, Nishio N, et al. Antioxidant role of astaxanthin in the green alga Haematococcus pluvialis. *Appl Microbiol Biotechnol* 1997;48:351-6.

4335 Jyonouchi H, Sun S, Tomita Y, et al. Astaxathin, a carotenoid without vitamin A activity, augments antibody responses in cultures including T-helper cell clones and suboptimal doses of antigen. *J Nutr* 1995;125:2483-92.

4336 Chew BP, Wong MW, Park JS, et al. Dietary beta-carotene and astaxanthin but not canthaxanthin stimulate splenocyte function in mice. *Anticancer Res* 1999;19;5223-8.

4337 Chew BP, Park JS, Wong MW, et al. A comparison of the Anticancer activities of dietary beta-carotene, canthaxanthin and astaxanthin in mice in vivo. *Anticancer Res* 1999;19:1849-54.

4338 Tanaka T, Morishita Y, Suzui M, et al. Chemoprevention of mouse urinary bladder carcinogenesis by the naturally occurring carotenoid astaxanthin. *Carcinogenesis* 1994;15:15-9.

4339 Tanaka T, Makita H, Oshnishi M, et al. Chemoprevention of rat oral carcinogenesis by naturally occurring xanthophylls, astaxanthin, and canthaxanthin. *Cancer Res* 1995;55:4059-64.

4340 Gradelet S, Le Bon AM, Berges R, et al. Dietary carotenoids inhibit aflatoxin B1-induced liver preneoplastic foci and DNA damage in the rat: role of the modulation of aflatoxin B1 metabolism. *Carcinogenesis* 1998;19:403-11.

4341 Bennedsen M, Wang X, Willen R, et al. Treatment of H. pylori infected mice with antioxidant astaxanthin reduces gastric inflammation, bacterial load and modulates cytokine release by splenocytes. *Immunol Lett* 1999;70:185-9.

4342 Bensky D, Gamble A, Kaptchuk T. Chinese Herbal Medicine Materia Medica. Seattle, WA: Eastland Press, 1996:214-6.

4343 Huang KC. The Pharmacology of Chinese Herbs. 2nd ed. Boca Raton, FL: CRC Press LLC., 1999:258.

4344 Chevallier A. The Encyclopedia of Medicinal Plants. New York, NY: DK Publishing. 1996:170.

4345 Yamamoto M, Ogawa K, Morita M, et al. The herbal medicine Inchin-ko-to inhibits liver cell apoptosis induced by transforming growth factor beta 1. *Hepatology* 1996;23(3):552-9.

4346 Yamamoto M, Miura N, Ohtake N, et al. Genipin, a metabolite derived from the herbal medicine Inchin-ko-to, and suppression of fas-induced lethal liver apoptosis in mice. *Gastroenterol* 2000;118:380-9.

4347 Saavedra J. Probiotics and infectious diarrhea. *Am J Gastroenterol* 2000;95:S16-8.

4348 Castagliuolo I, Riegler MF, Valenick L, et al. Saccharomyces boulardii protease inhibits the effects of clostridium difficile toxins A and B in human colonic mucosa. *Infection and Immun* 1999;67:302-7.

4349 Bleichner G, Blehaut H, Mentec H, et al. Saccharomyces boulardii prevents diarrhea in critically ill tube-fed patients. *Intensive Care Med* 1997;23:517-23.

4350 Lewis SJ, Potts LF, Barry RE. The lack of therapeutic effect of Saccharomyces boulardii in the prevention of antibiotic-related diarrhea in elderly patients. *J Infect* 1998;36:171-4.

4351 Elmer GW, McFarland LV. Comment on the lack of therapeutic effect of Saccharomyces boulardii in the prevention of antibiotic-related diarrhea in elderly patients. *J Infect* 1998;37:307-8.

4352 McFarland LV, Surawicz CM, Greenberg RN, et al. A randomized placebo-controlled trial of Saccharomyces boulardii in combination with standard antibiotics for Clostridium difficile disease. *JAMA* 1994;271:1913-8.

4353 McFarland LV, Surawicz CM, Greenberg RN, et al. Prevention of beta-lactam associated diarrhea by Saccharomyces boulardii compared with placebo. *Am J Gastroenterol* 1995;90:439-48.

4354 Surawicz CM, McFarland LV, Elmer G, et al. Treatment of recurrent clostridium difficile colitis with vancomycin and Saccharomyces boulardii. *Am J Gastroenterol* 1989;84:1285-7.

4355 Surawicz CM, Elmer GW, Speelman P, et al. Prevention of antibiotic-associated diarrhea by Saccharomyces boulardii: a prospective study. *Gastroenterol* 1989;96:981-8.

4356 Buts JP, Corthier G, Delmee M. Saccharomyces boulardii for Clostridium difficile-associated enteropathies in infants. *J Pediatr Gastroenterol Nutr* 1993;16:419-25.

4357 Pletinex M, Legein J, Vandenplas Y. Fungemia with Saccharomyces boulardii in a 1-year-old girl with protracted diarrhea. *J Pediatr Gastroenterol Nutr* 1995;21:113-5.

4358 Fredenucci I, Chomarat M, Boucaud C, et al. Saccharomyces boulardii fungemia in a patient receiving ultra-levure therapy. *CID* 1998;27:222-3.

4359 Hennequin C, Kauffmann-Lacroix C, Jobert A, et al. Possible role of catheters in Saccharomyces boulardii fungemia. *Eur J Clin Microbiol Infect Dis* 2000;19:16-20.

4360 Elmer GW, McFarland LV, Surawicz CM, et al. Behaviour of Saccharomyces boulardii in recurrent Clostridium difficile disease patients. *Aliment Pharmacol Ther* 1999;13:1663-8.

4361 Czerucka D, Roux I, Rampal P. Saccharomyces boulardii inhibits secretagogue-mediated adenosine 3',5'-cyclic monophosphate induction in intestinal cells. *Gastroenterol* 1994;106:65-72.

4362 Krammer M, Karbach U. Antidiarrheal action of the yeast Saccharomyces boulardii in the rat small and large intestine by stimulating chloride absorption. *Z Gastroenterol* 1993;31:73-7.

4363 Lewis SJ, Freedman AR. Review article: the use of biotherapeutic agents in the prevention and treatment of gastrointestinal disease. *Aliment Pharmacol Ther* 1998;12:807-22.

4366 Steiner M, Li W. Aged garlic extract, a modulator of cardiovascular risk factors: a dose-finding study on the effects of AGE on platelet functions. *J Nutr* 2001;131:980S-4S.

4367 Gorbach SL. Probiotics and gastrointestinal health. *Am J Gastroenterol* 2000;95:S2-S4.

4368 Schultz M, Sartor RB. Probiotics and inflammatory bowel diseases. *Am J Gastroenterol* 2000;95:S19-21.

4369 deRoos NM, Katan MB. Effects of probiotic bacteria on diarrhea, lipid metabolism, and carcinogenesis: a review of papers published between 1988 and 1998. *Am J Clin Nutr* 2000;71:405-11.

4370 Guandalini S, Pensabene L, Zikri MA, et al. Lactobacillus GG administered in oral rehydration solution to children with acute diarrhea: a multicenter European trial. *J Pediatr Gastroenterol Nutr* 2000;30:54.

4371 Vanderhoof JA, Whitney DB, Antonson DL, et al. Lactobacillus GG in the prevention of antibiotic-associated diarrhea in children. *J Pediatr* 1999;135:564-8.

4372 Arvola T, Laiho K, Torkkeli S, et al. Prophylactic Lactobacillus GG reduces antibiotic-associated diarrhea in children with respiratory infections: a randomized study. *Pediatrics* 1999;104:e64.

4373 Oberhelman RA, Gilman RH, Sheen P, et al. A placebo-controlled trial of Lactobacillus GG to prevent diarrhea in undernourished Peruvian children. *J Pediatr* 1999;134:15-20.

4374 Hilton E, Kolakowski P, Singer C, et al. Efficacy of Lactobacillus GG as a Diarrheal Preventative in Travelers. *J Travel Med* 1997;4:41-3.

4375 Vanderhoof JA, Young RJ, Murray N, et al. Treatment strategies for small bowel bacterial overgrowth in short bowel syndrome. *J Pediatr Gastroenterol Nutr* 1998;27:155-60.

4376 El-Nezami H, Kankaanpaa P, Salminen S, et al. Ability of dairy strains of lactic acid bacteria to bind a common food carcinogen, aflatoxin B1. *Food Chem Toxicol* 1998;36:321-6.

4377 Guarino A, Canani RB, Spagnuolo MI, et al. Oral bacterial therapy reduces the duration of symptoms and of viral excretion in children with mild diarrhea. *J Pediatr Gastroenterol Nutr* 1997;25:516-9.

4378 Hudault S, Lievin V, Bernet-Camard MF, et al. Antagonistic activity exerted in vitro and in vivo by Lactobacillus casei (strain GG) against Salmonella typhimurium C5 infection. *Appl Environ Microbiol* 1997;63:513-8.

4379 Sutas Y, Hurme M, Isolauri E. Down-regulations of anti-CD3 antibody-induced IL-4 production by bovine caseins hydrolyzed with Lactobacillus GG-derived enzymes. *Scand J Immunol* 1996;43:687-9.

4380 Saxelin M, Chuang NH, Chassy B, et al. Lactobacilli and bacteremia in southern Finland 1989-1992. *Clin Infect Dis* 1996;22:564-6.

4381 Malin M, Suomalainen H, Saxelin M, et al. Promotion of IgA immune response in patients with Crohn's disease by oral bacteriotherapy with Lactobacillus GG. *Ann Nutr Metab* 1996;40:137-45.

4382 Goldin BR, Gualtieri LJ, Moore RP. The effect of Lactobacillus GG on the initiation and promotion of DMH-induced intestinal tumors in the rat. *Nutr Cancer* 1996;25:197-204.

4383 Whiting PW, Clouston A, Kerlin P. Black cohosh and other herbal remedies associated with acute hepatitis. *Med J Aust* 2002;177:440-3.

4387 McIntosh GH, Royle PJ, Playne MJ. A probiotic strain of L. acidophilus reduces DMH-induced large intestinal tumors in male Sprague-Dawley rats. *Nutr Cancer* 1999;35:153-9.

4388 Mack DR, Michail S, Shu W, et al. Probiotics inhibit enteropathogenic E. coli adherence in vitro by inducing intestinal mucin gene expression. *Clin Exp Immunol* 1999;116:276-82.

4389 Tynkkynen S, Singh KV, Varmanen P. Vancomycin resistance factor of Lactobacillus rhamnosus GG in relation to enterococcal vancomycin resistance (van) genes. *Int J Food Microbiol* 1998;41:195-204.

4390 Klein G, Zill E, Schindler R, et al. Peritonitis associated with vancomycin-resistant Lactobacillus rhamnosus in a continuous ambulatory peritoneal dialysis patient; organism identification, antibiotic therapy, and case report. *J Clin Microbiol* 1998;36:1781-3.

4391 Kalima P, Masterton RG, Roddie PH, et al. Lactobacillus rhamnosus infection in a child following bone marrow transplant. *J Infect* 1996;32:165-7.

4392 Pochapin M. The effect of probiotics on Clostridium difficile diarrhea. *Am J Gastroenterol* 2000;95:S11-3.

4393 Goldin BR. Health Benefits of probiotics. *Br J Nutr* 1998;80:S203-7.

4394 Biller JA, Katz AJ, Flores AF, et al. Treatment of recurrent Clostridium difficile colitis with Lactobacillus GG. *J Pediatr Gastroenterol Nutr* 1995;21:224-6.

4397 Hilton E, Rindos P, Isenberg HD. Lactobacillus GG Vaginal Suppositories and Vaginitis. *J Clin Microbiol* 1995;33:1433.

4398 Rautio M, Jousimies-Somer H, Kauma H, et al. Liver abscess due to Lactobacillus rhamnosus strain indistinguishable from L. rhamnosus strain GG. *Clin Infect Dis* 1999;28:1159-60.

4399 Pelto L, Ioslauri E, Lilius EM, et al. Probiotic bacteria down-regulate the milk-induced inflammatory response in milk-hypersensitive subjects but have an immunostimulatory effect in healthy subjects. *Clin Exp Allergy* 1998;28:1474-9.

4400 Spencer H, Menaham L. Adverse effects of aluminum-containing antacids on mineral metabolism. *Gastroenterology* 1979;76:603-6.

4404 Folkers K, Langsjoen P, Willis R, et al. Lovastatin decreases coenzyme Q levels in humans. *Proc Natl Acad Sci U S A* 1990;87:8931.

4405 Mortensen SA, Leth A, Agner E, et al. Dose-related decrease of serum coenzyme Q10 during treatment with HMG-CoA reductase inhibitors. *Mol Aspects Med* 1997;18:S137-44.

4406 Ghirlanda G, Oradei A, Manto A, et al. Evidence of plasma CoQ10-lowering effect by HMG-CoA reductase inhibitors: A double blind, placebo-controlled study. *J Clin Pharmacol* 1993;33:226-9.

4407 De Pinieux G, Chariot P, Ammi-Said M, et al. Lipid-lowering drugs and mitochondrial function: Effects of HMG-CoA Reductase inhibitors on serum ubiquinone and blood lactate/pyruvate ratio. *Br J Clin Pharmacol* 1996;42:333-7.

4408 Bargossi AM, Grossi G, Fiorella PL, et al. Exogenous CoQ10 supplementation prevents plasma ubiquinone reduction induced by HMG-CoA reductase inhibitors. *Mol Aspects Med* 1994;15:187-93.

4409 Watts GF, Castelluccio C, Rice-Evans C, et al. Plasma coenzyme Q (ubiquinone) concentrations in patients treated with simvastatin. *J Clin Pathol* 1993;46:1055-7.

4410 Hanaki Y, Sugiyama S, Ozawa T, et al. Coenzyme Q10 and coronary artery disease. *Clin Investig* 1993;71:112-5.

4411 Ritsema GH, Ellers G. Potassium supplements prevent serious hypokalemia in colon cleansing. *Clin Radiol* 1994;49(12);874-6.

4412 Murry JJ, Healy MD. Drug-mineral interactions: a new responsibility for the hospital dietician. *J Am Diet Assoc* 1991;91:66-73.

4425 Garabedian-Ruffalo SM, Ruffalo RL. Drug and nutrient interactions. *AFP* 1986;33:165-74.

4426 Kishi T, Fujita N, Eguchi T, et al. Mechanism for reduction of serum folate by antiepileptic drugs during prolonged therapy. *J Neurol Sci* 1997;145:109-12.

4427 Froscher W, Maier V, Laage M, et al. Folate deficiency, anticonvulsant drugs, and psychiatric morbidity. *Clin Neuropharmacol* 1995;18:165-82.

4428 Hendel J, Dam M, Gram L, et al. The effects of carbamazepine and valproate on folate metabolism in man. *Acta Neurol Scan* 1984;69:226-31.

4429 Traccis S, Monaco F, Sechi GP, et al. Long-term therapy with carbamazepine: Effects on nerve conduction velocity. *Eur Neurol* 1983;22:410-6.

4430 Hoikka V, Alhava EM, Karjalainen P, et al. Carbamazepine and bone mineral metabolism. *Acta Neurol Scand* 1984;70:77-80.

4431 Rajantie J, Lamberg-Allardt C, Wilska M. Does carbamazepine treatment lead to a need of extra vitamin D in some mentally retarded children? *Acta Paediatr Scand* 1984;73:325-8.

4434 Cummings JH, Macfarlane G. Role of intestinal bacteria in nutrient metabolism. *J Parenter Enteral Nutr* 1997;21:357-65.

4435 Honma N. The effect of lactic acid bacteria, Part 1: biological significance. *New Medicines and Clinics* 1986;35:1-3.

4436 Gorbach SL. Bengt E. Gustafsson memorial lecture. Function of the normal human microflora. *Scand J Infect Dis Suppl* 1986;49:17-30.

4437 Hill MJ. Intestinal flora and endogenous vitamin synthesis. *Eur J Cancer Prev* 1997;6:S43-5.

REFERENCES

4438 Conly J, Stein K. Reduction of vitamin K2 concentrations in human liver associated with the use of broad spectrum antimicrobials. *Clin Invest Med* 1994;17:531-9.

4439 Conly JM, Stein K, Worobetz L, Rutledge-Harding S. The contribution of vitamin K2 (menaquinones) produced by the intestinal microflora to human nutritional requirements for vitamin K. *Am J Gastroenterol* 1994;89:915-23.

4440 Cordes I, Buchmann S, Scheffner D. [Vitamin K deficiency with erythromycin. Observation of a boy treated with valproate]. [Article in German]. *Monatsschr Kinderheilkd* 1990 Feb;138(2):85-7.

4441 Lipsky JJ. Antibiotic-associated hypoprothrombinemia. *J Antimicrob Chemother* 1988;21:281-300.

4442 Alitalo R, Ruutu M, Valtonen V, et al. Hypoprothrombinemia and bleeding during administration of cefamandole and cefoperazone. Report of three cases. *Ann Clin Res* 1985;17:116-9.

4443 Shimada K, Matsuda T, Inamatsu T, et al. Bleeding secondary to vitamin K deficiency in patients receiving parenteral cephem antibiotics. *J Antimicrob Chemother* 1984;14:325-30.

4445 Jandourek A, Vaishampayan JK, Vazquez JA. Efficacy of melaleuca oral solution for the treatment of fluconazole refractory oral candidiasis in AIDS patients. *AIDS* 1998;12:1033-7.

4446 Hammer KA, Carson CF, Riley TV. In-vitro activity of essential oils, in particular Melaleuca alternifolia (tea tree) oil and tea tree oil products, against Candida spp. *J Antimicrob Chemother* 1998;42:591-5.

4447 Atta-ur-Rahman, Choudhary MI, Naz S, et al. New steroidal alkaloids from the roots of buxus sempervirens. *J Nat Prod* 1999;62:665-9.

4448 Elsom GF, Hyde D. Susceptibility of methicillin-resistant Staphylococcus aureus to tea tree oil and mupirocin. *J Antimicrob Chemother* 1999;43:427-8.

4449 Robertson JI. Diuretics, potassium depletion and risk of arrhythmias. *Eur Heart J* 1984;5(Suppl A):25-8.

4450 Hammer KA, Carson CF, Riley TV. In vitro activities of ketoconazole, econazole, miconazole, and Melaleuca alternifolia (tea tree) oil against Malassezia species. *Antimicrob Agents Chemother* 2000;44:467-9.

4451 Nelson RR. Selection of resistance to the essential oil of Melaleuca alternifolia in Staphylococcus aureus. *J Antimicrob Chemother* 2000;45:549-50.

4452 Mountokalakis T, Dourakis S, Karatzas N, et al. Zinc deficiency in mild hypertensive patients treated with diuretics. *J Hypertens Suppl* 1984;2(3):S571-2.

4453 Campbell IA, Elmes PC. Ethambutol and the eye: zinc and copper (letter). *Lancet* 1975;2:711.

4454 Hathcock JN. Metabolic mechanisms of drug-nutrient interactions. *Fed Proc* 1985;44:124-9.

4455 West RJ, Lloyd JK. The effect of cholestyramine on intestinal absorption. *Gut* 1975;16:93-8.

4456 Cywes C, Millar AJ. Assessment of the nutritional status of infants and children with biliary atresia. *S Afr Med J* 1990;77:131-5.

4457 Elinder LS, Hadell K, Johansson J, et al. Probucol treatment decreases serum concentrations of diet-derived antioxidants. *Arterioscler Throm Vasc Biol* 1995;15:1057-63.

4458 Knodel LC, Talbert RL. Adverse effects of hypolipidaemic drugs. *Med Toxicol* 1987;2:10-32.

4459 Matsui MS, Rozovski SJ. Drug-nutrient interaction. *Clin Ther* 1982;4:423-40.

4460 Schwarz KB, Goldstein PD, Witztum JL, et al. Fat-soluble vitamin concentrations in hypercholestrolemic children treated with colestipol. *Pediatrics* 1980;65:243-50.

4461 Tonstad S, Silverstein M, Aksnes L, Ose L. Low dose colestipol in adolescents with familial hypercholesterolemia. *Arch Dis Child* 1996;74:157-60.

4462 Lems WF, Van Veen GJ, Gerrits MI, et al. Effect of low-dose prednisolone (with calcium and calcitriol supplementation) on calcium and bone metabolism in healthy volunteers. *Br J Rheumatol* 1998;37:27-33.

4463 Reid DM, Kennedy NS, Smith MA, et al. Total body calcium in rheumatoid arthritis: Effects of disease activity and corticosteroid treatment. *Br Med J* (Clin Res Ed) 1982;285:330-2.

4464 Lems WF, Jacobs JW, Netelenbos JC, et al. [Pharmacological prevention of osteoporosis in patients on corticosteroid medication]. [Article in Dutch]. *Ned Tijdschr Geneeskd* 1998;142:1904-8.

4465 Gennari C. Differential effect of glucocorticoids on calcium absorption and bone mass. *Br J Rheumatol* 1993;32:11-4.

4466 Need AG, Philcox JC, Hartley TF, et al. Calcium metabolism and osteoporosis in corticosteroid-treated postmenopausal women. *Aust N Z J Med* 1986;16:341-6.

4467 Reid IR, Ibbertson HK. Calcium supplements in the prevention of steroid-induced osteoporosis. *Am J Clin Nutr* 1986;44:287-90.

4468 Kahn SB, Fein SA, Brodsky I. Effects of trimethoprim on folate metabolism in man. *Clin Pharmacol Ther* 1968;9:550-60.

4469 Kline RM, Kline JJ, Di Palma J, Barbero GJ. Enteric-coated, pH-dependent peppermint oil capsules for the treatment of irritable bowel syndrome in children. *J Pediatr* 2001;138:125-8.

4470 Blum M, Kitai E, Ariel Y, et al. [Oral contraceptive lowers serum magnesium]. [Article in Hebrew]. Harefuah 1991;121(10):363-4.

4471 Lewis DP, Van Dyke DC, Willhite LA, et al. Phenytoin-folic acid interaction. *Ann Pharmacother* 1995;29:726-35.

4472 Berg MJ, Stumbo PJ, Chenard CA, et al. Folic acid improves phenytoin pharmacokinetics. *J Am Diet Assoc* 1995;95:352-6.

4473 Berg MJ, Fincham RW, Ebert BE, et al. Phenytoin pharmacokinetics: Before and after folic acid administration. *Epilepsia* 1992;33:712-20.

4474 Zerwekh JE, Homan R, Tindall R, et al. Decreased serum 24,25-dihydroxy vitamin D concentration during long-term anticonvulsant therapy in adult epileptics. *Ann Neurol* 1982;12(2):184-6.

4475 Bell RD, Pak CY, Zerwekh J, et al. Effect of phenytoin on bone and mineral density in ambulatory epileptic children. *Brain Dev* 1994;16:382-5.

4476 Badmaev V, Majeed M, Conte AA. Garcinia cambogia for weight loss. *JAMA* 1999;282:233-4; discussion 235.

4477 Shafer RB, Nuttall FQ. Calcium and folic acid absorption in patients taking anticonvulsant drugs. *J Clin Endocrinol Metab* 1975;41:1125-9.

4478 Schaller JL. Garcinia cambogia for weight loss. *JAMA* 1999;282:234; discussion 235.

4479 Kishi T, Kishi H, Watanabe T, et al. Bioenergetics in clinical medicine. XI. Studies on coenzyme Q and diabetes mellitus. *J Med* 1976;7:307-21.

4480 Firenzuoli F, Gori L. Garcinia cambogia for weight loss. *JAMA* 1999;282:234; discussion 235.

4481 Pellock JM, Howell J, Kendig EI Jr, et al. Pyridoxine deficiency in children treated with isoniazid. *Chest* 1985;87:658-61.

4482 Snider DE Jr. Pyridoxine supplementation during isoniazid therapy. *Tubercle* 1980;61:191-6.

4483 Termanini B, Gibril F, Sutliff VE, et al. Effect of long-term gastric acid suppressive therapy on serum vitamin B12 levels in patients with Zollinger-Ellison syndrome. *Am J Med* 1998;104:422-30.

4484 Bellou A, Aimone-Gastin I, De Korwin JD, et al. Cobalamin deficiency with megaloblastic anaemia in one patient under long-term omeprazole therapy. *J Intern Med* 1996;240:161-4.

4485 Saltzman JR, Kemp JA, Golner BB, et al. Effect of hypochlorhydria due to omeprazole treatment or atrophic gastritis on protein-bound vitamin B12 absorption. *J Am Coll Nutr* 1994;13:584-91.

4486 Marcuard SP, Albernaz L, Khazaine PG. Omeprazole therapy causes malabsorption of cyanocobalamin. *Ann Intern Med* 1994;120:211-5.

4487 Ishihara K, Oyaizu S, Onuki K, et al. Chronic (-)-hydroxycitrate administration spares carbohydrate utilization and promotes lipid oxidation during exercise in mice. *J Nutr* 2000;130:2990-5.

4488 Wiesel LL, Barritt AS, Stumpe WM. The synergistic action of para-aminobenzoic acid and cortisone in the treatment of rheumatoid arthritis. *Am J Med Sci* 1951;243-8.

4490 Carpentier JL, Bury J, Luyckx A, et al. Vitamin B12 and folic acid serum levels in diabetics under various therapeutic regimens. *Diabete Metab* 1976;2:187-90.

4491 Bristol-Myers Squibb Company. Glucophage package insert. Princeton, NJ; January 1999.

4492 Leeb BF, Witzmann G, Ogris E, et al. Folic acid cyanocobalamin levels in serum and erythrocytes during low-dose methotrexate therapy in rheumatoid arthritis and psoriatic arthritis patients. *Clin Exp Rheumatol* 1995;13:459-63.

4493 Morgan SL, Baggott JE, Lee JY, et al. Folic acid supplementation prevents deficient blood folate levels and hyperhomocysteinemia during long-term, low dose methotrexate therapy for rheumatoid arthritis: Implications for cardiovascular disease prevention. *J Rheumatol* 1998;25:441-6.

4494 Dijkmans BA. Folate supplementation and methotrexate. *Br J Rheumatol* 1995;34:1172-4.

4495 Becker GL. The case against mineral oil. *Am J Digestive Dis* 1953;19:344-7.

4496 Clark JH, Russell GJ, Fitzgerald JF, et al. Serum beta-carotene, retinol, and alpha-tocopherol levels during mineral oil therapy for constipation. *Am J Dis Child* 1987;141:1210-2.

4498 Prasad AS, Lei KY, Moghissi KS, et al. Effect of oral contraceptives on nutrients. III. Vitamins B6, B12 and folic acid. *Am J Obstet Gynecol* 1976;125:1063-9.

4500 Hocking GM. A dictionary of natural products. 2nd ed. Medford, OR: Plexus Publishing, 1997.

4502 Duke JA. CRC handbook of medicinal herbs. 1st ed. Boca Raton, FL: CRC Press, 1985.

4504 Weiss RF. Herbal medicine. 5th ed. Beaconsfield: Beaconsfield Publishers Ltd, 1998.

4505 DeSmet P, ed. Adverse effects of herbal drugs. 1st ed. Berlin, Heidelberg: Springer-Verlag, 1993.

4506 Miller LG, Wallace JM, eds. Herbal medicinals a clinician's guide. 1st ed. New York, NY: Pharmaceutical Prod Press, 1998.

4511 Palva IP, Salokannel SJ, Timonen T, et al. Drug-induced malabsorption of vitamin B12. IV. Malabsorption and deficiency of B12 during treatment with slow-release potassium chloride. *Acta Med Scand* 1972;191:355-7.

4512 Salokannel SJ, Palva IP, Takkunen JT, et al. Malabsorption of vitamin B12 during treatment with slow-release potassium chloride. Preliminary report. *Acta Med Scand* 1970;187:431-2.

4513 Mai I, Kruger H, Budde K, et al. Hazardous pharmacokinetic interaction of Saint John's wort (Hypericum perforatum) with the immunosuppressant cyclosporin. *Int J Clin Pharmacol Ther* 2000;38:500-2.

4514 D'Erasmo E, Ragno A, Raejntroph N, et al. Drug-induced osteomalacia. *Recenti Prog Med* 1998;89:529-33.

4515 Krogh-Jensen M, Ekelund S, Svendsen L. Folate and homocysteine status and haemolysis in patients treated with sulphasalazine for arthritis. *Scand J Clin Lab Invest* 1996;56:421-9.

4516 Logan EC, Williamson LM, Ryrie DR. Sulphasalazine associated pancytopenia may be caused by acute folate deficiency. *Gut* 1986;27:868-72.

4517 Grieco A, Caputo S, Bertoli A, et al. Megaloblastic anemia due to sulphasalazine responding to drug withdrawal alone. *Postgrad Med J* 1986;62:307-8.

4518 Whiskey E, Werneke U, Taylor D. A systematic review and meta-analysis of Hypericum perforatum in depression: a comprehensive clinical review. *Int Clin Psychopharmacol* 2001;16:239-52.

4519 Agrosi M, Mischiatti S, Harrasser PC, Savio D. Oral bioavailability of active principles from herbal products in humans. A study on Hypericum perforatum extracts using the soft gelatin capsule technology. *Phytomedicine* 2000;7:455-62.

4520 Jakovljevic V, Popovic M, Mimica-Dukic N, et al. Pharmacodynamic study of Hypericum perforatum L. *Phytomedicine* 2000;7:449-53.

4521 Jensen AG, Hansen SH, Nielsen EO. Adhyperforin as a contributor to the effect of Hypericum perforatum L. in biochemical models of antidepressant activity. *Life Sci* 2001;68:1593-605.

4522 Delport R, Ubbink JB, Serfontein WJ, et al. Vitamin B6 nutritional status in asthma. The effect of theophylline therapy on plasma pyridoxal-5-phosphate and pyridoxal levels. *Int J Vitam Nutr Res* 1988;58:67-72.

4523 Van Wouwe JP. Carnitine deficiency during valproic acid treatment. *Int J Vitam Nutr Res* 1995;65:211-4.

4524 Matsuda I, Ohtani Y, Ninomiya N. Renal handling of carnitine in chlidren with carnitine deficiency and hyperammonemia associated with valproate therapy. *J Pediatr* 1986;109:131-4.

4525 Ohtani Y, Endo F, Matsuda I. Carnitine deficiency and hyperammonemia associated with valproic acid therapy. *J Pediatr* 1982;101(5):782-5.

4526 Opala G, Winter S, Vance C, et al. The effect of valproic acid on plasma carnitine levels. *Am J Dis Child* 1991;145:999-1001.

4527 Melegh B, Kerner J, Kispal G, et al. Effect of chronic valproic acid treatment on plasma and urine carnitine levels in children: Decreased urinary excretion. *Acta Paediatr Hung* 1987;28(2):137-42.

4528 De Vivo DC, Bohan TP, Coulter DL, et al. L-carnitine supplementation in childhood epilepsy: Current perspectives. *Epilepsia* 1998;39:1216-25.

4529 Coulter DL. Carnitine, valproate, and toxicity. *J Child Neurol* 1991;6:7-14.

4530 Taliani U, Camellini A, Bernardi P, et al. A clinical case of severe megaloblastic anemia during treatment with primidone. *Acta Biomed Ateneo Parmense* 1989;60:245-8.

4531 Segal S, Kaminski S. Drug-nutrient interactions. *American Druggist* 1996;42-8.

4532 Glaxo-Wellcome, Inc. Daraprim package insert. Research Triangle Park, NC; August, 1996.

4533 Raskin HN, Fishman RA. Pyridoxine-deficiency neuropathy due to hydralazine. *N Engl J Med* 1965;273:1182-5.

4534 Seelig MS. Auto-immune complications of D-penicillamine - A possible result of zinc and magnesium depletion and of pyridoxine inactivation. *J Am Coll Nutr* 1982;1:207-14.

4535 Kozak SF, Inderlied CB, Hsu HY, et al. The role of copper on ethambutol's antimicrobial action and implications for ethambutol-induced optic neuropathy. *Diag Microbiol Infect Dis* 1998;30:83-7.

4536 Lambie DG, Johnson RH. Drugs and folate metabolism. *Drugs* 1985;30:145-55.

4537 Joosten E, Pelemans W. Megaloblastic anaemia in an elderly patient treated with triamterene. *Neth J Med* 1991;38:209-11.

4538 Hubner WD, Kirste T. Experience with St. John's Wort (Hypericum perforatum) in children under 12 years with symptoms of depression and psychovegetative disturbances. *Phytother Res* 2001;15:367-70.

4539 Aymard JP, Aymard B, Netter P, et al. Haematological adverse effects of histamine H2-receptor antagonists. *Med Toxicol Adverse Drug Exp* 1988;3:430-48.

4540 Belaiche J, Zittoun J, Marquet J, et al. Effect of ranitidine on secretion of gastric intrinsic factor and absorption of vitamin B12. *Gastroenterol Clin Biol* 1983;7:381-4.

4541 Salom IL, Silvis SE, Doscherholmen A. Effect of cimetidine on the absorption of vitamin B12. *Scand J Gastroenterol* 1982;17:129-31.

4542 Schempp CM, Muller K, Winghofer B, et al. Single-dose and steady-state administration of Hypericum perfotatum extract (St. John's wort) does not influence skin sensitivity to UV radiation, visible light, and solar-stimulated radiation. *Arch Dermatol* 2001;137:512-3.

4543 Race TF, Paes IC, Faloon WW. Intestinal malabsorption induced by oral colchicine. Comparison with neomycin and cathartic agents. *Am J Med Sci* 1970;259:32-41.

4544 Faloon WW, Chodos RB. Vitamin B12 absorption studies using cochicines, neomycin and continuous 57Co B12 administration. *Gastroenterolgy* 1969;56:1251.

4545 Webb DI, Chodos RB, Mahar CQ, et al. Mechanism of vitamin B12 malabsorption in patients receiving colchicine. *N Engl J Med* 1968;279:845-50.

4546 Amer College of Rheumatology ad hoc committee on clinical guidelines. Guidelines for monitoring drug therapy in rheumatoid arthritis. *Arthritis Rheum* 1996;39:723-31.

4547 Hielt K, Brynskov J, Hippe E, et al. Oral contraceptives and the cobalamin (vitamin B12) metabolism. *Acta Obstet Gynecol Scand* 1985;64:59-63.

4548 Sanpitak N, Chayutimonkul L. Oral contraceptives and riboflavin nutrition. *Lancet* 1974;1:836-7.

4549 Leyden JJ. Absorption of minocycline hydrochloride and tetracycline hydrochloride. Effect of food, milk, and iron. *J Am Acad Dermatol* 1985;12(2 Pt 1):308-12.

4550 Neuvonen PJ, Pentikainen PJ, Gothoni G. Inhibition of iron absorption by tetracycline [letter]. *Br J Clin Pharmacol* 1975;2(1):94-6.

4556 Schwinger RH, Eromann E. Heart failure and electrolyte disturbances. *Methods Find Exp Clin Pharmacol* 1992;14:315-25.

4557 Paaby P, Norvin E. The absorption of vitamin B12 during treatment with paraminosalicylic acid. *Acta Med Scand* 1966;180:561-4.

4558 Toskes PP, Deren JJ. Selective inhibition of vitamin B12 absorption by para-aminosalicylic acid. *Gastroenterology* 1972;62:1232-7.

4559 Longsreth GF, Newcomer AD, Westbrook PR. Para-aminosalicylic acid-induced malabsorption. *Am J Dig Dis* 1972;17:731-4.

4560 Zimmerman J. Drug interactions in intestinal transport of folic acid and methotrexate. Further evidence for the heterogeneity of folate transport in the human small intestine. *Biochem Pharmacol* 1992;44:1839-42.

4561 Nimmo WS. Drugs, diseases, and altered gastric emptying. *Clin Pharmacokinet* 1967;1(3):189-203.

4562 Andrews R, Greenhaff P, Curtis S, et al. The effect of dietary creatine supplementation on skeletal muscle metabolism in congestive heart failure. *Eur Heart J* 1998;19:617-22.

4563 Gordon A, Hultman E, Kaijser L, et al. Creatine supplementation in chronic heart failure increases skeletal muscle creatine phosphate and muscle performance. *Cardiovasc Res* 1995;30:413-8.

4564 Tarnopolsky M, Martin J. Creatine monohydrate increases strength in patients with neuromuscular disease. *Neurology* 1999;52:854-7.

4565 Tarnopolsky MA, Roy BD, MacDonald JR. A randomized, controlled trial of creatine monohydrate in patients with mitochondrial cytopathies. *Muscle Nerve* 1997;20:1502-9.

4566 Klivenyi P, Ferrante RJ, Matthews RT, et al. Neuroprotective effects of creatine in a transgenic animal model of amyotrophic lateral sclerosis. *Nat Med* 1999;5:347-50.

4567 Matthews RT, Yang L, Jenkins BG, et al. Neuroprotective effects of creatine and cyclocreatine in animal models of Huntington's disease. *J Neurosci* 1998;18:156-63.

4568 Matthews RT, Ferrante RJ, Klivenyi P, et al. Creatine and cyclocreatine attenuate MPTP neurotoxicity. *Exp Neurol* 1999;157:142-9.

4569 Mihic S, MacDonald JR, McKenzie S, Tarnopolsky MA. Acute creatine loading increases fat-free mass, but does not affect blood pressure, plasma creatinine, or CK activity in men and women. *Med Sci Sports Exerc* 2000;32:291-6.

4570 Rawson ES, Clarkson PM. Acute creatine supplementation in older men. *Int J Sports Med* 2000;21:71-5.

4571 Bermon S, Venembre P, Sachet C, et al. Effects of creatine monohydrate ingestion in sedentary and weight-trained older adults. *Acta Physiol Scand* 1998;164:147-55.

4572 Rawson ES, Wehnert ML, Clarkson PM. Effects of 30 days of creatine ingestion in older men. *Eur J Appl Physiol* 1999;80:139-44.

4573 Earnest CP, Almada AL, Mitchell TL. High-performance capillary electrophoresis-pure creatine monohydrate reduces blood lipids in men and women. *Clin Sci* (Colch) 1996;91:113-8.

4574 Demant TW, Rhodes EC. Effects of creatine supplementation on exercise performance. *Sports Med* 1999;28:49-60.

4575 Williams MH, Branch JD. Creatine supplementation and exercise performance: an update. *J Am Coll Nutr* 1998;17:216-34.

4576 Juhn MS. Oral creatine supplementation. Separating fact from hype. *Phys Sportsmed* 1999;27:47-50,53-54,56,61,89.

4577 Heinanen K, Nanto-Salonen K, Komu M, et al. Creatine corrects muscle 31P spectrum in gyrate atrophy with hyperornithinaemia. *Eur J Clin Invest* 1999;29:1060-5.

4578 Sipila I, Rapola J, Simell O, Vannas A. Supplementary creatine as a treatment for gyrate atrophy of the choroid and retina. *N Engl J Med* 1981;304:867-70.

4579 Ingwall JS, Morales MF, Stockdale FE, Wildenthal K. Creatine: a possible stimulus skeletal cardiac muscle hypertrophy. *Recent Adv Stud Cardiac Struct Metab* 1975;8:467-81.

4580 Vandenberghe K, Van Hecke P, Van Leemputte M, et al. Phosphocreatine resynthesis is not affected by creatine loading. *Med Sci Sports Exerc* 1999;31:236-42.

4581 Baerheim A, Larsen E, Digranes A. Vaginal application of lactobacilli in the prophylaxis of recurrent lower urinary tract infection in women. *Scand J Prim Health Care* 1994;12:239-43.

4582 Febbraio MA, Flanagan TR, Snow RJ, et al. Effect of creatine supplementation on intramuscular TCr, metabolism and performance during intermittent, supramaximal exercise in humans. *Acta Physiol Scand* 1995;155:387-95.

4583 Harris RC, Soderlund K, Hultman E. Elevation of creatine in resting and exercised muscle of normal subjects by creatine supplementation. *Clin Sci* (Colch) 1992;83:367-74.

4584 Juhn MS, O'Kane JW, Vinci DM. Oral creatine supplementation in male collegiate athletes: a survey of

dosing habits and side effects. *J Am Diet Assoc* 1999;99:593-5.
4586 Cisowski M, Bochenek A, Kucewicz E, et al. The use of exogenous creatine phosphate for myocardial protection in patients undergoing coronary artery bypass surgery. *J Cardiovasc Surg* (Torino) 1996;37:75-80.
4587 Chambers DJ, Haire K, Morley N, et al. St. Thomas' Hospital cardioplegia: enhanced protection with exogenous creatine phosphate. *Ann Thorac Surg* 1996;61:67-75.
4588 Francaux M, Poortmans JR. Effects of training and creatine supplement on muscle strength and body mass. *Eur J Appl Physiol* 1999;80:165-8.
4589 Green AL, Hultman E, Macdonald IA, et al. Carbohydrate ingestion augments skeletal muscle creatine accumulation during creatine supplementation in humans. *Am J Physiol* 1996;271:E821-6.
4590 Lamartiniere CA. Protection against breast cancer with genistein: a component of soy. *Am J Clin Nutr* 2000;71:1705S-7S.
4591 Balsom PD, Soderlund K, Sjodin B, Ekblom B. Skeletal muscle metabolism during short duration high-intensity exercise: influence of creatine supplementation. *Acta Physiol Scand* 1995;154:303-10.
4592 Birch R, Noble D, Greenhaff PL. The influence of dietary creatine supplementation on performance during repeated bouts of maximal isokinetic cycling in man. *Eur J Appl Physiol* 1994;69:268-76.
4593 Dawson B, Cutler M, Moody A, et al. Effects of oral creatine loading on single and repeated maximal short sprints. *Aust J Sci Med Sport* 1995;27:56-61.
4594 Prevost MC, Nelson AG, Morris GS. Creatine supplementation enhances intermittent work performance. *Res Q Exerc Sport* 1997;68:233-40.
4595 Barnett C, Hinds M, Jenkins DG. Effects of oral creatine supplementation on multiple sprint cycle performance. *Aust J Sci Med Sport* 1996;28:35-9.
4596 Cooke WH, Barnes WS. The influence of recovery duration on high-intensity exercise performance after oral creatine supplementation. *Can J Appl Physiol* 1997;22:454-67.
4597 Vanakoski J, Kosunen V, Meririnne E, Seppala T. Creatine and caffeine in anaerobic and aerobic exercise: effects on physical performance and pharmacokinetic considerations. *Int J Clin Pharmacol Ther* 1998;36:258-62.
4598 Cooke WH, Grandjean PW, Barnes WS. Effect of oral creatine supplementation on power output and fatigue during bicycle ergometry. *J Appl Physiol* 1995;78:670-3.
4599 Odland LM, MacDougall JD, Tarnopolsky MA, et al. Effect of oral creatine supplementation on muscle [PCr] and short-term maximum power output *Med Sci Sports Exerc* 1997;29:216-9.
4600 Snow RJ, McKenna MJ, Selig SE, et al. Effect of creatine supplementation on sprint exercise performance and muscle metabolism. *J Appl Physiol* 1998;84:1667-73.
4601 Leenders NM, Lamb DR, Nelson TE. Creatine supplementation and swimming performance. *Int J Sport Nutr* 1999;9:251-62.
4602 Jones AM, Atter T, Georg KP. Oral creatine supplementation improves multiple sprint performance in elite ice-hockey players. *J Sports Med Phys Fitness* 1999;39:189-96.
4603 Theodorou AS, Cooke CB, King RF, et al. The effect of longer-term creatine supplementation on elite swimming performance after an acute creatine loading. *J Sports Sci* 1999;17:853-9.
4604 Kamber M, Koster M, Kreis R, et al. Creatine supplementation - part I: performance, clinical chemistry, and muscle volume. *Med Sci Sports Exerc* 1999;31:1763-9.
4605 McNaughton LR, Dalton B, Tarr J. The effects of creatine supplementation on high-intensity exercise performance in elite performers. *Eur J Appl Physiol* 1998;78:236-40.
4606 McKenna MJ, Morton J, Selig SE, Snow RJ. Creatine supplementation increases muscle total creatine but not maximal intermittent exercise performance. *J Appl Physiol* 1999;87:2244-52.
4607 Rossiter HB, Cannell ER, Jakeman PM. The effect of oral creatine supplementation on the 1000-m performance of competitive rowers. *J Sports Sci* 1996;14:175-9.
4608 Uc A, Bishop WP, Sanders KD. Camphor Hepatotoxicity. *South Med J* 2000;93(6):596-8.
4609 South M. Neonatal seizures after pyridoxine use -- reply. *Lancet* 1999;354:2083.
4610 Parry GJ, Bredesen DE. Sensory neuropathy with low-dose pyridoxine. *Neurology* 1985;35:1466-8.
4611 Grebe HB, Gregory PJ. Inhibition of warfarin anticoagulation associated with chelation therapy. *Pharmacotherapy* 2002;22:1067-9.
4612 Enzymatic Therapy. "Remifemin". Available at: http://www.enzy.com/products/individual/eprod141.html (Accesssed 21 March 2000).
4613 Phytopharmica. "Remifemin". Available at: http://www.phytopharmica.com/consumer/products/1855-BP-remifemin.html (Accesssed 21 March 2000).
4614 Liske E, Wustenberg P. Therapy of climacteric complaints with Cimicifuga racemosa: herbal medicine with clinically proven evidence. *Menopause* 1998;5:250.
4615 Pepping J. Black cohosh: Cimicifuga racemosa. *Am J Health Syst Pharm* 1999;56:1400-2.
4616 Liske E. Therapeutic efficacy and safety of Cimicifuga racemosa for gynecologic disorders. *Adv Ther* 1998;15:45-53.
4618 Kruse SO, Lohning A, Pauli GF, et al. Fukiic and piscidic acid esters from the rhizome of Cimicifuga racemosa and the in vitro estrogenic activity of fukinolic acid. *Planta Med* 1999;65:763-4.
4619 Einer-Jensen N, Zhao J, Andersen KP, Kristoffersen K. Cimicifuga and Melbrosia lack oestrogenic effects in mice and rats. *Maturitas* 1996;25:149-53.
4620 Lehmann-Willenbrock E, Riedel HH. [Clinical and endocrinologic studies of the treatment of ovarian insufficiency manifestations following hysterectomy with intact adnexa]. [Article in German]. *Zentralbl Gynakol* 1988;110:611-8.
4621 Sen BH, Akdeniz BG, Denizci AA. The effect of ethylenediamine-tetraacetic acid on Candida albicans. *Oral Surg Oral Med Oral Pathol Oral Radiol Endod* 2000;90:651-5.
4623 Spencer H, Fuller H, Norris C, Williams D. Effect of magnesium on the intestinal absorption of calcium in man. *J Am Coll Nutr* 1994;15:485-92.
4624 Xu SS, Cai ZY, Qu ZW, et al. Huperzine-A in capsules and tablets for treating patients with Alzheimer disease. *Zhongguo Yao Li Xue Bao* 1999;20:486-90.
4625 Camps P, Cusack B, Mallender WD, et al. Huprine X is a novel high-affinity inhibitor of acetylcholinesterase that is of interest for treatment of Alzheimer's disease. *Mol Pharmacol* 2000;57:409-17.
4626 Sun QQ, Xu SS, Pan JL, et al. Huperzine-A capsules enhance memory and learning performance in 34 pairs of matched adolescent students. *Chung Kuo Yao Li Hsueh Pao* 1999;20:601-3.
4627 Horwitt MK. My valedictory on the differences in biological potency between RRR-alpha-tocopheryl and all-rac-alpha-tocopheryl acetate. *Am J Clin Nutr* 1999;69:341-2.
4628 Schempp CM, Ludtke R, Winghofer B, Simon JC. Effect of topical application of hypericum perforatum extract on skin

sensitivity to solar simulated radiation. *Photodermatol Photoimmunol Photomed* 2000;16:125-8.

4629 Shan MD, Hu LH, Chen ZL. Three new hyperforin Analogues from Hypericum perforatum. *J Nat Prod* 2001;664:127-30.

4630 Laakmann G, Dienel A, Kieser M. Clinical significance of hyperforin for the efficacy of Hypericum extracts on depressive disorders of different severities. *Phytomedicine* 998;6:435-42.

4631 Jacobson JM, Feinman L, Liebes L, et al. Pharmacokinetics, safety, and antiviral effects of hypericin, a derivative of St. John's Wort plant, in patients with chronic hepatitis C virus infection. *Antimicrob Agents Chemother* 2001;45:517-24.

4632 Khalifa AE. Hypericum perforatum as a nootropic drug: enhancement of retrieval memory of a passive avoidance conditioning paradigm in mice. *J Ethnopharmacol* 2001;76:49-57.

4633 Zhang W, Hinton D, Surnock A, et al. Malignant glioma sensitivity to radiotherapy, high-dose tamoxifen, and hypericin: corroborating clinical response in vitro: case report. *Neurosurger* 1996;38:587-590, discussion 590-1.

4634 Neunteufl T, Priglinger U, Heher S, et al. Effects of vitamin E on chronic and acute endothelial dysfunction in smokers. *J Am Coll Cardiol* 2000;35:277-83.

4635 Sano M, Ernesto C, Thomas RG, et al. A controlled trial of selegiline, alpha-tocopherol, or both as treatment for Alzheimer's disease. The Alzheimer's Disease Cooperative Study. *N Engl J Med* 1997;336:1216-22.

4636 Masaki KH, Losonczy KG, Izmirlian G, et al. Association of vitamin E and C supplement use with cognitive function and dementia in elderly men. *Neurology* 2000;54:1265-72.

4637 Socci DJ, Crandall BM, Arendash GW. Chronic antioxidant treatment improves the cognitive performance of aged rats. *Brain Res* 1995;693:88-94.

4638 Yamada K, Tanaka T, Han D, et al. Protective effects of idebenone and alpha-tocopherol on beta-amyloid-(1-42)-induced learning and memory deficits in rats: implication of oxidative stress in beta-amyloid-induced neurotoxicity in vivo. *Eur J Neurosci* 1999;11:83-90.

4639 Joseph JA, Shukitt-Hale B, Denisova NA, et al. Long-term dietary strawberry, spinach, or vitamin E supplementation retards the onset of age-related neuronal signal-transduction and cognitive behavioral deficits. *J Neurosci* 1998;18:8047-55.

4640 Nemeth I, Turi S, Haszon I, Bereczki C. Vitamin E alleviates the oxidative stress of erythropoietin in uremic children on hemodialysis. *Pediatr Nephrol* 2000;14:13-7.

4641 Inal M, Kanbak G, Sen S, et al. Antioxidant status and lipid peroxidation in hemodialysis patients undergoing erythropoietin and erythropoietin-vitamin E combined therapy. *Free Rad Res* 1999;31:211-6.

4642 Suthutvoravut U, Hathirat P, Sirichakwal P, et al. Vitamin E status, glutathione peroxidase activity and the effect of vitamin E supplementation in children with thalassemia. *J Med Assoc Thai* 1993;76:146-52.

4643 Hartman TJ, Albanes D, Pietinen P, et al. The association between baseline vitamin E, selenium, and prostate cancer in the alpha-tocopherol, beta-carotene cancer prevention study. *Cancer Epidemiol Biomarkers Prev* 1998;7:335-40.

4644 Deneo-Pellegrini H, De Stefani E, Ronco A, Mendilaharsu M. Foods, nutrients and prostate cancer: a case-control study in Uruguay. *Br J Cancer* 1999;80:591-7.

4645 Kristal AR, Stanford JL, Cohen JH, et al. Vitamin and mineral supplement use is associated with reduced risk of prostate cancer. *Cancer Epidemiol Biomarkers Prev* 1999;8:887-92.

4646 Chan JM, Stampfer MJ, Ma J, et al. Supplemental vitamin E intake and prostate cancer risk in a large cohort of men in the United States. *Cancer Epidemiol Biomarkers Prev* 1999;8:893-9.

4647 Cristol JP, Bosc JY, Badiou S, et al. Erythropoietin and oxidative stress in haemodialysis: beneficial effects of vitamin E supplementation. *Nephrol Dial Transplant* 1997;12:2312-7.

4648 Zipursky A, Brown EJ, Watts J, et al. Oral vitamin E supplementation for the prevention of anemia in premature infants: a controlled trial. *Pediatrics* 1987;79:61-8.

4649 Ferns G, Williams J, Forster L, et al. Cholesterol standardized plasma vitamin E levels are reduced in patients with severe angina pectoris. *Int J Exp Pathol* 2000;81:57-62.

4650 Motoyama T, Kawano H, Kugiyama K, et al. Vitamin E administration improves impairment of endothelium-dependent vasodilation in patients with coronary spastic angina. *J Am Coll Cardiol* 1998;32:1672-9.

4651 Rapola JM, Virtamo J, Ripatti S, et al. Effects of alpha tocopherol and beta carotene supplements on symptoms, progression, and prognosis of angina pectoris. *Heart* 1998;79:454-8.

4652 Spencer AP, Carson DS, Crouch MA. Vitamin E and coronary artery disease. *Arch Intern Med* 1999;159:1313-20.

4653 Poutaraud A, DiGregorio F, Tin VC, Girardin P. Effect of light on hypericins contents in fresh flowering top parts and in an extract of St. John's Wort (Hypericum perforatum). *Planta Med* 2001;67:254-9.

4655 Fish WH, Cohen M, Franzek D, et al. Effect of intramuscular vitamin E on mortality and intracranial hemorrhage in neonates of 1000 grams or less. *Pediatrics* 1990;85:578-84.

4656 Chiswick M, Gladman G, Sinha S, et al. Vitamin E supplementation and periventricular hemorrhage in the newborn. *Am J Clin Nutr* 1991;53:370S-2S.

4657 Watts JL, Milner R, Zipursky A, et al. Failure of supplementation with vitamin E to prevent bronchopulmonary dysplasia in infants less than 1,500 g birth weight. *Eur Resp J* 1991;4:188-90.

4658 Hunter DJ, Manson JE, Colditz GA, et al. A prospective study of the intake of vitamins C, E, and A and the risk of breast cancer. *N Engl J Med* 1993;329:234-40.

4659 Rohan TE, Howe GR, Friedenreich CM, et al. Dietary fiber, vitamins A, C, and E, and risk of breast cancer: a cohort study. *Cancer Causes Control* 1993;4:29-37.

4660 Ernster VL, Goodson WH III, Hunt TK, et al. Vitamin E and benign breast disease: a double-blind, randomized clinical trial. *Surgery* 1985;97:490-4.

4661 Meyer EC, Sommers DK, Reitz CJ, Mentis H. Vitamin E and benign breast disease. *Surgery* 1990;107:549-51.

4662 London RS, Sundaram GS, Murphy L, et al. The effect of vitamin E on mammary dysplasia: a double-blind study. *Obstet Gynecol* 1985;65:104-6.

4663 Leske MC, Chylack LT Jr, He Q, et al. Antioxidant vitamins and nuclear opacities: the longitudinal study of cataract. *Ophthalmol* 1998;105:831-6.

4664 Seddon JM, Christen WG, Manson JE, et al. The use of vitamin supplements and the risk of cataract among US male physicians. *Am J Publ Health* 1994;84:788-92.

4665 Tavani A, Negri E, La Vecchia C. Food and nutrient intake and risk of cataract. *Ann Epidemiol* 1996;6:41-6.

4666 Teikari JM, Rautalahti M, Haukka J, et al. Incidence of cataract operations in Finnish male smokers unaffected by alpha tocopherol or beta carotene supplements. *J Epidemiol Community Health* 1998;52:468-72.

4667 Teikari JM, Laatikainen L, Virtamo J, et al. Six-year supplementation with alpha-tocopherol and beta-carotene and age-related maculopathy. *Acta Ophthalmol Scand* 1998;76:224-9.

4668 Ludwig CU, Stoll HR, Obrist R, Obrecht JP. Prevention of cytotoxic drug induced skin ulcers with dimethyl sulfoxide (DMSO) and alpha-tocopherol. *Eur J Cancer Clin Oncol* 1987;23:327-9.

4670 Raju GB, Behari M, Prasad K, Ahuja GK. Randomized, double-blind, placebo-controlled, clinical trial of D-alpha-tocopherol (vitamin E) as add-on therapy in uncontrolled epilepsy. *Epilepsia* 1994;35:368-72.

4671 Ogunmekan AO, Hwang PA. A randomized, double-blind, placebo-controlled, clinical trial of D-alpha-tocopheryl acetate (vitamin E), as add-on therapy, for epilepsy in children. *Epilepsia* 1989;30:84-9.

4672 Delanian S, Balla-Mekias S, Lefaix JL. Striking regression of chronic radiotherapy damage in a clinical trial of combined pentoxifylline and tocopherol. *J Clin Oncol* 1999;17:3283-90.

4673 Delanian S. Striking regression of radiation-induced fibrosis by a combination of pentoxifylline and tocopherol. *Br J Radiol* 1998;71:892-4.

4675 Tahzib M, Frank R, Gauthier B, et al. Vitamin E treatment of focal segmental glomerulosclerosis: results of an open-label study. *Pediatr Nephrol* 1999;13:649-52.

4676 Varis K, Taylor PR, Sipponen P, et al. Gastric cancer and premalignant lesions in atrophic gastritis: a controlled trial on the effect of supplementation with alpha-tocopherol and beta-carotene. The Helsinki Gastritis Study Group. *Scand J Gastroenterol* 1998;33:294-300.

4677 Bukin YV, Draudin-Krylenko VA, Kuvshinov YP, et al. Decrease of ornithine decarboxylase activity in premalignant gastric mucosa and regression of small intestinal metaplasia in patients supplemented with high doses of vitamin E. *Cancer Epidemiol Biomarkers Prev* 1997;6:543-6.

4678 Dawsey SM, Wang GQ, Taylor PR, et al. Effects of vitamin/mineral supplementation on the prevalence of histological dysplasia and early cancer of the esophagus and stomach: results from the Dysplasia Trial in Linxian, China. *Cancer Epidemiol Biomarkers Prev* 1994;3:167-72.

4679 Wang GQ, Dawsey SM, Li JY, et al. Effects of vitamin/mineral supplementation on the prevalence of histological dysplasia and early cancer of the esophagus and stomach: results from the General Population Trial in Linxian, China. *Cancer Epidemiol Biomarkers Prev* 1994;3:161-6.

4681 Goldstein RK, Zillikens D, Miller K, et al. Local treatment of disseminated granuloma anulare with a vitamin E emulsion. *Hautarzt* 1991;42:176-8.

4682 Eldamhougy S, Elhelw Z, Yamamah G, et al. The vitamin E status among glucose-6 phosphate dehydrogenase deficient patients and effectiveness of oral vitamin E. *Int J Vita Nutr Res* 1988;58:184-8.

4683 Hafez M, Amar ES, Zedan M, et al. Improved erythrocyte survival with combined vitamin E and selenium therapy in children with glucose-6-phosphate dehydrogenase deficiency and mild chronic hemolysis. *J Pediatr* 1986;108:558-561.

4684 Johnson GJ, Vatassery GT, Finkel B, Allen DW. High-dose vitamin E does not decrease the rate of chronic hemolysis in glucose-6-phosphate dehydrogenase deficiency. *N Engl J Med* 1983;308:1014-7.

4685 Chan AC, Chow CK, Chiu D. Interaction of antioxidants and their implication in genetic anemia. *Proc Soc Exp Biol Med* 1999;222:274-82.

4686 Peyser CE, Folstein M, Chase GA, et al. Trial of d-alpha-tocopherol in Huntington's disease. *Am J Psychiatry* 1995;152:1771-5.

4687 Meydani SN, Meydani M, Blumberg JB, et al. Vitamin E supplementation and in vivo immune response in healthy elderly subjects. A randomized controlled trial. *JAMA* 1997;277:1380-6.

4688 Ravaglia G, Forti P, Maioli F, et al. Effect of micronutrient status on natural killer cell immune function in healthy free-living subjects aged >/=90 y. *Am J Clin Nutr* 2000;71:590-8.

4689 Pallast EG, Schouten EG, de Waart FG, et al. Effect of 50- and 100-mg vitamin E supplements on cellular immune function in noninstitutionalized elderly persons. *Am J Clin Nutr* 1999;69:1273-81.

4690 de la Fuente M, Ferrandez MD, Burgos MS, et al. Immune function in aged women is improved by ingestion of vitamins C and E. *Can J Physiol Pharmacol* 1998;76:373-80.

4691 Buzina-Suboticanec K, Buzina R, Stavljenic A, et al. Aging, nutritional status and immune response. *Int J Vita Nutr Res* 1998;68:133-41.

4692 De Waart FG, Portengen L, Doekes G, et al. Effect of 3 months vitamin E supplementation on indices of the cellular and humoral immune response in elderly subjects. *Br J Nutr* 1997;78:761-74.

4693 Kessopoulou E, Powers HJ, Sharma KK, et al. A double-blind, randomized, placebo, cross-over, controlled trial using the antioxidant vitamin E to treat reactive oxygen species associated male infertility. *Fertil Steril* 1995;64:825-31.

4695 Suleiman SA, Ali ME, Zaki ZM, et al. Lipid peroxidation and human sperm motility: protective role of vitamin E. *J Androl* 1996;17:530-7.

4696 Rolf C, Cooper TG, Yeung CH, Nieschlag E. Antioxidant treatment of patients with asthenozoospermia or moderate oligoasthenozoospermia with high-dose vitamin C and vitamin E: a randomized, placebo-controlled, double-blind study. *Hum Reprod* 1999;14:1028-33.

4697 Yau TM, Weisel RD, Mickle DA, et al. Vitamin E for coronary bypass operations. A prospective, double-blind, randomized trial. *J Thorac Cardiovasc Surg* 1994;108:302-10.

4698 Westhuyzen J, Cochrane AD, Tesar PJ, et al. Effect of preoperative supplementation with alpha-tocopherol and ascorbic acid on myocardial injury in patients undergoing cardiac operations. *J Thorac Cardiovasc Surg* 1997;113:942-8.

4699 Sisto T, Paajanen H, Metsa-Ketela T, et al. Pretreatment with antioxidants and allopurinol diminishes cardiac onset events in coronary artery bypass grafting. *Ann Thorac Surg* 1995;59:1519-23.

4700 Riley JD, Antony SJ. Leg cramps: differential diagnosis and management. *Am Fam Physician* 1995;52:1794-8.

4701 Roca AO, Jarjoura D, Blend D, et al. Dialysis leg cramps. Efficacy of quinine versus vitamin E. *ASAIO J* 1992;38:M481-5.

4702 Connolly PS, Shirley EA, Wasson JH, Nierenberg DW. Treatment of nocturnal leg cramps. A crossover trial of quinine vs vitamin E. *Arch Intern Med* 1992;152:1877-80.

4703 Fenichel GM, Brooke MH, Griggs RC, et al. Clinical investigation in Duchenne muscular dystrophy: penicillamine and vitamin E. *Muscle Nerve* 1988;11:1164-8.

4704 Orndahl G, Grimby G, Grimby A, et al. Functional deterioration and selenium-vitamin E treatment in myotonic dystrophy. A placebo-controlled study. *J Intern Med* 1994;235:205-10.

4705 Watanabe H, Kakihana M, Ohtsuka S, Sugishita Y. Randomized, double-blind, placebo-controlled study of supplemental vitamin E on attenuation of the development of nitrate tolerance. *Circulation* 1997;96:2545-50.

4706 Honegger UE, Scuntaro I, Wiesmann UN. Vitamin E reduces accumulation of amiodarone and desethylamiodarone and inhibits phospholipidosis in

REFERENCES

cultured human cells. *Biochem Pharmacol* 1995;49:1741-5.

4707 Kachel DL, Moyer TP, Martin WJ II. Amiodarone-induced injury of human pulmonary artery endothelial cells: protection by alpha-tocopherol. *J Pharmacol Exp Ther* 1990;254:1107-12.

4708 Benner SE, Winn RJ, Lippman SM, et al. Regression of oral leukoplakia with alpha-tocopherol: a community clinical oncology program chemoprevention study. *J Natl Cancer Inst* 1993;85:44-7.

4709 The Parkinson Study Group. Effects of tocopherol and deprenyl on the progression of disability in early Parkinson's disease. *N Engl J Med* 1993;328:176-83.

4710 Kieburtz K, McDermott M, Como P, et al. The effect of deprenyl and tocopherol on cognitive performance in early untreated Parkinson's disease. Parkinson Study Group. *Neurology* 1994;44:1756-9.

4711 Parkinson Study Group. Impact of deprenyl and tocopherol treatment on Parkinson's disease in DATATOP patients requiring levodopa. *Ann Neurol* 1996;39:37-45.

4712 de Rijk MC, Breteler MM, den Breeijen JH, et al. Dietary antioxidants and Parkinson disease. The Rotterdam Study. *Arch Neurol* 1997;54:762-5.

4713 Dreher F, Gabard B, Schwindt DA, Maibach HI. Topical melatonin in combination with vitamins E and C protects skin from ultraviolet-induced erythema: a human study in vivo. *Br J Dermatol* 1998;139:332-9.

4714 Dreher F, Denig N, Gabard B, et al. Effect of topical antioxidants on UV-induced erythema formation when administered after exposure. *Dermatol* 1999;198:52-5.

4715 Fuchs J, Kern H. Modulation of UV-light-induced skin inflammation by D-alpha-tocopherol and L-ascorbic acid: a clinical study using solar simulated radiation. *Free Radic Biol Med* 1998;25:1006-12.

4716 Eberlein-Konig B, Placzek M, Przybilla B. Protective effect against sunburn of combined systemic ascorbic acid (vitamin C) and d-alpha-tocopherol (vitamin E). *J Am Acad Dermatol* 1998;38:45-8.

4718 Gulmezoglu AM, Hofmeyr GJ, Oosthuisen MM. Antioxidants in the treatment of severe pre-eclampsia: an explanatory randomised controlled trial. *Br J Obstet Gynaecol* 1997;104:689-96.

4719 London RS, Murphy L, Kitlowski KE, Reynolds MA. Efficacy of alpha-tocopherol in the treatment of the premenstrual syndrome. *J Reprod Med* 1987;32:400-4.

4720 London RS, Sundaram GS, Murphy L, Goldstein PJ. The effect of alpha-tocopherol on premenstrual symptomatology: a double-blind study. *J Am Coll Nutr* 1983;2:115-22.

4721 Baumann LS, Spencer JS. The Effects of Topical Vitamin E on the Cosmetic Appearance of Scars. *Dermatol Surg* 1999;25:311-5.

4722 Jenkins M, Alexander JW, MacMillan BG, et al. Failure of topical steroids and vitamin E to reduce postoperative scar formation following reconstructive surgery. *J Burn Care Rehabil* 1986;7:309-12.

4723 Edmonds SE, Winyard PG, Guo R, et al. Putative analgesic activity of repeated oral doses of vitamin E in the treatment of rheumatoid arthritis. Results of a prospective placebo controlled double blind trial. *Ann Rheum Dis* 1997;56:649-55.

4724 Tutuncu NB, Bayraktar M, Varli K. Reversal of defective nerve conduction with vitamin E supplementation in type 2 diabetes: a preliminary study. *Diabetes Care* 1998;21:1915-8.

4725 Bursell SE, Clermont AC, Aiello LP, et al. High-dose vitamin E supplementation normalizes retinal blood flow and creatinine clearance in patients with type 1 diabetes. *Diabetes Care* 1999;22:1245-51.

4726 Paolisso G, D'Amore A, Giugliano D, et al. Pharmacologic doses of vitamin E improve insulin action in healthy subjects and non-insulin-dependent diabetic patients. *Am J Clin Nutr* 1993;57:650-6.

4727 Paolisso G, Di Maro G, Galzerano D, et al. Pharmacological doses of vitamin E and insulin action in elderly subjects. *Am J Clin Nutr* 1994;59:1291-6.

4730 van Rooij J, Schwartzenberg SG, Mulder PG, Baarsma SG. Oral vitamins C and E as additional treatment in patients with acute anterior uveitis: a randomised double masked study in 145 patients. *Br J Ophthalmol* 1999;83:1277-82.

4732 Tornwall ME, Virtamo J, Haukka JK, et al. The effect of alpha-tocopherol and beta-carotene supplementation on symptoms and progression of intermittent claudication in a controlled trial. *Atherosclerosis* 1999;147:193-7.

4733 Liede KE, Haukka JK, Saxen LM, Heinonen OP. Increased tendency towards gingival bleeding caused by joint effect of alpha-tocopherol supplementation and acetylsalicylic acid. *Ann Med* 1998;30:542-6.

4735 Setchell KD, Gosselin SJ, Welsh MB, et al. Dietary estrogens--a probable cause of infertility and liver disease in captive cheetahs. *Gastroenterol* 1987;93:225-33.

4736 Evans AM. Influence of dietary components on the gastrointestinal metabolism and transport of drugs. *Ther Drug Monit* 2000;22:131-6.

4737 Anon. Phytoestrogens. *Med Lett Drugs Ther* 2000;42:17-8.

4738 Hodgson JM, Puddey IB, Beilin LJ, et al. Supplementation with isoflavonoid phytoestrogens does not alter serum lipid concentrations: a randomized controlled trial in humans. *J Nutr* 1998;128:728-32.

4739 Hodgson JM, Puddey IB, Beilin LJ, et al. Effects of isoflavonoids on blood pressure in subjects with high-normal ambulatory blood pressure levels: a randomized controlled trial. *Am J Hypertens* 1999;12:47-53.

4740 Yanagihara K, Ito A, Toge T, Numoto M. Antiproliferative effects of isoflavones on human cancer cell lines established from the gastrointestinal tract. *Cancer Res* 1993;53:5815-21.

4741 Le Bail JC, Champavier Y, Chulia AJ, Habrioux G. Effects of phytoestrogens on aromatase, 3beta and 17beta-hydroxysteroid dehydrogenase activities and human breast cancer cells. *Life Sci* 2000;66:1281-91.

4742 Cassady JM, Zennie TM, Chae YH, et al. Use of a mammalian cell culture benzo(a)pyrene metabolism assay for the detection of potential anticarcinogens from natural products: inhibition of metabolism by biochanin A, an isoflavone from Trifolium pratense L. *Cancer Res* 1988;48:6257-61.

4743 Kurzer MS, Xu X. Dietary phytoestrogens. *Annu Rev Nutr* 1997;17:353-81.

4744 ARS-GRIN. Dr. Duke's Phytochemical and Ethnobotanical Databases. Available at: www.ars-grin.gov (Accessed 24 April 2000).

4746 Gambacciani M, Cappagli B, Piaggesi L, et al. Ipriflavone prevents the loss of bone mass in pharmacological menopause induced by GnRH-agonists. *Calcif Tissue Int* 1997;61:S15-8.

4747 Yamazaki I, Shino A, Shimizu Y, et al. Effect of ipriflavone on glucocorticoid-induced osteoporosis in rats. *Life Sci* 1986;38:951-8.

4748 Cecchettin M, Bellometti S, Cremonesi G, et al. Metabolic and bone effects after administration of ipriflavone and salmon calcitonin in postmenopausal osteoporosis. *Biomed Pharmacother* 1995;49:465-8.

4749 Nozaki M, Hashimoto K, Inoue Y, et al. Treatment of bone loss in oophorectomized women with a combination of ipriflavone and conjugated equine estrogen. *Int J Gynaecol Obstet* 1998;62:69-75.

4750 Xu X, Wang HJ, Murphy PA, Hendrich S. Neither background diet nor type of soy food affects short-term isoflavone bioavailability in women. *J Nutr* 2000;130:798-801.

4751 Scambia G, Mango D, Signorile PG, et al. Clinical effects of a standardized soy extract in postmenopausal women: a pilot study. *Menopause* 2000;7:105-11.

4752 Albertazzi P, Pansini F, Bottazzi M, et al. Dietary soy supplementation and phytoestrogen levels. *Obstet Gynecol* 1999;94:229-31.

4753 Kurzer MS, Xu X. Dietary phytoestrogens. *Annu Rev Nutr* 1997;17:353-81.

4755 Sirtori CR, Pazzucconi F, Colombo L, et al. Double-blind study of the addition of high-protein soya milk v. cows' milk to the diet of patients with severe hypercholesterolemia and resistance to or intolerance of statins. *Br J Nutr* 1999;82:91-6.

4756 Maugeri D, Panebianco P, Russo MS, et al. Ipriflavone-treatment of senile osteoporosis: results of a multicenter, double-blind clinical trial of 2 years. *Arch Gerontol Geriatr* 1994;19:253-63.

4757 Scali G, Mansanti P, Zurlo A, et al. Analgesic effect of ipriflavone versus sCalcitonin in the treatment of osteoporotic vertebral pain. *Curr Ther Res* 1991;49:1004-10.

4759 Mares-Perlman JA, Brady WE, Klein BE, et al. Serum carotenoids and tocopherols and severity of nuclear and cortical opacities. *Invest Ophthalmol Vis Sci* 1995;36:276-88.

4761 Graham DY, Anderson SY, Lang T. Garlic or jalapeno peppers for treatment of Helicobacter pylori infection. *Am J Gastroenterol* 1999;94:1200-2.

4762 Ernst E. Is garlic an effective treatment for Helicobacter pylori infection? *Arch Intern Med* 1999;159:2484-5.

4763 Aydin A, Ersoz G, Tekesin O, et al. Garlic oil and Helicobacter pylori infection. *Am J Gastroenterol* 2000;95:563-4.

4764 O'Gara EA, Hill DJ, Maslin DJ. Activities of Garlic Oil, Garlic Powder, and Their Diallyl Constituents against Helicobacter pylori. *Appl Environ Microbiol* 2000;66:2269-73.

4765 Calvet X, Carod C, Gene E. Re: Peppers at treatment for Helicobacter pylori infection. *Am J Gastroenterol* 2000;95:820-1.

4766 Ledezma E, DeSousa L, Jorquera A, et al. Efficacy of ajoene, an organosulphur derived from garlic, in the short-term therapy of tinea pedis. *Mycoses* 1996;39:393-5.

4767 Ledezma E, Lopez JC, Marin P, et al. Ajoene in the topical short-term treatment of tinea cruris and tinea corporis in humans. Randomized comparative study with terbinafine. *Arzneimittelforschung* 1999;49:544-7.

4768 Ankri S, Mirelman D. Antimicrobial properties of allicin from garlic. *Microbes Infect* 1999;1:125-9.

4769 Weber ND, Andersen DO, North JA, et al. In vitro virucidal effects of Allium sativum (garlic) extract and compounds. *Planta Med* 1992;58:417-23.

4770 Steinmetz KA, Kushi LH, Bostick RM, et al. Vegetables, fruit, and colon cancer in the Iowa Women's Health Study. *Am J Epidemiol* 1994;139:1-15.

4771 Witte JS, Longnecker MP, Bird CL, et al. Relation of vegetable, fruit, and grain consumption to colorectal adenomatous polyps. *Am J Epidemiol* 1996;144:1015-25.

4772 Le Marchand L, Hankin JH, Wilkens LR, et al. Dietary fiber and colorectal cancer risk. *Epidemiology* 1997;8:658-65.

4773 Dorant E, van den Brandt PA, Goldbohm RA. A prospective cohort study on the relationship between onion and leek consumption, garlic supplement use and the risk of colorectal carcinoma in The Netherlands. *Carcinogenesis* 1996;17:477-84.

4774 You WC, Zhang L, Gail MH, et al. Helicobacter pylori infection, garlic intake and precancerous lesions in a Chinese population at low risk of gastric cancer. *Int J Epidemiol* 1998;27:941-4.

4775 You WC, Blot WJ, Chang YS, et al. Allium vegetables and reduced risk of stomach cancer. *J Natl Cancer Inst* 1989;81:162-4.

4776 Takezaki T, Gao CM, Ding JH, et al. Comparative study of lifestyles of residents in high and low risk areas for gastric cancer in Jiangsu Province, China; with special reference to allium vegetables. *J Epidemiol* 1999;9:297-305.

4777 Key TJ, Silcocks PB, Davey GK, et al. A case-control study of diet and prostate cancer. *Br J Cancer* 1997;76:678-87.

4778 Dorant E, van den Brandt PA, Goldbohm RA. A prospective cohort study on Allium vegetable consumption, garlic supplement use, and the risk of lung carcinoma in The Netherlands. *Cancer Res* 1994;54:6148-53.

4779 Dorant E, van den Brandt PA, Goldbohm RA. Allium vegetable consumption, garlic supplement intake, and female breast carcinoma incidence. *Breast Cancer Res Treat* 1995;33:163-70.

4780 Mostafa MG, Mima T, Ohnishi ST, Mori K. S-allylcysteine ameliorates doxorubicin toxicity in the heart and liver in mice. *Planta Med* 2000;66:148-51.

4782 Holzgartner H, Schmidt U, Kuhn U. Comparison of the efficacy and tolerance of a garlic preparation vs. bezafibrate. *Arzneimittelforschung* 1992;42:1473-7.

4783 Jain AK, Vargas R, Gotzkowsky S, McMahon FG. Can garlic reduce levels of serum lipids? A controlled clinical study. *Am J Med* 1993;94:632-5.

4784 Mader FH. Treatment of hyperlipidaemia with garlic-powder tablets. Evidence from the German Association of General Practitioners' multicentric placebo-controlled double-blind study. *Arzneimittelforschung* 1990;40:1111-6.

4785 Rotzsch W, Richter V, Rassoul F, Walper A. [Postprandial lipemia under treatment with Allium sativum. Controlled double-blind study of subjects with reduced HDL2-cholesterol]. [Article in German]. *Arzneimittelforschung* 1992;42:1223-7.

4786 Silagy C, Neil A. Garlic as a lipid lowering agent--a meta-analysis. *J R Coll Physicians Lond* 1994;28:39-45.

4787 Vorberg G, Schneider B. Therapy with garlic: results of a placebo-controlled, double-blind study. *Br J Clin Pract Symp Suppl* 1990;69:7-11.

4788 Warshafsky S, Kamer RS, Sivak SL. Effect of garlic on total serum cholesterol. A meta-analysis. *Ann Intern Med* 1993;119:599-605.

4789 Adler AJ, Holub BJ. Effect of garlic and fish-oil supplementation on serum lipid and lipoprotein concentrations in hypercholesterolemic men. *Am J Clin Nutr* 1997;65:445-50.

4790 Morcos NC. Modulation of lipid profile by fish oil and garlic combination. *J Natl Med Assoc* 1997;89:673-8.

4791 Kenzelmann R, Kade F. Limitation of the deterioration of lipid parameters by a standardized garlic-ginkgo combination product. A multicenter placebo-controlled double-blind study. *Arzneimittelforschung* 1993;43:978-81.

4792 Superko HR, Krauss RM. Garlic powder, effect on plasma lipids, postprandial lipemia, low-density lipoprotein particle size, high-density lipoprotein subclass distribution and lipoprotein(a). *J Am Coll Cardiol* 2000;35:321-6.

4793 Simons LA, Balasubramaniam S, von Konigsmark M, et al. On the effect of garlic on plasma lipids and lipoproteins in mild hypercholesterolaemia. *Atherosclerosis* 1995;113:219-25.

4794 Luley C, Lehmann-Leo W, Moller B, et al. Lack of efficacy of dried garlic in patients with hyperlipoproteinemia. *Arzneimittelforschung* 1986;36:766-8.

4795 Neil HA, Silagy CA, Lancaster T, et al. Garlic powder in the treatment of moderate hyperlipidaemia: a controlled trial and meta-analysis. *J R Coll Physicians Lond* 1996;30:329-34.

4796 McCrindle BW, Helden E, Conner WT. Garlic extract therapy in children with hypercholesterolemia. *Arch Pediatr Adolesc Med* 1998;152:1089-94.

4797 Breithaupt-Grogler K, Ling M, Boudoulas H, Belz GG. Protective effect of chronic garlic intake on elastic properties of aorta in the elderly. *Circulation* 1997;96:2649-55.

4798 Koscielny J, Klussendorf D, Latza R, et al. The antiatherosclerotic effect of Allium sativum. *Atherosclerosis* 1999;144:237-49.

4799 Chutani SK, Bordia A. The effect of fried versus raw garlic on fibrinolytic activity in man. *Atherosclerosis* 1981;38:417-21.

4800 Blumenthal M, Goldberg A, Brinckmann J, eds. Herbal Medicine Expanded Commission E Monographs. Newton, MA: Integrative Medicine Communications, 2000.

4801 Kiesewetter H, Jung F, Jung EM, et al. Effects of garlic coated tablets in peripheral arterial occlusive disease. *Clin Investig* 1993;71:383-6.

4802 Kiesewetter H, Jung F, Jung EM, et al. Effect of garlic on platelet aggregation in patients with increased risk of juvenile ischaemic attack. *Eur J Clin Pharmacol* 1993;45:333-6.

4803 Legnani C, Frascaro M, Guazzaloca G, et al. Effects of a dried garlic preparation on fibrinolysis and platelet aggregation in healthy subjects. *Arzneimittelforschung* 1993;43:119-22.

4804 Ali M, Bordia T, Mustafa T. Effect of raw versus boiled aqueous extract of garlic and onion on platelet aggregation. *Prostaglandins Leukot Essent Fatty Acids* 1999;60:43-7.

4805 Morris J, Burke V, Mori TA, et al. Effects of garlic extract on platelet aggregation: a randomized placebo-controlled double-blind study. *Clin Exp Pharmacol Physiol* 1995;22:414-7.

4807 Arora RC, Arora S. Comparative effect of clofibrate, garlic and onion on alimentary hyperlipemia. *Atherosclerosis* 1981;39:447-52.

4808 Sasaki J, Kita T, Ishita K, et al. Antibacterial activity of garlic powder against Escherichia coli O-157. *J Nutr Sci Vitaminol* (Tokyo) 1999;45:785-90.

4809 Jepson RG, Kleijnen J, Leng GC. Garlic for peripheral arterial occlusive disease (Cochrane Review). In: The Cochrane Library, Issue 2, 2000. Oxford: Update Software.

4810 Gebhardt R, Beck H. Differential inhibitory effects of garlic-derived organosulfur compounds on cholesterol biosynthesis in primary rat hepatocyte cultures. *Lipids* 1996;31:1269-76.

4811 Qureshi AA, Din ZZ, Abuirmeileh N, et al. Suppression of avian hepatic lipid metabolism by solvent extracts of garlic: impact on serum lipids. *J Nutr* 1983;113:1746-55.

4812 Pedraza-Chaverri J, Tapia E, Medina-Campos ON, et al. Garlic prevents hypertension induced by chronic inhibition of nitric oxide synthesis. *Life Sci* 1998;62:71-7.

4813 Dirsch VM, Kiemer AK, Wagner H, Vollmar AM. Effect of allicin and ajoene, two compounds of garlic, on inducible nitric oxide synthase. *Atherosclerosis* 1998;139:333-9.

4814 American Academy Of Pediatrics Policy Statement. Camphor Revisited: Focus on Toxicity (RE9422). *Pediatrics* 1994;94:127-8. Available at: http://www.aap.org/policy/00300.html

4815 Ip C, Lisk DJ. Efficacy of cancer prevention by high-selenium garlic is primarily dependent on the action of selenium. *Carcinogenesis* 1995;16:2649-52.

4816 Anibarro B, Fontela JL, De La Hoz F. Occupational asthma induced by garlic dust. *J Allergy Clin Immunol* 1997;100:734-8.

4817 Zema MJ. Gemfibrozil, nicotinic acid and combination therapy in patients with isolated hypoalphalipoproteinemia: a randomized, open-label, crossover study. *J Am Coll Cardiol* 2000;35:640-6.

4818 Guyton JR, Blazing MA, Hagar J, et al. Extended-release niacin vs gemfibrozil for the treatment of low levels of high-density lipoprotein cholesterol. Niaspan-Gemfibrozil Study Group. *Arch Intern Med* 2000;160:1177-84.

4819 Alberts DS, Martinez ME, Roe DJ, et al. Lack of effect of a high-fiber cereal supplement on the recurrence of colorectal adenomas. Phoenix Colon Cancer Prevention Physicians' Network. *N Engl J Med* 2000;342:1156-62.

4820 Schatzkin A, Lanza E, Corle D, et al. Lack of effect of a low-fat, high-fiber diet on the recurrence of colorectal adenomas. Polyp Prevention Trial Study Group. *N Engl J Med* 2000;342:1149-55.

4821 Fuchs CS, Giovannucci EL, Colditz GA, et al. Dietary fiber and the risk of colorectal cancer and adenoma in women. *N Engl J Med* 1999;340:169-76.

4822 Iso H, Stampfer MJ, Manson JE, et al. Prospective study of calcium, potassium, and magnesium intake and risk of stroke in women. *Stroke* 1999;30:1772-9.

4823 Cueto-Manzano AM, Konel S, Freemont AJ, et al. Effect of 1,25-dihydroxyvitamin D3 and calcium carbonate on bone loss associated with long-term renal transplantation. *Am J Kidney Dis* 2000;35:227-36.

4824 Zittermann A, Bock P, Drummer C, et al. Lactose does not enhance calcium bioavailability in lactose-tolerant, healthy adults. *Am J Clin Nutr* 2000;71:931-6.

4825 Chan JM, Giovannucci E, Andersson SO, et al. Dairy products, calcium, phosphorous, vitamin D, and risk of prostate cancer. *Cancer Causes Control* 1998;9:559-66.

4826 Moschella C, Jaber BL. Interaction between cyclosporine and Hypericum perforatum (St. John's wort) after organ transplantation. *Amer J Kidney Dis* 2001;38:1105-7.

4828 Mennella JA, Johnson A, Beauchamp GK. Garlic ingestion by pregnant women alters the odor of amniotic fluid. *Chem Senses* 1995;20:207-9.

4829 Mennella JA, Beauchamp GK. Maternal diet alters the sensory qualities of human milk and the nursling's behavior. *Pediatrics* 1991;88:737-44.

4830 Mennella JA, Beauchamp GK. The effects of repeated exposure to garlic-flavored milk on the nursling's behavior. *Pediatr Res* 1993;34:805-8.

4831 Karliova M, Treichel U, Malago M, et al. Interaction of Hypericum perforatum (SJW) with cyclosporin A metabolism in a patient after liver transplantation. *J Hepatol* 2000;33:853-5.

4832 Cronin E. Dermatitis of the hands in caterers. *Contact Dermatitis* 1987;17:265-9.

4833 Lee TY, Lam TH. Contact dermatitis due to topical treatment with garlic in Hong Kong. *Contact Dermatitis* 1991;24:193-6.

4834 Mandelbaum A, Pertzborn F, Martin-Facklam M, Wiesel M. Unexplained decrease of cyclosporin trough levels in a compliant renal transplant patient. *Nephrol Dial Transplant* 2000;15:1473-4.

4835 Wang Z, Gorski JC, Hamman MA, et al. The effects of St. John's wort (Hyericum perforatum) on human cytochrome P450 activity. *Clin Pharmacol Ther* 2001;70:317-26.

4836 Assalian P. Sildenafil for SJW-induced sexual dysfunction. *J Sex Marital Ther* 2000;26:357-8.

4837 de Maat M, Hoetelmans R, Mathot R, et al. Drug interaction between St. John's wort and nevirapine. *AIDS* 2001;15:420-1.

4838 Vera JC, Rivas CI, Zhang RH, et al. Human HL-60 myeloid leukemia cells transport dehydroascorbic acid via the glucose transporters and accumulate reduced ascorbic acid. *Blood* 1994;84:1628-34.

4839 Spielholz C, Golde DW, Houghton AN, et al. Increased facilitated transport of dehydroascorbic acid without changes in sodium-dependent ascorbate transport in human melanoma cells. *Cancer Res* 1997;57:2529-37.

4840 Vera JC, Rivas CI, Zhang RH, Golde DW. Colony-stimulating factors signal for increased transport of vitamin C in human host defense cells. *Blood* 1998;91:2536-46.

4841 Agus DB, Vera JC, Golde DW. Stromal cell oxidation: a mechanism by which tumors obtain vitamin C. *Cancer Res* 1999;59:4555-8.

4842 Moertel CG, Fleming TR, Creagan ET, et al. High-dose vitamin C versus placebo in the treatment of patients with advanced cancer who have had no prior chemotherapy. A randomized double-blind comparison. *N Engl J Med* 1985;312:137-41.

4843 Creagan ET, Moertel CG, O'Fallon JR, et al. Failure of high-dose vitamin C (ascorbic acid) therapy to benefit patients with advanced cancer. A controlled trial. *N Engl J Med* 1979;301:687-90.

4844 Food and Nutrition Board, Institute of Medicine. Dietary Reference Intakes for Vitamin C, Vitamin E, Selenium, and Carotenoids. Washington, DC: National Academy Press, 2000. Available at: http://www.nap.edu/books/0309069351/html/

4846 Jolliet P, Simon N, Barre J, et al. Plasma coenzyme Q10 concentrations in breast cancer: prognosis and therapeutic consequences. *Int J Clin Pharmacol Ther* 1998;36:506-9.

4847 Canner PL, Berge KG, Wenger NK, et al. Fifteen year mortality in Coronary Drug Project patients: long-term benefit with niacin. *J Am Coll Cardiol* 1986;8:1245-55.

4848 Zhao XQ, Brown BG, Hillger L, et al. Effects of intensive lipid-lowering therapy on the coronary arteries of asymptomatic subjects with elevated apolipoprotein B. *Circulation* 1993;88:2744-53.

4850 Park YK, Sempos CT, Barton CN, et al. Effectiveness of food fortification in the United States: the case of pellagra. *Am J Public Health* 2000;90:727-38.

4851 Gibbons LW, Gonzalez V, Gordon N, Grundy S. The prevalence of side effects with regular and sustained-release nicotinic acid. *Am J Med* 1995;99:378-85.

4852 Whelan AM, Price SO, Fowler SF, Hainer BL. The effect of aspirin on niacin-induced cutaneous reactions. *J Fam Pract* 1992;34:165-8.

4853 Jungnickel PW, Maloley PA, Vander Tuin EL, et al. Effect of two aspirin pretreatment regimens on niacin-induced cutaneous reactions. *J Gen Intern Med* 1997;12:591-6.

4854 Capuzzi DM, Guyton JR, Morgan JM, et al. Efficacy and safety of an extended-release niacin (Niaspan): a long-term study. *Am J Cardiol* 1998;82:74-81;disc. 85U-6U.

4855 Gray DR, Morgan T, Chretien SD, Kashyap ML. Efficacy and safety of controlled-release niacin in dyslipoproteinemic veterans. *Ann Intern Med* 1994;121:252-8.

4856 McKenney JM, Proctor JD, Harris S, Chinchili VM. A comparison of the efficacy and toxic effects of sustained- vs immediate-release niacin in hypercholesterolemic patients. *JAMA* 1994;271:672-7.

4857 Knopp RH, Alagona P, Davidson M, et al. Equivalent efficacy of a time-release form of niacin (Niaspan) given once-a-night versus plain niacin in the management of hyperlipidemia. *Metabolism* 1998;47:1097-104.

4858 Knopp RH. Clinical profiles of plain versus sustained-release niacin (Niaspan) and the physiologic rationale for nighttime dosing. *Am J Cardiol* 1998;82:24U-28U;discussion 39U-41U.

4859 Crouse JR III. New developments in the use of niacin for treatment of hyperlipidemia: new considerations in the use of an old drug. *Coron Artery Dis* 1996;7:321-6.

4860 Garg A, Grundy SM. Nicotinic acid as therapy for dyslipidemia in non-insulin-dependent diabetes mellitus. *JAMA* 1990;264:723-6.

4861 Misra MC, Parshad R. Randomized clinical trial of micronized flavonoids in the early control of bleeding from acute internal haemorrhoids. *Br J Surgery* 2000;87:868-72.

4862 Leighton RF, Gordon NF, Small GS, et al. Dental and gingival pain as side effects of niacin therapy. *Chest* 1998;114:1472-4.

4863 American Society of Health-System Pharmacists. ASHP Therapeutic Position Statement on the safe use of niacin in the management of dyslipidemias. *Am J Health Syst Pharm* 1997;54:2815-9.

4864 Goldberg AC. Clinical trial experience with extended-release niacin (Niaspan): dose-escalation study. *Am J Cardiol* 1998;82:35U-38U;discussion 39U-41U.

4865 Ishii N, Nishihara Y. Pellagra encephalopathy among tuberculous patients: its relation to isoniazid therapy. *J Neurol Neurosurg Psychiatry* 1985;48:628-34.

4866 Darvay A, Basarab T, McGregor JM, Russell-Jones R. Isoniazid induced pellagra despite pyridoxine supplementation. *Clin Exp Dermatol* 1999;24:167-9.

4867 National Cholesterol Education Program. Cholesterol Lowering in the Patient with Coronary Heart Disease. 1997. Available at: http://www.nhlbi.nih.gov/health/prof/heart/chol/chol_low.pdf.

4868 Rabbani GH, Butler T, Bardhan PK, Islam A. Reduction of fluid-loss in cholera by nicotinic acid: a randomized controlled trial. *Lancet* 1983;2:1439-42.

4869 Briend A, Nath SK, Heyman M, Desjeux JF. Comparative effects of nicotinic acid and nicotinamide on cholera toxin-induced secretion in rabbit ileum. *J Diarrhoeal Dis Res* 1993;11:97-100.

4870 Hudson CJ, Lin A, Cogan S, et al. The niacin challenge test: clinical manifestation of altered transmembrane signal transduction in schizophrenia? *Biol Psychiatry* 1997;41:507-13.

4871 Johansson JO, Egberg N, Asplund-Carlson A, Carlson LA. Nicotinic acid treatment shifts the fibrinolytic balance favourably and decreases plasma fibrinogen in hypertriglyceridaemic men. *J Cardiovasc Risk* 1997;4:165-71.

4872 Kolb H, Burkart V. Nicotinamide in type 1 diabetes. Mechanism of action revisited. *Diabetes Care* 1999;22:B16-20.

4873 Gale EA. Theory and practice of nicotinamide trials in pre-type 1 diabetes. *J Pediatr Endocrinol Metab* 1996;9:375-9.

4874 Elliott RB, Pilcher CC, Fergusson DM, Stewart AW. A population based strategy to prevent insulin-dependent diabetes using nicotinamide. *J Pediatr Endocrinol Metab* 1996;9:501-9.

4875 Lampeter EF, Klinghammer A, Scherbaum WA, et al. The Deutsche Nicotinamide Intervention Study: an attempt to prevent type 1 diabetes. DENIS Group. *Diabetes* 1998;47:980-4.

4876 Reimers JI, Andersen HU, Pociot F. [Nicotinamide and prevention of insulin-dependent diabetes mellitus. Rationale, effects, toxicology and clinical experiences. ENDIT Group]. [Article in Danish]. *Ugeskr Laeger* 1994;156:461-5.

4877 Pozzilli P, Visalli N, Cavallo MG, et al. Vitamin E and nicotinamide have similar effects in maintaining residual beta cell function in recent onset insulin-dependent diabetes. *Eur J Endocrinol* 1997;137:234-9.

4878 Visalli N, Cavallo MG, Signore A, et al. A multi-centre randomized trial of two different doses of nicotinamide in patients with recent-onset type 1 diabetes (the IMDIAB VI). *Diabetes Metab Res Rev* 1999;15:181-5.

4879 Pozzilli P, Visalli N, Signore A, et al. Double blind trial of nicotinamide in recent-onset IDDM (the IMDIAB III study). *Diabetologia* 1995;38:848-52.

4880 Pozzilli P, Browne PD, Kolb H. Meta-analysis of nicotinamide treatment in patients with recent-onset IDDM. The Nicotinamide Trialists. *Diabetes Care* 1996;19:1357-63.

4881 Greenbaum CJ, Kahn SE, Palmer JP. Nicotinamide's effects on glucose metabolism in subjects at risk for IDDM. *Diabetes* 1996;45:1631-4.

4882 Polo V, Saibene A, Pontiroli AE. Nicotinamide improves insulin secretion and metabolic control in lean type 2 diabetic patients with secondary failure to sulphonylureas. *Acta Diabetol* 1998;35:61-4.

4883 Jonas WB, Rapoza CP, Blair WF. The effect of niacinamide on osteoarthritis: a pilot study. *Inflamm Res* 1996;45:330-4.

4884 McCarty MF, Russell AL. Niacinamide therapy for osteoarthritis--does it inhibit nitric oxide synthase induction by interleukin 1 in chondrocytes? *Med Hypotheses* 1999;53:350-60.

4885 Sperduto RD, Hu TS, Milton RC, et al. The Linxian cataract studies. Two nutrition intervention trials. *Arch Ophthalmol* 1993;111:1246-53.

4886 Illingworth DR, Stein EA, Mitchel YB, et al. Comparative effects of lovastatin and niacin in primary hypercholesterolemia. A prospective trial. *Arch Intern Med* 1994;154:1586-95.

4887 Vacek JL, Dittmeier G, Chiarelli T, et al. Comparison of lovastatin (20 mg) and nicotinic acid (1.2 g) with either drug alone for type II hyperlipoproteinemia. *Am J Cardiol* 1995;76:182-4.

4888 Vega GL, Grundy SM. Lipoprotein responses to treatment with lovastatin, gemfibrozil, and nicotinic acid in normolipidemic patients with hypoalphalipoproteinemia. *Arch Intern Med* 1994;154:73-82.

4889 Guyton JR, Goldberg AC, Kreisberg RA, et al. Effectiveness of once-nightly dosing of extended-release niacin alone and in combination for hypercholesterolemia. *Am J Cardiol* 1998;82:737-43.

4890 Lal SM, Hewett JE, Petroski GF, et al. Effects of nicotinic acid and lovastatin in renal transplant patients: a prospective, randomized, open-labeled crossover trial. *Am J Kidney Dis* 1995;25:616-22.

4891 Peikert A, Wilimzig C, Kohne-Volland R. Prophylaxis of migraine with oral magnesium: results from a prospective, multi-center, placebo-controlled and double-blind randomized study. *Cephalalgia* 1996;16:257-63.

4892 Richter O. Several countries issue restrictions on St. John's wort. Richter's Herb Letter 7/30/00. Available at: www.richters.com (Accessed 01 March 2002).

4893 Wilson JL. Topical shark cartilage subdues psoriasis: research review and preliminary clinical results. *Altern Complement Ther* 2000;6:291.

4894 Neovastat clinical trial abstracts. Presented at the American Association for Cancer Research 92nd annual meeting. March 27, 2001.

4895 Taubert K. [Magnesium in migraine. Results of a multicenter pilot study]. [Article in German]. *Fortschr Med* 1994;112:328-30.

4897 Schrader E. Equivalence of St. John's wort extract (Ze 117) and fluoxetine: a randomized, controlled study in mild-moderate depression. *Int Clin Psychopharmacol* 2000;15:61-8.

4898 Thanapongsathorn W, Vajrabukka T. Clinical trial of oral diosmin (Daflon) in the treatment of hemorrhoids. *Dis Colon Rectum* 1992;35:1085-8.

4899 Linde K, Mulrow CD. St. John's wort for depression. *Cochrane Database Syst Rev* 2000;2:CD000448.

4900 Cospite M. Double-blind, placebo-controlled evaluation of clinical activity and safety of Daflon 500 mg in the treatment of acute hemorrhoids. *Angiology* 1994;45:566-73.

4901 Mero A, Miikkulainen H, Riski J, et al. Effects of bovine colostrum supplementation on serum IGF-I, IgG, hormone, and saliva IgA during training. *Appl Physiol* 1997;83:1144-51.

4903 Sarker SA, Casswall TH, Mahalanabis D, et al. Successful treatment of rotavirus diarrhea in children with immunoglobulin from immunized bovine colostrum. *Pediatr Infect Dis J* 1998;17:1149-54.

4904 Mitra AK, Mahalanabis D, Ashraf H, et al. Hyperimmune cow colostrum reduces diarrhoea due to rotavirus: a double-blind, controlled clinical trial. *Acta Paediatr* 1995;84:996-1001.

4905 Greenberg PD, Cello JP. Treatment of severe diarrhea caused by Cryptosporidium parvum with oral bovine immunoglobulin concentrate in patients with AIDS. *J Acquir Immune Defic Syndr Hum Retrovirol* 1996;13:348-54.

4906 Plettenberg A, Stoehr A, Stellbrink HJ, et al. A preparation of bovine colostrum in the treatment of HIV-positive patients with chronic diarrhea. *Clin Invest* 1993;71:42-5.

4907 Rump JA, Arndt R, Arnold A, et al. Treatment of diarrhea in human immunodeficiency virus-infected patients with immunoglobulins from bovine colostrum. *Clin Invest* 1992;70:588-94.

4908 Nord J, Ma P, DiJohn D, et al. Treatment with bovine hyperimmune colostrum of cryptosporidial diarrhea in AIDS patients. *AIDS* 1990;4:581-4.

4909 Ylitalo S, Uhari M, Rasi S, et al. Rotaviral antibodies in the treatment of acute rotaviral gastroenteritis. *Acta Paediatr* 1998;87:264-7.

4911 Playford RJ, Floyd DN, Macdonald CE, et al. Bovine colostrum is a health food supplement which prevents NSAID induced gut damage. *Gut* 1999;44:653-8.

4912 FDA. Center for Food Safety and Applied Nutrition, Office of Premarket Approval, EAFUS: A food additive database. Available at: vm.cfsan.fda.gov/~dms/eafus.html.

4913 Sargent EV, Adolph J, Clemmons MK, et al. Evaluation of flu-like symptoms in workers handling xanthan gum powder. *Occup Med* 1990;32(7):625-30.

4914 Wade A, Weller PJ, eds. Handbook of Pharmaceutical Excipients. 2nd ed. Washington, DC: Am Pharmaceutical Assn, 1994.

4915 van der Reijden WA, van der Kwaak H, Vissink A, et al. Treatment of xerostomia with polymer-based saliva substitutes in patients with Sjogren's syndrome. *Arthritis Rheum* 1996; 39:57-63.

4916 Osilesi O, Trout DL, Glover EE, et al. Use of xanthan gum in dietary management of diabetes mellitus. *Am J Clin Nutr* 1985; 42(4): 597-603.

4917 Eastwood MA, Brydon WG, Anderson DM. The dietary effects of xanthan gum in man. *Food Addit Contam* 1987;4:17-26.

4918 Daly J, Tomlin J, Read NW. The effect of feeding xanthan gum on colonic function in man: correlation with in vitro determinants of bacterial breakdown. *Br J Nutr* 1993; 69(3): 897-902.

4919 Di Carlo G, Mascolo N, Izzo AA, Capasso F. Flavonoids: Old and new aspects of a class of natural therapeutic drugs. *Life Sci* 1999;65:337-53.

4920 van der Reijden WA, Buijs MJ, Damen JJ, et al. Influence of polymers for use in saliva substitutes on de- and remineralization of enamel in vitro. *Caries Res* 1997;31(3):216-23.

4926 Bounous G, Baruchel S, Falutz J, et al. Whey proteins as a food supplement in HIV-seropositive individuals. *Clin Invest Med* 1993;16:204-9.

4927 Vandenplas Y, Hauser B, Van den Borre C, et al. Effect of a whey hydrolysate prophylaxis of atopic disease. *Ann Allergy* 1992;68:419-24.

4928 McIntosh GH. Colon cancer: dietary modifications required for a balanced protective diet. *Prev Med* 1993;22:767-74.

4929 Fukushima Y, Kawata Y, Onda T, Kitagawa M. Long-term consumption of whey hydrolysate formula by lactating women reduces the transfer of beta-lactoglobulin into human milk. *Nutr Sci Vitaminol* (Tokyo) 1997;43:673-8.

4930 Kennedy RS, Konok GP, Bounous G, et al. The use of a whey protein concentrate in the treatment of patients with metastatic carcinoma: a phase I-II clinical study. *Anticancer Res* 1995;15:2643-9.

4932 Salomon SB, Jung J, Voss T, et al. An elemental diet containing medium-chain triglycerides and enzymatically hydrolyzed protein can improve gastrointestinal tolerance in people infected with HIV. *J Am Diet Assoc* 1998;98:460-2.

4933 Papenburg R, Bounous G, Fleiszer D, Gold P. Dietary milk proteins inhibit the development of dimethylhydrazine-induced malignancy. *Tumor Biol* 1990;11:129-36.

4934 Fayer R, Guidry A, Blagburn BL. Immunotherapeutic efficacy of bovine colostral immunoglobulins from a hyperimmunized cow against cryptosporidiosis in neonatal mice. *Infect Immun* 1990;58:2962-5.

4935 Vergel NR, Salvato P, Mooney M. Anabolic steroids, resistance exercise and protein supplementation effect on lean body mass in HIV+ patients. *Int Conf AIDS* 1998;12:557 (abstract # 32185).

4936 Voss T, Rowe B, Graf L, et al. Management of HIV-related weight loss and diarrhea with an enteral formula containing whey peptides and medium-chain triglycerides. *Int Conf AIDS* 1991;7(:223 (abstract # WB2165).

4937 Baruchel S, Olivier R, Wainberg M. Anti-HIV and anti-apoptotic activity of the whey protein concentrate: IMMUNOCAL. *Int Conf AIDS* 1994;10:32 (abstract # 421A).

4938 Hillman JD, Peng AT, Gilliam AC, et al. Treatment of Kaposi Sarcoma with oral administration of shark cartilage in a Human Herpes virus 8-seropositive, Human Immunodeficiency Virus-Seronegative homosexual man. *Arch Dermatol* 2001;137:1149-52.

4939 Wong CW, Liu AH, Regester GO, et al. Influence of whey and purified whey proteins on neutrophil functions in sheep. *J Dairy Res* 1997;64:281-8.

4940 Wong CW, Watson DL. Immunomodulatory effects of dietary whey proteins in mice. *J Dairy Res* 1995;62:359-68.

4941 Engelson ES, et al. Effect of a high protein diet upon protein metabolism in HIV-infected men and women. *Int Conf AIDS* 1998;12:553 (abstract #32166).

4942 Laoprasert N, Wallen ND, Jones RT, et al. Anaphylaxis in a milk-allergic child following ingestion of lemon sorbet containing trace quantities of milk. *J Food Prot* 1998;61:1522-4.

4943 Bounous G, Batist G, Gold P. Whey proteins in cancer prevention. *Cancer Lett* 1991;7:91-4.

4944 Semla TP, Beizer JL, Higbee MD. Geriatric Dosage Handbook. 4th ed. Hudson, OH: Lexicomp, 1998.

4945 Neuvonen PJ. Interactions with the absorption of tetracyclines. *Drugs* 1976;11:45-54.

4946 Moufida S, Marzouk B. Biochemical characterization of blood orange, sweet orange, lemon, bergamot and bitter orange. *Phytochemistry* 2003;62:1283-9.

4947 Gaullier JM, Halse J, Hoye K, et al. Conjugated linoleic acid supplementation for 1 y reduces body fat mass in healthy overweight humans. *Am J Clin Nutr* 2004;79:1118-25.

4948 FDA. Center for drug evaluation and research. Generic drug List. 2003. Available at: http://www.fda.gov/cder/ogd/approvals/1stgen0103.htm

4949 FDA. List of All Orphan Products Designations and Approvals. Levocarnitine. Available at: http://www.fda.gov/orphan/designat/alldes.rtf

4950 Morin S. Isoflavones and bone health. *Menopause* 2004;11:239-41.

4951 Chen YM, Ho SC, Lam SS, et al. Beneficial effect of soy isoflavones on bone mineral content was modified by years since menopause, body weight, and calcium intake: a double-blind, randomized, controlled trial. *Menopause* 2004;11246-54.

4952 Gallagher JC, Satpathy R, Rafferty K, Haynatzka V. The effect of soy protein isolate on bone metabolism. *Menopause* 2004;11:290-98.

4953 FDA Fact Sheet. I. FDA's New Interim Final Rule Prohibiting Use of Certain Cattle Materials that May Carry the Risk of Bovine Spongiform Encephalopathy in Human Foods and Cosmetics. July 9, 2004. Available at: www.www.cfsan.fda.gov/~comm/bsefact2.html

4954 Villa P, Cova D, De Francesco L, et al. Protective effect of diosmetin on in vitro cell membrane damage and oxidative stress in cultured rat hepatocytes. *Toxicology* 1992;73:179-89.

4956 Koyuncu H, Berkarda B, Baykut F, et al. Preventive effect of hesperidin against inflammation in CD-1 mouse skin caused by tumor promoter. *Anticancer Res* 1999;19:3237-41.

4959 Craig WJ. Health-promoting properties of common herbs. *Am J Clin Nutr* 1999;70:491-9.

4960 FDA Talk Paper. FDA Allows Whole Oat Foods to make Claim on Reducing the Risk of Heart Disease. 1997. Available at: vm.cfsan.fda.gov/~lrd/tpoats.html

4961 Wursch P, Pi-Sunyer FX. The role of viscous soluble fiber in the metabolic control of diabetes. A review with special emphasis on cereals rich in beta-glucan. *Diabetes Care* 1997;20:1774-80.

4962 Pietinen P, Rimm EB, Korhonen P, et al. Intake of dietary fiber and risk of coronary heart disease in a cohort of Finnish men. The alpha-tocopherol, beta-carotene cancer prevention study. *Circulation* 1996;94:2720-7.

4963 Van Horn L. Fiber, lipids, and coronary heart disease. A statement for healthcare professionals from the Nutr Committee, Am Heart Assn. *Circulation* 1997;95:2701-4.

4964 Rimm EB, Ascherio A, Giovannucci E, et al. Vegetable, fruit, and cereal fiber intake and risk of coronary heart disease among men. *JAMA* 1996;275:447-51.

4965 He J, Klag MJ, Whelton PK, et al. Oats and buckwheat intakes and cardiovascular disease risk factors in an ethnic minority of China. *Am J Clin Nutr* 1995;61:366-72.

4966 Khaw KT, Barrett-Connor E. Dietary fiber and reduced ischemic heart disease mortality rates in men and women: a 12-year prospective study. *Am J Epidemiol* 1987;126:1093-102.

4967 Morris JN, Marr JW, Clayton DG. Diet and heart: a postscript. *Br Med J* 1977;2:1307-14.

4968 Kromhout D, de Lezenne C, Coulander C. Diet, prevalence and 10-year mortality from coronary heart disease in 871 middle-aged men. The Zutphen Study. *Am J Epidemiol* 1984;119:733-41.

4969 American Dietetic Association Website. Available at: www.eatright.org/adap1097.html (Accessed 16 July 1999).

4970 Chen HL, Haack VS, Janecky CW, et al. Mechanisms by which wheat bran and oat bran increase stool weight in humans. *Am J Clin Nutr* 1998;68:711-9.

4972 Kwiterovich PO Jr. The role of fiber in the treatment of hypercholesterolemia in children and adolescents. *Pediatrics* 1995;96:1005-9.

4973 Romero AL, Romero JE, Galaviz S, Fernandez ML. Cookies enriched with psyllium or oat bran lower plasma LDL cholesterol in normal and hypercholesterolemic men from Northern Mexico. *J Am Coll Nutr* 1998;17:601-8.

4974 Marlett JA, Hosig KB, Vollendorf NW, et al. Mechanism of serum cholesterol reduction by oat bran. *Hepatol* 1994;20:1450-7.

4975 Poulter N, Chang CL, Cuff A, et al. Lipid profiles after the daily consumption of an oat-based cereal: a controlled crossover trial. *Am J Clin Nutr* 1994;59:66-9.

4976 Braaten JT, Wood PJ, Scott FW, et al. Oat beta-glucan reduces blood cholesterol concentration in hypercholesterolemic subjects. *Eur J Clin Nutr* 1994;48:465-74.

4977 Ripsin CM, Keenan JM, Jacobs DR Jr, et al. Oat products and lipid lowering. A meta-analysis. *JAMA* 1992;267:3317-25.

4979 Cooper SG, Tracey EJ. Small-bowel obstruction caused by oat-bran bezoar. *N Engl J Med* 1989;320:1148-9.

4980 Pick ME, Hawrysh ZJ, Gee MI, et al. Oat bran concentrate bread products improve long-term control of diabetes: a pilot study. *J Am Diet Assoc* 1996;96:1254-61.

4981 Wood PJ, Braaten JT, Scott FW, et al. Effect of dose and modification of viscous properties of oat gum on plasma glucose and insulin following an oral glucose load. *Br J Nutr* 1994;72:731-43.

4982 Braaten JT, Scott FW, Wood PJ, et al. High beta-glucan oat bran and oat gum reduce postprandial blood glucose and insulin in subjects with and without type 2 diabetes. *Diabet Med* 1994;11:312-8.

4983 Braaten JT, Wood PJ, Scott FW, Riedel KD, et al. Oat gum lowers glucose and insulin after an oral glucose load. *Am J Clin Nutr* 1991;53:1425-30.

4984 Arffmann S, Hojgaard L, Giese B, Krag E. Effect of oat bran on lithogenic index of bile and bile acid metabolism. *Digestion* 1983;28:197-200.

4985 Rosario PG, Gerst PH, Prakash K, Albu E. Dentureless distention: oat bran bezoars cause obstruction. *J Am Geriatr Soc* 1990;38:608.

4986 Baum MK, Javier JJ, Mantero-Atienza E, et al. Zidovudine-associated adverse reactions in a longitudinal study of asymptomatic HIV-1-infected homosexual males. *J Acquir Immune Defic Syndr* 1991;4:1218-26.

5000 Langford SD, Boor PJ. Oleander toxicity: an examination of human and animal toxic exposures. *Toxicology* 1996;109:1-13.

5001 Ferrea G, Canessa A, Sampietro F, Cruciani M, Romussi G, Bassetti D. In vitro activity of a Combretum micranthum extract against herpes simplex virus types 1 and 2. *Antiviral Res* 1993;21(4):317-25.

5002 Centers for Disease Control and Prev. Ostrich fern poisoning New York and western Canada, 1994. *JAMA* 1995;273:912-3.

5003 Makino T, Ono T, Muso E, Honda G. Inhibitory effect of Perilla frutescens and its phenolic constituents on cultured murine mesangial cell proliferation. *Planta Med* 1998;64:541-45.

5004 Bruynzeel DP. Bulb dermatitis. Dermatological problems in the flower bulb industries. *Contact Dermatitis* 1997;37(2):70-7.

5005 Bruynzeel DP, de Boer EM, Brouwer EJ, et al. Dermatitis in bulb growers. *Contact Dermatitis* 1993;29(1):11-5.

5006 Middleton E. Some biological properties of plant flavonoids. *Ann Allergy* 1988;61:53-7.

5007 Moraes-Cerdeira RM, Burandt CL Jr, Bastos JK, et al. Evaluation of four Narcissus cultivars as potential sources for galanthamine production.

5009 Murray M, Pizzorno J, eds. Encyclopedia of Natural Medicine, 2nd ed. Rocklin, CA: Prima Health, 1998.

5010 Murray M. The Healing Power of Herbs, 2nd ed. Rocklin, CA: Prima Health, 1995.

5011 Lininger S. The Natural Pharmacy. Prima Health. Rocklin, CA: 1998.

5013 Moore M. Herbal Materia Medica fifth edition, Southwest School of Botanical Medicine: Bisbee, AZ 1995.

5014 Manufacturer: Aubrey Organics. Tampa, FL.

5016 Manufacturer: Schiff Pharmaceuticals. Salt Lake City, UT.

5017 Manufacturer: Country Life.

5019 Manufacturer: Nature's Way. Springville, UT.

5020 Manufacturer: Twinlab. Ronkonkoma, NY.

5022 Manufacturer: Earthrise. Petaluma, CA.

5023 Manufacturer: Nature's Answer. Hanppange, NY.

5024 Manufacturer: Walgreens. Deerfield, IL.

5025 Manufacturer: Natrol. Chatsworth, CA

5026 Manufacturer: Solaray.

5027 Manufacturer: Atkins Nutritionals.

5029 Cockerham MB, Weinberger BB, Lerchie SB. Oral glutamine for the prevention of oral mucositis associated with high-dose paclitaxel and melphalan for autologous bone marrow transplantation. *Ann Pharmacother* 2000;34:300-3.

5030 Schardt D. Stevia, A Bittersweet Tale. *Nutrition Action Healthletter* April 2000- U.S. Edition. Available at: www.cspinet.org/nah/4_00/stevia.html (Accessed 25 June 2004).

5031 Melis MS, Sainati AR. Effect of calcium and verapamil on renal function of rats during treatment with stevioside. *J Ethnopharmacol* 1991;33:257-622.

5032 Jeppesen PB, Gregersen S, Poulsen CR, Hermansen K. Stevioside acts directly on pancreatic beta cells to secrete insulin: actions independent of cyclic adenosine monophosphate and adenosine triphosphate-sensitive K+-channel activity. *Metabolism* 2000;49:208-14.

5033 Melis MS. Effects of chronic administration of Stevia rebaudiana on fertility in rats. *J Ethnopharmacol* 1999;67:157-61.

5034 Toskulkao C, Chaturat L, Temcharoen P, Glinsukon T. Acute toxicity of stevioside, a natural sweetener, and its metabolite, steviol, in several animal species. *Drug Chem Toxicol* 1997;20:31-44.

5035 Toskulkao C, Sutheerawatananon M, Wanichanon C, et al. Effects of stevioside and steviol on intestinal glucose absorption in hamsters. *J Nutr Sci Vitaminol* (Tokyo) 1995;41:105-13.

5036 Wasuntarawat C, Temcharoen P, Toskulkao C, et al. Developmental toxicity of steviol, a metabolite of stevioside, in the hamster. *Drug Chem Toxicol* 1998;21:207-22.

5037 Stevia: Not Ready For Prime Time. Ctr for Sci in the Public Interest. Available at: www.cspinet.org/additives/stevia (Accessed 28 March 2000).

5038 Hartter S, Grozinger M, Weigmann H, et al. Increased bioavailability of oral melatonin after fluvoxamine coadministration. *Clin Pharmacol Ther* 2000;67:1-6.

5039 Ravina A, Slezak L, Mirsky N, et al. Reversal of corticosteroid-induced diabetes mellitus with supplemental chromium. *Diabet Med* 1999;16:164-7.

5040 Roeback JR Jr, Hla KM, Chambless LE, Fletcher RH. Effects of chromium supplementation on serum high-density lipoprotein cholesterol levels in men taking beta-blockers. A randomized, controlled trial. *Ann Intern Med* 1991;115:917-24.

5041 National Collegiate Athletic Association. List of banned drug classes for 2004-2005. Available at: www.ncaa.org

5043 Magainin Presents Neuroblastoma Data for Squalamine at AACR Meeting. Available at: www.prnewswire.com (Accessed 3 April 2000).

5044 Iron chefs get nutritional boost cooking vegetables. American Chemical Society website. Available at: center.acs.org/applications/news//story.cfm?story=347 (Accessed 6 April 2000).

5047 FDA announces the availability of new Ephedrine and street drug alternative docs. Available at: www.fda.gov (Accessed 6 April 2000).

5049 Findling RL, Maxwell K, Scotese-Wojtila L, et al. High-dose pyridoxine and magnesium administration in children with autistic disorder: an absence of salutary effects in a double-blind, placebo-controlled study. *J Autism Dev Disord* 1997;27:467-78.

5050 Coleman M. Infantile spasms associated with 5-hydroxytryptophan administration in patients with Down's syndrome. *Neurology* 1971;21:911-9.

5051 Hagg S, Spigset O, Mjorndal T, Dahlqvist R. Effect of caffeine on clozapine pharmacokinetics in healthy volunteers. *Br J Clin Pharmacol* 2000;49:59-63.

5052 Vadoud-Seyedi J, de Dobbeleer G, Simonart T. Treatment of haemodialysis-associated pseudoporphyria with N-acetylcysteine: report of two cases. *Br J Dermatol* 2000;142:580-1.

5053 Lynch SR, Dassenko SA, Cook JD, et al. Inhibitory effect of a soybean-protein--related moiety on iron absorption in humans. *Am J Clin Nutr* 1994;60:567-72.

5054 Eberhard P, Gall HM, Muller I, Moller R. Dramatic augmentation of a food allergy by acetylsalicylic acid. *J Allergy Clin Immunol* 2000;105:844.

5055 Mundell EJ. Mussel extract helps arthritic dogs. Available at: www.reutershealth.com (Accessed 18 April 2000).

5056 Ohnishi ST, Ohnishi T, Ogunmola GB. Sickle cell anemia: a potential nutritional approach for a molecular disease. *Nutrition* 2000;16:330-8.

5058 Aro A, Mannisto S, Salminen I, et al. Inverse association between dietary and serum conjugated linoleic acid and risk of breast cancer in postmenopausal women. *Nutr Cancer* 2000;38:151-7.

5059 Almada A, Harvey P, Platt K. Effects of chronic oral glucosamine sulfate on fasting insulin resistance index (FIRI) in non-diabetic individuals. *FASEB J* 2000;14:A750.

5060 Awoke S, Lawrence GD. Cimetidine and hyperparathyroidism [letters]. *Lancet* 1980;1:1134.

5061 Antioxidant lozenge could help ward off flu. Available at: www.reutershealth.com (Accessed 19 April 2000).

5063 Chaturvedi A, Sarojini G, Devi NL. Hypocholesterolemic effect of amaranth seeds (Amaranthus esculantus). *Plant Foods Hum Nutr* 1993;44:63-70.

5064 Oesterheld J, Kallepalli BR. Grapefruit juice and clomipramine: shifting metabolitic ratios. *J Clin Psychopharmacol* 1997;17:62-3.

5065 van Agtmael MA, Gupta V, van der Wosten TH, et al. Grapefruit juice increases the bioavailability of artemether. *Eur J Clin Pharmacol* 1999;55:405-10.

5066 van Agtmael MA, Gupta V, van der Graaf CA, van Boxtel CJ. The effect of grapefruit juice on the time-dependent decline of artemether plasma levels in healthy subjects. *Clin Pharmacol Ther* 1999;66:408-14.

5067 Damkier P, Hansen LL, Brosen K. Effect of diclofenac, disulfiram, itraconazole, grapefruit juice and erythromycin on the pharmacokinetics of quinidine. *Br J Clin Pharmacol* 1999;48:829-38.

5068 Takanaga H, Ohnishi A, Murakami H, et al. Relationship between time after intake of grapefruit juice and the effect on pharmacokinetics and pharmacodynamics of nisoldipine in healthy subjects. *Clin Pharmacol Ther* 2000:67:201-14.

5069 Takanaga H, Ohnishi A, Matsuo H, et al. Pharmacokinetic analysis of felodipine-grapefruit juice interaction based on an irreversible enzyme inhibition model. *Br J Clin Pharmacol* 2000;49:49-58.

5070 Dresser GK, Spence JD, Bailey DG. Pharmacokinetic-pharmacodynamic consequences and clinical relevance of cytochrome P450 3A4 inhibition. *Clin Pharmacokinet* 2000;38:41-57.

5071 Coreg monograph. In: Gillis MC, Ed. Compendium of Pharmaceuticals and Specialities (CPS). 34th ed. Ottawa, Ontario, CAN:Canadian Pharmacists Assn, 1999:395.

5072 He K, Iyer KR, Hayes RN, et al. Inactivation of cytochrome P450 3A4 by bergamottin, a component of grapefruit juice. *Chem Res Toxicol* 1998;11:252-9.

5073 Ernst E, Rand JI, Barnes J, Stevinson C. Adverse effects profile of the herbal antidepressant St. John's wort (Hypericum perforatum L.). *Eur J Clin Pharmacol* 1998;54:589-94.

5074 Lantz MS, Buchalter E, Giambanco V. St. John's wort and antidepressant drug interactions in the elderly. *J Geriatr Psychiatry Neurol* 1999;12:7-10.

5075 Taylor LH, Kobak KA. An open-label trial of St. John's wort (Hypericum perforatum) in obsessive-compulsive disorder. *J Clin Psychiatry* 2000;61:575-8.

5076 Fed Trade Comm. Marketers of Vitamin O settles FTC charges of making false health claims. 2000. Available at: www.ftc.gov/opa/2000/05/rosecreek2.htm.

5080 McCrory DC, Matchar DB, Gray RN, et al. Evidence-based guidelines for migraine headache: overview of program description and methodology. US Headache Consortium, April 2000. www.aan.com/cgi-bin/whatsnewlink.pl?loc=/public/practiceguidelines (Accessed 3 May 2000).

5081 Butner LE, Fulco PP, Feldman G, et al. Calcium carbonate-induced hypothyroidism. *Ann Intern Med* 2000:132:595.

5082 Schneyer CR. Calcium carbonate and reduction of levothyroxine efficacy. *JAMA* 1998;279:750.

5084 Codina R, Ardusso L, Lockey RF, et al. Sensitization to soybean hull allergens in subjects exposed to different levels of soybean dust inhalation in Argentina. *J Allergy Clin Immunol* 2000;105:570-6.

5085 Anto JM, Sunyer J, Rodriguez-Roisin R, et al. Community outbreaks of asthma associated with inhalation of soybean dust. Toxicoepidemiological Committee. *N Engl J Med* 1989;320:1097-1102.

5086 White MC, Etzel RA, Olson DR, Goldstein IF. Re-examination of epidemic asthma in New Orleans, Louisianna, in relation to the presence of soy at the harbor. *Am J Epidemiol* 1997;145:432-8.

5087 Snow V, Lascher S, Mottur-Pilson C. Pharmacologic treatment of acute major depression and dysthymia. *Ann Intern Med* 2000;132:738-42.

5088 Schedules of controlled substances: addition of gamma-hydroxybutyric acid to Schedule I. *Fed Regist* 2000;65:13235-8.

5089 Kachhi PN, Henderson SO. Priapism after androstenedione intake for athletic performance enhancement. *Ann Emerg Med* 2000;35:391-3.

5090 Khatta M, Alexander BS, Krichten CM, et al. The effect of coenzyme Q10 in patients with congestive heart failure. *Ann Intern Med* 2000;132:636-40.

5091 Ferrara LA, Raimondi AS, d'Episcopo L, et al. Olive oil and reduced need for antihypertensive medications. *Arch Intern Med* 2000;160:837-42.

5092 McEvoy AW, Kitchen ND, Thomas DG. Intracerebral haemorrhage in young adults: the emerging importance of drug misuse. *BMJ* 2000;320:1322-4.

5093 Marks L, Partin AW, Epstein JI, et al. Effects of a saw palmetto herbal blend in men with symptomatic benign prostatic hyperplasia. *J Urol* 2000;163:1451-6.

5094 Gerber GS. Saw palmetto for the treatment of men with lower urinary tract symptoms. *J Urol* 2000;163:1408-12.

5095 Goepel M, Hecker U, Krege S, et al. Saw palmetto extracts potently and noncompetitively inhibit human alpha1-adrenoceptors in vitro. *Prostate* 1999;38:208-15.

5096 Shelton RC, Keller MB, Gelenberg A, et al. Effectiveness of St. John's wort in major depression: A randomized, placebo-controlled trial. *JAMA* 2001;285:1978-86.

5097 Harel Z, Gascon G, Riggs S, et al. Fish oil vs olive oil in the management of recurrent headaches in adolescents. Advancing Children's Health 2000. Joint Meeting of Pediatric Academic Soc and Am Acad of Pediatrics; Abstract 30.

5098 Murray MT, Pizzorno JE Jr. Melaleuca alternifolia. In: Textbook of Natural Medicine. New York, NY: Churchill Livingstone, 1999:817-20.

5103 Bennett WG, Cerda JJ. Benefits of dietary fiber. Myth or medicine? *Postgrad Med* 1996;99(2):153-6, 166-8, 171-2 passim.

5104 Reddy BS. Role of dietary fiber in colon cancer: an overview. *Am J Med* 1999;106:16S-9S.

5105 Almy TP. Fiber and the gut. *Am J Med* 1981;71(2):193-5.

5106 Almy TP, Howell DA. Medical progress; Diverticular disease of the colon. *N Engl J Med* 1980;302:324-31.

5107 Kritchevsky D. Dietary fibre and cancer. *Eur J Cancer Prev* 1997;6(5):435-41.

5108 Dwyer JT, Goldin B, Gorbach S, Patterson J. Drug therapy reviews: dietary fiber and fiber supplements in the therapy of gastrointestinal disorders. *Am J Hosp Pharm* 1978;35:278-87.

5109 Kalant H, Roschlau WHE, Eds. Principles of Med. Pharmacology. New York, NY: Oxford Univ Press, 1998.

5110 Bloom FE, Kupfer DJ. Psychopharmacology: The Fourth Generation of Progress. New York, NY: Raven Press, Ltd., 1995.

5111 www.betterbodz.com.

5112 www.thewayup.com.

5113 Cocito L, Bianchetti A, Bossi L, et al. GABA and phosphatidylserine in human photosensitivity: a pilot study. *Epilepsy Res* 1994;17(1):49-53.

5114 Cavagnini F, Pinto M, Dubini A, et al. Effects of gamma aminobutyric acid (GABA) and muscimol on endocrine pancreatic function in man. *Metabolism* 1982;31(1):73-7.

5115 Cavagnini F, Invitti C, Pinto M, Maraschini C, Di Landro A, Dubini A, Marelli A. Effect of acute and repeated administration of gamma aminobutyric acid (GABA) on growth hormone and prolactin secretion in man. *Acta Endocrinol* (Copenh) 1980;93(2):149-54.

5116 Nurnberger JI Jr, Berrettini WH, Simmons-Alling S, et al. Intravenous GABA administration is anxiogenic in man. *Psychiatry Res* 1986;19:113-7.

5119 Brown D. Encyclopedia of herbs and their uses. 1st ed. New York, NY: Dorland Kindersley Publ. Inc., 1995.

5121 Duke JA. The Green Pharmacy. Emmaus, PA: Rodale Press, 1997.

5122 Moyad MA, Pienta KJ, Montie JE. Use of PC-SPES, a commercially available supplement for prostate cancer, in a patient with hormone-naive disease. *Urology* 1999;54:319-28.

5129 Accatino L, Pizarro M, Solis N, Koenig CS. Effects of diosgenin, a plant-derived steroid, on bile secretion and hepatocellular cholestasis induced by estrogens in the rat. *Hepatology* 1998;28:129-40.

5130 Aradhana AR, Rao AS, Kale RK. Diosgenin-a growth stimulator of mammary gland of ovariectomized mouse. *Indian J Exp Biol* 1992;30:367-70.

5131 Yamada T, Hoshino M, Hayakawa T, et al. Dietary diosgenin attenuates subacute intestinal inflammation associated with indomethacin in rats. *Am J Physiol* 1997;273:G355-64.

5133 Beltz SD, Doering PL. Efficacy of nutritional supplements used by athletes. *Clin Pharm* 1993;12:900-8.

5136 Wagner JC. Use of chromium and cobamamide by athletes. *Clin Pharm* 1989;8:832-4.

5137 Williams MH. Vitamin and mineral supplements to athletes: do they help? *Clin Sports Med* 1984;3:623-37.

5139 Gilman AG, et al, eds. Goodman and Gilman's The Pharmacological Basis of Therapeutics. 8th ed. New York, NY: Pergamon Press, 1990.

5140 Buchman AL, Dubin M, Jenden D, et al. Lecithin increases plasma free choline and decreases hepatic steatosis in long-term total parenteral nutrition patients. *Gastroenterology* 1992;102:1363-70.

5141 Wagenmakers A. Muscle amino acid metabolism at rest and during exercise: role in human physiology and metabolism. *Exerc Sport Sci Rev* 1998;26:287-314.

5142 Tuzhilin SA, Dreiling DA, Narodetskaja RV, Lukash LK. The treatment of patients with gallstones by lecithin. *Am J Gastroenterol* 1976;65:231-5.

5143 Chan H, Abraham G, Oreopoulos DG. Oral lecithin improves ultrafiltration in patients on peritoneal dialysis. *Perit Dial Int* 1989;9:203-5.

5144 Lieber CS. Alcohol and the liver: 1994 update. *Gastroenterol* 1994;106:1085-105.

5145 Cohen BM, Lipinski JF, Altesman RI. Lecithin in the treatment of mania: double-blind, placebo-controlled trials. *Am J Psychiatry* 1982;139:1162-4.

5146 Harris CM, Dysken MW, Fovall P, et al. Effect of lecithin on memory in normal adults. *Am J Psychiatry* 1983;140:1010-2.

5147 Simons LA, Hickie JB, Ruys J. Treatment of hypercholesterolaemia with oral lecithin. *Aust N Z J Med* 1977;7:262-6.

5148 Oosthuizen W, Vorster HH, Vermaak WJ, et al. Lecithin has no effect on serum lipoprotein, plasma fibrinogen and macro molecular protein complex levels in hyperlipidaemic men in a double-blind controlled study. *Eur J Clin Nutr* 1998;52(6):419-24.

5149 Brinkman SD, Smith RC, Meyer JS, et al. Lecithin and memory training in suspected Alzheimer's disease. *J Gerontol* 1982;37:4-9.

5150 Brinkman SD, Pomara N, Goodnick PJ, et al. A dose-ranging study of lecithin in the treatment of primary degenerative dementia (Alzheimer disease). *J Clin Psychopharmacol* 1982;2:281-5.

5151 Pomara N, Domino EF, Yoon H, et al. Failure of single-dose lecithin to alter aspects of central cholinergic activity in Alzheimer's disease. *J Clin Psychiatry* 1983;44:293-5.

5152 Etienne P, Dastoor D, Gauthier S, et al. Alzheimer disease: lack of effect of lecithin treatment for 3 months. *Neurol* 1981;31:1552-4.

5153 Facts and Comparisons, loose leaf edition. St. Louis, MO: Wolters Kluwer Co., 1999.

5155 Holan KR, Holzbach RT, Hsieh JY, et al. Effect of oral administration of essential phospholipid, beta-glycerophosphate, and linoleic acid on biliary lipids in patients with cholelithiasis. *Digestion* 1979;19:251-8.

5156 Maltby N, Broe GA, Creasey H, et al. Efficacy of tacrine and lecithin in mild to moderate Alzheimer's disease: double-blind trial. *BMJ* 1994;308:879-83.

5158 Portakal O, Ozkaya O, Erden Inal M, et al. Coenzyme Q10 concentrations and antioxidant status in tissues of breast cancer patients. *Clin Biochem* 2000;33:279-84.

5159 Lund EL, Quistorff B, Spang-Thomsen M, Kristjansen PE. Effect of radiation therapy on small-cell lung cancer is reduced by ubiquinone intake. *Folia Microbiol* (Praha) 1998;43:505-6.

5160 Grunewald KK, Bailey RS. Commercially marketed supplements for bodybuilding athletes. *Sports Med* 1993;15:90-103.

5161 Sehested P, Lund HI, Kristensen O. Oral choline in cerebellar ataxia. *Acta Neurol Scand* 1980;62:124-6.

5162 McNamara JO, Carwile S, Hope V, et al. Effects of oral choline on human complex partial seizures. *Neurology* 1980;30:1334-6.

5163 Shronts EP. Essential nature of choline with implications for total parenteral nutrition. *J Am Diet Assoc* 1997;97:639-46.

5164 Spector SA, Jackman MR, Sabounjian LA, et al. Effect of choline supplementation on fatigue in trained cyclists. *Med Sci Sports Exerc* 1995;27:668-73.

5165 Gupta SK, Gaur SN. A placebo controlled trial of two dosages of LPC antagonist-choline in the management of bronchial asthma. *Indian J Chest Dis Allied Sci* 1997;39:149-56.

5166 Gaur SN, Agarwal G, Gupta SK. Use of LPC antagonist, choline, in the management of bronchial asthma. *Indian J Chest Dis Allied Sci* 1997;39:107-13.

5170 Mohs RC, Davis KL, Tinklenberg JR, Hollister LE. Choline chloride effects on memory in the elderly. *Neurobiol Aging* 1980;1:21-5.

5171 Davis KL, Berger PA. Pharmacological investigations of the cholinergic imbalance hypotheses of movement disorders and psychosis. *Biol Psychiatry* 1978;13:23-49.

5172 Davis KL, Hollister LE, Berger PA. Choline chloride in schizophrenia. *Am J Psychiatry* 1979;136:1581-4.

5173 Lawrence CM, Millac P, Stout GS, Ward JW. The use of choline chloride in ataxic disorders. *J Neurol Neurosurg Psychiatry* 1980;43:452-4.

5174 Buchman AL, Dubin MD, Moukarzel AA, et al. Choline deficiency: a cause of hepatic steatosis during parenteral nutrition that can be reversed with intravenous choline supplementation. *Hepatology* 1995;22:1399-403.

5175 Tan J, Bluml S, Hoang T, et al. Lack of effect of oral choline supplement on the concentrations of choline metabolites in human brain. *Magn Reson Med* 1998;39:1005-10.

5177 Hay IC, Jamieson M, Ormerod AD. Randomized trial of aromatherapy. Successful treatment for alopecia areata. *Arch Dermatol* 1998;134:1349-52.

5178 Albright CD, Liu R, Mar MH, et al. Diet, apoptosis, and carcinogenesis. *Adv Exp Med Biol* 1997;422:97-107.

5179 Yen CL, Mar MH, Zeisel SH. Choline deficiency-induced apoptosis in PC12 cells is associated with diminished membrane phosphatdylcholine and sphingomyelin, accumulation of ceramide and diacylglycerol, and activiation of a caspase. *FASEB J* 1999;13:135-42.

5180 Zeisel SH. Choline: an important nutrient in brain development, liver function and carcinogenesis. *J Am Coll Nutr* 1992;11:473-81.

5184 Fava M, Giannelli A, Rapisarda V, et al. Rapidity of onset of the antidepressant effect of parenteral S-adenosyl-L-methionine. *Psychiatry Res* 1995;56:295-7.

5188 Bradley JD, Flusser D, Katz BP, et al. A randomized, double blind, placebo controlled trial of intravenous loading with S-adenosylmethionine (SAM) followed by oral SAM therapy in patients with knee osteoarthritis. *J Rheumatol* 1994;21:905-11.

5189 Bressa GM. S-adenosyl-l-methionine (SAMe) as antidepressant: meta-analysis of clinical studies. *Acta Neurol Scand Suppl* 1994;154:7-14.

5190 Bell KM, Potkin SG, Carreon D, Plon L. S-adenosylmethionine blood levels in major depression: changes with drug treatment. *Acta Neurol Scand Suppl* 1994;154:15-8.

5191 Lambert J, Cormier J. Potential interaction between warfarin and boldo-fenugreek. *Pharmacotherapy* 2001;21:509-12.

5192 Salmaggi P, Bressa GM, Nicchia G, et al. Double-blind, placebo-controlled study of S-adenosyl-L-methionine in depressed postmenopausal women. *Psychother Psychosom* 1993;59:34-40.

5193 Berlanga C, Ortega-Soto HA, Ontiveros M, Senties H. Efficacy of S-adenosyl-L-methionine in speeding the onset of action of imipramine. *Psychiatry Res* 1992;44:257-62.

5195 Kagan BL, Sultzer DL, Rosenlicht N, Gerner RH. Oral S-adenosylmethionine in depression: a randomized, double-blind, placebo-controlled trial. *Am J Psychiatry* 1990;147:591-5.

5196 Rosenbaum JF, Fava M, Falk WE, et al. The antidepressant potential of oral S-adenosyl-l-methionine. *Acta Psychiatr Scand* 1990;81:432-6.

5197 Heartwire. Antioxidants get a vote of confidence in cardiac transplant patients. Available at: http://www.theheart.org/viewEntityDispatcherAction.do?primaryKey=174806 (Accessed 13 December 2001).

5198 Chawla RK, Bonkovsky HL, Galambos JT. Biochemistry and pharmacology of S-adenosyl-L-methionine and rationale for its use in liver disease. *Drugs* 1990;40:98-110.

5199 Domljan Z, Vrhovac B, Durrigl T, Pucar I. A double-blind trial of ademetionine vs naproxen in activated gonarthrosis. *Int J Clin Pharmacol Ther Toxicol* 1989;27:329-33.

5200 Bell KM, Plon L, Bunney WE Jr, Potkin SG. S-adenosylmethionine treatment of depression: a controlled clinical trial. *Am J Psychiatry* 1988;145:1110-4.

5201 Vahora SA, Malek-Ahmasi P. S-adenosylmethionine in the treatment of depression. *Neurosci Biobehav Rev* 1988;12:139-41.

5202 Baldessarini RJ. Neuropharmacology of S-adenosyl-L-methionine. *Am J Med* 1987;83:95-103.

5203 Konig B. A long-term (two years) clinical trial with S-adenosylmethionine for the treatment of osteoarthritis. *Am J Med* 1987;83:78-80.

5204 Berger R, Nowak H. A new medical approach to the treatment of osteoarthritis. Report of an open phase IV study with ademetionine (Gumbaral). *Am J Med* 1987;83:84-8.

5205 Muller-Fassbender H. Double-blind clinical trial of S-adenosylmethionine versus ibuprofen in the treatment of osteoarthritis. *Am J Med* 1987;83:81-3.

5206 Vetter G. Double-blind comparative clinical trial with S-adenosylmethionine and indomethacin in the treatment of osteoarthritis. *Am J Med* 1987;83:78-80.

5207 Maccagno A, Di Giorgio EE, Caston OL, Sagasta CL. Double-blind controlled clinical trial of oral S-adenosylmethionine versus piroxicam in knee osteoarthritis. *Am J Med* 1987;83:72-7.

5208 Caruso I, Pietrogrande V. Italian double-blind, multicenter study comparing S-adenosylmethionine, naproxen, and placebo in the treatment of degenerative joint disease. *Am J Med* 1987;83:66-71.

5209 di Padova C. S-adenosylmethionine in the treatment of osteoarthritis. Review of the clinical studies. *Am J Med* 1987;83:60-5.

5210 Palumbo G, Avanzini F, Alli C, et al. Effects of vitamin E on clinic and ambulatory blood pressure in treated hypertensive patients. Collaborative Group of the Primary

REFERENCES

REFERENCES

Prevention Project (PPP)--Hypertension study. *Am J Hypertens* 2000;13:564-7.

5211 Tavoni A, Vitali C, Bombardieri S, Pasero G. Evaluation of S-adenosylmethionine in primary fibromyalgia. A double-blind crossover study. *Am J Med* 1987;83:107-10.

5213 Laudanno OM. Cytoprotective effect of S-adenosylmethionine compared with that of misoprostol against ethanol-, aspirin-, and stress-induced gastric damage. *Am J Med* 1987;83(5A):43-7.

5215 Glorioso S, Todesco S, Mazzi A, et al. Double-blind, multicentre study of the activity of S-adenosylmethionine in hip and knee osteoarthritis. *Int J Clin Pharmacol Res* 1985;5:39-49.

5216 Lipinski JF, Cohen BM, Frankenburg F, et al. Open trial of S-adenosylmethionine for treatment of depression. *Am J Psychiatry* 1984;141:448-50.

5217 Castagna A, Le Grazie C, Accordini A, et al. Cerebrospinal fluid S-adenosylmethionine (SAMe) and glutathione concentrations in HIV infection: effect of parenteral treatment with SAMe. *Neurol* 1995;45:1678-83.

5218 Tan SV, Guiloff RJ. Hypothesis on the pathogenesis of vacuolar myelopathy, dementia, and peripheral neuropathy in AIDS. *J Neurol Neurosurg Psychiatry* 1998;65:23-8.

5219 Almasio P, Bortolini M, Pagliaro L, Coltorti M. Role of S-adenosyl-L-methionine in the treatment of intrahepatic cholestasis. *Drugs* 1990;40:111-23.

5221 Volkmann H, Norregaard J, Jacobsen S, et al. Double-blind, placebo-controlled cross-over study of intravenous S-adenosyl-L-methionine in patients with fibromyalgia. *Scand J Rheumatol* 1997;26:206-11.

5222 Chan PC, Tam SC, Robinson JD, et al. Effect of phosphatidylcholine on ultrafiltration in patients on continuous ambulatory peritoneal dialysis. *Nephron* 1991;59:100-3.

5223 Domino EF, May WW, Demetriou S, et al. Lack of clinically significant improvement of patients with tardive dyskinesia following phosphatidylcholine therapy. *Biol Psychiatry* 1985;20:1189-96.

5224 Jenkins PJ, Portmann BP, Eddleston AL, Williams R. Use of polyunsaturated phosphatidyl choline in HBsAg negative chronic active hepatitis: results of prospective double-blind controlled trial. *Liver* 1982;2:77-81.

5225 Guan R, Ho KY, Kang JY, et al. The effect of polyunsaturated phosphatidyl choline in the treatment of acute viral hepatitis. *Aliment Pharmacol Ther* 1995;9:699-703.

5226 Niederau C, Strohmeyer G, Heintges T, et al. Polyunsaturated phosphatidyl-choline and interferon alpha for treatment of chronic hepatitis B and C: a multi-center, randomized, double-blind, placebo-controlled trial. Leich Study Group. *Hepatogastroenterol* 1998;45:797-804.

5228 Ladd SL, Sommer SA, LaBerge S, Toscano W. Effect of phosphatidylcholine on explicit memory. *Clin Neuropharmacol* 1993;16:540-9.

5229 Aronson PJ, Lorincz AL. Promotion of palmar sweating with oral phosphatidylcholine. *Acta Derm Venereol* 1985;65:19-24.

5231 Friedel HA, Goa KL, Benfield P. S-adenosyl-L-methionine. A review of its pharmacological properties and therapeutic potential in liver dysfunction and affective disorders in relation to its physiological role in cell metabolism. *Drugs* 1989;38:389-416.

5232 Bottiglieri T, Hyland K, Reynolds EH. The clinical potential of ademetionine (S-adenosylmethionine) in neurological disorders. *Drugs* 1994;48:137-52.

5233 Moyad MA. Alternative therapies for advanced prostate cancer. What should I tell my patients? *Urologic Clinics of North America* 1999;26:413-7.

5234 U.S. Department of Agriculture, Agricultural Research Service. USDA Nutrient Database for Standard Reference, Release 14. Nutrient Data Laboratory. Available at: http://www.nal.usda.gov/fnic/foodcomp

5235 Diaz BA, Dominguez HR, Uribe AF. Parenteral S-adenosylmethionine compared to placebos in the treatment of alcoholic liver diseases. *An Med Interna* 1996;13:9-15.

5236 Loguercio C, Nardi G, Argenzio F, et al. Effect of S-adenosyl-L-methionine administration on red blood cell cysteine and glutathione levels in alcoholic patients with and without liver disease. *Alcohol* 1994;29:597-604.

5238 Podymova SD, Nadinskaia M. [Clinical trial of heptral in patients with chronic diffuse liver disease with intrahepatic cholestasis syndrome]. [Article in Russian]. *Klin Med* (Mosk) 1998;76:45-8.

5239 Frezza M, Surrenti C, Manzillo G, et al. Oral S-adenosylmethionine in the symptomatic treatment of intrahepatic cholestasis. A double-blind, placebo-controlled study. *Gastroenterology* 1990;99:211-5.

5240 Frezza M, Centini G, Cammareri G, et al. S-adenosylmethionine for the treatment of intrahepatic cholestasis of pregnancy. Results of a controlled clinical trial. *Hepatogastroenterology* 1990;37:122-5.

5241 Jacobsen S, Danneskiold-Samsoe B, Andersen RB. Oral S-adenosylmethionine in primary fibromyalgia. Double-blind clinical evaluation. *Scand J Rheumatol* 1991;20:294-302.

5243 Heyman JA, et al. Failure of long term high-dose lecithin to retard progression of early-onset Alzheimer's disease. *Neural Transm Suppl* 1987;24:279-86.

5244 Botanical Dermatological Database. Annonaceae (Custard apple family). http://archive.uwcm.ac.uk/uwcm/dm/BoDD/BotDermFolder/BotDermA/ANNO.html. (Accessed 17 August 2001).

5245 Cavaliere H, Floriano I, Medeiros-Neto G. Gastrointestinal side effects of orlistat may be prevented by concomitant prescription of natural fibers (psyllium mucilloid). *Int J Obes Relat Metab Disord* 2001;25:1095-9.

5246 Washington N, Harris M, Mussellwhite A, Spiller RC. Moderation of lactulose-induced diarrhea by psyllium: effects on motility and fermentation. *Am J Clin Nutr* 1998;67:317-21.

5247 Coniglio SJ, Lewis JD, Lang C, et al. A randomized, double-blind, placebo-controlled trial of single-dose intravenous secretin as treatment for children with autism. *J Pediatr* 2001;138:649-55.

5248 Azuma J, Sawamura A, Awata N. Usefulness of taurine in chronic congestive heart failure andits prospective application. *Jpn Circ J* 1992;56:95-9.

5249 Laird RD, Webb M. Psychotic episode during use of St. John's wort. *J Herb Pharmacother* 2001;1:81-7.

5250 Castleman M. The healing herbs, the ultimate guide to the curative power of nature's medicines. 2nd ed. New York, NY:Bantam Books, 1995.

5251 Reid D. A handbook of Chinese healing herbs. Boston, MA:Shambhala, 1995.

5252 Sifton D, ed. The PDR family guide to natural medicines & healing therapies. New York, NY:Three Rivers Press, 1999.

5253 Hoffman D. The herbal handbook: a user's guide to medical herbalism. rev ed. Rochester, VT:Healing Arts Press, 1998.

5254 Weiner MA, Weiner JA. Herbs that heal: prescription for herbal healing. Mill Valley, CA:Quantum Books, 1999.

5255 Raintree tropical plant database, Amazon plants. www.rain-tree.com/plants.htm (Accessed 30 July 1999).

5260 Zakay-Rones Z, Varsano N, Zlotnik M, et al. Inhibition of several strains of influenza virus in vitro and reduction of symptoms by an elderberry extract (Sambucus nigra L.) during an outbreak of influenza B Panama. *J Altern Complement Med* 1995;1:361-9.

5263 Lust J. The herb book. New York, NY: Bantam Books, 1999.

5264 Brand C, Snaddon J, Bailey M, Cicuttini F. Vitamin E is ineffective for symptomatic relief of knee osteoarthritis: a six month double blind, randomised, placebo controlled study. *Ann Rheum Dis* 2001;60:946-9.

5267 Botanical.Com A Modern Herbal. www.botanical.com (Accessed 31 July 1999).

5269 Herbal Monographs. Healthlink. www.healthline.com (Accessed 1 August 1999).

5271 Azuma J, Sawamura A, Awata N, et al. Therapeutic effect of taurine in congestive heart failure: a double-blind crossover trial. *Clin Cardiol* 1985;8:276-82.

5274 GHS Gold. Gerovital Direct Prod. www:gerivital.co.uk (Accessed 3 August 1999).

5275 Fogarty A, Lewis S, Weiss S, Britton J. Dietary vitamin E, IgE concentrations, and atopy. *Lancet* 2000;356:1573-4.

5276 Herbal Materia Medica 4.0. website: www.herb.com/materia.htm (Acessed 6 August 1999).

5277 Aubourg P, Adamsbaum C, Lavallard-Rousseau MC, et al. A two-year trial of oleic and erucic acids (Lorenzo's oil) as treatment for adrenomyeloneuropathy. *N Engl J Med* 1993;329(11):745-52.

5278 DiGregorio VY, Schroeder DJ. Lorenzo's oil therapy of adrenoleukodystrophy. *Ann Pharmacother* 1995;29(3):312-3.

5279 Brown D. Encyclopedia of herbs and their uses. New York, NY:Dorland Kindersley Publ., Inc., 1995.

5280 Chesney RW. Taurine: its biological role and clinical implications. *Adv Pediatr* 1985;32:1-42.

5286 Rauma AL, Nenonen M, Helve T, et al. Effect of a strict vegan diet on energy and nutrient intakes by Finnish rheumatoid patients. *Eur J Clin Nutr* 1993;47:747-9.

5290 Lowe FC, Dreikorn K, Borkowski A, et al. Review of recent placebo-controlled trials utilizing phytotherapeutic agents for treatment of BPH. *Prostate* 1998;37(3):187-93.

5292 Buck AC, Cox R, Rees RW, et al. Treatment of outflow tract obstruction due to benign prostatic hyperplasia with the pollen extract, cernilton. A double-blind, placebo-controlled study. *Br J Urol* 1990;66(4):398-404.

5293 Rugendorff EW, Weidner W, Ebeling L, Buck AC. Results of treatment with pollen extract (Cernilton N) in chronic prostatitis and prostatodynia. *Br J Urol* 1993;71:433-8.

5294 Yasumoto R, Kawanishi H, Tsujino T, et al. Clinical evaluation of long-term treatment using cernitin pollen extract in patients with benign prostatic hyperplasia. *Clin Ther* 1995;17(1):82-7.

5295 Lowe FC, Ku JC. Phytotherapy in treatment of benign prostatic hyperplasia: a critical review. *Urol* 1996;48(1):12-20.

5296 Buck AC, Rees RW, Ebeling L. Treatment of chronic prostatitis and prostatodynia with pollen extract. *Br J Urol* 1989;64:496-9.

5297 Habib FK, Ross M, Lewenstein A, et al. Identification of a prostate inhibitory substance in a pollen extract. *Prostate* 1995;26:133-9.

5298 Loschen G, Ebeling L. [Inhibition of arachidonic acid cascade by extract of rye pollen]. [Article in German]. *Arzneimittelforschung* 1991;41:162-7.

5301 Al-Assmar SE. The seeds of the Hawaiian baby woodrose are a powerful hallucinogen. *Arch Intern Med* 1999;159:2090.

5304 Shawcross WE. Recreational use of ergoline alkaloid from Argyreia nervosa. *J Psychoactive Drugs* 1983;15:251-9.

5305 Chou CT, Chang SC. The inhibitory effect of common traditional anti-rheumatic herb formulas on prostaglandin E and interleukin 2 in vitro: a comparative study with Tripterygium wilfordii. *J Ethnopharmacol* 1998;62:167-71.

5306 Azuma J, Hasegawa H, Sawamura A, et al. Therapy of congestive heart failure with orally administered taurine. *Clin Ther* 1983;5:398-408.

5308 Jeppsson A, Ekroth R, Friberg P, et al. Renal effects of alpha-ketoglutarate early after coronary operations. *Ann Thorac Surg* 1998;65(3):684-90.

5309 Wernerman J, Hammarqvist F, Vinnars E. Alpha-ketoglutarate and postoperative muscle catabolism. *Lancet* 1990;335(8691):701-3.

5310 Blomqvist BI, Hammarqvist F, von der Decken A, et al. Glutamine and alpha-ketoglutarate prevent the decrease in muscle free glutamine concentration and influence protein synthesis after total hip replacement. *Metabolism* 1995;44(9):1215-22.

5311 Riedel E, Nundel M, Hampl H. Alpha-Ketoglutarate application in hemodialysis patients improves amino acid metabolism. *Nephron* 1996;74(2):261-5.

5312 Kjellman U, Bjork K, Ekroth R, et al. Alpha-ketoglutarate for myocardial protection in heart surgery. *Lancet* 1995;345(8949):552-3.

5313 Kjellman UW, Bjork K, Ekroth R, et al. Addition of alpha-ketoglutarate to blood cardioplegia improves cardioprotection. *Ann Thorac Surg* 1997;63(6):1625-33.

5314 Aussel C, Coudray-Lucas C, Lasnier E, et al. Alpha-Ketoglutarate uptake in human fibroblasts. *Cell Biol Int* 1996;20(5):359-63.

5315 Huxtable RJ, Chubb J, Azari J. Physiological and experimental regulation of taurine content in the heart. *Fed Proc* 1980;39:2685-90.

5318 Stabilized Oxygen. Portal Market. www.portalmarket.com/earthportals/Portal_Market/eathportals/portal_Ma_/oxygen.htm (Accessed 7 October 1999).

5320 Oxygen caps. Lifeplus vitamins. www.lifeplusvitamins.simpletnet.com/1p27p.html (Accessed 7 October 1999).

5321 How to use Oxy boost. O2oxyboost. www.o2xyboost.com/howto.htm (Accessed 7 October 1999).

5326 Salen G, Shefer S, Nguyen L, et al. Sisterolemia. *J Lipid Res* 1992;33:945-55.

5327 Berges RR, Windeler J, Trampisch HJ, et al. Randomised, placebo-controlled, double-blind clinical trial of beta-sitosterol in patients with benign prostatic hyperplasia. Beta-sitosterol Study Group. *Lancet* 1995;345:1529-32.

5328 Klippel KF, Hiltl DM, Schipp B. A multicentric, placebo-controlled, double-blind clinical trial of beta-sitosterol (phytosterol) for the treatment of benign prostatic hyperplasia. *Br J Urol* 1997;80:427-32.

5329 Wilt TJ, MacDonald R, Ishani A. beta-sitosterol for the treatment of benign prostatic hyperplasia: a systematic review. *BJU Int* 1999;83:976-83.

5330 Becker M, Staab D, Von Bergmann K. Treatment of severe familial hypercholesterolemia in childhood with sitosterol and sitostanol. *J Pediatr* 1993;122:292-6.

5331 Oster P, Schlierf G, Heuck CC, et al. [Sitosterol in familial hyperlipoproteinemia type II. A randomized, double-blind, cross-over study]. [Article in German]. *Dtsch Med Wochenschr* 1976;101:1308-11.

5332 Schlierf G, Oster P, Heuck CC, et al. Sitosterol in juvenile type II hyperlipoproteinemia. *Atherosclerosis* 1978;30:245-8.

5333 Schwartzkopff W, Jantke HJ. [Dose-effect of beta-sitosterin in type IIa and IIb hypercholesterolemias]. [Article in German]. *MMW Munch Med Wochenschr* 1978;120:1575-8.

5334 Becker M, Staab D, Von Bergman K. Long-term treatment of severe familial hypercholesterolemia in children: effect of sitosterol and bezafibrate. *Pediatrics* 1992;89:138-42.

5335 Bouic PJ, Clark A, Lamprecht J, et al. The effects of B-sitosterol (BSS) and B-sitosterol glucoside (BSSG) mixture

REFERENCES

on selected immune parameters of marathon runners: inhibition of post marathon immune suppression and inflammation. *Int J Sports Med* 1999;20:258-62.
5336 Weststrate JA, Meijer GW. Plant sterol-enriched margarines and reduction of plasma total- and LDL-cholesterol concentrations in normocholesterolaemic and mildly hypercholesterolaemic subjects. *Eur J Clin Nutr* 1998;52:334-43.
5337 Donald PR, Lamprecht JH, Freestone M, et al. A randomised placebo-controlled trial of the efficacy of beta-sitosterol and its glucoside as adjuvants in the treatment of pulmonary tuberculosis. *Int J Tubercul Lung Dis* 1997;1:518-22.
5338 Gerolami A, Sarles H. Letter: Beta-sitosterol and chenodeoxycholic acid in the treatment of cholesterol gallstones. *Lancet* 1975;2:721.
5339 Tangedahl TN, Thistle JL, Hofmann AF, et al. Effect of beta-sitosterol alone or in combination with chenic acid on cholesterol saturation of bile and cholesterol absorption in gallstone patients. *Gastroenterol* 1979;76:1341-6.
5340 Anon. Cholesterol-lowering Margarines. *Med Lett Drugs Ther* 1999;41:56-8.
5342 Bouic PJ, Lamprecht JH, Plant sterols and sterolins: a review of their immune-modulating properties. *Altern Med Rev* 1999;4:170-7.
5343 Vutyavanich T, Kraisarin T, Ruangsri R. Ginger for nausea and vomiting in pregnancy: randomized, double-masked, placebo-controlled trial. *Obstet Gynecol* 2001;97:577-82.
5344 Lomaestro BM, Malone M. Glutathione in health and disease: pharmacotherapeutic issues. *Ann Pharmacother* 1995;29:1263-73.
5345 Flagg EW, Coates RJ, Jones DP, et al. Dietary glutathione intake and the risk of oral and pharyngeal cancer. *Am J Epidemiol* 1994;139(5):453-65.
5346 Walsh SW, Wang Y. Deficient glutathione peroxidase activity in preeclampsia is associated with increased placental production of thromboxane and lipid peroxides. *Am J Obstet Gynecol* 1993;169:1456-61.
5347 Knapen MF, Mulder TP, Van Rooij IA, et al. Low whole blood glutathione levels in pregnancies complicated by preeclampsia or the hemolysis, elevated liver enzymes, low platelets syndrome. *Obstet Gynecol* 1998;92:1012-5.
5348 Knapen MF, Peters WH, Mulder TP, et al. Glutathione and glutathione-related enzymes in decidua and placenta of controls and women with pre-eclampsia. *Placenta* 1999;20:541-6.
5349 Marshall KA, Reist M, Jenner P, et al. The neuronal toxicity of sulfite plus peroxynitrite is enhanced by glutathione depletion: implications for Parkinson's disease. *Free Radic Biol Med* 1999;27:515-20.
5350 Jenner P, Olanow CW. Understanding cell death in Parkinson's disease. *Ann Neurol* 1998;44(3 Suppl 1):S72-84.
5351 Jenner P. Oxidative mechanisms in nigral cell death in Parkinson's disease. *Mov Disord* 1998;(13 Suppl)1:24-34.
5352 Pearce RK, Owen A, Daniel S, et al. Alterations in the distribution of glutathione in the substantia nigra in Parkinson's disease. *J Neural Transm* 1997;104(6-7):661-77.
5353 Merad-Boudia M, Nicole A, Santiard-Baron D, et al. Mitochondrial impairment as an early event in the process of apoptosis induced by glutathione depletion in neuronal cells: relevance to Parkinson's disease. *Biochem Pharmacol* 1998;56:645-55.
5354 Sechi G, Deledda MG, Bua G, et al. Reduced intravenous glutathione in the treatment of early Parkinson's disease. *Prog Neuropsychopharmacol Biol Psychiatry* 1996;20(7):1159-70.
5357 De Mattia G, Bravi MC, Laurenti O, et al. Influence of reduced glutathione infusion on glucose metabolism in patients with non-insulin-dependent diabetes mellitus. *Metabolism* 1998;47(8):993-7.
5358 Ciuchi E, Odetti P, Prando R. The effect of acute glutathione treatment on sorbitol level in erythrocytes from diabetic patients. *Diabetes Metab* 1997;23(1):58-60.
5359 Usberti M, Lima G, Arisi M, et al. Effect of exogenous reduced glutathione on the survival of red blood cells in hemodialyzed patients. *J Nephrol* 1997;10(5):261-5.
5360 Amano J, Suzuki A, Sunamori M. Salutary effect of reduced glutathione on renal function in coronary artery bypass operation. *J Am Coll Surg* 1994;179:714-20.
5361 Cook GC, Sherlock S. Results of a controlled clinical trial of glutathione in cases of hepatic cirrhosis. *Gut* 1965; 6(5):472-6.
5362 Witschi A, Reddy S, Stofer B, et al. The systemic availability of oral glutathione. *Eur J Clin Pharmacol* 1992;43(6):667-9.
5363 Hagen TM, Wierzbicka GT, Bowman BB, et al. Fate of dietary glutathione: disposition in the gastrointestinal tract. *Am J Physiol* 1990;259(4 Pt 1):G530-5.
5364 Aw TY, Wierzbicka G, Jones DP. Oral glutathione increases tissue glutathione in vivo. *Chem Biol Interact* 1991;80(1):89-97.
5367 Roum JH, Borok Z, McElvaney NG, et al. Glutathione aerosol suppresses lung epithelial surface inflammatory cell-derived oxidants in cystic fibrosis. *J Appl Physiol* 1999;87(1):438-43.
5368 Holroyd KJ, Buhl R, Borok Z, et al. Correction of glutathione deficiency in the lower respiratory tract of HIV seropositive individuals by glutathione aerosol treatment. *Thorax* 1993;48(10):985-9.
5369 Borok Z, Buhl R, Grimes GJ, et al. Effect of glutathione aerosol on oxidant-antioxidant imbalance in idiopathic pulmonary fibrosis. *Lancet* 1991;338(8761):215-6.
5372 Marrades RM, Roca J, Barbera JA, et al. Nebulized glutathione induces bronchoconstriction in patients with mild asthma. *Am J Respir Crit Care Med* 1997;156(2 Pt 1):425-30.
5373 Smyth JF, Bowman A, Perren T, et al. Glutathione reduces the toxicity and improves quality of life of women diagnosed with ovarian cancer treated with cisplatin: results of a double-blind, randomised trial. *Ann Oncol* 1997;8(6):569-73.
5374 Cascinu S, Cordella L, Del Ferro E, et al. Neuroprotective effect of reduced glutathione on cisplatin-based chemotherapy in advanced gastric cancer: a randomized, double-blind, placebo-controlled trial. *J Clin Oncol* 1995;13(1):26-32.
5375 Links M, Lewis C. Chemoprotectants: a review of their clinical pharmacology and therapeutic efficacy. *Drugs* 1999;57(3):293-308.
5376 Leone R, Fracasso ME, Soresi E, et al. Influence of glutathione administration on the disposition of free and total platinum in patients after administration of cisplatin. *Cancer Chemother Pharmacol* 1992;29(5):385-90.
5377 Graziano F, Cardarelli N, Marcellini M, et al. A pilot clinical trial of postoperative intensive weekly chemotherapy using cisplatin, epi-doxorubicin, 5-fluorouracil, 6S-leucovorin, glutathione and filgrastim in patients with resected gastric cancer. *Tumori* 1998;84(3):368-71.
5378 Plaxe S, Freddo J, Kim S, et al. Phase I trial of cisplatin in combination with glutathione. *Gynecol Oncol* 1994;55:82-6.
5379 Locatelli MC, D'Antona A, Labianca R, et al. A phase II study of combination chemotherapy in advanced ovarian carcinoma with cisplatin and cyclophosphamide plus

reduced glutathione as potential protective agent against cisplatin toxicity. *Tumori* 1993;79(1):37-9.

5380 Di Re F, Bohm S, Oriana S, et al. High-dose cisplatin and cyclophosphamide with glutathione in the treatment of advanced ovarian cancer. *Ann Oncol* 1993;4(1):55-61.

5381 Parnis FX, Coleman RE, Harper PG, et al. A randomised double-blind placebo controlled clinical trial assessing the tolerability and efficacy of glutathione as an adjuvant to escalating doses of cisplatin in the treatment of advanced ovarian cancer. *Eur J Cancer* 1995;31A(10):1721.

5382 Cascinu S, Frontini L, Comella G, et al. Intensive weekly chemotherapy is not effective in advanced pancreatic cancer patients: a report from the Italian Group for the Study of Dig. Tract Cancer (GISCAD). *Br J Cancer* 1999;79(3-4):491-4.

5383 Cascinu S, Labianca R, Alessandroni P, et al. Intensive weekly chemotherapy for advanced gastric cancer using fluorouracil, cisplatin, epi-doxorubicin, 6S-leucovorin, glutathione, and filgrastim: a report from the Italian Group for the Study of Digestive Tract Cancer. *J Clin Oncol* 1997;15(11):3313-9.

5384 Lenzi A, Culasso F, Gandini L, Placebo-controlled, double-blind, cross-over trial of glutathione therapy in male infertility. *Hum Reprod* 1993;8:1657-62.

5385 Coppola L, Grassia A, Giunta R, et al. Glutathione (GSH) improved haemostatic and haemorheological parameters in atherosclerotic subjects. *Drugs Exp Clin Res* 1992;18(11-12):493-8.

5386 Powers SK, Hamilton K. Antioxidants and exercise. *Clin Sports Med* 1999;18(3):525-36.

5387 Anderson ME. Glutathione: an overview of biosynthesis and modulation. *Chem Biol Interact* 1998;24;111-112:1-14.

5388 Lu SC. Regulation of hepatic glutathione synthesis: current concepts and controversies. *FASEB J* 1999;13(10):1169-83.

5389 Amores-Sanchez MI, Medina MA. Glutamine, as a precursor of glutathione, and oxidative stress. *Mol Genet Metab* 1999;67(2):100-5.

5392 Ruffmann R, Wendel A. GSH rescue by N-acetylcysteine. *Klin Wochenschr* 1991;69(18):857-62.

5393 Droge W, Holm E. Role of cysteine and glutathione in HIV infection and other diseases associated with muscle wasting and immunological dysfunction. *FASEB J* 1997;11(13):1077-89.

5394 Herzenberg LA, De Rosa SC, Dubs JG, et al. Glutathione deficiency is associated with impaired survival in HIV disease. *Proc Natl Acad Sci U S A* 1997;94(5):1967-72.

5395 Samiec PS, Drews-Botsch C, Flagg EW, et al. Glutathione in human plasma: decline in association with aging, age-related macular degeneration, and diabetes. *Free Radic Biol Med* 1998;24(5):699-704.

5396 Bains JS, Shaw CA. Neurodegenerative disorders in humans: the role of glutathione in oxidative stress-mediated neuronal death. *Brain Res Brain Res Rev* 1997;25:335-58.

5397 Loguercio C, Di Pierro M. The role of glutathione in the gastrointestinal tract: a review. *Ital J Gastroenterol Hepatol* 1999;31(5):401-7.

5398 Powers SK, Ji LL, Leeuwenburgh C. Exercise training-induced alterations in skeletal muscle antioxidant capacity: a brief review. *Med Sci Sports Exerc* 1999;31(7):987-97.

5429 Gylling H, Miettinen TA. Cholesterol reduction by different plant stanol mixtures and with variable fat intake. *Metabolism* 1999;48:575-80.

5430 Gylling H, Puska P, Vartiainen E, et al. Serum sterols during stanol ester feeding in a mildly hypercholesterolemic population. *J Lipid Res* 1999;40(4):593-600.

5431 Gylling H, Radhakrishnan R, Miettinen TA. Reduction of serum cholesterol in postmenopausal women with previous myocardial infarction and cholesterol malabsorption induced by dietary sitostanol ester margarine: women and dietary sitostanol. *Circulation* 1997;96:4226-31.

5432 Gylling H, Miettinen TA. Serum cholesterol and cholesterol and lipoprotein metabolism in hypercholesterolaemic NIDDM patients before and during sitostanol ester-margarine treatment. *Diabetologia* 1994;37(8):773-80.

5433 Gylling H, Miettinen TA. Effects of inhibiting cholesterol absorption and synthesis on cholesterol and lipoprotein metabolism in hypercholesterolemic non-insulin-dependent diabetic men. *J Lipid Res* 1996;37(8):1776-85.

5434 Gylling H, Puska P, Vartiainen E, et al. Retinol, vitamin D, carotenes and alpha-tocopherol in serum of a moderately hypercholesterolemic population consuming sitostanol ester margarine. *Am J Cardiol* 1999;145(2):279-85.

5435 Hallikainen MA, Uusitupa MI. Effects of 2 low-fat stanol ester-containing margarines on serum cholesterol concentrations as part of a low-fat diet in hypercholesterolemic subjects. *Am J Clin Nutr* 1999;69(3):403-10.

5436 Heinemann T, Kullak-Ublick GA, Pietruck B, et al. Mechanisms of action of plant sterols on inhibition of cholesterol absorption. Comparison of sitosterol and sitostanol. *Eur J Clin Pharmacol* 1991;40 Suppl 1:S59-63.

5437 Jones PJ, Ntanios FY, Raeini-Sarjaz M, et al. Cholesterol-lowering efficacy of a sitostanol-containing phytosterol mixture with a prudent diet in hyperlipidemic men. *Am J Clin Nutr* 1999;69(6):1144-50.

5438 Gylling H, Siimes MA, Miettinen TA. Sitostanol ester margarine in dietary treatment of children with familial hypercholesterolemia. *J Lipid Res* 1995;36(8):1807-12.

5439 Miettinen TA, Puska P, Gylling H, et al. Reduction of serum cholesterol with sitostanol-ester margarine in a mildly hypercholesterolemic population. *N Engl J Med* 1995;333(20):1308-12.

5440 Lutjohann D, von Bergmann K. Phytosterolaemia: diagnosis, characterization and therapeutical approaches. *Ann Med* 1997;29(3):181-4.

5441 Vanhanen HT, Kajander J, Lehtovirta H. Serum levels, absorption efficiency, faecal elimination and synthesis of cholesterol during increasing doses of dietary sitostanol esters in hypercholesterolaemic subjects. *Clin Sci* (Colch) 1994;87(1):61-7.

5443 Cholesterol-lowering margarines. *Medical Letter* 1999;41:56-8.

5444 Cowley G, Underwood A. *Newsweek*. July 5, 1999; pp. 46-50.

5446 Czap A. Beware the son of SAMe. *Altern Med Rev* 1999;4:73.

5447 Whyte RI, Schork MA, Sloan H, et al. Adjuvant treatment using transfer factor for bronchogenic carcinoma: long-term follow-up. *Ann Thorac Surg* 1992;53:391-6.

5448 Powell-Tuck J, Jamieson CP, Bettany GE, et al. A double blind, randomised, controlled trial of glutamine supplementation in parenteral nutrition. *Gut* 1999;45:82-8.

5449 Houdijk AP, Rijnsburger ER, Jansen J, et al. Randomised trial of glutamine-enriched enteral nutrition on infectious morbidity in patients with multiple trauma. *Lancet* 1998;352:772-6.

5450 Jones C, Palmer TE, Griffiths RD. Randomized clinical outcome study of critically ill patients given glutamine-supplemented enteral nutrition. *Nutrition* 1999;15:108-15.

5451 Schloerb PR, Skikne BS. Oral and parenteral glutamine in bone marrow transplantation: a randomized, double-blind study. *JPEN J Parenter Enteral Nutr* 1999;23:117-22.

5452 Brown SA, Goringe A, Fegan C, et al. Parenteral glutamine protects hepatic function during bone marrow transplantation. *Bone Marrow Transplant* 1998;22:281-4.

5453 Ziegler TR, Bye RL, Persinger RL, et al. Effects of glutamine supplementation on circulating lymphocytes after bone marrow transplantation: a pilot study. *Am J Med Sci* 1998;315:4-10.

5454 Wilmore DW, Schloerb PR, Ziegler TR. Glutamine in the support of patients following bone marrow transplantation. *Curr Opin Clin Nutr Metab Care* 1999;2:323-7.

5455 Rohde T, Asp S, MacLean DA, et al. Competitive sustained exercise in humans, lymphokine activated killer cell activity, and glutamine--an intervention study. *Eur J Appl Physiol* 1998;78:448-53.

5456 Rohde T, MacLean DA, Pedersen BK. Effect of glutamine supplementation on changes in the immune system induced by repeated exercise. *Med Sci Sports Exerc* 1998;30:856-62.

5457 Bowtell JL, Gelly K, Jackman ML, et al. Effect of oral glutamine on whole body carbohydrate storage during recovery from exhaustive exercise. *J Appl Physiol* 1999;86(6):1770-7.

5458 Decker-Baumann C, Buhl K, Frohmuller S, et al. Reduction of chemotherapy-induced side-effects by parenteral glutamine supplementation in patients with metastatic colorectal cancer. *Eur J Cancer* 1999;35:202-7.

5460 Niihara Y, Zerez CR, Akiyama DS, et al. Oral L-glutamine therapy for sickle cell anemia: I. Subjective clinical improvement and favorable change in red cell NAD redox potential. *Am J Hematol* 1998;58(2):117-21.

5461 Noyer CM, Simon D, Borczuk A, et al. A double-blind placebo-controlled pilot study of glutamine therapy for abnormal intestinal permeability in patients with AIDS. *Am J Gastroenterol* 1998;93:972-5.

5462 Okuno SH, Woodhouse CO, Loprinzi CL, et al. Phase III controlled evaluation of glutamine for decreasing stomatitis in patients receiving fluorouracil (5-FU)-based chemotherapy. *Am J Clin Oncol* 1999;22:258-61.

5464 Castell LM, Newsholme EA. Glutamine and the effects of exhaustive exercise upon the immune response. *Can J Physiol Pharmacol* 1998;76:524-32.

5465 Antonio J, Street C. Glutamine: a potentially useful supplement for athletes. *Can J Appl Physiol* 1999;24:1-14.

5466 Walsh NP, Blannin AK, Robson PJ, et al. Glutamine, exercise and immune function. Links and possible mechanisms. *Sports Med* 1998;26:177-91.

5467 Griffiths RD. Glutamine: establishing clinical indications. *Curr Opin Clin Nutr Metab Care* 1999;2:177-82.

5468 Sacks GS. Glutamine supplementation in catabolic patients. *Ann Pharmacother* 1999;33:348-54.

5469 Miller AL. Therapeutic considerations of L-glutamine: a review of the literature. *Altern Med Rev* 1999;4:239-48.

5470 Amores-Sanchez MI, Medina MA. Glutamine, as a precursor of glutathione, and oxidative stress. *Mol Genet Metab* 1999;67:100-5.

5473 Reishi. Mothernature encyclopedia. www.mothernature.com/ency/herb/reishi.asp. (Accessed 7 November 1999).

5476 Tao J, Feng KY. Experimental and clinical studies on inhibitory effect of ganoderma lucidum on platelet aggregation. *J Tongji Med Univ* 1990;10(4):240-3.

5477 Wasser SP, Weis AL. Therapeutic effects of substances occurring in higher Basidiomycetes mushrooms: a modern perspective. *Crit Rev Immunol* 1999;19:65-96.

5478 Gau JP, Lin CK, Lee SS, et al. The lack of antiplatelet effect of crude extracts from ganoderma lucidum on HIV-positive hemophiliacs. *Am J Chin Med* 1990;18:175-9.

5479 Singh AB, Gupta SK, Pereira BM, et al. Sensitization to Ganoderma lucidum in patients with respiratory allergy in India. *Clin Exp Allergy* 1995;25:440-7.

5480 Min BS, Nakamura N, Miyashiro H, et al. Triterpenes from the spores of Ganoderma lucidum and their inhibitory activity against HIV-1 protease. *Chem Pharm Bull* (Tokyo) 1998;46:1607-12.

5481 el-Mekkawy S, Meselhy MR, Nakamura N, et al. Anti-HIV-1 and anti-HIV-1-protease substances from Ganoderma lucidum. *Phytochem* 1998;49:1651-7.

5482 Kim RS, Kim HW, Kim BK. Suppressive effects of Ganoderma lucidum on proliferation of peripheral blood mononuclear cells. *Mol Cells* 1997;7:52-7.

5483 Wang SY, Hsu ML, Hsu HC, et al. The anti-tumor effect of Ganoderma lucidum is mediated by cytokines released from activated macrophages and T lymphocytes. *Int J Cancer* 1997;70:699-705.

5484 Kim HS, Kacew S, Lee BM. In vitro chemopreventive effects of plant polysaccharides (Aloe barbadensis miller, Lentinus edodes, Ganoderma lucidum and Coriolus versicolor). *Carcinogenesis* 1999;20:1637-40.

5485 Hijikata Y, Yamada S. Effect of Ganoderma lucidum on postherpetic neuralgia. *Am J Chin Med* 1998;26:375-81.

5486 Komoda Y, Shimizu M, Sonoda Y, et al. Ganoderic acid and its derivatives as cholesterol synthesis inhibitors. *Chem Pharm Bull* (Tokyo) 1989;37:531-3.

5487 Hikino H, Ishiyama M, Suzuki Y, et al. Mechanisms of hypoglycemic activity of ganoderan B: a glycan of Ganoderma lucidum fruit bodies. *Planta Med* 1989;55:423-8.

5488 Lee SY, Rhee HM. Cardiovascular effects of mycelium extract of Ganoderma lucidum: inhibition of sympathetic outflow as a mechanism of its hypotensive action. *Chem Pharm Bull* (Tokyo) 1990;38:1359-64.

5489 Kim DH, Shim SB, Kim NJ, et al. Beta-glucuronidase-inhibitory activity and hepatoprotective effect of Ganoderma lucidum. *Biol Pharm Bull* 1999;22:162-4.

5490 Yoon SY, Eo SK, Kim YS, et al. Antimicrobial activity of Ganoderma lucidum extract alone and in combination with some antibiotics. *Arch Pharm Res* 1994;17:438-42.

5491 Chen K, Li C. Recent advances in studies on traditional Chinese anti-aging materia medica. *J Tradit Chin Med* 1993;13:223-6.

5492 van der Hem LG, van der Vliet JA, Bocken CF, et al. Ling Zhi-8: studies of a new immunomodulating agent. *Transplantation* 1995;60:438-43.

5494 Wang HX, Ng TB, Liu WK, et al. Polysaccharide-peptide complexes from the cultured mycelia of the mushroom Coriolus versicolor and their culture medium activate mouse lymphocytes and macrophages. *Int J Biochem Cell Biol* 1996;28:601-7.

5500 Alander M, Satokari R, Korpela R, et al. Persistence of colonization of human colonic mucosa by a probiotic strain, Lactobacillus rhamnosus GG, after oral consumption. *Appl Environ Microbiol* 1999;65:351-4.

5501 Bensky D, Gamble A, Kaptchuk T. Chinese Herbal Medicine Materia Medica. Seattle, WA: Eastland Press. 1996;483-5.

5502 Huang KC. The pharmacology of Chinese herbs. 2nd ed. Boca Raton, LA: CRC Press LLC. 1999;266-7.

5503 Kim HS, Lim HK, Park WK. Antinarcotic effects of the velvet antler water extract on morphine in mice. *J Ethnopharmacol* 1999;66:41-9.

5504 Goldsmith LA. The velvet case. *Arch Dermatol* 1988;124:768.

5505 Anon. Human clinical trials show significant results for New Zealand deer antler velvet's effect on sports performance. www.prnewswire.com (Accessed 7 March 2000).

5518 Ko KM, Yip TT, Tsao SW, et al. Epidermal growth factor from deer (Cervus elaphus) submaxillary gland and velvet antler. *Gen Comp Endocrinol* 1986;3(3):431-40.

5524 Department of Health and Human Services. 21 CFR Part 310.548 Drug products containing colloidal silver ingredients. *Federal Register*: August 17, 1999. Available

at: http://frwebgate2.access.gpo.gov/cgi-bin. waisgate.cgi?WAIS.
5525 Fung MC, Bowen DL. Silver products for medical indications: risk-benefit assessment. *J Toxicol Clin Toxicol* 1996;34:119-26.
5526 Fung MC, Weintraub M, Bowen DL. Colloidal silver proteins marketed as health supplements. *JAMA* 1995;274:1196-7.
5531 Daly JM, Lieberman MD, Goldfine J, et al. Enteral nutrition with supplemental arginine, RNA, and omega-3 fatty acids in patients after operation: immunologic, metabolic and clinical outcome. *Surgery* 1992;112:56-67.
5532 Senkal M, Kemen M, Homann HH, et al. Modulation of postoperative immune response by enteral nutrition with a diet enriched with arginine, RNA, and omega-3 fatty acids in patients with upper gastrointestinal cancer. *Eur J Surg* 1995;161:115-22.
5533 Kemen M, Senkal M, Homann HH, et al. Early postoperative enteral nutrition with arginine-omega-3 fatty acids and ribonucleic acid-supplemented diet vs placebo in cancer patients: an immunologic evaluation of impact. *Crit Care Med* 1995;23:652-9.
5534 Gianotti L, Braga M, Fortis C, et al. A prospective, randomized clinical trial on perioperative feeding with an arginine, omega-3-fatty acid, and RNA-enriched enteral diet: effect on host response and nutritional status. *Journal of Parenteral and Enteral Nutrition* 1999;23(6):314-20.
5535 Saffle JR, Wiebke G, Jennings K, et al. Randomized trial of immune-enhancing enteral nutrition in burn patients. *J Trauma* 1997;42(5):793-802.
5536 Bower RH, Cerra FB, Bershadsky B, et al. Early enteral administration of a formula (Impact) supplemented with arginine, nucleotides, and fish oil in intensive care unit patients: results of a multicenter, prospective, randomized clinical trial. *Crit Care Med* 1995;23(3):436-49.
5538 Li L. Erythematous skin reaction to subcutaneous injection of ribonucleic acid. *Contact Dermatitis* 1999;41:239.
5539 Schubert R, Hohlweg U, Renz D, Doefler W. On the fate of orally ingested foreign DNA in mice: chromosomal association and placental transmission o the fetus. *Mol Gen Genet* 1998;259:569-76.
5541 Huang KC. The pharmacology of Chinese herbs. 2nd ed. New York, NY: CRC Press LLC. 1999;385-6, 400-1.
5543 Van Buren CT, Rudolph F. Dietary nucleotides: a conditional requirement. *Nutr* 1997;13:470-2.
5544 Bensky D, Gamble A, Kaptchuk T. Chinese Herbal Medicine Materia Medica. Seattle, WA: Eastland Press 1996:107-8.
5545 Huang KC. The Pharmacology of Chinese Herbs. 2nd ed. New York: CRC Press LLC. 1999:113-114, 417.
5546 Chen SH, Yen YP, Chen XS. Effect of jiantangkang on blood glucose, sensitivity of insulin, and blood viscosity in non-insulin dependent diabetes mellitus. *Chung Kuo Chung His I Chieh Ho Tsa Chih* 1997;17:666-8.
5547 Wang HK, Xia Y, Yang ZY, et al. Recent advances in the discovery and development of flavonoids and their analogues as antitumor and anti-HIV agents. *Adv Exp Med Biol* 1998;439:191-225.
5548 DiPaola RS, Zhang H, Lambert GH, et al. Clinical and biologic activity of an estrogenic herbal combination (PC-SPES) in prostate cancer. *N Engl J Med* 1998;339:785-91.
5549 Smol'ianinov ES, Gol'dberg VE, Matiash MG, et al. Effect of Scutellaria baicalensis extract on the immunologic status of patients with lung cancer receiving antineoplastic chemotherapy. *Eksp Klin Farmakol* 1997;60(6):49-51.
5550 Gol'dberg VE, Ryzhakov VM, Matiash MG, et al. Dry extract of Scutellaria baicalensis as a hemostimulant in antineoplastic chemotherapy in patients with lung cancer. *Eksp Klin Farmakol* 1997;60(6):28-30.
5551 Zhang H, Huang J. Preliminary study of traditional Chinese medicine treatment of minimal brain dysfunction: analysis of 100 cases. *Chung Hsi I Chieh Ho Tsa Chih* 1990;10:278-9, 260.
5552 Kuno Y, Kawabe Y, Sakakibara S. Allergic contact dermatitis associated with photosensitivity, from alantolactone in a chrysanthemum farmer. *Contact Dermatitis* 1999;40:224-5.
5553 Paulsen E, Sogaard J, Andersen KE. Occupational dermatitis in Danish gardeners and greenhouse workers (III). Compositae-related symptoms. *Contact Dermatitis* 1998;38:140-6.
5554 deJong NW, Vermeulen AM, van Wijik RG, deGroot H. Occupational allergy caused by flowers. *Allergy* 1998;53:204-9.
5555 Yu XY. [A prospective clinical study on reversion of 200 precancerous patients with hua-sheng-ping]. [Article in Chinese]. *Chung Kuo Chung His I Chieh Ho Tsa Chih* 1993;13:147-9.
5556 Camplimi P, Sertoli A, Fabbri P, Panconesi E. Alantolactone sensitivity in chrysanthemum contract dermatitis. *Contact Dermatitis* 1978;4(2):93-102.
5557 Bleumink E, Mitchell JC, Geismann TA, Towers GH. Contact hypersensitivity to sesquiterpene lactones in Chrysanthemum dermatitis. *Contact Dermatitis* 1976;2(2):81-8.
5558 Huang KC. The Pharmacology of Chinese Herbs. 2nd ed. New York: CRC Press LLC. 1999:101-102.
5559 Bensky D, Gamble A, Kaptchuk T. Chinese Herbal Medicine Materia Medica. Seattle, WA: Eastland Press, 1996:359-60.
5598 Wangen TE, Duncan AM, Merz-Demlow BE, et al. Effects of soy isoflavones on markers of bone turnover in premenopausal and postmenopausal women. *J Clin Endocrinol Metab* 2000;85:3043-8.
5599 Lutz M, Bonilla S, Concha J, et al. Effect of dietary oils, cholesterol and antioxidant vitamin supplementation on liver microsomal fluidity and xenobiotic-metabolizing enzymes in rats. *Annals of Nutr and Metabolism* 1998;42(6):350-9.
5600 Farber JM, Carter AO, Varughese PV, et al. Listeriosis traced to the consumption of alfalfa tablets and soft cheese. [Letter to the Editor] *N Engl J Med* 1990;322:338.
5601 Sullivan JB Jr, Rumack BH, Thomas H Jr, et al. Pennyroyal oil poisoning and hepatotoxicity. *JAMA* 1979;242:2873-4.
5602 Anon. Toxic hypoglycemic syndrome - Jamaica, 1989-91. *MMWR Morb Mortal Wkly Rep* 1992;41:53-5.
5603 Sinn LE, Porterfield JF. Fatal taxine poisoning from yew leaf ingestion. *J Forensic Sci* 1991;36(2):599-601.
5604 Van IG, Visser R, Peltenburg H, et al. Sudden unexpected death due to Taxus poisoning. A report of five cases, with review of the literature. *Forensic Sci Int* 1992;56(1):81-7.
5605 Krenzelok EP, Jacobsen TD, Aronis J. Is the yew really poisonous to you? *J Toxicol Clin Toxicol* 1998;36(3):219-23.
5606 Fox DW, Hart MC, Bergeson PS, et al. Pyrrolizidine (Senecio) intoxication mimicking Reye syndrome. *J Pediatr* 1978;93:980-2.
5607 Sullivan G, Chavez PI. Mexican good-luck charm potentially dangerous. *Vet Hum Toxicol* 1981;23:259-60.
5608 Niyogi SK. Deadly crab's eye: Abrus precatorius poisoning. *N Engl J Med* 1969;281(1):51-2.
5609 Sherratt HS, Turnbull DM. Methylene blue and fatal encephalopathy from ackee fruit poisoning. *Lancet* 1999;353(9164):1623-4.
5610 Lebo DB, Ditto AM, Boxer MB, et al. Anaphylaxis to ackee fruit. *J Allergy Clin Immunol* 1996;98(5Pt1):997-8.
5611 Challoner KR, McCarron MM. Castor bean intoxication. *Ann Emerg Med* 1990;19:1177-83.

5612 Palatnick W, Tenenbein M. Hepatotoxicity from castor bean ingestion in a child. *J Toxicol Clin Toxicol* 2000;38(1):67-9.

5613 Aplin PJ, Eliseo T. Ingestion of castor oil plant seeds. *Med J Aust* 1997;167(5);260-1.

5614 McGee J, Patrick RS, Wood CB, Blumgart LH. A case of veno-occlusive disease of the liver in Britain associated with herbal tea consumption. *J Clin Pathol* 1976;29:788-94.

5617 Cassidy DE, Drewry J, Fanning JP. Podophyllum toxicity: a report of a fatal case and a review of the literature. *J Toxicol Clin Toxicol* 1982;19:35-44.

5618 Rosenstein G, Rosenstein H, Freeman M, Weston N. Podophyllum-a dangerous laxative. *Pediatrics* 1976;57:419-21.

5619 Cohle SD, Trestrail JD III, Graham MA, et al. Fatal pepper aspiration. *Am J Dis Child* 1988;142(6):633-6.

5620 Sheahan K, Page DV, Kemper T, Suarez R. Childhood sudden death secondary to accidental aspiration of black pepper. *Am J Forensic Med Pathol* 1988;9(1):51-3.

5621 Anon. Plant Poisonings - New Jersey. *MMWR Morb Mortal Wkly Rep* 1981;30:65-7.

5622 Urich RW, Bowerman DL, Levisky JA, Pflug JL. Datura stramonium: a fatal poisoning. *J Forensic Sci* 1982;27:948-54.

5623 Anon. Jimson weed poisoning- Texas, New York, and California, 1994. *MMWR Morb Mortal Wkly Rep* 1995;44(3):41-4.

5624 McHenry LE, Hall RC. Angel's trumpet. Lethal and psychogenic aspects. *J Fla Med Assoc* 1978;65(3):192-6.

5625 Hall RC, Popkin MK, Mchenry LE. Angel's Trumpet psychosis: a central nervous system anticholinergic syndrome. *Am J Psychiatry* 1977;134(3):312-4.

5626 Greene GS, Patterson SG, Warner E. Ingestion of angel's trumpet: an increasingly common source of toxicity. *South Med J* 1996;89(4):365-9.

5627 Francis PD, Clarke CF. Angel trumpet lily poisoning in five adolescents: clinical findings and management. *J Paediatr Child Health* 1999;35:93-5.

5628 Anon. FDA Import Alert #53-03, 1991. Availble at: http://www.fda.gov/ora/fiars/ora_import_ia5303.html

5629 Pine, D. Cool tips for a hot season. FDA/CFSAN Cosmetics 1992. Available at: http://vm.cfsan.fda.gov/~dms/cos-815.html

5631 Jackson R. Quick suntan pills in Canada. *J Am Acad Dermatol* 1981;4(2):233.

5632 Lober CW. Canthaxanthin- the "tanning" pill. *J Am Acad Dermatol* 1985;13:660.

5633 Anon. A suntan in capsules - orobronze. *Drug Ther Bull* 1983;21:57.

5634 Rock GA, Decary F, Cole RS. Orange plasma from tanning capsules. *Lancet* 1981;1(8235):1419-20.

5635 Bluhm R, Branch R, Johnston P, Stein R. Aplastic anemia associated with canthaxanthin ingested for 'tanning' purposes. *JAMA* 1990;264(9):1141-2.

5636 Harnois C, Samson J, Malenfant M, Rousseau A. Canthaxanthin retinopathy. Anatomic and funtional reversibility. *Arch Ophthalmol* 1989;107(4):538-40.

5637 Herbert V. Canthaxanthin toxicity. *Am J Clin Nutr* 1991;53(2):573-4.

5638 White GL Jr, Beesley R, Thiese SM, Murdock RT. Retinal crystals and oral tanning agents. *Am Fam Physician* 1988;37(3):125-6.

5639 Chang TS, Aylward W, Clarkson JG, Gass JD. Asymmetric canthaxanthin retinopathy. *Am J Ophthalmol* 1995;119(6):801-2.

5640 Leyon H, Ros AM, Nyberg S, Algvere P. Reversibility of canthaxanthin deposits within the retina. *Acta Ophthalmol* (Copenh) 1990;68(5):607-11.

5641 Espaillat A, Aiello LP, Arrigg PG, et al. Canthaxanthine retinopathy. *Arch Ophtahalmol* 1999;117:412-3.

5642 Anon. Permitted colouring agents for use in medicinal products - E 161 Canthaxanthine. Health and Consumer Protection - The European Commission 1998. Available at: http://europa.eu.int/comm/food/index_en.htm

5643 Durant J, Chantre P, Gonzalez G, et al. Efficacy and safety of Buxus sempervirens L. preparations (SPV30) in HIV-infected asymptomatic patients: a multicentre, randomized, double-blind, placebo-controlled trial. *Phytomedicine* 1998;5:1-10.

5644 Anon. Porphyria information for patients and their families. University of Cape Town / Medical Research Council - Liver Research Center 2000. Available at: http://web.uct.ac.za/depts/porphyria/

5646 Clarke R. Prevention of vitamin B-12 deficiency in old age. *Am J Clin Nutr*. 2001;73:151-152.

5647 Vainio H, Rautalahti M. An international evaluation of the cancer preventive potential of carotenoids. *Cancer Epidemiol Biomarkers Prev* 1998;7(8):725-8.

5648 Huang DS, Odeleye OE, Watson RR. Inhibitory effects of canthaxanthin on in vitro growth of murine tumor cells. *Cancer Lett* 1992;65(3):209-13.

5649 Stahl W, Sies H. The role of carotenoids and retinoids in gap junctional communication. *Int J Vitam Nutr Res* 1998;68:354-9.

5650 Segal S, Foley J. The metabolism of D-ribose in man. *J Clin Invest* 1958;37:719-35.

5651 Foker JE, Einzig S, Wang T. Adenosine metabolism and myocardial preservation. Consequences of adenosine catabolism on myocardial high-energy compounds and tissue blood flow. *J Thorac Cardiovasc Surg* 1980;80:506-16.

5652 Pasque MK, Spray TL, Pellom GL, et al. Ribose-enhanced myocardial recovery following ischemia in the isolated working rat heart. *J Thorac Cardiovasc Surg* 1982;83:390-8.

5653 Pasque MK, Wechsler AS. Metabolic intervention to affect myocardial recovery following ischemia. *Ann Surg* 1984;200(1):1-12.

5654 Ward HB, St Cyr JA, Cogordan JA. Recovery of adenine nucleotide levels after global myocardial ischemia in dogs. *Surgery* 1984;96(2):248-55.

5655 Compston JE, Horton LW. Oral 25-hydroxyvitamin D3 in treatment of osteomalacia associated with ileal resection and cholestyramine therapy. *Gastroenterol* 1978;74:900-2.

5656 Stathis CG, Febbraio MA, Carey MF, et al. Influence of sprint training on human skeletal muscle purine nucleotide metabolism. *J Appl Physiol* 1994;76(4):1802-9.

5657 Tullson PC, Bangsbo J, Hellsten Y, et al. IMP metabolism in human skeletal after exhaustive exercise. *J Appl Physiol* 1995;78(1):146-52.

5658 Hellsten-Westing Y, Norman B, Balsom PD, et al. Decreased resting levels of adenine nucleotides in human skeletal muscle after high-intensity training. *J Appl Physiol* 1993;74:2523-8.

5659 Chatham JC, John Challiss RA, Radda GK, et al. Studies of the protective effect of ribose in myocardial ischaemia by using P31-nuclear-magnetic-resonance spectroscopy. *Biochem Soc Trans* 1985;13:885-6.

5660 St Cyr JA, Bianco RW, Schneider JR, et al. Enhanced high energy phosphate recovery with ribose infusion after global myocardial ischemia in a canine model. *J Surg Res* 1989;46:157-62.

5662 Perlmutter NS, Wilson RA, Angello DA, et al. Ribose facilitates thallium-201 redistribution in patients with coronary artery disease. *J Nucl Med* 1991;32:193-200.

5663 Hegewald MG, Palac RT, Angello DA, et al. Ribose infusion accelerates thallium redistribution with early imaging compared with late 24-hour imaging without ribose. *J Am Coll Cardiol* 1991;18:1671-81.

5664 Pliml W, von Arnim T, Stalein A, et al. Effects of ribose on excercise-induced ischaemia in stable coronary artery disease. *Lancet* 1992;340:507-10.

5665 Geisbuhler TP, Schwager TL. Ribose-enhanced synthesis of UTP, CTP, and GTP from parent nucleosides in cardiac myocytes. *J Mol Cell Cardiol* 1998;30:879-87.

5666 Muller C, Zimmer HG, Gross M, et al. Effect of ribose on cardiac adenine nucleotides in a donor model for heart transplantation. *Eur J Med Res* 1998;3:554-8.

5667 Burke ER. D-Ribose What You Need To Know. Garden City Park, NY: Avery Publishing Group 1999;1-43.

5676 Gross M, Reiter S, Zollner N. Metabolism of D-ribose administered continuously to healthy persons and to patients with myoadenylate deaminase deficiency. *Klin Wochenschr* 1989;67:1205-13.

5677 Zollner N, Reiter S, Gross M, et al. Myoadenylate deaminase deficiency: successful symptomatic therapy by high dose oral administration of ribose. *Klin Wochenschr* 1986;64:1281-90.

5678 Steele IC, Patterson VH, Nicholls DP. A double blind, placebo controlled, crossover trial of D-ribose in McArdle's disease. *J Neurol Sci* 1996;136:174-7.

5679 Wagner DR, Gresser U, Zollner N. Effects of oral ribose on muscle metabolism during bicycle ergometer in AMPD-deficient patients. *Ann Nutr Metab* 1991;35:297-302.

5680 Wagner DR, Felbel J, Gresser U, et al. Muscle metabolism and red cell ATP/ADP concentration during bicycle ergometer in patients with AMPdeficiency. *Klin Wochneschr* 1991;69:251-5.

5682 Fox IH, Kelley WN. Phosphoribosylpyrophosphate in man: biochemical and clinical significance. *Ann Intern Med* 1971;74:424-33.

5683 Lan EL, Ugwu SO, Blanchard J, et al. Preformulation studies with melanotan II: a potential skin cancer chemopreventive peptide. *J Pharm Sci* 1994;83:1081-4.

5684 Pinsuwan S, Myrdal PB, Yalkowsky SH. Systemic delivery of melanotan II through the ocular route in rabbits. *J Pharm Sci* 1997;86:396-7.

5685 Dorr RT, Lines R, Levine N, et al. Evaluation of melanotan-II, a superpotent cyclic melanotropic peptide in a pilot phase-I clinical study. *Life Sci* 1996;58:1777-84.

5686 Hadley ME, Hruby VJ, Blanchard J, et al. Discoverdevelopment of novel melanogenic drugs. Melanotan-I and -II. *Pharm Biotechnol* 1998;11:575-95.

5687 Wessells H, Fuciarelli K, Hansen J, et al. Synthetic melanotropic peptide initiates erections in men with psychogenic erectile dysfunction; double-blind, placebo controlled crossover study. *J Urol* 1998;160:389-93.

5688 Wessells H, Gralnek DR, Dorr RT, et al. Erectogenic properties of melanotan II in men with organic erectile dysfunction. 1999. Abstract Info-American Urological Association, Inc.

5691 Wisniowski LA. FDA Import Alert #62-06 1992. Available at: http://www.fda.gov/ora/fiars/ora_import_ia6206.html.

5692 Sant GR, LaRock DR. Standard intravesical therapies for interstial cystitis. *Urol Clin North Am* 1994;21(1):73-83.

5693 Birder LA, Kanai AJ, de Groat WC. DMSO: effect on bladder afferent neurons and nitric oxide release. *J Urol* 1997;158:1989-95.

5694 Sant GR. Intravesical 50% dimethyl sulfoxide (Rimso-50) in treatment of interstitial cystitis. *Urology* 1987;29(4 Suppl):17-21.

5695 Barker SB, Matthews PN, Philip PF, Williams G. Prospective study of intravesical dimethyl sulphoxide in the treatment of chronic inflammatory bladder disease. *Br J Urol* 1987;59(2):142-4.

5696 Fowler JE Jr. Prospective study of intravesical dimthyl sulfoxide in treatment of suspected early interstitial cystitis. *Urology* 1981;18(1):21-6.

5697 Shirley SW, Stewart BH, Mirelman S. Dimethyl sulfoxide in treatment of inflammatory genitourinary disorders. *Urology* 1978;11(3):215-20.

5698 Bertelli G. Prevention and management of extravasation of cytotoxic drugs. *Drug Saf* 1995;12(4):245-55.

5699 Dorr RT. Antidotes to vesicant chemotherapy extravasations. *Blood Rev* 1990;4(1):41-60.

5701 Barber MD, Ross JA, Voss AC, et al. The effect of an oral nutritional supplement enriched with fish oil on weight-loss in patients with pancreatic cancer. *Br J Cancer* 1999;81:80-6.

5702 Goodfellow J, Bellamy MF, Ramsey MW, et al. Dietary supplementation with marine omega-3 fatty acids improve systemic large artery endothelial function in subjects with hypercholesterolemia. *J Am Coll Cardiol* 2000;35:265-70.

5703 Fenton WS, Hibbeln J, Knable M. Essential fatty acids, lipid membrane abnormalities, and the diagnosis and treatment of schizophrenia. *Biol Psychiatry* 2000;47:8-21.

5704 Nordoy A, Bonaa KH, Sandset PM, et al. Effect of omega-3 fatty acids and simvastatin on hemostatic risk factors and postprandial hyperlipemia in patients with combined hyperlipemia. *Arterioscler Thromb Vasc Biol* 2000;20:259-65.

5705 Hsu HC, Lee YT, Chen MF. Effect of n-3 fatty acids on the composition and binding properties of lipoproteins in hypertriglyceridemic patients. *Am J Clin Nutr* 2000;71:28-35.

5706 Roche HM, Gibney MJ. Effect of long-chain n-3 polyunsaturated fatty acids on fasting and postprandial triacylglycerol metabolism. *Am J Clin Nutr* 2000;71:232S-7S.

5707 Nestel PJ. Fish oil and cardiovascular disease: lipids and arterial function. *Am J Clin Nutr* 2000;71:228S-31S.

5708 Stordy BJ. Dark adaptation, motor skills, docosahexaenoic acid, and dyslexia. *Am J Clin Nutr* 2000;71:323S-6S.

5709 Belluzzi A, Boschi S, Brignola C, et al. Polyunsaturated fatty acids and inflammatory bowel disease. *Am J Clin Nutr* 2000;71:339S-42S.

5710 Navarro E, Esteve M, Olive A, et al. Abnormal fatty acid pattern in rheumatoid arthritis. A rationale for treatment with marine and botanical lipids. *J Rheumatol* 2000;27:298-303.

5711 Burgess JR, Stevens L, Zhang W, Peck L. Long-chain polyunsaturated fatty acids in children with attention-deficit hyperactivity disorder. *Am J Clin Nutr* 2000;71:327S-30S.

5713 Su KP, Shen WW, Huang SY. Are omega3 fatty acids beneficial in depression but not mania? *Arch Gen Psychiatry* 2000;57:716-7.

5714 Siegers CP. Cytotoxicity of alkylphenols from Ginkgo biloba. *Phytomedicine* 1999;6:281-3.

5715 Ranchon I, Gorrand JM, Cluzel J, et al. Functional protection of photoreceptors from light-induced damage by dimethylurea and Ginkgo biloba extract. *Invest Ophthalmol Vis Sci* 1999;40:1191-9.

5716 Gardiner P, Wornham W. Recent review of complementary and alternative medicine used by adolescents. *Curr Opin Pediatr* 2000;12:298-302.

5717 Brautigam MR, Blommaert FA, Verleye G, et al. Treatment of age-related memory complaints with Gingko biloba extract: a randomized double blind placebo-controlled study. *Phytomedicine* 1998;5:425-34.

5718 Mix JA, Crews WD Jr. An examination of the efficacy of Ginkgo biloba extract EGb761 on the neuropsychologic functioning of cognitively intact older adults. *J Altern Complement Med* 2000;6:219-29.

REFERENCES

5719 Kudolo GB. The effect of 3-month ingestion of Ginkgo biloba extract on pancreatic beta-cell function in response to glucose loading in normal glucose tolerant individuals. *J Clin Pharmacol* 2000;40:647-54.

5720 van Dongen MC, van Rossum E, Kessels AG, et al. The efficacy of ginkgo for elderly people with dementia and age-associated memory impairment: new results of a randomized clinical trial. *J Am Geriatr Soc* 2000;48:1183-94.

5721 Diamond BJ, Shiflett SC, Reiwel N, et al. Ginkgo biloba extract: mechanisms and clinical indications. *Arch Phys Med Rehabil* 2000;81:668-78.

5723 Marcilhac A, Dakine N, Bourhim N, et al. Effect of chronic administration of Gingko biloba extract or Ginkgolide on the hypothalamic-pituitary-adrenal axis in the rat. *Life Sci* 1998;62:2329-40.

5724 Amri H, Ogwuegbu SO, Boujrad N, et al. In vivo regulation of peripheral-type benzodiazepine and glucocorticoid synthesis by Gingko biloba extract EGb 761 and isolated ginkgolides. *Endocrinology* 1996;137:5707-18.

5728 Heimbach J, Rieth S, Mohamedshah F, et al. Safety assessment of iron EDTA [sodium iron (Fe(3+)) ethylenediaminetetraacetic acid]: summary of toxological fortification and exposure data. *Food Chem Toxicol* 2000;38:99-111.

5729 Schubert J. Chelation in medicine. *Sci Am* 1966;214:40-50.

5730 Zatlin GS, Senaldi EM, Bruckheim AH. Adult lead poisoning. *Am Fam Physician* 1985;32:137-43.

5731 Chisolm JJ Jr. BAL, EDTA, DMSA and DMPS in the treatment of lead poisoning in children. *J Toxicol Clin Toxicol* 1992;30:493-504.

5732 Lin JL, Ho HH, Yu CC. Chelation therapy for patients with elevated body lead burden and progressive renal insufficiency. A randomized, controlled trial. *Ann Intern Med* 1999;130:7-13.

5733 Mortensen ME, Walson PD. Chelation therapy for childhood lead poisoning. The changing scene in the 1990s. *Clin Pediatr* (Phila) 1993;32:284-91.

5734 Mehbod H. Treatment of lead intoxication. Combined use of peritoneal dialysis and edetate calcium disodium. *JAMA* 1967;201:972-4.

5735 Shrand H. Treatment of lead poisoning with intramuscular edathamil calcium-disodium. *Lancet* 1961;1:310-2.

5736 Gordon RA, Roberts G, Amin Z, et al. Aggressive approach in the treatment of acute lead encephalopathy with an extraordinarily high concentration of lead. *Arch Pediatr Adolesc Med* 1998;152:1100-4.

5737 Grier MT, Meyers DG. So much writing, so little science: a review of 37 years literature on edetate sodium chelation therapy. *Ann Pharmacother* 1993;27:1504-9.

5738 Chappell LT, Janson M. EDTA chelation therapy in the treatment of vascular disease. *J Cardiovasc Nurs* 1996;10:78-86.

5739 Kidd PM. Integrative cardiac revitalization: bypass surgery, angioplasty, and chelation. Benefits, risks, and limitations. *Altern Med Rev* 1998;3:4-17.

5740 Ernst E. Chelation therapy for coronary heart disease: An overview of all clinical investigations. *Am Heart J* 2000;140:139-41.

5741 Elihu N, Anandasbapathy S, Frishman WH. Chealtion therapy in cardiovascular disease: ethylenediaminetetraacetic acid, deferoxamine, and dexrazoxane. *J Clin Pharmacol* 1998;38:101-5.

5742 Ernst E. Chelation therapy for peripheral arterial occlusive disease: a systematic review. *Circulation* 1997;96:1031-3.

5743 Chappell LT. EDTA chelation therapy should be more commonly used in the treatment of vascular disease. *Altern Ther Health Med* 1995;1:53-7.

5744 Christensen K, Theilade D. Edta chelation therapy: an ethical problem. *Med Hypothesis* 1999;53:69-70.

5746 Gundling K, Ernst E. Complementary and alternative medicine in cardiovascular disease: what is the evidence it works? *West J Med* 1999;171:191-4.

5747 Soffer A. Chelation therapy for arteriosclerosis. *JAMA* 1975;233:1206-7.

5749 Green S. Chelation therapy: unproven claims and unsound theories. Quackwatch 2000. Available at: http://www.quackwatch.org (Accessed 17 November 2000).

5750 Kitchell JR, Palmon F, Aytan N, Meltzer LE. The treatment of coronary artery disease with disodium EDTA. A reappraisal. *Am J Cardiol* 1963;11:501-6.

5751 Olszewer E, Carter JP. EDTA chelation therapy in chronic degenerative disease. *Med Hypotheses* 1998;27:41-9.

5752 Sloth-Nielsen J, Guldager B, Mouritzen C, et al. Arteriographic findings in EDTA chelation therapy on peripheral arteriosclerosis. *Am J Surg* 1991;162:122-5.

5753 Guldager B, Jelnes R, Jorgensen SJ, et al. EDTA treatment of intermittent claudication--a double-blind, placebo-controlled study. *J Intern Med* 1992;231:261-7.

5754 van Rij AM, Solomon C, Packer SG, Hopkins WG. Chelation therapy for intermittent claudication. A double-blind, randomized, controlled trial. *Circulation* 1994;90:1194-9.

5756 Anon. Questions and Answers about chelation therapy. American Heart Association 2000. Available at: www.americanheart.org. (Accessed 17 November 2000).

5757 Neldner KH, Winkelmann RK, Perry HO. Scleroderma An evaluation of treatment with disodium edetate. *Arch Dermatol* 1962;86:95-9.

5758 Fuleihan FJ, Kurban AK, Abboud RT, et al. An objective evaluation of the treatment of systemic scleroderma with disodium EDTA, pyridoxine and reserpine. *Br J Dermatol* 1968;80:184-9.

5759 Barnett AJ, Coventry DA. Scleroderma. 1. Clinical features, course of illness and response to treatment in 61 cases. *Med J Aust* 1969;1:992-1001.

5760 Keech MK, McCann DS, Boyle AJ, Pinkus H. Effect of ethylenediaminetetra-acetic acid (EDTA) and tetrahyroxyquinone on sclerodermatous skin. Histologic and chemical studies. *J Invest Dermatol* 1966;47:235-46.

5761 Lyon AF, DeGraff AC. Reappraisal of digitalis. X. Treatment of digitalis toxicity. *Am Heart J* 1967;73:835-7.

5762 Surawica B. Use of the chelating agent, EDTA, in digitalis intoxication and cardiac arrhthymias. *Prog Cardiovasc Dis* 1960;2:432-43.

5763 Popovici A, Geschickter CF, Reinovsky A, Rubin M. Experimental control of serum calcium levels in vivo. *Proc Soc Exp Biol Med* 1950;74:415-7.

5764 Taweechaisupapong S, Doyle RJ. Sensitivity of bacterial coaggregation to chelating agents. *FEMS Immunol Med Microbiol* 2000;28:343-6.

5765 Beasley R, Fishwick D, Miles JF, Hendeles L. Preservatives in nebulizer solutions: risks without benefit. *Pharmacother* 1998;18:130-9.

5768 Lamas GA, Ackermann A. Clinical evaluation of chelation therapy: is there any wheat amidst the chaff? *Am Heart J* 2000;140:4-5.

5769 Chappell LT, Wilson J, Ernst E. Chelation therapy for vascular disease. *Circulation* 1999; 99:164-5.

5770 Margolis S. Chelation therapy is ineffective for the treatment of peripheral vascular disease. *Altern Ther Health Med* 1995;1:53-6.

5771 Lacy CF, Armstrong LL, Ingrim NB, et al. Drug Information Handbook. 6th ed. Hudson, OH:Lexi-Comp Inc 1998:439-41.

5772 Ellsworth AJ, Witt DM, Dugdale DC, et al. Medical Drug Reference. Saint Louis, MO: Mosby-Year Book Inc 1998:302-3.

5773 Golan A, Savir H, Bar-Meir S, et al. Band keratopathy due to hyperparathyroidism. *Ophthalmologica* 1975;171:119-22.

5774 Yanoff M, Duker JS. Ophthalmology. Saint Louis, MO: Mosby-Year Book Inc., 1999.

5775 Carey CF, Lee HH, Woeltje KF. The Washington Manual of Medical Therapeutics. Philadelphia, PA: Lippincott-Raven Publishers, 1998.

5784 Melchoir J, Spasov AA, Ostrovskij OV, et al. Double-blind, placebo-controlled pilot and phase III study of activity of standardized Andrographis paniculata Herba Nees extract fixed combination (Kan Jang) in the treatment of uncomplicated upper-respiratory tract infection. *Phytomedicine* 2000;7:341-50.

5786 Davidson MH, Dugan LD, Burns JH, et al. The hypocholesterolemic effects of beta-glucan in oatmeal and oat bran. *JAMA* 1991;265(14):1833-9.

5787 Ripsen CM, Keenan JM, Jacobs DR, et al. Oat products and lipid lowering. A meta-analysis. *JAMA* 1992;267:3317-25.

5788 Brown L, Rosner B, Willett WW, et al. Cholesterol-lowering effects of dietary fiber: a meta-analysis. *Am J Clin Nutr* 1999;69:30-42.

5789 Lia A, Hallmans G, Sandberg AS, et al. Oat beta-glucan increases bile acid excretion and a fiber-rich barley fraction increases cholesterol excretion in ileostomy subjects. *Am J Clin Nutr* 1995;62:1245-51.

5790 Lovegrove JA, Clohessy A, Milon H, et al. Modest doses of beta-glucan do not reduce concentrations of potentially atherogenic lipoproteins. *Am J Clin Nutr* 2000;72(1):49-55.

5792 Food and Drug Administration. Food labeling: health claims: oats and coronary heart disease. *Fed Regist* 1996;61:296-313.

5794 Van Horn LV, Liu K, Parker D, et al. Serum lipid response to oat product intake with a fat-modified diet. *J Am Diet Assoc* 1986;86:759-64.

5795 Anderson JW, Gilinsky NH, Deakins DA, et al. Lipid responses of hypocholesterolemic men to oat-bran and wheat-bran intake. *Am J Clin Nutr* 54:678-83.

5796 Braaten JT, Wood PJ, Scott FW, et al. Oat beta-glucan reduces blood cholesterol concentration in hypercholesterolemic subjects. *Eur J Clin Nutr* 1994;48:465-74.

5797 Foulke J. FDA Allows Whole Oat Foods To Make Health Claim on Reducing the Risk of Heart Disease. FDA Talk Paper. 1997. Available at: http://www.fda.gov/bbs/topics/ANSWERS/ANS00782.html.

5798 Raskind JY, El-Chaar GM. The role of carnitine supplementation during valproic acid therapy. *Ann Pharmacother* 2000;34:630-8.

5799 Murakami K, Sugimoto T, Woo M, et al. Effect of L-carnitine supplementation on acute valproate intoxication. *Epilepsia* 1996;37:687-9.

5800 Cash CD. Gamma-hydroxybutyrate: an overview of the pros and cons for it being a neurotransmitter and/or a useful therapeutic agent. *Neurosci Biobehav Rev* 1994;18:291-304.

5801 Maitre M. The gamma-hydroxybutyrate signaling system in brain: organization and functional implications. *Prog Neurobiol* 1997;51:337-61.

5802 Feigenbaum JJ, Howard SG. Gamma hydroxybutyrate is not a GABA agonist. *Prog Neurobiol* 1996;50:1-7.

5803 Mamelak M. Gammahydroxybutyrate: an endogenous regulator of energy metabolism. *Neurosci Biobehav Rev* 1989;13:187-98.

5804 Van Cauter E, Plat L, Scharf MB, et al. Simultaneous stimulation of slow-wave sleep and growth hormone secretion by gamma-hydroxybutyrate in normal young Men. *J Clin Invest* 1997;100:745-53.

5805 Cash CD. What is the role of the gamma-hydroxybutyrate receptor? *Med Hypotheses* 1996;47(6):455-9.

5806 Gerra G, Caccavari R, Fontanesi B, et al. Naloxone and metergoline effects on growth hormone response to gamma-hydroxybutyric acid. *Int Clin Psychopharmacol* 1995;10:245-50.

5807 Ferrara SD, Tedeschi L, Frison G, Rossi A. Fatality due to gamma-hydroxybutyric acid (GHB) and heroin intoxication. *J Forensic Sci* 1995;40:501-4.

5808 Holoye PY, Duelge J, Hansen RM, et al. Prophylaxis of Ifosamide toxicity with oral acetylcysteine. *Semin Oncol* 1983;10:66-71.

5809 Compston JE, Thompson RP. Intestinal absorption of 25-hydroxyvitamin D and osteomalacia in primary biliary cirrhosis. *Lancet* 1977;1:721-4.

5810 Ellinwood EH Jr, Gonzalez AE, Dougherty GG Jr. Gamma-Butyrolactone effects on behavior induced by dopamine agonists. *Biol Psychiatry* 1983;18:1023-32.

5811 Dougherty GG, Ellinwood EH Jr. Influence of gamma-butyrolactone on behavior due to dopaminergic drugs. *Physiol Behav* 1983;30:607-12.

5812 Snead OC III, Bearden LJ. Naloxone overcomes the dopaminergic, EEG, and behavioral effects of gamma-hydroxybutyrate. *Neurol* 1980;30:832-8.

5813 Kohrs FP, Porter WH, et al. Gamma-hydroxybutyrate intoxication and overdose. [Letter and responses]. *Ann Emerg Med* 1999;33:475-6.

5814 Law M. Plant sterol and stanol margarines and health. *BMJ* 2000;320:861-4.

5816 Molgaard J, von Schenck H, Olsson AG. Alfalfa seeds lower low density lipoprotein cholesterol and apolipoprotein B concentrations in patients with type II hyperlipoproteinemia. *Atherosclerosis* 1987;65:173-9.

5819 Bolman WM, Richmond JA. A double-blind, placebo-controlled, crossover pilot trial of low dose dimethylglycine in patients with autistic disorder. *J Autism Dev Disord* 1999;29(3):191-4.

5820 Reap EA, Lawson JW. Stimulation of the immune response by dimethylglycine, a nontoxic metabolite. *J Lab Clin Med* 1990;115(4):481-6.

5821 Tonda ME, Hart LL. N,N-dimthylglycine and L-carnitine as performance enhancers in athletes. *Ann Pharmacother* 1992;26:935-7.

5822 Weiss RC. Immunologic responses in healthy random-source cats fed N,N-dimethylglycine-supplemented diets. *Am J Vet Res* 1992;53(5):829-33.

5823 Gascon G, Patterson B, Yearwood K, Slotnick H. N,N-dimethylglycine and epilepsy. *Epilepsia* 1989;30(1):90-3.

5824 Freed WJ. Prevention of strychnine-induced seizures and death by the N-methylated glycine derivatives betaine, dimethylglycine and sarcosine. *Pharmacol Biochem Behav* 1985;22(4):641-3.

5825 Graber CD, Goust JM, Glassman AD, et al. Immunomodulating properties of dimethylglycine in humans. *J Infect Dis* 1981;143(1):101-5.

5826 Roach ES, Carlin L. N,N dimethylglycine for epilepsy [letter]. *N Engl J Med* 1982;307:1081-2.

5827 Herbert V. N,N-dimethylglycine for epilepsy [letter]. *N Engl J Med* 1983;308:527-8.

5828 Freed WJ. N,N-dimethylglycine, betaine and seizures [letter]. *Arch Neurol* 1984;41:1129-30.

5829 Ward TN, Smith EB, Reeves AG. Dimethylglycine and reduction of mortality in penicillin-induced seizures [letter]. *Ann Neurol* 1985;17:213.

REFERENCES

5830 Kendall RV. Comment: N,N-dimethylglycine and L-carnitine as performance enhancers in athletes [letter]. *Ann Pharmacother* 1994;28:973.

5837 Lardy H, Partridge B, Kneer N, Wei Y. Ergosteroids: induction of thermogenic enzymes in liver of rats treated with steroids derived from dehydroepiandrosterone. *Proc Natl Acad Sci U S A* 1995;92:6617-9.

5838 Heaton KW, Lever JV, Barnard RE. Osteomalacia associated with cholestyramine therapy for post-ileectomy diarrhea. *Gastroenterol* 1972;62:642-6.

5839 Shi J, Schulze S, Lardy HA. The effect of 7-oxo-DHEA acetate on memory in young and old C57BL/6 mice. *Steroids* 2000;65:124-9.

5840 Davidson MH, Weeks C, Lardy H, et al. Clinical Safety and Endocrine Effects of 7-KETO-DHEA. Abstract presented at: Experimental Biology 98, April 19-22, 1998, San Francisco, CA. Abstract obtained from Humanetics Corporation website.

5841 Nelson R, Herron M, Weeks C, Lardy H. Dehydroepiandrosterone and 7-KETO-DHEA augment Interleukin 2 (IL2) Production by Human Lymphocytes In Vitro. Abstract presented at: The 5th Conference on Retroviruses and Opportunistic Infections, February 1-5, 1998, Chicago, IL. Abstract obtained from Humanetics Corporation.

5842 Colker CM, Torina GC, Swain MA, Kalman DS. Double-Blind Study Evaluating the Effects of Exercise Plus 3-Acetyl-7-oxo-dehydroepiandrosterone on Body Composition and the Endocrine System in Overweight Adults. Abstract presented at 2nd ASEP Annual Meeting, October 14-16, 1999, and published in *Journal of Exercise Physiology* online, Volume 2 Number 4 October 1999.

5847 Ng TP, Tan WC, Lee YK. Occupational asthma in a pharmacist induced by chlorella, a unicellular algae preparation. Resp Med 1994;88:555-7.

5848 Ruama AL, Torronen R, Hanninen O, Mykkanen H. Vitamin B12 status of long-term adherents of a strict uncooked vegan diet ("living food diet") is compromised. *J Nutr* 1995;125:2511-5.

5849 Davis DR. Some algae are potentially adequate sources of vitamin B-12 for vegans (letter, comment). *J Nutr* 1997;127:378,380.

5850 Morimoto T, Nagatsu A, Murakami N, et al. Anti-tumor-promoting glyceroglycolipids from the green alga, Chlorella vulgaris. *Phytochemistry* 1995;40:1433-7.

5851 Tyml R. Present state and possibilities of the medical use of chlorococcal algae. *Acta Univ Palacki Olomuc Fac Med* 1982;103:273-9.

5852 Jitsukawa K, Suizu R, Hidano A. Chlorella photosensitization. New phytophotodermatosis. *Int J Dermatol* 1984;23:263-8.

5853 Nelson AM, Neafie RC. Protothecosis. In: Strickland GT. Hunter's Tropical Medicine and Emerging Infectious Disease. 8th edition. WB Saunders Co., Philadelphia, PA. 2000:547.

5854 Lissoni P, Barni S, Cazzaniga M, et al. Efficacy of the concomitant administration of the pineal hormone melatonin in cancer immunotherapy with low-dose IL-2 in patients with advanced solid tumors who had progressed on Il-2 alone. *Oncology* 1994;51:344-7.

5855 Lissoni P, Barni S, Tancini G, et al. A randomised study with subcutaneous low-dose interleukin 2 alone vs. interleukin 2 plus the pineal neurohormone melatonin in advanced solid neoplasms other than renal cancer and melanoma. *Br J Cancer* 1994;69:196-9.

5856 Bubis M, Zisapel N. Modulation by melatonin of protein secretion from melanoma cells: is cAMP involved? *Molecular and Cellular Endocrinology* 1995;112:169-73.

5857 Lissoni P, Paolorossi F, Tancini G, et al. A phase II study of tamoxifen plus melatonin in metastatic solid tumour patients. *Br J Cancer* 1996;74:1466-8.

5862 Xiong H, Li Y, Slavik MF, Walker JT. Spraying chicken skin with selected chemicals to reduce attached Salmonella typhimurium. *J Food Prot* 1998;61:272-5.

5863 Sakamoto S, Sato K, Maitani T, Yamada T. [Analysis of components in natural food additive "grapefruit seed extract" by HPLC and LC/MS]. [Article in Japanese]. *Eisei Shikenjo Hokoku* 1996;(114):38-42.

5864 Calori-Domingues MA, Fonseca H. Laboratory evaluation of chemical control of aflatoxin production in unshelled peanuts (Arachis hypogaea L.). *Food Addit Contam* 1995;12(3):347-50.

5865 Ranzani MR, Fonseca H. Mycological evaluation of chemically-treated unshelled peanuts. *Food Addit Contam* 1995;12(3):343-6.

5866 Ionescu G, Kiehl F, Wichmann-Kunz F, et al. Oral citrus seed extract in atopic eczema: in vitro and in vivo studies on intestinal microflora. *J Orthomolec Med* 1990;5(3):155-7.

5867 Von Woedtke T, Schluter B, Pflegel P, et al. Aspects of the antimicrobial efficacy of grapefruit seed extract and its relation to preservative substances contained. *Pharmazie* 1999;54(6):452-6.

5868 Reiter WJ, Pycha A, Schatzl G, et al. Serum dehydroepiandrosterone sulfate concentrations in men with erectile dysfunction. *Urology* 2000;55:755-8.

5869 Hayashi T, Teiji Esaki T, Emiko Muto E, et al. Dehydroepiandrosterone retards atherosclerosis formation through its conversion to estrogen: the possible role of nitric oxide. *Arterioscler Thromb Vasc Biol* 2000;20:782-92.

5870 Kline MD, Jaggers ED. Mania onset while using dehydroepiandrosterone (letter). *Am J Psychiatry* 1999;156:971.

5871 Moriyama Y, Yasue H, Yoshimura M, et al. The plasma levels of dehydroepiandrosterone sulfate are decreased in patients with chronic heart failure in proportion to the severity. *J Clin Endocrinol Metab* 2000;85:1834-40.

5872 Barry NN, McGuire JL, van Vollenhoven RF. Dehydroepiandrosterone in systemic lupus erythematosus: relationship between dosage, serum levels, and clinical response. *J Rheumatol* 1998;25:2352-6.

5873 Mainous AG, Hueston WJ, Connor MK. Serum vitamin C levels and use of health care resources for wheezing episodes. *Arch Fam Med* 2000;9:241-5.

5874 Moffat SD, Zonderman AB, Harman M, et al. The relationship between longitudinal declines in dehydroepiandrosterone sulfate concentrations and cognitive performance in older men. *Arch Intern Med* 2000;160:2193-8.

5875 Lykkesfeldt J, Christen S, Wallock LM, et al. Ascorbate is depleted by smoking and replaced by moderate supplementation: a study in male smokers and nonsmokers with matched dietary antioxidant intakes. *Am J Clin Nutr* 2000;71:530-6.

5876 Riemersma RA, Carruthers KF, Elton RA, Fox KA. Vitamin C and the risk of acute myocardial infarction. *Am J Clin Nutr* 2000;71:1181-6.

5877 Simon JA, Hudes ES. Serum ascorbic acid and gallbladder disease prevalence among US adults. *Arch Intern Med* 2000;160:931-6.

5878 Loria CM, Klag MJ, Caulfield LE, Whelton PK. Vitamin C status and mortality in US adults. *Am J Clin Nutr* 2000;72:139-45.

5879 Sherman DL, Keaney JF, Biegelsen ES, et al. Pharmacological concentrations of ascorbic acid are required for the beneficial effect on endothelial vasomotor function in hypertension. *Hypertension* 2000;35:936-41.

5880 Daels-Rakotoarison DA, Seidel V, Gressier B, et al. Neurosedative and antioxidant activities of phenylpropanoids from Ballota nigra. *Arzneimittelforschung* 2000;50(1):16-23.

5881 McAlindon TE, Jacques P, Zhang Y, et al. Do antioxidant micronutrients protect against the development and progression of knee osteoarthritis? *Arthritis Rheum* 1996;39:648-56.

5882 Blumenthal RD, Lew W, Reising A, et al. Antioxidant vitamins reduce normal tissue toxicity induced by radio-immunotherapy. *Int J Cancer* 2000;86:276-80.

5883 Chan TY. Drug interactions as a cause of overanticoagulation and bleedings in Chinese patients receiving warfarin. *Int J Clin Pharmacol Ther* 1998;36:403-5.

5884 Izzat MB, Yim APC, El-Zufari MH. A taste of Chinese medicine! *Ann Thorac Surg* 1998;66:941-2.

5885 Millqvist E. Cough provocation with capsaicin is an objective way to test sensory hyperreactivity in patients with asthma-like symptoms. *Allergy* 2000;55:546-50.

5886 Sharma A, Gautam S, Jadhav SS. Spice extracts as dose-modifying factors in radiation inactivation of bacteria. *J Agric Food Chem* 2000;48:1340-4.

5887 Galve-Roperh I, Sanchez C, Cortes ML, et al. Anti-tumoral action of cannabinoids: involvement of sustained ceramide accumulation and extracellular signal-regulated kinase activation. *Nat Medicine* 2000;6(3):313-9.

5888 Piomelli D. Pot of gold for glioma therapy. *Nat Medicine* 2000;6(3):255-6.

5889 Baker D, Pryce G, Croxford JL, et al. Cannabinoids control spasticity and tremor in a multiple sclerosis model. *Nature* 2000;404:84-7.

5890 Merchant RE, Carmack CA, Wise CM. Nutritional supplementation with Chlorella pyrenoidosa for patients with fibromyalgia syndrome: a pilot study. *Phytother Res* 2000;14:167-73.

5891 Konishi F, Tanaka K, Himeno K, et al. Antitumor effect induced by a hot water extract of Chlorella vulgaris (CE): resistance to Meth-A tumor growth mediated by CE-induced polymorphonuclear leukocytes. *Cancer Immunol Immunother* 1985;19:73-8.

5892 Miyazawa Y, Murayama T, Ooya N, et al. Immunomodulation by a unicellular green algae (Chlorella pyrenoidosa) in tumor-bearing mice. *J Ethnopharmacol* 1988;24:135-46.

5893 Haggans CJ, Hutchins AM, Olson BA, et al. Effect of flaxseed consumption on urinary estrogen metabolites in postmenopausal women. *Nutr Cancer* 1999;33:188-95.

5894 Nesbitt PD, Lam Y, Thompson LU. Human metabolism of mammalian lignan precursors in raw and processed flaxseed. *Am J Clin Nutr* 1999;69:549-55.

5895 Sung MK, Lautens M, Thompson LU. Mammalian lignans inhibit the growth of estrogen-independent human colon tumor cells. *Anticancer Res* 1998;18:1405-8.

5896 Nestel PJ, Pomeroy SE, Sasahara T, et al. Arterial compliance in obese subjects is improved with dietary plant n-3 fatty acid from flaxseed oil despite increased LDL oxidizability. *Arterioscler Thromb Vasc Biol* 1997;17(6):1163-70.

5897 Thompson LU, Rickard SE, Cheung F, et al. Variability in anticancer lignan levels in flaxseed. *Nutr Cancer* 1997;27:26-30.

5898 Nordstrom DC, Honkanen VE, Nasu Y, et al. Alpha-linolenic acid in the treatment of rheumatoid arthritis. A double-blind, placebo-controlled and randomized study: flaxseed vs. safflower seed. *Rheumatol Int* 1995;14:231-4.

5899 Cunnane SC, Ganguli S, Menard C, et al. High alpha-linolenic acid flaxseed (Linum usitatissimum): some nutritional properties in humans. *Br J Nutr* 1993;69:443-53.

5900 Rudolph FB, Van Buren CT. The metabolic effects of enterally administered ribonucleic acids. *Curr Opin Clin Nutr Metab Care* 1998;1:527-30.

5902 Kenny FS, Pinder SE, Ellis IO, et al. Gamma linolenic acid with tamoxifen as primary therapy in breast cancer. *Int J Cancer* 2000;85:643-8.

5910 Duke J. The Green Pharmacy. Emmaus: Rodale Press, 1997

5911 Lhotta K, Hofle G, Gasser R, Finkenstedt G. Hypokalemia, hyperreninemia, and osteoporosis in a patient ingesting large amounts of cider vinegar. *Nephron* 1998;80:242-3.

5912 Nutrition Search. Nutrition Almanac, Revised Edition. New York: McGraw-Hill Book Company. 1979.

5913 Burton TM. In trials, potion of herbs slows prostate cancer. *Wall Street Journal* May 17, 2000, p.B-1.

5914 Coutinho EM. Gossypol: a contraceptive for men. *Contraception* 2002;65:259-63.

5915 Coyle T, Levante S, Shetler M, Winfield J. In vitro and in vivo cytotoxicity of gossypol against central nervous system tumor cell lines. *J Neurooncol* 1994;19:25-35.

5916 Jacobson ED, Faloon WW. Malasorptive effects of neomycin in commonly used doses. *JAMA* 1961;175:187-90.

5919 Matsui MS, Rozovski SJ. Drug-nutrient interaction. *Clin Ther* 1982;4:423-40.

5921 Ehrenfeld M, Levy M, Sharon P, et al. Gastrointestinal effects of long-term colchicine therapy in patients with recurrent polyserositis (Familial Mediterranean Fever). *Dig Dis Sci* 1982;27:723-7.

5922 Seddon JM, Ajani UA, Sperduto R, et al. Dietary carotenoids, vitamins A, C, and E, and advanced age-related macular degeneration. *JAMA* 1994;272:1413-20.

5923 Lopez A, Sims DE, Ablett RF, et al. Effect of emu oil on auricular inflammation with croton oil in mice. *Am J Vet Res* 1999;60:1558-61.

5924 Pariza M, Park Y, Cook ME. Conjugated linoleic acid and the control of cancer and obesity. *Toxicol Sci* 1999;52:107-10.

5925 Jiang J, Wolk A, Vessby B. Relation between the intake of milk fat and the occurrence of conjugated linoleic acid in human adipose tissue. *Am J Clin Nutr* 1999;70:21-7.

5926 O'Shea M, Stanton C, Devery R. Antioxidant enzyme defense responses of human MCF-7 and SW480 cancer cells to conjugated linoleic acid. *Anticancer Res* 1999;19:1953-60.

5927 Cesano Al, Visonneau S, Scimeca JA, et al. Opposite effects of linoleic acid and conjugated linoleic acid on human prostatic cancer in SCID mice. *Anticancer Res* 1998;18:1429-34.

5928 West DB, Delany JP, Camet PM, et al. Effects of conjugated linoleic acid on body fat and energy metabolism in the mouse. *Am J Physiol* 1998;275:R667-72.

5929 DeLany JP, Blohm F, Truett AA, et al. Conjugated linoleic acid rapidly reduced body fat content in mice without affecting energy intake. *Am J Physiol* (Regulatory Integrative Comp Physiol) 1999;276:45:R1172-9.

5930 Clement I, Banni S, Andioni E, et al. Conjugated linoleic acid-enriched butter fat alters mammary gland morphogenesis and reduces cancer risk in rats. *J Nutr* 1999;129:2135-42.

5931 Banni S, Angioni E, Casu V, et al. An increase in vitamin A status by the feeding of conjugated linoleic acid. *Nutr Cancer* 1999;33:53-7.

5932 Kelly ML, Berry JR, Dwyer DA, et al. Dietary fatty acid sources affect conjugated linoleic acid concentrations in milk from lactating dairy cows. *J Nutr* 128:881-5.

5933 Herbel BK, McGuire MK, McGuire MA, Shultz TD. Safflower oil consumption does not increase plasma

REFERENCES

REFERENCES

conjugated linoleic acid concentrations in humans. *Am J Clin Nutr* 1998;67:332-7.

5934 Sebedio JL, Gnaedig S, Chardigny JM. Recent advances in conjugated linoleic acid research. *Curr Opin Clin Nutr Metab Care* 1999;2:499-506.

5935 Scimeca JA. Toxicological evaluation of dietary conjugated linoleic acid in male Fischer 344 rats. *Food Chem Toxicol* 1998;36(5);391-5.

5936 McCarty MF. Toward a wholly nutritional therapy for type 2 diabetes. *Med Hypotheses* 2000;54(3):483-7.

5937 Izumi T, Piskula MK, Osawa S, et al. Soy isoflavone aglycones are absorbed faster and in higher amounts than their glucosides in humans. *J Nutr* 2000;130:1695-9.

5939 Murkies A, Dalais FS, Briganti EM, et al. Phytoestrogens and breast cancer in postmenopausal women: a case control study. *Menopause* 2000;7:289-96.

5940 Shalita AR, Smith JG, Parish LC, et al. Topical nicotinamide compared with clindamycin gel in the treatment of inflammatory acne vulgaris. *Int J Dermatol* 1995;34:434-7.

5941 Birch EE, Garfield S, Hoffman DR, et al. A randomized controlled trial of early dietary supply of long-chain polyunsaturated fatty acids and mental development in term infants. *Dev Med Child Neurol* 2000;42:174-81.

5942 Berges RR, Windeler J, Trampisch HJ, et al. Randomized, placebo-controlled, double-blind clinical trial of beta-sitosterol in patients with benign prostatic hyperplasia. *Lancet* 1995;345:1529-32.

5944 Fleming T, ed. PDR for Herbal Medicines, 2nd ed. Montvale: Medical Economics 2000.

5954 Bwititi P, Musabayane CT, Nhachi CF. Effects of Opuntia megacantha on blood glucose and kidney function in streptozotocin diabetic rats. *J Ethnopharmacol* 2000;69:247-52.

5955 Trejo-Gonzalez A, Gabriel-Ortiz G, Puebla-Perez A, et al. A purified extract from prickly pear cactus (Opuntia fuliginosa) controls experimentally induced diabetes in rats. *J Ethnopharmacol* 1996;55:27-33.

5956 Ahmad A, Davies J, Randall S, Skinner GR. Antiviral properties of extract of Opuntia streptacantha. *Antiviral Res* 1996;30:75-85.

5957 Roman-Ramos R, Flores-Saenz JL, Alarcon-Aguilar FJ. Anti-hyperglycemic effect of some edible plants. *J Ethnopharmacol* 1995;48:25-32.

5958 Fernandez ML, Lin EC, Trejo A, McNamara DJ. Prickly pear (Opuntia sp.) pectin alters hepatic cholesterol metabolism without affecting cholesterol absorption in guinea pigs fed a hypercholesterolemic diet. *J Nutr* 1994;124:817-24.

5959 Frati AC, Xilotl Diaz N, Altamirano P, et al. The effect of two sequential doses of Opuntia streptacantha upon glycemia. *Arch Invest Med* (Mex) 1991;22:333-6.

5960 Frati-Munari AC, Licona-Quesada R, Araiza-Andraca CR, et al. Activity of Opuntia streptocantha in healthy individuals with induced hyperglycemia. *Arch Invest Med* (Mex) 1990;21:99-102.

5961 Frati-Munari AC, Altamirano-Bustamante E, Rodrigues-Barcenas N, et al. Hypoglycemic action of Opuntia streptacantha Lemaire: study using raw extracts. *Arch Invest Med* (Mex) 1989;20:321-5.

5962 Frati-Munari AC, Del Valle-Martinez LM, Ariza-Andraca CR, et al. Hypoglycemic action of different doses of nopol (Opuntia streptacantha) in patients with type II diabetes mellitus. *Arch Invest Med* (Mex) 1989;20:197-201.

5963 Frati Munari AC, Quiroz Lazaro JL, Alramirano Bustamante P, et al. The effect of various doses of nopal (Opuntia streptacantha Lemaire) on the glucose tolerance test in healthy individuals. *Arch Invest Med* (Mex) 1988;19:143-8.

5964 Frati-Munari AC, Gordillo BE, Altamirano P, Ariza CR. Hypoglycemic effect of Opuntia streptacantha Lemaire in NIDDM. *Diabetes Care* 1988;11:63-6.

5968 Meckes-Lozyoa M, Roman-Ramos R. Opuntia streptacantha; a coadjutor in the treatment of diabetes mellitus. *Am J Chin Med* 1986;14:116-8.

5969 Frati-Munari AC, Roca-Vides RA, Lopez-Perez RJ, et al. The glycemic index of some foods common in Mexico. *Gac Med Mex* 1991;127:163-70.

5970 Frati Munari AC, Vera Lastra O, Ariza Andraca CR. Evaluation of nopol capsules in diabetes mellitus. *Gac Med Mex* 1992;128:431-6.

5971 Medical Economic. Physician's Desk Reference. Montvale:Medical Economics, 1999:1289.

5973 McCalla CX. Instantaneous cure of acute frontal cephalalgia. Manufacturer information from High Chemical Company; 1995.

5975 Manufacturer Information. Sarapin. Injection technique in pain control. High Chemical Company. Information not dated.

5979 Spencer H, Kramer L, Norris C, Osis D. Effect of small doses of aluminum-containing antacids on calcium and phosphorus metabolism. *Am J Clin Nutr* 1982;36:32-40.

5991 Asero R. Detection and clinical characterization of patients with oral allergy syndrome caused by stable allergens in Rosaceae and nuts. *Ann Allergy Asthma Immunol* 1999;83:377-83.

5992 Durak I, Kacmaz M, Buyukkocak S, et al. Hazelnut supplementation enhances plasma antioxidant potential and lowers plasma cholesterol levels [letter]. *Clin Chim Acta* 1999;284:113-5.

5993 Caballero T, Pascual C, Garcia-Ara MC, et al. IgE crossreactivity between mugwort pollen (Artemisia vulgaris) and hazelnut (Abellana nux) in sera from patients with sensitivity to both extracts. *Clin Exp Allergy* 1997;27:1203-11.

5994 Pumphrey RS, Wilson PB, Faragher EB, Edwards SR. Specific immunoglobulin E to peanut, hazelnut and brazil nut 731 patients: similar patterns found at all ages. *Clin Exp Allergy* 1999;29:1256-9.

5995 Savage GP, McNeil DL. Chemical composition of hazelnuts (Corylus avellana) grown in New Zealand. *Int J Food Sci Nutr* 1998;49:199-203.

5996 Caballero T, Martin-Esteban M. Association between pollen hypersensitivity and edible vegetable allergy: a review. *J Investig Allergol Clin Immunol* 1998;8:6-16.

5997 Sutherland MF, O'Hehir RE, Czarny D, Suphioglu C. Macadamia nut anaphylaxis: demonstration of specific IgE reactivity and partial cross-reactivity with hazelnut. *J Allergy Clin Immunol* 1999;104:889-90.

5998 Munoz MF, Lopez-Cazana JM, Villas F, et al. Exercise-induced anaphylactic reaction to hazelnut. *Allergy* 1994;49:314-6.

5999 O'Mahony M, Mitchell E, Gilbert RJ, Hutchinson DN, et al. An outbreak of foodborne botulism associated with contaminated hazelnut yoghurt. *Epidemiol Infect* 1990;104:389-95.

6000 King DS, Sharp RL, Vukovich MD, et al. Effect of oral androstenedione on serum testosterone and adaptations to resistance training in young men. A randomized controlled trial. *JAMA* 1999;281:2020-8.

6001 Roche Laboratories, Inc. Package insert for Xenical. April 1999.

6002 Fetrow CW, Avila JR. Professional's Handbook of Complementary & Alternative Medicines. 1st ed. Springhouse, PA: Springhouse Corp., 1999.

6004 Rabinowitz MB, Gonick HC, Levin SR, Davidson MB. Effects of chromium and yeast supplements on carbohydrate and lipid metabolism in diabetic men. *Diabetes Care* 1983;6:319-27.

6006 Mother Nature Products website: www.mothernature.com (Accessed 23 July 1999).

6007 Kehoe WA. Secretin for the treatment of autism. *Pharmacist's Letter/Prescriber's Letter* 1998;14:141212.

6008 Gurley BJ, Gardner SF, Hubbard MA. Content versus label claims in ephedra-containing dietary supplements. *Am J Health Syst Pharm* 2000;57:963-9.

6009 White LM, Gardner SF, Gurley BJ, et al. Pharmacokinetics and Cardiovascular Effects of Ma-Huang (Ephedra sinica) in Normotensive Adults. *J Clin Pharmacol* 1997;37:116-22.

6010 Arlt W, Haas J, Callies F, et al. Biotransformation of oral dehydroepiandrosterone in elderly men: significant increase in circulating estrogens. *J Clin Endocrinol Metab* 1999;84:2170-6.

6011 Barnhart KT, Freeman E, Grisso JA, et al. The effect of dehydroepiandrosterone supplementation to symptomatic perimenopausal women on serum endocrine profiles, lipid parameters, and health-related quality of life. *J Clin Endocrinol Metab* 1999;84:3896-902.

6012 Callies F, Arlt W, Siekmann L, et al. Influence of oral dehydroepiandrosterone (DHEA) on urinary steroid metabolites in males and females. *Steroids* 2000;65:98-102.

6013 Tilvis RS, Kahonen M, Harkonen M. Dehydroepiandrosterone sulfate, diseases and mortality in a general aged population. *Aging* (Milano) 1999;11:30-4.

6014 Mazza E, Maccario M, Ramunni J, et al. Dehydroepiandrosterone sulfate levels in women. Relationships with age, body mass index and insulin levels. *J Endocrinol Invest* 1999;22:681-7.

6015 Rossouw F, Kruger PE, Rossouw J. The effect of creatine monohydrate loading on maximal intermittent exercise and sport-specific strength in well trained power-lifters. *Nutr Res* 2000;20:505-14.

6016 Timby N, Eriksson A. Gamma-Hydroxybutyrate-Associated Deaths. *Am J Med* 2000;108:518.

6017 Connor WE. Harbingers of coronary heart disease: dietary saturated fatty acids and cholesterol. Is chocolate benign because of its stearic acid content? *Am J Clin Nutr* 1999;70:951-2.

6018 Arts IC, Hollman PC, Kromhout D. Chocolate as a source of tea flavonoids (Letter). *Lancet* 1999;354:488.

6019 Bruinsma K, Taren DL. Chocolate: Food or Drug? *J Am Diet Assoc* 1999;99:1249-58.

6020 Mustad VA, Kris-Etherton PM, Derr J, et al. Comparison of the effects of diets rich in stearic acid versus myristic acid and lauric acid on platelet fatty acids and excretion of thromboxane A2 and PGI2 metabolites in healthy young men. *Metabolism* 1993;42:463-9.

6022 Ross GW, Abbott RD, Petrovitch H, et al. Association of coffee and caffeine intake with the risk of parkinson disease. *JAMA* 2000;283:2674-9.

6023 Tobias JD. Caffeine in the treatment of apnea associated with respiratory syncytial virus infection in neonates and infants. *South Med J* 2000;93:297-304.

6024 Watson JM, Jenkins EJ, Hamilton P, et al. Influence of caffeine on the frequency and perception of hypoglycemia in free-living patients with type 1 diabetes. *Diabetes Care* 2000;23:455-9.

6025 Lloyd T, Johnson-Rollings N, Eggli DF, et al. Bone status among postmenopausal women with different habitual caffeine intakes: a longitudinal investigation. *J Am Coll Nutr* 2000;19:256-61.

6026 American Academy of Pediatrics. The transfer of drugs and other chemicals into human milk (RE9403). Available at: www.aap.org/policy/00026.html (Accessed 13 June 2000).

6027 Hu FB, Stampfer MJ, Manson JE, et al. Dietary saturated fats and their food sources in relation to the risk of coronary heart disease in women. *Am J Clin Nutr* 1999;70:1001-8.

6028 Hambrecht R, Hilbrich L, Erbs S, et al. Correction of endothelial dysfunction in chronic heart failure: additional effects of exercise training and oral L-arginine supplementation. *J Am Coll Cardiol* 2000;35:706-13.

6029 Setchell KD, Cassidy A. Dietary isoflavones: biological effects and relevance to human health. *J Nutr* 1999;129:758S-67S.

6030 Lissin LW, Cooke JP. Phytoestrogens and cardiovascular health. *J Am Coll Cardiol* 2000;35:1403-10.

6031 Nemecz G. Green tea. *U.S. Pharmacist* 2000;May:67-70.

6032 Leenen R, Roodenburg AJ, Tijburg LB, et al. A single dose of tea with or without milk increases plasma antioxidant activity in humans. *Eur J Clin Nutr* 2000;54:87-92.

6033 Hodgson JM, Puddey IB, Croft KD, et al. Acute effects of ingestion of black and green tea on lipoprotein oxidation. *Am J Clin Nutr* 2000;71:1103-7.

6034 Hardy ML. Herbs of special interest to women. *J Am Pharm Assoc* 2000;40:234-42.

6036 Belch J, Hill A. Evening primrose oil and borage oil in rheumatologic conditions. *Am J Clin Nutr* 2000;71:352S-6S.

6037 Watson PS, Scalia GM, Galbraith A, et al. Lack of effect of coenzyme Q on left ventricular function in patients with congestive heart failure. *J Am Coll Cardiol* 1999;33:1549-52.

6038 Permanetter B, Rossy W, Klein G, et al. Ubiquinone (coenzyme Q10) in the long-term treatment of idiopathic dilated cardiomyopathy. *Eur Heart J* 1992;13:1528-33.

6039 Vick JA, Shipman WH. Effects of whole bee venom and its fractions (apamin and melittin) of plasma cortisol levels in the dog. *Toxicon* 1972;10:377-80.

6040 Vick JA, Mehlman B, Brooks R, et al. Effect of bee venom and melittin on plasma cortisol in the unanesthetized monkey. *Toxicon* 1972;10:581-6.

6041 Hider RC. Honeybee venom: A rich source of pharmacologically active peptides. *Endeavour* 1988;12(2):60-5.

6042 Subbalakshmi C, Nagaraj R, Sitaram N. Biological activities of C-terminal 15-residue synthetic fragment of melittin: design of an analog with improved antibacterial activity. *FEBS Lett* 1999;448:62-6.

6043 de Jong NW, Vermeulen AM, de Groot H. Allergy to bumblebee venom. III. Immunotherapy follow-up study (safety and efficacy) in patients with occupational bumblebee-venom anaphylaxis. *Allergy* 1999;54:980-4.

6044 Cuende E, Fraguas J, Pena JE, et al. Beekeepers' arthropathy. *J Rheumatol* 1999;26:2684-90.

6045 Caldwell JR. Venoms, copper, and zinc in the treatment of arthritis. *Rheum Dis Clin North Am* 1999;25(4):919-28.

6046 Petroianu G, Liu J, Helfrich U, et al. Phosholipase A2-induced coagulation abnormalities after bee sting. *Am J Emerg Med* 2000;18:22-7.

6047 Langsjoen PH, Langsjoen PH, Folkers K. Long-term efficacy and safety of coenzyme Q10 therapy for idiopathic dilated cardiomyopathy. *Am J Cardiol* 1990;65:521-3.

6048 Heck AM, DeWitt BA, Lukes AL. Potential interactions between alternative therapies and warfarin. *Am J Health Syst Pharm* 2000;57:1221-7.

6049 Forastiere F, Pistelli R, Sestini P, et al. Consumption of fresh fruit rich in vitamin C and wheezing symptoms in children. *Thorax* 2000;55:283-8.

6050 Haderslev KV, Jeppesen PB, Mortensen PB, Staun M. Absorption of calcium and magnesium in patients with intestinal resections treated with medium chain fatty acids. *Gut* 2000;46:819-23.

6051 Rani PU, Naidu MU. Subjective and polysomnographic evaluation of a herbal preparation in insomnia. *Phytomedicine* 1998;5:253-7.

6052 Terjung RL, Clarkson P, Eichner ER, et al. The American College of Sports Medicine Roundtable on the physiological and health effects of oral creatine supplementation. *Med Sci Sports Exerc* 2000;32:706-17.

6053 Rico-Sanz J, Marco MT. Creatine enhances oxygen uptake and performance during alternating intensity exercise. *Med Sci Sports Exerc* 2000;32(2):379-85.

6054 Hatch GE. Asthma, inhaled oxidants, and dietary antioxidants. *Am J Clin Nutr* 1995;61:625S-30S.

6055 Carey IM, Strachan DP, Cook DG. Effects of changes in fresh fruit consumption on ventilatory function in healthy British adults. *Am J Respir Crit Care Med* 1998;158:728-33.

6056 Schwartz J, Weiss ST. Relationship between dietary vitamin C intake and pulmonary function in the First National Health and Nutrition Examination Survey (NHANES I). *Am J Clin Nutr* 1994;59:110-4.

6057 Butland BK, Fehily AM, Elwood PC. Diet, lung function, and lung function decline in a cohort of 2512 middle aged men. *Thorax* 2000;55:102-8.

6058 Troisi RJ, Willett WC, Weiss ST, et al. A prospective study of diet and adult-onset asthma. *Am J Respir Crit Care Med* 1995;151:1401-8.

6059 Griessen M, Ammann P, Selz L, et al. Comparison of the effect of medium-chain and long-chain triacylglycerols on calcium absorption in healthy subjects. *Am J Clin Nutr* 1999:69(6):1237-42.

6060 Wobenzym N media kit. Naturally Vitamins (Marlyn Nutraceuticals, Inc.): Scottsdale, AZ.

6061 Stricker PR. Other ergogenic agents. *Clin Sports Med* 1998;17:283-97.

6062 Keller KL, Fenske NA. Uses of vitamins A, C, and E and related compounds in dermatology: A review. *J Am Acad Dermatol* 1998;39:611-25.

6064 Kligman AM. Topical treatments for photoaged skin. Separating the reality from the hype. *Postgrad Med* 1997;102:115-26.

6065 Katiyar SK, Ahmad N, Mukhtar H. Green Tea and Skin. *Arch Dermatol* 2000;136:989-94.

6066 Caspi O, Greenfield RH, Gurgevich S. Case report in integrative medicine: a 24-year-old male with medically intractable seizures. *Int Med* 1998;1:173-6.

6067 Itil TM, Eralp E, Ahmed I, Kunitz A, et al. The pharmacological effects of ginkgo biloba, a plant extract, on the brain of dementia patients in comparison with tacrine. *Psychopharmacol Bull* 1998;34:391-7.

6068 Mease PJ, Merrill JT, Lahita RG, et al. GL701 (prasterone, dehydroepiandrosterone) improves systemic lupus erythematosus. 2000 American College of Rheumatology Meeting. Philadelphia, PA. October 29-November 2. Abstract 1230.

6069 Mazzanti G, Mascellino MT, Battinelli L, Coluccia D, et al. Antimicrobial investigation of semipurified fractions of Ginkgo biloba leaves. *J Ethnopharmacol* 2000;71:83-8.

6070 Birnbaum J, Charpin D, Vervloet D. Rapid hymenoptera venom immunotherapy: comparative safety of three protocols. *Clin Exp Allergy* 1993;23:226-30.

6071 Bomalaski JS, Ford T, Hudson AP, Clark MA. Phospholipase A2-activating protein induces the synthesis of IL-1 and TNF in human monocytes. *J Immunol* 1995;154:4027-31.

6072 Somerfield SD. Bee venom and arthritis: magic, myth, or medicine? *N Z Med J* 1986;99:281-3.

6073 Nortier JL, Martinez MC, Schmeiser HH, et al. Urothelial carcinoma associated with the use of a Chinese herb (Aristolochia fangchi). *N Engl J Med* 2000;342:1686-92.

6074 Hollister-Stier Laboratories LLC. Instructions and dosing schedule for allergenic extracts hymenoptera venom prodcts. No. 355120-HD1.

6075 Li JT, Yunginger JW. Management of insect sting hypersensitivity. *Mayo Clin Proc* 1992;67(2):188-94.

6076 Golden DB, Kagey-Sobotka A, Lichtenstein LM. Survey of patients after discontinuing venom immunotherapy. *J Allergy Clin Immunol* 2000;105(2 Pt 1):385-90.

6077 Bousquet J, Muller UR, Dreboro S, et al. Immunotherapy with hymenoptera venoms. *Allergy* 1987;42:401-13.

6078 Ewan PW. ABC of allergies. Venom allergy. *BMJ* 1998;316:1365-8.

6079 Anon. Alpha Hydroxy Acids in Cosmetics. July 31, 1997. FDA. www.fda.gov/opacom/backgrounders/alphabg.html.

6080 Kurtzweil P. Alpha-hydroxy acids for skin care: Smooth sailing or rough seas? FDA 1999. www.fda.gov. (Accessed 18 August 2000).

6081 Sullivan RJ, Allen JS, Otto C, et al. Effects of chewing betel nut (Areca catechu) on the symptoms of people with schizophrenia in Palau, Micronesia. *Br J Psychiatry* 2000;177:174-8.

6082 Werbach MR. Nutritional strategies for treating chronic fatigue syndrome. *Altern Med Rev* 2000;5:93-108.

6083 Jacobson W, Saich T, Borysiewicz LK, et al. Serum folate and chronic fatigue syndrome. *Neurol* 1993;43:2645-7.

6084 Borchers AT, Keen CL, Stern JS, Gershwin ME. Inflammation and Native American medicine: the role of botanicals. *Am J Clin Nutr* 2000;72:339-47.

6085 Dietrich R, Paglieroni TG, Wun T, et al. Cocoa inhibits platelet activation and function. *Am J Clin Nutr* 2000;72:30-5.

6086 Darouiche RO, Hull RA. Bacterial interference for prevention of urinary tract infection: an overview. *J Spinal Cord Med* 2000;23:136-40.

6087 Gionchetti P, Rizzello F, Venturi A, et al. Oral bacteriotherapy as maintenance treatment in patients with chronic pouchitis: a double-blind, placebo-controlled trial. *Gastroenterology* 2000;119:305-9.

6088 Reid G, Bruce AW, Cook RL, et al. Effect on urogenital flora of antibiotic therapy for urinary tract infection. *Scand J Infec Dis* 1990;22:43-7.

6089 McGroarty JA. Probiotic use of lactobacilli in the human female urogenital tract. *FEMS Immunol Med Microbiol* 1993;6:251-64.

6090 Velraeds MM, Van der Mei HC, Reid G, et al. Inhibition of initial adhesion of uropathogenic Enterococcus faecalis by biosurfactants from Lactobacillus isolates. *Appl Environ Microbiol* 1996;62:1958-63.

6091 Reid G, Cook RL, Bruce AW. Examination of strains of Lactobacilli for properties that may influence bacterial interference in the urinary tract. *J Urol* 1987;138:330-5.

6092 Chan RCY, Reid G, Irvin RT, et al. Competitive exclusion of uropathogens from human uroepithelial cells by Lactobacillus whole cells and cell wall fragments. *Infect Immun* 1985;47:84-9.

6093 Herthelius M, Gorbach SL, Mollby R, et al. Elimination of vaginal colonization with Escherichia coli by administration of indigenous flora. *Infect Immun* 1989;57:2447-51.

6094 Bruce AW, Reid G. Intravaginal instillation of Lactobacilli for prevention of recurrent urinary tract infections. *Can J Microbiol* 1988;34:339-43.

6095 Reid G, Bruce AW, Taylor M. Influence of three-day antimicrobial therapy and Lactobacillus vaginal suppositories on recurrence of urinary tract infections. *Clin Ther* 1992;14:11-6.

6096 Gupta K, Stapleton AE, Hooton TM, et al. Inverse association of H2O2-producing Lactobacilli and vaginal Escherichia coli colonization in women with recurrent urinary tract infections. *J Infect Dis* 1998;178:446-50.

6097 Mease PJ, Ginzler EM, Gluck OS, et al. Improvement in bone mineral density in steroid-treated SLE patients during treatment with GL701 (prasterone, dehydroepiandrosterone). 2000 American College of Rheumatology Meeting. Philadelphia, PA. October 29-November 2. abstract 835.

6098 van Vollenhoven RF. Dehydroepiandrosterone in systemic lupus erythematosus. *Rheum Dis Clin North Am* 2000;26:349-62.

6099 Roberfroid MB. Prebiotics and probiotics: are they functional foods? *Am J Clin Nutr* 2000;71:1682S-7S.

6101 Jarrar D, Wang P, Cioffi WG, et al. Mechanisms of the salutary effects of dehydroepiandrosterone after trauma-hemorrhage. Direct or indirect effects on cardiac and hepatocellular functions? *Arch Surg* 2000;135:416-23.

6102 Markowitz JS, Carson WH, Jackson CW. Possible dihydroepiandrosterone-induced mania. *Biol Psychiatry* 1999;45:241-2.

6103 Israel RJ, Sonis ST. Topical dehydroascorbic acid (DHA) reduces moderate to severe mucositis in the hamster acute radiation model. 36th Am Soc Clin Oncol Ann Mtg Prog Proceedings/Abstracts: Abstract 2367.

6104 Zavaleta N, Caulfield LE, Garcia T. Changes in iron status during pregnancy in peruvian women receiving prenatal iron and folic acid supplements with or without zinc. *Am J Clin Nutr* 2000;71:956-61.

6105 Gossage C, Deyhim M, Moser-Veillon PB, et al. Effect of beta-carotene supplementation and lactation on carotenoid metabolism and mitogenic T-lymphocyte proliferation. *Am J Clin Nutr* 2000;71(4):950-5.

6106 Thijs C, van Houwelingen A, Poorterman I, et al. Essential fatty acids in breast milk of atopic mothers: comparison with non-atopic mothers, and effect of borage oil supplementation. *Eur J Clin Nutr* 2000;54:234-8.

6107 Agrawal A. Potato peel extract holds potential as antiboitic. Reuters Health May 23, 2000. www.medscape.com (Accessed 23 May 2000).

6110 Mares-Perlman JA, Brady WE, Klein R, et al. Serum antioxidants and age-related macular degeneration in a population-based case-control study. *Arch Ophthalmol* 1995;113:518-23.

6112 Breidenbach T, Hoffmann MW, Becker T, et al. Drug interaction of St John's wort with ciclosporin. *Lancet* May 2000;355:1912.

6114 Miller MJ, Vergnolle N, Wallace JL, et al. Sangre de grado is a potent and unique inhibitor of neurogenic inflammation and promotes healing in experimental necrotizing enterocolitis. Pediatric Academic Soc and Acad Pediatrics Joint Mtg, May 12-6 2000:Abstract 979.

6116 Blumenthal M, Goldberg A, Brinckmann J (eds). Herbal Medicine Expanded Commission E Monographs. Newton,MA;Integrative Medicine Communications, 2000.

6118 Lewis CJ, Alpert S. Letter to health care professionals -- FDA concerned about botanical products, including dietary supplements, containing aristolochic acid. Office of Nutritional Products, Labeling, Dietary Supplements. Center for Food Safety and Applied Nutrition. May 31, 2000.

6122 Abramowicz M, ed. Calcium supplements. *Med Lett* 2000;42:29-31.

6123 Beall DP, Scofield RH. Milk-alkali syndrome associated with calcium carbonate consumption. Report of 7 patients with parathyroid hormone levels and an estimate of prevalence among patients hospitalized with hypercalcemia. *Medicine* (Baltimore) 1995;74:89-96.

6124 Moser LR, Smythe MA, Tisdale JE. The use of calcium salts in the prevention and management of verapamil-induced hypotension. *Ann Pharmacother* 2000;34:622-9.

6126 Holmes-McNary M, Baldwin AS, Jr. Chemopreventive properties of trans-resveratrol are associated with inhibition of activation of the IkappaB kinase. *Cancer Res* 2000;60:3477-83.

6127 Atkinson C, Compston JE, Robins SP, Bingham SA. The effects of isoflavone phytoestrogens on bone; preliminary results from a large randomized, controlled trial. Endocrine Soc 82nd Ann Mtg, Toronto, CAN 2000;Jun 21-4:abstract 196.

6128 Gerber G, Lowe FC, Spigelman S. The use of a standardized extract of red clover isoflavones for the alleviation of BPH symptoms. Endocrine Soc 82nd Ann Mtg, Toronto, CAN 2000;Jun 21-4:abstract 2359.

6129 Mitchell S. Plant modification may enhance public consumption of omega-3 fatty acids. Reuters Health 2000;Jun 8. www.medscape.com/reuters/prof/2000/06/06.08/20000608publ001.html (Accessed 8 June 2000).

6131 Whitehouse MW. Turmeric has anti-inflammatory effects. 9th Asia Pacific League of Associations for Rheumatology Congress, 2001.

6132 Kulkarni PM, Schuman PC, Merlino NS, Kinzie JL. Lactic acidosis and hepatic steatosis in HIV seropositive patients treated with nucleoside analogues. Natl AIDS Treatment Advocacy Project. Dig Disease Week Liver Conf, San Diego,CA. 2000;May 21-4:Rep11.

6133 Roodenburg AJ, Leenen R, van het Hof KH, et al. Amount of fat in the diet affects bioavailability of lutein esters but not of alpha-carotene, beta-carotene, and vitamin E in humans. *Am J Clin Nutr* 2000;71:1187-93.

6134 Stahl W, Heinrich U, Jungmann H, et al. Carotenoids and carotenoids plus vitamin E protect against ultraviolet light-induced erythema in humans. *Am J Clin Nutr* 2000;71:795-8.

6135 Zhu M, Wong PY, Li RC. Effect of oral administration of fennel (Foeniculum vulgare) on ciprofloxacin absorption and disposition in the rat. *J Pharm Pharmacol* 1999;51:1391-6.

6136 Sandler AD, Sutton KA, DeWeese J, et al. Lack of benefit of a single dose of synthetic human secretin in the treatment of autism and pervasive developmental disorder. *N Engl J Med* 1999;341(24):1801-6.

6137 Singh N, Singh PN, Hershman JM. Effect of calcium carbonate on the absorption of levothyroxine. *JAMA* 2000;283:2822-5.

6138 Nusko G, Schneider B, Schneider I, et al. Anthranoid laxative use is not a risk factor for colorectal neoplasia: results of a prospective case control study. *Gut* 2000;46:651-5.

6140 NCAA prohibits schools from supplying creatine to students. Reuters Heath 2000;Jun 13. www.medscape.com/reuters/prof/2000/06/06.13/20000613publ004.html (Accessed 13 June 2000).

6143 Mori TA, Burke V, Puddey IB, et al. Purified eicosapentaenoic and docosahexaenoic acids have differential effects on serum lipids and lipoproteins, LDL particle size, glucose, and insulin in mildly hyperlipidemic men. *Am J Clin Nutr* 2000;71:1085-94.

6144 Lewin PK. Temporary henna tattoo with permanent scarification. *CMAJ* 1999;160:310.

6145 Lestringant GG, Bener A, Frossard PM. Cutaneous reactions to henna and associated additives. *Br J Dermatol* 1999;141:598-600.

6146 Etienne A, Piletta P, Hauser C, Pasche-Koo F. Ectopic contact dermatitis from henna. *Contact Dermatitis* 1997;:183.

6147 Wantke F, Gotz M, Jarisch R. Contact dermatitis due to henna, solvent red 1 and solvent red 3, a case report. *Contact Dermatitis* 1992;27:346-7.

6148 Nigam PK, Saxena AK. Allergic contact dermatitis from henna. *Contact Dermatitis* 1988;18:55-6.

6149 Gupta BN, Mathur AK, Agarwal C, Singh A. Contact sensitivity to henna. *Contact Dermatitis* 1986;15:303-4.

6150 Pasricha JS, Gupta R, Panjwani S. Contact dermatitis to henna (Lawsonia). *Contact Dermatitis* 1980;6:288-9.

6151 Cronin E. Immediate type hypersensitivity to henna. *Contact Dermatitis* 1979;5:198-9.

6152 Katz J, West KP Jr, Khatry SK, et al. Maternal low-dose vitamin A or {beta}-carotene supplementation has no effect on fetal loss and early infant mortality: a randomized, cluster trial in Nepal. *Am J Clin Nutr* 2000;71:1570-6.

6153 West KP Jr, Katz J, Khatry SK, et al. Double-blind cluster, randomised trial of low dose supplementation with vitamin A or beta carotene on mortality related to pregnancy in Nepal. The NNIPS-2 Study Group. *BMJ* 1999;318:570-5.

6154 Christian P, West KP Jr, Khatry SK, et al. Vitamin A or beta-carotene supplementation reduces but does not eliminate maternal night blindness in Nepal. *J Nutr* 1998;128:1458-63.

6155 Traikovich SS. Use of topical ascorbic acid and its effects on photodamaged skin topography. *Arch Otolaryngol Head Neck Surg* 1999;125:1091-8.

6166 Cellex-C product information for professionals. Cellex-C. www.cellex-c.com/pro_side/navigator.html (Accessed 14 June 2000).

6167 Vutyavanich T, Wongtra-ngan S, Ruangsri R. Pyridoxine for nausea and vomiting of pregnancy: a randomized, double-blind, placebo-controlled trial. *Am J Obstet Gynecol* 1995;173:881-4.

6168 Sahakian V, Rouse D, Sipes S, et al. Vitamin B6 is effective therapy for nausea and vomiting of pregnancy: a randomized, double-blind, placebo-controlled study. *Obstet Gynecol* 1991;78:33-6.

6169 Sandler B, Aronson P. Yohimbine-induced cutaneous drug eruption, progressive renal failure, and lupus-like syndrome. *Urol* 1993;41(4):343-5.

6170 Wang ZQ, Zhang XH, Baldor LC, et al. Chromium picolinate enhances insulin sensitivity in an animal model for the metabolic syndrome: the obese, insulin resistant JCR:LA-corpulent rat. Am Diabetes Assn's 60th Sci Sessions & Expo, San Antonio, TX 2000;Jun 9-13: abstract 291.

6171 Nelson L, Rao A, Olson P. Unique hydrolyzed whey protein isolates with antihypertensive activity. Institute of Food Tech 2000 Ann Mtg & Food Expo:abstract 38-6. Available at: ift.confex.com/ift/2000/techprogram/paper_5129.htm

6172 Ajani UA, Hennekens CH, Spelsberg, A, et al. Alcohol consumption and risk of type 2 diabetes mellitus among US male physicians. *Arch Intern Med* 2000;160:1025-30.

6173 Shaper AG, Wannamethee SG. Alcohol intake and mortality in middle aged men with diagnosed coronary heart disease. *Heart* 2000;83:394-9.

6174 Vally H, de Klerk N, Thompson PJ. Alcoholic drinks: important triggers for asthma. *J Allergy Clin Immunol* 2000;105:462-7.

6175 Lanthony P, Cosson JP. [The course of color vision in early diabetic retinopathy treated with ginkgo biloba extract. A preliminary, double-blind versus placebo study]. [Article in French]. *J Fr Ophtalmol* 1988;11:671-4.

6176 Grandjean EM, Berthet P, Ruffmann R, Leuenberger P. Efficacy of oral long-term N-acetylcysteine in chronic bronchopulmonary disease: a meta-analysis of published double-blind, placebo-controlled clinical trials. *Clin Ther* 2000;22:209-21.

6177 Puig L. Pharmacodynamic interaction with phototoxic plants during PUVA therapy. *Br J Dermatol* 1997;136:973-4.

6178 Gral N, Beani JC, Bonnot D, et al. [Plasma levels of psoralens after celery ingestion]. [Article in French]. *Ann Dermatol Venereol* 1993;120:599-603.

6179 Desperate remedies. *New Scientist* 1999;Nov 27:34-6.

6180 Eagon PK, Elm MS, Hunter DS, et al. Medicinal herbs: modulation of estrogen action. Era of Hope Mtg, Dept Defense; Breast Cancer Res Prog, Atlanta, GA 2000;Jun 8-11.

6181 Joss JD, LeBlond RF. Potentiation of warfarin anticoagulation associated with topical methyl salicylate. *Ann Pharmacother* 2000;34(6):729-33.

6182 Walter MC, Lochmuller H, Reilich P, et al. Creatine monohydrate in muscular dystrophies: A double-blind, placebo-controlled clinical study. *Neurology* 2000;54:1848-50.

6183 Gilliam JD, Hohzorn C, Martin D, Trimble MH. Effect of oral creatine supplementation on isokinetic torque production. *Med Sci Sports Exerc* 2000;32:993-6.

6185 Hallikainen MA, Sarkkinen ES, Uusitupa MI. Plant stanol esters affect serum cholesterol concentrations of hypercholesterolemic men and women in a dose-dependent manner. *J Nutr* 2000;130(4):767-76.

6186 Rome LA, Lippmann ML, Dalsey WC, et al. Prevalence of cocaine use and its impact on asthma exacerbation in an urban population. *Chest* 2000;117(5):1324-9.

6187 Potter SM, Zelazo PR, Stack DM, Papageorgiou AN. Adverse effects of fetal cocaine exposure on neonatal auditory information processing. *Pediatrics* 2000;105:E40. Available at: www.pediatrics.org/cgi/content/full/105/3/e40.

6188 Maier SM, Turner ND, Lupton JR. Serum lipids in hypercholesterolemic men and women consuming oat bran and amaranth products. *Cereal Chem* 2000:77(3);297-302.

6190 Gobel H, Fresenius J, Heinze A, et al. [Effectiveness of Oleum menthae piperitae and paracetamol in therapy of headache of the tension type]. [Article in German]. *Nervenarzt* 1996;67:672-81.

6191 Umeta M, West CE, Haidar J, et al. Zinc supplementation and stunted infants in Ethiopia: a randomised controlled trial. *Lancet* 2000;355:2021-6.

6192 Khanna VJ, Shieh S, Benjamin J, et al. Necrolytic acral erythema associated with hepatitis C effective treatment with interferon alfa and zinc. *Arch Dermatol* 2000;136:755-7.

6193 Booth SL, Tucker KL, Chen H, et al. Dietary vitamin K intakes are associated with hip fracture but not with bone mineral density in elderly men and women. *Am J Clin Nutr* 2000;71:1201-8.

6196 Armanini D, De Palo CB, Mattarello MJ, et al. Effect of licorice on reduction of body fat mass in healthy subjects. *J Endocrinol Invest* 2003;26:646-50.

6197 Blanco C, Diaz-Perales A, Collada C, et al. Class I chitinases as potential panallergens involved in the latex-fruit syndrome. *J Allergy Clin Immunol* 1999;103(3 Pt 1):507-13.

6198 Varnell MA. Enhanced herb may help female sexual dysfunction. Reuters Health 2000;Jun 27. www.reutershealth.com/frame/eline.html Accessed 28 June 2000).

6199 Landbo C, Almdal TP. [Interaction between warfarin and coenzyme Q10]. [Article in Danish]. *Ugeskr Laeger* 1998;160:3226-7.

6200 Rey JM, Walter G. Hypericum perforatum (St. John's wort) in depression: pest or blessing? *Med J Aust* 1998;169:583-6.

6201 Brown TM. Acute St. John's wort toxicity. *Am J Emerg Med* 2000;18:231-2.

6203 Bremme K, Eneroth P, Nordstrom L, Nilsson B. Effects of infusion of the beta-adrenoceptor agonist terbutaline on serum magnesium in pregnant women. *Magnesium* 1986;5:85-94.

6204 Kehoe WA. Vitamin E and heart disease. *Pharmacist's Letter/Prescriber's Letter* 2000;16:160307.

6205 Khilnani G, Parchani H, Toshniwal G. Hypomagnesemia due to beta 2-agonist use in bronchial asthma. *J Assoc Physicians India* 1992;40:346.

6206 Szolomicki S, Samochowiec L, Wojcicki J, Drozdzik M. The influence of active components of Eleutherococcus senticosus on cellular defense and physical fitness in man. *Phytother Res* 2000;14:30-5.

6208 Diamond BJ, Shiflett SC, Feiwel N, et al. Ginkgo biloba extract: mechanisms and clinical indications. *Arch Phys Med Rehabil* 2000;81:668-78.

6209 Bos WJ, Postma DS, van Doormaal JJ. Magnesiuric and calciuric effects of terbutaline in man. *Clin Sci* 1988;74:595-7.

6210 Gustafson T, Boman K, Rosenhall L, et al. Skeletal muscle magnesium and potassium in asthmatics treated with oral beta-2-agonists. *Eur Resp J* 1996;9:237-40.

6211 Pittler MH, Ernst E. Ginkgo biloba extract for the treatment of intermittent claudication: a meta-analysis of randomized trials. *Am J Med* 2000,108:276-81.

6212 Li AL, Shi YD, Landsmann B, et al. Hemorheology and walking of peripheral arterial occlusive diseases patients during treatment with Ginkgo biloba extract. *Chung Kuo Yao Li Hsueh Pao* 1998;19:417-21.

6213 Peters H, Kieser M, Holscher U. Demonstration of the efficacy of ginkgo biloba special extract EGb 761 on intermittent claudication - a placebo-controlled, double-blind multicenter trial. *Vasa* 1998;27:106-10.

6214 Rigney U, Kimber S, Hindmarch I. The effects of acute doses of standardized Ginkgo biloba extract on memory and psychomotor performance in volunteers. *Phytother Res* 1999;13:408-15.

6215 Subhan Z, Hindmarch I. The psychopharmacological effects of Ginkgo biloba extract in normal healthy volunteers. *Int J Clin Pharmacol Res* 1984;4:89-93.

6216 Rai GS, Shovlin C, Wesnes KA. A double-blind, placebo-controlled study of Ginkgo biloba extract ('tanakan') in elderly outpatients with mild to moderate memory impairment. *Curr Med Res Opin* 1991;12:350-5.

6217 Lipworth BJ, McDevitt DG. Beta-adrenoceptor responses to inhaled salbutamol in normal subjects. *Eur J Clin Pharmacol* 1989;36:239-45.

6218 Holgers KM, Axelsson A, Pringle I. Ginkgo biloba extract for the treatment of tinnitus. *Audiol* 1994;33:85-92.

6219 Meyer B. [Multicenter, randomized, double-blind drug vs. placebo study of the treatment of tinnitus with Ginkgo biloba extract]. [Article in French]. *Presse Med* 1986;15:1562-4.

6220 Cesarani A, Meloni F, Alpini D, et al. Ginkgo biloba (EGb 761) in the treatment of equilibrium disorders. *Adv Ther* 1998;15:291-304.

6221 Haguenauer JP, Cantenot F, Koskas H, Pierart H. [Treatment of equilibrium disorders with Ginkgo biloba extract. A multicenter, double-blind drug vs. placebo study]. [Article in French]. *Presse Med* 1986;15:1569-72.

6222 Hopfenmuller W. [Evidence for a therapeutic effect of Ginkgo biloba special extract. Meta-analysis of 11 clinical studies in patients with cerebrovascular insufficiency in old age]. [Article in German]. *Arzneimittelforschung* 1994;44:1005-13.

6223 Kleijnen J, Knipschild P. Ginkgo biloba for cerebral insufficiency. *Br J Clin Pharmacol* 1992;34:352-8.

6224 Wettstein A. Cholinesterase inhibitors and Gingko extracts-are they comparable in the treatment of dementia? Comparison of published, placebo-controlled efficacy studies of at least six months duration. *Phytomedicine* 2000;6:393-401.

6225 Kanowski S, Herrmann WM, Stephan K, et al. Proof of efficacy of the ginkgo biloba special extract (EGb 761) in outpatients suffering from mild to moderate primary degenerative dementia of the Alzheimer type or multi-infarct dementia. *Pharmacopsych* 1996;29:47-56.

6226 National Institutes of Health. Clinical trials. www.clinicaltrials.gov/ct/gui/c/r (Accessed 15 June 2000).

6227 Lebuisson DA, Leroy L, Rigal G. [Treatment of senile macular degeneration with Ginkgo biloba extract. A preliminary double-blind drug vs. placebo study]. [Article in French]. *Presse Med* 1986;15:1556-8.

6228 Evans JR. Ginkgo biloba extract for age-related macular degeneration. *Cochrane Database Syst Rev* 2000;CD001775.

6229 Tamborini A, Taurelle R. [Value of standardized Ginkgo biloba extract (EGb 761) in the management of congestive symptoms of premenstrual syndrome]. [Article in French]. *Rev Fr Gynecol Obstet* 1993;88:447-57.

6230 Roncin JP, Schwartz F, D'Arbigny P. Ginkgo biloba (EGb 761) in control of acute mountain sickness and vascular reactivity to cold exposure. *Aviat Space Environ Med* 1996;67:445-52.

6231 Fowler JS, Wang GJ, Volkow ND et al. Evidence that gingko biloba extract does not inhibit MAO A and B in living human brain. *Life Sci* 2000;66:141-6.

6232 Porsolt RD, Roux S, Drieu K. Evaluation of a ginkgo biloba extract (EGb 761) in functional tests for monoamine oxidase inhibition. *Arzneimittelforschung* 2000;50:232-5.

6233 White HL, Scates PW, Cooper BR. Extracts of Ginkgo biloba leaves inhibit monoamine oxidase. *Life Sci* 1996;58:1315-21.

6234 Snowdon DA, Tully CL, Smith CD, et al. Serum folate and the severity of atrophy of the neocortex in Alzheimer disease: findings from the Nun study. *Am J Clin Nutr* 2000;71:993-8.

6235 Chao CL, Chien KL, Lee YT. Effect of short-term vitamin (folic acid, vitamins B6 and B12) administration on endothelial dysfunction induced by post-methionine load hyperhomocysteinemia. *Am J Cardiol* 1999;84:1359-61.

6236 Usui M, Matsuoka H, Miyazaki H, et al. Endothelial dysfunction by acute hyperhomocyst(e)inaemia: restoration by folic acid. *Clin Sci* (Colch) 1999;96:235-9

6237 Nelen WL, Blom HJ, Steegers EA, et al. Homocysteine and folate levels as risk factors for recurrent early pregnancy loss. *Obstet Gynecol* 2000;95:519-24.

6238 Ortega RM, Manas LR, Andres P, et al. Functional and psychic deterioration in elderly people may be aggravated by folate deficiency. *J Nutr* 1996;126:1992-9.

6239 Fava M, Borus JS, Alpert JE, et al. Folate, vitamin B12, and homocysteine in major depressive disorder. *Am J Psychiatry* 1997;154:426-8.

6240 Norton SA, Ruze P. Kava dermopathy. *J Am Acad Dermatol* 1994;31:89-97.

6241 Suitor CW, Bailey LB. Dietary folate equivalents: interpretation and application. *J Am Diet Assoc* 2000;100:88-94.

6242 Suitor CW, Bailey LB. Food folate vs synthetic folic acid: a comparison. *J Am Diet Assoc* 1999;99:285.

6243 Food and Nutrition Board, Institute of Medicine. Dietary Reference Intakes for Thiamin, Riboflavin, Niacin, Vitamin B6, Folate, Vitamin B12, Pantothenic Acid, Biotin, and Choline (2000). Washington, DC: National Academy Press, 2000. Available at: http://books.nap.edu/books/0309065542/html/.

6244 Winther K, Randlov C, Rein E, Mehlsen J. Effects of ginkgo biloba extract on cognitive function and blood pressure in elderly subjects. *Curr Ther Res* 1998;59:881-8.

REFERENCES

6245 Nardini M, De Stefano R, Iannuccelli M, et al. Treatment of depression with L-5-hydroxytryptophan combined with chlorimipramine, a double-blind study. *Int J Clin Pharmacol Res* 1983;3:239-50.

6246 Steinberg S, Annable L, Young SN, Liyanage N. A placebo-controlled study of the effects of L-tryptophan in patients with premenstrual dysphoria. *Adv Exp Med Biol* 1999;467:85-8.

6247 Ghadirian AM, Murphy BE, Gendron MJ. Efficacy of light versus tryptophan therapy in seasonal affective disorder. *J Affect Disord* 1998;50:23-7.

6248 Leathwood PD, Chauffard F, Heck E, Munoz-Box R. Aqueous extract of valerian root (Valeriana officinalis L.) improves sleep quality in man. *Pharmacol Biochem Behav* 1982;17:65-71.

6249 Donath F, Quispe S, Diefenbach K, et al. Critical evaluation of the effect of valerian extract on sleep structure and sleep quality. *Pharmacopsych* 2000;33:47-53.

6250 Bourin M, Bougerol T, Guitton B, Broutin E. A combination of plant extracts in the treatment of outpatients with adjustment disorder with anxious mood: controlled study vs placebo. *Fundam Clin Pharmacol* 1997;11:127-32.

6251 Fisher AA, Purcell P, Le Couteur DG. Toxicity of Passiflora incarnata L. *J Toxicol Clin Toxicol* 2000;38:63-6.

6252 Klein G, Kullich W. Short-term treatment of painful osteoarthritis of the knee with oral enzymes. *Clin Drug Invest* 2000;19:15-23.

6253 Kane S, Goldberg MJ. Use of bromelain for mild ulcerative colitis. *Ann Intern Med* 2000;132:680.

6254 Caso MA, Vargas RR, Salas VA, Begona IC. Double-blind study of a multivitamin complex supplemented with ginseng extract. *Drugs Exp Clin Res* 1996;22:323-9.

6255 Hill AJ, Peikin SR, Ryan CA, Blundell JE. Oral administration of proteinase inhibitor II from potatoes reduces energy intake in man. *Physiol Behav* 1990;48:241-6.

6256 Akobeng AK, Miller V, Stanton J, et al. Double-blind, randomized, controlled trial of glutamine-enriched polymeric diet in the treatment of active Crohn's disease. *J Pediatr Gastroenterol Nutr* 2000;30:78-84.

6257 Belluzzi A, Brignola C, Campieri M, et al. Effect of an enteric-coated fish-oil preparation on relapses in Crohn's disease. *N Engl J Med* 1996;334:1557-60.

6258 Belluzzi A, Brignola C, Campieri M, et al. Effects of new fish oil derivative on fatty acid phospholipid-membrane pattern in a group of Crohn's disease patients. *Dig Dis Sci* 1994;39:2589-94.

6259 Lorenz-Meyer H, Bauer P, Nicolay C, et al. Omega-3 fatty acids and low carbohydrate diet for maintenance of remission in Crohn's disease. A randomized controlled multicenter trial. Study Group Members (German Crohn's Disease Study Group). *Scand J Gastroenterol* 1996;31:778-85.

6260 Smith W, Mitchell P, Leeder SR. Dietary fat and fish intake and age-related maculopathy. *Arch Ophthalmol* 2000;118:401-4.

6261 Anderson JW, Davidson MH, Blonde L, et al. Long-term cholesterol-lowering effects of psyllium as an adjunct to diet therapy in the treatment of hypercholesterolemia. *Am J Clin Nutr* 2000;71:1433-8.

6262 Davidson MH, Maki KC, Kong JC, et al. Long-term effects of consuming foods containing psyllium seed husk on serum lipids in subjects with hypercholesterolemia. *Am J Clin Nutr* 1998;67:367-76.

6263 Olson BH, Anderson SM, Becker MP, et al. Psyllium-enriched cereals lower blood total cholesterol and LDL cholesterol, but not HDL cholesterol, in hypercholesterolemic adults: results of a meta-analysis. *J Nutr* 1997;127:1973-80.

6264 FDA, Ctr Food Safety, Applied Nutr. FDA allows foods containing psyllium to make health claim on reducing risk of heart disease. Available at: http://vm.cfsan.fda.gov/~lrd/tpsylliu.html.

6265 McRorie J, Kesler J, Bishop L, et al. Effects of wheat bran and Olestra on objective measures of stool and subjective reports of GI symptoms. *Am J Gastroenterol* 2000;95:1244-52.

6266 Chandalia M, Garg A, Lutjohann D, et al. Beneficial effects of high dietary fiber intake in patients with type 2 diabetes mellitus. *N Engl J Med* 2000;342:1392-8.

6269 Kuroki F, Iida M, Tominaga M, et al. Multiple vitamin status in Crohn's disease. Correlation with disease activity. *Dig Dis Sci* 1993;38:1614-8.

6270 Lashner BA, Provencher KS, Seidner DL, et al. The effect of folic acid supplementation on the risk for cancer or dysplasia in ulcerative colitis. *Gastroenterology* 1997;112:29-32.

6271 Lashner BA. Red blood cell folate is associated with the development of dysplasia and cancer in ulcerative colitis. *J Cancer Res Clin Oncol* 1993;119:549-54.

6278 Maherzi A, Galan P, Cezard JP, et al. Assessment of iron status in children and adolescents with Crohn's disease: value of basic red cell ferritin. *Ann Nutr Metab* 1996;40:331-5.

6279 Gasche C, Reinisch W, Lochs H, et al. Anemia in Crohn's disease. Importance of inadequate erythropoietin production and iron deficiency. *Dig Dis Sci* 1994;39:1930-4.

6280 Galland L. Magnesium and inflammatory bowel disease. *Magnesium* 1988;7:78-83.

6281 Geerling BJ, Badart-Smook A, Stockbrugger RW, Brummer RJ. Comprehensive nutritional status in patients with long-standing Crohn disease currently in remission. *Am J Clin Nutr* 1998;67:919-26.

6282 Englisch W, Beckers C, Unkauf M, et al. Efficacy of Artichoke dry extract in patients with hyperlipoproteinemia. *Arzneimittelforschung* 2000;50:260-5.

6284 de la Taille A, Hayek OR, Buttyan R, et al. Effects of a phytotherapeutic agent, PC-SPES, on prostate cancer: a preliminary investigation on human cell lines and patients. *BJU Int* 1999;84:845-50.

6285 Kubota T, Hisatake J, Hisatake Y, et al. PC-SPES: a unique inhibitor of proliferation of prostate cancer cells in vitro and in vivo. *Prostate* 2000;42:163-71.

6286 Pfeifer BL, Pirani JF, Hamann SR, Klippel KF. PC-SPES, a dietary supplement for the treatment of hormone-refractory prostate cancer. *BJU Int* 2000;85:481-5.

6287 Porterfield H. Survey of Us Too members and other prostate cancer patients to evaluate the efficacy and safety of PC-SPES. *Mol Urol* 1999;3(3):333-6.

6289 Chan P, Tomlinson B. Antioxidant effects of Chinese traditional medicine: focus on trilinolein isolated from the Chinese herb sanchi. *J Clin Pharmacol* 2000;40:457-61.

6290 Hui KM, Wang XH, Xue H. Interaction of flavones from the roots of Scutellaria baicalensis with the benzodiazepine site. *Planta Med* 2000;66:91-3.

6291 Liao JF, Wang HH, Chen MC, et al. Benzodiazepine binding site-interactive flavones from Scutellaria baicalensis root. *Planta Med* 1998;64:571-2.

6292 Nishioka T, Kawabata J, Aoyama Y. Baicalein, an alpha-glucosidase inhibitor from Scutellaria baicalensis. *J Nat Prod* 1998;61:1413-5.

6293 Gao Z, Huang K, Yang X, Xu H. Free radical scavenging and antioxidant activities of flavonoids extracted from the radix of Scutellaria baicalensis Georgi. *Biochim Biophys Acta* 1999;1472:643-50.

6294 Lee BH, Lee SJ, Kang TH, et al. Baicalein: an in vitro antigenotoxic compound from Scutellaria baicalensis. *Planta Med* 2000;66:70-1.

6295 Blaszczyk T, Krzyzanowska J, Lamer-Zarawska E. Screening for antimycotic properties of 56 traditional Chinese drugs. *Phytother Res* 2000;14:210-2.

6297 Goransson K, Liden S, Odsell L. Oral zinc in acne vulgaris: a clinical and methodological study. *Acta Derm Venereol* 1978;58:443-8.

6298 Hillstrom L, Pettersson L, Hellbe L, et al. Comparison of oral treatment with zinc sulphate and placebo in acne vulgaris. *Br J Dermatol* 1977;97:681-4.

6299 Meynadier J. Efficacy and safety study of two zinc gluconate regimens in the treatment of inflammatory acne. *Eur J Dermatol* 2000 May;10:269-73.

6300 Marshall LF, Camp PE, Bowers SA. Dimethyl sulfoxide for the treatment of intracranial hypertension: a preliminary trial. *Neurosurg* 1984;14(6):659-63.

6301 Karaca M, Bilgin UY, Akar M, de la Torre JC. Dimethyl sulphoxide lowers ICP after head trauma. *Eur J Clin Pharmacol* 1991;40(1):113-4.

6302 de la Torre JC. Role of dimethyl sulfoxide in prostaglandin-thromboxane and platelet systems after cerebral ischemia. *Ann N Y Acad Sci* 1983;411:293-308.

6303 Rosenstein ED. Topical agents in the treatment of rheumatic disorders. *Rheum Dis Clin North Am* 1999;25(4):899-918.

6304 Trice JM, Pinals RS. Dimethyl sulfoxide: a review of its use in the rheumatic disorders. *Semin Arthritis Rheum* 1985;15(1):45-60.

6306 Merlini G. Treatment of primary amyloidosis. *Semin Hematol* 1995;32(1):60-79.

6307 Rand-Luby L, Pommier RF, Williams ST, et al. Improved outcome of surgical flaps treated with topical dimethylsulfoxide. *Ann Surg* 1996;224(4):583-9.

6308 Thiers BH. Unusual treatments for herpesvirus infections II, herpes zoster. *J Am Acad Dermatol* 1983;8(3):433-6.

6309 Burton WJ, Gould PW, Hursthouse MW, et al. A multicentre trial of Zostrum (5 percent idoxuridine in dimethyl sulphoxide) in herpes zoster. *N Z Med J* 1981;94(696):384-6.

6310 MacCallum FO, Juel-Jensen BE. Herpes simplex virus skin infection in man treated with idoxuridine in dimethyl sulphoxide. Results of double-blind controlled trial. *Br Med J* 1966;2:805-7.

6311 Juel-Jensen BE, MacCallum FO, Mackenzie AM, Pike MC. Treatment of zoster with idoxuridine in dimethyl sulphoxide. Results of two double-blind controlled trials. *Br Med J* 1970;4:776-80.

6312 Wildenhoff KE, Esmann V, Ipsen J, et al. Treatment of trigeminal and thoracic zoster with idoxuridine. *Scand J Infect Dis* 1981;13(4):257-62.

6313 Williams HJ, Furst DE, Dahl SL, et al. Double-blind, multicenter controlled trial comparing topical dimethyl sulfoxide and normal saline for treatment of hand ulcers in patients with systemic sclerosis. *Arthritis Rheum* 1985;28:308-14.

6314 Torres MA, Furst DE. Treatment of generalized systemic sclerosis. *Rheum Dis Clin North Am* 1990;16(1):217-41.

6315 Takacs T, Montet JC. In vitro dissolution of cholesterol biliary stones. *Gut* 1995;37(1):157-8.

6317 Kingery WS. A critical review of controlled clinical trials for peripheral neuropathic pain and complex regional pain syndromes. *Pain* 1997;73(2):123-39.

6318 Rowley SD. Hematopoietic stem cell processing and cryopreservation. *J Clin Apheresis* 1992;7(3):132-4.

6320 Zambelli A, Poggi G, Da Prada G, et al. Clinical toxicity of cryopreserved circulation progenitor cells infusion. *Anticancer Res* 1998;18:4705-8.

6321 Salim AS. The relationship between Helicobacter pylori and oxygen-derived free radicals in the mechanism of duodenal ulceration. *Intern Med* 1993;32(5):359-64.

6323 Prior D, Mitchell A, Nebauer M, Smith M. Oncology nurses' experience of dimethyl sulfoxide odor. *Cancer Nurs* 2000;23:134-40.

6324 Rubin LF. Toxicologic update of dimethyl sulfoxide. *Ann N Y Acad Sci* 1983;411:6-10.

6325 Wolf P, Simon M. Dimethyl sulphoxide (DMSO) induced serum hyperosmolality. *Clin Biochem* 1983;16(4):261-2.

6326 Brayton CF. Dimethyl sulfoxide (DMSO): a review. *Cornell Vet* 1986;76(1):61-90.

6327 Spremulli EN, Dexter DL. Polar solvents: a novel class of antineoplastic agents. *J Clin Oncol* 1984;2(3):227-41.

6328 Toren A, Rechavi G. What really cures in autologous bone marrow transplantation? A possible role for dimethylsulfoxide. *Med Hypothesis* 1993;41(6):495-8.

6329 Evans MS, Reid KH, Sharp JB Jr. Dimethylsuloxide (DMSO) blocks conduction in peripheral nerve C fibers: a possible mechanism of analgesia. *Neurosci Lett* 1993;150(2):145-8.

6330 Jacob SW, Herschler R. Pharmacology of DMSO. *Cryobiology* 1986;23:14-27.

6331 Neulieb RL, Neulieb MK. The diverse actions of dimtheyl sulphoxide: an indicator of membrane transport activity. *Cytobios* 1990;63(254-255):139-65.

6332 Fitzgerald P, Moss N, O'Mahony S, Whelton MJ. Accidental hemlock poisoning. *Br Med J* (Clin Res Ed) 1987;295(6613):1657.

6334 Mitchell MI, Routledge PA. Hemlock water dropwort poisoning-a review. *Clin Toxicol* 1978;12(4):417-26.

6335 Ball MJ, Flather ML, Forfar JC. Hemlock water dropwort poisoning. *Postgrad Med J* 1987;63(739):363-5.

6336 Mitchell MI, Routledge PA. Poisoning by hemlock water dropwort [letter]. *Lancet* 1977;1(8008):423-4.

6337 Anger JP, Anger F, Chauvel Y, et al. [Fatal poisoning by water dropwort]. [Article in French]. *Eur J Toxicol Environ Hyg* 1976;9(2):119-25.

6338 Lopez TA, Cid MS, Bianchini ML. Biochemistry of hemlock (Conium maculatum L.) alkaloids and their acute and chronic toxicity in livestock. A review. *Toxicon* 1999;37(6):841-65.

6339 Panter KE, Keeler RF, Baker DC. Toxicosis in livestock from the hemlocks (Conium and Cicuta spp.). *J Anim Sci* 1988;66(9):2407-13.

6340 Drummer OH, Roberts AN, Bedford PJ, et al. Three deaths from hemlock poisoning. *Med J Aust* 1995;162:592-3.

6341 Frank BS, Panter KE. Ingestion of poison hemlock (Conium maculatum). *West J Med* 1995;163:573-4.

6344 Krenzelok EP, Jacobsen TD, Aronis JM. Hemlock ingestions: the most deadly plant exposures. NACCT Abstracts 1996: Abstract #131.

6346 Starreveld E, Hope E. Cicutoxin poisoning (water hemlock). *Neurol* 1975;25(8):730-4.

6347 Costanza DJ, Hoversten VW. Accidental ingestion of water hemlock. Report of two patients with acute and chronic effects. *Calif Med* 1973;119(2):78-82.

6348 Knutsen OH, Paszkowski P. New aspects in the treatment of water hemlock poisoning. *J Toxicol Clin Toxicol* 1984;22(2):157-66.

6349 Anon. Water hemlock poisoning-Maine, 1992. *MMWR Morb Mortal Wkly Rep* 1994;43(13):229-31.

6350 Applefeld JJ, Caplan ES. A case of water hemlock poisoning. *JACEP* 1979;8(10):401-3.

6351 Carlton BE, Tufts E, Girard DE. Water hemlock poisoning complicated by rhabdomyolysis and renal failure. *Clin Toxicol* 1979;14(1):87-92.

6352 Robson P. Water hemlock poisoning. *Lancet* 1965;2(7425):1274-5.

6353 Landers D, Seppi K, Blauer W. Seizures and death on a white river float trip. Report of water hemlock poisoning. *West J Med* 1985;142:637-40.

6354 Mutter L. Poisoning by western water hemlock. *Can J Public Health* 1976;67:386.

6355 Withers LM, Coler FR, Nelson RB. Water-hemlock poisoning. *N Engl J Med* 1969;281:566-7.

6356 Guillemant J, Le HT, Accarie C, et al. Mineral water as a source of dietary calcium: acute effects on parathyroid function and bone resorption in young men. *Am J Clin Nutr* 2000;71:999-1002.

6357 Penninx BW, Guralnik JM, Ferrucci L, et al. Vitamin B(12) deficiency and depression in physically disabled older women: epidemiologic evidence from the Women's Health and Aging Study. *Am J Psychiatry* 2000;157:715-21.

6358 Benito-Leon J, Porta-Etessam J. Shaky-leg syndrome and vitamin B12 deficiency. *N Engl J Med* 2000;342:981.

6359 Prabhala A, Garg R, Dandona P. Severe myopathy associated with vitamin D deficiency in western New York. *Arch Intern Med* 2000;160:1199-203.

6360 Suzuki Y, Oishi Y, Yamazaki H, et al. How to avoid bone loss in patients with prostatic carcinoma receiving long-term LHRH-analogue. 2000 AbstractInfo-Am Urol Assn, Inc.

6362 Minne HW, Pfeifer M, Begerow B, et al. Vitamin D and calcium supplementation reduces falls in elderly women via improvement of body sway and normalization of blood pressure: a prospective, randomized, and double-blind study. Abstracts World Congress on Osteoporosis 2000.

6366 Kauwell GP, Lippert BL, Wilsky CE, et al. Folate status of elderly women following moderate folate depletion responds only to a higher folate intake. *J Nutr* 2000;130:1584-90.

6367 Riddell LJ, Chisholm A, Williams S, Mann JI. Dietary strategies for lowering homocysteine concentrations. *Am J Clin Nutr* 2000;71:1448-54.

6368 Chatelain C, Autet W, Brackman F. Comparison of once and twice daily dosage forms of Pygeum africanum extract in patients with benign prostatic hyperplasia: a randomized, double-blind study, with long-term open label extension. *Urology* 1999;54:473-8.

6369 Niyogi SK. The toxicology of Abrus precatorius linnaeus. *J Forensic Sci* 1970;15:529-36.

6370 Sinclair CJ, Geiger JD. Caffeine use in sports. A pharmacological review. *J Sports Med Phys Fitness* 2000;40:71-9.

6371 Erenberg A, Leff RD, Haack DG, et al. Caffeine citrate for the treatment of apnea of prematurity: a double-blind, placebo-controlled study. *Pharmacother* 2000;20:644-52.

6372 Suleman A, Siddiqui NH. Haemodynamic and cardiovascular effects of caffeine. Medicine On Line Int J Medicine 2000. www.priory.com/pharmol/caffeine.htm (Accessed 14 April 2000).

6373 Bolla KI, Funderburk FR, Cadet JL. Differential effects of cocaine and cocaine alcohol on neurocognitive performance. *Neurology* 2000;54(12):2285-92.

6374 Heesch CM, Wilhelm CR, Ristich J, et al. Cocaine activates platelets and increases the formation of circulating platelet containing microaggregates in humans. *Heart* 2000;83:688-95.

6376 Fawzi WW, Msamanga G, Hunter D, et al. Randomized trial of vitamin supplements in relation to vertical transmission of HIV-1 in Tanzania. *J Acquir Immune Defic Syndr* 2000;23:246-54.

6377 Russell RM. The vitamin A spectrum: from deficiency to toxicity. *Am J Clin Nutr* 2000;71:878-84.

6378 Cumming RG, Mitchell P, Smith W. Diet and cataract: the Blue Mountains Eye Study. *Ophthalmology* 2000;10:450-6.

6379 van Zandwijk N, Dalesio O, Pastorino U, et al. EUROSCAN, a randomized trial of vitamin A and N-acetylcysteine in patients with head and neck cancer or lung cancer. For the European Organization for Research and Treatment of Cancer Head and Neck and Lung Cancer Cooperative Groups. *J Natl Cancer Inst* 2000;92(12):977-86.

6380 Sporn MB. Retinoids and demethylating agents-looking for partners. *J Natl Cancer Inst* 2000;92:780-1.

6381 Widschwendter M, Berger J, Hermann M, et al. Methylation and silencing of the retinoic acid receptor-beta2 gene in breast cancer. *J Natl Cancer Inst* 2000;92:826-32.

6382 Omenn GS, Goodman GE, Thornquist MD, et al. Risk factors for lung cancer and for intervention effects in CARET, the Beta-Carotene and Retinol Efficacy Trial. *J Natl Cancer Inst* 1996;88:1550-9.

6384 Lindenmuth GF, Lindenmuth EB. The efficacy of echinacea compound herbal tea preparation on the severity and duration of upper respiratory and flu symptoms: a randomized, double-blind, placebo-controlled study. *J Altern Complement Med* 2000;6:327-34.

6385 Dorn M, Knick E, Lewith G. Placebo-controlled, double-blind study of Echinaceae pallidae radix in upper respiratory tract infections. *Complement Ther Med* 1997;5:40-2.

6386 Melchart D, Walther E, Linde K, et al. Echinacea root extracts for the prevention of upper respiratory tract infections: a double-blind, placebo-controlled randomized trial. *Arch Fam Med* 1998;7:541-5.

6387 Parnham MJ. Benefit-risk assessment of the squeezed sap of the purple coneflower (Echinacea purpurea) for long-term oral immunostimulation. *Phytomedicine* 1996;3:95-102.

6388 Luettig B, Steinmuller C, Gifford GE, et al. Macrophage activation by the polysaccharide arabinogalactan isolated from plant cell cultures of Echinacea purpurea. *J Natl Cancer Inst* 1989;81:669-75.

6389 Stimpel M, Proksch A, Wagner H, et al. Macrophage activation and induction of macrophage cytotoxicity by purified polysaccharide fractions from the plant Echinacea purpurea. *Infect Immun* 1984;46:845-9.

6390 Binns SE, Purgina B, Bergeron C. Light-mediated antifungal activity of Echinacea extracts. *Plant Med* 2000;66:241-4.

6391 Perry NB, van Klink JW, Burgess EJ, et al. Alkamide levels in Echinacea purpurea: effects of processing, drying and storage. *Planta Med* 2000;66:54-6.

6392 Henneicke-von Zepelin H, Hentschel C, Schnitker J, et al. Efficacy and safety of a fixed combination phytomedicine in the treatment of the common cold (acute viral respiratory tract infection): results of a randomised, double blind, placebo-controlled, multicentre study. *Curr Med Res Opin* 1999;15:214-27.

6393 Pryor WA, Stahl W, Rock CL. Beta carotene: from biochemistry to clinical trials. *Nutr Rev* 2000;58:39-53.

6394 Westphal S, Orth M, Ambrosch A, et al. Postprandial chylomicrons VLDLs in severe hypertriacylglycerolemia are lowered more effectively than are chylomicron remnants after treatment with n-3 fatty acids. *Am J Clin Nutr* 2000;71:914-20.

6395 Norrish AE, Skeaff CM, Arribas GL, et al. Prostate cancer risk and consumption of fish oils: a dietary biomarker-based, case-control study. *Br J Cancer* 1999;81:1238-42.

6396 Kinrys G. Hypomania associated with omega3 fatty acids. *Arch Gen Psychiatry* 2000;57:715-6.

6397 Baxter P, Aicardi J. Neonatal seizures after pyridoxine use. *Lancet* 1999;354:2082-3.

6398 Ogilvie GK, Fettman MJ, Mallinckrodt CH, et al. Effect of fish oil, arginine, and doxorubicin chemotherapy on remission and survival time for dogs with lymphoma: a double-blind, randomized, placebo-controlled study. *Cancer* 2000;88:1916-28.

6399 Stark KD, Park EJ, Maines VA, Holub BJ. Effect of a fish-oil concentrate on serum lipids in postmenopausal women receiving and not receiving hormone replacement therapy in a placebo-controlled, double-blind trial. *Am J Clin Nutr* 2000;72:389-94.

6400 Brenner R, Azbel V, Madhusoodanan S, et al. Comparison of an extract of Hypericum (LI 160) and sertraline in the treatment of depression: A double-blind, randomized pilot study. *Clin Ther* 2000;22:411-9.

6401 Pizzorno JE, Murray MT, eds. Textbook of Natural Medicine. 2nd ed. Edinburgh:Churchill Livingstone, 1999.

6402 Mathews JD, Riley MD, Fejo L, et al. Effects of heavy usage of kava on physical health: Summary of a pilot survey in an aboriginal community. *Med J Aust* 1988;148:548-55.

6403 Imai K. Nakachi K. Cross-sectional study of effects of drinking green tea on cardiovascular and liver diseases. *BMJ* 1995;310:693-6.

6404 Hegarty VM, May HM, Khaw K. Tea drinking and bone mineral density in older women. *Am J Clin Nutr* 2000;71:1003-7.

6405 Iuliano L, Micheletta F, Maranghi M, et al. Bioavailability of vitamin E as function of food intake in healthy subjects: effects on plasma peroxide-scavenging activity and cholesterol-oxidation products. *Arterioscler Thromb Vasc Biol* 2001;21:E34-7.

6406 Pye JK, Mansel RE, Hughes LE. Clinical experience of drug treatments for mastalgia. *Lancet* 1985;2:373-7.

6407 Morisco C, Trimarco B, Condorelli M. Effect of coenzyme Q10 therapy in patients with congestive heart failure: A long-term, multicenter, randomized study. *Clin Investig* 1993;71:S134-6.

6408 Hofman-Bang C, Rehnqvist N, Swedberg K, et al. Coenzyme Q10 as an adjunctive treatment of congestive heart failure. *J Card Fail* 1995;1:101-7.

6409 Baggio E, Gandini R, Plauncher AC, et al. Italian multicenter study on the safety and efficacy of coenzyme Q10 as adjunctive therapy in heart failure. CoQ10 Drug Surveillance Investigators. *Mol Aspects Med* 1994;15 Suppl:S287-94.

6410 Pizzorno JE, Murray MT, eds. Textbook of Natural Medicine. 2nd ed. New York: Churchill Livingston, 1999.

6412 Teixeira SR, Potter SM, Weigel R, et al. Effects of feeding 4 levels of soy protein for 3 and 6 wk on blood lipids and apolipoproteins in moderately hypercholesterolemic men. *Am J Clin Nutr* 2000;71:1077-84.

6413 Merz-Demlow BE, Duncan AM, Wangen KE, et al. Soy isoflavones improve plasma lipids in normocholesterolemic, premenopausal women. *Am J Clin Nutr* 2000;71:1462-9.

6414 Heaney RP, Dowell MS, Rafferty K, et al. Bioavailability of the calcium in fortified soy imitation milk, with some observations on method. *Am J Clin Nutr* 2000;71:1166-9.

6415 White LR, Petrovitch H, Ross GW, et al. Brain aging and midlife tofu consumption. *J Am Coll Nutr* 2000;19:242-55.

6416 Grodstein F, Mayeux R, Stampfer MJ. Tofu and cognitive function: food for thought. *J Am Coll Nutr* 2000;19:207-9.

6417 Giles JT, Palat CT III, Chien SH, et al. Evaluation of Echinacea for treatment of the common cold. *Pharmacother* 2000;20:690-7.

6418 Pepping J. Echinacea. *Am J Health Syst Pharm* 1999;56:121-3.

6420 Anon. Horse Chestnut. The Natural Pharmacist 2000. www.tnp.com/substance.asp?ID=62. (Accessed 24 June 2000).

6423 Galluzzi S, Zanetti O, Binetti G, et al. Coma in a patient with Alzheimer's disease taking low dose trazodone and Ginkgo biloba. *J Neurol Neurosurg Psychiatry* 2000;68:679-80.

6424 Carraro JC, Raynaud JP, Koch G, et al. Comparison of phytotherapy (Permixon) with finasteride in the treatment of benign prostate hyperplasia: a randomized international study of 1,098 patients. *Prostate* 1996;29:231-40.

6425 Roby CA, Anderson GD, Kantor E, et al. St. John's wort: Effect on CYP3A4 activity. *Clin Pharmacol Ther* 2000;67:451-7.

6426 Schempp CM, Winghofer B, Ludtke R, et al. Topical application of St. John's wort (Hypericum perforatum L.) and its metabolite hyperforin inhibits the allostimulatory capacity of epidermal cells. *Br J Dermatol* 2000;142:979-84.

6427 Kleber E, Obry T, Hippeli S, et al. Biochemical activities of extracts from Hypericum perforatum L. *Arzneimittelforschung* 1999;49:106-9.

6428 Williams JW, Mulrow CD, Chiquette E, et al. A systematic review of newer pharmacotherapies for depression in adults: Evidence report summary. *Ann Intern Med* 2000;132:743-56.

6429 Stevinson C, Ernst E. A pilot study of Hypericum perforatum for the treatment of premenstrual syndrome. *BJOG* 2000;107:870-6.

6430 Anderson PO, Knoben JE. Handbook of Clinical Drug Data. 8th ed. Stamford, CT: Appleton & Lange, 1997.

6431 Zambon D, Sabate J, Munoz S, et al. Substituting walnuts for monounsaturated fat improves the serum lipid profile of hypercholesterolemic men and women. *Ann Intern Med* 2000;132:538-46.

6432 Kovacs DJ, Berk T. Recurrent Clostridium difficile-associated diarrhea and colitis treated with saccharomyces cerevisiae (baker's yeast) in combination with antibiotic therapy. A case report. *J Am Board Fam Pract* 2000;13(2):138-40.

6433 Savarese D, Boucher J, Corey B, et al. Glutamine treatment of paclitaxel-induced myalgias and arthralgias [letter]. *J Clin Oncol* 1998;16:3918-9.

6434 Woelk H. Comparison of St. John's wort and imipramine for treating depression: randomized controlled trial. *BMJ* 2000;321:536-9.

6435 Barone GW, Gurley BJ, Ketel BL, et al. Drug interaction between St. John's wort and cyclosporin. *Ann Pharmacother* 2000;34:1013-6.

6436 Lusardi P, et al. Cardiovascular effects of melatonin in hypertensive patients well controlled by nifedipine: a 24-hour study. *Br J Clin Pharmacol* 2000;49:423-7.

6437 Mitwalli A, Ayiomamitis A, Grass L, et al. Control of hyperoxaluria with large doses of pyridoxine in patients with kidney stones. *Int Urol Nephrol* 1988;20:353-9.

6438 Gill HS, Rose GA. Mild metabolic hyperoxaluria and its response to pyridoxine. *Urol Int* 1986;41:393-6.

6439 Yendt ER, Cohanim M. Response to physiologic dose of pyridoxine in type I primary hyperoxaluria. *N Engl J Med* 1985;312:953-7.

6440 Revusova V, Gratzlova J, Zvara V, et al. The evaluation of some biochemical parameters in pyridoxine-treated calcium oxalate renal stone formers. *Urol Int* 1977;32:348-52.

6441 Curhan GC, Willet WC, Speizer FE, et al. Intake of vitamin B6 and C and the risk of kidney stones in women. *J Am Soc Nephrol* 1999;10:840-5.

6442 Curhan GC, Willet WC, Rimm EB, et al. A prospective study of the intake of vitamins C and B6, and the risk of kidney stones in men. *J Urol* 1996;155:1847-51.

6443 Arnold LE, Kleykamp D, Votolato NA, et al. Gamma-linolenic acid for attention-deficit hyperactivity disorder: Placebo-controlled comparison to D-amphetamine. *Biol Psychiatry* 1989;25:222-8.

6444 Haslam RHA, et al. Is there a role for megavitamin therapy in attention deficit hyperactivity disorder? *Adv Neurol* 1992;58:303-10.

6445 Stoll BA. Dietary supplements of dehydroepiandrosterone in relation to breast cancer risk. *Eur J Clin Nutr* 1999;53:771-5.

6446 Baulieu EE, Thomas G, Legrain S, et al. Dehydroepiandrosterone (DHEA), DHEA sulfate, and aging. Contribution of the DHEAge study to a sociobiomedical issue. *Proc Natl Acad Sci U S A* 2000;97:4279-84.

6447 van Vollenhoven RF, Park JL, Genovese MC, et al. A double-blind, placebo-controlled, clinical trial of dehydroepiandrosterone in severe lupus erythematosus. *Lupus* 1999;8:181-7.

6448 Jameson S. Statistical data support prediction of death within 6 months on low levels of coenzyme Q10 and other entities. *Clin Investig* 1993;71(8 Suppl):S137-9.

6449 Alekel DL, St. Germain A, Peterson CT et al. Isoflavone-rich soy protein isolate attenuates bone loss in the lumbar spine of perimenopausal women. *Am J Clin Nutr* 2000;72:844-52.

6450 Budzinski JW, Foster BC, Vandenhoek S, et al. An in vitro evaluation of human cytochrome P450 3A4 inhibition by selected commercial herbal extracts and tinctures. *Phytomedicine* 2000;7:273-82.

6451 Houston JB, Levy G. Drug biotransformation interactions in man VI: Acetaminophen and ascorbic acid. *J Pharm Sci* 1976;65:1218-21.

6452 Owen CA, Tyce GM, Flock EV, et al. Heparin-ascorbic acid antagonism. *Mayo Clin Proc* 1970;45:140-5.

6453 Dresser GK, Bailey DG, Carruthers SG. Grapefruit juice-felodipine interaction in the elderly. *Clin Pharmacol Ther* 2000;68:28-34.

6455 Upmalis DH, Lobo R, Bradley L, et al. Vasomotor symptom relief by soy isoflavone extract tablets in postmenopausal women: A multicenter, double-blind, randomized, placebo-controlled study. *Menopause* 2000;7:236-42.

6456 Chrubasik S, Eisenberg E, Balan E, et al. Treatment of low back pain exacerbations with willow bark extract: a randomized double-blind study. *Am J Med* 2000;109:9-14.

6457 Stevinson C, Pittler MH, Ernst E. Garlic for treating hypercholesterolemia: a meta-analysis of randomized clinical trials. *Ann Intern Med* 2000;133:420-9.

6458 Douglas RM, Chalker EB, Treacy B. Vitamin C for preventing and treating the common cold. *Cochrane Database Syst Rev* 2000;2:CD000980.

6459 Ross EA, Szabo NJ, Tebbett IR. Lead content of calcium supplements. *JAMA* 2000;284:1425-29.

6460 Heaney RP. Lead in calcium supplements. Cause for alarm or celebration? *JAMA* 2000;284:1432-3.

6461 Vuksan V, Stavro MP, Sievenpiper JL, et al. Similar postprandial glycemic reductions with escalation of dose and administration time of American ginseng in type 2 diabetes. *Diabetes Care* 2000;23:1221-6.

6462 Aman MG, Mitchell EA, Turbott SH. The effects of essential fatty acid supplementation by Efamol in hyperactive children. *J Abnorm Child Psychol* 1987;15:75-90.

6463 Moore LB, Goodwin B, Jones SA, et al. St. John's wort induces hepatic drug metabolism through activation of the pregnane X receptor. *Proc Natl Acad Sci U S A* 2000;97:7500-2.

6464 Cats A, Scholten P, Meuwissen SGM, et al. Acute Fasciola hepatica infection attributed to chewing khat. *Gut* 2000;47:584-5.

6465 Garlic: Effects on cardiovascular risks and disease, protective effects against cancer, and clinical adverse effects. Summary, evidence report/technol assessment: no 20. AHRQ Publ No. 01-E022, 2000;Oct. Agency for Healthcare Res and Quality. Rockville, MD.

6466 Divi RL, Chang HC, Doerge DR. Anti-thyroid isoflavones from soybean: isolation, characterization, and mechanisms of action. *Biochem Pharmacol* 1997;54:1087-96.

6468 Anon. Herbal Rx for prostate problems. *Consumer Reports* 2000;Sep:60-2.

6470 Alvarez-Arroyo MV, Traba ML, Rapado TA, et al. Correlation between 1.25 dihydroxyvitamin D serum levels and fractional rate of intestinal calcium absorption in hypercalciuric nephrolithiasis. Role of phosphate. *Urol Res* 1992;20:96-7.

6471 Hirt M, Nobel S, Barron E. Zinc nasal gel for the treatment of common cold symptoms: A double-blind, placebo-controlled trial. *Ear Nose Throat J* 2000;79:778-82.

6472 Chantre P, Cappelaere A, Leblan D, et al. Efficacy and tolerance or Harpagophytum procumbens versus diacerhein in treatment of osteoarthritis. *Phytomedicine* 2000;7:177-84.

6473 Cheng TO. St. John's wort interaction with digoxin [letter]. *Arch Intern Med* 2000;160:2548.

6474 Vormfelde SV, Poser W. Hyperforin in extracts of St. John's wort (Hypericum perforatum) for depression [letter]. *Arch Intern Med* 2000;160:2548.

6475 Wentworth JM, Agostini M, Love J, et al. St. John's wort, a herbal antidepressant, activates the steroid X receptor. *J Endocrinol* 2000;166:R11-6.

6476 Obach RS. Inhibition of human cytochrome P450 enzymes by constituents of St. John's wort, an herbal preparation used in the treatment of depression. *J Pharmacol Exp Ther* 2000;294:88-95.

6477 Lane-Brown MM. Photosensitivity associated with herbal preparations of St. John's wort (Hypericum perforatum). *Med J Aust* 2000;172:302.

6478 Lal S, Iskandar H. St. John's wort and schizophrenia. *CMAJ* 2000;163:262-3.

6479 Carey CF, Lee HH, Woeltje KF (eds). Washington Manual of Medical Therapeutics. 29th ed. New York, NY: Lippincott-Raven, 1998.

6480 Dorn M. [Efficacy and tolerability of Baldrian versus oxazepam in non-organic and non-psychiatric insomniacs: a randomized, double-blind, clinical, comparative study]. [Article in German]. *Forsch Komplementarmed Klass Naturheilkd* 2000;7:79-84.

6481 Parsons M, Simpson M, Ponton T. Raspberry leaf and its effects on labour: safety and efficacy. *Aust Coll Midwives Inc J* 1999;12:20-5.

6482 Heliovaara M, Aho K, Knekt P, et al. Coffee consumption, rheumatoid factor, and the risk of rheumatoid arthritis. *Ann Rheum Dis* 2000;59:631-5.

6483 de la Taille A, Buttyan R, Hayek O, et al. Herbal therapy PC-SPES: In vitro effects and evaluation of its efficacy in 69 patients with prostate cancer. *J Urol* 2000;164:1229-34.

6484 Small EJ, Frohlich MW, Bok R, et al.Prospective trial of the herbal supplement, PC-SPES, in patients with pregressive prostate cancer. *J Clin Oncol* 2000;18:3595-603.

6485 Wen HY, Davis RL, Shi B, et al. Bioavailability of selenium from veal, chicken, beef, lamb, flounder, tuna, selenomethionine, and sodium selenite assessed in selenium-deficient rats. *Biol Trace Elem Res* 1997;58:43–53.

6486 Haller CA, Benowitz NL. Adverse cardiovascular and central nervous system events associated with dietary supplements containing ephedra alkaloids. *N Engl J Med* 2000;343:1833-8.

6487 Leikin JB, Klein L. Ephedra causes myocarditis. *Clin Toxicol* 2000;38:353-4.

6488 Gurley B. Extract versus herb: Effect of formulation on the absorption rate of botanical ephedrine from dietary supplements containing ephedra (ma huang). *Ther Drug Monit* 2000;22:497.

6490 Le Bars PL, Kieser M, Itil KZ. A 26-week analysis of a double-blind, placebo-controlled trial of the Ginkgo biloba extract EGb 761 in dementia. *Dement Geriatr Cogn Disord* 2000;11:230-7.

6491 Forstl H. Clinical issues in current drug therapy for dementia. *Alzheimer Dis Assoc Disord* 2000;14:S103-S108.

6492 Campos-Toimil M, Lugnier C, Droy-Lefaix M, et al. Inhibition of type 4 phosphodiesterase by rolipram and Ginkgo biloba extract (EGb 761) decreases agonist-induced rises in internal calcium in human endothelial cells. *Arterioscler Thromb Vasc Biol* 2000;20:e34-e40.

6493 Ritch R. Potential role for Ginkgo biloba extract in the treatment of glaucoma. *Med Hypotheses* 2000;54:221-35.

6494 Bastianetto S, Ramassamy C, Dore S, et al. The ginkgo biloba extract (EGb 761) protects hippocampal neurons against cell death induced by beta-amyloid. *Eur J Neurosci* 2000;12:1882-90.

6495 Thal LJ, Calvani M, Amato A, et al. A 1-year controlled trial of acetyl-l-carnitine in early onset AD. *Neurol* 2000;55:805-10.

6496 Spitzer RL, Terman M, Williams JBW, et al. Jet lag: Clinical features, validation of a new syndrome-specific scale, lack of response to melatonin in a randomized, double-blind trial. *Am J Psychiatry* 1999;156:1392-6.

6497 Drago F, Busa L. Acute low doses of melatonin restore full sexual activity in impotent male rats. *Brain Res* 2000;878:98-104.

6498 von Bahr C, Ursing C, Yasui N, et al. Fluvoxamine but not citalopram increases serum melatonin in healthy subjects – an indication that cytochrome P450 CYP1A2 and CYP2C19 hydroxylate melatonin. *Eur J Clin Pharmacol* 2000;56:123-7.

6499 Grozinger M, Hartter S, Wang X, et al. Fluvoxamine strongly inhibits melatonin metabolism in a patient with low-amplitude melatonin profile. *Arch Gen Psychiatry* 2000 Aug;57:812-3.

6500 Mills S, Bone K. Principles and Practice of Phytotherapy. London: Churchill Livingstone, 2000.

6501 Michaelsson G, Juhlin L, Vahlquist A. Effects of oral zinc and vitamin A in acne. *Arch Dermatol* 1977;113:31-6.

6502 Dreno B, Amblard P, Agache P, et al. Low doses of zinc gluconate for inflammatory acne. *Acta Derm Venereol* 1989;69:541-3.

6503 Orris L, Shalita AR, Sibulkin D, et al. Oral zinc therapy of acne. Absorption and clinical effect. *Arch Dermatol* 1978;114:1018-20.

6504 Weismann K, Wadskov S, Sondergaard J. Oral zinc sulphate therapy for acne vulgaris. *Acta Derm Venereol* 1977;57:357-60.

6505 Cunliffe WJ, Burke B, Dodman B, Gould DJ. A double-blind trial of a zinc sulphate/citrate complex and tetracycline in the treatment of acne vulgaris. *Br J Dermatol* 1979;101:321-5.

6506 Michaelsson G, Juhlin L, Ljunghall K. A double-blind study of the effect of zinc and oxytetracycline in acne vulgaris. *Br J Dermatol* 1977;97:561-6.

6507 Amer M, Bahgat MR, Tosson Z, et al. Serum zinc in acne vulgaris. *Int J Dermatol* 1982;21:481-4.

6508 Michaelsson G, Vahlquist A, Juhlin L. Serum zinc and retinol-binding protein in acne. *Br J Dermatol* 1977;96:283-6.

6509 Michaelsson G, Ljunghall K. Patients with dermatitis herpetiformis, acne, psoriasis and Darier's disease have low epidermal zinc concentrations. *Acta Derm Venereol* 1990;70:304-8.

6510 Huang X, Cuajungco MP, Atwood CS, et al. Alzheimer's disease, beta-amyloid protein and zinc. *J Nutr* 2000;130:1488S-92S.

6511 Lovell MA, Robertson JD, Teesdale WJ, et al. Copper, iron and zinc in Alzheimer's disease senile plaques. *J Neurol Sci* 1998;158:47-52.

6512 Lovell MA, Xie C, Markesbery WR. Protection against amyloid beta peptide toxicity by zinc. *Brain Res* 1999;823:88-95.

6513 Burrows NP, Turnbull AJ, Punchard NA, et al. A trial of oral zinc supplementation in psoriasis. *Cutis* 1994;54:117-8.

6514 Leibovici V, Statter M, Weinrauch L, et al. Effect of zinc therapy on neutrophil chemotaxis in psoriasis. *Isr J Med Sci* 1990;26:306-9.

6515 Clemmensen OJ, Siggaard-Andersen J, Worm AM, et al. Psoriatic arthritis treated with oral zinc sulphate. *Br J Dermatol* 1980;103:411-5.

6516 Dixon JS, Bird HA, Martin MF, et al. Biochemical and clinical changes occurring during the treatment of rheumatoid arthritis with novel antirheumatoid drugs. *Int J Clin Pharmacol Res* 1985;5:25-33.

6517 Rasker JJ, Kardaun SH. Lack of beneficial effect of zinc sulphate in rheumatoid arthritis. *Scand J Rheumatol* 1982;11:168-70.

6518 Zoli A, Altomonte L, Caricchio R, et al. Serum zinc and copper in active rheumatoid arthritis: correlation with interleukin 1 beta and tumour necrosis factor alpha. *Clin Rheumatol* 1998;17:378-82.

6519 Simkin PA. Oral zinc sulphate in rheumatoid arthritis. *Lancet* 1976;2:539-42.

6520 Berger MM, Spertini F, Shenkin A, et al. Trace element supplementation modulates pulmonary infection rates after major burns: a double-blind, placebo-controlled trial. *Am J Clin Nutr* 1998;68:365-71.

6521 Marshall I. Zinc for the common cold. *Cochrane Database Syst Rev* 2000;CD001364.

6522 Jackson JL, Lesho E, Peterson C. Zinc and the common cold: a meta-analysis revisited. *J Nutr* 2000;130:1512S-5S.

6523 Guide to Clinical Preventive Services. 2nd ed. Natl Institute of Health, 1996. Available at: http://hstat2.nlm.nih.gov/download/409812772438.html

6524 Schaeken MJ, Van der Hoeven JS, Saxton CA, Cummins D. The effect of mouthrinses containing zinc and triclosan on plaque accumulation, development of gingivitis and formation of calculus in a 28-week clinical test. *J Clin Periodontol* 1996;23:465-70.

6525 Stephen KW, Saxton CA, Jones CL, et al. Control of gingivitis and calculus by a dentifrice containing a zinc salt and triclosan. *J Periodontol* 1990;61:674-9.

6526 Svatun B, Saxton CA, Rolla G. Six-month study of the effect of a dentifrice containing zinc citrate and triclosan on plaque, gingival health, and calculus. *Scand J Dent Res* 1990;98:301-4.

6527 Svatun B, Saxton CA, Huntington E, Cummins D. The effects of a silica dentifrice containing Triclosan and zinc citrate on supragingival plaque and calculus formation and the control of gingivitis. *Int Dent J* 1993;43:431-9.

6528 Williams C, McBride S, Mostler K, et al. Efficacy of a dentifrice containing zinc citrate for the control of plaque and gingivitis: a 6-month clinical study in adults. *Compend Contin Educ Dent* 1998;19:4-15.

6529 Polenik P. Zinc in etiology of periodontal disease. *Med Hypotheses* 1993;40:182-5.

6530 Cunningham JJ, Fu A, Mearkle PL, Brown RG. Hyperzincuria in individuals with insulin-dependent diabetes mellitus: concurrent zinc status and the effect of high-dose zinc supplementation. *Metabolism* 1994;43:1558-62.

6531 Rauscher AM, Fairweather-Tait SJ, Wilson PD, et al. Zinc metabolism in non-insulin dependent diabetes mellitus. *J Trace Elem Med Biol* 1997;11:65-70.

REFERENCES

6532 Blostein-Fujii A, DiSilvestro RA, Frid D, et al. Short-term zinc supplementation in women with non-insulin-dependent diabetes mellitus: effects on plasma 5'-nucleotidase activities, insulin-like growth factor I concentrations, and lipoprotein oxidation rates in vitro. *Am J Clin Nutr* 1997;66:639-42.

6533 Faure P, Benhamou PY, Perard A, et al. Lipid peroxidation in insulin-dependent diabetic patients with early retina degenerative lesions: effects of an oral zinc supplementation. *Eur J Clin Nutr* 1995;49:282-8.

6534 Mahajan PM, Jadhav VH, Patki AH, et al. Oral zinc therapy in recurrent erythema nodosum leprosum: a clinical study. *Indian J Lepr* 1994;66:51-7.

6535 Mathur NK, Bumb RA, Mangal HN. Oral zinc in recurrent Erythema Nodosum Leprosum reaction. *Lepr India* 1983;55:547-52.

6536 Mathur NK, Bumb RA, Mangal HN, Sharma ML. Oral zinc as an adjunct to dapsone in lepromatous leprosy. *Int J Lepr Other Mycobact Dis* 1984;52:331-8.

6537 George J, Bhatia VN, Balakrishnan S, Ramu G. Serum zinc/copper ratio in subtypes of leprosy and effect of oral zinc therapy on reactional states. *Int J Lepr Other Mycobact Dis* 1991;59:20-4.

6538 Brody I. Topical treatment of recurrent herpes simplex and post-herpetic erythema multiforme with low concentrations of zinc sulphate solution. *Br J Dermatol* 1981;104:191-4.

6539 Eby GA, Halcomb WW. Use of topical zinc to prevent recurrent herpes simplex infection: review of literature and suggested protocols. *Med Hypotheses* 1985;17:157-65.

6540 Kneist W, Hempel B, Borelli S. [Clinical, double-blind trial of topical zinc sulfate for herpes labialis recidivans]. [Article in German]. *Arzneimittelforschung* 1995;45:624-6.

6541 Arens M, Travis S. Zinc salts inactivate clinical isolates of herpes simplex virus in vitro. *J Clin Microbiol* 2000;38:1758-62.

6542 Heyneman CA. Zinc deficiency and taste disorders. *Ann Pharmacother* 1996;30:186-7.

6543 Abu-Hamdan DK, Desai H, Sondheimer J, et al. Taste acuity and zinc metabolism in captopril-treated hypertensive male patients. *Am J Hypertens* 1988;1:303S-8S.

6544 Henkin RI, Martin BM, Agarwal RP. Efficacy of exogenous oral zinc in treatment of patients with carbonic anhydrase VI deficiency. *Am J Med Sci* 1999;318:392-405.

6545 Henkin RI, Martin BM, Agarwal RP. Decreased parotid saliva gustin/carbonic anhydrase VI secretion: an enzyme disorder manifested by gustatory and olfactory dysfunction. *Am J Med Sci* 1999;318:380-91.

6546 Henkin RI, Schecter PJ, Friedewald WT, et al. A double-blind study of the effects of zinc sulfate on taste and smell dysfunction. *Am J Med Sci* 1976;272:285-99.

6547 Ripamonti C, Zecca E, Brunelli C, et al. A randomized, controlled clinical trial to evaluate the effects of zinc sulfate on cancer patients with taste alterations caused by head and neck irradiation. *Cancer* 1998;82:1938-45.

6548 Mahajan SK, Prasad AS, Lambujon J, et al. Improvement of uremic hypogeusia by zinc: a double-blind study. *Am J Clin Nutr* 1980;33:1517-21.

6549 Watson AR, Stuart A, Wells FE, et al. Zinc supplementation and its effect on taste acuity in children with chronic renal failure. *Hum Nutr Clin Nutr* 1983;37:219-25.

6550 Sprenger KB, Bundschu D, Lewis K, et al. Improvement of uremic neuropathy and hypogeusia by dialysate zinc supplementation: a double-blind study. *Kidney Int Suppl* 1983;16:S315-8.

6551 Shankar AH, Prasad AS. Zinc and immune function: the biological basis of altered resistance to infection. *Am J Clin Nutr* 1998;68:447S-63S.

6552 Prasad AS. Zinc and immunity. *Mol Cell Biochem* 1998;188:63-9.

6553 Girodon F, Galan P, Monget AL, et al. Impact of trace elements and vitamin supplementation on immunity and infections in institutionalized elderly patients: a randomized, controlled trial. MIN. VIT. AOX. geriatric network. *Arch Intern Med* 1999;159:748-54.

6554 Bjorksten B, Back O, Gustavson KH, et al. Zinc and immune function in Down's syndrome. *Acta Paediatr Scand* 1980;69:183-7.

6555 Licastro F, Chiricolo M, Mocchegiani E, et al. Oral zinc supplementation in Down's syndrome subjects decreased infections and normalized some humoral and cellular immune parameters. *J Intellect Disabil Res* 1994;38:149-62.

6556 Cahill DJ, Fox R, Wardle PG, et al. Multiple follicular development associated with herbal medicine. *Hum Reprod* 1994;9:1469-70.

6557 McCaleb RS, Leigh E, Morien K. The Encyclopedia of Popular Herbs. Roseville, CA: Prima Health, 2000.

6558 Heiman SW. Pycnogenol for ADHD? *J Am Acad Child Adolesc Psychiatry* 1999;38:357-8.

6559 Greenblatt J. Nutritional supplements in ADHD. *J Am Acad Child Adolesc Psychiatry* 1999;38:1209-11.

6562 Maes M, De Vos N, Demedts P, et al. Lower serum zinc in major depression in relation to changes in serum acute phase proteins. *J Affect Disord* 1999;56:189-94.

6563 Provinciali M, Montenovo A, Di Stefano G, et al. Effect of zinc or zinc plus arginine supplementation on antibody titre and lymphocyte subsets after influenza vaccination in elderly subjects: a randomized controlled trial. *Age Ageing* 1998;27:715-22.

6564 Kelly P, Musonda R, Kafwembe E, et al. Micronutrient supplementation in the AIDS diarrhea-wasting syndrome in Zambia: a randomized controlled trial. *AIDS* 1999;13:495-500.

6565 Tang AM, Graham NM, Saah AJ. Effects of micronutrient intake on survival in human immunodeficiency virus type 1 infection. *Am J Epidemiol* 1996;143:1244-56.

6566 Mocchegiani E, Veccia S, Ancarani F, et al. Benefit of oral zinc supplementation as an adjunct to zidovudine (AZT) therapy against opportunistic infections in AIDS. *Int J Immunopharmacol* 1995;17:719-27.

6568 Brook AC, Johnston DG, Ward MK, et al. Absence of a therapeutic effect of zinc in the sexual dysfunction of haemodialysed patients *Lancet* 1980;2:618-20.

6569 Goldiner WH, Hamilton BP, Hyman PD, Russell RM. Effect of the administration of zinc sulfate on hypogonadism and impotence in patients with chronic stable hepatic cirrhosis. *J Am Coll Nutr* 1983;2:157-62.

6570 Khedun SM, Naicker T, Maharaj B. Zinc, hydrochlorothiazide and sexual dysfunction. *Cent Afr J Med* 1995;41:312-5.

6571 Mahajan SK, Abbasi AA, Prasad AS, et al. Effect of oral zinc therapy on gonadal function in hemodialysis patients. A double-blind study. *Ann Intern Med* 1982;97:357-61.

6572 Rodger RS, Sheldon WL, Watson MJ, et al. Zinc deficiency and hyperprolactinaemia are not reversible causes of sexual dysfunction in uraemia. *Nephrol Dial Transplant* 1989;4:888-92.

6573 Fuse H, Kazama T, Ohta S, Fujiuchi Y. Relationship between zinc concentrations in seminal plasma and various sperm parameters. *Int Urol Nephrol* 1999;31:401-8.

6574 Henkel R, Bittner J, Weber R, et al. Relevance of zinc in human sperm flagella and its relation to motility. *Fertil Steril* 1999;71:1138-43.

6575 Chia SE, Ong CN, Chua LH, et al. Comparison of zinc concentrations in blood and seminal plasma and the various sperm parameters between fertile and infertile men. *J Androl* 2000;21:53-7.

REFERENCES

6576 Hunt CD, Johnson PE, Herbel J, Mullen LK. Effects of dietary zinc depletion on seminal volume and zinc loss, serum testosterone concentrations, and sperm morphology in young men. *Am J Clin Nutr* 1992;56:148-57.

6577 Mohan H, Verma J, Singh I, et al. Inter-relationship of zinc levels in serum and semen in oligospermic infertile patients and fertile males. *Indian J Pathol Microbiol* 1997;40:451-5.

6578 Omu AE, Dashti H, Al-Othman S. Treatment of asthenozoospermia with zinc sulphate: andrological, immunological and obstetric outcome. *Eur J Obstet Gynecol Reprod Biol* 1998;79:179-84.

6579 Mares-Perlman JA, Klein R, Klein BE, et al. Association of zinc and antioxidant nutrients with age-related maculopathy. *Arch Ophthalmol* 1996;114:991-7.

6580 Smith W, Mitchell P, Webb K, Leeder SR. Dietary antioxidants and age-related maculopathy: the Blue Mountains Eye Study. *Ophthalmology* 1999;106:761-77.

6581 VandenLangenberg GM, Mares-Perlman JA, Klein R, et al. Associations between antioxidant and zinc intake and the 5-year incidence of early age-related maculopathy in the Beaver Dam Eye Study. *Am J Epidemiol* 1998;148:204-14.

6582 Evans JR, Henshaw K. Antioxidant vitamin and mineral supplementation for preventing age-related macular degeneration. *Cochrane Database Syst Rev* 2000;(2):CD000253.

6583 Newsome DA, Swartz M, Leone NC, et al. Oral zinc in macular degeneration. *Arch Ophthalmol* 1988;106:192-8.

6584 Stur M, Tittl M, Reitner A, Meisinger V. Oral zinc and the second eye in age-related macular degeneration. *Invest Ophthalmol Vis Sci* 1996;37:1225-35.

6585 Sack RL, Brandes RW, Kendall AR, et al. Entrainment of free-running circadian rhythms by melatonin in blind people. *N Engl J Med* 2000;343:1070-7.

6586 Grazioso CF, Isalgue M, de Ramirez I, et al. The effect of zinc supplementation on parasitic reinfestation of Guatemalan schoolchildren. *Am J Clin Nutr* 1993;57:673-8.

6587 Sharquie KE, Najim RA, Farjou IB. A comparative controlled trial of intralesionally-administered zinc sulphate, hypertonic sodium chloride and pentavalent antimony compound against acute cutaneous leishmaniasis. *Clin Exp Dermatol* 1997;22:169-73.

6588 Rodriguez de la Serna A, Diaz-Rubio M. Multicenter clinical trial of zinc acexamate in the prevention of nonsteroidal antiinflammatory drug induced gastroenteropathy. Spanish Study Group on NSAID Induced Gastroenteropathy Prevention. *J Rheumatol* 1994;21:927-33.

6589 Jimenez E, Bosch F, Galmes JL, Banos JE. Meta-analysis of efficacy of zinc acexamate in peptic ulcer. *Digestion* 1992;51:18-26.

6590 Garcia-Plaza A, Arenas JI, Belda O, Diago A, et al. [A multicenter, clinical trial. Zinc acexamate vs famotidine in the treatment of acute duodenal ulcer. Study group of zinc acexamate]. [Article in Spanish]. *Rev Esp Enferm Dig* 1996;88:757-62.

6591 Frommer DJ. The healing of gastric ulcers by zinc sulphate. *Med J Aust* 1975;2:793-6.

6592 Wray D. A double-blind trial of systemic zinc sulfate in recurrent aphthous stomatitis. *Oral Surg Oral Med Oral Pathol* 1982;53:469-72.

6593 Merchant HW, Gangarosa LP, Glassman AB, Sobel RE. Zinc sulfate supplementation for treatment of recurring oral ulcers. *South Med J* 1977;70:559-61.

6594 Gupta VL, Chaubey BS. Efficacy of zinc therapy in prevention of crisis in sickle cell anemia: a double blind, randomized controlled clinical trial. *J Assoc Physicians India* 1995;43:467-9.

6595 Leonard MB, Zemel BS, Kawchak DA, et al. Plasma zinc status, growth, and maturation in children with sickle cell disease. *J Pediatr* 1998;132:467-71.

6596 Prasad AS, Beck FW, Kaplan J, et al. Effect of zinc supplementation on incidence of infections and hospital admissions in sickle cell disease (SCD). *Am J Hematol* 1999;61:194-202.

6597 Aydinok Y, Coker C, Kavakli K, et al. Urinary zinc excretion and zinc status of patients with beta-thalassemia major. *Biol Trace Elem Res* 1999;70:165-72.

6598 Uysal Z, Akar N, Kemahli S, et al. Desferrioxamine and urinary zinc excretion in beta-thalassemia major. *Pediatr Hematol Oncol* 1993;10:257-60.

6599 Benso L, Gambotto S, Pastorin L, et al. Growth velocity monitoring of the efficacy of different therapeutic protocols in a group of thalassaemic children. *Eur J Pediatr* 1995;154:205-8.

6600 Sigurjonsdottir HA, Manhem K, Wallerstedt S. Liquorice-induced hypertension- a linear, dose-response relationship. Endocrine Soc 82nd Ann Mtg, Toronto, CAN, 2000; Jun 21-4:abstract 2279.

6601 Anon. Roasting process to pump up cancer fighting properties of coffee unveiled by oncology sciences corp. PRNewswire 2000; Jun 30. www.prnewswire.com (Accessed 3 July 2000).

6602 Szmeja Z, Kulczynski B, Sosnowski Z, Konopacki K. [Therapeutic value of flavonoids in Rhinovirus infections]. [Article in Polish]. *Otolaryngol Pol* 1989;43(3):180-4.

6603 Pennell MM. One to two drinks a day may reduce risk of Alzheimer dementia. Reuters Health. www.medscape.com/reuters/prof/2000/07/07.11/20000711epid005.html (Accessed 11 July 2000).

6604 Takahashi J, Kawakatsu K, Wakayama T, Sawaoka H. Elevation of serum theophylline levels by ipriflavone in a patient with chronic obstructive pulmonary disease. *Eur J Clin Pharmacol* 1992;43(2):207-8.

6606 Goldschmidt RH, Dong BJ. Treatment of AIDS and HIV-related conditions: 2000. *J Am Board Fam Pract* 2000;13:274-98. Full text available at www.medscape.com/viewarticle/405799_print.

6607 Watzl B, Bub A, Blockhaus M, et al. Prolonged tomato juice consumption has no effect on cell-mediated immunity of well-nourished elderly men and women. *J Nutr* 2000;130:1719-23.

6608 Anon. FDA Grants orphan drug designation to Tishcon Corp UbiQGel (Coenzyme Q10). PRNewswire 2000; Jul 25. www.prnewswire.com (Accessed 25 July 2000).

6610 Anon. Court backs Food & Drug Administration's check of cholestin. NewsExcite.com. news.excite.com/news/ap/000723/19/cholesterol-dispute (Accessed 25 July 2000).

6611 Tepel M, van der Giet M, Schwarzfeld C, et al. Prevention of radiographic-contrast-agent-induced reductions in renal function by acetylcysteine. *N Engl J Med* 2000;343:180-4.

6612 Galloway GP, Frederick SL, Staggers FE Jr, et al. Gamma-hydroxybutyrate: an emerging drug of abuse that causes physical dependence. *Addiction* 1997;92(1):89-96.

6613 Price G. In-patient detoxification after GHB dependence. *Br J Psychiatry* 2000;177:181.

6614 Murray MT. Encyclopedia of Nutritional Supplements. Rocklin, CA: Prima Health, 1996.

6620 Nationwide alert on hallmark labs injectable adrenal cortex extract. FDA. Available at: www.fda.gov/bbs/topics/NEWS/NEW00539.html

6624 Fowler JF Jr. Systemic contact dermatitis caused by oral chromium picolinate. *Cutis* 2000;65:116.

6625 Pérez C, Domínguez E, Canal JR, et al. Hypoglycaemic activity of an aqueous extract from Ficus carica (fig tree) leaves in streptozotocin diabetic rats. *Pharmaceutical Biology* 2000;38:181-6.

REFERENCES

6627 La Marca G, Pumilia G, Martino A. [Effectiveness of mesoglycan topical treatment of leg ulcers in subjects with chronic venous insufficiency]. [Article in Italian]. *Minerva Cardioangiol* 1999;47:315-9.

6628 Laurora G, Cesarone MR, Belcaro G, et al. [Control of the progress of arteriosclerosis in high risk subjects treated with mesoglycan. Measuring the intima media]. [Article in Italian]. *Minerva Cardioangiol* 1998;46:41-7.

6629 Raso AM, Maggio D, Trogolo M, et al. [Effectiveness of mesoglycan therapy in patients with ischemia of the lower limbs. Preliminary results of a new therapeutic protocol]. [Article in Italian]. *Minerva Cardioangiol* 1997;45:383-92.

6630 Scondotto G, Catena G, Aloisi D. [Use of mesoglycan in venous pathology]. [Article in Italian]. *Minerva Med* 1997;88:537-41.

6631 Blardi P, Messa G, Puccetti L, et al. [Effects on the coagulation-fibrinolysis system of a single oral dose of mesoglycan at the beginning and at the end of a prolonged treatment in man]. [Article in Italian]. *Recenti Prog Med* 1995;86:282-9.

6632 Lightdale JR, Hayer C, Duer A, et al. Effects of intravenous secretin on language and behavior of children with autism and gastrointestinal symptoms: a single-blinded, open-label pilot study. *Pediatrics* 2001;108:90.

6633 Vecchio F, Zanchin G, Maggioni F, et al. Mesoglycan in treatment of patients with cerebral ischemia: effects on hemorheologic and hematochemical parameters. *Acta Neurol* (Napoli) 1993;15:449-56.

6634 Lotti T, Celasco G, Tsampau D, et al. Mesoglycan treatment restores defective fibrinolytic potential in cutaneous necrotizing venulitis. *Int J Dermatol* 1993;32:368-71.

6635 Ambrosio LA, Marchese G, Filippo A, et al. The effect of mesoglycan in patients with cerebrovascular disease: a psychometric evaluation. *J Int Med Res* 1993;21:138-46.

6637 Orlandi G, Viapiano F, Massetani R, et al. Clinical-instrumental evaluation of the effects of mesoglycan sulphate in chronic vascular encephalopathy. *Acta Neurol* (Napoli) 1991;13:255-60.

6638 Agrati AM, De Bartolo G, Palmieri G. [Heparan sulfate: efficacy and safety in patients with chronic venous insufficiency]. [Article in Italian]. *Minerva Cardioangiol* 1991;39:395-400.

6639 Abate G, Berenga A, Caione F, et al. [Controlled multicenter study on the therapeutic effectiveness of mesoglycan in patients with cerebrovascular disease]. [Article in Italian]. *Minerva Med* 1991;82:101-5.

6640 Prandoni P, Cattelan AM, Carta M. [Long-term sequelae of deep venous thrombosis of the legs. Experience with mesoglycan]. [Article in Italian]. *Ann Ital Med Int* 1989;4:378-85.

6641 Cazzato G, Zorzon M, Mase G, et al. [Mesoglycan in acute focal cerebral ischemia]. [Article in Italian]. *Riv Neurol* 1989;59:121-6.

6642 Vittoria A, Messa GL, Frigerio C, et al. Effect of a single dose of mesoglycan on the human fibrinolytic system, and the profibrinolytic action of nine daily doses. *Int J Tissue React* 1988;10:261-6.

6643 Andreozzi GM, Signorelli S, Lo Duca S, et al. Effects of mesoglycan sulfate on the arterial elastic module. *Angiology* 1987;38:593-600.

6644 Petruzzellis V, Velon A. [Therapeutic action of oral mesoglycan in the pharmacologic treatment of the varicose syndrome and its complications]. [Article in Italian]. *Minerva Med* 1985;76:543-8.

6645 Scondotto G, De Fabritiis A, Guastarobba A, et al. [Use of a minor fibrinolytic drug (mesoglycan) in phlebitis]. [Article in Italian]. *Minerva Med* 1984;75:1733-8.

6646 Postiglione A, De Simone B, Rubba P, et al. Effect of oral mesoglycan on plasma lipoprotein concentration and on lipoprotein lipase activity in primary hyperlipoproteinemia. *Pharmacol Res Commun* 1984;16:1-8.

6650 Fukuda Y, Sawata M, Washizuka M, et al. [Effect of liver hydrolysate on hepatic proliferation in regenerating rat liver]. [Article in Japanese]. *Nippon Yakurigaku Zasshi* 1999;114:233-8.

6651 Betz JM. Guidance for industry: labeling for dietary supplement products containing St. John's wort and saw palmetto. American Herbal Products Association, August 2000.

6652 Brown BT. Treating cancer with coffee enemas and diet. *JAMA* 1993;269:1635-6.

6653 Gerson M. The cure of advanced cancer by diet therapy: a summary of 30 years of clinical experimentation. *Physiol Chem Phys* 1978;10:449-64.

6654 Wagner SL. Fatal asthma in a child after use of an animal shampoo containing pyrethrin. *West J Med* 2000;173(2):86-7.

6655 Carl W, Emrich LS. Management of oral mucositis during local radiation and systemic chemotherapy: a study of 98 patients. *J Prosthet Dent* 1991;66:361-9.

6656 Fidler P, Loprinzi CL, O'Fallon JR, et al. Prospective evaluation of a chamomile mouthwash for prevention of 5-FU-induced oral mucositis. *Cancer* 1996;77:522-5.

6657 Rostler S. Spoonful of cinnamon may help insulin go into cells. Reuters Health. www.reutershealth.com/frame2/eline.html (Accessed 25 August 2000).

6660 Fridkin M, Najjar VA. Tuftsin: its chemistry, biology, and clinical potential. *Crit Rev Biochem Mol Biol* 1989;24(1):1-40.

6661 Volk HD, Eckert R, Diamantstein T, Schmitz H. [Immunorestitutive action of hydrolysates and ultrafiltrates of bovine spleen]. [Article in German]. *Arzneimittelforschung* 1991;41(12):1281-5.

6662 Corazza GR, Zoli G, Ginaldi L, et al. Tuftsin deficiency in AIDS. *Lancet* 1991;337(8732):12-3.

6668 Anon. FDA authorizes new coronary heart disease health claim for plant sterol and plant stanol esters. FDA. 2000. Available at: www.fda.gov/bbs/topics/ANSWERS/ANS01033.html.

6669 Anon. FDA takes action against firms marketing unapproved drugs. FDA. 2000. www.fda.gov/bbs/topics/ANSWERS/ANS01032.html.

6670 Anon. Vitamin E can relieve sleep disorder that affects millions, medical specialists report. PRNewswire www.prnewswire.com (Accessed 7 September 2000).

6672 Anon. Postscript on laetrile. FDA. 1987. Available at: www.fda.gov/bbs/topics/ANSWERS/ANS00309.html.

6673 Anon. Laetrile (Amygdalin, other Names). FDA. 1987. www.fda.gov/ora/fiars/ora_import_ia6201.html.

6675 Anon. FDA warns against consuming dietary supplements containing tiratricol. FDA. 2000. Available at: www.fda.gov/bbs/topics/ANSWERS/ANS01057.html.

6677 Skotnicki AB. Therapeutic application of calf thymus extract (TFX). *Med Oncol Tumor Pharmacother* 1989;6(1):31-43.

6678 Aiuti F, Sirianni MC, Fiorilli M, et al. A placebo-controlled trial of thymic hormone treatment of recurrent herpes simplex labialis infection in immunodeficient host: results after a 1-year follow-up. *Clin Immunol Immunopathol* 1984;30(1):11-8.

6679 De Martino M, Rossi ME, Muccioli AT, Vierucci A. T lymphocytes in children with recurrent respiratory infections: effect of the use of thymostimulin on the alterations of T-cell subsets. *Int J Tissue React* 1984;6(3):223-8.

6680 Iaffaioli RV, Frasci G, Tortora G, et al. Effect of thymic extract thymostimulin on the incidence of infections and myelotoxicity during adjuvant chemotherapy for breast cancer. *Thymus* 1988-89;12(2):69-75.

6681 Banos V, Gomez J, Garcia A, et al. Effectiveness of immunomodulating treatment (thymostimulin) in chronic obstructive pulmonary disease. *Respiration* 1997;64(3):220-3.

6682 Lin CY, Hsu HC, Chen CL, Shen EY. Treatment of combined immunodeficiency with thymic extract (Thymostimulin). *Ann Allergy* 1987;58(5):379-84.

6683 Lin CY, Hsu CH, Liu KC, et al. Serial immunologic and histopathologic studies in the treatment of necrotizing fasciitis with combined immunodeficiency by a bovine thymic extract (thymostimulin). *J Pediatr Surg* 1986;21(11):1000-4.

6684 De Mattia D, Decandia P, Ferrante P, et al. Effectiveness of thymostimulin and study of lymphocyte-dependent antibacterial activity in children with recurrent respiratory infections. *Immunopharmacol Immunotoxicol* 1993;15:447-59.

6685 Aiuti F, Ammirati P, Fiorilli M, et al. Immunologic and clinical investigation on a bovine thymic extract. Therapeutic applications in primary immunoedificiencies. *Pediatr Res* 1979;13(7):797-802.

6686 Hegarty JE, Nouri Aria KT, Eddleston AL, Williams R. Controlled trial of a thymic hormone extract (Thymostimulin) in autoimmune chronic active hepatitis. *Gut* 1984;25(3):279-83.

6687 Kenady DE, Chretien PB, Potvin C, Simon RM. Thymosin reconstitution of T-cell deficits in vitro in cancer patients. *Cancer* 1977;39(2):575-80.

6688 Armerding D, Katz DH. Activation of T and B lymphocytes in vitro. IV. Regulatory influence on specific T cell functions by a thymus extract factor. *J Immunol* 1975;114(4):1248-54.

6689 Kouttab NM, Prada M, Cazzola P. Thymomodulin: biological properties and clinical applications. *Med Oncol Tumor Pharmacother* 1989;6(1):5-9.

6690 Burger O, Ofek I, Tabak M, et al. A high molecular mass constituent of cranberry juice inhibits helicobacter pylori adhesion to human gastric mucus. *FEMS Immunol Med Microbiol* 2000;29:295-301.

6691 Calsini P, Mocchegiani E, Fabris N. The pharmacodynamics of thymomodulin in elderly humans. *Drugs Exp Clin Res* 1985;11(9):671-4.

6693 Anon. Can vitamin E supplementation forestall muscle-damaging effects of a single bout of resistance training? Amer Physiological Soc press release. www.faseb.org/aps/meetings/mtg_pressrel6.htm (Accessed 26 September 2000).

6694 Genova R, Guerra A. [A thymus extract (thymomodulin) in the prevention of childhood asthma]. [Article in Italian]. *Pediatr Med Chir* 1983;5(5):395-402.

6695 Bagnato A, Brovedani P, Comina P, et al. Long-term treatment with thymomodulin reduces airway hyperresponsiveness to methacholine. *Ann Allergy* 1989;62(5):425-8.

6696 Maiorano V, Chianese R, Fumarulo R, et al. Thymomodulin increases the depressed production of superoxide anion by alveolar macrophages in patients with chronic bronchitis. *Int J Tissue React* 1989;11(1):21-5.

6697 Fiocchi A, Borella E, Riva E, et al. A double-blind clinical trial for the evaluation of the therapeutical effectiveness of a calf thymus derivative (Thymomodulin) in children with recurrent respiratory infections. *Thymus* 1986;8(6):331-9.

6698 Longo F, Lepore L, Agosti E, Panizon F. [Evaluation of the effectiveness of thymomodulin in children with recurrent respiratory infections]. [Article in Italian]. *Pediatr Med Chir* 1988;10(6):603-7.

6699 Galli L, de Martino M, Azzari C, et al. [Preventive effect of thymomodulin in recurrent respiratory infections in children]. [Article in Italian]. *Pediatr Med Chir* 1990;12(3):229-32.

6700 Douglas RM, Miles HB, Moore BW, et al. Failure of effervescent zinc acetate lozenges to alter the course of upper respiratory tract infections in Australian adults. *Antimicrob Agents Chemother* 1987;31:1263-5.

6703 Prasad AS, Fitzgerald JT, Bao B, et al. Duration of symptoms and plasma cytokine levels in patients with the common cold treated with zinc acetate. A randomized, double-blind, placebo-controlled trial. *Ann Intern Med* 2000;133:245-52.

6705 Petrus EJ, Lawson KA, Bucci LR, Blum K. Randomized, double-masked, placebo-controlled clinical study of the effectiveness of zinc acetate lozenges on common cold symptoms in allergy-tested subjects. *Curr Ther Res* 1998;59:595-607.

6706 Desbiens NA. Lessons learned from attempts to establish the blind in placebo-controlled trials of zinc for the common cold. *Ann Intern Med* 2000;133:302-3.

6708 Antoniou LD, Shalhoub RJ, Sudhakar T, Smith JC Jr. Reversal of uraemic impotence by zinc. *Lancet* 1977;2:895-8.

6709 Berbari P, Thibodeau A, Germain L, et al. Antiangiogenic effects of the oral administration of liquid cartilage extract in humans. *J Surg Res* 1999;87:108-13.

6711 Pittler MH, Vogler BK, Ernst E. Feverfew for preventing migraine. *Cochrane Database Syst Rev* 2000;3:CD002286.

6712 Brun J, Claustrat B, Saddier P, Chazot G. Nocturnal melatonin excretion is decreased in patients with migraine without aura attacks associated with menses. *Cephalalgia* 1995;15:136-9.

6713 Pugh WJ, Sambo K. Prostaglandin synthetase inhibitors in feverfew. *J Pharm Pmarmacol* 1988;40:743-5.

6714 Natl Cancer Institute CancerNet. Cartilage website: www.cancernet.nci.nih.gov/cam/cartilage.htm (Accessed 18 August 2000).

6716 Leitner SP, Rothkopf MM, Haverstick L, et al. Two phase II studies of oral dry shark cartilage powder (SCP) in patients (pts) with either metastatic breast or prostate cancer refractory to standard treatment. *Proceedings of Amer Soc Clinical Oncol* 1998;17:A240.

6717 Rosenbluth RJ, Jennis AA, Cantwell S, DeVries J. Oral shark cartilage in the treatment of patients with advanced primary brain tumors. A phase II pilot study. *Proceedings of Amer Soc Clinical Oncol* 1999;18:A554.

6718 Evans WK, Latreille J, Batist G, et al. AE-941, an inhibitor of angiogenesis: rationale for development in combination with induction chemotherapy/radiotherapy in patients with non small cell lung cancer (NSCLC). *Proceedings of Amer Soc of Clinical Oncol* 1999;18:A1938.

6719 Patnaik A, Rowinsky E, Hammond L, et al. A phase I and pharmacokinetic (PK) study of the unique angiogenesis inhibitor, squalamine lactate (MSI-1256F). *Proceedings of Amer Soc of Clinical Oncol* 1999;18:A622.

6720 Kalidas M, Hammond LA, Patnaik P, et al. A phase I and pharmacokinetic (PK) study of the angiogenesis inhibitor, squalamine lactate (MSI-1256F). Proceedings of Amer Soc of Clinical Oncol 2000;19:A698.

6721 Bhargava P, Trocky N, Marshall J, et al. A phase I safety, tolerance and pharmacokinetic study of rising dose, rising duration continuous infusion of MSI-1256F (Squalamine Lactate) in patients with advanced cancer. *Proceedings of Amer Soc Clinical Oncol* 1999;18:A698.

6722 Mathews J. Media feeds frenzy over shark cartilage as cancer treatment. *J Natl Cancer Inst* 1993;85:1190-1.

6723 Gomes EM, Souto PR, Felzenszwalb I. Shark-cartilage containing preparation protects cells against hydrogen peroxide induced damage and mutagenesis. *Mutat Res* 1996;367:204-8.

6724 Fontenele JB, Araujo GB, de Alencar JW, Viana GS. The analgesic and anti-inflammatory effects of shark cartilage are due to a peptide molecule and are nitric oxide (NO) system dependent. *Biol Pharm Bull* 1997;20:1151-4.

6725 Fontenele JB, Viana GS, Xavier-Filho J, de-Alencar JW. Anti-inflammatory and analgesic activity of a water-soluble fraction from shark cartilage. *Braz J Med Biol Res* 1996;29:643-6.

6726 Sheu JR, Fu CC, Tsai ML, Chung WJ. Effect of U-995, a potent shark cartilage-derived angiogenesis inhibitor, on anti-angiogenesis and anti-tumor activities. *Anticancer Res* 1998;18:4435-41.

6727 Anon. AEterna announces the commencement of patient enrollment for the NIH - sponsored phase III clinical trial of AE-941/Neovastat in the treatment of lung cancer. Aeterna 2000 News Release 2000 May 17.

6729 Herb.com. Herbal Materia Medica 4.0 website. URL: http://herb.com/materia.htm (Accessed 22 August 2000).

6733 Colorado State Univ. Colorado AES project COL00271. 1999-2000 website. www.colostate.edu/depts/aes/projs/271.htm (Accessed 22 August 2000).

6734 Coulombe RA. Improve food safety through discovery and control of natural and induced toxicants and antitoxicants. Fedrip database, Natl Technical Info Svc (Ntis). Fedrip/1999/07801368.

6735 United Plant Savers. United Plant Savers at risk forum website. www.plantsavers.org/endanger2.html (Accessed 5 August 2000).

6736 Beck JJ, Stermitz FR. Addition of methyl thioglycolate and benzylamine to (Z)-ligustilide, a bioactive unsaturated lactone constituent of several herbal medicines. An improved synthesis of (Z)-ligustilide. *J Nat Prod* 1995;58:1047-55.

6738 Pipitone VR. Chondroprotection with chondroitin sulfate. *Drugs Exp Clin Res* 1991;17:3-7 .

6739 Sparks MJ, O'Sullivan P, Herrington AA, Morcos SK. Does peppermint oil relieve spasm during barium enema? *Br J Radiol* 1995;68:841-3.

6740 Madisch A, Heydenreich CJ, Wieland V, et al. Treatment of functional dyspepsia with a fixed peppermint oil and caraway oil combination preparation as compared to cisapride. A multicenter, reference-controlled, double-blind equivalence study. *Arzneimittelforschung* 1999;49:925-32.

6741 May B, Kuntz HD, Kieser M, Kohler S. Efficacy of a fixed peppermint oil/caraway oil combination in non-ulcer dyspepsia. *Arzneimittelforschung* 1996;46:1149-53.

6742 Micklefield GH, Greving I, May B. Effects of peppermint oil and caraway oil on gastroduodenal motility. *Phytother Res* 2000;14:20-3.

6743 Morton CA, Garioch J, Todd P, et al. Contact sensitivity to menthol and peppermint in patients with intra-oral symptoms. *Contact Dermatitis* 1995;32:281-4.

6744 Beesley A, Hardcastle J, Hardcastle PT, Taylor CJ. Influence of peppermint oil on absorptive and secretory processes in rat small intestine. *Gut* 1996;39:214-9.

6745 Shwaireb MH. Caraway oil inhibits skin tumors in female BALB/c mice. *Nutr Cancer* 1993;19:321-5.

6746 Herb Info Canada. Caraway website. www.herb.plant.org/caraway.htm (Accessed 11 September 2000).

6749 Leicester RJ, Hunt RH. Peppermint oil to reduce colonic spasm during endoscopy. *Lancet* 1982;2:989.

6750 Champault G, Patel JC, Bonnard AM. A double-blind trial of an extract of the plant Serenoa repens in benign prostatic hyperplasia. *Br J Clin Pharmacol* 1984;18:461-2.

6751 Braeckman J. The extract of serenoa repens in the treatment of benign prostatic hyperplasia: a multicenter open study. *Curr Ther Res* 1994;55:776-85.

6752 Reece-Smith H, Memon A, Smart CJ, Dewbury K. The value of permixon in benign prostatic hypertrophy. *Br J Urol* 1986;58:36-40.

6753 Lee YL, Owens J, Thrupp L, Cesario TC. Does cranberry juice have antibacterial activity? *JAMA* 2000;283:1691.

6754 Pedersen CB, Kyle J, Jenkinson AM, et al. Effects of blueberry and cranberry juice consumption on the plasma antioxidant capacity of healthy female volunteers. *Eur J Clin Nutr* 2000;54:405-8.

6755 Foo LY, Lu Y, Howell AB, Vorsa N. The structure of cranberry proanthocyanidins which inhibit adherence of uropathogenic P-fimbriated Escherichia coli in vitro. *Phytochemistry* 2000;54:173-81.

6756 Jepson RG, Mihaljevic L, Craig J. Cranberries for preventing urinary tract infections. *Cochrane Database Syst Rev*. 2001;(3):CD001321.

6757 Ofek I, Goldhar J, Zafriri D, et al. Anti-Escherichia coli adhesin activity of cranberry and blueberry juices. *N Engl J Med*. 1991;324:1599.

6758 Haverkorn MJ, Mandigers J. Reduction of bacteriuria and pyuria using cranberry juice. *JAMA* 1994;272:590.

6759 Foda MMR, Middlebrook PF, Gatfield CT, et al. Efficacy of cranberry in prevention of urinary tract infection in a susceptible pediatric population. *Can J Urol* 1995;2:98-102.

6760 Walker EB, Barney DP, Mickelsen JN, et al. Cranberry concentrate: UTI prophylaxis. *J Fam Pract* 1997;45:167-8.

6762 Wilt T, Ishani A, Stark G, et al. Serenoa repens for benign prostatic hyperplasia (Cochrane Review). In: The Cochrane Library, Issue 3, 2000. Oxford: Update Software.

6763 Sokeland J. Combined sabal and urtica extract compared with finasteride in men with benign prostatic hyperplasia: analysis of prostate volume and therapeutic outcome. *BJU Int* 2000;86:439-42.

6764 Boyle P, Robertson C, Lowe F, Roehrborn C. Meta-analysis of clinical trials of permixon in the treatment of symptomatic benign prostatic hyperplasia. *Urology* 2000;55:533-9.

6765 Di Silverio F, Monti S, Sciarra A, et al. Effects of long-term treatment with Serenoa repens (Permixon) on the concentrations and regional distribution of androgens and epidermal growth factor in benign prostatic hyperplasia. *Prostate* 1998;37:77-83.

6766 Di Silverio F, D'Eramo G, Lubrano C, et al. Evidence that Serenoa repens extract displays an antiestrogenic activity in prostatic tissue of benign prostatic hypertrophy patients. *Eur Urol* 1992;21:309-14.

6767 Calabrese C, Berman SH, Babish JG, et al. A phase I trial of andrographolide in HIV positive patients and normal volunteers. *Phytother Res* 2000;14:333-8.

6769 Levin RM, Das AK. A scientific basis for the therapeutic effects of Pygeum africanum and Serenoa repens. *Urol Res* 2000;28:201-9.

6770 Bayne CW, Ross M, Donnelly F, Habib FK. The selectivity and specificity of the actions of the lipido-sterolic extract of serenoa repens (permixon) on the prostate. *J Urol* 2000;164:876-81.

6771 Strauch G, Perles P, Vergult G, et al. Comparison of finasteride (Proscar) and Serenoa repens (Permixon) in the inhibition of 5-alpha reductase in healthy male volunteers. *Eur Urol* 1994;26:247-52.

6772 Stepanov VN, Siniakova LA, Sarrazin B, Raynaud JP. Efficacy and tolerability of the lipidosterolic extract of Serenoa repens (Permixon) in benign prostatic hyperplasia: a double-blind comparison of two dosage regimens. *Adv Ther* 1999;16:231-41.

6773 Bayne CW, Donnelly F, Ross M, Habib FK. Serenoa repens (Permixon): a 5 alpha-reductase types I and II inhibitor-new evidence in a coculture model of BPH. *Prostate* 1999;40:232-41.

6774 Sokeland J, Albrecht J. [Combination of Sabal and Urtica extract vs. finasteride in benign prostatic hyperplasia (Aiken stages I to II). Comparison of therapeutic effectiveness in a one year double-blind study]. [Article in German]. *Urologe A* 1997;36:327-33.

6775 Grasso M, Montesano A, Buonaguidi A, et al. Comparative effects of alfuzosin versus Serenoa repens in the treatment of symptomatic benign prostatic hyperplasia. *Arch Esp Urol* 1995;48:97-103.

6776 Adriazola-Semino M, Lozano-Ortega JL, Garcia-Cobo E, et al. [Symptomatic treatment of benign hypertrophy of the prostate. Comparative study of prazosin and serenoa repens]. [Article in Spanish]. *Arch Esp Urol* 1992; 45:211-3.

6777 Carbin BE, Larsson B, Lindahl O. Treatment of benign prostatic hyperplasia with phytosterols. *Br J Urol* 1990;66:639-41.

6778 Descotes JL, Rambeaud JJ, Deschaseaux P, Faure G. Placebo-controlled evaluation of the efficacy and tolerability of Permixon in benign prostatic hyperplasia after exclusion of placebo responders *Clin Drug Invest* 1995; 9:291-7.

6779 Paubert-Braquet M, Mencia Huerta JM, Cousse H, Braquet P. Effect of the lipidic lipidosterolic extract of Serenoa repens (Permixon) on the ionophore A23187-stimulated production of leukotriene B4 (LTB4) from human polymorphonuclear neutrophils. *Prostaglandins Leukot Essent Fatty Acids* 1997;57:299-304.

6780 Gutierrez M, Garcia de Boto MJ, Cantabrana B, Hidalgo A. Mechanisms involved in the spasmolytic effect of extracts from Sabal serrulata fruit on smooth muscle. *Gen Pharmacol* 1996;27:171-6.

6781 Roberts KL. A comparison of chilled cabbage leaves and chilled gelpaks in reducing breast engorgement. *J Hum Lact* 1995;11:17-20.

6782 Roberts KL, Reiter M, Schuster D. A comparison of chilled and room temperature cabbage leaves in treating breast engorgement. *J Hum Lact* 1995;11:191-4.

6783 Roberts KL, Reiter M, Schuster D. Effects of cabbage leaf extract on breast engorgement. *J Hum Lact* 1998;14:231-6.

6784 Nikodem VC, Danziger D, Gebka N, et al. Do cabbage leaves prevent breast engorgement? A randomized, controlled study. *Birth* 1993;20:61-4.

6785 Shifer P. Cabbage leaf enzymes. *J Hum Lact* 1995;11:264.

6786 Corrieri D. Cabbage leaves: an effective treatment for swollen tissues. *J Hum Lact* 1992;8:126-7.

6788 Lampe JW, King IB, Li S, et al. Brassica vegetables increase and apiaceous vegetables decrease cytochrome P450 1A2 activity in humans: changes in caffeine metabolite ratios in response to controlled vegetable diets. *Carcinogenesis* 2000;21:1157-62.

6789 Lust KD, Brown JE, Thomas W. Maternal intake of cruciferous vegetables and other foods and colic symptoms in exclusively breast-fed infants. *J Am Diet Assoc* 1996;96:46-8.

6790 Stoewsand GS. Bioactive organosulfur phytochemicals in Brassica oleracea vegetables-a review. *Food Chem Toxicol* 1995;33:537-43.

6791 Isbir T, Yaylim I, Aydin M, et al. The effects of Brassica oleraceae var capitata on epidermal glutathione and lipid peroxides in DMBA-initiated-TPA-promoted mice. *Anticancer Res* 2000;20:219-24.

6792 van Poppel G, Verhoeven DT, Verhagen H, Goldbohm RA. Brassica vegetables and cancer prevention. Epidemiology and mechanisms. *Adv Exp Med Biol* 1999;472:159-68.

6793 Yurtsever E, Yardimci KT. The in vivo effect of a Brassica oleracea var. capitata extract on Ehrlich ascites tumors of MUS musculus BALB/C mice. *Drug Metabol Drug Interact* 1999;15:215-22.

6794 Ballantyne CS, Phillips SM, MacDonald JR, et al. The acute effects of androstenedione supplementation in healthy young males. *Can J Appl Physiol* 2000;25:68-78.

6796 Weber B, Lewicka S, Deuschle M, et al. Testosterone, androstenedione and dihydrotestosterone concentrations are elevated in female patients with major depression. *Psychoneuroendocrinology* 2000;25:765-71.

6797 Douglas AS, Robins SP, Hutchison JD, et al. Carboxylation of osteocalcin in post-menopausal osteoporotic women following vitamin K and D supplementation. *Bone* 1995;17:15-20.

6798 Knapen MH, Hamulyak K, Vermeer C. The effect of vitamin K supplementation on circulating osteocalcin (bone Gla protein) and urinary calcium excretion. *Ann Intern Med* 1989;111:1001-5.

6799 Yonemura K, Kimura M, Miyaji T, Hishida A. Short-term effect of vitamin K administration on prednisolone-induced loss of bone mineral density in patients with chronic glomerulonephritis. *Calcif Tissue Int* 2000;66:123-8.

6800 Bierenbaum ML, Reichstein R, Watkins TR. Reducing atherogenic risk in hyperlipemic humans with flaxseed supplementation: a preliminary report. *J Am Coll Nutr* 1993;12:501-4.

6801 Lampe JW, Martini MC, Kurzer MS, et al. Urinary lignan and isoflavonoid excretion in premenopausal women consuming flaxseed powder. *Am J Clin Nutr* 1994;60:122-8.

6802 Clark WF, Parbtani A, Huff MW, et al. Flaxseed: a potential treatment for lupus nephritis. *Kidney Int* 1995;48:475-80.

6803 Cunnane SC, Hamadeh MJ, Liede AC, et al. Nutritional attributes of traditional flaxseed in healthy young adults. *Am J Clin Nutr* 1995;61:62-8.

6804 Merchant RE, Rice CD, Young HF. Dietary Chlorella pyrenoidosa for patients with malignant glioma: effects on immunocompetence, quality of life, and survival. *Phytother Res* 1990;4:220-31.

6805 Thompson LU, Rickard SE, Orcheson LJ, Seidl MM. Flaxseed and its lignan and oil components reduce mammary tumor growth at a late stage of carcinogenesis. *Carcinogenesis* 1996;17:1373-6.

6806 Prasad K. Dietary flax seed in prevention of hypercholesterolemic atherosclerosis. *Atherosclerosis* 1997;132:69-76.

6807 Prasad K, Mantha SV, Muir AD, Westcott ND. Reduction of hypercholesterolemic atherosclerosis by CDC-flaxseed with very low alpha-linolenic acid. *Atherosclerosis* 1998;136:367-75.

6808 Jenkins DJ, Kendall CWC, Vidgen E, et al. Health aspects of partially defatted flaxseed, including effects on serum lipids, oxidative measures, and ex vivo androgen and progestin activity: a controlled, crossover trial. *Am J Clin Nutr* 1999;69:395-402.

6809 Alonso L, Marcos ML, Blanco JG, et al. Anaphylaxis caused by linseed (flaxseed) intake. *J Allergy Clin Immunol* 1996;98:469-70.

6810 Brouwer IA, Verhoef P, Urgert R. Betaine supplementation and plasma homocysteine in healthy volunteers (letter). *Arch Intern Med* 2000;160:2546-7.

6811 Mar MH, Zeisel SH. Betaine in wine: answer to the French paradox? *Med Hypotheses* 1999;53:383-5.

6812 Soderling E, Le Bell A, Kirstila V, Tenovuo J. Betaine-containing toothpaste relieves subjective symptoms of dry mouth. *Acta Odontol Scand* 1998;56:65-9.

6813 Barak AJ, Beckenhauer HC, Tuma DJ. Betaine, ethanol, and the liver: a review. *Alcohol* 1996;13:395-8.

REFERENCES

6814 FDA News. Dietary Supplement Firms, Seasilver USA, Inc., and Americaloe, Inc., Sign Consent Decree With FDA TO Stop Selling Product Claiming To Cure "Over 650" Diseases. March 17, 2004.

6815 Lee B, Sue D. Xylitol for prevention of dental caries. *DICP* 1989;23:691-2.

6816 Uhari M, Kontiokari T, Koskela M, Niemela M. Xylitol chewing gum in prevention of acute otitis media: double-blind, randomized trial. *BMJ* 1996;313:1180-4.

6817 Uhari M, Kontiokari T, Niemela M. A novel use of xylitol sugar in preventing acute otitis media. *Pediatrics* 1998;102:879-84.

6818 Soderling E, Isokangas P, Pienihakkinen K, Tenovuo J. Influence of maternal xylitol consumption on acquisition of mutans streptococci by infants. *J Dent Res* 2000;79(3):882-7.

6819 Makinen KK. Can the pentitol-hexitol theory explain the clinical observations made with xylitol? *Med Hypotheses* 2000;54:603-13.

6820 Crapo PA. Use of alternative sweeteners in diabetic diet. *Diabetes Care* 1988;11:174-82.

6821 Makinen KK. The rocky road of xylitol to its clinical application. *J Dent Res* 2000;79:1352-5.

6822 Gales MA, Nguyen TM. Sorbitol compared with xylitol in prevention of dental caries. *Ann Pharmacother* 2000;34:98-100.

6823 Gronbaek M, Becker U, Johnasen D, et al. Type of alcohol consumed and mortality from all causes, coronary heart disease, and cancer. *Ann Intern Med* 2000;133:411-9.

6824 Galanis DJ, Joseph C, Masaki KH, et al. A longitudinal study of drinking and cognitive performance in elderly Japanese American men: the Honolulu-Asia aging study. *Am J Publ Health* 2000;90:1254-9.

6825 Ganry O, Baudoin C, Fardellone P. Effect of alcohol intake on bone mineral density in elderly women. *Am J Epidemiol* 2000;151:773-80.

6826 Caccetta RA, Croft KD, Beilin LJ, Puddey IB. Ingestion of red wine significantly increases plasma phenolic acid concentrations but does not acutely affect ex vivo lipoprotein oxidizability. *Am J Clin Nutr* 2000;71:67-74.

6827 Cooper HA, Exner DV, Domanski MJ. Light-to-moderate alcohol consumption and prognosis in patients with left ventricular systolic dysfunction. *J Am Coll Cardiol* 2000;35:1753-9.

6828 Durak I, Burak Cimen MY, Buyukkocak S, et al. The effect of red wine on blood antioxidant potential. *Curr Med Res Opin* 1999;15:208-13.

6829 Cervilla JA, Prince M, Joels S, et al. Long-term predictors of cognitive outcome in a cohort of older people with hypertension. *Br J Psychiatry* 2000;177:66-71.

6832 Van der Gaag MS, Ubbink JB, Sillanaukee P, et al. Effect of consumption of red wine, spirits, and beer on serum homocysteine. *Lancet* 2000;355:1522.

6833 Arimoto-Kobayashi S, Sugiyama C, Harada N, et al. Inhibitory effects of beer and other alcoholic beverages on mutagenesis and DNA adduct formation induced by several carcinogens. *J Agric Food Chem* 1999;47:221-30.

6834 Berger K, Ajani UA, Kase CS, et al. Light-to-moderate alcohol consumption and risk of stroke among US male physicians. *N Engl J Med* 1999;341:1557-64.

6835 Boffetta P, Garfinkel L. Alcohol drinking and mortality among men enrolled in an American Cancer Society prospective study. *Epidemiology* 1990;1:342-8.

6836 Feskanich D, Korrick SA, Greenspan SL, et al. Moderate alcohol consumption and bone density among postmenopausal women. *J Womens Health* 1999;8:65-73.

6837 Friedman LA, Kimball AW. Coronary heart disease mortality and alcohol consumption in Framingham. *Am J Epidemiol* 1986;124:481-9.

6838 Gaziano JM, Buring JE, Breslow JL, et al. Moderate alcohol intake, increased levels of high-density lipoprotein and its subfractions, and decreased risk of myocardial infarction. *N Engl J Med* 1993;329:1829-34.

6839 Gorinstein S, Zemser M, Berliner M, et al. Moderate beer consumption and positive biochemical changes in patients with coronary atherosclerosis. *J Intern Med* 1997;242:219-24.

6840 Kannel WB, Ellison RC. Alcohol and coronary heart disease: the evidence for a protective effect. *Clin Chim Acta* 1996;246:59-76.

6841 Langer RD, Criqui MH, Reed DM. Lipoproteins and blood pressure as biological pathways for effect of moderate alcohol consumption on coronary heart disease. *Circulation* 1992;85:910-5.

6842 Sacco RL, Elkind M, Boden-Albala B, et al. The protective effect of moderate alcohol consumption on ischemic stroke. *JAMA* 1999;281:53-60.

6843 Thun MJ, Peto R, Lopez AD, et al. Alcohol consumption and mortality among middle-aged and elderly US adults. *N Engl J Med* 1997;337:1705-14.

6844 Swain R, Kaplan-Machlis B. Magnesium for the next millennium. *South Med J* 1999;92:1040-7.

6845 Meyer KA, Kushi LH, Jacobs DR, et al. Carbohydrates, dietary fiber, and incident type 2 diabetes in older women. *Am J Clin Nutr* 2000;71:921-30.

6846 Crosby V, Wilcock A, Corcoran R. The safety and efficacy of a single dose (500 mg or 1 g) of intravenous magnesium sulfate in neuropathic pain poorly responsive to strong opioid analgesics in patients with cancer. *J Pain Symptom Manage* 2000;19:35-9.

6847 Bendich A. The potential for dietary supplements to reduce premenstrual syndrome (PMS) symptoms. *J Am Coll Nutr* 2000;19:3-12.

6848 Tramer MR, Schneider J, Marti RA, Rifat K. Role of magnesium sulfate in postoperative analgesia. *Anesthesiology* 1996;84:340-7.

6849 Vanpee D, Delgrange E, Gillet JB, Donckier J. Ingestion of antacid tablets (Rennie) and acute confusion. *J Emerg Med* 2000;19:169-71.

6850 Castelo-Branco C, Pons F, Vicente JJ, et al. Preventing postmenopausal bone loss with ossein-hydroxyapatite compounds. Results of a two-year, prospective trial. *J Reprod Med* 1999;44:601-5.

6851 Wolf RL, Cauley JA, Baker CE, et al. Factors associated with calcium absorption efficiency in pre- and perimenopausal women. *Am J Clin Nutr* 2000;72:466-71.

6852 Jorde R, Bonaa KH. Calcium from dairy products, vitamin D intake, and blood pressure: the Tromso study. *Am J Clin Nutr* 2000;71:1530-5.

6853 Dawson-Hughes B, Harris SS, Krall EA, Dallal GE. Effect of withdrawal of calcium and vitamin D supplements on bone mass in elderly men and women. *Am J Clin Nutr* 2000;72:745-50.

6854 Need AG, Horowitz M, Morris HA, Nordin BEC. Vitamin D status: effects on parathyroid hormone and 1,25-dihydroxyvitamin D in postmenopausal women. *Am J Clin Nutr* 2000;71:1577-81.

6855 Gesensway D. Vitamin D. *Ann Intern Med* 2000;133:318.

6856 Wortsman J, Matsuoka LY, Chen TC, et al. Decreased bioavailability of vitamin D in obesity. *Am J Clin Nutr* 2000;72:690-3.

6857 Shah M, Salhab N, Patterson D, Seikaly MG. Nutritional rickets still afflict children in north Texas. *Tex Med* 2000;96:64-8.

6858 Liu VJ, Abernathy RP. Chromium and insulin in young subjects with normal glucose tolerance. *Am J Clin Nutr* 1982;35:661-7.

6859 Anderson RA, Polansky MM, Bryden NA, et al. Effects of supplemental chromium on patients with symptoms of reactive hypoglycemia. *Metabolism* 1987;36:351-5.

6860 Trent LK, Thieding-Cancel D. Effects of chromium picolinate on body composition. *J Sports Med Phys Fitness* 1995;35:273-80.

6861 Lukaski HC, Bolonchuk WW, Siders WA, Milne DB. Chromium supplementation and resistance training: effects on body composition, strength, and trace element status of men. *Am J Clin Nutr* 1996;63:954-65.

6862 Hallmark MA, Reynolds TH, DeSouza CA, et al. Effects of chromium and resistive training on muscle strength and body composition. *Med Sci Sports Exerc* 1996;28:139-44.

6863 Stearns DM, Belbruno JJ, Wetterhahn KE. A prediction of chromium (III) accumulation in humans from chromium dietary supplements. *FASEB J* 1995;9:1650-7.

6864 Kaats GR, Blum K, Fisher JA, Adelman JA. Effects of chromium picolinate supplementation on body composition: a randomized, double-masked, placebo-controlled study. *Curr Ther Res* 1996;57:747-56.

6865 Campbell WW, Beard JL, Joseph LJ, et al. Chromium picolinate supplementation and resistive training by older men: effects on iron status and hematologic indexes. *Am J Clin Nutr* 1997;66:944-9.

6866 McCarty MF. Chromium supplementation and iron metabolism [letter]. *Am J Clin Nutr* 1997;65:890-2.

6867 Anderson RA, Cheng N, Bryden NA, et al. Elevated intakes of supplemental chromium improve glucose and insulin variables in individuals with type 2 diabetes. *Diabetes* 1997;46:1786-91.

6868 Kaats GR, Blum K, Pullin D, et al. A randomized, double-masked, placebo-controlled study of the effects of chromium picolinate supplementation on body composition: a replication and extension of a previous study. *Curr Ther Res* 1998;59:379-88.

6869 Vincent JB. The biochemistry of chromium. *J Nutr* 2000;130:715-8.

6871 Mahan LK, Escott-Stump S. Krause's Food, Nutrition, and Diet Therapy. 9th edition. W.B.Saunders Co., Philadelphia, PA, 1996.

6874 Yetiv JZ. Clinical applications of fish oils. *JAMA* 1988;260:665-70.

6875 Israel DH, Gorlin R. Fish oils in the prevention of atherosclerosis. *J Am Coll Cardiol* 1992;19:174-85.

6876 Mueller BA, Talbert RL. Biological mechanisms and cardiovascular effects of omega omega-3 fatty acids. *Clin Pharm* 1988;7:795-807.

6877 Darbinyan V, Kteyan A, Panossian A, et al. Rhodiola rosea in stress induced fatigue - a double blind cross-over study of a standardized extract SHR-5 with a repeated low-dose regimen on the mental performance of healthy physicians during night duty. *Phytomedicine* 2000;7(5):365-71.

6878 Force M, Sparks WS, Ronzio RA. Inhibition of enteric parasites by emulsified oil of oregano in vivo. *Phytother Res* 2000:14:213-4.

6879 Anon. Milk thistle: Effects on liver disease and cirrhosis and clinical adverse effects. Summary, Evidence Report/ Technology Assessment: Number 21, September 2000. Agency for Healthcare Research and Quality, Rockville, MD. Available at: www.ahrq.gov/clinic/milktsum.htm.

6880 Liberto M, Cobrinik D. Growth-factor dependent induction of p21(CIP1) by the green tea polyphenol, epigallocatechin gallate. *Cancer Lett* 2000;154(2):151-61.

6881 Srivastava RC, Husain MM, Hasan SK, Athar M. Green tea polyphenols and tannic acid act as potent inhibitors of phorbol ester-induced nitric oxide generation in rat hepatocytes independent of their antioxidant properties. *Cancer Lett* 2000;153(1-2):1-5.

6882 Kao Y, Hiipakka RA, Liao S. Modulation of obesity by green tea catechin. *Am J Clin Nutr* 2000;72:1232-41.

6883 Booth GL, Wang EE. Preventive health care, 2000 update: screening and management of hyperhomocysteinemia for the prevention of coronary artery disease events. The Canadian Task Force on Preventive Health Care. *CMAJ* 2000;163:21-9.

6884 Tremblay R, Bonnardeaux A, Geadah D, et al. Hyperhomocystinemia in hemodialysis patients: effects of 12-month supplementation with hydrosoluble vitamins. *Kidney Int* 2000;58:851-8.

6885 Boyde TRC. Pyridoxine supplements in the carpal tunnel syndrome (letter). *BMJ* 1995;311:631.

6886 Mukhtar H, Ahmad N. Tea polyphenols: prevention of cancer and optimizing health. *Am J Clin Nutr* 2000;71:1698S-1702S.

6887 Brinkhaus B, Lindner M, Schuppan D, Hahn EG. Chemical, pharmacological and clinical profile of the east Asian medical plant Centella asiatica. *Phytomedicine* 2000;7:427-48.

6888 Camargo CA, Stampfer MJ, Glynn RJ, et al. Moderate alcohol consumption and risk for angina pectoris or myocardial infarction in U.S. male physicians. *Ann Intern Med* 1997;126:372-5.

6889 Pearson TA. What to advise patients about drinking alcohol. The clinician's conundrum. *JAMA* 1994;272:967-8.

6890 Rehm JT, Bondy SJ, Sempos CT, Vuong CV. Alcohol consumption and coronary heart disease morbidity and mortality. *Am J Epidemiol* 1997;146:495-501.

6891 Rimm EB, Chan J, Stampfer MJ, et al. Prospective study of cigarette smoking, alcohol use and the risk of diabetes in men. *Br Med J* 1995;310:555-9.

6892 Goldberg I, Mosca L, Piano MR, Fisher EA. AHA Science Advisory: Wine and your heart: a science advisory for healthcare professionals from the Nutrition Committee, Council on Epidemiology and Prevention, and Council on Cardiovascular Nursing of the American Heart Association. *Circulation* 2001;103:472-5.

6893 Malarcher AM, Giles WH, Croft JB, et al. Alcohol intake, type of beverage, and the risk of cerebral infarction in young women. *Stroke* 2001;32:77-83.

6894 Ridker PM, Vaughan DE, Stampfer MJ, et al. Association of moderate alcohol consumption and plasma concentration of endogenous tissue-type plasminogen activator. *JAMA* 1994;272:929-33.

6895 Nadir A, Reddy D, Van Thiel DH. Cascara-sagrada induced intrahepatic cholestasis causing portal hypertension: case report and review of herbal hepatotoxicity. *Am J Gastroenterol* 2000;95:3634-7.

6896 Feskens EJM, Oomen CM, Hogendoorn E, et al. Arginine intake and 25-year CHD mortality: the seven countries study (letter). *Eur Heart J* 2001;22:611-2.

6897 Ackermann RT, Mulrow CD, Ramirez G, et al. Garlic shows promise for improving some cardiovascular risk factors. *Arch Intern Med* 2001;161:813-24.

6898 Anon. Epidemiological notes and reports: Macuna pruriens-associated pruritus, New Jersey. *MMWR Morb Mortal Wkly Rep* 1985;34(48):732-3.

6899 Nagashayana N, Sankarankutty P, Nampoothiri MRV, et al. Association of l-DOPA with recovery following Ayurveda medication in Parkinson's Disease. *J Neurol Sci* 2000;176:124-7.

6900 Houang ET, Ahmet Z, Lawrence AG. Successful treatment of four patients with recalcitrant vaginal trichomoniasis with a combination of zinc sulfate douche and metronidazole therapy. *Sex Transm Dis* 1997;24:116-9.

6901 Stromberg HE, Agren MS. Topical zinc oxide treatment improves arterial and venous leg ulcers. *Br J Dermatol* 1984;111:461-8.

REFERENCES

6902 Wilkinson EA, Hawke CI. Oral zinc for arterial and venous leg ulcers. *Cochrane Database Syst Rev* 2000;2:CD001273.

6903 Sandstrom B, Kivisto B, Cederblad A. Absorption of zinc from soy protein meals in humans. *J Nutr* 1987;117:321-7.

6905 Birmingham CL, Goldner EM, Bakan R. Controlled trial of zinc supplementation in anorexia nervosa. *Int J Eat Disord* 1994;15:251-5.

6906 Katz RL, Keen CL, Litt IF, et al. Zinc deficiency in anorexia nervosa. *J Adolesc Health Care* 1987;8:400-6.

6908 Lagiou P, Wuu J, Trichopoulou A, et al. Diet and benign prostatic hyperplasia: a study in Greece. *Urology* 1999;54:284-90.

6909 Zaichick VYe, Sviridova TV, Zaichick SV. Zinc in the human prostate gland: normal, hyperplastic and cancerous. *Int Urol Nephrol* 1997;29:565-74.

6910 Zaichick VY, Sviridova TV, Zaichick SV. Zinc concentration in human prostatic fluid: normal, chronic prostatitis, adenoma and cancer. *Int Urol Nephrol* 1996;28:687-94.

6911 Ewing CI, Gibbs AC, Ashcroft C, David TJ. Failure of oral zinc supplementation in atopic eczema. *Eur J Clin Nutr* 1991;45:507-10.

6912 David TJ, Wells FE, Sharpe TC, et al. Serum levels of trace metals in children with atopic eczema. *Br J Dermatol* 1990;122:485-9.

6913 Mulder TP, van der Sluys Veer A, Verspaget HW, et al. Effect of oral zinc supplementation on metallothionein and superoxide dismutase concentrations in patients with inflammatory bowel disease. *J Gastroenterol Hepatol* 1994;9:472-7.

6914 Sjogren A, Floren CH, Nilsson A. Evaluation of zinc status in subjects with Crohn's disease. *J Am Coll Nutr* 1988;7:57-60.

6915 Van de Wal Y, Van der Sluys Veer A, Verspaget HW, et al. Effect of zinc therapy on natural killer cell activity in inflammatory bowel disease. *Aliment Pharmacol Ther* 1993;7:281-6.

6916 Dronfield MW, Malone JD, Langman MJ. Zinc in ulcerative colitis: a therapeutic trial and report on plasma levels. *Gut* 1977;18:33-6.

6917 Naber TH, van den Hamer CJ, Baadenhuysen H, Jansen JB. The value of methods to determine zinc deficiency in patients with Crohn's disease. *Scand J Gastroenterol* 1998;33:514-23.

6918 Relea P, Revilla M, Ripoll E, et al. Zinc, biochemical markers of nutrition, and type I osteoporosis. *Age Ageing* 1995;24:303-7.

6920 Atik OS. Zinc and senile osteoporosis. *J Am Geriatr Soc* 1983;31:790-1.

6921 Paaske PB, Pedersen CB, Kjems G, Sam IL. Zinc in the management of tinnitus. Placebo-controlled trial. *Ann Otol Rhinol Laryngol* 1991;100:647-9.

6923 Allen LH, Rosado JL, Casterline JE, et al. Lack of hemoglobin response to iron supplementation in anemic Mexican preschoolers with multiple micronutrient deficiencies. *Am J Clin Nutr* 2000;71:1485-94.

6924 Mujika I, Padilla S, Ibanez J, et al. Creatine supplementation and sprint performance in soccer players. *Med Sci Sports Exerc* 2000;32:518-25.

6925 Francaux M, Demeure R, Goudemant JF, Poortmans JR. Effect of exogenous creatine supplementation on muscle PCr metabolism. *Int J Sports Med* 2000;21:139-45.

6926 Rico-Sanz J, Mendez Marco MT. Creatine enhances oxygen uptake and performance during alternating intensity exercise. *Med Sci Sports Exerc* 2000;32:379-85.

6927 Rico-Sanz J. Creatine reduces human muscle PCr and pH decrements and P(i) accumulation during low-intensity exercise. *J Appl Physiol* 2000;88:1181-91.

6928 Becque MD, Lochmann JD, Melrose DR. Effects of oral creatine supplementation on muscular strength and body composition. *Med Sci Sports Exerc* 2000;32:654-8.

6929 Willer B, Stucki G, Hoppeler H, et al. Effects of creatine supplementation on muscle weakness in patients with rheumatoid arthritis. *Rheumatology* (Oxford) 2000;39:293-8.

6930 Checking in on creatine: three studies shed light on physiological response to popular supplement. NCAA. 2000 Apr24. www.ncaa.org/news/20000424/active/3709n45.html (Accessed 19 July 2000).

6931 Ead RD. Oral zinc sulphate in alopacia areata- a double-blind trial. *Br J Dermatol* 1981;104:483-4.

6932 Camacho FM, Garcia-Hernandez MJ. Zinc aspartate, biotin, and clobetasol propionate in the treatment of alopecia areata in childhood. *Pediatr Dermatol* 1999;16:336-8.

6933 Pattrick M, Heptinstall S, Doherty M. Feverfew in rheumatoid arthritis: a double-blind, placebo-controlled study. *Ann Rheum Dis* 1989;48:547-9.

6935 Awang DVC. Prescribing therapeutic feverfew [Tancetum pathrnium (L.) Schultz Bip., syn. Chrysanthemumparthenium (L.) Bernh.]. *Int Med* 1998;1:11-3.

6936 Heptinstall S, Groenewegen WA, Spangenberg P, Loesche W. Extracts of feverfew may inhibit platelet behaviour via neutralization of sulphydryl groups. *J Pharm Pharmacol* 1987;39:459-65.

6937 Wong HC. Is feverfew a pharmacologic agent? *CMAJ* 1999;160:21-2.

6938 de Weerdt GJ, Bootsman HPR, Hendriks H. Herbal medicines in migraine prevention. Randomized double-blind, placebo-controlled, crossover trial of a feverfew preparation. *Phytomedicine* 1996;3:225-30.

6939 Sumner H, Salan U, Knight DW, Hoult JR. Inhibition of 5-lipoxygenase and cyclo-oxygenase in leukocytes by feverfew. Involvement of sesquiterpene lactones and other components. *Biochem Pharmacol* 1992;43:2313-20.

6941 Williams CA, Hoult JR, Harborne JB, et al. A biologically active lipophilic flavonol from Tanacetum parthenium. *Phytochemistry* 1995;38:267-70.

6942 Heptinstall S, White A, Williamson L, Mitchell JR. Extracts of feverfew inhibit granule secretion in blood platelets and polymorphonuclear leucocytes. *Lancet* 1985;1:1071-4.

6943 Makheja AN, Bailey JM. A platelet phospholipase inhibitor from the medicinal herb feverfew (Tanacetum parthenium). *Prostaglandins Leukot Med* 1982;8:653-60.

6944 Groenewegen WA, Heptinstall S. A comparison of the effects of an extract of feverfew and parthenolide, a component of feverfew, on human platelet activity in-vitro. *J Pharm Pharmacol* 1990;42:553-7.

6945 Heptinstall S, Groenewegen WA, Spangenberg P, Losche W. Inhibition of platelet behaviour by feverfew: a mechanism of action involving sulphydryl groups. *Folia Haematol Int Mag Klin Morphol Blutforsch* 1988;115:447-9.

6946 Williams CA, Harborne JB, Geiger H, Hoult JR. The flavonoids of Tanacetum parthenium and T. vulgare and their anti-inflammatory properties. *Phytochemistry* 1999;51:417-23.

6947 Jain NK, Kulkarni SK. Antinociceptive and anti-inflammatory effects of Tanacetum parthenium L. extract in mice and rats. *J Ethnopharmacol* 1999;68:251-9.

6948 Barsby R, Salan U, Knight DW, Hoult JR. Irreversible inhibition of vascular reactivity by feverfew. *Lancet* 1991;338:1015.

6949 Barsby RW, Salan U, Knight DW, Hoult JR. Feverfew and vascular smooth muscle: extracts from fresh and dried plants show opposing pharmacological profiles, dependent upon sesquiterpene lactone content. *Planta Med* 1993;59:20-5.

6950 Barsby RW, Salan U, Knight DW, Hoult JR. Feverfew extracts and parthenolide irreversibly inhibit vascular responses of the rabbit aorta. *J Pharm Pharmacol* 1992;44:737-40.

6951 Biggs MJ, Johnson ES, Persaud NP, Ratcliffe DM. Platelet aggregation in patients using feverfew for migraine. *Lancet* 1982;2:776.

6953 Makheja AN, Bailey JM. The active principle in feverfew. *Lancet* 1981;2:1054.

6954 Collier HO, Butt NM, McDonald-Gibson WJ, Saeed SA. Extract of feverfew inhibits prostaglandin biosynthesis. *Lancet* 1980;2:922-3.

6955 Heptinstall S, Awang DV, Dawson BA, et al. Parthenolide content and bioactivity of feverfew (Tanacetum parthenium (L.) Schultz-Bip.). Estimation of commercial and authenticated feverfew products. *J Pharm Pharmacol* 1992;44:391-5.

6956 Groenewegen WA, Heptinstall S. Amounts of feverfew in commercial preparations of the herb. *Lancet* 1986;1:44-5.

6957 Ross JJ, Arnason JT, Birnboim HC. Low concentrations of the feverfew component parthenolide inhibit in vitro growth of tumor lines in a cytostatic fashion. *Planta Med* 1999;65:126-9.

6958 Lamminpaa A, Estlander T, Jolanki R, Kanerva L. Occupational allergic contact dermatitis caused by decorative plants. *Contact Dermatitis* 1996;34:330-5.

6959 Johnson ES, Kadam NP, Hylands DM, Hylands PJ. Efficacy of feverfew as prophylactic treatment of migraine. *Br Med J* (Clin Res Ed) 1985;291:569-73.

6960 Murphy JJ, Heptinstall S, Mitchell JR. Randomized, double-blind, placebo-controlled trial of feverfew in migraine prevention. *Lancet* 1988;2:189-92.

6961 Palevitch D, Earon G, Carasso R. Feverfew (tanacetum parthenium) as a prophylactic treatment for migraine- a double-blind, placebo-controlled study. *Phytotherapy Res* 1997;11:508-11.

6962 Anderson D, Jenkinson PC, Dewdney RS, et al. Chromosomal aberrations and sister chromatid exchanges in lymphocytes and urine mutagenicity of migraine patients: a comparison of chronic feverfew users and matched non-users. *Hum Toxicol* 1988;7:145-52.

6964 Waller PC, Ramsay LE. Efficacy of feverfew as prophylactic treatment of migraine. *Br Med J* (Clin Res Ed) 1985;291:1128.

6965 Vogler BK, Pittler MH, Ernst E. Feverfew as a preventive treatment for migraine: a systematic review. *Cephalalgia* 1998;18:704-8.

6969 Calapai G, Firenzuoli F, Saitta A, et al. Antiobesity and cardiovascular toxic effects of Citrus aurantium extracts in the rat: A preliminary report. *Fitoterapia* 1999;70:586-92.

6971 Carnat A, Carnat AP, Fraisse D, Lamaison JL. [Standardization of the sour orange flower and leaf]. [Article in French]. *Ann Pharm Fr* 1999;57:410-4.

6972 Ramadan W, Mourad B, Ibrahim S, Sonbol F. Oil of bitter orange: new topical antifungal agent. *Int J Dermatol* 1996;35:448-9.

6973 Mwaiko GL. Citrus peel oil extracts as mosquito larvae insecticides. *East Afr Med J* 1992;69:223-6.

6974 Satoh Y, Tashiro S, Satoh M, et al. [Studies on the bioactive constituents of Aurantii Fructus Immaturus]. [Article in Japanese]. *Yakugaku Zasshi* 1996;116:244-50.

6975 Huang YT, Wang GF, Chen CF, et al. Fructus aurantii reduced portal pressure in portal hypertensive rats. *Life Sci* 1995;57:2011-20.

6976 Kim DH, Song MJ, Bae EA, Han MJ. Inhibitory effect of herbal medicines on rotavirus infectivity. *Biol Pharm Bull* 2000;23:356-8.

6977 Hernandez L, Munoz RA, Miro G, et al. Use of medicinal plants by ambulatory patients in Puerto Rico. *Am J Hosp Pharm* 1984;41:2060-4.

6978 Zhao XW, Li JX, Zhu ZR, et al. Anti-shock effects of synthetic effective compositions of fructus aurantii immaturus. Experimental study and clinical observation. *Chin Med J* (Engl) 1989;102:91-3.

6979 Keogh AM, Baron DW. Sympathomimetic abuse and coronary artery spasm. *Br Med J* 1985;291:940.

6981 Quackwatch. Unconventional cancer treatments: dietary treatments. www.quackwatch.com/01QuackeryRelatedTopics/OTA/ota03.html.

6982 Nenonen MT, Helve TA, Rauma AL, Hanninen OO. Uncooked, lactobacilli-rich, vegan food and rheumatoid arthritis. *Br J Rheumatol* 1998;37:274-81.

6983 Bargossi AM, Battino M, Gaddi A, et al. Exogenous CoQ10 preserves plasma ubiquinone levels in patients treated with 3-hydroxy-3-methylglutaryl coenzyme A reductase inhibitors. *Int J Clin Lab Res* 1994;24:171-6.

6984 Folkers K, Langsjoen P, Willis R, et al. Lovastatin decreases coenzyme Q levels in humans. *Proc Natl Acad Sci U S A* 1990;87:8931-4.

6985 Ghirlanda G, Oradei A, Manto A, et al. Evidence of plasma CoQ10-lowering effect by HMG-CoA reductase inhibitors: a double-blind, placebo-controlled study. *J Clin Pharmacol* 1993;33:226-9.

6986 Mortensen SA, Leth A, Agner E, Rohde M. Dose-related decrease of serum coenzyme Q10 during treatment with HMG-CoA reductase inhibitors. *Mol Aspects Med* 1997;18:S137-S144.

6987 Georgetown Univ Med Center. Cytochrome P450 interaction table. Available at: www. dml.georgetown.edu/depts/pharmacology.davetab.html.

6988 Wang J, Lu A, Chi J. Multicenter clinical trial of the serum lipid-lowering effects of a monascus purpureus (red yeast) rice preparation from traditional Chinese medicine. *Cur Ther Res* 1997;58:964-78.

6990 Am Heart Assn. Am Heart Assn meeting report: Chinese condiment cuts blood cholesterol. www.americanheart.org/Whats_News/AHA_News_Releases/03-25-99-chinese.html (Accessed 2 August 2000).

6991 Am Heart Assn. Comment: the Am Heart Assn urges caution on cholestin. www.americanheart.org/Whats_News/AHA_News_Releases/03-25-99-comment.htm (Accessed 2 August 2000).

6993 Kou W, Lu Z, Guo J. [Effect of xuezhikang on the treatment of primary hyperlipidemia]. [Article in Chinese]. *Chung Hua Nei Ko Tsa Chih* 1997;36:529-31.

6994 US Dept Health, Human Services, FDA. Pharmanex, Inc, administrative proceeding, public docket #97P-0441: final decision. Available at: www.fda.gov/ohrms/dockets/dockets/97p0441/ans0002.pdf .

6995 Havel R. Dietary supplement or drug? The case of Cholestin. *Am J Clin Nutr* 1000;69:175-6.

6996 Bliznakov EG. More on the Chinese red-yeast-rice supplement and its cholesterol-lowering effect. *Am J Clin Nutr* 2000;71:152-7.

6997 Wigger-Alberti W, Bauer A, Hipler UC, Elsner P. Anaphylaxis due to Monascus purpureus-fermented rice (red yeast rice). *Allergy* 1999;54:1330-1.

6998 Jacobs KM, Hirsch KA. Psychiatric complications of Ma-huang. *Psychosomatics* 2000;41:58-62.

6999 Federal Trade Commission. FTC Action against Lane Laboratories. Available at: www.ftc.gov/opa/2000/06/lanelabs.htm.

7000 Greenberg S, Frishman WH. Co-enzyme Q10: a new drug for cardiovascular disease. *J Clin Pharmacol* 1990;30:596-608.

7001 Deenstra M, Haalboom JRE, Struyvenberg A. Decrease of plasma potassium due to inhalation of beta-2-agonists: absence of an additional effect of intravenous theophylline. *Eur J Clin Invest* 1988;18:162-5.

7002 Stockley I. Drug Interactions, 4th ed. London, UK: Pharmaceut Press, 1996.

7005 Locock RA. Capsicum. *Can Pharm J* 1985;118:517-9.

7006 Visudhiphan S, Poolsuppasit S, Piboonnukarintr O, Timliang S. The relationship between high fibrinolytic activity and daily capsicum ingestion in Thais. *Am J Clin Nutr* 1982;35:1452-8.

7007 Cordell GA, Araujo OE. Capsaicin: identification, nomenclature, and pharmacotherapy. *Ann Pharmacother* 1993;27:330-6.

7008 Avorn J, Manone M, Gurwitz JH, et al. Reduction of bacteriuria and pyuria after ingestion of cranberry juice. *JAMA* 1994;271:751-4.

7010 Brown D. Herbal Prescriptions for Better Health. Rocklin, CA: Prima Publishing, 1996.

7011 Amann W. [Akne vulgaris und agnus castus (Agnolyt)]. [Article in German]. *Z Allgemeinmed* 1975;14:1645-7.

7012 Du Mee C. Vitex agnus castus. *Aust J Med Herb* 1993;5:63-5.

7013 Brown D. Vitex agnus castus clinical monograph. *Qtrly Rev Natural Med* 1994;2:111-21.

7014 Wuttke W. Dopaminergic action of extracts of Agnus Castus. *Forschende Komplementarmedizen* 1996;3:329-30.

7015 Jarry H, Leonhardt S., Gorkow C, Wuttke W. In vitro prolactin but not LH and FSH release is inhibited by compounds in extracts of Agnus Castus: direct evidence for a dopaminergic principle by the dopamine receptor assay. *Exp Clin Endocrinol* 1994;102:448-54.

7016 Merz P, Gorkow C, Schroder A, et al. The effects of a special Agnus castus extract (BP1095el) on prolactin secretion in healthy male subjects. *Exp Clin Endocrinol Diabetes* 1996;104:447-53.

7020 HP-200 in Parkinson's Disease study group. An alternative medicine treatment for Parkinson's disease: Results of a multicenter clinical trial. *J Altern Complement Med* 1995;1(3):249-55.

7021 Infante ME, Perez AM, Simao MR, et al. Outbreak of acute toxic psychosis attributed to Mucuna pruriens. *Lancet* 1990;336:1129.

7022 Helbling A, Brander KA, Pichler WJ. Anaphylactic shock after subcutaneous injection of mandragora D3, a homeopathic drug. *J Allergy Clin Immunol* 2000;106 (5 pt 1):989-90.

7023 Dean CE. Prasterone (DHEA) and mania. *Ann Pharmacother* 2000;34:1419-22.

7024 Escher M, Desmeules J, Giostra E, Mentha G. Drug Points: hepatitis associated with kava, a herbal remedy for anxiety. *BMJ* 2001;322:139.

7025 Zhang SY, Robertson D. A study of tea tree oil ototoxicity. *Audiol Neurootol* 2000;5:64-8.

7026 Reginster JY, Deroisy R, Rovati LC, et al. Long-term effects of glucosamine sulfate on osteoarthritis progression: a randomized, placebo-controlled trial. *Lancet* 2001;357:251-6.

7027 Piscitelli SC, Burstein AH, Welden N, et al. The effect of garlic supplements on the pharmacokinetics of saquinavir. *Clin Infect Dis* 2002;34:234-8.

7028 Rayburn K, Martinez R, Escobedo M, et al. Glycemic effects of various species of nopal (Opuntia sp.) in type 2 diabetes mellitus. *Texas J Rural Health* 1998;26:68-76.

7029 Malhotra S, Bailey DG, Paine MF, Watkins PB. Seville orange juice-felodipine interaction: comparison with dilute grapefruit juice and involvement of furocoumarins. *Clin Pharmacol Ther* 2001;69:14-23.

7030 Gregory PJ. Seizure associated with Ginkgo biloba? *Ann Intern Med* 2001;134:344.

7031 Buck DS, Nidorf DM, Addino JG. Comparison of two topical preparations for the treatment of onychomycosis: Melaleuca alternifolia (Tea Tree) oil and clotrimazole. *J Fam Pract* 1994;38:601-5.

7032 Syed TA, Qureshi ZA, Ali SM, et al. Treatment of toenail onychomycosis with 2% butenafine and 5% Melaleuca alternifolia (tea tree) oil in cream. *Trop Med Int Health* 1999;4:284-7.

7033 Tsubono Y, Nishino Y, Komatsu S, et al. Green tea and the risk of gastric cancer in Japan. *N Engl J Med* 2001;344:632-6.

7034 Sano T, Sasako M. Green tea and gastric cancer. *N Engl J Med* 2001;344:675-6.

7035 Mittman P. Randomized, double-blind study of freeze-dried Urtica dioica in the treatment of allergic rhinitis. *Planta Med* 1990;56:44-7.

7038 McCarty DJ, Csuka M, McCarthy G, et al. Treatment of pain due to fibromyalgia with topical capsaicin: A pilot study. *Semin Arthr Rheum* 1994;23:41-7.

7039 Natl Cancer Inst. Mistletoe (PDQ). CancerNet. www.cancernet.nci.nih.gov/cam/mistletoe.htm#7 (Accessed 30 March 2001).

7040 Lissoni P, Barni S, Mandala M, et al. Decreased toxicity and increased efficacy of cancer chemotherapy using the pineal hormone melatonin in metastatic solic tumor patients with poor clinical status. *Eur J Cancer* 1999;35:1688-92.

7041 Kliukiene J, Tynes T, Andersen A. Risk of breast cancer among Norwegian women with visual impairment. *Br J Cancer* 2001;84:397-9.

7042 Erren TC, Piekarski C. Does winter darkness in the arctic protect against cancer? The melatonin hypothesis revisited. *Med Hypotheses* 1999;53:1-5.

7043 Lissoni P, Barni S, Meregalli S, et al. Modulation of cancer endocrine therapy by melatonin: a phase II study of tamoxifen plus melatonin in metastatic breast cancer patients progressing under tamoxifen alone. *Br J Cancer* 1995;71:854-6.

7044 Kaegi E. Unconventional therapies for cancer: 3. Iscador. *CMAJ* 1998;158:1157-9.

7045 Grossarth-Matichek R, Kiene H, Baumgartner SM, et al. Use of Iscador, an extract of European mistletoe (Viscum album), in cancer treatment: prospective nonrandomized and randomized matched-pair studies nested within a cohort study. *Alt Thera* 2001;7:57-78.

7046 Bailey DG, Dresser GK, Munoz C, et al. Reduction of fexofenadine bioavailability by fruit juices. *Clin Pharmacol Ther* 2001;69:P21.

7047 Sindrup SH, Madsen C, Bach FW, et al. St. John's wort has no effect on pain in polyneuropathy. *Pain* 2000;91:361-5.

7048 Bliddal H, Rosetzsky A, Schlichting P, et al. A randomized, placebo-controlled, cross-over study of ginger extracts and ibuprofen in osteoarthritis. *Osteoarthritis Cartilage* 2000;8:9-12.

7049 Holtmann G, Madisch A, Juergen H, et al. A double-blind, randomized, placebo-controlled trial on the effects of an herbal preparation in patients with functional dyspepsia [Abstract]. Ann Mtg Digestive Disease Week 1999 May.

7050 Fabre N, Urizzi P, Souchard JP, et al. An antioxidant sinapic acid ester isolated from Iberis amara. *Fitoterapia* 2000;71:425-8.

7051 Steimer P. Iberogast therapy in gastroenterology. *Der Krankenhaus Arzt* 1983;56:1005-8.

7052 Roberts W, Weaver L, Brian J, et al. Repeated doses of porcine secretin in the treatment of autism: A randomized, placebo-controlled trial. *Pediatrics* 2001;107:e71.

7053 Mulvihill SJ, Debas HT. Regulatory peptides in the gut. In: Greenspan FS, Strewler GJ, Eds. Basic & Clinical

Endocrinology. 5th ed. Stamford, CT: Appleton & Lange, 1997:581.
7054 Jacobson JS, Troxel AB, Evans J, et al. Randomized trial of black cohosh for the treatment of hot flashes among women with a history of breast cancer. *J Clin Oncol* 2001;19:2739-45.
7055 Schellenberg R. Treatment for the premenstrual syndrome with agnus castus fruit extract: prospective, randomized, placebo-controlled study. *Br Med J* 2001;322:134-7.
7056 Gallo M, Sarkar M, Au W, et al. Pregnancy outcome following gestational exposure to echinacea: A prospective controlled study. *Arch Intern Med* 2000;160:3141-3.
7057 Soon SL, Crawford RI. Recurrent erythema nodosum associated with echinacea herbal therapy. *J Am Acad Dermatol* 2001;44:298-9.
7058 Davies S, Howard JM, Hunnisett A, et al. Age-related decreases in chromium levels in 51,665 hair, sweat, and serum samples from 40,872 patients – implications for the prevention of cardiovascular disease and type II diabetes. *Metabolism* 1997;46:469-73.
7059 Melchart D, Linde K, Fischer P, Kaesmayr J. Echinacea for preventing and treating the common cold. *Cochrane Database Syst Rev* 2000;2:CD000530.
7060 Abraham AS, Brooks BA, Eylath U. The effects of chromium supplementation on serum glucose and lipids in patients with and without non-insulin dependent diabetes. *Metabolism* 1992;41:768-71.
7061 Gregory PJ. Minerals for diabetes. *Pharmacist's Letter/ Prescriber's Letter* 2000;16:160212.
7062 Steben RE, Boudroux P. The effects of pollen and pollen extracts on selected blood factors and performance of athletes. *J Sports Med Phys Fitness* 1978;18:271-8.
7063 Maughan RJ, Evans SP. Effects of pollen extract upon adolescent swimmers. *Br J Sports Med* 1982;16:142-5.
7064 Sur S, Camara M, Buchmeier A, et al. Double-blind trial of pyridoxine (vitamin B6) in the treatment of steroid-dependent asthma. *Ann Allergy* 1993;70:147-52.
7065 Collipp PJ, Goldzier S III, Weiss N, et al. Pyridoxine treatment of childhood bronchial asthma. *Ann Allergy* 1975;35:93-7.
7066 Shimizu T, Maeda S, Mochizuki H, et al. Theophylline attenuates circulating vitamin B6 levels in children with asthma. *Pharmacology* 1994;49:392-7.
7067 FDA. Information paper on L-tryptophan and 5-hydroxy-L-tryptophan. Office of Nutritional Products, Labeling, Dietary Supplements. Center for Food Safety and Applied Nutrition. February 2001.
7068 Russmann S, Lauterberg BH, Hebling A. Kava hepatotoxicity [letter]. *Ann Intern Med* 2001;135:68.
7069 Hu X, et al. Antilipemic effect of Gynostemma pentaphyllum in patients. *Fujian Med J* 1988;10:4-6.
7070 Zhou H, et al. Treatment of hyperlipidemia with Gynostemma pentaphyllum jiaogulan. *Hunan Med J* 1991;8:259-60.
7071 Tan H, Liu ZL, Liu MJ. Antithrombotic effect of Gynostemma pentaphyllum. *Zhongguo Zhong Xi Yi Jie He Za Zhi* 1993;13:278-80.
7072 de Lemos ML. Effects of soy phytoestrogens genistein and daidzein on breast cancer growth. *Ann Pharmacother* 2001;35:1118-21.
7073 Massey LK, Palmer RG, Horner HT. Oxalate content of soybean seeds (Glycine max. Leguminosae), soyfoods, and other edible legumes. *J Agric Food Chem* 2001;49:4262-6.
7074 Terris MK, Issa MM, Tacker JR. Dietary supplementation with cranberry concentrate tablets may increase the risk of nephrolithiasis. *Urology* 2001;57:26-9.
7075 Gregory PJ. Does glucosamine increase serum lipid levels and blood pressure? *Pharmacist's Letter/Prescriber's Letter* 2001;17:171115.
7076 Lauritzen CH, Reuter HD, Repges R, et al. Treatment of premenstrual tension syndrome with Vitex agnus castus: Controlled-double blind versus pyridoxine. *Phytomedicine* 1997;4:183-9.
7077 Gerhard II, Patek A, Monga B, et al. Mastodynon for female infertility. *Forsch Komplementarmed* 1998;5:272-8.
7078 Berger D. Schaffner W, Schrader E, et al. Efficacy of Vitex agnus castus L. extract Ze 440 in patients with premenstrual syndrome (PMS). *Arch Gynecol Obstet* 2000;264:150-3.
7079 Loch EG, Selle H, Boblitz N. Treatment of premenstrual syndrome with a phytopharmaceutical formulation containing Vitex agnus castus. *J Womens Health Gend Based Med* 2000;9:315-20.
7080 Shaver K. Potassium iodide for nuclear exposure. *Pharmacist's Letter/Prescriber's Letter* 2001;17:171214.
7081 Zhdanova IV, Wurtman RJ, Regan MM, et al. Melatonin treatment for age-related insomnia. *J Clin Endocrinol Metab* 2001;86:4727-30.
7082 Shamir E, Barak Y, Shalman I, et al. Melatonin treatment for tardive dyskinesia: A double-blind, placebo-controlled, crossover study. *Arch Gen Psychiatry* 2001;58:1049-52.
7083 Backon J. Ginger in preventing nausea and vomiting of pregnancy: a caveat due to its thromboxane synthetase activity and effect on testosterone binding. *Eur J Obstet Gynecol Reprod Biol* 1991;42:163-4.
7084 Altman RD, Marcussen KC. Effects of ginger extract on knee pain in patients with osteoarthritis. *Arthritis Rheum* 2001;44:2531-38.
7085 Marcus DM, Suarez-Almazor ME. Is there a role for ginger in the treatment of osteoarthritis? *Arthritis Rheum* 2001;44:2461-2.
7086 Shaver K. Liver toxicity with kava. *Pharmacist's Letter/ Prescriber's Letter* 2001;18:180115.
7087 Vonau B, Chard S, Mandalia S, et al. Does the extract of the plant Echinacea purpurea influence the clinical course of recurrent genital herpes? *Int J STD AIDS* 2001;12:154-8.
7088 Lee SH, Oe T, Blair IA. Vitamin C-induced decomposition of lipid hydroperoxides to endogenous genotoxins. *Science* 2001;292:2083-4.
7089 Beckmann-Knopp S, Rietbrock S, Weyhenmeyer R, et al. Inhibitory effects of silibinin on cytochrome P-450 enzymes in human liver microsomes. *Pharmacol Toxicol* 2000;86:250-6.
7090 Granger AS. Ginkgo biloba precipitating epileptic seizures. *Age Ageing* 2001;30:523-5.
7091 Favreau JT, Ryu Ml, Braunstein G, et al. Severe hepatotoxicity associated with the dietary supplement LipoKinetix. *Ann Intern Med* 2002;136:590-5.
7092 Mathijssen RHJ, Verweij J, De Bruijn P, et al. Modulation of irinotecan (CPT-11) metabolism by St. John's wort in cancer patients. American Association for Cancer Research Annual Meeting, San Francisco, April 2002. Abstract 2443.
7093 Health Canada warns public not to use Hua Fo (DIN 02243366). Health Canada Online April 5, 2002. Available at: http://www.hc.sc.gc.ca/english/protestion/warnings/2002/2002_26e.htm (Accessed 5 April 2002).
7094 Hypericum Depression Trial Study Group. Effect of Hypericum perforatum (St. John's wort) in major depressive disorder: A randomized controlled trial. *JAMA* 2002;287:1807-14.
7095 Mai I, Bauer S, Krueger H, et al. Wechselwirkungen von Johaniskraut mit tacrolismus bei nierentransplantierten patienten. Symposium Phytopharmaka VII. Forschung und Klinische Anwendung, Berlin, October, 2001.
7096 Consultation letter MLX 286: Proposals to prohibit the herbal ingredient Kava-Kava (Piper methysticum) in unlicensed medicines. Medicines Control Agency, United Kingdom, July 19, 2002.

7100 Gorman JF. The vitamin C controversy. *Postgrad Med* 1980;67:64,69.

7101 Hemila H. Vitamin C intake and susceptibility to the common cold. *Br J Nutr* 1997;77:59-72.

7102 Gorton HC, Jarvis K. The effectiveness of vitamin C in preventing and relieving the symptoms of virus-induced respiratory infections. *J Manipulative Physiol Ther* 1999;22:530-3.

7103 Plat J, van Onselen EN, van Heugten MM, Mensink RP. Effects on serum lipids, lipoproteins and fat soluble antioxidant concentrations of consumption frequency of margarines and shortenings enriched with plant stanol esters. *Eur J Clin Nutr* 2000;54:671-7.

7104 Hallikainen MA, Sarkkinen ES, Uusitupa MI. Effects of low-fat stanol ester enriched margarines on concentrations of serum carotenoids in subjects with elevated serum cholesterol concentrations. *Eur J Clin Nutr* 1999;53:966-9.

7105 Hallikainen MA, Sarkkinen ES, Gylling H, et al. Comparison of the effects of plant sterol ester and plant stanol ester-enriched margarines in lowering serum cholesterol concentrations in hypercholesterolaemic subjects on a low-fat diet. *Eur J Clin Nutr* 2000;54:715-25.

7106 Huber R, Barth H, Schmitt-Graff A, Klein R. Hypereosinophilia induced by high-dose intratumoral and peritumoral mistletoe application to a patient with pancreatic carcinoma. *J Altern Complement Med* 2000;6:305-10.

7107 Buckle J. Use of aromatherapy as a complementary treatment for chronic pain. *Altern Ther Health Med* 1999;5:42-51.

7110 Irikura B, Kennelly E. American Health Consultants. Blue Cohosh: a word of caution. 1999. Available at: www.ahcpub.com/ahc_root_html/hot/archive/atwh1099.html.

7111 May J, Chan CH, King A, et al. Time-kill studies of tea tree oils on clinical isolates. *J Antimicrob Chemother* 2000;45:639-43.

7113 Maggioni M, Picotti GB, Bondiolotti GP, et al. Effects of phosphatidylserine therapy in geriatric patients with depressive disorders. *Acta Psychiatr Scand* 1990;81:265-70.

7114 Funfgeld EW, Baggen M, Nedwidek P, et al. Double-blind study with phosphatidylserine (PS) in parkinsonian patients with senile dementia of Alzheimer's type (SDAT). *Prog Clin Biol Res* 1989;317:1235-46.

7115 Blokland A, Honig W, Brouns F, Jolles J. Cognition-enhancing properties of subchronic phosphatidylserine (PS) treatment in middle-aged rats: comparison of bovine cortex PS with egg PS and soybean PS. *Nutrition* 1999;15:778-83.

7116 Pepping J. Phosphatidylserine. *Am J Health-Syst Pharm* 1999;56:2038,2043-4.

7117 Kidd PM. Attention Deficit/Hyperactivity disorder (ADHD) in children: rationale for its integrative management. *Altern Med Rev* 2000;5:402-28.

7118 Amaducci L. Phosphatidylserine in the treatment of Alzheimer's disease: results of a multicenter study. *Psychopharmacol Bull* 1988;24:130-4.

7119 Villardita C, Grioli S, Salmeri G, et al. Multicentre clinical trial of brain phosphatidylserine in elderly patients with intellectual deterioration. *Clin Trials J* 1987;24:84-93.

7120 Palmieri G, Palmieri R, Inzoli MR, et al. Double-blind controlled trial of phosphatidylserine in patients with senile mental deterioration. *Clin Trials J* 1987;24:73-83.

7121 Kidd PM. Phosphatidylserine; Membrane nutrient for memory. A clinical and mechanistic assessment. *Altern Med Rev* 1996;1:70-84.

7122 Chevallier A. Encyclopedia of Herbal Medicine. 2nd ed. New York, NY: DK Publ, Inc., 2000.

7123 Agricultural Research Service. Dr. Duke's phytochemical and ethnobotanical databases. www.ars-grin.gov/cgi-bin/duke/farmacy2.pl?575 (Accessed 31 January 2001).

7124 Cao GW, Yang WG, Du P. [Observation of the effects of LAK/IL-2 therapy combining with Lycium barbarum polysaccharides in the treatment of 75 cancer patients]. [Article in Chinese]. *Chung Hua Chung Liu Tsa Chih* 1994;16:428-31.

7125 Kim SY, Lee EJ, Kim HP, et al. LCC, a cerebroside from lycium chinense, protects primary cultured rat hepatocytes exposed to galactosamine. *Phytother Res* 2000;14:448-51.

7126 Huang KC. The Pharmacology of Chinese Herbs, KC Huang, 2nd ed. Boca Raton, FL: CRC Press,1999.

7127 Das SC, Isichei CO, Okwuasaba FK, et al. Chemical, pathological and toxicological studies of the effects of RICOM-1013-J of Ricinus communis var minor on women volunteers and rodents. *Phytother Res* 2000;14:15-9.

7128 Isichei CO, Das SC, Ogunkeye OO, et al. Preliminary clinical investigation of the contraceptive efficacy and chemical pathological effects of RICOM-1013-J of Ricinus communis var minor on women volunteers. *Phytother Res* 2000;14:40-2.

7129 Rodriguez J, Crespo JF, Lopez-Rubio A, et al. Clinical cross-reactivity among foods of the Rosaceae family. *J Allergy Clin Immunol* 2000;106:183-189.

7130 Price PA. Vitamin K nutrition and postmenopausal osteoporosis. *J Clin Invest* 1993;91:1268.

7131 Weber P. Management of osteoporosis: is there a role for vitamin K? *Int J Vitam Nutr Res* 1997;67:350-356.

7132 Tamatani M, Morimoto S, Nakajima M, et al. Decreased circulating levels of vitamin K and 25-hydroxyvitamin D in osteopenic elderly men. *Metabolism* 1998;47:195-9.

7133 Shearer MJ. The roles of vitamins D and K in bone health and osteoporosis prevention. *Proc Nutr Soc* 1997;56:915-37.

7134 Jamal SA, Browner WS, Bauer DC, Cummings SR. Warfarin use and risk for osteoporosis in elderly women. Study of Osteoporotic Fractures Research Group. *Ann Intern Med* 1998;128:829-832.

7135 Food and Nutrition Board, Institute of Medicine. Dietary Reference Intakes for Vitamin A, Vitamin K, Arsenic, Boron, Chromium, Copper, Iodine, Iron, Manganese, Molybdenum, Nickel, Silicon, Vanadium, and Zinc. Washington, DC: National Academy Press, 2002. Available at: www.nap.edu/books/0309072794/html.

7136 Rubin MA, Miller JP, Ryan AS, et al. Acute and chronic resistive exercise increase urinary chromium excretion in men as measured with an enriched chromium stable isotope. *J Nutr* 1998;128:73-78.

7137 Rabinovitz H, Leibovitz A, Madar Z, et al. Blood glucose and lipid levels following chromium supplementation in diabetic elderly patients on a rehabilitation program. Program Abstracts, 53rd Annual Scientific Meeting, Gerontological Society of America. *Gerontologist* 2000;40:38.

7139 Leo MA, Lieber CS. Alcohol, vitamin A, and beta-carotene: adverse interactions, including hepatotoxicity and carcinogenicity. *Am J Clin Nutr* 1999;69:1071-85.

7140 Weber G, Adamczyk A, Freytag S. Treatment of acne with a yeast preparation. *Fortschr Med* 1989;107:563-6.

7141 Crawford M, Galli C, Visioli F, et al. Role of Plant-Derived Omega-3 Fatty Acids in Human Nutrition. *Ann Nutr Metab* 2000;44:263-5.

7142 Connor WE. Alpha-linolenic acid in health and disease. *Am J Clin Nutr* 1999;69:827-8.

7143 Connor WE. Importance of n-3 fatty acids in health and disease. *Am J Clin Nutr* 2000;71:171S-5S.

7144 Eritsland J. Safety considerations of polyunsaturated fatty acids. *Am J Clin Nutr* 2000;71:197S-201S.

REFERENCES

7145 Gibson RA, Makrides M. n-3 polyunsaturated fatty acid requirements of term infants. *Am J Clin Nutr* 2000;71:251S-5S.

7146 Pang D, Allman-Farinelli MA, Wong T, et al. Replacement of linoleic acid with alpha-linolenic acid does not alter blood lipids in normolipidaemic men. *Br J Nutr* 1998;80:163-7.

7147 De Stefani E, Deneo-Pellegrini H, Boffetta P, et al. Alpha-linolenic acid and risk of prostate cancer: a case-control study in Uruguay. *Cancer Epidemiol Biomarkers Prev* 2000;9:335-8.

7148 Simopoulos AP. Essential fatty acids in health and chronic disease. *Am J Clin Nutr* 1999;70:560S-9S.

7149 Li D, Sinclair A, Wilson A, et al. Effect of dietary alpha-linolenic acid on thrombotic risk factors in vegetarian men. *Am J Clin Nutr* 1999;69:872-82.

7150 de Lorgeril M, Renaud S, Mamelle N, et al. Mediterranean alpha-linolenic acid-rich diet in secondary prevention of coronary heart disease. *Lancet* 1994;343:1454-9.

7151 Bemelmans WJ, Muskiet FA, Feskens EJ, et al. Associations of alpha-linolenic acid and linoleic acid with risk factors for coronary heart. *Eur J Clin Nutr* 2000;54:865-71.

7152 Ascherio A, Rimm EB, Giovannucci EL, et al. Dietary fat and risk of coronary heart disease in men: cohort follow up study in the United States. *BMJ* 1996;313:84-90.

7153 Hu FB, Stampfer MJ, Manson JE, et al. Dietary intake of alpha-linolenic acid and risk of fatal ischemic heart disease among women. *Am J Clin Nutr* 1999;69:890-7.

7154 Hu FB, Stampfer MJ, Manson JE, et al. Frequent nut consumption and risk of coronary heart disease in women: prospective cohort study. *BMJ* 1998;317:1341-5.

7155 Pedersen JI, Ringstad J, Almendingen K, et al. Adipose tissue fatty acids and risk of myocardial infarction-a case-control study. *Eur J Clin Nutr* 2000;54:618-25.

7156 Christensen JH, Christensen MS, Toft E, et al. Alpha-linolenic acid and heart rate variability. *Nutr Metab Cardiovasc Dis* 2000;10:57-61.

7157 Cunnane SC. The Canadian Society for Nutritional Sciences 1995 Young Scientist Award Lecture. Recent studies on the synthesis, beta-oxidation, and deficiency of linoleate and alpha-linolenate: are essential fatty acids more aptly named indispensable or conditionally dispensable fatty acids? *Can J Physiol Pharmacol* 1996;74:629-39.

7158 Lam AY, Elmer GW, Mohutsky MA. Possible interaction between warfarin and Lycium Barbarum. *Ann Pharmacother* 2001;35:1199-201.

7161 Chevallier A. Encyclopedia of Herbal Medicine. 2nd ed. New York, NY: DK Publ, Inc., 2000.

7162 Dr. Duke's Phytochemical and Ethnobotanical Databases. www.ars-grin.gov/cgi-bin/duke/farmacy2.pl.

7165 de Deckere EA, Korver O, Verschuren PM, Katan MB. Health aspects of fish and n-3 polyunsaturated fatty acids from plant and marine origin. *Eur J Clin Nutr* 1998;52:749-53.

7166 Allman-Farinelli MA, Hall D, Kingham K, et al. Comparison of the effects of two low fat diets with different alpha-linolenic:linoleic acid ratios on coagulation and fibrinolysis. *Atherosclerosis* 1999;142:159-68.

7167 Freeman VL, Meydani M, Yong S, et al. Prostatic levels of fatty acids and the histopathology of localized prostate cancer. *J Urol* 2000;164:2168-72.

7168 Klein V, Chajes V, Germain E, et al. Low alpha-linolenic acid content of adipose breast tissue is associated with an increased risk of breast cancer. *Eur J Cancer* 2000;36:335-40.

7169 Das A Jr, Hammad TA. Efficacy of a combination of FCHG49 glucosamine hydrochloride, TRH122 low molecular weight sodium chondroitin sulfate and manganese ascorbate in the management of knee osteoarthritis. *Osteoarthritis Cartilage* 2000;8:343-50.

7170 Natl Inst Health, Natl Inst Environmental Health Sci. Indole-3-carbinol. Available at: http://ntp-server.niehs.nih.gov.

7171 Dashwood RH. Indole-3-carbinol: anticarcinogen or tumor promoter in brassica vegetables? *Chem Biol Interact* 1998;110:1-5.

7172 Rosen CA, Woodson GE, Thompson JW, et al. Preliminary results of the use of indole-3-carbinol for recurrent respiratory papillomatosis. *Otolaryngol Head Neck Surg* 1998;118:810-5.

7173 Bell MC, Crowley-Nowick P, Bradlow HL, et al. Placebo-controlled trial of indole-3-carbinol in the treatment of CIN. *Gynecol Oncol* 2000;78:123-9.

7174 Wong GY, Bradlow L, Sepkovic D, et al. Dose-ranging study of indole-3-carbinol for breast cancer prevention. *J Cell Biochem Suppl* 1997;28-29:111-6.

7175 Michnovicz JJ. Increased estrogen 2-hydroxylation in obese women using oral indole-3-carbinol. *Int J Obes Relat Metab Disord* 1998;22:227-9.

7176 Balk JL. Indole-3-carbinol for cancer prevention. *Altern Med Alert* 2000; 3:105-7.

7177 Michnovicz JJ, Bradlow HL. Induction of estradiol metabolism by dietary indole-3-carbinol in humans. *J Natl Cancer Inst* 1990;82:947-9.

7178 Telang NT, Katdare M, Bradlow HL, et al. Inhibition of proliferation and modulation of estradiol metabolism: novel mechanisms for breast cancer prevention by the phytochemical indole-3-carbinol. *Proc Soc Exp Biol Med* 1997;216:246-52.

7179 Bradlow HL, Michnovicz J, Telang NT, Osborne MP. Effects of dietary indole-3-carbinol on estradiol metabolism and spontaneous mammary tumors in mice. *Carcinogenesis* 1991;12:1571-4.

7180 Grubbs CJ, Steele VE, Casebolt T, et al. Chemoprevention of chemically-induced mammary carcinogenesis by indole-3-carbinol. *Anticancer Res* 1995;15:709-16.

7181 Kojima T, Tanaka T, Mori H. Chemoprevention of spontaneous endometrial cancer in female Donryu rats by dietary indole-3-carbinol. *Cancer Res* 1994;54:1446-9.

7182 Yuan F, Chen DZ, Liu K, et al. Anti-estrogenic activities of indole-3-carbinol in cervical cells: implication for prevention of cervical cancer. *Anticancer Res* 1999;19:1673-80.

7183 Jin L, Qi M, Chen DZ, et al. Indole-3-carbinol prevents cervical cancer in human papilloma virus type 16 (HPV16) transgenic mice. *Cancer Res* 1999;59:3991-7.

7184 Kim DJ, Han BS, Ahn B, et al. Enhancement by indole-3-carbinol of liver and thyroid gland neoplastic development in a rat medium-term multiorgan carcinogenesis model. *Carcinogenesis* 1997;18:377-81.

7185 Pence BC, Buddingh F, Yang SP. Multiple dietary factors in the enhancement of dimethylhydrazine carcinogenesis: main effect of indole-3-carbinol. *J Natl Cancer Inst* 1986;77:269-76.

7186 Bailey GS, Dashwood RH, Fong AT, et al. Modulation of mycotoxin and nitrosamine carcinogenesis by indole-3-carbinol: quantitative analysis of inhibition versus promotion. *IARC Sci Publ* 1991;105:275-80.

7187 He YH, Friesen MD, Ruch RJ, Schut HA. Indole-3-carbinol as a chemopreventive agent in 2-amino-1-methyl-6-phenylimidazo[4,5-b]pyridine (PhIP) carcinogenesis: inhibition of PhIP-DNA adduct formation, acceleration of PhIP metabolism, and induction of cytochrome P450 in female F344 rats. *Food Chem Toxicol* 2000;38:15-23.

7188 Bradlow HL, Sepkovic DW, Telang NT, Osborne MP. Multifunctional aspects of the action of indole-3-carbinol as an antitumor agent. *Ann N Y Acad Sci* 1999;889:204-13.

REFERENCES

7189 Srivastava B, Shukla Y. Antitumour promoting activity of indole-3-carbinol in mouse skin carcinogenesis. *Cancer Lett* 1998;134:91-5.

7190 Exon JH, South EH. Dietary indole-3-carbinol alters immune functions in rats. *J Toxicol Environ Health A* 2000;59:271-9.

7191 Garry D, Figueroa R, Guillaume J, Cucco V. Use of castor oil in pregnancies at term. *Altern Ther Health Med* 2000;6:77-9.

7192 Lokkevik E, Skovlund E, Reitan JB, et al. Skin treatment with bepanthen cream versus no cream during radiotherapy-a randomized, controlled trial. *Acta Oncol* 1996;35:1021-6.

7193 Williams CL, Bollella MC, Strobino BA, et al. Plant stanol ester and bran fiber in childhood: effects on lipids, stool weight and stool frequency in preschool children. *J Am Coll Nutr* 1999;18:572-81.

7194 Tammi A, Ronnemaa T, Gylling H, et al. Plant stanol ester margarine lowers serum total and low-density lipoprotein cholesterol concentrations of healthy children: the STRIP project. Spec Turku Coronary Risk Factors Intervention Project. *J Pediatr* 2000;136:503-10.

7195 Lichtenstein AH, Deckelbaum RJ. Stanol/sterol ester-containing foods and blood cholesterol levels: a statement for healthcare professionals from Nutrition Committee, Council on Nutrition, Physical Activity, Metabolism of American Heart Association. *Circulation* 2001;103:1177-9.

7196 Jones PJ, Raeini-Sarjaz M, Ntanios FY, et al. Modulation of plasma lipid levels and cholesterol kinetics by phytosterol versus phytostanol esters. *J Lipid Res* 2000;41:697-705.

7198 Berges RR, Kassen A, Senge T. Treatment of symptomatic benign prostatic hyperplasia with beta-sitosterol: an 18-month follow-up. *BJU Int* 2000;85:842-6.

7201 Granerus AK, Jagenburg R, Svanborg A. Kaliuretic effect of L-dopa treatment in parkinsonian patients. *Acta Med Scand* 1977;210(4):291-7.

7202 Stoll AL, Severus WE, Freeman MP, et al. Omega 3 fatty acids in bipolar disorder: A preliminary double-blind, placebo-controlled trial. *Arch Gen Psychiatry* 1999;56:407-12.

7203 Vaidya AB, Rajagopalan TG, Mankodi NA, et al. Treatment of Parkinson's disease with the cowhage plant-Mucuna pruriens Bak. *Neurol India* 1978;26:171-6.

7204 Pras N, Woerdenbag HJ, Batterman S, et al. Mucuna pruriens: improvement of the biotechnological production of the anti-Parkinson drug L-dopa by plant cell selection. *Pharm World Sci* 1993;15:263-8.

7205 Vadivel V, Janardhanan K. Nutritional and anti-nutritional composition of velvet bean: an under-utilized food legume in south India. *Int J Food Sci Nutr* 2000;51:279-87.

7206 Vaidya RA, Aloorkar SD, Sheth AR, Pandya SK. Activity of bromoergocryptine, Mucuna pruriens and L-dopa in the control of hyperprolactinaemia. *Neurol India* 1978;26:179-182.

7207 Vaidya RA, Sheth AR, Aloorkar SD, et al. The inhibitory effect of the cowhage plant-Mucuna pruriens-and L-dopa on chlorpromazine-induced hyperprolactinaemia in man. *Neurol India* 1978;26:177-8.

7208 Gelenberg AJ, Wojcik JD, Falk WE, et al. Tyrosine for depression: a double-blind trial. *J Affect Disord* 1990;19:125-32.

7209 Eisenberg J, Asnis GM, van Praag HM, Vela RM. Effect of tyrosine on attention deficit disorder with hyperactivity. *J Clin Psychiatr* 1988;49:193-5.

7210 Reimherr FW, Wender PH, Wood DR, Ward M. An open trial of L-tyrosine in the treatment of attention deficit disorder, residual type. *Am J Psychiatr* 1987;144:1071-3.

7211 Wood DR, Reimherr FW, Wender PH. Amino acid precursors for the treatment of attention deficit disorder, residual type. *Psychopharmacol Bull* 1985;21:146-9.

7212 van Spronsen FJ, van Rijn M, Bekhof J. Phenylketonuria: tyrosine supplementation in phenylalanine-restricted diets. *Am J Clin Nutr* 2001;73:153-7.

7213 Poustie VJ, Rutherford P. Tyrosine supplementation for phenylketonuria. *Cochrane Database Syst Rev* 2000;2:CD001507.

7214 Roberts SA, Thorpe JM, Ball RO, Pencharz PB. Tyrosine requirement of healthy men receiving a fixed phenylalanine intake determined by using indicator amino acid oxidation. *Am J Clin Nutr* 2001 Feb;73:276-82.

7215 Neri DF, Wiegmann D, Stanny RR, et al. The effects of tyrosine on cognitive performance during extended wakefulness. *Aviat Space Environ Med* 1995;66:313-9.

7217 Food and Nutrition Board, Institute of Medicine. The Role of Protein and Amino Acids in Sustaining and Enhancing Performance. Washington, DC: National Academy Press, 1999. Available at: http://www.nap.edu/books/0309063469/html.

7219 Horning MS, Blakemore LJ, Trombley PQ. Endogenous mechanisms of neuroprotection: role of zinc, copper, and carnosine. *Brain Res* 2000;852:56-61.

7220 Grover JK, Vats V, Rathi SS, Dawar R. Traditional Indian anti-diabetic plants attenuate progression of renal damage in streptozotocin induced diabetic mice. *J Ethnopharmacol* 2001;76:233-8.

7221 Akhtar MS, Qureshi AQ, Iqbal J. Antidiabetic evaluation of Mucuna pruriens, Linn seeds. *J Pak Med Assoc* 1990;40:147-50.

7222 Guerranti R, Aguiyi JC, Errico E, et al. Effects of Mucuna pruriens extract on activation of prothrombin by Echis carinatus venom. *J Ethnopharmacol* 2001;75:175-80.

7223 Manyam BV. Paralysis agitans and levodopa in "Ayurveda": ancient Indian medical treatise. *Mov Disord* 1990;5:47-8.

7224 Sheng Y, Pero RW, Amiri A, Bryngelsson C. Induction of apoptosis and inhibition of proliferation in human tumor cells treated with extracts of Uncaria tomentosa. *Anticancer Res* 1998;18:3363-8.

7225 Sandoval M, Charbonnet RM, Okuhama NN, et al. Cat's claw inhibits TNFalpha production and scavenges free radicals: role in cytoprotection. *Free Radic Biol Med* 2000;29:71-78.

7226 Mohamed AF, Matsumoto K, Tabata K, et al. Effects of Uncaria tomentosa total alkaloid and its components on experimental amnesia in mice: elucidation using the passive avoidance test. *J Pharm Pharmacol* 2000;52:1553-1561.

7227 Santa Maria A, Lopez A, Diaz MM, et al. Evaluation of the toxicity of Uncaria tomentosa by bioassays in vitro. *J Ethnopharmacol* 1997;57:183-7.

7229 Anon. Petasites hybridus. *Altern Med Rev* 2001;6:207-9.

7230 Grossmann WM, Schmidramsl H. An extract of Petasites hybridus is effective in the prophylaxis of migraine. *Int J Clin Pharmacol Ther* 2000;38:430-5.

7231 Mauz C, Candrian U, Luthy J, et al. [Method for the reduction of pyrrolizidine alkaloids from medicinal plant extracts]. [Article in German; English abstract]. *Pharm Acta Helv* 1985;60:256-9.

7232 NIH Consensus Statements. Phenylketonuria: Screening and Management. http://odp.od.nih.gov/consensus/cons/113/113_statement.htm#3 (Accessed 6 September 2001).

7233 Bozzetti F, Biganzoli L, Gavazzi C, et al. Glutamine supplementation in cancer patients receiving chemotherapy: a double-blind randomized study. *Nutrition* 1997;13:748-51.

7234 Yamasaki K, Nakano M, Otake T, et al. Anti-HIV-1 activity of Labiatae plants, especially aromatic plants. *Int Conf AIDS* 1996;11(1):65.

7235 Savarese D, Al-Zoubi A, Boucher J. Glutamine for irinotecan diarrhea. *J Clin Oncol* 2000;18:450-1.

7236 Brown GA, Vukovich MD, Martini ER, et al. Endocrine responses to chronic androstenedione intake in 30- to 56-year-old men. *J Clin Endocrinol Metab* 2000;85:4074-80.

7237 Ross GD, Vetvicka V, Yan J, et al. Therapeutic intervention with complement and beta-glucan in cancer. *Immunopharmacology* 1999;42:61-74.

7238 Muller A, Rice PJ, Ensley HE, et al. Receptor binding and internalization of a water-soluble (1-->3)-beta-D-glucan biologic response modifier in two monocyte/macrophage cell lines. *J Immunol* 1996;156:3418-25.

7239 Yan J, Vetvicka V, Xia Y, et al. Beta-glucan, a "specific" biologic response modifier that uses antibodies to target tumors for cytotoxic recognition by leukocyte complement receptor type 3 (CD11b/CD18). *J Immunol* 1999;163:3045-52.

7240 Penna C, Dean PA, Nelson H. Pulmonary metastases neutralization and tumor rejection by in vivo administration of beta glucan and bispecific antibody. *Int J Cancer* 1996;65:377-382.

7241 Williams DL, Pretus HA, McNamee RB, et al. Development, physicochemical characterization and preclinical efficacy evaluation of a water soluble glucan sulfate derived from Saccharomyces cerevisiae. *Immunopharmacology* 1991;22:139-55.

7242 Mueller A, Raptis J, Rice PJ, et al. The influence of glucan polymer structure and solution conformation on binding to (1-->3)-beta-D-glucan receptors in a human monocyte-like cell line. *Glycobiology* 2000;10:339-46.

7243 Sherwood ER, Williams DL, McNamee RB, et al. Enhancement of interleukin-1 and interleukin-2 production by soluble glucan. *Int J Immunopharmacol* 1987;9:261-7.

7244 Patchen ML, Liang J, Vaudrain T, et al. Mobilization of peripheral blood progenitor cells by Betafectin PGG-Glucan alone and in combination with granulocyte colony-stimulating factor. *Stem Cells* 1998;16:208-17.

7245 Turnbull JL, Patchen ML, Scadden DT. The polysaccharide, PGG-Glucan, enhances human myelopoiesis by direct action independent of an additive to early-acting cytokines. *Acta Haematol* 1999;102:66-71.

7246 Portera CA, Love EJ, Memore L, et al. Effect of macrophage stimulation on collagen biosynthesis in the healing wound. *Am Surg* 1997;63:125-31.

7247 Bowers GJ, Patchen ML, MacVittie TJ, et al. Glucan enhances survival in an inraabdominal infection model. *J Surg Res* 1989;47(2):183-188.

7248 Liang J, Melican D, Cafro L, et al. Enhanced clearance of a multiple antibiotic resistant Staphylococcus aureus in rats treated with PGG-glucan is associated with increased leukocyte counts and increased neutrophil oxidative burst activity. *Int J Immunopharmacol* 1998;20:595-614.

7249 Wakshull E, Brunke-Reese D, Lindermuth J, et al. PGG-Glucan, a soluble beta-(1,3)-glucan, enhances the oxidative burst response, microbicidal activity, and activates an NF-kappa B-like factor in human PMN: evidence for a glycosphingolipid beta-(1,3)-glucan receptor. *Immunopharmacology* 1999;4:89-107.

7250 Tsiapali E, Whaley S, Kalbfleisch J, et al. Glucans exhibit weak antioxidant activity, but stimulate macrophage free radical activity. *Free Radic Biol Med* 2001;30:393-402.

7251 Williams DL, Sherwood ER, Browder IW, et al. Pre-clinical safety evaluation of soluble glucan. *Int J Immunopharmacol* 1988;10;405-14.

7252 Duvic M, Reisman M, Finley V, et al. Glucan-induced keratoderma in acquired immunodeficiency syndrome. *Arch Dermatol* 1987;123:751-6.

7253 Wan G, Li C, Guo S, et al. An airborne mold-derived product, beta-1,3-D-glucan, potentiates airway allergic responses. *Eur J Immunol* 1999;29(8):2491-2497.

7254 Yoshioka S, Ohno N, Miura T, et al. Immunotoxicity of soluble beta-glucans induced by indomethacin treatment. *FEMS Immunol Med Microbiol* 1998;21(3):171-179.

7255 Lissoni P, Cazzaniga M, Tancini G, et al. Reversal of clinical resistance to LHRH analogue in metastatic prostate cancer by the pineal hormone melatonin: efficacy of LHRH analogue plus melatonin in patients progressing on LHRH analogue alone. *Eur Urol* 1997;31:178-81.

7256 Mazieres B, Combe B, Phan Van A, et al. Chondroitin sulfate in osteoarthritis of the knee: a prospective, double blind, placebo controlled multicenter clinical study. *J Rheumatol* 2001;28:173-81.

7258 Amin AH, Subbaiah TV, Abbasi KM. Berberine sulfate: antimicrobial activity, bioassay, and mode of action. *Can J Microbiol* 1969;15:1067-76.

7259 Sun D, Courtney HS, Beachey EH. Berberine sulfate blocks adherence of Streptococcus pyogenes to epithelial cells, fibronectin, and hexadecane. *Antimicrob Agents Chemother* 1988;32:1370-4.

7260 Nishino H, Kitagawa K, Fujiki H, Iwashima A. Berberine sulfate inhibits tumor-promoting activity of teleocidin in two-stage carcinogenesis on mouse skin. *Oncology* 1986;43:131-4.

7261 Okamura K, Suzuki M, Chihara T, et al. Clinical evaluation of schizophyllan combined with irradiation in patients with cervical cancer. A randomized controlled study. *Cancer* 1986;58:865-72.

7262 Mansell PW, Ichinose H, Reed RJ, et al. Macrophage-mediated destruction of human malignant cells in vivo. *J Natl Cancer Inst* 1975;54:571-80.

7263 Kimura Y, Tojima H, Fukase S, Takeda K. Clinical evaluation of sizofilan as assistant immunotherapy in treatment of head and neck cancer. *Acta Otolaryngol Suppl* 1994;511:192-5.

7264 Miyazaki K, Mizutani H, Katabuchi H, et al. Activated (HLA-DR+) T-lymphocyte subsets in cervical carcinoma and effects of radiotherapy and immunotherapy with sizofiran on cell-mediated immunity and survival. *Gynecol Oncol* 1995;56:412-40.

7265 Arinaga S, Karimine N, Takamuku K, et al. Enhanced induction of lymphokine-activated killer activity after lentinan administration in patients with gastric carcinoma. *Int J Immunopharmac* 1992;14:535-539.

7266 Matsuoka H, Seo Y, Wakasugi H, et al. Lentinan potentiates immunity and prolongs the survival time of some patients. *Anticancer Res.* 1997 Jul-Aug;17:2751-5.

7267 Gordon M, Bihari B, Goosby E, et al. A placebo-controlled trial of the immune modulator, lentinan, in HIV-positive patients: a phase I/II trial. *J Med* 1998;29:305-30.

7268 Browder W, Williams D, Pretus H, et al. Beneficial effect of enhanced macrophage function in the trauma patient. *Ann Surg* 1990;211:605-12; discussion 612-3.

7269 Babineau TJ, Marcello P, Swails W, et al. Randomized phase I/II trial of a macrophage-specific immunomodulator (PGG-glucan) in high-risk surgical patients. *Ann Surg* 1994;220:601-9.

7270 Babineau TJ, Hackford A, Kenler A, et al. A phase II multicenter, double-blind, randomized, placebo-controlled study of three dosages of an immunomodulator (PGG-glucan) in high-risk surgical patients. *Arch Surg* 1994;129:1204-10.

7271 Dellinger EP, Babineau TJ, Bleicher P, et al. Effect of PGG-glucan on the rate of serious postoperative infection or death observed after high-risk gastrointestinal operations. Betafectin Gastrointestinal Study Group. *Arch Surg* 1999;134:977-83.

7272 Nicolosi R, Bell SJ, Bistrian BR, et al. Plasma lipid changes after supplementation with beta-glucan fiber from yeast. *Am J Clin Nutr* 1999;70:208-12.

7273 Bell S, Goldman VM, Bistrian BR, et al. Effect of beta-glucan from oats and yeast on serum lipids. *Crit Rev Food Sci Nutr* 1999;39:189-202.

7275 Genest K, Hughes DW. Natural products in Canadian pharmaceuticals IV. Hydrastis canadensis. *Can J Pharm Sci* 1969;4(2):41-5.

7277 Ammon HP, Muller AB. Forskolin: From a ayurvedic remedy to a modern agent. *Planta Med* 1985;6:473-7.

7278 Baumann G, Felix S, Sattelberger U, Klein G. Cardiovascular effects of forskolin (HL-362) in patients with idiopathic congestiv cardiomyopathy. A comparative study with dobutamine and sodium nitroprusside. *J Cardiovasc Pharmacol* 1990;16(1):93-100.

7279 Kramer W, Thormann J, Kindler M, Schlepper M. Effects of forskolin on left ventricular function in dilated cardiomyopathy. *Arzneimittleforschung* 1987;37:364-7.

7280 Lichey J, Friedrich T, Priesnitz M, et al. Effect of forskolin on methacholine-induced bronchoconstriction in extrinsic asthmatics. *Lancet* 1984;2:167.

7281 Bauer K, Dietersdorfer F, Kaspar S, et al. Pharmacodynamic effects of inhaled dry powder formulations of fenoterol and colforsin in asthma. *Clin Pharmacol Ther* 1993;53(1):76-83.

7282 Meyer BH, Stulting AA, Muller FO, et al. The effects of forskolin eye drops on intra-ocular pressure. *S Afr Med J* 1987;71:570-1.

7283 Brubaker RF, Carlson KH, Kullerstrand LJ, et al. Topical forskolin (colforsin) and aqueous flow in humans. *Arch Ophthalmol* 1987;105:637-41.

7284 Seto C, Eguchi S, Araie M, et al. Acute effects of topical forskolin on aqueous humor dynamics in man. *Jpn J Ophthalmol* 30(3):238-44.

7285 Daniele B, Perrone F, Gallo C, et al. Oral glutamine in the prevention of fluorouracil induced intestinal toxicity: a double blind, placebo controlled, randomised trial. *Gut* 2001;48:28-33.

7286 John JF, Kuk R, Rosenthal A et al. Synergistic antiretroviral activities of the herb, Prunella vulgaris, with AZT, ddI, and ddC. *Abstr Gen Meet Am Soc Microbiol* 1994;94:481.

7288 Petit RG, French C. Phase III Clinical Trial Design Considerations for Oral Treatments of Chemotherapy-Induced Mucositis: AES-14 (Uptake-Facilitated L-Glutamine) Pivotal Studies.

7289 Manns B, Hyndman E, Burgess E, et al. Oral vitamin B(12) and high-dose folic acid in hemodialysis patients with hyper-homocyst(e)inemia. *Kidney Int* 2001;59:1103-1109.

7291 Mebane AH. L-Glutamine and mania. *Am J Psychiatry* 984;141:1302-3.

7292 Meldrum BS. Glutamate as a neurotransmitter in the brain: review of physiology and pathology. *J Nutr* 2000;130:1007S-15S.

7293 Garlick PJ. Assessment of the safety of glutamine and other amino acids. *J Nutr* 2001;131:2556S-61S.

7294 Chapman AG. Glutamate and epilepsy. *J Nutr* 2000;130:1043S-5S.

7295 van Zaanen HC, van der Lelie H, Timmer JG, et al. Parenteral glutamine dipeptide supplementation does not ameliorate chemotherapy-induced toxicity. *Cancer* 1994;74:2879-84.

7296 Coghlin Dickson TM, Wong RM, Negrin RS, et al. Effect of oral glutamine supplementation during bone marrow transplantation. *JPEN J Parenter Enteral Nutr* 2000;24:61-6.

7297 Zoli G, Care M, Falco F, et al. Effect of oral glutamine on intestinal permeability and nutritional status in Crohn's disease [abstract]. *Gastroenterology* 1995;108:A766.

7298 Ribeiro Junior H, Ribeiro T, Mattos A, et al. Treatment of acute diarrhea with oral rehydration solutions containing glutamine. *J Am Coll Nutr* 1994;13:251-5.

7299 van der Hulst RR, van Kreel BK, von Meyenfeldt MF, et al. Glutamine and the preservation of gut integrity. *Lancet* 1993;341:1363-5.

7300 Jian ZM, Cao JD, Zhu XG, et al. The impact of alanyl-glutamine on clinical safety, nitrogen balance, intestinal permeability, and clinical outcome in postoperative patients: a randomized, double-blind, controlled study of 120 patients. *JPEN J Parenter Enteral Nutr* 1999;23:S62-6.

7303 Age-Related Eye Disease Study Research Group. A randomized, placebo-controlled, clinical trial of high-dose supplementation with vitamins C and E, beta carotene, and zinc for age-related macular degeneration and vision loss. AREDS report no. 8. *Arch Ophthalmol* 2001;119:1417-36.

7304 Age-Related Eye Disease Study Research Group. A randomized, placebo-controlled, clinical trial of high-dose supplementation with vitamins C and E and beta carotene for age-related cataract and vision loss: AREDS report no. 9. *Arch Ophthalmol* 2001;119:1439-52.

7305 Jampol LM. Antioxidants, zinc, age-related macular degeneration: results and recommendations. *Arch Ophthalmol.* 2001;119:1533-4.

7306 Thomas MR, Litin SC, Osmon DR, et al. Lack of effect of Lactobacillus GG on antibiotic-associated diarrhea: a randomized, placebo-controlled trial. *Mayo Clin Proc* 2001;76:883-9.

7307 Lee SC, Park SW, Kim DK, et al. Iron supplementation inhibits cough associated with ACE inhibitors. *Hypertension* 2001;38:166-170.

7308 Hallberg L. Does calcium interfere with iron absorption? *Am J Clin Nutr* 1998;68:3-4.

7309 Chuntrasakul C, Siltharm S, Sarasombath S, et al. Metabolic and immune effects of dietary arginine, glutamine and omega-3 fatty acids supplementation in immunocompromised patients. *J Med Assoc Thai* 1998;81:334-43.

7310 Clark RH, Feleke G, Din M, et al. Nutritional treatment for acquired immunodeficiency virus-associated wasting using beta-hydroxy beta-methylbutyrate, glutamine, and arginine: a randomized, double-blind, placebo-controlled study. *JPEN J Parenter Enteral Nutr* 2000;24:133-9.

7311 Wahed A, Dasgupta A. Positive and negative in vitro interference of Chinese medicine dan shen in serum digoxin measurement. Elimination of interference by monitoring free digoxin concentration. *Am J Clin Pathol* 2001;116:403-408.

7312 Bhopal JS. St John's wort-induced sexual dysfunction. *Can J Psychiatry* 2001;46:456-457.

7313 Albert S, Bhattacharya D, Klaudiny J, et al. The family of major royal jelly proteins and its evolution. *J Mol Evol* 1999;49:290-297.

7314 Leung R, Ho A, Chan J, et al. Royal jelly consumption and hypersensitivity in the community. *Clin Exp Allergy* 1997;27:333-6.

7315 Harwood M, Harding S, Beasley R, Frankish PD. Asthma following royal jelly. *N Z Med J* 1996;109:325.

7316 Laporte JR, Ibaanez L, Vendrell L, Ballarin E. Bronchospasm induced by royal jelly. *Allergy* 1996;51:440.

7317 Piscoya J, Rodriguez Z, Bustamante SA, et al. Efficacy and safety of freeze-dried cat's claw in osteoarthritis of the knee: mechanisms of action of the species Uncaria guianensis. *Inflamm Res* 2001;50:442-448.

7318 Venkataramanan R, Ramachandran V, Komoroski BJ, et al. Milk thistle, a herbal supplement, decreases the activity of CYP3A4 and uridine diphosphoglucuronosyl transferase in human hepatocyte cultures. *Drug Metab Dispos* 2000;28:1270-3.

7319 Zhu W, Zhang JS, Young CY. Silymarin inhibits function of the androgen receptor by reducing nuclear localization of the receptor in the human prostate cancer cell line LNCaP. *Carcinogenesis* 2001;22:1399-403.

7320 Sonnenbichler J, Scalera F, Sonnenbichler I, Weyhenmeyer R. Stimulatory effects of silibinin and silicristin from the milk thistle Silybum marianum on kidney cells. *J Pharmacol Exp Ther* 1999;290:1375-83.

7321 Bunout D, Hirsch S, Petermann M. [Controlled study of the effect of silymarin on alcoholic liver disease.] [Article in Spanish]. *Rev Med Chil* 1992;120:1370-5.

7322 Trinchet JC, Coste T, Levy VG. [Treatment of alcoholic hepatitis with silymarin. A double-blind comparative study in 116 patients]. [Article in French]. *Gastroenterol Clin Biol* 1989;13:120-4.

7323 Paulova J, Dvorak M, Kolouch F, et al. [Verification of the hepatoprotective and therapeutic effect of silymarin in experimental liver injury with tetrachloromethane in dogs]. [Article in Czech] *Vet Med* (Praha) 1990;35:629-35.

7325 Malsch U, Kieser M. Efficacy of kava-kava in the treatment of non-psychotic anxiety, following pretreatment with benzodiazepines. *Psychopharmacology* (Berl) 2001;157:277-83.

7326 Blasiak J, Kowalik J. A comparison of the in vitro genotoxicity of tri- and hexavalent chromium. *Mutat Res* 2000;469:135-45.

7327 Genazzani AD, Stomati M, Strucchi C, et al. Oral dehydroepiandrosterone supplementation modulates spontaneous and growth hormone-releasing hormone-induced growth hormone and insulin-like growth factor-1 secretion in early and late postmenopausal women. *Fertil Steril* 2001;76:241-8.

7328 Robinzon B, Cutolo M. Should dehydroepiandrosterone replacement therapy be provided with glucocorticoids? *Rheumatology* (Oxford) 1999;38:488-95.

7329 Cesaro S, Chinello P, Rossi L, Zanesco L. Saccharomyces cerevisiae fungemia in a neutropenic patient treated with Saccharomyces boulardii. *Support Care Cancer* 2000;8:504-5.

7330 Setchell KD, Brown NM, Desai P, et al. Bioavailability of pure isoflavones in healthy humans and analysis of commercial soy isoflavone supplements. *J Nutr* 2001;131:1362S-75S.

7331 Strom BL, Schinnar R, Ziegler EE, et al. Exposure to soy-based formula in infancy and endocrinological and reproductive outcomes in young adulthood. *JAMA* 2001;286:807-14.

7332 Setchell KD, Zimmer-Nechemias L, Cai J, Heubi JE. Exposure of infants to phyto-oestrogens from soy-based infant formula. *Lancet* 1997;350:23-7.

7333 Clarkson TB, Anthony MS, Morgan TM. Inhibition of postmenopausal atherosclerosis progression: a comparison of the effects of conjugated equine estrogens and soy phytoestrogens. *J Clin Endocrinol Metab* 2001;86:41-7.

7334 Nomura A, Henderson BE, Lee J. Breast cancer and diet among the Japanese in Hawaii. *Am J Clin Nutr* 1978;31:2020-5.

7335 Lee HP, Gourley L, Duffy SW, et al. Dietary effects on breast-cancer risk in Singapore. *Lancet* 1991;337:1197-200.

7336 Shu XO, Jin F, Dai Q, et al. Soyfood intake during adolescence and subsequent risk of breast cancer among Chinese women. *Cancer Epidemiol Biomarkers Prev* 2001;10:483-88.

7337 Messina M, Barnes S, Setchell KD. Phyto-oestrogens and breast cancer. *Lancet* 1997;350:971-2.

7338 Goodman MT, Wilkens LR, Hankin JH, et al. Association of soy and fiber consumption with the risk of endometrial cancer. *Am J Epidemiol* 1997;146:294-306.

7339 Nagata C, Inaba S, Kawakami N, et al. Inverse association of soy product intake with serum androgen and estrogen concentrations in Japanese men. *Nutr Cancer* 2000;36:14-8.

7340 Wu AH, Yang D, Pike MC. A meta-analysis of soyfoods and risk of stomach cancer: the problem of potential confounders. *Cancer Epidemiol Biomarkers Prev* 2000;9:1051-8.

7341 Ji BT, Chow WH, Yang G, et al. Correspondence re: AH Wu et al, A meta-analysis of soyfoods and risk of stomach cancer: the problem of potential confounders. *Cancer Epidemiol Biomarkers Prev* 2001;10:570.

7342 Somekawa Y, Chiguchi M, Ishibashi T, Aso T. Soy intake related to menopausal symptoms, serum lipids, and bone mineral density in postmenopausal Japanese women. *Obstet Gynecol* 2001;97:109-15.

7343 Weaver CM, Elmore D, Spence LA, et al. Effects of soy isoflavones on calcium metabolism and bone resorption in postmenopausal women. *Altern Ther Health Med* 2001;7:S35.

7344 Vincent A, Fitzpatrick LA. Soy isoflavones: are they useful in menopause? *Mayo Clin Proc* 2000;75:1174-84.

7345 Lichtenstein AH. Got soy? *Am J Clin Nutr* 2001;73:667-8.

7346 Gardner CD, Newell KA, Cherin R, Haskell WL. The effect of soy protein with or without isoflavones relative to milk protein on plasma lipids in hypercholesterolemic postmenopausal women. *Am J Clin Nutr* 2001;73:728-35.

7347 Ashton EL, Dalais FS, Ball MJ. Effect of meat replacement by tofu on CHD risk factors including copper induced LDL oxidation. *J Am Coll Nutr* 2000;19:761-7.

7348 Stephenson TJ, Anderson JW, Fanti P. Soy protein use in early diabetic nephropathy. *Altern Ther Health Med* 2001;7:S31-2.

7349 US Department of Justice, Drug Enforcement Agency, Diversion Control Program. Drugs and Chemicals of Concern: Salvia Divinorum, ska Maria Pastora, Salvia (Salvinorin A, Divinorin A). 2002. Available at: http://www.deadiversion.usdoj.gov/drugs_concern/salvia_d/summary.htm.

7350 Valdes LJ 3rd, Diaz JL, Paul AG. Ethnopharmacology of ska Maria Pastora (Salvia divinorum, Epling and Jativa-M.). *J Ethnopharmacol* 1983;7:287-312.

7351 Valdes LJ 3rd. Salvia divinorum and the unique diterpene hallucinogen, Salvinorin (divinorin) A. *J Psychoactive Drugs* 1994;26:277-83.

7352 Siebert DJ. Salvia divinorum and salvinorin A: new pharmacologic findings. *J Ethnopharmacol* 1994;43:53-6.

7353 Hennequin C, Thierry A, Richard GF, et al. Microsatellite typing as a new tool for identification of Saccharomyces cerevisiae strains. *J Clin Microbiol* 2001;39:551-9.

7354 Kim DH, Jin YH, Park JB, Kobashi K. Silymarin and its components are inhibitors of beta-glucuronidase. *Biol Pharm Bull* 1994;17:443-5.

7355 Pares A, Planas R, Torres M, et al. Effects of silymarin in alcoholic patients with cirrhosis of the liver: results of a controlled, double-blind, randomized and multicenter trial. *J Hepatol* 1998;28:615-21.

7356 Buzzelli G, Moscarella S, Giusti A, et al. A pilot study on the liver protective effect of silybin-phosphatidylcholine complex (IdB1016) in chronic active hepatitis. *Int J Clin Pharmacol Ther Toxicol* 1993;31:456-60.

7357 Whittaker P. Iron and zinc interactions in humans. *Am J Clin Nutr* 1998;68:442S-6S.

7358 Foth D, Cline JM. Effects of mammalian and plant estrogens on mammary glands and uteri of macaques. *Am J Clin Nutr* 1998;68:1413S-7S.

7359 Burr ML, Fehily AM, Gilbert JF, et al. Effects of changes in fat, fish, and fibre intakes on death and myocardial reinfarction: diet and reinfarction trial (DART). *Lancet* 1989;2:757-61.

7360 Sellmayer A, Witzgall H, Lorenz RL, Weber PC. Effects of dietary fish oil on ventricular premature complexes. *Am J Cardiol* 1995;76:974-7.

7361 Nilsen DW, Albrektsen G, Landmark K, et al. Effects of a high-dose concentrate of n-3 fatty acids or corn oil introduced early after an acute myocardial infarction on serum triacylglycerol and HDL cholesterol. *Am J Clin Nutr* 2001;74:50-6.

7362 Billman GE, Hallaq H, Leaf A. Prevention of ischemia-induced ventricular fibrillation by omega 3 fatty acids. *Proc Natl Acad Sci U S A* 1994;91:4427-30.

7363 Billman GE, Kang JX, Leaf A. Prevention of sudden cardiac death by dietary pure omega-3 polyunsaturated fatty acids in dogs. *Circulation* 1999;99:2452-7.

7364 Kromhout D, Bosschieter EB, de Lezenne Coulander C. The inverse relation between fish consumption and 20-year mortality from coronary heart disease. *N Engl J Med* 1985;312:1205-9.

7365 Kromhout D, Feskens EJ, Bowles CH. The protective effect of a small amount of fish on coronary heart disease mortality in an elderly population. *Int J Epidemiol* 1995;24:340-5.

7366 Sorensen NS, Marckmann P, Hoy CE, et al. Effect of fish-oil-enriched margarine on plasma lipids, low-density-lipoprotein particle composition, size, and susceptibility to oxidation. *Am J Clin Nutr* 1998;68:235-41.

7367 Rissanen T, Voutilainen S, Nyyssonen K, et al. Fish oil-derived fatty acids, docosahexaenoic acid and docosapentaenoic acid, and the risk of acute coronary events: the Kuopio ischaemic heart disease risk factor study. *Circulation* 2000;102:2677-9.

7368 Sirtori CR, Crepaldi G, Manzato E, et al. One-year treatment with ethyl esters of n-3 fatty acids in patients with hypertriglyceridemia and glucose intolerance: reduced triglyceridemia, total cholesterol and increased HDL-C without glycemic alterations. *Atherosclerosis* 1998;137:419-27.

7369 Luo J, Rizkalla SW, Vidal H, et al. Moderate intake of n-3 fatty acids for 2 months has no detrimental effect on glucose metabolism and could ameliorate the lipid profile in type 2 diabetic men. Results of a controlled study. *Diabetes Care* 1998;21:717-24.

7370 Gillum RF, Mussolino ME, Madans JH. The relationship between fish consumption and stroke incidence. The NHANES I Epidemiologic Follow-up Study (National Health and Nutrition Examination Survey). *Arch Intern Med* 1996;156:537-42.

7371 Keli SO, Feskens EJ, Kromhout D. Fish consumption and risk of stroke. The Zutphen Study. *Stroke* 1994;25:328-32.

7372 Yamori Y, Nara Y, Mizushima S, et al. Nutritional factors for stroke and major cardiovascular diseases: international epidemiological comparison of dietary prevention. *Health Rep* 1994;6:22-7.

7373 Iso H, Rexrode KM, Stampfer MJ, et al. Intake of fish and omega-3 fatty acids and risk of stroke in women. *JAMA* 2001;285:304-12.

7374 Orencia AJ, Daviglus ML, Dyer AR, et al. Fish consumption and stroke in men. 30-year findings of the Chicago Western Electric Study. *Stroke* 1996;27:204-9.

7375 Morris MC, Manson JE, Rosner B, et al. Fish consumption and cardiovascular disease in the physicians' health study: a prospective study. *Am J Epidemiol* 1995;142:166-75.

7377 van Dam M, Stalenhoef AFH, Wittekoek J. Efficacy of concentrated n-3 fatty acids in hypertriglyceridaemia: a comparison with gemfibrozil. *Clin Drug Invest* 2001;21:175-81.

7378 Terry P, Lichtenstein P, Feychting M, et al. Fatty fish consumption and risk of prostate cancer. *Lancet* 2001;357:1764-6.

7379 Consumer Lab. Product Review: Omega-3 Fatty Acids (EPA and DHA) from Fish/Marine Oils. website: http://www.consumerlab.com/results/omega3.asp (Accessed 30 November 2001).

7380 Deslypere JP. Influence of supplementation with N-3 fatty acids on different coronary risk factors in men--a placebo controlled study. *Verh K Acad Geneeskd Belg* 1992;54:189-16.

7381 Hwang DH, Chanmugam PS, Ryan DH, et al. Does vegetable oil attenuate the beneficial effects of fish oil in reducing risk factors for cardiovascular disease? *Am J Clin Nutr* 1997;66:89-96.

7382 Vogel RA, Corretti MC, Plotnick GD. The postprandial effect of components of the Mediterranean diet on endothelial function. *J Am Coll Cardiol* 2000;36:1455-60.

7383 Kelley DS, Rudolph IL. Effect of individual fatty acids of omega-6 and omega-3 type on human immune status and role of eicosanoids. *Nutrition* 2000;16:143-5.

7384 Meydani SN, Dinarello CA. Influence of dietary fatty acids on cytokine production and its clinical implications. *Nutr Clin Pract* 1993;8:65-72.

7386 Klipstein-Grobusch K, Geleijnse JM, den Breeijen JH, et al. Dietary antioxidants and risk of myocardial infarction in the elderly: the Rotterdam Study. *Am J Clin Nutr* 1999;69:261-6.

7387 Todd S, Woodward M, Tunstall-Pedoe H, Bolton-Smith C. Dietary antioxidant vitamins and fiber in the etiology of cardiovascular disease and all-causes mortality: results from the Scottish Heart Health Study. *Am J Epidemiol* 1999;150:1073-80.

7388 Brown BG, Zhao XQ, Chait A. Simvastatin and niacin, antioxidant vitamins, or the combination for the prevention of coronary disease. *N Engl J Med* 2001;345:1583-93.

7389 Bordia A, Verma SK, Srivastava KC. Effect of ginger (Zingiber officinale Rosc.) and fenugreek (Trigonella foenumgraecum L.) on blood lipids, blood sugar and platelet aggregation in patients with coronary artery disease. *Prostaglandins Leukot Essent Fatty Acids* 1997;56:379-84.

7390 Yochum LA, Folsom AR, Kushi LH. Intake of antioxidant vitamins and risk of death from stroke in postmenopausal women. *Am J Clin Nutr* 2000;72:476-83.

7394 Joshipura KJ, Ascherio A, Manson JE, et al. Fruit and vegetable intake in relation to risk of ischemic stroke. *JAMA* 1999;282:1233-39.

7400 Grontved A, Brask T, Kambskard J, Hentzer E. Ginger root against seasickness: a controlled trial on the open sea. *Acta Otolaryngol* 1998;105:45-9.

7401 Srivastava KC, Mustafa T. Ginger (Zingiber officinale) and rheumatic disorders. *Medical Hypotheses* 1989;29:25-8.

7402 Caprioli J, Sears M. Forskolin lowers intraocular pressure in rabbits, monkeys, and man. *Lancet* 1983;1:958-60.

7403 Caprioli J, Sears M, Bausher L, et al. Forskolin lowers intraocular pressure by reducing aqueous inflow. *Invest Ophthalmol Vis Sci* 1984;25(3):268-77.

7404 Sultana D, Peindl KS, Wisner KL. Rash associated with St. John's wort treatment in premenstrual dysphoric disorder. *Arch Women Ment Health* 2000;3:99-101.

7405 Burstein NL, Sears ML, Mead A. Aqueous flow in human eyes is reduced by forskolin, a potent adenylate cyclase activator. *Exp Eye Res* 1984;39(6):745-9.

7406 Metzger H, Lindner E. The positive inotropic-acting forskolin, a potent adenylatecyclase activator. *Arzneimittelforschung* 1981;31(8):1248-50.

7407 Lindner E, Metzger H. The action of forskolin on muscle cells is modified by hormones, calcium ions and calcium antagonists. *Arzneimittelforschung* 1983;33(10):1436-41.

7408 Seamon KB, Daly JW. Forskolin: a unique diterpene activator of cyclic AMP-generating systems. *J Cyclic Nucleotide Res* 1981;7(4):201-24.

7409 Kreutner W, Chapman RW, Gulbenkian A, Tozzi S. Bronchodilator and antiallergy activity of forskolin. *Eur J Pharmacol* 1985;111(1):1-8.

7410 Christenson JT, Thulesius O, Nazzal MM. The effect of forskolin on blood flow, platelet metabolism, aggregation and ATP release. *Vasa* 1995;24:56-61.

7411 Agarwal KC, Zielinski BA, Maitra RS. Significance of plasma adenosine in the antiplatelet activity of forskolin: potentiation by dipyridamole and dilazep. *Thromb Haemost* 1989;61:106-10.

7412 Agarwal KC, Parks RE. Forskolin: a potential antimetastatic agent. *Int J Cancer* 1983;32(6):801-4.

7413 Tzanakakis GN, Agarwal KC, Vezeridis MP. Inhibition of hepatic metastasis from a human pancreatic adenocarcinoma (RWP-2) in the nude mouse by prostacyclin, forskolin, and ketoconazole. *Cancer* 1990;65(3):446-51.

7501 Williams CA, Harborne JB, Newman M, et al. Chrysin and other leaf exudate flavonoids in the genus Pelargonium. *Phytochemistry* 1997;46:1349-53.

7502 Galijatovic A, Otake Y, Walle UK, Walle T. Extensive metabolism of the flavonoid chrysin by human Caco-2 and Hep G2 cells. *Xenobiotica* 1999;29:1241-56.

7503 Lee H, Yeom H, Kim YG, et al. Structure-related inhibition of human hepatic caffeine N3-demethylation by naturally occurring flavonoids. *Biochem Pharmacol* 1998;55:1369-75.

7504 Galijatovic A, Walle UK, Walle T. Induction of UDP-glucuronosyltransferase by the flavonoids chrysin and quercetin in Caco-2 cells. *Pharm Res* 2000;17:21-6.

7505 Walle UK, Galijatovic A, Walle T. Transport of the flavonoid chrysin and its conjugated metabolites by the human intestinal cell line Caco-2. *Biochem Pharmacol* 1999;58:431-8.

7506 Kellis JT Jr, Vickery LE. Inhibition of human estrogen synthetase (aromatase) by flavones. *Science* 1984;225:1032-4.

7507 Kao YC, Zhou C, Sherman M, et al. Molecular basis of the inhibition of human aromatase (estrogen synthetase) by flavone and isoflavone phytoestrogens: A site-directed mutagenesis study. *Environ Health Perspect* 1998;106:85-92.

7508 Jeong HJ, Shin YG, Kim IH, Pezzuto JM. Inhibition of aromatase activity by flavonoids. *Arch Pharm Res* 1999;22:309-12.

7509 Breinholt V, Lauridsen ST, Dragsted LO. Differential effects of dietary flavonoids on drug metabolizing and antioxidant enzymes in female rat. *Xenobiotica* 1999;29:1227-40.

7510 Nagao A, Seki M, Kobayashi H. Inhibition of xanthine oxidase by flavonoids. *Biosci Biotechnol Biochem* 1999;63:1787-90.

7511 Steerenberg PA, Garssen J, Dortant P, et al. Protection of UV-induced suppression of skin contact hypersensitivity: a common feature of flavonoids after oral administration? *Photochem Photobiol* 1998;67:456-61.

7512 Critchfield JW, Coligan JE, Folks TM, Butera ST. Casein kinase II is a selective target of HIV-1 transcriptional inhibitors. *Proc Natl Acad Sci U S A* 1997;94:6110-5.

7513 Walle T, Otake Y, Galijatovic A, et al. Induction of UDP-glucuronosyltransferase UGT1A1 by the flavonoid chrysin in the human hepatoma cell line hep G2. *Drug Metab Dispos* 2000;28:1077-82.

7514 Brown GA, Vukovich MD, Reifenrath TA, et al. Effects of anabolic precursors on serum testosterone concentrations and adaptations to resistance training in young men. *Int J Sport Nutr Exerc Metab* 2000;10:340-59.

7517 World Health Organization. Guidelines for Iodine Prophylaxis following Nuclear Accidents: www.who.int/environmental_information/ Information_resources/on_line_radiation.htm. (Accessed 11 January 2002).

7518 Center for Drug Evaluation and Research. Guidance. Potassium iodide as a thyroid blocking agent in radiation emergencies. Food and Drug Administration December 2001. Available at: http://www.fda.gov/cder/guidance/4825fnl.htm.

7520 Vissers MN, Zock PL, Meijer GW, Katan MB. Effect of plant sterols from rice bran oil and triterpene alcohols from sheanut oil on serum lipoprotein concentrations in humans. *Am J Clin Nutr* 2000;72:1510-5.

7521 Sugano M, Koba K, Tsuji E. Health benefits of rice bran oil. *Anticancer Res* 1999;19:3651-7.

7522 Dowling EA, Redondo DR, Branch JD, et al. Effect of Eleutherococcus senticosus on submaximal and maximal exercise performance. *Med Sci Sports Exerc* 1996;28:482-9.

7523 Shang SY, Ma YS, Wang SS. [Effect of eleutherosides on ventricular late potential with coronary heart disease and myocarditis]. [Article in Chinese] *Zhong Xi Yi Jie He Za Zhi* 1991;11:280-1, 261.

7524 Shi Z, Liu C, Li R. [Effect of a mixture of Acanthopanax senticosus and Elsholtzia splendens on serum-lipids in patients with hyperlipemia]. [Article in Chinese] *Zhong Xi Yi Jie He Za Zhi* 1990r;10:155-6, 132.

7525 Hacker B, Medon PJ. Cytotoxic effects of Eleutherococcus senticosus aqueous extracts in combination with N6-(delta 2-isopentenyl)-adenosine and 1-beta-D-arabinofuranosylcytosine against L1210 leukemia cells. *J Pharm Sci* 1984;73:270-2.

7526 Glatthaar-Saalmuller B, Sacher F, Esperester A. Antiviral activity of an extract derived from roots of Eleutherococcus senticosus. *Antiviral Res* 2001;50:223-8.

7527 Sui DY, Lu ZZ, Li SH, Cai Y. [Hypoglycemic effect of saponin isolated from leaves of Acanthopanax senticosus (Rupr. et Maxin.) Harms]. [Article in Chinese] *Zhongguo Zhong Yao Za Zhi* 1994;19:683-5, 703.

7528 Sui DY, Lu ZZ, Ma LN, Fan ZG. [Effects of the leaves of Acanthopanax senticosus (Rupr. et Maxim.) Harms. On myocardial infarct size in acute ischemic dogs]. [Article in Chinese]. *Zhongguo Zhong Yao Za Zhi* 1994;19:746-7, 764.

7529 Han L, Cai D. [Clinical and experimental study on treatment of acute cerebral infarction with Acanthopanax Injection]. [Article in Chinese] *Zhongguo Zhong Xi Yi Jie He Za Zhi* 1998;18:472-4.

7530 Shen ML, Zhai SK, Chen HL, Immunomopharmacological effects of polysaccharides from Acanthopanax senticosus on experimental animals. *Int J Immunopharmacol* 1991;13:549-54.

7531 Medon PJ, Ferguson PW, Watson CF. Effects of Eleutherococcus senticosus extracts on hexobarbital metabolism in vivo and in vitro. *J Ethnopharmacol* 1984;10:235-41.

7532 Harkey MR, Henderson GL, Zhou L, et al. Effects of Siberian ginseng (Eleutherococcus senticosus) on c-DNA-expressed P450 drug metabolizing enzymes. *Alt Ther* 2001;7:S14.

7533 Harkey MR, Henderson GL, Gershwin ME, et al. Variability in commercial ginseng products: an analysis of 25 preparations. *Am J Clin Nutr* 2001;73:1101-6.

7538 Naseem MZ, Patil SR, Patil SR, et al. Antispermatogenic and androgenic activities of Momordica charantia (Karela) in albino rats. *J Ethnopharmacol* 1998;61:9-16.

7539 Schreiber CA, Wan L, Sun Y, et al. The antiviral agents, MAP30 and GAP31, are not toxic to human spermatozoa and may be useful in preventing the sexual transmission of

REFERENCES

human immunodeficiency virus type 1. *Fertil Steril* 1999;72:686-90.

7540 Bourinbaiar AS, Lee-Huang S. The activity of plant-derived antiretroviral proteins MAP30 and GAP31 against herpes simplex virus in vitro. *Biochem Biophys Res Commun* 1996;219:923-9.

7541 Jiratchariyakul W, Wiwat C, Vongsakul M, et al. HIV inhibitor from Thai bitter gourd. *Planta Med* 2001;67:350-3.

7542 Lee-Huang S, Huang PL, Huang PL, et al. Inhibition of the integrase of human immunodeficiency virus (HIV) type 1 by anti-HIV plant proteins MAP30 and GAP31. *Proc Natl Acad Sci U S A* 1995;92:8818-22.

7543 Lee-Huang S, Huang PL, Nara PL, et al. MAP 30: a new inhibitor of HIV-1 infection and replication. *FEBS Lett* 1990;272:12-8.

7555 Food and Nutrition Board, Institute of Medicine. Dietary Reference Intakes for Calcium, Phosphorus, Magnesium, Vitamin D, and Fluoride. Washington, DC: National Academy Press, 1999. Available at: http://books.nap.edu/books/0309063507/html/index.html.

7556 Cox IM, Campbell MJ, Dowson D. Red blood cell magnesium and chronic fatigue syndrome. *Lancet* 1991;337:757-60.

7557 Hinds G, Bell NP, McMaster D, McCluskey DR. Normal red cell magnesium concentrations and magnesium loading tests in patients with chronic fatigue syndrome. *Ann Clin Biochem* 1994;31:459-61.

7558 Kuratsune H, Yamaguti K, Sawada M, et al. Dehydroepiandrosterone sulfate deficiency in chronic fatigue syndrome. *Int J Mol Med* 1998;1:143-6.

7559 Himmel PB, Seligman TM. A Pilot Study Employing Dehydroepiandrosterone (DHEA) in the Treatment of Chronic Fatigue Syndrome. [Abstract] *J Clin Rheumatol* 1999:5:56-9.

7561 Kaslow JE, Rucker L, Onishi R. Liver extract-folic acid-cyanocobalamin vs placebo for chronic fatigue syndrome. *Arch Intern Med* 1989;149:2501-3.

7562 Lloyd AR, Hickie I, Brockman A, et al. Immunologic and psychologic therapy for patients with chronic fatigue syndrome: a double-blind, placebo-controlled trial. *Am J Med* 1993 Feb;94(2):197-203.

7563 Behan PO, Behan WM, Horrobin D. Effect of high doses of essential fatty acids on the postviral fatigue syndrome. *Acta Neurol Scand* 1990;82:209-16.

7564 Warren G, McKendrick M, Peet M. The role of essential fatty acids in chronic fatigue syndrome. A case-controlled study of red-cell membrane essential fatty acids (EFA) and a placebo-controlled treatment study with high dose of EFA. *Acta Neurol Scand* 1999;99:112-6.

7565 Hederos CA, Berg A. Epogam evening primrose oil treatment in atopic dermatitis and asthma. *Arch Dis Child* 1996;75:494-7.

7566 Berth-Jones J, Graham-Brown RA. Placebo-controlled trial of essential fatty acid supplementation in atopic dermatitis. *Lancet* 1993;341:1557-60.

7567 Whitaker DK, Cilliers J, de Beer C. Evening primrose oil (Epogam) in the treatment of chronic hand dermatitis: disappointing therapeutic results. *Dermatology* 1996;193:115-20.

7568 Bordoni A, Biagi PL, Masi M, et al. Evening primrose oil (Efamol) in the treatment of children with atopic eczema. *Drugs Exp Clin Res* 1988;14:291-7.

7569 Schalin-Karrila M, Mattila L, Jansen CT, Uotila P. Evening primrose oil in the treatment of atopic eczema: effect on clinical status, plasma phospholipid fatty acids and circulating blood prostaglandins. *Br J Dermatol* 1987;117:11-9.

7570 Biagi PL, Bordoni A, Hrelia S, et al. The effect of gamma-linolenic acid on clinical status, red cell fatty acid composition and membrane microviscosity in infants with atopic dermatitis. *Drugs Exp Clin Res* 1994;20:77-84.

7571 Clark WF, Parbtani A, Naylor CD, et al. Fish oil in lupus nephritis: clinical findings and methodological implications. *Kidney Int* 1993;44:75-86.

7572 Walton AJ, Snaith ML, Locniskar M, et al. Dietary fish oil and the severity of symptoms in patients with systemic lupus erythematosus. *Ann Rheum Dis* 1991;50:463-6.

7573 DiGiacomo RA, Kremer JM, Shah DM. Fish-oil dietary supplementation in patients with Raynaud's phenomenon: a double-blind, controlled, prospective study. *Am J Med* 1989;86:158-64.

7574 Harel Z, Biro FM, Kottenhahn RK, Rosenthal SL. Supplementation with omega-3 polyunsaturated fatty acids in the management of dysmenorrhea in adolescents. *Am J Obstet Gynecol* 1996;174:1335-8.

7575 Deutch B, Jorgensen EB, Hansen JC. Menstrual discomfort in Danish women reduced by dietary supplements of omega-3 PUFA and B12 (fish oil or seal oil capsules). *Nut Res* 2000;20:621-31.

7585 Bonithon-Kopp C, Kronborg O, Giacosa A, et al. Calcium and fibre supplementation in prevention of colorectal adenoma recurrence: a randomised intervention trial. European Cancer Prevention Organisation Study Group. *Lancet* 2000;356:1300-6.

7591 Hikino H, Takahashi M, Otake K, Konno C. Isolation and hypoglycemic activity of eleutherans A, B, C, D, E, F, and G: glycans of Eleutherococcus senticosus roots. *J Nat Prod* 1986;49:293-7.

7592 Yun-Choi HS, Kim JH, Lee JR. Potential inhibitors of platelet aggregation from plant sources, III. *J Nat Prod* 1987;50:1059-64.

7593 Asano K, Takahashi T, Miyashita M, et al. Effect of Eleutherococcus senticosus extract on human physical working capacity. *Planta Med* 1986:175-7.

7594 Krahwinkel T, Willershausen B. The effect of sugar-free green tea chew candies on the degree of inflammation of the gingiva. *Eur J Med Res* 2000;5:463-7.

7595 Schapowal A. Petasites Study Group. Randomised controlled trial of butterbur and cetirizine for treating seasonal allergic rhinitis. *BMJ* 2002;324:144-6.

7596 Ziolo G, Samochowiec L. Study on clinical properties and mechanisms of action of Petasites in bronchial asthma and chronic obstructive bronchitis. *Pharm Acta Helv* 1998;72:378-80.

7597 Scheidegger C, Dahinden C, Wiesmann U. Effects of extracts and of individual components from Petasites on prostaglandin synthesis in cultured skin fibroblasts and on leucotriene synthesis in isolated human peripheral leucocytes. *Pharm Acta Helv* 1998;72:376-8.

7598 Jariwalla RJ. Rice-bran products: phytonutrients with potential applications in preventive and clinical medicine. *Drugs Exp Clin Res* 2001;27:17-26.

7599 Voigt RG, Llorente AM, Jensen CL, et al. A randomized, double-blind, placebo-controlled trial of docosahexaenoic acid supplementation in children with attention-deficit/hyperactivity disorder. *J Pediatr* 2001;139:189-96.

7600 Dusman K, Plowman SA, McCarthy K, et al. The effects of Endurox on the physiological responses to stair-stepping exercise. *Med Sci Sports Exerc* 1998;30 Suppl:S323.

7601 Cheuvroni SN, Moffatt RF, Biggerstaff KD, et al. Effects of Endurox on various metabolic responses to exercise. *Med Sci Sports Exerc* 1998;30 Suppl:S32.

7602 Luo P, Wang L. Peripheral blood mononuclear cell production of TNF-alpha in response to North American ginseng stimulation [abstract]. *Alt Ther* 2001;7:S21.

7603 Caicoya M. Fish consumption and stroke: a community case-control study in Asturias, Spain. *Neuroepidemiology* 2002;21:107-14.

7604 Williams CM. Effects of inulin on lipid parameters in humans. *J Nutr* 1999 Jul;129(7 Suppl):1471S-3S.

7605 Roberfroid MB, Van Loo JA, Gibson GR. The bifidogenic nature of chicory inulin and its hydrolysis products. *J Nutr* 1998;128:11-9.

7606 Menne E, Guggenbuhl N, Roberfroid M. Fn-type chicory inulin hydrolysate has a prebiotic effect in humans. *J Nutr* 2000;130:1197-9.

7607 Hoeger WW, Harris C, Long EM, Hopkins DR. Four-week supplementation with a natural dietary compound produces favorable changes in body composition. *Adv Ther* 1998;15:305-14.

7608 Gay-Crosier F, Schreiber G, Hauser C. Anaphylaxis from inulin in vegetables and processed food. *N Engl J Med* 2000;342:1372.

7610 Diez-Tejedor E, Fuentes B. Fish consumption and stroke: benefit or risk? *Neuroepidemiology* 2002;21:105-6.

7611 Kruger MC, Coetzer H, de Winter R, et al. Calcium, gamma-linolenic acid and eicosapentaenoic acid supplementation in senile osteoporosis. *Aging* (Milano) 1998;10:385-94.

7612 Pinsky C, Bose R. Pharmacological and toxicological investigations of cesium. *Pharmacol Biochem Behav* 1984;21:17-23.

7613 Sartori HE. Cesium therapy in cancer patients. *Pharmacol Biochem Behav* 1984;21:11-3.

7614 Hunt PJ, Gurnell EM, Huppert FA, et al. Improvement in mood and fatigue after dehydroepiandrosterone replacement in Addison's disease in a randomized, double blind trial. *J Clin Endocrinol Metab* 2000;85:4650-6.

7615 Trivedi DP, Khaw KT. Dehydroepiandrosterone sulfate and mortality in elderly men and women. *J Clin Endocrinol Metab* 2000;85:4650-6.

7616 Beer NA, Jakubowicz DJ, Matt DW, et al. Dehydroepiandrosterone reduces plasma plasminogen activator inhibitor type 1 and tissue plasminogen activator antigen in men. *Am J Med Sci* 1996;311:205-10.

7617 Araghiniknam M, Chung S, Nelson-White T, et al. Antioxidant activity of dioscorea and dehydroepiandrosterone (DHEA) in older humans. *Life Sci* 1996;59:PL147-57.

7618 Legrain S, Massien C, Lahlou N, et al. Dehydroepiandrosterone replacement administration: pharmacokinetic and pharmacodynamic studies in healthy elderly subjects. *J Clin Endocrinol Metab* 2000;85:3208-17.

7619 Strandberg TE, Jarvenpaa AL, Vanhanen H, McKeigue PM. Birth outcome in relation to licorice consumption during pregnancy. *Am J Epidemiol* 2001;153:1085-8.

7620 Sigurjonsdottir HA, Franzson L, Manhem K, et al. Liquorice-induced rise in blood pressure: a linear dose-response relationship. *J Hum Hypertens* 2001;15:549-52.

7621 Phillips S, Hutchinson S, Ruggier R. Zingiber officinale does not affect gastric emptying rate. A randomised, placebo-controlled, crossover trial. *Anaesthesia* 1993;48:393-5.

7622 Srivastava KC. Effect of onion and ginger consumption on platelet thromboxane production in humans. *Leukot Essent Fatty Acids* 1989;35:183-5.

7623 Grontved A, Hentzer E. Vertigo-reducing effect of ginger root. A controlled clinical study. *Orl J Otorhinolaryngol Relat Spec* 1986;48:282-6.

7624 Stewart JJ, Wood MJ, Wood CD, Mims ME. Effects of ginger on motion sickness susceptibility and gastric function. *Pharmacology* 1991;42:111-20.

7625 Wood CD, Manno JE, Wood MJ, et al. Comparison of efficacy of ginger with various antimotion sickness drugs. *Clin Res Pr Drug Regul Aff* 1988;6:129-36.

7626 Park GJ, Mann SP, Ngu MC. Acute hepatitis induced by Shou-Wu-Pian, a herbal product derived from Polygonum multiflorum. *J Gastroenterol Hepatol* 2001;16:115-7.

7627 But PP, Tomlinson B, Lee KL. Hepatitis related to the Chinese medicine Shou-wu-pian manufactured from Polygonum multiflorum. *Vet Hum Toxicol* 1996;38:280-2.

7628 Langner E, Greifenberg S, Gruenwald J. Ginger: history and use. *Adv Ther* 1998;15:25-44.

7629 Gadek JE, DeMichele SJ, Karlstad MD, et al. Effect of enteral feeding with eicosapentaenoic acid, gamma-linolenic acid, and antioxidants in patients with acute respiratory distress syndrome. Enteral Nutrition in ARDS Study Group. *Crit Care Med* 1999;27:1409-20.

7630 Tollesson A, Frithz A. Borage oil, an effective new treatment for infantile seborrhoeic dermatitis. *Br J Dermatol* 1993;129:95.

7631 Parvals O, Vander Stricht B, Vanhaeten-Fastre R, Vanhaeten M. TLC detection of pyrrolizidine alkaloids in oil extracted from the seed of borago officinalis. *Journal of Planar Chromatography* 1994;7:80-2.

7632 Henz BM, Jablonska S, van de Kerkhof PC, et al. Double-blind, multicentre analysis of the efficacy of borage oil in patients with atopic eczema. *Br J Dermatol* 1999;140:685-8.

7633 Henz BM. Efficacy of borage oil in patients with atopic eczema - reply from author. *Br J Dermatol* 2000;143:201.

7634 Engler MM, Engler MB, Erickson SK, Paul SM. Dietary gamma-linolenic acid lowers blood pressure and alters aortic reactivity and cholesterol metabolism in hypertension. *J Hypertens* 1992;10:1197-204.

7635 Fisher BAC, Harbige LS. Effect of omega-6 lipid-rich borage oil feeding on immune function in healthy volunteers (abstract). *Biochemical Society Transactions* 1997;25:343S.

7636 St-Onge MP, Farnworth ER, Savard T, et al. Kefir consumption does not alter plasma lipid levels or cholesterol fractional synthesis rates relative to milk in hyperlipidemic men: a randomized controlled trial [ISRCTN10820810]. *BMC Complement Altern Med* 2002;2(1):1.

7637 Monauni T, Zenti MG, Cretti A, et al. Effects of glucosamine infusion on insulin secretion and insulin action in humans. *Diabetes* 2000;49:926-35.

7638 Pouwels MJ, Jacobs JR, Span PN, et al. Short-term glucosamine infusion does not affect insulin sensitivity in humans. *J Clin Endocrinol Metab* 2001;86:2099-103.

7639 Yun J, Tomida A, Nagata K, Tsuruo T. Glucose-regulated stresses confer resistance to VP-16 in human cancer cells through a decreased expression of DNA topoisomerase II. *Oncol Res* 1995;7:583-90.

7640 Olszewski AJ, Szostak WB, McCully KS. Plasma glucosamine and galactosamine in ischemic heart disease. *Atherosclerosis* 1990;82:75-83.

7641 Nowak A, Szczesniak L, Rychlewski T, et al. Glucosamine levels in people with ischaemic heart disease with and without type II diabetes. *Pol Arch Med Wewn* 1998;100:419-25.

7642 Bagasra O, Whittle P, Heins B, Pomerantz RJ. Anti-human immunodeficiency virus type 1 activity of sulfated monosaccharides: comparison with sulfated polysaccharides and other polyions. *J Infect Dis* 1991;164:1082-90.

7645 Alic M. Baker's yeast in Crohn's disease—can it kill you? *Am J Gastroenterol* 1999;94:1711.

7646 Plein K, Hotz J. Therapeutic effects of Saccharomyces boulardii on mild residual symptoms in a stable phase of Crohn's disease with special respect to chronic diarrhea – a pilot study. *Gastroenterol* 1993;31:129-34.

REFERENCES

7652 Muller J, Remus N, Harms KH. Mycoserological study of the treatment of paediatric cystic fibrosis patients with Saccharomyces boulardii (Saccharomyces cerevisiae Hansen CBS 5926). *Mycoses* 1995;38:119-23.

7653 Nagata C, Takatsuka N, Kawakami N, Shimizu H. Soy product intake and hot flashes in Japanese women: results from a community-based prospective study. *Am J Epidemiol* 2001;153:790-3.

7654 Duncan AM, Merz BE, Xu X, et al. Soy isoflavones exert modest hormonal effects in premenopausal women. *J Clin Endocrinol Metab* 1999;84:192-7.

7655 Glazier MG, Bowman MA. A review of the evidence for the use of phytoestrogens as a replacement for traditional estrogen replacement therapy. *Arch Intern Med* 2001;161:1161-72.

7656 Chen C, Wang X, Chen D, et al. Tofu consumption and blood lead levels in young Chinese adults. *Am J Epidemiol* 2001;153:1206-12.

7657 Morito K, Hirose T, Kinjo J, et al. Interaction of phytoestrogens with estrogen receptors alpha and beta. *Biol Pharm Bull* 2001;24:351-6.

7658 Van Patten CL, Olivotto IA, Chambers GK, et al. Effect of soy phytoestrogens on hot flashes in postmenopausal women with breast cancer: a randomized, controlled clinical trial. *J Clin Oncol* 2002;20:1449-55.

7659 Scheiber MD, Liu JH, Subbiah MT, et al. Dietary inclusion of whole soy foods results in significant reductions in clinical risk factors for osteoporosis and cardiovascular disease in normal postmenopausal women. *Menopause* 2001;8:384-92.

7660 Mei J, Yeung SS, Kung AW. High dietary phytoestrogen intake is associated with higher bone mineral density in postmenopausal but not premenopausal women. *J Clin Endocrinol Metab* 2001;86:5217-21.

7661 Busby MG, Jeffcoat AR, Bloedon LT, et al. Clinical characteristics and pharmacokinetics of purified soy isoflavones: single-dose administration to healthy men. *Am J Clin Nutr* 2002;75:126-36.

7662 Horn-Ross PL, Hoggatt KJ, Lee MM. Phytoestrogens and thyroid cancer risk: the San Francisco Bay Area thyroid cancer study. *Cancer Epidemiol Biomarkers Prev* 2002;11:43-9.

7663 Wu AH, Stanczyk FZ, Hendrich, S et al. Effects of soy foods on ovarian function in premenopausal women. *Br J Cancer* 2000;82:1879-86 .

7664 Riby JE, Chang GHF, Firestone GL, Bjeldanes LF. Ligand-independent activation of estrogen receptor function by 3,3'-diindolylmethane in human breast cancer cells. *Biochem Pharmacol* 2000;60:167-77.

7665 McDougal A, Gupta MS, Ramamoorthy K, et al. Inhibition of carcinogen-induced rat mammary tumor growth and other estrogen-dependent responses by symmetrical dihalo-substituted analogs of diindolylmethane. *Cancer Lett* 2000;151:169-79.

7666 Chen I, McDougal A, Wang F, Safe S. Aryl hydrocarbon receptor-mediated antiestrogenic and antitumorigenic activity of diindolylmethane. *Carcinogenesis* 1998 Sep;19:1631-9.

7667 Lake BG, Tredger JM, Renwick AB, et al. 3'3-diindolylmethane induces CYP1A2 in cultured precision-cut human liver slices. *Xenobiotica* 1998;28:803-11.

7668 Ge X, Yanni S, Rennert G, et al. 3'3-diindolylmethane induces apoptosis in human cancer cells. *Biochem Biophys Res Commun* 1996;228:153-8.

7669 Chen I, Safe S, Bjeldanes L. Indole-3-carbinol and diindolylmethane as aryl hydrocarbon (Ah) receptor agonists and antagonists in T47D human breast cancer cells. *Biochem Pharmacol* 1996;51:1069-76.

7670 Sartori HE. Nutrients and cancer: an introduction to cesium therapy. *Pharmacol Biochem Behav* 1984;21:7-10.

7671 Neulieb R. Effect of oral intake of cesium chloride: a single case report. *Pharmacol Biochem Behav* 1984;21:15-6.

7672 Healon Prescribing Information. Pharmacia & Upjohn, Kalamazoo, MI, 2002.

7673 Igea JM, Cuesta J, Cuevas M, et al. Adverse reaction to pomegranate ingestion. *Allergy* 1991;46:472-4.

7674 Gaig P, Bartolome B, Lleonart R, et al. Allergy to pomegranate (Punica granatum). *Allergy* 1999;54:287-8.

7685 Kakuda T, Yanase H, Utsunomiya K, et al. Protective effect of gamma-glutamylethylamide (theanine) on ischemic delayed neuronal death in gerbils. *Neurosci Lett* 2000;289:189-92.

7686 Kimura R, Murata T. Effect of theanine on norepinephrine and serotonin levels in rat brain. *Chem Pharm Bull* 1986;34:3053-57.

7687 Yokogoshi H, Kobayashi M. Hypotensive effect of gamma-glutamylethylamide in spontaneously hypertensive rats. *Life Sci* 1998;62:1065-8.

7688 Sugiyama T, Sadzuka Y, Tanaka K, Sonobe T. Inhibition of glutamate transporter by theanine enhances the therapeutic efficacy of doxorubicin. *Toxicol Lett* 2000:121:89-96.

7689 Sadzuka Y, Sugiyama T, Sonobe T. Improvement of idarubicin induced antitumor activity and bone marrow suppression by theanine, a component of tea. *Cancer Lett* 2000;158:119-24.

7690 Sadzuka Y, Sugiyama T, Sonobe T. Efficacies of tea components on doxorubicin induced antitumor activity and reversal of multidrug resistance. *Toxicol Lett* 2000;114:155-62.

7691 Cheng CL, Koo MWL. Effects of Centella asiatica on ethanol induced gastric mucosal lesions in rats. *Life Sci* 2000;67:2647-53.

7692 Babu TD, Kuttan G, Padikkala J. Cytotoxic and anti-tumour properties of certain taxa of Umbelliferae with special reference to Centella asiatica (L.) Urban. *J Ethnopharmacol* 1995;48:53-7.

7693 Koch R. Comparative study of venostatin and pycnogenol in chronic venous insufficiency. *Phytother Res* 2002:16:S1-S5.

7694 Jialal I, Devaraj S, Hirany S, et al. The effect of pycnogenol supplementation on markers of inflammation. *Alternative Therapies* 2001;7:S17.

7695 Cheshier JE, Ardestani-Kaboudanian S, Liang B, et al. Immunomodulation by pycnogenol in retrovirus-induced or ethanol-fed mice. *Life Sci* 1996;58:87-96.

7696 Saliou C, Rimbach G, Molni H, McLaughlin L, Hosseini S, Lee J, et al. Solar ultraviolet-induced erythema in human skin and nuclear factor-kappa-b-dependent gene expression in keratinocytes are modulated by a French Maritime pine bark extract. *Free Radic Biol Med* 2001;30:154-60.

7697 Park YC, Rimbach G, Saliou C, et al. Activity of monomeric, dimeric, and trimeric flavonoids on NO production, TNF-alpha secretion, and NF-KB-dependent gene expression in RAW 264.7 macrophages. *FEBS Letters* 2000:465;93-7.

7698 Virgili F, Kim D, Packer L. Procyanidins extracted from pine bark protect alpha-tocopherol in ECV 304 endothelial cells challenged by activated RAW 264.7 macrophages: role of nitric oxide and peroxynitrite. *FEBS Letters* 1998;431:315-8.

7699 Liu F, Lau BHS, Peng Q, Shah V. Pycnogenol protects vascular endothelial cells from beta-amyloid-induced injury. *Biol Pharm Bull* 2000;23:735-737.

7700 Vikrant V, Grover JK, Tandon N, et al. Treatment with extracts of Momordica charantia and Eugenia jambolana prevents hyperglycemia and hyperinsulinemia in fructose fed rats. *J Ethnopharmacol* 2001;76:139-43.

7701 Leventhal LJ, Boyce EG, Zurier RB. Treatment of rheumatoid arthritis with gammalinolenic acid. *Ann Intern Med* 1993;119:867-73.

7702 Zurier RB, Rossetti RG, Jacobson EW, et al. Gamma-linolenic acid treatment of rheumatoid arthritis. A randomized, placebo-controlled trial. *Arthritis Rheum* 1996;39:1808-17.

7703 Schwick HG, Heide K. Immunochemistry and immunology of collagen and gelatin. *Bibl Haematol* 1969;33:111-25.

7704 Moskowitz RW. Role of collagen hydrolysate in bone and joint disease.*Semin Arthritis Rheum* 2000;30:87-99.

7706 Brown KE, Leong K, Huang CH, et al. Gelatin/chondroitin 6-sulfate microspheres for the delivery of therapeutic proteins to the joint. *Arthritis Rheum* 1998;41:2185-95.

7707 Kakimoto K, Kojima Y, Ishii K, et al. The suppressive effect of gelatin-conjugated superoxide dismutase on disease development and severity of collagen-induced arthritis in mice. *Clin Exp Immunol* 1993;94:241-6.

7708 Kelso JM. The gelatin story. *J Allergy Clin Immunol* 1999;103:200-2.

7709 Nakayama T, Aizawa C, Kuno-Sakai H. A clinical analysis of gelatin allergy and determination of its causal relationship to the previous administration of gelatin-containing acellular pertussis vaccine combined with diphtheria and tetanus toxoids. *J Allergy Clin Immunol* 1999;103:321-5.

7710 Sakaguchi M, Inouye S. Anaphylaxis to gelatin-containing rectal suppositories. *J Allergy Clin Immunol* 2001;108:1033-4.

7711 PDR Electronic Library. Montvale, NJ: Medical Economics Company, Inc., 2001.

7712 Feskanich D, Singh V, Willett WC, Colditz GA. Vitamin A intake and hip fractures among postmenopausal women. *JAMA* 2002;287:47-54.

7713 Melhus H, Michaelsson K, Kindmark A, et al. Excessive dietary intake of vitamin A is associated with reduced bone mineral density and increased risk for hip fracture. *Ann Intern Med* 1998;129:770-8.

7714 Gey KF, Stahelin HB, Eichholzer M. Poor plasma status of carotene and vitamin C is associated with higher mortality from ischemic heart disease and stroke: Basel Prospective Study. *Clin Investig* 1993;71:3-6.

7715 Knekt P, Reunanen A, Jarvinen R, et al. Antioxidant vitamin intake and coronary mortality in a longitudinal population study. *Am J Epidemiol* 1994;139:1180-9.

7716 Keli SO, Hertog MG, Feskens EJ, Kromhout D. Dietary flavonoids, antioxidant vitamins, and incidence of stroke: the Zutphen study. *Arch Intern Med* 1996;156:637-42.

7717 Food and Drug Administration, Center for Food Safety and Applied Nutrition. Consumer Questions and Answers About BSE. March 2001 Available at: http://vm.cfsan.fda.gov/~comm/bsefaq.html.

7718 Brown P. Afterthoughts about Bovine Spongiform Encephalopathy and Variant Creutzfeldt-Jakob Disease. Emerging Infectious Diseases 2001:7. Website: http://www.cdc.gov/ncidod/eid/vol7no3_supp/brown.htm (Accessed 1 April 2002).

7722 Elsayed NM, Bendich A. Dietary antioxidants: potential effects on oxidative products in cigarette smoke. *Nut Res* 2001;21:551-67.

7724 Watkins ML, Erickson JD, Thun MJ, et al. Multivitamin use and mortality in a large prospective study. *Am J Epidemiol* 2000;152:149-62.

7725 Title LM, Cummings PM, Giddens K, et al. Effect of folic acid and antioxidant vitamins on endothelial dysfunction in patients with coronary artery disease. *J Am Coll Cardiol* 2000;36:758-65.

7726 Hertog MG, Feskens EJ, Hollman PC, et al. Dietary antioxidant flavonoids and risk of coronary heart disease: the Zutphen Elderly Study. *Lancet* 1993;342:1007-1011.

7727 Meseguer E, Taboada R, Sanchez V, et al. Life-threatening parkinsonism induced by kava-kava. *Mov Disord* 2002;17:195-6.

7728 Ruze P. Kava-induced dermopathy: a niacin deficiency? *Lancet* 1990;335:1442-5.

7729 Shabert JK, Winslow C, Lacey JM, Wilmore DW. Glutamine-antioxidant supplementation increases body cell mass in AIDS patients with weight loss: a randomized, double-blind controlled trial. *Nutrition* 1999;15:860-4.

7730 Scolapio JS, McGreevy K, Tennyson GS, Burnett OL. Effect of glutamine in short-bowel syndrome. *Clin Nutr* 2001;20:319-23.

7731 Alverdy JC. Effects of glutamine-supplemented diets on immunology of the gut. *JPEN J Parenter Enteral Nutr* 1990;14:109S-13S.

7732 Mertes N, Schulzki C, Goeters C, et al. Cost containment through L-alanyl-L-glutamine supplemented total parenteral nutrition after major abdominal surgery: a prospective randomized double-blind controlled study. *Clin Nutr* 2000;19:395-401.

7733 Reeds PJ, Burrin DG. Glutamine and the bowel. *J Nutr* 2001;131:2505S-8S.

7734 Newsholme P. Why is L-glutamine metabolism important to cells of the immune system in health, postinjury, surgery or infection? *J Nutr* 2001;131:2515S-22S.

7735 Wilmore DW. The effect of glutamine supplementation in patients following elective surgery and accidental injury. *J Nutr* 2001;131:2543S-9S.

7736 Kusumoto I. Industrial production of L-glutamine. *J Nutr* 2001;131:2552S-5S.

7737 Furst P. New developments in glutamine delivery. *J Nutr* 2001;131:2562S-8S.

7738 Ziegler TR. Glutamine supplementation in cancer patients receiving bone marrow transplantation and high dose chemotherapy. *J Nutr* 2001;131:2578S-84S.

7739 Medina MA. Glutamine and cancer. *J Nutr* 2001;131:2539S-42S.

7740 Neu J. Glutamine in the fetus and critically ill low birth weight neonate: metabolism and mechanism of action. *J Nutr* 2001;131:2585S-9S.

7741 Szajewska H, Kotowska M, Mrukowicz JZ, et al. Efficacy of Lactobacillus GG in prevention of nosocomial diarrhea in infants. *J Pediatr* 2001;138:361-5.

7742 Chandra RK. Effect of Lactobacillus on the incidence and severity of acute rotavirus diarrhoea in infants. A prospective placebo-controlled double-blind study. *Nut Res* 2001;22:65-9.

7743 Rautava S, Kalliomaki M, Isolauri E. Probiotics during pregnancy and breast-feeding might confer immunomodulatory protection against atopic disease in the infant. *J Allergy Clin Immunol* 2002;109:119-21.

7744 Halpern GM, Prindiville T, Blankenburg M, et al. Treatment of irritable bowel syndrome with Lacteol Fort: a randomized, double-blind, cross-over trial. *Am J Gastroenterol* 1996;91:1579-85.

7745 Maggi L, Mastromarino P, Macchia S, et al. Technological and biological evaluation of tablets containing different strains of lactobacilli for vaginal administration. *Eur J Pharm Biopharm* 2000;50:389-95.

7746 Wagner RD, Pierson C, Warner T, et al. Biotherapeutic effects of probiotic bacteria on candidiasis in immunodeficient mice. *Infect Immun* 1997;65:4165-4172.

7747 Mao Y, Nobaek S, Kasravi B, et al. The effects of Lactobacillus strains and oat fiber on methotrexate-induced enterocolitis in rats. *Gastroenterology* 1996;111:334-44.

REFERENCES

7748 Palmfeldt J, Hahn-Hagerdal B. Influence of culture pH on survival of Lactobacillus reuteri subjected to freeze-drying. *Int J Food Microbiol* 2000;55:235-8.

7749 Alak JI, Wolf BW, Mdurvwa EG, et al. Effect of Lactobacillus reuteri on intestinal resistance to Cryptosporidium parvum infection in a murine model of acquired immunodeficiency syndrome. *J Infect Dis* 1997;175:218-21.

7750 Kasravi FB, Adawi D, Molin G, et al. Effect of oral supplementation of lactobacilli on bacterial translocation in acute liver injury induced by D-galactosamine. *J Hepatol* 1997;26:417-24.

7751 Shornikova AV, Casas IA, Isolauri E, et al. Lactobacillus reuteri as a therapeutic agent in acute diarrhea in young children. *J Pediatr Gastroenterol Nutr* 1997;24:399-404.

7752 Wolf BW, Wheeler KB, Ataya DG, Garleb KA. Safety and tolerance of Lactobacillus reuteri supplementation to a population infected with the human immunodeficiency virus. *Food Chem Toxicol* 1998;36:1085-94 .

7753 Shornikova AV, Casas IA, Mykkanen H, et al. Bacteriotherapy with Lactobacillus reuteri in rotavirus gastroenteritis. *Pediatr Infect Dis J* 1997;16:1103-7.

7754 Madsen KL, Doyle JS, Jewell LD, et al. Lactobacillus species prevents colitis in interleukin 10 gene-deficient mice. *Gastroenterology* 1999;116:1107-14.

7755 Casas IA, Dobrogosz WJ. Validation of the probiotic concept: Lactobacillus reuteri confers broad-spectrum protection against disease in humans and animals. *Microbial Ecology in Health and Disease* 2000;12:247-85.

7756 Gill HS, Rutherfurd KJ. Probiotic supplementation to enhance natural immunity in the elderly: effects of a newly characterized immunostimulatory strain of Lactobacillus rhamnosus HN001 (DR20) on leucocyte phagocytosis. *Nutr Res* 2001;21:183-9.

7757 Sheih YH, Chiang BL, Wang LH, et al. Systemic immunity-enhancing effects in healthy subjects following dietary consumption of the lactic acid bacterium Lactobacillus rhamnosus HN001. *J Am Coll Nutr* 2001;20:149-56.

7758 Kishi A, Uno K, Matsubara Y, et al. Effect of the oral administration of Lactobacillus brevis subsp. coagulans on interferon-alpha producing capacity in humans. *J Am Coll Nutr* 1996;15:408-12.

7759 Doncheva NI, Antov GP, Softove EB, Nyagolov YP. Experimental and clinical study on the hypolipidemic and antisclerotic effect of Lactobacillus bulgaricus strain GB N 1 (48). *Nutr Res* 2002;22:393-403.

7760 Fujisawa T, Benno Y, Yaeshima T, Mitsuoka T. Taxonomic study of the Lactobacillus acidophilus group, with recognition of Lactobacillus gallinarum sp. nov. and Lactobacillus johnsonii sp. nov. and synonymy of Lactobacillus acidophilus group A3 (Johnson et al. 1980) with the type strain of Lactobacillus amylovorus (Nakamura 1981). *Int J Syst Bacteriol* 1992;42:487-91.

7771 Kucuk O, Sarkar FH, Sakr W, et al. Phase II randomized clinical trial of lycopene supplementation before radical prostatectomy. *Cancer Epidemiol Biomarkers Prev* 2001;10:861-8.

7772 Giovannucci E, Rimm EB, Liu Y, et al. A prospective study of tomato products, lycopene, and prostate cancer risk. *J Natl Cancer Inst* 2002;94:391-8.

7773 Lu QY, Hung JC, Heber D, et al. Inverse associations between plasma lycopene and other carotenoids and prostate cancer. *Cancer Epidemiol Biomarkers Prev* 2001;10:749-56.

7774 Matlaga BR, Hall MC, Stindt D, Torti FM. Response of hormone refractory prostate cancer to lycopene. *J Urol* 2001;166:613.

7775 Popp W, Horak F, Jager S, et al. Horse chestnut (Aesculus hippocastanum) pollen: a frequent cause of allergic sensitization in urban children. *Allergy* 1992;47:380-3.

7776 Lilja JJ, Kivisto KT, Backman JT, Neuvonen PJ. Effect of grapefruit juice dose on grapefruit juice-triazolam interaction: repeated consumption prolongs triazolam half-life. *Eur J Clin Pharmacol* 2000;56:411-5.

7777 Erlund I, Meririnne E, Alfthan G, Aro A. Plasma kinetics and urinary excretion of the flavanones naringenin and hesperetin in humans after ingestion of orange juice and grapefruit juice. *J Nutr* 2001;131:235-41.

7778 Chan WK, Nguyen LT, Miller VP, Harris RZ. Mechanism-based inactivation of human cytochrome P450 3A4 by grapefruit juice and red wine. *Life Sci* 1998;62:PL135-42.

7779 Ho PC, Ghose K, Saville D, Wanwimolruk S. Effect of grapefruit juice on pharmacokinetics and pharmacodynamics of verapamil enantiomers in healthy volunteers. *Eur J Clin Pharmacol* 2000;56:693-8.

7780 Uno T, Ohkubo T, Sugawara K, et al. Effects of grapefruit juice on the stereoselective disposition of nicardipine in humans: evidence for dominant presystemic elimination at the gut site. *Eur J Clin Pharmacol* 2000;56:643-9.

7781 Bailey DG, Dresser GK. Grapefruit juice-lovastatin interaction. *Clin Pharmacol Ther* 2000;67:690.

7782 Lilja JJ, Kivisto KT, Neuvonen PJ. Duration of effect of grapefruit juice on the pharmacokinetics of the CYP3A4 substrate simvastatin. *Clin Pharmacol Ther* 2000;68:384-90.

7783 Geliebter J, Mittelman A, Tiwari RK. PC-SPES and prostate cancer. *J Nutr* 2001;131:164S-166S.

7784 Ades T, Gansler T, Miller M, Rosenthal DS. PC-SPES: current evidence and remaining questions. *CA Cancer J Clin* 2001;51:199-204.

7785 Oh WK, George DJ, Hackmann K, et al. Activity of the herbal combination, PC-SPES, in the treatment of patients with androgen-independent prostate cancer. *Urology* 2001;57:122-6.

7786 de la Taille A, Hayek OR, Burchardt M, et al. Role of herbal compounds (PC-SPES) in hormone-refractory prostate cancer: two case reports. *J Altern Complement Med* 2000;6:449-51.

7787 Schiff JD, Ziecheck WS, Choi B. Pulmonary embolus related to PC-SPES use in a patient with PSA recurrence after radical prostatectomy. *Urology* 2002;59:444.

7788 Wilson GB, Paddock GV, Fudenberg HH. Bovine 'transfer factor': an oligoribonucleopeptide which initiates antigen-specific lymphocytes responsiveness. *Thymus* 1982;4:335-50.

7789 Rozzo SJ, Merryman CF, Kirkpatrick CH. Murine transfer factor. IV. Studies with genetically regulated immune responses. *Cell Immunol* 1988;115:130-45.

7790 Mikula I, Pistl J, Rosocha J. Stabilization of Salmonella-specific dialyzable leukocyte extracts. *Vet Immunol Immunopathol* 1992;32:103-21.

7791 Burger DR, Klesius PH, Vandenbark AA, et al. Transfer of keyhole limpet hemocyanin dermal reactivity to man with bovine transfer factor. *Cell Immunol* 1979;43:192-6.

7792 Wilson GB, Newell RT, Burdash NM. Bovine dialyzable lymph node extracts have antigen-dependent and antigen-independent effects on human cell-mediated immunity in vitro. *Cell Immunol* 1979;47:1-18.

7793 Kirkpatrick CH. Transfer factors: identification of conserved sequences in transfer factor molecules. *Mol Med* 2000;6:332-41.

7794 Spitler LE. Transfer factor therapy in the Wiskott-Aldrich syndrome. Results of long-term follow-up in 32 patients. *Am J Med* 1979;67:59-66.

7795 Jonas S, Wichter M, Spitler L. Amyotrophic lateral sclerosis: failure of transfer factor therapy. *Ann Neurol* 1979;6:84.

7797 Roda E, Viza D, Pizza G, et al. Transfer factor for the treatment of HBsAg-positive chronic active hepatitis. *Proc Soc Exp Biol Med* 1985;178:468-75.

7798 Basten A, McLeod JG, Pollard JD, et al. Transfer factor in treatment of multiple sclerosis. *Lancet* 1980;2:931-4.

7799 Fog T, Pedersen L, Raun NE, et al. Long-term transfer-factor treatment for multiple sclerosis. *Lancet* 1978;1:851-3.

7800 Fujisawa T, Yamaguchi Y, Kimura H, et al. Adjuvant immunotherapy of primary resected lung cancer with transfer factor. *Cancer* 1984;54:663-9.

7801 St Germain A, Peterson CT, Robinson JG, Alekel DL. Isoflavone-rich or isoflavone-poor soy protein does not reduce menopausal symptoms during 24 weeks of treatment. *Menopause* 2001;8:17-26.

7802 Han KK, Soares JM Jr, Haidar MA, et al. Benefits of soy isoflavone therapeutic regimen on menopausal symptoms. *Obstet Gynecol* 2002;99:389-94.

7803 Ho SC, Woo JL, Leung SS, et al. Intake of soy products is associated with better plasma lipid profiles in the Hong Kong Chinese population. *J Nutr* 2000;130:2590-3.

7804 Goodman-Gruen D, Kritz-Silverstein D. Usual dietary isoflavone intake is associated with cardiovascular disease risk factors in postmenopausal women. *J Nutr* 2001;131:1202-6.

7805 Lu LJ, Anderson KE, Grady JJ, Nagamani M. Effects of an isoflavone-free soy diet on ovarian hormones in premenopausal women. *J Clin Endocrinol Metab* 2001;86:3045-52.

7806 Persky VW, Turyk ME, Wang L, et al. Effect of soy protein on endogenous hormones in postmenopausal women. *Am J Clin Nutr* 2002;75:145-53.

7807 de los Reyes GC, Koda RT. Determining hyperforin and hypericin content in eight brands of St. John's wort. *Am J Health Syst Pharm* 2002;59:545-7.

7808 Schulz V. Incidence and clinical relevance of the interactions and side effects of Hypericum preparations. *Phytomedicine* 2001;8:152-60.

7809 Gorski JC, Hamman MA, Wang Z, et al. The effect of St. John's wort on the efficacy of oral contraceptives (abstract MPI-80). *Clin Pharmacol Ther* 2001;71:P25.

7810 Hennessy M, Kelleher D, Spiers JP, et al. St Johns wort increases expression of P-glycoprotein: implications for drug interactions. *Br J Clin Pharmacol* 2002;53:75-82.

7811 Parker V, Wong AH, Boon HS, Seeman MV. Adverse reactions to St John's Wort. *Can J Psychiatry* 2001;46:77-9.

7812 Patel S, Robinson R, Burk M. Hypertensive crisis associated with St. John's Wort. *Am J Med* 2002;112:507-8.

7813 Kanaya Y, Nakamura M, Kobayashi N, Hiramori K. Effects of L-arginine on lower limb vasodilator reserve and exercise capacity in patients with chronic heart failure. *Heart* 1999;81:512-7.

7814 Park KG. The immunological and metabolic effects of L-arginine in human cancer. *Proc Nutr Soc* 1993;52:387-401.

7815 Maxwell AJ, Zapien MP, Pearce GL, et al. Randomized trial of a medical food for the dietary management of chronic, stable angina. *J Am Coll Cardiol* 2002;39:37-45.

7816 Ceremuzynski L, Chamiec T, Herbaczynska-Cedro K. Effect of supplemental oral L-arginine on exercise capacity in patients with stable angina pectoris. *Am J Cardiol* 1997;80:331-3.

7817 Blum A, Hathaway L, Mincemoyer R, et al. Oral L-arginine in patients with coronary artery disease on medical management. *Circulation* 2000;101:2160-4.

7818 Siani A, Pagano E, Iacone R, et al. Blood pressure and metabolic changes during dietary L-arginine supplementation in humans. *Am J Hypertens* 2000;13:547-51.

7819 Tepaske R, Velthuis H, Oudemans-van Straaten HM, et al. Effect of preoperative oral immune-enhancing nutritional supplement on patients at high risk of infection after cardiac surgery: a randomised placebo-controlled trial. *Lancet* 2001;358:696-701.

7820 Wu G, Meininger CJ. Arginine nutrition and cardiovascular function. *J Nutr* 2000;130:2626-9.

7821 Mullen MJ, Wright D, Donald AE, et al. Atorvastatin but not L-arginine improves endothelial function in type I diabetes mellitus: a double-blind study. *J Am Coll Cardiol* 2000;36:410-6.

7822 Cheng JW, Balwin SN. L-arginine in the management of cardiovascular diseases. *Ann Pharmacother* 2001;35:755-64.

7823 Giovannucci E, Rimm EB, Colditz GA, et al. A prospective study of dietary fat and risk of prostate cancer. *J Natl Cancer Inst* 1993;85:1571-9.

7824 Newcomer LM, King IB, Wicklund KG, Stanford JL. The association of fatty acids with prostate cancer risk. *Prostate* 2001;47:262-8.

7825 El-Bayoumy K. The protective role of selenium on genetic damage and on cancer. *Mutat Res* 2001;475:123-39.

7826 Fleshner NE, Kucuk O. Antioxidant dietary supplements: Rationale and current status as chemopreventive agents for prostate cancer. *Urology* 2001;57:90-4.

7827 Stewart MS, Spallholz JE, Neldner KH, Pence BC. Selenium compounds have disparate abilities to impose oxidative stress and induce apoptosis. *Free Radic Biol Med* 1999;26:42-8.

7828 Liu S, Shia D, Liu G, et al. Roles of Se and NO in apoptosis of hepatoma cells. *Life Sci* 2000;68:603-10.

7829 Baum MK, Miguez-Burbano MJ, Campa A, Shor-Posner G. Selenium and interleukins in persons infected with human immunodeficiency virus type 1. *J Infect Dis* 2000;182 Suppl 1:S69-73.

7830 Constans J, Delmas-Beauvieux MC, Sergeant C, et al. One-year antioxidant supplementation with beta-carotene or selenium for patients infected with human immunodeficiency virus: a pilot study. *Clin Infect Dis* 1996;23:654-6.

7831 Wuyi W, Linsheng Y, Shaofan H, et al. Prevention of endemic arsenism with selenium. *Current Science* 2001;81:1215-8.

7832 Shiobara Y, Yoshida T, Suzuki KT. Effects of dietary selenium species on Se concentrations in hair, blood, and urine. *Toxicol Appl Pharmacol* 1998;152:309-14.

7833 Finley JW, Davis CD, Feng Y. Selenium from high selenium broccoli protects rats from colon cancer. *J Nutr* 2000;130:2384-9.

7834 Schrauzer GN. Selenomethionine: a review of its nutritional significance, metabolism and toxicity. *J Nutr* 2000;130:1653-6.

7835 Bogye G, Alfthan G, Machay T, Zubovics L. Enteral yeast-selenium supplementation in preterm infants. *Arch Dis Child Fetal Neonatal Ed* 1998;78:F225-6.

7836 Schrauzer GN. Nutritional selenium supplements: product types, quality, and safety. *J Am Coll Nutr* 2001;20:1-4.

7837 King JC. Effect of reproduction on the bioavailability of calcium, zinc and selenium. *J Nutr* 2001;131:1355S-8S.

7838 Trafikowska U, Zachara BA, Wiacek M, et al. Selenium supply and glutathione peroxidase activity in breastfed Polish infants. *Acta Paediatr* 1996;85:1143-5.

7839 Zapletal C, Heyne S, Golling M, et al. Influence of selenium therapy on liver microcirculation after warm ischemia/ reperfusion: an intravital microscopy study. *Transplant Proc* 2001;33:974-5.

7840 Ustundag Y, Boyacioglu S, Haberal A, et al. Plasma and gastric tissue selenium levels in patients with Helicobacter pylori infection. *J Clin Gastroenterol* 2001;32:405-8.

7841 Shen CL, Song W, Pence BC. Interactions of selenium compounds with other antioxidants in DNA damage and apoptosis in human normal keratinocytes. *Cancer Epidemiol Biomarkers Prev* 2001;10:385-90.

7842 Fartasch M, Teal J, Menon GK. Mode of action of glycolic acid on human stratum corneum: ultrastructural and functional evaluation of the epidermal barrier. *Arch Dermatol Res.* 1997;289:404-9.

7843 Grace E, Emans SJ, Drum DE. Hematologic abnormalities in adolescents who take oral contraceptive pills. *J Pediatr* 1982;101:771-4.

7844 Green TJ, Houghton LA, Donovan U, et al. Oral contraceptives did not affect biochemical folate indexes and homocysteine concentrations in adolescent females. *J Am Diet Assoc* 1998;98:49-55.

7845 Facchinetti F, Nappi RE, Sances MG, et al. Effects of a yeast-based dietary supplementation on premenstrual syndrome. A double-blind placebo-controlled study. *Gynecol Obstet Invest* 1997;43:120-4.

7846 Sinai Y, Kaplun A, Hai Y, Halperin B. Enhancement of resistance to infectious diseases by oral administration of brewer's yeast. *Infect Immun* 1974;9:781-7.

7847 Postmes T, van den Bogaard AE, Hazen M. Honey for wounds, ulcers, and skin graft preservation. *Lancet* 1993;341:756-7.

7848 Subrahmanyam M. Early tangential excision and skin grafting of moderate burns is superior to honey dressing: a prospective randomised trial. *Burns* 1999;25:729-31.

7849 Efem SE. Clinical observations on the wound healing properties of honey. *Br J Surg* 1988;75:679-81.

7850 Bose B. Honey or sugar in treatment of infected wounds? *Lancet* 1982;1:963.

7851 Lancaster S, Krieder RB, Rasmussen C, et al. Effects of honey on glucose, insulin and endurance cycling performance. Abstract presented 4/4/01 at Experimental Biology 2001, Orlando, FL.

7852 Hamzaoglu I, Saribeyoglu K, Durak H, et al. Protective covering of surgical wounds with honey impedes tumor implantation. *Arch Surg* 2000;135:1414-7.

7853 Diaz-Perales A, Collada C, Blanco C, et al. Cross-reactions in the latex-fruit syndrome: A relevant role of chitinases but not of complex asparagine-linked glycans. *J Allergy Clin Immunol* 1999;104:681-7.

7854 Caparros-Lefebvre D, Elbaz A. Possible relation of atypical parkinsonism in the French West Indies with consumption of tropical plants: a case-control study. Caribbean Parkinsonism Study Group. *Lancet* 1999;354:281-6.

7855 Padma P, Pramod NP, Thyagarajan SP, Khosa RL. Effect of the extract of Annona muricata and Petunia nyctaginiflora on Herpes simplex virus. *J Ethnopharmacol* 1998;61:81-3.

7856 Roman G. Tropical myeloneuropathies revisited. *Curr Opin Neurol* 1998;11:539-44.

7857 Oberlies NH, Chang CJ, McLaughlin JL. Structure-activity relationships of diverse Annonaceous acetogenins against multidrug resistant human mammary adenocarcinoma (MCF-7/Adr) cells. *J Med Chem* 1997;40:2102-6.

7858 Jaramillo MC, Arango GJ, Gonzalez MC, et al. Cytotoxicity and antileishmanial activity of Annona muricata pericarp. *Fitoterapia* 2000;71:183-6.

7859 Manna SK, Mukhopadhyay A, Van NT, Aggarwal BB. Silymarin suppresses TNF-induced activation of NF-kappa B, c-Jun N-terminal kinase, and apoptosis. *J Immunol* 1999;163:6800-9.

7860 Amato P, Christophe S, Mellon PL. Estrogenic activity of herbs commonly used as remedies for menopausal symptoms. *Menopause* 2002;9:145-50.

7861 Schneider Y, Vincent F, Duranton B, et al. Anti-proliferative effect of resveratrol, a natural component of grapes and wine, on human colonic cancer cells. *Cancer Lett* 2000;158:85-91.

7862 Kozuki Y, Miura Y, Yagasaki K. Resveratrol suppresses hepatoma cell invasion independently of its anti-proliferative action. *Cancer Lett* 2001;167:151-6.

7863 Laden BP, Porter TD. Resveratrol inhibits human squalene monooxygenase. *Nutrition Research* 2001;21:747-53.

7864 Piver B, Berthou F, Dreano Y, Lucas D. Inhibition of CYP3A, CYP1A and CYP2E1 activities by resveratrol and other non volatile red wine components. *Toxicol Lett* 2001;125:83-91.

7865 Bowers JL, Tyulmenkov VV, Jernigan SC, Klinge CM. Resveratrol acts as a mixed agonist/antagonist for estrogen receptors alpha and beta. *Endocrinology* 2000;141:3657-67.

7866 Docherty JJ, Fu MM, Stiffler BS, et al. Resveratrol inhibition of herpes simplex virus replication. *Antiviral Res* 1999;43:145-55.

7867 Shuster S, McArthur CA, Arnott N, Schapowal A. Treating seasonal allergic rhinitis. *BMJ* 2002;324:1277.

7868 Behr J, Maier K, Degenkolb B, et al. Antioxidative and clinical effects of high-dose N-acetylcysteine in fibrosing alveolitis. Adjunctive therapy to maintenance immunosuppression. *Am J Respir Crit Care Med* 1997;156:1897-901.

7869 Tenenbein PK, Sitar DS, Tenenbein M. Interaction between N-acetylcysteine and activated charcoal: implications for the treatment of acetaminophen poisoning. *Pharmacotherapy* 2001;21:1331-6.

7870 Adair JC, Knoefel JE, Morgan N. Controlled trial of N-acetylcysteine for patients with probable Alzheimer's disease. *Neurology* 2001;57:1515-7.

7871 Molnar Z, Shearer E, Lowe D. N-Acetylcysteine treatment to prevent the progression of multisystem organ failure: a prospective, randomized, placebo-controlled study. *Crit Care Med* 1999;27:1100-4.

7872 Arstall MA, Yang J, Stafford I, et al. N-acetylcysteine in combination with nitroglycerin and streptokinase for the treatment of evolving acute myocardial infarction. Safety and biochemical effects. *Circulation* 1995;92:2855-62.

7873 Estensen RD, Levy M, Klopp SJ, et al. N-acetylcysteine suppression of the proliferative index in the colon of patients with previous adenomatous colonic polyps. *Cancer Lett* 1999;147:109-14.

7874 Weinbroum AA, Rudick V, Ben-Abraham R, Karchevski E. N-acetyl-L-cysteine for preventing lung reperfusion injury after liver ischemia-reperfusion: a possible dual protective mechanism in a dose-response study. *Transplantation* 2000;69:853-9.

7875 Pastorino U, Infante M, Maioli M, et al. Adjuvant treatment of stage I lung cancer with high-dose vitamin A. *J Clin Oncol* 1993;11:1216-22.

7876 Lannuzel A, Michel PP, Caparros-Lefebvre D, et al. Toxicity of Annonaceae for dopaminergic neurons: potential role in atypical parkinsonism in Guadeloupe. *Mov Disord* 2002;17:84-90.

7877 Kanwar U, Kaur R, Chadha S, Sanyal S. Gossypol-induced inhibition of glucose uptake in human ejaculated spermatozoa may be mediated by lipid peroxidation. *Contraception* 1990;42:573-87.

7878 Mock DM, Quirk JG, Mock NI. Marginal biotin deficiency during normal pregnancy. *Am J Clin Nutr* 2002;75:295-9.

7879 Zempleni J, Helm RM, Mock DM. In vivo biotin supplementation at a pharmacologic dose decreases proliferation rates of human peripheral blood mononuclear cells and cytokine release. *J Nutr* 2001;131:1479-84.

7880 Coggeshall JC, Heggers JP, Robson MC, et al. Biotin status and plasma glucose in diabetics. *Annals New York Academy of Sciences*, 389-92.

7881 Beaulieu AJ, Gohh RY, Han H, et al. Enhanced reduction of fasting total homocysteine levels with supraphysiological versus standard multivitamin dose folic acid supplementation in renal transplant recipients. *Arterioscler Thromb Vasc Biol* 1999;19:2918-21.

7882 Kramer K, Senninger N, Herbst H, Probst W. Effective prevention of adhesions with hyaluronate. *Arch Surg* 2002;137:278-82.

7883 Dougados M. Sodium hyaluronate therapy in osteoarthritis: arguments for a potential beneficial structural effect. *Semin Arthritis Rheum* 2000;30(2 Suppl 1):19-25.

7884 Altman RD. Intra-articular sodium hyaluronate in osteoarthritis of the knee. *Semin Arthritis Rheum* 2000;30(2 Suppl 1):11-8.

7885 Altman RD, Moskowitz R. Intraarticular sodium hyaluronate (Hyalgan) in the treatment of patients with osteoarthritis of the knee: a randomized clinical trial. Hyalgan Study Group. *J Rheumatol* 1998;25:2203-12.

7886 Frizziero L, Govoni E, Bacchini P. Intra-articular hyaluronic acid in the treatment of osteoarthritis of the knee: clinical and morphological study. *Clin Exp Rheumatol* 1998;16:441-9.

7887 Petrella RJ, DiSilvestro MD, Hildebrand C. Effects of hyaluronate sodium on pain and physical functioning in osteoarthritis of the knee: a randomized, double-blind, placebo-controlled clinical trial. *Arch Intern Med* 2002;162:292-8.

7888 Felson DT, Anderson JJ. Hyaluronate sodium injections for osteoarthritis: hope, hype, and hard truths. *Arch Intern Med* 2002;162:245-7.

7889 Palacioz K. New Product: Gelclair Concentrated Oral Gel. *Pharmacist's Letter/Prescriber's Letter* 2002;18:180711.

7890 Hyalgan Prescribing Information. Sanofi-Synthelabo, Inc. New York, NY, 2002.

7891 Synvisc Prescribing Information. Wyeth-Ayerst Pharmaceuticals, Philadelphia, PA, 2000.

7892 Gelclair Prescribing Information. Cell Pathways, Inc. Horsham, PA, 2002.

7893 Duperre J, Grenier B, Lemire J, et al. Effect of timolol vs. acetazolamide on sodium hyaluronate-induced rise in intraocular pressure after cataract surgery. *Can J Ophthalmol* 1994;29:182-6.

7894 Kavouni A, Stanec JJ. Human antihyaluronic acid antibodies. *Dermatol Surg* 2002;28:359-60.

7895 Norrish AE, Jackson RT, Sharpe SJ, Skeaff CM. Prostate cancer and dietary carotenoids. *Am J Epidemiol* 2000;151:119-23.

7896 Arab L, Steck S. Lycopene and cardiovascular disease. *Am J Clin Nutr* 2000;71:1691S-5S.

7897 Kohlmeier L, Kark JD, Gomez-Gracia E, et al. Lycopene and myocardial infarction risk in the EURAMIC Study. *Am J Epidemiol* 1997;146:618-26.

7898 Neuman I, Nahum H, Ben-Amotz A. Reduction of exercise-induced asthma oxidative stress by lycopene, a natural antioxidant. *Allergy* 2000;55:1184-9.

7899 Richelle M, Bortlik K, Liardet S, et al. A food-based formulation provides lycopene with the same bioavailability to humans as that from tomato paste. *J Nutr* 2002;132:404-8.

7900 Campbell N, Paddock V, Sundaram R. Alteration of methyldopa absorption, metabolism, and blood pressure control by ferrous sulfate and ferrous gluconate. *Clin Pharmacol Ther* 1988;43:381-6.

8000 Loprinzi CL, Goldberg RM, Burnham NL. Cancer-associated anorexia and cachexia. Implications for drug therapy. *Drugs* 1992;43:499-506.

8001 Loprinzi CL, Goldberg RM, Su JQ, et al. Placebo-controlled trial of hydrazine sulfate in patients with newly diagnosed non-small-cell lung cancer. *J Clin Oncol* 1994;12:1126-9.

8002 Loprinzi CL, Kuross SA, O'Fallon JR, et al. Randomized, placebo-controlled evaluation of hydrazine sulfate in patients with advanced colorectal cancer. *J Clin Oncol* 1994;12:1121-5.

8003 Kosty MP, Fleishman SB, Herndon JE II, et al. Cisplatin, vinblastine, and hydrazine sulfate in advanced, non-small-cell lung cancer: a randomized, placebo-controlled, double-blind phase III study of the cancer and leukemia Group B. *J Clin Oncol* 1994;12:1113-20.

8004 Chlebowski RT, Bulcavage L, Grosvenor M, et al. Hydrazine sulfate in cancer patients with weight loss. A placebo-controlled clinical experience. *Cancer* 1987;59:406-10.

8005 Kaegi E. Unconventional therapies for cancer: 4. Hydrazine sulfate. Task Force on Alternative Therapies of the Canadian Breast Cancer Research Initiative. *CMAJ* 1998;158:1327-30.

8006 Poyares DR, Guilleminault C, Ohayon MM, Tufik S. Can valerian improve the sleep of insomniacs after benzodiazepine withdrawal? *Prog Neuropsychopharmacol Biol Psychiatry* 2002;26:539-45.

8007 Akhondzadeh S, Naghavi HR, Shayeganpour A, et al. Passionflower in the treatment of generalized anxiety: a pilot double-blind randomized controlled trial with oxazepam. *J Clin Pharm Ther* 2001;26:363-7.

8008 Schnyder G, Roffi M, Pin R, et al. Decreased rate of coronary restenosis after lowering of plasma homocysteine levels. *N Engl J Med* 2001;345:1593-600.

8009 Schnyder G, Roffi M, Pin R, et al. Decreased rate of coronary stenosis after lowering of plasma homocysteine levels. *N Engl J Med* 2001;345:1593-600.

8010 Office of Public Affairs. State health director warns consumers about prescription drugs in herbal products. California Department of Health Services 2002. http://www.applications.dhs.ca.gov/pressreleases/store/pressreleases/02-03.html (Accessed 8 Feb 2002).

8011 Smith WP. Epidermal and dermal effects of topical lactic acid. *J Am Acad Dermatol* 1996;35:388-91.

8012 Scazzocchio F, Corneta MF, Tomassini L, Palmery M. Antibacterial activity of Hydrastis canadensis extract and its major isolated alkaloids. *Planta Med* 2001;67:561-4.

8013 Fan YY, Chapkin RS. Importance of dietary gamma-linolenic acid in human health and nutrition. *J Nutr* 1998;128:1411-4.

8014 Chin-Dusting JP, Kaye DM, Lefkovits J, et al. Dietary supplementation with L-arginine fails to restore endothelial function in forearm resistance arteries of patients with severe heart failure. *J Am Coll Cardiol* 1996;27:1207-13.

8015 Wallace AW, Tom WL. Interaction of L-arginine and phosphodiesterase inhibitors in vasodilation of the porcine internal mammary artery. *Anesth Analg* 2000;90:840-6.

8016 Katz SD, Khan T, Zeballos GA, et al. Decreased activity of the L-arginine-nitric oxide metabolic pathway in patients with congestive heart failure. *Circulation* 1999;99:2113-7.

8017 Ali M, Thomson M, Afzal M. Garlic and onions: their effect on eicosanoid metabolism and its clinical relevance. *Prostaglandins Leukot Essent Fatty Acids* 2000;62(2):55-73.

8018 Lamm DL, Riggs DR. The potential application of allium sativum (garlic) for the treatment of bladder cancer. *Urol Clin North Am* 2000;27:157-62.

8019 Ledezma E, Marcano K, Jorquera A. Efficacy of ajoene in the treatment of tinea pedis: A double-blind and comparative study with terbinafine. *J Am Acad Dermatol* 2000;43:829-32.

REFERENCES

8020 Haggans CJ, Travelli EJ, Thomas W, et al. The effect of flaxseed and wheat bran consumption on urinary estrogen metabolites in premenopausal women. *Cancer Epidemiol Biomarker Prev* 2000;9:719-25.

8021 Clark WF, Kortas C, Heidenheim P, et al. Flaxseed in lupus nephritis: a two-year nonplacebo-controlled crossover study. *J Am Coll Nutr* 2001;20:143-8.

8022 Serraino M, Thompson LU. The effect of flaxseed supplementation on early risk markers for mammary carcinogenesis. *Cancer Lett* 1991;60:135-42.

8023 Rickard SE, Yuan YV, Thompson LU. Plasma insulin-like growth factor I levels in rats are reduced by dietary supplementation of flaxseed or its lignan secoisolariciresinol diglycoside. *Cancer Lett* 2000;161:47-55.

8024 Adlercreutz H. Diet, breast cancer, and sex hormone metabolism. *Ann N Y Acad Sci* 1990;595:281-90.

8025 Adlercreutz H, Heikkinen R, Woods M, et al. Excretion of the lignans enterolactone and enterodiol and of equol in omnivorous and vegetarian postmenopausal women and in women with breast cancer. *Lancet* 1982;2:1295-9.

8026 Kilkkinen A, Stumpf K, Pietinen P, et al. Determinants of serum enterolactone concentration. *Am J Clin Nutr* 2001;73:1094-100.

8027 McHugh CP. Garlic as a tick repellent. *JAMA* 2001;285:41,42.

8028 Ali M, Afzal M. A potent inhibitor of thrombin stimulated platelet thromboxane formation from unprocessed tea. *Prostaglandins Leukot Med* 1987;27:9-13.

8029 Ardlie NG, Glew G, Schultz BG, Schwartz CJ. Inhibition and reversal of platelet aggregation by methyl xanthines. *Thromb Diath Haemorrh* 1967;18:670-3.

8030 Samarrae WA, Truswell AS. Short-term effect of coffee on blood fibrinolytic activity in healthy adults. *Atherosclerosis* 1977;26:255-60.

8031 Leitzmann MF, Willett WC, Rimm EB, et al. A prospective study of coffee consumption and the risk of symptomatic gallstone disease in men. *JAMA* 1999;281:2106-12.

8032 Ruhl CE, Everhart JE. Association of coffee consumption with gallbladder disease. *Am J Epidemiol* 2000;152:1034-8.

8033 Klag MJ, Wang NY, Meoni LA, et al. Coffee intake and risk of hypertension: The John Hopkins precursors study. *Arch Intern Med* 2002;162:657-62.

8034 Brenner H, Rothenbacher D, Bode G, Adler G. Relation of smoking and alcohol and coffee consumption to active Helicobacter pylori infection: cross sectional study. *BMJ* 1997;315:1489-92.

8035 Olthof MR, Hollman PC, Zock PL, Katan MB. Consumption of high doses of chlorogenic acid, present in coffee, or of black tea increases plasma total homocysteine concentrations in humans. *Am J Clin Nutr* 2001;73:532-8.

8036 Jee SH, He J, Appel LJ, et al. Coffee consumption and serum lipids: a meta-analysis of randomized controlled clinical trials. *Am J Epidemiol* 2001:153:353-62.

8037 de Roos B, Caslake MJ, Stalenhoef AF, et al. The coffee diterpene cafestol increases plasma triacylglycerol by increasing the production rate of large VLDL apolipoprotein B in healthy normolipidemic subjects. *Am J Clin Nutr* 2001;73:45-52.

8038 Michaud DS, Giovannucci E, Willett WC, et al. Coffee and alcohol consumption and risk of pancreatic cancer in two prospective United States cohorts. *Cancer Epidemiol Biomarkers Prev* 2001;10:429-37.

8039 Tavani A, Pregnolato A, La Vecchia C, et al. Coffee consumption and the risk of breast cancer. *Eur J Cancer Prev* 1998;7:77-82.

8040 Tavani A, La Vecchia C. Coffee and cancer: a review of epidemiological studies, 1990-1999. *Eur J Cancer Prev* 2000;9:241-56.

8041 Hartman TJ, Tangrea JA, Pietinen P, et al. Tea and coffee consumption and risk of colon and rectal cancer in middle-aged Finnish men. *Nutr Cancer* 1998;31:41-8.

8042 Anon. Filtering the news about coffee. *UC Berkeley Wellness Letter* 2001:17:1-2.

8043 Ferrini RL, Barrett-Connor E. Caffeine intake and endogenous sex steroid levels in postmenopausal women. The Rancho Bernardo Study. *Am J Epidemiol* 1996:144:642-4.

8044 Hickenbottom SJ, Follett JR, Lin Y, et al. Variability in conversion of beta-carotene to vitamin A in men as measured by using a double-tracer study design. *Am J Clin Nutr* 2002;75:900-7.

8045 Prakash P, Russell RM, Krinsky NI. In vitro inhibition of proliferation of estrogen-dependent and estrogen-independent human breast cancer cells treated with carotenoids or retinoids. *J Nutr* 2001;131:1574-80.

8046 Kumar B, Cole WC, Prasad KN. Alpha tocopheryl succinate, retinoic acid and polar carotenoids enhanced the growth-inhibitory effect of a cholesterol-lowering drug on immortalized and transformed nerve cells in culture. *J Am Coll Nutr* 2001;20:628-36.

8047 Benvenga S, Ruggeri RM, Russo A, et al. Usefulness of L-carnitine, a naturally occurring peripheral antagonist of thyroid hormone action, in iatrogenic hyperthyroidism: a randomized, double-blind, placebo-controlled clinical trial. *J Clin Endocrinol Metab* 2001;86:3579-94.

8048 Sole MJ, Jeejeebhoy KN. Conditioned nutritional requirements and the pathogenesis and treatment of myocardial failure. *Curr Opin Clin Nutr Metab Care* 2000;3:417-24.

8049 Famularo G, De Simone C, Cifone G. Carnitine stands on its own in HIV infection treatment. *Arch Intern Med* 1999;159:1143-4.

8050 Hudson JI, Pope HG, Daniels SR, Horwitz RI. Eosinophilia-myalgia syndrome or fibromyalgia with eosinophilia? *JAMA* 1993;269:3108-9.

8051 Shapiro S. L-tryptophan and eosinophilia-myalgia syndrome. *Lancet* 1994;344:817-9.

8052 Hatch DL, Goldman LR. Reduced severity of eosinophilia-myalgia syndrome associated with consumption of vitamin-containing supplements before illness. *Arch Intern Med* 1993;153: 2368-73.

8053 Sullivan EA, Kamb ML, Jones JL, et al. The natural history of eosinophilia-myalgia syndrome in a tryptophan-exposed cohort in South Carolina. *Arch Intern Med* 1996;156:973-9.

8054 Philen RM, HIll RH, Flanders WD, et al. Tryptophan contaminants associated with eosinophilia-myalgia syndrome. *Am J Epidemiol* 1993;138:154-9.

8055 Bohme A, Wolter M, Hoelzer D. L-tryptophan-related eosinophilia-myalgia syndrome possibly associated with a chronic B-lymphocytic leukemia. *Ann Hematol* 1998;77:235-8.

8056 Singhal AB, Caviness VS, Begleiter AF, et al. Cerebral vasoconstriction and stroke after use of serotonergic drugs. *Neurology* 2002;58:130-3.

8057 Morgan MS, Arlian LG, Vyszenski-Moher DL, et al. English plantain and psyllium: lack of cross-allergenicity by crossed immunoelectrophoresis. *Ann Allergy Asthma Immunol* 1995;75:351-9.

8058 Pastors JG, Blaisdell PW, Balm TK, et al. Psyllium fiber reduces rise in postprandial glucose and insulin concentrations in patients with non-insulin-dependent diabetes. *Am J Clin Nutr* 1991;53:1431-5.

8059 Rigaud D, Paycha F, Meulemans A, et al. Effect of psyllium on gastric emptying, hunger feeling and food intake in normal volunteers: a double blind study. *Eur J Clin Nutr* 1998;52:239-45.

8060 Anderson JW, Riddell-Mason S, Gustafson NJ, et al. Cholesterol-lowering effects of psyllium-enriched cereal as an adjunct to a prudent diet in the treatment of mild to moderate hypercholesterolemia. *Am J Clin Nutr* 1992;56:93-8.

8061 Roberts DC, Truswell AS, Bencke A, et al. The cholesterol-lowering effect of a breakfast cereal containing psyllium fibre. *Med J Aust* 1994;161:660-4.

8062 Wolever TM, Jenkins DJ, Mueller S, et al. Method of administration influences the serum cholesterol-lowering effect of psyllium. *Am J Clin Nutr* 1994;59:1055-9.

8064 Wolever TM, Vuksan V, Eshuis H, et al. Effect of method of administration of psyllium on glycemic response and carbohydrate digestibility. *J Am Coll Nutr* 1991;10:364-71.

8065 Jenkins DJ, Kendall CW, Axelsen M, et al. Viscous and nonviscous fibres, nonabsorbable and low glycaemic index carbohydrates, blood lipids and coronary heart disease. *Curr Opin Lipidol* 2000;11:49-56.

8066 Bell LP, Hectorne K, Reynolds H, et al. Cholesterol-lowering effects of psyllium hydrophilic mucilloid. Adjunct therapy to a prudent diet for patients with mild to moderate hypercholesterolemia. *JAMA* 1989;261:3419-23.

8067 Jenkins DJ, Wolever TM, Vidgen E, et al. Effect of psyllium in hypercholesterolemia at two monosaturated fatty acid intakes. *Am J Clin Nutr* 1997;65:1524-33.

8068 Segawa K, Kataoka T, Fukuo Y. Cholesterol-lowering effects of psyllium seed associated with urea metabolism. *Biol Pharm Bull* 1998;21:184-7.

8069 Gelissen IC, Brodie B, Eastwood MA. Effect of Plantago ovata (psyllium) husk and seeds on sterol metabolism: studies in normal and ileostomy subjects. *Am J Clin Nutr* 194;59:395-400.

8070 Anderson JW, Jones AE, Riddell-Mason S. Ten different dietary fibers have significantly different effects on serum and liver lipids of cholesterol-fed rats. *J Nutr* 1994;124:78-83.

8071 Wolever TM, ter Wal P, Spadafora P, Robb P. Guar, but not psyllium, increases breath methane and serum acetate concentrations in human subjects. *Am J Clin Nutr* 1992;55:719-22.

8072 Jensen CD, Spiller GA, Gates JE, et al. The effect of acacia gum and a water-soluble dietary fiber mixture on blood lipids in humans. *J Am Coll Nutr* 1993;12:147-54.

8073 Kwiterovich PO. The role of fiber in the treatment of hypercholesterolemia in children and adolescents. *Pediatrics* 1995;96:1005-9.

8074 Dennison BA, Levine DM. Randomized, double-blind, placebo-controlled, two-period crossover clinical trial of psyllium fiber in children with hypercholesterolemia. *J Pediatr* 1993;123:24-9.

8075 Davidson MH, Dugan LD, Burns JH, et al. A psyllium-enriched cereal for the treatment of hypercholesterolemia in children: a controlled, double-blind, crossover study. *Am J Clin Nutr* 1996;63:96-102.

8076 Williams CL, Bollella M, Spark A, Puder D. Soluble fiber enhances the hypocholesterolemic effect of the step I diet in childhood. *J Am Coll Nutr* 1995;14:251-7.

8077 Ho Y, Tan M, Seow-Choen F. Micronized purified flavonidic fraction compared favorably with rubber band ligation and fiber alone in the management of bleeding hemorrhoids. *Dis Colon Rectum* 2000;43:66-9.

8078 Anon. The scoop on psyllium. *UC Berkeley Wellness Letter* 2001;17:2.

8079 Lantner RR, Espiritu BR, Zumerchik P, Tobin MC. Anaphylaxis following ingestion of a psyllium-containing cereal. *JAMA* 1990;264:2534-6.

8080 Schneider RP. Perdiem causes esophageal impaction and bezoars. *South Med J* 1989;82:1449-50.

8081 Shulman LM, Minagar A, Weiner WJ. Perdiem causing esophageal obstruction in Parkinson's disease. *Neurology* 1999;52:670-1.

8082 Gerber M. Fiber and breast cancer: another piece of the puzzle--but still an incomplete picture. *J Natl Cancer Inst* 1996;88:857-8.

8083 Alabaster O, Tang ZC, Frost A, Shivapurkar N. Potential synergism between wheat bran and psyllium: enhanced inhibition of colon cancer. *Cancer Lett* 1993;75:53-8.

8084 Clague JE, Edwards RH, Jackson MJ. Intravenous magnesium loading in chronic fatigue syndrome. *Lancet* 1992;340:124-5.

8085 Young IS, Trimble ER. Magnesium and chronic fatigue syndrome. *Lancet* 1991;337;1094-5.

8086 Gantz NM. Magnesium and chronic fatigue. *Lancet* 1991;338:66.

8087 Deulofeu R, Gascon J, Gimenez N, Corachan M. Magnesium and chronic fatigue syndrome. *Lancet* 1991;338:641.

8088 Douban S, Brodsky MA, Whang DD, Whang R. Significance of magnesium in congestive heart failure. *Am Heart J* 1996;132:664-71.

8089 Costello RB, Moser-Veillon PB, DiBianco R. Magnesium supplementation in patients with congestive heart failure. *J Am Coll Nutr* 1997;16:22-31.

8090 Seelig M, Altura BM. How best to determine magnesium requirement: need to consider cardiotherapeutic drugs that affect its retention. *J Am Coll Nutr* 1997;16:4-6.

8091 Teragawa H, Kato M, Yamagata T, et al. The preventive effect of magnesium on coronary spasm in patients with vasospastic angina. *Chest* 2000;118:1690-5.

8092 Kosch M, Hausberg M, Westermann G, et al. Alterations in calcium and magnesium content of red cell membranes in patients with primary hypertension. *Am J Hypertens* 2001;14:254-8.

8093 Grether JK, Hoogstrate J, Walsh-Greene E, Nelson KB. Magnesium sulfate for tocolysis and risk of spastic cerebral palsy in premature children born to women without preeclampsia. *Am J Obstet Gynecol* 2000;183:717-25.

8094 Cohen JS. High-dose oral magnesium treatment of chronic, intractable erythromelalgia. *Ann Pharmacother* 2002;36:255-60.

8095 Birrer RB, Shallash AJ, Totten V. Hypermagnesemia-induced fatality following epsom salt gargles. *J Emerg Med* 2002;22:185-8.

8096 Frankel BL, Patten BM, Gillin JC. Restless leg syndrome. Sleep-electroencephalographic and neurologic findings. *JAMA* 1974;230:1302-3.

8097 Ettinger B, Citron JT, Livermore B, Dolman LI. Chlorthanlidone reduces calcium oxalate calculous recurrence but magnesium hydroxide does not. *J Urol* 1988;139:679-84.

8098 Sacks FM, Willett WC, Smith A, et al. Effect on blood pressure of potassium, calcium, and magnesium in women with low habitual intake. *Hypertension* 1998;31:131-8.

8099 Sabatier M, Arnaud MJ, Kastenmayer P, et al. Meal effect on magnesium bioavailability from mineral water in healthy women. *Am J Clin Nutr* 2002;75:65-71.

8100 Dufour MC. If you drink alcoholic beverages do so in moderation: what does this mean? *J Nutr* 2001;131:552S-61S.

8101 Koehler KM, Baumgartner RN, Garry PJ, et al. Association of folate intake and serum homocysteine in elderly persons according to vitamin supplementation and alcohol use. *Am J Clin Nutr* 2001;73:628-37.

8102 Thadhani R, Camargo CA, Stampfer MJ, et al. Prospective study of moderate alcohol consumption and risk of hypertension in young women. *Arch Intern Med* 2002;162:569-74.

8103 Klatsky AL. Should patients with heart disease drink alcohol. *JAMA* 2001;285:2004-6.

8104 Abramson JL, Williams SA, Krumholz HM, Vaccarino V. Moderate alcohol consumption and risk of heart failure among older persons. *JAMA* 2001;285:1971-7.

8105 Delgado O, Romano EL, Belfort E, et al. Dialyzable leukocyte extract therapy in immunodepressed patients with cutaneous leishmaniasis. *Clin Immunol Immunopathol* 1981;19:351-9.

8110 Samman S, Sandstrom B, Toft MB, et al. Green tea or rosemary extract added to foods reduces nonheme-iron absorption. *Am J Clin Nutr* 2001;73:607-12.

8111 Bartley GB, Hilty MD, Andreson BD, et al. "Maple-syrup" urine odor due to fenugreek ingestion. *N Engl J Med* 1981;305:467.

8112 Broca C, Manteghetti M, Gross R, et al. 4-Hydroxyisoleucine: effects of synthetic and natural analogues on insulin secretion. *Eur J Pharmacol* 2000;390:339-45.

8113 Shaw JC. Green tea polyphenols may be useful in the treatment of androgen-mediated skin disorders. *Arch Dermatol* 2001;137:664.

8114 Chantre P, Lairon D. Recent findings of green tea extract AR25 (Exolise) and its activity for the treatment of obesity. *Phytomedicine* 2002;9:3-8.

8115 Cronin JR. Green tea extract stokes thermogenesis: will it replace ephedra? *Altern Comp Ther* 2000;6:296-300.

8116 Wu CH, Yang YC, Yao WJ, et al. Epidemiological evidence of increased bone mineral density in habitual tea drinkers. *Arch Intern Med* 2002;162:1001-6.

8117 Pisters KM, Newman RA, Coldman B, et al. Phase I trial of oral green tea extract in adult patients with solid tumors. *J Clin Oncol* 2001;19:1830-8.

8118 Chung LY, Cheung TC, Kong SK, et al. Induction of apoptosis by green tea catechins in human prostate cancer DU145 cells. *Life Sci* 2001;68:1207-14.

8119 Geleijnse JM, Launer LJ, Van der Kuip DA, et al. Inverse association of tea and flavonoid intakes with incident myocardial infarction: the Rotterdam Study. *Am J Clin Nutr* 2002;75:880-6.

8120 Mukamal KJ, Maclure M, Muller JE, et al. Tea consumption and mortality after acute myocardial infarction. *Circulation* 2002;105:2476-81.

8121 Peters U, Poole C, Arab L. Does tea affect cardiovascular disease? A meta-analysis. *Am J Epidemiol* 2001;154:495-503.

8122 Geleijnse JM, Witteman JC, Launer LJ, et al. Tea and coronary heart disease: protection through estrogen-like activity? *Arch Intern Med* 2000;160:3328-9.

8123 Shahrzad S, Aoyagi K, Winter A, et al. Pharmacokinetics of gallic acid and its relative bioavailability from tea in healthy humans. *J Nutr* 2001;131:1207-10.

8124 Esimone CO, Adikwu MU, Nwafor SV, Okolo CO. Potential use of tea extract as a complementary mouthwash: comparative evaluation of two commercial samples. *J Altern Complement Med* 2001;7:523-7.

8125 Morrison LM, Bajwa GS, Alfin-Slater RB, Ershoff BH. Prevention of vascular lesions by chondroitin sulfate A in the coronary artery and aorta of rats induced by a hypervitaminosis D, cholesterol-containing diet. *Atherosclerosis* 1972;16:105-18.

8126 Morrison LM. Treatment of coronary arteriosclerotic heart disease with chondroitin sulfate-A: preliminary report. *J Am Geriatr Soc* 1968;16:779-85.

8127 Cao LC, Boeve ER, de Bruijn WC, et al. Glycosaminoglycans and semisynthetic sulfated polysaccharides: an overview of their potential application in treatment of patients with urolithiasis. *Urology* 1997;50:173-83.

8128 Adebowale AO, Cox DS, Liang Z, et al. Analysis of glucosamine and chondroitin sulfate content in marketed products and the Caco-2 permeability of chondroitin sulfate raw materials. *JANA* 2000;3:37-44.

8129 Horrobin DF. Evening primrose oil and premenstrual syndrome. *Med J Aust* 1990;153:630-1.

8131 Fernandez-Jarne E, Martinez-Losa E, Prado-Santamaria M, et al. Risk of first non-fatal myocardial infarction negatively associated with olive oil consumption: a case-control study in Spain. *Int J Epidemiol* 2002;31:474-80.

8132 Madigan C, Ryan M, Owens D, et al. Dietary unsaturated fatty acids in type 2 diabetes: higher levels of postprandial lipoprotein on a linoleic acid-rich sunflower oil diet compared with an oleic acid-rich olive oil diet. *Diabetes Care* 2000;23:1472-7.

8133 Menendez JA, del Mar Barbacid M, Montero S, et al. Effects of gamma-linolenic acid and oleic acid on paclitaxel cytotoxicity in human breast cancer cells. *Eur J Cancer* 2001;37:402-13.

8134 Zurier RB, Furse RK, Rosetti RG. Gamma-linolenic acid (GLA) prevents amplification of interleukin-1-beta (IL-1-beta). *Altern Ther* 2001;7:112.

8135 Rozen TD, Oshinsky ML, Gebeline CA, et al. Open label trial of coenzyme Q10 as a migraine preventive. *Cephalalgia* 2002;22:137-41.

8136 Burton TM. Maker of herbal cancer therapy shuts its operations, citing recall. *Wall Street Journal* May 2002.

8137 Oh WK, George DJ, Kantoff PW. Rapid rise of serum prostate specific antigen levels after discontinuation of the herbal therapy PC-SPES in patients with advanced prostate carcinoma: report of four cases. *Cancer* 2002;94:686-9.

8138 Brown GA, Vukovich MD, Martini ER, et al. Effects of androstenedione-herbal supplementation on serum sex hormone concentrations in 30- to 59-year-old men. *Int J Vitam Nutr Res* 2001;71:293-301.

8139 Muth ER, Laurent JM, Jasper P.The effect of bilberry nutritional supplementation on night visual acuity andcontrast sensitivity. *Altern Med Rev* 2000;5:164-73.

8140 Lietti A, Forni G. Studies on Vaccinium myrtillus anthocyanosides. II. Aspects of anthocyanins pharmacokinetics in the rat. *Arzneimittelforschung* 1976;26:832-5.

8141 Lietti A, Cristoni A, Picci M. Studies on Vaccinium myrtillus anthocyanosides. I. Vasoprotective and antiinflammatory activity. *Arzneimittelforschung* 1976;26:829-32.

8142 Shi M, Chang L, He G. [Stimulating action of Carthamus tinctorius L., Angelica sinensis (Oliv.) Diels and Leonurus sibiricus L. on the uterus]. [Article in Chinese]. *Zhongguo Zhong Yao Za Zhi* 1995;20:173-5, 192.

8143 Martorano JT, Ahlgrimm M, Colbert T. Differentiating between natural progesterone and synthetic progestins: clinical implications for premenstrual syndrome and perimenopause management. *Compr Ther* 1998;24:336-9.

8144 Fitzpatrick LA, Pace C, Wiita B. Comparison of regimens containing oral micronized progesterone or medroxyprogesterone acetate on quality of life in postmenopausal women: a cross-sectional survey. *J Womens Health Gend Based Med* 2000;9:381-7.

8145 Koh KK, Jin DK, Yang SH, et al. Vascular effects of synthetic or natural progestagen combined with conjugated equine estrogen in healthy postmenopausal women. *Circulation* 2001;103:1961-6.

8146 Rosano GM, Webb CM, Chierchia S, et al. Natural progesterone, but not medroxyprogesterone acetate, enhances the beneficial effect of estrogen on exercise-induced myocardial ischemia in postmenopausal women. *J Am Coll Cardiol* 2000;36:2154-9.

8147 Fernandez JC, Mas R, Castano G, et al. Comparison of the efficacy, safety and tolerability of policosanol versus fluvastatin in elderly hypercholesterolaemic women. *Clin Drug Invest* 2001;21:103–13.

8148 Fung MC, Weintraub M, Bowen DL. Colloidal silver proteins marketed as health supplements. *JAMA* 1995;274:1196-7.

8149 Gulbranson SH, Hud JA, Hansen RC. Argyria following the use of dietary supplements containing colloidal silver protein. *Cutis* 2000;66:373-4.

8150 Singh BB, Mishra L, Aquilina N, Kohlbeck F. Usefulness of guggul (Commiphora mukul) for osteoarthritis of the knee: An experimental case study. *Altern Ther Health Med* 2001;7:120,112-4.

8151 Singh BB, Mishra L, Aquilina N, Kohlbeck F. Effectiveness of Commiphora mukul as an adjunctive therapy for osteoarthritis of the knee. *Alt Ther* 2001;7:S30.

8152 Antonio J, Colker CM, Torina GC, et al. Effects of a standardized guggulsterone phosphate supplement on body composition in overweight adults: a pilot study. *Curr Ther Res* 1999;60:220-7.

8153 Tripathi YB, Tripathi P, Malhotra OP, Tripathi SN. Thyroid stimulatory action of (Z)-guggulsterone: mechanism of action. *Planta Med* 1988;54:271-7.

8154 Kaul S, Kapoor NK. Cardiac sarcolemma enzymes & liver microsomal cytochrome P450 in isoproterenol treated rats. *Indian J Med Res* 1989;90:62-8.

8155 Agarwal RC, Singh SP, Saran RK, et al. Clinical trial of gugulipid – a new hypolipidemic agent of plant origin in primary hyperlipidemia. *Indian J Med Res* 1986;84:626-34.

8156 Panda S, Kar A. Gugulu (Commiphora mukul) induces triiodothyronine production: possible involvement of lipid peroxidation. *Life Sci* 1999;65:PL137-41.

8158 Malhotra SC, Ahuja MM, Sundaram KR. Long term clinical studies on the hypolipidaemic effect of Commiphora mukul (Guggulu) and clofibrate. *Indian J Med Res* 1977;65:390-5.

8159 Chan A, Reichmann H, Kogel A, et al. Metabolic changes in patients with mitochondrial myopathies and effects of coenzyme Q10 therapy. *J Neurol* 1998;245:681-5.

8160 Sobreira C, Hirano M, Shanske S, et al. Mitochondrial encephalomyopathy with coenzyme Q10 deficiency. *Neurology* 1997;48:1238-43.

8161 Boitier E, Degoul F, Desguerre I, et al. A case of mitochondrial encephalomyopathy associated with a muscle coenzyme Q10 deficiency. *J Neurol Sci* 1998;156:41-6.

8162 Chen RS, Huang CC, Chu NS. Coenzyme Q10 treatment in mitochondrial encephalomyopathies. Short-term double-blind, crossover study. *Eur Neurol* 1997;37:212-8.

8163 Bresolin N, Doriguzzi C, Ponzetto C, et al. Ubidecarenone in the treatment of mitochondrial myopathies: a multi-center double-blind trial. *J Neurol Sci* 1990;100:70-8.

8164 Brown GA, Vukovich MD, Martini ER, et al. Endocrine and lipid responses to chronic androstenediol-herbal supplementation in 30 to 58 year old men. *J Am Coll Nutr* 2001;20:520-8.

8165 Zanoli P, Avallone R, Baraldi M. Behavioral characterisation of the flavonoids apigenin and chrysin. *Fitoterapia* 2000;71:S117-S23.

8166 Wolfman C, Viola H, Paladini A, et al. Possible anxiolytic effects of chrysin, a central benzodiazepine receptor ligand isolated from Passiflora coerulea. *Pharmacol Biochem Behav* 1994;47:1-4.

8167 Medina JH, Paladini AC, Wolfman C, et al. Chrysin (5,7-di-OH-flavone), a naturally-occurring ligand for benzodiazepine receptors, with anticonvulsant properties. *Biochem Pharmacol* 1990;40:2227-31.

8168 Walle T, Otake Y, Brubaker JA, et al. Disposition and metabolism of the flavonoid chrysin in normal volunteers. *Br J Clin Pharmacol* 2001;51:143-6.

8169 Shin JS, Kim KS, Kim MB, et al. Synthesis and hypoglycemic effect of chrysin derivatives. *Bioorg Med Chem Lett* 1999;9:869-74.

8170 Galijatovic A, Otake Y, Walle UK, Walle T. Induction of UDP-glucuronosyltransferase UGT1A1 by the flavonoid chrysin in Caco-2 cells--potential role in carcinogen bioinactivation. *Pharm Res* 2001;18:374-9.

8171 Wang HK, Xia Y, Yang ZY, et al. Recent advances in the discovery and development of flavonoids and their analogues as antitumor and anti-HIV agents. *Adv Exp Med Biol* 1998;439:191-225.

8172 Lautraite S, Musonda AC, Doehmer J, et al. Flavonoids inhibit genetic toxicity produced by carcinogens in cells expressing CYP1A2 and CYP1A1. *Mutagenesis* 2002;17:45-53.

8175 Steiner GG. The correlation between cancer incidence and kava consumption. *Hawaii Med J* 2000;59:420-2.

8176 MacDonald R, Ishani A, Rutks I, Wilt TJ. A systematic review of Cernilton for the treatment of benign prostatic hyperplasia. *BJU Int* 2000;85:836-41.

8177 Maekawa M, Kishimoto T, Yasumoto R, et al. [Clinical evaluation of Cernilton on benign prostatic hypertrophy--a multiple center double-blind study with Paraprost]. [Article in Japanese]. *Hinyokika Kiyo* 1990;36:495-516.

8178 Habersang S, Leuschner F, Isaac O, Thiemer K. [Pharmacological studies with compounds of chamomile. IV. Studies on toxicity of (-)-alpha-bisabolol (author's transl)]. [Article in German]. *Planta Med* 1979;37:115-23.

8179 Grover JK, Vats V, Rathi SS, Dawar R. Traditional Indian anti-diabetic plants attenuate progression of renal damage in streptozotocin induced diabetic mice. *J Ethnopharmacol* 2001;76:233-8.

8180 Anila L, Vijayalakshmi NR. Beneficial effects of flavonoids from Sesamum indicum, Emblica officinalis and Momordica charantia. *Phytother Res* 2000;14:592-5.

8181 Aslam M, Stockley IH. Interaction between curry ingredient (karela) and drug (chlorpropamide). *Lancet* 1979:1:607.

8182 Holecek M. Relation between glutamine, branched-chain amino acids, and protein metabolism. *Nutrition* 2002;18:130-3.

8183 Khogali SE, Pringle SD, Weryk BV, Rennie MJ. Is glutamine beneficial in ischemic heart disease? *Nutrition* 2002;18:123-6.

8184 Ziegler TR, Bazargan N, Galloway JR. Glutamine supplemented nutrition support: saving nitrogen and saving money? *Clin Nutr* 2000;19:375-7.

8185 Szkudlarek J, Jeppesen PB, Mortensen PB. Effect of high dose growth hormone with glutamine and no change in diet on intestinal absorption in short bowel patients: a randomised, double blind, crossover, placebo controlled study. *Gut* 2000;47:199-205.

8186 Umpleby AM, Carroll PV, Russell-Jones DL, et al. Glutamine supplementation and GH/IGF-I treatment in critically ill patients: effects on glutamine metabolism and protein balance. *Nutrition* 2002;18:127-9.

8187 Secondary Direct Food Additives Permitted in Food for Human Consumption. Safe use of ozone when used as a gas or dissolved in water as an antimicrobial agent on food, including meat and poultry. *Federal Register* 66 http://www.fda.gov/OHRMS/Dockets/98fr/062601a.htm (Accessed 26 June 2001).

8188 Konno S, Tortorelis DG, Fullerton SA, et al. A possible hypoglycaemic effect of maitake mushroom on Type 2 diabetic patients. *Diabet Med* 2001;18:1010.

8189 Adachi K, Nanba H, Kuroda H. Potentiation of host-mediated antitumor activity in mice by beta-glucan obtained

REFERENCES

from Grifola frondosa (maitake). *Chem Pharm Bull* (Tokyo) 1987;35:262-70.

8190 Nanba H. Activity of maitake D-fraction to inhibit carcinogenesis and metastasis. *Ann N Y Acad Sci* 1995;768:243-5.

8191 Nanba H, Kubo K. Effect of Maitake D-fraction on cancer prevention. *Ann N Y Acad Sci* 1997;833:204-7.

8192 This P, De La Rochefordiere A, Clough K, et al. Phytoestrogens after breast cancer. *Endocr Relat Cancer* 2001;8:129-34.

8193 Howes J, Waring M, Huang L, Howes LG. Long-term pharmacokinetics of an extract of isoflavones from red clover (Trifolium pratense). *J Altern Complement Med* 2002;8:135-42.

8194 Tice J, Cummings SR, Ettinger B, et al. Few adverse effects of two red clover extracts rich in phytoestrogens: a multicenter, placebo-controlled trial. *Alt Ther* 2001;7:S33.

8195 Bendich A, Cohen M. Vitamin B6 safety issues. *Ann N Y Acad Sci* 1990;585:321-30.

8196 Schaumburg H, Kaplan J, Windebank A. Sensory neuropathy from pyridoxine abuse. A new megavitamin syndrome. *N Engl J Med* 1983;309:445-8.

8197 Gordon N. Pyridoxine dependency: an update. *Dev Med Child Neurol* 1997;39:63-5.

8198 Bernstein AL. Vitamin B6 in clinical neurology. *Ann N Y Acad Sci* 1990;585:250-60.

8199 Fuhr JE, Farrow A, Nelson HS Jr. Vitamin B6 levels in patients with carpal tunnel syndrome. *Arch Surg* 1989;124:1329-30.

8200 Smith GP, Rudge PJ, Peters TJ. Biochemical studies of pyridoxal and pyridoxal phosphate status and therapeutic trial of pyridoxine in patients with carpal tunnel syndrome. *Ann Neurol* 1984;15:104-7.

8201 Folkers K, Ellis J. Successful therapy with vitamin B6 and vitamin B2 of the carpal tunnel syndrome and need for determination of the RDAs for vitamins B6 and B2 for disease states. *Ann N Y Acad Sci* 1990;585:295-301.

8202 Ellis J, Folkers K, Watanabe T, et al. Clinical results of a cross-over treatment with pyridoxine and placebo of the carpal tunnel syndrome. *Am J Clin Nutr* 1979;32:2040-6.

8203 Stransky M, Rubin A, Lava NS, Lazaro RP. Treatment of carpal tunnel syndrome with vitamin B6: a double-blind study. *South Med J* 1989;82:841-2.

8204 Lewis PJ. Pain in the hand and wrist. Pyridoxine supplements may help patients with carpal tunnel syndrome. *BMJ* 1995;310:1534.

8205 Goldenberg RM, Girone JA. Oral pyridoxine in the prevention of oxalate kidney stones. *Am J Nephrol* 1996;16:552-3.

8217 Azuma J, Hasegawa H, Awata N, et al. Taurine for the treatment of congestive heart failure in humans. *Prog Clin Biol Res* 1983;125:61-72.

8218 Azuma J, Hasegawa H, Awata N, et al. Taurine for treatment of congestive heart failure. *Int J Cardiol* 1982;2:303-4.

8219 Paasonen MK, Penttila O, Himberg JJ, et al. Platelet taurine in patients with arterial hypertension, myocardial failure or infarction. *Acta Med Scand Suppl* 1980;642:79-84.

8220 Anon. Taurine involvement in retinal and heart muscle function. *Nutr Rev* 1975;33:343-7.

8221 Azuma J. Long-term effect of taurine in congestive heart failure: Preliminary report. *Adv Exp Med Biol* 1994;359:425-33.

8222 Azuma J, Takihara K, Awata N, et al. Taurine and failing heart: experimental and clinical aspects. *Prog Clin Biol Res* 1985;179:195-213.

8223 Hutter JA, Salman M, Stavinoha WB, et al. Antiinflammatory C-glucosyl chromone from Aloe barbadensis. *J Nat Prod* 1996;59:541-3.

8224 Reynolds T, Dweck AC. Aloe vera leaf gel: a review update. *J Ethnopharmacol* 1999;68:3-37.

8225 Mullins RJ, Heddle R. Adverse reactions associated with echinacea: the Australian experience. *Ann Allergy Asthma Immunol* 2002;88:42-51.

8226 Percival SS. Use of echinacea in medicine. *Biochem Pharmacol* 2000;60:155-8.

8227 Facino RM, Carini M, Aldini G, et al. Echinacoside and caffeoyl conjugates protect collagen from free radical-induced degradation: a potential use of echinacea extracts in the prevention of skin photodamage. *Planta Med* 1995;61:510-4.

8228 Turner RB, Riker DK, Gangemi JD. Ineffectiveness of echinacea for prevention of experimental rhinovirus colds. *Antimicrob Agents Chemother* 2000;44:1708-9.

8229 Food and Drug Administration, HHS. Status of certain additional over-the counter drug category II and III active ingredients. Final rule. *Fed Regist* 2002;67:31125-7.

8231 Kajiyama Y, Fujii K, Takeuchi H, Manabe Y. Ginkgo seed poisoning. *Pediatrics* 2002;109:325-7.

8232 Miwa H, Iijima M, Tanaka S, Mizuno Y. Generalized convulsions after consuming a large amount of gingko nuts. *Epilepsia* 2001;42:280-1.

8233 Lingaerde O, Foreland AR, Magnusson A. Can winter depression be prevented by Ginkgo biloba extract? A placebo-controlled trial. *Acta Psychiatr Scand* 1999;100:62-6.

8234 Piscitelli SC, Formentini E, Burstein AH, et al. Effect of milk thistle on the pharmacokinetics of indinavir in healthy volunteers. *Pharmacotherapy* 2002;22:551-6.

8235 Lyon MR, Cline JC, Totosy de Zepetnek J, et al. Effect of the herbal extract combination Panax quinquefolium and Ginkgo biloba on attention-deficit hyperactivity disorder: a pilot study. *J Psychiatry Neurosci* 2001;26:221-8.

8236 Kennedy DO, Scholey AB, Wesnes KA. The dose-dependent cognitive effects of acute administration of Ginkgo biloba to healthy young volunteers. *Psychopharmacology* (Berl) 2000;151:416-23.

8238 Jones MP, Melan MA, Witt-Enderby PA. Melatonin decreases cell proliferation and transformation in a melatonin receptor-dependent manner. *Cancer Lett* 2000;151:133-43.

8239 Kovacs J, Brodner W, Kirchlechner V, et al. Measurement of urinary melatonin: a useful tool for monitoring serum melatonin after its oral administration. *J Clin Endocrinol Metab* 2000;85:666-70.

8240 Shilo L, Dagan Y, Smorjik Y, et al. Effect of melatonin on sleep quality of COPD intensive care patients: a pilot study. *Chronobiol Int* 2000;17:71-6.

8241 Kumar AM, Tims F, Cruess DG, et al. Music therapy increases serum melatonin levels in patients with Alzheimer's disease. *Altern Ther Health Med* 1999;5:49-57.

8242 Pavelka K, Gatterova J, Gollerova V, et al. A 5-year randomized controlled, double-blind study of a glycosaminoglycan polysulphuric acid complex (Rumalon) as a structure modifying therapy in osteoarthritis of the hip and knee. *Osteoarthritis Cartilage* 2000;8:335-42.

8243 MacGregor FB, Abernethy VE, Dahabra S, et al. Hepatotoxicity of herbal remedies. *BMJ* 1989;299:1156-7.

8244 Nagtegaal JE, Laurant MW, Kerkhof GA, et al. Effects of melatonin on the quality of life in patients with delayed sleep phase syndrome. *J Psychosom Res* 2000;48:45-50.

8245 Shamir E, Laudon M, Barak Y, et al. Melatonin improves sleep quality of patients with chronic schizophrenia. *J Clin Psychiatry* 2000;61:373-7.

8246 Salti R, Galluzzi F, Bindi G, et al. Nocturnal melatonin patterns in children. *J Clin Endocrinol Metab* 2000;85:2137-44.

8247 Mishima K, Okawa M, Shimizu T, Hishikawa Y. Diminished melatonin secretion in the elderly caused by insufficient environmental illumination. *J Clin Endocrinol Metab* 2001;86:129-34.

8248 Sheldon SH. Pro-convulsant effects of oral melatonin in neurologically disabled children. *Lancet* 1998;351:1254.

8249 Bazil CW, Short D, Crispin D, Zheng W. Patients with intractable epilepsy have low melatonin, which increases following seizures. *Neurology* 2000;55:1746-8.

8250 Bent S, Patterson M, Garvin D. Valerian for sleep: a systematic review and meta-analysis. *Alternative Therapies* 2001;7:S4.

8251 Hartter S, Grozinger M, Weigmann H, et al. Increased bioavailability of oral melatonin after fluvoxamine coadministration. *Clin Pharmacol Ther* 2000;67:1-6.

8252 Lowe FC, Fagelman E. Cranberry juice and urinary tract infections: what is the evidence? *Urology* 2001;57:407-13.

8253 Kontiokari T, Sundqvist K, Nuutinen M, et al. Randomised trial of cranberry-lingonberry juice and Lactobacillus GG drink for the prevention of urinary tract infections in women. *BMJ* 2001;322:1571.

8254 DuGan CR, Cardaciotto PS. Reduction of ammoniacal urinary odors by the sustained feeding of cranberry juice. *J Psychiatr Nurs* 1966;467-70.

8256 De Bellis L, Gonzali S, Alpi A, et al. Purification and characterization of a novel pumpkin short-chain acyl-coenzyme A oxidase with structural similarity to acyl-coenzyme A dehydrogenases. *Plant Physiol* 2000;123:327-34.

8257 Younis YM, Ghirmay S, al-Shihry SS. African Cucurbita pepo L.: properties of seed and variability in fatty acid composition of seed oil. *Phytochemistry* 2000;54:71-5.

8260 Bushehri N, Jarrell ST, Lieberman S, et al. Oral reduced B-nicotinamide adenine dinucleotide (NADH) affects blood pressure, lipid peroxidation, and lipid profile in hypertensive rats (SHR). *Geriatr Nephrol Urol* 1998;8:95-100.

8262 Sivan Y, Laudon M, Kuint J, Zisapel N. Low melatonin production in infants with a life-threatening event. *Dev Med Child Neurol* 2000;42:487-91.

8263 Wurtman RJ. Age-related decreases in melatonin secretion--clinical consequences. *J Clin Endocrinol Metab* 2000;85:2135-6.

8265 Wright KP Jr, Myers BL, Plenzler SC, et al. Acute effects of bright light and caffeine on nighttime melatonin and temperature levels in women taking and not taking oral contraceptives. *Brain Res* 2000;873:310-7.

8266 Naylor S, Gleich GJ. Over-the-counter melatonin products and contamination. *Am Fam Physician* 1999;59:284, 287-8.

8267 Forsyth LM, Preuss HG, MacDowell AL, et al. Therapeutic effects of oral NADH on the symptoms of patients with chronic fatigue syndrome. *Ann Allergy Asthma Immunol* 1999;82:185-91.

8268 Lissoni P, Paolorossi F, Ardizzoia A, et al. A randomized study of chemotherapy with cisplatin plus etoposide versus chemoendocrine therapy with cisplatin, etoposide and the pineal hormone melatonin as a first-line treatment of advanced non-small cell lung cancer patients in a poor clinical state. *J Pineal Res* 1997;23:15-9.

8269 Herxheimer A, Petrie KJ. Melatonin for preventing and treating jet lag. *Cochrane Database Syst Rev* 2001;1:CD001520.

8270 Djeridane Y, Touitou Y. Chronic diazepam administration differentially affects melatonin synthesis in rat pineal and Harderian glands. *Psychopharmacology* (Berl) 2001;154:403-7.

8271 Briggs, Freeman, Yafee. Update Drugs in Pregnancy and Lactation. Lippincott Williams & Wilkins, 2001.

8272 Nishiyama K, Yasue H, Moriyama Y, et al. Acute effects of melatonin administration on cardiovascular autonomic regulation in healthy men. *Am Heart J* 2001;141:E9.

8273 Suhner A, Schlagenhauf P, Johnson R, et al. Comparative study to determine the optimal melatonin dosage form for the alleviation of jet lag. *Chronobiol Int* 1998;15:655-66.

8274 Lewy AJ, Ahmed S, Jackson JM, Sack RL. Melatonin shifts human circadian rhythms according to a phase-response curve. *Chronobiol Int* 1992;9:380-92.

8275 Rainer M, Kraxberger E, Haushofer M, et al. No evidence for cognitive improvement from oral nicotinamide adenine dinucleotide (NADH) in dementia. *J Neural Transm* 2000;107:1475-81.

8277 Politis MJ, Dmytrowich A. Promotion of second intention wound healing by emu oil lotion: comparative results with furasin, polysporin, and cortisone. *Plast Reconstr Surg* 1998;102:2404-7.

8278 Fukushima M, Ohashi T, Sekikawa M, Nakano M. Comparative hypocholesterolemic effects of five animal oils in cholesterol-fed rats. *Biosci Biotechnol Biochem* 1999;63:202-5.

8279 Schmidt U, Kuhn U, Ploch M, Hubner WD. Efficacy of the Hawthorne (Crataegus) Preparation LI 132 in 78 patients with chronic congestive heart failure defined as NYHA functional class II. *Phytomedicine* 1994;1:17-24.

8280 Zapfe jun G. Clinical efficacy of crataegus extract WS 1442 in congestive heart failure NYHA class II. *Phytomedicine* 2001;8:262-6.

8281 Tauchert M. Efficacy and safety of crataegus extract WS 1442 in comparison with placebo in patients with chronic stable New York Heart Association class-III heart failure. *Am Heart J* 2002;143:910-5.

8282 Castro N, Jung H, Medina R, et al. Interaction between grapefruit juice and praziquantel in humans. *Antimicrob Agents Chemother* 2002;46:1614-6.

8283 Jetter A, Kinzig-Schippers M, Walchner-Bonjean M, et al. Effects of grapefruit juice on the pharmacokinetics of sildenafil. *Clin Pharmacol Ther* 2002;71:21-9.

8284 Ebert U, Oertel R, Kirch W. Influence of grapefruit juice on scopolamine pharmacokinetics and pharmacodynamics in healthy male and female subjects. *Int J Clin Pharmacol Ther* 2000;38:523-31.

8285 Fuhr U, Muller-Peltzer H, Kern R, et al. Effects of grapefruit juice and smoking on verapamil concentrations in steady state. *Eur J Clin Pharmacol* 2002;58:45-53.

8286 Kanazawa S, Ohkubo T, Sugawara K. The effects of grapefruit juice on the pharmacokinetics of erythromycin. *Eur J Clin Pharmacol* 2001;56:799-803.

8287 Teng CS. Reversible changes in the content of cellular and microtubular tubulin in spermatogenic cells after gossypol treatment. *Contraception* 1997;55:183-8.

8288 Guo J, Reidenberg MM. Inhibition of 11beta-hydroxysteroid dehydrogenase by bioflavonoids and their interaction with furosemide and gossypol. *J Lab Clin Med* 1998;132:32-8.

8289 Shelley MD, Hartley L, Fish RG, et al. Stereo-specific cytotoxic effects of gossypol enantiomers and gossypolone in tumour cell lines. *Cancer Lett* 1999;135:171-80.

8290 Coutinho EM, Athayde C, Atta G, et al. Gossypol blood levels and inhibition of spermatogenesis in men taking gossypol as a contraceptive. A multicenter, international, dose-finding study. *Contraception* 2000;61:61-7.

8291 Shidaifat F, Canatan H, Kulp SK, et al. Inhibition of human prostate cancer cells growth by gossypol is associated with

REFERENCES

stimulation of transforming growth factor-beta. *Cancer Lett* 1996;107:37-44.

8292 Herve JC, Pluciennik F, Bastide B, et al. Contraceptive gossypol blocks cell-to-cell communication in human and rat cells. *Eur J Pharmacol* 1996;313:243-55.

8294 Gilbert NE, O'Reilly JE, Chang CJ, et al. Antiproliferative activity of gossypol and gossypolone on human breast cancer cells. *Life Sci* 1995;57:61-7.

8295 Liang XS, Rogers AJ, Webber CL, et al. Developing gossypol derivatives with enhanced antitumor activity. *Invest New Drugs* 1995;13:181-6.

8296 Leathwood PD, Chauffard F. Aqueous extract of valerian reduces latency to fall asleep in man. *Planta Med* 1985;2:144-8.

8300 Bredle DL, et al. Phosphate supplementation, cardiovascular function, and exercise performance in humans. *J Appl Physiol* 1988;65(4):1821-6.

8301 Duffy DJ, Conlee RK. Effects of phosphate loading on leg power and high intensity treadmill exercise. *Med Sci Sports Exerc* 1986;18(6):674-7.

8302 Perreault MM, Ostrop NJ, Tierney MG. Efficacy and safety of intravenous phosphate replacement in critically ill patients. *Ann Pharmacother* 1997;31(6):683-8.

8303 Rosen GH, et al. Intravenous phosphate repletion regimen for critically ill patients with moderate hypophosphatemia. *Crit Care Med* 1995;23(7):1204-10.

8304 Androstenediol 4AD. Vitanet. URL: store.yahoo.com/vitanet/vitan.html (Accessed 8 December 1999).

8305 Pittler MH, Ernst E. Guar gum for body weight reduction: Meta-analysis of randomized trials. *Am J Med* 2001;110:724-30.

8307 Hasegawa N. Inhibition of lipogenesis by pycnogenol. *Phytother Res* 2000;14:472-3.

8308 Noda Y, Kaneyuki T, Mori A, Packer L. Antioxidant activities of pomegranate fruit extract and its anthocyanidins: delphinidin, cyanidin, and pelargonidin. *J Agric Food Chem* 2002;50:166-71.

8309 Kaplan M, Hayek T, Raz A, et al. Pomegranate juice supplementation to atherosclerotic mice reduces macrophage lipid peroxidation, cellular cholesterol accumulation and development of atherosclerosis. *J Nutr* 2001;131:2082-9.

8310 Aviram M, Dornfeld L. Pomegranate juice consumption inhibits serum angiotensin converting enzyme activity and reduces systolic blood pressure. *Atherosclerosis* 2001;158:195-8.

8311 Moneam NM, el Sharaky AS, Badreldin MM. Oestrogen content of pomegranate seeds. *J Chromatogr* 1988;438:438-42.

8312 Sugiyama T, Sadzuka Y. Combination of theanine with doxorobucin inhibits hepatic metastasis of M5076 ovarian sarcoma. *Clin Cancer Res* 1999;5:413-6.

8313 Murai A, Miyahara T, Tanaka T, et al. The effects of pantethine on lipid and lipoprotein abnormalities in survivors of cerebral infarction. *Artery* 1985;12:234-43.

8314 Maggi GC, Donati C, Criscuoli G. Pantethine: a physiological lipomodulating agent in the treatment of hyperlipidemias. *Curr Ther Res* 1982;32:380-6.

8315 Da Col PG, Cattin L, Fonda M, et al. Pantethine in the treatment of hypercholesterolemia: a randomized double-blind trial versus tiadenol. *Curr Ther Res* 1984;36:314-22.

8316 Rubba P, Postaiglione B, De Simone F, et al. Comparative evaluation of the lipid-lowering effects of fenofibrate and pantethine in type II hyperlipoproteinemia. *Curr Ther Res* 1985;38:719-27.

8317 Angelica M, Pinto G, Ciaccheri C, et al. Improvement in serum lipid profile in hyperlipoproteinemia patients after treatment with pantethine: a cross-over double-blind trial versus placebo. *Curr Ther Res* 1983;33:1091-7.

8318 Gaddi A, Descovich GC, Noseda G, et al. Controlled evaluation of pantethine, a natural hypolipidemic compound, in patients with different forms of hyperlipoproteinemia. *Atherosclerosis* 1984;50:73-83.

8319 Prisco D, Rogasi PG, Matucci M, et al. Effect of oral treatment with pantethine on platelet and plasma phospholipids in IIa hyperlipoproteinemia. *Angiology* 1987;38:241-7.

8320 McCarty MF. Inhibition of acetyl-CoA carboxylase by cystamine may mediate the hypotriglyceridemic activity of pantethine. *Med Hypotheses* 2001;56:314-7.

8321 Cighetti G, Del Puppo M, Paroni R, et al. Modulation of HMG-CoA reductase activity by pantetheine/pantethine. *Biochim Biophys Acta* 1988;963:389-93.

8322 Carrara P, Matturri L, Galbussera M, et al. Pantethine reduces plasma cholesterol and the severity of arterial lesions in experimental hypercholesterolemic rabbits. *Atherosclerosis* 1984;53:255-64.

8323 Congdon NT, West ST, Duncan DT, et al. The effect of pantethine and ultraviolet-B radiation on the development of lenticular opacity in the emory mouse. *Curr Eye Res* 2000;20:17-24.

8324 Hiraoka T, Clark JI, LI XY, Thurston GM. Effect of selected anti-cataract agents on opacification in the selenite cataract model. *Exp Eye Res* 1996;62:11-9.

8325 Clark JI, Livesey JC, Steele JE. Delay or inhibition of rat lens opacification using pantethine and WR-77913. *Exp Eye Res* 1996;62:75-84.

8329 Gales MA, Nguyen TM. Sorbitol compared with xylitol in prevention of dental caries. *Ann Pharmacother* 2000 Jan;34(1):98-100.

8330 Romics I, Schmitz H, Frang D. Experience in treating benign prostatic hypertrophy with Sabal serrulata for one year. *Int Urol Nephrol* 1993;25:565-9.

8407 Yeh YY, Liu L. Cholesterol-lowering effect of garlic extracts and organosulfur compounds: human and animal studies. *J Nutr* 2001;131:989S-93S.

8408 Lau BH. Suppression of LDL oxidation by garlic. *J Nutr* 2001;131:985S-8S.

8409 Luk JM, Lai W, Tam P, Koo MW. Suppression of cytokine production and cell adhesion molecule expression in human monocytic cell line THP-1 by Tripterygium wilfordii polysaccharide moiety. *Life Sci* 2000;67:155-63.

8413 Wu D, Yu L, Nair MG, et al. Cyclooxygenase enzyme inhibitory compounds with antioxidant activities from Piper methysticum (kava kava) roots. *Phytomedicine* 2002;9:41-7.

8414 Singh YN. Kava: an overview. *J Ethnopharmacol* 1992;37:13-45.

8415 Bilia AR, Gallori S, Vincieri FF. Kava-kava and anxiety: growing knowledge about the efficacy and safety. *Life Sci* 2002;70:2581-97.

8416 Boonen G, Pramanik A, Rigler R, Haberlein H. Evidence for specific interactions between kavain and human cortical neurons monitored by fluorescence correlation spectroscopy. *Planta Med* 2000;66:7-10.

8417 Wooltorton E. Herbal kava: reports of liver toxicity. *CMAJ* 2002;166:777.

8418 Blanco C, Diaz-Perales A, Collada C, et al. Class I chitinases as potential panallergens involved in the latex-fruit syndrome. *J Allergy Clin Immunol* 1999;103:507-13.

8419 Eherer AJ, Santa Ana CA, Porter J, Fordtran JS. Effect of psyllium, calcium polycarbophil, and wheat bran on secretory diarrhea induced by phenolphthalein. *Gastroenterology* 1993;104:1007-12.

8420 Bliss DZ, Jung HJ, Savik K, et al. Supplementation with dietary fiber improves fecal incontinence. *Nurs Res* 2001;50:203-13.

8421 Marlett JA, Kajs TM, Fischer MH. An unfermented gel component of psyllium seed husk promotes laxation as a lubricant in humans. *Am J Clin Nutr* 2000;72:784-9.

8422 Qvitzau S, Matzen P, Madsen P. Treatment of chronic diarrhoea: loperamide versus ispaghula husk and calcium. *Scand J Gastroenterol* 1988;23:1237-40.

8423 Heather DJ, Howell L, Montana M, et al. Effect of a bulk-forming cathartic on diarrhea in tube-fed patients. *Heart Lung* 1991;20:409-13.

8424 Marlett JA, Li BU, Patrow CJ, Bass P. Comparative laxation of psyllium with and without senna in an ambulatory constipated population. *Am J Gastroenterol* 1987;82:333-7.

8425 Longstreth GF, Fox DD, Youkeles L, et al. Psyllium therapy in the irritable bowel syndrome. A double-blind trial. *Ann Intern Med* 1981;95:53-6.

8426 Prior A, Whorwell PJ. Double blind study of ispaghula in irritable bowel syndrome. *Gut* 1987;28:1510-3.

8427 Kumar A, Kumar N, Vij JC, et al. Optimum dosage of ispaghula husk in patients with irritable bowel syndrome: correlation of symptom relief with whole gut transit time and stool weight. *Gut* 1987;28:150-5.

8428 Misra SP, Thorat VK, Sachdev GK, Anand BS. Long-term treatment of irritable bowel syndrome: results of a randomized controlled trial. *Q J Med* 1989:73:931-9.

8429 Bobrove AM. Misoprostol, diarrhea, and psyllium mucilloid. *Ann Intern Med* 1990;112:386.

8430 Jenkins DJ, Kendal CW, Vuksan V. Viscous fibers, health claims, and strategies to reduce cardiovascular disease risk. *Am J Clin Nutr* 2000;71:401-2.

8431 Jensen CD, Haskell W, Whittam JH. Long-term effects of water-soluble dietary fiber in the management of hypercholesterolemia in healthy men and women. *Am J Cardiol* 1997;79:34-7.

8432 Spence JD, Huff MW, Heidenheim P, et al. Combination therapy with colestipol and psyllium mucilloid in patients with hyperlipidemia. *Ann Intern Med* 1995;123:493-9.

8433 Wolever TM, Jenkins DJ, Mueller S, et al. Psyllium reduces blood lipids in men and women with hyperlipidemia. *Am J Med Sci* 1994;307:269-73.

8434 Jacobson ED, Faloon WW. Malabsorptive effects of neomycin in commonly used doses. *JAMA* 1961;175:187-90.

8437 Matsui MS, Rozovski SJ. Drug-nutrient interaction. *Clin Ther* 1982;4(6):423-40.

8440 Boonen G, Pramanik A, Rigler R, Haberlein H. Evidence for specific interactions between kavain and human cortical neurons monitored by fluorescence correlation spectroscopy. *Planta Med* 2000;66:7-10.

8441 Russell RM, Golner BB, Krasinski SD, et al. Effect of antacid and H2 receptor antagonists on the intestinal absorption of folic acid. *J Lab Clin Med* 1988;112:458-63.

8442 Allen J. Choice of laxatives for constipation. *Pharmacist's Letter/Prescriber's Letter* 2002;18:180614.

8443 Cascara sagrada, aloe laxatives, O-9 contraceptives are category II-FDA. *The Tan Sheet* 2002;May:5.

8444 Bocchi EA, Vilella de Moraes AV, Esteves-Filho A, et al. L-arginine reduces heart rate and improves hemodynamics in severe congestive heart failure. *Clin Cardiol* 2000;23:205-10.

8445 Valsecchi R, Reseghetti A, Leghissa P, et al. Immediate contact hypersensitivity to pomegranate. *Contact Dermatitis* 1998;38:44-5.

8446 West S, Vitale S, Hallfrisch J, et al. Are antioxidants or supplements protective for age-related macular degeneration? *Arch Ophthalmol* 1994;112:222-7.

8447 Roberfroid MB. Functional effects of food components and the gastrointestinal system: chicory fructo-oligosaccharides. *Nutr Rev* 1996;54:S38-42.

8448 Kok N, Roberfroid M, Delzenne N. Dietary oligofructose modifies the impact of fructose on hepatic triacylglycerol metabolism. *Metabolism* 1996;45:1547-50.

8449 Dysseler P, Hoffem D. Inulin, an alternative dietary fibre. Properties and quantitative analysis. *Eur J Clin Nutr* 1995;49:S145-52.

8450 Pedersen A, Sandstrom B, Van Amelsvoort JM. The effect of ingestion of inulin on blood lipids and gastrointestinal symptoms in healthy females. *Br J Nutr* 1997;78:215-22.

8451 Abrams SA, Griffin IJ. Calcium absorption is increased in adolescent girls receiveing enriched inulin. World Congress of Pediatric Gastroenterology, Hepatology, & Nutrition, Boston, MA, August 5-9, 2000: Abstract 821.

8452 Agerbaek M, Gerdes LU, Richelsen B. Hypocholesterolaemic effect of a new fermented milk product in healthy middle-aged men. *Eur J Clin Nutr* 1995;49:346-52.

8453 Jyonouchi H, Sun S, Iijima K, Gross MD. Antitumor activity of astaxanthin and its mode of action. *Nutr Cancer* 2000;36:59-65.

8454 Kang JO, Kim SJ, Kim H. Effect of astaxanthin on the hepatotoxicity, lipid peroxidation and antioxidative enzymes in the liver of CCl4-treated rats. *Methods Find Exp Clin Pharmacol* 2001;23:79-84.

8455 Espaillat A, Aiello LP, Arrig PG, et al. Canthaxanthin retinopathy. *Arch Ophthalmol* 1999;117:412-3.

8456 van den Berg H. Carotenoid interactions. *Nutr Rev* 1999;57:1-10.

8457 Richelsen B, Kristensen K, Pedersen SB. Long-term (6 months) effect of a new fermented milk product on the level of plasma lipoproteins--a placebo-controlled and double blind study (abstract). *Eur J Clin Nutr* 1996;50:811-5.

8458 Leventhal LJ, Boyce EG, Zurier RB. Treatment of rheumatoid arthritis with gammalinolenic acid. *Ann Intern Med* 1993;119:867-73.

8459 Kast RE. Boarge oil reduction of rheumatoid arthritis activity may be mediated by increased cAMP that suppresses tumor necrosis factor-alpha. *Int Immunopharmacol* 2001;1:2197-9.

8462 Polsky B, Segal SJ, Baron PA, et al. Inactivation of human immunodeficiency virus in vitro by gossypol. *Contraception* 1989;39:579-87.

8463 Wu D. An overview of the clinical pharmacology and therapeutic potential of gossypol as a male contraceptive agent and in gynaecological disease. *Drugs* 1989;38:333-41.

8464 de Peyster A, Wang YY. Genetic toxicity studies of gossypol. *Mutat Res* 1993;297:293-312.

8465 Johansen RL, Misra HP. Effects of gossypol on the hepatic drug metabolizing system in rats. *Contraception* 1990;42:683-90.

8466 Taylor GT, Griffin MG, Bardgett M. Search for a male contraceptive: the effect of gossypol on sexual motivation and epididymal sperm. *J Med* 1991;22:29-44.

8467 Astaxanthin biochemical properties website. URL: http://www.astaxanthin.org. (Accessed 5 June 2002).

8468 Koutsikos D, Agroyannis B, Tzanatos-Exarchou H. Biotin for diabetic peripheral neuropathy. *Biomed Pharmacother* 1990;44:511-4.

8469 Keipert JA. Oral use of biotin in seborrhoeic dermatitis of infancy: a controlled trial. *Med J Aust* 1976;1:584-5.

8470 Barre DE. Potential of evening primrose, borage, black currant, and fungal oils in human health. *Ann Nutr Metab* 2001;45:47-57.

8472 Houghton JL, Philbin EF, Strogatz DS, et al. The presence of African American race predicts improvement in coronary endothelial function after supplementary L-arginine. *J Am Coll Cardiol* 2002;39:1314-22.

8473 Ohtsuka Y, Nakaya J. Effect of oral administration of L-arginine on senile dementia. *Am J Med* 2000;108:439.

8474 Amin HJ, Zamora SA, McMillan DD, et al. Arginine supplementation prevents necrotizing enterocolitis in the premature infant. *J Pediatr* 2002;140:425-31.

8475 Parker JO, Parker JD, Caldwell RW, et al. The effect of supplemental L-arginine on tolerance development during continuous transdermal nitroglycerin therapy. *J Am Coll Cardiol* 2002;39:1199-203.

8476 Chisholm A, Mann J, Skeaff M, et al. A diet rich in walnuts favourably influences plasma fatty acid profile in moderately hyperlipidaemic subjects. *Eur J Clin Nutr* 1998;52:12-6.

8477 Sabate J, Fraser GE, Burke K, et al. Effects of walnuts on serum lipid levels and blood pressure in normal men. *N Engl J Med* 1993;328:603-7.

8478 Feldman EB. The scientific evidence for a beneficial health relationship between walnuts and coronary heart disease. *J Nutr* 2002;132:1062S-101S.

8479 Asero R. Detection and clinical characterization of patients with oral allergy syndrome caused by stable allergens in Rosaceae and nuts. *Ann Allergy Asthma Immunol* 1999;83:377-83.

8480 Schaafsma G, Meuling WJ, van Dokkum W, Bouley C. Effects of a milk product, fermented by Lactobacillus acidophilus and with fructo-oligosaccharides added, on blood lipids in male volunteers. *Eur J Clin Nutr* 1998;52:436-40.

8481 Murofushi M, Mizuguchi J, Aibara K, Matuhasi T. Immunopotentiative effect of polysaccharide from kefir grain, KGF-C, administered orally in mice. *Immunopharmacology* 1986;12:29-35.

8482 Shiomi M, Sasaki K, Murofushi M, Aibara K. Antitumor activity in mice of orally administered polysaccharide from Kefir grain. *Jpn J Med Sci Biol* 1982;35:75-80.

8483 Rimada PS, Abraham AG. Polysaccharide production by kefir grains during whey fermentation. *J Dairy Res* 2001;68:653-61.

8484 De Vrese M, Keller B, Barth CA. Enhancement of intestinal hydrolysis of lactose by microbial beta-galactosidase (EC 3.2.1.23) of kefir. *Br J Nutr* 1992;67:67-75.

8485 Simova E, Beshkova D, Angelov A, et al. Lactic acid bacteria and yeasts in kefir grains and kefir made from them. *J Ind Microbiol Biotechnol* 2002;28:1-6.

8486 Alm L. Effect of fermentation on lactose, glucose, and galactose content in milk and suitability of fermented milk products for lactose intolerant individuals. *J Dairy Sci* 1982;65:346-52.

8487 Marquina D, Santos A, Corpas I, et al. Dietary influence of kefir on microbial activities in the mouse bowel. *Lett Appl Microbiol* 2002;35:136-40.

8488 Thoreux K, Schmucker DL. Kefir milk enhances intestinal immunity in young but not old rats. *J Nutr* 2001;131:807-12.

8489 Murofushi M, Shiomi M, Aibara K. Effect of orally administered polysaccharide from kefir grain on delayed-type hypersensitivity and tumor growth in mice. *Jpn J Med Sci Biol* 1983;36:49-53.

8490 O'Connor I, O'Brien N. Modulation of UVA light-induced oxidative stress by beta-carotene, lutein and astaxanthin in cultured fibroblasts. *J Dermatol Sci* 1998;16:226-230.

8491 Aruffo A, Stamenkovic I, Melnick M, et al. CD44 is the principal cell surface receptor for hyaluronate. *Cell* 1990;61:1303-13 .

8492 Culty M, Miyake K, Kincade PW, et al. The hyaluronate receptor is a member of the CD44 (H-CAM) family of cell surface glycoproteins. *J Cell Biol* 1990;111(6 Pt 1):2765-74 .

8493 Soderberg O, Hellstrom S. Consequences of using hyaluronan-coated tympanostomy tubes. *Acta Otolaryngol Suppl* 1987;442:50-3.

8494 Ruusuvaara P, Pajari S, Setala K. Effect of sodium hyaluronate on immediate postoperative intraocular pressure after extracapsular cataract extraction and IOL implantation. *Acta Ophthalmol* (Copenh) 1990;68:721-7.

8495 Percival SP. Complications from use of sodium hyaluronate (Healonid) in anterior segment surgery. *Br J Ophthalmol* 1982;66:714-6.

8496 Stamper RL, DiLoreto D, Schacknow P. Effect of intraocular aspiration of sodium hyaluronate on postoperative intraocular pressure. *Ophthalmic Surg* 1990;21:486-91.

8497 King SR, Hickerson WL, Proctor KG. Beneficial actions of exogenous hyaluronic acid on wound healing. *Surgery* 1991;109:76-84.

8498 Percival SP. Sodium hyaluronate in perspective: experiences from a four-year clinical trial. *Trans Ophthalmol Soc U K* 1985;104:616-20.

8499 Stearns V, Hayes DF. Cooling off hot flashes. *J Clin Oncol* 2002;20:1436-8.

8501 Said HM. Biotin: the forgotten vitamin. *Am J Clin Nutr* 2002;75:179-80.

8502 Simons LA, von Konigsmark M, Simons J, Celermajer DS. Phytoestrogens do not influence lipoprotein levels or endothelial function in healthy, postmenopausal women. *Am J Cardiol* 2000;85:1297-301.

8503 Vincent A, Ruan M, Fitzpatrick LA. Genistein, a Phytoestrogen, Inhibits Proliferation of Vascular Smooth Muscle Cells: A Possible Cardioprotective Mechanism. *Fertil Steril* 74:3:S25.

8504 Arjmandi BH. The role of phytoestrogens in the prevention and treatment of osteoporosis in ovarian hormone deficiency. *J Am Coll Nutr* 2001;20:398S-402S.

8505 Chen HL, Lu YH, Lin JJ, Ko LY. Effects of fructooligosaccharide on bowel function and indicators of nutritional status in constipated elderly men. *Nutr Res* 2000;20:1725-33.

8506 Pierre F, Perrin P, Bassonga E, et al. T cell status influences colon tumor occurrence in min mice fed short chain fructo-oligosaccharides as a diet supplement. *Carcinogenesis* 1999;20:1953-6 .

8507 Menne E, Guggenbuhl N, Roberfroid M. Fn-type chicory inulin hydrolysate has a prebiotic effect in humans. *J Nutr* 2000;130:1197-9.

8508 Bouhnik Y, Ouarne FF, Riottot M et al. Effects of prolonged ingestion of fructo-oligosaccharides (FOS) on colonic bifidobacteria, fecal enzymes and bile acids in humans. *Gastroenterol* 1994;106:A598.

8509 Cummings JH, Macfarlane GT, Englyst HN. Prebiotic digestion and fermentation. *Am J Clin Nutr* 2001;73:415S-420S.

8510 Uesugi T, Fukui Y, Yamori Y. Beneficial effects of soybean isoflavone supplementation on bone metabolism and serum lipids in postmenopausal Japanese women: a four-week study. *J Am Coll Nutr* 2002;21:97-102.

8511 D'Souza AL, Rajkumar C, Cooke J, Bulpitt CJ. Probiotics in prevention of antibiotic associated diarrhoea: meta-analysis. *BMJ* 2002;324:1361.

8512 Isolauri E, Sutas Y, Kankaanpaa P et al. Probiotics: effects on immunity. *Am J Clin Nutr* 2001;73:444S-450S.

8513 Deplancke B, Gaskins HR. Microbial modulation of innate defense: goblet cells and the intestinal mucus layer. *Am J Clin Nutr* 2001;73:1131S-41S.

8514 Reid G. Probiotic agents to protect the urogenital tract against infection. *Am J Clin Nutr* 2001;73:437S-443S.

8515 Kalliomaki M, Salminen S, Arvilommi H et al. Probiotics in primary prevention of atopic disease: a randomised placebo-controlled trial. *Lancet* 2001;357:1076-1079.

8516 Lu L, Walker WA. Pathologic and physiologic interactions of bacteria with the gastrointestinal epithelium. *Am J Clin Nutr* 2001;73;1124S-1130S.

8517 de Vrese M, Stegelmann A, Richter B, et al. Probiotics--compensation for lactase insufficiency. *Am J Clin Nutr* 2001;73:421S-9S.

8520 Dutkiewicz S. Usefulness of Cernilton in the treatment of benign prostatic hyperplasia. *Int Urol Nephrol* 1996;28:49-53.

8521 Van Horn L, Liu K, Gerber J, et al. Oats and soy in lipid-lowering diets for women with hypercholesterolemia: is there synergy? *J Am Diet Assoc* 2001;101:1319-25.

8522 Roemheld-Hamm B, Dahl NV. Herbs, menopause, and dialysis. *Semin Dial* 2002;15:53-9.

8523 Melchart D, Clemm C, Weber B, et al. Polysaccharides isolated from Echinacea purpurea herba cell cultures to counteract undesired effects of chemotherapy--a pilot study. *Phytother Res* 2002;16:138-42.

8524 Lenn J, Uhl T, Mattacola C, et al. The effects of fish oil and isoflavones on delayed onset muscle soreness. *Med Sci Sports Exerc* 2002;34:1605-13.

8525 Sheu BS, Wu JJ, Lo CY, et al. Impact of supplement with Lactobacillus- and Bifidobacterium-containing yogurt on triple therapy for Helicobacter pylori eradication. *Aliment Pharmacol Ther* 2002;16:1669-75.

8526 Martini MC, Kukielka D, Savaiano DA. Lactose digestion from yogurt: influence of a meal and additional lactose. *Am J Clin Nutr* 1991;53:1253-8.

8527 Kapiotis S, Hermann M, Held I, et al. Genistein, the dietary-derived angiogenesis inhibitor, prevents LDL oxidation and protects endothelial cells from damage by atherogenic LDL. *Arterioscler Thromb Vasc Biol* 1997;17:2868-74.

8528 Matvienko OA, Lewis DS, Swanson M, et al. A single daily dose of soybean phytosterols in ground beef decreases serum total cholesterol and LDL cholesterol in young, mildly hypercholesterolemic men. *Am J Clin Nutr* 2002;76:57-64.

8529 Nicholls J, Lasley BL, Nakajima ST, et al. Effects of soy consumption on gonadotropin secretion and acute pituitary responses to gonadotropin-releasing hormone in women. *J Nutr* 2002;132:708-14.

8530 Tonstad S, Smerud K, Hoie L. A comparison of the effects of 2 doses of soy protein or casein on serum lipids, serum lipoproteins, and plasma total homocysteine in hypercholesterolemic subjects. *Am J Clin Nutr* 2002;76:78-84.

8531 Jayagopal V, Albertazzi P, Kilpatrick ES, et al. Beneficial effects of soy phytoestrogen intake in postmenopausal women with type 2 diabetes. *Diabetes Care* 2002;25:1709-14.

8532 Anderson JJ, Chen X, Boass A, et al. Soy isoflavones: no effects on bone mineral content and bone mineral density in healthy, menstruating young adult women after one year. *J Am Coll Nutr* 2002;21:388-93.

8533 Tofler OB, Foy S, Ng K, et al. Coffee and coronary heart disease. *Heart Lung and Circulation* 2001;10:116-20.

8535 Jacobsen BK, Heuch I. Coffee, K-ras mutations and pancreatic cancer: a heterogeneous aetiology or an artefact? *J Epidemiol Community Health* 2000;54:654-5.

8536 Porta M, Malats N, Alguacil J, et al. Coffee, pancreatic cancer, and K-ras mutations: updating the research agenda. *J Epidemiol Community Health* 2000;54:656-9.

8537 Kuper HE, Mucci LA, Trichopoulos D. Coffee, pancreatic cancer, and the question of causation. *J Epidemiol Community Health* 2000;54:650-1.

8538 Kleemola P, Jousilahti P, Pietinen P, et al. Coffee consumption and the risk of coronary heart disease and death. *Arch Intern Med* 2000;160:3393-400.

8539 Urgert R, Meyboom S, Kuilman M, et al. Comparison of effect of cafetiere and filtered coffee on serum concentrations of liver aminotransferases and lipids: six month randomised controlled trial. *BMJ* 1996;313:1362-6.

8540 Avisar R, Avisar E, Weinberger D. Effect of coffee consumption on intraocular pressure. *Ann Pharmacother* 2002;36:992-5.

8541 Petty HR, Fernando M, Kindzelskii AL, et al. Identification of colchicine in placental blood from patients using herbal medicines. *Chem Res Toxicol* 2001;14:1254-8.

8542 Li W, Fitzloff JF, Farnsworth NR, Fong HH. Evaluation of commercial Ginkgo biloba dietary supplements for the presence of colchicine by high-performance liquid chromatography. *Phytomedicine* 2002;9:442-6.

8543 Burschka MA, Hassan HA, Reineke T, et al. Effect of treatment with Ginkgo biloba extract EGb 761 (oral) on unilateral idiopathic sudden hearing loss in a prospective randomized double-blind study of 106 outpatients. *Eur Arch Otorhinolaryngol* 2001;258:213-9.

8544 Polich J, Gloria R. Cognitive effects of a Ginkgo biloba/vinpocetine compound in normal adults: systematic assessment of perception, attention and memory. *Hum Psychopharmacol* 2001;16:409-16.

8545 Wolfe ML, Vartanian SF, Ross JL, et al. Safety and effectiveness of Niaspan when added sequentially to a statin for treatment of dyslipidemia. *Am J Cardiol* 2001;87:476-9,A7.

8546 Wink J, Giacoppe G, King J. Effect of very-low-dose naicin on high-density lipoprotein in patients undergoing long-term statin therapy. *Am Heart J* 2002;143:514-8.

8547 Chesney CM, Elam MB, Herd JA, et al. Effect of niacin, warfarin, and antioxidant therapy on coagulation parameters in patients with peripheral arterial disease in the Arterial Disease Multiple Intervention Trial (ADMIT). *Am Heart J* 2000;140:631-6.

8548 Gershoff SN, Prien EL. Effect of daily MgO and vitamin B6 administration to patients with recurring calcium oxalate kidney stones. *Am J Clin Nutr* 1967;20:393-9.

8549 Will EJ, Bijvoet OL. Pyridoxine therapy of adult primary oxalosis. *Proc Eur Dial Transplant Assoc* 1979;16:727-8.

8550 Amato M, Donzelli S, Lombardi M, et al. Primary hyperoxaluria: effect of treatment with vitamin B6 and shock waves. *Contrib Nephrol* 1987;58:190-2.

8551 Kanig SP, Conn RL. Kidney stones. Medical management and newer options for stone 'removal'. *Postgrad Med* 1985;78:38-44, 47-51.

8552 Collipp PJ, Chen SY, Sharma RK, et al. Tryptophane metabolism in bronchial asthma. *Ann Allergy* 1975;35:153-8.

8554 McCarty MF. High-dose pyridoxine as an 'anti-stress' strategy. *Med Hypotheses* 2000;54:803-7.

8555 De Souza MC, Walker AF, Robinson PA, Bolland K. A synergistic effect of a daily supplement for 1 month of 200 mg magnesium plus 50 mg vitamin B6 for the relief of anxiety-related premenstrual symptoms: a randomized, double-blind, crossover study. *J Womens Health Gend Based Med* 2000;9:131-9.

8556 Hansen CM, Shultz TD, Kwak HK, et al. Assessment of vitamin B-6 status in young women consuming a controlled diet containing four levels of vitamin B-6 provides an estimated average requirement and recommended dietary allowance. *J Nutr* 2001;131:1777-86.

8557 Cattaneo M, Lombardi R, Lecchi A, et al. Low plasma levels of vitamin B(6) are independently associated with a heightened risk of deep-vein thrombosis. *Circulation* 2001;104:2442-6.

REFERENCES

8558 Lerner V, Miodownik C, Kaptsan A, et al. Vitamin B(6) in the treatment of tardive dyskinesia: a double-blind, placebo-controlled, crossover study. *Am J Psychiatry* 2001;158:1511-4.

8559 St-Onge MP, Farnworth ER, Jones PJ. Consumption of fermented and nonfermented dairy products: effects on cholesterol concentrations and metabolism. *Am J Clin Nutr* 2000;71:674-81.

8560 Cadieux P, Burton J, Gardiner G, et al. Lactobacillus strains and vaginal ecology. *JAMA* 2002;287:1940-1941.

8561 MacGregor G, Smith AJ, Thakker B, Kinsella J. Yoghurt biotherapy: contraindicated in immunosuppressed patients? *Postgrad Med J* 2002;78:366-7.

8562 Canducci F, Armuzzi A, Cremonini F, et al. A lyophilized and inactivated culture of Lactobacillus acidophilus increases Helicobacter pylori eradication rates. *Aliment Pharmacol Ther* 2000;14:1625-1629.

8563 Losada MA, Olleros T. Towards a healthier diet for the colon: the influence of fructooligosaccharides and lactobacilli on intestinal health. *Nut Res* 2002;22:71-84.

8564 Friend BA, Shahani KM. Nutritional and therapeutic aspects of lactobacilli. *J Appl Nut* 1984;36:125-153.

8565 Hatakka K, Savilahti E, Ponka A, et al. Effect of long term consumption of probiotic milk on infections in children attending day care centres: double blind, randomised trial. *BMJ* 2001;322:1327.

8566 Rosenfeldt V, Michaelsen KF, Jakobsen M, et al. Effect of probiotic Lactobacillus strains on acute diarrhea in a cohort of nonhospitalized children attending day-care centers. *Pediatr Infect Dis J* 2002;21:417-419.

8567 Rosenfeldt V, Michaelsen KF, Jakobsen M, et al. Effect of probiotic Lactobacillus strains in young children hospitalized with acute diarrhea. *Pediatr Infect Dis J* 2002;21:411-416.

8568 Van Niel CW, Feudtner C, Garrison MM, Christakis DA. Lactobacillus therapy for acute infectious diarrhea in children: a meta-analysis. *Pediatrics* 2002;109:678-684.

8569 Ferko N, Levine MA. Evaluation of the association between St. John's wort and elevated thyroid-stimulating hormone. *Pharmacotherapy* 2001;21:1574-8.

8570 Hauben M. The association of St. John's wort with elevated thyroid-stimulating hormone. *Pharmacotherapy* 2002;22:673-5.

8571 Hasegawa N. Garcinia extract inhibits lipid droplet accumulation without affecting adipose conversion in 3T3-L1 cells. *Phytother Res* 2001;15:172-3.

8572 Westerterp-Plantenga MS, Kovacs EMR. The effect of (-)-hydroxycitrate on energy intake and satiety in overweight humans. *Int J Obes Relat Metab Disord* 2002;26:870-2.

8573 Bassett IB, Pannowitz DL, Barnetson RS. A comparative study of tea-tree oil versus benzoyl peroxide in the treatment of acne. *Med J Aust* 1990;153:455-8.

8574 Barrager E, Veltmann JR Jr, Schauss AG, Schiller RN. A multicentered, open-label trial on the safety and efficacy of methylsulfonylmethane in the treatment of seasonal allergic rhinitis. *J Altern Complement Med* 2002;8:167-73.

8575 Jacob S, Lawrence RM, Zucker M. The Miracle of MSM: The Natural Solution for Pain. New York: Penguin-Putnam, 1999.

8576 Murav'ev IuV, Venikova MS, Pleskovskaia GN, et al. Effect of dimethyl sulfoxide and dimethyl sulfone on a destructive process in the joints of mice with spontaneous arthritis. [Article in Russian]. *Patol Fiziol Eksp Ter* 1991;37-9.

8577 Allen LV. Methyl sulfonylmethane for snoring. *US Pharmacist* 2000;92-4.

8578 Lawrence RM. Methyl-sulfonyl-methane (MSM): a double blind study of its use in degenerative arthritis. *Int J of Anti-Aging Med* 1998;1:50.

8579 Tolbert L, Haigler T, Waits MM, Dennis T. Brief report: lack of response in an autistic population to a low dose clinical trial of pyridoxine plus magnesium. *Autism Dev Disord* 1993;23:193-9.

8581 Miller LG, Freeman B. Possible subdural hematoma associated with Ginkgo biloba. *J Herb Pharmacotherapy* 2002;2:57-63.

8582 Spinella M, Eaton LA. Hypomania induced by herbal and pharmaceutical psychotropic medicines following mild traumatic brain injury. *Brain Inj* 2002;16:359-67.

8583 Kudolo G. Ingestion of Ginkgo biloba extract significantly inhibits collagen-induced platelet aggregation and thromboxane A2 synthesis. *Alt Ther* 2001;7:105.

8584 Kressmann S, Muller WE, Blume HH. Pharmaceutical quality of different Ginkgo biloba brands. *J Pharm Pharmacol* 2002;54:661-9.

8585 Stough C, Clarke J, Lloyd J, Nathan PJ. Neuropsychological changes after 30-day Ginkgo biloba administration in healthy participants. *Int J Neuropsychopharmacol* 2001;4:131-4 .

8586 Solomon PR, Adams F, Silver A, et al. Ginkgo for memory enhancement: a randomized controlled trial. *JAMA* 2002;288:835-40.

8587 Nathan PJ, Ricketts E, Wesnes K, et al. The acute nootropic effects of Ginkgo biloba in healthy older human subjects: a preliminary investigation. *Hum Psychopharmacol* 2002;17:45-9.

8588 Mix JA, Crews WD. A double-blind, placebo-controlled, randomized trial of Ginkgo biloba extract EGb 761 in a sample of cognitively intact older adults: neuropsychological findings. *Hum Psychopharmacol* 2002;17:267-277.

8589 Stotzer PO, Blomberg L, Conway PL, et al. Probiotic treatment of small intestinal bacterial overgrowth by Lactobacillus fermentum KLD. *Scand J Infect Dis* 1996;28:615-9 .

8590 Kang BJ, Lee SJ, Kim MD, Cho MJ. A placebo-controlled, double-blind trial of Ginkgo biloba for anitdepressant-induced sexual dysfunction. *Hum Psychopharmacol* 2002;17:279-284.

8591 Scholey AB, Kennedy DO. Acute, dose-dependent cognitive effects of Ginkgo biloba, Panax ginseng and their combination in healthy young volunteers: differential interactions with cognitive demand. *Hum Psychopharmacol* 2002;17:35-44.

8592 Pepping J. DHEA: dehydroepiandrosterone. *Am J Health Syst Pharm* 2000;57:2048-50, 2053-4, 2056.

8593 Johannsson G, Burman P, Wiren L, et al. Low dose dehydroepiandrosterone affects behavior in hypopituitary androgen-deficient women: a placebo-controlled trial. *J Clin Endocrinol Metab* 2002;87:2046-52.

8594 Meston CM, Heiman JR. Acute dehydroepiandrosterone effects on sexual arousal in premenopausal women. *J Sex Marital Ther* 2002;28:53-60.

8595 Kim SS, Brody KH. Dehydroepiandrosterone replacement in Addison's disease. *Eur J Obstet Gynecol Reprod Biol* 2001;97:96-7.

8596 Reiter WJ, Schatzl G, Mark I, et al. Dehydroepiandrosterone in the treatment of erectile dysfunction in patients with different organic etiologies. *Urol Res* 2001;29:278-81.

8597 Mazat L, Lafont S, Berr C, et al. Prospective measurements of dehydroepiandrosterone sulfate in a cohort of elderly subjects: relationship to gender, subjective health, smoking habits, and 10-year mortality. *Proc Natl Acad Sci U S A* 2001;98:8145-50.

8598 Piketty C, Jayle D, Gonzalez-Canali G, et al. Low plasma levels of dehydroepiandrosterone (DHEA) and incidence of lipodystrophy. *HIV Med* 2001;2:136-8.

8599 Rowland NE, Marshall M, Robertson K. Anorectic effect of dehydroepiandrosterone combined with dexfenfluramine or thionisoxetine. *Eur J Pharmacol* 2001;419:61-64.

8600 Dharmananda S. The nature of ginseng: traditional use, modern use, and the question of dosage. *Herbalgram* 2002;54:34-51.

8601 Ellis JM, Reddy P. Effects of Panax ginseng on quality of life. *Ann Pharmacother* 2002;36:375-9.

8602 Kim YK, Guo Q, Packer L. Free radical scavenging activity of red ginseng aqueous extracts. *Toxicology* 2002;172:149-56.

8603 Ng TB, Wang H. Panaxagin, a new protein from Chinese ginseng possesses anti-fungal, anti-viral, translation-inhibiting and ribonuclease activities. *Life Sci* 2001;68:739-49.

8604 Cheng TO. Panax (ginseng) is not a panacea. *Arch Intern Med* 2000;160:3329.

8605 Pan SJ, Ding Z, Ivy JL. Ginseng's effects on glucose tolerance and mRNA profiles in a animal model of Type II diabetes. *Altern Ther* 2001;7:S26.

8608 Chrubasik S, Thanner J, Kunzel O, et al. Comparison of outcome measures during treatment with the proprietary Harpagophytum extract doloteffin in patients with pain in the lower back, knee or hip. *Phytomedicine* 2002;9:181-94.

8609 Circosta C, Occhiuto F, Ragusa S, et al. A drug used in traditional medicine: Harpagophytum procumbens DC. II. Cardiovascular activity. *J Ethnopharmacol* 1984;11:259-74.

8610 Costa De Pasquale R, Busa G, et al. A drug used in traditional medicine: Harpagophytum procumbens DC. III. Effects on hyperkinetic ventricular arrhythmias by reperfusion. *J Ethnopharmacol* 1985;13:193-9 .

8611 Soulimani R, Younos C, Mortier F, Derrieu C. The role of stomachal digestion on the pharmacological activity of plant extracts, using as an example extracts of Harpagophytum procumbens. *Can J Physiol Pharmacol* 1994;72:1532-6.

8612 Chrubasik S, Sporer F, Dillmann-Marschner R, et al. Physicochemical properties of harpagoside and its in vitro release from Harpagophytum procumbens extract tablets. *Phytomedicine* 2000;6:469-73.

8613 Grahame R, Robinson BV. Devils's claw (Harpagophytum procumbens): pharmacological and clinical studies. *Ann Rheum Dis* 1981;40:632.

8614 Lanhers MC, Fleurentin J, Mortier F, et al. Anti-inflammatory and analgesic effects of an aqueous extract of Harpagophytum procumbens. *Planta Med* 1992;58:117-23 .

8615 Baghdikian B, Lanhers MC, Fleurentin J, et al. An analytical study, anti-inflammatory and analgesic effects of Harpagophytum procumbens and Harpagophytum zeyheri. *Planta Med* 1997;63:171-6.

8616 Fiebich BL, Heinrich M, Hiller KO, Kammerer N. Inhibition of TNF-alpha synthesis in LPS-stimulated primary human monocytes by Harpagophytum extract SteiHap 69. *Phytomedicine* 2001;8:28-30..

8617 Whitehouse LW, Znamirowska M, Paul CJ. Devil's Claw (Harpagophytum procumbens): no evidence for anti-inflammatory activity in the treatment of arthritic disease. *Can Med Assoc J* 1983;129:249-51.

8618 Greenberg JE, Lynn M, Kirsner RS, et al. Mucocutaneous pigmented macule as a result of zinc deposition. *J Cutan Pathol* 2002;29:613-5.

8619 Freake HC, Govoni KE, Guda K, et al. Actions and interactions of thyroid hormone and zinc status in growing rats. *J Nutr* 2001;4:1135-41.

8620 Tang X, Shay NF. Zinc has an insulin-like effect on glucose transport mediated by phosphoinositol-3-kinase and Akt in 3T3-L1 fibroblasts and adipocytes. *J Nutr* 2001;131:1414-20.

8621 Grahn BH, Paterson PG, Gottschall-Pass KT, Zhang Z. Zinc and the eye. *J Am Coll Nutr* 2001;20:106-18.

8622 The Age-Related Eye Disease Study (AREDS) Research Group. The effect of five-year zinc supplementation on serum zinc, serum cholesterol and hematocrit in persons randomly assigned to treatment group in the age-related eye disease study: AREDS Report No. 7. *J Nutr* 2002;132:697-702.

8623 Godfrey HR, Godfrey NJ, Godfrey JC, Riley D. A randomized clinical trial on the treatment of oral herpes with topical zinc oxide/glycine. *Altern Ther Health Med* 2001;7:49-56.

8624 Bianchi GP, Marchesini G, Brizi M, et al. Nutritional effects of oral zinc supplementation in cirrhosis. *Nut Res* 2000;20:1079-89.

8625 Siberry GK, Ruff AJ, Black R. Zinc and human immunodeficiency virus infection. *Nut Res* 2002;22:527-38.

8626 Zemel BS, Kawchak DA, Fung EB, et al. Effect of zinc supplementation on growth and body composition in children with sickle cell disease. *Am J Clin Nutr* 2002;75:300-7.

8627 Prasad AS. Zinc deficiency in patients with sickle cell disease. *Am J Clin Nutr* 2002;75:181-2.

8628 Turner RB. Ineffectiveness of intranasal zinc gluconate for prevention of experimental rhinovirus colds. *Clin Infect Dis* 2001;33:1865-70.

8629 Belongia EA, Berg R, Liu K. A randomized trial of zinc nasal spray for the treatment of upper respiratory illness in adults. *Am J Med* 2001;111:103-8.

8630 Christian P, Khatry SK, Yamini S, et al. Zinc supplementation might potentiate the effect of vitamin A in restoring night vision in pregnant Nepalese women. *Am J Clin Nutr* 2001;73:1045-51.

8631 Sian L, Krebs NF, Westcott JE, et al. Zinc homeostasis during lactation in a population with a low zinc intake. *Am J Clin Nutr* 2002;75:99-103.

8632 King JC. Enhanced zinc utilization during lactation may reduce maternal and infant zinc depletion. *Am J Clin Nutr* 2002;75:2-3.

8633 Bhutta ZA, Bird SM, Black RE, et al. Therapeutic effects of oral zinc in acute and persistent diarrhea in children in developing countries: pooled analysis of randomized controlled trials. *Am J Clin Nutr* 2000;72:1516-22.

8634 Brown KH, Peerson JM, Rivera J, Allen LH. Effect of supplemental zinc on the growth and serum zinc concentrations of prepubertal children: a meta-analysis of randomized controlled trials. *Am J Clin Nutr* 2002;75:1062-71.

8635 Martorell R. Benefits of zinc supplementation for child growth. *Am J Clin Nutr* 2002;75:957-8.

8636 Rahman MM, Wahed MA, Fuchs GJ, et al. Synergistic effect of zinc and vitamin A on the biochemical indexes of vitamin A nutrition in children. *Am J Clin Nutr* 2002;75:92-8.

8637 Bhandari N, Bahl R, Taneja S, et al. Effect of routine zinc supplementation on pneumonia in children aged 6 months to 3 years: randomised controlled trial in an urban slum. *BMJ* 2002;324:1358.

8638 Muller O, Becher H, van Zweeden AB, et al. Effect of zinc supplementation on malaria and other causes of morbidity in west African children: randomised double blind placebo controlled trial. *BMJ* 2001;322:1567.

8639 California State Senate. SB1750 Dietary Supplements. Website: http://info.sen.ca.gov/pub/bill/sen/sb_1701-1750/sb_1750_bill_20020808_amended_asm.pdf (Accessed 5 September 2002).

8640 Atkinson RL. The herbal ephedra and caffeine debate continues. *Int J Obes Relat Metab Disord* 2002;26:589.

8641 Dulloo AG. Herbal simulation of ephedrine and caffeine in treatment of obesity. *Int J Obes Relat Metab Disord* 2002;26:590-2.

8642 Lindsay BD. Are serious adverse cardiovascular events an unintended consequence of the Dietary Supplement Health and Education Act of 1994? *Mayo Clin Proc* 2002;77:7-9.

8643 Samenuk D, Link MS, Homoud MK, et al. Adverse cardiovascular events temporally associated with ma huang, an herbal source of ephedrine. *Mayo Clin Proc* 2002;77:12-6.

8644 Haller CA, Jacob P 3rd, Benowitz NL. Pharmacology of ephedra alkaloids and caffeine after single-dose dietary supplement use. *Clin Pharmacol Ther* 2002;71:421-32.

8645 Greenway FL, Raum WJ, DeLany JP. The effect of an herbal dietary supplement containing ephedrine and caffeine on oxygen consumption in humans. *J Altern Complement Med* 2000;6:553-5.

8646 Bell DG, Jacobs I, Ellerington K. Effect of caffeine and ephedrine ingestion on anaerobic exercise performance. *Med Sci Sports Exerc* 2001;33:1399-403.

8647 Boozer CN, Daly PA, Homel P, et al. Herbal ephedra/ caffeine for weight loss: a 6-month randomized safety and efficacy trial. *Int J Obes Relat Metab Disord* 2002;26:593-604.

8648 Sesso HD, Stampfer MJ, Rosner B, et al. Seven-year changes in alcohol consumption and subsequent risk of cardiovascular disease in men. *Arch Intern Med* 2000;160:2605-12.

8649 Baer DJ, Judd JT, Clevidence BA, et al. Moderate alcohol consumption lowers risk factors for cardiovascular disease in postmenopausal women fed a controlled diet. *Am J Clin Nutr* 2002;75:593-9.

8650 Mukamal KJ, Maclure M, Muller JE, et al. Prior alcohol consumption and mortality following acute myocardial infarction. *JAMA* 2001:285:1965-70.

8651 Mukamal KJ, Longstreth WT, Mittleman MA. Alcohol consumption and subclinical findings on magnetic resonance imaging of the brain in older adults: the cardiovascular health study. *Stroke* 2001;32:1939-46.

8652 Liu Y, Tanaka H, Sasazuki S, et al. Alcohol consumption and severity of angiographically determined coronary artery disease in Japanese men and women. *Atherosclerosis* 2001;156:177-83.

8653 Ajani UA, Gaziano JM, Lotufo PA, et al. Alcohol consumption and risk of coronary heart disease by diabetes status. *Circulation* 2000;102:500-5.

8654 Solomon CG, Hu FB, Stampfer MJ, et al. Moderate alcohol consumption and risk of coronary heart disease among women with type 2 diabetes mellitus. *Circulation* 2000;102:494-9.

8655 Rapuri PB, Gallagher JC, Balhorn KE, Ryschon KL. Alcohol intake and bone metabolism in elderly women. *Am J Clin Nutr* 2000;72:1206-13.

8656 Mukherjee S, Sorrell MF. Effects of alcohol consumption on bone metabolism in elderly women. *Am J Clin Nutr* 2000;72:1073.

8657 Chen LC, Chou MH, Lin MF, Yang LL. Effects of Paeoniae Radix, a traditional Chinese medicine, on the pharmacokinetics of phenytoin. *J Clin Pharm Ther* 2001;26:271-8.

8658 Chou WC, Wu CC, Yang PC, Lee YT. Hypovolemic shock and mortality after ingestion of Tripterygium wilfordii hook F: a case report. *Int J Cardiol* 1995;49:173-7.

8659 Cheema P, El-Mefty O, Jazieh AR. Intraoperative haemorrhage associated with the use of extract of Saw Palmetto herb: a case report and review of literature. *J Intern Med* 2001;250:167-9.

8660 Salazar EL, Jayme V. Depletion of specific binding sites for estrogen receptor by Uncaria tomentosa. *Proc West Pharmacol Soc* 1998;41:123-4.

8661 Mur E, Hartig F, Eibl G, Schirmer M. Randomized double blind trial of an extract from the pentacyclic alkaloid-chemotype of uncaria tomentosa for the treatment of rheumatoid arthritis. *J Rheumatol* 2002;29:678-81.

8662 Ylisastigui L, Bakri Y, Amzazi S, et al. Soluble glycosaminoglycans Do not potentiate RANTES antiviral activity on the infection of primary macrophages by human immunodeficiency virus type 1. *Virology* 2000;278:412-22.

8663 Gregory SR, Piccolo N, Piccolo MT, et al. Comparision of propolis skin cream to silver sulfadiazine: a naturopathic alternative to antibiotics in treatment of minor burns. *J Altern Complement Med* 2002;8:77-83.

8664 Santos FA, Bastos EM, Uzeda M, et al. Antibacterial activity of Brazilian propolis and fractions against oral anaerobic bacteria. *J Ethnopharmacol* 2002;80:1-7.

8665 Kakuda T, Nozawa A, Unno T, et al. Inhibiting effects of theanine on caffeine stimulation evaluated by EEG in the rat. *Biosci Biotechnol Biochem* 2000;64:287-93.

8666 Yokozawa T, Oura H, Nakagawa H, et al. Effects of a component of green tea on the proliferation of vascular smooth muscle cells. *Biosci Biotechnol Biochem* 1995;59:2134-6.

8667 Yokozawa T, Dong E. Influence of green tea and its three major components upon low-density lipoprotein oxidation. *Exp Toxicol Pathol* 1997;49:329-35.

8668 Sadzuka Y, Sugiyama T, Miyagishima A, et al. The effects of theanine, as a novel biochemical modulator, on the antitumor activity of adriamycin. *Cancer Lett* 1996;105:203-9.

8669 Sugiyama T, Sadzuda Y. Enhancing effects of green tea components on the antitumor activity of adriamycin against M5076 ovarian sarcoma. *Cancer Lett* 1998;133:19-26.

8670 Yokogoshi H, Mochizuki M, Saitoh K. Theanine-induced reduction of brain serotonin concentration in rats. *Biosci Biotechnol Biochem* 1998;62:816-7.

8671 Leaf A. On the reanalysis of the GISSI-Prevenzione. *Circulation* 2002;105:1874-5.

8672 Bigger JT, El-Sherif T. Polyunsaturated fatty acids and cardiovascular events. *Circulation* 2001;103:623-5.

8673 Bucher HC, Hengstler P, Schindler C, Meier G. N-3 polyunsaturated fatty acids in coronary heart disease: a meta-analysis of randomized controlled trials. *Am J Med* 2002;112:298-304.

8674 Dewailly E, Blanchet C, Gingras S, et al. Relations between n-3 fatty acid status and cardiovascular disease risk factors among Quebecers. *Am J Clin Nutr* 2001;74:603-11.

8675 Tavani A, Pelucchi C, Negri E, et al. N-3 polyunsaturated fatty acids, fish, and nonfatal acute myocardial infarction. *Circulation* 2001:104:2269-72.

8676 Christensen JH, Skou HA, Fog L, et al. Marine n-3 fatty acids, wine intake, and heart rate variability in patients referred for coronary angiography. *Circulation* 2001;103:651-7.

8677 Holub BJ. Clinical nutrition: 4. Omega-3 fatty acids in cardiovascular care. *CMAJ* 2002:166:608-15.

8678 Dewailly E, Blanchet C, Lemieux S, et al. n-3 Fatty acids and cardiovascular disease risk factors among the Inuit of Nunavik. *Am J Clin Nutr* 2001;74:464-73.

8679 Connor WE. n-3 Fatty acids from fish and fish oil: panacea or nostrum? *Am J Clin Nutr* 2001;74;415-6.

8680 Maresta A, Balduccelli M, Varani E, et al. Prevention of postcoronary angioplasty restenosis by omega-3 fatty acids: main results of the Esapent for Prevention of Restenosis Italian Study (ESPRIT). *Am Heart J* 143:E5.

8681 Angerer P, Kothny W, Stork S, von Schacky C. Effect of dietary supplementation with omega-3 fatty acids on

progression of atherosclerosis in carotid arteries. *Cardiovasc Res* 2002;54:183-90.
8682 Oakenfull D. Soy protein, saponins and plasma cholesterol. *J Nutr* 2001;131:2971-2.
8683 Minihane AM, Khan S, Leigh-Firbank EC, et al. ApoE polymorphism and fish oil supplementation in subjects with an atherogenic lipoprotein phenotype. *Arterioscler Thromb Vasc Biol* 2000;20:1990-7.
8684 Schmitz PG, McCloud LK, Reikes ST, et al. Prophylaxis of hemodialysis graft thrombosis with fish oil: double-blind, randomized, prospective trial. *J Am Soc Nephrol* 2002;13:184-90.
8685 Jones WL, Kaiser SP. Pilot study; an emulsified fish oil supplement can significantly improve C-reactive protein, hemoglobin, albumin and urine output in chronic hemodialysis volunteers. *JANA* 2002;5:46-50.
8686 Donadio JV, Larson TS, Bergstralh EJ, Grande JP. A randomized trial of high-dose compared with low-dose omega-3 fatty acids in severe IgA nephropathy. *J Am Soc Nephrol* 2001;12:791-9.
8687 Holm T, Andreassen AK, Aukrust P, et al. Omega-3 fatty acids improve blood pressure control and preserve renal function in hypertensive heart transplant recipients. *Eur Heart J* 2001;22:428-36.
8688 Darbu S. Whitley E, Doll R, et al. Diet, smoking and lung cancer: a case-control study of 1000 cases and 1500 controls in South-West England. *Br J Cancer* 2001;84:728-35 .
8689 Aronson WJ, Glaspy JA, Reddy ST, et al. Modulation of omega-3/omega-6 polyunsaturated ratios with dietary fish oils in men with prostate cancer. *Urology* 2001;58:283-8.
8690 Terry P, Wolk A, Vainio H, Weiderpass E. Fatty fish consumption lowers the risk of endometrial cancer: a nationwide case-control study in Sweden. *Cancer Epidemiol Biomarkers Prev* 2002;11:143-5.
8691 Yam D, Peled A, Shinitzky M. Suppression of tumor growth and metastasis by dietary fish oil combined with vitamins E and C and cisplatin. *Cancer Chemother Pharmacol* 2001;47:34-40.
8692 Mabile S, Piolot A, Boulet L, et al. Moderate intake of n-3 fatty acids is associated with stable erythrocyte resistance to oxidative stress in hypertriglyceridemic subjects. *Am J Clin Nutr* 2001;74:449-56.
8693 Schoene NW. Vitamin E and omega-3 fatty acids: effectors of platelet responsiveness. *Nutrition* 2001;17:793-6.
8694 Deutch B, Jorgensen EB, Hansen JC. n-3 PUFA from fish or seal oil reduce atherogenic risk indicators in Danish women. *Nutr Res* 2000;20:1065-77.
8695 Higgins S, McCarthy SN, Corridan BM, et al. Measurement of free cholesterol, cholesteryl esters and cholesteryl linoleate hydroperoxide in copper-oxidised low density lipoprotein in healthy volunteers supplemented with a low dose of n-3 polyunsaturated fatty acids. *Nutr Res* 2000;20:1091-102.
8696 Calder PC. N-3 polyunsaturated fatty acids, inflammation and immunity: pouring oil on troubled waters or another fishy tale? *Nutr Res* 2001;21:309-41.
8697 Wallace JM, McCabe AJ, Roche HM, et al. The effect of low-dose fish oil supplementation on serum growth factors in healthy humans. *Eur J Clin Nutr* 2000;54:690-4.
8698 Lacaille B, Julien P, Deshaies Y, et al. Responses of plasma lipoproteins and sex hormones to the consumption of lean fish incorporated in a prudent-type diet in normolipidemic men. *J Am Coll Nutr* 2000;19:745-53.
8699 Pedersen HS, Mulvad G, Seidelin KN, et al. N-3 fatty acids as a risk factor for haemorrhagic stroke. *Lancet* 1999;353:812-3.
8700 Higdon JV, Du SH, Lee YS, et al. Supplementation of postmenopausal women with fish oil does not increase overall oxidation of LDL ex vivo compared to dietary oils rich in oleate and linoleate. *J Lipid Res* 2001;42:407-18.
8701 Engstrom K, Wallin R, Saldeen T. Effect of low-dose aspirin in combination with stable fish oil on whole blood production of eicosanoids. *Prostaglandins Leukot Essent Fatty Acids* 2001;64:291-7.
8702 Su KP, Shen WW, Huang SY. Omega-3 fatty acids as a psychotherapeutic agent for a pregnant schizophrenic patient. *Eur Neuropsycholpharmacol* 2001;11:295-9.
8704 Moriguchi T, Greiner RS, Salem N Jr. Behavioral deficits associated with dietary induction of decreased brain docosahexaenoic acid concentration. *J Neurochem* 2000;75:2563-73.
8705 Wainwright P. Nutrition and behaviour: the role of n-3 fatty acids in cognitive function. *Br J Nutr* 2000;83:337-9.
8706 Olsen SF, Sorensen JD, Secher NJ, et al. Randomised controlled trial of effect of fish-oil supplementation on pregnancy duration. *Lancet* 1992;339:1003-7.
8707 Sorensen JD, Olsen SF, Pedersen AK, et al. Effects of fish oil supplementation in the third trimester of pregnancy on prostacyclin and thromboxane production. *Am J Obstet Gynecol* 1993;168:915-22.
8708 Bittiner SB, Tucker WF, Cartwright I, Bleehen SS. A double-blind randomised placebo-controlled trial of fish oil in psoriasis. *Lancet* 1988;1:378-80.
8709 Ito Y, Suzuki K, Imai H, et al. Effects of polyunsaturated fatty acids on atrophic gastritis in a Japanese population. *Cancer Lett* 2001;163:171-8.
8710 Meier R, Wettstein A, Drewe J, et al. Fish oil (Eicosapen) is less effective than metronidazole, in combination with pantoprazole and clarithromycin, for Helicobacter pylori eradication. *Aliment Pharmacol Ther* 2001;15:851-5.
8711 Donadio JV, Grande JP, Bergstralh EJ, et al. The long-term outcome of patients with IgA nephropathy treated with fish oil in a controlled trial. *J Am Soc Nephrol* 1999;10:1772-7.
8712 Harel Z, Gascon G, Riggs S, et al. Supplementation with omega-3 polyunsaturated fatty acids in the management of recurrent migraines in adolescents. *J Adolesc Health* 2002;31:154-61.
8713 Pradalier A, Baudesson G, Delage A, et al. Failure of omega-3 polyunsaturated fatty acids in prevention of migraine: a double-blind study versus placebo. *Cephalalgia* 2001;21:818-22.
8714 Petersen M, Pedersen H, Major-Pedersen A, et al. Effect of fish oil versus corn oil supplementation on LDL and HDL subclasses in type 2 diabetes. *Diabetes Care* 2002;25:17048.
8715 Gamoh S, Hashimoto M, Sugioka K, et al. Chronic administration of docosahexaenoic acid improves reference memory-related learning ability in young rats. *Neuroscience* 1999;93:237-41.
8716 van den Ham EC, van Houwelingen AC, Hornstra G. Evaluation of the relation between n-3 and n-6 fatty acid status and parity in nonpregnant women from the Netherlands. *Am J Clin Nutr* 2001;73:622-7.
8717 Zuijdgeest-Van Leeuwen SD, Dagnelie PC, Wattimena JL, et al. Eicosapentaenoic acid ethyl ester supplementation: in cachectic cancer patients and healthy subjects: effects on lipolysis and lipid oxidation. *Clin Nutr* 2000;19:417-23.
8718 Thies F, Nebe-von-Caron G, Powell JR, et al. Dietary supplementation with eicosapentaenoic acid, but not with other long-chain n-3 or n-6 polyunsaturated fatty acids, decreases natural killer cell activity in healthy subjects aged >55 y. *Am J Clin Nutr* 2001;73:539-48.
8719 Nemets B, Stahl Z, Belmaker RH. Addition of omega-3 fatty acid to maintenance medication treatment for recurrent unipolar depressive disorder. *Am J Psychiatry* 2002;159:477-9.

8720 Emsley R, Myburgh C, Oosthuizen P, van Rensburg SJ. Randomized, placebo-controlled study of ethyl-eicosapentaenoic acid as supplemental treatment in schizophrenia. *Am J Psychiatry* 2002;159:1596-8.

8734 Yoshizawa K, Willett WC, Morris SJ, et al. Study of prediagnostic selenium level in toenails and the risk of advanced prostate cancer. *J Natl Cancer Inst* 1998;90:1219-24.

8735 Nomura AM, Lee J, Stemmermann GN, Combs GF. Serum selenium and subsequent risk of prostate cancer. *Cancer Epidemiol Biomarkers Prev* 2000;9:883-7.

8736 Brooks JD, Metter EJ, Chan DW, et al. Plasma selenium level before diagnosis and the risk of prostate cancer development. *J Urol* 2001;166:2034-8.

8737 Moyad MA. Selenium and vitamin E supplements for prostate cancer: evidence or embellishment? *Urology* 2002;59:9-19.

8738 Nelson MA, Reid M, Duffield-Lillico AJ, Marshall JR. Prostate cancer and selenium. *Urol Clin North Am* 2002;29(1):67-70.

8739 Antony AC. Megaloblastic Anemias. In: Hoffman R, Benz Jr EJ, Shattil SJ, et al. Hematology: Basic Principles and Practice. 3rd ed. New York, NY: Churchill Livingstone 2000: 451-79.

8740 Seitz U, Schule A, Gleitz J. [3H]-monoamine uptake inhibitition properties of kava pyrones. *Planta Med* 1997;63:548-549.

8741 Anon. Health Canada is advising consumers not to use any products containing kava. Health Canada Online 2002. http://www.hcsc.gc.ca/english/protection/warnings/2002/2002_02e.htm. (Accessed 9 July 2002).

8742 Anon. Hepatic toxicity possibly associated with kava-containing products-United States, Germany, Switzerland, 1999-2002. *MMWR Morb Mortal Wkly Rep* 2002;51(47):1065-7.

8743 Mathews JM, Etheridge AS, Black SR. Inhibition of human cytochrome P450 activities by kava extract and kavalactones. *Drug Metab Dispos* 2002;30:1153-1157.

8744 Reif S, Nicolson M, Bisset D, et al. Effect of grapefruit juice intake on etoposide bioavailability. *Eur J Clin Pharmacol* 2002;58:491-4.

8745 Freedman JE, Parker C, Li L, et al. Select flavonoids and whole juice from purple grapes inhibit platelet function and enhance nitric oxide release. *Circulation* 2001;103:2792-8.

8746 Stein JH, Keevil JG, Wiebe DA, et al. Purple grape juice improves endothelial function and reduces the susceptibility of LDL cholesterol to oxidation in patients with coronary artery disease. *Circulation* 1999;100:1050-5.

8758 Zempleni J, Mock DM. Bioavailability of biotin given orally to humans in pharmacologic doses. *Am J Clin Nutr* 1999;69:504-8.

8800 Richardson AJ, Puri BK. A randomized double-blind, placebo-controlled study of the effects of supplementation with highly unsaturated fatty acids on ADHD-related symptoms in children with specific learning difficulties. *Prog Neuropsychopharmacol Biol Psychiatry* 2002;26:233-9.

8801 Bender NK, Kraynak MA, Chiquette E, et al. Effects of marine fish oils on the anticoagulation status of patients receiving chronic warfarin therapy. *J Thromb Thrombolysis* 1998;5:257-61.

8803 Neuringer M, Reisbick S, Janowsky J. The role of n-3 fatty acids in visual and cognitive development: current evidence and methods of assessment. *J Pediatr* 1994;125:S39-47.

8805 Grekas D, Kassimatis E, Makedou A, et al. Combined treatment with low-dose pravastatin and fish oil in post-renal transplantation dislipidemia. *Nephron* 2001;88:329-33.

8807 Chan DC, Watts GF, Barrett PH, et al. Regulatory effects of HMG CoA reductase inhibitor and fish oils on apolipoprotein B-100 kinetics in insulin-resistant obese male subjects with dyslipidemia. *Diabetes* 2002;51:2377-86.

8808 Koo SI, Noh SK. Phosphatidylcholine inhibits and lysophosphatidylcholine enhances the lymphatic absorption of alpha-tocopherol in adult rats. *J Nutr* 2001;131:717-22.

8809 Lieber CS, Leo MA, Aleynik S, et al. Increased circulating level of dilinoleoylphosphatidylcholine is associated with protection against alcohol induced oxidative stress and liver fibrosis in man. *Hepatology* 2000;32(4Pt2):386A.

8811 Dhawan K, Kumar S, Sharma A. Anxiolytic activity of aerial and underground parts of Passiflora incarnata. *Fitoterapia* 2001;72:922-6.

8812 Kreydiyyeh SI, Usta J, Kaouk I, et al. The mechanism underlying the laxative properties of parsley extract. *Phytomedicine* 2001 Sep;8(5):382-8.

8813 Hong B, Ji YH, Hong JH, et al. A double-blind crossover study evaluating the efficacy of Korean red ginseng in patients with erectile dysfunction: a preliminary report. *J Urol* 2002;168:2070-3.

8814 Scaglione F, Weiser K, Alessandria M. Effects of the standardized ginseng extract G115 (Reg.) in patients with chronic bronchitis: A nonblinded, randomized, comparative pilot study. *Clin Drug Invest* 2001;21:41-5.

8815 Gandolfo M, Baeza M, De Barrio M, Anaphylaxis after eating figs. *Allergy* 2001;56:462-3.

8816 Krall EA, Wehler C, Garcia RI, et al. Calcium and vitamin D supplements reduce tooth loss in the elderly. *Am J Med* 2001;111:452-6.

8817 McCarron DA, Reusser ME. Are low intakes of calcium and potassium important causes of cardiovascular disease? *Am J Hypertens* 2001;14:206S-12S.

8818 Chapuy MC, Pamphile R, Paris E, et al. Combined calcium and vitamin D3 supplementation in elderly women: confirmation of reversal of secondary hyperparathyroidism and hip fracture risk: the Decalyos II study. *Osteoporos Int* 2002;13:257-64.

8819 Uusi-Rasi K, Sievanen H, Pasanen M, et al. Associations of calcium intake and physical activity with bone density and size in premenopausal and postmenopausal women: a peripheral quantitative computed tomography study. *J Bone Miner Res* 2002;17:544-52.

8820 Terry P, Baron JA, Bergkvist L, et al. Dietary calcium and vitamin D intake and risk of colorectal cancer: a prospective cohort study in women. *Nutr Cancer* 2002;43:39-46.

8821 Heaney RP, Nordin BE. Calcium effects on phosphorus absorption: implications for the prevention and co-therapy of osteoporosis. *J Am Coll Nutr* 2002;21:239-44.

8822 Roughead ZK, Zito CA, Hunt JR. Initial uptake and absorption of nonheme iron and absorption of heme iron in humans are unaffected by the addition of calcium as cheese to a meal with high iron bioavailability. *Am J Clin Nutr* 2002;76:419-25.

8823 Heller HJ, Poindexter JR, Adams-Huet B. Effect of estrogen treatment and vitamin D status on differing bioavailabilities of calcium carbonate and calcium citrate. *J Clin Pharmacol* 2002;42:1251-6.

8824 Heaney RP, Davies KM, Barger-Lux MJ. Calcium and weight: clinical studies. *J Am Coll Nutr* 2002;21:152S-5S.

8825 Zemel MB. Regulation of adiposity and obesity risk by dietary calcium: mechanisms and implications. *J Am Coll Nutr* 2002;21:146S-51S.

8826 Borghi L, Schianchi T, Meschi T, et al. Comparison of two diets for the prevention of recurrent stones in idiopathic hypercalciuria. *N Engl J Med* 2002;346:77-84.

8827 Ebeling PR, Wark JD, Yeung S, et al. Effects of calcitriol or calcium on bone mineral density, bone turnover, and fractures in men with primary osteoporosis: a two-year randomized, double blind, double placebo study. *J Clin Endocrinol Metab* 2001;86:4098-103.

8828 Niromanesh S, Laghaii S, Mosavi-Jarrahi A. Supplementary calcium in prevention of pre-eclampsia. *Int J Gynaecol Obstet* 2001;74:17-21.

8830 Lin YC, Lyle RM, McCabe LD, et al. Dairy calcium is related to changes in body composition during a two-year exercise intervention in young women. *J Am Coll Nutr* 2000;19:754-60.

8831 Bendich A. Calcium supplementation and iron status of females. *Nutrition* 2001;17:46-51.

8832 Heller HJ, Greer LG, Haynes SD, et al. Pharmacokinetic and pharmacodynamic comparison of two calcium supplements in postmenopausal women. *J Clin Pharmacol* 2000;40:1237-44.

8833 Pattanaungkul S, Riggs BL, Yergey AL, et al. Relationship of intestinal calcium absorption to 1,25-dihydroxyvitamin D [1,25(OH)2D] levels in young versus elderly women: evidence for age-related intestinal resistance to 1,25(OH)2D action. *J Clin Endocrinol Metab* 2000;85:4023-7.

8834 Bauman WA, Shaw S, Jayatilleke E, et al. Increased intake of calcium reverses vitamin B12 malabsorption induced by metformin. *Diabetes Care* 2000;23:1227-31.

8835 Fujita T, Ohgitani S, Nomura M. Fall of blood ionized calcium on watching a provocative TV program and its prevention by active absorbable algal calcium (AAA Ca). *J Bone Miner Metab* 1999;17:131-6.

8836 Bohmer H, Muller H, Resch KL. Calcium supplementation with calcium-rich mineral waters: a systematic review and meta-analysis of its bioavailability. *Osteoporos Int* 2000;11:938-43.

8837 Jackson KA, Savaiano DA. Lactose maldigestion, calcium intake and osteoporosis in African-, Asian-, and Hispanic-Americans. *J Am Coll Nutr* 2001;20:198S-207S.

8838 Heaney RP. Calcium needs of the elderly to reduce fracture risk. *J Am Coll Nutr* 2001;20:192S-197S.

8839 Anderson JJ. Calcium requirements during adolescence to maximize bone health. *J Am Coll Nutr* 2001;20:186S-91S.

8840 Jung ML, Baudino S, Ribereau-Gayon G, et al. Characterization of cytotoxic proteins from mistletoe (Viscum album L.). *Cancer Lett* 1990;51:103-8.

8841 Olsnes S, Stirpe F, Sandvig K, et al. Isolation and characterization of viscumin, a toxic lectin from Viscum album L. (mistletoe). *J Biol Chem* 1982;257:13263-70.

8842 Steuer-Vogt MK, Bonkowsky V, Ambrosch P, et al. The effect of an adjuvant mistletoe treatment programme in resected head and neck cancer patients: a randomised controlled clinical trial. *Eur J Cancer* 2001;37:23-31.

8843 Timoshenko AV, Cherenkevich SN, Gabius HJ. Viscum album agglutinin-induced aggregation of blood cells and the lectin effects on neutrophil function. *Biomed Pharmacother* 1995;49:153-8.

8844 Bussing A, Regnery A, Schweizer K. Effects of Viscum album L. on cyclophosphamide-treated peripheral blood mononuclear cells in vitro: sister chromatid exchanges and activation/proliferation marker expression. *Cancer Lett* 1995;94:199-205.

8845 Kuttan G, Vasudevan DM, Kuttan R. Isolation and identification of a tumour reducing component from mistletoe extract (Iscador). *Cancer Lett* 1988;41:307-14.

8846 Kuttan G, Kuttan R. Immunological mechanism of action of the tumor reducing peptide from mistletoe extract (NSC 635089) cellular proliferation. *Cancer Lett* 1992;66:123-30.

8847 Kuttan G, Vasudevan DM, Kuttan R. Presence of a receptor for the active component of Iscador in ascites fluid of tumour bearing mice. *Cancer Lett* 1989;48:223-7.

8848 Schaefermeyer G, Schaefermeyer H. Treatment of pancreatic cancer with Viscum album (Iscador): a retrospective study of 292 patients 1986-1996. *Complement Ther Med* 1998;6:172-7.

8849 Stirpe F, Sandvig K, Olsnes S, et al. Action of viscumin, a toxic lectin from mistletoe, on cells in culture. *J Biol Chem* 1982;257:13271-7.

8850 Koop H, Bachem MG. Serum iron, ferritin, and vitamin B12 during prolonged omeprazole therapy. *J Clin Gastroenterol* 1992;14:288-92.

8851 Monteleone P, Beinat L, Tanzillo C, et al. Effects of phosphatidylserine on the neuroendocrine response to physical stress in humans. *Neuroendocrinology* 1990;52:243-8.

8852 Monteleone P, Maj M, Beinat L, et al. Blunting by chronic phosphatidylserine administration of the stress-induced activation of the hypothalamo-pituitary-adrenal axis in healthy men. *Eur J Clin Pharmacol* 1992;42:385-8.

8853 Yamazaki M, Inoue A, Koh CS, et al. Phosphatidylserine suppresses Theiler's murine encephalomyelitis virus-induced demyelinating disease. *J Neuroimmunol* 1997;75:113-22.

8854 Monastra G, Cross AH, Bruni A, et al. Phosphatidylserine, a putative inhibitor of tumor necrosis factor, prevents autoimmune demyelination. *Neurology* 1993;43:153-63.

8855 Mallat Z, Benamer H, Hugel B, et al. Elevated levels of shed membrane microparticles with procoagulant potential in the peripheral circulating blood of patients with acute coronary syndromes. *Circulation* 2000;101:841-3.

8856 O'Brien KO, Zavaleta N, Caulfield LE, et al. Prenatal iron supplements impair zinc absorption in pregnant Peruvian women. *J Nutr* 2000 130:2251-5.

8857 Kim HY, Akbar M, Lau A, et al. Inhibition of neuronal apoptosis by docosahexaenoic acid (22:6n-3). Role of phosphatidylserine in antiapoptotic effect. *J Biol Chem* 2000;275:35215-23.

8858 Zanotti A, Valzelli L, Toffano G. Chronic phosphatidylserine treatment improves spatial memory and passive avoidance in aged rats. *Psychopharmacology* (Berl) 1989;99:316-21.

8859 Kelly GS. Nutritional and botanical interventions to assist with the adaptation to stress. *Altern Med Rev* 1999;4:249-65.

8860 Butler JD, Zatz M. Pantethine depletes cystinotic fibroblasts of cystine. *J Pediatr* 1983;102:796-8.

8861 Anonymous. Pantethine. *Altern Med Rev* 1998;3:379-81.

8862 Coronel F, Tornero F, Torrente J, et al. Treatment of hyperlipemia in diabetic patients on dialysis with a physiological substance. *Am J Nephrol* 1991;11:32-6.

8863 Wittwer CT, Graves CP, Peterson MA, et al. Pantethine lipomodulation: evidence for cysteamine mediation in vitro and in vivo. *Atherosclerosis* 1987;68:41-9.

8864 Bon GB, Cazzolato G, Zago S, et al. Effects of pantethine on in-vitro peroxidation of low density lipoproteins. *Atherosclerosis* 1985;57:99-106.

8865 Ranganathan S, Jackson RL, Harmony JA. Effect of pantethine on the biosynthesis of cholesterol in human skin fibroblasts. *Atherosclerosis* 1982;44:261-73.

8866 Davidsson L, Almgren A, Sandstrom B, Hurrell RF. Zinc absorption in adult humans: the effect of iron fortification. *Br J Nutr* 1995;74:417-25.

8867 Serraino M, Thompson LU. The effect of flaxseed supplementation on the initiation and promotional stages of mammary tumorigenesis. *Nutr Cancer* 1992;17:153-9.

8868 Mousavi Y, Adlercreutz H. Enterolactone and estradiol inhibit each other's proliferative effect on MCF-7 breast cancer cells in culture. *J Steroid Biochem Mol Biol* 1992;41:615-9.

8869 Gearhart MO, Sorg TB. Foscarnet-induced severe hypomagnesemia and other electrolyte disturbances. *Ann Pharmacother* 1993;27:285-9.

8870 Miller GD, Jarvis JK, McBean LD. The importance of meeting calcium needs with foods. *J Am Coll Nutr* 2001;20:168S-85S.

8871 Scopacasa F, Wishart JM, Need AG, et al. The effects of divided dose calcium on bone resorption in early postmenopausal women. *Bone* 2000;27:45S.

8872 Shah GM, Alvarado P, Kirschenbaum MA. Symptomatic hypocalcemia and hypomagnesemia with renal magnesium wasting associated with pentamidine therapy in a patient with AIDS. *Am J Med* 1990;89:380-2.

8873 Ebeling PR, Wark JD, Yeung S, et al. Effects of calcium and calcitriol on bone mass over three years in men with primary osteoporosis- A prospective cross-over study. *Bone* 2000;27:54S.

8874 Kozeny GA, Nicolas JD, Creekmore S, et al. Effects of interleukin-2 immunotherapy on renal function. *J Clin Oncol* 1988;6:1170-6.

8875 Hallberg L, et al. Calcium and iron absorption: mechanism of action and clinical importance. *Eur J Clin Nutr* 1992;46:317-27.

8876 Skikne BS, Lynch SR, Cook JD. Role of gastric acid in food iron absorption. *Gastroenterol* 1981;81:1068-71.

8877 Food and Drug Administration Science Background: Safety of Sodium Phosphates Oral Solution. September 17, 2001. Available at: http://www.fda.gov/cder/drug/safety/sodiumphospate.htm

8880 Braden GL, von Oeyen PT, Germain MJ, et al. Ritodrine- and terbutaline-induced hypokalemia in preterm labor: mechanisms and consequences. *Kidney Intl* 1997;51:1867-75.

8881 Shrestha M, Bidadi K, Gourlay S, Hayes J. Continuous vs intermittent albuterol, as high and low doses, in the treatment of severe acute asthma in adults. *Chest* 1996;110:42-7.

8882 Rahman ARA, McDevitt DG, Struthers AD, Lipworth BJ. The effects of enalapril and spironolactone on terbutaline-induced hypokalemia. *Chest* 1992;102:91-5.

8883 Clifton GD, Hunt BA, Patel RC, Burki NK. Effects of sequential doses of parenteral terbutaline on plasma levels of potassium and related cardiopulmonary responses. *Am Rev Respir Dis* 1990;141:575-9.

8884 Haalboom JRE, Deenstra M, Struyvenberg A. Effect of fenoterol on plasma potassium and cardiac ectopic activity (letter). *Lancet* 1989;2:45.

8885 Raimondi GA, Rodriguez-Moncalvo JJ. Effects of beta-adrenergic agents on hypokalemia (letter). *Chest* 1987;91(2):288-9.

8886 Gelmont DM, Balmes JR, Yee A. Hypokalemia induced by inhaled bronchodilators. *Chest* 1988;94:763-6.

8887 Morck TA, Lynch SR, Cook JD. Inhibition of food iron absorption by coffee. *Am J Clin Nutr* 1983;37:416-20.

8888 Black DA, Fraser CM. Iron deficiency anaemia and aspirin use in old age. *Br J Gen Pract* 1999;49:729-30.

8889 Kung M, White JR, Burki NK. The effect of subcutaneously administered terbutaline on serum potassium in asymptomatic adult asthmatics. *Am Rev Respir Dis* 1984;129:329-32.

8890 Rohr AS, Spector SL, Rachelefsky GS, et al. Efficacy of parenteral albuterol in the treatment of asthma: Comparison of its metabolic side effects with subcutaneous epinephrine. *Chest* 1986;89:348-51.

8891 Lipworth BJ, Clark RA, Dhillon DP, McDevitt DG. Comparison of the effects of prolonged treatment with low and high doses of inhaled terbutaline on beta-adrenoceptor responsiveness in patients with chronic obstructive pulmonary disease. *Am Rev Respir Dis* 1990;142:338-42.

8892 Kaufman G. Pyridoxine against amiodarone-induced photosensitivity (letter). *Lancet* 1984;1:51-2.

8893 Mulrow JP, Mulrow CD, McKenna WJ. Pyridoxine and amiodarone-induced photosensitivity. *Ann Intern Med* 1985;103:68-9.

8894 Bass JB, Farer LS, Hopewell PC, et al. Treatment of tuberculosis and tuberculosis infection in adults and children. *Am J Respir Crit Care Med* 1994;149:1359-74.

8895 Olness KN. Nutritional consequences of drugs used in pediatrics. *Clin Pediatr* 1985;24(8):417-20.

8896 Mydlik M, Derzsiova K, Zemberova E. Metabolism of vitamin B6 and its requirement in chronic renal failure. *Kidney Int* 1997;52, suppl.62:s56-9.

8897 Pool KD, Feit H, Kirkpatrick J. Penicillamine-induced neuropathy in rheumatoid arthritis. *Ann Intern Med* 1981;95:457-8.

8898 Ubbink JB, Delport R, Becker PJ, Bissport S. Evidence of a theophylline-induced vitamin B6 deficiency caused by noncompetitive inhibition of pyridoxal kinase. *J Lab Clin Med* 1989;113:15-22.

8899 Bartel PR, Ubbink JB, Delport R, et al. Vitamin B6 supplementation and theophylline-related effects in humans. *Am J Clin Nutr* 1994;60:93-9.

8900 Lote CJ, Thewles A, Wood JA, Zafar T. The hypomagnesaemic action of FK506: urinary excretion of magnesium and calcium and the role of parathyroid hormone. *Clin Sci* 2000;99:285-92.

8901 Glemain P, Coulange C, Grapin FN, Muszynski RC. No benefit in combining tamsulosin with Serenoa repens versus tamsulosin alone on storage/filling and voiding lower urinary tract symptoms. [Abstract]. *J Urol* 2001;167:374.

8902 Goldmann WH, Sharma AL, Currier SJ, et al. Saw palmetto berry extract inhibits cell growth and Cox-2 expression in prostatic cancer cells. *Cell Biol Int* 2001;25:1117-24.

8903 Setiawan VW, Zhang ZF, Yu GP, et al. Protective effect of green tea on the risks of chronic gastritis and stomach cancer. *Int J Cancer* 2001;92:600-4.

8904 Zijp IM, Korver O, Tijburg LB. Effect of tea and other dietary factors on iron absorption. *Crit Rev Food Sci Nutr* 2000;40:371-98.

8905 Duffy SJ, Vita JA, Holbrook M, et al. Effect of acute and chronic tea consumption on platelet aggregation in patients with coronary artery disease. *Arterioscler Thromb Vasc Biol* 2001;21:1084-9.

8906 Ratsula K, Haukkamaa M, Wichmann K, Luukkainen T. Vaginal contraception with gossypol: a clinical study. *Contraception* 1983;27:571-6.

8907 Burke BE, Neuenschwander R, Olson RD. Randomized, double-blind, placebo-controlled trial of coenzyme Q10 in isolated systolic hypertension. *South Med J* 2001;94:1112-7.

8908 Lonnrot K, Porsti I, Alho H, et al. Control of arterial tone after long-term coenzyme Q10 supplementation in senescent rats. *Br J Pharmacol* 1998;124:1500-6.

8909 Soja AM, Mortensen SA. Treatment of congestive heart failure with coenzyme Q10 illuminated by meta-analyses of clinical trials. *Mol Aspects Med* 1997;18:S159-68.

8910 Mortensen SA. Coenzyme Q10 as an adjunctive therapy in patients with congestive heart failure. *J Am Coll Cardiol* 2000;36:304-5.

8911 Bonetti A, Solito F, Carmosino G, et al. Effect of ubidecarenone oral treatment on aerobic power in middle-aged trained subjects. *J Sports Med Phys Fitness* 2000;40:51-7.

8912 Musumeci O, Naini A, Slonim AE, et al. Familial cerebellar ataxia with muscle coenzyme Q10 deficiency. *Neurology* 2001;56:849-55.

8913 Crane FL. Biochemical functions of coenzyme Q10. *J Am Coll Nutr* 2001;20:591-8.

8914 de Rijke YB, Bredie SJ, Demacker PN, et al. The redox status of coenzyme Q10 in total LDL as an indicator of in vivo oxidative modification. Studies on subjects with familial combined hyperlipidemia. *Arterioscler Thromb Vasc Biol* 1997;17:127-33.

8915 Bleske BE, Willis RA, Anthony M, et al. The effect of pravastatin and atorvastatin on coenzyme Q10. *Am Heart J* 2001;142:E2.

8916 Iwamoto Y, Nakamura R, Folkers K, Morrison RF. Study of periodontal disease and coenzyme Q. *Res Commun Chem Pathol Pharmacol* 1975;11:265-71.

8917 Wilkinson EG, Arnold RM, Folkers K, et al. Bioenergetics in clinical medicine. II. Adjunctive treatment with coenzyme Q in periodontal therapy. *Res Commun Chem Pathol Pharmacol* 1975;12:111-23.

8918 Wilkinson EG, Arnold RM, Folkers K. Bioenergetics in clinical medicine. VI. Adjunctive treatment of periodontal disease with coenzyme Q10. *Res Commun Chem Pathol Pharmacol* 1976;14:715-9.

8919 el Darouti M, Abu el Ela M. Necrolytic acral erythema: a cutaneous marker of viral hepatitis C. *Int J Dermatol* 1996;35:252-6.

8920 Sazawal S, Black RE, Menon VP, et al. Zinc supplementation in infants born small for gestational age reduces mortality: a prospective, randomized, controlled trial. *Pediatrics* 2001;108:1280-6.

8921 Girodon F, Lombard M, Galan P, et al. Effect of micronutrient supplementation on infection in institutionalized elderly subjects: a controlled trial. *Ann Nutr Metab* 1997;41:98-107.

8922 Jarvinen R, Knekt P, Hakulinen T, Aromaa A. Prospective study on milk products, calcium and cancers of the colon and rectum. *Eur J Clin Nutr* 2001;55:1000-7.

8923 FDA. Center for Devices and Radiological Health. StaarVisc. Sodium Hyaluronate. http://www.fda.gov/cdrh/pdf/P960033c.pdf. (Accessed 11 October 2002).

8924 Hesslink R Jr, Armstrong D 3rd, Nagendran MV, et al. Cetylated fatty acids improve knee function in patients with osteoarthritis. *J Rheumatol* 2002;29:1708-12.

8925 van de Weijer P, Barentsen R. Isoflavones from red clover (Promensil) significantly reduce menopausal hot flush symptoms compared with placebo. *Maturitas* 2002;42:187-93.

8926 Keen H, Payan J, Allawi J, et al. Treatment of diabetic neuropathy with gamma-linolenic acid. The gamma-Linolenic Acid Multicenter Trial Group. *Diabetes Care* 1993;16:8-15.

8927 Althius MD, Jordon NE, Ludington EA, Wittes JT. Glucose and insulin responses to dietary chromium supplements: a meta-analysis. *Am J Clin Nutr* 2002;76:148-55.

8928 Gunton JE, Hams G, Hitchman R, McElduff A. Serum chromium does not predict glucose tolerance in late pregnancy. *Am J Clin Nutr* 2001;73:99-104.

8929 Attenburrow MJ, Odontiadis J, Murray BJ, et al. Chromium treatment decreases the sensitivity of 5-HT2A receptors. *Psychopharmacology* (Berl) 2002;159:432-6.

8930 Holme SA, Roberts DL. Erythroderma associated with St John's wort. *Br J Dermatol* 2000;143:1127-8.

8931 Irefin S, Sprung J. A possible cause of cardiovascular collapse during anesthesia: long-term use of St. John's Wort. *J Clin Anesth* 2000;12:498-9.

8932 Kumar V, Jaiswal AK, Singh PN, Bhattacharya SK. Anxiolytic activity of Indian Hypericum perforatum Linn: an experimental study. *Indian J Exp Biol* 2000;38:36-41.

8933 Martonfi P, Repcak M, Ciccarelli D, Garbari F. Hypericum perforatum L. - chemotype without rutin from Italy. *Biochem Syst Ecol* 2001;29:659-61.

8934 Southwell IA, Bourke CA. Seasonal variation in hypericin content of Hypericum perforatum L. (St. John's Wort). *Phytochemistry* 2001;56:437-41.

8935 Bilia AR, Bergonzi MC, Morgenni F, et al. Evaluation of chemical stability of St. John's wort commercial extract and some preparations. *Int J Pharm* 2001;213:199-208.

8936 Calapai G, Crupi A, Firenzuoli F, et al. Serotonin, norepinephrine and dopamine involvement in the antidepressant action of hypericum perforatum. *Pharmacopsychiatry* 2001;34:45-9.

8937 Jacobson MD, Plancher KD, Kleinman WB. Vitamin B6 (pyridoxine) therapy for carpal tunnel syndrome. *Hand Clin* 1996;12:253-7.

8938 Shults CW, Oakes D, Kieburtz K, et al. Effects of coenzyme Q10 in early Parkinson disease: evidence of slowing of the functional decline. *Arch Neurol* 2002;59:1541-50.

8939 Shults CW, Beal MF, Fontaine D, et al. Absorption, tolerability, and effects on mitochondrial activity of oral coenzyme Q10 in parkinsonian patients. *Neurology* 1998;50:793-5.

8940 The Huntington Study Group. A randomized, placebo-controlled trial of coenzyme Q10 and remacemide in Huntington's disease. *Neurology* 2001;57:397-404.

8941 Ferrante RJ, Andreassen OA, Dedeoglu A, et al. Therapeutic effects of coenzyme Q10 and remacemide in transgenic mouse models of Huntington's disease. *J Neurosci* 2002;22:1592-9.

8942 Pavelka K, Gatterova J, Olejarova M, et al. Glucosamine sulfate use and delay of progression of knee osteoarthritis: A 3-year, randomized, placebo-controlled, double-blind study. *Arch Intern Med* 2002;162:2113-23.

8943 Rizkalla SW, Luo J, Kabir M, et al. Chronic consumption of fresh but not heated yogurt improves breath-hydrogen status and short-chain fatty acid profiles: a controlled study in healthy men with or without lactose maldigestion. *Am J Clin Nutr* 2000;72:1474-9.

8944 Du XL, Edelstein D, Dimmeler S, et al. Hyperglycemia inhibits endothelial nitric oxide synthase activity by post-translational modification at the Akt site. *J Clin Invest* 2001;108:1341-8.

8945 Kazzi GM, Bottoms SF, Rosen MG. Efficacy and safety of Laminaria digitata for preinduction ripening of the cervix. *Obstet Gynecol* 1982;60:440-3.

8946 Segermann J, Hotze A, Ulrich H, Rao GS. Effect of alpha-lipoic acid on the peripheral conversion of thyroxine to triiodothyronine and on serum lipid-, protein- and glucose levels. *Arzneimittelforschung* 1991;41:1294-8.

8948 Ringe JD, Rovati LC. Treatment of osteoporosis in men with fluoride alone or in combination with bisphosphonates. *Calcif Tissue Int* 2001;69:252-5.

8949 Gutteridge DH, Stewart GO, Prince RL, et al. A randomized trial of sodium fluoride (60 mg) +/- estrogen in postmenopausal posteoporotic vertebral fractures: increased vertebral fractures and peripheral bone loss with sodium fluoride; concurrent estrogen prevents peripheral loss, but not vertebral fractures. *Osteoporos Int* 2002;13:158-70.

8950 Position of the American Dietetic Association: the impact of fluoride on health. *J Am Diet Assoc* 2001;101:126-32.

8951 Zarafonetis CJ, Horrax TM. Treatment of peyronie's disease with para-aminobenzoacidic potassium (POTOBA). *J Urol* 1959;81:770-2.

8952 Pathak MA. Sunscreens: Topical and systemic approaches for protection of human skin against harmful effects of solar radiation. *J Am Acad Dermatol* 1982;7:285-312.

8953 Zarafonetis CJ. Darkening of gray hair during para-amino-benzoic acid therapy. *J Invest Dermatol* 1950;399-401.

8954 Sieve BF. The clinical effects of a new B Complex Factor, para-aminobenzoic acid, on pigmentation and fertility. *Southern Medicine & Surgery* 1942;135-9.

8955 Anderson KJ, Teuber SS, Gobeille A, et al. Walnut polyphenolics inhibit in vitro human plasma and LDL oxidation. *J Nutr* 2001;131:2837-42.

8956 Boerth J, Strong KM. The clinical utility of milk thistle (Silybum marianum) in cirrhosis of the liver. *Journal of Herbal Pharmacotherapy* 2002;2:11-7.

8957 Flora K, Hahn M, Rosen H, Benner K. Milk thistle (Silybum marianum) for the therapy of liver disease. *Am J Gastroenterol* 1998;93:139-43.

8958 Pepping J. Coenzyme Q10. *Am J Health-Syst Pharm* 1999;56:519-21.

8959 Kishi T, Makino K, Okamoto T, et al. Inhibition of myocardial respiration by psychotherapeutic drugs and prevention by coenzyme Q. In: Yamamura Y, Folkers K, Ito Y (eds). Biomedical and clinical aspects of coenzyme Q. Amsterdam: Elsevier/North-Holland Biomedical Press 1980;2:139-54.

8961 Luyckx VA, Ballantine R, Claeys M, et al. Herbal remedy-associated acute renal failure secondary to Cape aloes. *Am J Kidney Dis* 2002;39:E13.

8962 Ricciardelli C, Quinn DI, Raymond WA, et al. Elevated levels of peritumoral chondroitin sulfate are predictive of poor prognosis in patients treated by radical prostatectomy for early-stage prostate cancer. *Cancer Res* 1999;59:2324-8.

8963 Teede HJ, Dalais FS, Kotsopoulos D, et al. Dietary soy has both beneficial and potentially adverse cardiovascular effects: a placebo-controlled study in men and postmenopausal women. *J Clin Endocrinol Metab* 2001;86:3053-60.

8964 Simons LA, von Konigsmark M, Simons J, Celermajer DS. Phytoestrogens do not influence lipoprotein levels or endothelial function in healthy, postmenopausal women. *Am J Cardiol* 2000;85:1297-301.

8965 Tanos V, Brzezinski A, Drize O, et al. Synergistic inhibitory effects of genistein and tamoxifen on human dysplastic and malignant epithelial breast cells in vitro. *Eur J Obstet Gynecol Reprod Biol* 2002;102:188-94.

8966 Ju YH, Doerge DR, Allred KF, et al. Dietary Genistein Negates the Inhibitory Effect of Tamoxifen on Growth of Estrogen-dependent Human Breast Cancer (MCF-7) Cells Implanted in Athymic Mice. *Cancer Res* 2002;62:2474-7 .

8968 Paddon-Jones D, Keech A, Jenkins D. Short-term beta-hydroxy-beta-methylbutyrate supplementation does not reduce symptoms of eccentric muscle damage. *Int J Sport Nutr Exerc Metab* 2001;11:442-50.

8969 Rizzi R, Re F, Bianchi A, et al. Mutagenic and antimutagenic activities of Uncaria tomentosa and its extracts. *J Ethnopharmacol* 1993 Jan;38(1):63-77.

8970 Lai H, Lai S, Shor-Posner G, et al. Plasma zinc, copper, copper:zinc ratio, and survival in a cohort of HIV-1-infected homosexual men. *J Acquir Immune Defic Syndr Human Retrovirol* 2001;27:56-62.

8971 Cole A, May PM, Williams DR. Metal binding by pharmaceuticals. Part 1. Copper(II) and zinc(II) interactions following ethambutol administration. *Agents and Actions* 1981;11:296-305.

8972 Bosetti C, La Vecchia C, Negri E, Franceschi S. Wine and other types of alcoholic beverages and the risk of esophageal cancer. *Eur J Clin Nutr* 2000;54:918-20.

8974 Singletary KW, Gapstur SM. Alcohol and breast cancer: review of epidemiologic and experimental evidence and potential mechanisms. *JAMA* 2001;286:2143-51.

8976 de Vries JH, Hollman PC, van Amersfoort I, et al. Red wine is a poor source of bioavailable flavonols in men. *J Nutr* 2001;131:745-8.

8977 Tsunoda SM, Harris RZ, Christians U, et al. Red wine decreases cyclosporine bioavailabity. *Clin Pharmacol Ther* 2001;70:462-7.

8978 Klemola T, Vanto T, Juntunen-Backman K, et al. Allergy to soy formula and to extensively hydrolyzed whey formula in infants with cow's milk allergy: a prospective, randomized study with a follow-up to the age of 2 years. *J Pediatr* 2002;140:219-24.

8979 Ju YH, Allred CD, Allred KF, et al. Physiological concentrations of dietary genistein dose-dependently stimulate growth of estrogen-dependent human breast cancer (MCF-7) tumors implanted in athymic nude mice. *J Nutr* 2001;131:2957-62.

8980 Goldman LR, Newbold R, Swan SH. Exposure to soy-based formula in infancy. *JAMA* 2001;286:2402-3.

8982 Chiechi L, Secreto G, D'Amore M, et al. Efficacy of a soy rich diet in preventing postmenopausal osteoporosis: the Menfis randomized trial. *Maturitas* 2002;42:295.

8983 Trock B, Clarke R, Hilakivi-Clarke L. Soy intake and breast cancer risk: Results of a meta-analysis. Poster Presentation: International Scientific Conference on Complementary, Alternative, and Integrative Medicine Research, 2002.

8984 Dewell A, Hollenbeck CB, Bruce B. The effects of soy-derived phytoestrogens on serum lipids and lipoproteins in moderately hypercholesterolemic postmenopausal women. *J Clin Endocrinol Metab* 2002;87:118-21.

8985 Chiechi LM, Secreto G, Vimercati A, et al. The effects of a soy rich diet on serum lipids: the Menfis randomized trial. *Maturitas* 2002;41:97-104.

8986 Maskarinec G, Williams AE, Inouye JS, et al. A randomized isoflavone intervention among premenopausal women. *Cancer Epidemiol Biomarkers Prev* 2002;11:195-201.

8987 Kurzer MS. Hormonal effects of soy in premenopausal women and men. *J Nutr* 2002;132:570S-573S.

8988 Jenkins DJ, Kendall CW, Jackson CJ, et al. Effects of high- and low-isoflavone soyfoods on blood lipids, oxidized LDL, homocysteine, and blood pressure in hyperlipidemic men and women. *Am J Clin Nutr* 2002;76:365-72.

8989 Setchell KD, Brown NM, Zimmer-Nechemias L, et al. Evidence for lack of absorption of soy isoflavone glycosides in humans, supporting the crucial role of intestinal metabolism for bioavailability. *Am J Clin Nutr* 2002;76:447-53.

8990 Puska P, Korpelainen V, Hoie LH, et al. Soy in hypercholesterolaemia: a double-blind, placebo-controlled trial. *Eur J Clin Nutr* 2002;56:352-7.

8991 de Kleijn MJ, van der Schouw YT, Wilson PW, et al. Dietary intake of phytoestrogens is associated with a favorable metabolic cardiovascular risk profile in postmenopausal U.S. women: the Framingham study. *J Nutr* 2002;132:276-82.

8992 Barnes S, Grubbs C, Setchell KD, Carlson J. Soybeans inhibit mammary tumors in models of breast cancer. *Prog Clin Biol Res* 1990;347:239-53.

8993 Burow ME, Boue SM, Collins-Burow BM, et al. Phytochemical glyceollins, isolated from soy, mediate antihormonal effects through estrogen receptor alpha and beta. *J Clin Endocrinol Metab* 2001;86:1750-8.

8994 Smerzer KD, Gretebeck PJ. Effect of radix Acanthopanax senticosus on submaximal running peformance. *Med Sci Sports Excerc* 1998;30 Suppl:S278.

8995 Jepson RG, Mihaljevic L, Craig J. Cranberries for treating urinary tract infections. *Cochrane Database Syst Rev* 2000;2:CD001322.

8996 Horner NK, Lampe JW. Potential mechanisms of diet therapy for fibrocystic breast conditions show inadequate evidence of effectiveness. *J Am Diet Assoc* 2000;100:1368-80.

8997 MacDonald HB. Conjugated linoleic acid and disease prevention: a review of current knowledge. *J Am Coll Nutr* 2000 Apr;19:111S-8S.

8998 Altura BT, Memon ZI, Zhang A, et al. Low levels of serum ionized magnesium are found in patients early after stroke which result in rapid elevation in cytosolic free calcium and spasm in cerebral vascular muscle cells. *Neurosci Lett* 1997;230:37-40.

8999 Bhargava B, Chandra S, Agarwal VV, et al. Adjunctive magnesium infusion therapy in acute myocardial infarction. *Int J Cardiol* 1995;52:95-9.

9000 Muir KW, Lees KR. A randomized, double-blind, placebo-controlled pilot trial of intravenous magnesium sulfate in acute stroke. *Stroke* 1995;26:1183-8.

9001 Suter PM. The effects of potassium, magnesium, calcium, and fiber on risk of stroke. *Nutr Rev* 1999;57:84-8.

9002 Ascherio A, Rimm EB, Hernan MA, et al. Intake of potassium, magnesium, calcium, and fiber and risk of stroke among US men. *Circulation* 1998;98:1198-204.

9003 Muir KW, Lees KR. Dose optimization of intravenous magnesium sulfate after acute stroke. *Stroke* 1998;29:918-23.

9004 Bosetti C, La Vecchia C, Negri E, Franceschi S. Wine and other types of alcoholic beverages and the risk of esophageal cancer. *Eur J Clin Nutr* 2000;54:918-20.

9005 Kato H, Yoshikawa M, Miyazaki T, et al. Expression of p53 protein related to smoking and alcoholic beverage drinking habits in patients with esophageal cancers. *Cancer Lett* 2001;167:65-72.

9006 Singletary KW, Gapstur SM. Alcohol and breast cancer: review of epidemiologic and experimental evidence and potential mechanisms. *JAMA* 2001;286:2143-51.

9007 Duncan BB, Chambless LE, Schmidt MI, et al. Association of the waist-to-hip ratio is different with wine than with beer or hard liquor consumption. *Am J Epidemiol* 1995;142:1034-8.

9100 American Dental Association. "ADA Statement on FDA Toothpaste Warning Labels" http://www.ada.org/prof/prac/issues/statements/fluoride.html (Accessed 18 November 2002).

9101 Centers for Disease Control. National Center for Chronic Disease Prevention and Health Promotion. "Dietary Fluoride Supplement Schedule." http://www.cdc.gov/OralHealth/factsheets/fl-supplements.htm (Accessed 18 November 2002).

9102 Phipps KR, Orwoll ES, Mason JD, Cauley JA. Community water fluoridation, bone mineral density, and fractures: prospective study of effects in older women. *BMJ* 2000;321:860-4.

9103 Rubin CD, Pak CY, Adams-Huet B, et al. Sustained-release sodium fluoride in the treatment of the elderly with established osteoporosis. *Arch Intern Med* 2001;161:2325-33.

9104 Stendig-Lindberg G, Tepper R, Leichter I. Trabecular bone density in a two year controlled trial of peroral magnesium in osteoporsis. *Mag Res* 1993;6:155-63.

9105 Montgomery SA, Thal LJ, Amrein R. Meta-analysis of double blind randomized controlled clinical trials of acetyl-L-carnitine versus placebo in the treatment of mild cognitive impairment and mild Alzheimer's disease. *Int Clin Psychopharmacol* 2003;18:61-71.

9106 Gur A, Colpan L, Nas K, et al. The role of trace minerals in the pathogenisis of postmenopausal osteoporosis and a new effect of calcitonin. *J Bone Miner Metab* 2002;20:39-43.

9107 Anon. FDA approved potassium health claim notification for potassium containing foods. FDA www.cfsan.fda.gov/~dms/hclm-k.html (Accessed 5 July 2002).

9108 Hardy M, Coulter I, Morton SC, et al. S-Adenosyl-L-Methionine for Treatment of Depression, Osteoarthritis, and Liver Disease. Evidence Report/Technology Assessment Number 64. Agency for Healthcare Research and Quality, US Dept of Health and Human Services; 2002. AHRQ publication 02-E033. Rockville, Md. Available at: http://www.ahrq.gov/clinic/tp/sametp.htm.

9109 Delle Chiaie R, Pancheri P, Scapicchio P. Efficacy and tolerability of oral and intramuscular S-adenosyl-Lmethionine 1,4-butanedisulfonate (SAMe) in the treatment of major depression: comparison with imipramine in multicenter studies. *Am J Clin Nutr* 2002;76:1172S-6S.

9110 Bottiglieri T. S-Adenosyl-L-methionine (SAMe): from the bench to the bedside--molecular basis of a pleiotrophic molecule. *Am J Clin Nutr* 2002;76:1151S-7S.

9111 Soeken KL, Lee WL, Bausell RB, et al. Safety and efficacy of S-adenosylmethionine (SAMe) for osteoarthritis. *J Fam Pract* 2002;51:425-30.

9112 Lieber CS, Packer L. S-Adenosylmethionine: molecular, biological, and clinical aspects—an introduction. *Am J Clin Nutr* 2002;76:1148S-50S.

9113 Mischoulon D, Fava M. Role of S-adenosyl-L-methionine in the treatment of depression: a review of the evidence. *Am J Clin Nutr* 2002;76:1158S-61S.

9114 Saletu B, Anderer P, Di Padova C. Electrophysiological neuroimaging of the central effects of S-adenosyl-L-methionine by mapping of electroencephalograms and event-related potentials and low-resolution brain electromagnetic tomography. *Am J Clin Nutr* 2002;76:1162S-71S.

9115 Martinez-Chantar ML, Garcia-Trevijano ER, Latasa MU, et al. Importance of a deficiency in S-adenosyl-L-methionine synthesis in the pathogenesis of liver injury. *Am J Clin Nutr* 2002;76:1177S-82S.

9116 Lieber CS. S-Adenosyl-L-methionine: its role in the treatment of liver disorders. *Am J Clin Nutr* 2002;76:1183S-17S.

9117 Rahman MA, Ing TS. Cyclosporine and magnesium metabolism. *J Lab Clin Med* 1989;114:213-4.

9118 Cibere J, Esdaile JM, Thorne A, et al. Multicenter Randomized Double-Blind Placebo-Controlled Glucosamine Discontinuation Trial in Osteoarthritis. American College of Rheumatology Meeting; October 25-29, 2002. Abstract 1549.

9119 Ganu VA, Hu SI, Strassman J, et al. Inhibitors of N-glycosylation Reduce Cytokine-induced Production of Matrix Metalloproteinases, Nitric oxide, and PGE2 from Articular Chondrocytes: A Candidate Mechanism for the Chondroprotective Effects of d-Glucosamine. American College of Rheumatology Meeting; October 25-29, 2002. Abstract 616.

9121 Alvarez-Soria MA, Largo R, Diez-Ortego E, et al. Glucosamine Inhibits IL-1ß-induced NF-kappa B Activation in Human Osteoarthritic chondrocytes. American College of Rheumatology Meeting; October 25-29, 2002. Abstract 118.

9122 Tiku ML, Narla H, Karry SK, et al. Glucosamine Inhibits Advanced Lipoxidation Reaction and Chemical Modification of Lipoproteins by Scavenging Reactive Carbonyl Intermediates. American College of Rheumatology Meeting; October 25-29, 2002. Abstract 11.

9123 Agrati AM, Ambrosi G, Ferraro G, et al. Gemfibrozil efficacy vs pantethine in dyslipoproteinemic patients: a controlled study. *Curr Ther Res* 1989;45:650-63.

9124 Reginster JY, Meurmans L, Zegels B, et al. The effect of sodium monofluorophosphate plus calcium on vertebral fracture rate in postmenopausal women with moderate osteoporosis. A randomized, controlled trial. *Ann Intern Med* 1998;129:1-8.

9125 Alexandersen P, Riis BJ, Christiansen C, et al. Monofluorophosphate combined with hormone replacement therapy induces a synergistic effect on bone mass by dissociating bone formation and resorption in postmenopausal women: a randomized study. *J Clin Endocrinol Metab* 1999;84:3013-20.

9126 Chen WY, Abatangelo G. Functions of hyaluronan in wound repair. *Wound Repair Regen* 1999;7:79-89.

9127 Brown JP, Josse RG, et al. 2002 clinical practice guidelines for the diagnosis and management of osteoporosis in Canada. *CMAJ* 2002;167:S1-S34.

9128 Marinho VC, Higgins JP, Logan S, Sheiham A. Fluoride gels for preventing dental caries in children and adolescents. *Cochrane Database Syst Rev* 2002;2:CD002280.

9129 Haguenauer D, Welch V, Shea B, et al. Fluoride for treating postmenopausal osteoporosis.(Cochrane Review). *Cochrane Database Syst Rev* 2002;4:CD002825.

9130 Adachi JD, Bell MJ, Bensen WG, et al. Fluoride therapy in prevention of rheumatoid arthritis induced bone loss. *J Rheumatol* 1997;24:2308-13.

9132 Guanabens N, Farrerons J, Perez-Edo L, et al. Cyclical etidronate versus sodium fluoride in established postmenopausal osteoporosis: a randomized 3 year trial. *Bone* 2000;27:123-8.

9133 Meunier PJ, Sebert JL, Reginster JY, et al. Fluoride salts are no better at preventing new vertebral fractures than calcium-vitamin D in postmenopausal osteoporosis: the FAVOStudy. *Osteoporos Int* 1998;8:4-12.

9134 von Tirpitz C, Klaus J, Bruckel J, et al. Increase of bone mineral density with sodium fluoride in patients with Crohn's disease. *Eur J Gastroenterol Hepatol* 2000;12:19-24.

9139 Goa KL, Benfield P. Hyaluronic acid. A review of its pharmacology and use as a surgical aid in ophthalmology, and its therapeutic potential in joint disease and wound healing. *Drugs* 1994;47:536-66.

9140 US Food and Drug Administration. Center for Food Safety & Applied Nutrition. Office of Premarket Approval. Agency Response Letter GRAS Notice No. GRN 00056. December 4, 2000 Available at: http://vm.cfsan.fda.gov/~rdb/opa-g056.html.

9141 Lanca S, Alves A, Vieira AI, et al. Chromium-induced toxic hepatitis. *Eur J Intern Med* 2002;13:518-20.

9142 Maki KC, Davidson MH, Tsushima R, et al. Consumption of diacylglycerol oil as part of a reduced-energy diet enhances loss of body weight and fat in comparison with consumption of a triacylglycerol control oil. *Am J Clin Nutr* 2002;76:1230-6.

9143 Yamamoto K, Asakawa H, Tokunaga K, et al. Long-term ingestion of dietary diacylglycerol lowers serum triacylglycerol in type II diabetic patients with hypertriglyceridemia. *J Nutr* 2001;131:3204-7.

9144 Nagao T, Watanabe H, Goto N, et al. Dietary diacylglycerol suppresses accumulation of body fat compared to triacylglycerol in men in a double-blind controlled trial. *J Nutr* 2000;130:792-7.

9145 Taguchi H, Watanabe H, Onizawa K, et al. Double-blind controlled study on the effects of dietary diacylglycerol on postprandial serum and chylomicron triacylglycerol responses in healthy humans. *J Am Coll Nutr* 2000;19:789-96.

9146 Watanabe H, Onizawa K, Naito S, et al. Fat-soluble vitamin status is not affected by diacylglycerol consumption. *Ann Nutr Metab* 2001;45:259-64.

9148 Agteresch HJ, Dagnelie PC, van den Berg JW, Wilson JH. Adenosine triphosphate: established and potential clinical applications. *Drugs* 1999;58:211-32.

9149 Agteresch HJ, Rietveld T, Kerkhofs LG, et al. Beneficial effects of adenosine triphosphate on nutritional status in advanced lung cancer patients: a randomized clinical trial. *J Clin Oncol* 2002;20:371-8.

9150 Sherlock CH, Corey L. Adenosine monophosphate for the treatment of varicella zoster infections: a large dose of caution. *JAMA* 1985;253:1444-5.

9151 Agteresch HJ, Dagnelie PC, van der Gaast A, et al. Randomized clinical trial of adenosine 5'-triphosphate in patients with advanced non-small-cell lung cancer. *J Natl Cancer Inst* 2000;92:321-8.

9152 Haskell CM, Wong M, Williams A, Lee LY. Phase I trial of extracellular adenosine 5'-triphosphate in patients with advanced cancer. *Med Pediatr Oncol* 1996;27:165-73.

9153 Jatoi A, Loprinzi CL. Adenosine triphosphate: does it help cancer patients "get bigger and stronger"? *J Clin Oncol* 2002;20:362-3.

9154 Haskell CM, Mendoza E, Pisters KM, et al. Phase II study of intravenous adenosine 5'-triphosphate in patients with previously untreated stage IIIB and stage IV non-small cell lung cancer. *Invest New Drugs* 1998;16:81-5.

9155 Sklar SH, Blue WT, Alexander EJ, Bodian CA. Herpes zoster. The treatment and prevention of neuralgia with adenosine monophosphate. *JAMA* 1985;253:1427-30.

9156 Blommers J, de Lange-De Klerk ES, Kuik DJ, et al. Evening primrose oil and fish oil for severe chronic mastalgia: a randomized, double-blind, controlled trial. *Am J Obstet Gynecol* 2002;187:1389-94.

9157 Eisenach JC, Curry R, Hood DD. Dose response of intrathecal adenosine in experimental pain and allodynia. *Anesthesiology* 2002;97:938-42.

9158 Agteresch HJ, Dagnelie PC, Rietveld T, et al. Pharmacokinetics of intravenous ATP in cancer patients. *Eur J Clin Pharmacol* 2000;56:49-55.

9159 Leij-Halfwerk S, Agteresch HJ, Sijens PE, Dagnelie PC. Adenosine triphosphate infusion increases liver energy status in advanced lung cancer patients: an in vivo 31P magnetic resonance spectroscopy study. *Hepatology* 2002;35:421-4.

9160 Kichenin K, Seman M. Chronic oral administration of ATP modulates nucleoside transport and purine metabolism in rats. *J Pharmacol Exp Ther* 2000;294:126-33.

9161 Spak CJ, Ekstrand J, Zylberstein D. Bioavailability of fluoride added by baby formula and milk. *Caries Res* 1982;16:249-56.

9162 Reginster JY, Rovati LC, Setnikar I. Correct regimen of fluoride and calcium reduces the risk of vertebral fractures in postmenopausal osteoporosis [letter]. *Osteoporos Int* 2001;12:800.

9163 Schrauzer GN. Lithium: occurrence, dietary intakes, nutritional essentiality. *J Am Coll Nutr* 2002;21:14-21.

9164 Smith DF, Schou M. Kidney function and lithium concentrations of rats given an injection of lithium orotate or lithium carbonate. *J Pharm Pharmacol* 1979;31:161-3.

9165 Perlis RH, Sachs GS, Lafer B, et al. Effect of abrupt change from standard to low serum levels of lithium: a reanalysis of double-blind lithium maintenance data. *Am J Psychiatry* 2002;159:1155-9.

9166 Pinelli JM, Symington AJ, Cunningham KA, Paes BA. Case report and review of the perinatal implications of maternal lithium use. *Am J Obstet Gynecol* 2002;187:245-9.

9167 Morgenstern LB, Viscoli CM, Kernan WN, et al. Use of Ephedra-containing products and risk for hemorrhagic stroke. *Neurology* 2003;60:132-5.

9170 Bent S, Tiedt TN, Odden MC, Shilpak MG. The relative safety of ephedra compared with other herbal products. *Ann Intern Med* 2003;138. http://www.acponline.org/journals/annals/ephedra.htm (Accessed 4 February 2003).

9171 Gilroy DJ, Kauffman KW, Hall RA, et al. Assessing potential health risks from microcystin toxins in blue-green algae dietary supplements. *Environ Health Perspect* 2000;108:435-439.

9172 Iwasa M, Yamamoto M, Tanaka Y, et al. Spirulina-associated hepatotoxicity. *Am J Gastroenterol* 2002;97:3212-13.

9173 Kim HM, Lee EH, Cho HH, Moon YH. Inhibitory effect of mast cell-mediated immediate-type allergic reactions in rats by spirulina. *Biochem Pharmacol* 1998;55:1071-6.

9174 Goldberg DM, Yan J, Soleas GJ. Absorption of three wine-related polyphenols in three different matrices by healthy subjects. *Clin Biochem* 2003;36:79-87.

9175 Sesink AL, O'Leary KA, Hollman PC. Quercetin glucuronides but not glucosides are present in human plasma after consumption of quercetin-3-glucoside or quercetin-4'-glucoside. *J Nutr* 2001;131:1938-41.

9176 Otsuka H, Inaba M, Fujikura T, Kunitomo M. Histochemical and functional characteristics of metachromatic cells in the nasal epithelium in allergic rhinitis: studies of nasal scrapings and their dispersed cells. *J Allergy Clin Immunol* 1995;96:528-36.

9181 Herxheimer A, Petrie KJ. Melatonin for the prevention and treatment of jet lag. *Cochrane Database Syst Rev* 2002;2:CD001520.

9182 Bernstein DI, Bernstein CK, Deng C, et al. Evaluation of the clinical efficacy and safety of grapeseed extract in the treatment of fall seasonal allergic rhinitis: a pilot study. *Ann Allergy Asthma Immunol* 2002;88:272-8.

9183 Hale LP, Greer PK, Sempowski GD. Bromelain treatment alters leukocyte expression of cell surface molecules involved in cellular adhesion and activation. *Clin Immunol* 2002;104:183-90.

9184 Nettis E, Napoli G, Ferrannini A, Tursi A. IgE-mediated allergy to bromelain. *Allergy* 2001;56:257-8.

9185 Takeshita K, Saisho Y, Kitamura K, et al. Pneumonitis induced by ou-gon (scullcap). *Intern Med* 2001;40:764-8.

9186 Harrison EH, Hussain MM. Mechanisms involved in the intestinal digestion and absorption of dietary vitamin A. *J Nutr* 2001;131:1405-8.

9187 Zimmerman CL, Han S, Wiedmann TS. The absorption of retinoic acids from the gastrointestinal tract is dependent upon chemical structure. *Cancer Chemother Pharmacol* 2001;47:27-33.

9188 Semba RD, Kumwenda N, Taha TE, et al. Impact of vitamin A supplementation on anaemia and plasma erythropoietin concentrations in pregnant women: a controlled clinical trial. *Eur J Haematol* 2001;66:389-95.

9189 Denke MA. Dietary retinol--a double-edged sword. *JAMA* 2002;287:102-4.

9190 Michaelsson K, Lithell H, Vessby B, Melhus H. Serum retinol levels and the risk of fracture. *N Engl J Med* 2003;348:287-94.

9191 Lips P. Hypervitaminosis A and fractures. *N Engl J Med* 2003;348:347-9.

9192 Johansson S, Lind PM, Hakansson H, et al. Subclinical hypervitaminosis A causes fragile bones in rats. *Bone* 2002;31:685-9.

9193 Fairfield KM, Hankinson SE, Rosner BA, et al. Risk of ovarian carcinoma and consumption of vitamins A, C, and E and specific carotenoids: a prospective analysis. *Cancer* 2001;92:2318-26.

9194 Botterweck AA, van den Brandt PA, Goldbohm RA. Vitamins, carotenoids, dietary fiber, and the risk of gastric carcinoma: results from a prospective study after 6.3 years of follow-up. *Cancer* 2000;88:737-48.

9195 Schunemann HJ, Grant BJ, Freudenheim JL, et al. The relation of serum levels of antioxidant vitamins C and E, retinol and carotenoids with pulmonary function in the general population. *Am J Respir Crit Care Med* 2001;163:1246-55.

9196 Ballew C, Bowman BA, Russell RM, et al. Serum retinyl esters are not associated with biochemical markers of liver dysfunction in adult participants in the third National Health and Nutrition Examination Survey (NHANES III), 1988--1994. *Am J Clin Nutr* 2001;73:934-40.

9197 Ross AC. Addressing research questions with national survey data-the relation of vitamin A status to infection and inflammation. *Am J Clin Nutr* 2000;72:1069-70.

9198 Ahn WS, Lee JM, Namkoong SE, et al. Effect of retinoic acid on HPV titration and colposcopic changes in Korean patients with dysplasia of the uterine cervix. *J Cell Biochem Suppl* 1997;28-29:133-9.

9199 Meyskens FL Jr, Graham V, Chvapil M, et al. A phase I trial of beta-all-trans-retinoic acid delivered via a collagen sponge and a cervical cap for mild or moderate intraepithelial cervical neoplasia. *J Natl Cancer Inst* 1983;71:921-5.

9201 Ziaei S, Hantoshzadeh S, Rezasoltani P, Lamyian M. The effect of garlic tablet on plasma lipids and platelet aggregation in nulliparous pregnants at high risk of preeclampsia. *Eur J Obstet Gynecol Reprod Biol* 2001;99:201-6.

9202 Senapati SK, Dey S, Dwivedi SK, Swarup D. Effect of garlic (Allium sativum L.) extract on tissue lead level in rats. *J Ethnopharmacol* 2001;76:229-32.

9203 Staba EJ, Lash L, Staba JE. A commentary on the effects of garlic extraction and formulation on product composition. *J Nutr* 2001;131:1118S-9S.

9204 Henderson L, Yue QY, Bergquist C, et al. St John's wort (Hypericum perforatum): drug interactions and clinical outcomes. *Br J Clin Pharmacol* 2002;54:349-56.

9205 Schempp CM, Kirkin V, Simon-Haarhaus B, et al. Inhibition of tumour cell growth by hyperforin, a novel anticancer drug from St. John's wort that acts by induction of apoptosis. *Oncogene* 2002;21:1242-50.

9206 Mathijssen RH, Verweij J, de Bruijn P, et al. Effects of St. John's wort on irinotecan metabolism. *J Natl Cancer Inst* 2002;94:1247-9.

9207 Fleischauer AT, Arab L. Garlic and cancer: a critical review of the epidemiologic literature. *J Nutr* 2001;131:1032S-40S.

9208 Horie T, Awazu S, Itakura Y, Fuwa T. Alleviation by garlic of antitumor drug-induced damage to the intestine. *J Nutr* 2001;131:1071S-4S.

9209 Gardner CD, Chatterjee LM, Carlson JJ. The effect of a garlic preparation on plasma lipid levels in moderately hypercholesterolemic adults. *Atherosclerosis* 2001;154:213-20.

9219 Sunder-Plassmann G, Fodinger M, Buchmayer H, et al. Effect of high dose folic acid therapy on hyperhomocysteinemia in hemodialysis patients: results of the Vienna multicenter study. *J Am Soc Nephrol* 2000;11:1106-16.

9220 Rosado JL, Solomons NW, Allen LH. Lactose digestion from unmodified, low-fat and lactose-hydrolyzed yogurt in adult lactose-maldigesters. *Eur J Clin Nutr* 1992;46:61-7.

9222 Inoue M, Tajima K, Hirose K, et al. Tea and coffee consumption and the risk of digestive tract cancers: data from a comparative case-referent study in Japan. *Cancer Causes Control* 1998;9:209-16.

9223 Tajima K, Tominaga S. Dietary habits and gastro-intestinal cancers: a comparative case-control study of stomach and large intestinal cancers in Nagoya, Japan. *Jpn J Cancer Res* 1985;76:705-16.

9224 Choi YT, Jung CH, Lee SR, et al. The green tea polyphenol (-)-epigallocatechin gallate attenuates beta-amyloid-induced neurotoxicity in cultured hippocampal neurons. *Life Sci* 2001;70:603-14.

9225 Kono S, Ikeda M, Tokudome S, Kuratsune M. A case-control study of gastric cancer and diet in northern Kyushu, Japan. *Jpn J Cancer Res* 1988;79:1067-74.

9226 Ji BT, Chow WH, Yang G, et al. The influence of cigarette smoking, alcohol, and green tea consumption on the risk of carcinoma of the cardia and distal stomach in Shanghai, China. *Cancer* 1996;77:2449-57.

9227 Yu GP, Hsieh CC. Risk factors for stomach cancer: a population-based case-control study in Shanghai. *Cancer Causes Control* 1991;2:169-74.

9228 Zhang M, Binns CW, Lee AH. Tea consumption and ovarian cancer risk: a case-control study in China. *Cancer Epidemiol Biomarkers Prev* 2002;11:713-8.

9229 Locher R, Emmanuele L, Suter PM, et al. Green tea polyphenols inhibit human vascular smooth muscle cell proliferation stimulated by native low-density lipoprotein. *Eur J Pharmacol* 2002;434:1-7.

9230 Hodgson JM, Croft KD, Mori TA, et al. Regular ingestion of tea does not inhibit in vivo lipid peroxidation in humans. *J Nutr* 2002;132:55-8.

9231 de Maat MP, Pijl H, Kluft C, Princen HM. Consumption of black and green tea had no effect on inflammation, haemostasis and endothelial markers in smoking healthy individuals. *Eur J Clin Nutr* 2000;54:757-63.

9232 Leung LK, Su Y, Chen R, et al. Theaflavins in black tea and catechins in green tea are equally effective antioxidants. *J Nutr* 2001;131:2248-51.

9233 Terry P, Wolk A. Tea consumption and the risk of colorectal cancer in Sweden. *Nutr Cancer* 2001;39:176-9.

9234 Su LJ, Arab L. Tea consumption and the reduced risk of colon cancer -- results from a national prospective cohort study. *Public Health Nutr* 2002;5:419-25.

9235 Michels KB, Holmberg L, Bergkvist L, Wolk A. Coffee, tea, and caffeine consumption and breast cancer incidence in a cohort of Swedish women. *Ann Epidemiol* 2002;12:21-6.

9236 Checkoway H, Powers K, Smith-Weller T, et al. Parkinson's disease risks associated with cigarette smoking, alcohol consumption, and caffeine intake. *Am J Epidemiol* 2002;155:732-8.

9237 Temme EH, Van Hoydonck PG. Tea consumption and iron status. *Eur J Clin Nutr* 2002;56:379-86.

9238 Traitler H, Winter H, Richli U, Ingenbleek Y. Characterization of gamma-linolenic acid in Ribes seed. *Lipids* 1984;19:923-8.

9239 Declume C. Anti-inflammatory evaluation of a hydroalcoholic extract of black currant leaves (Ribes nigrum). *J Ethnopharmacol* 1989;27:91-8.

9241 Upton R, Petrone C, eds. Black Haw Bark, Viburnum prunifolium: Analytical, quality control, and therapeutic monograph. American Herbal Pharmacopoeia and Therapeutic Compendium. Santa Cruz, CA: American Herbal Pharmacopoeia. 2000.

9242 Kushak RI, Drapeau C, Winter HS. The effect of blue-green algae Aphanizomenon flos-Aquae on nutrient assimilation in rats. *JANA* 2001;3:35-39.

9243 Heaney RP, Weaver CM. Effect of psyllium on absorption of co-ingested calcium. *J Am Geriatr Soc* 1995;43:261-3.

9244 James JM, Cooke SK, Barnett A, Sampson HA. Anaphylactic reactions to a psyllium-containing cereal. *J Allergy Clin Immunol* 1991;88:402-8.

9245 Arlian LG, Vyszenski-Moher DL, Lawrence AT, et al. Antigenic and allergenic analysis of psyllium seed components. *J Allergy Clin Immunol* 1992;89:866-76.

9246 Kaplan MJ. Anaphylactic reaction to "Heartwise." *N Engl J Med* 1990;323:1072-3.

9247 Schaller DR. Anaphylactic reaction to "Heartwise." *N Engl J Med* 1990;323:1073.

9248 Little P, Trafford L. Dietary fibre and renal failure: comparison of sterculia and ispaghula. *Clin Nephrol* 1991;36:309.

9249 Jarjis HA, Blackburn NA, Redfern JS, Read NW. The effect of ispaghula (Fybogel and Metamucil) and guar gum on glucose tolerance in man. *Br J Nutr* 1984;51:371-8.

9250 Alabaster O, Tang Z, Shivapurkar N. Dietary fiber and the chemopreventive modelation of colon carcinogenesis. *Mutat Res* 1996;350:185-97.

9300 Gregory JF. Case study: folate bioavailability. *J Nutr* 2001;131:1376S-1382S.

9301 Fohr IP, Prinz-Langenohl R, Bronstrup A, et al. 5,10-Methylenetetrahydrofolate reductase genotype determines the plasma homocysteine-lowering effect of supplementation with 5-methyltetrahydrofolate or folic acid in healthy young women. *Am J Clin Nutr* 2002;75:275-82.

9302 Rasmussen LB, Ovesen L, Bulow I, et al. Folate intake, lifestyle factors, and homocysteine concentrations in younger and older women. *Am J Clin Nutr* 2000;72:1156-63.

9303 Murua AL, Quintana I, Janson J, et al. Plasmatic homocysteine response to vitamin supplementation in elderly people. *Thromb Res* 2000;100:495-500.

9304 de Bree A, Verschuren WM, Blom HJ, Kromhout D. Association between B vitamin intake and plasma homocysteine concentration in the general Dutch population aged 20-65 y. *Am J Clin Nutr* 2001;73:1027-33.

9305 McKay DL, Perrone G, Rasmussen H, et al. Multivitamin/mineral supplementation improves plasma B-vitamin status and homocysteine concentration in healthy older adults consuming a folate-fortified diet. *J Nutr* 2000;130:3090-6.

9306 Vos E. Multivitamin supplements are effective and inexpensive agents to lower homocysteine levels. *Arch Intern Med* 2001;161:774-5.

9307 Wald DS, Bishop L, Wald NJ, et al. Randomized trial of folic acid supplementation and serum homocysteine levels. *Arch Intern Med* 2001;161:695-700.

9308 Nallamothu BK, Fendrick M, Rubenfire M, et al. Potential clinical and economic effects of homocyst(e)ine lowering. *Arch Intern Med* 160:3406-12.

9309 Koebnick C, Heins UA, Hoffman I, et al. Folate status during pregnancy in women is improved by long-term high vegetable intake compared with the average western diet. *J Nutr* 2001;131:733-9.

9310 Mangoni AA, Jackson SH. Homocysteine and cardiovascular disease: current evidence and future prospects. *Am J Med* 2002;112:556-65.

9311 Loria CM, Ingram DD, Feldman JJ, et al. Serum folate and cardiovascular disease mortality among US men and women. *Arch Intern Med* 2000;160:3258-62.

9312 Voutilainen S, Rissanen TH, Virtanen J, et al. Low dietary folate intake is associated with an excess incidence of acute coronary events. *Circulation* 2001;103:2674-80.

9313 Thambyrajah J, Landray MJ, Jones HJ, et al. A randomized double-blind placebo-controlled trial of the effect of homocysteine-lowering therapy with folic acid on endothelial function in patients with coronary artery disease. *J Am Coll Cardiol* 2001;37:1858-63.

9314 Woo KS, Chook P, Chan LL, et al. Long-term improvement in homocysteine levels and arterial endothelial function after 1-year folic acid supplementation. *Am J Med* 2002;112:535-9.

9315 Pullin CH, Ashfield-Watt PA, Burr ML, et al. Optimization of dietary folate or low-dose folic acid supplements lower homocysteine but do not enhance endothelial function in healthy adults, irrespective of the methylenetetrahydrofolate reductase (C677T) genotype. *J Am Coll Cardiol* 2001;38:1799-805.

9316 Gori T, Burstein JM, Ahmed S, et al. Folic acid prevents nitroglycerin-induced nitric oxide synthase dysfunction and nitrate tolerance. *Circulation* 2001:104;1119-23.

9317 Loscalzo J. Folate and nitrate-induced endothelial dysfunction. A simple treatment for a complex pathobiology. *Circulation* 2001;104:1086-8.

9318 Bazzano LA, He J, Ogden LG, et al. Dietary intake of folate and risk of stroke in US men and women: NHANES I epidemiolgic follow-up study. *Stroke* 2002;33:1183-8.

9319 Mayer O, Simon J, Rosolova H, et al. The effects of folate supplementation on some coagulation parameter and oxidative status surrogates. *Eur J Clin Pharmacol* 2002;58:1-5.

9320 Stehouwer CD. Clinical relevance of hyperhomocysteinaemia in atherothrombotic disease. *Drugs and Aging* 2000;16:251-60.

9321 Stulc T, Melenovsky V, Grauova B, et al. Folate supplementation prevents plasma homocysteine increase after fenofibrate therapy. *Nutrition* 2001;17:721-3.

9322 Thambyrajah J, Landray MJ, McGlynn FJ, et al. Does folic acid decrease plasma homocysteine and improve endothelial function in patients with predialysis renal failure? *Circulation* 2000;102:871-5.

9324 van der Dijs FP, Fokkema MR, Dijck-Brouwer DA, et al. Optimization of folic acid, vitamin B12, and vitamin B6 supplements in pediatric patients with sickle cell disease. *Am J Hematol* 2002;69:239-46.

9325 Su LJ, Arab L. Nutritional status of folate and colon cancer risk: evidence from NHANES I epidemiologic follow-up study. *Ann Epidemiol* 2001;11:65-72.

9326 Fuchs CS, Willett WC, Colditz GA, et al. The influence of folate and multivitamin use on the familial risk of colon cancer in women. *Cancer Epidemiol Biomarkers Prev* 2002;11:227-34.

9327 Stolzenberg-Solomon RZ, Pietinen P, Barrett MJ, et al. Dietary and other methyl-group availability factors and pancreatic cancer risk in a cohort of male smokers. *Am J Epidemiol* 2001;153:680-7.

9328 Shrubsole MJ, Jin F, Dai Q, et al. Dietary folate intake and breast cancer risk: results from the Shanghai Breast Cancer Study. *Cancer Res* 2001;61:7136-41.

9329 Huang RF, Ho Y, Lin H, et al. Folate deficiency induces a cell cycle-specific apoptosis in HepG2 cells. *J Nutr* 1999;129:25-31.

9330 Duthie SJ, Whalley LJ, Collins AR, et al. Homocysteine, B vitamin status, and cognitive function in the elderly. *Am J Clin Nutr* 2002;75:908-13.

9331 Smith AD. Homocysteine, B vitamins, and cognitive deficit in the elderly. *Am J Clin Nutr* 2002;75:785-6.

9332 Botez MI, Cadotte M, Beaulieu R, et al. Neurologic disorders responsive to folic acid therapy. *Can Med Assoc J* 1976;115:217-23.

9333 Botez MI, Peyronnard J, Berube L, Labrecque R. Relapsing neuropathy, cerebral atrophy and folate deficiency. *Appl Neurophysiol* 1979;42:171-83.

9334 Wong WY, Merkus HM, Thomas CM, et al. Effects of folic acid and zinc sulfate on male factor subfertility: a double-blind, randomized, placebo-controlled trial. *Fertil Steril* 2002;77:491-8.

9335 Garcia A, Pombo-Paris A, Evans L, et al. Is low-dose oral cobalamin enough to normalize cobalamin function in older people? *J Am Geriatr Soc* 2002;50:1401-4.

9336 Russman S, Junker E, Lauterburg BH. Remethylation and transsulfuration of methionine in cirrhosis: studies with L-[H3-methyl-1-C]methionine. *Hepatology* 2002;36:1190-6.

9337 Niculescu MD, Zeisel SH. Diet, methyl donors and DNA methylation: interactions between dietary folate, methionine and choline. *J Nutr* 2002;132:2333S-5S.

9338 Btaiche IF, Khalidi N. Parenteral nutrition-associated liver complications in children. *Pharmacotherapy* 2002;22:188-211.

9339 Cottington EM, LaMantia C, Stabler SP, et al. Adverse event associated with methionine loading test: a case report. *Arterioscler Thromb Vasc Biol* 2002;22:1046-50.

9340 Anon. Should methionine be added to paracetamol formulations? *Drug Ther Perspect* 1997;10:11-3.

9341 Epner DE, Morrow S, Wilcox M, Houghton JL. Nutrient intake and nutritional indexes in adults with metastatic cancer on a phase I clinical trial of dietary methionine restriction. *Nutr Cancer* 2002;42:158-66.

9342 Epner DE. Can dietary methionine restriction increase the effectiveness of chemotherapy in treatment of advanced cancer? *J Am Coll Nutr* 2001;20:443S-9S.

9343 Ward M, McNulty H, Pentieva K, et al. Fluctuations in dietary methionine intake do not alter plasma homocysteine concentrations in healthy men. *J Nutr* 2000;130:2653-7.

9344 Kokko JP. Fluids and electrolytes. In: Goldman L, Bennett JC. Cecil Textbook of Medicine. 21st ed. Philadelphia, PA: W.B. Saunders Co. 2000:59.

9345 Barshop BA. Homocystiniuria. In: Goldman L, Bennett JC. Cecil Textbook of Medicine. 21st ed. Philadelphia, PA: W.B. Saunders Co. 2000:1115-6.

9346 Anon. The role of isoflavones in menopausal health: consensus opinion of the North American Menopause Society. *Menopause* 2000;7:215-29.

9347 Gonzalez Begne M, Yslas N, Reyes E, et al. Clinical effect of a Mexican sanguinaria (Polygonum aviculare L.) on gingivitis. *J Ethnopharmacol* 2001;74(1):45-51.

9348 la Cour B, Molgaard P, Yi Z. Traditional Chinese medicine in treatment of hyperlipidaemia. *J Ethnopharmacol* 1995;46(2):125-9.

9349 Lin L, Lau BH. Protection of vascular endothelial cells from hydrogen peroxide-induced oxidant injury by gypenosides, saponins, of Gynostemma pentaphyllum. *Phytother Res* 1993;7:299-304.

9350 Takagi J, Imada T, Kikuchi T, et al. A new platelet aggregation factor from gynostemma pentaphyllum Makino. *Chem Pharm Bull* (Tokyo) 1985;33:5568-71.

9351 Lawrence VA, Loewenstein JE, Eichner ER. Aspirin and folate binding: in vivo and in vitro studies of serum binding and urine excretion of endogenous folate. *J Lab Clin Med* 1984;103:944-8.

9352 Butterworth CE, Hatch KD, Gore H, et al. Improvement in cervical dysplasia associated with folic acid therapy in users of oral contraceptives. *Am J Clin Nutr* 1982;35:73-82.

9353 Halsted CH, Gandhi G, Tamura T. Sulfasalazine inhibits the absorption of folates in ulcerative colitis. *N Engl J Med* 1981;305:1513-7.

9354 Hiilesmaa VK, Teramo K, Granstrom ML, Bardy AH. Serum folate concentrations during pregnancy in women with epilepsy: relation to antiepileptic drug concentrations, number of seizures, and fetal outcome. *Br Med J* 1983;287:577-9.

9355 Dansky LV, Rosenblatt DS, Andermann E. Mechanisms of teratogenesis: folic acid and antiepileptic therapy. *Neurology* 1992;42:32-42.

9356 Lewis DP, Van Dyke DC, Stumbo PJ, Berg MJ. Drug and environmental factors associated with adverse pregnancy outcomes. Part I: antiepileptic drugs, contraceptives, smoking, and folate. *Ann Pharmacother* 1998;32:802-17.

9357 Reynolds EH. Neurological aspects of folate and vitamin B12 metabolism. *Clinics in Haematology* 1976;5:661-96.

9358 Reynolds EH. Folate metabolism and anticonvulsant therapy. *Proc R Soc Med* 1974;67:68.

9359 Reynolds EH, Trimble MR. Adverse neuropsychiatric effects of anticonvulsant drugs. *Drugs* 1985;29:570-81.

9360 Alter HJ, Zvaifler NJ, Rath CE. Interrelationship of rheumatoid arthritis, folic acid and aspirin. *Blood* 1971;38:405-16.

9361 Baggott JE, Morgan SL, Ha T, et al. Inhibition of folate-dependent enzymes by non-steroidal anti-inflammatory drugs. *Biochem J* 1992;282:197-202.

9362 Frequin ST, Wevers RA, Braam M, et al. Decreased vitamin B12 and folate levels in cerebrospinal fluid and serum of multiple sclerosis patients after high-dose intravenous methylprednisolone. *J Neurol* 1993;240:305-8.

9363 Klipstein FA, Berlinger FG, Reed LJ. Folate deficiency associated with drug therapy for tuberculosis. *Blood* 1967;29:697-712.

9364 Russell RM, Krasinski SD, Samloff IM, et al. Folic acid malabsorption in atrophic gastritis: possible compensation by bacterial folate synthesis. *Gastroenterol* 1986;91:1476-82.

9366 Buysschaert M, Wallemacq PE, Dramais AS, Hermans MP. Hyperhomocysteinemia in type 2 diabetes. *Diabetes Care* 2000;23:1816-22.

9367 Aarsand AK, Carlsen SM. Folate administration reduces circulating homocysteine levels in NIDDM patients on long-term metformin treatment. *J Intern Med* 1998;244:169-74.

9368 Berchtold P, Dahlqvist A, Gustafson A, Asp NG. Effects of a biguanide (metformin) on vitamin B12 and folic acid absorption and intestinal enzyme activities. *Scand J Gastroenterol* 1971;6:751-4.

9369 Ortiz Z, Shea B, Suarez Almazor M, et al. Folic acid and folinic acid for reducing side effects in patients receiving methotrexate for rheumatoid arthritis (Cochrane Review). *Cochrane Database Syst Rev* 2000;2:CD000951.

9370 Check WA. Folate for oral contraceptive users may reduce cervical cancer risk. *J Am Med Assoc* 1980;244:633-4.

9371 Shojania AM. Oral contraceptives: effect on folate and vitamin B12 metabolism. *Can Med Assoc J* 1982;126:244-7.

9372 Barone C, Bartoloni C, Ghirlanda G, Gentiloni N. Megaloblastic anemia due to folic acid deficiency after oral contraceptives. *Haematologica* 1979;64:190-5.

9373 Mooij PN, Thomas CM, Doesburg WH, Eskes TK. Multivitamin supplementation in oral contraceptive users. *Contraception* 1991;44:277-88.

9374 Russell RM, Dutta SK, Oaks EV, et al. Impairment of folic acid absorption by oral pancreatic extracts. *Dig Dis Sci* 1980;25:369-73.

9375 Corcino J, Waxman S, Herbert V. Mechanism of triamterene-induced megaloblastosis. *Ann Intern Med* 1970;73:419-24.

9376 Prouse PJ, Shawe D, Gumpel JM. Macrocytic anemia in patients treated with sulfasalazine for rheumatoid arthritis. *BMJ* 1986;293:1407.

9377 Longstreth GF, Green R. Folate status in patients receiving maintenance doses of sulfasalazine. *Arch Intern Med* 1983;143:902-4.

9378 Drake S, Lampasona V, Nicks HL, Schwarzmann SW. Pentamidine isethionate in the treatment of Pneumocystis carinii pneumonia. *Clin Pharm* 1985;4:507-16.

9379 Lashner BA, Heidenreich PA, Su GL, et al. Effect of folate supplementation on the incidence of dysplasia and cancer in chronic ulcerative colitis. *Gastroenterol* 1989;97:255-9.

9380 Van Delden C, Hirschel B. Folinic acid supplements to pyrimethamine-sulfadiazine for Toxoplasma encephalitis are associated with better outcome (letter). *J Infect Dis* 1996;173:1294-5.

9381 Pelliniemi TT, Kasanen A, Sundquist H. Lack of haematological side effects during prophylactic use of trimethoprim over four years. *Curr Ther Res* 1983;34:436-40.

9382 Kobrinsky NL, Ramsay NKC. Acute megaloblastic anemia induced by high-dose trimethoprim-sulfamethoxazole. *Ann Intern Med* 1981;94:780-1.

9383 Naderer O, Nafziger AN, Bertino JS. Effects of moderate-dose versus high-dose trimethoprim on serum creatinine and creatinine clearance and adverse reactions. *Antimicrob Agents Chemother* 1997;41:2466-70.

9384 Kinzie BJ, Taylor JW. Trimethoprim and folic acid (letter). *Ann Intern Med* 1984;101:565.

9385 Hollander H. Leukopenia, trimethoprim-sulfamethoxazole, and folinic acid (letter). *Ann Intern Med* 1985;102:138.

9386 Stock C. Trimethoprim-sulfamethoxazole and folinic acid (letter). *Ann Intern Med* 1985;102:277.

9387 Safrin S, Lee BL, Sande MA. Adjunctive folinic acid with trimethoprim-sulfamethoxazole for Pneumocystis carinii pneumonia in AIDS patients is associated with an increased risk of therapeutic failure and death. *J Infect Dis* 1994;170:912-7.

9388 Thompson JB, Hess DR, Poley JR, et al. Intestinal malabsorption induced by paraminosalicylic acid (abstract). *Gastroenterol* 1970;58:1001.

9389 Milne DB, Canfield WK, Mahalko JR, Sandstead HH. Effect of oral folic acid supplements on zinc, copper, and iron absorption and excretion. *Am J Clin Nutr* 1984;39:535-9.

9390 Kakar F, Henderson MM. Potential toxic side effects of folic acid (letter). *J Natl Cancer Inst* 1985;74:2638.

9391 Butterworth CE, Hatch K, Cole P, et al. Zinc concentration in plasma and erythrocytes of subjects receiving folic acid supplementation. *Am J Clin Nutr* 1988;47:484-6.

9392 Fuller NJ, Bates CJ, Evans PH, Lucas A. High folate intakes related to zinc status in preterm infants. *Eur J Pediatr* 1992;151:51-3.

9393 Kauwell GPA, Baily LB, Gregory JF, et al. Zinc status is not adversely affected by folic acid supplementation and zinc intake does not impair folate utilization in human subjects. *J Nutr* 1995;125:66-72.

9394 Koutts J, Van der Weyden MB, Cooper M. Effect of trimethoprim on folate metabolism in human bone marrow. *Aust N Z J Med* 1973;3:245-50.

9395 Line DH, Seitanidis B, Morgan JO, Hoffbrand AV. The effects of chemotherapy on iron, folate, and vitamin B12 metabolism in tuberculosis. *Quart J Med* 1971;40:331-40.

9396 Evans DI, Attock B. Folate deficiency in pulmonary tuberculosis: relationship to treatment and to serum vitamin A and beta carotene. *Tubercle* 1971;52:288-94.

9397 Halsted CH, McIntyre PA. Intestinal malabsorption caused by aminosalicylic acid therapy. *Arch Intern Med* 1972;130;935-9.

9398 Bygbjerg IC, Lund JT, Hording M. Effect of folic and folinic acid on cytopenia occurring during cotrimoxazole treatment of Pneumocystis carinii pneumonia. *Scand J Infect Dis* 1988;20:685-6.

9399 Nunn PP, Allistone JC. Resistance to trimethoprim-sulfamethoxazole in the treatment of Pneumocystis carinii pneumonia. Implication of folinic acid. *Chest* 1984;86:149-50.

9400 Homocysteine Lowering Trialists' Collaboration. Lowering blood homocysteine with folic acid based supplements: meta-analysis of randomized trials. *BMJ* 1998;316:894-8.

9401 Bronstrup A, Hages M, Prinz-Langenohl R, Pietrzik K. Effects of folic acid and combinations of folic acid and vitamin B12 on plasma homocysteine concentrations in healthy young women. *Am J Clin Nutr* 1998;68:1104-10.

9402 Ueland PM, Refsum H, Beresford SAA, Vollset SE. The controversy over homocysteine and cardiovascular risk. *Am J Clin Nutr* 2000;72:324-32.

9403 Holven KB, Holm T, Aukrust P, et al. Effect of folic acid treatment on endothelium-dependent vasodilation and nitric oxide-derived end products in hyperhomocysteinemic subjects. *Am J Med* 2001;110:536-42.

9404 Bostom AG, Selhub J, Jacques PF, Rosenberg IH. Power shortage: clinical trials testing the "homocysteine hypothesis" against a background of folic acid-fortified cereal grain flour. *Ann Intern Med* 2001;135:133-7.

9405 Clarke R, Armitage J. Vitamin supplements and cardiovascular risk: review of the randomized trials of homocysteine-lowering vitamin supplements. *Semin Thromb Hemost* 2000;26:341-8.

9406 van der Griend R, Biesma DH, Haas FJLM, et al. The effect of different treatment regimens in reducing fasting and postmethionine-load homocysteine concentrations. *J Intern Med* 2000;248:223-9.

9407 Selhub J, Jacques PF, Bostom AG, et al. Relationship between plasma homocysteine and vitamin status in the Framingham study population. Impact of folic acid fortification. *Public Health Rev* 2000;28:117-45.

9408 Keebler ME, De Souza C, Fonesca V. Diagnosis and treatment of hyperhomocysteinemia. *Curr Atheroscler Rep* 2001;3:54-63.

9409 Sunder-Plassmann G, Winkelmayer WC, Fodinger M. Therapeutic potential of total homocysteine-lowering drugs on cardiovascular disease. *Expert Opin Investig Drugs* 2000;9:2637-51.

9410 den Heijer M, Brouwer IA, Bos GMJ, et al. Vitamin supplementation reduces blood homocysteine levels. A controlled trial in patients with venous thrombosis and healthy volunteers. *Arterioscler Thromb Vasc Biol* 1998;18:356-61.

9411 Boushey CJ, Beresford SA, Omenn GS, Motulsky AG. A quantitative assessment of plasma homocysteine as a risk factor for vascular disease. Probable benefits of increasing folic acid intakes. *JAMA* 1995;274:1049-57.

9412 Schnyder G, Roffi M, Flammer Y, et al. Effect of homocysteine-lowering therapy with folic acid, vitamin B12, and vitamin B6 on clinical outcome after percutaneous coronary intervention. The Swiss Heart Study: A randomized controlled trial. *JAMA* 2002;288:973-9.

9413 Sunder-Plassmann G, Fodinger M, Buchmayer H, et al. Effect of high dose folic acid therapy on hyperhomocysteinemia in hemodialysis patients: results of the Vienna Multicenter Study. *J Am Soc Nephrol* 2000;11:1106-16.

9414 Bostom A, Shemin D, Gohh R, et al. Treatment of mild hyperhomocysteinemia in renal transplant recipients versus hemodialysis patients. *Transplantation* 2000;69:2128-31.

9415 Dierkes J, Domrose U, Bosselmann P, et al. Homocysteine lowering effect of different multivitamin preparations in patients with end-stage renal disease. *J Ren Nutr* 2001;11:67-72.

9416 Bostom AG, Shemin D, Gohh RY, et al. Treatment of hyperhomocysteinemia in hemodialysis patients and renal transplant recipients. *Kidney Intl* 2001;59:s246-s252.

9417 Dierkes J, Domrose U, Ambrosch A, et al. Response of hyperhomocysteinemia to folic acid supplementation in patients with end-stage renal disease. *Clin Nephrol* 1999;51:108-15.

9418 Griffith SM, Fisher J, Clarke S, et al. Do patients with rheumatoid arthritis established on methotrexate and folic acid 5 mg daily need to continue folic acid supplements long term? *Rheumatology* 2000;39:1102-9.

9419 Endresen GK, Husby G. Folate supplementation during methotrexate treatment of patients with rheumatoid arthritis. An update and proposal for guidelines. *Scand J Rheumatol* 2001;30:129-34.

9420 Schroder H, Clausen N, Ostergard E, Pressler T. Folic acid supplements in vitamin tablets: a determinant of hematological drug tolerance in maintenance therapy of childhood acute lymphoblastic leukemia. *Pediatr Hematol Oncol* 1986;3:241-7.

9421 Keating JN, Wada L, Stokstad ELR, King JC. Folic acid: effect on zinc absorption in humans and in the rat. *Am J Clin Nutr* 1987;46:835-9.

9422 Belknap D, Davidson LJ, Smith CR. The effects of psyllium hydrophilic mucilloid on diarrhea in enterally fed patients. *Heart Lung* 1997;26:229-37.

9423 Cheskin LJ, Kamal N, Crowell MD, et al. Mechanisms of constipation in older persons and effects of fiber compared with placebo. *J Am Geriatr Soc* 1995;43:666-9.

9424 Maciejko JJ, Brazg R, Shah A, et al. Psyllium for the reduction of cholestyramine-associated gastrointestinal symptoms in the treatment of primary hypercholesterolemia. *Arch Fam Med* 1994;3:955-60.

9425 Everson GT, Daggy BP, McKinley C, Story JA. Effects of psyllium hydrophilic mucilloid on LDL-cholesterol and bile acid synthesis in hypercholesterolemic men. *J Lipid Res* 1992;33:1183-92.

9426 Daggy BP, O'Connell NC, Jerdack GR, et al. Additive hypocholesterolemic effect of psyllium and cholestyramine in the hamster: influence on fecal sterol and bile acid profiles. *J Lipid Res* 1997;38:491-502.

9427 Hiraishi K, Narabayashi I, Fujita O, et al. Blueberry juice: preliminary evaluation as an oral contrast agent in gastrointestinal MR imaging. *Radiology* 1995;194:119-23.

9429 Joseph JA, Denisova N, Fisher D, et al. Membrane and receptor modifications of oxidative stress vulnerability in aging. Nutritional considerations. *Ann N Y Acad Sci* 1998;854:268-76.

9431 Kennelly EJ, Baggett S, Nuntanakorn P, et al. Analysis of thirteen populations of black cohosh for formononetin. *Phytomedicine* 2002;9:461-7.

9432 Loser B, Kruse SO, Melzig MF, Nahrstedt A. Inhibition of neutrophil elastase activity by cinnamic acid derivatives from Cimicifuga racemosa. *Planta Med* 2000;66:751-3.

9434 Hayashi O, Hirahashi T, Katoh T, et al. Class specific influence of dietary Spirulina platensis on antibody production in mice. *J Nutr Sci Vitaminol* (Tokyo) 1998;44:841-51.

9435 Bodinet C, Freudenstein J. Influence of Cimicifuga racemosa on the proliferation of estrogen receptor-positive human breast cancer cells. *Breast Cancer Res Treat* 2002;76:1-10.

9436 Freudenstein J, Dasenbrock C, Nisslein T. Lack of promotion of estrogen-dependent mammary gland tumors in vivo by an isopropanolic Cimicifuga racemosa extract. *Cancer Res* 2002;62:3448-52.

9437 Liske E, Hanggi W, Henneicke-von Zepelin HH, et al. Physiological investigation of a unique extract of black cohosh (Cimicifugae racemosae rhizoma): a 6-month clinical study demonstrates no systemic estrogenic effect. *J Womens Health Gend Based Med* 2002;11:163-74.

9439 Tavani A, Negri E, La Vecchia C. Food and nutrient intake and risk of cataract. *Ann Epidemiol* 1996;6:41-6.

9442 Erlund I, Kosonen T, Alfthan G, et al. Pharmacokinetics of quercetin from quercetin aglycone and rutin in healthy volunteers. *Eur J Clin Pharmacol* 2000;56:545-53.

9443 Walle T, Otake Y, Walle UK, Wilson FA. Quercetin glucosides are completely hydrolyzed in ileostomy patients before absorption. *J Nutr* 2000;130:2658-61.

9444 Koga T, Meydani M. Effect of plasma metabolites of (+)-catechin and quercetin on monocyte adhesion to human aortic endothelial cells. *Am J Clin Nutr* 2001;73:941-8.

9445 Ellis JM, Kishi T, Azuma J, Folkers K. Vitamin B6 deficiency in patients with a clinical syndrome including the carpal tunnel defect. Biochemical and clinical response to therapy with pyridoxine. *Res Commun Chem Pathol Pharmacol* 1976;13:743-57.

9446 Ellis JM, Azuma J, Watanabe T, et al. Survey and new data on treatment with pyridoxine of patients having a clinical syndrome including the carpal tunnel and other defects. *Res Commun Chem Pathol Pharmacol* 1977;17:165-77.

9447 Ellis J, Folkers K, Levy M, et al. Therapy with vitamin B6 with and without surgery for treatment of patients having the idiopathic carpal tunnel syndrome. *Res Commun Chem Pathol Pharmacol* 1981;33:331-44.

9448 Franzblau A, Rock CL, Werner RA, et al. The relationship of vitamin B6 status to median nerve function and carpal tunnel syndrome among active industrial workers. *J Occup Environ Med* 1996;38:485-91.

9449 Folkers K, Ellis J, Watanabe T, et al. Biochemical evidence for a deficiency of vitamin B6 in the carpal tunnel syndrome based on a crossover clinical study. *Proc Natl Acad Sci U S A* 1978;75:3410-2.

9450 Gerritsen AA, de Krom MC, Struijs MA, et al. Conservative treatment options for carpal tunnel syndrome: a systematic review of randomised controlled trials. *J Neurol* 2002;249:272-80.

9451 McKinley MC, McNulty H, McPartlin J, et al. Low-dose vitamin B-6 effectively lowers fasting plasma homocysteine in healthy elderly persons who are folate and riboflavin replete. *Am J Clin Nutr* 2001;73:759-64.

9452 Friso S, Jacques PF, Wilson PW, et al. Low circulating vitamin B(6) is associated with elevation of the inflammation marker C-reactive protein independently of plasma homocysteine levels. *Circulation* 2001;103:2788-91.

9453 Byers CM, DeLisa JA, Frankel DL, Kraft GH. Pyridoxine metabolism in carpal tunnel syndrome with and without peripheral neuropathy. *Arch Phys Med Rehabil* 1984;65:712-6.

9454 Hartman TJ, Woodson K, Stolzenberg-Solomon R, et al. Association of the B-vitamins pyridoxal 5'-phosphate (B6), B12, and folate with lung cancer risk in older men. *Am J Epidemiol* 2001;153:688-94.

9455 Favier R, Caceres E, Guillon L, et al. Coca chewing for exercise: hormonal and metabolic responses of nonhabitual chewers. *J Appl Physiol* 1996;81:1901-7.

9456 Favier R, Caceres E, Sempore B, et al. Fluid regulatory hormone response to exercise after coca-induced body fluid shifts. *J Appl Physiol* 1997;83:376-82.

9457 Sauvain M, Rerat C, Moretti C, et al. A study of the chemical composition of Erythroxylum coca var. coca leaves collected in two ecological regions of Bolivia. *J Ethnopharmacol* 1997;56:179-91.

9458 Buck AA, Sasaki TT, Hewitt JJ, Macrae AA. Coca chewing and health. An epidemiologic study among residents of a Peruvian village. *Am J Epidemiol* 1968;88:159-77.

9459 Roldan CA, Aliabadi D, Crawford MH. Prevalence of heart disease in asymptomatic chronic cocaine users. *Cardiology* 2001;95:25-30.

9460 Engelke BF, Gentner WA. Determination of cocaine in "Mate de Coca" herbal tea. *J Pharm Sci* 1991;80:96.

9461 Bedford JA, Nail GL, et al. Comparative stimulus properties of two fractions of the coca leaf (E. coca). *Pharmacol Biochem Behav* 1981;15:907-9.

9462 Bedford JA, Lovell DK, Turner CE, et al. The anorexic and actometric effects of cocaine and two coca extracts. *Pharmacol Biochem Behav* 1980;13:403-8.

9463 ElSohly MA, Brenneisen R, Jones AB. Coca paste: chemical analysis and smoking experiments. *J Forensic Sci* 1991;36:93-103.

9465 Jee SH, Miller ER 3rd, Guallar E, et al. The effect of magnesium supplementation on blood pressure: a meta-analysis of randomized clinical trials. *Am J Hypertens* 2002;15:691-6.

9466 Hornyak M, Voderholzer U, Hohagen F, et al. Magnesium therapy for periodic leg movements-related insomnia and restless legs syndrome: an open pilot study. *Sleep* 1998;21:501-5.

9467 Dagnelie PC, van Staveren WA, van den Berg H. Vitamin B-12 from algae appears not to be bioavailable. *Am J Clin Nutr* 1991;53:695-7.

9468 Romay C, Ledon N, Gonzalez R. Further studies on anti-inflammatory activity of phycocyanin in some animal models of inflammation. *Inflamm Res* 1998;47:334-8.

9469 Romay C, Armesto J, Remirez D, et al. Antioxidant and anti-inflammatory properties of C-phycocyanin from blue-green algae. *Inflamm Res* 1998;47:36-41.

9470 Shastri D, Kumar M, Kumar A. Modulation of lead toxicity by Spirulina fusiformis. *Phytother Res* 1999;13:258-60.

9472 Popoviciu L, Asgian B, Delast-Popoviciu D, et al. Clinical, EEG, electromyographic and polysomnographic studies in restless legs syndrome caused by magnesium deficiency (abstract). *Rom J Neurol Psychiatry* 1993;31:55-61.

9473 Belfort MA, Anthony J, Saade GR, Allen JC Jr. A comparison of magnesium sulfate and nimodipine for the prevention of eclampsia. *N Engl J Med* 2003;348:304-11.

9474 Ladner DP, Klein SD, Steiner RA, Walt H. Synergistic toxicity of delta-aminolaevulinic acid-induced protoporphyrin IX used for photodiagnosis and hypericum extract, a herbal antidepressant. *Br J Dermatol* 2001;144:916-8.

9475 Keithley JK, Swanson B, Sha BE, et al. A pilot study of the safety and efficacy of cholestin in treating HIV-related dyslipidemia. *Nutrition* 2002;18:201-4.

9476 Volz HP, Murck H, Kasper S, Moller HJ. St John's wort extract (LI 160) in somatoform disorders: results of a placebo-controlled trial. *Psychopharmacology* (Berl) 2002;164:294-300.

9477 Dagnelie PC. Some algae are potentially adequate sources of vitamin B-12 for vegans. *J Nutr* 1997;2:379.

9478 Bernstein AL, Dinesen JS. Brief communication: effect of pharmacologic doses of vitamin B6 on carpal tunnel syndrome, electroencephalographic results, and pain. *J Am Coll Nutr* 1993;12:73-6.

9479 Kawada A, Kashima A, Shiraishi H, et al. Pyridoxine-induced photosensitivity and hypophosphatasia. *Dermatology* 2000;201:356-60.

9480 Delport R, Ubbink JB, Vermaak WJ, Becker PJ. Theophylline increases pyridoxal kinase activity independently from vitamin B6 nutritional status. *Res Commun Chem Pathol Pharmacol* 1993;79:325-33.

9481 Badner NH, Freeman D, Spence JD. Preoperative oral B vitamins prevent nitrous oxide-induced postoperative plasma homocysteine increases. *Anesth Analg* 2001;93:1507-10.

9482 Keniston RC, Nathan PA, Leklem JE, Lockwood RS. Vitamin B6, vitamin C, and carpal tunnel syndrome. A cross-sectional study of 441 adults. *J Occup Environ Med* 1997;39:949-59.

9483 Ellis JM, Folkers K, Levy M, et al. Response of vitamin B-6 deficiency and the carpal tunnel syndrome to pyridoxine. *Proc Natl Acad Sci U S A* 1982;79:7494-8.

9484 Jackson GF, Saady JJ, Poklis A. Urinary excretion of benzoylecgonine following ingestion of Health Inca Tea. *Forensic Sci Int* 1991;49:57-64.

9492 Gunn TR, Wright IM. The use of black and blue cohosh in labour. *N Z Med J* 1996;109:410-1.

9493 Baillie N, Rasmussen P. Black and blue cohosh in labour. *N Z Med J* 1997;110:20-1.

9494 Kronenberg F, Fugh-Berman A. Complementary and alternative medicine for menopausal symptoms: a review of randomized, controlled trials. *Ann Intern Med* 2002;137:805-13.

9495 Schenk P, Vonbank K, Schnack B, et al. Intravenous magnesium sulfate for bronchial hyperreactivity: a randomized, controlled, double-blind study. *Clin Pharmacol Ther* 2001;69:365-71.

9496 Ciarallo L, Brousseau D, Reinert S. Higher-dose intravenous magnesium therapy for children with moderate to severe acute asthma. *Arch Pediatr Adolesc Med* 2000;154:979-83.

9497 Ceremuzynski L, Gebalska J, Wolk R, Makowska E. Hypomagnesemia in heart failure with ventricular arrhythmias. Beneficial effects of magnesium supplementation. *J Intern Med* 2000;247:78-86.

9498 Demirkaya S, Dora B, Topcuoglu MA, et al. A comparative study of magnesium, flunarizine and amitriptyline in the prophylaxis of migraine. *J Headache Pain* 2000;1:179-86.

9499 Rossier P, van Erven S, Wade DT. The effect of magnesium oral therapy on spasticity in a patient with multiple sclerosis. *Eur J Neurol* 2000;7:741-4.

9500 Pere AK, Lindgren L, Tuomainen P, et al. Dietary potassium and magnesium supplementation in cyclosporine-induced hypertension and nephrotoxicity. *Kidney Int* 2000;58:2462-72.

9501 Cohen AC. Pyridoxine in the prevention and treatment of convulsions and neurotoxicity due to cycloserine. *Ann N Y Acad Sci* 1969;166:346-9.

9502 Goldin BR, Lichtenstein AH, Gorbach SL. Nutritional and metabolic roles of intestinal flora. In: Shils ME, Olson JA, Shike M, eds. Modern Nutrition in Health and Disease, 8th ed. Malvern, PA: Lea & Febiger, 1994.

9503 Ubbink JB, Vermaak WJ, Delport R, et al. The relationship between vitamin B6 metabolism, asthma, and theophylline therapy. *Ann N Y Acad Sci* 1990;585:285-94.

9504 Butterworth CE. Interactions of nutrients with oral contraceptives and other drugs *J Am Diet Assoc* 1973;62:510-4.

9505 Tyrer LB. Nutrition and the pill. *J Reprod Med* 1984;29:547-50.

9506 Haspels AA, Bennink HJ, Schreurs WH. Disturbance of tryptophan metabolism and its correction during oestrogen treatment in postmenopausal women. *Maturitas* 1978;1(1):15-20.

9507 Rolla G, Bucca C, Bugiani M, et al. Hypomagnesemia in chronic obstructive lung disease: effect of therapy. *Magnes Trace Elem* 1990;9:132-6.

9508 Lund B, Storm TL, Lund B, et al. Bone mineral loss, bone histomorphometry and vitamin D metabolism in patients with rheumatoid arthritis on long-term glucocorticoid treatment. *Clin Rheumatol* 1985;4:143-9.

9509 Rickers H, Deding A, Christiansen C, Rodbro P. Mineral loss in cortical and trabecular bone during high-dose prednisone treatment. *Calcif Tissue Int* 1984;36:269-73.

9510 van der Vange N, van der Berg H, Kloosterboer HJ, Haspels AA. Effects of seven low-dose combined contraceptives on vitamin B6 status. *Contraception* 1989;40(3):377-84.

9511 Herbert V, Jacob E. Destruction of vitamin B12 by ascorbic acid. *JAMA* 1974;230:241-2.

9512 Mezzano D, Kosiel K, Martinez C, et al. Cardiovascular risk factors in vegetarians: normalization of hyperhomocysteinemia with vitamin B12 and reduction of platelet aggregation with n-3 fatty acids. *Thromb Res* 2000;100:153-60.

9513 Ruscin JM, Page RL, Valuck RJ. Vitamin B12 deficiency associated with histamine-2-receptor antagonists and a proton-pump inhibitor. *Ann Pharmacother* 2002;36:812-6.

9514 Force RW, Nahata MC. Effect of histamine H2 receptor antagonists on vitamin B12 absorption. *Ann Pharmacother* 1992;26:1283-6.

9515 Morris AJ, Murray L, Sturrock RD, et al. Short report: the effect of misoprostol on the anaemia of NSAID enteropathy. *Aliment Pharmacol Ther* 1994;8:343-6.

9516 Selby PL, Peacock M, Bambach CP. Hypomagnesemia after small bowel resection: treatment with 1-alpha-hydroxylated vitamin D metabolites. *Br J Surg* 1984;71:334-7.

9517 Whyte KF, Addis GJ, Whitesmith R, Reid JL. Adrenergic control of plasma magnesium in man. *Clin Sci* 1987;72:135-8.

9518 Fishman SM, Christian P, West KP. The role of vitamins in the prevention and control of anemia. *Public Health Nutr* 2000;3:125-50.

9519 Isaac G, Holland OB. Drug-induced hypokalamia: A cause for concern. *Drugs & Aging* 1992;2(1):35-41.

9520 Callaghan TS, Hadden DR, Tomkin GH. Megaloblastic anemia due to vitamin B12 malabsorption associated with longterm metformin treatment. *Br Med J* 1980;280:1214-5.

9521 Gilligan MA. Metformin and vitamin B12 deficiency (letter). *Arch Intern Med* 2002;162:484-5.

9522 Andres E, Noel E, Goichot B. Metformin-associated vitamin B12 deficiency (letter). *Arch Intern Med* 2002;162:2251-2.

9523 Bauman WA, Spungen AM, Shaw S, et al. Increased intake of calcium reverses vitamin B12 malabsorption induced by metformin. *Diabetes Care* 2000;23:1227-31.

9524 De Simone C, Famularo G, Tzantzoglou S, et al. Carnitine depletion in peripheral blood mononuclear cells from patients with AIDS: effect of oral L-carnitine. *AIDS* 1994;8:655-60.

9525 Mydlik M, Derzsiova K, Zemberova E. Influence of water and sodium diuresis and furosemide on urinary excretion of vitamin B6, oxalic acid and vitamin C in chronic renal failure. *Miner Electrolyte Metab* 1999;25(4-6):352-6.

9526 Hanauer SB, Sandborn W, and Practice Parameters Committee of the American College of Gastroenterology. Management of Crohn's disease in adults. *Am J Gastroenterol.* 2001;96:635-43.

9527 Marie RM, Le Biez E, Busson P, et al. Nitrous-oxide anesthesia-associated myelopathy. *Arch Neurol* 2000;57:380-2.

9528 Force RW, Meeker AD, Cady PS, et al. Increased vitamin B12 requirement associated with chronic acid suppression therapy. *Ann Pharmacother* 2003;37:490-3.

9529 Nielsen FH. Biochemical and physiologic consequences of boron deprivation in humans. *Environ Health Perspect* 1994;102:59-63.

9530 McCormick DB. Riboflavin. In: Shils ME, Olson JA, Shike M, Ross AC, eds. Modern Nutrition in Health and Disease. 9th ed. Baltimore, MD: Williams & Wilkins, 1999. pg.391-9.

9531 Beloosesky Y, Grinblat J, Weiss A, et al. Electrolyte disorders following oral sodium phosphate administration for bowel cleansing in elderly patients. *Arch Intern Med* 2003;163:803-8.

9532 Kinsella LJ, Green R. Anesthesia paresthetica: nitrous oxide-induced cobalamin deficiency. *Neurology* 1995;45:1608-10.

9533 Pinto J, Raiczyk GB, Huang YP, Rivlin RS. New approaches to the possible prevention of side effects of chemotherapy by nutrition. *Cancer* 1986;58:1911-4.

9534 Crane J, Burgess CD, Graham AN, Maling TJB. Hypokalemic and electrocardiographic effects of aminophylline and salbutamol in obstructive airways disease. *N Z Med J* 1987;100:309-11.

9535 Tanphaichitr V. Thiamin. In: Shils ME, Olson JA, Shike M, Ross AC, Eds. Modern Nutrition in Health and Disease. 9th ed. Baltimore, MD: Williams & Wilkins, 1999. pg.381-9.

9536 Alston TA. Does metformin interfere with thiamine? (letter) *Arch Intern Med* 2003;163:983.

9537 Zantvoort FA, Derkx FHM, Boomsma F, et al. Theophylline and serum electrolytes (letter). *Ann Intern Med* 1986;104:134-5.

9538 Braat MCP, Jonkers RE, Bel EH, Van Boxtel CJ. Quantification of theophylline-induced eosinopenia and hypokalamia in healthy volunteers. *Clin Pharmacokinet* 1992;22(3):231-7.

9539 Flack JM, Ryder KW, Strickland D, Whang R. Metabolic correlates of theophylline therapy: a concentration-related phenomenon. *Ann Pharmacother* 1994;28:175-9.

9540 Patterson AJ, Brown WJ, Roberts DC, Seldon MR. Diteray treatment of iron deficiency in women of childbearing age. *Am J Clin Nutr* 2001;74:650-6.

9541 Heath AL, Skeaff CM, O'Brien SM, et al. Can dietary treatment of non-anemic iron deficiency improve iron status? *J Am Coll Nutr* 2001;20:477-85.

9542 Schumann K, Borch-Iohnsen B, Hentze MW, Marx JJ. Tolerable upper intakes for dietary iron set by the US Food and Nutrition Board (commentary). *Am J Clin Nutr* 2002;76:499-500.

9543 Sempos CT. Do body iron stores increase the risk of developing coronary heart disease? (commentary). *Am J Clin Nutr* 2002;76:501-3.

9544 Tuomainen TP, Punnonen K, Nyyssonen K, Salonen JT. Association between body iron stores and the risk of acute myocardial infarction in men. *Circulation* 1998;97:1461-6.

9545 Salonen JT, Nyyssonen K, Korpela H, et al. High stored iron levels are associated with excess risk of myocardial infarction in Eastern Finnish men. *Circulation* 1992;86:803-11.

9546 Ascherio A, Willett WC, Rimm EB, et al. Dietary iron intake and risk of coronary disease among men. *Circulation* 1994;89:969-74.

9547 Stampfer MJ, Grodstein F, Rosenberg I, et al. A prospective study of plasma ferritin and risk of myocardial infarction in US physicians (abstract). *Circulation* 1993;87:688.

9548 Serum ferritin is not a risk factor for coronary artery disease in men and women aged > or = 62 years. *Am J Cardiol* 1993;72:347-8.

9549 Sempos CT, Looker AC, Gillum RF, Makuc DM. Body iron stores and the risk of coronary heart disease. *N Engl J Med* 1994;330:1119-24.

9550 Danesh J, Appleby P. Coronary heart disease and iron status: Meta-analyses of prospective studies. *Circulation* 1999;99:852-4.

9552 Ingram DM, Hickling C, West L, et al. A double-blind randomized controlled trial of isoflavones in the treatment of cyclical mastalgia. *Breast* 2002;11:170-4.

9553 Nelsen J, Barrette E, Tsouronix C, et al. Red clover (Trifolium pratense) monograph: A clinical decision support tool. *J Herbal Pharmacotherapy* 2002;2:49-72.

9554 Kathan RH. Kelp extracts as antiviral subatances. *Ann N Y Acad Sci* 1965;130:390-7.

9555 Harrell BL, Rudolph AH. Letter: Kelp diet: A cause of acneform eruption. *Arch Dermatol* 1976;112:560.

9556 Eliason BC. Transient hyperthyroidism in a patient taking dietary supplements containing kelp. *J Am Board Fam Pract* 1998;11:478-80.

9557 Mester L, Mester M, Nityanand S. Inhibition of platelet aggregation by "guggulu" steroids. *Planta Med* 1979;37:367-9.

9558 Dhawan K, Kumar S, Sharma A. Anti-anxiety studies on extracts of Passiflora incarnata Linneaus. *J Ethnopharmacol* 2001;78:165-70.

9559 Russell RL, Pacelli KA, Kennedy KA. The development of multiple drug resistance in EMT6 cells after treatment with Brefeldin A (B), Tunicamycin (T), Hypoxia (H), 2-deoxyglucose (D), or Glucosamine (G). *FASEB J* 1993;7:A690.

9560 Tikkanen MJ, Wahala K, Ojala S, et al. Effect of soybean phytoestrogen intake on low density lipoprotein oxidation resistance. *Proc Natl Acad Sci U S A* 1998;95:3106-10.

9561 Kerry N, Abbey M. The isoflavone genistein inhibits copper and peroxyl radical mediated low density lipoprotein oxidation in vitro. *Atherosclerosis* 1998;140:341-7.

9562 Iso H, Sato S, Umemura U, et al. Linoleic acid, other fatty acids, and the risk of stroke. *Stroke* 2002;33(8):2086-93.

9563 Starvic B. Quercetin in our diet: from potent mutagen to probable anticarcinogen. *Clin Biochem* 1994;27:245-8.

9564 Ferry DR, Smith A, Malkhandi J, et al. Phase I clinical trial of the flavonoid quercetin: Pharmacokinetics and evidence for in vivo tyrosine kinase inhibition. *Clin Cancer Res* 1996;2:659-67.

9565 Jensen GS, Ginsberg DI, Drapeau C. Blue-green algae as an immuno-enhancer and biomodulator. *JANA* 2001;3:24-30.

9566 Watkins DW, Khalafi R, Cassidy MM, Vahouny GV. Alterations in calcium, magnesium, iron, and zinc metabolism by dietary cholestyramine. *Dig Dis Sci* 1985;30:477-82.

9567 Campbell NRC, Hasinoff B. Ferrous sulfate reduces levodopa bioavailability: Chelation as a possible mechanism. *Clin Pharmacol Ther* 1989;45:220-5.

9568 Campbell NRC, Hasinoff BB, Stalts H, et al. Ferrous sulfate reduces thyroxine efficacy in patients with hypothyroidism. *Ann Intern Med* 1992;117:1010-3.

9569 Garcia-Casal MN, Layrisse M, Solano L, et al. Vitamin A and beta-carotene can improve nonheme iron absorption from rice, wheat and corn by humans. *J Nutr* 1998;128:646-50.

9570 Cook JD. Food iron availability: back to the basics. *Am J Clin Nutr* 1998;67:593-4.

9571 Fleming DJ, Jacques PF, Dallal GE, et al. Dietary determinants of iron stores in a free-living elderly population: The Framingham Heart Study. *Am J Clin Nutr* 1998;67:722-33.

9572 Cook JD, Reddy MB. Effect of ascorbic acid intake on nonheme-iron absorption from a complete diet. *Am J Clin Nutr* 2001 Jan;73:93-8.

9573 Hallberg L, Hulthen L. Prediction of dietary iron absorption: an algorithm for calculating absorption and bioavailability of dietary iron. *Am J Clin Nutr* 2000;71:1147-60.

9574 Package insert for Paser granules. Jacobus Pharmaceutical Co., Inc. Princeton, NJ. July 1996.

9575 Zempsky WT, Rosenstein BJ, Carroll JA, Oski FA. Effect of pancreatic enzyme supplements on iron absorption. *Am J Dis Child* 1989;143:969-72.

9576 Upadhyay R, Torley HI, McKinlay AW, et al. Iron deficiency anaemia in patients with rheumatic disease receiving non-steroidal anti-inflammatory drugs: the role of upper gastrointestinal lesions. *Ann Rheum Dis* 1990;49:359-62.

9577 Davies NM. Toxicity of nonsteroidal anti-inflammatory drugs in the large intestine. *Dis Colon Rectum* 1995;38:1311-21.

9578 Stewart CA, Termanini B, Sutliff VE, et al. Iron absorption in patients with Zollinger-Ellison Syndrome treated with long-term gastric acid antisecretory therapy. *Aliment Pharmacol Ther* 1988;12:83-98.

9579 Valberg LS, Flanagan PR, Chamberlain MJ. Effects of iron, tin, and copper on zinc absorption in humans. *Am J Clin Nutr* 1984;40:536-41.

9580 Crofton RW, Gvozdanovic D, Gvozdanovic S, et al. Inorganic zinc and the intestinal absorption of ferrous iron. *Am J Clin Nutr* 1989;50:141-4.

9581 Rossander-Hulten L, Brune M, Sandstrom B, et al. Competitive inhibition of iron absorption by manganese and zinc in humans. *Am J Clin Nutr* 1991;54:152-6.

9582 O'Brien KO, Zavaleta N, Caulfield LE, et al. Influence of prenatal iron and zinc supplements on supplemental iron absorption, red blood cell iron incorporation, and iron status in pregnant Peruvian women. *Am J Clin Nutr* 1999;69:509-15.

9583 Donangelo CM, Woodhouse LR, King SM, et al. Supplemental zinc lowers measures of iron status in young women with low iron reserves. *J Nutr* 2002;132:1860-4.

9584 Solomons NW, Jacob RA. Studies on the bioavailability of zinc in humans: effects of heme and nonheme iron on the absorption of zinc. *Am J Clin Nutr* 1981;34:475-82.

9585 Dietze F, Bruschke G. Inhibition of iron absorption by pancreatic extracts (letter). *Lancet* 1970;1:424.

9586 Lynch SR. Interaction of iron with other nutrients. *Nutr Rev* 1997;55:102-10.

9587 Prasad GV, Wong T, Meliton G, Bhaloo S. Rhabdomyolysis due to red yeast rice (Monascus purpureus) in a renal transplant recipient. *Transplantation* 2002;74:1200-1.

9588 Heber D, Lembertas A, Lu QY, et al. An analysis of nine proprietary Chinese red yeast rice dietary supplements: implications of variability in chemical profile and contents. *J Altern Complement Med* 2001;7:133-9.

9589 Mahalanabis D, Chowdhury A, Jana S, et al. Zinc supplementation as adjunct therapy in children with measles accompanies by pneumonia: a double-blind, randomized controlled trial. *Am J Clin Nutr* 2002;76:604-7.

9590 Sklar SH, Buimovici-Klein E. Adenosine in the treatment of recurrent herpes labialis. *Oral Surg Oral Med Oral Pathol* 1979;48:416-7.

9591 Wang C, Makela T, Hase T, et al. Lignans and flavonoids inhibit aromatase enzyme in human preadipocytes. *J Steroid Biochem Mol Biol* 1994;50:205-12.

9592 Adlercreutz H, Fotsis T, Bannwart C, et al. Determination of urinary lignans and phytoestrogen metabolites, potential antiestrogens and anticarcinogens, in urine of women on various habitual diets. *J Steroid Biochem* 1986;25:791-7.

9593 Rose DP. Dietary fiber and breast cancer. *Nutr Cancer* 1990;13:1-8.

9594 Hak AE, Stampfer MJ, Campos H, et al. Plasma carotenoids and tocopherols and risk of myocardial infarction in a low-risk population of US male physicians. *Circulation* 2003;108:802-7.

9595 McDuffie JR, Calis KA, Booth SL, et al. Effects of orlistat on fat-soluble vitamins in obese adolescents. *Pharmacotherapy* 2002;22:814-22.

9596 Ernst E. St. John's Wort supplements endanger the success of organ transplantation. *Arch Surg* 2002;137:316-9.

9597 Kasper S, Dienel A. Cluster analysis of symptoms during antidepressant treatment with Hypericum extract in mildly to moderately depressed out-patients. A meta-analysis of data from three randomized, placebo-controlled trials. *Psychopharmacology* (Berl) 2002;164:301-8.

9598 Barrett S. Coral Calcium. June 12, 2003. http://www.quackwatch.org/01QuackeryRelatedTopics/DSH/coral.html (Accessed 26 June 2003).

9599 Smith SR, Kendall MJ. Metabolic responses to beta-2 stimulants. *J R Coll Physicians Lond* 1984;18:190-4.

9600 Jaffe IA. The antivitamin B6 effect of penicillamine. Clinical and immunological implications. *Adv Biochem Psychopharmacol* 1972;4:217-26.

9601 Callies F, Fassnacht M, van Vlijmen JC, et al. Dehydroepiandrosterone replacement in women with adrenal insufficiency: effects on body composition, serum leptin, bone turnover, and exercise capacity. *J Clin Endocrinol Metab* 2001;86:1968-72.

9602 Research abstract. American Association of Cancer Research. Annual meeting, July 2003.

9603 Bertelli A, Cerrati A, Giovannini L, et al. Protective action of L-carnitine and coenzyme Q10 against hepatic triglyceride infiltration induced by hyperbaric oxygen and ethanol. *Drugs Exp Clin Res* 1993;19:65-8.

9604 Dr. Duke's Phytochemical and Ethnobotanical Databases. www.ars-grin.gov/cgi-bin/duke/farmacy2.pl.

9605 Health Canada warns public not to use Vigor-Max. Health Canada Online May 27, 2003. http://www.hc-sc.gc.ca/english/protection/warnings/2003/2003_35.htm (Accessed 28 June 2003).

9606 Bracken MB, Triche EW, Belanger K, et al. Association of maternal caffeine consumption with decrements in fetal growth. *Am J Epidemiol* 2003;157:456-66.

9607 Bara AI, Barley EA. Caffeine for asthma. *Cochrane Database Syst Rev* 2001;4:CD001112.

9608 Ueno H, Mori T, Fujinaga T. Topical formulations and wound healing applications of chitosan. *Adv Drug Deliv Rev* 2001;52:105-15.

9609 Tsujikawa T, Kanauchi O, Andoh A, et al. Supplement of a Chitosan and ascorbic acid mixture for Crohn's disease. A pilot study. *Nutrition* 2003;19:137-9.

9610 Giustina A, Ventura P. Weight-reducing regimens in obese subjects: effects of a new dietary fiber integrator. *Acta Toxicol Ther* 1995;16:199-214.

9611 Campos Y, Arenas J. Muscle carnitine deficiency associated with zidovudine-induced mitochondrial myopathy. *Ann Neurol* 1994;36:680-1.

9612 Hirose S, Mitsudome A, Yasumoto S, et al. Valproate therapy does not deplete carnitine levels in otherwise healthy children. *Pediatrics* 1998;101:E9 (abstract). Full text at: www.pediatrics.org/cgi/content/full/101/5/e9.

9613 Ryan MP. Diuretics and potassium/magnesium depletion: directions for treatment. *Am J Med* 1987;82:38-47.

9614 Hollifield JW. Magnesium depletion, diuretics, and arrhythmias. *Am J Med* 1987;82:30-7.

9615 Schwarz RE, Zagala-Nevarez K. Significant hypomagnesemia after celiotomy: implications of preoperative bowel cleansing with sodium phosphate purgative. *Surgery* 2002;131:236.

9616 Ehrenpreis ED, Wieland JM, Cabral J, et al. Symptomatic hypocalcemia, hypomagnesemia, and hyperphosphatemia sceondary to Fleet's Phospho-Soda colonoscopy preparation in a patient with a jejunoileal bypass. *Dig Dis Sci* 1997;42:858-60.

9617 Palestine AG, Polis MA, De Smet MD, et al. A randomized, controlled trial of foscarnet in the treatment of cytomegalovirus retinitis in patients with AIDS. *Ann Intern Med* 1991;115:665-73.

9618 Burnett RJ, Reents SB. Severe hypomagnesemia induced by pentamidine. *DICP* 1990;24:239-40.

9619 Gradon JD, Fricchione L, Sepkowitz D. Severe hypomagnesemia associated with pentamidine therapy. *Rev Infect Dis* 1991;13:511-2.

9620 Niederstadt C, Steinhoff J, Erbsloh-Moller B, et al. Effect of FK506 on magnesium homeostasis after renal transplantation. *Transplant Proc* 1997;29:3161-2.

9621 Seelig MS. Increased need for magnesium with the use of combined oestrogen and calcium for osteoporosis treatment. *Magnes Res* 1990;3:197-215.

9622 Heidenreich O. Mode of action of conventional and potassium-sparing diuretics--aspects with relevance to Mg-sparing effects. *Magnesium* 1984;3:248-56.

9623 Nielsen FH, Hunt CD, Mullen LM, Hunt JR. Effect of dietary boron on mineral, estrogen, and testosterone metabolism in postmenopausal women. *FASEB J* 1987;1:394-7.

9624 Spencer H, Norris C, Williams D. Inhibitory effects of zinc on magnesium balance and magnesium absorption in man. *J Am Coll Nutr* 1994;13:479-84.

9625 Hirschel-Scholz S, Paunier L, Bonjour JP. Interference of WR-2721 with magnesium metabolism: mechanism of action. *Miner Electrolyte Metab* 1988;14:114-20.

REFERENCES

9626 Martin M, Diaz-Rubio E, Casado A, et al. Intravenous and oral magnesium supplementation in the prophylaxis of cisplatin-induced hypomagnesemia. Results of a controlled trial. *Am J Clin Oncol* 1992;15:348-51

9627 Runeberg L, Miettinen TA, Nikkila EA. Effect of cholestyramine on mineral excretion in man. *Acta Med Scand* 1972;192:71-6.

9628 Quamme GA. Renal handling of magnesium: drug and hormone interactions. *Magnesium* 1986;5:248-72.

9629 Kleeman CR, Levi J, Better O. Kidney and adrenocortical hormones. *Nephron* 1975;15:261-78.

9630 Cantilena LR, Klaassen CD. The effect of chelating agents on the excretion of endogenous metals. *Toxicol Appl Pharmacol* 1982;63:344-50.

9631 Gottlieb SS. Importance of magnesium in congestive heart failure. *Am J Cardiol* 1989;63:39G-42G.

9632 Thompson CB, Sullivan KM, June CH, Thomas ED. Association between cyclosporine neurotoxicity and hypomagnesemia. *Lancet* 1984;2:1116-20.

9633 Allen RD, Hunnisett AG, Morris PJ. Cyclosporine and magnesium. *Lancet* 1985;1:1283-4.

9634 Hardwick LL, Jones MR, Brautbar N, Lee DB. Magnesium absorption: mechanisms and the influence of vitamin D, calcium and phosphate. *J Nutr* 1991;121:13-23.

9635 Charles P, Mosekilde L, Sondergard K, Jensen FT. Treatment with high-dose oral vitamin D2 in patients with jejunoileal bypass for morbid obesity. Effects on calcium and magnesium metabolism, vitamin D metabolites and faecal lag time. *Scand J Gastroenterol* 1984;19:1031-8.

9636 Fukumoto S, Matsumoto T, Tanaka Y, et al. Renal magnesium wasting in a patient with short bowel syndrome with magnesium deficiency: effect of 1-alpha-hydroxyvitamin D3 treatment. *J Clin Endocrinol Metab* 1987;65:1301-4.

9637 Krejs GJ, Nicar MJ, Zerwekh JE, et al. Effect of 1,25-dihydroxyvitamin D3 on calcium and magnesium absorption in the healthy human jejunum and ileum. *Am J Med* 1983;75:973-6.

9638 Muneyyirci-Delale O, Nacharaju VL, Dalloul M, et al. Serum ionized magnesium and calcium in women after menopause: inverse relation of estrogen with ionized magnesium. *Fertil Steril* 1999;71:869-72.

9639 Seelig MS. Interrelationship of magnesium and estrogen in cardiovascular and bone disorders, eclampsia, migraine, and premenstrual syndrome. *J Am Coll Nutr* 1993;12:442-58.

9640 Stanton MF, Lowenstein FW. Serum magnesium in women during pregnancy, while taking contraceptives, and after menopause. *J Am Coll Nutr* 1987;6:313-9.

9641 Rolla G, Bucca C. Magnesium, beta-agonists, and asthma. *Lancet* 1988;1:989.

9671 File SE, Jarrett N, Fluck E, et al. Eating soya improves human memory. *Psychopharmacology* (Berl) 2001;157:430-6.

9672 Cambria-Kiely JA. Effect of soy milk on warfarin efficacy. *Ann Pharmacother* 2002;36:1893-6.

9673 Shelnutt SR, Cimino CO, Wiggins PA, et al. Pharmacokinetics of the glucuronide and sulfate conjugates of genistein and daidzein in men and women after consumption of a soy beverage. *Am J Clin Nutr* 2002;76:588-94.

9674 Ziegler RG, Hoover RN, Pike MC, et al. Migration patterns and breast cancer risk in Asian-American women. *J Natl Cancer Inst* 1993;85:1819-27.

9675 Salleng K, Pan Y, Anthony MS, et al. Interactive effects of estradiol and dietary soy on the uteri of rats (abstract). *Alternative Therapies* 2001;7:S29.

9676 Brown BD, Thomas W, Hutchins A, et al. Types of dietary fat and soy minimally affect hormones and biomarkers associated with breast cancer risk in premenopausal women. *Nutr Cancer* 2002;43:22-30.

9677 Sun CL, Yuan JM, Arakawa K, et al. Dietary soy and increased risk of bladder cancer: the Singapore Chinese Health Study. *Cancer Epidemiol Biomarkers Prev* 2002;11:1674-7.

9678 Yildirir A, Tokgozoglu SL, Oduncu T, et al. Soy protein diet significantly improves endothelial function and lipid parameters. *Clin Cardiol* 2001;24:711-6.

9679 Dent SB, Peterson CT, Brace LD, et al. Soy protein intake by perimenopausal women does not affect circulating lipids and lipoproteins or coagulation and fibrinolytic factors. *J Nutr* 2001;131:2280-7.

9680 Engel PA. New onset migraine associated with use of soy isoflavone supplements. *Neurology* 2002;59:1289-90.

9681 Phipps WR, Wangen KE, Duncan AM, et al. Lack of effect of isoflavonic phytoestrogen intake on leptin concentrations in premenopausal and postmenopausal women. *Fertil Steril* 2001;75:1059-64.

9682 Lee YS, Chen X, Anderson JJB. Physiological concentrations of genistein stimulate the proliferation and protect against free radical-induced oxidative damage of MC3T3-E1 osteoblast-like cells. *Nutr Res* 2001;21:1287-98.

9683 Gardner-Thorpe D, O'Hagen C, Young I, Lewis SJ. Dietary supplements of soya flour lower serum testosterone concentrations and improve markers of oxidative stress in men. *Eur J Clin Nutr* 2003;57:100-6.

9684 Jones G, Dwyer T, Hynes K, et al. A randomized controlled trial of phytoestrogen supplementation, growth and bone turnover in adolescent males. *Eur J Clin Nutr* 2003;57:324-7.

9685 Wang Z, Hamman MA, Huang SM, et al. Effect of St. John's wort on the pharmacokinetics of fexofenadine. *Clin Pharmacol Ther* 2002;71:414-20.

9686 Wheatley D. Hypericum in seasonal affective disorder (SAD). *Curr Med Res Opin* 1999;15:33-7.

9687 Chan LY, Chiu PY, Lau TK. A study of hypericin-induced teratogenicity during organogenesis using a whole rat embryo culture model. *Fertil Steril* 2001;76:1073-4.

9690 Dias MF, Sousa E, Cabrita S, et al. Chemoprevention of DMBA-induced mammary tumors in rats by a combined regimen of alpha-tocopherol, selenium, and ascorbic Acid. *Breast J* 2000;6:14-19.

9691 Wit JM, Langenhorst VJ, Jansen M, et al. Dehydroepiandrosterone sulfate treatment for atrichia pubis. *Horm Res* 2001;56:134-9.

9692 Strous RD, Maayan R, Lapidus R, et al. Dehydroepiandrosterone augmentation in the management of negative, depressive, and anxiety symptoms in schizophrenia. *Arch Gen Psychiatry* 2003;60:133-41.

9693 Meno-Tetang GM, Blum RA, Schwartz KE, Jusko WJ. Effects of oral prasterone (dehydroepiandrosterone) on single-dose pharmacokinetics of oral prednisone and cortisol suppression in normal women. *J Clin Pharmacol* 2001;41:1195-205.

9694 Arlt W, Callies F, Koehler I, et al. Dehydroepiandrosterone supplementation in healthy men with an age-related decline of dehydroepiandrosterone secretion. *J Clin Endocrinol Metab* 2001;86:4686-92.

9695 Munoz-Hoyos A, Sanchez-Forte M, Molina-Carballo A, et al. Melatonin's role as an anticonvulsant and neuronal protector: experimental and clinical evidence. *J Child Neurol* 1998;13:501-9.

9696 Schapel GJ, Beran RG, Kennaway DL, et al. Melatonin response in active epilepsy. *Epilepsia* 1995;36:75-8.

9697 Sandyk R, Tsagas N, Anninos PA. Melatonin as a proconvulsive hormone in humans. *Int J Neurosci* 1992;63:125-35.

9698 Sandyk R. Melatonin and petit-mal epilepsy: an hypothesis. *Int J Neurosci* 1992;65:83-90.

9699 Peled N, Shorer Z, Peled E, Pillar G. Melatonin effect on seizures in children with severe neurologic deficit disorders. *Epilepsia* 2001;42:1208-10.

9700 Papezova H, Yamamotova A, Nedvidkova J. Pain modulation role of melatonin in eating disorders. *Eur Psychiatry* 2001;16:68-70.

9701 Citera G, Arias MA, Maldonado-Cocco JA, et al. The effect of melatonin in patients with fibromyalgia: a pilot study. *Clin Rheumatol* 2000;19:9-13.

9702 Pringsheim T, Magnoux E, Dobson CF, et al. Melatonin as adjunctive therapy in the prophylaxis of cluster headache: a pilot study. *Headache* 2002;42:787-92.

9703 Golombek DA, Escolar E, Burin LJ, et al. Chronopharmacology of melatonin: inhibition by benzodiazepine antagonism. *Chronobiol Int* 1992;9:124-31.

9704 Cagnacci A, Zanni AL, Veneri MG, et al. Influence of exogenous melatonin on catecholamine levels in postmenopausal women prior and during oestradiol replacement. *Clin Endocrinol* (Oxf) 2000;53:367-72.

9705 Williams G, Waterhouse J, Mugarza J, et al. Therapy of circadian rhythm disorders in chronic fatigue syndrome: no symptomatic improvement with melatonin or phototherapy. *Eur J Clin Invest* 2002;32:831-7.

9706 Stone BM, Turner C, Mills SL, Nicholson AN. Hypnotic activity of melatonin. *Sleep* 2000;23:663-9.

9707 Dodge NN, Wilson GA. Melatonin for treatment of sleep disorders in children with developmental disabilities. *J Child Neurol* 2001;16:581-4.

9708 Smits MG, Nagtegaal EE, van der Heijden J, et al. Melatonin for chronic sleep onset insomnia in children: a randomized placebo-controlled trial. *J Child Neurol* 2001;16:86-92.

9709 Andrade C, Srihari BS, Reddy KP, Chandramma L. Melatonin in medically ill patients with insomnia: a double-blind, placebo-controlled study. *J Clin Psychiatry* 2001;62:41-5.

9710 Poeggeler B, Miravalle L, Zagorski MG, et al. Melatonin reverses the profibrillogenic activity of apolipoprotein E4 on the Alzheimer amyloid Abeta peptide. *Biochemistry* 2001;40:14995-5001.

9711 Hill SM, Collins A, Kiefer TL. The modulation of oestrogen receptor-alpha activity by melatonin in MCF-7 human breast cancer cells. *Eur J Cancer* 2000;36(Suppl 4):117-8.

9712 Cuzzocrea S, Reiter RJ. Pharmacological action of melatonin in shock, inflammation and ischemia/reperfusion injury. *Eur J Pharmacol* 2001;426:1-10.

9713 Cagnacci A, Arangino S, Renzi A, et al. Influence of melatonin administration on glucose tolerance and insulin sensitivity of postmenopausal women. *Clin Endocrinol* (Oxf) 2001;54:339-46.

9714 Burgess HJ, Sletten T, Savic N, et al. Effects of bright light and melatonin on sleep propensity, temperature, and cardiac activity at night. *J Appl Physiol* 2001;91:1214-22.

9715 Williamson BL, Tomlinson AJ, Naylor S, Gleich GJ. Contaminants in commercial preparations of melatonin. *Mayo Clin Proc* 1997;72:1094-5.

9716 Williamson BL, Tomlinson AJ, Mishra PK, et al. Structural characterization of contaminants found in commercial preparations of melatonin: similarities to case-related compounds from L-tryptophan associated with eosinophilia-myalgia syndrome. *Chem Res Toxicol* 1998;11:234-40.

9717 Thomson CD, Robinson MF. Urinary and fecal excretions and absorption of a large supplement of selenium: superiority of selenate over selenite. *Am J Clin Nutr* 1986;44:659-63.

9718 Combs GF Jr. Selenium in global food systems. *Br J Nutr* 2001;85:517-47.

9719 Schrauzer GN, Sacher J. Selenium in the maintenance and therapy of HIV-infected patients. *Chem Biol Interact* 1994;91:199-205.

9720 Baeten JM, Mostad SB, Hughes MP, et al. Selenium deficiency is associated with shedding of HIV-1--infected cells in the female genital tract. *J Acquir Immune Defic Syndr* 2001;26:360-4.

9721 Djujic IS, Jozanov-Stankov ON, Milovac M, et al. Bioavailability and possible benefits of wheat intake naturally enriched with selenium and its products. *Biol Trace Elem Res* 2000;77:273-85.

9722 Duffield-Lillico AJ, Reid ME, et al. Baseline characteristics and the effect of selenium supplementation on cancer incidence in a randomized clinical trial: a summary report of the Nutritional Prevention of Cancer Trial. *Cancer Epidemiol Biomarkers Prev* 2002;11:630-9.

9723 Finley JW, Ip C, Lisk DJ, et al. Cancer-protective properties of high-selenium broccoli. *J Agric Food Chem* 2001;49:2679-83.

9724 Sher L. Role of selenium depletion in the etiopathogenesis of depression in patient with alcoholism. *Med Hypotheses* 2002;59:330-3.

9725 Berger MM, Reymond MJ, Shenkin A, et al. Influence of selenium supplements on the post-traumatic alterations of the thyroid axis: a placebo-controlled trial. *Intensive Care Med* 2001;27:91-100.

9726 Milde D, Novak O, Stu ka V, et al. Serum levels of selenium, manganese, copper, and iron in colorectal cancer patients. *Biol Trace Elem Res* 2001;79:107-14.

9727 Navarrete M, Gaudry A, Revel G, et al. Urinary selenium excretion in patients with cervical uterine cancer. *Biol Trace Elem Res* 2001;79:97-105.

9728 Beck MA, Nelson HK, Shi Q, et al. Selenium deficiency increases the pathology of an influenza virus infection. *FASEB J* 2001;15:1481-3.

9729 Hawkes WC, Turek PJ. Effects of dietary selenium on sperm motility in healthy men. *J Androl* 2001;22:764-72.

9730 Khan Z, Macdonald C, Wicks AC, et al. Use of the 'nutriceutical', bovine colostrum, for the treatment of distal colitis: results from an initial study. *Aliment Pharmacol Ther* 2002;16:1917-22.

9731 Playford RJ, Macdonald CE, Johnson WS. Colostrum and milk-derived peptide growth factors for the treatment of gastrointestinal disorders. *Am J Clin Nutr* 2000;72:5-14.

9732 Sievenpiper JL, Arnason JT, Leiter LA, Vuksan V. Variable effects of American ginseng: a batch of American ginseng (Panax quinquefolius L.) with a depressed ginsenoside profile does not affect postprandial glycemia. *Eur J Clin Nutr* 2003;57:243-8.

9733 Li J, Huang M, Teoh H, Man RY. Panax quinquefolium saponins protects low density lipoproteins from oxidation. *Life Sci* 1999;64:53-62.

9734 Yuan CS, Attele AS, Wu JA, et al. Panax quinquefolium L. inhibits thrombin-induced endothelin release in vitro. *Am J Chin Med* 1999;27:331-8.

9735 Wang X, Sakuma T, Asafu-Adjaye E, Shiu GK. Determination of ginsenosides in plant extracts from Panax ginseng and Panax quinquefolius L. by LC/MS/MS. *Anal Chem* 1999;71:1579-84.

9736 Benishin CG, Lee R, Wang LC, Liu HJ. Effects of ginsenoside Rb1 on central cholinergic metabolism. *Pharmacology* 1991;42:223-9.

9737 Rao CV, Wang CQ, Simi B, et al. Chemoprevention of colon cancer by a glutathione conjugate of 1,4-phenylenebis(methylene)selenocyanate, a novel organoselenium compound with low toxicity. *Cancer Res* 2001;61:3647-52.

9738 Zadok D, Levy Y, Glovinsky Y, et al. The effect of anthocyanosides on night vision (abstract). *Invest Ophthalmol Vis Sci* 1997;38:S633.

9739 Levy Y, Glovinsky Y. The effect of anthocyanosides on night vision. *Eye* 1998;12:967-9.

9740 Shekelle PG, Hardy ML, Morton SC, et al. Efficacy and safety of ephedra and ephedrine for weight loss and athletic performance: a meta-analysis. *JAMA* 2003;289:1537-45.

9741 Anon. Ephedra and ephedrine for weight loss and athletic performance enhancement: clinical efficacy and side effects. *Evid Rep Technol Assess* (Summ) 2003;76:1-4.

9744 Stewart LS. Endogenous melatonin and epileptogenesis: facts and hypothesis. *Int J Neurosci* 2001;107:77-85.

9745 Fauteck J, Schmidt H, Lerchl A, et al. Melatonin in epilepsy: first results of replacement therapy and first clinical results. *Biol Signals Recept* 1999;8:105-10.

9746 Molina-Carballo A, Munoz-Hoyos A, Reiter RJ, et al. Utility of high doses of melatonin as adjunctive anticonvulsant therapy in a child with severe myoclonic epilepsy: two years' experience. *J Pineal Res* 1997;23:97-105.

9747 Nathan PJ, Wyndham EL, Burrows GD, Norman TR. The effect of gender on the melatonin suppression by light: a dose response relationship. *J Neural Transm* 2000;107:271-9.

9748 Tooley GA, Armstrong SM, Norman TR, Sali A. Acute increases in night-time plasma melatonin levels following a period of meditation. *Biol Psychol* 2000;53:69-78.

9749 Sener G, Satiroglu H, Kabasakal L, et al. The protective effect of melatonin on cisplatin nephrotoxicity. *Fundam Clin Pharmacol* 2000;14:553-60.

9750 Nickelsen T, Lang A, Bergau L. The effect of 6-, 9- and 11-hour time shifts on circadium rhythms: adaptation of sleep parameters and hormonal patterns following the intake of melatonin or placebo. *Advances Pineal Res* 1991;5:303-6.

9751 Leman ES, Sisken BF, Zimmer S, Anderson KW. Studies of the interactions between melatonin and 2 Hz, 0.3 mT PEMF on the proliferation and invasion of human breast cancer cells. *Bioelectromagnetics* 2001;22:178-84.

9759 Wesnes KA, Ward T, McGinty A, Petrini O. The memory enhancing effects of a Ginkgo biloba/Panax ginseng combination in healthy middle-aged volunteers. *Psychopharmacology* (Berl) 2000;152:353-61.

9760 Kudolo GB, Dorsey S, Blodgett J. Effect of the ingestion of Ginkgo biloba extract on platelet aggregation and urinary prostanoid excretion in healthy and Type 2 diabetic subjects. *Thromb Res* 2002;108:151-60.

9761 Van Dael P, Davidsson L, Munoz-Box R, et al. Selenium absorption and retention from a selenite- or selenate-fortified milk-based formula in men measured by a stable-isotope technique. *Br J Nutr* 2001;85:157-63.

9762 Robinson MF, Thomson CD, Jenkinson CP, et al Long-term supplementation with selenate and selenomethionine: urinary excretion by New Zealand women. *Br J Nutr* 1997;77:551-63.

9763 Peretz A, Siderova V, Neve J. Selenium supplementation in rheumatoid arthritis investigated in a double blind, placebo-controlled trial. *Scand J Rheumatol* 2001;30:208-12.

9764 Bogye G, Alfthan G, Machay T. Bioavailability of enteral yeast-selenium in preterm infants. *Biol Trace Elem Res* 1998;65:143-51.

9765 Viola H, Wasowski C, Levi de Stein M, et al. Apigenin, a component of Matricaria recutita flowers, is a central benzodiazepine receptors-ligand with anxiolytic effects. *Planta Med* 1995;61:213-6.

9766 van Ketel WG. Allergy to Matricaria chamomilla. *Contact Dermatitis* 1982;8:143.

9767 Maiche AG, Grohn P, Maki-Hokkonen H. Effect of chamomile cream and almond ointment on acute radiation skin reaction. *Acta Oncol* 1991;30:395-6.

9768 van Ketel WG. Allergy to Matricaria chamomilla. *Contact Dermatitis* 1987;16:50-1.

9769 Deliorman D, Calis I, Ergun F. A new acyclic monoterpene glucoside from Viscum album ssp. album. *Fitoterapia* 2001;72:101-5.

9770 Tusenius KJ, Spoek JM, Kramers CW. Iscador Qu for chronic hepatitis C: an exploratory study. *Complement Ther Med* 2001;9:12-6.

9771 Suzukawa M, Abbey M, Howe PR, Nestel PJ. Effects of fish oil fatty acids on low density lipoprotein size, oxidizability, and uptake by macrophages. *J Lipid Res* 1995;36:473-84.

9772 Pawlosky RJ, Hibbeln JR, Lin Y, et al. Effects of beef- and fish-based diets on the kinetics of n-3 fatty acid metabolism in human subjects. *Am J Clin Nutr* 2003;77:565-72.

9773 Augustsson K, Michaud DS, Rimm EB, et al. A prospective study of intake of fish and marine fatty acids and prostate cancer. *Cancer Epidemiol Biomarkers Prev* 2003;12:64-7.

9774 Terry PD, Rohan TE, Wolk A. Intakes of fish and marine fatty acids and the risks of cancers of the breast and prostate and of other hormone-related cancers: a review of the epidemiologic evidence. *Am J Clin Nutr* 2003;77:532-43.

9775 Arjmandi BH, Khalil DA, Smith BJ, et al. Soy protein has a greater effect on bone in postmenopausal women not on hormone replacement therapy, as evidenced by reducing bone resorption and urinary calcium excretion. *J Clin Endocrinol Metab* 2003;88:1048-54.

9776 Nagata C, Shimizu H, Takami R, et al. Soy product intake is inversely associated with serum homocysteine level in premenopausal Japanese women. *J Nutr* 2003;133:797-800.

9777 Jenkins DJ, Kendall CW, D'Costa MA, et al. Soy consumption and phytoestrogens: effect on serum prostate specific antigen when blood lipids and oxidized low-density lipoprotein are reduced in hyperlipidemic men. *J Urol* 2003;169:507-11.

9780 Pedersen A, Baumstark MW, Marckmann P, et al. An olive oil-rich diet results in higher concentrations of LDL cholesterol and a higher number of LDL subfraction particles than rapeseed oil and sunflower oil diets. *J Lipid Res* 2000;41:1901-11.

9781 Yalcin SS, Tekinalp G, Ozalp I. Peculiar odor of traditional food and maple syrup urine disease. *Pediatr Int* 1999;41:108-9.

9782 Sewell AC, Mosandl A, Bohles H. False diagnosis of maple syrup urine disease owing to ingestion of herbal tea. *N Engl J Med* 1999;341:769.

9783 Sowmya P, Rajyalakshmi P. Hypocholesterolemic effect of germinated fenugreek seeds in human subjects. *Plant Foods Hum Nutr* 1999;53:359-65.

9784 Pathak P, Srivastava S, Grover S. Development of food products based on millets, legumes and fenugreek seeds and their suitability in the diabetic diet. *Int J Food Sci Nutr* 2000;51:409-14.

9785 Fam A. Use of titrated extract of Centella asiatica (TECA) in bilharzial bladder lesions. *Int Surg* 1973;58:451-2.

9786 Belcaro GV, Rulo A, Grimaldi R. Capillary filtration and ankle edema in patients with venous hypertension treated with TTFCA. *Angiology* 1990;41:12-8.

9789 Eun HC, Lee AY. Contact dermatitis due to madecassol. *Contact Dermatitis* 1985;13:310-3.

9790 Hurot JM, Cucherat M, Haugh M, Fouque D. Effects of L-carnitine supplementation in maintenance hemodialysis patients: a systematic review. *J Am Soc Nephrol* 2002;13:708-14.

9791 Vicari E, La Vignera S, Calogero AE. Antioxidant treatment with carnitines is effective in infertile patients with prostatovesiculoepididymitis and elevated seminal leukocyte concentrations after treatment with nonsteroidal anti-inflammatory compounds. *Fertil Steril* 2002;78:1203-8.

9792 Akhondzadeh S, Kashani L, Fotouhi A, et al. Comparison of Lavandula angustifolia Mill. tincture and imipramine in the treatment of mild to moderate depression: a double-blind, randomized trial. *Prog Neuropsychopharmacol Biol Psychiatry* 2003;27:123-7

9794 Cheung KL. Management of cyclical mastalgia in oriental women: pioneer experience of using gamolenic acid (Efamast) in Asia. *Aust N Z J Surg* 1999;69:492-4.

9796 Simpson M, Parsons M, Greenwood J, Wade K. Raspberry leaf in pregnancy: its safety and efficacy in labor. *J Midwifery Womens Health* 2001;46:51-9.

9797 Gartner R, Gasnier BC, Dietrich JW, et al. Selenium supplementation in patients with autoimmune thyroiditis decreases thyroid peroxidase antibodies concentrations. *J Clin Endocrinol Metab* 2002;87:1687-91.

9798 Reid ME, Duffield-Lillico AJ, Garland L, et al. Selenium supplementation and lung cancer incidence: an update of the nutritional prevention of cancer trial. *Cancer Epidemiol Biomarkers Prev* 2002;11:1285-91.

9800 French AL, Kirstein LM, Massad LS, et al. Association of vitamin A deficiency with cervical squamous intraepithelial lesions in human immunodeficiency virus-infected women. *J Infect Dis* 2000;182:1084-9.

9801 Fawzi WW, Msamanga GI, Hunter D, et al. Randomized trial of vitamin supplements in relation to transmission of HIV-1 through breastfeeding and early child mortality. *AIDS* 2002;16:1935-44.

9802 Kokkonen J, Mottonen M, Karttunen TJ, Lanning M. Mucosal pathology of the upper gastrointestinal tract associated with intensive chemotherapy in children: vitamin A supplements do not prevent lesions. *Pediatr Hematol Oncol* 2002;19:181-92.

9803 Schrauzer GN, Shrestha KP. Lithium in drinking water and the incidences of crimes, suicides, and arrests related to drug addictions. *Biol Trace Elem Res* 1990 May;25:105-13.

9804 Rosenthal G. Interaction of ascorbic acid and warfarin. *JAMA* 1971;215:1671.

9805 Hume R, Johnstone JM, Weyers E. Interaction of ascorbic acid and warfarin. *JAMA* 1972;219:1479.

9806 Smith EC, Skalski RJ, Johnson GC, Rossi GV. Interaction of ascorbic acid and warfarin. *JAMA* 1972;221:1166.

9807 Deckert FW. Ascorbic acid and warfarin. *JAMA* 1973;223:440.

9808 Kuo SM, Lin CP, Morehouse HF Jr. Dihydropyridine calcium channel blockers inhibit ascorbic acid accumulation in human intestinal Caco-2 cells. *Life Sci* 2001;68:1751-60.

9809 Padayatty SJ, Levine M. New insights into the physiology and pharmacology of vitamin C. *CMAJ* 2001;164:353-5.

9810 Johnston CS, Thompson LL. Vitamin C status of an outpatient population. *J Am Coll Nutr* 1998;17:366-70.

9811 Johnston CS, Bowling DL. Stability of ascorbic acid in commercially available orange juices. *J Am Diet Assoc* 2002;102:525-9.

9812 Carr AC, Zhu BZ, Frei B. Potential antiatherogenic mechanisms of ascorbate (vitamin C) and alpha-tocopherol (vitamin E). *Circ Res* 2000;87:349-54.

9813 Langlois M, Duprez D, Delanghe J, et al. Serum vitamin C concentration is low in peripheral arterial disease and is associated with inflammation and severity of atherosclerosis. *Circulation* 2001;103:1863-8.

9814 McQuillan BM, Hung J, Beilby JP, et al. Antioxidant vitamins and the risk of carotid atherosclerosis. The Perth Carotid Ultrasound Disease Assessment study (CUDAS). *J Am Coll Cardiol* 2001;38:1788-94.

9815 Lonn E. Do antioxidant vitamins protect against atherosclerosis? The proof is still lacking. *J Am Coll Cardiol* 2001;38:1795-8.

9816 Rossig L, Hoffmann J, Hugel B, et al. Vitamin C inhibits endothelial cell apoptosis in congestive heart failure. *Circulation* 2001;104:2182-7.

9817 Heart Protection Study Collaborative Group. MRC/BHF Heart Protection Study of antioxidant vitamin supplementation in 20,536 high-risk individuals: a randomised placebo-controlled trial. *Lancet* 2002;360:23-33.

9818 Raitakari OT, Adams MR, McCredie RJ, et al. Oral vitamin C and endothelial function in smokers: short-term improvement, but no sustained beneficial effect. *J Am Coll Cardiol* 2000;35:1616-21.

9819 Hirashima O, Kawano H, Motoyama T, et al. Improvement of endothelial function and insulin sensitivity with vitamin C in patients with coronary spastic angina: possible role of reactive oxygen species. *J Am Coll Cardiol* 2000;35:1860-6.

9820 Natali A, Sironi AM, Toschi E, et al. Effect of vitamin C on forearm blood flow and glucose metabolism in essential hypertension. *Arterioscler Thromb Vasc Biol* 2000;20:2401-6.

9821 Kim MK, Sasaki S, Sasazuki S, et al. Lack of long-term effect of vitamin C supplementation on blood pressure. *Hypertension* 2002;40:797-803.

9822 Mullan BA, Young IS, Fee H, McCance DR. Ascorbic acid reduces blood pressure and arterial stiffness in type 2 diabetes. *Hypertension* 2002;40:804-9.

9823 Flood V, Smith W, Wang JJ, et al. Dietary antioxidant intake and incidence of early age-related maculopathy: the Blue Mountains Eye Study. *Ophthalmology* 2002;109:2272-8.

9824 Laurin D, Foley DJ, Masaki KH, et al. Vitamin E and C supplements and risk of dementia. *JAMA* 2002;288:2266-8.

9825 Kennedy M, Bruninga K, Mutlu EA, et al. Successful and sustained treatment of chronic radiation proctitis with antioxidant vitamins E and C. *Am J Gastroenterol* 2001;96:1080-4.

9826 Prasad KN, Cole WC, Kumar B, Che Prasad K. Pros and cons of antioxidant use during radiation therapy. *Cancer Treat Rev* 2002;28:79-91.

9827 Evans AT, Husain S, Durairaj L, et al. Azithromycin for acute bronchitis: a randomised, double-blind, controlled trial. *Lancet* 2002;359:1648-54.

9828 Simon JA, Hudes ES. Relation of ascorbic acid to bone mineral density and self-reported fractures among US adults. *Am J Epidemiol* 2001;154:427-33.

9830 Batterham M, Gold J, Naidoo D, et al. A preliminary open label dose comparison using an antioxidant regimen to determine the effect on viral load and oxidative stress in men with HIV/AIDS. *Eur J Clin Nutr* 2001;55:107-14.

9831 Hemila H. Vitamin C and common cold incidence: a review of studies with subjects under heavy physical stress. *Int J Sports Med* 1996;17:379-83.

9832 Carr AB, Einstein R, Lai LY, et al. Vitamin C and the common cold: using identical twins as controls. *Med J Aust* 1981;2:411-2.

9833 Audera C, Patulny RV, Sander BH, Douglas RM. Mega-dose vitamin C in treatment of the common cold: a randomized controlled trial. *Med J Aust* 2001;175:359-62.

9834 Hemila H. Vitamin C supplementation and common cold symptoms: factors affecting the magnitude of the benefit. *Med Hypotheses* 1999;52:171-8.

9835 Hemila H. Vitamin C supplementation and the common cold--was Linus Pauling right or wrong? *Int J Vitam Nutr Res* 1997;67:329-35.

9836 Hemila H. Vitamin C supplementation and common cold symptoms: problems with inaccurate reviews. *Nutrition* 1996;12:804-9.

9837 Bachleitner-Hofmann T, Gisslinger B, Grumbeck E, Gisslinger H. Arsenic trioxide and ascorbic acid: synergy with potential implications for the treatment of acute myeloid leukaemia? *Br J Haematol* 2001;112:783-6.

9838 Mayne ST, Risch HA, Dubrow R, et al. Nutrient intake and risk of subtypes of esophageal and gastric cancer. *Cancer Epidemiol Biomarkers Prev* 2001;10:1055-62.

9839 Jacobs EJ, Henion AK, Briggs PJ, et al. Vitamin C and vitamin E supplement use and bladder cancer mortality in a large cohort of US men and women. *Am J Epidemiol* 2002;156:1002-10.

9840 FDA Orphan Drug List. http://www.fda.gov/ohrms/dockets/dailys/00/mar00/030100/lst0094.pdf (Accessed 2 May 2003).

9871 Morgenstern C, Biermann E. The efficacy of Ginkgo special extract EGb 761 in patients with tinnitus. *Int J Clin Pharmacol Ther* 2002;40:188-197.

9872 Hauns B, Haring B, Kohler S, et al. Phase II study of combined 5-fluorouracil/ Ginkgo biloba extract (GBE 761 ONC) therapy in 5-fluorouracil pretreated patients with advanced colorectal cancer. *Phytother Res* 2001;15:34-38.

9873 Sumioka I, Matsura T, Yamada K. Therapeutic effect of S-allylmercaptocysteine on acetaminophen-induced liver injury in mice. *Eur J Pharmacol* 2001;433:177-85.

9874 Bordia A, Verma SK, Srivastava KC. Effect of garlic (Allium sativum) on blood lipids, blood sugar, fibrinogen and fibrinolytic activity in patients with coronary artery disease. *Prostaglandins Leukot Essent Fatty Acids* 1998;58:257-63.

9875 Sheela CG, Kumud K, Augusti KT. Anti-diabetic effects of onion and garlic sulfoxide amino acids in rats. *Planta Med* 1995;61:356-7.

9876 Hsing AW, Chokkalingam AP, Gao YT, et al. Allium vegetables and risk of prostate cancer: a population-based study. *J Natl Cancer Inst* 2002;94:1648-51.

9878 Martinez E, Domingo P, Roca-Cusachs A. Potentiation of acenocoumarol action by L-carnitine. *J Intern Med* 1993;233:94.

9879 Lange HW, Dambrink JH, Pasalary M, et al. Folate therapy increases in-stent restenosis: results from the folate after coronary intervention trial (FACIT). American College of Cardiology 52nd Annual Scientific Session. Chicago March 30 - April 4, 2003. Abstract 31-7.

9880 Schwarz UI, Buschel B, Kirch W. Unwanted pregnancy on self-medication with St John's wort despite hormonal contraception. *Br J Clin Pharmacol* 2003;55:112-3.

9881 Anon. Final report on the safety assessment of Hypericum perforatum extract and Hypericum perforatum oil. *Int J Toxicol* 2001;20:31-9.

9882 The Medicines Control Agency (MCA), Epogam and Efamast (gamolenic acid) - withdrawal of marketing authorizations. http://www.mca.gov.uk/whatsnew/epogam.htm. (Accessed 2 June 2003).

9883 Moro GE, Warm A, Arslanoglu S, Miniello V. Management of bovine protein allergy: new perspectives and nutritional aspects. *Ann Allergy Asthma Immunol* 2002;89:91-6.

9885 Georges B, Galland S, Rigault C, et al. Beneficial effects of L-carnitine in myoblastic C2C12 cells. Interaction with zidovudine. *Biochem Pharmacol* 2003;65:1483-8.

9890 Hodgson JM, Watts GF, Playford DA, et al. Coenzyme Q10 improves blood pressure and glycaemic control: a controlled trial in subjects with type 2 diabetes. *Eur J Clin Nutr* 2002;56:1137-42.

9891 McGowan JD, Altman RE, Kanto WP Jr. Neonatal withdrawal symptoms after chronic maternal ingestion of caffeine. *South Med J* 1988;81:1092-4.

9892 Nehlig A, Debry G. Consequences on the newborn of chronic maternal consumption of coffee during gestation and lactation: a review. *J Am Coll Nutr* 1994;13:6-21.

9893 Cropley M, Cave Z, Ellis J, Middleton RW. Effect of kava and valerian on human physiological and psychological responses to mental stress assessed under laboratory conditions. *Phytother Res* 2002;16:23-7.

9894 Hadley S, Petry JJ. Valerian. *Am Fam Physician* 2003;67:1755-8.

9895 Kohnen R, Oswald WD. The effects of valerian, propranolol, and their combination on activation, performance and mood of healthy volunteers under social stress conditions. *Pharmacopsychiatry* 1988;21:447-8.

9896 Andreatini R, Sartori VA, Seabra ML, Leite JR. Effect of valepotriates (valerian extract) in generalized anxiety disorder: a randomized placebo-controlled pilot study. *Phytother Res* 2002;16:650-4.

9898 Kallio H, Yang B, Peippo P. Effects of different origins and harvesting time on vitamin C, tocopherols, and tocotrienols in sea buckthorn (Hippophae rhamnoides) berries. *J Agric Food Chem* 2002;50:6136-42.

9899 Warburton DM, Bersellini E, Sweeney E. An evaluation of a caffeinated taurine drink on mood, memory and information processing in healthy volunteers without caffeine abstinence. *Psychopharmacology* (Berl) 2001;158:322-8.

9900 Huxtable R, Bressler R. Elevation of taurine in human congestive heart failure. *Life Sci* 1974;14:1353-9.

9901 Eros E, Geher P, Gomor B, Czeizel AE. Epileptogenic activity of folic acid after drug induces SLE (folic acid and epilepsy). *Eur J Obstet Gynecol Reprod Biol* 1998;80:75-78.

9903 Tsitsimpikou C, Tsamis GD, Siskos PA, et al. Study of excretion of ecdysterone in human urine. *Rapid Commun Mass Spectrom* 2001;15:1796-801.

9904 Chermnykh NS, Shimanovskii NL, Shutko GV, Syrov VN. [The action of methandrostenolone and ecdysterone on the physical endurance of animals and on protein metabolism in the skeletal muscles]. [Article in Russian]. *Farmakol Toksikol* 1988;51:57-60.

9905 Syrov VN, Kurmukov AG. [Anabolic activity of phytoecdysone-ecdysterone isolated from Rhaponticum carthamoides (Willd.) Iljin]. [Article in Russian] *Farmakol Toksikol* 1976;39:690-3.

9906 Hackbert L, Heiman JR. Acute dehydroepiandrosterone (DHEA) effects on sexual arousal in postmenopausal women. *J Womens Health Gend Based Med* 2002;11:155-62.

9916 Burke GL, Legault C, Anthony M, et al. Soy protein and isoflavone effects on vasomotor symptoms in peri- and postmenopausal women: the Soy Estrogen Alternative Study. *Menopause* 2003;10:147-53.

9917 Balk JL, Whiteside DA, Naus G, et al. A pilot study of the effects of phytoestrogen supplementation on postmenopausal endometrium. *J Soc Gynecol Investig* 2002;9:238-42.

9919 Jenkins DJ, Kendall CW, Connelly PW, et al. Effects of high- and low-isoflavone (phytoestrogen) soy foods on inflammatory biomarkers and proinflammatory cytokines in middle-aged men and women. *Metabolism* 2002;51:919-24.

9920 Garner LF, Klinger JD. Some visual effects caused by the beverage kava. *J Ethnopharmacol* 1985;13:307-311.

9921 Denham A, McIntyre M, Whitehouse J. Kava--the unfolding story: report on a work-in-progress. *J Altern Complement Med* 2002;8:237-263.

9923 Baum SS, Hill R, Rommelspacher H. Effect of kava extract and individual kavapyrones on neurotransmitter levels in the nucleus accumbens of rats. *Prog Neuropsychopharmacol Biol Psychiatry* 1998;22:1105-1120.

9924 Singh YN. Effects of kava on neuromuscular transmission and muscle contractility. *J Ethnopharmacol* 1983;7:267-76.

9925 National Academy of Science. Lost Crops of the Incas Little-Known Plants of the Andes with Promise for Worldwide Cultivation (1989). Available at: http://books.nap.edu/books/030904264X/html/57.html.

9926 Ganzera M, Zhao J, Muhammad I, Khan IA. Chemical profiling and standardization of Lepidium meyenii (Maca) by reversed phase high performance liquid chromatography. *Chem Pharm Bull* (Tokyo) 2002;50:988-99.

9927 Piacente S, Carbone V, Plaza A, et al. Investigation of the tuber constituents of maca (Lepidium meyenii Walp.). *J Agric Food Chem* 2002;50:5621-25.

9928 Gonzales GF, Cordova A, Vega K, et al. Effect of Lepidium meyenii (MACA) on sexual desire and its absent relationship with serum testosterone levels in adult healthy men. *Andrologia* 2002;34:367-72.

9929 Li G, Ammermann U, Quiros CF. Gluconsinolate contents in Maca (Lepidium peruvianum Chacon) seeds, sprouts, mature plants, and several derived commercial products. *Economic Botany* 2001;55:255-62.

9930 Terano T, Hirai A, Hamazaki T, et al. Effect of oral administration of highly purified eicosapentaenoic acid on platelet function, blood viscosity and red cell deformability in healthy human subjects. *Atherosclerosis* 1983;46:321-31.

9931 Aquilani R, Iadarola P, Boschi F, et al. Reduced plasma levels of tyrosine, precursor of brain catecholamines, and of essential amino acids in patients with severe traumatic brain injury after rehabilitation. *Arch Phys Med Rehabil* 2003;84:1258-65.

9932 Vanscheidt W, Jost V, Wolna P, et al. Efficacy and safety of a Butcher's broom preparation (Ruscus aculeatus L. extract) compared to placebo in patients suffering from chronic venous insufficiency. *Arzneimittelforschung* 2002;52:243-250.

9933 Goldman LS, Genel M, Bezman RJ, Slanetz PJ. Diagnosis and treatment of attention-deficit/hyperactivity disorder in children and adolescents. Council on Scientific Affairs, American Medical Association. *JAMA* 1998;279:1100-7.

9934 Anon. Clinical practice guideline: diagnosis and evaluation of the child with attention-deficit/hyperactivity disorder. American Academy of Pediatrics. *Pediatrics* 2000;105:1158-70.

9935 Wender PH, Wolf LE, Wasserstein J. Adults with ADHD. An overview. *Ann N Y Acad Sci* 2001;931:1-16.

9936 Leibson CL, Katusic SK, Barbaresi WJ, et al. Use and costs of medical care for children and adolescents with and without attention-deficit/hyperactivity disorder. *JAMA* 2001;285:60-6.

9937 Milberger S, Biederman J, Faraone SV, et al. Is maternal smoking during pregnancy a risk factor for attention deficit hyperactivity disorder in children? *Am J Psychiatry* 1996;153:1138-42.

9938 Oades RD. Dopamine may be 'hyper' with respect to noradrenaline metabolism, but 'hypo' with respect to serotonin metabolism in children with attention-deficit hyperactivity disorder. *Behav Brain Res* 2002;130:97-102.

9939 No authors listed. Moderators and mediators of treatment response for children with attention-deficit/hyperactivity disorder: the Multimodal Treatment Study of children with Attention-deficit/hyperactivity disorder. *Arch Gen Psychiatry* 1999;56:1088-96.

9940 Jensen PS, Hinshaw SP, Swanson JM, et al. Findings from the NIMH Multimodal Treatment Study of ADHD (MTA): implications and applications for primary care providers. *J Dev Behav Pediatr* 2001;22:60-73.

9941 Anon. Clinical practice guideline: treatment of the school-aged child with attention-deficit/hyperactivity disorder. American Academy of Pediatrics. *Pediatrics* 2001;108:1033-44.

9942 Greenhill LL, Pliszka S, Dulcan MK, et al. Practice parameter for the use of stimulant medications in the treatment of children, adolescents, and adults. *J Am Acad Child Adolesc Psychiatry* 2002;41:26S-49S.

9943 Biederman J, Faraone SV, Monuteaux MC, et al. Growth deficits and attention-deficit/hyperactivity disorder revisited: impact of gender, development, and treatment. *Pediatrics* 2003;111:1010-6.

9944 Szymanski ML, Zolotor A. Attention-deficit/hyperactivity disorder: management. *Am Fam Physician* 2001;64:1355-62.

9945 Kehoe, WA. Atomoxetine (Strattera). *Pharmacist's Letter/Prescriber's Letter* 2003;19:190102

9946 Chan E, Rappaport LA, Kemper KJ. Complementary and alternative therapies in childhood attention and hyperactivity problems. *J Dev Behav Pediatr* 2003;24:4-8.

9948 Bornstein RA, Baker GB, Carroll A, et al. Plasma amino acids in attention deficit disorder. *Psychiatry Res* 1990;33:301-6.

9949 Baker GB, Bornstein RA, Rouget AC, et al. Phenylethylaminergic mechanisms in attention-deficit disorder. *Biol Psychiatry* 1991;29:15-22.

9950 Zametkin AJ, Karoum F, Rapoport JL. Treatment of hyperactive children with D-phenylalanine. *Am J Psychiatry* 1987;144:792-4.

9951 Wood DR, Reimherr FW, Wender PH. Treatment of attention deficit disorder with DL-phenylalanine. *Psychiatry Res* 1985;16:21-6.

9952 Ghose K. l-Tryptophan in hyperactive child syndrome associated with epilepsy: a controlled study. *Neuropsychobiology* 1983;10:111-4.

9954 Jellin JM, Gregory P, Batz F, Hitchens K, et al. *Pharmacist's Letter/Prescriber's Letter* Natural Medicines Comprehensive Database. Stockton, CA: Therapeutic Research Faculty; 2003. www.naturaldatabase.com (Accessed 9 July 2003).

9955 Mitchell EA, Aman MG, Turbott SH, Manku M. Clinical characteristics and serum essential fatty acid levels in hyperactive children. *Clin Pediatr* (Phila) 1987;26:406-11.

9956 Torrioli MG, Vernacotola S, Mariotti P, et al. Double-blind, placebo-controlled study of L-acetylcarnitine for the treatment of hyperactive behavior in fragile X syndrome. *Am J Med Genet* 1999;87:366-8.

9957 Haslam RH, Dalby JT, Rademaker AW. Effects of megavitamin therapy on children with attention deficit disorders. *Pediatrics* 1984;74:103-11.

9958 Arnold LE, Christopher J, Huestis RD, Smeltzer DJ. Megavitamins for minimal brain dysfunction. A placebo-controlled study. *JAMA* 1978;240:2642-43.

9959 Kershner J, Hawke W. Megavitamins and learning disorders: a controlled double-blind experiment. *J Nutr* 1979;109:819-26.

9960 Brenner A. The effects of megadoses of selected B complex vitamins on children with hyperkinesis: controlled studies with long-term follow-up. *J Learn Disabil* 1982;15:258-64.

9962 Beard J. Iron deficiency alters brain development and functioning. *J Nutr* 2003;133:1468S-72S.

9965 Bekaroglu M, Aslan Y, Gedik Y, et al. Relationships between serum free fatty acids and zinc, and attention deficit hyperactivity disorder: a research note. *J Child Psychol Psychiatry* 1996;37:225-7.

REFERENCES

9966 Toren P, Eldar S, Sela BA, et al. Zinc deficiency in attention-deficit hyperactivity disorder. *Biol Psychiatry* 1996;40:1308-10.

9967 Arnold LE, Votolato NA, Kleykamp D, et al. Does hair zinc predict amphetamine improvement of ADD/hyperactivity? *Int J Neurosci* 1990;50:103-7.

9969 Kozielec T, Starobrat-Hermelin B. Assessment of magnesium levels in children with attention deficit hyperactivity disorder (ADHD). *Magnes Res* 1997;10:143-8.

9970 Agricultural Research Service- Germplasm Resources Information Network. "Botanicals Generally Recognized As Safe" http://www.ars-grin.gov/duke/syllabus/gras.htm (Accessed 10 July 2003).

9972 Cala S, Crismon ML, Baumgartner J. A survey of herbal use in children with attention-deficit-hyperactivity disorder or depression. *Pharmacotherapy* 2003;23:222-30.

9973 Wolraich ML, Wilson DB, White JW. The effect of sugar on behavior or cognition in children. A meta-analysis. *JAMA* 1995;274:1617-21.

9974 Wolraich ML, Lindgren SD, Stumbo PJ, et al. Effects of diets high in sucrose or aspartame on the behavior and cognitive performance of children. *N Engl J Med* 1994;330:301-7.

9975 Milich R, Pelham WE. Effects of sugar ingestion on the classroom and playground behavior of attention deficit disordered boys. *J Consult Clin Psychol* 1986;54:714-8.

9976 Wolraich M, Milich R, Stumbo P, Schultz F. Effects of sucrose ingestion on the behavior of hyperactive boys. *J Pediatr* 1985;106:675-82.

9977 Dosreis S, Zito JM, Safer DJ, et al. Parental perceptions and satisfaction with stimulant medication for attention-deficit hyperactivity disorder. *J Dev Behav Pediatr* 2003;24:155-62.

9978 Barkley RA, Fischer M, Smallish L, Fletcher K. Does the treatment of attention-deficit/hyperactivity disorder with stimulants contribute to drug use/abuse? A 13-year prospective study. *Pediatrics* 2003;111:97-109.

9979 Wilens TE, Faraone SV, Biederman J, Gunawardene S. Does stimulant therapy of attention-deficit/hyperactivity disorder beget later substance abuse? A meta-analytic review of the literature. *Pediatrics* 2003;111:179-85.

9980 Tjon Pian Gi CV, Broeren JP, Starreveld JS, A Versteegh FG. Melatonin for treatment of sleeping disorders in children with attention deficit/hyperactivity disorder: a preliminary open label study. *Eur J Pediatr* 2003;162:554-5.

9981 Shekim WO, Antun F, Hanna GL, et al. S-adenosyl-L-methionine (SAM) in adults with ADHD, RS: preliminary results from an open trial. *Psychopharmacol Bull* 1990;26:249-53.

9984 Tenenbaum S, Paull JC, Sparrow EP, et al. An experimental comparison of Pycnogenol and methylphenidate in adults with Attention-Deficit/Hyperactivity Disorder (ADHD). *J Atten Disord* 2002;6:49-60.

9985 Yim TK, Wu WK, Pak WF, et al. Myocardial protection against ischaemia-reperfusion injury by a Polygonum multiflorum extract supplemented 'Dang-Gui decoction for enriching blood', a compound formulation, ex vivo. *Phytother Res* May;14:195-9.

9986 Ho SC, Tai ES, Eng PH, et al. In the absence of dietary surveillance, chitosan does not reduce plasma lipids or obesity in hypercholesterolaemic obese Asian subjects. *Singapore Med J* 2001;42:6-10.

9987 Guerciolini R, Radu-Radulescu L, Boldrin M, et al. Comparative evaluation of fecal fat excretion induced by orlistat and chitosan. *Obes Res* 2001;9:364-7.

9988 Milewicz A, Gejdel E, Sworen H, et al. [Vitex agnus castus extract in the treatment of luteal phase defects due to latent hyperprolactinemia. Results of a randomized placebo-controlled double-blind study]. [Article in German]. *Arzneimittelforschung* 1993;43:752-6.

9990 Dixon-Shanies D, Shaikh N. Growth inhibition of human breast cancer cells by herbs and phytoestrogens. *Oncol Rep* 1999;6:1383-7.

9991 Ohyama K, Akaike T, Hirobe C, Yamakawa T. Cytotoxicity and apoptotic inducibility of Vitex agnus-castus fruit extract in cultured human normal and cancer cells and effect on growth. *Biol Pharm Bull* 2003;26:10-18.

9993 Akhondzadeh S, Noroozian M, Mohammadi M, et al. Melissa officinalis extract in the treatment of patients with mild to moderate Alzheimer's disease: a double blind, randomised, placebo controlled trial. *J Neurol Neurosurg Psychiatry* 2003;74:863-6.

9994 Kennedy DO, Scholey AB, Tildesley NT, et al. Modulation of mood and cognitive performance following acute administration of Melissa officinalis (lemon balm). *Pharmacol Biochem Behav* 2002;72:953-64.

9995 Koytchev R, Alken RG, Dundarov S. Balm mint extract (Lo-701) for topical treatment of recurring herpes labialis. *Phytomedicine* 1999;6:225-30.

9996 Beck V, Unterrieder E, Krenn L, et al. Comparison of hormonal activity (estrogen, androgen and progestin) of standardized plant extracts for large scale use in hormone replacement therapy. *J Steroid Biochem Mol Biol* 2003;84:259-68.

9997 Dog TL, Powell KL, Weisman SM. Critical evaluation of the safety of Cimicifuga racemosa in menopause symptom relief. *Menopause* 2003;10:299-313.

9998 Liu J, Burdette JE, Xu H, et al. Evaluation of estrogenic activity of plant extracts for the potential treatment of menopausal symptoms. *J Agric Food Chem* 2001;49:2472-9.

9999 Davis VL, Jayo MJ, Hardy ML, et al. Effects of black cohosh on mammary tumor development and progression in MMTV-neu transgenic mice. 94th Annual Meeting of the American Association for Cancer Research, Washington, DC. July 11-14, 2003;abstract R910.

10000 Rockwell S, Fajolu O, Liu Y, et al. The herbal medicine black cohosh alters the response of breast cancer cells to some agents used in cancer therapy. Annual Meeting of the American Association for Cancer Research, Washington, DC. July 11-14, 2003;abstract 2721.

10002 Tallia AF, Cardone DA. Asthma exacerbation associated with glucosamine-chondroitin supplement. *J Am Board Fam Pract* 2002;15:481-4.

10003 Dulloo AG, Miller DS. Ephedrine, caffeine and aspirin: "over-the-counter" drugs that interact to stimulate thermogenesis in the obese. *Nutrition* 1989;5:7-9.

10004 Kalman D, Incledon T, Gaunaurd I, et al. An acute clinical trial evaluating the cardiovascular effects of an herbal ephedra-caffeine weight loss product in healthy overweight adults. *Int J Obes* 2002;26:1363-66.

10005 Schweinfurth J, Pribitkin E. Sudden hearing loss associated with ephedra use. *Am J Health Syst Pharm* 2003;60:375-7.

10006 Lemaitre RN, King IB, Mozaffarian D, et al. n-3 Polyunsaturated fatty acids, fatal ischemic heart disease, and nonfatal myocardial infarction in older adults: the Cardiovascular Health Study. *Am J Clin Nutr* 2003;77:319-25.

10007 Kris-Etherton PM, Harris WS, Appel LJ, et al. Fish consumption, fish oil, omega-3 fatty acids, and cardiovascular disease. *Circulation* 2002;106:2747-57.

10008 Bruera E, Strasser F, Palmer JL, et al. Effect of fish oil on appetite and other symptoms in patients with advanced cancer and anorexia/cachexia: a double-blind, placebo-controlled study. *J Clin Oncol* 2003;21:129-34.

10009 Koh KJ, Pearce AL, Marshman G, et al. Tea tree oil reduces histamine-induced skin inflammation. *Br J Dermatol* 2002;147:1212-7.
10010 Jacobs MR, Hornfeldt CS. Melaleuca oil poisoning. *J Toxicol Clin Toxicol* 1994;32:461-4.
10011 Elliott C. Tea tree oil poisoning. *Med J Aust* 1993;159:830-1.
10012 Carson CF, Riley TV. The antimicrobial activity of tea tree oil. *Med J Aust* 1994;160:236.
10013 Carson CF, Riley TV. Toxicity of the essential oil of Melaleuca alternifolia or tea tree oil. *J Toxicol Clin Toxicol* 1995;33:193-4.
10014 Carson CF, Cookson BD, Farrelly HD, Riley TV. Susceptibility of methicillin-resistant Staphylococcus aureus to the essential oil of Melaleuca alternifolia. *J Antimicrob Chemother* 1995;35:421-4.
10015 Knight TE, Hausen BM. Melaleuca oil (tea tree oil) dermatitis. *J Am Acad Dermatol* 1994;30:423-7.
10016 Moss A. Tea tree oil poisoning. *Med J Aust* 1994;160:236.
10017 Blackwell AL. Tea tree oil and anaerobic (bacterial) vaginosis. *Lancet* 1991;337:300.
10018 Kahela P, Anttila M, Tikkanen R, Sundquist H. Effect of food, food constituents and fluid volume on the bioavailability of sotalol. *Acta Pharmacol Toxicol* (Copenh) 1979;44:7-12.
10019 Eastwood GL. Pharmacologic prevention of colonic neoplasms. Effects of calcium, vitamins, omega fatty acids, and nonsteroidal anti-inflammatory drugs. *Dig Dis* 1996;14:119-28.
10020 Gades MD, Stern JS. Chitosan supplementation does not affect fat absorption in healthy males fed a high-fat diet, a pilot study. *Int J Obes* 2002;26:119-22.
10021 Thanou M, Verhoef JC, Junginger HE. Oral drug absorption enhancement by chitosan and its derivatives. *Adv Drug Deliv Rev* 2001;52:117-26.
10022 Colombo P, Sciutto AM. Nutritional aspects of chitosan employment in hypocaloric diet. *Acta Toxicol Ther* 1996;17:287-302.
10023 Macchi G. A new approach to the treatment of obesity: Chitosan's effects on body weight reduction and plasma cholesterol levels. *Acta Toxicol Ther* 1996;17:303-320.
10024 Sciutto AM, Colombo P. Lipid-lowering effect of Chitosan dietary integrator and hypocaloric diet in obese subjects. *Acta Toxicol Ther* 1995;16:215-29.
10025 Veneroni G, Veneroni F, Contos S, et al. Effect of a new chitosan dietary integrator and hypocaloric diet on hyperlipidemia and overweight in obese patients. *Acta Toxicol Ther* 1996;17:53-70.
10026 Hammer KA, Carson CF, Riley TV. Susceptibility of transient and commensal skin flora to the essential oil of Melaleuca alternifolia (tea tree oil). *Am J Infect Control* 1996;24:186-9.
10027 Chan CH, Loudon KW. Activity of tea tree oil on methicillin-resistant Staphylococcus aureus (MRSA). *J Hosp Infect* 1998;39:244-5.
10028 Cox SD, Mann CM, Markham JL, et al. The mode of antimicrobial action of the essential oil of Melaleuca alternifolia (tea tree oil). *J Appl Microbiol* 2000;88:170-5.
10029 Bruynzeel DP. Contact dermatitis due to tea tree oil. *Trop Med Int Health* 1999;4:630.
10030 Greig JE, Thoo SL, Carson CF, Riley TV. Allergic contact dermatitis following use of a tea tree oil hand-wash not due to tea tree oil. *Contact Dermatitis* 1999;41:354-5.
10031 Varma S, Blackford S, Statham BN, Blackwell A. Combined contact allergy to tea tree oil and lavender oil complicating chronic vulvovaginitis. *Contact Dermatitis* 2000;42:309-10.
10032 Khanna M, Qasem K, Sasseville D. Allergic contact dermatitis to tea tree oil with erythema multiforme-like id reaction. *Am J Contact Dermat* 2000;11:238-42.
10033 Satchell AC, Saurajen A, Bell C, Barnetson RS. Treatment of interdigital tinea pedis with 25% and 50% tea tree oil solution: a randomized, placebo-controlled, blinded study. *Australas J Dermatol* 2002;43:175-8.
10034 Lin CH, Chen TJ, Hsieh YL, et al. Kinetics of germanium dioxide in rats. *Toxicology* 1999;132:147-53.
10035 Budman DR, Schulman P, Vinciguerra V, Degnan TJ. Phase I trial of spirogermanium given by infusion in a multiple-dose schedule. *Cancer Treat Rep* 1982;66:173-5.
10037 Mainwaring MG, Poor C, Zander DS, Harman E. Complete remission of pulmonary spindle cell carcinoma after treatment with oral germanium sesquioxide. *Chest* 2000;117:591-3.
10038 Vogelzang NJ, Gesme DH, Kennedy BJ. A phase II study of spirogermanium in advanced human malignancy. *Am J Clin Oncol* 1985;8:341-4.
10039 Ettinger DS, Finkelstein DM, Donehower RC, et al. Phase II study of N-methylformamide, spirogermanium, and 4-demethoxydaunorubicin in the treatment of non-small cell lung cancer (EST 3583): an Eastern Cooperative Oncology Group study. *Med Pediatr Oncol* 1989;17:197-201.
10040 Higuchi I, Izumo S, Kuriyama M, et al. Germanium myopathy: clinical and experimental pathological studies. *Acta Neuropathol* (Berl) 1989;79:300-4.
10041 Matsusaka T, Fujii M, Nakano T, et al. Germanium-induced nephropathy: report of two cases and review of the literature. *Clin Nephrol* 1988;30:341-5.
10042 Hess B, Raisin J, Zimmermann A, et al. Tubulointerstitial nephropathy persisting 20 months after discontinuation of chronic intake of germanium lactate citrate. *Am J Kidney Dis* 1993;21:548-52.
10043 Luck BE, Mann H, Melzer H, et al. Renal and other organ failure caused by germanium intoxication. *Nephrol Dial Transplant* 1999;14:2464-8.
10044 Schauss AG. Nephrotoxicity and neurotoxicity in humans from organogermanium compounds and germanium dioxide. *Biol Trace Elem Res* 1991;29:267-80.
10045 Yanagisawa H, Yamazaki N, Sato G, Wada O. L-Arginine treatment may prevent tubulointerstitial nephropathy caused by germanium dioxide. *Kidney Int* 2000;57:2275-84.
10046 Yang MK, Kim YG. Protective role of germanium-132 against paraquat-induced oxidative stress in the livers of senescence-accelerated mice. *J Toxicol Environ Health A* 1999;58:289-97.
10047 Peng X, Lingxia Z, Schrauzer GN, Xiong G. Selenium, boron, and germanium deficiency in the etiology of Kashin-Beck disease. *Biol Trace Elem Res* 2000;77:193-7.
10048 Goodman S. Therapeutic effects of organic germanium. *Med Hypotheses* 1988;26:207-15.
10049 Schein PS, Slavik M, Smythe T, et al. Phase I clinical trial of spirogermanium. *Cancer Treat Rep* 1980;64:1051-6.
10050 Trope C, Mattsson W, Gynning I, et al. Phase II study of spirogermanium in advanced ovarian malignancy. *Cancer Treat Rep* 1981;65:119-20.
10051 Gerber GB, Leonard A. Mutagenicity, carcinogenicity and teratogenicity of germanium compounds. *Mutat Res* 1997;387:141-6.
10052 Asaka T, Nitta E, Makifuchi T, et al. Germanium intoxication with sensory ataxia. *J Neurol Sci* 1995;130:220-3.
10053 Wendakoon CN, Thomson AB, Ozimek L. Lack of therapeutic effect of a specially designed yogurt for the eradication of Helicobacter pylori infection. *Digestion* 2002;65:16-20.
10054 Zhu DP. Dong Quai. *Am J Chin Med* 1987;15:117-25.

REFERENCES

10055 Consumer Alert: FDA Plans Regulation Prohibiting Sale of Ephedra-Containing Dietary Supplements and Advises Consumers to Stop Using These Products. December 30, 2003. Available at: http://www.fda.gov/oc/initiatives/ephedra/december2003/advisory.html.

10056 Choy YM, Leung KN, Cho CS, et al. Immunopharmacological studies of low molecular weight polysaccharide from Angelica sinensis. *Am J Chin Med* 1994;22:137-45.

10057 Hoult JR, Paya M. Pharmacological and biochemical actions of simple coumarins: natural products with therapeutic potential. *Gen Pharmacol* 1996;27:713-22.

10058 Stough C, Lloyd J, Clarke J, et al. The chronic effects of an extract of Bacopa monniera (Brahmi) on cognitive function in healthy human subjects. *Psychopharmacology* 2001;156:481-4.

10059 Yadav SK, Jain AK, Tripathi SN, Gupta JP. Irritable bowel syndrome: therapeutic evaluation of indigenous drugs. *Indian J Med Res* 1989;90:496-503.

10060 Samiulla DS, Prashanth D, Amit A. Mast cell stabilising activity of Bacopa monnieri. *Fitoterapia* 2001;72:284-5.

10061 Kidd PM. A review of nutrients and botanicals in the integrative management of cognitive dysfunction. *Altern Med Rev* 1999 Jun;4(3):144-61.

10062 Jowko E, Ostaszewski P, Jank M, et al. Creatine and beta-hydroxy-beta-methylbutyrate (HMB) additively increase lean body mass and muscle strength during a weight-training program. *Nutrition* 2001;17:558-66.

10063 Green AL, Simpson EJ, Littlewood JJ, et al. Carbohydrate ingestion augments creatine retention during creatine feeding in humans. *Acta Physiol Scand* 1996;158:195-202.

10064 Preen D, Dawson B, Goodman C, et al. Effect of creatine loading on long-term sprint exercise performance and metabolism. *Med Sci Sports Exerc* 2001;33:814-21.

10065 Persky AM, Muller M, Derendorf H, et al. Single- and multiple-dose pharmacokinetics of oral creatine. *J Clin Pharmacol* 2003;43:29-37.

10066 Williams M, Jarvis MF. Purinergic and pyrimidinergic receptors as potential drug targets. *Biochem Pharmacol* 2000;59:1173-85.

10067 Sklar SH, Alexander EJ, Blue WT, Bodian CA. Herpes zoster: adenosine monophosphate for the prevention of post-neuralgia. *JAMA* 1985;254:912.

10068 Beltramino R, Penenory A, Buceta AM. An open-label, randomized multicenter study comparing the efficacy and safety of Cyclo 3 Fort versus hydroxyethyl rutoside in chronic venous lymphatic insufficiency. *Angiology* 2000;51:535-44.

10069 Redman DA. Ruscus aculeatus (butcher's broom) as a potential treatment for orthostatic hypotension, with a case report. *J Altern Complement Med* 2000;6:539-49.

10070 Cappelli R, Nicora M, Di Perri T. Use of extract of Ruscus aculeatus in venous disease in the lower limbs. *Drugs Exp Clin Res* 1988;14:277-83.

10071 Ivie GW, Holt DL, Ivey MC. Natural toxicants in human foods: psoralens in raw and cooked parsnip root. *Science* 1981;213:909-10.

10072 Sanai T, Okuda S, Onoyama K, et al. Germanium dioxide-induced nephropathy: a new type of renal disease. *Nephron* 1990;54:53-60.

10073 Krapf R, Schaffner T, Iten PX. Abuse of germanium associated with fatal lactic acidosis. *Nephron* 1992;62:351-6.

10074 Takeuchi A, Yoshizawa N, Oshima S, et al. Nephrotoxicity of germanium compounds: report of a case and review of the literature. *Nephron* 1992;60:436-42.

10075 May B, Kohler S, Schneider B. Efficacy and tolerability of a fixed combination of peppermint oil and caraway oil in patients suffering from functional dyspepsia. *Aliment Pharmacol Ther* 2000;14:1671-7.

10076 Biagiotti G, Cavallini G. Acetyl-L-carnitine vs tamoxifen in the oral therapy of Peyronie's disease: a preliminary report. *BJU Int* 2001;88:63-7.

10077 Aviram M, Brox J, Nordoy A. Effects of postprandial plasma and chylomicrons on endothelial cells. Differences between dietary cream and cod liver oil. *Acta Med Scand* 1986;219:341-8.

10078 Sidransky H. Tryptophan and carcinogenesis: review and update on how tryptophan may act. *Nutr Cancer* 1997;29:181-94

10079 Knoll Pharmaceutical Company. Meridia package insert. 2000. Mt. Olive, NJ USA.

10080 Hansen JB, Olsen JO, Wilsgard L, Osterud B. Effects of dietary supplementation with cod liver oil on monocyte thromboplastin synthesis, coagulation and fibrinolysis. *J Intern Med Suppl* 1989;225:133-9.

10081 al-Meshal MA, Lutfi KM, Tariq M. Cod liver oil inhibits indomethacin induced gastropathy without affecting its bioavailability and pharmacological activity. *Life Sci* 1991;48:1401-9.

10082 Landymore RW, MacAulay MA, Cooper JH, Sheridan BL. Effects of cod-liver oil on intimal hyperplasia in vein grafts used for arterial bypass. *Can J Surg* 1986;29:129-31.

10083 Brox JH, Killie JE, Osterud B, et al. Effects of cod liver oil on platelets and coagulation in familial hypercholesterolemia (type IIa). *Acta Med Scand* 1983;213:137-44.

10084 Johnson KL, Klarskov K, Benson LM, et al. Presence of peak X and related compounds: the reported contaminant in case related 5-hydroxy-L-tryptophan associated with eosinophilia-myalgia syndrome. *J Rheumatol* 1999;26:2714-7.

10085 Greenberg AS, Takagi H, Hill RH, et al. Delayed onset of skin fibrosis after the ingestion of eosinophilia-myalgia syndrome-associated L-tryptophan. *J Am Acad Dermatol.* 1996;35:264-6.

10086 Hallert C, Kaldma M, Petersson BG. Ispaghula husk may relieve gastrointestinal symptoms in ulcerative colitis in remission. *Scand J Gastroenterol* 1991;26:747-50.

10087 Adachi J, Asano M, Ueno Y. Tetrahydro-beta-carboline-3-carboxylic acids and contaminants of L-tryptophan. *J Chromatogr A* 2000;881:501-15.

10088 McRorie JW, Daggy BP, Morel JG, et al. Psyllium is superior to docusate sodium for treatment of chronic constipation. *Aliment Pharmacol Ther* 1998;12:491-7.

10089 Rossander L. Effect of dietary fiber on iron absorption in man. *Scand J Gastroenterol Suppl* 1987;129:68-72.

10090 Ejderhamn J, Hedenborg G, Strandvik B. Long-term double-blind study on the influence of dietary fibres on faecal bile acid excretion in juvenile ulcerative colitis. *Scand J Clin Lab Invest* 1992;52:697-706.

10091 Frati Munari AC, Benitez Pinto W, Raul Ariza Andraca C, Casarrubias M. Lowering glycemic index of food by acarbose and Plantago psyllium mucilage. *Arch Med Res* 1998;29:137-41.

10092 Ashraf W, Pfeiffer RF, Park F, et al. Constipation in Parkinson's disease: objective assessment and response to psyllium. *Mov Disord* 1997;12:946-51.

10093 DiPalma JA, Brady CE. Steakhouse spasm. *J Clin Gastroenterol* 1987;9:274-8.

10094 Roe DA, Kalkwarf H, Stevens J. Effect of fiber supplements on the apparent absorption of pharmacological doses of riboflavin. *J Am Diet Assoc* 1988;88:211-3.

10095 Anderson JW, Zettwoch N, Feldman T, et al. Cholesterol-lowering effects of psyllium hydrophilic mucilloid for hypercholesterolemic men. *Arch Intern Med* 1988;148:292-6.

10096 Marteau P, Flourie B, Cherbut C, et al. Digestibility and bulking effect of ispaghula husks in healthy humans. *Gut* 1994;35:1747-52.

10097 Strommen GL, Dorworth TE, Walker PR, et al. Treatment of suspected postcholecystectomy diarrhea with psyllium hydrophilic mucilloid. *Clin Pharm* 1990;9:206-8.

10098 Nordstrom M, Melander A, Robertsson E, Steen B. Influence of wheat bran and of a bulk-forming ispaghula cathartic on the bioavailability of digoxin in geriatric in-patients. *Drug Nutr Interact* 1987;5:67-9.

10099 Rodriguez-Moran M, Guerrero-Romero F, Lazcano-Burciaga G. Lipid- and glucose-lowering efficacy of Plantago Psyllium in type II diabetes. *J Diabetes Complications* 1998;12:273-8.

10101 Erbagci Z, Akcali C. Biweekly serial glycolic acid peels vs. long-term daily use of topical low-strength glycolic acid in the treatment of atrophic acne scars. *Int J Dermatol* 2000;39(10):789-94.

10102 Javaheri SM, Handa S, Kaur I, Kumar B. Safety and efficacy of glycolic acid facial peel in Indian women and melasma. *Int J Dermatol* 2001;40:354-7.

10103 Ghadishah D, Gorchynski J. Airway compromise after routine alpha-hydroxy facial peel administration. *J Emerg Med* 2002;22(4):353-5.

10104 Van Scott EJ, Yu RJ. Hyperkeratinization, corneocyte cohesion, and alpha hydroxy acids. *J Am Acad Dermatol* 1984;11(5Pt1):867-79.

10105 Hutson SM, Harris RA. Introduction. Symposium: Leucine as a nutritional signal. *J Nutr* 2001;131:839S-40S.

10106 Harris RA, Kobayashi R, Murakami T, Shimomura Y. Regulation of branched-chain alpha-keto acid dehydrogenase kinase expression in rat liver. *J Nutr* 2001;131:841S-5S.

10107 Hutson SM, Lieth E, LaNoue KF. Function of leucine in excitatory neurotransmitter metabolism in the central nervous system. *J Nutr* 2001;131:846S-50S.

10108 Anthony JC, Anthony TG, Kimball SR, Jefferson LS. Signaling pathways involved in translational control of protein synthesis in skeletal muscle by leucine. *J Nutr* 2001;131:856S-60S.

10109 Lynch CJ. Role of leucine in the regulation of mTOR by amino acids: revelations from structure-activity studies. *J Nutr* 2001;131:861S-5S.

10110 Kimball SR, Jefferson LS. Control of protein synthesis by amino acid availability. *Curr Opin Clin Nutr Metab Care* 2002;5:63-7.

10111 Lynch CJ, Hutson SM, Patson BJ, et al. Tissue-specific effects of chronic dietary leucine and norleucine supplementation on protein synthesis in rats. *Am J Physiol Endocrinol Metab* 2002; 283:E824-35.

10112 Proud CG. Regulation of mammalian translation factors by nutrients. *Eur J Biochem* 2002;269:5338-49.

10113 Anthony JC, Lang CH, Crozier SJ, et al. Contribution of insulin to the translational control of protein synthesis in skeletal muscle by leucine. *Am J Physiol Endocrinol Metab* 282:E1092-101.

10114 Kimball SR, Farrell PA, Jefferson LS. Invited review: Role of insulin in translational control of protein synthesis in skeletal muscle by amino acids or excercise. *J Appl Physiol* 2002;93:1168-80.

10115 Gietzen DW, Magrum LJ. Molecular mechanisms in the brain involved in the anorexia of branced-chain amino acid deficiency. *J Nutr* 2001;131:851S-5S.

10116 Layman DK. The role of leucine in weight loss diets and glucose homeostasis. *J Nutr* 2003;133:261S-7S.

10117 Scarna A, Gijsman HJ, McTavish SF, et al. Effects of a branched-chain amino acid drink in mania. *Br J Psychiatry* 2003;182:210-3.

10118 van Loon LJ, Kruijshoop M, Menheere PP, et al. Amino acid ingestion strongly enhances insulin secretion in patients with long-term type 2 diabetes. *Diabetes Care* 2003;26:625-30.

10120 Randall T. Khat abuse fuels Somali conflict, drains economy. *JAMA* 1993;269:12-13.

10121 Upton R, ed. Chaste Tree Fruit. American Herbal Pharmacopoeia and Therapeutic Compendium. Santa Cruz, CA; American Herbal Pharmacopoeia 2001:1-37.

10122 Meier B, Berger D, Hoberg E, et al. Pharmacological activities of Vitex agnuscastus extracts in vitro. *Phytomedicine* 2000;7:373-381.

10123 Gardyn J, Mittelman M, Zlotnik J, et al. Oral contraceptives can cause falsely low vitamin B12 levels. *Acta Haematol* 2000;104:22-4.

10124 Russell RM, Baik H, Kehayias JJ. Older men and women efficiently absorb vitamin B-12 from milk and fortified bread. *J Nutr* 2001;131:291-3.

10125 Louwman MW, van Dusseldorp M, van de Vijver FJ, et al. Signs of impaired cognitive function in adolescents with marginal cobalamin status. *Am J Clin Nutr* 2000;72:762-9.

10126 Seal EC, Metz J, Flicker L, Melny J. A randomized, double-blind, placebo-controlled study of oral vitamin B12 supplementation in older patients with subnormal or borderline serum vitamin B12 concentrations. *J Am Geriatr Soc* 2002;50:146-51.

10127 Ellis FR, Nasser S. A pilot study of vitamin B12 in the treatment of tiredness. *Br J Nutr* 1973;30:277-83.

10128 Di Castelnuovo A, Rotondo S, Iacoviello L, et al. Meta-analysis of wine and beer consumption in relation to vascular risk. *Circulation* 2002;105:2836-44.

10129 Rimm EB, Stampfer MJ. Wine, beer, and spirits: are they really horses of a different color? *Circulation* 2002;105:2806-7.

10130 Klipstein-Grobusch K, den Breeijen JH, Grobbee DE, et al. Dietary antioxidants and peripheral arterial disease: the Rotterdam study. *Am J Epidemiol* 2001;154:145-9.

10131 Luchsinger JA, Tang M, Shea S, Mayeux R. Antioxidant vitamin intake and risk of Alzheimer disease. *Arch Neurol* 2003;60:203-8.

10132 Kim MK, Ahn SH, Lee-Kim. Relationship of serum alpha-tocopherol, carotenoids and retinol with the risk of breast cancer. *Nutr Res* 2001;21:797-809.

10133 Cramer DW, Kuper H, Harlow BL, Titus-Ernstoff L. Carotenoids, antioxidants and ovarian cancer risk in pre- and postmenopausal women. *Int J Cancer* 94:128-34.

10134 Albanes D, Virtamo J, Taylor PR, et al. Effects of supplemental beta-carotene, cigarette smoking, and alcohol consumption on serum carotenoids in the Alpha-Tocopherol, Beta-Carotene Cancer Prevention Study. *Am J Clin Nutr* 1997;66:366-72.

10135 Erlinger TP, Guallar E, Miller ER, et al. Relationship between systemic markers of inflammation and serum beta-carotene levels. *Arch Intern Med* 2001;161:1903-8.

10136 Fuller CJ, Butterfoss DN, Failla ML. Relative bioavailability of beta-carotene from supplement sources. *Nutrition Research* 2001;21:1209-15.

10137 Gurudu S, Fiocchi C, and Katz JA. Inflammatory bowel disease. *Best Pract Res Clin Gastroenterol* 2002;16:77-90.

10139 Hypponen E, Laara E, Reunanen A, et al. Intake of vitamin D and risk of type 1 diabetes: a birth-cohort study. *Lancet* 2001;358:1500-3.

10140 Meyer H, Smedshaug GB, Kvaavik E, et al. Can vitamin D supplementation reduce the risk fracture in the elderly? A randomized controlled trial. *J Bone Miner Res* 2002;17:709-15.

10141 Devine A, Wilson SG, Dick IM, Prince RL. Effects of vitamin D metabolites on intestinal absorption and bone turnover in elderly women. *Am J Clin Nutr* 2002;75:283-8.

REFERENCES

10142 Koutkia P, Chen TC, Holick MF. Vitamin D intoxication associated with an over-the-counter supplement. *N Engl J Med* 2001;345:66-7.

10143 Oerter Klein KO, Janfaza M, Wong JA, Chang RJ. Estrogen bioactivity in Fo-Ti and other herbs used for their estrogen-like effects as determined by a recombinant cell bioassay. *J Clin Endocrinol Metab* 2003;88:4077-9.

10144 Pittler MH, Schmidt K, Ernst E. Hawthorn extract for treating chronic heart failure: meta-analysis of randomized trials. *Am J Med* 2003;114:665-74.

10145 Kerckhoffs DA, Hornstra G, Mensink RP. Cholesterol-lowering effect of beta-glucan from oat bran in mildly hypercholesterolemic subjects may decrease when beta-glucan is incorporated into bread and cookies. *Am J Clin Nutr* 2003;78:221-7.

10146 Richardson MA, Bevans ML, Read LL, et al. Efficacy of the branched-chain amino acids in the treatment of tardive dyskinesia in men. *Am J Psychiatry* 2003;160:1117-24.

10147 Hiroshige K, Sonta T, Suda T, et al. Oral supplementation of branched-chain amino acid improves nutritional status in elderly patients on chronic haemodialysis. *Nephrol Dial Transplant* 2001;16:1856-62.

10148 Ametov AS, Barinov A, Dyck PJ, et al. The sensory symptoms of diabetic polyneuropathy are improved with alpha-lipoic acid. *Diabetes Care* 2003;26:770-6.

10149 Verbruggen G, Goemaere S, Veys EM. Systems to assess the progression of finger joint osteoarthritis and the effects of disease modifying osteoarthritis drugs. *Clin Rheumatol* 2002;21:231-43.

10150 Henry-Launois B. Evaluation of the use of financial impact of Chondrosulf 400 in current medical practice. Part of the Proceedings of a Scientific Symposium held at the XIth EULAR Symposium: New approaches in OA: Chondroitin sulfate (CS 4&6) not just a symptomatic treatment. Geneva, 1998.

10151 Linday LA, Dolitsky JN, Shindledecker RD, Pippenger CE. Lemon-flavored cod liver oil and multivitamin-mineral supplement for the secondary prevention of otitis media in young children: pilot research. *Ann Otol Rhinol Laryngol* 2002:111:642-52.

10152 Singh RB, Neki NS, Kartikey K, et al. Effect of coenzyme Q10 on risk of atherosclerosis in patients with recent myocardial infarction. *Mol Cell Biochem* 2003;246:75-82.

10153 Tavani A, Pelucchi C, Parpinel M, et al. n-3 polyunsaturated fatty acid intake and cancer risk in Italy and Switzerland. *Int J Cancer* 2003;105:113-116.

10154 Dallongeville J, Yarnell J, Ducimetiere P, et al. Fish consumption is associated with lower heart rates. *Circulation* 2003;108:820-5.

10155 Madsen T, Christensen JH, Blom M, Schmidt EB. The effect of dietary n-3 acids on serum concentrations of C-reactive protein: a dose-response study. *Br J Nutr* 2003;89:517-22.

10156 Nuttall SL, Kendall MJ, Bombardelli E, Morazzoni P. An evaluation of the antioxidant activity of a standardized grape seed extract, Leucoselect. *J Clin Pharm Ther* 1998;23:385-89.

10157 Bagchi D, Bagchi M, Stohs SJ, et al. Cellular protection with proanthocyanidins derived from grape seeds. *Ann N Y Acad Sci* 2002;957:260-70.

10158 Hermans K, Stockman D, Van den Branden F. Grapefruit and tonic: a deadly combination in a patient with the long QT syndrome. *Am J Med* 2003;114:511-512.

10159 Greenblatt DJ, von Moltke LL, Harmatz JS. Time course of recovery of cytochrome P450 3A function after single doses of grapefruit juice. *Clin Pharmacol Ther* 2003;74:121-29 .

10160 de Luis DA, Izaola O, Cuellar L, et al. Effect of c-reactive protein and interleukins blood levels in postsurgery arginine-enhanced enteral nutrition in head and neck cancer patients. *Eur J Clin Nutr* 2003;57:96-9.

10161 Miyamoto H, Yeh S, Lardy H, et al. Delta5-androstenediol is a natural hormone with androgenic activity in human prostate cancer cells. *Proc Natl Acad Sci U S A* 1998;95:11083-88.

10162 Brown GA, Martini ER, Roberts BS, et al. Acute hormonal response to sublingual androstenediol intake in young men. *J Appl Physiol* 2002;92:142-6.

10163 Hardman JG, Limbird LE, eds. Goodman and Gilman's The Pharmacological Basis of Therapeutics, 10th ed. New York, NY: McGraw-Hill, 2001.

10164 Bobak M, Skodova Z, Marmot M. Beer and obesity: a cross-sectional study. *Eur J Clin Nutr* 2003;57:1250-53.

10165 Koh-Banerjee P, Chu N, Spiegelman D, et al. Prospective study of the association of changes in dietary intake, physicial activity, alcohol consumption, and smoking with 9-y gain in waist circumference among 16 587 US men. *Am J Clin Nutr* 2003;78:719-27.

10166 Keogh GF, Cooper GJ, Mulvey TB, et al. Randomized controlled crossover study of the effect of a highly beta-glucan-enriched barley on cardiovascular disease risk factors in mildly hypercholesterolemic men. *Am J Clin Nutr* 2003;78:711-18.

10201 Chen JF, Xu K, Petzer JP, et al. Neuroprotection by caffeine and A(2A) adenosine receptor inactivation in a model of Parkinson's disease. *J Neurosci* 2001;21:RC143.

10202 Massey LK. Is caffeine a risk factor for bone loss in the elderly? *Am J Clin Nutr* 2001;74:569-70.

10203 Greer F, Friars D, Graham TE. Comparison of caffeine and theophylline ingestion: exercise metabolism and endurance. *J Appl Physiol* 2000;89:1837-44.

10204 Dreher HM. The effect of caffeine reduction on sleep quality and well-being in persons with HIV. *J Psychosom Res* 2003;54:191-8.

10205 Kamimori GH, Penetar DM, Headley DB, et al. Effect of three caffeine doses on plasma catecholamines and alertness during prolonged wakefulness. *Eur J Clin Pharmacol* 2000;56:537-44.

10206 Grandjean AC, Reimers KJ, Bannick KE, Haven MC. The effect of caffeinated, non-caffeinated, caloric and non-caloric beverages on hydration. *J Am Coll Nutr* 2000;19:591-600.

10207 Francis AJ, Dempster RJ. Effect of valerian, Valeriana edulis, on sleep difficulties in children with intellectual deficits: randomised trial. *Phytomedicine* 2002;9:273-9.

10208 Johansson AK, Korte H, Yang B, et al. Sea buckthorn berry oil inhibits platelet aggregation. *J Nutr Biochem* 2000;11:491-5.

10209 Stevinson C, Ernst E. Valerian for insomnia: a systematic review of randomized clinical trials. *Sleep Med* 2000;1:91-9.

10210 Brownson C, Hipkiss AR. Carnosine reacts with a glycated protein. *Free Radic Biol Med* 2000;28:1564-1570.

10211 Guliaeva NV. Superoxide-scavenging activity of carnosine in the presence of copper and zinc ions. *Biokhimiia* 1987;52:1216-1220.

10212 Virgili F, Pagana G, Bourne L, et al. Ferulic acid excretion as a marker of consumption of a French maritime pine (Pinus maritima) bark extract. *Free Radic Biol Med* 2000;28:1249-56.

10213 Bito T, Roy S, Sen CK, Packer L. Pine bark extract pycnogenol downregulates IFN-gamma-induced adhesion of T cells to human keratinocytes by inhibiting inducible ICAM-1 expression. *Free Radic Biol Med* 2000;28:219-27.

10214 Hosseini S, Lee J, Sepulveda RT, et al. A randomized, double-blind, placebo-controlled, prospective, 16 week crossover study to determine the role of pycnogenol in modifying blood pressure in mildly hypertensive patients. *Nutr Res* 2001;21:1251-60.

10215 Peet M, Horrobin DF. A dose-ranging study of the effects of ethyl-eicosapentaenoate in patients with ongoing depression despite apparently adequate treatment with standard drugs. *Arch Gen Psychiatry* 2002;59:913-9.

10216 Oksanen PJ, Salminen S, Saxelin M, et al. Prevention of travellers' diarrhoea by Lactobacillus GG. *Ann Med* 1990;22:53-6.

10217 Dawson EB, Albers JH, McGanity WJ. The apparent effect of iron supplementation on serum selenium levels in teenage pregnancy. *Biol Trace Elem Res* 2000;77:209-17.

10218 Gonzales GF, Cordova A, Vega K, et al. Effect of Lepidium meyenii (Maca), a root with aphrodisiac and fertility-enhancing properties, on serum reproductive hormone levels in adult healthy men. *J Endocrinol* 2003;176:63-168.

10219 Zheng BL, He K, Kim CH, et al. Effect of a lipidic extract from lepidium meyenii on sexual behavior in mice and rats. *Urology* 2000;55:598-602.

10220 Berndt SI, Carter HB, Landis PK, et al. Calcium intake and prostate cancer risk in a long-term aging study: the Baltimore Longitudinal Study of Aging. *Urology* 2002;60:1118-23.

10221 Wollschlaeger B. Efficacy of vinpocetine in the management of cognitive impairment and memory loss. *JANA* 2001;4:25-30.

10222 Feigin VL, Doronin BM, Popova TF, et al. Vinpocetine treatment in acute ischaemic stroke: a pilot single-blind randomized clinical trial. *Eur J Neurol* 2001;8:81-5.

10223 Pataki T, Bak I, Kovacs P, et al. Grape seed proanthocyanidins improved cardiac recovery during reperfusion after ischemia in isolated rat hearts. *Am J Clin Nutr* 2002;75:894-9.

10224 Agarwal C, Sharma Y, Agarwal R. Anticarcinogenic effect of a polyphenolic fraction isolated from grape seeds in human prostate carcinoma DU145 cells: modulation of mitogenic signaling and cell-cycle regulators and induction of G1 arrest and apoptosis. *Mol Carcinog* 2000;28:129-38.

10225 Furukawa S, Saito H, Inoue T, et al. Supplemental glutamine augments phagocytosis and reactive oxygen intermediate production by neutrophils and monocytes from postoperative patients in vitro. *Nutrition* 2000;16:323-9.

10226 Jowell PS, Robuck-Mangum G, Mergener K, et al. A double-blind, randomized, dose response study testing the pharmacological efficacy of synthetic porcine secretin. *Aliment Pharmacol Ther* 2000;14:1679-84.

10227 Pecking AP, Fevrier B, Wargon C, Pillion G. Efficacy of Daflon 500 mg in the treatment of lymphedema (secondary to conventional therapy of breast cancer). *Angiology* 1997;48:93-8.

10228 Somekawa Y, Chiguchi M, Ishibashi T, et al. Efficacy of ipriflavone in preventing adverse effects of leuprolide. *J Clin Endocrinol Metab* 2001;86:3202-6.

10229 Guilhou JJ, Dereure O, Marzin L, et al. Efficacy of Daflon 500 mg in venous leg ulcer healing: a double-blind, randomized, controlled versus placebo trial in 107 patients. *Angiology* 1997;48:77-85.

10230 Zhen QS, Ye X, Wei ZJ. Recent progress in research on Tripterygium: a male antifertility plant. *Contraception* 1995;51:121-9.

10231 Huang L, Feng S, Wang H. Decreased bone mineral density in female patients with systemic lupus erythematosus after long-term administration of Tripterygium Wilfordii Hook. F. *Chin Med J* 2000;113:159-61.

10232 Kao NL, Richmond GW, Moy JN. Resolution of severe lupus nephritis associated with Tripterygium wilfordii hook F ingestion. *Arthritis Rheum* 1993;36:1751-2.

10233 Cibere J, Deng Z, Lin Y, et al. A Randomized Double Blind, Placebo Controlled Trial of Topical Tripterygium wilfordii in Rheumatoid Arthritis: Reanalysis Using Logistic Regression Analysis. *J Rheumatol* 2003;30:465-7.

10234 Salvatore S, Heuschkel R, Tomlin S, et al. A pilot study of N-acetyl glucosamine, a nutritional substrate for glycosaminoglycan synthesis, in paediatric chronic inflammatory bowel disease. *Aliment Pharmacol Ther* 2000;14:1567-79.

10235 Campbell FA, Tramer MR, Carroll D, et al. Are cannabinoids an effective and safe treatment option in the management of pain? A qualitative systematic review. *BMJ* 2001;323:13-6.

10237 Donati C, Barbi G, Cairo G, et al. Pantethine improves the lipid abnormalities of chronic hemodialysis patients: results of a multicenter clinical trial. *Clin Nephrol* 1986;25:70-4.

10238 Arsenio L, Bodria P, Magnati G, et al. Effectiveness of long-term treatment with pantethine in patients with dyslipidemia. *Clin Ther* 1986;8:537-45.

10239 Klein TW, Newton CA, Nakachi N, Friedman H. Delta 9-tetrahydrocannabinol treatment suppresses immunity and early IFN-gamma, IL-12, and IL-12 receptor beta 2 responses to Legionella pneumophila infection. *J Immunol* 2000;164:6461-6.

10240 Zhu LX, Sharma S, Stolina M, et al. Delta-9-tetrahydrocannabinol inhibits antitumor immunity by a CB2 receptor-mediated, cytokine-dependent pathway. *J Immunol* 2000;165:373-80.

10241 Tramer MR, Carroll D, Campbell FA, et al. Cannabinoids for control of chemotherapy induced nausea and vomiting: quantitative systematic review. *BMJ* 2001;323:16-21.

10242 Solowij N, Stephens RS, Roffman RA, et al. Cognitive functioning of long-term heavy cannabis users seeking treatment. *JAMA* 2002;287:1123-31.

10243 Yeum KJ, Ahn SH, Rupp de Paiva SA, et al. Correlation between carotenoid concentrations in serum and normal breast adipose tissue of women with benign breast tumor or breast cancer. *J Nutr* 1998;128:1920-6.

10244 Levi F, Pasche C, Lucchini F, La Vecchia C. Selected micronutrients and colorectal cancer: a case-control study from the canton of Vaud, Switzerland. *Eur J Cancer* 2000;36:2115-9.

10245 Johnson EJ, Hammond BR, Yeum KJ, et al. Relation among serum and tissue concentrations of lutein and zeaxanthin and macular pigment density. *Am J Clin Nutr* 2000;71:1555-62.

10246 Anon. Zinc Against Plasmodium Study Group. Effect of zinc on the treatment of Plasmodium falciparum malaria in children: a randomized controlled trial. *Am J Clin Nutr* 2002;76:805-12.

10247 Mossad SB. Effect of zincum gluconicum nasal gel on the duration and symptom severity of the common cold in otherwise healthy adults. *QJM* 2003;96:35-43.

10248 Baqui AH, Black RE, El Arifeen S, et al. Effect of zinc supplementation started during diarrhoea on morbidity and mortality in Bangladeshi children: community randomised trial. *BMJ* 2002;325:1059-62.

10249 Suzuki H, Rhim JH. Effect of samgyetang feeding on plasma lipids, glucose, glycosylated hemoglobin, and stress-induced gastric ulcers in mice. *Nutr Res* 2000;20:575-84.

10250 Javitt DC, Zylberman I, Zukin SR, et al. Amelioration of negative symptoms in schizophrenia by glycine. *Am J Psychiatry* 1994;151:1234-6.

10251 Heresco-Levy U, Javitt DC, Ermilov M, et al. Double-blind, placebo-controlled, crossover trial of glycine adjuvant therapy for treatment-resistant schizophrenia. *Br J Psychiatry* 1996;169:610-7.

10252 Heresco-Levy U, Javitt DC, Ermilov M, et al. Efficacy of high-dose glycine in the treatment of enduring negative symptoms of schizophrenia. *Arch Gen Psychiatry* 1999;56:29-36.

REFERENCES

10253 Potkin SG, Jin Y, Bunney BG, Costa J, Gulasekaram B. Effect of clozapine and adjunctive high-dose glycine in treatment-resistant schizophrenia. *Am J Psychiatry* 1999;156:145-7.

10254 de Koning TJ, Duran M, Dorland L, et al. Beneficial effects of L-serine and glycine in the management of seizures in 3-phosphoglycerate dehydrogenase deficiency. *Ann Neurol* 1998;44:261-5.

10255 Harvey SG, Gibson JR, Burke CA. L-cysteine, glycine and dl-threonine in the treatment of hypostatic leg ulceration: a placebo-controlled study. *Pharmatherapeutica* 1985;4:227-30.

10256 Fries MH, Rinaldo P, Schmidt-Sommerfeld E, et al. Isovaleric acidemia: response to a leucine load after three weeks of supplementation with glycine, L-carnitine, and combined glycine-carnitine therapy. *J Pediatr* 1996;129:449-52.

10257 Javitt DC, Balla A, Sershen H, Lajtha A. A.E. Bennett Research Award. Reversal of phencyclidine-induced effects by glycine and glycine transport inhibitors. *Biol Psychiatry* 1999;45:668-79.

10258 Thurman RG, Zhong Z, von Frankenberg M, et al. Prevention of cyclosporine-induced nephrotoxicity with dietary glycine. *Transplantation* 1997;63:1661-7.

10259 Zhong Z, Arteel GE, Connor HD, et al. Cyclosporin A increases hypoxia and free radical production in rat kidneys: prevention by dietary glycine. *Am J Physiol* 1998;275:F595-604.

10260 Yin M, Ikejima K, Arteel GE, Seabra V, et al. Glycine accelerates recovery from alcohol-induced liver injury. *J Pharmacol Exp Ther* 1998;286:1014-9.

10261 Rose ML, Madren J, Bunzendahl H, Thurman RG. Dietary glycine inhibits the growth of B16 melanoma tumors in mice. *Carcinogenesis* 1999;20:793-8.

10262 Rose ML, Cattley RC, Dunn C, et al. Dietary glycine prevents the development of liver tumors caused by the peroxisome proliferator WY-14,643. *Carcinogenesis* 1999;20:2075-81.

10263 Helzlsouer KJ, Huang HY, Alberg AJ, et al. Association between alpha-tocopherol, gamma-tocopherol, selenium, and subsequent prostate cancer. *J Natl Cancer Inst* 2000;92:2018-23.

10264 Park EJ, Pezzuto JM. Botanicals in cancer chemoprevention. *Cancer Metastasis Rev* 2002;21:231-55.

10265 Chiao JW, Chung FL, Kancherla R, et al. Sulforaphane and its metabolite mediate growth arrest and apoptosis in human prostate cancer cells. *Int J Oncol* 2002;20:631-6.

10266 Whittaker P, Vanderveen JE, Dinovi MJ, et al. Toxicological profile, current use, and regulatory issues on EDTA compounds for assessing use of sodium iron EDTA for food fortification. *Regul Toxicol Pharmacol* 1993;18:419-27.

10267 Hayashi O, Katoh T, Okuwaki Y. Enhancement of antibody production in mice by dietary Spirulina platensis. *J Nutr Sci Vitaminol* (Tokyo) 1994;40:431-41.

10268 Morgan LR, Holdiness MR, Gillen LE. N-acetylcysteine: its bioavailability and interaction with ifosfamide metabolites. *Semin Oncol* 1983;10:56-61.

10269 Morgan LR, Donley PJ, Harrison EF, Hunter HL. The control of ifosfamide-induced hematuria with N-acetylcysteine in patients with advanced carcinoma of the lung. *Semin Oncol* 1982;9:71-4.

10270 Loehrer PJ Sr, Birch R, Kramer BS, et al. Ifosfamide plus N-acetylcysteine in the treatment of small cell and non-small cell carcinoma of the lung: a Southeastern Cancer Study Group Trial. *Cancer Treat Rep* 1986;70:919-20.

10271 Loehrer PJ, Williams SD, Einhorn LH. N-acetylcysteine and ifosfamide in the treatment of unresectable pancreatic adenocarcinoma and refractory testicular cancer. *Semin Oncol* 1983;10:72-5.

10272 Anfossi G, Russo I, Massucco P, et al. N-acetyl-L-cysteine exerts direct anti-aggregating effect on human platelets. *Eur J Clin Invest* 2001;31:452-61.

10274 Teuri U, Karkkainen M, Lamberg-Allardt C, Korpela R. Addition of inulin to breakfast does not acutely affect serum ionized calcium and parathyroid hormone concentrations. *Ann Nutr Metab* 1999;43:356-64.

10275 Norman JA, Pickford CJ, Sanders TW, Waller M. Human intake of arsenic and iodine from seaweed-based food supplements and health foods available in the UK. *Food Addit Contam* 1988;5:103-9.

10276 Dutta T, Basu UP. Crude extract of Centella asiatica and products derived from its glycosides as oral antifertility agents. *Indian J Exp Biol* 1968;6:181-2.

10277 Hausen BM. Centella asiatica (Indian pennywort), an effective therapeutic but a weak sensitizer. *Contact Dermatitis* 1993;29:175-9.

10278 Bilbao I, Aguirre A, Zabala R, et al. Allergic contact dermatitis from butoxyethyl nicotinic acid and Centella asiatica extract. *Contact Dermatitis* 1995;33:435-6.

10279 Dagnelie G, Zorge IS, McDonald TM. Lutein improves visual function in some patients with retinal degeneration: a pilot study via the Internet. *Optometry* 2000;71:147-64.

10283 Madar Z, Abel R, Samish S, Arad J. Glucose-lowering effect of fenugreek in non-insulin dependent diabetics. *Eur J Clin Nutr* 1988;42:51-4.

10284 Bhardwaj PK, Dasgupta DJ, Prashar BS, Kaushal SS. Control of hyperglycaemia and hyperlipidaemia by plant product. *J Assoc Physicians India* 1994;42:33-5.

10285 Nicolodi M, Sicuteri F. Fibromyalgia and migraine, two faces of the same mechanism. Serotonin as the common clue for pathogenesis and therapy. *Adv Exp Med Biol* 1996;398:373-9.

10286 Caruso I, Sarzi Puttini P, Cazzola M, Azzolini V. Double-blind study of 5-hydroxytryptophan versus placebo in the treatment of primary fibromyalgia syndrome. *J Int Med Res* 1990;18:201-9.

10287 Priori R, Conti F, Luan FL, et al. Chronic fatigue: a peculiar evolution of eosinophilia myalgia syndrome following treatment with L-tryptophan in four Italian adolescents. *Eur J Pediatr* 1994;153:344-6.

10288 Klein R, Berg PA. A comparative study on antibodies to nucleoli and 5-hydroxytryptamine in patients with fibromyalgia syndrome and tryptophan-induced eosinophilia-myalgia syndrome. *Clin Investig* 1994;72:541-9.

10289 Simat TJ, Kleeberg KK, Muller B, Sierts A. Synthesis, formation, and occurrence of contaminants in biotechnologically manufactured L-tryptophan. *Adv Exp Med Biol* 1999;467:469-80.

10291 Qian ZM, Xu MF, Tang PL. Polysaccharide peptide (PSP) restores immunosuppression induced by cyclophosphamide in rats. *Am J Chin Med* 1997;25:27-35.

10292 Williams GM, Iatropoulos MJ, Whysner J. Safety assessment of butylated hydroxyanisole and butylated hydroxytoluene as antioxidant food additives. *Food Chem Toxicol* 1999;37:1027-38.

10293 Botterweck AA, Verhagen H, Goldbohm RA, et al. Intake of butylated hydroxyanisole and butylated hydroxytoluene and stomach cancer risk: results from analyses in the Netherlands Cohort Study. *Food Chem Toxicol* 2000;38:599-605.

10294 Freeman DJ, Wenerstrom G, Spruance SL. Treatment of recurrent herpes simplex labialis with topical butylated hydroxytoluene. *Clin Pharmacol Ther* 1985;38:56-9.

10295 Coohill TP, Babich M, Taylor WD, Snipes W. A comparison of herpes simplex virus plaque development after viral treatment with anti-DNA or antilipid agents. *Biophys J* 1980;30:517-21.

10296 Modlin M. Urinary phosphorylated inositols and renal stone. *Lancet* 1980;2:1113-4.

10297 Grases F, Costa-Bauza A. Phytate (IP6) is a powerful agent for preventing calcifications in biological fluids: usefulness in renal lithiasis treatment. *Anticancer Res* 1999;19:3717-22.

10298 Grases F, Garcia-Gonzalez R, Torres JJ, Llobera A. Effects of phytic acid on renal stone formation in rats. *Scand J Urol Nephrol* 1998;32:261-5.

10299 Cinatl J, Morgenstern B, Bauer G, et al. Glycyrrhizin, an active component of liquorice roots, and replication of SARS-associated coronavirus. *Lancet* 2003;361:2045-6.

10300 Kent UM, Aviram M, Rosenblat M, Hollenberg PF. The licorice root derived isoflavan glabridin inhibits the activities of human cytochrome P450S 3A4, 2B6, and 2C9. *Drug Metab Dispos* 2002;30:709-15.

10303 Shlian DM, Goldstone J. Toxicity of butylated hydroxytoluene. *N Engl J Med* 1986;314:648-9.

10305 Stalenhoef AF. Images in clinical medicine. Phytosterolemia and xanthomatosis. *N Engl J Med* 2003;349:51.

10306 Leitzmann MF, Stampfer MJ, Wu K, et al. Zinc supplement use and risk of prostate cancer. *J Natl Cancer Inst* 2003;95:1004-7.

10307 Kockler DR, McCarthy MW, Lawson CL. Seizure activity and unresponsiveness after hydroxycut ingestion. *Pharmacotherapy* 2001;21:647-51.

10309 Davidson JR, Abraham K, Connor KM, McLeod MN. Effectiveness of chromium in atypical depression: a placebo-controlled trial. *Biol Psychiatry* 2003;53:261-4.

10310 Richy F, Bruyere O, Ethgen O, et al. Structural and symptomatic efficacy of glucosamine and chondroitin in knee osteoarthritis: a comprehensive meta-analysis. *Arch Intern Med* 2003;163:1514-22.

10311 Scroggie DA, Albright A, Harris MD. The effect of glucosamine-chondroitin supplementation on glycosylated hemoglobin levels in patients with type 2 diabetes mellitus: a placebo-controlled, double-blinded, randomized clinical trial. *Arch Intern Med* 2003;163:1587-90.

10312 Braham R, Dawson B, Goodman C. The effect of glucosamine supplementation on people experiencing regular knee pain. *Br J Sports Med* 2003;37:45-9.

10313 Hoffer LJ, Kaplan LN, Hamadeh MJ, et al. Sulfate could mediate the therapeutic effect of glucosamine sulfate. *Metabolism* 2001;50:767-70.

10314 Cardinal BJ, Engels HJ. Ginseng does not enhance psychological well-being in healthy, young adults: results of a double-blind, placebo-controlled, randomized clinical trial. *J Am Diet Assoc* 2001;101:655-60.

10315 Baici A, Horler D, Moser B, et al. Analysis of glycosaminoglycans in human serum after oral administration of chondroitin sulfate. *Rheumatol Int* 1992;12:81-8.

10316 Setnikar I, Rovati LC. Absorption, distribution, metabolism and excretion of glucosamine sulfate. A review. *Arzneimittelforschung* 2001;51:699-725.

10317 Yu JG, Boies SM, Olefsky JM. The effect of oral glucosamine sulfate on insulin sensitivity in human subjects. *Diabetes Care* 2003;30:523-8.

10319 Logan JL, Ahmed J. Critical hypokalemic renal tubular acidosis due to Sjogren's syndrome: association with the purported immune stimulant echinacea. *Clin Rheumatol* 2003;22:158-9.

10320 Hoheisel O, Sandberg M, Bertram S, et al. Echinagard treatment shortens the course of the common cold: a double blind, placebo-controlled clinical trial. *Eur J Clin Res* 1997;9:261-268.

10321 Woodman RJ, Mori TA, Burke V, et al. Effects of purified eicosapentaenoic and docosahexaenoic acids on glycemic control, blood pressure, and serum lipids in type 2 diabetic patients with treated hypertension. *Am J Clin Nutr* 2002;76:1007-15.

10322 Erkkila AT, Lehto S, Pyorala K, Uusitupa MI. n-3 Fatty acids and 5-y risks of death and cardiovascular disease events in patients with coronary artery disease. *Am J Clin Nutr* 2003;78:65-71.

10323 Finnegan YE, Howarth D, Minihane AM, et al. Plant and marine derived (n-3) polyunsaturated fatty acids do not affect blood coagulation and fibrinolytic factors in moderately hyperlipidemic humans. *J Nutr* 2003;133:2210-3.

10324 Cho E, Hung S, Willet W, et al. Prospective study of dietary fat and the risk of age-related macular degeneration. *Am J Clin Nutr* 2001;73:209-18.

10325 Spapen H, Diltoer M, Van Malderen C, et al. Soluble fiber reduces the incidence of diarrhea in septic patients receiving total enteral nutrition: a prospective, double-blind, randomized, and controlled trial. *Clin Nutr* 2001;20:301-5.

10326 Parisi GC, Zilli M, Miani MP, et al. High-fiber diet supplementation in patients with irritable bowel syndrome (IBS): a multicenter, randomized, open trial comparison between wheat bran diet and partially hydrolyzed guar gum (PHGG). *Dig Dis Sci* 2002;47:1697-704.

10327 Cohen M, Wolfe R, Mai T, Lewis D. A randomized, double blind, placebo controlled trial of a topical cream containing glucosamine sulfate, chondroitin sulfate, and camphor for osteoarthritis of the knee. *J Rheumatol* 2003;30:523-8.

10328 Jenkins DJ, Kendall CW, Augustin LS, et al. Effect of wheat bran on glycemic control and risk factors for cardiovascular disease in type 2 diabetes. *Diabetes Care* 2002;25:1522-8.

10329 Mai I, Stormer E, Bauer S, et al. Impact of St John's wort treatment on the pharmacokinetics of tacrolimus and mycophenolic acid in renal transplant patients. *Nephrol Dial Transplant* 2003;18:819-22.

10332 Wyatt K, Dimmock P, Jones P, et al. Efficacy of progesterone and progestogens in management of premenstrual syndrome: systematic review. *BMJ* 2001;323:776-80.

10334 Perry NS, Bollen C, Perry EK, Ballard C. Salvia for dementia therapy: review of pharmacological activity and pilot tolerability clinical trial. *Pharmacol Biochem Behav* 2003;75:651-9.

10335 Markowitz JS, Devane CL, Chavin KD, et al. Effects of garlic (Allium sativum L.) supplementation on cytochrome P450 2D6 and 3A4 activity in healthy volunteers. *Clin Pharmacol Ther* 2003;74:170-7.

10336 Thomet OA, Schapowal A, Heinisch IV, et al. Anti-inflammatory activity of an extract of Petasites hybridus in allergic rhinitis. *Int Immunopharmacol* 2002;2:997-1006.

10337 Lee DK, Carstairs IJ, Haggart K, et al. Butterbur, a herbal remedy, attenuates adenosine monophosphate induced nasal responsiveness in seasonal allergic rhinitis. *Clin Exp Allergy* 2003;33:882-6.

10339 Pletz MW, Petzold P, Allen A, et al. Effect of calcium carbonate on bioavailability of orally administered gemifloxacin. *Antimicrob Agents Chemother* 2003;47:2158-60.

10340 Barch DH, Rundhaugen LM, Stoner GD, et al. Structure-function relationships of the dietary anticarcinogen ellagic acid. *Carcinogenesis* 1996;17:265-9.

10342 Constantinou A, Stoner GD, Mehta R, et al. The dietary anticancer agent ellagic acid is a potent inhibitor of DNA topoisomerases in vitro. *Nutr Cancer* 1995;23:121-30.

10343 Xu Y, Deng JZ, Ma J, et al. DNA damaging activity of ellagic acid derivatives. *Bioorg Med Chem* 2003;11:1593-6.

10344 Mullen W, Stewart AJ, Lean ME, et al. Effect of freezing and storage on the phenolics, ellagitannins, flavonoids, and antioxidant capacity of red raspberries. *J Agric Food Chem* 2002;508:5197-201.

10345 Oesser S, Seifert J. Stimulation of type II collagen biosynthesis and secretion in bovine chondrocytes cultured with degraded collagen. *Cell Tissue Res* 2003;311:393-9.

10346 Cirigliano MD, Szapary PO. Horny goat weed for erectile dysfunction. *Alt Med Alert* 2001;4:19-22.

10348 Zanarini MC, Frankenburg FR. Omega-3 Fatty acid treatment of women with borderline personality disorder: a double-blind, placebo-controlled pilot study. *Am J Psychiatry* 2003;160:167-9.

10349 Ostad SN, Soodi M, Shariffzadeh M, et al. The effect of fennel essential oil on uterine contraction as a model for dysmenorrhea, pharmacology and toxicology study. *J Ethnopharmacol* 2001;76:299-304.

10350 van der Griend R, Haas FJ, Biesma DH, et al. Combination of low-dose folic acid and pyridoxine for treatment of hyperhomocysteinaemia in patients with premature arterial disease and their relatives. *Atherosclerosis* 1999;143:177-83.

10351 Hilsden RJ, Scott CM, Verhoef MJ. Complementary medicine use by patients with inflammatory bowel disease. *Am J Gastroenterol* 1998;93:697-701.

10352 Engler MM, Engler MB, Malloy MJ, et al. Antioxidant Vitamins C and E Improve Endothelial Function in Children With Hyperlipidemia: Endothelial Assessment of Risk from Lipids in Youth (EARLY) Trial. *Circulation* 2003;108:1059-63.

10353 Brody S, Preut R, Schommer K, Schurmeyer TH. A randomized controlled trial of high dose ascorbic acid for reduction of blood pressure, cortisol, and subjective responses to psychological stress. *Psychopharmacology* 2002;159:319-24.

10354 Block G, Mangels AR, Norkus EP, et al. Ascorbic acid status and subsequent diastolic and systolic blood pressure. *Hypertension* 2001;37:261-7.

10355 Nishiguchi S, Shiomi S, Enomoto M, et al. Does ascorbic acid prevent retinopathy during interferon therapy in patients with chronic hepatitis C? *J Gastroenterol* 2001;36:486-91.

10356 Traxer O, Huet B, Poindexter J, et al. Effect of ascorbic acid consumption on urinary stone risk factors. *J Urol* 2003;170:397-401.

10357 Pohle T, Brzozowski T, Becker JC, et al. Role of reactive oxygen metabolites in aspirin-induced gastric damage in humans: gastroprotection by vitamin C. *Aliment Pharmacol Ther* 2001;15:677-87.

10358 Osganian SK, Stampfer MJ, Rimm E, et al. Vitamin C and risk of coronary heart disease in women. *J Am Coll Cardiol* 2003;42:246-52.

10359 Zullo A, Rinaldi V, Hassan C, et al. Ascorbic acid and intestinal metaplasia in the stomach: a prospective, randomized study. *Aliment Pharmacol Ther* 2000;14:1303-9.

10360 Yoshinaga M, Ohtani A, Harada N, et al. Vitamin C inhibits corpus gastritis in Helicobacter pylori-infected patients during acid-suppressive therapy. *J Gastroenterol Hepatol* 2001;16:1206-10.

10361 Ziaei S, Faghihzadeh S, Sohrabvand F, et al. A randomised placebo-controlled trial to determine the effect of vitamin E in treatment of primary dysmenorrhoea. *BJOG* 2001;108:1181-3.

10362 Pathak A, Roth P, Piscitelli J, Johnson L. Effects of vitamin E supplementation during erythropoietin treatment of the anaemia of prematurity. *Arch Dis Child Fetal Neonatal Ed* 2003;88:F324-8.

10363 Delanian S, Porcher R, Balla-Mekias S, Lefaix JL. Randomized, placebo-controlled trial of combined pentoxifylline and tocopherol for regression of superficial radiation-induced fibrosis. *J Clin Oncol* 2003;21:2545-50.

10364 Liu M, Wallmon A, Olsson-Mortlock C, et al. Mixed tocopherols inhibit platelet aggregation in humans: potential mechanisms. *Am J Clin Nutr* 2003;77:700-6.

10365 Vivekananthan DP, Penn MS, Sapp SK, et al. Use of antioxidant vitamins for the prevention of cardiovascular disease: meta-analysis of randomised trials. *Lancet* 2003;361:2017-23.

10366 Pace A, Savarese A, Picardo M, et al. Neuroprotective effect of vitamin E supplementation in patients treated with cisplatin chemotherapy. *J Clin Oncol* 2003;21:927-31.

10367 Traber MG, Schiano TD, Steephen AC, et al. Efficacy of water-soluble vitamin E in the treatment of vitamin E malabsorption in short-bowel syndrome. *Am J Clin Nutr* 1994;59:1270-4.

10368 Sokol RJ, Johnson KE, Karrer FM, et al. Improvement of cyclosporin absorption in children after liver transplantation by means of water-soluble vitamin E. *Lancet* 1991;338:212-4.

10369 Fryer MJ. Vitamin E as a protective antioxidant in progressive renal failure. *Nephrology* 2000;5:1-7.

10370 Calhoun KE, Pommier RF, Muller P, et al. Dehydroepiandrosterone sulfate causes proliferation of estrogen receptor-positive breast cancer cells despite treatment with fulvestrant. *Arch Surg* 2003;138:879-83.

10371 Szapary PO, Wolfe ML, Bloedon LT, et al. Guggulipid for treatment of hypercholesterolemia: a randomized controlled trial. *JAMA* 2003;290:765-72.

10372 Horn-Ross PL, John EM, Canchola AJ, et al. Phytoestrogen intake and endometrial cancer risk. *J Natl Cancer Inst* 2003;95:1158-64.

10373 Cummings JH, Christie S, Cole TJ. A study of fructo oligosaccharides in the prevention of travellers' diarrhoea. *Aliment Pharmacol Ther* 2001;15:1139-45.

10374 Durak I, Yilmaz E, Devrim E, et al. Consumption of aqueous garlic extract leads to significant improvement in patients with benign prostate hyperplasia and prostate cancer. *Nutr Res* 2003;23:199-204.

10375 Schneir AB, Ly BT, Clark RF. A case of withdrawal from the GHB precursors gamma-butyrolactone and 1,4-butanediol. *J Emerg Med* 2001;21:31-3.

10376 Sivilotti ML, Burns MJ, Aaron CK, Greenberg MJ. Pentobarbital for severe gamma-butyrolactone withdrawal. *Ann Emerg Med* 2001;38:660-5.

10377 Hormann HP, Korting HC. Evidence for the efficacy and safety of topical herbal drugs in dermatology: part I: anti-inflammatory agents. *Phytomedicine* 1994;1:161-71.

10378 Quaranta L, Bettelli S, Uva MG, et al. Effect of Ginkgo biloba extract on preexisting visual field damage in normal tension glaucoma. *Ophthalmology* 2003;110:359-62.

10379 dos Santos AF, Sant'Ana AE. Molluscicidal properties of some species of Annona. *Phytomedicine* 2001;8:115-20.

10381 Raupp P, Hassan JA, Varughese M, Kristiansson B. Henna causes life threatening haemolysis in glucose-6-phosphate dehydrogenase deficiency. *Arch Dis Child* 2001;85:411-2.

10382 Yates KM, O'Connor A, Horsley CA. "Herbal Ecstasy": a case series of adverse reactions. *N Z Med J* 2000;113:315-7.

10383 Comaish JS, Kersey PJ. Contact dermatitis to extract of horse chestnut (esculin). *Contact Dermatitis* 1980;6:150-1.

10384 Haier MI, Tsai N, Komura ST, Chiu CL. Fatal hepatorenal failure associated with hydrazine sulfate. *Ann Intern Med* 2000;133:877-80.

10385 Gershanovich ML, Danova LA, Ivin BA, Filov VA. Results of clinical study antitumor action of hydrazine sulfate. *Nutr Cancer* 1981;3:7-12.

10386 Shebek J, Rindone JP. A pilot study exploring the effect of kudzu root on the drinking habits of patients with chronic alcoholism. *J Altern Complement Med* 2000;6:45-8.

10387 Palatnik A, Frolov K, Fux M, Benjamin J. Double-blind, controlled, crossover trial of inositol versus fluvoxamine for the treatment of panic disorder. *J Clin Psychopharmacol* 2001;21:335-9.

10388 Halperin SA, Smith B, Nolan C, et al. Safety and immunoenhancing effect of a Chlorella-derived dietary supplement in healthy adults undergoing influenza vaccination: randomized, double-blind, placebo-controlled trial. *CMAJ* 2003;169:111-7.

10389 Suksamrarn A, Jankam A, Tarnchompoo B, Putchakarn S. Ecdysteroids from a Zoanthus sp. *J Nat Prod* 2002;65:1194-7.

10390 Bucci LR. Selected herbals and human exercise performance. *Am J Clin Nutr* 2000;72:624S-36S.

10391 Hudson S, Tabet N. Acetyl-L-carnitine for dementia. *Cochrane Database Syst Rev* 2003;2:CD003158.

10392 Boullata JI, McDonnell PJ, Oliva CD. Anaphylactic reaction to a dietary supplement containing willow bark. *Ann Pharmacother* 2003;37:832-5.

10393 Yoshida S, Takayama Y. Licorice-induced hypokalemia as a treatable cause of dropped head syndrome. *Clin Neurol Neurosurg* 2003;105:286-7.

10394 Hainer MI, Tsai N, Komura ST, Chiu CL. Fatal hepatorenal failure associated with hydrazine sulfate. *Ann Intern Med* 2000;133:877-80.

10395 Pettegrew JW, Levine J, McClure RJ. Acetyl-L-carnitine physical-chemical, metabolic, and therapeutic properties: relevance for its mode of action in Alzheimer's disease and geriatric depression. *Mol Psychiatry* 2000;5:616-32.

10396 Boivin D, Gendron S, Beaulieu E, et al. The antiangiogenic agent Neovastat (AE-941) induces endothelial cell apoptosis. *Mol Cancer Ther* 2002;1:795-802.

10397 Falardeau P, Champagne P, Poyet P, et al. Neovastat, a naturally occurring multifunctional antiangiogenic drug, in phase III clinical trials. *Semin Oncol* 2001;28:620-5.

10398 Gingras D, Renaud A, Mousseau N, et al. Matrix proteinase inhibition by AE-941, a multifunctional antiangiogenic compound. *Anticancer Res* 2001;21:145-55.

10399 Sauder DN, Dekoven J, Champagne P, et al. Neovastat (AE-941), an inhibitor of angiogenesis: Randomized phase I/II clinical trial results in patients with plaque psoriasis. *J Am Acad Dermatol* 2002;47:535-41.

10400 Donovan JL, DeVane CL, Chavin KD, et al. Siberian Ginseng (Eleutheroccus senticosus) Effects on CYP2D6 and CYP3A4 Activity in Normal Volunteers. *Drug Metab Dispos* 2003;31:519-22.

10401 Morris KT, Toth-Fejel S, Schmidt J, et al. High dehydroepiandrosterone-sulfate predicts breast cancer progression during new aromatase inhibitor therapy and stimulates breast cancer cell growth in tissue culture: a renewed role for adrenalectomy. *Surgery* 2001;130:947-53.

10403 Calhoun K, Pommier R, Cheek J, et al. The effect of high dehydroepiandrosterone sulfate levels on tamoxifen blockade and breast cancer progression. *Am J Surg* 2003;185:411-5.

10404 Davidson M, Marwah A, Sawchuk RJ, et al. Safety and pharmacokinetic study with escalating doses of 3-acetyl-7-oxo-dehydroepiandrosterone in healthy male volunteers. *Clin Invest Med* 2000;23:300-10.

10405 Sulcova J, Hill M, Masek Z, et al. Effects of transdermal application of 7-oxo-DHEA on the levels of steroid hormones, gonadotropins and lipids in healthy men. *Physiol Res* 2001;50:9-18.

10406 Percheron G, Hogrel JY, Denot-Ledunois S, et al. Effect of 1-year oral administration of dehydroepiandrosterone to 60- to 80-year-old individuals on muscle function and cross-sectional area: a double-blind placebo-controlled trial. *Arch Intern Med* 2003;163:720-7.

10407 Anon. FDA issue advisory on star anise "teas." FDA News P03-67; September 10, 2003.

10408 Danao-Camara T. Potential side effects of treatment with glucosamine and chondroitin. *Arthritis Rheum* 2000;43:2853.

10409 Guillaume MP, Peretz A. Possible association between glucosamine treatment and renal toxicity: comment on the letter by Danao-Camara. *Arthritis Rheum* 2001;44:2943-4.

10410 Mougios V, Matsakas A, Petridou A, et al. Effect of supplementation with conjugated linoleic acid on human serum lipids and body fat. *J Nutr Biochem* 2001;12:585-94.

10411 Thom E, Wadstein J, Gudmundsen O. Conjugated linoleic acid reduces body fat in healthy exercising humans. *J Int Med Res* 2001;29:392-6.

10412 Davidson MH, Maki KC, Synecki C, et al. Effects of dietary inulin on serum lipids in men and women with hypercholesterolemia. *Nutr Res* 1998;18:503-17.

10413 Brighenti F, Casiraghi MC, Canzi E, Ferrari A. Effect of consumption of a ready-to-eat breakfast cereal containing inulin on the intestinal milieu and blood lipids in healthy male volunteers. *Eur J Clin Nutr* 1999;53:726-33.

10414 Gibson GR, Beatty ER, Wang X, Cummings JH. Selective stimulation of bifidobacteria in the human colon by oligofructose and inulin. *Gastroenterology* 1995;108:975-82.

10415 Kleessen B, Sykura B, Zunft HJ, Blaut M. Effects of inulin and lactose on fecal microflora, microbial activity, and bowel habit in elderly constipated persons. *Am J Clin Nutr* 1997;65:1397-402.

10416 Stanislavov R, Nikolova V. Treatment of erectile dysfunction with pycnogenol and L-arginine. *J Sex Marital Ther* 2003;29:207-13.

10417 Heron S, Yarnell E. The safety of low-dose Larrea tridentata (DC) Coville (creosote bush or chaparral): a retrospective clinical study. *J Altern Complement Med* 2001;7:175-85.

10418 Sesso HD, Liu S, Gaziano JM, Buring JE. Dietary lycopene, tomato-based food products and cardiovascular disease in women. *J Nutr* 2003;133:2336-41.

10419 Nobaek S, Johansson ML, Molin G, et al. Alteration of intestinal microflora is associated with reduction in abdominal bloating and pain in patients with irritable bowel syndrome. *Am J Gastroenterol* 2000;95:1231-8.

10421 St-Onge MP, Jones PJ. Physiological effects of medium-chain triglycerides: potential agents in the prevention of obesity. *J Nutr* 2002;132:329-32.

10422 Burns A, Byrne J, Ballard C, Holmes C. Sensory stimulation in dementia. *BMJ* 2002;325:1312-3.

10423 Cerny A, Shmid K. Tolerability and efficacy of valerian/lemon balm in healthy volunteers (a double blind, placebo-controlled, multicentre study). *Fitoterapia* 1999;70:221-8.

10424 Glass JR, Sproule BA, Herrmann N, et al. Acute pharmacological effects of temazepam, diphenhydramine, and valerian in healthy elderly subjects. *J Clin Psychopharmacol* 2003;23:260-8.

10425 Ishani A, MacDonald R, Nelson D, et al. Pygeum africanum for the treatment of patients with benign prostatic hyperplasia: a systematic review and quantitative meta-analysis. *Am J Med* 2000;109:654-64.

10426 Wilt T, Ishani A, Mac Donald R, et al. Pygeum africanum for benign prostatic hyperplasia. *Cochrane Database Syst Rev* 2002;CD001044.

10427 DiCenzo R, Shelton M, Jordan K, et al. Coadministration of milk thistle and indinavir in healthy subjects. *Pharmacotherapy* 2003;23:866-70.

REFERENCES

10428 Shyu KG, Cheng JJ, Kuan P. Acetylcysteine protects against acute renal damage in patients with abnormal renal function undergoing a coronary procedure. *J Am Coll Cardiol* 2002;40:1383-8.

10429 Pela R, Calcagni AM, Subiaco S, et al. N-acetylcysteine reduces the exacerbation rate in patients with moderate to severe COPD. *Respiration* 1999;66:495-500.

10430 Tepel M, van der Giet M, Statz M, et al. The antioxidant acetylcysteine reduces cardiovascular events in patients with end-stage renal failure: a randomized, controlled trial. *Circulation* 2003;107:992-5.

10431 Waterhouse ET, Washington C, Washington N. An investigation into the efficacy of the pectin based anti-reflux formulation-Aflurax. *Int J Pharm* 2000;209:79-85.

10432 Webster MJ. Physiological and performance responses to supplementation with thiamin and pantothenic acid derivatives. *Eur J Appl Physiol Occup Physiol* 1998;77:486-91.

10433 Anon. Calcium pantothenate in arthritic conditions. A report from the General Practitioner Research Group. *Practitioner* 1980;224:208-11.

10434 Gaede P, Poulsen HE, Parving HH, Pedersen O. Double-blind, randomised study of the effect of combined treatment with vitamin C and E on albuminuria in Type 2 diabetic patients. *Diabet Med* 2001;18:756-60.

10435 Terry P, Lagergren J, Ye W, et al. Inverse association between intake of cereal fiber and risk of gastric cardia cancer. *Gastroenterology* 2001;120:387-91.

10436 Jiao DH, Ma YH, Chen SJ, et al. Resume of 400 cases of acute upper digestive tract bleeding treated by rhubarb alone. *Pharmacology* 1980;20 Suppl 1:128-30.

10437 Saller R, Buechi S, Meyrat R, Schmidhauser C. Combined herbal preparation for topical treatment of Herpes labialis. *Forsch Komplementarmed Klass Naturheilkd* 2001;8:373-82.

10438 Hilsden RJ, Verhoef MJ, Best A, Pocobelli G. Complementary and alternative medicine use by Canadian patients with inflammatory bowel disease: results from a national survey. *Am J Gastroenterol* 2003;98:1563-8.

10439 Vasile A, Goldberg R, Kornberg B. Pyridoxine toxicity: report of a case. *J Am Osteopath Assoc* 1984;83:790-1.

10440 Ardizzone S, Porro GB. Inflammatory bowel disease: new insights into pathogenesis and treatment. *J Intern Med* 2002;252:475-96.

10443 Attar A, Flourie B, Rambaud JC, et al. Antibiotic efficacy in small intestinal bacterial overgrowth-related chronic diarrhea: a crossover, randomized trial. *Gastroenterology* 1999;117:794-7.

10447 Chan LY, Chiu PY, Lau TK. An in-vitro study of ginsenoside Rb(1)-induced teratogenicity using a whole rat embryo culture model. *Hum Reprod* 2003;18:2166-8.

10448 Groning R, Breitkreutz J, Muller RS. Physico-chemical interactions between extracts of Hypericum perforatum L. and drugs. *Eur J Pharm Biopharm* 2003;56:231-6.

10450 Fong KC, Kinnear PE. Retrobulbar haemorrhage associated with chronic Ginkgo biloba ingestion. *Postgrad Med J* 2003;79:531-2.

10451 deVere White RW, Hackman RM, Soares SE, et al. Effects of a mushroom mycelium extract on the treatment of prostate cancer. *Urology* 2002;60:640-4.

10452 Anon. Possible interaction between warfarin and cranberry juice. *Current Problems in Pharmacovigilance* 2003;29:8.

10453 Sharma RA, McLelland HR, Hill KA, et al. Pharmacodynamic and pharmacokinetic study of oral Curcuma extract in patients with colorectal cancer. *Clin Cancer Res* 2001;7:1894-900.

10454 Matsuyama Y, Morita T, Higuchi M, Tsujii T. The effect of taurine administration on patients with acute hepatitis. *Prog Clin Biol Res* 1983;125:461-8.

10455 Smith LJ, Lacaille F, Lepage G, et al. Taurine decreases fecal fatty acid and sterol excretion in cystic fibrosis. A randomized double-blind trial. *Am J Dis Child* 1991;145:1401-4.

10456 Hiatt WR, Regensteiner JG, Creager MA, et al. Propionyl-L-carnitine improves exercise performance and functional status in patients with claudication. *Am J Med* 2001;110:616-22.

10457 Stalenhoef AF, Hectors M, Demacker PN. Effect of plant sterol-enriched margarine on plasma lipids and sterols in subjects heterozygous for phytosterolaemia. *J Intern Med* 2001;249:163-6.

10458 Burke V, Hodgson JM, Beilin LJ, et al. Dietary protein and soluble fiber reduce ambulatory blood pressure in treated hypertensives. *Hypertension* 2001;38:821-6.

10459 Wangen KE, Duncan AM, Xu X, Kurzer MS. Soy isoflavones improve plasma lipids in normocholesterolemic and mildly hypercholesterolemic postmenopausal women. *Am J Clin Nutr* 2001;73:225-31.

10460 Albert A, Altabre C, Baro F, et al. Efficacy and safety of a phytoestrogen preparation derived from Glycine max (L.) Merr in climacteric symptomatology: a multicentric, open, prospective and non-randomized trial. *Phytomedicine* 2002;9:85-92.

10461 Shao ZM, Shen ZZ, Fontana JA, Barsky SH. Genistein's "ER-dependent and independent" actions are mediated through ER pathways in ER-positive breast carcinoma cell lines. *Anticancer Res* 2000;20:2409-16.

10462 Conaway CC, Getahun SM, Liebes LL, et al. Disposition of glucosinolates and sulforaphane in humans after ingestion of steamed and fresh broccoli. *Nutr Cancer* 2000;38:168-78.

10463 Nestle M. Broccoli sprouts in cancer prevention. *Nutr Rev* 1998;56:127-30.

10464 Elmadfa I, Heinzle C, Majchrzak D, Foissy H. Influence of a probiotic yoghurt on the status of vitamins B(1), B(2) and B(6) in the healthy adult human. *Ann Nutr Metab* 2001;45:13-8.

10465 Purohit V, Russo D. Role of S-adenosyl-L-methionine in the treatment of alcoholic liver disease: introduction and summary of the symposium. *Alcohol* 2002;27:151-4.

10466 Charlton CG, Crowell B Jr. Parkinson's disease-like effects of S-adenosyl-L-methionine: effects of L-dopa. *Pharmacol Biochem Behav* 1992;43:423-31.

10467 Elson CO. Genes, microbes, and T cells - new therapeutic targets in Crohn's disease. *N Engl J Med* 2002;346:614-6.

10468 Dalton SD, Rahimi AR. Emerging role of riboflavin in the treatment of nucleoside analogue-induced type B lactic acidosis. *AIDS Patient Care STDS* 2001;15:611-4.

10472 Hamilton IM, Gilmore WS, Benzie IF, et al. Interactions between vitamins C and E in human subjects. *Br J Nutr* 2000;84:261-7.

10473 Salonen RM, Nyyssonen K, Kaikkonen J, et al. Six-year effect of combined vitamin C and E supplementation on atherosclerotic progression: the Antioxidant Supplementation in Atherosclerosis Prevention (ASAP) Study. *Circulation* 2003;107:947-53.

10501 Palva IP, Salokannel SJ, Palva HLA, et al. Drug-induced malabsorption of vitamin B12. VII Malabsorption of B12 during treatment with potassium citrate. *Acta Med Scand* 1974;196:525-6.

10502 Lees F. Radioactive vitamin B12 absorption in the megaloblastic anemia caused by anticonvulsant drugs. *Q J Med* 1961;30:231-48.

10503 Reynolds EH, Hallpike JF, Phillips BM, et al. Reversible absorptive defects in anticonvulsant megaloblastic anemia. *J Clin Pathol* 1965;18:593-8.

10504 Frenkel EP, McCall MS, Sheehan RG. Cerebrospinal fluid folate and vitamin B12 in anticonvulsant-induced megaloblastosis. *J Lab Clin Med* 1973;81:105-15.

10505 Reynolds EH. Schizophrenia-like psychoses of epilepsy and disturbances of folate and vitamin B12 metabolism induced by anticonvulsant drugs. *Br J Psychiatry* 1967;113:911-9.

10506 Levy WC, Soine LA, Huth MM, Fishbein DP. Thiamine deficiency in heart failure (letter). *Am J Med* 1992;93:705-6.

10507 Leslie D, Gheorghiade M. Is there a role for thiamine supplementation in the management of heart failure. *Am Heart J* 1996;131:1248-50.

10508 Saif MW. Is there a role for thiamine in the management of congestive heart failure? (letter) *South Med J* 2003;96:114-5.

10509 Lubetsky A, Winaver J, Seligmann H, et al. Urinary thiamine excretion in the rat: effects of furosemide, other diuretics, and volume load. *J Lab Clin Med* 1999;134:232-7.

10510 Botez MI, Botez T, Ross-Chouinard A, Lalonde R. Thiamine and folate treatment of chronic epileptic patients: a controlled study with the Wechsler IQ scale. *Epilepsy Res* 1993;16:157-63.

10511 Botez MI, Joyal C, Maag U, Bachevalier J. Cerebrospinal fluid and blood thiamine concentrations in phenytoin-treated epileptics. *Can J Neurol Sci* 1982;9:37-9.

10512 Patrini C, Perucca E, Reggiani C, Rindi G. Effects of phenytoin on the in vivo kinetics of thiamine and its phosphoesters in rat nervous tissues. *Brain Res* 1993;628:179-86.

10513 Levy G, Gibaldi M, Procknal JA. Effect of an anticholinergic agent on riboflavin absorption in man. *J Pharm Sci* 1972;61:798-9.

10514 Grundhofer B, Gibaldi M. Biopharmaceutic factors that influence effects of anticholinergic drugs: comparison of propantheline, hexocyclium, and isopropamide. *J Pharm Sci* 1977;66:1433-5.

10515 Yanagawa N, Shih RN, Jo OD, Said HM. Riboflavin transport by isolated perfused rabbit renal proximal tubules. *Am J Physiol Cell Physiol* 2000;279:C1782-6.

10516 Jusko WJ, Levy G. Effect of probenecid on riboflavin absorption and excretion in man. *J Pharm Sci* 1967;56:1145-9.

10517 Jusko WJ, Levy G, Yaffe SJ, Gorodischer R. Effect of probenecid on renal clearance of riboflavin in man. *J Pharm Sci* 1970;59:473-7.

10518 Pinto J, Huang YP, Rivlin RS. Inhibition of riboflavin metabolism in rat tissues by chlorpromazine, imipramine and amitriptyline. *J Clin Invest* 1981;67:1500-6.

10519 Pinto J, Huang YP, Pelliccione N, Rivlin RS. Cardiac sensitivity to the inhibitory effects of chlorpromazine, imipramine, and amitriptyline upon formation of flavins. *Biochem Pharmacol* 1982;31:3495-9.

10520 Pelliccione N, Pinto J, Huang YP, Rivlin RS. Accelerated development of riboflavin deficiency by treatment with chlorpromazine. *Biochem Pharmacol* 1983;32:2949-53.

10521 Raiczyk GB, Dutta P, Pinto J. Chlorpromazine and quinacrine inhibit flavin adenine dinucleotide biosynthesis in skeletal muscle. *Physiologist* 1985;28:322.

10522 Dutta P, Pinto J, Rivlin R. Antimalarial effects of riboflavin deficiency. *Lancet* 1985;2:1040-3.

10523 Ahmed F, Bamji MS, Iyengar L. Effect of oral contraceptive agents on vitamin nutrition status. *Am J Clin Nutr* 1975;28:606-15.

10524 Briggs M. Oral contraceptives and vitamin nutrition (letter). *Lancet* 1974;1:1234-5.

10525 Newman LJ, Lopez R, Cole HS, et al. Riboflavin deficiency in women taking oral contraceptive agents. *Am J Clin Nutr* 1978;31:247-9.

10526 Roe DA, Bogusz S, Sheu J, et al. Factors affecting riboflavin requirements of oral contraceptive users and non-users. *Am J Clin Nutr* 1982;35:495-501.

10527 Lewis CM, King JC. Effect of oral contraceptive agents on thiamin, riboflavin, and pantothenic acid status in young women. *Am J Clin Nutr* 1980;33:832-8.

10528 Ogura R, Ueta H, Hino Y, et al. Riboflavin deficiency caused by treatment with adriamycin. *J Nutr Sci Vitaminol* 1991;37:473-7.

10529 Raiczyk GB, Pinto J. Inhibition of flavin metabolism by adriamycin in skeletal muscle. *Biochem Pharmacol* 1988;37:1741-4.

10530 Pinto J, Huang YP, Pelliccione N, Rivlin RS. Adriamycin inhibits flavin synthesis in heart: possible relation to cardiotoxicity of anthracyclines (abstract). *Clin Res* 1983;31;467A.

10531 Richman DD, Fischl MA, Grieco MH, et al. The toxicity of azidothymidine (AZT) in the treatment of patients with AIDS and AIDS-related complex. *N Engl J Med* 1987;317:192-7.

10532 Falguera M, Perez-Mur J, Puig T, Cao G. Study of the role of vitamin B12 and folinic acid supplementation in preventing hematologic toxicity of zidovudine. *Eur J Haematol* 1995;55:97-102.

10533 Gharakhanian S, Navarette MS, Cardon B, Rozenbaum W. Vitamin B12 injections in patients treated with zidovudine. *AIDS* 1990;4:701-2.

10534 Ohkawa H, Ohishi N, Yagi K. Hydroxylation of the 7- and 8-methyl groups of riboflavin by the microsomal electron transfer system of rat liver. *J Biol Chem* 1983;258:5629-33.

10535 Hamajima S, Ono S, Hirano H, Obara K. Induction of the FAD synthetase system in rat liver by phenobarbital administration. *Int J Vit Nutr Res* 1979;49:59-63.

10536 Vir SC, Love AH. Riboflavin nutriture of oral contraceptive users. *Int J Vitam Nutr Res* 1979;49:286-90.

10537 Vimokesant S, Nakornchai S, Rungruangsak K, et al. Food habits causing thiamine deficiency in humans. *J Nutr Sci Vitaminol* 1976;22:1-2.

10538 Vimokesant S, Kunjara S, Rungruangsak K, et al. Beriberi caused by antithiamin factors in food and its prevention. *Ann N Y Acad Sci* 1982;378:123-36.

10539 Smidt LJ, Cremin FM, Grivetti LE, Clifford AJ. Influence of folate status and polyphenol intake on thiamin status in Irish women. *Am J Clin Nutr* 1990;52:1077-92.

10540 Hilker DM, Somogyi JC. Antithiamins of plant origin: their chemical nature and mode of action. *Ann N Y Acad Sci* 1982;378:137-44.

10541 Waldenlind L. Studies on thiamine and neuromuscular transmission. *Acta Physiologica Scandinavica. Supplementum* 1978;459:1-35.

10542 Coronato A, Glass GB. Depression of the intestinal uptake of radio-vitamin B12 by cholestyramine. *Proc Soc Exp Biol Med* 1973;142:1341-4.

10543 Leonard JP, Desager JP, Beckers C, Harvengt C. In vitro binding of various biological substances by two hypocholesterolemic resins. *Arzneimittel-Forschung* 1979;29:97-81.

10544 Somogyi JC, Nageli U. Antithiamine effect of coffee. *Int J Vit Nutr Res* 1976;46:149-53.

10545 Hathcock JN, Hattan DG, Jenkins MY, et al. Evaluation of vitamin A toxicity. *Am J Clin Nutr* 1990;52:183-202.

10546 Walters BN, Gubbay SS. Tetracycline and benign intracranial hypertension: report of five cases. *Br Med J* 1981;282:19-20.

10547 Pearson MG, Littlewood SM, Bowden AN. Tetracycline and benign intracranial hypertension (letter). *Br Med J* 1981;282:568-9.
10548 Thorp VJ. Effect of oral contraceptive agents on vitamin and mineral requirements. *J Am Diet Assoc* 1980;76:581-4.
10549 Domingo JL, Gomez M, Llobet JM, Richart C. Effect of ascorbic acid on gastrointestinal aluminum absorption (letter). *Lancet* 1991;338:1467.
10550 Domingo JL, Gomez M, Llobet JM, Corbella J. Influence of some dietary constituents on aluminum absorption and retention in rats. *Kidney Int* 1991;39:598-601.
10551 Partridge NA, Regnier FE, White JL, Hem SL. Influence of dietary constituents on intestinal absorption of aluminum. *Kidney Int* 1989;35:1413-7.
10552 Aksoy M, Basu TK, Brient J, Dickerson JW. Thiamin status of patients treated with drug combinations containing 5-fluorouracil. *Eur J Cancer* 1980;16:1041-5.
10553 Ulusakarya A, Vantelon JM, Munck JN, et al. Thiamine deficiency in a patient receiving chemotherapy for acute myeloblastic leukemia (letter). *Am J Hematol* 1999;61:155-6
10554 De Reuck JL, Sieben GJ, Sieben-Praet MR, et al. Wernicke's encephalopathy in patients with tumors of the lymphoid-hemopoietic systems. *Arch Neurol* 1980;37:338-41.
10555 Briggs MH, Briggs M. Thiamine status and oral contraceptives. *Contraception* 1975;11:151-4.
10556 Vir SC, Love AH. Effect of oral contraceptive agents on thiamin status. *Int J Vit Nutr Res* 1979;49:291-5.
10557 DiPalma JR, Ritchie DM. Vitamin Toxicity. *Annu Rev Pharmacol Toxicol* 1977;17:133-48.
10558 Bauernfeind JC, Newmark H, Brin M. Vitamins A and E nutrition via intramuscular or oral route. *Am J Clin Nutr* 1974;27:234-53.
10559 Kusin JA, Reddy V, Sivakumar B. Vitamin E supplements and the absorption of a massive dose of vitamin A. *Am J Clin Nutr* 1974;27:774-6.
10560 Bendich A, Langseth L. Safety of vitamin A. *Am J Clin Nutr* 1989;49:358-71.
10561 Willett WC, Stampfer MJ, Underwood BA, et al. Vitamins A, E and carotene: effects of supplementation on their plasma levels. *Am J Clin Nutr* 1983;38:559-66.
10562 Ayres S, Mihan R, Scribner MD. Synergism of vitamins A and E with dermatologic applications. *Cutis* 1979;23:600-3, 689-90.
10563 Jagadeesan V, Reddy V. Interrelationship between vitamin E and A: a clinical study. *Clin Chim Acta* 1978;90:71-4.
10564 Garrett-Laster M, Oaks L, Russell RM, Oaks E. A lowering effect of a pharmacological dose of vitamin E on serum vitamin A in normal adults. *Nutr Res* 1981;1:559-64.
10565 Barrowman JA, Broomhall J, Cannon AM, et al. Impairment of vitamin A absorption by neomycin. *Clin Sci* 1972;42:17P.
10566 Schade RWB, van't Laar A, Majoor CLH, Jansen AP. A comparative study of the effects of cholestyramine and neomycin in the treatment of type II hyperlipoproteinemia. *Acta Med Scand* 1976;199:175-80.
10567 Glueck CJ, Tsang RC, Fallat RW, Scheel D. Plasma vitamin A and E levels in children with familial type II hyperlipoproteinemia during therapy with diet and cholestyramine resin. *Pediatrics* 1974;54:51-5.
10568 Probstfield JL, Lin TL, Peters J, Hunninghake DB. Carotenoids and vitamin A: the effect of hypocholesterolemic agents on serum levels. *Metabolism* 1985;34:88-91.
10569 Lipid Research Clinics Program. The Lipid Research Clinics' Coronary Primary Prevention Trial Results: 1. Reduction in incidence of coronary heart disease. *J Am Med Assoc* 1984;251:351-64.
10570 Davidson MH, Hauptman J, DiGirolamo M, et al. Weight control and risk factor reduction in obese subjects treated for 2 years with orlistat. *JAMA* 1999;281:235-42.
10571 Sjostrom L, Rissanen A, Andersen T, et al. Randomised placebo-controlled trial of orlistat for weight loss and prevention of weight regain in obese patients. *Lancet* 1998;352:167-73.
10572 Mowat C, Carswell A, Wirz A, McColl KE. Omeprazole and dietary nitrate independently affect levels of vitamin C and nitrite in gastric juice. *Gastroenterol* 1999;116:813-22.
10573 Hamon NW, Awang DVC. Horsetail. *Can Pharm J* 1992:399-401.
10574 Bar-Or D, Yoel G. Calcium and calciferol antagonize effect of verapamil in atrial fibrillation. *Br Med J* 1981;282:1585-6.
10575 Grad JM, Bahlis NJ, Reis I, et al. Ascorbic acid enhances arsenic trioxide-induced cytotoxicity in multiple myeloma cells. *Blood* 2001;98(3):805-13.
10576 Bahlis NJ, McCafferty-Grad J, Jordan-McMurry I, et al. Feasability and correlates of arsenic trioxide combined with ascorbic acid-mediated depletion of intracellular glutathione for the treatment of relapsed/refractory multiple myeloma. *Clin Cancer Res* 2002;8:3658-68.
10577 Tannirandorn P, Epstein S. Drug-induced bone loss. *Osteoporosis Int* 2000;11(8):637-59.
10578 Collins N, Maher J, Cole M, et al. A prospective study to evaluate the dose of vitamin D required to correct low 25-hydroxyvitamin D levels, calcium, and alkaline phosphatase in patients at risk of developing antiepileptic drug-induced osteomalacia. *Q J Med* 1991;78:113-22.
10582 Davies VA, Rothberg AD, Argent AC, et al. Precursor prothrombin status in patients receiving anticonvulsant drugs. *Lancet* 1985;1:126-8.
10583 Briggs M, Briggs M. Vitamin C requirements and oral contraceptives. *Nature* 1972;238:277.
10585 Rivers JM. Oral contraceptives and ascorbic acid. *Am J Clin Nutr* 1975;28(5):550-4.
10586 Hudiburgh NK, Milner AN. Influence of oral contraceptives on ascorbic acid and triglyceride status. *J Am Diet Assoc* 1979;75:19-22.
10587 Kuo SM, Lin CP. 17Beta-estradiol inhibition of ascorbic acid accumulation in human intestinal Caco-2 cells. *Eur J Pharmacol* 1998;361:253-9.
10588 Mc Leod DC, Nahata MC. Inefficacy of ascorbic acid as a urinary acidifier (letter). *N Engl J Med* 1977;296:1413.
10589 Hansten PD, Hayton WL. Effect of antacid and ascorbic acid on serum salicylate concentration. *J Clin Pharmacol* 1980;20:326-31.
10590 Loh HS, Wilson CW. The interactions of aspirin and ascorbic acid in normal men. *J Clin Pharmacol* 1975;15:36-45.
10591 Sahud MA, Cohen RJ. Effect of aspirin ingestion on ascorbic-acid levels in rheumatoid arthritis. *Lancet* 1971;1:937-8.
10592 Wilson CW, Greene M. The relationship of aspirin to ascorbic acid metabolism during the common cold. *J Clin Pharmacol* 1978;18:21-8.
10593 Martineau P, Tawil N. Low-molecular-weight heparins in the treatment of deep-vein thrombosis. *Ann Pharmacother* 1998;32:588-98,601.
10594 Zimran A, Shilo S, Fisher D, Bab I. Histomorphometric evaluation of reversible heparin-induced osteoporosis in pregnancy. *Arch Intern Med* 1986;146:386-8.
10595 Dahlman TC. Osteoporotic fractures and the recurrence of thromboembolism during pregnancy and the puerperium in 184 women undergoing thromboprophylaxis with heparin. *Am J Obstet Gynecol* 1993;168:1265-70.

10596 Barbour LA, Kick SD, Steiner JF, et al. A prospective study of heparin-induced osteoporosis in pregnancy using bone densitometry. *Am J Obstet Gynecol* 1994;170:862-9.

10597 Aarskog D, Aksnes L, Lehmann V. Low 1,25-dihydroxyvitamin D in heparin-induced osteopenia (letter). *Lancet* 1980;2:650-1.

10598 Monreal M, Olive A, Lafoz E, del Rio L. Heparins, coumarin and bone density (letter). *Lancet* 1991;338:706.

10599 Pettila V, Leinonen P, Markkola A, et al. Postpartum bone mineral density in women treated for thromboprophylaxis with unfractionated heparin or LMW heparin. *Thromb Haemost* 2002;87:182-6.

10600 Offenbacher EG. Promotion of chromium absorption by ascorbic acid. *Trace Elements Electrolytes* 1994;11:178-81.

10601 Agency for Healthcare Research and Quality. "Evidence Report/Technology Assessment Number 54: Management of Allergic and Nonallergic Rhinitis" http://www.ahrq.gov/clinic/epcsums/rhinsum.pdf (Accessed 4 March 2003).

10602 Skoner DP. Allergic rhinitis: definition, epidemiology, pathophysiology, detection, and diagnosis. *J Allergy Clin Immunol* 2001;108:S2-8.

10603 Blanc PD, Trupin L, Earnest G, et al. Alternative therapies among adults with a reported diagnosis of asthma or rhinosinusitis: data from a population-based survey. *Chest* 2001;120:1461-1467.

10604 Zuckerman GB, Bielory L. Complementary and alternative medicine herbal therapies for atopic disorders. *Am J Med* 2002;113:47S-51S.

10605 Schapowal A. Petasites Study Group. Randomised controlled trial of butterbur and cetirizine for treating seasonal allergic rhinitis. *BMJ* 2002;324:144-6.

10606 Jellin J, Gregory PJ, Batz F, Hitchens K, et al. Natural Medicines Comprehensive Database. Stockton, CA: Therapeutic Research Faculty; 2002. www.naturaldatabase.com (Accessed 6 February 2003).

10607 Ziment I, Tashkin DP. Alternative medicine for allergy and asthma. *J Allergy Clin Immunol* 2000;106:603-614.

10608 Podoshin L, Gertner R, Fradis M. Treatment of perennial allergic rhinitis with ascorbic acid solution. *Ear Nose Throat J* 1991;70:54-55.

10609 Bucca C, Rolla G, Oliva A, Farina JC. Effect of vitamin C on histamine bronchial responsiveness of patients with allergic rhinitis. *Ann Allergy* 1990;65:311-314.

10610 Fortner BR Jr, Danziger RE, Rabinowitz PS, Nelson HS. The effect of ascorbic acid on cutaneous and nasal response to histamine and allergen. *J Allergy Clin Immunol* 1982;69:484-488.

10611 Johnston CS, Solomon RE, Corte C. Vitamin C depletion is associated with alterations in blood histamine and plasma free carnitine in adults. *J Am Coll Nutr* 1996;15:586-591.

10612 Jaber R. Respiratory and allergic diseases: from upper respiratory tract infections to asthma. *Prim Care* 2002;29:231-261.

10613 Food and Drug Administration Press Release. "Pacific Biologic Recalls Seven Herbal Products That Contain the Herb Akebia Trifoliata Caulis (Mu Tong) and the Herb Asarum Sieboldii Herba Cum Radix (Xi Xin) Because of a Possible Health Risk." http://www.fda.gov/oc/po/firmrecalls/pacificbio8_01.html (Accessed 10 February 2003).

10614 Ernst E. "Alternative" therapies for asthma: reason for concern? *Chest* 2001;120:1433-1434.

10615 Johnston CS, Bowling DL. Stability of ascorbic acid in commercially available orange juices. *J Am Diet Assoc* 2002;102:525-529.

10616 Di Caro A, Perola E, Bartolini B, et al. Fractions of chemically oversulphated galactosaminoglycan sulphates inhibit three enveloped viruses: human immunodeficiency virus type 1, herpes simplex virus type 1 and human cytomegalovirus. *Antivir Chem Chemother* 1999;10:33-8.

10617 Tamir S, Eizenberg M, Somjen D, et al. Estrogenic and antiproliferative properties of glabridin from licorice in human breast cancer cells. *Cancer Res* 2000;60:5704-9.

10618 Strandberg TE, Andersson S, Jarvenpaa AL, et al. Preterm birth and licorice consumption during pregnancy. *Am J Epidemiol* 2002;156:803-5.

10619 Hussain RM. The sweet cake that reaches parts other cakes can't! *Postgrad Med J* 2003;79:115-6.

10620 Johnson-Kozlow M, Kritz-Silverstein D, Barrett-Connor E, et al. Coffee consumption and cognitive function among older adults. *Am J Epidemiol* 2002;156:842-50.

10621 Wisborg K, Kesmodel U, Bech BH, et al. Maternal consumption of coffee during pregnancy and stillbirth and infant death in first year of life: prospective study. *BMJ* 2003;326:420.

10622 Stone MB, Merrick MA, Ingersoll CD, et al. Preliminary comparison of bromelain and Ibuprofen for delayed onset muscle soreness management. *Clin J Sport Med* 2002;12:373-8.

10623 Leung R, Thien FC, Baldo B, et al. Royal jelly-induced asthma and anaphylaxis: clinical characteristics and immunologic correlations. *J Allergy Clin Immunol* 1995;96:1004-7.

10624 Peacock S, Murray V, Turton C. Respiratory distress and royal jelly. *BMJ* 1995;311:1472.

10625 Hucker HB, Ahmad PM, Miller EA, et al. Metabolism of dimethyl sulphoxide to dimethyl sulphone in the rat and man. *Nature* 1966;209:619-20.

10627 Sugimoto K, Ohmori M, Tsuruoka S, et al. Different effects of St John's wort on the pharmacokinetics of simvastatin and pravastatin. *Clin Pharmacol Ther* 2001;70:518-24.

10628 Bauer S, Stormer E, Johne A, et al. Alterations in cyclosporin A pharmacokinetics and metabolism during treatment with St John's wort in renal transplant patients. *Br J Clin Pharmacol* 2003;55:203-11.

10629 Ernst E, Pittler MH. Yohimbine for erectile dysfunction: a systematic review and meta-analysis of randomized clinical trials. *J Urol* 1998;159:433-6.

10630 Kaziro GS. Metronidazole (Flagyl) and Arnica Montana in the prevention of post-surgical complications, a comparative placebo controlled clinical trial. *Br J Oral Maxillofac Surg* 1984;22:42-9.

10631 Abdelmalek MF, Angulo P, Jorgensen RA, et al. Betaine, a promising new agent for patients with nonalcoholic steatohepatitis: results of a pilot study. *Am J Gastroenterol* 2001;96:2711-7.

10633 Birketvedt GS, Travis A, Langbakk B, Florholmen JR. Dietary supplementation with bean extract improves lipid profile in overweight and obese subjects. *Nutrition* 2002;18:729-33.

10634 Naguib YM. Antioxidant activities of astaxanthin and related carotenoids. *J Agric Food Chem* 2000;48:1150-4.

10635 Zabihi E, Abdollahi M. Endocrinotoxicity induced by Coriandrum sativa: a case report. *WHO Drug Information* 2001;16:15.

10636 Huynh NT, Tayek JA. Oral arginine reduces systemic blood pressure in type 2 diabetes: its potential role in nitric oxide generation. *J Am Coll Nutr* 2002;21:422-7.

10637 Venho B, Voutilainen S, Valkonen VP, et al. Arginine intake, blood pressure, and the incidence of acute coronary events in men: the Kuopio Ischaemic Heart Disease Risk Factor Study. *Am J Clin Nutr* 2002;76:359-64.

10638 Neil HA, Meijer GW, Roe LS. Randomised controlled trial of use by hypercholesterolaemic patients of a vegetable oil sterol-enriched fat spread. *Atherosclerosis* 2001;156:329-37.

10639 Taussig SJ, Batkin S. Bromelain, the enzyme complex of pineapple (Ananas comosus) and its clinical application. An update. *J Ethnopharmacol* 1988;22:191-203.

10640 Zvosec DL, Smith SW, McCutcheon JR, et al. Adverse events, including death, associated with the use of 1,4-butanediol. *N Engl J Med.* 2001;344:87-94.

10641 Green GA, Catlin DH, Starcevic B. Analysis of over-the-counter dietary supplements. *Clin J Sport Med* 2001;11:254-9.

10642 Moussard C, Alber D, Toubin MM, et al. A drug used in traditional medicine, harpagophytum procumbens: no evidence for NSAID-like effect on whole blood eicosanoid production in human. *Prostaglandins Leukot Essent Fatty Acids* 1992;46:283-6.

10643 Zemtsov A, Gaddis M, Montalvo-Lugo VM, Zemstov A. Moisturizing and cosmetic properties of emu oil: a pilot double blind study. *Australas J Dermatol* 1996;37:159-61.

10644 Hipkiss AR, Preston JE, Himswoth DT, et al. Protective effects of carnosine against malondialdehyde-induced toxicity towards cultured rat brain endothelial cells. *Neurosci Lett* 1997;238:135-8.

10645 Preston JE, Hipkiss AR, Himsworth DT, et al. Toxic effects of beta-amyloid(25-35) on immortalised rat brain endothelial cell: protection by carnosine, homocarnosine and beta-alanine. *Neurosci Lett* 1998;242:105-8.

10646 Moses, G. Thyroxine interacts with celery seed tablets? *Australian Prescriber* 2001;24:6-7.

10647 Hori K, Martin TG, Rainey P, Robertson WO. Believe it or not--silver still poisons! *Vet Hum Toxicol* 2002;44:291-2.

10648 McKenna JK, Hull CM, Zone JJ. Argyria associated with colloidal silver supplementation. *Int J Dermatol* 2003;42:549.

10649 Wang N, Luo HW, Niwa M, Ji J. A new platelet aggregation inhibitor from Salvia miltiorrhiza. *Planta Med* 1989;55:390-1.

10650 Stander S, Luger T, Metze D. Treatment of prurigo nodularis with topical capsaicin. *J Am Acad Dermatol* 2001;44:471-8.

10651 Popper C. Do Vitamins or Minerals (Apart from Lithium) have mood-stabilizing effects? *J Clin Psychiatry* 2001;62:933-35.

10652 Cashman K, Baker A, Ginty F, et al. No effect of copper supplementation on biochemical markers of bone metabolism in healthy young adult females despite apparently improvedcopper status. *Eur J Clin Nutr* 2001;55:525-31.

10653 Goldfain D, Lavergne A, Galian A, et al. Peculiar acute toxic colitis after ingestion of colocynth: a clinicopathological study of three cases. *Gut* 1989;30:1412-18.

10654 Schneider-Gold C, Beck M, Wessig C, et al. Creatine monohydrate in DM2/PROMM. A double-blind placebo-controlled clinical study. *Neurology* 2003;60:500-2.

10655 Rees C, Oppong K, Mardini H, et al. Effect of L-Ornithine-L-Aspartate on patients with and without TIPS undergoing glutamine challenge: a double blind, placebo controlled trial. *Gut* 2000;47:571-4.

10656 Dyer J, Roth B, Hyma B. Gamma-Hydroxybutyrate withdrawal syndrome. *Ann Emerg Med* 2001;37:147-53.

10657 Ingels M, Rangan C, Bellezzo J, Clark R. Coma and respiratory depression following the ingestion of GHB and its precursors: Three cases. *J Emerg Med* 2000;19:47-50.

10658 Mason P, Kerns II W. Gamma Hydroxybutyric Acid (GHB) Intoxication. *Acad Emerg Med* 2002;9:730-39.

10659 Tzipori S, Roberton D, Chapman C. Remission of diarrhoea due to cryptosporidiosis in an immunodeficient child treated with hyperimmune bovine colostrum. *Br Med J* 1986;293:1276-7.

10660 Kaplan BJ, Simpson JS, Ferre RC, et al. Effective mood stabilization with a chelated mineral supplement: an open-label trial in bipolar disorder. *J Clin Psychiatry* 2001;62:936-44.

10661 Pfaffenrath V, Wessely P, Meyer C, et al. Magnesium in the prophylaxis of migraine--a double-blind placebo-controlled study. *Cephalalgia* 1996;16:436-40.

10663 Wang F, Van Den Eeden SK, Ackerson LM, et al. Oral magnesium oxide prophylaxis of frequent migrainous headache in children: a randomized, double-blind, placebo-controlled trial. *Headache* 2003;43:601-10.

10664 Rodriguez-Moran M, Guerrero-Romero F. Oral magnesium supplementation improves insulin sensitivity and metabolic control in type 2 diabetic subjects: A randomized double-blind controlled trial. *Diabetes Care* 2003;26:1147-52.

10665 Lee JW. Manganese intoxication. *Arch Neurol* 2000;57:597-9.

10666 Powers KM, Smith-Weller T, Franklin GM, et al. Parkinson's disease risks associated with dietary iron, manganese, and other nutrient intakes. *Neurology* 2003;60:1761-6.

10667 Subbotina MD, Timchenko VN, Vorobyov MM, et al. Effect of oral administration of tormentil root extract (Potentilla tormentilla) on rotavirus diarrhea in children: a randomized, double blind, controlled trial. *Pediatr Infect Dis J.* 2003;22:706-11.

10668 Lopez de Romana D, Lonnerdal B, Brown KH. Absorption of zinc from wheat products fortified with iron and either zinc sulfate or zinc oxide. *Am J Clin Nutr* 2003;78:279-83.

10669 Krone CA, Wyse EJ, Ely JT. Cadmium in zinc-containing mineral supplements. *Int J Food Sci Nutr* 2001;52:379-82.

10670 Lewy AJ, Bauer VK, Cutler NL, Sack RL. Melatonin treatment of winter depression: a pilot study. *Psychiatry Res* 1998;77:57-61.

10671 Pei Z, Pang SF, Cheung RT. Administration of melatonin after onset of ischemia reduces the volume of cerebral infarction in a rat middle cerebral artery occlusion stroke model. *Stroke* 2003;34:770-5.

10672 Ernst E, Schmidt K, Steuer-Vogt MK. Mistletoe for cancer? A systematic review of randomised clinical trials. *Int J Cancer* 2003;107:262-7.

10673 Togna GI, Togna AR, Franconi M, et al. Olive oil isochromans inhibit human platelet reactivity. *J Nutr* 2003;133:2532-6.

10674 Lipsky PE, Tao XL. A potential new treatment for rheumatoid arthritis: thunder god vine. *Semin Arthritis Rheum* 1997;26:713-23.

10675 Tao X, Younger J, Fan FZ, et al. Benefit of an extract of Tripterygium Wilfordii Hook F in patients with rheumatoid arthritis: a double-blind, placebo-controlled study. *Arthritis Rheum* 2002;46:1735-43.

10676 Tao X, Cush JJ, Garret M, Lipsky PE. A phase I study of ethyl acetate extract of the chinese antirheumatic herb Tripterygium wilfordii hook F in rheumatoid arthritis. *J Rheumatol* 2001;28:2160-7.

10677 Jiang X. Clinical observations on the use of the Chinese herb Tripterygium wilfordii Hook for the treatment of nephrotic syndrome. *Pediatr Nephrol* 1994;8:343-4.

10678 Brooks JD, Paton V. Potent induction of carcinogen defense enzymes with sulforaphane, a putative prostate cancer chemopreventive agent. *Prostate Cancer Prostatic Dis* 1999;2:S8.

10679 Vermeulen M, van Rooijen HJ, Vaes WH. Analysis of isothiocyanate mercapturic acids in urine: a biomarker for cruciferous vegetable intake. *J Agric Food Chem* 2003;51:3554-9.

10680 Zhang J, Svehlikova V, Bao Y, et al. Synergy between sulforaphane and selenium in the induction of thioredoxin reductase 1 requires both transcriptional and translational modulation. *Carcinogenesis* 2003;24:497-503.

10681 Zhang Y, Callaway EC. High cellular accumulation of sulphoraphane, a dietary anticarcinogen, is followed by rapid transporter-mediated export as a glutathione conjugate. *Biochem J* 2002;364:301-7.

10682 Heiss E, Herhaus C, Klimo K, et al. Nuclear factor kappa B is a molecular target for sulforaphane-mediated anti-inflammatory mechanisms. *J Biol Chem* 2001;276:32008-15.

10683 Miranda CL, Stevens JF, Helmrich A, et al. Antiproliferative and cytotoxic effects of prenylated flavonoids from hops (Humulus lupulus) in human cancer cell lines. *Food Chem Toxicol* 1999;37:271-85.

10684 Milligan SR, Kalita JC, Heyerick A, et al. Identification of a potent phytoestrogen in hops (Humulus lupulus L.) and beer. *J Clin Endocrinol Metab* 1999;84:2249-52.

10685 Milligan SR, Kalita JC, Pocock V, et al. The endocrine activities of 8-prenylnaringenin and related hop (Humulus lupulus L.) flavonoids. *J Clin Endocrinol Metab* 2000;85:4912-5.

10686 Henderson MC, Miranda CL, Stevens JF, et al. In vitro inhibition of human P450 enzymes by prenylated flavonoids from hops, Humulus lupulus. *Xenobiotica* 2000;30:235-51.

10687 Duffield-Lillico AJ, Slate EH, Reid ME, et al. Selenium supplementation and secondary prevention of nonmelanoma skin cancer in a randomized trial. *J Natl Cancer Inst* 2003;95:1477-81.

10688 Levisky JA, Karch SB, Bowerman DL, et al. False-positive RIA for methamphetamine following ingestion of an Ephedra-derived herbal product. *J Anal Toxicol* 2003;27:123-4.

10689 Walton R, Manos GH. Psychosis related to ephedra-containing herbal supplement use. *South Med J* 2003;96:718-20.

10690 Sandhu RS, Prescilla RP, Simonelli TM, Edwards DJ. Influence of goldenseal root on the pharmacokinetics of indinavir. *J Clin Pharmacol* 2003;43:1283-8.

10691 Reider N, Komericki P, Hausen BM, et al. The seamy side of natural medicines: contact sensitization to arnica (Arnica montana L.) and marigold (Calendula officinalis L.). *Contact Dermatitis* 2001;45:269-72.

10692 Lontos S, Jones RM, Angus PW, Gow PJ. Acute liver failure associated with the use of herbal preparations containing black cohosh. *Med J Aust* 2003;179:390-1.

10693 Maheu E, Mazieres B, Valat JP, et al. Symptomatic efficacy of avocado/soybean unsaponifiables in the treatment of osteoarthritis of the knee and hip: a prospective, randomized, double-blind, placebo-controlled, multicenter clinical trial with a six-month treatment period and a two-month followup demonstrating a persistent effect. *Arthritis Rheum* 1998;41:81-91.

10694 Lequesne M, Maheu E, Cadet C, Dreiser RL. Structural effect of avocado/soybean unsaponifiables on joint space loss in osteoarthritis of the hip. *Arthritis Rheum* 2002;47:50-8.

10695 Henrotin YE, Sanchez C, Deberg MA, et al. Avocado/soybean unsaponifiables increase aggrecan synthesis and reduce catabolic and proinflammatory mediator production by human osteoarthritic chondrocytes. *J Rheumatol* 2003;30:1825-34.

10696 Beckham SG, Earnest CP. Four weeks of androstenedione supplementation diminishes the treatment response in middle aged men. *Br J Sports Med* 2003;37:212-8.

10697 Reimund E. Butylated hydroxytoluene, lipid-enveloped viruses, and AIDS. *Med Hypotheses* 1987;23:39-42.

10698 Grogan MW. Toxicity from BHT ingestion. *West J Med* 1986;145:245-6.

10699 Shlian DM, Goldstone J. More on BHT toxicity. *West J Med* 1986;145:699.

10701 Jacobson M, Liebman B, Schmidt SB, eds. Defensive eating: staying lean in a fattening world. *Nutrition Action Healthletter* 2001;28:3-8.

10702 Blair SN, Nichaman MZ. The public health problem of increasing prevalence rates of obesity and what should be done about it. *Mayo Clin Proc* 2002;77:109-13.

10703 Young LR, Nestle M. The contribution of expanding portion sizes to the US obesity epidemic. *Am J Public Health* 2002;92:246-9.

10704 Dickerson L, Carek PJ. Drug therapy for obesity. *Am Fam Physician* 2000; 61:2131-43.

10705 Guidelines on Overweight and Obesity. National Heart, Lung, and Blood Institute 1998. http://www.nhlbi.nih.gov/guidelines/obesity (Accessed 11 Feb 2002).

10706 Palacioz K. Phenylpropanolamine withdrawal. *Pharmacist's Letter/Prescriber's Letter* 2000;12:161202.

10707 Allen J. New Drug: Sibutramine. *Pharmacist's Letter/Prescriber's Letter* 1998;3:140305.

10708 Kehoe WA. Bupropion for weight loss. *Pharmacist's Letter/Prescriber's Letter* 1999;15:150710.

10709 FDA. Information paper on L-tryptophan and 5-hydroxy-L-tryptophan. Feb 2001. Available at: http://vm.cfsan.fda.gov/~dms/ds-tryp1.html.

10710 Health Canada requests recall of certain products containing ephedra/ephedrine. Health Canada Online 2002. www.hc-sc.gc.ca/english/protection/warnings/2002/2002_01e.htm (Accessed 9 January 2002).

10711 Palacioz K. Meridia safety concerns. *Pharmacist's Letter/Prescriber's Letter* 2002;18:180408.

10712 Straus SE. History of chronic fatigue syndrome. *Rev Infect Dis* 1991;13:S2-S7.

10713 Reid S, Chalder T, Cleare A, et al. Chronic fatigue syndrome. *BMJ* 2000;320:292-6.

10714 CDC. National Center for Infectious Diseases. "Chronic Fatigue Syndrome" website: http://www.cdc.gov/ncidod/diseases/cfs/index.htm (Accessed 28 January 2002).

10715 Jason LA, Richman JA, Rademaker AW, et al. A community-based study of chronic fatigue syndrome. *Arch Intern Med* 1999;159:2129-37.

10716 Stevens DL. Chronic fatigue. *West J Med* 2001;175:315-19.

10717 Schluederberg A, Straus SE, Peterson P, et al. NIH conference. Chronic fatigue syndrome research. Definition and medical outcome assessment. *Ann Intern Med* 1992;117:325-31.

10718 Bates DW, Buchwald D, Lee J, et al. Clinical laboratory test findings in patients with chronic fatigue syndrome. *Arch Intern Med* 1995;155:97-103.

10719 Aaron LA, Buchwald D. A review of the evidence for overlap among unexplained clinical conditions. *Ann Intern Med* 2001;134:868-81.

10720 US Department of Health and Human Services. Chronic Fatigue Syndrome Coordinating Committee. "Chronic Fatigue Syndrome State of the Science Conference." http://www4.od.nih.gov/orwh/state-of-science.pdf (Accessed 12 February 2002).

10721 Whiting P, Bagnall AM, Sowden AJ, et al. Interventions for the treatment and management of chronic fatigue syndrome: a systematic review. *JAMA* 2001;286:1360-8.

10722 Wilson A, Hickie I, Lloyd A, et al. Longitudinal study of outcome of chronic fatigue syndrome. *BMJ* 1994;308:756-9.

10723 Natelson BH. Chronic fatigue syndrome. *JAMA* 2001;285:2557-9.

10724 Kavelaars A, Kuis W, Knook L, et al. Disturbed neuroendocrine-immune interactions in chronic fatigue syndrome. *J Clin Endocrinol Metab* 2000;85:692-6.

10725 See DM, Broumand N, Sahl L, Tilles JG. In vitro effects of echinacea and ginseng on natural killer and antibody-dependent cell cytotoxicity in healthy subjects and chronic fatigue syndrome or acquired immunodeficiency syndrome patients. *Immunopharmacology* 1997;35:229-35.

10726 Stewart JM. Autonomic nervous system dysfunction in adolescents with postural orthostatic tachycardia syndrome and chronic fatigue syndrome is characterized by attenuated vagal baroreflex and potentiated sympathetic vasomotion. *Pediatr Res* 2000;48:218-26.

10727 Rowe PC, Calkins H, DeBusk K, et al. Fludrocortisone acetate to treat neurally mediated hypotension in chronic fatigue syndrome: a randomized controlled trial. *JAMA* 2001;285:52-9.

10728 Grant JE, Veldee MS, Buchwald D. Analysis of dietary intake and selected nutrient concentrations in patients with chronic fatigue syndrome. *J Am Diet Assoc* 1996;96:383-6.

10729 Martin RW, Ogston SA, Evans, JR. Effects of vitamin and mineral supplementation symptoms associated with chronic fatigue syndrome with Coxsackie B antibodies. *J Nut Med* 1994;4:11-23.

10730 Soetekouw PM, Wevers RA, Vreken P, et al. Normal carnitine levels in patients with chronic fatigue syndrome. *Neth J Med* 2000;57:20-4.

10731 Fulle S, Mecocci P, Fano G, et al. Specific oxidative alterations in vastus lateralis muscle of patients with the diagnosis of chronic fatigue syndrome. *Free Radic Biol Med* 2000;29:1252-9.

10732 Afari N, Eisenberg DM, Herrell R, et al. Use of alternative treatments by chronic fatigue syndrome discordant twins. *Int Med* 1999;2:97-103.

10733 Hoechst Marion Roussel, Inc. Arava (leflunomide) product information. Kansas City, MO: September 1998.

10734 Pavelka K, Gatterova J, Olejarova M, et al. Glucosamine sulfate decreases progression of knee osteoarthritis in a long-term, randomized, placebo-controlled, independent, confirmatory trial. ACR Abstract Concurrent Session. OA-Advances in Management. November 1, 2000. Page S384, Abstract 1908.

10735 Topical Capsaicin NNTs. *Bandolier* 1996;29-36. www.jr2.ox.ac.uk:80/bandolier.

10736 Schulz A, Hilgers RD, Niedermeier W. The effect of splinting of teeth in combination with reconstructive periodontal surgery in humans. *Clin Oral Investig* 2000;4:98-105.

10737 Vuola J, Bohling T, Kinnunen J, et al. Natural coral as bone-defect-filling material. *J Biomed Mater Res* 2000;51:117-22.

10738 Thalgott JS, Klezl Z, Timlin M, Giuffre JM. Anterior lumbar interbody fusion with processed sea coral (coralline hydroxyapatite) as part of a circumferential fusion. *Spine* 2002;27:E518-25.

10739 Marchac D, Sandor G. Use of coral granules in the craniofacial skeleton. *J Craniofac Surg* 1994;5:213-7.

10740 Demers C, Hamdy CR, Corsi K, et al. Natural coral exoskeleton as a bone graft substitute: a review. *Biomed Mater Eng* 2002;12:15-35.

10741 Roux FX, Brasnu D, Menard M, et al. Madreporic coral for cranial base reconstruction. 8 years experience. *Acta Neurochir* (Wien) 1995;133:201-205.

10742 Federal Trade Commission. FTC and FDA Take New Actions in Fight Against Deceptive Marketing. http://www.ftc.gov/opa/2003/06/trudeau.htm (Accessed 28 July 2003).

10743 Ylitalo R, Lehtinen S, Wuolijoki E, et al. Cholesterol-lowering properties and safety of chitosan. *Arzneimittelforschung* 2002;52:1-7.

10748 Munshi NC, Loehrer PJ Sr, Williams SD, et al. Comparison of N-acetylcysteine and mesna as uroprotectors with ifosfamide combination chemotherapy in refractory germ cell tumors. *Invest New Drugs* 1992;10:159-163.

10749 Bhutta AT, Cleves MA, Casey PH, et al. Cognitive and behavioral outcomes of school-aged children who were born preterm: a meta-analysis. *JAMA* 2002;288:728-37.

10750 Milberger S, Biederman J, Faraone SV, et al. Pregnancy, delivery and infancy complications and attention deficit hyperactivity disorder: issues of gene-environment interaction. *Biol Psychiatry* 1997;41:65-75.

10751 Elia J, Ambrosini PJ, Rapoport JL. Treatment of attention-deficit-hyperactivity disorder. *N Engl J Med* 1999;340:780-8.

10752 Weiss M, Murray C. Assessment and management of attention-deficit hyperactivity disorder in adults. *CMAJ* 2003;168:715-22.

10753 Pliszka SR, McCracken JT, Maas JW. Catecholamines in attention-deficit hyperactivity disorder: current perspectives. *J Am Acad Child Adolesc Psychiatry* 1996;35:264-72.

10754 National Institutes of Health Consensus Development Conference Statement. Phenylketonuria: Screening and Management http://odp.od.nih.gov/consensus/cons/113/113_statement.htm (Accessed 15 August 2003).

10755 Schechter MD, Timmons GD. Objectively measured hyperactivity--II. Caffeine and amphetamine effects. *J Clin Pharmacol* 1985;25:276-80.

10756 Schnackenberg RC. Caffeine as a substitute for Schedule II stimulants in hyperkinetic children. *Am J Psychiatry* 1973;130:796-8.

10757 Garfinkel BD, Webster CD, Sloman L. Methylphenidate and caffeine in the treatment of children with minimal brain dysfunction. *Am J Psychiatry* 1975;132:723-8.

10758 Conners CK. The acute effects of caffeine on evoked response, vigilance, and activity level in hyperkinetic children. *J Abnorm Child Psychol* 1979;7:145-51.

10759 Arnold LE, Christopher J, Huestis R, Smeltzer DJ. Methylphenidate vs dextroamphetamine vs caffeine in minimal brain dysfunction: controlled comparison by placebo washout design with Bayes' analysis. *Arch Gen Psychiatry* 1978;35:463-73.

10760 Huestis RD, Arnold LE, Smeltzer DJ. Caffeine versus methylphenidate and d-amphetamine in minimal brain dysfunction: a double-blind comparison. *Am J Psychiatry* 1975;132:868-70.

10762 National Institute of Allergy and Infectious Diseases. The Common Cold. http://www.niaid.nih.gov/factsheets/cold.htm (Accessed 28 August 2003).

10763 Gwaltney JM Jr. The Common Cold. In: Principles and Practices of Infectious Diseases, 5th ed. Mandell GL, Bennett JE, Dolin R, eds. New York, NY: Churchill Livingstone; 2000. pgs. 651-6.

10764 National Institute of Allergy and Infectious Diseases. Flu. http://www.niaid.nih.gov/factsheets/flu.htm (Accessed 28 August 2003).

10765 Savolainen C, Blomqvist S, Hovi T. Human rhinoviruses. *Paediatr Respir Rev* 2003;4:91-8.

10766 Heikkinen T, Jarvinen A. The common cold. *Lancet* 2003;361:51-9.

10767 Treanor, JJ. Influenza virus. In: Principles and Practices of Infectious Diseases, 5th ed. Mandell GL, Bennett JE, Dolin R, eds. New York, NY: Churchill Livingstone; 2000. pgs. 1823-49.

10768 Gwaltney JM Jr, Hayden FG. Psychological stress and the common cold. *N Engl J Med* 1992;326:644-5.

10769 Bensenor IM, Cook NR, Lee IM, et al. Active and passive smoking and risk of colds in women. *Ann Epidemiol* 2001;11:225-31.

10770 National Institute of Allergy and Infectious Diseases. Is it a Cold or the Flu? http://www.niaid.nih.gov/publications/cold/sick.pdf (Accessed 29 August 2003).

10771 Cohen S, Tyrrell DA, Smith AP. Psychological stress and susceptibility to the common cold. *N Engl J Med* 1991;325:606-12.

10772 Takkouche B, Regueira C, Gestal-Otero JJ. A cohort study of stress and the common cold. *Epidemiology* 2001;12:345-9.

10773 Bridges CB, Harper SA, Fukuda K, et al. Prevention and control of influenza: Recommendations of the Advisory Committee on Immunization Practices (ACIP). *MMWR Recomm Rep* 2003:52(RR-8);1-34. Available at: http://www.cdc.gov/mmwr/preview/mmwrhtml/rr5208a1.htm (Accessed 30 August 2003).

10774 FDA News: First Nasal Mist Flu Vaccine Approved. June 17, 2003. http://www.fda.gov/bbs/topics/NEWS/2003/NEW00913.html (Accessed 30 August 2003).

10775 Couch RB. Prevention and treatment of influenza. *N Engl J Med* 2000;343:1778-87.

10776 Cooper NJ, Sutton AJ, Abrams KR, et al. Effectiveness of neuraminidase inhibitors in treatment and prevention of influenza A and B: systematic review and meta-analyses of randomised controlled trials. *BMJ* 2003;326:1235.

10777 Sun Y, Hersh EM, Lee SL, et al. Preliminary observations on the effects of the Chinese medicinal herbs Astragalus membranaceus and Ligustrum lucidum on lymphocyte blastogenic responses. *J Biol Response Mod* 1983;2:227-37.

10778 Carod-Artal FJ. Neurological syndromes linked with the intake of plants and fungi containing a toxic component (I). Neurotoxic syndromes caused by the ingestion of plants, seeds and fruits. *Rev Neurol* 2003;36:860-71.

10780 Takkouche B, Regueira-Mendez C, Garcia-Closas R, et al. Intake of vitamin C and zinc and risk of common cold: a cohort study. *Epidemiology* 2002;13:38-44.

10781 Jellin JM, Gregory P, Batz F, Hitchens K, et al. *Pharmacist's Letter/Prescriber's Letter* Natural Medicines Comprehensive Database. Stockton, CA: Therapeutic Research Faculty; 2003. www.naturaldatabase.com (Accessed 1 September 2003).

10782 Melchart D, Linde K, Fischer P, Kaesmayr J. Echinacea for preventing and treating the common cold. *Cochrane Database Syst Rev* 2000;2:CD000530.

10783 Turner RB. The treatment of rhinovirus infections: progress and potential. *Antiviral Res* 2001;49:1-14.

10784 Turner RB, Cetnarowski WE. Effect of treatment with zinc gluconate or zinc acetate on experimental and natural colds. *Clin Infect Dis* 2000;31:1202-8.

10785 Venuta A, Spano C, Laudizi L, et al. Essential fatty acids: the effects of dietary supplementation among children with recurrent respiratory infections. *J Int Med Res* 1996;24:325-30.

10786 Kew S, Banerjee T, Minihane AM, et al. Lack of effect of foods enriched with plant- or marine-derived n-3 fatty acids on human immune function. *Am J Clin Nutr* 2003;77:1287-95.

10787 Josling P. Preventing the common cold with a garlic supplement: a double-blind, placebo-controlled survey. *Adv Ther* 2001;18:189-93.

10788 Graat JM, Schouten EG, Kok FJ. Effect of daily vitamin E and multivitamin-mineral supplementation on acute respiratory tract infections in elderly persons: a randomized controlled trial. *JAMA* 2002;288:715-21.

10789 Bonham M, O'Connor JM, Alexander HD, et al. Zinc supplementation has no effect on circulating levels of peripheral blood leucocytes and lymphocyte subsets in healthy adult men. *Br J Nutr* 2003;89:695-703.

10791 Matheson NJ, Symmonds-Abrahams M, Sheikh A, et al. Neuraminidase inhibitors for preventing and treating influenza in children. *Cochrane Database Syst Rev* 2003;(3):CD002744.

10792 Sutter AI, Lemiengre M, Campbell H, Mackinnon HF. Antihistamines for the common cold. *Cochrane Database Syst Rev* 2003;3:CD001267.

10793 Hayden FG, Diamond L, Wood PB, et al. Effectiveness and safety of intranasal ipratropium bromide in common colds. A randomized, double-blind, placebo-controlled trial. *Ann Intern Med* 1996;125:89-97.

10794 Schroeder K, Fahey T. Over-the-counter medications for acute cough in children and adults in ambulatory settings. *Cochrane Database Syst Rev* 2001;(3):CD001831.

10795 Gabrielian ES, Shukarian AK, Goukasova GI, et al. A double blind, placebo-controlled study of Andrographis paniculata fixed combination Kan Jang in the treatment of acute upper respiratory tract infections including sinusitis. *Phytomedicine* 2002;9:589-97.

10796 Barak V, Halperin T, Kalickman I. The effect of Sambucol, a black elderberry-based, natural product, on the production of human cytokines: I. Inflammatory cytokines. *Eur Cytokine Netw* 2001;12:290-6.

10797 Schwarz E, Metzler J, Diedrich JP, et al. Oral administration of freshly expressed juice of Echinacea purpurea herbs fail to stimulate the nonspecific immune response in healthy young men: results of a double-blind, placebo-controlled crossover study. *J Immunother* 2002;25:413-20.

10798 Tragni E, Tubaro A, Melis S, Galli CL. Evidence from two classic irritation tests for an anti-inflammatory action of a natural extract, Echinacina B. *Food Chem Toxicol* 1985;23:317-9.

10799 Muller-Jakic B, Breu W, Probstle A, et al. In vitro inhibition of cyclooxygenase and 5-lipoxygenase by alkamides from Echinacea and Achillea species. *Planta Med* 1994;60:37-40.

10800 Barrett BP, Brown RL, Locken K, et al. Treatment of the common cold with unrefined echinacea. A randomized, double-blind, placebo-controlled trial. *Ann Intern Med* 2002;137:939-46.

10801 Hansson O, Sillanpaa M. Pyridoxine and serum concentration of phenytoin and phenobarbitone. *Lancet* 1976;1:256.

10802 Schulten B, Bulitta M, Ballering-Bruhl B, et al. Efficacy of Echinacea purpurea in patients with a common cold. A placebo-controlled, randomised, double-blind clinical trial. *Arzneimittelforschung* 2001;51:563-8.

10803 McElroy BH, Miller SP. Effectiveness of zinc gluconate glycine lozenges (Cold-Eeze) against the common cold in school-aged subjects: a retrospective chart review. *Am J Ther* 2002;9:472-5.

10804 Vickers AJ, Smith C. Homoeopathic Oscillococcinum for preventing and treating influenza and influenza-like syndromes. *Cochrane Database Syst Rev* 2000;(2):CD001957.

10805 Singh M. Heated, humidified air for the common cold. *Cochrane Database Syst Rev* 2001;(4):CD001728.

10806 Rennard BO, Ertl RF, Gossman GL, et al. Chicken soup inhibits neutrophil chemotaxis in vitro. *Chest* 2000;118:1150-7.

10807 Takkouche B, Regueira-Mendez C, Garcia-Closas R, et al. Intake of wine, beer, and spirits and the risk of clinical common cold. *Am J Epidemiol* 2002;155:853-8.

10808 Watzl B, Bub A, Briviba K, Rechkemmer G. Acute intake of moderate amounts of red wine or alcohol has no effect on the immune system of healthy men. *Eur J Nutr* 2002;41:264-70.

10809 Turk S, Bozfakioglu S, Ecder ST, et al. Effects of zinc supplementation on the immune system and on antibody response to multivalent influenza vaccine in hemodialysis patients. *Int J Artif Organs* 1998;21:274-278.

REFERENCES

10810 Akhondzadeh S, Noroozian M, Mohammadi M, et al. Salvia officinalis extract in the treatment of patients with mild to moderate Alzheimer's disease: a double blind, randomized and placebo-controlled trial. *J Clin Pharm Ther* 2003;28:53-9.

10811 Tildesley NT, Kennedy DO, Perry EK, et al. Salvia lavandulaefolia (Spanish Sage) enhances memory in healthy young volunteers. *Pharmacol Biochem Behav* 2003;75:669-74.

10812 Perry NB, Anderson RE, Brennan NJ, et al. Essential oils from dalmatian sage (Salvia officinalis l.): variations among individuals, plant parts, seasons, and sites. *J Agric Food Chem* 1999;47:2048-54.

10813 Broadhurst CL, Polansky MM, Anderson RA. Insulin-like biological activity of culinary and medicinal plant aqueous extracts in vitro. *J Agric Food Chem* 2000;48:849-52.

10814 Sahyoun NR, Jacques PF, Russell RM. Carotenoids, vitamins C and E, and mortality in an elderly population. *Am J Epidemiol* 1996;144:501-11.

10815 Nyyssonen K, Parviainen MT, Salonen R, et al. Vitamin C deficiency and risk of myocardial infarction: prospective population study of men from eastern Finland. *BMJ* 1997;314:634-8.

10816 Kritchevsky SB, Shimakawa T, Tell GS, et al. Dietary antioxidants and carotid artery wall thickness. The ARIC Study. Atherosclerosis Risk in Communities Study. *Circulation* 1995;92:2142-50.

10817 Ramirez J, Flowers NC. Leukocyte ascorbic acid and its relationship to coronary artery disease in man. *Am J Clin Nutr* 1980;33:2079-87.

10818 Hodis HN, Mack WJ, LaBree L, et al. Serial coronary angiographic evidence that antioxidant vitamin intake reduces progression of coronary artery atherosclerosis. *JAMA* 1995;273:1849-54.

10819 Byers T, Guerrero N. Epidemiologic evidence for vitamin C and vitamin E in cancer prevention. *Am J Clin Nutr* 1995;62:1385S-92S.

10821 Negri E, Franceschi S, Bosetti C, et al. Selected micronutrients and oral and pharyngeal cancer. *Int J Cancer* 2000;86:122-7.

10822 You WC, Zhang L, Gail MH, et al. Gastric dysplasia and gastric cancer: Helicobacter pylori, serum vitamin C, and other risk factors. *J Natl Cancer Inst* 2000;92:1607-12.

10823 Freudenheim JL, Marshall JR, Vena JE, et al. Premenopausal breast cancer risk and intake of vegetables, fruits, and related nutrients. *J Natl Cancer Inst* 1996;88:340-8.

10824 Gandini S, Merzenich H, Robertson C, Boyle P. Meta-analysis of studies on breast cancer risk and diet: the role of fruit and vegetable consumption and the intake of associated micronutrients. *Eur J Cancer* 2000;36:636-46.

10825 Michels KB, Holmberg L, Bergkvist L, et al. Dietary antioxidant vitamins, retinol, and breast cancer incidence in a cohort of Swedish women. *Int J Cancer* 2001;91:563-7.

10826 Wu K, Helzlsouer KJ, Alberg AJ, et al. A prospective study of plasma ascorbic acid concentrations and breast cancer (United States). *Cancer Causes Control* 2000;11:279-83.

10827 Szatmari SZ, Whitehouse PJ. Vinpocetine for cognitive impairment and dementia. *Cochrane Database Syst Rev* 2003;1:CD003119.

10828 Bereczki D, Fekete I. Vinpocetine for acute ischaemic stroke. *Cochrane Database Syst Rev* 2000;2:CD000480.

10829 Hitzenberger G, Sommer W, Grandt R. Influence of vinpocetine on warfarin-induced inhibition of coagulation. *Int J Clin Pharmacol Ther Toxicol* 1990;28:323-8.

10830 Markowitz JS, Donovan JL, DeVane CL, et al. Effect of St. John's wort on drug metabolism by induction of cytochrome P450 3A4 enzyme. *JAMA* 2003;290:1500-4.

10831 Whooley MA, Simon GE. Managing depression in medical outpatients. *N Engl J Med* 2000;343:1942-50.

10832 Kessler RC, Berglund P, Demler O, et al. The epidemiology of major depressive disorder: results from the National Comorbidity Survey Replication (NCS-R). *JAMA* 2003;289:3095-105.

10833 Remick RA. Diagnosis and management of depression in primary care: a clinical update and review. *CMAJ* 2002;167:1253-60.

10834 Bostwick JM, Pankratz VS. Affective disorders and suicide risk: a reexamination. *Am J Psychiatry* 2000;157:1925-32.

10835 Ruo B, Rumsfeld JS, Hlatky MA, et al. Depressive symptoms and health-related quality of life: the Heart and Soul Study. *JAMA* 2003;290:215-21.

10841 Kessler RC, Soukup J, Davis RB, et al. The use of complementary and alternative therapies to treat anxiety and depression in the United States. *Am J Psychiatry* 2001;158:289-94.

10842 Knaudt PR, Connor KM, Weisler RH, et al. Alternative therapy use by psychiatric outpatients. *J Nerv Ment Dis* 1999;187:692-5.

10843 Hypericum Depression Trial Study Group. Effect of Hypericum perforatum (St. John's wort) in major depressive disorder: a randomized controlled trial. *JAMA* 2002;287:1807-14.

10844 Findling RL, McNamara NK, O'Riordan MA, et al. An open-label pilot study of St. John's wort in juvenile depression. *J Am Acad Child Adolesc Psychiatry* 2003;42:908-914.

10845 Hammerness P, Basch E, Ulbricht C, et al. St. John's wort: a systematic review of adverse effects and drug interactions for the consultation psychiatrist. *Psychosomatics* 2003;44:271-82.

10846 Rayburn WF, Gonzalez CL, Christensen HD, Stewart JD. Effect of prenatally administered hypericum (St John's wort) on growth and physical maturation of mouse offspring. *Am J Obstet Gynecol* 2001;184:191-5.

10847 Gurley BJ, Gardner SF, Hubbard MA, et al. Cytochrome P450 phenotypic ratios for predicting herb-drug interactions in humans. *Clin Pharmacol Ther* 2002;72:276-87.

10848 Foster BC, Vandenhoek S, Hana J, et al. In vitro inhibition of human cytochrome P450-mediated metabolism of marker substrates by natural products. *Phytomedicine* 2003;10:334-42.

10849 Draves AH, Walker SE. Analysis of the hypericin and pseudohypericin content of commercially available St John's Wort preparations. *Can J Clin Pharmacol* 2003;10:114-118.

10850 Benjamin J, Agam G, Levine J, et al. Inositol treatment in psychiatry. *Psychopharmacol Bull* 1995;31:167-75.

10851 Nemets B, Mishory A, Levine J, Belmaker RH. Inositol addition does not improve depression in SSRI treatment failures. *J Neural Transm* 1999;106:795-8.

10852 McLean A, Rubinsztein JS, Robbins TW, Sahakian BJ. The effects of tyrosine depletion in normal healthy volunteers: implications for unipolar depression. *Psychopharmacology* (Berl) 2003 Sept 4 [Epub ahead of print].

10853 Shaw K, Turner J, Del Mar C. Tryptophan and 5-hydroxytryptophan for depression. *Cochrane Database Syst Rev* 2002;1:CD003198.

10854 Bell C, Abrams J, Nutt D. Tryptophan depletion and its implications for psychiatry. *Br J Psychiatry* 2001;178:399-405.

10855 Murphy FC, Smith KA, Cowen PJ, et al. The effects of tryptophan depletion on cognitive and affective processing in healthy volunteers. *Psychopharmacology* (Berl) 2002;163:42-53.

10856 Walinder J, Skott A, Carlsson A, et al. Potentiation of the antidepressant action of clomipramine by tryptophan. *Arch Gen Psychiatry* 1976;33:1384-89.

10857 van Praag HM. Management of depression with serotonin precursors. *Biol Psychiatry* 1981;16:291-310.

10858 Byerley WF, Judd LL, Reimherr FW, Grosser BI. 5-Hydroxytryptophan: a review of its antidepressant efficacy and adverse effects. *J Clin Psychopharmacol* 1987;7:127-37.

10859 Maes M, Christophe A, Delanghe J, et al. Lowered omega3 polyunsaturated fatty acids in serum phospholipids and cholesteryl esters of depressed patients. *Psychiatry Res* 1999;85:275-91.

10860 Tiemeier H, van Tuijl HR, Hofman A, et al. Plasma fatty acid composition and depression are associated in the elderly: the Rotterdam Study. *Am J Clin Nutr* 2003;78:40-6.

10861 Levine M, Beattie BL, McLean DM. Comparison of one- and two-dose regimens of influenza vaccine for elderly men. *CMAJ* 1987;137:722-6.

10862 Gross PA, Weksler ME, Quinnan GV Jr, et al. Immunization of elderly people with two doses of influenza vaccine. *J Clin Microbiol* 1987;25:1763-5.

10863 Widmer AF. Replace hand washing with use of a waterless alcohol hand rub? *Clin Infect Dis* 2000;31:136-43.

10864 Eby GA. Elimination of efficacy by additives in zinc acetate lozenges for common colds. *Clin Infect Dis* 2001 May 15;32(10):1520.

10865 Sattar SA, Abebe M, Bueti AJ, et al. Activity of an alcohol-based hand gel against human adeno-, rhino-, and rotaviruses using the fingerpad method. *Infect Control Hosp Epidemiol* 2000;21:516-9.

10866 Peet M, Horrobin DF. A dose-ranging study of the effects of ethyl-eicosapentaenoate in patients with ongoing depression despite apparently adequate treatment with standard drugs. *Arch Gen Psychiatry* 2002;59:913-9.

10867 Tanskanen A, Hibbeln JR, Hintikka J, et al. Fish consumption, depression, and suicidality in a general population. *Arch Gen Psychiatry* 2001;58:512-513.

10868 Hibbeln JR. Fish consumption and major depression. *Lancet* 1998;351:1213.

10869 Marangell LB, Martinez JM, Zboyan HA, et al. A double-blind, placebo-controlled study of the omega-3 fatty acid docosahexaenoic acid in the treatment of major depression. *Am J Psychiatry* 2003;160:996-8.

10870 Rapoport SI, Bosetti F. Do lithium and anticonvulsants target the brain arachidonic acid cascade in bipolar disorder? *Arch Gen Psychiatry* 2002;59:592-6.

10871 Su KP, Huang SY, Chiu CC, Shen WW. Omega-3 fatty acids in major depressive disorder. A preliminary double-blind, placebo-controlled trial. *Eur Neuropsychopharmacol* 2003;13:267-71.

10872 Nemets B, Stahl Z, Belmaker RH. Addition of omega-3 fatty acid to maintenance medication treatment for recurrent unipolar depressive disorder. *Am J Psychiatry* 2002;159:477-9.

10874 Tollefson GD, Haus E, Garvey MJ, et al. 24 hour urinary dehydroepiandrosterone sulfate in unipolar depression treated with cognitive and/or pharmacotherapy. *Ann Clin Psychiatry* 1990;2:39-45.

10875 Legrain S, Berr C, Frenoy N, et al. Dehydroepiandrosterone sulfate in a long-term care aged population. *Gerontology* 1995;41:343-51.

10876 Barrett-Connor E, von Muhlen D, Laughlin GA, Kripke A. Endogenous levels of dehydroepiandrosterone sulfate, but not other sex hormones, are associated with depressed mood in older women: the Rancho Bernardo Study. *J Am Geriatr Soc* 1999;47:685-91.

10877 Morrison MF, Katz IR, Parmelee P, et al. Dehydroepiandrosterone sulfate (DHEA-S) and psychiatric and laboratory measures of frailty in a residential care population. *Am J Geriatr Psychiatry* 1998;6:277-84.

10879 Bottiglieri T, Laundy M, Crellin R, et al. Homocysteine, folate, methylation, and monoamine metabolism in depression. *J Neurol Neurosurg Psychiatry* 2000;69:228-32.

10880 Alpert M, Silva RR, Pouget ER. Prediction of treatment response in geriatric depression from baseline folate level: interaction with an SSRI or a tricyclic antidepressant. *J Clin Psychopharmacol* 2003;23:309-13.

10881 Tiemeier H, van Tuijl HR, Hofman A, et al. Vitamin B12, folate, and homocysteine in depression: the Rotterdam Study. *Am J Psychiatry* 2002;159:2099-101.

10882 Morris MS, Fava M, Jacques PF, et al. Depression and folate status in the US Population. *Psychother Psychosom* 2003;72:80-7.

10883 Tolmunen T, Voutilainen S, Hintikka J, et al. Dietary folate and depressive symptoms are associated in middle-aged Finnish men. *J Nutr* 2003;133:3233-6.

10884 Taylor MJ, Carney S, Geddes J, Goodwin G. Folate for depressive disorders. *Cochrane Database Syst Rev* 2003;2:CD003390.

10885 Coppen A, Swade C, Jones SA, et al. Depression and tetrahydrobiopterin: the folate connection. *J Affect Disord* 1989;16:103-7.

10886 Passeri M, Cucinotta D, Abate G, et al. Oral 5'-methyltetrahydrofolic acid in senile organic mental disorders with depression: results of a double-blind multicenter study. *Aging* (Milano) 1993;5:63-71.

10887 Godfrey PS, Toone BK, Carney MW, et al. Enhancement of recovery from psychiatric illness by methylfolate. *Lancet* 1990;336:392-5.

10888 Bell IR, Edman JS, Morrow FD, et al. Brief communication. Vitamin B1, B2, and B6 augmentation of tricyclic antidepressant treatment in geriatric depression with cognitive dysfunction. *J Am Coll Nutr* 1992;11:159-63.

10889 Oren DA, Teicher MH, Schwartz PJ, et al. A controlled trial of cyanocobalamin (vitamin B12) in the treatment of winter seasonal affective disorder. *J Affect Disord* 1994;32:197-200.

10892 Clayton AH, Pradko JF, Croft HA, et al. Prevalence of sexual dysfunction among newer antidepressants. *J Clin Psychiatry* 2002;63:357-66.

10893 Kang BJ, Lee SJ, Kim MD, Cho MJ. A placebo-controlled, double-blind trial of Ginkgo biloba for antidepressant-induced sexual dysfunction. *Hum Psychopharmacol* 2002;17:279-84.

10894 Nurnberg HG, Hensley PL, Gelenberg AJ, et al. Treatment of antidepressant-associated sexual dysfunction with sildenafil: a randomized controlled trial. *JAMA* 2003;289:56-64.

10895 Collins TF, Welsh JJ, Black TN, et al. Study of the teratogenic potential of guar gum. *Food Chem Toxicol* 1987;25:807-814.

10896 Vuorinen-Markkola H, Sinisalo M, Koivisto VA. Guar gum in insulin-dependent diabetes: effects on glycemic control and serum lipoproteins. *Am J Clin Nutr* 1992;56:1056-1060.

10897 Superko HR, Haskell WL, Sawrey-Kubicek L, Farquhar JW. Effects of solid and liquid guar gum on plasma cholesterol and triglyceride concentrations in moderate hypercholesterolemia. *Am J Cardiol* 1988;62:51-55.

10898 Todd PA, Benfield P, Goa KL. Guar gum. A review of its pharmacological properties, and use as a dietary adjunct in hypercholesterolaemia. *Drugs* 1990;39:917-28.

10899 FDA List of Orphan Designations and Approvals. http://www.fda.gov/orphan/DESIGNAT/list.htm (Accessed 27 October 2003).

10900 Batist G, Patenaude F, Champagne P, et al. Neovastat (AE-941) in refractory renal cell carcinoma patients: report of a phase II trial with two dose levels. *Ann Oncol* 2002;13:1259-63.

10901 Bone RA, Landrum JT, Friedes LM, et al. Distribution of lutein and zeaxanthin stereoisomers in the human retina. *Exp Eye Res* 1997;64:211-8.
10902 Eye Disease Case-Control Study Group. Antioxidant status and neovascular age-related macular degeneration. *Arch Ophthalmol* 1993;111:104-9.
10903 Hammond BR Jr, Johnson EJ, Russell RM, et al. Dietary modification of human macular pigment density. *Invest Ophthalmol Vis Sci* 1997;38:1795-801.
10904 Wright JV, Ogle DJ, Hoare L. Improvement of vision in macular degeneration associated with intravenous zinc and selenium therapy: Two cases. *J Nutr Med* 1990;1:133-8.
10905 Thylefors B, Negrel A-D, Pararajasegaram R, Dazie KY. Global data on blindness. *Bull World Health Organ* 1995;73:115-21.
10906 Kahn HA, Leibowitz HM, Ganley JP et al. The Framingham Eye Study. 1. Outline and major prevalence findings. *Am J Epidemiol* 1977;106:17-32.
10907 Klein BE, Klein R, Lee KE. Incidence of age-related cataract. The Beaver Dam Eye Study. *Arch Ophthalmol* 1998;116: 219-25.
10908 Taylor A, Nowell T. Oxidative stress and antioxidant function in relation to risk for cataract. *Adv Pharmacol* 1997;38:515-36.
10909 Rao GN, Sadasivudu B, Cotlier E. Studies of glutathione s-transferase, glutathione peroxidase and glutathione reductase in human normal and cataractous lenses. *Ophthalmic Res* 1983;15:173-9.
10910 Jacques PF, Taylor A, Hankinson SE, et al. Long-term vitamin C supplement use and prevalence of early age-related opacities. *Am J Clin Nutr* 1997;66:911-6.
10911 Chylack LT, Brown NP, Bron A, et al. The Roche European American Cataract Trial (REACT): A randomized clinical trial to investigate the efficacy of an oral antioxidant micronutrient mixture to slow progression of age-related cataract. *Ophthalmic Epidemiol* 2002;9(1):49-80.
10912 Bhat KS. Nutritional status of thiamine, riboflavin and pyridoxine in cataract patients. *Nutr Rep Inter* 1987;36:685-92.
10913 Skalka HW, Prchal JT. Cataracts and riboflavin deficiency. *Am J Clin Nutr* 1981;34:861-3.
10914 Bravetti G. Preventative medical treatment of senile cataract with vitamin E and anthocyanosides: clinical evaluation. *Ann Ottalmol Clin Ocul* 1989; 115:109.
10915 Zenon GJ, Abobo CV, Carter BL, Ball DW. Potential use of aldose reductase inhibitors to prevent diabetic complications. *Clin Pharm* 1990;9:446-57.
10916 Nakai N, Fujii Y, Kobashi K, Nomura K. Aldose reductase inhibitors: flavonoids, alkaloids, acetophenones, benzophenones, and spirohydantoins of chroman. *Arch Biochem Biophys* 1985;239:491-6.
10917 Swamy-Mruthinti S, Carter AL. Acetyl-L-carnitine decreased glycation of lens proteins: in vitro studies. *Exp Eye Res* 1999;69:109-15.
10918 Varma SD, Devamanoharan PS, Rutzen AR, et al. Attenuation of galactose-induced cataract by pyruvate. *Free Radic Res* 1999;30:253-63.
10919 Arkell SM, Lightman DA, Sommer A, et al. The prevalence of glaucoma among Eskimos of northwest Alaska. *Arch Ophthalmol* 1987;105:482-5.
10920 Ginkgo may protect against stroke damage. www.medscape.com/reuters/prof/2000/05/05.03/20000503scie003.html (Accessed 3 May 2000).
10921 Chung HS, Harris A, Kristinsson JK, et al. Ginkgo biloba extract increases ocular blood flow velocity. *J Ocul Pharmacol Ther* 1999;15:233-40.
10922 Merte HJ, Merkle W. Long-term treatment with Ginkgo biloba extract of circulatory disturbances of the retina and optic nerve. *Klin Monatsbl Augenheilkd* 1980;177:577-83.
10923 La Rosa FA and Lee DA. Collagen degradation in glaucoma: will it gain a therapeutic value? *Current Opinion in Ophthalmology* 2000;11:90-3.
10924 Schachtschabel DO, Binninber E. Stimulatory effects of ascorbic acid in hyaluronic acid synthesis of in vitro cultured normal and glaucomatous trabecular meshwork cells of the human eye. *Z Gerontol* 1993;26:243-6.
10925 Linner E. Intraocular pressure regulation and ascorbic acid. *Acta Soc Med Ups* 1964;69:225-32.
10926 Linner E. The pressure lowering effect of ascorbic acid in ocular hypertension. *Acta Ophthalmol* (Copenh) 1969;47:685-9.
10927 Virno M, Bucci MG, Pecori-Giraldi J, Missiroli A. Oral treatment of glaucoma with vitamin C. *Eye Ear Nose Throat Monthly* 1967;46:1502-8.
10928 Green K. Marijuana smoking vs. cannabinoids for glaucoma therapy. *Archives of Ophthalmology* 1998;116:1433-7.
10929 Goldberg J, Flowerdew G, Smith E, et al. Factors assoicated with age-related macular degeneration. *Am J Epidemiol* 1988;128:700-10.
10930 Porcella A, Maxia C, Gessa GL, Pani L. The synthetic cannabinoid WIN55212-2 decreases the intraocular pressure in human glaucoma resistant to conventional therapies. *European Journal of Neuroscience* 2001;13:409-12.
10931 Varma SD, Mikuni I, Kinoshita JH. Flavonoids as inhibitors of lens aldose reductase. *Science* 1975;188:1215-6.
10932 NIH Consensus Development Panel on Osteoporosis Prevention, Diagnosis, and Therapy. Osteoporosis prevention, diagnosis, and therapy. *JAMA* 2001;285:785-95.
10933 Steinweg KK. Menopause, bone physiology, and osteoporosis prevention. *Clin Fam Prac* 2002;4:89-111.
10934 National Osteoporosis Foundation. "America's Bone Health: The State of Osteoporosis and Low Bone Mass." Website: http://www.nof.org/advocacy/prevalence/index.htm (Accessed 11 June 2002).
10935 National Institute of Health Osteoporosis and Related Bone Diseases National Resource Center. "Fast Facts on Osteoporosis." Website: http://www.osteo.org/osteofastfact.html (Accessed 11 June 2002).
10936 National Osteoporosis Foundation. "Osteoporosis in Men." Website: http://www.nof.org/men/strategies_men.htm (Accessed 11 June 2002).
10937 Prelevic GM. Osteoporosis in men. *J R Soc Med* 2001;94:620-3.
10938 Sakhaee K, Bhuket T, Adams-Huet B, et al. Meta-analysis of calcium bioavailability: A comparison of calcium citrate with calcium carbonate. *Am J Ther* 1999;6:313-21.
10940 Chapin RE, KU WW, Kenney MA, et al. The effect of dietary bone on bone strength in rats. *Fundam Appl Toxicol* 1997;35:205-15.
10941 Sheng MHC, Taper LJ, Viet H, et al. Dietary bone supplementation enhanced the action of estrogen, but not that of parathyroid hormone, to improve trabecular bone quality in ovariectomized rats. *Biol Trace Elem Res* 2001;82:109-23.
10942 Nielsen FH. Studies on the relationship between boron and magnesium which possibly affects the formation and maintenance of bones. *Magnes Trace Elem* 1990;9:61-9.
10943 Volpe SL, Taper LJ, Meacham S. The relationship between boron and magnesium status and bone mineral density in the human: a review. *Magnes Res* 1993;6:291-6.
10944 Rico H, Roca-Botran C, Hernandez ER, et al. The effect of supplemental copper on osteopenia induced by ovariectomy in rats. *Menopause* 2000;7:413-6.
10945 Yee CD, Kubena KS, Walker M, et al. The relationship of nutritional copper to the development of postmenopausal osteoporosis in rats. *Biol Trace Elem Res* 1995;48:1-11.

10946 Gillespie WJ, Avenell A, Henry DA, et al. Vitamin D and vitamin D analogues for preventing fractures associated with involutional and post-menopausal osteoporosis. *Cochrane Database Syst Rev* 2001;(1):CD000227.

10947 Kritz-Silverstein D, Goodman-Gruen DL. Usual dietary isoflavone intake, bone mineral density, and bone metabolism in postmenopausal women. *J Womens Health Gend Based Med* 2002;11:69-78.

10948 Clifton-Bligh PB, Baber RJ, et al. The effect of isoflavones extracted from red clover (Rimostil) on lipid and bone metabolism. *Menopause* 2001;8:259-65.

10949 Johnell O, Gullberg B, Kanis JA. Risk factors for hip fracture in European women: the MEDOS Study. Mediterranean Osteoporosis Study. *J Bone Miner Res* 1995;10:1802-15.

10950 Kanis J, Johnell O, Gullberg B et al. Risk factors for hip fracture in men from southern Europe: the MEDOS study. Mediterranean Osteoporosis Study. *Osteoporos Int* 1999;9:45-54.

10951 Kahn AJ, Halloran B. Dehydroepiandrosterone supplementation and bone turnover in middle-aged to elderly men. *J Clin Endocrinol Metab* 2002;87:1544-9.

10952 Lucas EA, Wild RD, Hammond LJ et al. Flaxseed improves lipid profile without altering biomarkers of bone metabolism in postmenopausal women. *J Clin Endocrinol Metab* 2002;87:1527-32.

10953 Adam M, Spacek P, Hulejova H. [Postmenopausal osteoporosis. Treatment with calcitonin and a diet rich in collagen proteins]. [Article in Czech]. *Cas Lek Cesk* 1996;135:74-8.

10954 Heaney RP. Protein and calcium: antagonists or synergists? *Am J Clin Nutr* 2002;75:609-10.

10955 Dawson-Hughes B, Harris SS. Calcium intake influences the association of protein intake with rates of bone loss in elderly men and women. *Am J Clin Nutr* 2002;75:773-9.

10956 Munger RG, Cerhan JR, Chiu BC. Prospective study of dietary protein intake and risk of hip fracture in postmenopausal women. *Am J Clin Nutr* 1999;69:147-52.

10957 Schurch MA, Rizzoli R, Slosman D, et al. Protein supplements increase serum insulin-like growth factor-I levels and attenuate proximal femur bone loss in patients with recent hip fracture. A randomized, double-blind, placebo-controlled trial. *Ann Intern Med* 1998;128(10):801-9.

10958 Grady D, Herrington D, Bittner V, et al. Cardiovascular disease outcomes during 6.8 years of hormone therapy: Heart and Estrogen/progestin Replacement Study follow-up (HERS II). *JAMA* 2002;288:49-57.

10959 Rossouw JE, Anderson GL, Prentice RL, et al. Risks and benefits of estrogen plus progestin in healthy postmenopausal women: principal results from the Women's Health Initiative randomized controlled trial. *JAMA* 2002;288:321-33.

10960 Hays J, Ockene JK, Brunner RL, et al. Effects of estrogen plus progestin on health-related quality of life. *N Engl J Med* 2003;348:1839-54.

10961 Wassertheil-Smoller S, Hendrix S, Limacher M, et al. Effect of estrogen plus progestin on stroke in postmenopausal women: The Women's Health Initiative: A randomized trial. *JAMA* 2003;289:2673-84.

10962 Shumaker SA, Legault C, Thal L, et al. Estrogen plus progestin and the incidence of dementia and mild cognitive impairment in postmenopausal women: The Women's Health Initiative Memory Study: A randomized controlled trial. *JAMA* 2003;289:2651-62.

10963 Steinauer JE, Subak LL, Grady D, et al. Hormone therapy for prevention of urinary incontinence: the HERS Study. *Obstet Gynecol* 2003;101(4 Suppl):10S-11S

10964 Hlatky MA, Boothroyd D, Vittinghoff E, et al. Quality-of-life and depressive symptoms in postmenopausal women after receiving hormone therapy: Results from the Heart and Estrogen/Progestin Replacement Study (HERS) trial. *JAMA* 2002;287:591-7.

10965 North American Menopause Society. Menopause Core Curriculum Study Guide. 2002. http://www.menopause.org/edumaterials/studyguide/sgtoc.html (Accessed 22 April 2003).

10966 Greendale GA, Lee NP, Arriola ER. The menopause. *Lancet* 1999;353:571-80.

10967 Whiteman MK, Staropoli CA, Langenberg PW, et al. Smoking, body mass, and hot flashes in midlife women. *Obstet Gynecol* 2003;101:264-72.

10968 Barnabei VM, Grady D, Stovall DW, et al. Menopausal symptoms in older women and the effects of treatment with hormone therapy. *Obstet Gynecol* 2002;100:1209-18.

10969 Grady D. Postmenopausal Hormones--therapy for symptoms only. *N Engl J Med* 2003;348:1835-7.

10970 Kass-Annese B. Alternative therapies for menopause. *Clin Obstet Gynecol* 2000;43:162-83.

10971 Newton KM, Buist DS, Keenan NL, et al. Use of alternative therapies for menopause symptoms: Results of a population-based survey. *Obstet Gynecol* 2002;100:18-25.

10972 Mahady GB, Parrot J, Lee C, et al. Botanical dietary supplement use in peri- and postmenopausal women. *Menopause* 2003;10:65-72.

10973 de Kleijn MJ, van der Schouw YT, Wilson PW, et al. Intake of dietary phytoestrogens is low in postmenopausal women in the United States: The Framingham study (1-4). *J Nutr* 2001;131:1826-32.

10974 Jellin JM, Gregory P, Batz F, Hitchens K, et al. *Pharmacist's Letter/Prescriber's Letter* Natural Medicines Comprehensive Database. Stockton, CA: Therapeutic Research Faculty; 2003. www.naturaldatabase.com (Accessed 16 April 2003).

10975 Baber RJ, Templeman C, Morton T, et al. Randomized placebo-controlled trial of an isoflavone supplement and menopausal symptoms in women. Climacteric 1999;2:85-92.

10976 Knight DC, Howes JB, Eden JA. The effect of Promensil, an isoflavone extract, on menopausal symptoms. *Climacteric* 1999;2:79-84.

10977 Puschner B, Galey FD, Holstege DM, et al. Sweet clover poisoning in dairy cattle in California. *J Am Vet Med Assoc* 1998;212:857-9.

10978 Lemay A, Dodin S, Kadri N, et al. Flaxseed dietary supplement versus hormone replacement therapy in hypercholesterolemic menopausal women. *Obstet Gynecol* 2002;100:495-504.

10979 Liu J, Burdette JE, Xu H, et al. Evaluation of estrogenic activity of plant extracts for the potential treatment of menopausal symptoms. *J Agric Food Chem* 2001;49:2472-9.

10980 Boue SM, Wiese TE, Nehls S, et al. Evaluation of the estrogenic effects of legume extracts containing phytoestrogens. *J Agric Food Chem* 2003;51:2193-9.

10981 Wiklund IK, Mattsson LA, Lindgren R, et al. Effects of a standardized ginseng extract on quality of life and physiological parameters in symptomatic postmenopausal women: a double-blind, placebo-controlled trial. *Int J Clin Pharmacol Res* 1999;19:89-99.

10982 Hammond TG, Whitworth JA. Adverse reactions to ginseng [letter]. *Med J Aust* 1981;1:492.

10983 Punnonen R, Lukola A. Oestrogen-like effect of ginseng. *Br Med J* 1980;281:1110.

10984 Lee YJ, Jin YR, Lim WC, et al. Ginsenoside-Rb1 acts as a weak phytoestrogen in MCF-7 human breast cancer cells. *Arch Pharm Res* 2003;26:58-63.

REFERENCES

REFERENCES

10985 Lasco A, Frisina N, Morabito N, et al. Metabolic effects of dehydroepiandrosterone replacement therapy in postmenopausal women. *Eur J Endocrinol* 2001;145:457-61.

10986 Stomati M, Monteleone P, Casarosa E, et al. Six-month oral dehydroepiandrosterone supplementation in early and late postmenopause. *Gynecol Endocrinol* 2000;14:342-63.

10987 Wuttke W, Seidlova-Wuttke D, Gorkow C. The Cimicifuga preparation BNO 1055 vs. conjugated estrogens in a double-blind placebo-controlled study: effects on menopause symptoms and bone markers. *Maturitas* 2003;44:S67-77.

10988 Huntley A, Ernst E. A systematic review of the safety of black cohosh. *Menopause* 2003;10:58-64.

10989 Komesaroff PA, Black CV, Cable V, et al. Effects of wild yam extract on menopausal symptoms, lipids and sex hormones in healthy menopausal women. *Climacteric* 2001;4:144-50.

10990 Waters DD, Alderman EL, Hsia J, et al. Effects of hormone replacement therapy and antioxidant vitamin supplements on coronary atherosclerosis in postmenopausal women: A randomized controlled trial. *JAMA* 2002;288:2432-40.

10991 Tice JA, Ettinger B, Ensrud K, et al. Phytoestrogen supplements for the treatment of hot flashes: the Isoflavone Clover Extract (ICE) study: a randomized controlled trial. *JAMA* 2003;290:207-14.

10992 National Institute of Neurological Disorders and Stroke. Headache: Hope through Research. http://www.ninds.nih.giv/healinfo/DISORDER/Headache/head.htm. Updated 11/19/98.

10993 Mauskop A, Altura BM. Role of magnesium in the pathogenesis and treatment of migraines. *Clinical Neuroscience* 1998;5:24-7.

10994 Adelman J, Adelman R. Current options for the prevention and treatment of migraine. *Clin Ther* 2001;23:772-88.

10995 Freitag F. What's new in migraine prevention? *NHF Headlines* 2001 July/Aug No. 121:1-2.

10996 Castelli S, Meossi C, Domenici R, et al. Magnesium in the prophylaxis of primary headache and other periodic disorders in children. *Pediatr Med Chir* 1993;15(5):481-8.

10997 Nagtegaal JE, Smits MG, Swart AC, et al. Melatonin-responsive headache in delayed sleep phase syndrome: preliminary observations. *Headache* Apr 1998;38(4):303-307.

10998 Jansen T, Romiti R, Kreuter A, Altmeyer P. Rosacea fulminans triggered by high-dose vitamins B6 and B12. *J Eur Acad Dermatol Venereol* 2001;15:484-5.

10999 Stevens LJ, Zentall SS, Deck JL, et al. Essential fatty acid metabolism in boys with attention-deficit hyperactivity disorder. *Am J Clin Nutr* 1995;62:761-8.

11000 Tardif JC. Probucol and multivitamins in the prevention of restenosis after coronary angioplasty. *N Engl J Med* 1997;337:365-372.

11001 Ness AR, Powles JW, Khaw KT. Vitamin C and cardiovascular disease: a systematic review. *J Cardiovasc Risk* 1996;3:513-521.

11002 Enstrom JE, Kanim LE, Klein MA. Vitamin C intake and mortality among a sample of the United States population. *Epidemiology* 1992;3:194-202.

11003 Slater GJ, Jenkins D. Beta-hydroxy-beta-methylbutyrate (HMB) supplementation and the promotion of muscle growth and strength. *Sports Med* 2000;30:105-16.

11004 Badiali D, Corazziari E, Habib FI, et al. Effect of wheat bran in treatment of chronic nonorganic constipation. A double-blind controlled trial. *Dig Dis Sci* 1995;40:349-56.

11005 Moon J, Yu SJ, Kim HS, Sohn J. Induction of G(1) cell cycle arrest and p27(KIP1) increase by panaxydol isolated from Panax ginseng. *Biochem Pharmacol* 2000;59:1109-16.

11006 Keum YS, Park KK, Lee JM, et al. Antioxidant and anti-tumor promoting activities of the methanol extract of heat-processed ginseng. *Cancer Lett* 2000;150:41-8.

11007 Tamaoki J, Nakata J, Kawatani K, et al. Ginsenoside-induced relaxation of human bronchial smooth muscle via release of nitric oxide. *Br J Pharmacol* 2000;130:1859-64.

11008 de Benito V, de Barrio M, de Lopez-Saez MP, et al. Anaphylactic shock caused by impurities in orgotein preparations. *Allergol Immunopathol* (Madr) 2001;29:272-5.

11009 Jiang L, Zhao N, Ni L. Retrospective study of adverse events in patients with rheumatoid arthritis treated with second-line drugs. *Zhonghua Liu Xing Bing Xue Za Zhi* 2002;23:213-7.

11010 Naveh E, Werman MJ, Sabo E, Neeman I. Defatted avocado pulp reduces body weight and total hepatic fat but increases plasma cholesterol in male rats fed diets with cholesterol. *J Nutr* 2002;132:2015-8.

11011 Kremery V Jr. Systemic chlorellosis, an emerging infection in humans caused by algae. *Int J Antimicrob Agents* 2000;15:235-7.

11012 National Institutes of Health (NIH). Glucosamine/Chondroitin Arthritis Intervention Trial (GAIT) Begins Patient Recruitment. National Center for Complementary and Alternative Medicine, 2000. Available at: http://nccam.nih.gov/news/19972000/121100/.

11013 Gupta MC, Garg SK, Badyal D, et al. Effect of grapefruit juice on the pharmacokinetics of theophylline in healthy male volunteers. *Methods Find Exp Clin Pharmacol* 1999;21:679-82.

11014 Frosst P, Blom HJ, Milos R, et al. A candidate genetic risk factor for vascular disease: a common mutation in methylenetetrahydrofolate reductase. *Nat Genet* 1995;10:111-3.

11016 Amabeoku GJ, Chikuni O, Akino C, Mutetwa S. Pharmacokinetic interaction of single doses of quinine and carbamazepine, phenobarbitone and phenytoin in healthy volunteers. *East Afr Med J* 1993;70:90-3.

11017 Dysken MW, Cumming RJ, Channon RA, Davis JM. Drug interaction between ascorbic acid and fluphenazine. *JAMA* 1979;241:2008.

11018 FDA Talk Paper. FDA Allows Foods Containing Psyllium To Make Health Claim On Reducing Risk Of Heart Disease. 1998. Available at: http://www.fda.gov/bbs/topics/ANSWERS/ANS00850.html.

11019 Naganuma M, Hirose S, Nakayama Y, et al. A study of the phototoxicity of lemon oil. *Arch Dermatol Res* 1985;278:31-6.

11020 Farnsworth N, Bingel A, Cordell G, et al. Potential value of plants as sources of new antifertility agents I. *J Pharm Sci* 1975;64:535-98.

11021 Anon. EPOGAM Capsules. G.D. Searle (South Africa) (Pty) Ltd. January 1990. Available at: http://home.intekom.com/pharm/searle/epogm.html.

11022 Nix D, Zelenitsky S, Symonds W, et al. The effect of fluconazole on the pharmacokinetics of caffeine in young and elderly subjects. *Clin Pharmacol Ther* 1992;51:183.

11023 FDA, HHS. Final Rule Declaring Dietary Supplements Containing Ephedrine Alkaloids Adulterated Because They Present An Unreasonable Risk. 21 CFR Part 119. February 11, 2004. Available at: http://www.fda.gov/OHRMS/DOCKETS/98fr/1995n-0304-nfr0001.pdf

11024 Akhondzadeh S, Fallah-Pour H, Afkham K, et al. Comparison of Crocus sativus L. and imipramine in the treatment of mild to moderate depression: A pilot double-blind randomized trial [ISRCTN45683816]. *BMC Complement Altern Med* 20042;4:12.

11101 Arroll B, Kenealy T. Antibiotics for the common cold. *Cochrane Database Syst Rev* 2002;(3):CD000247.

11102 Dowell SF, Marcy SM, Phillips WR, et al. Principles of judicious use of antimicrobial agents for pediatric upper respiratory tract infections. *Pediatrics* 1998;101:163-5.

11103 Gonzales R, Bartlett JG, Besser RE, et al. Principles of appropriate antibiotic use for treatment of acute respiratory tract infections in adults: background, specific aims, and methods. *Ann Intern Med* 2001;134:479-86.

11104 Sperber SJ, Hendley JO, Hayden FG, et al. Effects of naproxen on experimental rhinovirus colds. A randomized, double-blind, controlled trial. *Ann Intern Med* 1992;117:37-41.

11105 Gwaltney JM Jr. Combined antiviral and antimediator treatment of rhinovirus colds. *J Infect Dis* 1992;166:776-82.

11106 Winther B, Mygind N. The therapeutic effectiveness of ibuprofen on the symptoms of naturally acquired common colds. *Am J Rhinol* 2001;15:239-42.

11107 Dales RE, Lunau MA, Tierney MG, Schweitzer I. Chronic cough responsive to ibuprofen. *Pharmacotherapy* 1992;12:331-3.

11108 Papsin B, McTavish A. Saline nasal irrigation: Its role as an adjunct treatment. *Can Fam Physician* 2003;49:168-73.

11109 Adam P, Stiffman M, Blake RL Jr. A clinical trial of hypertonic saline nasal spray in subjects with the common cold or rhinosinusitis. *Arch Fam Med* 1998;7:39-43.

11110 Freestone C, Eccles R. Assessment of the antitussive efficacy of codeine in cough associated with common cold. *J Pharm Pharmacol* 1997;49:1045-9.

11111 Kimura S, Tamayama M, Minami M, et al. Docosahexaenoic acid inhibits blood viscosity in stroke-prone spontaneously hypertensive rats. *Res Commun Mol Pathol Pharmacol* 1998;100:351-61.

11112 Leng GC, Smith FB, Fowkes FG, et al. Relationship between plasma essential fatty acids and smoking, serum lipids, blood pressure and haemostatic and rheological factors. *Prostaglandins Leukot Essent Fatty Acids* 1994;51:101-108.

11113 Nelson GJ, Schmidt PS, Bartolini GL, et al. The effect of dietary docosahexaenoic acid on platelet function, platelet fatty acid composition, and blood coagulation in humans. *Lipids* 1997;32:1129-36.

11114 Karagas MR, Greenberg ER, Nierenberg D, et al. Risk of squamous cell carcinoma of the skin in relation to plasma selenium, alpha-tocopherol, beta-carotene, and retinol: a nested case-control study. *Cancer Epidemiol Biomarkers Prev* 1997;6:25-9.

11115 Hodek P, Trefil P, Stiborova M. Flavonoids-potent and versatile biologically active compounds interacting with cytochromes P450. *Chem Biol Interact* 2002;139:1-21.

11116 Griffenberg L, Morris M, Atkinson N, Levenback C. The effect of dietary fiber on bowel function following radical hysterectomy: a randomized trial. *Gynecol Oncol* 1997;66:417-24.

11117 Anti M, Pignataro G, Armuzzi A, et al. Water supplementation enhances the effect of high-fiber diet on stool frequency and laxative consumption in adult patients with functional constipation. *Hepatogastroenterology* 1998;45:727-32.

11118 Helton WS; SSAT, AGA, ASGE Consensus Panel. 2001 consensus statement on benign anorectal disease. *J Gastrointest Surg* 2002;6:302-3.

11119 Jensen SL, Harling H, Tange G, et al. Maintenance bran therapy for prevention of symptoms after rubber band ligation of third-degree haemorrhoids. *Acta Chir Scand* 1988;154:395-98.

11120 Food and Nutrition Board, Institute of Medicine. Dietary Reference Intakes for Energy, Carbohydrate, Fiber, Fat, Fatty Acids, Cholesterol, Protein, and Amino Acids (Macronutrients). Washington, DC: National Academy Press, 2002. Available at: http://www.nap.edu/books/0309085373/html/.

11121 Chaparral-induced toxic hepatitis-California and Texas, 1992. *MMWR Morb Mortal Wkly Rep* 1992;41:812-4.

11122 Estes JD, Stolpman D, Olyaei A, et al. High prevalence of potentially hepatotoxic herbal supplement use in patients with fulminant hepatic failure. *Arch Surg* 2003;138:852-8.

11123 Anesini C, Ferraro G, Lopez P, Borda E. Different intracellular signals coupled to the antiproliferative action of aqueous crude extract from Larrea divaricata Cav. and nor-dihydroguaiaretic acid on a lymphoma cell line. *Phytomedicine* 2001;8:1-7.

11124 McDonald RW, Bunjobpon W, Liu T, et al. Synthesis and anticancer activity of nordihydroguaiaretic acid (NDGA) and analogues. *Anticancer Drug Des* 2001;16:261-70.

11125 Lambert JD, Zhao D, Meyers RO, et al. Nordihydroguaiaretic acid: hepatotoxicity and detoxification in the mouse. *Toxicon* 2002;40:1701-8.

11126 Quiroga EN, Sampietro AR, Vattuone MA. Screening antifungal activities of selected medicinal plants. *J Ethnopharmacol* 2001;74:89-96.

11127 Gnabre JN, Brady JN, Clanton DJ, et al. Inhibition of human immunodeficiency virus type 1 transcription and replication by DNA sequence-selective plant lignans. *Proc Natl Acad Sci U S A* 1995;92:11239-43.

11128 Shasky DR. Contact dermatitis from Larrea tridentata (creosote bush). *J Am Acad Dermatol* 1986;15:302.

11129 Smith AY, Feddersen RM, Gardner KD Jr, Davis CJ Jr. Cystic renal cell carcinoma and acquired renal cystic disease associated with consumption of chaparral tea: a case report. *J Urol* 1994;152:2089-91.

11130 Qiu D, Kao PN. Immunosuppressive and anti-inflammatory mechanisms of triptolide, the principal active diterpenoid from the Chinese medicinal herb Tripterygium wilfordii Hook. f. *Drugs R D* 2003;4:1-18.

11131 Lue Y, Sinha Hikim AP, Wang C, et al. Triptolide: a potential male contraceptive. *J Androl* 1998;19:479-86.

11132 Shi YL, Bai JP, Wang WP. Ion-channels in human sperm membrane and contraceptive mechanisms of male antifertility compounds derived from Chinese traditional medicine. *Acta Pharmacol Sin* 2003;24:22-30.

11133 Qian SZ, Hu YZ, Wang SM, et al. Effects of Tripterygium hypoglaucum (Levl.) Hutch on male fertility. *Adv Contracept* 1988;4:307-10.

11134 Lupton JR, Robinson MC, Morin JL. Cholesterol-lowering effect of barley bran flour and oil. *J Am Diet Assoc* 1994;94:65-70.

11135 Jenkins DJ, Wesson V, Wolever TM, et al. Wholemeal versus wholegrain breads: proportion of whole or cracked grain and the glycaemic response. *BMJ* 1988;297:958-60.

11136 Hapke HJ, Strathmann W. [Pharmacological effects of hordenine]. [Article in German]. *Dtsch Tierarztl Wochenschr* 1995;102:228-32.

11137 Fasano A, Catassi C. Current approaches to diagnosis and treatment of celiac disease: an evolving spectrum. *Gastroenterology* 2001;120:636-51.

11138 Zhang F, Altorki NK, Mestre JR, et al. Curcumin inhibits cyclooxygenase-2 transcription in bile acid- and phorbol ester-treated human gastrointestinal epithelial cells. *Carcinogenesis* 1999;20:445-51.

11139 Surh YJ. Anti-tumor promoting potential of selected spice ingredients with antioxidative and anti-inflammatory activities: a short review. *Food Chem Toxicol* 2002;40:1091-7.

11140 Araujo CC, Leon LL. Biological activities of Curcuma longa L. *Mem Inst Oswaldo Cruz* 2001;96:723-8.

11141 Deeb D, Xu YX, Jiang H, et al. Curcumin (diferuloyl-methane) enhances tumor necrosis factor-related apoptosis-inducing ligand-induced apoptosis in LNCaP prostate cancer cells. *Mol Cancer Ther* 2003;2:95-103.

11142 Thaloor D, Singh AK, Sidhu GS, et al. Inhibition of angiogenic differentiation of human umbilical vein endothelial cells by curcumin. *Cell Growth Differ* 1998;9:305-12.

11143 Shah BH, Nawaz Z, Pertani SA. Inhibitory effect of curcumin, a food spice from turmeric, on platelet-activating factor- and arachidonic acid-mediated platelet aggregation through inhibition of thromboxane formation and Ca2+ signaling. *Biochem Pharmacol* 1999;58:1167-72.

11144 Thamlikitkul V, Bunyapraphatsara N, Dechatiwongse T, et al. Randomized double blind study of Curcuma domestica Val. for dyspepsia. *J Med Assoc Thai* 1989;72:613-20.

11145 Rasyid A, Rahman AR, Jaalam K, Lelo A. Effect of different curcumin dosages on human gall bladder. *Asia Pac J Clin Nutr* 2002;11:314-8.

11146 Hata M, Sasaki E, Ota M, et al . Allergic contact dermatitis from curcumin (turmeric). *Contact Dermatitis* 1997;36:107-8.

11147 Antony S, Kuttan R, Kuttan G. Immunomodulatory activity of curcumin. *Immunol Invest* 1999;28:291-303.

11148 Kuttan R, Sudheeran PC, Josph CD. Turmeric and curcumin as topical agents in cancer therapy. *Tumori* 1987;73:29-31.

11149 Deodhar SD, Sethi R, Srimal RC. Preliminary study on antirheumatic activity of curcumin (diferuloyl methane). *Indian J Med Res* 1980;71:632-4.

11150 Lal B, Kapoor AK, Asthana OP, et al. Efficacy of curcumin in the management of chronic anterior uveitis. *Phytother Res* 1999;13:318-22.

11151 Korting HC, Schafer-Korting M, Hart H, et al. Anti-inflammatory activity of hamamelis distillate applied topically to the skin. Influence of vehicle and dose. *Eur J Clin Pharmacol* 1993;44:315-8.

11152 Gol'dman II. [Anaphylactic shock after gargling with an infusion of Calendula]. [Article in Russian]. *Klin Med* (Mosk) 1974;52:142-3.

11153 Xu QF, Fang XL, Chen DF. Pharmacokinetics and bioavailability of ginsenoside Rb1 and Rg1 from Panax notoginseng in rats. *J Ethnopharmacol* 2003;84:187-92.

11154 Shelton RC. St John's Wort for the treatment of depression. *Lancet Neurol* 2002;1:275.

11155 Jafek BW, Linschoten M, Murrow BW. Zicam Induced Anosmia. American Rhinologic Society 49th Annual Fall Scientific Meeting abstract. Orlando, Florida. September 20, 2003. http://app.american-rhinologic.org/programs/2003ARSFallProgram071503.pdf (Accessed 24 November 2003).

11156 Uebayashi H, Hatanaka T, Kanemura F, Tonosaki K. Acute anosmia in the mouse: behavioral discrimination among the four basic taste substances. *Physiol Behav* 2001;72:291-6.

11157 Noor R, Mittal S, Iqbal J. Superoxide dismutase--applications and relevance to human diseases. *Med Sci Monit* 2002;8:RA210-5.

11158 Society of Surgery of the Alimentary Tract, Inc. Management of ulcerative colitis. SSAT patient care guidelines 2002. Available at: http://www.ssat.com/cgi-bin/colitis.cgi?affiliation

11159 Sojka J, Wastney M, Abrams S, et al. Magnesium kinetics in adolescent girls determined using stable isotopes: effects of high and low calcium intake. *Am J Physiol* 1997;273:R710-5.

11160 Product information for infliximab (Remicade). Centocor, Inc. Malvern, PA. April 2003.

11161 Vihtamaki T, Parantainen J, Koivisto AM, et al. Oral ascorbic acid increases plasma oestradiol during postmenopausal hormone replacement therapy. *Maturitas* 2002;42:129-35.

11162 Murphy LL, Lee TJ. Ginseng, sex behavior, and nitric oxide. *Ann N Y Acad Sci* 2002;962:372-7.

11163 Eadie MJ. Convulsive ergotism: epidemics of the serotonin syndrome? *Lancet Neurol* 2003;2:429-34.

11164 Etzel RA. Mycotoxins. *JAMA* 2002;287:425-7.

11165 Ben-Arye E, Golden E, Wengrower D, et al. Wheat grass juice in the treatment of active distal ulcerative colitis a randomized double-blind placebo-controlled trial. *Scand J Gastroenterol* 2002;4:444-9.

11166 Beal JE, Olson R, Laubenstein L, et al. Dronabinol as a treatment for anorexia associated with weight loss in patients with AIDS. *J Pain Symptom Manage* 1995;10:89-97.

11167 Consroe P, Musty R, Rein J, et al. The perceived effects of smoked cannabis on patients with multiple sclerosis. *Eur Neurol* 1997;38:44-8.

11168 Zajicek J, Fox P, Sanders H, et al. Cannabinoids for treatment of spasticity and other symptoms related to multiple sclerosis (CAMS study): multicentre randomised placebo-controlled trial. *Lancet* 2003;362:1517-26.

11215 Thorpe A, Neal D. Benign prostatic hyperplasia. *Lancet* 2003;361:1359-67.

11216 Emberton M, Andriole GL, de la Rosette J, et al. Benign prostatic hyperplasia: a progressive disease of aging men. *Urology* 2003;61:267-73.

11217 Verhamme KM, Dieleman JP, Bleumink GS, et al. Incidence and prevalence of lower urinary tract symptoms suggestive of benign prostatic hyperplasia in primary care--the Triumph project. *Eur Urol* 2002;42:323-8.

11218 Young JM, Muscatello DJ, Ward JE. Are men with lower urinary tract symptoms at increased risk of prostate cancer? A systematic review and critique of the available evidence. *BJU Int* 2000;85:1037-48.

11219 Medina JJ, Parra RO, Moore RG. Benign prostatic hyperplasia (the aging prostate). *Med Clin North Am* 1999;83:1213-29.

11221 AUA Practice Guidelines Committee. AUA guideline on management of benign prostatic hyperplasia (2003). Chapter 1: Diagnosis and treatment recommendations. *J Urol* 2003;170:530-47.

11224 Vela Navarrete R, Garcia Cardoso JV, Barat A, et al. BPH and Inflammation: pharmacological effects of Permixon on histological and molecular inflammatory markers. Results of a double blind pilot clinical assay. *Eur Urol* 2003;44:549-55.

11225 Markowitz JS, Donovan JL, Devane CL, et al. Multiple doses of saw palmetto (Serenoa repens) did not alter cytochrome P450 2D6 and 3A4 activity in normal volunteers. *Clin Pharmacol Ther* 2003;74:536-42.

11226 Santa Maria Margalef A, Paciucci Barzanti R, Reventos Puigjaner J, et al. [Antimitogenic effect of Pygeum africanum extracts on human prostatic cancer cell lines and explants from benign prostatic hyperplasia]. [Article in Spanish]. *Arch Esp Urol* 2003;56:369-78.

11227 Konrad L, Muller HH, Lenz C, et al. Antiproliferative effect on human prostate cancer cells by a stinging nettle root (Urtica dioica) extract. *Planta Med* 2000;66:44-7.

11228 Schottner M, Gansser D, Spiteller G, et al. Lignans from the roots of Urtica dioica and their metabolites bind to human sex hormone binding globulin (SHBG). *Planta Med* 1997;63:529-32.

11229 Lichius JJ, Muth C. The inhibiting effects of Urtica dioica root extracts on experimentally induced prostatic hyperplasia in the mouse. *Planta Med* 1997;63:307-10.

11230 Vontobel HP, Herzog R, Rutishauser G, Kres H. [Results of a double-blind study on the effectiveness of ERU (extractum radicis Urticae) capsules in conservative treatment of benign prostatic hyperplasia]. [Article in German]. (Abstract). *Urologe A* 1985;24:49-51.

11231 Friederich M, Theurer C, Schiebel-Schlosser G. [Prosta Fink Forte capsules in the treatment of benign prostatic hyperplasia. Multicentric surveillance study in 2245 patients]. [Article in German]. *Forsch Komplementarmed Klass Naturheilkd* 2000;7:200-4.

11232 Carbin BE, Larsson B, Lindahl O. Treatment of benign prostatic hyperplasia with phytosterols. *Br J Urol* 1990;66:639-41.

11233 Zhang X, Ouyang JZ, Zhang YS, et al. Effect of the extracts of pumpkin seeds on the urodynamics of rabbits: an experimental study. *J Tongji Med Univ* 1994;14:235-8.

11234 Kassen A, Berges R, Senge T, et al. Effect of beta-sitosterol on transforming growth factor-beta-1 expression and translocation protein kinase C alpha in human prostate stromal cells in vitro. *Eur Urol* 2000;37:735-41.

11235 Wan XS, Zhou Z, Kennedy AR, Kopelovich L. In vitro evaluation of chemopreventive agents using cultured human prostate epithelial cells. *Oncol Rep* 2003;10:2009-14.

11236 Mahomed IM, Ojewole JA. Hypoglycemic effect of Hypoxis hemerocallidea corm (African potato) aqueous extract in rats. *Methods Find Exp Clin Pharmacol* 2003;25:617-23.

11237 Obermuller-Jevic UC, Olano-Martin E, Corbacho AM, et al. Lycopene inhibits the growth of normal human prostate epithelial cells in vitro. *J Nutr* 2003;133:3356-60.

11238 Geller J, Sionit L, Partido C, et al. Genistein inhibits the growth of human-patient BPH and prostate cancer in histoculture. *Prostate* 1998;34:75-9.

11239 Jarred RA, McPherson SJ, Jones ME, et al. Anti-androgenic action by red clover-derived dietary isoflavones reduces non-malignant prostate enlargement in aromatase knockout (ArKo) mice. *Prostate* 2003;56:54-64.

11240 Risbridger GP, Wang H, Frydenberg M, Husband A. The in vivo effect of red clover diet on ventral prostate growth in adult male mice. *Reprod Fertil Dev* 2001;13:325-9.

11241 Preuss HG, Marcusen C, Regan J, et al. Randomized trial of a combination of natural products (cernitin, saw palmetto, B-sitosterol, vitamin E) on symptoms of benign prostatic hyperplasia (BPH). *Int Urol Nephrol* 2001; 33: 217-25.

11242 Lee M. Management of benign prostatic hyperplasia. Pharmacotherapy - A Pathophysiological Approach, 5th edition (1999). New, NY: McGraw-Hill Publishing Division.

11243 Debruyne F, Koch G, Boyle P, et al. [Comparison of a phytotherapeutic agent (Permixon) with an alpha-blocker (Tamsulosin) in the treatment of benign prostatic hyperplasia: a 1-year randomized international study]. [Article in French]. *Eur Urol* 2002;41:497-506.

11244 Lee HS, Ahn YJ. Growth-Inhibiting Effects of Cinnamomum cassia Bark-Derived Materials on Human Intestinal Bacteria. *J Agric Food Chem* 1998;46:8-12.

11245 Koh WS, Yoon SY, Kwon BM, et al. Cinnamaldehyde inhibits lymphocyte proliferation and modulates T-cell differentiation. *Int J Immunopharmacol* 1998;20:643-60.

11246 Kwon BM, Lee SH, Choi SU, et al. Synthesis and in vitro cytotoxicity of cinnamaldehydes to human solid tumor cells. *Arch Pharm Res* 1998;21:147-52.

11247 Anderson RA, Broadhurst CL, Polansky MM, et al. Isolation and Characterization of Polyphenol Type-A Polymers from Cinnamon with Insulin-like Biological Activity. *J Agric Food Chem* 2004;52:65-70.

11248 Jarvill-Taylor KJ, Anderson RA, Graves DJ. A hydroxychalcone derived from cinnamon functions as a mimetic for insulin in 3T3-L1 adipocytes. *J Am Coll Nutr* 2001;20:327-36.

11249 Imparl-Radosevich J, Deas S, Polansky MM, et al. Regulation of PTP-1 and insulin receptor kinase by fractions from cinnamon: implications for cinnamon regulation of insulin signalling. *Horm Res* 1998;50:177-82.

11250 Bravata DM, Sanders L, Huang J, et al. Efficacy and safety of low-carbohydrate diets: a systematic review. *JAMA* 2003;289:1837-50.

11251 Anon. The Atkins diet. *Med Lett Drugs Ther* 2000;42:52.

11252 Atkins RC, Ornish D, Wadden T. Low-carb, low-fat diet gurus face off. Interview by Joan Stephenson. *JAMA* 2003;289:1767-8, 1773.

11253 Foster GD, Wyatt HR, Hill JO, et al. A randomized trial of a low-carbohydrate diet for obesity. *N Engl J Med* 2003;348:2082-90.

11254 Samaha FF, Iqbal N, Seshadri P, et al. A low-carbohydrate as compared with a low-fat diet in severe obesity. *N Engl J Med* 2003;348:2074-81.

11255 Westman EC, Yancy WS, Edman JS, et al. Effect of 6-month adherence to a very low carbohydrate diet program. *Am J Med* 2002;113:30-6.

11256 Ludwig DS. The glycemic index: physiological mechanisms relating to obesity, diabetes, and cardiovascular disease. *JAMA* 2002;287:2414-23.

11257 Foster-Powell K, Holt SH, Brand-Miller JC. International table of glycemic index and glycemic load values: 2002. *Am J Clin Nutr* 2002;76:5-56.

11258 Brand-Miller JC, Holt SH, Pawlak DB, McMillan J. Glycemic index and obesity. *Am J Clin Nutr* 2002;76:281S-5S.

11259 Ellison S. The good, the bad and the high glycemic. *Wall Street Journal* November 24, 2003.

11260 Anon. Dietary fat consensus statements. *Am J Med* 2002;113 Suppl 9B:5S-8S.

11261 Pirozzo S, Summerbell C, Cameron C, Glasziou P. Advice on low-fat diets for obesity. *Cochrane Database Syst Rev* 2002;2:CD003640.

11262 St. Jeor ST, Howard BV, Prewitt TE, et al. Dietary protein and weight reduction: A statement for healthcare professionals from the Nutrition Committee of the Council on Nutrition, Physical Activity, and Metabolism of the American Heart Association. *Circulation* 2001;104:1869-74.

11263 Cheuvront SN. The Zone diet phenomenon: a closer look at the science behind the claims. *J Am Coll Nutr* 2003;22:9-17.

11264 Heshka S, Anderson JW, Atkinson RL, et al. Weight loss with self-help compared with a structured commercial program: a randomized trial. *JAMA* 2003;289:1792-8.

11265 FDA Center for Food Safety and Nutrition. What are some of the questionable weight loss products? http://www.cfsan.fda.gov/~dms/qa-nut4.html. (Accessed December 20, 2003).

11266 Yanovski SZ, Yanovski JA. Obesity. *N Engl J Med* 2002;346:591-602.

11267 Pellati F, Benvenuti S, Melegari M, Firenzuoli F. Determination of adrenergic agonists from extracts and herbal products of Citrus aurantium L. var. amara by LC. *J Pharm Biomed Anal* 2002;29:1113-9.

11268 Colker CM, Kalman DS, Torina GC, et al. Effects of Citrus aurantium extract, caffeine, and St. John's wort on body fat loss, lipid levels, and mood states in overweight healthy adults. *Curr Ther Res* 1999;60:145-153.

11269 Penzak SR, Acosta EP, Turner M, et al. Effect of Seville orange juice and grapefruit juice on indinavir pharmacokinetics. *J Clin Pharmacol* 2002;42:1165-70.

11270 Edwards DJ, Fitzsimmons ME, Schuetz EG, et al. 6',7'-Dihydroxybergamottin in grapefruit juice and Seville orange juice: effects on cyclosporine disposition, enterocyte CYP3A4, and P-glycoprotein. *Clin Pharmacol Ther* 1999;65:237-44.

11271 Food and Drug Administration, Center for Food Safety and Applied Nutrition. Letter to Health Care Professionals on Hazardous Dietary Supplement LipoKinetix. November 19,

2001. Available at: http://www.cfsan.fda.gov/~dms/ds-ltr25.html
11272 Abo-Khatwa AN, al-Robai AA, al-Jawhari DA. Lichen acids as uncouplers of oxidative phosphorylation of mouse-liver mitochondria. *Nat Toxins* 1996;4:96-102.
11273 Schmiedlin-Ren P, Edwards DJ, Fitzsimmons ME, et al. Mechanisms of enhanced oral availability of CYP3A4 substrates by grapefruit constituents. Decreased enterocyte CYP3A4 concentration and mechanism-based inactivation by furanocoumarins. *Drug Metab Dispos* 1997;25:1228-33.
11274 Rogers JD, Zhao J, Liu L, et al. Grapefruit juice has minimal effects on plasma concentrations of lovastatin-derived 3-hydroxy-3-methylglutaryl coenzyme A reductase inhibitors. *Clin Pharmacol Ther* 1999;66:358-66.
11275 Veronese ML, Gillen LP, Burke JP, et al. Exposure-dependent inhibition of intestinal and hepatic CYP3A4 in vivo by grapefruit juice. *J Clin Pharmacol* 2003;43:831-9.
11276 Bailey DG, Dresser GK, Bend JR. Bergamottin, lime juice, and red wine as inhibitors of cytochrome P450 3A4 activity: comparison with grapefruit juice. *Clin Pharmacol Ther* 2003;73:529-37 .
11277 Becquemont L, Verstuyft C, Kerb R, et al. Effect of grapefruit juice on digoxin pharmacokinetics in humans. *Clin Pharmacol Ther* 2001;70:311-6.
11278 Dresser GK, Bailey DG, Leake BF, et al. Fruit juices inhibit organic anion transporting polypeptide-mediated drug uptake to decrease the oral availability of fexofenadine. *Clin Pharmacol Ther* 2002;71:11-20.
11279 National Institute of Diabetes and Digestive and Kidney Diseases. Crohn's Disease. NIH Publication No. 03-3410 January 2003. Available at: http://digestive.niddk.nih.gov/ddiseases/pubs/crohns/index.htm.
11280 Shelton MJ, Wynn HE, Hewitt RG, DiFrancesco R. Effects of grapefruit juice on pharmacokinetic exposure to indinavir in HIV-positive subjects. *J Clin Pharmacol* 2001;41:435-42.
11281 National Institute of Diabetes and Digestive and Kidney Diseases. Ulcerative Colitis. NIH Publication No. 03-1597 April 2003. Available at: http://digestive.niddk.nih.gov/ddiseases/pubs/colitis/index.htm.
11282 Parker RB, Yates CR, Soberman JE, Laizure SC. Effects of grapefruit juice on intestinal P-glycoprotein: evaluation using digoxin in humans. *Pharmacotherapy* 2003;23:979-87.
11283 Scott CM, Verhoef MJ, Hilsden RJ. Inflammatory bowel disease patient's descision to use complementary therapies: links to existing models of care. *Complement Ther Med* 2003;11:22-7.
11284 Stenson WF, Korzenik J. Inflammatory Bowel Disease. In: Yamada T, ed. Textbook of Gastroenterology. 4th ed. Philadelphia, PA: Lippincott Williams & Wilkins; 2003.
11285 Bolton-Smith C, Price RJ, Fenton ST, et al. Compilation of a provisional UK database for the phylloquinone (vitamin K1) content of foods. *Br J Nutr* 2000;83:389-99.
11286 Stein JH, Carlsson CM, Papcke-Benson K, et al. The effects of lipid-lowering and antioxidant vitamin therapies on flow-mediated vasodilation of the brachial artery in older adults with hypercholesterolemia. *J Am Coll Cardiol* 2001;38:1806-13.
11287 Carlsson CM, Papcke-Benson K, Carnes M, et al. Health-related quality of life and long-term therapy with pravastatin and tocopherol (vitamin E) in older adults. *Drugs Aging* 2002;19:793-805.
11288 Rakel D. Prostate health. *Clin Fam Prac* 2002;4:967-971.
11289 McConnell JD, Roehrborn CG, Bautista OM, et al. The long-term effect of doxazosin, finasteride, and combination therapy on the clinical progression of benign prostatic hyperplasia. *N Engl J Med* 2003;349:2387-98.
11292 Katsukawa H, Imoto T, Ninomiya Y. Induction of salivary gurmarin-binding proteins in rats fed gymnema-containing diets. *Chem Senses* 1999;24:387-92.
11293 Henry DA, Mitchell AS, Aylward J, et al. Glucomannan and risk of oesophageal obstruction. *Br Med J* 1986;292:591-2.
11294 Passaretti S, Franzoni M, Comin U, et al. Action of glucomannans on complaints in patients affected with chronic constipation: a multicentric clinical evaluation. *Ital J Gastroenterol* 1991;23:421-5.
11295 Staiano A, Simeone D, Del Giudice E, et al. Effect of the dietary fiber glucomannan on chronic constipation in neurologically impaired children. *J Pediatr* 2000;136:41-5.
11296 Arenz A, Kelin M, Flehe K, et al. Occurrence of neurotoxic 4'-O-methylpyridoxine in ginkgo biloba leaves, ginkgo medications and Japanese ginkgo food. *Planta Med* 1996;62:548-51.
11297 Weidner MS, Sigwart K. Investigation of the teratogenic potential of a zingiber officinale extract in the rat. *Reprod Toxicol* 2001;15:75-80.
11298 Wilkinson JM. Effect of ginger tea on the fetal development of Sprague-Dawley rats. *Reprod Toxicol* 2000;14:507-12.
11299 Nagabhushan M, Amonkar AJ, Bhide SV. Mutagenicity of gingerol and shogaol and antimutagenicity of zingerone in Salmonella/microsome assay. *Cancer Lett* 1987;36:221-33.
11300 Slain D, Ansden J, Khakoo R, et al. Effects of High-Dose Vitamin C on the Steady State Pharmacokinetics of the Protease Inhibitor Indinavir in Healthy Volunteers. Interscience Conference on Antimicrobial Agents and Chemotherapy (ICAAC) Meeting. Poster A-1610. Chicago, Sept 13-17, 2003.
11301 Mishra LC, Singh BB, Dagenais S. Scientific basis for the therapeutic use of Withania somnifera (ashwagandha): a review. *Altern Med Rev* 2000;5:334-46.
11302 Darlington S, Williams G, Neale R, et al. A randomized controlled trial to assess sunscreen application and beta carotene supplementation in the prevention of solar keratoses. *Arch Dermatol* 2003;139:451-5.
11303 Virtamo J, Pietinen P, Huttunen JK, et al. Incidence of cancer and mortality following alpha-tocopherol and beta-carotene supplementation: a postintervention follow-up. *JAMA* 2003;290:476-85.
11304 Gann PH, Khachik F. Tomatoes or lycopene versus prostate cancer: is evolution anti-reductionist? *J Natl Cancer Inst* 2003;95:1563-5.
11305 Boileau TW, Liao Z, Kim S, et al. Prostate carcinogenesis in N-methyl-N-nitrosourea (NMU)-testosterone-treated rats fed tomato powder, lycopene, or energy-restricted diets. *J Natl Cancer Inst* 2003;95:1578-86.
11306 Barrett S. Zicam Marketers Sued. United States District Court Western District of Michigan Southern Division, Filed October 14, 2003, Case No. 4:03CV0146.
11307 Bokura H, Kobayashi S. Chitosan decreases total cholesterol in women: a randomized, double-blind, placebo-controlled trial. *Eur J Clin Nutr* 2003;57:721-5.
11308 Maron DJ, Lu GP, Cai NS, et al. Cholesterol-lowering effect of a theaflavin-enriched green tea extract: a randomized controlled trial. *Arch Intern Med* 2003;163:1448-53.
11309 Kemberling JK, Hampton JA, Keck RW, et al. Inhibition of bladder tumor growth by the green tea derivative epigallocatechin-3-gallate. *J Urol* 2003;170:773-6.
11310 Ahn WS, Yoo J, Huh SW, et al. Protective effects of green tea extracts (polyphenon E and EGCG) on human cervical lesions. *Eur J Cancer Prev* 2003;12:383-90.
11311 van Marle J, Aarsen PN, Lind A, van Weeren-Kramer J. Deglycyrrhizinised liquorice (DGL) and the renewal of rat stomach epithelium. *Eur J Pharmacol* 1981;72:219-25.

11312 Turpie AG, Runcie J, Thomson TJ. Clinical trial of deglydyrrhizinized liquorice in gastric ulcer. *Gut* 1969;10:299-302.

11313 Tewari SN, Wilson AK. Deglycyrrhizinated liquorice in duodenal ulcer. *Practitioner* 1973;210:820-3.

11314 Willetts KE, Clements MS, Champion S, et al. Serenoa repens extract for benign prostate hyperplasia: a randomized controlled trial. *BJU Int* 2003;92:267-70.

11315 Infante S, Baeza ML, Calvo M, et al. Anaphylaxis due to caffeine. *Allergy* 2003;58:681-2.

11316 Podolsky DK. Inflammatory bowel disease. *N Engl J Med* 2002;347:417-29.

11317 Massey LK, Whiting SJ. Caffeine, urinary calcium, calcium metabolism and bone. *J Nutr* 1993;123:1611-4.

11318 Panagiotakos DB, Pitsavos C, Chrysohoou C, et al. The J-shaped effect of coffee consumption on the risk of developing acute coronary syndromes: the CARDIO2000 case-control study. *J Nutr* 2003;133:3228-32.

11320 Gusev EI, Skvortsova VI, Dambinova SA, et al. Neuroprotective effects of glycine for therapy of acute ischaemic stroke. *Cerebrovasc Dis* 2000;10:49-60.

11321 Evins AE, Fitzgerald SM, Wine L, et al. Placebo-controlled trial of glycine added to clozapine in schizophrenia. *Am J Psychiatry* 2000;157:826-8.

11322 File SE, Fluck E, Fernandes C. Beneficial effects of glycine (bioglycin) on memory and attention in young and middle-aged adults. *J Clin Psychopharmacol* 1999;19:506-12.

11323 Hart AL, Stagg AJ, Kamm MA. Use of probiotics in the treatment of inflammatory bowel disease. *J Clin Gastroenterol* 2003;36:111-9.

11324 Behmanesh Y, Abdollahi M. Hemolysis after consumption of Viola tricolor. *WHO Drug Inf* (Iran) 2002;16:15-16.

11325 Carden SM, Good WV, Carden PA, Good RM. Garlic and the strabismus surgeon. Clin Experiment Ophthalmol 2002;30:303-4.

11326 Age-Related Eye Disease Study Research Group. Potential public health impact of age-related eye disease study results: AREDS report no. 11. *Arch Ophthalmol* 2003;121:1621-4.

11327 Kamphuis MM, Lejeune MP, Saris WH, Westerterp-Plantenga MS. Effect of conjugated linoleic acid supplementation after weight loss on appetite and food intake in overweight subjects. *Eur J Clin Nutr* 2003;57:1268-74.

11328 Chambers BK, Camire ME. Can cranberry supplementation benefit adults with type 2 diabetes? *Diabetes Care* 2003;26:2695-6.

11330 Benzi G. Is there a rationale for the use of creatine either as nutritional supplementation or drug administration in humans participating in a sport? *Pharmacol Res* 2000;41:255-64.

11331 Bosco C, Tihanyi J, Pucspk J, et al. Effect of oral creatine supplementation on jumping and running performance. *Int J Sports Med* 1997;18:369-72.

11332 Groeneveld GJ, Veldink JH, van der Tweel I, et al. A randomized sequential trial of creatine in amyotrophic lateral sclerosis. *Ann Neurol* 2003;53:437-45.

11333 Wheaton DH, Hoffman DR, Locke KG, et al. Biological safety assessment of docosahexaenoic acid supplementation in a randomized clinical trial for X-linked retinitis pigmentosa. *Arch Ophthalmol* 2003;121:1269-78.

11334 Wolkowitz OM, Kramer JH, Reus VI, et al. DHEA treatment of Alzheimer's disease: a randomized, double-blind, placebo-controlled study. *Neurology* 2003;60:1071-6.

11335 Priyadarsini KI, Khopde SM, Kumar SS, Mohan H. Free radical studies of ellagic acid, a natural phenolic antioxidant. *J Agric Food Chem* 2002;50:2200-6.

11336 Baker J, Zhang X, Boucher T, Keyler D. Investigation of quality in ephedrine-containing dietary supplements. *Journal of Herbal Pharmacotherapy* 2003;3:5-17.

11337 Liem A, Reynierse-Buitenwerf GH, Zwinderman AH, et al. Secondary prevention with folic acid: effects on clinical outcomes. *J Am Coll Cardiol* 2003;41:2105-13.

11338 van Oort FV, Melse-Boonstra A, Brouwer IA, et al. Folic acid and reduction of plasma homocysteine concentrations in older adults: a dose-response study. *Am J Clin Nutr* 2003;77:1318-23.

11339 Rose DP, Connolly JM, Liu XH. Effects of linoleic acid and gamma-linolenic acid on the growth and metastasis of a human breast cancer cell line in nude mice and on its growth and invasive capacity in vitro. *Nutr Cancer* 1995;24:33-45.

11340 Towheed TE. Current status of glucosamine therapy in osteoarthritis. *Arthritis Rheum* 2003;49:601-4.

11341 Takwale A, Tan E, Agarwal S, et al. Efficacy and tolerability of borage oil in adults and children with atopic eczema: randomised, double blind, placebo controlled, parallel group trial. *BMJ* 2003;327:1385.

11342 Williams HC. Evening primrose oil for atopic dermatitis. *BMJ* 2003;327:1358-9.

11343 Buckley M, Goff A, Knapp W. Fish oil interaction with warfarin. *Ann Pharmacother* 2004;38:50-2.

11344 Raitt M, Connor W, Morris C, et al. Antiarrhythmic effects of n-3 polyunsaturated fatty acids in survivors of ventricular tachyarrhythmias. *Circulation* 2003;108:1.

11345 Ng MK, Nakhla S, Baoutina A, et al. Dehydroepiandrosterone, an adrenal androgen, increases human foam cell formation: a potentially pro-atherogenic effect. *J Am Coll Cardiol* 2003;42:1967-74.

11346 Portnoi G, Chng LA, Karimi-Tabesh L, et al. Prospective comparative study of the safety and effectiveness of ginger for the treatment of nausea and vomiting in pregnancy. *Am J Obstet Gynecol* 2003;189:1374-7.

11347 Khan A, Safdar M, Ali Khan M, et al. Cinnamon improves glucose and lipids of people with type 2 diabetes. *Diabetes Care* 2003;26:3215-8.

11349 O'Mara NB. Ipecac for the Home Treatment of Poisonings. *Pharmacist's Letter/Prescriber's Letter* 2003;19:191201.

11350 Bilici M, Yildirim F, Kandil S, et al. Double-blind, placebo-controlled study of zinc sulfate in the treatment of attention deficit hyperactivity disorder. *Prog Neuropsychopharmacol Biol Psychiatry* 2004;28:181-90.

11351 McElhaney JE, Gravenstein S, Cole SK, et al. A Placebo-Controlled Trial of a Proprietary Extract of North American Ginseng (CVT-E002) to Prevent Acute Respiratory Illness in Institutionalized Older Adults. *J Am Geriatr Soc* 2004;52:13-9.

11352 Song Y, Manson JE, Buring JE, Liu S. Dietary magnesium intake in relation to plasma insulin levels and risk of type 2 diabetes in women. *Diabetes Care* 2004;27:59-65.

11353 Salazar-Martinez E, Willett WC, Ascherio A, et al. Coffee consumption and risk for type 2 diabetes mellitus. *Ann Intern Med* 2004;140:1-8.

11354 Kaplan SA, Volpe MA, Te AE. A prospective, 1-year trial using saw palmetto versus finasteride in the treatment of category III prostatitis/chronic pelvic pain syndrome. *J Urol* 2004;171:284-8.

11355 McBride BF, Karapanos AK, Krudysz A, et al. Electrocardiographic and hemodynamic effects of a multicomponent dietary supplement containing ephedra and caffeine: a randomized controlled trial. *JAMA* 2004;291:216-21.

11356 Munger KL, Zhang SM, O'Reilly E, et al. Vitamin D intake and incidence of multiple sclerosis. *Neurology* 2004;62:60-5.

REFERENCES

11357 Chen HL, Sheu WH, Tai TS, et al. Konjac supplement alleviated hypercholesterolemia and hyperglycemia in type 2 diabetic subjects--a randomized double-blind trial. *J Am Coll Nutr* 2003;22:36-42.

11358 Vuksan V, Sievenpiper JL, Owen R, et al. Beneficial effects of viscous dietary fiber from Konjac-mannan in subjects with the insulin resistance syndrome: results of a controlled metabolic trial. *Diabetes Care* 2000;23:9-14.

11359 Vuksan V, Jenkins DJ, Spadafora P, et al. Konjac-mannan (glucomannan) improves glycemia and other associated risk factors for coronary heart disease in type 2 diabetes. A randomized controlled metabolic trial. *Diabetes Care* 1999;22:913-9.

11360 Shima K, Tanaka A, Ikegami H, et al. Effect of dietary fiber, glucomannan, on absorption of sulfonylurea in man. *Horm Metab Res* 1983;15:1-3.

11361 Doi K, Matsuura M, Kawara A, Baba S. Treatment of diabetes with glucomannan (konjac mannan). *Lancet* 1979;1:987-8.

11362 Di Marco MP, Edwards DJ, Wainer IW, Ducharme MP. The effect of grapefruit juice and seville orange juice on the pharmacokinetics of dextromethorphan: the role of gut CYP3A and P-glycoprotein. *Life Sci* 2002;71:1149-60.

11363 Muir AH, Robb R, McLaren M, et al. The use of Ginkgo biloba in Raynaud's disease: a double-blind placebo-controlled trial. *Vasc Med* 2002;7:265-7.

11364 Ward E, Picton S, Reid U, et al. Oral glutamine in paediatric oncology patients: a dose finding study. *Eur J Clin Nutr* 2003;57:31-6.

11365 Shirai T, Hayakawa H, Akiyama J, et al. Food allergy to green tea. *J Allergy Clin Immunol* 2003;112:805-6.

11366 Jatoi A, Ellison N, Burch PA, et al. A phase II trial of green tea in the treatment of patients with androgen independent metastatic prostate carcinoma. *Cancer* 2003;97:1442-6.

11367 Yeh GY, Eisenberg DM, Kaptchuk TJ, Phillips RS. Systematic review of herbs and dietary supplements for glycemic control in diabetes. *Diabetes Care* 2003;26:1277-94.

11368 Herndon JE 2nd, Fleishman S, Kosty MP, Green MR. A longitudinal study of quality of life in advanced non-small cell lung cancer: Cancer and Leukemia Group B (CALGB) 8931. *Control Clin Trials* 1997;18:286-300.

11369 Teschke R, Gaus W, Loew D. Kava extracts: safety and risks including rare hepatotoxicity. *Phytomedicine* 2003;10:440-6

11370 Schmidt P, Boehncke WH. Delayed-type hypersensitivity reaction to kava-kava extract. *Contact Dermatitis* 2000;42:363-4.

11371 Schulze J, Raasch W, Siegers CP. Toxicity of kava pyrones, drug safety and precautions--a case study. *Phytomedicine* 2003;10:68-73.

11372 Pittler MH, Ernst E. Kava extract for treating anxiety. *Cochrane Database Syst Rev* 2003;1:CD003383.

11373 Cairney S, Maruff P, Clough AR, et al. Saccade and cognitive impairment associated with kava intoxication. *Hum Psychopharmacol* 2003;18:525-33.

11374 Samman S, Sivarajah G, Man JC, et al. A mixed fruit and vegetable concentrate increases plasma antioxidant vitamins and folate and lowers plasma homocysteine in men. *J Nutr* 2003;133:2188-93.

11375 Plotnick GD, Corretti MC, Vogel RA, et al. Effect of supplemental phytonutrients on impairment of the flow-mediated brachial artery vasoactivity after a single high-fat meal. *J Am Coll Cardiol* 2003;41:1744-9.

11376 Wise JA, Morin RJ, Sanderson R, et al. Changes in plasma carotenoid, alpha-tocopherol, and lipid peroxide levels in response to supplementation with concentrated fruit and vegetable extracts: A pilot study. *Curr Ther Res* 1996;57:445-61.

11377 Smith MJ, Inserra PF, Watson RR, et al. Supplementation with fruit and vegetable extracts may decrease DNA damage in the peripheral lymphocytes of an elderly population. *Nutr Res* 1999;19:1507-18.

11378 Wullt M, Hagslatt ML, Odenholt I. Lactobacillus plantarum 299v for the treatment of recurrent Clostridium difficile-associated diarrhoea: a double-blind, placebo-controlled trial. *Scand J Infect Dis* 2003;35:365-7.

11379 Kim HJ, Camilleri M, McKinzie S, et al. A randomized controlled trial of a probiotic, VSL#3, on gut transit and symptoms in diarrhoea-predominant irritable bowel syndrome. *Aliment Pharmacol Ther* 2003;17:895-904.

11380 Wei H, Loimaranta V, Tenovuo J, et al. Stability and activity of specific antibodies against Streptococcus mutans and Streptococcus sobrinus in bovine milk fermented with Lactobacillus rhamnosus strain GG or treated at ultra-high temperature. *Oral Microbiol Immunol* 2002;17:9-15.

11381 Kalliomaki M, Salminen S, Poussa T, et al. Probiotics and prevention of atopic disease: 4-year follow-up of a randomised placebo-controlled trial. *Lancet* 2003;361:1869-71.

11382 Sullivan A, Barkholt L, Nord CE. Lactobacillus acidophilus, Bifidobacterium lactis and Lactobacillus F19 prevent antibiotic-associated ecological disturbances of Bacteroides fragilis in the intestine. *J Antimicrob Chemother* 2003;52:308-11.

11383 Majamaa H, Isolauri E. Probiotics: a novel approach in the management of food allergy. *J Allergy Clin Immunol* 1997;99:179-85.

11384 Ize-Ludlow D, Ragone S, Bernstein JN, et al. Chemical composition of Chinese star anise (Illicium verum) and neurotoxicity in infants. *JAMA* 2004;291:562-3.

11386 Woo J, Lau E, Ho SC, et al. Comparison of Pueraria lobata with hormone replacement therapy in treating the adverse health consequences of menopause. *Menopause* 2003;10:352-61.

11387 Toole JF, Malinow MR, Chambless LE, et al. Lowering homocysteine in patients with ischemic stroke to prevent recurrent stroke, myocardial infarction, and death: the Vitamin Intervention for Stroke Prevention (VISP) randomized controlled trial. *JAMA* 2004;291:565-75.

11388 Hanley DF. The challenge of stroke prevention. *JAMA* 2004;291:621-2.

11389 Rozenfeld V, Crain JL, Callahan AK. Possible augmentation of warfarin effect by glucosamine-chondroitin. *Am J Health Syst Pharm* 2004;61:306-307.

11390 Zandi PP, Anthony JC, Khachaturian AS, et al. Reduced risk of Alzheimer disease in users of antioxidant vitamin supplements: the Cache County Study. *Arch Neurol* 2004;61:82-8.

11391 Keinan-Boker L, van Der Schouw YT, Grobbee DE, Peters PH. Dietary phytoestrogens and breast cancer risk. *Am J Clin Nutr* 2004;79:282-8.

11392 Meunier PJ, Roux C, Seeman E, et al. The effects of strontium ranelate on the risk of vertebral fracture in women with postmenopausal osteoporosis. *N Engl J Med* 2004;350:459-68.

11393 El-Hajj Fuleihan G. Strontium ranelate--a novel therapy for osteoporosis or a permutation of the same? *N Engl J Med* 2004;350:504-6.

11394 Verberckmoes SC, De Broe ME, D'Haese PC. Dose-dependent effects of strontium on osteoblast function and mineralization. *Kidney Int* 2003;64:534-43.

11395 Meunier PJ, Slosman DO, Delmas PD, et al. Strontium ranelate: dose-dependent effects in established postmenopausal vertebral osteoporosis--a 2-year randomized placebo controlled trial. *J Clin Endocrinol Metab* 2002;87:2060-6.

11396 Marie PJ, Ammann P, Boivin G, Rey C. Mechanisms of action and therapeutic potential of strontium in bone. *Calcif Tissue Int* 2001;69:121-9.
11397 Henrotin Y, Labasse A, Zheng SX, et al. Strontium ranelate increases cartilage matrix formation. *J Bone Miner Res* 2001;16:299-308.
11399 Brandi ML. New treatment strategies: ipriflavone, strontium, vitamin D metabolites and analogs. *Am J Med* 1993;95:69S-74S.
11400 Reeve J, Arlot M, Wootton R, et al. Skeletal blood flow, iliac histomorphometry, and strontium kinetics in osteoporosis: a relationship between blood flow and corrected apposition rate. *J Clin Endocrinol Metab* 1988;66:1124-31.
11401 Jenkins DJ, Kendall CW, Mehling CC, et al. Combined effect of vegetable protein (soy) and soluble fiber added to a standard cholesterol-lowering diet. *Metabolism* 1999;48:809-16.
11402 Skoryna SC. Effects of oral supplementation with stable strontium. *Can Med Assoc J* 1981;125:703-12.
11403 Donath A, Nordio S, Macagno F, Gatti R. The effect of hydrochlorothiazide and of sodium in the diet on calcium and strontium transport in intestine and kidney. *Isr J Med Sci* 1971;7:393.
11404 Gutteridge DH, Robinson CJ, Joplin GF. Delayed strontium absorption in post-menopausal osteoporosis and osteomalacia. *Clin Sci* 1968;34:351-63.
11405 Eisenberg E. Effects of androgens, estrogens and corticoids on strontium kinetics in man. *J Clin Endocrinol Metab* 1966;26:566-72.
11406 Verdon F, Burnand B, Stubi CL, et al. Iron supplementation for unexplained fatigue in non-anaemic women: double blind randomised placebo controlled trial. *BMJ* 2003;326:1124.
11407 Kovacs EM, Westerterp-Plantenga MS, Saris WH. The effects of 2-week ingestion of (--)-hydroxycitrate and (--)-hydroxycitrate combined with medium-chain triglycerides on satiety, fat oxidation, energy expenditure and body weight. *Int J Obes Relat Metab Disord* 2001;25:1087-94.
11408 Schule C, Baghai T, Ferrera A, Laakmann G. Neuroendocrine effects of Hypericum extract WS 5570 in 12 healthy male volunteers. *Pharmacopsychiatry* 2001;34:S127-33.
11409 Buyse G, Mertens L, Di Salvo G, et al. Idebenone treatment in Friedreich's ataxia: neurological, cardiac, and biochemical monitoring. *Neurology* 2003;60:1679-81.
11410 Mariotti C, Solari A, Torta D, et al. Idebenone treatment in Friedreich patients: one-year-long randomized placebo-controlled trial. *Neurology* 2003;60:1676-9.
11411 Filla A, Moss AJ. Idebenone for treatment of Friedreich's ataxia? *Neurology* 2003;60:1569-70.
11412 Geromel V, Darin N, Chretien D, et al. Coenzyme Q(10) and idebenone in the therapy of respiratory chain diseases: rationale and comparative benefits. *Mol Genet Metab* 2002;77:21-30.
11413 Hausse AO, Aggoun Y, Bonnet D, et al. Idebenone and reduced cardiac hypertrophy in Friedreich's ataxia. *Heart* 2002;87:346-9.
11414 Artuch R, Colome C, Vilaseca MA, et al. Monitoring of idebenone treatment in patients with Friedreich's ataxia by high-pressure liquid chromatography with electrochemical detection. *J Neurosci Methods* 2002;115:63-6.
11415 Schols L, Vorgerd M, Schillings M, et al. Idebenone in patients with Friedreich ataxia. *Neurosci Lett* 2001;306:169-72.
11416 Lerman-Sagie T, Rustin P, Lev D, et al. Dramatic improvement in mitochondrial cardiomyopathy following treatment with idebenone. *J Inherit Metab Dis* 2001;24:28-34.
11417 Anonymous. Idebenone - monograph. *Altern Med Rev* 2001;6:83-6.
11418 Rustin P, von Kleist-Retzow JC, Chantrel-Groussard K, et al. Effect of idebenone on cardiomyopathy in Friedreich's ataxia: a preliminary study. *Lancet* 1999;354:477-9.
11419 Rego AC, Santos MS, Oliveira CR. Influence of the antioxidants vitamin E and idebenone on retinal cell injury mediated by chemical ischemia, hypoglycemia, or oxidative stress. *Free Radic Biol Med* 1999;26:1405-17.
11420 Shivaram KN, Winklhofer-Roob BM, Straka MS, et al. The effect of idebenone, a coenzyme Q analogue, on hydrophobic bile acid toxicity to isolated rat hepatocytes and hepatic mitochondria. *Free Radic Biol Med* 1998;25:480-92.
11421 Weyer G, Babej-Dolle RM, Hadler D, et al. A controlled study of 2 doses of idebenone in the treatment of Alzheimer's disease. *Neuropsychobiology* 1997;36:73-82.
11422 Ikejiri Y, Mori E, Ishii K, et al. Idebenone improves cerebral mitochondrial oxidative metabolism in a patient with MELAS. *Neurology* 1996;47:583-5.
11423 Esposti MD, Ngo A, Ghelli A, et al. The interaction of Q analogs, particularly hydroxydecyl benzoquinone (idebenone), with the respiratory complexes of heart mitochondria. *Arch Biochem Biophys* 1996;330:395-400.
11424 Pisano P, Durand A, Autret E, et al. Plasma concentrations and pharmacokinetics of idebenone and its metabolites following single and repeated doses in young patients with mitochondrial encephalomyopathy. *Eur J Clin Pharmacol* 1996;51:167-9.
11425 Mashima Y, Hiida Y, Oguchi Y. Remission of Leber's hereditary optic neuropathy with idebenone. *Lancet* 1992;340:368-9.
11426 Ihara Y, Namba R, Kuroda S, et al. Mitochondrial encephalomyopathy (MELAS): pathological study and successful therapy with coenzyme Q10 and idebenone. *J Neurol Sci* 1989;90:263-71.
11427 Gutzmann H, Hadler D. Sustained efficacy and safety of idebenone in the treatment of Alzheimer's disease: update on a 2-year double-blind multicentre study. *J Neural Transm* 1998;54:301-10.
11428 Morris CR, Morris SM Jr, Hagar W, et al. Arginine therapy: a new treatment for pulmonary hypertension in sickle cell disease? *Am J Respir Crit Care Med* 2003;168:63-9.
11429 Marakis G, Walker AF, Middleton RW, et al. Artichoke leaf extract reduces mild dyspepsia in an open study. *Phytomedicine* 2002;9:694-9.
11430 Oldemeyer JB, Biddle WP, Wurdeman RL, et al. Acetylcysteine in the prevention of contrast-induced nephropathy after coronary angiography. *Am Heart J* 2003;146:E23.
11431 Fabjan N, Rode J, Kosir IJ, et al. Tartary buckwheat (Fagopyrum tataricum Gaertn.) as a source of dietary rutin and quercitrin. *J Agric Food Chem* 2003;51:6452-5.
11432 Gheldof N, Wang XH, Engeseth NJ. Buckwheat honey increases serum antioxidant capacity in humans. *J Agric Food Chem* 2003;51:1500-5.
11433 Yokozawa T, Kim HY, Nonaka G, Kosuna K. Buckwheat extract inhibits progression of renal failure. *J Agric Food Chem* 2002;50:3341-5.
11434 Tomotake H, Shimaoka I, Kayashita J, et al. Physicochemical and functional properties of buckwheat protein product. *J Agric Food Chem* 2002;50:2125-9.
11435 Schiffner R, Przybilla B, Burgdorff T, et al. Anaphylaxis to buckwheat. *Allergy* 2001;56:1020-1.
11436 Lee SY, Lee KS, Hong CH, Lee KY. Three cases of childhood nocturnal asthma due to buckwheat allergy. *Allergy* 2001;56:763-6.
11437 Wieslander G, Norback D. Buckwheat allergy. *Allergy* 2001;56:703-4.

11438 Skrabanja V, Liljeberg Elmstahl HG, Kreft I, Bjorck IM. Nutritional properties of starch in buckwheat products: studies in vitro and in vivo. *J Agric Food Chem* 2001;49:490-6.

11439 Dietrych-Szostak D, Oleszek W. Effect of processing on the flavonoid content in buckwheat (Fagopyrum esculentum Moench) grain. *J Agric Food Chem* 1999;47:4384-7.

11440 Thompson T. Case problem: questions regarding the acceptability of buckwheat, amaranth, quinoa, and oats from a patient with celiac disease. *J Am Diet Assoc* 2001;101:586-7.

11441 Kim CD, Lee WK, No KO, et al. Anti-allergic action of buckwheat (Fagopyrum esculentum Moench) grain extract. *Int Immunopharmacol* 2003;3:129-36.

11442 Bijlani RL, Gandhi BM, Gupta MC, et al. Effect of whole buckwheat (Fagopyrum esculentum) flour supplementation on lipid profile & glucose tolerance. *Indian J Med Res* 1985;81:162-8.

11443 Fritz SB, Gold BL. Buckwheat pillow-induced asthma and allergic rhinitis. *Ann Allergy Asthma Immunol* 2003;90:355-8.

11444 Mukoda T, Sun B, Ishiguro A. Antioxidant activities of buckwheat hull extract toward various oxidative stress in vitro and in vivo. *Biol Pharm Bull* 2001;24:209-13.

11445 Lee P. Should millet, buckwheat, and quinoa be included in a gluten-free diet? *J Am Diet Assoc* 1999;99:1361.

11446 Harkrader RJ, Reinhart PC, Rogers JA, et al. The history, chemistry and pharmacokinetics of Sanguinaria extract. *J Can Dent Assoc* 1990;56:7-12.

11447 Seifen E, Adams RJ, Riemer RK. Sanguinarine: a positive inotropic alkaloid which inhibits cardiac Na+,K+-ATPase. *Eur J Pharmacol* 1979;60:373-7.

11448 Becci PJ, Schwartz H, Barnes HH, Southard GL. Short-term toxicity studies of sanguinarine and of two alkaloid extracts of Sanguinaria canadensis L. *J Toxicol Environ Health* 1987;20:199-208.

11449 Degenring FH, Suter A, Weber M, Saller R. A randomised double blind placebo controlled clinical trial of a standardised extract of fresh Crataegus berries (Crataegisan) in the treatment of patients with congestive heart failure NYHA II. *Phytomedicine* 2003;10:363-9.

11450 Schwinger RH, Pietsch M, Frank K, Brixius K. Crataegus special extract WS 1442 increases force of contraction in human myocardium cAMP-independently. *J Cardiovasc Pharmacol* 2000;35:700-7.

11451 Jouad H, Lemhadri A, Maghrani M, et al. Hawthorn evokes a potent anti-hyperglycemic capacity in streptozotocin-induced diabetic rats. *Journal of Herbal Pharmacotherapy* 2003;3:19-29.

11452 Graham PH, Browne L, Cox H, Graham J. Inhalation aromatherapy during radiotherapy: results of a placebo-controlled double-blind randomized trial. *J Clin Oncol* 2003;21:2372-6.

11453 Buckley JD, Brinkworth GD, Abbott MJ. Effect of bovine colostrum on anaerobic exercise performance and plasma insulin-like growth factor I. *J Sports Sci* 2003;21:577-88

11454 Brinkworth GD, Buckley JD. Bovine colostrum supplementation does not affect nutrient absorptive capacity in healthy young men. *Nutr Res* 2003;23:1619-29.

11455 Kalvatchev Z, Walder R, Garzaro D. Anti-HIV activity of extracts from Calendula officinalis flowers. *Biomed Pharmacother* 1997;51:176-80.

11456 Wuttke W, Jarry H, Christoffel V, et al. Chaste tree (Vitex agnus-castus)--pharmacology and clinical indications. *Phytomedicine* 2003;10:348-57.

11457 Walker AF, Bundy R, Hicks SM, Middleton RW. Bromelain reduces mild acute knee pain and improves well-being in a dose-dependent fashion in an open study of otherwise healthy adults. *Phytomedicine* 2002;9:681-6.

11458 Paulsen E. Contact sensitization from Compositae-containing herbal remedies and cosmetics. *Contact Dermatitis* 2002;47:189-98.

11459 Hughes R, Carr A. A randomized, double-blind, placebo-controlled trial of glucosamine sulphate as an analgesic in osteoarthritis of the knee. *Rheumatology* 2002;41:279-84.

11460 Dell'Agli M, Parapini S, Basilico N, et al. In vitro studies on the mechanism of action of two compounds with antiplasmodial activity: ellagic acid and 3,4,5-trimethoxyphenyl(6'-O-aalloyl)-beta-D-glucopyranoside. *Planta Med* 2003;69:162-4.

11462 Brooks SM, Sholiton LJ, Werk EE Jr, Altenau P. The effects of ephedrine and theophylline on dexamethasone metabolism in bronchial asthma. *J Clin Pharmacol* 1977;17:308-18.

11463 Hallfrisch J, Scholfield DJ, Behall KM. Blood pressure reduced by whole grain diet containing barley or whole wheat and brown rice in moderately hypercholesterolemic men. *Nutr Res* 2003;23:1631-42.

11464 Genazzani AD, Stomati M, Bernardi F, et al. Long-term low-dose dehydroepiandrosterone oral supplementation in early and late postmenopausal women modulates endocrine parameters and synthesis of neuroactive steroids. *Fertil Steril* 2003;80:1495-501.

11465 Buvat J. Androgen therapy with dehydroepiandrosterone. *World J Urol* 2003;21:346-55.

11466 Andres, E. Does metformin interfere with thiamine?-author reply. *Arch Intern Med.* 2003;163:983..

11467 Babaei-Jadidi R, Karachalias N, Ahmed N, et al. Prevention of incipient diabetic nephropathy by high-dose thiamine and benfotiamine. *Diabetes* 2003;52:2110-20.

11468 Cederbaum S. Phenylketonuria: an update. *Curr Opin Pediatr* 2002;14:702-6.

11469 Wilson CJ, Van Wyk KG, Leonard JV, Clayton PT. Phenylalanine supplementation improves the phenylalanine profile in tyrosinaemia. *J Inherit Metab Dis.* 2000;23:677-83.

11470 Alford C, Cox H, Wescott R. The effects of red bull energy drink on human performance and mood. *Amino Acids* 2001;21:139-50.

11472 Klatte ET, Scharre DW, Nagaraja HN, et al. Combination therapy of donepezil and vitamin E in Alzheimer disease. *Alzheimer Dis Assoc Disord* 2003;17:113-6.

11473 Fernando C. Poisoning due to Abrus precatorius (jequirity bean). *Anaesthesia* 2001;56:1178-80.

11474 Kilbourne EM, Philen RM, Kamb ML, Falk H. Tryptophan produced by Showa Denko and epidemic eosinophilia-myalgia syndrome. *J Rheumatol Suppl* 1996;46:81-8.

11475 Horwitz RI, Daniels SR. Bias or biology: evaluating the epidemiologic studies of L-tryptophan and the eosinophilia-myalgia syndrome. *J Rheumatol Suppl* 1996;46:60-72.

11476 Shapiro S. Epidemiologic studies of the association of L-tryptophan with the eosinophilia-myalgia syndrome: a critique. *J Rheumatol Suppl* 1996;46:44-58.

11477 Mayeno AN, Gleich GJ. The eosinophilia-myalgia syndrome: lessons from Germany. *Mayo Clin Proc* 1994;69:702-4.

11478 Carr L, Ruther E, Berg PA, Lehnert H. Eosinophilia-myalgia syndrome in Germany: an epidemiologic review. *Mayo Clin Proc* 1994;69:620-5.

11479 Arosio E, Ferrari G, Santoro L, et al. A placebo-controlled, double-blind study of mesoglycan in the treatment of chronic venous ulcers. *Eur J Vasc Endovasc Surg* 2001;22:365-72.

11480 Xie HJ, Yasar U, Sandberg M, Rane A. Paeoniae Radix, a traditional Chinese medicine, and CYP2C9 activity. *J Clin Pharm Ther* 2002;27:229-30.

11481 Maitrejean M, Comte G, Barron D, et al. The flavanolignan silybin and its hemisynthetic derivatives, a novel series of

potential modulators of P-glycoprotein. *Bioorg Med Chem Lett* 2000;10:157-60.
11482 Bonham MJ, Galkin A, Montgomery B, et al. Effects of the herbal extract PC-SPES on microtubule dynamics and paclitaxel-mediated prostate tumor growth inhibition. *J Natl Cancer Inst* 2002;94:1641-7.
11485 Lam SK, Ng TB. Pananotin, a potent antifungal protein from roots of the traditional Chinese medicinal herb Panx notoginseng. *Planta Med* 2002;68:1024-8.
11486 Lam SK, Ng TB. A xylanase from roots of sanchi ginseng (Panax notoginseng) with inhibitory effects on human immunodeficiency virus-1 reverse transcriptase. *Life Sci* 2002;70:3049-58.
11487 Cicero AF, Vitale G, Savino G, Arletti R. Panax notoginseng (Burk.) effects on fibrinogen and lipid plasma level in rats fed on a high-fat diet. *Phytother Res* 2003;17:174-8.
11488 Chan RY, Chen WF, Dong A, et al. Estrogen-like activity of ginsenoside Rg1 derived from Panax notoginseng. *J Clin Endocrinol Metab* 2002;87:3691-5.
11490 Wilhelm KP, Biel S, Siegers CP. Role of flavonoids in controlling the phototoxicity of Hypericum perforatum extracts. *Phytomedicine* 2001;8:306-9.
11491 Ansari RA, Tripathi SC, Patnaik GK, Dhawan BN. Antihepatotoxic properties of picroliv: an active fraction from rhizomes of Picrorhiza kurrooa. *J Ethnopharmacol* 1991;34:61-8.
11492 Sharma ML, Rao CS, Duda PL. Immunostimulatory activity of Picrorhiza kurroa leaf extract. *J Ethnopharmacol* 1994;41:185-92.
11493 Bedi KL, Zutshi U, Chopra CL, Amla V. Picrorhiza kurroa, an ayurvedic herb, may potentiate photochemotherapy in vitiligo. *J Ethnopharmacol* 1989;27:347-52.
11494 Chander R, Kapoor NK, Dhawan BN. Picroliv, picroside-I and kutkoside from Picrorhiza kurrooa are scavengers of superoxide anions. *Biochem Pharmacol* 1992;44:180-3.
11501 Giraud DW, Martin HD, Driskell JA. Plasma and dietary vitamin C and E levels of tobacco chewers, smokers, and nonusers. *J Am Diet Assoc* 1995;95:798-800.
11502 Kaugars GE, Riley WT, Brandt RB, et al. The prevalence of oral lesions in smokeless tobacco users and an evaluation of risk factors. *Cancer* 1992;70:2579-85.
11503 Saadeh G, Bauer T, Licata A, Sheeler L. Antacid-induced osteomalacia. *Cleve Clin J Med* 1987;54:214-6.
11504 Shetty AK, Thomas T, Rao J, Vargas A. Rickets and secondary craniosynostosis associated with long-term antacid use in an infant. *Arch Pediatr Adolesc Med* 1998;152:1243-5.
11505 Nebeker HG, Coburn JW. Aluminum and renal osteodystrophy. *Annu Rev Med* 1986;37:79-95.
11506 Gesensway D. Vitamin D. *Ann Intern Med* 2000;133:319-20.
11507 Matsuoka LY, Ide L, Wortsman J, et al. Suncreens suppress cutaneous vitamin D3 synthesis. *J Clin Endocrinol Metab* 1987;64:1165-8.
11508 Matsuoka LY, Wortsman J, Hanifan N, Holick MF. Chronic suncreen use decreases circulating concentrations of 25-hydroxyvitamin D. *Arch Dermatol* 1988;124:1802-4.
11509 Prystowsky JH. Photoprotection and the vitamin D status of the elderly. *Arch Dermatol* 1988;124:1844-8.
11510 Marks R, Foley PA, Jolley D, et al. The effect of reular sunscreen use on vitamin D levels in an Australian population. *Arch Dermatol* 1995;131:415-21.
11511 Sollitto RB, Kraemer KH, DiGiovanna JJ. Normal vitamin D levels can be maintained despite rigorous photoprotection: six years' experience with xeroderma pigmentosum. *J Am Acad Dermatol* 1997;37:942-7.
11512 Dowd P, Zheng ZB. On the mechanism of the anticlotting action of vitamin E quinone. *Proc Natl Acad Sci U S A* 1995;92:8171-5.
11513 Haubenstock A, Schmidt P, Zazgornik J, Balcke P, Kopsa H. Hypoprothrombobinaemic bleeding associated with ceftriaxone. *Lancet* 1983;1:1215-6.
11514 Hooper CA, Haney BB, Stone HH. Gastrointestinal bleeding due to vitamin K deficiency in patients on parenteral cefamandole. *Lancet* 1980;1:39-40.
11515 Bhat RV, Deshmukh CT. A study of Vitamin K status in children on prolonged antibiotic therapy. *Indian Pediatr* 2003;40:36-40.
11516 Sattler FR, Weitekamp MR, Ballard JO. Potential for bleeding with the new beta-lactam antibiotics. *Ann Intern Med* 1986;105:924-31.
11517 Kobayashi K, Haruta T, Maeda H, et al. Cerebral hemorrhage associated with vitamin K deficiency in congenital tuberculosis treated with isoniazid and rifampin. *Pediatr Infect Dis J* 2002;21:1088-90.
11518 Van Steenbergen W, Vermylen J. Reversible hypoprothrombinemia in a patient with primary biliary cirrhosis treated with rifampicin. *Am J Gastroenterol* 1995;90:1526-8.
11519 Vroonhof K, van Rijn HJ, van Hattum J. Vitamin K deficiency and bleeding after long-term use of cholestyramine. *Neth J Med* 2003;61:19-21.
11520 MacWalter RS, Fraser HW, Armstrong KM. Orlistat enhances warfarin effect. *Ann Pharmacother* 2003;37:510-2.
11521 Cornelissen M, Steegers-Theunissen R, Kollee L, et al. Increased incidence of neonatal vitamin K deficiency resulting from maternal anticonvulsant therapy. *Am J Obstet Gynecol* 1993;168:923-8.
11522 Cornelissen M, Steegers-Theunissen R, Kollee L, et al. Supplementation of vitamin K in pregnant women receiving anticonvulsant therapy prevents neonatal vitamin K deficiency. *Am J Obstet Gynecol* 1993;168:884-8.
11523 Renzulli P, Tuchschmid P, Eich G, et al. Early vitamin K deficiency bleeding after maternal phenobarbital intake: management of massive intracranial haemorrhage by minimal surgical intervention. *Eur J Pediatr* 1998;157:663-5.
11524 Bleyer WA, Skinner AL. Fatal neonatal hemorrhage after maternal anticonvulsant therapy. *JAMA* 1976;235:626-7.
11525 Thorp JA, Gaston L, Caspers DR, Pal ML. Current concepts and controversies in the use of vitamin K. *Drugs* 1995;49:376-87.
11526 Basu TK. Vitamin C-aspirin interactions. *Int J Vitam Nutr Res Suppl* 1982;23:83-90.
11527 Johansson U, Akesson B. Interaction between ascorbic acid and acetylsalicylic acid and their effects on nutritional status in man. *Int J Vitam Nutr Res* 1985;55(2):197-204.
11528 Weininger J, King JC. Effect of oral contraceptives on ascorbic acid status of young women consuming a constant diet. *Nutr Rep Int* 1977;15(3):255-64.
11529 Demontis R, Leflon A, Fournier A, et al. 1 alpha(OH) vitamin D3 increases plasma aluminum in hemodialyzed patients taking AI(OH)3. *Clin Nephrol* 1986;26:146-9.
11530 Frier BM, Scott RD. Osteomalacia and arthropathy associated with prolonged abuse of purgatives. *Br J Clin Pract* 1977;31:17-9.
11531 Odes HS, Fraser GM, Krugliak P, et al. Effect of cimetidine on hepatic vitamin D metabolism in humans. *Digestion* 1990;46:61-4.
11532 Bengoa JM, Bolt MJ, Rosenberg IH. Hepatic vitamin D 25-hydroxylase inhibition by cimetidine and isoniazid. *J Lab Clin Med* 1984;104;546-52.
11533 Keith DA, Gundberg CM, Japour A, et al. Vitamin K-dependent proteins and anticonvulsant medication. *Clin Pharmacol Ther* 1983;34:529-32.

REFERENCES

11534 Tam DA Jr, Myer EC. Vitamin K-dependent coagulopathy in a child receiving anticonvulsant therapy. *J Child Neurol* 1996;11:244-6.

11535 Niki E, Noguchi N, Tsuchiharski H, Gotoh N. Interaction among vitamin C, vitamin E and beta-carotene. *Am J Clin Nutr* 1995;62:1322s-6s.

11536 Gey KF. Vitamins E plus C and interacting conutrients required for optimal health. *Biofactors* 1998;7:113-74.

11537 Cheung MC, Zhao XQ, Chait A, et al. Antioxidant supplements block the response of HDL to simvastatin-niacin therapy in patients with coronary artery disease and low HDL. *Arterioscler Thromb Vasc Biol* 2001;21:1320-6.

11538 Harris ED, Percival SS. A role for ascorbic acid in copper transport. *Am J Clin Nutr* 1991;54:1193s-7s.

11539 Crowe M, Wollner L, Griffiths RA. Hypercalcemia following vitamin D and thiazide therapy in the elderly. *Practitioner* 1984;228:312-3.

11540 Parfitt AM. Thiazide-induced hypercalcemia in vitamin D-treated hypoparathyroidism. *Ann Intern Med* 1972;77:557-63.

11541 O'Mara NB. Thiazide Diuretics and the Risk of Osteoporosis. *Pharmacist's Letter* 2003;19(11):191105.

11542 Ekvall S, Mitchell A. The effect of supplemental vitamin E on vitamin A serum levels in cystic fibrosis. *Int J Vit Nutr Res* 1978;48:325-32.

11543 Giugliano D, Marfella R. Antioxidants and nitrate tolerance (letter). *Circulation* 1998;98:1350-1.

11544 Watanabe H, Kakihana M, Ohtsuka S, Sugishita Y. Randomized, double-blind, placebo-controlled study of ascorbate on the preventive effect of nitrate tolerance in patients with congestive heart failure. *Circulation* 1998;97:886-91.

11545 Lehman J, Martin HL, Lashley EL, et al. Vitamin E in foods from high and low linoleic acid diets. *J Am Diet Assoc* 1986;86:1208-16.

11546 Kelly G. The interaction of cigarette smoking and antioxidants. Part III: ascorbic acid. *Altern Med Rev* 2003;8(1):43-54.

11547 Melhorn DK, Gross S. Relationships between iron-dextran and vitamin E in iron deficiency anemia in children. *J Lab Clin Med* 1969;74:789-802.

11548 Bredie SJ, de Bruin TW, Demacker PN, et al. Comparison of gemfibrozil versus simvastatin in familial combined hyperlipidemia and effects on apolipoprotein-B-containing lipoproteins, low-density lipoprotein subfraction profile, and low-density lipoprotein oxidizability. *Am J Cardiol* 1995;75:348-53.

11549 Wander RC, Du SH, Ketchum SO, Rowe KE. Effects of interaction of RRR-alpha-tocopheryl acetate and fish oil on low-density-lipoprotein oxidation in postmenopausal women with and without hormone-replacement therapy. *Am J Clin Nutr* 1996;63:184-93.

11550 American Academy of Dermatology press release. July 3, 2003. Vitamin D + Sunshine = Bad Medicine. American Academy of Dermatology urges public to practice sun safety. Available at: www.aad.org/PressReleases/VitD_Sunshine.html (accessed 3/31/04).

11555 Sivakumaran M, Ghosh K, Zaidi Y, Hutchinson RM. Osteoporosis and vertebral collapse following low-dose, low molecular weight heparin therapy in a young patient. *Clin Lab Haematol* 1996;18:55-7.

11561 Williams SE, Wardman AG, Taylor GA, et al. Long term study of the effect of rifampicin and isoniazid on vitamin D metabolism. *Tubercle* 1985;66:49-54.

11562 Kovacs CS, Jones G, Yendt ER. Primary hyperparathyroidism masked by antituberculous therapy-induced vitamin D deficiency. *Clin Endocrinol* (Oxf) 1994;41:831-8.

11563 Perry W, Erooga MA, Brown J, Stamp TC. Calcium metabolism during rifampicin and isoniazid therapy for tuberculosis. *J R Soc Med* 1982;75:533-6.

11564 Shah SC, Sharma RK, Hemangini, Chitle AR. Rifampicin induced osteomalacia. *Tubercle* 1981;62:207-9.

11565 Brodie MJ, Boobis AR, Hillyard CJ, et al. Effect of rifampicin and isoniazid on vitamin D metabolism. *Clin Pharmacol Ther* 1982;32:525-30.

11566 Feetam CL, Leach RH, Meynell MJ. Lack of a clinically important interaction between warfarin and ascorbic acid. *Toxicol Appl Pharmacol* 1975;31(3):544-7.

11567 Weintraub M, Griner PF. Warfarin and ascorbic acid: lack of evidence for a drug interaction. *Toxicol Appl Pharmacol* 1974;28(1):53-6.

11568 Prasad KN. Modulation of the effects of tumor therapeutic agents by vitamin C. *Life Sci* 1980;27(4):275-80.

11569 Weijl NI, Cleton FJ, Osanto S. Free radicals and antioxidants in chemotherapy induced toxicity. *Cancer Treat Rev* 1997;23:209-40.

11570 Lamson DW, Brignall MS. Antioxidants in cancer therapy; their actions and interactions with oncologic therapies. *Alt Med Rev* 1999;4:304-29.

11571 Sandstrom B. Micronutrient interactions: effects on absorption and bioavailability. *Br J Nutr* 2001;85Suppl2:S181-5.

11572 Prasad KN, Kumar A, Kochupillai V, Cole WC. High doses of multiple antioxidant vitamins: essential ingredients in improving the efficacy of standard cancer therapy. *J Am Coll Nutr* 1999;18:13-25.

11573 Valk EEJ, Hornstra G. Relationship between vitamin E requirement and polyunsaturated fatty acid intake in man: a review. *Int J Vit Nutr Res* 2000;70:31-42.

11574 Ogunmekan AO. Relationship between age and vitamin E level in epileptic children and normal children. *Am J Clin Nutr* 1979;32:2269-71.

11575 Kataoka K, Kanamori N, Oishi M, et al. Vitamin E status in pediatric patients receiving antiepileptic drugs. *Devel Pharmacol Ther* 1989;14:96-101.

11576 Ogunmekan AO. Plasma vitamin E (alpha-tocopherol) levels in normal children and in epileptic children with and without anticonvulsant drug therapy. *Trop Geogr Med* 1985;37:175-7.

11577 Higashi A, Ikeda T, Matsukura M, Matsuda I. Serum zinc and vitamin E concentrations in handicapped children treated with anticonvulsants. *Devel Pharmacol Ther* 1982;5:109-13.

11578 Higashi A, Tamari H, Ikeda T, et al. Serum vitamin E concentration in patients with severe multiple handicaps treated with anticonvulsants. *Pediatr Pharmacol* 1980;1:129-34.

11580 Schrogie JJ. Coagulopathy and fat-soluble vitamins (letter). *JAMA* 1975;232:19.

11581 Steiner M, Glantz M, Lekos A. Vitamin E plus aspirin compared with aspirin alone in patients with transient ischemic attacks. *Am J Clin Nutr* 1995;62:1381s-4s.

11582 Celestini A, Pulcinelli FM, Pignatelli P, et al. Vitamin E potentiates the antiplatelet activity of aspirin in collagen-stimulated platelets. *Haematologica* 2002;87:420-6.

11583 Stampfer MJ, Jakubowski JA, Faigel D, et al. Vitamin E supplementation effect on human platelet function, arachidonic acid metabolism, and plasma prostacyclin levels. *Am J Clin Nutr* 1988;47:700-6.

11584 Jandak J, Steiner M, Richardson PD. Alpha-tocopherol, an effective inhibitor of platelet adhesion. *Blood* 1989;73:141-9.

11585 Freedman JE, Farhat JH, Loscalzo J, Keaney JF. Alpha-tocopherol inhibits aggregation of human platelets by a protein kinase C-dependent mechanism. *Circulation* 1996;94:2434-40.

11586 Steiner M. Vitamin E, a modifier of platelet function: rationale and use in cardiovascular and cerebrovascular disease. *Nutr Rev* 1999;57:306-9.

11587 Yoshida H, Ishikawa T, Ayaori M, et al. Beneficial effect of gemfibrozil on the chemical composition and oxidative susceptibility of low density lipoprotein: a randomized, double-blind, placebo-controlled study. *Atherosclerosis* 1998;139:179-87.

11588 Weijl NI, Hopman GD, Wipkink-Bakker A, et al. Cisplatin combination chemotherapy induces a fall in plasma antioxidants of cancer patients. *Ann Oncol* 1998;9:1331-7.

11589 Ladas EJ, Jacobson JS, Kennedy DD, et al. Antioxidants and cancer therapy: a systematic review. *J Clin Oncol* 2004;22:517-28.

11701 Wang H, Ng TB. Ginkbilobin, a novel antifungal protein from Ginkgo biloba seeds with sequence similarity to embryo-abundant protein. *Biochem Biophys Res Commun* 2000;279:407-11.

11702 Yang X, Chen J, Qian Z, Guo T. [Study on the antibacterial activity of ginkgolic acids]. [Article in Chinese]. *Zhong Yao Cai* 2002;25:651-3.

11703 McBride K, Slotnick B, Margolis FL. Does intranasal application of zinc sulfate produce anosmia in the mouse? An olfactometric and anatomical study. *Chem Senses* 2003;28:659-70.

11704 Burd GD. Morphological study of the effects of intranasal zinc sulfate irrigation on the mouse olfactory epithelium and olfactory bulb. *Microsc Res Tech* 1993;24:195-213.

11705 Ducray A, Bondier JR, Michel G, et al. Recovery following peripheral destruction of olfactory neurons in young and adult mice. *Eur J Neurosci* 2002;15:1907-17.

11706 Mayer AD, Rosenblatt JS. Peripheral olfactory deafferentation of the primary olfactory system in rats using ZnSO4 nasal spray with special reference to maternal behavior. *Physiol Behav* 1993;53:587-92.

11707 DeCook CA, Hirsch AR. Anosmia due to inhalational zinc: a case report (abstract). *Chem Senses* 2000;25:659.

11708 Gardner SF, Franks AM, Gurley BJ, et al. Effect of a multicomponent, ephedra-containing dietary supplement (Metabolife 356) on Holter monitoring and hemostatic parameters in healthy volunteers. *Am J Cardiol* 2003;91:1510-3, A9.

11709 Girelli D, Martinelli N, Pizzolo F, et al. The interaction between MTHFR 677 C-->T genotype and folate status is a determinant of coronary atherosclerosis risk. *J Nutr* 2003;133:1281-5.

11711 Prasain JK, Jones K, Kirk M, et al. Profiling and quantification of isoflavonoids in kudzu dietary supplements by high-performance liquid chromatography and electrospray ionization tandem mass spectrometry. *J Agric Food Chem* 2003;51:4213-8.

11712 Kleijnen J, Knipschild P, Ter Riet G. Garlic, onions and cardiovascular risk factors: a review of the evidence from human experiments with emphasis on commercially available preparations. *Br J Clin Pharmacol* 1989;28:535-44.

11713 Tisdall FF, Brown A, Defries RD. Persistent anosmia following zinc sulfate nasal spraying. *JPed* 1938;18:60-2.

11714 Chobot V, Kremenak J, Opletal L. [Phytotherapeutic aspects of diseases of the circulatory system. 4. Chitin and chitosan]. [Article in Czech]. *Ceska Slov Farm* 1995;44:190-95.

11715 Piskun RP, Pentiuk AA, Serkova VK, et al. [Enterosorbents in the treatment of atherosclerosis]. [Article in Russian]. *Eksp Klin Farmakol* 1998;61:69-74.

11716 Wolk A, Manson J, Stampfer M, et al. Long-term Intake of Dietary Fiber and Decreased Risk of Coronary Heart Disease Among Women. *JAMA* 1999;281:1998-2004.

11717 *Federal Register* November 10, 1998;63(217):62977-63015.

11719 Scelfo GM, Flegal AR. Lead in calcium supplements. *Environ Health Perspect* 2000;108:309-19.

11720 Ingolfsdottir K. Usnic acid. *Phytochemistry* 2002;61:729-36.

11722 Kim RB. Drugs as P-glycoprotein substrates, inhibitors, and inducers. *Drug Metab Rev* 2002;34:47-54.

11723 Ruppin DC, Middleton WR. Clinical use of medium chain triglycerides. *Drugs* 1980;20:216-24.

11724 Bach AC, Babayan VK. Medium-chain triglycerides: an update. *Am J Clin Nutr* 1982;36:950-62.

11725 Babayan VK. Medium chain triglycerides and structured lipids. *Lipids* 1987;22:417-20.

11726 Christophe A, Matthys F, Verdonk G. Chylous-fluid triglycerides and lipoproteins in a patient with chylothorax put on a diet of butter or medium-chain triglyceride [proceeedings]. *Arch Int Physiol Biochim* 1980;88:B17-B19.

11727 Jalili F. Medium-chain triglycerides and total parenteral nutrition in the management of infants with congenital chylothorax. *South Med J* 1987;80:1290-3.

11728 Jensen GL, Mascioli EA, Meyer LP, et al. Dietary modification of chyle composition in chylothorax. *Gastroenterology* 1989;97:761-5.

11729 Fernandez Alvarez JR, Kalache KD, Grauel EL. Management of spontaneous congenital chylothorax: oral medium-chain triglycerides versus total parenteral nutrition. *Am J Perinatol* 1999;16:415-20.

11730 Gibert CL, Wheeler DA, Collins G, et al. Randomized, controlled trial of caloric supplements in HIV infection. *J Acquir Immune Defic Syndr* 1999;22:253-9.

11731 Tuomilehto J, Hu G, Bidel S, et al. Coffee Consumption and Risk of Type 2 Diabetes Mellitus Among Middle-aged Finnish Men and Women. *JAMA* 2004;291:1213-9.

11732 Arnlov J, Vessby B. Coffee consumption and insulin sensitivity. *JAMA* 2004;291:1199-201.

11733 Nawrot P, Jordan S, Eastwood J, et al. Effects of caffeine on human health. *Food Addit Contam* 2003;20:1-30.

11734 Food and Nutrition Board, Institute of Medicine. Nutrition during lactation. Washington, DC: National Academy Press, 1991. Available at: http://books.nap.edu/books/0309043913/html.

11735 Gertz BJ, Holland SD, Kline WF, et al. Studies of the oral bioavailability of alendronate. *Clin Pharmacol Ther* 1995;58:288-98.

11736 May DC, Jarboe CH, VanBakel AB, Williams WM. Effects of cimetidine on caffeine disposition in smokers and nonsmokers. *Clin Pharmacol Ther* 1982;31:656-61.

11737 Abernethy DR, Todd EL. Impairment of caffeine clearance by chronic use of low-dose oestrogen-containing oral contraceptives. *Eur J Clin Pharmacol* 1985;28:425-8.

11738 Brown NJ, Ryder D, Branch RA. A pharmacodynamic interaction between caffeine and phenylpropanolamine. *Clin Pharmacol Ther* 1991;50:363-71.

11739 Sanderink GJ, Bournique B, Stevens J, et al. Involvement of human CYP1A isoenzymes in the metabolism and drug interactions of riluzole in vitro. *J Pharmacol Exp Ther* 1997;282:1465-72.

11740 Wahllander A, Paumgartner G. Effect of ketoconazole and terbinafine on the pharmacokinetics of caffeine in healthy volunteers. *Eur J Clin Pharmacol* 1989;37:279-83.

11741 Carrillo JA, Benitez J. Clinically significant pharmacokinetic interactions between dietary caffeine and medications. *Clin Pharmacokinet* 2000;39:127-53.

11742 Stanek EJ, Melko GP, Charland SL. Xanthine interference with dipyridamole-thallium-201 myocardial imaging. *Pharmacother* 1995;29:425-7.

11743 Smith A. Effects of caffeine on human behavior. *Food Chem Toxicol* 2002;40:1243-55.

11744 Robert D, Jorgetti V, Leclercq M, et al. Does vitamin K excess induce ectopic calcifications in hemodialysis patients? *Clin Nephrol* 1985;24:300-4.

11745 Minkoff S, Axelrod S. Efficacy of strontium chloride in dental hypersensitivity. *J Periodontol* 1987;58:470-4.

11746 Kishore A, Mehrotra KK, Saimbi CS. Effectiveness of desensitizing agents. *J Endod* 2002;28:34-5.

11747 Gunawardana DH, Lichtenstein M, Better N, Rosenthal M. Results of strontium-89 therapy in patients with prostate cancer resistant to chemotherapy. *Clin Nucl Med* 2004;29:81-5.

11748 Oosterhof GO, Roberts JT, de Reijke TM, et al. Strontium(89) chloride versus palliative local field radiotherapy in patients with hormonal escaped prostate cancer: a phase III study of the European Organisation for Research and Treatment of Cancer, Genitourinary Group. *Eur Urol* 2003;44:519-26.

11749 Ashayeri E, Omogbehin A, Sridhar R, Shankar RA. Strontium 89 in the treatment of pain due to diffuse osseous metastases: a university hospital experience. *J Natl Med Assoc* 2002;94:706-11.

11750 Baziotis N, Yakoumakis E, Zissimopoulos A, et al. Strontium-89 chloride in the treatment of bone metastases from breast cancer. *Oncology* 1998;55:377-81.

11751 Quilty PM, Kirk D, Bolger JJ, et al. A comparison of the palliative effects of strontium-89 and external beam radiotherapy in metastatic prostate cancer. *Radiother Oncol* 1994;31:33-40.

11752 Robinson RG, Preston DF, Schiefelbein M, Baxter KG. Strontium 89 therapy for the palliation of pain due to osseous metastases. *JAMA* 1995;274:420-4.

11753 Dahl SG, Allain P, Marie PJ, et al. Incorporation and distribution of strontium in bone. *Bone* 2001;28:446-53.

11754 Grynpas MD, Hamilton E, Cheung R, et al. Strontium increases vertebral bone volume in rats at a low dose that does not induce detectable mineralization defect. *Bone* 1996;18:253-9.

11755 Metastron prescribing information. Medi-Physics, Inc., Amersham Healthcare, Arlington Heights, IL, 1998. http://www.cancerpaintherapy.com/METATECHPAGE.htm. (Accessed 13 March 2004).

11756 Canadian Advisory Board on Dentin Hypersensitivity. Consensus-based recommendations for the diagnosis and management of dentin hypersensitivity. *J Can Dent Assoc* 2003;69:221-6.

11757 Drug Enforcement Agency. Peyote and mescaline. http://www.usdoj.gov/dea/concern/peyote.html. (Accessed 14 March 2004).

11758 Gilmore HT. Petoye use during pregnancy. *S D J Med* 2001;54:27-9.

11759 Cabeza M, Bratoeff E, Heuze I, et al. Effect of beta-sitosterol as inhibitor of 5 alpha-reductase in hamster prostate. *Proc West Pharmacol Soc* 2003;46:153-5.

11761 Sakko AJ, Ricciardelli C, Mayne K, et al. Modulation of prostate cancer cell attachment to matrix by versican. *Cancer Res* 2003;63:4786-91.

11762 Hiroyuki F, Tomohide Y, Kazunori O. Efficacy and safety of Touchi extract, an alpha-glucosidase inhibitor derived from fermented soybeans, in non-insulin-dependent diabetic mellitus. *J Nutr Biochem* 2001;12:351-56.

11763 Sovak M, Seligson AL, Konas M, et al. Herbal composition of PC-SPES for management of prostate cancer: identification of active principles.*J Natl Cancer Inst* 2002;94:1275-81.

11764 de Lemos ML. Herbal supplement PC-SPES for prostate cancer. *Ann Pharmacother* 2002;36:921-6.

11765 Pirani JF. The effects of phytotherapeutic agents on prostate cancer: an overview of recent clinical trials of PC SPES. *Urology* 2001;58:36-8.

11767 Ochoa M Jr, Wittes RE, Krakoff IH. Trial of hydrazine sulfate (NSC-150014) in patients with cancer. *Cancer Chemother Rep* 1975:1151-4.

11768 Bergner A, Bergner RK. Pulmonary hypersensitivity associated with pancreatin powder exposure. *Pediatrics* 1975;55:814-7.

11769 Wiessmann KJ, Baur X. Occupational lung disease following long-term inhalation of pancreatic extracts. *Eur J Respir Dis* 1985;66:13-20.

11770 Underwood DA. Which medications should be held before a pharmacologic or exercise stress test? *Cleve Clin J Med* 2002;69:449-50.

11771 Aqel RA, Zoghbi GJ, Trimm JR, et al. Effect of caffeine administered intravenously on intracoronary-administered adenosine-induced coronary hemodynamics in patients with coronary artery disease. *Am J Cardiol* 2004;93:343-6.

11772 Zheng XM, Williams RC. Serum caffeine levels after 24-hour abstention: clinical implications on dipyridamole (201)Tl myocardial perfusion imaging. *J Nucl Med Technol* 2002;30:123-7.

11773 Pittler MH, Thompson CO, Ernst E. Artichoke leaf extract for treating hypercholesterolaemia. *Cochrane Database Syst Rev* 2002;3:CD003335.

11774 Pittler MH, White AR, Stevinson C, Ernst E. Effectiveness of artichoke extract in preventing alcohol-induced hangovers: a randomized controlled trial. *CMAJ* 2003;169:1269-73.

11775 Sagduyu K. Peppermint oil for irritable bowel syndrome. *Psychosomatics* 2002;43:508-9.

11776 Nolen HW 3rd, Friend DR. Menthol-beta-D-glucuronide: a potential prodrug for treatment of the irritable bowel syndrome. *Pharm Res* 1994;11:1707-11.

11777 Nash P, Gould SR, Bernardo DE. Peppermint oil does not relieve the pain of irritable bowel syndrome. *Br J Clin Pract* 1986;40:292-3.

11778 Dew MJ, Evans BK, Rhodes J. Peppermint oil for the irritable bowel syndrome: a multicentre trial. *Br J Clin Pract* 1984;38:394-98.

11779 Rees WD, Evans BK, Rhodes J. Treating irritable bowel syndrome with peppermint oil. *Br Med J* 1979;2:835-6.

11780 Somerville KW, Richmond CR, Bell GD. Delayed release peppermint oil capsules (Colpermin) for the spastic colon syndrome: a pharmacokinetic study. *Br J Clin Pharmacol* 1984;18:638-40.

11781 Davies SJ, Harding LM, Baranowski AP. A novel treatment of postherpetic neuralgia using peppermint oil. *Clin J Pain* 2002;18:200-2.

11782 Weston CF. Anal burning and peppermint oil. *Postgrad Med J* 1987;63:717.

11783 Dresser GK, Wacher V, Wong S, et al. Evaluation of peppermint oil and ascorbyl palmitate as inhibitors of cytochrome P4503A4 activity in vitro and in vivo. *Clin Pharmacol Ther* 2002;72:247-55.

11784 Wacher VJ, Wong S, Wong HT. Peppermint oil enhances cyclosporine oral bioavailability in rats: comparison with D-alpha-tocopheryl poly(ethylene glycol 1000) succinate (TPGS) and ketoconazole. *J Pharm Sci* 2002;91:77-90.

11785 Stuchlik M, Zak S. Lipid-based vehicle for oral drug delivery. *Biomed Pap Med Fac Univ Palacky Olomouc Czech Repub* 2001;145:17-26.

11786 Food Standards Agency. Medicines and Healthcare products Regulatory Agency (MHRA). Expert Group on Vitamins and Minerals. Available at: http://www.foodstandards.gov.uk/multimedia/pdfs/vitmin2003.pdf.

11787 Mouser JF, Hak EB, Helms RA, et al. Chromium and zinc concentrations in pediatric patients receiving long-term parenteral nutrition. *Am J Health Syst Pharm* 1999;56:1950-6.

11788 Vermeulen RC, Scholte HR. Exploratory open label, randomized study of acetyl- and propionylcarnitine in chronic fatigue syndrome. *Psychosom Med* 2004;66:276-82.

11789 Lawson MJ, Knight RE, Tran K, et al. Failure of enteric-coated peppermint oil in the irritable bowel syndrome: a randomized double-blind crossover study. *J Gastroenterol Hepatol* 1988;3:235-8.

11791 Menendez JA, Colomer R, Lupu R. Omega-6 polyunsaturated fatty acid gamma-linolenic acid (18:3n-6) is a selective estrogen-response modulator in human breast cancer cells: gamma-Linolenic acid antagonizes estrogen receptor-dependent transcriptional activity, transcriptionally represses estrogen receptor expression and synergistically enhances tamoxifen and ICI 182,780 (Faslodex) efficacy in human breast cancer cells. *Int J Cancer* 2004;10;109:949-54.

11792 Biesalski HK, Obermueller-Jevic UC. UV light, beta-carotene and human skin--beneficial and potentially harmful effects. *Arch Biochem Biophys* 2001;389:1-6.

11793 Mathews-Roth MM. Treatment of the cutaneous porphyrias. *Clin Dermatol* 1998;16:295-8.

11794 Moulds RF, Malani J. Kava: herbal panacea or liver poison? *Med J Aust* 2003;178:451-3.

11795 Gow PJ, Connelly NJ, Hill RL, et al. Fatal fulminant hepatic failure induced by a natural therapy containing kava. *Med J Aust* 2003;178:442-3.

11796 Rozen TD. Melatonin as treatment for idiopathic stabbing headache. *Neurology* 2003;61:865-6.

11797 Fies P, Dienel A. [Ginkgo extract in impaired vision--treatment with special extract EGb 761 of impaired vision due to dry senile macular degeneration]. [Article in German]. *Wien Med Wochenschr* 2002;152:423-6.

11798 Richer S, Stiles W, Statkute L, et al. Double-masked, placebo-controlled, randomized trial of lutein and antioxidant supplementation in the intervention of atrophic age-related macular degermation: the Veterans LAST study (Lutein Antioxidant Supplement Trial). *Optometry* 2004;75:216-30.

11799 Morris MC, Donoghue A, Markowitz JA, Osterhoudt KC. Ingestion of tea tree oil (Melaleuca oil) by a 4-year-old boy. *Pediatr Emerg Care* 2003;19:169-71.

11800 Siepmann M, Krause S, Joraschky P, et al. The effects of St John's wort extract on heart rate variability, cognitive function and quantitative EEG: a comparison with amitriptyline and placebo in healthy men. *Br J Clin Pharmacol* 2002;54:277-82.

11801 Dean AJ, Moses GM, Vernon JM. Suspected withdrawal syndrome after cessation of St. John's wort. *Ann Pharmacother* 2003;37:150.

11802 Morimoto T, Kotegawa T, Tsutsumi K, et al. Effect of St. John's wort on the pharmacokinetics of theophylline in healthy volunteers. *J Clin Pharmacol* 2004;44:95-101.

11803 Singh V, Kaul S, Chander R, Kapoor NK. Stimulation of low density lipoprotein receptor activity in liver membrane of guggulsterone treated rats. *Pharmacol Res* 1990;22:37-44.

11804 Bilia AR, Gallori S, Vincieri FF. St. John's wort and depression: efficacy, safety and tolerability-an update. *Life Sci* 2002;70:3077-96.

11805 Huntley AL, Ernst E. Soy for the treatment of perimenopausal symptoms--a systematic review. *Maturitas* 2004;47:1-9.

11806 Secreto G, Chiechi LM, Amadori A, et al. Soy isoflavones and melatonin for the relief of climacteric symptoms: a multicenter, double-blind, randomized study. *Maturitas* 2004;47:11-20.

11807 Yamamoto S, Sobue T, Kobayashi M, et al. Soy, isoflavones, and breast cancer risk in Japan. *J Natl Cancer Inst* 2003;95:906-13.

11808 FDA. Office of Regulatory Affairs. Automatic detention of stevia leaves, extract of stevia leaves, and food containing stevia. http://www.fda.gov/ora/fiars/ora_import_ia4506.html (Accessed 21 April 2004).

11809 Hsieh MH, Chan P, Sue YM, et al. Efficacy and tolerability of oral stevioside in patients with mild essential hypertension: a two-year, randomized, placebo-controlled study. *Clin Ther* 2003;25:2797-808.

11810 Chan P, Tomlinson B, Chen YJ, et al. A double-blind placebo-controlled study of the effectiveness and tolerability of oral stevioside in human hypertension. *Br J Clin Pharmacol* 2000;50:215-20.

11811 Geuns JM. Stevioside. *Phytochemistry* 2003;64:913-21.

11812 Gregersen S, Jeppesen PB, Holst JJ, Hermansen K. Antihyperglycemic effects of stevioside in type 2 diabetic subjects. *Metabolism* 2004;53:73-6.

11813 Lailerd N, Saengsirisuwan V, Sloniger JA, et al. Effects of stevioside on glucose transport activity in insulin-sensitive and insulin-resistant rat skeletal muscle. *Metabolism* 2004;53:101-7.

11814 Kenny AM, Biskup B, Robbins B, et al. Effects of vitamin D supplementation on strength, physical function, and health perception in older, community-dwelling men. *J Am Geriatr Soc* 2003;51:1762-7.

11815 Vieth R. Vitamin D supplementation, 25-hydroxyvitamin D concentrations, and safety. *Am J Clin Nutr* 1999;69:842-56.

11816 Seyrek N, Balal M, Karayaylali I, et al. Which parameter is more influential on the development of arteriosclerosis in hemodialysis patients? *Ren Fail* 2003;25:1011-8.

11817 Medline Plus. Laxatives, Oral. National Library of Medicine. Available at: http://www.nlm.nih.gov/medlineplus/druginfo/uspdi/202319.html.

11818 DiMeglio LA, White KE, Econs MJ. Disorders of phosphate metabolism. *Endocrinol Metab Clin North Am* 2000;29:591-609.

11819 Clarke BL, Wynne AG, Wilson DM, Fitzpatrick LA. Osteomalacia associated with adult Fanconi's syndrome: clinical and diagnostic features. *Clin Endocrinol* (Oxf) 1995;43:479-90.

11820 Marx SJ. Hyperparathyroid and hypoparathyroid disorders. *N Engl J Med* 2000;343:1863-75.

11821 Rouillard S, Lane NE. Hepatic osteodystrophy. *Hepatology* 2001;33:301-7.

11822 Linden KG, Weinstein GD. Psoriasis: current perspectives with an emphasis on treatment. *Am J Med* 1999;107:595-605.

11823 Malluche HH, Monier-Faugere MC, Koszewski NJ. Use and indication of vitamin D and vitamin D analogues in patients with renal bone disease. *Nephrol Dial Transplant* 2002;17 Suppl 10:6-9.

11824 Prince RL, Glendenning P. 8: Disorders of bone and mineral other than osteoporosis. *Med J Aust* 2004;180:354-9.

11825 Mellibovsky L, Diez A, Perez-Vila E, et al. Vitamin D treatment in myelodysplastic syndromes. *Br J Haematol* 1998;100:516-20.

11826 Chevrel G, Meunier PJ. Osteogenesis imperfecta: lifelong management is imperative and feasible. *Joint Bone Spine* 2001;68:125-9.

11827 American College of Obstetricians and Gynecologists, ACOG practice bulletin. Clinical management guidelines for obstetrician-gynecologists. Number 50, January 2003. *Obstet Gynecol* 2004;103:203-16.

REFERENCES

11828 Staff AC, Berge L, Haugen G, et al. Dietary supplementation with L-arginine or placebo in women with pre-eclampsia. *Acta Obstet Gynecol Scand* 2004;83:103-7.

11829 Endres S, De Caterina R, Schmidt EB, et al. N-3 polyunsaturated fatty acids: update 1995. *Eur J Clin Invest* 1995;25:629-38.

11830 Resnick DJ, Softness B, Murphy AR, et al. Case report of an anaphylactoid reaction to arginine. *Ann Allergy Asthma Immunol* 2002;88:67-8.

11831 Weimann G, Lubenow N, Selleng K, et al. Glucosamine sulfate does not crossreact with the antibodies of patients with heparin-induced thrombocytopenia. *Eur J Haematol* 2001;66:195-9.

11832 Institute of Medicine. Caffeine for the Sustainment of Mental Task Performance: Formulations for Military Operations. Washington, DC: National Academy Press, 2001. Available at: http://books.nap.edu/books/0309082587/html/index.html.

11833 Castellanos FX, Rapoport JL. Effects of caffeine on development and behavior in infancy and childhood: a review of the published literature. *Food Chem Toxicol* 2002;40:1235-42.

11834 Heseltine D, Dakkak M, woodhouse K, et al. The effect of caffeine on postprandial hypotension in the elderly. *J Am Geriatr Soc* 1991;39:160-4.

11835 Rakic V, Beilin LJ, Burke V. Effect of coffee and tea drinking on postprandial hypotension in older men and women. *Clin Exp Pharmacol Physiol* 1996;23:559-63.

11836 Howell LL, Coffin VL, Spealman RD. Behavioral and physiological effects of xanthines in nonhuman primates. *Psychopharmacology* (Berl) 1997;129:1-14.

11837 Chou T. Wake up and smell the coffee. Caffeine, coffee, and the medical consequences. *West J Med* 1992;157:544-53.

11838 Holmgren P, Norden-Pettersson L, Ahlner J. Caffeine fatalities--four case reports. *Forensic Sci Int* 2004;139:71-3.

11839 Dews PB, O'Brien CP, Bergman J. Caffeine: behavioral effects of withdrawal and related issues. *Food Chem Toxicol* 2002;40:1257-61.

11840 Beach CA, Mays DC, Guiler RC, et al. Inhibition of elimination of caffeine by disulfiram in normal subjects and recovering alcoholics. *Clin Pharmacol Ther* 1986;39:265-70.

11841 Toeller M, Buyken AE, Heitkamp G, et al. Fiber intake, serum cholesterol levels, and cardiovascular disease in European individuals with type 1 diabetes. EURODIAB IDDM Complications Study Group. *Diabetes Care* 1999;22 Suppl 2:B21-8.

11842 Youngkin EQ, et al, eds. Pharmacotherapeutics - a primary care clinical guide. Stamford, CT: Appleton & Lange. 1999.

11844 Durrant KL. Known and hidden sources of caffeine in drug, food, and natural products. *J Am Pharm Assoc* 2002;42:625-37.

11845 Cannon ME, Cooke CT, McCarthy JS. Caffeine-induced cardiac arrhythmia: an unrecognised danger of healthfood products. *Med J Aust* 2001;174:520-1.

11847 Jia Q, Hong MF, Minter D. Pikuroside: a novel iridoid from Picrorhiza kurroa. *J Nat Prod* 1999;62:901-3.

11848 Vaidya AB, Antarkar DS, Doshi JC, et al. Picrorhiza kurroa (Kutaki) Royle ex Benth as a hepatoprotective agent--experimental & clinical studies. *J Postgrad Med* 1996;42:105-8.

11849 Rajeshkumar NV, Kuttan R. Protective effect of Picroliv, the active constituent of Picrorhiza kurroa, against chemical carcinogenesis in mice. *Teratog Carcinog Mutagen* 2001;21:303-13.

11850 Rastogi R, Srivastava AK, Rastogi AK. Long term effect of aflatoxin B(1) on lipid peroxidation in rat liver and kidney: effect of picroliv and silymarin. *Phytother Res* 2001;15:307-10.

11851 Rajeshkumar NV, Kuttan R. Inhibition of N-nitrosodiethylamine-induced hepatocarcinogenesis by Picroliv. *J Exp Clin Cancer Res* 2000;19:459-65.

11852 Saraswat B, Visen PK, Patnaik GK, Dhawan BN. Ex vivo and in vivo investigations of picroliv from Picrorhiza kurroa in an alcohol intoxication model in rats. *J Ethnopharmacol* 1999;66:263-9.

11853 Baruah CC, Gupta PP, Nath A, et al. Anti-allergic and anti-anaphylactic activity of picroliv--a standardised iridoid glycoside fraction of Picrorhiza kurroa. *Pharmacol Res* 1998;38:487-92.

11854 Chander R, Singh K, Visen PK, et al. Picroliv prevents oxidation in serum lipoprotein lipids of Mastomys coucha infected with Plasmodium berghei. *Indian J Exp Biol* 1998;36:371-4.

11855 Mittal N, Gupta N, Saksena S, et al. Protective effect of Picroliv from Picrorhiza kurroa against Leishmania donovani infections in Mesocricetus auratus. *Life Sci* 1998;63:1823-34.

11856 Dwivedi Y, Rastogi R, Garg NK, Dhawan BN. Effects of picroliv, the active principle of Picrorhiza kurroa, on biochemical changes in rat liver poisoned by Amanita phalloides. *Zhongguo Yao Li Xue Bao* 1992;13:197-200.

11857 Dorsch W, Stuppner H, Wagner H, et al. Antiasthmatic effects of Picrorhiza kurroa: androsin prevents allergen- and PAF-induced bronchial obstruction in guinea pigs. *Int Arch Allergy Appl Immunol* 1991;95:128-33.

11858 Doshi VB, Shetye VM, Mahashur AA, Kamat SR. Picrorrhiza kurroa in bronchial asthma. *J Postgrad Med* 1983;29:89-95.

11859 Van den Worm E, Beukelman CJ, Van den Berg AJ, et al. Effects of methoxylation of apocynin and analogs on the inhibition of reactive oxygen species production by stimulated human neutrophils. *Eur J Pharmacol* 2001;433:225-30.

11860 't Hart BA, Simons JM, Knaan-Shanzer S, et al. Antiarthritic activity of the newly developed neutrophil oxidative burst antagonist apocynin. *Free Radic Biol Med* 1990;9:127-31.

11862 Sato J, Nakata H, Owada E, et al. Influence of usual intake of dietary caffeine on single-dose kinetics of theophylline in healthy human subjects. *Eur J Clin Pharmacol* 1993;44:295-8.

11863 Goldenberg D, Golz A, Joachims HZ. The beverage mate: a risk factor for cancer of the head and neck. *Head Neck* 2003;25:595-601.

11864 Sewram V, De Stefani E, Brennan P, Boffetta P. Mate consumption and the risk of squamous cell esophageal cancer in uruguay. *Cancer Epidemiol Biomarkers Prev* 2003;12:508-13.

11865 Esmelindro AA, Girardi Jdos S, Mossi A, et al. Influence of agronomic variables on the composition of mate tea leaves (Ilex paraguariensis) extracts obtained from CO2 extraction at 30 degrees C and 175 bar. *J Agric Food Chem* 2004;52:1990-5.

11866 Andersen T, Fogh J. Weight loss and delayed gastric emptying following a South American herbal preparation in overweight patients. *J Hum Nutr Diet* 2001;14:243-50.

11867 Saldana MD, Zetzl C, Mohamed RS, Brunner G. Extraction of methylxanthines from guarana seeds, mate leaves, and cocoa beans using supercritical carbon dioxide and ethanol. *J Agric Food Chem* 2002;50:4820-6.

11868 Stone NJ. Fish consumption, fish oil, lipids, and coronary heart disease. *Circulation* 1996;94:2337-40.

11869 Picado C, Castillo JA, Schinca N, et al. Effects of a fish oil enriched diet on aspirin intolerant asthmatic patients: a pilot study. *Thorax* 1988;43:93-7.

11872 Sandor PS, Di Clemente L, Coppola G, et al. A randomized controlled trial of coenzyme Q10 in migraine prophylaxis. 56th Annual Meeting, American Academy of Neurology; April 24-May 1, 2004; San Francisco, CA. Abstract S43.004.

11873 FDA. List of Orphan Designations and Approvals. http://www.fda.gov/orphan/DESIGNAT/list.htm (Accessed 19 June 2004).

11874 Gray J, ed. Therapeutic Choices, second ed. Ottawa: Canadian Pharmacists Association, 1998.

11875 McLeroy VJ, Schendel HE. Influence of oral contraceptives on ascorbic acid concentrations in healthy, sexually mature women. *Am J Clin Nutr* 1973;26:191-6

11876 Rivers JM, Devine MM. Plasma ascorbic acid concentrations and oral contraceptives. *Am J Clin Nutr* 1972;25:684-9.

11877 Playford DA, Watts GF, Croft KD, Burke V. Combined effect of coenzyme Q10 and fenofibrate on forearm microcirculatory function in type 2 diabetes. *Atherosclerosis* 2003;168:169-79.

11878 Mennella J. Alcohol's effect on lactation. *Alcohol Res Health* 2001;25:230-4.

11879 Mukamal KJ, Conigrave KM, Mittleman MA, et al. Roles of drinking pattern and type of alcohol consumed in coronary heart disease in men. *N Engl J Med* 2003;348:109-18.

11880 Departments of Health and Human Services and Agriculture. Dietary Guidelines for Americans, 5th edition. Available at: http://www.health.gov/dietaryguidelines/dga2000/document/choose.htm#alcohol.

11881 Sharma OP. Hypercalcemia in granulomatous disorders: a clinical review. *Curr Opin Pulm Med* 2000;6:442-7.

11882 Stedman C. Herbal hepatotoxicity. *Semin Liver Dis* 2002;22:195-206.

11883 FDA. Pyrrolizidine Alkaloids. Center for Food Safety & Applied Nutrition Foodborne Pathogenic Microorganisms and Natural Toxins Handbook. Available at: http://vm.cfsan.fda.gov/~mow/chap42.html.

11884 Das UN. The lipids that matter from infant nutrition to insulin resistance. *Prostaglandins Leukot Essent Fatty Acids* 2002;67:1-12.

11885 Schmidt EB, Dyerberg J. Omega-3 fatty acids. Current status in cardiovascular medicine. *Drugs* 1994;47:405-24.

11886 Pfrunder A, Schiesser M, Gerber S, et al. Interaction of St John's wort with low-dose oral contraceptive therapy: a randomized controlled trial. *Br J Clin Pharmacol* 2003;56:683-90.

11887 Hall SD, Wang Z, Huang SM, et al. The interaction between St John's wort and an oral contraceptive. *Clin Pharmacol Ther* 2003;74:525-35.

11888 Frye RF, Fitzgerald SM, Lagattuta TT, Egorin MJ. Effect of St. John's wort on imatinib mesylate pharmacokinetics (abstract PDII-B-4). ASCPT Annual Meeting 2004;75:P96.

11889 Komoroski BJ, Zhang S, Cai H, et al. Induction and inhibition of cytochromes p450 by the St. John's wort constituent hyperforin in human hepatocyte cultures. *Drug Metab Dispos* 2004;32:512-8.

11890 Jiang X, Williams KM, Liauw WS, et al. Effect of St John's wort and ginseng on the pharmacokinetics and pharmacodynamics of warfarin in healthy subjects. *Br J Clin Pharmacol* 2004;57:592-9.

11891 Yun YP, Do JH, Ko SR, et al. Effects of Korean red ginseng and its mixed prescription on the high molecular weight dextran-induced blood stasis in rats and human platelet aggregation. *J Ethnopharmacol* 2001;77:259-64.

11892 Turunen M, Olsson J, Dallner G. Metabolism and function of coenzyme Q. *Biochim Biophys Acta* 2004;1660:171-99.

11893 American Association of Clinical Endocrinologists. American Association of Clinical Endocrinologists medical guidelines for the clinical use of dietary supplements and nutraceuticals. *Endocr Pract* 2003;9:417-70.

11894 Tran MT, Mitchell TM, Kennedy DT, Giles JT. Role of coenzyme Q10 in chronic heart failure, angina, and hypertension. *Pharmacotherapy* 2001;21:797-806.

11895 Ishii N, Senoo-Matsuda N, Miyake K, et al. Coenzyme Q10 can prolong C. elegans lifespan by lowering oxidative stress. *Mech Ageing Dev* 2004;125:41-6.

11896 Lee CK, Pugh TD, Klopp RG, et al. The impact of alpha-lipoic acid, coenzyme Q10 and caloric restriction on life span and gene expression patterns in mice. *Free Radic Biol Med* 2004;36:1043-57.

11897 Welch KM. Current opinions in headache pathogenesis: introduction and synthesis. *Curr Opin Neurol* 1998;11:193-7.

11898 Thompson PD, Clarkson P, Karas RH. Statin-associated myopathy. *JAMA* 2003;289:1681-90.

11899 Thibault A, Samid D, Tompkins AC, et al. Phase I study of lovastatin, an inhibitor of the mevalonate pathway, in patients with cancer. *Clin Cancer Res* 1996;2:483-91.

11900 Kim WS, Kim MM, Choi HJ, et al. Phase II study of high-dose lovastatin in patients with advanced gastric adenocarcinoma. *Invest New Drugs* 2001;19:81-3.

11901 Snider S. Octacosanol in parkinsonism. *Ann Neurol* 1984;16:723.

11902 Chello M, Mastroroberto P, Romano R, et al. Protection by coenzyme Q10 of tissue reperfusion injury during abdominal aortic cross-clamping. *J Cardiovasc Surg* (Torino) 1996;37:229-35.

11903 Chello M, Mastroroberto P, Romano R, et al. Protection by coenzyme Q10 from myocardial reperfusion injury during coronary artery bypass grafting. *Ann Thorac Surg* 1994;58:1427-32.

11904 Taggart DP, Jenkins M, Hooper J, et al. Effects of short-term supplementation with coenzyme Q10 on myocardial protection during cardiac operations. *Ann Thorac Surg* 1996;61:829-33.

11905 Engelsen J, Nielsen JD, Winther K. Effect of coenzyme Q10 and Ginkgo biloba on warfarin dosage in stable, long-term warfarin treated outpatients. A randomised, double blind, placebo-crossover trial. *Thromb Haemost* 2002;87:1075-6.

11906 O'Connor AM, Merel NH, Te HS, Cohen SM. A case of autoimmune hepatitis associated with the use of black cohosh (abstract). *Am J Gastroenterol* 2003;98:S165.

11909 Vitetta L, Thomsen M, Sali A. Black cohosh and other herbal remedies associated with acute hepatitis. *Med J Aust* 2003;178:411-2.

11910 Thomsen M, Vitetta L, Schmidt M, Sali A. Acute liver failure associated with the use of herbal preparations containing black cohosh. *Med J Aust* 2004;180:598-600.

11911 Bodinet C, Freudenstein J. Influence of marketed herbal menopause preparations on MCF-7 cell proliferation. *Menopause* 2004;11:281-9.

11912 Einbond LS, Shimizu M, Xiao D, et al. Growth inhibitory activity of extracts and purified components of black cohosh on human breast cancer cells. *Breast Cancer Res Treat* 2004;83:221-31.

11913 American College of Obstetricians and Gynecologists Committee on Practice Bulletins--Gynecology. ACOG Practice Bulletin. Clinical Management Guidelines for Obstetrician-Gynecologists. Use of botanicals for management of menopausal symptoms. *Obstet Gynecol* 2001;97:suppl 1-11 .

11915 De Benito V, Alzaga R. Occupational allergic contact dermatitis from cassia (Chinese cinnamon) as a flavouring agent in coffee. *Contact Dermatitis* 1999;40:165.

11916 Bischoff-Ferrari HA, Dawson-Hughes B, Willett WC, et al. Effect of Vitamin D on falls: a meta-analysis. *JAMA* 2004;291:1999-2006.

11917 Flicker L, Mead K, MacInnis RJ, et al. Serum vitamin D and falls in older women in residential care in Australia. *J Am Geriatr Soc* 2003;51:1533-8.

11918 Dhesi JK, Moniz C, Close JC, et al. A rationale for vitamin D prescribing in a falls clinic population. *Age Ageing* 2002;31:267-71.

11919 Janssen HC, Samson MM, Verhaar HJ. Vitamin D deficiency, muscle function, and falls in elderly people. *Am J Clin Nutr* 2002;75:611-5.

11920 Drake TE, Maibach HI. Allergic contact dermatitis and stomatitis caused by a cinnamic aldehyde-flavored toothpaste. *Arch Dermatol* 1976;112:202-3.

11921 Bischoff-Ferrari HA, Borchers M, Gudat F, et al. Vitamin D receptor expression in human muscle tissue decreases with age. *J Bone Miner Res* 2004;19:265-9.

11922 Pfeifer M, Begerow B, Minne HW. Vitamin D and muscle function. *Osteoporos Int* 2002;13:187-94.

11923 Prabhala A, Garg R, Dandona P. Severe myopathy associated with vitamin D deficiency in western New York. *Arch Intern Med* 2000; 160:1199–203.

11924 Pfeifer M, Begerow B, Minne HW, et al. Effects of a short-term vitamin D and calcium supplementation on body sway and secondary hyperparathyroidism in elderly women. *J Bone Miner Res* 2000;15:1113-8.

11925 Dhesi JK, Bearne LM, Moniz C, et al. Neuromuscular and psychomotor function in elderly subjects who fall and the relationship with vitamin D status. *J Bone Miner Res* 2002;17:891-7.

11926 Graafmans WC, Ooms ME, Hofstee HM, et al. Falls in the elderly: a prospective study of risk factors and risk profiles. *Am J Epidemiol* 1996;143:1129-36.

11927 Meyer HE, Smedshaug GB, Kvaavik E, et al. Can vitamin D supplementation reduce the risk of fracture in the elderly? A randomized controlled trial. *J Bone Miner Res* 2002;17:709-15.

11928 Lips P, Graafmans WC, Ooms ME, et al. Vitamin D supplementation and fracture incidence in elderly persons. A randomized, placebo- controlled clinical trial. *Ann Intern Med* 1996;124:400-6.

11930 Chapuy MC, Arlot ME, Duboeuf F, et al. Vitamin D3 and calcium to prevent hip fractures in the elderly women. *N Engl J Med* 1992;327:1637-42.

11931 Trivedi DP, Doll R, Khaw KT. Effect of four monthly oral vitamin D3 (cholecalciferol) supplementation on fractures and mortality in men and women living in the community: randomised double blind controlled trial. *BMJ* 2003;326:469.

11932 Dukas L, Bischoff HA, Lindpaintner LS, et al. Alfacalcidol reduces the number of fallers in a community-dwelling elderly population with a minimum calcium intake of more than 500 mg daily. *J Am Geriatr Soc* 2004;52:230-6.

11933 Heaney RP, Dowell MS, Hale CA, Bendich A. Calcium absorption varies within the reference range for serum 25-hydroxyvitamin D. *J Am Coll Nutr* 2003;22:142-6.

11935 Holick MF. Vitamin D: importance in the prevention of cancers, type 1 diabetes, heart disease, and osteoporosis. *Am J Clin Nutr* 2004;79:362-71.

11936 Holick MF. Sunlight and vitamin D: both good for cardiovascular health. *J Gen Intern Med* 2002;17:733-5.

11937 Arnas LAG, Heaney RP, Hollis BW. Vitamin D2 is much less effective than vitamin D3 in humans (abstract OR22-2). The Endocrine Society 86th Annual Meeting, June 16-19, New Orleans, LA.

11938 Trang HM, Cole DE, Rubin LA, et al. Evidence that vitamin D3 increases serum 25-hydroxyvitamin D more efficiently than does vitamin D2. *Am J Clin Nutr* 1998;68:854-8.

11939 Bischoff HA, Stahelin HB, Dick W, et al. Effects of vitamin D and calcium supplementation on falls: a randomized controlled trial. *J Bone Miner Res* 2003;18:343-51.

11940 L'Abbe MR, Whiting SJ, Hanley DA. The Canadian health claim for calcium, vitamin D and osteoporosis. *J Am Coll Nutr* 2004;23:303-8.

11941 Lee DK, Gray RD, Robb FM, et al. A placebo-controlled evaluation of butterbur and fexofenadine on objective and subjective outcomes in perennial allergic rhinitis. *Clin Exp Allergy* 2004;34:646-9.

11942 Gray RD, Haggart K, Lee DK, Cull S, Lipworth BJ. Effects of butterbur treatment in intermittent allergic rhinitis: a placebo-controlled evaluation. *Ann Allergy Asthma Immunol* 2004;93:56-60.

11943 Estruch R, Sacanella E, Badia E, et al. Different effects of red wine and gin consumption on inflammatory biomarkers of atherosclerosis: a prospective randomized crossover trial. Effects of wine on inflammatory markers. *Atherosclerosis* 2004;175:117-23.

11944 Wang MY, West BJ, Jensen CJ, et al. Morinda citrifolia (Noni): a literature review and recent advances in Noni research. *Acta Pharmacol Sin* 2002;23:1127-41.

11945 Wang SM, Lee LJ, Huang YT, et al. Magnolol stimulates steroidogenesis in rat adrenal cells. *Br J Pharmacol* 2000;131:1172-8.

11946 Kuribara H, Kishi E, Hattori N, et al. The anxiolytic effect of two oriental herbal drugs in Japan attributed to honokiol from magnolia bark. *J Pharm Pharmacol* 2000;52:1425-9.

11947 Maruyama Y, Kuribara H, Kishi E, et al. Confirmation of the anxiolytic-like effect of dihydrohonokiol following behavioural and biochemical assessments. *J Pharm Pharmacol* 2001;53:721-5.

11948 Kuribara H, Kishi E, Maruyama Y. Does dihydrohonokiol, a potent anxiolytic compound, result in the development of benzodiazepine-like side effects? *J Pharm Pharmacol* 2000;52:1017-22.

11949 Zhong WB, Wang CY, Ho KJ, et al. Magnolol induces apoptosis in human leukemia cells via cytochrome c release and caspase activation. *Anticancer Drugs* 2003;14:211-7.

11950 Nakazawa T, Yasuda T, Ohsawa K. Metabolites of orally administered Magnolia officinalis extract in rats and man and its antidepressant-like effects in mice. *J Pharm Pharmacol* 2003;55:1583-91

11951 Hou YC, Chao PD, Chen SY. Honokiol and magnolol increased hippocampal acetylcholine release in freely-moving rats. *Am J Chin Med* 2000;28:379-84.

11952 Tachikawa E, Takahashi M, Kashimoto T. Effects of extract and ingredients isolated from Magnolia obovata thunberg on catecholamine secretion from bovine adrenal chromaffin cells. *Biochem Pharmacol* 2000;60:433-40 .

11953 Jung KY, Kim DS, Oh SR, et al. Magnone A and B, novel anti-PAF tetrahydrofuran lignans from the flower buds of Magnolia fargesii. *J Nat Prod* 1998;61:808-11.

11954 Judy WV, Hari SP, Stogsdill WW, et al. Antidiabetic activity of a standardized extract (Glucosol) from Lagerstroemia speciosa leaves in Type II diabetics. A dose-dependence study. *J Ethnopharmacol* 2003;87:115-7.

11955 Kakuda T, Sakane I, Takihara T, et al. Hypoglycemic effect of extracts from Lagerstroemia speciosa L. leaves in genetically diabetic KK-AY mice. *Biosci Biotechnol Biochem* 1996;60:204-8.

11956 Hayashi T, Maruyama H, Kasai R, et al. Ellagitannins from Lagerstroemia speciosa as activators of glucose transport in fat cells. *Planta Med* 2002;68:173-5.

11957 Hattori K, Sukenobu N, Sasaki T, et al. Activation of insulin receptors by lagerstroemin. *J Pharmacol Sci* 2003;93:69-73.

11958 Unno T, Sugimoto A, Kakuda T. Xanthine oxidase inhibitors from the leaves of Lagerstroemia speciosa (L.) Pers. *J Ethnopharmacol* 2004;93:391-5.

11959 Suzuki Y, Unno T, Ushitani M, et al. Antiobesity activity of extracts from Lagerstroemia speciosa L. leaves on female KK-Ay mice. *J Nutr Sci Vitaminol* (Tokyo) 1999;45:791-5.

11960 Zheng G, Sayama K, Okubo T, et al. Anti-obesity effects of three major components of green tea, catechins, caffeine and theanine, in mice. *In Vivo* 2004;18:55-62.

11961 Peters EM, Anderson R, Nieman DC, et al. Vitamin C supplementation attenuates the increases in circulating cortisol, adrenaline and anti-inflammatory polypeptides following ultramarathon running. *Int J Sports Med* 2001;22:537-43.

11962 Pittler MH, Stevinson C, Ernst E. Chromium picolinate for reducing body weight: meta-analysis of randomized trials. *Int J Obes Relat Metab Disord* 2003;27:522-9.

11963 Benton D, Donohoe RT, Sillance B, Nabb S. The influence of phosphatidylserine supplementation on mood and heart rate when faced with an acute stressor. *Nutr Neurosci* 2001;4:169-78.

11964 McClatchey W. From Polynesian healers to health food stores: changing perspectives of Morinda citrifolia (Rubiaceae). *Integr Cancer Ther* 2002;1:110-20.

11965 Hornick CA, Myers A, Sadowska-Krowicka H, et al. Inhibition of angiogenic initiation and disruption of newly established human vascular networks by juice from Morinda citrifolia (noni). *Angiogenesis* 2003;6:143-9.

11966 Zhang ZQ, Yuan L, Yang M, et al. The effect of Morinda officinalis How, a Chinese traditional medicinal plant, on the DRL 72-s schedule in rats and the forced swimming test in mice. *Pharmacol Biochem Behav* 2002;72:39-43.

11967 Clinicaltrials.gov. Phase I Study of Noni in Cancer Patients. http://www.clinicaltrials.gov/ct/show/NCT00033878?order=1 (Accessed 17 September 2004).

11968 Ferguson DM, Steidle CP, Singh GS, et al. Randomized, placebo-controlled, double blind, crossover design trial of the efficacy and safety of Zestra for Women in women with and without female sexual arousal disorder. *J Sex Marital Ther* 2003;29:33-44.

11969 Fourcroy JL. Female sexual dysfunction: potential for pharmacotherapy. *Drugs* 2003;63:1445-57.

11970 Yale SH, Liu K. Echinacea purpurea therapy for the treatment of the common cold: a randomized, double-blind, placebo-controlled clinical trial. *Arch Intern Med* 2004;164:1237-41 .

11971 Wiwanikit V, Taungjarwinai W. A case report of suspected ginseng allergy. *Medscape General Medicine* 6 (3), 2004. http://www.medscape.com/viewarticle/482833 (Accessed 17 September 2004).

11972 Allan SJ, Kavanagh GM, Herd RM, Savin JA. The effect of inositol supplements on the psoriasis of patients taking lithium: a randomized, placebo-controlled trial. *Br J Dermatol* 2004;150:966-9.

11973 Onderoglu S, Sozer S, Erbil KM, et al. The evaluation of long-term effcts of cinnamon bark and olive leaf on toxicity induced by streptozotocin administration to rats. *J Pharm Pharmacol* 1999;51:1305-12.

11976 Bailey DG, Dresser GK, Bend JR. Bergamottin, lime juice, and red wine as inhibitors of cytochrome P450 3A4 activity: comparison with grapefruit juice. *Clin Pharmacol Ther* 2003;73:529-37.

11977 Soni MG, Burdock GA, Preuss HG, et al. Safety assessment of (-)-hydroxycitric acid and Super CitriMax, a novel calcium/potassium salt. *Food Chem Toxicol* 2004;42:1513-29.

11978 Azais-Braesco V, Pascal G. Vitamin A in pregnancy: requirements and safety limits. *Am J Clin Nutr* 2000;71:1325S-33S.

11979 Burns CP, Halabi S, Clamon G, et al. Phase II study of high-dose fish oil capsules for patients with cancer-related cachexia. *Cancer* 2004;101:370-8.

11980 Waites KB, Canupp KC, Armstrong S, DeVivo MJ. Effect of cranberry extract on bacteriuria and pyuria in persons with neurogenic bladder secondary to spinal cord injury. *J Spinal Cord Med* 2004;27:35-40.

11981 Kurz A, Van Baelen B. Ginkgo biloba compared with cholinesterase inhibitors in the treatment of dementia: a review based on meta-analyses by the Cochrane collaboration. *Dement Geriatr Cogn Disord* 2004;18:217-26.

11982 Schmidt JM, Greenspoon JS. Aloe vera dermal wound gel is associated with a delay in wound healing. *Obstet Gynecol* 1991;78:115-7.

11983 Rajasekaran S, Sivagnanam K, Ravi K, Subramanian S. Hypoglycemic effect of Aloe vera gel on streptozotocin-induced diabetes in experimental rats. *J Med Food* 2004;7:61-6.

11984 Langmead L, Feakins RM, Goldthorpe S, et al. Randomized, double-blind, placebo-controlled trial of oral aloe vera gel for active ulcerative colitis. *Aliment Pharmacol Ther* 2004;19:739-47.

11985 Salen G, von Bergmann K, Lutjohann D, et al. Ezetimibe effectively reduces plasma plant sterols in patients with sitosterolemia. *Circulation* 2004;109:966-71.

11986 Behall KM, Scholfield DJ, Hallfrisch J. Lipids significantly reduced by diets containing barley in moderately hypercholesterolemic men. *J Am Coll Nutr* 2004;23:55-62.

11987 Stewart MJ, Steenkamp V. Pyrrolizidine poisoning: a neglected area in human toxicology. *Ther Drug Monit* 2001;23:698-708.

11988 Food and Drug Administration. FDA Advises Dietary Supplement Manufacturers to Remove Comfrey Products From the Market. July 6, 2001. Available at: http://www.cfsan.fda.gov/~dms/dspltr06.html.

11989 Sudhop T, Lutjohann D, Kodal A, et al. Inhibition of intestinal cholesterol absorption by ezetimibe in humans. *Circulation* 2002;106:1943-8.

11990 Stickel F, Seitz HK. The efficacy and safety of comfrey. *Public Health Nutr* 2000;3:501-8.

11991 Huxtable RJ, Awang DV. Pyrrolizidine poisoning. *Am J Med* 1990;89:547-8.

11992 Koll R, Klingenburg S. [Therapeutic characteristance and tolerance of topical comfrey preparations. Results of an observational study of patients]. [Article in German]. *Fortschr Med Orig* 2002;120:1-9.

11993 Nahas EP, Neto JN, DeLuca L, et al. Benefits of soy germ isoflavone in postmenopausal women with contraindication for conventional hormone replacement therapy. *Maturitas* 2004;48:372-80.

11994 Crisafulli A, Marini H, Bitto A, et al. Effects of genistein on hot flushes in early postmenopausal women: a randomized, double-blind EPT- and placebo-controlled study. *Menopause* 2004;11:400-4.

11995 Visentin V, Morin N, Fontana E, et al. Dual action of octopamine on glucose transport into adipocytes: inhibition via beta3-adrenoceptor activation and stimulation via oxidation by amine oxidases. *J Pharmacol Exp Ther* 2001;299:96-104.

11996 D'Andrea G, Terrazzino S, Leon A, et al. Elevated levels of circulating trace amines in primary headaches. *Neurology* 2004;62:1701-5,

11997 Kennedy DD, Tucker KL, Ladas ED, et al. Low antioxidant vitamin intakes are associated with increases in adverse effects of chemotherapy in children with acute lymphoblastic leukemia. *Am J Clin Nutr* 2004;79:1029-36.

11998 Brodkin RH, Bleiberg J. Sensitivity to topically applied vitamin E. *Arch Dermatol* 1965;92:76-7.

11999 Booth SL, Golly I, Sacheck JM, et al. Effect of vitamin E supplementation on vitamin K status in adults with normal coagulation status. *Am J Clin Nutr* 2004;80:143-8.

12000 Gaby AR. Methylsulfonylmethane as a treatment for seasonal allergic rhinitis: more data needed on pollen counts and questionnaire. *J Altern Complement Med* 2002;8:229.

12001 Health and Human Services. HHS launches crackdown on products containing Andro. March, 2004.

12002 Mangold T. Sampling the Kalahari cactus diet. BBC News; May 30, 2003.

12003 Pfizer returns rights of P57. Phytopharm Press Release; July 30, 2003.

12004 Phytopharm plc successful completion of proof of principle clinical study of P57 for Obesity. Phytopharm Press Release; December 5, 2001.

12005 FDA Warns Distributors of Dietary Supplements Promoted Online for Weight Loss. FDA Press Release; April 1, 2004.

12006 Cohen B, Schardt D. Center for Science in the Public Interest. Letter to Food and Drug Administration. Commissioner Mark McClellan, MD, PhD. March 4, 2004.

12008 Winther K, Hedman C. Assessment of the Effects of the Herbal Remedy Femal on the Symptoms of Premenstrual Syndrome: A Randomized, Double-Blind, Placebo-Controlled Study. *Curr Ther Res Clin Exp* 2002;63:344-53..

12009 Asao T, Kuwano H, IDE M, et al. Spasmolytic effect of peppermint oil in barium during double-contrast barium enema compared with Buscopan. *Clinical Radiology* 2003;58:301-5.

12010 Henmi H, Endo T, Kitajima Y, et al. Effects of ascorbic acid supplementation on serum progesteron levels in patients with luteal phase defect. *Fertil Steril* 2003;80:459-61.

12011 Neinhuys JW. The True Story of Oscillococcinum. HomeoWatch 2003. http://www.homeowatch.org/history/oscillo.html (Accessed 21 April 2004).

12012 Durackova Z, Trebaticky B, Novotny V, et al. Lipid metabolism and erectile function improvement by Pycnogenol, extract from the bark of Pinus pinaster in patients suffering from erectile dysfunction-a pilot study. *Nutr Res* 2003;23:1189-98..

12013 Matsumoto K, Akao Y, Kobayashi E, et al. Induction of aptosis by xanthones from mangosteen in human leukemia cell lines. *J Nat Prod* 2003;66:1124-7.

12014 Suksamrarn S, Suwannapoch N, Phakhodee W, et al. Antimycobacterial activity of prenylated xanthones from the fruits of Garcinia mangostana. *Chem Pharm Bull* (Tokyo) 2003;51:857-9.

12015 Ho CK, Huang YL, Chen CC. Garcinone E, a xanthone derivative, has potent cytotoxic effect against hepatocellular carcinoma cell lines. *Planta Med* 2002;68:975-9.

12016 Nilar, Harrison LJ. Xanthones from the heartwood of Garcinia mangostana. *Phytochemistry* 2002;60:541-8.

12017 Chairungsrilerd N, Furukawa K, Ohta T, et al. Histaminergic and serotonergic receptor blocking substances from the medicinal plant Garcinia mangostana. *Planta Med* 1996;62:471-2.

12018 Yu RJ, Van Scott EJ. Hydroxycarboxylic Acids, N-Acetylamino Sugars, and N-Acetylamino Acids. *SKINmed* 2002;2:117-22.

12019 Phillips TJ, Gottlieb AB, Leyden JJ, et al. Efficacy of 0.1% tazarotene cream for the treatment of photodamage: A 12-month multicenter, randomized trail. *Arch Dermatol* 2002;138:1486-93.

12020 Gheresitich I, Brazzini B, Perris K, et al. Pyruvic acid peels for the treatment of photoaging. *Dermatol Surg* 2004;30:32-6.

12021 Beitner H. Randomized, placebo controlled, double-blind study on the clinical efficacy of a cream containing 5% alpha-lipoic acid related to photoaging of facial skin. *Br J Dermatol* 2003;149:841-9.

12022 Rattan SI, Clark BF. Kinetin delays onset of aging characteristics in human fibroblasts. *Biochem Biophys Res Commun* 1994;201:665-72.

12023 Uhoda I, Faska N, Robert C, et al. Split face study on the cutaneous tensile effect of 2-dimethylaminoethanol (deanol) gel. *Skin Res Technol* 2002;8:164-7.

12024 Executive Summary of The Third Report of The National Cholesterol Education Program (NCEP) Expert Panel on Detection, Evaluation, And Treatment of High Blood Cholesterol In Adults (Adult Treatment Panel III). *JAMA* 2001;285:2486-97.

12026 Boehringer S. Raising HDL and niacin use. *Pharmacist's Letter* 2004;20:200504.

12027 O'Mara N. New drug: Ezetimide (Zetia). *Pharmacist's Letter* 2003:18:181202.

12028 Shields K. Heart healthy foods. *Pharmacist's Letter* 2003;19:191205.

12030 Nykamp DL, Fackih MN, Compton AL. Possible association of acute lateral-wall myocardial infarction and bitter orange supplement. *Ann Pharmacother* 2004;38:812-6.

12031 Kubo I, Fujita K, Kubo A, et al. Antibacterial activity of coriander volatile compounds against Salmonella choleraesuis. *J Agric Food Chem* 2004;52:3329-32.

12032 Yuan CS, Wei G, Dey L, et al. American ginseng reduces warfarin's effect in healthy patients: a randomized, controlled trial. *Ann Intern Med* 2004;141:23-7.

12033 McKenney J. New perspectives on the use of niacin in the treatment of lipid disorders. *Arch Intern Med* 2004;164:164:697-705.

12034 Kreijkamp-Kaspers S, Kok L, Grobbee DE, et al. Effect of soy protein containing isoflavones on cognitive function, bone mineral density, and plasma lipids in postmenopausal women: A randomized controlled trial. *JAMA* 2004;292:65-74.

12035 Hansen TM, Lerche A, Kassis V, et al. Treatment of rheumatoid arthritis with prostaglandin E1 precursors cis-linoleic acid and gamma-linolenic acid. *Scand J Rheumatol* 1983;12:85-8.

12036 Belch JJ, Ansell D, Madhok R, et al. Effects of altering dietary essential fatty acids on requirements for non-steroidal anti-inflammatory drugs in patients with rheumatoid arthritis: A double blind placebo controlled study. *Ann Rheum Dis* 1988;47:96-104.

12037 Oxholm P, Manthorpe R, Prause JU, Horrobin D. Patients with primary Sjogren's syndrome treated for two months with evening primrose oil. *Scand J Rheumatol* 1986;15:103-8.

12038 McKendry RJ. Treatment of Sjogren's syndrome with essential fatty acids, pyridoxine and vitamin C. *Prostaglandins Leukot Med* 1982;8:403-8.

12039 File SE, Jarrett N, Fluck E, et al. Eating soya improves human memory. *Psychopharmacology* (Berl) 2001;157:430-6.

12040 Kritz-Silverstein D, Von Muhlen D, Barrett-Connor E, Bressel MA. Isoflavones and cognitive function in older women: the SOy and Postmenopausal Health In Aging (SOPHIA) Study. *Menopause* 2003;10:196-202.

12041 Haselkorn T, Stewart SL, Horn-Ross PL. Why are thyroid cancer rates so high in southeast Asian women living in the United States? The Bay Area Thyroid Cancer Study. *Cancer Epidemiol Biomarkers Prev* 2003;12:144-50.

12042 Grundy SM, Cleeman JI, Merz, CN, et al. Implications of recent clinical trials for the National Cholesterol Education Program Adult Treatment Panel III guidelines. *Circulation* 2004;110:227-39.

12044 Setchell KDR, Lydeking-Olsen E. Dietary phytoestrogens and their effect on bone: evidence from in vitro and in vivo, human observational, and dietary intervention studies. *Am J Clin Nutr* 2003;78:593S-609S.

12045 Imataka G, Mikami T, Yamanouchi H, et al. Vitamin D deficiency rickets due to soybean milk. *J Paediatr Child Health* 2004;40:154-5.

12046 Cummings JL. Alzheimer's disease. *N Engl J Med* 2004;351:56-67.

12047 Finkel RS, Zarlengo KM. Blue cohosh and perinatal stroke. *N Engl J Med* 2004;351:302-3.

12048 Duffy R, Wiseman H, File SE. Improved cognitive function in postmenopausal women after 12 weeks of consumption of a soya extract containing isoflavones. *Pharmacol Biochem Behav* 2003;75:721-9.

12049 Setchell KDR, Brown NM, Lydeking-Olsen E. The clinical importance of the metabolite equol - A clue to the effectiveness of soy and its isoflavones. *J Nutr* 2002;132:3577-84.

12050 Barr SI. Increased dairy product of calcium intake: Is body weight or composition affected in humans? *J Nutr* 2003;133:245S-8S.

12051 Zemel MB. Role of calcium and dairy products in energy partitioning and weight management. *Am J Clin Nutr* 2004;79:907S-12S.

12052 Shapses SA, Heshka S, Heymsfield SB. Effect of calcium supplementation on weight and fat loss in women. *J Clin Endocrinol Metab* 2004;89:632-7.

12053 Kang JY, Yeoh KG, Chia HP, et al. Chili - protective factor against peptic ulcer? *Dig Dis Sciences* 1995;40:576-9.

12054 Najm WI, Reinsch S, Hoehler F, et al. S-adenosyl methionine (SAMe) versus celecoxib for the treatment of osteoarthritis symptoms: A double-blind crossover trial. *BMC Musculoskelet Disord* 2004;5:6.

12055 Mozaffarian D, Psaty BM, Rimm EB, et al. Fish intake and risk of incident atrial fibrillation. *Circulation* 2004;110:368-73.

12056 Lee A, Patterson V. A double blind study of L-threonine in patients with spinal spasticity. *Acta Neurol Scand* 1993;88:334-8.

12057 Blin O, Pouget J, Aubrespy G, et al. A double-blind placebo controlled trial of L-threonine in amyotrophic lateral sclerosis. *J Neurol* 1992;239:79-81.

12058 Roufs JB. L-threonine as a symptomatic treatment for amyotrophic lateral sclerosis (ALS). *Med Hypotheses* 1991;34:20-3.

12059 Growdon JH, Nader TM, Schoenfeld J, Wortman RJ. L-threonine in the treatment of spasticity. *Clin Neuropharmacol* 1991;14:403-12.

12060 Akhondzadeh S, Mohammadi MR, Khademi M. Zinc sulfate as an adjunct to methylphenidate for the treatment of attention deficit hyperactivity disorder in children :a double blind and randomized trial. *BMC Psychiatry* 2004;4:9.

12061 Gaudineau C, Beckerman R, Welbourn S, Auclair K. Inhibition of human P450 enzymes by multiple constituents of the Ginkgo biloba extract. *Biochem Biophys Res Comm* 2004;318:1072–8.

12062 Bartle WR. Grapefruit juice might still be a factor in warfarin response. *Am J Health-Syst Pharm* 1999;56:676.

12063 Sullivan DM, Ford MA, Boyden TW. Grapefruit juice and the response to warfarin. *Am J Health-Syst Pharm* 1998;55:1581-3.

12064 Seidlova-Wuttke D, Hesse O, Jarry H, et al. Evidence for selective estrogen receptor modulator activity in a black cohosh (Cimicifuga racemosa) extract: comparison with estradiol-17beta. *Eur J Endocrinol* 2003;149:351-62

12069 FDA. U.S. District Judge Issues Permanent Injunction Against Lane Labs-USA, Inc. and Orders Firm to Refund Money to Purchasers of Illegally Marketed Unapproved Drugs. FDA News; July 13, 2004. Available at: www.fda.gov/bbs/topics/news/2004/NEW01086.html (Accessed 3 August 2004).

12070 Suzuki Y, Kondo K, Matsumoto Y, et al. Dietary supplementation of fermented soybean, natto, suppresses intimal thickening and modulates the lysis of mural thrombi after endothelial injury in rat femoral artery. *Life Sci* 2003;73:1289-98.

12071 Suzuki Y, Kondo K, Ichise, H, et al. Dietary supplementation with fermented soybeans suppresses intimal thickening. *Nutrition* 2003;19:261–4.

12072 Sumi H, Hamada H, Tsushima H, et al. A novel fibrinolytic enzyme (nattokinase) in the vegetable cheese Natto; a typical and popular soybean food in the Japanese diet. *Experientia* 1987;43:1110-1.

12073 Sumi H, Hamada H, Nakanishi K, Hiratani H. Enchancement of fibrinolytic activity in plasma by oral administration of nattokinase. *Acta Haematol* 1990;84:139-43.

12074 Fujita M, Hong K, Ito Y, et al. Thrombolytic effect of nattokinase on a chemically induced thrombosis model in a rat. *Biol Pharm Bull* 1995;18:1387-91.

12075 Cesarone MR, Belcaro G, Nicolaides AN, et al. Prevention of venous thrombosis in long-haul flights with Flite Tabs: The LONFLIT-FLITE randomized, controlled trial. *Angiology* 2003;54:531-9.

12076 Kraemer WJ, Ratamess NA, Anderson JM, et al. Effect of a cetylated fatty acid topical cream on functional mobility and quality of life of patients with osteoarthritis. *J Rheumatol* 2004;31:767-74.

12077 Morris MC, Evans DA, Bianias JL, et al. Dietary niacin and the risk of incident Alzheimer's disease and of cognitive decline. *J Neurol Neurosurg Psychiatry* 2004;75:1093-99.

12078 Middleton E, Kandaswami C, Theoharides TC. The effects of plant flavonoids on mammalian cells: implications for inflammation, heart disease, and cancer. *Pharmacol Rev* 2000;52:673-751.

12079 Robbins RC. Effect of methoxylated flavones on erythrocyte aggregation and sedimentation in blood of normal subjects: Evidence of a dietary role for flavonoids. *Int J Vitam Nutr Res* 1973;43:494-503.

12080 Robbins RC. Stabilization of flow properties of blood with phenylbenzo-y-pyrone derivatives (Flavonoids). *Int J Vitam Nutr Res* 1977;47:373-82.

12081 Robbins RC. Action in human blood of methoxylated flavones which confer disease resistance on both plants and animals: Concept of a dietary conditioned mechanism of defense against disease. *Int J Vitam Nutr Res* 1975;45:51-60.

12082 Robbins RC. Specificities between blood cell adhesion in human diseases and antiadhesion action in vitro of methoxylated flavones. *J Clin Pharmacol* 1973;13:401-7.

12083 Robbins RC. In vitro effects of penta-, hexa-, and hepta-methoxylated flavones on aggregation of cells in blood from hospitalized patients. *J Clin Pharmacol* 1973;13:271-5.

12084 Manthey JA, Guthrie N. Antiproliferative effects of citrus flavonoids against six human cancer cell lines. *J Agric Food Chem* 2002;50:5837-43.

12085 Wiese J, McPherson S, Odden MC, Shlipak MG. Effect of Opuntia ficus indica on symptoms of the alcohol hangover. *Arch Intern Med* 2004;164:1334-40.

12086 Tesoriere L, Butera D, Pintaudi AM, et al. Supplementation with cactus pear (Opuntia ficus-indica) fruit decreases oxidative stress in healthy humans: a comparative study with vitamin C. *Am J Clin Nutr* 2004;80:391-5.

12087 Vinson JA, Teufel K, Wu N. Green and black teas inhibit atherosclerosis by lipid, antioxidant, and fibrinolytic mechanisms. *J Agric Food Chem* 2004;52:3661-5.

12088 DeLuca P, Rothman D, Zurier RB. Marine and botanical lipids as immunomodulatory and therapeutic agents in the

REFERENCES

treatment of rheumatoid arthritis. *Rheum Dis Clin North Am* 1995;21:759-77.

12089 Rothman D, DeLuca P, Zurier RB. Botanical lipids: effects on inflammation, immune responses, and rheumatoid arthritis. *Semin Arthritis Rheum* 1995;25:87-96.

12090 Fujita M, Nomura K, Hong K, et al. Purification and characterization of a strong fibrinolytic enzyme (nattokinase) in the vegetable cheese natto, a popular soybean fermented food in Japan. *Biochem Biophys Res Commun* 1993;197:1340-7.

12091 Urano T, Ihara H, Umemura K, et al. The Profibrinolytic Enzyme Subtilisin NAT Purified from Bacillus subtilis Cleaves and Inactivates Plasminogen Activator InhibitorType 1. *J Biol Chem* 2001;276:24690-6.

12092 Cohen LE, Spurlock R, Salem A, Mercado E. Argyria in the silver state. *Federal Practitioner* 2004;April:9-17.

12093 Garba M, Yakasai IA, Bakare MT, Munir HY. Effect of Tamarindus indica. L on the bioavailability of ibuprofen in healthy human volunteers. *Eur J Drug Metab Pharmacokinet* 2003;28:179-84.

12094 Meydani SN, Leka LS, Fine BC, et al. Vitamin E and respiratory tract infections in elderly nursing home residents. *JAMA* 2004;292:828-36.

12095 Parcell AC, Smith JM, Schulthies SS, et al. Cordyceps sinensis (CordyMax Cs-4) supplementation does not improve endurance exercise performance. *Int J Sport Nutr Exerc Metab* 2004;14:236-42.

12096 Syed TA, Ahmad SA, Holt AH, et al. Management of psoriasis with Aloe vera extract in a hydrophilic cream: a placebo-controlled, double-blind study. *Trop Med Int Health* 1996;1:505–9.

12097 Muller MJ, Hollyoak MA, Moaveni Z, et al. Retardation of wound healing by silver sulfadiazine is reversed by Aloe vera and nystatin. *Burns* 2003;28:834-6.

12098 Heggie S, Bryant GP, Tripcony L, et al. A phase III study on the efficacy of topical aloe vera gel on irradiated breast tissue. *Cancer Nurs* 2002;25:442-51.

12099 Rundek T, Naini A, Sacco R, et al. Atorvastatin decreases the coenzyme Q10 level in the blood of patients at risk for cardiovascular disease and stroke. *Arch Neurol* 2004;61:889-92.

12100 Gatti G, Barzaghi N, Acuto G, et al. A comparative study of free plasma choline levels following intramuscular administration of L-alpha-glycerylphosphorylcholine and citocholine in normal volunteers. *Int J Clin Pharmacol Ther Toxicol* 1992;30:331-5.

12101 Di Perri R, Coppola G, Ambrosio LA, et al. A multicentre trial to the evaluate the efficacy and tolerability of alpha-glycerylphosphorylcholine versus cytosine diphosphocholine in patients with vascular dementia. *J Int Med Res* 1991;19:330-41.

12102 Barbagallo Sangiorgi G, Barbagallo M, Giordano M, et al. Alpha-glycerophosphocholine in the mental recovery of cerebral ischemic attacks: An Italian multicenter clinical trial. *Ann N Y Acad Sci* 1994;717:253-69.

12103 Canal N, Franceschi M, Alberoni M, et al. Effect of L-alpha-glyceryl-phosphorylcholine on amnesia caused by scopolamine. *Int J Clin Pharmacol Ther Toxicol* 1991;29:103-7.

12104 Gafner S, Bergeron C, Batcha LL, et al. Inhibitor of [3H]-LSD binding to 5-HT7 receptors by flavonoids from Scutellaria lateriflora. *J Nat Prod* 2003;66:535-7.

12105 Unfer V, Casini ML, Costabile L, et al. Endometrial effects of long-term treatment with phytoestrogens: a randomized, double-blind, placebo-controlled study. *Fertil Steril* 2004;82:145-8.

12106 Ziegler D, Nowak H, Kemplert P, et al. Treatment of symptomatic diabetic polyneuropathy with the antioxidant alpha-lipoic acid: A meta-analysis. *Diabet Med* 2004;21:114-21.

12107 Tannis AJ, Barban J, Conquer JA. Effect of glucosamine supplementation on fasting and non-fasting plasma glucose and serum insulin concentrations in healthy individuals. *Osteoarthritis Cartilage* 2004;12:506-11.

12108 Pirotta M, Gunn J, Chondros P, et al. Effect of lactobacillus in preventing post-antibiotic vulvovaginal candidiasis: a randomized, controlled trial. *BMJ* 2004;329(7465):548. Epub 2004 Aug 27.

12110 Ghafar MA, Golliday E, Bingham J, et al. Regression of prostate cancer following administration of genistein combined polysaccharide (GCP), a nutritional supplement: A case report. *J Altern Complement Med* 2002;8:493-7.

12111 Belobrajdic DP, McIntosh GH, Owens JA. A high-whey-protein diet reduces body weight gain and alters insulin sensitivity relative to red meat in Wister rats. *J Nutr* 2004;134:1454-8.

12112 Kurowska EM, Manthey JA. Hypolipidemic Effects and Absorption of Citrus Polymethoxylated Flavones in Hamsters with Diet-Induced Hypercholesterolemia. *J Agric Food Chem* 2004;52:2879-86.

12113 Pittler MH, Ernst E. Horse chestnut seed extract for chronic venous insufficiency (Cochrane Review). In: The Cochrane Library, Issue 3, 2004. Chichester, UK: John Wiley & Sons, Ltd..

12114 Kohler S, Funk P, Kieser M. Influence of a 7-day treatment with Ginkgo biloba special extract EGb 761 on bleeding time and coagulation: a randomized, placebo-controlled, double-blind study in healthy volunteers. *Blood Coagul Fibrinolysis* 2004;15:303–9.

12115 Lilja JJ, Juntti-Patinen L, Neuvonen PJ. Orange juice substantially reduces the bioavailability of the beta-adrenergic-blocking agent celiprolol. *Clin Pharmacol Ther* 2004;75:184-90.

12116 Tian R, Koyabu N, Takanaga H, et al. Effects of grapefruit juice and orange juice on the intestinal efflux of P-glycoprotein substrates. *Pharm Res* 2002;19:802-9.

12117 Cifuentes M, Riedt CS, Brolin RE, et al. Weight loss and calcium intake influence calcium absorption in overweight postmenopausal women. *Am J Clin Nutr* 2004;80:123–30.

12118 Grau MV, Baron JA, Sandler RS, et al. Vitamin D, calcium supplementation, and colorectal adenomas: Results of a randomized trial. *J Natl Cancer Inst* 2003;95:1765-71.

12119 Zemel MB, Miller SL. Dietary calcium and dairy modulation of adiposity and obesity risk. *Nutr Rev* 2004;62:125-31.

12120 Cho E, Smith-Warner SA, Spiegelman D, et al. Dairy foods, calcium, and colorectal cancer: A pooled analysis of 10 cohort studies. *J Natl Cancer Inst* 2004;96:1015-22.

12121 Zemel MB, Shi H, Greer B, et al. Regulation of adiposity by dietary calcium. *FASEB J* 2000;14:1132-8.

12122 McCarron DA. Calcium and magnesium nutrition in human hypertension. *Ann Intern Med* 1983;98:800-5.

12124 Buchowski MS, Semenya J, Johnson AO. Dietary calcium intake in lactose maldigesting intolerant and tolerant African-American women. *J Am Coll Nutr* 2002;21:47-54.

12125 Tanasescu M, Ferris AM, Himmelgreen DA, et al. Biobehavioral factors are associated with obesity in Puerto Rican children. *J Nutr* 2000;130:1734–42.

12126 Jacqmain M, Doucet E, Després JP, et al. Calcium intake, body composition, and lipoprotein-lipid concentrations in adults. *Am J Clin Nutr* 2003;77:1448–52.

12127 Davies KM, Heaney RP, Recker RR, et al. Calcium intake and body weight. *J Clin Endocrinol Metab* 2000;85:4635-8.

12128 Zemel MB, Thompson W, Milstead A, et al. Calcium and dairy acceleration of weight and fat loss during energy restriction in obese adults. *Obes Res* 2004;12:582–90.

12129 Babb SM, Appelmans KE, Renshaw PF, et al. Differently effect of CDP-choline on brain cytosolic choline levels in younger and older subjects as measured by magnetic resonance spectroscopy. *Psychopharmacology* (Berl) 1996;127:88-94.

12130 Spiers PA, Myers D, Hochanadel GS, et al. Citicoline improves verbal memory in aging. *Arch Neurol* 1996;53:441-8.

12131 Fioravanti M, Yanagi M. Cytidinephosphoholine (CDP choline) for cognitive and behavioural disturbances associated with chronic cerebral disorders in the elderly (Cochrane Review). In: The Cochrane Library, Issue 3, 2004. Chichester, UK: John Wiley & Sons, Ltd.

12132 Conant R, Schauss AG. Therapeutic applications of citicoline for stroke and cognitive function in the elderly: A review of the literature. *Altern Med Rev* 2004;9:17-31.

12133 Barrachina M, Dominguez I, Ambrosio S, et al. Neuroprotective effect of citicoline in 6-hydroxydopamine-lesioned rats and in 6-hydroxydopamine-treated SH-SY5Y human neuroblastoma cells. *J Neurol Sci* 2003;215:105-10.

12134 Adibhatla RM, Hatcher JF. Citicoline decreases phospholipase A2 stimulation and hydroxyl radical generation in transient cerebral ischemia. *J Neurosci Res* 2003;73:308-15.

12135 Cohen RA, Browndyke JN, Moser DJ, et al. Long-term citicoline (cytidine diphosphate choline) use in patients with vascular dementia: Neuroimaging and neuropsychological outcomes. *Cerebrovasc Dis* 2003;16:199-204.

12136 Savci V, Goktalay G, Cansev M, et al. Intravenously injected citicoline increases blood pressure and reverses hypotension in haemorrhagic shock: effect is mediated by central cholinergic activation. *Eur J Pharmacol* 2003;468:129-39.

12137 Dempsey RJ, Raghavendra Rao VL. Cytidinediphosphocholine treatment to decrease traumatic brain injury-induced hippocampal neuronal death, cortical contusion volume, and neurological dysfunction in rats. *J Neurosurg* 2003;98:867-73.

12138 Sobrado M, Lopez MG, Carceller F, et al. Combined nipodimine and citicoline reduce infarct size, attenuate apoptosis, and increase BCL-2 expression after focal cerebral ischemia. *Neuroscience* 2003;118:107-13.

12139 Davalos A, Castillo J, Alvarez-Sabin J, et al. Oral citicoline in acute ischemic stroke: An individual patient date pooling analysis of clinical trials. *Stroke* 2002;33:2850-7.

12140 Adibhatla RM, Hatcher JF. Citicoline mechanisms and clinical efficacy in cerebral ischemia. *J Neurosci Res* 2002;70:133-9.

12141 FDA Warning Letter to Mr. Stephen Cheng, Window Rock Enterprises. August 19, 2004. Available at: http://www.fda.gov/foi/warning_letters/g4945d.htm. (Accessed 17 September 2004).

12142 Kris-Etherton PM, Lichtenstein AH, Howard BV, et al. AHA Science Advisory: Antioxidant vitamin supplements and cardiovascular disease. *Circulation* 2004;110:637-41.

12143 Maki T, Takahashi K, Shibata S. An anti-emetic principle of Pinellia ternata tuber. *Planta Med* 1987;53:410-4.

12144 Chen D, Wu CF, Huang L, Ning Z. Effect of the aqueous extract of Xiao-Ban-Xia-Tang on gastric emptying in mice. *Am J Chin Med* 2002;30:207-14.

12145 Kim SH, Jeong H, Kim YK, et al. IgE-mediated occupational asthma induced by herbal medicine, Bahna (Pinellia ternata). *Clin Exp Allergy* 2000;31:779-81.

12146 Nagai T, Kiyohara H, Munakata K, et al. Pinellic acid from the tuber of Pinellia ternata Breitenbach as an effective oral adjuvant for nasal influenza vaccine. *Int Immunopharmacol* 2002;2:1183-93.

12147 FDA, HHS. Final rule declaring dietary supplements containing ephedrine alkaloids adulterated because they present an unreasonable risk. *Fed Regist* 2004;69:6787-6854.

12148 Uebelhart D, Malaise M, Marcolongo R, et al. Intermittent treatment of knee osteoarthritis with oral chondroitin sulfate: A one-year, randomize, double-blind, multicenter study versus placebo. *Osteoarthritis Cartilage* 2004;12:269-76.

12149 Peres MFP, Zukerman E, da Cunha Tanuri F, et al. Melatonin, 3 mg, is effective for migraine prevention. *Neurology* 2004;63:757.

12150 Lange H, Suryapranata H, De Luca G, et al. Folate therapy and in-stent restenosis after coronary stenting. *N Engl J Med* 2004; 350:2673-81.

12151 Herrmann H. Prevention of cardiovascular events after percutaneous coronary intervention. *N Engl J Med* 2004;350:2708-10.

12152 Sauer J, Tabet N, Howard R. Alpha lipoic acid for dementia (Cochrane Review). In: The Cochrane Library, Issue 3, 2004. Chichester, UK: John Wiley & Sons, Ltd.

12153 Pittler MH, Ernst E. Feverfew for preventing migraine (Cochrane Review). In: The Cochrane Library, Issue 3, 2004. Chichester, UK: John Wiley & Sons, Ltd.

12154 Vanapalli SR, Chen Y, Ellingrod VL, et al. Orange juice decreases the oral bioavailability of ivermectin in health volunteers. *Clin Pharmacol Ther* 2003;73 (Abstract PDII-A-10):P94.

12155 Gorski JC, Huang S, Zaheer NA, et al. The effect of Echinacea on CYP3A activity in vivo. *Clin Pharmacol Ther* 2003;73 (Abstract PDII-A-8):P94.

12156 Norris FH, Denys EH. Nutritional supplements in amyotrophic lateral sclerosis. *Adv Exp Med Biol* 1987;209:183-9.

12158 Langmead L, Makins RJ, Rampton DS. Anti-inflammatory effects of aloe vera gel in human colorectal mucosa in vitro. *Aliment Pharmacol Ther* 2004;19:521-7.

12159 Olsen DL, Raub W, Bradley C, et al. The effect of aloe gel/mild soap versus mild soap alone in preventing skin reactions in patients undergoing radiation therapy. *Oncol Nurs Forum* 2001;28:543-7.

12160 Gallagher J, Gray M. Is aloe vera effective for healing chronic wounds? *J Wound Ostomy Continence Nurs* 2003;30:68-71.

12161 Kaufman T, Kalderon N, Ullmann Y, Berger J. Aloe vera gel hindered wound healing of experimental second-degree burns: a quantitative controlled study. *J Burn Care Rehabil* 1988;9:156-9.

12162 Miller MB, Koltai PJ. Treatment of experimental frostbite with pentoxifylline and aloe vera cream. *Arch Otolaryngol Head Neck Surg* 1995;121:678-80.

12163 Williams MS, Burk M, Loprinzi CL, et al. Phase III double-blind evaluation of an aloe vera gel as a prophylactic agent for radiation-induced skin toxicity. *Int J Radiat Oncol Biol Phys* 1996;36:345-9.

12164 Vogler BK, Ernst E. Aloe vera: a systematic review of its clinical effectiveness. *Br J Gen Pract* 1999;49:823-8.

12165 Bachmann HU, Hoffmann A. Interaction of food supplement L-carnitine with oral anticoagulant acenocoumarol. *Swiss Med Wkly* 2004;134:385.

12166 Lin Y, Rudrum M, van der Wielen RPJ, et al. Wheat germ policosanol failed to lower plasma cholesterol in subjects with normal to mildly elevated cholesterol concentrations. *Metabolism* 2004;53:1309-14.

12167 Numazawa M, Mutsumi A, Asano N, Ito Y. A time-dependent inactivation of aromatase by 19-substituted androst-4-ene-3,6,,17-triones. *Steroids* 1993;58:40-6.

12168 Covey DF, Hood WF. Enzyme-generated intermediates derived from 4-androstene-3,6,17-trione and 1,4,6-androstatriene-3,17-dione cause a time-dependent decrease

in human placental aromatase activity. *Endocrinology* 1981;108:1597-9.
12169 Balercia G, Mosca F, Mantero F, et al. Coenzyme Q10 supplementation in infertile men with idiopathic asthenozoospermia: an open, uncontrolled pilot study. *Fertil Steril* 2004;81:93-8.
12170 Berman M, Erman A, Ben-Gal T, et al. Coenzyme Q10 in patients with end-stage heart failure awaiting cardiac transplantation: a randomized, placebo-controlled study. *Clin Cardiol* 2004;27:295–9.
12171 Lee AN, Werth VP. Activation of autoimmunity following use of immunostimulatory herbal supplements. *Arch Dermatol* 2004;140:723-7.
12172 Oshio H, Tsukui M, Matsuoka T. Isolation of L-ephedrine from "Pinelliae Tuber." *Chem Pharm Bull* 1978;26:2096-7.
12173 Rejdak R, Toczolowski J, Krukowski J, et al. Oral citicoline treatment improves visual pathway function in glaucoma. *Med Sci Monit* 2003;9:PI24-8.
12175 Palevitch D, Earon G, Levin I. Treatment of benign prostatic hypertrophy with Opuntia ficus-indica (L.) Miller. *Int J Comp Alt Med* 1994;Sept:21-2.
12176 Moreno MDM. Cognitive improvement in mild to moderate Alzheimer's dementia after treatment with the acetylcholine precursor choline alfoscerate: A multicenter, double-blind, randomized, placebo-controlled trial. *Clin Ther* 2003;25:178-93
12177 Sedjo RL, Papenfuss MR, Craft NE, Guiliano AR. Effect of plasma micronutrients on clearance of oncogenic human papillomavirus (HPV) infection (United States). *Cancer Causes Control* 2003;14:319-26.
12178 Lyon AW, Mayhew WJ. Cesium toxicity: A case of self-treatment by alternate therapy gone awry. *Ther Drug Monit* 2003;25:114-6.
12179 Fukazawa I, Uchida N, Uchida E, Yasuhara H. Effects of grapefruit juice on the pharmacokinetics of atorvastatin and pravastatin in Japanese. *Br J Clin Pharmacol* 2003;57:448-55.
12251 Stratigos AJ, Arndt KA, Dover JS. Advances in cutaneous aesthetic surgery. *JAMA* 1998;280:1397-98.
12252 Anon. Dermatologists can help consumers find the best products to rejuvenate their skin. American Academy of Dermatology, 1999. Available at: http://www.aad.org/PressReleases/rejuvenate.html.
12253 Anon. Skin trauma: A tan is an early warning sign. American Academy of Dermatology, 1996. Available at: www.aad.org.PressReleases/PHOTOAGE.html.
12254 Drake LA, Dinehart SM, Farmer ER, et al. Guidelines of care for photoaging/photodamage. American Academy of Dermatology, 2000. Available at: www.aad.org/Guidelines/Photoagingdamage.html.
12255 Young LY, Koda-Kimble MA, eds. Photosensitivity and Burns. Applied Therapeutics: The Clinical Use of Drugs. 6th ed. Vancouver, WA: Applied Thera Inc., 1995.
12256 Davis WM. Antiaging products and tactics. *Drug Topics* 1997;17:92-101.
12257 McEvoy GK, ed. AHFS Drug Information. Bethesda, MD: American Society of Health-system Pharmacists, 2000.
12258 Anon. Cosmetic dermatology handbook. American Academy of Dermatology, 2000. Available at: www.aad.org/ss00/cosmetic.html.
12259 Song KH. Botulinum toxin type A injection for the treatment of frown lines. *Ann Pharmacother* 1998;32:1365-67.
12260 Anon. Alpha-hydroxy acids appear effective in improving skin appearance. American Academy of Dermatolog. 1997. Available at: www.aad.org/PressReleases/alpha.html.
12261 Anon. Adding vitamins to the mix: Skin care products that can benefit the skin. American Academy of Dermatology, 2000. Available at: www.aad.org/PressReleases/skincare.html.
12262 Anon. All dried out. American Academy of Dermatology, 2000. Available at: www.aad.org/ss98driedou.html.
12263 Anon. Mature skin. American Academy of Dermatology, 2000. Available at: www.aad.org/pamphlets/mature.html.
12264 Anon. Skin tips. American Academy of Dermatology, 1999. Available at: www.aad.org/ss99/stips.html.
12265 Katiyar SK, Mukhtar H. Tea antioxidants in cancer chemoprevention. *J Cell Biochem Suppl* 1997;27:59-67.
12276 Gray JA, Enz A, Spiegel R. Muscarinic agonists for senile dementia: past experience and future trends. *Trends Pharmacol Sci* 1989;Suppl:85-8.
12277 Harbaugh RE, Roberts DW, Coombs DW, et al. Preliminary report: intracranial cholinergic drug infusion in patients with Alzheimer's disease. *Neurosurgery* 1984;15:514-8.
12278 Harbaugh RE, Reeder TM, Senter HJ, et al. Intracerebroventricular bethanechol chloride infusion in Alzheimer's disease. Results of a collaborative double-blind study. *J Neurosurg* 1989;71:481-6.
12279 Bodick NC, Offen WW, Levey AI, et al. Effects of xanomeline, a selective muscarinic receptor agonist, on cognitive function and behavioral symptoms in Alzheimer disease. *Arch Neurol* 1997;54:465-73.
12280 Ott BR, Owens NJ. Complementary and alternative medicines for Alzheimer's disease. *J Geriatr Psychiatry Neurol* 1998;11:163-73..
12281 Higgins JP, Flicker L. Lecithin for dementia and cognitive impairment. *Cochrane Database Syst Rev* 2000;4:CD001015.
12282 Marsh GR, Linnoila M. The effects of deanol on cognitive performance and electrophysiology in elderly humans. *Psychopharmacology* (Berl) 1979;66:99-104.
12283 Behl C. Alzheimer's disease and oxidative stress: implications for novel therapeutic approaches. *Prog Neurobiol* 1999;57:301-23.
12284 Markesbery WR, Carney JM. Oxidative alterations in Alzheimer's disease. *Brain Pathol* 1999;9:133-46.
12285 Floyd RA. Neuroinflammatory processes are important in neurodegenerative diseases: an hypothesis to explain the increased formation of reactive oxygen and nitrogen species as major factors involved in neurodegenerative disease development. *Free Radic Biol Med* 1999;26:1346-55.
12286 Rosler M, Retz W, Thome J, Riederer P. Free radicals in Alzheimer's dementia: currently available therapeutic strategies. *J Neural Transm* Suppl 1998;54:211-9.
12287 Perrig WJ, Perrig P, Stahelin HB. The relation between antioxidants and memory performance in the old and very old. *J Am Geriatr Soc* 1997;45:718-24.
12288 McCaddon A, Davies G, Hudson P, et al. Total serum homocysteine in senile dementia of Alzheimer type. *Int J Geriatr Psychiatry* 1998;13:235-9.
12289 Clarke R, Smith AD, Jobst KA, et al. Folate, vitamin B12, and serum total homocysteine levels in confirmed Alzheimer disease. *Arch Neurol* 1998;55:1449-55.
12290 Ebly EM, Schaefer JP, Campbell NR, Hogan DB. Folate status, vascular disease and cognition in elderly Canadians. *Age Ageing* 1998;27:485-91.
12291 Wynn M, Wynn A. The danger of B12 deficiency in the elderly. *Nutr Health* 1998;12:215-26.
12292 Schumacher M, Robel P, Baulieu EE. Development and regeneration of the nervous system: a role for neurosteroids. *Dev Neurosci* 1996;18:6-21.
12293 Baulieu EE. Neurosteroids: of the nervous system, by the nervous system, for the nervous system. *Recent Prog Horm Res* 1997;52:1-32.
12294 Danenberg HD, Haring R, Fisher A, et al. Dehydroepiandrosterone (DHEA) increases production and

release of Alzheimer's amyloid precursor protein. *Life Sci* 1996;59:1651-7.
12295 Majewska MD. Neuronal actions of dehydroepiandrosterone. Possible roles in brain development, aging, memory, and affect. *Ann N Y Acad Sci* 1995;774:111-20.
12296 Sunderland T, Merril CR, Harrington MG, et al. Reduced plasma dehydroepiandrosterone concentrations in Alzheimer's disease. *Lancet* 1989;2:570.
12297 Nasman B, Olsson T, Backstrom T, et al. Serum dehydroepiandrosterone sulfate in Alzheimer's disease and in multi-infarct dementia. *Biol Psychiatry* 1991;30:684-90.
12298 Leblhuber F, Neubauer C, Peichl M, et al. Age and sex differences of dehydroepiandrosterone sulfate (DHEAS) and cortisol (CRT) plasma levels in normal controls and Alzheimer's disease (AD). *Psychopharmacology* (Berl) 1993;111:23-6.
12299 Kleijnen J, Knipschild P. Ginkgo biloba. *Lancet* 1992;340:1136-9.
12300 Tamaki N, Kusunoki T, Matsumoto S. The effect of vinpocetine on cerebral blood flow in patients with cerebrovascular disorders. *Ther Hung* 1985;33:13-21.
12301 Brown D, Gaby A, Reichert R, et al. Dementia and age-related cognitive decline. *Journal of Naturopathic Medicine* 1998;8:26-41.
12302 Dysken M. A review of recent clinical trials in the treatment of Alzheimer's dementia. *Psychiatric Annals* 1987;17: 178.
12303 Lobay D. Alzheimer's disease: an overview for clinical practice. *Journal of Naturopathic Medicine* 1998;6:77-84.
12304 Chen CL, Muller DC, Andres R, et al. A prospective study of plasma levels of alpha-tocopherol (vitamin E), beta-carotene, and ascorbic acid (vitamin C) and risk of developing Alzheimer's disease in the Baltimore Longitudinal Study of Aging. *Neurology* 1998;50:A231-32.
12305 Kwok T, Tang C, Woo J, et al. Randomized trial of the effect of supplementation on the cognitive function of older people with subnormal cobalamin levels. *Int J Geriatr Psychiatry* 1998;13:611-6.
12306 Leblhuber F, Neubauer C, Peichl M, et al. Age and sex differences of dehydroepiandrosterone sulfate (DHEAS) and cortisol (CRT) plasma levels in normal controls and Alzheimer's disease (AD). *Psychopharmacology* 1993;111:23-6.
12307 Otomo E, Atarashi J, Araki G, et al. Comparison of Vinpocetin with ifenprodil tartrate and dihydroergotoxine mesylate treatment and results of long-term treatment with Vinpocetine. *Curr Therapeutic Res* 1985;37:811-821.
12309 Foster S. Ginkgo Biloba. Austin: American Botanical Council, 1996.
12310 Rosenwasser LJ. Treatment of allergic rhinitis. *Am J Med* 2002;113:17S-24S.
12351 Lin A, Nguy CH, Shic F, Ross BD. Accumulation of methylsulfonylmethane in the human brain: identification by multinuclear magnetic resonance spectroscopy. *Toxicol Lett* 2001;123:169-77.
12352 Lenzi A, Sgro P, Salacone P, et al. A placebo-controlled double-blind randomized trial of the use of combined l-carnitine and l-acetyl-carnitine treatment in men with asthenozoospermia. *Fertil Steril* 2004;81:1578-84.
12353 Cavallini G, Caracciolo S, Vitali G, et al. Carnitine versus androgen administration in the treatment of sexual dysfunction, depressed mood, and fatigue associated with male aging. *Urology* 2004;63:641-6.
12354 Sperber SJ, Shah LP, Gilbert RD, et al. Echinacea purpurea for prevention of experimental rhinovirus colds. *Clin Infect Dis* 2004;38:1367-71.
12355 Goel V, Lovlin R, Barton R, et al. Efficacy of a standardized echinacea preparation (Echinilin) for the treatment of the common cold: a randomized, double-blind, placebo-controlled trial. *J Clin Pharm Ther* 2004;29:75-83.
12356 George SA, Bilsland DJ, Wainwright NJ, Ferguson J. Failure of coconut oil to accelerate psoriasis clearance in narrow-band UVB phototherapy or photochemotherapy. *Br J Dermatol* 1993;128:301-5.
12357 Laureles LR, Rodriguez FM, Reano CE, et al. Variability in fatty acid and triacylglycerol composition of the oil of coconut (Cocos nucifera L.) hybrids and their parentals. *J Agric Food Chem* 2002;50:1581-6.
12358 Mendis S, Samarajeewa U, Thattil RO. Coconut fat and serum lipoproteins: effects of partial replacement with unsaturated fats. *Br J Nutr* 2001;85:583-9.
12359 Teuber SS, Peterson WR. Systemic allergic reaction to coconut (Cocos nucifera) in 2 subjects with hypersensitivity to tree nut and demonstration of cross-reactivity to legumin-like seed storage proteins: new coconut and walnut food allergens. *J Allergy Clin Immunol* 1999;103:1180-5.
12360 Tella R, Gaig P, Lombardero M, et al. A case of coconut allergy. *Allergy* 2003;58:825-6.
12361 Reiser R, Probstfield JL, Silvers A, et al. Plasma lipid and lipoprotein response of humans to beef fat, coconut oil and safflower oil. *Am J Clin Nutr* 1985;42:190-7.
12362 Alexaki A, Wilson TA, Atallah MT, et al. Hamsters fed diets high in saturated fat have increased cholesterol accumulation and cytokine production in the aortic arch compared with cholesterol-fed hamsters with moderately elevated plasma non-HDL cholesterol concentrations. *J Nutr* 2004;134:410-5.
12363 Muller H, Lindman AS, Blomfeldt A, et al. A diet rich in coconut oil reduces diurnal postprandial variations in circulating tissue plasminogen activator antigen and fasting lipoprotein (a) compared with a diet rich in unsaturated fat in women. *J Nutr* 2003;133:3422-7.
12366 Latha M, Pari L. Antihyperglycaemic effect of Cassia auriculata in experimental diabetes and its effects on key metabolic enzymes involved in carbohydrate metabolism. *Clin Exp Pharmacol Physiol* 2003;30:38-43.
12367 Pari L, Latha M. Effect of Cassia auriculata flowers on blood sugar levels, serum and tissue lipids in streptozotocin diabetic rats. *Singapore Med J* 2002;43:617-21.
12368 Sabu MC, Subburaju T. Effect of Cassia auriculata Linn. on serum glucose level, glucose utilization by isolated rat hemidiaphragm. *J Ethnopharmacol* 2002;80:203-6.
12369 Abesundara KJ, Matsui T, Matsumoto K. alpha-Glucosidase inhibitory activity of some Sri Lanka plant extracts, one of which, Cassia auriculata, exerts a strong antihyperglycemic effect in rats comparable to the therapeutic drug acarbose. *J Agric Food Chem* 2004;52:2541-5.
12370 Pari L, Ramakrishnan R, Venkateswaran S. Antihyperglycaemic effect of Diamed, a herbal formulation, in experimental diabetes in rats. *J Pharm Pharmacol* 2001;53:1139-43.
12371 Latha M, Pari L. Preventive effects of Cassia auriculata L. flowers on brain lipid peroxidation in rats treated with streptozotocin. *Mol Cell Biochem* 2003;243:23-8.
12372 Kumar Rajagopal S, Manickam P, Periyasamy V, Namasivayam N. Activity of Cassia auriculata leaf extract in rats with alcoholic liver injury. *J Nutr Biochem* 2003;14:452-8.
12373 Thabrew I, Munasinghe J, Chackrewarthi S, Senarath S. The effects of Cassia auriculata and Cardiospermum halicacabum teas on the steady state blood level and toxicity of carbamazepine. *J Ethnopharmacol* 2004;90:145-50.
12374 Lane JD, Barkauskas CE, Surwit RS, Feinglos MN. Caffeine impairs glucose metabolism in type 2 diabetes. *Diabetes Care* 2004;27:2047-8.
12375 Petrie HJ, Chown SE, Belfie LM, et al. Caffeine ingestion increases the insulin response to an oral-glucose-tolerance

test in obese men before and after weight loss. *Am J Clin Nutr* 2004;80:22-8.

12376 Kim KW, Kim HD, Jung JS, et al. Characterization of antidepressant-like effects of p-synephrine stereoisomers. *Naunyn Schmiedebergs Arch Pharmacol* 2001;364:21-6.

12377 Song DK, Suh HW, Jung JS, et al. Antidepressant-like effects of p-synephrine in mouse models of immobility tests. *Neurosci Lett* 1996;214:107-10.

12378 Suzuki O, Matsumoto T, Oya M, Katsumata Y. Oxidation of synephrine by type A and type B monoamine oxidase. *Experientia* 1979;35:1283-4.

12379 Andrew R, Best SA, Watson DG, et al. Analysis of biogenic amines in plasma of hypertensive patients and a control group. *Neurochem Res* 1993;18:1179-82.

12380 Poolsup N, Suthisisang C, Prathanturarug S, et al. Andrographis paniculata in the symptomatic treatment of uncomplicated upper respiratory tract infection: systematic review of randomized controlled trials. *J Clin Pharm Ther* 2004;29:37-45.

12381 Spasov AA, Ostrovskij OV, Chernikov MV, Wikman G. Comparative controlled study of Andrographis paniculata fixed combination, Kan Jang and an Echinacea preparation as adjuvant, in the treatment of uncomplicated respiratory disease in children. *Phytother Res* 2004;18:47-53.

12382 Amaryan G, Astvatsatryan V, Gabrielyan E, et al. Double-blind, placebo-controlled, randomized, pilot clinical trial of ImmunoGuard--a standardized fixed combination of Andrographis paniculata Nees, with Eleutherococcus senticosus Maxim, Schizandra chinensis Bail. and Glycyrrhiza glabra L. extracts in patients with Familial Mediterranean Fever. *Phytomedicine* 2003;10:271-85.

#100 Abc Acidophilus/Bifidum Complex **-** Systemic Formulas
Each capsule contains: A minimum of one billion Lactobacillus acidophilus (NAS strain) and one billion Bifidobacterium bifidum (Malyoth strain) uniquely suspended in an anaerobic, sunflower oil matrix containing vitamin E as a natural antioxidant.

#101 ACP Vitamin ACP **-** Systemic Formulas
Rose Hips • Orange peel • Bone Meal • Vitamin C • RNA/DNA Liver Factors • Lemon Bioflavonoid • Vitamin E • RNA/DNA Thymus Factors • Pedra Hume Ca • Acacia Gum flower • Vitamin A.
See Editor's Note No. 14, page 2055.

#102 ACX Vitamin Detox **-** Systemic Formulas
Rose Hips • Vitamin C • RNA/DNA Liver Factors • Lemon Bioflavonoid • Pimiento • Vitamin E • Damiana • Pedra Hume Ca • RNA/DNA Thymus Factors • Vitamin A • Acacia Gum Flower • Hesperidin • RNA/DNA Spleen Factors • Peach Bark • Sun Dew.
See Editor's Note No. 14, page 2055.

#111 AZV Multi-Vitamin and Mineral Supplement **-** Systemic Formulas
RNA/DNA Liver Factors • Rose Hips • Kelp • Linseed Oil • Vitamin A • Vitamin D • Vitamin E • Vitamin C • Calcium • Niacin • Phosphorus • Iron • Vitamin B1 (Thiamine) • Vitamin B2 (Riboflavin) • Magnesium • Vitamin B6 (Pyridoxine HCl) • Pantothenic Acid • Potassium • Zinc • Manganese • Vitamin B12 (Cyanocobalamin) • Lemon Bioflavonoid • Autolyzed RNA/DNA .
See Editor's Note No. 14, page 2055.

#115 BSV Vitamin B Stress Complex **-** Systemic Formulas
Abutua • Centaury • Red Bone Marrow • Nettle • Poke Root • Spearmint • RNA/DNA Liver Factors and Parotid Factors • Guarana • Vitamin B2 • Fringe Tree • Choline Bitartrate • Inositol • Niacinamide • PABA • Vitamin B1 • Calcium Pantothenate • Vitamin B6 • Niacin • Vitamin B12 • Folic Acid • Biotin.
See Editor's Note No. 14, page 2055.

#12 B Brain **-** Systemic Formulas
RNA/DNA Brain Factors • Italian Pimiento • L-Alanine • Stevia • Tayuya • Vitamin B2 • Rutin • Niacin • Vitamin B6 • L-Glutamic Acid • Hydroxyproline • L-Proline • RNA/DNA Pituitary Factors • RNA/DNA Thalamus Factors.
See Editor's Note No. 14, page 2055.

#120 CAL Calcium Plus **-** Systemic Formulas
Calcium (from Citrate, Lactate, Hydroxide, Bone Meal, Bone Ash, Carbonate, Oyster Shell, Lysinate, Methionate, and Aspartate) • Lecithin • Magnesium Oxide • Vitamin C • Vitamin E • Trace Minerals • Iron Chelate • Copper Carbonate • Vitamin D • Betaine HCl • Boron Chelate.

#126 CTV Vitamin C Therapeutic **-** Systemic Formulas
Ascorbic Acid • Sodium Ascorbate • Beta-carotene (source of Vit. A) • Sago Palm • Calcium Ascorbate • Calcium Carbonate • Bioflavonoids • Potassium Bitartrate • Hesperidin • Rose Hips • Thymol Iodide.

#130 EZV 200 IU Vitamin E **-** Systemic Formulas
Lactose • Fructose • Vitamin E • Honey Bake.

#132 FLX Vegetable Omega-3 Flaxseed Oil **-** Systemic Formulas
Superunsaturate (Alphalinolenic Acid, Omega-3) • Polyunsaturate (Linoleic Acid, Omega-6) • Monounsaturate (Oleic Acid) • Saturated Fatty Acid • Beta Carotene • Vitamin E • Phytosterols • Lecithin • Traces of Fiber.

#134 LEV Lecithin **-** Systemic Formulas
Lecithin • Inositol • Choline • Phospholipids.

#14 Colon **-** Systemic Formulas
Psyllium Husks • Cascara Sagrada • Licorice Root • Peach Bark • Stillingia • Dolomite • Calcium Carbonate • Citric Acid • Potassium Bicarbonate.

#140 Min Multi-Mineral Plus **-** Systemic Formulas
Great Salt Lake Water • Calcium Carbonate • Horse Tail • Magnesium Oxide • Calcium Lactate • Calcium Citrate • Irish Moss • Magnesium Chloride • Red Root • Zinc Chelate • Kelp • Manganese Chelate • Iron Chelate • Vitamin C • Iron Aspartate • Potassium Bitartrate • Copper Chelate • Manganese Picolinate • Zinc Picolinate • Molybdenum Chelate • Vanadium Chelate • Chromium Chelate • Selenium Chelate.

#150 PRO Nutro Protein **-** Systemic Formulas
Whey Protein • Pasteurized Saccharomyces Cerevisiae • Rice Protein • Green Lipped Mussel • RNA/DNA Trachea Factors • Dolomite • Dulse • Pimiento • Choline • Papain • Horse Tail (source of silica) • Niacin • Pancreatin Enzyme • Vitamin C • Tyrosine • Valine • Aspartic Acid • Cystine • Methionine • Vitamin B6 • Vitamin E • RNA/DNA Thalamus Factors.
See Editor's Note No. 14, page 2055.

#155 PTM Potassium Stabilizer **-** Systemic Formulas
Potassium Bitartrate • Potassium Chloride • Magnesium Oxide • Boldo • Pfaffia • Kelp • Maracuja • Chamomile.

#17 D Digestive **-** Systemic Formulas
Pancrelipase Enzyme • Golden Seal • RNA/DNA Oxbile Factors • Aspartic Acid • Betaine HCl • L-Glutamic Acid • Echinacea • Lipase • Amylase • Protease • Pepsin • Ammonium Chloride.
See Editor's Note No. 14, page 2055.

#18 DS Digestive Stabilizer **-** Systemic Formulas
Kola Nut • Pancrelipase Enzyme • RNA/DNA Oxbile Factors • Betaine HCl • Echinacea • Glutamic Acid • Spearmint • RNA/DNA Liver Factors • Calcium • Papaya leaves • Golden Seal • Aspartic Acid • Ammonium Chloride • Pancreatin Enzyme • Gentian root • Guava powder • Bromelain • Pepsin 1/3000.
See Editor's Note No. 14, page 2055.

#22 F+ Female Plus **-** Systemic Formulas
Sarsaparilla • Blue Cohosh • Dong Quai • Tayuya • False Unicorn • Cana do Brejo • Carrapichinho • Pfaffia • Motherwort • Balm Mint • Agoniada.

#31 GA Adrenal **-** Systemic Formulas
RNA/DNA Adrenal Factors • Echinacea • Vitamin C • D-Calcium Pantothenate • Inositol • Ma Huang • Sete Sangrias • RNA/DNA Spleen Factors • Zinc Chelate • Selenium Aspartate.
See Editor's Note No. 30, page 2056.

#32 GB Pituitary **-** Systemic Formulas
RNA/DNA Brain Factors • Whey Protein • RNA/DNA Pituitary Factors • Peach Bark • Jaborandi • RNA/DNA Orchic Factors • L-Methionine • Vitamin B6 • Superoxidedismutase.
See Editor's Note No. 14, page 2055.

#39 GF Thyroid **-** Systemic Formulas
Irish Moss • Thyroid-6x dilution • Pata de Vaca • Abutua Kelp • Cucurbita Pepo • RNA/DNA Lung Factors • RNA/DNA Thymus Factors.
See Editor's Note No. 14, page 2055.

#400 APHA pH Control **-** Systemic Formulas
Rhubarb Root • Spearmint • Calcium Carbonate • Nettle • Seaweed • Hyssop • Shave Grass • RNA/DNA Adrenal Factors • Potassium Bitartrate.
See Editor's Note No. 14, page 2055.

#402 ARTA Arthro Support **-** Systemic Formulas
Chapu de Couro • Spearmint Leaves • Pomegranate • Vitamin B2 • RNA/DNA Adrenal Factors • Potassium Bitartrate • Magnesium Sulfate • Vitamin B6 • Niacin • Chaparral • Mistletoe • Yucca • Tayuya • Burdock Seed • Lysine • Isoleucine • Methionine •

Magnesium Chelate • RNA/DNA Pituitary Factors • Zinc Chelate • Chromium Chelate.
See Editor's Note No. 14, page 2055.

#403 ATAK Shield Rejuvenator - Systemic Formulas
Pau d'Arco • Yarrow • Stevia • Calcium Carbonate • Betaine HCl • Tayuya • Gravel Root • Pimpinella Root • Yellow Dock • Echinacea • Rose Hips.

#405 BLDB Blood Builder - Systemic Formulas
RNA/DNA Blood Factors • Burdock • RNA/DNA Liver Factors • Wahoo • RNA/DNA Spleen Factors • L-Cystine • L-Leucine • Chlorophyll.
See Editor's Note No. 14, page 2055.

#408 CLNZ Toxin Chelator - Systemic Formulas
Dandelion Root • Pfaffia • Cinquefoil • Milk Thistle • Mountain Mahogany • Yucca • Vitamin E • Wahoo • RNA/DNA Liver Factors • L-Methionine.
See Editor's Note No. 14, page 2055.

#41 GT Thymus - Systemic Formulas
Vitamin C • Sweet Basil • Golden Seal • RNA/DNA Thymus Factors • Poke Root • Pau d'Arco • RNA/DNA Liver Factors and Lung Factors • Calcium Carbonate • Zinc Aspartate • RNA/DNA Spleen Factors • Magnesium Chloride • Bitter Root • Beta Carotene • Thymol Iodide • RNA/DNA Stomach Factors • Selenium Yeast • Chromium Chelate • Vitamin B2 • Inositol • Niacinamide • PABA • Vitamin B1 • Calcium Pantothenate • Vitamin B6 • Niacin • Vitamin B12 • Folic Acid • Biotin.
See Editor's Note No. 14, page 2055.

#425 DIJS Stomach Antacid - Systemic Formulas
Oregon Grape • Golden Seal • Spearmint • Sodium Bicarbonate • Potassium Bitartrate • Sodium Chloride • Spearmint Oil • Anise Oil • Potassium Bicarbonate • Sodium Citrate • Malt Diastase • Chlorophyll.

#428 DSIR Digestant Internal Regenerator - Systemic Formulas
RNA/DNA Stomach and Duodenal Factors • Echinacea • Rose Hips • Ma Huang • Stevia • Allantoin • RNA/DNA Thymus Factors • Hesperidin • Vitamin C • L-Methionine • Senna Pod • L-Glutamic Acid • Vitamin A • Pau d'Arco • Vitamin B6 • Spearmint Oil • Aloe Vera • Sodium Copper Chlorophyll.
See Editor's Note No. 30, page 2056.

#435 Gold Shield Plus - Systemic Formulas
Golden Seal • Niacin • Vitamin B6 • Rose Hips • Vitamin C • Fenugreek • Garlic • Vitamin B1 • Elder Berry • Spearmint Oil • Lomatium Dissecutim.

#44 H Heart - Systemic Formulas
RNA/DNA Heart Factors • Lecithin • Chromium Chelate • Phenylalanine • Sete Sangrias • Tayuya • RNA/DNA Thymus Factors • Woodruff • RNA/DNA Spleen Factors • Tyrosine • Vitamin B2 • Carnitine • Vitamin B1 • Niacin • Vitamin B6 • Calcium (from Pantothenate) • Folic Acid • Biotin.
See Editor's Note No. 14, page 2055.

#45 HCV Heart Cardio Vascular - Systemic Formulas
Sete Sangrias • RNA/DNA Heart Factors • Pimiento • Cassia Bark • Stevia • Hawthorne berries • Potassium Bitartrate.

#450 KDIR Diuretic - Systemic Formulas
Manganese Chelate • Ch de Bugre • Juniper berry • Peach bark • Saw Palmetto • Zinc Aminoate • Magnesium Sulfate • Peach leaves • Uva Ursi.

#46 HN Heart Nerve - Systemic Formulas
RNA/DNA Brain and Spleen Factors • Hesperidin • RNA/DNA Lung Factors • Calcium Pantothenate • Niacin • Tayuya • Vitamin B2 • L-Threonine • RNA/DNA Aorta Factors • L-Methionine • Selenium Chelate • RNA/DNA Heart Factors • Beta Carotene • Chromium Chelate.
See Editor's Note No. 14, page 2055.

#460 KYRO Muscle/Ligament/Tissue Strengthener - Systemic Formulas
Orange peel • Beta Carotene • Collagen • Bone Meal • Pfaffia • Vitamin C • Manganese Chelate • Slippery Elm • RNA/DNA Liver Factors • Vitamin B12 • Sete Sangrias • Vitamin E • Lemon Bioflavonoid • Pimiento • RNA/DNA Heart Factors • Hesperidin • Stevia • Cassia bark • Potassium Bitartrate • Vitamin A • Hawthorne berry.

#481 OXAA Cell Organizer - Systemic Formulas
Centaury herb • Red Clover blossom • Peach bark • Stillingia • Buckthorn bark • Oregon Grape • Cascara Sagrada • Prickly Ash bark • Cinquefoil • Saw Palmetto • Burdock root.

#482 OXCC Cell Cleanser - Systemic Formulas
Choke Cherry • Irish Moss • Pimiento • Blessed Thistle • Peach Bark • Oregon Grape • Fringe Tree • Red Clover • Burdock root.

#483 OXOX Cell Activator - Systemic Formulas
Fenugreek • Cyani Petals • Pulsatilla • Mandrake • Myrrh Gum • Gentian Root • Primrose • Pfaffia • Bugleweed • Barberry • Prickly Ash • Golden Seal • Blue Vervain • Catnip • Allantoin • Comfrey Root.

#486 SENG Red Ginseng Plus - Systemic Formulas
Red Ginseng • Pasteurized Saccharomyces Cerevisiae • Potassium Phosphate • Yucca • Chaparral.

#488 VIVI Anti Viro - Systemic Formulas
Pau D'Arco • Lomatium Dissecutim Oil • Vitamin E.

#491 VRM1 Large Pathogens - Systemic Formulas
Pau d'Arco • Rose Hips • Garlic • Valerian Root • Hops • Bromelain • Zapilopatle Beans • Hojas de Jalapa • Dolomite • Worm Seed Oil.

#492 VRM2 Small Pathogens - Systemic Formulas
Black Walnut Husks • Wormseed Herb • Kamala • Quassia Chips • Bromelain Enzyme • Bethyl Nut.

#493 VRM3 Micro Pathogens - Systemic Formulas
Black Walnut Husks • Carrapichinho • Erva Tostao • Aniz Estrelado • Bromelain Enzyme • Worm Seed Oil • Yerba Santa.

#494 VRM4 Cellular Pathogens - Systemic Formulas
Kamala • Guarana • Carrapichinho • Maracuj • Wormseed Herb • Papain • Alfazema.

#50 I Eyes - Systemic Formulas
Rue Herb • Eye Bright • Vitamin A • Vitamin E • Chap'u de Couro • Proline • Cystine • RNA/DNA Eye Factors • Vitamin B6 • Valine • Niacin • RNA/DNA Brain Factors.
See Editor's Note No. 14, page 2055.

#58 Ks Kidney Stabilizer - Systemic Formulas
Rose Hips • Gelatin • RNA/DNA Kidney Factors • Magnesium Sulfate • Juniper Berries • Vitamin C • Sete Sangrias • Spearmint Herb • Calcium Carbonate, Hesperidin Complex • Serine • Phenylalanine • RNA/DNA Adrenal and Thalamus Factors • Tyrosine • Vitamin A • Sodium Copper Chlorophyll.
See Editor's Note No. 14, page 2055.

#60 L Liver - Systemic Formulas
RNA/DNA Liver Factors • Mountain Mahogany • Spearmint Leaves • Vitamin A • Vitamin D • Ragweed • Golden Seal • Quince Seed • Boldo • Vitamin C • Vitamin E.
See Editor's Note No. 14, page 2055.

#61 LB Liver Normalizer - Systemic Formulas
Red Beet • Betaine HCl • Choline Bitartrate • Lipase 24.

#62 LS Liver Stimulant - Systemic Formulas
Rose Hips • Vitamin C • Chromium Chelate • Magnesium Chelate • Red Beet • Sete Sangrias • Ch de Bugre • Potassium Chelate • RNA/DNA Adrenal Factors • Choline Bitartrate • Iron Chelate • RNA/DNA Thymus Factors • Vitamin A • RNA/DNA Pituitary and Liver Factors.
See Editor's Note No. 14, page 2055.

#70 M+ Male Endocrine - Systemic Formulas
RNA/DNA Orchic Factors • Hops • Boldo (from Chile) • Cipó Caboclo • Abacateiro • Agoniada • Chinese Bamboo • Cipó Cravo • RNA/DNA Prostate Factors • African Yohimbe • Eucalyptus • Catuaba • Muirapuama.
See Editor's Note No. 14, page 2055.

#72 Mpc Prostata Corrector - Systemic Formulas
Cucurbita Pepo Oil • Pau D'Arco • RNA/DNA Prostate Factors • Gingko Leaves • Pau D'Alho • RNA/DNA Orchic, Thymus, Pituitary & Hypothalamus Factors • Golden Seal • Echinacea Purpurea • Thyme.
See Editor's Note No. 14, page 2055.

#73 Mpr Prostata Ovatum - Systemic Formulas
Cucurbita Pepo Oil.

#75 N3 Anti-Tensive - Systemic Formulas
Tayuya • Blue Vervain • Valerian Root Extract • Senna Leaves • L-Methionine • Passion Flower Extract • Calcium Chelate • Saw Palmetto • Sete Sangrias • Mandrake Root • Ephedra • Tyrosine.
See Editor's Note No. 30, page 2056.

#77 NC Calm - Systemic Formulas
Calcium Carbonate • Dulse • Passion Flowers • Muirapuama • RNA/DNA Brain Factors • Tayuya • Boldo • Selenium Chelate • RNA/DNA Spleen and Lung Factors • Valerian • Niacin • Vitamin B12 • Vitamin B2 • Vitamin B1.
See Editor's Note No. 14, page 2055.

#78 P Pancreas - Systemic Formulas
RNA/DNA Pancreas Factors • Catuaba • Cynita Cactus • Japecanga • Pata de Vaca • Pedra Hume Ca • Zinc Oxide.
See Editor's Note No. 14, page 2055.

#79 Ps Pancreas Stabilizer - Systemic Formulas
RNA/DNA Pancreas Factors • Catuaba • Cynita Cactus • Japecanga • Pata de Vaca • Pedra Hume Ca • Zinc Oxide.
See Editor's Note No. 14, page 2055.

#80 R Lung - Systemic Formulas
Golden Seal • RNA/DNA Lung Factors • Pancreatin 4x • RNA/DNA Thymus Factors • L-Lysine • Aspartic Acid • Allantoin • Tayuya • Aloe Vera.
See Editor's Note No. 14, page 2055.

#82 S Spleen - Systemic Formulas
RNA/DNA Spleen Factors • Pedra Hume Ca • Nettle • Sweet Gum Tree • RNA/DNA Liver Factors and Pancreas Factors • Lysine • L-Methionine • Leucine • Isoleucine.
See Editor's Note No. 14, page 2055.

#FPMS Female Premenses Syndrome - Systemic Formulas
Vitamin B6 • Cystine • Vitamin A • Magnesium Sulfate • Vitamin E • L-Thionine • Muirapuama • Blue Malva • Pata de Vaca • RNA/DNA Pituitary Factors • L-Methionine • RNA/DNA Duodenal Factors • Choline • Motherwort • Angelica • Cyani Blossoms • Niacin • Inositol • Histidine • Superoxidedismutase • Dong Quai • Zinc Chelate • Vitamin B12 • Octacosanol.
See Editor's Note No. 14, page 2055.

@zit.gone - Pacific BioLogic
Kochia fruit • Licorice root • Phellodendron bark • Coptis rhizome • Chrysanthemum flower • Forsythia fruit • Ophiopogonis tuber • Rehmannia root (fresh) • Trichosanthis root • Scrophularia root.

10 Mushroom Combination - Olympia Nutrition
Contains: Cordyceps, Reishi, Maitake, Shitake, Poria, Polyporus, Coriolus, Tremella, Hericium, and Wood Ear mushrooms.

10% Plus Nighttime Cream - Jason
Alpha Hydroxy Acids.

100% ANY WHEY Protein - Optimum Nutrition
Each scoop (20.5 g) contains: Protein Blend: Whey Protein Isolate, Whey Protein Concentrate, Whey Protein Hydrosylate • Natural Flavor.

100% Egg Protein - Healthy 'N Fit Nutritionals
100% pure extracted egg albumen (with a protein efficiency ratio of 3.9 or greater), enzymatic digest of egg albumia containing naturally occurring amino acids, vanilla flavoring, bromelain and papain.

100% Egg Protein - Optimum Nutrition
Each scoop (29.4 g) contains: Egg Albumen • Cocoa • Artificial Flavor • Lecithin • Sucralose.

100% Natural Vitamin E - Basic Nutrition - GNC
Each capsule contains: Vitamin E (as d-alpha Tocopheryl Acetate) 400 IU. Other Ingredients: Soybean oil, Gelatin, Glycerin.

100% Natural Whey Protein - Optimum Nutrition
Each scoop (31.4 g) contains: Stevia leaf extract (stevia rebaudiana, standardized to 90% steviosides) 70 mg • Enzyme Blend 10 mg: Aminogen, Lactase (standardized to 100,000 FCC units/g) • Protein Blend: Whey Protein Isolate, Whey Protein Concentrate, Whey Peptides • Cocoa • Fructose • Lecithin • Natural Flavor.

100% Whey Protein - Optimum Nutrition
Each scoop (28.4 g) contains: Enzyme Blend 10 mg: Aminogen, Lactase (standardized to 100,000 FCC units/g) • Protein Blend: Whey Protein Concentrate, Whey Protein Isolate, Whey Peptides • Natural and Artificial Flavor, Lecithin, Acesulfame Potassium • Salt.

1000 mg MSM, Bones and Joints - CVS Pharmacy
Each tablet contains: MSM 1000 mg. Other Ingredients: Cellulose, Stearic Acid, Magnesium Stearate, Silicon Dioxide.

1000-K Alternative Formula - Douglas Laboratories
Each caplet contains: Proprietary Blend >1000 mg: Alpha-Carotene, Beta-Carotene, Bioflavonoids, Burdock, Astragalus, Echinacea Angustifolia, Echinacea Purpurea, Evening Primrose oil (dry), Ellagic Acid (cherries), GLA (borage seed oil, dry), Genistein (isoflavone), Ginger root, L-Glutathione, Grape seed extract, Green Tea extract, Glycyrrhetinic Acid, Lignans, Ligusticum, Lutein, Lycopene, Maitake, Shitake, and Reishi Mushrooms, Quercetin, Pectin (apple), Nucleic acids (RNA and DNA), Cartilage powder (bovine and shark), Sesame seed powder, Cruciferous Vegetables (broccoli, cabbage, cauliflower, kale), Solanaceous Foods (tomatoes, peppers, eggplant), Umbelliferous Vegetables (carrots, celery, parsnips).
See Editor's Note No. 14, page 2055.

12-1/2% Plus with SPF 12-1/2 Protective Moisturizer - Jason
Antioxidant Ester-C • Vita`min E.

19-Nor 250 - AST Sports Science
Each capsule contains: 19-Norandrostenedione 250 mg.

19-Nor Andro 100 - Metabolic Response Modifiers
Each capsule contains: 19-norandrostenedione (19-nor-4-androstene-3, 17-dione) 100 mg.

19-Nor - Metabolic Response Modifiers
Two capsules contain: 19-norandrostenedione 100 mg • 19-nor-4-androstene-3, 17-diol 100 mg • 5-androstenediol 50 mg.

19-Nor-3-Andro - AST Sports Science
Each capsule contains: 19-Norandrostenedione 100 mg • Androstenediol 100 mg • Androstenedione 100 mg.
See Editor's Note No. 47, page 2058.

BRAND NAMES

1-AD **-** ErgoPharm
Each capsule contains: 1-Androstene-3beta, 17beta-diol 100 mg. Other Ingredients: Gelatin, Microcrystalline Cellulose, Modified Cornstarch, Magnesium Stearate, Silica.

1-Testabolin **-** BSN Inc.
Each capsule contains: 17-Hydroxy-5-Alpha-Androst-1-ene-3-one-ECMM (ether carbon molecular modification) 75 mg • Clomitrophin-Q (cissus quadragularis) 150 mg • Kre-Alkalyn 334 mg. Other Ingredients: Magnesium Stearate, Magnesium Silicate, Gelatine, Syloid, White Rice.

1-TU **-** Nutrex, Inc.
Each liqui-cap contains: 1-TU Proprietary Blend 50 mg: 5-Androst-1-Ene-3-One-17-8-Undecanoate, Oleic Acid. Other Ingredients: Sesame Oil, Gelatin.

200 mg of Zen **-** Allergy Research Group
Two capsules contain: GABA (gamma-aminobutyric acid) 550 mg • L-Theanine 200 mg. Other Ingredients: Silicon Dioxide, Carbowax.

21 Grain Lecithin **-** Schiff
Each softgel contains: Lecithin Proprietary Blend 1.36 g: Choline Phosphatides, Inositol Phosphatides, Cephalin, Linoleic Acid. Other Ingredients: Gelatin, Glycerin.

25,000 IU Natural Vitamin A & Beta Carotene **-** Progressive Labs
Each softgel capsule contains: Vitamin A (as beta carotene) 15,000 IU • Vitamin A (from fish liver oil) 10,000 IU • Alfalfa 5 mg • Cranberry juice concentrate 5 mg • Carrot oil 6 mg • Lecithin 5 mg. Other Ingredients: Gelatin.

2DaySlimDown **-** Momentum
Vitamin C • Vitamin B6 • Vitamin B12 • Vitamin B3 (niacin) • Chromium Polynicotinate • Aloe Vera gel • Garcinia Cambogia • Ginseng tea • Burdock root tea • Licorice root tea • Fennel seed tea • Sumac tea • Pau d'Arco tea • Ginkgo Biloba tea • Peppermint tea.

2nd Wind **-** Resource Wellness
Two capsules contain: Proprietary Blend 698 mg: Flammulina Velutipes, Eleutherococcus Senticosus (siberian ginseng root extract), Citrus Reticulata (peel extract), Ganoderma lucidum, Panax Ginseng (root extract) • Cordyceps sinensis. Other Ingredients: Gelatin, Maltodextrin, Magnesium Stearate, Silicon Dioxide, Sodium Lauryl Sulfate, Polysorbate 80.

2nd Wind **-** The Sports Nutrition Source, Inc.
Each scoop contains: Vitamin C 180 mg • Caffeine 20 mg • Ginseng powdered root 10 mg • Chromium Picolinate 200 mcg.

3 mg Biotin Forte - Vitaline Formulas **-** Integrative Therapeutics
Each tablet contains: Vitamin C (as ascorbic acid) 200 mg • Thiamin (as thiamine mononitrate) 10 mg • Riboflavin 10 mg • Niacin (as niacinamide) 40 mg • Vitamin B6 (as pyridoxine HCl) 25 mg • Folic Acid 800 mcg • Vitamin B12 (as cyanocobalamin) 10 mcg • Biotin 3 mg • Pantothenic Acid (as calcium pantothenate) 10 mg • Zinc (as zinc acetate) 30 mg. Other Ingredients: Microcrystalline Cellulose, Cellulose, Sodium Starch Glycolate, Silicon Dioxide, Vegetable Stearine, Calcium Stearate, Hydroxypropyl Methylcellulose, Titanium Dioxide.

30 Day Beauty Secret **-** Futurebiotics
Formula I - Two tablets contain: • Royal Jelly (freeze dried) 50 mg • Horsetail (extract equivalent to) 300 mg • Dong Quai (extract equivalent to) 100 mg • Polygonum Multiflorum (extract equivalent to) 140 mg • Peony Root (extract equivalent to) 120 mg • Betaine HCl 75 mg • Selenium (Amino Acid Chelate) 50 mcg • Iodine (Kelp) 175 mcg • Iron (Amino Acid Chelate) 8 mg • Magnesium (Oxide, Amino Acid Chelate) 150 mg • Manganese (Amino Acid Chelate) 10 mg • Boron 3 mg • Zinc (Gluconate) 15 mg • Calcium (Carbonate, Phosphate, Casein) 300 mg • Phosphorus (Calcium Phosphate) 150 mg • Collagen 100 mg • Ribonucleic Acid (RNA) 50 mg • Sodium Phosphate 1 mg • Gelatin 200 mg • Papain 25 mg • Keratin 30 mg • Formula II - Each caplet contains: Beta Carotene 10,000 IU • Vitamin C 150 mg • Vitamin B1 (Thiamin) 10 mg • Vitamin B2 (Riboflavin) 10 mg • Niacinamide 60 mg • Vitamin D (Fish Liver Oil) 200 IU • Vitamin E (Natural Mixed Tocopherols) 30 IU • Vitamin B6 (Pyridoxine) 10 mg • Vitamin B12 (Cyanocobalamin) 16 mcg • Folic Acid 400 mcg • Biotin 300 mcg • Pantothenic Acid 30 30 mg • Inositol 50 mg • Para Amino Benzoic Acid (PABA) 50 mg • Choline (Bitartrate) 150 mg.

30 Day Value Pack **-** Nature's Life
Mega-Vita-Min Vitamin C, 500 mg. Each tablet contains: Beta Carotene (Vitamin A equivalent to 5000 IU) 3 mg • Vitamin B1 (Thiamine HCl) 10 mg • Vitamin B2 (Riboflavin) 10 mg • Vitamin B6 (Pyridoxine HCl) 10 mg • Vitamin B12 (Cobalamin concentrate) 100 mcg • Niacin 10 mg • Pantothenic Acid (d-Calcium Pantothenate) 20 mg • Folic Acid 400 mcg • Choline (Bitartrate) 90 mg • Biotin (d-Biotin) 50 mcg • PABA (Para Aminobenzoic Acid) 20 mg • Lemon Bioflavonoids Complex (TESTLAB) 15 mg • Vitamin C 100 mg • Vitamin E (d-Alpha Tocopheryl with mixed Tocopherols) 10 IU • Boron (Full-Range Amino Acid Chelated) 25 mcg • Calcium (Full-Range Amino Acid Chelated) 50 mg • Chromium (Nutrition 21 Picolinate) 50 mcg • Copper (Full-Range Amino Acid Chelated) 200 mcg • Iodine (Icelandic Kelp) 225 mcg • Magnesium (Full-Range Amino Acid Chelated) 50 mg • Manganese (Full-Range Amino Acid Chelated) 2 mg • Molybdenum (Proteinate) 25 mcg • Phosphorus (Full-Range Amino Acid Chelated & Complexed) 19 mcg • Potassium (Proteinate) 15 mg • Selenium (Nutrition 21 Selenomethionine) 25 mcg • Silicon (Dioxide) 25 mcg • Vanadium (Full-Range Amino Acid Chelated) 25 mcg • Zinc (Nutrition 21 Picolinate) 2 mg • Betaine HCl 30 mg • Nuclei Acids (RNA & DNA from Yeast) 30 mg • Co Q10 (Co-enzyme Ubiquinone) 500 mcg • Essential Fatty Acids (Soy, Spirulina) 25 mg • Super Green Pro 96 (Soy Protein Super Food) 330 mg. In a natural base containing: Rose Hips concentrate, Acerola, Rutin, Hesperidin, Lecithin, Milk-Free Lactobacillus Acidophilus, Alfalfa Leaf, Watercress, Parsley, "72 Trace Minerals", Rice Bran, Spirulina, Barley Green, Psyllium, Apple Pectin, Oat Bran, Bromelain, Papain, Chlorella & Chlorophyll.

3A Calcium **-** LaneLabs
Three capsules contain: Calcium (as calcium hydroxide, calcium oxide, combined with algae amino acid extract) 450 mg. Other Ingredients: Gelatin, Water, Glycerin.

3-Daily **-** The Vitamin Shoppe
Three capsules contain: Vitamin A Activity 25000 IU • Vitamin E 400 IU • Green Tea extract 50 mg • L-Glutathione 10 mg • Vitamin D 400 IU • Vitamin C 500 mg • CoQ10 100 mcg • Selenium 50 mcg • Pycnogenol 100 mcg • N-Acetyl Cysteine 15 mg • Molybdenum 50 mcg • Vitamin B1 50 mg • Vitamin B2 50 mg • Niacinamide 50 mg • Vitamin B6 50 mg • Vitamin B12 500 mcg • Folic Acid 800 mcg • Inositol 50 mg • Choline 50 mg • PABA 50 mg • Vitamin K 30 mcg • Biotin 50 mcg • Pantothenic Acid 50 mg • Calcium 100 mg • Magnesium 50 mg • Zinc 15 mg • Iron 10 mg • Iodine 150 mcg • Potassium 50 mg • Manganese 5 mg • Chromium 100 mcg • Boron 3 mg • Apple Pectin 50 mg • Betaine HCl 25 mg • Glutamic Acid 25 mg • Papain 25 mg • Pepsin 25 mg • Amylase 10 mcg • Lipase 10 mcg • Chlorophyll 10 mg • Spirulina 45 mg • Chlorella 45 mg • Barley Grass 45 mg • Alfalfa concentrate 45 mg • Bee Pollen 45 mg • Rutin 50 mg • Bioflavonoids 50 mg • Shark Cartilage 50 mg • Siberian Ginseng 45 mg • Royal Jelly 15 mg • Echinacea/Golden Seal 50 mg • Shiitake/Reishi Mushrooms 45 mg • RNA/DNA 45 mg. A concentrated blend of: broccoli, tomato, garlic, onions, cauliflower, brussel sprouts, carrots, parsley, watercress, and pure dry cold-pressed borage.

4-Diol 250 **-** AST Sports Science
Each capsule contains: 4-Androstenediol 250 mg.

4-in-1 Body Slim - Pro Health
Three capsules contain: Chromium (50% picolinate, 50% polynicotinate) 150 mcg • Psyllium husk fiber 600 mg • Konjak Glucomannan 450 mg • Guar Gum 300 mg • Oat Bran fiber 300 mg • Chitosan (93% deacetylate) 300 mg • Apple Pectin 300 mg • Gymnema Sylvestre extract (2.5% gymnemic acids) 75 mg • L-Carnitine (tartrate) 30 mg. Other Ingredients: Gelatin, Dicalcium Phosphate Anhydrous, Silica, Magnesium Stearate.

5 HTP Plus - Olympian Labs
Each capsule contains: 5-HTP (L-5 hydroxytryptophan) 100 mg • Vitamin B-6 10 mg • Magnesium Citrate 40 mg • Valerian powder 100 mg • Hops 50 mg • Calcium Citrate 80 mg.

50+ - Futurebiotics
Three capsules contain: Beta-carotene 10,000 IU • Vitamin C (buffered ascorbate) 300 mg • Vitamin E (natural) 100 IU • Vitamin D (as Vitamin D3) 400 IU • Vitamin B1 25 mg • Vitamin B2 25 mg • Vitamin B3 (niacinamide) 25 mg • Vitamin B6 25 mg • Vitamin B12 100 mcg • Pantothenic Acid 25 mg • Biotin 300 mcg • Folic Acid 400 mcg • PABA 25 mg • Choline Bitartrate 50 mg • Inositol 25 mg • Calcium (ascorbate, carbonate, chelate) 200 mg • Magnesium (oxide, chelate) 3 mg • Potassium (chloride, iodide) 20 mg • Zinc (gluconate) 15 mg • Copper (gluconate) 2 mg • Manganese (amino acid chelate) 3 mg • Iodine (potassium iodide) 150 mcg • Selenium (amino acid chelate) 150 mcg • Chromium (amino acid chelate) 200 mcg • Molybdenum (amino acid chelate) 50 mcg • Siberian Ginseng 50 mg • Ginkgo Biloba 25 mg • Turmeric 25 mg • Garlic (Pure-Gar 1500 deodorized concentrate) 200 mg • Cayenne 25 mg • Gotu Kola 100 mg • Alfalfa 50 mg.

5-Diol 250 - AST Sports Science
Each capsule contains: 5-Androstenediol 250 mg.

5-HTP - Metabolic Response Modifiers
Each capsule contains: 5-HTP (5-hydroxytryptophan) 100 mg.

5HTP - Pro Health
Each capsule contains: 5HTP (5-hydroxy-l-tryptophan, from griffonia seed) 50 mg. Other Ingredients: Rice Flour, Gelatin, Water.

5-HTP - Swanson
Each capsule contains: L-5 HTP (L-5 hydroxytryptophan) 50 mg.

5HTP 50 mg - Vital Nutrients
Each capsule contains: 5HTP 50 mg • Pyridoxine HCl 5 mg • Pyridoxal-5-Phosphate 2 mg.

5-HTP Plus Formula - Douglas Laboratories
Each vegetarian capsule contains: L-5-Hydroxytryptophan 75 mg • Pyridoxal-5-Phosphate 7.5 mg • Proprietary Blend 50 mg: L-Tyrosine, L-Glutamine.

5HTP, 5-L-Hydroxytryptophan - NutriCology
Each capsule contains: 5HTP (5-L-hydroxytryptophan) 50 mg. Other Ingredients: Cellulose, Stearic Acid, Silicon Dioxide.

5-Hydroxy L-Tryptophan - Progressive Labs
Each capsule contains: 5-Hydroxy L-Tryptophan 100 mg.

6-OXO - ErgoPharm
Three capsules contain: 6-OXO (3;6;17-androstenetrione) 300 mg. Other Ingredients: Microcrystalline Cellulose.

7 Day Smoke Away - Aromatherapy Formula - The Quit Smoking Co.
Active Ingredients: Ylang Ylang • Rosemary • Peppermint • Eucalyptus • Virgin Olive Oil • Alcohol.
See Editor's Note No. 1, page 2053.

7 Day Smoke Away - Calming Dietary Supplement - The Quit Smoking Co.
Each capsule contains: Avena Sativa (Oats) 10:1 Concentration • Lobelia Inflata (lobelia leaf) 1% lobeline • Capsicum Annuum (cayenne fruit) • Glycyrrhiza Glabra (deglycerized licorice root) • Zingiber Officinale (ginger root) 5% • Piper Methysticum (kava kava leaf) 30% kavalactones • Myristica Fragrans (nutmeg fruit).

7 day Smoke Away - Cleanse and Calm Formula - The Quit Smoking Co.
Each capsule contains: Proprietary Blend 575 mg: Avena Sativa (Oats) 10:1 Concentration, Lobelia Inflata (lobelia leaf) 1% lobeline, Capsicum Annuum (cayenne fruit), Glycyrrhiza Glabra (deglycerized licorice root), Zingiber Officinale (ginger root) 5%, Piper Methysticum (kava kava leaf) 30% kavalactones, Myristica Fragrans (nutmeg fruit).

7 Day Smoke Away - Craving Control Formula - The Quit Smoking Co.
Each tablet contains: Plantain major 3X • Caladium seguinum 6X • Daphne indica 6X.
See Editor's Note No. 1, page 2053.

7 Day Smoke Away - Lung Saver - The Quit Smoking Co.
Each capsule contains: Vitamin C • Vitamin B6 • Picrorhiza Kurroa • Boswellia Serrata • Piper Longum extract • Lobelia • Adhtoda Vasica • Licorice • Ginger • Piper Nigrum fruit • Tylophora Asmatica • N-Acetyl-Cysteine (NAC) • Marshmallow (Althea Officinalis).

7 Herb Formula - Daniel Chapter One
Cat's Claw (Una de Gato) • Sheep Sorrel • Siberian Ginseng • Slippery Elm • Burdock root • Turkey Rhubarb • Watercress.

7 Keto DHEA - Pro Health
Each capsule contains: 7-Keto DHEA (3-acetyl-7-oxo-dehydroepiandrosterone, synthetic) 25 mg. Other Ingredients: Rice Flour, Gelatin, Water.

7 Vitamin Treatment Cream - Orjene
Vitamin A • Vitamin B5 • Vitamin C • Vitamin D • Vitamin E • Vitamin F • Vitamin H • Antioxidants. Fortified with Beta Carotene.

707 Wei Yao Gastropathy Capsules - Zhengjiang Chinese Medicine Works
Yuan Hu • Wu Zei Gu • Qing Ma Ziang • Zhen Hu Mu • Ming Fan • Fen Huang Yi.
See Editor's Note No. 46, page 2058.

714X - CERBE Distribution Inc.
Each 6.5 mL vial contains: Camphor or a nitrogenated derivative 0.09 mg/mL • NaCl 8.2 mg/mL • Aluminum <0.5 ppm • Antimony <1.0 ppm • Arsenic <1.0 ppm • Barium 0.7 ppm • Bore <0.05 ppm • Cadmium <0.05 ppm • Calcium 0.5 ppm • Chromium <0.1 ppm • Cobalt <1.0 ppm • Copper 0.01 ppm • Iron <0.1 ppm • Lead <1.0 ppm • Magnesium 6.5 ppm • Mercury <1.0 ppm • Molybdenum <1.0 ppm • Nickel <0.1 ppm • Phosphorus <5.0 ppm • Zinc 2.0 ppm.

7-Keto - Enzymatic Therapy/PhytoPharmica
Each capsule contains: DHEA (dehydroepiandrosterone; as 7-Keto) 25 mg.

7-Keto DHEA - PhysioLogics
Each softgel contains: 7-Keto Dehydroepiandrosterone Acetate 25 mg. Other Ingredients: Soybean Oil, Gelatin, Lecithin, Beeswax / Soybean Oil Mixture, Glycerin, Titanium Dioxide Color.

7-Keto Fuel - TwinLab
Each capsule contains: 7-Keto DHEA (3-Acetyl-7-Oxo-Dehydroepiandrosterone) 50 mg.

7-Keto Lean - PhytoPharmica
Each capsule contains: Iodine (potassium iodide) 100 mcg • Copper (gluconate) 500 mcg • Manganese (Krebs cycle chelate) 500 mcg • 7 KETO DHEA 100 mg • L-Tyrosine 100 mg • Asparagus root/rhizome extract (asparagus officinalis, standardized to contain 4.0%-8.0% asparagosides) 100 mg • Choline Bitartrate 50 mg • Inositol (rice) 50 mg.

7-Keto Naturalean **-** Enzymatic Therapy
Each capsule contains: 7-Keto DHEA 100 mg • L-Tyrosine 100 mg • Asparagus root extract (Asparagus officinalis) standardized to contain 4.0-8.0% asparagosides 100 mg • Choline Bitartrate FCC 50 mg • Inositol 50 mg • Copper (Gluconate) 500 mcg • Manganese (Krebs Cycle Chelate) 500 mcg • Iodine (Potassium Iodine) 100 mcg. Other Ingredients: Magnesium stearate, Colloidal Silicon dioxide, and Gelatin capsule.

8 Billion Acidophilus & Bifidus **-** Now
Each capsule contains: A guaranteed potency of: Lactobacillus Acidophilus 4 billion • Bifidobacterium Bifidum 3.2 billion • Bifidobacterium Longum 0.8 billion.

8% Plus Antioxidant Cuticle Cream **-** Jason
Vitamin A • Vitamin C • Vitamin E.

90% Protein Powder **-** Puritan's Pride
Two tablespoons (20 g) contain: L-Isoleucine 850 mg • L-Leucine 1122 mg • L-Lysine 1092 mg • L-Methionine 225 mg • L-Threonine 659 mg • L-Phenylalanine 902 mg • L-Valine 867 mg • L-Histidine 451 mg • L-Arginine 1318 mg • L-Aspartic Acid 2012 mg • L-Cysteine 225 mg • L-Serine 902 mg • L-Glutamic Acid 3312 mg • L-Tryptophan 225 mg • L-Proline 884 mg • L-Glycine 728 mg • L-Alanine 746 mg • L-Tyrosine 659 mg.

911 Caps **-** Global Health Trax
Each capsule contains: Chitosan 600 mg • Garcinia (whole plant) 375 mg • Gymnema Sylvestre root 250 mg • Kidney Bean (phaseo vulgaris) 250 mg. Other Ingredients: Methylcellulose, Gelatin.

A & D Natural Capsules **-** Progressive Labs
Each softgel contains: Vitamin A (from fish liver oil, Skip Jack liver oil) 10,000 IU • Vitamin D (from fish liver oil, Skip Jack liver oil) 400 IU.

A & D Vitamins **-** Puritan's Pride
Each softgel contains: Vitamin A 5,000 IU • Vitamin D 400 IU.

A & E Mulsion **-** Aspen Group, Inc.
Each drop contains: Emulsified Vitamin A (palmitate) 5000 IU • Vitamin E (dl-alpha tocopheryl acetate) 10 IU.

A Bonanza of B Vitamins **-** Swanson
Each capsule contains: Thiamin (as thiamin HCl)(vitamin B-1) 100 mg • Riboflavin (vitamin B-2) 100 mg • Niacinamide USP 100 mg • Vitamin B-6 USP (as pyridoxine HCl) 100 mg • Folic Acid 400 mcg • Vitamin B-12 (as cyanocobalamin) 100 mcg • Biotin USP 100 mcg • Pantothenic Acid (as d-calcium pantothenate) 100 mg • Choline (as choline bitartrate) 100 mg • Inositol 100 mg • PABA (para-aminobenzoic acid) 100 mg.

A Kid's Companion High Potency Chewable Multi-Vitamin Mineral Formula **-** Natrol
Two wafers contain: Vitamins/Minerals: Vitamin A Activity (Palmitate) 2500 IU • Vitamin A (Beta Carotene) 2500 IU • Vitamin D (Calciferol) 400 IU • Vitamin E (d-Alpha Tocopheryl Succinate) 30 IU • Vitamin C (Ascorbic Acid) 60 mg • Vitamin B1 (Thiamine HCl) 2.5 mg • Vitamin B2 (Riboflavin) 2.5 mg • Vitamin B6 (Pyridoxine HCl) 2.5 mg • Vitamin B12 (Cyanocobalamin) 10 mcg • Niacinamide 20 mg • Calcium (Carbonate) 200 mg • Iron (Gluconate) 5 mg • Folic Acid 400 mcg • Biotin 150 mcg • Pantothenic Acid (Calcium d-Pantothenate) 12.5 mg • Choline (Bitartrate) 10 mg • Inositol 10 mg • PABA (Para Amino Benzoic Acid) 5 mg • Iodine (Kelp) 150 mcg • Magnesium (Oxide) 50 mg • Zinc (Gluconate) 2.5 mg • Copper (Gluconate) 200 mcg • Vitamin K 25 mcg • Selenium, organically bound concentrate 5 mcg • Chromium (ChromeMate) 10 mcg • Manganese (Gluconate) 1 mg • Potassium (Chloride) 1 mg • Silica from standardized Horsetail extract 1.5 mg • Glycine 200 mg • Lemon Bioflavonoids 25 mg • Bee Pollen 25 mg • Acerola 25 mg • Black Currant 25 mg. Flavored with natural fruit extracts (Lemon, Orange) natural flavors (Butterscotch, Vanilla) & sweetened with Fructose.

A Perfect You Bar, Chocolate Peanut **-** Advocare International
Each bar contains: L-Glutamine 500 mg • Choline 5 mg • Inositol 5 mg • Bromelain 50 mg • Papain 50 mg • Carrot root powder 100 mg. Other Ingredients: Any Protein Blend (calcium caseinate, whey protein isolate, L-glutamine), Milk Chocolate Flavored Coating (sugar, fractionated palm kernel oil, nonfat milk, lactose, cocoa processed with alkali, dextrose, soy lecithin, natural flavor), High Fructose Corn Syrup, Maltitol Syrup, Cocoa Processed with Alkali, Toasted Soy Pieces, Ground Peanuts, Crisped Rice (rice flour, malt extract, rice bran), Natural Flavors, Calcium Phosphate, Canola Oil, Malt Extract, Barley Extract, Medium Chain Triglycerides, Carrot Powder, Magnesium Oxide, Sucratose, Bromelain, Papain, Ascorbic Acid, Maltodextrin, Choline Bitartrate, Ferric Orthophosphate, Vitamin E Acetate, Inositol, Niacinamide, Zinc Oxide, Manganese Sulfate, Copper Gluconate, Calcium Pantothenate, Pyridoxine HCl, Riboflavin, Thiamine Mononitrate, Vitamin A Palmitate, Chromium Citrate, Folic Acid, Sodium Molybdate, Sodium Selenite, Biotin, Phytonadione, Potassium Iodide, Cholecalciferol, Cyanocobalamin.

A Perfect You Energy Drink **-** Advocare International
Each packet contains: Vitamin A (as beta-carotene and vitamin A palmitate) 2500 IU • Vitamin C (as ascorbic acid) 180 mg • Vitamin E (as alpha tocopheryl acetate) 30 IU •Thiamine (as HCl) 3 mg • Riboflavin 3.4 mg • Niacin (as niacinamide and niacin) 60 mg • Pyridoxine (as HCl) 15 mg • Vitamin B12 (as cyanocobalamin) 45 mcg • Pantothenic Acid (as calcium pantothenate) 50 mg • Zinc (as monomethionine - OptiZinc) 3 mg • Copper (as amino acid chelate) 200 mcg • Chromium (as polynicotinate - ChromeMate) 24 mcg • L-Carnitine (as HCl) 10 mg • Taurine 200 mg • Gamma Aminobutyric Acid (GABA) 100 mg • L-Glycine 100 mg • L-Phenylalanine 500 mg • Ribonucleic Acid 2 mg • Ubiquinone (coenzyme Q-10) 100 mcg • Choline (as citrate and bitartrate) 450 mg • Caffeine 100 mg • Green Orange extract (pericarp - citrus aurantium) 125 mg. Other Ingredients: Maltodextrin, Natural Flavor, Citric Acid, Xanthan Gum, Sucralose.
See Editor's Note No. 40, page 2058.

A Perfect You Meal Replacement Shake (Chocolate) **-** Advocare International
APY Protein Concentrate: Whey Protein concentrate, Calcium Caseinate, Sodium Caseinate, Milk Protein Isolate, Soy Protein Isolate, L-Glutamine, L-Lysine Hydrochloride, L-Leucine, L-Isoleucine, L-Valine • Fructose • Maltodextrin • Cocoa (processed with alkali) • Vitamin/Mineral Mix: Calcium Phosphate, Magnesium Oxide, Potassium Citrate, Potassium Chloride, Ascorbic Acid, Ferrous Fumarate, Vitamin E Acetate, Choline Bitartrate, Inositol, Niacinamide, Zinc Oxide, Manganese Sulfate, Calcium Pantothenate, Copper Sulfate, Vitamin A Palmitate, Pyridoxine Hydrochloride, Riboflavin, Thiamine Mononitrate, Chromium Chloride, Folic Acid, Sodium Molybdate, Biotin, Potassium Iodide, Sodium Selenite, Phytonadione, Cholecalciferol, Cyanocobalamin • Natural and Artificial Flavors • Gum Acacia • Guar Gum • Medium-Chain Triglycerides • Apple powder • Soy Fiber • Oat Fiber • Cellulose • Soy Lecithin • Rice Syrup solids • Corn Syrup solids • Lactobacillus Acidophilus • Bifidobacterium Bifidum • Sucralose • Bromelain • Papain.

A Perfect You Nutritional Supplements **-** Advocare International
Two white packets contain: Vitamin A (as palmitate) 2500 IU • Vitamin A (as beta-carotene) 12,500 IU • Vitamin C (as ascorbic acid/mineral ascorbates) 600 mg • Vitamin D (as ergocalciferol) 400 IU • Vitamin E (as d-alpha tocopheryl succinate) 150 IU • Thiamine 9 mg • Riboflavin 10.2 mg • Niacin / Niacinamide 120 mg • Vitamin B6 12 mg • Folic Acid 800 mcg • Vitamin B12 (as cyanocobalamin) 36 mcg • Biotin 300 mcg • Pantothenic Acid 40 mg • Calcium (as amino acid chelate) 150 mg • Phosphorus (as amino acid chelate) 100 mg • Iodine (from kelp) 150 mcg • Magnesium (as amino acid chelate) 200 mg • Zinc (as monomethionine - Opti Zinc) 15 mg • Selenium (as selenomethionine) 80 mcg • Copper (as amino acid chelate) 2 mg •

Manganese (as amino acid chelate) 4 mg • Chromium (as polynicotinate - ChromeMate) 100 mcg • Molybdenum (as amino acid chelate) 50 mcg • Potassium (as amino acid chelate/phosphate) 100 mg • Boron (as amino acid chelate) 300 • Vanadium (as bis-maltolato-oxovanadium) 50 mcg • Silicon (as amino acid chelate) 500 mg • Inositol 6 mg • Choline (as bitartrate) 60 mg • Coenzyme Q-10 150 mcg • Octacosanol 2000 mcg • Ribonucleic Acid (RNA) 2000 mcg • Odorless Garlic (bulb powder - allium sativum) 50 mg • L-Glutathione 5 mg • Gamma-Oryzanol 5 mg • Citrus Bioflavonoids 100 mg • Red Wine Polyphenols 5 mg • Milk Thistle extract (fruit - silybum marianum) 5 mg • Ginkgo extract (leaf - ginkgo biloba) 10 mg • L-Methionine 100 mg • Eicosapentaenoic Acid (from marine lipids) 360 mg • Docosahexaenoic Acid (from marine lipids) 240 mg • 5-Hydroxytryptophan (seed - griffonia simplicifolia) 25 mg • D-Limonene powder 300 mg • Grapefruit juice powder 200 mg. Two silver packets contain: Garcinia extract (fruit - garcinia cambogia) 2000 mg • Tulsi extract (leaf - ocimum sanctum) 50 mg • Taurine 50 mg • L-Carnitine 25 mg • Beta-Sitosterol 25 mg • Gymnema extract (leaf - gymnema sylvestre) 10 mg • Green Orange extract (pericarp - citrus aurantium) 1000 mg • Guarana extract (seed - paullinia cupana) 550 mg • Green Tea extract (leaf - camellia sinensis) 20 mg • Oolong Tea extract (leaf - camellia sinensis) 200 mg • Siberian Ginseng extract (root - eleutherococcus senticosus) 50 mg • Lactobacillus Acidophilus 0.5 billion • Bifidobacterium Bifidus 0.5 billion • Fructooligosaccharides 250 mg • Moomiyo 25 mg • Aloe Vera powder 50 mg. Other Ingredients: Dicalcium Phosphate, Silicon Dioxide, Cellulose, Stearic Acid, Magnesium Stearate, Vanillin, Gelatin, Water, Beet Root Powder (for color).
See Editor's Note No. 40, page 2058.

A.H.C.C. - AHCC - Quality of Life Labs
Two capsules contain: Proprietary Blend 500 mg: Mushroom Mycelia extract, Candelilla Wax, Cyclodextrin, Microcrystalline Cellulose. Other Ingredients: Silica, Gelatin, Glycerin.

A.M.P. - Molo-Cure Research, Inc.
Each capsule contains: Freeze-dried Aloe Vera 125 mg • Soy Lecithin 375 mg.

A.S.A.P. - The Herbalist
Black Cohosh root • Passionflower herb • Scullcap herb • Valerian root • Lobelia leaf • Prickly Ash bark.

A+Zinc - Nutrilite
Each tablet contains: Vitamin A 10000 IU • Zinc Oxide 15 mg • Zinc Gluconate 15 mg.

A-25 Plex - Progressive Labs
Each softgel contains: Vitamin A (beta carotene) 15,000 IU • Vitamin A (from fish liver oil) 10,000 IU • Alfalfa 5 mg • Cranberry juice concentrate 5 mg • Carrot oil 6 mg • Lecithin 5 mg.

A-25,000 IU Fish Oil - Rexall - Sundown
Each softgel contains: Vitamin A (from fish liver oil) 25,000 IU. Inactive Ingredients: Soybean Oil, Gelatin, Glycerin.

AARP Pharmacy Service Formula 502 (Seniors Vitamins) - Retired Persons Services, Inc.
Each caplet contains: Vitamin A (as vitamin A acetate and 3% as beta carotene) 5200 IU • Vitamin C (as ascorbic acid) 60 mg • Vitamin D (as cholecalciferol) 200 IU • Vitamin E (as DL-alpha tocopheryl acetate) 15 IU • Thiamin (vitamin B1 as thiamine mononitrate) 1.2 mg • Riboflavin 1.4 mg • Niacin (as niacinamide) 16 mg • Vitamin B6 (as pyridoxine hydrochloride) 2.2 mg • Folic Acid (folate) 400 mcg • Vitamin B12 (as cyanocobalamin) 3 mcg • Pantothenic Acid (as D-calcium pantothenate) 10 mg • Calcium (as dicalcium phosphate and calcium carbonate) 100 mg • Iron (as ferrous fumarate) 10 mg • Phosphorous (as dicalcium phosphate) 77 mg • Iodine (as potassium iodide) 150 mcg • Magnesium (as magnesium oxide) 30 mg • Zinc (as zinc oxide) 15 mg • Copper (as cupric sulfate) 2 mg • Manganese (as manganese sulfate) 1 mg • Potassium (as potassium sulfate) 5 mg.

Abana - The Himalaya Drug Company (Himalaya Heal
Each tablet contains: Arjuna (terminalia arjuna) 30 mg • Ashvagandha (withania somnifera) 20 mg • Badranj Boya (nepeta hindostana) 20 mg • Dashamoola 20 mg: Aegle Marmelos root, Gmelina Arborea root, Oroxylum Indicum root, Clerodendrum Phlomidis root, Stereospermum Chelonoides root, Desmodium Gangeticum root, Uraria Picta root, Solanum Indicum root, Solanum Surattense root, Tribulus Terrestris root • Guduchi (tinospora cordifolia) 10 mg • Amalaki (emblica officinalis) 10 mg • Haritaki (terminalia chebula) 10 mg • Bhringaraja (eclipta alba syn. e.prostrata) 10 mg • Yashti-Madhu (glycyrrhiza glabra) 10 mg • Shatavari (asparagus racemosus) 10 mg • Punarnava (boerhaavia diffusa) 10 mg • Guggulu (balsamodendron mukul syn. commiphora wightii, purified) 30 mg • Shilajeet (mineral pitch, purified) 20 mg • Mandukaparni (centella asiatica) 10 mg • Shankhapushpi (convolvulus pluricaulis syn. c.microphyllus) 10 mg • Vishnu Priya (ocimum sanctum syn. o.tenuiflorum) 10 mg • Jatamansi (nardostachys jatamansi) 10 mg • Pippali (piper longum) 10 mg • Yawani (carum copticum syn. trachyspermum ammi) 10 mg • Sunthi (zingiber officinale) 10 mg • Nagapashana Bhasma (calx serpentine, magnesium silicate) 10 mg • Shankh Bhasma (conch shell/ash) 10 mg • Makardwaj (sulphide of mercury) 10 mg • Musta (cyperus rotundus) 5 mg • Vacha (acorus calamus) 5 mg • Vidanga (embelia ribes) 5 mg • Lavanga (syzygium aromaticum) 5 mg • Jyotishmati (celastrus paniculatus) 5 mg • Chandana (santalum album) 5 mg • Ela (elettaria cardamomum) 5 mg • Shatapuspha (foeniculum vulgare) 5 mg • Satapatrika (rosa damascena syn. r.centifolia) 5 mg • Tvak Patra (cinnamomum cassia) 5 mg • Abhrak Bhasma (powdered talc, biotite calx) 5 mg • Mukta Pishti (processed pearl) 5 mg • Akik Pishti (processed agate) 5 mg • Yeshab Pishti (processed vyomashma) 5 mg • Yakut Pishti (processed manikya) 5 mg • Praval Pishti (processed coral) 5 mg • Kumkuma (crocus sativus) 2 mg.

ABC Dophilus - Solgar
Each 1/2 tsp serving contains: ABC Dophilus powder complex (supplying 1 billion live microorganisms) 1 g: B. Bifidum 350 million viable organisms, S. Thermophilus 350 million viable microorganisms, B. Infantis 350 million viable microorganisms. Other Ingredients: Maltodextrin, Silica, Casein (a milk derivative).

ABC Plus SENIOR - Puritan's Pride
Each tablet contains: Vitamin A (as vitamin A acetate and beta carotene) 3500 IU • Vitamin C (as ascorbic acid) 60 mg • Vitamin D (as cholecalciferol) 400 IU • Vitamin E (as DL-alpha tocopheryl acetate) 45 IU • Vitamin K (as phytonadione) 10 mcg • Thiamin (vitamin B1 as thiamin mononitrate) 1.5 mg • Riboflavin (vitamin B2) 1.7 mg • Niacin (as niacinamide) 20 mg • Vitamin B6 (as pyridoxine hydrochloride) 3 mg • Folic Acid 400 mcg • Vitamin B12 (as cyanocobalamin) 25 mcg • Biotin (as D-biotin) 30 mcg • Pantothenic Acid (as D-calcium pantothenate) 10 mg • Calcium (as calcium carbonate and dicalcium phosphate) 200 mg • Phosphorus (as dicalcium phosphate) 48 mg • Iodine (as potassium iodide) 150 mcg • Magnesium (as magnesium oxide) 100 mg • Zinc (as zinc oxide) 15 mg • Selenium (as sodium selenate) 20 mcg • Copper (as cupric oxide) 2 mg • Manganese (as manganese sulfate) 2 mg • Chromium (as chromium chloride) 150 mcg • Molybdenum (as sodium molybdate) 75 mcg • Chloride (as potassium chloride) 72 mg • Potassium (as potassium chloride) 80 mg • Boron (as sodium borate) 150 mcg • Nickel (as nickel sulfate) 5 mcg • Silica (as silicon dioxide) 2 mg • Vanadium (as sodium metavanadate) 10 mcg • Lycopene (from tomato fruit extract) 300 mcg • Lutein (from marigold flower extract) 250 mcg. Other Ingredients: Cellulose (plant origin), Croscarmellose, Vegetable Stearic Acid, Vegetable Magnesium Stearate, Mannitol, Cellulose Coating, Starch, FD&C Blue No. 2 Lake, Titanium Dioxide Color, FD&C Yellow No. 6 Lake, FD&C Red No. 40 Lake.

ABC Plus with Lutein & Lycopene - Puritan's Pride
Each tablet contains: Vitamin A (as retinyl acetate and beta carotene) 3500 IU • Vitamin C (as ascorbic acid) 60 mg • Vitamin D (as cholecalciferol) 400 IU • Vitamin E (as DL-alpha tocopheryl acetate)

30 IU • Vitamin K (as phytonadione) 25 mcg • Thiamin (vitamin B1, as thiamin mononitrate) 1.5 mg • Riboflavin (vitamin B2) 1.7 mg • Niacin (as niacinamide) 20 mg • Vitamin B6 (as pyridoxine hydrochloride) 2 mg • Folic Acid 400 mcg • Vitamin B12 (as cyanocobalamin) 6 mcg • Biotin (as D-biotin) 30 mcg • Pantothenic Acid (as D-calcium pantothenate) 10 mg • Calcium (as dicalcium phosphate and calcium carbonate) 162 mg • Iron (as ferrous fumarate) 18 mg • Phosphorus (as dicalcium phosphate) 109 mg • Iodine (as potassium iodide) 150 mcg • Magnesium (as magnesium oxide) 100 mg • Zinc (as zinc oxide) 15 mg • Selenium (as sodium selenite) 20 mcg • Copper (as cupric oxide) 2 mg • Manganese (as manganese sulfate) 2 mg • Chromium (as chromium chloride) 120 mcg • Molybdenum (as sodium molybdate) 75 mcg • Chloride (as potassium chloride) 72 mg • Potassium (as potassium chloride) 80 mg • Boron (as sodium borate) 150 mcg • Nickel (as nickel sulfate) 5 mcg • Silica (as silicon dioxide) 2 mg • Tin (as tin chloride) 10 mcg • Vanadium (as sodium metavanadate) 10 mcg • Lutein (from marigold flower extract) 250 mcg • Lycopene (from tomato fruit extract) 300 mcg. Other Ingredients: Cellulose (plant origin), Croscarmellose, Vegetable Stearic Acid, Vegetable Magnesium Stearate, Mannitol, Cellulose Coating, Starch, FD&C Yellow No. 6 Lake, Titanium Dioxide Color.

AbGone **-** Albion Medical
Two capsules contain: Vitamin C (ascorbic acid) 175 mg • Zinc (zinc citrate) 7.5 mg • Chromium 100 mcg • Dandelion root/leaf powder 150 mg • AbGone Proprietary Blend 820 mg: Phosphatidylserine, CLA, L-Leucine, L-Isoleucine, L-Valine. Other Ingredients: Soybean Oil, Beeswax, Kosher Gelatin, Glycerin, Titanium Dioxide, Purified Water, FD&C Red #40, FD&C Blue #1, FD&C Blue #6.

Absorbable Calcium **-** PhysioLogics
Two softgels contain: Vitamin D (as cholecalciferol) 100 IU • Calcium (as calcium carbonate) 1000 mg. Other Ingredients: Soybean Oil, Gelatin, Glycerin, Lecithin, Titanium Dioxide Color.

Absorbable Calcium with Vitamin D **-** Nature's Bounty
Two softgels contain: Vitamin D (as Cholecalciferol) 100 IU • Calcium (as Calcium Carbonate) 1000 mg. Other Ingredients: Soybean Oil, Gelatin, Glycerin, Lecithin, Titanium Dioxide Color.

Absorbable Calcium with Vitamin D **-** Puritan's Pride
Two softgels contain: Vitamin D (as cholecalciferol) 100 IU • Calcium (as calcium carbonate) 1000 mg. Other Ingredients: Soybean Oil, Gelatin, Glycerin, Lecithin, Titanium Dioxide Color.

Absorbable Iron with Hematinic Factors **-** The Vitamin Shoppe
Each tablet contains: Iron 50 mg • Heme Iron 25 mg • Vitamin C 75 mg • Copper 1 mg • Folic Acid 200 mcg • Vitamin B12 12.5 mcg.

AbsorbAid **-** Nature's Sources
Two capsules contain: Lipase 1145 LU • Amylase 8316 SKBU • Protease (from Bromelain) 36 GDU • Cellulase 299 CU • Lactase 900 LacU.

Absorbitol Fat Binder **-** Natrol
Two capsules contain: Chitosan Complex 900 mg. Other Ingredients: Magnesium Stearate, Gelatin.

Accel Dietary Supplement **-** Atkins Nutritionals, Inc.
Each capsule contains: Niacin (B3) 15 mg • Chromium (as chromium polynicotinate) 100 mcg • Glucomannan (konjac flour) 350 mg • Green Tea leaf extract (providing caffeine 50 mg, epigallocatechin gallate 90 mg) 350 mg. Other Ingredients: Gelatin, Magnesium Stearate.

Acceleration **-** PhytoPharmica
Each capsule contains: Cola Nut extract (cola nitida) 250 mg (contains 35 mg of caffeine) • Green Tea extract (Camellia sinensis) 250 mg (contains 15 mg of caffeine) • Ma Huang extract (Ephedra sinensis) 250 mg (contains 15 mg of ephedrine).
See Editor's Note No. 21 and No. 30, page 2056.

Acceleration (Ephedra Free!) **-** PhytoPharmica
Each capsule contains: Bitter Orange fruit extract (citrus x aurantium, standardized to contain 6% synephrine) 250 mg • Cola nut extract (cola nitida, standardized to contain 35 mg caffeine) 250 mg • Green Tea leaf extract (camellia sinensis, containing 15 mg caffeine) 110 mg. Other Ingredients: Gelatin, Cellulose, Magnesium Stearate, Silicon Dioxide, Titanium Dioxide Color.
See Editor's Note No. 40, page 2058.

Accu-Mind & Memory **-** Leiner Health Products
Each caplet contains: Ginkgo Biloba extract (Ginkgo biloba) leaf 60 mg • Vinpocetine 5 mg. Other Ingredients: Dicalcium Phosphate, Cellulose, Silicon Dioxide, Croscarmellose Sodium, Stearic Acid, Dextrin, Crospovidone, Magnesium Stearate, Dextrose, Lecithin, Sodium Carboxymethylcellulose, Sodium Citrate.

ACE Antioxidant Complex **-** Nature's Life
Each tablet contains: Beta Carotene (Vitamin A equivalent to 5000 IU) 3 mg • Vitamin C 500 mg • Vitamin E (d-Alpha Tocopheryl Succinate) 200 IU • Selenium (Selenomax Selenomethionine) 25 mcg. In a natural base of Rose Hips powder & Nature's Life Greens (A proprietary blend of 24 vegetables & herbs, microalgae, sea vegetables & sprouts).

ACE Ultimate Antioxidant Plus **-** Nature's Life
Two capsules contain: Antioxidant Nutrients: Beta Carotene (vitamin A equivalent to 25,000 IU) 15 mg • Vitamin C 1000 mg • Vitamin E (D-alpha tocopheryl succinate) 300 IU • Vitamin B2 (riboflavin, riboflavin-5-phosphate) 10 mg • Selenium (selenite, methionine) 200 mcg • Glutathione (glutamine/cysteine / glycine tripeptide) 100 mg • Superoxide Dismutase - inducing Minerals: Zinc (citrate, picolinate) 10 mg • Manganese (citrate) 10 mg • Copper (citrate, gluconate) 1 mg • Antioxidant Flavonoids: Lemon Bioflavonoids Complex (TESTLAB 50% total bioflavonoids as flavanones, hesperidin, naringenin & eriocitrin = 50%) 25 mg • Quercetin (dimorphandra pod) 25 mg • Rutin (saphora japonica) 25 mg • Hesperidin (citrus) 25 mg • Pine bark Proanthocyanidins (pinus maritima extract) 5 mg • Epigallocatechin Gallate (camellia sinensis (green tea) extract) 5 mg.

Acerola Chewable C 120 mg **-** Source Naturals
Each tablet contains: Vitamin C (as ascorbic acid & sodium ascorbate) 120 mg • Bioflavonoids 20 mg • Rutin 20 mg • Acerola Cherry 5 mg • Rosehips 4 mg.

Acerola Chewable C 500 mg **-** Source Naturals
Each tablet contains: Vitamin C (as ascorbic acid & sodium ascorbate) 500 mg • Bioflavonoids 20 mg • Rutin 20 mg • Acerola Cherry 5 mg • Rosehips 4 mg.

Acetabolan **-** MuscleTech
Six capsules contain: Acetyl-L-Carnitine 1000 mg • Glutamine 2000 mg • L-Leucine 1000 mg • L-Valine 250 mg • L-Isoleucine 250 mg • OKG 100 mg • Zinc 60 mg • Taurine 1000 mg.

Acetabolan II **-** MuscleTech
Six capsules contain: NAC (as N-Acetyl-Cysteine Hydrochloride) 400 mg. Ingredients: Acetyl-L-Carnitine • Tribulus terrestris • ZincTech: a unique blend of Chelated Zinc, Magnesium, & Vitamin B6.

Acetyl L-Carnitine **-** NSI - Nutraceutical Sciences Institute
Each tablet contains: Acetyl L-Carnitine 500 mg.

Acetyl L-Carnitine **-** Optimum Nutrition
Each capsule contains: Acetyl L-Carnitine 1000 mg. Other Ingredients: Gelatin, Magnesium Stearate.

Acetyl L-Carnitine **-** PhysioLogics
Each capsule contains: Acetyl L-Carnitine (as acetyl l-carnitine hydrochloride) 250 mg. Other Ingredients: Dicalcium Phosphate, Gelatin, Vegetable Magnesium Stearate.

Some Brand Name Natural Products - What they Contain

www.NaturalDatabase.com contains MANY more listings than appear here.

Acetyl L-Carnitine **-** Pro Health
Each capsule contains: Acetyl L-Carnitine 500 mg. Other Ingredients: Rice Flour, Gelatin, Magnesium Stearate.

Acetyl L-Carnitine **-** Source Naturals
Each tablet contains: Acetyl-l-Carnitine 500 mg.

Acetyl L-Carnitine 500 mg with Alpha Lipoic Acid 200 mg **-** Vitamin World
Each capsule contains: Acetyl L-Carnitine 500 mg • Alpha Lipoic Acid 200 mg. Other Ingredients: Gelatin, Marnesium Silicate, Vegetable Magnesium Stearate.

Acetyl L-Carnitine Powder **-** Vital Nutrients
Each 1/4 teaspoon contains: Acetyl-L-Carnitine HCl 1500 mg.

Acetyl-L-Carnitine **-** Douglas Laboratories
Each capsule contains: Acetyl-L-Carnitine 500 mg.

Acetyl-L-Carnitine (250 mg) **-** Allergy Research Group
Each capsule contains: Acetyl-L-Carnitine 250 mg. Other Ingredients: Cellulose, Silicon Dioxide, Stearic Acid.

Acetyl-L-Carnitine (250 mg) **-** NutriCology
Each capsule contains: Acetyl-L-Carnitine 250 mg. Other Ingredients: Cellulose, Silicon Dioxide, Stearic Acid.

Acetyl-L-Carnitine (500 mg) **-** Allergy Research Group
Each capsule contains: Acetyl-L-Carnitine 500 mg. Other Ingredients: Cellulose, Silicon Dioxide, Stearic Acid.

Acetyl-L-Carnitine (500 mg) **-** NutriCology
Each capsule contains: Acetyl-L-Carnitine 500 mg. Other Ingredients: Cellulose, Silicon Dioxide, Stearic Acid.

Acetyl-L-Carnitine 500 - GNC A-Z **-** GNC
Each capsule contains: Acetyl-L-Carnitine Hydrochloride 500 mg. Other Ingredients: Gelatin, Cellulose.

ACF 223 **-** Gero Vita International
Each capsule contains: Vitamin A (as beta-carotene) 900 IU • Vitamin B3 (as niacinamide) 60 mg • Zinc (as gluconate) 7.6 mg • Selenium 13.6 mcg • Copper (as copper gluconate) 0.6 mg • Manganese 0.136 mg • Chromium 28 mcg • Molybdenum 15.2 mcg • L-Carnitine Fumarate 100 mg • MultiMins 78 mg • Uncaria Tomentosa bark extract 50 mg • Tocotrienols 30 mg • CoQ10 10 mg. Other Ingredients: Silica, Magnesium Stearate, Gelatin, Cellulose, Dicalcium Phosphate.

Acid Defense Nature's Acid Relief Formula **-** Garden of Life, Inc.
Each tablespoon (12 g) contains: Mineral Matrix from Goat's Milk Whey 10,060 mg • Potassium 411 mg • Calcium 146 mg • Chloride 130 gm • Phosphorus 116 mg • Sodium 88 mg • Zinc 370 mcg • Iron 240 mcg • Molybdenum 29 mcg • Chromium 5.5 mcg • Selenium 1 mcg • Copper 8 mcg • Manganese 0.7 mcg • Beet juice concentrate (33:1) 600 mg • Carrot juice concentrate (33:1) 600 mg • Barley Grass juice concentrate (33:1) 600 mg • Stomach Soothe Enzyme Blend 150 mg: Amylase 9000 DU, Glucoamylase 20 AGU, Lipase 400 LU, Alpha Galactosidase 150 GalU, Malt Diastase 950 DP, Cellulose 800 CU, Sucrose 675 SU, Lactose 650 ALU.

Acid Redux **-** Now
Each lozenge contains: Vitamin C (as ascorbic acid) 12 mg • Vitamin D (as cholecalciferol) 150 IU • Calcium (as calcium carbonate) 116 mg • Magnesium (from magnesium hydroxide) 11 mg • Potassium (from potassium hydroxide) 4 mg • Acid Redux 373 mg: Calcium Carbonate, Magnesium Hydroxide, Potassium Hydroxide • Stevia Rebaudiana leaf extract (enzyme-treated, min. 80% glycosylsteviosides). Other Ingredients: Fructose, Maltodextrin, Sorbitol, Stearic Acid, Natural Peppermint Flavor, Gum Acacia (food grade).

Acid-A-Cal **-** Enzymatic Therapy
Each capsule contains: Calcium Chloride 96 mg • Calcium Phosphate 90 mg • Magnesium Glycerophosphate 51 mg • Vitamin C (Ascorbic Acid/Rose Hips) 50 mg • Vitamin B6 (Pyridoxine HCL) 25 mg • Betaine HCL 96 mg • Ammonium Chloride 96 mg • Raw Kidney Tissue 30 mg • Citrus Bioflavonoids 30 mg. All organs & glands derived from bovine sources.
See Editor's Note No. 14, page 2055.

Acida-Zyme **-** Progressive Labs
Each capsule contains: Betaine HCl 200 mg • Glutamic Acid HCl 100 mg • Ammonium Chloride 35 mg • Pepsin USP/NF 25 mg • Protease (from plant enzymes) 150 Units.

Acid-Ease **-** Enzymatic Therapy
Two capsules contain: Slippery Elm bark (ulma fulva) 200 mg • Marshmallow root extract (althaea officinalis, 4.25:1) 200 mg • Gamma-Oryzanol (from rice bran oil) 150 mg • Pure Plant Enzymes Blend 109 mg: Amylase (USP XXI [pH6.8]) 27,500 USP (FCC IV [pH4.8]) 11,900 DU, Lipase II (FCC III [pH6.5]) 54 LU, Cellulase I (FCC IV [pH4.5]) 19 CU.

AcidFree **-** Performance Labs
Each tablet contains: Calcium (precipitated calcium, carbonated) 200 mg • FOS (fructooligosaccharides) 40 mg • Proprietary Digestive Enzyme Blend 15 mg: Amylase, Neutral Protease, Lactase, Lipase, Cellulase. Other Ingredients: Sorbitol, Sucrose, Mannitol, Pregelatinized Starch, Cellulose Gum, Natural Flavor, Sodium Potassium Polyphosphate, Stearic Acid, Magnesium Stearate.

Acidophilase **-** Wakunaga of America
Each caspule contains: Lactobacillus acidophilus 1 billion live cells • Food Enzyme complex 155 mg: Protease, Amylase, & Lactase in a vegetable starch complex.

Acidophilus - Lactobacillus **-** Jamieson
Each capsule contains: Minimum two billion active cells of Lactobacillus acidophilus and probiotic cultures.

Acidophilus **-** Nature Made
Each tablet contains: L. Acidophilus cells 500 million.

Acidophilus **-** PhysioLogics
Each softgel contains: Lactobacillus Acidophilus (contains over 100 million active lactobacillus acidophilus, including naturally occurring metabolic product produced by lactobacilli, at time of manufacture) 10 mg. Other Ingredients: Soybean Oil, Gelatin, Glycerin, Beeswax / Soybean Oil Mixture, Lecithin, Titanium Dioxide Color.

Acidophilus **-** PhytoPharmica
Each capsule contains: Proprietary blend of active cultures 4 billion. Contains a specific mixture of Lactobacillus acidophilus, Lactobacillus rhamnosus, Bifidobacteria longum, Bifidobacteria breve.
See Editor's Note No. 21, page 2056.

Acidophilus - Super Blue Green **-** Cell Tech
Two capsules contain: Vitamin K 6.8 mcg • Proprietary Blend 410 mg: Lactobacillus Acidophilus, Blue-Green Algae (aph. flos-aquae) 170 mg. Other Ingredients: Maltodextrin, Plant Cellulose, Gelatin Capsule.

Acidophilus - Super Strain **-** Jamieson
Each capsule contains: Lactobacillus Acidophilus 10% • Lactobacillus Rhamnosus 50% • Streptococcus Thermophilus 20% • Bifidobacterium Longum 10% • Bifidobacterium Bifidum 10%.

Acidophilus E.C. **-** Progressive Labs
Each high potency capsule contains 2.8 billion live organisms from specially selected strains of lactobacillus acidophilus and lactobacillus casei subsp. Rhamnosus in a base of maltodextrin.

Some Brand Name Natural Products - What they Contain

www.NaturalDatabase.com contains MANY more listings than appear here.

Acidophilus Pearls - Enzymatic Therapy
Each pearle capsule contains: Proprietary Probiotic Blend 1 Billion: Lactobacillus Acidophilus, Bifidobacterium Longum. Other Ingredients: Palm Oil, Gelatin, Glycerin, Lecithin, Pectin.

Acidophilus XTRA - Rexall - Sundown
Each two caplets contain: Proprietary Blend (40,000 CFU) 40 mg: Lactobacillus acidophilus • Lactobacillus bulgaricus • Streptococcus thermophilus • Bifidobacterium bifidum. Inactive Ingredients: Rice Maltodextrin, Cellulose, Croscarmellose Sodium, Magnesium Stearate, Silica, Stearic Acid.

Acidophilus, Milk Free - Schiff
Each tablet contains: Calcium (as dicalcium phosphate anhydrous) 47 mg • Lactobacillus Acidophilus 1,000,000,000 CFU. Other Ingredients: Cellulose, Silicon Dioxide, Modified Cellulose Gum, Magnesium Stearate.

Acidophilus/Bifidobacter/FOS - Vital Nutrients
Each capsule contains: Lactobacillus Acidophilus 2 billion • Bifidobacter Lactis 2 billion • FOS (fructooligosaccharides) 150 mg.

Ack-Nee with MAT - Olympian Labs
Two capsules contain: Vitamin A 10000 IU • Beta Carotene (pro-vitamin A) 500 IU • Vitamin E (d-a-tocopheryl acetate) 120 IU • L-Carnitine Fumarate 200 mg • Vitamin C 60 mg • Pantothenic Acid 20 mg • Vitamin B-6 (pyridoxine HCl) 5 mg • Chromium (picolinate, Cromax) 100 mcg • Selenium (l-selenomethionine) 70 mcg • Proprietary Blend 500 mg: Goldenseal, Curcumin extract, Enzyme blend (protease, lipase, amylase), MAT.

Acktiva 100% Pure Coral Calcium - Progressive Health Nutraceuticals
Two capsules contain: Coral Calcium 2000 mg: Yielding Calcium 480 mg, Magnesium 240 mg • Vitamin D 800 IU. Other Ingredients: Rice Powder, Gelatin.

Acti-Flex - FreeLife International
Six caplets contain: Proprietary Blend 1350 mg: Bromelain (80 GDU), Ashwagandha root (withania somnifera), Yucca root extract (yucca schidigera, standardized 10% saponins) • Glucosamine Hydrochloride 1200 mg • Turmeric Rhizome standardized extract (curcuma longa, 92% curcuminoids) 1200 mg • Ginger root standardized (zingiber officinale, 0.8% essential oils, 0.4% amino acids) 1200 mg • Feverfew herb standardized extract (chrysanthemum parthenium, 0.4% parthenolide) 600 mg • Pregnenolone (pharmeceutical-grade) 50 mg • Boron (chelated) 1 mg.

Actilife Super Antioxidant - Crystal Springs
Two tablets contain: Red Grape extract seeds 100 mg • Polygonum cuspidatum extract root 100 mg • Trans-Resveratrol 20 mg • Total Resveratrols 24 mg • Emodin 10 mg • Zinc 30 mg.

Actisyn - SportPharma
Each packet contains: Actipro Protein Substrate: Ion Exchanged Whey Protein Isolate, Whey Protein Concentrate, Enzymatically Hydrolyzed Whey Protein, Pepti-Lean Select Micro-Peptides •Actiplex: Specific Ratios of L-Glutamine, Taurine, L-Leucine, & N-Acetyl-L-Cysteine • Anticell Vitamins & Minerals: Ascorbic Acid, DL- Alpha Tocopheryl Acetate, Vitamin A Palmitate, Potassium Chloride, Magnesium Aspartate, Magnesium Fumerate, Magnesium Oxide, Pyridoxine HCl, Niacinamide, Calcium Phosphate, Magnesium Orotate, Sodium Chloride, Alpha Lipoic Acid, Calcium Alpha-Ketoglutarate, Zinc Gluconate, L-Selenomethionine • Maltodextrin •Actigen: Tri-Methyl Glycine, Specific Nucleotides including: Purine and Pyrimidine Isolates, RNA Hydrolysates •natural & artificial Vanilla & Cream Flavors • CMC Gum • Aspartame •Sunett Brand Sweetener (Acesulfame K).

Activated Fiber Tablets - Herbalife
Each tablet contains: Sodium Choleate • L-Carnitine.

Activated Quercetin - Source Naturals
Three tablets contain: Quercetin 1000 mg • Vitamin C (magnesium ascorbate) 600 mg • Magnesium (magnesium ascorbate) 47 mg • Bromelain (2000 GDU per g) 300 mg.

Active A - Source Naturals
Each tablet contains: Beta Carotene (pro-vitamin A) 15,000 IU • Vitamin A (palmitate) 10,000 IU.

Active Aloe brand - Aloecorp
Aloe Vera.
See Editor's Note No. 44, page 2058.

Active B-50 - The Vitamin Shoppe
Each capsule contains: Vitamin B1 (Thiamin) 50 mg • Vitamin B2 (Riboflavin) 50 mg • Vitamin B6 (Pyridoxine HCl) 50 mg • Vitamin B12 (Cobalamin Concentrate) 50 mcg • Niacinamide 50 mg • Folic Acid 400 mcg • Pantothenic Acid (d-Calcium Pantothenate) 50 mg • Biotin 50 mcg • Choline 50 mg • Inositol 50 mg • PABA (Para Amino Benzoic Acid) 50 mg. In a base of Alfalfa, Watercress, Parsley, Lecithin, and Rice Concentrate.

Active Booster Compound - Starlight International
Each caplet contains: Potassium (as Potassium Gluconate) 8.3 mg • Uva Ursi extract, 4:1 (Arctostaphylos uva ursi, leaf) 300 mg • Corn Silk Pistils extract, 4:1 (Zea mays, flower) 300 mg • Citric Acid 200 mg • Parsley leaf extract (Petroselinum crispum, leaf) 50 mg. Other Ingredients: Dicalcium Phosphate, Microcystalline Cellulose, Stearic Acid, Sodium Starch Glycolate, Croscarmellose Sodium, Magnesium Stearate, Silicon Dioxide, Pharmaceutical Shellac, Hydroxypropylmethylcellulose, Carbowax Powder, Calcium Carbonate, Mono & Diglycerides, Gum Acacia.

Active Calcium - USANA Health Sciences
Four tablets contain: Calcium (as Citrate and Carbonate) 800 mg • Magnesium (as Citrate, Amino Acid Chelate and Oxide) 400 mg • Vitamin K (as Phylloquinone) 60 mcg • Vitamin D (Vitamin D3 as Cholecalciferol) 400 IU • Boron (as Citrate) 1.32 mg • Silicon (as Amino Acid Complex) 9 mg. Other Ingredients: Microcrystalline Cellulose, Pregelatinized Starch, Ascorbyl Palmitate, Dextrin, Croscarmellose Sodium, Dextrose.

Active Calcium Chewable - USANA Health Sciences
Each tablent contains: Vitamin D (Vitamin D3 as Cholecalciferol) 100 IU • Calcium (as Citrate and Carbonate) 200 mg • Magnesium (as Oxide and Citrate) 100 mg • Boron (as Amino Acid Complex) 0.33 mg • Silicon (as Amino Acid Complex) 2 mg. Other Ingredients: Xylitol, Maltodextrin, Dextrose, Lecithin, Vegetable-Derived Stearic Acid, Natural Flavor Blend, Natural Flavors, Citric Acid, Guar Gum, Malic Acid, Natural Carmine Color.

Active Enzymes - Global Health Trax
Each capsule contains: Digeseb Plus Proprietary Blend 450 mg: Protease, Carbohydrases, Lipase • Cellulase 75 mg • Proprietary Enzyme Blend 75 mg: Xylanase, Beta-Glucanases, Phytase, Hemicellulases • Probiotic Blend 75 mg: Lactobacillus Biffidum, Lactobacillus Longum.

Active Joints - Health Smart Vitamins
Each caplet contains: Vitamin C (ascorbic acid) 60 mg • Manganese (as manganese glycinate) 2 mg • Glucosamine Sulfate 500 mg • Sea Cucumber 100 mg • Chondroitin Sulfate 400 mg.
See Editor's Note No. 15, page 2055.

Active One Senior Multivitamin - Rainbow Light
Each tablet contains: Vitamin A (50% beta-carotene, 50% palmitate) 5000 IU • Vitamin C (ascorbic acid) 120 mg • Vitamin D (D3, cholecalciferol) 400 IU • Vitamin E (D-alpha tocopheryl succinate) 100 IU • Thiamin (vitamin B1) 10 mg • Riboflavin (vitamin B2) 10 mg • Niacinamide (vitamin B3) 30 mg • Pyridoxine (vitamin B6) 15 mg • Folic Acid 800 mcg • Cyanocobalamin (vitamin B12) 200 mcg • Biotin 150 mcg • Pantothenic Acid (vitamin B5) 20 mg • Calcium (carbonate) 200 mg • Magnesium (oxide) 100 mg • Zinc (citrate)

15 mg • Selenium (amino acid chelate, selenomethionine) 15 mg • Copper (amino acid chelate) 1.5 mg • Manganese (citrate) 2 mg • Chromium (amino nicotinate) 200 mcg • Molybdenum (amino acid chelate) 100 mcg • Potassium (citrate) 10 mg • Plant-Source Enzymes: Protease 664 HUT, Amylase 226 DU, Lipase 3 LU, Cellulase 2 CU • Citrus Bioflavonoids 25 mg • Betaine HCl 20 mg • Choline (bitartrate) 30 mg • Inositol 10 mg • Boron (glycinate) 1 mg • Lutein (esters) 1 mg • Lycopene (from tomato extract) 500 mcg • Green Foods/Superfoods: Spirulina 20 mg, 4:1 Organic Vegetable Juice Extract 50 mg: Alfalfa, Kamut, Barley grass, Oat grass, Stinging Nettle leaf, Kale, Broccoli, Cabbage, Parsley • Rosemary leaf essential oil 2 mg. Other Ingredients: Cellulose, Modified Cellulose Gum, Stearic Acid (vegetable), Silica, Magnesium Stearate, Vegetable Food Glaze.

***ActiveCal Caramel Chews* - GNC**
Each chew contains: Vitamin D 100 IU • Vitamin K 40 mcg • Calcium 500 mg. Ingredients: Corn syrup, Calcium Carbonate, Sugar, Sweetened Condensed Skim Milk, Partially Hydrogenated Soybean oil, Whey, Mono & Diglycerides, Soy Lecithin, Artificial Flavor, Vitamin D, Vitamin K.

***ActiveCal Chocolate Chews* - GNC**
Each chew contains: Vitamin D 100 IU • Vitamin K 40 mcg • Calcium 500 mg. Ingredients: Corn syrup, Calcium Carbonate, Sugar, Sweetened Condensed Skim Milk, Partially Hydrogenated Soybean oil, Whey, Cocoa (processed with alkali), Mono & Diglycerides, Soy Lecithin, Artificial Flavor, Vitamin D, Vitamin K.

***Activin 50 Mg Grape Seed Extract* - Natrol**
Each tablet contains: ActiVin (Grape Seed extract) 50 mg. Other Ingredients: Dicalcium Phosphate, Microcrystalline Cellulose, Mono & Di-Glycerides, Stearic Acid, Silicon Dioxide, Magnesium Stearate.

***Acti-Zyme* - Nature's Plus**
Two capsules contain: Live Food Enzymes: Aminogen (Aspergillus niger & Aspergillus oryzae proteolytic enzyme complex) 100 mg • Lugamase (Saccharamyces cerevisae & Aspergillus oryzae oligosaccharide enzyme complex) 100 mg • Amylase (30000 units/gram) 50 mg • Lactase (1000 units/gram) 50 mg • Lipase (5000 units/gram) 50 mg • Cellulase (5000 units/gram) 50 mg • Protease (100000 units/gram) 50 mg • Oxidase (5000 units/gram) 50 mg • Bromelain (2000 GDU/gram) 50 mg • Diastase (1000 units/gram) 5 mg • Maltase (1000 units/gram) 5 mg. Lactic Flora and Growth Accelerants: FOS (Fructooligosaccharides), lactic flora growth accelerant 100 mg • Lactospor, micro-encapsulated pure culture of B. Coagulans, provides 300 million viable cells 50 mg. Bioavailability Enhancing Phytonutrient: Bioperine (Piper nigrum fruit) standardized 95% 1-piperoylpiperidine 5 mg.

***ActoTherm* - Advocare International**
Each caplet contains: Niacin 20 mg • Vitamin A (as beta-carotene) 1000 IU • Magnesium (as phosphate) 50 mg • Potassium (as phosphate) 100 mg • Guarana seed extract (paullinia cupana) 200 mg • Green Tea leaf extract (camellia sinensis) 10 mg • Capsicum fruit extract (capsicum annuum) 16 mg • Proprietary Blend Thermogen-HC 112 mg: Gotu Kola extract, Cinnamon Ramulus extract, Peppermint extract, Lemon Verbana extract, Chamomile extract, Ginger extract, Chinese Licorice root extract, Sweet Citrus peel extract, Chicory extract. Other Ingredients: Calcium Sulfate, Dicalcium Phosphate, Silicon Dioxide, Cellulose, Stearic Acid, Magnesium Stearate.

***Acutrim 16-Hour Steady Control* - Ciba Self-Medication, Inc.**
Each tablet contains: Phenylpropanolamine HCl 75 mg. Other Ingredients: Cellulose Acetate, Hydroxypropyl Methylcellulose, Stearic Acid.

***Acutrim Maximum Strength* - Ciba Self-Medication, Inc.**
Each tablet contains: Phenylpropanolamine HCl 75 mg. Other Ingredients: Acacia, Calcium Carbonate, FD&C Yellow #10 Aluminum Lake, FD&C Yellow #6 Aluminum Lake, Guar Gum, Hydroxypropyl Methylcellulose, Microcrystalline Cellulose, Silicon Dioxide, Stearic Acid.

***Acutrim Natural A.M.* - Heritage Consumer Products**
Two tablets contain: Orange extract (4% synephrine) 100 mg • Niacin 100 mg • Guarana seed extract 300 mg • Polygonum cuspidatum root extract 25 mg • L-Arginine 450 mg • Guar Gum 200 mg • Citrus Pectin 50 mg.
See Editor's Note No. 40, page 2058.

***Acutrim Natural P.M.* - Heritage Consumer Products**
Two tablets contain: Niacin 180 mg • L-Arginine 450 mg • Polygonum cuspidatum 30 mg • Inositol Hexanicotinate 100 mg • L-Glutamine 40 mg • Guar Gum 250 mg • Citrus Pectin 50 mg.

***Adagin* - Dazzle, Inc.**
Each tablet contains: Calcium (as calcium carbonate) 36 mg • Proprietary Blend 520 mg: L-Arginine, Mucuna Pruriens 15% L-dopa, Ashwaganda, Alpha GPC, Tribulis Terrestris Extract 40%, Cordyceps Sinensis Extract, Optizine. Other Ingredients: Silicon Dioxide, Magnesium, Gelatin.

***Adam's Equalizer* - Zeller**
Purified Water • Natural Glycerin • Stearal Konium Chloride • D-Alpha Tocopherol (vitamin E) • Avocado oil • Jojoba oil • Saw Palmetto • Pygeum Africanum • Ginseng • Uva-Ursi • Pumpkin seed extract • Sarsaparilla • Natural Progesterone • Vitamin C (acerola) • OptiZinc Zinc • Rosemary extract • Carrot oil • Lemon Grass oil.

***Adaptrin* - Pacific BioLogic**
Each capsule contains: Proprietary Blend 500 mg: Iceland Moss • Red Sandalwood • Hardy Orange • Vetiver • Margosa • Spiral Flag • White Sandalwood • Cloves • Columbine • Wild Lettuce • Marigold • Knotgrass • Licorice • Valerian • Camphor bark • Gypsum • Cardamom • Jamaican Pepper • Ribwort (plantain) • Heartleaved Sida Cordifolia • Myrobalan • Blackthorn • Golden Cinquefoil • Gingerlily • Homeopathic Monkshood.
See Editor's Note No. 39, page 2058.

***Adenergy* - Optimum Nutrition**
Each caplet contains: Calcium 20 mg • Adenosine 5'-Triphosphate Disodium (peak ATP) 125 mg • Proprietary Adenergizing Blend 406 mg: ATP, Caffeine, Theophylline, Polyphenols (including EGCG). Other Ingredients: Enteric Coating (enteric polymer (methacrylic acid/methlmethacrylate), titanium dioxide, triethyl citrate, talc), Calcium Citrate, Microcystalline Cellulose, Dicalcium Phosphate, Solutab, Stearic Acid, Magnesium Stearate, Silica.

***Adipokinetix* - Syntrax Innovations**
Each capsule or tablet contains: Caffeine 100 mg • Phenylpropanolamine (PPA) 25 mg • Yohimbine HCl 3 mg.

***Adipoxil* - I Force**
Three capsules contain: Vitamin B5 (D-cal pantothenate) 50 mg • Green Tea extract 500 mg • Guarana extract (22% caffeine) 450 mg • Citrus Aurantium (6.9% synephrine) 400 mg • Lecithin (phosphatidyl choline 105 mg) 300 mg • L-Carnitine L-Tartrate 300 mg • White Willow bark extract (15% salicin) 105 mg • 2,3-Aminomutase 100 mg • 5-Methyl-7-Methoxy-Isoflavone 60 mg • 7-Isopropoxyisoflavone 55 mg • Coleus Forskohlii (95% forskolin) 50 mg • Ginger root powder 50 mg. Other Ingredients: Gelatin, Microcrystalline Cellulose, Magnesium Stearate, Silica.
See Editor's Note No. 40, page 2058.

***ADR Complex* - Professional Botanicals**
Each caplet contains: Vitamin C 100 mg • Vitamin B6 25 mg • Pantothenic Acid 250 mg • Adrenal 150 mg • Pituitary 30 mg • Barberry 150 mg • Blessed Thistle 100 mg.

***Adrenal 100* - Professional Botanicals**
Each tablet contains: Raw Adrenal substance (freeze-dried) 100 mg. Base: Thymus, Lymph, Duodenal Substance.

Some Brand Name Natural Products - What they Contain

www.NaturalDatabase.com contains MANY more listings than appear here.

BRAND NAMES

Adrenal Chelate **-** Atrium Inc.
Each tablet contains: Raw Adrenal concentrate (not an extract) 80 mg • L-Leucine 10 mg • L-Isoleucine 20 mg • D-Calcium Pantothenate 60 mg • Sodium Ascorbate 120 mg • Potassium Aspartate 30 mg • Hesperidin Complex 150 mg • Bioflavonoid Complex 75 mg • Chlorophyll 10 mg. In a base of Alfalfa, Celery & Parsley.
See Editor's Note No. 14, page 2055.

Adrenal Cortex 75 **-** Professional Botanicals
Each tablet contains: Raw Adrenal Cortex substance (freeze-dried) 75 mg. Base: Thymus, Lymph, Duodenal Substances.

Adrenal Cortex Extract **-** BioMax Limited
Each dropper (0.166 ml) contains: Adrenal Cortex extract (bovine) 66.66 mcg. Other Ingredients: Glycerin, Alcohol, Stevia.

Adrenal Cortex, Organic Glandular **-** NutriCology
Each capsule contains: Adrenal Cortex tissue (bovine) 250 mg. Other Ingredients: Cellulose, Magnesium Stearate.
See Editor's Note No. 14, page 2055.

Adrenal Energy **-** Pro Health
Two capsules contain: Vitamin C (as ascorbic acid) 250 mg • Pantothenic Acid 50 mg • Licorice root (glycyrrhiza glabra) 250 mg • L-Tyrosine 250 mg • Eleuthero root (eleutherococcus senticosus) 200 mg • Pregnenolone 50 mg • CoQ10 30 mg • DHEA 10 mg. Other Ingredients: Gelatin (capsule shell), Silica, Rice Flour, Magnesium Stearate.

Adrenal Health - Wellzymes **-** Enzymes, Inc.
Two capsules contain: n-zimes Proprietary Enzyme Blend 65 mg: pHysioProtease (177,600 pHysio-U), CereCalase Plus • Panax Ginseng root extract (standardized to contain 8% ginsenosides) 160 mg • Bupleurum root extract (equivalent to 400 mg raw herb) 100 mg • Rice Bran 65 mg • Siberian Ginseng root extract (standardized to contain 0.8% eleutherosides) 40 mg. Other Ingredients: Plant Cellulose, Water.

Adrenal Plus **-** Futurebiotics
Raw Adrenal concentrate 80 mg • Vitamin C (Ascorbic Acid) 150 mg • Pantothenic Acid 60 mg • Zinc (Gluconate) 5 mg • Manganese (Amino Acid Chelate) 1 mg • Schizandra (6:1) 20 mg • Chinese Licorice (10:1) 12 mg • Niacinamide 80 mg.
See Editor's Note No. 14, page 2055.

Adrenal Support **-** PhytoPharmica
Two capsules contain: Vitamin C (ascorbic acid/rose hip fruit) 125 mg • Vitamin B6 (pyridoxine HCl) 25 mg • Pantothenic Acid (calcium D-pantothenate) 125 mg •L-Tyrosine 250 mg •Betaine 125 mg • Pituitary extract 60 mg • Adrenal extract (predigested soluble concentrate) 50 mg • Ginger (Zingiber officinale) root (rhizome) extract 6.5:1 50 mg • Adrenal cortex extract 17 mg.
See Editor's Note No. 14 and No. 21, pages 2055 and 2056.

Adrenal Support **-** Vital Nutrients
Two capsules contain: Adrenal (whole, bovine) 300 mg • Adrenal (cortex, bovine) 150 mg • Eleuthero extract (eleutherococcus senticosus, 28:1) 200 mg • Ashwagandha extract (5:1) 200 mg • Cordyceps Sinensis extract (4:1) 100 mg • Pantothenic Acid 100 mg.
See Editor's Note No. 14, page 2055.

Adrenal Trophic **-** Progressive Labs
Each capsule contains: Pantothenic Acid (as d-calcium panothenate) 50 mg • Raw Porcine Adrenal concentrate 80 mg. Other Ingredients: Rice Flour, Magnesium Stearate.

Adrenal, Desiccated **-** Standard Process, Inc.
Two tablets contain: Proprietary Blend 444 mg: Bovine Adrenal, Carrot root. Other Ingredients: Calcium Lactate, Honey, Arabic Gum, Calcium Stearate.
See Editor's Note No. 14, page 2055.

Adrenal, Organic Glandular **-** NutriCology
Each capsule contains: Adrenal tissue (bovine) 300 mg. Other Ingredients: Cellulose, Silicon Dioxide, Stearic Acid.
See Editor's Note No. 14, page 2055.

Adrenal-Cortex Complex **-** Enzymatic Therapy
Each capsule contains: Adrenal-Cortex Complex 250 mg • Multi-Glandular Complex: Raw Liver, Raw Lung, Raw Pancreas, Raw Heart, Raw Kidney, Raw Spleen, & Raw Brain 100 mg.
See Editor's Note No. 14, page 2055.

Adrenal-Cortex Fractions **-** PhytoPharmica
Each capsule contains: Adrenal-Cortex Complex 250 mg • Multi-Glandular Complex 100 mg: Raw Liver, Raw Lung, Raw Pancreas, Raw Heart, Raw Kidney, Raw Spleen, Raw Brain. All organs & glands derived from bovine sources except raw pancreas (porcine).
See Editor's Note No. 31, page 2056.

Adren-Comp **-** Enzymatic Therapy
Each capsule contains: Chinese Thoroughwax extract (Bupleurum falcatum) 150 mg • Korean Ginseng root extract 3:1 (Panax ginseng) 100 mg • Siberian Ginseng extract (Eleutherococcus senticosus) (standardized to contain greater than 1% eleutheroside E) 100 mg • Mexican Yam extract 10:1 (Dioscorea spinosa) (standardized to contain 10% Diosgenin) 100 mg • Licorice root extract (Glycyrrhiza glabra) (standardized to contain 5% Glycyrrhizic acid) 50 mg • Curcuma root extract 10:1 (Curcuma longa) 50 mg.

Adrenerlin **-** Bodyonics, Ltd.
Two capsules contain: Maca Pure (Lepidum meyenii) (standardized to contain 0.6% macamides and macanes) 450 mg • Jeevani Botanical Complex (Tricopus zylanicus, Ashwanga (Withania somnifera), Piper Longum, Vishnukranthi (Evolvus alsinoies) 150 mg • Peptide GPX 250 mg • D-Ribose 10 mg • Acetyl-L-Carnitine 10 mg • Bitter Orange (standardized 4% synephrine) 83.3 mg • Yerba Mate and Guarana Extract (standardized) 200 mg Methylxanthines/ Caffeine 910 mg • Mucuna Pruriens (standardized 15% L-Dopa) 33.3 mg • Calcium Pyruvate 10 mg. Other Ingredients: Magnesium Stearate, Gelatin.
See Editor's Note No. 40, page 2058.

Adreno Chelate **-** Progressive Labs
Each capsule contains: Calcium (Proteinate) 27 mg • Chloride (Proteinate) 50 mg • Sodium (Proteinate) 20 mg • Potassium (Proteinate) 20 mg • Raw Bovine Adrenal concentrate 40 mg • L-Isoleucine 10 mg • L-Leucine 10 mg.
See Editor's Note No. 14, page 2055.

Adreno Trophic **-** Progressive Labs
Each capsule contains: Pantothenic Acid (calcium pantothenate) 50 mg • Raw Bovine Adrenal concentrate 80 mg.
See Editor's Note No. 14, page 2055.

Adreno-Cortex **-** Atrium Inc.
Each tablet contains: Adrenal Cortex • Pituitary Anterior 20 mg • Pineal, bovine source 10 mg • Vitamin C (Calcium Ascorbate) 25 mg.
See Editor's Note No. 14, page 2055.

Adreno-Medulla Plus **-** Atrium Inc.
Each tablet contains: Adrenal Medulla 100 mg • Hypothalamus 15 mg • Pituitary Posterior Bovine Source 10 mg • Vitamin C (Calcium Ascorbate) 25 mg.
See Editor's Note No. 14, page 2055.

Adren-Plus **-** PhytoPharmica
Each capsule contains: Bupleurum Chinense root 150 mg • Eleuthero root extract (eleutherococcus senticosus, standardized to contain a minimum of 0.5% eleutheroside E) 100 mg • Licorice root and rhizome extract (glycyrrhiza glabra, standardized to contain 5% glycyrrhizic acid) 50 mg • Panax Ginseng root extract (standardized to contain minimum of 7% ginsenosides) 100 mg • Tumeric rhizome

extract (curcuma longa, standardized to contain 85-100% curcumin) 15 mg • Wild Yam root extract (dioscorea villosa, standardized to contain 10% diosgenin) 100 mg.

Adult Echinacea+C+Zinc Cherry Flavor - LiFizz Effervescent Vitamins
Each tablet contains: Vitamin C (Ascorbic Acid) 1500 mg • Zinc 15 mg • Echinacea extract (Echinacea purpurea) 100 mg. Other Ingredients: Citric Acid, Sodium Bicarbonate, Sorbitol, Mannitol, Polyethylene Glycol 6000, Cherry Flavor, Povidone, Aspartame, Acesulfame Potassium, Magnesium Stearate, Silicon Dioxide, Simethicone.

Adult Echinacea+C+Zinc Lemon/Lime Flavor - LiFizz Effervescent Vitamins
Each tablet contains: Vitamin C (Ascorbic Acid) 1500 mg • Zinc 15 mg • Echinacea extract (Echinacea purpurea) 100 mg. Other Ingredients: Citric Acid, Sodium Bicarbonate, Sorbitol, Mannitol, Polyethylene Glycol 6000, Lemon Flavor, Povidone, Aspartame, Acesulfame Potassium, Lemon/Lime Flavor, Magnesium Stearate, Silicon Dioxide, Simethicone.

Adult Multivitamin Chewable - Nature Made
Two tablets contain: Vitamin A (2% as beta carotene) 5000 IU • Vitamin C 250 mg • Vitamin D 400 IU • Vitamin E 30 IU • Thiamin 1.5 mg • Riboflavin 1.7 mg • Niacin 20 mg • Vitamin B6 2 mg • Folic Acid 400 mcg • Vitamin B12 6 mcg • Biotin 40 mcg • Pantothenic Acid 10 mg • Calcium 200 mg • Phosphorus 100 mg • Iodine 150 mcg • Magnesium 20 mg • Zinc 15 mg • Copper 2 mg • Sodium 15 mg. Other Ingredients: Dibasic Calcium Phosphate, Sorbitol, Fructose, Xylitol, Stearic Acid, Mono and Diglycerides of Fatty Acids, Carrageenan, Gelatin, Aspartame, Yellow 6 Lake, Corn Starch, Silicon Dioxide, Magnesium Stearate, Natural and Artificial Flavors, Modified Food Starch, Red 40 Lake.
See Editor's Note No. 45, page 2058.

Adult Multi-Vitamin Orange Flavor - LiFizz Effervescent Vitamins
Each tablet contains: Vitamin A (Palmitate and Beta Carotene) 5000 IU • Vitamin C 60 mg • Vitamin D 400 IU • Vitamin E 15 IU • Thiamin 1.5 mg • Riboflavin 1.7 mg • Niacinamide 20 mg • Vitamin B6 2 mg • Folic Acid 400 mcg • Vitamin B12 6 mcg • Biotin 300 mcg • Pantothenic Acid 10 mg • Calcium 200 mg • Iron 6 mg • Magnesium 80 mg • Zinc 5 mg.

Adult-C-Vitamin Pink Grapefruit Flavor - LiFizz Effervescent Vitamins
Each tablet contains: Vitamin C (Ascorbic Acid) 500 mg. Other Ingredients: Citric Acid, Sorbitol, Potassium Bicarbonate, Sodium Bicarbonate, Mannitol, Grapefruit Flavor, Polyethylene Glycol 6000, Orange Flavor, Aspartame, Acesulfame Potassium, Wild Berry Powder, Silicon Dioxide, Lemon/Lime flavor, Magnesium Stearate.

Adult-C-Vitamin Raspberry Flavor - LiFizz Effervescent Vitamins
Each tablets contains: Vitamin C (Ascorbic Acid) 500 mg. Other Ingredients: Citric Acid, Sodium Bicarbonate, Potassium Bicarbonate, Sorbitol, Mannitol, Polyethylen Glycol 6000, Red Beet Powder, Raspberry Flavor, Aspartame, Acesulfame Potassium, Magnesium Stearate.

Adults 50 + Vita-Vim - Jamieson
Each caplet contains: Vitamin A (Acetate) 3000 IU • Beta Carotene 3000 IU • Vitamin D 400 IU • Vitamin C 90 mg • Vitamin E 75 IU • Vitamin B1 2.25 mg • Vitamin B2 3.2 mg • Vitamin B3 (No Flush Niacinamide) 40 mg • Vitamin B5 10 mg • Vitamin B6 8 mg • Vitamin B12 25 mcg • Folic Acid 600 mcg • Biotin 45 mcg • Calcium 200 mg • Copper (from Oxide) 2 mg • Iodine 0.15 mg • Magnesium 50 mg • Zinc (from Zinc Oxide) 15 mg • Potassium (Non Citrate form) 80 mg • Manganese (Sulfate Source) 5 mg • Chromium (Non Chelated) 100 mcg • Selenium (Non Chelated) 25 mcg • Vanadium 10 mcg • Molybdenum 1 mcg • Nickel 5 mcg • Tin 10 mcg • Phosphorus 125 mcg • Silicon 10 mcg • Ginkgo Biloba 250 mg • Lutein 300 mcg • Lycopene 300 mcg • Digestive Enzyme Absorption Factors: derived from Peppermint, Bromelain, Papain, Amylase, Lipase, Cellulose 2000 mcg.

AdvaCal - LaneLabs
Three capsules contain: Elemental Calcium (as calcium hydroxide, calcium oxide, combined with algae amino acid extract) 450 mg. Other Ingredients: Citric Acid, Gelatin, Water, Glycerine.

Advanced B Heart Health Formula - Nature Made
Each tablet contains: Vitamin B6 (pyridoxine hydrochloride) 10 mg • Natural Folate (Metafolin, L-methylfolate) 400 mcg • Vitamin B12 (cyanocobalamin) 200 mcg • Phytonutrient Blend 100 mg: Green Tea extract, Grape seed extract, Blueberry, Strawberry, Blackberry, Raspberry, Cranberry, Sour Cherry fruit, Blueberry extract. Other Ingredients: Cellulose Gel, Dibasic Calcium Phosphate, Talc, Gelatin, Silicon Dioxide, Croscarmellose Sodium, Magnesium Stearate, Hydroxypropyl Methylcellulose, Polyethylene Glycol.

Advanced Chromium HCA - Health Smart Vitamins
Each capsule contains: Calcium (as calcium salt of hydroxy citric acid) 79 mg • Chromium (as chromium picolinate) 100 mcg • Garcinia cambogia fruit (50% (-) hydroxycitric acid [HCA], 250 mg) 500 mg.

Advanced C-Jointin - Puritan's Pride
Three softgels contain: Vitamin C (as Ascorbic Acid) 60 mg • Vitamin E (as d-Alpha-Tocopherol) 10 IU • Manganese (as Manganese Aspartate) 1 mg • Boron (as Boron Citrate) 1.5 mg • Evening Primrose Oil 250 mg • MSM (Methylsulfonylmethane) 750 mg • Chondroitin Sulfate 200 mg • Glucosamine Sulfate 1,000 mg.
See Editor's Note No. 15, page 2055.

Advanced C-Jointin - Vitamin World
Three softgels contain: Vitamin C (as ascorbic acid) 60 mg • Vitamin E (as d-alpha tocopherol) 10 IU • Manganese (as manganese aspartate) 1 mg • Glucosamine Sulfate (2KCl) 1000 mg • MSM (methylsulfonylmethane) 750 mg • Chondroitin Sulfate 200 mg • Evening Primrose Oil 250 mg • Boron (as boron citrate) 1.5 mg. Other Ingredients: Soybean Oil, Gelatin, Glycerin, Beeswax / Soybean Oil Mixture, Lecithin, Caramel Color.
See Editor's Note No. 15, page 2055.

Advanced Colloidal Chromium/Vanadium - Futurebiotics
Each 1 tsp serving contains: Chromium 0.18 ppm • Vanadium 0.18 ppm. Other Ingredients: Deionized Water.

Advanced CoQ10 - Changes International, Inc.
Each capsule contains: Coenzyme Q10 50 mg.

Advanced E + Grape Seed Extract - Leiner Health Products
Each softgel contains: Vitamin E (dl-Alpha Tocopherol) 400 IU • Grape Seed extract 20 mg. Other Ingredients: Gelatin, Vegetable Oil, Glycerin, Yellow Beeswax, Unbleached Lecithin, Titanium Dioxide, Carmine.

Advanced E with Alpha Lipoic Acid - Leiner Health Products
Each softgel contains: Vitamin C (Ascorbic Acid) 20 mg • Vitamin E (dl-Alpha Tocopherol, d-Alpha Tocopherol) 400 IU • Alpha Lipoic Acid 30 mg • Rice Bran oil 5 mg. Other Ingredients: Gelatin, Glycerin, Yellow Beeswax, Soybean Oil, Lecithin, Titanium Dioxide, Turmeric.

Advanced Formula - Biotech Corp.
Each tablet contains: Folate 400 mg • Pantothenic Acid 100 mg • Biotin 700 mcg • Iodine 75 mcg • Zinc 75 mg • Shen Min 225 mg • Shen Min (He Shou Wu root powder) 435 mg • Isoflavones 10 mg • Saw Palmetto berries standardized extract 160 mg • Silica 20 mg • Black Pepper extract 2.5 mg.

Advanced Formula Shen Min For Men - Biotech Corp.
Two tablets contain: Folate (as folic acid) 800 mcg • Pantothenic Acid (as dicalcium pantothenate) 200 mg • Biotin 1400 mcg • Iodine (from

kelp) 150 mcg • Zinc (as zinc monomethionine) 15 mg • Shen Min Herb Blend 1320 mg: He Shou Wu (12:1 extract, standardized for chrysophanics and resveratrol), He Shou Wu root powder (polygonum multiflorum) • Shen Min Botanical Blend 450 mg: Saw Palmetto berries (sabal serrulata), Beta Sitosterol, Isoflavones (from pueraria lobata root and soybeans) • Silica (from colloidals) 40 gm • BioPerine Piper Nigrum standardized extract 5 mg. Other Ingredients: Microcrystalline Cellulose, Croscarmellose Sodium, Stearic Acid, Magnesium Stearate, Pharmaceutical Glaze.

Advanced Formula Shen Min For Women - Biotech Corp.
Two tablets contain: Vitamin A (as retinyl palmitate) 5000 IU • Vitamin B6 (pyridoxine HCl) 10 mg • Niacin (as nicotinic acid) 20 mg • Pantothenic Acid 200 mg • Biotin 1400 mcg • Shen Min (polygonum multiflorum, 12:1 standardized extract) 450 mg • He Shou Wu root powder 870 mg • Soy Isoflavones (glycine max, from 50 mg 40% standardized soybean extract) 20 mg • Black Cohosh root (cimicifuga racemosa, 2.5% sesquiterpene lactones) 40 mg • Horse Chestnut standardized extract (20% escin) 50 mg • Hydrolyzed Collagen 250 mg • Silica (from plant sources) 100 mg • Ginkgo Biloba leaf 100 mg • Uva Ursi root standardized extract (10% arbutin) 50 mg • Burdock root (4:1 extract) 25 mg • Cayenne pepper (80,000 scoville heat units) 25 mg • BioPerine Black pepper (piper nigrum standardized extract) 2 mg. Other Ingredients: Microcrystalline Cellulose, Croscarmellose Sodium, Stearic Acid, Magnesium Stearate, Dicalcium Phosphate, Pharmaceutical Glaze.

Advanced Geri-Max - Puritan's Pride
Each tablet contains: Vitamin A 10,000 IU • Vitamin C 250 mg • Vitamin D 400 IU • Vitamin E 150 IU • Thiamin 50 mg • Riboflavin 50 mg • Niacin 100 mg • Vitamin B6 50 mg • Folic Acid 400 mcg • Vitamin B12 50 mcg • Biotin 300 mcg • Pantothenic Acid 100 mg • Calcium 10 mg • Iron 1 mg • Iodine 150 mcg • Magnesium 1.54 mg • Zinc 1.15 mg • Copper 0.25 mg • Manganese 0.61 mg • Potassium 1 mg • PABA 50 mg • Inositol 250 mg • Choline Bitartrate 250 mg • Rutin 25 mg • Citrus Bioflavonoid complex 25 mg • Hesperidin complex 25 mg • Betaine Hydrochloride 25 mg • L-Glutamic Acid 25 mg • Omega-3 EPA / DHA 50 mg. In a natural base of Alfalfa, Watercress, Parsley, Lecithin, and Rice Polishings.

Advanced Ginkgo 24% - Doctor's A-Z
Each softgel contains: Ginkgo Biloba leaf extract (24% flavone glycosides, 6% terpene lactones) 60 mg.

Advanced Joint Support - Futurebiotics
Four capsules contain: Glucosamine Sulfate 1000 mg • Vitamin C (Buffered Ascorbate) 750 mg • Vitamin E (natural) 400 IU • Calcium (Ascorbate) 185 mg • Selenium (Amino Acid Chelate) 100 mcg • Zinc (Amino Acid Chelate) 15 mg • Bovine Cartilage 200 mg • Pancreatin 4X (Quadruple Strength) 100 mg containing: (Lipase 1600 USP units, Amylase 10000 USP units, Protease 10000 USP units) • Papain 60 mg • Bromelain 50 mg • Turmeric (standardized Curcumin) 250 mg • Cayenne powder 15 mg • Ginger powder 100 mg • Boswellin (standardized for 65% Boswellic Acid) 100 mg • Devil's Claw 50 mg • Rutin 50 mg.
See Editor's Note No. 14, page 2055.

Advanced Lutein & Bilberry - Doctor's A-Z
Each softgel contains: Bilberry extract (25% anthocyanidins) 20 mg • FloraGLO Lutein extract (from marigold) 6 mg.

Advanced Prostate Formula - Rx Vitamins
Three capsules contain: Saw Palmetto fruit 320 mg • Stinging Nettle root 100 mg • African Pygeum bark 50 mg • Zinc 50 mg • Glycine 50 mg • Alanine 50 mg • Glutamic Acid 50 mg • Vitamin B6 50 mg • Vitamin E 100 IU in Borage seed oil.

Advanced Strength Ginkgo Biloba - Leiner Health Products
Each caplet contains: Ginkgo Biloba extract (Ginkgo biloba) leaf 75 mg • Lecithin 15 mg. Other Ingredients: Dicalcium phosphate, Cellulose, Silicon Dioxide, Stearic Acid, Croscarmellose Sodium, Dextrin, Magnesium Stearate, Dextrose, Sodium Carboxymethylcellulose, Sodium Citrate.

Advanced Strength Kava Kava - Leiner Health Products
Each caplet contains: Kava Kava extract (Piper methysticum) root 400 mg. Other Ingredients: Dicalcium Phosphate, Cellulose, Talc, Stearic Acid, Croscarmellose Sodium, Silicon Dioxide, Magnesium Stearate, Crospovidone, Hydroxypropyl Methylcellulose, Hydroxypropyl Cellulose, Polysorbate 80, Polyethylene Glycol 3350.

Advanish cream - Gero Vita International
Active Ingredient: Hydroquinone 2.0%. Inactive Ingredients: Deionized Water, Glycolic Acid, Triethanolamine, Glycerin, Petrolatum, Cetyl Alcohol, Glyceryl Stearate, Stearic Acid, DEA-Cetyl Phosphate, Octyl Methoxycinnamate, Sodium Bisulfite, Kojic Dipalmitate, Mulberry extract, Licorice root extract, Ascorbic acid, Tocopheryl Acetate, Dimethicone, Sodium Lauroyl Oat Amino Acids, Phenoxyethanol, Disodium EDTA, Xanthan Gum, Fragrance, Methylparaben, Propylparaben.

Advantage - Metabolic Nutrition
Each packet (62 g) contains: Vitamin A • Vitamin B6 • Vitamin B12 • Vitamin C • Vitamin D • Vitamin E • Biotin • Calcium • Copper • Folic Acid • Iodine • Iron • Magnesium • Niacin • Pantothenic Acid • Phosphorus • Riboflavin • Thiamine • Zinc • Enzyme Additives: Betaine HCl, Pancreatin, Pepsin, Papain, Amylase.

AdvantaSoy brand - Cargill Health & Food Technologies
Soy.
See Editor's Note No. 44, page 2058.

Advantin - Advocare International
Each capsule contains: Ginger extract (root - zingiber officinale) 200 mg • Boswellia extract (gum resin - boswellia serrata) 150 mg • Curcumin powder (root - Curcuma longa) 100 mg • Whole Papaya powder (fruit - carica papaya) 50 mg • Papain 50 mg • Bromelain 50 mg. Other Ingredients: Silicon Dioxide, Magnesium Stearate, Gelatin.

Advantra Z (Advantra-Z, AdvantraZ) brand - Nutratech
Citrus Aurantium.
See Editor's Note No. 44, page 2058.

AdvoKids Spark - Advocare International
Each pouch contains: Vitamin A (as beta-carotene from D. satina mixed carotenoids) 2500 IU • Vitamin C (as ascorbic acid) 180 mg • Vitamin E (as D-alpha-tocopheryl acetate) 30 IU • Thiamine 3 mg • Riboflavin 3.4 mg • Niacin (as niacin and niacinamide) 60 mg • Vitamin B6 (as pyridoxine HCl) 6 mg • Vitamin B12 (as cyanocobalamin) 45 mcg • Pantothenic Acid (as calcium pantothenate) 30 mg • Zinc (as monomethionine - OptZinc) 3 mg • Copper (as glycinate) 200 mcg • Chromium (as polynicotinate - ChromeMate) 60 mcg • Sodium (as phosphate) 20 mg • L-Tyrosine 500 mg • Choline (as citrate and bitartrate) 400 mg • Taurine 200 mg • Glycine 100 mg • Gamma-Aminobutyric Acid 100 mg • Caffeine 60 mg • L-Carnitine (as tartrate) 10 mg • Coenzyme Q-10 100 mcg. Other Ingredients: Maltodextrin, Citric Acid, Natural Flavor, Artificial Flavor, Sodium Phosphate, Sucralose, Silicon Dioxide.

Aflexa - McNeil Consumer Healthcare
Each tablet contains: Glucosamine 340 mg (Glucosamine Sulfate, Glucosamine Hydrochloride). Other Ingredients: Cellulose, Hydroxypropyl, Methylcellulose, Polyethylene Glycol, Silicon Dioxide, Propylene Glycol, Crospovidone, Hydroxypropyl Cellulose, Titanium Dioxide, Magnesium Stearate, Polysorbate 80, Povidone.

After Max - Optimum Nutrition
Three scoops (97 g) contain: Proprietary Protein Blend: Whey Protein Concentrate, Glutamine Peptides, Whey Protein Isolate, Hydrolyzed Whey Peptides • Maltodextrin • Cocoa • Natural and Artificial Flavors • Salt • Acesulfame Potassium • Vitamin/Mineral Blend: Ascorbic Acid, D-Alpha Tocopheryl Succinate, Maltoxextrin, Niacinamide, D-Calcium Pantothenate, Pyridoxine Hydrochloride, Chromium Polynicotinate, Riboflavin, Vitamin A Palmitate, Biotin, Folic Acid, Cholecalciferol, Cyanocobalamin • Sucralose.

Some Brand Name Natural Products - What they Contain

www.NaturalDatabase.com contains MANY more listings than appear here.

AfterFX Bar - Bavarian Mint - Nutripeak
Each bar contains: Protein 34 g • Vitamin A (Retinyl Palmitate) 5000 IU • Vitamin C (Ascorbic Acid) 120 mg • Vitamin D (Cholecalciferol) 400 IU • Vitamin E (dl-Alpha Tocopheryl Acetate) 60 IU • Thiamin Mononitrate (Vitamin B1) 1.5 mg • Riboflavin (Vitamin B2) 1.7 mg • Niacin (Niacinamide) 20 mg • Vitamin B6 (Pyridoxine Hydrochloride) 2 mg • Folic Acid 400 mcg • Vitamin B12 (Cyanocobalamin) 6 mcg •Biotin 300 mcg •Pantothenic Acid (Calcium D-Pantothenate) 10 mg •Calcium (Tricalcium Phosphate and Monocalcium Phosphate) 500 mg •Iron (Ferrous Fumarate) 18 mg •Phosphorus 300 mg •Iodine (Potassium Iodide) 150 mcg •Magnesium Oxide 100 mg •Zinc Amino Acid Chelate 15 mg •Copper Gluconate 2 mg •Sodium 75 mg •Potassium 250 mg • HMB (as calcium-b-hydroxy-b-methylbutyrate) 585 mg •L-Glutamine 3 mg. Other Ingredients: Metamyosyn Protein Blend: Bovine Hydrolyzed Collagen, Calcium Caseinate, Milk Protein Concentrate, Whey Protein Isolate, Whey Protein Concentrate, Dried Egg Albumen; Coating: Maltitol, Salatrim, Cocoa (processed with alkali), Butter Oil, Soy Lecithin, Acesulfame K, Vanilla; Glycerin; Water; Natural and Artificial Flavors; Brown Rice Syrup; Medium Chain Triglycerides; Cocoa (processed with alkali); Cocoa extract; Polydextrose; Potassium Sorbate (preservative); Salt; Sucralose; Partially Hydrogenated Soybean Oil; Partially Hydrogenated Cottonseed Oil. May contain traces of peanuts and/or other nuts.

Age Right Formula - Nature's Way
Four capsules contain: Acetylcarnitine 50 mcg • Acetylcysteine 50 mcg • Betaine Anhydrous 50 mg • Biotin (Biotin Triurate) 500 mcg • Boron (Amino Acid Chelate) 500 mcg • Calcium 43 mg • Calcium Pantethonate 175 mg • Caromix (Mixed Carotenoids) 2000 IU • Chromium Picolinate 100 mcg • Citrus Bioflavonoids 250 mg • Coenzyme Q10 (Ubiquinone) 15 mg • Copper (Amino Acid Chelate) 500 mcg • Fizyme Enzyme Formula 65 mg • Folic Acid (Folate) 250 mcg • Grape seed dried extract 15 mg • Green Tea (Polyphenol Catechin extract) 75 mg • Inositol 15 mg • Kelp (whole Thallus) 25 mcg • Manganese (Amino Acid Chelate) 2.5 mg • Molybdenum Triuturate 25 mcg • Niacinamide 47.5 mg • Potassium (Aspartate, Chloride) 25 mg • Riboflavin (Vitamin B2) 25 mg • Selenium (l-Selenomethione) 25 mcg • Thiamine (Vitamin B1) 25 mg • Vitamin A (Retinol Palmitate) 2530 IU • Vitamin B12 (Cyanocobalamin) 250 mcg • Vitamin B6 (Pyridoxine HCL) 25 mg • Vitamin C (Ascorbic Acid) 250 mg • Vitamin D (as Vitamin D3) (Cholecalciferol) 200 IU • Vitamin E (d-Alpha Tocopheryl) 200 IU • Vitamin K (Phytonadione) 30 mcg • Zinc (Amino Acid Chelate) 5 mg. Other Ingredients: Gelatin, Magnesium Stearate, Millet.

AgeErasers SAMe - Bodyonics, Ltd.
Each tablet contains: Vitamin B12 50 mcg • Folic Acid 100 mcg • SAMe 200 mg. Other Ingredients: Calcium Phosphate, Stearic Acid, Croscarmellose, Magnesium Strearate.

Ageless - Oasis Wellness Network
Four capsules contain: Vitamin B3 (as niacin, niacinamide) 35 mg • Vitamin B6 (as pyridoxal-5-phosphate) 8 mg • Serenix Corn extract 1000 mg • Energetix 3-Ginseng Complex 750 mg: Panax Ginseng extract, Rhodiola extract, Eleuthero extract • Green Tea extract (70% polyphenols/25% EGCG, 5% theanine) 440 mg • Ornithine Ketoglutarate 300 mg • Protectin Proprietary Blend 300 mg: Catechu bark, Scullcap root • MaxCell Proprietary Blend 30 mg: Zisyphus Jujube, Piper Nigrum, Aloe Vera, Glycyrrhiza Glabra. Other Ingredients: Magnesium Stearate, Cellulose.

AHA (Alpha Hydroxy Acids) 2oz - Derma E
Purified Water • Glycolic Acid • Glycerin • Caprylic Triglyceride • Jojoba Oil • Cetearyl Alcohol • Cetearate 20 • Stearic Acid • Glyceryl Stearate • Peg 100 Stearate • Cetyl Alcohol • Xanthan Gum • Green Tea extract • Lemon extract • Passion Fruit extract • Dimethicone • Methylparaben • Sodium Hydroxide • I. Urea.

AHCC - Source Naturals
Two capsules contain: AHCC Proprietary Blend 1 g: Mushroom mycelia extract, Candelilla wax, Cyclodextrin, Microcrystalline Cellulose • Bioperine Black Pepper extract 6 mg. Other Ingredients: Gelatin, Magnesium Stearate.

Air Power - Enzymatic Therapy
Each tablet contains: Glycerol Guaiacolate 200 mg • Fenugreek powder 4:1 (trigonella foenum-graecum) 350 mg • Marshmallow extract 4:1 mucilage content 30-40% (althaea officinalis) 125 mg • PABA (para-aminobenzoic Acid) 50 mg • Mullein leaf (verbascum nigrum) 50 mg.

Airborne - Knight-McDowell Labs
Each tablet contains: Vitamin A 5000 IU • Vitamin C 1000 mg • Vitamin E 30 IU • Magnesium 40 mg • Zinc 8 mg • Selenium 15 mcg • Manganese 3 mg • Potassium 75 mg • Organic Herbal Extracts 350 mg: Lonicera, Forsythia, Schizonepeta, Ginger, Chinese Vitex, Isatis root, Echinacea • Amino Acids 50 mg (Glutamine, Lysine). Other Ingredients: Citric Acid, Sorbitol, Sodium Bicarbonate, Natural Orange Flavor, Polyethylene Glycol, Aspartame, Mineral and Canola Oil, Riboflavin.

AirDefense - NaturalCare
Active Ingredients: Pink Root (spigelia anthelmia) 3X • Origanum Vulgare (oregano) 3X, 6X • Luffa Operculata (luffa fruit) 6X • Hydrastis Canadensis (golden seal) 3X, 6X, 12X • Echinacea Angustifolia (cone flower) 3X, 6X, 12X • Zinc Gluconate (zincum gluconicum) 2X, 6X • Euphorbium Officinarum 4X, 6X, 12X • Silver (argentum metallicum) 8X • Potassium Sulfate (kali sulphuricum) 3X, 6X, 12X • Allium Cepa (red onion) 6X • Ragweed (ambrosia artemisiaefolia) 6X • Calcium Sulfide (hepar sulphuris calcareum) 8X • Potassium Dichromate (kali bichromicum) 6X, 10X • Sanguinaria Canadensis (blood root) 6X • Lemna Minor (duckweed) 3X • Pulsatilla (windflower) 3X • Sabadilla (cevadilla seed) 6X • Silicea (silicon dioxide) 8X. Other Ingredients: Aloe Vera Extract, Bitter Melon Fruit Extract (momordica charantia), Colloidal Silver, D-Mannose (natural saccharide), Grapefruit Seed Extract, Green Tea Extract, Licorice Extract (root), Tea Tree Oil.
See Editor's Note No. 1, page 2053.

AKG Fuel - TwinLab
Three capsules contain: Alpha-Ketoglutaric Acid (from Magnesium Alpha-Ketoglutarate) 1250 mg • Magnesium (from Magnesium Alpha-Ketoglutarate) 210 mg • L-Glutamine 1000 mg.

AKN Skin Care - Nature's Way
Two capsules contain: Proprietary Blend 930 mg: Burdock root, Capsicum root, Dandelion root, Echinacea Purpurea root, Kelp (whole thallus), Licorice root, Plantain root, Sarsaparilla root, Yellow Dock root. Other Ingredients: Gelatin.

ALC Fuel - TwinLab
Each capsule contains: Acetyl-L-Carnitine (ALC) 1000 mg.

Alert - PhytoPharmica
Each capsule contains: Cola Nut extract (Cola nitida; contains 35 mg caffeine) 250 mg • Green Tea extract (Camellia sinensis; contains 15 mg caffeine) 250 mg • Oat Straw extract 10:1 (Avena sativa) 50 mg • Schisandra extract (standardized to contain 9% schizandrin) 50 mg • Siberian Ginseng extract (Eleutherococcus senticosus; (standardized to contain greater than 1% eleutheroside E) 50 mg • Ginger root extract 6.5:1 (Zingiber officinale) 25 mg • Korean Ginseng root extract (Panax ginseng; standardized to contain 7% saponis calculated as ginsenoside Rg1) 10 mg • Chromium (Polynicotinate) 100 mcg.

Alert Vitalizing Formula - Starlight International
Two capsules contain: Potassium (as potassium glycerophosphate) 35 mg • Schisandra extract 4:1 (schisandra chinensis, berry) 250 mg • Oriental Ginseng (panax ginseng, root) 300 mg • Guarana extract 6:1 (paulina cupana, seed) 600 mg • Caffeine 132 mg • Adrenal Substance 150 mg • Coenzyme Q10 5.0 mg • Siberian Ginseng (eicutherococcus senticosus, root) 1.0 mg • Spirulina 1.0 mg. Other Ingredients: Dicalcium Phosphate, Magnesium Stearate, Silicon

Dioxide, Gelatin.
See Editor's Note No. 14, page 2055.

Alertis Compound **-** The Herbalist
False Unicorn root • Squaw Vine herb • Cramp bark • Blue Cohosh root • Ginger root.

Alfalfa **-** Quest
Each tablet contains: Organic Alfalfa 650 mg. Other Ingredients: Terra Alba, Silica, Magnesium Stearate (vegetable source).

Alfalfa **-** Puritan's Pride
Three tablets contain: Alfalfa leaf (Medicago sativa) 1,500 mg. Other Ingredients: Dicalcium Phosphate, Vegetable Stearic Acid, Vegetable Magnesium Stearate, Croscarmellose.

Alfalfa Complex **-** Shaklee
Ten tablets contain: Calcium 300 mg • Iron 0.36 mg • Phosphorus 150 mg • Magnesium 10 mg • Sodium 10 mg • Alfalfa powder (Medicago sativa) leaf 2.85 g. Other Ingredients: Dicalcium Phosphate, Maltodextrin, Fructose, Tricalcium Phosphate, Spearmint Oil (Mentha spicata) Leaf.

Alfalfa Concentrate **-** Marlyn
Each tablet contains: Vegetarian Organically Grown Alfalfa 648 mg.

Alfalfa Leaves **-** Nature's Way
Three capsules contain: Alfalfa leaf 1.22 g • Vitamin C 1.46 mg.

Alfalfa-Devil's Claw Formula **-** Quest
Each caplet contains: Alfalfa leaf powder (Medicago sativa) 70 mg • Alfalfa seed powder 70 mg • Burdock root powder (Arctium lappa) 70 mg • Celery seed powder (Apium graveolens) 70 mg • Devil's Claw root powder (Herpagophytum procumbens) 70 mg • Cayenne powder (Capsicum) 35 mg • Kelp powder (Fucus versiculosis) 35 mg • Queen of the Meadow root powder (Filipendula ulmaria) 5 mg • Sarsaparilla root powder (Smilax officinalis) 5 mg. Other Ingredients: Calcium Phosphate, Microcrystalline Cellulose, Vegetable Stearin, Croscarmellose Sodium, Magnesium Stearate (vegetable source).

Alfa-Max **-** Nature's Way
Each capsule contains: Alfalfa leaf 420 mg.

Alive! Whole Food Energizer (Iron Free) Veggie Cap **-** Nature's Way
Six capsules contain: Amino Acids Blend 225 mg: Glutamine, Asparagine, Leucine, Alanine, Arginine, Lysine, Threonine, Valine, Glycine, Isoleucine, Serine, Proline, Phenylalanine, Tyrosine, Histidine, Methionine, Tryptophan, Cysteine • Biotin Triurate 300 mcg • Boron Amino Acid Chelate 1 mg • Calcium (citrate, carbonate) 250 mg • Chlorophyll (from spirulina) 4 mg • Choline Bitartrate 30 mg • Chromium Polynicotinate 120 mcg • Citrus Bioflavonoid Complex 60 mg: Eriocitrin 600 mcg, Naringin/Narirutin/other Flavonones 1.8 mg, Flavonols 600 mcg, Flavones/related Phenolic compounds 600 mcg • Copper Amino Acid Chelate 2 mg • Digestive Enzyme Blend 100 mg: Protease I, Protease II, Peptizyme SP, Amylase, Lactase, Invertase, Lipase, Cellulase, Alpha Galactosidase, Betaine HCl, Bromelain (from pineapple), Papain (from papaya) • DNA (from spirulina, chlorella) 4 mg • Eleuthero root 50 mg • Folic Acid (folate) 400 mcg • Garden Veggies Juice Powder Blend 500 mg: Parsley, Kale, Spinach, Wheat Grass, Brussels Sprouts, Asparagus, Broccoli, Cauliflower, Beet, Carrot, Cabbage, Garlic • Green Food/Spirulina Blend 500 mg: Spirulina (microalgae), Alfalfa (leaf, stem), Barley Grass, Dandelion (leaf), Wheat Grass, Spinach (leaf), Lemon Grass, Nettle (leaf), Blessed Thistle (stem, leaf, flower), Chlorella (broken-cell microalgae), Chickweed (stem, leaf, flower), Blue Green Algae (microalgae), Cilantro (leaf) • Hesperidin 2 mg • Inositol 50 mg • Iodine 150 mcg • Lutein (from marigold) 200 mcg • Magnesium (as citrate, oxide) 125 mg • Manganese Amino Acid Chelate 4 mg • Molybdenum Triurate 75 mcg • MycoDefense Mushroom Blend 100 mg: Cordyceps, Reishi, Shiitake, Hiratake, Maitake, Ymabushitake, Mimembatsutake, Kawaratake, Chaga, Zhu Ling, Agarikon, Mesima • Niacinamide 125 mg • Omega Fatty Acid Seed Blend 100 mg: Flax seed powder, Sunflower seed powder, providing: Alpha-Linoleic Acid, Oleic Acid, Linoleic Acid, Palmitic Acid, Stearic Acid, Behenic Acid, Gadoleic Acid, Palmitoleic Acid, Eicosanoic Acid, Lignoceric Acid • Orchard Fruits Juice Powder blend 100 mg: Plum, Cranberry, Blueberry, Strawberry, Blackberry, Bilberry, Cherry, Apricot, Papaya, Orange, Grape, Pineapple • PABA (para aminobenzoic acid) 25 mg • Pantothenic Acid 125 mg • Potassium Amino Acid Chelate 50 mg • Riboflavin (vitamin B2) 25 mg • RNA (from spirulina, chlorella) 14 mg • Rutin 25 mg • Selenium Monomethionine 70 mcg • Sodium 15 mg • Thiamine (vitamin B1) 25 mg • Vitamin A (retinol, palmitate) 15,000 IU • Vitamin B12 (cyanocobalamin) 200 mcg • Vitamin B6 (pyridoxine HCl) 50 mg • Vitamin C (ascorbic acid) 1 g • Vitamin D (D3, cholecalciferol) 400 IU • Vitamin E (d-alpha tocopheryl succinate) 200 IU • Vitamin K (phytonadione) 80 mcg • Zinc Amino Acid Chelate 15 mg. Other Ingredients: Plant-Derived Cellulose, Vegetable Magnesium Stearate.

Alive! Whole Food Energizer (Iron-free) **-** Nature's Way
Three tablets contain: Amino Acids Blend 225 mg: Glutamine, Asparagine, Leucine, Alanine, Arginine, Lysine, Threonine, Valine, Glycine, Isoleucine, Serine, Proline, Phenylalanine, Tyrosine, Histidine, Methionine, Tryptophan, Cysteine • Beta Carotene 10,000 IU • Biotin Triurate 300 mcg • Boron Amino Acid Chelate 1 mg • Calcium (citrate, carbonate) 250 mg • Chlorophyll (from spirulina) 4 mg • Choline Bitartrate 30 mg • Chromium Polynicotinate 120 mcg • Citrus Bioflavonoid Complex 60 mg: Eriocitrin 600 mcg, Naringin/Narirutin/other Flavonones 1.8 mg, Flavonols 600 mcg, Flavones/related Phenolic compounds 600 mcg • Copper Amino Acid Chelate 2 mg • Digestive Enzyme Blend 100 mg: Protease I, Protease II, Peptizyme SP, Amylase, Lactase, Invertase, Lipase, Cellulase, Alpha Galactosidase, Betaine HCl, Bromelain (from pineapple), Papain (from papaya) • DNA (from spirulina, chlorella) 4 mg • Eleuthero root 50 mg • Folic Acid (folate) 400 mcg • Garden Veggies Juice Powder Blend 500 mg: Parsley, Kale, Spinach, Wheat Grass, Brussels Sprouts, Asparagus, Broccoli, Cauliflower, Beet, Carrot, Cabbage, Garlic • Green Food/Spirulina Blend 500 mg: Spirulina (microalgae), Alfalfa (leaf, stem), Barley Grass, Dandelion (leaf), Wheat Grass, Spinach (leaf), Lemon Grass, Nettle (leaf), Blessed Thistle (stem, leaf, flower), Chlorella (broken-cell microalgae), Chickweed (stem, leaf, flower), Blue Green Algae (microalgae), Cilantro (leaf) • Hesperidin 2 mg • Inositol 50 mg • Iodine 150 mcg • Lutein (from marigold) 200 mcg • Magnesium (as citrate, oxide) 125 mg • Manganese Amino Acid Chelate 4 mg • Molybdenum Triurate 75 mcg • MycoDefense Mushroom Blend 100 mg: Cordyceps, Reishi, Shiitake, Hiratake, Maitake, Ymabushitake, Mimembatsutake, Kawaratake, Chaga, Zhu Ling, Agarikon, Mesima • Niacinamide 125 mg • Omega Fatty Acid Seed Blend 100 mg: Flax seed powder, Sunflower seed powder, providing: Alpha-Linoleic Acid, Oleic Acid, Linoleic Acid, Palmitic Acid, Stearic Acid, Behenic Acid, Gadoleic Acid, Palmitoleic Acid, Eicosanoic Acid, Lignoceric Acid • Orchard Fruits Juice Powder Blend 100 mg: Plum, Cranberry, Blueberry, Strawberry, Blackberry, Bilberry, Cherry, Apricot, Papaya, Orange, Grape, Pineapple • PABA (para aminobenzoic acid) 25 mg • Pantothenic Acid 125 mg • Potassium Amino Acid Chelate 50 mg • Riboflavin (vitamin B2) 25 mg • RNA (from spirulina, chlorella) 14 mg • Rutin 25 mg • Selenium Monomethionine 70 mcg • Sodium 15 mg • Thiamine (vitamin B1) 25 mg • Vitamin A (retinol, palmitate) 5000 IU • Vitamin B12 (cyanocobalamin) 200 mcg • Vitamin B6 (pyridoxine HCl) 50 mg • Vitamin C (ascorbic acid) 1 g • Vitamin D (D3, cholecalciferol) 400 IU • Vitamin E (d-alpha tocopheryl succinate) 200 IU • Vitamin K (phytonadione) 80 mcg • Zinc Amino Acid Chelate 15 mg. Other Ingredients: Glycerin, Vegetable Magnesium Stearate, Vegetable Modified Cellulose, Vegetable Modified Cellulose Gum, Vegetable Stearic Acid.

Alive! Whole Food Energizer (with Iron) **-** Nature's Way
Three tablets contain: Amino Acids blend 225 mg: Glutamine, Asparagine, Leucine, Alanine, Arginine, Lysine, Threonine, Valine, Glycine, Isoleucine, Serine, Proline, Phenylalanine, Tyrosine, Histidine, Methionine, Tryptophan, Cysteine • Beta Carotene 10,000

IU • Biotin Triurate 300 mcg • Boron Amino Acid Chelate 1 mg • Calcium (citrate, carbonate) 250 mg • Chlorophyll (from spirulina) 4 mg • Choline Bitartrate 30 mg • Chromium Polynicotinate 120 mcg • Citrus Bioflavonoid Complex 60 mg: Eriocitrin 600 mcg, Naringin/Narirutin/other Flavonones 1.8 mg, Flavonols 600 mcg, Flavones/related Phenolic compounds 600 mcg • Copper Amino Acid Chelate 2 mg • Digestive Enzyme blend 100 mg: Protease I, Protease II, Peptizyme SP, Amylase, Lactase, Invertase, Lipase, Cellulase, Alpha Galactosidase, Betaine HCl, Bromelain (from pineapple), Papain (from papaya) • DNA (from spirulina, chlorella) 4 mg • Eleuthero root 50 mg • Folic Acid (folate) 400 mcg • Garden Veggies Juice Powder Blend 500 mg: Parsley, Kale, Spinach, Wheat Grass, Brussels Sprouts, Asparagus, Broccoli, Cauliflower, Beet, Carrot, Cabbage, Garlic • Green Food/Spirulina Blend 500 mg: Spirulina (microalgae), Alfalfa (leaf, stem), Barley Grass, Dandelion (leaf), Wheat Grass, Spinach (leaf), Lemon Grass, Nettle (leaf), Blessed Thistle (stem, leaf, flower), Chlorella (broken-cell microalgae), Chickweed (stem, leaf, flower), Blue Green Algae (microalgae), Cilantro (leaf) • Hesperidin 2 mg • Inositol 50 mg • Iodine 150 mcg • Iron Amino Acid Chelate 18 mg • Lutein (from marigold) 200 mcg • Magnesium (as citrate, oxide) 125 mg • Manganese Amino Acid Chelate 4 mg • Molybdenum Triurate 75 mcg • MycoDefense Mushroom Blend 100 mg: Cordyceps, Reishi, Shiitake, Hiratake, Maitake, Ymabushitake, Mimembatsutake, Kawaratake, Chaga, Zhu Ling, Agarikon, Mesima • Niacinamide 125 mg • Omega Fatty Acid Seed Blend 100 mg: Flax seed powder, Sunflower seed powder, providing: Alpha-Linoleic Acid, Oleic Acid, Linoleic Acid, Palmitic Acid, Stearic Acid, Behenic Acid, Gadoleic Acid, Palmitoleic Acid, Eicosanoic Acid, Lignoceric Acid • Orchard Fruits Juice Powder Blend 100 mg: Plum, Cranberry, Blueberry, Strawberry, Blackberry, Bilberry, Cherry, Apricot, Papaya, Orange, Grape, Pineapple • PABA (para aminobenzoic acid) 25 mg • Pantothenic Acid 125 mg • Potassium Amino Acid Chelate 50 mg • Riboflavin (vitamin B2) 25 mg • RNA (from spirulina, chlorella) 14 mg • Rutin 25 mg • Selenium Monomethionine 70 mcg • Sodium 15 mg • Thiamine (vitamin B1) 25 mg • Vitamin A (retinol, palmitate) 5000 IU • Vitamin B12 (cyanocobalamin) 200 mcg • Vitamin B6 (pyridoxine HCl) 50 mg • Vitamin C (ascorbic acid) 1 g • Vitamin D (D3, cholecalciferol) 400 IU • Vitamin E (d-alpha tocopheryl succinate) 200 IU • Vitamin K (phytonadione) 80 mcg • Zinc Amino Acid Chelate 15 mg. Other Ingredients: Glycerin, Vegetable Magnesium Stearate, Vegetable Modified Cellulose, Vegetable Modified Cellulose Gum, Vegetable Stearic Acid.

***Alive! Whole Food Energizer (with Iron) Veggie Cap* - Nature's Way**

Six capsules contain: Amino Acids blend 225 mg: Glutamine, Asparagine, Leucine, Alanine, Arginine, Lysine, Threonine, Valine, Glycine, Isoleucine, Serine, Proline, Phenylalanine, Tyrosine, Histidine, Methionine, Tryptophan, Cysteine • Biotin Triurate 300 mcg • Boron Amino Acid Chelate 1 mg • Calcium (citrate, carbonate) 250 mg • Chlorophyll (from spirulina) 4 mg • Choline Bitartrate 30 mg • Chromium Polynicotinate 120 mcg • Citrus Bioflavonoid Complex 60 mg: Eriocitrin 600 mcg, Naringin/Narirutin/other Flavonones 1.8 mg, Flavonols 600 mcg, Flavones/related Phenolic compounds 600 mcg • Copper Amino Acid Chelate 2 mg • Digestive Enzyme Blend 100 mg: Protease I, Protease II, Peptizyme SP, Amylase, Lactase, Invertase, Lipase, Cellulase, Alpha Galactosidase, Betaine HCl, Bromelain (from pineapple), Papain (from papaya) • DNA (from spirulina, chlorella) 4 mg • Eleuthero root 50 mg • Folic Acid (folate) 400 mcg • Garden Veggies Juice Powder Blend 500 mg: Parsley, Kale, Spinach, Wheat Grass, Brussels Sprouts, Asparagus, Broccoli, Cauliflower, Beet, Carrot, Cabbage, Garlic • Green Food/Spirulina Blend 500 mg: Spirulina (microalgae), Alfalfa (leaf, stem), Barley Grass, Dandelion (leaf), Wheat Grass, Spinach (leaf), Lemon Grass, Nettle (leaf), Blessed Thistle (stem, leaf, flower), Chlorella (broken-cell microalgae), Chickweed (stem, leaf, flower), Blue Green Algae (microalgae), Cilantro (leaf) • Hesperidin 2 mg • Inositol 50 mg • Iodine 150 mcg • Iron Amino Acid Chelate 18 mg • Lutein (from marigold) 200 mcg • Magnesium (as citrate, oxide) 125 mg • Manganese Amino Acid Chelate 4 mg • Molybdenum Triurate 75 mcg • MycoDefense Mushroom Blend 100 mg: Cordyceps, Reishi, Shiitake, Hiratake, Maitake, Ymabushitake, Mimembatsutake, Kawaratake, Chaga, Zhu Ling, Agarikon, Mesima • Niacinamide 125 mg • Omega Fatty Acid Seed Blend 100 mg: Flax seed powder, Sunflower seed powder, providing: Alpha-Linoleic Acid, Oleic Acid, Linoleic Acid, Palmitic Acid, Stearic Acid, Behenic Acid, Gadoleic Acid, Palmitoleic Acid, Eicosanoic Acid, Lignoceric Acid • Orchard Fruits Juice Powder Blend 100 mg: Plum, Cranberry, Blueberry, Strawberry, Blackberry, Bilberry, Cherry, Apricot, Papaya, Orange, Grape, Pineapple • PABA (para aminobenzoic acid) 25 mg • Pantothenic Acid 125 mg • Potassium Amino Acid Chelate 50 mg • Riboflavin (vitamin B2) 25 mg • RNA (from spirulina, chlorella) 14 mg • Rutin 25 mg • Selenium Monomethionine 70 mcg • Sodium 15 mg • Thiamine (vitamin B1) 25 mg • Vitamin A (retinol, palmitate) 15,000 IU • Vitamin B12 (cyanocobalamin) 200 mcg • Vitamin B6 (pyridoxine HCl) 50 mg • Vitamin C (ascorbic acid) 1 g • Vitamin D (D3, cholecalciferol) 400 IU • Vitamin E (d-alpha tocopheryl succinate) 200 IU • Vitamin K (phytonadione) 80 mcg • Zinc Amino Acid Chelate 15 mg. Other Ingredients: Plant-Derived Cellulose, Vegetable Magnesium Stearate.

***AlkaSlim (Alka-Slim, Alka Slim, AlkaSlim)* - Dr. M.T. Morter**

Barley malt • Soy Protein complex • Fiber Complex: Psyllium, Guar, Apple Pectin • Alkalizing Complex: Bee Pollen, Barley grass, Alfalfa juice concentrate, Spinach, Parsley, Celery, Spirulina • Barley grass juice • Natural Fruit and Vanilla Flavors • Lecithin • Bromelain (pineapple enzyme) • Methionine • RNA - DNA complex • Schizandra • Siberian Ginseng • Foti • Bioflavonoid - Hesperidin complex • Beta Sitosterol plant lipid complex • Gamma Oryzanol (brown rice extract) • Octacosonal.

***All Purpose Multivitamin/Mineral* - Leiner Health Products**

Each tablet contains: Vitamin E (dl-Alpha Tocopheryl Acetate) 15 IU • Magnesium Oxide 100 mg • Calcium 160 mg • Phosphorus 125 mg • Folate (Folic Acid) 400 mcg • Iodine 150 mcg • Iron (Ferrous Fumarate) 18 mg • Niacin (Niacinamide) 20 mg • Riboflavin (Vitamin B2) 1.7 mg • Thiamin Mononitrate (Vitamin B1) 1.5 mg • Vitamin A Palmitate 5000 • Vitamin B12 (Cyanocobalamin - USP Method 2) 6 mcg • Vitamin B6 (Pyridoxine Hydrochloride) 2 mg • Vitamin C (Ascorbic Acid) 60 mg • Vitamin D (Ergocalciferol) 400 IU. Other Ingredients: Dicalcium Phosphate, Gelatin, Hydroxypropyl Methylcellulose, Croscarmellose Sodium, Sodium Starch Glycolate, Niacinamide, dl-Alpha Tocopheryl Acetate, Cellulose, Tricalcium Phosphate, Silicon Dioxide, Titanium Dioxide, Starch, Polyethylene Glycol 3350, Hydroxypropyl Cellulose, Magnesium Stearate, Yeast, Pyridoxine Hydrochloride, Polysorbate 80, Pharmaceutical Glaze, Resin, Povidone, Potassium Iodide.

***All-Day Complete* - Swanson**

Each rounded scoop (15 g) contains: Vitamin A (as palmitate) 8000 IU • Vitamin A (as beta-carotene) 1000 IU • Vitamin C (as ascorbic acid) 1 g • Vitamin D (as cholecalciferol) 500 IU • Vitamin E (as d-alpha tocopheryl acetate) 400 IU • Vitamin K 5 mcg • Thiamin (as thiamin HCl; vitamin B-1) 25 mg • Riboflavin (vitamin B-2) 25 mg • Niacin (as niacinamide) 100 mg • Vitamin B-6 (as pyridoxine HCl) 25 mg • Folic Acid 400 mcg • Vitamin B-12 (as cyanocobalamin) 25mcg • Biotin 300 mcg • Pantothenic Acid (as d-calcium pantothenate) 100 mg • Calcium (from calcium carbonate and dicalcium phosphate) 500 mg • Iron (as ferrous gluconate) 18 mg • Phosphorus (from d-calcium phosphate) 200 mg • Iodine (from potassium iodide) 150 mcg • Magnesium (from magnesium oxide) 200 mg • Zinc (from zinc oxide) 15 mg • Selenium (as proteinate) 50 mcg • Copper (from copper gluconate) 1 mg • Manganese (from manganese sulfate) 4 mg • Chromium (as chromium proteinate complex) 50 mcg • Molybdenum (as amino acid chelate) 50 mcg • Potassium (as potassium citrate) 99 mg • Lecithin 750 mg • Lemon Bioflavonoid complex 400 mg • Hesperidin complex 25 mg • PABA (para-aminobenzoic acid) 25 mg • Rutin (from buckwheat) 25 mg • Choline (from lecithin) 20 mg • Inositol (from lecithin) 15 mg • Betaine HCl 2 mg • Papain (from papaya) 2 mg • Kelp 1.5 mg.

Some Brand Name Natural Products - What they Contain

www.NaturalDatabase.com contains MANY more listings than appear here.

All-Day Complete (for Seniors) **-** Swanson
Each rounded scoop (15 g) contains: Vitamin A (as palmitate) 8000 IU • Vitamin A (as beta-carotene) 1000 IU • Vitamin C (as ascorbic acid) 1 g • Vitamin D (as cholecalciferol) 500 IU • Vitamin E (as d-alpha tocopheryl acetate) 400 IU • Vitamin K 5 mcg • Thiamin (as thiamin HCl; vitamin B-1) 25 mg • Riboflavin (vitamin B-2) 25 mg • Niacin (as niacinamide) 100 mg • Vitamin B-6 (as pyridoxine HCl) 25 mg • Folic Acid 400 mcg • Vitamin B-12 (as cyanocobalamin) 25 mcg • Biotin 300 mcg • Pantothenic Acid (as d-calcium pantothenate) 100 mg • Calcium (from calcium carbonate and dicalcium phosphate) 500 mg • Iron (as ferrous gluconate) 18 mg • Phosphorus (from d-calcium phosphate) 200 mg • Iodine (from potassium iodide) 150 mcg • Magnesium (from magnesium oxide) 200 mg • Zinc (from zinc oxide) 15 mg • Selenium (as proteinate) 50 mcg • Copper (from copper gluconate) 1 mg • Manganese (from manganese sulfate) 4 mg • Chromium (as chromium proteinate complex) 50 mcg • Molybdenum (as amino acid chelate) 50 mcg • Potassium (as potassium citrate) 99 mg • Lecithin 1.4 g • Fructooligosaccharides (FOS) 1 g •Lemon Bioflavonoid complex 400 mg • Inositol (from inositol and lecithin) 100 mg • Choline (from lecithin) 50 mg • Ginkgo Biloba powder 25 mg • Hesperidin complex 25 mg • PABA (para-aminobenzoic acid) 25 mg •Rutin (from buckwheat) Coenzyme Q10 20 mg • Reishi Mushroom extract 5 mg • Betaine HCl 2 mg • Papain (from papaya) 2 mg • Kelp 1.5 mg.

Aller-Aid Formula II **-** NutriCology
Each capsule contains: Iodine (from kelp) 30 mcg • Selenium (from kelp) 200 mcg • Macrocystis Pyrifera (kelp) 200 mg. Other Ingredients: Silicon Dioxide, Magnesium Stearate.

Aller-B **-** Progressive Labs
Each capsule contains: Thiamin (Vitamin B1) 50 mg • Riboflavin (Vitamin B2) 50 mg • Niacinamide 50 mg • Vitamin B6 50 mg • Folate (Folic Acid) 400 mcg • Vitamin B12 60 mcg • Biotin 50 mcg • Pantothenic Acid 100 mg • Choline Bitartrate 50 mg • Inositol 25 mg • PABA (Para Aminobenzioc Acid) 50 mg.

Aller-C **-** Vital Nutrients
Each capsule contains: Vitamin C (pure ascorbic acid) 450 mg • Quercetin 250 mg • Citrus Bioflavonoids (60%) 150 mg • Bromelain (2400 gdu, pure uncut) 50 mg.

Aller-C Support Formula **-** The Vitamin Factory
Each tablet contains: Vitamin C (Calcium Ascorbate) 500 mg • Calcium (Ascorbate, Citrate, Pantothenate) 100 mg • Vitamin B5 (Calcium Pantothenate) 50 mg • Pycnogenol (Maritime Pine bark extract) 15 mg.

Aller-Cal **-** Atrium Inc.
Each tablet contains: Adrenal 80 mg • Pituitary 10 mg • Liver Substance 6 mg • Parathyroid 5 mg • Calcium 20.4 mg • Pantothenic Acid 26 mg • Folic Acid 130 mcg • Ammonium Chloride 30 mg • Choline Bitartrate 25 mg • Methionine 14 mg • Inositol 12 mg • Glutamic Acid HCL 12 mg • Betaine HCL 3.6 mg • Hydrolized Amino Acids 150 mg • Dulse 50 mg • Persic oil 36 mg • Linseed oil 12 mg.
See Editor's Note No. 14, page 2055.

AllerClear **-** Enzymatic Therapy
Active Ingredient: Ephedra Sinensis (providing pseudophedrine HCl 60 mg). Other Ingredients: Vitamin E (DL-alpha tocopherol) 75 IU • Vitamin C (ascorbic acid) 150 mg • Pantothenic Acid (D-calcium pantothenate) 150 mg • Choline (bitartrate) 150 mg • Macrocystis Pyrifera 150 mg • Lung extract 90 mg • Adrenal extract 80 mg • Methionine 75 mg • Pancreatic Enzymes (3X) 65 mg • Ammonium Chloride 50 mg • Calcium Chloride 50 mg • Glutamic Acid HCl 50 mg • Betaine HCl 50 mg • Pepsin (1:10000) 49 mg • Magnesium Glycerophosphate 30 mg • Spleen extract 25 mg • Pancreas extract 15 mg • Thymus extract 15 mg • Niacinamide 10 mg • Liver Fractions 10 mg • Vitamin B6 (Pyridoxine HCl) 5 mg.
See Editor's Note No. 21 and No. 30, page 2056.

Aller-G Formula 25 **-** Olympian Labs
Two capsules contain: Vitamin C 200 mg •Histidine 60 mg •Citrus Aurantium extract 200 mg •Bee Pollen 75 mg •Propolis 25 mg •Pantothenic Acid 75 mg • Citrus Bioflavonoid Complex 30 mg •Niacin 20 mg •Goldenseal 25 mg •Echinacea 50 mg •Garlic 25 mg •Yerba Santa 50 mg •Nettle 80 mg •Mullein 40 mg •White Willow Bark 6 mg.
See Editor's Note No. 40, page 2058.

Allergia **-** HerbaSway
Bitter Orange • Ginger • Panax Ginseng • Blackberry • Kudzu • HerbaSwee (Cucurbitaceae fruit).
See Editor's Note No. 40, page 2058.

allergy & hayfever **-** nelsons - Nelson Bach USA Ltd.
Active Ingredients: Allium Cepa 30C HPUS • Euphrasia 30C HPUS • Sabadilla 30C HPUS. Inactive Ingredients: Lactose, Sucrose.
See Editor's Note No. 1, page 2053.

Allergy Essentials **-** Swanson
Three capsules contain: Vitamin C (as calcium ascorbate) 100 mg • Zinc (from zinc chelate and zinc gluconate) 15 mg • Ma Huang extract (6% ephedra) 250 mg • Bromelain (2400 GDU) 100 mg • Licorice root extract (1% glycyrrhizic acid) 100 mg • N-Acetyl-Cysteine 100 mg • Nettle extract (5:1) 100 mg • Quercetin 100 mg • White Willow Bark 100 mg • Cayenne pepper 100,000 HU 50 mg • Echinacea root extract (4% echinacosides) 50 mg • Goldenseal root 50 mg • Grapeseed extract (95% proanthocyanidins) 30 mg.
See Editor's Note No. 30, page 2056.

Allergy Eye Drops **-** Natural Ophthalmics
Active Ingredients: Apis HPUS 6x • Sabadilla HPUS 6x • Allium Cepa HPUS 6x • Eyebright (euphrasia) HPUS 4x. Inactive Ingredients: Sterile Water, Sodium Chloride, Sodium Citrate, Citrate, Polysorbate 80.

Allergy MD **-** Long Life, Inc.
Amylase • Cellulase • Fenugreek • Licorice • Methionine • Lipase • Mullein • Niacinamide • Pantothenic Acid • Protease • Sida Cordifolia extract • Vitamin A • Vitamin C • Yerba Santa.
See Editor's Note No. 39, page 2058.

Allergy Relief **-** Futurebiotics
Three capsules contain: Vitamin A (as beta-carotene) 5000 IU • Vitamin C 1000 mg • Pantothenic Acid 100 mg • Zinc (as OptiZinc zinc monomethionine) 15 mg • MSM (methyl-sulfonyl-methane) 500 mg • Citrus Bioflavonoids 100 mg • Quercetin 25 mg • Rutin 25 mg • Bitter Orange (Citrus aurantium) peel powder extract (standardized for 4% synephrine, 4 mg) 100 mg • Grape Seed extract powder (standardized for 95% polyphenols, 29 mg) 30 mg • Stinging Nettle extract powder (leaf) (standardized for 2% plant silica, 2 mg) 100 mg • N-Acetyl-Cysteine (NAC) 100 mg • L-Histidine 200 mg. Other Ingredients: Gelatin, Cellulose, Magnesium stearate, Water.
See Editor's Note No. 40, page 2058.

Allergy Shield **-** NSI - Nutraceutical Sciences Institute
Each four capsules contain: MSM 1.5 g • Bioflavoniod as Quercetin 500 mg • Bioflavonoid as Rutin 150 mg • Bioflavonoid as Hesperin 350 mg • Protease 50,000 HUT • Vitamin C (as magnesium ascorbate, Ester C) 1 g.

Allergy Support **-** Olympia Nutrition
Quercetin • Nettle • Licorice • Vitamin C.

AllergyCare **-** Nature's Way
Each capsule contains: Pseudoephedrine HCl 60 mg. Other Ingredients: Brigham Tea Herb, Elder Flowers, Eyebright (stem, leaf, flower), Ginger, Golden Rod Herb, Licorice Root.

AllerPlus **-** PhytoPharmica
Two capsules contain: Pseudoephedrine HCl (from Ephedra sinensis) 60 mg • Vitamin E (DL-Alpha Tocopherol) 75 IU • Vitamin C (Ascorbic Acid) 150 mg • Pantothenic Acid (D-Calcium Pantothenate) 150 mg • Choline (Bitartrate) 150 mg • Macrocystis Pyrifera

BRAND NAMES

150 mg • Lung extract 90 mg • Adrenal extract 80 mg • Methionine 75 mg • Pancreatic Enzymes (3X) 65 mg (Treated for enteric activity) • Ammonium Chloride 50 mg • Calcium Chloride 50 mg • Glutamic Acid HCL 50 mg • Betaine HCL 50 mg • Pepsin (1:10000) 49 mg • Magnesium Glycerophosphate 30 mg • Spleen extract 25 mg • Pancreas extract 15 mg • Thymus extract 15 mg • Niacinamide 10 mg • Liver Fractions 10 mg • Vitamin B6 (Pyridoxine HCl) 5 mg.
See Editor's Note No. 21 and No. 30, page 2056.

Aller-Response **-** Source Naturals
Three tablets contain: Quercetin 600 mg • Vitamin C (ascorbic acid and zinc ascorbate) 500 mg • Bitter orange standardized extract 500 mg • Bromelain (2000 GDU per g) 300 mg • Nettle root extract 100 mg • Ginkgo Biloba standardized leaf extract 75 mg • Licorice root extract 50 mg • Magnesium (amino acid chelate) 50 mg • Vitamin A (palmitate) 2500 IU • Vitamin B-6 (pyridoxine HCl) 5 mg • Vitamin B-12 (cyanocobalamin) 12 mcg • Zinc (ascorbate) 10 mg.
See Editor's Note No. 40, page 2058.

Aller-Sin Caps **-** Douglas Laboratories
Each capsule contains: Proprietary Blend 440 mg: Boneset herb, Fenugreek seeds, Horseradish root, Mullein leaves, Fennel seeds.

AllerZinc **-** Quantum, Inc.
Each drop contains: Zinc 9 mg • Ephedrine from Ephedra Extract 2 mg • Quercetin 80 mg • Lobelia 15 mg • Licorice 15 mg. Other Ingredients: Sugar, Corn Syrup, Natural Flavor.
See Editor's Note No. 21 and No. 30, page 2056.

Allicin Rich Garlic Powder 1,500 mg **-** Jamieson
Each caplet contains: Allicin Garlic (equivalent to 2 cloves of garlic) 1500 mg.

Allicin Rich Garlic Powder 300 mg **-** Jamieson
Each caplet contains: Garlic bulb powder (containing 750 mcg Allicon and 5000 mcg Alliin) 300 mg.

Allisyn Garlic Cinnamon Oil **-** Genestra - Seroyal
Each capsule contains: Garlic extract (yielding allicin, no less than 5 mg) 500 mg • Cinnamon bark oil (yielding cinnamaldehyde, no less than 40 mg) 200 mg.

Allorganic Trace Minerals-B12 **-** Standard Process, Inc.
Each tablet contains: Proprietary Blend 173 mg: Kelp, Alfalfa, Magnesium Citrate, Dried Pea (vine) juice, Bovine Orchic extract, Bovine Bone, Dried Buckwheat (leaf) juice, Buckwheat (seed), Defatted Wheat (germ), Oat Flour, Dicalcium Phosphate, Carrot (root), Peanut (bran) • Manganese Lactate 16 mg • Potassium Para-Aminobenzoate 10 mg • Honey • Iron Liver Chelate 1.4 mg • Calcium Stearate • Prolamine Iodine (zein) 145 mcg • Cyanocobalamin 5 mcg.

Alluna **-** SmithKline Beecham
Two tablets contain: Valerian root extract 500 mg • Hops extract 120 mg. Other Ingredients: Microcrystalline Cellulose, Soy Polysaccharide, Hydrogenated Castor oil, Hydroxypropyl Methylcellulose, Titanium Dioxide (less than 20%), Propylene Glycol, Magnesium Stearate, Silica, Polyethylene Glycol (400, 6000, 20000), Blue 2 Lake, Artificial flavoring.

Allurex Female **-** Allurex
Each 300 mg capsule contains: Avena Sativa 1X • Sabal Serrulata 2X.
See Editor's Note No. 1, page 2053.

Allurex Male **-** Allurex
Each 300 mg capsule contains: Avena Sativa 1X.
See Editor's Note No. 1, page 2053.

Almond Amaretto - Revival **-** Physicians Laboratories
Eight fluid ounces contain: Certified Isoflavone 15 mg. Other Ingredients: Whole Roasted Soybeans, Natural and Artificial Flavors.

Aloe & Chamomile Skin Soothing Moisturizer 4oz **-** Derma E
Purified Water • Stearic Acid • Jojoba oil • Cetyl Alcohol • Stearyl Alcohol • Aloe Vera Gel • Glyceryl Stearate SE • Caprylic Triglyceride • Glycerin • Almond oil • Chamomile extract • Tocopheryl Acetate (vitamin E) • Retinyl Palmitate (vitamin A) • Ergocalciferol (vitamin D) • Allantoin • Panthenol • Methylparaben • TEA • I. Urea • Fragrant Oils.

Aloe & Chamomile Skin Toner 8oz **-** Derma E
Purified Water • Herbal Extracts Blend: Aloe Vera, Chamomile, Cucumber, Lavender, Rose Hips, Rosemary • NAPCA • Sodium Citrate • DL-Panthenol • Polysorbate 20 • Natural Color • Methylparaben • I. Urea • Fragrant Oils.

Aloe & E Moisturizing Lotion 10.1oz **-** Derma E
Purified Water • Aloe Vera Gel • Safflower oil • Cetyl Alcohol • Glyceryl Stearate • PEG 100 Stearate • Stearic Acid • Glycerin • Tocopheryl Acetate (vitamin E) • Retinyl Palmitate (vitamin A) • Ergocalciferol (vitamin D) • Allantoin • Panthenol • Methylparaben • TEA • I. Urea • Fragrant Oils.

Aloe & E with Allantoin **-** Derma E
Aloe Vera gel • Vitamin E.

Aloe Gold **-** Oasis Wellness Network
Each ounce (30 mL) contains: FOS (fructo-oligosaccharide) 1.7 g • Active Aloe (200:1) 280 mg • Carragel 95 mg • Pine Needle leaf extract 28 mg • Citric Acid 11 mg • Green Tea root extract 2.8 mg • MaxCell Proprietary Blend 25 mg: Jujube fruit extract, Black Pepper extract, Aloe Vera (dried gel), Chinese Licorice root. Other Ingredients: Sodium Benzoate, Potassium Sorbate.

Aloe Immune - 150 mg **-** 4R Health Products
Each capsule contains: Aloe Vera gel 150 mg. Other Ingredients: Rice Flower.

Aloe Immune - 500 mg **-** 4R Health Products
Each capsule contains: Aloe Vera gel 500 mg. Other Ingredients: Magnesium Stearate.

Aloe Isolate **-** Progressive Labs
Each capsule contains: Aloe Vera Mucilaginous Polysaccharide (freeze-dried) 30 mg.

Aloe Seltzer C **-** Nutraceutics Corp.
Each tablet contains: Vitamin C (as l-ascorbic acid) 1000 mg • Lyopilized whole Aloe Vera gel (betamannin) 50 mg • Other Ingredients: Sodium Bicarbonate, Citric Acid, Glucose, Orange Flavor, Magnesium Carbonate, Polyethylene Glycol, Calcium Carbonate, Sodium Carbonate.

Aloe Vera **-** Leiner Health Products
Each softgel contains: Aloe Vera gel 25 mg. Other Ingredients: Vegetable Oil, Gelatin, Hydrogenated Soybean and Cottonseed Oil, White Beeswax.

Aloe Vera **-** Puritan's Pride
Each capsule contains: Aloe Vera (Aloe barbadensis, leaf) 470 mg. Other Ingredients: Gelatin, Silica, Vegetable Magnesium Stearate.

Aloe Vera 200 **-** New Chapter, Inc.
Two tablets contain: Freeze dried Aloe Vera juice concentrate (200:1) 300 mg.

Aloe Vera Capsules **-** Indiana Botanic Gardens
Each capsule contains: Aloe Vera leaf powder 500 mg. Other Ingredients: Gelatin, Water.

Aloe Vera Deep Skin Moisturizer Vitamin D Cell Refining Cream **-** Orjene
85% pure Aloe Vera • Bee Pollen • Vitamin F Complex • PABA-free sunblock.

Aloe Vera Gel **-** Jamieson
Contains: Purified Water • Carrageenan (gelling agent from red seaweed) • 100% Aloe Vera Concentrate.

Aloe Vera Gel **-** Nature's Bounty
Each softgel contains: Aloe Vera Gel (200:1 extract: Equivalent to 5,000 mg or approximately one teaspoonful of 100% pure aloe vera inner leaf gel) 25 mg. Other Ingredients: Beeswax/Soybean Oil Mixture, Gelatin, Glycerin, Cottonseed Oil.

Aloe Vera Gel **-** Puritan's Pride
Each softgel contains: Premium Concentrated Aloe Vera Gel 200:1 (Equivalent to 5000 mg or approximately one teaspoonful of 100% pure aloe vera inner leaf gel) 25 mg.

Aloe Vera Juice **-** Progressive Labs
Aloe Vera gel (98.94% pure, naturally processed, cold stabilized) • Fructose • Citric Acid • Ascorbic Acid.

Aloe Vera Moisture Cream **-** Jamieson
Contains: 200 Biologically Active Compounds of Aloe Vera Concentrate • Almond Oil • Avocado Oil • Cactus • Yucca.

Aloe Vera Moisturizing Gel 8oz **-** Derma E
Aloe Vera Gel • Purified Water • Glycerine • Carbomer • Potassium Sorbate • Triethanolamine • Polysorbate 20 • Methylparaben • Fragrant Oils • Plant Extracts.

Aloe Vera Soothing Moisturizing Gel **-** Jamieson
Contains: Aloe Vera Concentrate • Cactus • Yucca.

Aloe Vital **-** Source Naturals
Each tablet contains: Organic whole leaf aloe vera powder (200:1 concentrate) 200 mg.

Alozone-M **-** T-Up Biosystems
Each teaspoon (5mL) contains: Proprietary Blend 670 mg: Aloe Vera • Iron • Boron • Lithium • Fluoride • Copper • Zinc • Selenium • Chromium • Valadium • Cobalt • Nickel • All Natural Ultra-Wide Mineral System.

Alpha betic **-** Abkit
Each caplet contains: Vitamin A 5000 IU • Vitamin C (ascorbic acid) 120 mg • Vitamin D (as cholecalciferol) 400 IU • Vitamin E (as D-alpha tocopheryl succinate) 60 IU • Thiamin (vitamin B1) 1.5 mg • Riboflavin (vitamin B2) 1.7 mg • Niacin 20 mg • Vitamin B6 (as pyridoxine hydrochloride) 2 mg • Folic Acid 400 mcg • Vitamin B12 (as cyanocobalamin) 6 mcg • Biotin 150 mcg • Pantothenic Acid (as D-calcium pantothenate) 10 mg • Calcium (as calcium sulfate) 200 mg • Iodine (as sodium iodide) 150 mcg • Magnesium (as magnesium oxide) 200 mg • Zinc (as zinc citrate) 15 mg • Selenium (as selenomethionine) 50 mcg • Manganese (as manganese sulfate) 5 mg • Chromium (as chromium picolinate) 200 mcg • Potassium (as potassium chloride) 100 mg • Vanadium (as vanadium sulfate) 100 mcg • Lutein (as lutein ester) 500 mcg • Alpha Lipoic Acid 60 mg. Other Ingredients: Stearic Acid, Cellulose, Magnesium Stearate, Beta Carotene.

Alpha CF Liquid - 1 oz **-** Boericke & Tafel
Aconitum Napellus 4X • Bryonia Alba 3X • Eupatorium Perfoliatum 2X • Gelsemium Sempervirens 4X • Ipecacuanha 3X • Phosphorus 5X • Eucalyptus Globulus 1X.
See Editor's Note No. 1, page 2053.

Alpha Lipoderm & Green Tea Extract 2oz **-** Derma E
Purified Water • Green Tea extract • Stearic Acid • Alpha Lipoic Acid • Allantoin • Pantehnol • Caprylic Triglyceride • Jojoba Oil • Cetyl Alcohol • Polysorbate 20 • Glyceryl Stearate • PEG 100 Stearate • Tocopheryl Acetate (vitamin E) • Ascorbyl Palmitate (vitamin C) • Dimethicone • Allantoin • TEA • Retinyl Palmitate (vitamin A) • Ergocalciferol (vitamin D) • Methylparaben • Citricidal • Phenoxyethanol.

Alpha Lipoic Acid 100 MG **-** PhysioLogics
Each capsule contains: Alpha Lipoic Acid 100 mg. Other Ingredients: Dicalcium Phosphate, Gelatin, Silica, Vegetable Magnesium Stearate.

Alpha Lipoic Acid **-** Leiner Health Products
Each tablet contains: Alpha Lipoic Acid 50 mg. Other Ingredients: Cellulose, Calcium Carbonate, Croscarmellose Sodium, Stearic Acid, Magnesium Stearate, Silicon Dioxide, Hydroxypropyl Methylcellulose, Polyethylene Glycol, Hydroxypropyl Cellulose.

Alpha Lipoic Acid **-** Life Extension
Each capsule contains: Alpha Lipoic Acid (100% pharmaceutically pure) 100 mg.

Alpha Lipoic Acid **-** Metabolic Response Modifiers
Each capsule contains: Alpha Lipoic acid 100 mg.

Alpha Lipoic Acid **-** Now
Each Vcap contains: Vitamin C (as ascorbic acid) 250 mg • Vitamin E (as d-alpha tocopheryl succinate) 30 IU • Alpha Lipoic Acid 100 mg. Other Ingredients: Rice Flour, Cellulose (capsule).

Alpha Lipoic Acid **-** NSI - Nutraceutical Sciences Institute
Each capsule contains: Alpha Lipoic Acid 300 mg.

Alpha Lipoic Acid **-** Olympian Labs
Each capsule contains: Crystalline Alpha Lipoic Acid 100 mg.

Alpha Lipoic Acid **-** Optimum Nutrition
Each capsule contains: Alpha Lipoic Acid 100 mg. Other Ingredients: Microcrystalline Cellulose, Gelatin, Magnesium Stearate.

Alpha Lipoic Acid **-** Progressive Labs
Each capsule contains: Alpha Lipoic Acid 100 mg • Bioperine Piper Nigrum extract (piperine) 5 mg. Other Ingredients: Rice Flour, Gelatin.

Alpha Lipoic Acid **-** Swanson
Each capsule contains: Alpha Lipoic Acid 50 mg.

Alpha Lipoic Acid 100 - GNC A-Z **-** GNC
Each capsule contains: Alpha Lipoic Acid 100 mg. Other Ingredients: Soybean oil, Gelatin, Glycerin, Corob extract, Titanium Dioxide.

Alpha Lipoic Acid 100 mg **-** Puritan's Pride
Each capsule contains: Alpha Lipoic Acid 100 mg.

Alpha Lipoic Acid 100 mg **-** Vitamin World
Each capsule contains: Alpha Lipoic Acid 100 mg. Other Ingredients: Rice Powder, Gelatin, Silica, Vegetable Magnesium Stearate.

Alpha Lipoic Acid 200 mg **-** Puritan's Pride
Each capsule contains: Alpha Lipoic Acid 200 mg.

Alpha Lipoic Acid 200 MG **-** PhysioLogics
Each capsule contains: Alpha Lipoic Acid 200 mg. Other Ingredients: Cellulose (plant origin), Dicalcium Phosphate, Gelatin, Vegetable Magnesium Stearate, Silica.

Alpha Lipoic Acid 200 mg **-** Vitamin World
Each capsule contains: Alpha Lipoic Acid 200 mg. Other Ingredients: Rice Powder, Gelatin, Silica, Vegetable Magnesium Stearate.

Alpha Lipoic Acid 30 mg **-** Puritan's Pride
Each capsule contains: Alpha Lipoic Acid 30 mg.

Alpha Lipoic Acid 30 mg **-** Vitamin World
Each capsule contains: Alpha Lipoic Acid 30 mg. Other Ingredients: Dicalcium Phosphate, Gelatin, Silica, Vegetable Magnesium Stearate.

Alpha Lipoic Acid 300 mg **-** Vitamin World
Each capsule contains: Alpha Lipoic Acid 300 mg. Other Ingredients: Soybean Oil, Soy Lecithin, Gelatin, Glycerin, Caramel Color.

Alpha Lipoic Acid 400 **-** Pure Encapsulations
Each vegetarian capsule contains: Alpha Lipoic Acid (thioctic acid) 400 mg • Vitamin C (as ascorbyl palmitate) 16 mg. Inactive Ingredients: Hypo-allergenic Plant Fiber, Vegetable Capsule.

Alpha Lipoic Acid 50 - GNC A-Z **-** GNC
Each capsule contains: Alpha Lipoic Acid 50 mg. Other Ingredients: Soybean oil, Gelatin, Glycerin, Carob extract, Titanium Dioxide.

Alpha Lipoic Acid Extra Strength with MAT **-** Olympian Labs
Each capsule contains: Crystalline Alpha Lipoic Acid 200 mg. Other Ingredients: MAT (a proprietary blend of nutritional ingredients).

Alpha Male Plus+ **-** Albert M. O'Connor, M.D.
Each capsule contains: Thiamin 1 mg • Riboflavin 1 mg • Niacin 1 mg • Vitamin B6 1 mg • Folic Acid 1 mg • Vitamin B12 1 mcg • Biotin 1 mg • Pantothenic Acid 1 mg • Zinc 15 mg • Elk Velvet Antler 250 mg • Nettle root powder 100 mg • Oriental Ginseng 80 mg • Oligomeric Proanthocyanidins 50 mg • Cnidium Monnier 25 mg • Saw Palmetto extract 25 mg • Inositol 1 mg • Choline (bitartrate) 1 mg • PABA 1 mg.

Alpha Sun Capsules **-** Cell Tech
Four capsules contain: Vitamin K 40 mcg • Blue-Green Algae (aph. flos-aquae) 1 g. Other Ingredients: Plant Fiber, Water.

Alpha Sun Tablets **-** Cell Tech
Four tablets contain: Vitamin K 40 mcg • Blue-Green Algae (aph. flos-aquae) 1 g. Other Ingredients: Croscarmellose Sodium, Stearic Acid, Maltodextrin, Calcium Carbonate.

Alpha-Lipoic Acid **-** Source Naturals
Each tablet contains: Alpha-Lipoic acid 50 mg.

Alpha-Lipoic Acid **-** Pro Health
Each tablet contains: Alpha Lipoic Acid 100 mg. Other Ingredients: Cellulose, Stearic Acid, Silica, Magnesium Stearate.

Alpha-Lipoic Acid **-** Rexall - Sundown
Each caplet contains: Alpha-Lipoic Acid 50 mg. Inactive Ingredients: Maltodextrin, Microcrystalline Cellulose, Crospovidone, Hydrogenated Cottonseed Oil, Silica, Turmeric, Natural & Artificial Flavors, Magnesium Stearate.

Alphastat Rx-Prostate **-** Nature's Plus
Each softgel contains: Zinc 15 mg • Alphastat complex 200 mg: Serenoa Repens fruit extract and Haematococcus pluvialis algae extract providing free fatty acids and astaxanthin.

Alternecal-Rx **-** Alternecare Health Products
Each tablet contains: Tri- Calcium Phosphate 1000 mg • Magnesium 500 mg • Zinc 10 mg • Copper 3 mg • Oat Straw 25 mg • Boron 3 mg • Vitamin C 30 mg • Vitamin D 400 IU • Ashwagandha 25 mg • Silica 25 mg.

Alticort **-** PhytoPharmica
Contains: 1.8% Salicylic Acid. Other Ingredients: Purified Water • Organic Fatty Acid Complex (C11-C18), Glyceryl Stearate, Chamomile extract (0.5% Flavonoid Content) • 18-Beta-Glycyrrhetinic Acid (from Licorice root extract) • Allantoin 2.0% from Comfrey root extract • Dimethicone, Vitamin E (Antioxidant). Hypoallergenic Fragrance.

Altovis **-** Wagner Nutraceuticals
Each caplet contains: Altovis Proprietary Blend 906 mg: Green Tea leaf extract (provides caffeine 100 mg), Cordyceps extract (mycelium), Eleutherococcus Senticosus root standardized extract, Panax Ginseng root standardized extract, Vinpocetine (from vocanga tree seeds), Octacosanol. Other Ingredients: Dicalcium Phosphate, Microcrystalline Cellulose, Croscarmellose Sodium, Stearic Acid, Silica, Magnesium Stearate, Film Coat (hypromellose, hydroxypropyl cellulose, polyethylene glycol, propylene glycol, titanium dioxide, FD&C yellow #6 lake, riboflavin, FD&C blue #2 lake).

AM Herbal Maximizer **-** Slimlife
Three caplets contain: Chromium (as picolinate) 200 mcg • Bladderwrack powder 5 mg • Goldenrod leaf powder 5 mg • Corn Silk pistils powder 5 mg • Hawthorn berries powder 20 mg • Licorice root powder 20 mg • Marshmallow root powder 25 mg • Guarana extract 25 mg • Kola nut extract 30 mg • Cayenne Pepper powder • Chitosan 180 mg • Garcinia Cambogia powder 50 mg. Other Ingredients: Dicalcium Phosphate, Cellulose, Stearic Acid, Magnesium Stearate, Silicone Dioxide, Croscarmellose Sodium, Pharmaceutical Glaze, Talc USP.

AM Menopause Formula **-** PhytoPharmica
Each tablet contains: Green Tea (Camellia sinesis) leaf extract (standardized to contain 14% caffeine) 250 mg • Panax Ginseng root phytosome (bound to phosphatidylcholine under patent) 50 mg •Black Cohosh (Cimicifuga racemosa) root and rhizome extract 20 mg.

AM Plus (Brain 111 Formula) AM Super Capsule **-** Alpha Zebra
Two capsules contain: Beta Carotene 25 IU • Thiamine HCl (vitamin B1) 50 mg • Riboflavin (vitamin B2) 50 mg • Niacin (vitamin B3) 20 mg • Pantothenic Acid (vitamin B5) 75 mg • Pyridoxine HCl (vitamin B6) 50 mg • Cyanocobalamin concentrate (vitamin B12/Sorbitol) 500 mcg • Vitamin C 55 mg • Bioflavonoids with Rose Hips 45 mg • Vitamin E (dry, DL-alpha tocopherol) 25 IU • Biotin 300 mcg • Choline Bitartrate (phosphatidyl) 75 mg • Soy Lecithin (phospholipids) 50 mg • Folic Acid 500 mcg • Inositol 50 mg • Inosine 40 mg • Para-Aminobenzioc Acid (PABA) 30 mg • Calcium Phosphate (chelated) 40 mg • Chromium Picolinate (chelated) 200 mcg • Copper (oxide, chelated) 1 mg • Magnesium (oxide, chelated) 25 mg • Manganese (oxide, chelated) 45 mg • Phosphorus (oxide, chelated)12 mg • Potassium (oxide, chelated) 50 mg • Zinc (oxide, chelated) 50 mg • Boron (chelated) 1 mg • Molybdenum (oxide, chelated) 100 mcg • Selenium (oxide, chelated) 200 mcg • Silicon 400 mcg • L-Aspartic Acid 25 mg • L-Cysteine 15 mg • L-Glutamine 115 mg • L-Glycine 15 mg • L-Leucine 50 mg • L-Lysine 15 mg • L-Methionine 70 mg • L-Tyrosine 70 mg • L-Phenylalanine 100 mg • L-Serine 25 mg • A-Ketoglutaric Acid 15 mg • Raw Adrenal freeze dried concentrate 25 mg • Gamma Aminobutyric Acid - GABA 25 mg • Glutamic Acid 5 mg • RNA/DNA (complex) 25 mg • Beta Hydrochloride 5 mg • Bromelain 3 mg • Pancreatin 10 mg • Papain 10 mg • Pepsin 10 mg • Protease Enzyme 3 mg • Bee Pollen 40 mg • Royal Jelly 35 mg • Ginkgo Biloba (50:1, contains 24% ginkgolides heterosides) 50 mg • Ginkgo Biloba (8:1, contains 24% ginkgolides) 160 mg • Gotu Kola 128 mg • Panax Korean Ginseng 88 mg • Ginger root 80 mg • Mexican Yam 80 mg • Echinacea Angustifolia 76 mg • Spirulina Algae 75 mg • Fo-Ti 60 mg • Oat Straw 60 mg • Siberian Ginseng 60 mg • Beet root powder 60 mg • Alfalfa 50 mg • Peppermint leaves 60 mg • Eyebright (euphrasia herb) 60 mg • Licorice root (de-glycyrrhiznated) 56 mg • Passionflower 48 mg • Capsicum 40 mg • Dandelion root 40 mg • Hawthorn berry 40 mg • Mexican Damiana leaves 32 mg • Kelp 28 mg • Aloe Vera 28 mg • Fennel 28 mg • Sarsaparilla 28 mg • Cabbage seed 24 mg • Sea Plant concentrate 20 mg • Saw Palmetto berry 20 mg • Burdock root 20 mg • Chamomile 20 mg • Slippery Elm 20 mg • Kava Kava 16 mg • Horseradish 16 mg • Suma 12 mg.

AM Plus (Brain 111 Formula) Energizer Formula **-** Alpha Zebra
Each capsule contains: Niacinamide (vitamin B3) 40 mg • Pyridoxine HCl (vitamin B6) 25 mg • Cyanocobalamin concentrate (vitamin B12, sorbitol) 500 mcg • Bioflavonoids (including rose hips) 30 mg • L-Glutamine 50 mg • L-Phenylalanine 50 mg • L-Methionine 30 mg • L-Tyrosine 25 mg • L-Aspartic Acid 10 mg • L-Taurine 10 mg • L-Asparigne 10 mg • L-Alanine 10 mg • L-Glycine 10 mg • Pancreatin 20 mg • Gamma Aminobutyric Acid (GABA) 10 mg • Soy Lecithin (phospholipids) 10 mg • Royal Jelly 25 mg • Beet root powder 80 mg • Cantaloupe 80 mg • Yucca 60 mg • American Cenuary 60 mg • Mexican Yam 60 mg • Bissy Nut 60 mg • Kava Kava root 56 mg • Fo-Ti 48 mg • Oat Straw 48 mg • Capsicum / Cayenne 44 mg • Bee Pollen 40 mg • Dandelion root 40 mg • Brigham Tea 40 mg • Artichoke 40 mg • Wild Lettuce 40 mg • Rosemary leaves 40 mg • Yerba Mate 32 mg • Peppermint leaves 32 mg • Sarsaparilla 25 mg • Ginger root 24 mg • Suma 24 mg • Hawthorn berry 16 mg • American

Ginseng 16 mg • Cabbage seed 16 mg • Parsley 16 mg • Fenugreek 16 mg • Gotu Kola 16 mg • Muira Puama 12 mg • Spirulina Algae 12 mg.

AM/PM Menopause Formula - PhytoPharmica
AM Formula: Each yellow tablet contains: Green Tea leaf extract (camellia sinensis, standardized to contain 35 mg caffeine) 250 mg • Panax Ginseng root phytosome (one part panax ginseng extract, standardized to contain 37.5% ginsenosides, bound to two parts phosphatidylcholine) 50 mg • Black Cohosh root and rhizome extract (standardized to contain 2.5% triterpene glycosides calculated as 27-deoxyactein) 20 mg. Other Ingredients: Cellulose, Modified Cellulose, Modified Cellulose Gum, Titanium Dioxide Color, Magnesium Stearate, Lecithin, Carnauba Wax.

AM/PM PeriMenopause Formula - PhytoPharmica
AM Formula: Each yellow tablet contains: Green Tea leaf extract (camellia sinensis, standardized to contain 35 mg caffeine) 250 mg • Rhodiola root extract (rhodiola rosea, standardized to contain 3% rosavins and 1% salidroside) 205 mg • Chaste Tree berry extract (vitex agnus-castus, standardized to contain 0.5% agnusides) 40 mg • Black Cohosh root and rhizome extract (standardized to contain 2.5% triterpene glycosides calculated as 27-deoxyactein) 20 mg. Other Ingredients: Cellulose, Modified Cellulose, Modified Cellulose Gum, Titanium Dioxide Color, Magnesium Stearate, Lecithin, Carnauba Wax. PM Formula: Each purple tablet contains: Valerian root extract (valeriana officinalis, standardized to contain a minimum of 0.8% valerenic acids) 200 mg • Hops flower 6.6:1 extract (humulus lupulus) 100 mg • L-Theanine 50 mg • Black Cohosh root and rhizome extract (standardized to contain 2.5% triterpene glycosides calculated as 27-deoxyactein) 20 mg. Other Ingredients: Cellulose, Modified Cellulose, Modified Cellulose Gum, Magnesium Stearate, Carrot and Paprika Extract Color, Lecithin, Carnauba Wax.

Amazon A-F - Raintree Nutrition, Inc.
Each capsule contains: Proprietary Blend 650 mg: Jatoba, Fedegoso, Brazilian Peppertree, Pau d'Arco, Clavillia, Anamu.

Amazon A-P - Raintree Nutrition, Inc.
Each capsule contains: Proprietary Blend 650 mg: Epazote, Graviola, Fedegoso, Anama, Simarouba, Carqueja, Guaco, Amargo, Erva Tostao, Cat's Claw.

Amazon Athletic Support - Raintree Nutrition, Inc.
Each capsule contains: Proprietary Blend 650 mg: Suma, Sarsaparilla, Maca, Chuchuhuasi, Muria Puama, Yerba Mate, Tayuya, Iporuru.

Amazon A-V - Raintree Nutrition, Inc.
Each capsule contains: Proprietary Blend 600 mg: Bitter Melon, Clavillia, Mullaca, Macela, Vassourinha, Chanca Piedra, Jergon Sacha, Corqueja.

Amazon Blood Support - Raintree Nutrition, Inc.
Each capsule contains: Proprietary Blend 600 mg: Artichoke, Suma, Cat's Claw, Bitter Melon, Yerba Mate, Sarsaparilla, Vassourinha, Maca.

Amazon Bowel Support - Raintree Nutrition, Inc.
Each capsule contains: Proprietary Blend 650 mg: Cat's Claw, Macela, Boldo, Jurubeba, Simarouba, Tayuya, Anamu.

Amazon Calm Support - Raintree Nutrition, Inc.
Each capsule contains: Proprietary Blend 650 mg: Graviola, Manaca, Mulungu, Passionflower, Catuaba, Muira Puama, Damiana, Chamomile.

Amazon C-F - Raintree Nutrition, Inc.
Each capsule contains: Proprietary Blend 650 mg: Picao Preto, Fedegoso, Amor Seco, Bitter Melon, Clavillia, Mullaca, Gervao, Cat's Claw, Simarouba, Brazillian Peppertree.

Amazon CNS Support - Raintree Nutrition, Inc.
Each capsule contains: Proprietary Blend: 650 mg: Iporuru, Tayuya, Manaca, Pau d'Arco, Amor Seco, Mulungu.

Amazon Detox Support - Raintree Nutrition, Inc.
Each capsule contains: Proprietary Blend 600 mg: Boldo, Amor Seco, Artichoke, Sarsaparilla, Cat's Claw, Carqueja, Nettles.

Amazon Digestion Support - Raintree Nutrition, Inc.
Each capsule contains: Proprietary Blend 650 mg: Boldo, Carqueja, Espinheira Santa, Picao Preto, Jurubeba, Gervao, Cat's Claw.

Amazon Energy Support - Raintree Nutrition, Inc.
Each capsule contains: Proprietary Blend 650 mg: Jatoba, Guarana, Yerba Mate, Maca, Suma.

Amazon F-Tonic Support - Raintree Nutrition, Inc.
Each capsule contains: Proprietary Blend 650 mg: Abuta, Suma, Simarouba, Sarsaparilla, Chuchuhuasi, Damiana, Pau d'Arco.

Amazon Gallbladder Support - Raintree Nutrition, Inc.
Each capsule contains: Proprietary Blend 600 mg: Chanca Piedra, Boldo, Artichoke, Erva Tostao, Carqueja, Jurubeba.

Amazon Hair Support - Raintree Nutrition, Inc.
Each capsule contains: Proprietary Blend 650 mg: Nettles, Mutamba, Muira Puama, Sarsaparilla, Avenco, Gervao, Catuaba, Chuchuhuasi.

Amazon Heart Support - Raintree Nutrition, Inc.
Each capsule contains: Proprietary Blend 650 mg: Abuta, Hawthorn, Chanca Piedra, Picao Preto, Stevia, Brazilian Peppertree, Erva Tostao.

Amazon Hypertension Support - Raintree Nutrition, Inc.
Each capsule contains: Abuta • Artichoke • Bitter Melon • Chanca Piedra • Graviola • Jurubeba • Mullaca • Suma • Periwinkle • Stevia • Pedra hume caa.
See Editor's Note No. 21, page 2056.

Amazon Immune Support - Raintree Nutrition, Inc.
Each capsule contains: Proprietary Blend 650 mg: Cat's Claw, Mullaca, Erva Tostao, Sarsaparilla, Anamu, Fedegoso.

Amazon Joint-Muscle Support - Raintree Nutrition, Inc.
Each capsule contains: Proprietary Blend 650 mg: Amor Seco, Cat's Claw, Chuchuhuasi, Tayuya, Iporuru, Picao Preto, Guaco, Sarsaparilla.

Amazon Kidney Support - Raintree Nutrition, Inc.
Each capsule contains: Proprietary Blend 650 mg: Chanca Piedra, Boldo, Cipo Cabeludo, Erva Tostao, Abuta.

Amazon Liver Support - Raintree Nutrition, Inc.
Each capsule contains: Proprietary Blend 600 mg: Carqueja, Picao Preto, Erva Tostao, Artichoke, Boldo, Chanca Piedra, Guaco.

Amazon Lung Support - Raintree Nutrition, Inc.
Each capsule contains: Proprietary Blend 650 mg: Amor Seco, Embauba, Samambaia, Mullaca, Mutamba, Jatoba, Avenca.

Amazon Menopause Support - Raintree Nutrition, Inc.
Each capsule contains: Proprietary Blend 650 mg: Muira Puama, Suma, Damiana, Maca, Dong Quai, Black Cohosh, Sarsaparilla, Passionflower.

Amazon Menstrual Support - Raintree Nutrition, Inc.
Each capsule contains: Proprietary Blend 650 mg: Abuta, Chuchuhuasi, Tayuya, Iporuru, Cramp Bark, Periwinkle, Erva Tostao.

Amazon Mood Support - Raintree Nutrition, Inc.
Each capsule contains: Proprietary Blend 650 mg: Tayuya, Damiana, Muira Puama, Passion Flower, Chamomile, Graviola, Mulungu.

Amazon M-Tonic Support - Raintree Nutrition, Inc.
Each capsule contains: Proprietary Blend 650 mg: Muira Puama, Catuaba, Chuchuhuasi, Suma, Maca, Nettles, Sarsaparilla, Jatoba.

Some Brand Name Natural Products - What they Contain

www.NaturalDatabase.com contains MANY more listings than appear here.

Amazon Prostate Support - Raintree Nutrition, Inc.
Each capsule contains: Proprietary Blend 650 mg: Mutamba, Brazilian Peppertree, Jatoba, Nettles, Pau d'Arco, Graviola, Cipo Cabeludo.

Amazon Sinus Support - Raintree Nutrition, Inc.
Each capsule contains: Proprietary Blend 650 mg: Nettles, Yerba Mate, Jatoba, Gervao, Pau d'Arco, Picao Preto, Carqueja.

Amazon Skin-A Support - Raintree Nutrition, Inc.
Each capsule contains: Proprietary Blend 650 mg: Abuta, Bitter Melon, Chuchuhuasi, Espinheira Santa, Fedegoso, Sarsaparilla, Tayuya.

Amazon Skin-P Support - Raintree Nutrition, Inc.
Each capsule contains: Proprietary Blend 650 mg: Samambaia, Cat's Claw, Suma, Sarsaparilla, Fedegoso, Boldo, Pau d'Arco.

Amazon Urinary Support - Raintree Nutrition, Inc.
Each capsules contains: Proprietary Blend 650 mg: Chanca Piedra, Anamu, Jatoba, Brazilian Peppertree, Pau d'Arco, Erva Tostao.

Amazon Weight Loss Support - Raintree Nutrition, Inc.
Each capsule contains: Proprietary Blend 650 mg: Cha de Bugre, Carqueja, Guarana, Jurubeba, Picao Preto, Yerba Mate, Annatto.

AmbroDerm Lotion - Mannatech
Water • Emu Oil • Glycereth-26 • Sorbitol • Glycerin • Germaben II (propylene glycol, diazolidinyl urea, methylparaben, propylparaben) • Polysorbate 80 • Tocopherol Acetate • Ambrotose Complex (patent pending; naturally occurring plant saccharides, including freeze-dried Aloe Vera gel extract - manapol powder) •Carbomer • Aminomethyl Propanol • Retinyl Palmitate • Fragrance • Allantoin.

AmbroStart Drink Mix, Orange - Mannatech
Each tablespoon contains: Vitamin A (100% as beta-carotene) 400 IU • Proprietary Blend Energy Complex 5.9 g: Fructose, Citric Acid, Medium Chain Triglycerides, Calcium Citrate, Magnesium Aspartate, Magnesium Succinate, Potassium Aspartate, Potassium Succinate, Choline Bitartrate, Lecithin • Mannatech 2001 Fiber (Arabinogalactan) 3.0 g • Ambrotose Complex (patent pending) 697 mg: Arabinogalactan (larix decidua gum), Manapol Aloe Vera gel extract (inner leaf gel), Gum Ghatti, Gum Tragacanth • Stevia extract (leaf). Other Ingredients: Silicon Dioxide, Natural Flavors, Calcium Pyruvate.

Ambrotose AO - Mannatech
Each capsule contains: Vitamin E (as mixed d-alpha-, d-beta-, d-delta-, and d-gamma-tocopherols) 18 IU • Proprietary Blend MTech AO 113 mg: Quercetin Dihydrate, Grape skin extract (fruit), Green Tea extract (leaves), Australian Bush Plum (terminalia ferdinandiana fruit) • Ambrotose Phyto Formula 333 mg: Gum Arabic, Xanthan Gum, Gum Tragacanth, Gum Ghatti, Aloe Vera gel extract (inner leaf gel - manapol powder) • Phyt•Aloe Complex: Broccoli, Brussels Sprout, Cabbage, Carrot, Cauliflower, Garlic, Kale, Onion, Tomato, Turnip, Papaya, Pineapple. Other Ingredients: Vegetable-Based Cellulose Capsules.

Ambrotose Complex, Capsules - Mannatech
Each capsule contains: Proprietary Blend Ambrotose Complex (patent pending) 150 mg: Arabinogalactan (larix decidua gum), Manapol Aloe Vera gel extract (inner leaf gel), Gum Ghatti, Gum Tragacanth. Other Ingredients: Brown Rice Flour, Silicon Dioxide, Magnesium Stearate.

Ambrotose Complex, Powder - Mannatech
Each 1/4 tsp serving contains: Proprietary Blend Ambrotose Complex (patent pending) 0.44 g: Arabinogalactan (larix decidua gum), Rice Starch, Manapol Aloe Vera gel extract (inner leaf gel), Gum Ghatti, Glucosamine HCl, Gum Tragacanth.

Ambrotose with Lecithin - Mannatech
Each capsule contains: Calcium 70 mg • Proprietary Blend Ambrotose Complex (patent pending) 150 mg: Arabinogalactan (larix decidua gum), Manapol Aloe Vera gel extract (inner leaf gel), Gum Ghatti, Gum Tragacanth • Lecithin powder 50 mg. Other Ingredients: Calcium Carbonate, Dibasic Calcium Phosphate, Gelatin, Brown Rice Flour, Cellulose, Silicon Dioxide, Magnesium Stearate.

Ameal S - Calpis USA
Three tablets contain: Lactotripeptide (derived from milk protein) 6 mg. Other Ingredients: Whey Powder, Sorbitol, Corn Starch, Maltodextrin, Natural & Artificial Flavors, Cellulose, Polyglycerol Esters of Fatty Acids, Anhydride Citric Acid, Aspartame, Calcium Triphosphate.

American Ginseng - Nature's Way
Two capsules contain: American Ginseng root 1.1 g. Other Ingredients: Gelatin, Magnesium stearate.

American Ginseng (500 mg) - Vital Nutrients
Each capsule contains: Panax Quinquefolius (American ginseng, minimum 4% ginsenosides) 500 mg.

American Ginzing - Traditional Medicinals
Contains: American Ginseng root • Licorice root • Ginger rhizome • Cinnamon bark • Sarsaparilla root • Dong Quai root.

Amino 1000 - Puritan's Pride
Three tablets contain: Vitamin C (as ascorbyl palmitate) 30 mg • Hydrolyzed Protein 3000 mg • L-Alanine 210 mg • L-Arginine 189 mg • L-Aspartic Acid 114 mg • L-Cysteine 9.9 mg • L-Glutamic Acid 114 mg • L-Glycine 588 mg • L-Histidine 23.4 mg • L-Hydroxyproline 378 mg • L-Isoleucine 40.8 mg • L-Leucine 66.6 mg • L-Lysine 99 mg • L-Methionine 22.8 mg • L-Phenylalanine 45 mg • L-Proline 303 mg • L-Serine 106.8 mg • L-Threonine 38.4 mg • L-Tyrosine 17.1 mg • L-Valine 57.3 mg.

Amino 1000 (Now Sports) - Now
Four capsules contain: Vitamin B6 13 mg • Proprietary Blend 4 g: Amino Acids from Soy Protein Isolate, Predigested Casei, Predigested Lactalbumin, Carnitine, Ornithine and Gelatin. Other Ingredients: Gelatin (capsule), Magnesium Stearate.

Amino 1500 - Puritan's Pride
Six tablets contain: L-Ornithine HCl 161.1 mg • L-Lysine 836.2 mg • L-Histidine 198.6 mg • L-Arginine 329.2 mg • L-Aspartic Acid 861.3 mg • L-Threonine 376.3 mg • L-Serine 629.2 mg • L-Glutamic Acid 1259.7 mg • L-Proline 635.6 mg • L-Glycine 162.0 mg • L-Alanine 388.8 mg • L-Cystine 250.9 mg • L-Valine 445.3 mg • L-Methionine 203.8 mg • L-Isoleucine 543.5 mg • L-Leucine 977.4 mg • L-Tyrosine 339.7 mg • L-Phenylalanine 376.3 mg.

Amino 1500 (Now Sports) - Now
Three chewable tablets contain: Vitamin B6 (as pyridoxine HCl) 3.2 mg • Proprietary Blend 4.5 g: Amino Acids, Proteins sourced from Whey Protein • Stevia Rebaudiana leaf extract. Other Ingredients: Magnesium Stearate, Cellulose, Stearic Acid, Cellulose, Magnesium Stearate, Fructose, Natural Flavor.

Amino 2000 - Puritan's Pride
Each tablet contains: L-Lysine 282.4 mg • L-Histidine 61.6 mg • L-Arginine 84.6 mg • L-Aspartic Acid 326.0 mg • L-Threonine 211.8 mg • L-Serine 164.6 mg • L-Proline 190.4 mg • L-Alanine 127.2 mg • L-Glycine 59.2 mg • L-Glutamic Acid 275.4 mg • L-Cysteine 80.4 mg • L-Valine 173.6 mg • L-Methionine 64.2 mg • L-Isoleucine 187.6 mg • L-Leucine 321.8 mg • L-Tyrosine 90.4 mg • L-Phenylalanine 97.6 mg • L-Tryptophan 52.2 mg • L-Carnitine 10.0 mg.

Amino 2222 Capsules - Optimum Nutrition
Two capsules contain: Pharmaceutical Grade 3Amino Acids2 (derived from Predigested Lactalbumen, Soy Protein Isolate & Whey Protein concentrate) 2222 mg • L-Ornithine • L-Carnitine.

Amino Acid 1000 mg - Nature's Life
Ten capsules contain: Casein Hydrolysate • Glycine • L-Proline • L-Arginine • L-Alanine • Pyridoxine HCl • L-Ornithine • L-Serine • L-Cystine • Whole Egg powder. Providing, based on a typical analysis:

L-Alanine 663 mg • L-Arginine 665 mg • L-Aspartic Acid 447 mg • L-Cystine 4 mg • L-Glutamic Acid 1222 mg • Glycine 1806 mg • L-Histidine 157 mg • L-Isoleucine (esssential amino acid) 313 mg • L-Leucine (essential amino acid) 512 mg • L-Ornithine 250 mg • L-Lysine (essential amino acid) 471 mg • L-Methionine (essential amino acid) 166 mg • L-Phenylalanine (essential amino acid) 313 mg • L-Proline 1640 mg • L-Serine 505 mg • L-Threonine (essential amino acid) 262 mg • L-Tryptophan (essential amino acid) 70 mg • L-Tyrosine 200 mg • L-Valine (essential amino acid) 408 mg.

Amino Acid Complex **-** Pro Health
Each tablet contains: Vitamin C (as ascorbic acid) 15 mg • Vitamin B6 (as pyridoxine HCl) 5 mg • Proprietary Blend 1 g: L-Lysine, L-Glutamic Acid base, L-Leucine, L-Tyrosine, L-Aspartic Acid, L-Alanine, L-Glutamine, Glycine, L-Methionine, L-Threonine, L-Serine, L-Valine, L-Proline, L-Phenylalanine, L-Ornithine, L-Isoleucine, L-Arginine base, L-Histidine, L-Cysteine HCl, L-Cystine base, Taurine, L-Carnitine, L-Tartrate, L-Citruline. Other Ingredients: Stearic Acid, Dibasic Calcium Phosphate, Colloidal Silicon Dioxide, Modified Cellulose Gum, Magnesium Stearate, Calcium Ascorbate.

Amino Acids from Whey Protein **-** Rexall - Sundown
Two tablets contain: Calcium 178 mg • Whey Protein concentrate 200 mg • Glutamic Acid 12.3 mg • Aspartic Acid 7.6 mg • Leucine 7.3 mg • Lysine 6.5 mg • Threonine 4.6 mg • Proline 4.2 mg • Isoleucine 3.9 mg • Serine 3.9 mg • Valine 3.9 mg • Alanine 3.4 mg • Phenylalanine 2.3 mg • Cystine 2.1 mg • Arginine 1.7 mg • Histidine 1.5 mg • Glycine 1.4 mg • Tyrosine 1.3 mg • Methionine 1.2 mg • Tryptophan 1.1 mg. Other Ingredients: Dicalcium Phosphate, Microcrystalline Cellulose, Croscarmellose Sodium, Silica, Magnesium Stearate.

Amino Athlete **-** Source Naturals
Each tablet contains: Vitamin B6 5 mg • Vitamin C (ascorbic acid) 15 mg.

Amino Blend **-** Progressive Labs
Three capsules contain: L-Alanine 147 mg • L-Arginine 138 mg • L-Cysteine 23 mg • L-Cystine 26 mg • L-Glutamine 28 mg • Glycine 95 mg • L-Histidine 73 mg • L-Isoleucine 71 mg • L-Leucine 203 mg • L-Lysine 203 mg • L-Methionine 55 mg • L-Ornithine 23 mg • L-Proline 77 mg • L-Serine 95 mg • L-Threonine 91 mg • L-Tyrosine 77 mg • L-Valine 120 mg • Taurine 48 mg • L-Aspartic Acid 206 mg • L-Phenylalanine 102 mg • L-Glutamic Acid 349 mg.

Amino Complex **-** Puritan's Pride
Each tablet contains: L-Arginine 50 mg • L-Cysteine 50 mg • L-Histidine 50 mg • L-Isoleucine 50 mg • L-Leucine 50 mg • L-Lysine Hydrochloride 50 mg • L-Methionine 50 mg • L-Ornithine Hydrochloride 50 mg • L-Phenylalanine 50 mg • L-Threonine 50 mg • L-Tyrosine 50 mg • L-Valine 50 mg.

Amino Day **-** Source Naturals
Each tablet contains: Vitamin B6 5 mg • Vitamin C (ascorbic acdi) 15 mg.

Amino Fuel (Anabolic Amino Acid Drink) **-** TwinLab
Peptide Bonded & Free Amino Acids (derived from the natural Pancreatic digests of Whey Protein & Egg White Protein) 20 g • Protein-sparing Carbohydrates (predominantly from Glucose Polymers) 50 g. Other Ingredients: L-Carnitine, Branched Chain Amino Acids (L-Leucine, L-Isoleucine & L-Valine), Essential Vitamins & Minerals, Zinc Picolinate, Boron, GTF Chromium, Chromium Picolinate & Chromium Polynicotinate.

Amino Fuel (Mega Anabolic Chewable Wafers) 7500 mg **-** TwinLab
Two wafers contain: Peptide Bonded & Free Amino Acids 7500 mg (7.5 g). Each wafer contains: L-Carnitine • Branched Chain Amino Acids (L-Leucine, L-Isoleucine & L-Valine) • Pharmaceutical Grade Peptide Bonded & Free Amino Acids derived from the natural Pancreatic digests of Whey Protein (Lactalbumin) & Egg White (Albumin).

Amino Fuel (Peptide Bonded Amino Acid Liquid Concentrate) **-** TwinLab
L-Carnitine • Branched Chain Amino Acids (L-Leucine, L-Isoleucine & L-Valine) • Pharmaceutical Grade, Peptide Bonded & Free Amino Acids • Stress B Complex Vitamins • Lipotropic Factors: Choline & Inositol • Complex Carbohydrates (Glucose Polymers) • Pure Crystalline Fructose. Each serving contains: Peptide Bonded & Free Amino Acids [derived from the natural Pancreatic digests of Whey Protein (Lactalbumin), Egg Protein (Albumin), Liver Protein & other Animal Proteins] 15 g.

Amino Fuel (Peptide Bonded Amino Acid Tablets) **-** TwinLab
L-Carnitine • Branched Chain Amino Acids (L-Leucine, L-Isoleucine & L-Valine) • Peptide Bonded Amino Acids [derived from Pharmaceutical Grade Pancreatic (Enzymatic) digests of Whey Protein (Lactalbumin) & Egg White Protein (Albumin)].

Amino Fuel 1000 Tabs **-** TwinLab
L-Carnitine • Branched Chain Amino Acids (L-Leucine, L-Isoleucine & L-Valine) • Peptide Bonded Amino Acids [derived from Pharmaceutical Grade Pancreatic (Enzymatic) digests of Whey Protein (Albumin)].

Amino Fuel 1500 Tablets **-** TwinLab
Each tablet contains: Peptide Bonded Amino Acids & Branched Chain Amino Acids [derived from Pharmaceutical Grade Pancreatic digests of Whey Protein (Lactalbumin) & Egg White Protein (Albumin)] 1500 mg. No lower quality amino acid sources are present, such as soy or casein.

Amino Fuel 2000 (Extra Strength Amino Acid Tablets) **-** TwinLab
Each tablet contains: Protein (as Peptide Bonded Amino Acids) derived from Pharmaceutical Grade Pancreatic digests of Whey Protein (Lactalbumin) & Egg White Protein 2000 mg.

Amino Fuel Stack **-** TwinLab
Six capsules contain: HMB (B-Hydroxy B-Methylbutyrate Monohydrate) 3000 mg • L-Glutamine 2000 mg • Acetyl-L-Carnitine 1000 mg • Taurine 200 mg • N-Acetyl-Cysteine (NAC) 200 mg.

Amino Mass **-** Source Naturals
Four tablets contain: L-Arginine Pyroglutamate 1,000 mg • L-Lysine HCl 1,000 mg • ChromeMate Chromium GTF (Chromium Polynicotinate) 100 mcg.

Amino Night **-** Source Naturals
Four tablets contain: Arginine Pyroglutamate 816 mg • L-Lysine HCl 816 mg • L-Ornithine (from 469 mg of L-ornithine HCl) 368 mg.

Amino Strength **-** Source Naturals
Each tablet contains: Arginine Pyroglutamate 330 mg • l-Ornithine (from 382 mg of L-Ornithine HCl) 300 mg.

Amino Ty **-** Genestra - Seroyal
Each capsule contains: L-Tyrosine 403 mg • Amino Acids 100 mg.

Amino-BC **-** ANS - Applied Nutrition Sciences
Branched Chain Amino Acids.

AminoBuild: Chocolate Flavor **-** Pharmanex
Three scoops (45 g) contain: Vitamin A (as Vitamin A Palmitate) 1000 IU • Vitamin C (as Ascorbic Acid) 60 mg • Vitamin D (as Vitamin D3) (as Cholecalciferol) 40 IU • Vitamin E (as d-Alpha Tocopheryl Acetate) 30 IU • Thiamin (as Thiamin Mononitrate) 0.3 mg • Riboflavin (as Riboflavin) 0.34 mg • Niacin (as Niacinamide) 4 mg • Vitamin B6 (as Pyridoxine Hydrochloride) 0.4 mg • Folate (as Folic Acid) 80 mcg • Vitamin B12 (as Cyanocobalamin) 1.2 mcg • Biotin (as Biotin) 60 mcg • Pantothenic Acid (as d-Calcium Pantothenate) 2 mg • Calcium (as Dicalcium Phosphate) 540 mg • Phosphorus (as Dicalcium Phosphate) 400 mg • Iodine (as Calcium Iodate) 15 mcg • Magnesium (as Magnesium Citrate) 80 mg • Zinc (as Zinc Gluconate) 3 mg • Selenium (as Sodium Selenate) 14 mcg • Copper (as Copper Gluconate) 0.2 mg • Manganese (as Manganese

Gluconate) 0.4 mg • Chromium (as Chromium Polynicotinate 24 mcg • Molybdenum (as Sodium Molybdate) 15 mcg • Sodium (as Sodium Chloride, Soy Protein Isolate) 250 mg • Potassium (from Soy Protein Isolate) 360 mg • Stevia (Stevia Rebaudiana) (Leaves) 50 mg. Other Ingredients: Protein Blend (Supro7 Soy Protein Isolate, Cross Flow Microfiltration Whey Protein Isolate, Whey Protein Hydrolysate), Crystalline Fructose, Natural Flavors, Alkalized Cocoa Powder, Magnesium Citrate, Sodium Chloride, Dicalcium Phosphate, Ascorbic Acid, dl-Alpha Tocopheryl Acetate, Stevia, Medium Chain Triglycerides, Zinc Gluconate, Chromium Polynicotinate, Biotin, Vitamin A Palmitate, Niacinamide, Manganese Gluconate, Copper Gluconate, d-Calcium Pantothenate, Pyridoxine Hydrochloride, Cholecalciferol, Riboflavin, Thiamin Mononitrate, Cyanocobalamin, Folic Acid, Calcium Iodate, Sodium Molybdate, Sodium Selenate.

AminoBuild: Vanilla Flavor **-** Pharmanex
Three scoops (45 g) contain: Vitamin A (as Vitamin A Palmitate) 1000 IU • Vitamin C (as Ascorbic Acid) 60 mg • Vitamin D3 (as Cholecalciferol) 40 IU • Vitamin E (as d-Alpha Tocopheryl Acetate) 30 IU • Thiamin (as Thiamin Mononitrate) 0.3 mg • Riboflavin (as Riboflavin) 0.34 mg • Niacin (as Niacinamide) 4 mg • Vitamin B6 (as Pyridoxine Hydrochloride) 0.4 mg • Folate (as Folic Acid) 80 mcg • Vitamin B12 (as Cyanocobalamin) 1.2 mcg • Biotin (as Biotin) 60 mcg • Pantothenic Acid (as d-Calcium Pantothenate) 2 mg • Calcium (as Dicalcium Phosphate) 540 mg • Phosphorus (as Dicalcium Phosphate) 400 mg • Iodine (as Calcium Iodate) 15 mcg • Magnesium (as Magnesium Citrate) 80 mg • Zinc (as Zinc Gluconate) 3 mg • Selenium (as Sodium Selenate) 14 mcg • Copper (as Copper Gluconate) 0.2 mg • Manganese (as Manganese Gluconate) 0.4 mg • Chromium (as Chromium Polynicotinate 24 mcg • Molybdenum (as Sodium Molybdate) 15 mcg • Sodium (as Sodium Chloride, Soy Protein Isolate) 250 mg • Potassium (from Soy Protein Isolate) 360 mg • Stevia (Stevia Rebaudiana) (Leaves) 50 mg. Other Ingredients: Protein Blend (Supro7 Soy Protein Isolate, Cross Flow Microfiltration Whey Protein Isolate, Whey Protein Hydrolysate), Crystalline Fructose, Natural Vanilla Flavors, Magnesium Citrate, Sodium Chloride, Dicalcium Phosphate, Ascorbic Acid, Stevia, Medium Chain Triglycerides, dl-Alpha Tocopheryl Acetate, Zinc Gluconate, Chromium Polynicotinate, Biotin, Vitamin A Palmitate, Niacinamide, Manganese Gluconate, Copper Gluconate, d-Calcium Pantothenate, Pyridoxine Hydrochloride, Cholecalciferol, Riboflavin, Thiamin Mononitrate, Cyanocobalamin, Folic Acid, Calcium Iodate, Sodium Molybdate, Sodium Selenate.

Amino-Cartilage **-** Nutri-Quest Rx
Six tablets contain: Natural Hydrolyzed Protein 6000 mg. Typically Providing: Isoleucine 66 mg • Leucine 174 mg • Lysine 216 mg • Methionine 30 mg • Phenylalanine 126 mg • Threonine 120 mg • Valine 168 mg • Arginine 468 mg • Histidine 36 mg • Alanine 546 mg • Tyrosine 24 mg • Serine 198 mg • Aspartic Acid 336 mg • Glutamic Acid 582 mg • Glycine 1362 mg • Hydroxlysine 60 mg • Hydroxyproline 654 mg • Proline 834 mg.

Aminogen **-** Herbalife
Each tablet contains: Aminogen 250 mg.

Amino-Gram Forte **-** Douglas Laboratories
Each tablet contains: L-Lysine 148 mg • L-Histidine 30 mg • L-Arginine 39 mg • L-Aspartic 74 mg • L-Threonine 41 mg • L-Serine 53 mg • L-Glutamic Acid 230 mg • L-Proline 110 mg • L-Alanine 34 mg • L-Cystine 9.4 mg • L-Valine 71.5 mg • L-Methionine 32 mg • L-Isoleucine 59 mg • L-Tyrosine 16 mg • L-Leucine 102.1 mg • L-Phenylalanine 22 mg • L-Tryptophan (naturally occurring) 13 mg • L-Cysteine 10 mg • L-Glutamine 15.3 mg • Taurine 10.7 mg. In a base of Carnitine.

Aminologic **-** PhysioLogics
Three capsules contain: L-Glutamine 185 mg • L-Aspartic Acid 107 mg • L-Tyrosine 103 mg • L-Leucine 97 mg • L-Valine 97 mg • Taurine 90 mg • L-Phenylalanine 88 mg • L-Proline 82 mg • L-Lysine 77 mg • L-Isoleucine 71 mg • L-Serine 71 mg • L-Alanine 60 mg • L-Threonine 59 mg • L-Methionine 55 mg • L-Arginine 54 mg • Papain NF 50 mg • Bromelain 50 mg • Glycine 48 mg • L-Histidine 41 mg • Pancreatin 4X 25 mg • L-Cystine 23 mg.
See Editor's Note No. 14, page 2055.

AminoZyme **-** Nature's Plus
Each capsule contains: AMINOGEN (Aspergillus niger & Aspergillus oryzae proteolytic complex) 250 mg • Vitamin B6 (Pyridoxine HCL) 10 mg • CoQ10 (Ubiquinone) 2.5 mg • Chromium (Polynicotinate) 25 mcg • Vanadium (Sulfate) 10 mcg.

Amore Plus-Rx **-** H Enterprise
Vitamin E • Calcium • Arginine • Saw Palmetto • Damiana • Celery • Chinese Cinnamon • Pygeum Africanum bark • Gotu Kola • Rice flour • Magnesium Stearate • Silica.

Amp Energy Drink **-** PepsiCo, Inc
Carbonated Water • High Fructose Corn Syrup and/or Sugar • Citric Acid • Orange juice from concentrate • Natural Flavors • Guarana • Sodium Benzoate • Sodium Polyphosphates • Maltodextrin • Caffeine • Gum Arabic • Erythoric Acid • Taurine • Panax Ginseng • Calcium Disodium EDTA • Potassium Benzoate • Brominated Vegetable oil • Yellow 5.

Amplify **-** NDS Nutrition
Each level scoop contains: Proprietary Blend 908 g: Cold-Filtered Whey Protein concentrate, Whey Protein isolate, Hydrolyzed Whey Protein (producing di, tri-oligo and poly-peptides from speically filtered and ion-exchanged whey protein concentrate (comprising B-lactoglobulin [approx. 46%], A-lactobumin [approx. 24%], immunoglobin [approx. 10%], lactoferrin)), Natural Flavors.

AmyNex-I **-** Global Life Laboratory Corp.
Each capsule contains: Turmeric (Curcuma longa) 200 mg • Ginger (Zingiber officinale) 190 mg • Ginkgo (Ginkgo biloba) 120 mg. Other Ingredients: Gelatin, Magnesium.

Anabolic Complex **-** The Kutting Edge
Two capsules contain: 10-Norandrosenedione 100 mg • 5-Andro-3B-17B Diol 100 mg • Androstenedione 100 mg • Phosphatidylserine 100 mg • Tribulus 150 mg • Chrysin 50 mg.
See Editor's Note No. 47, page 2058.

Anabolic Fuel **-** TwinLab
Four capsules contain: L-Leucine 2000 mg • L-Valine 500 mg • L-Isoleucine 500 mg.

Anabolic Max - Biochem **-** Country Life
Four tablets contain: L-Glutamine 1000 mg • L-Arginine (pyroglutamate) 900 mg • Creatine Monohydrate 500 mg • L-Citrulline 300 mg • Taurine 300 mg • Betaine HCl 300 mg • Cinnamon extract 250 mg • Green Tea extract 100 mg • DHA (docosahexaenoic acid) 100 mg • Ginseng (panax ginseng) 50 mg • PAK (pyridoxine, alpha-ketoglutarate) 25 mg • Niacin 25 mg • Pantothenic Acid / Pantethine 90/10 25 mg.

Andro Heat - Substrate Solutions **-** ErgoPharm
Four capsules contain: Caffeine (naturally occuring in 2000 mg of Kola Nut herb) 200 mg • Ephedrine (naturally occuring in 250 mg of Ma Huang herb) 20 mg • 4-Androstenediol 100 mg.
See Editor's Note No. 30, page 2056.

Andro Infusion **-** Mass Quantities, Inc.
Each capsule contains: 4-Androstenediol 100 mg • 5-Androstenediol 50 mg • Silymarin 20 mg • Niacin 10 mg • Zinc 5 mg.

Andro Stack - Substrate Solutions **-** ErgoPharm
Each capsule contains: 4-Androstenediol 100 mg • 4-Androstenedione 100 mg.

Andro Surge **-** Country Life
Each capsule contains: Tribulus Terrestris 100 mg • Moomiyo 50 mg • Dehydroepiandrosterone 50 mg • Vitamin E 25 IU.
See Editor's Note No. 47, page 2058.

Some Brand Name Natural Products - What they Contain

www.NaturalDatabase.com contains MANY more listings than appear here.

BRAND NAMES

Andro Surge - MRM
Each capsule contains: Androstenedione 100 mg.
See Editor's Note No. 47, page 2058.

Andro-150 Poppers - Pinnacle
Two tabs contain: Balanced Andro Complex 150 mg: 4-AD 128 mg, 4-AD-EC 15 mg, NOR-4-AD 5 mg, A1-E 2 mg. Other Ingredients: Fructose, Sorbitol, Natural Flavor, Stearic Acid, Magnesium Stearate, Cellulose, Croscarmellose, Sucralose.
See Editor's Note No. 47, page 2058.

Andro-6 - EAS
Four tablets contain: DHEA 50 mg • Androstenedione 100 mg • Tribulus terrestris 250 mg • Chrysin 150 mg • Saw Palmetto extract 180 mg • Indole-3-Carbinol 50 mg • Zinc Glycinate 8 mg.
See Editor's Note No. 47, page 2058.

Androbolic - ProLab
Each two tablets contain: 19-Norandrostenedione 100 mg • 4-Androstene-3,17 Diol 100 mg • 5-Androstene-3,17 Diol 50 mg • Tribulus Terrestris 250 mg • Saw Palmetto 180 mg • Chrysin 150 mg • Indole 3 Carbinol 50 mg.

Andro-Diol - New Hope Health Products
Each capsule contains: 4-androstene-3, 17-diol 100 mg.

Androdiol Select 300 - ErgoPharm
Each capsule contains: 4-Androstenediol (androdiol) 300 mg. Other Ingredients: Corn Starch.

Androdyne - Cytodyne Technologies
Three capsules contain: 19-Norandrostenedione 100 mg • 5-Androstene-3B, 17b-Diol 50 mg • 4-Androstene-3,17-dione 50 mg • AA-t3 Anti-Aromatase Complex 100 mg: Chrysin, Indole 3-Carbinol, 7-IsoPropoxyIsoflavone • Zinc Gluconate 20 mg • B3 Nicotinic Acid 50 mg.

Andro-Edge - Aarisse Health Care
Each 1.75 oz pump contains: 4-Androstene-3, 17-Dione Androstenediol • Tribulus Terrestris • Chrysin • Damiana extract • Vitamin E • Zinc.

Andro-Plex - Ortho Molecular Products
Each tablet contains: Vitamin A (fish liver oil) 2500 IU • Vitamin C 100 mg • Vitamin E (d-alpha tocopherol) 50 IU • Calcium (amino acid chelate) 50 mg • Magnesium (amino acid chelate) 25 mg • Zinc (amino acid chelate) 15 mg • Orchic (testicle substance) 100 mg • Raw Adrenal Tissue 10 mg • Raw Pituitary Tissue 5 mg • Raw Prostate Tissue 100 mg • Proprietary Blend Base 123.5 mg: Saw Palmetto (serenoa repens), Damiana leaves (turmera aphrodesiaca), Licorice root (glycyrrhiza glabra), Sarsparilla (smilax medica), Ginseng (panax ginseng), Hibisucs, DNA, RNA.
See Editor's Note No. 14, page 2055.

AndroPlex 700 - AST Sports Science
Two capsules contain: Tribulus Terrestris 500 mg • Androstenedione 100 mg • DHEA 100 mg.
See Editor's Note No. 47, page 2058.

Andro-Stack 850 - Optimum Nutrition
Two capsules contain: pharmaceutical grade Androstenedione (Delta-4-androstene-3-17-dione) 100 mg • pharmaceutical grade DHEA (Dehydroepiandrosterone) 100 mg • Tribulus terrestris 650 mg.
See Editor's Note No. 47, page 2058.

AndrosteDERM - MedLean
2 ml contain: 4-Androstenediol (Androdiol from Pat Arnold's LPJ Research) 90 mg • Androstenedione 30 mg.
See Editor's Note No. 47, page 2058.

Androstene Power - Olympian Labs
Each capsule contains: 4-Androstene 3, 17-dione 50 mg.

Androstenediol 300 - Higher Power
Each capsule contains: Androstenediol (4-Androstene,17-diol) 300 mg.

Androstenedione with Yohimbe - Puritan's Pride
Each capsule contains: Androstenedione 100 mg • Yohimbe bark extract (standardized for 8 mg Yohimbine) 400 mg.
See Editor's Note No. 47, page 2058.

Androstenetrione Powder - ErgoPharm
Each 1/4 tsp serving contains: Androstenetrione 440 mg.

Andro-Surge - Metabolic Response Modifiers
Each capsule contains: Androstenedione (4-androstene-3, 17-dione) 100 mg.
See Editor's Note No. 47, page 2058.

Andro-Surge - New Hope Health Products
Each capsule contains: Androstenedione (4-androstene-3, 17-dione) 100 mg.
See Editor's Note No. 47, page 2058.

Andro-Xtreme - Metabolic Response Modifiers
Two capsules contain: Dehydroepiandrosterone (DHEA) 100 mg • Androstenedione (4-androstene-3, 17-dione) 100 mg • 5-androstenediol (5-androstene 3, 17- diol) 50 mg • Tribulus terrestris 500 mg • Chrysin 250 mg.
See Editor's Note No. 47, page 2058.

ANDRO-Xtreme - New Hope Health Products
Each capsule contains: Dehydroepiandrosterone (DHEA) 100 mg • Androstenedione (4-androstene-3, 17-dione) 100 mg • 5-androstenediol (5-androstene-3, 17-diol) 50 mg • Tribulus terrestris 500 mg • Chrysin 250 mg.
See Editor's Note No. 47, page 2058.

Androzyme - Progressive Labs
Each capsule contains: Vitamin E (d-alpha tocopheryl succinate) 50 IU • Zinc (as zinc aspartate) 15 mg • Raw Orchic concentrate (bovine) 100 mg • Siberian Ginseng (Eleutherococcus senticosus) 100 mg • L-Carnitine 30 mg.
See Editor's Note No. 14, page 2058.

Angel Hair - Revival - Physicians Laboratories
Two ounces contain: Certified Isoflavone 15 mg. Other Ingredients: Soy Protein Isolate, Niacin, Iron (ferrous sulfate), Thiamin Mononitrate, Riboflavin, Folic Acid.

AngioBlock - NutriCology
Four capsules contain: Convolvulus Arvensis leaves extract 1000 mg. Other Ingredients: Maltodextrin.

Animal Chews - Puritan's Pride
Two tablets contain: Vitamin A (as retinyl palmitate & beta carotene) 5,000 IU • Vitamin C (as calcium ascorbate) 120 mg • Vitamin D (as cholecalciferol) 400 IU • Vitamin E (as d-alpha tocopheryl acid succinate) 30 IU • Vitamin K (as phytonadione) 2 mcg • Thiamin (Vitamin B1; as thiamine mononitrate) 1.5 mg • Riboflavin (Vitamin B2) 1.7 mg • Niacin (as niacinamide) 20 mg • Vitamin B6 (as pyridoxine hydrochloride) 2 mg • Folic Acid 400 mcg • Vitamin B12 (as cyanocovalamin) 6 mcg • Biotin (as d-biotin) 300 mcg • Pantothenic Acid (as d-calcium pantothenate) 10 mg • Calcium (as calcium carbonate, calcium citrate, and calcium ascorbate) 250 mg • Iron (as ferrous fumarate) 4 mg • Iodine (as potassium iodide and kelp) 75 mcg • Magnesium (as magnesium ascorbate and magnesium oxide) 100 mg • Zinc (as zinc amino acid chelate) 7.5 mg • Selenium (as L-Selenomethionine) 15 mcg • Copper (as cupric gluconate) 1 mg • Manganese (as manganese gluconate) 1 mg • Chromium (as chromium polynicotinate) 15 mcg • Molybdenum (as sodium molybdate) 10 mcg • Boron (sodium borate) 10 mcg • Vanadium (as vanadyl sulfate) 5 mcg • Nickel (as nickelous sulfate) 2 mcg • Tin (as stannous chloride) 2 mcg • Choline Phosphatides (as lecithin) 2 mg • Inositol Phosphatides (as lecithin) 5 mg • Rutin 5 mg • Green Barley

juice powder 3 mg • Chlorella powder 3 mg • Spirulina powder 5 mg • Alfalfa juice powder 5 mg • Rice Bran powder 10 mg • Carrot juice powder 5 mg • Natural Licorice root 4 mg.

Animal Chews with Calcium **-** Puritan's Pride
Two tablets contain: Vitamin A (50% as retinyl palmitate and 50% as beta-carotene) 5,000 IU • Vitamin C (as calcium ascorbate) 120 mg • Vitamin D (as cholecalciferol) 400 IU • Vitamin E (as d-alpha tocopheryl acid succinate) 30 IU • Thiamin (as thiamine mononitrate) 1.5 mg • Riboflavin 1.7 mg • Niacin (as niacinamide) 20 mg • Vitamin B6 (as pyridoxine hydrochloride) 2 mg • Folic Acid 0.4 mg • Vitamin B12 (as cyanocobalamin) 6 mcg • Biotin 100 mcg • Pantothenic Acid (as d-calcium pantothenate) 10 mg • Calcium (as calcium carbonate, calcium citrate, and calcium ascorbate) 250 mg. In a base containing Raspberry Juice Concentrate, Rose Hips, Acerola, Black Currant Juice, Fructose, Fruit Juice Solids, Dried Dates, Dried Apricots, and Dried Peaches.

Animal Cuts Free **-** Universal
Each pack contains: Niacin (as niacinamide) 15 mg • Vitamin B6 (as pyridoxine HCl) 2 mg • Thermogenic Complex 575 mg: Synephrine, Octopamine, Tyramine, EGCG (epigallocatechin gallate), L-Theanine, PEA (phenylethylamine) • Lipotropic Complex 75 mg: Choline Citrate, Betaine HCl, Inositol Monophosphate • Metabolic Complex 900 mg: Guarana (22% caffeine), L-Carnitine • Diuretic Complex 750 mg: Dandelion extract (taraxol, taraxerol), Uva Ursi extract (arbutin, methyl-arbutin) • Thyroid Complex 175 mg: Guggul (2.5% guggulsterones), Soy Isoflavones • Insulin Potentiators 100 mg: Alpha Lipoic Acid, Chromium Polynicotinate, Chromium Picolinate • Nucleotide Regulators 300 mg: Phospate, Inosine, Phosphatidylcholine • Neurotransmitter Regulators 250 mg: St. John's Wort (0.3% hypericin), L-Tyrosine • Animal Cuts Complex 812 mg: Citriline Hydroxycitric Acid, Grapefruit extract (naringin, naringenin), White Willow bark, Phenylalanine (as L-phenylalanine), Ginger root extract (gingerols, shoagols). Other Ingredients: Bitter Orange Extract, Green Tea Extract, Cocoa Extract, Potassium Phosphate, Magnesium Phosphate, Magnesium Stearate, Gelatin, Stearic Acid.
See Editor's Note No. 40, page 2058.

Animal Mix **-** Professional Complementary Health Formul
Adrenal 3X, 4X • ACTH 6X, 30X • Histamine 12X • Liver 6X, 12X • Camel, Cat (short and long haired), Chicken, Cow, Dog (short and long haired), Duck, Fish Scale (fresh and salt water), Goat (angora/mohair), Goose, Guinea Pig Hog, Horse, Llama, Mouse, Pheasant, Quail, Rabbit, Rat, Sheep (wool), Turkey 6X, 12X, 60X, 100X • Purified Water • 20% USP Alcohol.
See Editor's Note No. 1, page 2053.

Animal Pak **-** Universal
Two paks (22 tablets) contain: Vitamin A (as acetate & 66% as beta-carotene) 9900 IU • Vitamin C (as ascorbic acid) 1 g • Vitamin D (as ergocalciferol) 680 IU • Vitamin E (as D-A-tocopheryl acetate) 300 IU • Thiamin (as thiamin HCl) 76 mg • Riboflavin 76 mg • Niacin (as niacinamide) 82 mg • Vitamin B6 (as pyridoxine HCl) 72 mg • Folic Acid 400 mcg • Vitamin B12 (as cyanocobalamin) 6 mcg • Biotin 300 mcg • Pantothenic Acid (as calcium pantothenate) 76 mg • Calcium (as citrate, carbonate) 2 g • Phosphorus (as calcium phosphate) 228 mg • Iodine (from kelp) 150 mcg • Magnesium (as oxide) 133 mg • Zinc (as oxide) 30 mg • Selenium (as selenite) 50 mcg • Copper (as sulfate) 600 mcg • Manganese (as sulfate) 11 mg • Chromium (as picolinate) 6 mcg • Potassium (as sulfate) 200 mg • Amino Acid Blend: Lysine (from lactalbumin) 300 mg, Methionine (from lactalbumin) 500 mg, Leucine (from lactalbumin) 100 mg, Valine (from lactalbumin) 760 mg, Threonine (from lactalbumin) 48 mg, Glutamic Acid (from lactalbumin) 700 mg, Phenylalanine (from lactalbumin) 560 mg, Arginine (as L-arginine) • Performance Optimizers: Siberian Ginseng root 2 g, Oriental Ginseng root 250 mg, Smilax Officinalis root 500 mg, Protogen A (as thioctic acid) 200 mg, Inosine (as hypoxanthine riboside) 500 mg, Pyridoxine A-Ketoglutarate (PAK) 200 mg, Carnitine (as L-carnitine) 25 mg, Chromium Picolinate 50 mcg, Coenzyme A 20 mg, Coenzyme B12 10 mg, Phosphatidylcholine 200 mg, Para-Aminobenzoic Acid (PABA) 400 mg, Colostrum (bovine) 25 mg, Argentine Liver (bovine) 3.9 g, Shark Cartilage 1 g, Choline Complex 1.2 g, Citrus Bioflavonoids 1 g • Essential Fatty Acid Complex: Linoleic Acid 200 mg, Oleic Acid 100 mg • Digestive Enzymes: Betaine HCl 200 mg, Pepsin 64 mg, Papain 64 mg, Ox Bile (bovine) 120 mg, Pancreatin 700 mg, Mycozyme 64 mg. Other Ingredients: Maltodextrin, Calcium Sulfate, Choline Citrate, Magnesium Stearate, Stearic Acid, Parsley, Goldenseal, Dong Quai, Burdock, Alfalfa, Watercress, Rice Bran, Cellulose, Rose Hips.
See Editor's Note No. 14, page 2055.

Animal Stak **-** Universal
Each pak contains: Vitamin C (as ascorbic acid) 50 mg • Vitamin B6 (as pyridoxine HCl) 10 mg • Calcium (as sulfate, phosphate) 200 mg • Zinc (as picolinate) 15 mg • Chromium (as picolinate) 100 mcg • Prohormone Complex: 19-Nor-5-Androstenedione 100 mg, 5-Androxydiol 100 mg, Dehydroepiandrosterone 50 mg • LH Boosters: Tribulus extract (standardized to 20-29% steroidal saponins) 250 mg, Acetyl-L-Carnitine 250 mg, L-Carnitine 100 mg • Growth Hormone Secretagogues: L-Arginine Pyroglutamate 2.5 g, L-Ornithine Alpha-Ketoglutarate 1.3 g, L-Taurine 750 mg, Colostrum (bovine) 250 mg • Anti-Aromatase Inhibitors: Chrysin 250 mg, Kudzu extract (isoflavones) 150 mg • DHT Blockers: Beta Sitosterol 250 mg, Saw Palmetto fruit 200 mg, Pygeum Africanum Hook f. bark 50 mg • Thermogenic Factors: Guarana extract (standardized for 20-29% steroidal saponins) 570 mg, Bitter Orange extract (standardized for 4% synephrine) 500 mg, Coleus Forskohlii extract (standardized for 20% forskohlin) 50 mg • Liver Detoxifiers: Lysolphosphatidylcholine 100 mg, Milk Thistle seed 75 mg.
See Editor's Note No. 40, page 2058.

Anise Star Galaxy **-** RedSafari
100% Pure Anise Star essential oil.

Anorex **-** Klein-Becker
Two capsules contain: Calcium (amino acid chelate) 264 mg • Vitamin B6 25 mg • Anorex (Leptoprin) Proprietary Blend 989 mg: Acetylsalicylic Acid 324 mg, Caffeine (34 mg from standardized kola nut) (280 mg) 200 mg, Green Tea leaf extract (standardized for polyphenols/catechins content), L-Tyrosine, Kelp (0.155 Iodine [100 mg]), Ephedrine Alkaloids from Ma Huang (10% extract from whole plant 200 mg), Cayenne (fruit).
See Editor's Note No. 21 and No. 30, page 2056.

Anorex-SF **-** Klein-Becker
Two capsules contain: Calcium (amino acid chelate) 132 mg • Anorex (Leptoprin S-F) Proprietary Blend 1493.5 mg: Calcium Phosphate, Commiphora Mukul extract, Garcinia Cambogia (HCA 125 mg), L-Tyrosine, Acetylsalicylic Acid (162.5 mg), Dipotassium Phosphate, Sodium Phosphate, Disodium Phosphate, Phosphatidyl Choline, Scutellaria root, Bupleurum root, Epimedium herb. Other Ingredients: Rice Flour.
See Editor's Note No. 21, page 2056.

Anotesten **-** MuscleTech
Six capsules contain: 4-Androstenediol 150 mg • Androstenedione 250 mg • DHEA 100 mg • Tribulus Terrestris 1000 mg • Chrysin 150 mg • Indole-3-Carbinol (I3C) 50 mg • Saw Palmetto (standardized for 25% fatty acids) 320 mg.
See Editor's Note No. 47, page 2058.

Antacid **-** Progressive Labs
Each tablet contains: Calcium Carbonate 500 mg which supplies: Calcium (from calcium carbonate) 200 mg. Other Ingredients: Dextrose, Mannitol, Cellulose, Magnesium Stearate, Glycine and Spearmint oil. Free of Sodium & Aluminum.

Anthocyan **-** PhytoPharmica
Two capsules contain: Vitamin A (beta-carotene) 10,000 IU • Vitamin C (ascorbic acid) 200 mg • Riboflavin (vitamin B2) 10 mg •Bilberry (Vaccinium myrtillus fruit berry) extract (standardized to contain 25% anthocyanosides [40 mg per 2 capsules] calculated as anthocyanidins) 160 mg.
See Editor's Note No. 21, page 2056.

Anti **-** Grandma's Herbs
Each capsule contains: Proprietary Blend 0.451 g: Garlic herb, Goldenseal root, Echinacea Angustifolia root, Myrrh gum, Plantain leaves, Propolis herb. Other Ingredients: Gelatin.

Anti-Age/Energy Formula **-** Body Language Vitamin Co.
Each capsule contains: Alpha Lipoic Acid 150 mg • Acetyl L-Carnitine 150 mg • Coenzyme Q10 60 mg • Glutathione 30 mg.

Anti-Aging **-** Vidafit
Each serving contains: Biotin 30 mcg • Folate 400 mcg • Niacin 20 mg • Pantothenic Acid 10 mg • Riboflavin 1.7 mg • Thiamine 1.5 mg • Vitamin A 3300 IU • Vitamin B12 6 mcg • Vitamin B6 10 mg • Vitamin C 120 mg • Vitamin D 400 IU • Vitamin E 30 IU • Boron 1 mg • Calcium 500 mg • Magnesium 250 mg • Phosphorus 500 mg • Selenium 70 mcg • Zinc 15 mg • Acetyl-L-Carnitine 50 mg • Coenzyme Q10 20 mg • Quercetin 20 mg • Bilberry 50 mg • Ginkgo extract 50 mg • Grape Seed extract 50 mg • Soy Protein 2 grams.

Anti-Anxiety **-** PhytoPharmica
Twenty drops contain: Cicuta virosa 4x • Gaultheria 4x • Ignatia 4x • Staphysagria 4x • Asa foetida 3x • Corydalis formosa 3x • Hyoscyamus 3x • Sumbulus 3x • Valeriana officianalis 3x • Avena sativa 1x. In a base of 40% USP alcohol by volume.
See Editor's Note No. 1 and No. 21, see pages 2053 and 2056.

Anti-Arthritis Glucosamine Chondroitin **-** Crystal Springs
Each tablet contains: Glucosamine (Sulfate) 600 mg • Chondroitin Sulfate 400 mg.
See Editor's Note No. 15, page 2055.

AntiBetic Pancreas Tonic **-** Gero Vita International
Each capsule contains: Pterocarpus Marsupium (Indian kino tree, fabaceae family) 195 mg • Gymnema Sylvestre (gymnema) 175 mg • Momordica Charantia (bitter melon) 40 mg • Azadirachta Indica (neem) 20 mg • Tinospora Cordifolia (heart leaved moonseed) 30 mg • Aegle Marmelos (bael) 40 mg • Syzygium Cumini (jambolan) 50 mg • Cinnamonum Tamala (cinnamon leaf) 20 mg • Trigonella Foenum-Graecum (fenugreek) 65 mg • Ficus Racemosa (cluster fig) 15 mg.

AntiBio 1 **-** Dial Herbs
Echinacea • Goldenseal • Poke root • Cayenne.

AntiBio 2 **-** Dial Herbs
Echinacea • Myrrh • Poke root • Cayenne.

Anti-Catabolic Fuel **-** TwinLab
Four capsules contain: L-Leucine 1000 mg • L-Valine 225 mg • L-Isoleucine 225 mg • Ketoisocaproate (KIC) 100 mg • L-Ornithine, Alpha-Ketoglutarate 1000 mg • L-Glutamine 250 mg.

Anti-Cholesterol Formula **-** Body Language Vitamin Co.
Three tablets contain: Artichoke (Cynara scolymnus, 15% caffeoylquinic/chlorogenic acids) 100 mg • Chitosan 300 mg • Garlic 300 mg • Chinese Red Yeast Rice 500 mg • Garcinia fruit 100 mg • Myristica fragrans 100 mg • Grapefruit Pectin 400 mg • Gugulipid 200 mg • Beta-sitosterol 200 mg • Hyaluronic Acid 200 mg • EDTA 200 mg • Milk Thistle 250 mg • Policosanol 10 mg • Vitamin B12 mcg • Folate 400 mcg.

Anti-Depressant Formula With St. John's Wort **-** Life Extension
Each capsule contains: Standardized Herbal Blend 0.450 mg: St. John's Wort (standardized for 0.3% hypericin), Kava Kava, Ginkgo Biloba.

Anti-Fatigue **-** PhytoPharmica
Twenty drops contain: Zincum muriaticum 8x • Gelsemium sempervirens 6x • Picricum acidum 6x • Acidum phosphoricum 3x • Valeriana officinalis 1x. In a base of 45% USP alcohol by volume.
See Editor's Note No. 1 and No. 21, pages 2053 and 2056.

Anti-Fungal **-** The Herbalist
Thuja leaf • Usnea lichen • Spilanthes herb • Pau D'Arco inner bark • Echinacea root • Calendula flower • Cayenne pepper.

Anti-Fungal Salve **-** Blessed Herbs
Jewelweed • Black Walnut hulls • Pau d'Arco bark • Usnea lichen • Calendula flowers • Spilanthes • Echinacea Angustifolia root • Goldenseal root • Myrrh Gum • Organic Cold-Pressed Olive oil • Beeswax • Essential oils of Tea Tree & Thyme linalol.

Anti-HangOver **-** Jamieson
Each capsule contains: Botanical Complex AK280 (Perilla Frutescens, Agastache Rugosa) 243 mg • Taurine 37 mg.

Anti-Insom **-** Dial Herbs
Hops • Lobelia • Valerian • Cayenne.

Anti-Nausea Ginger Gum **-** Sea-Band LTD
Each piece contains: Ginger oil (equivalent to 8 g fresh ginger root) 25 mg.

AntiOx, Cysteine Free **-** NutriCology
Each capsule contains: Vitamin A (40% as retinyl palmitate and 60% as beta-carotene) 12,500 IU • Vitamin C (as ascorbyl palmitate) 4 mg • Vitamin E (as DL-alpha-tocopheryl acetate) 100 IU • Thiamin (as thiamin hydrochloride) 10 mg • Riboflavin (80% as riboflavin and 20% as riboflavin-5-phosphate) 12.5 mg • Niacin (50% as niacinamide) 10 mg • Vitamin B6 (80% as pyridoxine hydrochloride and 20% as pyridoxal-5-phosphate) 12.5 mg • Folic Acid 100 mcg • Vitamin B12 (as cyanocobalamin) 100 mcg • Pantothenic Acid (as calcium pantothenate) 25 mg • Zinc (as zinc citrate) 7.5 mg • Selenium (87% as sodium selenite and 13% as selenomethionine) 75 mcg • Copper (as copper sebacate) 0.5 mg • Manganese (as manganese citrate) 5 mg • Glutathione (reduced) 50 mg • L-Methionine 75 mg • Taurine 75 mg • Trimethylglycine 50 mg • Coenzyme Q10 10 mg • Proanthocyanidins, as Grape seed extract 1.25 mg. Other Ingredients: Magnesium Stearate, Silicon Dioxide.

Anti-Ox: Herbal Antioxidant **-** The Herbalist
Pau D'Arco inner bark • Astragalus root • Ginkgo leaf • Milk Thistle seed • Licorice root • Cayenne pepper.

Antioxidant **-** Oasis Wellness Network
Each tablet contains: Vitamin C (as ascorbic acid) 125 mg • Vitamin E (as d-alpha-tocopheryl acetate) 50 IU • Niacin (as niacinamide ascorbate) 25 mg • Folate (as folic acid) 100 mcg • Calcium (as calcium sulfate) 15 mg • MaxCell Proprietary Blend 125 mg: Zisyphus Jujube, Aloe Vera gel, Piper Nigrum, Glycyrrhiza Glabra • L-Cysteine (base) 50 mg • Bioflavonoid Complex 25 mg • Green Tea leaf extract 25 mg • Rosemary leaf extract 25 mg • Turmeric rhizome extract 25 mg • Carotenoid mixture 10 mg • Grape seed extract 10 mg. Other Ingredients: Calcium Sulfate, Stearic Acid, Cellulose, Silica, Magnesium Stearate.

Antioxidant - Wellzymes **-** Enzymes, Inc.
Three capsules contain: Vitamin A (as Beta-Carotene from Dunaliella Algae) 7500 IU • Vitamin C (from Acerola Cherries) 45 mg • Vitamin E (from d-Alpha Tocopheryl Acid Succinate) 90 IU • Zinc (from Zinc Citrate) 9 mg • Selenium (from Selenium Citrate) 45 mcg • Copper (from Copper Citrate) 0.75 mg • Manganese (from Manganese Citrate) 3 mg • n-zimes Proprietary Enzyme Blend 36 mg: pHysioProtease (88,800 pHysio-U), CereCalase Plus • Proprietary Herbal Blend 159 mg: Quercetin, Rutin, Hesperidin extract, Citrus Bioflavonoids, Rice Bran, Green Tea leaf extract, Lutein extract, Lycopenes extract, Grape seed extract, Lipoic Acid, Milk Thistle seed extract, Ginkgo Biloba leaf extract, Bilberry fruit extract, conc. of Brococoli, Cabbage, Brussel sprouts, Cauliflower, Kale, Watercress. Other Ingredients: Plant Cellulose, Water.

Antioxidant - Bioset **-** Enzymes, Inc.
Each capsule contains: Vitamin A (100% as Beta-Carotene from Dunaliella) 5000 IU • Vitamin C (100% from Acerola Cherries) 47 mg • Vitamin E (100% from d-Alpha Tocopheryl Succinate) 100 IU •

Zinc (100% from Zinc Citrate) 5 mg • Selenium (100% from SeaSel Kelp) 15 mcg • Manganese (100% from Manganese Citrate) 3 mg • Proprietary Enzyme Blend 81 mg: pHysioProtease, Catalase • Proprietary Herbal Blend 81 mg: Turmeric root extract, Green Tea leaf extract, Quercetin, Lutein extract, Bilberry fruit extract, Grape seed extract, Alpha-Lipoic Acid. Other Ingredients: Plant Cellulose, Water.

***Anti-oxidant* - Douglas Laboratories**
Three capsules contain: Vitamin C (as ascorbic acid/ascorbyl palmitate complex) 200 mg • Bioflavonoids 200 mg • L-Cysteine 200 mg • Choline Bitartrate 200 mg • Inositol 200 mg • Vitamin E 150 IU • L-Methionine 20 mg • Vitamin A (as beta carotene) 12,500 IU • Vitamin B1 40 mg • Vitamin B2 20 mg • Niacinamide 20 mg • Pantothenic Acid 20 mg • Vitamin B6 (as pyridoxal-5-phosphate) 20 mg • DMG (dimethylglycine) 20 mg • Glutathione 15 mg • Selenium (as selenium Krebs) 50 mcg.

***Antioxidant 4000 Vitamins & Mineral* - Nature's Bounty**
Two softgels contain: Vitamin A (as Beta Carotene) 20000 IU • Vitamin C (as Ascorbic Acid) 400 mg • Vitamin E (as dl-Alpha Tocopheryl Acetate) 250 IU • Selenium (as Selenium Yeast) 50 mcg • Proprietary Blend: Carrot powder, Broccoli powder, Spinach powder 6 mg. Other Ingredients: Gelatin, Soy Lecithin, Glycerin, Vegetable Oil.

***Antioxidant Booster* - Advocare International**
Two caplets contain: Vitamin E (as d-alpha tocopheryl succinate) 250 IU • Vitamin C (as ascorbic acid & ascorbyl palmitate) 1000 mg • Beta-Carotene 15,000 IU • Selenium (as selenomethionine) 35 mcg • Zinc (as monomethionine - OptiZinc) 5 mg • Manganese (as amino acid chelate) 1 mg • Green Tea extract (leaf - camellia sinensis) 50 mg • Milk Thistle extract (fruit - silybum marianum) 50 mg • Grape extract (seed/skin - vitis vinifera Activin) 100 mg. Other Ingredients: Dicalcium Phosphate, Silicon Dioxide, Cellulose, Stearic Acid, Magnesium Stearate.

***Antioxidant Caps* - Now**
Two capsules contain: Vitamin A (from 15 mg Beta-Carotene) 25000 IU • Vitamin C (from Calcium Ascorbate) 500 mg • Vitamin E (natural d-Alpha Succinate) 300 IU • Calcium (Ascorbate) 50 mg • Zinc (Picolinate) 5 mg • Selenium (L-Selenomethionine) 25 mcg • N-Acetyl-Cysteine 100 mg • L-Glutathione 25 mg • Alfalfa juice concentrate (Green Superfood) 250 mg • Wheat Sprout concentrate (Enzyme active) 100 mg.

***Anti-Oxidant Caps* - Vital Nutrients**
Each capsule contains: Natural Mixed Carotenes 10,000 IU • Vitamin C (ascorbic acid 100%) 250 mg • Vitamin E (natural source) 200 IU • Selenium (selenomethionine) 50 mcg • Selenium (sodium selenite) 50 mcg • N-Acetyl-Cysteine 100 mg • Ginkgo extract (50:1, 24%/6%) 25 mg • Green Tea extract (80% catechins) 25 mg.

***Antioxidant Cocktail Custom Paks* - The Vitamin Shoppe**
Each packet contains: Vitamin A (as 100% beta-carotene) 15 mg (25000 IU) • Vitamin C (as ascorbic acid) 2000 mg • Vitamin E (as d-alpha, d-gamma, d-beta, d-delta tocopherol) 400 IU • Selenium (as selenomethionine) 200 mcg • Alpha-carotene 1 mg (833 IU) • Lycopene (LYC-O-MATO) 5 mg • Lutein 5 mg • Zeaxanthin 0.24 mg • Phytoene 0.055 mg • Phytofluene 0.026 mg • Citrus Bioflavonoids 1000 mg • Hesperidin 100 mg • Rutin 100 mg • Rose Hips (Rosa canina) fruit 160 mg • Acerola 20 mg.

***Antioxidant Cocktail II* - The Vitamin Shoppe**
Two capsules contain: Pine bark extract (Pycnogenol) 30 mg • Grape Seed Extract (vitis vinifera, Activin) 50 mg • Alpha Lipoic Acid 50 mg • Green Tea leaves (camellia sinensis, standardized to 75% polyphenols) 50 mg.

***Antioxidant Formula* - Nature's Way**
Two capsules contain: Beta Carotene 25,000 IU • Coenzyme Q10 (ubiquinone) 5 mg • Copper amino acid chelate 2 mg • Green Tea, polyphenol catechin extract 10 mg • L-Cysteine 100 mg • Quercetin (eucalyptus) 100 mg • Selenium (l-selenomethione) 200 mcg • Vitamin C 500 mg • Vitamin E (d-alpha tocopheryl) 400 IU • Zinc amino acid chelate 15 mg. Other Ingredients: Gelatin, Magnesium stearate, Maltodextrin, Silica.

***Antioxidant Formula* - Body Language Vitamin Co.**
Two tablets contain: N-Acetyl-L-Cysteine 100 mg • Vitamin E (d-alpha) 400 IU • Beta Carotene 12,000 IU • Vitamin C 800 mg • L-Glutathione 60 mg • Chromium Picolinate 120 mcg • Niacinamide 100 mg • Selenium (methionate) 200 mcg • Vitamin B12 100 mcg • Folic Acid 800 mcg • Manganese (glycinate) 5 mg • Zinc (monomethionate) 30 mg • Ginkgo Biloba (24% ginkgo flavoglycosides) 60 mg • Korean Ginseng (25% ginsenosides) 25 mg • Grape Seed extract 45 mg • Green Tea extract 25 mg • Alpha Lipoic Acid 25 mg • Coenzyme Q10 10 mg • Citrus Bioflavonoids 100 mg • Lutein 5 mg • dl-Methionine 60 mg.

***Anti-Oxidant Formula #1* - Olympian Labs**
Two capsules contain: Cat's Claw (uncaria tomentosa) 500 mg • Ginkgo Biloba extract 60 mg • Crystalline CoQ10 30 mg • Grape Seed extract 50 mg.

***Antioxidant Fuel* - TwinLab**
Three capsules contain: Beta-Carotene (pro-Vitamin A) 25000 IU • Vitamin C 1000 mg • Natural Vitamin E (Succinate) 800 IU • CoQ10 (Coenzyme Q10) 30 mg • N-Acetyl Cysteine (NAC) 200 mg • L-Glutathione 100 mg • Selenium (from Selenomethionine & Selenate 50/50 mixture) 100 mcg • Alpha-Lipoic Acid (reduced) 100 mcg.

***Antioxidant Tablet* - Leiner Health Products**
Each tablet contains: Vitamin E (d-Alpha Tocopherol Acid Succinate and dl-Alpha Tocopheryl Acetate) 200 IU • Vitamin C (Ascorbic Acid) 250 mg • Selenium 70 mcg • Lutein 0.5 mg • Pine bark extract (Pycnogenol brand) 1 mg. Inactive Ingredients: Calcium Carbonate, Gelatin, Cellulose, Maltodextrin, Crospovidone, Croscarmellose Sodium, Silicon Dioxide, Spinach, Magnesium Stearate, Tricalcium Phosphate, Starch, Dicalcium Phosphate, Hydroxypropyl Methylcellulose, Pharmaceutical Glaze, Vegetable Oil, Ethylcellulose, Hydroxypropyl Cellulose, Sorbitol, Polysorbate 80, Ascorbyl Palmitate, Sodium Selenate, Polyethylene Glycol, Tocopherols, Zeaxanthin.

***AntioxidEnz* - Enzymes, Inc.**
Each capsule contains: Vitamin A (from dualiella algae) 3000 IU • Vitamin C (from acerola cherries extract) 50 mg • Vitamin E (from d-alpha tocopheryl acid succinate) 100 IU • Zinc (from zinc citrate) 7.5 mg • Selenium (from kelp) 30 mcg • n-zimes Proprietary Blend 166 mg: pHysioprotease, Catalase • Proprietary Blend 130 mg: Turmeric root extract, Quercetin, Green Tea leaf extract, Lycopenes, Grape Seed extract, Bilberry fruit extract, Alpha-Lipoic Acid, Lutein. Other Ingredients: Cellulose, Water.

***AntioxidEnz* - Advanced Formula**
Each vegetarian capsule contains: Vitamin A (from dunaliella algae) 3000 IU • Vitamin C (from acerola cherries extract) 50 mg • Vitamin E (from d-alpha tocopheryl acid succinate) 100 IU • Zinc (from zinc citrate) 7.5 mg • Selenium (from kelp) 30 mcg • Enzyme Blend 166 mg: pHysioProtease, Catalase • Proprietary Blend 130 mg: Turmeric root extract, Quercetin, Green Tea leaf extract, Lycopenes, Grape seed extract, Bilberry fruit extract, Alpha-Lipoic Acid, Lutein. Other Ingredients: Vegetarian Capsule (cellulose, water).

***AntiSpasmodic* - Dial Herbs**
Scullcap • Skunk Cabbage • Black Cohosh • Myrrh • Lobelia • Cayenne

***Anti-Stress* - Oasis Wellness Network**
Each tablet contains: Ashwagandha root extract 150 mg • MaxCell Proprietary Blend 125 mg: Zisyphus Jujube, Aloe Vera gel, Piper Nigrum, Glycyrrhiza Glabra • Gotu Kola extract (whole plant) 100 mg • Taurine 100 mg • Jujube seed extract (zisyphus spinosa) 100 mg • Kava Kava root extract 50 mg. Other Ingredients: Calcium Sulfate, Stearic Acid, Cellulose, Silica, Magnesium Stearate.

Anxiety Control - Pain & Stress Center
Four capsules contain: GABA 800 mg • Glycine 200 mg • Glutamine 280 mg • Magnesium 200 mg • Passion Flower 300 mg • Primula officinalis 300 mg • Vitamin B6 20 mg.

Anxiety-X - Olympian Labs
Two capsules contain: GABA (gamma aminobutyric acid) 150 mg • Niacinamide 150 mg • L-Tyrosine 40 mg • Glycine 40 mg • L-Glutamine 40 mg • Inositol 150 mg • Kava Kava 20 mg • Motherwort 20 mg • Wintergreen 30 mg.

Aorta-Glycan - Enzymatic Therapy
Each capsule contains: Aorta-Glycan (Mesoglycan) 50 mg, a mixture of highly-purified bovine-derived glycosaminoglycans (GAGs) naturally present in the aorta including: Dermatan Sulfate, Heparan Sulfate, Hyaluronic Acid, Chondroitin Sulfate, & related Hexosaminoglycans.
See Editor's Note No. 15, page 2055.

Aphrodesia - Life Extension
Each tablet contains: Yohimbine 25 mg • Kelp 10 mg • Zinc Orotate 120 mg • Niacin 20 mg • Selenium 200 mcg • Siberian Ginseng 60 mg • Damiana leaf 20 mg • Bee Pollen 75 mg • Lecithin 25 mg • L-Lysine 20 mg • Calcium Gluconate 90 mg • Pituitary Gland extract 35 mg.

APM 60 - Double-Shot Chocolate - Nutripeak
Each packet contains: Protein 60 g • Vitamin A (Retinyl Palmitate and Beta Carotene) 4500 IU • Vitamin C (Ascorbic Acid) 60 mg • Vitamin D (Cholecalciferol) 240 IU • Vitamin E (dl-Tocopheryl Acetate) 45 IU • Vitamin K (Phytonadione) 40 mcg • Thiamin (Vitamin B1) 0.9 mcg • Riboflavin (Vitamin B2) 1 mg • Niacin (Niacinamide) 20 mg • Vitamin B-6 (Pyridoxine Hydrochloride) 1 mg • Folic Acid 400 mcg • Vitamin B-12 (Cyanocobalamin) 3 mcg • Biotin 180 mcg • Pantothenic Acid (Calcium D-Pantothenate) 4 mg • Calcium Lactate 2 g • Iron (Ferrous Fumarate) 7.2 mg • Phosphorus (Tricalcium Phosphate and Dicalcium Phosphate) 1.3 mg • Iodine (Potassium Iodide) 52 mg • Magnesium (Trimagnesium Phosphate and Magnesium Oxide) 440 mg • Zinc Oxide 5.2 mg • Selenium (Sodium Molybdate) 31 mcg • Copper (Cupric Sulfate) 0.7 mg • Manganese Sulfate 1 mg • Chromium 48 mcg • Molybdenum (Sodium Molybdate) 60 mcg • Sodium 340 mcg • Potassium Chloride and Citrate 1 g • ARS Proprietary Blend: L-Glutamine, Potassium Bicarbonate, Monosodium Orthophosphate, Sodium Citrate Dihydrate, L-Carnosine, Trans-Ferulic Acid 1.6 g • TNA Proprietary Blend: DL-Phenylalanine, L-Tyrosine, Taurine 800 mg • Proulin Proprietary Blend: Myo-Inositol, Alpha-Lipoic Acid, Vanadium, Chromium 201 mg. Other Ingredients: Metamyosyn Protein Blend: Milk Protein Concentrate, Calcium Sodium Caseinate, Whey Protein Concentrate, Dried Egg Albumen, Whey Protein Isolate, Bovine lactoferrin; Cocoa (processed with alkali); Xanthan Gum; Sodium Carboxymethylcellulose; Maltodextrin; Sucralose; Acesulfame Potassium; Natural and Artificial Flavors.

Appetite Control - The Council On Natural Health
Two tablets contain: Vitamin C (as ascorbic acid) 50 mg • Chromium (as patented chromium dinicotinate glycinate) 200 mcg • Garcinia Cambogia fruit extract (50% [-] hydroxycitric acid) 250 mg • Chitosan 500 mg • 5-HTP (from griffonia simplicifolia seed extract) 12.5 mg • Capsicum (cayenne) Pepper 30 mg • Ginger root 15 mg. Other Ingredients: Dicalcium Phosphate, Microcrystalline Cellulose, Croscarmellose Sodium, Stearic Acid, Magnesium Stearate, Silica, Pharmaceutical Glaze.

Apple Cider Vinegar - American Health
Two tablets contain: Apple Cider Vinegar (equivalent to pure cider vinegar 1 tsp) 600 mg. Other Ingredients: Dicalcium Phosphate, Cellulose (plant origin), Vegetable Stearic Acid, Croscarmellose, Silica, Vegetable Magnesium Stearate.

Apple Cider Vinegar - Chroma Slim
Two caplets contain: Vitamin B6 (as pyridoxine HCl) 20 mg • Calcium 70 mg • Chromium (as chromium polynicotinate) 120 mcg • Apple Cider Vinegar Complex 600 mg • Grapefruit powder 400 mg • Premium Herbal Blend 300 mg: Buchu leaf extract, Parsley leaf/stem, Juniper berry, Uva-Ursi leaf, Dandelion root • Soy Lecithin 100 mg. Other Ingredients: Microcrystalline Cellulose, Maltodextrin, Dicalcium Phosphate, Crospovidone, Modified Food Starch, Hydroxypropyl Methylcellulose, Calcium Silicate, Silica, Magnesium Stearate, PEG.

Apple Cider Vinegar - Natural Brand
Two tablets contain: Apple Cider Vinegar 600 mg • Cayenne Pepper fruit powder (capsicum frutescens) 100 mg • Ginger root powder (zingiberis officinale) 100 mg • Garcinia Cambogia fruit extract (50% hydroxycitric acid 50 mg) 100 mg. Other Ingredients: Cellulose, Dicalcium Phosphate.

Apple Cider Vinegar - Only Natural, Inc.
Each capsule contains: Apple Cider Vinegar 500 mg.

Apple Cider Vinegar - Source Naturals
Each tablet contains: Apple Cider Vinegar (concentrated to 35% acetic acid) 500 mg. Other Ingredients: Sorbitol, Stearic Acid, Modified Cellulose Gum, Colloidal Silicon Dioxide, Magnesium Stearate.

Apple Cider Vinegar 500 mg - Natural Factors
Each caplet contains: Apple Cider Vinegar 500 mg. Other Ingredients: Gelatin Capsule (gelatin, purified water), Maltodextrin, Food Starch, Magnesium Stearate (vegetable grade).

Apple Cider Vinegar Plus - Only Natural, Inc.
Each capsule contains: Apple Cider Vinegar 500 mg • Cayenne Pepper 100 mg • Grapefruit rind 100 mg.

Apple Cinnamon Celebration - Revival - Physicians Laboratories
Each bar contains: Certified Isoflavone 160 mg. Other Ingredients: Soy Protein Isolate, Rice Flour, Malt, Salt, Corn Syrup, Sugar, Corn Starch, Water, Gelatin, Artificial Flavoring, Dried Apples, Glycerin, Sunflower Oil, Natural Flavors, Soy Lecithin, Ground Cinnamon.

Appleheart Chondroitin Sulfate - Appleheart
Each capsule contains: Chondroitin Sulfate 300 mg. Other Ingredients: Cellulose, Gelatin, Vegetable Stearate.
See Editor's Note No. 15, page 2055.

Appleheart Echinacea - Appleheart
Each capsule contains: standarized Echinacea Angustifolia and Echinacea Purpurea 250 mg • Rice Protein • Gelatin • Cellulose • Vegetable Stearate.

Appleheart Glucosamine Sulfate - Appleheart
Each capsule contains: Glucosamine Sulfate (from Glucosamine Sulfate Potassium) 500 mg • Potassium 65 mg. Other Ingredients: Gelatin, Cellulose, Vegetable Stearate.

Appleheart Melatonin - Appleheart
Each capsule contains: Melatonin 3mg.
See Editor's Note No. 16 and No. 21, pages 2055 and 2056.

Appleheart Saw Palmetto - Appleheart
Each capsule contains: Saw Palmetto berry 160 mg • Olive Oil • Water • Gelatin.

Appleheart St. John's Wort - Appleheart
Each capsule contains: standardized St. John's Wort 250 mg • Gelatin • Rice Protein • Cellulose • Magnesium Stearate (Vegetable Source).

Apple-Honey Lactobacillus Acidophilus - Nature's Life
Unfiltered Apple juice • Purified Water • Pasteurized Honey • Soy Protein Isolate • Lactobacillus Acidophilus Culture.

AppSignal - Pharmanex
Two wafers contain: Sucrose • Cocoa Powder • Microcrystalline Cellulose • Protein Complex (Hydrolyzed Soy Protein, Soy Protein Isolate, Egg Albumin) • L-Tyrosine • AbsorbaLean Fiber Complex:

Apple Pectin, Fructooligosaccharides, Locust Bean Gum, Carrageenan, Microcrystalline Cellulose • Stearic Acid • Lecithin Powder • Natural and Artificial Flavors • Sorbitol • L-Histidine Hydrochloride • Pyridoxine Hydrochloride • Magnesium Stearate • Folic Acid.

Aqua Ban **-** Thompson Medical Co.
Each tablet contains: Active Ingredient: Pamabrom 50 mg (Diuretic). Other Ingredients: Carnauba Wax • Croscarmellose Sodium • FD&C Blue No. 1 Aluminum Lake • Hydroxypropyl Methylcellulose • Lactose • Magnesium Stearate • Microcrystalline Cellulose • Polyethylene Glycol • Polysorbate 80 • Starch • Titanium Dioxide.

Aqua Greens **-** Futurebiotics
Twelve tablets contain: Chlorella 1000 mg • Spirulina 2500 mg • Klamath Blue/Green Algae 500 mg • Kelp 250 mg • D. Salina 100 mg.

AquaActin **-** Nature's Plus
Two capsules contain: Chinese Green Tea [(Camellia sinensis leaf) decaffeinated, standardized 50% Polyphenols] 250 mg • Horsetail [(Equisetum arvense stem) standardized 10% Silicic Acid, 7% Silica] 150 mg • Uva Ursi [(Arctostaphylos uva-ursi leaf) standardized 20-25% Arbutin] 100 mg • Vitamin B6 (Pyridoxine HCl) 75 mg • Goldenseal [(Hydrastis canadensis root & rhizome) standardized 10% Alkaloids, 5% Hydrastine] 50 mg • Artichoke [(Cynara scolymus flower) standardized 2.5-5% Caffeylquinic Acids] 50 mg.

Aqua-Action **-** Nature's Plus
Each capsule contains: Buchu leaves 125 mg • Couchgrass 100 mg • Juniper berries 100 mg • Parsley leaves 100 mg • Corn Silk 75 mg • Uva Ursi leaves 50 mg • Celery seed 50 mg.

Aqua-Flow **-** Enzymatic Therapy
Two capsules contain: Potassium Citrate 200 mg • Magnesium (Oxide) 50 mg • Vitamin B6 (Pyridoxine HCL) 25 mg • Other Ingredients: Bearberry extract (Uva Ursi) contains 10% Arbutin 200 mg • Lespedeza extract (Lespedeza capitatae) contains 8% Flavonoids 100 mg • Boldo extract (Peumus boldo) contains 1.52% essential oils 100 mg • Goldenrod extract (Solidago virgaurea) contains 5% flavonoids 100 mg.

Aqua-Lim **-** Aspen Group, Inc.
Each tablet contains: Buchu leaves 70 mg • Couch Grass 70 mg • Hydrangea root 35 mg • Corn Silk 35 mg • Uva Ursi 10 mg • Hypothalamus 30 mg • Raw Kidney concentrate 30 mg • Vitamin B6 16 mg • Bladder Wrack 100 mg • Magnesium: Protein Chelated 50 mg.
See Editor's Note No. 14, page 2055.

Aquatone **-** PharmAssure
Two tablets contain: Vitamin B6 (as Pyridoxine Hydrochloride) 15 mg • Magnesium (as Magnesium Gluconate) 25 mg • Potassium (as Potassium Gluconate) 99 mg • Uva Ursi Extract (Arctostaphylos uva ursi;20% Arbutin=150 mg) 750 mg. Other Ingredients: Cellulose, Calcium Carbonate.

Arbu-Tone **-** PhytoPharmica
Two capsules contain: Boldo leaf 2:1 extract (peumus boldus) 100 mg • Dandelion root 4:1 extract (taraxacum officinale) 100 mg • Early Goldenrold aerial part extract (solidago serotina, standardized to contain 5% flavonoids) 100 mg • Magnesium (as magnesium oxide) 50 mg • Potassium (as potassium citrate) 70 mg • Uva-Ursi leaf extract (arctostaphylos uva-ursi, standardized to contain 20% arbutin) 200 mg • Vitamin B6 (as pyridoxine HCl) 25 mg.

Arctic Root **-** Swedish Herbal Institute
Each tablet contains: Rhodiola Rosea extract SHI-Rr5 180 mg.

A-Retic **-** Douglas Laboratories
Each tablet contains: Proprietary Blend 480 mg: Juniper berry dried powder, Buchu leaves, Uva-Ursi, Cubeb, Asparagus.

Arginine **-** Vital Nutrients
Each capsule contains: Arginine (l-form, from pure 100% l-arginine base) 750 mg.

Arginine & Ornithine **-** Olympian Labs
Each capsule contains: L-Arginine 500 mg • L-Ornithine 250 mg.

Arginine + Ornithine **-** Jarrow Formulas
Each capsule contains: L-Arginine 500 mg • L-Ornithine (from 319 mg l-ornithine hydrochloride) 250 mg. Inactive Ingredients: Cellulose, Magnesium Stearate, Gelatin.

Arginine 1000 - GNC A-Z **-** GNC
Each tablet contains: L-Arginine 1000 mg. Other Ingredients: Cellulose.

Arginine Plus with ActiFolate 120T **-** Metagenics
Two tablets contain: Folate (as folic acid, l-5-methyl tetrahydrofolate, 5-formyl tetrahydrofolate) 400 mcg • L-Arginine 1500 mg • L-Glycine 10 mg.

Arginine Pyroglutamate/Lysine **-** Ultimate Nutrition
Each capsule contains: L-Arginine Pyroglutamate 500 mg • L-Lysine 250 mg.

Arginine Ultra **-** FreeLife International
Two caplets contain: Calcium as Calcium carbonate and Calcium hydrogen phosphate 100 mg • L-Arginine Hydrochloride 1500 mg. Other Ingredients: Galactomannan, Cellulose, Fractionated Vegetable oil, Fruit Pectin, Vita-Coat: vegetable resin, alpha-lipoic acid.

Arginine-Ornithine 1500 **-** Puritan's Pride
Two capsules contain: L-Arginine 1000 mg • L-Ornithine 500 mg • Chromium picolinate 6.2 mcg.

ArginMax for Female Sexual Fitness **-** The Daily Wellness Company
Six tablets contain: Vitamin A (as palmitate) 5000 IU • Vitamin C (as ascorbic acid) 60 mg • Vitamin E (as d-alpha-tocopherol) 30 IU • Thaimin (B1, as thiamin mononitrate) 1.7 mg • Riboflavin (B2) 1.7 mg • Niacin (B3, as niacinamide) 20 mg • Vitamin B6 (as pyridoxine hydrochloride) 2 mg • Folate, Folic Acid, Folacin (as folic acid) 400 mcg • Vitamin B12 (as cyanocobalamin) 6 mcg • Biotin 300 mcg • Pantothenic Acid (as calcium d-pantothenate) 10 mg • Calcium (as carbonate) 500 mg • Iron (as gluconate) 9 mg • Zinc (as gluconate) 7.5 mg • Proprietary Blend: L-Arginine 2500 mg, Korean Ginseng root extract (panax ginseng, root/aerial parts) 100 mg, Ginkgo Biloba leaf extract 50 mg • Damiana leaf (turnera aphrodisiaca) leaf 50 mg. Other Ingredients: Microcrystalline Cellulose, Hydroxypropyl Methylcellulose, Pharmaceutical Glaze, Silica, Titanium Dioxide (color), Magnesium Stearate, PEG, Polysorbate 80.

ArginMax for Men **-** The Daily Wellness Company
Six capsules contain: L-Arginine 3000 mg •American Ginseng 100 mg • Korean Ginseng 100 mg • Ginkgo Biloba 50 mg •Vitamin A 5000 IU •Vitamin C 60 mg •Vitamin E 30 IU •Thiamin 1.5 mg •Riboflavin 1.7 mg • Niacin 20 mg •Vitamin B6 2 mg • Folate 400 mcg •Vitamin B12 6 mcg • Biotin 300 mcg •Pantothenic Acid 10 mg • Calcium 500 mg • Iron 9 mg • Zinc 7.5 mg.

Arko-Lesterol **-** Arkopharma
Each capsule contains: Gugulon (commiphora mukul) 170 mg • Chrysanthellum (chrysanthellum americanum) 170 mg.

Arnica Gel **-** Jamieson
Contains: Arnica Montana Flowers Tincture 1.5% w/w (European Arnica Equivalent to 7.5% of a 20% NFXI).

Arnica Oil **-** Blessed Herbs
Arnica flower & leaf • Organic Cold-Pressed Olive oil.

ArnicAid **-** Hyland's
Three tablets contain: Arnica Montana 30X • Hypericum Perfoliatum 6X • Ruta Graveolens 6X • Ledum Palustre 6X • Bellis Perennis 6X.

Base: Lactose N.F.
See Editor's Note No. 1, page 2053.

ArniSport **-** Hyland's
Three tablets contain: Arnica Montana 30X • Hypericum Perfoliatum 6X • Ruta Graveolens 6X • Ledum Palustre 6X • Bellis Perennis 6X • Hyland's Bioplasma: Calcarea Fluorica 6X, Calcarea Phosphorica 3X, Calcarea Sulphurica 3X, Ferrum Phosphoricum 3X, Kali Muriaticum 3X, Kali Phosphoricum 3X, Kali Sulphuricum 3X, Magnesia Phosphorica 3X, Natrum Nuriaticum 6X, Natrum Phosphoricum 3X, Natrum Sulphuricum 3X, Silicea 6X. Base: Lactose N.F.
See Editor's Note No. 1, page 2053.

Aromadex **-** VPX Sports
Each 8 cc serving contains: 3;6; 17-Androstenetrione 100 mg • 4-Androsten-4-ol-3Beta-dione 50 mg. Other Ingredients: Lipoject Technologies Proprietary Liposomal Matrix, Vegetable Gum, Sucralose, Potassium Sorbate, Artificial Flavors, Natural Colors.

Aromasaurus Rex **-** Abra Therapeutics
Sodium Borate • Sodium Carbonate • Vegetable Glycerin • Sodium Sesquicarbonate • Sodium Laurel Sulfoacetate • Sweet Almond oil • Wheatgerm oil • Hop flower extract • Valerian root extract • Essential oils of Sweet Orange, Tangerine, Lime, Lavender, Cedarwood.

ArteClear **-** Pacific BioLogic
Rhubarb rhizome • Salvia root • Sea Weed • Polygonum root • Polygonatum rhizome • Cassia seeds • Aucklandia root • Hawthorn fruit • Pseudoginseng root.

Artemisinin **-** EcoNugenics
Each capsule contains: Artemisinin 100 mg. Other Ingredients: Gelatin, Maltodextrin, Magnesium Stearate.

Arth Rx **-** Symmetry
Each packet contains: Glucosamine • Chondroitin Sulfate • Hydrolyzed gelatin • Boswellia • Curcumin • Bilberry • Grape Seed extract • Grape Skin extract • Tumeric extract.
See Editor's Note No. 15, page 2055.

Arth-9 **-** Rx Vitamins
Four capsules contain: Glucosamine Sulfate (Aminomonosaccharide) 1000 mg • Vitamin C (Ascorbic Acid) 250 mg • Bromelain 250 mg • Calcium (Citrate) 250 mg • Boswellin 250 mg • Curcumin 100 mg • Zinc (L-Monomethionine) 30 mg • Chondroitin Sulfate A (CSA) 25 mg • Copper (Glycinate) 2 mg.
See Editor's Note No. 15, page 2055.

Artho-Health Formula **-** Youngevity
Cosamin (Glucosamine Sulfate 200 mg, Chondroitin Sulfate 160 mg) • Vitamin C 15 mg • Manganese 500 mcg • Vilcabamba Mineral Essence: Potassium, Calcium, Magnesium, Zinc, Chromium, Selenium, Iron, Copper, Molybdenum, Vanadium, Iodine, Cobalt, Manganese.
See Editor's Note No. 15, page 2055.

Artho-Therapy **-** PhytoPharmica
Each tablet contains: Capsaicin 0.025%. Other Ingredients: Purified water, Alcohol, Glycerin, Triethanolamine, Escin (Horse chestnut extract), Glory Lily, Methylparaben, Lavender essential oil.
See Editor's Note No. 21, page 2056.

Arthred brand **-** Degussa Food Ingredients/BL BioActives
Hydrolyzed Collagen.
See Editor's Note No. 44, page 2058.

Arthred Collagen Formula **-** NutriCology
Two level scoops (approx. 10.5 g) contain: Hydrolyzed Collagen 10.5 g.
See Editor's Note No. 14, page 2055.

Arthred-G - Richardson Labs **-** Rexall - Sundown
Each rounded scoop contains: Arthred (enzymatically hydrolyzed collagen protein) 7 g • Glucosamine & Chondroitin Complex: Glucosamine HCl, Glucosamine Sulfate (potassium salt, sodium free), Chondroitin Sulfate.
See Editor's Note No. 15, page 2055.

Arth-Rid Us **-** The Herbalist
Devil's Claw root bark • Yucca root • Yerba Mansa root • Black Cohosh root • Wild Yam root.

Arthri-Gesic Liquid Glucosamine **-** Quantum, Inc.
Each 10 mL serving contains: Glucosamine HCl 500 mg • White Willow Bark extract 50 mg • Devil's Claw extract 25 mg • Curcumin extract 500 mcg. Other Ingredients: Glycerin, Water, Potassium Sorbate, Stevia, Natural Beet Color, Tangerine Oil.

Arthrimin Glucosamine Sulfate **-** Jamieson
Each capsule contains: Glucosamine Sulfate (from Potassium Chloride Complex) 500 mg.

Arthrimin GS - Zinaxin **-** Jamieson
Each capsule contains: Ginger Extract (Zinaxin Ev. Ext 77 standardized equivalent to 3500 dried ginger) 255 mg.

Arthrimin GS Glucosamine Sulfate 500 mg **-** Jamieson
Each capsule contains: Glucosamine Sulfate (from Potassium Chloride Complex) 500 mg. Other Ingredients: Peppermint Leaf, and Betaine Hydrochloride.

Arthrimin Joints + Bones - Glucosamine Chondroitin Complex **-** Jamieson
Each capsule contains: Glucosamine HCl 250 mg • Chondroitin Sulfate 200 mg.
See Editor's Note No. 15, page 2055.

Arthrimin Joints + Bones - Glucosamine MSM Complex **-** Jamieson
Each capsule contains: Glucosamine HCl 333 mg • MSM (Methylsulfonylmethane) 250 mg • Turmeric Extract 25 mg.
See Editor's Note No. 15, page 2055.

Arthrimin Joints + Bones - Glucosamine/Chondroitin/ MSM/ Hyaluronic Acid - Effervescent Drink Crystals Complex **-** Jamieson
Each pouch contains: Glucosamine Complex (Derived from Sulfate and HCl) 1500 mg • Hyaluronic Acid (Derived from Glucosamine Complex) 300 mg • Chondroitin Sulfate 1200 mg • MSM (Methylsulfonylmethane) 1000 mg.
See Editor's Note No. 15, page 2055.

Arthrimin Joints + Bones - MSM 1000 mg **-** Jamieson
Each caplet contains: MSM (methylsulfonylmethane) 1000 mg.

ArthritiCare **-** Aarisse Health Care
CMO (cis-9-cetylmyristoleate) • Shea Butter • Speedwell • Glucosamine sulfate • Chondroitin sulfate • MSM (methyl-sulfonylmethane) • Pregnenolone • Comfrey • Ginger • Primrose Oil • Dong Quai • Citric Acid • Vitamin A • Vitamin E • Panthenol (vitamin B5) • Glycerine • Allantoin.
See Editor's Note No. 15, page 2055.

Arthritis Guardian **-** Clinician's Choice
Three tablets contain: Shark Cartilage 1500 mg • Glucosamine Sulfate 450 mg • Linoleic Acid, Gamma Linolenic Acid (sunflower oil, borage oil) 150 mg • Boswellia 30 mg • Cayenne Fruit 30 mg • Glycosaminoglycan 30 mg • White Willow Bark 30 mg • Proprietary blend: Carrot Powder, Citrus Bioflavonoids Complex, Grape Powder 9 mg.

arthritis pain **-** nelsons - Nelson Bach USA Ltd.
Active Ingredients: Berber vulg 30c HPUS • Calc fluor 30c HPUS • Causticum 30c HPUS • Dulcamara 30c HPUS • Rhus tox 30c HPUS • Bryonia 30c HPUS • Rhododendron 30c HPUS • Nux vom 30c HPUS • Actaea 30c HPUS • Pulsatilla 30c HPUS. Inactive Ingredients: Lactose, Sucrose.
See Editor's Note No. 1, page 2053.

Arthritis Pain Formula **-** Hyland's
Two tablets contain: Arnica Montana 6X • Cimicifuga Racemosa 3X • Guaiacum 3X • Bryonia 3X • Rhus Toxicodendron 6X. Base: Lactose USP.
See Editor's Note No. 1, page 2053.

Arthritis Relief **-** Dr. Mike's Vitamins
Four vegetarian capsules contain: Glucosamine Sulfate Potassium (from shellfish) 1500 mg • Methylsulfonylmethane (MSM, natural organic sulfur compound) 750 mg • Shark Cartilage 150 mg • Ginger root 120 mg • Curcumin (turmeric root extract) 115 mg. Other Ingredients: Cellulose (plant derivative), Magnesium Stearate (vegetable oil derivative).

Arthritis Remedy **-** PhytoPharmica
Each tablespoon contains: Aurum muriaticum natronatum 8x • Mercurius corrosivus 6x •Silicea 6x • Sulphur 4x • Bryonia 3x • Colchicum 3x • Natrum salicylicum 3x • Viscum album 3x • Dulcamara 2x • Kalium iodatum 2x •Betula 1x •Rubia tinctorum 1x. In a base of 20% USP alcohol by volume.
See Editor's Note No. 1 and No. 21, pages 2053 and 2056.

Arthro Herbal-Rx **-** Alternecare Health Products
Two capsules contain: Chondroitin Sulfate (Bovine Cartilage) 150 mg • Glucosamine Sulfate 350 mg • Cat's Claw 25 mg • Quercetin 50 mg • Bromelain 50 mg • Alfalfa 25 mg • Devil's Claw 10 mg • Yucca 20 mg • Pycnogenol 5 mg • Grape seed 5 mg • Suma 25 mg • Siberian Ginseng 25 mg • Lipoic Acid 25 mg.
See Editor's Note No. 15, page 2055.

Arthro-7 **-** Gero Vita International
Each capsule contains: Chicken Collagen type II 400 mg • Methylsulfonylmethane (MSM) 50 mg • Cetyl Myristoleate (CMO) 50 mg • Bromelain (2400 GDU) 15 mg • Curcuma Longa Extract (root, 95% Curcumin) • Vitamin C (as Ascorbic Acid) 70 mg • Lipase (30 USP units) 50 mg.
See Editor's Note No. 14, page 2055.

Arthro-7 Topical Gel **-** Gero Vita International
Active Ingredient: 1.26% Menthol. Other Ingredients: Purified Water, Methylsulfonylmethane (MSM), Glycerine, Hyaluronic Acid, Carbomer, Ginger root extract (10% total gingerols), Cetyl Myristoleate (CMO), Triethanolamine, Polysorbate 20, Methylparaben, FD&C Blue #1.

ArthroColl brand **-** Cyvex Nutrition, Inc.
Chicken Collagen Type II.
See Editor's Note No. 44, page 2058.

Arthro-Glucosamine **-** Nutri-Quest Rx
Each tablet supples: Glucosamine Sulfate 100 mg • N-Acetyl Glucosamine 50 mg • L-Glutathione 2 mg • N-Acetyl Cysteine 5 mg • L-Cysteine 50 mg • L-Glutamic Acid 50 mg • L-Glycine 50 mg • L-Taurine 25 mg • Vitamin C 50 mg • Vitamin E (Succinate) 25 IU • Pantothenic Acid 50 mg • Soluble Trachea (16% Chondroitin Sulfate-A) 25 mg • Silymarin 5 mg • Milk Thistle 100 mg • Green Lipped Mussel 25 mg (natural source of Mucopolysaccharides & Superoxide Dismutase).
See Editor's Note No. 15, page 2055.

Arthro-HCP - MET-Rx **-** Rexall - Sundown
Fourteen grams contain: Arthred (Hydrolyzed Collagen Protein) 10 g • Maltodextrin • Glucosamine Hydrochloride & Glucosamine Sulfate 1.5 g.
See Editor's Note No. 21, page 2056.

ArthroPlex **-** Aidan Products, LLC
Each capsule contains: Methylsulfonylmethane 250 mg • Glucosamine Sulfate 325 mg • Chondroitin Sulfate 300 mg • Bromelain (600 GDU) 25 mg. Other Ingredients: Gelatin (capsule), Maltodextrin.
See Editor's Note No. 15, page 2055.

ArthroPro System **-** Life Extension
Four capsules contain: Nettle leaf extract (super-concentrate) 1125 mg • Chondroitin Sulfate 2450 mg • N-Acetyl-D-Glucosamine 500 mg • Glucosamine Sulfate (from shellfish) 500 mg • Nexrutine 750 mg • Ginger (powdered extract, 5% gingerols) 60 mg • Chondroitin Sulfate 1650 mg. Other Ingredients: Gelatin, Water.
See Editor's Note No. 15, page 2055.

Arthro-SYN **-** Douglas Laboratories
Four capsules contain: Vitamin A 2500 IU • Vitamin B1 (thiamin) 40 mg • Vitamin B2 (riboflavin) 20 mg • Niacin / Niacinamide 100 mg • Vitamin B5 (pantothenic acid) 50 mg • Vitamin B6 50 mg • Vitamin C 500 mg • Hesperidin Complex 25 mg • Rutin 25 mg • Bioflavonoids 150 mg • Folic Acid 200 mcg • Vitamin E 100 IU • Choline Bitartrate 20 mg • Inositol 20 mg • PABA (para-aminobenzoic acid) 10 mg • Calcium (citrate complex) 125 mg • Magnesium (aspartate complex) 125 mg • Manganese (sulfate) 100 mg • Zinc (amino acid chelate) 25 mg • Potassium (aspartate complex) 25 mg • Selenomethionine 50 mcg • Copper (sebacate complex) 2 mg • Chromium (GTF) 100 mcg • L-Cystine 75 mg • L-Histidine 25 mg • DL-Phenylalanine 100 mg • Omega-3 Fatty Acids (DHA/EPA) 100 mg • Trypsin 25 mg • Chymotrypsin 25 mcg • Bromelain 150 mcu • Bovine Tracheal Cartilage (BTC) 100 mg • Papain 25 mg • Raw Veal Bone 25 mg • Yucca extract 100 mg.
See Editor's Note No. 14, page 2055.

Arthrovedic **-** Gero Vita International
Two capsules contain: Herbal Proprietary Blend 830 mg: Commiphora Mukul gum extract (24% lipids), Withania Somnifera root extract (0.5% alkaloids), Boswellia Serrate gum extract (basalic acid 4.5%), Cyperus Rotundus tuber extract (0.45% alkaloids), Paederia Foetida leaf extract (0.45% alkaloids), Vitex Negundo leaf extract (0.10% alkaloids), Holarrhena Antidysenterica bark extract (0.10% alkaloids), Smilax China root extract (60% water-soluble extractive), Boerhoavia Diffusa root extract (0.8% alkaloids), Tribulus Terrestris root extract (7% saponins), Apium Graveolens seed extract (60% water-soluble extractive), Sida Cordifolia root extract (50% water-soluble extractive), Trachyspermum Ammi fruit extract (60% water-soluble extractive), Trigonella Foenum-Graecum seed extract (10% saponins) • Proprietary Phytominerals Blend 200 mg. Other Ingredients: Dicalcium Phosphate, Silicon Dioxide, Vegetable Magnesium Stearate, Gelatin, ACF 223.
See Editor's Note No. 39, page 2058.

Arth-Support Formula **-** Douglas Laboratories
Four tablets contain: Proprietary Blend 500 mg: Turmeric (curcuma longa), Pancreatin 8X (providing protease, amylase, lipase activity), Licorice (glycyrrhiza glabra), Quercetin, Betaine HCl / Glutamic Acid HCl, Shark Cartilage powder, Glucosamine Sulfate, Pepsin, Bromelain (minimum 2000 m.c.u.), SOD / Glutathione Peroxidase (young wheat sprouts), Feverfew, Devil's Claw, Proanthocyanidins (red wine grapes), Ginseng (panax), Skullcap, N-Acetyl-L-Cysteine / L-Cysteine HCl, L-Methionine • Beta-Carotene (vitamin A activity) 15,000 IU • Vitamin A (palmitate, water dispersible) 5000 IU • Vitamin D (D3) 50 IU • Vitamin E (succinate) 200 IU • Vitamin C (ascorbic acid) 1000 mg • Vitamin B1 (thiamine HCl) 50 mg • Vitamin B2 (riboflavin) 25 mg • Niacin 20 mg • Niacinamide 100 mg • Pantothenic Acid (as d-calcium pantothenate) 150 mg • Vitamin B6 (as pyridoxine HCl/pyridoxal-5-phosphate complex) 25 mg • Vitamin B12 100 mcg • Folic Acid 800 mcg • Biotin 300 mcg • Choline (from choline citrate/bitartrate) 20 mg • Inositol 25 mg • Citrus Bioflavonoid Complex 100 mg • PABA (para-aminobenzoic acid) 300 mg • Calcium (citrate/ascorbate complex) 300 mg • Magnesium (aspartate/ascorbate complex) 300 mg • Potassium (aspartate complex) 75 mg • Zinc (aspartate complex) 50 mg • Copper (amino acid chelate) 2 mg • Manganese (aspartate complex) 15 mg • Chromium GTF (organically bound with GTF activity-low allergenicity) 200 mcg • Selenium (organic selenium in Krebs Cycle (citrate, fumarate, malate, glutarate, succinate complex) and kelp) 300 mcg • Molybdenum (Krebs) 50 mcg • Vanadium (Krebs) 25 mcg • Boron (aspartate/citrate complex) 1 mg • Trace Elements (sea vegetation) 100 mg.

Some Brand Name Natural Products - What they Contain

www.NaturalDatabase.com contains MANY more listings than appear here.

BRAND NAMES

Arthur - Children's Chewable Multivitamins - Jamieson
Each tablet contains: Vitamin A 5000 IU • Vitamin D (as Vitamin D3) 3 400 IU • Vitamin E 10 IU • Vitamin C 40 mg • Vitamin B1 1.5 mg • Vitamin B2 1.7 mg • Niacinamide 20 mg • Pantothenic Acid 10 mg • Vitamin B6 2 mg • Vitamin B12 4 mcg • Folic Acid 0.1 mg • Biotin 30 mcg • Calcium 162 mg • Phosphorus 125 mg • Copper 1 mg • Iodine 0.15. Blended in a base of concentrated fruits and vegetables derived from: Tomato, Broccoli, Carrot, Orange Fiber, Cranberry, and Lemon Bioflavonoids.

Artichoke - Arkopharma
Each capsule contains: Artichoke (cynara scolymus) 400 mg.

Artichoke Extract - PhytoPharmica
Two capsules contain: Artichoke (Cynara scolymus leaf extract 5:1) 320 mg.

Artichoke Extract - Nature's Way
Two capsules contain: Artichoke dried extract 600 mg • Milk Thistle seed 300 mg. Other Ingredients: Gelatin, Magnesium stearate, Maltodextrin, Silica.

As-Comp - Enzymatic Therapy
Each capsule contains: Ephedrine from Ma Huang extract (Ephedra sinensis) 200 mg] 12 mg. Other Ingredients: Ginger root extract 6.5:1 (Zingiber officinale) 65 mg • Licorice root extract (Glycyrrhiza glabra) standardized to contain 5% Glycyrrhizic acid) 50 mg • Marshmallow root extract 4:1 (Althaea officinalis) (Mucilage content 30-40%) 50 mg • Sundew Herb extract 4:1 (Drosera rotundifolia) 40 mg • Euphorbia Herb extract 4:1 (Euphorbia hirta) 40 mg • Senega root extract 4:1 (Polygala senega) 40 mg • Goldenseal root extract (Hydrastis canadensis) standardized to contain 5% total Alkaloids including Berberine, Hydrastine & Canadine 20 mg.
See Editor's Note No. 21 and No. 30, page 2056.

Ascorbate-C - Atrium Inc.
Each teaspoon (5 gm) contains: Vitamin C (Calcium Ascorbate) 2000 mg • Rose Hips 1450 mg • Acerola 1000 mg • Lemon Bioflavonoids 500 mg • Rutin 25 mg • Hesperidin 25 mg • Calcium (from Calcium Ascorbate) 230 mg.

Ascorbplex 1,000 (Buffered) - Douglas Laboratories
Each tablet contains: Vitamin C (ascorbates) 1000 mg • Calcium 90 mg • Magnesium 125 mcg • Potassium 60 mg • Pectin 100 mg • Bioflavonoid complex 100 mg.

Ascorbyl Palmitate (500 mg) - Now
Each capsule contains: Vitamin C (from ascorbyl palmitate) 200 mg • Ascorbyl Palmitate 500 mg. Other Ingredients: Cellulose (vegetable source), Magnesium Stearate (vegetable source), Silica.

Asotas Plus for HER - Unknown
Each two tablets contain: Niacin (as niacinamide) 10 mg • Dong Quai (1% extract) 200 mg • Avena Sativa (4:1 extract) 200 mg •Yohimbe (2% extract) 100 mg • Sarsaparilla (root) 600 mg • Siberian Ginseng (8% extract) 300 mg • Panax Ginseng (10% extract) 300 mg • Maca (herb powder) 100 mg •Damiana (4:1 extract) 100 mg • Black Cohosh (2.5% extract) 40 mg • False Unicorn (root) 40 mg • Asparagus 60 mg • Artichoke 40 mg • Wild Yam (6% extract) 50 mg. Other Ingredients: Magnesium Stearate, Stearic Acid, Microcrystalline Cellulose.

Asotas Plus for HIM - Unknown
Each two tablets contain: Niacin (as niacinamide) 10 mg • Yohimbe bark (as 2% extract) 250 mg • Avena Sativa (as 10:1 extract) 150 mg • Androstenedione 100 mg • Saw Palmetto (as 4:1 extract) 100 mg • Guarana (as 22% extract) 300 mg • Taurine (as l-taurine HCl) 200 mg • Siberian Ginseng (as 40% extract) 30 mg • Panax Ginseng (as 40% extract) 30 mg • Tribulus Terrestris (as 40% extract) 50 mg •Rhodiola Rosea (as extract) 10 mg • Wild Yam (as 10:1 extract) 250 mg • Maca (as powder) 100 mg • Arginine (as l-arginine HCl) 100 mg. Other Ingredients: Di-calcium Phosphate, Magnesium Stearate, Stearic Acid.
See Editor's Note No. 47, page 2058.

Asparagus Extract - Enzymatic Therapy/PhytoPharmica
Each capsule contains: Asparagus rhizome extract (asparagus officinalis, standardized to contain 4-8% asparagosides) 170 mg. Other Ingredients: Cellulose, Gelatin, Magnesium Stearate, Titanium Dioxide Color.

Aspen - Body Booster with Power - Aspen Group, Inc.
Each tablet contains: Raw Testicular concentrate (not an extract) of Bovine sources 300 mg • Multiple Glans Raw Gland concentrate (not an extract) containing Raw Liver Duodenum, Pancreas (porcine sources) & Raw Heart , Pituitary, Kidney, Spleen, Thymus & Adrenal concentrates of Bovine sources 225 mg • Cayenne 25 mg • Gotu Kola 25 mg • Fo-Ti 25 mg • Damiana 32 mg • Guarana 50 mg.
See Editor's Note No. 14, page 2055.

Aspen - Candida - Aspen Group, Inc.
Each capsule contains: Pau D'Arco 4:1 extract 100 mg • Calcium Caprylate 100 mg • Goldenseal root extract 100 mg • Garlic extract (odorless) 50 mg • Licorice root extract 50 mg • Caprilic Acid 25 mg • Oregano 25 mg • Tea Tree oil 5 mg.

Aspen - Cardio- Health - Aspen Group, Inc.
Each caplet contains: Vitamin E (d-alpha tocopheryl acetate) 200 IU • Vitamin C 50 mg • Garlic extract (allium sativum) 300 mg • Hawthorn extract of leaf & flower (crategus laevigata) 50 mg • Co-Enzyme Q10 (ubiquinone) 5 mg.

Aspen - Daily Essentials - Aspen Group, Inc.
Three tablets contain: Vitamin E (d-alpha) 200 IU • Vitamin A 5000 IU • Beta Carotene 5000 IU • Vitamin D 400 IU • Vitamin C 400 mg • Folic Acid 400 mcg • Thiamine 1.5 mg • Riboflavin 1.7 mg • Niacin 20 mg • Vitamin B6 2 mg • Vitamin B12 6 mcg • Biotin 300 mcg • Pantothenic Acid 10 mg • Calcium (citrate) 600 mg • Phosphorus 450 mg • Iodine (kelp) 150 mcg • Magnesium (carbonate) 200 mg • Copper (gluconate) 2 mg • Zinc (gluconate) 15 mg • Vitamin K 100 mcg • Selenium (yeast) 75 mcg • Manganese (gluconate) 5 mg • Chromium (aspartate) 200 mcg • Molybdenum 150 mcg • Nickel 15 mcg • Tin 15 mcg • Vanadium 5 mg • Boron (citrate) 2 mg • Potassium (gluconate) 100 mg • Grape seed extract 10 mg • CoQ10 10 mg.

Aspen - Flexile Plus - Aspen Group, Inc.
Three capsules contain: Glucosamine HCl 99% 1500 mg • Chondroitin Sulfate (purified chondroitin sulfate 95%, mixed glycosominoglycans 5%) 1200 mg • Manganese Ascorbate 240 mg • Bromelain 100 mg • Boswellia Serrata extract 100 mg.
See Editor's Note No. 15, page 2055.

Aspen - Imun- Comp - Aspen Group, Inc.
Two tablets contain: Vitamin C (Ascorbic Acid) 250 mg • Vitamin B1 (Thiamin HCl) 30 mg • Vitamin E (d-Alpha Tocopherol) 200 IU • Beta Carotene 5000 IU • Copper (Gluconate) 300 mcg • Selenium Chelate 25 mcg • Zinc (Gluconate) 15 mg • Bone Marrow 65 mg • Lymph 65 mg • Papain 50 mg • Pituitary Whole 15 mg • Spleen 130 mg • Thymus 550 mg • Bromelain 50 mg • Echinacea extract 300 mg • L-Lysine HCl 250 mg • Trypsin 1:75 25 mg • Blue Flag 130 mg • Fennel 70 mg • Goldenseal herb 70 mg.
See Editor's Note No. 14, page 2055.

Aspen - Maximal Sterol Complex - Aspen Group, Inc.
Six tablets contain: Fucosterol 6963 mcg • Beta Sitosterol 5148 mcg • Campestrol 3069 mcg • Stigmatero 1749 mcg • Other Naturally Occuring Sterols 9174 mcg (26103 mcg of Sterols) • Liver 2600 mg • Orchic 1000 mg • Thymus 200 mg • Heart 200 mg • Lung 200 mg • Kidney 200 mg • Adrenal 150 mg • Prostate 120 mg • Pituitary 150 mg • Hypothalamus 60 mg • Pancreas 120 mg • Bee pollen 1000 mg • Korean Ginseng 100 mg • Royal Jelly 30 mg • Calcium 200 mg • Magnesium 100 mg • Potassium 99 mg • Octacosanol 1650 mcg • RNA 60 mg • DNA 30 mg • Linoleic Acid 1040 mg • Oleic Acid

698 mg • Palmitic Acid 263 mg • Linolenic Acid 109 mg • Stearic Acid 56 mg • Lignoceric Acid 14 mg • Arachidonic Acid 13 mg • Elcoanoic Acid 11 mg • Behenic C Acid 6 mg • Myristic Acid 5 mg • Capsicum 100 mg • Alfalfa 100 mg • Dandelion root 100 mg • Garlic 100 mg • Yellow Dock 100 mg • Gota Kola 100 mg • Licorice root 100 mg • Arginine 1200 mg • Lysine 600 mg • Ornithine 600 mg • Leucine 40 mg • Valine 38 mg • Lysine 34 mg • Isoleucine 30 mg • Phenylalanine 30 mg • Theronine 24 mg • Methionine 20 mg • Tryptophan 8 mg • Trace Minerals.
See Editor's Note No. 14, page 2055.

Aspen - Mega Max - Aspen Group, Inc.
Each tablet contains: Vitamin C 250 mg • Vitamin E 150 IU • Vitamin A 25,000 USP Units • Vitamin D 1000 USP Units • Vitamin B1 75 mg • Vitamin B2 75 mg • Vitamin B6 75 mg • Vitamin B12 75 mg • Niacinamide 75 mg • Choline 75 mg • Inositol 75 mg • Para Aminobenzoic Acid 75 mg • Pantothenic Acid 75 mg • Biotin 75 mg • Folic Acid 400 mcg • Rutin 25 mg • Citrus Bioflavonoids Complex 25 mg • Hesperidin Complex 5 mg • Betaine HCl 25 mg • Glutamic Acid 25 mg • Iodine 15 mg • Calcium 50 mg • Potassium 10 mg • Iron 10 mg • Magnesium 7.2 mg • Manganese 6.1 mg • Zinc 15 mg • Selenium 10 mcg • Amino Acids: Arginine, Aspartic Acid, Alanine, Cystine, Glutamic Acid, Glycine, Histidine, Isoleucine, Lucine, Lysine, Methionine, Ornithine, Phenylalanine, Proline, Serine, Threonine, Tyrosine, Tryptophan, Valine. Natural Base of: Alfalfa, Parsley, Golden Seal root, Buckthorn root, Rosemary, Watercress, Mandrake root, Spinach, Lovage, Kelp, Kale, Ginseng, Rhubarb root.

Aspen - Mid-Life Plus - Aspen Group, Inc.
Each caplet contains: Vitamin E (as natural d-alpha tocopherol succinate) 30 IU • Vitamin C 60 mg • Thiamin (as thiamin mononitrate) 2 mg • Riboflavin 2 mg • Niacin (niacinamide) 20 mg • Vitamin B6 (as pyridoxine HCl) 10 mg • Vitamin B12 (as cyanocobalamin) 6 mcg • Folate (as folic acid) 400 mcg • Calcium (from calcium carbonate) 150 mg • Selenium (from L-Selenomethionine) 70 mcg • Boron (chelate) 1.5 mg • Purified Isoflavones from soybean & pueraria root 50 mg • Kava Kava root standardized extract (30% kavalactones) 100 mg • Black Cohosh root 40 mg.

Aspen - Muscle Builder - Aspen Group, Inc.
Four tablets contain: Gamma Oryzanol 50 mg • Inosine 200 mg • Testicular Glan 600 mg • L-Ornithine 700 mg • Beta-Sitosterol 200 mg • Adrenal 400 mg • Thymus 400 mg.
See Editor's Note No. 14, page 2055.

Aspen - Osteo - Aspen Group, Inc.
Each tablet contains: Calcium Orotate 376 mg • Magnesium Orotate 200 mg • Calcium Aspartate 24 mg • Vitamin D 400 mg.

Aspen - Primrose - Aspen Group, Inc.
Each softgel contains: Evening Primrose oil 500 mg • Vitamin E (d-alpha tocopherol) 10 IU • Gamma Linolenic Acid 40 mg • Linoleic Acid 350 mg.

Aspen - Soy Special - Aspen Group, Inc.
Each tablet contains: Soy isoflavones 50 mg.

AspirActin - Nature's Plus
Three capsules contain: White Willow bark [(Salix alba) standardized 7-9% Salicin] 500 mg • Kava Kava [(Piper methysticum root) standardized 29-31% Kavalactones] 50 mg • Inositol Hexanicotinate (Flush-Free Niacin) 50 mg • Cayenne [(Capsicum frutescens fruit) standardized 100000 STU] 25 mg • Ginkgo Biloba leaf (standardized 24% Ginkgo Flavone-Glycosides, 6% Terpene Lactones) 10 mg.

Astaxanthin 4 mg - Now
Each softgel contains: Vitamin A (100% as natural beta-carotene) 105 IU • Vitamin E (as natural D-alpha tocopherol) 50 IU • BioAstin Natural Astaxanthin (from haematococcus pluvialis extract) 4 mg • Lutein 40 mcg. Other Ingredients: Safflower Oil, Gelatin, Glycerin, Water, Carob Extract (natural color).

Astaxanthin Complex - Solgar
Each softgel contains: Proprietary Blend 4 mg: Astaxanthin (from h. pluvialis, 3.4 mg), Lutein, Beta Carotene, Canthaxanthin, Other Carotenoids. Inactive Ingredients: Safflower oil, Gelatin, Glycerin, Yellow Beeswax, Lecithin, Caramel.

AstaZANTHIN - La Haye Labs
Astaxanthin.
See Editor's Note No. 44, page 2058.

AstaZanthin - Source Naturals
Marine Algae (Haematococcus pluvialis) 10 mg. Natural concentrate (AstaZanthin) yielding Astaxanthin complex 1 mg.

Astazanthin & Pycnogenol Age Protection Creme 2oz - Derma E
Purified Water • Glycerin • Caprylic Triglyceride • Stearic Acid • Jojoba oil • Glyceryl Stearate • Cetyl Alcohol • Stearyl Alcohol • Astazanthin Astaxanthin (1%) • Pycnogenol (1%) • Tocopheryl Acetate (vitamin E) • Ergocalciferol (vitamin D) • Retinyl Palmitate (vitamin A) • TEA • Polysorbate 20 • Titanium Dioxide • Methylparaben • Ethylparaben • I. Urea • Fragrant Oils.

Asthma & Allergy Remedy - PhytoPharmica
Twenty to fifty drops contain: Adrenalinum 6x •Stramonium 6x •Belladonna 4x • Ephedra vulgaris 4x • Ipecacuanha 4x •Lobelia 3x •Solidago virgaurea 3x •Yerba santa 3x •Sambucus 1x. In a base of 40% USP alcohol by volume.
See Editor's Note No. 1 and No. 21, pages 2053 and 2056.

Asthma-X5 - Olympian Labs
Each capsule contains 500 mg: Proprietary Blend: Schisandra Berries, Green Tea, Mormon Tea, Coleus Forskohlii, Lobelia, Feverfew, Skullcap, Licorice root, Ginger.

Astragalus - Jamieson
Each caplet contains: Astragalus Root Formula (T-Cell 7) 3000 mg.

Astragalus - Nature's Way
Three capsules contain: Astragalus root 1.41 g. Other Ingredients: Gelatin, Magnesium stearate.

Astragalus - Now
Two capsules contain: Total Carbohydrate 0.7 g • Dietary Fiber 0.5 g • Astragalus root powder (a. membranaceus) 1.0 g. Other Ingredients: Stearic Acid.

Astragalus - Pharmanex
Each capsule contains: Astragalus root extract(Astragalus membranaceus)(10:1) 250 mg. Other Ingredients: Rice Flour, Gelatin, Magnesium Stearate, Silicon Dioxide.

Astragalus - Pro Health
Each capsule contains: Astragalus root powder (A. membranaceus) 500 mg. Other Ingredients: Stearic Acid.

Astragalus Plus - The Herbalist
Astragalus root • Echinacea root • Lomatium root • Myrrh Gum • Poke root • Wild Indigo root • Yarrow flower • Cayenne pepper.

Astragalus Root Extract - 300 mg - Vital Nutrients
Each capsule contains: Astragalus Membranaceus root extract (15:1) 300 mg.

Astragalus-Shitake Virtue - Blessed Herbs
Astragalus root • Echinacea angustifolia root • Licorice root • Shitake mycelium • Grain alcohol & Distilled Water.

A-Team: Adrenal Support - The Herbalist
Siberian Ginseng fresh-dried root (Eleuthero sent) • Oats fresh milky seed (Avena sativa) • Licorice fresh-dried root (Glycyrrhiza glabra) • Gotu Kola fresh herb (Hydrocotyle asiatica) • Cayenne fresh-dried pepper (Capsicum anuum).

BRAND NAMES

Athero Chelates **-** PhytoPharmica
Twelve tablets contain: Ammonium Chloride 291 mg • Betaine HCl 300 mg • Bromelain (1800 MCU/g) 150 mg • Calcium (as monocalcium phosphate) 150 mg • Copper (as copper gluconate) 113 mcg • Iodine (from kelp) 600 mcg • L-Methionine 600 mcg • Magnesium (as magnesium orotate and magnesium ascorbate) 146 mg • Manganese (as manganese ascorbate) 6 mg • Mucopolysaccharide (soluble) 300 mg • Niacin (as niacinamide and niacin) 630 mg • Potassium (as potassium orotate, potassium aspartate, potassium chloride, and potassium phosphate) 75 mg • Proprietary Phytosterol Blend 450 mg: Beta Sitosterol, Campesterol, Stigmasterol, other Plant Sterols • Selenium (as selenium ascorbate) 300 mcg • Taurine 300 mg • Vitamin B6 (as pyridoxine HCl) 150 mg • Vitamin C (ascorbic acid) 1.5 g • Zinc (as zinc ascorbate) 9 mg.

Athero-Plus **-** Atrium Inc.
Two film coated tablets contain: Vitamin A Palmitate 3334 IU • Vitamin D (as Vitamin D3) (Fish oil) 67 IU • Vitamin B1 (Thiamine Mononitrate) 34 mg • Vitamin B2 (Riboflavin) 17 mg • Vitamin B6 (Pyridoxine HCL) 34 mg • Vitamin B12 (Cyanocobalamin) 34 mcg • Vitamin C (Ascorbic Acid, Sago Palm) 400 mg • Vitamin E Succinate 134 IU • Beta Carotene 5000 IU • Biotin 100 mcg • Niacin/ Niacinamide 67 mg • D-Calcium Pantothenate 167 mg • Folic Acid 267 mcg • Calcium Orotate 170 mg • Chromium Aspartate 67 mcg • Copper Gluconate 0.67 mg • Iodine (Kelp) 40 mcg • Iron (Ferrous Fumerate) 6.67 mg • Magnesium Orotate 170 mg • Magnesium Aspartate 6.67 mg • Molybdenum (Kelp) 34 mcg • Potassium Orotate 34 mg • Selenium Aspartate 67 mcg • Zinc Orotate 6.67 mg • Bromelain 50 mg • Choline Bitartrate 34 mg • L-Methionine 20 mg • PABA 17 mg • Rutin 17 mg.

Athle-Peak **-** The Herbalist
Jamaican Sarsaparilla root • Siberian Ginseng root • American Ginseng root • Licorice root • Wild Yam root • Cinnamon bark • Cayenne pepper.

Athletic Performance **-** Vidafit
Each serving contains: Niacin 6 mg • Pantothenic Acid 4 mg • Riboflavin 1.3 mg • Thiamine 1.2 mg • Vitamin B12 2.4 mcg • Vitamin B6 1.3 mg • Vitamin C 75 mg • Vitamin E 10 IU • Complex Carbohydrates 12 grams • Soy Protein 4 grams • Whey Protein 8 grams.

Athletic Performance Plus **-** Vidafit
Each serving contains: Niacin 6 mg • Pantothenic Acid 4 mg • Riboflavin 1.2 mg • Thiamine 1.1 mg • Vitamin B12 2.4 mcg • Vitamin B6 1.5 mg • Vitamin C 75 mg • Vitamin E 10 IU • Complex Carbohydrates 15 grams • Creatine Monohydrate 1000 mg • Siberian Ginseng 150 mg • Guarana Extract 100 mg • Soy Protein 5 grams • Whey Protein 10 grams.

Athletic Recovery **-** Vidafit
Each serving contains: Vitamin C 75 mg • Vitamin E 10 IU • Calcium 100 mg • Copper 0.5 mg • Magnesium 120 mg • Phosphorus 100 mg • Potassium 700 mg • Zinc 5 mg • Complex Carbohydrates 15 grams • Soy Protein 3 grams • Whey Protein 7 grams.

Athletic Strength **-** Vidafit
Each serving contains: Niacin 10 mg • Riboflavin 1.3 mg • Thiamine 1.2 mg • Vitamin B12 2.4 mcg • Vitamin B6 1.3 mg • Vitamin C 75 mg • Vitamin E 10 IU • Chondroitin Sulfate 250 mg • Glucosamine 500 mg • Siberian Ginseng 150 mg • Soy Protein 7 grams • Whey Protein 18 grams.
See Editor's Note No. 15, page 2055.

Athletica **-** HerbaSway
Bitter Orange • Kudzu • Panax Ginseng • Siberian Ginseng • Astragalus • Schisandra • Ginger • Knotweed • Blackberry • Licorice • HerbaSwee (Cucurbitaceae fruit).
See Editor's Note No. 40, page 2058.

Atkins Allergy **-** Atkins Nutritionals, Inc.
Six tablets contain: Pantethine (co-enzyme A precursor) 360 mg • Bioperine (Piperine) 5 mg • Citrus Bioflavonoids 1000 mg • Grape seed extract (Activin) 60 mg • Vitamin B12 (Cyanocobalamin) 1000 mcg • Vitamin B6 (Pyridoxine) 50 mg • Vitamin C (buffered) 2000 mg • Vitamin A (Acetate) 10000 IU • Quercetin (Flavonoid) 840 mg • Calcium (3-Phosphate, Ascorbate) 700 mg • Magnesium (Carbonate) 200 mg.

Atkins Basic #3 **-** Atkins Nutritionals, Inc.
Each tablet contains: Magnesium Oxide 8 mg • Copper Sulfate 200 mcg • Vitamin E (d Alpha Tocopherol) 20 IU • Cyanocobalamin (Vitamin B12) 30 mcg • Biotin 75 mcg • Folic Acid 100 mcg • Pyridoxine (HCL) (Vitamin B6) 20 mg • Pyridoxal 5-Phosphate 2 mg • Calcium Pantothenate (Vitamin B5) 25 mg • Pantethine (80%) 25 mg • Niacinamide 5 mg • Niacin (Vitamin B3) 2 mg • Vitamin C (Calcium Ascorbate) 120 mg • Riboflavin (Vitamin B2) 4 mg • Thiamine (HCL) (Vitamin B1) 5 mg • Vitamin D (as Vitamin D2) 15 IU • Beta Carotene 500 IU • Vitamin A 200 IU • L-Glutathione (reduced) 5 mg • N-Acetyl-L-Cysteine 20 mg • Octacosanol 150 mcg • Selenium 40 mcg • Vanadyl Sulfate 15 mcg • Molybdenum (Sodium) 10 mcg • Chromium (Polynicotinate) 50 mcg • Zinc (Chelate) 10 mg • Manganese (Chelate) 4 mg • PABA 100 mg • Inositol 80 mg • Choline Bitartrate 100 mg.

Atkins Blood Pressure **-** Atkins Nutritionals, Inc.
Six tablets contain: Taurine 1500 mg • Bioperine (Piperine) 5 mg • Hawthorn (1.5% Vitexin conc.) 300 mg • Calcium (from Ascorbate) 75 mg • Magnesium (Carbonate, Glycinate) 600 mg • Vitamin C (buffered) 600 mg • Pantethine (co-enzyme A precursor) 35 mg • L-Arginine base 100 mg • Inositol 600 mg • N-Acetyl-L-Cysteine 150 mg • Chromium (Picolinate) 200 mcg • Garlic 600 mg • Vitamin B6 (Pyridoxine) 150 mg • Potassium (Citrate) 99 mg.

Atkins Blood Sugar Tablets **-** Atkins Nutritionals, Inc.
Six tablets contain: Chromium (Picolinate) 500 mcg • Bioperine (Piperine) 5 mg • Folic Acid (Folate) 800 mcg • Vitamin E natural 150 IU • Manganese (Glycinate) 30 mg • Selenium (Selenomethionine) 120 mcg • Inositol 900 mg • Niacinamide 300 mg • Vitamin C (buffered) 1200 mg • Bis-Glycinato Oxovanadium Complex (BGOV) 15 mg • Biotin 4 mg • Taurine 600 mg • Alpha-Lipoic Acid 240 mg • Magnesium (Glycinate, Carbonate) 600 mg • Zinc (Monomethionine) 50 mg.

Atkins Cholesterol **-** Atkins Nutritionals, Inc.
Three tablets contain: Calcium (as phosphate) approx. 200 mg • Phosphorus (as calcium phosphate) approx. 115 mg • Inositol Hexanicotinate 1600 mg • Guggul Lipids 100 mg • Beta-, Stigma-, Campa-Sterol 225 mg • Garlic 300 mg • Pantethine (as a co-enzyme A precursor) 100 mg • L-Arginine 100 mg • Absorb Best Tablet Base (an exclusive all natural digestion-supporting base) 345 mg. Other Ingredients: Cellulose, Lecithin extracts, Croscarmellose Sodium, Magnesium Stearate, Silica, Natural Food Glaze. Includes: Pantethine, Garlic, Arginine, DGL Licorice, Lactoferrin, Spirulina, Bromelain, Inulin, Bioperine, Acidophilus (lactal and bifido bacterium).

Atkins Cold & Flu **-** Atkins Nutritionals, Inc.
Four tablets contain: natural Beta-Carotene 20000 IU • Bioperine (Piperine) 5 mg • Copper (Chelate) 4 mg • Vitamin B6 (Pyridoxine) 16 mg • Vitamin B3 (Niacinamide) 60 mg • Vitamin B2 (Riboflavin) 8 mg • Dimethylglycine (DMG) 80 mg • Folic Acid (Folate) 800 mcg • Garlic 640 mg • Magnesium (Ascorbate) 60 mg • Selenium (Selenate) 120 mcg • Citrus Bioflavonoids 320 mg • Calcium Pantothenate (Vitamin B5) 320 mg • Vitamin C buffered 2000 mg • Zinc (Monomethionine) 100 mg • Quercetin (Flavonoid) 320 mg • Vitamin A (Acetate) 13333 IU.

Atkins Dieters Advantage **-** Atkins Nutritionals, Inc.
Four tablets contain: Citrin (55% Hydroxycitric Acid) 450 mg • Chromium (Polynicotinate) 200 mcg • Soy extract (containing active Saponins) 1500 mg • Methionine 250 mg • L-Carnitine Peptide

Complex 500 mg • Vitamin B6 (Pyridoxine) 20 mg • Pantethine (Coenzyme A precursor) 20 mg • Asparagus concentrate 50 mg • Parsley concentrate 50 mg • Kelp 20 mg • Spirulina 50 mg • Potassium (Citrate) 99 mg • Magnesium (Citrate/Carbonate) 60 mg • L-Glutamine 75 mg • DL-Phenylalanine 150 mg • L-Tyrosine 75 mg • Bioperine (Piperine) 5 mg.

Atkins Essential Oils **-** Atkins Nutritionals, Inc.
Each capsule contains: Flaxseed oil 400 mg • Vitamin E 5 IU • Fish oil (50% Omega-3 potency) 400 mg • Borage seed oil 400 mg.

Atkins Heart Care **-** Atkins Nutritionals, Inc.
Eight tablets contain: Magnesium (Glycinate, Carbonate) 400 mg • Bioperine (Piperine) 5 mg • Cayenne 500 mg • Bromelain (Proteolytic Enzyme) 500 mg • Vitamin B6 (Pyridoxine) 10 mg • Folic Acid (Folate) 800 mcg • Selenium (Methionate) 150 mcg • Hawthorn (1.5% Vitexin conc.) 100 mg • Ginkgo Biloba (6% Terpene conc.) 60 mg • natural Beta-Carotene (Dunaliella salina) 12000 IU • Chromium (Picolinate) 200 mcg • Vitamin C (buffered) 1000 mg • Vitamin E natural 400 IU • Taurine 500 mg • Calcium (3-Phosphate) 500 mg.

Atkins Memory **-** Atkins Nutritionals, Inc.
Eight tablets contain: Phosphatidylserine (PS) 160 mg • Bioperine (Piperine) 5 mg • Folic Acid (Folate) 800 mcg • Vitamin B12 (Cyanocobalamin) 1000 mcg • Vitamin B1 (Thiamine) 100 mg • N-Acetyl-L-Cysteine 1000 mg • Octacosanol 6 mg • Ginkgo Biloba (6% Terpene lactone conc.) 60 mg.

Atkins Menopause **-** Atkins Nutritionals, Inc.
Four tablets contain: Black Cohosh (Cimicifuga rademosal) (2.5% Triterpenes) 25 mg • Vitamin E (d-Alpha-Tocopheryl) 200 IU • Bioperine (Piperine) 5 mg • Vitamin K 50 mg • Folic Acid 800 mcg • Tocotrienols mixed 3 mg • Boron (Boroglutamate) 3 mg • Alpha Lipoic Acid 10 mg • Pantethine (co-enzyme A precursor) 25 mg • Vitamin B6 (Pyridoxine) 50 mg • Calcium (Sulfate) 65 mg • Magnesium (Sulfate) 70 mg • Beta-Sitosterol 50 mg • Gamma Oryzanol 150 mg • Garlic (PurGar) 250 mg • Soy Phosphatidylcholine 400 mg • PABA (Para Amino Benzoic Acid) 500 mg • Soy Isoflavones concentrate (23.6% Genistein/Genistin; 3.8% Daidzin/Daldzein) 100 mg.

Atkins Shake Mix - Cappuccino **-** Atkins Nutritionals, Inc.
Cappuccino shake mix contains: Lipo-Pro Blend (special formulation containing: Calcium Caseinate, Milk Protein concentrate, Egg Whites, Glutamine Peptides, Hydrolyzed Whey Protein concentrate & Whey Protein Isolate) • High Oleic Sunflower oil • Lecithin • Enzyme Modified Soy Protein • Carmel Color • Guar Gum • Vitamins & Minerals • Natural & Artificial Flavors • Acesulfame Potassium • Beta-Carotene.

Atkins Shake Mix - Chocolate **-** Atkins Nutritionals, Inc.
Chocolate shake mix contains: Lipo-Pro Blend (special formulation containing: Calcium Caseinate, Milk Protein concentrate, Egg Whites, Glutamine Peptides, Hydrolyzed Whey Protein concentrate & Whey Protein Isolate) • Dutch Cocoa • High Oleic Sunflower oil • Polydextrose • Lecithin • Guar Gum • Vitamins & Minerals • Vanillin • Acesulfame Potassium • Beta-Carotene.

Atkins Shake Mix - Vanilla **-** Atkins Nutritionals, Inc.
Vanilla Shake Mix contains: Lipo-Pro Blend (special formulation containing: Calcium Caseinate, Milk Protein concentrate, Egg Whites, Glutamine Peptides, Hydrolyed Whey Protein concentrate & Whey Protein Isolate) • High Oleci Sunflower oil • Lecithin • Guar Gum • Vitamins & Minerals • Natural & Artificial Flavors • Acesulfame Potassium • Beta-Carotene.

ATP Fuel **-** TwinLab
Each three capsules contains: Creatine Monohydrate & Creatine Pyruvate 3000 mg • Potassium Phosphate 300 mg • ATP (Adenosine Triphosphate) 60 mg.

ATP Plus **-** Progressive Labs
Six tablets contain: Magnesium (as magnesium hydroxide) 300 mg • Malic Acid 1200 mg.

Atri A.S.F **-** Atrium Inc.
Each tablet contains: Raw Tissue concentrates (not extracts) of Bovine source of the following 200 mg: Thymus 80 mg • Partoid 80 mg • Adrenal 20 mg • Spleen 20 mg.
See Editor's Note No. 14, page 2055.

Atri CU- Chelate **-** Atrium Inc.
Each tablet contains: Spleen 28.5 mg • Brain 7.5 mg • Liver 5 mg • Heart 3.5 mg • Kidney 3.5 mg • Thymus 2 mg • Adrenal 2 mg • Pituitary 1 mg • Pancreas 1 mg • Duodenum 1 mg • Copper (Protein Chelated) 2 mg.
See Editor's Note No. 31, page 2056.

Atri E-Derm **-** Atrium Inc.
Each gram contains: Natural Vitamin E (d-Alpha Tocopheryl Acetate) 30 IU. In an absorbent base containing unsaturated fatty acids from Flax & Beet Lipids, Natural Vitamin A & Lecithin.

Atri Flexile **-** Atrium Inc.
Each capsule contains: Glucosamine Sulfate 500 mg • Uncaria tomentosa 200 mg • Curcumin 50 mg • Bromelain 25 mg.

Atri Free Amino **-** Atrium Inc.
Each capsule contains: Free Form Amino Acids: L- Alanine • L-Arginine • L-Aspartic Acid • L-Citruline • L-Cystine • L-Glutamic Acid • L-Glutamine • L-Glysine • L-Histidine HCl • L-Hydroxproline • L-Isoleucine • L-Leucine • L-Lysine • L-Methionine • L-Phenylalanine • L-Proline • L-Serine • L-Threonine • L-Tyrosine • L-Valine • L-Taurine.

Atri K-Chelate **-** Atrium Inc.
Each tablet contains: As chelated proteinates (Amino Acid Chelated Minerals): Potassium 100 mg • Raw Tissue concentrate from the following: (Spleen 28.5 mg, Brain 7.5 mg, Liver 5 mg, Heart 3.5 mg, Kidney 3.5 mg, Thymus 2 mg, Adrenal 2 mg, Pituitary 1 mg, Pancreas 1 mg & Duodenum 1 mg) 55 mg.
See Editor's Note No. 31, page 2056.

Atri Multi-Hypo **-** Atrium Inc.
Three tablets contain: Vitamin A (from Fish Liver oil) 10000 IU • Vitamin D (as Vitamin D3) 400 IU • Vitamin B 10 mg • Vitamin B2 10 mg • Vitamin B6 10 mg • Vitamin B12 50 mcg • Niacinamide 100 mg • Pantothenic Acid 50 mg • Folic Acid 400 mcg • Vitamin C 120 mg • Vitamin E (d-Alpha Tocopherol Succinate) 15 mg • Biotin 30 mcg • Calcium 97 mg • Magnesium 72 mg • Manganese 15 mg • Potassium 53 mg • Zinc 15 mg • Iron (from Iron Sulfate) 18 mg • Iodine (from Kelp) 150 mcg • Choline Bitartrate 30 mg • Inositol 30 mg • PABA (Para Amino Benzoic Acid) 30 mg • Citrus Bioflavonoids 100 mg • Hesperidin 25 mg • Rutin 20 mg • Glutamic Acid 18 mg • L-Lysine (Monohydrochloride) 30 mg • L-Methionine 30 mg.

Atri Zinc Plus **-** Atrium Inc.
Each tablet contains: Ascorbic Acid & Sodium Ascorbate 125 mg • Zinc Gluconate 25 mg • Rutin 25 mg.

Atri-770 **-** Atrium Inc.
Each capsule contains: Cold Pressed concentrated Wheat Germ oil 770 mg.

Atri-A + E Mulsion High concentrate **-** Atrium Inc.
Each drop contains: Emulsified Vitamin A Palmitate 15000 IU • Vitamin E (d-Alpha Tocopheryl Acetate) 10 IU.

Atri-A + E Mulsion Regular concentrate **-** Atrium Inc.
Each drop contains: Emulsified Vitamin A Palmitate 5000 IU • Vitamin E (d-Alpha Tocopheryl Acetate) 10 IU.

Atri-Acidic **-** Atrium Inc.
Each tablet contains: Raw Stomach concentrate (Bovine) 50 mg • Raw Duodenum concentrate (Bovine) 50 mg • Betaine HCL 460 mg •

Glutamic Acid HCL 200 mg • Pepsin 1:20000 25 mg • Potassium Chloride 25 mg.
See Editor's Note No. 14, page 2055.

Atri-Aloe-Lax **-** Atrium Inc.
Each capsule contains: Aloe 450 mg.

Atri-Aloe-V **-** Atrium Inc.
Each capsule contains: Aloe ferox (Aloe Vera resin) 430 mg • Aloe barbadensis (Aloe Vera leaf) 100 mg.

Atri-Amino **-** Atrium Inc.
Six tablets contain: Isoleucine 90 mg • Leucine 216 mg • Lysine 270 mg • Methionine 54 mg • Phenylalanine 132 mg • Threonine 132 mg • Valine 156 mg • Arginine 528 mg • Histidine 48 mg • Alanine 660 mg • Tyrosine 18 mg • Serine 252 mg • Aspartic Acid 402 mg • Cystine 18 mg • Glutamic Acid 684 mg • Glycine 1650 mg • Hydroxylysine 54 mg • Hydroxyproline 846 mg • Proline 984 mg.

Atri-Arthritis Spray **-** Atrium Inc.
Four fluid ounces contains: Oil of Wintergreen (Methyl Salicylate) 15% • Menthol 6% • IPA Alcohol. In a specially formulated, non-greasy base.

Atri-Bio-C **-** Atrium Inc.
Each tablet contains: Calcium Ascorbate 500 mg • Bioflavonoids 500 mg • Acerola 10 mg • Hesperidin 10 mg • Rutin 10 mg.

Atri-BLP **-** Atrium Inc.
Each capsule contains: Cayenne 200 mg • Parsley 90 mg • Ginger root 50 mg • Goldenseal root 40 mg • Garlic 35 mg • Siberian Ginseng 30 mg.

Atri-Cal Chelate **-** Atrium Inc.
Three tablets contain: As Chelated Proteinates (Amino Acid Chelated Minerals) Calcium 450 mg • Raw Tissue concentrate from: (Spleen 74.1 mg, Brain 19.5 mg, Liver 13 mg, Heart 9.1 mg, Kidney 9.1 mg, Thymus 2 mg, Adrenal 2 mg, Pituitary 1 mg, Pancreas 2.6 mg, Duodenum 2.6 mg) 135 mg.
See Editor's Note No. 31, page 2056.

Atri-C-Flu **-** Atrium Inc.
Each capsule contains: Garlic 300 mg • Parsley 60 mg • Rose Hips 60 mg • Rosemary 25 mg • Watercress 20 mg.

Atri-Daily Essentials **-** Atrium Inc.
Three tablets contain: Vitamin E (d-Alpha) 200 IU • Beta Carotene 5000 IU • Vitamin D 400 IU • Folic Acid 400 mcg • Thiamine 1.5 mg • Riboflavin 1.7 mg • Niacin 20 mg • Vitamin B6 2 mg • Vitamin B12 6 mcg • Biotin 300 mcg • Pantothenic Acid 10 mg • Calcium Citrate 600 mg • Phosphorous 450 mg • Iodine (Kelp) 150 mcg • Magnesium (Carbonate) 200 mg • Copper (Gluconate) 2mg • Zinc (Gluconate) 15 mg • Vitamin K 100 mcg • Selenium (yeast) 75 mcg • Manganese (Gluconate) 5 mg • Chromium (Aspartate) 200 mcg • Molybdenum 150 mcg • Nickel 15 mcg • Tin 15 mcg • Vanadium 5 mg • Boron (Citrate) 2 mg • Potassium (Gluconate) 100 mg • Grape seed extract 10 mg • CoQ10 10 mg.

Atri-Detox **-** Atrium Inc.
Each capsule contains: Red Clover Blossoms 150 mg • Chaparral 80 mg • Licorice root 50 mg • Peach bark 50 mg • Oregon Grape root 40 mg • Stillingia 35 mg • Cascara Sagrada bark 30 mg • Sarsaparilla root 30 mg • Burdock root 15 mg • Buckthorn bark 10 mg.

Atri-Disco **-** Atrium Inc.
Each tablet contains: First Phase (in Stomach) Manganese Sulfate 200 mg • Calcium Ascorbate 100 mg • Magnesium Aspartate 50 mg. Second Phase (in Duodenum) Alpha-Chymotrypsin 4 mg • Papain 100 mg • Bromelain 100 mg • Pancreatin 5x 50 mg.
See Editor's Note No. 14, page 2055.

Atri-DMG Plus **-** Atrium Inc.
Each tablet contains: NN Dimethyl Glycine 19.3 mg • Calcium Gluconate 30.7 mg • Glycine 25 mg • Lysine 25 mg.

Atri-EPA Plus **-** Atrium Inc.
Each capsule contains: Salmon oil [containing EPA Eicosapentaenoic Acid 180 mg & DHA Docosahexaenoic Acid 120 mg] 1000 mg • Vitamin A (Fish oil) 100 IU • Vitamin E (Fish oil) 5 IU.

Atri-F **-** Atrium Inc.
Each capsule contains: Cold Processed Persic oil (yielding the following Lipid Acids referred to as Vitamin F factors: Oleic 192 mg, Linoleic 109 mg, Palmitic 18 mg, Stearic 4 mg, Linolenic 701 mcg, Heptodecanoic 400 mcg, Arachadic 330 mcg, Arachidonic 111 mcg) 370 mg • Potassium 113 mcg • Sodium 14 mcg • Magnesium 7 mcg • Phosphorus 4 mg • Calcium 4 mcg • "trace amounts of: Manganese, Chromium, Zinc, Iron, Copper, Boron & Barium" • Palmitoleic 5 mg.

Atri-Fem-Reg **-** Atrium Inc.
Each capsule contains: Goldenseal root 120 mg • Blessed Thistle 100 mg • Cramp bark 80 mg • Uva Ursi leaves 70 mg • False Unicorn 50 mg • Raspberry leaves 30 mg • Squaw Vine 20 mg • Ginger root 10 mg.

Atri-Flav-1000 **-** Atrium Inc.
Three tablets contain: Vitamin C 1000 mg • Citrus Bioflavonoids 1000 mg • Rutin 100 mg. Other Ingredients: Rose Hips & Acerola, in a base containing Raw Spleen concentrate 4 mg.
See Editor's Note No. 14, page 2055.

Atri-FM-H **-** Atrium Inc.
Each capsule contains: Black Cohosh 200 mg • Sarsaparilla root 150 mg • Siberian Ginseng 40 mg • Licorice root 35 mg • False Unicorn 30 mg • Blessed Thistle 25 mg • Squaw Vine 20 mg.

Atri-Gastro **-** Atrium Inc.
Each capsule contains: Colloidal Silica 200 mg • Irish Moss 50 mg • Beef Duodenum 20 mg • Pepsin 20 mg • Stomach Mucosa 10 mg • Di-Sodium Phosphate 10 mg.
See Editor's Note No. 14.

Atri-GE-132 **-** Atrium Inc.
Each capsule contains: Germanium Sesquioxide 150 mg.

Atri-GE-132 Sub **-** Atrium Inc.
Each tablet contains: Germanium Sesquioxide 25 mg.

Atri-Gesic **-** Atrium Inc.
Three ounces contain: Lanolin • Menthol • Methyl Salicylate • Oil of Cassia • Stearic Acid • Spermwax • GMS • Tea • Methyl Gluceth E 10 • Camphor • Methyl Nicotinate • Propyl Parasept • Deionized Water.

Atri-Glucomannan **-** Atrium Inc.
Each capsule contains: Glucomannan Dietary Fiber (Konjac root source) 500 mg.

Atri-Greens Plus **-** Atrium Inc.
Each tablet contains: Vitamin A (Palmitate) 5000 IU • Vitamin C (Ascorbic Acid) 240 mg • Vitamin E (Acetate) 45 mg • Beta Carotene 150 mg • Selenium (Yeast) 50 mcg • Spirulina 25 mg • Chlorophyll 2 mg. In a base of cruciferous vegetables: Broccoli, Brussels Sprouts, Cabbage, Carrot, Cauliflower, Kale, Mustard Greens, Pumpkin, Spinach & Turnip Greens.

Atri-Herb-CLS **-** Atrium Inc.
Each capsule contains: Gentian root 50 mg • Valerian root 50 mg • Catnip 40 mg • Goldenseal root 40 mg • Barberry bark 30 mg • Cascara Sagrada 30 mg • Irish Moss 30 mg • Fenugreek seed 30 mg • Bugleweed 25 mg • Yellow Dock root 25 mg • St. John's Wort 25 mg • Brigham Tea 25 mg • Red Clover Blossoms 25 mg • Chickweed 25 mg.

Atri-IBC **-** Atrium Inc.
Each capsule contains: Eyebright 100 mg • Goldenseal root • Barberry bark 100 mg • Red Raspberry leaves 100 mg • Cayenne 100 mg.

Atri-INF - Atrium Inc.
Each capsule contains: Plantain 200 mg • Black Walnut leaves 100 mg • Goldenseal root 60 mg • Marshmallow root 50 mg • Bugleweed 40 mg.

Atri-Kid-Uri - Atrium Inc.
Each capsule contains: Juniper berries 200 mg • Parsley 120 mg • Uva Ursi leaves 50 mg • Marshmallow root 45 mg • Ginger root 40 mg • Goldenseal root 20 mg.

Atri-Lacto - Atrium Inc.
Each capsule contains: Lactobacillus Acidophilus & Bulgaras culture 400 mg. Contains a minimum two million total bacteria count.

Atri-Lax - Atrium Inc.
Each capsule contains: Psyllium husks 100 mg • Cascara Sagrada bark 100 mg • Prune concentrate 100 mg • Senna leaves 100 mg • Licorice root 45 mg • Chlorophyll 10 mg.

Atri-LB-CLS - Atrium Inc.
Each capsule contains: Cascara Sagrada 150 mg • Bayberry root bark 75 mg • Cayenne 75 mg • Ginger root 50 mg • Goldenseal root 50 mg • Lobelia 30 mg • Red Raspberry leaves 30 mg • Turkey Rhubarb root 30 mg • Fennel seed 20 mg.

Atri-Lipotropic - Atrium Inc.
Three capsules contain: Choline Bitartrate 1000 mg • Inositol 1000 mg • Methionine 300 mg.

Atri-Liv-GLB - Atrium Inc.
Each capsule contains: Barberry root bark 120 mg • Wild Yam 80 mg • Cramp bark 60 mg • Fennel seed 50 mg • Yellow Dock 40 mg • Ginger root 35 mg • Catnip 30 mg • Peppermint leaves 30 mg.

Atri-Ly Poll - Atrium Inc.
Each tablet contains: Raw Bovine Tissue concentrate (not extracts) 20 mg: (Pituitary 5 mg • Adrenal 15 mg) • special blend of Bee Pollen 250 mg. In a base of L-Lysine 400 mg (an Amino Acid known to be essential in human nutrition).
See Editor's Note No. 14, page 2055.

Atri-Lym-Inf - Atrium Inc.
Each capsule contains: Cayenne 150 mg • Echinacea 120 mg • Myrrh Gum 100 mg • Hawthorn berries 100 mg • Licorice root 30 mg.

Atri-Mag Chelate Plus - Atrium Inc.
Each tablet contains: Amino Acid Chelated Minerals as: Magnesium 300 mg. Raw Tissue concentrates (Bovine source) from: Spleen 29 mg • Brain 8 mg • Liver 5 mg • Heart 4 mg • Kidney 4 mg • Thymus 2 mg • Adrenal 2 mg • Pituitary 1 mg • Duodenum 1 mg • Pancreas 1 mg.
See Editor's Note No. 31, page 2056.

Atri-Medicated Psoriasis Shampoo - Atrium Inc.
Eight fluid ounces contain: Active Ingredients: Coal Tar solution USP 5% • Colloidal Sulfur 2% • Salicylic Acid 2%. In a special base of Surface Active Cleansers, Wetting Agents & Lanolin.

Atri-Mega Plus - Atrium Inc.
Four tablets contain: Vitamin A Acetate 25000 IU • Vitamin D (as Vitamin D3) Cholecalciferol 1000 IU • Vitamin E Acetate 100 IU • Vitamin C (with Rose Hips) 500 mg • Folic Acid 0.1 mg • Thiamine (Vitamin B1) 50 mg • Riboflavin (Vitamin B2) 50 mg • Niacin 100 mg • Vitamin B6 50 mg • Vitamin B12 50 mcg • Biotin 50 mcg • Pantothenic Acid 50 mg • Choline Bitartrate 50 mg • Calcium (as Oyster Shell & Calcium Carbonate) 700 mg • Iodine (Kelp) 225 mcg • Iron (Ferrous Fumerate) 30 mg • Magnesium (as Oxide) 200 mg • Zinc (as Sulfate) 36 mg • Manganese (as Carbonate) 3mg • Potassium (Chloride & Kelp) 99 mg • Chromium (as Chelate) 20 mcg • Selenium (Yeast) 60 mcg • Betaine HCl 50 mg • Papain 200 mg • Para Aminobenzoic Acid 50 mg • Citrus Bioflavonoids 50 mg • Inositol 50 mg • Ribonucleic Acid (Yeast extract) 200 mg.

Atri-Mega-Lacto - Atrium Inc.
Each capsule contains: Lactobacillus Acidophilus with Bifidus Four Billion CFU (Colony Forming Units).

Atri-Min 74 - Atrium Inc.
Each tablet contains: Sea Bed Montmorillonite (also known as Mineral 74100 mg Volcanic Montmorillonite) 900 mg.

Atri-Multi - Atrium Inc.
Each tablet contains: Vitamin A (from Fish Liver oil) 3333 IU • Vitamin D (as Vitamin D3) 133 IU • Vitamin B1 4 mg • Vitamin B2 3 mg • Vitamin B6 3 mg • Vitamin B12 11 mcg • Niacinamide 34 mg • Pantothenic Acid 17 mg • Folic Acid 134 mcg • Vitamin C 40 mg • Vitamin E (d-Alpha Tocopherol) 5 mg • Biotin 10 mcg • Calcium 32 mg • Magnesium 24 mg • Manganese 5 mg • Potassium 18 mg • Zinc 5 mg • Iron (from Sulfate) 6 mg • Iodine (from Kelp) 50 mcg • Choline Bitartrate 10 mg • PABA 9 mg • Citrus Bioflavonoids 100 mg • Hesperidin 9 mg • Rutin 7 mg • Glutamic Acid 6 mg • L-Lysine 10 mg • L-Methionine 10 mg • RNA (from Yeast) 15 mg. In a base of Watercress, Kelp, Alfalfa, Parsley.

Atri-Nerv - Atrium Inc.
Each capsule contains: Black Cohosh 100 mg • Cayenne 100 mg • Hops Flowers 80 mg • Scullcap 70 mg • Wood Betony 50 mg • Passiflora 40 mg • Valerian root 20 mg • Ladys Slipper 10 mg.

Atri-Neuro - Atrium Inc.
Each tablet contains: Choline (Choline Bitartrate) 200 mg • L-Histidine 50 mg • L-Phenylalanine 50 mg • GABA (Amino Buteric Acid) 50 mg • L-Tyrosine 50 mg • Raw Brain concentrate 25 mg • Niacin 15 mg • Pyridoxine HCl 50 mg.
See Editor's Note No. 31, page 2056.

Atri-NTL-CA - Atrium Inc.
Each capsule contains: Horsetail grass 300 mg • Oat Straw 100 mg.

Atri-Ortho-Phos - Atrium Inc.
Each drop contains: Ortho Phosphoric Acid 13 mg • Inositol 0.57 mg • Choline Bitartrate 0.27 mg. Thirty drops contain: Ortho Phosphoic Acid 390 mg • Inositol 17 mg • Choline Bitartrate 8 mg.

Atri-Oxy - Atrium Inc.
Two tablets contain: Vitamin A (Beta Carotene) 25000 IU • Vitamin E (d-Alpha Tocopherol) 400 IU • Vitamin C 1000 mg • Bioflavonoid Complex 150 mg • Superoxide Dismutase 100 mg • Selenium 100 mcg • Zinc 25 mg • Copper 2 mg • Astragalus 50 mg • Rosemary 50 mg • Milk Thistle (Slymarin) 50 mg • Spirulina 100 mg • Chromium Picolinate 25 mcg • Grape seed extract 50 mg • CoEnzyme Q-10 10 mg • L-Glutathione 10 mg • L-Cysteine 100 mg • Reishi Mushroom 50 mg • Curcumin 50 mg.

Atri-PMS - Atrium Inc.
Three tablets contain: Vitamin A Acetate 5000 IU • Vitamin B6 (Pyridoxine HCL) 100 mg • Adrenal concentrate 50 mg • Hypothalamus concentrate 10 mg • Ovary concentrate 50 mg • Pituitary concentrate 10 mg • Passion Flower 75 mg • Dong Quai 50 mg • Cramp bark 50 mg • Chionanthus 50 mg • Valerian 75 mg • Magnesium (Oxide) 200 mg • Iron (Peptonate) 20 mg • Red Raspberry 50 mg.
See Editor's Note No. 14, page 2055.

Atri-Pros - Atrium Inc.
Each capsule contains: Cayenne 160 mg • Uva Ursi leaves 70 mg • Parsley 60 mg • Goldenseal root 50 mg • Gravel root 50 mg • Juniper berries 30 mg • Marshmallow root 25 mg • Ginger root 20 mg • Siberian Ginseng 15 mg.

Atri-Psoriasis Ointment - Atrium Inc.
Four ounces contains: Sulfur ppt 1.5% • Salicylic Acid 1.5% • Coal Tar Solution USP 2%.

Atri-Res - Atrium Inc.
Each capsule contains: Marshmallow root 200 mg • Mullein 120 mg • Comfrey leaves 100 mg • Chickweed 50 mg. Professional Formula.

Atri-RNA/DNA **-** Atrium Inc.
Each tablet contains: RiboNucleic Acid (RNA) 180 mg • DeoxyNucleic Acid (DNA) 40 mg.

Atri-SDT **-** Atrium Inc.
Each tablet contains: Trypsin 4 mg • Chymotrypsin 2 mg • Pancreatin 2 mg • Bromelain 3 mg • Papayotin 4 mg • Thymus concentrate (Bovine) 2 mg • Mannitol 13 mg. In a specially prepared natural spearmint flavored slow dissolving tablet base.
See Editor's Note No. 14, page 2055.

Atri-Selenium+E **-** Atrium Inc.
Each tablet contains: Vitamin C (Ascorbic Acid) 250 mg • Vitamin E (d-Alpha Tocopherol) 200 IU • Vitamin B1 (Thiamine HCL) 4 mg • Vitamin B2 (Riboflavin) 4 mg • Vitamin B6 (Pyridoxine HCL) 4 mg • Niacin 10 mg • Pantothenic Acid 50 mg • Selenium (Selenium Yeast) 50 mcg • Raw Heart concentrate 10 mg. In a base of Bone Meal.
See Editor's Note No. 14, page 2055.

Atri-S-G-V **-** Atrium Inc.
Each tablet contains: Selenium 50 mcg • Germanium 225 mcg • Vanadium 225 mcg, as Protein Chelates.

Atri-Statin **-** Atrium Inc.
Each tablet contains: Caprylic Acid 110 mg.

Atri-Stress-B+C **-** Atrium Inc.
Two tablets contain: Vitamin C (Ascorbic Acid) 500 mg • Vitamin B1 (Thiamine HCL) 100 mg • Vitamin B2 (Riboflavin) 100 mg • Vitamin B6 (Pyridoxine HCL) 100 mg • Vitamin B12 (Cyanocobalamin) 500 mcg • Niacinamide 100 mg • Pantothenic Acid 100 mg • Folic Acid 400 mcg • Biotin 100 mcg • Lemon Bioflavonoids 250 mg • Choline (Choline Bitartrate) 100 mg • Inositol 100 mg • PABA 50 mg.

Atri-Thy-Kelp **-** Atrium Inc.
Each capsule contains: Mullein 140 mg • Parsley 90 mg • Watercress 80 mg • Kelp (Norwegian) 70 mg • Irish Moss 60 mg • Iceland Moss 40 mg.

Atri-Trace **-** Atrium Inc.
Three tablets contain: Calcium (Egg & Oyster Shells) 250 mg • Magnesium (Gluconate) 50 mg • Manganese (Gluconate) 10 mg • Potassium (Gluconate) 50 mg • Zinc (Gluconate)15 mg • Vitamin D (as Vitamin D3) 133 IU • Vitamin B6 50 mg • Glutamic Acid HCL 325 mg.

Atri-V&M+Complete **-** Atrium Inc.
Six tablets contains: Vitamin A (Fish oil) 10000 IU • Vitamin D (Fish oil) 400 IU • Vitamin C (Calcium Ascorbate, Acerola, Rose Hips) 400 mg • Vitamin E 60 IU • Vitamin B1 • Vitamin B2 10 mg • Vitamin B6 10 mg • Vitamin B12 25 mcg • Niacin 60 mg • Calcium (Bone Meal & Calcium Carbonate) 750 mg • Magnesium (Oxide) 375 mg • Phosphorus (Bone Meal) 700 mg • Iron (Amino Acid Chelate) 20 mg • Iodine (Kelp) 150 mcg • Potassium (Proteinate) 20 mg • Zinc (Amino Acid Chelate) 20 mg • Manganese (Amino Acid Chelate) 15 mg • Choline (Bitartrate) 50 mg • Inositol 500 mg • Lecithin 50 mg • Pantothenic Acid 50 mg • Folic Acid 400 mcg • PABA 30 mg • RNA-DNA 15 mg • Betaine HCL 25 mg • Biotin 100 mcg. In a base of Alfalfa, Kelp, Rose Hips, Acerola, Fish Liver oils, Bone Meal, Citrus Bioflavonoids, Papaya, Bromelain Enzymes & Essential Amino Acids.

Atri-Vana **-** Atrium Inc.
Each capsule contains: Vanadyl Sulfate 25 mg.

Atri-Verm **-** Atrium Inc.
Each capsule contains: Pumpkin seed 100 mg • Culver's root 70 mg • Violet leaves 60 mg • Cascara Sagrada bark 50 mg • Slippery Elm bark 45 mg • Witch Hazel bark 40 mg • Mullein 30 mg • Echinacea 20 mg.

Atri-Yeast **-** Atrium Inc.
Four tablets contain: Protein from a Special Yeast 1200 mg • Niacin 66 mg • Pantothenic Acid 13 mg • Vitamin B1 13 mg • Vitamin B2 13 mg • Vitamin B6 3 mg • Chromium 25 mcg • Selenium 7.5 mcg.

Atri-Zinc Chelate Plus **-** Atrium Inc.
Each tablet contains: Amino Acid Chelated Minerals as: Zinc 29 mg. Raw Tissue concentrates (Bovine source) from: Spleen 29 mg • Brain 8 mg • Liver 5 mg • Heart 4 mg • Kidney 4 mg • Thymus 2 mg • Adrenal 2 mg • Pituitary 1 mg • Duodenum 1 mg.
See Editor's Note No. 31, page 2056.

Attend **-** Vaxa International
Each capsule contains: Proprietary Blend 715 mg: L-Isoleucine, L-Leucine, L-Valine, L-Tyrosine, L-Cysteine, L-Cystine, DL-Methionine, DLPA, L-Glutamic Acid, GABA, L-Glycine, L-Glutathione, Catechol, Pregnenolone, Trifolium Pratense (trans-cis-cloramide), Flax Seed powder, Pyridoxine, Calcium Pantothenate, Magnesium Aspartate, Zinc (OptiZinc), Niacinamide, Radix Heraclei, Gotu Kola, Ginkgo Biloba, Chromium (ChromeMate GTF), DMAE, Pycnogenol, Pine Bark extract, NADH, Sodium Bicarbonate, Phosphatidylcholine, Phosphatidylethanolamine, Phosphatidylserine, Phosphatidylinositol, Medium Chain Triglycerides, Caprylic Acid, Lauric Acid, Myristic Acid, Palmitic Acid, Stearic Acid, Oleic Acid, Linoleic Acid, Linolenic Acid, Arachidic Acid, EPA (Eicosapentaenoic Acid), Ecicosatrienoic Acid, Arachidonic Acid, Gamma Linolenic Acid, DHA (Decosahexaenoic Acid), Agaricus muscarius, Argentum nitricum, Avena sativa, Caffeinum, Cimicifuga racemosa, Fluoricum acidum, Humulus lupulis, Hyoscyamus niger, Ignatia amara, Iodum, Kali bromatum, Kali phosphoricum, Lithium bromatum, Lithium carbonicum, Natrum muriaticum, Hypothalamus, Corticohypothalmic Axis, Diopside, Parasympathetic Ganglia, Rhodonite.

Attention! **-** Olympia Nutrition
Contains DHA 250 mg • Phosphatidylserine 20 mg • DMAE 100 mg • Choline 100 mg • TMG.

Avacor nutricap DHT Blocker **-** Global Vision
Active Ingredients: Maidenhair Tree • Vaccinium Myrtillus • Equisetum • Sabal Serrulata.

Avena Sativa Complex **-** Puritan's Pride
Each capsule contains: Avena Sativa 300 mg • Siberian Ginseng 150 mg • Nettle 50 mg.

Avlimil **-** Warner Health Care
Each tablet contains: Avlimil Proprietary Blend 756 mg: Salvia Officinalis (sage leaf), Rubus Idaeus (red raspbery leaf), Isoflavones (from pueraria montana (kudzu) root extract/ trifolium pratense (red clover) extract), Capsicum Annuum (capsicum pepper), Glycyrrhiza Glabra (licorice root), Morella Cerifera (bayberry fruit), Turnera Diffusa (damiana leaf), Valeriana Officinalis (valeriana root), Zingiber Officinale (ginger root), Actaea Caremosa (black cohosh root). Other Ingredients: Dicalcium Phosphate, Microcrystalline Cellulose, Croscarmellose Sodium, Stearic Acid, Magnesium Stearate, Silica, Hypromellose, Titanium Dioxide, Propylene Glycol, FD&C Blue #1 Lake, FD&C Red #3.

Avocado & E Dry Skin Relief Creme 4oz **-** Derma E
Purified Water • Safflower oil • Stearic Acid • Cetyl Alcohol • Glyceryl Stearate • Avocado oil • Glycerin • Tocopheryl Acetate (vitamin E) • Retinyl Palmitate (vitamin A) • Ergocalciferol (vitamin D) • Panthenol • Sunflower oil • Wheat Germ oil • Allantoin • Methylparaben • TEA • I. Urea • Natural Plant extract • Fragrant oils.

B Complex **-** Nature's Sunshine
Each capsule contains: Vitamin B1 (thiamine) 33 mg • Vitamin B2 (riboflavin) 33 mg • Niacinamide 33 mg • Vitamin B6 (pyridoxine HCl) 33 mg • Folic Acid 133 mcg • Vitamin B12 (cyanocobalamin) 33 mcg • Biotin 100 mcg • Pantothenic Acid (d-calcium pantothenate) 33 mg • Choline (bitartrate) 33 mg •Inositol 33 mg.

B Complex **-** Shaklee
Each two capsules contain: Thiamin (as Thiamin mononitrate) 20.25 mg • Riboflavin 22.95 mg • Niacin (as Niacinamide) 270 mg • Vitamin B6 (as Pyridoxine hydrochloride) 27 mg • Folate (as Folic acid) 400 mcg • Vitamin B12 (as Cyanocobalamin) 81 mcg • Biotin (as D-Biotin) 300 mcg • Pantothenic acid (as D-Calcium pantothenate) 135 mg. Other Ingredients: Microcrystalline Cellulose, Torula Yeast, Brewer's Yeast, Hydroxypropyl Methylcellulose, Croscarmellose Sodium, Hydroxylated Soy Lecithin.

B Complex 100 with Iron **-** Schiff
Each tablet contains: Vitamin B1 (as thiamin mononitrate) 100 mg •Vitamin B2 (as riboflavin) 100 mg • Vitamin B3 (as niacinamide) 100 mg • Vitamin B6 (as pyridoxine hydrochloride) 100 mg • Folate (as folic acid) 200 mcg • Vitamin B12 (as cyanocobalamin) 100 mcg • Biotin 100 mcg • Pantothenic Acid (as d-calcium pantothenate) 100 mg • Calcium (as calcium carbonate and dicalcium phosphate) 145 mg • Iron (as ferrous fumarate) 18 mg • Proprietary Blend 5 mg: Alfalfa Herb powder, Lecithin powder, Parsley leaf powder, Watercress leaf extract, Whole Brown Rice concentrate • Choline Bitartrate 100 mcg •Inositol 100 mcg •PABA (para-aminobenzoic acid) 100 mcg. Other Ingredients: Cellulose, Stearic Acid, Cellulose Gum, Silicon Dioxide, Magnesium Stearate, Coating (hydroxypropyl methylcellulose, polyethylene glycol).

B Complex 100% RDA **-** Rexall - Sundown
Each tablet contains: Thiamin (vitamin B1, from thiamin mononitrate) 1.5 mg • Riboflavin (vitamin B2) 1.7 mg • Niacin (as niacinamide) 20 mg • Vitamin B6 (as pyridoxine HCl) 2 mg • Folic Acid 400 mcg • Vitamin B12 (as cyanocobalamin) 6 mcg • Calcium 35 mg. Other Ingredients: Dicalcium Phosphate, Microcrystalline Cellulose, Croscarmellose Sodium, Hydroxypropyl Methylcellulose, Magnesium Stearate, Thiethyl Citrate.

B Complex Maxi **-** Rexall - Sundown
Each two softgels contain: Thiamin (vitamin B1, as thiamin mononitrate) 15 mg • Riboflavin (vitamin B2) 17 mg • Niacin (as niacinamide) 200 mg • Vitamin B6 (as pyridoxine HCl) 20 mg • Folic Acid 400 mcg • Vitamin B12 (as cyanocobalamin) 60 mcg • Pantothenic Acid (as calcium d-pantothenate) 100 mg • B Complex Base Blend 600 mcg: Choline Bitartrate, Inositol, Para-Aminobenzoic Acid (PABA). Other Ingredients: Soybean Oil, Gelatin, Glycerin, Soy Lecithin, Silica, Caramel, Magnesium Stearate, Dicalcium Phosphate, Titanium Dioxide, D-alpha-tocopherol.

B Complex Vitamins **-** Nature's Bounty
Each tablet contains: Thiamin (vitamin B1, as thiamin hydrochloride) 5 mg • Riboflavin (as vitamin B2) 5 mg • Niacin (as niacinamide) 40 mg • Vitamin B6 (as pyridoxine hydrochloride) 1 mg • Vitamin B12 (as cyanocobalamin) 1 mcg • Pantothenic Acid (as D-calcium pantothenate) 4.6 mg • Inositol 10 mg • Choline Bitartate 20 mg • Desiccated Liver powder 100 mg • Brewer's Yeast 50 mg. Other Ingredients: Dicalcium Phosphate, Celullose (plant origin), Vegetable Stearic Acid, Croscarmellose, Cellulose Coating, Silica, Vegetable Magnesium Stearate, Mannitol.
See Editor's Note No. 14, page 2055.

B Complex Vitamins plus B-12 **-** Nature's Bounty
Each tablet contains: Thiamin (vitamin B1, as thiamin hydrochloride and brewer's yeast) 7 mg • Riboflavin (vitamin B2, as riboflavin and brewer's yeast) 14 mg • Niacin (as niacin and brewer's yeast) 4.5 mg • Vitamin B12 (as cyanocobalamin and brewer's yeast) 25 mcg • Protease (as papain powder) 10 mg. Other Ingredients: Dicalcium Phosphate, Cellulose (plant origin), Vegetable Stearic Acid, Croscarmellose, Silica, Mannitol, Vegetable Magnesium Stearate.

B Complex Vitamins plus Iron **-** Nature's Bounty
Each tablet contains: Thiamin (vitamin B1, as thiamin hydrochloride) 5 mg • Riboflavin (vitamin B2) 5 mg • Niacin (as niacinamide) 50 mg • Vitamin B6 (as pyridoxine hydrochloride) 1 mg • Vitamin B12 (as cyanocobalamin) 1 mcg • Pantothenic Acid (as D-calcium pantothenate) 4.6 mg • Iron (as ferrous sulfate) 10 mg • Choline Bitartrate 20 mg • Inositol 10 mg • Dessicated Liver 100 mg • Brewer's Yeast 50 mg. Other Ingredients: Cellulose (plant origin), Dicalcium Phosphate, Vegetable Stearic Acid, Silica, Croscarmellose, Cellulose Coating, Vegetable Magnesium Stearate, Mannitol.
See Editor's Note No. 14, page 2055.

B Complex with Vitamin C **-** Jamieson
Each tablet contains: Vitamin B1 5 mg • Vitamin B2 5 mg • Niacinamide 50 mg • Vitamin B6 5 mg • Vitamin B12 10 mcg • Biotin 10 mcg • Pantothenic Acid 25 mg • Folic Acid 0.05 mg • Vitamin C 250 mg • Lipotropic Factors: Choline Bitartrate 50 mg • Inositol 50 mg. Also contains Para-Aminobenzoic Acid.

B Healthy **-** iVillage Inc.
Each tablet contains: Thiamin 16.67 mg • Riboflavin 16.67 mg • Niacin 16.67 mg • Vitamin B6 16.67 mg • Folic Acid 133.33 mcg • Vitamin B12 16.67 mcg • Biotin 100 mcg • Pantothenic Acid 16.67 mg • Calcium 110 mg • iVillage Blend 5 mg: Spinach leaf, Acerola fruit extract (malpighia glabra), Broccoli floweret. Other Ingredients: Microcrystalline Cellulose, Maltodextrin, Acacia, Magnesium Stearate, Sodium Carboxymethylcellulose, Hydroxypropyl Methylcellulose, Glycerin.

B-1 100 mg **-** Puritan's Pride
Each tablet contains: Vitamin B-1 (Thiamine Hydrochloride) 100 mg.

B-1 250 mg **-** Puritan's Pride
Each tablet contains: Vitamin B-1 (Thiamine Hydrochloride) 250 mg.

B100 Complex **-** Natrol
Each tablet contains: Vitamin B1 (Thiamine) 100 mg • Vitamin B2 (Riboflavin) 100 mg • Vitamin B6 (Pyroxidoxine) 100 mg • Vitamin B12 (Cobalamin) 100 mcg • Niacinamide 100 mg • Folic Acid 400 mcg • Biotin 100 mcg • Pantothenic Acid 100 mg • Choline 100 mg • Inositol 100 mg • PABA 100 mg • ULTRAGREEN 150 mg. Other Ingredients: Microcrystalline Cellulose, Calcium Carbonate, Croscarmellose Sodium, Stearic Acid, Silicon Dioxide, Magnesium Stearate.

B-100 Complex **-** Rexall - Sundown
Each tablet contains: Thiamin (vitamin B1, as thiamin HCl) 1.5 mg • Riboflavin (vitamin B2) 1.7 mg • Niacin (as niacinamide) 20 mg • Vitamin B6 (as pyridoxine HCl) 2 mg • Folic Acid 400 mcg • Vitamin B12 (as cyanocobalamin) 6 mcg • Pantothenic Acid (as calcium d-pantothenate) 10 mg • Calcium 120 mg • Vitamin Co-Factor Blend 1 mg: Choline Bitartrate, Para-Aminobenzoic Acid (PABA), Inositol. Other Ingredients: Dicalcium Phosphate, Microcrystalline Cellulose, Croscarmellose Sodium, Magnesium Stearate.

B100 Complex - Timed Release **-** Jamieson
Each caplet contains: Vitamin B1 100 mg • Vitamin B2 100 mg • Vitamin B3 100 mg • Vitamin B6 100 mg • Vitamin B12 100 mcg • Biotin 100 mcg • Pantothenic Acid 100 mg • Folic Acid 0.4 mg • Lipotropic Factors: Choline Bitartrate 100 mg, Inositol 100 mg. Also contains Para-Aminobenzoic Acid.

B-100 Complex Yeast Free **-** Rexall - Sundown
Each caplet contains: Thiamin (vitamin B1, as thiamin mononitrate) 100 mg • Riboflavin (vitamin B2) 100 mg • Niacin (as niacinamide) 100 mg • Vitamin B6 (as pyridoxine HCl) 100 mg • Folic Acid 400 mcg • Vitamin B12 (as cyanocobalamin) 100 mcg • Biotin 100 mg • Pantothenic Acid (as calcium d-pantothenate) 100 mg • Calcium 60 mg • B-Factor Blend 3.4 mg: Alfalfa (aerial parts), Choline Bitartrate, Para-Aminobenzoic Acid (PABA), Inositol, Parsley (aerial parts), Rice Bran, Watercress (aerial parts). Other Ingredients: Microcrystalline Cellulose, Dicalcium Phosphate, Croscarmellose Sodium, Stearic Acid, Soy Polysaccharides, Hydroxypropyl Methylcellulose, Silica, Magnesium Stearate, Hydroxypropyl Cellulose, PEG.

B-100 Complex Yeast Free **-** Vitamin World
Each capsule contains: Thiamin (vitamin B1, as thiamin mononitrate) 100 mg • Riboflavin (vitamin B2) 100 mg • Niacin (as niacinamide)

100 mg • Vitamin B6 (as pyridoxine hydrochloride) 100 mg • Folic Acid 400 mcg • Vitamin B12 (as cyanocobalamin) 100 mcg • Biotin 100 mcg • Pantothenic Acid (as D-calcium pantothenate) 100 mg • Choline Bitartrate 100 mg • PABA (para-aminobenzoic acid) 100 mg • Inositol 100 mg • Proprietary Blend 7.5 mg: Alfalfa, Watercress, Parsley, Lecithin, Rice Bran. Other Ingredients: Gelatin, Vegetable Magnesium Stearate, Silica.

B-100 Mg Complex Timed **-** Rexall - Sundown
Each caplet contains: Thiamin (vitamin B1, as thiamin mononitrate) 100 mg • Riboflavin (vitamin B2) 100 mg • Niacin (as niacinamide) 100 mg • Vitamin B6 (as pyridoxine HCl) 100 mg • Folic Acid 400 mcg • Vitamin B12 (as cyanocobalamin) 100 mcg • Biotin 100 mcg • Pantothenic Acid (as calcium d-pantothenate) 100 mg • Calcium 90 mg • Base Complex Blend 4.4 mg: Alfalfa (leaves), Choline Bitartrate, Para-Aminobenzoic Acid (PABA), Soy Lecithin, Inositol, Parsley (aerial parts), Rice Bran, Watercress (aerial parts). Other Ingredients: Dicalcium Phosphate, Cellulose, Methylcellulose, Hydrogenated Vegetable Oil, Stearic Acid, Hydroxypropyl Methylcellulose, Silica, Magnesium Stearate, Hydroxypropyl Cellulose, PEG.

B-100 Ultra B-Complex **-** Puritan's Pride
Each tablet contains: Thiamin (Vitamin B1; as thiamine mononitrate) 100 mg • Riboflavin (Vitamin B2) 100 mg • Niacin (as niacinamide) 100 mg • Vitamin B6 (as pyridoxine hydrochloride) 100 mg • Folic Acid 400 mcg • Vitamin B12 (as cyanocobalamin) 100 mcg • Biotin (as d-biotin) 100 mcg • Pantothenic Acid (as d-calcium pantothenate) 100 mg • Inositol 100 mg • PABA (para-aminobenzoic acid) 100 mg • Choline Bitartrate 100 mg • Proprietary Blend: Parsley leaves powder, Rice Bran defatted powder, Watercress leaves powder, Alfalfa leaves powder, Lecithin granules 5 mg.

B-12 100 mcg **-** Puritan's Pride
Each tablet contains: Vitamin B-12 (Cyanocobalamin) 100 mcg.

B-12 1000 mcg **-** Puritan's Pride
Each tablet contains: Vitamin B-12(Cyanocobalamin) 1000 mcg.

B-12 1000 mcg **-** Rexall - Sundown
Each tablet contains: Vitamin B12 (as cyanocobalamin) 1 mg • Calcium 26 mg. Other Ingredients: Dextrose Direct Compression, Dicalcium Phosphate, Croscarmellose Sodium, Magnesium Stearate.

B-12 1500 mcg **-** Puritan's Pride
Each tablet contains: Vitamin B-12 (Cobalamin concentrate) 1500 mcg.

B-12 1500 mcg **-** Rexall - Sundown
Each caplet contains: Vitamin B12 (as cyanocobalamin) 1.5 mg • Calcium 150 mg. Other Ingredients: Dicalcium Phosphate, Calcium Sulfate, Hydroxypropyl Methylcellulose, Hydrogenated Cottonseed Oil, Stearic Acid, Silica, Magnesium Stearate.

B-12 250 mcg **-** Puritan's Pride
Each tablet contains: Vitamin B-12 (Cyanocobalamin) 250 mcg.

B-12 500 mcg **-** Puritan's Pride
Each tablet contains: Vitamin B-12 (Cyanocobalamin) 500 mcg.

B-12 500 mcg **-** Rexall - Sundown
Each caplet contains: Vitamin B12 (as cyanocobalamin) 500 mcg • Calcium 50 mg. Other Ingredients: Dicalcium Phosphate, Croscarmellose Sodium, Magnesium Stearate.

B-12 Lingual **-** Progressive Labs
Each tablet contains: Vitamin B12 1000 mcg • Folate (folic acid) 400 mcg, in a base of Mannitol and Natural Cherry flavor.

B-12 Neurobolic **-** Pharmalogic
Four sprays contain: Vitamin B12 500 mcg • Dibencozide (coenzyme B12) 500 mcg • ATP (adenosine triphosphate) 10,000 mcg • Alpha-glycerylphosphorylcholine 10,000 mcg. Other Ingredients: Purified Water, Sodium Benzoate, Potassium Sorbate, Glycerin, Citric Acid, Sodium Citrate (to adjust the pH to approximately 6.2).

B12-Active **-** PhytoPharmica
Each tablet contains: Vitamin B12 (methylcobalamin) 1,000 mcg.

B-150 **-** Puritan's Pride
Each tablet contains: Thiamin (Vitamin B1; as thiamine mononitrate) 150 mg • Riboflavin (Vitamin B2) 150 mg • Niacin (as niacinamide) 150 mg • Vitamin B6 (as pyridoxine hydrochloride) 150 mg • Folic Acid 150 mcg • Vitamin B12 (as cyanocobalamin) 150 mcg • Biotin (as d-biotin) 150 mcg • Pantothenic Acid (as d-calcium pantothenate) 150 mg • Choline Bitartrate 150 mg • PABA (para-aminobenzoic acid) 150 mg • Inositol 150 mg • Proprietary Blend 7.5 mg: Alfalfa, Watercress, Parsley, Lecithin, and Rice Bran.

B-2 **-** Puritan's Pride
Each tablet contains: Vitamin B-2 (Riboflavin) 100 mg.

B-2 (100 mg) **-** Marlyn
Each tablet contains: Riboflavin (vitamin B2) 100 mg.

B4 - Skin Formula **-** Life Extension
Each tablet contains: Polysaccharides (marine protein fractions) 50 mg • L- Ascorbic Acid 30 mg • Silicon Dioxide 7 mg • L-Cysteine 5 mg • Zinc Gluconate 2 mg • Calcium Gluconate 1.8 mg • Selenomethionine 50 mcg • Vitamin A 2600 IU • D-Alpha Acetate 6 IU.

B-50 B-Complex Vitamin **-** Puritan's Pride
Each tablet contains: Thiamin (vitamin B1, as thiamin mononitrate) 50 mg • Riboflavin (vitamin B2) 50 mg • Niacin (as niacinamide) 50 mg • Vitamin B6 (as pyridoxine hydrochloride) 50 mg • Folic Acid 400 mcg • Vitamin B12 (as cyanocobalamin) 50 mcg • Biotin (as D-biotin) 50 mcg • Pantothenic Acid (as D-calcium pantothenate) 50 mg • PABA (para-aminobenzoic acid) 50 mg • Inositol 50 mg • Choline Bitartrate 50 mg • Proprietary Blend 2.5 mg: Alfalfa, Watercress, Parsley, Lecithin, Rice Bran. Other Ingredients: Cellulose (plant origin), Dicalcium Phosphate, Vegetable Stearic Acid, Croscarmellose, Cellulose Coating, Silica, Mannitol, Vegetable Magnesium Stearate.

B-50 Caps With C **-** Now
Each capsule contains: Vitamin B1 (Thiamine) 50 mg • Vitamin B2 (Riboflavin) 50 mg • Vitamin B3 (Niacinamide) 50 mg • Vitamin B6 (Pyridoxine) 50 mg • Vitamin B12 100 mcg • Biotin 100 mcg • Folic Acid 400 mcg • Pantothenic Acid 100 mg • Vitamin C (Ascorbic Acid) 250 mg • PABA 50 mg • Choline (Bitartrate) 50 mg • Inositol 50 mg.

B50 Complex **-** Jamieson
Each caplet contains: Vitamin B1 50 mg • Vitamin B2 50 mg • Vitamin B3 50 mg • Vitamin B6 50 mg • Vitamin B12 mcg • Biotin 50 mcg • Pantothenic Acid 50 mg • Folic Acid 0.4 mg. Lipotropic Factors: Choline Bitartrate 50 mg, Inositol 50 mg. Also contains Para-Aminobenzoic Acid.

B-50 Complex **-** Now
Each capsule contains: Vitamin B1 (Thiamine HCL) 50 mg • Vitamin B2 (Riboflavin) 50 mg • Vitamin B3 (Niacinamide) 50 mg • Vitamin B5 Pantothenic Acid 50 mg • Vitamin B6 (Pyridoxine HCL) 50 mg • Vitamin B12 (Cyanocobalamin) 50 mcg • Biotin 50 mcg • Folic Acid 400 mcg • PABA 50 mg • Choline (Bitartrate) 50 mg • Inositol 50 mg.

B-50 Complex **-** Rexall - Sundown
Each caplet contains: Thiamin (vitamin B1, as thiamin mononitrate) 50 mg • Riboflavin (vitamin B2) 50 mg • Niacin (as niacinamide) 50 mg • Vitamin B6 (as pyridoxine HCl) 50 mg • Folic Acid 400 mcg • Vitamin B12 (as cyanocobalamin) 50 mg • Biotin 50 mg • Pantothenic Acid (as calcium d-pantothenate) 50 mg • Calcium 36 mg • PABA (Para-Aminobenzoic Acid) 50 mg • Choline Bitartrate 50 mg • Inositol 5 mg • Alfalfa Base Complex 222 mcg: Alfalfa (leaves), Parsley (aerial parts), Watercress (aerial parts), Rice Bran. Other Ingredients: Dicalcium Phosphate, Microcrystalline Cellulose,

Croscarmellose Sodium, Hydrogenated Vegetable Oil, Hydroxypropyl Methylcellulose, Silica, Magnesium Stearate, Titanium Dioxide.

B-50 Vitamin B-Complex **-** Puritan's Pride
Each capsule contains: Thiamin (Vitamin B1; as thiamine mononitrate) 50 mg • Riboflavin (Vitamin B-2) 50 mg • Niacin (as niacinamide) 50 mg • Vitamin B6 (as pyridoxine hydrochloride) 50 mg • Folic Acid 100 mcg • Vitamin B12 (as cyanocobalamin) 50 mcg • Biotin (as d-biotin) 50 mcg • Pantothenic Acid (as d-calcium pantothenate) 50 mg • PABA (as para-aminobenzoic acid) 50 mg • Inositol 50 mg • Choline Bitartrate 50 mg • Proprietary Blend 2.5 mg: Alfalfa, Watercress, Parsley, Lecithin, Rice Bran.

B-6 100 mg **-** Puritan's Pride
Each tablet contains: Vitamin B-6 (Pyridoxine Hydrochloride) 100 mg.

B-6 100 mg **-** Progressive Labs
Each capsule contains: Vitamin B6 (pyridoxine HCl) 100 mg. Other Ingredients: Rice Flour, Magnesium Stearate, Gelatin.

B-6 100 mg **-** Rexall - Sundown
Each tablet contains: Vitamin B6 (as pyridoxine HCl) 100 mg • Calcium 38 mg. Other Ingredients: Dicalcium Phosphate, Croscarmellose Sodium, Magnesium Stearate.

B-6 200 mg **-** Puritan's Pride
Each tablet contains: Vitamin B-6 (Pyridoxine Hydrochloride) 200 mg.

B-6 50 mg **-** Puritan's Pride
Each tablet contains: Vitamin B-6 (Pyridoxine Hydrochloride) 50 mg.

B6 Min **-** Atrium Inc.
Each capsule contains: Vitamin B6 (Pyridoxine HCL) 200 mg • Magnesium Gluconate 120 mg • Potassium Gluconate 120 mg.

B-6 Timed Release **-** Source Naturals
Each tablet contains: Vitamin B6 (as pyridoxine HCl, from vegetables) 100 mg • Calcium 31 mg. Other Ingredients: Dibasic Calcium Phosphate, Microcrystalline Cellulose, Stearic Acid, Modified Cellulose Gum, Colloidal Silicon Dioxide, Magnesium Stearate.

B6+B Complex **-** Vital Nutrients
Each capsule contains: Thiamine HCl (vitamin B1) 50 mg • Riboflavin (vitamin B2) 20 mg • Riboflavin 5' Phosphate 5 mg • Niacinamide (vitamin B3) 100 mg • Pyridoxine HCl (vitamin B6) 250 mg • Pyridoxal 5 Phosphate 15 mg • Folic Acid 400 mcg • Hydrocobalamin (vitamin B12) 200 mcg • Biotin 200 mcg • Calcium Pantothenate (vitamin B5) 75 mg.

B75 Complex **-** Jamieson
Each tablet contains: Vitamin B1 75 mg • Vitamin B2 75 mg • Niacinamide 75 mg • Vitamin B6 75 mg • Vitamin B12 75 mcg • Biotin 75 mcg • Pantothenic Acid 75 mg • Folic Acid 0.6 mg. Lipotropic Factors: Choline Bitartrate 75 mg, Inositol 75 mg. Also contains Para-Aminobenzoic Acid.

Ba Wei Di Huang Wan (Rehmannia Eight Formula) **-** Qualiherb
Six honey-pills contain: Poria Cocos Rx. (fu ling) 39 mg • Moutan Radicis Cx. (mu dan pi) 39 mg • Alismatis Rz. (ze xie) 39 mg • Rehmanniae Rx. Prep. (shou di huang) 104 mg • Corni Fr. (shan zhu yu) 52 mg • Dioscoreae Rz. (shan yao) 52 mg • Fu Zi B. 13 mg • Cinnamomi Cx. (rou gui) 13 mg • Honey 249 mg.

Baby-Cal Syrup **-** Hadas Natural Products
Natural Citrus flavored Fructose-Glucose syrup • Fennel 200 mg • Chamomile 200 mg • Caraway 200 mg.

Baby's Bliss Gripe Water **-** MOM Enterprises, Inc.
Ingredients: Ginger • Fennel • Sodium Bicarbonate • Fructose • Deionized Water.

BackAche with Arnica **-** Hyland's
Two tablets contain: Benzoicum Acidum 3X • Colchicum Autumnale 3X • Sulphur 3X • Arnica Montana 6X • Rhus Toxicodendron 6X. Base: Lactose N.F.
See Editor's Note No. 1, page 2053.

Back-Relief **-** Futurebiotics
Four capsules contain: Magnesium (as magnesium amino acid chelate) 300 mg • Alfalfa whole juice 225 mg • Yucca root powder 200 mg • Cayenne fruit powder extract 25 mg • Valerian root powder extract 12 mg • Pancreatin 4X quadruple strength (supplying 1600 USP units lipase, 10000 USP units amylase, 1000 USP protease) 125 mg • DL-Phenylalanine 250 mg. Other Ingredients: Magnesium stearate, Gelatin, Water.
See Editor's Note No. 14, page 2055.

Bakol - Basikol **-** Arkopharma
Each capsule contains: Non-esterfied Phytosterols 200 mg • Vitamin E 2.5 mg.

Balance Meal Neutralizer **-** Legacy for Life
Two capsules contain: Betasanne Chitosan, Betaine HCl complex 450 mg.

BALANCE Shake (cafe mocha) **-** Legacy for Life
Protein blend: Whey Protein Isolate, Whey Protein Concentrate, Soy Protein Isolate, Egg Powder with immune components • Inulin • Decaffeinated Coffee • Natural and Artificial flavors • Cocoa (processed with alkali) • L-Taurine • Glucomannan • Cellulose Gum • Potassium Citrate • Calcium Carbonate • Dipotassium Phosphate • Soy Lecithin • Magnesium Oxide • Psyllium • Maltodextrin • Enzyme Blend: Proteases, Amylase, Lactase, Cellulase • Acesulfame Potassium • Sucralose.

BALANCE Shake (Dutch chocolate) **-** Legacy for Life
Protein blend: Whey Protein Isolate, Whey Protein Concentrate, Soy Protein Isolate, Egg Powder with immune components • Cocoa (processed with alkali) • Inulin • Natural and Artificial flavors • L-Taurine • Glucomannan • Cellulose Gum • Potassium Citrate • Calcium Carbonate • Dipotassium Phosphate • Soy Lecithin • Magnesium Oxide • Psyllium • Maltodextrin • Enzyme Blend: Proteases, Amylase, Lactase, Cellulase • Acesulfame Potassium • Sucralose.

BALANCE Shake (vanilla creme) **-** Legacy for Life
Protein Blend: Whey Protein Isolate, Whey Protein Concentrate, Soy Protein Isolate, Egg powder with immune components • Inulin • Natural and Artificial flavors • Potassium Citrate • L-Taurine • Glucomannan • Cellulose Gum • Calcium Carbonate • Dipotassium Phosphate • Soy Lecithin • Magnesium Oxide • Psyllium • Maltodextrin • Enzyme Blend: Proteases, Amylase, Lactase, Cellulase • Acesulfame Potassium • Sucralose.

Balanced B-100 Timed Release **-** Nature Made
Each tablet contains: Thiamin (thiamin mononitrate) 100 mg • Riboflavin 100 mg • Niacin (niacinamide) 100 mg • Vitamin B6 (pyridoxine hydrochloride) 100 mg • Folic Acid 400 mcg • Vitamin B12 (cyanocobalamin) 100 mcg • Biotin 100 mcg • Pantothenic Acid (D-calcium pantothenate) 100 mg. Other Ingredients: Dibasic Calcium Phosphate, Cellulose, Hydroxypropyl Methylcellulose, Stearic Acid, Silicon Dioxide, Magnesium Stearate, Croscarmellose Sodium, Polyethylene Glycol, Carnauba Wax.

Balanced B-50 Timed Release **-** Nature Made
Each tablet contains: Thiamin (thiamin mononitrate) 50 mg • Riboflavin 50 mg • Niacin (niacinamide) 50 mg • Vitamin B6 (pyridoxine hydrochloride) 50 mg • Folic Acid 400 mcg • Vitamin B12 (cyanocobalamin) 50 mcg • Biotin 50 mcg • Pantothenic Acid (D-calcium pantothenate) 50 mg. Other Ingredients: Dibasic Calcium Phosphate, Cellulose, Hydroxypropyl Methylcellulose, Stearic Acid, Silicon Dioxide, Magnesium Stearate, Polyethylene Glycol, Carnauba Wax.

Some Brand Name Natural Products - What they Contain

www.NaturalDatabase.com contains MANY more listings than appear here.

BRAND NAMES

Bao He Wan Plus **-** Secara
Three tablets contain: Chinese Hawthorn fruit 5:1 extract (shan zha) 516 mg • Organic Artichoke leaf 354 mg • Pinellia rhizome 5:1 extract (ban xia) 231 mg • Hoelen Sclerotium 5:1 extract (fu ling) 231 mg • Organic Gentian root (qin jiao) 192 mg • Massa Fermentata 5:1 extract (shen qu) 192 mg • Tangerine peel 4:1 extract (chen pi) 153 mg • Papain 135 mg • Radish seed 5:1 extract (lai fu zi) 96 mg • Forsythia fruit 5:1 extract (lian qiao) 93 mg • Bromelain 2400 GDU/ gram 45 mg • Lactase 12 mg.

Barlean's Flax Oil **-** The Vitamin Shoppe
Each 1 tsp serving provides: Omega-3 7.7 g • Omega-6 2.3 g • Omega 9 2.2 g • VitaLox [a natural protectant blend of Ascorbic Acid and Rosemary extracts] 30 mg.

Barlean's Flax Oil High Lignin Formula **-** The Vitamin Shoppe
Each tablespoon provides: Omega-3 6.1 g • Omega-6 1.8 g • Omega 9 1.7 g • Flaxseed Particles 2.6 g • VitaLox [a natural protectant blend of ascorbic acid and rosemary extracts] 30 mg.

Barlean's Vita-Flax **-** The Vitamin Shoppe
Certified Organic Flax Seed Powder containing: Protein (NX6.25) 34.7% • Fat 14.7% • Energy 435 Kcal/100 g. Vitamin E 0.01% • Dietary Fiber 34.2%. Total Fiber: Soluble Fiber 38%, Insoluble Fiber 62%.

BarleyGreen Premium **-** AIM USA
Ten caplets contain: Vitamin A (as beta-carotene) 1000 IU • Vitamin C 9 mg • Calcium 35 mg • Iron 0.5 mg • Sodium 50 mg • Magnesium 12 mg • Potassium 240 mg • Iodine 20 mcg • Chlorophyll 13 mg. Ingredients: Organic Young Barley Grass Juice, Organic Maltodextrin, Organic Brown Rice, Kelp (Kombu), Magnesium Stearate.

BarleyLife **-** AIM USA
Each tablespoon (5 g) contains: Vitamin A (beta-carotene) 1370 IU • Vitamin B1 (thiamin) 0.04 mg • Vitamin B2 (riboflavin) 0.0895 mg • Vitamin B6 0.0635 mg • Vitamin B12 0.0385 mg • Folic Acid 5.3 mg • Niacin 0.4295 mg • Pantothenic Acid 0.11 mg • Vitamin C 1.39 mg • Vitamin E 0.505 IU • Vitamin K 121.5 mcg • Calcium 45.25 mg • Chromium 1.1 mcg • Copper 0.0255 mg • Iodine 22 mcg • Iron 0.745 mg • Magnesium 11 mg • Manganese 0.1595 mg • Molybdenum 0.0015 mg • Phosphorous 20.7 mg • Zinc 0.1135 mg. Ingredients: Green Barley Juice, Maltodextrin, Brown Rice, Kelp.

Basic Antioxidant **-** GNC
Each capsule contains: Vitamin A (as Natural beta-Carotene) 5000 IU •Vitamin C (as Ascorbic Acid) 300 mg • Vitamin E (as d-alpha Tocopherol) 200 IU • Selenium (as Selenium Yeast) 200 mcg. Other Ingredients: Soybean Oil, Gelatin, Glycerin, Caramel Color, Titanium Dioxide.

Basic Vita-Vim - Level 1 Potency Multivitamin **-** Jamieson
Each caplet contains: Vitamin A (Acetate) 2000 IU • Beta Carotene 3000 IU • Vitamin D 400 IU • Vitamin C 90 mg • Vitamin E 25 IU • Vitamin B1 2.25 mg • Vitamin B2 3.2 mg • Vitamin B3 (No Flush Niacinamide) 40 mg • Vitamin B5 10 mg • Vitamin B6 3 mg • Vitamin B12 14 mcg • Folic Acid 400 mcg • Biotin 45 mcg • Calcium 175 mg • Iron (from Fumarate) 10 mg • Copper 2 mg • Iodine 0.15 mg • Magnesium 50 mg • Phosphorus 125 mg • Lutein 300 mcg.

B-Assure **-** The Vitamin Shoppe
Each capsule contains: 100 mg Champignon (Agaricus bisporus) stem and cap.

B-Basic **-** PhysioLogics
Each capsule contains: Vitamin B6 (as pyridoxine hydrochloride) 25 mg • Folic Acid 800 mcg • Vitamin B12 (as cyanocobalamin) 100 mcg • Betaine Hydrochloride 50 mg. Other Ingredients: Rice Powder, Gelatin, Vegetable Magnesium Stearate, Silica.

BCAA 1000 Caps **-** Optimum Nutrition
Two capsules contain: L-Leucine 500 mg • L-Isoleucine 250 mg • L-Valine 250 mg. Other Ingredients: Gelatin, Magnesium Stearate.

BCAA 5000 Powder **-** Optimum Nutrition
Each 1 tsp (5 g) serving contains: L-Valine 1250 mg • L-Leucine 2500 mg • L-Isoleucine 1250 mg.

B-Com **-** Professional Botanicals
Each capsule contains: Thiamin (vitamin B1) 50 mg • Riboflavin (vitamin B2) 50 mg • Niacin (as niacinamide) 50 mg • Vitamin B6 50 mg • Folate (folic acid) 100 mcg • Vitamin B12 50 mcg • Pantothenic Acid 100 mg • D-Biotin 50 mcg • Choline Bitartrate 50 mg • Inositol 50 mg • PABA (para amino benzoic acid) 50 mg. Other Ingredients: Alfalfa, Watercress, Parsley, Lecithin, Rice Bran, EDS Enzymes/ Cofactors.

B-Complex **-** Vital Nutrients
Each capsule contains: Thiamine HCl (vitamin B1) 100 mg • Riboflavin (vitamin B2) 25 mg • Riboflavin 5' Phosphate (activated vitamin B2) 10 mg • Pyridoxine HCl (vitamin B6) 25 mg • Pyridoxal 5' Phosphate (activated vitamin B6) 15 mg • Calcium Pantothenate (vitamin B5) 200 mg • Hydroxocobalamin (vitamin B12, pure powder) 500 mcg • Inositol Hexaniacinate (no-flush niacin) 25 mg • Niacinamide 75 mg • Folic Acid (pure powder) 800 mcg • Biotin (pure powder) 400 mcg.

B-Complex **-** Health Smart Vitamins
Each caplet contains: Thiamin (as thiamin mononitrate) 100 mg • Riboflavin 100 mg • Niacin (as niacinamide) 100 mg • Vitamin B6 (as pyridoxine hydrochloride) 100 mg • Folate (folic acid) 400 mcg • Vitamin B12 (as cyanocobalamin) 100 mcg • Biotin 300 mcg • Pantothenic acid (as calcium pantothenate) 100 mg • Calcium (as dicalcium phosphate, calcium pantothenate, calcium stearate) 100 mg • Phosphorus (as dicalcium phosphate) 70 mg • Choline (as choline bitartrate) 100 mg • Inositol 100 mg • Para-aminobenzoic acid 100 mg.

B-Complex **-** Nutri-Quest Rx
Two tablets contain: Vitamin B1 100 mg • Vitamin B2 100 mg • Vitamin B6 50 mg • Niacinamide 100 mg • Pantothenic Acid 100 mg • Vitamin B12 100 mcg • Folic Acid 300 mcg • Biotin 100 mcg • Choline Bitartrate 100 mg • Inositol 100 mg • PABA 50 mg.

B-Complex & B-12 **-** Puritan's Pride
Each tablet contains: Thiamin (Vitamin B1; as Thiamine Hydrochloride and Brewer's Yeast) 7 mg • Riboflavin (Vitamin B2) (as Riboflavin and Brewer's Yeast) 14 mg • Niacin (as Niacin and Brewer's Yeast) 4.5 mg • Vitamin B12 (as Cyanocobalamin and Brewer's Yeast) 25 mcg • Protease (as Papain Powder) 10 mg.

B-Complex 100 **-** The Vitamin Shoppe
Each capsule contains: Vitamin B1 100 mg • Vitamin B2 100 mg • Vitamin B6 100 mg • Vitamin B12 100 mcg • Niacinamide 100 mg • Folic Acid 400 mcg • Pantothenic Acid 100 mg • D-Biotin 100 mcg • Choline Bitartrate 100 mg • Inositol 100 mg • PABA 100 mg.

B-Complex 125 - GNC A-Z **-** GNC
Each tablet contains: Vitamin C (as Ascorbic Acid) 125 mg • Thiamin (as Thiamin Mononitrate) 125 mg • Riboflavin 125 mg • Niacin (as Niacinamide) 125 mg • Vitamin B6 (Pyridoxine Hydrochloride) 125 mg • Folate, Folic Acid, Folacin 400 mcg • Vitamin B12 (as Cyanocobalamin) 125 mcg • Biotin 125 mcg • Pantothenic Acid (as Calcium d-Pantothenate) 125 mg • Choline Bitartrate 125 mg • Inositol 125 mcg • Para-aminobenzoic Acid (PABA) 75 mg. Other Ingredients: Cellulose, Dicalcium Phosphate, Vegetable Acetoglycerides, Rose Hips powder (Rosina canina), Brewer's Yeast, Lecithin, Alfalfa leaf powder (Medicago sativa), Watercress herb powder (Nasturtium officinale), Parsley herb powder (Petroselinum sativum), Whole Brown Rice (Oryza sativa).

Some Brand Name Natural Products - What they Contain

www.NaturalDatabase.com contains MANY more listings than appear here.

B-Complex 50 - GNC A-Z - GNC
Each capsule contains: Thiamin (as Thiamin Mononitrate) 50 mg • Riboflavin (vitamin B2) 50 mg • Niacin (as Niacinamide) 50 mg • Vitamin B6 (as Pyridoxine Hydrochloride) 50 mg • Folate, Folic Acid, Folacin 400 mcg • Vitamin B12 (as Cyanocobalamin) 50 mcg • Biotin 50 mcg • Pantothenic acid (as Calcium d-Pantothenate) 50 mg • Choline Bitartrate 50 mg • Inositol 50 mg • Para-aminobenzoic Acid (PABA) 50mg. Other Ingredients: Gelatin, Mono- & Diglycerides, Whole Brown rice powder (Oryza sativa), Brewer's Yeast, Lecithin, Alfalfa leaf powder (Medicago sativa), Watercress herb powder (Nasturcium officinale), Parsley herb powder (Petroselinum sativum).

B-Complex 50 mg - Nature's Life
Each tablet contains: Vitamin B1 (Thiamine HCl) 50 mg • Vitamin B2 (Riboflavin) 50 mg • Vitamin B6 (Pyridoxine HCl) 50 mg • Vitamin B12 (Cobalamin concentrate) 50 mcg • Niacinamide 50 mg • Pantothenic Acid (d-Calcium Pantothenate) 50 mg • Choline (Bitartrate) 50 mg • Inositol 50 mg • Biotin 50 mcg • Folic Acid 400 mcg • PABA (Para Aminobenzioc Acid) 50 mg • Lecithin 8 mg. In a natural base of Alfalfa, Parsley, Rice Bran & Watercress.

B-Complex 75 Complete - GNC A-Z - GNC
Two tablets contain: Vitamin A (50% as beta-Carotene and 50% as Retinyl Acetate) 10,000 IU • Vitamin C (as Ascorbic Acid) 500 mg • Vitamin D (as Cholecalciferol) 400 IU • Vitamin E (as d-alpha tocopheryl succinate) 100 IU • Thiamin (as Thiamin Mononitrate) 75 mg • Riboflavin 75 mg • Niacin (as Niacinamide and Niacin) 75 mg • Vitamin B6 (as Pyridoxine Hydrochloride) 75 mg • Folate, Folic Acid, Folacin 400 mcg • Vitamin B12 (as Cyanocobalamin) 250 mcg • Biotin 75 mcg • Pantothenic acid (as Calcium d-Pantothenate) 100 mg • Iron (as Ferrous Fumarate) 18 mg • Selenium (as Hydrolyzed Rice Protien Chelate) 50 mcg • Copper (as Copper Gluconate) 2 mg • Chromium (as Hydrolyzed Rice Protien chelate) 25 mcg • Citrus Bioflavonoid Complex 100 mg • Bee Pollen 50 mg • Valerian root powder (Valeriana officinalis) 25 mg • Licorice root powder (Glycyrrhiza glabra) 25 mg • Goldenseal herb powder (Hydrastis Canadensis) 50 mg • Korean Ginseng root powder (Panax Ginseng) 50 mg • Guarana seed extract (Paullinia cupana) 50 mg. Other Ingredients: Dicalcium Phosphate, Cellulose, Food Glaze.

B-Complex Sublingual Liquid - Puritan's Pride
Each 1 dropper serving (1.0 cc) contains: Vitamin C (as Ascorbic Acid) 60 mg • Riboflavin (Vitamin B2; as Riboflavin 5-Phosphate Sodium) 1.7 mg • Niacin (as Niacinamide) 20 mg • Vitamin B6 (as Pyridoxine Hydrochloride) 2 mg • Vitamin B12 (as Cyanocobalamin) 1,200 mcg • Pantothenic Acid (as Dexpanthenol) 30 mg.

B-Complex Supplement - Leiner Health Products
Each tablet contains: Thiamin Mononitrate (Vitamin B1) 10 mg • Riboflavin (Vitamin B2) 10 mg • Vitamin B6 (Pyridoxine Hydrochloride) 10 mg • Niacin (Niacinamide) 10 mg • Biotin (USP Method 2) 10 mcg • Folate (Folic Acid) 100 mcg • Vitamin B12 (Cyanocobalamin - USP Method 2) 10 mcg • Pantothenic Acid 10 mg. Other Ingredients: Calcium Carbonate, Maltodextrin, Hydroxypropyl Methycellulose, d-Calcium Pantothenate, Cellulose, Starch, Para-Aminobenzoic Acid, Croscarmellose Sodium, Sodium Starch Glycolate, Silicon Dioxide, Hydroxypropyl Cellulose, Red 40 Lake, Polyethylene Glycol 3350, Magnesium Stearate, Resin, Dicalcium Phosphate, Polysorbate 80, Titanium Dioxide, Povidone, Pharmaceutical Glaze.

B-Complex with B-12 Sublingual Liquid - Nature's Bounty
Each dropperful (1 mL) contains: Riboflavin (vitamin B2, as riboflavin 5'-phosphate sodium) 1.7 mg • Niacin (as niacinamide) 20 mg • Vitamin B6 (as pyridoxine hydrochloride) 2 mg • Vitamin B12 (as cyanocobalamin) 1200 mcg • Pantothenic Acid (as dexpanthenol) 30 mg. Other Ingredients: Purified Water, Sorbitol, Glycerin, Citric Acid, Potassium Sorbate, Natural Flavors.

B-Complex with Folic Acid - Biodelivery Nutritional Systems - Nutritional Therapeutics, Inc.
Two tablets contain: Choline Bitartrate 250 mg • D-Calcium Pantothenate 100 mg • Inositol 100 mg • Niacinamide 100 mg • PABA 50 mg • Riboflavin 50 mg • Thiamine HCL 50 mg • Pyridoxine HCL 45 mg • Pantethine 25 mg • Pyridoxal -5-Phosphate 5 mg • Biotin 200 mcg • Folic Acid 800 mcg • Cyanocobalamin 200 mcg • NT Factor tablet base 355 mg.

B-Complex with Vitamin C - Nature Made
Each caplet contains: Vitamin C (from ascorbic acid) 300 mg • Thiamin (from thiamin mononitrate) 15 mg • Riboflavin 10.2 mg • Niacin (from niacinamide ascorbate) 50 mg • Vitamin B6 (from pyridoxine hydrochloride) 5 mg • Pantothenic Acid (from D-calcium pantothenate) 10 mg. Other Ingredients: Dibasic Calcium Phosphate, Cellulose Gel, Croscarmellose Sodium, Hydroxypropyl Methylcellulose, Magnesium Stearate, Polyethylene Glycol.
See Editor's Note No. 45, page 2058.

BCQ - Vital Nutrients
Each capsule contains: Boswellia Serrata (65% boswellic acids) 200 mg • Bromelain (2400 gdu/2600 mcu) 100 mg • Curcuma Longa (curcumin 95%) 200 mg • Quercetin 100 mg.

Be Sure - Wakunaga of America
Two caplets contain: Aspergillus Enzyme Complex 300 mg. Other Ingredients: Cellulose, Silica, Magnesium Stearate (vegetable source).

Bean & Vegi Formula - Enzymatic Therapy
Two capsules contain: Pure Plant Enzymes Blend 235 mg: Alpha-Galactosidase (FCC IV [pH5.5]) 900 GalU, Amylase (USP XXI [pH6.8]) 16,500 USP (FCC IV [pH4.8]) 7140 DU, Cellulase I, II (FCC IV [Ph4.5]) 332 CU, Protease I,II,III (USP XXIII [Ph7.5]) 6550 USP (FCC IV [Ph7.0] 10,500 PC.. FCC IV [Ph4.7] 11,900 HUT, Lipase II (FCC III [Ph6.5]) 54 LU.

Bean Pods - Arkopharma
Each capsule contains: White Kidney Bean pods (phaseolus vulgaris) 320 mg.

beCalm'd - Neurogenesis Inc.
Each capsule contains: D / L-Phenylalanine 300 mg • L-Glutamine 150 mg • 5-HTP 5 mg • Vitamin B6 (pyridoxine HCl) 1 mg • Calcium (chelate, citrate) 50 mg • Magnesium (chelate, oxide) 25 mg • Folic Acid 0.01 mg.

Bedwetting Tablets - Hyland's
Each tablet contains: Equisetum hyemale as Scouring Rush 3X HPUS • Rhus aromatica (Fragrant Sumac) 3X HPUS • Belladonna 3X HPUS (0.0003% Allkaloids). In a base of Lactose NF (Milk Sugar).
See Editor's Note No. 1, page 2053.

Bee Complete - Futurebiotics
Two tablets contain: Bee Pollen 1,000 mg • Royal Jelly 25 mg • Bee Propolis 500 mg.

Bee Pollen - Source Naturals
Each tablet contains: Whole nugget Bee Pollen 500 mg.

Bee Pollen Chewable - Atrium Inc.
Each tablet contains: Bee Pollen 300 mg.

Bee Pollen Complex - Puritan's Pride
Each tablet contains: Bee Pollen 1000 mg • Bee Propolis 10 mg • Royal Jelly 10 mg.

Beef Liver 1500 mg - Nature's Life
Six tablets contain: Argentine Beef Liver (defatted, desicated, pesticide free) 9000 mg • Vitamin B12 (cobalamin concentrate) 1000 mcg • Vitamin B2 457 mcg • Vitamin B6 224 mcg • Vitamin B12 1 mg • Niacin 2.2 mg • Choline 94 mg • Calcium 2.7 mg • Copper 90 mcg • Iron 6.3 mg • Manganese 90 mcg • Potassium 94 mg • Sodium 28 mg • Zinc 1.3 mg • Amino Acids (naturally occurring): Alanine 747 mg • Arginine 297 mg • Aspartic Acid 99 mg • Cysteine 351 mg • Cystine 103 mg • Glutamic Acid 108 mg • Glysine 792 mg • Histidine (essential amino acid) 198 mg • Isoleucine (essential amino acid) 207 mg • Leucine (essential amino acid) 198 mg • Lysine (essential amino acid) 558 mg • Methionine (essential amino acid)

315 mg • Phenylalanine (essential amino acid) 369 mg • Proline 99 mg • Serine 441 mg • Threonine (essential amino acid) 306 mg • Tyrosine 396 mg • Tryptophan (essential amino acid) 36 mg • Valine (essential amino acid) 90 mg.
See Editor's Note No. 14, page 2055.

Bee-Happy Plus **-** Bee-Alive Inc.
Each capsule contains: Rhodiola Rosea root extract (standardized to 1% rosavins 0.5 mg) 50 mg • St. John's Wort flowering tops extract (standardized to 0.3% hypericin 0.45 mg) 150 mg • Siberian Ginseng root (eleutherococcus senticosus) 25 mg • Honey (dried) 25 mg. Other Ingredients: Microcrystalline Cellulose, Stearic Acid, Magnesium Stearate, Calcium Silicate, Gelatin (capsule shell).

Beelith **-** Beach Pharmaceuticals
Each tablet contains: Magnesium Oxide (equivalent to 362 mg of magnesium) 600 mg • Pyridoxine Hydrochloride (equivalent of Vitamin B6) 20 mg.

beeSatisfied Fruit Bar (Blueberry) **-** Bee-Alive Inc.
Each bar (35 g) contains: Apples • Honey • Blueberries • Natural Flavor • Ascorbic Acid • Non-Freeze Dried Royal Jelly.

beeSatisfied Fruit Bar (Raspberry) **-** Bee-Alive Inc.
Each bar (35 g) contains: Apples • Honey • Raspberries • Natural Flavor • Ascorbic Acid • Non-Freeze Dried Royal Jelly.

beeSatisfied Fruit Bar (Strawberry) **-** Bee-Alive Inc.
Each bar (35 g) contains: Apples • Honey • Strawberries • Natural Flavor • Ascorbic Acid • Non-Freeze Dried Royal Jelly.

Bend & Flex **-** Gero Vita International
Two capsules contain: Glucosamine Sulfate 500 mg • Turmeric rhizome extract (95% curcumin) 400 mg • Nexrutine (phellodendron bark extract) 250 mg • Exclzyme (proprietary blend of enzymes) 200 mg • Black Pepper fruit extract (10% volatile oil) 20 mg • Piper Longum fruit extract (2.5% piperine) 20 mg • Ginger rhizome extract (5% volatile oils) 20 mg. Other Ingredients: Gelatin, Silicon Dioxide, Magnesium Stearate.

BeneCardia **-** Natrol
Each tablet contains: Niacin (as inositol hexa-nicotinate) 600 mg • Bovine Protein Hydrolysate 25 mg • Policosanol (from rice bran, carnauba and candelilla wax) 5 mg. Other Ingredients: Cellulose, Stearic Acid, Silica, Cellulose Gum, Magnesium Stearate, Methylcellulose, Glycerin.

Benecol **-** McNeil Consumer Healthcare
Three softgels contain: Plant Stanol Esters 1.5 g. Other Ingredients: Gelatin, Glycerin, Sunflower Oil, Titanium Dioxide, Soybean Oil, Annatto Extract, Red 40, Yellow 8, Blue 1, Yellow 5.

Benecol Light Spread **-** McNeil Consumer Healthcare
Liquid Canola oil • Water • Partially Hydrogenated Soybean oil • Liquid Soybean oil • Plant Stanol Esters • Salt • Emulsifiers (vegetable mono- and diglycerides, soy lecithin, polyglycerol esters of fatty acids) • Potassium Sorbate • Citric Acid • Calcium Disodium EDTA • Artificial Flavor • DL-Alpha Tocopheryl Acetate • Vitamin A Palmitate • Beta Carotene.

Benecol Regular Spread **-** McNeil Consumer Healthcare
Liquid Canola oil • Water • Partially Hydrogenated Soybean oil • Liquid Soybean oil • Plant Stanol Esters • Salt • Emulsifiers (vegetable mono- and diglycerides, soy lecithin, polyglycerol esters of fatty acids) • Potassium Sorbate • Citric Acid • Calcium Disodium EDTA • Artificial Flavor • DL-Alpha Tocopheryl Acetate • Vitamin A Palmitate • Beta Carotene.

Benecol Smart Chews **-** McNeil Consumer Healthcare
Each chew contains: Plant Stanol Esters 0.85 g.

Benefiber **-** Novartis
Partially hydrolyzed Guar Gum.

BeneFin Caplets **-** LaneLabs
Four caplets contain: BeneFin Organically Processed Whole Shark Cartilage 750 mg • Calcium 591 mg • Phosphorous 315 mg • Magnesium 8 mg • Zinc 135 mcg • Sodium 18 mg • Potassium 1 mg. Other Ingredients: Carnauba Wax, Hypromellose, Magnesium Stearate, Microcrystalline Cellulose, Tragacanth Gum.
See Editor's Note No. 9 and No. 21, pages 2054 and 2056.

Benejoint **-** LaneLabs
Menthol (1.25%) • Aloe Vera • Apricot kernal oil • BeneFin Shark Cartilage (providing glucosamine, collagen, chondroitin sulfate) • Capsaicin • Carbomer • Cetyl Esters Wax • Citrus seed extract • Imidazolidinyl Urea • Jojoba oil • Lanolin Anhydrous • Lavender oil • Lemon • Methylhydroxybenzoate • Polawax GP200 • Propylhydroxybenzoate • Soft White Parafin • Water.

Benzo Berries **-** Unknown
Two tablets contain: 5-HTP extract 10X • Phenepropaloxamine • Valerian root extract 10X • Wild Berry extract 10X • Kava Kava extract 10X • Bioperine Black Pepper extract.

Berberine Complex **-** PhytoPharmica
Two capsules contain: Berberis Vulgaris bark of root 6:1 extract (barberry) 400 mg • Oregon Grape root 6:1 extract (berberis aquifolium) 400 mg • Goldenseal root and rhizome 4:1 extract (hydrastis canadensis, standardized to contain 5% total alkaloids including berberine, hydrastine, and canadine) 100 mg.

Berberis Formula **-** Genestra - Seroyal
Each capsule contains: Barberry extract 4:1 (equivalent to 800 mg) 200 mg • Oregon Grape extract 4:1 (equivalent to 800 mg) 200 mg • Goldenseal extract (standardized 5%) 50 mg • Barberry 25 mg • Oregon Grape 25 mg. Contains no less than 4,500 mcg Hydrastine and Berberine.

Berry Barley Essence **-** Green Foods Corp.
Each 5.3 oz jar contains: Proprietary Blend 150 g: Young Barley Grass powdered juice, Maltodextrin, Raspberry, Strawberry, Other Natural Flavors, Chicory root extract (contains FOS), Brown rice, Stevia Extract.

BerryVida brand **-** Cyvex Nutrition, Inc.
High ORAC Berries with Polyphenols, Anthocyanin and Ellagic Acid.
See Editor's Note No. 44, page 2058.

Best Defense High-Potency Herbal Defense Complex **-** Pro Health
Three tablets contain: Vitamin A (as palmitate 4000 IU, beta carotene 1000 IU) 5000 IU • Vitamin C (from ascorbic acid, zinc, calcium, magnesium ascorbates) 1278 mg • Calcium 47 mg • Zinc (as zinc ascorbate) 23 mg • Selenium (as sodium selenate) 25 mcg • Copper (as copper sebacate) 300 mcg • Garlic Clove 360 mg • Propolis 324 mg • Boneset leaf 238 mg • Polygonum Odoratum rhizome 200 mg • Echinacea root 196 mg • Echinacea extract 164 mg • Isatis root/leaf 159 mg • Isatis root/leaf 159 mg • Horehound stems 150 mg • Propolis extract 126 mg • Bioflavonoids 120 mg • Astragalus root 90 mg • Angelica root 87 mg • Mullein leaf 80 mg • Goldenseal root 75 mg • Eleutherococcus Senticosus root 65 mg • Hawthorn berry 55 mg • Oregon Grape root 55 mg • Eleutherococcus Senticosus root extract 54 mg • Pau D'Arco bark extract 36 mg • Cayenne fruit 30 mg. Other Ingredients: Modified Cellulose Gum, Stearic Acid, Colloidal Silicon Dioxide, Calcium, Magnesium Ascorbate, Magnesium Stearate.

Best Friends **-** Changes International, Inc.
Each tablet contains: Vitamin A (as Alpha- and Beta-Carotene with mixed Carotenoids from D. Salina algae) 5000 IU • Vitamin C (as Ascorbic Acid with Sodium and Calcium Ascorbates) 100 mg • Vitamin D (as Cholecalciferol) 400 IU • Vitamin E (as mixed natural D-Alpha and DL-Alpha-Tocopherol Acetate) 80 IU • Thiamin (as Thiamin HCl) 1.5 mg • Riboflavin 1.7 mg • Niacin (as Niacinamide) 2 mg • Vitamin B6 (as Pyridoxine HCl) 2 mg • Folate (as Folic Acid) 400 mcg • Vitamin B12 (as Cyanocobalamin) 12 mcg • Biotin

75 mcg • Pantothenic Acid (as D-Calcium Pantothenate) 10 mg • Calcium (as Calcium Carbonate and Citrate) 125 mg • Iron (as Ferrous Fumarate) 5 mg • Iodine (as Potassium Iodide) 75 mcg • Magnesium (as Magnesium Oxide, Glycinate, and Citrate) 40 mg • Zinc (as Zinc Citrate and Glycinate) 5 mg • Selenium (as Selenomethionine) 25 mcg • Copper (as Copper Oxide, Citrate, Gluconate, and Glycinate) 2 mg •Manganese (as Manganese Sulfate, Citrate, Gluconate, and Glycinate) 1 mg • Chromium (as Chromium Dinicotinate Glycinate) 50 mcg • Molybdenum (as natural Molybdic Acid) 50 mcg • Fruit and vegetable phytonutrient concentrates 1500 mg: Dunaliela salina algae, Parsley, Tomato, Spinach, Kale, Yellow Squash, Turmeric, Orange, Cranberry, Lemon, Tangerine, Grapefruit, Red Grape, Strawberry, Cherry, Peach, Raspberry, Onion, Garlic, Leek, Broccoli, Cauliflower, Mustard Greens, Cabbage. Other Ingredients: Fructose, Sorbitol, Natural and Artificial flavors, Microcrystalline Cellulose, Stearic Acid, Carrageenan, Glycine, Maltodextrin, Citric Acid, Magnesium Stearate, Silica, Fractionated vegetable oil, Salt, and Carmine red.

BestCafe - NutriCology
Each 2 mL (60 drops) serving contains: Proprietary Blend 2 mL: Ginkgo Biloba, Catechins, Resveratrol, Ginsenoside. Other Ingredients: Natural Coffee Flavor, Vegetable Glycerin, Purified Water.

Beta 1,3 Glucan - PhysioLogics
Each tablet contains: Beta 1,3 Glucan (saccharomyces cerevisiae, from cell wall concentrate). Other Ingredients: Cellulose (plant origin), Dicalcium Phosphate, Acacia Gum, Vegetable Stearic Acid, Croscarmellose, Silica, Cellulose Coating, Vegetable Magnesium Stearate.

Beta 1,3 Glucans - Solgar
Each tablet contains: Beta 1,3 Glucans (from yeast cell wall concentrate Saccaromyces cerevisiae) 200 mg. Inactive Ingredients: Microcrystalline Cellulose, Vegetable Cellulose, Vegetable Stearic Acid, Titanium Dioxide, Vegetable Glycerin, Silica, Vegetable Magnesium Stearate, Caramel.

Beta Carotene - Olympian Labs
Each softgel contains: Beta Carotene 25000 IU.

Beta Carotene - Puritan's Pride
Each softgel contains: Beta Carotene (25,000 IU) 15 mg.

Beta Carotene 10,000 IU - Jamieson
Each caplet contains: Beta Carotene 10,000 IU.

Beta Carotene 25,000 IU - Rexall - Sundown
Each softgel contains: Vitamin A (100% as beta-carotene) 25,000 IU. Inactive Ingredients: Soybean Oil, Gelatin, Glycerin, Water.

Beta Carotene 25,000 IU - Jamieson
Each caplet contains: Beta Carotene (Pro-Vitamin A) 25,000 IU (15 mg).

Beta Carotene 25,000 IU - Nature Made
Each softgel contains: Vitamin A (100% as beta carotene) 25,000 IU. Other Ingredients: Soybean Oil, Gelatin, Glycerin, Partially Hydrogenated Cottonseed Oil and Soybean Oil, Water.
See Editor's Note No. 45, page 2058.

Beta Carotene 25,000 IU with Vitamin C & E - Jamieson
Each caplet contains: Beta Carotene 25,000 IU (15 mg) • Vitamin C (Ascorbic Acid) 250 mg • Vitamin E (Succinate) 100 IU.

Beta Carotene 5000 IU Chewable - Jamieson
Each tablet contains: Beta Carotene (Pro-Vitamin A) 5000 IU (3 mg).

Beta Carotene 6 - GNC A-Z - GNC
Each capsule contains: Vitamin A (as beta-Carotene 6 mg) 10,000 IU. Other Ingredients: Soybean oil, Gelatin, Glycerin, Partially Hydrogenated Corn oil.

Beta Carotene Provitamin A - Nature's Bounty
Each softgel contains: Vitamin A (as 100% Beta Carotene) 10000 IU. Other Ingredients: Soybean Oil, Gelatin, Beeswax, Glycerin, Lecithin.

Beta Carotene Provitamin A - Puritan's Pride
Each softgel contains: Beta Carotene (10000 IU) 6 mg.

Beta Carotene with Vitamin D - Puritan's Pride
Each softgel contains: Beta Carotene (25,000 IU) 15 mg • Vitamin D 400 IU.

Beta Fast GXR - Informulab
Each tablet contains: Gymnema Sylvestre (25% standardized extract) 400 mg.

Beta Glucan - Pro Health
Each capsule contains: Saccharomyces Cerevisiae Glucan-A extract (cell wall, providing 70-75% polysacharrides as beta 1-3-glucans 350-375 mg) 500 mg. Other Ingredients: Gelatin, Magnesium Stearate, Water.

Beta Glucan - Source Naturals
Each capsule contains: Purified beta-1, 3-glucan (derived from baker's yeast cell wall) 7.5 mg.

Beta Glucans - Natrol
Two capsules contain: Oat Bran extract Seed (Avena sativa) 1500 mg, supplying Beta Glucan 185 mg. Other Ingredients: Oat Bran powder, Magnesium Stearate, Gelatin.

Beta Sitosterol - Source Naturals
Three tablets contain: Soybean Hull 750 mg (yielding total sterols 660 mg, 324 mg as beta-sitosterol). Other Ingredients: Microcrystalline Cellulose, Dibasic Calcium, Phosphate, Sorbitol, Stearic Acid, Colloidal Silicon Dioxide, Magnesium Stearate, Modified Cellulose Gum.

BETA-C - Pharmagel
Beta Hydroxy Acid • Stabilized Vitamin C.

Beta-Carotene 15 - GNC A-Z - GNC
Each capsule contains: Vitamin A (100% as beta-Carotene 15mg) 25,000 IU. Other Ingredients: Soybean Oil, Gelatin, Partially Hydrogenated Corn Oil, Glycerin.

Beta-Carotene 25 - GNC
Each tablet contains: Vitamin A (as beta-Carotene) 41,666 IU. Other Ingredients: Dicalcium Phosphate, Cellulose.

Beta-Carotene 25,000 IU - Schiff
Each softgel contains: Vitamin A (100% as beta carotene) 25,000 IU. Other Ingredients: Carrot Oil, Softgel (soybean oil, gelatin, glycerin), Purified Water.

BetaGen - EAS
Each 6.6 gram serving contains: Ca HMB Monohydrate 1000 mg • Creatine Monohydrate 2000 mg • Potassium Phosphate 50 mg • L-Glutamine 400 mg • Taurine 200 mg. Ingredients: Dextrose, Phosphagen (HPCE pure Creatine Monohydrate) • Calcium b-Hydroxy b-Methylbutyrate Monohydrate • Citric Acid • L-Glutamine • Natural Flavors • Taurine • Potassium Phosphate • Aspartame • Beta-Carotene for color. Contains Phenylalanine.

Betaine HCl/Pepsin & Gentian - Vital Nutrients
Each capsule contains: Betaine HCl 520 mg • Pepsin (1:15,000, pure un-cut pepsin, lactose free) 21 mg • Gentian root extract (5:1, equivalent to gentian root powder 250 mg) 50 mg.

BetaLean Ephedra Free - EAS
Two tablets contain: Calcium (from calcium carbonate) 360 mg • Chromium (from chromium polynicotinate) 150 mcg • Green Tea leaf extract (50% polyphenols, 150mg; 35% catechins, 105%; 9% epigallocatechin gallate, EGCG, 27 mg) 300 mg • Bitter Orange fruit (6% synephrine, 18 mg) 300 mg • Proprietary Blend 225 mg: L-Tyrosine, Potassium Phosphate, White Willow bark, L-Carnitine

(tartate) • Caffeine (from caffeine anhydrous, green tea leaf) 200 mg • Naringin (from grapefruit) 75 mg. Other Ingredients: Stearic Acid, Microcrystalline Cellulose, Magnesium Stearate, Silicon dioxide, Coating.
See Editor's Note No. 40, page 2058.

Betalin-7-EC **-** BSN Inc.
Two capsules contain: 20-Hydroxy-Beta-Ecdysterone (96% extract from rhaponticum carthamoides) 100 mg • 7-Hydroxy-ECMM (5-methyl-7-hydroxy isoflavone ethyl carbonate molecular modification) 267 mg • 4-Hydroxyisoleucine (extracted from fenugreek) 50 mg. Other Ingredients: Cellulose, Magnesium Stearate, Gelatin.

Beta-mannan **-** Alotek Supplement Company
Two capsules contain: Vitamin E (as d-alpha-tocopherol) 100 IU • Proprietary blend of freeze-dried Aloe vera gel concentrates and extracts containing beta-mannans and beta-glucans 600 mg • IP6 (inositol hexaphosphate, derived from grains) 184 mg. Other Ingredients: defatted rice bran flour.

Beta-Sea 10,000 IU **-** Holista
Each capsule contains: Beta Carotene (from Dunaliella salina algae) 10000 IU. Other Ingredients: Carotenoids.

Beta-Sea 25,000 IU **-** Holista
Each capsule contains: Beta Carotene (from Dunaliella salina algae) 25000 IU. Other Ingredients: Carotenoids.

Better BodyEnergy for Life **-** HealthWatchers System
Ma Huang • Chromium Picolinate • Brindel Berry • White Willow Bark • Ginger Root • Hawthorn Berry • Licorice Root • Gotu Kola • Passion Flower • Siberian Ginseng • Guarana • Rhemannia Root • Bladderwrack • Reishi Mushroom • Astragalus.
See Editor's Note No. 30, page 2056.

Better Living Multi Vitamins **-** Health Center for Better Living
Each tablet contains: Vitamin A (Natural Fish Liver Oil) 10,000 IU• Beta Carotene (6 mg) 10000 mg • Vitamin B1 (Thiamine HCL) 75 mg • Vitamin B2 (Riboflavin) 75 mg • Vitamin B3 (Niacinamide) 75 mg • Vitamin B5 (Pantothenic) 75 mg • Vitamin B6 (as pyridoxine HCl) 75 mg • Vitamin B12 (as cyanocobalamin) 100 mcg • Biotin 100 mcg• Folic Acid 400 mcg • Vitamin C (Ascorbic Acid) 250 mg • Vitamin D (Natural FLO) 400 IU • Vitamin E (100% Natural d-alpha) 150 IU • Calcium (Ostershell) 100 mg • Magnesium (Oxide, amino acid chelate) 60 mg • Zinc (Amino acid chelate) 1 mg • Iodine (Kelp) 150 mcg • Iron (Amino acid chelate) • Chromium (Yeast Free GFT) 50 mcg • Boron (Amino acid chelate) 500 mcg • Molybdenum (Amino acid chelate) 50 mcg • Nucleic 50 mg.

BetterMan **-** Interceuticals
Each capsule contains: Proprietary Blend: Radix Ginseng, Rhizoma Dioscoreae, Radix Paeonia Alba, Herba Epimedii, Cornu Cervi Pantotrichum, Radix Astragali, Poria Cocos, Radix Morindae Officinalis, Fructus Corni, Cortex Eucommiae, Radix Angelicae Sinensis, Fructus Lycii, Radix Rehmanniae, Rhizoma Chuanxiong, Fructus Schisandrae, Acanthopanax Senticosus, Cynomorium Songaricum Rupr, Cortex Cinnamomi.

BetterWOMAN **-** Interceuticals
Each capsule contains: Proprietary Blend 400 mg: Asian Ginseng root, Chinese Yam rhizome, Chinese Peony root, Deer Antler velvet, Astragalus root, Poria Sclerotium, Morinda root, Asiatic Dogwood fruit, Eucommia stem, Dong Quai root, Bupleurum root, Lycium fruit, Rehmannia root, Epimedium leaf, Szechuan Lovage root, Schisandra fruit, Eleuthero root, Cynomorium stem, Cassia bark, Palm-leaf Raspberry fruit. Other Ingredients: Gelatin, Microcrystalline Celluose, Water, Magnesium Stearate, Silicon Dioxide.

Beyond Basics **-** Metabolic Response Modifiers
Three tablets contain: Vitamin A (as Beta-Carotene Palmitate) 15,000 IU • Vitamin C (as Ascorbic acid) 500 mg • Vitamin E (as d-Alpha Tocopherol Acetate) 200 IU • Vitamin B1 (as Thiamine HCl) 20 mg • Vitamin B2 (as Riboflavin) 30 mg • Vitamin D (as Cholecalciferol) 400 IU • Vitamin K1 (as Phylloquinine) 60 mcg • Niacin (Niacinamide 1:1) 30 mg • Pantothenic Acid (as Calcium d-Pantothenate) 25 mg • Vitamin B6 (as Pyridoxine HCl) 20 mg • Vitamin B12 (as Cyanocobalamin) 200 mcg • Biotin 75 mcg • Folic Acid 400 mcg • Calcium (as Calcium Carbonate Citrate 4:1) 200 mg • Magnesium (as Oxide Glycinate 4:1) 125 mg • Zinc (as Zinc Citrate) 10 mg • Copper (as Copper Citrate) 2 mg • Potassium (as Potassium Citrate) 75 mg • Molybdenum (as Molybdate) 100 mcg • Iodine (as Kelp) 150 mcg • Selenium (as l-Selenomethionine) 50 mcg • Chromium (as Chromium Chelate) 200 mcg • Boron (as Potassium Borate) 3 mg • Silica (as Colloidal Silica) 10 mg • Organic Horsetail 275 mg • Vanadium (as Vanadyl Sulfate) 50 mcg • Choline (as Choline Bitartrate) 25 mg • Inositol 30 mg.

Beyond Echinacea **-** Flora, Inc.
Echinacea • Balsam root • Peruvian Cat's Claw bark.

BF & SC **-** MMS Pro
Each capsule contains: Calendula flowers • White Oak bark • Marshmallow root • Mullein leaves • Black Walnut hulls • Gravel root • Slippery Elm bark • Wormwood • Scullcap.

Bicreatol XS **-** BSN Inc.
Two scoops contain: Calcium 310 mg • Magnesium 400 mg • Phosphorus 200 mg • Folic Acid 800 mcg • Vitamin B12 (cyanocobalamin) 500 mcg • Vitamin B6 (pyridoxine HCl) 50 mg • Bicreaplex 11 g: Micronized Creatine - Magnesium Hydrate, Glycovol Glycocyamine, Betapure Trimethylglycine • L-Glutamine & Glutamine Peptides 5 mg • Phosphoplexx 600 mg: Di-Potassium Phosphate, Sodium Bi-Phosphate, Calcium Phosphate • Nitrolen-4 300 mg: 4-Hydroxyisoleucine from Fenugreek and Vanadyl Sulfate. Other Ingredients: Micro-Filtered Whey Protein Concentrate, Rice Protein Concentrate, Maltodextrin, Canola Oil, MCT Oil, Natural & Artificial Flavors, Corn Syrup Solids, Sucralose, Sodium Caseinate, Mono and Diglycerides, Sodium Alginate, Lecithin.

Bifidus - Super Blue Green **-** Cell Tech
Two capsules contain: Vitamin K 6.8 mcg • Proprietary Blend 470 mg: Bifidobacterium Bifidum, Blue-Green Algae (aphanizomenon flos-aquae) 170 mg. Other Ingredients: Maltodextrin, rice bran, gelatin capsule (gelatin, water), vegetable magnesium stearate (encapsuling aid).

Bifidus Balance +FOS **-** Jarrow Formulas
Each capsule contains: FOS (Fructo-Oligo-Saccharides) 210 mg • Bifidobacterium Breve R070 40% 800 million • Bifidobacterium Longum R023 40% 800 million • Bifidobacterium Bifidum R071 15% 300 million • Bifidobacterium Infantis R033 5% 100 million. Other Ingredients: Maltodextrin, Magnesium Stearate, Ascorbic Acid.

Bifoviden ID **-** Metagenics
Each capsule contains: Proprietary Blend 15 billion live organisms: Bifidobacterium Lactis BI-07, Bifidobacterium Lactis BI-01, Streptococcus Thermophilus St-21.

Big 100 - GNC A-Z **-** GNC
Each tablet contains: Thiamin (as Thiamin Mononitrate) 100 mg • Riboflavin 100 mg • Niacin (as Niacinamide) 100 mg • Vitamin B6 (as Pyridoxine Hydrochloride) 100 mg • Folate, Folic Acid, Folacin 400 mcg • Vitamin B12 (as Cyanocobalamin) 100 mcg • Biotin 100 mcg • Pantothenic Acid (as Calcium d-Pantothenate) 100 mg • Choline Bitartrate 100 mg • Inositol 100 mcg • Para-Aminobenzoic Acid (PABA) 30 mg. Other Ingredients: Cellulose, Dicalcium Phosphate, Vegetable Acetoglycerides.

Big 150 - GNC A-Z **-** GNC
Each tablet contains: Thiamin (as Thiamin Mononitrate) 150 mg • Riboflavin 150 mg • Niacin (as Niacinamide) 150 mg • Vitamin B6 (as Pyridoxine Hydrochloride) 150 mg • Folate, Folic Acid, Folacin 400 mcg • Vitamin B12 (as Cyanocobalamin) 150 mcg • Biotin 150 mcg • Pantothenic acid (as Calcium d-Pantothenate) 150 mg

• Choline Bitartrate 150 mg • Inositol 150 mcg • Para-aminobenzoic Acid (PABA) 150 mg. Other Ingredients: Dicalcium Phosphate, Cellulose, Whole Brown Rice Powder (oryza sativa).

Big 50 Timed Release - GNC A-Z - GNC
Each tablet contains: Thiamin (as thiamin mononitrate) 50 mg • Riboflavin 50 mg • Niacin (as niacinamide) 50 mg • Vitamin B6 (as pyridoxine hydrochloride) 50 mg • Folate, Folic Acid, Folacin 400 mcg • Vitamin B12 (as cyanocobalamin) 50 mcg • Biotin 50 mcg • Pantothenic Acid (as calcium d-pantothenate) 50 mg • Choline Bitartrate 50 mg • Inosotil 50 mg • Para Amino Benzoic Acid (PABA) 30 mg. Other Ingredients: Dicalcium Phosphate, Cellulose, Brewer's Yeast, Lecithin, Alfalfa leaf powder (medicago sativa), Watercress herb powder (nasurtium officinale), Parsley herb powder (petroselinium sativum), Whole Brown Rice (oryza powder), Vegetable Acetoglycerides.

Big Daddy - The Sports Nutrition Source, Inc.
Each 225 gram serving contains: Sodium 50 mg • Potassium 145 mg • Protein 40 g.

Bilberry - Basic Nutrition - GNC
Each capsule contains: Bilberry fruits powder (Vaccinium myrtillus) 500 mg. Other Ingredients: Gelatin, Cellulose.

Bilberry - Jamieson
Each capsule contains: Bilberry fruit 2500 mg.

Bilberry - Leiner Health Products
Each caplet contains: Bilberry extract (Vaccinium myrtillus) berry 80 mg. Other Ingredients: Calcium Carbonate, Cellulose, Maltodextrin, Hydroxypropyl Methylcellulose, Silicon Dioxide, Polyethylene Glycol 3350, Croscarmellose Sodium, Hydroxypropyl Cellulose, Pharmaceutical Glaze, Yellow 5 Lake, Blue 1 Lake, Crospovidone, Magnesium Stearate, Polysorbate 80, Titanium Dioxide.

Bilberry - Progressive Labs
Each all-vegetable capsule contains: Bilberry leaf powder (Vaccinum myrtillus) 370 mg • Bilberry extract (Vaccinum myrtillus) 80 mg • Anthocyanids (from above) 25 mg.

Bilberry - Rexall - Sundown
Each two capsules contain: Bilberry Extract 4:1 (fruit) 80 mg. Other Ingredients: Gelatin, Natural Vegetable Fiber.

Bilberry - Solaray - Nutraceutical Corp.
Each capsule contains: Bilberry berry extract 60 mg. Inactive Ingredients: Cellulose, Gelatin, Magnesium Stearate.

Bilberry 1000 mg, Concentrated - GNC Herbal Plus - GNC
Each capsule contains: Bilberry Fruits (vaccinum myrtillus; from 10 mg bilberry fruit extract 100:1) 1000 mg. Other Ingredients: Soybean Oil, Gelatin, Glycerin, Caramel Color, Titanium Dioxide (natural mineral whitener).

Bilberry Complex w/Lutein - Pro Health
Each capsule contains: Vitamin A (as beta carotene) 10,000 IU • Riboflavin (vitamin B2) 10 mg • Bilberry extract (vaccinium myrtillus, standardized for 25% anthocyanidins 20 mg) 80 mg • Carrot root powder (daucus carota sativa) 300 mg • Citrus Bioflavonoid complex (35% hesperidin 40 mg) 114 mg • Floraglo Lutein extract (from marigold flowers, standardized for 5% lutein 3 mg, 0.22% zeaxanthin 132 mcg) 60 mg. Other Ingredients: Rice Flour, Gelatin, Maltodextrin, Water.

Bilberry Extract - Nature's Way
Each capsule contains: Bilberry fruit (dried extract 25% anthocyanins) 80 mg • Elderberry 125 mg • Other Ingredients: Gelatin, Millet.

Bilberry Extract - NSI - Nutraceutical Sciences Institute
Each capsule contains: Bilberry extract (standardized to 25% anthocyanosides) 160 mg.

Bilberry Extract - PhytoPharmica
Two capsules contain: Bilberry berry extract (vaccinium myrtillus fructus, standardized to contain 25% anthocyanosides [40 mg] calculated as anthocyanidins) 160 mg.

Bilberry Extract - Source Naturals
Each tablet contains: Bilberry (Vaccinium myrtillus, standardized extract, yielding 18.5 mg Anthocyanosides) 50 mg.

Bilberry Extract - Swanson
Each capsule contains: Bilberry extract (25% anthocyanidins) 60 mg • Bilberry powder 360 mg • Citrus Bioflavonoids 50 mg.

Bilberry Formula - Quest
Each caplet contains: Bilberry (Vaccinium myrtillus) (provided by 50 mg P.E. 1:100 standardized to contain 25% anthocyanosides) 5000 mg • Citrus Bioflavonoids (providing Hesperidin 50 mg) 200 mg • Carrot powder (Daucus carota) 100 mg. Other Ingredients: Calcium Phosphate, Microcrystalline Cellulose, Vegetable Stearin, Croscarmellose Sodium, Magnesium Stearate (vegetable source).

Bilberry Fruit - PhysioLogics
Each capsule contains: Bilberry fruit extract (vaccinium myrtillus, standardized to contain 25% anthocyanosides 15 mg) 60 mg. Other Ingredients: Cellulose (plant origin), Beet Root Concentrate, Gelatin, Dicalcium Phosphate, Vegetable Magnesium Stearate, Silica.

Bilberry i sight - Nature's Life
Each two capsules contain: Vitamin A (100% as beta carotene from dunaliella salina algae) 15,000 IU • Vitamin E (as d-alpha tocopheryl succinate) 400 IU • Vitamin C (from calcium ascorbate) 300 mg • Riboflavin (vitamin B2) 3 mg • Niacin 40 mg • Calcium (from calcium ascorbate) 30 mg • Bilberry fruit extract (vaccinium myrtillus, standardized to 25% anthocyanosides) 360 mg • Alpha Carotene (from D. salina algae) 288 mcg • Cryptoxanthin (from D. salina algae) 70 mcg • Zeaxanthin (from D. salina algae) 58 mcg • Lutein (from D. salina algae) 45 mcg. Other Ingredients: Cellulose, Vegetarian Magnesium Stearate.

Bilberry-Go! - Wakunaga of America
Each caplet contains: Bilberry standardized extract (fruit) 120 mg. Other Ingredients: Cellulose, Starch, Magnesium Stearate (vegetable source), Silica.

Bile-Gest - Atrium Inc.
Each tablet contains: Ox Bile concentrate 195 mg • Collinsonia root 310 mg • Glycine 50 mg • Pepsin 30 mg • Raw Liver concentrate 30 mg.
See Editor's Note No. 14, page 2055.

Binge Breaker - Enforma Natural Products
Two capsules contain: St. John's Wort (.2 -.3 Hypericin) • Kava Kava (70% Kavalactones) • Vitamin C (Ascorbic Acid) • Vitamin B1 (Thiamine) • Vitamin B2 (Riboflavin) • Vitamin B6 (Pyridoxine) • Vitamin B3 (Niacin).

Bio Berry Grape Seed Extract Plus - Flora, Inc.
Grape Seed Extract 50 mg • Bilberry 10 mg. In a base of Cranberry powder.

Bio C Plus - Nutrilite
Each tablet contains: Vitamin C (30 mg from acerola cherries) 250 mg • Lemon Bioflavonoid concentrate (from lemon pulp and peel) 35 mg. Other Ingredients: Corn Starch, Microcrystalline Cellulose, Modified Cellulose Gum, Hydroxypropyl Methylcellulose, Magnesium Stearate, Acacia, Maltodextrin, Glycerin.

Bio C-Complex 1000 - The Vitamin Shoppe
Each capsule contains: Pure Crystalline Vitamin C (fortified with Rose Hips) 1000 mg • Citrus Bioflavonoids Complex 100 mg.

Bio C-Complex 500 - The Vitamin Shoppe
Vitamin C (fortified with Rose Hips Conc.) 500 mg • Citrus Bioflavonoids Complex 250 mg.

Bio Q-Gel Mega 100 - Solanova
Each softsule contains: Vitamin E (d-alpha tocopherol concentrate) 150 IU • Coenzyme Q10 (Ubidecarenone USP) 100 mg. Other Ingredients: Gelatin, Sorbitol, Glycerin, Purified Water, Hydroxylated Lecithin, Medium Chain Triglycerides, Annato Seed Extract, Soybean Oil.

Bio Rejuvenate - Windspirit Productions, Inc.
Each two softgets contain: Astaxanthin 5 mg. Ingredients: Algal Meal extract (haematococcus pluvialis), Rice Bean oil, Gelatin, Vegetable Glycerin Water, Beta-carotene, Lutein.

Bio St. John's - Pharmanex
Each capsule contains: Cordyceps Sinensis (CordyMax Cs-4, standardized to adenosine & mannitol content) 375 mg • St. John's Wort (hypericum extract, standardized to 0.3% hypericin) 225 mg.

Bio Trim - Dial Herbs
Ma Huang • Kola Nut • Ginger • White Willow • Ginkgo Biloba • Bladderwrack • Fo-Ti • Hawthorn berries • Saw Palmetto • Beet Powder • Chromium Proteinate • Zinc Picolinate • Boron Proteinate • Chromium Picolinate • Kola Nut extract.
See Editor's Note No. 30, page 2056.

Bioactive B12 - Enzymatic Therapy
Each tablet contains: Vitamin B12 (as methylcobalamin) 1 mg. Other Ingredients: Fructose, Mannitol, Stearic Acid, Cellulose, Natural Cherry Flavor, Magnesium Stearate, Silicon Dioxide.

BioAstin Brand - Nutrex, Inc.
Natural Astaxanthin from Microalgae.
See Editor's Note No. 44, page 2058.

Bio-Balanced Calcium Magnesium - Pro Health
Each tablet contains: Calcium (amino acid chelate, from oyster shells) 250 mg • Magnesium (amino acid chelate) 125 mg • Vitamin D (cholecalciferol) 200 IU. Other Ingredients: Calcium Phosphate Dibasic, Stearic Acid, Hydroxypropyl Cellulose, Croscarmellose Sodium, Magnesium Stearate, Silicon Dioxide, Sodium Lauryl Sulfate.

BioBeads - Natrol
Each bead contains: Proprietary Blend 1 Billion: Lactobacillus Acidophilus, Bifidobacterium Bifidum, Bifidobacterium Longum, Lactobacillus Rhamnosus. Other Ingredients: Vegetable Oil, Gelatin, Glycerine, Lecithin, Pectin.

BioCalth Caplets - Nature's Solution
Three caplets contain: Calcium L-Threonate 2325 mg • Calcium (element) 300 mg. Other Ingredients: Microcrystalline Cellulose, Carboxymenthylcellulose, Magnesium Silicate, Magnesium Stearate, Maltodextrin.

BioCalth Kids - Nature's Solution
Each piece of gum contains: Vitamin A (as vitamin A palmitate) 2500 IU • Vitamin C (as calcium ascorbate) 30 mg • Vitamin D (as cholecalciferol) 200 • Vitamin E (as d-alpha tocopheryl acetate) 19 IU • Vitamin K (as phytonadione) 40 mcg • Thiamin (as thiamine mononitrate) 0.75 mg • Riboflavin 0.85 mg • Niacin (as niacinamide) 10 mg • Vitamin B6 (as pyridoxine hydrochloride) 1 mg • Folic Acid 200 mcg • Vitamin B12 (as cyanocobalamin) 3 mcg • Biotin 25 mcg • Pantothenic Acid (as d-calcium) 5 mg • Calcium D-Threonate (BioCalth) 200 mg. Other Ingredients: Pharmagums, Tutti-Frutti (natural), Natural Color, Citric Acid, Sucralose, Magnesium Stearate.

BioCalth Powder - Nature's Solution
Two packets contain: Calcium L-Threonate 2320 mg • Calcium (element) 300 mg.

Biochem Aller-Max - Country Life
Each two capsules contain: Quercetin 250 mg • N-Acetyl Cysteine 200 mg • Bromelain 100 mg • L-Histidine 200 mg • Vitamin A (Palmitate) 2500 IU • Vitamin C (Calcium Ascorbate) 250 mg • Pantothenic Acid 200 mg • Zinc 10 mg • Grape seed extract 5 mg • Stinging Nettle 100 mg • Cayenne 20 mg.

Biochem Chrom-Adyl Surge - Country Life
Each capsule contains: Chromium 500 mcg • BMOV (Bis-Maltol OXO Vandium) 5 mg • Vanadyl Sulfate 5 mg.

Biochem Prosta-Max for Men - Country Life
Each two tablets contain: Glycine 250 mg • L-Glutamic Acid 250 mg • Bromelain 100 mg • Vitamin A (beta carotene) 10,000 IU • Vitamin E 200 IU • Vitamin C 250 mg • Vitamin B1 (thiamin) 25 mg • Vitamin B2 (riboflavin) 20 mg • Vitamin B6 (pyridoxine) 20 mg • Zinc 50 mg • Saw Palmetto 100 mg • Pygeum 100 mg • Parsley 75 mg.

Biochem Ultimate Athlete's Pain Formula - Country Life
Three softgel capsules contain: Boswellia Serrata extract 500 mg • Omega-3 Fish oil concentrate 400 mg • Glucosamine HCl 250 mg • Glucosamine Sulfate 250 mg • Chondroitin Sulfate 200 mg • Poly-NAG (N-acetyl glucosamine) 50 mg • Vitamin C (ascorbyl palmitate) 50 mg • Green Lipped Mussel extract 50 mg • CMO (cetyl myristoleate) 50 mg • Gamma-Linolenic Acid (borage seed oil) 50 mg • Vitamin E (d-alpha tocopheryl acetate) 25 IU • Manganese (sulfate) 5 mg • Boron (borogluconate) 1.5 mg.
See Editor's Note No. 15, page 2055.

Biochem Ultimate Fat Metabolizer - Country Life
Each three tablets contain: Choline Bitartrate 500 mg • Inositol 500 mg • L-Carnitine 500 mg • L-Methionine 500 mg • Taurine 500 mg • Phosphatidyl Choline 200 mg • Betaine HCL 200 mg • Dandelion 100 mg • Milk Thistle 100 mg • Barberry 100 mg • Artichoke extract 50 mg • Vitamin B6 (Pyridoxine • Alpha-Ketoglutarate/Pyridoxal-5-Phosphate) 10 mg • Chromium 400 mcg.

Biochem Ultimate Sports Multiple - Country Life
Each four tablets contain: Vitamin A (Carotene Complex) 5000 IU • Vitamin D (Ergocalciferol) 200 IU • Vitamin E (d-Alpha Tocopheryl Succinate) 400 IU • Vitamin C (Ascorbic Acid) 1000 mg • Grape seed extract/Grape skin 100 mg • Vitamin B1 (Thiamine HCL/Thiamine Cocarboxylase) 100 mg • Vitamin B2 (Riboflavin/Riboflavin 5 Phosphate) 100 mg • Vitamin B3 (Niacin/Niacinamide) 200 mg • Vitamin B5 (d-Calcium Pantothenate/Pantethine) 200 mg • Vitamin B6 (Pyridoxine HCL/Pyridoxal 5 Phosphate) 100 mg • Folic Acid 400mcg • Vitamin B12 (Cyanocobalamine/Didencozide) 200 mcg • d-Biotin 300 mcg • PABA 200 mcg • Selenium 100 mcg • Molybdenum 10 mcg • Choline Bitartrate 200 mg • Inositol 100 mg • Bromelain 100 mg • Betaine HCL 200 mg • L-Methionine 50 mg • Taurine 50 mg.

BioChoice Immune Support - Chocolate - Legacy for Life
Each packet (27 g) contains: Sodium 160 mg • Potassium 55 mg • Protein 7 g • Vitamin A 5000 IU • Vitamin C 60 mg • Vitamin D (as Vitamin D3) 400 IU • Vitamin E 30 IU • Niacin 20 mg • Folic Acid 0.4 mg • Pantothenic Acid 10 mg • Vitamin B6 2 mg • Vitamin B2 (Riboflavin) 1.7 mg • Vitamin B1 (Thiamin) 1.5 mg • Vitamin B12 6 mcg • Biotin 0.3 mg • Calcium 100 mg • Copper 0.6 mg • Iodine 45 mcg • Iron 5.4 mg • Magnesium 10 mg • Phosphorus 120 mg • Zinc 4.5 mg • Vitamin K (as Vitamin K1) 80 mcg • Manganese 0.6 mg • Chromium 36 mcg. Other Ingredients: Protein blend (Egcel [egg powder], soy protein isolate, milk protein), Maltodextrin, Oat fiber, Cocoa, Natural Chocolate and Vanilla flavor, Soy lecithin, Guar Gum, Xanthan Gum.

BioChoice Immune Support - Strawberry - Legacy for Life
Each packet (24 g) contains: Sodium 160 mg • Potassium 55 mg • Protein 7 g • Vitamin A 5000 IU • Vitamin C 60 mg • Vitamin D (as Vitamin D3) 400 IU • Vitamin E 30 IU • Niacin 20 mg • Folic Acid 0.4 mg • Pantothenic Acid 10 mg • Vitamin B6 2 mg • Vitamin B2 (Riboflavin) 1.7 mg • Vitamin B1 (Thiamin) 1.5 mg • Vitamin B12 6 mcg • Biotin 0.3 mg • Calcium 100 mg • Copper 0.6 mg • Iodine 45 mcg • Iron 5.4 mg • Magnesium 10 mg • Phosphorus 120 mg • Zinc 4.5 mg • Vitamin K (as Vitamin K1) 80 mcg • Manganese 0.6 mg • Chromium 36 mcg. Other Ingredients: Protein Blend (Egcel [egg

powder], Soy protein isolate, milk protein), Maltodextrin, Oat fiber, artificial Strawberry flavor, Beet extract, Soy lecithin, Guar Gum, Xanthan Gum.

BioChoice Immune Support - Vanilla - Legacy for Life
Each packet (24 g) contains: Vitamin A 5000 IU • Vitamin C 60 mg • Vitamin D (Vitamin D3) 400 IU • Vitamin E 30 IU • Niacin 20 mg • Folic Acid 0.4 mg • Pantothenic Acid 10 mg • Vitamin B6 2 mg • Vitamin B2 (Riboflavin) 1.7 mg • Vitamin B1 (Thiamin) 1.5 mg • Vitamin B12 6 mcg • Biotin 0.3 mg • Calcium 100 mg • Copper 0.6 mg • Iodine 45 mcg • Iron 5.4 mg • Magnesium 10 mg • Phosphorus 120 mg • Zinc 4.5 mg • Vitamin K (as Vitamin K1) 80 mcg • Manganese 0.6 mg • Chromium 36 mcg. Other Ingredients: Protein blend (Egcel [egg powder], soy protein isolate, milk protein), Maltodextrin, Oat fiber, Natural Vanilla flavor, Soy lecithin, Guar Gum, Xanthan Gum.

BioChoice Immune Support Drink Mix (chocolate) - Legacy for Life
Each 27 g serving contains: Vitamin A 5000 IU • Vitamin C 60 mg • Vitamin D (D3) 400 IU • Vitamin E 30 IU • Niacin 20 mg • Folic Acid 0.4 mg • Pantothenic Acid 10 mg • Vitamin B6 2 mg • Vitamin B2 (riboflavin) 1.7 mg • Vitamin B1 (thiamin) 1.5 mg • Vitamin B12 6 mcg • Biotin 0.3 mg • Calcium 100 mg • Copper 0.6 mg • Iodine 45 mcg • Iron 5.4 mg • Magnesium 10 mg • Phosphorus 120 mg • Zinc 4.5 mg • Vitamin K (K1) 80 mcg • Manganese 0.6 mg • Chromium 26 mcg. Other Ingredients: Protein Blend (Egcel egg powder, soy protein isolate, milk protein), Maltodextrin, Oat Fiber, Cocoa, Natural Chocolate and Vanilla Flavor, Soy Lecithin, Guar Gum Xanthan Gum.

BioChoice Immune Support Drink Mix (strawberry) - Legacy for Life
Each 24 g serving contains: Vitamin A 5000 IU • Vitamin C 60 mg • Vitamin D (D3) 400 IU • Vitamin E 30 IU • Niacin 20 mg • Folic Acid 0.4 mg • Pantothenic Acid 10 mg • Vitamin B6 2 mg • Vitamin B2 (riboflavin) 1.7 mg • Vitamin B1 (thiamin) 1.5 mg • Vitamin B12 6 mcg • Biotin 0.3 mg • Calcium 100 mg • Copper 0.6 mg • Iodine 45 mcg • Iron 5.4 mg • Magnesium 10 mg • Phosphorus 120 mg • Zinc 4.5 mg • Vitamin K (K1) 80 mcg • Manganese 0.6 mg • Chromium 26 mcg. Other Ingredients: Protein Blend (Egcel egg powder, soy protein isolate, milk protein), Maltodextrin, Oat Fiber, Artificial Strawberry Flavor, Beet Extract, Soy Lecithin, Guar Gum Xanthan Gum.

BioChoice Immune Support Drink Mix (vanilla) - Legacy for Life
Each 24 g serving contains: Vitamin A 5000 IU • Vitamin C 60 mg • Vitamin D (D3) 400 IU • Vitamin E 30 IU • Niacin 20 mg • Folic Acid 0.4 mg • Pantothenic Acid 10 mg • Vitamin B6 2 mg • Vitamin B2 (riboflavin) 1.7 mg • Vitamin B1 (thiamin) 1.5 mg • Vitamin B12 6 mcg • Biotin 0.3 mg • Calcium 100 mg • Copper 0.6 mg • Iodine 45 mcg • Iron 5.4 mg • Magnesium 10 mg • Phosphorus 120 mg • Zinc 4.5 mg • Vitamin K (K1) 80 mcg • Manganese 0.6 mg • Chromium 26 mcg. Other Ingredients: Protein Blend (Egcel egg powder, soy protein isolate, milk protein), Maltodextrin, Oat Fiber, Cocoa, Natural Vanilla Flavor, Soy Lecithin, Guar Gum Xanthan Gum.

BioChoice Immune26 capsules - Legacy for Life
Each capsule contains: Hyperimmune Egg powder (Egcel).

BioChoice Immune26 packets - Legacy for Life
Each 4.5 g packet contains: Hyperimmune Egg powder (Egcel).

BioChoice Immune26 powder - Legacy for Life
Each 4.5 g scoop contains: Hyperimmune Egg powder (Egcel).

Biochol - Ketopharm USA
Each capsule contains: Fenugreek seed 305 mg • Garlic bulb 55 mg • Cloves 55 mg • Cinnamon bark 55 mg • Ginger root 55 mg • Costus root 55 mg.

BioCosanol brand - Cyvex Nutrition, Inc.
Policosanol.
See Editor's Note No. 44, page 2058.

Bio-Directed Antioxidant - Nikken Inc.
Two capsules contain: Vitamin A (as d. salina, beta carotene, spirulina pacifica, chlorella vulgaris) 10,000 IU • Vitamin C (as ascorbic acid, calcium ascorbate, acerola cherry) 300 mg • Vitamin E (as d-alpha tocopheryl succinate, d-alpha tocopheryl acetate, alpha, beta, gamma, delta tocopherols) 150 IU • Zinc (as zinc citrate) 15 mg • Selenium (l-selenomethionine) 140 mcg • Green Tea polyphenol extract (camellia sinensis) 500 mg • Alpha Lipoic Acid 50 mg • N-Acetyl L-Cysteine 50 mg • Grape Seed extract (vitis vinifera l.) 25 mg • Glutathione (reduced) 20 mg • Lycopenes 2 mg. Other Ingredients: Gelatin, Maltodextrin, Magnesium Stearate, Silicon Dioxide.

Bio-Directed Digestion - Nikken Inc.
Three capsules contain: Protease (from papaya) 450 mg • Fructooligosaccharides (100% fiber) 375 mg • Amylase 150 mg • Cellulase 75 mg • Lactase 75 mg • Broccoli sprout powder 45 mg • Tomato fruit powder 45 mg • Wheat Grass powder 45 mg • Lactobacillus Sporogenes 45 mg • Papaya fruit powder 45 mg • Fiber 375 mg. Other Ingredients: Gelatin, Magnesium Stearate.

Bio-Directed Fat Metabolism - Nikken Inc.
Two tablets contain: Vitamin C (as ascorbic acid) 30 mg • Vitamin B1 (as thiamine mononitrate) 1.5 mg • Vitamin B2 (as riboflavin) 1.7 mg • Vitamin B6 (as pyridoxine hydrochloride) 2 mg • Folate (as folic acid) 200 mcg • Vitamin B12 (as cyanocobalamin) 6 mcg • Chromium (as chromium picolinate, chromium chelate) 180 mcg • Garcinia Cambogia fruit 500 mg • L-Carnitine (as l-carnitine tartrate) 250 mg • Inositol (as myo-inositol) 25 mg • Bioperine Piperine extract (from black pepper) 2.5 mg. Other Ingredients: Croscarmellose Sodium, Cellulose, Stearic Acid, Calcium Carbonate, Silicon Dioxide, Magnesium Stearate, Dextrin, Dextrose, Lecithin, Sodium Carboxymethylcellulose, Sodium Citrate.

Bio-Directed For Men - Nikken Inc.
Two tablets contain: Vitamin C (as ascorbic acid) 120 mg • Vitamin E (as d-alpha tocopheryl succinate, alpha, beta, gamma, delta tocopherols) 120 IU • Vitamin B6 (as pyridoxine hydrochloride)5 mg • Folate (as folic acid) 400 mcg • Vitamin B12 (as cyanocobalamin) 30 mcg • Calcium (as calcium carbonate) 300 mg • Zinc (as zinc citrate) 15 mg • Selenium (as l-selenomethionine) 140 mcg • Saw Palmetto fruit extract (serenoa repens, 25% phytosterols) 250 mg • Echinacea Purpurea leaf 50 mg • Taurine 50 mg • Ginkgo Biloba leaf extract (standardized to 24% ginkgoflavoneglycosides, 6% terpene lactones) 30 mg • Curcumin root extract complex (curcuma longa) 25 mg • Garlic bulb (allium sativum) 25 mg • Green Tea polyphenol extract (camellia sinensis) 25 mg • Glycine 25 mg • L-Glutamine 25 mg • Pygeum Africanum root extract 25 mg • Glutathione (reduced) 10 mg • Alpha Lipoic Acid 5 mg • Lycopenes 0.25 mg. Other Ingredients: Dextrose, Cellulose, Dicalcium Phosphate, Croscarmellose Sodium, Stearic Acid, Silicon Dioxide, Dextrin, Magnesium Stearate, Lecithin, Sodium Carboxymethylcellulose, Sodium Citrate.

Bio-Directed For Women - Nikken Inc.
Four tablets contain: Vitamin C (as ascorbic acid, ascorbyl palmitate) 250 mg • Vitamin D (as cholecalciferol) 200 IU • Vitamin E (as d-alpha tocopheryl succinate, alpha, beta, gamma tocopherols) 30 IU • Vitamin B6 (as pyridoxine hydrochloride, pyridoxal 5 phosphate) 10 mg • Folate (as folic acid) 210 mcg • Vitamin B12 (as cyanocobalamin) 12 mcg • Calcium (as calcium carbonate, calcium citrate) 750 mg • Iron (as iron amino acid chelate) 18 mg • Magnesium (magnesium oxide, magnesium citrate) 100 mg • Cranberry fruit powder 250 mg • IsoflavonePlus complex 210 mg: Fenugreek whole plant, N-Acetyl L-Cysteine, Dong Quai root, Soy Isoflavones, Black Cohosh root • Grape Seed extract (vitis vinifera l.) 25 mg • Lutein 1.5 mg • Melatonin 0.1 mg. Other Ingredients: Cellulose, Dextrose,

Croscarmellose Sodium, Stearic Acid, Silicon Dioxide, Magnesium Stearate, Dextrin, Lecithin, Sodium Carboxymethylcellulose, Sodium Citrate.

Bio-Directed Immunity **-** Nikken Inc.
Each capsule contains: Proprietary Blend 500 mg: Cordyceps Sinensis, Agaricus Blazei, Maitake (grifolia frondosa), Reishi (ganoderma lucidum), Trametes Versicolor, Shiitake (lentinula edodes), Hericium Erinaceus, Tremella Mesenterica, Phellinus Linteus, Pleurotus Tuber-Regium, Oyster (pleurotus ostreatus), Chaga (inonotus obliques), Lepiota Prorera, Enoki (flammulina velutipes). Other Ingredients: Magnesium Stearate, Hydroxypropyl Methylcellulose (vegetarian capsule).

Bio-Directed Joint **-** Nikken Inc.
Three softgels contain: Glucosamine Hydrochloride 300 mg • Methylsulfonylmethane (MSM) 150 mg • High Potency CM Complex 1125 mg: Cetyl Myristoleate complex 900 mg, EPA (eicosapentaenoic acid) 135 mg, DHA (docosahexaenoic acid) 90 mg. Other Ingredients: Gelatin, Glycerin,Titanium Dioxide, Chlorophyll.

Bio-Directed Liver Support **-** Nikken Inc.
Three capsules contain: Maximum Purifying Blend 1260 mg: Artichoke leaf extract (cynara floridanum), Sarsaparilla root extract (smilax aristolochaiefolii). Other Ingredients: Gelatin, Cellulose, Magnesium Stearate.

Bio-Directed Mental Clarity **-** Nikken Inc.
Two capsules contain: Vitamin C (as ascorbic acid, ascorbyl palmitate) 150 mg • Vitamin E (as d-alpha tocopheryl succinate, d-alpha tocopheryl acetate, alpha, beta, gamma, delta tocopherols) 100 IU • Green Tea polyphenol extract (camellia sinensis) 500 mg • L-Glutamine 250 mg • L-Tyrosine 250 mg • Cordyceps Sinensis 200 mg • Ginkgo Biloba leaf extract (standardized to 24% ginkgoflavoneglycosides, 6% terpene lactones) 60 mg • Alpha Lipoic Acid 50 mg • N-Acetyl L-Cysteine 25 mg • Grape Seed extract (vitis vinifera l.) 20 mg • Glutathione (reduced) 10 mg. Other Ingredients: Gelatin, Silicon Dioxide, Magnesium Stearate.

Bio-Directed Multi-Vitamin/Mineral **-** Nikken Inc.
Four tablets contain: Vitamin A Palmitate (100% as beta carotene, d. salina) 12,500 IU • Vitamin C (as ascorbic acid, calcium ascorbate, ascorbyl palmitate) 500 mg • Vitamin D (as cholecalciferol) 200 IU • Vitamin E (as d-alpha tocopheryl succinate, alpha, beta, gamma tocopherols) 180 IU • Vitamin K (as phytonadione) 20 mcg • Thiamin (vitamin B1) 4.5 mg • Riboflavin (vitamin B2) 5.1 mg • Niacin (as niacinamide) 60 mg • Vitamin B6 (as pyridoxine hydrochloride, pyridoxal 5 phosphate) 10 mg • Folate (as folic acid) 400 mcg • Vitamin B12 (as cyanocobalamin) 18 mcg • Biotin 300 mcg • Pantothenic Acid (as d-calcium pantothenate) 30 mg • Iodine (as potassium iodide) 150 mcg • Magnesium (as magnesium oxide, magnesium citrate) 100 mg • Zinc (as zinc citrate) 15 mg • Selenium (as yeast, sodium selenate) 70 mcg • Copper (as copper citrate) 2 mg • Manganese (as manganese citrate) 2 mg • Chromium (as chromium picolinate, yeast) 120 mcg • Potassium (as chloride) 50 mg • Nikkomannan Glucomannan root (amorphophallus konjac, 100% fiber) 250 mg • Taurine 250 mg • L-Glutamine 100 mg • Deep Sea Mineral Complex Trace Minerals 100 mg • L-Tyrosine 100 mg • Bromelain 50 mg • N-Acetyl-L-Cysteine 50 mg • Alpha Lipoic Acid 10 mg • Choline (choline bitartrate, choline dihydrogen citrate) 200 mg. Other Ingredients: Cellulose, Dextrose, Starch, Stearic Acid, Silicon Dioxide, Magnesium Stearate, Dextrin, Lecithin, Sodium Carboxymethylcellulose, Sodium Citrate, Chromium Picolinate.

Bio-Directed Restful Night **-** Nikken Inc.
Two tablets contain: Vitamin C (as ascorbic acid, ascorbyl palmitate) 60 mg • Calcium (as calcium carbonate, calcium citrate) 500 mg • Vitamin D (as cholecalciferol) 200 IU • Vitamin E (as d-alpha tocopheryl succinate, alpha, beta, gamma, delta tocopherols) 30 IU • Vitamin K (as phytonadione) 40 mcg • Magnesium (as magnesium oxide, magnesium citrate) 200 mg • Manganese (as manganese citrate) 2 mg • Alpha Lipoic Acid 10 mg • Chamomile flower extract 10 mg • Hops leaf extract 10 mg • Valerian root extract 10 mg • Grape Seed extract (vitis vinifera l.) 10 mg • Melatonin 0.1 mg. Other Ingredients: Gelatin, Silicon Dioxide, Magnesium Stearate, Cellulose.

Bio-EFA Borage Oil 90 **-** Health From The Sun
Each capsule contains: Cis- Linoleic Acid (Omega-6) 190 mg • Gamma Linolenic Acid (GLA) (Omega-6) 90 mg • Oleic Acids (Omega-9) 75 mg. Ingredients: 100% Pure Borage oil 500 mg.

BioEFA with CLA **-** 4 Life
Two softgels contain: Vitamin E (as D-alpha, beta, delta and gamma tocopherols) 15 IU • Alpha Linolenic Acid (ALA, from organic flax seed oil, linum usitatissimum seed) 275 mg • Conjugated Linoleic Acid (CLA, from sunflower seed, helianthus annuus seed) 244 mg • Gamma Linolenic Acid (from borage seed oil, boraga officinalis seed) 69 mg • Eicosapentaenoic Acid (EPA, from fish oil) 66 mg • Docosahexaenoic Acid (DHA, from fish oil) 44 mg. Other Ingredients: Gelatin, Glycerin, Purified Water.

Bio-Energy **-** Oasis Wellness Network
Each tablet contains: Magnesium (as potassium magnesium aspartate) 100 mg • Chromium (as chromium polynicotinate) 100 mcg • Alpha-Ketoglutaric Acid 100 mg • MaxCell Proprietary Blend 83 mg: Zisyphus Jujube, Piper Nigrum, Aloe Vera gel, Glycyrrhiza Glabra • Siberian Ginseng root extract 67 mg • Panax Ginseng root extract 17 mg • Coenzyme Q10 6 mg. Other Ingredients: Calcium Sulfate, Stearic Acid, Cellulose, Silica, Magnesium Stearate.

Bioflora **-** PhysioLogics
Each caplet contains: Fructooligosaccharides (FOS) 500 mg • Lactobacillus Acidophilus (providing 1.02 billion active cells) 255 mg • Lactobacillus Bifidus (providing 0.12 billion active cells) 30 mg • Lactobacillus Bulgaricus (providing 0.12 billion active cells) 30 mg • Turmeric root (curcurma longa) 10.8 mg. Other Ingredients: Cellulose (plant origin), Vegetable Stearic Acid, Croscarmellose, Silica, Vegetable Magnesium Stearate, Cellulose Coating.

BioGenistein Plus **-** 4 Life
Each capsule contains: Proprietary Blend 400 mg: Soy isoflavone extract (contains 35 mg of genistein and genistin and 40 mg of total isoflavones, Glycine max., seeds), Broccoli powder extract (contains highly concentrated sulforaphane compounds, Brassica oleracea, sprouts), Quercitin, Curcumin (from turmeric, Curcum long L.), Dietary indoles (including Indole-3-carbinol). Other Ingredients: Gelatin Capsule, Peppermint Leaf, and Vegetable Oil.

BioGinkgo 27/7 **-** Pharmanex
Each tablet contains: Ginkgo leaf extract (ginkgo biloba, 50:1) 60 mg. Other Ingredients: Lactose Anhydrous, Microcrystaline Cellulose, Corn Starch, Sodium Starch Glycolate, Opadry Colors (containing yellow lake 5, blue lake 1), Colloidal Silicon Dioxide, Magnesium Stearate.

Biogra **-** Olympian Labs
Each capsule contains: DHEA 10 mg •Thymus Gland 20 mg •Octacosanol 600 mg •Raw Orchic 20 mg •L-Tyrosine 250 mg •Vitamin C 30 mg •Vitamin B-6 10 mg •Damiana 80 mg •Wild Yam 20 mg •Yohimbe Bark 20 mg •Gotu Kola 20 mg •Siberian Ginseng 20 mg •Licorice root powder 20 mg •Jamaican Ginger 20 mg • Dong Quai 20 mg •Sarsaparilla 20 mg •Zinc Gluconate 20 mg.
See Editor's Note No. 14, page 2055.

Biogra for Women **-** Olympian Labs
Each capsule contains: Proprietary Blend: Damiana, Wild Yam, Gotu Kola, Sarsaparilla, Saw Palmetto, Siberian Ginseng, Dong Quai, Kelp, L-Tyrosine, L-Phenylalanine, Fo-Ti, Para-Aminobenzoic Acid, Bee Propolis 685 mg.

BioGreens **-** The Vitamin Shoppe
Three teaspoons contain: Organically grown wheatgrass, alfalfa 1923 mg • Soy Lecithin (99% oil-free, 97% phosphatides) 1862 mg • Royal Jelly, Bee Pollen, Honey Extract 1070 mg • Spirulina, Chlorella 700 mg • Vegetable Concentrate (carrot, spinach, bean sprout, celery,

tomato, daikon) 700 mg • High Pectin Fruit Fibers (apple, banana, pineapple, papaya) 500 mg • Fructooligosaccharides from Chicory root 400 mg • Dairy-Free Probiotic Cultures (Lactobacillus acidophilus, L. bifidus, L. plantarum, L. rhamnosus, S. thermopilus) 360 mg • Wheat Germ Extract 350 mg • Vitamin E 120 IU • Acerola Berry Powder 120 mg • Licorice Root Extract 120 mg • Brown Rice 112 mg • Red Beet Extract 90 mg • Lipase 0.5 units • Amylase 0.5 skb units • Protease 10 hut • Aloe Vera 50 mg • Green Tea extract 30 mg • Reishi Mushroom 30 mg • Cat's Claw Extract 30 mg • Yucca Root Extract 30 mg • Ginger Root 30 mg • Ginkgo Biloba 20 mg • Bilberry Extract (25% anthocyanidins) 20 mg • Garcinia Extract 20 mg • Konjac Yam extract 20 mg • Maltodextrin 900 mg. Plus 60 mg of the following herbal extracts: Milk Thistle, Siberian Ginseng, Echinacea, American Ginseng.

Bio-Guard **-** Progressive Labs
Micellized antioxidant formula. Two mL contain: Vitamin A 10000 IU • Beta Carotene 2500 IU • Vitamin C 50 mg • Vitamin E 100 IU • Selenium (as selenomethionine) 50 mcg.

BioLax **-** Body Wise International, Inc.
Two caplets contain: Aloe Vera leaf extract 200:1 500 mg • Senna leaf 400 mg • Prune fruit 250 mg • Fig fruit 200 mg • Psyllium whole husks 100 mg • Celery seed 100 mg • Green Barley Grass 100 mg • Cruciferous Vegetables 100 mg • Lactobacillus Acidophilus 100 mg • Anise Seed 20 mg.

BioLean **-** Wellness International Network, Ltd.
Each AM serving of 2 tablets and 1 capsule contains: Calcium (as calcium carbonate, dicalcium phosphate anhydrous) 317 mg • Proprietary Blend 1300 mg: Ephedra Alkaloids (25 mg, as ma huang), Caffeine (12 mg, as green tea leaf), Schisandrae berry, Rehmannia root, Hawthorne berry, Jujube seed, Alisma root, Angelicae Dahuricae root, Epimedium, Poria Cocos, Rhizoma Rhei, Stephania root, Angelicae Sinensis root, Codonopsis root, Euconium bark, Notoginseng root • L-Phenylalanine 196 mg • L-Tyrosine 196 mg • L-Carnitine 9.42 mg. Inactive Ingredients: Cellulose, Stearic Acid, Starch, Sodium Lauryl Sulfate, Hydroxypropyl Cellulose, Magnesium Stearate, Croscarmelose Sodium, Silicon Dioxide.
See Editor's Note No. 30, page 2056.

BioLean Accelerator **-** Wellness International Network, Ltd.
Each caplet contains: Proprietary Blend 250 mg: Microcrystalline Cellulose, Black Sesame seed, Raw Chinese Foxglove root, Chinese Wolfberry root, Achyranthes root, Cornelian Cherry fruit, Chinese Yam, Eclipta herb, Rose Hips, Privet fruit, Mulberry fruit spike, Polygonat rhizome, Cooked Chinese Foxglove root, Poria Cocos, Cuscuta seed, Foxnut seed, Alisma rhizome, Moutan bark, Phellodendron bark, Anemarrhena rhizome, Schisandra berry, Royal Jelly • L-Phenylalanine 200 mg • L-Tyrosine 200 mg. Other Ingredients: Calcium Carbonate, Calcium Phosphate Dibasic, Partially Hydrogenated Vegetable Oil, Hydroxypropyl Cellulose, Croscarmellose Sodium, Magnesium Stearate, Silicon Dioxide, Sodium Lauryl Sulfate.

BioLean Free **-** Wellness International Network, Ltd.
Four caplets contain: Niacin (as niacinamide) 40 mg • Vitamin B6 (as pyridoxine HCl) 16 mg • Chromium (as chromium Chelavite, dinicolinate glycinate) 400 mcg • Potassium (as potassium citrate) 100 mg • Standardized Botanical Extracts 2972 mg: Green Tea leaf extract (10% methylxanthines), Yerba Mate leaf extract (10% methylxanthines), Korean Ginseng root extract (4% ginsenosides), Uva Ursi leaf (20% arbutin), Guarana seed (22% methylxanthines), Quebracho bark extract (10% quebrachine) • Non-Irradiated Pure Herbs and Thermogenic Spices 1440 mg: Gotu Kola leaf (centella asiatica), Ceylon Cinnamon bark, Chinese Horseradish root, Jamaican Ginger root, Tumeric rhizome, Nigerian Cayenne Pepper (fruit), English Mustard seed, Ho Shou Wu root, Ginkgo Biloba leaf (24% ginkgoflavoneslycosides and 6% bilobalides) • L-Tyrosine 500 mg • DL-Methionine 100 mg • Vanadium (as BMOV) 400 mcg. Other Ingredients: Dicalcium Phosphate, Cellulose, Cellulose Gum, Vegetable Stearic Acid, Silica, Vegetable Magnesium Stearate, Vegetable Resin Glaze.

BioLean LipoTrim **-** Wellness International Network, Ltd.
Each capsule contains: Chromium (as chromium polynicotinate, ChromeMate) 100 mcg • Garcinia Cambogia fruit (as hydroxycitrate CitriMax) 500 mg. Inactive Ingredients: Gelatin, Calcium Sulfate, Talc, Magnesium Stearate, Silicon Dioxide.

BiOmega-3 **-** USANA Health Sciences
Each capsule contains: Mixed Natural Tocopherols 1 mg • EPA (as Fish Oil) 180 mg • DHA (as Fish Oil) 120 mg • Total Omega-3 (as Fish Oil) 330 mg. Other Ingredients: Gelatin and Glycerin.

Bio-Organics Breathe-Eze **-** Bullivant's Natural Health Products (May
Each capsule contains: Inula helenium (Elecampane) root & rhiz dry 500 mg • Grindelia robusta (Grindelia) herb fl. dry 400 mg • Thymus vulgaris (Thyme) herb fl. dry 300 mg • Glycyrrhiza glabra (Licorice) root & stolon dry 250 mg • Euphorbia hirta (Euphorbia) herb dry 40 mg.

BioPectin **-** Flora, Inc.
Modified citrus pectin.

Bioperine **-** Source Naturals
Each tablet contains: Bioperine (95% pure piperine extracted from black pepper) 10 mg.

Bioperine brand **-** Sabinsa Corporation
Black Pepper extract.
See Editor's Note No. 44, page 2058.

Bio-Phoria **-** Olympian Labs
Two capsules contain: Proprietary Blend: St. John's Wort extract, Phosphatidyl Serine, Acetyl L-Carnitine, Gotu Kola 700 mg.

BioPro **-** PhytoPharmica
Two capsules contain: Vitamin A (fish liver oil) 3,000 IU •Vitamin B6 (pyridoxine HCl) 20 mg •Zinc (chelate) 40 mg • Essential fatty acids (unrefined vegetable lipids) 1,260 mg •Amino acid complex 300 mg •Prostate extract (freeze-dried) 300 mg • Saw Palmetto berry extract (4:1) 200 mg.
See Editor's Note No. 21, page 2056.

Biopure E 400 **-** Dial Herbs
Natural Vitamin E (soy-free d-alpha tocopherol) • Medium Chain Triglycerides (coconut) • Oleic Acid (canola oil). Capsule Shell: Gelatin, Vegetable Glycerine, Water.

Bios Life 2 **-** Unicity International, Inc.
Each packet contains: Vitamin A (from beta-carotene) 1000 IU • Vitamin C 60 mg • Vitamin E 30 IU • Thiamin (B1) 2.7 mg • Riboflavin (B2) 3.06 mg • Niacinamide (B3) 36 mg • Pyridoxine (B6) 3.6 mg • Biotin (B7) 30 mcg • Folic Acid (B9) 120 mcg • Cyanocobalamin (B12) 10.8 mcg • Calcium 100 mg • Chromium (as polynicotinate) 45 mcg • Selenium 5.5 mcg • Zinc 0.9 mg. Ingredients: Guar Gum, Gum Arabic, Locust Bean Gum, Pectin, Oat Fiber, Calcium Carbonate, Natural Orange Flavor, Ascorbic Acid, Stevia, Niacinamide, dl-Alpha-Tocopheryl Acetate, Natural Cream Flavor, Maltodextrin, Zinc Gluconate, Pyridoxine HCl, Riboflavin, Thiamin HCI, Beta-Carotene, Chromium Polynicotinate (ChromeMate), Folic Acid, Biotin, Sodium Selenite, Cyanocobalamin.

BioSculpt **-** 4 Youthful Health
Each 1 oz serving (30 mL) contains: Vitamin B5 60 mg • Vitamin B6 4 mg • Hydrolyzed Collagen 3000 mg • BioSculpt Complex 8500 mg: Aloe Vera gel, Garcinia Cambogia fruit (standardized to 50% hydroxycitric acid), Potassium Pyruvate, CLA, L-Carnitine • Proprietary Blend 1000 mg: L-Alanine, L-Lysine, L-Proline, L-Glutamine, L-Leucine, Hydroxyproline, Dimethyl Glycine.

BioShape – Royal BodyCare
Four caplets contain: Vitamin C (from ascorbyl palmitate) 40 mg • Calcium (from Super CitriMax Full Strength brand) 200 mg • Chromium (polynicotinate) 160 mcg • Potassium (From Super CitriMax Full Strength brand) 290 mg • Garcinia Cambogia fruit extract (Super CitriMax brand, providing (-) hydroxycitric acid 1120 mg) 1867 mg • Gymnema Sylvestre leaves extract (providing gymnemic acids 40 mg) 160 mg • Proprietary Amino Acid Blend 2000 mg: Isoleucine (as L-isoleucine), L-Lysine (as L-lysine HCl), Phenylalanine (as L-phenylalanine), Arginine (as L-arginine HCl), Glutamine (as L-glutamine), Leucine (as L-leucine), Methionine (as L-methionine), Threonine (as L-threonine), Valine (as L-valine), Histidine (as L-histidine HCl), L-5 Hydroxytryptophan. Other Ingredients: Microcrystalline Cellulose, Stearic Acid, Cellulose Gum, Silicon Dioxide.

Biosorb Silymarin - Metabolic Response Modifiers
Each capsule contains: Biosorb Silymarin (yielding 80 mg silymarin) 250 mg.

Biospec Muscle Builder - BioTherapies, Inc.
Two rounded tablespoons (28.4 g) contain: Riboflavin 0.136 mg • Niacin 0.8 mg • Calcium 200 mg • Phosphorus 150 mg • Iron 1.44 mg. Typical Amino Acid Profile: Alanine 1000 mg, Arginine 1490 mg, Aspartic Acid 2390 mg, Cystine 360 mg, Glycine 840 mg, Histidine 700 mg, Isoleucine 1490 mg, Leucine 2400 mg, Lysine 1900 mg, Methionine 590 mg, Phenylalanine 1370 mg, Proline 2160 mg, Serine 1420 mg, Threonine 1080 mg, Tryptophan 380 mg, Tyrosine 1260 mg, Valine 1000 mg.

Biotic Buddies - Advocare International
Each packet contains: Lactobacillus Acidophilus 1 billion • Bifidobacterium Bifidus 1 billion • Fructooligosaccharides 500 mg. Other Ingredients: Dextrose, Maltodextrin, Inulin, Natural Strawberry Flavor, Silicon Dioxide.

Biotin - Jamieson
Each tablet contains: Biotin 250 mcg.

Biotin - Nature's Bounty
Each tablet contains: Biotin 300 mcg. Other Ingredients: Dicalcium Phosphate, Cellulose, Vegetable Stearic Acid, Vegetable Magnesium Stearate.

Biotin - Source Naturals
Each tablet contains: Biotin 600 mcg.

Biotin - Basic Nutrition - GNC
Each tablet contains: Biotin 600 mcg. Other Ingredients: Dicalcium Phosphate, Cellulose, Magnesium Stearate.

Biotin 1000 mcg Vegetarian Formula - Vitamin World
Each tablet contains: Biotin (D-biotin) 1000 mcg. Other Ingredients: Dicalcium Phosphate, Cellulose (plant origin) Vegetable Stearic Acid, Croscarmellose, Cellulose Coating, Silica, Vegetable Magnesium Stearate.

Biotin 300 - GNC A-Z - GNC
Each tablet contains: Biotin 300 mg. Other Ingredients: Dicalcium Phosphate, Cellulose, Whole Brown Rice powder (Oryza sativa).

Biotin 300 mcg - Vitamin World
Each tablet contains: Biotin 300 mcg. Other Ingredients: Dicalcium Phosphate, Cellulose (plant origin), Vegetable Stearic Acid, Croscarmellose, Silica, Vegetable Magnesium Stearate.

Biotin 600 - GNC A-Z - GNC
Each tablet contains: Biotin 600 mcg. Other Ingredients: Dicalcium Phosphate, Cellulose.

Biotin 800 mcg - Rexall - Sundown
Each tablet contains: Biotin 800 mcg • Calcium 20 mg. Other Ingredients: Dextrose, Dicalcium Phosphate, Croscarmellose Sodium, Magnesium Stearate.

BioVin brand - Cyvex Nutrition, Inc.
Grape extract.
See Editor's Note No. 44, page 2058.

BioVin Plus brand - Cyvex Nutrition, Inc.
Grape seed extract.
See Editor's Note No. 44, page 2058.

BioVinca brand - Cyvex Nutrition, Inc.
Vinpocetine.
See Editor's Note No. 44, page 2058.

Biovital Plus - Enzymatic Therapy
Vitamin A (Beta Carotene) non-toxic form of Vitamin A 40000 IU • Vitamin A Fish Liver oil 25000 IU • Vitamin E (D-Tocopherol Succinate) 800 IU • Vitamin D Fish Liver oil 600 IU • Vitamin C (Ascorbic Acid/Rose Hips) 3000 mg • Calcium (Carbonate, Citrate, Aspartate, Gluconate) 625 mg • Potassium Aspartate 375 mg • Magnesium Aspartate 375 mg • Pantothenic Acid (D-Calcium Pantothenate) 250 mg • Thiamine HCL (Vitamin B1) 250 mg • Niacin/Niacinamide 250 mg • Manganese (Aspartate) 186 mg • Vitamin B6 (Pyridoxine HCL) 150 mg • Riboflavin (Vitamin B2/ Liver) 100 mg • Zinc (Aspartate) 92 mg • Iron (Aspartate) 60 mg • Copper (Aspartate) 2 mg • Biotin 1 mg • Folic Acid 800 mcg • Chromium Aspartate 428 mcg • Iodine (Kelp) 225 mcg • Selenium (Aspartate) 120 mcg • Vitamin B12 /Liver (Cyanocobalamin) 100 mcg • Other ingredients: Choline Bitartrate /Liver 750 mg • Bromelain (600 MCU) 400 mg • Pancreatic Enzymes (10X) 400 mg • PABA (Para Aminobenzoic Acid) 250 mg • Citrus Bioflavonoids 250 mg • Lipase 200 mg • L-Methionine 200 mg • Trace Mineral Complex "Containing 72 trace minerals" 200 mg • Alfalfa juice concentrate 200 mg • Liver concentrate (20X) 200 mg • Multi-Glandular concentrate 200 mg • Adrenal extract freeze-dried 200 mg • Thymus extract freeze-dried 200 mg • Saw Palmetto Berry extract 4:1 (Serenoa repens) 125 mg • Ma Huang extract (Ephedra sinensis) standardized to contain 6% Ephedrine 125 mg • Sarsaparilla root 4:1 (Smilax officinalis) 125 mg • Inositol 100 mg.
See Editor's Note No. 21 and No. 30, page 2056.

Bio-Zyme - PhytoPharmica
Two tablets contain: Amylase 10 mg • Bromelain (1200 MCU/g) 50 mg • Chymotrypsin 2 mg • Lipase 10 mg • Lysozyme 10 mg • Pancreatic Enzymes 10X 325 mg • Papain 50 mg • Trypsin 75 mg.

Biting Insect Mix - Professional Complementary Health Formul
Adrenal 3X, 4X • ACTH 6X, 30X • Histamine 12X • Liver 6X, 12X • Ant (black/fire/red), Bedbug, Bee (five types), Chigger, Cockroach, Deerfly, Flea, Horsefly, House Fly, Lice (head and body), Mosquito, Moth, Spider (five types), Tick, Wasp 6X, 12X, 60X, 100X • Purified Water • 20% USP Alcohol.
See Editor's Note No. 1, page 2053.

Bitters Virtue - Blessed Herbs
Aloe • Myrrh Gum • Senna • Camphor • Turkey Rhubarb root • Zedoary root • Manna • Carline Thistle • Angelica root • Licorice root • Fennel seed • Anise seed • Pomeranz peel • Gentian root • Galangal root & Peach brandy.

Black Cohosh - Source Naturals
Each tablet contains: Black Cohosh standardized extract 2.5% (Cimicifuga racemosa roots and rhizome) (yielding 2 mg of Triterpene Glycosides) (containing 27-deoxyactein) 80 mg.

Black Cohosh - Enzymatic Therapy
Each tablet contains: Black Cohosh root/rhizome extract (cimicifuga racemosa, standardized to contain 2.5% triterpene glycosides calculated as 27-deoxyactein) 20 mg. Other ingredients: Cellulose, Modified Cellulose, Magnesium Stearate, Lecithin, Peppermint Leaf, Carnauba Wax.

Some Brand Name Natural Products - What they Contain

www.NaturalDatabase.com contains MANY more listings than appear here.

Black Cohosh **-** Jamieson
Each caplet contains: Black Cohosh Root 40 mg.

Black Cohosh **-** Leiner Health Products
Each caplet contains: Black Cohosh extract powder (Cimicifuga racemosa) root 40 mg • Lecithin 25 mg. Other Ingredients: Calcium Carbonate, Dicalcium Phosphate, Cellulose, Maltodextrin, Stearic Acid, Croscarmellose Sodium, Silicon Dioxide, Magnesium Stearate, Dextrin, Hydroxypropyl Methylcellulose, Polyethylene Glycol 3350.

Black Cohosh **-** Nature's Way
Each capsule contains: Black Cohosh root 515 mg. Other Ingredients: Gelatin, Magnesium stearate, Millet.

Black Cohosh **-** PhysioLogics
Two softgels contain: Black Cohosh root/rhizome extract (cimicifuga racemosa, standardized to contain 2.5% triterpene glycosides conatining 27-deoxyactein, 2 mg) 80 mg. Other Ingredients: Soybean Oil, Gelatin, Glycerin, Beeswax / Soybean Oil Mixture, Lecithin, Caramel Color, Titanium Dioxide Color.

Black Cohosh 1000 mg, Concentrated - GNC Herbal Plus **-** GNC
Each capsule contains: Black Cohosh Root (cimicifuga racemosa; from 250 mg black cohosh root extract 4:1) 1000 mg. Other Ingredients: Soybean Oil, Gelatin, Glycerin, Partially Hydrogenated Soybean Oil, Caramel Color, Titanium Dioxide (natural mineral whitener).

Black Cohosh Extract **-** Nature's Way
Each tablet contains: Black Cohosh dried extract 40 mg. Other Ingredients: Cellulose, Maltodextrin, Modified Cellulose Gum, Silica, Stearic Acid.

Black Cohosh Root **-** Now
Two capsules contain: Black Cohosh (Cimicifuga Racemosa) root 1100 mg. Other Ingredients: Gelatin (capsule), Stearic Acid.

Black Cohosh Standardized Extract **-** Now
Two capsules contain: Black Cohosh root & rhizome 160 mg • Cimicfuga racemosa (standardized to contain 2.5% total triterpene Glycosides, calculated as 27-Deoxyactein) 4 mg • Licorice root 250 mg • Dong Quai root (Angelica sinensis) 250 mg.

Black Cohosh Whole Herb **-** Rexall - Sundown
Each capsule contains: Black Cohosh (root) 540 mg. Other Ingredients: Gelatin.

Black Cohosh-Blue Cohosh Virtue **-** Blessed Herbs
Black Cohosh root • Blue Cohosh root • Ginger root • Beth root • Grain alcohol & Distilled Water.

Black Currant 1000 **-** Health From The Sun
Each capsule contains: Alpha-Linolenic Acid (ALA) (Omega-3) 130 mg • Gamma Linolenic Acid (Omega-6) 170 mg • Linoleic Acid (Omega-6) 430 mg • Oleic Acid (Omega-9) 90 mg • Stearidonic Acid (Omega -3) 25 mg. Ingredients: Black Currant seed oil, Gelatin, Glycerine, Water.

Black Currant 500 **-** Health From The Sun
Each capsule contains: Alpha-Linolenic Acid (ALA)(Omega-3) 65 mg • Gamma Linolenic Acid (GLA)(Omega-6) 85 mg • Linoleic Acid (Omega-6) 215 mg • Oleic Acid (Omega-9) 45 mg • Stearidonic Acid (Omega-3) 12 mg. Ingredients: Black Currant seed oil, Gelatin, Glycerine, Water.

Black Currant Oil **-** Puritan's Pride
Each softgel contains: Black Currant oil 460 mg.

Black Currant seed oil **-** Nutri-Quest Rx
Each capsule contains: Black Currant seed oil 250 mg • Fatty Acid composition: Gamma Linolenic acid 16.9% • Linoleic 45.2% • Oleic 12.7% • Alpha Linolenic 11.7% • Palmitic 7.4% • Stearidonic 2.9% • Stearic 1.6% • Eicosenoic Acid 1.1%. Other Ingredients: Myristic, Arachidic, Behenic, Lignoceric, Palmitoleic Acids with natural Vitamin E 5 IU.

Black Currant Seed Oil **-** Vital Nutrients
Each capsule contains: Black Currant seed oil 460 mg (containing gamma linolenic acid 70 mg).

Black Ointment **-** 1st Herb Source
Chaparral herb • Lobelia herb • Comfrey herb • Red Clover herb • Plantain root • Golden Seal root • Myrrh gum • Marshmallow root • Mullein herb • Chickweed herb. In a base of Olive oil, Beeswax, Pine Tar, Vitamin E oil.

Black Seed & Green Tea Blend **-** Amazing Herbs
Thirty grams (1.06 ounces) contain: Proprietary Blend: Black Cumin Seed powder, Green Tea leaves.

Black Seed & Peppermint Tea **-** Amazing Herbs
Thirty grams (1.06 ounces) contain: Proprietary Blend: Black Cumin Seed powder, Peppermint leaves.

Black Seed Female Energy Tea **-** Amazing Herbs
Thirty grams (1.06 ounces) contain: Proprietary Blend: Black Cohosh, Ginseng, Ginkgo, Black Cumin Seed, St. John's Wort, Gotu Kola, Green Tea, Red Raspberry leaf, Rose Hips.

Black Seed Ground Herb **-** Amazing Herbs
Three ounces contain: Black Cumin Seed herb (100% pure, non-iradiated, untreated, unwashed, finely ground).

Black Seed Herbal Honey: Energizing Blend **-** Amazing Herbs
Sixteen ounces contain: Proprietary Blend: Black Seed oil (100% pure), Ginger, Ginseng, Ginkgo Biloba, Raw Natural Honey.

Black Seed Herbal Honey: Immune Boost **-** Amazing Herbs
Sixteen ounces contain: Proprietary Blend: Black Seed oil (100% pure), Echinacea, Elderberry, Garlic, Raw Natural Honey.

Black Seed Herbal Honey: Soothing Blend **-** Amazing Herbs
Sixteen ounces contain: Proprietary Blend: Black Seed oil (100% pure), Hyssop, Chamomile, Thyme, Raw Natural Honey.

Black Seed Male Energy Tea **-** Amazing Herbs
Thirty grams (1.06 ounces) contain: Proprietary Blend: Ginseng, Ginkgo, Yohimbe, Saw Palmetto, Green Tea, Black Cumin Seed, Echinacea, Mint, Rose Hips.

Black Seed Original Plain **-** Amazing Herbs
Each capsule contains: Pure Black Seed herb (black cumin, nigella sativa) 500 mg.

Black Seed Relaxing Blend **-** Amazing Herbs
Thirty grams (1.06 ounces) contain: Proprietary Blend: Black Cumin Seed powder, Hops, Valerian, Passion Flower, Mint, Orange peel, Chamomile, Stevia.

Black Seed Rooibos Tea Blend **-** Amazing Herbs
Thirty grams (1.06 ounces) contain: Proprietary Blend: Black Cumin Seed powder, South African Rooibos.

Black Seed Whole Herb **-** Amazing Herbs
Four ounces contain: Black Cumin Seed herb (100% pure, non-iradiated, untreated, unwashed).

Blackstrap Molasses with Iron **-** Swanson
Each tablet contains: Blackstrap Molasses with 29 mg of Iron.

Bladderwrack-Dandelion Virtue **-** Blessed Herbs
Ma Huang • Guarana seed • Dandelion blend of flower, leaf & root • Bladderwrack • Grain alcohol & Distilled Water.
See Editor's Note No. 30, page 2056.

Blast of Grass **-** Green Foods Corp.
Active Ingredient: Barley Grass Essence.

BLF # Breathe Easy Without Stimulants - Health Center for Better Living
Two tablets contain: Siberian Ginseng root extract (0.8% eleutherosides) 250 mg • American Ginseng root 250 mg • Ginger root standardized extract (5% gingerols) • Peppermint leaf 75 mg • Chickweed herb (aerial parts) 50 mg • Myrrh resin 50 mg • Mullein leaf 50 mg • Yerba Mate leaf (20% alkaloids) • MSM (methyisulforaimethan, 36% organic sulfur) 1,000 mg.

BLF #1 Clear Complexion - Health Center for Better Living
Each capsule contains: Burdock Root 84 mg • Dandelion Root 84 mg • Red Clover tops 84 mg • Echinacea root 56 mg • Yellow Dock root 56 mg • Capsicum 28 mg • Alfalfa Leaf 28 mg • Valerian Root 28 mg.

BLF #12 Cholest-A Ingredients - Health Center for Better Living
Each capsule contains: Hawthorn Berry 113 mg • Fenugreek Seed 75 mg • Capsicum 75 mg • Plantain Herb 75 mg • Red Clover Blossom 75 mg • Black Cohosh Root 38 mg.

BLF #125 Woman's Balance - Health Center for Better Living
Each capsule contains: Dong Quai Root 102 mg • Damiana Leaf 61 mg • Kelp Atlantic 61 mg • Sarsaparilla Root 61 mg • Saw Palmetto Berry 41 mg • Chickweed Herb 41 mg • Capsicum 41 mg • Black Cohosh Root 41 mg.

BLF #13 Body Circulation - Health Center for Better Living
Each capsule contains: Capsicum 84 mg • Bayberry Bark 34 mg • Hyssop Leaf 17 mg • Skullcap 17 mg • Witch Hazel Bark 17 mg.

BLF #16 Colon Helper - Health Center for Better Living
Each capsule contains: Slippery Elm Bark 145 mg • Aloe 145 mg • White Oak Bark 73 mg • Blue Vervain Herb 73 mg • Gentain Root 36 mg • Goldenseal Herb 15 mg.

BLF #17 Regularity Ingredients - Health Center for Better Living
Each capsule contains: Buckthorn Bark 113 mg • Cascara Sagrada Bark 113 mg • Chickweed Herb 75 mg • Elder Flower 75 mg • Oregon Grape Root 38 mg • Mandrake Root 38 mg.

BLF #2 Allergy First Aid - Health Center for Better Living
Each caplet contains: Allergy Herbal Blend 200 mg: Hyssop whole plant, Mullein leaves, Thyme whole plant, Chrysanthemum flower, Magnolia flower, Angelica root, Vitex fruit, Atractylodes Rhizome, Bellflower root, Field Mint, Immature Tangerine peel, Ledebouriella root, Moutan bark, Perilla leaf and Schizonepeta stem • Boswellia Gum resin (40% boswellic acid) 100 mg • Yerba Mate leaf (20% alkaloids) 50 mg • Meadowsweet 4:1 extract 50 mg • Eucalyptus leaf extract 25 mg • Fennel seed 25 mg.

BLF #21 Endless Energy - Health Center for Better Living
Each capsule contains: Ginseng Root 75 mg • Foti Root • Bee Pollen Granules 75 mg • Damiana Leaf 75 mg • Capsicum 50 mg • Kola Nut 50 mg • Echinacea Root 25 mg • Licorice Root 25 mg.

BLF #225 Man's Rejuvenator - Health Center for Better Living
Each capsule contains: Saw Palmetto Berry 75 mg • Cornsilk 75 mg • Gota Kola Herb 75 mg • Damiana Leaf 75 mg • Juniper Berry 38 mg • Kelp Atlantic 38 mg • Parsley Leaf 38 mg • Uva Ursi Leaf 38 mg.

BLF #23 Vision Booster - Health Center for Better Living
Vitamin A [as retinyl palmitate and 75% as beta-carotene with natural mixed carotenoids (alpha-carotene, beta-carotene, cryptoxanthin, zeaxanthin and lutein)] 10,000 IU • Vitamin C (as ascorbic acid) 250 mg • Vitamin E (as d-alpha-tocopheryl succinate and 50% as dl-alpha-tocopheryl acetate) 100 IU • Selenium (as selenomethionine) 100 mcg • Bilberry Herb blend [Bilberry leaf and Bilberry fruit standardized extract (25% anthocyanins)] 75 mg • Eyebright herb blend [Eyebright herb and eyebright herb 4:1 extract (whole plant)] 75 mg • Lutein (from marigold flower) 5 mg • L-Glutathione 5 mg • Taurine 5 mg • Quercetin dihydrate 75 mg • Lycium berry 5:1 extract 50 mg.

BLF #24 Fresh Start - Health Center for Better Living
Alfalfa • Hyssop • Chamomile • Cornsilk • "Vitamins and minerals with antioxidant and diuretic qualities."

BLF #3 Love Formula - Health Center for Better Living
Two caplets contain: Tribulus terrestris extract (20% furanosterois) fruit and root 400 mg • Damiana leaf 125 mg • Fo-ti root 125 mg • Gota Kola leaf extract (10% total asiaticosides) 50 mg • Saw Palmetto berry extract (85-95% sterols and fatty acid) 150 mg • Korean Ginseng root extract (10% ginsenosides) 200 mg.

BLF #30 Head-X - Health Center for Better Living
Each capsule contains: Fenugreek seed 107 mg • Feverfew herb 107 mg • Passion Flower herb 43 mg • Rosemary leaf 43 mg • Peppermint leaf 43 mg • Thyme leaf 21 mg • Marjoram leaf 21 mg • Blue Violet leaf 21 mg • Wood Betony herb 21 mg • Lobelia herb 21 mg.

BLF #31 Healthy Heart - Health Center for Better Living
Each capsule contains: Angelica root 45 mg • Blue Cohosh root 45 mg • Borage herb 45 mg • Capsicum 45 mg • Blue Vervain herb 45 mg • Peppermint leaf 45 mg • Wood Betony herb 45 mg • Sheep Sorrel herb 23 mg • Garlic Bulb 23 mg • Barberry Bark 23 mg • Goldenseal root 23 mg • Motherwort herb 23 mg • Scullcap herb 23 mg.

BLF #35 Sleep Like a Baby - Health Center for Better Living
Each capsule contains: Hops flower 113 mg • Passion flower 113 mg • Scullcap herb 75 mg • Catnip leaf 38 mg • Peppermint leaf 38 mg • Rosemary leaf 38 mg • Mullein leaf 38 mg.

BLF #38 Kidney Flush - Health Center for Better Living
Each caplet contains: Vitamin B6 (as pyridoxine HCl) 5 mg • Magnesium (as magnesium oxide) • Potassium (as potassium citrate) • Uva Ursi Leaf standardized extract (20% arbutin) 100 mg • Chokeberry fruit standardized extract (35% quinic acid) 100 mg • Cranberry juice 10:1 concentrate 50 mg • Dandelion root standardized extract (20% taraxasterol) 50 mg • Aloe Vera 200x gel 25 mg • Herbal Blend 200 mg: Couchgrass (whole plant), Buchu leaf, Uva Ursi leaf, Juniper berry, Hydrangea root, Cornsilk stylus.

BLF #41 Liver De-Tox - Health Center for Better Living
Each capsule contains: Fennel seed 107 mg • Chicory root 107 mg • Angelica root 54 mg • Cleavers herb 54 mg • Dandelion root 27 mg • Gentian root 27 mg • Hops flower 27 mg • Elder flower 27 mg • Wormwood herb 11 mg • Lobelia herb 11 mg.

BLF #42 Prime Lung - Health Center for Better Living
Each capsule contains: Mullein leaf 101 mg • Coltsfoot herb 101 mg • Chickweed herb 67 mg • Fenugreek seed 34 mg • Pennyroyal leaf 34 mg • Myrrh Gum 34 mg • Yarrow flower 34 mg • Nettle leaf 34 mg • Lobelia herb 13 mg.

BLF #43 Bone & Nail Builder - Health Center for Better Living
Each capsule contains: Bee Pollen Granules 87 mg • Horsetail 43 mg • Oatstraw 43 mg • Kelp Atlantic 43 mg • Ginseng root 43 mg • Foti root 43 mg • Chamomile flower 43 mg • Rose hips 43 mg • Red Clover blossom 43 mg • Lobelia Herb 17 mg.

BLF #44 Woman's Change - Health Center for Better Living
Two tablets contain: Black Cohosh root extract (2.5% triterpene glycosides) 160 mg • Dong Quai root extract (1% lingustilide) 200 mg • Chaste Tree berry extract (5% vitexi cacpin) 100 mg • Licorice root extract (13% glycyrrhizin) 100 mg • Soybean and Kudzu root extract (20% total isoflavones) 150 mg • Damiana leaf 100 mg • Wild Yam root extract (5% diosgenin) 150 mg • Red Clover flowers 100 mg.

BLF #47 Rest Ease Ingredients - Health Center for Better Living
Each capsule contains: Valerian root 101 mg • Wintergreen leaf 67 mg • Peppermint leaf 67 mg • Spearmint leaf 67 mg • Sassafras root bark 34 mg • Capsicum 34 mg • Burdock root 34 mg • Buckthorn bark 34 mg • Lobelia herb 13 mg.

BLF #48 Anti-Stress - Health Center for Better Living
Each capsule contains: Hops flower 99 mg • Valerian root 99 mg • Scullcap herb 66 mg • Catnip leaf 66 mg • Passion Flower herb 66 mg • Red Clover herb 33 mg • Black Cohosh root 20 mg.

BLF #49 Stable Sugar - Health Center for Better Living
Each capsule contains: Juniper Berries 94 mg • Uva Ursi leaf 94 mg • Garlic Bulb 94 mg • Dandelion root 47 mg • Capsicum 47 mg • Mullein leaf 47 mg • Licorice root 28 mg.

BLF #52 Fatigue Fighter - Health Center for Better Living
Prime Ingredients: Capsicum • Ginseng.

BLF #53 Male Vigor - Health Center for Better Living
Two caplets contain: Yohimbe bark extract (2% yohimbe, 4% total alkaiods) 500 mg • Tribulus terrestris extract (20% furanosterols) fruit and root • Korean Ginseng root extract (10% ginsenosides) 200 mg • Yerba Mate leaf extract (20% total alkaloids) 125 mg • Saw Palmetto berry extract (85-95% sterols and fatty acid) 160 mg • Male support blend of Damiana leaf, Fo-ti root, Gota Kola leaf, and Pumpkin Seed concentrate 250 mg.

BLF #54 Sinus & Hayfever Ingredients - Health Center for Better Living
Each capsule contains: Myrrh Gum 148 mg • Echinacea Root 74 mg • Bayberry Bark 74 mg • Plantain Herb 74 mg • Saw Palmetto Berry 22 mg • Licorice Root 22 mg • Goldenseal Herb.

BLF #55 Pro Skin Enhancer - Health Center for Better Living
Each capsule contains: Red Clover blossom 115 mg • Spikenard root 115 mg • Dandelion root 58 mg • Chickweed herb 29 mg • Plantain herb 29 mg • Blue Vervain herb 29 mg • Sarsaparilla root 29 mg • Buckthorn bark 29 mg • Goldenseal root 17 mg.

BLF #57 Vein Vanish - Health Center for Better Living
Each capsule contains: White Oak bark 87 mg • Witch Hazel bark 87 mg • Bayberry bark 87 mg • Capsicum 87 mg • Kelp Atlantic 43 mg • Goldenseal root 43 mg • Lobelia herb 17 mg.

BLF #59 Weight Loss - Health Center for Better Living
Each capsule contains: Nettle leaf 139 mg • Chickweed herb 93 mg • Seawrack 93 mg • Kelp Atlantic 35 mg • Fennel seed 23 mg • Hawthorn berry 23 mg • Dandelion root 12 mg • Echinacea root 12 mg • Burdock root 12 mg • Licorice root 5 mg • Chia seed 5 mg.

BLF #6 Healthy Joints - Health Center for Better Living
Burdock • Alfalfa • Kelp • Vitamin C • Vitamin E • Vitamin B6.

BLF #61 P.M.S. Stop - Health Center for Better Living
Each capsule contains: Black Cohosh Root 82 mg • Dong Quai Root 82 mg • Red Raspberry Leaf 82 mg • Chaste Tree Berry 57 mg • Ginger Root 49 mg • Dandelion Root 41 mg • Motherwort Herb 33 mg • Valerian Root 25 mg.

BLF #75 Prostate Support - Health Center for Better Living
Two tablets contain: Zinc (as zinc glycinate) 15 mg • Saw Palmetto berry extract (85-95% sterols and fatty acid) 320 mg • Pygeum bark 4:1 extract 100 mg • Pumpkin seed 10:1 concentrate 100 mg • Tomato lycopene concentrate (10,000 lycopene) 100 mg • Urinary tract support blend [Chokeberry extract (35% quinic acid), Cranberry juice 10:1 concentrate, Uva-Ursi leaf extract (20% arbutin)].

BLF #9: 120 Over 80 - Health Center for Better Living
Two tablets contain: Calcium (as calcium carbonate and calcium citratemalate-glycinate) 500 mg • Magnesium (as magnesium oxide and magnesium amino acid chelate) 200 mg • Potassium (as postassium citrate) • Ginger root extract (5% gingerols) 100 mg • Odor-controlled Garlic extract (10,000 ppm allicin) 300 mg • Hawthorn berry extract (5% flavonoid glycosides) 250 mg • Capsicum pepper 50 mg • Panax Ginseng root extract (10% ginsenosides) 100 mg • Onion bulb 50 mg • Parsley leaf 50 mg.

Block It - PotentHerbs
Two capsules contain: Proprietary Blend 1000 mg: Chromium Polynicotinate 200 mcg, Phaseolus Vulgaris L (Phase 2), Chitosan (Quik-o-san), Gymnema Sylvestre. Other Ingredients: Certified Kosher Gel Caps.
See Editor's Note No. 37, page 2057.

Blood Pressure - Grandma's Herbs
Each capsule contains: Proprietary Blend 0.477 g: Cayenne Pepper fruit, Garlic clove, Black Cohosh root, Mistletoe leaf, Sassafras root, Ginko leaf, Valerian root, Wild Yam root, Nettle leaf, Horsetail grass, Bladderwrack leaf, Hyssop herb, Ginseng root, Bladder Pod herb, Dong Quai root, Bayberry bark. Other Ingredients: Gelatin.

Blood Pressure - Nutrivention
Three tablets contain: Vitamin B6 100 mg • Calcium 50 mg • Potassium 45 mg • Magnesium 30 mg • Manganese 15 mg • Vitamin D 50 IU • Hawthorne berries 500 mg • Apple Pectin 500 mg • Garlic powder concentrate 500 mg • Cayenne pepper 500 mg • Black Cohosh 300 mg • Valerian root (Star root) 200 mg • Hops 200 mg • L-Taurine 100 mg.

Blood Pressure Control - TwinLab
Two tablets contain: C-12 Peptide (enzymatically hydrolyzed casein) 100 mg. Other Ingredients: Maltodextrin, Cellulose, Vegetable Stearic Acid, Calcium Phosphate, Croscarmellose Sodium, Silica, Magnesium Stearate, Polyethylene Glycol, Carrageenan, Water.

Blood Sugar - Bioset - Enzymes, Inc.
Each capsule contains: Vitamin E (100% from d-Alpha Tocopheryl Acid Succinate) 30 mg • Zinc (100% from Zinc Citrate) 5 mg • Manganese (100% from Manganese Citrate) 1 mg • Chromium (50% from Chromium Picolinate, 50% from Chromium GTF Polynicotinate) 1 mg • Proprietary Herbal Blend 415 mg: Gymnema leaf extract, Bitter Melon extract, Jambolan seed extract, Garlic bulb conc., Green Tea leaf extract, Black Currant seed extract • Lipase 25 mg. Other Ingredients: Plant Cellulose, Water.

Blood Sugar Balance - ProHerbs - Mason Vitamins, Inc.
Two tablets contain: Biotin 600 mcg • Magnesium (as Oxide) 200 mg • Zinc (as Sulfate) 30 mg • Gymnema Sylvestre leaves (standardized to 24% Gymnemic Acid) 300 mg • Bitter Melon powder (Momordica charantia fruit) 200 mg • Ginkgo Biloba leaf (standardized to 24% flavonoids glycosides & 6% terpene lactones) 120 mg • Chromium Picolinate 400 mcg • Alpha Lipoic Acid 150 mg • Quercetin 50 mg • Vanadium (as Vanadyl Pentoxide) 40 mcg. Other Ingredients: Dicalcium Phosphate, Microcrystalline Cellulose, Croscarmellose Sodium, Hydroxypropylmethylcellulose, Magnesium Stearate, Mineral Oil, Polyethylene Glycol, Stearic Acid, Titanium Dioxide, Sodium Lauryl Sulfate, FD&C Yellow #6 Lake, Red #40 Lake, Iron Oxide.

Blood Sugar Balance - Wellzymes - Enzymes, Inc.
Two capsules contain: Vitamin E (from d-Alpha Tocopheryl Acid Succinate) 40 IU • Chromium (from Chromium GTF Polynicolinate) 100 mcg • n-zimes Proprietary Enzyme Blend 20 mg: Lipase, CereCalase Plus • Proprietary Herbal Blend 330 mg: Gymnema leaf extract (standardized to contain 25% gymnemic acid), Fenugreek seed extract (equivalent to 400 mg raw herb), Rice Bran, Quercetin. Other Ingredients: Plant Cellulose, Water.

Blood Sugar Blues - The Herbalist
Devil's Club root bark • Blueberry leaf • Dandelion root • Oregon Grape root • Uva Ursi leaf • Juniper berry • Licorice root • Elecampane root.

Blood Sugar Essentials **-** Swanson
Each tablet contains: Vitamin C (as calcium ascorbate) 100 mg • Vitamin E (as d-alpha tocopheryl succinate) 133.3 IU • Magnesium (from magnesium oxide) 66.7 mg • Biotin 333.3 mcg • Zinc (OptiZinc®) 5 mg • Chromium (from Chromax® chromium picolinate) 66.7 mcg • Gymnema Sylvestre powder 134 mg • Momordica Charantia (2.5%) 100 mg • Fenugreek seed powder 67 mg • Inositol 50 mg • Vanadyl Sulfate 4 mg.

Blood Sugar Formula **-** Nature's Way
Three capsules contain: Bilberry leaf 255 mg • Bitter Melon dried extract 150 mg • Caromix (Mixed Carotenoids) 30 mg • Chromium Polynicotinate 300 mcg • Fenugreek dried extract 210 mg • Gymnema sylvestre dried extract 66 mg • Prickly Pear leaf pad 420 mg. Other Ingredients: Gelatin, Magnesium Stearate, Millet.

Bloussant **-** WellQuest International, Inc.
Each tablet contains: Saw Palmetto extract (Serenoa Repens) leaf 150 mg • Fennel Seed (Foeniculum Vulgare) fruit 50 mg • Dong Quai leaf 50 mg • Damiana (Tumera Diffusa) leaf 100 mg • Blessed Thistle (Cnicus Benedictus) leaf 40 mg • Dandelion (Taraxaci Herba) root 40 mg • Watercress (Nasturtium Officinale) leaf 40 mg • Black Cohosh (Cimicifuga Racemosa) root 50 mg • Wild Yam (Dioscorea Villosa) root 40 mg. Other Ingredients: Silicon Dioxide, Magnesium Stearate, Titanium Dioxide, Gelatin, and Water.

Blubberwack **-** The Herbalist
Bladderwrack • Gotu Kola herb • Kelp • Echinacea root • Kola Nut • Licorice root.

Blue Green Algae **-** PhysioLogics
Each capsule contains: Klamath Lake Blue Green Algae (aphanizomenon flos-aquae) 500 mg. Other Ingredients: Gelatin, Vegetable Magnesium Stearate, Silica.

Blue Green Algae **-** Rexall - Sundown
Each two capsules contain: Blue Green Algae Blend: Spirulina Blue-Green Algae (spirulina platensis), Watercress (aerial parts), Klamath Blue-Green Algae (aphanizomenon flos-aquae) 750 mg. Other Ingredients: Gelatin.

Blue Green Algae from Upper Klamath Lake **-** Futurebiotics
Blue-Green algae 500 mg.

Blue Green Micro Algae **-** Olympian Labs
Each capsule contains: Blue Green Micro Algae 380 mg.

Blue Joint Soother **-** Biorganics, Inc.
Aloe Vera Gel • Emu Oil • SD-Alcohol 40-B • Glucosamine Sulfate (from shellfish) • Dimethyl Sulfone (MSM) • Oleoresin of Capsicum • Arnica extract • Sorbitol • Chondroitin Sulfate • Menthol • White Nettle extract • Witch Hazel • Coriander Oil • Kava Kava extract • Willow bark extract • Propylene Glycol • Methylparaben • Propylparaben • Diazolidinyl Urea • Carbomer • Chamomile • Marigold extract • Triethanolamine • Ascorbyl Palmitate (vitamin C) • Tocopherol Acetate (vitamin E) • Fragrance • FD&C Blue #1. See Editor's Note No. 15, page 2055.

Blue-Green Connection **-** HealthWatchers System
Spirulina • Chlorella • Klamath Lake Algae • Ginkgo Biloba • CoQ10 • Wheatgrass • Alfalfa • Chlorophyll.

Blue-Green Stuff **-** Blue Stuff, Inc.
Each gel cap contains: Organic Wheatgrass juice powder • Barley Grass juice powder • organic Oatgrass juice powder • organic Spirulina.

B-Nase **-** Nutraceutics Corp.
Four sprays contain: Vitamin B12 500 mcg • Dibencozide (coenzyme B12) 500 mcg • ATP (adenosine triphosphate) 10,000 mcg • Alpha Glycerylphosphorylcholine 10,000 mcg. Other Ingredients: Purified Water, Sodium Benzoate, Potassium Sorbate, Glycerin, Citric Acid, Sodium Citrate.

Body Answers Grapefruit Diet **-** GNC
Each capsule contains: CitraSens Grapefruit extract 500 mg. Other Ingredients: Gelatin, Cellulose.

Body Balance **-** Life Force International
Each 30 mL contains: Proprietary Blend: Aloe Vera juice, Black Cherry, Raw Honey, Pure Water, Fucus Gardneri, Ulva Latuca, Alaria Valida, Nerecocystis Leutkeana, Laminaria, Ulva Linza, Gigartina, Costaria Costata, Phodymenia Pertusa.

Body Contouring Cream **-** Herbalife
Water • Cetyl Esters • Isopropyl Myristate • Stearyl Alcohol • Hydrogenated Coco-glycerides • Steareth-20 • Caffeine • Propylene Glycol • Lecithin • Aminophylline • Imidazolidinyl • Urea • Methylparaben • Carbomer • Propylparaben • Triethanolamine • Algae • Magnolia Bark extract • Fragrance • Horsetail extract • Rose Hips extract • Mate.

Body Fortress Hardcore Formula Creatine Powder **-** U.S. Nutrition
Each scoop (5 g) contains: HPLC Pure Creatine Monohydrate 5000 mg.

Body Guard **-** Jamieson
Chlorhexidine Gluconate • Glycerin • Nonoxynol-9 • Witch Hazel Herbal Extract.

Body Octane **-** MAN
Each level 1 tsp (8 grams) serving contains: Citruline Malate 3500 mg • L-Carnitine L-Tartrate 1500 mg • Beta-Alanine 1000 mg • Histidine 500 mg. Other Ingreients: Maltodextrin, Citric Acid, Natural Orange Flavor, Natural Vanilla, Sucralose, Sodium Chloride.

Body Rewards Daily Multiple **-** Enzymatic Therapy
Each tablet contains: Vitamin A (50% as beta carotene and as retinyl acetate) 5000 IU • Vitamin C (ascorbic acid) 200 mg • Vitamin D (as cholecalciferol) 400 IU • Vitamin E (as d-alpha tocopheryl acid succinate) 100 IU • Vitamin K (as phytonadione) 80 mcg • Thiamin (as thiamin HCl, vitamin B1) 15 mg • Riboflavin (vitamin B2) 17 mg • Niacin (as niacin and niacinamide) 20 mg • Vitamin B6 (as pyridoxine HCl) 20 mg • Folic Acid 800 mcg • Vitamin B12 (as cyanocobalamin) 60 mcg • Biotin 300 mcg • Pantothenic Acid (as calcium D-pantothenate) 10 mg • Calcium (from tricalcium phosphate) 200 mg • Phosphorus (as tricalcium phosphate) 100 mg • Iodine (as potassium iodide) 150 mcg • Magnesium (as magnesium oxide and magnesium aspartate) 1000 mg • Zinc (as zinc ascorbate) 15 mg • Selenium (as L-selenomethionine) 70 mcg • Manganese (as manganese citrate) 2 mg • Chromium (as chromium picolinate) 120 mcg • Molybdenum (as sodium molybdate) 75 mcg • Green Tea leaf extract (camellia sinensis, standardized to contain 4.2 mg caffeine) 30 mg • Boron (as sodium borate) 1 mg • Vanadium (as vanadyl sulfate) 16 mcg. Other Ingredients: Cellulose, Modified Cellulose, Modified Cellulose Gum, Magnesium Stearate, Lecithin, Riboflavin Color, Carnauba Wax.

Body Rewards Digestion Formula **-** Enzymatic Therapy
Each capsule contains: Proprietary Plant Enzyme Blend 156 mg: Protease, Amylase, Lipase, Lactase, Phytase, Cellulase, Sucrase, Maltase. Other Ingredients: Gelatin, Cellulose, Titanium Dioxide Color.

Body Rewards Fruit & Veggie 5 **-** Enzymatic Therapy
Eight capsules contain: Vitamin A (as beta carotene) 11,822 IU • Vitamin C (ascorbic acid) 480 mg • Psyllium husk (plantago ovata) 2665 mg • Pectin (from citrus fruits) 16 mg • Proprietary PhytoRedoxin Blend 19 mg: Lutein 5% (from calendula officinalis), Lycopene, Quercetin. Other Ingredients: Cellulose, Gelatin, Titanium Dioxide Color, Magnesium Stearate, Silicon Dioxide.

Body Rewards Healthy Skin **-** Enzymatic Therapy
Three softgels contain: Proprietary Essential Oils Blend 2402 mg: Fish oil, Borage seed oil (borago officinalis), Flax seed oil (linum

usitatissimum). Other Ingredients: Gelatin, Glycerin, Mixed Tocopherols (preservative).

Body Rox **-** USANA Health Sciences
Each tablet contains: Vitamin A (as Beta Carotene) 3000 IU • Vitamin C (as Calcium Ascorbate) 167 mg • Vitamin D (Vitamin D3 as Cholecalciferol) 133 IU • Vitamin E (as D-Alpha Tocopheryl Succinate) 66.7 IU • Vitamin K (as Phylloquinone) 12 mcg • Thiamine (as Thiamine HCl) 3 mg • Riboflavin 3 mg • Niacin (as Niacin and Niacinamide) 5 mg • Vitamin B6 (as Pyridoxine HCl) 3 mg • Folate (as Folic Acid) 267 mcg • Vitamin B12 (as Cyanocobalamin) 20 mcg • Biotin 100 mcg • Pantothenic Acid (as D-Calcium Pantothenate) 10 mg • Calcium (as Ascorbate and Citrate) 50 mg • Iodine (as Potassium Iodide) 50 mcg • Magnesium (as Amino Acid Chelate) 25 mg • Zinc (as Citrate) 4 mg • Selenium (as Amino Acid Complex) 40 mcg • Copper (as Gluconate) 0.33 mg • Manganese (as Amino Acid Chelate) 1 mg • Chromium (as Amino Acid Chelate) 50 mcg • Molybdenum (as Amino Acid Chelate) 10 mcg • Bioflavonoid Complex 30 mg: Rutin, Hesperidin (Citrus SPP. L. fruit), Green Tea Extract Decaffeinated (Camellia Sinensis Hunt leaf) • Inositol 10 mg • Choline Bitartrate 15 mg • Cruciferous Extract (Brassica Oleracea L.) 25 mg • N-Acetyl-L-Cysteine 10 mg • Boron (as Amino Acid Complex) 0.33 mg. Other Ingredients: Microcrystalline Cellulouse, Croscarmellose Sodium, Maltodextrin, Ascorbyl Palmitate, Sodium Citrate, Collodial Silicon Dioxide, Lecithin.

Body Shape **-** Hydroderm
Organic Kukui nut oil • Organic Caffeine • Organic Lecithin (liposomes). Other Ingredients: Water, Potassium Sorbate, Peg 8 Stearate, Cetyl Alcohol, Stearic Acid, Polysorbate 80, Decamethyltetrasiloxane, Silicone Resin Dimethicone, Green Tea Extract, Carbomer, Triethanolamine, Silicone Glycol Copolymer, Propylene Glycol, Sodium Chloride, Tocopheryl Acetate Dl-a, Disodium EDTA, Glycolic Acid, Fragrance Tropical, Propylparaben, Methylparaben.

Body Solutions - Evening Formula **-** Mark Nutritionals, Inc.
Each tablespoon contains: Chromium (as chromium picolinate, chromium polynicotinate, and chromium cruciferate) 15 mcg • Proprietary Blend of Aloe Vera Gel, Collmark, Fosmark, Leanmark, Conjugated Linoleic Acid, Stevia 6 mL. Other Ingredients: Purified Water, Glycerin, Natural Kiwi Flavor, Natural Strawberry Flavor, Xanthan Gum, Sodium benzoate, Potassium sorbate.

Body Stuff **-** Blue Stuff, Inc.
Each 8 oz bottle contains: Whole leaf Aloe Vera concentrate • Purified Water • Squalene • Emu oil • Glyceryl Stearate • Lanolin Alcohol • Propylene Glycol • Sorbitan Sesquioleate • Stearic Acid • Dimethicone • PEG-75 Lanolin • Allantoin • Polysorbate-60 • Apricot Kernel oil • Sesame Seed oil • Jojoba oil • Carbomer-940 • Treithanolamine • Methylparaben • Fragrance • Imidazolidinyl Urea • Proylparaben.

BodyLean Bars **-** Advocare International
Maltitol Syrup • BodyLean Protein Blend (whey protein isolate, calcium caseinate, soy protein isolate, milk protein isolate) • Dark Chocolate flavored coating (sugar, fractionated palm kernel oil, cocoa [processed with alkali], lactose, dextrose, soy lecithin, natural flavor) • High Fructose Corn Syrup • Rice Syrup • Partially Defatted Peanut Flour • Crisp Grain (soy protein isolate, rice flour, malt, salt) • Ground Peanuts • Natural Flavor • Honey • Salt • Magnesium Oxide • Glycerin • Potassium Chloride • L-Leucine • Sucralose • Ascorbic Acid • L-Valine • L-Isoleucine • Maltodextrin • Niacinamide • Calcium Pantothenate • Bromelain • Papain • Manganese Sulfate • Pyridoxine HCl • Riboflavin • Thiamine Mononitrate • Biotin • Cyanocobalamin.

BodyLean Shake, Vanilla **-** Advocare International
Metabolically Balanced Protein Isolate (containing total milk protein, calcium, sodium caseinate, whey protein concentrate, soy protein concentrate, branched chain amino acids [L-leucine, L-isoleucine, L-valine]) • Fructose • Natural Flavors • Artificial Flavors • Magnesium Oxide • Ascorbic Acid • Acesulfame Potassium • Pyridoxine Hydrochloride • Calcium Pantothenate • Niacin • Manganese Sulfate • Papain • Bromelain • Thiamine Hydrochloride • Riboflavin • Biotin • Cyanocobalamin.

BodySynergy Anti-Craving Formula **-** Rexall - Sundown
Two tablets contain: Vitamin B-6 (from pyridoxine HCl and pyridoxal-5-phophate) 12 mg • Calcium 125 mg • Chromium (from chromium polynicotinate) 133 mcg • Sodium 10 mg • BodySynergy proprietary blend: DL-Phenylalanine, L-Tyrosine, Stinging Nettle leaf, L-Glutamine, L-Carnitine 1237 mg. Other Ingredients: Dicalcium Phosphate, Cellulose, Croscarmellose Sodium, Silica, Stearic Acid, Calcium Citrate, Hydroxypropyl Methylcellulose, Magnesium Stearate, PEG.

BodySynergy Meal Replacement Drink Mix - Chocolate **-** Rexall - Sundown
Each packet contains: Sodium 100 mg • Protein 18 g • Vitamin A (Retinyl Palmitate) 1250 IU • Vitamin C (Ascorbic Acid) 15 mg • Calcium 500 mg • Electrolytic Iron 4.5 mg • Vitamin D (Cholecalciferol) 100 IU • Vitamin E (dl-Alpha Tocopheryl Acetate) 7.5 IU • Thiamin Mononitrate 0.375 mg • Riboflavin 0.425 mg • Niacin (Niacinamide) 5 mg • Vitamin B6 (Pyridoxine Hydrochloride) 0.5 mg • Folate (Folic Acid) 100 mcg • Vitamin B12 (Cyanocobalamin) 1.5 mg • Biotin 75 mcg • Pantothenic Acid (Calicum D-Pantothenate) 2.5 mg • Phosphorous (Dicalcium Phosphate) 700 mg • Iodine (Potassium Iodide) 37.5 mcg • Magnesium 8 mg • Zinc Oxide 3.75 mg • Copper Gluconate 0.5 mg. Other Ingredients: Fructose, Maltodextrin, Soy Protein isolate, Whey Protein isolate, Whey Protein concentrate, Cocoa Processed with Alkali, Dicalcium Phosphate, Natural and Artificial Chocolate flavor, Carrageenan, Dipotassium Phosphate, Natural Cream flavor, Xanthan Gum, Stevia extract.

BodySynergy Meal Replacement Drink Mix - Vanilla **-** Rexall - Sundown
Each packet contains: Sodium 100 mg • Protein 18 g • Potassium 340 mg • Vitamin A (Retinyl Palmitate) 1250 IU • Vitamin C (Ascorbic Acid) 15 g • Calcium 500 mg • Electrolytic Iron 4.5 mg • Vitamin D (Cholecalciferol) 100 IU • Vitamin E (dl-Alpha Tocopheryl Acetate) 7.5 IU • Thiamin Mononitrate 0.375 mg • Riboflavin 0.425 mg • Niacin (Niacinamide) 5 mg • Vitamin B6 (Pyridoxine Hydrochloride) 0.5 mg • Folate (Folic Acid) 100 mcg • Vitamin B12 (Cyanocobalamin) 1.5 mcg • Biotin 75 mcg • Pantothenic Acid (Calcium D-Pantothenate) 2.5 mg • Phosphorus (Dicalcium Phosphate) 700 mg • Iodine (Potassium Iodide) 37.5 mcg • Magnesium 8 mg • Zinc Oxide 3.75 mg • Copper Gluconate 0.5 mg. Other Ingredients: Fructose, Maltodextrin, Soy Protein isolate, Whey Protein isolate, Whey Protein concentrate, Cocoa Processed with Alkali, Natural and Artificial Chocolate Flavor, Carrageenan, Dipotassium Phosphate, Natural Cream Flavor, Xanthan Gum, Stevia extract.

Bold BBQ Soynuts - Revival **-** Physicians Laboratories
Each 1/6 cup contains: Certified Isoflavone 10 mg. Other Ingredients: Soy Protein (whole roasted soybeans), Soybean Oil, Salt, Dextroxe, Spices, Malto Dextrin, Smoke Flavor, Paprika, Extractives of Spice and Paprika.

Bone - Bioset **-** Enzymes, Inc.
Two capsules contain: Calcium (100% from Calcium Citrate) 114 mg • Magnesium (100% from Magnesium Aspartate) 76 mg • Manganese (100% from Manganese Citrate) 2 mg • Proprietary Herbal Blend 125 mg: Horsetail herb extract, Oat straw extract, Soy Isoflavones • Proprietary Enzyme Blend 73 mg: pHysioProtease, Phytase • Boron Citrate 10 mg. Other Ingredients: Plant Cellulose, Water.

Bone & Joint Care **-** Natrol
Three capsules contain: Vitamin D (as cholecalciferol) 20 IU • Vitamin K (as Phytonadione) 10 mcg • Calcium (as calcium carbonate & calcium citrate) 250 mg • Magnesium (as Magnesium oxide) 125 mg • Zinc (as zinc citrate) 5 mg • Copper (as copper gluconate) 100 mcg • Glucosamine Sulfate 250 mg • MSM (Methyl Sulfonyl Methane) 250 mg • Ipriflavone 100 mg • Sea Cucumber •

100 mg Mucopolysaccarides (26%) 26 mg • Horsetail grass 100 mg • Silica (8%) 8 mg • Bamboo 100 mg • Salicylic Acid 10 mg • Boron 2 mg. Other Ingredients: Silicon Dioxide, Magnesium Stearate, Gelatin.

Bone & Joint Defense System **-** Puritan's Pride
Each tablet contains: Vitamin A 208.34 IU • Vitamin C 8.33 mg • Vitamin D 66.67 IU • Vitamin E 8.33 IU • Vitamin K 8.33 mcg • Vitamin B6 1.33 mg • Folic Acid 100 mcg • Vitamin B12 8.33 mcg • Pantothenic Acid 8.33 mg • Calcium 333.33 mg • Magnesium 83.33 mg • Zinc 6 mg • Selenium 2 mcg • Copper 1 mg • Manganese 3.67 mg • Molybdenum 83.33 mcg • Potassium 33 mg • Silica 667 mcg • Boron 1.33 mg • Vanadium 66.67 mcg • Glucosamine Sulfate 41.67 mg • N-Acetyl Cysteine 4.3 mg • Pycnogenol Pine bark extract 80 mcg • Coenzyme Q-10 84 mcg • DL-Phenylalanine 4.33 mg • L-Proline 4.33 mg • Glycine 16.67 mg • S.O.D. 8.33 mcg • Mucopolysaccharide complex 21 mg • Hydrolyzed Collagen Protein 21 mg • Herbal Support Complex 36.67 mg. Other Ingredients: Milk Thistle, Alfalfa, Garlic, Young Barley Grass, Spirulina, Kelp, Devil's Claw, Hydrangea Root, Irish Moss, Yucca Root, White Willow Bark, Slippery Elm Bark.

Bone & Joint Formula **-** Oasis Wellness Network
Two tablets contain: Vitamin C 100 mg • Vitamin D (D3) 100 IU • Calcium (as aspartate, phosphate) 95 mg • Magnesium (as citrate) 24 mg • Manganese (as amino acid chelate) 2.5 mg • Glucosamine Sulfate 250 mg • Microcrystalline Hydroxyapatite (MCHC) 200 mg • Chondroitin Sulfate 150 mg • Horsetail stems/leaf extract (4:1) 10 mg • MaxCell Proprietary Blend 50 mg: Zisyphus Jujube, Aloe Vera gel, Piper Nigrum, Glycyrrhiza Glabra • Boron (as citrate) 1.5 mg. Other Ingredients: Stearic Acid, Cellulose, Magnesium Stearate, Silica.
See Editor's Note No. 15, page 2055.

Bone 350 Plus **-** Atrium Inc.
Each tablet contains: Raw Calf Bone concentrate 350 mg • Equisetum (Horsetail Rush) 150 mg.
See Editor's Note No. 14, page 2055.

Bone Assure **-** Life Extension
Six capsules contain: Calcium (from bis-glycinate, supplying elemental calcium) 1000 mg • Magnesium Oxide (supplying elemental magnesium) 320 mg • Zinc Citrate (supplying elemental zinc 12 mg) 35 mg • Manganese Citrate (supplying elemental manganese 3 mg) 10 mg • Boron (from amino acid chelate) 2 mg • Copper Sulfate (supplying elemental copper 1.5 mg) 3.7 mg • Oat Straw (10:1 silica source) 40 mg • Vitamin D (D3) 400 IU • Folic Acid 200 mcg • TMG (trimethylglycine/betaine) 100 mg • Vitamin B6 15 mg.

Bone Balance **-** Source Naturals
Each tablet contains: Vitamin C (as magnesium & calcium ascorbates, ascorbic acid & manganese ascorbate) 72 mg • Vitamin D (as cholecalciferol) 50 IU • Vitamin B6 (as pyridoxine HCl) 5 mg • Folate (as folic acid) 150 mg • Calcium (as calcium citrate, carbonate, malate, fumarate, ethanolamine phosphate & ascorbate) 150 mg • Magnesium (as magnesium oxide, citrate, fumarate, malate, & ascorbate) 150 mg • Zinc (as zinc chelate) 2 mg • Copper (as copper sebacate) 250 mcg • Manganese (as manganese ascorbate) 2 mg • genistein-rich Soy concentrate (SoyLife, yielding 6.4 mg total isoflavones) 208 mg • L-Lysine (HCl) 15 mg • Silica (from horsetail silica extract) 3 mg • Boron (as amino acid chelate) 750 mcg.

Bone Builder **-** Schiff
Three tablets contain: Calcium (carbonate, chelate, citrate-malate) 1000 mg • Magnesium (oxide, chelate) 400 mg • Vitamin D (as vitamin D3, cholecalciferol) 400 IU • Vitamin C (ascorbic acid) 150 mg • Vitamin K (phytonadione) 25 mcg • Vitamin B6 (pyridoxine, coenzyme pyridoxal-5-phosphate) 10 mg • Vitamin B12 (cyanocobalamin, coenzyme dibencozide) 25 mcg • Folic Acid (folic acid, coenzyme tetrahydrafolate) 200 mcg • Boron (chelate) 1 mg • Zinc (Optizinc) 7.5 mg • Copper (lysinate) 1 mg • Manganese (glycinate) 10 mg • Molybdenum (chelate) 50 mcg • Silica (magnesium trisillicate) 25mg • Strontium (chloride) 100 mcg • Vanadium (vanadyl sulfate) 50 mcg • Sulphur (vanadyl sulfate) 30 mcg • Betaine HCl 50 mg • Glucose Polymers (maltodextrin) 50 mcg • Citrus Bioflavonoids Complex 250 mg • Fennel (4:1 extract) 100 mg • Black Cohosh (4:1 extract) 100 mg • Blessed Thistle (4:1 extract) 100 mg. Natural base: Cellulose, Vegetable Sterates, Silica.

Bone Building Hair Teeth & Nails Formula **-** Youngevity
Calcium 250 mg • Magnesium 100 mg • Manganese 0.5 mg • Boron 240 mg • Vitamin D (as Vitamin D3) 150 IU • Horsetail grass 25 mg • Rose Hips 25 mg • Vilcabamba Mineral Essence: Potassium, Calcium, Magnesium, Zinc, Chromium, Selenium, Iron, Copper, Molybdenum, Vanadium, Iodine, Cobalt, Manganese.

Bone Calcium **-** Now
Four tablets contain: Calcium (from 4000 mg Microcrystalline Hydroxyapatite) 1000 mg • Magnesium (from 835 mg Magnesium Oxide) 500 mg • Phosphorus (Hydroxyapatite) 500 mg • Zinc (Amino Acid Chelate) 15 mg • Copper (Amino Acid Chelate) 2 mg • Vitamin D (Cholecalciferol) 200 IU • Manganese (Amino Acid Chelate) 7 mg • Boron (Amino Acid Chelate) 3 mg.

Bone Calcium Complex **-** NutriCology
Three capsules contain: Vitamin C (as ascorbic acid) 67 mg • Vitamin D (as cholecalciferol) 130 IU • Vitamin K (as phytonadione) 67 mcg • Vitamin B6 (as pyridoxine hydrochloride and pyridoxal-5'-phosphate) 4.3 mg • Folic Acid 130 mg • Calcium (as calcium hydroxyapatite) 270 mg • Magnesium (as magnesium citrate) 170 mg • Zinc (as zinc citrate) 3.3 mg • Copper (as copper sebacate) 0.17 mg • Manganese (as manganese citrate) 2 mg • Chromium (as chromium nitrate) 50 mcg • Boron (as glycerol borate) 1 mg • Chondroitin Sulfate 130 mg • Horsetail dried stems extract (equisetum arvense) 8.3 mg • Dong Quai dried root extract (angelica sinensis) 83 mg • Licorice dried root extract (glycyrrhiza glabra) 83 mg • Alfalfa dried leaves extract (medicago sativa) 83 mg. Other Ingredients: Cellulose, Silicon Dioxide.
See Editor's Note No. 15, page 2055.

Bone Care **-** Puritan's Pride
Two tablets contain: Vitamin D (as Cholecalciferol) 800 IU • Vitamin K (as Phytonadione) 100 mcg • Calcium (as Calcium Carbonate and Calcium Gluconate) 1,200 mg • Magnesium (as Magnesium Oxide and Magnesium Gluconate) 300 mg. Other Ingredients: Cellulose (Plant Origin), Croscarmellose, Cellulose Coating, Vegetable Magnesium Stearate, Mannitol.

Bone Enrich with Ostivone **-** Pro Health
Two caplets contain: Vitamin D (cholecalciferol) 200 IU • Calcium (citrate, carbonate) 600 mg • Ostivone Ipriflavone (7-isopropoxyisoflavone) 300 mg • SoyLife Soy extract (3% isoflavones) 100 mg • Boron (citrate, glycinate, aspartate) 1.5 mg. Other Ingredients: Microcrystalline Cellulose (plant fiber), Stearic Acid, Magnesium Stearate, Croscarmellose Sodium, Glaze.

Bone Essentials **-** Swanson
Two capsules contain: Vitamin D (as cholecalciferol) 400 IU • Vitamin K (as phytonadione) 100 mcg • Calcium (from citrate/citrate maleate) 350 mg • Magnesium (from glycinate/oxide) 174 mg • Zinc (from zinc oxide) 30 mg • Copper (from copper gluconate) 2 mg • Manganese (from manganese gluconate) 3.6 mg • SoyLife Soy extract (3% soy isoflavones) 50 mg • Lactose 5 mg • L-Arginine 5 mg • L-Lysine (HCl) 5 mg • Silica (horsetail herb) 5 mg • Boron (from gluconate) 3 mg • Strontium Chloride 20 mcg.

Bone Formula **-** Pharmanex
Two capsules contain: Vitamin C (as Calcium Ascorbate Complex - Ester C) 60 mg • Vitamin D (as Vitamin D3) (as Cholecalciferol) 50 IU • Vitamin K (as Vitamin K1) (as Phytonadione) 20 mcg • Calcium (as Calcium Carbonate, Calcium Propionate) 250 mg • Magnesium (as Magnesium Asparate, Magnesium Oxide) 125 mg • Isoflavones - from Soy extract 12.5 mg • Silicon (as Sodium Metasilicate) 5 mg • Boron (as Boron Citrate) 1.5 mg. Other Ingredients: Magnesium Stearate, Sodium Carboxymethylcellulose.

Some Brand Name Natural Products - What they Contain

www.NaturalDatabase.com contains MANY more listings than appear here.

Bone Health - Enzymes, Inc.
Two capsules contain: Manganese (from Manganese Citrate) 1.5 mg • Boron (from Boron Citrate) 2 mg • Proprietary Enzyme Blend 84 mg: Protease Blend (alkaline, neutral and acid proteases), CereCalase Plus • Proprietary Herbal Blend 310 mg: Chlorella Algae (cracked-wall), Red Clover flower extract (equivalent to 300 mg raw herb), Almond concentrate, Horsetail herb extract (equivalent to 160 mg raw herb), Oat straw extract (equivalent to 400 mg raw herb), Rice Bran. Other Ingredients: Plant Cellulose, Water.

Bone Maximizer - Metabolic Response Modifiers
Six capsules contain: Hydroxyapatite (MCHC) 4,000 mg • Calcium (from MCHC) 1,000 mg • Protein (from MCHC) 1,000 mg • Phosphorus (from MCHC) 500 mg • Magnesium oxide glycinate 300 mg • Zinc (citrate) 18 mg • Boron (citrate) 2 mg • Vitamin D (as Vitamin D3 cholecalciferol) 480 IU • Vitamin K (as Vitamin K1, phylloquinone) 120 mcg • Vitamin C (ascorbic acid) 72 mg • MSM (methyl-sulfonyl-methane) 120 mg • Glucosamine (HCl) 120 mg • Horsetail extract (silica) 25 mg • Pregnenolone 10 mg.

Bone Maximizer II - Metabolic Response Modifiers
Six capsules contain: Hydroxyapatite (MCHC) 4,000 mg • Calcium (from MCHC) 1,000 mg • Protein (from MCHC) 1,000 mg • Phosphorus (from MCHC) 500 mg • Magnesium Glycinate 200 mg • Zinc (citrate) 18 mg • Boron (citrate) 2 mg • Vitamin D (as Vitamin D3 cholecalciferol) 480 IU • Vitamin K1 (phylloquinone) 120 mcg • Vitamin C (ascorbic acid) 72 mg • MSM (methyl-sulfonyl-methane) 120 mg • Glucosamine (HCl) 120 mg • Horsetail extract (silica) 25 mg.

Bone Meal with Natural Vitamin D - Puritan's Pride
Four tablets contain: Vitamin D (as Cholecalciferol) 400 IU • Calcium (as Bone Meal) 880 mg • Iron (as Ferrous Sulfate) 1.8 mg • Phosphorus (as Bone Meal) 400 mg • Magnesium (as Magnesium Gluconate) 3.7 mg • Zinc (as Zinc Gluconate) 0.080 mg • Copper (as Copper Gluconate) 0.013 mg • Manganese (as Manganese Gluconate) 0.011 mg • Red Beef Bone Marrow 15 mg.

Bone Protector with Ostivone - Natrol
Six capsules contain: Calcium (as calcium citrate) 1200 mg • 7-Isopropoxy-Isoflavone 600 mg. Other Ingredients: Rice powder, Magnesium Stearate, Gelatin.

Bone Reinforcer with Hydroxyapatite - Puritan's Pride
Four tablets contain: Vitamin C 60 mg • Vitamin D 400 IU • Calcium 1200 mg • Magnesium 400 mg • Zinc 15 mg • Copper 2 mg • Manganese 2.5 mg • Boron 3 mg • Silica 20 mg • Betaine Hydrochloride 100 mg.

Bone Renew with Ostivone - Source Naturals
Four tablets contain: Calcium (as Calcium Citrate, Ethanolamine Phosphate and Malate) 800 mg • Ipriflavone (Ostivone) 600 mg.

Bone Review - Source Naturals
Four tablets contain: Calcium (as Calcium Citrate, Ethanolamine Phosphate and Malate) 800 mg • Ipriflavone (Ostivone) 600 mg.

Bone Support - TwinLab
Four tablets contain: Vitamin D (from Cholecalciferol) 800 IU • Calcium (from Calcium Citrate & Carbonate) 1500 mg • Magnesium (from Magnesium Aspartate & Oxide) 750 mg •Ostivone (Ipriflavone) (7-Isopropoxy Isoflavone) 600 mg • Novasoy Phytoestrogen extract (containing 40 mg of Soy Isoflavones) 100 mg • Boron (from Boron Citrate, Glycinate & Aspartate) 3 mg. Other Ingredients: Pharmaceutical Glaze, Cellulose, Stearic Acid Sodium Lauryl Sulfate, Magnesium Stearate, Colloidal Silicon Dioxide.

Bone Support - Zone Labs
Three softgels contain: Vitamin D (cholecalciferol) 200 IU • Vitamin K (phytonadione) 10 mcg • Calcium (as carbonate, citrate, gluconate, aspartate, malate, micronized hydroxyapatite) 750 mg • Magnesium (as oxide, aspartate, citrate) 400 mg • Boron (as calcium borogluconate) 1 mg • Horsetail extract (equisetum arvense) 25 mg. Other Ingredients: Gelatin, High Oleic Safflower Oil, Glycerin, Purified Water, Titanium Dioxide, Lecithin, Silicon Dioxide.

Bone Support Formula with Vitamin D - Health Smart Vitamins
Four caplets contain: Vitamin A (as beta-carotene) 25,000 IU • Vitamin D (cholecalciferol) 4 mg • Vitamin K (phytonadione) 0.08 mg • Calcium (as 50% calcium carbonate, 25% calcium citrate, 25% calcium glycinate) 1000 mg • Magnesium (as 75% magnesium oxide, 25% magnesium glycinate) 400 mg • Zinc (as zinc citrate) 15 mg • Copper (as copper asparate) 1.50 mg • Boron (as sodium borate) 1.50 mg.

Bones & Joints Body Benefits Pak - Leiner Health Products
Each packet contains: Magnesium 233 mg • Calcium Carbonate 498 mg • Iron 8 mg • Manganese 7.5 mg • Riboflavin (Vitamin B2) 5.1 mg • Thiamin (Vitamin B1) 4.5 mg • Vitamin B12 18 mcg • Vitamin B6 6 mg • Selenium 200 mcg • Molybdenum 208 mcg • Niacin 40 mg • Biotin 60 mcg • Chloride 72 mg • Potassium 80 mg • Copper 3.5 mg • Chromium 200 mcg • Vitamin E 460 IU • Vitamin A 7500 IU • Zinc 20 mg • Phosphorus 130 mg • Vitamin C 620 mg • Folate 400 mcg • Iodine 150 mcg • Pantothenic Acid 10 mg • Vitamin D 400 IU • Vitamin K 80 mcg • Boron 200 mcg • Citrus Bioflavonoids complex 10 mg • Ginkgo Biloba leaf 25 mg • Grape Seed extract (Vitis vinefera) seed 1 mg • Hesperidin complex 5 mg • Kelp powder (Macrocystis pyrifera) frond 5 mg • Lecithin 10 mg • Mixed Carotenoids complex 10 mg • Nickel 6.5 mcg • Siberian Ginseng powder (Eleutherococcus senticosus) root 25 mg • Silicon Dioxide 2 mg • Tin 13 mcg • Tocotrienol complex 5 mg • Trace Mineral complex 10 mg • Vanadium 13 mcg. Other Ingredients: Glucosamine Sulfate, Glucosamine Hydrochloride, Cellulose, Methylcellulose, Maltodextrin, Hydroxypropyl Methylcellulose, Polyethylene Glycol 3350, Propylene Glycol, Starch, Crospovidone, Croscarmellose Sodium, Acacia.

Bonnisan Drops - The Himalaya Drug Company (Himalaya Heal
Each 1 mL serving contains: Dill oil (anethum sowa) 0.00162 mL • Guduchi (tinospora cordifolia) 0.45 mg • Himsra (caparis spinosa) 0.45 mg • Pippali (piper longum) 0.45 mg • Amalaki (emblica officinalis) 0.45 mg • Kasani (cichorium intybus) 0.45 mg • Kasamarda (cassia occidentalis) 0.45 mg • Haritaki (terminalia chebula) 0.45 mg • Ela (elattaria cardamomum) 0.45 mg • Biranjasipha (achillea millefolium) 0.45 mg • Jhavuka (tamarix gallica) 0.45 mg • Gokshura (tribulus terrestris) 0.45 mg • Punarnava (boerhaavia diffusa) 0.45 mg.

Bonnisan Liquid - The Himalaya Drug Company (Himalaya Heal
Each 1 tsp serving contains: Dill oil (anethum sowa) 0.0018 mL • Guduchi (tinospora cordifolia) 0.5 mg • Himsra (capparis spinosa) 0.5 mg • Pippali (piper longum) 0.5 mg • Amalaki (emblica officinalis) 0.5 mg • Kasani (cichorium intybus) 0.5 mg • Kasamarda (cassia occidentalis) 0.5 mg • Haritaki (terminalia chebula) 0.5 mg • Ela (elattaria cardamomum) 0.5 mg • Biranjasipha (achillea millefolium) 0.5 mg • Jhavuka (tamarix gallica) 0.5 mg • Gokshura (triblus terrestris) 0.5 mg • Punarnava (boerhaavia diffusa) 0.5 mg.

Borage Oil - PhysioLogics
Each softgel contains: Borage (borago officinalis seed oil) 1000 mg containing: Gamma Linolenic Acid (GLA) 240 mg, Linoleic Acid (LA) 360 mg. Other Ingredients: Gelatin, Glycerin.

Borage Oil - Vital Nutrients
Each capsule contains: Borage oil (extracted without chemicals, contains gamma linolenic acid 240 mg) 1000 mg.

Borage Oil - Rexall - Sundown
Each two softgels contain: Vitamin E (as d-alpha-tocopherol) 30 IU • Borage (seed oil) 1 g • Gamma Linolenic Acid (GLA) 200 mg. Other Ingredients: Gelatin, Glycerin, Water.

Borage Oil 240 **-** Health From The Sun
Each capsule contains: Gamma Linolenic Acid (GLA) (Omega-6) 240 mg • Linoleic Acid (Omega-6) 370 mg • Oleic Acid (Omega-9) 15 mg. Other Ingredients: Borage seed oil, Gelatin, Glycerine, Water.

Borage Oil 300 **-** Health From The Sun
Each capsule contains: Gamma Linolenic Acid (GLA) (Omega-6) 300 mg • Linoleic Acid (Omega-6) 480 mg • Oleic Acid (Omega-9) 190 mg. Ingredients: Borage seed oil, Gelatin, Glycerine, Water.

Borage-Licorice Virtue **-** Blessed Herbs
Borage • Astragalus root • Licorice root • Siberian Ginseng root • Wild American Ginseng root • Suma root • Reishi mycelium • Ginger root • Grain alcohol & Distilled water.

Boron **-** Nature's Way
Each capsule contains: Boron amino acid chelate 3 mg. Other Ingredients: Cellulose, Gelatin, Maltodextrin, Millet.

Boron Complex Plus **-** The Vitamin Shoppe
Four capsules contain: Boron 3 mg • Calcium 1000 mg • Magnesium 500 mg • Vitamin D (as Vitamin D3) 400 IU • Zinc 15 mg • Manganese 5 mg • Copper 500 mcg • Betaine HCl 324 mg.

Boswellia Extract **-** Source Naturals
Three tablets contain: Boswellia serrata extract (yielding 788 mg of Boswellic Acids) 1,125 mg.

Boswellia Extract - 400 mg **-** Vital Nutrients
Each veg capsule contains: Boswellia Serrata extract (65% boswellic acids as organic acids, true boswellic acids 30%-40% by HPLC, alpha and beta boswellic acids, 3-acetyl-beta boswellic acid, 3-acetyl alpha boswellic acid, 11-keto-beta-boswellic acid, 3-acetyl-11-ketone-beta boswellic acid) 400 mg.

Boswellin **-** Now
Each capule contains: Boswellin (Boswellia serrata; extract of gum resins standardized to contain 65% [162 mg] Boswellic Acids) 250 mg • Curcumin extract (Curcuma longa; min 90% standardized extract of turmeric root powder) 100 mg • Turmeric root powder 150 mg. Other Ingredients: Rice Flour, Magnesium Stearate, Silica.

Botanaflor **-** Pharmanex
Each capsule contains: Jerusalem Artichoke with Fructooligosaccharides 100 mg • Cellulose Powder 100 mg • Citrus Pectin 98 mg • Apple Pectin Fiber 66 mg • Konjac Root (Glucomannan) 59 mg • Date Fiber 52 mg • Prune Fiber 48 mg • Soybean Fiber 43 mg • Papaya Powder with Papain 30 mg • Pineapple Powder with Bromelain 30 mg • Bifidobacterium Bifidum 30 mg • Lactobacillus Acidophilus.

Botaname **-** Pharmanex
Two capsules contain: Garcinia Cambogia 500 mg • Peppermint powder 104 mg • Brewer's Yeast 100 mg • Cinnamon Ramulus powder 86 mg • Lemon Verbena powder 86 mg • Chamomile flower powder 69 mg • Ginger root powder 69 mg • Chinese Licorice root extract 35 mg • Sweet Citrus Peel 35 mg • Chicory powder 16 mg.

Botanical Chi **-** Naturally Safe Technologies
Lycium berry • Cassia bark • Aloe Vera barbadensis • Schisandra berry • Dandelion root • Passion flower • Chinese Wild Yam • Kudzu root • Rosemary • American Ginseng • Rhodiola crenulata • Fo-Ti • Astragalus • Rosehips • Bee Pollen • Lemon Balm • Grapefruit seed extract • Phytonutrients.

Botopical the Botanical Instant Wrinkle Eraser Eye Repair **-** pH Beauty Labs LLC
Water (aqua) • Stearic Acid • Ethylene/Acrylic Acid Copolymer • Glyceryl Stearate • PEG-100 Stearate • Caprylic/Capric Triglyceride • Sodium Polystyrene Sulfonate • Propylene Glycol • Phytonadione (vitamin K1) • Green Coffee extract • Cucumis Sativus fruit extract (cucumber) • Algae extract • Artemisia Vulgaris extract • Polyquaternium-10 • Hyaluronic Acid • Aloe Barbadensis leaf juice • Glycerin • Propylene Glycol • Diazolidinyl Urea • Methylparaben • Propylparaben • Cyclopentasiloxane • C30-45 Alkyl Dimethicone/Polycyclohexane Oxide • Crosspolymer • Acrylates/Acrylamide Copolymer • Mineral oil • Polysorbate 85 • Carbomer • Triethanolamine • Trisodium EDTA • Propylparaben • Methylparaben • Fragrance (parfum).

Botopical the Botanical Instant Wrinkle Eraser Forehead Smoother **-** pH Beauty Labs LLC
Water (aqua) • Stearic Acid • Ethylene/Acrylic Acid Copolymer • Glyceryl Stearate • PEG-100 Stearate • Caprylic/Capric Triglyceride • Sodium Polystyrene Sulfonate • Propylene Glycol • Camellia Sinensis seed extract (green tea) • Saccharomyces-Copper-Ferment • Glycerin • Carbomer • Propylene Glycol • Diazolidinyl Urea • Methylparaben • Propylparaben • Aloe Barbadensis leaf juice • Chamomilla Recutita flower extract (matricaria) • Algae extract • Artemisia Vulgaris extract • Cyclopentasiloxane • C30-45 Alkyl Dimethicone/Polycyclohexane Oxide • Triethanolamine • Crosspolymer • Trisodium EDTA • Propylparaben • Methylparaben • Fragrance (parfum).

Botopical the Botanical Instant Wrinkle Eraser Lip Treatment **-** pH Beauty Labs LLC
Water (aqua) • Stearic Acid • Ethylene/Acrylic Acid Copolymer • Glyceryl Stearate • PEG-100 Stearate • Caprylic/Capric Triglyceride • Sodium Polystyrene Sulfonate • Propylene Glycol • Olea Europaea extract (olive) • Glycerin • Carbomer • Aloe Barbadensis leaf juice • Algae extract • Artemisia Vulgaris extract • Cyclopentasiloxane • C30-45 Alkyl Dimethicone/Polycyclohexane Oxide • Propylene Glycol • Diazolidinyl Urea • Methylparaben • Propylparaben • Crosspolymer • Triethanolamine • Trisodium EDTA • Propylparaben • Methylparaben • Fragrance (parfum).

Bounty Bears Plus Extra C **-** Nature's Bounty
Each tablet contains: Vitamin A (as Retinyl Acetate and Beta Carotene) 2500 IU • Vitamin C (as Ascorbic Acid and Sodium Ascorbate) 250 mg • Vitamin D (as Cholecalciferol) 400 IU • Vitamin E (as d-Alpha Tocopheryl Acetate) 15 IU • Thiamin (as Thiamine Mononitrate) 1.05 mg • Riboflavin (Vitamin B-2) 1.2 mg • Niacin (as Niacinamide) 13.5 mg • Vitamin B-6 (as Pyridoxine Hydrochloride) 1.05 mg • Folic Acid 300 mg • Vitamin B-12 (as Cyanocobalamin) 4.5 mcg. Other Ingredients: Sugar, Vegetable Stearic Acid, Natural Orange Flavor, Vegetable Magnesium Stearate, Silica, Mannitol, FD&C Red No. 40, FD&C Yellow No. 6, FD&C Blue No. 2.

Bovine Cartilage Plus **-** Atrium Inc.
Each capsule contains: Freeze Dried Bovine Cartilage 600 mg • Freeze Dried Soluble Trachea Substance 150 mg.
See Editor's Note No. 14, page 2055.

BowelSoothe **-** Vita Pharmica - formerly Neopharmica
Each packet contains: Herbal Concentrate 10 g: White Peony Root, Atractylodes Rhizome, Cardamon Seed, Paederia Scandens stem, Sonchus Brachyotus, Chinese Licorice root.

Brain **-** Enzymes, Inc.
Each capsule contains: Proprietary Herbal Blend 460 mg: Ginkgo Biloba leaf extract, Ginseng root extract, Gotu Kola extract, Rice Bran, Bacopin, Schizandra extract, Grape seed extract, Lecithin • pHysioProtease 40 mg. Other Ingredients: Plant Cellulose, Water.

Brain & Eye Nutritional Fertilizer **-** Life Extension
Each softgel contains: DHA (docosahexaenoic acid, from microalgae) 200 mg • EPA (eicosapentanoic acid) 180 mg • Lecithin 800 mg • Vitamin E 5 IU. Other Ingredients: Soybean Oil, Purified Water, Glycerin.

Brain Actives **-** VitaStore
Six tablets contain: Ginkgo Biloba (24% Flavoneglycosides, 6% Terpene Lactones) 100 mg • Phosphatidylserine 300 mg • L-Methionine 300 mg • OPC Complex (Pine Bark & Grapeseed Extracts) 100 mg • Vitamin B1 (Thiamine) 1.5 mg • Vitamin B2 (Riboflavin) 1.5 mg • Vitamin B3 (Niacin) 20 mg • Vitamin B5 (Pantothenic Acid) 10 mg • Vitamin B6 (Pyridoxine) 2 mg • Vitamin

B12 6 mcg • Lecithin 1000 mcg • Acetyl L-Carnitine 500 mg • L-Glutamine 250 mg • Manganese 35 mg.

Brain Aid **-** NutriCology
Each tablet contains: Vitamin A (as beta-carotene) 1000 IU • Vitamin C (as ascorbic acid) 5 mg • Vitamin E (as D-alpha-tocopheryl acid succinate) 5 IU • Thiamin (67% as thiamin hydrochloride and 33% as TTFD) 7.5 mg • Riboflavin (67% as riboflavin hydrochloride and 33% as riboflavin-5-phosphate) 7.5 mg • Niacin (86% as niacinamide) 17.5 mg • Vitamin B6 (75% as pyridoxine hydrochloride and 25% as pyridoxal-5-phosphate) 10 mg • Folic Acid 50 mcg • Vitamin B12 (as dibencoside) 25 mcg • Biotin 50 mcg • Pantothenic Acid (as calcium pantothenate) 20 mg • Zinc (as zinc citrate) 5 mg • Selenium (90% as sodium selenite and 10% as selenomethionine) 25 mcg • Copper (as copper sebacate) 0.5 mg • Chromium (as chromium nicotinate) 25 mcg • Molybdenum (as sodium molybdate) 25 mcg • Boron (as boron citrate) 250 mcg • Ginkgo Biloba extract 15 mg • Siberian Ginseng extract 15 mg • Korean Ginseng extract 20 mg • Gotu Kola extract 50 mg • L-Glutamine 125 mg • L-Tyrosine 100 mg • Acetyl-L-Carnitine 25 mg • Choline Bitartrate 40 mg • Inositol 25 mg • DMAE (dimethylaminoethanol) 125 mg • Phosphatidylcholine 125 mg • Phosphatidylserine 10 mg • Quercetin 25 mg • Cayenne pepper 25 mg. Other Ingredients: Dicalcium Phosphate, Cellulose, Magnesium Stearate, Silicon Dioxide, Stearic Acid.

Brain Alert **-** Nutrapathic
Two tablets contain: Vitamin B1 10 mg • Vitamin B6 20 mg • Vitamin B12 40 mcg • Niacin 10 mg • Niacinamide 10 mg • Biotin 30 mcg • Choline Bitartrate 20 mg • Inositol 10 mg • PABA 20 mg • Vitamin F 4 mg • Calcium 20 mg • Chloride 4 mg • Copper 4 mg • Magnesium 10 mg • Manganese 6 mg • Phosphorus 10 mg • Potassium 10 mg • Selenium 10 mcg • Silica 4 mg • Zinc 20 mg. Other Ingredients: Brain, Egg Lecithin, Rye Green, Red Clover, Peppermint leaves, L-Tyrosine, L-Arginine, Lecithin granules, Barley Green, Bee Pollen, Gotu Kola, Ginkgo, Glutamic Acid, L-Phenylalanine, L-Glutamine, DNA, RNA, Hypothalamus, Pineal, Pituitary, Valerian, Ginseng, Spirulina, Wood Betony, Bupleurum root, Chondroitin Sulfate, CoQ10.
See Editor's Note No. 31, page 2056.

Brain Booster **-** Optimum Nutrition
Each capsule contains: Ginkgo Biloba Extract (standardized for 24% flavone glycosides and 6% terpene lactones) 60 mg • Siberian Ginseng Extract (standardized for Eleutheroside B 400 mcg and D 300 mcg) 150 mg • Gotu Kola 250 mg. In a base of Bee Pollen and Ginkgo biloba leaf powders.
See Editor's Note No. 21, page 2056.

Brain Care **-** Quantum, Inc.
Two tablets contain: Vitamin E (d-Alpha Tocopherol) 100 IU • Phosphatidylserine complex 100 mg • Phosphatidyl Choline 95 mg • Ginkgo leaf (Ginkgo Biloba) (24% Ginkgo Flavone Glycosides) 60 mg • Alpha-Linolenic Acid (Borage Oil) 50 mg • Coenzyme Q10 30 mg • DHA (Docosahexaenoic Acid) 10 mg • EPA (Eicosahexaenoic Acid) 10 mg. Other Ingredients: Stearic Acid, Guar Gum, Magnesium Stearate.

Brain Essentials **-** PhytoPharmica
Three tablets contain: Vitamin C (Ascorbic Acid) 300 mg • Magnesium Aspartate 100 mg • Potassium Aspartate 100 mg • Zinc Aspartate 30 mg • Manganese (Chelate) 15 mg • Folic Acid 800 mcg • Vitamin B12 (Cyanocobalamin) 500 mcg • L-Glutamine 300 mg • L-Phenylalanine 300 mg • Brain extract freeze-dried 300 mg • Choline (Bitartrate) 200 mg • Gamma-Aminobutyric Acid (GABA) 100 mg • Alpha-Ketoglutaric Acid 100 mg • Glycine 100 mg • L-Tyrosine 100 mg • Pituitary extract freeze-dried 65 mg • L-Methionine 50 mg • RNA/DNA Complex 50 mg • L-Cysteine 50 mg • Pyridoxal Phosphate 15 mg.
See Editor's Note No. 21 and No. 31, page 2056.

Brain Essentials **-** Swanson
Each capsule contains: Vitamin E (as d-alpha tocopheryl succinate) 100 IU • Vitamin B-6 (as pyridoxine HCl) 25 mg • Vitamin B-12 (as cyanocobalamin) 250 mcg • Pantothenic Acid (as d-calcium pantothenate) 25 mg • Gotu Kola extract (10% asiaticosides) 150 mg • L-Glutamine 100 mg • L-Tyrosine 100 mg • Phosphatidylcholine (from lecithin) 100 mg • Ginkgo Biloba leaf extract (24% flavone glycosides, 6% terpene lactones) 60 mg • DHA (docosahexaenoic acid) 30 mg • Alpha Lipoic Acid 25 mg • DMAE Bitartrate 2 mg • Phosphatidylserine 1 mg.

Brain Fuel **-** Futurebiotics
Three tablets contain: Ginkgo Biloba (24% standardized extract) 45 mg • Korean Ginseng (7% ginsenoside extract) 15 mg • American Ginseng (7% ginsenoside extract) 10 mg • Gotu Kola extract (4:1 extract equivalent to) 150 mg • Ginkgo Biloba leaves 200 mg • Gotu Kola leaves 250 mg • Chinese Licorice extract (glycyrrhiza) 150 mg • Tyrosine 150 mg • Glutamine 275 mg • Phosphatidyl Choline (55% strength) 250 mg • Vitamin C 60 mg • Vitamin E (natural succinate) 5 IU • Vitamin B6 25 mg • Folic Acid 400 mcg • Vitamin B12 25 mcg • Vitamin B5 35 mg • Potassium 200 mg • Betaine HCl 50 mg • Bromelain 50 mg • Para Amino Benzoic Acid (PABA) 75 mg • L-Methionine 75 mg • Ribonucleic Acid (RNA) 50 mg.

Brain Fuel II **-** Futurebiotics
Two capsules contain: Vitamin E (as d-alpha tocopheryl acetate) 100 IU • Vitamin B6 (as pyridoxine hydrochloride) 25 mg • Vitamin B12 (as Cyanocobalamin) 25 mcg • Pantothenic acid (as calcium pantothenate) 25 mg • DHA (decosahexaenoic acid) 100 mg • Phosphatidylcholine (supplying 55% (110 g) choline) 200 mg • Alpha Lipoic Acid 100 mg • Ginkgo biloba leaf powder extract [standardized for 24% (11 g) ginkgo heterosides] 45 mg • Korean ginseng root powder extract [standardized for 7% (1 mg) ginsenosides] 15 mg • Gotu Kola leaf 4:1 powder extract 38 mg. Other Ingredients: Gelatin, Water.

Brain Lightning **-** Novus Research
Three capsules contain: Vitamin E 100 IU • Vitamin B-1 (Thiamin) 25 mg • Vitamin B-3 (Niacin, non-flushing, as niacinamide) 10 mg • Vitamin B-5 (Pantothenic Acid) 25 mg • Vitamin B-6 (Pyridoxine 5-Phosphate) 25 mg • Vitamin B-12 (as Cyanocobalamin) 250 mcg • Magnesium 50 mg • Zinc (as Amino Acid Chelate) 10 mg • Manganese (as Manganese Chelate) 5 mg • Selenium (as Amino Acid Chelate) 200 mcg • Proprietary Synergistic Blend: [DMAE (dimethylaminoethanol), Pregnenolone, Trimethylglycine (TMG), L-Tyrosine, Huperzine A (pure molecular alkaloid), Vinpocetine, DL Phenylalanine (DLPA), GABA (gamma aminobutyric acid), Ginkgo Biloba] 1490 mg. Other Ingredients: Magnesium Silicate, Calcium Carbonate, Silicon Dioxide, Cellulose (non-reactive mixing agents).

Brain Link Complex **-** Pain & Stress Center
Five tablespoons contain: Vitamin A • Vitamin C • Calcium • Iron • Vitamin D • Vitamin E • Thiamin • Riboflavin • Niacin • Vitamin B6 • Folate •Vitamin B12 • Biotin • Pantothenic Acid • Iodine • Magnesium • Zinc • Selenium • Copper • Manganese • Chromium • Molybdenum • Amino Acid Profile: Alanine 290 mg • Arginine 149 mg • Aspartic Acid 573 mg • Cystine/Cysteine 167 mg • Glutamic Acid 837 mg • Glycine 2101 mg • Histidine 103 mg • Isoleucine 485 mg • Leucine 852 mg • Lysine 521 mg • Methionine 149 mg • Phenylalanine 335 mg • Proline 242 mg • Serine 202 mg • Threonine 252 mg • Tryptophan (from natural milk, egg protein) 111 mg • Tyrosine 898 mg • Valine 478 mg • Taurine 1500 mg • GABA 1500 mg • L-Glutamine 3000 mg • Inositol 50 mg • Choline 50 mg • PABA 2 mg.

Brain Nutrition **-** Enzymatic Therapy
Three tablets contain: Vitamin C (Ascorbic Acid) 300 mg • Magnesium Aspartate 100 mg • Potassium Aspartate 100 mg • Zinc Aspartate 30 mg • Manganese (Chelate) 15 mg • Folic Acid 800 mcg • Vitamin B12 (Cyanocobalamin) 500 mcg • Other Ingredients: L-Glutamine 300 mg • L-Phenylalanine 300 mg • Brain extract freeze-dried 300 mg • Choline (Bitatrate) 200 mg • Gamma-Aminobutyric

Acid (GABA) 100 mg • Alpha-Ketoglutaric Acid 100 mg • Glycine 100 mg • L-Tyrosine 100 mg • Pituitary extract freeze-dried 65 mg • L-Methionine 50 mg • RNA-DNA Complex 50 mg • L-Cysteine 50 mg • Pyridoxal Phosphate 15 mg.
See Editor's Note No. 21 and No. 31, page 2056.

Brain Pep **-** Pep Products, Inc.
Each capsule contains: Ginkgo Biloba • Kola Nut • Gotu Kola • Siberian Ginseng • Schizandra • Ginger • L-Glutamine 130 mg.

Brain Plus **-** Progressive Labs
Each capsule contains: Raw Porcine Brain concentrate 100 mg • Choline (bitartrate) 100 mg • Inositol 100 mg. This product contains naturally occuring RNA/DNA qualitatively from the brain concentrate.
See Editor's Note No. 14, page 2055.

Brainpower **-** Gero Vita International
Each capsule contains: Vitamin C (as ascorbic acid) 60 mg • Vitamin E (as dl-alpha-tocopheryl acetate) 30 IU • Thiamin (as thiamin mononitrate) 3 mg • Riboflavin 1.7 mg • Niacin 15 mg • Vitamin B6 (as pyridoxine hydrochloride) 1.2 mg • Folic Acid 200 mcg • Vitamin B12 (as cyanocobalamin) 7.5 mcg • Pantothenic Acid (as calcium pantothenate) 15 mg • Pyroglutamic Acid 125 mg • L-Tyrosine 75 mg • Choline (as choline bitartrate) 37.5 mg • Acetyl-L-Carnitine 32 mg • Cola seed extract 32 mg • L-Glutamine 18 mg • Ginkgo leaf extract (ginkgo biloba, 24% ginkgo flavoneglycosides, 6% terpene lactones) 15 mg • Vinpocetine 10 mg • L-Phenylalanine 3 mg • L-Cysteine 3 mg. Other Ingredients: Silicon Dioxide, Magnesium Stearate, Purified Talc, Gelatin.

Brainwash Shampoo **-** Evergreen Research
Active Ingredients: Ginkgo Biloba • Grape seed extract. Other Ingredients: Peppermint Oil, Calendula Oil, Arnica.

BrainWave Plus **-** Allergy Research Group
Each capsule contains: Acetyl-L-Carnitine 100 mg • L-Glutamine 80 mg • Choline Bitartrate 40 mg • Phosphatidylserine 30 mg • Ginkgo Biloba extract (standardized to 24% ginkgo flavonglycosides and 6% terpene lactones) 24 mg • Siberian Ginseng extract (15:1) 20 mg • Panax Ginseng extract (standardized to 7% ginsenosides) 20 mg • Ashwaganda extract 20 mg • Gotu Kola, powdered 10 mg • Royal Jelly 20 mg • Bacopa Monniera extract (standardized to 30% bacosides) 20 mg • Vinpocetine 2 mg • CDP-Choline 50 mg • Huperzine A 20 mcg • Thymus 20 mg • DMAE (dimethylaminoethanol) 20 mg. Other Ingredients: Cellulose, Magnesium Stearate, Silicon Dioxide.

BrainWave Plus **-** NutriCology
Each capsule contains: Acetyl-L-Carnitine 100 mg • L-Glutamine 80 mg • Choline Bitartrate 40 mg • Phosphatidylserine 30 mg • Ginkgo Biloba extract (standardized to 24% ginkgo flavonglycosides and 6% terpene lactones) 24 mg • Siberian Ginseng 15:1 extract 20 mg • Panax Ginseng extract (standardized to 7% ginsenosides) 20 mg • Ashwaganda extract 20 mg • Gotu Kola (powdered) 10 mg • Royal Jelly 20 mg • Bacopa Monniera extract (standardized to 30% bacosides) 20 mg • Vinpocetine 2 mg • CDP - Choline 50 mg • Huperzine A 20 mcg • Thymus 20 mg • DMAE (dimethylaminoethanol) 20 mg. Other Ingredients: Cellulose, Magnesium Stearate, Silicon Dioxide.

Brave Hart Deer Velvet Capsules **-** Hart Products
Deer Velvet 300 mg.

Breakfast Blend - Revival **-** Physicians Laboratories
Eight fluid ounces contain: Certified Isoflavone 15 mg. Other Ingredients: Whole Roasted Soybeans, Natural and Artificial Flavors.

Breast Care System-3 **-** Natrol
Calcium 24 mg • Calcium D-Glucarate 200 mg. Breast Care Formula: Selenium 50 mcg • Green Tea Extract 50 mg • Garlic 50 mg • Grape Seed Extract 20 mg. Ultra Green Breast Care Ingredients: Rice Powder, Silica, Magnesium Stearate, Gelatin.
See Editor's Note No. 21, page 2056.

Breast Enhance **-** NewLibido
Each six tablets contain: Saw Palmetto extract (30% sterols) 300 mg • Kava Kava (10% kava lactones) 300 mg • Dandelion (4:1 extract) 150 mg • Dong Quai extract (.08% ligustilide) 150 mg • Wild Yam extract 10:1 (4%-7% std) 150 mg • Chasteberry extract (4:1) 150 mg • Oat Bran 300 mg • Motherwort 500 mg • Blessed Thistle 500 mg • Folic Acid (as folate) 300 mcg • Biotin 300 mcg • Zinc (as amino acid chelate) 12 mg • Selenium (as amino acid chelate) 120 mcg. Other Ingredients: Di-calcium Phosphate, Magnesium Stearate, Stearic Acid.

Breast Essentials **-** Swanson
Two capsules contain: Calcium (from calcium d-glucarate) 24 mg • Selenium (as selenomethionine) 100 mcg • SoyLife Soy extract (3% soy isoflavones) 400 mg • Calcium D-Glucarate 200 mg • Green Tea extract (48% polyphenols) 200 mg • Rosemary leaf extract (6% rosemaric acid) 200 mg • Citrus Bioflavonoids (Citrus aurantium; 25% bioflavonoids) 100 mg • Boron (from boron aspartate) 3 mg.
See Editor's Note No. 40, page 2058.

Breast Health **-** Schiff
Two capsules contain: Calcium (as calcium d-gluconate and calcium borogluconate) 37 mg • Selenium (as selenium yeast) 100 mcg • Calcium D-Gluconate 200 mg • Green Tea leaf extract (carnellia sinensis) 200 mg • Polyphenols 100 mg • Rosemary leaf extract (rosmarinus officinalis) 155 mg • Rosmarinic Acid 14 mg • Soy Isoflavones concentrate 31 mg • Isoflavones 12 mg • Citrus Bioflavonoids 25 mg • Boron (as calcium boroglucarate) 3 mg. Other Ingredients: Maltodextrin, Gelatin, Silicon Dioxide, Magnesium Stearate.

Breast Health Formula **-** Great American Nutrition
Two capsules contain: Calcium (as calcium d-glucarate) 24 mg • Selenium (as selenomethionine, from SelenoMax) 100 mcg • Calcium D-Glucarate 200 mg • Green Tea leaf extract (Ccellia sinensis, standardized to 48% polyphenols) 200 mg • Rosemary folia extract (rosemarinus officialis, standardized to 6% rosemaric acid) 200 mg • Soy extract (standardized to 3% isoflavones) 400 mg • Citrus peel bioflavonoids (citrus aurantium, standardized to 25% bioflavonoids) 100 mg • Boron Aspartate 3 mg. Other Ingredients: White Rice powder.
See Editor's Note No. 40, page 2058.

BreastSuccess **-** EyeFive, Inc.
Three capsules contain: Fenugreek seed 219 mg • Fennel Seed 162 mg • L-Tyrosine 135 mg • Mexican Wild Yam root 96 mg • Pacific Kelp 90 mg • Damiana leaf 51 mg • Dong Quai root 48 mg • Mother's Wort herb 48 mg • Black Cohosh root extract 45 mg • Oat grass 42 mg • Blessed Thistle herb 39 mg • Hops flower 30 mg.

Breath Aid **-** D & E Pharmaceuticals
Each tablet contains: Ephedrine 12.5 mg • Guaifenesin 100 mg.

Breathe Easy **-** Traditional Medicinals
Each brewed cup contains: Pseudoephedrine (ephedra sinisa, naturally occurring in whole ma huang herb) 0.5 mg Other Ingredients: Peppermint leaf, Licorice root, Fennel seed, Eucalyptus leaf, Pleurisy root, Calendula flower, Ginger rhizome.
See Editor's Note No. 30, page 2056.

Breathe Easy Tea **-** Traditional Medicinals
Each brewed cup contains: Manganese 0.04 mg • Licorice root 300 mg • Eucalyptus leaf 285 mg • Bitter Fennel seed 255 mg • Proprietary Blend 255 mg: Peppermint leaf, Calendula flower, Pleurisy root, Ginger rhizome.

Breathe Well **-** Gero Vita International
Each capsule contains: Vitamin E (as dl-alpha-tocopheryl acetate) 50 IU • Proprietary Herbal Blend 390 mg: Adhatoda Vasika leaf extract, Glycyrrhiza Globra root extract (25% glycyrrhizine), Alpinia Golango

root extract (30% ASE 90), Inula Racemosa root extract (30% ASE 90), Phyllanthus Emblica fruit extract (5% tannins), Myrica Nagi bark extract, Sida Cordifolia root extract, Clerodendrum Indicum root extract (0.5% active principle), Hedychium Spicatum root extract (0.5% volatile oil), Pistacia Integerrima gall extract (0.5% tannins), Picrorhiza Kurroa root extract (1% bitter), Zingiber Officinale rhizome extract (0.5% volatile oil), Ocimum Sanctum leaf extract, Abies Webbiana leaf extract • Quercetin 75 mg • PhytoSel 30 mg. Other Ingredients: Gelatin, Magnesium Stearate, Silica, Rice Flour. See Editor's Note No. 39, page 2058.

Breathe-Aid Formula - Nature's Way
Two capsules contain: Proprietary Formula: Chickweed leaf & stem • Ephedra HCL • Guafinesin • Lobelia herb • Marshmallow root • Mullein leaf. Other Ingredients: Gelatin, Magnesium Stearate, Millet. See Editor's Note No. 30, page 2056.

BreatheSmart - Health Smart Vitamins
Each capsule contains: Vitamin C (ascorbic acid) 150 mg • Piper Longum fruit (1.5% piperine, 1.5 mg) 100 mg • Picrorhiza Kurroa root (4%-5% kutkin, 2 mg - 2.5 mg) 50 mg • Quercetin 50 mg • Ginkgo leaf (24% ginkgo flavonglycosides, 9.6 mg; 6% terpene lactones, 2.4 mg) 40 mg • Tylophora asthmatica leaf (0.1%- 0.25% tylophorine alkaloids, 0.03 mg - 0.075 mg) 30 mg • Serratiopeptidase 7.5 mg.

Breath-EZ - Indiana Botanic Gardens
Two capsules contain: Breath EZ Herbal Blend 900 mg: Licorice root powder, Echinacea Purpurea powder, Saw Palmetto berry powder, Bayberry root bark powder, Myrrh gum powder, Plantain herb powder, Goldenseal root powder. Other Ingredients: Gelatin, Rice Flour, Water.

Brevail - Lignan Research
Each capsule contains: Vitamin D (as vitamin D3) 400 IU • Lignan extract from Flaxseed (Brevail) 200 mg • Secoisolariciresinol Diglycoside (from Brevail) 50 mg. Other Ingredients: Rice Powder, Maltodextrin, Magnesium Stearate, Silica, Gelatin, Titanium Dioxide, Vanilla Extract.

Brewer's Yeast - Nature's Life
Twelve tablets contain: Vitamin B1 1 mg • Vitamin B2 1 mg • Vitamin B6 240 mg • Choline 23 mg • Folic Acid 120 mcg • Niacin 3 mg • Inositol 23 mg • Pantothenic Acid 600 mcg • Calcium 360 mcg • Chromium 9 mcg • Copper 300 mcg • Iodine 18 mcg • Iron 2 mg • Magnesium 6 mg • Manganese 30 mcg • Phosphorus 8 mg • Potassium 10 mg • Selenium 12 mcg • Sodium 460 mcg • Zinc 600 mcg • Protein Profile 2.9 g: Alanine 216 mg, Arginine 155mg, Aspartic Acid 302 mg, Cysteine 72 mg, Glycine 148 mg, Glutamic Acid 402 mg, Histidine (essential amino acid) 78 mg, Isoleucine (essential amino acid) 140 mg, Leucine (essential amino acid) 222 mg, Lysine (essential amino acid) 234 mg, Methionine (essential amino acid) 43 mg, Phenylalanine (essential amino acid) 135 mg, Proline 140 mg, Serine 150 mg, Threonine (essential amino acid) 143 mg, Tryptophan (essential amino acid) 50 mg, Tyrosine 81 mg, Valine (essential amino acid) 179 mg.

Brewer's Yeast - The Vitamin Shoppe
Six tablets contain: Vitamin B1 48 mg • Vitamin B2 16 mg • Niacin 1.6 mg • Folic Acid 13 mcg • Vitamin B6 160 mcg • Choline 15 mg • Pantothenic Acid 200 mcg • Biotin 20 mcg • Inositol 15 mg.

Brewer's Yeast 500 - GNC A-Z - GNC
Eight tablets contain: Thiamin .4 mg • Riboflavin .1 mg • Niacin 1.2 mg. Ingredients: Dry Debittered Brewer's Yeast.

Brewer's Yeast Powdered - GNC A-Z - GNC
Two tablespoons contain: Thiamin 1.05 mg • Riboflavin 1.36 mg • Niacin 9 mg • Vitamin B6 0.7 • Folate, Folic Acid, Folacin 40 mcg • Vitamin B12 0.12 mcg • Biotin 12 mcg • Pantothenic Acid 0.6 mg • Iron 1.8 mg • Phosphorus 20 mg • Magnesium 32 mg • Zinc 3 mg • Copper 1 mg. Ingredients: Brewer's Yeast.

Brigham Tea - Nature's Way
Two capsules contain: Brigham Tea herb 830 mg. Other Ingredients: Gelatin, Magnesium stearate, Millet.

Bright Eyes - Grandma's Herbs
Each capsule contains: Proprietary Blend 0.450 g: Eyebright herb, Fennel seed, Rue herb, Chamomile flower, Goldenseal root, Red Raspberry leaf/seed, Blue Vervain herb, Bayberry bark, Cayenne Pepper (40,000 HU).

Brighten-Up - Changes International, Inc.
Two caplets contain: St. John's Wort standardized extract aerial parts (0.3% hypericin) 300 mg • Panax Ginseng root standardized extract (4% ginsenosides) 200 mg • Ashwagandha root (Withania somnifera) 200 mg • Green Tea leaf standardized extract (20% methylxanthines) 150 mg • Kava Kava root standardized extract (30% kavalactones) 50 mg • Siberian Ginseng root standardized extract (0.8% eleutherosides) 50 mg • Schizandra berry standardized extract (9% schizandrins) 50 mg. Other Ingredients: Dicalcium Phosphate, Vegetable Cellulose, Fractionated vegetable oil, Soy polysaccharides, Silica, and Vegetable resin glaze.

Bright-Eyes - Futurebiotics
Three tablets contain: Bilberry extract (standardized for 25% anthocyanidins) 10 mg • Eyebright (extract equivalent to) 500 mg • Chamomile (extract equivalent to) 250 mg • Rosemary (extract equivalent to) 200 mg • Beta Carotene 20,000 IU • Vitamin A 5000 IU • Quercetin 100 mg • Citrus bioflavonoids 100 mg • Vitamin C 1000 mg • Natural Vitamin E (d-alpha succinate) 200 IU • Vitamin B2 (riboflavin) 40 mg • Rutin 100 mg • Selenium (from selenomethionine) 100 mcg • Zinc (monomethionine) 15 mg • Vitamin B6 5 mg • Niacinamide 10 mg • Pantothenic Acid (B5) 40 mg • Chromium (GTF) 200 mcg • L-Cysteine 100 mg • L-Glutamine 75 mg. In a base of: Alfalfa, Carrot, Parsley & Dandelion.

BRIO Adult Multivitamin - Functional Products
Each wafer contains: Vitamin A (Retinol Palmitate) 2667 IU • Vitamin C (Ascorbic Acid) 60 mg • Vitamin D (Calciferol D3) 0.005 mg • Vitamin E (dl-alpha tocopherol) 10 mg • Vitamin B1 (Thiamine) 1.4 mg • Vitamin B2 (Riboflavin) 1.6 mg • Niacin 18 mg • Vitamin B6 (Pyridoxine) 2 mg • Folic Acid 0.2 mg • Vitamin B12 (Cyanocobalamin) 0.001 mg • Biotin 0.15 mg • Pantothenic Acid 6 mg • Calcium (Calcium Carbonate) 1200 mg • Magnesium (Magnesium Oxide) 45 mg • Zinc (Zinc Sulfate) 3 mg. Ingredients: Citric Acid, Sodium Carbonate, Potassium Carbonate, Corn Starch, Natural Orange Flavor, Mannitol, Potassium Chloride, Beet Root Color, Aspartame, Acesulfame K, Maltodextrin.

BRIO Children's Multivitamin - Functional Products
Each wafer contains: Vitamin A (Retinol Palmitate) 1333 IU • Vitamin C (Ascorbic Acid) 30 mg • Vitamin D (Calciferol D3) 0.0025 mg • Vitamin E (dl-Alpha Tocopherol) 5 mg • Vitamin B1 (Thiamine) 0.7 mg • Vitamin B2 (Riboflavin) 0.8 mg • Niacin 9 mg • Vitamin B6 (Pyridoxine) 1 mg • Folic Acid 0.1 mg • Vitamin B12 (Cyanocobalamin) 0.0005 mg • Biotin 0.075 mg • Pantothenic Acid 3 mg • Calcium (Calcium Carbonate) 250 mg. Ingredients: Citric Acid, Sodium Carbonate, Potassium Hydrogen Carbonate, Beet Root Color, Maltodextrin, Rice Starch, Artificial Strawberry Flavor, Potassium Chloride, Aspartame, Acesulfame K.

BRIO Echinacea - Functional Products
Each wafer contains: Vitamin C (Ascorbic Acid) 200 mg • Echinacea (Dried Juice) 200 mg. Ingredients: Citric Acid, Sodium Hydrogen Carbonate, Potato Starch, Aspartame, Acesulfame K, Natural Lemon Flavor.

Brite-Life - Advocare International
Each caplet contains: Pyridoxine (as HCl) 100 mg • St. John's Wort extract (leaf/flower - hypericum perforatum) 450 mg • L-Tyrosine 300 mg. Other Ingredients: Dicalcium Phosphate, Silicon Dioxide, Cellulose, Stearic Acid, Magnesium Stearate.

Some Brand Name Natural Products - What they Contain

www.NaturalDatabase.com contains MANY more listings than appear here.

BroccoPhane brand - Cyvex Nutrition, Inc.
Standardized Broccoli sprout powder.
See Editor's Note No. 44, page 2058.

BroccoSinolate brand - Cyvex Nutrition, Inc.
Broccoli extract.
See Editor's Note No. 44, page 2058.

Bromelain - Source Naturals
Each tablet contains: Bromelain (2000 GDU per g) 500 mg.

Bromelain 2400 - Vitaline Formulas
Each capsule contains: Bromelain (2400 mcu/gm) 500 mg.

Bromelain 2400gdu - Vital Nutrients
Each capsule contains: Bromelain (2400 gdu/3600 mcu per gram, pure uncut bromelain) 375 mg.

Bromelain Complex - PhytoPharmica
Two capsules contain: Vitamin C (calcium ascorbate) 225 mg • Pantothenic Acid (calcium D-pantothenate) 125 mg • Bromelain (1800 MCU/g, enzymes derived from pineapple stems) 750 mg.

Bromelain Forte - Ortho Molecular Products
Each capsule contains: Bromelain 1200 GDU • Papain 110 MCU.

Bromelain Joint-Ease - Nature's Life
Four capsules contain: Bromelain [an enzyme from Pineapple fruit (Ananassa sativa) activity of 1500 mg = 3000 GDU (4500 MCU)] 1500 mg • Quercetin (Dimorphandra pod) 400 mg • Vitamin C (Ascorbic Acid) 750 mg • Zinc (Picolinate, Gluconate, Citrate) 15 mg • Copper (Gluconate, Citrate) 1 mg • Manganese (Citrate, Aspartate) 3 mg.

Bromelain Plus - Enzymatic Therapy
Each tablet contains: Vitamin C (Calcium Ascorbate) 225 mg • Pantothenic Acid (D-Calcium Pantothenate) 125 mg. Other Ingredients: Bromelain (1800 MCU) pineapple enzyme 750 mg.

Bromezyme - Progressive Labs
Each capsule contains: Bromelain 50 mg • Papain 20 mg • Raw Spleen concentrate 20 mg • Raw Calf Thymus 10 mg.
See Editor's Note No. 14, page 2055.

Bronchitis Remedy - PhytoPharmica
Twenty drops contain: Antimonium tartaricum 4x • Ipecacuanha 4x • Pimpinella saxifraga 2x • Cetraria islandica 1x • Eucalyptus globulus 1x. In a base of 45% USP alcohol by volume.
See Editor's Note No. 1 and No. 21, pages 2053 and 2056.

Bronchoril - PhytoPharmica
Each tablet contains: Glycerol Guaiacolate 200 mg • Fenugreek seed powder 4:1 (trigonella foenum-graecum) 350 mg • Marshmallow 4:1 extract (althaea officinalis, mucilage content 30%-40%) 125 mg • PABA (para-aminobenzoic acid) 50 mg • Mullein leaf (verbascum nigrum) 50 mg.

B-Stress with Siberian Ginseng and Coenzymes - Nature's Way
Two capsules contain: Biotin (biotin triurate) 300 mcg • Calcium Pantethonate 150 mg • Choline Bitartrate 50 mg • Chromium Picolinate 200 mcg • Folic Acid (folate) 400 mcg • Inositol 100 mg • Niacin (Vitamin B3) 25 mg • Niacinamide 100 mg • PABA (para aminobenzoic acid) 50 mg • Pyridoxine HCl 100 mg • Riboflavin (Vitamin B2) 40 mg • Siberian Ginseng root 250 mg • Thiamine (Vitamin B1) 50 mg • Vitamin B12 (Cyanacobalamin) 100 mcg • Vitamin C (Ascorbic Acid) 500 mg.

Bu Zhong Yi Qi Tang Plus - Secara
Three tablets contain: Organic Ginger rhizome (gan jiang) 405 mg • Organic Gentian root (qin jiao) 300 mg • Astragalus root 5:1 extract (huang qi) 300 mg • Shiitake fruit body (20% polysaccharides (40 mg)) 201 mg • Atractylodes root 5:1 extract (bai zhu) 198 mg • Dong Quai root 5:1 extract (dang gui) 198 mg • Asian Ginseng root (ren shen, 5% ginsenosides (10 mg)) 198 mg • Tangerine peel 4:1 extract (chen pi) 141 mg • Bupleurum root 5:1 extract (chai hu) 120 mg • Licorice root 5:1 extract (gan cao) 99 mg • Chinese Cimicifuga rhizome 5:1 extract (sheng ma) 60 mg.

Buckley's Mixture Cough Suppresant - W.K. Buckley Limited
Each teaspoon (5 mL) contains: Dextromethorphan Hydrobromide 12.5 mg • Ammonium Carbonate • Camphor • Canada Balsam • Carrageenan • Glycerine • Menthol • Pine Needle Oil • Sodium Butylparaben • Sodium Propylparaben • Sodium Saccharin • Tincture of Capsicum • Water.

Buffered C 500 mg - Vital Nutrients
Each capsule contains: Buffered Vitamin C (from calcium ascorbate 367 mg) 300 mg • Buffered Vitamin C (from magnesium ascorbate 145 mg) 100 mg • Buffered Vitamin C (from potassium ascorbate 112 mg) 100 mg • Calcium (ascorbate) 34 mg • Magnesium (ascorbate) 7 mg • Potassium (ascorbate) 22 mg.

Buffered C Powder 2000 mg - The Vitamin Shoppe
Each teaspoon contains: Vitamin C (calcium ascorbate) 2000 mg • Rose Hips 1450 mg • Acerola 1000 mg • Lemon Bioflavonoids 500 mg • Rutin 25 mg • Hesperidin 25 mg • Calcium (ascorbate) 230 mg.

Buffered TLC - Jarrow Formulas
Two teaspoons contain: Vitamin C 3000 mg • Calcium 450 mg • Magnesium 250 mg • Potassium 99 mg • L-Taurine 1,000 mg • L-Lysine 250 mg • L-Proline 250 mg • Bromelain (2,000 mcu) 300 mg. Other Ingredients: Ribose, Mannitol, L-Glycine, Natural Lime and Mandarin flavors.

Buffered Vitamin C - Bee-Alive Inc.
Each capsule contains: Vitamin C (from calcium ascorbate, magnesium ascorbate, potassium ascorbate, zinc and rose hips fruit) 500 mg • Calcium 45 mg • Proprietary Blend 200 mg: Citrus Bioflavonoid complex, Rose Hips fruit, Hesperidin, Rutin, Acerola fruit. Other Ingredients: Cellulose, Calcium Phosphate, Gelatin, Vegetable Stearate, Silica.

Buffered Vitamin C 500 with Rose Hips - Schiff
Each tablet contains: Vitamin C (as calcium ascorbate) 500 mg • Calcium (as calcium ascorbate) 31 mg • Rose Hips fruit (rosa canina) 25 mg. Other Ingredients: Cellulose, Hydroxypropyl Methylcellulose, Coating (hydroxypropyl methylcellulose, maltodextrin, polyethylene glycol), Magnesium Stearate.

Buffered Vitamin C Capsules - NutriCology
Two capsules contain: Vitamin C (as ascorbic acid) 1000 mg • Calcium (as calcium carbonate) 190 mg • Magnesium (as magnesium carbonate) 104 mg • Potassium (as potassium carbonate) 16 mg. Other Ingredients: Cellulose, Stearic Acid.

Buffered Vitamin C Powder - NutriCology
Each 1 tsp (4.7 g) serving contains: Vitamin C (as ascorbic acid) 2135 mg • Calcium (as calcium carbonate) 405 mg • Magnesium (as magnesium carbonate) 215 mg • Potassium (as potassium carbonate) 90 mg. Other Ingredients: Cellulose.

Bug Off! Kids Biting Insect Repelling Wrist Band - Kaz, Inc.
Active Ingredients: Citronella Oil • Geraniol Oil • Lemongrass Oil (15.75%). Inactive Ingredient: Polyethylene (84.25%).

Burdock - Nature's Way
Two capsules contain: Burdock root 1.08 g. Other Ingredients: Gelatin, Magnesium stearate.

Burdock-Dandelion Formula - Quest
Each caplet contains: Burdock root powder (Arctium lappa) 90 mg • Dandelion root powder (Taraxacum officinale) 90 mg • Oregon Grape root powder (Mahonia aquifolium) 90 mg • Red Clover blossoms powder (Trifolium praetense) 90 mg • Echinacea angustifolia root powder (Echinacea angustifolia) 30 mg • Yellow Dock root powder (Rhumex) 30 mg • Cayenne powder (Capsicum) 20 mg • Kelp powder (Fucus vesiculosis) 20 mg • Licorice root powder (Glycirrhiza

glabra) 5 mg. Other Ingredients: Calcium Phosphate, Microcrystalline Cellulose, Vegetable Stearin, Croscarmellose Sodium, Magnesium Stearate (vegetable source).

Burn Gel **-** Nature's Way
Calendula Officinalis (marigold) 1X • Cantharis (cantharides) 3X • Sulphur (sulfur) 6X • Urtica Dioica (stinging nettle) 1X.
See Editor's Note No. 1, page 2053.

Burn It **-** ANS - Applied Nutrition Sciences
Chromium Picolinate • Vitamin E • Selenium • Zinc.

BustPro **-** HealthMinded
Four capsules contain: BustPro Proprietary Blend 2000 mg: Saw Palmetto berry, Wild Yam extract, Damiana, Dong Quai extract, Fennel seed, Black Cohosh extract, Dandelion root, Blessed Thistle, Watercress leaf. Other Ingredients: Stearic Acid, Magnesium Stearate.

Butcher's Broom **-** Now
Two capsules contain: Butchers Broom 5:1 extract (rascus aculeatus) (root) 200 mg. Other Ingredients: Rice Flour.

Butcher's Broom **-** Nature's Way
Two capsules contain: Butchers Broom root 940 mg. Other Ingredients: Gelatin, Magnesium stearate.

Butcher's Broom **-** Source Naturals
Each tablet contains: Butcher's Broom 500 mg.

Butt It Out - Stop Smoking **-** Paradise
Each capsule contains: Lobelia Inflata leaf 130 mg. In Base of Organic Brown Rice Flour.

ButyrEn **-** NutriCology
Each tablet contains: Calcium (as calcium/magnesium butyrate) 100 mg • Magnesium (as calcium/magnesium butyrate) 100 mg • Butyrate 815 mg. Other Ingredients: Dicalcium Phosphate, Celluose, Magnesium Stearate, Silicon Dioxide.

Bye Mygrain **-** DreamPharm
Two capsules contain: Bay (laurus nobilis) 60 mg • Feverfew (tanacetum parthenium) 80 mg • Evening Primrose herb (oenothera biennis) 60 mg • Willow bark (salix species) 50 mg • Ligusticum Chuan Xiang root 100 mg • Angelica Dahurica root 100 mg • Gastrodia Elata rhizome 50 mg.

C + Herbs **-** Jarrow Formulas
Each tablet contains: Silymarin (Silybum marianum) 30:1 Concentrate (standardized to 80% silybin) 75 mg • PicroLiv (3.5- 4% Kutkin from Picrorrhiza kurroa) 50 mg • Astragalus Root 6:1 Concentrate 150 mg • Schisandra 5:1 Concentrate 75 mg • Scutelluria root (Skullcap) 4:1 concentrate 150 mg • Vitamin C (Ascorbic Acid) 500 mg. Other Ingredients: Magnesium Stearate.

C All Inclusive 1000 mg **-** Rexall - Sundown
Each tablet contains: Vitamin C 600 mg • Calcium 74 mg • Bioflavonoid Complex 48 mg: Rose Hips & Seeds, Citrus Bioflavonoids, Rutin, Hesperidin, Acerola Fruit Extract 4:1. Other Ingredients: Ascorbic Acid, Calcium Sulfate, Microcrystalline Cellulose, Croscarmellose Sodium, Magnesium Stearate, Hydroxypropyl Methylcellulose, Sweet Orange (peel and fruit), Bitter Orange (fruit), PEG.
See Editor's Note No. 40, page 2058.

C Aspa Scorb **-** Progressive Labs
Each teaspoon (5100 mg) supplies: Vitamin C 4000 mg • Magnesium (from magnesium ascorbate and magnesium aspartate) 250 mg • Zinc (from zinc ascorbate) 30 mg • Selenium (from selenium ascorbate) 50 mcg • Manganese (from manganese ascorbate) 4.2 mg • Potassium (from potassium ascorbate and potassium aspartate) 96 mg.

C Every Day **-** Hadas Natural Products
Each 5 mL serving contains: Orange flavored Sorbitol syrup • Rose Hip extract with Vitamin C 300 mg.

C&E **-** Nature's Bounty
Each softgel contains: Vitamin C (as ascorbic acid and rose hips) 500 mg • Vitamin E (as D-alpha tocopherol plus D-beta, D-gamma and D-delta tocopherols) 400 IU. Other Ingredients: Gelatin, Glycerin, Soybean Oil, Soy Lecithin, Caramel Color, Yellow Beeswax.

C&F Formula **-** Dial Herbs
Vinegar • Glycerine • Honey • the Tinctures of Garlic, Comfrey, Wormwood, Marshmallow, White Oak bark, Black Walnut, Mullein, Scullcap, Uva Ursi, Lobelia.

C-1000 **-** Source Naturals
Each tablet contains: Vitamin C (as ascorbic acid) 1000 mg. Other Ingredients: Microcrystalline Cellulose, Stearic Acid, Hydroxypropyl Cellulose, Modified Gum, Magnesium Stearate, Colloidal Silicon Dioxide.

C-1000 **-** PhysioLogics
Each capsule contains: Vitamin C (as ascorbic acid) 1000 mg • Citrus Bioflavonoids (citrus spp., fruit) 30 mg. Other Ingredients: Gelatin, Vegetable Magnesium Stearate, Titanium Dioxide Color.

C-1000 - Biodelivery Nutritional Systems **-** Nutritional Therapeutics, Inc.
Each tablet contains: Vitamin C (Calcium Ascorbate-Niascorbate) 1000 mg • Bioflavonoids 100 mg • Pantethine 5 mg • NT Factor tablet base 50 mg.

C-1000 mg Ascorbic Acid **-** Rexall - Sundown
Each caplet contains: Vitamin C (as ascorbic acid) 1 g. Other Ingredients: Cornstarch, Crospovidone, Magnesium Stearate, Hydroxypropyl Methylcellulose, PEG.

C-1000 mg Rosehip Timed **-** Rexall - Sundown
Each caplet contains: Vitamin C 1 g • Calcium 35 mg • Bioflavonoid Complex 19 mg: Rose Hips & Seeds, Citrus Bioflavonoids, Rutin, Acerola Fruit Extract 4:1. Other Ingredients: Hydrogenated Cottonseed Oil, Dicalcium Phosphate, Hydroxypropyl Methylcellulose, Silica, Magnesium Stearate, Orange (fruit), Bitter Orange (fruit).
See Editor's Note No. 40, page 2058.

C-1000 with Rosehips **-** Rexall - Sundown
Each caplet contains: Vitamin C 1 g • Bioflavonoid Complex 17 mg: Rose Hips & Seeds, Citrus Bioflavonoids, Rutin, Acerola Fruit Extract 4:1. Other Ingredients: Microcrystalline Cellulose, Stearic Acid, Silica, Croscarmellose Sodium, Magnesium Stearate, Orange (fruit), Bitter Orange (fruit).
See Editor's Note No. 40, page 2058.

C-1000-TR **-** Atrium Inc.
Each tablet contains: Vitamin C 1000 mg • Naturally Associated Bioflavonoid Complex 100 mg.

C-250 mg Ascorbic Acid **-** Rexall - Sundown
Each tablet contains: Vitamin C (as ascorbic acid) 250 mg. Other Ingredients: Dicalcium Phosphate, Microcrystalline Cellulose, Stearic Acid, Croscarmellose Sodium, Magnesium Stearate.

C-500 - Biodelivery Nutritional Systems **-** Nutritional Therapeutics, Inc.
Each tablet contains: Vitamin C (Calcium Ascorbate-Niascorbate) 500 mg • Bioflavonoids 100 mg • Pantethine 5 mg • NT Factor tablet base 50 mg.

C-500 mg Ascorbic Acid **-** Rexall - Sundown
Each tablet contains: Vitamin C (as ascorbic acid) 500 mg. Other Ingredients: Cornstarch, Crospovidone, Magnesium Stearate.

C-500 mg Chew w/Rosehips **-** Rexall - Sundown
Each tablet contains: Vitamin C (as sodium ascorbate, ascorbic acid & rose hips with seeds) 500 mg • Sodium 40 mg. Other Ingredients: Compressible Sugar, Hydrogenated Cottonseed Oil, Stearic Acid, Natural Orange Flavor (with other natural flavors), Magnesium Stearate, Yellow 6 Lake.

Some Brand Name Natural Products - What they Contain
www.NaturalDatabase.com contains MANY more listings than appear here.

BRAND NAMES

C-500 mg Time Release **-** Rexall - Sundown
Each capsule contains: Vitamin C (as ascorbic acid) 500 mg. Other Ingredients: Gelatin, Pharmaceutical Glaze, Sucrose, Starch, Talc, Titanium Dioxide, Yellow 5 (tartrazine), Yellow 6, Red 40.

C-500 Timed Colorfree **-** Rexall - Sundown
Each capsule contains: Vitamin C (as ascorbic acid) 500 mg. Other Ingredients: Gelatin, Pharmaceutical Glaze, Sucrose, Talc, Food Starch.

C-500 with Rosehips **-** Rexall - Sundown
Each caplet contains: Vitamin C 500 mg • Bioflavonoid Complex 9 mg: Rose Hips & Seeds, Citrus Bioflavonoids, Rutin, Acerola Fruit Extract 4:1. Other Ingredients: Microcrystalline Cellulose, Stearic Acid, Silica, Croscarmellose Sodium, Magnesium Stearate, Orange (fruit), Bitter Orange (fruit).
See Editor's Note No. 40, page 2058.

C-500 XTRA **-** Rexall - Sundown
Each tablet contains: Vitamin C 500 mg • Zinc (as zinc oxide) 5 mg • Selenium (as selenium yeast chelate) 33 mcg • Orange Peel Extract 100 mg • Citrus Bioflavonoids 25 mg • Rutin 50 mg • XTRA Premium Blend 5.25 mg: Alfalfa (leaf), Rose Hips & Seeds, Parsley (aerial parts), Acerola Fruit Extract 1:4. Other Ingredients: Ascorbic Acid, Dicalcium Phosphate, Croscarmellose Sodium, Hydroxypropyl Methylcellulose, Magnesium Stearate, PEG.

CAC Tabs **-** Dial Herbs
Cascara Sagrada • Buckthorn • Burdock • Chaparral • Dandelion • Licorice root • Barberry • Red Clover.

Cacao **-** Nature's Way
Two capsules contain: Cacao (whole fruit) 1.1 g. Other Ingredients: Cellulose, Gelatin.

Cactus (Nopal) **-** Natural Dynamics
Each capsule contains: Nopal 650 mg.

Cactus Diet **-** Cactu-Life
Each capsule contains: Opuntia Streptacantha 500 mg.

Caffeine Mix **-** Professional Complementary Health Formul
Adrenal 3X, 4X • ACTH 6X, 30X • Histamine 12X • Liver 6X, 12X • Methylxanthine-bearing foods: Caffeine, Chocolate (milk, dark, white), Coffee (five types), Decaffeinated Coffee, Cola, Espresso, Tea 6X, 12X, 60X, 100X • Purified Water • 20% USP Alcohol.
See Editor's Note No. 1, page 2053.

Cal Apatite Forte Capsules **-** Metagenics
Three capsules contain: MCHC (microcrystalline hydroxyapatite concentrate) 3036 mg • Calcium (as MCHC) 684 mg • Phosphorus (as MCHC) 357 mg • Vitamin D (as cholecalciferol) 600 IU • Boron (as boron citrate) 300 mcg.

Cal Mag Liquid **-** Genestra - Seroyal
Each tablespoon contains: Calcium Carbonate 600 mg • Magnesium Oxide 300 mg • Vitamin D (as vitamin D3) 100 IU. Other Ingredients: Natural Spearmint Flavor.

Cal/Mag Balance **-** Nutri-Quest Rx
Each tablet contains: Calcium Aspartate 175 mg • Calcium Citrate 175 mg • Magnesium Aspartate 175 mg • Magnesium Glycinate 175 mg • Vitamin C 25 IU • Vitamin D 20 mg of HCL.

Cal/Mag Citrate with Vitamin D **-** Country Life
Each four softgels contain: Calcium (citrate, carbonate) 400 mg • Magnesium (carbonate, citrate) 400 mg • Vitamin D (cholecalciferol) 100 IU. Inactive Ingredients: Soybean Oil, Lecithin, Gelatin, Glycerin, Purified Water, Titanium Dioxide.

Cal/Mag Complex **-** Country Life
Each tablet contains: Calcium (as calcium hydroxyapatite, citrate, asparate, alpha-ketoglutartate, lysinate) 1000 mg • Phosphorous (from calcium hydroxyapatite) 500 mg • Magnesium (as magnesium oxide, citrate, taurinate, alpha-ketoglutarate, magnesium aspartate) 500 mg.

Cal-1000 Complete **-** Puritan's Pride
Two tablets contain: Vitamin A (as Retinyl Acetate) 5,000 IU • Vitamin C (as Ascorbic Acid) 60 mg • Vitamin C (as Cholecalciferol) 400 IU • Vitamin E (as dl-Alpha Tocopheryl Acetate) 30 IU • Thiamin (Vitamin B-1; as Thiamine Mononitrate) 1.5 mg • Riboflavin (Vitamin B-2) 1.7 mg • Niacin (as Niacinamide) 20 mg • Vitamin B-6 (as Pyridoxine Hydrochloride) 2 mg • Folic Acid 400 mcg • Vitamin B-12 (as Cyanocobalamin) 6 mcg • Biotin (as d-Biotin) 300 mcg • Pantothenic Acid (as d-Calcium Pantothenate) 10 mg • Calcium (as Calcium Carbonate) 1,000 mg • Iron (as Ferrous Fumarate) 18 mg.

Cal-Acid Complex **-** Atrium Inc.
Four tablets contain: Calcium (from Oyster Shell, Oyster Shell-Citrus Juice Complex, & Calcium Caseinate) 750 mg • Magnesium (from Magnesium Citrus Juice Complex & Oxide) 210 mg • Manganese (Manganese-Citrus Carbonate Juice Complex) 5 mg • Copper (as Gluconate) 0.1 mg • Vitamin D (Fish oil) 400 USP IU • Vitamin C with Rose Hips 40 mg • Vitamin E 10 IU • Betaine HCL & Glutamic Acid HCL sufficient to provide dilute HCL10 min. Amino Acids, Peptides, & Polypeptides from Hydrolized Soy Protein with Lecithin & Alfalfa juice concentrate.

Cal-Acid Maxi **-** Atrium Inc.
Four tablets contain: Calcium (Calcium Citrate, Calcium Caseinate & Oyster Shell) 1500 mg • Magnesium (Magnesium Citrus Juice Complex & Oxide) 500 mg • Manganese (Manganese Citrus Carbonate Juice) 10 mg • Vitamin D (Fish oil) 500 IU • Vitamin C with Rose Hips 100 mg • Vitamin E (d-Alpha Tocopherol) 20 IU • Horsetail (Silica) 250 mg • Boron (Citrate) 3 mg. Betaine HCL & Glutamic Acid HCL sufficient to provide dilute HCL. Amino acids, peptids & polypeptids from hydrolyzed soy protein with Lecithin & Alfalfa juice concentrate.

Calamacin **-** MMS Pro
Each capsule contains: Scullcap herb • Wood Betony • Black Cohosh root • Hops flowers • Valerian root • Cayenne.

Calcet Triple Calcium **-** Mission Pharmacal
Two tablets contain: Vitamin D (Vitamin D3; as cholecalciferol) 200 IU • Calcium (as calcium carbonate, calcium gluconate, calcium lactate) 300 mg. Other Ingredients: Polyethylene Glycol, HPMC, Croscarmellose Sodium, Color, Magnesium Stearate, FD & C Yellow 5 Lake, Magnesium Silicate, Carnauba Wax.

Cal-Chew Calcium 350 mg **-** Jamieson
Each tablet contains: Calcium (as Calcium Carbonate, Calcium Citrate, Calcium Malate, Calcium Succinate, Calcium Aspartate, Calcium Glutamate, Calcium Fumarate) 350 mg • Iron 0.4 mg.

Calci-Lean **-** Gero Vita International
Two capsules contain: Vitamin C (as magnesium ascorbate) 77 mg • Calcium (as calcium gluconate) 19 mg • Magnesium (as magnesium ascorbate) 10 mg • Proprietary Herbal Blend 890 mg: Guggul gum extract (24% lipids), Nut Grass tuber extract (0.15% alkaloids), Plumbago Zeylanica root extract (0.01% alkaloids), Embelia Ribes fruit extract, Operculina Turpenthurn root extract (2.5% resins), Picorhiza Kurroa root extract (1% bitter), Emblic fruit extract (5% tannins), Tropical Almond fruit extract (7.5% tannins), Belleric Myrobalan fruit extract (5% tannins), Piper Longum fruit extract (0.5% volatile oil), Black Pepper fruit extract (1% volatile oil), Ginger rhizome extract (0.5% volatile oils) • Proprietary Enzyme Blend 100 mg: Bromelain, Amylase, HermiSeb, Peptizyme SP, Catalase, Lipase, Amla. Other Ingredients: Gelatin, Silicon Dioxide, Magnesium Stearate.

Calcimate **-** GNC
Two tablets contain: Vitamin D (as cholecalciferol) 200 IU • Calcium (as calcium citrate malate) 500 mg • Magnesium (as magnesium oxide) 125 mg • Zinc (as zinc oxide) 8 mg • Copper (as cupric oxide) 1 mg • Boron (as boron citrate) 1 mg. Other Ingredients: Cellulose.

Some Brand Name Natural Products - What they Contain

www.NaturalDatabase.com contains MANY more listings than appear here.

***Calcimate 400* - GNC**
Three tablets contain: Vitamin D (as Cholecalciferol) 200 IU • Calcium (as Calcium Citrate Malate) 400 mg. Other Ingredients: Cellulose.

***Calcimate Plus 800* - GNC**
Four tablets contain: Vitamin D (as Cholecalciferol) 200 IU • Calcium (as Calcium Citrate Malate) 800 mg • Magnesium (as Magnesium Oxide) 100 mg • Potassium (as Potassium Chloride) 99 mg. Other Ingredients: Cellulose, Titanium Dioxide, Vegetable Acetoglycerides.

***Calcium - Animal Parade* - Nature's Plus**
Two tablets contain: Calcium (as aminoate complex) 250 mg • Magnesium (as aminoate complex) 50 mg.

***Calcium - Basic Nutrition* - GNC**
Each tablet contains: Calcium (as Calcium Carbonate) 600 mg. Other Ingredients: Gelatin, Cellulose, Soy Fiber, Titanium Dioxide, Vegetable Acetoglycerides, Magnesium Stearate.

***Calcium* - Natrol**
Three tablets contain: Calcium 500 mg • Magnesium 200 mg • Fruitbase 640 mg. Other Ingredients: Mono- and Di-Glycerides, Croscarmellose Sodium, Silicon Dioxide, Stearic Acid, Magnesium Stearate.

***Calcium* - PhytoPharmica**
Each tablet contains: Calcium (from tricalcium phosphate and calcium citrate) 333 mg &#8226 Magnesium (as magnesium oxide and magnesium aspartate) 133 mg &#8226 Phosphorus (from tricalcium phosphate) 150 mg &#8226 Sodium 5 mg &#8226 Vitamin D (as cholecalciferol) 133 IU.

***Calcium & Magnesium* - Nature's Way**
Three capsules contain: Calcium (citrate, carbonate, malate) 500 mg • Magnesium (oxide, aspartate) 250 mg •Sodium 5 mg. Other Ingredients: Cellulose, Gelatin, Magnesium Stearate.

***Calcium & Magnesium* - NSI - Nutraceutical Sciences Institute**
Each four capsules contain: Calcium (from 2,227 mg calcium citrate malate) 500 mg • Magnesium (from 1,190 mg magnesium citrate) 250 mg.

***Calcium & Magnesium* - Source Naturals**
Each tablet contains: Calcium (from 1,250 mg of Amino Acid Chelate) 250 mg • Magnesium (from 625 mg of Amino Acid Chelate) 125 mg • Vitamin D (Cholecalciferol) 500 IU.

***Calcium & Magnesium Complex* - Health Smart Vitamins**
Three caplets contain: Calcium (as 80% calcium citrate, 19% calcium carbonate, 1% calcium stearate) 503 mg • Magnesium (as 50% magnesium citrate, 50% magnesium glycinate) 250 mg.

***Calcium & Magnesium Complex* - Nature's Way**
Three capsules contain: Calcium (citrate, carbonate, malate) 500 mg • Magnesium (oxide, aspartate) 250 mg • Sodium 5 mg. Other Ingredients: Cellulose, Gelatin, Magnesium-Stearate.

***Calcium (Citrate/Malate)* - Vital Nutrients**
Each capsule contains: Calcium (citrate/malate) 150 mg.

***Calcium + D, Natural Source* - Leiner Health Products**
Each tablet contains: Calcium Carbonate 600 mg • Vitamin D (Cholecalciferol) 200 IU. Other Ingredients: Maltodextrin, Hydroxypropyl Methylcellulose, Talc, Croscarmellose Sodium, Acacia, Hydroxypropyl Cellulose, Titanium Dioxide, Silicon Dioxide, Starch, Magnesium Stearate, Polysorbate 80, Polyethylene Glycol 3350, Sodium Citrate, Yellow 6 Lake.

***Calcium +D* - Rexall - Sundown**
Three tablets contain: Vitamin D (as cholecalciferol) 400 IU • Calcium (from oyster shell) 1 g. Other Ingredients: Maltodextrin, Cellulose, Mineral Oil, Croscarmellose Sodium, Hydroxypropyl Methylcellulose, Carboxymethylcellulose Sodium, PEG, Carnauba Wax, Crospovidone, Magnesium Stearate, Stearic Acid.

***Calcium +D 500 mg* - Rexall - Sundown**
Each caplet contains: Vitamin D (as cholecalciferol) 200 IU • Calcium (from oyster shell) 500 mg. Other Ingredients: Maltodextrin, Microcrystalline Cellulose, Mineral Oil, Hydroxypropyl Methylcellulose, Soy Poly-Saccharides, Titanium Dioxide, PEG, Polysorbate 80, Yellow 5 Lake (tartrazine), Blue 1 Lake, Carnauba Wax, Stearic Acid, Magnesium Stearate, Crospovidone.

***Calcium 1000 Magnesium 400 - GNC A-Z* - GNC**
Three tablets contain: Calcium (as Calcium Carbonate) 1000 mg • Magnesium (as Magnesium Oxide) 400 mg • Zinc (as Zinc Oxide) 15 mg • Copper (as Cupric Oxide) 1 mg. Other Ingredients: Cellulose.

***Calcium 1200 with D* - Rexall - Sundown**
Two softgels contain: Vitamin D (as cholecalciferol) 200 IU • Calcium (as calcium carbonate) 1.2 g. Other Ingredients: Soybean Oil, Gelatin, Glycerin, Soy Lecithin, Water, Titanium Dioxide (color).

***Calcium 500 mg* - Rexall - Sundown**
Each caplet contains: Calcium (from oyster shell) 500 mg. Other Ingredients: Maltodextrin, Cellulose, Hydroxypropyl Methylcellulose, Mineral Oil, Titanium Dioxide (color), PEG, Yellow 5 Lake, Polysorbate 80, Blue 1 Lake, Stearic Acid, Magnesium Stearate, Crospovidone.

***Calcium 500 mg* - Nature Made**
Each tablet contains: Calcium (from calcium carbonate) 500 mg. Other Ingredients: Maltodextrin, Cellulose, Hydroxypropyl Methylcellulose, Soy Polysaccharides, Polyethylene Glcyol.
See Editor's Note No. 45, page 2058.

***Calcium 600* - Pro Health**
Each tablet contains: Vitamin D (as cholecalciferol) 400 IU • Calcium (as carbonate, citrate, mined from earth deposits) 600 mg. Other Ingredients: Stearic Acid, Microcrystalline Cellulose, Croscarmellose Sodium, Magnesium Stearate, Pharmaceutical Glaze.

***Calcium 600 / Magnesium 300 - GNC A-Z* - GNC**
Three capsules contain: Vitamin D (as cholecalciferol) 100 IU • Calcium (as calcium carbonate) 600 mg • Magnesium (as magnesium oxide) 300 mg. Other Ingredients: Gelatin, Cellulose.

***Calcium 600 +D* - Rexall - Sundown**
Each caplet contains: Vitamin D (as cholecalciferol) 200 IU • Calcium (as calcium carbonate) 600 mg. Other Ingredients: Maltodextrin, Cellulose, Hydroxypropyl Methylcellulose, Titanium Dioxide (color), Mineral Oil, PEG, Polysorbate 80, Stearic Acid, Magnesium Stearate, Crospovidone.

***Calcium 600 mg* - Nature Made**
Each tablet contains: Vitamin D 200 IU • Calcium 600 mg. Other Ingredients: Maltodexrin, Cellulose, Hydroxypropyl Methylcellulose, Soy Polysacchardies, Polyethylene Glycol.
See Editor's Note No. 45, page 2058.

***Calcium and Magnesium with Zinc* - Nature Made**
Each tablet contains: Calcium (from calcium carbonate) 333 mg • Magnesium (from magnesium oxide) 133 mg • Zinc (from zinc sulfate) 5 mg. Other Ingredients: Maltodextrin, Croscarmellose Sodium, Silicon Dioxide, Magnesium Stearate, Hydroxypropyl Methylcellulose, Cellulose, Polyethylene Glycol.
See Editor's Note No. 45, page 2058.

***Calcium Ascorbate* - Atrium Inc.**
Each tablet contains: Vitamin C (Ascorbic Acid) 1000 mg.

***Calcium Ascorbate* - Source Naturals**
Each half-rounded teaspoon contains: Vitamin C (as calcium ascorbate) 2150 mg • Calcium (as calcium ascorbate) 245 mg.

Some Brand Name Natural Products - What they Contain

www.NaturalDatabase.com contains MANY more listings than appear here.

BRAND NAMES

Calcium Ascorbate C-Complex 1000 mg **-** The Vitamin Shoppe
Each 1000 mg capsule contains: Vitamin C as calcium ascorbate 750 mg • Citrus Bioflavonoids 100 mg • Hesperidin 50 mg • Rutin 25 mg • Calcium 75 mg.

Calcium Ascorbate Crystals **-** Nature's Life
Each teaspoon contains: Vitamin C (Calcium Ascorbate) 3240 mg • Calcium (Calcium Ascorbate) 360 mg.

Calcium Citrate **-** NutriCology
Each capsule contains: Calcium (as calcium citrate) 150 mg. Other Ingredients: Stearic Acid.

Calcium Citrate (250 mg) **-** Pro Health
Each tablet contains: Calcium (as calcium citrate) 250 mg. Other Ingredients: L-Glutamic Acid, Cellulose, Modified Cellulose Gum, Stearic Acid, Silica, Magnesium Stearate.

Calcium Citrate 1000 - GNC A-Z **-** GNC
Four tablets contain: Calcium (as calcium citrate) 1000 mg. Other Ingredients: Cellulose.

Calcium Citrate Capsules **-** Optimum Nutrition
Two capsules contain: Vitamin D (as cholecalciferol) 200 IU • Calcium (as calcium citrate) 300 mg • Magnesium (as magnesium oxide, aspartate) 150 mg. Other Ingredients: Gelatin, Magnesium Stearate.

Calcium Citrate Malate **-** Rexall - Sundown
Two caplets contain: Vitamin D (as cholecalciferol) 200 IU • Calcium (as calcium citrate malate) 500 mg. Other Ingredients: Microcrystalline Cellulose, Stearic Acid, Titanium Dioxide (color), Dextrose, Silica, Magnesium Stearate, Hydroxypropyl Methylcellulose, PEG, Sodium Carboxymethylcellulose, Carnauba Wax, Mineral Oil, Sodium Citrate, Polysorbate 80, Dextrin.

Calcium Citrate Plus - GNC A-Z **-** GNC
Four tablets contain: Vitamin D (as cholecalciferol) 100 IU • Calcium (as calcium citrate) 800 mg • Magnesium (as magnesium oxide) 400 mg • Casein Phosphopeptide 75 mg. Other Ingredients: Cellulose, Titanium Dioxide, Vegetable Acetoglycerides.

Calcium Citrate Plus Vitamin D **-** Progressive Labs
Four tablets contain: Calcium (as calcium citrate) 3240 mg • Calcium (Calcium Ascorbate) 360 mg.

Calcium Citrate with Vitamin D **-** Nature Made
Three tablets contain: Vitamin D 300 IU • Calcium (from calcium citrate) 750 mg. Other Ingredients: Cellulose Gel, Stearic Acid, Hydroxypropyl Methylcellulose, Croscarmellose Sodium, Titanium Dioxide Artificial Color, Magnesium Stearate, Polyethylene Glycol, Triethyl Citrate, Polysorbate 80, Sodium Citrate, Corn Starch.
See Editor's Note No. 45, page 2058.

Calcium Citrate with Zinc & Magnesium **-** Now
Two tablets contain: Vitamin D (Fish oil) 100 IU • Calcium (Citrate) 600 mg • Magnesium (Oxide, Aspartate) 300 mg • Zinc (Amino Acid Chelate) 15 mg • Manganese (Amino Acid Chelate) 5 mg • Copper (Amino Acid Chelate) 1 mg.

Calcium Citrate/Malate Complex **-** Nature's Way
Two capsules contain: Calcium (citrate, carbonate, malate) 500 mg. Other Ingredients: Cellulose, Gelatin, Magnesium Stearate, Silica.

Calcium Complete Capsules GNC A-Z **-** GNC
Two capsules contain: Calcium (as Cacium Carbonate) 600 mg • Magnesium (as Magnesium Oxide) 300 mg. Other Ingredients: Soybean Oil, Gelatin, Glycerin, Titanium Dioxide.

Calcium Complete Tablets - GNC A-Z **-** GNC
Three tablets contain: Vitamin C (as ascorbic acid) 300 mg • Calcium (as calcium carbonate) 1200 mg • Magnesium (as magnesium oxide) 600 mg • Betaine hydrochloride 50 mg. Other Ingredients: Cellulose, Soy fiber, Titanium Dioxide, Rose Hips powder (rosina canina).

Calcium Complex 750 **-** Optimum Nutrition
Each tablet contains: Vitamin D (as cholecalciferol) 200 IU • Calcium (as calcium carbonate, citrate) 500 mg • Magnesium (as magnesium oxide, aspartate) 250 mg. Other Ingredients: Pharmaceutical Glaze, Stearic Acid, Magnesium Stearate, Croscarmellose Sodium (disintegrant), Silica.

Calcium Complex Bone Formula **-** Nature's Way
Three capsules contain: Boron Amino Acid Chelate 1.5 mg • Calcium (citrate, carbonate, malate) 500 mg • Copper Amino Acid Chelate 500 mcg • Folic Acid (folate) 100 mcg • Horsetail Grass 12.6 mg • Magnesium (oxide, aspartate) 2.5 mg • Manganese Aspartate 2.5 mg • Vitamin B6 (as pyridoxine HCl) 12.5 mg • Vitamin D (D3, cholecalciferol) 100 IU • Vitamin K (phytonadione) 37.5 mcg • Zinc Amino Acid Chelate 5 mg. Other Ingredients: Cellulose, Gelatin, Magnesium-Stearate.

Calcium D-Glucarate **-** Source Naturals
Each two tablets contain: Calcium from 1000 mg Calcium d-Glucarate 1230 mg.

Calcium D-Glucarate - Tyler **-** Integrative Therapeutics
Three capsules contain: Calcium (as calcium d-glucarate) 180 mg • Calcium D-Glucarate USP 1.5 g. Other Ingredients: Microcrystalline Cellulose, Gelatin, Water.

Calcium Effervescent **-** Progressive Labs
Two tablets contain: Calcium (from calcium carbonate) 1000 mg • Vitamin D (as cholecaciferol) 400 IU. Ingredients: Citric Acid, Calcium Carbonate, Sorbitol, Sodium Bicarbonate, Sodium Carbonate, Magnesium Carbonate, Aspartame, Mineral oil, Natural Orange flavor, Cholecalciferol. Contains Phenylalanine.

Calcium Lactate **-** Puritan's Pride
Three tablets contain: Calcium (as calcium lactate trihydrate) 250 mg.

Calcium Magnesium Citrate **-** NutriCology
Each capsule contains: Calcium (as calcium citrate) 100 mg • Magnesium (as magnesium citrate) 100 mg. Other Ingredients: Stearic Acid, Cellulose.

Calcium Magnesium Phosphorus Superabsorbeze **-** Nature's Life
Each tablespoon contains: Calcium (Calcium Phosphate) 600 mg • Magnesium (Hydroxide, Carbonate) 300 mg • Vitamin D (as Vitamin D3) (Cholecalciferol) 200 IU. In a natural base of Purified Water, Citric Acid, Sorbital, natural Orange flavor & Cellulose.

Calcium Magnesium Superabsorbeze **-** Nature's Life
Each tablespoon contains: Calcium (Citrate, Lactate/ Gluconate) 600 mg • Phosphorus (Calcium Phosphate) 600 mg • Magnesium (Hydroxide, Carbonate) 300 mg • Vitamin D (as Vitamin D3) (Cholecalciferol) 200 IU. In a natural base of Purified Water, Citric Acid, Fructose, natural Orange flavor, Cellulose & Ascorbic Acid.

Calcium Magnesium Zinc **-** Nature's Life
Three tablets contain: Calcium (Carbonate, Citrate/Malate) 1000 mg • Magnesium (Oxide, Citrate) 600 mg • Zinc (Picolinate, Citrate) 15 mg • Copper (Gluconate, Citrate) 1 mg • Silicon (Dioxide) 20 mg • Boron (Citrate) 100 mcg • Glutamic Acid HCl 100 mg. In a natural base of Springtime Horsetail Herb (Equisetum arvense).

Calcium Night **-** Source Naturals
Four tablets contain: Calcium (Citrate, Malate, Carbonate, Fumarate and Ascorbate) 600 mg • Magnesium (Oxide, Malate, Citrate, Fumarate and Ascorbate) 600 mg • Vitamin C (Magnesium and Calcium Ascorbate, Ascorbic Acid, and Manganese Ascorbate) 275 mg • Vitamin B-6 (Pyridoxine HCl) 20 mg • Vitamin D-3 (Cholecalciferol) 200 IU • Folic Acid 200 mcg • Silica (Horsetail Silica extract) 9 mg • Manganese (Ascorbate) 6 mg • Boron (Amino Acid Chelate) 3 mg • Copper Sebacate 1 mg.

Calcium Oyster Shell 1000 mg **-** Rexall - Sundown
Three tablets contain: Vitamin D (as cholecalciferol) 400 IU • Calcium (from oyster shell) 1 g. Other Ingredients: Maltodextrin, Cellulose, Mineral Oil, Croscarmellose Sodium, Hydroxypropyl Methylcellulose, Carboxymethylcellulose Sodium, PEG, Carnauba Wax, Crospovidone, Magnesium Stearate, Stearic Acid.

Calcium Plus 1000 - GNC A-Z **-** GNC
Three tablets contain: Vitamin A (as retinyl palmitate) 4000 IU • Vitamin C (as ascorbic acid) 100 mg • Vitamin D (as cholecalciferol) 400 IU • Calcium (as calcium carbonate) 1000 mg • Iron (as ferrous gluconate) 10 mg • Magnesium (as magnesium oxide) 500 mg. Other Ingredients: Cellulose, Rose Hips Powder (rosina canina).

Calcium Plus Soy **-** Rexall - Sundown
Each tablet contains: Vitamin D 200 IU • Calcium 600 mg • Magnesium 50 mg • Soy Isoflavones 25 mg • Trans-Resveratrol 2 mg. Other Ingredients: Calcium Carbonate, Magnesium Oxide, Soybean Extract, Microcrystalline Cellulose, Lactose, Hydroxypropyl Methylcellulose, Magnesium Stearate, Titanium Dioxide (color), Silica, Croscarmellose Sodium, Tricetin, Polygonum Cuspidatum Siebold & Zucc. Extract (root), Stearic Acid, Cholecalciferol.

Calcium Plus Vitamin D & Minerals **-** Leiner Health Products
Each tablet contains: Manganese Sulfate 1.8 mg • Calcium Carbonate 600 mg • Copper (Cupric Oxide) 1 mg • Vitamin D (Cholecalciferol) 200 IU • Zinc Oxide 7.5 mg • Magnesium Oxide 40 mg • Boron 250 mcg. Other Ingredients: Maltodextrin, Hydroxypropyl Methylcellulose, Titanium Dioxide, Magnesium Stearate, Sodium Borate, Red 40 Lake, Yellow 6 Lake, Blue 1 Lake, and may contain less than 2% of Cellulose, Talc, Starch, Mineral Oil, Croscarmellose Sodium, Hydroxypropyl Cellulose, Silicon Dioxide, Polyethylene Glycol 8000, Polysorbate 80, Sodium Lauryl Sulfate, Polyethylene Glycol 3350, Crospovidone, Gelatin, Stearic Acid.

Calcium Pyruvate **-** Allergy Research Group
Each capsule contains: Calcium (as calcium pyruvate) 110 mg • Pyruvate 530 mg. Other Ingredients: Stearic Acid.

Calcium Pyruvate **-** Natrol
Each capsule contains: Calcium (as calcium pyruvate) 122 mg • Pyruvate (as calcium pyruvate) 528 mg • Cayenne Pepper 50 mg. Inactive Ingredients: Magnesium Stearate, Silica, Gelatin.

Calcium Pyruvate **-** NutriCology
Each capsule contains: Calcium (as calcium pyruvate) 110 mg • Pyruvate 530 mg. Other Ingredients: Stearic Acid.

Calcium with Vitamin D 500 mg **-** Nature Made
Each tablet contains: Vitamin D 200 IU • Calcium (from calcium carbonate) 500 mg. Other Ingredients: Maltodextrin, Cellulose Gel, Soy Polysaccharides, Hydroxypropyl Methylcellulose, Corn Starch, Polyethylene Glycol.
See Editor's Note No. 45, page 2058.

Calcium with Vitamin D 600 mg **-** Nature Made
Each tablet contains: Vitamin D 200 IU • Calcium (from calcium carbonate) 600 mg. Other Ingredients: Maltodextrin, Cellulose, Hydroxypropyl Methylcellulose, Soy Polysaccharides, Polyethylene Glycol, Carnauba Wax.
See Editor's Note No. 45, page 2058.

Calcium Xtra **-** Puritan's Pride
Three tablets contain: Vitamin A (as Retinyl Acetate) 4,000 IU • Vitamin C (as Ascorbic Acid) 100 mg • Vitamin D (as Cholecalciferol) 400 IU • Calcium (as Calcium Carbonate) 1,000 mg • Iron (as Ferrous Gluconate) 10 mg • Magnesium (as Magnesium Oxide) 500 mg.

Calcium, Magnesium & Vitamin D **-** Nature's Way
Three capsules contain: Calcium (citrate, carbonate, malate) 500 mg • Magnesium (oxide, aspartate) 250 mg • Vitamin D (D3, cholecalciferol) 400 IU. Other Ingredients: Cellulose, Gelatin, Magnesium-Stearate.

Calcium/Magnesium **-** Vital Nutrients
Each capsule contains: Calcium (50% succinate and carbonate) 200 mg • Magnesium (40% citrate and 60% oxide) 100 mg.

Calcium/Magnesium (Citrate) **-** Vital Nutrients
Each capsule contains: Calcium (citrate/malate) 90 mg • Magnesium (citrate) 90 mg.

Calcium/Magnesium with Vitamin D **-** Jamieson
Each caplet contains: Vitamin D (as Cholecalciferol) 133 IU • Calcium (as Calcium Carbonate, Calcium Citrate, Calcium Succinate, Calcium Asparate, Calcium Glutamate, Calcium Furmarate) 333 mg • Magnesium (as Magnesium Oxide, Magnesium Citrate, Magnesium Malate, Magnesium Succiante, Magnesium Asparate, Magnesium Glutamate, Magnesium Fumarate) 167 mg.

Calcium-Magnesium - Biodelivery Nutritional Systems **-** Nutritional Therapeutics, Inc.
Each tablet contains: Calcium (Citrate) 250 mg • Magnesium (Oxide) 250 mg • NT Factor tablet base 200 mg.

Calcium-Magnesium Complex **-** The Vitamin Shoppe
Four tablets contain: Calcium 1500 mg • Magnesium 420 mg • Vitamin D 1000 IU • Vitamin E 20 IU • Vitamin C 80 mg • Manganese 10 mg. Plus Betaine HCl and Glutamic Acid HCl. In a base containing: Hydrolyzed Soy Protein, Lecithin, and Alfalfa Powder.

Calcium-Magnesium for Children **-** The Vitamin Shoppe
Each tablet contains: Calcium 200 mg • Magnesium 100 mg.

Calcium-Magnesium with Vitamin D **-** Schiff
Two softgels contain: Vitamin D (from fish liver oil and as cholecalciferol) 100 IU • Calcium (as calcium carbonate) 600 mg • Magnesium (as magnesium oxide) 300 mg. Other Ingredients: Vegetable Oil, Lecithin, Softgel (gelatin, glycerin, titanium dioxide for color), Silicon Dioxide.

Calcium-Magnesium-Zinc **-** The Vitamin Shoppe
Three tablets contain: Elemental Calcium 1500 mg • Elemental Magnesium 750 mg • Elemental Zinc 45 mg.

CalciWise **-** Resource Wellness
Each chew contains: Vitamin A 1,000 IU • Vitamin D 200 IU • Vitamin K 40 mcg • Riboflavin 0.8 mg • Calcium 600 mg • Sodium 10 mg. Other Ingredients: Corn Syrup, High Fructose Corn Syrup, Sweetened Condensed Skim Milk, Sugar, Chocolate Liqueur, High Oleic Sunflower Oil, Cocoa (Processed with Alkali), Glycerol Monostearate, Salt, Artificial Flavor, Maltodexrin, Soy Lecithin.

Calendula Oil **-** Blessed Herbs
Calendula flower & Organic Cold-Pressed Olive oil.

Calendula Salve **-** Dial Herbs
Calendula • Chamomile • Mullein. In a base of Beeswax, Glycerine & Cold Pressed Olive oil.

Calgest **-** PhytoPharmica
Two capsules contain: Vitamin C (ascorbic acid/rose hips) 100 mg • Vitamin B6 (pyridoxine HCl) 50 mg • Calcium chloride 192 mg • Calcium phosphate 180 mg • Magnesium glycerophosphate 104 mg • Betaine HCl 192 mg •Ammonium chloride 192 mg •Kidney extract (freeze-dried) 60 mg •Mixed bioflavonoids (citrus) 60 mg.
See Editor's Note No. 14, page 2055.

Calm (Stress Relief) Herbal Transdermal 1/4oz **-** Derma E
Jojoba oil • Sweet Almond oil • Tocopheryl Acetate (vitamin E) • Champaca Absolute • Jonquil.

Calm Aid Formula **-** Nature's Way
Two capsules contain: Blue Vervain stem, leaf, flower, fruit 150 mg • Chamomile flower 75 mg • Kava (dried extract 30% Kavalactones)

350 mg • L-5 Hydroxytryptophan (Griffonia bean extract) 5 mg • Niacin (Vitamin B3) 6.66 mg • Passion flower stem, leaf, flower, fruit 75 mg • Riboflavin (Vitamin B2) 568 mcg • Scullcap herb 60 mg • Thiamine (Vitamin B1) 500 mcg • Vitamin B12 (Cyanocobalamin) 2 mcg • Vitamin B6 (Pyridoxine HCL) 660 mcg • Wood Betony stem, leaf, flower 100 mg. Other Ingredients: Gelatin, Magnesium Stearate, Millet.

Calm Colon **-** Samra Health and Beauty
Each capsule contains: Proprietary Blend 500 mg: Yin Chen, Atractylodes root, Schisandra fruit, Job's Tears seed, Codonopsis, Huo Xiang, Chinese Thoroughwax root, Raxinus Chinensis bark, Polyporus, Asian Psyllium seed, Phellodendron bark, Licorice root, Ginger root, Magnolia bark, Fang Feng root, Tangerine peel, White Peony root, Costus root, Chinese Goldthread root, Fragrant Angelica root. Other Ingredients: Gelatin, Silicon Dioxide, Magnesium Stearate.

Calm Thoughts **-** Source Naturals
Three tablets contain: Kava root extract (Piper methysticum) (Standardized to 30% kavalactones yielding 105 mg of kavalactones) 350 mg • Siberian Ginseng root 200 mg • Bacopa Monniera leaf extract (Standardized to 20% bacosides yielding 20 mg of bacosides) 100 mg • Lemon Balm herb 100 mg • St. John's Wort extract (Hypericum perforatum) (50 mg Standardized to 0.3% hypericin and 50 mg 4:1 extract) 100 mg • Valerian root 60 mg • Ashwagandha root 50 mg • Ginger root 50 mg • Licorice root extract (4:1) 50 mg • Ginkgo Biloba leaf extract (50:1) (Standardized to 24% Ginkgo flavone glycosides and 6% terpene lactones) 30 mg • Schizandra fruit 30 mg • Vitamin C (as Ascorbic Acid) 100 mg • Vitamin B1 (Thiamin) 25 mg • Vitamin B2 (Riboflavin) 25 mg • Niacinamide 25 mg • Vitamin B6 (Pyridoxine HCl) 25 mg • Vitamin B12 (Cyanocobalamin) 25 mcg • Vitamin B5 (Pantothenic Acid) 50 mg • Calcium (as Calcium Citrate) 100 mg • Magnesium (275 mg Magnesium Oxide and 25 mg Magnesium Taurinate) 300 mg • Zinc (as Zinc Citrate) 15 mg • Manganese (as Manganese Citrate) 3 mg • GABA (Gamma Amino Butyric Acid) 500 mg • Taurine (as Magnesium Taurinate) 300 mg • L-Tyrosine (200 mg as L-Tyrosine and 50 mg N-Acetyl L-Tyrosine) 250 mg.

Calm Thoughts Kava **-** Source Naturals
Three tablets contain: Kava root extract (Piper methysticum) standardized to 30% Kavalactones, Yielding 105 mg to Kavalactones 350 mg • Siberian Ginseng root 200 mg • Bacopa monniera leaf extract, standardized to 20% Bacosides, Yielding 20 mg of Bacosides 100 mg • Lemon Balm herb 100 mg • St. John's wort extract (Hypericum perforatum) 50 mg standardized to 0.3 % Hypericin and 50 mg 4:1 extract 100 mg • Valerian root 60 mg • Ashwagandha root 50 mg • Ginger root 50 mg • Licorice root extract (4:1) 50 mg • Ginkgo Biloba leaf extract (50:1) standardized to 24% Ginkgo Flavone Glycosides and 6% Terpene Lactones 30 mg • Schizandra fruit 30 mg • Vitamin C (as Ascrobic Acid) 100 mg • Vitamin B1 (Thiamin) 25 mg • Vitamin B2 (Riboflavin) 25 mg • Niacinamide 25 mg • Vitamin B6 (Pyridoxine HCl) 25 mg • Vitamin B12 (Cyanocobalamin) 25 mcg • Vitamin B5 (Pantothenic Acid) 50 mg • Calcium (as Calcium Citrate) 100 mg • Magnesium (275 mg Magnesium Oxide and 25 mg Magnesium Taurinate) 300 mg • Zinc (as Zinc Citrate) 15 mg • Manganese (as Manganese Citrate) 3 mg • GABA (Gamma Amino Butyric Acid) 500 mg • Taurine (as Magnesium Taurinate) 300 mg • L-Tyrosine (200 mg as L-Tyrosine and 50 mg N-Acetyl-l-Tyrosine) 250 mg.

CAL-MAG **-** The Vitamin Shoppe
Each tablet contains: Calcium 500 mg • Magnesium 250 mg.

Cal-Mag Boron **-** Puritan's Pride
Three tablets contain: Calcium (as Calcium Carbonate, Calcium Citrate and Calcium Gluconate) 1,000 mg • Magnesium (as Magnesium Oxide, Magnesium Citrate, and Magnesium Gluconate) 400 mg • Boron (as Boron Citrate) 3 mg.

Cal-Mag Chewable **-** Quest
Each tablet contains: Elemental Calcium (Citrate, Phosphate) 300 mg • Elemental Magnesium (Citrate, Oxide) 150 mg • Vitamin D (as Vitamin D3) 100 IU. Other Ingredients: Sorbitol, Silicon Dioxide, Magnesium Stearate, Sucralose and Spearmint Flavor.

Cal-Mag Citrate **-** Puritan's Pride
Four tablets contain: Calcium (as Calcium Carbonate, Calcium Aspartate) 1,000 mg • Magnesium (as Magnesium Oxide and Magnesium Citrate) 500 mg.

Cal-Mag Fizz **-** Baywood International
Each scoop contains: Vitamin D 200 IU • Vitamin B1 (Thiamin HCL) 750 mcg • Vitamin B2 (Riboflavin) 850 mcg • Vitamin B3 (Niacinamide) 10 mg • Vitamin B6 (Pyridoxine HCL) 1 mg • Vitamin B12 (Cyanocobalamin) 3 mcg • Vitamin B5 (Pantothenic Acid) 5 mg • Calcium 500 mg • Magnesium 200 mg • Proprietary Blend 12 mg: Selenium, Potassium, Boron.

Cal-Mag Potassium **-** Puritan's Pride
Two tablets contain: Calcium (carbonate, citrate, asparate) 500 mg • Magnesium (oxide, citrate, aspartate) 500 mg • Potassium (gluconate, aspartate, citrate) 99 mg.

CAL-MAG w/Zinc and Vitamin D **-** Dial Herbs
Vitamin D • Calcium from Gluconate & Lactate • Magnesium • Zinc • Aqueous Extracts from: Hibiscus, Chamomile, Fennel, Spinach • Fructose • Mango Juice • Orange Juice • Natural Flavor • Locust Seed Flour.

Cal-Mag-Zinc **-** Puritan's Pride
Three tablets contain: Calcium (as Calcium Carbonate and Calcium Gluconate) 1,000 mg • Magnesium (as Magnesium Oxide and Magnesium Gluconate) 400 mg • Zinc (as Zinc Gluconate and Zinc Citrate) 25 mg.

Cal-Mag-Zinc **-** Schiff
Two tablets contain: Vitamin D (as cholecalciferol) 100 IU • Calcium (as calcium carbonate) 500 mg • Magnesium (as magnesium oxide) 250 mg • Zinc (as zinc citrate) 25 mg • Proprietary Blend 56 mg: Citrates, Fumarates, Succinates, Gluconates, Aspartates, Ascorbates, Amino Acid Chelates, Ketoglutarates. Other Ingredients: Cellulose, Stearic Acid, Croscarmellose Sodium, Coating (methylcellulose titanium dioxide, polyethylene glycol), Magnesium Stearate.

Cal-Mag-Zinc Liquid **-** Metabolic Response Modifiers
Each tablespoon contains: Vitamin D (as Vitamin D3 cholecalciferol) 400 IU • Calcium (tri-calcium phosphate citrate, gluconate, lactate) 600 mg • Magnesium (hydroxide, carbonate) 300 mg • Phosphate (tri-calcium phosphate) 300 mg • Zinc (citrate) 22.5 mg • Potassium (citrate) 50 mg.

CalmEz **-** Allergy Research Group
Three tablets contain: Proprietary Blend 1800 mg: Ramulus Uncariae hook extract, Ziziphus Spinosa seed extract, Albisia Julibrissin bark extract. Other Ingredients: Rice Starch.

Cal-Min **-** Progressive Labs
Each tablet contains: Calcium (as calcium proteinate) 300 mg. In a base of mixed vegetable concentrate from: Cultured Peas, Lentils, Buckwheat, Millet, and Chlorophyll, carefully dried to preserve their natural trace nutrient and enzyme content.

CalmingBlend **-** Rexall - Sundown
Each capsule contains: Ashwaganda root extract (standardized to 1.5% withanolides, 3 mg; standardized to 1% alkaloids, 2 mg) 200 mg • Valerian root extract (standardized to 0.8% valerenic acid, 0.5 mg) 67 mg • Proprietary Blend: Kava Kava root, German Chamomile flower head, Hops (strobiles) 133 mg. Other Ingredients: Gelatin.

Calms Forte **-** Hyland's
Each tablet contains: Passiflora 1X • Avena Sativa 1X • Chamomilla 2X • Calcarea Phosphorica 2X HPUS • Ferrum Phosphoricum 3X

HPUS • Kali Phosphoricum 3X HPUS • Natrum Phosphoricum 3X HPUS • Magnesia Phosphoricum 3X HPUS.

***CalmTabs* - Puritan's Pride**
Four tablets contain: Valerian root 258 mg • Passiflora flower 258 mg • Celery seed 258 mg • Catnip leaf 258 mg • Hops flower 129 mg • Dried Orange Peel 129 mg.

***Calorad* - Essentially Yours Industries Corp.**
Demineralized Water • Collagen Hydrolysat • Aloe Vera • Vegetal Glycerin • Potassium Sorbate • Citrus Extracts • Natural Peach Flavor.

***Calotren* - Formula Master Botanicals**
Each 500 mL bottle contains: Purified Water • Collagen Hydrolysate • Aloe Vera • Glycerin • Potassium Sorbate • Natural Flavoring • Methyl Paraben.

***Cal-Para* - Atrium Inc.**
Each tablet contains: Alkalinizing Calcium Lactate 325 mg • Calcium Aspartate (supplying Elemental Calcium 52) 80 mg • Magnesium Aspartate 75 mg • Magnesium Citrate (supplying Elemental Magnesium 21 mg) 70 mg.

***Calsorb* - PhysioLogics**
Three caplets contain: Calcium (as 80% calcium citrate, 19% calcium carbonate, 1% calcium stearate) 500 mg • Magnesium (as 50% magnesium citrate, 50% magnesium glycinate) 250 mg. Other Ingredients: Microcrystalline Cellulose, Stearic Acid, Croscarmellose Sodium, Hydroxypropyl Methylcellulose, Silicon Dioxide, Magnesium Silicate, Polyethylene Glycol.

***Calsure* - Rexall - Sundown**
Each tablet contains: Calcium 250 mg. Other Ingredients: Stearic Acid, Titanium Dioxide, Silica, Magnesium Stearate, Hydroxypropyl Methylcellulose, Microcrystalline Cellulose.

***Cal-Sym* - Atrium Inc.**
Each tablet contains: Acidifying Calcium Phosphate 100 mg • Calcium Ascorbate 50 mg • Calcium Aspartate (supplies Elemental Calcium 34 mg compounded to insure acidic pH) 35 mg • Ammonium Chloride 100 mg • Betaine HCL 12 mg • Glutamic Acid HCL120 mg.

***Caltrate 600 + Soy* - Wyeth**
Each two tablets contain: Soy Isoflavones 50 mg • Calcium 1200 mg • Vitamin D 400 IU.

***Caltrate Plus* - Wyeth**
Each tablet contains: Vitamin D 200 IU • Calcium 600 mg • Magnesium 40 mg • Zinc 7.5 mg • Copper 1 mg • Manganese 1.8 mg • Boron 250 mcg. Other Ingredients: Maltodextrin, Cellulose, Mineral Oil, Hydroxypropyl Methylcellulose, Titanium Dioxide, Sodium Lauryl Sulfate, Cupric Oxide, FD&C Red No. 40, FD&C Yellow No. 6, FD&C Blue No. 1, Gelatin, Crospovidone, Stearic Acid, Magnesium Stearate.

***Canadian Ginseng* - Jamieson**
Each capsule contains: Canadian Ginseng whole root (Panax quinquefolium, containing a minimum of 5% Ginsenosides) 250 mg.

***Candex* - Pure Essence Labs**
Two capsules contain: Cellulase 74,000 CU • Hemicellulase 30,000 HCU • Amylase 4000 DU • Invertase 1000 SU • Malt Diastase 200 DP • Glucoamylase 100 AGU. Other Ingredients: Cellulose, Rice Bran, Water, Soya Lecithin Oil.

***Candicidal* - Source Naturals**
Each capsule contains: Brevibacterium linens 2 billion cells • Vitamin B-6 (pyridoxine HCl) 10 mg • Methionine 200 mg.

***Candicin* - Genestra - Seroyal**
Each capsule contains: Oregano oil • Clove oil • Wormwood extract • Ginger extract • Evening Primrose oil.

***Candid Care* - Natrol**
Two capsules contain: Zinc 9 mg • FOS 500 mg • Garlic 100 mg • Undecylenic Acid (as Zinc undecylenate acid) 50 mg • Citrus extract, dried powder from grapefruit Seed 25 mg. Other Ingredients: Microcrystalline Cellulose, Silicon Dioxide, Magnesium Stearate, Gelatin.

***Candida Formula* - Enzymatic Therapy**
Each capsule contains: Oregano oil extract (Origanum vulgare) 0.1 ml • Thyme oil extract (Thymus vulgaris) 0.05 ml • Peppermint oil extract (Mentha piperta) 0.05 ml • Goldenseal root (Hydrastis canadensis) standardized to contain 5% total Alkaloids including: Berberine, Hydrastine, & Canadine 50 mg.

***Candida Forte* - Nature's Plus**
Two softgels contain: Safflower oil 1000 mg • Vitamin C (ascorbate) 500 mg • L-Cysteine free-form amino acid 100 mg • Zinc (ascorbate) 50 mg • Pau D'Arco 50 mg • Vitamin B6 (pyridoxine HCl) 50 mg • Acidophilus (lactobacillus) supplying 80 million viable cells 20 mg • Vitamin A (fish liver oil) 10,000 IU • Beta Carotene (supplying 15,000 IU Vitamin A activity) 9 mg • Garlic (equivalent to 500 mg of fresh garlic) 1 mg • Biotin 100 mcg • Free-Form Amino Acid Complex 198.08 mg: L-Glutamine 40.8 mg, L-Lysine 25 mg, L-Leucine 20.2 mg, L-Proline 16.2 mg, L-Valine 14 mg, L-Serine 12.6 mg, L-Isoleucine 11 mg, L-Phenylalanine 9.32 mg, L-Threonine 8.64 mg, L-Arginine 7.3 mg, L-Alanine 6.28 mg, L-Aspartic Acid 7 mg, L-Methionine 6.08 mg, L-Histidine 5.74 mg, L-Glycine 3.52 mg, L-Tyrosine 3 mg, L-Cysteine 1.4 mg. In a Base of Black Walnut.

***candida/yeast* - nelsons - Nelson Bach USA Ltd.**
Active Ingredients: Candida alb 30c HPUS • Kreosotum 30c HPUS • Thuja occ 30c HPUS. Inactive Ingredients: Lactose, Sucrose.
See Editor's Note No. 1, page 2053.

***Candistatin* - PhysioLogics**
Two capsules contain: Calcium (as calcium caprylate) 58 mg • Magnesium (as magnesium caprylate) 46 mg • Caprylic Acid 800 mg • Goldthread root (coptis groenlandica, standardized to contain 10% alkaloids) 100 mg • Pau D'Arco herb (tabebuia impetiginosa) 60 mg. Other Ingredients: Gelatin, Vegetable Magnesium Stearate, Silica.

***Candistroy* - Nature's Secret**
Two tablets contain: Zinc tannates • Barberry root extract • Goldenseal root • Pau d'Arco bark • Oregon Grape root • Peppermint oil • Orange peel • Licorice root • Cinnamon bark • Clove buds • Thyme leaf • Allicin.

***Cappuccino Comfort Fructose - Revival* - Physicians Laboratories**
Each packet contains: Certified Isoflavone 160 mg. Other Ingredients: Soy Protein Isolate, Fructose, Sucrose, Real Coffee Powder, Natural and Artificial Flavor, Dutch Processed Cocoa, Soy Lecithin, Calcium Phosphate, Potassium Chloride, Sodium Chloride, Xanthan Gum, Carboxymethylcellulose, Undegraded Carrageenan.

***Cappuccino Comfort Splenda - Revival* - Physicians Laboratories**
Each packet contains: Certified Isoflavone 160 mg. Ingredients: Soy Protein Isolate, Cocoa, Maltodextrin, Caclium Phosphate, Soy Lecithin, Salt, Potassium Chloride, Artificial Flavor, Carrageenan, Carboxymethylcellulose, Xanthan Gum, Sucralose.

***Cappuccino Comfort Unsweetened - Revival* - Physicians Laboratories**
Each packet contains: Certified Isoflavone 160 mg. Other Ingredients: Soy Protein Isolate, Real Coffee Powder, Natural and Artificial Flavor, Dutch Processed Cocoa, Soy Lecithin, Calcium Phosphate, Potassium Chloride, Sodium Chloride, Xanthan Gum, Carboxymethylcellulose, Undegraded Carrageenan.

Some Brand Name Natural Products - What they Contain

www.NaturalDatabase.com contains MANY more listings than appear here.

Caprylate Complex **-** Progressive Labs
Three capsules contain: Caprylic Acid (as caprylate) 1290 mg • Calcium (as caprylate) 100 mg • Magnesium (as caprylate) 50 mg • Zinc (as caprylate) 5 mg.

Caprylic Acid Complex **-** Jamieson
Each capsule contains: Caprylic Acid (from calcium and magnesium caprilate) 200 mg • Garlic (odour controlled allicin-rich) 150 mg • Thyme 100 mg • Black Walnut Hulls 50 mg • Borage Oil 50 mg.

CapsiCool Cayenne **-** Nature's Way
Two capsules contain: Proprietary Formula: Cayenne pepper fruit • Ginger • Glucomannan root. Other ingredients: Gelatin.

Caramel Corn - Revival **-** Physicians Laboratories
Eight fluid ounces contain: Certified Isoflavone 15 mg. Ingredients: Roasted Whole Soybeans, Natural and Artificial Flavors.

Cararthron **-** Chalmers Dale
Each tablet contains: Extract Blend: Trichosanthes Kirilowii root (Chinese snakegourd) 4 g • Clematis Siinensis root (wellingxian) 2 g • Prunella Vulgaris flower (self heal) 2 g.

Caratomax **-** Shaklee
Each capsule contains: Vitamin A 5000 IU • Lycopene 5 mg • Lutein 5 mg • Zeaxanthin 200 mcg • Alpha Carotene 1.5 mg • CaratoMax Proprietary Blend 70 mg: Quercitin, Grapeseed extract (Vitis vinifera) seed/skin, Broccoli Sprouts extract (Brassica oleracea italica) whole sprout. Other Ingredients: Soybean Oil, Beeswax, Palm Oil, Soy Lecithin, Gelatin, Glycerine, Water, Annatto.

Carb Cutter with Phase 2 Starch Neutralizer **-** Health and Nutrition Systems
Each tablet contains: Phase 2 Starch Neutralizer from White Kidney Bean (Phaseolus vulgaris) extract 500 mg • Proprietary Carb Free Blend 50 mg: Gymnema Sylvestre leaf, Fenugreek seed, Garcinia Cambogia fruit extract (50% hydroxycitric acid), Vanadium (as vanadyl sulfate). Other Ingredients: Dicalcium Phosphate, Microcrystalline Cellulose, Croscarmellose Sodium, Stearic Acid, Magnesium Stearate, Silica, Pharmaceutical Glaze.

Carb Defense **-** Dynamic Nutritional Products
Each vegetarian tablet contains: Chromium (as chromium polynicotinate) 100 mcg • Vanadium (as vanadyl sulfate) 100 mcg • Northern White Kidney Bean extract (phaseolus vulgaris) 750 mg. Other Ingredients: Cellulose, Calcium Phosphate, Stearic Acid, Vegetable Magnesium Stearate, Modified Cellulose Gum, Silicon Dioxide.

Carb Explosion - Orange **-** Rexall - Sundown
Each scoop contains: Vitamin A 3000 IU • Vitamin C (Ascorbic Acid) 6 mg • Vitamin D (Cholecalciferol) 40 IU • Vitamin E (dl-Alpha Tocopheryl Acetate) 3 IU • Thiamin Mononitrate (Vitamin B-1) 0.15 mg • Riboflavin (Vitamin B-2) 0.17 mg • Niacin (Niacinamide) 2 mg • Vitamin B-6 (Pyridoxine HCl) 0.2 mg • Folic Acid 40 mcg • Vitamin B-12 (Cyanocobalamin) 0.6 mcg • Biotin 30 mcg • Pantothenic Acid (Calcium D-Pantothenate) 1 mg • Electrolytic Iron 1.8 mg • Phosphorus 50 mg • Iodine 0.15 mg • Magnesium Phosphate Dibasic 40 mg • Zinc Oxide 1.5 mg • Copper Gluconate 0.2 mg • Chromium Polynicotinate 90 mcg • Sodium Chloride 100 mg • Potassium Chloride 75 mg • Carb Explosion Enzyme Blend: Glucoamylase, Malt Diastase, Amylase, Phytase, Hemicellulase, Beta-Glucanase 250 mg. Other Ingredients: Crystalline Fructose, Maltodextrin, Dextrose, Natural and Artificial Orange Flavor, Citric Acid, Malic Acid, Dicalcium Phosphate, Beta-Carotene, Potassium Iodide.

****Carb Intercept with Phase 2 Starch Neutralizer*** **-** Natrol
Two capsules contain: White Kidney Bean extract (phaseolamin vugaris) 1 g. Other Ingredients: Gelatin, Silica, Magnesium Stearate.
See Editor's Note No. 37, page 2057.

Carb Zapper **-** New Sun
Two tablets contain: Magnesium (as oxide) 50 mg • Phaseolin EX Phaseolus Vulgaris extract 750 mg • Gymnemalin Gymnema Sylvestre extract 100 mg • Alpha Lipoic Acid 25 mg • Chromium Picolinate 150 mcg • Chromium Polynicotinate 50 mcg • Vanadium (as BMOV) 100 mcg. Other Ingredients: Magnesium Stearate, Stearic Acid.
See Editor's Note No. 37, page 2057.

Carba-E-A-C **-** Atrium Inc.
Each rounded teaspoon contains approximately: Vitamin A Acetate 4000 IU • Vitamin C from Ascorbic Acid 100 mg • Vitamin E 33 IU. In a carrier of Carbamide (food grade).

Carbo Fuel (Complex Carbohydrate Peak Performance Energy Drink) **-** TwinLab
Each serving contains: Carbohydrates (from Glucose Polymers & Crystalline Pure Fructose) (no high fructose corn syrups are present) 80 grams. Other Ingredients: Vitamin B1, Vitamin B2, Vitamin B3, Vitamin B6, Pantothenic Acid, Biotin, Potassium, Magnesium, Yeast-Free GTF Chromium, Inosine, L-Carnitine, CoQ10, Lipoic Acid, Pantetheine, Pyridoxine-Alpha-Ketoglutarate, Soluble Potassium (Phosphate & Succinates), Citrates, Aspartates, Fumarates, Malates, Alpha-Ketoglutarates.

CarbohydrEnz **-** Enzymes, Inc.
Each capsule contains: n-zimes Proprietary Blend 512 mg: Amylase, Protease blend, alpha-Galactosidase, CereCalase Plus, Glucoamylase, Malt Diatase, Lipase, Pectinase, Invertase, Cellulase, Lactase, Xylanase • Proprietary Blend 190 mg: Ginger root extract, Fennel seed extract. Other Ingredients: Cellulose, Water.

Carbolin **-** Phytobase, Inc.
Two vegetable capsules contain: Magnesium (citrate) 14 mg • Chromium (polynicotinate) 42 mcg • Proprietary Blend 1180 mg: Phaseolamine complex (phaseolamine, phaseolamine 2250), Citrin HCA, American Ginseng, Cassia Nomame 10:1 extract, Green Tea 50% extract, Vanadyl Sulfate.

Carbo-Meta **-** Atrium Inc.
Each tablet contains: Pyridoxal-5-Phosphate 20 mg • Pyridoxine HCL 50 mg • Chromium Aspartate 500 mcg • Magnesium 50 mg • Manganese 5 mg • Zinc Aspartate 15 mg.

Carbonyl Iron 25 mg **-** Rexall - Sundown
Two tablets contain: Calcium 117 mg • Iron (as carbonyl iron) 50 mg. Other Ingredients: Dicalcium Phosphate, Maltodextrins, Corn Syrup Solids, Croscarmellose Sodium, Magnesium Stearate.

CarbOut 255 **-** Unknown
Each tablet contains: Phaseolus Vulgaris extract (kidney bean) 500 mg. Other Ingredients: Gelatin, Glycerin, Water, Cellulose, Magnesium Stearate, Vegetable Stearin, Silica.

Carbs Away **-** FreeLife International
Each caplet contains: Chromium (as patented Chelavite chromium dinicotinate glycinate) 200 mcg • Carbohydrate Reducing Blend 125 mg: Phaseolus Vulgaris seed (2500 units/gm), Gymnema Sylvestre leaf standardized extract (25% gymnemic acid), Banaba leaf standardized extract (lagerstoemia speciosa, 1% corosolic acid), Momordica Charantia fruit (2.5% bitter principles) • Proprietary Blend 25 mg: Purified Methylsulfonylmethane, Piper Nigrum fruit standardized extract (95% piperine) • Vanadium (from glycinate chelate) 100 mcg. Other Ingredients: Calcium Hydrogen Phosphate, Cellulose, Cellulose Gum, Fractionated Vegetable Oil, Colloidal Silica, Vita-Coat (vegetable resin, alpha-lipoic acid).

Carctol **-** IvyComm Systems
Each capsule contains: Hemidesmus Indicus 20 mg • Tribulus Terrestris 20 mg • Piper Cubeba Linn 120 mg • Ammani Vesicatoria 20 mg • Lepidium Sativum Linn 20 mg • Blepharis Edulis 200 mg • Smilax China Linn 80 mg • Rheumemodi Wall 20 mg.

Some Brand Name Natural Products - What they Contain

www.NaturalDatabase.com contains MANY more listings than appear here.

Cardio 150 - Atrium Inc.
Each tablet contains: Raw Heart concentrate (not an extract) of Bovine source 150 mg.
See Editor's Note No. 14, page 2055.

Cardio 20 - Futurebiotics
Six capsules contain: Beta-carotene 25,000 IU • Vitamin C (buffered ascorbate)1000 mg • Vitamin E (natural) 400 IU • Niacin (timed release, flush-free) 250 mg • Choline Bitartrate 150 mg • Inositol 75 mg • Calcium (ascorbate) 250 mg • Magnesium (oxide, chelate) 400 mg • Potassium (gluconate) 99 mg • Coenzyme Q10 15 mg • L-Carnitine 100 mg • Taurine 100 mg • Procyanidol 35 mg • Hawthorn berries (4:1 extract) 250 mg • Soy Isoflavone extract 100 mg • Cholestatin Beta-sitosterol complex 250 mg • Garlic (pure-gar 1500 deodorized concentrate) 400 mg • Cayenne 100 mg • Ginger 50 mg • Chlorella 250 mg.

Cardio Care - Vidafit
Each serving contains: Biotin 30 mcg • Folate 400 mcg • Niacin 16 mg • Pantothenic Acid 5 mg • Riboflavin 1.3 mg • Thiamine 1.2 mg • Vitamin A 3300 IU • Vitamin B12 2.4 mcg • Vitamin B6 1.7 mg • Vitamin C 100 mg • Vitamin D 200 IU • Vitamin E 10 IU • Calcium 500 mg • Chromium 50 mcg • Copper 2 mg • Iodine 70 mcg • Magnesium 320 mg • Phosphorus 500 mg • Potassium 700 mg • Zinc 15 mg • Coenzyme Q10 25 mg • Bilberry 50 mg • Garlic 10 mg • Ginkgo extract 100 mg • Grape Seed extract 50 mg • Soy Protein 5 grams.

Cardio Chelate - Nutri-Quest Rx
Six tablets contain: Vitamin A (Palmitate) 3000 IU • Beta Carotene 7500 IU • Vitamin D (as Vitamin D3) 100 IU • Vitamin C (Sago) 300 mg • Vitamin B1 30 mg • Vitamin B2 30 mg • Vitamin B6 75 mg • Vitamin B12 500 mcg • Biotin 200 mcg • Niacin 60 mg • D-Calcium Pantothenate (Pantothenic Acid) 150 mg • Folic Acid 300 mcg • Vitamin E (Succinate) 300 IU • Iodine (Kelp) 100 mcg • PABA 100 mg • Lecithin 120 mg • Choline Bitartrate 250 mg • Cysteine HCL 250 mg • L-Methionine 75 mg • L-Lysine 100 mg • Bromelaine 30 mg • Lemon Bioflavonoid 900 mg • Rutin 30 mg • Inositol 75 mg • Garlic 120 mg • Cayenne 30 mg • Hawthorne berries 100 mg • Pancreatin 6X 25 mg • Thymus 30 mg • Spleen 30 mg • Heart 30 mg • Adrenal (Nutritrophic) 30 mg • Whole Pituitary 30 mg • Papain 30 mg • L-Glycine 75 mg • Calcium Gluconate 37 mg • Manganese Chelate 2.5 mg • Copper Gluconate 7.8 mcg • Molybdenum Chelate 12 mcg • Chromium Chelate 102 mcg • Selenium Chelate 30 mcg • Calcium Ascorbate 100 mg • Calcium Aspartate 100 mg • Potassium Aspartate 25 mg • Magnesium Ascorbate 75 mg • Magnesium Aspartate 75 mg • Ferrous Gluconate 15 mg • Zinc Aspartate 15 mg. In a base containing: Calcium Phosphate, Magnesium Phosphate, Calcium Flouride, Ferric Phosphate, Kali Phosphate, Silica, Chiorinum, Peppermint leaves, Black Cohosh, Scullcap, Licorice root, Watercress, Siberian Ginseng, Red Beet root, Parsley.
See Editor's Note No. 14, page 2055.

Cardio Cholestamax - Biotech Corp.
Two tablets contain: Shen Min (he shou wu, 12:1 extract standardized to 10% chrysophanics and 1.9% resveratrol) 100 mg • Natural Vitamin E (dl-alpha tocopherol succinate) 400 IU • Folic Acid 800 mcg • Selenium (as organic selenomethionine) 150 mcg • Chromium (as patented dinicotinate glycinate) 200 mcg • Potassium (citrate) 50 mg • Aged Garlic (5:1 extract, equivalent to one clove of fresh garlic) 360 mg • Guggulipid Commiphora Mukul standardized extract 100 mg • Inula root (inula racemose, standardized to 2% analactones) 100 mg • Cholestatin purified Plant Phytosterols 100 mg • Tomato concentrate (a source of lycopene) 100 mg • Hawthorne berry (crutageous oxycantha, standardized to 5% vitexin-2' rhamnoside) 100 mg. Other Ingredients: Dicalcium Phosphate, Microcrystalline Cellulose, Croscarmellose Sodium, Stearic Acid, Magnesium Stearate, Pharmaceutical Glaze.

Cardio Complex - Leiner Health Products
Each softgel contains: Vitamin E (dl-Alpha Tocopherol and d-Alpha Tocopherol) 400 IU • Folate (Folic Acid) 400 mcg • Vitamin B12 (Cyanocobalamin) 6 mcg • Vitamin B6 (Pyridoxine Hydrochloride) 2 mg. Other Ingredients: Gelatin, Vegetable Oil, Glycerin, Yellow Beeswax, Unbleached Lecithin, Titanium Dioxide, Dicalcium Phosphate, Red 40.

Cardio EDTA Chelate - Olympia Nutrition
EDTA 400 mg • MSM 100 mg • NAC 50 mg • Vitamin C 100 mg.

Cardio Essentials - Royal Numico
Six capsules contain: Coenzyme Q10 100 mg • Proprietary Blend 3.5 g: L-Carnitine, L-Taurine, Hawthorn berry (standardized to 1.8% vitexin). Other Ingredients: Gelatin (capsules), Stearic Acid, Calcium Silicate, Silicon Dioxide.

Cardio Flow - Progressive Labs
Six capsules contain: Vitamin A (retinyl palmitate) 10,000 IU • Vitamin C (ascorbic acid and zinc ascorbate) 640 mg • Elemental Potassium (from Potassium Aspartate 684 mg, from Potassium Orotate 300 mg) 210 mg • Elemental Magnesium (from Magnesium Aspartate 1400 mg, from Magnesium Orotate 714 mg) 330 mg • Elemental Zinc (from Zinc Ascorbate 168 mg) 25 mg • Elemental Selenium (Selenium Ascorbate 70 mg) 70 mcg • Sodium 28 mg • EDTA (Ethylenediamine tetra-acetic acid) 800 mg • Disodium EDTA 200 mg • L-Glutathione, reduced 20 mg • Bromelain (2000 GDU) 300 mg • Papain (525 TU/mg) 30 mg • Cilantro (coriander) 500 mg • Butcher's Broom 150 mg • Cardio Flow 600 mg: a proprietary blend of the following extracts: [Inula racemosa (root), Saussurea lappa (root), Terminalia arjuna (root), Desmodium gingatic (leaves), Commiphora mukul (resin), Bacopa monniera (leaves), Convolvulous pluricaulis (leaves)]. Other Ingredients: Rice flour, Magnesium Stearate.

Cardio Formula - Pharmanex
Three capsules contain: Vitamin E (D-alpha tocopherol) 100 IU • Vitamin B6 (as pyridoxine hydrochloride) 20 mg • Folate (as folic acid) 400 mcg • Vitamin B12 (as cyanocobalamin) 60 mcg • Marine Fish Oil (providing omega-3 fatty acids) 2000 mg • EPA 360 mg • DHA 240 mg • Garlic powder (allium sativum) 325 mg • White Willow bark (salix alba) 250 mg • Rosemary leaf extract (rosarinus officinalis) 12 mg • Policosanol (beeswax extract) 10 mg.

Cardio Guardian - Clinician's Choice
Three tablets contain: Vitamin C (ascorbic acid) 180 mg • Vitamin E (dl-alpha tocopheryl acetate) 400 IU • Niacin (niacinamide) 300 mg • Niacin 100 mg • Vitamin B6 (pyridoxine hydrochloride) 23 mg • Folate (folic acid) 600 mcg • Vitamin B12 (cyanocobalmin) 150 mcg • Magnesium (glycinate) 15 mg • Zinc (gluconate) 15 mg • Selenium (aspartate) 120 mcg • RoseOx (patented, standardized process for an extract of Rosemary) 150 mg • Hawthorn 4:1 Extract 150 mg • Triphala Extract (Sstd. 40% tannin) 90 mg • White Willow Bark 60 mg • Motherwort 4:1 Extract 30 mg • L-Carnitine 30 mg • Seacol 30 mg • Linoleic Acid, Gamma Linolenic Acid (sunflower oil, borage oil) 30 mg • Proprietary blend 45 mg: Grape Powder, Cayenne Fruit, Coenzyme Q10.

Cardio Plus - Atrium Inc.
Three tablets contain: Vitamin E Acetate 300 IU • Vitamin C (with Rose Hips) 60 mg • Thiamine Mononitrate 15 mg • Vitamin B2 Riboflavin 2 mg • Niacin 100 mg • Vitamin B6 15 mg • Vitamin B12 2 mcg • Magnesium (as Citrus Juice Complex & Oxide) 100 mg • Zinc (as Gluconate) 5 mg • Potassium (as Citrus Juice Complex & Chloride) 99 mg • Chromium (amino acid complex) 10 mcg • Selenium (in yeast) 48 mcg • Choline Bitartrate 66 mg. In a base containing Lecithin 80 mg, Para Aminobenzoic Acid 30 mg, Inositol 4 mg, Cold Processed Heart Protein 90 mg.
See Editor's Note No. 14, page 2055.

Cardio ProtoChol - Fields of Nature - Inverness Medical Innovations, Inc.
Each capsule contains: Vitamin E (as D-Alpha Tocopheryl Acid Succinate) 10 IU • Niacin Powder 3 mg • Soybean Isoflavones extract (Novasoy) (Isoflavones 13 mg) 33 mg • Garlic bulb extract (Allicin 333 mcg) 33 mg • Guggulipids Extract (Guggulsterones 0.8 mg) 33

mg • Red Rice Yeast Extract (Lovastain 134 mcg) 33 mg • Lemon Bioflavonoids Complex 10 mg • Chitosan Powder 50 mg. Other Ingredients: Calcium Carbonate, Hydroxymethyl Propylcellulose, Magnesium Stearate, Silicon Dioxide.

Cardio Q10 - Health Smart Vitamins
Two capsules contain: Vitamin E (as d-alpha tocopheryl acetate) 542 IU • Calcium (as dicalcium phosphate) 3 mg • Selenium (as selenonmethionine) 50 mcg • Coenzyme Q10 60 mg.

Cardio Q10 - PhysioLogics
Each capsule contains: Vitamin E (as d-Alpha Tocopherol) 200 IU • Calcium (as Dicalcium Phosphate) 2 mg • Selenium (as Selenomethionine) 25 mcg • Coenzyme Q10 30 mg.

Cardio Results - Changes International, Inc.
Two caplets contain: Vitamin B6 (as Pyridoxine HCl) 15 mg • Folate (as Folic acid) 400 mcg • Vitamin B12 (as Cyanocobalamin) 250 mcg • Red Yeast rice (from fermentation of Monascus pupureus Went) 600 mg • Purified Soy phytosterols (45-55% Beta-Sitosterol) 50 mg. Other Ingredients: Dicalcium phosphate, Vegetable cellulose, Fractionated vegetable oil, Soy polysaccharides, Silica, and Vita-Lok vegetable resin glaze.

Cardio Stack - Maruda Nutrition
Three capsules contain: Vitamin B6 10 mg • Folate 400 mcg • Vitamin B12 50 mcg • Carnitine blend 1000 mg • Rhodiola Rosea 200 mg • Green Tea / Guarana (200 mg total active caffeine) 500 mg • Lipotropic Blend 100 mg: DL-Methionine, Choline Bitartrate, Inositol • Electrolyte Replenishing Blend 100 mg: Calcium Citrate, Magnesium Oxide, Potassium Gluconate • Krebs Cycle blend 100 mg.

Cardio Support Formula - The Vitamin Factory
Each tablet contains: Vitamin E (d-Alpha Tocopheryl-Succinate) 100 IU • Folic Acid 100 mcg • White Willow bark extract 4:1 100 mg • Hawthorne berry extract 50 mg • Coenzyme Q10 30 mg • Oat Beta Glucan powder (min 18%) 25 mg • Pycnogenol (Maritime Pine bark extract) 15 mg.

Cardio Support with Q-Gel - Zone Labs
Each softgel contains: Natural Vitamin E (D-alpha tocopheryl acetate) 22 IU • Natural Coenzyme Q-10 (ubidecarenone) 15 mg. Other Ingredients: Gelatin, Sorbitol, Glycerin, Purified Water, Polysorbate 80, Hydroxylated Lecithin, Medium Chain Triglycerides, Annatto Seed Extract.

Cardio Tonic - Puritan's Pride
Three caplets contain: Coenzyme Q10 20 mg • Vitamin E 100 IU • Vitamin C 300 mg • Folic Acid 400 mcg • Niacin (Vitamin B3) 20 mg • Vitamin B6 (pyridoxine) 50 mg • Calcium 100 mg • Magnesium 100 mg • Potassium 99 mg • Selenium Proteinate 150 mcg • L-Carnitine 50 mg • L-Taurine 300 mg • Garlic 100 mg • Hawthorn berry 5:1 50 mg • Lecithin 50 mg • Ginger 25 mg.

Cardioace - Vitabiotics
Two capsules contain: Omega-3 Fish oil 800 mg • Vitamin D 5 mcg • Vitamin E 80 mg • Vitamin C 60 mg • Vitamin B1 (thiamin) 10 mg • Vitamin B2 (riboflavin) 1.6 mg • Vitamin B6 (pyridoxine HCl) 10 mg • Folic Acid 500 mcg • Vitamin B12 (cyanocobalamin) 20 mcg • Zinc 10 mg • Manganese 3 mg • Copper 2 mg • Chromium 100 mcg • Selenium 160 mcg • Natural Mixed Carotenoids 4 mg • Garlic 200 mg • Lecithin 40 mg.

CardioAntioxidant - Advocare International
Four capsules contain: Vitamin A (as beta-carotene from D. salina mixed carotenoids) 10,000 IU • Vitamin C (as magnesium ascorbate) 600 mg • Vitamin E (as d-alpha-tocopheryl succinate) 400 IU • Thiamine 1.5 mg • Niacin (as inositol hexanicotinate) 60 mg • Vitamin B6 (as pyridoxine HCl) 20 mg • Folic Acid 1000 mg • Vitamin B12 (as cyanocobalamin) 60 mcg • Zinc (as monomethionine OptiZinc) 5 mg • Selenium (as selenomethionine) 35 mcg • Manganese (as gluconate) 0.5 mg • Taurine 600 mg • Coenzyme Q-10 100 mg • Golden Root extract (root - rhodiola rosea) 50 mg • Green Tea extract (leaf - camellia sinensis Sinensa) 50 mg • Lipoic Acid 50 mg • L-Carnitine 50 mg • Ascorbyl Palmitate 15 mg. Other Ingredients: Silicon Dioxide, Magnesium Stearate, Gelatin.

CardioBALANCE - Mannatech
Each capsule contains: Vitamin C (as ascorbic acid, acerola [fruit], camu-camu [fruit]) 60 mg • Vitamin E (as d-alpha tocopheryl acetate, mixed d-alpha-, d-beta-, d-delta-, and d-gamma-tocopherols and mixed tocotrienols) 15 IU • Folate (as folic acid) 200 mcg • Vitamin B6 (as pyridoxine hydrochloride and pyridoxal 5-phosphate) 2 mg • Vitamin B12 (as cyanocobalamin) 16.7 mcg • Magnesium (as magnesium oxide, magnesium citrate and magnesium glycinate) 34 mg • L-Arginine 333.3 mg • Proprietary Herbal Blend 88 mg: Garlic extract (root), Grape extract (seed & skin), Hawthorn extract (crataegus pinnatifida fruit), Carambola (fruit) • Taurine 100 mg • Trimethylglycine 83.3 mg • Alpha-Lipoic Acid 20 mg • N-Acetyl-L-Cysteine 16.7 mg • Ambrocosanol Complex 8.3 mg: Ambrotose Complex (patent pending) [arabinogalactan (larix decidua gum), Aloe Vera gel extract (inner leaf gel), Manapol powder, Gum Ghatti, Gum Tragacanth], Octacosanol, Triacontanol, Hexacosanol, Tetracosanol, Heptacosanol • Coenzyme Q10 1.67 mg. Other Ingredients: Gelatin, Magnesium Stearate.

Cardio-Basics - Rexall - Sundown
Each two tablets contain: Vitamin A (100% as beta-carotene) 2500 IU • Vitamin C (as ascorbyl palmitate and ascorbic acid) 300 mg • Vitamin D (as cholecalciferol) 200 IU • Vitamin E (as d-alpha-tocopheryl acid succinate) 200 IU • Thiamin (as thiamin mononitrate) 10 mg • Riboflavin (Vitamin B-2) 10 mg • Niacin (as niacinamide and niacin) 65 mg • Vitamin B-6 (as pyridoxine HCl) 15 mg • Folic Acid 130 mcg • Vitamin B-12 (as cyanocobalamin) 30 mcg • Biotin 100 mcg • Pantothenic Acid (as calcium d-pantothenate) 60 mg • Calcium 50 mg • Phosphorus 20 mg • Magnesium (as magnesium oxide) 60 mg • Zinc (as zinc oxide) 10 mg • Selenium (as sodium selenate) 30 mcg • Copper (as cupric oxide) 0.5 mg • Manganese (as manganese sulfate) 2 mg • Chromium (as chromium amino acid chelate) 15 mcg • Molybdenum (as molybdenum yeast chelate) 6 mcg • Sodium 5 mg • Potassium (as potassium chloride) 30 mg • L-Proline 150 mg • L-Lysine HCl 150 mg • L-Arginine HCl 50 mg • L-Carnitine Tartrate 50 mg • L-Cysteine HCl 50 mg • Inositol 50 mg • Coenzyme Q-10 10 mg • Pycnogenol Pine Bark extract 10 mg. Inactive Ingredients: Cellulose, Tricalcium Phosphate, Croscarmellose Sodium, Stearic Acid, Povidone, Dicalcium Phosphate, Silica, Pharmaceutical Glaze, Magnesium Stearate, Hydroxypropyl Methylcellulose, Hydroxypropyl Cellulose, PEG.

Cardio-Chelate - Metabolic Response Modifiers
Each capsule contains: EDTA (Ethylenediamine-Tetra-Acetic acid) 400 mg • MSM (Methyl-Sulfonyl-Methane) 100 mg • NAC (N-Acetyl-Cysteine) 50 mg • Vitamin C (ascorbic acid) 100 mg.

Cardiogarl - Olympian Labs
Three capsules contain: Ginkgo Biloba leaf extract 120 mg • Garlic extract 600 mg • Bilberry extract 150 mg • Coenzyme Q10 60 mg • Hawthorn Berry extract 210 mg.

Cardio-Glycan - PhytoPharmica
Each capsule contains: Glycosaminoglycans (GAGs) 50 mg.
See Editor's Note No. 14, page 2055.

CardioLogics with Policosanol - PhysioLogics
Two softgels contain: Vitamin E (as d-alpha tocopherol) 200 IU • Vitamin B6 (as pyridoxine hydrochloride) 20 mg • Folic Acid 400 mcg • Vitamin B12 (as cyanocobalamin) 50 mcg • Fish Oil 1000 mg containing: EPA (eicosapentaenoic acid) 180 mg, DHA (docosahexaenoic acid) 120 mg • Policosanol (oryza sp., from rice wax) 10 mg • Co-Enzyme Q-10 30 mg. Other Ingredients: Gelatin, Glycerin, Yellow Beeswax, Lecithin, Caramel Color, Mannitol.

CardioMate - FreeLife International
Each softgel conains: Natural Vitamin E (from mixed tocopherols) 60 IU • Coenzyme Q10 60 mg • Hawthorne flower and leaf standardized

extract (1.8-2.2% vitexin) 200 mg • Aged Garlic (from standardized 70:1 exract) 200 mg • Capsicum standardized extract (2500 SHU) 5 mg • Parsley seed oil (2000:1 concentrate) 7 mg. Other Ingredients: Rice Bran Oil, Gelatin, Glycerin, Water, Yellow Beeswax, Annatto, Carob, Other Natrual Coloring Agents.

Cardio-Natto **-** Gero Vita International
Each capsule contains: Nattokinase (fermented soybean extract) 150 mg. Other Ingredients: Gelatin, Silicon Dioxide, Magnesium Stearate.

CardiOptima **-** Advocare International
Each pouch contains: Vitamin C (as potassium/calcium ascorbates) 1000 mg • Vitamin E (as d-alpha tocopheryl acetate) 150 IU • Niacin (as inositol hexanicotinate) 70 mg • Vitamin B6 (as pyridoxine HCl) 20 mg • Folic Acid 400 mcg • Vitamin B12 (as cyanocobalamin) 60 mcg • Calcium (as ascorbate and citrate) 100 mg • Magnesium (as citrate) 60 mg • Sodium 10 mg • Potassium (as ascorbate) 170 mg • L-Lysine (as HCl) 800 mg • L-Proline 200 mg • Taurine 500 mg • L-Carnitine 100 mg • Coenzyme Q-10 5 mg • Turmeric extract 50 mg • Grape extract (seed/skin, vitis vinifera, Activin brand) 100 mg • Proprietary Blend 375 mg: Hawthorn leaf and flower extract, Hibiscus flower extract, Hawthorn Berry extract, Gotu Kola extract, Golden Root extract. Other Ingredients: Fructose, Maltodextrin, Citric Acid, Gum Arabic, Natural Flavors, Artificial Flavors, Beet Root Powder, Sucralose, Silicon Dioxide.

CardioSupport **-** Aidan Products, LLC
Each tablet contains: Vitamin A (25% palmitate/75% carotenoids) 4000 IU • Vitamin C (ascorbic acid) 250 mg • Vitamin D (D3) 50 IU • Vitamin E (d-alpha tocopheryl succinate) 65 IU • Thiamine (mononitrate, vitamin B1) 20 mg • Riboflavin (vitamin B2) 20 mg • Niacin (vitamin B3) 35 mg • Pyridoxine (hydrochloride, vitamin B6) 20 mg • Folic Acid 40 mcg • Cyanocobalamin (vitmain B12) 20 mcg • D-Biotin 30 mcg • Pantothenic Acid (CA salt) 20 mg • Calcium (carbonate) 50 mg • Iodine (kelp) 15 mcg • Magnesium (oxide, granular) 40 mg • Zinc (monomethionine) 3 mg • Selenium (amino acid chelate) 25 mcg • Copper (gluconate) 20 mcg • Manganese (gluconate) 0.5 mg • Chromium (picolinate, Nutrition 21) 30 mcg • Potassium (amino acid chelate, 20%) 10 mg • Choline (bitartrate) 72 mg • Inositol 4 mg • L-Carnitine 20 mg • DL-Methionine 20 mg • Citric Acid 15 mg • Para Aminobenzoic Acid 20 mg • Bioflavonoids (lemon) 150 mg • Bromelain (1200 MCU/GM) 10 mg • Coenzyme Q-10 (ubiquinone) 5 mg • EDTA (disodium salt) 15 mg. Other Ingredients: Silicon Dioxide, Hydrogenated Vegetable Oil, Magnesium Stearate (vegetable source).

Cardiotrate **-** Progressive Labs
Each capsule contains: Raw Bovine heart concentrate 140 mg prepared by a special process which does not exceed physiological temperature (37° C). Guaranteed to be free of chemical pesticides and synthetic hormones.
See Editor's Note No. 14, page 2055.

Cardiovascular Health - Wellzymes **-** Enzymes, Inc.
Two capsules contain: Vitamin E (from d-Alpha Tocopheryl Acid Succinate) 50 IU • Coenzyme Q10 (Ubiquinone) 25 mg • n-zimes Proprietary Enzyme Blend 72 mg: pHysioProtease (177,600 pHysio-U), CereCalase Plus • Proprietary Herbal Blend 300 mg: Hawthorne leaf and flower extract (standardized to contain 1.8% vitexin), Garlic bulb concentrate, Grape seed extract (standardized to contain 95% proanthocyanidins), Rice Bran. Other Ingredients: Plant Cellulose, Water.

Cardio-Vite **-** Atrium Inc.
Each tablet contains: Vitamin B1 2.2 mg • Vitamin B2 2.2 mg • Vitamin B6 50 mg • Pantothenic Acid 50 mg • Niacinamide 15 mg • Magnesium 50 mg • Potassium 50 mg.

CardioZyme **-** VP Nutrition
Each capsule contains: Nattokinase NSK-SD 700 FU • Amylase 2525 DU • Protease 11,000 HUT • Minerals 40 mg • Glucoamylase 30 AGU • Lipase 450 FCCFIP • Cellulase 700 SU.

Cardiphenol Plus **-** Gero Vita International
Each capsule contains: Morinda Citrifolia fruit extract (4:1) 100 mg • Red Wine extract (30% polyphenols) 100 mg • Prune extract (60% polyphenols) • Blueberry extract (16% chlorogenic acid) 50 mg • Pomegranate extract (40% ellagic acid, 60% polyphenols) 50 mg • Apple extract (60% polyphenols, 5% chlorogenic acid) 50 mg • Proprietary Enzyme Blend 30 mg: Amylase, Cellulase, Hemicellulase, Protease, Xylanase, Beta-Glucanase. Other Ingredients: Gelatin, Silicon Dioxide, Magnesium Stearate, Rice Flour Powder.

Careseng **-** Blossom Portfolio Sdn Bhd
Active Ingredient: Wild American Ginseng 50 mL. Inactive Ingredient: Normal Saline 250 mL.

Careseng #1 Solution of Ginseng Extract (Ginsenoside Rh2 and Aglycon Sapogenins) **-** EcoNugenics
Each bottle contains: Ginsenosides, Sapogenins 600 mg.

Caribbean Tanning Secret **-** Futurebiotics
Each tablet contains: Vitamin C 13 mg • Vitamin B 625 mg • Copper Gluconate 0.7 mg • Para Amino Benzoic Acid (PABA) 13 mg. In a base containing: L-tyrosine, Aloe Vera, Carrot powder, & Yucca powder.

Carmidas **-** Hadas Natural Products
Each 5 mL serving contains: Natural Citrus flavored Sucrose syrup • Fennel 200 mg • Chamomile 200 mg • Caraway 200 mg.

Carni Fuel **-** TwinLab
Each capsule contains: Carni Fuel L-Carnitine Magnesium Citrate 500 mg • L-Carnitine 200 mg • Magnesium 30 mg.

Carni Fuel (L-Carnitine Liquid Concentrate) **-** TwinLab
Each tablespoonful (15 ml) contains: L-Carnitine 1000 mg.

Carni Lean **-** The Sports Nutrition Source, Inc.
Each capsule contains: L-Carnitine 1000 mg.

Carnitine 500 mg **-** Vital Nutrients
Each capsule contains: Carnitine (l-form, from carnitine tartrate 752 mg) 500 mg.

Carotenoid Complex **-** The Vitamin Shoppe
Each softgel contains: Phytofluene 0.033 mg • Lycopene (LYC-O-MATO) 5 mg • Lutein 5 mg • Beta-carotene (6251 IU Vitamin A) 3.75 mg • Alpha-carotene (1042 IU Vitamin A) 1.25 mg • Zeaxanthin 0.26 mg • Phytoene 0.098 mg. In a base of tomato and carrot concentrate.

Carpal-X **-** Olympian Labs
Two capsules contain: Vitamin C 120 mg • Vitamin B-6 (pyridoxine HCl) 100 mg • Vitamin B-2 (riboflavin) 10 mg • Zinc 5 mg • Copper 500 mcg • Proprietary Blend: Grape Seed extract, CoQ10, White Willow Bark extract, Horse Chestnut extract, Cayenne Pepper, Enzyme blend (protease, lipase, amylase), Sea Cucumber, Yucca, Devil's Claw, Boswellia Serrata extract, Curcumin extract 795 mg.

Carrot Essence **-** Green Foods Corp.
Each 6.8 oz jar contains: Proprietary Blend 192 g: Powdered Carrot juice, Maltodextrin, Acerola.

Cartilade **-** BioTherapies, Inc.
Shark Cartilage.

Cartilage Care **-** PhysioLogics
Each capsule contains: Vitamin C (as ascorbic acid) 60 mg • Manganese (as manganese glycinate) 2 mg • Sodium (from chondroitin sulfate) 10 mg • Glucosamine Sulfate KCl 200 mg • Chondroitin Sulfate 100 mg • Glucosamine Hydrochloride 100 mg • Sea Cucumber 100 mg. Other Ingredients: Rice Powder, Gelatin, Vegetable Magnesium Stearate, Silica.
See Editor's Note No. 15, page 2055.

***Cartilage Companion* - PhysioLogics**
Each capsule contains: Glucosamine Sulfate 200 mg • Chondroitin Sulfate 67 mg • Methylsulfonylmethane (MSM) 333 mg.
See Editor's Note No. 15, page 2055.

***Cartilage Companion HP* - PhysioLogics**
Three tablets contain: Glucosamine Sulfate 2KCl 1500 mg • Chondroitin Sulfate 1200 mg • Methylsulfonylmethane (msm) 500 mg. Other Ingredients: Cellulose (plant origin), Cellulose Coating, Vegetable Magnesium Stearate, Silica, Titanium Dioxide Color.
See Editor's Note No. 15, page 2055.

***Cartilage Companion With MSM* - PhysioLogics**
Each capsule contains: Methylsulfonylmethane (msm) 333 mg • Glucosamine Sulfate (2KCl) 200 mg • Chondroitin Sulfate 67 mg. Other Ingredients: Rice Powder, Gelatin, Silica, Vegetable Magnesium Stearate.
See Editor's Note No. 15, page 2055.

***Cartilage Formula* - Pharmanex**
Two capsules contain: Vitamin C (Ascorbic Acid) 100 mg • Vitamin E (d-Alpha Tocopheryl Succinate, Beta, Delta, Gamma Tocopherols) 50 IU • Zinc (Zinc Propionate) 7.5 mg • Boron (Boron Citrate) 3 mg • Glucosamine (Glucosamine Sulfate, Glucosamine Hydrochloride) 750 mg • Boswellia Serrata extract (Min. 95% Boswellic Acids) 150 mg • Tumeric extract (Min. 95% Curcumin) 100 mg • Quercetin 25 mg • Rutin 25 mg. Other Ingredients: Silicon Dioxide, Magnesium Stearate.

***Cascara Sagrada* - Nature's Way**
Two capsules contain: Cascara Sagrada bark 850 mg. Other Ingredients: Plant-derived Cellulose.

***Castor Oil* - Home Health Products, Inc.**
Castor Oil.

***Cata-Comp* - Enzymatic Therapy**
Two capsules contain: Vitamin A (Beta Carotene) non-toxic form of Vitamin A 10000 IU • Vitamin E (D-Alpha Tocopherol Succinate) 75 IU • Vitamin C (Ascorbic Acid) 500 mg • Zinc (Picolinate) 10 mg • Manganese (Picolinate) 2 mg • Riboflavin (Vitamin B2) 2 mg • Selenium selenomethionine 75 mcg • Other Ingredients: Hachimijiogan Herbal Complex 200 mg • Curcuma root extract (curcuma longa, standardized to contain 97% Curcumin) 100 mg • L-Cysteine 50 mg • L-Glutamine 50 mg • L-Glycine 50 mg.

***Catalyn* - Standard Process, Inc.**
Three tablets contain: Proprietary Blend 832 mg: Defatted Wheat (germ), Carrot (root), Calcium Lactate, Nutritional Yeast, Bovine Adrenal, Bovine Liver, Bovine Spleen, Bovine Kidney, Dried Pea (vine) juice, Dried Alfalfa juice, Ganoderma Lucidum (mushroom), Lentinula Edodes (mushroom) Oat Flour, Soy Bean Lecithin, Rice Bran extract • Honey • Magnesium Citrate • Glycerine • Arabic Gum • Ascorbic Acid 4 mg • Pyridoxine Hydrochloride 1 mg • Vitamin A Palmitate 1200 IU • Gelatin • Cocarboxylase • Riboflavin 0.2 mg • Cholecalciferol 312 IU.
See Editor's Note No. 14.

***Catalyn (Chewable)* - Standard Process, Inc.**
Three tablets contain: Proprietary Blend 468 mg: Cherry powder, defatted Wheat (germ), Carrot (root), Calcium Lactate, nutritional Yeast, Bovine Adrenal, Bovine Liver, Magnesium Citrate, Bovine Spleen, Bovine Kidney, Ganoderma Lucidum, Lentinula Edodes, dried Alfalfa juice, Soy Bean Lecithin, Rice Bran extract. Other Ingredients: Dried Cane Juice, Maltodextrine, Honey, Calcium Stearate, Natural Cherry Flavor, Glycerine, Arabic Gum, Ascorbic Acid, Pyridoxine Hydrochloride, Vitamin A Palmitate, Gelatin, Cocarboxylase, Riboflavin, Cholecalciferol.
See Editor's Note No. 14.

***Catalyst* - Advocare International**
Three capsules contain: L-Glutamine 1200 mg • L-Leucine 450 mg • L-Isoleucine 225 mg • L-Valine 225 mg. Other Ingredients: Silicon Dioxide, Magnesium Stearate, Gelatin.

***Cataplex A* - Standard Process, Inc.**
Each two tablets contain: Proprietary Blend 584 mg: Carrot root, Calcium Lactate, Defatted Wheat germ, Bovine Kidney, Oat flour, nutritional Yeast, Rice Bran extract, Magnesium Citrate, Alfalfa flour, Mixed Tocopherols, Ascorbic Acid, Carrot oil, Soy Bean Lecithin. Inactive Ingredients: Honey, Arabic Gum, Calcium Stearate, Vitamin A Palmitate, Gelatin.

***Cataplex E* - Standard Process, Inc.**
Each two tablets contain: Proprietary Blend 523 mg: Bovine Orchic extract, Inositol, Dried Pea (vine) juice, Ribonucleic Acid, Oat Flour, Bovine Adrenal, Beet (root), Bovine Spleen, Ovine Spleen, Beet (root) juice, Bovine Liver, Manganese Lactate, Ascorbic Acid • Honey • Selenium Yeast 11 mcg • Potassium Para-Aminobenzoate • Mixed Tocopherols 5 IU • Arabic Gum.

***Catnip* - Nature's Way**
Two capsules contain: Catnip (stem, leaf, flower) 760 mg. Other Ingredients: Gelatin.

***Catnip and Fennel* - Dial Herbs**
Catnip • Peppermint • Fennel • Lobelia.

***Catnip and Peppermint* - Dial Herbs**
Catnip • Peppermint • Lobelia.

***Cat's Claw* - Nature's Way**
Three capsules contain: Cat's Claw bark 1.45 g. Other Ingredients: Gelatin, Magnesium stearate, Millet.

***Cat's Claw* - Olympian Labs**
Each capsule contains: Cat's Claw (uncaria tomentosa) 500 mg.

***Cat's Claw 5000* - Now**
Each capsule contains: Cat's Claw (Uncaria tomentosa) (Inner bark) 15:1 standardized extract equivalent 333 mg. Other Ingredients: Stearic Acid.

***Cat's Claw Caplet* - Leiner Health Products**
Each caplet contains: Cat's Claw extract (Uncaria tomentosa) 250 mg. Other Ingredients: Calcium Carbonate, Cellulose, Maltodextrin, Hydroxypropyl Methylcellulose, Silicon Dioxide, Polyethylene Glycol 3350, Croscarmellose Sodium, Hyroxypropyl Cellulose, Pharmaceutical Glaze, Crospovidone, Magnesium Stearate, Yellow 5 Lake, Blue 1 Lake, Polysorbate 80, Titanium Dioxide.

***Cat's Claw Defense Complex* - Source Naturals**
Four tablets contain: Cat's Claw inner bark (Uncaria Tomentosa) 2000 mg • Whole-Leaf Aloe Vera powder (200:1 Concentrate) 200 mg • Proanthodyn (from Grape Seed extract) 60 mg • Quercetin 400 mg • Green Tea extract 40 mg • Turmeric root extract (Yielding 95% Curcumin) 400 mg • Silymarin (Milk Thistle seed extract) 50 mg • Reishi Mycelia biomass 200 mg • Shiitake Mycelia biomass 200 mg • Maitake Mycelia biomass 150 mg • Astragalus root 200 mg • St. John's Wort herb extract 100 mg • St. John's Wort herb powder 100 mg • Siberian Ginseng root 100 mg • Siberian Ginseng root extract 100 mg • Schizandra berries 200 mg • Pau d'Arco bark 100 mg • Pau d'Arco bark extract 100 mg • Isatis leaf 150 mg • Vitamin A (Beta Carotene) 10000 IU • Vitamin C (Ascorbic Acid, Magnesium and Zinc Ascorbates) 350 mg • Magnesium (Ascorbate) 10 mg • Zinc (Ascorbate) 12 mg • N-Acetyl Cysteine 600 mg.

***Cayenne* - Leiner Health Products**
Each softgel contains: Oleoresin Capsicum extract (Oleoresin capsicum) fruit 25 mg. Other Ingredients: Soybean Oil, Gelatin, Glycerin, Beeswax, Lecithin, Caramel, Titanium Dioxide, Red 40, Yellow 6, Blue 1.

Some Brand Name Natural Products - What they Contain

www.NaturalDatabase.com contains MANY more listings than appear here.

Cayenne **-** Nature's Way
Each capsule contains: Cayenne pepper fruit 450 mg. Other Ingredients: Gelatin.

Cayenne **-** Now
Each capsule contains: Cayenne Pepper (Capsium Frutescens) 500 mg.

Cayenne **-** Pharmanex
Each capsule contains: Cayenne (Capisicum Annum)(Pepper)(40000 Heat Units) 450 mg. Other Ingredients: Gelatin, Magnesium Stearate, Silicon Dioxide.

Cayenne Extra Hot **-** Nature's Way
Each capsule contains: Proprietary Formula: Cayenne pepper fruit • Ginger • Hawthorne berry. Other Ingredients: Gelatin.

Cayenne Garlic **-** Nature's Way
Two capsules contain: Proprietary Blend 1.06 g: Cayenne pepper fruit, Garlic bulb. Other Ingredients: Gelatin.

Cayenne Goldenseal (formerly B/P) **-** Nature's Way
Two capsules contain: Proprietary Blend 1000 mg: Cayenne pepper fruit, Eleuthero root, Garlic bulb, Ginger, Goldenseal stem/leaf/ flower, Parsley herb. Other Ingredients: Gelatin.

Cayenne Hawthorn with Vitamin E **-** Nature's Way
Two capsules contain: Proprietary Blend 1040 mg: Cayenne pepper fruit, Hawthorn berry, Lecithin, Vitamin E (d-alpha tocopheryl). Other Ingredients: Gelatin.

Cayenne Herbal Pain Relieving Ointment **-** Nature's Way
Primary Ingredients: Capsaicin • Menthol. Other Ingredients: Beeswax, Eucalyptus, Olive oil, Vitamin E (d-alpha tocopheryl).

Cayenne, Super **-** Swanson
Two capsules contain: Cayenne pepper (100,000 heating units) 450 mg • Ginger root powder 200 mg • Hawthorn berry powder 200 mg • Lecithin granules 50 mg.

C-Blast Lemon Lime **-** GNC
Each packet contains: Vitamin C (ascorbic acid) 1000 mg • Thiamin HCl 0.38 mg • Riboflavin 0.43 mg • Niacin (niacinamide) 5 mg • Vitamin B6 (pyridoxine HCl) 10 mg • Folate, Folic Acid, Folacin 12.5 mcg • Vitamin B12 (cyanocobalamin) 25 mcg • Pantothenic Acid 2.5 mg • Calcium (ascorbate) 50 mg • Magnesium (ascorbate) 60 mg • Zinc (ascorbate) 2 mg • Manganese (ascorbate) 1 mg • Chromium (ascorbate) 10 mcg. Other Ingredients: Fructose, Natural Lemon Lime Flavors, Potassium Bicarbonate, Citric Acid, Tartaric Acid, Malic Acid, Sodium Bicarbonate, Aspartic Acid, Quercetin, Calcium Pantothenate.

C-Blast Tangerine **-** GNC
Each packet contains: Vitamin C (ascorbic acid) 1000 mg • Thiamin HCl 0.38 mg • Riboflavin 0.43 mg • Niacin (niacinamide) 5 mg • Vitamin B6 (pyridoxine HCl) 10 mg • Folate, Folic Acid, Folacin 12.5 mcg • Vitamin B12 (cyanocobalamin) 25 mcg • Pantothenic Acid 2.5 mg • Calcium (ascorbate) 50 mg • Magnesium (ascorbate) 60 mg • Zinc (ascorbate) 2 mg • Manganese (ascorbate) 1 mg • Chromium (ascorbate) 10 mcg. Other Ingredients: Fructose, Natural Tangerine Flavors, Potassium Bicarbonate, Citric Acid, Tartaric Acid, Malic Acid, Sodium Bicarbonate, Aspartic Acid, Quercetin, Calcium Pantothenate.

CBlock **-** Absolute Nutrition
Two tablets contain: Chromium (as chormium dinicotinate glycinate) 200 mcg • Vanadium (as BMOV) 100 mg • Trim Plex Phaseolus Vulgaris (as white kidney bean extract) 700 mg. Other Ingredients: Dicalcium Phosphate, Cellulose, Cellulose Gum, Vegetable Stearic Acid, Silica, Vegetable Magnesium Stearate, Vegetable Resin Glaze.

C-B-R **-** Source Naturals
Each tablet contains: Vitamin C (as ascorbic acid) 500 mg • Citrus Bioflavonoid Complex 500 mg • Rutin 52 mg • Hesperidin Complex 50 mg • Acerola Cherry fruit 1 mg.

CCM Calcium **-** Source Naturals
Each tablet contains: Calcium (from Calcium Citrate and Calcium Malate) 300 mg.

C-Complex 1000 **-** Puritan's Pride
Each tablet contains: Vitamin C (as Ascorbic Acid and Rose Hips) 1000 mg • Citrus Bioflavonoids 100 mg • Rutin 50 mg • Hesperidin complex 25 mg • Acerola powder 1 mg • Alfalfa leaf powder 1 mg • Barley grass powder 1 mg.

C-Complex 500 **-** Puritan's Pride
Each tablet contains: Vitamin C (with Rose Hips and other natural sources) 500 mg • Citrus Bioflavonoids 100 mg • Rutin (Buckwheat) 50 mg • Hesperidin complex 25 mg • Acerola 1.0 mg • Alfalfa leaf 1 mg • Barley Grass 1 mg. Other Ingredients: Vegetable Stearic Acid, Cellulose Coating, Silica, Vegetable Magnesium Stearate.

C-Complex/ Bioflavonoids/ Rutin **-** Nature's Life
Each tablet contains: Vitamin C 500 mg • Lemon Bioflavonoids Complex (natural whole unaltered TESTLAB concentrate containing Hesperidin, Eriocitrin, Flavonols, & Flavones derived from freshly dejuiced Lemons) 500 mg • Acerola (Malpighia glabra) 50 mg • Hesperidin 50 mg • Rutin (Saphora japonica) 50 mg • Calcium (naturally buffering Calcium Carbonate) 12 mg. In a natural base of Bell Peppers & Rose Hips powder.

CDC Chondro Forte **-** Genestra - Seroyal
Each tablet contains: Vitamin C (ascorbic acid) 150 mg • Chondroitin Sulfate (collagen, 8:1) 100 mg • Glucosamine Sulfate 100 mg • Manganese Citrate 65 mg • Marine Mucopolysaccharides 50 mg • Papain 25 mg • Wild Yam (10:1, equivalent to 250 mg) 25 mg • L-Proline 25 mg • L-Glutamic Acid 20 mg • L-Cysteine 15 mg • Zinc (aspartate acid chelate) 10 mg • Non-citrus Bioflavonoids 15 mg • Hesperidin 15 mg.
See Editor's Note No. 15, page 2055.

CDP Choline **-** Jarrow Formulas
Each capsule contains: CDP Choline (from stabilized cytidine 5'diphosphocholine) 250 mg. Other Ingredients: Rice Powder, Silicon Dioxide, Magnesium Stearate.

CDP Choline Caps 250 MG **-** Life Extension
Each capsule contains: CDP-Choline (cytidine-5-diphosphocholine, elemental choline 51.25 per capsule) 250 mg. Other Ingredients: Rice Flour, Magnesium Stearate, Silica, Gelatin, Water.

CDP-Choline **-** Life Enhancement Products, Inc.
Each capsule contains: Citicoline 250 mg. Other Ingredients: Silicon Dioxide, Gelatin Capsule.

CDP-Choline Caps **-** Prolongevity
Each capsule contains: Cytidine 5-diphosphocholine 250 mg. Other Ingredients: Rice Flour, Magnesium Stearate, Silica, Gelatin, Water.

CDT CoQ10 **-** Olympian Labs
Each capsule contains: Crystalline Coenzyme Q10 60 mg.

Celasine **-** Aidan Products, LLC
Water • Aloe Barbadensis leaf juice • Cyclomethicone • Propylene Glycol • Arachidyl Propionate • Stearyl Alcohol • Glyceryl Stearate • Peg-100 Stearate • Glycine Soja (soybean) oil • Glycerin • Cetyl Alcohol • Cetearyl Alcohol • Ceteareth-20 • Tetrahexadecyl Ascorbate • L-Carnosine • Sodium Hyaluronate • Tocopheryl Acetate • Carbomer • Acrylates/C10-30 Alkyl Acrylate Crosspolymer • Triethanolamine • Dimethicone Copolyol • Tetrasodium EDTA • Methylparaben • Propylparaben • Imidazolidinyl Urea • DMDM Hydantoin.

Celebrity Diet Quickstart Peach Mango Juice - Celebrity Products Direct, Inc.
Purified Water • Juice Concentrates: Pear, Grape, Mango, Peach, Kiwi, Plum • Natural Flavoring • Potassium Citrate • Ascorbic Acid (vitamin C), D-Alpha-Tocopheryl Acetate (vitamin E) • Niacinamide (vitamin B3) • Calcium Pantothenate (vitamin B5) • Vitamin A Palmitate • Pyridoxine Hydrochloride (vitamin B6) • Riboflavin -5' Phosphate (vitamin B2) • Thiamine Mononitrate (vitamin B1) • Bilberry extract • Green Tea extract • Ginkgo Biloba extract • Grape Seed extract • Biotin • Cyanocobalamin (vitamin B12).

Celebrity Diet Quickstart Wild Berry Juice - Celebrity Products Direct, Inc.
Purified Water • Juice Concentrates: Pear, Cherry, Strawberry, Raspberry, Blueberry, Kiwi, Cranberry, Blackberry • Natural Flavoring • Potassium Citrate • Ascorbic Acid (vitamin C), D-Alpha-Tocopheryl Acetate (vitamin E) • Niacinamide (vitamin B3) • Calcium Pantothenate (vitamin B5) • Vitamin A Palmitate • Pyridoxine Hydrochloride (vitamin B6) • Riboflavin -5' Phosphate (vitamin B2) • Thiamine Mononitrate (vitamin B1) • Bilberry extract • Green Tea extract • Ginkgo Biloba extract • Grape Seed extract • Biotin • Cyanocobalamin (vitamin B12).

Celestial Seasonings - Saw Palmetto - Celestial Seasonings
Two capsules contain: Vitamin E (as d-alpha tocopherol acetate) 90 IU • Zinc (as gluconate) 15 mg • Proprietary Blend: Saw Palmetto berries, Saw Palmetto extract, Stinging Nettle root extract 1230 mg.

Celite Complex 75 - Jamieson
Two capsules contain: Concentrated Citrus Bioflavonoids (Vitamin P) 100 mg • Ginkgo Biloba extract flavoglycoside-rich JGB24 250 mg • Bilberry extract anthocyanoside-rich JMF25 750 mg • Oil of Madagascar Cinnamon 20 mg • South Pacific Sea Kelp extract 25 mg • Bromelain Enzyme (from Pineapple) 100 mg • Kola Nut extract 250 mg. Other Ingredients: Soybean Oil, Vegetable Oil, Gelatin, Glycerin, Lecithin, Purified Water.

Celite Complex 75 - Firming Gel - Jamieson
Water • Glycerin • Butylene Glycol • Kola Nut (Cola acuminata) extract • Coneflower (Echinacea purpurea) extract • Propylene Glycol • Butylene Glycol • Camellia oleifera extract • Arnica montana extract • Dimethylsilanol Hyaluronate • Jojoba Esters • Butcher's Broom (Rucus aculeatus) extract • Kelp (Macrocystis pyrifera) extract • Imidazolidinyl Urea • Triethanolamine • Carbomer • Methyl Paraben • Ethyl Paraben • Fragrance.

Celite Complex 75 - Smoothing & Firming Gel - Jamieson
Contains: Jojoba Esters (toning beads) • Kola Nut Extract • Echinacea Extract • Camellia Oleifera Extract • Arnica Montana Extract • Butcherbroom Extract • Kelp Extract.

Cell Boost with IP-6 - Ultimate Nutrition
Two capsules contain: Calcium 101 mg • Phosphorous 195 mg • Calcium Magnesium Phytate (Inositol Hexaphosphate) 1000 mg.

Cell Forte Max 3 Maitake - Enzymatic Therapy
Two capsules contain: Ip-6 (inositol hexaphosphate) 800 mg • Inositol 220 mg • Maitake Mushroom extract (grifola frondosa, standardized to contain pure d-fraction 9 mg) 30 mg • Poa Cat's Claw root extract (uncaria tomentosa, pentacyclic chemotype, standardized to contain a minimum of 1.3% pentacyclic oxindole alkaloids) 10 mg. Other Ingredients: Gelatin, Magnesium Stearate, Titanium Dioxide Color, Silicon Dioxide.

Cell Forte with IP-6 - Enzymatic Therapy
Each capsule contains: IP-6 (inositol hexaphosphate, from rice) 400 mg • Inositol (from rice) 110 mg.

Cell Guard - Source Naturals
Three tablets contain: Vitamin A (beta carotene 15000 IU and palmitate 10000 IU) 25000 IU • Vitamin B-1 (thiamin) 10 mg • Vitamin B-2 (riboflavin) 10 mg • Niacin 30 mg • Vitamin B-5 (calcium D-Pantothenate) 50 mg • Vitamin B-6 (pyridoxine HCl) 30 mg • Vitamin B-12 (cyanocobalamin) 100 mcg • Vitamin C (ascorbic acid, magnesium and calcium ascorbates) 2000 mg • Vitamin E D-alpha Tocopheryl (natural) 400 IU • Folic acid 800 mcg • Calcium (ascorbate) 30 mg • Copper (sebacate) 1 mg • Magnesium (ascorbate, citrate, succinate and oxide) 120 mg • Selenium (from high-selenium yeast and sodium selenite) 200 mcg • Zinc (OptiZinc zinc monomethionine) 30 mg. Other Ingredients: N-Acetyl Cysteine 300 mg, N,N-Dimethyl Glycine HCl 150 mg, Coenzyme Q10 (ubiquinone) 30 mg, Herbal blend (unique) 600 mg.

Cell Strength - Source Naturals
Four tablets contain: Phosphorus 460 mg • Calcium 300 mg.

Cell Strength - Source Naturals
Each tablet contains: Calcium ethanolamine phosphate 600 mg.

Cell U Less - Olympian Labs
Each capsule contains: Grape Seed extract 50 mg • Bladderwrack extract 100 mg • Gotu Kola extract 300 mg • Horse Chestnut extract 100 mg.

Cella Free - Bodyonics, Ltd.
Six tablets contain: Herbal BioModulators 1000 mg: Evening Primrose Oil (contains Gamma Linolenic Acid (GLA), Borage Seed Oil, Bladderwrack extract, dried Fucus Vesiculosus extract, Fish Oil [containing the Omega-3 polyunsaturated fatty acids EPA (eicosapentaenoic acid) and DHA (docosahezaenoic acid)], Grape Seed extract, Bioflavonoids, Soy Lecithin, Fatty Acids, dried Sweet Red Clover extract (Mellotus Officinals,Tri Folium pratense, standardized to 1% biochanina), dried Ginkgo Biloba extract (standardized to contain flavonglycosides) • Protein/Fiber BioModulators 1750 mg: A mixture of Bioactive Oligopeptides prepared from food grade proteins by means of enzymatic hydrolysis of Bovine Globin Proteins, Casein and Wheat Protein; Chitosan (Fibrabind) • Therma/ Fluid Balance BioModulators 1000 mg: Uva Ursi (standardized to contain 120 mg of yydroxyquinone), Yerba Mate (standardized to contain 300 mg methyl xanthines). Other Ingredients: Calcium Carbonate, Stearic Acid, Croscarmellose, Magnesium Stearate.
See Editor's Note No. 14.

Cellasene - Thompson Nutritional Products
Three softgels contain: Iodine 720 mcg • Cellasene Lipovascolen 702 mg • Cellasene support blend 1230 g. Other Ingredients: Bladderwrack extract, Grape seed extract, Sweet Clover extract, Ginko Biloba, Borage, Fish oil, Soya Lecithin.

Cellex-C Betaplex Clear Complexion Mask - Cellex-C International Inc.
Kaolin • Glycolic Acid • Echinacea • Peppermint • Rosemary • Olive leaf extract • Green Tea extract.
See Editor's Note No. 17, page 2055.

Cellex-C Betaplex Facial Firming Water - Cellex-C International Inc.
Witch Hazel • Glycolic Acid • Malic Acid • Willow Bark extract • Clover extract • Pomegranate extract.
See Editor's Note No. 17, page 2055.

Cellex-C Betaplex Fresh Complexion Mist - Cellex-C International Inc.
Witch Hazel • Rice Wine • Lactic Acid • Malic Acid • Willow bark extract • Cucumber extract • Horsetail extract • Lavender oil • Peppermint oil • Thyme oil.
See Editor's Note No. 17, page 2055.

Cellex-C Betaplex Gentle Cleansing Milk - Cellex-C International Inc.
Sunflower seed oil • Lactic Acid • Willow Bark extract • Aloe Barbadensis gel • Vitamin E • Allantoin • Sassafras extract • Chamomile extract • Ginseng extract • Milfoil extract • Lemongrass extract.
See Editor's Note No. 17, page 2055.

Some Brand Name Natural Products - What they Contain

www.NaturalDatabase.com contains MANY more listings than appear here.

Cellex-C Betaplex Gentle Foaming Cleanser - Cellex-C International Inc.
Aloe Barbadensis gel • Lactic Acid • Willow Bark extract • Cucumber extract • Clover extract.
See Editor's Note No. 17, page 2055.

Cellex-C Betaplex Line Smoother - Cellex-C International Inc.
Lactic Acid • Glycolic Acid • Malic Acid • Sodium Hyaluronate • Willow Bark extract.
See Editor's Note No. 17, page 2055.

Cellex-C Betaplex New Complexion Cream - Cellex-C International Inc.
Lactic Acid • Glycolic Acid • Malic Acid • Glycerin • Willow Bark extract • Aloe Barbadensis gel • Vitamin E • Allantoin • Evening Primrose Oil • Chamomile extract.
See Editor's Note No. 17, page 2055.

Cellex-C Betaplex Smooth Skin Complex - Cellex-C International Inc.
Lactic Acid • Glycolic Acid • Malic Acid • Vitamin E • Willow Bark extract • Aloe Barbadensis gel • Lecithin • Allantoin.
See Editor's Note No. 17, page 2055.

Cellex-C Bio-Botanical - Cellex-C International Inc.
Aloe Vera gel • Primrose oil • Sodium Hyaluronate • Phospholipids • Vitamin E • Chamomile extract • Allantoin • Lavandula Vera.
See Editor's Note No. 17, page 2055.

Cellex-C Bio-Tan - Cellex-C International Inc.
DHA • Tyrosine • Melanin • Erythrulose • Walnut extract • Phospholipids.
See Editor's Note No. 17, page 2055.

Cellex-C Body Smoothing Lotion - Cellex-C International Inc.
Ascorbic Acid • Vitamin E • Tomato extract • Evening Primrose oil • Tyrosine • Zinc • Hyaluronic Acid • Aloe Vera extract • Chamomile extract • Allantoin • Bioflavonoids.
See Editor's Note No. 17, page 2055.

Cellex-C Eye Contour Cream Plus - Cellex-C International Inc.
Ascorbic Acid • Tyrosine • Zinc • Bioflavonoids • Vitamin E • Sodium Hyaluronate • Evening Primrose Oil • Tomato oil • Aloe Barbadensis gel • Chamomile extract • Allantoin.
See Editor's Note No. 17, page 2055.

Cellex-C Eye Contour Gel - Cellex-C International Inc.
Ascorbic Acid • Tyrosine • Zinc • Bioflavonoids • Sodium Hyaluronate.
See Editor's Note No. 17, page 2055.

Cellex-C Fade Away Gel For Sun & Age Spots - Cellex-C International Inc.
Glucosamine • Ascorbic Acid • Tyrosine • Zinc • Green Tea extract • Sodium Hyaluronate • Cucumber extract • Thyme extract.
See Editor's Note No. 17, page 2055.

Cellex-C GLA. - Cellex-C International Inc.
Gamma Linolenic Acid • Evening Primrose Oil • Vitamin A Palmitate • Vitamin E • Wheat Germ Oil • Witch Hazel • Liposomes • Milk Thistle seed extract • Lemon oil flavonoids.
See Editor's Note No. 17, page 2055.

Cellex-C GLA. Extra Moist - Cellex-C International Inc.
Glycophospholipids • Evening Primrose Oil • Witch Hazel extract • Wheat Germ oil • Retinyl Palmitate • Vitamin E • Allantoin • Milk Thistle seed extract • Chamomile extract.
See Editor's Note No. 17, page 2055.

Cellex-C GLA. Eye Balm - Cellex-C International Inc.
Gamma Linolenic Acid • Evening Primrose Oil • Vitamin A Palmitate • Vitamin E • Wheat Germ oil • Witch Hazel • Liposomes • Milk Thistle seed extract • Lemon oil flavonoids.
See Editor's Note No. 17, page 2055.

Cellex-C High-Potency Serum - Cellex-C International Inc.
10% L-Ascorbic Acid • Tyrosine • Zinc • Sodium Hyaluronate • Bioflavonoids.
See Editor's Note No. 17, page 2055.

Cellex-C Hydra 5 B-Complex - Cellex-C International Inc.
Hyaluronic Acid • Pantothenic Acid.
See Editor's Note No. 17, page 2055.

Cellex-C Hydra Hand Cream SPF 15 - Cellex-C International Inc.
Kukui nut oil • Vitamin E • Lecithin • Shea Butter • Horse Chestnut extract • Hyaluronic Acid • Glycerin • Allantoin • Chamomile.
See Editor's Note No. 17, page 2055.

Cellex-C Sea Silk Oil-Free Moisturizer - Cellex-C International Inc.
Jojoba esters • Sodium Hyaluronate • Seasilk • Plankton extract • Sea Buckthorn extract • Watercress extract • Marine Algae extract • Seaweed extract.
See Editor's Note No. 17, page 2055.

Cellex-C Seline-E - Cellex-C International Inc.
Vitamin E • Bioflavonoids • Herbal essence.
See Editor's Note No. 17, page 2055.

Cellex-C Serum For Sensitive Skin - Cellex-C International Inc.
Ascorbic Acid • Tyrosine • Zinc • Sodium Hyaluronate • Pine Bark extract.
See Editor's Note No. 17, page 2055.

Cellex-C Skin Firming Cream Plus - Cellex-C International Inc.
Ascorbic Acid • Tyrosine • Vitamin E • Zinc • Bioflavonoids • Sodium Hyaluronate • Evening Primrose Oil • Tomato extract • Aloe Barbadensis gel • Chamomile extract • Allantoin.
See Editor's Note No. 17, page 2055.

Cellex-C Skin Firming Hand Cream - Cellex-C International Inc.
L- Ascorbic Acid • Tyrosine • Zinc • Chamomile.
See Editor's Note No. 17, page 2055.

Cellex-C Skin Perfecting Pen - Cellex-C International Inc.
Olive leaf • Rosemary • Lavender • Thyme • Eucalyptus extract • Peppermint extract • Zinc • Hyaluronic Acid.
See Editor's Note No. 17, page 2055.

Cellex-C Speed Peel & Polish Gel - Cellex-C International Inc.
Ficin Enzyme • Melon extract • Natural Bamboo extract (providing micro-cylinders of silica) • Jojoba oil • Hyaluronic Acid.
See Editor's Note No. 17, page 2055.

Cellex-C Sun Care SPF 15 - Cellex-C International Inc.
Octinoxate 7% • Octisalate 4% • Zinc Oxide 2% • Titanium Dioxide 2% • Total Hydroxy-Benzoates 0.17%.
See Editor's Note No. 17, page 2055.

Cellex-C Sun Care SPF 30+ - Cellex-C International Inc.
Octinoxate 7.5% • Octisalate 5% • Zinc Oxide 3% • Titanium Dioxide 2% • Total Hydroxybanzoates 0.17%.
See Editor's Note No. 17, page 2055.

Cellex-C Sun Rescue Gel **-** Cellex-C International Inc.
L- Ascorbic Acid • Tyrosine • Zinc • Green Tea extract • Glycine • Peppermint.
See Editor's Note No. 17, page 2055.

Cellex-C Under-Eye Toning Gel **-** Cellex-C International Inc.
Azulene • Cornflower • Nicotinic Acid • Beta 1,3 glucans • Witch Hazel • Glycosaminoglycans • Plant Tannins • Cucumber extract • Kigelia extract.
See Editor's Note No. 17, page 2055.

CellMend IP-6 **-** Nature's Way
Three tablets contain: C-Med-100 patented Cat's Claw extract 300 mg • Inositol 150 mg • IP-6 (inositol hexaphosphate from rice) 1.6 g • Ribose (as d-ribose) 90 mg.

CELL-Tech **-** MuscleTech
Each serving contains: Creatine Monohydrate 10 g • Insulin-releasing Dextrose 75 g • Insulin-potentiating Lipoic Acid 200 mg • Chromium Picolinate 300 mcg • Potassium 150 mg • Phosphates 100 mg • Taurine • Magnesium.

Celltrex Skin Hydrating Fluid (original) **-** Nu Skin Enterprises
Water • Aloe Vera gel • Propylene Glycol • Hydroxypropyl Methylcellulose • Avian Collagen • Hyaluronic Acid • Linoleic Acid • Linolenic Acid • Oleic Acid • Tocopherol • Citric Acid • Arachidonic Acid • Triethanolamine • Disodium EDTA • Methylparaben • Propylparaben.

Celltrex Ultra Recovery Fluid **-** Nu Skin Enterprises
Water • Glycerin • Guar Hydroxypropyl-Trimonium Chloride • Ethoxydigylcol • Olea Europaea oil (olive fruit) • PEG-60 Hydrogenated Castor oil • Tocopheryl Acetate • Retinyl Palmitate • Citrus Aurantium var. Dulcis oil (orange) • Lavandula Angustifolia oil (lavender) • Anthemis Nobilis flower oil • Isoceteth-20 • Oleth-10 • Sodium Hydroxide • Citric Acid • Sodium Chloride • Disodium EDTA • Methylparaben • Ethylparaben • Propylparaben.

Cellular Detox Bath **-** Abra Therapeutics
Sodium Borate • Sodium Sulfate • Sodium Chloride • Sodium Sesquicarbonate • Olive Oil • Essential Oils Blend: Grapefruit, Juniper, Lavender, Lemongrass, Cedar leaf, Fir, Peru Balsam • Herbal Extracts Blend: Dandelion root, Burdock root • Vitamin A • Vitamin C • Vitamin E • Chromium Oxide • Trace Mineral Salts.

Cellular Detox Salt Scrub **-** Abra Therapeutics
20% Volcanic ash • Natural Mineral Blend: Sodium Borate, Sodium Sulfate, Sodium Chloride • Organic Oils Blend: Almond oil, Olive oil, Sunflower oil, Jojoba oil, Grapefruit oil, Tea Tree oil, Juniper oil, Lime oil • Organic Comfrey • Dandelion • Burdock root • Natural Trace Minerals • Natural Vitamin E.

Cellular Fort MAX3 **-** PhytoPharmica
Two capsules contain: Calcium (from calcium magnesium phytate) 130 mg • Inositol 220 mg • IP-6 (inositol hexaphosphate, from calcium magnesium phytate) 800 mg • Magnesium (from calcium magnesium phytate) 40 mg • Maitake mushroom extract (grifola frondosa, standardized to contain 9 mg of pure D-fraction) 30 mg • Phosphorus (from calcium magnesium phytate) 190 mg • POA Cat's Claw root extract (uncaria tomentosa, pentacyclic chemotype, Saventaro brand, standardized to contain a minimum of 1.3% pentacyclic oxindole alkaloids (POAs) and to be free of tetracyclic oxindole alkaloids (TOAs)) 10 mg.

Cellular Forte with IP-6 and Inositol capsules **-** PhytoPharmica
Two capsules contain: Calcium (from calcium magneisum phytate) 130 mg • Inositol 220 mg • IP-6 (inositol hexaphosphate) 800 mg • Magnesium (from calcium magnesium phytate) 40 mg • Phosphorus (from calcium mangeisum phytate) 190 mg.

Cellular Forte with IP-6 and Inositol Powder **-** PhytoPharmica
Each heaping scoop contains: Calcium (from calcium magnesium phytate) 520 mg • Inositol 880 mg • IP-6 (inositol hexaphosphate, from calcium magnesium phytate) 3.2 g • Magnesium (from calcium magnesium phytate) 160 mg • Phosphorus (from calcium magnesium phytate) 760 mg • Stevia leaf 12:1 extract (stevia rebaudiana) 60 mg.

Cellular Support Advanced (No Iron) **-** Pro Health
Two tablets contain: Vitamin A (as beta carotene 7500 IU, palmitate 5000 IU) 12,500 IU • Vitamin C (as ascorbic acid, ascorbyl palmitate) 500 mg • Vitamin D (D3, as cholecalciferol) 200 IU • Vitamin E (as natural d-alpha tocopheryl) 200 IU • Thiamin (vitamin B1) 50 mg • Riboflavin (vitamin B2) 50 mg • Niacinamide 35 mg • Niacin 15 mg • Vitamin B6 (as pyridoxine HCl) 50 mg • Folate (as folic acid) 400 mcg • Vitamin B12 (as cyanocobalamin) 100 mcg • Biotin 150 mcg • Pantothenic Acid (as calcium d-pantothenate) 50 mg • Calcium (as calcium chelate, citrate, malate) 100 mg • Iodine (from kelp) 100 mcg • Magnesium (as magnesium chelate, citrate, oxide) 100 mg • Zinc (as zinc citrate, monomethionine) 15 mg • Selenium (as l-selenomethionine, sodium selenite) 100 mcg • Copper (as copper sebacate) 1 mg • Manganese (as manganese citrate) 3 mg • Chromium (as chromium polynicotinate) 100 mcg • Molybdenum (as molybdenum chelate) 100 mcg • Potassium (as potassium citrate) 50 mg • N-Acetyl Cysteine 100 mg • Hawthorn berry 75 mg • Milk Thistle seed extract (yielding silymarin 60 mg) 72 mg • L-Tyrosine 50 mg • Choline (as bitartrate) 50 mg • Inositol 50 mg • DMAE (as bitartrate) 30 mg • Alpha-Lipoic Acid 25 mg • MSM (methylsulfonylmethane) 25 mg • Grape Seed extract 25 mg • Coenzyme Q-10 20 mg • Ginkgo Biloba leaf 24% (50:1 extract) 20 mg • Turmeric rhizome extract (95%) 15 mg • Bilberry standardized extract 10 mg • Pepper fruit extract 3 mg • Boron Amino Acid Chelate 2 mg. Other Ingredients: Stearic Acid, Acacia Gum, Modified Cellulose Gum, Colloidal Silicon Dioxide, Magnesium Stearate.

Cellular Support Advanced (With Iron) **-** Pro Health
Two tablets contain: Vitamin A (as beta carotene 7500 IU, palmitate 5000 IU) 12,500 IU • Vitamin C (as ascorbic acid, ascorbyl palmitate) 500 mg • Vitamin D (D3, as cholecalciferol) 200 IU • Vitamin E (as natural d-alpha tocopheryl) 200 IU • Thiamin (vitamin B1) 50 mg • Riboflavin (vitamin B2) 50 mg • Niacinamide 35 mg • Niacin 15 mg • Vitamin B6 (as pyridoxine HCl) 50 mg • Folate (as folic acid) 400 mcg • Vitamin B12 (as cyanocobalamin) 100 mcg • Biotin 150 mcg • Pantothenic Acid (as calcium d-pantothenate) 50 mg • Calcium (as calcium chelate, citrate, malate) 100 mg • Iron (as iron fumarate) 6 mg • Iodine (from kelp) 100 mcg • Magnesium (as magnesium chelate, citrate, oxide) 100 mg • Zinc (as zinc citrate, monomethionine) 15 mg • Selenium (as l-selenomethionine, sodium selenite) 100 mcg • Copper (as copper sebacate) 1 mg • Manganese (as manganese citrate) 3 mg • Chromium (as chromium polynicotinate) 100 mcg • Molybdenum (as molybdenum chelate) 100 mcg • Potassium (as potassium citrate) 50 mg • N-Acetyl Cysteine 100 mg • Hawthorn berry 75 mg • Milk Thistle seed extract (yielding silymarin 60 mg) 72 mg • L-Tyrosine 50 mg • Choline (as bitartrate) 50 mg • Inositol 50 mg • DMAE (as bitartrate) 30 mg • Alpha-Lipoic Acid 25 mg • MSM (methylsulfonylmethane) 25 mg • Grape Seed extract 25 mg • Coenzyme Q-10 20 mg • Ginkgo Biloba leaf 24% (50:1 extract) 20 mg • Turmeric rhizome extract (95%) 15 mg • Bilberry standardized extract 10 mg • Pepper fruit extract 3 mg • Boron Amino Acid Chelate 2 mg. Other Ingredients: Stearic Acid, Acacia Gum, Modified Cellulose Gum, Colloidal Silicon Dioxide, Magnesium Stearate.

Cell-U-Loss **-** Herbalife
Each tablet contains: Vitamin C 250 mg • Potassium 297 mg • Iron 9 mg • Proprietary Blend 1000 mg: Buchu, Couch Grass, Cornsilk, Hydrangea, Juniper berry, Uva Ursi • Lecithin 50 mg • Kelp 100 mg • Cider Vinegar 100 mg.

Some Brand Name Natural Products - What they Contain

www.NaturalDatabase.com contains MANY more listings than appear here.

CelluPlex **-** Jamieson
Each capsule contains: Bilberry extract 750 mg • Kola Nut extract 250 mg • Ginkgo Biloba extract 250 mg • Concentrated Citrus Bioflavonoids PF 100 (vitamin P) 100 mg • Active PSP Bromelain Enzyme (from fresh pineapple) 100 mg • Mineral-Rich Pacific Sea Kelp Extract 25 mg • Oil of Madagascar Cinnamon Leaf 20 mg.

Cellu-Rid **-** Biotech Corp.
Two tablets contain: Vitamin C (ascorbic acid) 80 mg • Iron (as ferrous fumarate) 9 mg • HerbaCell! Proprietary Herb Blend 200 mg: Senna leaves (cassia angustifolia), Cascara Sagrada bark, Apple rind extract, Milk Thistle root extract (silybum marianum), BioPerine standardized Piper Nigrum tailed pepper extract, Cinnamon root extract (cinnamomum verum) • White Willow bark (salix alba) 100 mg • Kelp 33 mg • Apple Cider Vinegar 33 mg • Guarana seed (paullinia cupana) 20 mg • Soy Lecithin 16 mg • Rose Hips 10 mg • Buchu leaves (betulina bosma) 5 mg • Couch Grass (cynodon dactylon) 5 mg • Hydrangea Arborescens root 5 mg • Uva Ursi (arctostaphylos uva-ursi) 5 mg • Juniper berries (juniperus vulgaris) 5 mg. Other Ingredients: Gelatin, Silica, Potassium (as potassium chloride).

Cellu-Trim **-** Enforma Natural Products
Two capsules contain: White Willow bark • Vitamin C (ascorbic acid) • Hydragia root • Sida Cordifolia • Uva Ursi • Tinospora Cordifolia • Potassium Chloride.
See Editor's Note No. 39, page 2058.

Cellu-Var Capsules **-** Enzymatic Therapy/PhytoPharmica
Each capsule contains: Butchers Broom extract (Ruscus aculeatus) standardized to contain 10% Saponins calculated as Ruscogenin 100 mg • Gotu Kola extract (Centella asiatica) standardized to contain 70% of selected Triterpenic Acids: Asiaticoside, Asiatic Acid, & Madecassic Acid from Centella 30 mg • Escin extract (Aesculus hippocastanum) 10 mg.
See Editor's Note No. 21, page 2056.

Cellu-Var Cream **-** Enzymatic Therapy
Deionized Water • Horse Chestnut (Escin) extract • Sea Ware extract • Cola vera extract • Rosemary extract in a base of Cholestanol (Dihydrocholesterol), a natural emulsifying agent.

Censor **-** NDS Nutrition
Each capsule contains: Proprietary Blend 1000 mg: CLA (conjugated linoleic acid), GLA (gamma linoleic acid), ALA (alpha linoleic acid), EPA (eicosapentaenoic acid), DHA (docosahexaenoic acid), Omega 3-6-9 Blend.

Central-Vite Select Formula Plus **-** Leiner Health Products
Each tablet contains: Folate (Folic Acid) 200 mcg • Iron (Ferrous Fumarate) 9 mg • Phosphorus 48 mg • Vitamin B12 (Cyanocobalamin, USP Method 2) 25 mcg • Magnesium Oxide 100 mg • Molybdenum 160 mcg • Calcium Carbonate 200 mg • Chloride 72 mg • Potassium Chloride and Iodide 80 mg • Manganese Sulfate 3.5 mg • Vitamin A (Acetate) 7500 IU • Vitamin B6 (Pyridoxine Hydrochloride) 3 mg • Vitamin C (Ascorbic Acid) 90 mg • Vitamin E (dl-Alpha Tocopheryl Acetate) 45 IU • Zinc Oxide 22.5 mg • Vitamin K (Phytonadione) 10 mcg • Chromium Chloride 130 mcg • Copper Oxide 2 mg • Iodine 150 mcg • Niacin (Niacinamide) 20 mg • Pantothenic Acid 10 mg • Riboflavin (Vitamin B2) 1.7 mg • Selenium 70 mcg • Thiamin Mononitrate (Vitamin B1) 1.5 mg • Vitamin D 400 IU • Biotin (USP Method 2) 30 mcg • Boron 150 mcg • Nickel (Nickelous Sulfate) 5 mcg • Silicon Dioxide 10 mcg • Vanadium 10 mcg. Other Ingredients: Dicalcium Phosphate, Gelatin, Cellulose, Starch, Croscarmellose Sodium, Sodium Starch Glycolate, Hydroxypropyl Methylcellulose, Polyethylene Glycol 3350, Tricalcium Phosphate, Magnesium Stearate, Hydroxypropyl Cellulose, Resin, Beta Carotene, Polysorbate 80, Pharmaceutical Glaze, Sodium Metasilicate.

Centrum **-** Wyeth
Each tablet contains: Nickel (Nickelous Sulfate) 5 mcg • Vitamin A Acetate 5000 IU • Tin (Stannous Chloride) 10 mcg • Vitamin C (Ascorbic Acid) 60 mg • Vitamin D 400 IU • Vanadium (Sodium Metavanadate) 10 mcg • Silicon Dioxide 2 mg • Vitamin E (dl-Alpha Tocopheryl Acetate) 30 IU • Boron (Potassium Borate) 150 mcg • Vitamin K (Phytonadione) 25 mcg • Thiamin Mononitrate (Vitamin B1) 1.5 mg • Riboflavin (Vitamin B2) 1.7 mg • Niacin (Vitamin B3, Niacinamide) 20 mg • Vitamin B6 (Pyridoxine Hydrochloride) 2 mg • Folate (Folic Acid) 400 mcg • Vitamin B12 (Cyanocobalamin) 6 mcg • Biotin 30 mcg • Pantothenic Acid (Calcium Pantothenate) 10 mg • Calcium Carbonate 162 mg • Iron (Ferrous Fumarate) 18 mg • Phosphorus (Calcium Carbonate) 109 mg • Iodine 150 mcg • Magnesium Oxide 100 mg • Zinc Oxide 15 mg • Selenium (Sodium Selenate) 20 mcg • Copper (Cupric Acid) 2 mg • Manganese Sulfate 3.5 mg • Chromium 65 mcg • Molybdenum 160 mg • Chloride 72 mg • Potassium Chloride 80 mg. Other Ingredients: Microcrystalline Cellulose, Gelatin, Crospovidone, Hydroxypropyl Methylcellulose, Titanium Dioxide, Magnesium Stearate, Stearic Acid, Triethyl Citrate, Polysorbate 80, FD&C Yellow #6.

Centrum Focused Formula Stress **-** Wyeth
Each tablet contains: Vitamin C 150 mg • Vitamin E 22.5 IU • Thiamin (B1) 15 mg • Riboflavin (B2) 4.8 mg • Niacin (B3) 50 mg • Vitamin B6 5 mg • Folate, Folic Acid, Folacin 200 mcg • Vitamin B12 12.5 mcg • Biotin 15 mcg • Pantothenic Acid 12.5 mg • Zinc 7.5 mg • Copper 1 mg • Ginseng standardized root extract (Panax ginseng) 62.5 mg.
See Editor's Note No. 21, page 2056.

Centrum Focused Formulas - Energy **-** Wyeth
Each tablet contains: Supplement facts: Thiamin (Vitamin B1) 3 mg • Riboflavin (Vitamin B2) 0.85 mg • Niacin (Vitamin B3) 10 mg • Vitamin B6 1 mg • Vitamin B12 3 mcg • Biotin 15 mcg • Pantothenic Acid 5 mg • Taurine 100 mg • Panax Ginseng standardized extract (root) 62.5 mg. Ingredients: Dibasic Calcium Phosphate, Taurine, Ginseng standardized root extract (Panax Ginseng), Microcrystalline Cellulose, Crospovidone, Maltodextrin, Hydroxypropyl Methylcellulose, Niacinamide, Calcium Pantothenate, Magnesium Stearate, Titanium Dioxide, Polyethylene Glycol, Thiamin Mononitrate, Polysorbate 80, FD&C Yellow #6 Aluminum Lake, Pyridoxine Hydrochloride, Riboflavin, Starch, Biotin, Citric Acid, Sodium Citrate, Silicon Dioxide, Cyanocobalamin, Sodium Benzoate, Sorbic Acid.
See Editor's Note No. 21, page 2056.

Centrum Focused Formulas Bone Health **-** Wyeth
Each two tablets contain: Supplement facts: Vitamin D 200 IU • Calcium (Citrate) 500 mg • Magnesium 40 mg • Zinc 7.5 mg • Copper 1 mg • Manganese 1.8 mg • Boron 250 mcg • Lycopene 1.5 mg • Saw Palmetto (Standardized lipophilic fruit extract, Serenoa repens) 160 mg. Ingredients: Calcium Citrate, Magnesium Oxide, Talc, Hydroxypropyl Methylcellulose, Sodium Starch Glycolate, Titanium Dioxide, Magnesium Stearate, Zinc Oxide, Mineral Oil, Manganese Sulfate Monohydrate, Vitamin D (Cholecalciferol), Polysorbate 80, Sodium Borate, Polyethlene Glycol, Cupric Oxide, Gelatin, Sucrose, Starch, Carnauba Wax, Vegetable Oil, DL-Alpha-Tocopherol.
See Editor's Note No. 21, page 2056.

Centrum Focused Formulas Heart **-** Wyeth
Each tablet contains: Supplement facts: Vitamin E 200 IU • Vitamin B6 5 mg • Folate, Folic Acid, Folacin 200 mcg • Vitamin B12 200 mcg • Selenium 25 mcg • Manganese 1 mg • Garlic Powder (bulb) (Allium sativum) 300 mg • Taurine 33 mg • Coenzyme Q10 4 mg. Ingredients: DL-Alpha Tocopherol Acetate, Garlic powder (Bulb, Alium sativum), Microcrystalline Cellulose, Dibasic Calcium Phosphate, Calcium Silicate, Taurine, Croscarmellose sodium, Sodium Selenate, Gelatin, Hydroxypropyl methylcellulose, Silicon Doxide, Magnesium Stearate, Pyridoxine Hydrochloride, Ubidecarenone, Titanium Dioxide, Polyethylene Glycol, Polysorbate 80, Magnesium Sulfate Monohydrate, FD&C Red #40 Aluminum Lake, FD&C Blue #2 Aluminum Lake, Folic Acid, Cyanocobalamin, Citric Acid, Starch, Sodium Citrate, Sodium Benzoate, Sorbic Acid.
See Editor's Note No. 21, page 2056.

***Centrum Focused Formulas Mental Clarity* - Wyeth**
Each tablet contains: Supplement Facts: Vitamin E 20 IU • Thiamin (B1) 0.55 mg • Riboflavin (B2) 0.85 mg • Niacin (B3) 10 mg • Vitamin B6 1 mg • Folate, Folic Acid, Folacin 200 mcg • Vitamin B12 3 mcg • Biotin 5 mcg • Pantothenic Acid 7.5 mg • Ginkgo Biloba standardized leaf extract 60 mg • Choline 8 mg. Ingredients: Dibasic Calcium Phosphate, Microcrystalline Cellulose, Ginkgo Biloba standardized extract, Dl-alpha Tocopheryl Acetate, Choline Bitartrate, Hydroxypropyl methylcellulose Crospovidone, maltodextrin, Niacinamide, Zinc Oxide, Calcium Pantothenate, Calcium Silicate, Magnesium Stearate, Titanium Dioxide, Gelatin, Polyethylene Glycol, Polysorbate 80, Silicon Dioxide, FD&C Blue #2 Aluminum Lake, FD&C Red #40 Aluminum Lake, FD&C Yellow #6 Aluminum Lake, Pyridoxine Hydrochloride, Riboflavin, Thiamine Mononitrate, Folic Acid, Starch, Citric Acid, Sodium Citrate, Cyanocobalamin, Sodium Benzoate, Sorbic Acid.
See Editor's Note No. 21, page 2056.

***Centrum Focused Formulas Prostate* - Wyeth**
Each softgel contains: Vitamin A as Beta-carotene 5000 IU • Lycopene 1.5 mg • Saw Palmetto standardized Lipophilic fruit extract (Serenoa repens) 160 mg.
See Editor's Note No. 21, page 2056.

***Centrum Herbals Echinacea* - Wyeth**
Each capsule contains: Echinacea extract flower and root (Echinacea purpurea) 100 mg. Standardized to contain (based on extract weight): Total Phenols (marker) 3.0%, Cichoric Acid (natural active), Isobutyl Alkylamides (natural active), Activity Measure 15-lipoxygenase enzymatic assay. Other Ingredients: Dibasic Calcium Phosphate, Cellulose, Lactose Monohydrate, Hydroxypropyl Cellulose, Ethylcellulose, Castor Oil, Gelatin, Silicon Dioxide, Sodium Lauryl Sulfate, Propylene Glycol, Titanium Dioxide.
See Editor's Note No. 21, page 2056.

***Centrum Herbals Garlic* - Wyeth**
Each capsule contains: Garlic powder (bulb) Allium sativum 300 mg • Allin (marker) allicin potential 45% 1300 mcg. Standardized to contain: Gamma Glytamyl-S allyl-cysteine (natural active) • Gamma Glytamyl-S-trans-1-propenyl-cysteine (natural active) • Gamma glutamyl-phenylalanine (natural active) • Activity Measure Angiotensin converting enzyme assay.
See Editor's Note No. 21, page 2056.

***Centrum Herbals Ginkgo Biloba* - Wyeth**
Each capsule contains: Ginkgo Biloba leaf extract 60 mg. Standardized to contain (based on extract weight): Ginkgo Flavone glycosides (marker) 24%, Terpene Lactones (marker) 6%, ginkgolide A (natural active), Ginkgolide B (natural active), Amentoflavone (natural active). Activity measure: GABA Central binding assay. Other Ingredients: Sucrose, Cellulose, Lactose, Monohydrate, Dibasic Calcium Phosphate, Hydroxypropyl Cellulose, Ethylcellulose, Castor Oil, Flavor Extractives of St. John's Bread, Glucose, Caramel color, Silicon Dioxide, Sodium Lauryl Sulfate, Propylene Glycol, Tianium Dioxide.
See Editor's Note No. 21, page 2056.

***Centrum Herbals Ginseng* - Wyeth**
Each capsule contains: Ginseng root extract 100 mg. Standardized to contain (based on extract weight): Total Ginenosides (marker) 7.0%, Ginsenoside Rb1 (natural active), Ginsenoside Rg1 (natural active). Activity measure: Phospholipase A2 enzymatic assay. Other Ingredients: Dibasic Calcium Phosphate, Cellulose, Lactose, Monohydrate, Hydroxypropyl Cellulose, Ethylcellulose, Castor Oil, Gelatin, Silicon Dioxide, Sodium Lauryl Sulfate, Propylene Glycol, Titanium Dioxide.
See Editor's Note No. 21, page 2056.

***Centrum Herbals Saw Palmetto* - Wyeth**
Each softgel contains: Saw Palmetto berry extract (Serenoa repens) 160 mg. Total Fatty Acids (marker) 80% (Standardized to contain-based on extract weight): Linolenic Acid (natural active) • Lauric Acid, Ethyl Ester (natural active) • Linoleic Acid, Ethyl Ester (natural active) • Activity measure: Adrenergic alpha 1B binding assay. Inactive Ingredients: Corn Oil, Yellow Wax, Gelatin, Propylene Glycol, Hydroxypropyl Methylcellulose, Titanium Dioxide, Carmine.
See Editor's Note No. 21, page 2056.

***Centrum Herbals St. John's Wort* - Wyeth**
Each capsule contains: St. John's Wort (Hypericum perforatum) flower and leaves 300 mg. Standardized to contain (based on extract weight): Total Hypericin compounds (marker) 0.3%, Hyperforin (marker), Quercetin (natural active), Amentoflavone (natural active), Gaba & Proline (natural actives). Activity measure: Muscarinic M1 binding assay. Other Ingredients: Dibasic Calcium Phosphate, Maltodextrin, Cellulose, Lactose Monohydrate, Silicon Dioxide, Hydroxypropyl Cellulose, Ethycellulose, Castor Oil, Gelatin, Sodium Lauryl Sulfate, Propylene Glycol, Titanium Dioxide.
See Editor's Note No. 21, page 2056.

***Centrum Kids* - Wyeth**
Each tablet contains: Vitamin A Acetate 5000 IU • Sodium 14 mg • Vitamin C (Ascorbic Acid and Sodium Ascorbate) 250 mg • Vitamin D 400 IU • Vitamin E (dl-Alpha Tocopheryl Acetate) 15 IU • Thiamin Mononitrate (Vitamin B1) 1.5 mg • Riboflavin (Vitamin B2) 1.7 mg • Niacin (Niacinamide, Vitamin B3) 13.5 mg • Vitamin B6 (Pyridoxine Hydrochloride) 1 mg • Folate (Folic Acid) 300 mcg • Vitamin B12 (Cyanocobalamin) 5 mcg • Calcium Carbonate 108 mg • Phosphorus (Calicum Phosphate) 50 mg • Zinc Oxide 4 mg • Copper (Cupric Oxide) 0.5 mg. Other Ingredients: Sugar, Mannitol, Mono- and Diglycerides, Microcrystalline Cellulose, Modified Food Starch, Gelatin, Stearic Acid, FD&C Yellow #6 Lake, Food Starch, Aspartame, Carrageenan, Magnesium Stearate, Natural and Artificial Flavors, Guar Gum, FD&C Red #40 Lake, FD&C Blue #2 Lake, Silicon Dioxide, Partially Hydrogenated Coconut Oil, Dextrose, Beta Carotene, Lactose, Acacia.

***Centrum Liquid Supplement* - Wyeth**
Each 1 tbsp serving (15 mL) contains: Vitamin A Palmitate 2500 IU • Vitamin C (Ascorbic Acid) 60 mg • Vitamin D (as Vitamin D3) 400 IU • Vitamin E (dl-Alpha Tocopheryl Acetate) 30 IU • Thiamin Hydrochloride (Vitamin B1) 1.5 mg • Riboflavin 5-Phosphate Sodium (Vitamin B2) 1.7 mg • Niacin (Vitamin B3, Niacinamide) 20 mg • Vitamin B6 (Pyridoxine Hydrochloride) 2 mg • Vitamin B12 (Cyanocobalamin) 6 mcg • Biotin 300 mcg • Pantothenic Acid (D-Panthenol) 10 mg • Iron (Ferrous Gluconate) 9 mg • Iodine (Potassium Iodide) 150 mcg • Zinc Gluconate 3 mg • Manganese Chloride 2 mg • Chromium Chloride 25 mcg • Molybdenum (Sodium Molybdate) 25 mg. Other Ingredients: Water, Sucrose, Ethyl Aclohol 5.4% w/v, Glycerin, Polysorbate 80, Citric Acid, Sodium Benzoate, D-Panthenol, BHA, Natural and Artificial Flavor, Food Starch, Edetic Acid.

***Centrum Multivitamin/Multimineral* - Wyeth**
Each tablet contains: Vitamin A (29% as beta carotene) 3500 IU • Vitamin C 60 mg • Vitamin D 400 IU • Vitamin E 30 IU • Vitamin K 25 mcg • Thiamin (B1) 1.5 mg • Riboflavin (B2) 1.7 mg • Niacin (B3) 20 mg • Vitamin B6 2 mg • Folate, Folic Acid, Folacin 400 mcg • Vitamin B12 6 mcg • Biotin 30 mcg • Pantothenic Acid 10 mg • Calcium 162 mg • Iron 18 mg • Phosphorus 109 mg • Iodine 150 mcg • Magnesium 100 mg • Zinc 15 mg • Selenium 20 mcg • Copper 2 mg • Manganese 2 mg • Chromium 120 mcg • Molybdenum 75 mcg • Chloride 72 mg • Potassium 80 mg • Nickel 5 mcg • Tin 10 mcg • Silicon 2 mg • Vanadium 10 mcg • Boron 150 mcg • Lutein 250 mcg • Lycopene 300 mcg. Other Ingredients: Dibasic Calcium Phosphate, Magnesium Oxide, Potassium Chloride, Microcrystalline Cellulose, Gelatin, Acacia Senegal Gum, Butylated Hydroxytoluene, Crospovidone, FD&C Yellow 6, FD&C Yellow 6 Aluminum Lake, Hypromellose, Magnesium-Stearate, Polysorbate 80, Pregelatinized Starch, Purified Water, Starch, Sucrose, Titanium Dioxide, Calcium Stearate, Glucose, Lactose Monohydrate.

Some Brand Name Natural Products - What they Contain

www.NaturalDatabase.com contains MANY more listings than appear here.

Centrum Performance - Wyeth
Each tablet contains: Ginseng root extract 50 mg • Vitamin A 5000 IU • Ginkgo root extract 60 mg • Vitamin C 120 mg • Vitamin D 400 IU • Boron 60 mg • Vitamin E 60 IU • Nickel 5 mcg • Silicon 4 mg • Vitamin K 25 mcg • Tin 10 mg • Thiamin (B1) 4.5 mg • Vanadium 10 mcg • Riboflavin (B2) 5.1 mg • Niacin (B3) 40 mg • Vitamin B6 6 mg • Folate (Folic Acid) 400 mcg • Vitamin B12 18 mcg • Biotin 40 mcg • Pantothenic Acid 10 mg • Calcium 100 mg • Iron 18 mg • Phosphorus 48 mg • Iodine 150 mcg • Magnesium 40 mg • Zinc 15 mg • Selenium 70 mcg • Copper 2 mg • Manganese 4 mg • Chromium 120 mcg • Molybdenum 75 mg • Chloride 72 mg • Potassium 80 mg.

Centrum Silver - Wyeth
Each tablet contains: Nickel (Nickelous Sulfate) 5 mcg • Vitamin A Acetate 5000 IU • Silicon Dioxide 2 mg • Vitamin C (Ascorbic Acid) 60 mg • Vitamin D 400 IU • Vanadium (Sodium Metavanadate) 10 mcg • Boron (Borates) 150 mcg • Vitamin E (dl-Alpha Tocopheryl Acetate) 45 IU • Vitamin K (Phytonadione)10 mcg • Thiamin Mononitrate (Vitamin B1) 1.5 mg • Riboflavin (Vitamin B2) 1.7 mg • Niacin (Niacinamide, Vitamin B3) 20 mg • Vitamin B6 (Pyridoxine Hydrochloride) 3 mg • Folate (Folic Acid) 400 mcg • Vitamin B12 (Cyanocobalamin) 25 mcg • Biotin 30 mcg • Pantothenic Acid (Calcium Pantothenate) 10 mg • Calcium Carbonate 200 mg • Phosphorus 48 mg • Iodine (Potassium Iodide) 150 mcg • Magnesium Oxide 100 mg • Zinc Oxide 15 mg • Selenium (Sodium Selenate) 20 mcg • Copper (Cupric Oxide) 2 mg • Manganese Sulfate 2 mg • Chromium Chloride 150 mcg • Molybdenum (Sodium Molybdate) 75 mg • Chloride 72 mg • Potassium Chloride 80 mg. Other Ingredients: Microcrystalline Cellulose, Gelatin, Starch, Crospovidone, Hydroxypropyl Methylcellulose, Titanium Dioxide, Sucrose, Magnesium Stearate, Triethyl Citrate, Lactose, Polysorbate 80, Beta Carotene, Lutein, Glucose, FD&C Yellow No. 6 Lake, FD&C Blue No. 2 Lake, FD&C Red No. 40 Lake.

Centrum with Lutein - Wyeth
Each tablet contains: Boron (Borates) 120 mcg • Vitamin A Acetate 5000 IU • Nickel (Nickelous Sulfate) 5 mcg • Vitamin C (Ascorbic Acid) 60 mg • Silicon Dioxide 2 mcg • Vitamin D 400 IU • Vitamin E (dl-Alpha Tocopheryl Acetate) 30 IU • Tin (Stannous Chloride) 10 mcg • Vanadium (Sodium Metavanadate) 10 mcg • Vitamin K (Phytonadione) 25 mcg • Lutein 250.0 mcg • Thiamin Mononitrate (Vitamin B1) 1.5 mg • Riboflavin (Vitamin B2) 1.7 mg • Niacin (Vitamin B3, Niacinamide) 20 mg • Vitamin B6 (Pyridoxine HCl) 2 mg • Folate (Folic Acid) 400 mcg • Vitamin B12 (Cyanocobalamin) 6 mcg • Biotin 30 mcg • Pantothenic Acid (Calcium Pantothenate) 10 mg • Calcium Carbonate 162 mg • Iron (Ferrous Fumarate) 18 mg • Phosphorus 109 mg • Iodine (Potassium Iodide) 150 mcg • Magnesium Oxide 100 mg • Zinc Oxide 15 mg • Selenium (Sodium Selenate) 20 mcg • Copper (Cupric Oxide) 2 mg • Manganese Sulfate 2 mg • Chromium Chloride 120 mcg • Molybdenum (Sodium Molybdate) 75 mg • Potassium Chloride 80 mg. Other Ingredients: Calcium Phosphate, Microcrystalline Cellulose, Gelatin, Crospovidone, Hydroxypropyl Methylcellulose, Starch, Titanium Dioxide, Sucrose, Magnesium Stearate, Triethyl Citrate, Lactose, Polysorbate 80, Beta Carotene, Glucose, FD&C Yellow #6 Lake.

Century Formula - Swanson
Each tablet contains: Vitamin A (as acetate) 5000 IU • Vitamin C USP (as ascorbic acid) 90 mg • Vitamin D USP (as cholecalciferol) 400 IU • Vitamin E (as d-alpha tocopheryl acetate) 30 IU • Vitamin K (as phytonadione) 25 mcg • Thiamin USP (as thiamin mononitrate; vitamin B-1) 2.25 mg • Riboflavin USP (vitamin B-2) 2.6 mg • Niacinamide 20 mg • Vitamin B-6 (pyridoxine HCl) 3 mg • Folic Acid 400 mcg • Vitamin B-12 (as cyanocobalamin) 9 mcg • Biotin 25 mcg • Pantothenic Acid (as d-calcium pantothenate) 10 mg • Calcium (from dicalcium phosphate) 162 mg • Iron (as ferrous fumarate) 27 mg • Iodine (as potassium iodide) 150 mcg • Magnesium (from magnesium oxide) 100 mg • Zinc (from zinc fultate) 15 mg • Selenium (as sodium selenate) 25 mcg • Copper (from copper gluconate) 2 mg • Manganese (from manganese sulfate) 5 mg • Chromium (as chromium chloride) 25 mcg • Molybdenum (sodium molybdate) 25 mcg • Potassium (as potassium chloride) 57.2 mg.

Cerebra - Natrapharm, Inc.
Each tablet contains: Huperzine A (Chinese club moss) 50 mcg • Vitamin E.

Cerebrex - Gero Vita International
Each capsule contains: Vitamin B6 (as pyridoxol-5-phosphate) 6.7 mg • Folic Acid 300 mcg • Citrus Bioflavonoids (13% bioflavonoids) 300 mg • Phosphatidylserine 150 mg • Ginkgo Biloba leaf extract (24% ginkgo flavoneglycosides/6% terpene lactones) 50 mg • Mixed Tocopherols 20 IU • Methylcobalamin 100 mcg. Other Ingredients: Rice Flour, Silicon Dioxide, Magnesium Stearate, Gelatin Capsule, ACF 223.

Cernilton Flower Pollen - Cernitin America
Two tablets contain: Rye Grass Pollen (Cernitin Flower Pollen) Extract Water-Soluble Pollen Extract (T60) 120 mg • Cernitin Flower Pollen Extract Fat-Soluble Pollen Concentrate (GBX) 6 mg. Other Ingredients: Cellulose (plant fiber), Magnesium Stearate (vegetable source).

Cernilton T.S. Flower Pollen Triple Strength - Cernitin America
Two capsules contain: Rye Grass Pollen (Cernitin Flower Pollen) Extract Water-Soluble Pollen concentrate (T60) 360 mg • Cernitin Flower Pollen extract fat-soluble pollen concentrate (GBX) 18 mg. Other Ingredients: Cellulose (plant fiber), Magnesium Stearate (vegetable source).

Certain Sleep - Gero Vita International
Two capsules contain: Vitamin B6 (as pyridoxine hydrochloride) 0.5 mg • Magnesium (as magnesium aspartate) 18.74 mg • Zinc (as zinc monomethionine, aspartate) 1.26 mg • Proprietary Blend 900 mg: Jujube seed extract, Schisandra fruit extract (10% schisandrin), Polygala root extract, Anemorrhena rhizome extract (1% sarsosapogenin), Chinese Thoroughwax root extract, Uncaria Rhynchophylla stem extract • 5-Hydroxytryptophan 100 mg. Other Ingredients: Silicon Dioxide, Magnesium Stearate, Gelatin.

Cetyl Myristoleate Complex - PhysioLogics
Each capsule contains: Cetyl Myristoleate Complex 550 mg. Other Ingredients: Gelatin, Vegetable Magnesium Stearate, Silica.

CetylPure - Natrol
Two capsules contain: Cetyl Myristoleate proprietary blend (CetylPure) 1100 mg. Other Ingredients: Silica, Magnesium Stearate, Gelatin.

CFS/FM Energy Formula - Pro Health
Three capsules contain: Vitamin B12 (as cyanocobalamin) 500 mcg • Pantothenic Acid (as d-calcium pantothenate) 25 mg • Magnesium (as potassium magnesium aspartate, dihydrate) 98 mg • Potassium (as potassium magnesium aspartate, dihydrate) 98 mg • 7-Keto 1 DHEA (3-acetyl-7-oxo-dehydroepiandrosterone) 10 mg • Acetyl-L-Carnitine HCl 500 mg • Borage Oil (borago officinalis, spray-dried herb, 11.5% gamma linoleic acid 15 mg) 130.5 mg • Alpha Lipoic Acid 200 mg • Coenzyme Q10 (as ubidicarenone) 10 mg • D-ribose 50 mg • L-Taurine (free form amino acid) 500 mg • Malic Acid (from apples) 200 mg • Panax Ginseng root powder 200 mg. Other Ingredients: Gelatin, Calcium Silicate, Magnesium Stearate, Water.

CFS/FM Multi with Malic Acid - Pro Health
Each tablet contains: Vitamin A (natural fish liver oil) 7500 IU • Beta-Carotene 10,000 IU • Vitamin B1 (thiamine HCl) 50 mg • Vitamin B2 (riboflavin) 50 mg • Vitamin B3 (niacinamide) 50 mg • Vitamin B5 (pantothenic acid) 50 mg • Vitamin B6 (pyridoxine HCl) 50 mg • Vitamin B12 (cyanocobalamin) 250 mcg • Biotin 100 mcg • Folic Acid 400 mcg • Vitamin C (ascorbic acid) 250 mg • Vitamin D (natural fish liver oil) 400 IU • Vitamin E (100% d-alpha) 150 IU • Calcium (amino acid chelate, oystershell) 100 mg • Magnesium (oxide, amino acid chelate) 60 mg • Zinc (amino acid chelate) 15 mg

• Copper (amino acid chelate) 1 mg • Iodine (kelp) 150 mcg • Iron (amino acid chelate) 10 mg • Choline (bitartrate) 100 mg • Inositol 75 mg • PABA 30 mg • Rutin 25 mg • Citrus Bioflavonoids 100 mg • Betaine (HCl) 25 mg • Glutamic Acid 25 mg • Potassium (amino acid chelate) 10 mg • Manganese (amino acid chelate) 5 mg • Selenium (amino acid chelate) 200 mcg • Chromium (yeast-free gtf) 250 mcg • Boron (amino acid chelate) 500 mcg • Molybdenum (amino acid chelate) 50 mcg • Nucleic Acid 50 mg • Malic Acid 100 mg • Magnesium Hydroxide 25 mg • IP-6 100 mg • Nova Soy 50 mg. Other Ingredients: Alfalfa, Parsley, Lecithin, Rose Hips, Di-Calcium Phosphate, Cellulose, Stearic Acid, Silica.

CGP **-** Metabolic Nutrition
Each scoop (2 tsp) contains: Creatine - Glycerol - Phosphate 10 g • Potassium 720 mg • Alpha-Lipoic Acid 100 mg • Magnesium 75 mg • Calcium 50 mg • Sodium 30 mg.

C-Grams **-** Advocare International
Two caplets contain: Vitamin C (as potassium/magnesium/calcium ascorbates and ascorbic acid) 1000 mg • L-Lysine 300 mg • Mixed Citrus Flavonoids 100 mg • Alpha-Ketoglutaric Acid 50 mg. Other Ingredients: Dicalcium Phosphate, Silicon Dioxide, Cellulose, Stearic Acid, Magnesium Stearate.

CGT10 **-** Optimum Nutrition
Each 2 tsp (20 g) serving contains: Creatine Monohydrate 5 g • L-Glutamine 3 g • Taurine 2 g. Other Ingredients: Dextrose, Citric Acid, Beet Color, Artificial Flavor, Acesulfame Potassium.

Chamomile **-** Nature's Way
Two capsules contain: Chamomile flower 700 mg. Other Ingredients: Gelatin.

Chamomile & Ylang Ylang Body Lotion 8oz **-** Derma E
Purified Water • Jojoba Oil • Safflower oil • Glycerin • Octylpalmitate • Glyceryl Stearate • PEG 100 Stearate • Cetyl Alcohol • Tocopheryl Acetate (vitamin E) • Lavender oil • Geranium oil • Panthenol • Allantoin • Retinyl Palmitate (vitamin A) • Ergocalciferol (vitamin D) • Methylparaben • I. Urea • Fragrant Oils.

Chamomile Calm **-** Botanical Laboratories
Each 1 mL serving contains: Skullcap herb • Chamomile flowers • Fennel seed • Hops strobiles • Catnip herb. Other Ingredients: Kosher Coconut and/or Palm Kernal Glycerine, Purified Water, Citric Acid.

Change-O-Life 7 Herb Blend Formula **-** Nature's Way
Three capsules contain: Proprietary Blend 1320 mg: Black Cohosh root, Blessed Thistle, Eleuthero root, False Unicorn root, Licorice root, Sarsaparilla root, Squaw Vine (vine, leaf, fruit). Other Ingredients: Gelatin, Magnesium Stearate.

Changes Now **-** Changes International, Inc.
Two capsules contain: Vitamin C (Ascorbic acid) 50 mg • Lipase 300 LU • Calcium sulfate 100 mg • Multi-Source Fiber Complex 650 mg: Chitosan (Deacylated cellulose biopolymer), Glucomannan, Citrus Pectin, and Oat fiber. Other Ingredients: Gelatin, Magnesium stearate, and Silica.

Changes Relief **-** Changes International, Inc.
Three caplets contain: Vitamin C (as Ascorbic Acid) 100 mg • Calcium (as Calcium Monohydrogen Phosphate) 300 mg • Phosphorus (as Calcium Monohydrogen Phosphate) 225 mg • Zinc (as Zinc Monomethionine) 13.75 mg • Copper (as Copper Gluconate) 500 mcg • Manganese (as Manganese Sulfate) 5 mg • Glucosamine Hydrochloride/Glucosamine Sulfate/N-Acetyl Glucosamine blend (with Chondroitin precursors) 750 mg • Turmeric rhizome standardized extract (12x) 300 mg • Boswellia serrata gum-resin 300 mg • Devil's Claw root standardized extract (5% harpagosides) 125 mg • Bromelain (80 GDU/g) 125 mg • White Willow bark 4:1 extract 150 mg • Ginger root standardized extract (5% gingerols) 125 mg • Alpine Snow Rose leaf (50% active polyphenolic proanthocyanidins) 213 mg. Other Ingredients: Vegetable cellulose, Fractionated vegetable oil, Soy polysaccharides, Silica, and Vegetable resin glaze. See Editor's Note No. 15, page 2055.

Changing Times **-** Nature's Plus
Two tablets contain: Wild Brazilian SUMA (Pfaffia paniculata [Martius] Kuntze) 300 mg • Calcium amino acid chelate/complex 200 mg • Magnesium amino acid chelate/complex 100 mg • Vitamin B6 (Pyridoxine HCL) 100 mg • Pantothenic Acid 100 mg • Phosphatidylcholine 100 mg • Siberian Ginseng (Eleutherococcus senticosus) 100 mg • Niacinamide 25 mg • Vitamin E natural 200 IU • Vitamin B12 from Cobalamin 200 mcg • Selenium yeast free, amino acid complex 50 mcg. Yeast free. Sugar & starch free.

Chaparral and Red Clover **-** Dial Herbs
Chaparral • Red Clover • Echinacea • Buchu leaves • Blood root.

Charcoal **-** Country Life
Each capsule contains: Activated Charcoal 520 mg.

Charcoal **-** Source Naturals
Each capsule contains: Charcoal 260 mg.

Charcoal **-** Nature's Way
Two capsules contain: Activated Charcoal 560 mg. Other Ingredients: Gelatin.

Charco-Zyme **-** Atrium Inc.
Each capsule contains: Papaya leaf 65 mg • Papain 32.5 mg • Mycozyme 32.5 mg • Rennin NF 3.75 mg • Activated Charcoal 130 mg. In a base of Alfalfa & Peppermint.

Chase Kolic Gripe Water **-** Stella Pharmaceutical Canada, Inc.
Each 5 mL contains: Alcohol Anhydrous 0.1945 mL • Ginger 0.05 mL • Dill Oil 0.002 mL • Sodium Bicarbonate 50 mg.

Chase Kolik Alcohol Free Gripe Water **-** Stella Pharmaceutical Canada, Inc.
Each 150 mL contains: Fennel Oil 0.05% • Sodium Bicarbonate 1%.

Chaser - Freedom From Hangovers **-** Living Essentials
Each two capsules contain: Activated Calcium Carbonate 618 mg • Vegetable Carbon 332 mg.

Chaser - Wine **-** Living Essentials
Each two caplets contains: Activated Calcium Carbonate 650 mg • Vegetable Carbon 350 mg • Vitamin B2 1 mg. Other Ingredients: Croscarmellose Sodium, Sucrose, Cellulose, Stearic Acid, Magnesium Citrate.

Chaste Tree-Siberian Ginseng Virtue **-** Blessed Herbs
Chaste Tree berry • Siberian Ginseng root • Hawthorn berry, leaf & flower • Lavender flower • Wild Yam root • Licorice root • Grain alcohol & Distilled Water.

Chasteberry Extract **-** Enzymatic Therapy
Each capsule contains: Chaste Tree berry extract (vitex agnus-castus, standardized to contain 0.5% agnusides) 225 mg. Other Ingredients: Gelatin, Cellulose, Magnesium Stearate, Silicon Dioxide, Titanium Dioxide Color.

Cheat Tabs **-** Fizogen
Three tablets contain: Enzytrox (calorie intercepting agent) 2000 mg: Glucomannan, Phaseolus Vulgaris extract, Platycodi radix extract, Garcinia Cambogia extract, Pandalidus Biopolymer extract • Neurotrol (appetite controlling blend) 130 mg: Hoodia Gordonii cactus extract, Caralluma cactus extract, Simthin Jojoba seed extract, Griffonia Simplicifolia seed extract • Digestol (hyper digestive fusion) 75 mg: Terminalia Chebula fruit extract, Terminlais Belerica fruit extract, Emblica Officinalis fruit extract. Other Ingredients: Di Calcium Phosphate, Magnesium Stearate, Stearic Histrene, Maltodextrin, Plasdone, Acesulfame-K.

Chelated Calcium **-** Puritan's Pride
Six tablets contain: Calcium (as Calcium Amino Acid Chelate) 900 mg.

Some Brand Name Natural Products - What they Contain

www.NaturalDatabase.com contains MANY more listings than appear here.

Chelated Calcium Magnesium **-** Nature's Bounty
Two tablets contain: Calcium (as calcium carbonate, oyster shell, and calcium gluconate) 1000 mg • Magnesium (as magnesium oxide and magnesium gluconate) 500 mg. Other Ingredients: Cellulose (plant origin), Croscarmellose, Titanium Dioxide Color, Cellulose Coating, Vegetable Magnesium Stearate.

Chelated Calcium Magnesium Zinc **-** Nature's Bounty
Three tablets contain: Calcium (as Calcium Carbonate and Calcium Gluconate) 1000 mg • Magnesium (as Magnesium Oxide and Magnesium Gluconate) 400 mg • Zinc (as Zinc Gluconate and Zinc Citrate) 25 mg. Other Ingredients: Cellulose, Croscarmellose, Acacia Gum, Maltodextrin, Titanium Dioxide Color, Cellulose Coating, Vegetable Magnesium Stearate.

Chelated Calcium-Magnesium **-** Schiff
Six tablets contain: Calcium (as calcium glycinate from rice protein chelate) 780 mg • Magnesium (as magnesium glycinate from rice protein chelate) 468 mg. Other Ingredients: Citric Acid, Cellulose, Croscarmellose Sodium, Magnesium Stearate.

Chelated CAL-MAG **-** Puritan's Pride
Each tablet contains: Calcium 500 mg • Magnesium 250 mg.

Chelated Potassium 99 mg (Inspired By Nature) **-** Puritan's Pride
Each caplet contains: Potassium (as potassium gluconate) 99 mg. Other Ingredients: Crospovidone, Vegetable Stearic Acid, Silica, Vegetable Magnesium Stearate, Cellulose Coating.

Chelated Zinc 100 mg **-** Puritan's Pride
Each tablet contains: Zinc (from Zinc Gluconate) 100 mg.

Chelated Zinc 25 mg **-** Puritan's Pride
Each tablet contains: Zinc (from Zinc Gluconate) 25 mg.

Chelated Zinc 50 mg **-** Puritan's Pride
Each tablet contains: Zinc (from Zinc Gluconate) 50 mg.

Chelated Zinc Lozenges 23 mg (Inspired By Nature) **-** Puritan's Pride
Each lozenge contains: Zinc (as zinc citrate and zinc gluconate) 23 mg. Other Ingredients: Fructose, Sorbitol, Honey Powder, Vegetable Stearic Acid, Citric Acid, Silica, Vegetable Magnesium Stearate, Natural Lemon Flavor, Orange Flavor.

Chem-Defense **-** Source Naturals
Each tablet contains: Molybdenum (aspartate, citrate) 120 mcg • Glutathione 50 mg • Coenzymated Vitamin B-2 (flavin mononucle-otide) 2.25 mg.

Chem-Ex **-** Enzymatic Therapy
Two capsules contain: Pantothenic Acid (D-Calcium Pantothenate) 80 mg • Zinc (Chelate) 40 mg • L-Cysteine 300 mg • L-Methionine 200 mg • Alpha-Ketoglutarate 60 mg • Taurine 50 mg • Glycine 40 mg. This exclusive formula also contains Licorice root extracts (Glycyrrhiza glabra).

Cherry Fruit Extract **-** Enzymatic Therapy/PhytoPharmica
Two capsules contain: Sweet Cherry fruit 10:1 extract (prunus avium) 1000 mg.

Chew Chew Vites Multiple **-** Nature's Life
Two tablets contain: Vitamin A (Fish Liver oil) 5000 IU • Vitamin D (as Vitamin D3) (Cholecalciferol) 400 IU • Vitamin E (d-Alpha Tocopheryl with Beta, Gamma, & Delta Tocopherols) 30 IU • Vitamin B1 (Thiamine HCl) 5 mg • Vitamin B2 (Riboflavin) 5 mg • Vitamin B6 Pyridoxine HCl) 5 mg • Vitamin B12 (Cyanocobalamin) 10 mcg • Niacinamide 10 mg • Pantothenic Acid (d-Calcium Pantothenate) 10 mg • Folic Acid 0.1 mg • Choline (Bitartrate) 25 mcg • Inositol 25 mcg • PABA (Para Aminobenzoic Acid) 300 mcg • Biotin 75 mcg • Vitamin C (with Rose Hips) 150 mg • Calcium (Carbonate, Gluconate, Citrate) 28 mg • Chromium (Picolinate Nutrition 21) 50 mcg • Copper (Full ranged Amino Acid Chelate) 0.1 mg • Iodine (Kelp) 0.1 mg • Iron (Full ranged Amino Acid Chelate) 5 mg • Magnesium (Full ranged Amino Acid Chelate)15 mg • Manganese (Full ranged Amino Acid Chelate) 0.3 mg • Phosphorus (Proteinate) 4 mg • Potassium (Proteinate) 11.5 mg • Silicon (Dioxide) 5 mg • Zinc (Picolinate) 2 mcg • Essential Fatty Acids 5 mg • Hawaiian Spirulina 10 mg • Chlorophyll, Alfalfa 10 mg • Chlorella algae 10 mg. In a natural base of low Glycemic pure Crystalline Fructose, pasteurized Honey powder, natural Lemon flavor, Vegetarian Acidophilus powder, natural Pineapple flavor, Rose Hips powder, Lecithin, Lemon Bioflavonoids, Barley Grass, Sunflower Seed powder, Rice Bran, Wheat Germ, Alfalfa leaf, Watercress & Parsley.

Chewable Acerola C Complex 500 mg **-** The Vitamin Shoppe
Each wafer contains: Vitamin C (fortified with Acerola extract & Rose Hips Concentrate) 500 mg • Bioflavonoid complex 50 mg. Sweetened exclusively with fructose, a naturally occurring sweetener found in fruit, and all-natural Acerola cherry flavoring.

Chewable C 500 Cherry Flavor - GNC A-Z **-** GNC
Each tablet contains: Vitamin A (100% as beta-carotene) 1000 IU • Vitamin C (as ascorbic acid and sodium ascorbate) 500 mg • Vitamin E (as dl-alpha tocopheryl acetate) 5 mg. • Citrus Bioflavonoids Complex 5 mg. Other Ingredients: Sorbitol, Cellulose, Artificial and Natural Flavors, Stevia leaves powder.

Chewable C 500 Fruit Flavor - GNC A-Z **-** GNC
Each tablet contains: Vitamin C (as ascorbic acid) 500 mg • Citrus Bioflavonoids Complex 5 mg. Other Ingredients: Dextrose, Turbinado Sugar, Cellulose, Artificial Flavor, Rose Hips powder (Rosina Canina), Acerola, Black Currant powder, Green Pepper powder, Hesperidin Complex, Rutin powder, Citrus Pectin, Potassium Chloride, Magnesium Oxide.

Chewable C 500 Orange Flavor - GNC A-Z **-** GNC
Each tablet contains: Vitamin C (as ascorbic acid and sodium ascorbate with other natural sources of Vitamin C) 500 mg • Vitamin E (as dl-alpha tocopheryl acetate) 5 IU • Citrus Bioflavonoids Complex (from 12.5 mg of citrus bioflavonids complex 4X) 50 mg. Other Ingredients: Sorbitol, Natural Color (annatto), Natural Flavors, Magnesium Stearate, Cellulose, Acrola, Black Currant, Green Pepper.

Chewable C-500 mg with Rose Hips **-** Puritan's Pride
Each tablet contains: Vitamin C with Rose Hips 500 mg.

Chewable Cal Mag Plus **-** Shaklee
Four tablets contain: Vitamin D (as Cholecalciferol) 200 IU • Calcium (as Calcium carbonate and Calcium citrate) • 1000 mg • Magnesium (as Magnesium oxide) 100 mg • Zinc (as Zinc gluconate) 1.5 mg • Copper (as Copper gluconate) 0.2 mg • Manganese (as Manganese gluconate) 0.2 mg • Boron (as Boron protein hydrolysate) 1.0 mg. Other Ingredients: Dextrose, Mannitol, Sorbitol, Acacia Gum, Natural Berry, Other Flavors, Citric Acid.

Chewable Calcium **-** Rexall - Sundown
Each tablet contains: Vitamin D (as cholecalciferol) 100 IU • Calcium (as calcium carbonate) 600 mg. Other Ingredients: Dicalcium Phosphate, Microcrystalline Cellulose, Hydroxypropyl Merthylcellulose, Hydrogenated Cottonseed Oil, Magnesium Stearate, PEG.

Chewable Calcium + D **-** Leiner Health Products
Each tablet contains: Calcium Carbonate 300 mg • Vitamin D (Ergocalciferol) 100 IU • Calories 5. Other Ingredients: Sorbitol, Stearic Acid, Cocoa, Magnesium Stearate, Maltodextrin, Silicon Dioixde, Natural Vanilla, Maltol, Gelatin.

Chewable Calcium 600 Cherry Flavor - GNC A-Z **-** GNC
Each tablet contains: Vitamin D (as cholecalciferol) 200 IU • Calcium (as calcium carbonate, tricalcium phosphate and calcium citrate) 600 mg • Boron (as boron gluconate) 1 mg. Other Ingredients: Sorbitol, Mannitol, Natural Flavor.

Some Brand Name Natural Products - What they Contain

www.NaturalDatabase.com contains MANY more listings than appear here.

Chewable Calcium with Vitamin D **-** Nature's Bounty
Four wafers contain: Vitamin D (as Ergocalciferol) 400 IU • Calcium (as Calcium Carbonate and Dicalcium Phosphate) 560 mg • Phosphorus (as Dicalcium Phosphate) 100 mg • Buckwheat (Fagopyrum esculentum) seed 10.4 mg • Corn Bran (Zea mays) seed 10.4 mg. Other Ingredients: Sucrose, Dextrose, Cellulose, Acacia Gum, Cottonseed Oil, Artificial Flavor, Silica, Vegetable Magnesium Stearate, Sodium Chloride.

Chewable Cellular Forte with IP-6 and Inositol **-** PhytoPharmica
Each tablet contains: Calcium (from calcium magnesium phytate) 130 mg &#8226 Inositol 220 mg &#8226 IP-6 (inositol hexaphosphate from calcium magnesium phytate) 800 mg &#8226 Magnesium (from calcium magnesium phytate) 40 mg &#8226 Phosphorus (from calcium magnesium phytate) 190 mg.

Chewable Digestion **-** Enzymes, Inc.
Each chewable tablet contains: Proprietary Enzyme Blend 209 mg: Amylase, Invertase, Glucoamylase, Protease, Lipase, Malt Diastase, Lactase, Cellulase, Pectinase, CereCalase, alpha-Galactosidase, Peptidase. Other Ingredients: Dextrose (Corn Sugar), Fructose (Fruit Sugar), Natural Raspberry Flavor, Silica (Mineral), Plant Cellulose, Citric Acid, Veg. Magnesium Stearate, Proprietary Plant-derived Sweetener.

Chewable E **-** Country Life
Each wafer contains: Vitamin E (D-alpha tocopheryl succinate) 450 IU.

Chewable E 400 - GNC A-Z **-** GNC
Each tablet contains: Vitamin E (as d-alpha Tocopheryl Succinate) 400 IU. Other Ingredients: Dextron, Sorbitol, Fructose, Cellulose, Natural Flavors.

Chewable Echinacea **-** Leiner Health Products
Two tablets contain: Vitamin C (Ascorbic Acid) 60 mg • Total Carbohydrates 2 g • Echinacea Purpurea root powder 25 mg. Other Ingredients: Dextrose, Natural Raspberry Flavor, Magnesium Stearate, Silicon Dioxide, Carmine.

Chewable Ester-C 300 **-** GNC
Each tablet contains: Vitamin C (as Ester-C Calcium Ascorbate) 300 mg. Other Ingredients: Sorbitol, Sucrose, Dextrose, Fructose, Carrageenan, Citric Acid, Natural Wildberry Flavor, Sucralose.

Chewable Glucosamine Sulfate **-** J. R. Carlson Laboratories, Inc.
Each tablet contains: Glucosamine Sulfate (providing sulfur 4 g) 500 mg.

Chewable Orange Juice C 500 mg **-** The Vitamin Shoppe
Each chewable tablet contains: 500 mg Vitamin C, blend of natural Orange Juice concentrate, Orange Juice pulp, Orange peels, and natural fruit sugar.

Chewable Q-60 + Creatine **-** Jarrow Formulas
Each tablet contains: Coenzyme Q10 (from biologically fermented soy) 60 mg • Creatine (from sarcosine) 500 mg. Other Ingredients: Xylitol, Fibersol (maltodextrin), Magnesium Stearate (vegetable source), Lo Han Quo, Microcrystalline Cellulose, Silicon Dioxide, Stearic Acid (veggie), Natural Orange Cream Flavor.

Chewable Vita C **-** Shaklee
Each tablet contains: Vitamin C (as Ascorbic acid) 100 mg. Other Ingredients: Sorbitol, Rosehips Powder, Natural Lemon Flavor, Lemon Bioflavonoid, Hesperidin Complex, Orange Bioflavonoid, Grapefruit Bioflavonoid, Grapefruit Oil.

Chewable Vitamin C - Basic Nutrition **-** GNC
Each tablet contains: Vitamin C (as Ascorbic Acid and other natural sources of Vitamin C) 100 mg • Citrus Bioflavonoids Complex 5 mg. Other Ingredients: Dextrose, Turbinado Sugar, Stearic Acid, Magnesium Stearate, Artificial Flavor, Rose hips, Acerola, Black Currant, Green Pepper, Hesperidin, Rutin, Citrus pectin, Potassium Chloride, Magnesium Oxide.

Chewable Vitamin C - YourLife **-** Leiner Health Products
Each tablet contains: Vitamin C (Ascorbic Acid) 500 mg • Sodium 40 mg. Other Ingredients: Sucrose, Sodium Ascorbate, Stearic Acid, Starch, Natural flavor, Magnesium Stearate, Silicon Dioxide, Sorbitol, Yellow 6 Lake, Lactose, Ethylmaltol.

Chewable Vitamin C 500 mg **-** Nature Made
Each tablet contains: Vitamin C (from sodium ascorbate, ascorbic acid, lemon bioflavonoids) 500 mg. Other Ingredients: Sugar, Fructose, Stearic Acid, Dextrose, Maltodextrin, Corn Starch, Magnesium Stearate, Natural Orange Flavors with Other Natural Flavors, Silica Gel.
See Editor's Note No. 45, page 2058.

Chewable Vitamin C 500MG **-** Nature Made
Each tablet contains: Vitamin C 500 mg • Sodium 40 mg.
See Editor's Note No. 45, page 2058.

Chewable Vitamin C with Acerola **-** Leiner Health Products
Each wafer contains: Vitamin C 500 mg • Other Ingredients: Sugar, Ascorbic Acid, Stearic Acid, Cellulose, Silicon Dioxide, Artificial Flavor, Acerola, Magnesium Stearate, Starch, Rose Hips, Lemon Bioflavonoids Complex, Hesperidin Complex, Buckwheat, Caramel, Rutin, Green Pepper Extract, Black Currant Extract.

Chewy C 500 Orange **-** GNC
Each chew contains: Vitamin C 500 mg. Ingredients: Corn syrup, Sugar, Partially Hydrogenated Soybean oil, Ascorbic Acid, Mono & Diglycerides, Soy Lecithin, Salt, Natural Flavor, FD&C Yellow #6.

CHI Chinese Herbal Bar **-** Nature's Plus
Each 1.5 oz. bar contains: Ancient Chinese Herbs: Huang Qi (Astragalus root) 312 mg • Dang Shen (Relative root) 228 mg • Ling Zhi (Reishi mushroom) 192 mg • Bai Zhu (Attractylodes root) 144 mg • Ji Xue Teng (Millettia stem) 144 mg • Tu Si Zi (Dodder seed) 144 mg • Shan Yao (Chinese Yam root) 144 mg • Nu Zhen zi (Privet fruit) 144 mg • Di Huang (Rehmannia root) 138 mg • Bei Sha Shen (Sand root) 136 mg • Wu Wei Zi (Schisandra fruit) 114 mg • Jiang (Ginger root) 114 mg • Suan Zao Ren (Jujube seed) 114 mg • Chieh Keng (Balloon Flower root) 114 mg • Gan Cao (Licorice root) 108 mg • Peony root (bai shoa) 72 mg • Ju Luo (Tangerine peel) 72 mg.

Chickweed Formula **-** Quest
Each caplet contains: Chickweed powder (Stellaria media) 120 mg • Fennel seed powder (Foeniculum vulgare) 80 mg • Burdock root powder (Actium lappa) 80 mg • Chia seeds powder (Salvia columbariae) 70 mg • Bladderwrack powder (Fucus Vesiculosis) 30 mg • Kelp powder (Fucus Vesiculosis) 30 mg. Other Ingredients: Calcium Phosphate, Microcrystalline Cellulose, Vegetable Stearin, Croscarmellose Sodium, Magnesium Stearate (vegetable source).

Child Lax **-** Dial Herbs
Senna • Fennel • Rhubarb.

Children Immu-C **-** Nutri-Quest Rx
Each tablet contains: Vitamin C (Sago Palm) 125 mg • Biotin 20 mcg • Folic Acid 10 mcg • Vitamin A (Palmitate) 1500 IU • Rutin 7.5 mg • Lemon Bioflavonoids 10 mg • Hesperidin Complex 7.5 mg • Propolis 1 mg • Lymph 1 mg • Thymus 1 mg • Spleen 1 mg. In a base of Fructose & Maltodextrin, with pleasant tasting Tropical Fruit Flavoring.
See Editor's Note No. 14.

Children's Chewable Vita-Bear **-** The Vitamin Shoppe
Each tablet contains: Vitamin C 200 mg • Citrus Bioflavonoid Complex 20 mg.

Children's Chewable Vitamin C **-** Health Smart Vitamins
Each tablet contains: Vitamin C (as ascorbic acid) 250 mg.

Some Brand Name Natural Products - What they Contain

www.NaturalDatabase.com contains MANY more listings than appear here.

Children's Chewable Vitamins with Minerals - Schiff
Each tablet contains: Vitamin A (as palmitate) 5000 IU • Vitamin C (as ascorbic acid) 60 mg • Vitamin D (as cholecalciferol) 400 IU • Vitamin E (as d-alpha tocopheryl succinate) 30 IU • Thiamin (as mononitrate) 1.5 mg • Riboflavin 1.7 mg • Niacin (as niacinamide) 20 mg • Vitamin B-6 (as pyridoxine hydrochloride) 2 mg • Folic Acid 400 mcg • Vitamin B-12 (as cyanocobalamin) 6 mcg • Calcium (as calcium phosphate) 41 mg • Iron (as ferrous fumarate) 18 mg • Phosphorus (as calcium phosphate) 31 mg • Magnesium (as oxide) 6 mg • Zinc (as oxide) 2 mg. Other Ingredients: Fructose, Cellulose, Sorbitol, Stearic Acid, Natural Flavor, Silica, Magnesium Stearate, Citric Acid.

Children's Chewables - Swanson
Each tablet contains: Vitamin A (as acetate, beta-carotene) 2500 IU • Vitamin C USP (as ascorbic acid) 60 mg • Vitamin D (as cholecalciferol) 400 IU • Vitamin E (as d-alpha tocopheryl acetate) 15 IU • Thiamin USP (as thiamin HCl; vitamin B-1) 1.05 mg • Riboflavin USP (vitamin B-2) 1.2 mg • Niacinamide 13.5 mg • Vitamin B-6 (pyridoxine HCl) 1.05 mg • Folic Acid 300 mcg • Vitamin B-12 (cyanocobalamin) 4.5 mcg.

Children's Echinacea+C+Zinc Raspberry Flavor - LiFizz Effervescent Vitamins
Each tablet contains: Vitamin C 400 mg • Zinc (Zinc Oxide, Zinc Sulfate) 10 mg • Echinacea extract (Echinacea purpurea) 67 mg. Other Ingredients: Citric Acid, Sodium Bicarbonate, Sorbitol, Mannitol, Red Beet Powder, Raspberry Flavor, Polyethylene Glycol 6000, Aspartame, Acesulfame Potassium, Wild Berry Powder, Magnesium Stearate, Silicon Dioxide.

Children's Multi Vitamins - Jamieson
Each tablet contains: Vitamin A 5000 IU • Vitamin D (as Vitamin D3) 400 IU • Vitamin C 100 mg • Vitamin E 5 IU • Vitamin B1 1.5 mg • Vitamin B2 1.2 mg • Vitamin B6 1 mg • Vitamin B12 6 mcg • Pantothenic Acid 10 mg • Niacinamide 10 mg • Iron 5 mg.

Children's Multi-Vi-Min - NutriCology
Each capsule contains: Vitamin A (as retinyl palmitate) 800 IU • Vitamin E (as DL-alpha-tocopheryl-acetate) 16 IU • Thiamin (as thiamin hydrochloride) 4 mg • Riboflavin (as riboflavin-5-phosphate) 2 mg • Niacin (as niacinamide) 2 mg • Vitamin B6 (as pyridoxine hydrochloride and pyridoxal-5-phosphate) 6.2 mg • Folic Acid 12 mcg • Vitamin B12 32 mcg • Biotin 16 mcg • Pantothenic Acid (as calcium pantothenate) 20 mg • Iron (as ferric ammonium citrate) 0.7 mg • Magnesium (as magnesium citrate) 10 mg • Zinc (as zinc citrate) 1.1 mg • Selenium (as sodium selenite) 8 mcg • Copper (as copper citrate) 60 mcg • Manganese (as manganese citrate) 0.6 mcg • Chromium (as amino acid complex) 16 mcg • Molybdenum (as sodium molybdate) 8 mcg • Potassium (as potassium chloride) 4 mg • Vanadium (as vanadium pentoxide) 8 mcg • PABA (para-aminobenzoic acid) 8 mg • Glutamic Acid 8 mg. Other Ingredients: Cellulose, Magnesium Stearate, Silicon Dioxide.

Children's Multivitamin Liquid - Schiff
Two teaspoons (10 ml) contain: Vitamin A (as vitamin a acetate) 2500 IU • Vitamin C (as ascorbic acid) 40 mg • Vitamin D (as cholecalciferol) 400 IU • Vitamin E (as alpha tocopheryl acetate) 10 IU • Thiamin (as thiamin hydrochloride) 0.7 mg • Riboflavin (as riboflavin-5-phosphate) 0.8 mg • Niacin (as niacinamide) 9 mg • Vitamin B6 (as pyridoxine hydrochloride) 0.7 mg • Folate (as folic acid) 200 mcg • Vitamin B12 (as cyanocobalamin) 3 mcg • Biotin 150 mcg • Pantothenic Acid (as d-calcium pantothenate) 5 mg • Iron (as ferrous sulfate) 10 mg • Zinc (as zinc sulfate) 8 mg. Other Ingredients: Malitol, Water, Glycerin, Prepylene Glycol, Natural Flavor, Carrageenan, Citric Acid.

Children's Multi-Vitamins - LiFizz Effervescent Vitamins
Each tablet contains: Vitamin A 2500 IU • Vitamin C 60 mg • Vitamin D 200 IU • Vitamin E 9 IU • Thiamin 1.05 mg • Riboflavin 1.19 mg • Niacinamide 14 mg • Vitamin B6 1.4 mg • Folic Acid 280 mcg • Vitamin B12 4.2 mcg • Biotin 210 mcg • Pantothenic Acid 7.9 mg • Calcium 200 mg. Available in Grape, Bubblegum, Orange, and Fruit Punch flavors.

Children's Vita-Gels - Nature's Plus
Each softgel contains: Vitamin A (as beta carotene) 5000 IU • Vitamin C (as ascorbic acid) 50 mg • Vitamin D (as ergocalciferol) 200 IU • Vitamin E (as d-alpha tocopheryl acetate) 25 IU • Vitamin B1 (as thiamine HCl) 5 mg • Vitamin B2 (as riboflavin) 5 mg • Niacin (as niacinamide) 10 mg • Vitamin B6 (as pyridoxine HCl) 5 mg • Folate (as folic acid) 10 mcg • Vitamin B12 (as cyanocobalamin) 10 mcg • Biotin 50 mcg • Pantothenic Acid (as calcium pantothenate) 10 mg • Calcium (as gluconate) 10 mg • Iron (as gluconate) 5 mg • Iodine (from kelp) 100 mcg • Magnesium (as gluconate) 0.25 mg • Zinc (as gluconate) 0.25 mg • Manganese (as gluconate) 0.05 mg • Potassium (as gluconate) 1 mg • Choline (as bitartrate) 2 mg • Inositol 1 mg • PABA (para-aminobenzoic acid) 0.6 mg.

Child's Chewable Vitamins + Iron - Penwel
Each tablet contains: Vitamin A (Acetate & Beta Carotene) 2500 IU • Vitamin D (Ergocalciferol) 400 IU • Vitamin E (dl-Alpha tocopheryl Acetate) 15 IU • Vitamin C (Ascorbic Acid & Sodium Ascorbate) 60 mg • Folic Acid 0.3 mcg • Thiamine Mononitrate (Vitamin B1) 1.05 mg • Riboflavin (Vitamin B2) 1.2 mg • Niacin (Niacinamide) 13.5 mg • Vitamin B6 (Pyridoxine HCl) 1.05 mg • Vitamin B12 (Cyanocobalamin) 4.5 mcg • Iron (Ferrous Fumarate) 15 mg. Other Ingredients: Sugar, Corn Syrup Solids, Partially Hydrogenated Vegetable Oil, Stearic Acid, Maltodextrin, Natural and Artificial Flavorings, Starch, Tartaric Acid, Artificial Colors (Red #40, Blue #2, Yellow #6), Magnesium Stearate, and Gelatin.

Chill Out - Pacific BioLogic
Gotu Kola • Peony root • Polygoni vine • Valerian root • Passion flower • Skullcap • Lemon Balm • Sweetflag rhizome • Polygala root • Citrus peel (unripened) • Salvia root • Schizandra fruit.

Chill Pill - Futurebiotics
Three tablets contain: Vitamin B1 (thiamin) 5 mg • Vitamin B2 (riboflavin) 5 mg • Niacinamide 200 mg • Calcium (carbonate, phosphate, amino acid chelate) 150 mg • Vitamin B6 5 mg. In a balanced formula of Herbal extracts & powders: Valerian root, Chamomile, Avena Sativa, Kava Kava, Hops, Skullcap, Spearmint, Nettles, Hawthorn, Fennel, Horsetail, Peppermint, Motherwort.

China Chlorella 200 Mg - Natrol
Fifteen tablets contain: Protein 2 mg • Vitamin A 1665 mg • Vitamin C 500 mg • Thiamine (B1) 45 mcg • Riboflavin (B2) 140 mcg • Niacin 714 mcg • Calcium 6.2 mg • Iron 5 mg • Vitamin E 0.03 IU • Vitamin B6 51 mcg • Folic Acid 0.8 mcg • Vitamin B12 4 mcg • Phosphorus 30 mg • Iodine 18 mcg • Potassium 27.3 mg • Magnesium 10 mg • Zinc 2.2 mg • Copper 3 mcg • Biotin 6 mcg • Pantothenic Acid 40 mcg • Chlorophyll 90.1 mg • RNA 89.1 mg • DNA 8.5 mg • Germanium 76 ppm.

Chinese - Futurebiotics
Four tablets contain: Proprietary Blend of extracts and powders equivalent to a minumum of 7000 mg: Siberian Ginseng, Foti, Astragalus, Schizandra, LEM, Shiitake - Ganoderma Mushroom Complex, Chinese Licorice, Codonopsis, Echinacea • Beta Carotene 10,000 IU • Vitamin E (mixed tocopherols) 100 IU • Vitamin C 1000 mg • Selenium 100 mcg.

Chinese Red Ginseng 550 mg - Vitamin World
Each capsule contains: Chinese Red Ginseng root (Panax ginseng) 550 mg. Other Ingredients: Gelatin, Vegetable Magnesium Stearate, Silica.

Chisukit Syrup - Hadas Natural Products
Each 5 mL serving contains: Fructose-Glucose syrup with Sorbitol • Echinacea Angustifolia & Purpurea standardized organic extract 250 mg • Propolis standardized extract 250 mg • Rose Hip extract with Vitamin C 300 mg.

Some Brand Name Natural Products - What they Contain

www.NaturalDatabase.com contains MANY more listings than appear here.

BRAND NAMES

Chito Block 2000 Plus C - Tiffin International, Inc.
Three capsules contain: Chitosan 990 mg • Iron 0.5 mg • Vitamin C 60 mg. Other Ingredients: Microcrystalline Cellulose, Gelatin, Sodium Lauryl Sulfate, Colloidal Silicon Dioxide, Purified Water, Stearic Acid, Hydrogenated Vegetable Oil.
See Editor's Note No. 37, page 2057.

Chitodrene - Sterling-Grant Laboratories
Two tables contain: Vitamin C (as ascorbic acid) 100 mg • Chitosan (marine fiber concentrate) 1000 mg • Calcium 200 mg • Vegetable Cellulose 200 mg. Other Ingredients: Gelatin, Dicalcium Phosphate, Magnesium Stearate, Silica.

Chitoplex - Gero Vita International
Each teaspoon contains: Vitamin B6 (as pyridoxine hydrochloride) 10 mg • Chromium (as chromium polynicotinate) 500 mcg • Vitamin C (from acerola) 30 mg • Chitosan (15%) 3000 mg. Other Ingredients: Purified Water, Glycerine, Fructose, Natural Flavor, Citric Acid, Potassium Sorbate, Grapefruit Seed Extract.

Chitosan - Leiner Health Products
Two tablets contain: Chromium (Chromium picolinate) 100 mcg • Vitamin C 120 mg • Chitosan 1000 mg. Other Ingredients: Calcium Carbonate, Cellulose, Sodium Ascorbate, Maltodextrin, Acacia, Stearic Acid, Hydroxypropyl Methylcellulose, Magnesium Stearate, Hydroxypropyl Cellulose, Starch, Polysorbate 80, Polyethylene Glycol 3350.

Chitosan - NutriCology
Two capsules contain: Chitosan 1 g. Other Ingredients: Stearic Acid.

Chitosan - Olympian Labs
Two capsules contain: Chitosan 1000 mg.

Chitosan - Puritan's Pride
Two tablets contain: Chitosan 1000 mg.

Chitosan - PhysioLogics
Two tablets contain: Chitosan 1000 mg. Other Ingredients: Dicalcium Phosphate, Cellulose (plant origin), Vegetable Stearic Acid, Croscarmellose, Silica, Cellulose Coating, Vegetable Magnesium Stearate.

Chitosan - Swanson
Two capsules contain: LipoSan Ultra Chitosan (90%-93% deacetylated) 1 g.

Chitosan - The Vitamin Shoppe
Each capsule contains: Chitosan, minimum 90% Deacetylated Chitin 250 mg • Aloe Vera 50 mg.

Chitosan 500 mg - Natrol
Two capsules contain: Chitosan (95% deacetylated) 1000 mg.
See Editor's Note No. 37, page 2057.

Chitosan Diet Formula - Optimum Nutrition
Two capsules contain: Vitamin C (ascorbic acid) 200 mg • Chitosan (fiber, 90-95% deacetylated) 1 g. Other Ingredients: Gelatin, Microcrystalline Cellulose, Magnesium Stearate.

Chitosan Plus - Progressive Labs
Each capsule contains: Chitosan (marine fiber concentrate) 250 mg • Citric Acid 75 mg • Lipase (3000 units) 25 mg.

Chitosan-C with Biozan - Richardson Labs - Rexall - Sundown
Four caplets contain: BioZan 2500: Purified Chitosan, Betaine HCl, Oat Bran, Aloe, Beta Glucan • Chromium (picolinate) 200 mcg.

Chit-O-Slim Plus - Aspen Group, Inc.
Each capsule contains: Chitosan 500 mg • Chromium (picolinate) 50 mcg.

Chitosol - Sheldon Marketing
Four capsules contain: Chitosan 2000 mg • Vitamin C 400 mg.

Chizukit Forte For Adults - Hadas Natural Products
Each tablet contains: Echinacea Angustifolia & Purpurea standardized extract 500 mg • Propolis standardized extract 500 mg • Astragalus standardized extract 100 mg • Cat's Claw standardized extract 100 mg • Vitamin C 15 mg • Vitamin E 1 mg • Beta-Carotene 0.8 mg.

Chizukit Gold - Hadas Natural Products
Each tablet contains: Echinacea Angustifolia & Purpurea standardized extract 500 mg • Propolis standardized extract 330 mg • Astragalus standardized extract 150 mg • Cat's Claw standardized extract 150 mg • Panax Ginseng standardized extract 20 mg • Green Tea standardized extract 12.5 mg • Vitamin C 30 mg • Vitamin E 4 mg • Beta Carotene 0.4 mg.

Chizukit Syrup - Hadas Natural Products
Each 5 mL serving contains: Echinacea Angustifolia/Purpurea extract 250 mg • Propolis standardized extract 250 mg • Vitamin C 30 mg • Rose Hip extract 30 mg. Other Ingredients: Fructose-Glucose Syrup.

Chlorella - Earthrise Nutritionals, Inc.
Fifteen tablets contain: Sodium 3 mg • Vitamin A (100% Beta Carotene) 1500 IU • Calcium 4 mg • Iron 2 mg • Niacin 0.75 mg • Riboflavin 0.15 mg • Protein 1.8 g • Total Carb. 0.4 g • Potassium 35 mg • Vitamin C 4 mg • Vitamin E 0.7 IU • Magnesium 8.0 mg • Thiamin 0.05 mg • Vitamin B6 0.05 mg • Vitamin B12 0.12 mcg • Chlorophyll 80 mg • Mixed Carotenoids 8 mg.

Chlorella - Nature's Way
Three capsules contain: Chlorella Microalgae 1.23 g. Other Ingredients: Gelatin.

Chlorella - Pro Health
Three tablets contain: Vitamin A (100% as beta carotene) 3000 IU • Vitamin B12 3 mcg • Iron 3 mg • Zinc 2 mg • Chlorella 3000 mg • Chlorophyll 60 mg • RNA 89 mg • DNA 8.3 mg. Other Ingredients: Cellulose, Croscarmellose Sodium, Magnesium Stearate.

Chlorella - Source Naturals
Six tablets contain: Vitamin A (Beta Carotene) 1,665 IU • Vitamin B1 (Thiamin) 45 mcg • Vitamin B2 (Riboflavin) 140 mcg • Vitamin B3 (Niacin) 710 mcg • Vitamin B6 (Pyridoxine) 50 mcg • Vitamin B12 (Cyanocobalamin) 3.75 mcg • Biotin 5.7 mcg • Vitamin C (Ascorbic Acid) 460 mcg • Calcium 6 mg • Iodine 18 mcg • Iron 5 mg • Magnesium 9.45 mg • Phosphorus 29 mg • Zinc 2.1 mg • Chlorella Growth Factor (CGF) 60 mg • Chlorophyll 60 mg.

Chlorella Regularis - New Chapter, Inc.
Six capsules contain: Chlorella regularis 2340 mg.

Chlorofresh Liquid - Nature's Way
Each tablespoon conatins: Chlorophyll Copper complex 50 mg. Other Ingredients: Glycerin, Oil Of Mint, Water.

Chlorofresh Softgels - Nature's Way
Each softgel contains: Chlorophyll Copper complex 50 mg. Other Ingredients: Oil Of Mint.

Chlorophyll Complex - Standard Process, Inc.
Each two perles contain: Proprietary Blend 754 mg: Fat Soluble Extract from Sesame seed, Alfalfa, Tillandsia Usneoides, Buckwheat, Pea (vine), & Carrot; Soy Bean Lecithin. Inactive Ingredients: Gelatin, Glycerine, Water, Carob.

Chlorophyll Concentrate - Puritan's Pride
Each softgel contains: Chlorophyllin Copper 50 mg.

Chlorophyll Liquid - Dial Herbs
Chlorophyllin Copper complex • Water • Oil of Mint • Glycerine, vegetable derived.

Chlorophyll Softgels - Dial Herbs
Chlorophyllin Copper complex • Water • Oil of Mint • Glycerine, vegetable derived.

Chloroplex **-** Progressive Labs
Each softgel contains: Chlorophyllin 50 mg.

Chloroplus **-** Atrium Inc.
Each capsule contains: Vitamin A 11000 IU • Vitamin D (as Vitamin D3) 250 IU • Chlorophyll (oil soluble) 10 mg • Vitamin E (d-Alpha Tocopherol) 3 IU • Lecithin (Raw Unbleached) 210 mg • Pumpkin seed oil 45 mg • Sesame seed oil 22 mg • Halibut Liver oil • Skip Jack Liver oil.

Chocolate Daydream Fructose - Revival **-** Physicians Laboratories
Each packet contains: Certified Isoflavone 160 mg. Other ngredients: Soy Protein Isolate, Fructose, Sucrose, Cocoa, Calcium Phosphate, Maltodextrin, Soy Lecithin, Salt, Potassium Chloride, Artificial Flavor, Carrageenan, Carboxymethylcellulose, Xanthan Gum.

Chocolate Daydream Splenda - Revival **-** Physicians Laboratories
Each packet contains: Certified Isoflavone 160 mg. Other Ingredients: Soy Protein Isolate, Cocoa, Maltodextrin, Calcium Phosphate, Soy Lecithin, Salt, Potassium Chloride, Artificial Flavor, Carrageenan, Carboxymethylcellulose, Xanthan Gum, Sucralose.

Chocolate Daydream Unsweetened - Revival **-** Physicians Laboratories
Each packet contains: Certified Isoflavone 160 mg. Other Ingredients: Soy Protein Isolate, Cocoa, Maltodextrin, Calcium Phosphate, Soy Lecithin, Salt, Potassium Chloride, Artificial Flavor, Carrageenan, Carboxymethylcellulose, Xanthan Gum.

Chocolate Temptation - Revival **-** Physicians Laboratories
Each bar contains: Certified Isoflavone 160 mg. Other Ingredients: Corn syrup, Corn starch, Water, Gelatin, Soy Protein Isolate, Rice flour, Malt, Salt, Glycerin, Chocolate Liquor, Cocoa butter and dextrose, Soy Lecithin, Sunflower oil, Natural and Artificial Flavors, Cocoa powder.

Chocolate-covered Soynuts - Revival **-** Physicians Laboratories
Each 1/6 cup contains: Certified Isoflavone 10 mg. Other Ingredients: Milk Chocolate (sugar, whole milk powder, cocoa butter, chocolate liquor, lecithin), Soy Protein (whole roasted soybeans), Vanillin, Corn Syrup, Starch Gum, Soybean Oil, Confectioner's Glaze.

Cholarest SC **-** Metagenics
Each tablet contains: Policosanol [from sugar cane wax (Saccharum officinarum)] 10 mg.

CholesFiber **-** Source Naturals
Three heaping scoops contain: Dietary Fiber 15 g • Soluble Fiber 15 g • Protein 15 g • Soy Isoflavones 60 mg. Other Ingredients: Soy Protein, Apple Pectin, Grapefruit Pectin, Mixed Gums: Guar Gum, Arabic Gum, Xanthan Gum.

Cholesta Balance **-** PhysioLogics
Each softgel contains: Pantethine (80% purity, 307 mg) 384 mg • Gamma Oryzanol (from Rice Bran) 100 mg.

Cholestaid **-** Omni Nutraceuticals
Two tablets contain: Esterin extract of Alfalfa 900 mg • Citric Acid 100 mg. Other Ingredients: Microcrystalline, Croscarmellose Sodium, Stearic Acid, Silica.

Cholesta-Lo **-** Futurebiotics
Three tablets contain: Cholestatin 600 mg • Niacin (flush free) 200 mg • Chromium (polynicotinate) 100 mcg • Garlic (odorless) concentrate (2:1) 350 mg • Siberian Ginseng extract (10:1) 75 mg • Parsley 250 mg • Chickweed 200 mg • Hawthorn 150 mg • Ginger 200 mg • Cayenne 200 mg. ("75 mg of 10:1 Siberian Ginseng extract is equal to 750 mg of raw Siberian Ginseng. 350 mg of 2:1 Garlic is equal to 875 mg of raw Garlic.")

CholesTame **-** Jarrow Formulas
Four tablets contain: Red Yeast Rice Extract (Monascus purpureus) (Xie Zhi Kang) 4% Statins 2400 mg • Coenzyme Q10 (Ubiquinone) 30 mg • Artichoke Leaf Extract (Cynara scolymus) 2% cynarine 400 mg • Guggul (Commiphora mukul) 4% guggulsterones 500 mg • Alpha Lipoic Acid 100 mg • Grape Seed Extract (Vitis vinifera) 95% polyphenols 50 mg • Pantethine 200 mg • Lutein 10 mg • Taurine 250 mg.

CholesTame (New Formula with Sytrinol!) **-** Jarrow Formulas
Four tablets contain: Sytrinol (polymethoxylated flavonoid-tocotrienol complex) 300 mg • Plant Sterols (phytosterols) 2000 mg • Coenzyme Q10 (ubiquinone) 30 mg • Artichoke leaf extract (cynara scolymus, 2.5% cynarine) 400 mg • Alpha Lipoic Acid 100 mg • Grape seed extract (vitus vinifera, 95% polyphenols) 50 mg • Pantethine (coenzyme vitamin B5) 200 mg • Lutein (tagetes erecta, from 20 mg lutein esters) 10 mg • Taurine 250 mg • Lecithin (35% phosphatidylcholine) 200 mg. Other Ingredients: Dicalcium Phosphate, Silicon Dioxide, Modified Cellulose Gum, Stearic Acid, Magnesium Stearate, Modified Cellulose.

Cholestatin **-** Futurebiotics
Each tablet contains: Beta Sitosterol 200 mg • Campesterol 100 mg • Stigmasterol 80 mg. Other Ingredients: Dicalcium phosphate, Cellulose, Magnesium Stearate, Silica.

Cholestatin brand **-** Degussa Food Ingredients/BL BioActives
Phytosterols complex.
See Editor's Note No. 44, page 2058.

Cholesterol Essentials **-** Swanson
Two tablets contain: Vitamin C (ascorbic acid) 500 mg • Thiamin (as thiamin HCl; vitamin B-1) 7 mg • Riboflavin (vitamin B-2) 7 mg • Niacin (100 mg as flush-free inositol hexanicotinate and 7 mg as niacinamide) 107 mg • Vitamin B-6 (as pyridoxine HCl) 7 mg • Folic Acid 200 mcg • Vitamin B-12 (as cyanocobalamin) 200 mcg • Biotin 6.24 mcg • Pantothenic Acid (as d-calcium pantothenate) 6.24 mg • Chromium (from Chromax® chromium picolinate) 200 mcg • Gugulipid® (Commiphora mukul, 2.5% guggulsterones) 500 mg • Lecithin 300 mg • Oat Bran fiber 300 mg • Phosphatidylcholine (from lecithin and phosphatidylcholine) 200 mg • Odor-Controlled Garlic bulb (PureGar® 10,000 ppm allicin potential) 150 mg • Beta Sitosterol 50 mg • Citrus Bioflavonoids 50 mg • Choline Bitartrate 6.4 mg • Inositol 6.4 mg • PABA (para-aminobenzoic acid) 6.4 mg.

Cholesterol Metabolism **-** Nutrivention
Six tablets contain: Choline 500 mg • Inositol 500 mg • Niacinamide 200 mg Unsaturated Fatty Acids (7% GAMA Linolenic Acid • 64% Linoleic Acid) 500 mg • Pantothenic Acid 200 mg • Magnesium 200 mg • Vitamin B6 100 mg • Vitamin D 600 IU • Lecithin 600 mg • Hawthorne berries 400 mg • Garlic powder concentrate 400 mg • Apple Pectin 360 mg • L-Methionine 340 mg • Capsicum 200 mg • Ginger root 200 mg • Butcher's Broom 100 mg • Betaine HCL 100 mg.

Cholesterol Regulation Complex **-** Shaklee
Six tablets contain: Protein 2 g • Sodium 60 mg • Hydrolyzed Soy Protein Blend 3000 mg: Phytopeptides with bound phospholipids • N-acetylcysteine 200 mg. Other Ingredients: Dicalcium Phosphate, Croscarmellose Sodium.

Cholesterol Success **-** TwinLab
Each two tablets contain: Phytosterols (Reducol) 900 mg.

Cholesterol Support **-** Zone Labs
Three capsules contain: Garlic (odor reduced, 10,000 ppm allicin) 500 mg • Policosanol 10 mg • Phytosterols Complex (a source of plant sterols including beta sitosterol, capesterol and stigmasterol) 900 mg • Citrus Pectin 5 mg • Apple Pectin 5 mg • Ginger extract 5 mg. Other Ingredients: Gelatin, Microcrystalline Cellulose, Magnesium Stearate, Silica, Sodium Lauryl Sulfate.

CholesteSoy **-** FreeLife International
Two caplets contain: Niacin (from flush-free inositol hexanicotinate 250 mg) 200 mg • Vitamin B6 (as pyridoxine HCl) 10 mg • Folate (as folic acid) 200 mcg • Vitamin B12 (as cyanocobalamin) 100 mcg • Red Yeast Rice (from fermentation of monascus purpureus went) 1200 mg • Proprietary Blend 100 mg: Octadecanoic Acid, Magnesium Octadecanoate (from vegetable oil), Soy Phytosterols (beta-sitosterol, campesterol, stigamasterol), 2.5% Guggulsterone extract (commiphora mukul). Other Ingredients: Calcium Hydrogen Phosphate, Cellulose, Cellulose Gum, Silica, Vita-Coat (vegetable resin, alpha-lipoic acid).

Cholestin **-** Pharmanex
Each capsule contains: Policosanol (Beeswax extract 5:1) 15 mg. Other Ingredients: Soybean Oil, Lecithin, Gelatin, Glycerin, Purified Water, Carmine (for color).

Cholest-Off **-** Nature Made
Each tablet contains: Proprietary Blend 450 mg: Plant Sterols, Plant Stanols, Cellulose Gel, Gum Acacia, Magnesium Silicate, Croscarmellose Sodium, Silica Gel, Hydroxypropyl Methylcellulose, Titanium Dioxide (artificial color), Magnesium Stearate, Polyethylene Glycol, Triethyl Citrate, Polysorbate 80, Sodium Citrate.

Cholestoril **-** Enzymatic Therapy
Each tablet contains: Pantethine 300 mg.

Cholestoril Plus **-** Enzymatic Therapy
Each tablet contains: Proprietary Phytosterol Blend 400 mg: Beta Sitosterol, Campesterol, Stigmasterol, Brassicasterol, Other Plant Sterols • Pantethine 200 mg. Other Ingredients: Cellulose, Modified Cellulose Gum, Modified Cellulose, Silicon Dioxide, Magnesium Stearate, Lecithin, Carnauba Wax.

Cholestra **-** HerbaSway
Soy • Hawthorn berry • Green Tea • He Shou Wu • Cassia tora • Blackberry • HerbaSwee (Cucurbitaceae fruit).

Cholestrex **-** Source Naturals
Nine tablets contain: Niacin 480 mg • Vitamin C (Calcium Ascorbate, Ascorbic Acid and Zinc Ascorbate) 900 mg • Vitamin E (D-Alpha Tocopheryl) (Natural) 100 IU • Calcium (Calcium Ascorbate) 100 mg • Zinc (Zinc Ascorbate) 6 mg • Copper (Copper Sevacate) 2 mg • Chromium (ChromeMate GTF Chromium Polynicotinate) 300 mcg • Oats (bran and fiber) 2500 mg • Grapefruit Pectin 1400 mg • Psyllium seed husk 1100 mg • Lecithin (with 24% Phosphatidyl Choline) 900 mg • Alfalfa seed 600 mg • Beta Sitosterol 300 mg • L-Arginine 300 mg.

Cholest-Rite **-** Nu-Creations
Each capsule contains: Niacin 20 mg • Red Yeast 600 mg. Other Ingredients: Hawthorn extract, Artichoke extract, Gelatin, Magnesium Stearate.

Choline **-** Nature's Bounty
Each tablet contains: Choline Bitartrate 650 mg. Other Ingredients: Cellulose, Vegetable Stearic Acid, Food Glaze, Silica, Vegetable Magnesium Stearate, Magnesium Silicate, Croscarmellose.

Choline **-** Puritan's Pride
Each tablet contains: Choline (from Choline Bitartrate) 650 mg.

Choline & Inositol **-** Puritan's Pride
Each tablet contains: Choline Bitartrate 250 mg • Inositol 250 mg.

Choline & Inositol 250 mg & 250 mg **-** Nature's Way
Two capsules contain: Choline Bitartrate 500 mg • Inositol 500 mg. Other Ingredients: Cellulose, Magnesium Stearate, Silica.

Choline/Inositol 250/250 **-** Solgar
Each capsule contains: Choline (as choline bitartrate) 250 mg • Inositol 250 mg. Other Ingredients: Vegetable Cellulose, Silica, Vegetable Magnesium Stearate, Water, Vegetable Glycerin.

Choline/Inositol Tablets **-** Solgar
Each tablet contains: Calcium (as dicalcium phosphate) 25 mg • Choline (as choline bitartrate) 103 mg • Inositol 250 mg. Other Ingredients: Microcrystalline Cellulose, Dicalcium Phosphate, Vegetable Cellulose, Silica, Titanium Dioxide, Vegetable Stearic Acid, Vegetable Magnesium Stearate, Vegetable Glycerin.

Chondroitin Complex **-** Puritan's Pride
Each capsule contains: Glucosamine Sulfate (2KCl) 250 mg • Chondroitin Sulfate 200 mg • Vitamin C (Ascorbic Acid) 100 mg • Manganese 1 mg.
See Editor's Note No. 15, page 2055.

Chondroitin Plus **-** Atrium Inc.
Two capsules contain: Calcium Ascorbate 60 mg • Magnesium Ascorbate 60 mg • Vitamin C Content 100 mg • Thiamine HCL 25 mg • Pyridoxine HCL 10 mg • Niacinamide 60 mg • Manganese (Sulfate) 65 mg • Potassium (Citrate) 25 mg • Zinc (Citrate) 25 mg • Chondroitin Sulfates 125 mg • Mocopoly Saccharides 65 mg • Bioflavonoid Complex 50 mg • Betaine HCL 15 mg • Rutin 10 g • Black Cohosh 75 mg • Passiflora 75 mg • Valerian root 75 mg • Equestium 65 mg.
See Editor's Note No. 15, page 2055.

Chondroitin Sulfate **-** Jamieson
Each caplet contains: Chondroitin Sulfate (Equivalent to 400 mg Sodium Chondroitin Sulfate) 360 mg.
See Editor's Note No. 15, page 2055.

Chondroitin Sulfate **-** Leiner Health Products
Each tablet contains: Chondroitin Sulfate 600 mg. Other Ingredients: Cellulose, Dicalcium Phosphate, Stearic Acid, Croscarmellose Sodium, Magnesium Stearate, Silicon Dioxide, Titanium Dioxide, Hydroxypropyl Methylcellulose, Talc, Polyethylene Glycol 3350, Wax, Polysorbate 80.
See Editor's Note No. 15, page 2055.

Chondroitin Sulfate **-** Olympian Labs
Each capsule contains: Chondroitin Sulfate 400 mg.
See Editor's Note No. 15, page 2055.

Chondroitin Sulfate **-** PhysioLogics
Each capsule contains: Chondroitin Sulfate 250 mg. Other Ingredients: Rice Powder, Gelatin.
See Editor's Note No. 15, page 2055.

Chondroitin Sulfate - Swanson **-** Swanson
Each capsule contains: Chondroitin Sulfate 500 mg.
See Editor's Note No. 15, page 2055.

Chondroitin Sulfate 250 MG **-** Puritan's Pride
Each capsule contains: Chondroitin Sulfate 250 mg. Other Ingredients: Cellulose (plant origin), Gelatin, Dicalcium Phosphate, Vegetable Stearic Acid, Vegetable Magnesium Stearate.
See Editor's Note No. 15, page 2055.

Chondroitin Sulfate 400 - GNC A-Z **-** GNC
Each capsule contains: Chondroitin Sulfate Sodium 400 mg. Other Ingredients: Cellulose, Gelatin, Calcium Carbonate.
See Editor's Note No. 15, page 2055.

Chondroitin Sulfate 90% **-** Vital Nutrients
Each capsule conatins: Chondroitin Sulfate 90% 400 mg.
See Editor's Note No. 15, page 2055.

Chondroitin Sulfate/Glucosamine Sulfate **-** Metabolic Response Modifiers
Each capsule contains: Glucosamine sulfate KCl 500 mg • Chondroitin sulfate 400 mg.
See Editor's Note No. 15, page 2055.

Chondroytamine HCl **-** Olympian Labs
Each capsule contains: Chondroitin Sulfate 200 mg •Glucosamine HCl 250 mg.
See Editor's Note No. 15, page 2055.

Chondroytamine HCl (Double Strength) **-** Olympian Labs
Each capsule contains: Chondroitin Sulfate 400 mg • Glucosamine HCl 500 mg • Cat's Claw 30 mg • White Willow Bark 30 mg.
See Editor's Note No. 15, page 2055.

Chroma Slim Biozan - Richardson Labs **-** Rexall - Sundown
Four caplets contain: BioZan 2500 mg: Purified Chitosan, Betaine HCl, Oat bran, Aloe, Beta Glucan] 2500 mg • Chromium (Picolinate) 250 mcg.

Chroma Slim for Men - Richardson Labs **-** Rexall - Sundown
Four caplets contain: Trace Mineral Blend: Chromium Picolinate 400 mcg, Vanadium 120 mcg, Manganese Picolinate 2.5 mg • Proprietary Lipotropic Blend 3000 mg: Choline Bitartrate, L-Carnitine, Inositol, L-Methionine • Essential Nutrient & Amino Acid Blend 500 mg: Ferulic Acid Esters, Taurine, L-Lysine HCl, L-Glutamic Acid, Base, Glycine USP, Cernitin flower pollen extract 500 mg • Vitamin Blend: Pantothenic Acid 10 mg, Vitamin B6 5 mg • Thermogenic Herbal Blend 424 mg: Panax Ginseng powdered extract • Cayenne • Mustard seed powder • Cinnamon powder • Ginger root powdered extract • Uva Ursi • Standardized White Willow bark powder. In a base of Natural Peppermint, Saw Palmetto berries, Juniper berries, Spirulina.

Chroma Slim Plus - Richardson Labs **-** Rexall - Sundown
Four caplets contain: Trace Mineral Blend: Chromium Picolinate 400 mcg, Vanadium 120 mcg, Manganese Picolinate 2.5 mg • Proprietary Lipotropic & Lipid Transport Blend 3000 mg: Choline Bitartrate, L-Carnitine, Inositol, L-Methionine • Essential Nutrient & Amino Acid Blend 500 mg: Ferulic Acid Esters, Taurine, L-Lysine HCl, L-Glutamic Acid, Base, Glycine USP, Cernitin flower pollen extract • Vitamin Blend: Potassium Chloride USP, Pantothenic Acid 10 mg, Vitamin B6 5 mg. In a base of natural Peppermint and Bromelain.

Chromax brand **-** Nutrition 21
Chromium Picolinate.
See Editor's Note No. 44, page 2058.

Chromemate **-** Natrol
Each capsule contains: Chromium (polynicotinate) 200 mcg • L-Arginine 50 mg • L-Lysine 50 mg • Vitamin B6 (pyridoxine) 10 mg. Other Ingredients: Microcrystalline Cellulose, Magnesium Stearate, Gelatin.

ChromeMate GTF 200 **-** Pure Encapsulations
Each vegetarian capsule contains: Chromium (from chromium polynicotinate) 200 mg • Niacin (from chromium polynicotinate) 1.1-1.2 mg.

Chromic Fuel (Chromium Picolinate) **-** TwinLab
Pure Crystalline Chromium Picolinate (supplying of Trivalent Chromium 200 mcg) 1.67 mg.

Chromium **-** Source Naturals
Each tablet contains: Chromium (amino acid chelate) 200 mcg.

Chromium - Basic Nutrition **-** GNC
Each capsule contains: Chromium (as Chromium Picolinate) 200 mcg. Other Ingredients: Soybean oil, Gelatin, Glycerin, Magnesium Stearate, Caramel color, Titanium Dioxide.

Chromium (polynicotinate) 200 mcg **-** Vital Nutrients
Each capsule contains: Chromium (polynicotinate) 200 mcg.

Chromium Chelated 200 mcg **-** Jamieson
Each tablet contains: Chromium (vegetable protein chelate) 200 mcg.

Chromium Complex with ChromeMate **-** NutriCology
Each capsule contains: Niacin 50 mg • Vitamin B6 (as pyridoxine hydrochloride) 20 mg • Chromium (as chromium nicotinate) 250 mcg • L-Glutathione (reduced) 2.5 mg • Guar Gum (cyamopsis tetragonolobus, galactomannan) 450 mg. Other Ingredients: Cellulose, Magnesium Stearate, Silicon Dioxide.

Chromium GTF **-** Source Naturals
Each tablet contains: Chromium GTF (polynicotinate) 200 mcg • Niacin (polynicotinate) 1.8 mg.

Chromium GTF **-** Nature's Sunshine
Each tablet contains: Calcium (di-calcium phosphate) 80 mg • Phosphorus (dicalcium phosphate) 61 mg • Chromium (chromium amino acid chelate, chromium nicotinate) 500 mcg • Proprietary Blend 60 mg: Horsetail (equisetum arvense), Red Clover tops (trifolium pratense), Yarrow flower (achillea millefolium).

Chromium GTF **-** Quest
Each capsule contains: Chromium (HVP Chelate) 200 mcg. Other Ingredients: Microcrystalline Cellulose, Magnesium Stearate (vegetable source).

Chromium GTF **-** Pro Health
Two tablets contain: Chromium GTF (as polynicotinate, from chromate [niacin bound to chromium]) 400 mcg. Other Ingredients: Dicalcium Phosphate, Dextrose, Magnesium Stearate, Stearic Acid.

Chromium HCA **-** PhysioLogics
Each capsule contains: Calcium (as Calcium Salt of Hydroxy Citric Acid) 79 mg • Chromium (as Chromium Picolinate) 100 mcg • Garcinia cambogia [50% (-)- Hydroxy Citric Acid (HCA) 250 mg] 500 mg.

Chromium Nicotinate Complex **-** Progressive Labs
Each capsule contains: Niacin (as polynicotinate) 1300 mcg • Chromium (as polynicotinate) 200 mcg • Glutathione 250 mcg • Glycine 50 mcg • Cysteine 100 mcg • Aspartic Acid 100 mcg.

Chromium Picolinate - Basic Nutrition **-** GNC
Each tablet contains: Chromium (as Chromium Picolinate) 400 mcg. Other Ingredients: Dicalcium Phosphate, Cellulose, Stearic Acid, Silica, Magnesium Stearate.

Chromium Picolinate **-** Great American Nutrition
Each tablet contains: Chromium (picolinate) 200 mcg. Other Ingredients: Calcium Carbonate, Cellulose, Magnesium Stearate.

Chromium Picolinate **-** Metabolic Response Modifiers
Each capsule contains: Chromium (picolinate) 200 mcg.

Chromium Picolinate **-** Nature's Way
Each capsule contains: Chromium Picolinate 200 mcg. Other Ingredients: Cellulose, Maltodextrin, Millet.

Chromium Picolinate **-** Olympian Labs
Each capsule contains: Chromium (picolinate) 200 mcg.

Chromium Picolinate **-** Optimum Nutrition
Each capsule contains: Chromium (as chromium picolinate) 200 mcg. Other Ingredients: Gelatin, Microcrystalline Cellulose, Magnesium Stearate, Silica.

Chromium Picolinate **-** PhysioLogics
Each tablet contains: Chromium (as chromium picolinate) 200 mcg. Other Ingredients: Dicalcium Phosphate, Cellulose (plant origin), Vegetable Stearic Acid, Croscarmellose, Silica, Vegetable Magnesium Stearate.

Chromium Picolinate **-** PhytoPharmica
Each capsule contains: Chromium (picolinate) 200 mcg.

Chromium Picolinate **-** Pro Health
Each capsule contains: Chromium (as chromax chromium picolinate, from white rice) 200 mcg. Other Ingredients: Rice Flour, Gelatin, Water.

Chromium Picolinate - Richardson Labs - Rexall - Sundown
Each tablet contains: Chromium (Picolinate), derived from 3.2 mg of pure crystalline Chromium Picolinate.

Chromium Picolinate - Source Naturals
Each tablet contains: Trivalent Chromium (from Chromax brand of yeast-free Chromium Picolinate) 200 mcg.

Chromium Picolinate - Swanson
Each capsule contains: Chromium (from chromax chromium picolinate) 200 mcg.

Chromium Picolinate - The Vitamin Shoppe
Each softgel contains: Chromium Picolinate (compound of yeast-free trivalent chromium and picolinic acid) 200 mcg.

Chromium Picolinate 200 Capsules - GNC A-Z - GNC
Each capsule contains: Chromium (as chromax chromium picolinate) 200 mcg. Other Ingredients: Soybean oil, Gelatin, Glycerin, Titanium Dioxide.

Chromium Picolinate 200 mcg - Kroger - Kroger
Each tablet contains: Chromium (as chromium picolinate) 200 mcg. Other Ingredients: Calcium Carbonate, Maltodextrin, Cellulose, Croscarmellose Sodium, Silicon Dioxide, Magnesium Stearate, Dextrin, Dextrose, Lecithin, Sodium Carboxymethylcellulose, Sodium Citrate.

Chromium Picolinate 200 mcg - Nature Made
Each tablet contains: Chromium 200 mcg. Other Ingredients: Dibasic Calcium Phosphate, Cellulose, Magnesium Stearate.
See Editor's Note No. 45, page 2058.

Chromium Picolinate 200 mcg - Puritan's Pride
Each tablet contains: Chromium (as chromium picolinate) 200 mcg. Other Ingredients: Dicalcium Phosphate, Cellulose (plant origin), Vegetable Stearic Acid, Silica, Vegetable Magnesium Stearate.

Chromium Picolinate 200 mcg - Rexall - Sundown
Each tablet contains: Calcium 120 mg • Chromium (as chromium picolinate) 200 mcg. Other Ingredients: Dicalcium Phosphate, Microcrystalline Cellulose, Croscarmellose Sodium, Magnesium Stearate.

Chromium Picolinate 200 Tablets - GNC A-Z - GNC
Each tablet contains: Chromium (as chromax chromium picolinate) 200 mcg. Other Ingredients: Dicalcium Phosphate, Cellulose.

Chromium Picolinate 400 mcg XTRA - Rexall - Sundown
Each tablet contains: Calcium 128 mg • Chromium (as chromium picolinate) 400 mcg • Grapefruit Extract (fruit) 1 mg • Weight Loss Complement Blend 76 mg: Inositol, Soy Lecithin, Choline Bitartrate. Other Ingredients: Dicalcium Phosphate, Microcrystalline Cellulose, Croscarmellose Sodium, Silica, Magnesium Stearate.

Chromium Picolinate 500 - GNC A-Z - GNC
Each tablet contains: Chromium (as chromium picolinate) 500 mcg. Other Ingredients: Cellulose, Dicalcium Phosphate, Red Beet juice powder.

Chromium Picolinate GTF - Atrium Inc.
Each capsule contains: Chromium (Chromium Picolinate) 200 mcg.

Chromium Picolinate High Potency - Optimum Nutrition
Each tablet contains: Chromium (as Chromium Picolinate) 200 mcg. Other Ingredients: Gelatin, Microcrystalline Cellulose, Magnesium Stearate, Silica.

Chromium Picolinate Plus - Life Extension
Each capsule contains: Chromium Picolinate 300 mcg • Lipase 20 mg (blended in natural herb base).

Chromium Picolinate Plus - Progressive Labs
Each capsule contains: Chromium 200 mcg (from chromium picolinate 1640 mg) • Gamma Oryzanol 15 mg • Boron (as boron aspartate) 2 mg.

Chromium Plus with Oxidative Factors - The Vitamin Shoppe
Each tablet contains: Zinc 30 mg • Chromium 100 mcg • Selenium 100 mcg.

ChronFS-X - Olympian Labs
Each capsule contains: Raw Adrenal 50 mg • Licorice Rhizome 150 mg • Shitake Mushrooms 30 mg • Maitake Mushrooms 30 mg • Malic Acid 200 mg • Magnesium Glycinate 50 mg • Manganese Glycinate 10 mg • Potassium Gluconate 30 mg • Zinc Gluconate 20 mg.
See Editor's Note No. 14.

Chronic Red Eye Drops - Natural Ophthalmics
Active Ingredients: Argentum Nitricum HPUS 10x • Hepar Sulphur HPUS 10x • Eyebright (euphrasia) HPUS 6x • Pulsatilla HPUS 6x • Rhus Toxicodendron HPUS 12x. Inactive Ingredients: Sterile Water, Sodium Chloride, Sodium Citrate, Citrate, Polysorbate 80.

Chrysin - ProLab
Each capsule contains: Chrysin (5,7-Dihydroxyflanone) 250 mg.

Chrysin - Metabolic Response Modifiers
Each capsule contains: Chrysin (5,7-dihydroxyflavone) 500 mg.

Chrysin Deluxe - Mass Quantities, Inc.
Each capsule contains: Chrysin 250 mg • Daidzein 25 mg.

Cider Source - Nature's Health Connection
Six caplets contain: Apple Cider Vinegar 60,000 mg • Calcium 144 mg • Magnesium 54 mg.

Cider Vinegar - Naturally Vitamins
Each tablet contains: Apple Cider Vinegar (equivalent to apple cider vinegar 5 ml) 100 mg. Other Ingredients: Dicalcium Phosphate, Colloidal Silica, Modified Cellulose Gum, Cholesterol Free Magnesium Stearate, Stearic Acid.

Cider Vinegar Diet Formula - Now
Each capsule contains: Vitamin B6 (pyridoxine HCl) 3.5 mg • Chromium (as amino acid chelate) 100 mcg • Apple Cider Vinegar powder 250 mg • Lecithin 100 mg • Glucomannan tuber fiber (amorphophallus rivieri) 50 mg • Kelp algae (ascophyllum nodosum) 37 mg • Grapefruit fiber 15 mg. Other Ingredients: Gelatin (capsule), Silica, Magnesium Stearate.

CigNo - M.E. Cody Products, Inc.
Plantain (plantago major) 1X, Alchohol 18-22%.
See Editor's Note No. 1, page 2053.

Cimi-Fem - Source Naturals
Each table contains: Black Cohosh root (Cimi-Pure, standardized extract 2.5% yielding 2 mg triterpene glycosides, containing 27-deoxyactein) 80 mg.

Cineraria Eye Drops - Natural Ophthalmics
Active Ingredients: Cineraria Maritima 5x • Eyebright (euphrasia) 5x. Inactive Ingredients: Sterile Water, Sodium, Citrates, Polysorbate 80.

Cinnamon Quills 1:2 - Standard Process, Inc.
Each 5 mL serving contains: Cinnamon quills stem bark 1:2 extract (from cinnamomum zeylanicum 2.5 g) 5 mL. Other Ingredients: Purified Water, 70% Alcohol.

Cinnulor - Dr. Mark's
Each capsule contains: Cinnulin PF Cinnamomum Mairei extract 250 mg.

Circulate Dietary Supplement Tablets - HealthWatchers System
Vitamin B6 • Vitamin B2 • Vitamin B12 • Vitamin B15 • Vitamin D • OrthoPhosphoric Acid • EDTA • Fenugreek Seed • Superoxide Dismutase • Rutin • Catalase • Beet Leaf • Phosphatidyl Choline • Alfalfa • Spanish Moss • Urea • Orchick Hyaluridase • Beta Carotene

• Protomorphagens Pituitary • Heart • Liver • Kidney • Brain.
See Editor's Note No. 31, page 2056.

Circuleg **-** Puritan's Pride
Each tablet contains: Horse Chestnut Seed extract (aesculus hippocastanum: Standardized to 20% Aescin) 300 mg • Proprietary Herbal Blend 200 mg: Butcher's Broom (Ruscus aculeatus) root, Bilberry (Vaccinium myrtillus) fruit, Cayenne (Capsicum annum) fruit, Ginger (Zingiber officinale) fruit, Ginkgo leaf extract (Ginkgo biloba).

Circulite Oil **-** The Herbalist
Oils of Sweet Almond, Eucalyptus, Camphor, St. John's Wort flower, Calendula flower, French Lavender, Peppermint, Sage & Extracts of Prickly Ash bark, Ginger root, Lobelia leaf.

Circuplex **-** Futurebiotics
Two tablets contain: Vitamin C 100 mg • Vitamin B1 (thiamin) 8 mg • Niacinamide 414 mg • Vitamin B2 (riboflavin) 8 mg • Niacin 20 mg • Vitamin B6 20 mg • Vitamin B12 10 mcg • Zinc (gluconate) 5 mg • Manganese (amino acid chelate) 5 mg. In a tablet base of: Betaine HCl 20 mg, Citrus Bioflavonoids 50 mg, Alfalfa seed meal 200 mg, Oyster Shell Calcium 50 mg, Cayenne 10 mg, Ginger 200 mg, Prickly Ash bark 200 mg, Peppermint 100 mg.

Circusome **-** Jamieson
Horse Chestnut 5% • Arnica Flower 5% • Calendula 5% • Witch Hazel 4% • Butcher's Broom 2.5% • Peppermint Oil • Aloe Vera.

Circutone **-** The Herbalist
Prickly Ash bark • Hawthorn berry, leaf & flower • Bayberry root bark • Ginger root • Yarrow flower • Cayenne pepper.

Citicoline **-** QualiCeutix
Each capsule contains: Citicoline 500 mg. Other Ingredients: Gelatin, Microcrystalline Cellulose, Magnesium Stearate, Silicon Dioxide.

Citra Garcinia Cambogia **-** Olympian Labs
Each capsule contains: Garcinia (Hydroxycitrate) 500 mg.

Citracal Calcium Citrate 250 mg + D **-** Mission Pharmacal
Two tablets contain: Vitamin D (as vitamin D3; as cholecalciferol) 125 IU • Calcium (as Ultradense calcium citrate) 500 mg. Other Ingredients: Polyethylene Glycol, Citric Acid, Microcrystalline Cellulose, HPMC, Croscarmellose Sodium, Color, Magnesium Silicate, Magnesium Stearate.

Citracal Calcium Citrate caplets **-** Mission Pharmacal
Two caplets contain: Vitamin D (D3, as cholecalciferol) 400 IU • Calcium (as Ultradense calcium citrate) 630 mg. Other Ingredients: Polyethylene Glycol, Croscarmellose Sodium, HPMC, Color Added, Magnesium Silicate, Magnesium Stearate.

Citracal Calcium Citrate Caplets + D **-** Mission Pharmacal
Two caplets contain: Vitamin D (as Vitamin D3; as cholecalciferol) 400 IU • Calcium (as Ultradense calcium citrate) 630 mg. Other Ingredients: Polyethylene Glycol, Croscarmellose Sodium, HPMC, Color, Magnesium Silicate, Magnesium Stearate.

Citracal Calcium Citrate Liquitab **-** Mission Pharmacal
Each dissolved tablet contains: Calcium (as calcium citrate) 500 mg. Other Ingredients: Citric Acid, Adipic Acid, Saccharin Sodium, Orange Flavor, Cellulose Gum, Aspartame. This Product contains Nutrasweet. Phenylketonurics: contains 6 mg Phenylalanine per tablet.

Citracal Calcium Citrate tablets **-** Mission Pharmacal
Two tablets contain: Calcium (as Ultradense calcium citrate) 400 mg. Other Ingredients: Polyethylene Glycol, Croscarmellose Sodium, HPMC, Color, Magnesium Silicate, Magnesium Stearate.

Citracal Plus **-** Mission Pharmacal
Two tablets contain: Vitamin D (as vitamin D3; as cholecalciferol) 250 IU • Vitamin B6 (as pyridoxine hydrochloride) 10 mg • Calcium (as Ultradense calcium citrate) 500 mg • Magnesium (as magnesium oxide) 80 mg • Zinc (as zinc oxide) 10 mg • Copper (as copper gluconate) 1 mg • Manganese (as manganese gluconate) 1 mg • Boron (as sodium borate) 1 mg. Other Ingredients: Polyethylene Glycol, Povidone, Croscarmellose Sodium, HPMS, Color, Magnesium Stearate, Magnesium Silicate, Maltodextrin, Carnauba Wax.

Citracal Prenatal Rx **-** Mission Pharmacal
Each tablet contains: Vitamin A (Vitamin A palmitate) 2700 IU • Vitamin C (Ascorbic acid) 120 mg • Calcium (Calcium citrate) 125 mg • Iron (Carbonyl iron, Ferrous gluconate) 27 mg • Vitamin D (as Vitamin D3) (Cholecalciferol) 400 IU • Vitamin E (dl Alpha Tocopheryl acetate) 30 IU • Thiamin (Vitamin B1) 3 mg • Riboflavin (Vitamin B2) 3.4 mg • Niacinamide (Vitamin B3) 20 mg • Vitamin B6 (Pyridoxine HCl) 20 mg • Folic Acid 1 mg • Iodine (Potassium iodide) 150 mcg • Zinc (Zinc oxide) 25 mg • Copper (Cupric oxide) 2 mg • Docusate Sodium 50 mg.

Citramannan **-** The Vitamin Shoppe
Each capsule contains: Citrimax (Hydroxy Citric Acid) 400 mg • Glucomannan (Konjac) root 400 mg.

Citratherm **-** MetPro
Citrus aurantium • Chromium Picolinate • Vitamin C • Niacin • St. John's Wort.
See Editor's Note No. 40, page 2058.

Citri-Caps **-** Progressive Labs
Each capsule contains: Malibar Tamarind [Garcinia cambogia, standardized to contain 50% (-) hydroxycitric acid] 333 mg • Atractylodes (Atractylodes lancea) 50 mg • Seville Orange flower (Citrus aurantii) 50 mg • Chromium (as chromium picolinate) 50 mcg • Chromium (as chromium arginate) 15 mcg.
See Editor's Note No. 40, page 2058.

Citri-Caps Plus **-** Progressive Labs
Each capsule contains: Malibar Tamarind [Garcinia cambogia, standardized to contain 50% (-) hydroxycitric acid] 333 mg • Ma Huang Extract (Ephedra sinica) 200 mg • Yerba Mate 75 mg • Atractylodes (Atractylodes lancea) 50 mg • Seville Orange flower (Citrus Aurantii) 50 mg • Chromium (as chromium picolinate) 50 mcg • Chromium (as chromium arginate) 15 mcg.
See Editor's Note No. 30, page 2056.

CitriChrome **-** Swanson
Each capsule contains: Chromium (from Chromax® chromium picolinate) • CitriMax™ (Garcinia cambogia fruit extract) 500 mg, (-) Hydroxycitric Acid 250 mg.

CitriGenics **-** Roex
Six tablets contain: Citrimax Garcinia Cambogia 1500 mg • L-Carnitine 300 mg • Choline Bitartrate 100 mg • Inositol 100 mg • Betaine HCl 50 mg • Chromium 200 mcg • Green Tea extract 150 mg • Kola Nut extract 150 mg • Yerba Mate 100 mg • Ginger 100 mg • Spirulina 100 mg • Kelp with Trace Minerals 100 mg • Vitamin C 100 mg • Vitamin E 30 IU • Potassium 25 mg • Biotin 300 mcg • Niacinamide 50 mg • Vitamin A 5000 IU • Vitamin B6 20 mg • Vitamin B2 20 mg • Vitamin B12 6 mcg • Folic Acid 400 mcg • Iodine 150 mcg • Selenium 50 mcg.

CitriLean **-** Enzymatic Therapy
Each capsule contains: Garcinia cambogia extract (CitriMax) standardized to contain 50% (-) hydroxycitrate (125 mg/capsule) 250 mg • Ginger root extract 6.5:1 (Zingiber officinale) 50 mg • Fenugreek seed extract 4:1 (Trigonella foenum-graecum) 50 mg • Curcuma root extract (Curcuma longa) standardized to contain 4% curcumin 50 mg • Chromium Polynicotinate (ChromeMate) 25 mcg.

CiTrim **-** E'OLA
Each tablet contains: Garcinia Cambogia (CitriMax) 500 mg • Proprietary Blend 97 mg: Triphala, Cayenne Pepper, Piper Longum, Vanadyl Sulfate. Other Ingredients: DiCalcium Phosphate, Microcrystalline Cellulose, Calcium Stearate, Vegetable Stearine, Cros Carmellose Sodium.

CiTrim 250 - E'OLA
0.75 ml (Approx. 15 drops) contains: Chromium 50 mcg • CitriMax Garcinia Cambogia 543 mg • L-Carnitine 125 mg • DMAE Bitartrate 20 mg. Other Ingredients: Purified Water, Sodium Benzoate.

Citrimate - Nature's Plus
Each tablet contains: Standardized Garcinia cambogia extract supplying 50% [-] Hydroxycitrate 500 mg • Chromium (Polynicotinate) 100 mcg.

Citrimax - Nature's Plus
Each tablet contains: Standardized Garcinia cambogia extract supplying 50% [-] Hydroxycitrate 1000 mg.

CitriMax brand - InterHealth Nutraceuticals
Hydroxycitric Acid (HCA, extracted from garcinia cambogia fruit).
See Editor's Note No. 44, page 2058.

Citrimax Fat Burners - Optimum Nutrition
Citrimax (H.C.A).

Citrimax Plus ChromeMate - Pro Health
Each capsule contains: Calcium (from citrimax) 83 mg • Iodine (from kelp) 150 mcg • ChromeMate Chromium (from chromium polynicotinate) 100 mcg • Potassium 120 mg • Super Citrimax Garcinia Cambogia fruit extract (containing (-) hydroxycitric acid 450 mg) 750 mg • Panax Ginseng powder 100 mg. Other Ingredients: Gelatin (capsule), Cellulose, Magnesium Stearate, Silica.

CitrimaxPlus with ChromeMate - Natrol
Each capsule contains: Chromium (Polynicotinate) 100 mcg • (-) Hydroxycitric Acid 250 mg • Uva Ursi 100 mg • Cascara Sagrada 75 mg. Other Ingredients: Gelatin, Magnesium Stearate.

Citrin + Chromium - Olympia Nutrition
Hydroxycitrate (-) HCA • Chromium Picolinate.

CitriSate - Advocare International
Each caplet contains: D-Limonene powder 300 mg • Grapefruit juice powder 200 mg • 5-Hydroxytryptophan (seed - griffonia simplicifolia) 25 mg. Other Ingredients: Dicalcium Phosphate, Silicon Dioxide, Cellulose, Stearic Acid, Magnesium Stearate.

CitriThin - PhytoPharmica
Two capsules contain: Garcinia Cambogia extract (CitriMax) 500 mg standardized to contain 50% (-)hydroxycitrate (125 mg per capsule) • Ginger root extract 6.5:1 (Zingiber officinale) 100 mg • Fenugreek seed extract 4:1 (Trigonella foenum-graecum) 100 mg • Curcuma root extract (Curcuma longa) 100 mg standardized to contain 4% curcumin • Chromium Polynicotinate (ChromeMate) 50 mcg.

Citrus Bioflavonoids Complex 1000 - GNC A-Z - GNC
Each tablet contains: Citrus Bioflavonoids 1000 mg. Other Ingredients: Dicalcium Phosphate, Povidine.

Citrus Slender - Nature's Way
Each 14 g scoop contains: Arabinogalactan 2 g • Chromium Polynicotinate 100 mcg • Citrin 1.5 g • L-Carnitine L-Tartrate 800 mg. Other Ingredients: Citric Acid, Fructose, Lemon Crystals, Lemon/Lime Crystals, Lime Crystals, Sodium Chloride, Sorbitol, Stevia, dried extract.

C-Jointin With Glucosamine, MSM, Chondroitin And Other Joint Nutrition Factors - Puritan's Pride
Three softgels contain: Vitamin C (as ascorbic acid) 60 mg • Vitamin E (as d-alpha tocopherol) 10 IU • Manganese (as manganese aspartate) 1 mg • Glucosamine Sulfate (2KCl) 1000 mg • MSM (methylsulfonylmethane) 750 mg • Chondroitin Sulfate 200 mg • Evening Primrose Oil 250 mg • Boron (as boron citrate) 1.5 mg. Other Ingredients: Soybean Oil, Gelatin, Glycerin, Lecithin, Yellow Beeswax, Caramel Color.
See Editor's Note No. 15, page 2055.

CLA (1000 mg) - Pro Health
Each softgel contains: Sunflower Oil, Safflower Oil (high linoleic acid) 1000 mg • Conjugated Linoleic Acid (CLA) 700 mg • Cis-9 Trans-11 Isomer 330 mg • Trans-10 Cis-12 Isomer 330 mg. Other Ingredients: Gelatin, Glycerin, Water, Carob.

CLA - EAS
Each capsule contains: Vegetable Oil 1000 mg: 60% Conjugated Linoleic Acid (CLA), 40% other Monounsaturated & Saturated Fatty Acid. Other Ingredients: 0.02% TBHQ.

CLA - Now
Three softgels contain: Safflower oil (high linoleic acid) 3 g • Conjugated Linoleic Acid (CLA) 2.25 g • Cis-9, Trans-11 Isomer 1.05 g • Trans-10, Cis-12 Isomer 1.08 g • Other Isomers 120 mg. Other Ingredients: Gelatin, Glycerin, Water, Natural Color.

CLA 1000 - AST Sports Science
Each two softgels contain: Conjugated Linoleic Acid 80% 800 mg.

CLA 1000 - Human Development Technologies (HDT)
Each softgel capsule contains: Tonalin 1000 mg yielding Conjugated Linoleic Acid 700 mg.

CLA 1000 mg - Vitamin World
Two softgels contain: Tonalin CLA (from safflower oil, 74-82% conjugated linoleic acid) 2000 mg. Other Ingredients: Gelatin, Glycerin, Caramel Color, Titanium Dioxide Color.

CLA One brand - Pharmanutrients
Conjugated Linoleic Acid.
See Editor's Note No. 44, page 2058.

CLA Softgels - Optimum Nutrition
Each softgel contains: CLA One 1000 mg • CLA (conjugated linoleic acid) 750 mg. Other Ingredients: Gelatin, Glycerin, Water, Natural Caramel Color, Titanium Dioxide.

Clarina Cream - The Himalaya Drug Company (Himalaya Heal
Kumari (aloe barbadensis syn. a.vera) 200 mg • Badama (prunus amygdalus) 10 mg • Matsyakshi (alternathera sessilis) 10 mg • Manjishtha (rubia cordifolia) 5 mg • Tankana (sodium biborate) 12.5 mg • Yashad Bhasma (zinc calx) 12.5 mg • Base q.s. ad. 750 mg.

Classic Perfor-Max - Changes International, Inc.
Each capsule contains: Proanthocyanidin Blend (85% Proanthocyanidins) Grape seed extract and Pine Bark 4:1 extract 50 mg • Turmeric rhizome extract 25 mg. Other Ingredients: Maltodextrin, Calcium Sulfate, Gelatin, Cellulose, Magnesium Stearate, Silica, and Riboflavin color.

Classic Thermo-Lift (Classic ThermoLift) - Changes International, Inc.
Each capsule contains: Chromium (as Chromium picolinate) 200 mcg • MaHuang extract (aerial parts) (Standardized for 25 mg Ephedrine alkaloids) 310 mg • Proprietary herbal blend 260 mg: Guarana seed extract (39 mg Caffeine), White Willow bark, Siberian Ginseng root, Astragalus root, Bee Pollen, Bladderwrack kelp (Fucus vesiculosus), Ginger root, Gotu Kola leaf, Licorice root, Rehmannia root, and Reishi mushroom (fruiting body). Other Ingredients: Gelatin, Maltodextrin, Magnesium stearate, Wheat Germ, Silica, and Turmeric extract.
See Editor's Note No. 30, page 2056.

Clay Pack - Nu Skin Enterprises
Water (aqua) • Aloe Barbadensis • Kaolin • Butylene Glycol • Glycerin • Bentonite • Sodium PCA • RNA • Tocopheryl Acetate • Retinyl Palmitate • Royal Jelly • Honey (mel) • Hypnea Musciformis extract • Gelidiela Acerosa extract • Sargassum Filipendula extract • Sorbitol • Carbomer • Cellulose Gum • Triethanolamine • Methylparaben • Propylparaben • Disodium EDTA.

Some Brand Name Natural Products - What they Contain

www.NaturalDatabase.com contains MANY more listings than appear here.

CleanseSMART I - RenewLife
Artichoke leaf • Ashwaganda root • Beet leaf (green rind) • Bupleurum root • Burdock root • Celandine • Chlorella • Corn silk • Dandelion root • Hawthorne berry • Larch gum • Milk Thistle seed • Mullein leaf • Red clover leaf and stem • Turmeric root.

CleanseSMART II - RenewLife
Magnesium Hydroxide • Cape aloe gel • Rhubarb • Slippery Elm bark • Marshmallow root • Fennel seed • Triphalia • Ginger root.

Cleansing Herbs - Youngevity
Vitamin B2 • Cascara sagrada • Fennel • Peppermint • Yucca root • Pau d'Arco • Yellow Dock root • Vilcabamba Mineral Essence: Potassium, Calcium, Magnesium, Zinc, Chromium, Selenium, Iron, Copper, Molybdenum, Vanadium, Iodine, Cobalt, Manganese.

Cleansing Laxative - Zand
Each tablet contains: Cascara Sagrada bark 150 mg. Other Ingredients: Chinese Rhubarb Root, Frangula Bark, Gentian Root, Goldenseal Root, Fennel Seed, Kaolin Clay, Anise Seed, Oregon Grape Root.

Clear Energy Mind and Muscle Power - Garden of Life, Inc.
Three caplets contain: Poten-Zyme Adaptogen Blend 2700 mg: Eleutherococcus Senticosus, American Ginseng (panax quinquefolium), Cordyceps Sinensis, Reishi (ganoderma lucidum), Codonopsis root, Astragalus root, Polygonum Multiflorum, Schizandra berry, Lycium fruit, Licorice root, Aralia Racemosa, Black Diamond truffle, Maca extract • Rhodiola Rosea extract (3% rosavin) 300 mg • 5% Ecdysterone (from rhaponticum carthamoides) 100 mg. Other Ingredients: Cellulose, Stearates (vegetable source).

Clear Headache - Clear Products
Each capsule contains: Aconitum Napellus 3X • Belladonna 6X • Bryonia 6X • Gelsemium 3X • Hypericum 3X • Kali Phosphoricum 3X • Natrum Muriaticum 6X. Other Ingredients: Angelica Dahuricae Root, Chrysanthemum Flower, Ligustici Root, Notopterygium Root, Pueraria Root, Vitex Fruit, Mint Herb, Ginger Root, Sesame Seed, Tangarine Peel, Licorice Root.
See Editor's Note No. 1, page 2053.

Clear Migraine - Clear Products
Three capsules contain: Aconitum Napellus 3X • Belladonna 6X • Bryonia 6X • Cimicifuga Racemose 3X • Hypericum 3X • Iris Versicolor 6X • Kali Bichromicum 3X • Natrum Muriaticum 6X • Sanguinaria 3X • Spigellia 6X. Other Ingredients: Corydalis Tuber, Angelica Sinensis Root, Ligustici Root, Peony Root, Pueraria Root, Angelica Dahurica Root, Chrysanthemum Flower, Gastrodia Tuber, Rehmannia Root, Siler Root, Ginger, Root, Lycium Fruit, Tangerine Peel, Licorice Root.
See Editor's Note No. 1, page 2053.

Clear Sinus & Ear - Clear Products
Each capsule contains: Herbal Blend: Pueraria root, Angelica root, Peony root, Magnolia flower, Platycodon root, Coix seed, Ginger root, Perilla leaf, Silver root, Scutellaria root, Cinnamon bark, Licorice root. Other Ingredients: Magnesium Stearate, Gelatin, Silacone Dioxide.
See Editor's Note No. 1, page 2053.

Clear Skin - PhytoPharmica
Twenty drops contain: Cantharis 8x • Croton tiglium 8x • Arsenicum album 6x • Mercurius currosivus 6x • Pulsatilla 4x • Cistus canadensis 3x • Natrum phosphoricum 2x • Echinacea 1x • Juglans 1x • Viola tricolor 1x. In a base of 45% USP alcohol by volume.
See Editor's Note No. 1, page 2053.

Clear Skin 1 - Problem Skin Cleanser 6oz - Derma E
Purified Water • Tea Tree oil • Glycerin • Glyceryl Stearate • PEG 100 Stearate • Stearic Acid • Caprylic Triglyceride • Willow bark • Cetyl Alcohol • Cocobetaine • Lavender oil • Rosewood oil • Chamomile • Polysorbate-20 • Methylparaben • Ethylparaben • I. Urea.

Clear Skin 2 - Spot Blemish Treatment 1/2oz - Derma E
Purified Water • Glycerin • Tea Tree oil • Willow bark • Xanthan Gum • Chamomile • Rosewood oil • Lavender oil • Methylparaben • Ethylparaben • I. Urea.

Clear Skin 3 - Problem Skin Moisturizer 2oz - Derma E
Purified Water • Tea Tree oil • Lavender oil • Rosewood oil • Chamomile • Stearic Acid • Glyceryl Stearate • PEG 100 Stearate • Xanthan Gum • Glycerin • Caprylic Triglyceride • Willow bark • Cetyl Alcohol • Methylparaben • Ethylparaben • I. Urea.

Clear Thoughts - Rexall - Sundown
Two capsules contain: Vitamin E (as dl-alpha-tocopheryl acetate and d-alpha-tocopheryl succinate) 30 IU • Niacin (as niacinamide) 20 mg • Folic Acid 400 mcg • Vitamin B-12 (as cyanocobalamin) 60 mcg • Zinc (as zinc amino acid chelate) 15 mg • Ginkgo Biloba extract (standardized to 24% ginkgo flavonol glycosides, 14.4 mg; standardized to 6% terpene lactones, 3.6 mg) 60 mg • Gotu Kola aerial parts 150 mg • L-Glutamine 200 mg • L-Tyrosine 100 mg • Choline (as choline bitartrate) 50 mg • Phosphatidylserine complex (standardized to 30% phosphatidylserine, 15 mg) 50 mg • Damiana leaf 50 mg. Other Ingredients: Gelatin, Maltodextrin, Silica, Talc, Magnesium Stearate.

Clear Tinnitus - Clear Products
Each capsule contains: Calcarea Carbonica 6X • Cinchona Officinalis 3X • Chininum Sulphuricum 3X • Graphites 3X • Kali Carbonicum 6X • Lycopodium 3X • Salicylicium Acidum 3X • Proprietary Herbal Extracts Blend 500 mg: Pueraria root (ge gen), Platycodon root (jie geng), Angelica root (bai zhi), Coix seed (yi yi ren), Ginger root (sheng jiang), Ligustici root (chuan xiong), Peony root (bai shao), Perillia leaf (zi su ye), Magnolia flower (zin yi hua), Asarum leaf (xi xin), Cinnamon bark (gui zhi), Huang Qin (scutallaria root), Licorice root (gan cao). Other Ingredients: Magnesium Stearate, Gelatin, Silicon Dioxide.
See Editor's Note No. 1, page 2053.

Clear Vein Creme/Spider Vein & Bruise Solution 2oz - Derma E
Purified Water • Horse Chestnut extract • Witch Hazel extract • Grape skin extract • White Oak extract • Glycerin • Stearic Acid • Jojoba oil • Green Tea extract • Caprylic Triglyceride • Polysorbate 20 • Dimethicone • Glyceryl Stearate • PEG 100 Stearate • Pycnogenol • Cetyl Alcohol • Stearyl Alcohol • Tocopheryl Acetate (vitamin E) • Methylparaben • I. Urea.

ClearAc - Hyland's
Two tablets contain: Echinacea Angustifolia 6X • Berberis Vulgaris 6X • Sulphur Lod. 6X • Hepar Sulph. 6X. Base: Lactose.
See Editor's Note No. 1, page 2053.

CLENbutical - NutraBolics
Two capsules contain: Coleus Forskohlii 175 mg • Guarana extract (22% caffeine) 300 mg • White Kidney bean extract 400 mg • Green Tea extract (50% polyphenols) 200 mg • Citrus Aurantium (6% synephrine) 200 mg • Cayenne 100 mg • Ginger root 100 mg.
See Editor's Note No. 40, page 2058.

Clensa-Herb - Dial Herbs
Red Clover • Burdock • Echinacea • Chaparral • Mullein • Uva Ursi • Parsley • Marshmallow • Cascara Sagrada.

Clif BAR Apricot - Clif Bars
Brown Rice Syrup • Rolled Oats • Evaporated Cane Juice • Soy Protein Isolate • Rice Flour • Oat Flour • Soy Flour • Soybean • Dried Apricots (sulfured) • Apple Fiber • Oat Fiber • Milled Flaxseed • Soy Fiber • Chicory Extract • Lemon Fiber • Psyllium • Dried Apples • Prunes • Brown Rice • Malt Extract • Natural Flavor • Citric Acid • Sea Salt • Baking Soda • Decaffeinated Green Tea Extract.

Clif BAR Carrot Cake - Clif Bars
Brown Rice Syrup • Rolled Oats • Evaporated Cane Juice • Soy Protein Isolate • Rice Flour • Oat Flour • Soy Flour • Soybean • Dried

Apples • Apple Fiber • Oat Fiber • Milled Flaxseed • Soy Fiber • Chicory Extract • Lemon Fiber • Psyllium • Cocoa Butter • Soy Milk • Soy Lecithin • Dried Carrots • Brown Rice • Malt Extract • Soy Butter • Raisins • Coconut • Sea Salt • Natural Flavors • Spices • Baking Soda • Decaffeinated Green Tea Extract.

Clif BAR Chocolate Almond Fudge **-** Clif Bars
Brown Rice Syrup • Rolled Oats • Soy Protein Isolate • Rice Flour • Oat Flour • Soy Flour • Soybean • Evaporated Cane Juice • Soy Butter • Unsweetened Chocolate • Cocoa Butter • Soy Lecithin • Fig Paste • Almonds • Apple Fiber • Oat Fiber • Milled Flaxseed • Soy Fiber • Chicory Extract • Lemon Fiber • Psyllium • Natural Flavors • Sea Salt • Baking Soda • Decaffeinated Green Tea Extract.

Clif BAR Chocolate Brownie **-** Clif Bars
Brown Rice Syrup • Rolled Oats • Soy Protein Isolate • Rice Flour • Oat Flour • Soy Flour • Soybean • Evaporated Cane Juice • Unsweetened Chocolate • Cocoa Butter • Soy Lecithin • Fig Paste • Soy Butter • Dutch Process Cocoa • Apple Fiber • Oat Fiber • Milled Flaxseed • Soy Fiber • Chicory Extract • Lemon Fiber • Psyllium • Natural Flavors • Sea Salt • Baking Soda • Decaffeinated Green Tea Extract.

Clif BAR Chocolate Chip **-** Clif Bars
Brown Rice Syrup • Rolled Oats • Soy Protein Isolate • Rice Flour • Oat Flour • Soy Flour • Soybean • Evaporated Cane Juice • Unsweetened Chocolate • Cocoa Butter • Soy Lecithin • Soy Butter • Apple Fiber • Oat Fiber • Milled Flaxseed • Soy Fiber • Chicory Extract • Lemon Fiber • Psyllium • Fig Paste • Raisins • Brown Rice • Malt Extract • Natural Flavors • Sea Salt • Baking Soda • Cinnamon • Decaffeinated Green Tea Extract.

Clif BAR Chocolate Chip Peanut Crunch **-** Clif Bars
Unsweetened Chocolate • Cocoa Butter • Soy Lecithin • Peanut Butter • Peanut Flour • Apple Fiber • Oat Fiber • Milled Flaxseed • Soy Fiber • Chicory Extract • Lemon Fiber • Psyllium • Fig Paste • Peanuts • Natural Flavors • Sea Salt • Baking Soda • Decaffeinated Green Tea Extract.

Clif BAR Cookies 'N Cream **-** Clif Bars
Brown Rice Syrup • Rolled Oats • Soy Protein Isolate • Rice Flour • Oat Flour • Soy Flour • Soybean • Evaporated Cane Juice • Dutch Cocoa • Cocoa Butter • Chocolate Liquor • Oat Flour • Gum Arabic • Brown Rice • Malt Extract • Apple Fiber • Oat Fiber • Milled Flaxseed • Soy Fiber • Chicory Extract • Lemon Fiber • Psyllium • Soy Milk • Soy Lecithin • Almond Butter • Fig Paste • Natural Flavors • Cocoa • Sea Salt • Baking Soda • Decaffeinated Green Tea Extract.

Clif BAR Crunchy Peanut Butter **-** Clif Bars
Brown Rice Syrup • Rolled Oats • Soy Protein Isolate • Rice Flour • Oat Flour • Soy Flour • Soybean • Evaporated Cane Juice • Peanut Butter • Peanut Flour • Apple Fiber • Oat Fiber • Milled Flaxseed • Soy Fiber • Chicory Extract • Lemon Fiber • Psyllium • Fig Paste • Peanuts • Natural Flavor • Sea Salt • Baking Soda • Decaffeinated Green Tea Extract.

Clif BAR GingerSnap **-** Clif Bars
Brown Rice Syrup • Rolled Oats • Soy Protein Isolate • Rice Flour • Oat Flour • Soy Flour • Soybean • Evaporated Cane Juice • Ginger in cane syrup • Apple Fiber • Oat Fiber • Milled Flaxseed • Soy Fiber • Chicory Extract • Lemon Fiber • Psyllium • Soy Butter • Molasses • Fig Paste • Brown Rice • Malt Extract • Natural Flavors • Ground Ginger • Sea Salt • Baking Soda • Decaffeinated Green Tea Extract.

Clif SHOT Mmm...CHOCOLATE **-** Clif Bars
Brown Rice Syrup • Cocoa Powder • Chocolate Liquor • Natural Flavors • Sea Salt • Potassium Citrate • Magnesium Oxide.

Clif SHOT Mocha Mocha with Caffeine **-** Clif Bars
Brown Rice Syrup • Natural Flavors • Cocoa Powder • Kola Nut Extract (contains caffeine) • Sea Salt • Potassium Citrate • Magnesium Oxide.

Clif SHOT Razz Sorbet **-** Clif Bars
Brown Rice Syrup • Raspberry Puree • Sea Salt • Potassium Citrate • Magnesium Oxide.

Clif SHOT Sonic Strawberry with Caffeine **-** Clif Bars
Brown Rice Syrup • Strawberry Puree • Natural Flavor • Kola Nut Extract (contains caffeine) • Sea Salt • Potassium Citrate • Magnesium Oxide.

Clif SHOT Viva Vanilla **-** Clif Bars
Brown Rice Syrup • Natural Flavors • Sea Salt • Potassium Citrate • Magnesium Oxide.

Clinical Nutrients Antioxidant **-** PhytoPharmica
Three capsules contain: Vitamin A (beta-carotene) 10,000 IU • Vitamin C (ascorbic acid) 500 mg • Vitamin E (D-alpha tocopheryl succinate) 200 IU • Riboflavin (vitamin B2) 6 mg • Zinc (picolinate) 15 mg • Selenium (L-selenomethionine) 200 mcg • Manganese (gluconate) 2 mg • N-Acetylcysteine 100 mg • Red Cabbage (brassica oleracea) leaf extract 4:1 100 mg • Garlic (Allium sativum) bulb extract (deodorized) 100 mg • Ginger root/rhizome extract (zingiber officinale) 100 mg • Green Tea leaf extract (camellia sinensis) 100 mg • Blue-Green Algae 100 mg • Turmeric root extract (curcuma longa, standardized to contain 85%-100% curcumin) 50 mg • Grape seed extract (vitis vinifera, PCO, standardized to contain 95% procyanidolic oligomers [PCOs]) 10 mg.

Clinical Nutrients Eye Formula **-** PhytoPharmica
Three tablets contain: Bilberry fruit extract (vaccinium myrtillus, standardized to contain 25% anthocyanosides calculated as anthocyanidins) 160 mg • Copper (as copper gluconate) 1 mg • Grape seed extract (vitis vinifera, standardized to contain 95% procyanidolic oligomers (PCOs)) 50 mg • Hachimijiogan Herbal Complex 400 mg: Rehmannia root (rehmannia glutinosa), Poria whole plant (wolfiporia cocos), Chinese Yam root (dioscorea oppositafolia), Asiatic Dogwood aerial part (cornus officinalis), Barrenwort aerial part (epimedium grandiflorum), Water Plantain aerial part (alisma plantago-aquatica), Astragalus root (astragalus membranaceus), Cassia bark (cinnamomum aromaticum) • Lutein 5% (from calendula officinalis) 2 mg • Riboflavin (vitamin B2) 1.5 mg • Selenium (as L-selenomethionine) 50 mcg • Turmeric rhizome extract (curcuma longa, standardized to contain 85-100% curcumin) 50 mg • Vitamin A (50% as beta carotene and as retinyl acetate) 5000 IU • Vitamin C (ascorbic acid) 600 mg • Vitamin E (as D-alpha tocopheryl acid succinate) 60 IU • Zinc (as zinc picolinate) 9 mg.

Clinical Nutrients Flax Oil **-** PhytoPharmica
Each 1 tbsp serving (14 mL) contains: Flaxseed Oil 11 mL • Pumpkin Seed oil 2 mL • Borage seed oil 1 mL.

Clinical Nutrients Flax Oil Capsules **-** PhytoPharmica
Seven softgels contain: Flaxseed oil 5250 mg • Pumpkin seed oil 1050 mg • Borage seed oil 700 mg.

Clinical Nutrients for 45-Plus Women **-** PhytoPharmica
Six tablets contain: Betain HCl 25 mg • Bilberry fruit 4:1 extract (vaccinium myrtillus) 10 mg • Biotin 600 mcg • Black Tea leaf 5:1 extract (camellia sinensis) 50 mg • Boron (as sodium borate) 3 mg • Calcium (as calcium carbonate, tricalcium phosphate, and calcium citrate) 800 mg • Choline Bitartrate 215 mg • Chromium (as chromium picolinate) 200 mcg • Copper (as copper gluconate) 2 mg • Cranberry fruit extract (vaccinium macrocarpon, standardized to contain 5% anthocyanidins and 30% organic acids (quinic, malic, and citric acid) 25 mg • Folic Acid 800 mcg • Ginger rhizome extract (zingiber officinale) 60 mg • Grape seed 4:1 extract (vitis vinifera) 20 mg • Green Tea leaf 3:1 extract (camellia sinensis) 30 mg • Inositol 30 mg • Iodine (as potassium iodide) 450 mcg • Lipase 5 mg • Lutein (from calendula officinalis) 1.5 mg • Magnesium (as magnesium aspartate and magnesium oxide) 300 mg • Manganese (as manganese citrate) 2 mg • Molybdenum (as sodium molybdate) 75 mcg • Niacin (as niacinamide and niacin) 90 mg • Pantothenic Acid (as calcium D-pantothenate) 50 mg • Papain 15 mg • Pepsin (acid-stable protease) 5 mg • Phosphorus (from tricalcium phosphate) 180 mg • Potassium (as

potassium aspartate) 100 mg • Riboflavin (vitamin B2) 60 mg • Selenium (as L-selenomethionine) 200 mcg • Silicon (as magnesium trisilicate) 1 mg • Sour Cherry fruit 10:1 extract (prunus cerasus) 50 mg • Soy (glycine max) 30 mg • Thiamin (as thiamin HCl, vitamin B1) 60 mg • Vanadium (as vanadyl sulfate) 100 mcg • Vitamin A (75% as beta carotene and as retinyl acetate) 10,000 IU • Vitamin B12 (as cyanocobalamin) 800 mcg • Vitamin B6 (as pyridoxine HCl) 60 mg • Vitamin C (ascorbic acid) 300 mg • Vitamin D (as cholecalciferol) 400 IU • Vitamin E (as D-alpha tocopheryl acid succinate) 200 IU • Vitamin K (as phytonadione) 120 mcg • Zeaxanthin (from calendula officinalis) 60 mcg • Zinc (as zinc gluconate) 15 mg.

Clinical Nutrients for 50-Plus Men **-** PhytoPharmica
Four tablets contain: Betaine HCl 25 mg • Bilberry fruit 4:1 extract (vaccinium myrtillus) 10 mg • Biotin 600 mcg • Black Tea leaf 5:1 extract (camellia sinensis) 50 mg • Boron (as sodium borate) 3 mg • Bromelain (1200 MCU/g) 15 mg • Calcium (as calcium carbonate and calcium citrate) 400 mg • Choline Bitartrate 275 mg • Chromium (as chromium picolinate) 200 mcg • Copper (as copper gluconate) 2 mg • Folic Acid 800 mcg • Ginger rhizome extract (zingiber officinale) 40 mg • Grape seed 4:1 extract (vitis vinifera) 20 mg • Green Tea leaf 3:1 extract (camellia sinensis) 30 mg • Inositol 30 mg • Lipase 5 mg • Lutein (from calendula officinalis) 1.5 mg • Lycopene 2 mg • Magnesium (as magnesium aspartate and magnesium oxide) 250 mg • Manganese (as manganese citrate) 2 mg • Molybdenum (as sodium molybdate) 75 mcg • Niacin (as niacinamide and niacin) 120 mg • Panax Ginseng root extract (standardized to contain a minimum of 7% ginsenosides) 15 mg • Pantothenic Acid (as calcium D-pantothenate) 100 mg • Papain 15 mg • Pepsin (acid-stable protease) 5 mg • Potassium (as potassium aspartate) 100 mg • Riboflavin (vitamin B2) 60 mg • Saw Palmetto berry 4:1 extract (serenoa repens) 80 mg • Selenium (as L-selenomethionine) 200 mcg • Sodium 15 mg • Sour Cherry fruit 10:1 extract (prunus cerasus) 50 mg • Thiamin (as thiamin HCl, vitamin B1) 60 mg • Vanadium (as vanadyl sulfate) 100 mcg • Vitamin A (75% as beta carotene and as retinyl acetate) 10,000 IU • Vitamin B12 (as cyanocobalamin) 800 mcg • Vitamin B6 (as pyridoxine HCl) 60 mg • Vitamin C (ascorbic acid) 300 mg • Vitamin D (as cholecalciferol) 400 IU • Vitamin E (as D-alpha tocopheryl acid succinate) 200 IU • Vitamin K (as phytonadione) 120 mcg • Zeaxanthin (from calendula officinalis) 60 mcg • Zinc (as zinc gluconate) 30 mg.

Clinical Nutrients for Bone Health **-** PhytoPharmica
Three tablets contain: Vitamin C (ascorbic acid) 100 mg • Vitamin D (fish liver oil) 300 IU • Vitamin K (phytonadione) 300 mcg • Folic Acid 800 mcg • Vitamin B12 (cyanocobalamin) 800 mcg • Calcium (Krebs cycle chlelate/carbonate) 600 mg • Magnesium (Krebs cycle chelate) 150 mg • Zinc (picolinate) 15 mg • Copper (picolinate) 1 mg • Sodium 5 mg • Mixed flavonoids (citrus) 100 mg • Betaine HCl 30 mg • Soy (Glycine Max.) bean extract 20 mg • Boron (sodium tetrahydroborate) 3 mg • Silicon (sodium metasilicate) 1 mg • Strontium (chloride) 500 mcg.

Clinical Nutrients for Glucose Regulation **-** PhytoPharmica
2 tablets contain: Bilberry (vaccinium myrtillus extract standardized to contain 25% anthocyanosides calculated as anthocyanidins) 40 mg &#8226 Biotin 1 mg &#8226 Bitter Melon 2:1 extract (momordica charantia) 200 mg &#8226 Chromium (as chromium picolinate) 200 mcg &#8226 Copper (as copper gluconate) 0.5 mg &#8226 Fenugreek seed 4:1 extract (trigonella foenum-graceum) 100 mg &#8226 Folic Acid 400 mcg &#8226 Gymnema leaf extract (gymnema sylvestre, standardized to contain 25% gymnemic acids) 200 mg &#8226 Magnesium (as magnesium Krebs cycle chelates) 100 mg &#8226 Manganese (as manganese Krebs cycle chelates) 3.5 mg &#8226 Mixed Citrus Bioflavonoids 50% (from citrus fruits) 25 mg &#8226 Selenium (as L-selenomethionine) 50 mcg &#8226 Sodium 20 mg &#8226 Vanadium (as vanadyl sulfate) 1.6 mg &#8226 Vitamin B12 (as cyanocobalamin) 400 mcg &#8226 Vitamin B6 (as pyridoxine HCl) 10 mg &#8226 Vitamin C 300 mg &#8226 Vitamin E (as mixed tocopherols) 100 IU &#8226 Zinc (as zinc picolinate) 7.5 mg.

Clinical Nutrients for Heart Health **-** PhytoPharmica
Two tablets contain: Vitamin C (ascorbic acid) 100 mg • Vitamin E (D-alpha tocopheryl acetate) 100 IU • Niacin 100 mg • Vitamin B6 (pyridoxine HCl) 10 mg • Folic Acid 200 mcg • Vitamin B12 (cyanocobalamin) 200 mcg • Calcium pangamate 20 mg • Magnesium (oxide) 150 mg • Potassium (chloride) 75 mg • Hawthorn (Crataegus oxyacantha) leaf and flower extract (standardized to contain 1.8% vitexin-2-rhamnoside) 150 mg • Super seven complex mixture of herbs: Hydrangea (Hydrangea arborescens) root, Black Cohosh (Cimicifuga racemosa) root, (Rhizome) extract, Buchu (Barosma crenata) leaf extract, Couch Grass (Elytrigia repens) rhizome extract, Cornsilk (Zea mays) extract, Dandelion (Taraxacum officinale) leaf, Ginger (Zingiber officinale) root] 150 mg • Khella (ammi visnaga) fruit extract (standardized to contain a minimum of 10% pyrones calculated as khellin) 100 mg • L-Cysteine 100 mg • Carbamide 100 mg.

Clinical Nutrients for Joint Health - Capsules **-** PhytoPharmica
Four capsules contain: Vitamin C (ascorbic acid) 100 mg • Niacin/Niacinamide 330 mg • Vitamin B6 (pyridoxine HCl) 20 mg • Pantothenic Acid (calcium D-pantothenate) 100 mg • Magnesium (oxide) 100 mg • Zinc (picolinate) 3 mg • Copper (gluconate) 200 mcg • Manganese (chelate) 10 mg • Chloride (from glucosamine sulfate) 78 mg • Sodium 60 mg • Stabilized Glucosamine Sulfate 500 mg • Boswellia Serrata (gum resin) standardized to contain 65% boswellic acids 400 mg • Bio-Min T.R. 8 (a source of trace minerals) 100 mg • Chlorophyll 10 mg • Boron (sodium borate) 3 mg.

Clinical Nutrients for Joint Health - Tablets **-** PhytoPharmica
Two tablets contain: Vitamin C (ascorbic acid) 100 mg • Niacin/Niacinamide 330 mg • Vitamin B6 (pyridoxine HCl) 20 mg • Pantothenic Acid (calcium D-pantothenate) 100 mg • Magnesium (oxide) 100 mg • Zinc (picolinate) 3 mg • Copper (gluconate) 200 mcg • Manganese (chelate) 10 mg • Chloride (from glucosamine sulfate) 78 mg • Stabilized Glucosamine Sulfate 500 mg • Boswellia Serrata (gum resin) standardized to contain 65% boswellic acids 400 mg • Bio-Min T.R. 8 (a source of trace minerals) 100 mg • Chlorophyll 10 mg • Boron (sodium borate) 3 mg.

Clinical Nutrients for Male Teens **-** PhytoPharmica
Four tablets contain: Vitamin A (86% beta-carotene and 14% retinol) 17,500 IU • Vitamin C (ascorbic acid) 300 mg • Vitamin D (cholecalciferol) 100 IU • Vitamin E (D-alpha tocoptheryl succinate) 200 IU • Vitamin K (phytonadione) 60 mcg • Thiamin (thiamin HCl; vitamin B1) 30 mg • Riboflavin (vitamin B2) 30 mg • Niacin/Niacinamide 45 mg • Vitamin B6 (pyridoxine HCl) 30 mg • Folic Acid 800 mcg • Vitamin B12 (cyanocobalamin) 800 mcg • Biotin 300 mcg • Pantothenic Acid (calcium D-pantothenate) 30 mg • Calcium (citrate, carbonate) 400 mg • Iodine (kelp) 300 mcg • Magnesium (aspartate) 200 mg • Zinc (picolinate) 30 mg • Selenium (L-selenomethionine) 100 mcg • Copper (gluconate) 1.5 mg • Manganese (citrate) 15 mg • Chromium (polynicotinate) 200 mcg • Molybdenum (sodium molybdate) 25 mcg • Sodium 30 mg • Potassium (aspartate) 99 mg • Mixed flavonoids (citrus) 100 mg • Alfalfa leaf and stem juice concentrate (medicago sativa) 60 mg • Dandelion root 4:1 extract (taraxacum officinale) 60 mg • Ginger root/rhizome extract (zingiber officinale) 60 mg • Sarsaparilla root 4:1 extract (smilax officinalis) 60 mg • Choline Bitartrate 30 mg • Inositol 30 mg • Boron (sodium tetraborate decahydrate) 2 mg • Vanadium (sulfate) 50 mcg.

Clinical Nutrients for Men **-** PhytoPharmica
Three tablets contain: Bilberry fruit 4:1 extract (vaccinium myrtillus) 10 mg • Biotin 600 mcg • Black Tea leaf 5:1 extract 50 mg • Boron (as sodium borate) 2 mg • Calcium (as calcium carbonate and calcium citrate) 300 mg • Choline Bitartrate 215 mg • Chromium (as chromium picolinate) 200 mcg • Copper (as copper gluconate) 2 mg • Folic Acid 800 mcg • Ginger rhizome extract (zingiber officinale) 30 gm • Grape seed 4:1 extract (vitis vinifera) 20 mg • Green Tea leaf 3:1 extract (camellia sinensis) 30 mg • Inositol 30 mg • Iodine (as potassium iodide) 300 mcg • Lutein (from calendula officinalis)

1.5 mg • Lycopene 2 mg • Magnesium (as magnesium aspartate and magnesium oxide) 250 mg • Manganese (as manganese citrate) 2 mg • Molybdenum (as sodium molybdate) 75 mcg • Muira Puama root 6:1 extract (ptychopetalum olacoides) 30 mg • Niacin (as niacinamide and niacin) 90 mg • Panax Ginseng root extract (standardized to contain a minimum of 7% ginsenosides) 15 mg • Pantothenic Acid (as calcium D-pantothenate) 60 mg • Potassium (as potassium aspartate) 100 mg • Riboflavin (vitamin B2) 60 mg • Selenium (as L-selenomethionine) 200 mcg • Sodium 15 mg • Sour Cherry fruit 10:1 extract (prunus cerasus) 50 mg • Thiamin (as thiamin HCl, vitamin B1) 60 mg • Vanadium (as vanadyl sulfate) 100 mcg • Vitamin A (75% as beta carotene and as retinyl acetate) 10,000 IU • Vitamin B12 (as cyanocobalamin) 500 mcg • Vitamin B6 (as pyridoxine HCl) 60 mg • Vitamin C (ascorbic acid) 300 mg • Vitamin D (as cholecalciferol) 400 IU • Vitamin E (as D-alpha tocopheryl acid succinate) 200 IU • Vitamin K (as phytonadione) 80 mcg • Zeaxanthin (from calendula officinalis) 60 mcg • Zinc (as zinc gluconate) 30 mg.

Clinical Nutrients for Teens: Female Formula - PhytoPharmica
Four tablets contain: Vitamin A (88% beta-carotene and 12% retinol) 17,000 IU •Vitamin C (ascorbic acid) 300 mg • Vitamin D (ergocalciferol) 100 IU • Vitamin E (d-alpha tocopheryl succinate) 200 IU • Vitamin K (phytonadione) 60 mcg •Thiamin (thiamin HCl; vitamin B1) 30 mg •Riboflavin (vitamin B2) 30 mg • Niacin/Niacinamide 45 mg •Vitamin B6 (pyridoxine HCl) 90 mg •Folic Acid 800 mcg •Vitamin B12 (cyanocobalamin) 800 mcg • Biotin 300 mcg • Pantothenic Acid (calcium D-pantothenate) 30 mg • Calcium (citrate, carbonate) 500 mg • Iron (ferrous succinate) 30 mg •Iodine (kelp) 300 mcg • Magnesium (aspartate) 200 mg • Zinc (picolinate) 20 mg •Selenium (L-selenomethionine) 100 mcg • Copper (gluconate) 1.5 mg • Manganese (citrate) 15 mg •Chromium (polynicotinate) 200 mcg • Molybdenum (sodium molybdate) 25 mcg • Sodium 30 mg • Potassium (aspartate) 99 mg • Mixed flavonoids (citrus) 100 mg • Alfalfa (Medicago sativa) leaf and stem juice concentrate 60 mg • Choline Bitartrate 60 mg •Inositol 60 mg • Ginger (Zingiber officinale) root (rhizome) extract 60 mg •Dandelion (Taraxacum officinale) root extract 4:1 60 mg •Licorice (Glycyrrhiza glabra) root extract (standardized to contain 5% glycyrrhizic acid) 30 mg•Boron (sodium tetraborate decahydrate) 2 mg • Silica (sodium metasilicate) 1 mg • Vanadium (sulfate) 50 mcg.

Clinical Nutrients for Women - PhytoPharmica
Three tablets contain: Bilberry fruit 4:1 extract (vaccinium myrtillus) 10 mg • Biotin 600 mcg • Black Tea leaf 5:1 extract (camellia sinensis) 50 mg • Boron (as sodium borate) 3 mg • Calcium (as calcium carbonate, tricalcium phosphate, and calcium citrate) 500 mg • Chaste Tree berry extract (vitex agnus-castus, standadized to contain 0.5% agnusides) 20 mg • Choline Bitartrate 215 mg • Chromium (as chromium picolinate) 200 mcg • Copper (as copper gluconate) 2 mg • Cranberry fruit extract (vaccinium macrocarpon, standardized to contain 5% anthocyanidins and 30% organic acids (quinic, malic, and citric acid) 25 mg • Folic Acid 800 mcg • Ginger rhizome extract (zingiber officinale) 30 mg • Grape seed 4:1 extract (vitis vinifera) 20 mg • Green Tea leaf 3:1 extract (camellia sinensis) 30 mg • Inositol 30 mg • Iodine (as potassium iodide) 300 mcg • Iron (as ferrous succinate) 18 mg • Lutein (from calendula officinalis) 1.5 mg • Magnesium (as magnesium aspartate and magnesium oxide) 300 mg • Manganese (as manganese citrate) 2 mg • Molybdenum (as sodium molybdate) 75 mcg • Niacin (as niacinamide and niacin) 90 mg • Pantothenic Acid (as calcium D-pantothenate) 30 mg • Phosphorus (from tricalcium phosphate) 113 mg • Potassium (as potassium aspartate) 100 mg • Riboflavin (vitamin B2) 60 mg • Selenium (as L-selenomethionine) 200 mcg • Silicon (as magnesium trisilicate) 1 mg • Sour Cherry fruit 10:1 extract (prunus cerasus) 50 mg • Thiamin (as thiamin HCl, vitamin B1) 60 mg • Vanadium (as vanadyl sulfate) 100 mcg • Vitamin A (75% as beta carotene and as retinyl acetate) 10,000 IU • Vitamin B12 (as cyanocobalamin) 800 mcg • Vitamin B6 (as pyridoxine HCl) 95 mg • Vitamin C (ascorbic acid) 300 mg • Vitamin D (as cholecalciferol) 400 IU • Vitamin E (as D-alpha tocopheryl acid succinate) 200 IU • Vitamin K (as phytonadione) 90 mcg • Zeaxanthin (from calendula officinalis) 60 mcg • Zinc (as zinc gluconate) 20 mg.

Clinical Nutrients Prenatal Formula - PhytoPharmica
Four tablets contain: Biotin 600 mcg • Boron (as sodium borate) 1 mg • Calcium (as calcium carbonate, tricalcium phosphate, and calcium citrate) 1 g • Choline Bitartrate 90 mg • Chromium (as chromium polynicotinate) 200 mcg • Copper (as copper gluconate) 1.5 mg • Dandelion root 4:1 extract (taraxacum officinale) 60 mg • Folic Acid 800 mcg • Inositol 90 mg • Iodine (as potassium iodide) 300 mcg • Iron (as ferrous succinate) 30 mg • Magnesium (as magnesium citrate and magnesium oxide) 400 mg • Manganese (as manganese citrate) 2 mg • Mixed Citrus Bioflavonoids 50% (from citrus fruits) 90 mg • Molybdenum (as sodium molybdate) 25 mcg • Niacin (as niacin and niacinamide) 45 mg • Pantothenic Acid (as calcium D-pantothenate) 100 mg • Phosphorus (from tricalcium phosphate) 225 mg • Potassium (as potassium aspartate) 100 mg • Riboflavin (vitamin B2) 60 mg • Selenium (as L-selenomethionine) 100 mcg • Silicon (as magnesium trisilicate) 1 mg • Thiamin (as thiamin HCl, vitamin B1) 60 mg • Vanadium (as vanadyl sulfate) 50 mcg • Vitamin A (as beta carotene) 10,000 IU • Vitamin B12 (as cyanocobalamin) 800 mcg • Vitamin B6 (as pyridoxine HCl) 100 mg • Vitamin C (as ascorbic acid) 300 mg • Vitamin D (as cholecalciferol) 200 IU • Vitamin E (as D-alpha tocopheryl acid succinate) 200 IU • Vitamin K (as phytonadione) 500 mcg • Zinc (as zinc picolinate) 30 mg.

Clinical Nutrients to Retain Healthy Cholesterol Levels - PhytoPharmica
Each capsule contains: Red Yeast (Monascus purpureus) rice 475 mg • Artichoke (Cynara scolymus) leaf extract (standardized to contain 13%-18% caffeylquinic acids calculated as chlorogenic acid) 50 mg • Ginger (Zingiber officinale) root (rhizome) extract 50 mg • Coenzyme Q10 (CoQ10) 8 mg.
See Editor's Note No. 21, page 2056.

CM Complex - Source Naturals
Three 500 mg softgels contain: Cetyl Myristoleate 180 mg • Cetyl Oleate (base of mixed fatty acid esters, olive oil and vitamin E) 375 mg.

CM Source - Now
Each 500 mg capsule contains: Cetyl Myristoleate 100 mg.

CM+ - Metabolic Response Modifiers
Each softgel contains: Cetylmyristoleate (CMO) complex (Yielding 100 mg CMO) 500 mg.

CMG - Natrol
Two capsules contain: Cetyl Myristoleate Proprietary Blend (CetylPure) 500 mg • MSM (Methyl Sulfonyl Methane) 500 mg • Glucosamine Sulfate 500 mg • Sea Cucumber 25 mg. Other Ingredients: Silica, Magnesium stearate, Gelatin.

C-M-K Citrate - Progressive Labs
Each capsule contains: Calcium (as calcium citrate) 100 mg • Magnesium (as magnesium citrate) 100 mg • Potassium (as potassium citrate) 25 mg.

Co Enzyme Q10 - Jamieson
Each capsule contains: Co-Enzyme Q10 30 mg.

Co Q10 - Pharmanex
Each softgel contains: Vitamin E (from Mixed Tocopherols) 30 IU • Coenzyme Q10 (Ubiquinone) 30 mg. Other Ingredients: Rice Bran Oil, Gelatin, Glycerin, Yellow Beeswax, Annatto Extract, Titanium Dioxide.

Coagulase Oxygenation Formula, Fibrenase II - NutriCology
Each tablet contains: Proprietary Blend 500 mg: Panax Notoginseng root, Crataegus Oxyacantha fruit, Centella Asiatica leaves, Salvia Miltiorrhiza root. Other Ingredients: Cellulose, Stearic Acid.

Some Brand Name Natural Products - What they Contain

www.NaturalDatabase.com contains MANY more listings than appear here.

Cobra Powerful Men's Performance Enhancer **-** Natural Balance
Two capsules contain: Proprietary Blend 986 mg: Kola nut seed extract (contains caffeine), Yohimbe bark extract/powder, Oatstraw aerial portion extract, Nettles leaf extract, Eleuthero root, Horny Goat Weed aerial portion (epimedium), Catuaba bark, Muira Puama root, Korean Ginseng root/rhizome, Damiana leaf, Saw Palmetto fruit. Other Ingredients: Gelatin, Magnesium Stearate.

Cocoa Butter & E Replenishing Creme 4oz **-** Derma E
Purified Water • Safflower oil • Stearic Acid • Cetyl Alcohol • Glyceryl Stearate • PEG 100 Stearate • Cocoa butter • Glycerin • Tea • Tocopheryl Acetate (vitamin E) • Retinyl Palmitate (vitamin A) • Ergocalciferol (vitamin D) • Panthenol • Sunflower oil • Wheat Germ oil • Allantoin • Methylparaben • I. Urea • Annatto • Fragrant oils.

Cocoon GH Liquid Spray **-** Cocoon Nutrition
Each 1 oz dropper contains: Growth Hormone 600 ng. Other Ingredients: Purified Water, Sodium Citrate.

Cod Liver Oil - GNC A-Z **-** GNC
Each capsule contains: Vitamin A (as cod liver oil) 1250 IU • VItamin D (as cod liver oil) 135 IU. Other Ingredients: Gelatin, Soybean oil, Glycerin.

Cod Liver Oil **-** Jamieson
Each capsule contains: Vitamin A (Retinol) 1250 IU • Vitamin D 100 IU (Natural Vitamin A & D from North Atlantic Cod Liver Oils).

Cod Liver Oil **-** Nature's Way
Each softgel contains: Cod Liver Oil 1000 mg • Vitamin A (from cod liver oil) 1250 IU • Vitamin D (from cod liver oil) 135 IU. Other Ingredients: Gelatin, Glycerin, Water.

Cod Liver Oil **-** Puritan's Pride
Each softgel contains: Natural Vitamin A 2,664 IU • Natural Vitamin D (from 1,000 mg of Cod Liver Oil) 200 IU. Provides a rich source of Omega 3 fatty acids, EPA and DHA.

Cod Liver Oil & Evening Primrose Oil **-** Puritan's Pride
Each softgel contains: Natural Vitamin A 2,664 IU • Natural Vitamin D (from 500 mg of Cod Liver Oil) 200 IU • Evening Primrose Oil 500 mg. Provides a rich source of Omega-3 fatty acids, EPA and DHA.

Cod Liver Oil (A-2500, D-270) **-** Rexall - Sundown
Each softgel contains: Vitamin A (from cod liver oil) 2500 IU • Vitamin D (from cod liver oil) 270 IU • Cod Liver Oil 650 mg • Docosahexaenoic Acid (DHA) 52 mg • Eicosapentaenoic Acid (EPA) 52 mg. Other Ingredients: Gelatin, Glycerin, Water.

Cod Liver Oil with Omega-3 Fatty Acids - GNC A-Z **-** GNC
Each capsule contains: Vitamin A (as cod liver oil) 1250 IU • Vitamin D (as cod liver oil) 135 IU • Vitamin E (as d-alpha Tocopherol) 1 IU • EPA (Eicosapentaenoic Acid) 50 mg • DHA (Docosahexaenoic Acid) 40 mg. Other Ingredients: Gelatin, Soybean oil, Glycerin, Peppermint oil.

CoenZest **-** Holista
Each capsule contains: CoEnzyme Q10 (ubiquinone) 30 mg. Other Ingredients: Organic Flax Seed Oil.

Coenzymated B-1 **-** Source Naturals
Each tablet contains: Coenzyme Vitamin B1 (Cocarboxylase) (Yielding 16.25 mg of activated Vitamin B1) 25 mg. In a base of Mannitol, Sorbitol, Natural Peppermint, and Sodium Citrate.

Coenzyme Q10 **-** CVS Pharmacy
Each softgel contains: Coenzyme Q10 100 mg. Other Ingredients: Soybean Oil, Gelatin, Glycerin, Yellow Beeswax, Lecithin, Titanium Dioxide, Annatto, D-Alpha Tocopheryl, Turmeric.

Coenzyme Q10 **-** DreamPharm
Each capsule contains: Coenzyme Q10 30 mg • Radix Salviae Miltiorrhizae 170 mg • Angelica Sinensis 100 mg • Cinnamomi Ramulus 100 mg • Sclerotium Poriae Cocos 100 mg.

Coenzyme Q-10 - Fields of Nature **-** Inverness Medical Innovations, Inc.
Each capsule contains: Coenzyme Q-10 30 mg. Other Ingredients: Microcrystalline Cellulose, Gelatin, Magnesium Stearate.

Coenzyme Q-10 - GNC Preventive Nutrition **-** GNC
Each capsule contains: Coenzyme Q-10 30 mg. Other Ingredients: Dicalcium Phosphate, Cellulose, Gelatin, Stearic Acid.

Coenzyme Q-10 **-** Natrol
Each capsule contains: CoEnzyme Q10 30 mg. Other Ingredients: Rice Powder, Magnesium Stearate, Gelatin.

Coenzyme Q10 **-** Optimum Nutrition
Each capsule contains: Coenzyme Q10 100 mg. Other Ingredients: Microcrystalline Cellulose, Gelatin, Magnesium Stearate.

Coenzyme Q-10 **-** Puritan's Pride
Each softgel contains: Coenzyme Q-10 10 mg. Other Ingredients: Ricebran Oil, Gelatin, Glycerin, Yellow Beeswax.

Coenzyme Q10 **-** Solanova
Each softsule contains: Vitamin E (d-alpha tocopherol concentrate) 150 IU • Coenzyme Q-10 (ubidecarenone Hydrosoluble) 60 mg. Other Ingredients: Gelatin, Glycerin, Purified Water, Titanium Dioxide, Annato seed extract, plus a proprietary Bio-Solv base (polysorbate 80, lecithin, sorbitan monoleate, medium chain triglycerides).

Coenzyme Q10 **-** Source Naturals
Each sublingual tablet contains: Coenzyme Q10 30 mg.

Coenzyme Q-10 **-** The Vitamin Shoppe
Each capsule contains: Co-Enzyme Q10 75 mg. Other Ingredients: Cellulose, Magnesium Stearate, Water.

Coenzyme Q10 - YourLife **-** Leiner Health Products
Each softgel contains: Coenzyme Q10 30 mg. Other Ingredients: Hydrogenated Vegetable Oil, Refined Soybean Oil, Gelatin, Glycerin, Lecithin, Titanium Dioxide, Red 40 Lake, d-Alpha Tocopherol, Yellow 6 Lake, Blue 1 Lake.

Coenzyme Q10 & L-Carnitine **-** PhysioLogics
Each softgel contains: Vitamin C (as ascorbyl palmitate) 12 mg • Vitamin E (as d-alpha tocopherol) 75 IU • Gamma Tocopherol 10 mg • L-Carnitine (as l-carnitine fumarate) 250 mg • Coenzyme Q10 30 mg. Other Ingredients: Polysorbate 80, Gelatin, Glycerin, Lecithin, Oleyl Lactylic Acid, Titanium Dioxide Color, Beeswax (yellow), Annato Color.

Coenzyme Q10 (100 mg) **-** Pro Health
Each capsule contains: Coenzyme Q10 100 mg. Other Ingredients: Microcrystalline Cellulose, Gelatin, Magnesium Stearate, Silicon Dioxide.

Coenzyme Q10 (100 mg) with Vitamin E **-** Pro Health
Each softgel contains: Vitamin A (beta carotene, D. salina) 2000 IU • Vitamin E (d-alpha-tocopherol with mixed tocopherols) 100 IU • Coenzyme Q10 (from soy) 100 mg • Beta Carotene 1.18 mg. Other Ingredients: Rice Bran Oil, Yellow Beeswax, Gelatin, Glycerin, Water, Annatto Extract, Titanium Dioxide.

Coenzyme Q10 (30 mg) **-** Pro Health
Each Vcap contains: Coenzyme Q10 (from vegetable/plant lipids) 30 mg. Other Ingredients: White Rice Powder, Cellulose.

Coenzyme Q10 (400 mg) **-** Pro Health
Each softgel contains: Vitamin E (d-alpha-tocopherol) 30 IU • Coenzyme Q10 400 mg • Soy Lecithin 50 mg. Other Ingredients:

Rice Bran Oil, Gelatin, Glycerine (vegetable source), Lecithin, Purified Water, Beeswax, Annatto Extract (natural colorant).

Coenzyme Q10 (50 mg) **-** Pro Health
Each softgel contains: Vitamin E (d-alpha tocopherol acetate) 30 IU • Selenium (l-selenomethionine) 70 mcg • Coenzyme Q10 (from soy) 50 mg. Other Ingredients: Rice Bran Oil, Beeswax, Lecithin, Gelatin, Glycerine, Water, Annatto (natural color).

Coenzyme Q10 100 mg **-** Leiner Health Products
Each capsule contains: Coenzyme Q10 100 mg. Other Ingredients: Maltodextrin, Gelatin, Magnesium Stearate.

Coenzyme Q10 100 MG **-** PhysioLogics
Each capsule contains: Coenzyme Q10 100 mg. Other Ingredients: Rice Powder, Gelatin, Vegetable Magnesium Stearate.

Coenzyme Q10 100 mg with Vitamin E - Vitaline Formulas **-** Integrative Therapeutics
Each wafer contains: Vitamin E (as dl-alpha tocopheryl acetate, d-alpha tocopheryl acetate, mixed tocopherols) 300 IU • Coenzyme Q10 (ubiquinone) 100 mg. Other Ingredients: Fructose, Dextrates, Silicone Dioxide, Vanilla Flavor, Maple Nut Flavor, Licorice Extract, Vegetable Fatty Acids, Magnesium Sulfate.

Coenzyme Q-10 100MG **-** Nature Made
Each softgel contains: Coenzyme Q-10 100 mg.

Coenzyme Q10 200 mg - Vitaline Formulas **-** Integrative Therapeutics
Each tablet contains: Coenzyme Q10 (ubiquinone) 200 mg. Other Ingredients: Vegetable Fatty Acids, Silicon Dioxide, Magnesium Sulfate, Microcrystalline Cellulose, Stearic Acid, Croscarmellose Sodium, Magnesium Stearate.

Coenzyme Q10 200 mg with Vitamin E - Vitaline Formulas **-** Integrative Therapeutics
Each wafer contains: Vitamin E (from dl-alpha tocopheryl acetate, d-alpha tocopheryl acetate, and mixed tocopherols) 400 IU • Coenzyme Q10 (ubiquinone) 200 mg. Other Ingredients: Fructose, Dextrates, Silicon Dioxide, Calcium Silicate, Magnesium Stearate, Natural Vanilla flavor, Maple Nut Flavor, Licorice Root Extract, Vegetable Fatty Acids, Magnesium Sulfate.

Coenzyme Q-10 200mg **-** Nature Made
Each softgel contains: Coenzyme Q-10 200 mg.

Coenzyme Q10 30 mg **-** Leiner Health Products
Each softgel contains: Coenzyme Q10 30 mg. Other Ingredients: Hydrogenated Vegetable Oil, Refined Soybean Oil, Gelatin, Glycerin, Lecithin, Titanium Dioxide, Red 40 Lake, d-Alpha Tocopherol, Yellow 6 Lake, Blue 1 Lake.

Coenzyme Q10 30 MG **-** PhysioLogics
Each capsule contains: Coenzyme Q10 30 mg. Other Ingredients: Rice Powder, Gelatin, Silica, Vegetable Magnesium Stearate.

CoEnzyme Q10 30 mg **-** Vital Nutrients
Each capsule contains: CoEnzyme Q10 30 mg.

Coenzyme Q-10 30MG **-** Nature Made
Each softgel contains: Coenzyme Q-10 30 mg.

Coenzyme Q10 50 mg **-** Pro Health
Two capsules contain: Coenzyme Q10 50 mg. Other Ingredients: Microcrystalline Cellulose, Gelatin, Magnesium Stearate, Silicon Dioxide.

Coenzyme Q10 60 mg - Vitaline Formulas **-** Integrative Therapeutics
Each tablet contains: Coenzyme Q10 60 mg. Other Ingredients: Vegetable Fatty Acids, Silicon Dioxide, Magnesium Sulfate, Microcrystalline Cellulose, Stearic Acid, Magnesium Stearate.

Coenzyme Q10 Lozenges (200 mg) **-** Pro Health
Each lozenge contains: Vitamin E (as d-alpha tocopheryl succinate) 100 IU • CoQ10 (coenzyme Q10 as ubidecarenone, from plant lipids) 200 mg • Non-GE Soy Lecithin 50 mg. Other Ingredients: Fructose, Cellulose, Sorbitol, Stearic Acid (vegetable source), Silica, Citric Acid, Natural Orange Flavor, Magnesium Stearate (vegetable source).

CoEnzyme Q10 Powder **-** Vital Nutrients
Each 1/4 teaspoon contains: CoEnzyme Q10 300 mg.

Coenzyme Q10 Q-Sorb 120 MG **-** PhysioLogics
Each softgel contains: Q-Sorb Coenzyme Q10 120 mg. Other Ingredients: Rice Bran Oil, Gelatin, Glycerin, Lecithin, Beeswax / Soybean Oil Mixture, Titanium Dioxide Color.

Coenzyme Q10 Q-Sorb 200 MG **-** PhysioLogics
Each softgel contains: Q-Sorb Coenzyme Q10 200 mg. Other Ingredients: Rice Bran Oil, Gelatin, Glycerin, Lecithin, Titanium Dioxide Color, Beeswax / Soybean Oil Mixture.

Coenzyme Q10 Q-Sorb 75 MG **-** PhysioLogics
Each softgel contains: Coenzyme Q10 75 mg. Other Ingredients: Rice Bran oil, Gelatin, Glycerin, Lecithin, Beeswax / Soybean Oil Mixture, Titanium Dioxide Color.

Coffeccino **-** Advocare International
Each packet contains: Garcinia Cambogia extract 500 mg • Caffeine 120 mg • L-Tyrosine 800 mg. Other Ingredients: Fructose, Sugar, Polydextrose, Canola Oil, Corn Syrup Solids, Modified Casein, Coffee Powder, L-Tyrosine, Garcinia Cambogia Extract, Cocoa Powder, Caffeine, Natural Flavors, Artificial Flavors, Xanthan Gum, Ascorbic Acid, Calcium Pantothenate, Pyridoxine Hydrochloride, Chromium Polynicotinate (ChromeMate), Folic Acid.

Cognicine **-** Pacific BioLogic
DMAE • Bacopin • Ashwagandha extract • Black Pepper extract (bioperine).

Cognita (Preventive Nutrition) **-** GNC
Three capsules contain: Vitamin E (as natural D-alpha tocopheryl acetate) 272 IU • Thiamin (B1, as thiamin mononitrate) 100 mg • Folate, Folic Acid, Folacin 200 mcg • Vitamin B12 (as cyanocobalamin) 25 mcg • Phosphatidyl Choline (as soy lecithin) 250 mg • Ginkgo Biloba leaf extract 120 mg • EPA (eicosapentaenoic acid, as fish body oil) 75 mg • DHA (docosahexaenoic acid, as fish body oil) 50 mg • Coenzyme Q10 10 mg • Huperzine A 100 mg. Other Ingredients: Soybean Oil, Gelatin, Glycerin, Caramel Color, Titanium Dioxide (natural mineral whitener).

Cognizin brand **-** Kyowa Hakko U.S.A., Inc.
Citicoline.
See Editor's Note No. 44, page 2058.

CognoBlend **-** Unicity International, Inc.
Two capsules contain: Bacopa monniera leaf extract (standardized to 20% bacosides A&B, 30 mg) 150 mg • Ginkgo Biloba leaf extract (standardized to 24% ginkgo flavone glycosides, 14.4 mg; standardized to 6% terpene lactones, 3.6 mg) 60 mg • Cognitive Proprietary Blend 600 mg: Cat's Claw bark PTI-00703 (uncaria tomentosa), Gotu Kola leaf, Rosemary leaf. Other Ingredients: Gelatin.

Cold & Flu (Cold and Flu) Capsules **-** Quantum, Inc.
Three capsules contain: Vitamin C 25 mg • Echinacea angustifolia standardized to 4% phenolic compounds 100 mg • Elderberry (10:1 extract) 100 mg • Goldenseal root (3:1 extract) 25 mg. Other Ingredients: Vegetable Sterine, Magnesium stearate, Micro Crystalline Cellulose.

Cold & Flu (Cold and Flu) Liquid Extract **-** Quantum, Inc.
Each two ounces contain: Fresh undried Echinacea purpurea whole plant 30% • Goldenseal root 20% • Elderberry 40% • Echinacea angustifolia 10%. In a base of Alcohol (approximately 20%), Distilled Water.

Some Brand Name Natural Products - What they Contain

www.NaturalDatabase.com contains MANY more listings than appear here.

Cold & Flu Bath - Abra Therapeutics
Sodium Borate • Sodium Sulfate • Sodium Chloride • Sodium Sesquicarbonate • Olive Oil • Essential Oils Blend: Eucalyptus oil, Peppermint oil, Rosemary oil, Tea Tree oil • Herbal Extracts Blend: Echinacea, Sage leaves, Melissa, Dandelion, Berberry, Pepperwood • Chromium Oxide • Trace Mineral Salts.

Cold & Flu Remedy - PhytoPharmica
Twenty-five drops contain: Gelsemium sempervirens 6x • Aconitum napellus 4x • Arnica montana 4x • Belladonna 4x • Cinchona officinalis 4x • Bryonia 3x • Drosera rotundifolia 3x • Eupatorium 3x • Senega officinalis 3x • Eucalyptus globulus 1x. In a base of 50% USP alcohol by volume.
See Editor's Note No. 1, page 2053.

Cold and Flu Formula - Body Language Vitamin Co.
Each capsule contains: Vitamin C (ascorbic acid) 333 mg • Zinc 12 mg • Proprietary Blend 425 mg: Echinacea purpurea, Echinacea pallida, Goldenseal, Astragalus, Elder Flower, Linden Flower, Meadowsweet, L-Arginine, Quercetin, Bioflavonoids.

Cold Care P.M. - Traditional Medicinals
Active Ingredient: Menthol: 5 mg per cup as it naturally occurs in the Peppermint leaf (Mentha x piperia) present in the blend. Other Herbal Ingredients: Licorice root, Chamomile flower, Tilla Starflower, Yarrow flower, Passion flower herb, Eucalyptus leaf, Elder flower.

Cold Cayenne - Olympian Labs
Each capsule contains: Cayenne (40000 h.u.) 500 mg.

Cold Fusion NO2 - Legal Gear
Each 1 tsp serving contains: Arginine Complex: Arginine AKG 2:1 / Diarginine Malate 3500 mg, Taurine 1000 mg, Ornithine 250 mg, Acetyl-L-Carnitine 250 mg. Other Ingredients: Filtered Water, Glycerine, Sugar, Citric Acid, Natural and Artificial Flavors, Red no 40, Blue no 1, Sodium Saccharin, Sodium Benzoate.

Cold Relief - Jamieson
Each capsule contains: Ephedra (Ma Huang) 63.75 mg • Grindelia 2 mg • Andrographis 10 mg • Echinacea Purpurea 8.33 mg • Picrorrhiza 2.5 mg.
See Editor's Note No. 30, page 2056.

Cold Season Formula - Nature's Way
Three capsules contain: Echinacea purpurea (stem, leaf, flower) 450 mg • Ester-C (patented form of Vitamin C) 200 mg • Isatis 150 mg • Ligustrum fruits 70 mg • Sambucol (patented Black Elderberry extract) 100 mg • Siberian Ginseng root 150 mg • Usnea Barbata 100 mg • Vitamin A (retinol palmitate) 6,722 IU • Zinc amino acid chelate 25 mg. Other Ingredients: Cellulose, Gelatin, Magnesium stearate.

Cold Season Nutrition Booster - Advocare International
Each capsule contains: Echinacea root extract (echinacea purpurea) 200 mg • Astragalus root extract (astragalus membranaceus) 50 mg • Goldenseal root extract (hydrastis canadensis) 25 mg • Shiitake mushroom mycelium extract (lentinus edodes) 100 mg • Elderberry flower/fruit extract (sambucus canedensis) 10 mg • Quercetin 50 mg. Other Ingredients: Silicon Dioxide, Magnesium Stearate, Gelatin.

Cold Season Plus+ Zinc Lozenges - Quantum, Inc.
Each lozenge contains: Zinc acetate 14 mg • Vitamin A acetate 500 IU • Slippery Elm bark (Ulmus fulva) 20 mg • Propolis 5 mg. In a base of Goldenseal, Sugar, Dextrose, Fructose.

Cold Sore Relief - PhytoPharmica
Allantoin (1%), Lemon Balm leaf 65-75:1 extract (melissa officinalis), White Soft Paraffin, Benzyl Alcohol.

Cold-Eeze - Quigley Co.
Each lozenge contains: Zinc Gluconate 11.5 mg. Other Ingredients: Glycine, corn syrup, sucrose, and natural flavors.

Cold-Eezer Plus - Quigley Co.
Each lozenge contains: Zinc Gluconate 14.5 mg. Other Ingredients: Glycerine, corn syrup, sucrose, and natural flavors.

Coldflua - HerbaSway
Bitter Orange • Kudzu • Ginger • Echinacea • Astragalus • Knotweed • Schisandra • Blackberry • Licorice • Skullcap • Cayenne pepper • HerbaSwee (Cucurbitaceae fruit).
See Editor's Note No. 40, page 2058.

colds & flu - nelsons - Nelson Bach USA Ltd.
Active Ingredients: Anas barbariae 30C HPUS • Arsenicum Iod 30C HPUS • Gelsemium 30C HPUS • Eupatorium perf 30C HPUS. Inactive Ingredients: Lactose, Sucrose.
See Editor's Note No. 1, page 2053.

Cold-X10 - Olympian Labs
Three capsules contain: Ester C 180 mg • Zinc Gluconate 15 mg • Garlic 500 mg • Cat's Claw 250 mg • Echinacea 500 mg • Gotu Kola 100 mg • Proteolytic Enzymes 100 mg.

Colest-Oil - Aboca USA, Inc
Three capsules contain: Fish Oil 720 mg (eicosapentaenoic acid 150 mg, docosahexaenoic acid 370 mg) • Guggul Olec-Gum-Resin extract in Flaxseed oil (1:10) 330 mg • Garlic bulb extract in Flaxseed oil (1:10) 110 mg. Other Ingredients: Gelatin (capsule), Essential Oil Of Rosemary.

Coleus forskohlii - Vital Nutrients
Each capsule contains: Coleus Forskohlii extract (standardized to 10% forskolin) 90 mg.

Coleus Forskohlii extract - Enzymatic Therapy
Each capsule contains: Coleus Forskohlii extract standardized to contain 18% Forskolin (9 mg per capsule) 50 mg.

Colic Tablets - Hyland's
Each tablet contains: Dioscorea as Wild Yam 2X HPUS • Chamomilla as Chamomile 3X HPUS • Colocynth as Bitter Apple 3X HPUS. In a base of Lactose NF (Milk Sugar).
See Editor's Note No. 1, page 2053.

Colic-Ease Gripe Water - Colic-Ease, Inc.
Active Ingredients: Dill Oil • Caraway Oil • Cinnamon bark oil • Clove oil (clove bud) • Cardamon Oil. Inactive Ingredients: Deionized Water, Fructose.

Collagen Type II - Swanson
Six capsules contain: Hydrolyzed Type II Collagen (certified 100% chicken sternal cartilage) 3 g.
See Editor's Note No. 14.

Colloidal Magnesium Plus - Progressive Labs
Each capsule contains: Colloidal Calcium 25 mg • Colloidal Magnesium 50 mg • Colloidal Zinc 1.5 mg • Colloidal Copper 1 mg • Colloidal Manganese 0.1 mg • Colloidal Chromium 0.03 mg • Colloidal Molybdenum 0.012 mg.

Colloidal Minerals - Progressive Labs
Each 1/2 oz serving contains: Calcium 109 mg • Iron 0.24 mg • Phosphorus 109 mg • Iodine 180 mcg • Magnesium 56.9 mg • Zinc 16.3 mg • Selenium 0.09 mcg • Copper 1.24 mg • Manganese 2.8 mg • Chromium 0.4 mcg • Molybdenum 0.01 mcg • Chloride 0.1 mg • Sodium 0.74 mg • Potassium 171 mg • Sulfur 0.08 mg • Aluminum 2.15 mg • Silicon 0.4 mg • Lanthanum 0.1 mg • Thallium 0.02 mg • Cesium 0.4 mcg • Strontium 5.8 mcg • Vanadium 5.4 mcg • Boron 4.62 mcg • Nickel 4.45 mcg • Scandium 3.3 mcg • Ruthenium 3.13 mcg • Lithium 2.15 mcg • Titanium 1.57 mcg • Neodynium 0.15 mcg • Antimony 1.3 mcg • Cobalt 1.06 mcg • Flouride 0.94 mcg • Bismuth 0.33 mcg • Thallium 0.28 mcg • Zirconium 0.23 mcg • Beryllium 0.2 mcg • Cerium 0.2 mcg • Erbium 0.2 mcg • Bromine 0.16 mcg • Indium 0.13 mcg • Rubidium 0.13 mcg • Silver 0.1 mcg • Tin 0.1 mcg • Yttrium 0.1 mcg • Gallium 0.08 mcg • Tellurium 0.07 mcg • Praseodymium 0.05 mcg • Samarium 0.05 mcg • Barium 0.02 mcg •

BRAND NAMES

Cadmium 0.02 mcg • Dysprosium 0.02 mcg • Germanium 0.01 mcg • Gold < 0.01 mcg • Europium < 0.01 mcg • Niobium < 0.01 mcg • Palladium < 0.01 mcg • Ytterbium < 0.01 mcg • Hafnium < 0.01 mcg • Iridium < 0.01 mcg • Rhodium < 0.01 mcg • Terbium < 0.01 mcg • Holmium < 0.01 mcg • Lutetium < 0.01 mcg • Rhenium < 0.01 mcg • Tantalum < 0.01 mcg • Thorium < 0.01 mcg • Tungsten < 0.01 mcg • Plantium < 0.01 mcg • Carbon 7.8%. Other Ingredients: Water, Glycerine, Natural Flavor, Grapefruit seed extract, Stevia.

Colloidal Silver **-** Changes International, Inc.
Four droppers (4 mL) contain: Colloidal Silver 20 mcg. Other Ingredients: Demineralized water.

Colloidal Trace Minerals **-** Source Naturals
Two droppers (approximately 2.5 ml) contain: Boron, Calcium, Chromium, Copper, Iodine, Iridium, Iron, Lithium, Magnesium, Manganese, Molybdenum, Phosphorus, Potassium, Rhodium, Selenium, Silica, Silver, Sulfur, Vanadium, Zinc, Electrolyte complex (from colloidally suspended minerals, desalinated seawater, methylparaben).

Colloidal Vitamins **-** Progressive Labs
Each 1/2 oz serving contains: Vitamin A (as beta carotene) 5000 IU • Vitamin C (ascorbic acid) 300 mg • Vitamin D 400 IU • Vitamin E 60 IU • Vitamin K 300 mcg • Thiamin (Vitamin B1) 3 mg • Riboflavin (Vitamin B2) 3.4 mg • Niacin (as niacinamide) 40 mg • Vitamin B6 4 mg • Folate (folic acid) 400 mcg • Vitamin B12 3 mcg • Biotin 300 mcg • Pantothenic Acid 20 mg • Choline Bitartrate 50 mg • Myonositol (inositol) 50 mg • Essential Fatty Acid complex 10 mg • Amino Acid complex 10 mg • Aloe powder 3 mg. Other Ingredients: Water, Glycerine, Natural Flavor, Grapefruit seed extract, Stevia.

Coloklysis **-** PhysioLogics
Each scoop (12 g) contains: Dietary Fiber 9 g • Calcium (as tricalcium phosphate) 25 mg • Sodium 10 mg • Potassium 10 mg • Psyllium seed husk (plantago ovata) 9.1 g • Oat fiber (avena sativa) 1 g • Rice Bran 500 mg • Fructooligosaccharides 250 mg • Stevia leaf extract (stevia rebaudiana) 72 mg • Alfalfa (medicago sativa) 38 mg • Barley leaf (hordium vulgare) 38 mg • Apple Pectin (malus sylvestris) 38 mg • Buckthorn bark (frangula alnus) 38 mg • Papain (from carica papaya) 38 mg • Cascara Sagrada (rhamnus purshiana) 38 mg • Goldenseal (hydrastis canadensis) 38 mg • Triphala Blend 30 mg: Belleric Myrobalan fruit (terminalia bellerica), Emblic Myrobalan fruit (emblica officinalis), Tropical Almond fruit (terminalia chebula). Other Ingredients: Natural Flavors, Maltodextrin, Potato Starch, Acacia Gum.

Coloklysis Daily **-** PhysioLogics
Each scoop (13 g) contains: Dietary Fiber 10 mg • Calcium (as tricalcium phosphate) 30 mg • Sodium 10 mg • Psyllium seed husk (plantago ovata) 3.4 g • Oat fiber (avena sativa) 2.5 g • Guar Gum seed (cyamopsis tetragonolobus) 2.5 g • Acacia Gum 1.2 g • Apple Pectin 1 g • Rice Bran 500 mg • Fructooligosaccharides (FOS) 250 mg • L-Glutamine 100 mg • Aloe Vera leaf (aloe barbadensis) 100 mg • Licorice root extract (glycyrrhiza glabra) 100 mg • Ginger root (zingiber officinale) 100 mg • Stevia leaf extract (stevia rebaudiana) 59 mg. Other Ingredients: Maltodextrin, Natural Flavors, Acesulfame Potassium, Annatto, Riboflavin, Cornstarch.

Colon Cleanse **-** Nature's Rx
Each capsule contains: Bentonita Clay • Micro-Crystalline Cellulose • Psyllium Seed • Senna Leaf • Citrus Pectin • Oat Bran • Nutra Flora FOS • Acidophilus Blend • Barley Grass • Golden Seal • Prune Concentrate • Slippery Elm Bark • Aloe Vera Leaf Extract • Bio-Perine • Cascara Sagrada.

Colon Cleanser Daily **-** Health Smart Vitamins
Each scoop contains: Dietary Fiber 11 g • Blonde Psyllium (seed husks) 3 g • Oat Fiber 3 g • Guar Gum 3 g • Acacia Gum 1 mg • Apple Pectin 1 g • Rice Bran 500 mg • Fructooligosaccharides (FOS; from chicory root) 250 mg • Aloe Vera leaf 100 mg • Ginger root 100 mg • L-Glutamine 100 mg • Licorice root 100 mg • Stevia leaf 10 mg.

Colon Clear **-** Metabolic Response Modifiers
Each capsule contains: AG (Arabinogalactan) 200 mg • Cascara Sagrada bark 100 mg • Fennel seed 75 mg • Licorice root 50 mg • Ginger root 50 mg • Senna leaf 50 mg • Peppermint leaf 25 mg • Celery seed 25 mg • Triphala (Anala, Behada, Harada) 25 mg.

Colon Green **-** Futurebiotics
Six capsules contain: Psyllium seed husk powder 2490 mg • Alfalfa leaf powder 600 mg • Alfalfa juice powder 180 mg • Lactobacillus acidophilus (supplying 12 billion cells) 60 mg • Pau D'Arco bark powder 120 mg • Echinacea leaf powder extract 120 mg • Black Walnut hull powder extract 120 mg • Fenugreek seed powder 120 mg • Watercress powder 120 mg • Parsley leaf powder 120 mg • Rosemary leaf powder 120 mg • Clove flower powder 120 mg • Bayberry bark powder 120 mg • Cayenne fruit powder 120 mg • Lipase 114 LU* • Protease 1380 HUT* • Amylase 114 DU*. Other Ingredients: LU are Lipase Units, HUT are Hemoglobin Units-Tyrosine basis, DU are Alpha-Amylase Dextrinizing Units.

Colon Health - Wellzymes **-** Enzymes, Inc.
Each capsule contains: Proprietary Blend 225 mg: Lactobacillus Acidophilus, Lactobacillus Plantarum, Bifidobacterium Bifidum, Lactobacillus Casei, Lactobacillus Salivarius. Other Ingredients: Plant Cellulose, Water.

Colostrum **-** Jamieson
Each capsule contains: Concentrated Colostrum 250 mg.

Colostrum **-** Olympian Labs
Two capsules contain: Colostrum 1000 mg.

Colostrum **-** PhysioLogics
Each tablet contains: Colostrum (standardized to contain 30% (195 mg) of naturally occurring immunoglobins) 650 mg. Other Ingredients: Cellulose (plant origin), Povidone, Croscarmellose, Silica, Cellulose Coating, Vegetable Magnesium Stearate.

Colostrum **-** Pro Health
Two capsules contain: Colostrum (20% IGG, bovine source) 800 mg. Other Ingredients: Cellulose, Magnesium Stearate, Silicon Dioxide.

Colostrum 80/40 **-** Proper Nutrition - PNI
Three capsules contain: Immunoglobulin G 600 mg. Other Ingredients: Gelatin.

Colostrum FM Capsules **-** Global Health Trax
Four capsules contain: Vitamin A 873 IU • Vitamin C 10 mg • Calcium 59 mg • Bovine Colostrum 2000 mg. Other Ingredients: Gelatin Capsules.

Colostrum Lozenges **-** Olympian Labs
Two lozenges contain: Colostrum 1000 mg.

Comfrey and Fenugreek **-** Dial Herbs
Comfrey • Fenugreek.

Comfrey Ointment **-** Nature's Way
Beeswax • Comfrey leaves • Olive oil • Soybean oil • Tallow.

Comfrey/Aloe Capsules **-** Aloe Farms
Comfrey powder 100 mg • Aloe Vera powder 50 mg.

Commando 2000 **-** Nature's Plus
Two tablets contain: Vitamin C (fortified with rose hips) 1000 mg • Vitamin E (natural) 200 IU • Zinc (monomethionine) 20 mg • Selenium (selenomethionine) 100 mcg • Citrus Bioflavonoid Complex (active flavonols, flavonones, flavones, & naringen - 44%) 200 mg • Beta Carotene (carrot, Dunaliella salina, supplying 10000 IU vitamin A activity) 60 mg • Echinacea (Echinacea purpurea root/rhizome) 250 mg • Astragalus (Astragalus membranoceus root) 150 mg • Garlic (Allium sativum clove) 70 mg • Ginkgo biloba leaf (50:1, standardized 24% ginkgo flavone-glycosides, 6% terpene lactones) 5 mg • NAC (N-acetyl-cysteine) 20 mg • L-Methionine (free form amino acid) 15 mg • L-Glutathione (free form amino acid) 10 mg.

Compete **-** Mission Pharmacal
Each tablet contains: Vitamin A 5,000 IU • Vitamin C 90 mg • Vitamin D (as Vitamin D3) 400 IU • Vitamin E 43 IU • Thiamine 2 mg • Riboflavin 2.6 mg • Niacin 30 mg • Vitamin B6 20 mg • Folate 0.4 mg • Vitamin B12 9 mcg • Iron 27 mg • Zinc 25 mg. Other Ingredients: Microcrystalline Cellulose, Sugar, Calcium Carbonate, Color, Croscarmellose Sodium, Povidone, Food Glaze, Cyanocobalamin, Magnesium Stearate, Yellow 6 Lake, Carnauba Wax, White Beeswax, Sodium Benzoate.

Complete B **-** Puritan's Pride
Two tablets contain: Thiamin (Vitamin B1: as thiamine mononitrate) 10 mg • Riboflavin (Vitamin B2) 15 mg • Niacin (as niacinamide) 25 mg • Vitamin B6 (as pyridoxine hydrochloride) 10 mg • Folic Acid 400 mcg • Vitamin B12 (as cyancobalamin) 25 mcg • Biotin (as d-biotin) 100 mcg • Pantothenic Acid (as d-calcium pantothenate) 100 mg • PABA (para-aminobenzoic acid) 50 mg • Choline Bitartrate 250 mg • Inositol 250 mg.

Complete Cleanse **-** PhysioLogics
Two caplets contain: Calcium (from di-calcium phosphate) 260 mg • Phosphorous (from di-calcium phosphate) 200 mg • Enzyme-Activated Herbal Digestive Extract Blend 500 mg: Cellulose, Beet fiber root, Fenugreek seed, Licorice root, Fennel seed, Lipase (from Aspergullus cryzae), Date fruit, Fig fruit, Ginger root, Prune fruit • Herbal Detox Extract Blend 250 mg: Green Tea leaf, Grapefruit seed, Burdock root, Chickweed aerial parts, Gentian root, Milk Thistle seed, Red Clover blossom, Dandelion root, Marshmallow root, Rosemary leaf, Yarrow flower, Yellow Dock root • Enzyme-Activated Cleansing Fiber and Herb Blend 250 mg: Butternut bark, Beet fiber root, Licorice root, Flax seed, Peppermint Oil • Probiotic Flora Replenishment Complex 75 million cells: Fructooligosaccharides, Inulides (from dahlia tuber and chicory root), Lactic Culture of B. Coagulins • Intestinal Tract Immune Complex 250 mg: Black Walnut leaf, Methylsulfonylmethane (MSM), Garlic bulb. Inactive Ingredients: Stearic Acid, Vegetable Stearine, Silica, Croscarmellose Sodium, Magnesium Stearate, Spirulina, Lac-Resin.

Complete Cleanse - Fiber Formula **-** PhysioLogics
Each tablet contains: Proprietary Blend 588 mg: Cascara Sagrada bark (rhamnus purshiana), Fennel seed (foeniculum vulgare), Psyllium seed husk (plantago ovata), Ginger root (zingiber officinale), Acacia Gum sap (acacia senegal), Apple Pectin (malus sylvestris), Apple Powder (malus sylvestris), Alfalfa leaf (medicago sativa), Barley Rice seed (hardeum vulgare), Beet root (beta vulgaris), Glucomannan root (amorphophallus riviori), Karaya Gum sap (sterculia urens), Lemon Fiber (citrus limon), Peppermint leaf (mentha piperita), Oat Bran seed (avena sativa), Red Raspberry leaf (rubus idaeus), Slippery Elm bark (ulmus fulva), Chlorella Algae plant (chlorella pyrenoidosa), Lactobacillus Acidophilus, Guar Gum seed (cyamopsis tetragonolobus). Other Ingredients: Calcium Carbonate, Cellulose (plant origin), Vegetable Stearic Acid, Croscarmellose, Silica, Cellulose Coating.

Complete Cleanse - Herb Formula **-** PhysioLogics
Each tablet contains: Proprietary Blend 588 mg: Ginger root (zingiber officinale), Dandelion root (taraxacum officinale), Fenugreek seed (trigonella foenum-graecum), Alfalfa leaf (medicago sativa), Fennel seed (foeniculum vulgare), Yarrow flower (achillea millefolium), Hawthorn berry (crataegus laevigata), Horsetail (equisetum arvense, aerial parts), Marshmallow root (althaea officinalis), Licorice root (glycyrrhiza glabra), Peppermint leaf (mentha piperita), Skullcap (scutellaria baicalensis, aerial parts), Red Clover flower (trifolium pratense), Safflower seed oil (carthamus tinctorius), Red Raspberry leaf (rubus idaeus), Chickweed (stellaria media, aerial parts), Papaya leaf (carica papaya), Mullein leaf (lychnis coronaria), Burdock root (arctium lappa), Cayenne Pepper fruit (capsicum annuum), Irish Moss (chondrus crispus), Black Cohosh root (cimicufuga racemosa), Kelp (macrocystis pyrifera), Milk Thistle seed (silybum marianum), Slippery Elm bark (ulmus rubra), Ginkgo Biloba leaf (ginkgo biloba), Echinacea (echinacea angustifolia, aerial parts), Plantain seed (plantago lanceolata), Yellow Dock root (rumex crispus). Other Ingredients: Calcium Carbonate, Cellulose (plant origin), Vegetable Stearic Acid, Acacia Gum, Croscarmellose, Silica, Cellulose Coating.

Complete Diet Boost **-** Optimum Nutrition
Two capsules contain: Vitamin A (as mixed carotenoids) 1000 IU • Vitamin C (as ascorbic acid) 30 mg • Vitamin E (as D-alpha tocopheryl succinate) 30 IU • Vitamin B6 (as pyridoxine hydrochloride) 2 mg • Folic Acid 400 mcg • Vitamin B12 (as cyanocobalamin) 6 mcg • Pantothenic Acid (as D-calcium pantothenate) 10 mg • Magnesium (as magnesium aspartate) 5 mg • Chromium (as chromium GTF polynicotinate) 120 mcg • Proprietary Diet Boost Blend 1418 mg: Guarana seed extract (paullinia cupana, 30% caffeine), Green Tea leaf extract (camellia sinensis L., 40% EGCG/ 22% caffeine), Phase 2 - Brand Bean fruit extract (phaseolus vulgaris), Yerba Mate leaf (ilex paraguayensis, 20% caffeine), Kola Nut fruit extract (cola acuminata, 20% caffeine), Advantra-Z Citrus Aurantium fruit (citrus aurantium L., 30% synephrine), Metabromine-G (cocoa/guarana extract, 5% caffeine/5% theobromine), Ginger root powder, Cayenne fruit powder, DL-Methionine, Dandelion root powder, White Willow bark powder, DL-Phenylalanine, DMAE (2-dimethylaminoethanol), L-Tyrosine, Grape Seed extract (vitis vinifera L., 95% polyphenols), Acetyl-L-Tyrosine. Other Ingredients: Gelatin, Dicalcium Phosphate, Microcrystalline Cellulose, Magnesium Stearate, Stearic Acid, Silica.
See Editor's Note No. 40, page 2058.

Complete Energy **-** Rexall - Sundown
Each caplet contains: Vitamin A (25% [1250 IU] as beta-carotene) 5000 IU • Vitamin C (as ascorbic acid) 120 mg • Vitamin D (as cholecalciferol) 400 IU • Vitamin E (as dl-alpha-tocopheryl acetate) 60 IU • Vitamin K (as phytonadione) 25 mcg • Thiamin (as thiamin mononitrate) 4.5 mg • Riboflavin (vitamin BC) 5.1 mg • Niacin (as niacinamide) 35 mg • Vitamin B6 (as pyridoxine HCl) 6 mg • Folic Acid 400 mcg • Pantothenic Acid (as calcium d-pantothanate) 10 mg • Calcium (as dicalcium phosphate and calcium carbonate) 100 mg • Iron (as carbonyl iron) 18 mg • Phosphorus 48 mg • Iodine (as potassium iodide) 150 mcg • Magnesium (as magnesium oxide) 40 mg • Zinc (as zinc oxide) 15 mg • Selenium (as sodium selenate) 70 mcg • Copper (as cupric oxide) 2 mg • Manganese (as manganese sulfate) 4 mg • Chromium (chromium chloride) 120 mcg • Molybdenum (as sodium molybdate) 75 mcg • Chloride 75 mg • Potassium (as potassium chloride) 80 mg • Lutein 250 mcg • Ginkgo Biloba Extract (leaf) 60 mg • Citrus Bioflavonoids 25 mg • Guarana Extract (seed) 45 mg • American Ginseng (root) 50 mg • Nickel (as nickel sulfate) 5 mcg • Tin 10 mcg • Silicon 4 mg • Vanadium 10 mcg • Boron 150 mcg. Other Ingredients: Microcrystalline Cellulose, Croscarmellose Sodium, Hydroxypropyl Methylcellulose, Magnesium Stearate, Yellow 6 Lake, Caffeine, Corn Starch, PEG, Titanium Dioxide (color), Retinyl Acetate, Red 40 Lake, Polysorbate 80.

Complete Essential Fatty Acids **-** Source Naturals
Each three softgels contain: Vitamin E (as mixed tocopherols) 30 IU • Alpha-Linolenic Acid (ALA, omega-3) 636 mg • Linoleic Acid (omega-6) 522 mg • Oleic Acid (omega-9) 402 mg • Eicosapentaenoic Acid (EPA, omega-3) 360 mg • Docosahexaenoic Acid (DHA, omega-3) 240 mg • Gamma-Linolenic Acid (GLA, omega-6) 228 mg. Inactive Ingredients: Borage Seed Oil (non-GMO), Fish Oil (non-GMO), Flaxseed Oil (non-GMO), Gelatin, Glycerin, Purified Water.

Complete Heart **-** NutriCology
Each scoop (20 g) contains: Vitamin A (as beta-carotene) 2000 IU • Vitamin C (as ascorbic acid) 500 mg • Vitamin D (D3) 100 IU • Vitamin E (as D-alpha-tocopherol) 320 IU • Vitamin K 80 mcg • Thiamin (vitamin B1) 30 mg • Riboflavin (vitamin B2) 30 mg • Niacin 160 mg • Vitamin B6 16 mg • Folic Acid 320 mg • Vitamin B12 80 mcg • Biotin 240 mcg • Pantothenic Acid 100 mg • Calcium (as calcium citrate/gluconate) 280 mg • Magnesium (as magnesium glycinate/gluconate) 160 mg • Zinc (as zinc arginate) 12 mg • Selenium (as sodium selenite/selenomethionine) 80 mcg • Copper (as copper glycinate) 0.8 mg • Manganese (as manganese glycinate) 1 mg

BRAND NAMES

• Chromium (as chromium polynicotinate) 160 mcg • Molybdenum (as sodium molybdate) 40 mcg • Potassium (as potassium gluconate) 40 mg • Boron (as boron citrate) 0.4 mg • Vanadium (as vanadium pentoxide) 80 mcg • Alpha-Carotene 8 mg • Pregnenolone 6 mg • Dehydroepiandrosterone (DHEA) 6 mg • Coenzyme Q10 60 mg • Inositol 50 mg • Choline 50 mg • Para-Aminobenzoic Acid (PABA) 20 mg • Lecithin (26% phosphatidylcholine) 500 mg • L-Alanine 30 mg • L-Arginine 480 mg • L-Aspartic Acid 85 mg • L-Carnitine 200 mg • L-Cystine 10 mg • L-Glutamine 600 mg • Glycine 30 mg • L-Histidine 20 mg • L-Isoleucine 35 mg • L-Leucine 60 mg • L-Lysine 45 mg • L-Methionine 160 mg • L-Ornithine 200 mg • L-Phenylalanine 38 mg • L-Proline 38 mg • L-Serine 38 mg • Taurine 500 mg • L-Threonine 28 mg • L-Tyrosine 220 mg • L-Valine 40 mg • N-Acetyl-L-Cysteine 200 mg • Glutathione 100 mg • Pancreatin 10 mg • Papain 16 mg • Bromelain 20 mg • Grape skin extract 200 mg • Hawthorn berry extract 200 mg • Garlic (1% allicin) 100 mg • Lutein 2 mg • Lycopene 0.4 mg • Tocotrienols 20 mg • Trimethylglycine 200 mg • Methylsulfonylmethane 80 mg • Eicosapentaenoic Acid (EPA) 145 mg • Docosahexaenoic Acid (DHA) 95 mg • Gamma-Linolenic Acid 90 mg • Linolenic Acid 220 mg • Oleic Acid 85 mg • Palmitic Acid 65 mg • Stearic Acid 25 mg • Flax Seed oil 400 mg • Lipoic Acid 30 mg. Other Ingredients: Oat Bran, Honey Powder, Rice Bran, Psyllium Bran, Apple Fiber, Lemon Flavor, Stevia.

Complete Heart II without Hormones **-** NutriCology
Each scoop (20 g) contains: Vitamin A (as beta-carotene) 2000 IU • Vitamin C (as ascorbic acid) 500 mg • Vitamin D (D3) 100 IU • Vitamin E (as D-alpha-tocopherol) 320 IU • Vitamin K 80 mcg • Thiamin (vitamin B1) 30 mg • Riboflavin (vitamin B2) 30 mg • Niacin 160 mg • Vitamin B6 16 mg • Folic Acid 320 mg • Vitamin B12 80 mcg • Biotin 240 mcg • Pantothenic Acid 100 mg • Calcium (as calcium citrate/gluconate) 280 mg • Magnesium (as magnesium glycinate/gluconate) 160 mg • Zinc (as zinc arginate) 12 mg • Selenium (as sodium selenite/selenomethionine) 80 mcg • Copper (as copper glycinate) 0.8 mg • Manganese (as manganese glycinate) 1 mg • Chromium (as chromium polynicotinate) 160 mcg • Molybdenum (as sodium molybdate) 40 mcg • Potassium (as potassium gluconate) 40 mg • Boron (as boron citrate) 0.4 mg • Vanadium (as vanadium pentoxide) 80 mcg • Alpha-Carotene 8 mg • Coenzyme Q10 60 mg • Inositol 50 mg • Choline 50 mg • Para-Aminobenzoic Acid (PABA) 20 mg • Lecithin (26% phosphatidylcholine) 500 mg • L-Alanine 30 mg • L-Arginine 480 mg • L-Aspartic Acid 85 mg • L-Carnitine 200 mg • L-Cystine 10 mg • L-Glutamine 600 mg • Glycine 30 mg • L-Histidine 20 mg • L-Isoleucine 35 mg • L-Leucine 60 mg • L-Lysine 45 mg • L-Methionine 160 mg • L-Ornithine 200 mg • L-Phenylalanine 38 mg • L-Proline 38 mg • L-Serine 38 mg • Taurine 500 mg • L-Threonine 28 mg • L-Tyrosine 220 mg • L-Valine 40 mg • N-Acetyl-L-Cysteine 200 mg • Glutathione 100 mg • Pancreatin 10 mg • Papain 16 mg • Bromelain 20 mg • Grape skin extract 200 mg • Hawthorn berry extract 200 mg • Garlic (1% allicin) 100 mg • Lutein 2 mg • Lycopene 0.4 mg • Tocotrienols 20 mg • Trimethylglycine 200 mg • Methylsulfonylmethane 80 mg • Eicosapentaenoic Acid (EPA) 145 mg • Docosahexaenoic Acid (DHA) 95 mg • Gamma-Linolenic Acid 90 mg • Linolenic Acid 220 mg • Oleic Acid 85 mg • Palmitic Acid 65 mg • Stearic Acid 25 mg • Flax Seed oil 400 mg • Lipoic Acid 30 mg. Other Ingredients: Oat Bran, Honey Powder, Rice Bran, Psyllium Bran, Apple Fiber, Lemon Flavor, Stevia.

Complete Immune **-** NutriCology
Each serving scoop (20 g) provides: Co-Enzyme Q10 75 mg • Grape seed extract (95%) 250 mg • Alpha Carotene 5 mg • Beta Carotene (from mixed carotenoids) 7500 IU • Lycopene 1.5 mg • Vitamin E (mixed tocopherols) 200 IU • Vitamin C 1175 mg • Folic Acid 400 mcg • Vitamin A 2500 IU • Vitamin B1 23 mg • Vitamin B2 23 mg • Vitamin B3 (niacinamide) 150 mg • Vitamin B3 (niacin) 10 mg • Vitamin B5 150 mg • Vitamin B6 25 mg • Vitamin B12 200 mcg • Biotin 200 mcg • Inositol hexaphosphate 175 mg • Choline 63 mg • Germanium Sesquioxide 50 mg • N-Acetyl Cysteine 375 mg • Glutathione 175 mg • L-Carnitine 100 mg • Calcium (carbonate, glycinate) 50 mg • Magnesium (carbonate, glycinate) 75 mg • Vitamin D (as Vitamin D3) 200 IU • Zinc (arginate) 15 mg • Copper (glycinate) 1 mg • Potassium (ascorbate) 50 mg • Chromium (picolinate) 100 mcg • Molybdenum 125 mcg • Manganese 1.25 mg • Selenium 100 mcg • EPA 500 mg • Iron (aspartate) 1.5 mg • Iodine 75 mcg • MSM 100 mg • Borage oil 150 mg • Genistein from soy isolate 5 mg • Tocotrienol 25 mg • Biofavonoid complex 50 mg • Trimethyl Glycine 250 mg • Sulforaphane (broccoli) 50 mg • Beta Glucan (1-3) 25 mg • Green Tea extract 50 mg • Mushroom extract 1500 mg • Bromelain 163 mg • Turmeric 100 mg • Panax Ginseng 50 mg • Astragalus 50 mg • Taurine 250 mg • Lactoferrin 50 mg • In a base of Wheat bran, Hydrolized Whey protein, Oat bran, Rice bran, Psyllium bran, Apple fiber, Lemon flavor, Stevia, Lemon oil & Lime oil.

Complete La Femme Capsules **-** Baywood International
Four capsules contain: 2272 mg Proprietary Blend: Saw Palmetto berry, Pueraria Mirifica leaf, Dong Quai root, Damiana leaf, Hops flower, Fenugreek seed, Blessed Thistle leaf, Wild Yam root. Other Ingredients: Gelatin.

Complete La Femme Liquid **-** Baywood International
Each two mL serving contains: Proprietary Blend 565 mg: Saw Palmetto berry, Pueraria Mirifica leaf, Dong Quai root, Damiana leaf, Hops flower, Fenugreek seed, Blessed Thistle leaf, Wild Yam root. Other Ingredients: Distilled Water, Glycerin.

Complete Multi 50+ **-** Rexall - Sundown
Each caplet contains: Vitamin A (25% [1500 IU] as beta-carotene) 6000 IU • Vitamin C (as ascorbic acid) 120 mg • Vitamin D (as cholecalciferol) 400 IU • Vitamin E (as dl-alpha-tocopherol acetate) 60 IU • Vitamin K (as phytonadione) 10 mcg • Thiamin (as thiamin mononitrate) 1.5 mg • Riboflavin (vitamin B2) 1.7 mg • Niacin (as niacinamide) 20 mg • Vitamin B6 (as pyridoxine HCl) 3 mg • Folic Acid 400 mg • Vitamin B12 (as cyanocobalamin) 30 mcg • Biotin 30 mcg • Pantothenic Acid (as calcium d-pantothenate) 15 mg • Calcium (as calcium carbonate and dicalcium phosphate) 200 mg • Phosphorus 48 mg • Iodine (as potassium iodide) 150 mg • Magnesium (as magnesium oxide) 100 mg • Zinc (as zinc oxide) 22.5 mg • Selenium (as sodium selenate) 95 mcg • Copper (as cupric oxide) 2 mg • Manganese (as manganese sulfate) 4 mg • Chromium (chromium chloride) 120 mcg • Molybdenum (as sodium molybdate) 75 mcg • Chloride 75 mg • Potassium (as potassium chloride) 8 mg • Lutein 300 mcg • Citrus Bioflavonoids (from orange peel extract) 25 mg • Billberry (fruit) 10 mg • Blueberry (fruit) 10 mg • Elderberry (fruit) 10 mg • Nickel (as nickel sulfate) 5 mcg • Tin (as stannous chloride) 10 mcg • Silicon (as silica) 2mg • Vanadium (as sodium metavanadate) 10 mcg • Boron (as sodium borate and potassium borate) 150 mcg. Other Ingredients: Microcrystalline Cellulose, Croscarmellose Sodium, Hydroxypropyl Methylcellulose, Titanium Dioxide (color), Magnesium Stearate, Corn Starch, PEG, Retinyl Acetate, Blue 2 Lake, Polysorbate 80, Red 40 Lake, Yellow 6 Lake.

Complete Multi Daily **-** Rexall - Sundown
Each caplet contains: Vitamin A (40% [2000 IU] as beta-Carotene) 5000 IU • Vitamin C (as ascorbic acid) 120 mg • Vitamin D (as cholecalciferol) 400 IU • Vitamin E (as dl-alpha-tocopherol acetate) 45 IU • Vitamin K (as phytonadione) 25 mcg • Thiamin (as thiamin mononitrate) 1.9 mg • Riboflavin (vitamin B2) 2.1 mg • Niacin (as niacinamide) 25 mg • Vitamin B6 (as pyridoxine HCl) 2.5 mg • Folic Acid 400 mcg • Vitamin B12 (as cyanocobalamin) 7.5 mcg • Biotin 37.5 mcg • Pantothenic Acid (as calcium d-pantothenate) 12.5 mg • Calcium (as dicalcium phosphate and calcium carbonate) 162 mg • Iron (as carbonyl iron) 18 mg • Phosphorus 77 mg • Iodine (as potassium iodide) 150 mcg • Magnesium (as magnesium oxide) 100 mg • Zinc (as zinc oxide) 15 mg • Selenium (as sodium selenate) 70 mcg • Copper (as cupric oxide) 2 mg • Manganese (as manganese sulfate) 2.5 mg • Chromium (chromium chloride) 120 mcg • Molybdenum (as sodium molybdate) 75 mcg • Chloride 75 mg • Potassium (as potassium chloride) 80 mg • Lutein 300 mcg • Citrus Bioflavonoids (from orange peel extract) 25 mg • Nickel (as nickel sulfate) 5 mcg • Tin (as stannous chloride) 10 mcg • Silicon (as silica) 2 mg • Vanadium (as sodium metavanadate) 10 mcg • Boron (as sodium borate and potassium borate) 150 mcg. Other Ingredients: Microcrystalline Cellulose, Croscarmellose Sodium, Hydroxypropyl

Methylcellulose, Titanium Dioxide (color), Magnesium Stearate, Corn Starch, PEG, Retinyl Acetate, Polysorbate 80, Yellow 5 Lake, Yellow 6 lake, Blue 2 lake.

Complete Multi Women **-** Rexall - Sundown
Each caplet contains: Vitamin A (25% [1250 IU] as beta-carotene) 5000 IU • Vitamin C (as ascorbic acid) 120 mg • Vitamin D (as cholecalciferol) 400 IU • Vitamin E (as dl-alpha-tocopherol acetate) 45 IU • Vitamin K (as phytonadione) 80 mg • Thiamin (as thiamin mononitrate) 1.9 mg • Riboflavin (vitamin B2) 2.1 mg • Niacin (as niacinamide) 25 mg • Vitamin B6 (as pyridoxine HCl) 2.5 mg • Folic Acid 400 mcg • Vitamin B12 (as cyanocobalamin) 7.5 mcg • Biotin 37.5 mcg • Pantothenic Acid (as calcium d-pantothenate) 12.5 mg • Calcium (as dicalcium phosphate and calcium carbonate) 250 mg • Iron (as carbonyl iron) 27 mg • Phosphorus 77 mg • Iodine (as potassium iodide) 150 mcg • Magnesium (as magnesium oxide) 100 mg • Zinc (as zinc oxide) 15 mg • Selenium (as sodium selenate) 70 mcg • Copper (as cupric oxide) 2 mg • Manganese (as manganese sulfate) 2 mg • Chromium (chromium chloride) 120 mcg • Molybdenium (as sodium molybdate) 75 mcg • Chloride 37 mg • Potassium (as potassium chloride) 40 mg • Lutein 300 mcg • Citrus Bioflavonoids (from orange peel extract) 25 mg • Soy Isoflavones (from soybean extract) 10 mg • Blueberry (fruit) 10 mg • Cranberry (fruit) 10 mg • Elderberry (fruit) 10 mg • Nickel (as nickel sulfate) 5 mcg • Tin (as stannous chloride) 10 mcg • Vanadium (as sodium metavanadate) 10 mcg • Boron (as sodium borate and potassium borate) 150 mcg. Other Ingredients: Microcrystalline Cellulose, Croscarmellose Sodium, Hydroxypropyl Methylcellulose, Titanium Dioxide (color), Magnesium Stearate, Corn Starch, Triacetin, Retinyl Acetate, Yellow 6 Lake.

Complete Nerve **-** NutriCology
Each scoop (20 g) contains: Vitamin A (as beta-carotene) 1680 IU • Vitamin C (as ascorbic acid) 440 mg • Vitamin D (D3) 130 IU • Vitamin E (as mixed tocopherols) 360 IU • Vitamin K 45 mcg • Thiamin (vitamin B1) 22 mg • Riboflavin (vitamin B2) 22 mg • Niacin (as inositol hexanicotinate) 180 mg • Vitamin B6 22 mg • Folic Acid 350 mcg • Vitamin B12 22 mcg • Biotin 130 mcg • Pantothenic Acid 110 mg • Calcium (as calcium citrate/gluconate) 310 mg • Magnesium (as magnesium glycinate/gluconate) 130 mg • Zinc (as zinc arginate) 13 mg • Selenium (as sodium selenite/ selenomethionine) 90 mcg • Copper (as copper glycinate) 0.9 mg • Chromium (as chromium picolinate) 180 mcg • Potassium (as potassium gluconate) 45 mg • Alpha-Carotene 7 mg • Dehydroepiandrosterone (DHEA) 7 mg • Coenzyme Q10 67 mg • Inositol 22 mg • Choline 22 mg • Para-Aminobenzoic Acid 22 mg • Lecithin (26% phosphotidylcholine) 1440 mg • L-Alanine 35 mg • L-Arginine 110 mg • L-Aspartic Acid 95 mg • L-Carnitine 110 mg • L-Cystine 11 mg • L-Glutamine 67 mg • Glycine 67 mg • L-Histidine 22 mg • L-Isoleucine 45 mg • L-Lysine 50 mg • L-Methionine 180 mg • L-Ornithine Hydrochloride 220 mg • L-Phenylalanine 45 mg • L-Proline 45 mg • L-Serine 42 mg • Taurine 670 mg • L-Threonine 45 mg • L-Tyrosine 440 mg • N-Acetyl-L-Cysteine 440 mg • Glutathione (reduced) 110 mg • Pancreatin 13 mg • Papain 22 mg • Bromelain 22 mg • Grape skin extract 220 mg • Garlic (1% allicin) 45 mg • Lutein 1.8 mg • Lycopene 1.3 mg • Eicosapentaenoic Acid (EPA) 160 mg • Docosahexaenoic Acid (DHA) 110 mg • Palmitic Acid 130 mg • Stearic Acid 40 mg • Flax Seed Oil 440 mg • Lipoic Acid 45 mg • Methylsulfonylmethane 45 mg. Other Ingredients: Oat Bran, Rice Bran, Psyllium Bran, Stevia, Apple Fiber, Flavoring.

Complete Protein Diet **-** Optimum Nutrition
Each serving contains: Vanilla flavor Ingredients: Proprietary Protein Blend of Calcium Caseinate, Whey Protein Concentrate, Egg Albumen, Hydrolyzed Whey Peptides, Whey Protein Isolate, L-Glutamine • Canola oil • Artificial Flavor • Complete Vitamin Mineral Blend: di-Potassium Phosphate, Magnesium Oxide, Potassium Chloride, Ascorbic Acid, dl-Alpha Tocopherol Acetate, Niacinamide, Vitamin A Palmitate, Zinc Oxide, Potassium Iodide, Vitamin K, D-Calcium Pantothenate, Copper Sulfate, Manganese Sulfate, Vitamin D (as Vitamin D3), Pyridoxine Hydrochloride, Thiamine Mononitrate, Riboflavin, Selenium Glycinate, Molybdenum Glycinate, Chromium Picolinate, Folic Acid, Biotin, Cyanocobalamin • Lecithin • Cellulose Gum • Xanthan Gum • Aspartame • Acesulfame Potassium • Salt • FD&C Yellow #5 • FD&C Yellow #6.

Complete Protein Diet Bars **-** Optimum Nutrition
Each bar (50 g) contains: Protein Blend: Calcium Caseinate, Whey Protein Isolate, Soy Protein Isolate • Glycerine • Maltitol • Coating: Maltitol, Palm Kernal Oil, Non Fat Dry Milk Solids, Cocoa, Whole Milk Solids, Lecithin, Salt, Natural Flavor • Filtered Water • Natural and Artificial Flavor • Peanut Flour • Lecithin • Gum Arabic • Salt • Sucralose.

Complete Ultra **-** Rexall - Sundown
Each caplet contains: Vitamin A (as beta carotene) 5000 IU • Vitamin C (as ascorbic acid) 200 mg • Vitamin D (as cholecalciferol) 400 IU • Vitamin E (as dl-alpha tocopheryl acetate) 150 IU • Vitamin K (as phytonadione) 40 mcg • Thiamin (as thiamin mononitrate) 50 mg • Riboflavin (vitamin B2) 50 mg • Niacin (as niacinamide) 35 mg • Vitamin B6 (as pyridoxine HCl) 50 mg • Folic Acid 400 mcg • Vitamin B12 (as cyanocobalamin) 50 mcg • Biotin 50 mcg • Pantothenic Acid (as calcium d-pantothenate) 50 mg • Calcium (as dicalcium carbonate and calcium carbonate) 100 mg • Iron (as carbonyl iron) 9 mg • Phosphorous 35 mcg • Iodine (as potassium iodide) 150 mcg • Magnesium (as magnesium oxide) 25 mg • Zinc (as zinc oxide) 15 mg • Selenium (as sodium selenate) 70 mcg • Copper (as cupric acid) 2 mg • Manganese (as manganese sulfate) 2 mg • Chromium (as chromium chloride) 120 mcg • Molybdenum (as sodium molybdate) 75 mcg • Chloride 38 mg • Potassium (as potassium chloride) 40 mg • Bilberry extract (4:1, fruit) 15 mg • Blueberry (fruit) 15 mg • Citrus Bioflavonoids (from orange peel extract) 25 mg • Nickel (as nickel sulfate) 5 mcg • Tin (as stannous chloride) 10 mcg • Vanadium (as sodium metavanadate) 10 mcg • Boron (as sodium borate and potassium borate) 150 mcg. Other Ingredients: Microcrystalline Cellulose, Croscarmellose Sodium, Silica, Dextrin, Hydroxypropyl Methylcellulose, Titanium Dioxide, Corn Starch, Magnesium Stearate, PEG, Blue 1 Lake, Dextrose, Soy Lecithin, Retinyl Acetate.

CompleteGest **-** PhytoPharmica
Each capsule contains: Proprietary Plant Enzyme Blend 305 mg: Amylase, Protease, Lipase, Lactase, Phytase, Cellulase, Sucrase, Maltase. Other Ingredients: Modified Cellulose, Cellulose, Titanium Dioxide Color.

Completia Diabetic Multivitamin **-** Nature's Way
Two tablets contain: Alpha Lipoic Acid 50 mg • Beta Carotene 1000 IU • Betaine HCl 25 mg • Biotin, Biotin Triurate 300 mcg • Boron Amino Acid Chelate 1 mg • Calcium (calcium ascorbate, d-calcium pantothenate) 45 mg • Choline Bitartrate 50 mg • Chromium Polynicotinate 300 mcg • Cinnamon bark 300 mg • Citrus Bioflavonoid complex 25 mg • Copper Amino Acid Chelate 1 mg • Fenugreek seed 50 mg • Folic Acid (folate) 400 mcg • Hesperidin 1 mg • Inositol 100 mg • Iodine 10 mcg • L-Carnitine L-Tartrate 20 mg • Lutein (from marigold) 200 mcg • Magnesium (as citrate, oxide) 300 mg • Manganese Amino Acid Chelate 5 mg • Molybdenum Triturate 50 mcg • Neem leaf 50 mg • Niacinamide 20 mg • PABA (para aminobenzoic acid) 25 mg • Pantothenic Acid 100 mg • Potassium Amino Acid Chelate 10 mg • Quercetin, Eucalyptus 50 mg • Riboflavin (vitamin B2) 100 mg • Rutin 25 mg • Selenium Monomethionine 200 mcg • Taurine 100 mg • Thiamine (vitamin B1) 100 mg • Vanadium Triturate 10 mcg • Vitamin A (retinol palmitate) 5000 IU • Vitamin B12 (cyanocobalamin) 100 mcg • Vitamin B6 (as pyridoxine HCl) 100 mg • Vitamin C (ascorbic acid, calcium ascorbate) 500 mg • Vitamin D (D3, cholecalciferol) 400 IU • Vitamin E (d-alpha tocopheryl) 200 IU • Zinc Amino Acid Chelate 15 mg. Other Ingredients: Silica, Vegetable Magnesium Stearate, Vegetable Modified Cellulose, Vegetable Modified Cellulose Gum, Vegetable Stearic Acid, Vegetarian Glycerin.

Completia Healthy Heart Multi (Iron free) - Nature's Way
Each tablet contains: Beta Carotene 10,000 IU • Betaine HCl 25 mg • Biotin Triurate 75 mcg • Boron Amino Acid Chelate 500 mcg • Calcium (citrate, carbonate) 20 mg • Choline Bitartrate 25 mg • Chromium Polynicotinate 25 mcg • Citrus Bioflavonoid complex 25 mg • Copper Amino Acid Chelate 500 mcg • Folic Acid (folate) 800 mcg • Heart Herbal Blend 100 mg • Hesperidin 1 mg • Inositol 25 mg • Iodine 150 mcg • Lutein (from marigold) 100 mcg • Magnesium (as citrate, oxide) 10 mg • Manganese Amino Acid Chelate 1 mg • Molybdenum Triurate 25 mcg • Niacinamide 100 mg • PABA (para amionbenzoic acid) 25 mg • Pantothenic Acid 50 mg • Potassium Amino Acid Chelate 2 mg • Riboflavin (vitamin B2) 25 mg • Selenium Monomethionine 200 mcg • Sodium 10 mg • Thiamine (vitamin B1) 25 mg • Vitamin A (retinol, palmitate) 5000 IU • Vitamin B12 (cyanocobalamin) 400 mcg • Vitamin B6 (as pyridoxine HCl) 25 mg • Vitamin C (ascorbic acid) 150 mg • Vitamin D (D3, cholecalciferol) 400 IU • Vitamin E (d-alpha tocopheryl) 150 IU • Zinc Amino Acid Chelate 15 mg. Other Ingredients: Silica, Vegetable Magnesium Stearate, Vegetable Modified Cellulose, Vegetable Modified Cellulose Gum, Vegetable Stearic Acid, Vegetarian Glycerin.

Completia Prenatal Multivitamin - Nature's Way
Two tablets contain: Beta Carotene 8000 IU • Biotin Triurate 300 mcg • Calcium (citrate, carbonate) 600 mg • Choline Bitartrate 4 mg • Chromium Polynicotinate 50 mcg • Copper Amino Acid Chelate 2 mg • Dandelion root 50 mg • DHA (docosahexaenoic acid) 100 mg • Diatomaceous plant 10 mg • Folic Acid (folate) 800 mcg • Inositol 10 mg • Iodine 150 mcg • Iron Gluconate 45 mg • Magnesium (citrate, oxide) 300 mg • Manganese Amino Acid Chelate 2 mg • Nettle herb 50 mg • Niacinamide 20 mg • PABA (para aminobenzoic acid) 2 mg • Pantothenic Acid 10 mg • Peppermint leaves 50 mg • Peppermint oil 86 mg • Potassium Amino Acid Chelate 50 mg • Red Raspberry leaves 50 mg • Riboflavin (vitamin B2) 2 mg • Selenium Monomethionine 25 mcg • Sodium 10 mg • Thiamine (vitamin B1) 1.7 mg • Vitamin B12 (cyanocobalamin) 8 mcg • Vitamin B6 (pyridoxine HCl) 2.5 mg • Vitamin C (calcium ascorbate) 120 mg • Vitamin D (D3, cholecalciferol) 400 IU • Vitamin E (d-alpha tocopheryl) 30 IU • Vitamin K (phytonadione) 90 mcg • Zinc Amino Acid Chelate. Other Ingredients: Silica, Vegetable Cellulose, Vegetable Magnesium Stearate, Vegetable Modified Cellulose, Vegetable Modified Cellulose Gum, Vegetable Stearic Acid, Vegetarian Glycerin.

Completia Ultra Energy Multi (Iron-free) - Nature's Way
Each tablet contains: Beta Carotene 10,000 IU • Betaine HCl 25 mg • Biotin Triurate 75 mcg • Boron Amino Acid Chelate 500 mcg • Calcium (citrate, carbonate) 20 mg • Choline Bitartrate 31 mg • Chromium Polynicotinate 25 mcg • Citrus Bioflavonoid complex 25 mg • Copper Amino Acid Chelate 1 mg • Energizing Herbal Blend 100 mg • Folic Acid (folate) 400 mcg • Hesperidin 1 mg • Inositol 25 mg • Iodine 150 mcg • Magnesium (as citrate, oxide) 10 mg • Manganese Amino Acid Chelate 2 mg • Molybdenum Amino Acid Chelate 25 mcg • Niacinamide 100 mg • PABA (para aminobenzoic acid) 25 mg • Pantothenic Acid 100 mg • Potassium Amino Acid Chelate 1.8 mg • Riboflavin (vitamin B2) 100 mg • Rutin 25 mg • Selenium Monomethionine 25 mcg • Thiamine (vitamin B1) 100 mg • Vitamin A (retinol palmitate) 5000 IU • Vitamin B12 (cyanocobalamin) 100 mcg • Vitamin B6 (as pyridoxine HCl) 100 mg • Vitamin C (ascorbic acid) 150 mg • Vitamin D (D3, cholecalciferol) 400 IU • Vitamin E (d-alpha tocopheryl) 100 IU • Zinc Amino Acid Chelate 10 mg. Other Ingredients: Silica, Vegetable Magnesium Stearate, Vegetable Modified Cellulose, Vegetable Modified Cellulose Gum, Vegetable Stearic Acid, Vegetable Glycerin.

Complexion Perfect - Aspen Group, Inc.
Four tablets contain: Vitamin A 5000 IU • Beta Carotene 5000 IU • Vitamin B1 (thiamine) 25 mg • Vitamin B2 (riboflavin) 25 mg • Vitamin B3 (niacin) 50 mg • Vitamin B5 (pantothenic acid) 25 mg • Vitamin B6 (pyridoxine HCl) 50 mg • Biotin 300 mcg • Vitamin C (calcium ascorbate) 500 mg • Vitamin E (succinate) 400 IU • Magnesium Oxide 200 mg • Zinc (gluconate) 12 mg • Burdock root 600 mg • L-Lysine HCl 500 mg • L-Proline 500 mg • Yellow Dock 500 mg • Silica (derived from horsetail extract) 400 mg • Grape seed extract (proanthodyn) 50 mg • Selenomethionine 200 mcg • Chromium Picolinate 50 mcg • GTF Chromium 25 mcg.

Composition 1 - Dial Herbs
Bayberry • White Pine bark • Clove • Cinnamon • Ginger • Cayenne.

Concentrate - Enzymatic Therapy
Two capsules contain: DMAE (as 2-dimethylaminoethanol bitartrate) 100 mg • Phosphatidylserine (from soy) 60 mg • Taurine 25 mg • N-Acetylcysteine 25 mg • L-Theanine 25 mg. Other Ingredients: Gelatin, Cellulose, Magnesium Stearate.

Concentrated Broccoli - Jamieson
Each caplet contains: Concentrated Broccoli florets (Equivalent to 25000 mg fresh Broccoli) 450 mg • Concentrated Kale leaf and Radish root (Standardized to Active Isothiocyanates 450 mcg) 10 mg.

Concentrated Garlic - Leiner Health Products
Two tablets contain: Garlic (Allium sativum) clove powder 300 mg. Other Ingredients: Dicalcium Phosphate, Cellulose, Starch, Silicon Dioxide, Vanilla Flavor, Magnesium Stearate, Ethylcellulose, may contain less than 2% of Croscarmellose Sodium.

Concentrated Lung-Tan-Xie-Gan pills - China Beijing Tong-Ren Tang
Unknown.
See Editor's Note No. 46, page 2058.

Concentrated Saw Palmetto - GNC Herbal Plus - GNC
Each capsule contains: Saw Palmetto berries (serenoa repens) (from 38.5 mg of saw palmetto berries extract 26:1) 1000 mg. Other Ingredients: Soybean Oil, Gelatin, Glycerin, Caramel Color, Titanium Dioxide.

Confido (Speman forte) - The Himalaya Drug Company (Himalaya Heal
Each tablet contains: Salabmisri (orchis mascula) 78 mg • Kokilaksha (astercantha longifolia syn. hygophila auriculata) 38 mg • Vanya Kahu (lactuca scariola syn. l.serriola) 20 mg • Kapikachchhu (mucuna pruriens) 20 mg • Suvarnavang (mosaic gold, unsublimed tin preparation) 20 mg • Sarpagandha (rauwolfia serpentina, standardised to contain 1.5 mg of the total alkaloids) • Vriddadaru (argyreia speciosa syn. a.nervosa) 38 mg • Gokshura (tribulus terrestris) 38 mg • Jeevanti (leptadenia reticulata) 38 mg • Shaileyam (parmelia perlata) 20 mg.

Congaplex - Standard Process, Inc.
Three capsules contain: Proprietary Blend 673 mg: Bovine Thymus Cytosol extract, Carrot root, Ribonucleic Acid, Bovine Bone, Nutritional Yeast, Defatted Wheat germ, Bovine Adrenal, Dried Alfalfa juice, Oat flour, Alfalfa flour, Bovine Kidney, Veal Bone Meal, Veal Bone PMG extract, Reishi / Shiitake Mushroom blend, Dried Buckwheat leaf juice, Buckwheat seed, Peanut bran, Soy bean Lecithin, Mixed Tocopherols, Carrot oil. Other Ingredients: Calcium Lactate, Gelatin, Magnesium Citrate, Water, Ascorbic Acid, Colors, Calcium Stearate, Vitamin A Palmitate.

Congaplex (Chewable) - Standard Process, Inc.
Three tablets contain: Proprietary Blend 320 mg: Raspberry powder, Bovine Thymus Cytosol extract, Carrot root, Ribonucleic Acid, Bovine Bone, Defatted Wheat germ, Bovine Adrenal, Dried Alfalfa juice, Nutritional Yeast, Oat flour, Alfalfa flour, Bovine Kidney, Veal Bone meal, Veal Bone PMG extract, Reishi / Shiitake Mushroom blend, Dried Buckwheat leaf juice, Buckwheat seed, Peanut bran, Soy Bean Lecithin, Carrot oil, Mixed Tocopherols. Other Ingredients: Dehydrated Cane Juice, Cellulose, Maltodextrine, Calcium Lactate, Magnesium Citrate, Natural Flavor, Calcium Stearate, Ascorbic Acid, Vitamin A Palmitate.

Some Brand Name Natural Products - What they Contain

www.NaturalDatabase.com contains MANY more listings than appear here.

Congest-Away - Rainbow Light
Two tablets contain: Vitamin A (from beta-carotene, palmitate 1:1) 5000 IU • Vitamin C (ascorbic acid) 1000 mg • Zinc (citrate) 5 mg • Copper (amino acid chelate) 500 mcg • Spirulina 100 mg • Herbal Extract Blend (equivalent to 4824 mg of herbal powder) 1200 mg: Magnolia flower 4:1 extract (magnolia liliflorae), Yerba Santa leaves 4:1 extract, HoreHound herb 4:1 extract, Mullein herb 4:1 extract, Iceland Moss lichen 4:1 extract, Chinese Goldthread rhizome 4:1 extract, Ligusticum root 4:1 extract, Pinellia rhizome 4:1 extract (pinelliae ternata), Platycodon 4:1 extract (platycodi grandiflorum), Chinese Licorice root 4:1 extract, Tangerine peel 5:1 extract (standardized to 3% synephrine). Other Ingredients: Stearic Acid (vegetable), Modified Cellulose Gum, Silica, Magnesium Stearate, Vegetable Food Glaze.
See Editor's Note No. 40, page 2058.

Conjugated Linoleic Acid - PhysioLogics
Two softgels contain: Tonalin CLA (from safflower oil, contains 74-82% conjugated linoleic acid) 2000 mg. Other Ingredients: Gelatin, Glycerin, Caramel Color, Titanium Dioxide Color.

Conjugated Linoleic Acid (CLA) 500MG - Nature Made
Two softgels contain: Vitamin E 2 IU • Conjugated Linoleic Acid 500 mg.

Conjugated Linoleic Acid 1000 mg - 70% - Now
Each softgel contains: Sunflower/Safflower Oil (high linoleic acid) 1000 mg •Conjugated Linoleic Acid (CLA) 700 mg • Cis, Trans-11 Isomer 330 mg • Trans-10, Cis-12 Isomer 330 mg. Other Ingredients: Gelatin, Glycerin, Water, Carob.

Connect-All - Nature's Plus
Two tablets contain: Glucosamine Sulfate (Aminomonosaccharide) 300 mg • Bromelain, proteolytic enzyme 600 GDU/gram, 200 mg • Calcium (Aminoate) 200 mg • Vitamin C corn free 60 mg • Aloe Vera leaf naturally rich in Mucopolysaccharide 50 mg • Chondroitin Sulfate A (CSA) 50 mg • Zinc (Monomethionine) 15 mg • Chinese Sea Cucumber (Microchele nobilis) 10 mg • Copper (Aminoate) 1 mg. In a highly active base of Alfalfa, Chlorella, Spirulina & low temperature dried Barley Grass juice, supplying naturally occuring chlorophyll & trace minerals.
See Editor's Note No. 15, page 2055.

Connection - NutriCology
Two capsules contain: Vitamin C (as ascorbic acid) 33 mg • Vitamin E (as D-alpha-tocopheryl acid succinate) 55 IU • Calcium (as calcium citrate) 27 mg • Magnesium (as magnesium citrate) 40 mg • Zinc (as zinc citrate) 4 mg • Selenium (as sodium selenite/selenomethionine) 33 mcg • Copper (as copper sebacate) 0.27 mg • Manganese (as manganese citrate) 4.7 mg • Molybdenum (as sodium molybdate) 330 mcg • Boron (as boron citrate) 1.2 mg • N-Acetyl-D-Glucosamine 67 mg • Chondroitin Sulfate 130 mg • Glucosamine Sulfate 500 mg • L-Lysine 67 mg • L-Proline 107 mg • Hawthorne dried extract (crataegus oxyacantha) 295 mg • Horsetail dried extract (equisetum arvense) 6.7 mg • Bromelain 10 mg. Other Ingredients: Cellulose, Magnesium Stearate, Ethyl Vanillin.
See Editor's Note No. 15, page 2055.

Controlled-Release Melatonin - Douglas Labs/AMNI
Each tablet contains: Melatonin 2 mg.
See Editor's Note No. 16, page 2055.

Control-X - Gero Vita International
Each capsule contains: Asian Ginseng root extract (20% ginsenosides) 100 mg • Astragalus root extract (1% isoflavones, 10% amino acids) 100 mg • Psoralea fruit extract (8:1) 100 mg • Sharp-leaf Galongal fruit extract (8:1) 100 mg • Palm-leaf Raspberry fruit extract (12% organic acids) 100 mg • Cherokee Rose fruit extract (8:1) 100 mg • Cassia bark extract (5% cinnamaldehdyde) 50 mg • Chinese Cimicifuga rhizome extract (5% ferulic acid) 25 mg • Ginger rhizome extract (5% gingerols) 25 mg • Vinpocetine 5 mg. Other Ingredients: Gelatin, Dicalcium Phosphate, Magnesium Stearate, Silicon Dioxide.

Copper - GNC A-Z - GNC
Each tablet contains: Copper (as copper gluconate) 2mg. Other Ingredients: Dicalcium Phosphate, Cellulose.

Copper Sebacate - Source Naturals
Each tablet contains: Copper sebacate 22 mg.

Copper Sebacate - NutriCology
Each capsule contains: Copper (as copper sebacate) 4 mg. Other Ingredients: Cellulose, Dicalcium Phosphate, Magnesium Stearate, Silicon Dioxide.

CoQ Absorb - Pro Health
Each softgel contains: Vitamin A (beta carotene from D. salina) 1630 IU • Natural Vitamin E (d-alpha tocopherol with mixed tocopherols) 60 IU • Coenzyme Q10 (CoQsol) 60 mg. Other Ingredients: Rice Bran Oil, Gelatin, Glycerin, Water, Beeswax, Annato Extract, Titanium Oxide.

CoQ Heart - Shaklee
Each capsule contains: Coenzyme Q10 30 mg • Mixed tocopherols 5 mg • Resveratrol (Polygonum cuspidatum) root 640 mcg. Other Ingredients: Soybean Oil, Glyceryl Palmitostearate, Polyglyceryl Dioleate, Gelatin, Glycerine, Water, Annatto, Titanium Dioxide.

Co-Q10 - J. R. Carlson Laboratories, Inc.
Each softgel contains: Vitamin E (as d-Alpha Tocopherol) 1 IU • Co-Q10 (as Coenzyme Q10 50 mg).

CoQ10 - 100 mg - Nature's Way
Each capsule contains: Coenzyme Q10 (ubiquinone) 100 mg • Vitamin E (d-alpha tocopheryl) 5 IU. Other Ingredients: Annatto Oil, Gelatin, Glycerin, Rice Bran Oil, Titanium Dioxide, Water.

CoQ10 - Enzymatic Therapy
Each softgel contains: Coenzyme Q10 (CoQ10, ubiquinone 10) 50 mg. Other Ingredients: Soybean Oil, Gelatin, Beeswax, Lecithin.

CoQ-10 - Metabolic Response Modifiers
Each capsule contains: Ubiquinone (Coenzyme Q-10) 30 mg.

CoQ10 - Nature's Way
Each capsule or softgel contains: Coenzyme Q10 (ubiquinone) 60 mg. Other Ingredients: Gelatin, Millet, Turmeric Root.

CoQ10 - Now
Each capsule contains: Coenzyme Q10 30 mg. Other Ingredients: White Rice Powder.

CoQ-10 - Schiff
Each capsule contains: Coenzyme Q-10 30 mg. Other Ingredients: Rice Powder, Silica.

CoQ-10 - Solgar
Each capsule contains: CoEnzyme Q-10 (ubiquinone) 30 mg. Other Ingredients: Microcrystalline Cellulose, Gelatin, Vegetable Cellulose, Silica, Vegetable Magnesium Stearate, Water.

CoQ10 100 mg - PhytoPharmica
Each capsule contains: Coenzyme Q10 (CoQ10) verified by HPLC 100 mg.

COQ10 100 mg PLUS E - Progressive Labs
Each capsule contains: Co-Enzyme Q10 100 mg • Vitamin E (dl-alpha tocopheryl acetate) 100 IU.

CoQ-10 100mg - Sundown
Each softgel contains: Vitamin E (as D-alpha tocopherol) 5 IU • Coenzyme Q-10 100 mg. Other Ingredients: Soybean Oil, Gelatin, Glycerin, Water, Yellow Beeswax, Titanium Dioxide, Yellow 6 Lake, Red 40 Lake, Blue 1 Lake.

CoQ10 30 mg - PhytoPharmica
Each capsule contains: Coenzyme Q10 (CoQ10) verified by HPLC 30 mg.

Some Brand Name Natural Products - What they Contain

www.NaturalDatabase.com contains MANY more listings than appear here.

CoQ-10 30 mg **-** Rexall - Sundown
Each softgel contains: Vitamin E (as d-alpha-tocopherol) 5 IU • Coenzyme Q-10 30 mg. Other Ingredients: Soybean Oil, Gelatin, Glycerin, Water, Titanium Dioxide, Yellow 6 Lake, Yellow Beeswax, Red 40 Lake, Blue 1 Lake.

CoQ10 30 mg **-** Swanson
Each capsule contains: Coenzyme Q10 30 mg.

CoQ10 50 mg **-** PhytoPharmica
Each capsule contains: Coenzyme Q10 (CoQ10) verified by HPLC 50 mg.

CoQ-10 50 mg **-** Rexall - Sundown
Each softgel contains: Vitamin E (as d-alpha-tocopherol) 5 IU • Coenzyme Q-10 50 mg. Other Ingredients: Soybean Oil, Gelatin, Glycerin, Water, Yellow Beeswax, Titanium Dioxide, Yellow 6 Lake, Red 40 Lake, Blue 1 Lake.

CoQ-10 75 mg **-** Rexall - Sundown
Each softgel contains: Vitamin E (as d-alpha-tocopherol) 5 IU • Coenzyme Q-10 75 mg. Other Ingredients: Soybean Oil, Gelatin, Glycerin, Water, Yellow Beeswax, Titanium Dioxide, Yellow 6 Lake, Red 40 Lake, Blue 1 Lake.

CoQ10 Extra Strength **-** Olympian Labs
Each capsule contains: Crystalline Coenzyme Q10 150 mg.

CoQ10 Spray **-** Nature's Plus
Each spray contains: CoQ10 pharmaceutical grade Ubiquinone 30 mg. In a proprietary Liposomal Complex of Essential Metabolic Factors, Purified Water, Vegetable Glycerine, Purified Lecithin, Citrus Seed Extract (Citrus sinensis), Vitamin E & Natural Mandarin Tangerine Flavor.

CoQsol brand **-** Soft Gel Technologies, Inc.
CoQ10.
See Editor's Note No. 44, page 2058.

CoQuinone 30 **-** USANA Health Sciences
Each capsule contains: Coenzyme Q10 30 mg • Alpha Lipoic Acid 12.5 mg. Inactive Ingredients: Medium Chain Triglycerides, Gelatin, Glycerin Monooleate, Lecithin, Glycerin, Purified Water, Annatto seed extract, Titanium Dioxide.

Coral Calcium **-** Bob Barefoot's Best
Three caplets contain: Vitamin A (as Beta carotene) 5000 IU • Vitamin C (as Ascorbic acid) 60 mg • Vitamin D (as Cholecalciferol) 2000 IU • Vitamin E (as D-alpha-tocopherol) 30 IU • Thiamin (as Thiamin HCl) 1.5 mg • Riboflavin 1.7 mg • Niacin (as Niacinamide) 20 mg • Vitamin B6 (as Pyridoxine HCl) 2 mg • Folic acid 800 mcg • Vitamin B12 (as Cyanocobalamin) 6 mcg • Pantothenic Acid (as Calcium pantothenate) 10 mg • Calcium (from Coral calcium) 500 mg • Calcium 95 mg • Iron (as Amino acid chelate) 18 mg • Iodine (from Kelp) 108 mcg • Magnesium (from Coral calcium) 250 mg • Magnesium (from Citrate) 42 mg • Magnesium 7 mg • Zinc (as Amino acid chelate) 15 mg • Selenium (as Amino acid chelate) 30 mcg • Copper (as Amino acid chelate) 2 mg • Manganese (as Amino acid chelate) 1.44 mg • Chromium (as Amino acid chelate) 120 mcg • Coral Calcium 2000 mg • Cesium (as Chloride) 3 mg • Boron (as Amino acid chelate) 1000 mcg • Strontium (from Coral calcium) 3200 mcg. Other Ingredients: Cellulose, Croscarmellose Sodium, Maltodextrin, Microcrystalline Cellulose, Magnesium Stearate, Silica, Stearic Acid.
See Editor's Note No. 28, page 2056.

Coral Calcium **-** DreamPharm
Three capsules contain: Vitamin A (as palmitate) 300 IU • Vitamin C (as ascorbic acid) 80 mg • Vitamin D (vitamin D3) 820 IU • Vitamin E (d-alpha tocopheryl succinate) 60 IU • Calcium (from 1475 mg of coral calcium) 530 mg • Magnesium (from 1475 coral calcium & magnesium oxide) 265 mg • Zinc (as zinc oxide) 15 mg • Copper (as copper oxide) 3 mg • Coral Calcium (in proprietary base) 1475 mg. Other Ingredients: Cellulose, Silicon Dioxide, Magnesium Stearate.

Coral Calcium **-** Elation Therapy
Two capsules contain: Coral Calcium 1000 mg • Calcium 240 mg • Magnesium 120 mg • Vitamin D 400 IU.

Coral Calcium **-** GNC
Two capsules contain: Vitamin D (as Cholecalciferol) 200 IU • Calcium (as Coral calcium 1100 mg) 400 mg • Magnesium (as Magnesium oxide) 200 mg. Other Ingredients: Gelatin, Polyalditol, Titanium Dioxide.

Coral Calcium **-** Natrol
Three capsules contain: Vitamin D (as Cholecalciferol) 400 IU • Calcium (as Coral Calcium) 400 mg • Magnesium (from Coral and Amino Acid Chelate) 200 mg. Other Ingredients: Rice Powder, Gelatin, Silica, Magnesium Stearate.

Coral Calcium **-** NSI - Nutraceutical Sciences Institute
Three capsules contain: Beta Carotene 2500 IU • Vitamin C (as Magnesium ascorbate) 86 mg • Vitamin D (D3, as Cholecalciferol) 869 IU • Vitamin E (as D-alpha tocopherol succinate) 50 IU • Vitamin K (as Phytonadione) 18 mcg • Thiamine (as Vitamin B1) 1.5 mg • Riboflavin (as Vitamin B2) 1.7 mg • Niacinamide (as Vitamin B3) 20 mg • Pyridoxine HCl (as Vitamin B6) 2 mg • Folic Acid 400 mcg • Methylcobalamin (Vitamin B12) 6 mcg • Pantothenic Acid (Vitamin B5) 10 mg • Calcium (from Coral mineral powder) 400 mg • Iodine (from Kelp) 100 mcg • Magnesium (from Coral mineral powder) 24 mg • Magnesium (as Ascorbate) 5 mg • Magnesium (as Oxide) 169 mg • Zinc 8 mg • Selenium (as Selenomethionine) 70 mcg • Manganese (as Citrate) 2 mg • Chromium (as Polynicotinate) 100 mcg • L-Lysine (as HCl) 100 mg • Boron (as Citrate) 1.5 mg • Horsetail extract (standardized to 7% Silica) 29 mg. Other Ingredients: Magnesium Searate, Cellulose, Gelatin.

Coral Calcium **-** PhysioLogics
Two capsules contain: Calcium (from coral calcium 1000 mg) 370 mg. Other Ingredients: Gelatin, Rice Powder, Silica, Vegetable Magnesium Stearate.

Coral Calcium **-** Pro Health
Two Vcaps contain: Vitamin D (as ergocalciferol) 400 IU • Calcium (from fossilized coral calcium 35%) 500 mg • Magnesium (from magnesium oxide, citrate, aspartate 17%) 250 mg • Fossilized Coral Calcium (gross weight) 1430 mg. Other Ingredients: Cellulose, Maltodextrin, Mixed Tocopherols.

Coral Calcium **-** Pure Source
Two capsules contain: Vitamin A (as beta-carotene) 1945 IU • Vitamin C (as ascorbic acid) 47 mg • Vitamin D (as cholecalciferol) 544 IU • Vitamin E (as dl-alpha tocopheryl) 23 IU • Calcium (from coral calcium) 167 mg • Iodine (kelp) 100 mcg • Magnesium (from coral calcium) 83 mg • Magnesium (as magnesium citrate) 39 mg • Zinc (as amino acid chelate)10.9 mg • Selenium (as amino acid chelate) 20 mcg • Copper (as amino acid chelate) 1.6 mg • Manganese (as amino acid chelate) 0.96 mg • Chromium (as amino acid chelate) 57 mcg • Coral Calcium (70+ trace minerals with natural variability) 667 mg • Cesium 2 mg • Strontium (from coral calcium) 1.9 mg • Boron (as amino acid chelate) 43 mcg. Other Ingredients: Gelatin.

Coral Calcium **-** Source Naturals
Two capsules contain: Vitamin D (D3, as Cholecalciferol) 400 IU • Calcium 420 mg • Magnesium 8 mg • Coral Calcium 1.2 g. Other Ingredients: Gelatin, Dibasic Calcium Phosphate, Colloidal Silicon.

Coral Calcium 1 **-** PhysioLogics
Two capsules contain: Proprietary Blend of Coral Calcium 1000 mg: Calcium (from coral calcium) 240 mg, Magnesium (from coral calcium magnesium citrate) 120 mg, Vitamin D3 (as cholecalciferol) 800 IU • Trace Minerals. Other Ingredients: Cellulose, Modified Cellulose, Stearic Acid.

Coral Calcium 1000 mg Plus **-** Nature's Bounty
Two capsules contain: Vitamin C 5 mg • Vitamin D 400 IU • Calcium 370 mg • Magnesium 56 mg. Other Ingredients: Rice Powder, Gelatin, Vegetable Magnesium Stearate, Silica.

Coral Calcium 500 mg **-** Puritan's Pride
Two capsules contain: Calcium (from 1000 mg of coral calcium) 370 mg. Other Ingredients: Rice Powder, Gelatin, Silica, Vegetable Magnesium Stearate.

Coral Calcium Complex **-** PhysioLogics
Two capsules contain: Vitamin C (as ascorbic acid) 5 mg • Vitamin D (as cholecalciferol) 400 IU • Calcium (from coral calcium 1000 mg) 370 mg • Magnesium (as magnesium oxide, magnesium citrate) 56 mg. Other Ingredients: Rice Powder, Gelatin, Vegetable Magnesium Stearate, Silica.

Coral Calcium Factor **-** Coral Calcium Factor
Three capsules contain: Okinawa Marine Coral Calcium 1500 mg • Calcium (from coral) 360 mg • Magnesium (from coral) 180 mg • Vitamin D 800 mg. Also contains 75 other trace minerals and nutrients. Other Ingredients: Gelatin, Rice Powder.

Coral Calcium Factor Plus **-** Nature's Solution
Two capsules contain: Vitamin D 400 IU • Calcium 240 mg • Magnesium 120 mg • Coral Calcium 1000 mg. Other Ingredients: Silicon Dioxide, Cellulose, Magnesium Stearate, Gelatin.

Coral Calcium Mineral Complex **-** Nature's Rx
Each capsule contains: Coral Calcium 600 mg • Calcium (from coral) 230 mg • Vitamin D (D3, as cholecalciferol) 50 IU • Magnesium (from coral & 50 mg gluconate) 9 mg • Boron (chelate) 1 mg.

Coral Calcium with Magnesium **-** Source Naturals
Three tablets contain: Sodium 5 mg • Vitamin D (D3,as Cholecalciferol) 400 IU • Calcium (from Coral) 1200 mg • Magnesium (as Magnesium oxide, Chelate, Citrate from Coral) 600 mg • Coral Calcium 3.4 g. Other Ingredients: Stearic Acid, Acacia Gum, Magnesium Stearate, Modified Cellulose, Colloidal Silicon Dioxide.

Coral Complete **-** Global Health Trax
Two capsules contain: Vitamin C (as ascorbic acid) 10 mg • Vitamin D (as cholecalciferol) 800 IU • Calcium (from coral) 460 mg • Magnesium (from coral) 116 mg • Proprietary Blend 30 mg: Trace Minerals From Coral, Malic Acid, Betaine HCl. Other Ingredients: Gelatin, Magnesium Stearate (from vegetable source), Silica, Cellulose (from rice bran).

CORALadvantage Coral Calcium **-** Advanced Nutritional Innovations
Three capsules contain: Vitamin A (as beta carotene) 2500 IU • Vitamin C (as ascorbic acid) 86 mg • Vitamin D (D3) 869 IU • Vitamin E (as d-alpha tocopherol) 43 IU • Vitamin K (as phytonadione) 18 mcg • Thiamin (B1) 960 mcg • Riboflavin (B2) 1.09 mg • Niacinamide (B3) 12.8 mg • Vitamin B6 (as pyridoxine HCl) 4 mg • Folic Acid 256 mcg • Vitamin B12 (as cyanocobalamin) 3.84 mcg • Pantothenic Acid (B5) 6.4 mg • Calcium (from marine coral) 230 mg • Calcium (from calcium citrate) 136 mg • Iodine (from kelp) 96 mcg • Magnesium (from marine coral) 110 mg • Magnesium (from magnesium citrate) 88 mg • Zinc (amino acid chelate) 8 mg • Selenium (amino acid chelate) 70 mcg • Copper (amino acid chelate) 1 mg • Manganese (citrate) 2 mg • Chromium (amino acid chelate) 77 mcg • Lysine HCl 100 mg • Red Algae powder (Lithothamnium coralloides, yeilding 2 cups of elemental silicon) 29 mg • Malic Acid 15 mg • Boron (citrate) 1.5 mg • Strontium 1.6 mg • Cesium 1 mg. Other Ingredients: Plant Cellulose Capsules, Titanium Dioxide, At least 49 Trace Elements from Marine Coral and Red Algae.

CoralCalcium 1 **-** Vision Enterprises
Two capsules contain: Proprietary Blend 1000 mg: Coral Calcium, Calcium (from coral calcium) 240 mg, Magnesium (from coral calcium magnesium citrate) 120 mg, Vitamin D (D3, as cholecalciferol) 800 IU. Other Ingredients: Cellulose, Modified Cellulose, Stearic Acid.

CoraLife brand **-** BI Nutraceuticals
Sea Coral Calcium.
See Editor's Note No. 44, page 2058.

Cordephrine XC **-** HealthDesigns International
Each vegicap contains: Cordyceps Mycelia (Cordyceps sinensis) 450 mg. Other Ingredients: Pure plant cellulose (vegicaps). Does not contain ephedra or ephedrine.

Cordyceps **-** Metabolic Response Modifiers
Each capsule contains: Cordyceps mycelia (Cordyceps sinensis) 750 mg.

Cordyceps (Caterpillar Fungus) **-** Olympia Nutrition
Caterpillar fungus 500 mg.

Cordyceps Power 800 mg **-** Planetary Formulas
Two capsules contain: Cordyceps Proprietary Blend 1600 mg. Other Ingredients: Dibasic Calcium Phosphate, Colloidal Silicon Dioxide, Magnesium Stearate, Modified Cellulose Gum, Stearic Acid.

Cordyceps with Siberian Ginseng **-** Natrol
Each capsule contains: Cordyceps 300 mg • Siberian Ginseng 50 mg. Other Ingredients: Rice powder, silica, & gelatin.

CordyMax Cs-4 **-** Pharmanex
Two capsules contain: Cordyceps Cs-4 Mushroom Mycelia (cordyceps sinensis [berk.] sacc.) 1050 mg. Other Ingredients: Gelatin.

CorEnergy **-** Shaklee
Three capsules contain: Cordyceps 4:1 extract (Cordyceps sinensis) mushroom 750 mg • Ginseng root extract (Panax ginseng standardized to contain 10% ginsenosides) 200 mg • Green Tea extract (Camellia sinensis standardized to contain 50% polyphenols) leaf 200 mg. Other Ingredients: Microcrystalline Cellulose, Gelatin, Water, Titanium Dioxide.

CorePlex **-** Advocare International
Three caplets contain: Vitamin A (as palmitate) 2500 IU • Vitamin A (as beta-carotene) 12,500 IU • Vitamin C (as ascorbic acid) 600 mg • Vitamin D (as ergocalciferol) 400 IU •Vitamin E (as d-alpha tocopheryl succinate) 150 IU •Thiamine 9 mg • Riboflavin 10.2 mg • Niacin/Niacinamide 120 mg • Pantothenic Acid 40 mg • Vitamin B6 (pyridoxine HCl) 12 mg • Vitamin B12 (as cyanocobalamin) 36 mcg • Folic Acid 800 mcg • Biotin 300 mcg • Inositol 6 mg •Choline (as bitartrate) 60 mg •Calcium (as amino acid chelate) 150 mg • Magnesium (as amino acid chelate) 200 mg • Zinc (as monomethionine - OptiZinc) 15 mg • Iodine (from kelp) 150 mcg • Selenium (as selenomethionine) 80 mcg • Manganese (as amino acid chelate) 4 mg •Chromium (as polynicotinate - ChromeMate) 100 mcg • Molybdenum (as amino acid chelate) 50 mcg • Copper (as amino acid chelate) 2 mg • Potassium (as amino acid chelate) 100 mg • Boron (as amino acid chelate) 300 mcg • Vanadium (as bis-maltolato-oxovanadium) 50 mcg • Phosphorus (as amino acid chelate) 100 mg • Silicon (as amino acid chelate) 500 mcg • Coenzyme Q-10 150 mcg • Octacosanol 2 mg • Ribonucleic Acid (RNA) 2 mg • Odorless Garlic bulb powder (allium sativum) 50 mg •L-Glutathione 5 mg •Gamma-Oryzanol 5 mg •Citrus Flavonoids 100 mg •Red Wine Polyphenols 5 mg • Milk Thistle fruit extract (silybum marianum) 5 mg • Ginkgo Biloba leaf extract (ginkgo biloba) 10 mg • L-Methionine 100 mg. Other Ingredients: Dicalcium Phosphate, Silicon Dioxide, Cellulose, Stearic Acid, Magnesium Stearate, Peppermint Extract.

Coreplex **-** Flora, Inc.
Hawthorn blossoms & leaves • Passion Flower Herb • Hibiscus flowers • Hawthorn berry extract (1:4).

Coromega Orange Flavor **-** European Reference Botanical Laboratorie
Each packet contains: Vitamin C 45 mg • Vitamin E 7 IU • Folic Acid

100 mcg • Omega-3 fatty acids (EPA 350 mg, DHA 230 mg) 650 mg • Stevia Leaf extract 5 mg. Other Ingredients: Water, Egg Yolk, Natural Orange Flavor, Citric Acid, Sodium Benzoate, Vanillin, Beta Carotene, Potassium Sorbate, Menthol, Folic Acid.

Cort-Block **-** Muscle-Link
Two capsules contain: Phosphatidylserine 200 mg • Glutamine peptide 800 mg. Other Ingredients: Gelatin, Magnesium Stearate.

CortiDrene (Vitopril) **-** Wellspring Laboratories
Two capsules contain: Niacin (niacinamide, B3) 20 mg • Green Tea extract PE (40% (EGCG & polyphenols) 150 mg • Epimedium 100 mg • L-Theanine 66.7 mg • Citrus Aurantium 4% extract (synephrine) 55 mg • Beta Sitosterol complex 40 mg • Phosphatidylserine (20% extract) 8.3 mg • Grape seed extract 95% 30 mg • Chromium (picolinate) 50 mcg • St. John's Wort (powder) 50 mg • Valerian root (powder) 20 mg. Other Ingredients: Gelatin, Dicalcium Phosphate, Magnesium Stearate, Silica.
See Editor's Note No. 40, page 2058.

CortiSlim **-** Window Rock Health Laboratories
Each capsule contains: Vitamin C (as calcium ascorbate) 100 mg • Calcium (as calcium carbonate, calcium ascorbate) 150 mg • Chromium (as chromium polynicotinate) 50 mg • Cortiplex Proprietary Blend 155 mg: Magnolia bark extract (magnolia officinalis, 1.5% honokiol), Beta-Sitosterol, L-Theanine (Suntheanine) • Leptiplex Proprietary Blend 125 mg: Green Tea leaf extract (camellia sinensis, 50% EGCG), Bitter Orange peel extract (citrus aurantium, 5% synephrine) • Insutrol Proprietary Blend 16.5 mg: Banaba leaf extract (lagerstroemia speciosa, 1% corosolic acid), Vanadyl Sulfate (providing 5 mcg vanadium). Other Ingredients: Gelatin, Microcrystalline Cellulose, Water, Silicon Dioxide, Magnesium Stearate (vegetable derived).
See Editor's Note No. 33, page 2057.

Cortistat-PS **-** Champion Nutrition
Four capsules contain: Phosphatidylserine 100 mg • Phosphatidylcholine 105 mg • Phosphatidylethanolamine 70 mg • Phosphatidylinositol 30 mg • Arginine Aspartate 576 mg • Potassium Succinate 576 mg • Quercetin 100 mg • Feverfew 100 mg.

Cortitrol **-** Pharmanex
Each capsule contains: Magnolia 4:1 extract (magnolia officinalis) 133 mg • Epimedium water 6:1 extract (epimedium koreanum) 100 mg • L-Theanine 70:1 extract (from camillia sinensis) 66.7 mg • Beta-Sitosterol 40 mg • Phosphatidylserine 8.3 mg.

CortiZide **-** MedaBiotics
Two capsules contain: Calcium (chelate) 100 mg • Vitamin C (as ascorbic acid) 80 mg • Vitamin B6 (as pyridoxine HCl) 3 mg • Vitamin B12 (as cyanocobalamin) 500 mcg • Folic Acid (vitamin B9) 200 mcg • Chromium (as chromium dinicotinate glycinate) 100 mcg • Green Tea leaf extract (50% catechins and 35% polyphenols) 300 mg • Magnolia Officinalis bark 4:1 extract 70 mg • Suntheanine brand L-Theanine (100%) 60 mg • Phosphatidylserine 100 mg • Beta-Sitosterol 40 mg • Vanadium 60 mcg. Other Ingredients: Gelatin, Cellulose, Magnesium Stearate.

Cortiblock **-** Heaven Sent Naturals
Each tablet contains: Vitamin C 50 mg • Vitamin B1 1.25 mg • Vitamin B2 1.25 mg • Vitamin B6 2.5 mg • Vitamin B12 3 mcg • Folic Acid 200 mcg • Calcium (carbonate) 75 mg • Chromium (polynicotinate) 25 mcg • Biotin 75 mcg • Ridicort Blend 157.5 mg: Magnolia bark extract (1.5% honokiol), Beta-Sitosterol, Phosphatidylserine (20% extract), Valerian root, Rhodiola rosea, Suntheanine brand 100% L-Theanine • Synocet Blend 127.5 mg: Green Tea 50% extract (camellia sinensis), Bitter Orange peel 5% extract (citrus aurantium) • BAVA-K Blend 19.5 mg: Banaba leaf (lagerstromia speciosa, 1%), Vanadyl Sulfate (providing 2.5 mcg vanadium). Other Ingredients: Cellulose, Stearic Acid, Silica, Magnesium Stearate.
See Editor's Note No. 40, page 2058.

CortiBurn (adrenalzide) – MedaBiotics
Two capsules contain: Vitamin B6 (as pyridoxine HCl) 3 mg • Vitamin B12 (as cyanocobalamin) 25coryza0 mcg • Folic Acid (vitamin B9) 200 mcg • Advantra Z brand Citrus Aurantium 5% extract (contains 17.5 mg of synephrine) 350 mg • Green Tea leaf extract (50% catechins and 35% polyphenols) 300 mg • Guggulsterones 200 mg • Caffeine 150 mg • Phosphatidylserine 100 mg. Other Ingredients: Gelatin, Cellulose, Magnesium Stearate.
See Editor's Note No. 40, page 2058.

CortiCarb3000 (Phasisol) **-** Dynamic Nutritional Research
Two capsules contain: Chromium 100 mcg • Selenium 500 mcg • White Kidney bean extract 600 mg • Guggul 2.5% 300 mg • Green Tea extract 50% 250 mg • L-Tyrosine 150 mg • Citrus Aurantium extract 6% 85 mg • Alpha Lipoic Acid 60 mg • Valerian root powder 50 mg • St. John's Wort powder 50 mg. Other Ingredients: Gelatin, Dicalcium Phosphate, Magnesium Stearate, Silica.
See Editor's Note No. 40, page 2058.

CortiCept Rx **-** Nature's Rx
Each capsule contains: Vitamin C (as calcium ascorbate) 100 mg • Calcium (as calcium carbonate, calcium ascorbate) 100 mg • Magnesium (as magnesium chelate) 50 mg • Chromium (as chromium polynicotinate) 50 mg • Proprietary Blend 155 mg: Magnolia bark extract (magnolia officinalis, 1.5% honokiol), Beta-Sitosterol, Suntheanine brand 100% L-Theanine • Proprietary Blend 125 mg: Green Tea leaf extract (camellia sinensis, 50% EGCG), Bitter Orange peel extract (citrus aurantium, providing 5% synephrine) • Proprietary Blend 16.5 mg: Banaba leaf extract (lagerstroemia speicosa, 1% corosolic acid), Vanadyl Sulfate (providing 5 mcg vanadium).
See Editor's Note No. 40, page 2058.

CortiFast **-** AmerMed
Each capsule contains: Vitamin C (as calcium ascorbate) 120 mg • Coral Calcium 240 mg • Calcium (from coral calcium and calcium ascorbate) 100 mg • Chromium (as chromium polynicotinate) 50 mcg • Magnolia bark (magnolia officinalis, equivalent from 200 mg of 4:1 extract) 800 mg • Beta-Sitosterol 30 mg • Green Tea extract (camellia sinensis, 50% polyphenols) 175 mg • Hoodia cactus (equivalent from 25 mg of 4:1 extract) 100 mg • Banaba leaf extract (lagerstroemia speciosa, 1% corosolic acid) 25 mg • Vanadium (as amino acid chelate) 10 mcg. Other Ingredients: Gelatin Capsule, Maltodextrin.

Cortigen **-** Genetix Nutraceuticals
Two capsules contain: Vitamin B6 3 mg • Vitamin B12 500 mcg • Folic Acid 200 mcg • Vitamin C 80 mg • Calcium 100 mg • Chromium 100 mcg • Vanadium 60 mcg • Cortiol Proprietary Blend 530 mg: Green Tea extract, Magnolia bark extract, L-Theanine, Phosphatidylserine, Beta-Sitosterol.

CortiLess **-** Diet a Day, Inc.
Each capsule contains: Vitamin C (as calcium ascorbate) 100 mg • Calcium (as calcium carbonate and calcium ascorbate) 150 mg • Chromium (as ChromeMate brand chromium polynicotinate) 50 mcg • Blend 1 155 mg: Magnolia bark extract, Beta-Sitosterol, Suntheanine brand 100% L-Theanine • Blend 2 125 mg: Green Tea leaf extract (50% EGCG), Cocoa bean extract (12% theobromine) 125 mg • Blend 3 16.5 mg: Banaba leaf extract (1% corosolic acid), Vanadyl Sulfate (with 50 mcg vanadium). Other Ingredients: Gelatin, Cellulose, Magnesium Stearate, Silica.

Cortiloss **-** Delmar Labs
Each capsule contains: Vitamin C (as calcium ascorbate) 100 mg • Calcium (as calcium carbonate, calcium ascorbate) 150 mg • Chromium (as chromium polynicotinate) 50 mcg • Proprietary Blend 155 mg: Magnolia bark extract (magnolia officinalis, 1.5% honokiol), Beta-Sitosterol, Suntheanine brand 100% L-Theanine • Proprietary Blend 125 mg: Green Tea leaf extract (camellia sinensis, 50% EGCG), Bitter Orange peel extract (citrus aurantium, 5% synephrine) • Proprietary Blend 16.5 mg: Banaba leaf extract (lagerstroemia speciosa, 1% corosolic acid), Vanadyl Sulfate (providing 5 mcg

vanadium). Other Ingredients: Gelatin, Magnesium Stearate.
See Editor's Note No. 40, page 2058.

Cortipren - Window Rock Health
Each capsule contains: Proprietary Blend 155 mg: Magnolia bark (honokiol), Beta-Sitosterol, Suntheanine brand 100% L-Theanine • Proprietary Blend 125 mg: Green Tea extract (EGCG), Bitter Orange peel extract (synephrine) • Proprietary Blend 16.5 mg: Banaba leaf extract (corosolic acid), Vanadyl Sulfate • Vitamin C (as calcium ascorbate) 100 mg • Calcium (as calcium carbonate , calcium ascorbate) 150 mg • Chromium (as chromium polynicotinate) 50 mcg. Other Ingredients: Gelatin, Magnesium Stearate.
See Editor's Note No. 40, page 2058.

CortiPrep - Health Minded
Each capsule contains: Vitamin C (as calcium ascorbate) 100 mg • Calcium (as calcium carbonate, calcium ascorbate) 150 mg • Chromium (as chromium polynicotinate) 50 mg • CortiPrep Proprietary Blend 296.5 mg: Magnolia bark extract (magnolia officinalis, 1.5% honokiol), Beta-Sitosterol, Suntheanine brand 100% L-Theanine, Green Tea leaf extract (camellia sinensis, 50% EGCG), Bitter Orange peel extract (citrus aurantium, 5% synephrine), Banaba leaf extract (lagerstroemia speciosa, 1% corosolic acid), Vanadyl Sulfate (providing 5 mcg vanadium). Other Ingredients: Gelatin, Stearic Acid, Magnesium Stearate.
See Editor's Note No. 40, page 2058.

Coryza-Comp - Atrium Inc.
Each tablet contains: Vitamin A (Fish oil) 2000 IU • Vitamin C Ascorbic Acid 300 mg • Vitamin B6 Pyridoxine HCL 15 mg • Pantothenic Acid 25 mg • Calcium (Aspartate) 10 mg • Magnesium (Aspartate) 10 mg • Zinc (Aspartate) 2 mg • Citrus Bioflavonoids 150 mg • High RNA Yeast 50 mg • Bee Pollen 10 mg • Raw Spleen concentrate (Bovine) 10 mg • Raw Thymus concentrate (Bovine) 10 mg • Raw Adrenal concentrate 5 mg • Raw Lymph concentrate (Bovine) 5 mg. In a base of Alfalfa & Rose Hips.
See Editor's Note No. 14.

Coryza Forte - Progressive Labs
Each capsule contains: Vitamin A (as retinol & beta carotene) 4000 IU • Vitamin C (ascorbic acid) 300 mg • Vitamin B6 (pyridoxine HCl) 15 mg • Pantothenic Acid (as d-calcium pantothenate) 25 mg • Calcium (as calcium carbonate) 40 mg • Zinc (as zinc picolinate) 5 mg • Echinacea 50 mg • Citrus Bioflavonoid 5X complex (as undiluted hesperidin, naringin and rutin) 150 mg. Other Ingredients: Pollen, Raw Bovine Trachea, Raw Bovine Thymus, Raw Bovine Adrenal, Raw Bovine Lymph, Raw Bovine Spleen, RNA, Rose Hips, Whey, Cellulose, Magnesium Stearate, Gelatin.
See Editor's Note No. 14.

Cosamin - Nutramax Laboratories, Inc.
Each capsule contains: Glucosamine HCl (99%) 250 mg • Sodium Chondroitin Sulfate (95%) with Mixed Glycosaminoglycans (5%) 200 mg • Ascorbate (as manganese ascorbate) 33 mg • Manganese (as manganese ascorbate) 5 mg.
See Editor's Note No. 4, page 2053.

Cosamin DS Double Strength Capsules - Nutramax Laboratories, Inc.
Each tablet contains: Vitamin C (as manganese ascorbate) 16 mg • Manganese (as manganese ascorbate) 3 mg • High Purity FCHG-49 Glucosamine HCl 99% 500 mg • Low Molecular Weight TRH122 Sodium Chondroitin Sulfate 95% 400 mg.

Cosamin DS Double Strength Tablets - Nutramax Laboratories, Inc.
Each tablet contains: Vitamin C (as manganese ascorbate) 16 mg • Manganese (as manganese ascorbate) 3 mg • High Purity FCHG-49 Glucosamine HCl 99% 500 mg • Low Molecular Weight TRH122 Sodium Chondroitin Sulfate 95% 400 mg. Other Ingredients: Microcrystalline Cellulose, Croscarmellose Sodium, Magnesium Stearate.

Cosamin ProTek - Nutramax Laboratories, Inc.
Each capsule contains: Sodium 30 mg • Vitamin C 359 mg • Vitamin D3 400 IU • Vitamin E (d-alpha tocopherol) 35 IU • Manganese 1 mg • Glucosamine HCl 200 mg • Sodium Chondroitin Sulfate 95% and Mixed Glycosaminoglycans 5% 400 mg.
See Editor's Note No. 4, page 2053.

Cosamin ProTek Women's Formula - Nutramax Laboratories, Inc.
Each capsule contains: Sodium 30 mg • Vitamin C 9 mg • Vitamin D3 400 IU • Calcium 115 mg • Manganese 1 mg • Glucosamine HCl 200 mg • Sodium Chondroitin Sulfate 95% and Mixed Glycosaminoglycans 5% 400 mg.
See Editor's Note No. 4, page 2053.

CosaminDS (Cosamin DS) - Nutramax Laboratories, Inc.
Each capsule contains: Glucosamine HCl (99%) 500 mg • Sodium Chondroitin Sulfate (95%) with Mixed Glycosaminoglycans (5%) 400 mg • Ascorbate (as manganese ascorbate) 16 mg • Manganese (as manganese ascorbate) 3 mg.
See Editor's Note No. 15, page 2055.

Cosamine 500 mg - Kripps Pharmacy
Each capsule contains: Chondroitin Sulfate & Glucosamine powder (1:1 ratio) 500 mg.
See Editor's Note No. 15, page 2055.

Cositin - Life Extension
Each capsule contains: Glucosamine HCL 99+% 250 mg • Sodium Chondroitin Sulfate 95%/Mixed Glycosaminoglycans 5% 200 mg • Ascorbate (manganese ascorbate) 33 mg • Selenium (seleniomethionine) 25 mg • Bromelain 25 mg • Manganese (ascorbate) 5 mg.
See Editor's Note No. 15, page 2055.

Cosmopolitan Nutrition - Vitabiotics
Each capsule contains: Vitamin D (as vitamin D3 200 IU) 5 mcg • Vitamin E (natural source) 20 mg • Vitamin C 60 mg • Thiamin (vitamin B1) 10 mg • Riboflavin (vitamin B2) 5 mg • Niacin (vitamin B3) 18 mg • Pyridoxine Hydrochloride (vitamin B6) 25 mg • Folacin (as folic acid) 400 mcg • Cyanocobalamin (vitamin B12) 15 mcg • Biotin 0.15 mg • Pantothenic Acid 6 mg • Iron 14 mg • Magnesium 50 mg • Zinc 12 mg • Iodine 120 mcg • Manganese 2 mg • Copper 1.5 mg • Chromium (chelated) 100 mcg • Selenium 100 mcg • L-Carnitine 50 mg • Taurine 10 mg • Tyrosine 10 mg • Green tea extract (60% polyphenols) 40 mg • Cranberry extract 100 mg • Wheatgerm oil 200 mg • Natural Mixed Carotenoids 2 mg • Lecithin 15 mg.

Cough Syrup - Progressive Labs
Each 10 ml contains: Dextromethorphan Hydrobromide 10 mg • Guaifenesin 100 mg • Potassium Citrate 85 mg • Citric Acid 35 mg.

Cough Syrup with Honey - Hyland's
Ipecacuanha as Ipecac 6X HPUS • Aconitum napellus as Aconite 6X HPUS • Spongia tosta as Sponge 6X HPUS • Antimonium tartaricum as Potassium antimonium tartrate 6X HPUS. In simple syrup with Honey.
See Editor's Note No. 1, page 2053.

Cough-Eze Syrup - The Herbalist
Herbs of Marshmallow root, Slippery Elm bark, Elecampane root, Wild Cherry bark, Mullein leaf, Horehound leaf, Licorice root, Cubeb berry, Orange peel, Cinnamon bark & Ginger root, Extracts of Skunk Cabbage root & Lobelia leaf, Honey, Vegetable Glycerine & Peppermint Oil.

C-Plus Cold Tablets - Hyland's
Each tablet contains: Eupatorium perforliatum as Boneset 3X HPUS • Euphrasia officinalis as Eyebright 2X HPUS • Gelsemium sempervirens as Yellow Jasmine 3X HPUS • Kali iodatum as Potassium Iodide 3X HPUS. In a base of Lactose NF (Milk Sugar).
See Editor's Note No. 1, page 2053.

Some Brand Name Natural Products - What they Contain

www.NaturalDatabase.com contains MANY more listings than appear here.

BRAND NAMES

C-Plus-Citrus - Atrium Inc.
Each level teaspoon (3300 mg approx. wt.) contains: Vitamin C from: (Ascorbic Acid 900 mg & Sodium Ascorbate 625 mg) 1500 mg • Mannitol 1395 mg • Lemon Bioflavonoids 150 mg • Rose Hips 100 mg • Hesperidin Complex 50 mg • Rutin 30 mg. Contains natural Orange Juice flavor.

Cracked Skin Relief Creme 2oz - Derma E
Purified Water • Aloe Vera gel • Arnica extract • Bay leaf oil • Glycerin • Clove oil • Cetyl Alcohol • Caprylic Triglyceride • Glyceryl Stearate • PEG 100 Stearate • Stearic Acid • Allantoin • Panthenol • Jojoba oil • Dimethicone • Polysorbate 20 • Tocopheryl Acetate (vitamin E) • Retinyl Palmitate (vitamin A) • Methylparaben • Ethylparaben • Silica 3X • TEA • I. Urea.

Cramp Bark-Catnip Virtue - Blessed Herbs
Cramp bark • Catnip flower & herb • Motherwort • Scullcap • Yarrow flower & herb • Grain alcohol & Distilled Water.

Cramp Free - Health Center for Better Living
Calcium • Magnesium • Potassium • Other Herbs.

Cran Support - Natrol
Each capsule contains: Guaranteed Potency Cranberry extract supplying 90% solids 30-40% organic acids 400 mg • Uva Ursi leaves 115 mg • Vitamin C (Ascorbic Acid) 100 mg • FOS (Fruiti-Vin FructoOgligoSaccharides) 100 mg • Cat's Claw root 50 mg • Corn Silk 30 mg • Kava Kava root 8.5 mg. Other Ingredients: Silica, Magnesium Stearate, Annatto, Gelatin.

Cran-Aid - Traditional Medicinals
Roselle Hibiscus flower • Cranberry Fruit concentrate • German Chamomile flower • Rose Hip • Uva Ursi leaf • Cleavers herb • Althea root • Peppermint leaf • Stevia leaf.

Cranberry - Aspen Group, Inc.
Each tablet contains: Cranberry extract (25:1 extract) 250 mg • Vitamin C 60 mg • Echinacea (4:1 extract) 30 mg • Buchu (4:1 extract) 15 mg • Juniper berry (4:1 extract) 15 mg • Uva Ursi (4:1 extract) 15 mg.

Cranberry - Basic Nutrition - GNC
Each capsule contains: Cranberry fruit powder (Vaccinium Macrocarpon) 500 mg. Other Ingredients: Gelatin, Cellulose, Magnesium Stearate.

Cranberry - Leiner Health Products
Two caplets contain: Cranberry extract (Vaccinium macrocarpon) berry 600 mg. Other Ingredients: Calcium Carbonate, Cellulose, Maltodextrin, Croscarmellose Sodium, Talc, Silicon Dioxide, Polyethylene Glycol 3350, Crospovidone, Hyroxypropyl Methylcellulose, Magnesium Stearate, Hydroxypropyl Cellulose, Polysorbate 80.

Cranberry - Pharmanex
Each capsule contains: Cranberry fruit (15:1) concentrate (Vaccinium macrocarpon) 500 mg. Other Ingredients: Gelatin and Titanium Dioxide.

Cranberry + - PhysioLogics
Each softgel contains: Vitamin C (as ascorbic acid) 100 mg • Vitamin E (as d-alpha tocopherol acetate) 3 IU • Cranberry concentrate powder (vaccinium macrocarpon, from 12:1 concentrate, equivalent to fresh cranberries 1680 mg) 140 mg. Other Ingredients: Soybean Oil, Gelatin, Lecithin, Glycerin, Beeswax / Soybean Oil Mixture.

Cranberry 1000 mg, Concentrated - GNC Herbal Plus - GNC
Each capsule contains: Cranberry Juice (vaccinium macrocarpon; from 58.5 mg of cranberry juice concentrate 19:1) 1000 mg. Other Ingredients: Soybean Oil, Gelatin, Glycerin, Caramel Color, Titanium Dioxide (natural mineral whitener).

Cranberry Apple Cherry - Clif Bars
Brown Rice Syrup • Rolled Oats • Soy Protein Isolate • Rice Flour • Oat Flour • Soy Flour • Soybean • Evaporated Cane Juice • Dried Apples • Cranberries • Apple Juice • Prunes • Apple Fiber • Oat Fiber • Milled Flaxseed • Soy Fiber • Chicory Extract • Lemon Fiber • Psyllium • Brown Rice • Malt Extract • Dried Cherries • Natural Flavor • Sea Salt • Baking Soda • Decaffeinated Green Tea Extract.

Cranberry Concentrate - Now
Two capsules contain: Vitamin C (as ascorbic acid) 20 mg • Cranberry concentrate fruit (1400 mg of 8:1 concentrate) 1.4 g. Other Ingredients: Magnesium Stearate.

Cranberry Concentrate - Pro Health
Two capsules contain: Vitamin C (as ascorbic acid, from corn) 20 mg • Cranberry concentrate (1400 mg of 8:1 concentrate, from vaccinium macrocarpon) 1.4 g. Other Ingredients: Magnesium Stearate.

Cranberry Concentrate - Schiff
Two softgels contain: Vitamin C (as ascorbic acid) 10 mg • Cranberry fruit (vaccinium macrocarpon) 1 g. Other Ingredients: Soybean Oil, Softgel (gelatin, glycerin, water, caramel color), Lecithin, Silicon Dioxide.

Cranberry Juice - Maximum Concentrate - Jamieson
Each capsule contains: Cranberry Juice Concentrate 1:34 500 mg.

Cranberry Juice Concentrate 1000 mg - Jamieson
Each capsule contains: Vitamin C (as Ascorbic Acid) 10 mg • Cranberry juice concentrate 1000 mg.

Cranberry Plus - Futurebiotics
Cranberry Extract (25:1 extract) 250 mg • Vitamin C 50 mg • Echinacea (4:1 extract equivalent to) 25 mg • Buchu (4:1 extract equivalent to) 12.5 mg • Juniper Berry (4:1 extract equivalent to) 12.5 mg • Uva Ursi (4:1 extract equivalent to) 12.5 mg.

Cran-C - Holista
Each capsule contains: Vitamin C 100 mg • Concentrated Cranberries (Vaccinum macrocarpon) of 25:1 extract (equivalent to 1132 mg of fresh cranberry juice) 45.3 mg.

Cran-Caps - Progressive Labs
Three softgels contain: Vitamin C 30 mg • Cranberry juice concentrate 3000 mg • Phosphatide complex 90 mg. Free of sugar and artificial sweeteners.

CranExtra - Enzymatic Therapy
Each capsule contains: Vitamin C (Ascorbic Acid) 1000 mg. Other Ingredients: Cranberry extract (Vaccinium macrocarpon) standardized to contain 5% Anthocyanidins & 30% Organic Acids: Quinic, Malic, Citric & Hippuric Acid 100 mg • Uva Ursi (Arctostaphylos uva ursi) standardized to contain 20% Arbutin 100 mg.

CranGuard - PhytoPharmica
Two capsules contain: Vitamin C (ascorbic acid) 200 mg • Cranberry extract (vaccinium macrocarpon, standardized to contain 5% anthocyanidins & 30% organic acids (quinic, malic, citric & hippuric acid)) 200 mg • Uva Ursi (arctostaphylos uva ursi, standardized to contain 20% arbutin) 200 mg.

Cravex Capsules - Natrol
Two capsules contain: Calcium (from garcinia cambogia) 180 mg • Chromium (as chromium picolinate) 120 mcg • Garcinia Cambogia extract 1000 mg: Hydroxycitric Acid (HCA) 600 mg • Green Tea extract (25% polyphenols) 300 mg: Polyphenols 75 mg, Caffeine 60 mg. Other Ingredients: Gelatin Capsules, Silica, Magnesium Stearate.

Cravex Tablets - Natrol
Two tablets contain: Calcium 230 mg • Iodine (as Potassium Iodine) 150 mcg • Chromium (as Chromium Picolinate) 200 mcg • Gymnema Sylvestre powdered extract leaves 300 mg • Licorice root 250 mg Deglycyrrhizinated Licorice • powdered extract Glycerinic Acid (1%) 2.5 mg • L-Glutamine 250 mg • DL-Phenylalanine 250 mg • 5-

Hydroxytryptophan (5-HTP) 10 mg. Other Ingredients: Calcium Sulfate Dihydrate, Mono & Di-Glycerides, Microcrystalline Cellulose, Croscarmellose Sodium, Stearic Acid, Silicon Dioxide, Magnesium Stearate.

***CreActiv* - Metabolic Response Modifiers**
Two scoops (95.5 g) contains: Creatine monohydrate 12 g • L-Glutamine 5 g • BCAA blend 2 g • Alpha Lipoic Acid 300 mg • Dextrose 70 g • L-Taurine 1 g • L-Arginine 500 mg • Vitamin C 250 mg • Calcium 21 mg • Potassium 101 mg • Sodium 85 mg • Magnesium 100 mg • Phosphorus 160 mg • Chloride 122 mg • RNA 200 mg.

***Creagen* - ANS - Applied Nutrition Sciences**
Creatine Monohydrate.

***Creagen Plus* - ANS - Applied Nutrition Sciences**
Creatine Monohydrate • Dextrose • Taurine.

***Cream of Youth* - Life Extension**
Biologically Active Placenta Enzymes, Apricot kernal oil, Collagen, Elastin, Vitamin E, NaPCA, Aloe, Emollients, Fragrances.

***Creamy Cleansing Lotion (normal to dry skin)* - Nu Skin Enterprises**
Water (aqua) • Caprylic/Capric Triglycerides • Butylene Glycol • Isodecyl Neopentanoate • Glyceryl Stearate • PEG-100 Stearate • Disodium Cocoamphodiacetate • Limnanthes Alba seed oil (meadowfoam) • Glycine Soja lipds (soybean) • Dipotassium Glycyrrhizate • Artemisia Vulgaris extract (mugwort) • Laminaria Digitata extract (algae) • Glycerin • Carbomer • Stearyl Alcohol • Triethanolamine • Tetrasodium EDTA • Fragrance (parfum) • Phenoxyethanol • Chlorphenesin • Methylparaben • Benzoic Acid.

***Creamy Hydrating Masque* - Nu Skin Enterprises**
Water (aqua) • Isocetyl Stearate • Glycerin • Butylene Glycol • Decyl Oleate • Stearic Acid • Saccharide Isomerate • Cetearyl Ethylhexanoate • Cetyl Alcohol • Opuntia Tuna extract (cactus) • Pinus Strobus cone extract • PVM/MA Copolymer • Sodium Polyacrylate • Polyacrylamide • C13-14 Isoparaffin • Carbomer • Oleth-10 • Laureth-7 • Triethanolamine • Anthemis Nobilis flower oil • Lavandula Angustifolia oil (lavender) • Salvia Officinalis oil (sage) • Camellia Sinensis leaf extract • Disodium EDTA • Chlorphenesin • Ethylparaben • Methylparaben • Phenoxy-Ethanol • Propylparaben • Titanium Dioxide.

***Creapure brand* - Degussa Food Ingredients/BL BioActives**
Creatine Monohydrate.
See Editor's Note No. 44, page 2058.

***Creatine* - Life Extension**
Each teaspoon contains: Creatine Monohydrate (99% pure, crystallized) 5000 mg.

***Creatine* - Source Naturals**
Each tablet contains: Creatine Monohydrate 1,000 mg.

***Creatine 1000* - Higher Power**
Each 1 tsp (5 g) serving contains: 100% Pure Creatine Monohydrate 5 g.

***Creatine 2500 Caps* - Optimum Nutrition**
Two capsules contain: Creatine Monohydrate 2.5 g. Other Ingredients: Gelatin, Magnesium Stearate.

***Creatine 6000-ES* - MuscleTech**
Each teaspoon contains: Creatine Monohydrate 6000 mg • Proprietary blend 500 mg: Creatine Monohydrate, L-Methionine, L-Arginine, L-Glycine.

***Creatine 750 Caps* - Optimum Nutrition**
Each capsule contains: Creatine Monohydrate 750 mg. Other Ingredients: Gelatin, Calcium Phosphate, Magnesium Stearate, Silica.

***Creatine Blast* - Pharmanex**
Each scoop (42 g) contains: Phosphorus (as Dimagnesium Phosphate) 60 mg • Magnesium (as Dimagnesium Phosphate) 50 mg • Creatine Monohydrate 4 g • Taurine 1000 mg. Other Ingredients: Dextrose, Citric Acid, Natural Grape Flavor, Grape Skin Extract (color).

***Creatine Fuel* - TwinLab**
Each capsule contains: Creatine Monohydrate 700 mg. Each teaspoonful of powder contains: Creatine Monohydrate 5 g (5000 mg).

***Creatine Fuel Loading Drink* - TwinLab**
HPLC Pure Creatine Monohydrate with added Dextrose (a high glycemic carbohydrate) • Chromium • Taurine • Magnesium • Alpha Lipoic Acid. Other Ingredients: L-Glutamine 2 g.

***Creatine Fuel Plus* - TwinLab**
Creatine (Creatine Monohydrate) 7 g. It also contains muscle cell volumizers, insulin potentiators & anti-catabolic, lean body mass stimulators. Fat free.

***Creatine Fuel Stack* - TwinLab**
Six capsules contain: Creatine Monohydrate 5000 mg • L-Glutamine 2000 mg • Taurine 200 mg.

***Creatine Fuelchews* - TwinLab**
Each chew contains: Pure Creatine Monohydrate 1 g • Dextrose 3 g. No sucrose or fructose is present.

***Creatine Monohydrate* - Pro Health**
Five tablets contain: Creatine Monohydrate (from sarcosine [n; n dimethyl glycine]) 5000 mg. Other Ingredients: Stearic Acid, Dibasic Calcium Phosphate, Fiber (vegetable), Modified Cellulose Gum, Colloidal Silicon Dioxide, Magnesium Stearate.

***Creatine Monohydrate Powder* - ProLab**
Each teaspoon contains: Creatine Monohydrate 5 g.

***Creatine Now - Wild Cherry* - Rexall - Sundown**
Each packet contains: Vitamin C (Ascorbic Acid) 1000 mg • Thiamin Hydrochloride (Vitamin B-1) 15 mg • Riboflavin USP (Vitamin B-2) 20 mg • Niacin (Niacinamide) 50 mg • Vitamin B-6 (Pyridoxine Hydrochloride) 8.3 mg • Vitamin B-12 (Cyanocobalamin) 10 mcg • Biotin 150 mcg • Pantothenic Acid (Calcium D-Pantothenate) 25 mg • Calcium Citrate 175 mg • Sodium Bicarbonate 200 mg • Potassium Bicarbonate 180 mg • Creatine Citrate 5 g • Stevia extract 26 mg. Other Ingredients: Dextrose, Citric Acid, Natural and Artificial Cherry flavor, Cochineal extract.

***Creatine Plus* - Life Extension**
Two capsules contain: Pure Creatine Monohydrate 1500 mg • Sodium Phosphate (dibasic) 50 mg • Potassium Bicarbonate 50 mg.

***Creatine Powder* - Olympian Labs**
Each teaspoon contains: Creatine Monohydrate 5000 mg.

***Creatine Powder* - Optimum Nutrition**
Each 5 g serving (1 rounded tsp) contains: Creatine Monohydrate 5 g.

***Creatine Sport Gel* - Metabolic Response Modifiers**
Contains: Creatine monohydrate 6,000 mg • L-Glutamine 1,000 mg • L-Taurine 500 mg • Dextrose 25 g.

***CreaVATE* - ProLab**
Each capsule contains: Creatine Pyruvate 750 mg.

***Creavescent* - GEN - Genetic Evolutionary Nutrition**
Each serving contains: L-Glutamine 2 g • TCT TM (Total Creatine Transport) Proprietary Blend 5 g: Creatine Monohydrate. Ingredients: Creatine Monohydrate • Fructose • L-Glutamine • Mono Poly-Saccharide • 2-Hydroxy-1, 2, 3-Propanetricarboxylic Acid • Sodium Hydrogen Carbonate • Orange Solids • Calcium Phosphate • Vitamin A • Vitamin D • Riboflavin.

Some Brand Name Natural Products - What they Contain

www.NaturalDatabase.com contains MANY more listings than appear here.

BRAND NAMES

CreaVol ATP - SportPharma
Each 41 g serving contains: 99% pure microfine Crystalline Creatine 5 g • Adenine Mucleotides including ATP • Vanadyl Sulfate • Taurine • Disodium & Potassium Phosphate • Dextrose (about 35 g per serving).

C-Statin - Aidan Products, LLC
Each capsule contains: Convolvulus Arvensis leaves extract 250 mg. Other Ingredients: Gelatin Capsule, Maltodextrin.

C-Statin II - Aidan Products, LLC
Each capsule contains: Resveratrol 300 mg • Bromelain 125 mg • Curcumin 125 mg • Baikal Skullcap 50 mg • Quercetin 40 mg • Vitamin E (succinate) 30 IU. Other Ingredients: Gelatin Capsule, Maltodextrin.

C-Time 1000 with Rose Hips - Puritan's Pride
Each tablet contains: Vitamin C with Rose Hips 1000 mg.

C-Time 1500 with Rose Hips - Puritan's Pride
Each tablet contains: Vitamin C with Rose Hips 1500 mg.

C-Time 500 with Rose Hips - Puritan's Pride
Each tablet contains: Vitamin C with Rose Hips 500 mg.

CTR Support - PhysioLogics
Three capsules contain: Turmeric root (curcuma longa, standardized to contain 95% curcuminoids, 713 mg) 750 mg • Boswellia Serrate gum resin (frankincense, standardized to contain 60% boswellic acids, 300 mg) 500 mg • Bromelain (pineapple, from 600 (GDU) per gram) 250 mg • Ginger root (zingiber officinale, standardized to contain 5% gingerols, 5 mg) 100 mg • Devil's Claw root (harpagophytum procumbens, standardized to contain 2% harpagosides, 0.9 mg) 50 mg • Quercetin root (dimorphandra gardina) 50 mg • Yucca plant (yucca schidigera, standardized to contain 14% saponins, 7 mg) 50 mg. Other Ingredients: Gelatin, Rice Powder, Silica, Vegetable Magnesium Stearate.

Culturelle with Lactobacillus GG - Klaire Laboratories
Each capsule contains: Lactobacillus GG 10 billion cells. Other Ingredients: Gelatin, Inulin (plant carbohydrate).

Curazyme - Enzymatic Therapy
Each capsule contains: Vitamin C (Ascorbic Acid) 50 mg • Pantothenic Acid (D-Calcium Pantothenate) 25 mg • Magnesium (Oxide) 25 mg • Curcuma root extract (Curcuma longa) standardized to contain 97% Curcumin 200 mg • Bromelain (2000 MCU) 200 mg • Butchers Broom extract (Ruscus aculeatus) standardized to contain 10% Saponins calculated as Ruscogenin 100 mg • Pancreatic Enzymes (10X) 50 mg • L-Cysteine 25 mg.
See Editor's Note No. 14.

Curb Your Cravings Plus patch - Curb Your Cravings LLC
Fucus Vesiculosus • Guarana • 5-HTP • Zinc Pyruvate • DHEA • Yerba Mate • Lecithin • Flaxseed oil • L-Carnitine • Zinc Citrate.

CurcuMax - PhytoPharmica
Each capsule contains: Bromelain (2000 MCU/g) 200 mg • Butcher's Broom root and rhizome extract (ruscus aculeatus, standardized to contain 9-11% saponins calculated as ruscogenins) 100 mg • L-Cysteine (as L-cysteine HCl) 25 mg • Magnesium (as magnesium oxide) 50 mg • Pancreatic Enzymes (10X) 25 mg • Turmeric rhizome extract (curcuma longa, standardized to contain 85-100% curcumin) 200 mg • Vitamin C (ascorbic acid) 50 mg.
See Editor's Note No. 14.

Curcumin 95 - Jarrow Formulas
Each capsule contains: Curcumin (from turmeric root) 380 mg • Demethoxycurcumin 90 mg • Bisdemethoxycurcumin 15 mg • Other Turmeric substances 15 mg. Other Ingredients: Cellulose, Magnesium Stearate, Silicon Dioxide, Gelatin.

Curcumin Extract - 500 mg - Vital Nutrients
Each vegetarian capsule contains: Curcumin Longa extract (total curcuminoids minimum 90% by HPLC) 500 mg • Black Pepper extract (95%, bioperine piperine) 2.5 mg.

CV-10 (Cardiovascular Nutritional Support) - Rx Vitamins
Six capsules contain: L-Taurine 500 mg • L-Carnitine 500 mg • Magnesium (Taurate) 400 mg • Hawthorne berry 100 mg • Potassium (Citrate) 99 mg • CoQ10 30 mg • Vitamin B3 (Niacin) 25 mg • Vitamin B6 (Pyridoxine) 25 mg • Folic Acid 400 mcg • Vitamin E 200 IU.

CVS Echinacea - CVS Pharmacy
Three capsules contain: Echinacea 1140 mg. Other Ingredients: Echinacea Purpurea Herb powder, Gelatin, Maltodextrin, Cellulose, Calcium Carbonate, Magnesium Stearate, Silicon Dioxide, Dicalcium Phosphate, Microcrystalline Cellulose, Stearic Acid, Croscarmellose Sodium, Hydroxypropyl Methylcellulose, Hydroxypropyl Cellulose, Polyethylene Glycol.

CVS Saw Palmetto - CVS Pharmacy
Two capsules contain: Maltodextrin • Cellulose • Gelatin • Saw Palmetto extract • Calcium carbonate • Magnesium stearate • Silicon Dioxide.

CVS Saw Palmetto Softgels - CVS Pharmacy
Each softgel contains: Saw Palmetto extract (serenoa repens) fruit 160 mg. Other Ingredients: Olive Oil, Gelatin, Purified Water, Glycerin, FD&C Red #40, FD&C Yellow #6.

Cycla-Action - Nature's Plus
Each capsule contains: Blue Cohosh root 150 mg • Black Currant seed 125 mg • Mustard seed 75 mg • Red Raspberry leaves 75 mg • Cramp bark 75 mg • Squaw Vine 50 mg • False Unicorn 50 mg.

Cycl-A-Vites - Nature's Plus
Two tablets contain: whole Black Currant seeds naturally supplying GLA 300 mg • Magnesium amino acid chelate/complex 250 mg • Vitamin B6 (Pyridoxine HCL) 200 mg • Bromelain natural pineapple 150 mg • Calcium amino acid chelate/complex 125 mg • Iron amino acid chelate/complex 18 mg. In a natural base of Red Raspberry leaves, Strawberry Leaves, Dong Quai, Uva Ursi, & Peppermint. Yeast free. Sugar & starch free.

Cyclo 3 Fort - Unknown
Each capsule contains: Ruscus aculeatus root extract 150 mg • Trimethylhesperidin-chalcon 150 mg • Ascorbic acid 100 mg.

CycloDiol-4 (Sports One Cycloplex Pro-Hormone) - Sports One
Each lozenge contains: 4-Androstenediol Cycloplex (cyclodextrin complex) 25 mg.

CycloDiol-5 (Sports One Cycloplex Pro-Hormone) - Sports One
Each lozenge contains: 5-Androstenediol Cycloplex (cyclodextrin complex) 25 mg.

CycloDiol-XS (Sports One Cycloplex Pro-Hormone) - Sports One
Each lozenge contains: Nor-4-Androstenediol Cycloplex (cyclodextrin complex) 10 mg • 4-Androstenediol Cycloplex (cyclodextrin complex) 15 mg.

Cyclovar - Warner Laboratories
Proprietary Blend 250 mg: L-Arginine, Cnidium Monnier extract, Xanthoparmelia extract, ZMA, Gamma Amino Butyric acid, Narigen, Quebracho extract, Microcrystalline Cellulose, Lactose Solutab, Magnesium Stearate.

Cynara-SL Artichoke - Lichtwer Pharma
Each capsule contains: Artichoke extract (Dried leaf extract) 320 mg. Other Ingredients: Gelatin, Magnesium Stearate, Silicon Dioxide,

Talc, Titanium Dioxide, Sodium Lauryl Sulphate, FD&C Blue No. 1, FD&C Yellow No. 5.

Cystone **-** The Himalaya Drug Company (Himalaya Heal
Each tablet contains: Shilapuspha (didymocarpus pedicellata) 130 mg • Pasanabheda (saxifraga ligulata syn. bergenia ligulata/ciliata) 98 mg • Manjishtha (rubia cordifolia) 32 mg • Nagarmusta (cyperus scariosus) 32 mg • Apamarga (achyranthes aspera) 32 mg • Gojiha (onosma bracteatum) 32 mg • Sahadevi (vernonia cinerea) 32 mg • Shilajeet (mineral pitch, purified) 26 mg • Hajrul Yahood Bhasma (lime silicate calx) 32 mg.

Cytodrene **-** Weightlosscontrol
Each capsule contains: Proprietary Blend 700 mg: Sida cordifolia extract, Kola Nut extract, Green Tea extract, Yohimbe bark extract, White Willow bark, Chromium picolinate, Guggulsterones.
See Editor's Note No. 39, page 2058.

Cytodyne **-** Cytodyne Technologies
Six capsules contain: Acetyl L-Carnitine 1100 mg • Phosphatidylserine 175 mg • L-Alanine 200 mg • Alpha Ketoglutaric Acid 150 mg • L-Glutamine 2150 mg • Taurine 1050 mg • Ketoisocaporate 50 mg • Inositol 50 mg.

Cytomax **-** Champion Nutrition
Each 25 gram serving contains: Apple: Alpha-L-Polyactate • Energy 90 Kcal • Total Fat 0g • Sodium 100 mg • Potassium 120 mg • Total Carbohydrate 22 g • Sugars 10 g • Protein 0 g. Citrus: Energy 90 Kcal • Total Fat 0g • Sodium 100 mg • Potassium 120 mg • Total Carbohydrate 22 g • Sugars 10 g • Protein 0 g. Tangy-Orange: Energy 90 Kcal •Total Fat 0g • Sodium 100 mg • Potassium 120 mg • Total Carbohydrate 21 g • Sugars 11 g • Protein 0. Tropical: Energy 90 Kcal • Total Fat 0g • Sodium 100 mg • Potassium 100 mg • Total Carbohydrate 22 g • Sugars 11 g • Protein 0. Ingredients: Fructose • Alpha-L-Polyactate: our non-acidic patented L-Lactate formula combined with Sodium L-Lactate & Potassium L-Lactate •Metacarb (Champion Nutrition's original complex carbohydrate blend including Amylopectin Starches & Maltodextrins from Corn Hybrids) • Glucose • Citric Acid •Succinate ETF Our Exclusive Succinate Compound containing: Potassium Succinate, L-Glutamic Acid, Inosine, Magnesium Succinate, Calcium Succinate • Natural Flavoring • Malic Acid • L-Alanine • L-Glutamine • Ascorbic Acid • Natural Caramel Coloring • Potassium Citrate • Xanthan Gum • Sunett (Acesulfame-K) • Chromium Polynicotinate (Chromemate - GTF).

CytoPro **-** Cytodyne Technologies
Each rounded scoop contains: Cross Flow Micro/Ultra Filtered 100% pure Whey Protein Isolate (beta lactoglobulin 19,100 MW/50% alpha lactoalbumin 14,700 MW/20%, glycomacropeptides 16,200 MW/ 20%, glutamine peptides 6700 MW/5%, immunoglobulin 95,000 MW/3%, bovine serum albumin 65,000 MW/2%, protease peptone). CytoPro WPI (typical amino acid profile) 23.976 mg: L-Alanine 1071 mg, L-Arginine 538 mg, L-Aspartic Acid 2303 mg, L-Cysteine 276 mg, L-Glutamic Acid 3870 mg, L-Glutamine 548 mg, L-Glycine 522 mg, L-Histidine 393 mg, L-Isoleucine 1433 mg, L-Leucine 2341 mg, L-Lysine 1999 mg, L-Methionine 409 mg, L-Phenylalanine 768 mg, L-Proline 1553 mg, L-Serine 1184 mg, L-Taurine 1000 mg, L-Threonine 1409 mg, L-Tryptophan 464 mg, L-Tyrosine 567 mg, L-Valine 1328 mg.

CytoVol **-** EAS
Each 15 gram serving contains: L-Glutamine 2500 mg • Taurine 2000 mg • Manganese 50 mcg • Calcium AKG 1500 mg • Inositol 500 mg • Glycine 500 mg • RNA 250 mg • L-Alanine 2000 mg. Ingredients: Dextrose • L-Glutamine • Taurine • L-Alanine • Calcium Alpha-Ketoglutarate (AKG) • Citric Acid • Natural Flavors • Inositol • Glycine • Sodium Ribonucleic Acid (RNA) • Sodium Phosphate • Turmeric mixed with Maltodextrin for color • Aspartame • Manganese Glycinate. Contains Phenylalanine.

D-400 IU **-** Rexall - Sundown
Each softgel contains: Vitamin A (from fish liver oil) 700 IU • Vitamin D (from fish liver oil) 400 IU. Other Ingredients: Soybean Oil, Gelatin, Glycerin, Water.

Daily 3 Complete **-** The Vitamin Shoppe
Each tablet contains: Vitamin D 400 IU • Vitamin A Activity 25000 IU • Vitamin C 500 mg • Vitamin E 400 IU • Vitamin B1 50 mg • Vitamin B2 50 mg • Vitamin B6 50 mg • Vitamin B12 500 mcg • Niacinamide 50 mg • PABA 50 mg • Pantothenic Acid 50 mg • Choline Bitartrate 50 mg • Inositol 50 mg • Biotin 50 mcg • Folic Acid 800 mcg • Vitamin K 30 mcg • Selenium 50 mcg • Green Tea extract 50 mg • CoQ10 100 mcg • L-Glutathione 10 mg • Pycnogenol 100 mcg • N-Acetyl Cysteine 15 mg • Molybdenum 50 mcg • Calcium 100 mg • Magnesium 50 mg • Potassium 50 mg • Zinc 15 mg • Iodine 150 mcg • Iron 10 mg • Manganese 5 mg • Chromium 100 mcg • Boron 3 mg • Apple pectin 50 mg • Papain 25 mg • Lipase 10 mcg • Probiotics 10 mg • Betaine HCl 25 mg • Pepsin 25 mg • Protease 10 mcg • Glutamic Acid 25 mg • Amylase 10 mcg • Chlorophyll 10 mg • Spirulina 45 mg • Bee Pollen 45 mg • Echinacea / Golden Seal 50 mg • Shiitake / Reishi mushrooms 45 mg • Barley grass 45 mg • Royal Jelly 15 mg • Alfalfa concentrate 45 mg • Siberian Ginseng 45 mg • Chlorella 45 mg • RNA/DNA 45 mg. A concentrated blend of: broccoli, tomato, garlic, onions, cauliflower, brussel sprouts, carrots, parsley, watercress. Pure dry, cold-pressed borage, flaxseed, safflower oils providing the essential fatty acids, Omega 3-6-9.

Daily 3 with Antioxidant Factors **-** Puritan's Pride
Three capsules contain: Vitamin A (as Beta-Carotene) 25,000 IU • Vitamin C (as Calcium Ascorbate) 500 mg • Vitamin D (as Cholecalcifeol) 400 IU • Vitamin E (as d-Alpha Tocopherol Succinate) 400 IU • Vitamin K (as Phytonadione) 30 mcg • Thiamin (Vitamin B-1; as Thiamine Hydrochloride) 50 mg • Riboflavin (Vitamin B-2) 50 mg • Niacin (as Niacinamide) 50 mg • Vitamin B-6 (as Pyridoxine Hydrochloride) 50 mg • Folic Acid 800 mcg • Vitamin B-12 (as Coenzyme B-12) 500 mcg • Biotin 50 mcg • Pantothenic Acid (as d-Calcium Pantothenate) 50 mg • Calcium (as Calcium Carbonate) 100 mg • Iron (as Carbonyl Iron) 10 mg • Iodine (as Kelp) 150 mcg • Magnesium (as Magnesium Oxide) 50 mg • Zinc (as Zinc Picolinate) 15 mg • Selenium (as Selenomethionate) 50 mcg • Manganese (as Manganese Carbonate) 5 mg • Chromium (as GTF Chromium Yeast) 100 mcg • Potassium (as Potassium Chloride) 50 mg • Green Tea (Camellia sinensis) leaf 50 mg • N-Acetyl Cysteine 15 mg • L-Glutathione 10 mg • Coenzyme Q10 100 mcg • Pine bark extract (Pycnogenol) 100 mcg • Choline Bitartrate 50 mg • Inositol 50 mg • PABA (Para-Aminobenzoic Acid) 50 mg • Boron (as Boron Citrate) 3 mg • Spirulina (Spirulina plantensis) plant 20 mg • Chinese Chlorella (Chlorella pyrenoidosa) 20 mg • Barley Grass (plant) 20 mg • Alfalfa juice concentrate 20 mg • Octacosanol 100 mcg • Siberian Ginseng (Eleutherococcus senticosus) root 20 mg • Bee Pollen 20 mg • Citrus Bioflavonoids 20 mg • Rutin 20 mg • Echinacea / Goldenseal (Echinacea purpurea / Hydrastis canadensis) root 20 mg • Royal Jelly 15 mg • Reishi Mushroom (Ganoderma lucidum) aerial 15 mg • Shiitake Mushroom (Lentinus edodes) aerial 15 mg • Shark Cartilage 45 mg • Apple Pectin 20 mg • Betaine Hydrochloride 20 mg • L-Glutamic Acid 20 mg • Papain (Papaya) 20 mg • Pepsin Enzyme 20 mg • Lipase 10 mg • Amylase 10 mg • Chlorophyll (as Sodium Copper Chlorophyllin) 10 mg • Proprietary Blend: Broccoli, Tomato, Orange, Lemon, Blueberry, Cranberry, Garlic, Onion, Cauliflower, and Brussels Sprout Concentrates 20 mg.

Daily Antioxidant Packs **-** Puritan's Pride
Each pack (2 softgels, 3 tablets) contains: Beta Carotene 25,000 IU • Multi-Vitamin: Providing Vitamin A (as beta carotene), Vitamin D, and B-Complex Vitamins • Vitamin E 400 IU • Vitamin C with Rose Hips 500 mg • Multi-Mineral: A full accompaniment of major and trace minerals including Chromium, Calcium, Zinc, and the antioxidant Selenium.

Daily Balance Energy Vitalizer **-** Doctor's Preferred, Inc. (Phillips Healt

Each four capsules contains: L-Carnitine 200 mg • L-Tyrosine 500 mg • Coenzyme Q10 30 mg • Ginkgo Biloba 80 mg • Chromium Picolinate 100 mg • Sodium Bicarbonate 350 mg • Vitamin C 500 mg • Vitamin B 120 mg • Vitamin B2 25 mg • Vitamin B3 40 mg • Vitamin B5 250 mg • Vitamin B6 25 mg • Folic Acid 200 mcg • Vitamin B12 25 mg • Biotin 200 mcg • Choline 25 mg • Inositol 25 mg • PABA 25 mg • Calcium 100 mg • Magnesium 200 mg • Iodine 25 mcg • Zinc 7.5 mg • Selenium 70 mcg • Potassium 50 mg.

Daily Balance Hot Flash **-** Doctor's Preferred, Inc. (Phillips Healt

Each softgel contains: Vitamin E (as d-alpha tocopheryl) 200 mg • Soy Germ extract (providing 10% soy isoflavones 25 mg) 250 mg • Gamma Oryzan (from rice bran oil) 150 mg • Black Cohosh extract (providing 2.5% triterpine glycosides) 2 mg.

Daily Balance Iron **-** Doctor's Preferred, Inc. (Phillips Healt

Each capsule contains: Vitamin C (as ascorbic acid) 30 mg • Iron (as bisglynate) 25 mg.

Daily Balance Menorrhagia **-** Doctor's Preferred, Inc. (Phillips Healt

Each two capsules contain: Vitamin C (as ascorbic acid magnesium and calcium ascorbates) 350 mg • Vitamin E (as d-alpha tocopheryl succinate) 100 mg • Calcium (as ascorbate) 3 mg • Bromelain (from pineapples) 250 mg • Lemon Bioflavonoid complex 175 mg • Rutin (from buckwheat) 150 mg • Chaste Tree extract (from berry, providing 0.3% casticin 0.34 mg and 0.15% agnuside 0.17 mg) 112.5 mg • Chaste Tree powder (from berry) 25 mg • Quercetin (as dihydrate) 25 mg.

Daily Balance PMS **-** Doctor's Preferred, Inc. (Phillips Healt

Each two softgels contains: Vitamin E (as d-alpha tocopheryl) 100 mg • Calcium (as carbonate) 200 mg • Magnesium (as oxide, ascorbate) 112.5 mg • Chaste Tree extract (from berry, providing 0.3% casticin 0.34 mg and 0.15% agnuside 0.17 mg) 112.5 mg • GLA (from borage oil) 75 mg • Cramp Bark 30 mg • Grapeseed extract 25 mg.

Daily Balance Women's Multinutrient **-** Doctor's Preferred, Inc. (Phillips Healt

Each packet contains: Multinutrient (6 capsules): Vitamin A (as palmitate) 1000 IU • Vitamin C (as ascorbic crystals, mineral ascorbates) 600 mg • Vitamin D3 (as cholecalciferol) 400 IU • Vitamin K (as phytonadione) 30 mcg • Thiamine (as mononitrate) 40 mg • Riboflavin (vitamin B2) 40 mg • Niacin (as niacinamide, niacin) 50 mg • Vitamin B6 (as pyridoxine HCl) 100 mg • Folic Acid 400 mcg • Vitamin B12 (as cyanocabalamin) 100 mcg • Biotin 300 mcg • Pantothenic Acid (as calcium pantothenate) 150 mg • Calcium (as carbonate, malate, citrate, ascorbate) 700 mg • Magnesium (as oxide, ascorbate) 350 mg • Zinc (as chelate) 15 mg • Selenium (as methionine) 200 mcg • Copper (as gluconate) 2 mg • Manganese (as ascorbate) 5 mg • Chromium (as chelate) 200 mcg • Molybdenum (as ascorbate) 100 mcg • Potassium (as citrate) 100 mg • Lemon Bioflavonoid Complex 500 mg • Rutin (from buckwheat) 200 mg • Choline (as bitartrate) 50 mg • Para-Aminobenzoic Acid (PABA) 25 mg • Boron (from chelate) 2 mg • Inositol 25 mg. Essential Fatty Acids (2 softgels): Docosahexaenoic Acid (DHA) 300 mg • Eicosapentaenoic Acid (EPA) 200 mg • Other Omega-3 Fatty Acids 100 mg • Gamma-linolenic Acid (as borage oil) 50 mg • Proprietary Antioxidant B (ascorbyl palmitate, rosemary leaf extract, mixed tocopheryls) 6 mg. Antioxidant (2 softgels): Vitamin A (as beta-carotene) 10,000 IU • Vitamin C (as ascorbyl palmitate) 26 mg • Vitamin E (as d-alpha-tocopheryl acetate) 600 IU • Alpha Lipoic Acid 30 mg • Mixed Tocopherols 10 mg • Tocotrienols (from rice bran oil) 10 mg • Lycopene (from tomatoes) 5 mg • Lutein (from marigold extract) 4 mg.

Daily Basics - Original **-** Rexall - Sundown

Each packet contains: Vitamin A (100% as Beta-Carotene) 1,000 IU • Vitamin C (Ascorbic Acid) 60 mg • Vitamin E (dl-Alpha Tocopheryl Acetate) 30 IU • Niacin (Niacinamide) 36 mg • Vitamin B12 (Cyanocobalamin) 10.8 mcg • Selenium Chelate (Sodium Selenite) 4 mcg • Calcium Carbonate 100 mg • Thiamin HCl 2.7 mg • Vitamin B6 (Pyridoxine HCl) 3.6 mg • Biotin 29 mcg • Chromium Polynicotinate (ChromeMate) 52 mcg • Riboflavin 3 mg • Folate (Folic Acid) 120 mcg • Zinc Gluconate 0.9 mg. Other Ingredients: Guar Gum, Locust Bean Gum, Pectins, Oat Fiber, Maltodextrin, Gum Arabic, Natural and Artifical Orange Flavor, Aspartame, Artifical Vanilla Flavor.

Daily Detox **-** M.D. Labs

Sarsaparilla • Milk Thistle • Red Clover • Dandelion • Yellow Dock • Burdock • Hibiscus • Echinacea • Fenugreek • Ginger • Cascara Sagrada. Other Ingredients: All Natural Fruit & Spice extracts.

Daily Enzyme Complex **-** Futurebiotics

Pancreas* 235 mg • Ox bile 35 mg • Duodenum 20 mg • Papaya enzyme 125 mg • Betaine 20 mg • Liver 20 mg • Vitamin B1 (thiamin) 3 mg • Bromelain 50 mg • Niacinamide 10 mg • Vitamin B2 (riboflavin) 3 mg • Peppermint 25 mg • Anise 25 mg • Chamomile 25 mg. *Whole dried pancreas, a source of Pancreatin, Trypsin, Amylase, Lipase, Lisotozyme, Diatase & Chymosin.
See Editor's Note No. 14.

Daily Essentials **-** Aspen Group, Inc.

Each three tablets contain: Vitamin E (d-alpha) 200 IU • Vitamin A 5000 IU • Beta Carotene 5000 IU • Vitamin D 400 IU • Vitamin C 400 mg • Folic Acid 400 mcg • Thiamine 1.5 mg • Riboflavin 1.7 mg • Niacin 20 mg • Vitamin B6 2 mg • Vitamin B12 6 mcg • Biotin 300 mcg • Pantothenic Acid 10 mg • Calcium (citrate) 600 mg • Phosphorus 450 mg • Iodine (kelp) 150 mcg • Magnesium (carbonate) 200 mg • Copper (gluconate) 2 mg • Zinc (gluconate) 15 mg • Vitamin K 100 mcg • Selenium (yeast) 75 mcg • Manganese (gluconate) 5 mg • Chromium (aspartate) 200 mcg • Molybdenum 150 mcg • Nickel 15 mcg • Tin 15 mcg • Vanadium 5 mg • Boron (citrate) 2 mg • Potassium (gluconate) 100 mg • Grape seed extract 10 mg • CO Q10 10 mg.

Daily Essentials for Men **-** Health Smart Vitamins

Two caplets contain: Vitamin A (as 83% beta-carotene, 17% palmitate) 15,000 IU • Vitamin C (ascorbic acid) 250 mg • Vitamin D (as cholecalciferol) 400 IU • Vitamin E (as d-alpha tocopheryl) 200 IU • Vitamin K (as phytonadione) 25 mcg • Thiamin (as thiamin mononitrate) 25 mg • Riboflavin 25 mg • Niacin (as 50% nicotinic acid, 50% niacinamide) 50 mg • Vitamin B6 (as pyridoxine HCl) 25 mg • Folate (folic acid) 400 mcg • Vitamin B12 (as cyanocobalamin) 50 mcg • Biotin 300 mcg • Pantothenic acid (as calcium pantothenate) 25 mg • Calcium (as 87% calcium carbonate, 13% mixed calcium complexes) 258 mg • Iron (as iron sulfate) 6 mg • Iodine (as potassium iodide) 150 mcg • Magnesium (as 80% magnesium oxide, 10% magnesium citrate, 10% mangesium glycinate) 125 mg • Zinc (as zinc ascorbate) 30 mg • Selenium (as selenomethionine) 75 mcg • Copper (as copper citrate) 3 mg • Manganese (as manganese gluconate) 2 mg • Chromium (as chromium polynicotinate) 100 mcg • Molybdenum (as molybdenum amino acid chelate) 50 mcg • Oriental Ginseng root (Panax ginseng) 75 mg • Pumpkin seed 75 mg • Saw Palmetto berry 75 mg • Betaine HCl 25 mg • Citrus bioflavonoids 25 mg • Choline (as bitartrate) 25 mg • Insitol 25 mg • Lecithin (from soybean) 25 mg • Bromelain (from pineapple 6,000 PU/g, 120 PU) 20 mg • Lipase (from fermentation of Aspergillus niger) 10 mg • Papain (from latex of fruit) 10 mg • Para-aminobenzoic acid (PABA) 10 mg • Boron (as boron aspartate) 2 mg • Silicon (as silicon dioxide) 2 mg • Vanadium (as vanadium amino acid chelate) 10 mcg.

Daily Essentials for Women **-** Health Smart Vitamins

Two caplets contain: Vitamin A (as 83% beta-carotene, 17% palmitate) 15000 IU • Vitamin C (ascorbic acid) 250 mg • Vitamin D (as cholecalciferol) 400 IU • Vitamin E (as d-alpha-tocopherol)

200 IU • Vitamin K (as phytonadione) 25 mcg • Thiamin (as thiamin mononitrate) 25 mg • Riboflavin 25 mg • Niacin 50 mg • Vitamin B-6 (as pyridoxine HCl) 25 mg • Folate (folic acid) 400 mcg • Vitamin B-12 (cyanocobalamin) 100 mcg • Biotin 300 mcg • Pantothenic Acid (as calcium pantothenate) 25 mg • Calcium 507 mg • Iron (as iron glycinate) 18 mg • Magnesium 200 mg • Iodine (as potassium iodide) 150 mcg • Zinc (as zinc ascorbate) 15 mg • Selenium (as selenomethione) 75 mcg • Copper (as copper citrate) 2 mg • Manganese (as manganese gluconate) 2 mg • Chromium (as chromium polynicotinate) 100 mcg • Molybdenum 50 mcg • Dong Quai root 50 mg • Royal Jelly from bees 50 mg • Betaine HCl 25 mg • Bioflavonoids (from citrus) 25 mg • Choline (as choline bitartrate) 25 mg • Inositol 25 mg • Lecithin (from soybean) 25 mg • Bromelain 20 mg • Lipase 10 mg • Papain 10 mg • PABA (Para-Amino Benzoic Acid) 10 mg • Rutin 5 mg • Boron (as boron aspartate) 2 mg • Silicon (as silicon dioxide) 2 mg • Vanadium 10 mcg.

***Daily Multi-Vitamin & Mineral* - Swanson**
Each capsule contains: Vitamin A (from fish liver oil) 10000 IU • Vitamin C (Ester-C®, as calcium ascorbate) 200 mg • Vitamin D (from fish liver oil) 400 IU • Vitamin E (as d-alpha tocopheryl succinate) 15 IU • Thiamin (as thiamin mononitrate; vitamin B-1) 10 mg • Riboflavin USP (vitamin B-2) 10 mg • Niacinamide 100 mg • Vitamin B-6 (as pyridoxine HCl) 5 mg • Folic Acid 400 mcg • Vitamin B-12 (as cyanocobalamin) 5 mcg • Pantothenic Acid (as d-calcium pantothenate) 20 mg • Calcium (from bone meal and dolomite) 125 mg • Iron (from ferrous sulfate) 12 mg • Iodine (from kelp) 150 mcg • Magnesium (from magnesium oxide) 32.5 mg • Zinc (from zinc sulfate) 15 mg • Copper (from copper sulfate) 2 mg • Manganese (from manganese sulfate) 1 mg.

***Daily Therapy 7-Vitamin Foaming Cleansing Gel* - Orjene**
Vitamin-packed antioxidant formula with Sea Minerals.

***Daily Vita Plus* - Global Health Trax**
Each tablespoon (0.5 fl oz) contains: Vitamin A (as palmitate, natural carotenese) 5000 IU • Vitamin C (as ascorbic acid) 300 mg • Vitamin D (as cholecalciferol) 400 IU • Vitamin E (as d-alpha tocopherol) 60 IU • Vitamin K (K1, as phyto-menadione) 300 mcg • Thiamin (as thiamine HCl) 3 mg • Riboflavin (as riboflavin) 3.4 mg • Niacin (as niacinamide, niacin) 35 mg • Vitamin B6 (as pyridoxine HCl) 4 mg • Folic Acid 400 mcg • Vitamin B12 (as cyanocobalamin) 6 mcg • Biotin 300 mcg • Pantothenic Acid (as D-calcium pantothenate) 20 mg • Gluconodeltalactone 1 g • Choline Bitartrate 50 mg • Inositol 50 mg • Glucosamine Sulfate 30 mg • Essential Fatty Acid Complex 25 mg • Amino Acid Complex 25 mg • CMO (as cetyl myristoleate, cetyl oleate) 25 mg • Methylsulfonylmethane (MSM) 20 mg • PABA 20 mg • Coenzyme Q10 10 mg • Aloe Vera powder 10 mg. Other Ingredients: Purified Water, Glycerin, Citric Acid, Malic Acid, Pepper Extract (piper nigris), Natural Flavorings, Potassium Sorbate, Sodium Benzoate, Stevia.

***Daily Vita Plus, Vegetarian* - Global Health Trax**
Each tablespoon (0.5 fl oz) contains: Vitamin A (as palmitate, natural carotenese) 5000 IU • Vitamin C (as ascorbic acid) 300 mg • Vitamin D (as cholecalciferol) 400 IU • Vitamin E (as d-alpha tocopherol) 60 IU • Thiamin (as thiamine HCl) 3 mg • Riboflavin (as riboflavin) 3.4 mg • Niacin (as niacinamide, niacin) 35 mg • Vitamin B6 (as pyridoxine HCl) 4 mg • Folic Acid 400 mcg • Vitamin B12 (as cyanocobalamin) 6 mcg • Biotin 300 mcg • Pantothenic Acid (as D-calcium pantothenate) 20 mg • Gluconodeltalactone 1 g • Choline Bitartrate 50 mg • Inositol 50 mg • Astragalus (as astragalus membranaceus) 30 mg • Boswellin (as boswellia serrata) 30 mg • Milk Thistle (as silybum marianum) 30 mg • Essential Fatty Acid Complex 25 mg • Amino Acid Complex 25 mg • Methylsulfonylmethane (MSM) 20 mg • PABA 20 mg • Coenzyme Q10 10 mg • Aloe Vera powder 10 mg. Other Ingredients: Purified Water, Glycerin, Citric Acid, Malic Acid, Pepper Extract (piper nigris), Natural Flavorings, Potassium Sorbate, Sodium Benzoate, Stevia.

***Daily Vits One-A-Day Multiple* - Now**
Each tablet contains: Vitamin A (100% as Beta Carotene) 5000 IU • Vitamin B1 (Thiamine HCL) 1.5 mg • Vitamin B2 (Riboflavin) 1.7 mg • Vitamin B3 (Niacinamide) 20 mg • Vitamin B5 (Pantothenic Acid) 10 mg • Vitamin B6 (Pyridoxine HCL) 3 mg • Vitamin B12 (Cyanocobalamin) 9 mcg • Biotin 300 mcg • Folic Acid 400 mcg • Vitamin C (Ascorbic Acid) 90 mg • Vitamin D (Calciferol) 400 IU • Vitamin E (natural d-Alpha Tocopherol) 30 IU • Calcium (Carbonate, Phosphate) 100 mg • Magnesium (Oxide) 80 mg • Zinc (Amino Acid Chelate) 15 mg • Iron (Ferrochel Bisglycinate) 9 mg • Copper (Amino Acid Chelate) 1 mg • Iodine (Kelp) 150 mcg • Potassium (Chloride) 50 mg • Manganese (Amino Acid Chelate) 2 mg • Selenium (Amino Acid Chelate) 70 mcg • Chromium (Chelavite Chelate) 120 mcg • Molybdenum (Amino Acid Chelate) 50 mcg • Choline (Bitartrate) 10 mg • Inositol 10 mg • PABA 10 mg • Boron (Amino Acid Chelate) 500 mcg • Vanadium (Amino Acid Chelate) 50 mcg • Panax ginseng (5% Ginsenosides) 100 mg.

***Daily VM Caps* - The Vitamin Shoppe**
Each capsule contains: Vitamin A 10000 IU • Vitamin D 400 IU • Vitamin C 250 mg • Thiamin 8 mg • Riboflavin 8 mg • Niacin 25 mg • Vitamin B6 10 mg • Vitamin B12 25 mcg • Vitamin E 100 IU • Pantothenic Acid 25 mg • Biotin 300 mcg • Folate 400 mcg • Calcium 100 mg • Magnesium 50 mg • Iron 10 mg • Manganese 2 mg • Zinc 7 mg • Selenium 70 mcg • Chromium 50 mcg • Iodine 125 mcg • Citrus Bioflavonoids 25 mg • Para Aminobenzoic Acid 10 mg • Choline 10 mg • Inositol 10 mg • Potassium 10 mg • Betaine HCl 10 mg • Pepsin 10 mg • Papain 10 mg • Pancreatin 10 mg.
See Editor's Note No. 14.

***Dairy Digest* - Enzymes, Inc.**
Each capsule contains: n-zimes Proprietary Enzyme Blend 112 mg: Lactase, Invertase, Amylase, Glucoamylase, Malt Diastase, Lipase, Protease (alkaline, neutral and acid proteases plus peptidase), CereCalase, Cellulase, Xylanase, Pectinase • Proprietary Herbal Blend 385 mg: Ginger root extract (5% gingerols) plus whole root, Caraway seed, Blackberry leaf. Other Ingredients: Plant Cellulose, Water, Lecithin, Rice Bran.

***Dairy Enzyme Formula* - Enzymatic Therapy**
Two capsules contain: Pure Plant Enzymes Blend 183 mg: Protease I,II,III,IV (USP XXIII [pH7.5]) 29,250 USP (FCC IV [pH7.0]) 46,650 PC.. (FCC IV [pH4.7]) 36,200 HUT, Lactase I,II (FCC III pH4.5]) 3350 LacU, Amylase (USP XXI [pH6.8]) 5500 USP (FCC IV [pH4.8]) 2350 DU., Lipase II (FCC IV [pH6.5]) 54 LU.

***Dairy Mix* - Professional Complementary Health Formul**
Adrenal 3X, 4X • ACTH 6X, 30X • Histamine 12X • Liver 6X, 12X • Cheeses: American, Cheddar, Camembert, Cream, Brie, Swiss, Blue, Cottage, Parmesan, Ricotta, Edam • Milks: Cow, Goat, Human 6X, 12X, 60X, 100X • Purified Water • 20% USP Alcohol.
See Editor's Note No. 1, page 2053.

***DairyEnz* - Enzymes, Inc.**
Each capsule contains: n-zimes Proprietary Blend 213 mg: Lactase, Proteases, Invertase, Lipase. Other Ingredients: Gelatin, Water.

***Damiana Leaf 1000 mg, Concentrated - GNC Herbal Plus* - GNC**
Each capsule contains: Damiana Leaves (turnera aphrodisiaca; from 250 mg of damiana leaf extract 4:1) 1000 mg. Other Ingredients: Cellulose, Calcium Carbonate, Gelatin.

***Damiana/Ginseng Formula* - Nature's Way**
Two capsules contain: Proprietary Formula: Damiana leaves • Fo-Ti root • Gotu Kola stem, leaf • Licorice root • Sarsaparilla root • Saw Palmetto berry • Siberian Ginseng root • Wild Yam root • Other Ingredients: Gelatin.

***Damiana-Sarsaparilla Formula* - Quest**
Each caplet contains: Damiana leaf powder (Tunera aphrodisiaca) 120 mg • Sarsaparilla root powder (Smilax officinalis) 90 mg • Saw Palmetto berry powder (Serenoa serrulata) 90 mg • Siberian Ginseng

root powder (Eleutherococcus senticosus) 90 mg • Licorice root powder (Glycyrrhiza glabra) 60 mg • Kelp powder (Fucus versiculosis) 50 mg. Other Ingredients: Calcium Phosphate, Microcrystalline Cellulose, Vegetable Stearin, Croscarmellose Sodium, Magnesium Stearate (vegetable source).

Dandelion **-** Nature's Way
Three capsules contain: Dandelion root 1.62 g. Other Ingredients: Gelatin.

Dandelion Root **-** Now
Two capsules contain: Total Carbohydrate 0.7 g • Dandelion root (Taraxacom Officinale) 1.0 g. Other Ingredients: Magnesium Stearate.

Dandelion-Milk Thistle Virtue **-** Blessed Herbs
Dandelion blend of flower, leaf & root • Milk Thistle seed • Bladderwrack • Reishi mycelium • Scullcap • Licorice root • Prickly Ash bark • Grain alcohol & Distilled Water.

Dark Roast - Revival **-** Physicians Laboratories
Eight fluid ounces Contain: Certified Isoflavone 15 mg. Other Ingredients: Whole Roasted Soybeans, Natural and Artificial Flavors.

Dasimix Shiulit Herbal Extracts Syrup **-** Hadas Natural Products
Herb Extract Blend: Thyme, Echinacea, Elderberry, Sage, Anise.

DayBreak Instant Beverage **-** Starlight International
Each scoop contains: Vitamin A • Calcium • Vitamin D • Thiamin • Niacin • Folate • Biotin • Phosphorus • Selenium • Zinc • Chromium • Vitamin C • Iron • Vitamin E • Riboflavin • Vitamin B6 • Vitamin B12 • Pantothenic Acid • Iodine • Magnesium • Copper.

Deep Pore Cleanser **-** Jason
Vitamin C Complex • Alpha Lipoic Acid.

Defend & Resist Complex **-** Shaklee
Six tablets contain: Zinc (as Zinc gluconate) 15 mg • Echinacea extract (Echinacea purpurea) herb & root 168 mg • Larch tree extract (Larix sp.) heartwood 300 mg • Defend & Resist Proprietary Blend 480 mg: Elderberry extract & Juice concentrate (Sambucus nigra) fruit, Stevia (Stevia rebaudiana) leaf. Other Ingredients: Maltose, Microcrystalline Cellulose.

Defender **-** Health Factor
Each tablet contains: Beta Carotene 5000 IU • Vitamin C (Ascorbic Acid) 60 mg • Vitamin E (d-Alpha Tocopheryl) 30 IU • Zinc (Amino Acid Chelate) 20 mg • Copper (Citrate) 2 mg • Selenium (Amino Acid Chelate) 100 mcg • Manganese (Citrate) 2 mg • Chromium (Nicotinate) 100 mcg • Boron (Citrate) 100 mcg • Vanadium (Citrate) 50 mcg • Molybdenum (Citrate) 50 mcg • Silicon (Citrate) 20 mcg • Grape seed (95% Polyphenols) 20 mg • Bilberry (25% Anthocyanidins) 5 mg.

Defender BVM **-** PhysioLogics
Two caplets contain: Vitamin A (as Beta Carotene) 5000 IU • Vitamin C (as Ascorbic Acid) 100 mg • Vitamin E (as d-Alpha Tocopherol Succinate) 240 IU • Selenium (as Selenomethionine) 400 mcg • Manganese (as Manganese Glycinate) 1.75 mg • Tea Green leaf (50% Polyphenols, 75 mg) 150 mg • N-Acetyl L-Cysteine 50 mg • Resveratrol (8% Resveratrol, 4 mg) 50 mg • Alpha Lipoic Acid 25 mg.

Defender FX **-** PhysioLogics
Three capsules contain: Vitamin A (as beta carotene) 25,000 IU • Vitamin C (as ester-c calcium ascorbate) 500 mg • Vitamin E (as d-alpha tocopherol acetate) 400 IU • Calcium (as ester-c calcium ascorbate) 65.7 mg • Selenium (as l-selenomethionine) 50 mcg • Coenzyme Q10 3000 mcg • Pycnogenol 3000 mg • Citrus Bioflavonoid complex (citrus sinensis) 50 mg • Quercetin fruit (from dimorphandra mollis) 30 mg • L-Glutathione 1000 mcg • N-Acetyl-Cysteine 100 mg • Green Tea leaf extract (camellia sinensis, standardized to contain 50% polyphenols, 1.5 mg) 3 mg • Bilberry fruit (vaccinium myrtillus) 30 mg. Other Ingredients: Gelatin, Cellulose (plant origin), Silica, Vegetable Magnesium Stearate.

Defense Formula **-** Bee-Alive Inc.
Two half-droppers (2 mL) contain: Echinacea root extract (echinacea angustifolia) 0.8 ml • Goldenseal root extract 0.06 mgl • Royal Jelly (non-freeze dried) 50 mg. Other Ingredients: Vegetable Glycerin, Clover Honey, Deionized Water, Almond Extract.

Deferol **-** GeoDist, LLC
Each capsule contains: Pyridoxine HCl 50 mg • Folic Acid 0.4 mg • Proprietary Blend: Passiflora Coerulea leaf extract, Griffonia seed extract, Pyridoxyl 5-phosphate 125 mg. Other Ingredients: Magnesium Stearate, Rice Powder, Gelatin.

Defy Your Age **-** Pharmagel
10% Alpha Hydroxy Acids • Stabilized Oxygen.

Dental-Aid **-** Futurebiotics
Three capsules contain: Vitamin C (as ascorbic acid) 1000 mg • Calcium (as calcium citrate) 250 mg • MSM (methyl-sulfonyl methane) 200 mg • Citrus Bioflavonoids 110 mg • Hesperidin 55 mg • Rutin 55 mg • Quercetin 50 mg • CoEnzyme Q-10 15 mg • Ginger root powder 110 mg • Chamomile flower powder 35 mg • Prickly Ash bark powder 50 mg • Barberry fruit powder 35 mg • Cloves 17 mg • Lemon Grass 15 mg • Sage 12 mg • Angelica root 12 mg. Other Ingredients: Magnesium stearate, Gelatin, Water.

Dentalgel **-** NutriBiotic
Contains 0.4% Grapefruit extract.

Dentaplex **-** Collagenex Pharmaceuticals
Each tablet contains: Vitamin A (20% [1000 IU] as Beta Carotene, 80% [4000 IU] as Vitamin A Acetate) 5000 IU • Vitamin C (as Ascorbic Acid) 300 mg • Vitamin D 200 IU • Vitamin E (as dl-Alpha Tocopheryl Acetate) 30 IU • Thiamin (Vitamin B1) 7.5 mg • Riboflavin (Vitamin B2) 8.5 mg • Vitamin B6 (as Pyridoxine Hydrochloride) 10 mg • Folic Acid 400 mcg • Vitamin B12 (as Cyanocobalamin) 30 mcg • Calcium (as Calcium Carbonate) 333 mg • Magnesium (as Magnesium Oxide) 40 mg • Zinc (as Zinc Oxide) 20 mg • Selenium (as Sodium Selenate) 15 mcg • Copper (as Cupric Oxide) 2 mg • Molybdenum (as Sodium Molybdate) 25 mcg • Vanadium (as Sodium Metavanadate) 10 mcg.

Depremin **-** FreeLife International
Each tablet contains: St. John's Wort extract (Hypericum perforatum) patented St. John's Wort extract EV.EXT 119 300 mg. Other Ingredients: Calcium Hydrogen Phosphate, Potato Starch, Hydrous Magnesium Silicate, Silica Dioxide, Microcrystalline Cellulose, Magnesium Stearate.

Depress-X **-** Olympian Labs
Each capsule contains: 5-HTP 10 mg • Ginkgo Biloba extract 40 mg • Vitamin B-6 50 mg • Magnesium 120 mg • Vitamin B-3 (niacinamide) 20 mg.

Derma Beauty HA **-** Health Logics
Two capsules contain: Vitamin C (as calcium ascorbate) 120 mg • Vitamin E (as natural d-alpha tocopherol) 30 IU • Calcium (as calcium ascorbate) 20 mg • Hyaluronic Acid (from BioCell Collagen II) 100 mg • Bio-Optimized Proprietary Blend 1160 mg: BioCell Collagen II (patented collagen type II, hyaluronic acid, chondroitin sulfate), Citrus Bioflavonoids (fruit), Rosemary Antioxidant extract, Peppermint oil extract, Green Tea leaf extract (standardized for antioxidant epigallocatechin gallate, polyphenols), L-Leucine, Grape Seed extract (standardized for antioxidant oligomeric proanthocyanidins), Ascorbyl Palmitate, Alpha Lipoic Acid, DMAE Bitartrate. Other Ingredients: Kosher Gelatin.
See Editor's Note No. 15, page 2055.

Derma Care **-** PhytoPharmica
Two softgel capsules contain: Biotin 1 mg • Choline Bitartrate 100 mg • Folic Acid 100 mcg • Inositol 66 mg • Lecithin (from soy) 400 mg • Niacin (as niacinamide and niacin) 66 mg • Pantothenic Acid

BRAND NAMES

(as calcium D-pantothenate) 17 mg • Proprietary Omega Blend 700 mg: Wheat germ oil, Safflower seed oil • Riboflavin (vitamin B2) 3.4 mg • Vitamin A (from fish liver oil) 3332 IU • Vitamin B6 (as pyridoxine HCl) 20 mg • Vitamin C (ascorbic acid) 200 mg • Vitamin D (as cholecalciferol) 666 IU • Vitamin E (as D-alpha tocopherol) 66 IU • Zinc (as zinc chelate) 10 mg.

Derma Cleanse - Zenmed - Raging Creations, Ltd.
Each capsule contains: Flos Lonicerae (Jin yin hua) 70 mg • Fructus Forsythia (Lian Qiao) 70 mg • Yellow Dock (Radiz Rumicis) 84 mg • Fructus Gardenia Jasminoidis (Zhi zi) 56 mg • Radix Paeoniae Rubra (Chi shao yao) 56 mg • Cortex Moutan Radicis (Mu dan pi) 56 mg • Burdock Root seed (Fructus arttii) 84 mg • Chastetree Berry (Fructus Viticis angi-casti) 91 mg • Herba Schizsizonepetae (Jing jie) 42 mg • Dandelion root (Radix taraxici) 56 mg • Chamomile (Flos Anthemis seu Matricariae) 35 mg.

Derma Klear Healthy Skin - Enzymatic Therapy
Two capsules contain: Vitamin A (as retinyl acetate) 10,000 IU • Vitamin C (ascorbic acid) 200 mg • Niacin 10 mg • Vitamin B6 (as pyridoxine HCl) 8 mg • Vitamin B12 (as cyanocobalamin) 3 mcg • Pantothenic Acid (as calcium D-pantothenate) 10 mg • Calcium (as calcium lactate) 11 mg • Magnesium (as magnesium oxide) 72 mg • Zinc (as zinc chelate) 30 mg • Potassium (as potassium chloride) 200 mg • Sulfur (sublimed) 200 mg • Bromelain (1200 M.C.U./g) 200 mg • Thymus extract 25 mg • Ribonucleic Acid (RNA) 20 mg • Burdock root 4:1 extract (arctium lappa) 10 mg. Other Ingredients: Gelatin, Silicon Dioxide, Titanium Dioxide Color, Magnesium Stearate.
See Editor's Note No. 14.

Derma Q-Gel - Tishcon-GelTec
Active Ingredients: Coenzyme Q10 • Vitamin E • Vitamin C • Vitamin A (Retinyl palmitate) • Alpha-Lipoic Acid (Thioctic Acid) • Vitamin K (as Vitamin K1) • Vitamin D • Biotin • Panthenol • Grape Seed extract • Green Tea extract • Chamomile extract • GLA from Borage Oil, Evening Primrose Oil • Aloe Vera gel • Squalane • Kikui Nut oil • Jojoba oil • Sweet Almond oil • Wheat Germ oil • Avocado oil.

Derma Teen - Futurebiotics
MSM, combination of vitamins, minerals, and horsetail.

Derma-Klear Akne Treatment Cream - Enzymatic Therapy
Sulfur 2.5%. Other Ingredients: Purified Water, Zinc, Sage extract, Silymarin phytosome, Hawthorne extract, Chamomile extract, 18-Beta-Glycyrrhetinic Acid, essential oil of Rosemary, Urea, Vitamin E (tocopherol). Fragrance is natural & hypoallergenic.

DermaKlear Akne-Zyme - Enzymatic Therapy
Two capsules contain: Vitamin A (as retinyl acetate) 10,000 IU • Vitamin C (ascorbic acid) 200 mg • Niacin 10 mg • Vitamin B6 (as pyridoxine HCl) 8 mg • Vitamin B12 (as cyanocobalamin) 3 mcg • Pantothenic Acid (as calcium d-pantothenate) 10 mg • Calcium (from calcium lactate 60 mg) 11 mg • Magnesium (from magnesium oxide 120 mg) 72 mg • Zinc (as zinc chelate) 30 mg • Potassium (from potassium chloride 200 mg) 105 mg • Sulfur (sublimed) 200 mg • Bromelain (1200 M.C.U./G) 200 mg • Thymus extract 25 mg • Ribonucleic Acid (rna) 20 mg • Burdock root extract (acrtium lappa, 4:1) 10 mg. Other Ingredients: Gelatin, Silicon dioxide, Titanium Dioxide Color, Magnesium Stearate.
See Editor's Note No. 14.

Dermalin-APg - Klein-Becker
Lecithin • Octyl Palmitate • Water • Aminophylline • Isopropylparaben • Isobutylparaben • Butylparaben • Fragrance.

DermaSlim TD - Alvin Last
Abies Canadensis • Ammonium Bromatum • Ammonium Carbonicum • Antimonium Crudem • Argentum Metallicum • Argentum Nitircum • Calcarea Carbonica • Capsicum Annuum • Cinchona Officinalis • Fucus Vesiculosus • Graphites • Kali Bichromicum • Kali Carbonicum • Kali Phosphoricum • Lycopodium Clavatum • Natrum Muriaticum • Phosphorus • Pulsatilla • Silicea • Spongia Tosta • Staphsagria • Sulphur • Thyroidunum • Veratrum Album.

DermaVite Dietary Supplement - Stiefel Laboratories
Each tablet contains: Vitamin A (29% as beta carotene) 3500 IU • Vitamin C 120 mg • Vitamin E 60 IU • Riboflavin 8.5 mg • Vitamin B-6 10 mg • Folate 400 mcg • Biotin 600 mcg • Calcium 270 mg • Zinc 45 mg • Selenium 50 mcg • Copper 2 mg • Manganese 5 mg • Chromium 200 mcg • Lycopene 5 mg • Silicon 20 mg.

Desiccated Liver Tablets with B-12 and B-Complex - Puritan's Pride
Each tablet contains: Thiamin (Vitamin B-1; Thiamine Hydrochloride) 1 mg • Vitamin B-12 (as Cyanocobalamin) 1 mcg • Desiccated Liver 680 mg.

Designer Protein - Next Nutrition
Each level scoop contains: Designer Whey full spectrum Whey Peptides: Modified molecular weight and partially pre-digested Whey Protein concentrate, PDUF Whey Protein isolate, Whey Glutamine Peptides (including natural glutamine peptides), Taurine, L-Leucine, L-Phenylalanine • Cocoa (treated with alkali) • Whey Mineral complex • Lecithin • Natural and Artificial Chocolate flavor • Glutasynth: L-Glutamine, Oligofructose, Glutamine Peptides • Natural and Artificial Flavor Zinmag-6: Magnesium Oxide, Magnesium Asparate, Zinc Asparate, Pyridoxine • Artificial Peanut butter flavor • Salt • Cellulose Gum • Dried Cream extract • Xanthan Gum • Sodium Alginate • Artificial Caramel flavor • Acesulfame Potassium • Sucralose • Vanillin • Natural Vitamin E (as mixed tocopherols) • Lactoperoxidase.

Dessert Avert - Enforma Natural Products
Each lozenge contains: Gymnema Sylvestre • Clove oil (or Clove powder) • Fructose.

Detox - The Herbalist
Oregon Grape root • Yellow Dock root • Dandelion root • Burdock root • Fennel seed.

Detox Formula - Gary Null & Associates (GNA)
Each capsule contains: Apple Pectin 25 mg • Buckthorn bark 25 mg • Burdock root 25 mg • Cascara Sagrada bark 25 mg • Chrysanthemum 25 mg • Dandelion root 25 mg • Fennel seed 25 mg • Fiber 75 mg • Garlic 25 mg • Ginger root 25 mg • Goldenseal root 50 mg • Hibiscus 25 mg • Kelp 25 mg • Licorice root 25 mg • Marshmallow 25 mg • Orange peel 25 mg • Oregon Grape root 25 mg • Peppermint 25 mg • Prickly Ash bark 25 mg • Psyllium 50 mg • Red Clover 25 mg • Rose Hips 25 mg • Sarsaparilla root 25 mg • Stillingia 25 mg • Yellow Dock 25 mg.

Detox Formula - Pharmanex
Each capsule contains: Vitamin C (as calcium ascorbate) 150 mg • N-Acetyl-L-Cysteine 125 mg • Calcium D-Glucarate 125 mg • Silymarin (as milk thistle fruit extract 30:1 (silybum marianum L.)) 70 mg. Other Ingredients: Gelatin, Calcium Carbonate, Stearic Acid, Silicon Dioxide.

DeTox Formula - Vital Nutrients
Two capsules contain: Glutamine 250 mg • Glycine 250 mg • Taurine 250 mg • Milk Thistle extract (80%) 80 mg • Silybin A & B extract (80%) 20 mg • Curcumin extract (90%) 100 mg • N-Acetyl-Cysteine 100 mg • Alpha Lipoic Acid 100 mg • Grape seed extract (60:1) 50 mg • MSM 50 mg • Broccoli sprout extract 50 mg • Yellow Dock extract (4:1) 50 mg • Schisandra extract (30:1) 50 mg • Green Tea extract (80% catechins) 25 mg • Glutathione (reduced) 20 mg.

Detox Support - Now
Each capsule contains: Milk Thistle • Sodium Alginate • Chlorella • MSM as central ingredients.

Detoxene - Health Smart Vitamins
Two capsules contain: Vitamin C (as ascorbic acid) 50 mg • Vitamin E (as d-alpha tocopheryl acetate) 10 IU • Pectin (from citrus) 120 mg • Chlorella 60 mg • Algin (as alginic acid) 50 mg • Burdock root

50 mg • Red Clover flower 50 mg • Sarsaparilla root 50 mg • Cornsilk style and stigma 30 mg • Bromelain (from pineapple) 20 mg • Garlic bulb 20 mg • Goldenseal (whole herb) 20 mg • Juniper berry 20 mg • Kelp 20 mg • Turmeric root (95% curcumin; 19 mg) 20 mg • Dandelion root 10 mg • Milk Thistle seed (80% silymarin; 8 mg) 10 mg.

Detoxication Factors - Tyler - Integrative Therapeutics
Two capsules contain: Vitamin A (as natural beta-carotene with mixed carotenoids, palmitate) 6665 IU • Vitamin C (as magnesium ascorbate) 167 mg • Vitamin E (as d-alpha tocopheryl succinate) 83 IU • Thiamine (as thiamine HCl, thiamine pyrophosphate) 8.3 mg • Riboflavin (as riboflavin-5'-phosphate) 8.3 mg • Niacin 10 mg • Vitamin B6 (as pyridoxal-5'-phosphate) 10 mg • Folic Acid 200 mcg • Vitamin B12 (as cyanocobalamin, adenosylcobalamin) 41.6 mcg • Biotin 66.7 mcg • Pantothenic Acid (as calcium pantothenate) 33.3 mg • Magnesium (as magnesium citrate, ascorbate, malate) 78 mg • Zinc (as zinc picolinate) 10 mg • Selenium (as l-selenomethionine) 66.7 mcg • Copper (as copper sebicate) 66.7 mcg • Manganese (as manganese glycinate) 3.3 mg • Molybdenum (as molybdenum citrate) 50 mcg • Calcium d-Glucarate 66.7 mg • L-Methionine 66.7 mg • Glycine 66.7 mg • L-Glutamic Acid HCl 66.7 mg • Taurine 66.7 mg • L-Glutamine 66.7 mg • Choline (as choline bitartrate) 66.7 mg • NAC (n-acetyl cysteine) 66.7 mg • Quercetin 66.7 mg • Inositol 33.3 mg • L-Ornithine-L-Aspartate 33.3 mg • Broccoli aerial parts extract (Brassica oleracea, 0.7% total sulfur) 33.3 mg • Milk Thistle seed extract (Silybum marianium, 80% silymarin) 16.7 mg • L-Glutathione reduced 16.7 mg • L-Serine 16.7 mg • L-Histidine 16.7 mg • L-Carnitine (as l-carnitine tartrate) 16.7 mg • Coenzyme Q10 (ubiquinone) 8.3 mg • Proanthocyanidins (from grape seed extract, vinis vinifera) 3.3 mg • Superoxide Dismutase 33.3 mcg • Catalase 16.7 mcg. Other Ingredients: Microcrystalline Cellulose, Silicon Dioxide, Gelatin, Water.

Detoxil - Vitabiotics
Two tablets contain: Vitamin A (1333 IU) 400 mcg • Vitamin D (as D3 200 IU) 5 mcg • Vitamin E (natural source) 30 mg • Vitamin C 120 mg • Vitamin B1 (thiamin) 12 mg • Vitamin B2 (riboflavin) 5 mg • Vitamin B3 (niacin) 27 mg • Vitamin B6 (pyridoxine HCl) 30 mg • Folacin (as folic acid) 400 mcg • Vitamin B12 (cyanocobalamin) 20 mcg • Biotin 0.03 mg • Pantothenic Acid 50 mg • Iron 5 mg • Magnesium 50 mg • Zinc 15 mg • Manganese 8 mg • Copper 2 mg • Iodine 200 mcg • Selenium 120 mcg • Natural Mixed Carotenoids 2 mg • N-Acetyl Cysteine 30 mg • Methionine 40 mg • Phosphatidylcholine 10 mg • Artichoke concentrate extract 50 mg • Grapefruit concentrate extract 50 mg • Dandelion root extract 50 mg.

Detoxinal - PhysioLogics
Two capsules contain: Vitamin C (as ascorbic acid) 200 mg • Chlorella 200 mg • Garlic bulb (allium sativum) 100 mg • Milk Thistle seed (silybum marianum, 80% silymarin, 80 mg) 100 mg • Sodium Alginate 50 mg • Bromelain (from 600 gelatin digestive units, GDU, per gram) 50 mg • Burdock root (arctium lappa) 50 mg • Cascara Sagrada bark (rhamnus purshiana) 50 mg • Dandelion root (taraxacum officinale) 50 mg • Citrus Pectin (citrus spp.) 50 mg • Red Clover (trifolium pratense) 50 mg. Other Ingredients: Gelatin, Rice Flower Powder, Silica, Vegetable Magnesium Stearate.

Detoxygen - Nature's Plus
Two tablets contain: Hibiscus (Hibiscus sabdariffa) 250 mg • Red Clover (Trifolium pratense) 200 mg • Dandelion (Taraxacum officinale) 200 mg • Shiitake Mushroom (Lentinus edodes) 150 mg • Reishi Mushroom (Ganoderma lucidum) 50 mg • Echinacea (Echinacea purpurea) 100 mg • Cayenne (Capsicum frutescens) 75 mg • Yellow Dock (Rumex crispus) 50 mg • Milk Thistle (standardized 80% Silymarin) 50 mg • Celery Seed (Apium graveolens) 25 mg • Ginger root (Zingiber officinale) 25 mg • Juniper berries (Juniperus communis) 20 mg • Creatine Monohydrate Energy Precursor 100 mg • Co-Enzyme Q10 (Ubiquinone) 10 mg • Vitamin B12 (Cobalamin concentrate) 250 mcg.

Devil's Claw Complex - PhytoPharmica
Two capsules contain: Devil's Claw (Harpagophytum procumbens) root extract (standardized to contain 1.8%-2.2% harpagoside) 500 mg • Nettle leaf (Urticae dioica) leaf extract (standardized to contain 1% silicic acid) 500 mg • Ginger (Zingiber officinale) root extract (standardized to contain a minimum of 4.5% pungent compounds) 200 mg.
See Editor's Note No. 21, page 2056.

Devil's Club-Bilberry Virtue - Blessed Herbs
Devil's Club Root bark • Bilberry leaf • Reishi mycelium • Siberian Ginseng root • Grain alcohol & Distilled Water.

Dexatrim - Chattem, Inc.
Each gelcap contains: Phenylpropanolamine HCl 75 mg. Other Ingredients: Carnauba wax, FD&C Yellow No. 10 Aluminum Lake, FD&C Yellow No. 6 Aluminum Lake, Hydroxypropyl Methylcellulose, Iron Oxide, Magnesium Stearate, Microcrystalline Cellulose, Polyethylene Glycol, Polysorbate 80, Povidone, Silicon Dioxide, Stearic Acid, Titanium Dioxide.
See Editor's Note No. 21, page 2056.

Dexatrim Natural Ephedrine-Free Formula - Chattem, Inc.
Each caplet contains: Calcium 23 mg • Chromium (as Chromium Dinicotinate Glycinate) 83 mcg • Bitter Orange Peel powder extract 120 mg • Proprietary Blend: Siberian Ginseng extract, Green Tea leaf with added Caffeine, Fenugreek seed extract, Guarana seed extract with added Caffeine, Kola Nut extract with added Caffeine, Ginger root, Licorice root, and Vanadium amino acid chelate 340 mg. Other Ingredients: Microcrystalline Cellulose, Maltodextrin, Dicalcium Phosphate, Croscarmellose Sodium, Stearic Acid, Silicon Dioxide, Hydroxypropyl Methylcellulose, Polyethylene Glycol.
See Editor's Note No. 40, page 2058.

Dexatrim Natural Green Tea Formula - Chattem, Inc.
Each caplet contains: Iodine (from kelp) 30 mcg • Chromium (as chromium dinicotinate glycinate) 250 mcg • Vanadium (as vanadium amino acid chelate) 100 mcg • Green Tea leaf standardized extract (40 mg caffeine) 200 mg • Heartleaf standardized extract (12 mg ephedrine alkaloids) 120 mg • Herbal Blend 150 mg: Panax Ginseng root standardized extract, Licorice root, Cinnamon bark, Ginger root, Sarsaparilla root, Kelp. Other Ingredients: Dicalcium Phosphate, Microcrystalline Cellulose, Croscarmellose Sodium, Stearic Acid, Silica, Magnesium Stearate, Hydroxypropyl Methylcellulose, Hydroxypropyl Cellulose, Polywthylene Glycol, Titanium Dioxide, Riboflavin, Caramel.
See Editor's Note No. 39, page 2058.

Dexatrim Natural No Caffeine Formula - Chattem, Inc.
Each caplet contains: Chromium (as chromium dinicotinate glycinate) 250 mcg • Vanadium (as vanadium amino acid chelate) 100 mcg • Heartleaf standardized extract (12 mg naturally ocurring ephedrine) 120 mg • Thermonutrient Blend 100 mg: Steatite, Atractylodes rhizome, Baikal Skullcap root, Balloon-Flower root, Licorice root, Terra Alba, Da Huang root, Mirabilite, Dong Quai root, Field Mint leaf, Forsythia fruit, Gardenia fruit, Ginger root, Lovage root, Schizonepeta stem, Siler root, White Peony root. Other Ingredients: Dicalcium Phosphate, Microcrystalline Cellulose, Croscarmellose Sodium, Stearic Acid, Hydroxypropyl Cellulose, Polyethylene Glycol.
See Editor's Note No. 39, page 2058.

Dexatrim No Caffeine - Chattem, Inc.
Each gelcap contains: Phenylpropanolamine HCl 75 mg. Other Ingredients: Carnauba wax, FD&C Yellow No. 10 Aluminum Lake, Edetate Disodium, FD&C Blue No. 1, FD&C Red No. 40 Aluminum Lake, FD&C Yellow No. 6 Aluminum Lake, Gelatin, Glycerin, Hydroxypropyl Methylcellulose, Magnesium Stearate, Microcrystalline Cellulose, Pharmaceutical Glaze, Polyethylene Glycol, Polysorbate 80, Povidone, Propylene Glycol, Silicon Dioxide, Stearic Acid, Titanium Dioxide.

Dexatrim Results **-** Chattem, Inc.
Each caplet contains: Proprietary Blend 185 mg: Ephedra stem, Yohimbe bark, Siberian Ginseng root, Licorice root, Rutin, Kelp, Fenugreek seed, Hesperidin complex • Proprietary Blend 130 mg: Cocogen, Caffeine, Green Tea extract • Vitamin C 10 mg • Vitamin E 5 IU • Vitamin B6 2 mg • Pantothenic Acid 5 mg • Calcium 97 mg • Iron 54 mcg • Phosphorus 70 mg • Magnesium 6.7 mg • Chromium 40 mcg.
See Editor's Note No. 21 and No. 30.

Dexatrim Results Ephedrine Free Formula **-** Chattem, Inc.
Each caplet contains: Vitamin C (as ascorbic acid) 10 mg • Vitamin E (as d-alpha tocopheryl succinate) 5 IU • Vitamin B6 (as pyridoxine Hydrochloride) 2 mg • Pantothenic Acid (as d-calcium pantothenate) 5 mg • Calcium (as dicalcium phosphate) 90 mg • Phosphorus (as dicalcium phosphate) 70 mg • Magnesium (as magnesium oxide) 6.7 mg • Zinc (as zinc oxide) 2.5 mg • Manganese (as amino acid chelate) 0.67 mg • Chromium (as amino acid chelate) 40 mcg • Proprietary Herbal Blend #1 202 mg: Bitter Orange peel extract, Yohimbe bark, Eleuthero root, Licorice root, Rutin, Kelp, Fenugreek seed, Hesperidin complex • Proprietary Blend #2 130 mg: Cocoa extract, Caffeine, Green Tea leaf extract. Other Ingredients: Gelatin, Microcrystalline Cellulose, Croscarmellose Sodium, Stearic Acid, Silicon Dioxide, Pharmaceutical Glaze, Carnauba Wax.
See Editor's Note No. 40, page 2058.

DGC **-** AST Sports Science
Four level teaspoons (46 g) contain: Pure Dextrorotatory Glucose Crystals.

DGL **-** Enzymatic Therapy
Each chewable tablet contains: Licorice root extract 4:1 Deglycyrrhizinated (Glycyrrhiza glabra) 380 mg • Glycine (Amino Acid) 50 mg. In a base of Fructose.

DGL Chewable Licorice **-** Puritan's Pride
Each tablet contains: Deglycyrrihizinated Licorice root (Glycyrrihiza glabra) extract (4:1) 380 mg • Glycine (Amino Acid) 50 mg.

DGL Plus **-** Progressive Labs
Two capsules contain: Licorice root (Glycyrrhiza glabra): Deglycyrrhizinated Licorice extract 400 mg • NAG (N-Acetyl Glucosamine) 60 mg • Parotid Gland 10 mg • Gamma Oryzanol 50 mg • Glycine 50 mg.

DGL Powder **-** Vital Nutrients
Each level 1/8 teaspoon contains: Deglycyrrhinzinated Licorice (DGL) powder 300 mg.

DHA - Brain Support Complex **-** Leiner Health Products
Each softgel contains: DHA (Docosahexaenoic Acid) 100 mg. Other Ingredients: High Oleic Sunflower Oil, Algal Oil, Gelatin, Glycerin, Vanillin, Ascorbyl Pamitate, Mixed Natural Tocopherols.

DHA **-** Nordic Naturals
Two softgels contain: Vitamin E (mixed tocopherols) 12 IU • Omega-3 Fatty Acids 740 mg • DHA (docosahexaenoic acid) 500 mg • EPA (eicosapentaenoic acid) 150 mg • Other Omega-3 90 mg. Other Ingredients: Purified Deep Sea Fish Oil, Softgel Capsule (gelatin, water, glycerine, strawberry essence), Antioxidant Blend (lecithin, ascorbyl palmitate).

DHA **-** PhysioLogics
Each softgel contains: DHA (docosahexaenoic acid, as algal oil) 100 mg. Other Ingredients: Sunflower oil, Gelatin, Glycerin.

DHA Chewable **-** Metagenics
Each softgel contains: DHA (docosahexaenoic acid) 100 mg • EPA (eicosapentaenoic acid) 55 mg • Other Omega-3 Fatty Acids 25 mg.

DHA Gold brand **-** OmegaTech
Docosahexaenoic Acid.
See Editor's Note No. 44, page 2058.

DHA Neuromins **-** Source Naturals
Each softgel contains: Docosahexaenoic acid 100 mg.

DHEA - Basic Nutrition **-** GNC
Each capsule contains: Dehydroepiandrosterone (DHEA) 25 mg. Other Ingredients: Cellulose, Calcium Carbonate, Gelatin, Magnesium Stearate.

DHEA **-** Body Wise International, Inc.
Each capsule contains: DHEA (dehydroepiandrosterone) 25 mg • Calcium (from dicalcium phosphate) 6 mg.

DHEA **-** DreamPharm
Each capsule contains: DHEA 30 mg • Korean Ginseng (Panax ginseng) 200 mg • Chinese Yam (dioscorea opposite) 200 mg • Poria Cocos 70 mg.

DHEA **-** Leiner Health Products
Each tablet contains: DHEA (dehydroepiandrosterone) 25 mg. Other Ingredients: Dicalcium Phosphate, Cellulose, Stearic Acid, Silicon Dioxide, Magnesium Stearate, Polyethylene Glycol 3350, Crospovidone, Croscarmellose Sodium, Hydroxypropyl Methylcellulose, Hydroxypropyl Cellulose, Polysorbate 80.

DHEA **-** NewLibido
Each capsule contains: DHEA 100 mg. Other Ingredients: Gelatin, Dicalcium Phosphate, Magnesium Stearate, Stearic Acid, Microcrystalline Cellulose.

DHEA **-** Olympian Labs
Each capsule contains: DHEA (dehydroepiandrosterone) 25 mg.

DHEA **-** Optimum Nutrition
Each tablet contains: Calcium 110 mg • Phosphorus 85 mg • Dehydroepiandrosterone (DHEA) 50 mg. Other Ingredients: Dicalcium Phosphate, Stearic Acid, Microcrystalline Cellulose, Magnesium Stearate, Silica, Croscarmellose Sodium (disintegrant).

DHEA - Pharmaceutically Pure **-** Life Extension
Each capsule contains: Dehydroepiandrosterone (DHEA, 100% pharmaceutical grade) 50 mg.

DHEA **-** Pro Health
Each capsule contains: DHEA (dehydroepiandrosterone, synthesized from wild yam) 25 mg. Other Ingredients: Dicalcium Phosphate, Cellulose, Gelatin (capsule shell), Magnesium Stearate, Silica.

DHEA **-** Schiff
Each tablet contains: Calcium (as calcium carbonate) 137 mg • DHEA (dehydroepiandrosterone) 25 mg • Trans-Ferolic Acid 1 mg. Other Ingredients: Cellulose, Magnesium Stearate, Croscarmellose Sodium.

DHEA **-** Swanson
Each capsule contains: DHEA (dehydroepiandrosterone) 25 mg.

DHEA (50 mg) **-** Olympian Labs
Each capsule contains: DHEA (dehydroepiandrosterone) 50 mg.

DHEA 25 - GNC A-Z **-** GNC
Each capsule contains: DHEA (dehydroepiandrosterone) 25 mg. Other Ingredients: Cellulose, Calcium Carbonate, Gelatin.

DHEA 25 mg **-** Nature's Bounty
Each tablet contains: DHEA (dehydroepiandrosterone) 25 mg. Other Ingredients: Cellulose (plant origin), Dicalcium Phosphate, Croscarmellose, Vegetable Stearic Acid, Vegetable Magnesium Stearate, Silica.

DHEA 25 mg **-** Vital Nutrients
Each capsule contains: DHEA (dehydroepiandrosterone) 10 mg.

DHEA 25 mg (Inspired by Nature) **-** Puritan's Pride
Each tablet contains: DHEA (dehydroepiandrosterone) 25 mg. Other Ingredients: Cellulose (plant origin), Dicalcium Phosphate,

Croscarmellose, Vegetable Stearic Acid, Vegetable Magnesium Stearate, Silica.

DHEA 25 Timed Release - GNC A-Z - GNC
Each tablet contains: DHEA (dehydroepiandrosterone) 25g. Other Ingredients: Dicalcium Phosphate, Cellulose, Vegetable Acetoglycerides.

DHEA 5 mg (Inspired by Nature) - Puritan's Pride
Each tablet contains: DHEA (dehydroepiandrosterone) 5 mg. Other Ingredients: Dicalcium Phosphate, Cellulose (plant origin), Silica, Vegetable Magnesium Stearate.

DHEA Fuel - TwinLab
Each hard gelatin capsule contains: Pharmaceutical Grade DHEA (dehydroepiandrosterone) 25 mg. Other Ingredients: Potato Starch, Cellulose, Gelatin, Purified Water, Magnesium Stearate, MCT.

DHEA MAX - Nutraceutics Corp.
Each caplet contains: DHEA (dehydroepiandrosterone) 25 mg. Other Ingredients: Microcrystalline Cellulose, Non-Pariel Beads, Magnesium Stearate, Stearic Acid, Pharmaceutical Glaze, Lactose, FD&C Lake Blue Lake #1, FD&C Yellow Lake #6.

DHEA PLUS - Nutraceutics Corp.
Two caplets contain: Vitamin C (as ascorbic acid) 25 mg • Vitamin B6 (as pyridoxine hydrochloride) 6 mg • Pantothenic Acid (as calcium pantothenate) 25 mg • Proprietary Blend 1350 mg: Pentasterone, Smilex Aristolochiafolii (dried root), Beta sitosterol, Adrenal Cortex.

DHEA SL - Nutraceutics Corp.
Each caplet contains: DHEA (dehydroepiandrosterone) 25 mg. Other Ingredients: Magnesium Stearate.

DHEA Ultra - FreeLife International
Each tablet contains: DHEA (micronized dehydroepiandrosterone - 100% pharmaceutical grade) 25 mg · Metabolic Activation System (an exclusive coenzyme complex of Nicotinamide, Pyridoxal-5'-phosphate, Riboflavin-5'-phosphate, Pantothenic Acid, Thiamine) 10 mg · Bioavailability Enhancing System (ancient herbal tricatu blend - 2.5 mg of Bioperine [Piper nigrum fruit standardized 95% 1-piperoylpiperidine], Piper longum fruit, Zingiber officinalis root) 12.5 mg.

DHEA X-TRA - Progressive Labs
Each capsule contains: DHEA (dehydroepiandrosterone) 50 mg • Herbal Base 250 mg: Green Tea leaf extract (Camellia sinensis) 35% polyphelols, Schizandra berry (Schizandra chinensis), Soybean extract (Glycine max) 1% isoflavones (hypoallergenic), Ginkgo Biloba leaf extract (24% ginkgoflavonglycosides), Grape seed extract (Vitis vinifera) 40% proanthocyanidins.

DHEA-25 - PhytoPharmica
Each capsule contains: DHEA (Dehydroepiandrosterone) pharmaceutical grade 25 mg.

DHEA-25-X-TRA - Progressive Labs
Each capsule contains: DHEA (dehydroepiandrosterone) 25 mg • Herbal Base 250 mg: Green Tea leaf extract (Camellia sinensis) 35% polyphenols, Schizandra berry (Schizandra chinensis), Soybean extract (Glycine max) 1% isoflavones (hypoallergenic), Ginkgo Biloba leaf extract (24% ginkgoflavonglycosides), Grape seed extract (Vitis vinifera) 40% proanthocyanidins.

DHEA-5 - PhytoPharmica
Each capsule contains: DHEA 5 mg.

DHEAX - HealthWatchers System
Dioscorea Villosa • Alpha Ketoglutaric Acid • Phosphatidyl Serine • Pantothenic Acid • Gotu Kola Powder • Ginkgo Biloba Powder • Siberian Ginseng Powder • L-Glutamine • L-Tyrosine • L-Glycine • L-Arginine-HCl • L-Ornithine • L-Lysine • Pantathine • Beta Sitosterol.

Diabecon - The Himalaya Drug Company (Himalaya Heal
Each tablet contains: Meshashringi (gymnema sylvestre) 30 mg • Pitasara (pterocarpus marsupium) 20 mg • Yashti-Madhu (glycyrrhiza glabra) 20 mg • Saptarangi (casearia esculenta) 20 mg • Jambu (eugenia jambolana syn. syzygium cumini) 20 mg • Shatavari (asparagus racemosus) 20 mg • Punarnava (boerhaavia diffusa) 20 mg • Mundatika (sphaeranthus indicus) 10 mg • Guduchi (tinospora cordifolia) 10 mg • Kairata (swertia chirata syn. s.chirayita) 10 mg • Gokshura (tribulus terrestris) 10 mg • Bhumyaamlaki (phyllanthus amarus) 10 mg • Gumbhari (gmelina arborea) 10 mg • Karpasa (gossypium herbaceum) 10 mg • Daru Haridra (berberis aristata) 5 mg • Kumari (aloe vera syn. a.barbadensis) 5 mg • Triphala 3 mg: Emblica Officinalis, Terminalia Chebula, Terminalia Bellirica • Guggul (commiphora wightii, purified) 30 mg • Shilajeet (mineral pitch, purified) 30 mg • Sushavi (momordica charantia) 20 mg • Maricha (piper nigrum) 10 mg • Vishnu Priya (ocimum sanctum syn. o.tenuiflorum) 10 mg • Atibala (abutilon indicum) 10 mg • Haridra (curcuma longa) 10 mg • Jungli Palak (rumex maritimus) 5 mg • Vidangadi Lauham 27 mg: Embelia Ribes, Cyperus Rotundus, Terminalia Chebula, Terminalia Bellirica, Emblica Officinalis, Cedrus Deodara, Piper Longum, Piper Chaba, Plumbago Zeylanica, Zingiber Officinalis, Piper Nigrum, Iron Calx • Vang Bhasma (tin calx) 5 mg • Abhrak Bhasma (powdered talc, biotite calx) 10 mg • Praval Bhasma (coral calx) 10 mg • Akik Pishti (processed agate) 5 mg • Shingraf (cinnabar) 5 mg • Yashad Bhasma (zinc calx) 5 mg • Trikatu 5 mg: Piper Nigrum, Piper Longum, Zingiber Officinale.

Diabest - PhysioLogics
Three tablets contain: Vitamin A (palmitate) 2500 IU • Vitamin E (d-alpha tocopherol) 300 IU • Vitamin C (ascorbic acid) 300 mg • Magnesium (glycinate) 300 mg • Niacin 150 mg • Zinc (glycinate) 23 mg • Vitamin B6 (pyridoxine HCl) 15 mg • Copper (glycinate) 3 mg • Biotin 900 mcg • Chromium (niacin/glycine chelate) 200 mcg • Selenium (as selenomethionine) 50 mcg • Quercetin 150 mg • Ginkgo leaf (24% ginkgo flavonglycosides 75 mg, 6% terpene lactones 4.5 mg) 75 mg • Vanadyl Sulfate 750 mcg. Other Ingredients: Cellulose (plant origin), Croscarmellose, Vegetable Stearic Acid, Silica, Vegetable Magnesium Stearate, Cellulose Coating.

Diabest 2 - PhysioLogics
Each capsule contains: Chromium (as 67% chromium amino acid chelate, 33% chromium picolinate) 300 mcg •Gymnema Sylvestre leaf (standardized to contain 25% gymnemic acid, 50 mg) 200 mg •Bitter Melon fruit (momordica charantia, standardized to contain 7% bitter principles, 7 mg) 100 mg •Bis-Glycinate-Oxovanadium (BGOV) 10 mg •Vanadyl Sulfate 10 mg. Other Ingredients: Gelatin, Dicalcium phosphate, Cellulose (plant origin), Silica, Vegetable Magnesium Stearate.

Diabetic Support Formula - Puritan's Pride
Each tablet contains: Vitamin C (as Ascorbic Acid) 100 mg • Vitamin E (as dl-Alpha Tocopheryl Acetate) 30 IU • Biotin 350 mcg • Calcium (as Dicalcium Phosphate) 85 mg • Magnesium (as Magnesium Oxide) 250 mg • Zinc (as Zinc Oxide) 7.5 mg • Selenium (as Sodium Selenate) 70 mcg • Manganese (as Manganese Sulfate) 2 mg • Chromium (as Chromium Picolinate) 500 mcg • Lipoic Acid 30 mg • Vanadyl Sulfate 10 mg • Ginkgo Biloba (24% flavone glycosides) 20 mg • Coenzyme Q-10 5 mg • Taurine 50 mg • L-Carnitine 125 mg.

Diabetica Tea - HerbaSway
Panax Ginseng • Siberian Ginseng • Astragalus • Kudzu • Blackberry • Licorice • HerbaSwee (Cucurbitaceae fruit).

Diabinil - Thorne Research Inc.
Two capsules contain: Chromium (Ultachrome) 100 mcg • Vanadyl sulfate 3 mg • Gymnena sylvestre extract leaf (25% Gymnemic acid) 200 mg • Bilberry extract fruit (Vaccinium myritillus) (25% Anthocyanocides) 80 mg • Bitter Melon extract fruit (mormordica charantia) (0.5% Charantin) 80 mg • Quercetin Chalcone 400 mg • Alpha Lipoic Acid 100 mg.

Diablo - NutraBolics
Each (4 cc) serving contains: L-Citruline Malate 3000 g • Designer Cell-Oxidizing Complex 1000 g: DiArginine Malate, Bis-Carboxyethyl Germanium Sesquioxide, Trimethyl-Aminoethanol, Nicotinamide Adenine Dinucleotide.

Dia-B-Tea - Raintree Nutrition, Inc.
Each rounded teaspoon contains: Pata de Vaca • Pedra Hume Caa • Bitter Melon • Chanca Piedra • Stevia.

Di-Acid Dim - Atrium Inc.
Each tablet contains: First Phase (in Stomach): Glycine 32 mg • Pepsin 100 mg • Papain 50 mg. Second Phase (in Duodenum): Pancreatin 100 mg • Pancrelipase 50 mg • Amylase 30 mg • Bromelain 30 mg • Ox Bile extract 65 mg.
See Editor's Note No. 14.

Di-Acid Stim - Atrium Inc.
Each tablet contains: First Phase (in Stomach): Betaine HCL 100 mg • Glutamic Acid HCL 110 mg • Pepsin 100 mg • Papain 50 mg. Second Phase (in Duodenum): Pancreatin 100 mg • Pancrelipase 50 mg. Amylase 30 mg • Bromelain 40 mg • Ox Bile extract 60 mg.
See Editor's Note No. 14.

Dia-Comp - Enzymatic Therapy
Two capsules contain: Vitamin E (Mixed Tocopherols) 50 IU • Magnesium (Chelate) 100 mg • Vitamin C (Ascorbic Acid) 100 mg • Vitamin B6 (Pyridoxine HCL) 10 mg • Manganese (Chelate) 10 mg • Zinc (Picolinate) 5 mg • Biotin 1000 mcg • Vitamin B12 (Cyanoco-balamin) 250 mcg • Chromium (Picolinate) 50 mcg • Selenium (Aspartate) 40 mcg • Other Ingredients: Blueberry extract 4:1 (Vaccinium myrtillus fructus) 300 mg • Gymnema sylvestre extract standardized to contain 24% Gymnemic Acid 150 mg • Bitter Melon extract (Momordica charanita) 100 mg • Fenugreek seed extract (4:1) (Trigonella foenum-Ggaecum) 100 mg.

Diakof - The Himalaya Drug Company (Himalaya Heal
Each 1 tsp (5 mL) serving contains: Guggulu (balsamodendron mukul syn. commiphora wightii, purified) 35 mg • Draksha (vitis vinifera) 35 mg • Bishnupriya (ocimum sanctum syn. o.tenuiflorum) 25 mg • Jufa (hyssopus officinalis) 25 mg • Guduchi (tinospora cordifolia) 20 mg • Vasaka (adhatoda vasica syn. a.zeylanica) 15 mg • Jaatipatree (myristica fragrans, mace) 15 mg • Yashti-Madhu (glycyrrhiza glabra) 15 mg • Gojihva (onosma bracteatum) 10 mg • Neelapuspha (viola odorata) 10 mg • Triphala 9 mg: Emblica Officinalis, Terminalia Chebula, Terminalia Bellirica • Trikatu 9 mg: Piper Nigrum, Piper Longum, Zingiber Officinale • Vidanga (embelia ribes) 8 mg • Kantakari (solanum xanthocarpum syn. s.surattense) 8 mg • Taja (cinnamomum cassia) 8 mg • Navasagara (ammonii chloridum) 3 mg.

Diaper Ointment - Hyland's
Calendula flowers extract (calendula officinalis) 1X HPUS. Base: Petrolatum USP, 5% Lanolin USP.
See Editor's Note No. 1, page 2053.

Diarex - The Himalaya Drug Company (Himalaya Heal
Each tablet contains: Kutaja (holarrhena antidysenterica) 245 mg • Guduchi (tinospora cordifolia) 16 mg • Bilva (aegle marmelos) 245 mg • Dadima (punica granatum) 82 mg • Shankh Bhasma (conch shell calx, conch shell ash) 61 mg • Musta (cyperus rotundus) 51 mg.

Dibencozide - Source Naturals
Each tablet contains: Dibencozide (Coenzyme Vitamin B12) 10,000 mcg.

Diene-O-Lean - Pharmanex
Two capsules contain: Sunflower Oil 2000 mg • Conjugated Linoleic Acid 1200 mg • Capsaicin 100 mg.

Diene-O-Lean - Pharmanex
Three capsules contain: Safflower oil 3000 mg • Conjugated Linoleic Acid 2250 mg • Capsaicin (from cayenne pepper) 150 mg.

Diet Chitosan - Source Naturals
Each capsule contains: Chitosan (minimum 80% Deacetylated Chitin) 250 mg.

Diet CitriMax - Source Naturals
Each tablet contains: Garcinia cambogia extract [yielding 500 mg of (-) Hydroxycitric Acid as Calcium Hydroxycitrate] 1,000 mg • Chromium (60 mcg ChromeMate Chromium Polynicotinate and 60 mcg of Chromium Picolinate) 120 mcg.

Diet CitriMax Complex - Source Naturals
Three tablets contain: Garcinia cambogia extract [yielding 1,000 mg of (-) Hydroxycitric Acid as Calcium Hydroxycitrate] 2,000 mg • L-Phenylalanine 200 mg • Chromium (200 mcg ChromeMate Chromium Polynicotinate and 200 mcg Chromium Picolinate) 400 mcg.

Diet Clear Cleanse Fiber Re:Fresh - Source Naturals
Each scoop (3.75 g) contains: Proprietary Concentrate 3300 mg: Psyllium Husk Powder, Rice Bran Fiber, Oat Bran Powder, Grapefruit Pectin, Flax Seed, Barley Bran, and Acacia Gum • Lipase 100 mg • Stevia rebaudiana 100 mg • NutraFlora FOS (Fructooligosaccharides) 74 mg • Ginger Root 74 mg • Lactobacillus Acidophilus (providing 3 billion cells at packaging) 30 mg • Green Citrus Peel 25 mg • Anise Seed 20 mg.

Diet Clear Cleanse Herbal Re:Store - Source Naturals
Three tablets contain: L-Glutamine 300 mg • Oregon Grape root 225 mg • Blessed Thistle root 180 mg • Plantain herb 180 mg • Red Clover blossom 180 mg • Cloves fruit 180 mg • Artemesia herb 150 mg • Black Walnut hull extract (4:1) 150 mg • Bupleurum root 150 mg • Burdock root 150 mg • Ginger root 150 mg • Grapefruit Seed extract (80:1) 150 mg • Licorice root 150 mg • Quercetin 150 mg • Slippery Elm bark 150 mg • Vitamin C (as ascorbic acid) 150 mg • Yellow Dock root 150 mg • Dandelion root 120 mg • Cat's Claw bark 100 mg • Dandelion root extract (4:1) 100 mg • Milk Thistle seed extract (standardized to 83% silymarin) 90 mg • Bioflavonoid Complex 75 mg • Garlic clove 75 g • Sarsaparilla root 75 mg • Turmeric root 75 mg.

Diet Esteem Plus - Esteem Products, Ltd
Two capsules contain: Super CitriMax brand Garcinia Cambogia 200 mg • L-Carnitine 25 mg • Bromelain 100 mg • GTF ChromeMate brand Chromium 100 mcg • Siberian Ginseng (25x1) 500 mg • Gymnema Sylvestre 100 mg • Choline 200 mg • Lecithin 100 mg • Lipase 125 mg • Inositol 35 mg • Biotin 200 mcg • Pacific Kelp 150 mcg • Pyridoxine (B-6) 25 mg • Cayenne 30 mg.

Diet Fuel - TwinLab
Three capsules contain: Chromium 200 mcg • Citrimax: Garcinia cambogia, Hydroxycitrate extract 500 mg • Guarana extract 909 mg • L-Carnitine 100 mg • Ma Huang extract 334 mg • Potassium & Magnesium Phosphate 100 mg.
See Editor's Note No. 30, page 2056.

Diet Fuel Ephedra Free - TwinLab
Two capsules contain: Guarana Seed Extract (22% caffeine) 800 mg • Proprietary Blend 685 mg: Citrus Aurantium Fruit Extract (standardized for 19.5 mg synephrine alkaloids), St. John's Wort Extract (aerial parts; standardized for 0.9 mg hypericin), L-Phenylalanine, Green Tea Leaf Extract (standardized for epigallocatechin gallate), Quercetin, Citrus Bioflavonoid Complex (containing naringin), Ginger Root, Cayenne Fruit. Other Ingredients: Gelatin, Purified Water, MCT, Magnesium Stearate, Silica.
See Editor's Note No. 40, page 2058.

Diet Fuel With Chitosan Formula - TwinLab
Two capsules contain: Chitosan (fiber) 1000 mg. Other Ingredients: Cellulose, Gelatin, Purified Water, Magnesium Stearate, MCT.

Diet Lean Carb Blocker - Naturade
Two tablets contain: Calcium (as dibasic calcium phosphate) 200 mg • Phase2 Phaseolus Vulgaris bean extract 1000 mg. Other Ingredients:

Croscarmellose Sodium, Vegetable Stearic Acid, Magnesium Stearate, Silicon Dioxide, Hydroxypropyl Methylcellulose, Water.

Diet Metabo-7 **-** Source Naturals
Each tablet contains: Vitamin C (as ascorbic acid) 80 mg • Niacinamide 30 mg • Vitamin B6 (as pyridoxine HCl) 30 mg • Pantothenic Acid (as calcium-d-pantothenate) 80 mg • Chromium (as picolinate & polynicotinate) 400 mcg • Potassium (as potassium citrate) 20 mg • Iodine (from kelp) 100 mcg • GABA (gamma-aminobutyric acid) 500 mg • Phenylalanine (as l-& dl-phenylalanine) 500 mg • Sida cordifolia extract (6% yielding 30 mg ephedrine alkaloids) 500 mg • Gymnema sylvestre extract (GS4) 400 mg • Green Tea leaf extract (20% yielding 60 mg of caffeine) 300 mg • Glutamine 200 mg • Yogaraj Guggul Gum Resin 200 mg • Kola Nut extract (20% yielding 30 mg of caffeine) 150 mg • Yerba Mate extract (8% yielding 10 mg of caffeine) 125 mg • Dandelion leaf 100 mg • Bupleurum root 100 mg • L-Tryosine 100 mg • Horse Chestnut extract (yielding 14 mg Aescin) 70 mg • Dandelion root extract (4:1) 50 mg • Bladderwrack extract 30 mg • Ginkgo Biloba leaf extract (50:1) 30 mg • Ginger root 30 mg • N-Acetyl-Cysteine 30 mg • Black Pepper fruit extract (Bioperine) 3 mg.
See Editor's Note No. 39, page 2058.

Diet Pyruva-Nectar **-** Source Naturals
Two scoops (32 g) contain: Calcium Pyruvate Monohydrate 5 g. Other Ingredients: Fructose, Natural Flavorings, Gum Arabic, Red Beet Root (natural color), and Citric Acid.

Diet Pyruvate - 500 mg **-** Source Naturals
Each capsule contains: Calcium Pyruvate Monohydrate 500 mg.

Diet Pyruvate - 750 mg **-** Source Naturals
Each capsule contains: Calcium Pyruvate Monohydrate 750 mg.

Diet Support Formula **-** Now
Two capsules contain: Vitamin B6 (pyridoxine HCL) 10 mg • Chromium (chelavite chelate) 300 mcg • Iodine (kelp extract) 300 mcg • Bitter Orange extract (Citrus aurantium) containing 6% synepherine 350 mg • L-Carnitine (from 365 mg l-carnitine tartrate) 250 mg • Super Citrimax as Garcinia cambogia extract containing 225 mg (-)hydroxycitric acid 375 mg • Uva Ursi (Uvae ursi folium) 4:1 extract 50 mg • Green Tea extract (Carmellia sinenis) 30% calechins 200 mg.
See Editor's Note No. 40, page 2058.

Diet System 6 **-** Applied Nutrition
Six capsules contain: Super Citrimax: Garcinia extract 1500 mg. Energizing Herbs (Thermogenic Herbs): Kola nut extract 550 mg, Guarana extract 100 mg, Ginger 100 mg. Three Lipotropics including: Choline Bitartrate 100 mg, Inositol 100 mg, Betaine HCL 25 mg. Chromium (Chromium Picolinate 150 mcg, ChromeMate 150 mcg). L-Carnitine (L-Carnitine Complex) 300 mg. Vitamins & Minerals: "72 Trace Mineral Complex" 100 mg: Vitamin B3 20 mg, Vitamin B6 2 mg, Vitamin B12 6 mcg, Vitamin B2 1.7 mg, Vitamin E 15 IU, Folic Acid 400 mcg, Selenium 50 mcg , Vitamin C 60 mg, Potassium 25 mg, Iodine 150 mcg.

Diet Tonalin **-** Source Naturals
Three softgels contain: Conjugated Linoleic Acid 1800 mg. Other Ingredients: Gelatin (capsule), Glycerin, Purified Water, Caramel, Carob, Titanium Dioxide.

Diet Ultra III **-** The Vitamin Shoppe
Three tablets contain: Vitamin A (as acetate, beta-carotene) 10000 IU • Vitamin C (as ascorbic acid) 100 mg • Vitamin D (cholecalciferol) 400 IU • Vitamin E (as d-alpha tocopherol) 50 IU • Vitamin B1 (as thiamin hydrochloride) 25 mg • Vitamin B2 (as riboflavin) 25 mg • Vitamin B12 (as cobalamin) 25 mcg • Niacin (as nicotinic acid) 25 mg • Folic Acid 100 mcg • Biotin 100 mcg • Pantothenic Acid (as d-calcium pantothenate) 20 mg • Iron (as chelate) 10 mg • Calcium (as citrate) 100 mg • Iodine (from kelp) 150 mcg • Magnesium (as citrate) 50 mg • Zinc (as chelate) 15 mg • Selenium (as chelate) 25 mcg • Chromium (as chelate) 300 mcg • Gotu Kola (Centella asiatica) 50 mg • Siberian Ginseng (Eleutherococcus senticosus) root 50 mg • L-Carnitine 50 mg • Choline 150 mg • Inositol 150 mg • Omega-3 (fish) 15 mg.

Dieter's Green Tea **-** Triple Leaves Brand
Malva verticillata • Loquat leaf.

DietEz Meal Replacement Powder **-** NutriCology
Two scoops (40 g) contain: Vitamin A (56% as beta-carotene, 22% as vitamin A palmitate, 22% as carotenoid (mix)) 9000 IU • Vitamin C (as magnesium ascorbate) 300 mg • Calcium (as calcium citrate and phosphate) 300 mg • Iron (as ferric ammonium citrate) 3 mg • Vitamin D (D3, as cholecalciferol) 130 IU • Vitamin E (as mixed tocopherols) 100 IU • Thiamin (as thiamin hydrochloride) 15 mg • Riboflavin (as riboflavin-5-phosphate) 10 mg • Niacin (as niacinamide) 15 mg • Vitamin B6 (as pyridoxine hydrochloride) 15 mg • Folic Acid 100 mcg • Vitamin B12 (as methylcobalamin) 50 mcg • Biotin 150 mcg • Pantothenic Acid 200 mg • Phosphorus (as calcium phosphate and potassium phosphate) 142 mg • Iodine (as potassium iodide) 25 mcg • Magnesium (as magnesium citrate) 200 mg • Zinc (as zinc picolinate) 10 mg • Selenium (as selenomethionine) 50 mcg • Copper (as copper gluconate) 1 mg • Manganese (as manganese gluconate) 1.3 mg • Chromium (as chromium polynicotinate) 75 mcg • Molybdenum (as sodium molybdate) 50 mcg • Potassium (as potassium iodide and potassium phosphate) 120 mg • Boron (as sodium borate) 250 mcg • Vanadium (as sodium vanadate) 1000 mcg • N-Acetyl-L-Cysteine 50 mg • L-Glutathione (reduced) 50 mg • Glycine 1800 mg • Taurine 200 mg • L-Glutamine 1000 mg • Alpha-Lipoic Acid 20 mg • MSM (methylsulfonylmethane) 100 mg • Quercetin 100 mg • Green Tea extract (standardized to 40% catechins) 15 mg • Grape seed & skin extract (standardized to 95% polyphenols) 25 mg • Lactobacillus Sporogenes 300 million. Other Ingredients: Rice Protein Concentrate, Rice Syrup Solids, Cellulose, Natural Cherry Flavor.

Diet-Phen **-** Source Naturals
Three tablets contain: St. John's Wort standardized extract (hypericum perforatum, 0.3%, yielding hypericin 2.7 mg) 900 mg • Vitamin B3 (niacinamide) 25 mg • Vitamin B6 (pyridoxine hydrochloride) 25 mg • Chromium (100 mcg chromium polynicotinate, 100 mcg chromium picolinate) 200 mcg • Acetyl L-Carnitine 50 mg • L-Phenylalanine 500 mg • Green Tea leaf extract (yielding 33 mg caffeine) 300 mg • Ginger root 50 mg • Bitter Orange peel extract (8%, yielding 24 mg synephrine) 300 mg. Other Ingredients: Sorbitol, Stearic Acid, Colloidal Silicon Dioxide, Magnesium Stearate.
See Editor's Note No. 40, page 2058.

Diet-Phen (New Formula) **-** Source Naturals
Three tablets contain: St. John's Wort extract (Hypericum perforatum standardized extract 0.3% yielding 2.7 mg of hypericin) 900 mg • L-Phenylalanine 750 mg • Green Tea 300 mg • Cayenne 100 mg • Mustard seed 100 mg • Ginger root 100 mg • Piper nigrum 100 mg • Acetyl L-Carnitine 50 mg • Niacinamide 25 mg • Vitamin B6 (Pyridoxine HCl) 25 mg • Chromium (100 mcg ChromeMate Polynicotinate, 100 mcg Chromium Picolinate) 200 mcg.

Diet-Phen Ephedra Free **-** Source Naturals
Three tablets contain: St. John's Wort (Hypericum perforatum standardized extract 0.3% yielding 2.7 g of Hypericin) 900 mg • L-Phenylalanine 750 mg • Green Tea 300 mg • Cayenne 100 mg • Mustard Seed 100 mg • Ginger Root 100 mg • Piper Nigrum 100 mg • Acetyl L-Carnitine 50 mg • Vitamin B3 (Niacinamide) 25 mg • Vitamin B6 (Pyridoxine HCl) 25 mg • Chromium (100 mcg ChromeMate Chromium Polynicotinate, and 100 mcg Chromium Picolinate) 200 mcg.

Diet-Phen Ephedra Free (New Formula) **-** Source Naturals
Three tablets contain: Niacinamide 25 mg • Calcium 135 mg • Vitamin B6 (as pyridoxine HCl) 25 mg • Chromium (as chromium picolinate 100 mcg and polynicotinate 100 mcg) 200 mcg • St. John's Wort leaf/flower standardized extract (0.3%, yielding 2.7 mg

hypericin) 900 mg • L-Phenylalanine 750 mg • Green Tea leaf extract 165 mg • Cayenne fruit 100 mg • Mustard seed 100 mg • Ginger root 100 mg • Piper Nigrum seed 100 mg • Acetyl L-Carnitine 50 mg. Other Ingredients: Dibasic Calcium Phosphate, Stearic Acid, Colloidal Silicon Dioxide, Modified Cellulose Gum, Magnesium Stearate.

Diet-Phen for Men **-** Source Naturals
Two tablets contain: Niacinamide 17 mg • Vitamin B6 (as pyridoxine HCl) 17 mg • Chromium (as ChromeMate chromium polynicotinate and picolinate) 270 mcg • St. John's Wort leaf/flower extract (yielding 1.8 mg hypericum) 600 mg • Bitter Orange peel extract (yielding 16 mg synephrine) 400 mg • L-Phenylalanine 333 mg • Creatine Monohydrate 330 mg • L-Glutamine 133 mg • Panax Ginseng root extract (standardized to 8% ginsenosides) 67 mg • L-Carnitine L-Tartrate 33 mg. Other Ingredients: Dibasic Calcium Phosphate, Stearic Acid, Modified Cellulose Gum, Colloidal Silicon Dioxide, Magnesium Stearate.
See Editor's Note No. 40, page 2058.

DietPlex **-** NutriCology
Three tablets contain: Vitamin B6 (as pyridoxal-5-phosphate and pyridoxine hydrochloride) 22.5 mg • Calcium (as calcium pyruvate and dicalcium phosphate) 68 mg • Chromium (as chromium nicotinate) 6 mcg • Chitosan 600 mg • L-Carnitine 150 mg • Arthred (hydrolyzed collagen) 450 mg • Garcinia Cambogia fruit extract (75% hydroxycitric acid) 300 mg • Pyruvate (as calcium pyruvate) 320 mg. Other Ingredients: Dicalcium Phosphate, Modified Cellulose, Stearic Acid, Magnesium Stearate, Silicon Dioxide, Ethyl Vanillin.

Diet-Tech **-** MuscleTech
Four capsules contain: Chromium (as chromium polynicotinate) 300 mcg • GLUCO-TECH 2.2 g: Glucomannan (amorphophallus konjac), Xanthan gum • METABO-TECH 843 mg: Green Tea leaf extract (standardized for 95% polyphenols (70% catechins, 45% epigallocatechins gallate - 300 mg EGCG)), Caffeine (as caffeine anhydrous), Guarana seed extract, Yerba Mate leaf (ilex paraguariensis, standardized for 200 mg of caffeine), Alpha Lipoic Acid. Other Ingredients: Gelatin, Magnesium Stearate, Silica, Cellulose.

Digest Chewables - Ness **-** Enzymes, Inc.
Each tablet contains: n-zimes Proprietary Enzyme Blend 204 mg: Protease, Lipase, Amylase, Glucoamylase, Malt Diastase, Lactase, Invertase, alpha-Galactosidase, CereCalase, Cellulase, Pectinase. Other Ingredients: Dextrose (Corn Sugar), Fructose (Fruit Sugar), Natural Raspberry Flavor, Silica (mineral), Plant Cellulose, Citric Acid, Veg. Magnesium Sterate, Proprietary Plant-derived Sweetener.

Digest Chewables - Nutri-Essence **-** Enzymes, Inc.
Each tablet contains: n-zimes Proprietary Enzyme Blend 204 mg: Protease (alkaline, neutral and acid proteases plus peptidase), Lipase, Amylase, Glucoamylase, Malt Diastase, Lactase, Invertase, alpha-Galactosidase, CereCalase, Cellulase, Pectinase. Other Ingredients: Dextrose (Corn Sugar), Fructose (Fruit Sugar), Natural Raspberry Flavor, Silica (Mineral) Plant Cellulose, Citric Acid, Veg. Magnesium Sterate, Proprietary Plant-derived Sweetener.

Digest RC **-** Life Extension Foundation
Each two capsules contain: Black Radish extract 75 • Linden Bark Charcoal 75 mg • Artichoke extract 47 mg • Calcium Phosphate 45 mg • Cholic Acid 40 mg • Peppermint 15 mg. Inactive Ingredients: Beet Sugar, Talcum, Vegetable Starch, Magnesium Stearate, Arabic Gum, Gelatin, Silicon Dioxide.

Digest Support **-** Natrol
Two capsules contain: Proteolytic Enzymes: Protease I (20000 HUT) 200 mg • Protease II (16600 FCC) 8 mg • Amylolytic Enzymes: Amylase (10200 DU) 408 mg • Cellulase (410 CMC) 100 mg • Lactase (200 LAC) 20 mg • Lipolytic Enzymes: Lipase (300 LU) 100 mg • Maltase (90 DU) 90 mg • Sucrase (200 SU) 20 mg • Anti Gas Factor: Alpha Galactosidase (54 GAL) 54 mg. Other Ingredients: TriCalcium Phosphate, Silica, Magnesium Stearate, Gelatin.

Digestabs **-** Puritan's Pride
Two tablets contain: Pancreatin 600 mg • Amylase 260 mg • Pepsin 130 mg • Papain 130 mg • Ox Bile 130 mg • Betaine HCl 130 mg • Duodenal substance 60 mg.
See Editor's Note No. 14.

DigestEase **-** Pacific BioLogic
Ginger • Rhubarb • Elecampane • Gentian • Long Pepper • Tropical Almond • Emblic Myrobalan • Beleric Myrobalan • Glauber's Salt • Kaolin.

DigestEnz **-** Enzymes, Inc.
Each capsule contains: n-zimes Proprietary Blend 652 mg: Proteases, Amylase, Lipase, CereCalase Plus, Glucoamylase, Malt Diastase, alpha-Galactosidase, Invertase, Lactase, Pectinase, Cellulase. Other Ingredients: Cellulose, Water.

Di-Gest-Eze **-** Nutri-Quest Rx
Each two-phase tablet contains: Phase One (Stomach): Betaine HCl 155 mg • L-Glutamic Acid HCl 100 mg • Pepsin 105 mg • Papain 50 mg. Phase Two (Duodenum): Pancreatin 100 mg • Pancrelipase 50 mg • Amylase 30 mg • Bromelain 30 mg • Ox Bile 65 mg • Parotid 2 mg.
See Editor's Note No. 14.

Digestion - BioSet **-** Enzymes, Inc.
Each capsule contains: Proprietary Enzyme Blend 460 mg: Amylase, Protease, Lipase, CereCalase, Invertase, Glucoamylase, alpha-Galactosidase, Malt Diastase, Lactase, Pectinase, Cellulase, Peptidase. Other Ingredients: Plant Cellulose, Water.

Digestion - Nutri-Essence **-** Enzymes, Inc.
Each capsule contains: n-zimes Proprietary Blend 364 mg: Protease (alkaline, neutral and acid proteases plus peptidase), Lipase, Amylase, Glucoamylase, Malt Diastase, Lactase, Invertase, alpha-Galactosidase, CereCalase Plus, Cellulase, Xylanase, Pectinase • Proprietary Herbal Blend 155 mg: Ginger root extract (5% gingerols) plus whole root, Gentian root, Caraway seed, Peppermint leaf extract (4:1) plus whole leaf. Other Ingredients: Plant Cellulose, Water, Lecithin, Rice Bran.

Digestion Formula **-** Nature's Way
Two capsules contain: Angelica root 90 mg • Barberry bark 135 mg • Beet root 100 mg • Cayenne pepper fruit 25 mg • Dandelion root 315 mg • Fizyme enzyme formula 100 mg • Gentian root 135 mg. Other Ingredients: Gelatin, Magnesium stearate, Millet.

Digestive Enzyme Complex **-** Nutrilite
Each capsule contains: Lipase 31 mg • Lactase 40 mg • Amylase 20 mg • Alpha-Galactosidase 10 mg • Ginger Root Extract 150 mg • NUTRILITE Parsley Concentrate with Phytofactors Plant Compounds.

Digestive Enzymes **-** Jamieson
Each caplet contains: Papain 50 mg • Bromelain 30 mg • Lipase 30 mg • Amylase 50 mg • Lactase 30 mg • Cellulase 15 mg • Calcium Gluconate • Peppermint Leaf • Fennel Complex.

Digestive Formula **-** 4 Life
Each capsule contains: Ginger root 180 mg • Turmeric root 65 mg • Digestive Proprietary Blend 45 mg: Milk Thistle leaf extract, Artichoke root extract, Dandelion root extract, Gentian root extract, Ginger root extract, Turmeric root extract • Milk Thistle seed 30 mg • Dandelion root 30 mg • Artichoke leaf 30 mg • Gentian leaf 20 mg. Other Ingredients: Gelatin, Rice Bran, Silicon Dioxide, Magnesium Stearate.

Digestive Formula **-** Pharmanex
Each capsule contains: Ginger root 5:1 extract (zingiber officinale) 200 mg • Proprietary Enzyme Blend 145 mg: Amylase, Protease, Bromelain, acid stable Protease, Lipase, Cellulase, Lactase • Artichoke leaf 5:1 extract (cynara scolymus) 135 mg. Other Ingredients: Gelatin, Stearic Acid, Corn Starch.

Some Brand Name Natural Products - What they Contain

www.NaturalDatabase.com contains MANY more listings than appear here.

BRAND NAMES

Digestive Health - Wellzymes **-** Enzymes, Inc.
Each capsule contains: n-zimes Proprietary Enzyme Blend 215 mg: Protease Blend (alkaline, neutral and acid proteases plus peptidase), Lipase, Amylase, Glucoamylase, Malt Diastase, Invertase, Lactase, alpha-Galactosidase, Cellulase, CereCalase Plus, Xylanase, Pectinase. Other Ingredients: Plant Cellulose, Water.

Digestive Health Formula - Chinac **-** Metabolife International, Inc.
Each caplet contains: Amomum longiligulare (Chinese Amomum) • Oryza sativa (Rice) •Artemisia annua (Sweet Wormwood) •Crataegus cuneata (Chinese Hawthorn) • Armeniaca amarum (Apricot) •Xanthium sibiricum (Xanthium) •Wolfiporia cocos (Poria) • Coix Lacryma-jobi (Job's Tears).

Di-Indolin - Substrate Solutions **-** ErgoPharm
Three tablets contain: Di-Indolin [proprietary blend of Diindolymethane, Vitamin E (as d-Alpha Tocopheryl Succinate), Phosphatidylcholine] 300 mg. Other Ingredients: Calcium Carbonate, Cellulose, Food Grade Starch, Magnesium Sterate, Tocophersolan, Silica.

DIM Bioavailable Diindolylmethane **-** PhysioLogics
Each capsule contains: Diindolylmethane 100 mg. Other Ingredients: Rice Powder, Gelatin, Silica, Vegetable Magnesium Stearate.

Diol Stack - Substrate Solutions **-** ErgoPharm
Each tablet contains: Nor-4-Androstenediol 100 mg • 4-Androstenediol 100 mg.

Disc/Joint **-** Enzymes, Inc.
Two capsules contain: Vitamin C (100% from Acerola Cherries) 8 mg • Copper (100% as Copper Gluconate) 0.2 mg • Manganese (100% as Manganese Citrate) 5 mg • Proprietary Herbal Blend 750 mg: Methylsulfonylmethane (MSM), Devil's Claw root extract, Boswellia Gum extract, Yucca root extract, Tumeric root extract, Celery seed extract, Grape seed extract • Proprietary Enzyme Blend 221 mg: pHysioProtease, Bromelain, Peptidase • Boron Citrate 10 mg. Other Ingredients: Plant Cellulose, Water.

Ditox **-** Ditox Limited
Each 5 mL bottle contains: Vitamin B1 0.4 mg • Vitamin B6 0.4 mg. Other Ingredients: Alcohol 18%.

Diurex Long Acting Water Capsules **-** Alva-Amco Pharmacal Cos., Inc.
Each capsule contains: Active Ingredients: Caffeine Anhydrous • Acetaminophen • Potassium Salicylate. Other Ingredients: Non-Pariell seeds, Magnesium Oxide, Titanium Dioxide, plus other coloring & coating ingredients.

Diurex Water Caplets **-** Alva-Amco Pharmacal Cos., Inc.
Each caplet contains: Active Ingredient: Pamabrom 50 mg. Other Ingredients: Dicalcium Phosphate, FD&C Blue #1, Hydroxypropyl Methylcellulose, Magnesium Stearate, Polyethylene Glycol, Potassium Gluconate, Riboflavin, Stearic Acid, Titanium Dioxide. May also contain: Calcium Sulfate, Croscarmellose Sodium, Microcrystalline Cellulose, Mineral Oil, Polysorbate, Silicon Dioxide, Sodium Lauryl Sulfate.

Diurex Water Pills **-** Alva-Amco Pharmacal Cos., Inc.
Each pill contains: Active Ingredients: Potassium Salicylate • Caffeine Anhydrous • Salicylamide. Other Ingredients: Calcium Sulfate, Dicalcium Phosphate, Magnesium Trisilicate, Microcrystalline Cellulose, Starch, Magnesium Stearate, Stearic Acid, plus other fillers, coloring & coating ingredients.

Diutrate **-** Atrium Inc.
Each tablet contains: Buchu leaves 70 mg • Couch grass 70 mg • Hydrangea root 35 mg • Corn Silk 35 mg • Uva Ursi 10 mg • Hypothalamus 30 mg • Raw Kidney concentrate 60 mg • Vitamin B6 16 mg • Magnesium (Protein Chelated) 50 mg.
See Editor's Note No. 14.

DL-Alpha Vitamin E - Basic Nutrition **-** GNC
Each capsule contains: Vitamin E (as dl-alpha Tocopheryl Acetate) 400 IU. Other Ingredients: Gelatin, Glycerin.

DMAE **-** Source Naturals
Each tablet contains: DMAE Bitartrate 351 mg. Other Ingredients: Stearic Acid, Dibasic Calcium Phosphate, Magneisum Stearate, Colloidal Silicon Dioxide, Modified Cellulose Gum.

DMAE **-** PhysioLogics
Each capsule contains: DMAE (as dimethylaminoethanol bitartrate) 100 mg. Other Ingredients: Cellulose (plant origin), Gelatin, Silica, Vegetable Magnesium Stearate.

DMAE Firming Fluid **-** Reviva Labs
Demineralized spring water • DMAE Bitartrate • Glycerin (veg.) • Polysorbate 20 • Sodium Chloride • Simethicone • Hydroxytethylcellulose • Methyl Paraben • Propyl Paraben.

D-Mannose Powder Plus **-** Nutrifactor
Each level teaspoon (4.7 g) contains: D-Mannose 1500 mg • Cranberry (vaccinium macrocarpon) 800 mg • Vitamin C (as ascorbic acid) 60 mg. Other Ingredients: Natural Mixed Berry Flavor, Xylitol, Citric Acid, Sucralose.

D-Mannose U-Tract X-Tra **-** Progressive Labs
Four capsules contain: D-Mannose 2000 mg • Cratavin bark standardized extract (crataeva nurbula) 40 mg • White Willow bark standardized extract (salix alba) 60 mg • Salicin (from white willow bark extract) 9 mg • Swedish Pollen extract (cernitin 63) 20 mg. Other Ingredients: Gelatin, Magnesium Stearate.

DMG-B15-Plus **-** Enzymatic Therapy
Each capsule contains: Potassium Aspartate 125 mg • Magnesium Aspartate 125 mg • Calcium Gluconate 31 mg • Other Ingredients: Trimethylglycine (TMG) 100 mg • N,N-Dimethylglycine 100 mg • Glycine 25 mg.

D-MNS **-** Dial Herbs
Mistletoe • Blessed Thistle • Witch Hazel • Nettle • Shepherd's Purse • Red Raspberry • Cayenne.

DN-24 Hydracreme **-** Pharmagel
Vitamin Retinyl-A 25000 IU.

DNE Ephedrana 12.5 **-** D & E Pharmaceuticals
Each tablet contains: Ephedrine HCL 12.5 mg. In a proprietary herbal base of Ephedra, Guarana, Chromium.
See Editor's Note No. 30, page 2056.

Doctor's Choice Antioxidant **-** Enzymatic Therapy
Three capsules contain: Vitamin A (Beta Carotene) non-toxic form of Vitamin A 10000 IU • Vitamin E (D-Alpha Tocopherol) 200 IU • Vitamin C (Ascorbic Acid) 500 mg • Zinc (Picolinate) 15 mg • Manganese (Gluconate) 15 mg • Riboflavin (Vitamin B2) 6 mg • Selenium (L-Selenomethionine) 200 mcg • N-Acetylcysteine 100 mg • Cabbage extract (Brassica oleracea) 100 mg • Garlic extract, deodorized 100 mg • Ginger root extract 6.5:1 (Zingiber officinale) 100 mg • Green Tea extract (Camellia sinensis) 100 mg • Klamath Blue-Green Algae 100 mg • Curcuma root extract (Curcuma longa) standardized to contain 97% Curcumin 50 mg • Grape seed (PCO) extract (Procyanidolic oligomers (PCO) from grape seed extract) 10 mg. Other Ingredients: Cellulose, Calcium Silicate, Silicon Dioxide, & Gelatin Capsule.

Doctor's Choice Eye Formula **-** Enzymatic Therapy
Three tablets contain: Vitamin A (Fish Liver oil) 2500 IU • Vitamin A (Beta Carotene) non-toxic form of Vitamin A 2500 IU • Vitamin C (Ascorbic Acid) 600 mg • Vitamin E (D-Alpha Tocopheryl Acetate) 60 IU • Vitamin B2 (Riboflavin) 1.5 mg • Zinc (Picolinate) 9 mg • Selenium (L Selenomethionine) 50 mcg • Copper (Picolinate) 1 mg • Hachimijiogan Herbal Complex 400 mg • Bilberry (Vaccinium myrtillus fructus) Berry extract standardized to contain 25% Anthocyanosides (calculated as Anthocyanidins) 160 mg • Curcuma

(Curcuma Longa) root extract standardized to contain 85-97% Curcumin) 50 mg • Grape (Vitis vinifera) seed (PCO) extract standardized to contain 95% Procyanidolic Oligomers (PCOs) 50 mg • Lutein (Marigold flower extract) 2 mg. Other Ingredients: Cellulose, Calcium Carbonate, Cellulose Gum, Stearic Acid, Silicon Dioxide & Magnesium Stearate.

***Doctor's Choice Flax Oil* - Enzymatic Therapy**
Seven softgels contain: Flaxseed Oil 1050 mg • Pumpkin seed oil 1050 mg • Borage seed oil (borago officinalis) 700 mg • Omega-3 (ALA) 2625 mg • Omega-6 (LA) 1313 mg • Omega-9 (oleic acid) 1300 mg • Gamma Linolenic Acid (GLA) 163 mg. Other Ingredients: Gelatin Capsule, Rosemary Leaf Antioxidant (rasemarinus officinalis) S-327.

***Doctor's Choice Flax Oil fortified with Borage & Pumpkin* - Enzymatic Therapy**
Flaxseed oil • Pumpkin seed oil • Borage seed oil • Rosemary Antioxidant S-327 • Average analysis per tablespoon: Omega-3 (LNA) 5250 mg • Omega-6 (LA) 2625 mg • Omega-9 (Oleic) 2600 mg • Gamma-Linolenic Acid (GLA) 325 mg.

***Doctor's Choice for 45-Plus Women* - Enzymatic Therapy**
Six tablets contain: Vitamin A (Beta Carotene) 15000 IU • Vitamin A (Retinol) 2500 IU • Vitamin D 400 IU • Vitamin E (D-Alpha Tocopherol Succinate) 200 IU • Vitamin D 400 IU • Calcium (Citrate, Carbonate) 600 mg • Vitamin C (Ascorbic Acid) 300 mg • Magnesium (Aspartate) 300 mg • Potassium (Aspartate) 99 mg • Vitamin B6 (Pyridoxine HCL) 60 mg • Thiamine HCL (Vitamin B1) 60 mg • Riboflavin (Vitamin B2) 60 mg • Pantothenic Acid (D-Calcium Pantothenate) 50 mg • Niacin/Niacinamide 45 mg • Zinc (Picolinate) 15 mg • Manganese (Citrate) 15 mg • Copper (Gluconate) 1.5 mg • Folic Acid 800 mcg • Vitamin B12 (Cyanocobalamin) 800 mcg • Biotin 600 mcg • Vitamin K (Phytonadione) 60 mcg • Iodine (Kelp) 300 mcg • Chromium (Polynicotinate) 200 mcg • Selenium (L-Selenomet hionine) 100 mcg • Molybdenum (Sodium Molybdate) 25 mcg • Flavonoids mixed 100 mg • Alfalfa juice concentrate 100 mg • Dong Quai extract 4:1 (Angelica sinensis) 90 mg • Ginger root extract 6.5:1 (Zingiber officinale) 15 mg • Green Tea extract (Camellia sinensis) 30 mg • Choline Bitartrate 30 mg • Fennel seed extract 6:1 (Foeniculum vulgare) 30 mg • Inositol 30 mg • PABA (Para-Aminobenzoic Acid) 30 mg • Betaine HCL 25 mg • Glutamic Acid HCL 25 mg • Bromelain 15 mg • Papain 15 mg • Protease acid stable 5 mg • Lipase 5 mg • Boron (Sodium Tetraborate Decahydrate 3 mg • Silica (Sodium Metasilicate) 1 mg • Vanadium (Sulfate) 50 mcg. Other Ingredients: Cellulose, Cellulose Gum, Stearic Acid, Silicon Dioxide & Magnesium Stearate.

***Doctor's Choice for 50-Plus Men* - Enzymatic Therapy**
Four tablets contain: Vitamin A (Beta Carotene) 15000 IU • Vitamin A (Retinol) 2500 IU • Vitamin E (d-Alpha Tocopherol Succinate) 200 IU • Vitamin D (Ergocalciferol) 100 IU • Vitamin C (Ascorbic Acid) 300 mg • Magnesium (Aspartate) 250 mg • Calcium (Citrate • Carbonate) 250 mg • Niacin/Niacinamide 120 mg • Pantothenic Acid (D-Calcium Pantothenate) 100 mg • Potassium (Aspartate) 99 mg • Thiamine HCL (Vitamin B1) 60 mg • Riboflavin (Vitamin B2) 60 mg • Vitamin B6 (Pyridoxine HCL) 60 mg • Zinc (Picolinate) 30 mg • Manganese (Citrate) 15 mg • Copper (Gluconate) 1.5 mg • Folic Acid 800 mcg • Vitamin B12 (Cyanocobalamin) 800 mcg • Biotin 600 mcg • Iodine (Kelp) 300 mcg • Chromium (Polynicotinate) 200 mcg • Selenium (L-Selenomethionine) 100 mcg • Vitamin K (Phytonadione) 60 mcg • Molybdenum (Sodium Molybdate) 25 mcg • Mixed Flavonoids citrus 100 mg • Saw Palmetto Berry extract 4:1 (Serenoa repens) 80 mg • Ginger root extract 6.5:1 (Zingiber officinale) 60 mg • Alfalfa juice concentrate 60 mg • Choline Bitartrate 30 mg • Inositol 30 mg • PABA (Para-Aminobenzoic Acid) 30 mg • Green Tea extract (Camellia sinensis) 30 mg • Betaine HCL 25 mg • Glutamic Acid HCL 25 mg • Korean Ginseng root extract (Panax ginseng) standardized to contain 7% Saponins (calculated as Rg1) 15 mg • Bromelain 15 mg • Papain 15 mg • Protease acid stable 5 mg • Lipase 5 mg • Boron (Sodium Tetraborate Decahydrate) 2 mg • Vanadium (Sulfate) 50 mcg. Other Ingredients: Cellulose, Stearic Acid, Cellulose Gum, Silicon Dioxide, & Magnesium Stearate.

***Doctor's Choice for Arthritics* - Enzymatic Therapy**
Two tablets contain: Niacin/Niacinamide 330 mg • Pantothenic Acid (D-Calcium Pantothenate) 100 mg • Magnesium (Oxide) 100 mg • Calcium Chloride 32 mg • Vitamin C (Ascorbic Acid) 30 mg • Zinc (Picolinate) 3 mg • Manganese (Chelate) 3 mg • Glucosamine Sulfate 500 mg • PABA (Para-Aminobenzoic Acid) 400 mg • Bio-Min TR8 a source of trace minerals 100 mg • Glutamic Acid HCL 40 mg • Ammonium Chloride 32 mg • Betaine HCL 20 mg • Chlorophyll 10 mg • Boron (Sodium Tetraborate Decahydrate) 3 mg. Other Ingredients: Cellulose, Cellulose Gum, Stearic Acid, Silicon Dioxide, Magnesium Stearate, Alfalfa (Medicago sativa) leaves & stems juice concentrate, Black Cohosh (Cimicituga racemosa) root, Licorice (Glycyrrhiza glabra) root extract & Scullcap (Scutellaria baicalensis) whole plant.

***Doctor's Choice for Bone Health* - Enzymatic Therapy**
Three tablets contain: Vitamin C (Ascorbic Acid) 100 mg • Vitamin D (Fish Liver oil) 300 IU • Vitamin K (Phytonadione) 300 mcg • Folic Acid 800 mcg • Vitamin B12 (Cyanocobalamin) 800 mcg • Calcium (Krebs Cycle Chelate) 600 mg • Magnesium (Krebs Cycle Chelate) 150 mg • Vitamin C (Ascorbic Acid) 100 mg • Zinc (Picolinate) 15 mg • Sodium 6 mg • Copper (Picolinate) 1 mg • Mixed Flavonoids (Citrus) 100 mg • Betaine HCL 30 mg • Soy Bean extract standardized to contain 25% Saponins & 13-17% Isoflavones calculated as Genistein 20 mg • Boron (Sodium Tetrahydroborate) 3 mg • Silicon (Sodium Metasilicate) 1 mg • Strontium (Chloride) 500 mcg. Other Ingredients: Cellulose, Cellulose Gum, Stearic Acid, Silicon Dioxide, Magnesium Stearate.

***Doctor's Choice for Diabetics* - Enzymatic Therapy**
Two tablets contain: Vitamin E (Mixed Tocopherols) 100 IU • Vitamin C (Ascorbic Acid) 300 mg • Magnesium (Krebs Cycle Chelate) 100 mg • Vitamin B6 (Pyridoxine HCL) 10 mg • Manganese (Krebs Cycle Chelate) 7.5 mg • Zinc (Picolinate) 7.5 mg • Copper (Picolinate) 0.5 mg • Biotin 1000 mcg • Folic Acid 400 mcg • Vitamin B12 (Cyanocobalamin) 400 mcg • Chromium (Picolinate) 200 mcg • Selenium (Aspartate) 50 mcg • Gymnema sylvestre leaves extract standardized to contain 25% Gymnemic Acid 200 mg • Bitter Melon extract (Momordica charantia) 200 mg • Fenugreek seed extract (4:1) (Trigonella foenum-graecum) 100 mg • Bilberry extract (Vaccinium myrtillus fructus) standardized to contain 25% Anthocyanosides calculated as Anthocyanidins) 40 mg • Mixed Bioflavonoids (Citrus) 25 mg • Vanadyl Sulfate 5 mg. Other Ingredients: Calcium Carbonate, Cellulose, Cellulose Gum, Silicon Dioxide, Dicalcium Phosphate, Magnesium Stearate & Calcium Silicate.

***Doctor's Choice for Female Teens* - Enzymatic Therapy**
Four tablets contain: Vitamin A (Beta Carotene) 15000 IU • Vitamin A (Retinol) 2500 IU • Vitamin E (D-Alpha Tocopherol Succinate) 200 IU • Vitamin D (Ergocalciferol) 100 IU • Calcium (Citrate, Carbonate) 500 mg • Vitamin C (Ascorbic Acid) 300 mg • Magnesium (Aspartate) 200 mg • Potassium (Aspartate) 99 mg • Vitamin B6 (Pyridoxine HCL) 90 mg • Niacin/Niacinamide 45 mg • Iron (Ferrous Succinate) 30 mg • Pantothenic Acid (D-Calcium Pantothenate) 30 mg • Thiamine HCL (Vitamin B1) 30 mg • Riboflavin (Vitamin B2) 30 mg • Zinc (Picolinate) 20 mg • Manganese (Citrate) 15 mg • Copper (Gluconate) 1.5 mg • Folic Acid 800 mcg • Vitamin B12 (Cyanocobalamin) 800 mcg • Biotin 300 mcg • Iodine (Kelp) 300 mcg • Chromium (Polynicotinate) 200 mcg • Selenium (L-Selenomethionine) 100 mcg • Vitamin K (Phytonadione) 60 mcg • Molybdenum (Sodium molybdate) 25 mcg • Mixed Flavonoids (Citrus) 100 mg • Alfalfa juice concentrate 60 mg • Choline Bitartrate 60 mg • Inositol 60 mg • Ginger root extract 6.5:1 (Zingiber officinale) 60 mg • 8 Dandelion root extract 4:1 (Taraxacum officinale) 60 mg • Licorice root extract (Glycyrrhiza glabra) standardized to contain 5% Glycyrrhizic Acid 30 mg • Boron (Sodium Tetraborate Decahydrate) 2 mg • Silica (Sodium Metasilicate) 1 mg • Vanadium (Sulfate) 50 mcg. Other Ingredients:

Cellulose, Cellulose Gum, Stearic Acid, Magnesium Stearate & Silicon Dioxide.

Doctor's Choice for Healthy Cholesterol Levels **-** Enzymatic Therapy
Each capsule contains: Red Yeast Rice (Standardized to contain 1% Mevinolin) 475 mg • Artichoke (Cynara scolymus) leaf extract 50 mg • Ginger (Zingiber officinale) root extract 50 mg • Coenzyme Q10 (CoQ10) 8 mg. Other Ingredients: Soybean oil, Vegetable oil, Beeswax, Lecithin, and Gelatin capsule.

Doctor's Choice for Heart Health **-** Enzymatic Therapy
Two tablets contain: Vitamin E (D-Alpha Tocopherol) 100 IU • Magnesium (Oxide) 150 mg • Niacin 100 mg • Vitamin C (Ascorbic Acid) 100 mg • Potassium (Chloride) 75 mg • Calcium Pangamate 20 mg • Vitamin B6 (Pyridoxine HCL) 10 mg • Sodium 6 mg • Folic Acid 200 mcg • Vitamin B12 (Cyanocobalamin) 200 mcg • Hawthorne berry extract (Crataegus oxyacantha) standardized to contain 1.8% Vitexin-2'-Rhamnoside 150 mg • Super Seven Complex Mixture of Herbs: Hydrangea, Black Cohosh (Cimicifuga racemosa), Buchu leaves, Couch Grass, Corn Silk, Dandelion leaf (Taraxacum officinale) & Ginger root (Zingiber officinale) 150 mg • Khella extract (Ammi visnaga) standardized to contain a minimum of 10% Pyrones calculated as Khellin 100 mg • L-Cysteine 100 mg • Carbamide 100 mg. Other Ingredients: Cellulose, Cellulose Gum, Stearic Acid, Sodium Starch, Glycolate, Silicon Dioxide, Magnesium Stearate & Vanillin.

Doctor's Choice for Joint Health Capsules **-** Enzymatic Therapy
Four capsules contain: Vitamin C (ascorbic acid) 100 mg • Niacin (as niacinamide, niacin) 330 mg • Vitamin B6 (as pyridoxine HCl) 20 mg • Pantothenic Acid (as calcium d-pantothenate) 100 mg • Magnesium (as magnesium oxide) 100 mg • Zinc (as zinc picolinate) 3 mg • Copper (as copper gluconate) 200 mcg • Manganese (as manganese chelate) 2.5 mg • Chloride (from glucosamine sulfate) 78 mg • Sodium 55 mg • Glucosamine Sulfate (stabilized) 500 mg • Boswellia Serrata gum resin extract (standardized to contain 65% boswellic acids) 400 mg • Proprietary Trace Mineral Blend 24 mg: Selenium (as selenium yeast), Silicon (as magnesium trisilicate), Boron (as sodium borate), Nickel (as nickel chelate), Tin (as tin chelate), Molybdenum (as sodium molybdate), Vanadium (as vanadyl sulfate) • Boron (as sodium borate) 3 mg. Other Ingredients: Cellulose, Gelatin, Magnesium Stearate, Titanium Dioxide Color, Silicon Dioxide, Alfalfa Aerial Part Extract 10:1, Black Cohosh Root Extract 4:1, Licorice Root/Rhizome Extract, Chinese Skullcap Root Extract 4:1.

Doctor's Choice for Joint Health Tablets **-** Enzymatic Therapy
Two tablets contain: Vitamin C (ascorbic acid) 100 mg • Niacin (as niacinamide, niacin) 330 mg • Vitamin B6 (as pyridoxine HCl) 20 mg • Pantothenic Acid (as calcium d-pantothenate) 100 mg • Magnesium (as magnesium oxide) 100 mg • Zinc (as zinc picolinate) 3 mg • Copper (as copper gluconate) 200 mcg • Manganese (as manganese chelate) 2.5 mg • Chloride (from glucosamine sulfate) 78 mg • Sodium 60 mg • Glucosamine Sulfate (stabilized) 500 mg • Boswellia Serrata gum resin extract (standardized to contain 65% boswellic acids) 400 mg • Proprietary Trace Mineral Blend 24 mg: Selenium (as selenium yeast), Silicon (as magnesium trisilicate), Boron (as sodium borate), Nickel (as nickel chelate), Tin (as tin chelate), Molybdenum (as sodium molybdate), Vanadium (as vanadyl sulfate) • Boron (as sodium borate) 3 mg. Other Ingredients: Cellulose, Modified Cellulose, Modified Cellulose Gum, Magnesium Stearate, Titanium Dioxide Color, Lecithin, Alfalfa Aerial Part Extract 10:1, Black Cohosh Root Extract 4:1, Licorice Root/Rhizome Extract, Chinese Skullcap Root Extract 4:1, Carnauba Wax.

Doctor's Choice for Male Teens **-** Enzymatic Therapy
Four tablets contain: Vitamin A (Beta Carotene) 15000 IU • Vitamin A (Retinol) 2500 IU • Vitamin E (D-Alpha Tocopherol Succinate) 200 IU • Vitamin D (Ergocalciferol) 100 IU • Calcium (Citrate, Carbonate) 400 mg • Vitamin C (Ascorbic Acid) 300 mg • Magnesium (Aspartate) 200 mg • Potassium (Aspartate) 99 mg • Niacin/ Niacinamide 45 mg • Pantothenic Acid (D-CalciumPantothenate) 30 mg • Vitamin B6 (Pyridoxine HCL) 30 mg • Thiamine HCL (Vitamin B1) 30 mg • Riboflavin (Vitamin B2) 30 mg • Zinc (Picolinate) 30 mg • Manganese (Citrate) 15 mg • Copper (Gluconate) 1.5 mg • Folic Acid 800 mcg • Vitamin B12 (Cyanocobalamin) 800 mcg • Iodine (Kelp) 300 mcg • Chromium (Polynicotinate) 200 mcg • Selenium (L-Selenomethionine) 100 mcg • Vitamin K (Phytonadione) 60 mcg • Molybdenum (sodium Molybdate) 25 mcg • Biotin 300 mcg • Mixed Flavonoids (Citrus) 100 mg • Alfalfa juice concentrate 60 mg • Dandelion root extract 4:1 (Taraxacum officinale) 60 mg • Ginger root extract 6.5:1 (Zingiber officinale) 60 mg • Sarsaparilla root extract 4:1 (Simlax officinalis) 60 mg • Choline Bitartrate 30 mg • Inositol 30 mg • Boron (Sodium Tetraborate Decahydrate) 2 mg • Vanadium (Sulfate) 50 mcg.

Doctor's Choice for Men **-** Enzymatic Therapy
Three tablets contain: Vitamin A (Beta Carotene) non-toxic form of Vitamin A 15000 IU • Vitamin A (Retinol) 2500 IU • Vitamin E (D-Alpha Tocopherol Succinate) 200 IU • Vitamin D 100 IU • Magnesium (Aspartate, Chloride) 400 mg • Vitamin C (Ascorbic Acid) 300 mg • Calcium (Citrate, Carbonate) 200 mg • Potassium (Aspartate) 99 mg • Niacin 90 mg • Thiamine HCL (Vitamin B1) 60 mg • Riboflavin (Vitamin B2) 60 mg • Vitamin B6 (Pyridoxine HCL) 60 mg • Pantothenic Acid (D-Calcium Pantothenate) 60 mg • Zinc (Picolinate) 30 mg • Manganese (Citrate) 5 mg • Copper (Gluconate) 1 mg • Folic Acid 800 mcg • Vitamin B12 (Cyanocobalamin) 800 mcg • Biotin 600 mcg • Iodine (Kelp) 300 mcg • Chromium (Polynicotinate) 200 mcg • Selenium (Selenomethionine) 200 mcg • Vitamin K (Phytonadione) 60 mcg • Molybdenum (Sodium Molybdate) 25 mcg • Flavonoids mixed 50 mg • Alfalfa juice concentrate 50 mg • Choline Bitartrate 30 mg • Inositol 30 mg • Ginger root extract 6.5:1 (Zingiber officinale) 30 mg • Green Tea extract (Camellia sinensis) standardized to contain 70% Polyphenols 30 mg • Muira Puama extract 6:1 (Ptychopetalum olacoides) 30 mg • PABA (Para-Aminobenzoic Acid) 30 mg • Saw Palmetto Berry extract 4:1 (Serenoa repens) 30 mg • Korean Ginseng root extract (Panax ginseng) standardized to contain 7% Saponins (calculated as Ginsenoside Rg1) 15 mg • Carotenes from natural sources 5 mg • Boron (Sodium Tetraborate Decahydrate) 2 mg • Vanadium (Sulfate) 50 mcg. Other Ingredients: Cellulose, Cellulose Gum, Stearic Acid, Silicon Dioxide & Magnesium Stearate.

Doctor's Choice for Women **-** Enzymatic Therapy
Four tablets contain: Vitamin A (Beta Carotene) non-toxic form of Vitamin A 15000 IU • Vitamin A (Retinol) 2500 IU • Vitamin E (D-Alpha Tocopherol Succinate) 200 IU • Vitamin D 100 IU • Calcium (Citrate, Carbonate) 400 mg • Vitamin C (Ascorbic Acid) 300 mg • Magnesium (Aspartate, Chloride) 300 mg • Potassium (Aspartate) 99 mg • Vitamin B6 (Pyridoxine HCL) 90 mg • Niacin/Niacinamide 90 mg • Thiamine HCL (Vitamin B1) 60 mg • Riboflavin (Vitamin B2) 60 mg • Pantothenic Acid (D-Calcium Pantothenate) 30 mg • Zinc (Picolinate) 20 mg • Iron (Ferrous Succinate) 18 mg • Manganese (Citrate) 5 mg • Vitamin B6 (Pyridoxal-5-Phosphate) 5 mg • Copper (Gluconate) 1 mg • Folic Acid 800 mcg • Vitamin B12 (Cyanocobalamin) 800 mcg • Biotin 600 mcg • Iodine (Kelp) 300 mcg • Chromium (Polynicotinate) 200 mcg • Selenium (Selenomethionine) 200 mcg • Vitamin K (Phytonadione) 60 mcg • Molybdenum (Sodium molybdate) 25 mcg • Flavonoids, mixed 50 mg • Alfalfa juice concentrate 50 mg • Choline Bitartrate 30 mg • Inositol 30 mg • Dong Quai extract 4:1 (Angelica sinensis) 30 mg • Ginger root extract (6.5:1) (Zingiber officinale) 30 mg • Licorice root extract (Glycyrrhiza glabra) standardized to contain 5% Glycyrrhizic Acid 30 mg • PABA (Para-Aminobenzoic Acid) 30 mg • Chaste Tree Berry extract 5:1 (Vitex agnus-castus) 15 mg • Fennel seed extract 6:1 (Foeniculum vulgare) 15 mg • Carotenes from natural sources 5 mg • Boron (Sodium Tetraborate Decahydrate) 3 mg • Silica (Sodium Metasilicate) 1 mg • Vanadium (Sulfate) 50 mcg. Other Ingredients: Cellulose, Cellulose Gum, Magnesium Stearate, Stearic Acid, & Silicon Dioxide.

Doctor's Choice Prenatal Supplement **-** Enzymatic Therapy
Four tablets contain: Vitamin A (Beta Carotene) 15000 IU • Vitamin E (D-Alpha Tocopherol Succinate) 200 IU • Vitamin D (Ergocalciferol) 100 IU • Calcium (Citrate, Carbonate) 800 mg • Magnesium (Citrate) 400 mg • Vitamin C (Ascorbic Acid) 300 mg • Vitamin B6 (Pyridoxine HCL) 120 mg • Pantothenic Acid (D-Calcium Pantothenate) 100 mg • Potassium (Aspartate) 99 mg • Thiamine HCL (Vitamin B1) 60 mg • Riboflavin (Vitamin B2) 60 mg • Niacin/Niacinamide 45 mg • Iron (Ferrous succinate) 30 mg • Zinc (Picolinate) 30 mg • Manganese (Citrate) 15 mg • Copper (Gluconate) 1.5 mg • Folic Acid 800 mcg • Vitamin B12 (Cyanocobalamin) 800 mcg • Biotin 600 mcg • Vitamin K (Phytonadione) 500 mcg • Iodine (Kelp) 300 mcg • Chromium (Polynicotinate) 200 mcg • Selenium (L-Selenomethionine) 100 mcg • Molybdenum (Sodium Molybdate) 25 mcg • Ginger root extract 6.5:1 (Zingiber officinale) 150 mg • Mixed Flavonoids (Citrus) 90 mg • Choline Bitartrate 90 mg • Inositol 90 mg • Dandelion root extract 4:1 (Taraxacum officinale) 60 mg • Red Raspberry leaves 60 mg • Boron (Sodium Tetraborate Decahydrate) 1 mg • Silica (Sodium Metasilicate) 1 mg • Vanadium (Sulfate) 50 mcg. Other Ingredients: Cellulose, Cellulose Gum, Stearic Acid, Silicon Dioxide & Magnesium Stearate.

Dolicoccil Flu Solution **-** Dolisos
Each single dose tube contains: Anas Barbariae Hepatis Et Cordis Extractum (HPUS) 9C • Cuprum Gluconicum 3C • Echinacea Angustifolia (HPUS) 3C. Other Ingredients: Lactose, Sucrose.
See Editor's Note No. 1, page 2053.

Dolomite **-** Puritan's Pride
One tablet contains: Calcium (as Dolomite) 130 mg • Magnesium (as Dolomite) 78 mg.

Dolomite **-** The Vitamin Shoppe
Four tablets contain: Calcium 520 mg • Magnesium 312 mg.

DONA Crystalline Glucosamine Sulfate **-** Rotta Pharmaceuticals
Each packet contains: Sodium 150 mg • Crystalline Glucosamine Sulfate 1884 mg • Glucosamine Sulfate 1500 mg.

Dona Glucosamine Sulfate **-** Rotta Pharmaceuticals
Each packet contains: Crystalline Glucosamine Sulfate 1500 mg.

Dong Quai **-** Nature's Way
Two capsules contain: Dong Quai root 1110 mg. Other Ingredients: Gelatin, Magnesium stearate.

Dong Quai **-** Olympian Labs
Each capsule contains: Dong Quai 500 mg.

Dong Quai **-** Leiner Health Products
Each caplet contains: Dong Quai extract (Angelica sinensis) root 200 mg • Ligustilides (Dong Quai extract) 2 mg. Other Ingredients: Cellulose, Calcium Carbonate, Stearic Acid, Croscarmellose Sodium, Silicon Dioxide, Magnesium Stearate.

Dong Quai - Fingerprint Botanicals **-** GNC
Each capsule contains: Dong Quai 500 mg.

Dong Quai & Royal Jelly **-** Puritan's Pride
Each capsule contains: Dong Quai root powder 200 mg • Royal Jelly powder (from Royal Jelly 2:1 150 mg) 300 mg.

Dong Quai and Royal Jelly **-** GNC
Each capsule contains: Dong Quai 300 mg • Agnus Castus berry 50 mg • Royal Jelly 50 mg • Wild Yam root 50 mg.

Dong Quai Extract **-** Montana Naturals, Inc.
Each capsule contains: Dong Quai 200 mg.

Dong Quai Extract in Vegetable Glycerin **-** Nature's Herbs
Each drop contains: Dong Quai 565 mg.

Dong Quai Root - GNC Herbal Plus **-** GNC
Each capsule contains: Dong Quai 250 mg.

Double G SuperPower **-** DreamPharm
Each capsule contains: Panax Ginseng 250 mg • Ginkgo Biloba leaf extract (standardized to 20%) 80 mg • Ligusticum Chuan Xiang root 100 mg • Angelica Sinensis root 70 mg.

Double Strength Glucosamine 500 MG Chondroitin 400 MG **-** Puritan's Pride
Three tablets contain: Glucosamine Hydrochloride 1500 mg • Chondroitin Sulfate 1200 mg. Other Ingredients: Povidone, Beet Juice Color, Vegetable Magnesium Stearate, Silica, Cellulose (plant origin).
See Editor's Note No. 15, page 2055.

Down Size **-** Dial Herbs
Purified Water • Hydrolyzed Collagen • Glycerine • Natural Flavors • Aloe concentrate • Acesulfame Potassium • Citric Acid • Potassium Sorbate • Sodium Benzoate • Potassium Iodide.

Dr. Art Ulene's Glucosamine Plus Dietary Supplement **-** Nature's Bounty
Two tablets contain: Niacin (B3) 100 mg • Curcumin 100 mg • Glucosamine Hydrochloride 730 mg • Frankincense Extract (boswellia serrata, roxb. excolabr, gum resin) 300 mg • Glucosamine Sulfate 50 mg • Quercetin 100 mg • Turmeric (Curcuma longa, rhizome powder) 100 mg.

Dr. Earl Mindell's 4-SIGHT **-** GEN - Genetic Evolutionary Nutrition
Two caplets contain: Vitamin A (100% as beta-carotene with natural mixed carotenoids) 5000 IU • Vitamin C (from Citri-C Complex) 60 mg • Vitamin E (as natural D-alpha tocopheryl succinate) 30 IU • Selenium (as selenomethionine) 50 mcg • Taurine 400 mcg • Bilberry fruit standardized extract (25% anthocyanosides) 160 mg • Citri-C Complex (ascorbic and isoascorbic acids with citrus glycosyl flavones) 100 mg • Vision Support Herbal Blend 100 mg: Eyebright aerial parts, Ginkgo Biloba leaf extract, Green Tea leaf extract, Grape seed extract • N-Acetylcysteine 50 mg • Quercetin Dihydrate 25 mg • Lutein (as mixed xanthophylls from marigold flower) 6 mg. Other Ingredients: Calcium Hydrogen Phosphate, Cellulose, Cellulose Gum, Vegetable Stearic Acid, Colloidal Silica, Vegetable Magnesium Stearate, Vita-Coat (vegetable resin, alpha-lipoic acid).

Dr. Harris' Original Snore **-** Baywood International
Each caplet contains: Calcium (as dicalcium phosphate) 105 mg •Phosphorus (as dicalcium phosphate) 65 mg • Proprietary Blend 415 mg: Protease, Amylase, Lipase, Cellulase, Acerola concentrate fruit, Cayenne fruit, Echinacea root & aerial parts, Rose Hips fruit, Fenugreek seed, Slippery Elm bark, Red Clover aerial part, Yarrow flower, Eucalyptus leaf, Elderberry flower, fruit, Yellow Dock. Other Ingredients: Microcrystalline Cellulose, Silica, Maltodetrin, Croscarmellose Sodium, Magnesium Stearate.

Dr. Howell's Original Formula 1 - Genuine Nzimes **-** Enzymes, Inc.
Two capsules contain: n-zimes Proprietary Enzyme Blend 400 mg: Protease, Amylase, Lipase, Cellulase. Other Ingredients: Plant Fiber, Gelatin, Water.

Dr. Howell's Original Formula 10 - Genuine Nzimes **-** Enzymes, Inc.
Two capsules contain: n-zimes Proprietary Enzyme Blend 400 mg: Protease, Amylase, Lipase, Cellulase. Other Ingredients: Plant Fiber, Gelatin, Water.

Dr. Howell's Original Formula 10 powder - Genuine Nzimes **-** Enzymes, Inc.
Each 1/4 tsp serving contains: n-zimes Proprietary Enzyme Blend 530 mg: Protease, Amylase, Lipase, Cellulase.

Dr. Morrow's Blood Formula **-** Nutrition Dynamics, Inc.
Ten drops contain: Hamamelis virginica 3C • Pulsatilla nigricans 3C • Echinacea angustifolia 3C • Acidum hydrofluoricum 3C • Viburnum

prunifolium 3C • Tussilago farfara 3C • Aesculus hippocastanum 3X. See Editor's Note No. 1, page 2053.

Dr. Morrow's Body Ache Formula **-** Nutrition Dynamics, Inc.
Ten drops contain: Aconite 3C • Bryonia alba 3C • Eupatorium perfoliatum 3C • Ferrum Phosphate 6C • Apis mellifica 3C • Mercurius dulcis 6C • Arnica 3C.
See Editor's Note No. 1, page 2053.

Dr. Morrow's Digestion Formula **-** Nutrition Dynamics, Inc.
Ten drops contain: Nux vomica 3C • Bryonia alba 3C • Argentum nitricum 3C • Condurango 3C • Abies nigra 3C • Robinia pseudacacia 3C • Solidago 3X.
See Editor's Note No. 1, page 2053.

Dr. Morrow's Hives, Allergies, Poison Ivy, Poison Oak Formula **-** Nutrition Dynamics, Inc.
Ten drops contain: Ammonium carbonate 12X • Apis mellifica 30X • Arsinucum album 30X • Gridelia robusta 30X • Echinacea 6X • Crotalus horridus 20X.
See Editor's Note No. 1, page 2053.

Dr. Morrow's Insomnia Formula **-** Nutrition Dynamics, Inc.
Ten drops contain: Passiflora 3X • Ignatia 4C • Coffee cruda 5C • Tellurium 6C • Acid phosphorica 7C • Palladium 6C • Magnesia phosphorica 6C.
See Editor's Note No. 1, page 2053.

Dr. Morrow's Liver Formula **-** Nutrition Dynamics, Inc.
Ten drops contain: Chelidonium 3X • Taraxacum 3X • Carduus marianus 3X • Solidago 3X • Hydrastis 3C • Magnesia muriatica 3C • Cinchona 3C.
See Editor's Note No. 1, page 2053.

Dr. Morrow's Motion Sickness Formula **-** Nutrition Dynamics, Inc.
Ten drops contain: Tabacum 3C • Cocculus indicus 3C • Arnica montana 3C • Petroleum 3C • Belladonna 3C • Ipecac 3C • Ignatia 3C.
See Editor's Note No. 1, page 2053.

Dr. Morrow's Overexertion Formula **-** Nutrition Dynamics, Inc.
Ten drops contain: Phosphoric Acid 3C • Kali phosphoricum 6C • Anacardium 3C • Arnica 3C • Gelsemium 3C • Selenium 6C • Argentum nitricum 3C • Avena sativa 3X.
See Editor's Note No. 1, page 2053.

Dr. Morrow's Pile Formula **-** Nutrition Dynamics, Inc.
Ten drops contain: Aesculus hippocastanum 10X • Hamamelis canadensis 10X • Hydrastis canadensis 10X • Viburnum prunifolium 10X.
See Editor's Note No. 1, page 2053.

Dr. Morrow's Runny Nose Formula **-** Nutrition Dynamics, Inc.
Ten drops contain: Allium cepa 3C • Belladonna 3C • Euphrasia 3C • Mercurius dulcis 6C • Hydrastis 3C • Kali bichromicum 3C • Sambucus nigra 3C.
See Editor's Note No. 1, page 2053.

Dr. Morrow's Skin Formula **-** Nutrition Dynamics, Inc.
Ten drops contain: Saponaria officinalis 3X • Fumaria officinalis 3X • Sarsaparilla 3X • Hydrocotyle asiatica 3X • Viola tricolor 3X • Rhus venenata 3C • Lappa major 3C • Berberis vulgaris 3C.
See Editor's Note No. 1, page 2053.

Dr. Morrow's Sore Muscle Formula **-** Nutrition Dynamics, Inc.
Ten drops contain: Rhus toxicodendron 3C • Urtica urens 3C • Benzoic Acid 3C • Formic Acid 3C • Berberis vulgaris 3C • Ranunculus bulbosus 3C • Lithium carbonate 3C.
See Editor's Note No. 1, page 2053.

Dr. Morrow's Stop Cough Formula **-** Nutrition Dynamics, Inc.
Ten drops contain: Drosera 3C • Arnica 3C • Belladonna 3C • Cina 3C • Coccus cacti 3C • Corallium rubrum 6C • Cuprum metallicum 6C • Ferrum Phosphate 6C • Ipecac 3C • Solidago 1C.
See Editor's Note No. 1, page 2053.

Dr. Nanba's Maitake Beta Factor 4 fl oz **-** Planetary Formulas
Twenty-seven drops (approximately 1.25 ml) contain: Vitamin C (as ascorbic acid) 37.5 mg • Maitake (beta-glucan) Fraction++ 12.5 mg. Other Ingredients: Distilled Water, Vegetable Glycerin.

Dr. Nanba's Maitake Beta-Factor 163 mg **-** Planetary Formulas
Two tablets contain: Vitamin C (as ascorbic acid) 20 mg • Calcium 326 mg • Maitake (beta-glucan) Fraction 6 mg • Maitake Blend 320 mg: Maitake Fruiting Body, Maitake Mycelia Biomass. Other Ingredients: Dibasic Calcium Phosphate, Stearic Acid, Colloidal Silicon Dioxide, Modified Cellulose Gum, Magnesium Stearate.

Dr. Nanba's Maitake-Pro **-** Planetary Formulas
Two tablets contain: Dietary Fiber 1 g • Protein 1 g • Vitamin C (as ascorbic acid) 20 mg • Calcium 32 mg • Maitake (beta-glucan) Fraction++ 12.5 mg • Maitake Blend 2.07 g: Maitake Fruiting Body, Maitake Mycelia Biomass. Other Ingredients: Acacia Gum, Stearic Acid, Dibasic Calcium Phosphate, Colloidal Silicon Dioxide, Modified Cellulose Gum, Magnesium Stearate.

Dr. Powers Liquid Colloidal Mineral Source with Trace Minerals **-** Puritan's Pride
Each 1 fl oz (30 mL) contains: Vitamin B12 1100 mcg • Biotin 200 mcg • Calcium 25 mg • Magnesium 100 mg • Zinc 10 mg • Selenium 50 mcg • Manganese 5 mg • Chromium 50 mcg • Potassium 10 mg • Silica 1000 mcg.

Dream Cream **-** Sensaquest
Deionized Water • L-Arginine Monohydrochloride • Dimethicone Copolyolmethyl Ether (edicol 421) • Squalene (fitoderm) • Ethoxydiglycol (polawax a) • Acrylate/Aminoacrylates/C10-30 Alkyl PEG20 Itaconate Copolymer (structure plus 3802) • Glycerin / Glyceryl Monostearate • Silwet-7087 (emulsifying wax) • Cremaphor RH40 (hydrogenated castor oil) • Carbopol 940 • Methyl Paraben • Imidazolidinyl Urea (germall 115) • Propyl Paraben.

Dream Sleep **-** The Herbalist
Hops blossom • Passionflower herb • Skullcap herb • Valerian root.

Dream Time **-** Health Smart Vitamins
Two capsules contain: Calcium (as calcium stearate) 1 mg • Valerian root (0.8% valernic acids, 3 mg) 380 mg • German Chamomile flowers 180 mg • Peppermint leaf 180 mg • Bee Propolis extract 90 mg • Passionflower aerial parts 90 mg • American Ginseng root 80 mg.

Dry Eyes **-** Natural Ophthalmics
Active Ingredients: Alumina • Arsenicum Album • Eyebright (euphrasia) 8x • Nux Moschata • Zincum Metalicum. Inactive Ingredients: Sterile Water, Sodium Chloride, Citrates, Polysorbate 80.

Dry Mouth Citrus Lozenges **-** Thayers Natural Pharmaceuticals
Each lozenge contains: Sorbitol (natural sugar-free sweetener derived from cherries, berries, pears, and plums) • Apple Pectin • Vitamin C (ascorbic acid) • Natural Lemonade Flavor • Potassium Chloride • Stearic Acid • Calcium Stearate.

Dry Mouth Spray, Citrus **-** Thayers Natural Pharmaceuticals
Glycerin • Tris Amino • Potassium Chloride • Natural Lemon Flavor • Natural Lime Flavor • Purified Water.

Some Brand Name Natural Products - What they Contain

www.NaturalDatabase.com contains MANY more listings than appear here.

Dry Mouth Spray, Menthol **-** Thayers Natural Pharmaceuticals
Vegetable Glycerin • Tris Amino • Potassium Chloride • Natural Peppermint Flavor • Purified Water.

Dry Vitamin D **-** Nature's Way
Each capsule contains: Vitamin D (as Vitamin D3) cholecalciferol 400 IU. Other Ingredients: Cellulose, Gelatin, Maltodextrin, Millet.

D-Snore **-** WellQuest International, Inc.
Sweet Almond Oil • Sesame Oil • Sunflower Oil • Olive Oil • Grape Seed Oil • Lecithin • Orange Seed Extract in a base of glycerin • Purified de-ionized Water • Natural Peppermint extract.

Dymetadrine 25 **-** AST Sports Science
Each tablet contains: Ephedrine HCL 25 mg • Guaifenesin 200 mg.

Dymetadrine Xtreme **-** AST Sports Science
Each capsule contains: Vitamin B6 5 mg • Vitamin C 30 mg • Magnesium (as magnesium salicylate) 50 mg • Ephedra extract (standardized for 24 mg ephedrine alkaloids) 300 mg • L-Phenylalanine 150 mg • L-Tyrosine 150 mg • Caffeine (as anhydrous caffeine) 100 mg • Yohimbine HCl 2 mg.
See Editor's Note No. 21 and No. 30.

Dymetadrine Xtreme (Ephedra Free) **-** AST Sports Science
Two capsules contain: Magnesium (as magnesium salicylate) 60 mg • Vitamin C 44 mg • Vitamin B6 18 mg • NGRX Green Tea leaf extract (standardized for epigallocatechin gallate EGCG, l-phenylalanine, l-tyrosine, caffeine as caffeine anhydrous, norsynephrine HCl, theobromine HCl and yohimbine HCl) 1393 mg.

E 400 I.U. **-** Nature's Bounty
Each softgel contains: Vitamin E (as DL-alpha tocopheryl acetate and D-alpha tocopherol plus D-beta, D-gamma and D-delta tocopherol) 400 IU. Other Ingredients: Gelatin, Glycerin, Soybean Oil.

E Vitamin 1,000 I.U. **-** Nature Made
Each softgel contains: Vitamin E 1000 IU. Other Ingredients: Soybean Oil, Gelatin, Glycerin, Water.
See Editor's Note No. 45, page 2058.

E Vitamin 100 I.U. **-** Nature Made
Each softgel contains: Vitamin E (from DL-alpha tocopherol acetate) 100 IU. Other Ingredients: Soybean Oil, Gelatin, Glycerin, Water, Polysorbate 80.
See Editor's Note No. 45, page 2058.

E Vitamin 200 I.U. **-** Nature Made
Each softgel contains: Vitamin E (DL-alpha tocopherol acetate) 200 IU. Other Ingredients: Gelatin, Glycerin, water.
See Editor's Note No. 45, page 2058.

E Vitamin 400 I.U. **-** Nature Made
Each softgel contains: Vitamin E (from DL-alpha tocopheryl acetate) 400 IU. Other Ingredients: Gelatin, Glcyerin, Polysorbate 80, Water.
See Editor's Note No. 45, page 2058.

E Vitamin 400 I.U. **-** Nature Made
Each softgel contains: Vitamin E 400 IU. Other Ingredients: Gelatin, Glycerin, Soybean Oil, Water.
See Editor's Note No. 45, page 2058.

E Vitamin 800 I.U. **-** Nature Made
Each softgel contains: Vitamin E 800 IU. Other Ingredients: Soybean Oil, Gelatin, Glycerin, Water.
See Editor's Note No. 45, page 2058.

E.T.- Essiac Tonic **-** The Herbalist
Burdock root • Sheep Sorrel leaf • Slippery Elm bark • Turkey Rhubarb root.

E-1000 Mixed **-** Rexall - Sundown
Each softgel contains: Vitamin E (as dl-alpha-tocopheryl acetate and d-alpha-tocopherol) 1000 IU. Other Ingredients: Gelatin, Glycerin, Water.

E-1000 Natural **-** Rexall - Sundown
Each softgel contains: Vitamin E (as d-alpha-tocopherol) 1000 IU. Other Ingredients: Gelatin, Glycerin, Water.

E-12 Super Enzymes **-** Cell Tech
Each capsule contains: Proprietary Blend 500 mg: Plant-Based Enzyme Blend 193 mg: Blue-Green Algae (aphanizomenon flos-aquae) 25 mg, Fennel seed, Ginger root, Cayenne Pepper fruit • Amylase 5750 DU • Glucoamylase 13.5 AG • Invertase 0.2 IAU • Lactase 1000 ALU • Pectinase (with phytase) 15 endo-PGU • Cellulase 100 CU • Lipase 150 LU • Protease (I) 13,500 HUT • Protease (II) 3000 HUT • Acid-Stable Protease 5.35 SAPU • Bromelain 25,600 FCC PU • Papain 50,000 FCC PU. Other Ingredients: Rice Bran, Gelatin Capsule (gelatin, water).

E-200 Mixed **-** Rexall - Sundown
Each softgel contains: Vitamin E (as dl-alpha-tocopheryl acetate and d-alpha-tocopherol) 200 IU. Other Ingredients: Gelatin, Glycerin, Water.

E-200 Natural **-** Rexall - Sundown
Each softgel contains: Vitamin E (as d-alpha-tocopherol) 200 IU. Other Ingredients: Soybean Oil, Gelatin, Glycerin, Water.

E-400 Caps **-** TwinLab
Each capsule contains: Vitamin E 400 IU. Other Ingredients: Cellulose, Magnesium, Silicate, Croscarmellose, Sodium, Gelatin, Crospovidone, Purified Water, Silica, Magnesium Stearate, MCT.

E-400 D-Alpha Water Soluble **-** Rexall - Sundown
Each softgel contains: Vitamin E (as dl-alpha-tocopheryl acetate) 400 IU. Other Ingredients: Gelatin, Polysorbate 80, Glycerin, Water.

E-400 Mixed **-** Rexall - Sundown
Each softgel contains: Vitamin E (as dl-alpha-tocopheryl acetate and d-alpha-tocopherol) 400 IU. Other Ingredients: Gelatin, Glycerin, Water.

E-400 Natural **-** Rexall - Sundown
Each softgel contains: Vitamin E (as d-alpha-tocopherol) 400 IU. Inactive Ingredients: Gelatin, Glycerin, Water.

E-400 Plus Selenium **-** The Vitamin Shoppe
Each softgel contains: Vitamin E (d-alpha, d-beta, d-delta tocopheryls) 400 IU • Selenium (Selenomethionine) 50 mcg.

E-400 Sesame **-** Progressive Labs
Each softgel capsule contains: Vitamin E (d-alpha tocopherol) 400 IU • Sesame oil 200 mg. With Natural, Unesterified Mixed Tocopherols.

E-400 with Folic Acid **-** Rexall - Sundown
Each softgel contains: Vitamin E (as dl-alpha-tocopheryl acetate and d-alpha-tocopherol) 400 IU • Vitamin B6 (as pyridoxine HCl) 2 mg • Folic Acid 400 mcg • Vitamin B12 (as cyanocobalamin) 6 mcg. Inactive Ingredients: Gelatin, Glycerin, Soybean Oil, Water, Yellow Beeswax, Soy Lecithin, Polysorbate 80.

Ear Drops **-** NutriBiotic
Contains 0.1% grapefruit extract in a base of tea tree oil and vegetable glycerin.

Ear Oil **-** Blessed Herbs
Calendula flower • St. John's Wort flower • Mullein flower • Garlic & Organic Cold-Pressed Olive oil.

Earache Tablets **-** Hyland's
Each tablet contains: Pulsatilla as Passion Flower 30C HPUS • Chamomilla as Chamomile 30C HPUS • Sulphur 30C HPUS • Calcarea carbonica as Carbonate of Lime 30C HPUS • Belladonna 30C HPUS (3x10-60% Alkaloids) • Lycopodium as Club Moss 30C

HPUS. In a base of Lactose NF (Milk Sugar). See Editor's Note No. 1, page 2053.

Earthmends Breast Health Program **-** Cancer Wellness Institute
Each packet (containing one softgel and four capsules) contains: Vitamin A (as natural beta-carotene and mixed carotenes from natural antioxidant blend) 9000 IU • Vitamin E (as natural vitamin E succiante and d-alpha tocopherol) 200 IU • Selenium (from selenium yeast) 150 mcg. Energizing Complex - Yellow: Glutamine (as L-glutamine polypeptides) 100 mg • Propolis 75 mg • Bee Pollen 75 mg • Ginger extract (root) (3.75 mg gingerols/shoagols) 75 mg • Turmeric extract (root) (71.25 mg curcumins) 75 mg • Oriental Ginseng extract (root) (3.5 mg ginsenosides) 50 mg • Garlic concentrate (bulb) 50 mg. Mushroom Complex - Speckled: Chinese Skullcap (aerial) 75 mg • Maitake Mushroom (aerial) 50 mg • Reishi Mushroom (mycelia) 50 mg • Shitake Mushroom (aerial) 50 mg • Agaricus Mushroom (aerial) 50 mg • Panax Pseudoginseng Wal. (root) 50 mg • Rabdosia Rubescens (Hemsl.) Hara. (aerial) 35 mg • Dyer's Woad (aerial) 35 mg • Licorice (root) 25 mg • Chrysanthemum (flower) 25 mg • Agaricus Mushroom extract (aerial) 25 mg • Maitaki Mushroom extract (6.25 mg polysaccharides) 25 mg • Shitake Mushroom Lenode extract mycelia (aerial) (0.375 mg) 25 mg • Reishi Mushroom extract (aerial) (3.125 mg polysaccharides) 25 mg. Antioxidant Complex - Burgundy: Broccoli concentrate (with natural sulforophanes) (aerial) 200 mg • Colostrum 200 mg • Green Tea extract (leaf) (50 mg polyphenols) 100 mg • Grape seed extract (45 mg gallic acid equivalent) (40 mg polyphenols) 100 mg • Quercetin (flavonoid) 50 mg • Indole-3-Carbinol 40 mg. Red Clover Complex - Brown: Red Clover extract (flower) (20 mg isoflavones) 200 mg • Black Cohosh extract (root) (2.83 mg triterpeneglycosides) 113 mg • Dong Quai extract (root)(0.042 mg ferulic acids) 83 mg • Tocotrienols 43 mg. Flax Seed Oil Complex - Red: Flax Oil (seed) 200 mg • Natural Antioxidant Blend 100 mg from Carrot oil (root), Palm (fruit), Marigold (flower), Tomato (fruit), supplying Lutein, Lycopene, Phytoene, Phytofluene, Tocotrienols/Tocopherols, Zeaxanthin • Beta Sitosterol Complex (90 mg free sterols) 100 mg • Natural Lycopene (from Tomato fruit) 5 mg • Astaxanthin 2 mg. Other Ingredients: Gelatin, Soybean Oil, Lecithin, Glycerin, Rice Flour, Magnesium Stearate, Silicon Dioxide, Natural Beeswax.

Earthmends Prostate Health Program **-** Cancer Wellness Institute
Each packet (containing two softgels and three capsules) contains: Vitamin A (as natural beta-carotene and mixed carotenes from natural antioxidant blend) 9000 IU • Vitamin E (as natural vitamin E succinate and d-alpha-tocopherol) 200 IU • Zinc (as zinc amino acid chelate) 15 mg • Selenium (from selenium yeast) 150 mcg. Energizing Complex - Yellow: Glutamine (as L-glutamine polypeptides) 100 mg • Propolis 75 mg • Bee Pollen 75 mg • Ginger extract (root) (3.75 mg gingerols/shoagols) 75 mg • Turmeric extract (root) (71.25 mg curcumins) 75 mg • Oriental Ginseng extract (root) (3.5 mg ginsenosides) 50 mg • Garlic concentrate (bulb) 50 mg. Mushroom Complex - Speckled: Chinese Skullcap (aerial) 75 mg • Maitake Mushroom (aerial) 50 mg • Reishi Mushroom (mycelia) 50 mg • Shitake Mushroom (aerial) 50 mg • Agaricus Mushroom (aerial) 50 mg • Panax Pseudoginseng Wall. (root) 50 mg • Rabdosia Rubescens (Hemsl.) Hara. (aerial) 50 mg • Dyer's Woad (aerial) 35 mg • Licorice (root) 25 mg • Chrysanthemum (flower) 25 mg • Agaricus Mushroom extract (aerial) 25 mg • Maitake Mushroom extract (6.25 mg polysaccharides) 25 mg • Shitake Mushroom Lenode extract mycelia (aerial) (0.375 mg) 25 mg • Reishi Mushroom extract (aerial) (3.125 mg polysaccharides) 25 mg. Antioxidant Complex - Burgundy: Broccoli concentrate (with natural sulforophanes) (aerial) 200 mg • Colostrum 200 mg • Green Tea extract (leaf) (50 mg polyphenols) 100 mg • Grape Seed extract (45 mg gallic acid equivalent) (40 mg polyphenols) 100 mg • Quercetin (flavonoid) 50 mg • Indole-3-Carbinol 40 mg. Saw Palmetto Complex - Brown: Red Clover (flower) 200 mg • Saw Palmetto berry extract (seed) (136 mg free fatty acids) 160 mg • Stinging Nettle extract (root) (0.96 mg beta sitosterol) 120 mg • Pygeum extract (Pygeum africanum bark) (6.5 mg sterols) 50 mg • Beta Sitosterol complex (45 mg free sterols) 50 mg. Flax Seed Complex - Red: Flax Oil (seed) 200 mg • Natural Antioxidant Blend 150 mg: Carrot oil (root), Palm (fruit), Marigold (flower), Tomato (fruit), supplying Lutein, Lycopene, Phytoene, Phytofluene, Tocotrienols/Tocopherols, Zeaxanthin • Beta Sitosterol Complex (90 mg free sterols) 100 mg • Natural Lycopene (from Tomato fruit) 5 mg • Astaxanthin 2 mg. Other Ingredients: Gelatin, Soybean Oil, Lecithin, Glycerin, Magnesium Stearate, Silicon Dioxide, Natural Beeswax.

Earthmends Total Health Program **-** Cancer Wellness Institute
Five capsules contain: Fruit extract blend 900 mg: Banana (fruit), New Jersey Tomato (fruit), Delicious Apple (fruit), Strawberry (fruit), Kiwi (fruit), Peach (fruit), Whole Red Wine Grape (fruit), Wild Blueberry (fruit), Mango (fruit), Cantaloupe Melon (fruit), Hawaiian Pineapple (fruit), Cranberry (fruit), Bing Cherry (fruit), Plum (fruit), Elderberry (fruit), Apricot (fruit), Red Raspberry (fruit), Red Pepper (fruit), Eggplant (fruit) • Root Vegetable Extract Blend 450 mg: Carrot (root), Ginger (root), Beet (root), Onion (bulb), Sweet Potato (root), Potato (root) • Cruciferous Vegetable Extract Blend 375 mg: Broccoli (aerial), Spinach (leaf), Kale (leaf), Brussel Sprout (bud), Cabbage (leaf) • Citrus Fruit Extract Blend 350 mg: Orange (fruit), Grapefruit (fruit), Lemon (fruit), Lime (fruit) • Micro-Algae Blend 250 mg: Spirulina (Spirulina planatensis whole cell), Broken Cell Wall Chlorella (Chlorella spp. broken cells) • Soy isolate protein extract (Soybeans)(seed) 250 mg • Whole Cereal Grains and Grass Extract Blend 100 mg: Alfalfa (aerial), Barley (whole plant), Wheat (whole plant), Rye (whole plant) • Vegetable Extract Blend 75 mg: Cauliflower (florets), Corn (seed). Other Ingredients: Malarin, Collagen, Silicon Dioxide, Magnesium Stearate.

Easy Iron **-** Puritan's Pride
Each capsule contains: Iron (as Ferrous Bis-Glycinate) 28 mg • Vitamin C (as Ascorbic Acid) 60 mg • Folate (as Folic Acid) 400 mcg • Vitamin B12 (as Cyanocobalamin) 8 mcg.

Easy Iron **-** Vitamin World
Each capsule contains: Vitamin C (as Ascorbic Acid) 60 mg • Folic Acid 400 mcg • Vitamin B12 (as Cyanocobalamin) 8 mcg • Iron (as Ferrous Bis-Glycinate) 28 mg. Other Ingredients: Gelatin, Maltodextrin, Vegetable Magnesium Stearate, Silica.

Easy Now **-** Traditional Medicinals
Peppermint leaf • Spearmint leaf • Passion flower herb • Valerian root • Licorice root • Catnip leaf • Chamomile flower • Rosemary leaf • Lavender flower • Natural flavors.

Easylax - R-U Ved USA **-** Ayush Herbs
Terminalia chebula • Fennel • Trychospermum • Senna extract (8% sennodides).

Eater's Digest **-** Traditional Medicinals
Peppermint leaf • Ginger rhizome • Fennel seed • Rose Hip • Papaya leaf • Alfalfa Herb • Cinnamon bark.

EB5 Age Spot Formula **-** Pharmacist Heldfond's eb5 Formulas for Y
Hydroquinone 2% • Deionized Water • Mineral Oil • Cetearyl Alcohol • Ceteary1 Phosphate • Glycerin • Petroleum • Steareth-2 • Stearyl Alcohol • Steareth-10 • Bilberry Extract • Sugar Cane Extract • Sugar Maple Extract • Orange Extract • Lemon Extract • Octyl Methoxcinnamate • Benzophenone-3 • Sodium Sulfite • Sodium Meta Bisulfite • Citric Acid • Propylene Glycol • Diazolidinyl Urea • Methylparaben • Propylparaben.

EB5 Body Formula **-** Pharmacist Heldfond's eb5 Formulas for Y
Purified Water • Methylsilanol Mannuronate • Mate Extract • Gotu Kola Extract • Thea Sinensis Extract • Butylene Glycol • Glyeryl Stearate • Stearic Acid • Cyclomehticome • Octyl Palmitate • Myristy Myristate • Dimethicone • Sunflower Oil • Isopropyl Lanolate • Soy Serol • Cetareth 20 • Tocopheryl Acetate • Choleth-24 • Ceteth 24 •

Panthenol • Ivy Extract • Horsetail Extract • Kelp Extract • Algae Extract • Ginkgo Extract • Arnica Extract • Triethanolamine • Carbomer • Hydroxykpropyl • Methylcellulose • Disodium EDTA • Methylparaben • Propylparaben • Imadazolidinyl Urea • Fragrance.

EB5 Body Lotion - Pharmacist Heldfond's eb5 Formulas for Y

Water • Tocopheryl Acetate • Stearic Acid • Propylene Glycol • Dicaprylate/Dicaprate • Mineral Oil • Butylene glycol • Clyeryl Stearate SE • Sorbitan Stearate • Polysorbate-60 • Squalane • Soy Sterol • Panthenol • Oat Flour • Lanolin Alcohol • Retinyl Palmitate • Ergocalciferol • Dimenthicone • Imidazolidinyl Urea • Disodium EDTA • Carbomer-940 • Polyamino Sugar • Condensate • Urea • Methylparaben • Propylparaben • Triethanolamine • Fragrance.

EB5 Cleansing Formula - Pharmacist Heldfond's eb5 Formulas for Y

Purified Water • Cycerin • Caprylic/Capric Triglyceride • Stearic Acid • Peg 8 • Glycol Distearate • Cetyl Alcohol • Triethanolamine • Tocopheryl Acetate • Lactic Acid • Polyquatemium-7 • Panthenol • Peg-10 • Soya Sterol • Oat Flour • Cetearyl Alcohol • Peg-40 Castor Oil • Sodium Cetearyl Sulfate • Cocamide DEA • Carbomer • Disodium • EDTA • BHA • Methylparaben • Propylparaben • Quantemium-15 • Fragrance.

EB5 Facial Creme - Pharmacist Heldfond's eb5 Formulas for Y

Water • Propylene Glycol • Tocopheryl Acetate • Stearic Acid • Mineral Oil • Cetyl Alcohol • Oat Flour • Retinyl Palmitate • Ergocalciferol • Propylparaben • Triethanolamine • Methylparaben • Potassium Sorbate • Allantoin • Imidazolidinyl • Urea • Panthenol • Cobomer-940 • Soluble Animal Collagen.

EB5 Footcare Formula - Pharmacist Heldfond's eb5 Formulas for Y

Deionized Water • Mineral Oil • Propylene Glycol • Stearic Acid • Microcystalline Wax • Cetyl Alcohol • PEG-100 Stearate • vitamin E Acetate • Oat Protein • Triethanolamine • Menthol • Eucalyptus Oil • Fragrance • DL Panthenol • Allantoin • Imidazolidiny Urea • Methylparaben • Propylparaben • Potassium Sorbate • Chamomile • Comfrey • Tea Tree Oil • White Lily Extract • Corn Flower Extract • Sandalwood Extract • Sunflower Extract • Basil Extract • Sage Extract • Jasmine Extract • Sugar Cane Extract • Maple Extract • Citrus Extract • Apple Extract • Vitamin A • Vitamin D (as Vitamin D3) • Dipotassium • Glycyrrhzinate • Soluble Collagen • FD&C Blue #1 • FD&C Yellow #5.

EB5 Men's Facial Formula - Pharmacist Heldfond's eb5 Formulas for Y

Water • Propylene Glycol • Tocopheryl Acetate • Stearic Acid • Mineral Oil • Cetyl Alcohol • Oat Flour • Sodium PCA • Retinyl Palmiate • Ergocalciferol • Allantoin • Panthenol • Soluble Animal Collagen • Propylparaben • Triethanolamine • Methylparaben • Potassium Sorbate • Imidazolidinyl Urea • Carbomer-940 • Fragrance • FD&C Blue No. 1 • FD&C Red No. 33.

EB5 Toning Formula - Pharmacist Heldfond's eb5 Formulas for Y

Purified Water • Hydrolyzed Wheat Protein • Arnica Extract • Barley Extract • Triethanolamine • Lactic Acid • Polysorbate 20 • Sodium PCA • Vitamin E Acetate • Allantoin • Panthenol • Witch Hazel Distillate • Sage Extract • Birch Leaf Extract • Comfrey Extract • Sambucus Extract • Blackberry Extract • Horsetail Extract • Tetrasodium EDTA • Methylparaben • Imidazolidinyl Uera • Quantemium-15 • Fragrance.

E'balance - E'OLA

Two capsules contain: Proprietary Blend 665 mg: Soy Isoflavones, Black Cohosh (root) (Cimicifuga Racemosa), St. John's Wort (herb), Dong Quai (herb), Licorice (root), Chaste Tree (berry), Fennel (seed). Other Ingredients: Rice Flour, Gelatin, Magnesium Stearate.

EB-C - MMS Pro

Each capsule contains: Eyebright • Golden Seal root • Bayberry root bark • Red Raspberry • Cayenne.

ECA Stack - Nutra Sport

Two capsules contain: Ephedrine alkaloids (from whole ma huang plant extract) 20 mg • Caffeine (32.2 mg from bissey nut) 200 mg • Acetylsalicylic Acid 324 mg. Other Ingredients: Rice flour.
See Editor's Note No. 30, page 2056.

EchinaCare Capsules - PhytoPharmica

Each capsule contains: Echinacea purpurea (aerial part) concentrate 50:1 50 mg.

EchinaCare Liquid - PhytoPharmica

Forty to sixty drops contain: Echinacea purpurea (fresh-pressed juice from stems, leaves, and flowers) 1.5 ml.
See Editor's Note No. 21, page 2056.

Echinacea - DreamPharm

Each capsule contains: Echinacea herb 400 mg • Glycyrrhizae radix (licorice root) 100 mg.

Echinacea - Elderberry Syrup - Planetary Formulas

Each 1/2 tsp serving contains: Proprietary Blend 2.5 mL: Elderberry, Echinacea purpurea root, Isatis root, Honeysuckle flower, Forsythia flower, Boneset leaf, Platycodon root, Licorice root, Apricot seed, Gastrodia Tuber. Inactive Ingredients: Vegetable Glycerine, Purified Water, Honey, 1/10th of 1% Potassium Sorbate added as a preservative.

Echinacea - Gaia Herbs

Echinacea standardized for 1% isobutylamides and 4% phenolic compounds. Standardized Full Spectrum 90 mg of extract per capsule. Guaranteed Potency 45 mg of extract per capsule.

Echinacea - Leiner Health Products

Each caplet contains: Echinacea extract (Echinacea angustifolia & Echinacea purpurea) root 125 mg. Other Ingredients: Calcium Carbonate, Cellulose, Maltodextrin, Hydroxypropyl Methylcellulose, Silicon Dioxide, Polyethylene Glycol 3350, Croscarmellose Sodium, Hydroxypropyl Cellulose, Red 40 Lake, Blue 2 Lake, Pharmaceutical Glaze, Crospovidone, Magnesium Stearate, Polysorbate 80, Titanium Dioxide.

Echinacea - Nature's Bounty

Each capsule contains: Echinacea (Echinacea purpurea) root 400 mg. Other Ingredients: Gelatin, Vegetable Stearic Acid.

Echinacea - Nature's Way

Three capsules contain: Echinacea Purpurea stem, leaf, flower 1.20 g. Other Ingredients: Gelatin.

Echinacea - Now

Two capsules contain: Total Carbohydrate 620 mg • Echinacea purpurea powder root 800 mg. Other Ingredients: Stearic Acid.

Echinacea - Pharmanex

Each capsule contains: Echinacea purpurea root 6:1 extract 225 mg. Other Ingredients: Rice Flour, Gelatin.

Echinacea - Puritan's Pride

Each capsule contains: Echinacea (Echinacea purpurea) root 400 mg. Other Ingredients: Gelatin, Vegetable Stearic Acid.

Echinacea & Elderberry - Leiner Health Products

Each softgel contains: Zinc Gluconate 8 mg • Echinacea extract (Echinacea angustifolia, Echinacea purpurea) root and aerial parts 150 mg • Elderberry extract (Sambucus nigra) fruit 100 mg • Golden Seal extract (Hydrastis canadensis) root 100 mg. Other Ingredients: Flaxseed Oil, Gelatin, Lecithin, Wax, Yellow Turmeric, Caramel Powder, Titanium Dioxide.

Some Brand Name Natural Products - What they Contain

www.NaturalDatabase.com contains MANY more listings than appear here.

BRAND NAMES

Echinacea & Golden Seal Combo - Optimum Nutrition
Each capsule contains: Horse Chestnut extract (Aesculus hippocastanum) root 250 mg • Butcher's Broom powdered root 145 mg • Ginger powdered root 145 mg. Other Ingredients: Gelatin, Magnesium Stearate.

Echinacea & Goldenseal - Leiner Health Products
Each caplet contains: Echinacea extract (Echinacea angustifolia & Echinacea purpurea) root 75 mg • Golden Seal extract (Hydrastis canadensis) root 100 mg • Hesperidin 40 mg • Quercetin 20 mg • Rutin 40 mg. Other Ingredients: Calcium Carbonate, Cellulose, Maltodextrin, Hydroxypropyl Methylcellulose, Stearic Acid, Silicon Dioxide, Polyethylene Glycol 3350, Croscarmellose Sodium, Talc, Magnesium Stearate, Hydroxypropyl Cellulose, Pharmaceutical Glaze, Crospovidone, Yellow 5 Lake, Red 40 Lake, Blue 2 Lake, Titanium Dioxide, Polysorbate 80.

Echinacea & Goldenseal 1000 mg, Concentrated - GNC Herbal Plus - GNC
Each capsule contains: Echinacea Root (echinacea angustifolia; from 72 mg of echinacea root extract 7:1) 500 mg • Goldenseal Root (hydrastis canadensis; from 72 mg of goldenseal root extract 7:1) 500 mg. Other Ingredients: Soybean Oil, Gelatin, Glycerin, Caramel Color, Titanium Dioxide (natural mineral whitener).

Echinacea & Goldenseal Combo - Atrium Inc.
Two fluid ounces contains: Echinacea • Goldenseal. In a synergistic base of Red Clover, Burdock, Parsley, Fennel, Ginger, Chamomile, Barberry & Cayenne. Contains 16-18% Grain Alcohol.

Echinacea & Goldenseal Root - Now
Two capsules contain: Echinacea Purpurea root powder 450 mg • Goldenseal root powder (hydrastis canadensis) 450 mg.

Echinacea & Goldenseal, Peppermint - GNC Herbal Plus - GNC
Each dropperful (1mL) contains: Echinacea Extract (echinacea angustifolia, root; standardized to contain 4% echinacosides = 6 mg) 150 mg • Goldenseal Dried Root Extract (hydrastis canadesis) 0.025 mg • Stevia Extract (stevia rebaudiana, leaf) 3 mg. Other Ingredients: Deionized Water, USP Alcohol, Fructose, Glycerin, Natural Peppermint Flavor, Natural Vanilla Flavor, Methylparaben (a preservative), Natural Wintergreen Flavor, Propylparaben (a preservative).

Echinacea 1000 mg - Jamieson
Each capsule contains: Echinacea root 1000 mg.

Echinacea 150 mg - Jamieson
Each capsule contains: Echinacea (Echinacea purpurea, powdered extract 1:3) 150 mg • Panax Ginseng (Standardized to 4% ginsenosides) 250 mg.

Echinacea 150 mg with Ginseng 250 mg - Jamieson
Each capsule contains: Echinacea Purpurea (powdered extract 1:3) 150 mg • Panax Ginseng 250 mg.

Echinacea 300 mg - Jamieson
Each capsule contains: Echinacea herb (Echinacea Purpurea, powdered 1:3) 300 mg • Allicin Rich Garlic bulb powder 300 mg • Ginger root (Zingiber Officinale, powdered Extract 1:6) 300 mg.

Echinacea 300 mg with Garlic and Ginger - Jamieson
Each capsule contains: Echinacea Purpurea (powdered extract 1:3) 300 mg • Allicin Rich Garlic Bulb Powder 300 mg • Ginger Root (Zingiber officinale, powdered extract 1:6) 300 mg.

Echinacea 350 mg - Jamieson
Each capsule contains: Echinacea Purpurea (1:3 powdered extract) 350 mg.

Echinacea 400 mg - Puritan's Pride
Each capsule contains: Echinacea (echinacea purpurea, aerial) 400 mg. Other Ingredients: Gelatin.

Echinacea and Golden Seal - Optimum Nutrition
Echinacea Angustifolia extract • Goldenseal powder.

Echinacea and Goldenseal - Dial Herbs
Echinacea • Goldenseal • Cayenne.

Echinacea and Goldenseal - Jamieson
Each capsule contains: Echinacea Root 740 mg • Goldenseal Root 90 mg.

Echinacea and Goldenseal Tincture - Jamieson
Each 15 drops (1 ml) contains: Echinacea Purpurea 375 mg • Echinacea Angustifolia 100 mg • Goldenseal Root 25 mg.

Echinacea Angustifolia - Now
Each 1 1/2 droppersful contains: Echinacea Angustifolia root extract 1.2 ml. Other Ingredients: Grain Alcohol, Water.

Echinacea Angustifolia - Optimum Nutrition
Each capsule contains: Echinacea Angustifolia root extract (standardized to 4% echinacosides) 125 mg • Echinacea Angustifola root, powdered 225 mg • Echinacea Purpurea aerial 10 mg. Other Ingredients: Gelatin, Magnesium Stearate.

Echinacea Angustifolia, Extract - Nature's Way
Each capsule contains: Echinacea Angustifolia, dried extract 250 mg • Echinacea Purpurea stem, leaf, flower 190 mg. Other Ingredients: Gelatin, Millet.

Echinacea Balance - HerbaSway
Echinacea • Green Tea • Ginger • Blackberry • HerbaSwee (Cucurbitaceae fruit).

Echinacea Complete Care - Celestial Seasonings
Two capsules contain: Vitamin C (as ascorbic acid) 180 mg • Zinc (as gluconate) 15 mg • Proprietary Blend 1000 mg: Echinacea (root, stem, leaf, flower), Echinacea (standardized extract), Arabinogalactan. Other Ingredients: Dicalcium phosphate, gelatin, rice flour, stearic acid, magnesium stearate and silicon dioxide.

Echinacea Extract - Jamieson
Each capsule contains: Echinacea herb (Echinacea purpurea 1:3 powdered extract) 350 mg. Other Ingredients: Dicalcium Phosphate, Micorcrystalline Cellulose, Magnesium Stearate, Silicon Dioxide.

Echinacea Extract - Ortho Molecular Products
Each capsule contains: Echinacea Angustifolia extract 200 mg • Echinacea Purpurea 200 mg.

Echinacea Extract - Progressive Labs
Each capsule contains: Echinacea 250 mg • Polysaccharides (from Echinacea) 37.5 mg • Phenolic compounds (from Echinacea) 10 mg.

Echinacea Goldenseal - Jamieson
Each capsule contains: Calcium (as Calcium Sulfate) 30 mg • Echinacea root extract 4:1 (Echinacea purpurea Moench.) (4% Phenolic Compounds) 185 mg • Goldenseal root extract 2:1 (Hydrastis canadensis L.) (5% Alkaloids and Hydrastine Compounds) 45 mg.

Echinacea Plus - Aboca USA, Inc
Each capsule contains: Echinacea Purpurea flowering top whole phytocomplex concentrate (WPC, standardized to 2% total polyphenols, yielding 2.48 mg per capsule) 124 mg • Echinacea Pallida root WPC (standardized to 1.1% echinacoside, yielding 1.36 mg per capsule) 124 mg • Echinacea Angustifolia root WPC (standardized to 0.9% echinacoside, yielding 0.38 mg per capsule) 42 mg. Other Ingredients: Gelatin (capsule).

Echinacea Plus - Traditional Medicinals
Echinacea purpurea herb • Lemongrass leaf • Spearmint leaf • Echinacea angustifolia herb • concentrated extract of E. Purpurea root.

Echinacea Root - Basic Nutrition - GNC
Each capsule contains: Echinacea root powder (Echinacea Angustifolia) 500 mg. Other Ingredients: Gelatin, Cellulose, Magnesium Stearate.

Echinacea Root - GNC Herbal Plus - GNC
Each dropperful (1 mL) Contains: Echinacea extract (echinacea angustifolia, root, standardized to contain 4% echinacosides = 6 mg) 150 mg • Stevia extract (as steavia rebaudiana, leaf) 3 mg. Other Ingredients: Deionized Water, USP Alcohol, Fructose, Glycerin, Natural Peppermint flavor, Natural Vanilla flavor, Methylparaben, Natural Wintergreen flavor, Propylparaben (a preservative).

Echinacea Root 1000 mg, Concentrated - GNC Herbal Plus - GNC
Each capsule contains: Echinacea Root Extract (echinacea angustifolia; from 142.9 mg of echinacea root extract 7:1) 1000 mg. Other Ingredients: Gelatin, Soybean Oil, Glycerin, Caramel Color, Titanium Dioxide (natural mineral whitener).

Echinacea Root Complex - Nature's Way
Two capsules contain: Echinacea Angustifolia root • Echinacea Purpurea stem, leaf, flower • Proprietary Blend 900 mg. Other Ingredients: Gelatin, Magnesium Stearate.

Echinacea Tincture - Jamieson
Each 2 mL (40 drops) contains: Echinacea angustifolia (1:2 pure tincture in 45% Ethanol) Derived from alcohol maceration of fresh plants (aerial parts) 1000 mg.

Echinacea Whole Herb, 350 mg - Nature Made
Each capsule contains: Echinacea Purpurea aerial part 350 mg: Cichoric Acid 2.5 mg.

Echinacea with Goldenseal Liquid Extract - Quantum, Inc.
Two ounces contain: Fresh undried Echinacea purpurea whole plant 70% • Echinacea angustifolia 10% • Goldenseal root 20% • Alcohol 50%.
See Editor's Note No. 21, page 2056.

Echinacea with Zinc - Aspen Group, Inc.
Each capsule contains: Echinacea Purpurea 380 mg • Zinc (citrate) 3 mg.

Echinacea, Propolis & Ester C - Futurebiotics
Two capsules contain: Vitamin C (as Ester-C ascorbate) 500 mg • Calcium (as calcium ascorbate) 59 mg • Echinacea angustifolia leaf powder extract [standardized for 4% (5 mg) echinacosides] 125 mg • Echinacea angustifolia leaf powder 150 mg • Echinacea purpurea leaf powder 150 mg • Citrus bioflavonoid peel powder 250 mg • Bee Propolis powder 100 mg • Acerola berry (Rose Hips) powder 50 mg. Other Ingredients: Magnesium stearate, Gelatin, Water.

Echinacea/Astragalus/Reishi Formula - Nature's Way
Three capsules contain: Proprietary Formula: Astragalus root • Echinacea Purpurea stem, leaf, flower • Reishi (dried extract 10% Polysaccharides). Other Ingredients: Gelatin.

Echinacea/Ester-C Formula - Nature's Way
Two capsules contain: Calcium 27 mg • Echinacea Purpurea stem, leaf, flower 722 mg • Ester-C (Patented form of Vitamin C) 207 mg. Other Ingredients: Gelatin.

Echinacea/Ginseng Formula - Nature's Way
Two capsules contain: Proprietary Formula: Echinacea Angustifolia root • Echinacea Purpurea stem, leaf, flower • Siberian Ginseng root . Other Ingredients: Gelatin, Magnesium Stearate, Millet.

Echinacea/Goldenseal - Gaia Herbs
Echinacea and Goldenseal standardized for 1% isobutylamides and 15% total alkaloids. Standardized Full Spectrum 100 mg of extract per capsule. Guaranteed Potency 50 mg of extract per capsule.

Echinacea/GSR Formula - Nature's Way
Three capsules contain: Proprietary Formula: Burdock root • Cayenne pepper fruit • Echinacea Angustifolia root • Echinacea Purpurea stem, leaf, flower • Gentain root • Goldenseal stem, leaf, flower • Wood Betony stem, leaf, flower. Other Ingredients: Gelatin.

Echinacea-Go! - Wakunaga of America
Each capsule contains: Echinacea standardized extract (angustifolia & purpurea blend) leaf/root, standardized to 4% phenolic compounds. Other Ingredients: Cellulose, Colloidal Silica, Magnesium Stearate (vegetable source).

Echinacea-Goldenseal Formula - Quest
Each caplet contains: Echinacea angustifolia powder (provided by 100 mg P.E. 1:7 standardized to contain 4% echinacosides) 700 mg • Goldenseal root powder (Hydrastis canadensis) (provided by 50 mg P.E. 1:6 standardized to contain 5% hydrastine) 300 mg • Echinacea purpurea powder (Provided by 50 mg P.E. 1:5 standardized to contain 0.7% flavonoids) 250 mg • Astragalus root powder (Astragalus membranaceus) 100 mg. Other Ingredients: Calcium Phosphate, Microcrystalline Cellulose, Vegetable Stearin, Croscarmellose Sodium, Magnesium Stearate (vegetable source).

Echinacea-Reishi Virtue - Blessed Herbs
Astragalus root • Echinacea Angustifolia root • Pau d'Arco bark • Suma root • Siberian Ginseng root • Reishi mycelium • Licorice root • German Chamomile flower • Calendula flower • Grain alcohol & Distilled Water.

Echinaforce - Bioforce AG
Two tablets contain: Echinacea purpurea extract (95% herb and 5% roots) 538 mg • Lactose 250 mg.

EchinaFresh - Enzymatic Therapy
Each capsule contains: Echinacea purpurea 50:1 concentration of powder from the fresh-pressed juice of stems, leaves, & flowers of organically grown Echinacea purpurea 50 mg.

EchinaGuard - Nature's Way
Each capsule contains: Echinacea purpurea (stem, leaf, flower) 250 mg • EchinaGuard (Echinacea purpurea dried extract) 85 mg. Other Ingredients: Gelatin, Silica.

EchinaGuard Flexitabs - Nature's Way
Each flexitab contains: EchinaGuard (Echinacea Purpurea dried extract) 88 mg. Other Ingredients: Cherry Flavor, Citric Acid, Corn Starch, Fructose, Gelatin, Glycerol, Guar Gum, Lecithin.

Echinamax - Progena
Each capsule contains: Echinacea purpurea herb (standardized to a minumum level of 4% phenolics, 0.1% alkylamides, and 15% minimum polysaccharides) 100 mg • Echinacea purpurea herb (standardized to a minimum level of 1.5% cichoric acid) 400 mg.

Echinex - Chattem, Inc.
Each tablet contains: Standardized extract of Echinacea purpurea root & herb (4% total phenolic compounds) 250 mg • Standardized extract of Siberian Ginseng root (0.8% eleutherosides) 100 mg • Standardized extract of Ginger root (5% gingerols) 100 mg. Other Ingredients: Cellulose, Croscarmellose Sodium, Stearic Acid, Magnesium Stearate, Silicon Dioxide, Hydroxypropyl Methylcellulose (aqueous film coating).

EchinKids - Health Smart Vitamins
Two drops contains: Zinc (as zinc glycinate) 4 mg • Copper (as copper glycinate) 0.50 mg • Echinacea (root, aerial parts) 150 mg.

EchinSeal - Health Smart Vitamins
Two capsules contain: Goldenseal root 800 mg • Echinacea purpurea aerial parts 400 mg.

Some Brand Name Natural Products - What they Contain

www.NaturalDatabase.com contains MANY more listings than appear here.

EcoGen Fermented Soy Drink - EcoNugenics
Each bottle (8 oz) contains: Soy Isoflavones 150 mg • Providing: Genistein 70%, Daidzein 23%, Glycitein 7% • Protein 5.7 g • Calcium 32 mg • Iron 1 mg.

EcoGen Soybean Isoflavone Concentrate Powder - EcoNugenics
Five teaspoons (10 g) contain: EcoGen Soy Isoflavone Concentrate 10 g • Soy Isoflavones 191 mg: Glyciteins 92 mg, Genisteins 31 mg, Daidzeins 68 mg • Protein 4 g • Iron 1 mg.

EcoGen Soybean Isoflavone Concentrate Tablets - EcoNugenics
Four tablets contain: EcoGen Soy Isoflavone Concentrate 3 g • Soy Isoflavones 77 mg: Glyciteins 27 mg, Genisteins 10 mg, Daidzeins 40 mg • Protein 1 g • Iron 0.3 g. Other Ingredients: Calcium Sulfate, Stearic Acid, Silica, Magnesium Sulfate, Cellulose.

Eco-Green Multi - Now
Two tablets contain: Vitamin A (Beta Carotene) (15 mg) 25000 IU • Vitamin B1 (Thiamine HCl) 50 mg • Vitamin B2 (Riboflavin) 50 mg • Vitamin B3 (Niacinamide) 50 mg • Vitamin B5 (Pantothenic Acid) 50 mg • Vitamin B6 (Pyridoxine HCl) 50 mg • Vitamin B12 (Cyanocobalamin) 200 mcg • Biotin 100 mcg • Folic Acid 800 mcg • Vitamin C (Calcium Ascorbate) 500 mg • Vitamin D (Calciferol) 200 IU • Vitamin E (d-Alpha Succinate) 200 IU • Vitamin K (from green foods) 70 mcg • Calcium (Ascorbate, Citrate, Carbonate) 100 mg • Magnesium (50% Citrate, 50% Oxide) 100 mg • Zinc (Picolinate) 15 mg • Copper (Amino Acid Chelate) 500 mcg • Iodine (Kelp) 150 mcg • Potassium (Chloride) 25 mg • Manganese (Amino Acid Chelate) 5 mg • Selenium (L-Selenomethionine) 50 mcg • Chromium (Picolinate) 100 mcg • Molybdenum (Amino Acid Chelate) 50 mcg • Spirulina US grown 250 mg • Barley grass organically grown 250 mg • Chlorella (broken cell wall) 100 mg • Wheat grass organically grown 100 mg • Alfalfa juice concentrate 100 mg • Green Tea extract (40% Catechins) 50 mg • Choline (Bitartrate) 50 mg • Inositol 50 mg • PABA 30 mg • Trace Mineral concentrate 100 mg • Boron (Amino Acid Chelate) 1 mg • Vanadium (Amino Acid Chelate) 50 mcg • Panax ginseng (5% Ginsenosides) 100 mg • Bioflavonoids (40%) 50 mg • Rutin 25 mg • Bromelain (2000 GDU from pineapple) 50 mg • Papain (140 MCU from papaya) 25 mg • Pepsin Enzymes (NF 1:10000) 25 mg • Lipase (3400 Usp Units) 25 mg • Amylase (20000 USP Units) 10 mg • Chlorophyll from green foods 8 mg • Amino Acids from green foods 350 mg. Vegetarian formula base ingredients contain: Di-Calcium Phosphate, Cellulose, Stearic Acid, Magnesium Stearate & Silica.

E-Complete 400 - GNC
Each capsule contains: Vitamin E (as d-alpha Tocopherol) 400 IU • Tocotrienols 40 mg. Other Ingredients: Gelatin, Glycerin.

Edemex - Gero Vita International
Each capsule contains: Alisma rhizome extract (alisma orientale) 70 mg • Zhu Ling sclerotium extract (polyporus umbellatus) 70 mg • White Mulberry root extract (morus alba) 70 mg • Betel nut palm seed extract (areca catechu) 70 mg • Winter Melon fruit rind extract (benincasa hispidum) 50 mg • Bai-Zhu Atractylodes rhizome extract (atractylodes macrocephala) 50 mg • Cassia bark extract (cinnamomum cassia) 50 mg • Corn style extract (zea mays) 50 mg • Ginger rhizome extract (zingiber officinale) 35 mg. Other Ingredients: Silica, Magnesium Stearate, Gelatin.

EFA Attention Formula - Health From The Sun
Each capsule contains: Vitamin E (as d-Alpha Tocopherol) 5 IU • Magnesium from Magnesium Oxide 55 mg • Zinc from Zinc Sulfate 0.5 mg • High DHA Fish oil (70 mg Omega-3 DHA) 175 mg • Arachidonic Acid (from Fish oil) 3 mg • Borage oil (16 mg Omega-6 GLA) 80 mg • Lecithin 50 mg • Ashwagandha root extract 25 mg • Bacopa Monnieri Whole Plant extract 25 mg. Other Ingredients: Gelatin, Glycerine, Beeswax (emulsifier), Water, Carob powder.

EFA Complex - PhysioLogics
Two soft gels contain: Vitamin E (as d-Alpha Tocopherol) 20 IU • Eicosapentaenoic Acid (from Marine Lipids) 120 mg • Docosahexaenoic Acid (from Marine Lipids) 80 mg • Gamma-linolenic Acid (from Borage oil) 30 mg.

EFA Complex - New Improved Formula - PhysioLogics
Each softgel contains: Vitamin E (as d-alpha tocopherol) 5 IU • Flaxseed oil 400 mg • Borage seed oil 400 mg • Fish oil (50% omega-3) 400 mg • Fatty Acid Profile: Oleic Acid 152 mg, Linoleic Acid 180 mg, Gamma Linolenic Acid (GLA) 96 mg, Alpha Linolenic Acid 220 mg, Eicosapentaenoic Acid (EPA) 120 mg, Docosahexaenoic Acid (DHA) 80 mg. Other Ingredients: Gelatin, Glycerin.

EFA Derma-Skin Formula - Health From The Sun
Each capsule contains: Vitamin A from Palmitate 3000 IU • Vitamin C from Ascorbic Acid 60 mg • Vitamin D as Cholecalciferol 100 IU • Vitamin E as d-Alpha Tocopherol 40 IU • Zinc from Zinc Sulfate 10 mg • Organic Flax seed oil (450 mg Omega-3 ALA) 800 mg • Borage seed oil (120 mg Omega-6 GLA) 600 mg • Burdock root extract 4:1 50 mg • Yellow Dock root extract 4:1 50 mg. Other Ingredients: Gelatin, Glycerine, Beeswax (emulsifier), Water, Carob powder, Lecithin.

EFA Heart Formula - Health From The Sun
Three capsules contain: Borage oil (180 mg GLA) 900 mg • Fish oil (18% EPA, 12% DHA) 1200 mg • Flax seed oil, organic 300 mg • Folic Acid 300 mcg • Garlic extract (0.8% Allicin) 300 mg • Gugulipid (10% Gugulsterone) 300 mg • Hawthorne extract (2% Vitexin) 105 mg • Tocopherols, mixed 3.9 mg • Tocotrienols 11 mg • Vitamin B6 from Pyridoxine Hydrochloride 1.2 mg.

EFA Joint Formula - Health From The Sun
Three capsules contain: Protein 1 g • Vitamin C as Ascorbic Acid 75 mg • Vitamin D (as Vitamin D3) as Cholecalciferol 100 IU • Vitamin E as d-Alpha Tocopherol 30 IU • Zinc from Zinc Sulfate 15 mg • Manganese from Manganese Gluconate 330 mcg • Borage seed oil 300 mg GLA 1500 mg • Glucosamine Sulfate 1200 mg • Organic Flax seed oil (250 mg ALA) 450 mg • Boswellic Acid from Boswellia Resin extract 100 mg. Ingredients: Gelatin, Glycerine, Beeswax (emulsifer), Water, Carob powder, Soy Lecithin.

Efalex - Efamol
Two capsules contain: Efamol Pure Evening Primrose Oil 280 mg •DHA 120 mg •GLA 24 mg •Arachidonic Acid 10.5 mg •Thyme Oil 2 mg •Vitamin E 15 IU. Other Ingredients: Tuna Oil, Gelatin, Glycerin.

Efalex Liquid - Efamol
Four teaspoons contain: Efamol Pure Evening Primrose Oil 1200 mg •DHA 480 mg •GLA 96 mg •Arachidonic Acid 42 mg • Thyme Oil 8 mg •Vitamin E 15 IU. Other Ingredients: Sunflower Oil, Tuna Oil, Flavoring: lemon oil, lime oil.
See Editor's Note No. 21, page 2056.

Efamol Fortify - Efamol
Two capsules contain: Efamol Pure Evening Primrose Oil 800 mg •EPA 14 mg •GLA 64 mg •Vitamin E 30 IU •Calcium 200 mg. Other Ingredients: Calcium Carbonate, Gelatin, Glycerin, Marine Fish Oil, Glyceryl Monostearate, Titanium Dioxide Color.
See Editor's Note No. 21, page 2056.

Efamol PMS Control - Efamol
Two capsules contain: Efamol Pure Evening Primrose Oil 500 mg •GLA 40 mg •Vitamin C 60 mg •Vitamin E 30 IU • Niacin 12 mg •Vitamin B6 40 mg •Biotin 80 mcg • Magnesium 40 mg •Zinc 4 mg. Other Ingredients: Gelatin, Sorbitol Syrup, Glyceryl Monostearate, Glycerin, Ascorbic Acid, Heavy Magnesium Oxide, Pyridoxine HCl, Lecithin, Nicotinamide, Zinc Sulphate Monohydrate, d-Biotin.

Efamol Pure Evening Primrose Oil - Efamol
Two capsules contain: Efamol Pure Evening Primrose Oil 1000 mg • Linoleic Acid 330 mg • Gamma Linolenic Acid 80 mg. Other Ingredients: Gelatin, Glycerin.

Some Brand Name Natural Products - What they Contain

www.NaturalDatabase.com contains MANY more listings than appear here.

Efanatal **-** Efamol
Two capsules contain: Efamol Pure Evening Primrose Oil 500 mg • DHA (Docosahexaenoic Acid) 107 mg • Arachidonic Acid 9.4 mg •GLA 40 mg •Vitamin E 15 IU. Inactive Ingredients: Fish Oil, Gelatin, Glycerol, Carmine Color, Titanium Dioxide Color, Ammonium Phosphatide, Ascorbyl Palmitate.

Effervescent Glucosamine / Chondroitin **-** GNC
Fructose • Glucosamine HCl • Chondroitin Sulfate • Sodium Bicarbonate • Methyl Sulfonyl Methane (MSM) • Ascorbic Acid • Ascorbic Acid • Potassium Bicarbonate • Natural Pineapple flavor • Artificial Pineapple flavor • Calcium Pantothenate • Pyridoxine HCl • Cyanocobalamin.
See Editor's Note No. 15, page 2055.

Effisoy **-** FermaHealth
Each capsule contains: AglyMax standardized fermented Soy germ extract (includes 40 mg of the isoflavone aglycones, daidzein, glycitein and genistein). Other Ingredients: Gelatin, Soybean Oil, Glycerin, Dextrin, Carob, D-Alpha Tocopherol, Lecithin, Titanium Dioxide.

E-Gems Vitamin E 400 IU **-** J. R. Carlson Laboratories, Inc.
Each softgel contains: Vitamin E (as d-alpha tocopheryl acetate) 400 IU.

Egg Fuel **-** TwinLab
Each serving contains: Pure egg white protein.

EgSENTIALS **-** Bio Tech Pharmacal
Each capsule contains: Vitamin B6 (pyridoxal 5'-phosphate) 9 mg • Proprietary Blend 670 mg: Alpha Ketoglutaric Acid, L-Leucine, L-Valine, L-Lysine, L-Isoleucine, L-Phenylalanine, L-Threonine, L-Methionine, L-Tryptophan.

El Toro Loco Lemon-Lime Loco **-** Avera Sport
Purified Water • Crystalline Fructose • Corn Syrup Solids • Natural and Artificial Flavors • Ascorbic Acid • Pyridoxine Hydrochloride • Taurine • Caffeine • Potassium Gluconate • Sodium Chloride • Sodium Gluconate • Acesulfame Potassium • FD&C Yellow No. 5 • FD&C Blue No. 1 • Xanthan Gum • Sodium Benzoate • Potassium Sorbate (as preservatives).

El Toro Loco Orange Stomp **-** Avera Sport
Purified Water • Crystalline Fructose • Corn Syrup Solids • Natural and Artificial Flavors • Ascorbic Acid • Pyridoxine Hydrochloride • Taurine • Caffeine • Potassium Gluconate • Sodium Chloride • Sodium Gluconate • Acesulfame Potassium • FD&C Yellow No. 5 • FD&C Blue No. 1 • Xanthan Gum • Sodium Benzoate • Potassium Sorbate (as preservatives).

Elan Vital Multiple **-** Source Naturals
Six tablets contain: Pro-Vitamin A (beta carotene) 25000 IU • Vitamin A (palmitate) 10000 IU • Total Vitamin A activity 35000 IU • Vitamin B-1 (thiamin nitrate) 100 mg • Vitamin B-2 (riboflavin) 100 mg • Inositol Hexanicotinate, Niacinamide and Niacin 200 mg • Vitamin B-5 (calcium D-pantothenate) 100 mg • Vitamin B-6 (pyridoxine HCl) 100 mg • Vitamin B-12 (cyanocobalamin) 200 mcg • Biotin 500 mcg • Folic acid 800 mcg • Vitamin C (magnesium, manganese and zinc ascorbates) 1800 mg • Fat-Soluble Vitamin C (from 476 mg of ascorbyl palmitate) 200 mg • Total Vitamin C activity 2000 mg • Vitamin D (as Vitamin D-3, cholecalciferol) 400 IU • Vitamin E D-alpha Tocopheryl (natural) 600 IU • Boron (amino acid chelate) 2 mg • Calcium (succinate, carbonate, malate) 200 mg • Chromium (ChromeMate yeast-free polynicotinate 150 mcg and yeast-free picolinate 150 mcg) 300 mcg • Copper (sebacate) 1 mg • Iodine (from kelp) 150 mcg • Magnesium (ascorbate, oxide, succinate) 300 mg • Manganese (ascorbate) 10 mg • Molybdenum (amino acid chelate) 300 mcg • Potassium (succinate, alpha-ketoglutarate) 99 mg • Selenium (L-selenomethionine and sodium selenite) 250 mcg • Zinc (OptiZinc zinc monomethionine and ascorbate) 30 mg. Other Ingredients: N-Acetyl Cysteine 600 mg, Succinic Acid (free form) 300 mg, Choline (bitartrate) 100 mg, Inositol (hexanicotinate and inositol) 100 mg, N-A-G (N-acetyl glucosamine) 200 mg, DMAE (bitartrate) 40 mg, N-Acetyl L-Tyrosine 80 mg, Coenzyme Q10 (ubiquinone) 40 mg, alpha-Lipoic acid (thioctic acid) 40 mg, Quercetin 300 mg, Silymarin (milk thistle seed extract) 200 mg, Proanthodyn (from grape seed extract) 100 mg, Ginkgo Biloba 24% (50:1 extract) 40 mg, Bilberry extract (37% anthocyanosides) 20 mg.

Elations Cranberry Apple Twist **-** Proctor & Gamble
Each 4 oz bottle contains: Glucosamine HCl 1500 • Calcium 300 mg • Vitamin C 60 mg. Ingredients: Water, fructose, 2% or less juices from concentrate (apple, pear, cranberry), Citric Acid, Malic Acid, Calcium Hydroxide, Ascorbic Acid (vitamin C), Calcium Disodium EDTA, Red 40, Blue 1, Natural and Artificial Flavors.

Elations Ruby Red Grapefruit Lift **-** Proctor & Gamble
Each 4 oz bottle contains: Glucosamine HCl 1500 • Calcium 300 mg • Vitamin C 60 mg. Ingredients: Water, fructose, 2% or less juices from concentrate (cranberry, apple, grapefruit), Citric Acid, Malic Acid, Calcium Hydroxide, Ascorbic Acid (vitamin C), Calcium Disodium EDTA, Red 40, Blue 1, Natural and Artificial flavors.

Ela-Vites L-Phenylalanine Complex **-** Nature's Plus
Two tablets contain: L-Phenylalanine free form amino acid 600 mg • Vitamin C with Rose Hips 400 mg • L-Tyrosine free form amino acid 200 mg • Vitamin B6 (Pyridoxine HCl) 100 mg. In a natural herbal base containing Ginseng, Gotu Kola & Fo-Ti.

Elderberry **-** Natrol
Each lozenge contains: Vitamin C (as Calcium Ascorbate) 50 mg • Zinc (as Zinc Gluconate) 7.5 mg • Echinacea angustfolia entire plant 10 mg • Bee Propolis 10 mg • Slippery Elm Bark 10 mg • Elderberry 10 mg • Bee Pollen 10 mg. Other Ingredients: Hydrogenated Starch, Hydrolysate, natural Elderberry flavor, Grape skin for color.

Elderberry - Extra Strength **-** Jamieson
Each capsule contains: Elderberry fruit (Sambucus Nigra L. 40 mg powdered extract 1:50) 2000 mg.

Elderberry Lozenges **-** Quantum, Inc.
Each lozenge contains: Elderberry extract standardized to 5% total flavonoids (Sambucus nigra) 200 mg • Vitamin C (ascorbic acid) 100 mg • Marshmallow Althea powder 50 mg • Echinacea angustifolia standardized powder extract 4% phenolic compounds 25 mg • Mullein powder 10 mg. Other Ingredients: Menthol Crystals, Eucalyptus Oil, Peppermint Oil, Stevia Leaves and Stevioside, Sorbitol, Raspberry Flavoring.

Elderberry Syrup **-** Planetary Formulas
Each 1 tsp serving contains: Proprietary Blend 1.5 mL: Elderberry (4:1). Other Ingredients: Honey, Grain Alcohol (20-25%), Purified Water.

Elder-Zinc Lozenges **-** Now
Two lozenges contain: Vitamin C (Ascorbic Acid • Sodium Ascorbate) 300 mg • Zinc (as Zinc Gluconate) 24 mg • Elderberry (Sambucus nigra) 10:1 extract 200 mg • Echinacea purpurea root 50 mg • Bee Propolis 50 mg • Slippery Elm bark (Ulmus fulva) 50 mg.

Electrolyte Balance **-** The Vitamin Shoppe
Two tablets contain: Potassium 99 mg • Magnesium 500 mg • Calcium 250 mg • Boron 3 mg • Vitamin D 100 IU.

Elemax **-** Naturodoc
Each capsule contains: L-Glycine 200 mg • L-Tyrosine 150 mg • St. John's Wort (hypericum perforatum extract, 0.3% hypericin) 150 mg • Niacin (niacinol) 100 mg • 5-HTP (5-hydroxytryptophan) 25 mg • Siberian Ginseng (eleutherococcus senticosus, 1.2% eleutherosides) 25 mg • Ginkgo Biloba Extract (24% ginkgo extract) 25 mg • Colecus Forskohlii Extract (5-10% forskolin) 25 mg • Coenzyme B6 (pyridoxal-5-phosphate) 5 mg • Folic Acid 500 mcg.

Eleuthero Extract - PhytoPharmica
Each capsule contains: Siberian Ginseng root extract (eleutherococcus senticosus, standardized to contain a minimum of 0.5% eleutheroside E) 200 mg.

Elo-Plex - Progressive Labs
Each capsule contains: Vitamin C 100 mg • Vitamin B6 10 mg • Pantothenic Acid 50 mg • Zinc (as zinc proteinate) 3.3 mg • Copper (as copper proteinate) 0.3 mg • L-Tyrosine 150 mg • DL-Phenylalanine 80 mg • Adrenal 10 mg • Hypothalamus 15 mg.
See Editor's Note No. 14.

Elusan Prostate - Plantes & Medecines Inc.
Each capsule contains: Serenoa Repens Lipidosterolic extract 160 mg.

EluSun - Plantes & Medecines Inc.
Two capsules contain: Vitamin C (ascorbic acid) 30 mg • Vitamin E (alpha tocopherol acetate) 5 IU • Natural Carotenes 20 mg • Borage Oil 20 mg. Ingredients: Carrot Oil Macerate, Sunflower Oil, Soy Bean Oil, Lecithin, Gelatin, Glycerin, Purified Water.

EM PACT Drink Mix, Citrus (EMPACT, EM-PACT, EMPACT) - Mannatech
Each tablespoon contains: Calcium 40 mg • Proprietary Blend Energy/Endurance Complex 16.1 g: Fructose, Medium Chain Triglycerides, Creatine Monohydrate, Calcium Citrate, Magnesium Aspartate, Magnesium Succinate, Choline Bitartrate, L-Carnitine, Lecithin • Ambrotose Complex (patent pending) 25 mg: Arabinogalactan (larix decidua gum), Manapol Aloe Vera gel extract (inner leaf gel), Gum Ghatti, Gum Tragacanth. Other Ingredients: Citric Acid, Silicon Dioxide, Natural Flavors.

E-mergen-C - Alacer
Each packet contains: Vitamin C 1000 mg • Vitamin B1 (thiamine HCl) 0.38 mg • Vitamin B2 (riboflavin) 0.43 mg • Special Niacin complexes 5 mg • Vitamin B6 (pyridoxine HCl) 10 mg • Folic Acid 12.5 mcg • Vitamin B12 (cyanocobalamin) 25 mcg • Pantothenic Acid 2.5 mg • Calcium 50 mg • Magnesium 20 mg • Zinc 2 mg • Sodium 60 mg • Potassium 200 mg • Manganese 1.5 mg • Chromium (ascorbate) 10 mg. In a base of Citric, Tartaric, Aspartic, & Malic (apple) Acids.

Emerita - Transitions for Health, Inc.
Aloe Vera gel • Distilled Water • D-Alpha Tocopherol • Mixed Tocopherols • Cetyl Alcohol • Almond oil • Octyl Palmitate • Panthenol • Peg 8 Stearate • Glycerine • Progesterone • Polysorbate 60 • Hyaluronic Acid, Oil of Lemon, Keratin, Carbomer 940 • Grapefruit seed extract.

Emerita Hot Flash Formula - Transitions for Health, Inc.
Each capsule contains: Vitamin C (sodium ascorbate) 400 mg • Vitamin E (as d-alpha tocopheryl succinate) 100 mg • Bioflavonoids (as citrus bioflavonoid complex) 200 mg • Para-aminobenzoic acid 20 mg • Pantothenic acid (as calcium pantothenate) 20 mg • Adrenal Complex 5 mg. Other Ingredients: Rice Bran, Gelatin, Water, and Glycerin.

Emerita Libido Formula - Transitions for Health, Inc.
Each caplet contains: Calcium (from dicalciumphosphate) 86 mg • Muira Puama extract (4:1, equivalent to 700 mg, providing ptychopetalum olacoides) 175 mg • Ginkgo Biloba extract (standardized 24% ginko flavone glycosides, 6% terpene lactones) 120 mg • Motherwort (leonurus cardiaca) 100 mg • Damiana extract (turnera diffusa, 6.5:1, equivalent to 200 mg) 31 mg • Panax Ginseng root extract (50:1, equivalent to 300 mg) 6 mg. Other Ingredients: Vegetable Sterols, Cellulose, Magnesium Stearate.

Emerita Menopause Plus Formula - Transitions for Health, Inc.
Two caplets contain: Red Clover extract (standardized 8% isoflavonoids, Trifolium pratense flowering tops) 500 mg • Siberian Ginseng root (Eleutherococcus senticosus) 100 mg • Dandelion root (Taraxacum officinale) 100 mg • Dandelion leaf (Taraxacum officinale) 100 mg • Alfalfa leaf (Medicago sativa) 100 mg • Black Cohosh extract (standardized 2.5% triterpene glycosides, Cimicifuga racemosa root) 80 mg • Chaste Tree berry extract (standardized 0.6% aucubins, vitex agnus castus berries) 80 mg. Other Ingredients: Dicalcium Phosphate, Vegetable Sterols, Cellulose, Magnesium Stearate.

Emerita Response Cream - Transitions for Health, Inc.
Water • Glycerine • L-Arginine • L-Phenylalanine • L-Tyrosine • Sorbitol • Sucrose Stearate • Ginger extract (zingiber officinale) • Rosemary oil (rosemarinus officinalis) • Niacin • L-Histidine • Ginseng extract (panax ginseng) • Natural L-Menthol • Cinnamon oil (cinnamomum cassia) • Bergamot (citrus bergamia) • Cetosteryl alcohol • Ascorbyl Palmitate • Isopropyl Myristate • Octyl Palmitate • Carbomer • Triethanolamine.

Emerita - Transitions for Health, Inc.
Each capsule contains: Valerian root 100 mg • Scullcap leaf and flower 100 mg • Wild Lettuce leaves 50 mg • Lavender flowers 50 mg • Oat Straw tops 50 mg • Lady's Mantle leaves 50 mg. Other Ingredients: Rice Bran, Gelatin, Water, and Glycerin.

Em-Pact - Mannatech
Energy Complex: Fructose, Medium chain triglycerides, Creatine monohydrate, Calcium citrate, Magnesium aspartate, Magnesium succinate, Potassium aspartate, Potassium succinate, Choline bitartrate, L-carnitine, Lecithin • Ambrotose Complex: naturally occurring plant polysaccharides including freeze-dried Aloe Vera inner leaf gel extract - Manapol powder. Other Ingredients: Citric Acid, Natural Flavors.
See Editor's Note No. 17, page 2055.

Empower Plus - Truehope
Three capsules contain: Vitamin A (as retinyl palmitate) 1067 IU • Vitamin C (as ascorbic acid) 111 mg • Vitamin D (as cholecalciferol) 267 IU • Vitamin E (as d-alpha tocopheryl succinate) 67 IU • Vitamin B1 (as thiamine mononitrate) 3.33 mg • Vitamin B2 (as riboflavin) 2.5 mg • Vitamin B3 (as niacinamide) 16.7 mg • Vitamin B5 (as d-calcium pantothenate) 4 mg • Vitamin B6 (as pyridoxine hydrochloride) 6.7 mg • Vitamin B9 (as folic acid) 267 mcg • Vitamin B12 (as cyanocobalamin) 167 mcg • Vitamin H (as biotin) 20 mcg • Calcium 244 mg • Phosphorous 155 mg • Magnesium 111 mg • Potassium 44 mg • Iodine (from Pacific kelp) 33 mcg • Zinc 9 mg • Selenium 44 mcg • Copper 1.33 mg • Manganese 1.77 mg • Chromium 110 mcg • Molybdenum 29 mcg • Iron 2.66 mg • CNS Proprietary Blend 414.45 mg: DL-Phenylalanine, Glutamine, Citrus Bioflavonoids, Grape Seed, Choline Bitartrate, Inositol, Ginkgo Biloba, Methionine, Germanium Sesquioxide, Boron, Vanadium, Nickel. Other Ingredients: Gelatin.

Emprizone Gel - Mannatech
Water • Polyglyceryl Methacrylate/Propylene Glycol • Glycerin • Sorbitol • Glycereth-26 • Polysorbate 80 • Carbomer • Germaben II (propylene glycol, diazolidinyl urea, methylparaben, propylparaben) • Aminomethyl Propanol • Ambrotose Complex (patent pending): Arabinogalacan, Manapol Aloe Vera gel extract, Gum Ghatti, Gum Tragacanth • Benzethonium Chloride • Sodium Hyaluronate • Retinyll Palmitate • Allantoin • Tocopheryl Acetate.

Emulsified A Complex - Nature's Life
Each capsule contains: Vitamin A (Fish Liver oil) 7500 IU • Beta Carotene (Vitamin A equivalent to 7500 IU) 4.5 mg.

Emulsified Vitamin A Complex with Vitamin D - Puritan's Pride
Each softgel contains: Vitamin A 10,000 IU • Vitamin D 400 IU • Apple Pectin.

ENADA NADH - Menuco Corp.
Each micro tab provides: NADH 5.0 mg • Baking Soda (sodium bicarbonate) 3.0 mg • Vitamin C (sodium ascorbate) 0.3 mg. Other Ingredients: D-Mannitol, Microcrystalline Cellulose, Magnesium Stearate.

ENADA NADH **-** Life Extension
Each tablet contains: NADH (reduced B-nicotinamide adenine dinucleotide) 5 mg. Other Ingredients: D-mannitol, Sodium Bicarbonate, Sodium Ascorbate, Microcrystalline Cellulose, Magnesium Stearate, Enteric Coating.

ENADAlert **-** Pro Health
Each tablet contains: NADH (reduced 6-beta-nicotinamide adenine dinudeotide) 10 mg. Other Ingredients: D-Mannitol, Sodium Bicarbonate, Microcrystalline Cellulose, Natural Flavoring, Magnesium Stearate.

ENADAlert (e-NAD-alert) **-** Menuco Corp.
Each tablet contains: NADH 10 mg. Other Ingredients: D-Mannitol, Sodium Bicarbonate, Microcrystalline Cellulose, Natural Flavoring, Magnesium Stearate.

EnadaNADH 2.5 Mg **-** Natrol
Each micro tab contains: NADH (reduced 5-nicotinamide adenine dinucleotide) 2.5 mg • Baking Soda (Sodium Bicarbonate) 0.3 mg • Vitamin C (Sodium Ascorbate) 0.3 mg. Other Ingredients: D-Mannitol, Microcrystalline Cellulose, Magnesium Stearate.

EnadaNADH 5 Mg **-** Natrol
Each microtab contains: NADH (reduced 5-nicotinamide adenine dinucleotide) 5 mg • Baking Soda (Sodium Bicarbonate) 0.3 mg • Vitamin C (Sodium Ascorbate) 0.3 mg. Other Ingredients: D-Mannitol, Microcrystalline Cellulose, Magnesium Stearate.

End Fatigue Adrenal Stress-End **-** PhytoPharmica
Two capsules contain: Adrenal cortex extract 33 mg • Adrenal Polypeptide Fractions 400 mg • Betaine 250 mg • Licorice root and rhizome extract (glycyrrhiza glabra standardized to contain 5% glycyrrhizic acid) • L-Tyrosine 250 mg • Pantothenic Acid (calcium D-pantothenate) 100 mg • Vitamin B6 (pyridoxine HCl) 50 mg • Vitamin C (ascorbic acid/rose hip fruit) 150 mg.
See Editor's Note No. 14.

End Fatigue Daily Energy B Complex **-** PhytoPharmica
Each capsule contains: Choline Bitartrate 100 mg • Folic Acid 800 mcg • Niacin (as niacinamide) 50 mg • Pantothenic Acid (as calcium D-pantothenate) 50 mg • Riboflavin (vitamin B2) 75 mg • Thiamin (vitamin B1, as thiamin HCl) 75 mg • Vitamin B12 (as cyanocobalamin) 500 mcg • Vitamin B6 (as pyridoxine HCl) 85 mg. Other Ingredients: Gelatin, Cellulose, Modified Cellulose Gum, Magnesium Stearate, and Titanium Dioxide Color.

End Fatigue Energy Revitalization System **-** PhytoPharmica
Each rounded scoop contains: Betaine 750 mg • Biotin 200 mcg • Boron (as sodium borate) 2 mg • Chromium (as chromium picolinate) 200 mcg • Copper (as copper gluconate) 500 mcg • Glycine 390 mg • Hesperidin 50% (from citrus fruits) 500 mg • Inositol 750 mg • Inulin (from chicory root) 750 mg • Iodine (as potassium iodide) 150 mcg • L-Serine 240 mg • L-Tyrosine 377 mg • Magnesium (as magnesium glycinate) 200 mg • Malic Acid 900 mg &#8226 Manganese (as manganese citrate) 4 mg • Molybdenum (as sodium molybdate) 250 mcg • N-Acetylcysteine (NAC) 250 mg • Potassium (from whey protein, guar gum, potassium citrate, and potassium iodide) 50 mg • Selenium (as L-selenomethionine) 200 mcg • Stevia leaf 15:1 extract (stevia rebaudiana) 150 mg • Taurine 500 mg • Vitamin A (as 50% beta carotene and as retinyl acetate) 7000 IU • Vitamin C (ascorbic acid) 750 mg • Vitamin D (as cholecalciferol) 600 IU • Vitamin E (as D-alpha tocopheryl acetate) 100 IU • Whey Protein 7 g • Zinc (as zinc sulfate) 15 mg. Other Ingredients: Guar Gum, Natural Flavors.

End Fatigue Revitalizing Sleep Formula **-** PhytoPharmica
Each capsule contains: Hops flower 6.6:1 extract (humulus lupulus) • Jamaica Dogwood root extract (piscidia piscipula) 12 mg • L-Theanine (Suntheanine brand) 50 mg • Passionflower leaf and flower 4:1 extract (passiflora incarnata) 90 mg • Valerian root extract (valeriana officinalis, standardized to contain a minimum of 0.8% valerenic acids) 200 mg • Wild Lettuce leaf extract (lactuca virosa) 18 mg • Wild Lettuce leaf (lactuca virosa) 10 mg. Other Ingredients: Gelatin, Magnesium Stearate, Titanium Dioxide Color, and Silicon Dioxide.

EndoKinase **-** Longevity Plus
Each VegeCap (vegetarian) capsule contains: Nattokinase (1000 fibrin units of activity per capsul, active enzyme at 20,000 FU/gram) 50 mg.

Endorphin+ **-** PhysioLogics
Each capsule contains: DL-Phenylalanine 450 mg • White Willow bark (7.5% Salicin, 1.9 mg) 25 mg • Feverfew flower, leaf (1.2% Parthenolide, 0.3 mg) 25 mg • Ginger root (5% Gingerols, 1.25 mg) 25 mg.

Endurox **-** PacificHealth Laboratories, Inc.
Two caplets contain: Ciwujia root extract 800 mg • Calcium (sulfate) 130 mg. Other Ingredients: Microcrystalline Cellulose, Stearic Acid, Hydroxypropyl Cellulose, Magnesium Stearate, Titanium Dioxide, P.E.G., Caramel Color, Beet juice powder & Annatto extract.

Endurox Excel **-** PacificHealth Laboratories, Inc.
Each two caplets contain: Endurox (standardized root extract of the herb ciwujia) 1200 mg • Vitamin E 60 IU.

Endurox R4 **-** PacificHealth Laboratories, Inc.
Two scoops contain: Vitamin C 470 mg • Vitamin E 400 IU • Calcium 100 mg • Iron 1.8 mg • Magnesium 250 mg • Chloride 270 mg • Ciwujia (Endurox) 600 mg • L-Glutamine 420 mg • L-Arginine 1420 mg. Other Ingredients: Glucose, Whey Protein Concentrate, Crystalline Fructose, L-Arginine, Vitamin E Acetate, Ciwujia, Ascorbic Acid, Sodium Chloride, Citric Acid, L-Glutamine, Magnesium Oxide, Artificial Flavor, Potassium Phosphate, FD&C Red #40.

Endurox R4 Performance/Recovery Drink **-** PacificHealth Laboratories, Inc.
Each two rounded scoops (74.08 g) contains: Vitamin C 470 mg • Vitamin E 400 IU • Calcium 100 mg • Magnesium 250 mg • Sodium 220 mg • Potassium 120 mg • L-Glutamine 2560 mg • Branched Chain Amino Acids 2719 mg • L-Arginine 1247 mg.

Enerblast **-** Nature's Plus
Each tablet contains: Potassium Glycero-Phosphate 250 mg • Pyridoxal Alpha Ketoglutarate (PAK) 50 mg • Trimethylglycine (TMG) 25 mg • Inosine (HXR-Hypoxanthine Riboside) 25 mg • Creatine Phosphate 50 mcg.

Ener-G One Per Day **-** Vitol
Each tablet contains: Dibencozide (coenzyme B12) 3000 mcg • Boron (chelate, citrate, aspartate) 1000 mcg • Chromium (picolinate-yeast free gtf) 100 mcg • Vitamin C (calcium ascorbate/rose hips) 300 mg • Vitamin E (d-alpha tocopherol) 200 IU • Vitamin A (as beta carotene) 15,000 IU • Vitamin A (as palmitate) 10,000 IU • Vitamin D (cholecalciferol) 1000 IU • Vitamin B1 (thiamine) 75 mg • Vitamin B2 (riboflavin) 75 mg • Vitamin B6 (pyridoxine HCl) 75 mg • Vitamin B12 (cobalamin) 75 mcg • Vitamin B3 (niacinamide, niacin) 75 mg • Choline Bitartrate 30 mg • Inositol 30 mg • Para Aminobenzoic Acid 30 mg • Pantothenic Acid 30 mg • Biotin 75 mcg • Folic Acid 400 mcg • Rutin 10 mg • Citrus Bioflavonoids, Hesperidin Complex 20 mg • Quercetin (saphora japonica) 20 mg • Betaine HCl (beet molasses) 10 mg • Papain, Bromelain, Amylase, Protease, Lipase 30 mg • Glutamic Acid 10 mg • Iodine (kelp) 150 mcg • Calcium Chelate, Citrate 60 mg • Potassium Chelate, Citrate 10 mg • Iron Chelate, Citrate 10 mg • Magnesium Chelate, Citrate 20 mg • Manganese Chelate, Aspartate 3 mg • Molybdenum Chelate, Aspartate 75 mcg • Vanadium (amino acid chelate) 50 mcg • Strontium (amino acid chelate) 10 mcg • Sulfur (amino acid chelate) 5 mg • Silicon (amino acid chelate) 10 mcg • Zinc Chelate, Picolinate 20 mg • Copper Chelate, Aspartate 5 mg • Selenium (l-selenomethionine) 10 mcg • 74 Minerals, Trace Minerals 50 mg • L-Glutathione 5 mg • Free Form Amino Acids 60 mg: L-Lysine, L-Histidine, L-Isoleucine, L-Leucine, L-Phenylalanine, L-Threonine, L-Carnitine, L-Valine, L-Methionine, L-Arginine, L-Glycine, L-Taurine

(5 mg each) • Dong Quai 20 mg • Echinacea Purpurea 20 mg • Suma 20 mg • Siberian Ginseng 20 mg • Gotu Kola 10 mg • Golden Seal root 10 mg.

Energel Ephedra Free - GNC Energy - GNC
Two capsules contain: Iodine (as kelp) 37.5 mcg • Ginger Root Extract 4:1 (zingiber officinale) 25 mg • Mustard Seed Powder (sinapsis alba) 75 mg • Meadowsweet Powder (filipendula ulmaria) 100 mg • Guarana Seed Extract (paullinia cupana; 36% caffeine = 90 mg) 250 mg • Schisandra Extract 6:1 (schisandra chinensis) 8.3 mg • Indian Turmeric Extract 10:1 (curcuma longa) 4 mg • Siberian Ginseng Powder (eleutherococcus senticosus) 25 mg. Other Ingredients: Soybean Oil, Gelatin, Glycerin, Caramel Color, Titanium Dioxide (natural mineral whitener).

Energiza - HerbaSway
Bitter Orange • Panax Ginseng • Siberian Ginseng • Schisandra • Astragalus • Ginger • Kudzu • Blackberry • Licorice • HerbaSwee (Cucurbitaceae fruit).
See Editor's Note No. 40, page 2058.

Energizer Formula - Nature's Way
Two capsules contain: Proprietary Formula: Bee Pollen • Cayenne pepper fruit • Coenzyme Q10 (Ubiquinone) • Magnesium Stearate • Siberian Ginseng root • Spirulina • Thiamine (Vitamin B1) • Vitamin B12 (Cyanocobalamin). Other Ingredients: Gelatin, Millet.

Energizing Soy Protein - Creamy Cocoa - Shaklee
Three tablespoons (28 g) contain: Sugars (as fructose) 8 g • Soy protein isolate 14 g • Thiamin (as thiamin mononitrate) 2 mg • Riboflavin 2 mg • Niacin (as niacinamide) 10 mg • Vitamin B6 (as pyridoxine hydrochloride) 0.5 mg • Pantothenic acid (as calcium pantothenate) 2 mg • Calcium (as tricalcium phosphate and calcium carbonate) 500 mg • Iron 2 mg • Phosphorus (as tricalcium phosphate) 250 mg • Sodium 160 mg • Histidine 340 mg • Isoleucine 540 mg • Leucine 1160 mg • Lysine 900 mg • Methionine 180 mg • Phenylalanine 730 mg • Threonine 530 mg • Tryptophan 190 mg • Valine 690 mg. Other Ingredients: Cocoa Processed With Alkali, Natural Cocoa Flavor, Soy Lecithin, Guar Gum, Potassium Chloride.

Energizing Soy Protein - Natural Vanilla - Shaklee
Three tablespoons (28 g) contain: Sugars (as fructose and dextrose) 9 g • Soy protein isolate 14 g • Thiamin (as thiamin mononitrate) 2 mg • Riboflavin 2 mg • Niacin (as niacinamide) 10 mg • Vitamin B6 (as pyridoxine hydrochloride) 0.5 mg • Pantothenic acid (as calcium pantothenate) 2 mg • Calcium (as tricalcium phosphate and calcium carbonate) 500 mg • Iron 2 mg • Phosphorus (as tricalcium phosphate) 250 mg • Sodium 170 mg • Histidine 340 mg • Isoleucine 630 mg • Leucine 1160 mg • Lysine 890 mg • Methionine 180 mg • Phenylalanine 720 mg • Threonine 520 mg • Tryptophan 180 mg • Valine 650 mg. Other Ingredients: Soy Lecithin, Natural Vanilla Flavor, Guar Gum.

Energy - Now
Two capsules contain: Vitamin E (as d-alpha tocopheryl succinate) 15 IU • Vitamin B1 (from Thiamine HCL) 10 mg • Riboflavin (Vitamin B2) 10 mg • Niacin (Vitamin B3) 25 mg • Vitamin B6 (from Pyridoxine HCL) 10 mg • Vitamin B12 (as Cyanocobalamin) 100 mg • Vitamin B5 (from Calcium Pantothenate) 10 mg • Iodine (from Kelp) 225 mg • Chromium (as Chromium Chelavite) 200 mg • Potassium (from Potassium Aspartate) 55 mg • Guarana standardized extract (Paullinia Cupane, seed extract contains 42 mg caffeine) 280 mg • Green Tea extract (Camellia Sinensis, leaf extract contains 8 mg caffeine) 200 mg • Bitter Orange extract (Citrus Aurantium) fruit (min. 3% Synephrine) 150 mg • Panax Ginseng (5% Ginsenosides) root 150 mg • Siberian Ginseng (Eleutherococcus Senticosus) root 150 mg • Licorice (Glycyrrhiza Glabra) root 100 mg • Gotu Kola (Centella Asiatica) whole plant 100 mg • Cayenne (Capsicum annuum: 40,000 SHU) fruit 50 mg • Alpha Lipoic Acid 25 mg • COQ10 10 mg • Octacosanol (Spinach) 30 mcg. Other Ingredients: Gelatin (capsule), Magnesium Stearate.
See Editor's Note No. 40, page 2058.

Energy - Nutrivention
Each tablet contains: Pantothenic Acid 100 mg • Vitamin B12 300 mcg • Folic Acid 200 mcg • Aspartic Acid 100 mg • Gotu Kola 100 mg • Licorice root 100 mg • Siberian Ginseng 100 mg.

Energy Body Benefits Pak - Leiner Health Products
Each packet contains: Thiamin Mononitrate (Vitamin B1) 100 mg • Riboflavin (Vitamin B2) 100 mg • Vitamin B6 (Pyridoxine Hydrochloride) 100 mg • Niacin (Niacinamide) 100 mg • Biotin 100 mcg • Vitamin B12 100 mcg • Pantothenic Acid (d-Calcium Pantothenate)100 mg • Folate 400 mcg • American Ginseng extract (Panax quinquefolius) root 70 mg • Chinese Panax Ginseng extract (Panax ginseng) root 60 mg • Damiana (Turnera diffusa) leaf 2 mg • Fo-Ti (Polygonum multiflorum) root 2 mg • Gotu Kola (Centella asiatica) leaf 78 mg • Green Tea extract (Camellia sinensis) leaf (50% catechins) 2 mg • Guarana extract (Paullinia cupana) seed 78 mg • Jamaican Ginger (Zingiber officinalis) rhizome 2 mg • Korean Ginseng extract (Panax ginseng) root 70 mg • Siberian Ginseng (Eleutherococcus senticosus) root 500 mg • Yerba Mate extract (Ilex paraguariensis) leaf 575 mg. Other Ingredients: Dicalcium Phosphate, Calcium Carbonate, Croscarmellose Sodium, Hydrogenated Vegetable Oil, Cellulose.

Energy Elixir - Nature's Plus
Each serving contains: Royal Jelly lyophilized 3X-4.2% 10-HDA 250 mg • Guarana seed 125 mg • Spanish Bee Pollen 125 mg • Korean Ginseng 50 mg • Siberian Ginseng 50 mg • American Ginseng 12.5 mg. In a natural base of Purified Water, Wild Clover Honey, Citric Acid & Potassium Sorbate added to maintain freshness.

Energy Endurance Formula - Hansen's
Each can (246 mL) contains: Vitamin C 60 mg • Vitamin B2 1.7 mg • Niacin 20 mg • Vitamin B6 2 mg • Vitamin B12 6 mcg • Sodium 210 mg • Taurine 100 mg • L-Carnitine 300 mg • Panax Ginseng 200 mg. Ingredients: Carbonated Water, Sucrose, Glucose, Citric Acid, Taurine, Natural Flavors, Sodium Citrate, L-Carnitine, Natural Color, Panax Ginseng, Ascorbic Acid, Caffeine, Sodium Chloride, Niacinamide, Riboflavin, Inositol, Glucatronalactone, Pyridoxine Hydrochloride, Guarana, Cyanocobalamin.

Energy Formula - Pharmanex
Each capsule contains: Ginseng, Panax root 4:1 extract (Panax ginseng c.a. meyer) 300 mg • Schisandra berry 10:1 extract (schisandra chinensis) 100 mg • Rhodiola root (sedum rosium) 100 mg.

Energy Reserve - Clinician's Choice
Two tablets contain: Thiamin (mononitrate) 20 mg • Riboflavin 20 mg • Vitamin B12 (cyanocobalamin) 20 mcg • Siberian Ginseng Root 400 mg • Panax Ginseng Leaves 400 mg • Brazilian Guarana Seeds 200 mg • Green Tea Leaves 200 mg • Wild American Ginseng Root 100 mg • Red Chinese Ginseng Root 100 mg • Tienchi Ginseng Root 100 mg • Cayenne Fruit 20 mg • Proprietary Blend 6 mg: Bee Pollen, Citrus Bioflavonoids, Soy Isoflavones.

Energy Rush Ephedra Free - GNC Energy - GNC
Two capsules contain: Cocoa Seed Extract (theobroma cacao) 750 mg • Guarana Seed Extract (paullinia cupana; 22% caffeine = 82.5 mg) 375 mg • Citrus Aurantium Fruit Exchange (4% synephrine = 4 mg). Other Ingredients: Cellulose, Gelatin.
See Editor's Note No. 40, page 2058.

Energy Tonic Bath - Abra Therapeutics
Sodium Borate • Sodium Sulfate • Sodium Chloride • Sodium Sesquicarbonate • Olive Oil • Essential Oils Blend: Rosemary, Peppermint, Lemon, Lime, Nutmeg, Fir, Peru Balsam • Herbal Extracts Blend: Ginseng root, Ginkgo leaves, St. John's Wort flower • Chromium Oxide • Trace Mineral Salts.

Ener-T - Atrium Inc.
Each tablet contains: Primary Yeast 705 mg. Specially grown & formulated because of its content of an accessory factor known as Termitin, Complex-T or Vitamin T. This yeast also typically contains

50% Protein, trace amounts of many B-Complex Vitamins & Inositol as well as trace amounts of many minerals.

EnerX - WellQuest International, Inc.
Niacin • Zinc • Yohimbe • Tribulus Terrestris • Panax Ginseng • Guarana • Ashwagandha • Arginine • Damiana • Muira Puama • Potent Herbal Blend.

Enhancer Skin Conditioning Gel - Nu Skin Enterprises
Water (aqua) • Aloe Barbadensis leaf juice • Propylene Glycol • Glycerin • Polysorbate 20 • Hyaluronic Acid • Sodium PCA • Zinc Amino Acid Chelate • Algae extract • Sorbitol • Allantoin • Panthenol • Royal Jelly • RNA • Octyl Methoxycinnamate • Carbomer • Fragrance (parfum) • Triethanolamine • Diaxolidinyl Urea • Methylparaben • Propylparaben • Chlorophyllin - Copper complex.

Enhance-Rx - Body Wise International, Inc.
Each three capsules contain: Niacin 20 mg • Muira Puama root extract (4:1) 450 mg • L-Arginine 250 mg • Ashwagandha root extract (1% alkaloids) 150 mg • Ginkgo Biloba leaf extract (8:1) 150 mg • Oat Straw concentrate (5:1) 150 mg • Damiana leaf extract (4:1) 100 mg • Mucuna Pruriens seed extract (10% L-DOPA) 100 mg • Nettle root extract (0.8% beta sitosterols) 100 mg • Tribulus Terrestris fruit extract (45% saponins) 100 mg • Korean Ginseng root extract (5% ginsenosides) 75 mg • Horny Goat Weed aerial parts 75 mg • Catuaba bark 60 mg • Siberian Ginseng root extract (5:1) 15 mg. Inactive Ingredients: Gelatin, Cellulose, Magnesium Stearate, Silicon Dioxide.

Enlargo - Unknown
Two tablets contain: Zinc (oxide) 10 mg • Proprietary Blend 1300 mg: Jujube dates (ziziphus jujuba), L-Arginine HCl, Oat straw powder, Muira Puama bark powder, Nettles leaf powder, Cayenne powder (40 mhu), Korean Ginseng powder, Siberian Ginseng root powder, Boron Citrate, Licorice root powder, Pumpkin seed powder, Sarsaparilla root powder, Maca root powder, Oyster meat extract (4:1).

Enova Oil - ADM Kao
Dicylglycerol Oil (made from Soybean Oil and Canola Oil) • Vitamin E • Vitamin C • Polyglycerol Esters of Fatty Acids.

EnraX - Herbal Technologies, LLC
Two capsules contain: Proprietary Blend 800 mg: Epimedium Sagittatum (horny goat weed), Damiana leaves, Muira Puama, Oat Straw extract, Panax Ginseng root, Ginkgo Biloba leaves, Soy Protein, Oyster Meat, Stinging Nettle leaves, Saw Palmetto berries, Cayenne fruit powder, Tribulus Terrestris fruit, Inosine, Velvet Deer Antler. Other Ingredients: Gelatin, Magnesium Stearate.

Entrox - Baywood International
Each softgel contains: Vitamin E 0.6 IU • Perilia Oil 500 mg • Omega 3-alpha linolenic acid (ALA) 270 mg • Omega 6-linoleic acid (LA) 70 mg • Omega 9-oleic acid (OA) 65 mg.

EnurAid - Hyland's
Two tablets contain: Belladonna 6X • Cantharis 6X • Apris Mell 6X • Arnica Mont 6X • Allium Cepa 6X • Rhus Arom 6X • Equisetum Hyem 6X. Base: Lactose.
See Editor's Note No. 1, page 2053.

EnVigor - Resource Wellness
Each caplet contains: Vitamin C 60 mg • Vitamin E 30 IU • Thiamin 1.5 mg • Riboflavin 1.7 mg • Niacin 20 mg • Vitamin B6 2 mg • Vitamin B12 6 mcg • Biotin 300 mcg • Pantothenic Acid 10 mg • Calcium 260 mg • Standardized Ginkgo Biloba extract leaves 120 mg • Standardized Panax Ginseng extract root 200 mg. Other Ingredients: Dicalcium Phosphate, Microcrystalline Cellulose, Croscarmellose Sodium, Calcium Silicate, Stearic Acid, Magnesium Stearate, Methylcellulose, Hydroxypropyl Cellulose, Polyethylene Glycol.

Enviro-Gard - Aspen Group, Inc.
Four tablets contain: Vitamin A Palmitate 8000 IU • Beta Carotene 16,000 IU • Vitamin C 800 mg • Vitamin E 320 IU • Quercetin 160 mg • Zinc (gluconate) 12 mg • Copper Gluconate 0.1 mg • Yellow Dock 364 mg • Bupleurum 192 mg • Poria Cocos 192 mg • Gentian root 192 mg • Goldenseal 192 mg • Myrrh Gum 192 mg • Echinacea extract 192 mg • Milk Thistle extract (83% silymarin) 192 mg • N-Acetyl Cysteine 160 mg • Rosemary extract 160 mg • Hawthorn Berry extract 80 mg • Wild Yam root 80 mg • Wild Yam extract 77 mg • Marshmallow root 58 mg • Magnesium Ascorbate 24 mg • Grape seed extract 20 mg • Ginkgo Biloba 4 mg • Manganese Ascorbate 4 mg • Selenomethionine 80 mcg.

Enymall - Schiff
Each tablet contains: Calcium (as dicalcium phosphate, calcium carbonate) 115 mg • Phosphorous (as dicalcium phosphate) 44 mg • Pancreatic Enzymes 50 mg • Cellulase 30 mg • Papain (from papaya) 15 mg • Amylase 10 mg. Other Ingredients: Cellulose, Stearic Acid, Acacia Powder, Whey Powder, Cellulose Gum, Silicon Dioxide, Vegetable Oil Powder, Magnesium Stearate, Annatto Seed Powder, Curcumin Powder.

Enzocaine - NutriCology
Two capsules contain: Zinc (as zinc methionate) 10 mg • Selenium (50% as sodium selenite and 50% as selenomethionine) 40 mcg • Copper (as coper sebacate) 1 mg • Molybdenum (as sodium molybdate) 300 mcg • MSM (methylsulfonylmethane) 500 mg • Boswellia Serrata gum extract (standardized to 70% boswellic acid) 200 mg • Turmeric (95% curcumin) 400 mg • Bromelain (3600 MCU/g) 400 mg • Ginger (5% gingerols) 40 mg • White Willow bark extract (salix alba, standardized to 15% salicin) 50 mg. Other Ingredients: Cellulose, Stearic Acid.

ENZOGENOL - Pharmacy Express Ltd.
Each tablet contains: Enzogenol (Pinus radiata bark extract) 50 mg • Citrus Bioflavonoids 100 mg • Beta carotene (ProVitA) 5 mg • Natural Vitamin E (80 IU) 66.7 mg • Ester C 250 mg • Selenium (from selenomethionine) 75 ug • Zinc (from OptiZinc) 7.5 mg • Pyridoxine Hydrochloride (Vitamin B6) 25 mg • Cysteine 50 mg • Methionine 50 mg • Folic Acid 100 ug.

Enzolen - Enzo Nutraceuticals Ltd.
Each capsule contains: Shiitake mushroom extract 250 mg • Vitamin C 120 mg.

Enzy-Derm - Atrium Inc.
Each gram contains: Pancreatin 12 mg • Papayotin 7 mg • Bromelain 6 mg • Trypsin 4 mg • Lipase 1.5 mg • Amylase 1.5 mg • Chymotrypsin 0.15 mg. In a base containing Vitamin A & Vitamin E.
See Editor's Note No. 14.

Enzygen - Rexall - Sundown
Each tablet contains: Calcium 100 mg • Enzyme Blend 200 mg: Lipase 2400 LU, Cellulase 250 CAU, Amylase 750 SKBU, Lactose 350 LacU, Protease 100 SAPU. Other Ingredients: Dicalcium Phosphate, Croscarmellose Sodium, Magnesium Stearate.

Enzyme Aid Digestive Support - Nature's Life
Each tablet contains: Pancreatin (concentrate 4X NF) containing: (Protease activity 50000 USP IU; Amylase activity 50000 USP IU, Lipase activity 4000 USP IU) 500 mg • Glutamic Acid Hydrochloride 200 mg • Ox Bile extract 200 mg • Pepsin (NF 10000X) 200 mg • Lipase (activity 425 USP IU) 50 mg • Cellulase (activity 10 CMC-ASE IU) 10 mg.
See Editor's Note No. 14.

Enzyme Digestant - Natural Brand
Each tablet contains: Pancreatin 400 mg • Alpha Amylase 130 mg • Betaine hydrochloride 65 mg • Pepsin 65 mg • Papain 65 mg • Ox Bile Extract (8:1) 8.1 mg. Other Ingredients: Dicalcium Phosphate, Cellulose, Food Glaze.
See Editor's Note No. 14.

Enzymes - Nutrivention
Each capsule contains: Pancreatin 100 mg • Papain 60 mg • Anise (Pimpinella anisum) 50 mg • Fennel (Foeniculum vulgare) 50 mg •

Rutin 50 mg • Bromelain (natural Pineapple Enzyme) 45 mg • Trypsin 24 mg • Amylase 10 mg • Lipase 10 mg • L-Chymotrypsin 1 mg.
See Editor's Note No. 14.

Enzyte - Lifekey Healthcare, Inc.
Each tablet contains: Niacin 30 mg • Zinc (as zinc oxide) 15 mg • Enzyte Proprietary Blend 1494 mg: Tribulus Terrestris extract (aerial), L-Arginine Base, Korean Ginseng, Maca root (lepidium meyenii), Orhcic Substance, Epimedium Sagitatum extract (aerial), Yohimbe bark (pausinystalia yohimba) extract, Muira Puama (aerial), Avena Sativa extract (aerial), Ginkgo Biloba leaf extract, Saw Palmetto berries (serenoa repens), Copper Gluconate, Octacosonal, Thymus Gland. Other Ingredients: Dicalcium Phosphate, Micro-Crystalline Cellulose, Croscarmellose Sodium, Stearic Acid, Magnesium Stearate, Silica, Hypromellose, Hydroxypropyl Cellulose, Polyethylene Glycol, Titanium Dioxide, Propylene Glycol, FD&C Blue #2 Lake.

E'OLA Pak - E'OLA
Seven capsules contain: Vitamin A (as Palmitate) 12500 IU • Vitamin C (as Ascorbic Acid) 1000 mg • Calcium (as Calcium Carbonate) 1000 mg • Iron (as Ferrous Fumarate) 10 mg • Vitamin D (as Cholecalciferol) 667 IU • Vitamin E (as dl-Alpha Tocopheryl Succinate) 400 IU • Vitamin K (as Phytonadione) 50 mcg • Thiamin (Vitamin B1) 75 mg • Riboflavin (Vitamin B2) 75 mg • Niacin (80% as Niacinamide) 150 mg • Vitamin B6 (as Pyridoxine HCl) 75 mg • Folic Acid 800 mcg • Vitamin B12 (as Cyanocobalamin) 1000 mcg • Biotin 200 mcg • Pantothenic Acid (as D-Calcium Pantothenate) 150 mg • Phosphorus (as Phosphorus Protienate) 30 mg • Iodine (as Potassium Iodide) 100 mcg • Magnesium (as Magnesium Oxide) 500 mg • Zinc (as Amino Acid Chelate) 10 mg • Selenium (as Amino Acid Chelate) 100 mcg • Copper (as Amino Acid Chelate) 1 mg • Manganese (as Amino Acid Chelate) 2 mg • Chromium (as Amino Acid Chelate) 100 mcg • Molybdenum (as Amino Acid Chelate) 10 mcg • Boron 2 mg • Pine bark extract 5 mg • Grape (Seed) Extract 40 mg • Green Tea Extract 100 mg • Alpha-Lipoic Acid 35 mg • E'OLA Mineral Blend 10 mg. Other Ingredients: Potassium Chloride, Silica, Magnesium Stearate.

EPA - Nordic Naturals
Two softgels contain: Vitamin E (mixed tocopherols) 22 IU • Omega-3 Fatty Acids 1200 mg • EPA (eicosapentaenoic acid) 900 mg • DHA (docosahexaenoic acid) 200 mg • Other Omega-3 100 mg. Other Ingredients: Purified Deep Sea Fish Oil, Softgel Capsule (gelatin, water, glycerin, natural lemon oil), Antioxidant Blend (lecithin, ascorbyl palmitate), Rosemary Extract.

EPA Natural Fish Oil - Puritan's Pride
Each softgel contains: EPA (Eicosapentaenoic Acid) 180 mg • DHA (Docosahexaenoic Acid) 120 mg.

EPA with Garlic - Puritan's Pride
Each softgel contains: Marine Lipid Concentrate 1000 mg • EPA (Eicosapentaenoic Acid) 180 mg • DHA (Docosahexaenoic Acid) 120 mg • Odorless Garlic powder 50 mg • Vitamin E (d-Alpha Tocopherol) 10 IU.

EPA-1000 - PhysioLogics
Each softgel contains: Vitamin E (d-Alpha Tocopherol) 10 IU • Marine Lipid concentrate (18% EPA, 12% DHA) 1000 mg.

EPA-DHA Liquid - Metagenics
Each 1 tsp (5 mL) serving contains: EPA (eicosapentaenoic acid) 630 mg • DHA (docosahexaenoic acid) 630 mg • Other Omega-3 Fatty Acids 240 mg.

EPAForte - Nature's Plus
Each softgel contains: Marine Lipid concentrate 900 mg supplying: Eicosapentaenoic Acid (EPA) 162 mg, Docosahexaenoic Acid (DHA) 108 mg, total Omega-3 Fatty Acids 270 mg • Magnesium Aspartate equivalent to 60 mg of elemental Magnesium 300 mg • Vitamin E natural 50 IU • Vitamin B6 (Pyridoxine HCL) 10 mg • Garlic equivalent to 500 mg of fresh garlic 1 mg • Selenium, Biotron yeast-free amino acid complex 25 mcg.

EPH 833 - AST Sports Science
Two capsules contain: Magnesium (as magnesium salicylate) 60 mg • TX-6 1460 mg: Green Tea leaf extract (standardized for epigallocatechin gallate EGCG), L-Phenylalanine, Caffeine (as caffeine anhydrous), Norsynephrine HCl, Theobromine HCl.

EPH-833 - AST Sports Science
Each capsule contains: standardized 8% Ephedra extract 750 mg.
See Editor's Note No. 30, page 2056.

Ephedra Plus - PhytoPharmica
Each capsule contains: Ephedrine from 200 mg of Ma Huang extract (Ephedra sinensis) 12 mg • Ginger root extract 6.5:1 (Zingiber officinale) 65 mg • Licorice root extract (Glycyrrhiza glabra) standardized to contain 5% glycyrrhizic acid 50 mg • Marshmallow root extract 4:1 (Althaea officinalis; Mucilage content of 30-40%) 50 mg • Sundew Herb extract 4:1 (Drosera rotundifolia) 40 mg • Euphorbia Herb extract 4:1 (Euphorbia hirta) 40 mg • Senega root extract 4:1 (Polygala senega) 40 mg • Goldenseal root extract (Hydrastis canadensis) standardized to contain 5% total alkaloids, including berberine, hydrastine, & canadine 20 mg.
See Editor's Note No. 30, page 2056.

Ephedra Super Cap - D & E Pharmaceuticals
Each capsule contains: 883 mg of pure Ephedra extract.
See Editor's Note No. 30, page 2056.

Ephedra-Free - GNC Total Lean - GNC
Two tablets contain: Proprietary Blend 1350 mg: Guarana Seed Extract (paullinia cupana), Black Tea Leaves Extract (camellia sinensis), Grape Skin Extract (vitis vinifera), Ginger Root Extract (zingiber officinale), Grape Seed Extract (vitis vinifera), Dill Weed Extract (anethum graveolens). Other Ingredients: Dextrose, Cellulose, Starch Caramel Color, Titanium Dioxide, Ethyl Vanillin.

Ephedrine Formula 100 - D & E Pharmaceuticals
Each tablet contains: Ephedrine HCL 25 mg • Guaifenesin 100 mg.

Ephedrine Formula 200 - D & E Pharmaceuticals
Each tablet contains: Ephedrine HCL 25 mg • Guaifenesin 200 mg.

Ephedrine HCL 25 mg - D & E Pharmaceuticals
Each tablet contains: Ephedrine HCL 25 mg.

Ephedrine Sulphate 25 mg - D & E Pharmaceuticals
Each tablet contains: Ephedrine Sulphate 25 mg.

Epidril Cutting Gel (100% Solution) - Nutra Sport
Lecithin • Octyl-Palmitate • Water • Aminophylline • Isopropylparaben • Isobutylparaben • Butylparaben • Fragrance.

Episilk hand & body lotion - Hyalogic LLC
De-Ionized Water • Emulsifying wax • Vitis Vinifera Grapeseed oil • Caprylic/Capric Glycerides • Soy wax • Hyaluronic Acid • Persea Gratissima (avocado oil) • Simmondsia Chinensis (jojoba seed oil) • Aloe Barbadensis leaf juice • Stearyl Alcohol • Limnanthes Alba (meadowfoam) seed oil • Glucose • Glucose Oxidase • Lactoperoxidase • Butyrospermum Parkii (shea butter) • Vegetable Glycerine • Sorbitol • Tocopherol (vitamin E) • Bees wax • Methyl Cellulose • Cyamopsis Tetragonoloba (guar) gum • Allantoin.

Episilk premium facial cream - Hyalogic LLC
De-Ionized Water • Emulsifying Wax • Grapeseed oil • Caprylic/Capric Glycerides • Soy Wax • Stearyl Alcohol • Avocado oil • Jojoba oil • Aloe Vera • Meadowfoam seed oil • Hyaluronic Acid • Shea Butter • Vegetable Glycerine • Sorbitol • Vitamin E • Bees Wax • Methyl Cellulose • Guar Gum • Lactoperoxidase • Glucose Oxidase • Allantoin.

EPO Evening Primrose Oil - NutriCology
Each softgel contains: Evening Primrose Oil 500 mg providing Gamma-Linolenic Acid (omega-6) 45 mg and Linoleic Acid (omega-6) 375 mg.

Some Brand Name Natural Products - What they Contain

www.NaturalDatabase.com contains MANY more listings than appear here.

Epoch Rare Earth Mineral Infusions Firming - Nu Skin Enterprises
Copper Gluconate • Diospyros Virginiana leaf powder (persimmon).

Epoch Rare Earths Mineral Infusions Clarifying - Nu Skin Enterprises
Calcium Carbonate • Citrus Aurantium Amara powder (bitter orange).

Epoch Rare Earths Mineral Infusions DeStressing - Nu Skin Enterprises
Mother of Pearl Powder • Cucumis Sativus fruit powder (cucumber).

Epogam - Pharmacia Corp.
Each capsule contains: Gamolenic Acid (GLA) 40 mg • Vitamin E (d-alpha tocopheryl acetate) 10 mg.
See Editor's Note No. 27, page 2056.

Epresat Multivitamin - Flora, Inc.
Each tablet contains: Vitamin A • Vitamin B1 • Vitamin B2 • Vitamin B6 • Vitamin C • Vitamin D • Vitamin E • Niacinamide

E-Prime - USANA Health Sciences
Each capsule contains: Vitamin E (as d-alpha tocopherol) 200 IU • D-Gamma Tocotrienol 7 mg • Mixed Tocopherols 3.4 mg. Other Ingredients: Medium Chain Glycerides, Gelatin, Purified Water, Lecithin.

EQ-10 - E'OLA
Ten drops contain: Proprietary Blend 149 mg: DMAE Bitartrate, Aloe Vera Juice, Ginseng Root, Co-Enzyme Q-10, Chromium Chelavite, Kelp, Licorice Root, Royal Jelly, White Willow Bark, L-Arginine, L-Tyrosine, Manganese Chelazome, Cyanocobalamin. Other Ingredients: Water, Glycerin, Sodium Benzoate.

Equal Ratio CAL-MAG - Quest
Each tablet contains: Calcium (HVP Chelate) 100 mg • Magnesium (HVP Chelate) 100 mg • Vitamin D (as Vitamin D3) 200 IU. Other Ingredients: Croscarmellose Sodium, Magnesium Stearate (vegetable source), Microcrystalline Cellulose, Vegetable Stearin.

Ericsson's Alka-Mine Coral Calcium - KingsWay, Inc.
Coral Calcium • Magnesium • Ascorbic Acid • Silver.

Erotikava - Pacific Sensuals
Each 1 oz. serving contains: Vanuatu Kava Kava • Honey • Ginger • Lycium • Epimedium • Polygala • Liquid Amber • Saigon Cinnamon bark • Licorice • Vegetable Glycerine • Cnidium seed.

Esberitox - Enzymatic Therapy/PhytoPharmica
Three tablets contain: Echinacea Purpurea and Pallida root 1:1 (coneflower root) 22.5 mg • Thuja leaf (thuja occidentalis/white cedar leaf) 6 mg • Wild Indigo root (baptisia tinctoria) 30 mg.

Escalation - Enzymatic Therapy
Each capsule contains: Cola Nut extract (Cola nitida) (contains Caffeine 35 mg) 250 mg • Green Tea extract (Camellia sinensis) (contains Caffeine 15 mg) 250 mg • Ma Huang extract (Ephedra sinensis) (contains Ephedrine 15 mg) 250 mg.
See Editor's Note No. 21 and No. 30.

Escalation (Ephedra-FREE!) - Enzymatic Therapy
Each capsule contains: Bitter Orange fruit extract (citrus x aurantium, standardized to contain 6% synephrine) 250 mg • Cola nut extract (cola nitida, standardized to contain 35 mg caffeine) 250 mg • Green Tea leaf extract (camellia sinensis, containing 15 mg caffeine) 110 mg. Other Ingredients: Gelatin, Cellulose, Magnesium Stearate, Silicon Dioxide, Titanium Dioxide Color.
See Editor's Note No. 40, page 2058.

Escalert - Enzymatic Therapy
Two capsules contain: Cola Nut extract (cola nitida, contains caffeine 35 mg) 250 mg • Green Tea extract (camellia sinensis, contains Caffeine 15 mg) 250 mg • Oat Straw extract 10:1 (avena sativa) 50 mg • Schisandra extract (standardized to contain 9% schizandrin) 50 mg • Siberian Ginseng extract (eleutherococcus senticosus, standardized to contain greater than 1% eleutherosides E) 50 mg • Ginger root extract 6.5:1 (zingiber officinale) 25 mg • Korean Ginseng root extract (panax ginseng, standardized to contain 7% saponins calculated as ginsenoside Rg1) 10 mg • Chromium (polynicotinate) 100 mcg.

Esiak Caps - Now
Each capsule contains: 450 mg Proprietary Blend: Burdock (Articum Lappa) root (4:1 extract) • Sheep Sorrel (Rumex Acetosella) leaf (4:1 extract) • Slippery Elm bark (Ulmus fulva) bark (4:1 extract) • Turkey Rhubarb (Rheum palmatum) root (4:1 extract). Other Ingredients: Maltodextrin, Magnesium Stearate.

Eskimo-3 - PhytoPharmica
Three softgel capsules contain: Eskimo-3 brand Fish Oil containing Omega-3 Fatty Acids including 210-270 mg EPA (eicosapentaenoic acid) and 125-175 mg DHA (docosahexaenoic acid) 1.5 g. Other Ingredients: Gelatin, Glycerin, Mixed Tocopherols, Natural Lime Flavor, Natural Rosemary Flavor, Lecithin, Ascorbyl Palmitate.

Eskimo-3 - Enzymatic Therapy
Each softgel contains: Omega-3 Fatty Acids (provides EPA [eicosapentaenoic acid] 260 mg, DHA [docosahexaenoic acid] 165 mg) 600 mg. Other Ingredients: Gelatin, Glycerin, Mixed Tocopherols, Lemon Oil, Rosemary, Lecithin, Ascorbyl Palmitate.

Eskimo-3 (capsules) - Tyler - Integrative Therapeutics
Three capsules contain: Vitamin E (mixed tocopherols) 6.7 IU • Omega-3 Fatty Acids 600 mg • EPA (eicosapentaenoic acid) 260 mg • DHA (docosahexaenoic acid) 166 mg. Ingredients: Fish Oil, Gelatin, Glycerin, Mixed Tocopherols, Lemon Oil, Rosemary, Lecithin, Ascorbyl Palmitate.

Eskimo-3 (liquid) - Tyler - Integrative Therapeutics
Each teaspoon (5 mL) contains: Vitamin E (as mixed tocopherols) 20 IU • Omega-3 Fatty Acids 1.8 g • EPA (eicosapentaenoic acid) 750 mg • DHA (docosahexaenoic acid) 500 mg. Ingredients: Fish Oil, Mixed Tocopherols, Lemon Oil, Rosemary, Lecithin, Ascorbyl Palmitate.

Especially for MEN - The Vitamin Shoppe
Two capsules contain: Vitamin A 5000 IU • Vitamin C 30 mg • Vitamin D 200 IU • Vitamin E 100 IU • Vitamin K 75 mcg • Niacin 30 mg • Vitamin B1 30 mg • Vitamin B2 30 mg • Vitamin B6 30 mg • Folic Acid 400 mcg • Vitamin B12 30 mcg • Biotin 250 mcg • Pantothenic Acid 30 mg • Calcium 200 mg • Iodine 150 mcg • Magnesium 100 mg • Zinc 25 mg • Selenium 100 mcg • Copper 2 mg • Manganese 5 mg • Chromium 50 mcg • Chloride 28 mg • Beta-carotene 3 mg • Potassium 30 mg • Silica 10 mcg • Choline 10 mg • Inositol 10 mg • PABA 10 mg • Citrus Bioflavonoids 25 mg • Korean Ginseng 70 mg • Damiana leaf 70 mg • Oat Straw 50 mg • Garlic 50 mg • Oyster extract 50 mg • Prostate Glandular 50 mg • Saw Palmetto 50 mg • L-Cysteine 50 mg • Nettles leaf 30 mg • Pumpkin seed 30 mg • L-Methionine 10 mg • Alpha Lipoic Acid 5 mg • Lycopene 1 mg.

Especially for Women - The Vitamin Shoppe
Three capsules contain: Vitamin A Activity 10000 IU • Vitamin E 200 IU • Vitamin D 200 IU • Vitamin C 250 mg • Selenium 50 mcg • Vitamin B1 25 mg • Vitamin B2 25 mg • Niacinamide 25 mg • Vitamin B6 25 mg • Vitamin B12 250 mcg • Pantothenic Acid 25 mg • Citrus Bioflavonoids 100 mg • Biotin 100 mcg • Folic Acid 400 mcg • Choline Bitartrate 25 mg • Inositol 25 mg • PABA 25 mg • Calcium 200 mg • Magnesium 100 mg • Potassium 25 mg • Phosphorus 50 mg • Manganese 15 mg • Zinc 15 mg • Iron 18 mg • Chromium 50 mcg • Iodine 225 mcg • Boron 3 mg • Silica 5 mg • Black Currant 100 mg • Dong Quai 50 mg • Royal Jelly 100 mg.

Especially Yours - Nature's Plus
Each tablet contains: Vitamin A (as beta carotene) 10,000 IU • Vitamin C (corn free) 300 mg • Vitamin D (calciferol) 400 IU • Vitamin E (natural) 400 IU • Vitamin B1 (as thiamine HCl) 10 mg •

Vitamin B2 (as riboflavin) 10 mg • Niacin 10 mg • Vitamin B6 (as pyridoxine HCl) 100 mg • Folate (as folic acid) 800 mcg • Vitamin B12 (as cyanocobalamin) 100 mcg • Biotin 200 mcg • Pantothenic Acid (as calcium pantothenate) 50 mg • Calcium (as aminoate) 150 mg • Iron (aspartate) 40 mg • Iodine (kelp) 225 mcg • Magnesium (as aminoate) 300 mg • Zinc (picolinate) 20 mg • Selenium (as aminoate) 10 mcg • Manganese (ascorbate) 6.1 mg • Chromium (as aminoate) 15 mcg • Potassium (citrate) 15 mg • Inositol 25 mg • Choline (as bitartrate) 11 mg • PABA (para-aminobenzoic acid) 10 mg • Lemon Bioflavonoid Complex (active flavnols, flavonones, flavones & naringen - 44%) 50 mg • Rutin (Saphora japonica leaf) 25 mg • Amylase 30,000 units • Lipase 5000 units • Flax Seed (naturally supplying linolenic, linoleic and oleic acids) 100 mg • Black Currant seed (naturally supplying GLA) 25 mg • SUMA 50 mg • Dong Quai 50 mg • Damiana 50 mg • Buchu leaves 25 mg.

Essential 50+ - Nature Made

Each tablet contains: Vitamin A (vitamin A acetate) 5000 IU • Vitamin C (ascorbic acid) 120 mg • Vitamin D 400 IU • Vitamin E (DL-alpha tocopherol acetate) 60 IU • Vitamin K (phylloquinone) 10 mcg • Thiamin (B1, thiamin mononitrate) 3 mg • Riboflavin (B2) 3.4 mg • Niacin (B3, niacinamide ascorbate) 20 mg • Vitamin B6 (pyridoxine hydrochloride) 4 mg • Folate, Folic Acid, Folacin 400 mcg • Vitamin B12 (cyanocobalamin) 25 mcg • Biotin 30 mcg • Pantothenic Acid (D-calcium pantothenate) 10 mg • Calcium (calcium carbonate) 200 mg • Phosphorus 48 mg • Iodine (potassium iodide, kelp) 150 mcg • Magnesium (magnesium oxide) 100 mg • Zinc (zinc oxide) 15 mg • Selenium (sodium selenate) 50 mcg • Copper (copper oxide) 2 mg • Manganese (manganese sulfate) 2 mg • Chromium (chromium chloride) 120 mcg • Molybdenum (sodium molybdate) 25 mcg • Chloride 72 mg • Potassium (potassium chloride) 80 mcg • Nickel (nickelous sulfate) 5 mcg • Silicon (sodium metasilicate) 2 mg • Boron (sodium borates) 150 mcg • Vanadium (sodium metavanadate) 10 mcg • Lutein 250 mcg. Other Ingredients: Dibasic Calcium Phosphate, Cellulose Gel, Crospovidone, Gelatin, Acacia, Hydroxypropyl Methylcellulose, Silicon Dioxide, Corn Starch, Magnesium Stearate, Corn Oil, Modified Food Starch, Polyethylene Glycol.

See Editor's Note No. 45, page 2058.

Essential B Complete - Rexall - Sundown

Each tablet contains: Thiamin (as thiamin mononitrate) 1.5 mg • Riboflavin (Vitamin B-2) 1.7 mg • Niacin (as niacinamide) 20 mg • Vitamin B-6 (as pyridoxine HCl) 2 mg • Folic Acid 400 mcg • Vitamin B-12 (as cyanocobalamin) 6 mcg • Calcium 35 mg. Other Ingredients: Dicalcium Phosphate, Cellulose, Croscarmellose Sodium, Hydroxypropyl Methylcellulose, Magnesium Stearate, Triethyl Citrate.

Essential Balance - Nature Made

Each tablet contains: Vitamin A (vitamin A acetate) 5000 IU • Vitamin C (ascorbic acid) 120 mg • Vitamin D (vitamin D3) 400 IU • Vitamin E (DL-alpha tocopherol acetate) 50 IU • Vitamin K (phylloquinone) 25 mcg • Thiamin (B1, thiamin mononitrate) 1.5 mg • Riboflavin (B2) 1.7 mg • Niacin (B3, niacinamide ascorbate) 20 mg • Vitamin B6 (pyridoxine hydrochloride) 2 mg • Folate, Folic Acid, Folacin 400 mcg • Vitamin B12 (cyanocobalamin) 6 mcg • Biotin 20 mcg • Pantothenic Acid (D-calcium pantothenate) 10 mg • Calcium (dibasic calcium phosphate) 100 mg • Iron (ferrous fumarate) 9 mg • Phosphorus 77 mg • Iodine (potassium iodide) 150 mcg • Magnesium (magnesium oxide) 100 mg • Zinc (zinc oxide) 15 mg • Selenium (sodium selenate) 25 mcg • Copper (copper oxide) 2 mg • Manganese (manganese sulfate) 2 mg • Chromium (chromium chloride) 120 mcg • Molybdenum (sodium molybdate) 25 mcg • Chloride 36 mg • Potassium (potassium chloride) 40 mg • Nickel (nickelous sulfate) 5 mcg • Tin (stannous chloride) 10 mcg • Silicon (sodium metasilicate) 2 mg • Vanadium (sodium metavanadate) 10 mcg • Boron (sodium borate) 150 mcg • Lutein 250 mcg. Other Ingredients: Cellulose Gel, Croscarmellose Sodium, Stearic Acid, Gelatin, Magnesium Stearate, Silicon Dioxdie, Corn Starch, Hydroxypropyl Methylcellulose, Polyethylene Glycol.

See Editor's Note No. 45, page 2058.

Essential Bodyguard - Rexall - Sundown

Two tablets contain: Vitamin A (from retinyl acetate and 25% as beta-carotene) 4000 IU • Vitamin C 600 mg • Vitamin D (from cholecalciferol) 160 IU • Vitamin E (from dl-alpha-tocopheryl acetate and d-alpha-tocopheryl acid succinate) 120 IU • Thiamin (from thiamin HCl) 4 mg • Riboflavin (Vitamin B2) 8 mg • Niacin (as niacinamide) 4 mg • Vitamin B-6 (from pyridoxine HCl) 40 mg • Folic Acid 160 mcg • Vitamin B-12 (as cyanocobalamin) 100 mcg • Biotin 100 mcg • Pantothenic Acid (from calcium d-pantothenate) 40 mg • Calcium 20 mg • Iron (from ferrous fumarate) 4 mg • Magnesium (from magnesium oxide) 80 mg • Zinc (from zinc gluconate) 20 mg • Selenium (from selenium amino acid chelate) 80 mcg • Copper (from copper gluconate) 0.8 mg • Manganese (from manganese gluconate) 2 mg • Sodium 5 mg • Whey Protein Concentrate 200 mg • Echinacea Purpurea root 120 mg • Rutin 30 mg • Choline Bitartrate 40 mg • Goldenseal aerial parts 24 mg • Garlic extract 15:1 bulb 8 mg. Other Ingredients: Croscarmellose Sodium, Cellulose, Stearic Acid, Sodium Starch Glycolate, Magnesium Stearate, Silica, Hydroxypropyl Methylcellulose, Hydroxypropyl Cellulose, PEG.

Essential Daily - Nature Made

Each tablet contains: Vitamin A (vitamin A acetate) 5000 IU • Vitamin C (ascorbic acid) 60 mg • Vitamin D 400 IU • Vitamin E (DL-alpha tocopherol acetate) 30 IU • Thiamin (B1, thiamine mononitrate) 1.5 mg • Riboflavin (B2) 1.7 mg • Niacin (B3, niacinamide ascorbate) 20 mg • Vitamin B6 (pyridoxine hydrochloride) 2 mg • Folate, Folic Acid, Folacin 400 mcg • Vitamin B12 (cyanocobalamin) 6 mcg • Pantothenic Acid (D-calcium pantothenate) 10 mg • Calcium (calcium carbonate) 450 mg • Iron (ferrous fumarate) 18 mg • Zinc (zinc oxide) 15 mg. Other Ingredients: Cellulose Gel, Croscarmellose Sodium, Glycerides of Fatty Acids, Acacia, Maltodextrin, Hydroxypropyl Methylcellulose, Magnesium Stearate, Corn Starch, Modified Food Starch, Polyethylene Glycol.

See Editor's Note No. 45, page 2058.

Essential E - PhysioLogics

Each softgel contains: Vitamin E (as d-alpha tocopheryl acetate) 400 IU. Other Ingredients: Gelatin, Soybean Oil, Glycerin.

Essential Enzymes - Source Naturals

Each capsule contains: Vegetal analog of Pancreatin with acid-stable Protease (28652 FCC) 298 mg • Lipase (375 FCC) 125 mg • Alpha Amylase (630 FCC) 52 mg • Amyloglucosidase (2 FCC) 12.5 mg • Cellulase (100 FCC) 5 mg • Hemicellulase (650 FCC) 3 mg • Lactase (40 FCC) 5 mg.

See Editor's Note No. 14.

Essential Fatty Acid Complex - Health Smart Vitamins

Three softgels contain: Vitamin E (as d-alpha tocopherol) 30 IU • Eicosapentaenoic Acid (EPA: from marine lipids) 180 mg • Docosahexaenoic Acid (DHA: from marine lipids) 120 mg • Gamma Linolenic Acid (GLA: from borage oil) 45 mg.

Essential Fatty Acids - Nutri-Quest Rx

Each capsule contains: Cod Liver 500 mg • Flaxseed oil 135 mg • Extra Virgin Olive oil 135 mg • Vitamin A 1190 IU • Vitamin D 124 IU. Also contains: Oleic, Linoleic, Palmitic, Arachidic & Linolenic, Eicosapentaenoic, & Docosahexaenoic.

Essential Fish Oil Concentrate - Rexall - Sundown

Three softgels contain: Vitamin E (as dl-alpha-tocopheryl acetate) 300 IU • Fish Oil (Eicosapentaenoic Acid 540 mg, Docosahexaenoic Acid 360 mg) 3 g. Other Ingredients: Gelatin, Glycerin, Water.

Essential Man - Nature Made

Each tablet contains: Vitamin C 120 mg • Vitamin K 25 mcg • Thiamin 1.5 mg • Riboflavin 1.7 mg • Niacin 20 mg • Vitamin B6 2 mg • Folic Acid 400 mcg • Vitamin B12 6 mcg • Biotin 30 mcg • Pantothenic Acid 10 mg • Calcium 100 mg • Phosphorus 77 mg •

Iodine 150 mcg • Magnesium 100 mg • Zinc 15 mg • Selenium 25 mcg • Copper 2 mg • Manganese 2 mg • Chromium 120 mcg • Molybdenum 25 mcg • Chloride 36 mg • Potassium 40 mg • Boron 150 mcg • Nickel 5 mcg • Silicon 2 mg • Tin 10 mcg • Lutein 250 mcg • Vanadium 10 mcg • Lycopene 2 mg. Other Ingredients: Dibasic Calcium Phosphate, Cellulose Gel, Croscarmellose Sodium, Gelatin, Sugar, Corn Starch, Magnesium Stearate, Hydroxypropyl Methylcellulose, Modified Food Starch, Polyethylene Glycol.
See Editor's Note No. 45, page 2058.

Essential Man 50+ **-** Nature Made
Each tablet contains: Vitamin C 120 mg • Vitamin K 10 mcg • Thiamin 2 mg • Riboflavin 3.4 mg • Niacin 20 mg • Vitamin B6 4 mg • Folic Acid 400 mcg • Vitamin B12 25 mcg • Biotin 30 mcg • Pantothenic Acid 10 mg • Calcium 2000 mg • Phosphorus 48 mg • Iodine 150 mcg • Magnesium 100 mg • Zinc 15 mg • Selenium 100 mcg • Copper 2 mg • Manganese 2 mg • Chromium 120 mcg • Molybdenum 25 mcg • Chloride 72 mg • Potassium 80 mg • Boron 150 mcg • Nickel 5 mg • Silicon 2 mg • Vanadium 10 mcg • Lutein 250 mcg • Lycopene 2 mg • Vitamin A 5000 IU • Vitamin D 400 IU • Vitamin E 60 IU. Other Ingredients: Dibasic Calcium Phosphate, Cellulose Gel, Croscarmellose Sodium, Gelatin, Sugar, Corn Starch, Acacia, Magnesium Stearate, Hydroxypropyl Methylcellulose, Modified Food Starch, Polyethylene Glycol.
See Editor's Note No. 45, page 2058.

Essential Meal **-** Gary Null & Associates (GNA)
Fortified with branched chain amino acids.

Essential Minerals **-** Futurebiotics
Four tablets contain: Calcium (carbonate, aspartate, citrate) 1000 mg • Magnesium (oxide, aspartate, citrate) 800 mg • Vitamin D 200 IU • Boron (citrate) 3 mg • Iron (gluconate) 9 mg • Manganese (amino acid chelate) 5 mg • Copper (gluconate) 1.5 mg • Zinc (gluconate) 15 mg • Betaine HCl 250 mg • Potassium (chloride, proteinate) 75 mg.

Essential Nutrients **-** Progressive Labs
Six capsules contain: Vitamin A (retinyl palmitate) 10,000 IU • Vitamin A (beta carotene) 15,000 IU • Vitamin C (ascorbic acid) 1000 mg • Vitamin D (cholecalciferol) 80 IU • Vitamin E (d-alpha tocopheryl succinate) 400 IU • Thiamin (Vitamin B1) 50 mg • Riboflavin-5-Phosphate (Vitamin B2) 20 mg • Niacin 25 mg • Niacinamide 125 mg • Vitamin B6 (pyridoxine HCl with pyridoxal-5'-phosphate) 20 mg • Folate (folic acid) 800 mcg • Vitamin B12 (cyanocobalamin with adenosylocobalamin) 500 mcg • Biotin 800 mcg • Pantothenic Acid (d-calcium pantothenate) 500 mg • Calcium (aspartate & carbonate) 500 mg • Iodine (potassium iodide) 225 mcg • Magnesium (aspartate and oxide) 500 mg • Zinc (picolinate) 25 mg • Selenium (selenomethionine) 200 mcg • Copper (glycinate & oxide) 2 mg • Manganese (aspartate & sulfate) 20 mg • Chromium (as chromium picolinate) 200 mcg • Molybdenum (sodium molybdate) 100 mcg • Potassium (aspartate and chloride) 99 mg • Boron (chelate) 3 mg • Vanadium (vanadyl sulfate) 100 mcg • Choline Citrate 250 mg.

Essential Oils **-** Puritan's Pride
Each softgel contains: Flaxseed oil 400 mg • Borage oil 400 mg • Super EPA 400 mg • Oleic Acid (Omega 9) 152 mg • Linoleic Acid (Omega 6) 180 mg • Gamma/Alpha Linolenic Acid (Omega 3) 260 mg • Eicosapentaenoic Acid (EPA) 120 mg • Docosahexaenoic Acid (DHA) 80 mg • Vitamin E (d-alpha tocopherol) 5 IU.

Essential Omega-3 Complex **-** Shaklee
Three capsules contain: Vitamin E 9 IU • EPA (Eicosapentaenoic acid) 545 mg • DHA (Docosahexaenoic acid) 235 mg • Omega-3 fatty acid blend 195 mg. Other Ingredients: Natural Marine Lipid Concentrate, Mixed Tocopherols Concentrate, Gelatin, Glycerin, Water.

Essential Stuff Gel Caps - 1000 mg **-** Blue Stuff, Inc.
Each gel cap contains: Proprietary Blend 1000 mg: Pure Emu oil • Gelatin • Vitamin E.

Essential Stuff Gel Caps - 750 mg **-** Blue Stuff, Inc.
Each gel cap contains: Proprietary Blend 750 mg: Pure Emu oil • Gelatin • Vitamin E.

Essential Stuff Liquid **-** Blue Stuff, Inc.
Each 16 oz bottle contains: Emu oil • Safflower oil • Natura & Artificial Flavor • Aloe Vera oil • Stevia • Tocopherol.

Essential Woman **-** Nature Made
Each tablet contains: Vitamin A 3000 IU • Vitamin C 120 mg • Vitamin D 400 IU • Vitamin E 50 IU • Vitamin K 100 mcg • Thiamin 1.5 mg • Riboflavin 1.7 mg • Niacin 20 mg • Vitamin B6 2 mg • Folic Acid 400 mcg • Vitamin B12 6 mcg • Biotin 30 mcg • Pantothenic Acid 10 mg • Calcium 250 mg • Iron 18 mg • Phosphorus 77 mg • Iodine 150 mcg • Magnesium 100 mg • Zinc 15 mg • Selenium 25 mcg • Copper 2 mg • Manganese 2 mg • Chromium 120 mcg • Molybdenum 25 mcg • Chloride 36 mg • Potassium 40 mg • Boron 150 mcg • Nickel 5 mcg • Silicon 2 mg • Tin 10 mcg • Vanadium 10 mcg • Lutein 250 mcg.
See Editor's Note No. 45, page 2058.

Essential Woman 50+ **-** Nature Made
Each tablet contains: Vitamin A 3000 IU • Vitamin C 120 mg • Vitamin D 400 IU • Vitamin E 60 IU • Vitamin K 50 mcg • Thiamin 3 mg • Riboflavin 3.4 mg • Niacin 20 mg • Vitamin B6 4 mg • Folic Acid 400 mcg • Vitamin B12 25 mcg • Biotin 30 mcg • Pantothenic Acid 10 mg • Calcium 250 mg • Phosphorus 48 mg • Iodine 150 mcg • Magnesium 120 mg • Zinc 22 mg • Selenium 50 mcg • Copper 2 mg • Manganese 2 mg • Chromium 120 mcg • Molybdenum 25 mcg • Chloride 72 mg • Potassium 80 mg • Boron 150 mcg • Nickel 5 mcg • Silicon 2 mg • Tin 10 mcg • Vanadium 10 mcg • Lutein 250 mcg. Other Ingredients: Dibasic Calcium Phosphate, Cellulose Gel, Crospovidone, Gelatin, Acacia, Maltodextrin, Magnesium Stearate, Hydroxypropyl Methylcellulose, Corn Starch, Corn Oil, Modified Food Starch, Polyethylene Glycol.
See Editor's Note No. 45, page 2058.

Essentials - Chelated Mineral **-** USANA Health Sciences
Three tablets contain: Calcium (as Calcium Citrate) 270 mg • Magnesium (as Magnesium Citrate, Amino Acid Chelate, and Oxide) 300 mg • Iodine (as Potassium Iodide) 225 mcg • Zinc (as Zinc Citrate) 20 mg • Selenium (as L-Selenomethionine and Amino Acid Complex) 200 mcg • Copper (as Copper Gluconate) 3 mg • Manganese (as Manganese Gluconate) 5.1 mg • Chromium (as Chromium Picolinate and Polynicotinate) 300 mcg • Molybdenum (as Molybdenum Citrate) 50 mcg • Boron (as Boron Citrate) 3 mg • Silicon (as Amino Acid Complex) 3 mg • Vanadium (as Vanadyl Sulfate) 30 mcg • Ultra Trace Minerals 3 mg. Other Ingredients: Microcrystalline Cellulose, Pregelatinized Starch, Croscarmellose Sodium, Collodial Silicon Dioxide, Ascorbyl Palmitate, Dextrin, Dextrose.

Essentials - Mega Antioxidant **-** USANA Health Sciences
Three tablets contain: Vitamin A (as Beta Carotene) 15000 IU • Vitamin C (as Calcium, Potassium, Magnesium, Zinc Ascorbates) 1300 mg • Vitamin D 450 IU • Vitamin E (as D-Alpha Tocopheryl Succinate) 450 IU • Vitamin K (as Phylloquinone) 60 mcg • Vitamin B1 (as Thiamine HCl) 27 mg • Riboflavin 27 mg • Niacin (as Niacin and Niacinamide) 40 mg • Vitamin B6 (as Pyridoxine HCl) 27 mg • Folate (as Folic Acid) 1000 mcg • Vitamin B12 (as Cyanocobalamin) 60 mcg • Biotin 300 mcg • Pantothenic Acid (as D-Calcium Pantothenate) 90 mg • Olive Extract (Olea Europaea L., fruit) 30 mg • Bioflavonoid Complex: Rutin, Quercetin, Hesperidin (Citrus Spp. L., fruit), Green Tea Extract - Decaffeinated (Camillia Sinensis Hunt, leaves), Bilberry Extract (Vaccinium Myrtillus L., fruit) 193 mg • Inositol 150 mg • Choline Bitartrate 100 mg • N-Acetyl L-Cysteine 65 mg • Bromelain 50 mg • Alpha Lipoic Acid 15 mg • Coenzyme Q10 12 mg • Glutathione 10 mg • Curcumin Extract (Curcuma Longa L., Root) 15 mg • Lutein (Tagetes Erecta L., flower) 600 mcg • Lycopene 1 mg • Broccoli Concentrate (Brassica Oleracea V. Botrytis L.) Flower 15 mg. Other Ingredients: Microcrystalline Cellulose,

Pregelatinized Starch, Croscarmellose Sodium, Ascorbyl Palmitate, Dextrin, Collodial Silicon Dioxide, Dextrose.

Essentum **-** Vital Living, Inc.
Two packets contain: Vitamin A (as palmitate) 2500 IU • Vitamin C (as ascorbic acid) 30 mg • Calcium (amino acid chelate, aac) 50 mg • Vitamin D (as cholecalciferol) 200 IU • Vitamin E (as d-alpha tocopherol) 20 IU • Vitamin B1 (as thiamin mononitrate) 750 mcg • Vitamin B2 (as riboflavin) 850 mcg • D-Biotin 0.15 mg • Vitamin B5 (as calcium d-pantothenate) 5 mg • Phosphorous (as di-calcium phosphate) 48 mg • Iodine (as potassium iodide) 750 mcg • Magnesium (aac) 50 mg • Zinc (aac) 7.5 mg • Selenium (aac) 35 mcg • Copper (aac) 1 mg • Manganese (aac) 1 mg • Chromium (as chromium picolinate) 0.06 mg • Molybdenum (aac) 37.5 mcg • Potassium (as potassium chloride) 80 mg • Vitamin B Homocysteine Blend: Vitamin B6 (as pyridoxine HCl) 12.5 mg, Vitamin B9 (as folic acid/folate) 400 mcg, Vitamin B12 (as cyanocobalamin) 500 mcg • Plant Sterols Proprietary Blend 900 mg • Omega 3 Fatty Acids (as ethyl esters) Proprietary Blend 550 mg • Vitamin B3 (as niacin) 250 mg.

Essiac **-** Dial Herbs
Burdock • Sheep Sorrel • Rhubarb • Slippery Elm.

Ester C **-** Derma E
Each tablet contains: Vitamin C • Vitamin E • Antioxidants and Skin Rejuvenators.

Ester C - Vitamin C 500 mg **-** Jamieson
Each caplet contains: Vitamin C (Ester C) 500 mg • Grape Seed 1200 mg.

Ester C 1000 mg **-** The Vitamin Shoppe
Each tablet contains: Vitamin C (Calcium Ascorbate) 1000 mg • Calcium (as Ascorbate, Threonate) 125 mg.

Ester C 1000 mg with Bioflavonoids **-** The Vitamin Shoppe
Each tablet contains: Vitamin C (Calcium Ascorbate) (from 1250 mg Ester C) 1000 mg, plus Bioflavonoids Complex.

Ester C 500 mg **-** The Vitamin Shoppe
Each tablet contains: Vitamin C (Calcium Ascorbate) 500 mg • Calcium (as Ascorbate, Threonate) 60 mg.

Ester C 500 mg with Bioflavonoids **-** The Vitamin Shoppe
Each tablet contains: Vitamin C (Calcium Ascorbate) (from 625 mg Ester C) 500 mg, plus Bioflavonoids Complex.

Ester C Caps **-** Progressive Labs
Each capsule contains: Vitamin C (as calcium polyascorbate) 500 mg • Calcium (as calcium polyascorbate) 50 mg.

Ester C Plus Bioflavonoids and Pycnogenol 500 mg **-** The Vitamin Shoppe
Each capsule contains: Vitamin C (Calcium Ascorbate) (from 625 mg Ester C) 500 mg • Calcium (Calcium Ascorbate) 60 mg • Quercetin 25 mg • Pycnogenol 2.5 mg • Citrus Bioflavonoid Complex with Hesperidin and Rutin 200 mg.

Ester C Powder 2000 mg with Bioflavonoids **-** The Vitamin Shoppe
Each teaspoon contains: Vitamin C (Calcium Ascorbate) 2000 mg, plus Bioflavonoids Complex.

Ester C with Bioflavonoids, Vitamin C **-** Leiner Health Products
Each tablet contains: Vitamin C 500 mg • Citrus Bioflavonoids complex 200 mg. Other Ingredients: Ester-C Calcium Ascorbate, Calcium Carbonate, Cellulose, Croscarmellose Sodium, Crospovidone, Silicon Dioxide, Maltodextrin, Polyethylene Glycol 3350, Talc, Magnesium Stearate, Hydroxypropyl Methylcellulose, Hydroxypropyl Cellulose, Polysorbate 80.

Ester-C **-** PhysioLogics
Each capsule contains: Vitamin C (as ester-c calcium ascorbate) 500 mg • Calcium (as ester-c calcium ascorbate) • Citrus Bioflavonoid (citrus spp.) 100 mg • Rutin fruit (dimorphandra mollis) 5 mg • Hesperidin fruit complex (as citrus aurantium, citrus spp.) 5 mg. Other Ingredients: Gelatin, Cellulose (plant origin), Silica, Vegetable Magnesium Stearate.
See Editor's Note No. 40, page 2058.

Ester-C 1000 Mg with Bioflavonoids **-** Natrol
Each tablet contains: Vitamin C (as calcium ascorbate) 1000 mg • Calcium (as calcium ascorbate) 100 mg • Lemon Bioflavonoid Complex consisting of extracts from lemon 200 mg. Other Ingredients: Mono & Di-Glycerides, Stearic Acid, Croscarmellose Sodium, Silicon Dioxide, Magnesium Stearate.

Ester-C 250 Mg with Bioflavonoids **-** Natrol
Each tablet contains: Vitamin C (as calcium ascorbate) 250 mg • Calcium (as calcium ascorbate) 25 mg • Lemon Bioflavonoid Complex consisting of extracts from lemon 100 mg. Other Ingredients: Microcrystalline Cellulose, Stearic Acid, Croscarmellose Sodium, Silicon Dioxide, Magnesium Stearate.

Ester-C 500 Mg with Bioflavonoids **-** Natrol
Each tablet contains: Vitamin C (as calcium ascorbate) 500 mg • Calcium (as calcium ascorbate) 50 mg • Lemon Bioflavonoid Complex consisting of extracts from lemon 200 mg. Other Ingredients: Mono & Di-Glycerides, Stearic Acid, Croscarmellose Sodium, Silicon Dioxide, Magnesium Stearate.

Ester-C 1000 **-** Now
Each tablet contains: Vitamin C 1000 mg • Citrus Bioflavonoids (40%) 200 mg • Acerola powder 25 mg • Rose Hips powder 25 mg • Rutin 20 mg • Calcium 125 mg.

Ester-C 1000 - GNC A-Z **-** GNC
Each tablet contains: Vitamin C (as calcium ascorbic) 1000 mg • Calcium (as calcium ascorbic) 94 mg • Citrus Bioflavonoids Complex (from 50 mg of cirtus bioflavoniods complex 4X) 200 mg. Other Ingredients: Cellulose, Calcium Carbonate.

Ester-C 1000 mg tablets **-** Source Naturals
Each tablet contains: Vitamin C (as calcium ascorbate [Ester-C]) 500 mg • Calcium (as bioflavonoids & calcium ascorbate [Ester-C]) 90 mg • Bioflavonoid Complex 130 mg • Rutin 36 mg • Hesperidin Complex 35 mg.

Ester-C 1000 Timed Release - GNC A-Z **-** GNC
Each tablet contains: Vitamin C (as calcium ascorbate) 1000 mg • Calcium (as calcium ascorbate) 94 mg • Citrus Bioflavonoids Complex (from 50 mg of citrus biofalvonoids complex 4X) 200 mg. Other Ingredients: Cellulose, Food Glaze.

Ester-C 250 Mg **-** Natrol
Each tablet contains: Vitamin C (as calcium ascorbate) 250 mg • Calcium (as calcium ascorbate) 25 mg. Other Ingredients: Microcrystalline Cellulose, Stearic Acid, Mono & Di-Glycerides, Croscarmellose Sodium, Magnesium Stearate.

Ester-C 250 Mg Chewable **-** Natrol
Each wafer contains: Vitamin C (as calcium ascorbate) 250 mg • Calcium (as calcium ascorbate) 25 mg. Other Ingredients: Fructose, Glycine, Mono & Di-Glycerides, Stearic Acid, natural Orange flavor, Citric Acid, Silicon Dioxide, Microcrystalline Cellulose, Gum Acacia, Magnesium Stearate.

Ester-C 500 Mg capsules **-** Natrol
Each capsule contains: Vitamin C (as calcium ascorbate) 500 mg • Calcium (as calcium ascorbate) 50 mg. Other Ingredients: Magnesium Stearate, Microcrystalline Cellulose, Gelatin.

Ester-C 500 Mg tablets **-** Natrol
Each tablet contains: Vitamin C (as calcium ascorbate) 500 mg • Calcium (as calcium ascorbate) 50 mg. Other Ingredients: Microcrys-

talline Cellulose, Stearic Acid, Croscarmellose Sodium, Magnesium Stearate, Silicon Dioxide.

Ester-C 500 mg tablets **-** Puritan's Pride
Each tablet contains: Vitamin C (as Ester-C calcium ascorbate) 500 mg • Calcium (as Ester-C calcium ascorbate) 55 mg • Citrus Bioflavonoid fruit complex (citrus spp.) 200 mg • Rutin fruit (dimorphandra mollis) 10 mg • Hesperidin fruit complex (citrus spp.) 10 mg. Other Ingredients: Cellulose (plant origin), Vegetable Stearic Acid, Croscarmellose, Silica, Cellulose Coating, Vegetable Magnesium Stearate.

Ester-C 500 mg With Bioflavonoids capsules **-** Puritan's Pride
Each capsule contains: Vitamin C (as Ester-C calcium ascorbate) 500 mg • Calcium (as Ester-C calcium ascorbate) 55 mg • Citrus Bioflavonoid fruit (citrus sinensis) 100 mg • Rutin fruit (dimorphandra mollis) 5 mg • Hesperidin fruit complex (citrus spp.) 5 mg. Other Ingredients: Gelatin, Cellulose (plant origin), Silica, Vegetable Magnesium Stearate.

Ester-C 500 Mg with Bioflavonoids Vegetarian capsules **-** Natrol
Each capsule contains: Vitamin C (as calcium ascorbate) 500 mg • Calcium (as calcium ascorbate) 50 mg • Citrus Bioflavonoid Complex consisting of extracts from: lemon, orange, grapefruit, lime, & tangerine 200 mg. Other Ingredients: Magnesium Stearate, Silicon Dioxide, Vegetable Carbohydrate Gum, Glycerine.

Ester-C 500 Mg with Echinacea **-** Natrol
Each tablet contains: Vitamin C (as calcium ascorbate) 500 mg • Calcium (as calcium ascorbate) 50 mg • Echinacea extract (Phenolic compounds 4%) 50 mg • Echinacea (angustifolia) leaf powder 80 mg • Echinacea (Purpurea) leaf powder 80 mg • Echinacea (angustifolia) root powder 20 mg • Echinacea (Purpurea) root powder 20 mg. Other Ingredients: Calcium Carbonate, Mono & Di-Glycerides, Croscarmellose Sodium, Stearic Acid, Silicon Dioxide, Magnesium Stearate.

Ester-C 500 Mg with Pycnogenol & Proanthocyanidins capsules **-** Natrol
Each capsule contains: Vitamin C (as calcium ascorbate) 500 mg • Calcium (as calcium ascorbate) 50 mg • Grape skin powder 50 mg • Rutin 50 mg • Hesperidin Complex 50 mg • Quercetin 25 mg • Pycnogenol (pine bark extract) 5 mg. Other Ingredients: Silicon Dioxide, Magnesium Stearate, Gelatin.

Ester-C 500 Mg with Pycnogenol & Proanthocyanidins tablets **-** Natrol
Each tablet contains: Vitamin C (as calcium ascorbate) 500 mg • Calcium (as calcium ascorbate-carbonate) 70 mg • Grape skin powder 50 mg • Rutin 50 mg • Hesperidin 50 mg • Quercetin 25 mg • Pycnogenol (pine bark extract) 5 mg. Other Ingredients: Mono & Di-Glycerides, Calcium Carbonate, Croscarmellose Sodium, Silicon Dioxide, Stearic Acid & Magnesium Stearate.

Ester-C 500 with Citrus Bioflavonoids - GNC A-Z **-** GNC
Each tablet contains: Vitamin C (as calcium ascorbate) 500 mg • Calcium (as calcium ascorbate and dicalcium phosphate) 110 mg • Citrus Bioflavonoids Complex (from 50 mg of Citrus Bioflavonoids Complex 4X) 200 mg. Other Ingredients: Cellulose Calcium Carbonate.

Ester-C 500mg **-** Nature's Bounty
Each tablet contains: Vitamin C (as Ester-C calcium ascorbate) 500 mg • Calcium (as Ester-C calcium ascorbate) 55 mg • Citrus Bioflavonoid fruit complex (citrus spp.) 200 mg • Rutin fruit (dimorphandra mollis) 10 mg • Hesperidin fruit complex (citrus spp.) 10 mg. Other Ingredients: Cellulose (plant origin), Vegetable Stearic Acid, Croscarmellose, Silica, Cellulose Coating, Vegetable Magnesium Stearate.

Ester-C Antioxidant **-** Natrol
Two tablets contain: Vitamin A (as d-Salina beta carotene) 5000 IU • Vitamin C (as calcium ascorbate) 500 mg • Vitamin E (as d-alpha tocopheryl succinate with mixed tocopherols) 200 IU • Calcium (as ascorbate) 50 mg • Lemon Bioflavonoid Complex consisting of extracts from lemon 25 mg • a-Lipoic Acid 25 mg. Other Ingredients: TriCalcium Phosphate, Microcrystalline Cellulose, Stearic Acid, Silicon Dioxide, Croscarmellose Sodium, Magnesium Stearate.

Ester-C brand **-** Zila Nutraceuticals
Vitamin C.
See Editor's Note No. 44, page 2058.

Ester-C Cold Season **-** Natrol
Two capsules contain: Vitamin C (as calcium ascorbate) 500 mg • Calcium (as calcium ascorbate) 50 mg • Zinc (chelate) 10 mg • Reishi/Shiitake/ Maitake Blend, powdered extract (mushrooms) 150 mg • Echinacea 50:50 (purpurea & angustifolia), powdered extract supplying Phenolic compounds (4%) 75 mg • Citrus Bioflavonoid Complex extracts of: lemon, orange, grapefruit, lime & tangerine 50 mg • Black Elderberry extract, powdered 30 mg • Garlic, powdered extract bulb 30 mg • Licorice root extract supplying 25 % Glycerenic Acid 25 mg • Astragalus 25 mg • Cayenne supplying 40000 SCU 10 mg • Beta Glucans, oats 5 mg. Other Ingredients: Silica, Magnesium Stearate, Rice powder, Gelatin.

Ester-C Complex **-** Pro Health
Each tablet contains: Vitamin C (from ester-c calcium ascorbate 675 mg) 500 mg • Calcium (from ester-c calcium ascorbate [calcium corn base] 675 mg) 57 mg • Citrus Bioflavonoid complex (37% total bioflavonoids as hesperidin 100 mg) 200 mg • Acerola fruit extract (malpighia punicifolia L. 1:4) 75 mg • Rose Hips seed powder (rosae pseudofructus) 75 mg • Rutin seeds (dimorphandra mollis) 50 mg. Other Ingredients: Microcrystalline Cellulose, Stearic Acid, Magnesium Stearate, Silicon Dioxide, Pharmaceutical Glaze.

Ester-C Complex **-** Olympian Labs
Each capsule contains: Vitamin C (Ester C) 500 mg • Citrus Bioflavonoid Complex 200 mg.

Ester-C Complex Extra Strength **-** Olympian Labs
Each tablet contains: Ester C (Vitamin C) 1000 mg • Calcium (from Ester-C) 80 mg • Citrus Bioflavonoid Complex 50 mg • Grape Skin extract 50 mg • Rose Hips 50 mg.

Ester-C Complex Plus Calcium **-** Olympian Labs
Each capsule contains: Ester C (Vitamin C) 500 mg • Calcium (from Ester-C) 40 mg • Citrus Bioflavonoid Complex 200 mg.

Ester-C For Kids **-** Natrol
Each wafer contains: Vitamin C (as calcium ascrobate) 100 mg • Calcium (as calcium ascorbate) 10 mg • Citrus Bioflavonoids consisting of extracts from lemon 25 mg. Other Ingredients: Fructose, Mono & Di-Glycerides, Glycine, Cellulose, natural Tropical fruit flavor, Stearic Acid, Silica, Magnesium Stearate, Guar Gum, Citric Acid.

Ester-C Magnesium **-** NutriCology
Each capsule contains: Vitamin C (as magnesium ascorbate) 500 mg • Magnesium (as magnesium ascorbate) 35 mg. Other Ingredients: Cellulose.

Ester-C Nightime Formula **-** Natrol
Each tablet contains: Vitamin C (as calcium ascrobate) 500 mg • Calcium (as calcium ascorbate) 50 mg • Kava Kava root supplying 30% Kavalactones 100 mg • Valerian root supplying 0.8% Valerenic Acid 100 mg • Melatonin 1 mg. Other Ingredients: TriCalcium Phosphate, Cellulose, Stearic Acid, Silica, Magnesium Stearate.
See Editor's Note No. 26, page 2056.

Ester-C Powder **-** Natrol
Each teaspoon contains: Vitamin C (as calcium ascorbate) 3200 mg • Calcium (as calcium ascorbate) 320 mg.

Ester-C Powder with Bioflavonoids **- Natrol**
Each teaspoon contains: Vitamin C (as calcium ascorbate) 3000 mg • Calcium (as calcium ascorbate) 300 mg • Citrus Bioflavonoid Complex consisting of extracts from: lemon, orange, grapefruit, lime, & tangerine 300 mg.

Ester-C with Bioflavonoids **- Natrol**
Each capsule contains: Vitamin C (as calcium ascorbate) 500 mg • Calcium (as calcium ascorbate) 50 mg • Citrus Bioflavonoid Complex consisting of extracts from: lemon, orange, grapefruit, lime & tangerine 200 mg. Other Ingredients: Magnesium Stearate, Gelatin.

Ester-C with Echinacea **- Natrol**
Each capsule contains: Vitamin C (as calcium ascorbate) 500 mg • Calcium (as calcium ascorbate) 50 mg Echinacea extract (Phenolic compounds 4%) 50 mg • Echinacea (angustifolia) leaf powder 80 mg • Echinacea (Purpurea) leaf powder 80 mg • Echinacea (angustifolia) root powder 20 mg • Echinacea (Purpurea) root powder 20 mg. Other Ingredients: Silicon Dioxide, Magnesium Stearate, Gelatin.

Ester-C with Echinacea & Goldenseal Root **- Puritan's Pride**
Each capsule contains: Ester C (Polysascorbate) 500 mg • Echinacea (Eachinacea angustifolia) 100 mg • Goldenseal root (Hydrastis canadensis) 50 mg.

Ester-C Zinc Lozenges **- Natrol**
Each lozenge contains: Vitamin C (as calcium ascorbate) 150 mg • Calcium (as calcium ascorbate) 15 mg • Citrus Bioflavonoids consisting of extracts from lemon 25 mg • Zinc (Gluconate) 4.5 mg. Other Ingredients: Fructose, Mono & Di-Glycerides, Glycine, Cellulose, Natural Fruit Flavors, Stearic Acid, Silica, Magnesium Stearate, Guar Gum, Citric Acid.

Ester-E brand **- Zila Nutraceuticals**
Vitamin E.
See Editor's Note No. 44, page 2058.

Esterol with Ester-C **- NutriCology**
Each capsule contains: Vitamin C (as calcium ascorbate) 675 mg • Calcium (as calcium ascorbate) 75 mg • Rutin 50 mg • quercetin 25 mg • Proanthocyanidins 2.5 mg. Other Ingredients: Magnesium Stearate, Silicon Dioxide.

EstrAttune **- Health Smart Vitamins**
Each capsule contains: Vitamin E (as d-alpha tocopheryl acetate) 50 IU • Vitamin B6 (as pyridoxine HCl) 25 mg • Folate (folic acid) 200 mcg • Magnesium (as magnesium oxide) 100 mg • Zinc (as zinc amino acid chelate) 3.75 mg • Copper (as copper amino acid chelate) 0.5 mg • Black Cohosh root 100 mg • Chastetree berry (5% flavonoids) 100 mg • Dong Quai root (>= 0.8% ligustilides, >= 0.8 mg) 100 mg • Soy bean (5% isoflavones, 2.5 mg) 50 mg • Kava Kava root (30% kavalactones, 7.5 mg) 25 mg.

Estrin D **- Klein-Becker**
Two capsules contain: Vitamin B6 25 mg • Magnesium (as oxide) 100 mg • Estrin D Proprietary Blend 1323 mg: Yerba Mate leaf SE (standardized extract), Caffeine, Guarana seed SE, Damiana leaf/stem SE, Green Tea leaf SE, Ginger root, Kola nut SE, DHEA, Schisandra fruit, Scutellaria root SE, Tibetan Ginseng root SE, Cocoa nut SE, Jujube fruit, Thea Sinensis leaf complex SE.

Estro - 2 OZ **- Young Living Essential Oils**
Black Cohosh Extract • Blue Cohosh Extract • Royal Jelly • Fennel Oil (Foeniculum Vulgare) • Lavender Oil (Lavandula Angustifolia • Clary Sage Oil (Salvia Sclarea).

Estro Balance **- Puritan's Pride**
Each tablet contains: Vitamin E 30 IU • Thiamin (Vitamin B1) 2 mg • Riboflavin (Vitamin B2) 2 mg • Niacin 20 mg • Vitamin B6 10 mg • Calcium 150 mg • Selenium 150 mg • Boron 1.5 mg • Soy Isoflavones 50 mg • Kava Kava root extract (30% kavalactones) 100 mg • Black Cohosh root (cimicifuga racemosa) 40 mg.

Estro Suppress **- SciFit**
Each capsule contains: 5,7-Chrysin (dihydroxy-flavone) 200 mg • 3,6,17-Androstenetrione 100 mg. Other Ingredients: Magnesium Stearate, Gelatin.

EstroFactors **- Metagenics**
Three tablets contain: Vitamin A (50% as Betatene mixed carotenoids and 50% retinyl palmitate) 2500 IU • Vitamin D (as cholecalciferol) 200 IU • Vitamin E (as d-alpha tocopheryl acetate) 200 IU • Vitamin K 40 mcg • Vitamin B6 (pyridoxine HCl) 50 mg • Folate [Metafolin (as l-5-methyl tetrahydrofolate), folic acid, and 5-formyl tetrahydrofolate] 800 mcg • Vitamin B12 (as methylcobalamin and cyanocobalamin) 30 mg • Proprietary Blend of Isoflavones 100 mg: Red Clover flowering top extract (Trifolium pratense), Kudzu root extract (Pueraria lobata) • Turmeric rhizome extract (Curcuma longa, standardized to 95% curcuminoids) 210 mg • Rosemary leaf extract (Rosmarinus officinalis, contains 5.1%-7.6% carnosic acid/carnosol) 200 mg • Resveratrol (from Polygonum cuspudatum root extract) 2 mg • Trimethylglycine 200 mg • Chrysin 90 mg.

EstroGentle **- Bodyonics, Ltd.**
Black Cohosh • Soy germ • Red Clover leaf extract • Licorice root • Wild Yam • Chaste Tree berry • Other botanicals.

Estrolean Fat Burner Supreme **- Bodyonics, Ltd.**
Two capsules contain: Apple Extract (standardized for 5% phloridzin) 100 mg • Pomegranate Extract (standardized for 2% estrone) 100 mg • Sea Vegetable Extract (standardized for 5% phloroglucinols and 150 mcg iodine) 150 mg • Plant Based Enzymes: Lipase 1000 FIP, Protease 50,000 HUT, Amylase 5000 SKB • Herbal Metabogenics 300 mg: Guarana Extract, Green Tea Extract, Yerba Mate Extract (standardized for 66.6 mg caffeine) • Proprietary Blend 100 mg: Ginger Root Extract (zingiber officinale), Black Pepper Extract (piper nigrum), Licorice (glycyrrhiza glabra) • Citrus Aurantium (bitter orange; standardized for 4% synephrine) 66.6 mg • Rhodiola Rosea Extract (standardized for 3% rosavins) 50 mg • Rhododendron Caucasicum Extract (standardized for 3% taxifolian) 50 mg • Herbal Modulators 200 mg: Chromium Polynicotinate, L-Carnitine Tartrate, Garcinia Cambogia Extract, Grapefruit Extract, Cinnamon Twig Bar, Dong Quai Extract, Barberry Extract, Chaste Berry Extract. Other Ingredients: Cellulose, Talc, Magnesium Stearate, Gelatin.
See Editor's Note No. 40, page 2058.

EstroSoy **- Nature's Way**
Two capsules contain: Fermented Soy extract 890 mg • Red Clover blossoms 100 mg.

EstroSoy Plus **- Nature's Way**
Two capsules contain: Black Cohosh dried extract 40 mg • Fermented Soy extract 890 mg • Red Clover Blossoms 100 mg.

Estrotone **- New Chapter, Inc.**
Two softgels contain: Dong Quai (Angelica sinensis) root, extract (1% lingustilide- .80 mg) 80 mg • Schizandra (wu-wei-zi) berry extract (2% schizandrins- 1.6 mg) 80 mg • Ginger rhizome, certified organic, extract (minimum 20% pungent compounds- 10 mg, 5% ziniberene- 2.5 mg) 50 mg • Black Cohosh root and rhizome, extract (8% triterpene glycoside- 3.2 mg) 40 mg • Chaste Tree berry, extract (0.6% aucubin- 2.4mg, % 0.5 agnuside- 20 mg) 40 mg • Rosemary leaf and essential oil, extract (23% total phenolic anitoxidants- 2.3 mg) 10 mg. Other Ingredients: Evening primrose oil, Olive Oil, Yellow Beeswax, Gelatin, Vegetable glycerin, Purified Water, Carob.

Estroven **- Amerifit Nutrition**
Each caplet contains: Vitamin E (as natural d-alpha tocopherol succinate) 30 IU • Thiamin (as thiamin mononitrate) 2 mg • Riboflavin 2 mg • Niacin (niacinamide) 20 mg • Vitamin B6 (as pyridoxine HCl) 10 mg • Vitamin B12 (as cyanocobalamin) 6 mcg • Folate (as folic acid) 400 mcg • Calcium (from calcium carbonate) 150 mg • Selenium (from l-selenomethionine) 70 mcg • Boron (chelate) 1.5 mg • Purified Isoflavones from soybean & other plants 55 mg • Estroven Calming Herbal Blend 150 mg: Date Seed extract (Zizyphus spinosa), Magnolia bark extract • Black Cohosh root

40 mg. Other Ingredients: Pueraria Lobata Root Extract, Cellulose, Croscarmellose Sodium, Silica, Vegetable Magnesium Stearate, Titamium Dioxide (natural mineral source), Vanilla, Caramel Color.

Estroven Joint & Bone **-** Amerifit Nutrition
Four caplets contain: Vitamin C (as ascorbic acid) 100 mg • Vitamin D (as cholecalciferol) 400 IU • Vitamin K (as phytonadione) 80 mcg • Folate (as folic acid) 400 mcg • Calcium (as calcium carbonate) 600 mg • Glucosamine HCl 1500 mg • Chondroitin Sulfate 1200 mg • Isoflavones (from pueraria lobata root and non-GMO soybeans) 25 mg. Other Ingredients: Microcrystalline Cellulose, Vegetable Stearic Acid, Silica, Vegetable Coating.
See Editor's Note No. 48, page 2059.

Estroven Memory **-** Amerifit Nutrition
Each tablet contains: Zinc 7.5 mg • Ginkgo Biloba leaf standardized extract 60 mg • Panax Ginseng root standardized extract 125 mg • Green Tea leaf standardized extract 250 mg • Isoflavones 10 mg • Grape skin standardized extract 75 mg.
See Editor's Note No. 21, page 2056.

Estroven PMS **-** Amerifit Nutrition
Two tablets contain: Thiamin (as thiamin mononitrate) 1.5 mg • Riboflavin 1.7 mg • Niacin (as niacinamide) 20 mg • Vitamin B-6 (as pyridoxine HCl) 25 mcg • Folate (as folic acid) 200 mcg • Vitamin B-12 (as cyanocobalamin) 6 mcg • Pantothenic Acid (as D-calcium pantothenate) 10 mg • Calcium (as calcium carbonate) 200 mg • Magnesium (as magnesium oxide) 50 mg • Anti-bloating Herbal Diuretic Blend 300 mg: Couch Grass plant (agropyron repens), Buchu leaf (agathosma betulina), Arctostaphylos Uva Ursi leaf, Juniper berry (juniperus communis), Hydrangea Arborescens root, Cornsilk stylus (zea mays) • Feverfew standardized extract (aerial parts, tanacetum parthenium) 125 mg • Estroven Calming Herbal Blend 200 mg: Date seed extract (zizyphus spinosa), Magnolia bark extract • Chaste Berry standardized extract (vitex agnus castus) 60 mg • Ginger root (zingiber officinalis) 50 mg • Cramp bark (viburnum opulus) 20 mg • Isoflavones (from pureria lobata root and non-GMO soybeans) 10 mg. Other Ingredients: Cellulose, Cellulose Gum, Fractionated Vegetable Oil, Silica, Natural Glaze, Titanium Dioxide, Vanilla.

E-TOCO 400 **-** Progressive Labs
Each softgel contains: Vitamin E (mixed tocopherols) 400 IU • Sesame seed oil 200 mg • Nutriene 100 mg.

Eucalyptus Salve **-** Dial Herbs
Eucalyptus • Camphor • Mint. In a base of Beeswax, Glycerine & Cold Pressed Olive Oil.

European Grape Seed Extract 50 mg **-** Jamieson
Each caplet contains: Calcium 30 mg • Grape Seed 60:1 extract (Vitis vinifera) (Standardized to 95% Oligomeric Procyanidins) 50 mg.

Evecare Capsules **-** The Himalaya Drug Company (Himalaya Heal
Each capsule contains: Ashoka (saraca indica syn. s.asoca) 85 mg • Dashamoola 35 mg: Aegle Marmelos root, Gmelina Arborea root, Oroxylum Indicum root, Clerodendrum Phlomidis root, Stereospermum Chelonoides root, Desmodium Gangeticum root, Uraria Picta root, Solanum Indicum root, Solanum Surattense root, Tribulus Terrestris root • Lodhra (symplocos racemosa) 35 mg • Guduchi (tinospora cordifolia) 35 mg • Kakamachi (solanum nigrum) 35 mg • Punarnava (boerhaavia diffusa) 35 mg • Shatavari (asparagus racemosus) 35 mg • Kumari (aloe vera) 25 mg • Chandana (santalum album) 25 mg • Musta (cyperus rotundus) 25 mg • Vasaka (adhatoda vasica syn. a.zeylanica) 20 mg • Triphala 20 mg: Emblica Officinalis, Terminalia Chebula, Terminalia Bellirica • Trikatu 20 mg: Piper Nigrum, Piper Longum, Zingiber Officinale • Shalmali (bombax malabaricum syn. b.ceiba) 15 mg • Kasisa Godanti Bhasma (ferrous sulphate, gypsum calx) 35 mg • Yashada Bhasma (zinc calx) 35 mg.

Evecare Syrup **-** The Himalaya Drug Company (Himalaya Heal
Each 1 tsp (5 mL) serving contains: Gandapushpa (saraca indica syn. s.asoca) 50 mg • Dashamoola 33 mg: Aegle Marmelos root, Gmelina Arborea root, Oroxylum Indicum root, Clerodendrum Phlomidis root, Stereospermum Chelonoides root, Desmodium Gangeticum root, Uraria Picta root, Solanum Indicum root, Solanum Surattense root, Tribulus Terrestris root • Lodhra (symplocos racemosa) 33 mg • Guduchi (tinospora cordifolia) 33 mg • Kakamachi (solanum nigrum) 33 mg • Punarnava (boerhaavia diffusa) 32 mg • Shatavari (asparagus racemosus) 32 mg • Narikela (cocos nucifera) 32 mg • Kumari (aloe barbadensis) 25 mg • Chandana (santalum album) 25 mg • Vabbula (acacia arabica syn. a.nilotica) 25 mg • Musta (cyperus rotundus) 25 mg • Anantamul (hemidesmus indicus) 25 mg • Triphala 20 mg: Emblica Officinalis, Terminalia Chebula, Terminalia Bellirica • Vasaka (adhatoda vasica syn. a.zeylanica) 20 mg • Manjishtha (rubia cordifolia) 20 mg • Trikatu 20 mg: Piper Nigrum, Piper Longum, Zingiber Officinalis • Shalmali (bombax malabaricum syn. b.ceiba) 12 mg • Shilajeet (mineral pitch, purified) 5 mg.

Evening Primrose Deluxe **-** Health From The Sun
Each capsule contains: Gamma Linolenic Acid (GLA) (Omega-6) 130 mg • Linoleic Acid (Omega-6) 950 mg • Oleic Acid (Omega-9) 80 mg. Other Ingredients: Evening Primrose seed oil, Gelatin, Glycerine, Water.

Evening Primrose Oil **-** Health From The Sun
Two capsules contain: Gamma-Linolenic Acid (GLA) (Omega-6) 100 mg • Linoleic Acid (Omega-6) 730 mg • Oleic Acid (Omega-9) 60 mg. Other Ingredients: Evening Primrose seed oil, Gelatin, Glycerine, Water.

Evening Primrose Oil **-** Olympian Labs
Each softgel contains: Evening Primrose Oil 500 mg.

Evening Primrose Oil **-** PhysioLogics
Each softgel contains: Evening Primrose Oil 500 mg • Cis-Linoleic Acid (LA) 365 mg • Gamma-Linolenic Acid (GLA) 45 mg. Other Ingredients: Gelatin, Glycerin.

Evening Primrose Oil **-** Pro Health
Three softgels contain: Evening Primrose Oil 1.5 g • Gamma Linolenic Acid (gla) 135 mg • Cis-Linoleic Acid (omega-6) 1.08 g • Cis-Oleic Acid (omega-9) 120 mg. Other Ingredients: Gelatin, Glycerin, Water.

Evening Primrose Oil **-** Leiner Health Products
Each softgel contains: Evening Primrose Oil (Oenothera biennis) seed 500 mg. Other Ingredients: Gelatin, Glycerin, Purified Water.

Evening Primrose Oil **-** Jamieson
Each capsule contains: Vitamin E (as D-Alpha Tocopheryl Acetate) 13.6 IU • Gamma Linolenic Acid (GLA) 50 mg.

Evening Primrose Oil **-** Optimum Nutrition
Each softgel contains: Evening Primrose Oil 500 mg • Cis-Linoleic Acid 350 mg • Gamma-Linolenic Acid (GLA) 45 mg. Other Ingredients: Gelatin, Glycerin.

Evening Primrose Oil 1300 mg **-** Nature's Way
Each capsule contains: Evening Primrose oil, cold pressed 1.3 g • Vitamin E d-alpha tocopheryl 6 IU. Other Ingredients: Gelatin, Glycerin, Water.

Evening Primrose Oil 500 mg **-** Nature's Way
Each softgel contains: Evening Primrose Oil (cold pressed) 500 mg • Vitamin E (d-alpha tocopheryl) 6 IU. Other Ingredients: Gelatin, Glycerin, Water.

Evening Primrose Oil 500 mg **-** Jamieson
Each capsule contains: Evening Primrose Oil 500 mg • Vitamin E Natural d-Alpha Tocopheryl Acetate 13.6 IU.

Evening Primrose Oil 500 mg **-** Nature's Bounty
Each softgel contains: Evening Primrose Oil 500 mg: Cis-Linoleic Acid (LA) 365 mg, Gamma-Linolenic Acid (GLA) 45 mg. Other Ingredients: Gelatin, Glycerin.

Evening Primrose Oil 500 mg **-** Puritan's Pride
Each softgel contains: Evening Primrose Oil 500 mg: Cis-Linoleic Acid (LA) 365 mg, Gamma-Linolenic Acid (GLA) 45 mg. Other Ingredients: Gelatin, Glycerin.

Evening Primrose Oil Extra Strength **-** Olympian Labs
Each softgel contains: Evening Primrose Oil 1300 mg.

Evening Primrose Oil, 500mg **-** Nature Made
Two softgels contain: Vitamin E 30 IU • Evening Primrose seed oil 1 g: Cis-Linoleic Acid 720 mg, Gamma-Linolenic Acid 90 mg.

Ever Thin **-** Dynamic Nutritional Products
Two tablets contain: Vitamin B6 (as pyridoxine HCl) 50 mg • Chromium (as chromium polynicotinate) 200 mcg • L-Carnitine (as l-carnitine fumarate) 250 mg • Alpha Lipoic Acid (thioctic acid) 25 mg • Kelp powder 200 mg • Ever Thin Proprietary Thermogenic Blend 600 mg: Natural Cocoa extract (theobroma cacao), Theobromine, Citrus Aurantium (6% synephrine), Green Tea extract (98% polyphenols, 70% catechins, 40% EGCG, 6% caffeine).
See Editor's Note No. 40, page 2058.

EverCLR **-** Halo Supply Co.
Each capsule contains: Burdock root • Ashwaganda root • Echinacea Angustifolia root • Echinacea Purpurea root • Hydrangea root.

Everyday Detox **-** Traditional Medicinals
Sweet Tea Vine herb (Gynostemma pentaphyllum) • Schisandra fruit dried aqueous extract • Licorice root • Ginger rhizome • Star Anise fruit • Lycium fruit dried aqueous extract • Schisandra fruit • Kukicha twig (Camellia sinensis).

Everyday Essentials **-** iVillage Inc.
Each tablet contains: Vitamin A (20% as beta carotene) 5000 IU • Vitamin C 90 mg • Vitamin D 400 IU • Vitamin E 30 IU • Vitamin K 80 mcg • Thiamin 2.3 mg • Riboflavin 2.6 mg • Niacin 20 mg • Vitamin B6 2 mg • Folic Acid 400 mcg • Vitamin B12 9 mcg • Biotin 300 mcg • Pantothenic Acid 10 mg • Calcium 200 mg • Iron 6 mg • Phosphorus 45 mg • Iodine 150 mcg • Magnesium 100 mg • Zinc 15 mg • Selenium 70 mcg • Copper 2 mg • Manganese 2 mg • Chromium 120 mcg • Molybdenum 75 mcg. Other Ingredients: Microcrystalline Cellulose, Corn Starch, Sodium Carboxymethylcellulose, Sucrose, Acacia, Maltodextrin, Magnesium Stearate, Hydroxypropyl Methylcellulose, Glycerin.

Evolution 2 - Element II **-** Viogenix Corp.
Each scoop (12 g) contains: Calcium (lactate) 25 mg • Magnesium (oxide) 7.2 mg • Zinc (oxide) 15 mg • Copper (gluconate) 2 mg • Manganese (gluconate) 5 mg • Chromium (amino nicotinate) 200 mcg • Iodine (postassium iodide) 150 mcg • Selenium (sodium) 200 mcg • Molybdenum (sodium molybdate) 150 mcg • Vitamin A (acetate) 10,000 IU • Vitamin E (d-alpha-tocopheryl acetate) 100 IU • Vitamin D (vitamin D3, cholecalciferol) 400 IU • Vitamin C (ascorbic acid) 500 mg • Vitamin B1 (thiamine HCl) 25 mg • Vitamin B2 (riboflavin) 25 mg • Vitamin B3 (niacin) 50 mg • Vitamin B3 (niacinamide) 50 mg • Vitamin B5 (calcium pantothenate) 50 mg • Vitamin B6 (pyridoxine HCl) 25 mg • Vitamin B12 (cyanocobalamin) 100 mcg • Folic Acid 400 mcg • Biotin 300 mcg • PABA (para amino benzoic acid) 25 mg • Choline Bitartrate 25 mg • Inositol 25 mg • N-Acetyl L-Cysteine 175 mg • Enzyme Premix 50 mg.
Inactive Ingredients: Fructose, Natural Orange Powder, Potassium Bicarbonate, Citric Acid, Natural Orange Flavor, Digestive Enzymes (blend containing amylase, papain, lipase, bromelain, lactase, cellulase, maltase, sucrase), Stevia, Cholecalciferol, Silicon Dioxide.

Evolution 2 - Element III **-** Viogenix Corp.
Each spray contains: Phosphatidylserine 75 mg • Vinpocetine 5 mg • Carnitine Fumerate 100 mg • Ginko Biloba 5 mg • L-Theanine 2 mg • 5-HTP 1 mg • Choline Bitartrate 5 mg. Inactive Ingredients: Deionized Water, Lecithin Phospholipids, Citric Acid, Sodium Citrate, Potassium Sorbate, Sodium Benzoate, Maltodextrin, Glycine, Natural & Artificial Flavors.

Evolution 2 - Element IV **-** Viogenix Corp.
Each spray contains: N-Acetyl L-Cysteine 50 mg • Ellogic Acid 50 mg • Calcium D-Glucarate 15 mg • Acetyl L-Carnitine 10 mg • Carnosine 10 mg • Alpha Lipoic Acid 5 mg • Magnesium Citrate 5 mg • Coenzyme Q10 2 mg • Proprietary Blend (IMMONOSEB) 2 mg: Bromelain, Peptizine, Lactoperoxidase, Catalase, Lysozyme, Lactoferrin. Inactive Ingredients: Deionized Water, Lecithin Phospholipids, Polysorbate 60, Glycine, Citric Acid, Sodium Citrate, Potassium Sorbate, Sodium Benzoate, Methylparaben, Natural & Artificial Flavors.

Evolution 2 - Element l **-** Viogenix Corp.
Each spray contains: Proprietary Blend 200 mg: Alpha GPC (alpha glycerlphosphoryl choline), GABA (gamma amino butyric acid), Mucuna Pruriens (l-dopa bean extract), Moomiyo extract (Russian Mumie) • Proprietary Blend 300 mg: Ornithine Alpha Ketoglutarate, L-Glutamine, L-Arginine, L-Lysine, L-Valine, L-Isoleucine, L-Tyrosine, Glycine. Inactive Ingredients: Deionized Water, Lecithin Phospholipids, Sodium Citrate, Citric Acid, Potassium Sorbate, Maltodextrin, Methyl-Paraben, Propylparaben, Natural & Artificial Flavors.

Evolution 2 - Element V **-** Viogenix Corp.
Each spray contains: Vitamin A 2500 IU • Vitamin E 15 IU • Green Tea extract 10 mg • Grape Seed extract 10 mg • Pine Bark extract 10 mg • Bilberry extract 5 mg • Citrus Bioflavonoids 5 mg • Glutathione 1 mg • Selenium Citrate 50 mcg. Inactive Ingredients: Deionized Water, Lecithin Phospholipids, Polysorbate 60, Stevia extract, Glycine, Citric Acid, Sodium Citrate, Potassium Sorbate, Sodium Benzoate, Methylparaben, Natural & Artificial Flavors.

Exandra Lean **-** The Kutting Edge
Two capsules contain: Citrus Aurantium 125 mg • Nor-Ephedrine 23 mg • L-Phenylalanine 300 mg • Citri Max 500 mg • Acetyl L-Carnitine 100 mg • L-Tyrosine 80 mg • Ginger Root 50 mg • Vitamin B5 40 mg.
See Editor's Note No. 40, page 2058.

Exec-U-Stress **-** Nature's Plus
Three tablets contain: Vitamin C with Rose Hips 600 mg • Niacinamide (Vitamin B3) 300 mg • Pantothenic Acid (Vitamin B5) 300 mg • L-Cysteine free form amino acid 200 mg • L-Glycine free form amino acid 200 mg • Vitamin B1 (Thiamine) 200 mg • Vitamin E natural 200 IU • Vitamin B6 (Pyridoxine HCl) 100 mg • Inositol 100 mg • PABA (Para-aminobenzoic acid) 75 mg • Zinc amino acid chelate/complex 50 mg • Vitamin B2 (Riboflavin) 50 mg • Choline (Bitartrate) 32 mg • Beta Carotene supplying 15000 IU Vitamin A activity 9 mg • Folic Acid 400 mcg • Vitamin B12 from Cobalamin 200 mcg • Selenium amino acid complex 100 mcg • Biotin 100 mcg.

Exercise In A Bottle **-** Enforma Natural Products
Two capsules contain: Calcium Pyruvate 300 mg • CitriMax [Providing 40 mg of (-)Hydroxycitric Acid] 60 mg • Chromium Picolinate 25 mcg • Ginkgo Biloba 10 mg.

Exfoliant Scrub **-** Nu Skin Enterprises
Water • Aloe Barbadensis • Stearic Acid • Diatomaceous Earth • Propylene Glycol Stearate SE • Cetyl Alcohol • Glycerin • Allantoin • Tocopheryl Acetate • Retinyl Palmitate • Dioctyl Adipate • Octyl Stearate • Octyl Palmitate • Triethanolamine • Diazolidinyl Urea • Fragrance • Methylparaben • Propylparaben • Disodium EDTA.

Expectorant **-** Dial Herbs
Garlic • Bayberry • Mullein • Blood root • Cayenne • Lobelia.

Some Brand Name Natural Products - What they Contain

www.NaturalDatabase.com contains MANY more listings than appear here.

Ex-Stress Formula - Nature's Way
Two capsules contain: Proprietary Formula: Black Cohosh root • Cayenne pepper fruit • Hops flower • Scullcap herb • Valerian root • Wood Betony stem, leaf, flower. Other Ingredients: Gelatin.

Extend Libido Booster for Men - Rbhealth
Each capsule contains: Zinc 50 mg • Orchic substance 75 mg • Yohimbe powder 500 mg • Oyster Shell powder 75 mg • L-Arginine Hydrochloride 250 mg • Cayenne pepper 50 mg • Maca powder 250 mg • Tribulus Terrestris powder 50 mg • Oat Straw powder 150 mg • Astragalus powder 25 mg • Ginseng blend powder 125 mg • Sarsaparilla powder 25 mg • Catuaba powder 100 mg • Licorice root powder 20 mg • Muira Puama stem powder 75 mg • Pumpkin seed powder 20 mg • Nettle leaf powder 75 mg • Boron 2 mg. Other Ingredients: Magnesium Stearate, Silicon Dioxide, Gelatin, Titanium Dioxide.

Ex-Tox - Progressive Labs
Three capsules contain: Vitamin C 600 mg • Bentonite 300 mg • L-Lysine 60 mg • DL-Methionine 600 mg • Sodium Alginate 450 mg • Chlorophyll 60 mg • Fruit pectin 150 mg • Garlic powder 30 mg.

Extra Strength Glucosamine Chondroitin - Source Naturals
Two tablets contain: Glucosamine (as glucosamine sulfate) 1.5 g • Chondroitin (as chondroitin sulfate) 1.2 g.
See Editor's Note No. 15, page 2055.

Extra Strength Joint Maintenance - Puritan's Pride
Three tablets contain: Vitamin C (as ascorbic acid) 500 mg • Manganese (as manganese glycinate) 5 mg • Glucosamine Sulfate 1500 mg • Chondroitin Sulfate 1200 mg. Other Ingredients: Cellulose (plant origin), Crospovidone, Vegetable Stearic Acid, Titanium Dioxide Color, Cellulose Coating, Vegetable Magnesium Stearate, Silica.
See Editor's Note No. 15, page 2055.

Extra Strength Joint Maintenance Gels - Puritan's Pride - Puritan's Pride
Three softgels contain: Glucosamine Sulfate 1500 mg • Chondroitin Sulfate 1200 mg • Citrus Bioflavonoids 45 mg • Manganese (as manganese aspartate) 1.02 mg.
See Editor's Note No. 15, page 2055.

Extra Strength Joint Maintenance Gels - Vitamin World
Three softgels contain: Manganese (as manganese aspartate) 1 mg • Glucosamine Sulfate (2KCl) 1500 mg • Chondroitin Sulfate 1200 mg • Citrus Bioflavonoids 45 mg. Other Ingredients: Soybean Oil, Gelatin, Glycerin, Lecithin, St. John's Bread extract, Beeswax & Soybean Oil Mixture.
See Editor's Note No. 15, page 2055.

Extra Strength Joint Maintenance tablets - Vitamin World
Three tablets contain: Vitamin C (as ascorbic acid) 500 mg • Manganese (as manganese glycinate) 5 mg • Glucosamine Sulfate (KCl) 1500 mg • Chondroitin Sulfate 1200 mg. Other Ingredients: Cellulose, Crospovidone, Vegetable Stearic Acid, Titanium Dioxide Color, Cellulose Coating, Vegetable Magnesium Stearate, Silica.
See Editor's Note No. 15, page 2055.

Extra Strength Prosta-Metto - Puritan's Pride
Each softgel contains: Saw Palmetto extract (Serenoa repens: standardized to contain 85-95% fatty acids and biologically active sterol compounds) 160 mg • Pumpkin Seed oil extract (Cucurbita pepo) 40 mg • Pygeum Africanum extract 10 mg • Bearberry extract (Uva Ursi) 5 mg • Zinc (as Zinc Gluconate) 15 mg • Vitamin B6 5 mg.

Extra Strength Shen Min - Biotech Corp.
Two tablets contain: Shen Min Proprietary Blend 1755 mg: 12:1 He Shou Wu root (fo ti) standardized extract, He Shou Wu root powder • Herbal Purification Blend 600 mg: Eclipta Prostrata root, Radix Rehmannia root, Discorea Villosa root, Pocos Cocos aerial parts, Frucus Mori Albae root and stems, Frucus Ligusti Lucidi whole plant • BioPerine Black Pepper extract (piper nigrum) 3 mg. Other Ingredients: Dicalcium Phosphate, Microcrystalline Cellulose, Croscarmellose Sodium, Stearic Acid, Magnesium Stearate, Pharmaceutical Glaze.

Extra Strength Water Pill - Puritan's Pride
Each tablet contains: Potassium (as Potassium Gluconate) 40 mg • Buchu (Barosma betulina) leaf (25 mg of 4:1 extract) 100 mg • Uva Ursi (Arctostaphylos uva-ursi) leaf (33.3 mg of 3:1 extract) 100 mg • Juniper (Juniperus communis) berry 20 mg • Parsley (Petroselinum crispum) leaf 100 mg.

Extract Alpha - Gero Vita International
Three capsules contain: Proprietary Herbal Blend 2070 mg: CLA, Momordica Charantia extract (10% bitter principle), Green Tea extract (50% polyphenols), Choline Bitartrate, Wheat extract alpha (50%), L-Methionine, Inositol. Other Ingredients: Gelatin, Silicon Dioxide, Magnesium Stearate.

Extreme Power Plus - Dutch International Products
Green Tea • Kola Nut • 72 Trace Mineral Complex • Siberian Ginseng • Royal Jelly • White Willow bark • Ginger • Fo-Ti • Hawthorn berries • Saw Palmetto • Beet root powder • Chromium Picolinate • Guarana • Ma Huang • Zi Chi • Kelp • Citrimax • Calcium Carbonate • Magnesium Carbonate • Korean Ginseng • American Ginseng • Yerba Mate • Vitamin B12 • Bee Pollen.
See Editor's Note No. 30, page 2056.

Eye Beaute Pads - Pharmagel
Chamomile • Cucumber • Cornflower • Rosemary • Yarrow • Birch leaf • Sage • Nettle • Clover blossom.

Eye Care Complex - Leiner Health Products
Each tablet contains: Selenium 40 mcg • Vitamin A (Acetate) 2500 IU • Vitamin C (Ascorbic Acid) 30 mg • Bilberry 30 mg • Lutein 8 mg • Spinach 70 mg • Zeaxanthin 640 mcg. Other Ingredients: Calcium Carbonate, Gelatin, Glycerol, Starch, Cellulose, Maltodextrin Hydroxypropyl Methylcellulose, Croscarmellose Sodium, Crospovidone, Silicon Dioxide, Ascorbyl Palmitate, Dicalcium Phosphate, Polyethylene Glycol 3350, Tocopherols, Hydroxypropyl Cellulose, Magnesium Stearate, Pharmaceutical Glaze, Riboflavin, Blue 1 Lake, Titanium Dioxide, Polysorbate 80, Sodium Selenate.

Eye Defense - Nature Made
Two tablets contain: Vitamin A (100% as beta carotene) 5000 IU • Vitamin C (as ascorbic acid) 350 mg • Vitamin E (as DL-alpha tocopheryl acetate) 100 IU • Zinc (as zinc oxide) 15 mg • Copper (as copper oxide) 0.4 mg • Lutein 5 mg • Zeaxanthin 1 mg. Other Ingredients: Cellulose Gel, Talc, Gelatin, Sugar, Hydroxypropyl Methylcellulose, Corn Starch, Croscarmellose Sodium, Titanium Dioxide Artificial Color, Silica Gel, Magnesium Stearate, Polyethylene Glycol, Triethyl Citrate, Polysorbate 80, Sodium Citrate.

Eye Firming Gel - Pharmagel
Ginseng and plant extracts.

Eye Formula - Pharmanex
Each capsule contains: Beta-Carotene (Dunaliella Salina) 2500 IU • Vitamin C (Calcium Ascorbate, Ascorbic Acid) 150 mg • Vitamin E (d-Alpha Tocopheryl Succinate, Beta, Delta, Gamma Tocopherols) 75 IU • Zinc (Zinc Propionate) 2.5 mg • Selenium (L-Selenomethionine) 35 mcg • N-Acetyl-L-Cysteine 100 mg • Taurine 100 mg • Tumeric extract (Min. 95% Curcumin) 50 mg • Ginkgo Biloba extract (Min. 95% Flavonglycosides, Min. 6% Terpene Lactones) 30 mg • Alpha-Lipoic Acid 10 mg • Lutein (from Marigold flower extract) 2.5 mg. Other Ingredients: Calcium Carbonate, Sodium Carboxymethylcellulose, Magnesium Stearate, Talc.

Eye Guard Plus - Puritan's Pride
Four capsules contain: Beta Carotene (pro-vitamin A) 40,000 IU • Natural Vitamin E (succinate) 400 IU • Vitamin C 1,500 mg • Citrus Bioflavonoids Complex 250 mg • Quercetin (bioflavonoid) 100 mg • Bilberry extract (standardized 25%) 10 mg • Rutin 100 mg • Zinc

(picolinate) 25 mg • Selenium (selenomethionine) 100 mcg • Taurine 200 mg • N-Acetyl-Cysteine 200 mg • L-Glutathione 10 mg • Vitamin B2 (Riboflavin) 50 mg • Chromium (GTF) 200 mcg • Lutein 20 mg.

Eye Support **-** Now
Three capsules contain: Vitamin A (natural Beta Carotene • D. salina) 15 mg/25 000 IU • Vitamin C (as Ascorbic Acid) 300 mg • Vitamin E (as d-Alpha-Tocopheryl Succinate) 200 IU • Riboflavin (Vitamin B2) 20 mg • Zinc (as L-OptiZinc) 25 mg • Selenium 100 mcg • Bilberry standardized extract (Vaccinum myrtillus) (25% Anthocyanidins) 100 mg • Lutein 10 mg • Green Tea extract (Camellia sinensis) (40% Catechins) 150 mg • N-Acetyl-Cysteine (NAC) 100 mg • Rutin 100 mg.

Eye Treatment **-** Jason
Complete Vitamin C Complex • Vitamin E • Aloe Vera gel • Rose Hips.

Eyebright Formula **-** Nature's Way
Two capsules contain: Proprietary Formula: Bayberry bark • Cayenne pepper fruit • Eyebright stem, leaf, flower • Goldenseal root • Red Raspberry leaves. Other Ingredients: Gelatin.

Eyebright Herb **-** Now
Two capsules contain: Total Carbohydrate 650 mg • Eyebright herb (Euphrasia Officinalis) leaves and stems 940 mg. Other Ingredients: Stearic Acid.

Eye-Vites **-** Nature's Bounty
Each tablet contains: Vitamin A (as Beta Carotene) 5000 IU • Vitamin C (as Ascorbic Acid) 60 mg • Vitamin E (as dl-Alpha Tocopheryl Acetate) 30 IU • Zinc (as Zinc Oxide) 40 mg • Selenium (as Sodium Selenate) 40 mcg • Copper (as Cupric Oxide) 2 mg. Other Ingredients: Whey, Calcium Carbonate, Cellulose, Gelatin, Dicalcium Phosphate, Vegetable Stearic Acid, Croscarmellose, Cellulose Coating, Crospovidone, Vegetable Magnesium Stearate.

EZ Lung **-** EZ QUIT
Two tablets contain: Vitamin A (as retinyl palmitate, 10% as beta-carotene) 5000 IU • Vitamin C (as ascorbic acid) 150 mg • Vitamin D (as cholecalciferol) 200 IU • Vitamin E (as d-alpha-tocopheryl acetate) 30 IU • Thiamin (as thiamin HCl) 5 mg • Riboflavin 5 mg • Niacin (as niacinamide) 20 mg • Vitamin B6 (as pyridoxine HCl) 5 mg • Folate (as folic acid) 400 mcg • Vitamin B12 (as cyanocobalamin) 10 mcg • Pantothenic Acid (as d-calcium pantothenate) 10 mg • Calcium (as calcium carbonate) 300 mg • Iodine (from kelp) 150 mcg • Magnesium (as magnesium oxide) 100 mg • Zinc (as zinc citrate) 20 mg • Selenium (as selenium l-methionine) 200 mcg • Copper (as copper sulfate) 2 mg • Manganese (as manganese citrate) 2.5 mg • Chromium (as chromium dinicotinate glycinate) 120 mcg • Molybdenum (as sodium molybdate) 75 mcg • Stress Fighting Complex 150 mg: Korean Ginseng root extract (4% ginsenosides), Chamomile (flowering tops), Eleuthero root extract (0.8% total eleutherosides), Hops (strobile), Passion flower (whole plant) • Stress Fighting Complex 100 mg: Orange Bioflavonoids (30-40% total flavanones, flavonols, flavones, calculated as hesperidin), MSM (methylsulfonylmethane), Green Tea leaf extract, Ginger root standardized extract (5% gingerols), Calcium D-Glucarate, Bilberry fruit standardized extract. Other Ingredients: Microcrystalline Cellulose, Croscarmellose Sodium, Stearic Acid, Magnesium Stearate, Silica, Pharmaceutical Glaze.

EZ QUIT Cleanser **-** EZ QUIT
Six tablets contain: Iodine (from kelp) 200 mcg • Crave Control Blend 2500 mg: Alfalfa leaf, Eleuthero root, Licorice root, Echinacea Purpurea (aerial parts), Ginger root, Peppermint leaf, Lobelia (whole plant), Safflower seed oil, Bioperine standardized black pepper extract (95-97% piperine) • Cleansing Blend 1200 mg: Dandelion root, Cayenne Pepper, Sarsaparilla root, Buckhorn bark, Cascara Sagrada bark, Hyssop (aerial parts), Oregon Grape root, Barley grass, Bayberry fruit, Golden Seal (aerial parts) Lemon Verbena leaf, Oxbile extract, Elderberry fruit 10:1 extract. Other Ingredients: Dicalcium Phosphate, Microcrystalline Cellulose, Croscarmellose Sodium, Stearic Acid, Magnesium Stearate, Silica, Pharmaceutical Glaze.

E-Z Vite Multiple **-** Nature's Life
Two tablets contain: Vitamin A (Fish Liver oil) 10000 IU • Vitamin D (as Vitamin D3, Cholecalciferol) 400 IU • Vitamin B1 (Thiamine HCl) 10 mg • Vitamin B2 (Riboflavin) 10 mg • Vitamin B6 Pyridoxine HCl) 10 mg • Vitamin B12 (Cobalamin) 100 mcg • Niacin 30 mg • Pantothenic Acid (d-Calcium Pantothenate) 20 mg • Folic Acid 400 mcg • PABA (Para Aminobenzoic Acid) 30 mg • Biotin (d-Biotin) 3.5 mcg • Choline (Choline Bitartrate) 3 mg • Inositol 50 mg • Vitamin E (d-Alpha tocopherol, with Beta, Gamma & Delta Tocopherols) 10 IU • Vitamin C 100 mg • Lemon Bioflavonoids (TESTLAB) 30 mg • Rutin (Saphora japonica) 20 mg • Hesperidin Complex 5 mg • Calcium (Bone Meal) 40 mg • Copper (Gluconate) 100 mcg • Phosphorus (Bone Meal) 25 mg • Iodine (Icelandic Kelp) 100 mcg • Iron (Ferrous Fumarate) 10 mg • Magnesium (Oxide) 10 mg • Zinc (Gluconate) 2 mg • Potassium (Chloride) 10 mg • Manganese (Gluconate) 2 mg • Betaine HCl 25 mg • Liver (Defatted & Desiccated) 100 mg • RNA powder (Torula Yeast) 25 mg • Pancreatin (4 X N.F.) 25 mg. In a natural base of Raw Pancreas, Sodium Alginate, Torula B Yeast, Rose Hips & Acerola berries. See Editor's Note No. 14.

Ezorb Capsules **-** Elixer Industry
Each capsule contains: Calcium Aspartate Anhydrous (CalAA) 560 mg.

EZorb Powder **-** Elixer Industry
Calcium Aspartate Anhydrous (CalAA) powder.

Face Lift Activator (original formula) **-** Nu Skin Enterprises
Water • Aloe Barbadensis • Bladderwrack extract (fucus vesiculosus) • Allantoin • Panthenol • Sodium PCA • RNA • Benzalkonium Chloride • Butylene Glycol • Methylparaben • Phenoxyethanol • Disodium EDTA.

Face Lift Activator (sensitive formula) **-** Nu Skin Enterprises
Water • Aloe Vera gel (aloe barbadensis) • Hydrolyzed Wheat Protein • Allantoin • Panthenol • Sodium PCA • Citric Acid • Methylparaben • Phenoxyethanol • Tetrasodium EDTA • Methylchloroisothiazolinone • Methylisothiazolinone.

Face Lift Powder (original formula) **-** Nu Skin Enterprises
Albumin • Corn starch (zea mays) • Aloe Barbadensis • Silica • Hydrolyzed Elastin • Allantoin • Panthenol • Methylparaben.

Face Lift Powder (sensitive formula) **-** Nu Skin Enterprises
Acacia powder • Corn starch • Aloe • Allantoin • Panthenol • Ascorbic Acid • Methylparaben.

Facial Cleansing Bar **-** Nu Skin Enterprises
Sodium Cocoyl Isethionate • Maltodextrin • Stearic Acid • Cetyl Alcohol • Water • Nu Skin Cleansing Lotion: Water, Aloe Vera gel, Stearic Acid, Glyceryl Stearate SE, Dioctyl Adipate, Octyl Stearate, Octyl Palmitate, Propylene Glycol, Sodium PCA, Allantoin, RNA, Fragrance, Bladderwrack extract, Retinyl Palmitate, Ergocalciferol, Royal Jelly, Caramel, Cetearyl Alcohol, Ceteareth-20, Triethanolamine, Disodium EDTA, Butylparaben, Isobutylparaben, Isopropylparaben, Methylparaben, Phenoxyethanol • Sodium Isosteroyl Lactylate • Methyl Gluceth-20 • Sodium Lactate • Lactic Acid • Glycerin • Tocopheryl Acetate • Jojoba oil • Polyacrylamide • Titanium Dioxide • Fragrance.

Facial Scrub **-** Nu Skin Enterprises
Water • Aloe Barbadensis • Stearic Acid • Walnut shell powder (juglans regina) • Propylene Glycol Stearate SE • Cetyl Alcohol • Glycerin • Allantoin • Tocopheryl Acetate • Retinyl Palmitate • Dioctyl Adipate • Octyl Stearate • Octyl Palmitate • Triethanolamine • Quaternium-15 • Diazolidinyl Urea • Fragrance • Methylparaben • Propylparaben.

***Fade-Out Creme* - Pharmagel**
Vitamin C • Licorice Extract • PABA-free sunblock.

***False Unicorn-Squaw Vine Virtue* - Blessed Herbs**
False Unicorn root • Squaw vine • Black Haw bark • Grain alcohol & Distilled Water.

***Fast Balance-G.I.* - FoodScience of Vermont**
Each capsule contains: Mannon Oligosaccharides (MOS) 450 mg • Proprietary Probiotic Blend 50 mg: Lactobacillus Acidophilus, Lactobacillus Rhamnosus, Bifidobacterium Tongum (300 million CFU).

***Fast Food* - The Sports Nutrition Source, Inc.**
Two scoops contain: Sodium 300 mg • Potassium 600 mg • Protein 38 g • Vitamin A 2500 IU • Vitamin C 30 mg • Calcium 500 mg • Iron 9 mg • Vitamin D 200 IU • Vitamin E 15 IU • Vitamin K 35 mcg • Vitamin B-1 75 mg • Vitamin B-2 85 mg • Vitamin B-3 10 mg • Vitamin B-6 1 mg • Vitamin B-12 3 mcg • Biotin 125 mcg • Zinc 7.5 mcg • Copper 1 mg.

***Fast-Acting Zinaxin* - FreeLife International**
Each softgel contains: Patented Extract EV.EXT 77 [highly standardized extracts of rhizomes of Ginger (Zungiber officinale and Alpinia galanga)] 255 mg. Other Ingredients: Sunflower Seed oil, Gelatin, Beeswax, Lecithin, Vegetable Glycerin, Purified Water, Natural Chlorophyll Complex, Titanium Dioxide (natural mineral color).

***Fat & Sugar Block* - E'OLA**
Two tablets contain: Vitamin C (as Ascorbic Acid) 75 mg • Proprietary Blend 1050 mg: Chitosan, Gymnema Sylvestre, Garcinia Cambogia. Other Ingredients: Dicalcium Phosphate, Microcrystalline Cellulose, Croscarmellose Sodium, Stearic Acid, Silicon Dioxide.

***Fat Binding Diet System 6* - Applied Nutrition**
Two capsules contain: Vitamin C (ascorbic acid) 14 mg • Vitamin E (dl-alpha tocopheryl acetate) 4 IU • Riboflavin 0.5 mg • Niacin (niacinamide) 5 mg • Vitamin B6 (pyridoxine hydrochloride) 0.54 mg • Folic Acid 107 mcg • Vitamin B12 (cyanocobalamin) 2 mcg • Iodine (potassium iodine) 40 mcg • Selenium (sodium selenite) 14 mcg • Chromium (picolinate & 50% as polynicotinate) ChromeMate 80 mcg • Potassium (chloride) 6 mg • Garcinia Cambogia fruit (Super CitriMax, 60% Hydroxycitric acid extract) 460 mg • Chitosan (82% Deacetylated) 190 mg • Kola nut seed kernel extract (10% caffeine) 146 mg • Guarana seed extract (15% guaranine) 26 mg • Choline (bitartrate) 26 mg • Inositol 26 mg • Carnitine (L-Carnitine fumarate) 20 mg • Betaine (hydrochloride) 7 mg • Proprietary blend: [Ginger root, "72 Trace Minerals", Bioperine fruit (Piper nigrum extract, 95% Piperine)] 60 mg. Other Ingredients: Gelatin, montnirollinite, silica & magnesium stearate.

***Fat Bloc Chitosan 1000* - Ultimate Nutrition**
Each capsule contains: Vitamin C 50 mg • Chitosan 1000 mg. Other Ingredients: Cellulose, Dicalcium Phosphate, Gelatin, Magnesium Stearate.

***Fat Bloc Chitosan 500* - Ultimate Nutrition**
Each capsule contains: Vitamin C 40 mg • Chitosan 500 mg. Other Ingredients: Cellulose, Dicalcium Phosphate, Gelatin, Magnesium Stearate.

***Fat Burner* - Swanson**
Three tablets contain: Vitamin B-6 (as pyridoxine HCl) 50 mg • Chromium (from chromax chromium picolinate) 200 mcg • CitriMax (garcinia cambogia fruit extract) 1 g • Hydroxycitric Acid 500 mg • Choline Bitartrate 500 mg • Inositol 250 mg • L-Methionine 200 mg • Cider Vinegar powder 100 mg • Grapefruit powder 100 mg • Lecithin 100 mg • Taurine 100 mg.

***Fat Burner Non-Ephedra* - Natrol**
Three capsules contain: Chromium (as chromium picolinate) 100 mcg • Mucuna Prurient extract (l-dopa root)15 mg • Bitter Orange rind extract 20 mg • Synephrine 1.2 mg • Caffeine 100 mg. Other Ingredients: Rice Powder, Gelatin Capsule, Silica, Magnesium Stearate.
See Editor's Note No. 40, page 2058.

***Fat Burners* - Amerifit Nutrition**
Two caplets contain: Vitamin B6 (as pyridoxine HCl) 10 mg • Iron (as ferrous fumarate) 4 mg • Chromium (chromium picolinate) 50 mcg • Choline Complex 1000 mg: Choline Citrate, Buchu leaves, Uva Ursi root & fiber • Inositol 250 mg • L-Carnitine (as carnitine tartrate, carnitine HCl) 50 mg • L-Lysine 100 mg • Methionine 200 mg • Lecithin (from glycine max) 100 mg • Betaine HCl 200 mg • Essential Fatty Acids: (Linoleic, Oleic) 100 mg. Other Ingredients: Dicalcium Phosphate, Microcrystalline Cellulose, Magnesium Stearate, Croscarmellose Sodium • Stearic Acid & Vegetable glaze.
See Editor's Note No. 21, page 2056.

***Fat Busters* - Nature's Plus**
Each tablet contains: Calcium (as aminoate) 120 mg • Chromium (as polynicotinate) 120 mcg • Coleus Forskohlii extract (standardized 10% [25 mg] forskolin) 250 mg • Green Tea (Camellia sinensis leaf, decaffeinated, standardized 50% [100 mg] polyphenols) 200 mg • Green Orange (from fructus immaturus Citrus aurantium exocarp, standardized 4% [5 mg] synephrine) 125 mg • Korean Ginseng (Panax ginseng root, standardized to 15% [15 mg] ginsenosides) 100 mg • Ginger (Zingiber officinale root, standardized 4% [4 mg] volatile oils) 100 mg.
See Editor's Note No. 40, page 2058.

***Fat Digestion* - Enzymes, Inc.**
Each capsule contains: Proprietary Enzyme Blend 381 mg: Amylase, Lipase, Protease, Glucoamylase, Peptidase, alpha-Galactosidase, Cellulase. Other Ingredients: Plant Cellulose, Water.

***Fat Enzyme Formula* - Enzymatic Therapy**
Two capsules contain: Pure Plant Enzymes Blend 221 mg: Lipase I/II (FIP (pH7.0)) 1500 LU, (FCC III (pH6.5)) 1400 LU, Protease I/II/III/IV, (USP XXIII (pH7.5)) 16,350 USP, (FCC IV (pH7.0)) 26,100 PC.. (FCC IV (pH4.7)) 22,350 HUT, Amylase (USP XXI (pH6.8)) 16,500 USP, (FCC IV (pH4.8)) 7140 DU, Cellulase I (FCC IV (pH4.5)) 47.5 CU.

***Fat Free Gainers Fuel 1000* - TwinLab**
Each serving contains: Chromium (from Chromic Fuel Chromium Picolinate) 400 mcg. Other Ingredients: Branched Chain Amino Acids (L-Leucine, L-Isoleucine, L-Valine), Milk & Egg White Proteins, L-Carnitine & Kreb's Cycle Mineral Complexes (including Citrates, Aspartates, Succinates & Alpha-Ketoglutarates).

***Fat Free Gainers Fuel 2500* - TwinLab**
Chromium (from patented Chromic Fuel Chromium Picolinate) 400 mcg • Kreb's Cycle Mineral Complexes (including Citrates, Aspartates, Succinates & Alpha-Ketoglutarates) •Milk & Egg White Proteins • Branched Chain Amino Acids (L-Leucine, L-Isoleucine & L-Valine), L-Carnitine.

***Fat Metabolism Factors* - Michael's Naturopathic Programs**
Three tablets contain: Vitamin B6 (as pyridoxine) 100 mg • Iodine (from kelp) 225 mcg • Chromium (as chromium polynicotinate) 200 mcg • Potassium (as potassium amino acid complex) 210 mg • Proprietary Blend: Lecithin (from soy), Choline (as choline bitartrate), Inositol, Chickweed leaf (stellaria media), Fucus Vesiculosus leaf (sea wrack), Guggul gum (from commiphora mukul, 2.5% guggulsterones, 2.5 mg), Methionine (as L-methionine hydrochloride), Phenylalanine (as L-phenylalanine), White Ash bark (fraxinus americana), Bitter Orange fruit (citrus aurantium). Other Ingredients: Dicalcium Phosphate, Maltodextrin, Stearic Acid, Magnesium Stearate.
See Editor's Note No. 40, page 2058.

***Fat Metabolizer 2000* - Youngevity**
Cat's Claw • Siberian Ginseng • Bee Pollen • Kelp • Ephedra Sinica herb • White Willow bark • Licorice root • Hops flowers • Valerian root • Pantothenic Acid • Chromium Chelavite • Manganese

Chelazome • Vilcabamba Mineral Essence: Potassium, Calcium, Magnesium, Zinc, Chromium, Selenium, Iron, Copper, Molybdenum, Vanadium, Iodine, Cobalt, Manganese.
See Editor's Note No. 21 and No. 30, page 2056.

Fat Metabolizer 2001+ **-** Youngevity
Cat's Claw • Ephedra Sinica herb • White Willow bark • Caffeine • Kelp • Pantothenic Acid • Chromium Chelavite • Manganese Chelazome • Vilcabamba Mineral Essence: Potassium, Calcium, Magnesium, Zinc, Chromium, Selenium, Iron, Copper, Molybdenum, Vanadium, Iodine, Cobalt, Manganese.
See Editor's Note No. 21 and No. 30, page 2056.

Fat Predator **-** Fat Predator Weight Loss Company, Inc.
Each capsule contains: Ephedra extract • Cola Nut extract • White Willow bark.
See Editor's Note No. 21 and No. 30, page 2056.

Fat Predator Diet Capsules (no ephedra) **-** Fat Predator Weight Loss Company, Inc.
Two capsules contain: Pantothenic Acid (as d-calcium pantothenate) 40 mg • Citrus Aurantium 255 mg • Guarana 910 mg • White Willow bark 101 mg • Proprietary Blend 355 mg: L-Tyrosine, Acetyl L-Carnitine, Bitter Orange, Green Tea extract, Grape seed extract.
See Editor's Note No. 40, page 2058.

Fat Snatcher **-** Youngevity
Chitosan • Aloe Vera leaf • Citric Acid • Iso-Ascorbic Acid (Vitamin C).

Fat Stopper Formula **-** Health Tech Industries (Dr. Bussan's)
Two capsules contain: Chitosan 250 mg • TAT Metabolite (a proprietary process of Dews Research Laboratories) 100 mg • Bile Salts Extract NF 50 mg • Vitamin C (polyascorbic acid) 50 mg • Acetyl Pyruvate Bile 12 mg • Niacin 5 mg • Chromium Picolinate 25 mcg. Other Ingredients: Magnesium trisilicate, Magnesium stearate, trace FD& C Yellow #5 and natural Gelatin capsules.

Fat Trap **-** The Sports Nutrition Source, Inc.
Each capsule contains: Chitosan shellfish 500 mg • Fiber 500 mg.

Fat Trapper **-** Enforma Natural Products
Two capsules contain: Psyllium seed husk 420 mg • Chitin 80 mg.

Fat Trapper Plus **-** Enforma Natural Products
Two capsules contain: Psyllium seed husk 420 mg • Chitin 80 mg. Other Ingredients: Gelatin, Magnesium Stearate, Vegetable Stearine, Glycerin.

Fat-B-Gone **-** Biotech Corp.
Two tablets contain: Natural Vitamin E (d-alpha tocopherol succinate) 10 IU • Vitamin C (ascorbic acid) 500 mg • Chitosan 500 mg • Explosive Proprietary Tablet Dissolution 120 mg: Croscarmellose Sodium, Soy Fibers. Other Ingredients: Dicalcium Phosphate, Microcrystalline Cellulose, Stearic Acid, Silica, Magnesium Stearate, Pharmaceutical Glaze.

FatBlast **-** E.V.A. Pharmaceutics
Three capsules contain: Chitosan (HD) 554 mg • Psyllium husk 150 mg • Malic Acid 28 mg • Lipase (vegetarian) 14 mg • Aloe Vera leaf (concentrate 1200) 14 mg. Other Ingredients: Rice Flour, Partially Hydrogenated Cottonseed Oil Kosher, NF, Gelatin Capsule.

FatFree **-** Starlight International
Each two tablets contain: Maitake Mushroom extract, 4:1 (grifola frondosa, plant) 50 mg • Platycodon grandiflorum extract 5:1 (root) 140 mg • Glucomannan (amorphophalius konjac, root) 1000 mg • Gymnema sylvestre leaf 100 mg. Inactive Ingredients: Dicalcium Phosphate, Microcrystalline Cellulose, Stearic Acid Croscarmellose Sodium, Magnesium Stearate, Silicon Dioxide, Food Glaze, Ethylcellulose, Dextrin, Dextrose, Lecithin, Sodium Citrate.

Fatigue-Aid **-** Futurebiotics
Two capsules contain: Vitamin C (as buffered calcium ascorbate) 120 mg • Thiamin (as thiamin HCl) 25 mg • Riboflavin 25 mg • Niacin (as niacinamide) 25 mg • Vitamin B6 (as pyridoxine hydrochloride) 25 mg • Vitamin B12 (as cyanocobalamin) 250 mcg • Folic Acid 400 mcg • Pantothenic Acid 25 mg • Selenium (as amino acid chelate) 100 mcg • Citrus Bioflavonoids 250 mg • MSM (methyl-sulfonyl-methane) 200 mg • St. John's Wort powder extract (standardized for 0.3% (0.75 mg) hypericin) 250 mg • Astragalus root powder 200 mg • Pancreatin 4x (quadruple strength) (supplying 1600 USP units Lipase, 10000 USP units Amylase, 10000 USP units Protease) 125 mg • Spirulina 100 mg • Blackstrap Molasses powder 25 mg • Red Beet powder 25 mg • Licorice root powder 25 mg • Siberian Ginseng (50:1) root powder 25 mg. Other Ingredients: Gelatin, Water.
See Editor's Note No. 14.

Fatigued to Fantastic! Daily Energy B Complex **-** Enzymatic Therapy
Each capsule contains: Thiamin (as thiamin HCl, vitamin B1) 75 mg • Riboflavin (vitamin B2) 75 mg • Niacin (as niacinamide) 50 mg • Vitamin B6 (as pyridoxine HCl) 85 mg • Folic Acid 800 mcg • Vitamin B12 (as cyanocobalamin) 500 mcg • Pantothenic Acid (as calcium D-pantothenate) 50 mg • Choline Bitartrate 100 mg. Other Ingredients: Gelatin, Cellulose, Modified Cellulose Gum, Magnesium Stearate, Titanium Dioxide Color.

Fatigued to Fantastic! Daily Energy Enfusion **-** Enzymatic Therapy
Each level scoop (17 g) contains: Vitamin A (as 50% beta carotene and as retinyl acetate) 3500 IU • Vitamin C (ascorbic acid) 750 mg • Vitamin D (as cholecalciferol) 600 IU • Vitamin E (as d-alpha tocopheryl acetate) 100 IU • Biotin 200 mcg • Iodine (as potassium iodide) 150 mcg • Magnesium (as magnesium glycinate) 200 mg • Zinc (as zinc oxide) 15 mg • Selenium (as L-selenomethionine) 200 mcg • Copper (as copper gluconate) 500 mcg • Manganese (as manganese citrate) 4 mg • Chromium (as chromium picolinate) 200 mcg • Molybdenum (as sodium molybdate) 250 mcg • Sodium 20 mg • Potassium (as potassium citrate) 50 mg • Whey Protein 7 g • Malic Acid 900 mg • Inositol 750 mg • Inulin (from chicory root) 750 mg • Hesperidin (50% from citrus fruits) 500 mg • Taurine 500 mg • Glycine 390 mg • L-Tyrosine 377 mg • N-Acetylcysteine (NAC) 250 mg • L-Serine 240 mg • Boron (as sodium borate 2 mg). Other Ingredients: Guar Gum, Natural Flavors, Stevia Leaf.

Fatigued to Fantastic! Revitalizing Sleep Formula **-** Enzymatic Therapy
Each capsule contains: Valerian (valeriana officinalis; root extract standardized to contain a minimum of 0.8% valerenic acids) 200 mg • Passionflower (passiflora incarnata; leaf and flower extract 4:1) 90 mg • L-Theanine (suntheanine brand) 50 mg • Hops (humulus lupulus; flower extract 6.6:1) 30 mg • Wild Lettuce (lactuca virosa; leaf extract) 18 mg • Jamaica Dogwood (piscidia piscipula; root extract) 12 mg. Other Ingredients: Gelatin, Magnesium Stearate, Titanium Dioxide Color, Silicon Dioxide.

FATmelt - with Gymnema Sylvestre **-** Slimming and Nutrition Consultancy
Each capsule contains: L-Carnitine • Gymnema Sylvestre • Chromium Picolinate • Forskolii (4:1 extract) • Bioperine. In a Maltodextrin and Magnesium stearate base.

FBL101 **-** FBL Sciences
Three capsules contain: Proprietary Blend 1379 mg: Soy, Dong Quai root, Black Cohosh root, Licorice root, Gamma Oryzanol, Red Clover blossoms powder.

FBlock Chitosan Caps **-** Absolute Nutrition
Two capsules contain: Vitamin C (as ascorbic acid) 100 mg • Chitosan (marine fiber concentrate) 1000 mg • Lipase 300 LU • Calcium Sulfate 150 mg • Vegetable Cellulose 100 mg.
See Editor's Note No. 37, page 2057.

Some Brand Name Natural Products - What they Contain

www.NaturalDatabase.com contains MANY more listings than appear here.

FBlock Xtra - Absolute Nutrition
Two capsules contain: Vitamin C (as ascorbic acid) 100 mg • Chitosan (marine fiber concentrate) 1000 mg • Lipase 300 LU • Calcium Sulfate 150 mg • Vegetable Cellulose 100 mg. Other Ingredients: Gelatin, Vegetable Magnesium Stearate, Silica.

Feel Good Formula - Bee-Alive Inc.
Each capsule contains: Royal Jelly (non-freeze dried) 150 mg.

Feelfine - Feelfine
Active Ingredients: Fructose • Glucose • Sodium Bicarbonate • Vitamin C • Potassium Citricity • L-Cysteine • Magnesium Oxide • L-Glutamine • Kolin • Vitamin B1 (thiamine) • Vitamin B6 (pyridoxine) • Tricalciumphosphate. Other Ingredients: Passion Fruit flavor.

Fem Balance - The Vitamin Shoppe
Each capsule contains: Black Cohosh 20 mg.

Fem EstroPlex - Metagenics
Three tablets contain: Rutin 800 mg • Vitamin C (as ascorbic acid) 300 mg • Pantothenic Acid (as d-calcium pantothenate) 300 mg • Vitamin B6 (as pyridoxine hydrochloride) 50 mg • Vitamin E (as d-alpha tocopheryl succinate) 100 IU • Proprietary Herbal Extract Blend 1050 mg: Dandelion root (taraxacum officinale, 4.5:1 extract), Chasteberry fruit (vitex agnus-castus), Valerian root (valeriana officinalis), Motherwort aerial parts (leonurus cardiaca, 6.5:1 extract), Nettle root (urtica dioica, 10:1 extract).

Fem Fit - The Sports Nutrition Source, Inc.
Two scoops contain: Sodium 200 mg • Potassium 400 mg • Protein 26 g • Vitamin A 1675 IU • Vitamin C 20 mg • Calcium 335 mg • Iron 6 mg • Vitamin D 134 IU • Vitamin E 10 IU • Vitamin K 23 mcg • Vitamin B-1 50 mg • Vitamin B-2 57 mg • Vitamin B-3 6.7 mg • Vitamin B-6 670 mcg • Vitamin B-12 3 mcg • Biotin 64 mcg • Zinc 5 mcg • Copper 670 mcg.

FemActin - Nature's Plus
Three capsules contain: Dong Quai [(Angelica sinensis root) standardized 0.9% Ligustilide] 100 mg • Evening Primrose [(Oenothera biennis seed) standardized 4% Gamma-Linolenic Acid] 100 mg • Uva Ursi [(Arctostaphylos uva-ursi leaf) standardized 20-25% Arbutin] 75 mg • Suma [(Pfaffia paniculata root) standardized 5% Beta-Ecdysterone] 50 mg • Butcher's Broom [(Ruscus aculeatus L. rhizome) standardized 10% Saponin Glycosides] 50 mg • Nettle [(Urtica dioica leaf) standardized 1-2% Plant Silica] 50 mg • Goldenseal [(Hydrastis canadensis root & rhizome) standardized 10% Alkaloids, 5% Hydrastine]50 mg • Chasteberry [(Vitex agnus-castus fruit) standardized 0.5% Agnuside, 0.6% Aucubin] 50 mg • Vitamin B6 (Pyridoxine HCl) 25 mg • Iron (Amino Acid Chelate) 12 mg.

Femal - Natumin Pharma
Each tablet contains: PI 82 Pollen Pistil extract 120 mg • GC FEM Pollen extract 36 mg • Royal Jelly (freeze dried) 6 mg • Vitamin E (50%) 20 mg. Other Ingredients: Microcrystalline Cellulose 87 mg, Dicalcium Phosphate 87 mg, Magnesium Stearate 4 mg.

Female Advantage - Body Wise International, Inc.
Each three capsules contain: Magnesium 15 mg • Zinc 10 mg • Soy Protein Concentrate 516 mg • Valerian root 300 mg • Kava Kava root 250 mg • Alpha-Ketoglutaric Acid 50 mg • Dong Quai root 200 mg • Mexican Yam root 100 mg • Flaxseed 100 mg • Korean Ginseng root 75 mg • Siberian Ginseng root 75 mg • Indole-3-Carbinol 50 mg • L-Arginine HCL 50 mg • L-Lysine HCL 50 mg • Black Cohosh root 50 mg • Evening Primrose seed oil 50 mg • Passion Flower whole plant 50 mg • Suma root 50 mg • Gotu Kola whole plant 50 mg • Bromelain 50 mg • Goldenseal root 50 mg • Echinacea Purpurea root 20 mg • Licorice root 10 mg. Inactive Ingredients: Gelatin, Magnesium Stearate NF, Cellulose.

Female Balance - Bioset - Enzymes, Inc.
Each capsule contains: Vitamin E (100% from d-Alpha Tocopheryl Acid Succinate) 30 IU • Proprietary Herbal Blend 408 mg: Black Cohosh root extract, Chaste Tree berry extract, Ginkgo Biloba leaf extract, Oat straw extract, Soy Isoflavones • pHysioProtease 40 mg. Other Ingredients: Plant Cellulose, Water.

Female Balance - Enzymatic Therapy
Three capsules contain: Vitamin A (Beta Carotene) (Non-toxic form of Vitamin A) 16665 IU • Vitamin E (D-Alpha Tocopherol Succinate) 200 IU • Vitamin C (Ascorbic Acid) 200 mg • Magnesium L-Aspartate 150 mg • Pantothenic Acid (D-Calcium Pantothenate) 100 mg • Thiamine HCL (Vitamin B1) 50 mg • Riboflavin (Vitamin B2) 50 mg • Calcium Citrate 50 mg • Iron (Ferrous Succinate) 18 mg • Zinc (Gluconate) 15 mg • Chromium (Polynicotinate) 250 mcg • Folic Acid 100 mcg • Vitamin B12 (Cyanocobalamin concentrate) 50 mcg • Selenium (L-Selenomethionine) 50 mcg • Dong Quai extract (4:1) (Angelica sinensis) 75 mg • Licorice root extract (Glycyrrhiza glabra) standardized to contain 5% Glycyrrhizic acid) 60 mg • Milk Thistle extract (Silybum Marianum) standardized to contain 70% Silymarin calculated as Silybin) 50 mg • Black Cohosh extract (4:1) (Cimicifuga racemosa) 30 mg • Chaste Berry extract (5:1) (Vitex agnus-castus) 20 mg • Pyridoxal-5'-Phosphate 10 mg.

Female Balance - Now
Three capsules contain: Vitamin B6 50 mg • Folic Acid 400 mcg • Borage oil powder (45 mg GLA) 325 mg • Wild Yam root extract (6% Diosgenin) 225 mg • Dong Quai root extract 5:1 150 mg • Vitex Agnus castus extract 10:1 150 mg.

Female Balance - Olympia Nutrition
Borage Oil powder • Wild Yam root • Dong Quai • Vitex Agnus • Vitamin B6.

Female Cycle - Enzymes, Inc.
Two capsules contain: Vitamin E (100% from d-alpha Tocopheryl Acid Succinate) 100 IU • Proprietary Herbal Blend 850 mg: Chaste Tree berry extract, Dong Quai Rhizome extract, Cramp bark extract, Black Currant seed extract, Damiana leaf extract, Dandelion leaf extract, Soy Isoflavones • pHysioProtease 80 mg. Other Ingredients: Cellulose, Water.

Female Formula - 4 Life
Each capsule contains: Fenugreek seed 85 mg • Black Cohosh root 68 mg • Dong Quai root 68 mg • Ginger root 68 mg • Female Proprietary Extract Blend 45 mg: Black Cohosh root extract, Red Raspberry leaf extract, Dong Quai root extract, Valerian root extract, Fenugreek seed extract, Ginger seed extract, Licorice root extract, Black Hawk bark extract • Red Raspberry leaf extract 33 mg • Licorice root 33 mg. Other Ingredients: Gelatin Capsule, Rice Bran, Magnesium Stearate.

Female Formula - Oasis Wellness Network
Each tablet contains: Vitamin D (as cholecalciferol) 100 IU • Calcium (as citrate/malate/carbonate) 100 mg • Iron (as glyco amino acid chelate) 15 mg • Dong Quai root extract 100 mg • Rehmannia Glutinosa root extract 100 mg • MaxCell Proprietary Blend 100 mg: Zisyphus Jujube, Aloe Vera gel, Piper Nigrum, Glycyrrhiza Glabra • Jujube fruit extract 100 mg • Soy Isoflavone extract. Other Ingredients: Stearic Acid, Cellulose, Magnesium Stearate, Silica, Modified Food Starch.

Female Multi Vitamin - Health Center for Better Living
Each tablet contains: Vitamin A (as retinyl palmitate and 50% from beta-carotene) 3000 IU • Vitamin C (as ascorbic acid) 100 mg • Vitamin D (as cholecalciferol) 200 IU • Vitamin E (as dl-alpha-tocopheryl acetate) 25 IU • Thiamin (as thiamin HCl) 7 mg • Riboflavin 7 mg • Niacin (as niacinamide) 25 mg • Vitamin B6 (as pyridoxine HCl) 25 mg • Folate (as folic acid) 200 mcg • Vitamin B12 (as cyanocobalamin) 50 mcg • Biotin 35 mcg • Pantothenic Acid (as D-calcium patothenate) 25 mg • Calcium (as dicalcium phosphate) 75 mg • Iron (as ferrous fumarate) 18 mg • Iodine (from Kelp) 25 mcg • Magnesium (as magnesium oxide) 75 mg • Zinc (as zinc citrate) 5 mg • Copper (as copper gluconate) 250 mcg • Manganese (as manganese gluconate) 1 mg • Chromium (as chromium dinicotinate glycinate) 50 mcg • Inositol 10 mg • Choline bitartrate 10 mg • Bioflavonoids Complex: Citrus Bioflavonoids, Hesperidin, Rutin, and Quercetin trace.

Female Sage **-** Traditional Medicinals
Each cup brewed tea contains: Calcium 10 mg • Magnesium 4 mg • Manganese 0.04 mg • Potassium 25 mg • Essential Oil (of sage leaf) 750 mg • Chaste Tree Fruit 75 mg • Chaste Tree Fruit Dry Extract (10:1) 75 mg • Proprietary Blend 600 mg: Blue Vervain Herb, Organic Oatstraw Herb, Organic Lemongrass Leaf, Organic Bitter Fennel Seed, Rosemary Leaf, Organic Blessed Thistle Herb, Organic Stevia Leaf.

Female Support **-** Nutripeak
Fifteen drops contains: Oophorinum Sarcode (Ovary Gland) 8X. Other Ingredients: Purified Water, 20% USP Alcohol.
See Editor's Note No. 1, page 2053.

Female Toner **-** Traditional Medicinals
Spearmint leaf • Rose Hip • Red Raspberry leaf • Licorice root • Strawberry Leaf • Lemongrass leaf • Lemon Verbena leaf • Nettle leaf • Ginger rhizome • Chamomile flower • Angelica root • Blessed Thistle herb • Cramp bark.

Femaprin **-** Nature's Way
Each capsule contains: Vitamin B6 (as pyridoxine HCl) 100 mg • Vitex Agnus Castus (fruit) 100 mg • Vitex Agnus Castus dried extract (fruit, 0.6% agnusides) 225 mg. Other Ingredients: Gelatin, Magnesium Stearate, Millet.

Femarelle **-** Se-Cure Pharmaceuticals/Ventiv Health
Each capsule contains: Tofu (powder form - DT56a) 322 mg • Flaxseed 108 mg. Other Ingredients: Kosher Gelatin.

Femarone 17 - Unknown
Purified Water • Wild Yam extract • Polyacrymide/Isoparrafin/ Laureth-7 • Emulsifying Wax • C 12-15 Alkyl Benzoate • Glyceryl Stearate/PEG-100 Stearate • Progesterone (from wild yam) • Chaste Tree berry extract (vitex) • Glycerin / Alcohol • Jojoba oil • Swalane • Allantoin • Water/Phospholipids • Retinyl Palmitate • Ascorbyl Palmitate • A-Alpha Tocopherol • Liposomes of Vitamin A, C & E • Dong Quai extract • Licorice extract • Black Cohosh extract • Grapefruit seed extract • Sorbic Acid.

Femdiol **-** PhytoPharmica
Each capsule contains: Vitamin E (D-Alpha Tocopherol) 150 IU • Barlean's Flaxseed oil 300 mg • Gamma-Oryzanol 100 mg • Pumpkin seed oil (Curcurbita pepo) 50 mg • Soy extract 20 mg.

FemEssence **-** Advocare International
Three capsules contain: Niacin 20 mg • Vitamin B6 30 mg • Iron (as ferrous glycinate Ferrochel) 13.5 mg • Glucosamine (as HCl) 500 mg • Moomiyo 100 mg • Wild Yam extract (root - Dioscorea floribunda) 100 mg • Saw Palmetto extract (fruit - serenoa repens) 60 mg • Ginkgo extract (leaf - ginkgo biloba) 75 mg • Cranberry extract (fruit - vaccinium macrocarpon) 200 mg • Raspberry extract (leaf - rubus idaeus) 50 mg • Resveratrol (from polygonum cuspidatum) 5 mg • Lactobacillus Acidophilus 200 MM. Other Ingredients: Silicon Dioxide, Magnesium Stearate, Gelatin.

FemFactor **-** HealthMinded
Each capsule contains: Proprietary Blend 550 mg: Sage leaf, Red Raspberry leaf, Pueraria root, Red Clover, Cayenne pepper, Licorice root, Bayberry fruit, Damiana leaf, Valerian root, Ginger root, Black Cohosh root.

FEMFOCUS **-** Solgar
Three tablets contain: Protein 1 g • Vitamin A (as palmitate 5000 IU, 75% as natural beta-carotene from D.salina) 20000 IU • Vitamin C (as L-ascorbic acid) 400 mg • Vitamin D (as cholecalciferol) 400 IU • Vitamin E (as D-alpha tocopheryl succinate) 400 IU • Vitamin K (as phytonadione) 20 mcg • Thiamin (as thiamin mononitrate) 50 mg • Riboflavin 50 mg • Niacin (as niacinamide) 60 mg • Vitamin B-6 (as pyridoxine HCl) 50 mg • Folic Acid 800 mcg • Vitamin B-12 (as cobalamin) 200 mcg • Biotin (as D-biotin) 300 mcg • Pantothenic Acid (as D-ca pantothenate) 80 mg • Calcium (as calcium carbonate, glycinate, citrate) 400 mg • Iron (as iron bisglycinate) 18 mg • Iodine (as kelp) 150 mcg • Magnesium (as magnesium oxide, glycinate, citrate) 400 mg • Zinc (as zinc glycinate, histidinate) 30 mg • Selenium (as L-selenomethionine) 200 mcg • Copper (as copper glycinate) 1.5 mg • Manganese (as manganese glycinate) 2 mg • Chromium (as chromium nicotinoglycinate) 200 mcg • Molybdenum (as molybdenum glycinate) 50 mcg • Sodium 25 mg • Potassium (as potassium glycinate complex) 99 mg • Citrus Bioflavonoids 100 mg • Choline (as choline bitartrate) 100 mg • Inositol 100 mg • Pantethine 7 mg • Cocarboxylase 6 mg • Pyridoxal-5-Phosphate 6 mg • Riboflavin-5-Phosphate 6 mg • Dibencozide 21 mcg • Boron (as boron glycinate complex) 500 mcg • Dong Quai extract root (angelica sinensis) 25 mg • Uva Ursi extract leaf (arcostaphylos uva ursi) 25 mg • Chaste berry extract (vitex agnus-castus) 25 mg • American Ginseng extract root 25 mg • Milk Thistle extract aerial (silybum marianum) 25 mg • Black Cohosh extract root (cimicifuga racemosa) 25 mg • Soy Isoflavone extract seed 25 mg • Carotenoid Mix (alpha carotene, lutein, zeaxanthin, cryptoxanthin) 172 mcg. Other Ingredients: Microcrystalline Cellulose, Vegetable Cellulose, Vegetable Stearic Acid, Red Beet Powder, Titanium Dioxide, Vegetable Glycerin, Silica, Vegetable Magnesium Stearate.

FEMFOCUS - Black Cohosh **-** Solgar
Each vegicap contains: Black Cohosh extract root (triterpine glycosides 5 mg as 27-deoxyactein) 200 mg • Raw Black Cohosh powder root 200 mg • Soy Isoflavone concentrate seed (isoflavone 6 mg) 200 mg. Other Ingredients: Microcrystalline Cellulose; Vegetable Cellulose; Vegetable Magnesium Stearate; Vegetable Glycerin; Phyt02X Blend: Vitamin E, Beta Carotene and other Carotenoids, Rosemary extract aerial, Vitamin C (L-Ascorbic Acid), Water.

FEMFOCUS - Bone Support **-** Solgar
Four tablets contain: Vitamin D (as cholecalciferol) 600 IU • Vitamin K (as phytonadione) 80 mcg • Calcium (as calcium carbonate, glycinate, citrate) 800 mg • Iron 0.7 mg • Magnesium (as magnesium glycinate, citrate, oxide) 400 mg • Zinc (as zinc glycinate, histidinate) 10 mg • Copper (as copper lysinate) 0.5 mg • Sodium 20 mg • Ipriflavone (as 7-isopropoxyisoflavone) 600 mg • Soy Isoflavone Concentrate seed 400 mg • Boron (as boron glycinate complex) 1.5 mg. Other Ingredients: Microcrystalline Cellulose; Vegetable Cellulose; Methacrylic Acid; Vegetable Magnesium Stearate; Vegetable Stearic Acid; Glyceryl Triacetate; Vegetable Glycerin; PhytO2X Blend: Vitamin E, Beta-Carotene and other Carotenoids, Rosemary extract aerial, Vitamin C (L-Ascorbic Acid), Annatto, Grapeskin.

FEMFOCUS - Calcium Citrate **-** Solgar
Four tablets contain: Vitamin D (as cholecalciferol) 600 IU • Calcium (as calcium citrate) 1000 mg. Other Ingredients: Microcrystalline Cellulose, Silica, Vegetable Magnesium Stearate, Titanium Dioxide, Vegetable Cellulose, Vegetable Glycerin.

FEMFOCUS - Cranberry Berry Extract **-** Solgar
Each vegicap contains: Cranberry extract berry (organic acids 30 mg) 100 mg • Cranberry concentrate powder berry 300 mg. Other Ingredients: Vegetable Cellulose; Microcrystalline Cellulose; Silica; Vegetable Magnesium Stearate; Vegetable Glycerin; PhytO2X Blend: Vitamin E, Beta-Carotene and other Carotenoids, Rosemary extract aerial, Vitamin C, Water.

FEMFOCUS - Cranberry Extract with Vitamin C **-** Solgar
Each vegicap contains: Vitamin C (as L-ascorbic acid) 60 mg • Cranberry extract berry 400 mg. Other Ingredients: Vegetable Cellulose, Silica, Vegetable Magnesium Stearate, Vegetable Glycerin, Water.

FEMFOCUS - Dong Quai **-** Solgar
Each vegicap contains: Dong Quai extract root 150 mg • Raw Dong Quai powder root 300 mg. Other Ingredients: Microcrystalline Cellulose; Vegetable Cellulose; Vegetable Magnesium Stearate; Vegetable Glycerin; Phyt02X Blend: Vitamin E, Beta Carotene and other Carotenoids, Rosemary extract aerial, Vitamin C (L-Ascorbic Acid), Water.

FEMFOCUS - Ester-C Plus - Solgar
Each vegicaps contain: Vitamin C (as Ester-C calcium ascorbate) 500 mg • Calcium (as calcium ascorbate) 62 mg • Citrus Bioflavonoids 25 mg • Acerola 10 mg • Rose Hips fruit 10 mg • Rutin 5 mg. Other Ingredients: Vegetable Cellulose, Vegetable Magnesium Stearate, Silica, L-Threonic Acid, Vegetable Glycerin, Water.

FEMFOCUS - Evening Primrose Oil - Solgar
Each softgel contains: Vitamin E (as D-alpha tocopheryl acetate) 14 IU • Linoleic Acid 360 mg • Gamma-Linolenic Acid 50 mg • Oleic Acid 50 mg • Other Fatty Acids 40 mg. Other Ingredients: Evening Primrose Oil, Gelatin, Glycerin, Water.

FEMFOCUS - Flaxseed Oil - Solgar
Two softgels contain: Linolenic Acid 1425 mg • Oleic Acid 450 mg • Linoleic Acid 400 mg • Palmitic Acid 150 mg • Stearic Acid 75 mg. Other Ingredients: Flaxseed Oil, Gelatin, Glycerin, Carob Flavor, Water.

FEMFOCUS - Folic Acid - Solgar
Each tablet contains: Folic Acid 400 mcg • Calcium (as dicalcium phosphate) 70 mg. Other Ingredients: Vegetable Stearic Acid, Silica, Vegetable Cellulose.

FEMFOCUS - Gentle Iron - Solgar
Each vegicap contains: Iron (as iron bisglycinate) 25 mg. Other Ingredients: Microcrystalline Cellulose, Vegetable Cellulose, Vegetable Magnesium Stearate, Vegetable Glycerin, Water.

FEMFOCUS - Herbal Female Complex - Solgar
Each vegicap contains: Iron 1 mg • Standardized Chaste berry extract 75 mg • Dong Quai extract root 75 mg • Soy Isoflavone extract seed 100 mg • Milk Thistle extract aerial, seed (silymarin 40 mg) 50 mg • Black Cohosh extract root 100 mg • Motherwort extract aerial 75 mg • Raw Astragalus powder root 75 mg • Raw Korean Ginseng powder root 50 mg • Raw Dong Quai powder root 50 mg. Other Ingredients: Microcrystalline Cellulose; Vegetable Cellulose; Vegetable Stearic Acid; Vegetable Magnesium Stearate; Vegetable Glycerin; Phyt02X Blend: Vitamin E, Beta-Carotene and other Carotenoids, Rosemary extract aerial, Vitamin C (L-Ascorbic Acid), Water.

FEMFOCUS - Ipriflavone - Solgar
Each vegicap contains: Ipriflavone (as 7-isopropoxyisoflavone) 200 mg. Other Ingredients: Microcrystalline Cellulose, Vegetable Cellulose, Vegetable Magnesium Stearate, Vegetable Glycerin, Water.

FEMFOCUS - Non-GMO Isoflavones - Solgar
Each tablet contains: Total Soy Isoflavones seed (from soy isoflavone extract) 38 mg. Other Ingredients: Microcrystalline Cellulose, Vegetable Cellulose, Silica, Vegetable Magnesium Stearate, Caramel, Titanium Dioxide, Vegetable Glycerin.

FEMFOCUS - Oceanic Silica - Solgar
Each vegicap contains: Calcium 30 mg • Silica (from red algae powder, 25 mg elemental silicon) 54 mg. Other Ingredients: Vegetable Cellulose, Microcrystalline Cellulose, Vegetable Magnesium Stearate, Vegetable Glycerin, Water.

FEMFOCUS - Prenatal Tablets - Solgar
Four tablets contain: Vitamin A (as palmitate 3000 IU, 63% as natural beta-carotene from d. salina) 8000 IU • Vitamin C (as l-ascorbic acid) 100 mg • Vitamin D (as cholecalciferol) 400 IU • Vitamin E (as d-alpha tocopheryl succinate) 30 IU • Thiamin (as thiamin mononitrate) 1.7 mg • Riboflavin 2 mg • Niacin (as niacinamide) 20 mg • Vitamin B6 (as pyridoxine HCl) 2.5 mg • Folic Acid 800 mcg • Vitamin B12 (as cobalamin) 8 mcg • Biotin 300 mcg • Pantothenic Acid (as d-ca pantothenate) 10 mg • Calcium (as calcium carbonate, calcium citrate) 1300 mg • Iron (as iron bisglycinate) 27 mg • Iodine (as kelp) 150 mcg • Magnesium (as magnesium oxide, magnesium citrate) 450 mg • Zinc (as zinc chelate, zinc oxide) 15 mg • Copper (as copper chelate, copper gluconate) 2 mg • Selenium (as l-selenomethionine) 25 mcg • Manganese (as manganese chelate, manganese gluconate) 2 mg • Chromium (as chromium picolinate) 25 mcg • Potassium (from potassium amino acid complex, potassium gluconate) 50 mg • Inositol 10 mg • Choline (as choline bitartrate) 4 mg • PABA (as para aminobenzoic acid) 2 mg • Alpha Carotene 114 mcg • Cryptoxanthin 28 mcg • Zeaxanthin 23 mcg • Lutein 18 mcg • Soy Protein Isolate/ Amino Acid Blend 160 mg: L-Glutamic Acid, L-Aspartic Acid, L-Leucine, L-Arginine, L-Lysine, L-Phenylalanine, L-Serine, L-Proline, L-Valine, L-Isoleucine, L-Alanine, Glycine, L-Threonine, L-Tyrosine, L-Histidine, L-Cysteine, L-Methionine, L-Ornithine, Taurine. Other Ingredients: Microcrystalline Cellulose, Vegetable Cellulose, Vegetable Stearic Acid, Grape skin, Titanium Dioxide, Silica, Vegetable Magnesium Stearate, Vegetable Glycerin.

FEMFOCUS - Red Clover - Solgar
Each vegicap contains: Standardized Red Clover extract leaf (biochanin A 3 mg) 250 mg • Raw Red Clover powder leaf 225 mg. Other Ingredients: Vegetable Cellulose; Vegetable Magnesium Stearate; Vegetable Glycerin; PhytO2X Blend: Vitamin E, Beta-Carotene and other Carotenoids, Rosemary extract aerial, Vitamin C (L-absorbic acid), Water.

FEMFOCUS - Super GLA - Solgar
Each softgel contains: Linoleic Acid 498 mg • Gamma-Linolenic Acid 300 mg • Other Fatty Acids 296 mg • Oleic Acid 206 mg • Borage Oil 1300 mg. Other Ingredients: Gelatin, Glycerin, Water.

FEMFOCUS - Vitamin B12 - Solgar
Each nugget contains: Vitamin B-12 (as cobalamin) 1000 mcg. Other Ingredients: Mannitol, Vegetable Magnesium Stearate, Vegetable Stearic Acid, Natural Cherry Flavor.

FEMFOCUS - Vitamin B-6 - Solgar
Each tablet contains: Vitamin B-6 (as pyridoxine HCl) 50 mg • Calcium (as dicalcium phosphate) 50 mg. Other Ingredients: Dicalcium Phosphate, Vegetable Stearic Acid, Vegetable Magnesium Stearate, Vegetable Cellulose.

FEMFOCUS - Vitamin K - Solgar
Each tablet contains: Calcium (as dicalcium phosphate) 90 mg • Vitamin K (as phytonadione) 100 mcg. Other Ingredients: Vegetable Cellulose, Vegetable Stearic Acid, Vegetable Magnesium Stearate.

Fem-Gest - Progressive Labs
Ingredients: Stabilized Aloe Vera gel • Mexican Yam extract • Chamomile extract • Chaste Tree berry • Tocopheryl Acetate • Lavender extract • Jojoba oil • Safflower oil • Progesterone 950 mg • Carbomer 940 • Glyceryl Stearate (and) PEG-100 Stearate • C12-15 Alkyl Benzoate • Stearic Acid • Octyl Palmitate • Triethanolamine • Cetyl Alcohol • Methylparaben • Tetrasodium EDTA • Dimethicone • Propylparaben • Diazolidyl Urea.

FemGest Cream - Home Health Products, Inc.
Water • Vitamin E Acetate • Stearic Acid • Cetyl Alcohol • Glyceryl Stearate • Grapefruit Extract • Octyl Palmitate • Cetyl Esters • Progesterone • Aloe Vera Gel • Glycerin • Keratin • Propylene Glycol • Polysorbate 80 • Diazolidinylurea • Carbomer • Sweet Almond Oil • Triethanolamine • Methylparaben • Panthenol • Sodium Hyaluronate • Propylparaben.

FEM-H - MMS Pro
Each capsule contains: Black Cohosh root • Sarsaparilla root • Siberian Ginseng root • Licorice root • Blessed Thistle herb • Squaw Vine • False Unicorn root.

Feminene Female Support Formula - Market America, Inc.
Two tablets contain: Thiamin HCl (vitamin B1) 20 mg • Riboflavin (vitamin B2) 20 mg • Niacin (vitamin B3) 20 mg • D-Calcium Pantothenate (vitamin B5) 11.8 mg • Pyridoxine HCl (vitamin B6) 10 mg • Folic Acid 400 mcg • Cyanocobalamin (vitamin B12) 200 mcg • D-Alpha-Tocopherol (vitamin E) 50 IU • Soy extract (soy isoflavones, 3%) 200 mg • Dong Quai root 1% extract 200 mg • Evening Primrose oil 200 mg • Wild Yam 180 mg • Black Cohosh root 2.5% extract 160 mg • Chaste berry extract (vitex agnus-castus) 150 mg • Horsetail

150 mg • Red Clover 140 mg • Passiflora 120 mg • Valerian root 120 mg • Sage 100 mg • St. John's Wort 70 mg. Other Ingredients: Dicalcium Phosphate, Microcrystalline Cellulose, Stearic Acid, Magnesium Stearate, Croscarmellose Sodium, Silicon Dioxide.

FeminEstra **-** Pacific BioLogic
Poria Plant Fungus (hoelen) • Polygonum root (thin) • Moutan Root bark • Chinese Yam • Cherry (cornelian asiatic) • Rehmannia root (fresh) • Rehmannia root (cooked in wine) • Curculigo rhizome • Alisma (water plantain rhizome) • Pearl No Concentration.

FeminiCare **-** DreamPharm
Two capsules contain: Proprietary Blend: Astragalus radix, Ginseng radix, Atractylodes rhizoma, Sclerotium Poriae Cocos, Ziziphi semen, Longanae Arillus, Angelica Sinensis radix, Polygala radix, Glycyrrhiza radix, Saussurea radix, Zingiberis radix, Zizyphi fructus.

FeminiMate **-** DreamPharm
Two capsules contain: Proprietary Blend: Myrrha, Forsythiae Suspensae fructus, Glycyrrhizae radix, Coisis semen, Gardeniae fructus, Talcum, Scirpi rhizoma, Mantidis Vagina Oyorum, Phellodentri cortex, Sargentodoxa Cuneata, Patrinia Scabiosaefolia, Bullrush pollen, Dandelion, Ailanthus Altissima.

Feminine Balance **-** Advocare International
Two capsules contain: Pantothenic Acid 30 mg • Pyridoxine (as HCl) 12 mg • Vitamin E (as d-alpha tocopheryl succinate) 10 IU • Red Clover extract (flower/leaf - trifolium pratense) 500 mg • Black Cohosh extract (root - cimicifuga racemosa) 75 mg • Dong Quai extract (root - angelica plymorpha) 50 mg • Chaste Tree extract (berry - vitex agnus-castus) 200 mg. Other Ingredients: Silicon Dioxide, Magnesium Stearate, Gelatin.

Femme Advantage Creatine Serum **-** Muscle Marketing USA
Each serving contains: Creatine Monohydrate • Vitamin B12 • Ginseng • Royal Jelly • Vitamin B5 • Soluable Bioflavonoids • Ginkgo extract • Wild Yam extract • Papain extract.

Femme Alzare **-** Alpha Male Nutrition
Each tablet contains: Yohimbe bark extract (15:1) 400 mg • Maca extract (6:1) 250 mg • Arginine Alpha Ketoglutarate 190 mg • Arginine Ketoisocaproate 10 mg • 4-Androstenediol 2 mg • Bioperine 10 mg • Deer Antler 100 mg • Proprietary Blend 45 mg: Korean Ginseng powder, Siberian Ginseng powder, Tribulus Terrestris powder, Dong Quai powder, White Peony root powder, Lycium powder, Wild Yam powder, Sarsaparilla powder, Black Cohosh powder, Damiana powder. Other Ingredients: Gelatin, Magnesium Stearate, Stearic Acid, Microcrystalline Cellulose.

Fem-Mend Formula **-** Nature's Way
Two capsules contain: Proprietary Formula: Blessed Thistle • Cayenne pepper fruit • Cramp bark • False Unicorn root • Ginger • Goldenseal stem, leaf, flower • Red Raspberry leaves • Squaw Vine vine, leaf, fruit • Uva Ursi leaves. Other Ingredients: Gelatin.

FemTone **-** PhytoPharmica
Two capsules contain: Black Cohosh root 4:1 extract (cimicifuga racemosa) 50 mg • Chaste Tree berry extract (vitex agnus-castus, standardized to contain 0.5% agnusides) 50 mg • Dong Quai root 3.2:1 extract (angelica sinensis) 250 mg • False Unicorn root 3:1 extract (chamaelirium luteum) 50 mg • Fennel seed 3.9:1 extract (foeniculum vulgare) 25 mg • Hesperidin 50% (from citrus fruits) 200 mg • Licorice root and rhizome extract (glycyrrhiza glabra, standardized to contin 5% glycyrrhizic acid) 50 mg • Vitamin C (ascorbic acid) 100 mg.

Femtrol **-** Enzymatic Therapy
Two capsules contain: Vitamin C (Ascorbic Acid) 100 mg. Other Ingredients: Dong Quai extract 4:1 (Angelica sinensis) 250 mg • Hesperidin Complex standardized to contain 50% Bioflavonoids 200 mg • Licorice root extract (Glycyrrhiza glabra) standardized to contain 5% Glycyrrhizic Acid 50 mg • Chaste Tree Berry extract 5:1 (Vitex agnus-castus) 50 mg • Black Cohosh root extract 4:1 (Cimicifuga racemosa) 50 mg • False Unicorn root extract 4:1 (Helonias opulus) 50 mg • Fennel seed extract 6:1 (Foeniculum vulgare) 25 mg.

Fennel-Yam **-** Atrium Inc.
Each capsule contains: Fennel 250 mg •Wild Yam 250 mg.

Fen-Tastic **-** The Vitamin Shoppe
Two tablets contain: St. John's Wort root standardized for 3% hypericin 400 mg • Citrus Aurantium fruit 600 mg • 5-HTP 150 mg • Yerba Santa • Mate leaves standardized 20% methylzanthine 250 mg • White Willow bark 400 mg.
See Editor's Note No. 40, page 2058.

Fenugreek **-** Nature's Way
Two capsules contain: Fenugreek seed 1.22 g. Other Ingredients: Gelatin.

Fenugreek Seed **-** Motherlove Herbal Co.
Each 2 oz bottle contains: Fenugreek seed. In a base of certified kosher alcohol and glycerin.

Fenu-Thyme Formula **-** Nature's Way
Two capsules contain: Proprietary Formula: Fenugreek seed • Thyme leaf. Other Ingredients: Gelatin.

Feosol **-** SmithKline Beecham
Each tablet contains: Iron 65 mg. Inactive Ingredients: Calcium Sulfate, Starch, Glucose, Hydroxypropyl Methylcellulose, Talc, Stearic Acid, Polyethylene Glycol, Sodium Lauryl Sulfate, Mineral Oil, Titanium Dioxide, FD&C Yellow #10, FD&C Blue #2.

Fermalac Vaginal **-** Rougier Pharma
Each capsule contains: Over 2 billion fully viable bacilli (lyophilized cultures): Lactobacillus acidophilus, Lactobacillus bulgaricus, Streptococcus lactic (var. thermophilus).

Feroglobin B12 Capsules **-** Vitabiotics
Each capsule contains: Iron 24 mg • Zinc 12 mg • Copper 2 mg • Folic Acid 500 mcg • Vitamin B12 10 mcg • Vitamin B6 5 mg.

Feroglobin B12 Liquid **-** Vitabiotics
Five milliliters contain: Vitamin B1 4 mg • Vitamin B2 1 mg • Vitamin B6 2 mg • Vitamin B12 5 mcg • Vitamin C 10 mg • Folic Acid 150 mcg • Pantothenic Acid 2 mg • Calcium Glycerophosphate 10 mg • Niacin (vitamin B3) 8 mg • Iron 7 mg • Zinc 5 mg • Copper 0.25 mg • Manganese 0.25 mg • Lysine 40 mg • Iodine 40 mcg • Honey 100 mg • Malt 500 mg.

FerroComp **-** PhytoPharmica
Each capsule contains: Vitamin C (Ascorbic Acid) 60 mg • Iron (Ferrous Succinate) 25 mg • Folic Acid 200 mcg • Vitamin B12 (Cyanocobalamin) 100 mcg • Liquid Liver Fractions (predigested soluble concentrate) 250 mg • Chlorophyll (Fat-Soluble) 5 mg.
See Editor's Note No. 14.

Ferro-Sequels **-** Inverness Medical Innovations, Inc.
Each tablet contains: Iron 50 mg. Inactive Ingredients: Lactose, Ferrous Fumarate (equivalent to 50 mg of Elemental Iron), Microcrystalline Cellulose, Hydroxypropyl Methylcellulose, Docusate Sodium, Magnesium Stearate, Sodium Benzoate, Silicon Dioxide, Sodium Triethyl Citrate, Titanium Dioxide, Yellow #10, Blue #1, Sodium Lauryl Sulfate.

Ferrous Gluconate 28 mg Iron **-** Nature's Bounty
Each tablet contains: Iron (from 246 mg of ferrous gluconate) 28 mg. Other Ingredients: Cellulose (plant origin), Dicalcium Phosphate, Vegetable Stearic Acid, Cellulose Coating, Croscarmellose, Vegetable Magnesium Stearate.

Ferrous Sulfate **-** Nature's Bounty
Each tablet contains: Iron (as Ferrous Sulfate, anhydrous) 28 mg. Inactive Ingredients: Dicalcium Phosphate, Calcium Carbonate, Cellulose (Plant Origin), Croscarmellose, Vegetable Stearic Acid, Vegetable Magnesium Stearate, Cellulose Coating.

Fertil Male - LaneLabs
Each capsule contains: Lepidium Meyenii g. root 500 mg • HAI (heated algal ingredient) Amino Acid extract (from sea algae) 1.2 mg. Other Ingredients: Gelatin, Magneisum Stearate, Cellulose.

Fertility Blend for Men - The Daily Wellness Company
Two capsules contain: Vitamin C as ascorbic acid 120 mg • Vitamin E as d-alpha tocopherol 150 mg • Vitamin B6 as pyridoxine hydrochloride 2 mg • Vitamin B12 as cyanocobalamin 6 mcg • Folate as folic acid 400 mcg • Zinc as gluconate 15 mg • Selenium as sodium selenate 70 mcg • Proprietary Blend 610 mg: L-Carnitine as tartrate, Dong Quai (standardized to .1% ferulic acid), Coenzyme Q10. Inactive Ingredients: Rice Flour Powder, Magnesium Stearate, Silica.

Fertility Blend for Women - The Daily Wellness Company
Three capsules contain: Vitamin E (as d-alpha tocopherol) 150 mg • Vitamin B6 (as pyridoxine hydrochloride) 6 mg • Vitamin B12 (as cyanocobalamin) 12 mcg • Folate (as folic acid) 400 mcg • Iron (as gluconate) 18 mg • Magnesium (as oxide) 400 mg • Zinc (as gluconate) • Selenium (as sodium selenate) 70 mcg • Proprietary Blend 1080 mg: Chasteberry (Vitex agnus castus standardized to .5% agnusides), Green Tea (Camellia sinensis standardized to 50% phenols), L-arginine. Inactive Ingredients: Rice Flour Powder, Magnesium Stearate, Silica.

Fevera - HerbaSway
Cassia tora • Kudzu • Skullcap • Knotweed • Licorice • Blackberry • HerbaSwee (Cucurbitaceae fruit).

Feverfew - Leiner Health Products
Each caplet contains: Feverfew extract (Tanacetum parhenium) leaf 100 mg • Feverfew leaf (Tanacetum parthenium) 20 mg. Other Ingredients: Calcium Carbonate, Cellulose, Maltodextrin, Mannitol, Hydroxypropyl Methylcellulose, Silicon Dioxide, Polyethylene Glycol 3350, Croscarmellose Sodium, Titanium Dioxide, Hydroxypropyl Cellulose, Pharmaceutical Glaze, Crospovidone, Magnesium Stearate, Polysorbate 80, Blue 1 Lake, Yellow 6 Lake.

Feverfew - Now
Each capsule contains: Feverfew 0.9% 400 mg.

Feverfew - Pharmanex
Each capsule contains: Feverfew leaves and flowers (12:1) extract (Tanacetum parthenium) 125 mg. Other Ingredients: Rice Flour, Gelatin.

Feverfew - PhytoPharmica
Each capsule contains: Feverfew flower and leaf (tanacetum parthenium, standardized to contain 600 mcg of parthenolide) 100 mg. Other Ingredients: Gelatin, Cellulose, Modified Cellulose Gum, Magnesium Stearate, Titanium Dioxide Color.

Feverfew - Source Naturals
Each tablet contains: Feverfew extract 200 mg • Feverfew whole herb 50 mg • Magnesium (Oxide) 70 mg • Calcium (Carbonate) 35 mg • Vitamin C (Ascorbic Acid) 10 mg.

Feverfew (Nomigraine) Caplets - Life Brand
Each caplet contains: Dried Feverfew leaf (Tanacetum parthenium) 125 mg. This product is guaranteed to contain a minimum of 0.2% Parthenolide. Other Ingredients: Dicalcium Phosphate, Microcrystalline Cellulose, Silicon Dioxide, Magnesium Stearate (plant source), Stearic Acid (plant source).

Fiber 10 - Advocare International
Each pouch (0.7 oz / 20 g) contains: Vitamin A (as beta-carotene) 1000 IU • Vitamin C (as ascorbic acid) 30 mg • Sodium 10 mg. Other Ingredients: Fructose, Maltodextrin, Citric Acid, Natural Flavors, Artificial Flavors, Acesulfame Potassium, Papaya Fruit Powder, Prune Powder, Rhubarb Root Extract, Black Walnut Hull Extract, Licorice Root Powder, Lactobacillus Acidophilus, Bifidobacterium Bifidum, Digestive Enzyme Complex: Lipase, Cellulase, Protease; Fiber Blend: Psyllium Husk, Oats (oat fiber), Carboxymethylcellulose, Guar Gum, Citrus Pectin, Butternut Bark Powder.

Fiber Clense - Nutri-Quest Rx
Three tablets contain: Vitamin C 300 mg • Apple Pectin 150 mg • Garlic 150 mg • Rice Bran 600 mg • Sodium Alginate 300 mg • L-Cysteine 200 mg • DL-Methionine 100 mg • L-Lysine 30 mg • Chlorophyll 10 mg • Oat Bran 600 mg • Red Beet root 100 mg.

Fiber Delights - Chocolate Flavor - PhytoPharmica
Two chewable tablets contain: Proprietary Fiber Blend 4.4 g: Enriched Inulin Fiber with Fructooligosaccharides (FOS) from Chicory root, Oat Bran Fiber (avena sativa). Other Ingredients: Fructose, Cocoa Powder, Stearic Acid, Natural Flavors, Lecithin

Fiber Delights - Vanilla Flavor - PhytoPharmica
Two chewable tablets contain: Proprietary Fiber Blend 4.4 g: Enriched Inulin Fiber with Fructooligosaccharides (FOS) from Chicory root, Oat Bran fiber (avena sativa). Other Ingredients: Fructose, Stearic Acid, Lecithin, Natural Flavor.

Fiber Digestion - Enzymes, Inc.
Each capsule contains: Proprietary Enzyme Blend 488 mg: Amylase, CereCalase, Protease, Glucoamylase, alpha-Galactosidase, Malt Diastase, Pectinase, Cellulase, Lipase, Peptidase. Other Ingredients: Plant Cellulose, Water.

Fiber Formula - PhytoPharmica
Eight capsules contain: Proprietary Fiber Blend 3455 mg: Psyllium husk (plantago ovata), Oat Bran (avena sativa), Guar Gum seed extract (cyamopsis tetragonoloba), Pectin (from citrus fruit), Marshmallow roo 3.5:1 extract (althaea officinalis). Other Ingredients: Cellulose, Gelatin, Magnesium Stearate, Silicon Dioxide.

Fiber Max - FreeLife International
Four caplets contain: Dietary Fiber 2 g • Calcium (as calcium hydrogen phosphate) 400 mg • Microencapsulated Active Lactobacillus Cells 300 million CFU • Lipase Enzyme 500 Units • Triphala standardized extract (45% tannins, from fuits of belleric myrobalan, emblic and tropical almond) 25 mg • Aloe Vera whole leaf 50 mg • Butternut bark 750 mg • Proprietary Blend 915 mg: Vegetable Cellulose, Oat Fiber, Alfalfa, Golden Pea Fiber, Scandinavian Beet Fiber, Barley Greens, Slippery Elm bark, Oat greens • Proprietary Blend 500 mg: Chicory and Jerusalem Artichoke Fructo-Oligosaccharides, Larch Tree Arabinogalactan, Mannan- Oligosaccharides and Champex Champignon extract. Other Ingredients: Vegetable Stearic Acid, Silica, Vegetable Magnesium Stearate, Vita-Coat (vegetable resin, alpha-lipoic acid).

Fiber Plan - Shaklee
2 teaspoons (5 g) contain: Dietary fiber 4 g • Vitamin C 48 mg. Other Ingredients: Psyllium Husk, Pectin, Guar Gum, Locust Bean Gum, Maltodextrin, Ascorbic Acid.

Fiber Plan Daily Crunch - Shaklee
15 g contain: Dietary fiber 5 g • Soluble fiber 2 g • Insoluble fiber 2 g • Protein 1 g • Calcium 60 mg • Iron 0.8 mg • Sodium 25 mg. Other Ingredients: Rice Flour, Soy Fiber, Oat Bran, Psyllium Husk, Acacia Gum, Brown Rice Syrup, Pectin, Fructose, Guar Gum, Calcium Carbonate, Trisodium Phosphate.

Fiber Plan Daily Mix - Shaklee
2 tablespoons (15 g) contain: Dietary fiber 5 g • Soluble fiber 2 g • Insoluble fiber 2 g • Sugars 1 g • Protein 1 g • Calcium 60 mg • Iron 0.8 mg • Sodium 25 mg. Other Ingredients: Rice Flour, Soy Fiber, Oat Bran, Psyllium Husk, Acacia Gum, Brown Rice Syrup, Pectin, Fructose, Guar Gum, Calcium Carbonate, Trisodium Phosphate.

Fiber Soy-Pro - The Vitamin Shoppe
SUPRO Soy Protein Isolate and BeneFiber Soluble Fiber. Orange citrus natural flavor.

Some Brand Name Natural Products - What they Contain

www.NaturalDatabase.com contains MANY more listings than appear here.

FiberChoice **-** CNS, Inc.
Each chewable tablet contains: Fructan 2 g • Magnesium Stearate 25 mg. Other Ingredients: Citric Acid and other natural flavors.

Fibergy Drink - Almond Creme **-** USANA Health Sciences
Two scoops contain: Fiber Blend: Soy Fiber, Gum Arabic, Oat Bran, Wheat Bran, Cellulose Gum, Pea Fiber, Xanthan Gum, Corn Bran, Locust Bean Gum, Carrageenan, Citrus Pectin, Oligofructose, Inulin, Apple Fiber • Crystalline • Fructose • Corn Syrup Solids • Rich Syrup Solids • Soy Protein Isolate • High Oleic Sunflower Oil • Natural and Artificial Flavors • Potassium Chloride • Dipotassium Phosphate • Salt • Beta Carotene (color) • Sodium Caseinate (a milk derivative) • Tricalcium Phosphate • Magnesium Oxide • Ascorbic Acid (Vitamin C) • Mono and Diglycerides • Soy Lecithin • Ferric Orthophosphate • Folic Acid • Thiamin Mononitrate (Vitamin B1).

Fibergy Drink - Peach Mango **-** USANA Health Sciences
Two scoops contain: Fiber Blend: Gum Arabic, Soy Fiber, Oat Bran, Wheat Bran, Inulin, Pea Fiber, Oat Fiber, Sugar Beet Fiber, Cellulose Gum, Xanthan Gum, Oligofructose, Citrus Pectin, Stabilized Rice Bran, Apple Fiber • Crystalline Fructose • Natural and Artificial Flavors • High Oleic Sunflower Oil • Corn Syrup Solids • Salt • Beet Juice Powder (color) • Sodium Caseinate (a milk derivative) • Beta Carotene (color) • Mono and Diglycerides • Dipotassium Phosphate • Soy Lecithin.

Fiberific **-** Nature's Plus
Each 1.4 oz. bar contains: Calories 120 • Calories from Fat 18 • Total Fat 2 g • Saturated Fat 0 g • Cholesterol 0 mg • Total Carbohydrate 23 g • Complex Carbohydrate 14 g • Sugars 9 g • Dietary Fiber 8 g • Soluble Fiber 3.6 g • Insoluble Fiber 4.4 g • Protein 3 g • Sodium 43 mg • Potassium 196 mg. Ingredients: Rolled Oats, Wheat Germ, Brown Rice, Apples, Prunes & Oat Bran. Naturally flavored with Fruit Juice & Honey. No tropical oils.

FiberPlus **-** PhytoPharmica
Two capsules contain: FiberPlus Proprietary Blend 1000 mg: Psyllium hydrophilic muciloid, Grapefruit pectin, Oat (Avena sativa) fiber, Beet fiber, Carrot fiber, Fructooligosaccharides (FOS; from Jerusalem artichoke), Prune fiber, Ginger (Zingiber officinale) root and rhizome extract, Fenugreek (Trigonella foenum-graecum) seed extract 4:1, Goldenseal (Hydrastis canadensis) root and rhizome extract (standardized to contain 5% total alkaloids including berberine, hydrastine, and canadine), Chamomile (Matricaria recutita) root extract, Marshmallow (Althaea officinalis) root extract 4.25:1, Aloe Vera (Aloe barbadensis) leaf extract, and Cascara sagrada (Rhamnus purshiana) bark, trunk, and branch extract.

Fibersol **-** TwinLab
Each rounded teaspoonful contains: Fiber Blend Concentrate [from Psyllium Seed Husks, Guar Gum, Apple Pectin] 4 g • Vitamin C 100 mg.

Fiber-Time **-** Atrium Inc.
Twelve ounces contain: Bran Fiber • Cascara Sagrada bark • Citrus Fiber • Karaya Gum • Apple Pectin • Prune powder • Psyllium Plantago Ovata Blond • Rhubarb root • Rice Fiber • Sweet Whey.

FiberWise **-** Melaleuca
Ingredients: Psyllium Husk • Rice Bran • Fructooligosaccharides • Maltodextrin • Apple fiber • Oat fiber • Lactobacillus Sporogenes (acidophilus) • Coenzyme Q10 • Green Tea extract • Grape Seed extract • Aloe Vera extract • Garlic • Ginger root • Licorice root • Burdock • Peppermint • Slippery Elm • Fructose • Soy Lecithin • Natural Flavor • Calcium Carbonate • Malic Acid • Calcium Silica • Beta Carotene • Acesulfame Potassium • Ascorbic Acid • D-Alpha Tocopheryl Acetate • Beet juice powder • Vitamin A Palmitate.

Fiberzyme **-** Young Living Essential Oils
Each capsule contains: Proprietary Blend: Cellulase, Bee Pollen, Tarragon (artemisia dracunculus) oil, Ginger (zingiber officinale) oil, Peppermint (mentha piperita) oil, Juniper (juniperus osteosperma and/or j. scopulorum) oil, Fennel (foeniculum vulgare) oil, Lemongrass (cymbopogon flexuosus) oil, Anise (pimpinella anisum) oil, Patchouli (pogostemon cablin) oil.

FiboTane **-** Advocare International
Three capsules contain: Vitamin E (as d-alpha tocopheryl succinate) 15 IU • Chromium (as polynicotinate - ChromeMate) 25 mcg • Chitosan 600 mg • Guar Gum 750 mg • Taurine 300 mg • Beta-Sitosterol 100 mg • Odorless Garlic (bulb - allium sativum) 100 mg • Yellow Dock extract (root - rumex crispus) 100 mg • Niacinamide Ascorbate 50 mg • Buckthorn extract (bark - frangula alnus) 30 mg •Ascorbyl Palmitate 15 mg. Other Ingredients: Silicon Dioxide, Magnesium Stearate, Gelatin.

Fibre System Plus **-** 4 Life
Each packet contains: Psyllium (plantago afra, seed) 600 mg • Black Walnut (juglans reglia, hulls) 400 mg • Cranberry (fruit) 250 mg • Cascara Sagrada (bark) 100 mg • Ginger (root) 100 mg • Apple (fruit) 100 mg • Gentian (root) 85 mg • Alder Buckthorn (bark) 75 mg • Slippery Elm (bark) 60 mg • Licorice (root) 50 mg • Sage (leaves) 50 mg • Parsley (leaf) 50 mg • Papain (from Papaya fruit) 50 mg • Bromelain (from Pineapple fruit) 50 mg • Prune (fruit) 50 mg • Red Wheat Fiber (seed) 50 mg • Marshmallow (root) 40 mg • Hops (flower) 30 mg • Frangula extract (bark) 25 mg • Irish Moss (Chondruscrispus, aerial parts) 25 mg • Bee Pollen 25 mg • English Chamomile (flower) 25 mg • Pineapple (fruit) 20 mg • Papaya (fruit) 20 mg • Hawaiian Spirulina Pacifica 10 mg • Goldenseal (root) 10 mg. Other Ingredients: Gelatin Capsule, Rice Bran, Xanthan Gum, Locust Bean Gum, Magnesium Stearate.

FibreNet **-** Pharmanex
Four capsules contain: Chitosan (from shellfish) PolmerPlex 1000 mg. Other Ingredients: Calcium Carbonate, Magnesium Stearate.

FibreNet Plus **-** Pharmanex
Each scoop contains: Vitamin A (85% Beta-Carotene) 6877 IU • Vitamin C 12 mg • Vitamin D 80 IU • Vitamin E 4 IU • Thiamin 0.30 mg • Riboflavin 0.34 mg • Niacin 4 mg • Vitamin B6 0.40 mg • Folate 80 mcg • Vitamin B12 1.2 mg • Biotin 60 mcg • Pantothenic Acid 2 mg • Calcium 187 mg • Iron 3.8 mg • Phosphorus 100 mg • Iodine 30 mcg • Magnesium 60 mg • Zinc 3 mg • Copper 0.40 mg • Sodium 60 mg • Potassium 190 mg • PolmerPlex 1000 mg. Ingredients: Crystalline Fructose, Oat Bran, Stabilized Rice Bran, Gum Arabic, Natural and Artificial Flavors, PolmerPlex, High Oleic Sunflower Oil, Corn Syrup Solids, Tricalcium Phosphate, Citric Acid, Beta-Carotene, Dipotassium Phosphate Cellulose Gum, Sugar Beet Fiber, Potassium Citrate, Sodium Caseinate, Magnesium Oxide, Soy Fiber, Salt, Pea Fiber, Xanthan Gum, Ground Psyllium Husks, Ascorbic Acid, dl-Alpha Tocopheryl Acetate, Dicalcium Phosphate, Soy Lecithin, Vitamin A Palmitate, Niacinamide, Zinc Oxide, Electric Iron, Copper Gluconate, d-Calcium Pantothenate, Cholecalciferol, Pyridoxine Hydrochloride, Riboflavin, Thiamine Mononitrate, Cyanocobalamin, Folic Acid, Biotin, Potassium Iodide.

Fibro Plus **-** Aspen Group, Inc.
Two capsules contain: Elemental Magnesium 200 mg • Malic Acid 300 mg • Glyciante 50 mg.

FibroLeve **-** PharmAssure
Four tablets contain: Vitamin B6 (as Pyridoxine Hydrochloride) 15 mg • Magnesium (as Magnesium Oxide) 400 mg • Manganese (as Manganese Sulfate) 10 mg • Malic Acid 1200 mg • Boswellin serrata Resin Extract (65% Boswellic Acid=75 mg) 115 mg. Other Ingredients: Cellulose.

Fibromyalgin **-** Olympia Nutrition
Glucosamine, Collagen, Mag. Malate.

Fibro-X **-** Olympian Labs
Two capsules contain: Malic Acid 600 mg • Shark Cartilage 600 mg • White Willow Bark 50 mg • Valerian root 20 mg • Grape Seed extract 40 mg • Magnesium Glycinate 100 mg • Manganese Glycinate 5 mg.

Finally... The Solution for Women Sensitivity Enhancement Cream - Capital Marketing Ent., LLC
Deionzied Water • Aloe Barbadensis gel • Glyceryl Stearate • PEG-100 Stearate • PPG-2 Myristyl Ether Propionate • Glycerine • Capryic/Capric Triglyceride • Propylene Glycol • Diazolidinyl Urea • Methylparaben • Propylparaben • Cetyl Alcohol • Triethanolamine • Carbomer • Dimethicone • Fragrance • Benzyl Nicotinate.

Fingerprinted Alfalfa - GNC Herbal Plus - GNC
Each capsule contains: Alfalfa herb powder (Medicago sativa) 500 mg. Other Ingredients: Gelatin.

Fingerprinted Astragalus - GNC Herbal Plus - GNC
Each capsule contains: Astragalus root powder (as astragalus membranceus) 250 mg. Other Ingredients: Cellulose, Gelatin, Calcium Carbonate.

Fingerprinted Bilberry - GNC Herbal Plus - GNC
Each capsule contains: Bilberry fruit powder (vaccinium myrtillus L.) 500 mg. Other Ingredients: Gelatin, Cellulose.

Fingerprinted Black Cohosh - GNC Herbal Plus - GNC
Each capsule contains: Black Cohosh root powder (cimicifuga racemosa) 200 mg. Other Ingredients: Cellulose, Gelatin.

Fingerprinted Black Walnut Hulls - GNC Herbal Plus - GNC
Each capsule contains: Black Walnut hulls powder (juglans nigra) 300 mg. Other Ingredients: Gelatin, Cellulose, Calcium Carbonate.

Fingerprinted Burdock Root - GNC Herbal Plus - GNC
Each capsule contains: Burdock root powder (arctium lappa) 500 mg. Other Ingredients: Gelatin.

Fingerprinted Butcher's Broom 100 mg - GNC Herbal Plus - GNC
Each capsule contains: Butcher's Broom root powder (ruscus aculaetus) 100 mg. Other Ingredients: Cellulose, Calcium Carbonate, Gelatin.

Fingerprinted Butcher's Broom 500 mg - GNC Herbal Plus - GNC
Each capsule contains: Butcher's Broom root powder (ruscus aculaetus) 500 mg. Other Ingredients: Gelatin, Cellulose.

Fingerprinted Cayenne - GNC Herbal Plus - GNC
Each capsule contains: Cayenne Pepper powder (capsicum frutescens) 500 mg. Other Ingredients: Gelatin, Cellulose.

Fingerprinted Chickweed - GNC Herbal Plus - GNC
Each capsule contains: Chickweed powder (stellaria media) 500 mg. Other Ingredients: Gelatin.

Fingerprinted Chlorophyll - GNC Herbal Plus - GNC
Each capsule contains: Soybean Oil 453 mg • Chlorophyll 60 mg. Other Ingredients: Gelatin, Glycerin, Caramel Color, Titanium Dioxide.

FinoCarbo Plus - Aboca USA, Inc
Two capsules contain: Vegetable Charcoal 174 mg • Fennel fruit Whole Phytocomplex Concentrate (WPC) (foeniculum vulgare, standardized to 2% essential oil) 116 mg • Cumin fruit powder (cuminum cyminum, standardized to 2% essential oil) 87 mg • Chamomile flower freeze-dried extract (matricaria recutita, flavonoids apigenin-like minimum 1%) 87 mg • Star Anise fruit powder (illcium verum, essential oil minimum 7%) 40.6 mg • Lemon Balm leaf freeze-dried extract (melissa officianlis, standardized to 14% rosmarinic acid) 29 mg • Caraway fruit powder (carum carvi, essential oil minimum 2.2%) 29 mg. Other Ingredients: Gelatin (capsule), Essential Oils Of Fennel, Peppermint, Marjoram.

Firm Foundation Calcium Blend - Physicians Laboratories
Four capsules contain: Calcium 500 mg • Boron Citrate 3 mg.

Firm Foundation Multivitamin & Multimineral - Physicians Laboratories
Six capsules contain: Vitamin A (as beta carotene/a acetate) 5000 IU • Vitamin C (as calcium ascorbate) 60 mg • Vitamin D (as D cholecalciferol) 400 IU • Vitamin E (as E succinate) 30 IU • Vitamin K (as K phytonadione) 80 mcg • Thiamin (as thiamin HCl) 1.5 mg • Riboflavin 1.7 mg • Niacin (as niacinamide, inositol hexaniacinate) 20 mg • Vitamin B12 (as cyanocobalamin) 2 mg • Biotin 400 mcg • Pantothenic Acid (as d-calcium pantothenate) 6 mcg • Iodine (as kelp) 150 mcg • Magnesium (as magnesium aspartate, malate, citrate) 400 mg • Zinc (as zinc monomethionine) 15 mg • Selenium (as selenomethionine) 70 mcg • Copper (as copper chelate, citrate) 2 mg • Manganese (as manganese citrate) 2 mg • Chromium (as chromium polynicotinate) 120 mcg • Molybdenum (as molybdenum chelate) 75 mcg • Calcium 24 mg • Silicon (as sodium meta silicate) 2 mg • Vanadium (as vanadyl sulfate) 10 mcg • Proprietary Enzyme Blend 25 mg: Amyloglecoside, Amylase, Protease, Acid Protease, Cellulase, Lipase, Lactase.

Firm Foundation Vitamin E - Physicians Laboratories
Each capsule contains: Vitamin E (as d-alpha tocopheryl acetate) 400 IU • Ginger rhizome, Supercritical CO2 extract (zingiber officinale) 4 mg.

Firm Lotion - Mannatech
Water • Parrafin • Caprylic/Capric Triglycerides • C 12-15 Alkyl Benzoate • Cetyl Alcohol • Propylene Glycol • Dimethicone • Germaben II (propylene glycol, diazolidinyl urea, methylparaben, propylparaben) • Amino Methylpropanol • Ambrotose Complex (patent pending; naturally occurring plant saccharides including freeze-dried aloe vera gel complex - manapol powder) • Lactic Acid • Niacinamide • Emu Oil • Stearic Acid • Cholesterol • Lavender Oil • Carbomer • Herbal Complex: Barley extract, Clover extract, Ivy extract, Butcherbroom extract, Camellia Oleifera extract, Lady's Thistle extract • Wild Yam extract.

Fish Body Oil - Health Center for Better Living
Each softgel contains: EPA 180 mg • DHA 120 mg • Vitamin E 5 IU.

Fish Body Oils 1000 - GNC A-Z - GNC
Each capsule contains: EPA (Eicosapentaenoic Acid) 180 mg • DHA (Docosahexaenoid Acid) 120 mg. Other Ingredients: Gelatin, Glycerin, Vitamin E.

Fish Body Oils 1000 Deodorized - GNC A-Z - GNC
Each capsule contains: EPA (Eicosapentaenoic Acid) 180 mg • DHA (Docosahexaenoic Acid) 120 mg. Other Ingredients: Gelatin, Glycerin.

Fish Body Oils with GLA - GNC
Each capsule contains: Vitamin E (as d-alpha Tocopherol) 3 IU • EPA (Eicosapentaenoic Acid) 180 mg • DHA (Docosahexaenoic Acid) 120 mg • GLA (gamma Linolenic Acid) 23 mg. Other Ingredients: Fish body oil, Gelatin, Glycerin, Borage Oil (Borago officinalis), Enteric Coating: Hydroxypropyl Methylcellulose Phthalate, Titanium Dioxide, Flax seed oil, triacetin.

Fish Oil - Optimum Nutrition
Each softgel contains: Fish Oil 1000 mg • EPA (eicosapentaenoic acid) 180 mg • DHA (docosahexaenoic acid) 120 mg. Other Ingredients: Gelatin, Glycerin.

Fisol - Nature's Way
Each softgel contains: Fish Oil 500 mg • Vitamin E (d-alpha tocopheryl) 1 IU. Other Ingredients: Aqueaous Coating Solution, Gelatin, Glycerin, Water.

Fizzees - Advocare International
Each wafer contains: Vitamin C (as ascorbic acid) 240 mg • Wild Schisandra extract (fruit - schisandra chinensis) 30 mg • Echinacea extract (root - echinacea purpurea) 30 mg • Licorice extract (root - glycyrrhiza glabra) 20 mg • Spikenard extract (root and rhizome -

Aralia mandshurica) 10 mg. Other Ingredients: Dextrose, Potassium Bicarbonate, Citric Acid, Sucralose, Natural Flavors.

Flash Fighters **-** Puritan's Pride
Three tablets contain: Soy concentrate (yielding 65 mg total Isoflavones) 2,100 mg • Black Cohosh extract (Cimicifuga racemosa) root (2.5% triterpene glycosides) 160 mg • Dong Quai (Angelica sinensis) root 150 mg • Licorice (Glycyrrhiza glabra) root 150 mg • Vitex extract (Vitex agnus-castus) fruit 100 mg.

Flavay **-** VMAH
Two capsules contain: Masquelier's Oligomeric Proanthocyanidins seed/bark standardzed complex • Macrozyme Active Enzyme Blend 20 mg: Amylase, Cellulase, Lactase, Lipase, Protease, Maltase, Invertase.

Flavay Plus **-** VMAH
Two capsules contain: Vitamin A (100% as beta-carotene) 5000 IU • Vitamin C (ester-c calcium ascorbate) 60 mg • Vitamin E (d-alpha tocopherol succinate) 100 IU • Vitamin B1 (thiamin) 3 mg • Vitamin B2 (riboflavin) 6 mg • Vitamin B6 (pyridoxine) 10 mg • Vitamin B12 (cyanocobalamin) 20 mcg • Zinc Orotate 10 mg • Selenium (organically bound) 20 mcg • Phosphatidyl Serine 100 mg • GABA (gamma amino butyric acid) 60 mg • Ginkgo Biloba leaf standardized extract (24% ginkgo flavone glycosides, 6% terpene lactones) 50 mg • Masquelier's Oligomeric Proanthocyanidins seed/bark extract 50 mg.

Flax 1000 mg **-** Jamieson
Each capsule contains: Alpha Linolenic Acid (ALA) 500 mg.

Flax Borage Combo **-** Health From The Sun
Three capsules contain: Alpha-Linolenic Acid (ALA)(Omega-3) 825 mg • Gamma-Linolenic Acid (Omega-6) 72 mg • Linoleic Acid (Omega-6) 320 mg • Oleic Acid (Omega-9) 260 mg. Other Ingredients: Certified Organic Flax seed oil, Borage seed oil, Gelatin, Glycerine, Water, Carob powder.

Flax Lignan Gold **-** Health From The Sun
Each 1 tsp serving contains: 100% Certified Organic Flax seed oil & Particulate with Rosemary extract • Mixed Tocopherols (Vitamin E) • Ascorbyl Palmitate (Vitamin C) • Citric Acid to protect freshness.

Flax Liquid Gold **-** Health From The Sun
Each 1 tsp serving contains: 100% Certified Organic Flax seed oil with Rosemary extract • Mixed Tocopherols (Vitamin E) • Ascorbyl Palmitate (Vitamin C) • Citric Acid to protect freshness.

Flax Oil **-** Swanson
Each softgel contains: Calories 10 • Calories from Fat 9 • Total Fat 1 g • Organic Flax Oil 1 g.

Flax Oil **-** Metabolic Response Modifiers
Each softgel contains: Flax oil 1,000 mg • Linolenic acid (Omega-3) 550 mg • Linoleic acid (Omega-6) 170 mg • Oleic acid (Omega-9) 170 mg • Mixed short chain fatty acids 110 mg.

Flax Seed Oil **-** Pro Health
Each softgel contains: Vitmain A (100% as beta-carotene) 430 IU • Organic Flax Seed Oil (unrefined, from Washington flax seed) 1000 mg • Omega-3 Fatty Acids (as alpha-linolenic acid) 560 mg • Omega-6 Fatty Acids (as linoleic acid) 170 mg • Omega-9 Fatty Acids (as oleic acid) 172 mg. Other Ingredients: Gelatin, Glycerin, Carob Powder, Water.

Flax Seed Oil **-** Mass Quantities, Inc.
Each tablespoon contains: Omega-3 Alpha Lineolic Acid 6.2 g • Omega-6 Lineolic Acid 1.8 g • Omega-9 Oleic Acid 2 g.

Flax Seed Oil 1000 mg **-** Jamieson
Each capsule contains: Alpha Linolenic Acid (ALA) (from Flax seed oil) 500 mg.

Flax Seed Oil Liquid **-** NutriCology
Each 1 tbsp (approx. 14 g) serving contains: Flax seed oil 14 g providing Alpha-Linolenic Acid (omega-3) 8.1 g, Linoleic Acid (omega-6) 2.3 g, Oleic Acid (omega-9) 2.2 g. Other Ingredients: Rosemary, Mixed Tocopherol, Ascorbyl Palmitate, Citric Acid.

Flax Seed Oil Softgels **-** NutriCology
Each softgel contains: Flax Seed Oil 1000 mg providing Alpha-Linolenic Acid (omega-3) 570 mg, Linoleic Acid (omega-6) 155 mg, Oleic Acid (omega-9) 185 mg.

Flax Seed Oil with Borage Oil **-** Pro Health
Each softgel contains: Flax Seed oil (from wheat) 840 mg • Borage Oil 160 mg • Gamma Linoleic Acid (GLA) 35 mg • Omega-3 Fatty Acids (as linolenic acid) 455 mg • Omega-6 Fatty Acids (as linoleic acid) 190 mg • Omega-9 Fatty Acids (as oleic acid) 175 mg. Other Ingredients: Gelatin, Water, Glycerin, Natural Carob Coating.

Flax Seed Powder **-** NutriCology
Each 1 tbsp (approx. 9 g) serving contains: Flax seed powder 9 g providing Lignans 43 mg, Omega-3 Fatty Acids 670 mg, Omega-6 Fatty Acids 190 mg, Omega-9 Fatty Acids 210 mg.

Flax-O-Mega **-** Flora, Inc.
Cold pressed Flax Seed oil 1000 mg.

Flaxseed & Cod Liver Oil **-** Puritan's Pride
Each softgel contains: Cold-Pressed Linseed oil 500 mg • Vitamin A (from Cod Liver Oil) 1250 IU • Vitamin D (from Cod Liver Oil) 135 IU.

Flaxseed Oil **-** Optimum Nutrition
Each softgel contains: Flaxseed Oil 1000 mg. Other Ingredients: Gelatin, Glycerin, St. John's Bread Extract.

Flaxseed Oil 1200 MG **-** PhysioLogics
Each softgel contains: Flaxseed Oil 1200 mg (typically contains alpha-linolenic acid 702 mg) • Linoleic Acid 180 mg • Oleic Acid 210 mg • Other Fatty Acids, Phytonutrients 108 mg. Other Ingredients: Gelatin, Glycerin.

Flex Able Advanced Bone & Joint **-** Amerifit Nutrition
Six caplets contain: Vitamin C (ascorbic acid) 100 mg • Calcium (as dicalcium phosphate) 650 mg • Phophorus (as dicalcium phosphate) 500 mg • Zinc (as zinc nitrate) 15 mg • Copper (as copper gluconate) 2 mg • Glucosamine Hydrochloride 1500 mg • Chondroitin Sulfate 1200 mg • Citrus Bioflavonoids 500 mg. Other Ingredients: Microcrystalline Cellulose, Croscarmellose Sodium, Vegetable Stearic Acid, Silica, Vegetable Magnesium Stearate, Natural Vegetable Coating.

Flex Able Advanced Formula with Curcumin **-** Amerifit Nutrition
Two caplets contain: Glucosamine HCl 850 mg • Curcumin extract (curcuma longa, turmeric rhizome providing 95% curcuminoids) 300 mg • MSM (methylsulfonylmethane) 250 mg • Ginger root standardized extract (zingiber officinalis, 5% gingerols) 100 mg • Bioperine Tailed Pepper (standardized piper nigrum extract) 2.5 mg. Other Ingredients: Microcrystalline Cellulose, Croscarmellose Sodium, Stearic Acid, Silica, Magneseium Stearate, Pharmaceutical Glaze. See Editor's Note No. 21, page 2056.

Flex Able Maximum Strength **-** Amerifit Nutrition
Each capsule contains: Glucosamine Hydrochloride 500 mg • Chondroitin Sulfate 400 mg. Other Ingredients: Gelatin (capsule) Silica, Magnesium Stearate.

Flex Able Natural Chewables **-** Amerifit Nutrition
Each chewable wafer contains: Vitamin C 30 mg • Glucosamine HCl 750 mg • Chondroitin Complex 600 mg: Hydrolyzed Gelatin 475 mg, Chondroitin Sulfate 125 mg. Other Ingredients: Natural Cane Sugar, Dried Vegetable Oil Complex, Vegetable Cellulose, Citric Acid, Vegetable Stearic Acid, Natural Fruit Flavors, Silica, Turmeric (color), Vegetable Magnesium Stearate, Methylsulfonylmethane (MSM).

Some Brand Name Natural Products - What they Contain

www.NaturalDatabase.com contains MANY more listings than appear here.

Flex Able Sugar-Free Chewables **-** Amerifit Nutrition
Each chewable wafer contains: Vitamin C 30 mg • Glucosamine HCl 750 mg • Chondroitin Complex 600 mg: Hydrolyzed Gelatin 475 mg, Chondroitin Sulfate 125 mg. Other Ingredients: Sorbitol, Citric Acid, Vegetable Stearic Acid, Cellulose, Natural Flavors, Turmeric (color), Vegetable Stearate, Silica, Methylsulfonlymethane, Acesulfame, Aspartame (contains phenylalanine).

Flex Able Sugar-Free Orange Drink Mix **-** Amerifit Nutrition
Each packet contains: Protein 1 g • Vitamin C 60 mg • Glucosamine HCl 1500 mg • Chondroitin Sulfate 250 mg • Hydrolyzed Gelatin 950 mg. Other Ingredients: Citric Acid, Natural Flavor, Aspartame (contains phenylalanine), Beta Carotene Color, Silica.

FLEXAGEN **-** New Vitality
Three softgels contain: Celadrin Proprietary Blend of Fatty Acid Esters 1050 mg. Other Ingredients: Soy Lecithin, Fish Oil.

FlexAgility **-** PhytoPharmica
Each softgel contains: EV.EXT 77 Extract Proprietary Blend 255 mg: Ginger rhizome extract (zingiber officinale), Greater Galangal rhizome extract (alpinia galanga). Other Ingredients: Gelatin, Medium Chain Triglycerides, Glycerin, Beeswax, Silicon Dioxide.

Flexa-Herb **-** Dial Herbs
Kava Kava • Cramp bark • Cayenne • Ginger • Lobelia • Lady Slipper • Red Clover.

Flex-A-Min **-** Puritan's Pride
Three capsules contain: Glucosamine Sulfate 500 mg • Vitamin C 250 mg • Bromelain (2400 GDU per gram) 250 mg • Boswellin (Boswellia Serrata) 250 mg • Curcumin (Curcuma Longa) 50 mg • Zinc (Amino Acid Chelate) 10 mg • Chondroitin Sulfate A 10 mg • White Willow Bark 100 mg • Shark Cartilage 500 mg • Vervain 100 mg.
See Editor's Note No. 15, page 2055.

FlexAnew **-** Natrol
Two tablets contain: Calcium (as Calcium Carbonate) 330 mg • Glucosamine Sulfate 750 mg • Chondroitin Sulfate 300 mg • Nexrutine (Phellodendron Amurense bark extract) 250 mg.
See Editor's Note No. 15, page 2055.

Flexanol **-** NorthStar Nutritionals
Each capsule contains: Glucosamine HCL 300 mg • Methylsulfonylmethane (MSM) 100 mg • Boswellia Serrata 100 mg • Vitamin C (ascorbyl palmitate) 2 mg • Vitamin E (d-alpha tocopheryl acetate) 2 IU • Vitamin D (cholecalciferol) 20 IU • Eicosapentaenoic Acid (EPA) 24 mg • Docosahexaenoic Acid (DHA) 16 mg • Borage Oil 6 mg • Ginger root 24 mg • Sea Cucumber 20 mg.

Flexaplex **-** Progressive Labs
Three capsules contain: Vitamin A 3000 IU • Vitamin B6 150 mg • Vitamin B12 300 mcg • Magnesium 300 mg • Copper 3 mg • Potassium 25 mg • Adrenal (Bovine) 30 mg • Valerian root 150 mg • Slippery Elm 30 mg • Gentian root 30 mg • Cape Aloes 30 mg • Skullcap 30 mg • Rue powder 30 mg.
See Editor's Note No. 14, page 2055.

Flexcin **-** Flexcin International
Three capsules contain: CM8 Cetyl Myristoleate 750 mg • Type II Collagen 120 mg • Glucosamine Sulfate Potassium 550 mg • MSM complex (methylsulfonylmethane) 150 mg • Enzyme Blend 52 mg. Other Ingredients: Manganese, Zinc, Copper, Vitamin C, Calcium, Boron, Bromelain.

FlexCreme **-** Pharmanex
Menthol 1.25% • Benzyl Alcohol • Butylparaben • Carbomer • Cetyl Myristate • Cetyl Oleate • Cetyl Laurate • Ethylparaben • Glycerin • Glyceryl Stearate • Isobutylparaben • Lecithin • Mentha Piperita (peppermint oil) • Methylparaben • Olea Europaea (olive fruit oil) • PEG-100 Phenoxyethanol • Potassium Hydroxide • Propylparaben • Tocopheryl Acetate • Aqua (water).

Flexi-Licious Glucosamine Chews **-** Bronson Laboratories
Each chew contains: Glucosamine 500 mg.

FlexTend **-** Nature's Way
Three caplets contain: Vitamin C (Ascorbic Acid) 180 mg • Vitamin E Acetate 60 IU • Iron 0.78 mg • Sodium 160 mg • Glucosamine Sulfate (sodium salt) 1.5 g. Other Ingredients: Microcrystalline Cellulose, Maltodextrin, Croscarmellose Sodium, Stearic Acid, Magnesium Stearate, Silicon Dioxide, Hydroxypropyl Methylcellulose, Titanium Dioxide, Polyethylene Glycol, Caramel, Polysorbate 80.

Flintstones Plus Iron Children's Multivitamin **-** Bayer
Each chewable tablet contains: Vitamin A 2500 IU • Vitamin C 60 mg • Vitamin D 400 IU • Vitamin E 15 IU • Thiamin 1.05 mg • Riboflavin 1.2 mg • Niacin 13.5 mg • Vitamin B-6 1.05 mg • Folic Acid 300 mcg • Vitamin B-12 4.5 mcg • Iron 15 mg.

Flite Tabs **-** Aidan Products, LLC
Each capsule contains: Pinokinase Proprietary Blend 250 mg: Pycnogenol, Nattokinase.

Flor*Essence **-** Flora, Inc.
Burdock root • Sheep Sorrel • Slippery Elm • Turkish Rhubarb • Watercress • Kelp • Blessed Thistle • Red Clover.

Flora Vision **-** Flora, Inc.
Bilberry extract 250mg • Blueberry.

Floradix Iron and Herbs **-** Dial Herbs
Vitamin B1 • Vitamin B2 • Vitamin B6 • Folic Acid • Vitamin B12 • Vitamin C • Iron • Aqueous Extract from Carrot • Nettle Worth • Spinach • Quitch roots • Angelica roots • Fennel • Ocean Kelp • African Allow blossom • Orange peel • Juice concentrates: Pear, Red Grape, Blackcurrant, Orange, Blackberry, Cherry, Beetroot • Yeast (Saccharomyces cerevisiae) Extract • Honey • Rose Hip extract • Wheat Germ Extract • Natural Flavor.

FloraGLO brand **-** Kemin Foods
Lutein.
See Editor's Note No. 44, page 2058.

FlorEnz **-** Enzymes, Inc.
Each capsule contains: Proprietary Blend 473 mg: Bifidobacterium longum, Lactobacillus plantarum, Lactobacillus salivarius, Lactobacillus acidophilus, Lactobacillus rhamnosis. Other Ingredients: Cellulose, Water.

Flower Mix **-** Professional Complementary Health Formul
Adrenal 3X, 4X • ACTH 6X, 30X • Histamine 12X • Liver 6X, 12X • Aster, Camellia, Carnation, Chrysantehmum, Daffodil, Daisy, Daphne, Gardenia, Gentian, Fladiola, Honeysuckle, Iris, Lilac, Lily, Larkspur, Lupine, Marigold, Oleander, Pansy, Petunia, Peony, Poppy, Rose, Snapdragon, Tulip 6X, 12X, 60X, 100X • Purified Water • 20% USP Alcohol.
See Editor's Note No. 1, page 2053.

Flu Guard Nasal Spray **-** Jamieson
Each 1 ml dose contains: 42 mg of active ingredients: Echinacea Angustifolia • Baptista Tinctoria • Thuja Occidentalis • Astragalus Membranaceaus • Plantago Lanceolata • Scutellaria Baicalensis.

Flu Resist **-** NatraBio
Active ingredients: Influenzinum 12X • Adrenalinum 6X • Aconitum Napellus 6X • Baptisia Tinctoria 6X • Eupatorium Perfoliatum 6X • Euphrasia Officinarum 6X • Gelsemium Sempervirens 6X • Sticta Pulmonaria 6X • Rhus Toxicodendron 12X. Inactive ingredients: Purified Water, Sodium Chloride, Sodium Phosphate, Benzalkonium Chloride, Benzyl Alcohol, Potassium Chloride, Potassium Phosphate.
See Editor's Note No. 1, page 2053.

FLUIDjoint **-** Patent Health, LLC
Two chewable tablets contain: Proprietary Blend 2000 mg: Milk Protein Concentrate, Fructose, Canola Oil, Stearic Acid, Natural

French Vanilla Flavor, Caramel Flavor, Magnesium Stearate, Sucrolose, Vitamin B1, Vitamin B2.

Flush Free Niacin **-** Puritan's Pride
Each capsule contains: Niacin 400 mg • Inositol 100 mg.

Flush Free Niacin Inositol Hexanicotinate 500 mg **-** Nature's Bounty
Each capsule contains: Niacin (as inositol hexanicotinate) 400 mg • Inositol (as inositol hexanicotinate) 100 mg. Other Ingredients: Gelatin, Vegetable Magnesium Stearate, Silica.

Flush-Free HexaNiacin **-** Enzymatic Therapy
Each capsule contains: Niacin (Inositol hexaniacinate) contains 500 mg elemental Niacin 650 mg.

Flush-Free Niacin **-** PhytoPharmica
Each capsule contains: Niacin (flush-free Inositol hexaniacinate) 590 mg.

Flush-Free Niacin 500 mg **-** Nature's Life
Each tablet contains: Niacin (Inositol, Hexaniacinate) 500 mg.

FM Herbal Complex **-** Pro Health
Each capsule contains: Proprietary Blend 700 mg: Angelica Sinensis, Citrus Sinensis, Typha Angustifolia, Ligusticum Sinense, Saussura Costus, Gentiana Macrophylla, Carthamus Tinctorius, Bupleurum Chinense, Rheum Palmatum, Alisma Plantago Aquatica, Rehmannia Glutinosa, Achyranthes Bidentata, Paeonia Obovata, Glycyrrhiza Glabra, Commiphora Myrrha, Cyperus Rotundus, Isatis Indigotica, Paeonia Lactiflora, Eleutherococcus, Sessiliflorus, Loranthus Parasiticus, Platycoden Grandiflorum, Notopterygium Forbesii, Belamcanda Chinensis, Sargassum Pallidum, Phellodendron Chinense, Andrographis Paniculata, Sanguisorba Officinalis, Mentha Canadensis.

FM Relief **-** Pro Health
Six capsules contain: White Willow bark extract (standardized to 15% salicin) 30 mg • 5 HTP 100 mg • Malic Acid 1200 mg • Magnesium Hydroxide 300 mg • Glucosamine Sulfate 1500 mg • Chondroitin 200 mg • MSM 1000 mg • Boswellin 150 mg • Curcumin (95% curcuminoids) 50 mg. Other Ingredients: Magnesium Stearate, Gelatin, Water.
See Editor's Note No. 15, page 2055.

Focus Child **-** Source Naturals
Two tablets contain: Magnesium (from Magnesium Aspartate and Oxide) 100 mg • Zinc (as Zinc Picolinate) 2 mg • L-Aspartate (from Magnesium Aspartate) 310 mg • DMAE (as DMAE Bitartrate) 100 mg • Standardized Soybean Lecithin (LECI-PS) 50 mg • Yielding 40% Phosphatidylserine 20 mg • Phosphatidylcholine 6 mg • Phosphatidylethanolamine 3.5 mg • Phosphatidylinositol 1 mg • DHA (Docosahexaenoic Acid (Neuromins)) 15 mg • Grape Seed extract 15 mg.

Focus DHA **-** Source Naturals
Each softgel contains: Docosahexaenoic Acid (DHA) (from Alga Oil [Neuromins]) 100 mg.

Focus Factor **-** Vital Basics, Inc.
Four tablets contain: Vitamin A (from natural beta-carotene and mixed carotenoids) 4,000 IU • Vitamin C (as ascorbic acid, sodium ascorbate, calcium ascorbate, potassium ascorbate, zinc ascorbate, and ascorbyl palmitate) 250 mg • Vitamin D (as cholecalciferol) 100 IU • Vitamin E (as natural d-alpha- tocopheryl succinate) 30 IU • Thiamin (as thiamin mononitrate) 3mg • Riboflavin 1.7 mg • Niacin (from inositol hexanicotinate and 50% as niacinamide) 25 mg • Vitamin B6 (as pyridoxal-alpha-ketoglutarate, pyridoxal 5-phosphate) 15 mg • Folate (as folic acid) 400 mcg • Vitamin B12 (as cyanocobalamin) 20 mcg • Biotin 300 mcg • Pantothenic acid (as D-calcium pantothenate) 12 mg • Calcium (as calcium citrate, calcium succinate and calcium ascorbate) 50 mg • Iron (as Ferronly carbonyl Iron) 5 mg • Iodine (as potassium iodide and kelp (Ascophyllum nodosum)) 15 mcg • Magnesium (as magnesium citrate, magnesium malate and magnesium taurinate) 100 mg • Zinc (as zinc citrate and zinc ascorbate) 10 mg • Selenium (as selenomethionine) 20 mcg • Copper (as copper citrate and copper Chelazome) 0.4 mg • Manganese (as manganese citrate) 2 mg • Chromium (as chromium polynicotinate) 100 mcg • Molybdenum (as molybdenum amino acid chelate) 10 mcg • Potassium (as potassium citrate, potassium aspartate, and potassium ascorbate) 50 mg • Synergistic and proprietary formulation: L-Glutamine, DMAE (as DMAE bitartrate), L-pyroglutamic acid, phosphatidylserine, DHA concentrate (15% DHA from fish body oil), choline (as choline bitartrate), inositol, pyridoxal-alpha-ketoglutarate, N-acetyltyrosine, Bacopin (Bacopa monnieri extract) (leaf), bilberry fruit standardized extract (25% anthocyansides), GABA, pine bark and Activin (grape seed extract), vinpocetine, Trace-Lyte Electrolyte concentrate, Huperzine (extract of Huperzia serrata) (whole plant), boron (as boron chelate), vanadium (as vanadyl sulfate) 471 mg. Other Ingredients: Dicalcium Phosphate, Microcrystalline Cellulose, Croscarmellose Sodium, Stearic Acid, Silica, Magnesium Stearate and Pharmaceutical Glaze.

Focus Factor - Children's Chewable **-** Vital Basics, Inc.
Four wafers contain: Vitamin A (from natural beta-carotene and mixed carotenoids) 4,000 UI • Vitamin C (as ascorbic acid, sodium ascorbate and zinc ascorbate) 250 mg • Vitamin D (as cholecalciferol) 100 UI • Vitamin E (as natural d-alpha-tocopheryl succinate) 30 UI • Thiamin (as thiamin mononitrate) 3 mg • Riboflavin 1.7 mg • Niacin (from inositol hexanicotinate and 50% as niacinamide) 25 mg • Vitamin B6 (as pyridoxal alpha ketoglutarate) 5 mg • Folate (as folic acid) 40 mcg • Vitamin B12 (as cyanocobalamin) 20 mcg • Biotin 300 mcg • Pantothenic Acid (as D-calcium pantothenate) 12 mg • Calcium (as calcium citrate, calcium ascorbate, calcium malate and calcium succinate) 100 mg • Iron (as ferrocus glycinate) 10 mg • Iodine (as potassium iodide and kelp) 15 mcg • Magnesium (as magnesium citrate, magnesium malate and magnesium taurinate) 100 mg • Zinc (as zinc aspartate and zinc ascorbate) 10 mg • Selenium (as selenomathionine) 20 mcg • Copper (as copper citrate and copper Chelazome) 400 mcg • Manganese (as manganese citrate) 2 mg • Chromium (as chromium polynicotinate) 100 mcg • Potassium (as potassium citrate, potassium ascorbate and potassium aspartate) 50 mg • Synergistic and proprietary formulation, Phosphatidyl serine / soya lecithin complex, DMAE (as DMAE birartrate), Neuromins (Martex Docosahexaenoic acid concentrate), L-glutamine, L-pyroglutamic acid, pyridoxial alpha ketoglutarate, trace mineral complex, N-acetyl-tyrosine, GABA, Inositol, Bilberry (from 100:1 concentrate), Proanthocyanidin blend from Pine Bark and Activin (grape seed extract), Bacopin (Bacopa monnieri extract), Coenzyme Q-10, Huperzine (extract of huperzia serrata), Boron (as boron citrate), Vanadium (as vanadyl sulfate) 640 mg. Other Ingredients: Simple and Complex Carbohydrates from corn, Organic Sucanat with honey, Mixed Fruit, and Cherry Crystals, Cellulose, Magnesium Stearate and Silica.

FolaPro **-** Metagenics
Each tablet contains: Folate (Metafolin as L-5-methyl tetrahydrofolate) 800 mcg.

Folgard **-** Upsher-Smith Laboratories
Each tablet contains: Folic Acid 800 mcg • Vitamin B-6 10 mg • Vitamin B-12 115 mcg.

Folic Acid **-** GNC
Each tablet contains: Folic Acid 400 mcg. Other Ingredients: Dextrose, Whole Brown Rice Powder (Oryza Sativa).

Folic Acid **-** Leiner Health Products
Each tablet contains: Folate (Folic Acid) 400 mcg. Other Ingredients: Dicalcium Phosphate, Cellulose, Stearic Acid, Croscarmellose Sodium, Magnesium Stearate.

Folic Acid **-** Pro Health
Each tablet contains: Folic Acid (from biologically fermented yeast) 800 mcg • Vitamin B12 (cyanocobalamin) 25 mcg. Other Ingredients: Cellulose, Stearic Acid, Magnesium Stearate.

***Folic Acid* -** Nature's Bounty
Each tablet contains: Folic Acid 400 mcg. Other Ingredients: Dicalcium Phosphate, Vegetable Stearic Acid, Croscarmellose, Silica, Vegetable Magnesium Stearate.

***Folic Acid* -** Source Naturals
Each tablet contains: Folate (as folic acid) 800 mcg.

***Folic Acid 0.4 mg* -** Jamieson
Each tablet contains: Folic Acid 0.4 mg (400 mcg).

***Folic Acid 1 mg* -** Jamieson
Each tablet contains: Folic Acid USP 1 mg.

***Folic Acid 400 mcg* -** Schiff
Each tablet contains: Folate (as folic acid) 400 mcg • Calcium (as dibasic calcium phosphate) 25 mg. Other Ingredients: Dextrose, Corn Syrup, Silicon Dioxide, Magnesium Stearate.

***Folic Acid 400 mcg - GNC A-Z* -** GNC
Each tablet contains: Folic Acid (50%) 400 mcg. Other Ingredients: Dextrose, Whole Brown Rice Powder (oryza sativa).

***Folic Acid 400 mcg* -** Nature Made
Each tablet contains: Folate (from folic acid) 400 mcg. Other Ingredients: Dibasic Calcium Phosphate, Croscarmellose Sodium, Magnesium Stearate.
See Editor's Note No. 45, page 2058.

***Folic Acid 800 - GNC A-Z* -** GNC
Each tablet contains: Folic Acid 800 mcg. Other Ingredients: Whole Brown Rice powder (Oryza Sativa).

***Folic Acid Capsules* -** Optimum Nutrition
Each capsule contains: Folic Acid 400 mcg. Other Ingredients: Microcrystalline Cellulose, Gelatin, Magnesium Stearate.

***Folic Acid Dophilus Plus B-12* -** Dial Herbs
Two wafers contain: Folic Acid 800 mcg • Vitamin B12 400 mcg • Lactobacillus acidophilus • Lactobacillus plantarum • Lactobacillus bulgaricus • Lactobacillus casei 200 mcg.

***Folic Acid Plus B12* -** Life Extension
Each tablet contains: Pure Folic Acid 800 mcg • Vitamin B12 300 mcg.

***Foltx* -** Pan American Laboratories, Inc.
Each tablet contains: Folic Acid USP (Folacin) 2.5 mg • Cyanocobalamin USP (B-12) 1 mg • Pyridoxine HCl (B-6) 25 mg.

***For Men Only* -** Doctor's Best
Each tablet contains: L-Glycine 135 mg • L-Alanine 135 mg • L-Glutamic Acid 135 mg • Raw Prostate concentrate 100 mg • Saw Palmetto 100 mg • Golden Rod 50 mg • Pumpkin seed concentrate 10 mg • Vitamin E 10 IU • Zinc 5 mg • Flax Seed Oil 3 mg.
See Editor's Note No. 14.

***Formula 1* -** Enzymes, Inc.
Two capsules contain: Protease 80,000 HUT • Amylase 9000 DU • Lipase 168 LU • Cellulase 160 CU. Other Ingredients: Plant Fiber, Gelatin, Water.

***Formula 10 - Ness* -** Enzymes, Inc.
Two capsules contain: Brewers Yeast 200 mg • Sucrase (Invertase) 3.6 IAU • Gotu Kola aerial part (Cantella Asiatica) 100 mg • Amylase 6000 DU • Protease 30,000 HUT • Rose Hips (Rosa Canina) 50 mg • Lipase 24 LU • Cellulase 200 CU. Other Ingredients: Gelatin, Plant Fiber, Water.

***Formula 100* -** Puritan's Pride
Each tablet contains: Vitamin A (as retinyl palmitate and 20% as beta carotene) 10,000 IU • Vitamin C (as ascorbic acid and rose hips) 250 mg • Vitamin D (as cholecalciferol) 400 IU • Vitamin E (as d-alpha tocopheryl acid succinate) 150 IU • Thiamin (Vitamin B1; as thiamine mononitrate) 100 mg • Riboflavin (Vitamin B2) 100 mg • Niacin (as niacinamide) 100 mg • Vitamin B6 (as pyridoxine hydrochloride) 100 mg • Folic Acid 300 mcg • Vitamin B12 (as cyanocobalamin) 100 mcg • Biotin 100 mcg • Pantothenic Acid (as d-calcium pantothenate) 100 mg • Calcium (as calcium carbonate) 100 mg • Iron (as ferrous fumarate) 18 mg • Iodine (as kelp) 150 mcg • Magnesium (as magnesium oxide) 50 mg • Zinc (as zinc oxide) 15 mg • Selenium (as sodium selenate) 25 mcg • Copper (as cupric oxide) 0.5 mg • Manganese (as manganese sulfate) 6.1 mg • Chromium (as GTF chromium yeast) 200 mcg • Potassium (as potassium citrate) 10 mg • PABA (para-aminobenzoic acid) 100 mg • Choline Bitartrate 100 mg • Inositol 100 mg • Rutin 25 mg • Lemon Bioflavonoids 50 mg • Hesperidin 12.5 mg • Betaine Hydrochloride 30 mg • Octacosanol 50 mcg • Proprietary Blend 5 mg: Alfalfa Leaf, Watercress, Parsley Leaf, Rice Bran, Lecithin.

***Formula 11* -** Enzymes, Inc.
Two capsules contain: Vitamin C (Ascorbic acid) 100 mg • Citrus Bioflavonoids 200 mg • Acerola Cherries (Malpighia punicifolia) 50 mg • Rose Hips (Rosa canina) 50 mg • Amylase 500 DU. Other Ingredients: Plant Fiber, Gelatin, Water.

***Formula 113* -** Enzymes, Inc.
Two capsules contain: Vitamin C (Ascorbic acid) 50 mg • Amylase 12,000 DU • Citrus Bioflavonoids 110 mg • Wheat Germ 100 mg • Protease 40,000 HUT • Acerola Cherries (Malpighia puncifolia) 25 mg • Rose Hips (Rosa canina) 25 mg • Sucrase (Invertase) 0.2 IAU • Malt Diastase 270 DP • Lipase 38 LU • Cellulase 320 CU • Lactase 480 ALU. Other Ingredients: Plant Fiber, Gelatin, Water.

***Formula 12* -** Enzymes, Inc.
Three capsules contain: Burdock root (Arctium lappa) 450 mg • Citrus Bioflavonoids 450 mg • Cellulase 1800 CU • Amylase 3600 DU • Protease 7500 HUT • Lipase 15 LU. Other Ingredients: Gelatin, Plant Fiber, Water.

***Formula 13* -** Enzymes, Inc.
Two capsules contain: Wheat Germ 200 mg • Lecithin 100 mg • Sea Kelp (Macrocystis pyrifera) 20 mg • Amylase 1400 DU • Lipase 38 LU • Protease 4000 HUT • Cellulase 20 CU. Other Ingredients: Plant Fiber, Gelatin, Water.

***Formula 14* -** Enzymes, Inc.
Two capsules contain: Kelp (Laminaria digitata) 200 mg • Irish Moss 100 mg • Protease 50,000 HUT • Amylase 3000 DU • Lipase 48 LU • Cellulase 400 CU • Potassium Iodide 0.6 mg. Other Ingredients: Plant Fiber, Gelatin, Water.

***Formula 15* -** Enzymes, Inc.
Two capsules contain: Spirulina Pratensis 150 mg • Alfalfa juice concentrate (Medicago sativa) 150 mg • Parsley leaf (Petroselinum crispum) 100 mg • Protease 21,400 HUT • Amylase 2100 DU • Lipase 16 LU • Cellulase 28 CU. Other Ingredients: Plant Fiber, Gelatin, Water.

***Formula 16* -** Enzymes, Inc.
Two capsules contain: Calcium (as Calcium Lactate) 60 mg • Protease 12,200 HUT • Amylase 2000 DU • Lipase 24 LU. Other Ingredients: Plant Fiber, Gelatin, Water.

***Formula 17* -** Enzymes, Inc.
Two capsules contain: Pau D'arco bark (Tabebuia spp.) 200 mg • Yellow Dock root (Rumex crispus) 200 mg • Echinacea root (Echinacea purpurea) 180 mg • Mullein leaf (Verbascum thapsus) 20 mg • Protease 10,000 HUT • Amylase 1600 DU • Lipase 36 LU • Cellulase 60 CU. Other Ingredients: Gelatin, Plant Fiber, Water.

***Formula 18* -** Enzymes, Inc.
Two capsules contain: Lipase 386 LU • Amylase 9000 DU • Protease 30,500 HUT • Glucoamylase 27 AG • Cellulase 120 CU. Other Ingredients: Plant Fiber, Gelatin, Water.

***Formula 19* -** Enzymes, Inc.
Two capsules contain: Calcium (as Calcium Gluconate) 41 mg • Magnesium (as Magnesium Gluconate) 9 mg • Protease 4060 HUT •

Amylase 666 DU • Lipase 16 LU. Other Ingredients: Plant Fiber, Gelatin, Water, Silica.

Formula 2 **-** Enzymes, Inc.
Two capsules contain: Amylase 12,000 DU • Protease 49,180 HUT • Glucoamylase 27 AG • Lactobacillus Acidophilus 27 mg • Lipase 96 LU • Cellulase 120 CU. Other Ingredients: Plant Fiber, Gelatin, Water.

Formula 20 **-** Enzymes, Inc.
Two capsules contain: Amylase 6800 DU • Protease 19,600 HUT • Lipase 72 LU • Cellulase 80 CU. Other Ingredients: Plant Fiber, Gelatin, Water.

Formula 21 **-** Enzymes, Inc.
Two capsules contain: Protease 40,000 HUT • Amylase 4000 DU • Malt Diastase 540 DP • Sucrase (Invertase) 0.4 IAU • Lipase 72 LU • Cellulase 400 CU • Lactase 900 ALU. Other Ingredients: Plant Fiber, Gelatin, Water, Silica.

Formula 3 **-** Enzymes, Inc.
Three capsules contain: Amylase 27,000 DU. Other Ingredients: Plant Fiber, Gelatin, Water.

Formula 301 **-** Enzymes, Inc.
Two capsules contain: Rose Hips (Rosa canina) 180 mg • Alfalfa juice concentrate (Medicago sativa) 130 mg • Echinacea root (Echinacea purpurea) 90 mg • Lipase 136 LU • Protease 16,394 HUT • Mullein leaf (Verbascum thapsus) 10 mg • Amylase 1000 DU • Cellulase 80 CU. Other Ingredients: Plant Fiber, Gelatin, Water.

Formula 4 **-** Enzymes, Inc.
Three capsules contain: Protease 240,000 HUT. Other Ingredients: Plant Fiber, Gelatin, Water.

Formula 401 **-** Enzymes, Inc.
Two capsules contain: Horsetail aerial part (Equisetum arvense) 80 mg • Lactobacillus Acidophilus 57 mg • Lipase 138 LU • Protease 20,000 HUT • Cellulase 80 CU. Other Ingredients: Plant Fiber, Gelatin, Water.

Formula 416 **-** Enzymes, Inc.
Four capsules contain: Calcium (as Calcium Lactate) 60 mg • Protease 332,000 HUT • Amylase 2000 DU • Lipase 24 LU. Other Ingredients: Plant Fiber, Gelatin, Water.

Formula 419 **-** Enzymes, Inc.
Four capsules contain: Calcium (as Calcium Gluconate) 20 mg • Magnesium (as Magnesium Gluconate) 4 mg • Protease 332,000 HUT • Amylase 400 DU • Lipase 8 LU. Other Ingredients: Plant Fiber, Gelatin, Water.

Formula 5 **-** Enzymes, Inc.
Three capsules contain: Lipase 360 LU. Other Ingredients: Plant Fiber, Gelatin, Water.

Formula 501 **-** Enzymes, Inc.
Two capsules contain: Yucca aerial part (Yucca spp.) 175 mg • Alfalfa juice concentrate (Medicago sativa) 175 mg • Safflower petals (Carthamus tinctorius) 150 mg • Oat straw (Avena sativa) 50 mg • Protease 10,000 HUT • Amylase 1500 DU • Cellulase 200 CU • Lipase 12 LU. Other Ingredients: Gelatin, Plant Fiber, Water.

Formula 560 **-** Immunity Today, LLC.
Each capsule contains: Vitamin C 30 mg • Coenzyme Q10 5 mg • Proprietary Blend of Transfer Factor derived from Bovine Colostrum 165 mg.

Formula 6 **-** Enzymes, Inc.
Two capsules contain: Marshmallow root (Althaea Officinalis) 450 mg • Rose Hips (Rosa Canina) 150 mg • Amylase 10,000 DU • Protease 37,000 HUT • Cellulase 400 CU • Lipase 24 LU. Other Ingredients: Gelatin, Water, Plant Fiber.

Formula 600 Plus for Men **-** Nature's Life
Two capsules contain: Saw Palmetto berry (Serenoa repens B.) 600 mg • Active Aminos (l-Glutamic Acid, Glycine & L-Alanine) 170 mg • Zinc (Picolinate) 15 mg • Pumpkin seed (Curcurbita pepo) 50 mg • Pygeum africanum H. bark extract [(150:1) equivalent to 300 mg whole herb] 2 mg • Burdock root (Arctium lappa L.) 5 mg • Cayenne fruit (Capsicum annuum L. var. annuum) 5 mg • Goldenseal root (Hydrastis canadensis L.) 5 mg • Gravel root (Eupatorium purpureum L.) 5 mg • Juniper berry (Juniperus oxycedrus L.) 5 mg • Marshmallow root (Althaea officinalis L.) 5 mg • Parsley leaf (Petroselinum crispum(Mill) Nym.ex. A.W. Hill) 5 mg • White Pond Lily root (Nymphaea odorata) 5 mg • Vitamin B6 (Pyridoxine HCl) 5 mg • Copper (Gluconate) 1 mg • Nature's Life Active Aminos is an exclusive free-form blend of l-Glutamic Acid, l-Alanine & Glycine.

Formula 601 **-** Enzymes, Inc.
Two capsules contain: Comfrey leaf (Symphytum officinale) 400 mg • Papaya leaf (Carica papaya) 200 mg • Amylase 10,000 DU • Cellulase 400 CU • Lipase 24 LU. Other Ingredients: Gelatin, Water, Plant Fiber.

Formula 7 **-** Enzymes, Inc.
Two capsules contain: Safflower petals (Carthamus Tinctorius) 300 mg • Amylase 7200 DU • Lipase 138 LU • Protease 11,400 HUT • Cellulase 40 CU. Other Ingredients: Plant Fiber, Gelatin, Water.

Formula 701s **-** Enzymes, Inc.
Two capsules contain: Collinsonia root part (Collinsonia canadensis) 200 mg • Hawthorn berry (Crataegus oxycanthus) 200 mg • Protease 24,242 HUT • Amylase 3000 DU • Lipase 48 LU • Cellulase 40 CU. Other Ingredients: Gelatin, Plant Fiber, Water.

Formula 75 **-** Futurebiotics
Vitamin C (Rose hips) 250 mg • Vitamin A (palmitate 10,000 IU, beta carotene 7500 IU) 17,500 IU • Vitamin E (natural) 150 IU • Vitamin D (cholecalciferol) 400 IU • Riboflavin 75 mg • Thiamin 75 mg • Vitamin B6 (pyridoxine HCl) 75 mg • Niacinamide 75 mg • Vitamin B12 (cyanocobalamin) 75 mcg • Folic Acid 400 mcg • Pantothenic Acid 75 mg • Biotin 75 mcg • Iron (chelate) 1.3 mg • Calcium (chelate) 20 mg • Magnesium (chelate) 10 mg • Iodine (kelp) 150 mcg • Selenium (chelate) 25 mcg • Zinc (chelate) 10 mg • Manganese (chelate) 1 mg • Copper (chelate) 1 mg • Molybdenum (chelate) 25 mcg • Chromium (picolinate) 25 mcg • Boron (chelate complex) 0.5 mg • Potassium (chelate complex) 1.8 mg • Inositol 75 mg • Choline (bitartrate) 31 mg • Rutin 25 mg • Para Amino Benzoic Acid (PABA) 75 mg • Hesperidin complex 5 mg • Citrus bioflavonoid complex 25 mg • Betaine HCl 25 mg. In a Green Foods base of: Alfalfa, Barley & Chlorella.

Formula 8 **-** Enzymes, Inc.
Two capsules contain: Lactobacillus Acidophilus 53 mg • Lactase 1500 ALU • Amylase 1000 DU. Other Ingredients: Plant Fiber, Gelatin, Water.

Formula 801 **-** Enzymes, Inc.
Each teaspoon contains: Cellulase 75,000 CU • Lactobacillus Acidophilus 900 mg • Bifidobacterium Longum 500 mg. Other Ingredients: Plant Fiber, Silica.

Formula 9 **-** Enzymes, Inc.
Two capsules contain: Alfalfa juice concentrate (Medicago Sativa) 280 mg • Parsley leaf (Petroselinum Crispum) 134 mg • Horsetail aerial part (Equisetum Arvense) 120 mg • Rose Hips (Rosa Canina) 100 mg • Protease 30,500 HUT • Amylase 3400 DU • Lipase 29 LU. Other Ingredients: Plant Fiber, Gelatin, Water.

Formula HGH **-** HealthMinded
Four capsules contain: Formula HGH 2715 mg: Amino Peptide complex, Colostrum, Tribulus Terrestris, Citrus complex, Chrysin, Phosphatidyl Serine, Phosphatidyl Choline. Other Ingredients: Stearic Acid, Magnesium Stearate.

Formula IV - GNLD International, LLC.
Two capsules contain: Vitamin A (from fish liver oil) 4000 IU • Vitamin C (as ascorbic acid and from acerola cherry fruit (malpighia punicifolia)) 90 mg • Vitamin D (from fish liver oil) 400 IU • Vitamin E (as D-alpha tocopherol) 10 IU • Thiamine (as thiamine mononitrate and from yeast) 10 mg • Riboflavin (as riboflavin and from yeast) 10 mg • Niacin (as niacinamide and from yeast) 50 mg • Vitamin B6 (as pyridoxine hydrochloride and from yeast) 10 mg • Folic Acid 400 mcg • Vitamin B12 (as cyanocobalamin) 10 mcg • Pantothenic Acid (as calcium pantothenate and from yeast) 12 mg • Iron (as iron peptonate and from parsley leaves (petroselinum crispum)) 25 mg • Iodine (from kelp and as potassium iodide) 100 mcg • Magnesium (as magnesium oxide) 35 mg • Copper (as copper gluconate and from kelp) 2 mg • Manganese (as manganese gluconate) 10 mg • Potassium (as potassium gluconate) 10 mg • Linoleic Acid (from safflower oil) 176 mg • Inositol (as inoitol and from soy lecithin) 65 mg • Lecithin (from soy) 30 mg • Para-Aminobenzoic Acid 30 mg • Betaine Hydrochloride 10 mg • Mixed Tocopherols (non-alpha) 1 mg • TRE-EN-EN Grain Concentrate Blend 450 mg: Rice bran oil, Soy bean oil, Wheat germ oil • Phyto Enzyme Blend 45 mg: Lipase, Protease, Diastate, Amylase. Other Ingredients: Gelatin, Glycerin, Wax, Water, Hydrolyzed Collagen Protein, Titanium Dioixde, Natural Color.

Formula IV Plus - GNLD International, LLC.
Each packette contains: Vitamin A (from retinyl palmitate) 4000 IU • Vitamin C (as ascorbic acid and from acerola cherry fruit (malpighia punicifolia)) 90 mg • Vitamin D (from fish liver oil) 400 IU • Vitamin E (as D-alpha tocopherol) 10 IU • Thiamine (as thiamine mononitrate and from yeast) 10 mg • Riboflavin (as riboflavin and from yeast) 10 mg • Niacin (as niacinamide and from yeast) 50 mg • Vitamin B6 (as pyridoxine hydrochloride and from yeast) 10 mg • Folic Acid 400 mcg • Vitamin B12 (as cyanocobalamin) 10 mcg • Pantothenic Acid (as calcium pantothenate and from yeast) 12 mg • Iodine (from kelp and as potassium iodide) 100 mcg • Magnesium (as magnesium oxide) 35 mg • Zinc (as zinc oxide) 15 mg • Selenium (as sodium selenite) 40 mcg • Copper (as copper gluconate and from kelp) 2 mg • Manganese (as manganese gluconate) 10 mg • Chromium (chelated) 20 mcg • Molybdenum (as molybdenum trioxide) 30 mcg • Potassium (as potassium gluconate) 10 mg • Inositol 65 mg • Lecithin (from soy) 30 mg • Betaine Hydrochloride 10 mg • Mixed Tocopherols (non-alpha) 2 mg • Tre-En-En Grain Concentrate Blend 675 mg: Rice Bran oil, Soy bean oil, Wheat Germ oil • Phyto Enzyme Blend 45 mg: Lipase, Protease, Diastase, Amylase. Other Ingredients: Microcrystalline Celluose, Gelatin, Glycerin, Yellow Beeswax, Sodium Croscarmellose, Hydroxypropyl Methylcellulose, Water, Rice Bran, Wheat Bran, Silicon Dioxide, Magnesium Stearate, Titanium Dioixde, Natural Color, Triacetin.

Formula NT-OX - Jamieson
Each caplet contains: Vitamin A (as Retiyl Palmitate (5000 IU) and 67% (10,000 IU) as Beta Carotene) 15,000 IU • Vitamin C (as Ascorbic Acid) 500 mg • Vitamin E (as D-Alpha Tocopheryl Succinate) 100 IU • Selenium (from Yeast) 50 mcg • In a base of Borage Oil, Sunflower Oil, Rosehips, Rutin, Hesperidin, Citrus Bioflavonoids, Acerola, Kelp, Parsley, Watercress, Alfalfa, Bromelain, Papain, Amylase, Lipase, Cellulase.

Formula SF722 - Thorne Research Inc.
Each gelcap contains: 10-Undecenoic Acid derived from castor bean oil 50 mg. Inactive Ingredients: Extra Virgin Olive Oil, Gelatin, Glycerin, Water.

Formu-Leane - SupraLife
Each capsule contains: ChromeMate Chromium Polynicotinate 75 mcg • Proprietary Blend 485 mg: Ma Huang rhizome/roots, Advantra-Z Citrus Aurantium extract (6%), Guarana seed, Ginkgo Biloba leaf, Gymnema Sylvestre leaf, Gotu Kola leaf extract, Ci Wu Jia root (eleutherococcus senticosus), Green Tea leaf extract, Bladderwrack herb (fucus versiculosus), RiboCell D-Ribose. Other Ingredients: Gelatin, Magnesium Stearate.
See Editor's Note No. 30, page 2056.

Formu-Leane Z - SupraLife
Each capsule contains: ChromeMate Chromium Polynicotinate 75 mcg • Proprietary Blend 697 mg: Advantra-Z Citrus Aurantium extract (6%), Guarana seed, Ginkgo Biloba leaf, Gymnema Sylvestre leaf, Gotu Kola leaf extract, Ci Wu Jia root (eleutherococcus senticosus), Green Tea leaf extract, Bladderwrack herb (fucus versiculosus), RiboCell D-Ribose, Porio Cocos extract, Creatine, Cayenne, Juniper berry extract, Dandelion root extract, Butcher's Broom extract (ruscus aculeatus), Uva Ursi leaf extract, Bioperine. Other Ingredients: Gelatin, Magnesium Stearate.
See Editor's Note No. 40, page 2058.

ForSight - Resource Wellness
Three caplets contain: Vitamin A (89% as Beta Carotene) 15,000 IU • Vitamin C (Ascorbis Acid) 300 mg • Vitamin E Acetate 400 IU • Calcium 650 mg • Iron 0.74 mg • Sodium 10 mg • Lutein/Zeaxanthin 6 mg • Alpha Carotene 2 mg • Grape Seed extract 50 mg. Other Ingredients: Dicalcium Phosphate, Microcrystalline Cellulose, Croscramellose Sodium, Calcium Silicate, Magnesium Stearate, Stearic Acid, Hydroxypropyl Methylcellulose, Propylene Glycol, Polyethylene Glycol, Titanium Dioxide, FD&C Yellow No. 6 Lake, FD&C Red No. 40 Lake, FD&C Blue No. 2 Lake.

Forskolin Extract - PhytoPharmica
Each capsule contains: Coleus Forskohlii extract (standardized to contain 18% forskolin [9 mg per capsule]) 50 mg.

ForsLean brand - Sabinsa Corporation
Coleus Forskohlii.
See Editor's Note No. 44, page 2058.

Forten-Zyme 550 - Atrium Inc.
Each tablet contains: Maxistrength Pancreatin 550 mg (which has been prepared by the lyophilization method to insure the preservation & concentration of natural occuring factors such as Amylase, Lipase & Protease enzyme activity. Proteolytic activity is ensured as specific Chymotrypsin & Trypsin content.). This formula is compounded in a buffered base of Amino Acids for maximum stability.
See Editor's Note No. 14.

Fortified Pycnogenol - Puritan's Pride
Three tablets contain: Vitamin A (100% as Beta-Carotene) 25,000 IU • Calcium 340 mg • Selenium (from Selenium Yeast Chelate) 100 mcg • Pine bark extract (Pinus maritmus) 25 mg • Coenzyme Q-10 10 mg • Grape Seed extract (Vitis vinifera) 100 mcg • Whole Food Phytonutrient Blend: Broccoli (entire plant), Carrot (root), Spinach (leaf), Tomato (fruit) 120 mg.

Forza-T - InStone Nutrition
Three capsules contain: Vitamin B6 3.5 mg • Magnesium 150 mg • Zinc 10 mg • 6-OXO 300 mg • Tribulus Terrestris (protodioscin 20%) 190 mg. Other Ingredients: Gelatin, Microcrystalline Cellulose, Magnesium Stearate.

FOS + Fiber Fructooligosaccharides - Nikken Inc.
Two tablets contain: Dietary Fiber (as cellulose, legume fiber, apple pectin) 1.5 g • FOS (fructooligosaccharides) 500 mg. Other Ingredients: Acacia Gum, Silicon Dioxide, Croscarmellose Sodium, Magnesium Stearate, Cellulose Coating (hydroxypropyl cellulose, ethyl cellulose, hydroxypropyl methylcellulose, guar gum, propylene glycol, vegetable oil), Brazil Wax.

FOS Daily - Health Smart Vitamins
Each caplet contains: Fructooligosaccharides (FOS) 500 mg • Lactobacillus acidophilus 180 mg • Lactobacillus bulgaricus 30 mg • Streptococcus thermophilus 30 mg.

Fosfree - Mission Pharmacal
Two tablets contain: Vitamin A 3,000 IU • Vitamin C 100 mg • Vitamin D (as Vitamin D3) 300 IU • Thiamine 9 mg • Riboflavin 4 mg • Niacin 21 mg • Vitamin B6 5 mg • Vitamin B12 4 mcg • Pantothenic Acid 2 mg • Calcium 351 mg • Iron 29 mg. Other Ingredients: Sugar, Polyethylene Glycol, Color, Croscarmellose

Sodium, Povidone, Food Glaze, Cyanocobalamin, Magnesium Stearate, Yellow 5 Lake, Carnauba Wax, White Beeswax, Sodium Benzoate.

Four-In-One **-** Changes International, Inc.
Each capsule contains: Vitamin C (as Calcium Ascorbate) 120 mg • Aloe 200:1 concentrate leaf gel 200 mg • Wild Yam root (Mexican Yam) 50 mg • Cat's Claw root bark (Uncaria tomentosa) 300 mg • DHEA (Dehydroepiandrosterone) 5 mg. Other Ingredients: Gelatin, Magnesium Stearate, Calcium Stearate, and Silica.

Free Amino **-** Atrium Inc.
Full Spectrum - Composed of 22 Free Form Pure Amino Acids.

Free Aminos **-** Allergy Research Group
Each capsule contains: L-Alanine 41 mg • L-Arginine 62 mg • L-Cysteine 14 mg • L-Cystine 62 mg • L-Glutamine 28 mg • Glycine 28 mg • L-Histidine 49 mg • L-Isoleucine 69 mg • L-Leucine 69 mg • L-Lysine 98 mg • L-Methionine 14 mg • L-Phenylalanine 7.5 mg • L-Serine 14 mg • Taurine 4 mg • L-Threonine 56 mg • L-Tyrosine 28 mg • L-Valine 28 mg. Other Ingredients: Cellulose, Magnesium Stearate, Silicon Dioxide.

Free Aminos **-** NutriCology
Each capsule contains: L-Alanine 41 mg • L-Arginine 62 mg • L-Cysteine 14 mg • L-Cystine 62 mg • L-Glutamine 28 mg • Glycine 28 mg • L-Histidine 49 mg • L-Isoleucine 69 mg • L-Leucine 69 mg • L-Lysine 98 mg • L-Methionine 14 mg • L-Phenylalanine 7.5 mg • L-Serine 14 mg • Taurine 4 mg • L-Threonine 56 mg • L-Tyrosine 28 mg • L-Valine 28 mg. Other Ingredients: Cellulose, Magnesium Stearate, Silicon Dioxide.

Free-B **-** Atrium Inc.
Each tablet contains: Vitamin B1 (Thiamine HCL) 100 mg • Vitamin B2 (Riboflavin) 50 mg • Vitamin B6 (Pyridoxine HCL) 50 mg • Vitamin B12 (Cyanocobalamin) 100 mcg • Niacinamide 150 mg • Pantothenic Acid 100 mg • Biotin 150 mcg • Calcium (Dicalcium Phosphate) 20 mg • Copper (Gluconate) 1 mg • Phosphorus (Dicalcium Phosphate) 20 mg • Zinc (Aspartate) 30 mg.

French Paradox (French Parad'ox) **-** Arkopharma
Each capsule contains: Red Wine Marc extract (standardized to 25% anthocyanosides (62.5 mg) and 0.02% resveratrol (50 mcg)) 250 mg. Other Ingredients: Cellulose Derivative, Magnesium Stearate, Silica.

French Vanilla - Revival **-** Physicians Laboratories
Eight fluid ounces contain: Certified Isoflavone 15 mg. Other Ingredients: Whole Roasted Soybeans, Natural and Artificial Flavors.

Fresh Green Black Walnut Wormwood Complex **-** Now
Two droppersful (16 ml) contain: Proprietary blend: Green Black Walnut hulls (Juglans species) 1.6 ml • Wormwood herb (Artemisia absinthium) • Clove buds (Carophyllus species) extracts. Other Ingredients: Grain Alcohol, Distilled Water.

Fresh Nettle Leaf **-** Gaia Herbs
Nettle leaf (2% caffeic acids and derivatives). Standardized Full Spectrum 100 mg of extract per capsule. Guaranteed Potency 50 mg of extract per capsule.

Friendly Fiber **-** NSI - Nutraceutical Sciences Institute
Each six capsules contain: Apple Pectin 2.1 g • Oat Bran 2.1 g.

Friendly Flora **-** Nutri-Quest Rx
Each capsule contains: Jerusalem Artichoke (rich source of Fructooligosaccarides) 200 mg • Cellulase 1200 CU • Lactobacillus Acidophilus 400 million • Acerola extract 25 mg • Rose Hips 25 mg • Bifidobacterium Bifidum 200 million • Bifidobacterium Longum 200 million • Protease 7500 HUT • Lipase 52 LU • Lactobacillus Casei 100 million • Lactobacillus Plantarum 100 million • Lactobacillus Rueteri 100 million • Lactobacillus Salicarius 100 million • Amylase 275 DU • EDS Mineral Mix: Kelp, Calcium Ascorbate, Magnesium Citrate, Zinc Gluconate, Manganese Gluconate. In a base of pure plant fiber.

From The Earth **-** The Vitamin Shoppe
Three tablets contain: Vitamin A 15000 IU • Vitamin D 400 IU • Vitamin E 200 IU • Vitamin C 1000 mg • Vitamin B1 25 mg • Vitamin B2 25 mg • Vitamin B6 25 mg • Vitamin B12 500 mcg • Vitamin B3 25 mg • Inositol 25 mg • Choline 50 mg • PABA 25 mg • Pantothenic Acid 25 mg • Biotin 50 mcg • Folic Acid 400 mcg • Citrus Bioflavonoids Complex 125 mg • Rutin 25 mg • Quercetin 25 mg • Hesperidin 25 mg • Calcium 200 mg • Magnesium 100 mg • Potassium 99 mg • Zinc 15 mg • Manganese 5 mg • Molybdenum 50 mcg • Iodine 150 mcg • Copper 500 mcg • Selenium 50 mcg • Chromium 200 mcg • Boron 1 mg • Silica 5 mg • RNA 35 mg • DNA 10 mg • Carotenoids 4 mg • Chlorophyll 4 mg • Borage, Flax Seed, and Sunflower Oils 200 mg • L-Glutathione 5 mg • Spirulina 1000 mg • Wheat Grass 100 mg • Barley Grass 100 mg • Chlorella 100 mg • Bee Pollen 100 mg • Korean Ginseng root 50 mg • Garlic 10 mg • Bee Propolis extract 10 mg • Royal Jelly 5 mg • Bromelain 50 mg • Betaine HCl 50 mg • Papain 50 mg • Amylase 5 mg • Lipase 5 mg • Cellulase 5 mg • Lactobacillus Acidophilus, B. bifidum, L-bulgaricus (dairy free) 50 mg • Oat Bran 50 mg • Apple Pectin 50 mg • A unique blend of: Echinacea, Milk Thistle, Goldenseal, Ginger root, Ginkgo Biloba, Capsicum 50 mg.

From The Sea **-** Puritan's Pride
Three capsules contain: Glucosamine Sulfate (Aminomonosaccharide) 1000 mg • Sea Cucumber (Beche De-Mer) 1000 mg • Shark Cartilage 500 mg.

Fruit Max **-** Swanson
Two tablets contain: Apple fruit powder 80 mg • Apricot fruit powder 80 mg • Cherry fruit powder 80 mg • Lemon peel powder 80 mg • Orange peel powder 80 mg • Papaya powder 80 mg • Peach fruit powder 80 mg • Strawberry fruit powder 80 mg • Freeze-Dried Grape juice 50 mg • Freeze-Dried Orange juice 50 mg • Freeze-Dried Pineapple juice 50 mg • Prune juice powder 40 mg • Cranberry juice concentrate 20 mg.

Fruit Punch Phosphagen HP **-** EAS
Each 43 gram serving contains: Phosphagen 5.25 g • Taurine 1000 mg. Ingredients: Dextrose • Phosphagen (HPCE pure Creatine Monohydrate), Taurine • Natural & Artificial Flavor • Citric Acid • Beet Powder for color • Magnesium Phosphate • Disodium Phosphate •Potassium Phosphate.

Fruit4Life **-** Swanson
Two tablets contain: Apple fruit powder 80 mg • Apricot fruit powder 80 mg • Cherry fruit powder 80 mg • Lemon peel powder 80 mg • Orange peel powder 80 mg • Papaya powder 80 mg • Peach fruit powder 80 mg • Strawberry fruit powder 80 mg • Freeze-Dried Grape juice 50 mg • Freeze-Dried Orange juice 50 mg • Freeze-Dried Pineapple juice 50 mg • Prune juice powder 40 mg • Cranberry juice concentrate 20 mg.

Fruit-Easy **-** Progressive Labs
Two tablets contain: A blend of the following 1400 mg: Apples • Cranberry powder • Orange juice powder • Pineapple juice powder • Siberian Ginseng • Ginkgo Biloba • Peaches • Dates • Bromelain • Papain • Lipase • Amylase • Protease • Cellulase • Powdered Cellulose • Apple pectin • Citris pectin • Prune powder • Glucomannan • Lactobacillus Acidophilus • Calcium Gluconate • Green Tea.

Fruitplex **-** HealthWatchers System
Apple • Lemon • Strawberry • Blueberry • Plum • Cantaloupe • Pear • Cherry • Grapefruit • Raspberry • Grape • Orange • Peach • Watermelon • Pineapple • Papaya

Fruits of Life Potent Cellular Protection **-** Garden of Life, Inc.
Each tablespoon (10 g) contains: Antioxidant Fruit Organic Concentrate Blend 3000 mg: Blueberry, Raspberry, Strawberry, Blackberry, Prune, Raisin • Mineral Matrix Proprietary Blend 7000 mg: biologically active Alkalinizing Minerals, Enzymes, Probiotics from Goat's Milk.

Fuel for Thought Neuro Nutrition **-** Nature's Plus
Two tablets contain: L-Glutamine free form amino acid 250 mg • Lecithin (Soya) 250 mg • RNA (Ribonucleic acid) 200 mg • L-Tyrosine free form amino acid 200 mg • L-Phenylalanine free form amino acid 100 mg • Phosphatidylcholine 100 mg • Raw Pituitary concentrate 25 mg • Vitamin B6 (Pyridoxine HCL) 10 mg. Sugar & starch free.
See Editor's Note No. 14.

Full Spectrum Cinnamon Extract **-** Planetary Formulas
Two tablets contain: Calcium 50 mg • Cinnamomum Aromaticum bark extract 10:1 (yielding 8% flavonoids) 300 mg • Cinnamomum Aromaticum bark 100 mg. Other Ingredients: Dibasic Calcium Phosphate, Stearic Acid, Modified Cellulose Gum, Colloidal Silicon Dioxide.

Full Spectrum Jiaogulan **-** Planetary Formulas
Each tablet contains: Calcium 127 mg • Jiaogulan extract (gynostemma pentaphyllum, standardized to 10% gypenosides) 375 mg. Other Ingredients: Dibasic Calcium Phosphate, Stearic Acid, Colloidal Silicon Dioxide, Modified Cellulose Gum, Magnesium Stearate.

Full Spectrum Life Minerals **-** Pro Health
Two tablets contain: Vitamin D (as cholecalciferol) 200 IU • Calcium (from carbonate, amino acid chelate, citrate) 1000 mg • Iron (as amino acid chelate) 20 mg • Iodine (from kelp) 150 mcg • Magnesium (from magnesium oxide, amino acid chelate, citrate) 500 mg • Chromium (yeast-free) 100 mcg • Molybdenum (as amino acid chelate) 50 mcg • Potassium (as amino acid chelate) 99 mg • Zinc (as amino acid chelate) 22.5 mg • Selenium (as selenomethionine) 50 mcg • Copper (as amino acid chelate) 1 mg • Manganese (as amino acid chelate) 5 mg • L-Glutamic Acid (HCl) 50 mg • Boron (as amino acid chelate) 3 mg • Vanadium (as amino acid chelate) 50 mcg. Other Ingredients: Cellulose, Silica, Magnesium Stearate.

Full Spectrum Mineral Caps **-** Now
Four capsules contain: Vitamin D (as Cholecalciferol) 4000 IU • Calcium (from Hydroxapatite) 500 mg • Phosphorus (from Hydroxapatite) 193 mg • Iodine (from Kelp) 225 mcg • Magnesium (as Magnesium Oxide and Citrate) 500 mg • Zinc (as Amino Acid Chelate) 15 mg • Selenium (as l-Selenomethionine) 100 mcg • Copper (as Amino Acid Chelate) 2 mg • Manganese (as Amino Acid Chelate) 5 mg • Chromium (as Chromium Chelavite) 200 mcg • Molybdenum (as Amino Acid Chelate) 100 mcg • Potassium (as Amino Acid Chelate) 99 mg • Boron (as Amino Acid Chelate) 3 mg • Vanadium (as Amino Acid Chelate) 50 mcg. Other Ingredients: Gelatin (capsule), Rice Flour, Magnesium Stearate.

Full Spectrum Minerals **-** Now
Each tablet contains: Calcium (Carbonate, Amino Acid Chelate, Citrate) 1000 mg • Magnesium (Oxide, Amino Acid Chelate, Citrate) 500 mg • Zinc (Amino Acid Chelate) 22.5 mg • Iron (Amino Acid Chelate) 20 mg • Copper (Amino Acid Chelate) 1 mg • Potassium (Proteinate) 99 mg • Manganese (Amino Acid Chelate) 5 mg • Selenium (L-Selenium Methionine) 50 mcg • Chromium (yeast-free, Proteinate) 100 mcg • Molybdenum (Amino Acid Chelate) 59 mcg • Vanadium (Amino Acid Chelate) 50 mcg • Iodine (Kelp) 150 mcg • L-Glutamic Acid (HCL) 50mg • Vitamin D (Cholecalciferol) 200 IU • Boron 3 mg.

Full Spectrum Pycnogenol **-** Life Extension
Each capsule contains: Pycnogenol 5 mg • Pine bark extract (4:1, source of high potency proanthocyanidins & leucocyanidins) 30 mg • Grape Seed extract 100 mg • Quercetin 5 mg.

Fungal Defense Candida & Yeast Cleanse **-** Garden of Life, Inc.
Each caplet contains: Wild Oregano concentrate (6% volatile oils) 342 mg • Fungal Defense N•Zime Blend 233 mg: Protease 20,000 HUT, Cellulase 20,000 CU • Poten-Zyme D. Salina extract 120 mg • Olive leaf extract (20% oleuropin) 100 mg • Poten-Zyme Garlic juice extract (20:1) 95 mg • Ionic Fulvic Acid mineral blend 80 mg • HSO Probiotic Blend 800 Million CFU: L. Acidophilus, L. Bulgaricus, L. Lactis, L. Plantarum, L. Caseii, S. Boulardii, B. Bifidum, B. Subtilis, B. Lichenformis • Poten-Zyme Yucca juice extract (20:1) 30 mg. Other Ingredients: Cellulose, Stearates (vegetable source).

FX-Chrysin **-** GEN - Genetic Evolutionary Nutrition
Each capsule contains: Chrysin 250 mg • LPC (lysophosphatidyl choline) 200 mg.

FYI For Your Inflammation **-** Garden of Life, Inc.
Three caplets contain: Chicken Collagen Type II 805 mg • Wild Oregano concentrate (6% volatile oils) 465 mg • Poten-Zyme Cat's Claw extract 375 mg • Systemic Enzyme Blend 350 mg: Bromelain 80,000 HUT, Papain 2,100,00 FCCPU, Protease blend 250,000 FCCPU, Amylase 4000 DU, Lipase 1750 FCCLU, Cellulase 500 CU • Rhododendron Caucasicum extract (40% polyphenols) 150 mg • Poten-Zyme Ginger extract 115 mg • Poten-Zyme Turmeric extract 115 mg • Poten-Zyme Green Barley juice extract 115 mg • Phytosterol blend 60 mg • Laminaria extract (5% algae phenolics) 50 mg • Ulva extract (5% algae phenolics) 50 mg • Bayberry bark extract (77% myricetin) 50 mg. Other Ingredients: Cellulose, Stearates (vegetable source).

GH.3. Romanian Youth Formula **-** TheraCeuticals
Each capsule contains: Vitamin A (as beta-carotene) 1200 IU • Thiamin (as thiamin mononitrate) 10 mg • Vitamin B3 (as niacinamide) 80 mg • Vitamin B6 (as pyridoxine hydrochloride) 20 mg • Zinc (as PhytoZinc and zinc gluconate) 2.6 mg • Copper (as copper gluconate) 0.8 mg • Procaine (dimethylaminoethanol bitartrate 200 mg, para-aminobenzoic acid 75 mg) • Ginkgo leaf extract (24% flavone glycosides, 6% terpenes) 50 mg. Other Ingredients: Gelatin, Silicon Dioxide, Magnesium Stearate.

GI. Gel: Gastro-Intestinal Tonic **-** The Herbalist
Slippery Elm bark • Marshmallow root.

GI. Support **-** Now
Three capsules contain: Vitamin A (as Retinol Palmitate) 5000 IU • Vitamin B3 (as Niacinamide) 40 mg • Vitamin B5 (as Calcium Pantothenate) 50 mg • Biotin 1000 mcg • Folic Acid (Folate) 400 mcg • Zinc (as Zn Monomethionine) 15 mg • Selenium (as Selenomethionine) 140 mcg • L-Glutamine 500 mg • Apple Pectin 300 mg • N-Acetyl Glucosamine (NAG) 250 mg • Methylsulfonylmethane (MSM) 250 mg • Deglycyrrhizinated Licorice (DGL) 100 mg • Licorice extract 4:1 root 100 mg • Cat's Claw extract 15:1 bark 100 mg • Ginger powder root 100 mg • Aloe Vera concentrate 200:1 leaf (equivalent to 5000 mg fresh Aloe Vera) 25 mg • Pepsin Enzymes NF 1:10000) 50 mg • Pepsin (2000 USP papaya) 50 mg.

G/C 1000 **-** Progressive Labs
Each capsule contains: Vitamin C (from manganese ascorbate) 60 mg • Manganese (from manganese ascorbate) 15 mg • Glucosamine Hydrochloride 750 mg • Chondroitin Sulfate 250 mg.
See Editor's Note No. 15, page 2055.

GABA **-** Enzymatic Therapy/PhytoPharmica
Each capsule contains: Gamma-Aminobutyric Acid (GABA) 250 mg. Other Ingredients: Gelatin, Cellulose, Magnesium Stearate, Silicon Dioxide, Titanium Dioxide Color.

GABA **-** Source Naturals
Each tablet contains: GABA (gamma amino butyric acid) 750 mg.

GABA Calm **-** Source Naturals
Each tablet contains: GABA (Gamma Amino Butyric Acid) 100 mg • Glycine 50 mg • Magnesium Taurinate (Yielding 3 mg of Elemental Magnesium) 40 mg • N-Acetyl-L-Tyrosine 25 mg.

Gabatein brand **-** Cyvex Nutrition, Inc.
Green Tea extract.
See Editor's Note No. 44, page 2058.

***GABA-Val* - Progressive Labs**
Each capsule contains: Gamma Amino Butyric Acid (GABA) 50 mg • Valerian root extract (Valeriana officinalis) 300 mg • Thiamine HCl (Vitamin B1) 25 mg • Niacinamide 25 mg • Magnesium (amino acid chelate) 25 mg • Inositol 175 mg • Lupulin (hops pollen) 50 mg • Passion flower (Passiflora incarnata) 25 mg • Glutamic Acid 25 mg • Brain tissue 25 mg.
See Editor's Note No. 31, page 2056.

***Gainers Fuel (Anabolic Weight Gain Formula)* - TwinLab**
Each serving contains: Calories 531. Each serving also contains Branched Chain Amino Acids (including Peptide Bonded & Free Amino Acids) 21 g, Essential Vitamins, Minerals, Trace Elements, Key Metabolic Optimizers & Lipotropic Factors.

***Gainers Fuel 1000 (Super Anabolic Weight Gain Formula)* - TwinLab**
Each serving contains: Predigested Proteins & Amino Acids (Complex Carbohydrates, Anabolic Branched Chain Amino Acids) • Vitamins & Minerals •Pharmaceutical Grade Pancreatic digests of Whey Protein (Lactalbumin) & Egg White Protein (Albumin) • Chromium 400 mcg • Boron • L-Carnitine • Beta-Carotene • Kreb's Cycle Mineral Complexes (including Citrates, Aspartates, Succinates & Alpha-Ketoglutarates).

***Gainers Fuel 2500* - TwinLab**
Whey & Egg White Proteins • Branched Chain Amino Acids (L-Leucine, L-Isoleucine & L-Valine) • Essential Vitamins & Minerals • Chromium Picolinate & L-Carnitine (100% predigested). Low in fat without high levels of medium chain triglycerides that may cause gastrointestinal upset.

***Galagen brand* - Proventra**
Colostrum.
See Editor's Note No. 44, page 2058.

***GalantaMind - Galanta Mind* - Life Enhancement Products, Inc.**
Each capsule contains: Vitamin B5 (from calcium pantothenate) 100 mg • Galantamine Hydrobromide extract (from Lycoris radiata) 8 mg • Choline (from choline dihydrogen citrate) 200 mg.

***Gall & Liver Tablets* - Life Brand**
Agrimony herb 100.1 mg • Goose Grass 100.1 mg • Horehound herb 72.8 mg • Senna leaf 18.2 mg • Woodruff herb 81.25 mg • Wormwood herb 18.2 mg • Yarrow 81.9 mg. Excipients: Corn Starch, Sodium Bicarbonate, Silicon Dioxide, Magnesium Stearate, Methyl Paraben, Propyl Paraben.

***Gallbladder* - Enzymes, Inc.**
Each capsule contains: Proprietary Herbal Blend 400 mg: Globe Artichoke leaf extract, Dandelion root extract, Turmeric root extract, Lecithin, Dandelion leaf extract • Lipase 100 mg. Other Ingredients: Plant Cellulose, Water.

***Gallexier Herbal Bitters* - Flora, Inc.**
Artichoke • Dandelion • "other bitter herbs".

***Gamma Oryzanol* - Source Naturals**
Each tablet contains: Gamma Oryzanol 30 mg.

***GammaFrac* - Source Naturals**
Each tablet contains: Famma Oryzanol 25 mg • FRAC (Ferulic Acid Complex) 50 mg.

***Gammalen - In Oil Of Primrose* - Life Extension**
Each 560 mg capsule contains: Linoleic Acid 350 mg • Gamma Linoleic Acid 40 mg • Gamma Linolenic Acid 40 mg • Vitamin E 13.6 IU.

***Garcinia 1000* - Source Naturals**
Two tablets contain: Citrin Garcinia cambogia extract [yielding 1,000 mg of (-) Hydroxycitric Acid as Calcium Hydroxycitrate] 2,000 mg • Chromium (150 mcg from ChromeMate GTF Yeast-Free Polynicotinate and 150 mcg from Yeast-Free Chromium Picolinate) 300 mcg.

***Garcinia Cambogia Plus* - Atrium Inc.**
Each capsule contains: Garcinia cambogia (standardized to contain 50% Hydroxycitric Acid) 340 mg • Atractylodes 80 mg • Citrus aurantii 80 mg • Chromium Picolinate 500 mcg • Chromium Arginate 160 mcg.

***Garcinia Plus* - Source Naturals**
Two tablets contain: Garcinia cambogia Extract (Citrin, yielding 1,000 mg of (-) hydroxycitric acid as calcium hydroxycitrate) 2,000 mg • L-Phenylalanine 200 mg • Chromium (100 mcg from ChromeMate GTF yeast-free polynicotinate and 100 mcg from yeast-free chromium picolinate) 200 mcg.

***Garlic* - Pharmanex**
Each caplet contains: Garlic clove powder (Allium sativum) 650 mg. Other Ingredients: Excipients, Binders, Caplet Coating.

***Garlic* - Olympian Labs**
Each capsule contains: Garlic 500 mg.

***Garlic - Plus* - Aspen Group, Inc.**
Each tablet contains: High Potency Garlic (standardized to contain 2500 mcg of allicin) 300 mg • Enzyme Complex 60 mg • Rice Protein-Calcium complex 40 mg.

***Garlic & Golden Seal* - Nutrivention**
Two fl oz contains: Garlic oil • Goldenseal root • Safflower oil • cold-pressed Olive oil • Tocopherol (natural Vitamin E).

***Garlic & Parsley* - Jamieson**
Each tablet contains: Garlic Oil (equivalent to 350 mg fresh garlic) 0.59 mg • Parsley Leaf Powder 50 mg.

***Garlic (Allicin-Rich)* - Life Brand**
Garlic extract powder 500 mg (equivalent to 1500 mg of fresh Garlic cloves). Contains Allicin potential yield of 1.5 mg/g, Thiosulphonates 1.6 mg/g, Allicin 10 mg/g, Gamma Glutamylcysteines 20 mg/g. Other Ingrendients: Cellulose, Calcium Phosphate, Stearic Acid, Magnesium Stearate, Aqueous base film coat.

***Garlic Complex* - Shaklee**
Two tablets contain: Garlic powder (Allium sativum) clove 1 g • Spearmint oil (Mentha spicata) leaf 3 mg • Rosemary extract (Rosmarinus officinalis) herb 50 mg. Other Ingredients: Maltodextrin, Microcrystallline Cellulose, Carbohydrate gum, Hydroxylated Soy Lecithin, Ascorbyl Palmitate, Mixed Tocopherols Concentrate, Rosemary Extract.

***Garlic EC* - USANA Health Sciences**
Each tablet contains: Garlic powder (standardized to 6,000 g allicin yield) 650 mg. Inactive Ingredients: Microcrystalline Cellulose, Dibasic Calcium Phosphate, Hydroxypropyl Methylcellulose Phthalate, Colloidal Silicon Dioxide, Magnesium Silicate, Glycerol Triacetate, Croscarmellose Sodium, Vegetable-derived Stearic Acid, Vegetable-derived Magnesium Stearate.

***Garlic Echinacea Goldenseal+* - Futurebiotics**
Two tablets contain: Echinacea angustifolia leaf powder extract (standardized for 4% (5 mg) echinacosides) 125 mg • Echinacea purpurea leaf powder 80 mg • Echinacea angustifolia leaf powder 20 mg • Goldenseal root powder 225 mg • Garlic bulb powder extract (odorless) 200 mg • Chinese Cinnamon root powder 30 mg • Black Pepper bud powder 20 mg • Clove flower powder 50 mg • Astragalus root powder 50 mg • Ginger root powder 50 mg • Peppermint leaf powder 10 mg • Parsley leaf powder 100 mg • Chamomile flower powder 100 mg • Bayberry bark powder 100 mg • Cayenne fruit powder 25 mg • Barberry bark powder 50 mg • Myrrh resin powder 50 mg. Other Ingredients: Dicalcium phosphate, Cellulose, Stearic acid, Magnesium stearate, Silica.

Garlic HP **-** PhysioLogics
Each tablet contains: Garlic bulb (10000 mcg Allicin/gram) 400 mg.

Garlic HP 650 MG **-** PhysioLogics
Each tablet contains: Garlic bulb powder (allium sativum) 650 mg (standardized to contain a minimum: allicin yield 6500 mcg, total thiosulfinates yield 6500 mcg, alliin yield 14,500 mcg, gamma-glutamylcysteines 5200 mcg). Other Ingredients: Cellulose (plant origin), Calcium Carbonate, Food Glaze, Vegetable Stearic Acid, Croscarmellose, Silica, Vegetable Magnesium Stearate, Cellulose Coating.

Garlic Oil - Basic Nutrition **-** GNC
Each capsule contains: Garlic Oil (Allium sativa) 0.65 mg. Other Ingredients: Soybean Oil, Gelatin, Glycerin, Corn Oil, Dill Oil, Wheat Germ Oil.

Garlic with High Allicin Complex **-** Nikken Inc.
Each caplet contains: Whole Garlic powdered extract 600 mg Providing: Gamma Glutamylcysteines 12,000 mcg, Alliin 6000 mcg, Sulfur 4800 mcg, Thiosulfinates 1200 mcg, Allicin Yield 1200 mcg. Other Ingredients: Dicalcium Phosphate, Microcrystalline Cellulose, Croscarmellose Sodium, Silicon Dioxide, Stearic Acid, Magnesium Stearate, Enteric Coating (cellulose acetate phthalate, diethyl phthalate).

Garlic/Parsley Formula **-** Nature's Way
Two capsules contain: Proprietary Formula: Garlic bulb • Parsley herb. Other Ingredients: Gelatin.

Garlic-Go! **-** Wakunaga of America
Each caplet contains: Aged Garlic extract powder (bulb) 1000 mg. Other Ingredients: Cellulose, Silica, Magnesium Stearate (vegetable source).

Garlic-Gold **-** Olympian Labs
Each caplet contains: Garlic extract (alium satium) 600 mg • Allicin 7200 mcg.

Garlicin **-** Nature's Way
Each tablet contains: Garlicin alliinaise-rich garlic powder 300 mg. Other Ingredients: Aqueous Coating Solution, Cellulose, Modified Cellulose Gum, Silica, Stearic Acid, Xylitol.

Garlicin HC **-** Nature's Way
Each tablet contains: Calcium 26 mg • Cayenne pepper fruit 15 mg • Garlic bulb 259 mg • Hawthorn dried extract (19% oligomeric procyanidins) 25 mg • Rutin 12 mg • Vitamin E (d-alpha tocopheryl) 15 IU. Other Ingredients: Aqueous Coating Solution, Cellulose, Maltodextrin, Modified Cellulose Gum, Silica, Stearic Acid.

Garlife **-** Life Extension
Each tablet contains: Pure Garlic extract (odor suppressed, standardized to 10,000 ppm allicin) 900 mg.

Garlinase 4000 **-** Enzymatic Therapy
Each tablet contains: Garlic extract, equal to 4000 mg of fresh garlic, standardized to contain a minimum of 3.4% (11000 mcg) of Allicin per tablet by a unique patented process to assure maximum Allicin production in your body 320 mg.

GarliPure Daily Formula **-** Natrol
Each vegetarian capsule contains: Garlic (Allium sativum) powdered extract bulb 600 mg containing: Gamma Glutamylcysteines 12000 mcg • Allicin 6000 mcg • Sulfur 4800 mcg • Thiosulfinates 1200 mcg • Allicin Yield 1200 mcg. Other Ingredients: 100% Vegetarian capsule Shell made of Kosher Vegetable Cellulose & Water, Magnesium Stearate.

GarliPure Formula 500 **-** Natrol
Two tablets contain: Garlic (Allium sativum) powdered extract bulb 1000 mg containing: Gamma Glutamylcysteines 20000 mcg • Allicin 10000 mcg • Sulfur 8000 mcg • Thiosulfinates 1600 mcg • Allicin Yield 1500 mcg. Other Ingredients: Dicalcium Phosphate, Microcrystalline Cellulose, Stearic Acid, Magnesium Stearate, aqueous base film coat.

GarliPure Maximum Allicin Formula **-** Natrol
Each caplet contains: Garlic (Allium sativum) powdered extract bulb 600 mg: Gamma Glutamylcysteines 12000 mcg • Allicin 4800 mcg • Sulfur 3900 mcg • Thiosulfinates 3800 mcg • Allicin Yield 3600 mcg. Other Ingredients: Microcrystalline Cellulose, Stearic Acid, Dicalcium Phosphate, Magnesium Stearate Silicon Dioxide, Aqueous base film coat.

GarliPure Once Daily Potency **-** Natrol
Each tablet contains: Garlic (Allium sativum) 600 mg Powdered extract bulb containing: Allicin 13800 mcg • Thiosulfinates 6060 mcg • Allicin Yield 6000 mcg • Gamma Glutamylcysteines 4800 mcg • Sulfur 3900 mcg. Other Ingredients: Dicalcium Phosphate, Microcrystalline Cellulose, Croscarmellose Sodium, Silicon Dioxide, Stearic Acid, Magnesium Stearate.

GarliPure Organic Formula **-** Natrol
Two capsules contain: Garlic (Alium sativum), organically grown powdered extract bulb 1000 mg containing: Gamma Glutamylcysteines 15000 mcg • Allicin 10000 mcg • Sulfur 7000 mcg • Thiosulfinates 1600 mcg • Allicin Yield 1500 mcg. Other Ingredients: 100% Vegetarian capsule Shell made of Kosher Vegetable Cellulose & Water, Silicon Dioxide, Magnesium Stearate.

GarliPure Selenium Plus Formula **-** Natrol
Each capsule contains: Selenium 67 mcg • Garlic (Allium sativum) powdered extract bulb 400 mg: Gamma Glutamylcysteines 8000 mcg • Allicin 4400 mcg • Sulfur 3200 mcg • Thiosulfinates 2040 mcg • Allicin Yield 2000 mcg. Other Ingredients: Gelatin.
See Editor's Note No. 21, page 2056.

Garlique **-** Chattem, Inc.
Each tablet contains: Garlic bulb powder (not less than 500 mcg of allicin yield) 400 mg. Other Ingredients: Dicalcium Phosphate, Microcrystalline Cellulose, Croscarmellose Sodium, Stearic Acid, Magnesium Stearate, Sodium Lauryl Sulfate, Colloidal Silicon Dioxide, Hydroxypropyl Methylcellulose Phthalate, Talc, Titanium Dioxide, Triacetin, Pharmaceutical glaze (214-112).

Garlite **-** Nature's Plus
Each Vegicap contains: Deordorized Garlic (equivalent to a minimum of 2.5 times its weight in fresh garlic) 500 mg.

Garlitrin 4000 **-** PhytoPharmica
Each tablet contains: Garlic extract (Allium sativum) bulb extract (standardized to contain a minimum of 3.4% [11,000 mcg] of alliin per tablet) 320 mg.

Gas **-** Hyland's
Two tablets contain: Nux Moshata 3X • Asafetida 3X • Ignatia Amara 3X • Lycopodium Clavatum 6X. Base: Lactose USP.
See Editor's Note No. 1, page 2053.

Gas Ease **-** Enzymes, Inc.
Each capsule contains: n-zimes Proprietary Enzyme Blend 239 mg: alpha-Galactosidase, Amylase, Glucoamylase, Malt Diastase, CereCalase Plus, Cellulase, Xylanase, Pectinase, Lipase, Protease (alkaline, neutral and acid proteases plus peptidase) • Proprietary Herbal Blend 260 mg: Peppermint leaf extract (4:1) plus whole leaf, Fennel seed extract (4:1) plus whole seed, Caraway seed. Other Ingredients: Plant Cellulose, Rice Bran, Water, Lecithin.

GastrEnz **-** Enzymes, Inc.
Each capsule contains: Proprietary Blend 450 mg: Marshmallow extract, Green Papaya concentrate, Deglycyrrhizinized Licorice root extract, Licorice root extract • n-zimes Proprietary Blend 251 mg: Lipase, Amylase, Peptidase, Catalase, CereCalase Plus, Glucoamylase, Papain, Malt Diastase, Cellulase, Pectinase, alpha-Galactosidase, Ivertase, Lactase. Other Ingredients: Cellulose, Water.

Gastric Ease - wellzymes **-** Enzymes, Inc.
Each capsule contains: n-zimes Proprietary Enzyme Blend 73 mg: Catalase, Peptidase, Lipase, Amylase, Glucoamylase, Malt Diastase, Invertase, Lactase, alpha-Galactosidase, Cellulase, CereCalase Plus, Xylanase, Pectinase • Proprietary Herbal Blend 145 mg: Marshmallow root, Marshmallow root extract (equivalent to 200 mg of raw herb), Aloe Vera gel extract (equivalent to 2000 mg of raw gel). Other Ingredients: Plant Cellulose, Water.

Gastricin **-** Gero Vita International
Each capsule contains: Proprietary Blend 510 mg: Codonopsis Pilosula root 4:1 extract, Atractylodes Macrocephala rhizome 8:1 extract, Citrus Sacrodactylus fruit 8:1 extract, Cyperus Rotundus rhizome 8:1 extract, Pinellia Ternata tuber 8:1 extract, Amomum Villosum fruit 8:1 extract, Gardenia Jasminoides fruit 8:1 extract • PhytoSel 30 mg. Other Ingredients: Gelatin, Tricalcium Phosphate, Silicon Dioxide, Magnesium Stearate, Rice Flour, ACF 223.

Gastritix Formula **-** Nature's Way
Two capsules contain: Chamomile flower 62.5 mg • Fennel seed 237.5 mg • Ginger 237.5 mg • Marshmallow root 50 mg • Slippery Elm bark 125 mg • Wild Yam root 237.5 mg. Other Ingredients: Gelatin, Magnesium Stearate, Maltodextrin.

Gastro Calm **-** Enzymes, Inc.
Each capsule contains: Proprietary Herbal Blend 355 mg: Marshmallow root extract, Deglycyrrhizinized Licorice root extract, Ginger root extract, Quercetin • Proprietary Enzyme Blend 146 mg: Amylase, Peptidase, Lipase, CereCalase, Invertase, Cellulase, Glucoamylase, Catalase, Malt Diastase, alpha-Galactosidase, Lactase, Pectinase. Other Ingredients: Plant Cellulose, Water.

Gastro-Ad **-** PhysioLogics
Two tablets contain: Gastro-Ad powder (lactobacillus delbrueckii fermented soy protein) 1000 mg. Other Ingredients: Fructose, Sorbitol, Cellulose (plant origin), Natural Pineapple Flavor, Vegetable Magnesium Stearate, Vegetable Stearic Acid, Silica.

Gastro-Relief **-** PhytoPharmica
Each chewable tablet contains: Calcium Carbonate 250 mg • Deglycyrrhizinated Licorice (DGL) root extract (Glycyrrhiza glabra) 380 mg • Glycine (Amino Acid) 50 mg.

GastroSoothe **-** Enzymatic Therapy
Each tablet contains: Calcium Carbonate 250 mg • Deglycyrrhizinated Licorice (DGL) root extract (Glycyrrhiza glabra) 380 mg • Glycine (Amino Acid) 50 mg.

GastroSoothe Chocolate-Mint **-** Enzymatic Therapy
Each tablet contains: Calcium Carbonate 250 mg • Deglycyrrhizinated Licorice (DGL) root extract (Glycyrrhiza glabra) 380 mg • Glycine (Amino Acid) 50 mg. Flavored with Dutch Cocoa powder, Creme Flavor, & Peppermint.

GBE 24/6 brand **-** Soft Gel Technologies, Inc.
Ginkgo Biloba leaf extract.
See Editor's Note No. 44, page 2058.

GBLVR **-** Nutri-Quest Rx
Proprietary blend 500 mg: Bayberry • Red Beet root • Yellow Dock • Dandelion root • Fennel seeds • Peppermint • Ginger root • Wild Yam • Blessed Thistle • Garlic 500 mg. In a base of 6X tissue salts: Calc Fluor.

Gelly-Bees Royal Jelly **-** Nikken Inc.
Two tablets contain: Royal Jelly powder 200 mg • Fructooligosaccharides 200 mg. Other Ingredients: Dextrin, Corn Starch, Crystalline Cellulose, Magnesium Stearate.

GelStat Migraine **-** GelStat Corporation
Each OraDose dispenser (2 mL) contains: Ginger 2X • Feverfew 3X. Other Ingredients: Ascorbic Acid, Glycerin, Potassium Sorbate, Purified Water, Sorbitol, Xanthan Gum.
See Editor's Note No. 1, page 2053.

GEN Andro*Gen **-** GEN - Genetic Evolutionary Nutrition
Each capsule contains: Androstenedione 100 mg.
See Editor's Note No. 47, page 2058.

GEN CM Relief **-** GEN - Genetic Evolutionary Nutrition
Each capsule contains: CMO (Cetyl-Myristoleate) 500 mg.

GEN Multi*GenX **-** GEN - Genetic Evolutionary Nutrition
Each six capsules contain: Antioxidants: Vitamin C (Ascorbic Acid) 1000 mg • Vitamin E (natural d-Alpha Tocopherol) 40 IU • Propanthocyanidins (Grape seed extract) 25 mg • Citrus bioflavonoids 100 mg • Lipoic Acid 50 mg. Vitamins: Vitamin A (Retinol Palmitate) 5000 IU • Vitamin A (Beta Carotene) 20000 IU • Vitamin D (as Vitamin D3, Cholecalciferol) 400 IU • Vitamin B1 (Thiamine HCL) 50 mg • Vitamin B2 (Riboflavin) 50 mg • Vitamin B3 (Niacinamide) 50 mg • Vitamin B5 (Calcium d-Pantothenate) 50 mg • Vitamin B6 (Pyroxine HCL) 50 mg • Vitamin B12 (Cyanocobalamin) 40 mcg • Folic Acid 400 mcg • Biotin 300 mcg. Minerals: Calcium (from Citrate) 400 mg • Magnesium (from Citrate) 200 mg • Iron (from Fe glycinate) 9 mg • Potassium (from Chloride) 150 mg • Zinc (from Monomethionate-OptiZinc) 15 mg • Manganese (from Citrate) 10 mg • Iodine (from Kelp) 100 mcg • Copper (from Co Gluconate) 270 mcg • Chromium (from Cr Nicotinate/Glycinate) 200 mcg • Molybdenum (from Sodium Molybdate) 150 mcg • Selenium (from Amino Acid Chelate) 200 mcg. Lean Muscle Enhancement: RNA (Sodium Ribonucleic Acid) 150 mg • Inositol 40 mg • L-Carnitine 35 mg • Taurine (HCL) 75 mg • L-Glutamine 25 mg • MSM (Methyl Sulfonylmethane) 100 mg • Coenzyme Q10 (Ubiquinone) 30 mg.

GEN Pyruvate Burn **-** GEN - Genetic Evolutionary Nutrition
Each capsule contains: MED-PRO licensed Pyruvate, from a Pyruvic Acid Complex with Dihydroxyacetone 500 mg. Pyruvic Acid is stabilized with Calcium, Sodium, Potassium or Magnesium to form Pyruvate.

GEN Thermogen **-** GEN - Genetic Evolutionary Nutrition
Two capsules contain: Ma Huang extract standardized at 6%: 334 (334 x .06 = 20 mg) • Caffeine 200 mg • Naringin 40 mg • White Willow bark extract 75 mg • Potassium (Phosphate) 50 mg • Cayenne 35 mg.
See Editor's Note No. 30, page 2056.

GeniKinoko **-** Quality of Life Labs
Six capsules contain: Proprietary Blend 2010 mg: Fermented Soybean Isoflavone extract, Polysaccharides from Basidiomycetes Mushrooms, Cyclodextrin • Genistein 540 mg. Other Ingredients: Gelatin.

Genistein **-** Source Naturals
Four tablets contain: Soybean powder 4000 mg • Genistein 11.6 mg • Daidzein 42.4 mg • Glycitein 32 mg • Total Isoflavones 86 mg.

Genix **-** Gero Vita International
Each capsule contains: Zinc (zinc gluconate) 5mg • Tribulus fruit extract (45% steriod sopanins, tribulus terrestris) 400 mg • Barrenwort herb extract (epimedium grandiflorum) 100 mg • Policios Fruticosum root extract 100 mg • English Walnut semen extract (juglans regia) 67 mg • Nutmeg fruit extract (1% essential oils, myristica fragrans) 33 mg. Other Ingredients: Silica, Magnesium Stearate.

Geriforte Syrup **-** The Himalaya Drug Company (Himalaya Heal
Each 1 tsp (5 mL) serving contains: Chyavanprash concentrate 100 mg: Aegle Marmelos, Clerodendrum Phlomidis, Oroxylum Indicum, Gmelina Arborea, Stereospermum Chelonoides, Sida Cordifolia, Desmodium Gangeticum, Uraria Picta, Phaseolus Trilobus, Teramnus Labialis, Piper Longum, Tribulus Terrestris, Solanum Indicum, Solanum Xanthocarpum, Pistacia Integerrima, Phyllanthus Amarus, Vitis Vinifera, Leptadenia Reticulata, Inula Racemosa, Aquilaria Malaccensis, Terminalia Chebula, Tinospora Cordifolia, Dioscorea Bulbifera, Microstylis Muscifera, Microstylis Wallichi, Hedychium Spicatum, Cyperus Rotundus, Boerhaavia Diffusa, Polygonatum

Cirrihfolium, Elettaria Cardamomum, Santalum Album, Nymphaea Stellata, Pueraria Tuberosa, Adhatoda Vasica, Lilium Polyphyllum, Pentatropsis Capensis, Emblica Officinalis • Shilajeet (mineral pitch, purified) 20 mg • Kumkuma (crocus sativus) 5 mg • Himsra (capparis spinosa) 20 mg • Kasani (cichorium intybus) 20 mg • Daruharidara (berberis aristata) 15 mg • Vasaka (adhatoda vasica syn. a.zeylanica) 15 mg • Kakamachi (solanum nigrum) 10 mg • Arjuna (terminalia arjuna) 10 mg • Ashvagandha (withania somnifera) 10 mg • Guduchi (tinospora cordifolia) 10 mg • Draksha (vitis vinifera) 10 mg • Punarnava (boerhaavia diffusa) 10 mg • Kharjura (phoenix dactylifera) 10 mg • Birangasipha (achillea millefolium) 5 mg • Jhavuka (tamarix gallica) 5 mg • Kasamarda (cassia occidentalis) 5 mg • Shatavari (asparagus racemosus) 5 mg • Yashti-Madhu (glycyrrhiza glabra) 5 mg • Mandukaparni (centella asiatica) 5 mg • Haritaki (terminalia chebula) 5 mg • Vidana (embelia ribes) 5 mg • Mundi (sphaeranthus indicus) 5 mg • Gokshura (tribulus terrestris) 5 mg • Kapikachchhu (mucuna pruriens) 2.5 mg • Jatiphalam (myristica fragrans) 2.5 mg • Pippali (piper longum) 2.5 mg • Jaatipatree (myristica fragrans, mace) 2.5 mg • Lavanga (syzygium aromaticum) 2.5 mg • Ela (elettaria cardamomum) 2.5 mg • Yawani (carum copticum syn. trachyspermum ammi) 2.5 mg • Haridra (curcuma longa) 2.5 mg • Musali (asparagus adscendens) 2.5 mg • Udakiryaka (caesalpinia digyna) 2.5 mg • Bhringaraja (eclipta alba syn. e.prostrata) 2.5 mg • Jyothishmati (celastrus paniculatus) 2.5 mg • Vriddadaru (argyreia nervosa) 2.5 mg.
See Editor's Note No. 39, page 2058.

Geriforte Tablets **-** The Himalaya Drug Company (Himalaya Heal
Each tablet contains: Chyavanprash concentrate 100 mg: Aegle Marmelos, Clerodendrum Phlomidis, Oroxylum Indicum, Gmelina Arborea, Stereospermum Chelonoides, Sida Cordifolia, Desmodium Gangeticum, Uraria Picta, Phaseolus Trilobus, Teramnus Labialis, Piper Longum, Tribulus Terrestris, Solanum Indicum, Solanum Xanthocarpum, Pistacia Integerrima, Phyllanthus Amarus, Vitis Vinifera, Leptadenia Reticulata, Inula Racemosa, Aquilaria Malaccensis, Terminalia Chebula, Tinospora Cordifolia, Dioscorea Bulbifera, Microstylis Muscifera, Microstylis Wallichi, Hedychium Spicatum, Cyperus Rotundus, Boerhaavia Diffusa, Polygonatum Cirrihfolium, Elettaria Cardamomum, Santalum Album, Nymphaea Stellata, Pueraria Tuberosa, Adhatoda Vasica, Lilium Polyphyllum, Pentatropsis Capensis, Emblica Officinalis • Himsra (capparis spinosa) 13.8 mg • Kasani (cichorium intybus) 13.8 mg • Daruharidra (berberis aristata) 10 mg • Vasaka (adhatoda vasica) 10 mg • Kakamachi (solanum nigrum) 6.4 mg • Arjuna (terminalia arjuna) 6.4 mg • Biranjasipha (achillea millefolium) 3.2 mg • Kasamarda (cassia occidentalis) 3.2 mg • Jhavuka (tamarix gallica) 3.2 mg • Ashvagandha (withania somnifera) 30 mg • Shatavari (asparagus racemosus) 20 mg • Yashti-Madhu (glycyrrhiza glabra) 20 mg • Mandukaparni (centella asiatica) 20 mg • Shilajeet (mineral pitch, purified) 20 mg • Haritaki (terminalia chebula) 15 mg • Makardhwaj (sulphide of mercury) 10 mg • Musali (asparagus adscendens) 10 mg • Udakiryaka (caesalpinia digyna) 10 mg • Kapikachchhu (mucuna pruriens) 10 mg • Jatiphalam (myristica fragrans) 10 mg • Pippali (piper longum) 10 mg • Jaatipatree (myristica fragrans, mace) 10 mg • Bhringaraja (eclipta alba syn. e.prostrata) 10 mg • Vriddadaru (argyreia speciosa) 10 mg • Abhrak Bhasma (powdered talc, biotite calx) 10 mg • Jasad Bhasma (zinc calx) 10 mg • Kumkuma (crocus sativus) 7 mg • Mandur Bhasma (ferric oxide calx) 5 mg • Lavanga (sysygium aromaticum) 5 mg • Ela (elettaria cardamomum) 5 mg • Yawani (carum copticum syn. trachyspermum ammi) 5 mg • Haridra (curcuma longa) 5 mg • Jyothishmati (celastrus paniculatus) 5 mg • Loh Bhasma (iron calx) 5 mg.
See Editor's Note No. 39, page 2058.

Geritol Complete **-** SmithKline Beecham
Each tablet contains: Vitamin A 6000 IU • Vitamin C 60 mg • Vitamin D 400 IU • Vitamin E 30 IU • Vitamin K 25 mcg • Thiamin (B1) 1.5 mg • Riboflavin (B2) 1.7 mg • Niacin (B3) 20 mg • Vitamin B6 2 mg • Folate, Folic Acid, Folacin 0.45 mcg • Vitamin B12 6 mcg • Biotin 0.045 mcg • Pantothenic Acid 10 mg • Calcium 162 mg • Iron 18 mg • Phosphorus 125 mg • Iodine 174 mcg • Magnesium 100 mg • Zinc 15 mg • Selenium 15 mcg • Copper 2 mg • Manganese 2.5 mg • Chromium 15 mcg • Molybdenum 15 mg • Chloride 35 mg • Potassium 40 mg • Nickel 5 mcg • Tin 10 mcg • Silicon 80 mg • Vanadium 10 mcg. Other Ingredients: Microcrystalline Cellulose, Gelatin, Hydrolyzed Protein, Beta Carotene, Stearic Acid, Crospovidone, Hydroxypopyl Methylcellulose, Hydroxypropyl Cellulose, Glycerides of Stearic and Palmitic Acid, Polyethylene Glycol, Magnesium Stearate, Silica, Titanium Dioxide, FD&C Blue #2, FD&C Red #40, FD&C Yellow #6.

Geritol Extend **-** SmithKline Beecham
Each tablet contains: Vitamin A (40% beta carotene) 3333 IU • Vitamin D 200 IU • Vitamin E 13 IU • Vitamin C 55 mg • Folic Acid 0.2 mg • Thiamin (B1) 1.2 mg • Riboflavin (B2) 1.3 mg • Niacin 15 mg • Vitamin B6 2 mg • Vitamin B12 2.5 mcg • Vitamin K 80 mcg • Iron 9.5 mg • Zinc 14 mg • Iodine 130 mg • Magnesium 32 mg • Calcium 126 mg • Phosphorus 98 mg • Potassium 0.054 mg • Selenium 35 mcg.

Geritol Tonic **-** SmithKline Beecham
Thiamin (B1) 2.5 mg • Riboflavin (B2) 2.5 mg • Niacin 50 mg • Pantothenic Acid 2 mg • Vitamin B6 0.5 mg • Methionine 25 mg • Choline Bitartrate 50 mg • Sugars 7 g • Iron 18 mg.

Gero-Vita GH.3. **-** Gero Vita International
Two tablets contain: Vitamin A (as beta-carotene) 4000 IU • Vitamin C (as ascorbyl palmitate) 42 mg • Vitamin E (as dl-alpha-tocopheryl acetate) 200 IU • Thiamin (as thiamin mononitrate) 100 mg • Riboflavin 100 mg • Vitamin B3 (as niacin) 20 mg • Vitamin B6 (as pyridoxine hydrochloride) 50 mg • Folic Acid 800 mcg • Vitamin B12 (as cyanocobalamin) 20 mcg • Calcium (as calcium carbonate) 76 mg • Magnesium (as magnesium oxide) 100 mg • Zinc (as zinc picolinate) 1.2 mg • Selenium (as selenium amino acid chelate) 100 mcg • Chromium (as chromium polynicotinate) 20 mcg • St. John's Wort extract (entire plant, 0.3% hypericin) 400 mg • Procaine (dimethylaminoethanol bitartrate 200 mg, para-aminobenzoic acid 100 mg) • Ginkgo Biloba leaf powder 50 mg • L-Glutathione 4 mg. Other Ingredients: Microcrystalline Cellulose, Vegetable Stearic Acid, Croscarmellose Sodium, Silicon Dioxide, Gum Acacia, Vegetable Magnesium Stearate.
See Editor's Note No. 20, page 2056.

Gest-Tonic **-** The Herbalist
Angelica root • Gentian root • Oregon Grape root • Bayberry root bark • Fennel seed • Prickly Ash bark • Ginger root.

GH Fuel **-** TwinLab
Six capsules contain: L-Ornithine Alpha-Ketoglutarate 3000 mg • Ma Huang extract (standardized for 6% Ephedrine) 334 mg • Kola extract (standardized for 12% Caffeine) 1000 mg • L-Carnitine 100 mg • Chromium (from Chromic Fuel patented Chromium Picolinate) 400 mcg.
See Editor's Note No. 30, page 2056.

GH Fuel Cocktail **-** TwinLab
Two tablespoonfuls contain: L-Arginine 6 g • L-Ornithine 1 g • Taurine 250 mg • L-Carnitine 200 mg • Beta-Carotene 10000 IU • Vitamin D 100 IU • Vitamin C 1000 mg • Natural Vitamin E 400 IU • Vitamin B1 1.5 mg • Vitamin B2 1.9 mg • Vitamin B6 2 mg • Niacinamide 20 mg • Vitamin B12 12 mcg • Pantothenic Acid 500 mg • Folic Acid 400 mcg • Biotin 300 mcg • Choline 700 mg • Inositol 250 mg • Calcium (from KrebMins Calcium) 250 mg • Magnesium (from KrebMins Magnesium) 100 mg • Potassium (from KrebMins Potassium) 325 mg • Zinc (from Zinc Picolinate & KrebMins Zinc) 15 mg • Manganese (from KrebMins Manganese) 2 mg • Copper (from KrebMins Copper) 1 mg • Iodine (from Kelp) 10 mcg • Molybdenum (from KrebMins Molybdenum) 50 mcg • Chromium (from Chromium Picolinate) 100 mcg • Selenium (from KrebMins Selenium) 50 mcg • Boron (from Tri-Boron citrate, Aspartate & Glycinate) 1.5 mg. Natural orange flavor 100%.

GH Release **-** Nature's Plus
Two capsules contain: L-Ornithine free form amino acid 500 mg • L-Arginine free form amino acid 150 mg • Raw Pituitary concentrate 100 mg • Vitamin B6 (Pyridoxine HCL) 50 mg.
See Editor's Note No. 14, page 2055.

GH3 (GH-3, GH 3) **-** Gero Vita International
Each tablet contains: Hypericum Perforatum extract (0.3% hypericin) 400 mg • Procaine (2-dimethyl aminoethanol bitartrate (DMAE) 100 mg, Para-aminobenzoic acid (PABA) 50 mg) • Calcium Carbonate 100 mg • Thiamine Mononitrate 50 mg • Riboflavin 50 mg • Ascorbyl Palmitate 50 mg • Ginkgo Biloba 50 mg • Pyridoxine HCl 25 mg • Niacin 10 mg • Zinc Picolinate 3 mg • L-Glutathione 2 mg • Chromium Polynicotinate 0.1 mg • Folic Acid 400 mcg • Selenium (amino acid chelated) 50 mcg • Cobalamin 10 mcg • Beta-Carotene 2000 IU • Vitamin E 100 IU.

GH3 Gerovital **-** Nutraceutics Corp.
Two caplets contain: Vitamin B6 5 mg • Folic Acid 400 mcg • Vitamin B12 20 mcg • Pantothenic Acid 50 mg • Procaine (p-aminobenzoic acid 400 mg, 2-dimethylaminoethanol bitartrate 200 mg) • Gingko Biloba extract 500 mg • Proprietary Blend 300 mg: Proteusterone, Schizandra berry, Panax Ginseng root, Gotu Kola leaves.

GH3 Natural Enhancer **-** Vitamin & Mineral Therapies Internationa
Two tablets contain: Vitamin A (as beta carotene) 5000 IU • Vitamin E (as d-alpha tocopheryl) 200 IU • Thiamin (vitamin B1, as thiamin mononitrate) 50 mg • Riboflavin (as vitamin B2) 50 mg • Folic Acid 800 mcg • Calcium (as carbonate) 200 mg • Zinc (as amino acid chelate) 10 mg • Selenium (as amino acid chelate) 10 mg • Chromium (as polynicotinate) 60 mcg • St. John's Wort leaf 4:1 extract (hypercium perforatum) 400 mg • Glutathione 6 mg. Other Ingredients: Cellulose, Magnesium Stearate, Vegetable Stearins.

GH3 Natural Formula **-** Vitamin & Mineral Therapies Internationa
Two tablets contain: Vitamin A 5000 IU • Ester C Calcium Ascorbate (vitamin C) 100 mg • Magnesium 100 mg • Folic Acid 800 mcg • Vitamin B12 (cyanocobalamin) 200 mcg • Vitamin B6 (pyridoxine) 30 mg • Vitamin E 90 IU • Glutamic Acid Base 200 mg • L-Tyrosine 200 mg • Procaine (DMAE (dimethylaminoethanol bitartrate) 200 mg, PABA (para amino benzoic acid) 100 mg) • Glucosamine HCl 130 mg • Choline Bitartrate 100 mg • L-Taurine 100 mg • Ginkgo Biloba powder 50 mg. Other Ingredients: Cellulose, Vegetable Stearins, Magnesium Stearate.

GH3 Original Formula **-** Millenium Health
Each tablet contains: Procaine Hydrochloride 100 mg • Benzoic Acid 6 mg • Potassium Metabisulphite 5 mg • Di-Sodium Phosphate 0.5 mg. Other Ingredients: Natural Orange Coloring.

GH3XL **-** HealthWatchers System
L-Glutamic Acid • L-Tyrosine • L-Taurine • Glucosamine HCL • Choline Bitartrate • Magnesium • Vitamin B6 • Vitamin Bee pollen • Kelp • Dulse • Irish Moss • Ginseng • Nettles • Alfalfa • Fo-Ti • Pau d'Arco • Fennel Seed • Schizandra • Barley Grass • Acacia Gum • Saussurea • Cat's Claw • Ginger • Licorice.

GHR (HGHR) Gold **-** Linda Wade Herbal Products
Four capsules contain: Anterior Pituitary (bovine source) 80 mg • Hypothalamus 20 mg • Amino Acids blend (essential amino acids) 1200 mg • Phytosterol Complex 40 mg: Beta Sitosterol, Campesterol, Stigmasterol • Soy Phospholipid Complex 80 mg: Phosphatidyl Serine 40%, Phosphatidyl Choline, Phosphatidyl Ethanolamine, Phosphatidylinositol • Panax Ginseng 80 mg • Vitamin B1 (thiamin) 20 mg • Vitamin B2 (riboflavin) 12 mg • Vitamin B6 (pyridoxine) 40 mg • Vitamin B12 (cobalamin) 100 mg.
See Editor's Note No. 14.

GHR-15 **-** BIE Health
Two scoops contain: Anterior Pituitary (bovine source) 56 mg • Hypothalamus 8 mg • Saccharides (mono, poly, & oligo) 2500. In a base of: L-Glutamine 100 mg, L-Arginine 100 mg, L-Pyroglutamate 100 mg, L-Glycine 300 mg, L-Lysine 200 mg, L-Tyrosine 200 mg, GABA 100 mg.
See Editor's Note No. 14.

Ginger **-** Leiner Health Products
Each softgel contains: Ginger extract (Zingiber officinale) root 125 mg. Other Ingredients: Canola Oil, Gelatin, Glycerin, Yellow Beeswax, Lecithin, Caramel, Turmeric, Titanium Dioxide, Red 40, Annatto, Blue 1.

Ginger **-** Nature's Way
Two capsules contain: Ginger 1.1 g. Other Ingredients: Gelatin.

Ginger **-** Pharmanex
Each capsule contains: Ginger (Zingiber officinalis, root extract, 20:1) 125 mg. Other Ingredients: Soybean Oil, Gelatin, Purified Water, Glycerin, Beeswax, Carob.

Ginger & Curcumin Joint-Ease **-** Nature's Life
Four capsules contain: Ginger root (Zingiber officinale) 1300 mg • Curcumin [from Turmeric root (Curcuma longa) providing 90-95% Curcuminoids] 1300 mg.

Ginger Aid **-** Traditional Medicinals
Ginger rhizome • Blackberry leaf • Stevia leaf • natural Lemon flavor.

Ginger Root Extract **-** Now
Each Vcap contains: Ginger root extract (zingiber officinale, standardized to min. 5% gingerols) 250 mg • Ginger root powder (zingiber officinale) 225 mg. Other Ingredients: Cellulose (capsule), Starch, Magnesium Oxide, Magnesium Carbonate, Stearic Acid (vegetable source), Silica, Magnesium Stearate (vegetable source).

Gingerall **-** Enzymatic Therapy
Each capsule contains: Ginger root extract (Zingiber officinale) standardized to contain 20% pungent compounds calculated as 6-Gingerol & 6-Shogaol 100 mg.

GingerMax **-** PhytoPharmica
Each capsule contains: Ginger (Zingiber officinale) root extract (standardized to contain 20% pungent compounds calculated as 6-Gingerol and 6-Shogaol) 100 mg.

Ginkai **-** Lichtwer Pharma
Each tablet contains: LI 1370 Ginkgo Biloba leaf extract, standardized to 25% ginkgo flavonoids & 6% terpenoids 50 mg.

Ginkgo 5 **-** Pharmline
Active Ingredients: Ginkgo Biloba extract 24/6, standardized to not less than 24% total Ginkgo flavone glycosides & not less than 6% total terpene lactones.

Ginkgo Alert Formula **-** PhysioLogics
Each capsule contains: Niacin 5 mg • Vitamin B6 (as pyridoxine hydrochloride) 5 mg • Vitamin B12 (as cyanocobalamin) 250 mcg • Calcium (as dicalcium phosphate) 7 mg • L-Tyrosine 100 mg • DMAE (dimethylaminoethanol) 56 mg • L-Glutamine 150 mg • L-Pyroglutamic Acid 100 mg • Choline (as choline bitartrate) 50 mg • Ginkgo Biloba leaf extract (standardized to contain 24% alkaloids, 9.6 mg) 40 mg • Korean Ginseng root extract (panax ginseng, standardized to contain 14% ginsenosides, 3.5 mg). Other Ingredients: Gelatin, Silica, Vegetable Magnesium Stearate.

Ginkgo B **-** Metabolic Response Modifiers
Each capsule contains: Ginkgo biloba extract (100:1) 60 mg.

Ginkgo Biloba **-** Celestial Seasonings
Two capsules contain: Proprietary Blend 1700 mg: Ginkgo Biloba (leaves), Ginkgo Biloba (standardized extract, standardized to 24% ginkgoflanonone glycosides, 6% ginkgolides). Other Ingredients:

Dicalcium Phosphate, Gelatin, Rice Flour, Stearic Acid, Magnesium Stearate, Silicon Dioxide.

Ginkgo Biloba **-** CVS Pharmacy
Each softgel contains: Ginkgo Biloba extract (standardized to 24% lavone glyosides; 6% terpene lactones) 60 mg. Other Ingredients: Soybean Oil, Gelatin, Purified Water, Glycerin, Yellow Beeswax, Lecithin, Annatto, Titanium Dioxide, FD&C Yellow #5, FD&C Blue #1, FD&C Red #40.

Ginkgo Biloba **-** DreamPharm
Each capsule contains: Ginkgo Biloba leaf 300 mg • Sclerotium Poriae Cocos 100 mg • Dioscorea Oppositae rhizoma 100 mg.

Ginkgo Biloba - Herbal Harvest **-** Nature's Bounty
Each tablet contains: Ginkgo Biloba extract (Standardized for a minimum of 24% Ginkgo Flavone Glycosides and 6% terpenes) 30 mg.

Ginkgo Biloba **-** Jamieson
Each tablet contains: Ginkgo extract (50:1) Ginkgo biloba leaf (24% flavoglycosides) 40 mg.

Ginkgo Biloba **-** Life Extension
Each capsule contains: Ginkgo Biloba extract 120 mg.

Ginkgo Biloba **-** Natrol
Each capsule contains: Ginkgo Biloba leaf 50:1 extract (24% ginkgo flavonglycosides) (6% terpene lactone) 120 mg.

Ginkgo Biloba **-** Nature's Bounty
Each tablet contains: Ginkgo Biloba extract 30 mg. Other Ingredients: Dicalcium Phosphate, Cellulose, Vegetable Stearic Acid, Cellulose Coating, Silica, Vegetable Magnesium Stearate.

Ginkgo Biloba - Now **-** Now
Each Vcaps contains: Ginkgo Biloba extract (50:1 standardized extract containing 24% ginkgoflavonglycosides) 120 mg • Gotu Kola (Centella asiatica) (leaf) 200 mg • Siberian Ginseng (Eleutherococcus senticosus) (root) 150 mg.

Ginkgo Biloba **-** Olympian Labs
Each capsule contains: Ginkgo Biloba extract 120 mg.

Ginkgo Biloba **-** Puritan's Pride
Each tablet contains: Ginkgo Biloba Extract (standardized for a minumum of 24% Ginkgo Flavone Glycosides and 6% terpenes) 60 mg. Other Ingredients: Dicalcium Phosphate, Cellulose (Plant Origin), Vegetable Stearic Acid, Cellulose Coating, Croscarmellose, Silica, Vegetable Magnesium Stearate.

Ginkgo Biloba **-** Rexall - Sundown
Two capsules contain: Ginkgo Biloba leaf extract 40 mg • Ginkgo Biloba leaf 400 mg.

Ginkgo Biloba (50:1 extract) **-** Atrium Inc.
Each capsule contains: Ginkgo Biloba, 50:1 extract (24% Ginkgocides) 60 mg.

Ginkgo Biloba 24% - Enzymatic Therapy **-** Enzymatic Therapy
Each capsule contains: Ginkgo Biloba leaf extract (ginkgo biloba folia, standardized to contain 24% ginkgoflavonglycosides, 6% terpene lactones, and 2% bilobalide) 40 mg.

Ginkgo Biloba 24% **-** Swanson
Each capsule contains: Ginkgo Biloba leaf extract (24% flavone glycosides, 6% terpene lactones) 60 mg.

Ginkgo Biloba 24% Standardized Extract **-** Now
Each capsule contains: Ginkgo Biloba leaf powder 300 mg • Ginkgo Biloba extract (50:1 standardized extract containing 24% ginkgoflavonglycosides) 60 mg. Other Ingredients: Stearic Acid.

Ginkgo Biloba 250 **-** Enzymatic Therapy
Each capsule contains: Ginkgo (ginkgo biloba, leaf powder and extract standardized to contain 6 mg ginkgoflavonglycosides) 250 mg.

Ginkgo Biloba 40 mg **-** Leiner Health Products
Each tablet contains: Ginkgo Biloba extract (Ginkgo biloba) leaf 40 mg. Other Ingredients: Calcium Carbonate, Maltodextrin, Cellulose, Hydroxypropyl Methylcellulose, Polyethylene Glycol 3350, Crospovidone, Silicon Dioxide, Hydroxypropyl Cellulose, Titanium Dioxide, Magnesium Stearate, Yellow 5 Lake, Polysorbate 80, Yellow 6 Lake, Blue 2 Lake, Sodium Citrate.

Ginkgo Biloba 60 mg **-** Leiner Health Products
Each caplet contains: Ginkgo Biloba leaf extract (ginkgo biloba) 60 mg. Other Ingredients: Calcium Carbonate, Cellulose, Maltodextrin, Hydroxypropyl Methylcellulose, Silicon Dioxide, Polyethylene Glycol 3350, Croscarmellose Sodium, Hydroxypropyl Cellulose, Yellow 5 Lake, Blue 1 Lake, Pharmaceutical Glaze, Crospovidone, Magnesium Stearate, Polysorbate 80, Titanium Dioxide.

Ginkgo Biloba 60 mg **-** Puritan's Pride
Each tablet contains: Ginkgo Biloba extract (standardized for a minimum of 24% ginkgo flavone glycosides and 6% terpenes) 60 mg. Other Ingredients: Dicalcium Phosphate, Cellulose (plant origin), Vegetable Stearic Acid, Cellulose Coating, Croscarmellose, Silica, Vegetable Magnesium Stearate.

Ginkgo Biloba Complex **-** Vitamin World
Each capsules contains: Ginkgo Biloba leaf extract (standardized to contain 24% flavone glycosides, 9.6 mg) 40 mg • Ginkgo Biloba leaf 400 mg • Herbal Complex 320 mg: Eleuthero root (eleutherococcus senticosus), Citrus Bioflavonoids, Bilberry fruit 4:1 extract (vaccinium myrtillus). Other Ingredients: Gelatin, Rice Powder, Silica, Vegetable Magnesium Stearate.

Ginkgo Biloba Double Strength **-** Now
Each Vcap contain: Ginkgo Biloba extract leaf (50:1 standardized extract containing 24% ginkgoflaconglycosides) 120 mg • Gotu Kola (Centella Asiatica) leaf 200 mg • Siberian Ginseng (Eleutherococcus Senticoscus) root 150 mg. Other Ingredients: Stearic Acid.

Ginkgo Biloba Extra Strength, 60mg **-** Nature Made
Each capsule contains: Ginkgo Biloba leaf extract 60 mg: Flavone Glycosides 14.4 mg, Terpene Lactones 3.6 mg.

Ginkgo Biloba Extract **-** Quest
Each caplet contains: Ginkgo Biloba leaf extract (Ginkgo biloba) (provided by 60 mg P.E. 1:50 standardized to contain 24% Ginkgosides) 3000 mg • Citrus Bioflavonoids 200 mg providing Hesperidin 50 mg. Other Ingredients: Calcium Phosphate, Microcrystalline Cellulose, Croscarmellose Sodium, Vegetable Stearin, Magnesium Stearate (vegetable source).

Ginkgo Biloba Extract 60 mg **-** The Vitamin Shoppe
Each capsule contains: Ginkgo Biloba leaf extract (ginkgoselect, standardized to 24% ginkgoflavoglycosides 14 mg, 6% terpene lactones 3.5 mg.) 60 mg.

Ginkgo Biloba Extract **-** Nature's Bounty
Each tablet contains: Ginkgo Biloba extract (standardized for a minimum of 24% ginkgoflavoneglycosides, 6% terpenes) 30 mg. Other Ingredients: Dicalcium Phosphate, Cellulose (plant origin), Vegetable Stearic Acid, Cellulose Coating, Silica, Vegetable Magnesium Stearate.

Ginkgo Biloba Extract **-** Now
Each dropperful (0.8 ml) contains: Ginkgo Biloba extract 0.8 ml. Other Ingredients: Gotu Kola (centella asiatica), Siberian Ginseng (eleutherococcus senticosus), in a base of Distilled Water, Vegetable Glycerine, and Grain Alcohol.

Ginkgo Biloba Extract **-** NSI - Nutraceutical Sciences Institute
Each capsule contains: Ginkgo Biloba extract (standardized to 24% ginkgoflavoneglycosides and 6% terpene lactones) 120 mg.

Ginkgo Biloba Leaf Extract 50:1 - Basic Nutrition **-** GNC
Each tablet contains: Ginkgo Biloba leaf extract 50:1 50 mg. Other Ingredients: Dicalcium Phosphate, Cellulose, Stearic Acid, Magnesium Stearate, Food Glaze.

Ginkgo Biloba Plus **-** Wakunaga of America
Each capsule contains: Aged Garlic bulb extract powder 200 mg • Siberian Ginseng root extract 5:1 80 mg • Ginkgo Biloba leaf 50:1 extract (standardized to 24% ginkgoflavonglycosides & 6% terpene lactones) 40 mg. Other Ingredients: Cellulose, Magnesium Stearate (vegetable source).

Ginkgo Biloba Tincture **-** Jamieson
Each 1 ml (15 drops) contains: Ginkgo Biloba Leaf 500 mg.

Ginkgo Biloba Xtra **-** Sundown
Each tablet contains: Ginkgo Biloba leaf extract (standardized to 24% flavonol glycosides, 14.4 mg, standardized to 6% terpene lacones, 3.6 mg) 60 mg • Xtra Premium Blend 90 mg: Ashwagandha root, Gotu Kola (aerial parts), Siberian Ginseng root (eleuthero). Other Ingredients: Maltodextrin, Cellulose, Croscarmellose Sodium, Silica, Magnesium Stearate, Dextrin, Titanium Dioxide, Hydroxypropyl Methylcellulose, PEG, Acacia Gum, Guar Gum, Hydroxypropyl Cellulose, Dextrose Monohydrate, Soya Lecithin, Riboflavin (colorant), Yellow 6 Lake, Blue 2 Lake.

Ginkgo Biloba/Gotu Kola **-** Futurebiotics
Each capsule contains: Ginkgo Biloba leaf powder extract (standardized for 24% (29 mg) ginkgo heterosides) 120 mg • Gotu Kola leaf powder extract (standardized for 16% (32 mg) triterpenes) 200 mg. Other Ingredients: Gelatin, Water.

Ginkgo Booster **-** Puritan's Pride
Two tablets contain: Ginkgo Biloba extract (24%) 60 mg • L-Glutamine 100 mg • Lecithin 100 mg • L-Tyrosine 50 mg • Choline (Bitartrate) 100 mg • DMAE (2-Di Methylaminothanol) 40 mg • Vitamin B1 (Thiamine HCl) 20 mg • Vitamin B2 (Riboflavin) 20 mg • Vitamin B12 (Sobalamin/Dibencozide) 50 mcg • Niacin 10 mg • Niacinamide 40 mg • Pantothenic Acid (Calcium d-Pantothenate) 50 mg • Folic Acid 200 mcg • Biotin 50 mcg • Inositol 20 mg • Vitamin C (Ascorbic Acid) 50 mg • Iodine 50 mcg • Betaine HCl 20 mg. In a base of Fo-Ti and Siberian Ginseng.

Ginkgo Complex **-** NutriCology
Each capsule contains: Vitamin B6 (as pyridoxal-5-phosphate) 5 mg • Folic Acid 400 mcg • Vitamin B12 (as cyanocobalamin) 400 mcg • L-Glutamine 200 mg • L-Phenylalanine 100 mg • L-Tyrosine 100 mg • Ribonucleic Acid (RNA) 18 mg • Ginkgo Biloba extract 70 mg. Other Ingredients: Magnesium Stearate, Silicon Dioxide.

Ginkgo DHA Mind **-** The Vitamin Shoppe
Each capsule contains: Ginkgo Biloba leaf 24% ginkgoflavoglycosides 6% terpene 60 mg • DHA 50 mg.

Ginkgo Energizer **-** The Vitamin Shoppe
Each capsule contains: Ginkgo Biloba leaf standardized to 24% ginkgoflavoglycosides 6% ginkgolides-bilobalides 60 mg • CoQ10 30 mg.

Ginkgo Max 120 **-** Jamieson
Each caplet contains: Ginkgo Biloba Leaf Extract (40 mg of 1:50 extract, equivalent to 2000 mg of whole herb. Standardized to 24% Flavoglycosides with minimum 10 % Quercitin. Other active marker compounds established are, but not standardized to, proanthocyanidins, kaempferol, ginkgolides, bilobalides) 2000 mg.

Ginkgo Neuro-Mind **-** The Vitamin Shoppe
Each tablet contains: Vitamin B12 (as cyanocobalamin) 0.25 mcg • Vitamin B6 (as pyridoxine HCl) 10 mg • Ginkgo Biloba (Ginkgo biloba) leaf standardized to 24% ginkgoflavoglycosides 6% terpene lactones 50 mg • Phosphatidylserine (LECI-PS) 50 mg • DHA (Docosahexaenoic acid) (Neuromins) 50 mg.

Ginkgo Phytosome **-** PhytoPharmica
Each softgel capsule contains: Ginkgo (ginkgo biloba leaf phytosome; one part ginkgo extract, standardized to contain 24% ginkgoflavonglycosides and 6% terpene lactones including 2% bilobalide, bound to two parts phosphatidylcholine) 80 mg. Other Ingredients: Soybean Oil, Gelatin, Glycerin, Beeswax, Lecithin.

Ginkgo Plus for Memory **-** Aboca USA, Inc
Two capsules contain: Ginkgo leaf freeze-dried extract (ginkgo biloba, standardized to 1% terpene lactones, 3% ginkgo flavone glycosides) 160 mg • Bacopa aerial part Whole Phytocomplex Concentrate (WPC)(bacopa monnieri) 160 mg • Siberian Ginseng root (eleutherococcus senticosus, standardized to 0.7% eleutherosides B+E, WPC) 155 mg • Zinc Yeast (saccharomices cerevisiae with zinc, 10%, organically bound) 25 mg. Other Ingredients: Gelatin (capsule).

Ginkgo Sharp **-** Celestial Seasonings
Two capsules contain: Vitamin B3 (as niacinamide) 40 mg • Proprietary Blend 930 mg: Ginkgo Biloba (leaf), Ginkgo Biloba (standardized to 24% ginkgoflavonone glycosides and 6% ginkgolides.), DHA (50 mg as docohexaenoic acid). Other Ingredients: Dicalcium Phosphate, Gelatin, Rice Flour, Stearic Acid, Magnesium Stearate, Silicon Dioxide.

Ginkgo/Gotu Kola **-** Gaia Herbs
Ginkgo and Gotu Kola standardized for 12% flavonoid glycosides & 2.5% triterpenoids. Standardized Full Spectrum 100 mg of extract per capsule. Guaranteed Potency 50 mg of extract per capsule.

Ginkgo-24 **-** Source Naturals
Each tablet contains: Ginkgo Biloba leaf extract (50:1) (Yielding 24% Ginkgo Flavone Glycosides and 6% Terpene Lactones from 2,000 mg of Ginkgo biloba leaf) 40 mg.

Ginkgo-Combo Ginkgo Biloba Complex in Vegetarian Capsules **-** Nature's Plus
Two vegicaps contain: Ginkgo Biloba (8:1 extract ginkgoaceae) 240 mg • Capsicum fruit 160 mg • Gotu Kola root 160 mg • Vitamin E (natural) 100 IU.

Ginkgo-Go! **-** Wakunaga of America
Each caplet contains: Ginkgo Biloba standardized extract 50:1 (leaf) standardized with 24% Ginkgo flavonglycosides & 6% Terpene lactones 120 mg. Inactive Ingredients: Cellulose, Vegetable Starch, Magnesium Stearate (vegetable source), Silica.

Ginkgold **-** Nature's Way
Each tablet contains: Egb 761 Ginkgo Biloba leaf extract; standardized to 24% Ginkgo flavone glycosides & 6% terpene lactones 60 mg.

Ginkgolidin **-** PhytoPharmica
Each capsule contains: Ginkgo Biloba leaves extract (Ginkgo biloba folia; standardized to contain 24% ginkgoflavonglycosides, 6% terpene lactones & 2% bilobalide) 40 mg.

Ginkgo-PS **-** USANA Health Sciences
Each tablet contains: Ginkgo Biloba (Standardized Leaf Extract) 25 mg • Lecithin Enriched with Phosphatidylserine 125 mg. Other Ingredients: Dextrose, Hydroxypropyl Methylcellulose, Titamium Dioxide, Ascorbyl Palmitate, Carnauba Wax, Collodial Silicon Dioxide, Croscarmellose Sodium.

Ginko Biloba **-** HealthWatchers System
Two capsules contain: Standard Ginkgo Biloba 120 mg • Ginko Biloba Powder equivalent to 6000 mg.

Ginkoba **-** Boehringer Ingelheim
Each tablet contains: Standardized Ginkgo Biloba leaf extract (50:1) 40 mg. Other Ingredients: Hydroxypropyl Methylcellulose, Lactose,

Talc, Polyethylene Glycol, Magnesium Stearate, Titanium Dioxide, Synthetic Iron Oxides.

Ginkoba M/E **-** Boehringer Ingelheim
Each capsule contains: Panax Ginseng Extract (standardized G115) 100 mg • Ginkgo Biloba Extract (standarized GK501) 60 mg. Other Ingredients: Mannitol, Gelatin, Sicon dioxide, Magnesium Stearate.

Ginsana **-** Pharmaton Natural Health Products
Each capsule contains: Standardized G115 Ginseng root extract (Panax Ginseng, C.A. Meyer) 100 mg. Other Ingredients: Sunflower oil, gelatin, glycerin, lecithin, beeswax, chlorophyll.

Ginsana Chewy Squares **-** Pharmaton Natural Health Products
Each chewy square contains: Vitamin C • Standardized G115 Ginseng root extract (Panax Ginseng, C.A. Meyer) 50 mg. Other Ingredients: Sucrose, Glucose, Palm kernel oil, Gelatin, Citric Acid, Ascorbic Acid, Lecithin, Natural Flavoring & Coloring.

Ginsana Gold Formula **-** Pharmaton Natural Health Products
Each tablet contains: Vitamin A (10% as beta carotene) 2500 IU • Vitamin C 60 mg • Vitamin D 400 IU • Vitamin E 30 IU • Vitamin K 80 mcg • Thiamine (vitamin B1) 1.5 mg • Riboflavin (vitamin B2) 1.7 mg • Niacin (vitamin B3) 20 mg • Vitamin B6 2 mg • Folic Acid 400 mcg • Vitamin B12 6 mcg • Calcium (carbonate) 200 mg • Iron 18 mg • Phosphorous 160 mg • Magnesium Oxide 20 mg • Zinc (oxide) 15 mg • Copper 2 mg • Manganese 2 mg • Panax Ginseng root extract 80 mg.

GinsanaSport **-** Pharmaton Natural Health Products
Each capsule contains: Standardized G-115 Panax Ginseng Extract (Panax Ginseng, C.A. Meyer) (root) 200 mg. Other Ingredients: Sunflower oil, gelatin, glycerin, beeswax, lecithin, turmeric, titanium dioxide, FD&C Green No. 3.

Ginseng **-** Celestial Seasonings
Two capsules contain: Proprietary Blend 180 mg: Panax Ginseng (root), Panax Ginseng (standardized to 7% ginsenosides). Other ingredients: Dicalcium phosphate, gelatin, rice flour, stearic acid, magnesium stearate and silicon dioxide.

Ginseng **-** Leiner Health Products
Each softgel contains: Ginseng extract (Panax ginseng) root 100 mg. Other Ingredients: Gelatin, Soybean Oil, Vegetable Oil, Lecithin, Palm Oil, Glycerin, Sorbitol, Yellow Beeswax, Hydrogenated Coconut Oil, Titanium Dioxide, Yellow 5, Blue 1, Red 40, Green 3, Chlorophyll.

Ginseng **-** Source Naturals
Each tablet contains: Panax Ginseng root 648 mg.

Ginseng Energy **-** Celestial Seasonings
Two capsules contain: Vitamin E (as d-alpha tocopherol acetate) 10 IU • Vitamin B12 (as cyanocobalamin) 30 mcg • Proprietary Blend 1590 mg: Siberian Ginseng (root), Siberian Ginseng (standardized extract), Panax Ginseng (root), Panax Ginseng (standardized extract) • Coenzyme Q10 (as ubiquinone) 10 mg. Other Ingredients: Dicalcium Phosphate, Gelatin, Rice Flour, Stearic Acid, Magnesium Stearate, Silicon Dioxide. One serving size is equivalent to: Panax Ginseng 200 mg standardized to 7% ginsenosides, Siberian Ginseng 250 mg standardized to 0.8% eleutherosides.

Ginseng Extract **-** The Vitamin Shoppe
Each softgel contains: 100 mg Panax Ginseng extract standardized for 8% ginsenosides.

Ginseng Phytosome **-** PhytoPharmica
Each capsule contains: Panax Ginseng root phytosome (bound to phosphatidylcholine under patent) 50 mg.

Ginseng, Korean White, 560mg **-** Nature Made
Two capsules contain: Korean White Ginseng root 1.12 g: Ginsenosides 22.4 mg.

Ginseng/Aloe Capsules **-** Aloe Farms
Siberian Ginseng powder 150 mg, Aloe Vera powder 100 mg.

Ginseng/Collagen Firming Creme **-** Derma E
Ginseng • Collagen (contains 22 amino acids).

Ginseng-Go! **-** Wakunaga of America
Each capsule contains: Korean Ginseng extract powder (root) 300 mg. Other Ingredients: Cellulose, Magnesium Stearate (vegetable source).

Ginseven **-** Leiner Health Products
Each caplet contains: American Ginseng extract (Panax quinquefolius) root 75 mg • Ashwagandha extract (Withania somnifera) root 50 mg • Notoginseng extract (Panax notoginseng) root 50 mg • Panax Ginseng extract (Panax ginseng) root 100 mg • Schisandra extract (Schisandra chinensis) fruit 75 mg • Siberian Ginseng extract (Eleutherococcus senticosus) root 75 mg • Suma extract (Pfaffia paniculata) root 100 mg. Other Ingredients: Cellulose, Dicalcium Phosphate, Stearic Acid, Magnesium Stearate, Silicon Dioxide, Sodium Starch Glycolate, Polyethylene Glycol 3350.

GinSting **-** Futurebiotics
Two tablets contain: Korean Ginseng 1000 mg • Bee Pollen 500 mg.

GinSwee Tea **-** HerbaSway
Ginger • Panax Ginseng • Blackberry • HerbaSwee (Cucurbitaceae fruit).

GKG **-** EAS
Each capsule contains: Alpha-Ketoglutaric Acid 250 mg • L-Glutamine 275 mg • Taurine 150 mg • Calcium 63 mg • Potassium 25 mg • Magnesium 25 mg • RNA 9.5 mg • Manganese 400 mcg.

GLA Borage Oil **-** NutriCology
Each softgel contains: Borage Oil 1.3 g • Gamma-Linolenic Acid (omega-6) 300 mg • Linoleic Acid (Omega-6) 480 mg.

GLA Complex **-** Shaklee
Each capsule contains: Vitamin E (as D-alpha tocopherol concentrate) 15 IU • Gamma-Linolenic acid (from borage seed oil (Borago officinalis)) 90 mg • Linoleic acid (from sunflower seed oil (Helianthus annus) and borage seed oil (Borago officinalis)) 216 mg. Other Ingredients: Ascorbyl Palmitate, Mixed Tocopherols Concentrate, Rosemary Extract, Gelatin, Glycerin, Water.

GLA Forte **-** Nature's Plus
Two softgels contain: GLA (Gamma Linolenic Acid) from Borage seed oil & Black Currant Seed oil, 100 mg • Vitamin E (d-Alpha Tocopherol) 200 IU • Vitamin C corn free 100 mg • Vitamin B6 (Pyridoxine HCL) 50 mg • Niacinamide 25 mg • Zinc (Gluconate) 5 mg. In a base containing safflower oil, octacosanol, lecithin & rapeseed.

GLA Mega-260 **-** Progressive Labs
Each softgel contains: Borage oil 1300 mg which supplies no less than Gamma Linolenic Acid (GLA) 260 mg and Vitamin E 1.5 IU. Fatty Acid Composition: Gamma Linolenic Acid 260 mg • Linoleic Acid 494 mg • Oleic Acid 221 mg.

Glan-Fem Plus **-** Atrium Inc.
Each tablet contains: Ovary 80 mg • Adrenal 20 mg • Thyroid (Thyroxin Free) 20 mg • Pituitary 10 mg • Vitamin B1 15 mg • Vitamin B2 17 mg • Vitamin B6 16 mg • Vitamin C 120 mg • Niacinamide 60 mg • Folic Acid 200 mcg • Vitamin E (d-Alpha Tocopherol) 60 IU • Manganese (Protein Chelated) 5 mg • Selenium 20 mcg.
See Editor's Note No. 14.

Glan-Male Plus **-** Atrium Inc.
Each tablet contains: Orchic 80 mg • Adrenal 20 mg • Pituitary 10 mg • Vitamin B1 15 mg • Vitamin B2 17 mg • Vitamin B6 16 mg • Vitamin C 120 mg • Niacinamide 60 mg • Folic Acid 200 mcg • Vitamin E (d-Alpha Tocopherol) 60 IU • Manganese (Protein

Chelated) 5 mg • Selenium 20 mcg.
See Editor's Note No. 14.

Gla-Plus **-** Atrium Inc.
Each capsule contains: Gamma Linolenic Acid (from Black Currant) 40 mg • Vitamin E (d-Alpha Tocopheryl Acetate) 10 IU.

Gluca-Herb **-** Dial Herbs
Cedar berries • Uva Ursi • Licorice • Mullein • Cayenne.

Glucobetic **-** Flourish The Wellness Company
Each capsule contains: Zinc (gluconate) 15 mg • Chromium GTF (polynicotinate) 240 mcg • Vanadyl Sulfate 10 mg • Gymnema Sylvestre extract 200 mg • Bitter Melon extract (momordica charantia) 200 mg • Fenugreek extract (trigonella foenum-graecum) 100 mg • Bilberry extract (vaccinium myritllus) 40 mg • Cinnamon extract (cinnamomum verum) 30 mg • Jambolan (syzgium cumini) 75 mg • Pterocarpus Marsupium 200 mg • Gulvel (tinospora cordifolia) 50 mg.

Gluco-Essentials **-** Viable Herbal Solutions
Two capsules contain: Proprietary Blend 1200 mg: Bilberry (vaccinium myrtillus), Bitter Melon (momordica charantia), Cinnamon (cinnamomum zeylanicum), Citrus Bioflavonoids, Fenugreek seed (trigonellum foenum-graecum), American Ginseng (panax quinquefolium), Korean Ginseng (panax ginseng), Glucomannan (amorphophallus konjac), Goldenseal root (hydrastis canadensis), Gymnema (gymnema sylvestre), Holy Basil (ocimum basilicum), Jerusalem Artichoke (cynara scolymus), Mistletoe (viscum album), Olive leaf (olea europaea), Psyllium (plantago ovata), Quercetin, Suma root (pfaffia paniculata), Uva Ursi (arctosatphylos uva-ursi).

GlucoFlex PM **-** Windmill Health Products
Two caplets contain: Calcium (as calcium carbonate) 250 mg • Magnesium (as magnesium oxide) 100 mg • Glucosamine HCl 500 mg • Herbal Pain Relief Blend 350 mg: Feverfew leaf extract (0.2% parthenolide), White Willow bark, Turmeric Rhizome, Ginger root extract (5% gingerols) • Valerian root extract (0.8% valerenic acid) 200 mg • Hops (strobile) 100 mg. Other Ingredients: Microcrystalline Cellulose, Croscarmellose Sodium, Stearic Acid, Magnesium Stearate, Pharmaceutical Glaze.

Glucogen Ace **-** ANS - Applied Nutrition Sciences
Glucose • Vitamin A • Vitamin C • Vitamin E.

Glucogen Sport **-** ANS - Applied Nutrition Sciences
"Vitamins & Minerals enriched Glucose Drink for Sports people."

GlucoLean **-** Nutripeak
Two tablets contain: Selenium (as selenium amino acid chelate) 50 mcg • Chromium (as chromium polynicotinate) 200 mcg • Guggul extract 1000 mg • Gymnema Sylvestre leaf 150 mg • Coleus Forskohlii extract 130 mg • Alpha-Lipoic Acid 100 mg • D-Pinitol 25 mg • Bitter Melon extract fruit, seed 18.8 mg. Other Ingredients: Cellulose, Stearic Acid, Magnesium Stearate, Silica.

Glucomannan 500 Mg **-** Natrol
Two capsules contain: Hemicellulose 913 mg • Cellulose 61 mg • Pectin Substance 25 mg • Lignin 1 mg. From Amorphophallus Konjac root.

Glucomannan+ **-** Swanson
Three capsules contain: Chromium (50% from Chromax® chromium picolinate, 50% from chromium polynicotinate) 150 mcg • Psyllium husk fiber 600 mg • Konjac Glucomannan 450 mg • Apple Pectin • 300 mg • Chitosan (93% deacetylated) 300 mg • Guar Gum 300 mg • Oat Bran fiber 300 mg • Gymnema sylvestre extract (25% gymnemic acids) 75 mg • L-Carnitine (as tartrate) 30 mg.

Glucomine **-** Body Wise International, Inc.
Three capsules contain: Glucosamine Sulfate 1500 mg • Chondroitin Sulfate 150 mg • Boswellia Gum Std. Extract (Boswellia serrata) 25 mg • White Willow Bark (Salix alba) 25 mg • Devils Claw-Inner Bark (Harpagophytum procumbens) 25 mg • Tea Tree Oil (Melaleuca alternifolia) 25 mg • Una de Gato (Uncaria tomentosa) 25 mg.
See Editor's Note No. 15, page 2055.

Gluco-Pro 900 **-** Thompson Nutritional Products
Each tablet contains: Glucosamine HCl 500 mg • Chondroitin Sulfate 400 mg.
See Editor's Note No. 15, page 2055.

Glucoril **-** PhytoPharmica
Two capsules contain: Vitamin C (ascorbic acid) 100 mg • Vitamin E (mixed tocopherols) 50 IU • Vitamin B6 (pyridoxine HCl) 10 mg • Vitamin B12 (cyanocobalamin) 250 mcg • Biotin 1,000 mcg • Magnesium (Krebs chelate) 100 mg • Zinc (picolinate) 5 mg • Selenium (L-selenomethionine) 40 mcg • Manganese (Krebs chelate) 10 mg • Chromium (picolinate) 50 mcg • Blueberry (Vaccinium myrtillus fructus) extract 5:1 300 mg • Gymnema Sylvestre leaf extract 6:1 (standardized to contain 24% gymnemic acid) 150 mg • Bitter Melon (Momordica charantia) whole fruit extract 100 mg • Fenugreek (Trigonella foenum-graecum) seed extract 4:1 100 mg.

Glucosalage SO4 **-** Olympian Labs
Each capsule contains: Shark Cartilage 200 mg • Cat's Claw (uncaria tomentosa) 200 mg • Glucosamine Sulfate 2 KCl 200 mg.

Glucosalage SO4 (Extra Strength) **-** Olympian Labs
Two capsules contain: Shark Cartilage 400 mg • Cat's Claw 400 mg • Glucosamine Sulfate 400 mg • Proprietary Blend: Protease, Amylase, Lipase 100 mg. In a base of White Willow Bark, Valerian Root, Devil's Claw, and Black Willow.

Glucosamine & Chondroitin 500/400 **-** Now
Each capsule contains: Sodium 40 mg • Potassium (as Potassium Chloride) 60 mg • Glucosamine Sulfate (from 500 mg Glusocamine Potassium Sulfate complex) 375 mg • Chondroitin Sulfate (min. 90%) (Bovine Source) 400 mg • MSM 100 mg.
See Editor's Note No. 15, page 2055.

Glucosamine & Chondroitin Combo **-** Swanson
Each capsule contains: Glucosamine Sulfate (2KCl) 500 mg • Chondroitin Sulfate 250 mg.
See Editor's Note No. 15, page 2055.

Glucosamine & MSM Complex **-** Puritan's Pride
Three tablets contain: Glucosamine Sulfate 1500 mg • MSM 1000 mg • Ginger (Standardized 4% Volatile Oil) 100 mg • Vitamin C (Ascorbic Acid) 60 mg • Manganese 5 mg • White Willow 100 mg.

Glucosamine & UC II Complex **-** PhysioLogics
Two capsules contain: Glucosamine 2KCl 1500 mg • Undenatured Type II Collagen (from UC II undenatured type II collagen complex 40 mg) 10 mg. Other Ingredients: Rice Powder, Gelatin, Potassium Chloride, Silica, Vegetable Magnesium Stearate.

Glucosamine 500 mg / Chondroitin 400 mg Capsules **-** GNC
Three capsules contain: D-Glucosamine HCl 1500 mg • Chondroitin Sulfate Sodium 1200 mg. Other Ingredients: Soybean Oil, Gelatin, Glycerin, Caramel Color, Titanium Dioxide.
See Editor's Note No. 15, page 2055.

Glucosamine 500 mg / Chondroitin 400 mg Tablets - GNC A-Z **-** GNC
Each tablet contains: D-Glucosamine Hydrochloride 500 mg • Chondroitin Sulfate, Sodium 400 mg. Other Ingredients: Red Beet root juice powder.
See Editor's Note No. 15, page 2055.

Glucosamine 750 mg / Chondroitin 600 mg Tablets **-** GNC
Each tablet contains: D-Glucosamine HCl 750 mg • Chondroitin Sulfate 600 mg. Other Ingredients: Red Beet root juice powder.
See Editor's Note No. 15, page 2055.

Some Brand Name Natural Products - What they Contain

www.NaturalDatabase.com contains MANY more listings than appear here.

Glucosamine and MSM **-** Now
Two capsules contain: Glucosamine HCl (vegetarian source) 1000 mg • MSM 1000 mg. Other Ingredients: Cellulose (capsule), Magnesium Stearate (vegetable source), Stearic Acid (vegetable source), Silica.

Glucosamine Chondroitin & MSM **-** Natrol
Three tablets contain: Glucosamine Sulfate 1500 mg • Chondroitin Sulfate 1200 mg • MSM (methylsulfonylmethane) 250 mg • Organic Sulfur 83 mg. Other Ingredients: Cellulose, Stearic Acid, Silica, Cellulose Gum, Magnesium Stearate, Methylcellulose, Glycerine.
See Editor's Note No. 15, page 2055.

Glucosamine Chondroitin & MSM **-** Puritan's Pride
Three tablets contain: Glucosamine Sulfate (2KCl) 1500 mg • Chondroitin Sulfate 1200 mg • Methylsulfonylmethane (MSM) 500 mg. Other Ingredients: Cellulose (plant origin), Cellulose Coating, Vegetable Magnesium Stearate, Silica, Titanium Dioxide Color.
See Editor's Note No. 15, page 2055.

Glucosamine Chondroitin Complex with MSM **-** Source Naturals
Three tablets contain: Vitamin C (as ascorbic acid) 250 mg • Molybdenum (as molybdenum chelate) 320 mcg • Glucosamine Sulfate 1,500 mg • Chondroitin Sulfate 1,200 mg • MSM (methylsulfonylmethane) 800 mg.
See Editor's Note No. 15, page 2055.

Glucosamine Chondroitin HP **-** PhysioLogics
Three tablets contain: Glucosamine Hydrochloride 1500 mg • Chondroitin Sulfate 1200 mg. Other Ingredients: Povidone, Beet Root Juice, Vegetable Magnesium Stearate, Silica, Cellulose (plant origin).
See Editor's Note No. 15, page 2055.

Glucosamine Chondroitin MSM and Astaxanthin TABS **-** TwinLab
Each tablet contains: MSM 500 mg • Glucosamine 750 mg • Chondroitin 600 mg • Bio-Astin Astaxanthin 8 mg.
See Editor's Note No. 15, page 2055.

Glucosamine Chondroitin Sulfate **-** HealthWatchers System
Glucosamine Sulfate • Chondroitin Sulfate • Vitamin C.
See Editor's Note No. 15, page 2055.

Glucosamine Complex **-** Natrol
Each capsule contains: Glucosamine Sulfate 100 mg • Glucosamine HCl 300 mg • Glucosamine N-Acetyl 100 mg. Other Ingredients: Rice powder, Silicon Dioxide, Magnesium Stearate, Gelatin.

Glucosamine Complex 1000 mg **-** Schiff
Two tablets contain: Proprietary Blend 2 g (2000 mg): D-Glucosamine Hydrochloride, D-Glucosamine Sulfate, N-Acetyl D-Glucosamine. Other Ingredients: Cellulose, Copolyvidone, Magnesium Stearate, Silicon Dioxide, Potassium Chloride.

Glucosamine Complex Syn-flex Liquid Formula **-** Activex America
Each 1/4 oz serving contains: Proprietary Blend 1250 mg: Glucosamine HCl, Glucosamine Sulfate • Shark Cartilage (20% chondroitin sulfate) 25 mg • Boswellin 8 mg • Yucca powder 3 mg • Manganese (ascorbate) 5 mg • Bromelain 1 mg • Vitamin C 5 mg • Omega 3 Fatty Acid 5 mg • Omega 6 Fatty Acid 5 mg • Vitamin A 80 IU • Vitamin E 2 IU.
See Editor's Note No. 15, page 2055.

Glucosamine Complex With Chondroitin **-** Puritan's Pride
Two capsules contain: Vitamin C (as ascorbic acid) 200 mg • Manganese (as manganese sulfate) 2 mg • Sodium (as chondroitin sulfate) 30 mg • Glucosamine Sulfate (KCl) 500 mg • Chondroitin Sulfate 400 mg. Other Ingredients: Gelatin, Cellulose (plant origin), Vegetable Magnesium Stearate, Silica.
See Editor's Note No. 15, page 2055.

Glucosamine Formula **-** Symmetry
Each packet contains: Glucosamine • Chondroitin Sulfate • Hydrolyzed gelatin • Boswellia • Curcumin • Bilberry • Grape Seed extract • Grape Skin extract • Tumeric extract.
See Editor's Note No. 15, page 2055.

Glucosamine Fuel **-** TwinLab
Two tablets contain: Glucosamine Sulfate (Pure Pharmaceutical Grade) 1500 mg • Chondroitin Sulfate (Pure Pharmaceutical Grade) 1200 mg • Glycerol Fuel (contains 99.7% Pure Pharmaceutical Grade Glycerol).
See Editor's Note No. 15, page 2055.

Glucosamine HCl, Chondroitin & MSM **-** Swanson
Three tablets contain: Glucosamine HCl 750 mg • Chondroitin Sulfate 600 mg • OptiMSM (methylsulfonylmethane) 450 mg.
See Editor's Note No. 15, page 2055.

Glucosamine MSM Complex Joint Support Formula **-** Puritan's Pride
Three tablets contain: Vitamin C (as ascorbic acid) 60 mg • Manganese (as manganese sulfate) 5 mg • Glucosamine Sulfate (2KCl) 1500 mg • MSM (mehtylsulfonylmethane, 340 mg organic sulfur) 1000 mg • Ginger root extract (zingiber officinale, standardized to contain 4% volatile oils) 100 mg • White Willow bark (salix alba) 100 mg. Other Ingredients: Cellulose (plant origin), Vegetable Stearic Acid, Croscarmellose, Silica, Cellulose Coating, Vegetable Magnesium Stearate.

Glucosamine Plus CSA **-** Optimum Nutrition
Two capsules contain: Glucosamine Sulfate 1000 mg • Chondroitin Sulfate 800 mg. Other Ingredients: Gelatin, Microcrystalline Cellulose, Magnesium Stearate.

Glucosamine Sulfate - 500 mg **-** Vitamin World
Each capsule contains: Glucosamine Sulfate (2 KCl) 500 mg. Other Ingredients: Cellulose, Gelatin, Hydroxypropyl Methycellulose, Vegetable Magnesium Stearate.

Glucosamine Sulfate **-** NutriCology
Each capsule contains: Glucosamine Sulfate (sodium) 250 mg • Glucosamine Sulfate (potassium) 250 mg. Other Ingredients: Cellulose, Stearic Acid.

Glucosamine Sulfate **-** Olympian Labs
Each capsule contains: Glucosamine Sulfate (yielding Glucosamine Sulfate 500 mg and Potassium Chloride 170 mg) 670 mg.

Glucosamine Sulfate **-** Optimum Nutrition
Each capsule contains: Glucosamine (as glucosamine sulfate potassium) 750 mg. Other Ingredients: Gelatin, Microcrystalline Cellulose, Magnesium Stearate.

Glucosamine Sulfate **-** PhytoPharmica
Each capsule contains: Glucosamine Sulfate 500 mg.

Glucosamine Sulfate **-** Swanson
Each capsule contains: Glucosamine Sulfate (2KCl) 500 mg.

Glucosamine Sulfate & Shark Cartilage **-** Swanson
Each tablet contains: Glucosamine Sulfate (2KCl) 500 mg • Shark Cartilage 250 mg.

Glucosamine Sulfate 1,000 mg - Basic Nutrition **-** GNC
Each tablet contains: Glucosamine Sulfate (as D-Glucosamine Sulfate.2.NaCl) 1000 mg. Other Ingredients: Cellulose, Dicalcium Phosphate, Stearic Acid, Food Glaze, Silica, Magnesium Stearate.

Glucosamine Sulfate 1000 - GNC A-Z **-** GNC
Each tablet contains: Glucosamine Sulfate (as D-Glucosamine Sulfate.2NaCl) 1000 mg. Other Ingredients: Cellulose, Dicalcium Phosphate, Food Glaze.

Glucosamine Sulfate 1000 MG - PhysioLogics
Each capsule contains: Glucosamine Sulfate 2KCl 1000 mg. Other Ingredients: Gelatin, Vegetable Magnesium Stearate, Silica.

Glucosamine Sulfate 500 MG - PhysioLogics
Each capsule contains: Glucosamine Sulfate 2KCl 500 mg. Other Ingredients: Calcium Phosphate, Gelatin, Vegetable Magnesium Stearate.

Glucosamine Sulfate 500 MG - Puritan's Pride
Each capsule contains: Glucosamine Sulfate (2KCl) 500 mg. Other Ingredients: Calcium Phosphate, Gelatin, Vegetable Magnesium Stearate, Silica.

Glucosamine Sulfate 550 - GNC A-Z - GNC
Each capsule contains: Glucosamine Sulfate (as D-Glucosamine Sulfate.2NaCl) 550 mg. Other Ingredients: Cellulose, Gelatin.

Glucosamine Sulfate 550 mg - Basic Nutrition - GNC
Each capsule contains: Glucosamine Sulfate (as D-Glucosamine Sulfate.2NaCl) 550 mg. Other Ingredients: Cellulose, Gelatin, Magnesium Stearate.

Glucosamine Sulfate Capsules - PhytoPharmica
Three capsules contain: Stabilized Glucosamine Sulfate 1500 mg • Chloride (from glucosamine sulfate) 234 mg.

Glucosamine Sulfate Chondroitin Sulfate - Progressive Natural Products
Each 1 tbsp serving contains: Glucosamine Sulfate 500 mg • Vitamin C 500 mg • Chondroitin Sulfate 150 mg • Shark Cartilage 50 mg • CMO 25 mg • Cherry extract 25 mg • Sea Cucumber 25 mg • Manganese Aspartate 5 mg • Zinc Citrate 5 mg • Boron Citrate 1 mg.
See Editor's Note No. 15, page 2055.

Glucosamine Sulfate Complex - PhytoPharmica
Three capsules contain: Vitamin C (ascorbic acid) 1,000 mg • Chloride (from glucosamine sulfate) 156 mg • Sodium 100 mg •Stabilized Glucosamine Sulfate 1,000 mg •L-Tyrosine 500 mg.
See Editor's Note No. 21, page 2056.

Glucosamine Sulfate Packets - PhytoPharmica
Each packet contains: Chloride (from glucosamine sulfate) 234 mg • Glucosamine Sulfate (stabilized) 1500 mg.

Glucosamine Sulfate Packets, Orange-flavored - PhytoPharmica
Each packet contains: Carbohydrate <1 gm • Chloride (from glucosamine sulfate) 234 mg • Sodium (from glucosamine sulfate) 150 mg •Stabilized Glucosamine Sulfate (equivalent to three, 500 mg capsules) 1,500 mg.

Glucosamine Sulfate-750 - PhytoPharmica
Two tablets contain: Chloride (from glucosamine sulfate) 234 mg • Glucosamine Sulfate (stabilized) 1500 mg • Sodium 150 mg. Other Ingredients: Cellulose, Modified Cellulose, Magnesium Stearate, Lecithin, Carnauba Wax.

Glucosamine With MSM - Nature's Way
Two tablets contain: Methylsulfonylmethane (MSM) 750 mg • Glucosamine Sulfate Potassium Chloride (providing glucosamine sulfate 750 mg) 1050 mg. Other Ingredients: Maltodextrin, Cellulose, Stearic Acid, Modified Cellulose, Silica, Glycerin.

Glucosamine, Chondroitin & MSM - Swanson
Each tablet contains: Glucosamine Sulfate (2KCl) 500 mg • Chondroitin Sulfate 400 mg • OptiMSM (methylsulfonylmethane) 200 mg.
See Editor's Note No. 15, page 2055.

Glucosamine/Chondroitin/MSM - Doctor's Best
Two capsules contain: Sodium (from chondroitin sulfate) 28 mg • Chondroitin Sulfate 600 mg • MSM (Lignisul MSM) 500 mg • Chloride (from glucosamine sulfate KCl) 84 mg • Glucosamine Sulfate KCl 750 mg • Potassium (from glucosamine sulfate KCl) 91 mg. Other Ingredients: Cellulose, Magnesium Stearate, Gelatin Capsule.
See Editor's Note No. 15, page 2055.

Glucosamine/MSM Complex - Vitamin World
Three tablets contain: Vitamin C (as ascorbic acid) 60 mg • Manganese (as manganese sulfate) 5 mg • Glucosamine Sulfate (2KCl) 1500 mg • MSM (methylsulfonylmethane, 340 mg organic sulfur) 1000 mg • Ginger extract (zingiber officinale root, standardized for 4% volatile oils) 100 mg • White Willow (salix alba bark) 100 mg. Other Ingredients: Cellulose, Food Glaze, Vegetable Stearic Acid, Croscarmellose, Silica, Vegetable Magnesium Stearate.

Glucosa-Plex - Progressive Labs
Each capsule contains: Vitamin C 50 mg • Vitamin E (succinate) 25 IU • Pantothenic Acid 50 mg • Glucosamine Sulfate 100 mg • N-Acetyl Glucosamine 50 mg • L-Glutathione 2 mg • N-Acetyl Cysteine 5 mg • L-Cysteine 50 mg • L-Glutamic Acid 50 mg • L-Glycine 50 mg • L-Taurine 25 mg • Soluble Trachea (16% pure chondroitin sulfate-A) 25 mg • Milk Thistle (silybum marianum) 100 mg • Silymarin 5 mg • Green Lipped Mussel 25 mg (natural source of mucopolysaccharides and superoxide dismutase).
See Editor's Note No. 15, page 2055.

Glucosatrin - Market America, Inc.
Three tablets contain: Vitamin C (ascorbic acid) 100 mg • Vitamin K (phytonadione) 100 mcg • Zinc (as zinc sulfate) 10 mg • Copper (as copper gluconate) 30 mcg • Manganese (as manganese sulfate) 5 mg • Glucosamine HCl 1500 mg • Scutellaria Baicalensis root (Chinese skullcap) 150 mg • Oleanolic Acid 150 mg • Boswellia Gum resin extract 200 mg • Hops strobile extract 350 mg. Other Ingredients: Microcrystalline Cellulose, Stearic Acid, Croscarmellose Sodium, Magnesium Stearate, Silica, Pharmaceutical Glaze.

Glucos-Bal - Nutri-Quest Rx
Each tablet contains: Vanadyl Sulfate 3 mg • Chromium (Picolinate) 200 mcg • Vitamin B1 10 mg • Vitamin B2 5 mg • Vitamin B6 5 mg • Vitamin B12 10 mcg • Folic Acid 200 mcg • Biotin 500 mcg • Pantothenic Acid (D-Calcium Pantothenate) 20 mg • Niacinamide 20 mg • Niacin 6 mg • Magnesium Aspartate 100 mg • Calcium Ascorbate 100 mg • Manganese Aspartate 4 mg • Zinc (Picolinate) 1 mg • Selenium (Chelate) 30 mcg.

Glucose Metabolism Factors - Michael's Naturopathic Programs
Nine tablets contain: Vitamin C (as calcium ascorbate) 300 mg • Thiamin 300 mg • Niacin (as niacinamide and 20% as nicotinic acid) 300 mg • Pantothenic Acid (as calcium pantothenate) 210 mg • Calcium (as calcium amino acid chelate) 150 mg • Iodine (from kelp) 675 mcg • Magnesium (as magnesium amino acid chelate) 300 mg • Zinc (as zinc monomethionine) 90 mg • Manganese (as manganese amino acid chelate) 60 mg • Chromium (as chromium polynicotinate) 450 mcg • Proprietary Blend 3900 mg: Essential Fatty Acids (from flax seed; 7% gamma linolenic acid, 64% linoleic acid), Nopales Opuntia cactus, Cedar berry (thuja occidentalis), Glutamine (as L-glutamine), Golden Seal root (hydrastis candensis), Gymnema Sylvestre leaf, Milk Thistle seed extract (silybum marianum, 80% silymarin, 240 mg), Blueberry leaf (vaccinium myrtillus), Bitter Melon seed (momordica charantia), Ginger root (zingiber officinale), Vanadium (vanadyl sulfate). Other Ingredients: Dicalcium Phosphate, Terra Alba (calcium sulfate), Maltodextrin, Magnesium Stearate, Stearic Acid.

Glucose Regulation Complex - Shaklee
Two capsules contain: Magnesium (as Magnesium oxide) 200 mg • Zinc (as Zinc gluconate) 5 mg • Chromium (as Chromium polynicotinate) 400 mcg • Taurine 500 mg • Vanadium (as Vanadium amino acid chelate) 100 mcg • Alpha Lipoic Acid 10 mg • Banaba leaf extract (Lagerstroemia speciosa, standardized to contain 1% colosolic acid). Other Ingredients: Maltodextrin, Gelatin, Water.

Glucose Tabs **-** PhytoPharmica
Each tablet contains: Dextrose • Cellulose • Natural Raspberry Flavor • Citric Acid • Magnesium Stearate.

Glucosol **-** Life Extension Foundation
Each softgel capsule contains: Corosolic Acid extract (from lagestroemia speciosa L.) 24 mg. Other Ingredients: Rice Bran oil, Gelatin, Glycerin, Silica, Carob extract, Water, Titanium Dioxide.

Glucosol **-** Now
Each softgel contains: Glucosol (lagerstroemia speciosa L. standardized to 1% corosolic acid) 24 mg. Other Ingredients: Gelatin, Glycerol, Carob extract, Water, Titanium Dioxide.

Glucosol **-** NSI - Nutraceutical Sciences Institute
Each capsule contains: Lagerstroemia speciosa L. extract (glucosol) 24 mg. Other Ingredients: Cellulose, Magnesium Stearate.

Glucosol **-** Olympian Labs
Each softgel contains: Glucosol 1% standardized extract (lagerstroemia speciosa L., yeilding 240 mcg of corosolic acid) 24 mg.

Glucosol brand **-** Soft Gel Technologies, Inc.
Corosolic Acid.
See Editor's Note No. 44, page 2058.

Glucotize **-** Medical Research Institute (MRI)
Each tablet contains: A-Lipoic Acid (thioctic acid) 300 mg. Other Ingredients: Calcium Phosphate, Cellulose Esthers & composites, Magnesium Stearate.

Glucovite **-** TheraNutria
Six tablets contain: Vitamin A (67% as Beta-Carotene, 33% as Vitamin A Palmitate) 7500 IU • Vitamin C (Calcium Ascorbate) 1000 mg • Vitamin D (as Vitamin D3) 400 IU • Vitamin E (natural d-alpha, d-beta, d-gamma, d-delta-tocopherols) 100 IU • Vitamin K (as Vitamin K1) (Phylloquinone) 40 mcg • Thiamine (Mononitrate) 4.5 mg • Riboflavin 3.4 mg • Niacin (50% Niacin, 50% Niacinamide) 40 mg • Vitamin B6 (Pyridoxine HCl) 10 mg • Folic Acid 600 mcg • Vitamin B12 (Cyanocobalamin) 60 mcg • Biotin 200 mcg • Pantothenic Acid (D-Calcium Pantothenate) 20 mg • Calcium (Ascorbate, Propionate, Carbonate) 300 mg • Magnesium (Amino Acid Chelate) 200 mg • Iron (Amino Acid Chelate) 3.6 mg • Iodine (Potassium Iodide) 150 mcg • Zinc (Amino Acid Chelate) 15 mg • Copper (Amino Acid Chelate) 2 mg • Manganese (Amino Acid Chelate) 2 mg • Selenium (50% L-Selenomethionine, 50% Sodium Selenite) 140 mcg • Chromium (Glycine-Niacin Chelate) 600 mcg • Molybdenum (Amino Acid Chelate) 75 mcg • Boron (Citrate) 3 mg • Silicon (Sodium Metasilicate) 3 mg • Vanadium (Vanadyl Sulfate) 100 mcg • Citrus Bioflavonoids 10 mg • Quercetin 10 mcg • Glucosol Banaba leaf extract (L. speciosa L., min. 1% corosolic acid) 2 mg • Alpha-Lipoic acid (Thioctic acid). Other Ingredients: Modified Cellulose Gum, Cellulose, Vegetable Stearine, Silicon Dioxide, Magnesium Stearate, Hydroxymethyl Propylcellulose, Titanium Dioxide, Chlorophyll.

Glutagen **-** ANS - Applied Nutrition Sciences
Pure Glutamine.

Glutamine Caps **-** Optimum Nutrition
Each capsule contains: L-Glutamine 1000 mg. Other Ingredients: Gelatin, Magnesium Stearate.

Glutamine Capsules **-** Universal
Each capsule contains: L-Glutamine 750 mg • Manganese Sulfate 400 mcg • Potassium Phosphate 30 mg.

Glutamine Flora **-** Nutri-Quest Rx
Each tablet contains: Combined stabilized microencapsulated freeze-dried Lactobacillus Acidophilus, Bulgaricus & Bifidus 4.5 million IU • L-Glutamine 500 mg • Chlorophyll 20 mg • natural Vitamin E Succinate 5 IU.

Glutamine Fuel Capsules **-** TwinLab
Two capsules contain: L-Glutamine 1500 mg.

Glutamine Fuel Powder **-** TwinLab
Each teaspoonful contains: L-Glutamine 4500 mg (4.5 g).

Glutamine Powder **-** ProLab
Each 1 tsp (4.5 g) serving contains: L-Glutamine 4500 mg.

Glutamine Powder **-** Optimum Nutrition
Each 1 tsp (4.5 g) serving contains: L-Glutamine 4.5 g.

Glutathione Plus **-** Atrium Inc.
Each capsule contains: L-Glutathione 50 mg • L-Glutamine 200 mg.

Glycentials Antioxidant **-** Mannatech
Two tablets contain: Vitamin A (as dunaliella salina isolate [alpha-, beta-carotene, cryptoxanthin, zeaxanthin, lutein] in PNC) 2500 IU • Vitamin C (as ascorbic acid in PNC) 250 mg • Vitamin D (as cholecalciferol in PNC) 200 IU • Vitamin E (as d-alpha tocopheryl succinate, mixed d-alpha-, d-beta-, d-delta-, d-gamma-tocopherols, tocotrienols PNC) 200 IU • Thiamin (as thiamin mononitrate in PNC) 750 mcg • Riboflavin (as riboflavin in PNC) 850 mcg • Niacin (as niacinamide in PNC) 10 mg • Vitamin B6 (as pyridoxine hydrochloride, pyridoxal 5-phosphate in PNC) 4 mg • Folate (as folic acid in PNC) 400 mcg • Vitamin B12 (as cyanocobalamin in PNC) 12 mcg • Biotin (as biotin in PNC) 150 mcg • Pantothenic Acid (as d-calcium pantothenate in PNC) 5 mg • Calcium (as calcium carbonate, calcium citrate-malate-glycinate in ambroglycin) 500 mg • Iodine (as potassium iodide in ambroglycin) 75 mcg • Magnesium (as magnesium oxide, magnesium glycinate in ambroglycin) 250 mg • Zinc (as zinc glycinate in ambroglycin) 7.5 mg • Selenium (as selenomethionine in ambroglycin) 100 mcg • Copper (as copper glycinate in ambroglycin) 1 mg • Manganese (as manganese glycinate in ambroglycin) 1 mg • Chromium (as chromium dinicotinate-glycinate in ambroglycin) 100 mcg • Molybdenum (as molybdenum glycinate in ambroglycin) 37.5 mcg • Boron (as boron glycinate in ambroglycin) 1 mg • Silica (as silica glycinate in ambroglycin) 1 mg • Vanadium (as vanadium glycinate in ambroglycin) 25 mcg • Proprietary Blend Ambroglycin 240 mg: Glycinated Multiminerals Combined with Watercress (leaves), Spinach (leaves), Green Peas (fruit), Ginger (root), Ambrotose Complex (patent pending), Arabinogalactan (larix decidua gum) Manapol Aloe Vera gel extract (inner leaf gel), Gum Ghatti, Gum Tragacanth • Phytonutrient Complex 2 (PNC) 25 mg: Acerola Cherry (fruit), Orange (peel), Rice Bran, Rose Hips, Soy Protein containing Isoflavones • Inositol 12.5 mg • Choline (as choline bitartrate) 11 mg • Alpha-Lipoic Acid 25 mg • Quercetin 5 mg • Coenzyme Q10 4.5 mg. Other Ingredients: Microcrystalline Cellulose, Silicon Dioxide, Croscarmellose Sodium, Stearic Acid, Magnesium Stearate, Dibasic Calcium Phosphate, Pharmaceutical Glaze.

GLYCO-8 **-** Pharmagel
Glycolic Acid • Alpha Hydroxy Acids • Antioxidants.

Glyco-B **-** Atrium Inc.
Each tablet contains: Vitamin B1 35 mg • Vitamin B2 35 mg • Vitamin B6 35 mg • Vitamin B12 35 mcg • Vitamin C 180 mg • Pantothenic Acid 80 mg • Niacinamide 180 mg • Folic Acid 135 mcg • Choline Bitartrate 25 mg • Inositol 10 mg • Biotin 10 mcg • L-Lysine HCL 10 mg • Brewer's Yeast 50 mg • Pancrelipase 20 mg • Selenium 2 mcg • Adrenal 4 mg • Brain 4 mg • Liver 7 mg • Pancreas 2 mg.
See Editor's Note No. 31, page 2056.

Glycobar: Chocolate Chip **-** Pharmanex
Each bar contains: Honey • Peanut Butter: Peanuts, Salt • Semi Sweet Chocolate Chips: Sugar, Chocolate Liquor, Cocoa Butter, Soy Lecithin, Vanilla • Brown Sugar • Date Puree • Prune Puree • Rolled Oats • Sugar Beet Fiber • Brown Crisp Rice: Rice Flour, Rice Bran, Rosemary Extract • Modified Guar Gum • Oat Bran • Peanuts • Barley Flakes • Rye Flakes • Soybean Oil • Soy Lecithin • Whey Powder.

Glycobar: Peanut Butter and Jelly **-** Pharmanex
Each bar contains: Honey • Peanut Butter: Peanuts, Salt • Brown Sugar • Date Puree • Prune Puree • Rolled Oats • Strawberry and Blueberry Fruit Chips: Sugar, Strawberries, Blueberries, Glucose, Pectin, Citric Acid, Sodium Citrate, Natural Flavor • Brown Crisp Rice: Rice Flour, Rice Bran, Rosemary Extract • Modified Guar Gum • Oat Bran • Peanuts • Yogurt Chips: Sugar, Hydrogenated Palm Kernel Oil, Milk Solids, Color (Titanium Dioxide), Soy Lecithin, Vanilla • Barley Flakes • Rye Flakes • Soybean Oil • Soy Lecithin • Whey Powder.

GlycoBears with Ambrotose Complex (GlycoBears, Glyco Bears, Glyco-Bears) **-** Mannatech
Two tablets contain: Vitamin A (as retinyl palmitate, beta carotene and dunaliella salina extract [alpha carotene cryptoxanthin zeaxanthin leutin] in PNC) 2500 IU • Vitamin C (as ascorbic acid, sodium ascorbate and acerola cherry in PNC) 30 mg • Vitamin D3 (as cholecalciferol in PNC) 200 IU • Vitamin E (as d-alpha-tocopherol succinate and mixed d-alpha-, d-beta-, d-delta-, and d-gamma-tocopherols in PNC) 15 IU • Thiamin (as thiamin mononitrate in PNC) 0.75 mg • Riboflavin 0.85 mg • Niacin (as niacinamide in PNC) 10 mg • Vitamin B6 (as pyridoxine hydrochloride in PNC) 1 mg • Folate (as folic acid in PNC) 200 mcg • Vitamin B12 (as cyanocobalamin in PNC) 3 mcg • Biotin 150 mcg • Pantothenic Acid (as d-calcium pantothenate in PNC) 5 mg • Calcium (as calcium carbonate and calcium citrate in PNC) 12.5 mg • Iodine (as potassium iodide and kelp in PNC [ascophyllum nodosum - whole plant]) 37.5 mcg • Magnesium (as magnesium glycinate in PNC) 2 mg • Zinc (as zinc citrate in PNC) 3.75 mg • Selenium (as selenomethionine in PNC) 17.5 mcg • Copper (as cupric oxide and copper glycinate) 0.5 mg • Manganese (as manganese citrate in PNC) 0.5 mg • Chromium (as chromium niacinate diglycinate) 30 mcg • Molybdenum (as sodium molybdate in PNC) 20 mcg • Potassium (as potassium citrate in PNC) 2 mg • Choline (as choline bitartrate in PNC) 0.4 mg • Inositol 1 mg • PABA (p-aminobenzoic acid in PNC) 200 mcg • Vanadium (as vanadium glycinate) 10 mcg • Bioflavonoids 10 mcg • Proprietary Blend Ambrotose Complex (patent pending) 12.5 mg: Arabinogalactan (larix decidua gum), Manapol Aloe Vera gel extract (inner leaf gel), Gum Ghatti, Gum Tragacanth • Phytonutrient Complex (PNC) 25 mg: Pineapple, Broccoli, Carrot, Apple, Orange, Tomato, Cauliflower, Brussels Sprout, Beet, Blueberry, Celery, Grape, Grapefruit, Kale, Plum, Raspberry, Spinach, Strawberry, Watermelon, Radish, Lemon, Lime, Cantaloupe, Cherry, Leek or Yellow Pepper, Onion, Papaya, Peach, Pear, Ginger, Green Peas. Other Ingredients: Sorbitol, Stearic Acid, Fructo-Oligosaccharides, Natural Flavors (berry burst only), Dibasic Calcium Phosphate, Turmeric (tropical zing only), Natural Flavors (tropical zing only), Citric Acid, Magnesium Stearate, Malic Acid (berry burst only), Silicon Dioxide, Rice Syrup Solids, Carmine (berry burst only).

GlycoLEAN Accelerator **-** Mannatech
Country Mallow (contains ephedrine) • Proprietary Blend of antioxidants, digestive enzymes, and nutrients.
See Editor's Note No. 17 and No. 39.

GlycoLEAN Accelerator 2 **-** Mannatech
Two capsules contain: Chromium (as chromium dinicotinate glycinate, chromium polynicotinate) 30 mcg • Proprietary Herbal/Botanical Blend 582 mg: Bitter Orange extract (fruit), Green Tea extract (leaves), American Ginseng (root), Guarana extract (seed), Gotu Kola (leaves), Eleutherococcus Senticosus extract (root), Cinnamon (bark), Curcumin (root), Milk Thistle extract (seed), Bladderwrack (whole plant), Dandelion root, Cayenne (fruit) • Ambrotose Complex (patent pending): Arabinogalactan (larix decidua gum), Manapol Aloe Vera gel extract (inner leaf gel), Gum Ghatti, Gum Tragacanth • Piperine 2.5 mg. Other Ingredients: Gelatin, Microcrystalline Cellulose, Silicon Dioxide, Magnesium Stearate, Stearic Acid.
See Editor's Note No. 40, page 2058.

GlycoLEAN Catalyst **-** Mannatech
Two tablets contain: Vitamin A (as dunaliella salina isolate [alpha-, beta-carotene, cryptoxanthin, zeaxanthin lutein] in PNC) 2500 IU • Vitamin C (as ascorbic acid in PNC) 180 mg • Vitamin D (as cholecalciferol in PNC) 200 IU • Vitamin E (as d-alpha tocopheryl succinate, mixed d-alpha-, d-beta-, d-delta-, d-gama-tocopherols, and tocotrienols in PNC) 30 IU • Thiamin (as thiamin mononitrate in PNC) 3 mg • Riboflavin (as riboflavin in PNC) 3.4 mg • Niacin (as niacinamide in PNC) 10 mg • Vitamin B6 (as pyridoxine hydrochloride, pyridoxine-5 phosphate in PNC) 4 mg • Folate (as folic acid in PNC) 200 mcg • Vitamin B12 (as cyanocobalamin in PNC) 12 mcg • Biotin (as biotin in PNC) 150 mcg • Pantothenic Acid (as d-calcium pantothenate in PNC) 20 mg • Calcium (as calcium carbonate, calcium citrate-malate-glycinate in ambroglycin) 500 mg • Iodine (as potassium iodide in ambroglycin) 75 mcg • Magnesium (as magnesium oxide, magnesium glycinate, in ambroglycin) 245 mg • Zinc (as zinc glycinate in ambroglycin) 7.5 mg • Selenium (as selenomethionine in ambroglycin) 100 mcg • Copper (as copper glycinate in ambroglycin) 1 mg • Manganese (as manganese glycinate in ambroglycin) 1 mg • Chromium (as chromium dinicotinate glycinate in ambroglycin) 200 mcg • Molybdenum (as molybdenum glycinate in ambroglycin) 37.5 mcg • Blue Green Algae (as spirulina pratensis) 100 mg • Proprietary Blend Ambroglycin 248 mg: Glycinated Multiminerals Combined with Watercress (leaves), Spinach (leaves), Green Peas (fruit), Ginger (root), Ambrotose Complex (patent pending), Arabinogalactan (larix decidua gum), Manapol Aloe Vera gel extract (inner leaf gel), Gum Ghatti, Gum Tragacanth • Choline (as choline bitartrate) 25 mg • Inositol 12.5 mg • Phytonutrient Complex 2 (PNC) 18 mg: Acerola Cherry (fruit), Orange (peel), Rice Bran, Rose Hips, Soy Protein Containing Isoflavones • Alpha-Lipoic Acid 7.5 mg • Coenzyme Q10 6 mg • Boron (as boron glycinate in ambroglycin) 1 mg • Vanadium (as vanadyl glycinate in ambroglycin) 100 mcg. Other Ingredients: Microcrystalline Cellulose, Croscarmellose Sodium, Stearic Acid, Silicon Dioxide, Magnesium Stearate, Dibasic Calcium Phosphate, Pharmaceutical Glaze.

GlycoLEAN Fiber Full **-** Mannatech
Each capsule contains: Magnesium (as magnesium aspartate, magnesium citrate, magnesium oxide) 50 mg • Proprietary Blend 450 mg: Glucomannan, Arabinogalactan (larix decidua), Aloe Vera gel extract (inner leaf gel) • Flax (seed) 50 mg • Spirulina Platensis 50 mg • Gotu Kola (leaves) 25 mg • Lactobacillus Sporogenes 25 mg • Lipase 5 mg. Other Ingredients: Gelatin, Magnesium Stearate, Silicon Dioxide, Cellulose.

GlycoLEAN GlycoSlim Drink Mix, Chocolate **-** Mannatech
Soy Protein Isolate • Fructose • Inulin • Safflower Oil (non-hydrogenated) • Corn Syrup solids (non-hydrogenated) • Cocoa • Fructo-Oligosaccharides • Natural Flavors • Dicalcium Phosphate • Gum Blend: Cellulose Gum, Xanthan Gum, Carrageenan • Ascorbic Acid • Ferrous Fumarate • Magnesium Oxide • Silicon Dioxide • Beta Carotene • Biotin • Sodium Caseinate • Monoglycerides • Diglycerides • Dipotassium Phosphate • Sodium Chloride • D-Alpha-Tocopheryl Acetate • Lecithin • Zinc Citrate • Sodium Molybdate • Niacinamide • D-Calcium Pantothenate • Rice Protein concentrate • Pea Protein concentrate • Manganese Sulfate • Folic Acid • Copper Citrate • Chromium Dinicotinate-Glycinate • Selenomethionine • Pyridoxine Hydrochloride • Cholecalciferol • Thiamin Hydrochloride • Riboflavin • Cyanocobalamin • Potassium Iodide.

GlycoLEAN GlycoSlim Drink Mix, French Vanilla **-** Mannatech
Soy Protein Isolate • Non-Dairy Creamer (safflower oil, corn syrup solids, sodium caseinate, dipotassium phosphate, monoglycerides, diglycerides, lecithin, tocopherols, natural flavors, silicon dioxide) • Fructose • Inulin • Natural Flavors • Fructo-Oligosaccharides • Dicalcium Phosphate • Gum Blend: Cellulose Gum, Xanthan Gum, Carrageenan • Magnesium Oxide • Beta Carotene • Silicon Dioxide • Rice Protein concentrate • Ascorbic Acid • Ferrous Fumarate • Zinc Citrate • D-Alpha-Tocopheryl Acetate • Sodium Molybdate • Biotin •

Niacinamide • Selenomethionine • D-Calcium Pantothenate • Pea Protein concentrate • Manganese Sulfate • Copper Citrate • Folic Acid • Chromium Dinicotinate-Glycinate • Cholecalciferol • Pyridoxine Hydrochloride • Thiamin Hydrochloride • Riboflavin • Cyanocobalamin • Potassium Iodide.

GlycoLEAN Manager **-** Mannatech
Bitter Orange (contains synephrine) • Proprietary Blend of antioxidants, digestive enzymes, and nutrients.
See Editor's Note No. 17 and No. 40.

GlycoLoad **-** Optimum Nutrition
Each heaping scoop (59 g) contains: Proprietary GlycoLoad Carbohydrate Blend: Dextrose, Maltodextrin, Fructose • Non-GMO Soy Protein Isolate • Citric Acid • Calcium Citrate • Natural Flavor • Potassium Chloride • Natural Beet Color • Salt • Magnesium Oxide • Ascorbic Acid • D-Alpha Tocopheryl Succinate (natural vitamin E) • Dicalcium Phosphate • Biotin • Zinc Oxide • Niacinamide • Vitamin A Palmitate • D-Calcium Pantothenate • Folic Acid • Pyridoxine Hydrochloride • Riboflavin • Selenomethionine • Thiamin Mononitrate • Cyanocobalamin.

Glycoplex **-** Progressive Labs
Three capsules contain: Vitamin C 500 mg • Thiamin (Vitamin B1) 100 mg • Riboflavin (Vitamin B2) 100 mg • Niacinamide 500 mg • Vitamin B6 100 mg • Folate (folic acid) 300 mcg • Vitamin B12 50 mcg • Biotin 15 mcg • Pantothenic Acid (calcium pantothenate) 250 mcg • Chromium (chromium picolinate) 200 mcg • Inositol 50 mg • Pancrelipase 50 mg • Choline Bitartrate 50 mg • Pyloric substance 45 mg • Para Amino Benzoic Acid (PABA) 60 mg • L-Lysine Monohydrochloride 30 mg. Other Ingredients: Raw Adrenal, Raw Pancreas, Raw Brain and Raw Liver concentrates.
See Editor's Note No. 31, page 2056.

GlyMordica **-** Amazing Herbs
Bitter Melon (Momordica Charantia).

GNC Men's ArginMax **-** GNC
Six tablets contain: Vitamin A (as retinyl palmitate) 5000 IU • Vitamin C (as ascorbic acid) 60 mg • Vitamin E (as d-alpha tocopherol succinate) 30 IU • Thiamin (as thiamin mononitrate) 1.5 mg • Riboflavin (B2) 1.7 mg • Niacin (as niacinamide) 20 mg • Vitamin B-6 (pyridoxine hydrochloride) 2 mg • Folic Acid 400 mcg • Vitamin B-12 (cyanocobalamin) 6 mcg • Biotin 300 mcg • Pantothenic Acid (as calcium d-pantothenate) 10 mg • Zinc (as zinc gluconate) 15 mg • Selenium 70 mcg • L-Arginine 3000 mg • Korean Ginseng extract aerial parts and roots 100 mg • American Ginseng root 100 mg • Ginkgo Biloba extract leaf 50 mg • Other Ingredients: Microcrystallin Cellulose, Magnesium Stearate, Hydroxypropyl Methylcellulose, Pharmaceutical Glaze, Silica, Titanium Dioxide, PEG, Polysorbate 80.

GNC Vitamin B-12 - GNC A-Z **-** GNC
Each tablet contains: Vitamin B12 (as cyanocobalamin) 1000 mcg. Other Ingredients: Dicalcium Phosphate, Cellulose, Vegetable Stearate, Food Glaze, Whole Brown Rice powder (oryza sativa).

GNC Women's Arginmax **-** GNC
Six tablets contain: Vitamin A (as retinyl palmitate) 5000 IU • Vitamin C (as ascorbic acid) 60 mg • Vitamin E (as d-alpha tocopherol succinate) 30 IU • Thiamin (as thiamin mononitrate) 1.5 mg • Riboflavin (B2) 1.7 mg • Niacin (as niacinamide) 20 mg • Vitamin B-6 (pyridoxine hydrochloride) 2 mg • Folic Acid 400 mcg • Vitamin B-12 (cyanocobalamin) 6 mcg • Biotin 300 mcg • Pantothenic Acid (as calcium d-pantothenate) 10 mg • Calcium (as calcium carbonate) 500 mg • Iron (as ferrous gluconate) 9 mg • Zinc (as zinc gluconate) 7.5 mg • L-Arginine 2500 mg • Korean Ginseng extract aerial parts and roots 100 mg • Ginkgo Biloba extract leaf 50 mg • Damiana leaf 50 mg. Other Ingredients: Microcrystalline Cellulose, Hydroxypropyl Methylcellulose, Pharmaceutical Glaze, Silica, Titanium Dioxide, Magnesium Stearate, PEG, Polysorbate 80.

Goatein IG **-** Garden of Life, Inc.
Five caplets contain: Poten-Zyme Pure Goat's Milk Protein 4550 mg • Pure Goat's Milk Colostrum 450 mg. Other Ingredients: Cellulose, Stearates (vegetable source).

Goatein Pure Goat's Milk Protein **-** Garden of Life, Inc.
Each heaping tablespoon (15 g) contains: Goat's Milk Protein concentrate, Pre-digested Goat's Milk Protein concentrate containing a proprietary probiotic blend, Natural Vanilla.

Goat's Rue **-** Motherlove Herbal Co.
Each 2 oz bottle contains: Goat's Rue. In a base of certified kosher alcohol and glycerin.

Gold Label Noni Juice **-** Global Health Trax
Two tablespoons (1 fl oz) contain: Vitamin C 10 mg. Other Ingredients: Purified Water, Noni Fruit Juice Concentrate, Raspberry Juice Concentrate, Natural Flavors, Citric Acid, Kelp.

Gold Quest **-** Nulab, Inc.
Three capsules contain: Vitamin A (as acetate) 5000 IU • Beta Carotene 1 mg • Vitamin D (as vitamin D3) 600 IU • Vitamin E (as dl-alpha tocopheryl acetate) 45 IU • Vitamin C (as ascorbic acid) 90 mg • Thiamine (vitamin B1) 3 mg • Riboflavin (as vitamin B2) 3 mg • Niacinamide (as vitamin B3) 30 mg • Vitamin B6 (as pyridoxine HCL) 4 mg • Folate (as folic acid) 400 mcg • Vitamin B12 (as cyanocobalamin) 6 mg • Biotin 300 mcg • Pantothenic Acid (as calcium pantethonate) 10 mg • Calcium (as dicalcium phosphate) 30 mg • Magnesium (from magnesium oxide) 15 mg • Zinc (zinc aminoate) 15 mg • Copper (copper gluconate) 2 mg • Manganese (manganese aminoate) 7 mg • Iodine (potassium iodine) 150 mcg • Selenium (selenium aspartate) 100 mcg • Protein Blend 300 mg: Rice Protein, Egg-White Protein • Proprietary Herb Blend 432 mg: Maral root extract (leuzea carthamoides), Oat Straw extract (avena sativa), Black Currant powder (ribes nigrum). Other Ingredients: Gelatin, Water.

Gold Specifics Cardio Support **-** Solgar
Each three tablets contain: Calcium 175 mg • Magnesium (glycinate, oxide) 200 mg • Taurine 800 mg • Trimethylglycine (TMG, from beets) 800 mg • Soy Isoflavone Concentrate (seed) 500 mg • L-Carnitine 300 mg • Standardized Hawthorne extract (leaf/flower, vitexin 2 mg, 1.8%) 125 mg • Cayenne Powder (fruit) 100 mg • Coenzyme Q-10 (as ubiquinone) 60 mg • Grape Seed extract (phenolics 48 mg, 95%) 50 mg. Inactive Ingredients: Microcrystalline Cellulose, Vegetable Stearic Acid, Vegetable Cellulose, Methacrylic Acid, Silica, Vegetable Magnesium Stearate, Titanium Dioxide, Grapeskin, Natural Vitamin E (mixed tocopherols), Natural Beta Carotene, Other Carotenoids, Rosemary extract (aerial), Vitamin C (l-ascorbic acid), Vegetable Glycerin, Glyceryl Triacetate.

Gold Specifics Prostate Support **-** Solgar
Each two vegicaps contain: Calcium 25 mg • Zinc (as zinc glycinate) 10 mg • Selenium (as l-selenomethionine) 25 mcg • Sodium 15 mg • Modified Citrus Pectin 200 mg • Standardized Pygeum Africanum extract (bark, phytoesterols 3-5 mg, 2-3%) 150 mg • Standardized Saw Palmetto extract (berry, free fatty acids 68-75 mg, 45-50%) 150 mg • Standardized Stinging Nettles extract (leaf, silic acid 2 mg, 1%) 150 mg • Pumpkin powder (seed) 100 mg • Soy Isoflavone Concentrate (seed) 100 mg • Lycopene (from tomato) 7 mg. Inactive Ingredients: Microcrystalline Cellulose, Vegetable Cellulose, Vegetable Magnesium Stearate, Titanium Dioxide, Natural Vitamin E (mixed tocopherols), Natural Beta Carotene, Other Carotenoids, Rosemary extract (aerial), Vitamin C (l-ascorbic acid), Vegetable Glycerin, Riboflavin, Caramel, Water.

Goldcare Capsules **-** Vitabiotics
Each capsule contains: Vitamin A 900 mcg • Vitamin D 10 mcg • Vitamin E 20 mg • Vitamin C 80 mg • Vitamin B1 (thiamin) 12 mg • Vitamin B2 (riboflavin) 5 mg • Vitamin B3 (niacin) 20 mg • Vitamin B6 (pyridoxine HCl) 20 mg • Folic Acid 500 mcg • Vitamin B12 (cyanocobalamin) 20 mcg • Pantothenic Acid 10 mg • Iron 6 mg • Magnesium 75 mg • Zinc 15 mg • Iodine 130 mcg • Manganese 2 mg

• Copper 1.2 mg • Boron 1 mg • Chromium 100 mcg • Selenium 150 mcg • Citrus Bioflavonoids 16 mg • Natural Mixed Carotenoids 3 mg • Ginkgo Biloba extract 10 mg.

Golden Ener-Z **-** DreamPharm
Two capsules contain: Proprietary Blend: Cornu Cervi Parvum, Cardamom, Atractylodes, Codonopsis Pilosula, Angelica root, Licorice, Peony White root, Dolichos nut, Poria Cocos, Oryza Sativae germinatus, Barley sprouts, Ligustrum seed, Euryale seed, Deer Antler, Ginseng root, Dioscorea root, Crataegus fruit, Massa Medicata fermentata, Rehmannia cooked, Cnidium root, Cornus fruit, Polygonatum root, Psoralea Sorylifolia fruit, Astragalus root.

Golden Flax Meal **-** Nature's Life
Two tablespoons (17 g) contain: Low fat Omegaflo Flax seed meal (certified organic by Farm Verified Organic). Naturally occuring fatty acids: Alpha Linolenic Acid (Omega-3) 1710 mg • Linoleic Acid (Omega-6) 480 mg • Oleic Acid (Omega-9) 50 mg • Lignin Fiber 1003 mg • Lignan 13.6 mg.

Golden Flax Oil **-** Nature's Life
Each 1 tbsp serving contains: Lipid profile, based on a typical analysis of : Omega-3 as Alpha-Linolenic Acid EFA 8.6 g •Omega-6 as Alpha- Linoleic Acid EFA 2.7 g • Omega-9 as Oleic (Monounsaturated Fatty Acid) 2.4 g.

Golden Flax Oil 1000 mg **-** Nature's Life
Each capsule contains: 100% pure Flax oil (Certified Organically Grown) (Omegaflo Process fresh, unrefined, unfiltered, unbleached, virgin seed oil; Organically grown & processed according to California Organic Foods Act of 1990; Farm Verified Organic). Lipid profile based on a typical analysis: Omega-3 EFA as Alpha-Lenolenic Acid 570 mg • Omega-6 EFA as Linoleic Acid 180 mg • Omega-9 as Oleic Acid 160 mg • Vitamin A (from naturally occuring Beta Carotene) 286 IU • Vitamin E (from naturally occuring Tocopherols) 1 IU.

Golden Flower Blood Cleanser **-** Grandma's Herbs
Each capsule contains: Proprietary Blend 0.480 g: Burdock root, Pau d'Arco bark, Cleavers herb, Slippery Elm bark, Licorice root, Buckthorn bark, Cascara, Black Walnut hulls, Canaigre herb, Calendula flower, Aloe herb.

Golden Oolong Tea - Tea's Tea **-** Ito En (North America)
Each 16.9 fl oz bottle contains: Purified Water, Oolong Tea, Vitamin C (ascorbic acid).

Golden Spleen 500 **-** Enzymatic Therapy
Each capsule contains: Spleen Polypeptides 375 mg: A mixture of highly purified bovine-derived spleen polypeptides naturally present in the spleen, including Tuftsin, Splenopentin, Splenin, & Leukokinin • Goldenseal root extract 125 mg: (Hydrastis canadensis) standardized to contain 5% total Alkaloids including: Berberine, Hydrastine, & Canadine.
See Editor's Note No. 14.

Goldenseal **-** Leiner Health Products
Each caplet contains: Golden Seal extract (Hydrastis canadensis) root 100 mg. Other Ingredients: Calcium Carbonate, Cellulose, Maltodextrin, Hydroxypropyl Methylcellulose, Silicon Dioxide, Polyethylene Glycol 3350, Croscarmellose Sodium, Hydroxypropyl Cellulose, Pharmaceutical Glaze, Crospovidone, Magnesium Stearate, Yellow 5 Lake, Red 40 Lake, Blue 2 Lake, Titanium Dioxide, Polysorbate 80.

Goldenseal **-** Olympian Labs
Each capsule contains: Goldenseal root 500 mg.

Goldenseal **-** Pharmanex
Each capsule contains: Goldenseal root extract (Hydrastis canadensis) (4:1) 250 mg. Other Ingredients: Rice Flour, Gelatin, Magnesium Stearate, Silicon Dioxide.

Goldenseal & Echinacea **-** Olympian Labs
Each capsule contains: Goldenseal 225 mg • Echinacea 225 mg.

Goldenseal and Myrrh **-** Dial Herbs
Goldenseal • Myrrh.

Goldenseal Root **-** Now
Two capsules contain: Goldenseal root powder (hydrastis canadensis) 1000 mg.

Goldenseal Salve **-** Dial Herbs
Goldenseal • Myrrh • Shavegrass • Echinacea • Comfrey • Slippery Elm • Lobelia. In a base of Bees Wax , Glycerine & Cold Pressed Olive oil.

Goldenseal-Myrrh Virtue **-** Blessed Herbs
Goldenseal root • Myrrh Gum • Propolis • Grain alcohol & Distilled Water.

GolfoFlex **-** Pharmessen
Each capsule contains: Rosemary oil (rosmarinus officinalis) 6.5 mg • Clove oil (eugenia caryophyllata, bud) 2.5 mg. Other Ingredients: Methylcellulose, Avicel, Olive Oil, Aerosil (food grade certified), Capsule (100% vegetarian, certified Kosher & Pareve, & Halal).

GO-lite/am (Appetite Manager) **-** Enviro- Tech Nutritionals
Griffonia simplicifolia (Containing 5-hydroxytryptophan) • St. John's Wort.

GO-lite/fm (Fat Metabolizer) **-** Enviro- Tech Nutritionals
Chitosan • Vitamin C • Iodine • Chromium • Thermal Herbal Blend: Sida Cordifolia, Bitter Orange Peel • Yerba Mate leaf • Chitosan.
See Editor's Note No. 39 and No. 40.

Good Dream **-** DreamPharm
Each capsule contains: Proprietary Blend: Semen Zizyphi Spinosae, Albizziae Julibrissin, Caulis Polygoni Multiflori, Rhizoma Coptidis, Fructus Mori Albae, Fructus Schisandrae Chinensis, Radix Salviae Miltiorrhizzae, Radix Glycyrrhizae, Melatonin.
See Editor's Note No. 16, page 2055.

Good Morning (Zetox) **-** Global Health Products
Two capsules contain: Zeolite 765 mg • Vitamin A 200 mcg • Vitamin C 15 mg • Vitamin D 1.25 mcg • Vitamin E 2.5 mg • Niacin 4.5 mg • Folic Acid 50 mcg • Pantothenic Acid 1.5 mg • Vitamin B6 0.5 mg • Riboflavin 0.4 mg • Thiamin 0.35 mg • Biotin 0.037 mg • Vitamin B12 0.25 mcg.

Good-Nite **-** Changes International, Inc.
Each caplet contains: Melatonin 3 mg • Kava Kava root standardized extract (30% kavalactones) 250 mg • Herbal Extract Blend 275 mg: Valerian root standardized extract (0.8% valerenic acids), Catnip aerial parts, Chamomile flower, Hops stobile, Passion flower aerial parts, Skullcap root. Other Ingredients: Dicalcium Phosphate, Vegetable cellulose, Fractionated vegetable oil, Silica, Soy polysaccharides, and Vegetable resin glaze.
See Editor's Note No. 16, page 2055.

Gotu Kola **-** DaVinci Laboratories
Each capsule contains: Gotu Kola (centella asiatica, yielding triterpenes 45 mg) 450 mg.

Gotu Kola **-** FoodScience of Vermont
Each capsule contains: Gotu Kola (centella asiatica, yielding triterpenes 45 mg) 450 mg.

Gotu Kola **-** Nature's Way
Two capsules contain: Gotu Kola (stem, leaf) 870 mg.

Gotu Kola **-** Now
Two capsules contain: Sodium 10 mg • Total Carbohydrate 540 mg • Gotu Kola leaf (Centella Asiatica) 900 mg. Other Ingredients: Stearic Acid.

Gotu Kola **-** Olympian Labs
Each capsule contains: Gotu Kola 450 mg.

Gram-Two Vitamin C **-** The Vitamin Shoppe
Two tablets contain: Vitamin C 2000 mg: as Ascorbic Acid and as mineral ascorbates of Calcium, Magnesium, Zinc, and Manganese • Bioflavonoids 250 mg: Hesperidin, Rose Hips, Acerola Cherry, Pectin, Orange, Grapefruit, Lemon, Rutin.

Grape Seed **-** Pharmanex
Each capsule contains: Grape seed extract (Vitis vinifera) (100:1) 75 mg. Other Ingredients: Rice Flour, Gelatin, Magnesium Stearate, Silicon Dioxide.

Grape Seed (PCO) Extract **-** PhytoPharmica
Each capsule contains: Grape Seed extract (standardized to contain 95% procyanidolic oligomers (PCOS)) 50 mg. Other Ingredients: Cellulose, Gelatin, Magnesium Stearate, Silicon Dioxide, Titanium Dioxide Color.

Grape Seed (PCO) Phytosome **-** PhytoPharmica
Each capsule contains: Grape seed phytosome (vitis vinifera, standardized to contain 95% procyanidolic oligomers [PCOs]) bound to Phosphatidylcholine 50 mg.

Grape Seed Antioxidant **-** Now
Each capsule contains: Grape seed extract (95%) 60 mg • Citrus Bioflavonoids (40%) 300 mg.

Grape Seed Extract **-** Leiner Health Products
Each tablet contains: Grape seed extract (Vitis vinifera) seed 100 mg. Other Ingredients: Calcium Carbonate, Maltodextrin, Cellulose, Silicon Dioxide, Polyethylene Glycol 3350, Croscarmellose Sodium, Crospovidone, Magnesium Stearate, Hydroxypropyl Methylcellulose, Hydroxypropyl Cellulose, Polysorbate 80.

Grape Seed Extract **-** Metabolic Response Modifiers
Each capsule contains: Grape Seed extract (85-95% OPC's - offering a minimum 100 mg of OPC's with 20 mg of other vital flavonoids) 120 mg.

Grape Seed Extract **-** Olympian Labs
Each capsule contains: Grape Seed extract (120:1, consists of 85% Oligomeric Procyanidins) 100 mg.

Grape Seed Extract Extra Strength with MAT **-** Olympian Labs
Each capsule contains: Grape Seed extract (120:1, consists of 85% Oligomeric Procyanidins) 200 mg. Other Ingredients: MAT (proprietary blend of nutritional ingredients).

Grape Seed Extract Formula **-** Quest
Each caplet contains: Grape Seed powder (Vitis vinffera) (Provided by 25 mg P.E. 1:100 standardized to contain not less than 95% leucoanthocyanins) 2500 mg • Citrus Bioflavonoids 200 mg providing Hesperidin 50 mg • Rutin powder 25 mg. Other Ingredients: Calcium Phosophate, Microcrystalline Cellulose, Vegetable Stearin, Croscarmellose Sodium, Magnesium Stearate (vegetable source).

Grape Seed Extract Plus **-** Atrium Inc.
Each capsule contains: Grape seed extract (Leucocyanidins) 50 mg • Bioflavonoids 200 mg.

Grape Seed PCO Phytosome 100 mg **-** Enzymatic Therapy/ PhytoPharmica
Each capsule contains: Grape Seed phytosome (vitis vinifera, standardized to contain 95% procyanidolic oligomers (PCOs) from grape-seed extract bound to phosphatidylcholine) 100 mg. Other Ingredients: Gelatin, Magnesium Stearate, Silicon Dioxide, Titanium Dioxide Color.

Grapefruit Concentrate With Fiber & Herbs **-** Natrol
Two capsules contain: Grapefruit concentrate 10:1 300 mg • Psyllium Husk fiber 100 mg • Rice Bran fiber 100 mg • Oat Bran fiber 100 mg • Licorice root 100 mg • Uva Ursi 100 mg • Apple Cider vinegar 50 mg • Deep Ocean Kelp 50 mg • Lecithin 50 mg • Spirulina 50 mg • Vitamin B6 (Pyridoxine HCL) 25 mg • L-Phenylalanine 25 mg • Cascara Sagrada 20 mg. This is a 10 time concentration of the equivalent of 3000 mg of Whole Grapefruit. Other Ingredients: Silicon Dioxide, Magnesium Stearate, Gelatin, Microcrystalline Cellulose.

Grapefruit Extract **-** NutriBiotic
Grapefruit extract.

Grapeseed Extract **-** PhysioLogics
Each capsule contains: Grapeseed extract 100 mg • Citrus Bioflavonoid (citrus sinensis) 300 mg. Other Ingredients: Gelatin, Vegetable Magnesium Stearate, Silica.

Grapeseed Extract **-** Swanson
Each capsule contains: Grapeseed extract (95% proanthocyanidins) 50 mg.

Grapeseed Extract 100 mg **-** Puritan's Pride
Each capsule contains: Grapeseed extract 100 mg • Citrus Bioflavonoids 300 mg.

Grapeseed Extract 50 mg **-** Puritan's Pride
Each capsule contains: Grapeseed extract 50 mg • Citrus Bioflavonoids 500 mg.

Green 15 **-** Grandma's Herbs
Each capsule contains: Proprietary Blend 0.448 g: Wheat Grass herb, Alfalfa root, Red Raspberry leaf/pulp, Parsley herb, Barley Green herb, Spirulina herb, Horsetail Grass herb, Yucca root, Oat Straw herb, Nettle herb, Chia seed, Bee Pollen, Canaigre root, Ginseng root, Cayenne Pepper, Bladderpod herb, Aloe Vera herb. Other Ingredients: Gelatin.

Green Black Walnut Wormwood Complex **-** Now
Two droppersful (16 mL) contains: 1.6 mL proprietary blend of Green Black Walnut hulls (Juglans species) • Wormwood herb (Artemisia absinthium) • Clove buds (Carophyllus species) extracts. Other Ingredients: Grain Alcohol, Distilled Water.

Green Hornet Liquid **-** Unknown
Unknown.
See Editor's Note No. 49, page 2059.

Green Magma **-** Green Foods Corp.
Each 5.3 oz box contains: Proprietary Blend 150 g: Young Barley Grass powdered juice, Maltodextrin, Brown Rice.

Green Max Powder **-** Swanson
Each tablespoon (8.5 grams) contains: Vitamin A (as beta-carotene 40 mg) 66,666 IU • Soy Lecithin 2,142 g • Spirulina powder 1,356 g • Apple Fiber 1.35 g • Wheat Grass powder 445 mg • Alfalfa leaf powder 435 mg • Barley bran powder 435 mg • Brown Rice powder 350 mg • Chlorella (broken cell wall) 350 mg • Soy sprout powder 350 mg • Beet powder 335 mg • Lactobacillus probiotic culture 200 mg • Bee Pollen powder 150 mg • Royal Jelly powder 150 mg • Acerola cherry powder 115 mg • Barley grass powder 97 mg • Licorice root powder 60 mg • Dulse Thallus powder 20 mg • Ginkgo Biloba leaf powder 20 mg • Grape Seed extract (90% proanthocyanidins) 20 mg • Green Tea extract (50% polyphenols) 20 mg • Milk Thistle seed extract (80% silymarin) 20 mg • Astragalus root powder 10 mg • Bilberry powder 10 mg • Echinacea root powder 10 mg • Siberian Ginseng root powder 10 mg.

Green Multi **-** Nature's Life
Three tablets contain: Beta Carotene (equivalent to 25000 IU Vitamin A) 15 mg • Vitamin C 1000 mg • Vitamin E (d-Alpha Tocopheryl Succinate) 300 IU • Vitamin B1 (Thiamine Mononitrate) 25 mg • Vitamin B2 (Riboflavin, Riboflavin 5'-Phosphate) 25 mg • Vitamin B3 (Niacin) 25 mg • Pantothenic Acid (Calcium Pantothenate, Pantetheine-5' -Phosphate) 25 mg • Vitamin B6 (Pyridoxine HCl, Pyridoxal-5'-Phosphate) 25 mg • Folic Acid (Folacin) 400 mcg • Vitamin B12 100 mcg • Biotin (d-Biotin) 60 mcg • Choline (Bitartrate) 14 mg • Inositol (Niacinate) 20 mg • PABA (Para

Aminobenzoic Acid) 25 mg • Boron (Citrate, Nature's Life Greens) 100 mg • Calcium (Carbonate, Citrate/Malate) 250 mg • Chromium (Picolinate, Polynicotinate) 100 mcg • Copper (Citrate, Gluconate) 1 mg • Iodine (Potassium Iodine, Nature's Life Greens) 75 mcg • Iron (Glycinate, Nature's Life Greens) 10 mg • Magnesium (Oxide, Nature's Life Greens) 125 mg • Manganese (Gluconate, Citrate) 6 mg • Molybdenum (Molybdate, Nature's Life Greens) 50mcg • Potassium (Gluconate, Iodide, Nature's Life Greens) 90 mg • Selenium (Selenite, Cysteine) 100 mcg • Vanadium (Vanadyl Sulfate) 25 mcg • Zinc (Picoliante, Monomethionine) 15 mg • Lemon Bioflavonoids Complex (50% active) 100 mg • Quercetin (Saphora japonica) 25 mg • Rutin (Sapora japonica) 25 mg • Hesperidin (Citrus fruit peel) 25 mg • Bromelain from Pineapple (2000 GDU/g) 25 mg • Papain from Papaya (2000 USP units/g) 25 mg • Betaine HCl, beets 25 mg • Amylase (30000 SKB IU/g) 6 mg • Lipase 10000 Usp IU/g) 6 mg • Cellulase (10000 USP IU/g) 6 mg • Nature's Life Greens powder 1000 mg.

Green Phytofoods - Now
Each nine gram serving contains: Lecithin fine powder 2000 mg • Spirulina (Hawaiian) 1000 mg • Alfalfa juice concentrate 700 mg • Wheat grass powder organic 500 mg • Barley grass powder organic 500 mg • Carrot powder 500 mg • Barley Malt powder 400 mg • Broccoli powder 350 mg • Brown Rice Bran 350 mg • Apple fiber 350 mg • Apple Pectin 300 mg • Oat Bran 300 mg • Chlorella powder 300 mg • Red Beet powder 300 mg • Panax ginseng root powder (min 5% Ginsenosides) 250 mg • Siberian Ginseng root powder (Eleutherococcus senticosus) 100 mg • Peppermint powder 150 mg • Green Tea extract (Camellia sinensis) (40% Catechins) 100 mg • Royal Jelly powder (min 5% 10-HDA) 100 mg • Fructo Oligo Saccharides (NutraFlora FOS) 100 mg • Trace Mineral concentrate 100 mg • Milk Thistle extract (80% Silymarin) 80 mg • Kelp powder 50 mg • Ginkgo Biloba extract (24% Ginkgo Flavonglycosides) 20 mg • Grape seed extract (95% Polyphenols) 20 mg • Bilberry extract (25% Anthocyanidins) 20 mg • Plant Based Enzymes 100 mg: Protease 12500 HUT, Lipase 200 LU, Lactase 200 LAC, Bromelain 5000 FCC, Amylase 2500 DU, Cellulase 500 CMC, Papain 6000 PU • Coenzyme Q10 10 mg • Alpha Lipoic Acid 10 mg • Stevia extract 10 mg.

Green Source - Puritan's Pride
Three tablets contain: Vitamin A (100% as Beta Carotene) 15,000 IU • Vitamin C 1000 mg • Vitamin D 400 IU • Vitamin E 250 IU • Thiamin (Vitamin B-1) 25 mg • Riboflavin (Vitamin B-2) 25 mg • Niacin 25 mg • Vitamin B-6 25 mg • Folic Acid 400 mcg • Vitamin B-12 25 mcg • Biotin 50 mcg • Pantothenic Acid 25 mg • Calcium 250 mg • Iron 15 mg • Iodine 150 mcg • Magnesium 125 mg • Zinc 15 mg • Selenium 25 mcg • Copper 500 mcg • Manganese 4 mg • Chromium 100 mcg • Molybdenum 50 mcg • Potassium 50 mg • Boron 1 mg • Choline Bitartrate 50 mg • Inositol 25 mg • PABA (Para-Aminobenzoic Acid) 25 mg • Citrus Bioflavonoids Complex (Orange) 100 mg • Quercetin 25 mg • Rutin 25 mg • Hesperidin (Orange) 10 mg • Bromelain (Pineapple-2000 GDU/gm) 20 mg • Betaine Hydrochloride 20 mg • Papain (Papaya) 20 mg • Amylase 5 mg • Lipase 5 mg • Protease 1 mg • Cellulase 2.5 mg • Proprietary Lactobacillus blend 25 mg: L. Acidophilus, L. Bifidus, L. Bulgaricus (Milk-Free: minimum 1 billion viable micro-organisms per gram) • Oat Bran 25 mg • Pectin (Apple) 25 mg • RNA 35 mg • DNA 10 mg • Carotenoids 10 mg • Chlorophyll 4 mg • Vegetable Oil as Borage and Sunflower (dry, cold-pressed - providing Essential Fatty Acids, GLA) 100 mg • L-Glutathione 5 mg • Spirulina 1000 mg • Wheat grass juice (dry) 100 mg • Sprouted Barley juice (dry) 100 mg • Flaxseed Oil (dry) 100 mg • Chlorella (broken cell wall) 100 mg • Bee Pollen 100 mg • Siberian Ginseng (Eleutherococcus senticosus) root 50 mg • Dehydrated Garlic (allium sativum) bulb 10 mg • Proprietary herbal blend 60 mg: Echinacea (Echinacea purpurea) aerial, Milk Thistle (Silybum marianum) seed, Goldenseal (Hydrastis canadensis) root, Ginger root (Zingiber officinale), Ginkgo Biloba (Ginkgo biloba) leaf, Cayenne Pepper (Capsicum annuum) fruit. Other Ingredients: Cellulose (plant origin), Acacia Gum, Croscarmellose, Vegetable Stearic Acid, Vegetable Magnesium Stearate, Cellulose Coating.

Green Source Iron Free - Vitamin World
Three tablets contain: Vitamin A (100% as Beta Carotene) 15,000 IU • Vitamin C 1000 mg • Vitamin D 400 IU • Vitamin E 250 IU • Thiamin (Vitamin B-1) 25 mg • Riboflavin (Vitamin B-2) 25 mg • Niacin 25 mg • Vitamin B-6 25 mg • Folic Acid 400 mcg • Vitamin B-12 25 mcg • Biotin 50 mcg • Pantothenic Acid 25 mg • Calcium 250 mg • Iodine 150 mcg • Magnesium 125 mg • Zinc 15 mg • Selenium 25 mcg • Copper 0.5 mg • Manganese 4 mg • Chromium 100 mcg • Molybdenum 50 mcg • Potassium 50 mg • Boron 1 mg • Choline Bitartrate 50 mg • Inositol 25 mg • PABA (Para-Aminobenzoic Acid) 25 mg • Citrus Bioflavonoids Complex (Orange) 100 mg • Quercetin 25 mg • Rutin 25 mg • Hesperidin (Orange) 10 mg • Bromelain (Pineapple-2000 GDU/gm) 20 mg • Betaine Hydrochloride 20 mg • Papain (Papaya) 20 mg • Amylase 5 mg • Lipase 5 mg • Protease 1 mg • Cellulase 2.5 mg • Proprietary Lactobacillus blend 25 mg: L. Acidophilus, L. Bifidus, L. Bulgaricus (Milk-Free: minimum 1 billion viable micro-organisms per gram) • Oat Bran 25 mg • Pectin (Apple) 25 mg • RNA 35 mg • DNA 10 mg • Carotenoids 10 mg • Chlorophyll 4 mg • Vegetable Oil as Borage and Sunflower (dry, cold-pressed - providing Essential Fatty Acids, GLA) 100 mg • L-Glutathione 5 mg • Spirulina 1000 mg • Wheat grass juice (dry) 100 mg • Sprouted Barley juice (dry) 100 mg • Flaxseed Oil (dry) 100 mg • Chlorella (broken cell wall) 100 mg • Bee Pollen 100 mg • Siberian Ginseng (Eleutherococcus senticosus) root 50 mg • Dehydrated Garlic (allium sativum) bulb 10 mg • Proprietary herbal blend 60 mg: Echinacea (Echinacea purpurea) aerial, Milk Thistle (Silybum marianum) seed, Goldenseal (Hydrastis canadensis) root, Ginger root (Zingiber officinale), Ginkgo Biloba (Ginkgo biloba) leaf, Cayenne Pepper (Capsicum annuum) fruit. Other Ingredients: Cellulose (plant origin), Acacia Gum, Croscarmellose, Vegetable Stearic Acid, Vegetable Magnesium Stearate, Cellulose Coating.

Green Stuff - Gary Null & Associates (GNA)
Green Mix: Green Kamut juice, Wheat Grass juice, Barley Green juice, Alfalfa leaf, Oat grass juice, Broccoli, Parsley, Kale • Flaxseed • Raw Brown Rice • Fruit Juice Mix: Pineapple, Lemon, Lime • Carrot juice • Earthrise Farms Spirulina • Yucca root • Black Licorice root extract.

Green Tea Antioxidant - Enzymatic Therapy
Each capsule contains: Green Tea leaf extract (camellia sinensis, standardized to contain 47-52% polyphenols [catechin, epicatechin, epicatechin gallate, epigallocatechin gallate], 5-10% caffeine) 250 mg. Other Ingredients: Cellulose, Gelatin, Magnesium Stearate, Silicon Dioxide, Titanium Dioxide Color.

Green Tea Barley Essence - Green Foods Corp.
Each 5.3 oz jar contains: Proprietary Blend 150 g: Young Barley Grass powdered juice, Maltodextrin, Green Tea, Brown Rice, Natural Flavors.

Green Tea Bath - Abra Therapeutics
Sodium Borate • Sodium Sulfate • Sodium Chloride • Sodium Sesquicarbonate • Olive Oil • Herbal Extract Blend: Organic Whole Leaf Green Tea, Calendula, Chamomile flowers • Essential Oils Blend: Lemongrass oil, Grapefruit oil, Sweet Orange oil, Sweet Marjoram oil.

Green Tea Body Lotion - Abra Therapeutics
Organic Green Tea tips in spring water • Aloe Vera juice • Apricot • Coconut • Jojoba oil • Vegetable Emulsifying wax • Vegetable Glycerin • Shea Butter • Extract of Organic Green Tea leaf • Calendula flowers • Chamomile flowers • Rosehips Bioflavonoids • Natural Vitamin E • Essential Oils Blend: Lemongrass oil, Grapefruit oil, Sweet Orange oil, Sweet Marjoram oil, Sweet Fennel oil, Sage oil.

Green Tea Complex - Leiner Health Products
Each tablet contains: Vitamin C (Ascorbic Acid) 120 mg • Green Tea extract (Camellia sinensis) leaf 100 mg. Other Ingredients: Calcium Carbonate, Cellulose, Hesperidin Complex, Rutin, Maltodextrin, Quercetin, Silicon Dioxide, Polyethylene Glycol 3350, Croscarmellose Sodium, Starch, Crospovidone, Magnesium Stearate,

Hydroxypropyl Methylcellulose, Hydroxypropyl Cellulose, Polysorbate 80.

Green Tea Diet **-** Schiff
Each tablet contains: Green Tea extract EGCG (epigallocatechin gallate) 270 mg • Caffeine 150 mg.

Green Tea Diet, Timed Release **-** Schiff
Each tablet contains: Green Tea leaf extract (camellia sinensis) 225 mg • EGCG epigallocalechin gallate) 90 mg • Caffeine (as caffeine anhydrous) 50 mg. Other Ingredients: Cellulose, Dextrose, Coating (dextrin, titanium dioxide [color], hydroxypropyl methylcellulose, polyethylene glycol, soy lecithin, caramel color, dextrose, riboflavin), Croscarmellose Sodium, Magnesium Stearate.

Green Tea Extract **-** HealthWatchers System
Green Tea Extract • Green Tea Powder. Each capsule is the equivalent of 700 mg of Green Tea Powder.

Green Tea Extract **-** Nature's Way
Each capsule contains: Green Tea dried extract 170 mg • Red Clover blossoms 315 mg. Other Ingredients: Gelatin.

Green Tea Extract **-** NSI - Nutraceutical Sciences Institute
Each capsule contains: Green Tea extract (standardized 98% polyphenols, 80% Catechins, and 45% EGCG) 500 mg.

Green Tea Extract **-** Olympian Labs
Each capsule contains: Green Tea extract 500 mg.

Green Tea Extract **-** PhytoPharmica
Each capsule contains: Green Tea leaf extract(camellia sinensis, standardized to contain 47%-52% polyphenols [catechin, epicatechin, epicatechin gallate, and epigallocatechin gallate] and 5%-10% Caffeine) 250 mg.

Green Tea Formula GT80 **-** Jamieson
Each capsule contains: Green Tea Phytosome (Camellia sinensis) 80 mg • Synergistic Antioxidant Nutrients Derived from Vitamin C, Grape Seed Extract, Bioflavonoids 30 mg.

Green Tea Phytosome **-** Enzymatic Therapy/PhytoPharmica
Each capsule contains: Green Tea leaf phytosome (camellia sinensis) bound to Phosphatidylcholine 100 mg. Other Ingredients: Cellulose, Gelatin, Modified Cellulose Gum, Titanium Dioxide Color, Magnesium Stearate.

Green Tea Remedy **-** Puritan's Pride
Each caplet contains: Green Tea extract 200 mg • Reishi mushroom 25 mg • Maitake mushroom 25 mg • Shiitake mushroom 25 mg • Astragalus 100 mg • Ligustrum 50 mg • Cat's Claw 100 mg • Vitamin C 60 mg • Selenium 50 mcg • Zinc 6 mg • Spirulina 50 mcg • Super-Oxide Dismutase 10 mg • N-acetyl Cysteine 25 mg.

Green Tea Salt Glow **-** Abra Therapeutics
Purified Water • Aloe Vera • Coconut oil • Olive oil • Kukui oil • Jojoba oil • Stearic Acid • Glycerin • Glyceryl Stearate • Cetyl Alcohol • St. John's Wort extract • Wild Yam extract • French Lavender essential oil • Boswellia Olibanum essential oil • Sodium PCA • Allantoin • Lecithin • Methylparaben • Propylparaben.

Green Tea Salt Scrub **-** Abra Therapeutics
20% Volcanic Ash • Natural Mineral Blend: Sodium Borate, Sodium Sulfate, Sodium Chloride • Organic Oils Blend: Almond, Olive, Sunflower, Jojoba, Lemongrass, Grapefruit, Sweet Orange, Sweet Marjoram • Organic whole leaf Green Tea.

Green-Lipped Mussel **-** Quest
Each capsule contains: Freeze-dried Green Lipped Mussel (Perna canaliculus) 625 mg.

Gripe Water - Alcohol Free **-** R.W. Packaging, Ltd.
Each 5 mL contains: Sodium Bicarbonate 50 mg.

Gripe Water Liquid **-** R.W. Packaging, Ltd.
Each 5 mL contains: Sodium Bicarbonate 50 mg.

Gro Pro **-** Universal
Ten capsules contain: Creatine Monohydrate 5000 mg • L-Glutamine 2000 mg • Acetyl L-Carnitine 500 mg • L-Leucine (BCAA) 250 mg • L-Isoleucine (BCAA) 250 mg • L-Valine (BCAA) 250 mg • N-Acetyl-Cysteine (NAC) 200 mg • Tribulus Terrestris L. 250 mg • DHEA 50 mg • Zinc 15 mg.

Gro Tropin **-** Pinnacle
Three capsules contain: Alpha GPC (alpha-glycerylphosphorylcholine) 500 mg • AminoGlutein Peptide Glutamine Peptide (30%) 500 mg • Colostrum (colostral isoform extract) 500 mg • Tribulus Terrestris (40% furostanol saponins) 500 mg • Phoshphatidylserine 500 mcg • Chrysin (98% pure 5,7 dehydroxyflavone) 750 mcg. Other Ingredients: Magnesium Stearate, Gelatin.

Growth Fuel **-** TwinLab
Nine capsules contain: B-Hydroxy B-Methylbutyrate Monohydrate (HMB) 3000 mg • L-Glutamine 2000 mg • Creatine Monohydrate 5000 mg • N-Acetyl-Cysteine (NAC) 200 mg • Acetyl-L-Carnitine 50 mg • Zinc (from Zinc Picolinate) 30 mg • DHEA (Dehydroepiandrosterone) 50 mg.

GS-500 **-** Enzymatic Therapy
Three capsules contain: Chloride (from glucosamine sulfate) 234 mg • Sodium (from glucosamine sulfate) 150 mg • Glucosamine Sulfate (stabilized) 1500 mg. Other Ingredients: Gelatin, Magnesium Stearate, Silicon Dioxide, Titanium Dioxide Color.

GS-500 and Chondroitin **-** Enzymatic Therapy
Three tablets contain: Chloride 234 mg • Sodium 250 mg • Glucosamine Sulfate 1500 mg • Chondroitin Sulfate 1200 mg.
See Editor's Note No. 15, page 2055.

GSC (Glandular Stress Complex) **-** Progressive Labs
Each capsule contains: Vitamin B12 24 mcg • Raw Bovine Adrenal 15 mg • Raw Bovine Liver 15 mg • Raw Bovine Thymus 60 mg • Raw Bovine Spleen 15 mg • Raw Bovine Stomach 15 mg.
See Editor's Note No. 14, page 2055.

GS-Complex **-** Enzymatic Therapy
Three capsules contain: Vitamin C (ascorbic acid) 1000 mg • Chloride (from glucosamine sulfate) 156 mg • Sodium 100 mg • Glucosamine Sulfate (stabilized) 1000 mg • L-Tyrosine 500 mg. Other Ingredients: Gelatin, Silicon Dioxide, Magnesium Stearate, Titanium Dioxide Color.

GTF Chromium 200 mcg **-** Jamieson
Each tablet contains: GTF Chromium (Derived from Brewer's Yeast) 200 mcg.

Guar Gum **-** Atrium Inc.
Each tablet contains: Pure Guar Gum 1000 mg.

Guarana Chai **-** Traditional Medicinals
Assam Black leaf Tea • Cardamom seed • Ginger rhizome • Roasted Chicory root • Nutmeg seed • Organic Black Peppercorn • Guarana seed dry extract • Stevia leaf • Vanilla Bean dry extract • Clove stem • Rose petal • Cinnamon bark oil.

Guarana Energizer **-** Source Naturals
Each tablet contains: Guarana 900 mg.

Guarana-Gotu Kola Virtue **-** Blessed Herbs
Ma Huang • Siberian Ginseng root • Guarana seed • Gotu Kola • Licorice root • Grain alcohol & Distilled Water.
See Editor's Note No. 30, page 2056.

Guggulbolic **-** Syntrax Innovations
Each capsule contains: Guggulsterones 30 mg.

Guggulbolic Extreme **-** Syntrax Innovations
Each capsule contains: Guggul EZ100 30 mg • Guggul Resin extract (standardized for 30 mg total guggulsteroids) 30 mg. Other

Ingredients: Microcrystalline Cellulose, Gelatin, Titanium Dioxide, Yellow #5, Red #40.

GugulPlex **-** PhytoPharmica
Each tablet contains: Niacin 250 mg • Vitamin C 100 mg • Chromium 50 mcg • Guggul extract 250 mg • Ginger root extract 200 mg.

GugulPlus **-** Enzymatic Therapy
Each tablet contains: Niacin (Inositol hexaniacinate) 250 mg • Vitamin C (Potassium Ascorbate) 100 mg • Chromium (Chromium Polynicotinate) (ChromeMate brand of patented Niacin-bound GTF Chromium) 50 mcg • Other Ingredients: Guggul extract (Commiphora Mukul) standardized to contain Guggulsterones 25 mg/gram) 250 mg • Ginger root extract 6.5:1 (Zingiber officinale) 200 mg.

Gum Weed Salve **-** Dial Herbs
Gum Weed • Licorice • Myrrh • Goldenseal • Arnica • Strawberry • Lobelia • Cayenne. In a base of Bees Wax, Glycerine & Cold Pressed Olive oil.

Gum-Ease **-** The Herbalist
Echinacea root • Myrrh Gum • Blood root • Bayberry root bark • Peppermint oil (essential) • Cinnamon oil (essential) • Clove oil (essential).

Gymnema Sylvestre **-** Puritan's Pride
Each tablet contains: Gymnema Sylvestre 400 mg • Citrus Fiber 200 mg.

Gynecrine **-** Progressive Labs
Each capsule contains: Vitamin A 1000 IU • Vitamin C 100 mg • Vitamin E (dl-alpha tocopherol) 50 IU • Thiamin (Vitamin B1) 10 mg • Riboflavin (Vitamin B2) 10 mg • Vitamin B6 (pyridoxine) 18 mg • Iodine (as potassium iodide) 150 mcg • Magnesium (as magnesium oxide) 100 mg • Manganese (as manganese gluconate) 10 mg • Ovary concentrate (bovine) 20 mg • Mammary concentrate 10 mg • Pancreas concentrate 10 mg • Adrenal concentrate 10 mg • Pituitary concentrate 10 mg • Lecithin 10 mg • Flax seed oil 10 mg.
See Editor's Note No. 14.

Gypsy Cold Care **-** Traditional Medicinals
Each 1 cup serving contains: Menthol 5 mg (as it naturally occurs in the peppermint leaf, mentha x piperita). Other Ingredients: Rose Hip, Cinnamon Bark, Yarrow Flower, Ginger Rhizome, Elder Flower, Safflower Petal, Clover Stem, Hyssop Herb, Licorice Root Dry Extract.

Hair & Skin Formula **-** Nature's Way
Four capsules contain: Biotin (Biotin Triurate) 1.6 mg • Calcium 50 mg • Cayenne pepper fruit 160 mg • Fizyme Enzyme Formula 100 mg • Fo-Ti root 160 mg • Glucosamine HCL 400 mg • Horsetail grass 160 mg • Kelp (whole Thallus) 160 mg • MSM (Methyl Sulfonyl Methane) 600 mg • Nettle herb 160 mg • Oatstraw stem, leaf 160 mg • Rosemary herb 160 mg. Other Ingredients: Gelatin, Magnesium Stearate, Millet.

Hair & Skin Nutrition **-** Enzymatic Therapy
Each capsule contains: Vitamin A (Fish Liver oil) 1666 IU • Vitamin D (Fish Liver oil) 333 IU • Vitamin E (D-Alpha Tocopherol) 33 IU • Vitamin C (Ascorbic Acid) 100 mg • Niacin/Niacinamide 33 mg • Zinc (Chelate) 15 mg • Vitamin B6 (Pyridoxine HCL) 10 mg • Pantothenic Acid (D-Calcium Pantothenate) 8.3 mg • Riboflavin (Vitamin B2) 1.7 mg • Biotin 333 mcg • Folic Acid 33 mcg • Other ingredients: Unsaturated Free Fatty Acids (Linoleic, Arachidonic & Linolenic from Unrefined Germ oil & Safflower seed oil) 300 mg • Lecithin (Soy) 200 mg • Choline Bitartrate 50 mg • Intrinsic Glandular Lipids 50 mg • Inositol 33 mg. In a base of L-Cysteine as a natural amino acid synergistic component.
See Editor's Note No. 14.

Hair Clean 1-2-3 Lice Remover **-** Quantum, Inc.
Coconut Oil • Anise Oil • Ylang Ylang Oil • Isopropyl Alcohol.

Hair Formula **-** Pharmanex
Each capsule contains: Vitamin E (as D-Alpha Tocopheryl Acetate) 3 IU • Riboflavin (as Riboflavin-5-Phosphate) 0.75 mg • Vitamin B6 (as Pyridoxine Hydrochloride) 3 IU • Biotin (as Biotin) 200 mcg • Pantothenic Acid (as Calcium Pantothenate) 25 mg • DL-Methionine 200 mg • L-Cysteine 105 mg • Lactalbumin Hydrolysate 25 mg • Millet Extract 20 mg. Other Ingredients: Gelatin, Maltodextrin, Starch, Vanillin, Stearic Acid (Vegetable Derived), Silicon Dioxide.

Hair Genesis **-** HairGenesis
Each softgel contains: Beta Sitosterol 50 mg • Saw Palmetto Berry extract (85/95% liposterolic standardized) 200 mg • Lecithin 50 mg • Inositol 100 mg • Phosphatidyl Choline 25 mg • Niacin 15 mg • Biotin 100 mcg. Other Ingredients: Alcohol SDA-40, Propylene Glycol, Deionized Water, Polysorbate-80, Isoceteth-20, Hydrolyzed Mucopolysaccharides, Beta-Sitosterol, Biotin, Citric Acid.

Hair Million **-** DreamPharm
Each capsule contains: Proprietary Blend: Radix Angelicae Sinensis, Radix Bupleuri Chinensis, Sclerotium Poriae Cocos, Atractylodes Rhizoma, Paeoniae Radix, Glycyrrhizae Radix, Fructus Ligustri Lucidi, Fructus Lycii Chinensis, Radix Polygoni Multiflori, Radix Paeoniae Rubra, Herba Artemisiae Capillaris, Cortex Cinnamomi Cassiae, Eucommiae Ulmoides Bark, Rhizoma Gastrodiae Elatae, Radix Morindae Officinalis, Rhizoma Ligustici, Codonopsitis Sinensis, Fructus Liquidambaris, Uncaria Sinensis, Fructus Chaenomelis, Vaccaria Pyramidata, Hedyotis Diffusa, Laminaria Japonica, Tulipa Edulis, Eisenia Bicyclis.

Hair Nutrients **-** Biotech Corp.
Three tablets contain: Shen Min [a proprietary blend of 12:1 standardized He Shou Wu (Fo Ti) root extract and He Shou Wu root powder] 1755 mg • BioPerine Black Pepper extract 3 mg.

Hair Support for Men **-** Futurebiotics
Two capsules contain: Vitamin A (5000 IU as fish liver oil, 5000 IU as beta carotene) 10000 IU • Vitamin C (ascorbic acid) 250 mg • Vitamin D (ergocalciferol) 200 IU • Vitamin E (d-alpha tocopherol succinate) 30 IU • Vitamin B1 (thiamine HCl) 10 mg • Vitamin B2 (riboflavin) 10 mg • Vitamin B6 (pyridoxine HCl) 10 mg • Vitamin B12 (cyanocobalamin) 16 mcg • Folic Acid 400 mcg • Biotin (d-biotin) 500 mcg • Pantothenic Acid (calcium pantothenate) 100 mg • Zinc (amino acid chelate) 25 mg • Selenium (amino acid chelate) 100 mcg • Para Aminobenzoic Acid (PABA) 30 mg • Boron (amino acid chelate) 3 mg • MSM (methyl-sulfonyl-methane) 500 mg • Horsetail leaf powder extract (4:1) 50 mg • Saw Palmetto berry extract (4:1) powder 50 mg • Hair Support Herbal Base 200 mg: Citrus Bioflavonoids, Saw Palmetto berry powder, Schizandra berry extract powder, Horsetail leaf powder. Other Ingredients: Gelatin, Water.

Hair, Skin & Nails **-** Health Factor
Each capsule contains: Choline Bitartrate 100 mg • DL Methionine 100 mg • Borage Seed 150 mg • Flax Seed 150 mg • Gelatin 150 mg • Lecithin 100 mg.

Hair, Skin & Nails Advanced MSM Formula **-** Solgar
Each two tablets contain: Vitamin C (as l-ascorbic acid) 120 mg • Calcium 90 mg • Zinc (as zinc citrate) 15 mg • Copper (as copper glycinate) 2 mg • MSM (as methylsulfonylmethane) 1000 mg • Silicon (as silica, as L-corallioides [red algae powder]) 50 mg • L-Proline 50 mg • L-Lysine (as l-lysine HCl) 50 mg. Inactive Ingredients: Microcrystalline Cellulose, Vegetable Cellulose, Silica, Vegetable Stearic Acid, Vegetable Magnesium Stearate, Vegetable Glycerin.

Hair, Skin & Nails for Men **-** Futurebiotics
Three tablets contain: Beta Carotene 10,000 IU • Vitamin C 120 mg • Vitamin B2 (Riboflavin) 10 mg • Vitamin B1 (Thiamin) 10 mg • Calcium 600 mg • Iron (Amino Acid Chelate) 6 mg • Vitamin D (Fish Liver Oil) 200 IU • Vitamin E (Natural Mixed Tocopherols) 30 IU • Vitamin B6 (Pyridoxine) 10 mg • Folic Acid 400 mcg • Vitamin B12 16 mcg • Phosphorus 300 mg • Iodine (Kelp) 225 mcg • Magnesium (Oxide) 200 mg • Zinc (Gluconate) 25 mg • Biotin 400 mcg •

Pantothenic Acid (Calcium Salt) 30 mg • Choline (Bitartrate) 150 mg • Inositol 60 mg • Para Amino Benzoic Acid (PABA) 50 mg • Selenium (Amino Acid Chelate) 25 mcg • Manganese (Amino Acid Chelate) 10 mg • Niacinamide 50 mg • In a special potentiating base containing: Gelatin, Cysteine, Methionine, Ribonucleic Acid (RNA), Bioflavonoids, Betaine HCl, Oat Straw, Horsetail Extract, Saw Palmetto Berry, Smilax Extract, Siberian Ginseng Extract, Standardized Panax Ginseng Extract & Rutin.

Hair, Skin & Nails for Women **-** Futurebiotics
Three tablets contain: Vitamin A (Beta Carotene) 10,000 IU • Vitamin C 120 mg • Thiamin (B1) 10 mg • Riboflavin 10 mg • Niacinamide 50 mg • Calcium 600 mg • Iron (Amino Acid Chelate) 6 mg • Vitamin D (Fish Liver Oil) 200 IU • Vitamin E (Natural Mixed Tocopherols) 30 IU • Vitamin B6 (Pyridoxine) 10 mg • Folic Acid 400 mcg • Vitamin B12 16 mcg • Phosphorus 300 mg • Iodine (Kelp) 225 mcg • Magnesium (Oxide) 200 mg • Zinc (Gluconate) 15 mg • Biotin 400 mcg • Pantothenic Acid (Calcium Salt) 30 mg • Choline (Bitartrate) 150 mg • Inositol 60 mg • Para Amino Benzoic Acid (PABA) 50 mg • Selenium (Amino Acid Chelate) 25 mcg • Manganese (Amino Acid Chelate) 10 mg • Ribonucleic Acid (RNA) 60 mg • Bioflavonoids 50 mg • Rutin 25 mg • Betaine HCl 50 mg • In a base containing L-Cysteine, L-Methionine, Gelatin, Papain, Oat Straw, Echinacea, Horsetail, Asparagus.

Hair, Skin & Nails Formula w/2500 mcg Biotin - GNC Women's **-** GNC
Two tablets contain: Vitamin A (as retinyl acetate) 5000 IU • Vitamin C (as ascorbic acid) 120 mg • Vitamin D (as cholecalciferol) 200 IU • Vitamin E (as d-alpha tocopheryl succinate) 60 IU • Thiamin B1 (as thiamin mononitrate) 1.5 mg • Riboflavin B2 (vitamin B2) 1.7 mg • Niacin B3 (as niacinamide) 20 mg • Folate (folic acid, folacin) 200 mcg • Biotin 2500 mcg • Calcium (as calcium citrate malate) 200 mg • Phosphorus (as dicalcium phosphate) 100 mg • Zinc (as zinc oxide) 15 mg • Boron (as boron citrate) 1 mcg • MSM (methylsulfonylmethane) 100 mg • Hydrolyzed Gelatin 100 mg • L-Cysteine 100 mg • L-Methionine 50 mg • Horsetail Rush Herb Extract (equisetum arvense) 2 mg • Lutein 500 mcg. Other Ingredients: Cellulose, Titanium Dioxide (natural mineral whitener), Vegetable Acetoglycerides, Chlorophyllin.

Hair, Skin, & Nails **-** Health Smart Vitamins
Each capsule contains: Vitamin A (as beta carotene) 5,000 IU • MSM (methylsulfonylmethane) 233 mg • Tea green leaf (50% polyphenols, 60 mg) 120 mg • Horsetail stem (7% silica, 3.15 mg) 45 mg • Gotu Kola whole plant (10% triterpenes, 4 mg) 40 mg • Blueberry fruit (5% anthocyanins, 1.5 mg) 30 mg • Dandelion root 10 mg.

Hangover Relief **-** Hangover Solutions Inc.
Each tablet contains: Sodium (carbonates) 333 mg • Magnesium (oxide) 20 mg • Vitamin C (ascorbic acid) 200 mg • Vitamin B-1 4.5 mg • Vitamin B-2 5.1 mg • Niacinamide 60 mg • Pantothenic Acid (d-calcium pantothenate) 30 mg • Vitamin B-6 (pyridoxine) 6 mg • Vitamin B-12 18 mcg • Biotin 200 mcg • Folic Acid 400 mcg • Choline (bitartrate) 100 mg • Inositol 1 mg • PABA 1 mg • Acerola Cherry extract 50 mg • Ginger extract 50 mg • White Willow Bark 100 mg • L-Glutamine 600 mg • Yerba Mate 50 mg. Other Ingredients: Citric Acid, Sorbitol, Natural Orange Flavor, Acosulfame Potassium, Canola Oil, Docusate Sodium.

Hapizen Daytime Formula **-** Newtell, Inc.
Each capsule contains: Proprietary Blend 200 mg: Valerian root, Hops, Catnip, Passionflower, Chamomile.

Hapizen Nighttime Formula **-** Newtell, Inc.
Each capsule contains: Proprietary Blend 250 mg: Passionflower, Hops, Catnip, L-Valine, L-Tyrosine, White Willow bark, Inositol.

Happy Camper **-** Natural Balance
Two capsules contain: Proprietary blend 840 mg: Passion Flower • Kava Kava • Siberian Ginseng • Gotu Kola • Schisandra • Wood Betony • Lavender.

Harmonex - SunSource **-** Chattem, Inc.
Each caplet contains: Standardized St. John's Wort flower extract (0.3% hypericin) 450 mg • Standardized Siberian Ginseng root extract (0.8% eleutherosides) 90 mg. Other Ingredients: Microcrystalline Cellulose, Croscarmellose Sodium, Hydroxypropyl Methylcellulose, Sodium Carboxymethyl Cellulose, Magnesium Stearate, Dextrin, Dextrose, Mineral oil, Polyethylene Glycol, Caramel, Polysorbate 80, Propylene Glycol, Riboflavin, Silicon Dioxide, Sodium Citrate, Titanium Dioxide.

HAS Original Formula **-** Nature's Way
Two capsules contain: Proprietary Formula: Brigham Tea herb • Burdock root • Cayenne pepper fruit • Cleavers herb • Elecampane • Goldenseal root • Marshmallow root • Parsley herb • Rosemary herb. Other Ingredients: Gelatin.

Hawaiian Noni Juice **-** Youngevity
Purified Water • Morinda citrifolia • Lecithin • Potassium Sorbate • Artificial Flavoring • Vilcabamba Mineral Essence: Potassium, Calcium, Magnesium, Zinc, Chromium, Selenium, Iron, Copper, Molybdenum, Vanadium, Iodine, Cobalt, Manganese.

Hawthorn **-** PhysioLogics
Each capsule contains: Hawthorn leaf, flower extract (crataegus oxyacantha, standardized to contain 2% vitexin, 3 mg) 150 mg. Other Ingredients: Maltodextrin, Gelatin, Vegetable Magnesium Stearate, Silica.

Hawthorn **-** Pharmanex
Each capsule contains: Hawthorn flowers & leaves (5.5:1) extract (Crategus oxyacantha) 125 mg. Other Ingredients: Rice Flour, Gelatin.

Hawthorn **-** Leiner Health Products
Each caplet contains: Hawthorn extract (Crataegus spp.) leaves and flowers 250 mg. Other Ingredients: Calcium Carbonate, Glucose, Cellulose, Maltodextrin, Silicon Dioxide, Hydroxypropyl Methylcellulose, Polyethylene Glycol 3350, Croscarmellose Sodium, Pharmaceutical Glaze, Crospovidone, Magnesium Stearate, Hydroxypropyl Cellulose, Red 40 Lake, Polysorbate 80, Titanium Dioxide, Povidone.

Hawthorn Phytosome **-** Enzymatic Therapy/PhytoPharmica
Two capsules contain: Hawthorn leaf/flower phytosome (crataegus oxyacantha) bound to Phosphatidylcholine 200 mg. Other Ingredients: Cellulose, Gelatin, Magnesium Stearate, Silicon Dioxide, Titanium Dioxide Color.

Hawthorne - Factor VR25 **-** Jamieson
Each caplet contains: Hawthorne Flower 1250 mg.

Hay Relief **-** Rainbow Light
Each caplet contains: Nettle tops 260 mg • Golden seal rhizome and root powder 40 mg • Licorice root 40 mg • Lemon thyme herb 30 mg • Dong Quai root 20 mg • Eyebright herb 8 mg. Other Ingredients: Cellulose or Gum Arabic, Vegetable Stearin, and Silica.

Hazelnut - Revival **-** Physicians Laboratories
Eight fluid ounces contain: Certified Isoflavone 15 mg. Other Ingredients: Whole Roasted Soybeans, Natural and Artificial Flavors.

H-Complex **-** Progressive Labs
Each capsule contains: Vitamin E 15 IU • Stone root (Collinsonia canadensis) 400 mg • Comfrey root (Symphytum officinale) 50 mg • Bayberry bark (Myrica cerifera) 50 mg • Goldenseal root (Hydrastis canadensis) 40 mg • Green Beet leaf powder 25 mg • Betony (Betonica officinalis) 10 mg.

HDT Andros-D 100 **-** Human Development Technologies (HDT)
Each capsule contains: Androstenedione 100 mg • Zinc 15 mg • Bioperine 2.5 mg.
See Editor's Note No. 47, page 2058.

HDT GLX-37.5 - Human Development Technologies (HDT)
Each capsule contains: Vanadyl Sulfate (yielding 7.5 mg elemental Vanadium) 37.5 mg • Taurine 600 mg • Magnesium 200 mg • Selenium 33 mcg • Ginger 20 mg • Cinnamon 20 mg • Chromium Picolinate 200 mcg.

Head Relief - Now
Two capsules contain: Feverfew leaf (Tanacetum parthenium) (min. 0.9% Parthenolide) 400 mg • Kava root extract (Piper methysticum) (30% Kavalactones) 100 mg • Ginger root extract (Zingiber officinale) 5% standardized 50 mg • Proprietary Blend of extracts 50 mg: Purple Willow Bark (Salix purpurea), Meadow Sweet (Filipendula ulmaria), Wintergreen (Gaultheria procumbens) to 25% standardized salicin content.

Headacha - HerbaSway
Ginkgo Biloba • Dong Quai • Ginger • Kudzu • Bupleurum • Coptis • Blackberry • HerbaSwee (Cucurbitaceae fruit).

Headache - Hyland's
Two tablets contain: Iris Versicolor 3X • Gelsemium Sempervirens 3X • Ipecac 3X • Belladonna 6X. Base: Lactose USP.
See Editor's Note No. 1, page 2053.

Headache Relief - New Chapter, Inc.
Each capsule contains: Feverfew stem, leaf & flower, supercritical extract (1% parthenolide- 1.25 mg) 125 mg • Green Tea leaf extract (50% polyphenols- 50 mg) (7% caffeine) 100 mg • Wintergreen leaf extract, salicylic acid derivatives 75 mg • Ginger (rhizome) certified organic (minimum 20% pungent compounds- 10 mg, 4% zingiberene- 2 mg) 50 mg • Meadowsweet herb, extract, salicylic acid derivatives 38 mg • Purple Willow bark (Salix purpurea) extract salicylic acid derivatives 38 mg • California Poppy whole plant, extract 5:1(leaf & essential oil), supercritical extract (23% total phenolic antioxidants - 2.3 mg) 20 mg • Rosemary leaf & essential oil, supercritical extract (23% total phenolic antioxidants - 2.3 mg) 10 mg • Ginger rhizome, certified organic (post - supercritical ethanolic extract) (3% pungent compounds - 0.3 mg) 10 mg • Lavender flower, supercritical extract (25% linalool - 2.5 mg) 10 mg • Hops strobiles, supercritical extract (35% humulones - 1.7 mg) (12% lupulones - 0.6 mg) 5 mg • Valerian root (Valeriana officinalis & Valerians mexicanus) supercritical extract (60% valepotrates - 3 mg) 5 mg. Other Ingredients: Olive Oil certified organic, Yellow Beeswax, Gelatin, Vegetable Glycerine, Purified Water, Carob.

Headache Remedy - Lehning Laboratories
Ruta graveolens 8X • Argentum nitricum 6X • Digitalis purpurea 6X • Cimicifuga racemosa 4X • Gelsemium sempervirens 4X • Sanguinaria canadensis 4X • Chelidonium majus 3X • Cyclamen europaeum 3X • Iris versicolor 3X • Melilotus 3X. In a base of 40% USP alcohol by volume.
See Editor's Note No. 1, page 2053.

Headache Remedy - PhytoPharmica
Twenty drops contain: Ruta graveolens 8x • Argentum nitricum 6x • Digitalis purpurea 6x • Cimicifuga racemosa 4x • Gelsemium sempervirens 4x • Sanguinaria canadensis 4x • Chelidonium majus 3x • Cyclamen europaeum 3x • Iris versicolor 3x • Melilotus 3x. In a base of 40% USP alcohol by volume.
See Editor's Note No. 1 and No. 21.

Headmed - Baywood International
Each capsule contains: Riboflavin (Vitamin B2) 850 mg • Proprietary Blend 275 mg: Petasites Hybridus extract (40:1), Ginkgo Biloba leaf.

Heal-All Salve - Blessed Herbs
Goldenseal root • Heal-All • Comfrey root • German Chamomile flower • Plantain leaf • Echinacea Angustifolia root • Yarrow flower • Gotu Kola • St. John's Wort flower • Calendula flower • Organic Cold-Pressed Olive oil & Essential oil of Lavender.

Health Fitness - Vidafit
Each serving contains: Folate 300 mcg • Niacin 16 mg • Pantothenic Acid 5 mg • Riboflavin 1.3 mg • Thiamine 1.2 mg • Vitamin A 3300 mg • Vitamin B12 2.4 mcg • Vitamin B6 1.3 mg • Vitamin C 75 mg • Vitamin D 200 IU • Vitamin E 10 IU • Calcium 500 mg • Chromium 50 mcg • Copper 1 mg • Iodine 150 mcg • Magnesium 420 mg • Phosphorus 500 mg • Potassium 100 mg • Selenium 50 mcg • Zinc 15 mg • Whey Protein 2 grams.

Health Pak - Optimum Nutrition
Each pak (4 capsules) contains: Vitamin A (as Betatene natural mixed carotenoids) 25,000 IU • Vitamin C (as ascorbic acid) 1000 mg • Vitamin D (as cholecalciferol) 400 IU • Vitamin E (as D-alpha tocopherol succinate) 400 IU • Thiamin (as thiamin hydrochloride) 50 mg • Riboflavin 50 mg • Niacin (as niacinamide) 50 mg • Vitamin B6 (as pyridoxine hydrochloride) 50 mg • Folic Acid 400 mcg • Vitamin B12 (as cyanocobalamin) 50 mcg • Biotin 300 mcg • Pantothenic Acid (as D-calcium pantothenate) 50 mg • Calcium (as calcium carbonate, citrate) 500 mg • Iron (as ferrous fumarate) 5 mg • Iodine (as kelp) 5 mg • Magnesium (as magnesium oxide, aspartate) 250 mg • Zinc (as zinc picolinate) 15 mg • Selenium (as selenomethionine) 200 mcg • Copper (as copper AA chelate) 1 mg • Manganese (as manganese gluconate) 5 mg • Chromium (as chromium GTF) 100 mcg • Molybdenum (as molybdenum AA chelate) 250 mcg • Potassium (as potassium citrate, aspartate) 50 mg • Choline (as choline bitartrate) 50 mg • Inositol 50 mg • PABA (as para-aminobenzoic acid) 50 mg • Alpha-Carotene 467 mcg • Zeaxanthin 97 mcg • Cryptoxanthin 119 mcg • Lutein 76 mcg. Other Ingredients: Gelatin, Magnesium Stearate, Silica.

HealthPak 100 - AM Packet - USANA Health Sciences
Each packet contains: Vitamin A (as Beta Carotene) 10000 IU • Vitamin C (as Calcium, Potassium, Magnesium, and Zinc Ascorbates) 1166 mg • Vitamin D (Vitamin D3 as Cholecalciferol) 350 IU • Vitamin E (as D-Alpha Tocopheryl Succinate) 300 IU • Vitamin K (as Phylloquinone) 40 mcg • Thiamine (as Thiamine HCl) 18 mg • Riboflavin 18 mg • Niacin (as Niacin and Niacinamide) 26.6 mg • Vitamin B6 (as Pyridoxine HCl) 18 mg • Folate (as Folic Acid) 666 mcg • Vitamin B12 (as Cyanocobalamin) 40 mcg • Biotin 200 mcg • Pantothenic Acid (as D-Calcium Pantothenate) 60 mg • Calcium (as Calcium Citrate) 225 mg • Iodine (as Potassium Iodide) 75 mcg • Magnesium (as Magnesium Citrate, Amino Acid Chelate) 190 mg • Zinc (as Zinc Citrate) 6.7 mg • Selenium (as L-Selenomethionine and Amino Acid Complex) 67 mcg • Copper (as Amino Acid Chelate) 1 mg • Manganese (as Manganese Gluconate) 1.7 mg • Chromium (as Chromium Picolinate and Polynicotinate) 100 mcg • Molybdenum (as Molybdenum Citrate) 16.7 mcg • Bioflavonoid Complex: Rutin, Quercetin, Hesperidin (Citrus SPP. L.) Fruit, Green Tea Extract - Decaffeinated (Camellia Sinensis Hunt)(Leaves), Bilberry Extract (Vaccinium Myrtillus L.) Fruit 129 mg • Inositol 100 mg • Choline Bitartrate 66.6 mg • N-Acetyl-L-Cysteine 43.4 mg • Bromelain 33.4 mg • Alpha Lipoic Acid 10 mg • Coenzyme Q10 8 mg • Turmeric Extract (Curcuma Longal)Root 10 mg • Glutathione 6.6 mg • Broccoli Concentrate (Brassica Oleracea V. Botrytis L.) Flower 10 mg • Lutein (Tagetes Erecta L., Flower) 400 mcg • Lycopene 700 mcg • Boron (as Boron Citrate) 1.33 mg • Silicon (as Amino Acid Complex) 3.25 • Vanadium (as Vanadyl Sulfate) 10 mcg • Ultra Trace Minerals 1 mg • Grape Seed Extract 90 mg • Olive Extract (Olea Europaea L., Fruit) 20 mg. Other Ingredients: Microcrystalline Cellulose, Pregelatinized Starch, Croscarmellose Sodium, Ascorbyl Palmitate, Dextrin, Collodial Silicon Dioxide, Dextrose.

HealthPak 100 - PM Pack - USANA Health Sciences
Each packet contains: Vitamin A (as Beta Carotene) 5000 IU • Vitamin C (as Calcium, Potassium, Magnesium, and Zinc Ascorbates) 433 mg • Vitamin D (Vitamin D3 as Cholecalciferol) 350 IU • Vitamin E (as D-Alpha Tocopheryl Succinate) 300 IU • Vitamin K (as Phylloquinone) 20 mcg • Thiamine (as Thiamine HCL) 9 mg • Riboflavin 9 mg • Niacin (as Niacin and Niacinamide) 13.3 mg • Vitamin B6 (as Pyridoxine HCl) 9 mg • Folate (as Folic Acid) 333 mcg • Vitamin B12 (as Cyanocobalamin) 20 mcg • Biotin 100 mcg •

Pantothenic Acid (as D-Calcium Pantothenate) 30 mg • Calcium (as Calcium Citrate) 315 mg • Iodine (as Potassium Iodide) 150 mcg • Magnesium (as Magnesium Citrate, Amino Acid Chelate) 290 mg • Zinc (as Zinc Citrate)13.4 mg • Selenium (as L-Selenomethionine and Amino Acid Complex) 134 mcg • Copper (as Amino Acid Chelate) 2 mg • Manganese (as Manganese Gluconate) 3.4 mg • Chromium (as Chromium Picolinate and Polynicotinate) 200 mcg • Molybdenum (as Molybdenum Citrate) 33.4 mcg • Bioflavonoid Complex: Rutin, Quercetin, Hesperidin (Citrus SPP. L.) Fruit, Green Tea Extract - Decaffeinated (Camellia Sinensis Hunt)(Leaves), Bilberry Extract (Vaccinium Myrtillus L.) Fruit 90 mg • Inositol 50 mg • Choline Bitartrate 33.3 mg • N-Acetyl L-Cysteine 21.7 mg • Bromelain 16.7 mg • Alpha Lipoic Acid 5 mg • Coenzyme Q10 4 mg • Turmeric Extract (Curcuma Longal)Root 130 mg • Glutathione 3.3 mg • Broccoli Concentrate (Brassica Oleracea V. Botrytis L.) Flower 5 mg • Lutein (Tagetes Erecta L., Flower) 200 mcg • Lycopene 350 mcg • Resveratrol (Polygonum Cuspidatum Sieb. & Zucc., Root and Rhizome) 1000 mcg • Rosemary Extract (Rosmarinus Officinalis L., Leaves) 50 mg • Boron (as Boron Citrate) 2.33 mg • Silicon (as Amino Acid Complex) 4.25 • Vanadium (as Vanadyl Sulfate) 20 mcg • Ultra Trace Minerals 2 mg • Olive Extract (Olea Europaea L., fruit) 10 mg. Other Ingredients: Microcrystalline Cellulose, Pregelatinized Starch, Croscarmellose Sodium, Ascorbyl Palmitate, Dextrin, Collodial Silicon Dioxide, Dextrose.

HealthSmiles **-** Health Smart Vitamins
Two tablets contain: Vitamin A (as beta-carotene) 5,000 IU • Vitamin C (as ascorbic acid) 60 mg • Vitamin D (as ergocalciferol) 400 IU • Vitamin E (d-alpha tocopheryl acetate) 30 IU • Thiamin (as thiamin HCl) 1.5 mg • Riboflavin 1.7 mg • Niacin (as niacinamide) 20 mg • Vitamin B6 (as pyridoxine HCl) 2 mg • Folate (as folic acid) 10 mcg • Vitamin B12 (cyanocobalamin) 6 mcg • Biotin 50 mcg • Pantothenic acid (as calcium pantothenate) 10 mg • Calcium (as calcium amino acid chelate) 20 mg • Iron (as iron amino acid chelate) 5 mg • Iodine (from kelp) 100 mcg • Magnesium (as magnesium amino acid chelate) 10 mg • Zinc (as zinc amino acid chelate) 3 mg • Copper (as copper amino acid chelate) 50 mcg • Manganese (as maganese amino acid chelate) 50 mcg • Potassium (as potassium amino acid chelate) 1 mg • Apple fruit 50 mg • Papaya fruit 50 mg • Pineapple fruit 50 mg • Lemon Bioflavonoids 20 mg • Spirulina 20 mg • Sunflower oil seed 20 mg • Rice bran 10 mg • Beet Greens leaf 5 mg • Broccoli aerial parts 5 mg • Brown rice 5 mg • Carrot root 5 mg • Dog Rose (rose hips) 5 mg • Mango fruit 5 mg • Spinach leaf 5 mg • West Indian Cherry (fruit, Malpighia pruncifolia) 5 mg • Para-aminobenzoic acid (PABA) 400 mcg • Choline (as choline bitartrate) 10 mcg • Inositol 10 mcg.

Healthy Antioxidants **-** Health Smart Vitamins
Three tablets contain: Vitamin A (as beta-carotene) 20,000 IU • Vitamin C (ascorbic acid) 60 mg • Vitamin E (as d-alpha tocopheryl acetate) 30 IU • Calcium (as dicalcium phosphate) 3.5 mg • Selenium (as selenomethionine) 60 mcg • Garlic bulb (>=10,000 mcg allicin/g, >=4 mg) 400 mg • Tomato fruit (1% lycopene, 3 mg) 300 mg • Oregano leaf 150 mg • Rosemary leaf (>=6% carnosic acid, >=9 mg) 150 mg.

Healthy Cells Breast **-** Enzymatic Therapy/PhytoPharmica
Each tablet contains: Folic Acid 200 mcg • Vitamin B12 (cyanocobalamin) 500 mcg • Calcium D-Glucarate 200 mg • Iodine (as potassium iodide) 213 mcg • Broccoli floret and stalk concentrate (brassica oleracea, standardized to contain a minimum of 125 mcg sulforaphane) 125 mg • Green Tea (camellia sinensis) leaf extract (decaffeinated; standardized to contain a minimum of 70% polyphenols) 50 mg • Maitake mushroom powder (grifola frondosa) 50 mg • Maitake mushroom extract (grifola frondosa, standardized to contain a minimum of 28% D-fraction compound) 5 mg.

Healthy Cells Prostate **-** Enzymatic Therapy/PhytoPharmica
Each tablet contains: Calcium D-Glucarate 200 mg • Selenium (L-selenomethionine) 200 mcg • Broccoli floret and stalk concentrate (brassica oleracea, standardized to contain a minimum of 125 mcg of sulforaphane) 125 mg • Green Tea leaf extract (camillia sinensis, decaffeinated) 50 mg • Maitake mushroom powder (grifola frondosa) 50 mg • Maitake mushroom extract (grifola frondosa, standardized to contain a minimum of 28% D-fraction compound) 5 mg • Lycopene 2.5 mg.

Healthy Cholesterol **-** NSI - Nutraceutical Sciences Institute
Each four capsules contain: Gamma Oryzanol 300 mg • Gugulipids (standardized for 2.5% guggul sterones) 1000 mg • Beta Sitosterol 150 mg • Green Tea extract (standardized 98% polyphenols, 80% catechins, 45% EGCG) 300 mg • Artichoke extract (standardized for 5% cynarine) 600 mg • Grape seed extract (Activinf) 200 mg • Chromium (as chromium polynicotinate, Chromemates) 400 mcg • Pantethine 450 mg • Policosanol 20 mg.

Healthy Digestion **-** Health Smart Vitamins
Each capsule contains: Digestive Enzyme Blend: Ox Bile, Protease, Amylase, Lipase, Cellulase, Bromelain, Papain 138 mg • Plant Fiber Base: Sugar Beet Fiber, Rice Bran, Beech cellulose, Spruce cellulose 77 mg.
See Editor's Note No. 14.

Healthy Eyes **-** Health Smart Vitamins
Each capsule contains: Vitamin A (as beta-carotene) 6,000 IU • Vitamin E (as dl-alpha-tocopheryl acetate) 50 IU • Zinc (as zinc citrate) 25 mg • Selenium (as selenomethionine) 40 mcg • Copper (as copper citrate) 2 mg • Bilberry fruit (36% anthocyanosides, 21.6 mg) 60 mg.

Healthy Hair, Skin, & Nails (60) **-** Rainbow Light
Each capsule contains: Beta-Carotene 5000 IU • Vitamin E natural 100 IU • Tomato Paste concentrate (Lycopene)300 mg • Vitamin C (Zinc & Copper Ascorbates) 180 mg • Rice Bran 150 mg • Inositol 150 mg • Horsetail herb 4:1 extract 150 mg • Nettles tops 4:1 extract 120 mg • Ginger rhizome 4:1 extract 120 mg • L-Cysteine 100 mg • Spirulina 100 mg • PABA (Para Aminobenzioc Acid) 75 mg • Red Pepper fruit 60 mg • Pantothenic Acid (Vitamn B5) 60 mg • Rosemary leaf 4:1 extract 50 mg • Maidenhair Fern 40 mg • Marine Mineral Complex 25 mg • Niacin (Vitamin B3) 20 mg • Zinc (Ascorbate)15 mg • Rosemary oil 3 mg • Pyridoxine (Vitamin B6) 2 mg • Biotin 1800 mcg • Copper (Ascorbate) 1500 mcg • Folic Acid 400 mcg • Cyanocobalamin (Vitamin B12) 6 mcg.

Healthy Hearing **-** Health Smart Vitamins
Each capsule contains: Vitamin B12 (as cyanocobalamin) 100 mcg • Magnesium (as magnesium aspartate) 50 mg • Black Cohosh root 50 mg • Ginkgo leaf (24% ginkgo flavonglycosides, 7.2 mg; 6% terpene lactones, 1.8 mg) 30 mg • Vinpocetine 5 mg.

Healthy Heart with Folic Acid and B6 **-** Discount, Inc.
Each tablet contains: Vitamin B6 5 mg • Pyridoxal 5 Phosphate 0.5 mg • Folic Acid 600 mcg • Folinic Acid 1 mcg.

Healthy Immunity **-** Health Smart Vitamins
Each capsule contains: Astragalus root (70% polysaccharides, 70 mg) 100 mg • Elderberry (European elder berry - 10% anthocyanins, 10 mg) 100 mg • Tea green leaf (90% polyphenols, 90 mg) 100 mg • Shiitake (Mycelia extract, LEM, fruiting body) 60 mg • Reishi mycelica 30 mg • Grifola frondosa (maitake mushroom, fruiting body) 25 mg.

Healthy Joints **-** Health Smart Vitamins
Each capsule contains: Vitamin C (ascorbic acid) 60 mg • Manganese (as manganese glycinate) 2 mg • Glucosamine Sulfate 200 mg • Chondroitin Sulfate 100 mg • Glucosamine Hydrochloride 100 mg • Sea Cucumber 100 mg.
See Editor's Note No. 15, page 2055.

Healthy Legs Horse Chestnut Seed Extract **-** Leiner Health Products
Each caplet contains: Citrus Bioflavonoids complex 15 mg • Ginger powder (Zingiber officinale) root 100 mg • Gotu Kola (Centella asiatica) leaf 33 mg • Grape Seed extract (Vitis vinifera) seed 2 mg • Horse Chestnut extract (Aesculus hippocastanum) seed 300 mg.

Other Ingredients: Dicalcium Phosphate, Hydroxypropyl Methylcellulose, Stearic Acid, Dextrin, Titanium Dioxide, Magnesium Stearate, Polyethylene Glycol 8000, Lecithin.

Healthy Liver **-** NSI - Nutraceutical Sciences Institute
Each six capsules contain: Vitamin C (as magnesium ascorbate) 750 mg • Vitamin E (as d-alpha tocopherols succinate and mixed tocopherols) 250 IU • Thiamine (vitamin B1) 500 mg • Riboflavin (vitamin B2) 10 mg • Niacinamide (vitamin B3) 100 mg • Pyridoxine HCl (vitamin B6) 50 mg • Folic Acid 800 mcg • Vitamin B12 (methylcobalamin) 2 mg • Biotin 3 mg • Pantothenic Acid (vitamin B5) 50 mg • Magnesium (as ascorbate, Ester C) 51 mg • Zinc (as Opti-Zinc) 15 mg • Selenium (selenomethionine) 400 mcg • Chromium (Chrimate, as chromium polynicotinate) 200 mg • Molybdenum (as chelate, AAC) 150 mcg • Potassium (as citrate) 99 mg • Co-enzyme Q10 30 mg • Alpha Lipoic Acid 600 mg • Milk Thistle extract (80% silymarin) 900 mg • N-Acetyl-Cysteine 300 mg • Phosphatidylcholine (LeciPC35P) 400 mg.

Healthy Meal **-** Vidafit
Each serving contains: Folate 300 mcg • Niacin 16 mg • Pantothenic Acid 5 mg • Riboflavin 1.3 mg • Thiamine 1.2 mg • Vitamin A 2600 IU • Vitamin B12 2.4 mcg • Vitamin B6 1.3 mg • Vitamin C 75 mg • Vitamin D 200 IU • Vitamin E 10 IU • Calcium 500 mg • Chromium 50 mcg • Copper 1 mg • Iodine 150 mcg • Magnesium 420 mg • Phosphorus 500 mg • Potassium 100 mg • Selenium 50 mcg • Zinc 15 mg • Capsicum 5 mg • Glucomannan 500 mg • Soy Protein 6 grams • Whey Protein 12 grams.

Healthy Mood Body Benefits Pak **-** Leiner Health Products
Each packet contains: Kava Kava extract (Piper methysticum) root 200 mg • Lecithin 45 mg • Licorice extract (Glycyrrhiza glabra) root 60 mg • Siberian Ginseng extract (Eleutherococcus senticosus) root 150 mg • Siberian Ginseng powder (Eleutherococcus senticosus) root 45 mg • St. John's Wort extract (Hypericum perforatum) aerial parts 900 mg. Other Ingredients: Cellulose, Dicalcium Phosphate, Calcium Carbonate, Croscarmellose Sodium, Silicon Dioxide, Stearic Acid, Maltodextrin, Magnesium.

Healthy Prostate **-** Health Smart Vitamins
Each softgel contains: Saw Palmetto berry (85-95% fatty acids and sterols, 136-152 mg)160 mg • Pygeum africanum bark (>13% total sterols, >6.5 mg) 50 mg • Pumpkin seed oil 40 mg.

Healthy Snack **-** Vidafit
Each serving contains: Folate 300 mcg • Niacin 16 mg • Pantothenic Acid 5 mg • Riboflavin 1.3 mg • Thiamine 1.2 mg • Vitamin A 2600 IU • Vitamin B12 2.4 mcg • Vitamin B6 1.3 mg • Vitamin C 75 mg • Vitamin D 200 IU • Vitamin E 10 IU • Calcium 500 mg • Chromium 50 mcg • Copper 1 mg • Iodine 150 mcg • Magnesium 420 mg • Phosphorus 500 mg • Potassium 100 mg • Selenium 50 mcg • Zinc 15 mg • Capsicum 5 mg • Glucomannan 300 mg • Soy Protein 3 grams • Whey Protein 6 grams.

Healthy Soy Chocolate **-** Nature's Life
Each scoop (35 g) contains: Supro Soy Protein Isolate (with less than 2% Lecithin) • Rice Syrup Solids • Fructose • Cocoa powder (with less than 2% Lecithin) • Fructooligosaccharides • Magnesium Citrate • Calcium Carbonate • Glycine • Apple Pectin • Ascorbic Acid • d-Alpha Tocopherol Acetate • Zinc Citrate • Niacinamide • Copper Gluconate • d-Calcium Pantothenate • Manganese Gluconate • Vitamin A Palmitate • l-Selenomethionine • Cholecalciferol • Chromium Niacinate • Pyridoxine HCl • Thiamine Mononitrate • Riboflavin • Folic Acid • Biotin • Potassium Iodide • Sodium Selenite • Sodium Molybdate • Cyanocobalamin.

Healthy Soy Formula **-** Health Smart Vitamins
Each capsule contains: Soy bean (10% isoflavones, 30 mg) 300 mg • Red Clover aerial parts (8% isoflavones, 16 mg) 200 mg.

Healthy Soy Vanilla **-** Nature's Life
Each scoop (33 g) contains: Supro Soy Protein Isolate (with less than 2% lecithin) • Maltodextrin • Rice Syrup Solids • Fructose • Fructooligosaccharides • Magnesium Citrate • Calcium Carbonate • Glycine • Apple Pectin • natural Flavors • Ascorbic Acid • d-Alpha Tocopherol Acetate • Zinc Citrate • Niacinamide • Copper Gluconate • d-Calcium Pantothenate • Manganese Gluconate • Vitamin A Palmitate • l-Selenomethionine • Cholecalciferol • Chromium Niacinate • Pyridoxine HCl • Thiamine Mononitrate • Riboflavin • Folic Acid • Biotin • Potassium Iodide • Sodium Selenite • Sodium Molybdate • Cyanocobalamin.

Healthy Vein Support **-** Health Smart Vitamins
Each capsule contains: Vitamin C (ascorbic acid) 50 mg • Horse Chestnut aerial parts (15% escin, 33.75 mg) 225 mg • Butcher's Broom root (10% ruscogennis, 16.7 mg) 167 mg • Rutin 90 mg • Hesperidin (35% bioflavonoids, 26.25 mg) 75 mg.

Healthy Weight **-** Health Smart Vitamins
Two capsules contain: Calcium (as calcium salt of hydroxy citric acid) 79 mg • Chromium (as chromium picolinate) 100 mcg • Garcinia cambogia fruit (50% (-) hydroxy citric acid [HCA], 250 mg) 500 mg • L-carnitine (as L-carnitine tartrate) 166 mg.

Healthy Whey **-** Nature's Life
Three tablespoons (or each rounded scoop, 23 g) contain: Whey Protein concentrate • Natural Flavor composed of Di, Tri, Oligo & Polypeptides (providing 58% B-lactoglobulin, 22% A-Lactalbumin, 10% Immunoglobulin, 10% Minor Proteins & Lactoferrin).

Healthy Woman Soy Menopause **-** Personal Products
Each tablet contains: Soy Standardized extract 320 mg • Includes Isoflavones 55 mg.

HearAll **-** NaturalCare
Two capsules contain: Thiamine (B1, as thiamine mononitrate) 1.5 mg • Riboflavin (B2) 1.7 mg • Niacin (B3, as inositol hexanicinate, non-flush) 20 mg • Vitamin B6 (as pyridoxine HCl) 2 mg • Folic Acid 800 mcg • Vitamin B12 (as methylcobalamin) 500 mcg • Magnesium (as amino acid chelate) 93 mg • Zinc (as amino acid chelate) 10 mg • Proprietary Blend 415 mg: Acetyl L-Carnitine, N-Acetylcysteine, Butcher's Broom root (at 10% ruscogenin), Ginkgo Biloba leaf (at 24% flavoglycosides/6% terpenes), Vinpocetine, CoQ10, Alpha Lipoic Acid. Other Ingredients: Gelatin, Purified Water, Glycerin, Titanium Dioxide.

Heart Actives **-** VitaStore
Six tablets contain: Coenzyme Q-10 5 mg • Chitosan 500 mg • Hawthorne 200 mg • Chromium 100 mcg • Green Tea Extract 200 mg • Fiber Complex (Oat Bran & Psyllium) 1000 mg • Lecithin 500 mg • Vitamin B3 (Niacin) 50 mg • Calcium 500 mg • L-Carnitine 250 mg • Ginger 200 mg • EFA Complex (Essential Fatty Acids) 500 mg • Selenium 150 mcg • Vitamin B1 (Thiamine) 1.5 mg.

Heart Bran **-** Gero Vita International
Three capsules contain: OatVantage 50% Oat Beta-Glucan 1.5 g • Blue-Max Vaccinium Angustifolium extract 90 mg • Bil-Max Vaccinium Myrtillus 90 mg • Grape-Max Vitis labrusco 90 mg • Apple-Max Mallus Pumila 90 mg. Other Ingredients: Gelatin, Rice Flour, Magnesium Stearate, Silicon Dioxide, Titanium Dioxide.

Heart Essentials **-** Health Smart Vitamins
Two caplets contain: Vitamin A (as 83% beta-carotene, 17% palmitate) 15,000 IU • Vitamin C (as ascorbic acid) 250 mg • Vitamin D (as cholecalciferol) 400 IU • Vitamin E (as d-alpha tocopheryl) 400 IU • Thiamin (as thiamin mononitrate) 25 mg • Riboflavin 25 mg • Niacin (as 50% nicotinic acid, 50% niacinamide) 50 mg • Vitamin B6 (as pyridoxine HCl) 25 mg • Folate (folic acid) 400 mcg • Vitamin B12 (as cyanocobalamin) 100 mcg • Biotin 300 mcg • Pantothenic Acid (as calcium pantothenate) 25 mg • Calcium (as 71% calcium carbonate, 24% dicalcium phosphate, 5% mixed calcium complexes) 269 mg • Phosphorus (as dicalcium phosphate) 10 mg • Iodine (as potassium iodide) 150 mcg • Magnesium (as 90% magnesium oxide, 5% magnesium citrate, 5% magnesium glycinate) 100 mg • Zinc (as zinc ascorbate) 15 mg • Selenium (as selenomethionine) 100 mcg • Copper (as copper citrate) 2 mg • Manganese (as manganese

gluconate) 2 mg • Chromium (as chromium polynicotinate) 200 mcg • Molybdenum (as molybdenum amino acid chelate) 50 mcg • Potassium (as potassium citrate) 99 mg • Chondroitin Sulfate 50 mg • Betaine HCl 25 mg • Bioflavonoids 25 mg • Choline (as bitartrate) 25 mg • Garlic bulb (250 mcg allicin) 25 mg • Hawthorn leaf, flower (1.8% vitexin - 2" - rhamnoside) 0.45 mg • Inositol 25 mg • L-Carnitine 25 mg • Lecithin (from soybean) 25 mg • Bromelain (from pineapple, 6,000 PU/g, 120 PU) 20 mg • Coenzyme Q10 10 mg • Lipase (from fermentation of Aspergillus niger) 10 mg • Alpha Lipoic acid 10 mg • Papain (from latex of fruit) 10 mg • Para-aminobenzoic acid (PABA) 10 mg • Rutin 5 mg • Boron (as boron asparate) 2 mg • Silicon (as silicon dioxide) 2 mg • Vanadium (as vanadium amino acid chelate) 10 mcg.
See Editor's Note No. 15, page 2055.

Heart Essentials **-** Swanson
Each tablet contains: Vitamin C (as ascorbic acid) 100 mg • Vitamin E (as d-alpha tocopheryl succinate) 33.3 IU • Niacin 9 mg • Vitamin B-6 (as pyridoxine HCl) 17 mg • Folic Acid 135 mcg • Vitamin B-12 (as cyanocobalamin) 33.3 mcg • Calcium (from amino acid chelate) 33.3 mg • Magnesium (from amino acid chelate) 33.3 mg • Selenium (as selenomethionine) 50 mcg • Chromium (ChromeMate™) 33 mcg • Potassium (from amino acid chelate) 33 mg • Taurine 100 mg • Trimethylglycine 84 mg • Odor-Controlled Garlic bulb (PureGar® 10,000 ppm allicin potential) 34 mg • Hawthorn berry extract (1.8% vitexin-2' rhamnosides) 17 mg • L-Carnitine 17 mg • Lecithin 17 mg • Coenzyme Q10 10 mg • Ginger root extract (5% gingerols) 8.4 mg.

Heart Formula **-** Nature's Way
Two capsules contain: Betaine Anhydrous 200 mg • Coenzyme Q10 (Ubiquinone) 15 mg • Folic Acid (Folate) 300 mc • Hawthorne dried extract (1.8%-2.2% Vitexin) 350 mg • Niacin (Vitamin B3) 20 mg • Potassium (Aspartate, Chloride) 20 mg • Pyridoxine HCL 50 mg • Reishi dried extract (10% Polysaccharides) 25 mg • Siberian Ginseng root 250 mg • Vitamin B12 (Cyanocobalamin) 400 mcg • Vitamin E (d-Alpha Tocopheryl) 50 IU. Other Ingredients: Gelatin, Magnesium Stearate, Millet.

Heart Health Essential Omega III **-** Market America, Inc.
Two capsules contain: 100% Natural Vitamin E (D-alpha tocopherol) 15 IU • Fish Body Oil (50% purity) 3000 mg: EPA (eicosapentaenoic omega-3 fatty acid) 900 mg, DHA (docosahexaenoic omega-3 fatty acid) 600 mg. Other Ingredients: Gelatin, Glycerin, Natural Lemon Flavor.

Heart Health LipiTrim Ultra **-** Market America, Inc.
Two capsules contain: Tocotrienol Complex (from 167 mg NuTriene 30% tocotrienol oil) 50 mg • Policosanol (from 11.2 mg Marcosanol 90% policosanol complex) 10 mg. Other Ingredients: Soybean Oil, Gelatin, Glycerin, Soy Lecithin, Beeswax, Chlorophyll, Titanium Dioxide.

Heart Health TriActive **-** Market America, Inc.
Two tablets contain: Thiamin (vitamin B1 as thiamin mononitrate) 2.6 mg • Riboflavin (vitamin B2) 3 mg • Niacin (vitamin B3 as niacinamide) 25 mg • Pantothenic Acid (vitamin B5 as calcium D-pantothenate) 12.5 mg • Vitamin B6 (as pyridoxine hydrochloride) 15 mg • Vitamin B12 (as cyanocobalamin) 500 mcg • Biotin 150 mcg • Folate (as Metafolin) 300 mcg • Zinc (as zinc oxide) 7.5 mg • Garlic (allium sativum, minimum 1% allicin) 450 mg • Beta-Sitosterol (from 637.5 mg 40% beta-sitosterol plant sterols, as Cholestatin) 250 mg • Hawthorn berry 75 mg • Cassia Nomame (minimum 6% flavonoids) 50 mg • Guggulsterones (from 95% guggulsterones granules) 5 mg. Other Ingredients: Calcium Carbonate, Croscarmellose Sodium, Calcium Silicate, Microcrystalline Cellulose, Magnesium Stearate, Crospovidone, Dextrose, Hydroxypropylmethyl Cellulose, Colloidal Silicon Dioxide, Carnauba Wax, Vegetable Acetoglycerides, Polyethylene Glycol, Polysorbate 80.

Heart Power **-** Gero Vita International
Each capsule contains: Acetyl-L-carnitine 500 mg • Coenzyme Q10 100 mg • Alpha Lipoic Acid 50 mg. Other Ingredients: Gelatin, Silicon Dioxide, Magnesium Stearate.

Heart ReNew **-** Now
Each 2 tbsp serving contains: Thiamine (vitamin B1 from thiamine HCl) 3 mg • Riboflavin (vitamin B2) 3 mg • Niacin (vitamin B3 from inositol nicotinate, flush-free) 100 mg • Vitamin B6 (from pyridoxine HCl) 3 mg • Folate (as folic acid) 400 mcg • Vitamin B12 (as cyanocobalamin) 20 mcg • Pantothenic Acid (vitamin B5 from calcium d-pantothenate) 10 mg • Calcium 20 mg • Sodium 35 mg • Potassium 210 mg • Soy based Phospholipids 10 g (typically provides phosphtidylcholine 2.2 g, phosphatidylethanolamine 2 g, phosphatidylinositol 1.4 g, other phospholipids 1.5 g) • Choline 300 mg • Inositol (from phospholipids/inositol nicotinate) 240 mg • Soy Protein isolate (non-GE) 4 g • L-Carnitine (from L-carnitine tartrate) 500 mg • Trimethylglycine (TMG) 40 mg • Stevia Rebaudiana leaf extract (standardized to min. 80% rebaudioside A) 42 mg. Other Ingredients: Fructose, Natural Orange and Vanilla Flavors.

Heart Science **-** Source Naturals
Six tablets contain: Vitamin A (Beta Carotene) 45000 IU • Vitamin B1 (Thiamin) 50 mg • Inositol Hexanicotinate 500 mg • Vitamin B6 (Pyridoxine HCl) 25 mg • Coenzymated B6 (Pyridoxal-5'-Phosphate)(Yielding 16.9 mg of Vitamin B6) 25 mg • Vitamin B12 (Cyanocobalamin) 500 mcg • Folic Acid 800 mcg • Vitamin C (Magnesium Ascorbate) 1500 mg • Vitamin E (D-Alpha Tocopheryl) (Natural) 400 IU • Chromium (ChromeMate Polynicotinate 150 mcg and Chromium Picolinate 150 mcg) 300 mcg • Copper (Sebacate) 750 mcg • Magnesium (Ascorbate, Taurinate and Oxide) 300 mg • Potassium (Citrate) 99 mg • Selenium (L-Selenomethionine) 200 mcg • Silica (from 400 mg of Horsetail Extract) 28 mg • Coenzyme Q10 (Ubiquinone) 60 mg • L-Carnitine L-Tartrate 500 mg • Hawthorn berry extract 400 mg • Proanthodyn (grape seed extract)(with a Proanthocyanidolic Value of 95) 100 mg • L-Proline 500 mg • L-Lysine (HCl) 500 mg • N-A-G (N-Acetyl Glucosamine) 500 mg • Bromelain (2000 GDU per g) 1200 mg • Taurine (Magnesium Taurinate) 500 mg • Inositol (Hexanicotinate) 50 mg.

Heart Source Bars, Honey Nut Crunch **-** Advocare International
Rice Syrup • Crisp Rice (rice flour, malt extract, rice bran) • Toasted Rolled Oats • Peanuts • Ground Peanuts • Sesame Seeds • Glycerin • Figs • Natural Flavor • Artificial Flavor • Beta Glucan extract (from yeast) • Phytosterol • High Fructose Corn Syrup • Flax (seed) Oil • Guar Gum • Soybean Oil • Salt • Honey • Sucralose • Mixed Tocopherols (vitamin E) • L-Carnitine • Beta-Carotene • Soy Lecithin • Lipoic Acid • Folic Acid • Chromium Polynicotinate • TBHQ (added to protect flavor).

Heart Support **-** Olympia Nutrition
CoQ10 • Alpha Lipoic Acid • Garlic • Hawthorn • Cayenne • Magnesium.

Heart Support **-** Nutri-Quest Rx
Each tablet contains: Heart 100 mg • Spleen 40 mg • Co-Enzyme Q-10 2 mg • Vitamin C (Sago Palm) 100 mg • Vitamin E (Succinate) 100 IU • L-Carnitine HCL 20 mg.
See Editor's Note No. 14.

Heart Support **-** Now
Three tablets contain: Vitamin B1 (Thiamine HCL) 50 mg • Vitamin B6 (Pyridoxine HCL) 50 mg • Vitamin B12 (Cyanocobalamin) 1000 mcg • Folic Acid 800 mcg • Magnesium (Oxide/Aspartate) 200 mg • Potassium (Chloride/Aspartate) 200 mg • Iodine (Kelp extract) 300 mcg • Selenium (Selenomethionine) 140 mcg • Coenzyme Q10, pure 30 mg • L-Carnitine 400 mg • Pure-Gar Garlic 1000 mg • Hawthorne berry extract (standardized to contain 1.25% Vitexin-4' Rhamnoside) 150 mg • Alpha Lipoic Acid 20 mg • Ginger root 250 mg • Cayenne pepper (40000 Heat units) 150 mg.

Heartburn Free - Enzymatic Therapy
Each softgel contains: Orange (citrus sinesis, peel extract standardized to contain 98.5% d-limonene) 1000 mg.

HeartCare - Nature's Way
Each tablet contains: Hawthorn dried extract (19% oligomeric procyanidins) 80 mg.

HeartOption - BioImmune, Inc.
Each 20 gram scoop contains: Vitamin A (as beta-carotene) 1000 IU • Vitamin C 600 mg • Vitamin D (D3) 80 IU • Vitamin E (mixed tocopherols) 200 IU • Thiamin (vitamin B1) 20 mg • Riboflavin (vitamin B2) 20 mg • Vitamin B3 (inositol hexaniacinate) 60 mg • Vitamin B3 (niacinamide) 100 mg • Folic Acid 800 mcg • Vitamin B6 50 mg • Vitamin B12 (hydroxycobalamin) 300 mcg • Biotin 150 mcg • Pantothenic Acid (calcium) 90 mg • Calcium (gluconate) 50 mg • Magnesium (glycinate) 200 mg • Zinc (arginate) 15 mg • Selenium (methionate) 70 mcg • Manganese (citrate) 1 mg • Chromium (picolinate) 100 mcg • Molybdenum (glycinate) 50 mcg • Potassium (gluconate) 50 mg • Boron 0.5 mg • Vanadium (pentoxide) 70 mcg • Germanium Sesquioxide 25 mg • Alpha-Carotene 10 mg • Pregnenolone 5 mg • DHEA 3 mg • CoEnzyme Q10 50 mg • Cordyceps Sinensis 200 mg • Inositol 30 mg • Choline 40 mg • Para Amino Benzoic Acid 15 mg • Lecithin 600 mg • L-Alanine 76 mg • L-Arginine 400 mg • L-Aspartic Acid 204 mg • L-Carnitine 200 mg • L-Cystine 200 mg • L-Glutamic Acid 3.4 mg • L-Glycine 74 mg • L-Histidine 46 mg • L-Isoleucine 86 mg • L-Leucine 144 mg • L-Lysine 910 mg • L-Methionine 154 mg • L-Ornithine HCl 150 mg • L-Phenylalanine 92 mg • L-Proline 390 mg • L-Serine 92 mg • L-Taurine 600 mg • L-Threonine 66 mg • L-Tyrosine 66 mg • L-Tryptophan 11 mg • L-Valine 88 mg • N-Acetyl-Cysteine 50 mg • Glutathione 50 mg • Pancreatin 8X 2.5 mg • Papain 10 mg • Bromelain 25 mg • Grape Skin Extract 150 mg • Hawthorne Berry Extract 175 mg • Garlic (1% alicin) 80 mg • Tocotrienols 15 mg • Trimethyl Glycine 600 mg • Methylsulfonylmethane 50 mg • Alpha Lipoic Acid 50 mg. In a base of Oat Bran, Rice Bran, ISO Malt, Freeze-dried Pineapple, Pineapple Flavoring, Stevia, Silicon Dioxide.

Heart's Ease - The Herbalist
Hawthorn berry, leaf & flower • Dandelion root, leaf & flower • Skullcap herb • Yarrow flower • Horsetail herb • Lemon Balm herb • Prickly Ash bark • Cayenne pepper.

Heat - The Sports Nutrition Source, Inc.
Each capsule contains: Ma Huang Concentrate aerial parts 24 mg • Caffeine USP 80 mg • Guarana Concentrate seed 75 mg • White Willow Bark Concentrate 75 mg • Cayenne fruit 60 mg • Ginger root 40 mg.
See Editor's Note No. 30, page 2056.

Heavenly Skin & Hair Care - Gary Null & Associates (GNA)
Whole leaf Aloe Vera concentrate, Jojoba oil, Licorice and Grape seed extracts, Tri-Silica complex, MSM, Antioxidant Botanical extracts, Liposomal Vitamins, Oat Bran glucan, Tissue Respiratory Factor, and more.

Heavyweight Gainer 900 - Champion Nutrition
Each serving contains: Metacarb-III (branching complex carbohydrates extracted from Corn Hybrids including Maltodextrins) • Peptol-III: pre-digested highly efficient protein blend consisting of Whey Protein Concentrate, Fat-Free, Cholesterol-Free, Red-Muscle Protein Complex, Debitterized Enzyme Digest of Lactalbumin, & Egg White Protein • extra grade Whey • Fructose • low-fat Cocoa powder • MCT's • Metavite-III [Champion Nutrition's advanced Vitamin/ Mineral formula consisting of di-Calcium Pantothenate, Potassium, Citrate, Magnesium Gluconate, Potassium Chloride, Choline Bitartrate, Inositol, Ascorbic Acid, D-Calcium Pantothenate, Niacin, Zinc Gluconate, d-Alpha Tocopherol Succinate, Molybdenum Aspartate, Selenium Aspartate, Manganese Gluconate, Chromemate-GTF (Chromium Polynicotinate), Copper Gluconate, Pyridoxal-5-Phosphate, Thiamine HCL, D-Biotin, Potassium Iodid, Ergocalciferol, Folic Acid, Cyanocobalamin] • Cellulose Gum • Xanthan • Natural & Artificial Flavors • Lecithin • Sunnette Brand of Acesulfame-K • Carrageenan • Aspartame. Contains Phenylalanine.

Hemaplex - Progressive Labs
Each capsule contains: Iron (from 200 mg iron peptonate) 32 mg • Vitamin C (ascorbic acid) 200 mg • Thiamin HCl (Vitamin B1) 2 mg • Riboflavin (Vitamin B2) 2 mg • Niacin 13 mg • Niacinamide 15 mg • Vitamin B6 (pyridoxine HCl) 2 mg • Folate (folic acid) 400 mcg • Vitamin B12 (cyanocobalamin) 50 mcg • Base 50 mg: Raw Duodenum, Raw Liver, Raw Stomach, Red Bone Marrow, Beef Peptone, Citrus Pectin, Betaine HCl, Bile Salts, Rose Hips, Alfalfa, Wheat Germ.
See Editor's Note No. 14.

Hem-Care - PhytoPharmica
Two capsules contain: Butcher's Broom root and rhizome extract (ruscus aculeatus, standardized to contain 9-11% saponins calculated as ruscogenins) 100 mg • Calcium (as calcium lactate) 20 mg • Choline Bitartrate 150 mg • Glycosaminoglycans (GAGs) 25 mg • Sophora Japonica flower bud (standardized to contain 95% rutin) 100 mg • Phosphorus (as tricalcium phosphate) 25 mg • Stone Root root and rhizome (collinsonia canadensis) 500 mg • Vitamin C (ascorbic acid) 100 mg • Vitamin E (as D-alpha tocopheryl acid succinate) 30 IU.
See Editor's Note No. 14.

Hem-Mend: Hemorrhoid Support - The Herbalist
Stone root fresh dried (Collinsonia canadensis) • Celandine fresh-flowering herb (Chaelidonium majus) • Witch Hazel fresh-dried leaf (Hamamelis virginiana) • Horse Chestnut fresh nut (Aesculus hippocastanum).

Hemo-Plus - Atrium Inc.
Each tablet contains: Vitamin C 300 mg • Vitamin B1 10 mg • Vitamin B2 10 mg • Vitamin B6 10 mg • Vitamin B12 250 mcg • Folic Acid 800 mcg • Niacinamide 20 mg • Iron Peptonate 113 mg • Manganese (Proteinate Chelated) 5 mg • Liver 75 mg.
See Editor's Note No. 14.

Hemorrhoid Remedy - PhytoPharmica
Twenty drops contain: Aloe socotrina 4x • Sulphur 4x • Collinsonia canadensis 3x • Narum nitricum 3x • Nux vomica 3x • Paeonia officinalis 3x • Teucrium scorodonia 3x • Verbascum thapsus 2x • Aesculus hippocastanum 1x • Boldo 1x • Hamamelis virginiana 1x. In a base of 45% USP alcohol by volume.
See Editor's Note No. 1, page 2053.

Hemorrhoids - Hyland's
Two tablets contain: Aesculus Hippocastanum 3X • Ratanhia 3X • Nux Vomica 3X (0.0012% alkaloids) • Calcarea Fluorica 6X. Base: Lactose USP.
See Editor's Note No. 1, page 2053.

HemoStream - DreamPharm
Two capsules contain: Proprietary Blend: Chitosan, Barley Grass, Rehmannia radix, Angelica Sinensis radix, Cinnamomi Ramulus, Ligustici Wallchii rhizoma, Carthami Flos, Mass Medicata Fermentata, Scirpi rhizoma, Salivae Miltiorrhizae rhizoma, Zedoaria, Malt, Licorice, Crataegus fructus, Mastic, Agrimony, Burdock.

Hem-Tone - Enzymatic Therapy
Two capsules contain: Vitamin E (D-Alpha Tocopherol Succinate) 30 IU • Calcium Lactate 130 mg • Vitamin C (Ascorbic Acid) 100 mg • Phosphorus (Tricalcium Phosphate) 25 mg • Other Ingredients: Colinsonia root (Stone root) 500 mg • Choline Bitartrate 150 mg • Butchers Broom extract (Ruscus aculeatus) standardized to contain 10% Saponins (calculated as Ruscogenin) 100 mg • Rutin (Buckwheat) 100 mg • Glycosaminoglycans 25 mg: A mixture of highly purified bovine-derived Glycosaminoglycans naturally present in the aorta including Dermatan Sulfate, Heparan Sulfate, Hyaluronic Acid, Chondroitin Sulfate, & related Hexosaminoglycans.
See Editor's Note No. 15, page 2055.

Some Brand Name Natural Products - What they Contain

www.NaturalDatabase.com contains MANY more listings than appear here.

Hepatic Factors - Michael's Naturopathic Programs
Three tablets contain: Vitamin A (as beta carotene) 1500 IU • Vitamin E (as D-alpha tocopheryl succinate) 150 IU • Vitamin K (as phylloquinone) 45 mcg • Thiamin (as thiamin hydrochloride) 30 mg • Niacin (as nicotinic acid) 30 mg • Vitamin B12 (as cyanocobalamin) 300 mcg • Pantothenic Acid (as D-calcium pantothenate) 30 mg • Proprietary Blend 2153 mg: Lecithin (from soy), Choline (as choline bitartrate), Inositol, Dandelion root 4:1 extract (taraxacum officinale), Methionine (as L-methionine hydrochloride), Threonine (as L-threonine), Butternut root bark (juglans cinerea), Milk Thistle seed 20:1 extract (silybum marianum, 80% silymarin, 60 mg), Yellow Dock root (rumex crispus), Burdock root 4:1 extract (arcitum lappa). Other Ingredients: Microcrystalline Cellulose, Calcium Carbonate, Stearic Acid, Magnesium Stearate.

Hepatic Support - Zone Labs
Six capsules contain: Vitamin C (ascorbic acid) 100 mg • Organic Spirulina 700 mg • Barley juice powder 100 mg • Alfalfa juice powder 100 mg • Chlorella powder 50 mg • Milk Thistle extract (silymarin) 50 mg • Lecithin 50 mg • Hesperidin complex 50 mg • Rutin 50 mg • Indole 3 Carbinol 100 mg • Alpha Lipoic Acid 100 mg • L-Methionine 50 mg • L-Cysteine 50 mg • L-Carnitine (as fumarate) 25 mg • Choline (as choline bitartrate) 55 mg • Glutathione 50 mg • NAC (N-acetyl cysteine) 100 mg. Other Ingredients: Gelatin, Microcrystalline Celluose, FOS, Magnesium Stearate, Silica, Purified Water, Broccoli Extract, Brussels Sprout Extract, Cabbage Extract, Maitake Mushrooms, Sodium Lauryl Sulfate.

Hepato-C - Pacific BioLogic
Salvia root • Heydyotis • Scutellaria (barbat skullcap) • Peony root (red) • Codonopsis root (natural) • Lycium fruit • Dryopteris rhizome • Rhodiole Sachelanensi root • Polygonum root (thin) • Magnolia bark • Knotweed rhizome (bushy) • Astragalus root (Grade 1) • Capillaris shoots & leaves • Bitter Orange (ripened fruit) • Polyporus Sclerotium.
See Editor's Note No. 40, page 2058.

Hepato-Detox - Pacific BioLogic
Salvia root • Codonopsis root (natural) • Lycium fruit • Polygonatum rhizome • Astragalus root (Grade 1) • Reishi Mushroom • Privet fruit (ligustrum) • Ginseng root (red ji lin) • Cherry (cornelian asiatic).

Hepatox - PhytoPharmica
Three tablets contain: Barberry bark of root 6:1 extract (berberis vulgaris) 150 mg • Beet root (beta vulgaris) 300 mg • Betaine HCl 75 mg • Biotin 200 mcg • Boldo leaf 2:1 extract (peumus boldus) 150 mg • Celandine aerial part (chelidonium majus) 135 mg • Choline Bitartrate 850 mg • Evening Primrose seed oil (oenothera biennis, standardized to contain 4.5% gamma-linoleic acid (GLA) 30 mg • Fringe Tree bark (chionanthus virginicus) 135 mg • Inositol 50 mg • Liver (desiccated) 40 mg • L-Methionine 250 mg • Niacin (as nicain and nicainamide) 40 mg • Ox Bile extract 90 mg • Vitamin A (as retinyl acetate) 4500 IU • Vitamin B12 (as cyanocobalamin) 3 mcg • Vitamin C (ascorbic acid and from rose hips) 25 mg.
See Editor's Note No. 14, page 2055.

Hepol - ProJoba
Each tablet contains: Botanical Glutathione Yeast extract YH 85 mg • Aloe Vera extract 45 mg • Polbax extract 40 mg. Other Ingredients: Lacrose Alfa, Microcrystalline Cellulose, Magnesium Stearate, Colloidal Silicon Dioxide, Talc, Natural Resin.

Her Pleasure Sexual Enhancing Gel - Eve's Accents
L-Arginine • Menthol • Epimedium • Guarana seed extract • Damiana • Wild Yam (Mexican) • Purified Water.

Her Stuff - Blue Stuff, Inc.
Each 4 oz bottle contains: Whole leaf Aloe Vera • Purified Water • Yam extract • Polyglycerylmethacylate • Propylene Glycol • Carbomer-940 • Safflower oil • Emu oil • Isopropyl Palmitate • Natural Progesterone extract • Laureth-4 • Gluceryl Stearate • PEG-100 Stearate • Siberian Ginseng root extract • Black Cohosh root extract • Burdock root extract • Licorice root extract • Hops extract • Alfalfa extract • Tansy extract • Dang Gui extract • Sweet Almond oil • Jojoba oil • Avocado oil • Triethanolamine • Rosemary oil • Fragrance • Chamomile extract • Tetrasodium EDTA • Sodium Hydroxymethylglycinate • Tocopherol.

Herba Fuel - TwinLab
Three capsules contain: Ma Huang extract (standardized for 6% Ephedrine) 334 mg • Chinese Green Tea extract (standardized for 7% Caffeine & 20% Polyphenols) 1500 mg. In a natural base of Siberian Ginseng (Eleutherococcus senticosus).
See Editor's Note No. 30, page 2056.

HerbaCoral Coral Calcium & 72 Coral Minerals - HerbaLab
Three capsules contain: Vitamin C (as ascorbic acid) 15 mg • Vitamin D (as cholecalciferol) 1200 IU • Calcium (from coral) 690 mg • Magnesium (amino acid chelate & coral) 168 mg • Coral Powder 672 mg • Malic Acid 30 mg • Betaine Hydrochloride 15 mg.

Herbal Aloe Drink - Herbalife
Water • Aloe Vera Juice • Sodium Citrate • Citric Acid • Potassium Sorbate • Chamomile • Sodium Benzoate.

Herbal Breath - DreamPharm
Two capsules contain: Rhizoma Polygonati Odoranti 100 mg • Herba Menthae Haplocalysis 100 mg • Herba Agastaches Seu Pogostemi 100 mg • Spearmint leaf 100 gm • Semen Pruni Armeniacae 50 mg • Fructus Amomi Kravanh 50 mg.

Herbal Cold - Puritan's Pride
Each tablet contains: Vitamin C (calcium ascorbate) 500 mg • Calcium (calcium ascorbate) 50 mg • Poplar Bud extract 25 mg • Senega extract 10 mg • Oil of Thyme 5 mg • Oil of Eucalyptus 5 mg • Hore Hound powdered 10 mg • Coltsfoot powdered 10 mg • Licorice root powdered 15 mg • Capsicum powdered 10 mg • Cubeb powdered 10 mg • Slippery Elm bark powdered 10 mg • Fennel powdered 10 mg • Jamaican Ginger powdered 10 mg • Honey 10 mg • Lemon Juice 1 mg • Rutin 10 mg • Bee Pollen 10 mg • Bee Propolis 50 mg.

Herbal Cold Relief - Jamieson
Each capsule contains: Ephedra stem extract (Ephedra sinensis, equivalent to 10.2 mg of ephedrine) 62.5 mg • Grindelia aerial parts 1:4 extract (Grindelia Camporum) 0.5 mg • Eucalyptus oil (Eucalypyus Globulus) 0.05 mg • Echinacea Root (Echinacea purpurea) 100 mg.
See Editor's Note No. 30, page 2056.

Herbal Cold Season Defense - Quantum, Inc.
Three capsules contain: Vitamin C 250 mg • Echinacea angustifolia standardized to 4% phenolic compounds 100 mg • Elderberry (10:1) extract 100 mg • Goldenseal root (3:1) extract 25 mg. Other Ingredients: Vegetable Sterine, Magnesium Stearate, Micro Crystalline Cellulose.
See Editor's Note No. 21, page 2056.

Herbal Colon Cleanser & Tonic - Grandma's Herbs
Each capsule contains: Proprietary Blend .450 g: Cascara Sagrada, Senna pods, Psyllium seeds/hulls, Licorice root, Aloes, Turkey Rhubarb, Buckthorn, Prunes, Dandelion, Barberry, Slippery Elm, Marshmallow, Alfalfa, Calmus root, Plantain, Black Walnut, Butternut, Gentian root, Red Clover, Flax Seed, Sage Brush, Chicory, Fennel, Ginger, Chamomile, Calendula, Wahoo, Blue Vervain, Blue Flag, Red Raspberry leaf, Yucca.

Herbal Decongestant Expectorant Capsules - Life Brand
Ma Huang (Ephedra) 50 mg as a standardized extract 1:10 (equivalent to 500 mg Ma Huang) with 4 mg of total Ephedrines • Wild Horehound leaf 150 mg • Thyme herb extract (1:4) 100 mg (equivalent to 400 mg of Thyme) • Coltsfoot leaf 50 mg • Mullein leaf 50 mg • Cayenne 1.125 mg • Marshmallow root 9 mg • Slippery Elm bark 9 mg. Other Ingredients: Gelatin, Water.
See Editor's Note No. 30, page 2056.

Herbal Diuretic - Progressive Labs
Each capsule contains: Proprietary blend 120 mg: Buchu leaves

(Barsoma crenata) • Couch Grass root (Triticum repens) • Proprietary blend 330 mg: Hydrangea root (Hydrangea arborescens), Corn Silk (Stigmata maidis), Juniper berry (Juniperus communis), Burdock root (Arctium lappa), Uva Ursi leaf (Arctostaphylos Uva-Ursi), Ginger root (Zingiber officinale) Parsley (Petroselium sativum), Marshmallow root (Althaea officinalis).

Herbal Diuretic **-** Jamieson
Each capsule contains: Uva Ursi 200 mg • Buchu Leaves 100 mg.

Herbal Diuretic Formula **-** Quest
Each caplet contains: Uva Ursi leaf (Arctostaphylos uva-ursi) (Provided by 50 mg P.E. 1:4) 200 mg • Juniper berry extract (Junuperus communis) (Provided by 80 mg P.E. 1:4) 320 mg • Parsley root (Petroselinum crispum) (Provided by 40 mg P.E. 1:4) 160 mg. Other Ingredients: Buchu leaves, Cayenne, Corn Silk, Kelp, Parsley leaf, Pumpkin seed, Saw Palmetto berries, Calcium Phosphate, Vegetable Stearin, Croscarmellose Sodium, Magnesium Stearate (vegetable source).

Herbal Diuretic Tablets **-** Life Brand
Buchu leaf extract (1:4) 25 mg (equivalent to 100 mg Buchu leaf) • Uva Ursi leaf extract (1:3) 33.3 mg (equivalent to 100 mg Uva Ursi leaf) • Juniper berry extract (1:2) 50 mg (equivalent to 100 mg of Juniper berries) • Celery seed 75 mg • Parsley root 75 mg. Excipients: Microcrystalline Cellulose, Tricalcium Phosphate, Corn Starch, Magnesium Stearate.

Herbal Douche **-** Dial Herbs
Mineral Water • Aloe Vera • White Oak bark • Slippery Elm • Uva Ursi • Cayenne.

Herbal Ecstacy **-** Global World Media
Each pill contains: Ephedra • Ma Huang • Guarana • Gingko biloba • Cola Nut • Gotu-Kola • Fo-Ti-Tient (Fo-Ti) • Green Tea • Rou Gui (Chinese Nutmeg).
See Editor's Note No. 5 and No. 30.

Herbal Enhancer **-** Pentabosol
Two tablets contain: Cinnamon bark 150 mg • Green Tea leaf extract (36% catechin and polyphenols) 100 mg • Cloves 50 mg • Brewer's Yeast 100 mg • Flax Seed 100 mg • Cumin seed 25 mg • Garlic extract (odor controlled) 25 mg • Gymnema Sylvestre leaf 150 mg • Fenugreek seed 150 mg • Coriander 50 mg • Bilberry leaf 10 mg. Other Ingredients: Dicalcium Phosphate, Microcrystalline Cellulose, Croscarmellose Sodium, Stearic Acid, Magnesium Stearate, Silica, Pharmaceutical Glaze.

Herbal Expector-Aid **-** Quantum, Inc.
Each softgel contains: Vitamin C (ascorbic acid) 200 mg • Elderberry extract berry standardized to 5% flavonoids 200 mg • Fenugreek powder seed (4:1) extract 100 mg • Horehound powder flower, leaf, stem (4:1) extract 100 mg • Anise seed (4:1) extract 100 mg • Marshmallow root (4:1) extract 60 mg • Anise seed oil 40 mg • Echinacea extract flower, leaf (4:1 PE) 40 mg • Menthol Crystals 20 mg • Eucalyptus Oil 10 mg. Other Ingredients: Gelatin Shell: Gelatin, Glycerin, St. John's Bread, Titanium Dioxide; Liquid Fill: Sunflower Seed Oil, Beeswax, Lecithin.
See Editor's Note No. 21, page 2056.

Herbal Fem **-** Nutri-Quest Rx
Golden Seal root, Dong Quai, Blessed Thistle, Red Raspberry leaves, Squaw Vine, Scullcap, Cayenne, Blue Cohosh, Licorice root, Wild Yam root, Passion Flower 408 mg. In a base of 6X tissue salts: Calc Fluor, Calc Phos, Calc Sulph, Kali Mur, Kali Phos, Kali Sulph, Mag Phos, Nat Mur, Nat Phos, Nat Sulph, Silica.

Herbal Gargle **-** Dial Herbs
Sage • Myrrh • Goldenseal • Bayberry • Cayenne • Ginger • pure Apple cider vinegar aged in wood.

Herbal GI **-** PhysioLogics
Each capsule contains: Glucosamine (HCl) 150 mg • Gamma Oryzanol 200 mg • Chamomile (1.2% Apigenin, 1.8 mg; 0.5% Essential oil, 0.75 mg) 150 mg • Aloe Vera 100 mg • Wild Yam (6% total Saponins, 4.5 mg) 75 mg.

Herbal Gold Cigarettes **-** Alternative Cigarettes Inc
Each cigarette contains: Marshmallow • Yerba Santa • Damiana • Passion Flower • Jasmine • Ginseng. Regular, menthol, vanilla, and cherry are available.
See Editor's Note No. 6, page 2053.

Herbal Grobust **-** HomeCure, Inc.
Sabal • Damiana • Dong Quai • Blessed Thistle • Kava Kava • Dandelion root • Oat Bran • Wild Yam • Mother's Wort.

Herbal Immune Complex **-** Solgar
Standardized Astragalus root (glucosides 0.5 mg [0.5%], polysaccharides 70 mg [70%]) 100 mg • Standardized Cat's Claw extract inner bark (mitraphylline 3 mg [3%], polyphenols 15 mg [15%]) 100 mg • Standardized Echinacea purpurea extract root, leaf (echinacosides 4 mg [4%], polysaccharides 15 mg [15%]) 100 mg • Standardized Deglycyrrhized Licorice extract root (glycyrrhizin<1 mg [1%]) 100 mg • Standardized Elderberry extract berry (polyphenols 30 mg [30%]) 100 mg • Standardized Olive Leaf extract leaf (oleuropein 6 mg [6%]) 100 mg • Raw Elderberry powder flower 20 mg • Raw Echinacea powder root, leaf 20 mg • Raw Licorice powder root 20 mg • Raw Olive Leaf powder 20 mg • Raw Astragalus powder root 20 mg. Other Ingredients: Vegetable Cellulose, Vegetable Stearic Acid, Vegetable Magnesium Stearate, Vegetable Glycerin, PhytO2X Blend containing: Natural Vitamin E (mixed tocopherols), Natural Beta Carotene and other Carotenoids, Rosemary extract aerial, Vitamin C (L-ascorbic-acid), Water.

Herbal Insomnia Tablets **-** Life Brand
Valerian root extract (1:4) 50 mg (equivalent to 200 mg Valerian root) • Passion Flower herb 80 mg • Chamomile flower extract (1:4) 15 mg (equivalent to 60 mg Chamomile flowers) • Mistletoe herb 50 mg • Hops flower 50 mg • Wild Lettuce leaf 40 mg. Excipients: Tricalcium Phosphate, Corn Starch, Silicon dioxide, Magnesium Stearate.

Herbal Klenz **-** Progressive Labs
Each capsule contains: Vitamin A 3500 IU • Echinacea (Echinacea angustifolia) 200 mg • Golden Seal (Hydrastis canadensis) 125 mg • Irish Moss (Chondrus crispus) 40 mg • Ginger root (Zingiber officinale) 35 mg • Burdock root (Arctium lappa) 35 mg • Peony root (Paeonia officinalis) 35 mg • Peony root skin (Paeonia officinalis) 35 mg • Licorice root (Glycyrrhiza glabra) 25 mg • Red Clover flower (Trifolium pratense) 20 mg.

Herbal Laxative **-** Holista
Each capsule contains: Cascara Sagrada extract 200 mg • Senna leaves 250 mg.

Herbal Laxative (Stomach-Ease) Tablets **-** Life Brand
Senna leaves 240 mg • Cascara Sagrada bark 150 mg • Licorice root 30 mg • Juniper berries 8 mg • Rhubarb root 8 mg • Gentian root 8 mg • Buchu leaves 4 mg. Excipients: Corn Starch, Sodium Bicarbonate, Silicon Dioxide, Magnesium Stearate, oil of Peppermint.

Herbal Laxative Formula **-** Quest
Each caplet contains: Cascara Sagrada bark (Rhamnus purshiana) (Provided by 50 mg P.E. 7:1) 350 mg • Rhubarb root (Rheum officinale L.) (Provided by 30 mg P.E. 1:4) 120 mg. Other Ingredients: Cayenne, Ginger root, Licorice root, Marshmallow root, Calcium Phosphate, Croscarmellose Sodium, Microcrystalline Cellulose, Magnesium Stearate (vegetable source), Vegetable Stearin.

Herbal Lite **-** BioTreasures
Each caplet contains: Calcium Pyruvate 1050 mg • L-Phenylalanine 116 mg • Manganese Chelate 6 mcg • Chromium Polynicotinate 500 mcg • Proprietary Herbal Blend 1830 mg: Citrus Aurantium, Garcinia Cambogia, St. John's Wort, Green Tea, Gotu Kola, Siberian Ginseng, Stevia.
See Editor's Note No. 40, page 2058.

Some Brand Name Natural Products - What they Contain

www.NaturalDatabase.com contains MANY more listings than appear here.

Herbal Liver Complex **-** Solgar
Each vegicap contains: Standardized Milk Thistle extract aerial, seed (silymarin 80 mg [80%]) 100 mg • Standardized Dandelion extract whole plant (vitexin 3 mg [3%]) 100 mg • Standardized Turmeric extract root (curcuminoids 71 mg [95%]) 75 mg • Standardized Schisandra extract fruit (schisandrins 0.5 mg [1%]) 50 mg • Standardized Picrorizha kurroavv extract Picroliv (kutkin 3 mg [3.5%]) 75 mg • Standardized Phyllanthus amarus extract leaf (sesquiterpenes>2 mg [4%]) 50 mg • Phosphatidylcholine 100 mg • Raw Milk Thistle powder aerial 75 mg • Raw Dandelion powder root 75 mg. Other Ingredients: Microcrystalline Cellulose; Vegetable Cellulose; Vegetable Stearic Acid; Vegetable Magnesium Stearate; Vegetable Glycerin; PhytO2X Blend containing Natural Vitamin E (mixed tocopherols), Natural Beta Carotene and other Carotenoids, Rosemary extract aerial, Vitamin C (L-ascorbic acid), Water.

Herbal Male Complex **-** Solgar
Each vegicap contains: Standardized Saw Palmetto extract berry (FFA 34 mg-38 mg [45%-50%]) 75 mg • Standardized Nettles extract leaf (silic acid 0.75 mg [1%]) 75 mg • Standardized Astragalus extract root (glucosides 0.38 mg [0.5%], polysaccharides 53 mg [70%]) 75 mg • Standardized Korean Panax Ginseng extract root (eleutherosides 0.6 mg [0.8%]) 75 mg • Soy Isoflavone extract seed 75 mg • Raw Astragalus powder root 50 mg • Raw Korean Ginseng powder root 25 mg • Raw Siberian Ginseng powder root 25 mg • Raw Nettles powder leaf 25 mg. Other Ingredients: Microcrystalline Cellulose; Vegetable Cellulose; Vegetable Stearic Acid; Vegetable Magnesium Stearate; Vegetable Glycerin; PhtO2X blend containing Natural Vitamin E (mixed tocopherols), Natural Beta Carotene and Other Carotenoids, Rosemary extract aerial, Vitamin C (L-ascorbic acid), Water.

Herbal Migraine Formula **-** Quest
Each caplet contains: Feverfew powder (Tanacetum parthenium) (contains no less than 0.2% parthenolides) 125 mg. Other Ingredients: Calcium Phosphate, Croscarmellose Sodium, Microcrystalline Cellulose, Vegetable Stearin, Magnesium Stearate (vegetable source).

Herbal Nerve Tablets **-** Life Brand
Valerian root extract (1:4) 50 mg (equivalent to 200 mg Valerian root) • Skullcap herb 100 mg • Hops flowers 50 mg. Excipients: Tricalcium Phosphate, Corn Starch, Magnesium Stearate, Silicon Dioxide.

Herbal Niagra **-** Young Again Nutrients
Three capsules contain: Bulgarian Tribulus Terrestris 750 mg • Ginseng Panax 500 mg • Yohimbe Bark 300 mg • Saw Palmetto (25%) 100 mg • Vitamin B3 (Niacinamide) 50 mg.

Herbal Nightcap **-** Trader Joe's
Passion flower 150 mg • Chamomile 4 mg • Hops 60 mg.

Herbal Pain and Fever Relief **-** Holista
Each capsule contains: White Willow bark powder 300 mg • Meadowsweet extract 250 mg.

Herbal Pain Relief Formula **-** Quest
Each caplet contains: White Willow bark (Salix alba) (Provided by 250 mg P.E. 1:12 standardized to contain 11% Salicin) 3000 mg. Other Ingredients: Blue Vervain, Kelp, Red Raspberry leaf, Skullcap and Wood Betony. Calcium Phosphate, Magnesium Stearate (vegetable source), Microcrystalline Cellulose, Vegetable Stearin.

Herbal Phen Fen Stage 2 **-** HPF L.L.C.
Two tablets contain: St. John's Wort 400 mg • Ma Huang 250 mg • Green Tea leaf extract 450 mg. Other Ingredients: Dicalcium Phosphate, Microcrystalline Cellulose, Croscarmellose Sodium, Stearic Acid, Silica, Magnesium Stearate, Pharmaceutical glaze. See Editor's Note No. 30, page 2056.

Herbal Regulator **-** VitaStore
Two tablets contain: Potassium (as gluconate) 25 mg • Hydrangea root 100 mg • Graminis Rhizoma root 50 mg • Cornsilk 50 mg • Parsley whole herb 25 mg • Uva Ursi leaves 75 mg.

Herbal Relaxant Formula **-** Quest
Each caplet contains: Valerian root (Valeriana officinalis) (Provided by 100 mg P.E. 1:5 standardized to contain 0.8% Valerenic Acid) 500 mg • Chamomile flower (Chamomilla recutita L.) (Provided by 50 mg P.E. 1:4 standardized to contain 1% Apigenin) 200 mg. Other Ingredients: Ginger root, Hops, Marshmallow root, Skullcap, Calcium Phosphate, Croscarmellose Sodium, Magnesium Stearate (vegetable source), Microcrystalline Cellulose, Vegetable Stearin.

Herbal Seltzer **-** Dial Herbs
Sodium • White Willow bark • Fever Few • Ginger • Mint • Stevia • Potassium Bicarbonate • Sodium Bicarbonate • Citric Acid. Flavored & sweetened with natural orange flavorings, natural fruit flavors & dextrose.

Herbal Slim **-** Nature's Way
Four capsules contain: Proprietary formula: Black Walnut hulls • Burdock root • Chickweed leaf & stem • Echinacea Purpurea stem, leaf, flower • Fennel seed • Hawthorne berry • Kelp (whole Thallus) • Licorice root • Papaya leaves • Parsley herb • Safflower flower. Other Ingredients: Gelatin.

Herbal Throat Lozenges Sugar Free **-** Natureworks
Two lozenges contain: Menthol 6 mg • Peppermint Oil 2 mg. Other Ingredients: Bee Propolis, Chlorophyll, Capsicum, Wild Cherry Bark, Horehound, Rose Hips, Cocillana Bark, Euphorbia, Echinacea, Slippery Elm, Mullein, Lemon Balm, Black Cherry Flavor, Magnesium Stearate, Calcium Stearate, Silica.

Herbal Tranquility **-** Optimum Nutrition
Valerian root • Passionflower extract.

Herbal Tranquility Complex **-** Solgar
Each vegicap contains: Standardized Kava Kava extract root (kavalactones 30 mg [30%]) 100 mg • Standardized Valerian extract root (valernic acid 0.8 mg [0.8%]) 100 mg • Standardized Passionflower extract aerial (isovitexin 2mg-3mg [3%-4%]) 75 mg • Standardized Schisandra extract fruit (schisandrins 0.75 mg [1%]) 75 mg • Standardized St. John's Wort extract aerial (hypericin 0.23 mg [0.3%]) 75 mg • Standardized American Ginseng extract root (ginsenosides 5 mg [10%]) 50 mg • Raw Kava Kava powder root 50 mg • Raw St. John's Wort powder aerial 50 mg • Raw Valerian powder root 50 mg. Other Ingredients: Microcrystalline Cellulose; Vegetable Cellulose; Vegetable Stearic Acid; Vegetable Magnesium Stearate; Vegetable Glycerin; PhytO2X Blend containing Natural Vitamin E (mixed tocopherols), Natural Beta Carotene and other Carotenoids, Rosemary extract aerial, Vitamin C (L-ascorbic acid), Water.

Herbal Treasures **-** BioTreasures
Each caplet contains: Kelp 40 mg • Reishi Mushroom 40 mg • Papain (from Papaya) 40 mg • Alfalfa 200 mg • Vitamin A (Beta Carotene) 5000 IU • Vitamin C (Ester-C Calcium Ascorbate) 75 mg • Vitamin E (D-Alpha Tocopheryl Acetate) 30 IU • Vitamin B1 (Thiamine) 1.5 mg • Vitamin B2 (Riboflavin) 1.7 mg • Vitamin B3 (Niacin) 20 mg • Vitamin B5 (Pantothenic Acid) 10 mg • Vitamin B6 (Pyridoxine) 2 mg • Vitamin B12 (Cyanocobalamin) 6 mcg • Folic Acid 400 mcg • Calcium (Calcium Chelate) 400 mg • Magnesium (Ascorbate) 150 mg • Zinc (Zinc Chelate) 74 mg • Chromium (Chromium Polynicotate) 1000 mcg • Proprietary Herbal Blend 610 mg: Grape Seed extract, Garlic extract, Ginkgo biloba extract, Green Tea extract, Siberian Ginseng, Silymarin (Milk Thistle extract), Astragalus extract, Hawthorne berries extract, Horsetail extract, Ashwaganda extract, Stevia extract.

Herbal Up Formula **-** Nature's Way
Two capsules contain: Bee Pollen • Cayenne pepper fruit • Gotu Kola stem, leaf • Proprietary Blend (840 mg) • Siberian Ginseng root. Other Ingredients: Gelatin.

Herbal UR-Kidney **-** Nutri-Quest Rx
Proprietary blend 430 mg: Juniper Berries • Parsley • Uva Ursi, Marshmallow • Ginger • Golden Seal root • Corn Silk • Cleavers root.

In a base of 6X tissue salts: Mag Phos, Nat Sulph, Calc Phos, Calc Sulph.

Herbal V **-** Ultra-V
Two tablets contain: Yohimbe extract 2% 250 mg • Avena Sativa extract 10:1 150 mg • Androstenedione 90 mg • Saw Palmetto extract 4:1 100 mg • Guarana extract 22% 300 mg • Taurine 200 mg • Siberian Ginseng extract 35:1 30 mg • Tribulus Terrestris extract 40% 50 mg. Other Ingredients: Dicalcium Phosphate, Microcrystalline Cellulose, Magnesium Sterate, Stearic Acid.
See Editor's Note No. 47, page 2058.

Herbal V: Women's Formula **-** VitaZip, Inc.
Avena Sativa 10:1 Extract • Kava Kava 30% • Muira Puama 4:1 Extract • St. John's Wort 3% • Ginkgo Biloba 24%/6%.

Herbal Vivid Maximum Gain **-** Unknown
Three tablets contain: Niacin 75 mg • Zinc (as zinc oxide) 40 mg • Yohimbe bark 700 mg • Maca tuber 500 mg • Catuaba bark 125 mg • Muira Puama bark 125 mg • Tribulus aerial 100 mg • L-Arginine HCl 100 mg • Cola seed 75 mg • Oatstraw grassy stalks 75 mg • Stinging Nettle leaves 75 mg • Pumpkin seed 75 mg • Cayenne fruit (25,000 HU) 60 mg • Ginger root 60 mg • American Ginseng root 50 mg • Eleuthero root 50 mg • Asian Ginseng root 50 mg • Sarsaparilla root 50 mg • Orchic substance (bovine) 30 gm • Boron citrate 10 mg. Other Ingredients: Cellulose, Modified Cellulose, Gum Arabic (acacia), Silicon Dioxide, Vegetable Magnesium Stearate, Vegetable Stearic Acid, FD&C Blue #2/Indigo Carmine Lake.
See Editor's Note No. 14.

Herbal Water Control **-** Jamieson
Two capsules contain: Calcium (as Calcium Sulfate) 54 mg • Uva Ursi leaf (Arctostaghylos uva-ursi (L) Spreng) 400 mg • Buchu leaf (Barosma Betulina Bartl. Et Wendl.) 200 mg.

Herbal Women's Formula **-** Quest
Each caplet contains: White Willow bark powder (Salix alba) (Provided by 85 mg P.E. 1:12 standardized to contain 11% Salicin) 1000 mg • Valerian root (Valeriana officinalis) (Provided by 40 mg P.E. 1:5 standardized to contain 0.8% Valerenic Acid) 200 mg • Chamomile flower (Chamomilla recutita L.) (Provided by 20 mg P.E. 1:4 standardized to contain 1% Apigenin) 80 mg • Uva Ursi leaf (Arctostaphylos uva-ursi) (Provided by 50 P.E. 1:4 standardized to contain 10% Arbutin) 200 mg • Juniper berry (Juniperus communis) (Provided by 80 mg P.E. 1:4) 320 mg • Parsley root (Petroselinum crispum) (Provided by 40 mg P.E. 1:4) 160 mg. Other Ingredients: Calcium Phosphate, Croscarmellose Sodium, Magnesium Stearate (vegetable source), Microcrystalline Cellulose, Silicon Dioxide.

Herbal World Ginseng Complex **-** Vitamin World
Each capsule contains: American Ginseng root (Panax quinquefolius) 200 mg • Korean Ginseng root (Panax ginseng) 200 mg • Red Chinese Ginseng root (Panax ginseng) 200 mg • Siberian Ginseng root (eleutherococcus senticosus) 200 mg • Royal Jelly (57.14 mg of a 3.5:1 extract) 200 mg. Other Ingredients: Gelatin, Vegetable Magnesium Stearate, Silica.

Herbalax **-** Health Factor
Each capsule contains: Cascara Sagrada (Rhamnus purshiana) 260 mg • Peppermint (Menta piperita) 90 mg.

Herbal-Biotic **-** The Herbalist
Oregon Grape Root • Golden Seal root • Yerba Mansa root.

Herbal-F **-** Progressive Labs
Each capsule contains: Vitamin B6 (as pyridoxine HCl) 20 mg • Magnesium (as magnesium oxide/soy protein complex) 15 mg • Damiana leaf (Turnera aphrodisiaca) 60 mg • Passion flower (Passiflora incarnata) 40 mg • Black Cohosh root (Cimicifuga racemosa) 20 mg • Blue Cohosh root (Caulophyllum thalictroides) 20 mg • Ginger root (Zingiber officinale) 60 mg • Cramp bark (Viburnum opulus) 75 mg • Wild Yam root (Dioscorea villosa) 40 mg • False Unicorn root (Chamaelirium luteum) 40 mg • Squaw vine (Mitchella repens) 40 mg • Blackhaw bark (Viburnum punifolium) 40 mg • Prickly Ash bark (Zanthoxylum americanum) 40 mg • White Birch bark (Betula alba) 40 mg • Ovarian substance 10 mg.
See Editor's Note No. 14.

Herbalist's Choice **-** The Herbalist
Gotu Kola herb • Guarana seed • Kola Nut • American Ginseng root • Licorice root • Damiana leaf • Echinacea root • Osha root • Cinnamon bark • Ginger root • Cayenne pepper.

Herbal-M **-** Progressive Labs
Each capsule contains: Vitamin E 30 IU • Zinc (as zinc oxide) 15 mg • Damiana leaf (Turnera aphrodesiaca) 60 mg • Siberian Ginseng/ Korean Ginseng blend (Eleutherococcus senticosus & Panax ginseng) • Cayenne (Capsicum annuum) 50 mg • Dong Quai (Angelica sinensis) 25 mg • Yohimbe (Pausinystalia johimbe) 10 mg • Muira Puama (Pytchopetalum olacoides) 10 mg • Goldenrod (Solidago virguarea) 10 mg • Orchic Substance 10 mg.
See Editor's Note No. 14.

Herbaretic **-** Suddenly Slender
Each tablet contains: Alfalfa 50 mg • Buchu 50 mg • Uva Ursi 50 mg • Couch Grass 50 mg • Parsley 50 mg • Juniper berries 50 mg • Asparagus 50 mg • Watermelon seed powder 50 mg • Cubebs 50 mg • Shave Grass 50 mg • Corn Silk 50 mg • Golden Rod 50 mg • Cranberries 50 mg.

HerbaSlim **-** HerbaSway
St. John's Wort • Bitter Orange • Green Tea • Cassia tora • Panax Ginseng • Kudzu • Knotweed • Lycium • Cayenne pepper • Blackberry • HerbaSwee (Cucurbitaceae fruit).
See Editor's Note No. 40, page 2058.

Herbetom Pulm **-** Bioserum Laboratory
Each 10 mL contains: Proprietary Blend: Aloe Vera juice, Propolis, Elder extract, Beta Carotene, Pine bud extract, Thyme, Plantain, Golden Sun, Echinacea, Eucalyptus.

Herb-Lax **-** Shaklee
Each four tablets contain: Dietary fiber 1 g • Calcium 20 mg • Iron 0.36 mg • Herb-Lax Proprietary Blend 1.7 g: (standardized to contribute 16 mg total sennosides) Senna powder (Cassia augustifolia) leaf, Buckthorn powder (Rhamnus frangula) bark, Licorice powder (Glycyrrhiza glabra) root, Alfalfa powder (Medicago sativa) leaf, Fennel powder (Foeniculum vulgare) seed, Anise powder (Pimpinella anisum) seed, Rhubarb powder (Rheum palmatum) root, Blue malva powder (Malva sylvestris) flower, Culver's root powder (Veronicastrum virginicum) root. Other Ingredients: Microcrystalline Cellulose, Karaya Gum, Corn Syrup Solids, Malt Extract, Barley Extract.

Herbolax **-** The Himalaya Drug Company (Himalaya Heal
Each capsule/tablet contains: Trivruth (ipomoea turpethum syn. operculina turpethum) 70 mg • Haritaki (terminalia chebula) 50 mg • Kasani (cichorium intybus) 50 mg • Kasamarda (cassia occidentalis) 50 mg • Kakamachi (solanum nigrum) 40 mg • Yashti-Madhu (glycyrrhiza glabra) 40 mg • Sunthi (zingiber officinale) 45 mg • Vidanga (embelia ribes) 10 mg.

Herbs & Prunes Formula **-** Nature's Life
Each tablet contains: Senna leaf (Senna alexandrina) 400 mg • Rhubarb root (Rheum officinale) 10 mg • Chinese Asparagus root (Tian dong, Asparagus cochinchinensis) 5 mg • Beet leaf (Beta vulgaris rubra) 5 mg • Buckthorn bark (Rhamnus frangula) 5 mg • Cabbage leaf (Brassica oleracea capitata) 5 mg • Cascara Sagrada (Rhamnus purshiana) 5 mg • Celery leaf (Apium graveolens) 5 mg • Cranberry (Vaccinium macrocarpon) 5 mg • Culvers root (Leptandra virginica) 5 mg • Dried Prune (Prunus aractus) 5 mg • Parsley leaf (Petroselinum crispum) 5 mg • Spinach leaf (Spinacia oleracea) 5 mg.

Herbs For Kids Echinacea/GoldenRoot Orange **-** Botanical Laboratories
Each 1 mL serving contains: Echinacea Purpurea root extract •

Oregon Grape root extract. Other Ingredients: Kosher Coconut and/or Palm Kernal Glycerine, Purified Water, Natural Orange extract, Citric Acid.

Herbs For Kids Feverfew Blend **-** Botanical Laboratories
Each 1 mL serving contains: Meadowsweet herb extract • Feverfew herb • Yarrow flowers • Echinacea Purpurea root • Skullcap herb • Lemon Balm herb • Wild Oat tops. Other Ingredients: Kosher Coconut and/or Palm Kernal Glycerine, Purified Water, Citric Acid.

Herbs For Kids St. John's Wort Blend **-** Botanical Laboratories
Each 1 mL serving contains: St. John's Wort flowering tops extract • Lemon Balm herb • Chamomile flowers • Wild Oat tops • Skullcap herb • Peppermint leaf • Lavender flowers. Other Ingredients: Kosher Coconut and/or Palm Kernal Glycerine, Purified Water, Citric Acid.

Herbs For Kids Sweet Echinacea **-** Botanical Laboratories
Each 1 mL serving contains: Echinacea Purpurea root. Other Ingredients: Kosher Coconut and/or Palm Kernal Glycerine, Purified Water, Citric Acid.

Herbs For Kids Valerian Extract **-** Botanical Laboratories
Each 1 mL serving contains: Valerian root extract. Other Ingredients: Kosher Coconut and/or Palm Kernal Glycerine, Purified Water, Citric Acid.

HerbTech AD-FX **-** CV Technologies
Each capsule contains: American Ginseng (standardized extract HT-1001containing >15% ginsenosides) 125 mg • Ginkgo biloba standardized extract 29 mg (containing >4% terpenelactones).

HerbTech Cell-FX **-** CV Technologies
Each capsule contains: Shark Cartilage extract 200 mg.

HerbTech Cell-FX (Bulk Powder) **-** CV Technologies
Water-soluble concentrated Shark Cartilage 227 mg.

HerbTech Cell-FX 500 mg **-** CV Technologies
Each capsule contains: Shark Cartilage extract 500 mg.

HerbTech Cold-FX **-** CV Technologies
Each capsule contains: Concentrated North American Ginseng (Panax quinquefolium) extract 200 mg.

HerbTech Menta-FX **-** CV Technologies
St. John's Wort 200 mg • HT-1001 (extract of American Ginseng) 100 mg • Ginkgo Biloba 25 mg.

HerbTech Pressure-FX **-** CV Technologies
Each capsule contains: Shark Cartilage 180 mg • Cordyceps extract 20 mg.

HerbTech Remember-FX **-** CV Technologies
North American Ginseng (Panax quinquefolium) 100 mg.

Herpanacine **-** Diamond Formulas
Six capsules contain: L-Lysine 1500 mg • A-Beta-Carotene 25,000 IU • L-Tyrosine 500 mg • E-D-Alpha 200 IU • Selenium 100 mcg • Dandelion leaf • Sarsaparilla • Astragalus • Ligustrum • Echinacea.

Herpe-Caps **-** Life Extension
Each capsule contains: L-Lysine 500 mg • L-Glysine 20 mg.

Herp-Eeze **-** Olympian Labs
Each capsule contains: Larreastat 50 mg • Ascorbic Acid 250 mg.

HerpeStat Cold Sore Lip Shield **-** Origin BioMedicinals
Shea Butter • Bees Wax • Polyphenon 70 Green Tea catechin extract • Avena Sativa Oil • Zinc Oxide • Peppermint Oil • Geranium Oil • Prunella Vulgaris extract • Tea Tree Oil • Bergamot Oil • Vitamin C • Vitamin E.

HerpeStat Medicated Cream **-** Origin BioMedicinals
Active Ingredient: Prunella vulgaris 1% extract.

Herpilyn **-** Enzymatic Therapy
Active ingredient: Allantoin 1%. Other Ingredients: Melissa extract (Lemon Balm) 70:1, White Soft Paraffin, Benzyl Alcohol.

HGH Activator **-** Gero Vita International
Six sprays contain: Excell Activator (micro molecular polypeptide complex) 3000 mg. Other Ingredients: Purified Water, Phospholipids, Glycerin, Wheat Germ Oil, Sodium Citrate, Citric Acid, Potassium Sorbate, Maltodextrin, Methylparaben, Propylparaben, Glycine, Orange-Mint Natural Flavor.

HGH at Night **-** Global Health Trax
Two tablespoons (1 fl oz) contain: Potassium (from potassium sorbate) 35 mg • Collagen Hydrosylate 2 g • Fructo Oligo Saccharides (FOS) 200 mg • Conjugated Linoleic Acid (CLA) 100 mg • Trace Element Complex 500 mg • Amino Acid Complex 1250 mg: Glutamic Acid, Glutathione, Arginine, L-Carnitine, Ornithine, Methionine, L-Glutamine. Other Ingredients: Purified Water, Citric Acid, Sodium Benzoate, Berry Flavoring, Glycerin.

HGH Booster **-** Life Extension
Three sprays contain: L-Arginine 200 mg • L-Ornithine 100 mg • DHEA 1000 mcg • Glutamine 5 mcg • L-Lysine 5 mcg • Polymer Matrix 2 mcg.

HGH Release **-** NewLibido
Each two capsules contain: Arginine (l-arginine HCl) 200 mg • Ornithine (l-ornithine HCl) 150 mg • Lysine (l-lysine HCl) 50 mg • Glutamine (l-glutamine HCl) 150 mg • Colostrum (bovine) 100 mg • Anterior Pituitary (extract) 50 mg • Orinthine Alphaketoglutarate 50 mg • Glycine (l-glysine HCl) 50 mg. Other Ingredients: Gelatin, Dicalcium Phosphate, Magnesium Stearate, Stearic Acid.
See Editor's Note No. 14.

hGH SecreatGAIN **-** I Force
Three capsules contain: B6 (pyridoxal 5' phosphate) 10 mg • Zinc Monomethionine 20 mg • 2-Amino-5-Guanidinopentanoic Acid-5 Oxo L-Proline 1000 mg • 2,6-Diaminohexanoic Acid 100 mg • 2-Amino-4-(methylthio) Butanoic Acid 500 mg • Alpha Glyceryl-Phosphorylcholine 200 mg • Coleus Forskohlii (95% forskolin) 50 mg. Other Ingredients: Gelatin, Microcrystalline Cellulose, Magnesium Stearate, Silica.

HGH15 **-** HealthMinded
Four capsules contain: HGH15 Complex 1500 mg: Anterior Pituitary, Hypothalamus, Amino Acid blend, Phytosterol complex, Beta Sitosterol, Campesterol, Stigmasterol, Soy Phosphatides complex, Phosphatidyl Serine, Phosphatidyl Choline, Phosphatidyl Ethanolamine, Phosphatidyl Inositol, Panax Ginseng. Other Ingredients: Stearic Acid, Magnesium Stearate.

Hi Energy Multi for Men **-** Futurebiotics
Three tablets contain: Beta Carotene 25,000 IU • Vitamin C • (Ascorbic Acid, Palmitate) 250 mg • Vitamin D 200 IU • Vitamin E 60 IU • Vitamin B1 (Thiamin) 25 mg • Vitamin B2 (Riboflavin) 25 mg • Niacinamide 50 mg • Pantothenic Acid 25 mg • Vitamin B6 25 mg • Vitamin B12 100 mcg • Biotin 300 mcg • Folic Acid 400 mcg • Phosphatidyl Choline 100 mg • Inositol 75 mg • Ribonucleic Acid (RNA) 75 mg • Para Amino Benzoic Acid (PABA) 75 mg • Zinc (Monomethionine) 30 mg • Calcium (Phosphate, Citrate, Amino Acid Chelate) 200 mg • Magnesium (Citrate, Amino Acid Chelate) 200 mg • Iron (Gluconate) 6 mg • Potassium (Citrate) 99 mg • Chromium (Polynicotinate) 200 mcg • Copper (Gluconate) 2 mg • Iodine (Kelp) 200 mcg • Manganese (Proteinate) 5 mg • Molybdenum (Amino Acid Chelate) 25 mcg • Selenium (Selenomethionine) 200 mcg. In a base of herbal extracts, powders & nutritional concentrates equivalent to 2,000 mg: Active Ginsenosides (from Standardized Ginseng Extract), Saw Palmetto, Avena Sativa, Ginseng, Hawthorn, Garlic (Odorless Extract), Bee Pollen, Foti, Adrenal Concentrate, Octacosanol (Wheat Free), Alfalfa Juice Concentrate, Spirulina.
See Editor's Note No. 14.

Hi-B 100 Complex - Vegetarian Formula - Nature's Life
Each tablet contains: Vitamin B1 (Thiamine Hydrochloride) 100 mg • Vitamin B2 (Riboflavin) 100 mg • Vitamin B6 (Pyridoxine Hydrochloride) 100 mg • Vitamin B12 (Cobalamin concentrate) 100 mcg • Folic Acid 400 mcg • Biotin 100 mcg • Niacinamide 100 mg • Pantothenic Acid (d-Calcium Pantothenate) 100 mg • Choline (Bitartrate) 100 mg • PABA (Para Aminobenzoic Acid) 100 mg • Inositol 100 mg. In a natural base of Alfalfa, Parsley, Rice Bran & Watercress.

Hi-B-100 Complex - Nature's Life
Each capsule contains: Vitamin B1 (Thiamine HCl) 100 mg • Vitamin B2 (Riboflavin) 100 mg • Vitamin B6 (Pyridoxine HCl) 100 mg • Vitamin B12 (Cobalamin concentrate) 100 mcg • Niacinamide 100 mg • Pantothenic Acid (d-Calcium Pantothenate) 100 mg • Choline (Bitartrate) 100 mg • Inositol 100 mg • Biotin 100 mcg • Folic Acid 400 mcg • PABA (Para-Aminobenzioc Acid) 100 mg. In a natural base of Rice Bran.

High Absorption Calcium - Doctor's Best
Each tablet contains: Vitamin D (as cholecalciferol) 100 IU • Calcium (as calcium bis-glycinate) 250 mg • Zinc (as zinc bis-glycinate) 3.75 mg • Copper (as copper bis-glycinate) 0.5 mg • Manganese (as manganese bis-glycinate) 0.5 mg • Boron (as boron glycinate) 125 mcg • Black Pepper extract (fruit, Bioperine) 2 mg. Inactive Ingredients: Stearic Acid, Cellulose, Croscarmellose Sodium, Magnesium Stearate, Silicon Dioxide.

High Five - Pharmanex
Each tablet contains: Boswellia Serrata Extract (stem) 125 mg • Fungal Protease (Aspergillus Oryzae) 100 mg • Bromelain (from Pineapple extract) 50 mg • Quercetin 25 mg • Papain (from Papaya extract) 10 mg. Other Ingredients: Dicalcium Phosphate, Microcrystalline Cellulose, Cellulose Powder, Silica, Magnesium Stearate.

High Gamma Tocopherol - PhysioLogics
Each softgel contains: Vitamin E (as d-alpha tocopherol) 200 IU • D-Gamma-Tocopherol 200 mg • Other Tocopherols (d-delta, d-beta tocopherol) 78 mg • Tocotrienols 2 mg. Other Ingredients: Gelatin, Glycerin, Non-GMO Soybean Oil.

High Performance Creatine - Puritan's Pride
Each serving contains: Creatine Monohydrate 5.25 g • Taurine 1000 mg.

High Potency Apple Cider Vinegar - Now
Two capsules contain: Apple Cider Vinegar powder 900 mg. Other Ingredients: Gelatin (capsule), Magnesium Stearate, Silica.

High Potency B-Complex with Vitamin C - Puritan's Pride
Each caplet contains: Vitamin C (as ascorbic acid) 300 mg • Thiamin (Vitamin B1; as thiamine mononitrate) 15 mg • Riboflavin (Vitamin B2) 10.2 mg • Niacin (as niacinamide) 50 mg • Vitamin B6 (as pyridoxine hydrochloride) 5 mg • Pantothenic Acid (as d-calcium pantothenate) 10 mg. Other Ingredients: Dicalcium Phosphate, Cellulose (Plant Origin), Cellulose Coating, Croscarmellose, Vegetable Magnesium Stearate, Silica, FD&C Yellow No.5 Aluminum Lake, Titanium Dioxide Color, Vegetable Stearic Acid, Guar Gum.

High Potency Cal-Mag Plus - Quest
Each tablet contains: Calcium (Citrate) 250 mg • Magnesium (Oxide) 250 mg • Vitamin C (Ascorbic Acid) 150 mg • Vitamin D (as Vitamin D3) 100 IU • Zinc (Citrate) 10 mg. Other Ingredients: Croscarmellose Sodium, Magnesium Stearate (vegetable source), Microcrystalline Cellulose, Silicon Dioxide, Vegetable Stearin.

High Potency Grapine - Nature's Sunshine
Each tablet contains: Calcium (di-calcium phosphate) 60 mg • Phosphorous (di-calcium phosphate) 50 mg • Grapine proanthocyanidins from Grape seed & Pine bark 60 mg. Inactive Ingredients: Cellulose (plant fiber), Stearic Acid, Silicon Dioxide (powdered silica), Magnesium Stearate (vegetable).

High Potency Iron from Ferrous Sulfate - Leiner Health Products
Each tablet contains: Iron (Ferrous Sulfate) 27 mg. Other Ingredients: Calcium Carbonate, Starch, Maltodextrin, Cellulose, Croscarmellose Sodium, Tricalcium Phosphate, Hydroxypropyl Methylcellulose, Polyethylene Glycol 3350, Silicon Dioxide, Talc, Magnesium Stearate, Hydroxypropyl Cellulose, Red 40 Lake, Polysorbate 80, Titanium Dioxide, Povidone.

High Potency Magnesium 500 mg - Puritan's Pride
Each tablet contains: Magnesium (as magnesium oxide) 500 mg. Other Ingredients: Cellulose (plant origin), Starch, Povidone, Magnesium Silicate, Cellulose Coating, Titanium Dioxide Color, Vegetable Magnesium Stearate, Propylene Glycol.

High Potency Soft Multiple - Swanson
Each softgel contains: Vitamin A (as beta-carotene) 5000 IU •Vitamin C USP (as ascorbic acid) 150 mg • Vitamin D (as cholecalciferol) 200 IU •Vitamin E (as d-alpha tocopherol) 100 IU •Thiamin USP (as thiamin mononitrate; vitamin B-1) 25 mg • Riboflavin USP (vitamin B-2) 25 mg • Niacin (as niacin 5 mg; as niacinamide 25 mg) 30 mg • Vitamin B-6 (as pyridoxine HCl) 25 mg • Folic Acid 200 mcg • Vitamin B-12 (as cyanocobalamin) 25 mcg • Biotin 25 mcg • Pantothenic Acid (as d-calcium pantothenate) 25 mg • Calcium (from calcium carbonate) 100 mg • Iron (as ferrous fumarate) 7.5 mg • Iodine (as potassium iodide) 75 mcg • Magnesium (from magnesium oxide) 50 mg • Zinc (from zinc oxide) 7.5 mg • Selenium (from selenomethionine) 12.5 mcg • Copper (from copper gluconate) 0.5 mg • Manganese (from manganese sulfate) 5 mg • Chromium (from Chromax chromium picolinate) 12.5 mcg • Molybdenum (sodium molybdate) 12.5 mcg. Lecithin 40 mg • Choline (as choline bitartrate) 25 mg • Inositol 25 mg • PABA (para-aminobenzoic acid) 25 mg, Boron (from calcium borogluconate) 0.5 mg • Silica (from silicon dioxide) 0.25 mg • Vanadium (from vanadyl sulfate) 5 mcg.

High Strength Aloe Vera - Puritan's Pride
Each tablet contains: Aloe Vera(200:1 Extract, Aloe Barbadensis Miller) 100 mg. Other Ingredients: Dicalcium Phosphate, Cellulose (Plant Origin), Vegetable Stearic Acid, Croscarmellose, Cellulose Coating, Silica, Vegetable Magnesium Stearate.

High Strength Cod Liver Oil - Nature's Bounty
Each softgel contains: Vitamin A (as Cod Liver Oil and Retinyl Palmitate) 2664 IU • Vitamin D (as Cod Liver Oil and Cholecalciferol) 200 IU • Cod Liver Oil 1000 mg • Eicosapentaenoic Acid 110 mg • Docosahexaenoic Acid 100 mg. Other Ingredients: Gelatin, Glycerin.

High Stress B & C - Source Naturals
Each four tablets contain: Vitamin C (ascorbic acid) 666 mg • Vitamin D (vitamin D3 from cholesalceferol) 68 IU • Thiamin (vitamin B1) 66 mg • Riboflavin (vitamin B2) 40 mg • Niacin (as niacinamide 133 mg and niacin 33 mg) 166 mg • Vitamin B6 (pyridoxide HCl) 53 mg • Folate (as folate acid) 560 mcg • Vitamin B12 (as cyanocobalamin) 133 mcg • Biotin 133 mcg • Pantothenic Acid (as calcium d-pantothenate) 333 mg • Calcium 133 mg • Magnesium (as magnesium oxide & taurinate) 323 mg • Potassium (as potassium citrate) 33 mg • Valerian Root 400 mg • Catnip Leaf 333 mg • Zizyphus Seed 266 • Hops Flower 233 mg • Skullcap Leaf and Stem 233 mg • Chamomile Flower 200 mg • Passion Flower 200 mg • GABA (gamma amino butyric acid) 200 mg • Spirulina 200 mg • Wood Betony Leaf, Stem, and Flower 166 mg • Inositol 133 mg • Ginger Root 100 mg • Phosphatidyl Choline (as lecithin) 89 mg • Licorice Root 66 mg • L-Tyrosine 66 mg • Choline (as bitartrate) 66 mg • PABA (para amino benzoic acid) 53 mg.

High Thyroid - Enzymes, Inc.
Each capsule contains: Proprietary Herbal Blend 270 mg: Bugleweed herb extract, Lemon Balm herb extract, Flaxseed, Passionflower herb extract • Proprietary Blend 57 mg: Protease, CereCalase. Other Ingredients: Cellulose, Water.

Some Brand Name Natural Products - What they Contain
www.NaturalDatabase.com contains MANY more listings than appear here.

Higher Mind **-** Source Naturals
Four tablets contain: Phosphatidyl Serine (Leci-PS) 150 mg • Vitamin B1 (Thiamin) 100 mg • Vitamin B2 (Riboflavin) 25 mg • Vitamin B3 (Inositol Hexanicotinate 100 mg and Niacin 50 mg) 150 mg • Vitamin B5 (Pantothenic Acid) 50 mg • Vitamin B6 (PAK and Pyridoxine HCl) 100 mg • Vitamin B12 50 mcg • Folic Acid 800 mcg • Biotin 50 mcg • Vitamin C (Calcium and Zinc Ascorbates) 200 mg • Calcium (Ascorbate, Carbonate, Malate, Succinate) 100 mg • Magnesium (Malate, Succinate, Taurinate, Oxide) 200 mg • Zinc (Ascorbate) 10 mg • Manganese (Citrate) 5 mg • L-Pyroglutamic Acid 750 mg • L-Glutamine 500 mg • Acetyl L-Carnitine 300 mg • DMAE (Bitartrate) 100 mg • Taurine (Magnesium Taurinate) 200 mg • DLPA (DL-Phenylalanine) 200 mg • Phosphatidyl Choline 157.5 mg • Phosphatidyl Ethanolamine 105 mg • N-Acetyl L-Tyrosine 100 mg • GABA (Gamma Amino Butyric Acid) 100 mg • PAK (Pyridoxine Alpha-Ketoglutarate) 100 mg • Ginkgo Biloba extract 24% (50:1) 50 mg • Phosphatidyl Inositol 45 mg • Alpha-Lipoic Acid (Thioctic Acid) 20 mg • Coenzyme Q10 (Ubiquinone) 10 mg • Inositol 10 mg.

Himalayan Goji Juice **-** Dr. Earl Mindell
Reconstitued Goji juice (from whole lycium barbarum fruit) • Grape juice concentrate • Pear juice concentrate • Apple juice concentrate • Pear puree • Natural flavor • Sodium Benzoate • Potassium Sorbate.

Himcocid **-** The Himalaya Drug Company (Himalaya Heal
Each 1 tsp (5 mL) serving contains: Varatika (syn. cowrie bhasma, cowrie shell calx/ash) 70 mg • Dugdhapashana (soft stone/magnesium silicate) 70 mg • Mouktika Sukti (syn. mouktika bhasma, pearl oyster shell calx) 15 mg • Yashtimadhu (glycyrrhiza glabra) 5 mg.

Himcolin Gel **-** The Himalaya Drug Company (Himalaya Heal
Each 1 gm serving contains: Jyotishmati oil (celastrus paniculatus) 200 mg • Lathakasthuri oil (hibiscus abelmoschus) 150 mg • Vathada oil (prunus amygdalus) 100 mg • Nirgundi oil (vitex negundo) 100 mg • Karpasa oil (gossypium herbaceum) 50 mg • Mukulaka oil (pistacia vera) 50 mg • Jatiphalam oil (myristica fragrans) 30 mg • Jaatipatree oil (myristica fragrans, mace) 30 mg • Lavanga oil (syzygium aromaticum) 30 mg • Taja oil (cinnamomum cassia) 3 mg.

Himcospaz **-** The Himalaya Drug Company (Himalaya Heal
Each capsule contains: Sati (curcuma zedoaria) 25.5 mg • Sunthi (zingiber officinale) 24 mg • Ajamoda (apium graveolens) 96 mg.

Himplasia **-** The Himalaya Drug Company (Himalaya Heal
Each tablet contains: Gokshura (tribulus terrestris) 140 mg • Putikaranja (caesalpinia bonducella) 120 mg • Puga (areca catechu) 100 mg • Shatavari (asparagus racemosus) 80 mg • Varuna (crataeva nurvala) 80 mg • Akika Pishti (processed agate) 80 mg.

Hi-Potent-C (powdered) **-** Nutri-Quest Rx
Each level teaspoonful contains: Vitamin C 1500 mg • Mannitol 1355 mg • Rose Hips 250 mg • Lemon Bioflavinoids 130 mg • Hesperidin Complex 50 mg • Rutin 35 mg • Acerola concentrate 35 mg • natural Flavor.

Hives **-** Hyland's
Two tablets contain: Apis Mellifica Ca 3X • Urtica Urens 3X • Natrum Muriaticum 6X • Arsenicum Album 6X. Base: Lactose.
See Editor's Note No. 1, page 2053.

HMB **-** EAS
Each 4 capsule serving contains: HMB 1000 mg • Potassium Phosphate 200 mg.

HMB Caps **-** Optimum Nutrition
Each capsule contains: Hydroxymethyl Butyrate (HMB, as calcium beta-hydroxy beta-methylbutyrate monohydrate) 1000 mg. Other Ingredients: Gelatin, Microcrystalline Cellulose, Magnesium Stearate.

HMF Forte **-** Genestra - Seroyal
Each capsule contains: L. Acidophilus 4 billion CFU • L. Bifidus 1 billion CFU • FOS (Fructo-oligo-saccharides) 100 mg.

HMF Powder **-** Genestra - Seroyal
Each quarter teaspoon (1 g) contains: L. Acidphilus 3 billion CFU • L. Bifidus 3 billion CFU • FOS (fructo-oligo-saccharides) 450 mg.

HMF Replete **-** Genestra - Seroyal
Each packet contains: L. Acidophilus 10 billion CFU • L. Bifidus 10 billion CFU • L. Bulgaricus 10 billion CFU • FOS (fructo-oligo-saccharides) 9 g.

Holista Echinacea **-** Holista
Each capsule contains: Echinacea angustifolia/purpurea (root) (16:1 extract) 500 mg.

Holista Echinacea Tincture **-** Holista
Each mL contains: Echinacea angustifolia dried root 1:1 standardized extract in alcohol 45% 200 mg.

Holista Evening Primrose Oil 1000 mg **-** Holista
Each capsule contains: Evening Primrose Oil 1000 mg, containing 10% gamma-linolenic acid and 70% linoleic acid.

Holista Evening Primrose Oil 500 mg **-** Holista
Each capsule contains: Evening Primrose Oil (not less than 50 mg of gamma-linolenic acid and 350 mg of lenoleic acid) standardized to 10% GLA 500 mg.

Holista Feverfew **-** Holista
Each capsule contains: Feverfew (Tanacetum parthenium) standardized to a minimum of 0.2% parthenolide 125 mg.

Holista Lactase enzyme **-** Holista
Each capsule contains: Food Chemical Codex Lactase 3000 units.

Holista Milk Thistle **-** Holista
Each capsule contains: Milk Thistle (Silybum marianum) standardized to silymarin 80% 150 mg.

Holista Milk Thistle Tincture **-** Holista
Each mL contains: Milk Thistle seed from 1:1 fluid extract in 65% alcohol 0.2 mg.

Holista Saw Palmetto **-** Holista
Each caplet contains: Saw Palmetto (Serenoa repens) extract from berries 10:1 160 mg.

Holista Saw Palmetto Tincture **-** Holista
Each mL contains: Saw Palmetto dried berries of Seronoa repens 1:1 in 45% alcohol 0.2 mg.

Holista Tea Tree Oil 20% Lotion **-** Holista
Tea Tree oil (Melaleuca alternifolia) 0.2 mL. Other Ingredients: Water, Alcohol.

Holista Valerian **-** Holista
Each capsule contains: Valerian Root Extract standardized to 0.8% Valerenic Acid 500 mg.

Holista Valerian Tincture **-** Holista
Each mL contains: Valerian Root from the rhizome and roots of Valeriana officianalis 1:1 in 60% alcohol 0.2 mg.

Holista Zinc Lozenges **-** Holista
Each lozenge contains: Zinc (citrate) 5 mg • Echinacea 50 mg • Vitamin C 50 mg.

Homeopathic Bug Bite Relief **-** Hyland's
Active Ingredients: Apis Mellifica 3X HPUS • Calendula Officinalis 3X HPUS • Echinacea Angustifolia 3X HPUS • Ledum Palustre 3X HPUS • Urtica Dioica 3X HPUS. Inactive Ingredients: Petrolatum USP, Beeswax USP, Citronella Oil, Methylparaben USP, Propylparaben USP.
See Editor's Note No. 1, page 2053.

Homocysteine Control **-** Nature's Way
Each capsule contains: Betaine Anhydrous 500 mg • Folic Acid (folate) 800 mcg • Pyridoxine HCl 20 mg • Vitamin B-12 (cyanoco-

balamin) 400 mcg. Other Ingredients: Cellulose, Gelatin, Magnesium stearate, Millet.

Homocysteine De-Crease **-** Nutri-Quest Rx
Each tablet contains: Trimethylglycine 300 mg • Pyridoxal 5 Phosphate 5 mg (enteric coated) • Vitamin B12 200 mcg • Dimethyl Gluyine 25 mg • Niacinamide 20 mg • Cysteine 15 mg • Molybdenum Chelate 30 mcg • Selenium Chelate 15 mcg • Vitamin B6 15 mg (enertic coated) • Folic Acid 275 mg • Vitamin E Succinate 10 IU • Red Beet root 25 mg • Choline Bitartrate 10 mg • Magnesium Chelate 100 mg • Zinc Chelate 10 mg.

Homocysteine Formula **-** Nature's Life
Each capsule contains: Vitamin B6 (Pyridoxine HCl) 10 mg • Folic Acid 800 mcg • Vitamin B12 400 mcg • Choline (Bitartrate) 50 mg • Betaine HCl 50 mg.

Homocysteine Regulators **-** Now
Each Vcap contains: Vitamin B6 (as Coenzyme Pyridoxyl-5-Phosphate) 20 mg • Vitamin B12 (as Cyanocobalamin) 250 mcg • Folic Acid 800 mcg • Trimethylglycine (Betaine) 400 mg.

HomocystexPlus with TMG & TroxeRutin **-** Natrol
Each capsule contains: Riboflavin (Vitamin B2) 25 mg • Vitamin B6 (as pyridoxine HCl) 25 mg • Folic Acid 800 mcg • Vitamin B12 (as cobalamin) 500 mcg • Betaine TMG (as betaine trimethylglycine) 500 mg • TroxeRutin 100 mg • Choline (as choline bitartrate) 25 mg. Other Ingredients: Silicon Dioxide, Magnesium Stearate, Gelatin.

Honey Apple Double Ginseng **-** Traditional Medicinals
Asian Ginseng root (Panax ginseng) • American Ginseng root (Panax quinquefolius) • Siberian Ginseng root (Eleutherococcus senticosus) • Chamomile flower • Licorice root • Orange peel • dried Apples • Prince Ginseng rootlets (Pseudostellada heterophylla) • Natural Honey & Apple flavors.

Honey C Chews Chewable C 100 mg **-** Nature's Life
Each wafer contains: Vitamin C (buffered) 100 mg • Rose Hips powder (Rosa canina) 50 mg • Acerola berry powder (Malpighia glabra) 25 mg.

Honey C Chews Chewable C 300 mg **-** Nature's Life
Each wafer contains: Vitamin C (buffered) 300 mg • Rose Hips powder (Rosa canina) 50 mg • Acerola berry powder (Malpighia glabra) 25 mg.

Honey-B-Anise "Old Tyme" Sore Throat Syrup **-** Thayers Natural Pharmaceuticals
Vegetable Glycerin • Honey • Purified Water • Propylene Glycol • Anise Oil • Bee Propolis.

Hoodia Diet Tabs **-** Nature's Rx
Each tablet contains: Hoodia Gordonii (20:1) 50 mg • Calcium Pyruvate 300 mg • Calcium (from calcium pyruvate) 48 mg • Citrus Pectin 40 mg • Prune 30 mg • Grapefruit seed extract 30 mg • Chromium 100 mcg.

Hoodia Gordoni Cactus **-** Planet Hoodia
Each capsule contains: Hoodia Gordonii 400 mg.

Hoodia Weight-Loss **-** VitaSalveo
Three tablets contain: Chromium Polynicotinate 10% 100 mcg • Calcium Pyruvate 48 mg • Hoodia Gordonii powder 50 mg • Citrus Pectin 40 mg • Grapefruit seed extract (4:1) 30 mg • Prune powder 30 mg. Other Ingredients: Rice Bran Powder, Magnesium Stearate (NF/FCC vegetable grade, kosher).

HoodiaLean **-** Phytobase, Inc.
Two vegetable capsules contain: Hoodia Gordonii 20:1 extract 850 mg • Proprietary Blend 250 mg: Standardized Cocoa Almond blend, Suma root, Gymnema Sylvestre extract, Naringin, Cayenne pepper extract.

Hoodoba Diet Pills **-** Hoodoba
Two capsules contain: Vitamin B6 (as pyridoxal-5-phosphate) 3 mg • Manganese (as manganese sulfate) 2 mg • Chromium (chelated) 150 mcg • Hoodoba Proprietary Blend 1529 mg: Garcinia Cambogia fruit extract (50% hydroxycitric acid), Hoodia Gordonii Cactus, Citrus Aurantium extract (immature peel), Green Tea leaf extract (20% polyphenols), Nut Grass extract, Banaba leaf extract (1% corosolic acid), Red Panax Ginseng root, Vanadium (vanadyl sulfate), Bioperine extract. Other Ingredients: Gelatin, Microcrystalline Cellulose, Magnesium Stearate, Silica.
See Editor's Note No. 40, page 2058.

Hops, Valerian & Scullcap **-** Dial Herbs
Hops • Valerian • Scullcap.

Hormogen **-** Atrium Inc.
Each capsule contains: Lecithin 200 mg • Safflower oil 200 mg • Wheat Germ oil (Cold Pressed) 66.667 mg • Rice Bran oil 66.667 mg • Soybean oil 66.667 mg.

Hormone Harmony **-** iVillage Inc.
Two softgels contain: Schizandra berry extract (wu-wei-zi, 2% schizandrins, 3.2 mg) 160 mg • Ginger rhizome supercritical extract (certified organic, 30% pungent compounds, 8.1 mg; 8% zingiberene, 2.1 mg; 23 mg post-supercritical ethanolic (PSE) extract, 2% pungent compounds, 0.46 mg) 50 mg • Black Cohosh berry root & rhizome extract (8% triterpene glycosides, 3.2 mg) 40 mg • Chastetree berry extract (vitus agnus-castus, 0.6% aucubin, 0.2 mg; 0.5% agnuside, 0.2 mg) 40 mg • Rosemary leaf supercritical extract (23% total phenolic antioxidants, 2.3 mg) 10 mg. Other Ingredients: Evening Primrose Seed Oil Supercritical Extract, Olive Oil - Extra Virgin, Maltodextrin, Yellow Beeswax, Gelatin, Vegetable Glycerine, Purified Water, Carob.

Hormone Nutrients **-** Wellness for Women
Each capsule contains: Vitamin B-6 (as pyridoxine HCl) 50 mg • Magnesium (from amino acid chelate) 75 mg • Motherwort (5:1 concentrate) 100 mg • Vitex Chasteberry extract (0.5% agnusides) 100 mg • Dong Quai extract (1% ligustilides) 75 mg • SoyLife® Soy protein extract (1% soy isoflavones) 75 mg • Black Cohosh extract (2.5% triterpene-glycosides) 50 mg.

Horse Chestnut **-** Jamieson
Each caplet contains: Horse Chestnut Seed 1100 mg.

Horse Chestnut Extract **-** Enzymatic Therapy/PhytoPharmica
Each capsule contains: Horse Chestnut seed extract (aesculus hippocastanum, standardized to contain 20% triterpene glycosides calculated as escin) 250 mg. Other Ingredients: Gelatin, Cellulose, Magnesium Stearate, Silicon Dioxide, Titanium Dioxide Color.

Horse Chestnut Herbal Balm **-** Nature's Life
Deionized Water • Horse Chestnut seed extract [(Aesculus hippocastanum L.) standardized to 2% aescin] • Phospholipids from Safflower & Sunflower seed oil • Caprylic/Capric Triglyceride • Apricot Kernel oil • Soy Lecithin • Glycerine (Vegetable) • Tocopherol (natural Vitamin E) • Arnica extract • Panthenol • Saccharide Isomerate • Xanthan Gum • Carrageenan (Irish Moss) • Dimethicone • Lauroyl Lysine • Natural Fragrant Essential Oils Blend • Sodium Hydroxymethylglycinate.

Horsetail Extract Formula **-** Quest
Each caplet contains: Horsetail powder (Equisetum arvense) (provided by 125 mg 1:4 Aqueous Extract) 500 mg • Rosehips powder (Rose canina) 50 mg • Burdock root powder (Arctium lappa) 30 mg • Marshmallow root powder (Althaea officinalis) 30 mg • Parsley leaf powder (Plantago major) 30 mg • Slippery Elm bark powder (Ulmus fulva) 30 mg. Other Ingredients: Calcium Phosphate, Microcrystalline Cellulose, Croscarmellose Sodium, Magnesium Stearate (vegetable source), Vegetable Stearin.

Horsetail Plus Fo-Ti **-** The Herbalist
Horsetail fresh-dried herb (Equisetum arvense) • Fo-Ti fresh-dried root (Polygonum multiforum) • Nettles fresh-dried leaf (Urtica dioica)

• Red Clover fresh-dried blossom (Trifolium pratense) • Burdock fresh-dried root (Arctium lappa).

Hot Flash **-** Source Naturals
Three tablets contain: Soy concentrate, yielding 65 mg Isoflavones 2100 mg • Black Cohosh 160 mg • Dong Quai extract 150 mg • Licorice root extract 150 mg • Vitex extract 100 mg.

Hot Flashex **-** Natrol
Each tablet contains: Vitamin E (as d-alpha tocopherol) 50 IU • Calcium (as tri-calcium phosphate) 70 mg • Licorice 100 mg • Black Cohosh root 60 mg, Triterpenes (2.5%) 15 mg • Chamomile extract 50 mg • Kava Kava root 30 mg, Kavalactones (30%) 9 mg. Other Ingredients: Mono & Di-Glycerides, Croscarmellose Sodium, Silicon Dioxide, Stearic Acid, Magnesium Stearate.

Hot Jalapeno & Cheddar Soynuts - Revival **-** Physicians Laboratories
Each 1/6 cup contains: Certified Isoflavone 10 mg. Other Ingredients: Soy Protein (whole roasted soybeans), Soybean Oil, Cheddar Cheese, Salt, Whey, Maltodextrin, Blue Cheese, Nonfat Milk, Citric Acid, Jalapeno Powder, Dextrose, Green Chile Pepper, Onion and Garlic Powder, Natural and Artificial Flavors, Artificial Color (FD&C yellow #6).

Hot Mommies Essential 3 **-** Changes International, Inc.
Four tablets contain: Chromium (as chromium dinicotinate glycinate) 400 mcg • Citrus Aurantium extract (bitter orange) 1300 mg • Green Tea leaf extract 600 mg • Kudzu root extract 100 mg • Rhubarb root extract 160 mg • Carthamus Tinctorius seed 70 mg • Siberian Ginseng (eleuthero) 38 mg • Gypenosides from Gynostema pentaphyllum plant extract 21 mg • Proprietary Blend 1413 mg: Polygonum Multiflorium root extract, Lycium berry extract, Lotus seed, Dong Quai root extract, Ligusticum Wallichi root, White Atractylodes rhizome, Astragalus root extract, White Peony root extract, Sicklepod Senna seed (cassia tora), Crataegus Oxyacantha berry and leaf extract, Gymnema Sylvestre leaf extract, Licorice root extract. Other Ingredients: Dicalcium Phosphate, Microcrystalline Cellulose, Croscarmellose Sodium, Stearic Acid, Anise Oil, Magnesium Stearate, Silica, Calcium Silicate, Pharmaceutical Glaze.
See Editor's Note No. 40, page 2058.

Hot-Rox **-** BioTest Laboratories, LLC
Two capsules contain: Thiamin (vitamin B1) 20 mg • Niacin (vitamin B3) 20 mg • Pantothenic Acid 20 mg • Pyridoxal-5-Phosphate 50 mg • Vitamin B12 (methylcobalamin) 995 mcg • HOT-ROX Thermogenic Formula 950 mg: N-Acetyl-L-Tyrosine, MDX complex: Androst-5-ene-7-one-317-diethl-carbonate, Sclaremax propreitary Salvia Sclarea extract, Guggulsterone Z, Guggulsterone E; Caffeine, 5-Hydroxy - L-Tryptophan.

Hoxsey Formula **-** The Herbalist
Red Clover fresh-dried blossoms (Trifolium pratense)• Chaparral fresh-dried leaf (Larrea tridentata)• Licorice fresh-dried root (Glycyrrhiza glabra)• Oregon Grape fresh-dried root (Berberis nervosa)• Burdock fresh-dried root (Arcticum lappa)• Sarsaparilla fresh-dried root (Smilax ornata)• Echinacea fresh root (Echinacea angustifolia)• Prickly Ash fresh-dried bark (Zanthoxylum americanum).

HPX Hydrating Gel **-** Nu Skin Enterprises
Water • Kukui nut oil • Propylene Glycol • Human Placental Protein • Tocopheryl Acetate • Phospholipids • Tocopherol • Carbomer • Triethanolamine • Methylparaben • Disodium EDTA • Phenoxyethanol • BHT.

Hua Fo **-** Shenlong Natural International, Inc.
Each tablet contains: Panax Ginseng 18 mg • Ligustrum lucidum fruit (Privet fruit) 72 mg • Curculigoo orchiodes (Golden-Eye Grass rhizome) 54 mg. Other Ingredients: Epimemdium grandiflorum (Licentious Goat Wort) 84 mg, Polygonium multiflorum (Black Haired Mr. He) 72 mg.
See Editor's Note No. 3, page 2053.

Human Growth Complex **-** Ultra Lab
Each tablet contains: Somatotrophine (GH) 12X • Insulin-Like Growth Factor-1 (IGF-1) 12X • Alfalfa 3X • Arnica Montana 15X • Arsenicum Album 15X • Baptisia 15X • Bryonia 15X • China Officinalis 15X • Gelsemium Sempervirens 15X • Lacticum Acidum 15X • Lycopodium Clavatum 15X • Phosphorus 15X • Rhus Toxicodendron 15X • Ruta Graveolens 10X.
See Editor's Note No. 1, page 2053.

Human Growth Hormone (HGH) **-** Youngevity
Each capsule contains: L-Lysine HCL • L-Arginine • L-Ornithine • L-Glutamine • L-Tyrosine • Vilcabamba Mineral Essence: Potassium, Calcium, Magnesium, Zinc, Chromium, Selenium, Iron, Copper, Molybdenum, Vanadium, Iodine, Cobalt, Manganese.

HumanoVar **-** GEN - Genetic Evolutionary Nutrition
Each capsule contains: Vitamin E 30 IU • Selenium (from amino acid chelate) 50 mcg • Proteic Embryo Extract (from fertilized chicken eggs) 100 mg. Inactive Ingredients: Gelatine, Magnesium Stearate, Silicon Dioxide.

Huperzine A Complex **-** Puritan's Pride
Each tablet contains: Folic Acid 200 mcg • Vitamin B12 (as cyanocobalamin) 6 mcg • DMAE (from DMAE bitartrate) (dimethylaminoethanol) 50 mg • Panax ginseng (root standardized extract: provides 5 mg ginsenosides) 125 mg • Huperzine A (from standardized Huperiza serrata) leaf extract 50 mcg • L-Tyrosine 75 mg • Bioperine (from standardized piperine) 2.5 mg.

Huperzine A Complex **-** PhysioLogics
Each tablet contains: Folic Acid 200 mg • Vitamin B12 (as cyanocobalamin) 6 mcg • DMAE (dimethylaminoethanol, from dmae bitartrate) 50 mg • Ginseng root (panax ginseng, standardized extract providing 5 mg ginsenosides) 100 mg • Huperzine A (from standardized extract of huperzia serrate leaf) 50 mcg • L-Tyrosine 75 mg • Piper Nigrum fruit (from standardized piperine) 2.5 mg. Other Ingredients: Silica, Vegetable Magnesium Stearate, Vegetable Stearic Acid, Dicalcium Phosphate, Cellulose (plant origin), Croscarmellose.

Huperzine A Ginkgo/Ginseng **-** Nutrapharm, Inc.
Each capsule contains: Huperzine A 50 mcg • Ginkgo biloba extract 60 mg • Panax ginseng extract 150 mg. Other Ingredients: Malto dextrin, magnesium stearate, microcrystalline cellulose, & silica. Free of sugar, yeast, milk, artificial colors, flavors & dyes.

Huperzine A w/Ginkgo **-** Nutrapharm, Inc.
Each capsule contains: Huperzine A 50 mcg • Ginkgo biloba extract 60 mg. Other Ingredients: Malto dextrin, magnesium stearate, microcrystalline cellulose, & silica. Free of sugar, yeast, corn, milk, artificial colors, flavors & dyes.

Huperzine A w/Ginseng **-** Nutrapharm, Inc.
Each capsule contains: Huperzine A 50 mcg • Panax ginseng extract (standardized to 8% ginsenosides) 150 mg. Other Ingredients: Malto dextrin, magnesium stearate, microcrystalline cellulose, & silica. Free of sugar, yeast, corn, milk products, artificial colors, flavors & dyes.

Huperzine A w/Vitamin E **-** Nutrapharm, Inc.
Each capsule contains: Huperzine A 50 mcg • Vitamin E (D-alpha tocopheryl acetate) 100 IU. Other Ingredients: Malto dextrin, magnesium stearate, & silica. Free of sugar, yeast, corn, milk, artificial colors, flavors & dyes.

HVP **-** Nature's Sunshine
Each capsule contains: Proprietary Blend 390 mg: Valerian root, Skullcap herb, Hops flowers.

HY 2 **-** Pacific BioLogic
St. John's Wort.

Hyaluronic Acid **-** Vitamin World
Each capsule contains: Hyaluronic Acid (sodium hyaluronate) 20 mg. Other Ingredients: Rice Powder, Gelatin, Silica.

Some Brand Name Natural Products - What they Contain

www.NaturalDatabase.com contains MANY more listings than appear here.

BRAND NAMES

Hyben Vital **-** Hyben Vital International
Wild Dog Rose Hips (hips and kernals, dried and powdered).

Hydra Cleanse **-** Pharmagel
Aloe Vera • a complex of marine-based extracts of Seaweed, Algae, and Spirulina • Oat extract • Beta Glucan • Panthenol.

Hydra Fuel **-** TwinLab
Glucose Polymers & Glucose (approximately 5%) • Fructose (about 2%). Replenishes important Electrolytes & Minerals: Sodium, Potassium, Magnesium, Chloride, Chromium, Phosphorus.

Hydra Joint BASIC **-** Renutra Natural Health Products
Purified Water • Glucosamine Sulfate • MSM • Vitamin C (as ascorbic acid) • Citric Acid • Carrageenan • Natural Flavors • Potassium Sorbate • Sodium Benzoate • Stevia leaf extract.

Hydra Joint TOTAL **-** Renutra Natural Health Products
Purified Water • Glucosamine Sulfate • Chondroitin Sulfate • Citric Acid • MSM • Vitamin C (as ascorbic acid) • Natural Flavors • Stevia leaf extract • Carrageenan • Potassium Sorbate • Sodium Benzoate.

Hydrating Cleanser **-** Abra Therapeutics
Deionized Water • Extract of Orange Blossom • Rose Bud • Bulgarian Chamomile • Horsetail • French Lavender • Vegetable Glycerine • Kukui nut • Macadamia nut • Glyceryl Stearate • Aloe Vera gel • Stearic Acid • Jojoba nut oil • Sorbital • Avocado seed oil • Cucumber extract • Allantoin • Panthenol • Borage seed oil • Vitamin E • Vitamin A • Vitamin C • Essential Oils of Geranium and Ylang-Ylang • Methylparaben • Propylparaben.

Hydravax **-** Metabolic Nutrition
Three capsules contain: Dandelion root (20%) 2010 mg • Uva Ursi (20% arbutin) 1050 mg • Green Tea leaf (50%/35%) 900 mg • Cranberry powder 300 mg • Magnesium Citrate 180 mg • Couch Grass 150 mg • Corn Silk 150 mg • Buchu leaf (4:1) 90 mg • Juniper berry (4:1) 90 mg • Hydrangea root (4:1) 90 mg.

Hydroderm **-** Life Extension
Collagen (marine) • Distilled Water/Igepal • Cephene • Methyl Paraben • Ethyl Paraben • Propyl Paraben • Butyl Paraben • Isobutyl Paraben • Synasol • Serum Protein • Purified Water • PRE complex • Sodium Methylparaben • Imidazolidinyl Urea • Trisodium EDTA • Potassium Sorbate • Citric Acid • Ascorbic Acid.

HydroEye SoftGels **-** ScienceBased Health
Two capsules contain: Vitamin A (from retinyl palmitate) 1040 IU • Vitamin C (from calcium ascorbate, ester-c) 90 mg • Vitamin B6 (from pyridoxal 5 phosphate) 6.3 mg • Magnesium (from magnesium sulfate) 20 mg • Black Currant seed oil (15.6% gamma linolenic acid, [GLA]) 750 mg • Mucin Complex (60% mucin) 250 mg • Cod Liver oil 1.6 mg. Other Ingredients: Gelatin, Water, Vegetable Shortening, Glycerine, Lecithin, Beeswax, Titanium Dioxide, Caramel Color.

HydroTest **-** NutraBolics
Six milliliters contain: Liquid German Tribulus Terrestris (80% proctodioscin) 40 mg • Designer Pro-Testosterone Complex 500 mg: Eurycoma Longifolia (50:1), Avena Sativa (10:1), Rhodiola Rosea (3% rosavins, 39% salidorosides), Fenugreek 4-Hydroxy Isoleucine (30%).

Hydroxy Ripped **-** Puritan's Pride
Four capsules contain: Chromium 300 mcg • Hydroripped 2000 (Garcinia cambogia) fruit rind (containing 1,000 of HCA) 1,667 mg • Guarana extract (Paullina cupana) seed (standardized for 22% caffeine) 1,000 mg • Ma Huang extract (Ephedra sinica) aerial (standardized for 21 mg of ephedra alkaloids) 360 mg • Salicin complex (from White Willow Bark) Salix alba (containing 15% salicin) 150 mg • L-Carnitine 150 mg.
See Editor's Note No. 21 and No. 30.

Hydroxycut **-** MuscleTech
Four capsules contain: Hydroxagen (supplying 100 mg of Hydroxycitric Acid) 2000 mg • MaHuang extract 334 mg • Guarana extract 910 mg • Willow bark extract 100 mg • L-Carnitine 100 mg • Chromium Picolinate 300 mcg.
See Editor's Note No. 21 and No. 30.

Hydroxycut Caffeine-Free **-** MuscleTech
Three capsules contain: Calcium (as calcium hydroxycitrate) 152 mg • Chromium (as polynicotinate) 133 mg • Potassium (as hydroxycitrate) 225 mg • Hydroxagen Plus Blend 1.71 g: Garcinia Cambogia fruit/rind extract (standardized for hydroxycitric acid), Gymnema Sylvestre leaf extract (standardized for gymnemic acid), Glucomannan (amorphophallus konjac), Alpha Lipoic Acid, Willow bark extract (purple & white, standardized for salicin), L-Carnitine (as tartrate) • Hydroxy Tea I Caffeine-free Green Tea leaf extract (standardized for 95% polyphenols, 70% catechins, 45% epigallocatechin gallate, 90 mg) 200 mg. Other Ingredients: Gelatin, Magnesium Stearate, Silica, Cellulose.

Hydroxycut Ephedra Free **-** MuscleTech
Three capsules contain: Calcium (as hydroxycitrate) 265 mg • Chromium (as polynicotinate) 133 mcg • Potassium (as chloride/hydroxycitrate) 249 mg • Hydroxagen Plus Proprietary Blend 1.7 g: Garcinia Camboga fruit & rind extract (standardized for (-) hydroxycitrate acid), Glucomannan (amorphallus konjac), Alpha Lipoic Acid, Willow Bark extract (purple & white, standardized for salicin), L-Carnitine (as tartarate) • Hydroxy Tea Proprietary Blend 406 mg: Green Tea Leaf extract (standardized for 95% polyphenols: 70% catechins: 45% epigallocatechin gallate - 90 mg EGCG), Caffeine (as caffeine anhydrous), Guarana seed extract (standardized for 200 mg of caffeine). Other Ingredients: Gelatin, Magnesium Stearate, Silica, Cellulose.

Hy-Gear - MET-Rx **-** Rexall - Sundown
Each 40 g serving contains: Creatine Monohydrate 5 g • Carbohydrate 34 g. Ingredients: Citrus Mist flavor: CeraSport (Rice Syrup Solids, Sodium Chloride, Potassium Chloride & Trisodium Citrate) • Fructose • Creatine Monohydrate • Glucose • Natural & Artificial Flavors • Citric Acid • Malic Acid • Beta Carotene & Beet juice powder for color. Strazzyberry Flavor: CeraSport (Rice Syrup Solids, Sodium Chloride, Potassium Chloride & Trisodium Citrate) • Fructose • Creatine Monohydrate • Glucose • Natural & Artificial Flavors • Beet juice powder for color.

Hype-Ade Capsules **-** Enzymatic Therapy
Two capsules contain: Vitamin A (53% as beta carotene, retinyl acetate) 5000 IU • Vitamin C (ascorbic acid) 200 mg • Thiamin (as thiamin HCl, vitamin B1) 25 mg • Riboflavin (vitamin b2) 25 mg • Niacin (as niacinamide, niacin) 115 mg • Vitamin B6 (as pyridoxine HCl) 25 mg • Vitamin B12 (as cyanocobalamin) 25 mcg • Pantothenic Acid (as calcium d-pantothenate) 100 mg • Zinc (as zinc gluconate) 10 mg • Manganese (as manganese gluconate) 2.3 mg • Chromium (as chromium picolinate) 267 mcg • Potassium (as potassium aspartate) 50 mg • Inositol 200 mg • Pancreas extract (freeze-dried) 150 mg • Choline Bitartrate 100 mg • L-Methionine 100 mg • Beet root (beta vulgaris) 100 mg • Adrenal extract (freeze-dried) 65 mg • Betaine HCl 50 mg • Wild Yam root (dioscorea villosa) 50 mg • Pituitary extract 40 mg • Barberry bark of root extract (berberis vulgaris, 6:1) 30 mg. Other Ingredients: Gelatin, Magnesium Stearate, Silicon Dioxide, Titanium Dioxide Color, Dandelion Leaf, Goldenseal Root, Liver, Lung, Pancreas, Heart, Kidney, Spleen.
See Editor's Note No. 14.

Hyperbalance **-** Gero Vita International
Each capsule contains: Uncaria rhynchophylla (Chinese cat's claw) extract 100 mg • Heal-All (Prunella vulgaris) extract (herb) 100 mg • Apocynum venetum (plant) extract 100 mg • Eucommia (bark) extract 100 mg • Sickle Pod Senna (seed) extract 100 mg • Gastrodia (rhizome) extract 50 mg • Wild Chrysanthemum (flower) extract 50 mg • Rauwolfia yunnanenis (root) extract 15 mg. Other Ingredients: Dicalcium Phosphate, Silicon Dioxide, Vegetable Magnesium Stearate, Gelatin.

Some Brand Name Natural Products - What they Contain

www.NaturalDatabase.com contains MANY more listings than appear here.

HyperiCalm **-** Enzymatic Therapy
Each capsule contains: St. John's Wort (Hypericum perforatum) extract standardized to 0.3% hypericins (900 mcg) & 4% hyperforin (12 mg), verified by HPLC 300 mg.

HyperiMed **-** PhytoPharmica
Each capsule contains: St. John's Wort extract (hypericum perforatum, standardized to 0.3% hypericins (900 mcg) & 4% hyperforin (12 mg)), 300 mg.

Hypo-Ade **-** Enzymatic Therapy
Two tablets contain: Vitamin A (fish liver oil) 5000 IU • Vitamin C (ascorbic acid) 200 mg • Niacin/Niacinamide 115 mg • Potassium Chloride 100 mg • Pantothenic Acid (d-calcium pantothenate) 100 mg • Thiamine HCl (vitamin B1) 25 mg • Riboflavin (vitamin B2) 25 mg • Vitamin B6 (pyridoxine HCl) 25 mg • Zinc (oxide) 10 mg • Manganese (gluconate) 10 mg • Chromium (polynicotinate) 267 mcg • Vitamin B12 (cyanocobalamin) 25 mcg • Other Ingredients: Inositol 200 mg, Pancreas Extract 150 mg, Choline Bitartrate 100 mg, L-Methionine 100 mg, Green Beet Leaf Powder 100 mg, Adrenal Extract 65 mg, Betaine HCl 50 mg, Wild Yam 50 mg, Pituitary Extract 40 mg, Barberry Bark Of Root Extract (berberis vulgaris 4:1) 30 mg, Dandelion (taraxacum officinale), Goldenseal (hydrastis canadensis), Raw Liver, Raw Lung, Raw Pancreas, Raw Heart, Raw Kidney, Raw Spleen, Raw Brain.
See Editor's Note No. 14.

HypoAllergenic Taurine **-** Kirkman Laboratories
Each capsule contains: Taurine 325 mg. Inactive Ingredients: Plant Cellulose.

Hyporil **-** PhytoPharmica
Two tablets contain: Adrenal extract 65 mg • Barberry bark of root 6:1 extract (berberis vulgaris) 30 mg • Beet root (beta vulgaris) 100 mg • Betaine HCl 50 mg • Choline Bitartrate 100 mg • Chromium (as chromium polynicotinate) 267 mg • Inositol 200 mg • L-Methionine 100 mg • Manganese (as manganese gluconate) 2.3 mg • Niacin (as niacinamide and niacin) 115 mg • Pancreas extract (freeze-dried) 150 mg • Pantothenic Acid (as calcium D-pantothenate) 100 mg • Potassium (as potassium aspartate) 50 mg • Riboflavin (vitamin B2)25 mg • Thiamin (as thiamin HCl, vitamin B1) 25 mg • Vitamin A (53% as beta carotene and as retinyl acetate) 5000 IU • Vitamin B12 (as cyanocobalamin) 25 mcg • Vitamin B6 (as pyridoxine HCl) 25 mg • Vitamin C (ascorbic acid) 200 mg • Wild Yam (dioscorea villosa) 50 mg • Zinc (as zinc gluconate) 10 mg.
See Editor's Note No. 14.

Iberogast **-** Enzymatic Therapy/PhytoPharmica
German Chamomile flower (matricaria recutita) • Clown's Mustard plant (iberis amara) • Angelica root and rhizome (angelica archangelica) • Caraway fruit (carum carvi) • Milk Thistle fruit (silybum marianum) • Lemon Balm leaf (melissa officinalis) • Celandine aerial part (chelidonium majus) • Licorice root (glycyrrhiza glabra) • Peppermint leaf (mentha x piperita).

ICaps AREDS Formula **-** Alcon Laboratories
Two tablets contain: Vitamin C 226 mg • Vitamin E 200 IU • Zinc 34.8 mg • Copper 0.8 mg • Vitamin A 14,320 IU. Other Ingredients: Microcrystalline Cellulose, Dicalcium Phosphate, Gelatin, Hydroxypropyl Methylcellulose, Silicon Dioxide, Magnesium Stearate, Stearic Acid, Polyethylene Glycol, Sucrose, Dextrin, Titanium Dioxide, Corn Starch, FD&C Red #40 Lake, Dextrose Monohydrate, Lecithin, Ascorbyl Palmitate, FD&C Yellow #6 Lake, dl-Alpha Tocopherol, Sodium Ascorbate, Sorbic Acid, Sodium Benzoate, Polysorbate 80.

ICaps Lutein & Zeaxanthin Formula **-** Alcon Laboratories
Two tablets contain: Vitamin A (as beta carotene) 6600 IU • Vitamin C (as ascorbic acid) 400 mg • Vitamin E 150 IU • Riboflavin (B2) 10 mg • Zinc (as zinc acetate) 60 mg • Selenium 40 mcg • Copper 4 mg • Manganese 10 mg • Lutein & Zeaxanthin 4 mg. Other Ingredients: Hydroxypropyl Methylcellulose, Gelatin, Microcrystalline Cellulose, Dicalcium Phosphate, Silicon Dioxide, Magnesium Stearate, Corn Starch, Titanium Dioxide, Polyethylene Glycol, Ascorbyl Palmitate, Sodium Ascorbate, Sorbic Acid, Polysorbate 80, Sodium Benzoate, Carnauba Wax.

Iced Lemon Fibergy Bar **-** USANA Health Sciences
Each bar contains: Rolled Oats, Dextrose, Oat Fiber, Fractionated Palm Kernel Oil, Oat Flour, Citric Acid, Lemon Oil, Gum Arabic, Soy Lecithin, Crystalline Fructose, Inulin (Natural Extract of Chicory), High Fructose Corn Syrup, Dehydrated Cane Juice, Oat Bran, Barley Flour, Date Puree, Brown Crisp Rice (Rice Flour, Rice Bran, Rosemary Extract), Vegetable Glycerin, Oat Flour, Rolled Barley, Flax Seed Meal, Soy Lecithin, Natural Flavors, Baking Soda, Corn Starch, Gelatin.

Ideas **-** Starlight International
Each four tablets contain: St. John's Wort, 0.3% (hypericum perforatum, flowering parts) 400 mg • Gingko biloba extract, 4:1 (leaf) 100 mg • Basil / Tulsi extract, 4:1 (ocimum sanctum, leaf) 150 mg • Lemon Balm (melissa officinalis, leaf) 150 mg • Siberian Ginseng extract, 4:1 (eleutherocecus senticosus, root) 200 mg • Gotu Kola extract, 4:1 (cantella asiatica, plant) 150 mg • Bacopa Monneria (water hyssop extract, 4:1, plant) 150 mg • Spirulina 5 mg • Rosemary (rosmarinus officinalis, leaf) 5 mg • English Lavender (lavandula officinalis, flower) 5 mg. Inactive Ingredients: Dicalcium Phosphate, Microcrystalline Cellulose, Stearic Acid, Croscarmellose Sodium, Magnesium Stearate, Silicon Dioxide, Dextrin, Dextrose, Lecithin, Carboxymethylcellulose Sodium, Sodium Citrate.

IGF Fuel **-** TwinLab
Two capsules contain: DHEA (dehydroepiandrosterone) 50 mg • Zinc (from zinc picolinate) 50 mg • L-Glutamine 2000 mg.

IgG Boost **-** Pharmanex
Two capsules contain: Colostrum MFT (minimum 50% IgG content) 250 mg.

Illumination **-** Amazon Herb
Ua de Gato • Jatoba • Pau d'Arco • Tayuya • Fucus • Suma • Star Anise • Pedra Hume Ca • Carqueja • Horsetail • Artichoke • Boldo • Bitter Orange • Alfalfa • Quebra Pedra • Jurubeba • Passion Flower • Mulungu • Espinhiera Santa • Cajueiro • Muira Puama • Catuaba • Yerba Mate • Cornsilk • Lemon Balm • Peppermint • Lemon Grass • Pata de Vaca • Sarsaparilla • Chamomile • Stevia • Chuchuhuasi • Sangre de Drago.
See Editor's Note No. 40, page 2058.

Image Recovery Cream **-** Life Extension
Aloe, D.I. Water, Fruit Citric Acid, Glycolic Acid, Emulsifying Wax, Collagen, Protein, Squalene, Soybean oil, Calendula oil, Jojoba oil, Lemon extract, Keratin, Germaben 2.

Imm-Kine **-** Aidan Products, LLC
Each capsule contains: Lactobacillus Fermentum extract 250 mg • Beta 1,3 Glucans (from saccharomyces cerevisiae) 50 mg.

Immortale for Men **-** Roex
Each tablet contains: Tribulus Terrestris 250 mg • Panax ginseng 50 mg • Damiana 50 mg • Avena sativa 100 mg • Sarsaparilla 50 mg.

Immortale for Women **-** Roex
Each tablet contains: Tribulus Terrestris 250 mg • Panax ginseng 50 mg • Damiana 50 mg • Avena sativa 100 mg • Dong Quai 50 mg.

ImmPower **-** American Biosciences
Two capsules contain: A.H.C.C. (active hexose correlated compound) Proprietary Blend 1 g: Mushroom Mycelia extract, Candelilla wax, Cyclodextrin, Microcrystalline Cellulose. Other Ingredients: VCap Plant-Derived Cellulose, Water, Silica, Glycerin.

IMMU-C **-** Nutri-Quest Rx
Each tablet contains: Vitamin C (Sago Palm) 500 mg • Rutin 15 mg • Lemon Bioflavonoids 15 mg • Hesperidin Complex 15 mg • Tissue concentrates (not extracts) of Bovine Source from Lymph, Thymus,

Spleen • 5X Propolis 2 mg.
See Editor's Note No. 14.

Immugel - 4.2 OZ **- Young Living Essential Oils**
Deionized Water • Methylcellulose • Hydrolized Vegetable Protein • German Chamomile Extract • Cinnamon Oil • Clove • Rosemary • Lemon • Thyme • Oregano.

Immuguard **- Optimum Nutrition**
Echinacea Angustifolia extract • Goldenseal root.

Immumax-Rx **- Alternecare Health Products**
Each tablet contains: Bee Propolis 50 mg •Shiitake Mushroom 50 mg • Reishi Mushroom 50 mg • Garlic 25 mg • Suma 25 mg •Red Clover 25 mg •Pau d'Arco 25 mg • Milk Thistle 25 mg • Shark Cartilage 15 mg •Golden Seal 25 mg • Siberian Ginseng 25 mg • Echinacea 25 mg • Astragalus 25 mg • N-Acetyl Cysteine 15 mg • Zinc 15 mg • L-Glutathione 15 mg • CO Q10 5 mg.

ImmunACE **- Nature's Plus**
Two tablets contain: Vitamin C corn free 1000 mg • Vitamin E natural 400 IU • Beta Carotene pro-vitamin A, supplying Vitamin A 20000 IU • Zinc Amino Acid Chelate 300 mg, supplying Elemental Zinc 30 mg • L-Cysteine free form amino acid 200 mg • Iron Amino Acid Chelate 180 mg, supplying Elemental Iron 18 m • Selenium Amino Acid Complex 100 mg, supplying Elemental Selenium 200 mcg • Folic Acid 200 mcg. In a natural base of Pau D'Arco, Chlorophyll, Echinacea, Thyme, Juniper berry, Korean Ginseng, Irish Moss, Rosemary.

Immunace (Immunance) **- Vitabiotics**
Two capsules contain: Vitamin A 800 mcg • Vitamin D 10 mcg • Vitamin E 110 mg • Vitamin C 300 mg • Vitamin B1 (thiamin) 14 mg • Vitamin B2 (riboflavin) 8 mg • Vitamin B6 20 mg • Folic Acid 500 mcg • Vitamin B12 14 mcg • Pantothenic Acid 20 mg • Vitamin K 95 mcg • Betacarotene 6 mg • Iron 6 mg • Magnesium 100 mg • Zinc 15 mg • Iodine 200 mcg • Copper 2 mg • Manganese 4 mg • Selenium 200 mcg • Chromium 100 mcg • Cystine 40 mg • Methionine 40 mg • Bioflavonoids 30 mg.

ImmunActin Throat Spray **- Nature's Plus**
Purified Water • Exclusive Liposomal Herbal Complex:Olivir (Olea europa leaf extract) (supplying purified Calcium Elenolate), Kava Kava extract (Piper methysticum root) (standardized 4% Kavalactones), Echinacea extract (Echinacea angustifolia root & rhizome) (standardized 4% Echinacosides), Elderberry extract (Sambucus canadensis fruit) (standardized 30% Flavonoids), Ginger (Zingiber officinale root) (standardized 4% Volatile oils) • Wild Clover Honey • Oil of Peppermint.

ImmunActin Throat Syrup **- Nature's Plus**
Vegetable Glycerine • Exclusive Liposomal Herbal Complex: Elderberry extract (Sambucus canadensis fruit) (standardized 30% Falvonoids), Echinacea extract (Echinacea angustifolia root & rhizome) (standardized 4% Echinacosides), Slippery Elm (Ulmus rubra bark) (naturally rich in Phytosterols, Sesquitepenes & Mucilage), Goldenseal extract (Hydrastis canadensis root) (standardized 10% Alkaloids, 5% Hydrastine), White Willow extract (Salix alba bark) (standardized 7-9% Salicin), Astragalus extract (Astragalus membranaceus root) (standardized 0.4% 4'-Hydroxy-3'-Methoxyisoflavone 7-Sug), Schisandra extract (Schisandra chinensis fruit) (standardized 9% schisandrins), Zinc Gluconate • Wild Clover • Honey • Methol • Natural Cherry flavor.

ImmunActinB **- Nature's Plus**
Two capsules contain: Vitamin C corn free 300 mg • Vitamin E natural 100 IU • Echinacea [(Echinacea angustifolia root & rhizome) standardized 4% Echinacosides] 50 mg • Astragalus [(Astragalus membranaceus root) standardized 0.4% 4'-Hydroxy-3'-Methoxyisoflavone 7-Sug] 50 mg • Chinese Green Tea [(Camellia sinensis leaf) decaffeinated, standardized 20% Polyphelols] 50 mg • Tumeric [(Curcuma longa rhizome) standardized 95% Curcumin] 50 mg • Garlic odor-modified [(Allium sativum clove) standardized 0.35% Allicin, 0.65% Allicin, 0.40% Thiosulfinates, 0.085% Allyl Mercaptan] 50 mg • Schisandra [(Schisandra chinensis fruit) standardized 9% Schisandrins] 25 mg • Pau D'Arco [(Tabebuia impetiginosa bark) standardized 3% Naphthoquinones] 25 mg • Goldenseal [(Hydrastis canadensis root & rhizome) standardized 10% Alkaloids, 5% Hydrastine] 25 mg • Shiitake Mushroom [(Lentinus edodes mycelia) standardized 3.2% KS-2 Polysaccharides (peptidomannan)] 15 mg • Zinc (Monomethionine) 15 mg • Beta Carotene (supplying 10000 IU of Vitamin A activity) 6 mg • Grape seed [(Vitis vinifera) standardized 95% Proanthocyanidins] 5 mg • Bioperine [(Piper nigrum fruit) standardized 95% 1-Piperoylpiperidine] 5 mg.

Immun'Age **- PhytoPharmica**
Each packet contains: Fermented Papaya 3 g.

ImmunAssure **- Schiff**
Two tablets contain: Vitamin C (as ascorbic acid) 60 mg • Immunoglobulin G 500 mg • Proprietary Blend 72.5 mg: Andrographis Paniculata extract (leaf), Echinacea Purpurea extract (herb). Other Ingredients: Cellulose, Croscarmellose Sodium, Coating (hydroxypropyl methylcellulose, maltodextrin, polyethylene glycol), Magnesium Stearate, Silicon Dioxide.

Immune - Bioset **- Enzymes, Inc.**
Each capsule contains: Proprietary Herbal Blend 375 mg: Astragalus root extract, Goldenseal root extract, Echinacea Angustifolia root extract, Echinacea Purpurea root extract, Reishi Mushroom extract, Shiitake Mushroom extract • pHysioProtease 150 mg. Other Ingredients: Plant Cellulose, Water.

Immune **- Orenda International**
Two capsules contain: Calcium d-Glucarate 300 mg • Lactobacillus fementum extract (muramyl peptides) 200 mg • Oat Straw extract (beta 1,3 glucan) 50 mg. Other Ingredients: Cellulose, Rice Bran, Magnesium Sillicate, Silicon Dioxide.

Immune 7-Keto - GNC A-Z **- GNC**
Each tabet contains: 7-Keto-DHEA 25 mg. Other Ingredients: Dicalcium Phosphate, Cellulose.

Immune Actives **- VitaStore**
Each tablet contains: Echinacea 500 mg • Goldenseal 250 mg • Beta Carotene (Vitamin A) 2500 IU • Zinc Gluconate 30 mg • Vitamin C 120 mg • Licorice 150 mg • Astragalus 145 mg • Grape Seed extract 50 mg • Green Tea 200 mg • Garlic 300 mg • L-Lysine 500 mg.

Immune Booster **- Vidafit**
Each serving contains: Biotin 30 mcg • Folate 400 mcg • Niacin 20 mg • Pantothenic Acid 10 mg • Riboflavin 1.7 mg • Thiamine 1.5 mg • Vitamin A 2600 IU • Vitamin B12 6 mcg • Vitamin B6 2 mg • Vitamin C 120 mg • Vitamin D 200 IU • Vitamin E 30 IU • Boron 1 mg • Calcium 500 mg • Chromium 120 mcg • Copper 2 mg • Iodine 150 mcg • Magnesium 400 mg • Phosphorus 500 mg • Potassium 100 mg • Selenium 70 mcg • Zinc 30 mg • Acidophilus 50 mg • Astragalus 300 mg • Echinacea Extract 75 mg • Garlic 10 mg • Siberian Ginseng 100 mg • Soy Protein 2 g.

Immune Booster Body Benefits Pak **- Leiner Health Products**
Each packet contains: Zinc Gluconate 50 mg • Vitamin C 740 mg • Echinacea extract (Echinacea augustifolia, Echinacea purpurea) root 200 mg • Garlic (Allium sativum) clove 200 mg • Propolis 100 mg. Other Ingredients: Ascorbic Acid, Dicalcium Phosphate, Starch, Hydroxypropyl Methylcellulose, Maltodextrin, Croscarmellose Sodium, Silicon Dioxide, Cellulose, Stearic Acid, Rose Hips, Sodium Starch Glycolate, Magnesium.

Immune Builder **- JHS Natural Products**
Each capsule contains: Coriolus Versicolor extract 75 mg • Reishi fruit body extract 75 mg • Maitake fruit body extract 75 mg • Shiitake (lentinula edodes) extract 75 mg • Cordyceps Sinensis Cs-4 Mycelial extract 75 mg.

Immune Building Complex - Shaklee
Two caplets contain: Mach-4 Proprietary Blend of Macrophage Activating Chinese Herbs 500 mg: Pumpkin seed extract (Cucurbita moschata), Safflower extract (Carthamus tinctorius) flower, Asian plantain extract (plantago asiatica) seed, Japanese Honeysuckle extract (Lonicera japonica) flower. Microcrystalline Cellulose, Dicalcium Phosphate, Silicon Dioxide, Croscarmellose Sodium, Hydroxypropyl Methylcellulose, Titanium Dioxide, Soy Lecithin, Caramel Color, Carnauba Wax.

Immune Defense - ProHerbs - Mason Vitamins, Inc.
Two tablets contain: Vitamin C (Ascorbic Acid) 500 mg • Vitamin E (Dl-Alpha Tocopherol Acetate) 400 IU • Zinc (as Sulfate) 15 mg • Selenium (as Selenomethionine) 200 mcg • ActiVin Grape Seed extract (Vitis vinifera seeds standardized to 95% polyphenols) 100 mg • Echinacea root (Echinacea purpurea) 100 mg • Alpha Lipoic Acid (standardized to 4% phenolic compounds) 50 mg. Other Ingredients: Dicalcium Phosphate, Croscarmellose Sodium, Hydroxypropylmethylcellulose, Magnesium Stearate, Microcrystalline Cellulose, Mineral Oil, Polyethylene Glycol, Silicon Dioxide, Stearic Acid, Titanium Dioxide, Sodium Lauryl Sulfate, FD&C Yellow #6 Lake, Yellow #10 Lake.

Immune Formula - 4 Life
Each capsule contains: Licorice (root) 54 mg • Echinacea Purpurea (aerial parts) 54 mg • Schizandra (fruit) 54 mg • Siberian Ginseng (root) 54 mg • Astragalus (root) 54 mg • Gotu Kola (aerial parts) 54 mg • Immune Proprietary Extract Blend 45 mg: Astragalus extract (root), Echinacea Purpurea extract (aerial parts), Schizandra extract (fruit), Korean Ginseng extract (root), Siberian Ginseng extract (root), Licorice extract (root), Gotu Kola extract (aerial parts) • Korean Ginseng (root) 31 mg.

Immune Formula - Nature's Life
Three tablets contain: Antioxidant Vitamins: Beta Carotene [(Dunaliella salina) equivalent to 25000 IU Vitamin A] 15 mg • Other naturally occurring carotenoids in D. salina: Alpha Carotene (equivalent to 393 IU Vitamin A) 473 mcg • Cryptoxanthin (equivalent to 96 IU Vitamin A) 116 mcg • Zeaxanthin 95 mcg • Lutein 74 mcg • Vitamin C (Calcium Ascorbate) 1000 mg • Vitamin E (d-Alpha Tocopheryl Succinate) 200 IU. Other Nutrients: Vitamin A (Retinyl Palmitate) 8000 IU • Vitamin B6 (Pyridoxine HCl) 50 mg • Vitamin B12 (Cobalamin) 100 mcg • Folic Acid 400 mcg • Selenium (I-Selenomethionine) 100 mcg • Zinc (Citrate) 25 mg • Copper (Citrate) 2 mg • Medical Herbs: Echinacea purpurea root (Trout Lake Farm Certified Organically Grown) 500 mg • Korean Ginseng root extract [(Panax ginseng) standardized to 10% ginsenosides] 100 mg • Natural Base: Lemon Bioflavonoid Complex (50% active flavonols) 100 mg.

Immune Formula - Pharmanex
Each capsule contains: Vitamin C (as calcium ascorbate) 200 mg • Echinacea root 6:1 extract (echinacea purpurea) 225 mg • Goldenseal root 4:1 extract (hydrastis canadensis) 125 mg • Arabinogalactan 100 mg • Beta-Sitosterol 30 mg. Other Ingredients: Gelatin, Microcrystalline Cellulose, Magnesium Stearate, Silicon Dioxide.

Immune Guardian - Clinician's Choice
Three tablets contain: Vitamin C (ascorbic acid, calcium ascorbate) 150 mg • Vitamin E (dl-alpha tocopheryl acetate) 90 IU • Zinc (amino acid chelate) 90 IU • Selenium (selenomethionine) 150 mcg • Echinacea Angustifolia 450 mg • Echinacea Purpurea root 300 mg • Golden Seal root 150 mg • Kudzu root 150 mg • Odor Modified Garlic Bulb 150 mg • Bee Pollen 150 mg • RoseOx (patented, standardized process for an extract of Rosemary) 90 mg • Ascorbyl Palmitate 75 mg • Schizandra fruit 75 mg • Proprietary Blend 15 mg: Beta-Carotene, Reishi Mushroom, Shiitake Mushroom, Cinnamon bark, Grape powder.

Immune Health - Wellzymes - Enzymes, Inc.
Two capsules contain: n-zimes Proprietary Enzyme Blend 82 mg: pHysioProtease (236,800 pHysio-U), CereCalase Plus • Proprietary Herbal Blend 360 mg: Astragalus root extract (equivalent to 640 mg raw herb), Reishi Mushroom extract (equivalent to 160 mg raw herb), Cat's Claw herb extract (standardized to contain 1% oxindole alkaloids), Burdock root extract (equivalent to 160 mg raw herb). Other Ingredients: Plant Cellulose, Water.

Immune Health Formula - Chinac - Metabolife International, Inc.
Each caplet contains: Forsythia Suspensa (forsythia) • Isatis Tinctoria (isatis) • Astragalus Membranaceus (astragalus) • Lonicera Dasystyla (honeysuckle) • Belamcanda Chinensis (blackberry lily) • Paeonia Veitchii (Chinese peony).

Immune Protectors - TwinLab
Four hard gelatin capsules contain: Dry Vitamin A (from vitamin A acetate) 5000 IU • Dry Beta-Carotene (pro-vitamin A) 20,000 IU • Zinc (from zinc gluconate) 50 mg • Copper (from copper gluconate) 2 mg • Dry Vitamin E (D-alpha tocopheryl succinate) 400 IU • Selenium (from selenomethionine & selenite) 200 mcg • CoQ10 (coenzyme Q10) 5 mg • Vitamin B6 100 mg • Vitamin C 2000 mg • Citrus Bioflavonoids 100 mg • Quercetin (non-citrus bio-active bioflavonoid) 25 mg • L-Glutathione (reduced) 50 mg • Vitamin B12 250 mcg • Folic Acid 800 mcg • Pantothenic Acid 50 mg • Biotin 100 mcg • Vitamin B2 10 mg • Manganese (from manganese gluconate) 10 mg • Vitamin B3 (niacinamide) 10 mg. Base: Pau d'Arco, Onion, Garlic, Black Walnut, Echinacea, Golden Seal root.

Immune System - Nutrivention
Each tablet contains: Vitamin A 5000 IU • Pantothenic Acid 25 mg • Vitamin B6 25 mg • Vitamin C 20 mg • Vitamin B1 18 mg • Vitamin B2 18 mg • Vitamin E 15 IU • Inositol 15 mg • Choline 8 mg • Magnesium 5 mg • Zinc 5 mg • Folic Acid 400 mcg • Selenium 50 mcg • Echinacea 100 mg • Astragalus 100 mg • L-Cysteine 100 mg • Suma 100 mg • Codonopsis 75 mg • Rei-Shi Mushroom 75 mg • White Astractylodes 50 mg • Schizandra berries 50 mg • Privet berries 50 mg • Watercress 50 mg • Shiitake Mushroom 50 mg • Juniper berries 50 mg.

Immune System Booster Formula - Cambridge Nutraceuticals
Each serving contains: Glutamine 10 g • Vitamin A (as mixed carotenoids) 6500 IU • Vitamin C 200 mg • Vitamin E 125 IU • Selenium 70 mcg • N-Acetyl-Cysteine 600 mg.

Immune26 Wellness Bar (almond delight) - Legacy for Life
Rice syrup • Organic Egg White Protein • Organic Almond Butter • Egg powder with immune components • Organic crispy brown rice • Sliced Almonds • Raisins • Pure Vanilla • Sesame seeds • Spirulina • Almond extract • Kosher Sea Salt.

Immune26 Wellness Bar (peppermint brownie) - Legacy for Life
Rice syrup • Organic Egg White Protein • Organic Almond Butter • Egg powder with immune components • Chocolate Liquor • Organic crispy brown rice • Sliced Almonds • Raisins • Natural Flavoring • Pure Vanilla • Sesame seeds • Spirulina • Almond extract • Kosher Sea Salt.

Immune-Action - Nature's Plus
Each capsule contains: Astragalus root 200 mg • Ligustrum berries 100 mg • Schisandra berries 100 mg • Shiitake Mushrooms 100 mg • Echinacea root 100 mg • Young Barley leaves 50 mg • Pau D'Arco bark 50 mg.

Immunectar - Nature's Plus
Two tablespoons contain: Egg Yolk Lecithin 2000 mg & Phosphatidylcholine 250 mg, The above combination supplies: Neutral Lipids 60%, Phosphatidylcholine 20%, Phosphatidylethanolamine 3% • Colostrum Whey, naturally rich in immunoglobulins, nucleotides, gamma interferon, enzymes & vitamins 150 mg • SUMA (Pfaffia paniculata [Martius] Kuntze root) 150 mg • Chlorella 150 mg • Astragalus (Astragalus membranaceus root) 75 mg • Ligustrum (Ligustrum lucidum berries) 75 mg • Echinacea (Echinacea

angustifolia root) 75 mg • Schisandra (Schisandra chinensis berries) 75 mg • Shiitake (Lentinus edodes mushrooms) 75 mg • Coenzyme Q10 15 mg.

Immun-Eeze **-** Allergy Limited
Each capsule and lozenge together contain: Vitamin C (as ascorbic acid) 250 mg • Thiamin (as thiamine mononitrate) 25 mg • Riboflavin 25 mg • Niacin (as niacinamide) 20 mg • Vitamin B6 (as pyridoxine HCl) 25 mg • Vitamin B12 (as cyanocobalamin) 3 mg • Manganese (as manganese citrate) 6 mg. Other Ingredients: Maltodextrin, Sucrose, Gelatin, Vegetable-derived Magnesium Stearate, Croscarmellose Sodium, Silicon Dioxide.

Immunene **-** PhysioLogics
Each capsule contains: Astragalus root (astragalus membranaceus, standardized to contain 0.5% flavonglycosides, 0.5 mg) 100 mg • Cat's Claw bark (uncaria tomentosa, standardized to contain 4% triterpenes, 2 mg) 50 mg • Reishi Mushroom extract aerial parts (ganoderma lucidum, standardized to contain 4% triterpenes, 2 mg) 50 mg • Shiitake Mushroom aerial parts (lentinula edodes) 50 mg • Maitake Mushroom aerial parts (grifola frondosa) 10 mg • Shiitake Mushroom extract (lentinula edodes, standardized to contain 1.5% PPPT 1/0.3% EP3). Other Ingredients: Rice Powder, Gelatin, Vegetable Magnesium Stearate, Silica.

BRAND NAMES

ImmunEnz **-** Enzymes, Inc.
Each capsule contains: Proprietary Blend 375 mg: Echinacea purpurea root extract, Ginkgo biloba leaf extract, Garlic concentrate, Thyme extract, Reishi Mushroom extract, Mullein leaf extract, Eucalyptus leaf extract, Wild Indigo root extract • pHysioProtease 322 mg. Other Ingredients: Cellulose, Water.

ImmuneTune **-** Young Living Essential Oils
Each capsule contains: Tumeric Extract • Magnesium Citrate • Yucca Root • Potassium Citrate • Echinacea Root • Calcium Citrate • Wild Yam • Pantothenic Acid • Grape Seed Extract • Selenium • Chromium • Alpha Lipoic Acid • Ginger Extract • Orange Oil • Pine Oil • Ravensara Oil • Lemon Oil • Fir Oil • Cistus Oil • Gelatin.

Immuno Chews **-** Global Health Trax
Three tablets contain: Vitamin A 294 IU • Vitamin C 3 mg • Calcium 66 mg • Iron 1 mg • Bovine Colostrum 1350 mg. Other Ingredients: Fructose, Pineapple Flavoring, Magnesium.

Immuno Complex **-** Quality of Life Labs
Two capsules contain: Astragalus 850 mg • Echinacea 450 mg • Vitamin C 120 mg • A.H.C.C. Mushroom Mycelia extract Proprietary Blend 50 mg. Other Ingredients: Gelatin, Silicon Dioxide, Magnesium Stearate.

Immuno Support Complex **-** Nutrition Dynamics, Inc.
Each capsule contains: Vitamin C 200 mg • Pantothenic Acid 10 mg • Vitamin A 10,000 IU • Vitamin B12 10 mcg • Calcium Chelate 60 mg • Zinc Chelate • RNA 60 mg • Thymus 50 mg · Lemon Bioflavonoids 40 mg • Lymph 25 mg • Spleen 25 mg • Bromelain 20 mg. Other Ingredients: Bee Pollen, Dehydrated Pineapple.
See Editor's Note No. 14.

ImmunoBlend **-** Rexall - Sundown
Each capsule contains: Turmeric Rhizome extract (standardized to 95% curcuminoids, 95 mg) 100 mg • Echinacea Purpurea extract (standardized to 4% phenolic compounds, 4 mg) 100 mg • Immuno Proprietary Blend: Garlic bulb, Astragalus root, Reishi Mushroom, Cat's Claw Bark 175 mg. Other Ingredients: Gelatin.

Immunoboost **-** Shawnee Moon
Peony root • Gotu Kola • Chrysanthemum • Astragalus • Licorice • Kelp • Suma • Pau d'arco • Red Clover.

Immunocal **-** Immunotec Research, Ltd.
100% Milk Whey Protein.

ImmunoFin **-** LaneLabs
G-E Lipids 50 mg • Shark Liver Oil 250 mg.

Immunogarl-1 **-** Olympian Labs
Three capsules contain: Garlic extract 600 mg • Ginkgo Biloba leaf extract 120 mg •Proprietary Blend 600 mg: Amylase, Protease, Lipase • Ascorbic Acid 240 mg •L-Glutamine 450 mg •Maitake Mushroom 30 mg.

ImmunoGuard **-** Advocare International
Four capsules contain: Vitamin C (as ascorbic acid) 240 mg • Maitake extract (d-fraction - grifola frondosa) 100 mg • Reishi extract (fruit - ganoderma lucidum) 150 mg • Shiitake extract (mycelium - lentinus edodes) 200 mg • Broccoli extract (stem/flower/leaf - brassica oleracea) 300 mg • Green Tea extract (leaf - camellia sinensis) 150 mg • Curcumin extract (root - curcuma longa) 100 mg • Astragalus extract (root - astragalus membranaceus) 50 mg • Mixed Citrus Flavonoids 200 mg. Other Ingredients: Silicon Dioxide, Magnesium Stearate, Gelatin.

ImmunoKinoko **-** Quality of Life Labs
Two capsules contain: Proprietary Blend 1000 mg: Mushroom Mycelia extract, Candelilla Wax, Cyclodextrin, Microcrystalline Cellulose. Other Ingredients: Silica, Gelatin, Glycerin.

ImmunoLin Extra Strength Day-Time Drink Mix **-** Schiff
Each packet contains: Immunoglobulins (derived from cow's blood) 1000 mg • Vitamin C 60 mg • Echinacea 132 mg • Andrographis 1 mg.

ImmunoLin Extra Strength Night-Time Drink Mix **-** Schiff
Each packet contains: Immunoglobulins (derived from cow's blood) 1000 mg • Vitamin C 60 mg • Echinacea 132 mg • Andrographis 1 mg • Melatonin 1 mg.
See Editor's Note No. 26, page 2056.

ImmunoLin Tablets **-** Schiff
Each two tablets contains: Immunoglobulins (derived from cow's blood) 500 mg • Vitamin C 60 mg • Echinacea 132 mg • Andrographis 1 mg.

ImmunoMax Allergy **-** NorthStar Nutritionals
Two capsules contain: Methylsulfonylmethane (MSM) 250 mg • Acerola berry extract 50 mg • Apple skin extract 50 mg • Rhododendron Caucasicum 50 mg • Magnesium 100 mg • Pantothenic Acid 50 mg.

ImmunoShield **-** PhytoPharmica
Each tablet contains: Vitamin A (as acetate) 10,000 IU • Vitamin C (ascorbic acid) 200 mg • Vitamin D (as cholecalciferol) 35 IU • Vitamin B12 (as cyanocobalamin) 50 mcg • Pantothenic Acid (as calcium D-pantothenate) 25 mg • Calcium (as calcium lactate) 41 mg • Magnesium (as magnesium citrate) 6.7 mg • Zinc (as zinc gluconate) 10.5 mg • European Elder berry 4:1 extract (sambucus nigra) 100 mg • Alfalfa (medicago sativa) aerial part extract 10:1 50 mg • Astragalus root(astragalus membranaceus, extract standardized to conatin a minimum of 0.5% 4'-hydroxy-3'-methoxyisoflavone-7-glucoside) 50 mg • Mixed Citrus Bioflavonoids 50% (from citrus fruits) 30 mg • Proprietary Trace Mineral Blend 24 mg: Selenium (as selenium yeast), Silicon (as magnesium trisilicate), Boron (as sodium borate), Nickel (as nickel chelate), Tin (as tin chelate), Molybdenum (as sodium molybdate), Vanadium (as vanadyl sulfate). Other Ingredients: Cellulose, Modified Cellulose, Magnesium Stearate, Carnauba Wax, Lecithin.

ImmunoSTART **-** Mannatech
Each tablet contains: Colostrum (bovine) 150 mg • Beta-1,3 / 1,6 Glucans 2 20 mg • Lactoferrin 10 mg • Citrus Pectin 5 mg. Other Ingredients: Glucose, Stearic Acid, Natural Flavors, Citric Acid, Magnesium Stearate, Silicon Dioxide.

ImmunPlex **-** Pro Health
Each scoop (approx. 10.2 g) contains: Provon Undenatured Whey Protein Isolate (typical protein composition: beta-lactoglobulin 51%, gamma-lactalbumin 23%, glycomacropeptides 18%, bovine serum

albumin and immunoglobulins 5%, lactoferrin, lactoperoxidase and others 2%) • Natural Vanilla flavor.

Immuplex **-** Standard Process, Inc.
Two capsules contain: Proprietary Blend 565 mg: Bovine Liver (PMG) extract, Veal Bone extract, Nutritional Yeast, Bovine Spleen (PMG) extract, Bovine Thymus (PMG) extract, Bovine Thymus (Cytosol) extract, Bovine Liver, Bovine Spleen, Ovine Spleen, Calcium Lactate. Other Ingredients: Gelatin, Zinc Liver Chelate, Ascorbic Acid, Iron Liver Chelate, Water, Chromium Yeast, Copper Liver Chleate, Selenium Yeast, Mixed Tocopherols, Natural Colors, Pyridoxine Hydrochloride, Calcium Stearate, Vitamin A Palmitate, Folic Acid, Cyanocobalamin.
See Editor's Note No. 14.

IMMU-Power **-** Nutri-Quest Rx
Each tablet contains: Tissue concentrate (not an extract) from Thymus 60 mg • Vitamin A (palmitate) 300 IU • Vitamin B6 15 mg • Niacin 10 mg • Pantothenic Acid 55.5 mg • Vitamin B12 200 mcg • Folic Acid 150 mcg • Vitamin C (sago palm) 150 mg • Natural Vitamin E (succinate) 70 IU • Suma 7 mg • ISB Complex 107 mg: Magnesium, Selenium, SOD Type G, Zinc, Echinacea purpurea, Goldenseal, L-Cysteine HCl, L-Ornithine, Ferric Phosphate, Garlic • L- Aspartic Acid • Natural Flavor.
See Editor's Note No. 14.

Immutol **-** Immunocorp
Each capsule contains: Beta Glucan 375 mg.

I-MNS **-** Dial Herbs
Black Cohosh • Blue Cohosh • Red Raspberry • Catnip • Wild Yam • Wild Carrot • Motherwort • Pennyroyal • St. John's Wort.

Imperial Garlic 6500 **-** Puritan's Pride
Each tablet contains: Garlic bulb powder (allium sativum) 650 mg standardized to contain a minimum: Allicin yeild 6500 mcg, total thiosulfinates yield 6500 mcg, Alliin yield 14,500 mcg, Gamma-Glutamylcysteines 5200 mcg. Other Ingredients: Dicalcium Phosphate, Cellulose (plant origin), Food Glaze, Calcium Carbonate, Croscarmellose, Vegetable Stearic Acid, Hydroxypropyl Methylcellulose, Titanium Dioxide Color, Magnesium Silicate, Anise Oil (pimpinella anisum, seed).

Imperial Green Tea **-** Jamieson
Each tea bag contains: Chinese Green Tea leaf (Camellia sinensis) • Ginger root (Singiber officinale) • Leechee fruit (Litchi chinensis).

Imucell WGP **-** Biopolymer Engineering, Inc.
Each capsule contains: Beta Glucan (naturally derived from Saccromyces cerevisae) 250 mg. Inactive Ingredients: Microcrystalline Cellolose, Gelatin, Water.

Imumax **-** FreeLife International
Each tablet contains: Patented EV.EXT 10 standardized American Feverfew (Parthenium integrifolium) root 75 mg • standardized Echinacea (Echinacea purpurea) root 25 mg. Other Ingredients: Calcium Hydrogen Phosphate, Microcrystalline Cellulose, Silica Dioxide, Hydrous Magnesium Silicate, Magnesium Stearate, Zein, Alginates.

Indigestion **-** Hyland's
Two tablets contain: Cinchona Officinalis 3X HPUS • Hydrastis Canasensis 3X HPUS • Phosphoricum Acidum 3X HPUS • Kali Bichrominum 3X HPUS. Base: Lactose USP.
See Editor's Note No. 1, page 2053.

Indigestion Remedy **-** PhytoPharmica
Twenty drops contain: Podophyllum peltatum 4x • Carduus marianus 3x • Dolichos pruriens 3x • Leptandra virginica 3x • Lycopodium clavatum 3x • Nux vomica 3x • Boldo 1x • Chelidonium majus 1x. In a base of 50% USP alcohol by volume.
See Editor's Note No. 1, page 2053.

Indium XL **-** East Park
Indium Sulfate Anhydrous (.9999% pure) • Distilled Water.

Indium-Energy **-** East Park
Each tablet contains: Indium Sulfate (.9999% pure) 24 mg • Trace Minerals: Zinc Oxide, Copper Oxide, Selenium, Chromium, Manganese, Potassium Iodide, Dicalcium Phosphate. Other Ingredients: Microcrystalline Cellulose, Stearic Acid, Silicon Dioxide, Magnesium Stearate.

Indole Pro **-** MMS Pro
Each three capsules contain: Vitamin A 100 IU • Vitamin E (as d-alpha tocopheryl succinate) 13 IU • Potassium 10 mg • Proprietary Blend (BioResponse-DIM containing 25% diindolylmethane) 150 mg: Starch, Diindolylmethane, Natural Vitamin E, Phosphatidylcholine, Silica • Proprietary Blend (Protectamins) 150 mg: Spinach powder, Cabbage powder, concentrated Broccoli powder. Inactive Ingredients: Cellulose, Gelatin, Chlorophyll.

IndoleGard **-** NutriCology
Four capsules contain: BioResponse DIM (a patented diindolylmethane complex), Starch, DIM (25% min.), Vitamin E Succinate, Phosphatidylcholine, Silica 300 mg. Other Ingredients: Cellulose, Carbowax, Silicon Dioxide.

Indolplex **-** PhytoPharmica
Each tablet contains: Diindolylmethane (DIM) 30 mg.
See Editor's Note No. 21, page 2056.

Indolplex - Tyler **-** Integrative Therapeutics
Four capsules contain: Vitamin E 22 IU • Indolplex Proprietary Blend 240 mg: Food Grade Starch, Diindolylmethane, Tocophersolan, Phosphatidylcholine, Silica. Other Ingredients: Microcrystalline Cellulose, Ascorbyl Palmitate, Gelatin, Water.

Indolplex with DIM **-** Enzymatic Therapy/PhytoPharmica
Each tablet contains: Proprietary Blend 120 mg: Modified Food Starch, 25% Diindolylmethane (DIM), D-Alpha-Tocopheryl Succinate, Silicon Dioxide, Phosphatidylcholine. Other Ingredients: Calcium Carbonate, Modified Cellulose Gum, Modified Cellulose, Titanium Dioxide Color, Lecithin, Carnauba Wax.

InflamActin **-** Nature's Plus
Two capsules contain: Boswellin (Boswellia serrata gum resin) (standardized 65% Boswellic Acids) 250 mg • Bromelain (standardized 90 GDU) 150 mg • DLPA (dl-Phenylalanine) (Free Form Amino Acid) 100 mg • Turmeric (Curcuma longa rhizome) standardized 95% Curcumin 75 mg • Vitamin C (corn free) 60 mg • St. John's Wort (Hypericum perforatum flower) (standardized 0.3-0.5% Hypericin) 50 mg • Chamomile (Matricaria recutita flower) (standardized 1% Apigenin, 0.5% Essential oil) 50 mg • Feverfew (Tanacetum parthenium leaf) (standardized 0.7% Parthenolide) 50 mg • Goldenseal (Hydrastis canadensis root & rhizome) (standardized 10% Alkaloids, 5% Hydrastine) 25 mg • Ginger (Zingiber officinale root) standardized 4% Volatile oils 25 mg.

InflamActin Cream **-** Nature's Plus
Active ingredient: Methyl Salicylate 18%. Other Ingredients: Exclusive Liposomal Herbal Complex: Boswellin (Boswellia serrata gum resin extract) (standardized 65% Boswellic Acids), Tumeric rhizome extract (Curcuma longa) (standardized 95% Curcumin), Gorgonian extract (Pseudopterogoria elisbethae leaf) (standardized 4% Pseudopterosin), Natural Vitamin E. In a vanishing Liposomal Cream Base.

Inflamase **-** Progressive Labs
Each capsule contains: Enteric release phase: Pancreatin 100 mg • Lipase 10 mg • Amylase 10 mg • Trypsin 200 mg • Alpha Chymotrypsin 2 mg. Gastric release phase: Bromelain 100 mg • Catalase 25 mcg • Superoxide Dismutase 25 mcg.
See Editor's Note No. 14.

***InflammEnz* - Enzymes, Inc.**
Each capsule contains: Vitamin C (from Calcium and Potassium Ascorbates) 150 mg • Calcium (from Calcium Ascorbate and Citrate) 30 mg • Potassium (from Potassium Ascorbate) 10 mg • n-zimes Proprietary Blend 442 mg: pHysioProtease, Bromelain • Proprietary Blend 90 mg: Rutin, Grape seed extract. Other Ingredients: Cellulose, Water.

***Inflamzyme* - PhytoPharmica**
Each tablet contains: Vitamin C (ascorbic acid) 100 mg • Magnesium (carbonate) 25 mg •Bromelain (1800 MCU/g) 125 mg • Quercetin 125 mg • Mixed Citrus Bioflavonoids complex (50% concentrate) 100 mg • L-Cysteine (HCl) 75 mg.

***Inflavonoid Intensive Care* - Metagenics**
Two tablets contain: Lemon Bioflavonoid complex (standardized to 50% (100 mg) full spectrum bioflavonoids) 200 mg • Quercetin 100 mg • Vitamin C (as ascorbic acid) 200 mg • Boswellia gum extract (boswellia serrata, standardized to 70% (280 mg) boswellic acids) 400 mg • Turmeric rhizome extract (curcuma longa, standardized to 95% (285 mg) curcuminoids) 300 mg • Ginger rhizome extract (zingiber officinale, standardized to 5% (10 mg) gingerols) 200 mg • Cayenne Pepper fruit (capsicum annuum) 50 mg.

***Inholtra* - Omni Nutraceuticals**
Two Quicksorb gels contain: Vitamin C (as ascorbyl palmitate) 1 mg • Vitamin E (as D-alpha tocopherol) 7 IU • Manganese (as manganese aspartate) 0.60 mg • Omega-3 fatty acid (eicosapentainoic acid 400 mg and docosahexaenoic acid 300 mg) 465 mg • D-Glucosamine Sulfate 335 mg • N-Acetyl D-Glucosamine 335 mg • Omega-6 fatty acid (as gamma-linolenic acid) 135 mg. Other Ingredients: Vegetable Oil, Fish Oil, Gelatin, Glycerin, Carob, Water.

***Inholtra Natural Pain Relief Formula* - Omni Nutraceuticals**
Three quicksorb gels contain: Glucosamine Sulfate 500 mg • N-Acetyl D-Glucosamine 500 mg • Chondroitin Sulfate (as Chondroitin Sulfates A & B) 200 mg • EPA 400 mg • DHA 300 mg • GLA 300 mg • Vitamin E 10 IU • Ascorbyl Palmitate 5 mg • Manganese 1 mg. See Editor's Note No. 15, page 2055.

***Inositol* - Puritan's Pride**
Each tablet contains: Inositol 650 mg.

***Inositol* - Nature's Bounty**
Each tablet contains: Inositol 650 mg. Other Ingredients: Cellulose, Vegetable Stearic Acid, Food Glaze, Talc, Magnesium Silicate, Vegetable Magnesium Stearate.

***Inositol* - Source Naturals**
Each 1/4 teaspoon contains: Inositol powder 600 mg.

***Inositol 650 mg* - Solgar**
Each tablet contains: Calcium (as dicalcium phosphate) 65 mg • Inositol 650 mg. Other Ingredients: Dicalcium Phosphate, Microcrystalline Cellulose, Vegetable Cellulose, Vegetable Stearic Acid, Titanium Dioxide, Silica, Vegetable Glycerin, Carnauba Wax.

***Inositol 650 mg* - Vitamin World**
Each tablet contains: Inositol 650 mg. Other Ingredients: Cellulose (plant orign), Vegetable Stearic Acid, Food Glaze, Magnesium Silicate, Vegetable Magnesium Stearate.

***Inositol Hexaphosphate* - Olympian Labs**
Two capsules contain: Inositol Hexaphosphate 1000 mg • Kelp 100 mg • Wheat Grass 60 mg.

***Inositol Powder - GNC A-Z* - GNC**
Each 1/4 teaspoon contains: Inositol 600 mg.

***Inositol Powder* - Optimum Nutrition**
Each 1/4 level tsp (600 mg) serving contains: Inositol 600 mg.

***Inositol Powder* - Puritan's Pride**
Each 1/4 teaspoon contains: Inositol powder 600 mg.

***Inositol Powder* - Vitamin World**
Each 1/4 tsp (1g) serving contains: Inositol 1000 mg.

***InosoPhate 6 (IP6-Inositol Complex)* - EcoNugenics**
Each capsule contains: Inositol 280 mg • Inositol Hexaphosphate 230 mg. Other Ingredients: Gelatin, Magnesium Stearate, Silica.

***Instant Brewer's Yeast - GNC A-Z* - GNC**
Two tablespoons contain: Thiamin 0.75 mg • Riboflavin 1.2 mg • Niacin 8 mg • Vitamin B6 1.8 mg • Folate, Folic Acid, Folacin 20 mcg • Vitamin B12 0.12 mcg • Biotin 12 mcg • Pantothenic acid 0.6 mg • Iron 1.8 mg • Phosphorus 20 mg • Magnesium 28 mg • Zinc 2.25 mg • Copper 0.9 mg. Ingredients: Brewer's Yeast, Psyllium husk powder, Guar Gum, Citrus Pectin powder.

***Instant Soy'n Whey* - Next Nutrition**
Water-Extracted Soy Protein concentrate • Non-Denatured Whey Protein concentrate • Fructose • Natural Vanilla flavoring • Lecithin • Modified Food starch • Malic acid • Cellulose gum • Kudzu extract • Momordica extract • Stevia • Vitamin E.

***InsuLeanR* - NutraBolics**
Two capsules contain: D-Pinitol 20 mg • R- ALA 200 mg • Gymnema Sylvestre 200 mg • Banaba leaf extract (1% corosolic acid (glucosol)) 40 mg.

***Intact Colostrum* - GNC**
Each packet (20.4 grams) contains: Bovine Colostrum powder (standardized for minumum 15% IgG content). Other Ingredients: Artificial Vanilla Flavoring, Acesulfame Potassium.

***IntakeLean* - InStone Nutrition**
Each scoop (30 g) contains: EssentialPro: Calcium Caseinate, Whey Protein concentrate, Milk Protein concentrate, Hydrolyzed Wheat Gluten (as a source of glutamine peptides), Whey Protein Isolate, Hydrolyzed Whey Protein Concentrate • Ultra W3 Fatty Acid Blend: High-Oleic Sunflower Creamer, Conjugated Linoleic Acid, Flax Seed powder, Vegetable DHA powder • Dutch processed Cocoa • FiberZyme: Fibersol-2 Fiber, Digestive Enzyme blend • Natural and Artificial Flavors • Inulin • Vitamin and Mineral blend • Cellulose Gum • Tri-Calcium Phosphate • Xanthan Gum • Guar Gum • Acesulfame Potassium • Sucralose.

***IntakePerformance* - InStone Nutrition**
Each packet contains: EssentialPro: Calcium Caseinate, Whey Protein concentrate, Milk Protein concentrate, Hydrolyzed Wheat Gluten (as a source of glutamine peptides), Whey Protein Isolate, Hydrolyzed Whey Protein Concentrate • Ultra W3 Fatty Acid Blend: High-Oleic Sunflower Creamer, Conjugated Linoleic Acid, Flax Seed powder, Vegetable DHA powder • Dutch processed Cocoa • FiberZyme: Fibersol-2 Fiber, Digestive Enzyme blend • Natural and Artificial Flavors • Inulin • Vitamin and Mineral blend • Cellulose Gum • Tri-Calcium Phosphate • Xanthan Gum • Guar Gum • Acesulfame Potassium • Sucralose.

***IntegritE Max Capsules* - E'OLA**
Four capsules contain: Glucosamine Sulfate 1500 mg • MSM (Methylsulfonylmethane) 750 mg • Proprietary Blend 480 mg: Boswellia (bark), Sea Cucumber, L-Cysteine, Horsetail (shoots), Bromelain. Other Ingredients: Rice Flour, Gelatin, Magnesium Stearate.

***Intelectol* - Memory Secret**
Each tablet contains: Vinpocetine (from periwinkle seed extract) 5 mg. Other Ingredients: Lactose, Hydroxypropylcellulose, Magnesium Stearate, Talc.

***IntelleQ* - Advocare International**
Two capsules contain: Niacin 20 mg • Vitamin C (as potassium ascorbate) 60 mg • Choline (as bitartrate) 100 mg • Taurine 200 mg • Boron (as amino acid complex) 700 mcg • Ribonucleic Acid 1 mg • Phospholipid Complex (standardized phosphatidylserine) 150 mg • Ginkgo Biloba extract (leaf - ginkgo biloba) 100 mg • Gotu Kola extract (leaf/stem/flower - centella asiatica) 150 mg • Grape extract

(seed/skin - vitis vinifera Activin) 5 mg • Bacopa extract (leaf/stem - Bacopa monniera) 400 mg. Other Ingredients: Silicon Dioxide, Magnesium Stearate, Gelatin.

Intensive Eye Complex **-** Nu Skin Enterprises
Water • Aloe Barbadensis gel • Propylene Glycol Stearate SE • Squalane • Butylene Glycol • Caprylic/Capric Triglyceride • Octyl Stearate • Glycerin • Cetearyl Alcohol • Biosaccharide Gum-1 • Stearic Acid • Ceteareth-20 • Barrier Repair Complex: Linoleic Acid, Soy Stearols, Soy Phospholipids, Tocopherol, Ascorbyl Palmitate • Carrot extract (daucus carota sativis) • Shea Butter (butyrospermem perkii) • Kukui nut oil (aleurites moluccana) • Stearyl Glycyrrhetinate • Ginkgo Biloba extract • Allantoin • Phospholiids • Octyl Palmitate • Dioctyl Adipate • Aminomethyl Propanol • Methylparaben • Phenoxyethanol • Chlorphenesin • Phenylethyl Alcohol • Propylparaben • Disodium EDTA • Chlorhexidine Gluconate.

Interex **-** Benson Pendant
Each capsule contains: Epimedium Grandiflorum extract 187.50 mg • Muira Puama 4:1 extract (ptychopetalum) 75 mg • Maca 75 mg • L-Arginine Hydrochloride USP 75 mg • Cnidium Monnier extract 37.50 mg • Xanthroparmelia Scabrosa extract 37.50 mg • Tribulus Terrestris extract 37.50 mg • Mucuna Pruriens extract (15% levo-dopa) 37.5 mg • Coleus Forskolin 10% (ForsLean) 37.5 mg. Other Ingredients: Microcrystalline Cellulose, Silica, Dicalcium Phosphate, Talcum, Magnesium Stearate, Gelatin.

Internal Sweep powder (World's Best Internal Klenz) **-** Nature's Medicine Corporation
Alfalfa powder • Aloe Vera • Althaea root powder • Buchu leaf • Burdock root powder • Capsicum fruit powder • Chickweed leaf • Cinnamon bark powder • Citrus Pectin • Clove seed powder • Corn Silk • Dandelion root powder • Echinacea root powder • Fenugreek seed powder • Fennel seed powder • Flax seed powder • Fructooligosaccharides • Garlic powder (odorless) • Ginger root powder • Goldenseal root • Grapefruit Pectin • Guar gum • Irish Moss • Licorice root • Peppermint leaf • Rhubarb root bark powder • Stevia Rebaudiana • Papaya fruit powder • Pumpkin seed powder • Psyllium husks • Red Clover • Rhubarb root • Slippery Elm • Uva Ursi leaf. Other Ingredients: Acidophilus, Natural Banana Flavor, Natural Lemon Flavor, Fructose.

IntestaLife **-** Holista
Each capsule contains: 4 billion active cells specially cultured strains of Lactobacillus Rhamnosus • Lactobacillus acidophilus • Bifido longum.

Intestamend **-** Health From The Sun
Three capsules contain: Protein 1 g • Calcium 24 mg • Glutamine 200 mg • Lysine 132 mg • Leucine 103 mg • Methionine 49 mg • Threonine 59 mg • Valine 69 mg • Trypophane 11 mg • Isoleucine 60 mg • Phenylalanine 48 mg. Ingredients: Deep-Ocean White Fish, Gelatin, Glycerine, Water, natural Rosemary flavor.

Intestinal Fortitude **-** Nutri-Quest Rx
Each tablet contains: L-Glutamine 150 mg • Buffered Vitamin C (Sago) 25 mg • N-Acetyl Glucosamine 75 mg • Vitamin E Succinate 10 IU • Lipoic Acid 2 mg • Ginkgo Biloba extract 2 mg • Deglycerrized Licorice 50 mg • Slippery Elm 100 mg • Lactobacillus Acidophilus 1 million IU • Cats Claw 15 mg • Ginkgo Biloba herb 50 mg • Jerusalem Artichoke 25 mg • Zinc Chelate 5 mg • Lactobacillus Bifidus 1 million IU.

Intestinal Rescue **-** The Herbalist
Psyllium seed & husk • Guar gum • Ginger root • Medical Grade Pectin • Bentonite clay • Rhubarb root • Cinnamon bark.

Intestive **-** Proper Nutrition - PNI
Four capsules contain: Vitamin B12 0.23 mcg • Sodium 5 mg • Potassium 30 mg • White Fish 1.8 g • Omega-3 19 mg • Colostrum (casein- & lactose-free, bovine) 160 mg • Boswellia 40 mg. Other Ingredients: Gelatin.

Intimate Response **-** Source Naturals
Each tablet contains: Vitamin B6 (as pyridoxine HCl) 5 mg • Folate (as folic acid) 50 mcg • Wild Oats 150 mg • L-Arginine 100 mg • Dong Quai root extract 75 mg • Yohimbe bark standardized extract (yielding 2.5 mg yohimbines) 63 mg • Ginkgo Biloba leaf (24%, 50:1 extract) 60 mg • Panax Ginseng root extract 38 mg • Nettle root extract 25 mg • Epimedium Bicorum leaf extract 15 mg • Boron (as boron chelate) 1.5 mg • Pregnenolone 1.25 mg.

Intlecs Huperzine A **-** Intlecs
Each tablet contains: Huperzine A (Chinese club moss, Huperzia serrata) 50 mcg.

Intrasound Cleanse Formula **-** TriStar Online
Each scoop contains: Maltodextrin • Calcium Citrate • Natural Flavors • Magnesium Citrate • Gum • Citric Acid • Beta Carotene Gum • Stevia • Rebaudiana Extract • Soy Lecithin • Beet Powder • Lactobacillus Acidophilus • Lactobacillus Bifidus • Fructooligosaccharides • Papaya Powder • Prune Powder • Ascorbic Acid • Barley Sprout Powder • Wheat Sprout Powder • Oat Sprout Powder • Fenugreek. Fiber blend: Oat Fiber, Cellulose Gel/Cellulose, Purified Cellulose, Partially Hydrolyzed Soy Fiber, Psyllium Husk, Rice Bran, Citrus Pectin.

Intrasound Energy Drink **-** TriStar Online
Whole leaf aloe • Purified water • Natural Flavor • Fructose • Kaolin Clay • Trace Minerals • Citric Acid • Stevia • Xanthan Gum • Fiber • Ginseng Extract • Sage Extract • Dandelion Extract • Potassium Gluconate • Sodium Benzoate • Potassium Sorbate.

Intrasound Enzyme Formulas **-** TriStar Online
Each capsule contains: Amylase • Lipase • Protease • Cellulase • Intervase or Sucrase • Lactase • Malt Diastase • Calcium Citrate • Kaolin Clay • Beef Gelatin Capsule.

Intrasound Gel **-** TriStar Online
Generic Conductive Gel • Kaolin Clay.

Intrasound Herbal Accelerator **-** TriStar Online
Each capsule contains: Lipase • Cellulase • Amylase • Protease • Chromium Picolinate • Chromium Polynicotinate • Garcinia Cambogia Extract • Sida Cordifolia Herb • Yerba Mate • Kola Nut • Bladderwrack Algae • Cayenne Pepper • Siberian Ginseng Root.
See Editor's Note No. 39, page 2058.

Intrasound Mouth Rinse **-** TriStar Online
Whole leaf aloe • Purified Water • Natural Flavor • Kaolin Clay • Chlorophyll • Stevia • Sodium Benzoate.

Intrasound Powder **-** TriStar Online
Kaolin Clay.

Intrasound Tooth Gel **-** TriStar Online
Whole Leaf Aloe • Purified Water • Glycerin • Carrageenan (seaweed) • Hydrated Silica • Sodium Lauroyl Sarcosinate • Chlorophyll • Kaolin Clay • Natural Flavor • Stevia • Potassium Sorbate.

Intrinsic Plus **-** Progressive Labs
Each capsule contains: Vitamin B12 (cyanocobalamin) 500 mcg • Folate (folic acid) 800 mcg • Pancreatic enzyme concentrate 50 mg • Porcine Stomach 250 mg • Pyloric Substance 60 mg.
See Editor's Note No. 14, page 2055.

Invigorate II **-** Unknown
Some ingredients include: Proprietary Blend: Kryukova, Water, Natural Fruit Flavor, Citric Acid, Acesulfame Potassium, FD&C Red.
See Editor's Note No. 49, page 2059.

Invigorex **-** Austin Research, Inc.
Two capsules contain: Vitamin B6 (as pyridoxine HCl) 12.5 mg • Niacin (as niacinamide) 10 mg • Natural Vitamin E 15 IU • Zinc (as oxide) 7.5 mg • L-Arginine HCl 750 mg • Tribulus Terrestris extract (20%) 200 mg • Muira Puama extract (4:1) 150 mg • Jujube dates (ziziphus jujuba) 100 mg • Avena Sativa extract 100 mg • Peruvian Maca root 50 mg • Stinging Nettle extract (5:1) 25 mg • Horny Goat

BRAND NAMES

Weed powder 100 mg • Siberian Ginseng powder 100 mg • Saw Palmetto powder 50 mg. Other Ingredients: Gelatin, Microcrystalline Cellulose, Magnesium Stearate, Water.

IP-6 **-** PhysioLogics
Two capsules contain: Inositol Hexaphosphate 1020 mg. Other Ingredients: Cellulose (plant origin), Gelatin, Silica, Vegetable Magnesium Stearate.

IP6 Capsule **-** Jarrow Formulas
Each capsule contains: Calcium-Magnesium Inositol Hexaphosphate 615 mg • IP6 50 mg • Calcium 85 mg • Magnesium 30 mg. Other Ingredients: Rice powder, Magnesium Stearate.

IP6 Powder **-** Jarrow Formulas
Each scoop contains: Calcium-Magnesium Inositol Hexaphosophate 1230 mg • IP6 (extracted from rice bran) 1000 mg • Calcium 170 mg • Magnesium 60 mg.

IpriBone **-** GNC
Two tablets contain: Vitamin D (as Cholecalciferol) 400 IU • Calcium (as Calcimate Calcium Citrate Malate) 200 mg • 7-Isopropoxy Isoflavone (Ostivone) 600 mg.

Irish Cream - Revival **-** Physicians Laboratories
Eight fluid ounces contain: Certified Isoflavone 15 mg. Other Ingredients: Whole Roasted Soybeans, Natural and Artificial Flavors.

Iromin-G **-** Mission Pharmacal
Each tablet contains: Vitamin A 4000 IU • Vitamin C 100 mg • Vitamin D (as Vitamin D3; Cholecalciferol) 400 IU • Vitamin B1 4.8 mg • Vitamin B2 (Cyanocobalamin) 2 mg • Vitamin B3 10 mg • Vitamin B6 20 mg • Folate 0.8 mg • Vitamin B12 2 mcg • Vitamin B5 1 mg • Calcium 57 mg • Iron 29.5 mg. Other Ingredients: Sugar, Microcrystalline Cellulose, Color, Croscarmellose Sodium, Magnesium Stearate, Povidone, Red 40 Lake, Food Glaze, Carnauba Wax, Sodium Benzoate, White Beeswax, Yellow 6 Lake.

Iron **-** Source Naturals
Each tablet contains: Iron (from 250 mg of Iron Amino Acid Chelate) 25 mg.

Iron 18 mg Timed Release - GNC A-Z **-** GNC
Each tablet contains: Iron (as ferrochel) 18 mg. Other Ingredients: Dicalcium Phosphate, Cellulose.

Iron 35 mg Timed Release **-** Jamieson
Each caplet contains: Elemental Iron 35 mg.

Iron 50 mg - Solaray **-** Nutraceutical Corp.
Each capsule contains: Iron (Iron Amino Acid Chelate) 50 mg. Other Ingredients: Herb Base: Parsley leaf, Yellow Dock root, Gelatin, Whole Rice Concentrate (including bran, germ, and polishings), Magnesium Stearate.

Iron 50 mg Timed Release **-** Jamieson
Each caplet contains: Elemental Iron 50 mg.

Iron 65MG **-** Nature Made
Each tablet contains: Iron 65 mg.
See Editor's Note No. 45, page 2058.

Iron All Organic Iron Plus Liver, B-Complex, Vitamin C **-** Puritan's Pride
Two tablets contain: Vitamin C (as ascorbic acid and rose hips) 67 mg • Thiamin (vitamin B1 as thiamin hydrochloride) 1.5 mg • Riboflavin (vitamin B2) 3 mg • Niacin (as niacinamide) 0.5 mg • Vitamin B6 (as pyridoxine hydrochloride) 17 mcg • Folic Acid 11 mcg • Vitamin B12 (as cyanocobalamin) 8 mcg • Biotin (as D-biotin) 0.5 mcg • Pantothenic Acid (as D-calcium pantothenate) 45 mcg • Iron (as ferrous gluconate) 38 mg • Desiccated Liver 67 mg • L-Lysine (as L-lysine hydrochloride) 20 mg • Inositol 2 mg • Choline (as choline bitartrate) 1.5 mg • PABA (para-aminobenzoic acid) 10 mcg. Other Ingredients: Dicalcium Phosphate, Cellulose (plant origin), Croscarmellose, Vegetable Stearic Acid, Cellulose Coating, Vegetable Magnesium Stearate, Silica.
See Editor's Note No. 14.

Iron Caps **-** TwinLab
Each capsule contains: Iron (from Chelated Ferrous Fumarate) 18 mg.

Iron Complex **-** Nature's Life
Each capsule contains: Iron (Peptonate) 25 mg • Vitamin C 20 mg • Niacinamide 10 mg • Vitamin B1 (Thiamine HCl) 1 mg • Vitamin B2 (Riboflavin) 1 mg • Vitamin B6 (Pyridoxine HCl) 1 mg • Folic Acid 30 mcg • Vitamin B12 (Cobalamin concentrate) 15 mcg • Copper (Gluconate) 100 mcg • Manganese (Gluconate) 1 mg • Betaine HCl 15 mg. In a natural base of Rose Hips concentrate.

Iron Complex **-** PhytoPharmica
Two capsules contain: Vitamin C (ascorbic acid) 120 mg • Folic Acid 400 mcg • Vitamin B12 (cyanocobalamin) 200 mcg • Iron (ferrous succinate) 50 mg • Liquid Liver fractions (predigested soluble concentrate) 500 mg • Chlorophyll (fat-soluble) 10 mg.
See Editor's Note No. 14.

Iron Plex **-** PhysioLogics
Each capsule contains: Vitamin C (as ascorbic acid) 60 mg • Folic Acid 400 mcg • Vitamin B12 (as cyanocobalamin) 8 mcg • Iron (as ferrous bis-glycinate) 28 mg. Other Ingredients: Maltodextrin, Gelatin, Vegetable Magnesium Stearate, Silica.

Iron Plus **-** Nutri-Quest Rx
Each tablet contains: Iron (Ferrous Fumurate) 50 mg • Vitamin C 100 mg • L-Glycine 100 mg • Niacinamide 15 mg • Betaine HCL 15 mg • Vitamin E (Succinate) 15 IU • D-Calcium Pantothenate (Pantothenic Acid) 13 mg • Vitamin B2 4 mg • Vitamin B1 3 mg • Vitamin B6 2 mg • Folic Acid 200 mcg • Vitamin B12 25 mcg • Choline Bitartrate 12.5 mg.

Iron Plus C Complex **-** Shaklee
Each tablet contains: Vitamin C (as Ascorbic acid) 60 mg • Calcium (as Dicalcium and Tricalcium phosphate) 130 mg • Iron (as Ferrous fumarate) 18 mg • Phosphorus (as Dicalcium and Tricalcium phosphate) 100 mg. Other Ingredients: Maltodextrin, Modified Cellulose Gum, Beet Powder, Acacia Gum, Spinach Powder, Barley Flour, Locust Bean Gum, Agar-Agar.

Iron Woman **-** Traditional Medicinals
Yellow Dock root • Burdock root • Dandelion root • Licorice root • Nettle leaf • Prune fruit • Astragalus root • Stevia leaf.

Ironchel 18 mg - GNC A-Z **-** GNC
Each capsule contains: Iron (as ferrochel) 18 mg. Other Ingredients: Cellulose, Dicalcium Phosphate, Gelatin.

Iron-Folic Plus **-** Nutrilite
Each tablet contains: Folate (folic acid) 133 mcg • Iron 15 mg • Calcium 40 mg.

Iron-Free MultiLogics **-** PhysioLogics
Each caplet contains: Vitamin A (as 83% beta carotene, vitamin a palmitate) 15,000 IU • Vitamin C (as acorbic acid) 250 mg • Vitamin D (as cholecalciferol) 400 IU • Vitamin E (as d-alpha tocopheryl acetate) 150 IU • Thiamine (vitamin B1, as thiamin mononitrate) 75 mg • Riboflavin (vitamin B2) 75 mg • Niacin (as niacinamide) 75 mg • Vitamin B6 (as pyridoxine hydrochloride) 75 mg • Folic Acid 400 mcg • Vitamin B12 (as cyanocobalamin) 75 mcg • Biotin 300 mcg • Pantothenic Acid (as d-calcium pantothenate) 75 mg • Calcium (as dicalcium phosphate, lithothamnium) 92 mg • Iodine (as potassium iodide) 150 mg • Magnesium Chelate 10 mg • Zinc Chelate 10 mg • Selenium (as selenomethionate) 25 mcg • Copper (as copper amino acid chelate) 1 mg • Manganese (as manganese amino acid chelate) 1 mg • Chromium (as chromium amino acid chelate) 25 mcg • Molybdenum (as molybdenum amino acid chelate) 27 mcg • Boron (as boron amino acid chelate) 500 mcg • Inositol 75 mg • PABA (para-aminobenzoic acid) 75 mg • Choline (as choline bitartrate) 31 mg • Betaine Hydrochloride 25 mg • Citrus Bioflavonoids (citrus spp., fruit) 25 mg • Rutin (dimorphandra mollis, fruit) 25 mg •

Hesperidin Complex (citrus aurantium, citrus spp., fruit) 5 mg. Other Ingredients: Cellulose (plant origin), Gelatin, Croscarmellose, Vegetable Stearic Acid, Silica, Vegetable Magnesium Stearate, Cellulose Coating.
See Editor's Note No. 40, page 2058.

IsoBolic **-** NutraBolics
Two scoops (55 g) contain: Isobolic Advanced Protein Matrix: Cross-Flow Micro-Filtrated Whey Protein Isolate, Micellar Casein, Egg Isolate (egg albumin), Whey Protein Concentrate • CLA • Bromazyme • Flaxseed powder • Sucralose • Natural/Artificial Flavors.

Isochrome **-** Market America, Inc.
Each capful (3.33 g) contains: Boron (chelate) 2 mg • L-Carnitine 20 mg • Chromium (picolinate) 100 mcg • Chromium (argininate) 115 mcg • Coenzyme Q10 60 mg • Lipase 5 mg • Vitamin B2 (riboflavin) 3 mg • Vitamin B6 (pyridoxine HCl) 2 mg • Potassium (bicarbonate) 95 mg. Other Ingredients: Fructose, Glucose, Citric Acid, Maltodextrin, Silica, Calcium Sulfate, Natural Lemon-Lime Flavor.

Isolase Enzymes **-** Physicians Laboratories
Each capsule contains: Xylanase, Beta-Glucanase (from trichderma longibrachiatum) 224 IsoU.

IsoPure **-** Nature's Best
Each serving contains: Creamy Vanilla Ingredients: Ion Exchanged Whey Protein Isolate, Maltodextrin, Vitamin, Mineral & Amino Acid Blend, Natural & Artificial Flavor, Xanthan Gum, Aspartame, Acesulfame K. Dutch Chocolate Ingredients: Ion Exchange Whey Protein Isolate, Maltodextrin, Vitamin, Mineral & Amino Acid Blend, Cocoa, Xanthan Gum, Natural & Artificial Flavor, Aspartame, Acesulfame K. Orange Creamsicle Ingredients: Ion Exchange Whey Protein Isolate, Maltodextrin, Vitamin, Mineral & Amino Acid Blend, Natural & Artificial Flavor, Xanthan Gum, Aspartame, Acesulfame K, Artificial Color (Yellow #6). Strawberries & Cream Ingredients: Ion Exchange Whey Protein Isolate, Maltodextrin, Vitamin, Mineral & Amino Acid Blend, Natural & Artificial Flavor, Freeze-Dried Strawberry Crystals, Xanthan Gum, Aspartame, Acesulfame K, Artificial Color (Red #3). Chocolate Peanut Butter Swirl Ingredients: Ion Exchange Whey Protein Isolate, Maltodextrin, Vitamin, Mineral & Amino Acid Blend, Cocoa, Natural & Artificial Flavor, Xanthan Gum, Aspartame, Acesulfame K.

Isotonix B-12 Special Formula **-** Market America, Inc.
Each capful contains: Vitamin B2 (riboflavin-5-phosphate) 3 mg • Vitamin B12 (cyanocobalamin) 120 mcg • Folic Acid 400 mcg • Magnesium (carbonate) 40 mg • Potassium (bicarbonate) 94 mg. Other Ingredients: Fructose, Glucose, Citric Acid, Maltodextrin, Silica, Pectin, Calcium Sulfate, Natural Lemon-Lime Flavor.

Isotonix Calcium Plus Formula **-** Market America, Inc.
Each capful contains: Calcium (gluconate) 166.6 mg • Calcium (chloride) 166.6 mg • Calcium (lactate) 166.6 mg • Magnesium (bicarbonate) 40 mg • Vitamin D (D3) 400 IU • Potassium (bicarbonate) 99 mg • Boron (chelate) 1 mg. Other Ingredients: Malic Acid, Citric Acid, Calcium Sulfate, Beta-Carotene (vitamin A precursor), Silica, Natural Lemon Lime Flavor.

Isotonix Coenzyme Q10 **-** Market America, Inc.
Each capful (3.33 g) contains: Coenzyme Q10 100 mg • Vitamin E (acetate) 200 IU • Lipase 5 mg • Vitamin B2 (riboflavin) 3 mg • Potassium (bicarbonate) 108 mg. Other Ingredients: Fructose, Glucose, Citric Acid, Silica, Calcium Sulfate, Maltodextrin, Natural Lemon-Lime Flavor.

Isotonix Digestive Enzyme Formula with Probiotics **-** Market America, Inc.
Each capful (3.33 g) contains: DigeZyme 100 mg: Amylase 2400 U, Protease 600 U, Cellulase 20 U, Lactase 400 U, Lipase 100 U • Maltase 125 MWU • Sucrase 400 SU • Magnesium (carbonate) 24 mg • Potassium (bicarbonate) 88 mg • Lactobacillus Sporogenes (Lactospore) 150,000,000 CFU. Other Ingredients: Fructose, Glucose, Citric Acid, Maltodextrin, Silica, Apple Pectin, Calcium Sulfate, Natural Lemon-Lime Flavor.

Isotonix Formula MultiTech **-** Market America, Inc.
Each capful (3.3 g) contains: Beta-Carotene 10,000 IU • Vitamin B1 2.6 mg • Vitamin B2 3 mg • Niacin 40 mg • Pantothenic Acid 20 mg • Vitamin B6 4 mg • Vitamin B12 75 mcg • Folic Acid 400 mcg • Biotin 300 mcg • Vitamin C 150 mg • Vitamin D (D3) 400 IU • Vitamin E (d-alpha-tocopheryl succinate) 60 IU • Vitamin K 100 mcg • Calcium 50 mg • Chromium 120 mcg • Copper 1000 mcg • Iodine 150 mcg • Magnesium 25 mg • Potassium 108 mg • Selenium 55 mcg • Silicon 2 mg • Zinc 7.5 mg. Other Ingredients: Fructose, Citric Acid, Orange Fruit Powder, Mandarin Fruit Powder, Malic Acid, Glucose, Natural Orange Flavor, Tricalcium Phosphate, Sucralose.

Isotonix Formula MultiTech with Iron **-** Market America, Inc.
Each capful (3.3 g) contains: Beta-Carotene 10,000 IU • Vitamin B1 2.6 mg • Vitamin B2 3 mg • Niacin 40 mg • Pantothenic Acid 20 mg • Vitamin B6 4 mg • Vitamin B12 75 mcg • Folic Acid 400 mcg • Biotin 300 mcg • Vitamin C 150 mg • Vitamin D (D3) 400 IU • Vitamin E (d-alpha-tocopheryl succinate) 60 IU • Vitamin K 100 mcg • Calcium 50 mg • Chromium 120 mcg • Copper 1000 mcg • Iodine 150 mcg • Iron 15 mg • Magnesium 25 mg • Potassium 108 mg • Selenium 55 mcg • Silicon 2 mg • Zinc 7.5 mg. Other Ingredients: Fructose, Citric Acid, Orange Fruit Powder, Mandarin Fruit Powder, Malic Acid, Glucose, Natural Orange Flavor, Tricalcium Phosphate, Sucralose.

Isotonix Maximum ORAC Formula **-** Market America, Inc.
Each capful (3.33 g) contains: Potassium (bicarbonate) 125 mg • Vitamin C (ascorbic acid) 100 mg • Cranberry 200 mg • Blueberry 100 mg • Grape 93 mg • Raspberry 90 mg • Elderberry 40 mg • Black Currant 40 mg • Pomegranate 40 mg • Plum 20 mg • Choke Cherry 20 mg • Natural Tocopherol (d-gamma 70%, d-delta 21%, d-alpha 7%, d-beta 2%) 30 mg • Tocotrienols (mixed isomers) 20 mg • Bioperine Black Pepper extract 56 mcg. Other Ingredients: Fructose, Citric Acid, Maltodextrin, Glucose, Silica.

Isotonix Might-a-Mins **-** Market America, Inc.
Each capful contains: Beta-Carotene (vitamin A precursor) 2500 IU • Vitamin B1 (thiamin HCl) 0.75 mg • Vitamin B2 (riboflavin) 0.85 mg • Vitamin B3 (niacin/niacinamide 1:4) 10 mg • Vitamin B5 (calcium d-pantothenate) 5 mg • Vitamin B6 (pyridoxine HCl) 1 mg • Vitamin B12 (cyanocobalamin) 3 mcg • Biotin 33 mcg • Vitamin C (ascorbic acid) 30 mg • Vitamin D (D3) 200 IU • Vitamin E (as d-alpha-tocopheryl succinate) 15 IU • Calcium (lactate, carbonate, sulfate, phosphate, citrate) 30 mg • Chromium (amino acid chelate) 10 mcg • Copper (gluconate) 182.2 mcg • Iodine (potassium iodide) 75 mcg • Magnesium (carbonate) 5 mg • Manganese (sulfate) 1 mg • Selenium (amino acid chelate) 20.6 mcg • Silicon (dioxide) 20 mg • Potassium (bicarbonate, citrate) 120 mg • Zinc (gluconate) 5.7 mg • Proprietary Phytonutrient Blend 1.04 g: Apple, Broccoli, Carrot, Cranberry, Grape, Kiwi, Lemon, Lime, Orange, Peach, Pineapple, Raspberry, Spinach, Strawberry, Tomato • Lactobacillus Sporogenes (Lactospore) 50,000,000 CFU. Other Ingredients: Fructose, Citric Acid, Malic Acid, Glucose, Natural Mandarin Orange Flavor, Sucralose.

Isotonix OPC-3 **-** Market America, Inc.
Each capful (3.33 g) contains: Grape seed extract 25 mg • Red Wine extract 30 mg • Pine bark extract (Pycnogenol) 25 mg • Bilberry extract 25 mg • Citrus Bioflavonoids extract 93 mg • Potassium (bicarbonate) 93 mg. Other Ingredients: Fructose, Glucose, Citric Acid, Maltodextrin, Silica, Calcium Sulfate, Pectin.

Isotonix Vision Formula with Lutein **-** Market America, Inc.
Each capful (3.33 g) contains: Beta Carotene 5000 IU • Vitamin C (ascorbic acid) 75 mg • Vitamin E (d, l-alpha-tocopheryl acetate) 33 IU • Potassium (bicarbonate) 150 mg • Zinc (lactate) 7 mg • Chromium (arginate) 100 mcg • Copper (gluconate) 100 mcg • Bilberry 50 mg • Taurine 42 mg • Quercetin 25 mg • Eyebright 10 mg • Lutein 7 mg • Lycopene 2 mg • Zeaxanthin 1.4 mg. Other

Ingredients: Fructose, Natural Orange Powder, Citric Acid, Natural Orange Flavor, Malic Acid, Calcium Phosphate, Glucose, Silica, Sucralose.

Isotonix Vitamin C Formula **-** Market America, Inc.
Each capful (3.33 g) contains: Vitamin C (ascorbic acid) 500 mg • Beta-Carotene (vitamin A precursor) 800 IU • Potassium (bicarbonate) 101 mg. Other Ingredients: Fructose, Glucose, Maltodextrin, Malic Acid, Natural Orange Flavor, Silica, Citric Acid.

IVC-Max **-** Aidan Products, LLC
Each capsule contains: Vitamin C 50 mg • Vitamin K (phytoquinone, from vitamin K1 1% on mannitol) 1.25 mg • Niacinamide 50 mg • Biotin 100 mcg • Selenium (from selenium amino acid chelate, 1% Se) 100 mcg • Alpha Lipoic Acid 150 mg • Quercetin 125 mg • Grape Seed Extract 25 mg.

Ivy Calm **-** PhytoPharmica
Each 2 tsp serving contains: English Ivy leaf extract (hedera helix, standardized to contain hedaracoside C 9 mg) 33 mg. Other Ingredients: Purified Water, Glycerol, Fructose, Natural Flavors, Sucrose Laurate, Potassium Sorbate, Citric Acid.

Ivy Extract **-** Enzymatic Therapy/PhytoPharmica
Two tablets contain: English Ivy leaf extract (hedera helix 4:1) 50 mg. Other Ingredients: Lactose, Cellulose, Stearic Acid, Magnesium Stearate, Silica.

Jambrulin **-** Unjha Ayurvedic Pharmacy
Each tablet contains: Jamungiri extract 20% • Tribung Bhasma 20% • Refined Shilajet (mineral pitch) 20% • Mamejave extract 10% • Bili Patra 10% • Gudmar 10% • Nim Patra 10%.

Jarro-Dophilus + Colostrum **-** Jarrow Formulas
Each capsule contains: Lactobacillus Rhamnosus R049 20% 672 million • Lactobacillus Casei R215 20 % 672 million • Lactobacillus Plantarum R202 20% 672 million • Lactobacillus Acidophilus R052 10% 336 million • Bifidobacterium Longum R023 20% 672 million • Bifidobacterium Breve R070 10% 336 million • Colostrum 500 mg. Other Ingredients: Ascorbic Acid, Magnesium Stearate.

Jarro-Dophilus + FOS **-** Jarrow Formulas
Each capsule Contains: FOS (Fructo-Oligo-Saccharides) 210 mg • Lactobacillus Rhamnosus R049 20% 672 million • Lactobacillus Casei R215 20 % 672 million • Lactobacillus Plantarum R202 20% 672 million • Lactobacillus Acidophilus R052 10% 336 million • Bifidobacterium Longum R023 672 million • Bifidobacterium breve R070 10% 336 million • Vitamin C 1 mg. Other Ingredients: Maltodextrin, Magnesium Stearate.

Jarro-Dophilus + FOS Powder **-** Jarrow Formulas
Each capsule Contains: FOS (Fructo-Oligo-Saccharides) 4000 mg • Lactobacillus Rhamnosus R049 20% 2.4 billion • Lactobacillus Casei R215 20 % 2.4 billion • Lactobacillus Plantarum R202 20% 2.4 billion • Lactobacillus Acidophilus R052 10% 1.2 billion • Bifidobacterium Longum R023 2.4 billion • Bifidobacterium Breve R070 10% 1.2 billion • Vitamin C 1 mg. Other Ingredients: Maltodextrin, Magnesium Stearate.

Jarro-Dophilus + Lactoferrin **-** Jarrow Formulas
Each capsule Contains: Lactobacillus Rhamnosus R049 20% 672 million • Lactobacillis Casei R215 20 % 672 million • Lactobacillus Plantarum R202 20% 672 million • Lactobacillus Acidophilus R052 10% 336 million • Bifidobacterium Longum R023 20% 672 million • Bifidobacterium Breve R070 10% 336 million • Lactoferrin 200 mg. Other Ingredients: Ascorbic Acid, Magnesium Stearate.

Jarsin 300 **-** Lichtwer Pharma
Each tablet contains: Dry St. John's Wort extract 300 mg. Other Ingredients: Lactose Monohydrate, Silicon Dioxide, Cellulose powder, Magnesium Stearate, Vanillin, Dimeticon Emulsion, Hypromellose, Macrogol 4000, Saccharin Sodium, Talcum, Titanium Dioxide, Iron Oxide Hydrate.

Jarsin 750 **-** Lichtwer Pharma
Each tablet contains: -arzneilich wirksamer Bestandteil: Trockenextrakt aus Johanniskraut (3-6:1) 750 mg • Auszugsmittel: Menthol 80% (V/V). Inactive Ingredients: Hochdisperses Siliciumdioxid, Mikrokristalline Cellulose, Vanillin, Hypromellose, Stearinsaure, Eisenoxid Gelb (E 172), Titandioxid (E 171), Lactose-Monohydrat, Hoherkettige, Partialglyceride, Sojapolysaccharid.

Jiaogulan **-** Solaray
Two capsules contain: Jiaogulan root/rhizome extract (gynostemma pentaphyllum, guaranteed 98% gypenosides) 804 mg • Jiaogulan aerial parts (gynostemma pentaphyllum) 200 mg.

Jiaogulan Gynostemma **-** Paradise Herbs
Each vcap contains: Gynostemma Pentaphyllum whole plant extract 12:1 (equivalent to whole plant 3000 mg) 250 mg • 30% Gypenosides 75 mg. Other Ingredients: Capsules (vegetable cellulose).

JIN-ZHI Thermo Drops **-** E'OLA
Fifteen drops contain: Zhi Shi (Citrus Aurantium) 250 mg • Proprietary Blend 18 mg: Caffeine, Guarana Herb, Ginseng Root, Licorice Root. Other Ingredients: Water, Glycerin, Citric Acid, Sodium Benzoate.
See Editor's Note No. 40, page 2058.

Joint & Muscle Pain Cream **-** Shaklee
Active Ingredients: Menthol (5%). Inactive Ingredients: Aloe Barbadensis leaf gel (aloe vera), Butylene Glycol, Carbomer, Cetyl Alcohol, Cyclomethicone, Dimethicone, Glyceryl Stearate, Imidazolidinyl Urea, Methylparaben, PEG-12 Glyceryl Distearate, PEG-100 Stearate, Phenoxyethanol, Propylparaben, Prunus Amygdalus dulcis oil (sweet almond), Purified Water, Triethanolamine, Xanthan Gum.

Joint Actives **-** VitaStore
Six tablets contain: Glucosamine HCl 1500 mg • Shark Cartilage 500 mg • Salix Alba 200 mg • Boswellia 250 mg • Green Lipped Mussel 250 mg • Quercetin 300 mg • Manganese 5 mg • L-Methionine 100 mg • Zinc Gluconate 25 mg • Turmeric 250 mg • Bromelain 200 mg • Vitamin C 300 mg • Vitamin E 90 IU.

Joint Aid **-** Optimum Nutrition
Six capsules contain: Vitamin C (as ascorbic acid) 1000 mg • Vitamin D (as cholecalciferol) 400 IU • Vitamin E (as DL-alpha tocopherol acetate) 200 IU • Calcium (as calcium carbonate, citrate) 500 mg • Magnesium (as magnesium oxide, aspartate) 250 mg • Zinc (as zinc picolinate) 20 mg • Glucosamine (as glucosamine sulfate potassium) 1500 mg • Chondroitin (as chondroitin sulfate) 150 mg • Turmeric rhizome extract (curcuma longa, standardized to 95% curcuminoids) 1500 mg • Quercetin (as quercetin dihydrate) 100 mg • Borage oil 50 mg • Marine Lipids 50 mg. Other Ingredients: Gelatin, Magnesium Stearate, Silica.

Joint Care Move Free Plus MSM **-** Schiff
Two tablets contain: Glucosamine Complex 500 mg: Glucosamine Hydrochloride, N-Acetyl D-Glucosamine, Glucosamine Sulfate • Chondroitin Sulfate 400 mg • MSM (methylsulfonylmethane) 750 mg.
See Editor's Note No. 15, page 2055.

Joint Complex **-** Puritan's Pride
Three capsules contain: Glucosamine Sulfate 500 mg • Vitamin C 250 mg • Bromelain (2400 GDU per gram) 250 mg • Boswellin (Boswellia Serrata) 250 mg • Curcumin (Curcuma Longa) 50 mg • Zinc (Amino Acid Chelate) 10 mg • Chondroitin Sulfate A 10 mg • White Willow Bark 100 mg • Shark Cartilage 500 mg • Vervain 100 mg.
See Editor's Note No. 15, page 2055.

Joint Cream **-** The Vitamin Shoppe
Glucosamine • Boswellin • Capsaicin.

Some Brand Name Natural Products - What they Contain

www.NaturalDatabase.com contains MANY more listings than appear here.

Joint Essentials **-** Swanson
Three capsules contain: Vitamin C (as ascorbic acid) 250 mg • Zinc (from amino acid chelate) 15 mg • Manganese 5 mg • Glucosamine Sulfate (2KCl) 500 mg • Boswellian Boswellia Serrata Resin (65% boswellic acid) 250 mg • Bromelain (2400 GDU) 250 mg • Chondroitin Sulfate 200 mg • OptiMSM (methylsulfonylmethane) 100 mg • White Willow Bark 100 mg • Curcumin 50 mg • Devil's Claw powder 25 mg • Quercetin 25 mg • Sea Cucumber 25 mg • Yucca root extract 25 mg.
See Editor's Note No. 15, page 2055.

Joint Fitness **-** Celestial Seasonings
Two capsules contain: Vitamin C (as ascorbic acid) 225 mg • Pantothenic Acid (as calcium pantothenate) 15 mg • Glucosamine Sulfate/HCl 150 mg • Flax Seed 225 mg • Turmeric (standardized to 95% curcuminoids) extract 185 mg. Other Ingredients: Dicalcium Phosphate, Gelatin, Rice Flour, Stearic Acid, Magnesium Stearate, Silicon Dioxide.

Joint Formula **-** PharmAssure
Two tablets contain: Sodium 140 mg • Vitamin C (as Ascorbic Acid) 60mg • Selenium (as Selenium Chelate) 100 mcg • D-Glucosamine Sulfate 750 mg • .2NaCl Chondroitin Sulfate, Sodium 600 mg • Boswellin serrate Resin Extract (65% Boswellic Acid=200 mg) 308 mg • Bromelain 200 GDU. Other Ingredients: Cellulose, Croscarmellose Sodium, Dicalcium Phosphate.
See Editor's Note No. 15, page 2055.

Joint Fuel **-** TwinLab
Six capsules contain: Glucosamine Sulfate 1500 mg • Chondroitin Sulfate A (CSA) 100 mg • Zinc (from Chelated Zinc Picolinate) 30 mg • Manganese (from Chelated Manganese Gluconate) 5 mg • Vitamin C 1000 mg • Natural Vitamin E (Succinate) 800 IU • Selenium (from Selenomethionine) 200 mcg • Turmeric extract (Curcuma longa) (standardized for 95% Curcumin) 1300 mg • Quercetin (Bioflavonoid) 100 mg • Bromelain 200 mg.
See Editor's Note No. 15, page 2055.

Joint Fuel Liquid Concentrate **-** TwinLab
Each tablespoon contains: Glucosamine HCl 500 mg • Chondroitin Sulfate 400 mg • Betaine 166 mg • Hydrolyzed Collagen 33 mg • Chicken Type II Collagen 33 mg • Vitamin B6 3.3 mg • Folic Acid 400 mcg • Vitamin B12 166 mcg.
See Editor's Note No. 15, page 2055.

Joint Health - One-A-Day **-** Bayer
Each tablet contains: Vitamin C 30 mg • Vitamin E 30 IU • Manganese 1.5 mg • Lecithin 10 mg • Glucosamine Sulfate powder (includes Dipotassium CI 125 mg) 500 mg • Devil's Claw Standardized extract (Harpagophytum procumbens) root 134 mg.
See Editor's Note No. 21, page 2056.

Joint Health - Wellzymes **-** Enzymes, Inc.
Two capsules contain: Zinc (from Zinc Citrate) 14 mg • Copper (from Copper Citrate) 1 mg • Manganese (from Manganese Citrate) 8 mg • Boron (from Boron Citrate) 0.4 mg • n-zimes Proprietary Enzyme Blend 108 mg: pHysioProtease (236,800 pHysio-U), Bromelain, CereCalase Plus • Proprietary Herbal Blend 235 mg: Boswellia resin extract (standardized to contain 60% boswellic acid), Horsetail herb extract (equivalent to 200 mg raw herb), Rice Bran, Turmeric root extract (standardized to 95% curcumin), White Willow bark extract (standardized to contain 12% salicin). Other Ingredients: Plant Cellulose, Water.

Joint Health Complex **-** Shaklee
Three capsules contain: Zinc (as Zinc gluconate) 1.5 mg • Copper (as Copper gluconate) 0.2 mg • Manganese (as Manganese gluconate) 0.2 mg • Glucosamine hydrochloride 1.4 g • Osteokinetics Enhanced Proprietary Blend 450 mg: Devil's Claw extract (Harpagophytum procumbens) root, Alfalfa concentrate (Medicago sativa) leaf • Boron (as Boron protein hydrolysate) 0.5 mg. Other Ingredients: Maltodextrin, Gelatin, Water.

Joint Health Formula - Chinac **-** Metabolife International, Inc.
Each caplet contains: Achryranthes bidentata (Achyranthes) • Wenyujin concisa (Wen Curcuma) • Erythrina variegata (Coral Tree) • Atractylodes macrocephala (Bai-Zhu Atractylodes) • Notopterygium incisum (Notopterygium) • Angelica pubescens (Pubescent Angelica).

Joint Juice (Lemon Iced Tea) **-** Joint Juice, Inc.
Each 8 fl oz serving contains: Vitamin C 60 mg • Glucosamine HCl 1500 mg.

Joint Juice (Orange-Tangerine) **-** Joint Juice, Inc.
Each 8 fl oz serving contains: Vitamin C 60 mg • Glucosamine HCl 1500 mg.

Joint Juice (Tropical) **-** Joint Juice, Inc.
Each 8 fl oz serving contains: Vitamin C 60 mg • Glucosamine HCl 1500 mg.

Joint Maintenance **-** Puritan's Pride
Three softgels contain: Manganese (from manganese aspartate) 1 mg • Glucosamine Sulfate (2KCl) 1500 mg • Chondroitin Sulfate 1200 mg • Citrus Bioflavonoids (citrus sinensis, fruit) 45 mg. Other Ingredients: Soybean Oil, Gelatin, Glycerin, Lecithin, Caramel Color, Beeswax (yellow).
See Editor's Note No. 15, page 2055.

Joint Movement Glucosamine & Chondrotin with MSM and Collagen **-** Symtec
Two tablespoons (30 mL) contain: Sodium 75 mg • Vitamin C (as ascorbic acid) 60 mg • Vitamin D (as vitamin D3-cholecalciferol) 400 IU • Glucosamine HCl 2000 mg • Chondroitin Sulfate (as chondroitin sulfate disodium) 1200 mg • MSM 500 mg • Collagen 50 mg.
See Editor's Note No. 15, page 2055.

Joint Performance **-** Metabolic Response Modifiers
Four capsules contain: Glucosamine Sulfate 1000 mg • MSM (Methyl-Sulfonyl-Methane) 500 mg • Noto-Gin (Panax Ginseng 45% saponins) 100 mg • Chondroitin complex 280 mg • Collagen complex 200 mg • Sea Cucumber 100 mg • CMO (25%) 100 mg • Boswellia 200 mg • Bromelain (2400 GDU) 100 mg • White Willow bark (0.1% salicylates) 80 mg • Tumeric (95% curcuminoids) 75 mg • Manganese (citrate) 8 mg.
See Editor's Note No. 15, page 2055.

Joint Rejuvenator **-** BioTreasures
Each caplet contains: Glucosamine Sulfate 1500 mg • Chondroitin Sulfate 750 mg • Turmeric 750 mg • Devil's Claw 400 mg • Bromelain 100 mg.
See Editor's Note No. 15, page 2055.

Joint Rescue **-** TwinLab
Three softgels contain: Vitamin E (from d-Alpha Tocopherols) 400 IU • Glucosamine HCl & Glucosamine Sulfate 750 mg • Chondroitin Sulfate 50 mg • Turmeric powder extract (standardized for 95% Curcumin) 650 mg • Boswellin (Boswellia serrata extract) (standardized for 65% Boswellic Acids) 13 mg • Ginger root extract 50 mg • EPA 750 mg • DHA 750 mg • Borage Oil 100 mg.
See Editor's Note No. 15, page 2055.

Joint Rescue Formula with Glucosamine+ **-** Health Tech Industries (Dr. Bussan's)
Each capsule contains: Glucosamine sulfate 500 mg • Herbal Extract Complex 125 mg: Wild Yam, Licorice root, Aloe Vera, Pfaffia root, Red Poppy flower, Tumeric, White Peony root, Yucca, Corydalis rhizome, Super Dioxide Dismutase (SOD), Catalase Oxidants • Methionine 75 mg • Malic Acid 50 mg • Polyascorbic Acid (vitamin c) 25 mg • Niacinamide 10 mg • Pantothenic Acid (vitamin B5) 5 mg • Manganese Gluconate Chelate 5 mg.

Joint Soother - Vitamin World
Three tablets contain: Glucosamine Sulfate (2KCl) 1500 mg • Chondroitin Sulfate 1200 mg • MSM (methylsulfonylmethane) 500 mg. Other Ingredients: Cellulose, Titanium Dioxide Color, Cellulose Coating, Vegetable Stearic Acid, Vegetable Magnesium Stearate, Silica.

Joint Support - Futurebiotics - Futurebiotics
Four tablets contain: Devil's Claw 400 mg • Yucca 300 mg • Horsetail 200 mg • Ginger 200 mg • Alfalfa juice concentrate 200 mg • Chinese Cinnamon 250 mg • Magnesium: (oxide, chloride, ascorbate) 400 mg • Beta Carotene 250 mg • Vitamin C (ascorbic acid, Rose hips) 120 mg • Niacin 8 mg • Niacinamide 250 mg • Vitamin D (Fish oils) 200 IU • Vitamin E (natural) 25 IU • Vitamin B6 (pyridoxine HCl) 8 mg • Vitamin B12 (cyanocobalamin) 12 mcg • Zinc (sulfate) 15 mg • Copper (gluconate) 750 mcg • Biotin 80 mcg • Pantothenic Acid 35 mg • Selenium (methionate) 120 mcg • Glutamic Acid HCl 100 mg • Lecithin 100 mg • Betaine HCl 75 mg • Para Amino Benzoic Acid (PABA) 25 mg • Potassium (sulfate) 20 mg.

Joint Support - Now
Three capsules contain: Vitamin B3 (Niacinamide) 100mg • Vitamin B5 (Pantothenic Acid) 100 mg • Vitamin B6 (Pyridoxine HCl) 50 mg • Vitamin C (Ascorbic Acid) 100 mg • Magnesium (Oxide) 200 mg • Zinc (Picolinate) 15 mg • Manganese (Amino Acid Chelate) 7 mg • Copper (Amino Acid Chelate) 3 mg • Glucosamine HCl 1000 mg • Boswellin standardized herbal extract of Boswellia serrata 300 mg • Sea Cucumber 300 mg • Bromelain (2000 GDU activity from pineapple) 150 mg • PABA (Para-Aminobenzoic Acid) 10 mg • Devil's Claw (Harpagophytum procumbens) 100 mg.

Joint Support - Olympia Nutrition
Glucosamine • Boswellin • Sea Cucumber • Bromelain • Yucca • Alfalfa.

Joint Support Formula - Health Smart Vitamins
Each capsule contains: Methylsulfonylmethane (MSM) 333 mg • Glucosamine Sulfate 200 mg • Chondroitin Sulfate 67 mg.
See Editor's Note No. 15, page 2055.

Joint Synergy - Olympia Nutrition
Glucosamine Sulfate • Sea Cucumber • MSM • Hydrolyzed Cartilage.

Joint Synergy + - Metabolic Response Modifiers
Four capsules contain: Glucosamine Sulfate (KCl) 1000 mg • MSM (methyl-sulfonyl-methane) 500 mg • Panax Pseudoginseng (noto-panax ginseng, 50-60% Saponins supplying 45% Ginsenosides) 100 mg • Chondroitin complex 280 mg • Collagen complex 200 mg • Sea Cucumber (25% mucopolysaccharides) 100 mg • CMO (25%) 100 mg • Boswellia serrata 200 mg • Bromelain (2400 GDU) 100 mg • White Willow bark (0.1% salicylates) 80 mg • Tumeric (95% curcuminoids) 75 mg • Manganese (citrate) 8 mg.
See Editor's Note No. 15, page 2055.

Jointace Capsules - Vitabiotics
Two capsules contain: Glucosamine Sulfate 400 mg • Omega-3 Fish Oil 400 mg • Cod Liver Oil 400 mg • Vitamin D 10 mcg • Vitamin E 80 mg • Vitamin C 60 mg • Folic Acid 500 mcg • Vitamin B12 20 mcg • Zinc 15 mg • Manganese 3 mg • Copper 2 mg • Selenium 160 mcg • Boron 1.5 mg • Lecithin 30 mg.

Jointace Fizz - Vitabiotics
Each tablet contains: Glucosamine Sulfate 675 mg • Chondroitin Sulfate 100 mg • Vitamin C 60 mg • Magnesium 25 mg • Ginger extract 40 mg.
See Editor's Note No. 15, page 2055.

Jointace Tablets - Vitabiotics
Two tablets contain: Glucosamine Sulfate 1000 mg • Chondroitin Sulfate 400 mg • Vitamin D 10 mcg • Vitamin E 40 mg • Vitamin C 60 mg • Folic Acid 400 mcg • Vitamin B12 20 mcg • Zinc 10 mg • Manganese 4 mg • Copper 1 mg • Selenium 120 mcg • Ginger root extract 80 mg.
See Editor's Note No. 15, page 2055.

JointFlex - SmartScience Laboratories, Inc.
Active Ingredient: Camphor (3.1%). Inactive Ingredients: Acetylated lanolin, acrylates/C10-30, alkyl acrylate, crosspolymer, aloe vera, C12-15 alkyl benzoate, chondroitin sulfate, purified water, diazolidnyl urea, dimethicone, dimethiconol stearate, disodium EDTA, dl panthenol, glucosamine sulfate, glycerin, glycerol stearate, glycosaminoglycans, hydroxylated lanolin, hydroxypropylene methylcellulose, lodopropynyl, butylcarbomate, methyl gluceth-20, methyl glucose, sesquistearate, peppermint oil, polysorbate 20, potassium carbomer, tocopheryl acetate.
See Editor's Note No. 15, page 2055.

JointPower - Trimedica
Six capsules contain: Glucosamine Sulfate 1500 mg • Vitamin C 1000 mg • natural Vitamin E (Succinate) 800 IU • Manganese (Chelated Manganese Gluconate) 5 mg • Zinc (Chelated Zinc Picolinate) 15 mg • Copper (Chelated Copper Gluconate) 1.5 mg • Tumeric (Curcuma longa) extract (standardized for 95% Curcumin) 1300 mg • Boswellia serrata extract (standardized for 60-65 Boswellic Acids) 100 mg • Bromelain 100 mg • Selenium (from Selenomethionine) 200 mcg.

Joint-Ritis - Naturopathic Labs Intl., Inc.
Active Ingredient: Natural Menthol 16%. Inactive Ingredients: Lanolin, Eucalyptus Oil, Copaiba Oil, Lavender Oil, Glucosamine Sulfate, Chondroitin Sulfate.
See Editor's Note No. 15, page 2055.

Joints Formula - Nature's Way
Three capsules contain: Alfalfa concentrate 125 mg • Boswellia dried extract 300 mg • Copper (Amino Acid Chelate) 1 mg • Glucosamine HCL 750 mg • Grape seed dried extract 48 mg • Manganese Amino Acid Chelate 5 mg • Nettle root 250 mg • Wild Yam root 75 mg • Zinc Amino Acid Chelate 7.5 mg. Other ingredients: Gelatin, Magnesium Stearate, Millet.

Jojoba & E Skin Oil - Derma E
90% Jojoba • 10% Vitamin E oil.

Juice Plus+ Garden Blend - NSA International
Two capsules contain: Proprietary Blend 1500 mg: Vegetable juice powder and pulp from Carrots, Parsley, Beets, Kale, Broccoli, Cabbage, Spinach, and Tomato; Lipase, Amylase, Protease, Cellulase, Beet Fiber, Barley Bran, Oat Bran, Cabbage Fiber, Glucomannan, Plant Cellulose, dried Plant Fiber, Lactobacillus Acidophilus, Anthocyanins, Allicin, Lycopene, Polyphenol Catechins, Dunaliella Salina, Indole Carbinols.
See Editor's Note No. 35, page 2057.

Juice Plus+ Orchard Blend - NSA International
Two capsules contain: Proprietary Blend 1500 mg: Fruit juice powder and pulp from Apple, Orange, Pineapple, Cranberry, Peach, Acerola Cherry, Papaya, Bromelain, Papain, Lipase, Amylase, Protease, Cellulase, Apple Pectin, Citrus Pectin, Date Fiber, Prune Powder, Glucomannan, Citrus Bioflavonoids, Dried Plant Fiber, Lactobacillus Acidophilus, Anthocyanins, Polyphenol Catechins, Dunaliella Salina, Indole Carbinoles.
See Editor's Note No. 36, page 2057.

JuiceRX - Harcourt & Johnston
100% pure whole leaf Aloe Vera juice, Honey, Eleuthero Ginseng, Wild Cherry, Cultivated Seaweed (alaria valida, costaria costata, fucus gardneri, gigartina, laminaria, nereocysts, phodympRhenia pertusa, ulva latuca, ulva linza), Citric Acid, Spirulina, Potassium Benzoate, Potassium Sorbate.

Jungamals - Pharmanex
Each capsule contains: Vitamin A (as vitamin A palmitate, 50% as beta-carotene) 2500 IU • Vitamin C (sodium ascorbate) 150 mg •

Vitamin D (D3, as cholecalciferol) 200 IU • Vitamin E (D-alpha tocopheryl acetate) 30 IU • Vitamin K (phytonadione) 20 mcg • Thiamin (thiamin mononitrate) 0.75 mg • Riboflavin (riboflavin) 0.85 mg • Niacin (niacinamide) 10 mg • Vitamin B6 (as pyridoxine hydrochloride) 1 mg • Folate (as folic acid) 200 mcg • Vitamin B12 (as cyanocobalamin) 3 mcg • Biotin (as biotin) 150 mcg • Pantothenic Acid (as D-calcium pantothenate) 5 mg • Calcium (calcium carbonate, calcium citrate) 150 mg • Iron (iron chelate) 4.5 mg • Iodine (as potassium iodide) 37.5 mcg • Magnesium (magnesium aspartate, magnesium oxide) 100 mg • Zinc (zinc chelate) 3.75 mg • Selenium (L-selenomethionine, sodium selenite) 35 mcg • Copper (as copper chelate, copper oxide) 0.5 mg • Manganese (as manganese chelate) 0.5 mg • Chromium (as chromium chelate) 60 mcg • Molybdenum (as molybdenum chelate) 37.5 mcg • Silicon (as sodium metasilicate) 1 mg. Other Ingredients: Fructose, Sorbitol, Sucrose, Natural Flavors, Citric Acid, Stearic Acid, Tumeric (for color), Carrageenan Gum, Microcrystalline Cellulose, Malic Acid, Carmine (for color).

Just An Ounce Calcium/Magnesium Lead Free **-** Trimedica
Each fluid ounce contains: Calcium 1200 mg • Magnesium 600 mg • Iron 5 mg • Zinc 5 mg • Manganese 5 mg • Copper 1 mg • Chromium 0.2 mg • Selenium 0.2 mg • Molybdenum 0.2 mg • Vanadium 0.1 mg • Potassium 90 mg • Iodine 0.15 mg • Boron 0.05 mg • Vitamin D 400 IU. Other Ingredients: Purified Water, Glycerine, Calcium, Carbonate, Magnesium Hydroxide, Mineral Extracts, Additional Trace Mineral Blend: Silver, Antimony, Barium, Beryllium, Bismuth, Bromine, Carbon, Cerium, Cesium, Chlorine, Cobalt, Dysprosium, Erbium, Europium, Fluorine, Gadolinium, Gallium, Gold, Hafnium, Holmium, Niobium, Nitrogen, Osmium, Oxygen, Palladium, Phosphorus, Platinum, Praseodymium, Rhenium, Ruthenium, Samarium, Scandium, Silicon, Sodium, Strontium, Sulfur, Tantalum, Tellurium, Terbium, Thallium, Thorium, Thulium, Tin, Titanium, Tungsten, Ytterbium, Zirconium.

Just Once B-Complete **-** Rainbow Light
Each tablet contains: Thiamin (vitamin B1) 50 mg • Riboflavin (vitamin B2) 50 mg • Niacinamide (vitamin B3) 50 mg • Pyridoxine HCl (vitamin B6) 50 mg • Folic Acid 400 mcg • Cyanocobalamin (vitamin B12) 50 mcg • Biotin 300 mcg • Pantothenic Acid (vitamin B5) 50 mg • Choline 42 mg • Inositol 50 mg • PABA (para-aminobenzoic acid) 50 mg • Rice Bran 50 mg • Rice Bran 4:1 extract (equivalent to 100 mg of rice bran powder) 25 mg • Spirulina 30 mg • Siberian Ginseng root 100 mg • Vegetables, Herbs & Greens 4:1 extracts (equivalent to 60 mg of whole food powder) 15 mg: Astragalus root, Beet, Broccoli, Carrot, Celery, Green Beans, Horsetail herb, Jujube fruit, Stinging Nettle tops, Parsley, Seaweed, Spinach. Inactive Ingredients: Vegetable Gum, Modified Cellulose, Cellulose, Silica, Stearic Acid (vegetable), Magnesium Stearate, Vegetable Food Glaze.

Just Once Daily Herbs **-** Rainbow Light
Each tablet contains: 2:1 Herbal extracts (equivalent to 900 mg of herbal powder) 450 mg: Reishi herb, Siberian Ginseng root, Milk Thistle seed, Ginger root, Schisandra fruit, Vegetarian Cordyceps herb, Gentian root • Siberian Ginseng root 400 mg • Spirulina 100 mg. Inactive Ingredients: Vegetable Gum, Microcrystalline Cellulose, Silica, Stearic Acid (vegetable), Magnesium Stearate, Vegetable Food Glaze.

Just Once Food-Based C-1000 **-** Rainbow Light
Each tablet contains: Vitamin C (ascorbic acid) 1000 mg • Citrus Bioflavonoids 50 mg • Whole Food Blend 40 mg: Orange, Guava, Broccoli • Elderberry fruit (2:1 extract, equivalent to 30 mg of herbal powder) 15 mg • Spirulina 10 mg. Inactive Ingredients: Cellulose, Stearic Acid (vegetable), Modified Cellulose, Silica, Magnesium Stearate, Vegetable Food Glaze.

Just Once Food-Based Calcium **-** Rainbow Light
Each tablet contains: Calcium (carbonate, amino acid chelate, citrate-malate) 500 mg • Magnesium (oxide, aspartate) 250 mg • Vitamin D 100 IU • Stinging Nettles tops 20 mg • Horsetail whole herb 20 mg • Spirulina 20 mg • Glutamic Acid HCl 20 mg. Inactive Ingredients: Cellulose, Stearic Acid (vegetable), Modified Cellulose Gum, Silica, Magnesium Stearate, Vegetable Food Glaze.

Just Once Food-Based Magnesium **-** Rainbow Light
Each tablet contains: Magnesium (oxide) 400 mg • Chlorella 20 mg • Spirulina 20 mg • 2:1 Herbal extracts (equivalent to 50 mg of herbal powder) 25 mg: Fennel seed, Peppermint leaf. Inactive Ingredients: Microcrystalline Cellulose, Stearic Acid (vegetable), Modified Cellulose Gum, Silica, Magnesium Stearate, Vegetable Food Glaze.

Just Once Iron-Free Multivitamin **-** Rainbow Light
Each tablet contains: Vitamin A (beta-carotene) 10,000 IU • Vitamin C (ascorbic acid, magnesium ascorbate) 200 mg • Vitamin D 100 IU • Vitamin E (dl-alpha tocopheryl succinate) 60 IU • Vitamin K (phytonadione) 30 mcg • Thiamin (vitamin B1) 6 mg • Riboflavin (vitamin B2) 6 mg • Niacinamide (vitamin B3) 30 mg • Pyridoxine (vitamin B6) 6 mg • Folic Acid 400 mcg • Cyanocobalamin (vitamin B12) 25 mcg • Biotin 300 mcg • Pantothenic Acid (vitamin B5) 30 mg • Calcium (amino acid chelate) 30 mg • Iodine (from kelp) 100 mcg • Magnesium (glycinate, ascorbate) 30 mg • Zinc (citrate, monomethionine) 5 mg • Selenium (selenomethionine) 25 mcg • Copper (glycinate) 500 mcg • Manganese (glycinate) 2.5 mg • Chromium (dinicotinate) 50 mcg • Molybdenum (aspartate) 12 mcg • Potassium (chloride, citrate) 20 mg • Boron (citrate, asparate, glycinate) 50 mcg • Vanadium (vanadyl sulfate) 8 mcg • Bioflavonoids (from lemon) 60 mg • Choline 15 mg • Inositol 15 mg • Rutin 15 mg • Hesperidin 10 mg • PABA (para-aminobenzoic acid) 5 mg • Protease 332 HUT • Amylase 113 DU • Lipase 1.2 LU • Cellulase 1.3 CU • Apple Pectin 20 mg • Green Papaya 12 mg • Spirulina 100 mg • Siberian Ginseng root 75 mg • Tomato Paste powder 40 mg • Ginkgo leaf 30 mg • Wheat Sprouts Complex 20 mg • Vegetable & Herbs Concentrates 20 mg: Horsetail herb, Jujube fruit, Carrots, Broccoli, Spinach, Parsley, Stinging Nettles tops, Celery, Astragalus root, Beets, Green Beans, Seaweed. Inactive Ingredients: Stearic Acid (vegetable), Modified Cellulose, Microcrystalline Cellulose, Silica, Magnesium Stearate, Vegetable Food Glaze.

Just Once Kid's One MultiStars **-** Rainbow Light
Each tablet contains: Vitamin A (as palmitate, beta-carotene) 400 IU • Vitamin C (ascorbic acid) 10 mg • Vitamin D (cholecalciferol) 400 IU • Vitamin E (d-alpha tocopheryl succinate) 10 IU • Vitamin K (phylloquinone) 20 mcg • Thiamin (vitamin B1) 2 mg • Riboflavin (vitamin B2) 2 mg • Niacinamide (vitamin B3) 13 mg • Pyridoxine (vitamin B6) 2 mg • Folic Acid 200 mcg • Cyanocobalamin (vitamin B12) 1 mcg • Biotin 25 mcg • Pantothenic Acid (vitamin B5) 4 mg • Calcium (carbonate) 100 mg • Iron (carbonyl) 5 mg • Iodine (kelp) 25 mcg • Magnesium (oxide) 50 mg • Zinc (oxide) 2.5 mg • Selenium (amino acid chelate) 20 mcg • Copper (amino acid chelate) 250 mcg • Mangenese (citrate) 1.5 mg • Chromium (glycinate, dinicotinate) 30 mcg • Molybdenum (amino acid chelate) 30 mcg • Potassium (citrate) 15 mg • Citrus Bioflavonoids 25 mg • PABA (para-aminobenzoic acid) 1 mg • Spirulina 10 mg • 2:1 Herbal extracts (equivalent to 100 mg of herbal powder) Proprietary Blend 50 mg: Stinging Nettles tops, Ginger rhizome, Peppermint herb, German Chamomile flowers • Organic Vegetables Extracts (equivalent to 50 mg of vegetable powder) Proprietary Blend 12.5 mg: Kamut leaf juice, Barley Grass juice, Oat Grass juice, Alfalfa leaf juice, Dandelion greens, Carrots, Collards, Cauliflower, Stinging Nettles, Parsley, Onions. Inactive Ingredients: Fructose, Dextrates, Natural Orange, Pineapple & Cherry Flavors, Vegetable Stearine, Silica, Magnesium Stearate, Citric Acid.

Just Once Men's One Multivitamin **-** Rainbow Light
Each tablet contains: Vitamin A (palmitate, beta-carotene) 10,000 IU • Vitamin C (ascorbic acid) 120 mg • Vitamin D (vitamin D3, cholecalciferol) 50 IU • Vitamin E (dl-alpha tocopheryl succinate) 100 IU • Vitamin K (phytonadione) 100 mcg • Thiamin (vitamin B1) 25 mg • Riboflavin (vitamin B2) 25 mg • Niacinamide (vitamin B3) 25 mg • Pyridoxine HCl (vitamin B6) 25 mg • Folic Acid 400 mcg • Cyanocobalamin (vitamin B12) 25 mcg • Biotin 150 mcg • Pantothenic Acid (vitamin B5) 25 mg • Calcium (citrate-malate) 50 mg • Magnesium (oxide) 25 mg • Zinc (citrate) 20 mg • Selenium

(selenomethionine, amino acid chelate) 200 mcg • Copper (amino acid chelate) 2 mg • Chromium (amino acid chelate) 200 mcg • Molybdenum (amino acid chelate) 75 mcg • Choline (bitartrate) 25 mg • PABA (para-aminobenzoic acid) 25 mg • Inositol 25 mg • Citrus Bioflavonoids 25 mg • Saw Palmetto berry (2:1 extract equivalent to 100 mg of herbal powder) 50 mg • Tomato Paste Concentrate (providing lycopene) 50 mg • Spirulina 50 mg • Protease 664 HUT • Amylase 226 DU • Lipase 2.4 LU • Cellulase 2.7 CU. Inactive Ingredients: Vegetable Cellulose, Microcrystalline Cellulose, Stearic Acid (vegetable), Magnesium Stearate, Silica, Vegetable Food Glaze.

Just Once Multivitamin **-** Rainbow Light
Each tablet contains: Vitamin A (beta-carotene) 10,000 IU • Vitamin C (ascorbic acid, magnesium ascorbate) 240 mg • Vitamin D 100 IU • Vitamin E (d-alpha tocopheryl) 60 IU • Vitamin K 30 mcg • Thiamin (vitamin B1) 6 mg • Riboflavin (vitamin B2) 6 mg • Niacinamide (vitamin B3) 30 mg • Pyridoxine (vitamin B6) 6 mg • Folic Acid 400 mcg • Cyanocobalamin (vitamin B12) 25 mcg • Biotin 300 mcg • Pantothenic Acid (vitamin B5) 30 mg • Calcium (amino acid chelate) 30 mg • Iron (glycinate) 2 mg • Iodine (from kelp) 100 mcg • Magnesium (glycinate, ascorbate) 30 mg • Zinc (citrate, monomethionine) 5 mg • Selenium (selenomethionine) 25 mcg • Copper (glycinate) 500 mcg • Manganese (glycinate) 2 mg • Chromium (dinicotinate) 50 mcg • Molybdenum (aspartate) 10 mcg • Potassium (chloride, citrate) 20 mg • Boron (glycinate) 50 mcg • Vanadium (vanadyl sulfate) 8 mcg • Bioflavonoids (from lemon) 60 mg • Rutin 15 mg • Choline 15 mg • Inositol 15 mg • Hesperidin 10 mg • PABA (para-aminobenzoic acid) 5 mg • Protease 1189 HUT • Amylase 93 DU • Lipase 1 LU • Cellulase 1 CU • Apple Pectin 20 mg • Green Papaya 10 mg • Spirulina 100 mg • Siberian Ginseng root 70 mg • Ginkgo leaf 30 mg • Wheat sprouts 20 mg • Stinging Nettles tops (4:1 extract) 10 mg • Carotene Complex 10 mg: Carrot root, Parsley leaf • Spinach leaf 10 mg. Inactive Ingredients: Microcrystalline Cellulose, Silica, Stearic Acid (vegetable), Modified Starch, Magnesium Stearate, Vegetable Food Glaze.

Just Once Prenatal One Multivitamin **-** Rainbow Light
Each tablet contains: Vitamin A (as palmitate 3500 IU, beta-carotene 2500 IU) 6000 IU • Vitamin C (ascorbic acid) 100 mg • Vitamin D (vitamin D3, cholecalciferol) 400 IU • Vitamin E (dl-alpha tocopheryl succinate) 100 IU • Thiamin (vitamin B1) 10 mg • Riboflavin (vitamin B2) 10 mg • Niacinamide (vitamin B3) 20 mg • Pyridoxine (vitamin B6) 15 mg • Folic Acid 800 mcg • Cyanocobalamin (vitamin B12) 25 mcg • Biotin 300 mcg • Pantothenic Acid (vitamin B5) 15 mg • Calcium (carbonate, citrate-malate) 200 mg • Iron (amino acid chelate) 30 mg • Iodine (kelp) 150 mcg • Magnesium (oxide) 100 mg • Zinc (citrate) 15 mg • Copper (amino acid chelate) 2 mg • Vitamin K (phytonadione) 65 mcg • Selenium (selenomethionine) 100 mcg • Manganese (citrate) 2 mg • Chromium (amino acid chelate) 120 mcg • Molybdenum (amino acid chelate) 75 mcg • Potassium (citrate) 10 mg • Citrus Bioflavonoids 25 mg • Choline (bitartrate) 10 mg • Inositol 10 mg • PABA (para-aminobenzoic acid) 10 mg • Boron (glycinate) 1 mg • Protease 660 HUT • Amylase 226 DU • Lipase 2.4 LU • Cellulase 2.8 CU • Spirulina 20 mg • Ginger root (fresh juice, 10:1 extract equivalent to 200 mg of herbal powder) 20 mg • Red Raspberry leaf (2:1 extract equivalent to 100 mg of herbal powder) 50 mg. Inactive Ingredients: Microcrystalline Cellulose, Stearic Acid (vegetable), Modified Cellulose, Magnesium Stearate, Silica, Vegetable Food Glaze.

Just Once Total Antioxidant Protection **-** Rainbow Light
Each tablet contains: Vitamin A (as beta-carotene from D. salina) 5000 IU • Vitamin C (ascorbic acid) 500 mg • Vitamin E (dl-alpha tocopheryl succinate) 100 IU • Zinc (citrate) 10 mg • Selenium (selenomethionine, amino acid chelate) 100 mcg • Copper (amino acid chelate) 1 mg • Dunaliella Salina 51 mg • 4:1 Herbal Extracts Proprietary Blend (equivalent to 280 mg of herb powder) 70 mg: Bilberry herb, Marigold flowers, Turmeric herb • Tomato Paste powder (providing lycopene) 50 mg • Vegetables, Herbs & Greens 4:1 extracts Proprietary Blend (equivalent to 300 mg of powder) 75 mg: Astragalus root, Beet, Broccoli, Carrot, Celery, Green Beans, Horsetail herb, Jujube herb, Stinging Nettle tops, Parsley, Seaweed, Spinach • Rosemary leaf oil 0.5 mg • Spirulina 40 mg. Other Ingredients: Cellulose, Stearic Acid (vegetable), Silica, Magnesium Stearate, Vegetable Food Glaze.

Just Once Veggies & Greens **-** Rainbow Light
Each tablet contains: Vitamin A beta-carotene from spirulina) 2338 IU • Vitamin C (from vegetables) 5 mg • Vitamin B12 (from spirulina) 1.1 mcg • Iron (from spirulina and vegetables) 0.7 mg • Spirulina 500 mg • Chlorella 50 mg • Barley Grass 50 mg • Wheat Grass 50 mg • Vegetables, Herbs & Greens 4:1 extracts (equivalent to 600 mg of powder) 150 mg: Astragalus root, Beet, Broccoli, Carrot, Celery, Green Beans, Horsetail herb, Jujube fruit, Stinging Nettles tops, Parsley, Seaweed, Spinach • Broccoli powder 125 mg • Cabbage powder 125 mg • Tomato Paste Concentrate (providing lycopene) 125 mg • Rosemary leaf oil 0.5 mg • Ginger root 50 mg. Inactive Ingredients: Stearic Acid (vegetable), Silica, Modified Cellulose, Cellulose, Magnesium Stearate, Vegetable Food Glaze.

Just Once Women's One Multivitamin **-** Rainbow Light
Each tablet contains: Vitamin A (palmitate, beta-carotene) 10,000 IU • Vitamin C (ascorbic acid) 120 mg • Vitamin D (vitamin D3, cholecalciferol) 100 IU • Vitamin E (d-alpha tocopheryl succinate) 100 IU • Vitamin K (phytonadione) 100 mcg • Thiamin (vitamin B1) 25 mg • Riboflavin (vitamin B2) 25 mg • Niacinamide (vitamin B3) 25 mg • Pyridoxine HCl (vitamin B6) 25 mg • Folic Acid 400 mcg • Cyanocobalamin (vitamin B12) 25 mcg • Biotin 150 mcg • Pantothenic Acid (vitamin B5) 25 mg • Calcium (carbonate, citrate-malate) 200 mg • Iron (amino acid chelate) 6 mg • Magnesium (oxide) 100 mg • Zinc (citrate) 10 mg • Selenium (selenomethionine, amino acid chelate) 200 mcg • Copper (amino acid chelate) 1 mg • Manganese (citrate) 2 mg • Chromium (amino acid chelate) 200 mcg • Molybdenum (amino acid chelate) 75 mcg • Choline (bitartrate) 25 mg • PABA (para-aminobenzoic acid) 25 mg • Inositol 25 mg • Boron (glycinate) 1 mg • Citrus Bioflavonoids 25 mg • Non-GMO Soy Isoflavones (2.5%) 25 mg • Red Clover blossoms (2:1 extract, equivalent to 50 mg of herbal powder) 25 mg • Dong Quai root (4:1 extract, equivalent to 200 mg of herbal powder) 50 mg • Spirulina 50 mg • Protease 664 HUT • Amylase 226 DU • Lipase 2.4 LU • Cellulase 2.7 CU. Inactive Ingredients: Vegetable Cellulose, Microcrystalline Cellulose, Stearic Acid (vegetable), Silica, Magnesium Stearate, Vegetable Food Glaze.

Just Peachy Fructose - Revival **-** Physicians Laboratories
Each packet contains: Certified Isoflavone 160 mg. Other Ingredients: Soy Protein Isolate, Fructose, Sucrose, Natural and Artificial Flavor, Soy Lecithin, Calcium Phosphate, Maltodextrin, Potassium Chloride, Sodium Chloride, Xanthan Gum, Beta-carotene, Real Peach powder, Carboxymethylcellulose, Undegraded Carrageenan.

Just Peachy Splenda - Revival **-** Physicians Laboratories
Each packet contains: Certified Isoflavone 160 mg. Other Ingredients: Soy Protein Isolate, Cocoa, Maltodextrin, Calcium Phosphate, Soy Lecithin, Salt, Potassium Chloride, Artificial Flavor, Carrageenan, Carboxymethylcellulose, Xanthan Gum, Sucralose.

Just Peachy Unsweetened - Revival **-** Physicians Laboratories
Each packet contains: Certified Isoflavone 160 mg. Other Ingredients: Soy Protein Isolate, Natural and Artificial Flavor, Soy Lecithin, Calcium Phosphate, Maltodextrin, Potassium Chloride, Sodium Chloride, Xanthan Gum, Beta-Carotene, Real Peach Powder, Carboxymethylcellulose, Undegraded Carrageenan.

Just-Whey **-** SportPharma
Each serving contains: Non-denatured specially filtered Whey Protein concentrate • Ion-exchanged Whey Protein • Natural & Artificial Vanilla Flavors • Acesulfame K.

Juven **-** MTI BioTech
Each 23 gram packet contains: Arginine (free-base) 7 g • Glutamine 7 g • HMB (calcium-beta-hydroxy-beta-methylbutyrate) 1.5 g. Inactive Ingredients: Citric Acid, Natural & Artificial Flavors, Sugar,

Dipotassium Phosphate, Aspartame, Acesulfame Potassium, FD&C Yellow #6 or FD&C Blue Lake #2 and FD&C Red #40.

Juvenon Energy Formula **-** Juvenon, Inc.
Each tablet contains: Calcium (from calcium carbonate) 78 mg • Alpha Lipoic Acid 200 mg • Acetyl-L-Carnitine HCl 500 mg. Inactive Ingredients: Calcium Carbonate, Stearic Acid, Sllicon Dioxide, Croscarmellose Sodium, Acacia, Magnesium Stearate, White Cellulose Film-coat containing Titanium Dioxide.

K & MG Aspartate **-** Atrium Inc.
Each tablet contains: Potassium Aspartate (which yields potassium 78 mg & l-aspartic acid 209 mg) 261 mg • Magnesium Aspartate (which yields magnesium 28 mg & l-aspartic acid 242 mg) 278 mg.

K & U **-** MMS Pro
Each capsule contains: Juniper berries • Parsley herb • Ginger root • Uva Ursi leaves • Marshmallow root • Cramp bark • Golden Seal root.

KAL Beyond Calcium **-** Nutraceutical Corp.
Each five tablets contain: Vitamin D (as Vitamin D3) (as natural Cholecalciferol) 400 IU • Calcium (as Calcium Citrate) 1000 mg • Magnesium (as Magnesium Citrate) 400 mg • Boron (as Boron Amino Acid Chelate) 6 mg • Horsetail 20 mg • Guaranteed Potency Soy Isoflavones (from NovaSoy supplying 25 mg (40%) Isoflavones and 12.5 mg (20%) Genistin) 62.5 • Ipriflavone (as 7-Isopropoxy - Isoflavone from Ostivone) 200 mg • ActiSorb Base 10 mg: Bioperine extract (Black Pepper - Piper longum), Cayenne (Capsicum frutecens), Turmeric (Curcuma longa), Rosemary (Rosmarinus officinalis), Ginger (Zingiber officinale). Other Ingredients: Cellulose, Stearic Acid, Silica, and Magnesium Stearate.

KAL Magnesium Glycinate 400 Vegetarian Formulation **-** Nutraceutical Corp.
Each tablet contains: Magnesium (as magnesium glycinate) 200 mg. Other Ingredients: Cellulose, Stearic Acid, Magnesium Stearate.

Kalm-Assure **-** Nature's Plus
Each tablet contains: Rapid Release Layer: Pantothenic Acid (Vitamin B5) 50 mg • GABA (Gamma Aminobutyric Acid) 25 mg • Magnesium (Citrate) 25 mg • Pyridoxal-5-Phosphate (P5P) 5 mg. Sustained Release Layer: Kava (Piper methysticum root) standardized 30% kavalactones 100 mg • Passion Flower (Passiflora incarnata) standardized 4% Isovitexin 75 mg • Hops fruit (Humulus lupulus) standardized 5.2% bitter acids 10 mg • Siberian Ginseng (Eleutherococcus senticosus) standardized 0.8% Eleutherosides 25 mg • Chamomile (Matricaria recutita flower) standardized 1% Apigenin 25 mg.

Kan Jang (Kanjang) **-** Swedish Herbal Institute
Each tablet contains: Standardized Andrographis paniculata root extract (4% Andrographolides) 300 mg. Other Ingredients: Mycrocrystalline, Sodium Starch Glyconate, Magnesium Stearate, Zien.

Kaprex **-** Metagenics
Each tablet contains: Proprietary Blend 440 mg: Luduxin (reduced iso-alpha acids from humulus lupulus extract, magnesium salt), Oleanolic Acid (from olive leaf extract, olea europaea), Rosemary leaf extract (rosmarinus officinalis).

Kava 30% **-** Nature's Way
Each capsule contains: Kava dried extract (30% kavalactones) 350 mg • Passion Flower stem, leaf, fruit & flower 500 mg.

Kava Extract **-** NSI - Nutraceutical Sciences Institute
Each softgel contains: Kava (Kaviar, kavalactones 84%) 75 mg.

Kava Kava **-** Gaia Herbs
Kava Kava standardized for 5% kavalactones. Standardized Full Spectrum 136 mg of extract per capsule. Guaranteed Potency 68 mg of extract per capsule.

Kava Kava **-** Olympian Labs
Each capsule contains: Kava extract 500 mg.

Kava Kava **-** Puritan's Pride
Each capsule contains: Kava Kava root (in a millet grain base) 300 mg.

Kava Kava **-** Leiner Health Products
Each caplet contains: Kava Kava extract (Piper methysticum) root 200 mg. Other Ingredients: Calcium Carbonate, Cellulose, Maltodextrin, Hydroxypropyl Methylcellulose, Silicon Dioxide, Polyethylene Glycol 3350, Croscarmellose Sodium, Hydroxypropyl Cellulose, Crospovidone, Magnesium Stearate, Yellow 6 Lake, Red 40 Lake, Blue 2 Lake, Pharmaceutical Glaze, Polysorbate 80, Titanium Dioxide.

Kava Kava **-** Quest
Each capsule contains: Kava Kava (provided by 150 mg P.E. 1:12 standardized to 30% Kavalactones) 1800 mg. Other Ingredients: Microcrystalline Cellulose, Magnesium Stearate (vegetable source).

Kava Kava **-** Pharmanex
Each softgel contains: Kava Kava root (11:1) extract (Piper methysticum) 175 mg. Other Ingredients: Soybean Oil, Gelatin, Glycerin, Maltodextrin, Beeswax, Lecithin, Carob.

Kava Kava 3000 mg **-** Jamieson
Each capsule contains: Kava Kava root (Piper methysticum, 250 mg powdered extract 1:12) 3000 mg. Other Ingredients: Gelatin, Calcium Sulfate, Maltodextrin, Cellulose, Magnesium Stearate, Silica.

Kava Kava Plus **-** The Herbalist
Kava Kava root • Siberian Ginseng root • St. John's Wort flowering tops • Oat seed • Skullcap herb.

Kava Kava Root Extract **-** Source Naturals
Each softgel contains: Kava Kava root extract (Piper methysticum) (standardized to 40% Kavalactones, yielding 70 mg of Kavalactones) 175 mg. In a base of Soybean Oil, Lecithin and Beeswax.

Kava Kava XTRA **-** Sundown
Each capsule contains: Kava Kava root extract (standardized to 30% kavalactones, 75 mg) 250 mg • XTRA Premium Blend 100 mg: Hops (strobiles), German Chamomile flower heads, Passionflower flowers/ fruit. Other Ingredients: Gelatin, Natural Vegetable Fiber.

Kava Kava-Valerian Virtue **-** Blessed Herbs
Kava Kava root • Scullcap • Valerian root • St. John's Wort flower • Lobelia • Arnica flower & herb • Grain alcohol & Distilled Water.

Kava Oasis **-** New Chapter, Inc.
Each softgel contains: Kava root, supercritical extract, (60% kavapyrones- 75 mg) 125 mg • Valerian root, (Valeriana officinalis & Valeriana mexicanus) supercritical extract, (60% valepotriates- 3 mg) 5 mg • Lavender flower, supercritical extract (25% Linalool- 1.2 mg) 5 mg • Passion Flower herb, extract, (3% vitexin- 0.15 mg) 5 mg • Chastetree berry, extract (0.6% aucubin- 0.03 mg) (0.5% agnuside- 0.025 mg) 5 mg • Gotu Kola leaf, extract, (10% asiaticoside- 0.5 mg) (3.% triterpenes- 1.5 mg) 5 mg • Ginger supercritical broad spectrum complex (rhizome), certified organic, (minimum 20% pungent compounds- 1 mg, 4% zingiberene- 0.2 mg) 5 mg • Chamomile flower, supercritical extract (minimum 25% alpha-bisabolol- 1.2 mg) 5 mg. Other Ingredients: Olive Oil (certified organic), Yellow Beeswax.

Kava-30 **-** PhytoPharmica
Each capsule contains: Kava (Piper methysticum) root and rhizome extract (standardized to contain 30% kavalactones [75 mg of kavalactones]) 250 mg.
See Editor's Note No. 21, page 2056.

Some Brand Name Natural Products - What they Contain

www.NaturalDatabase.com contains MANY more listings than appear here.

Kava-55 - PhytoPharmica
Each capsule contains: Kava (Piper methysticum) root (rhizome) extract (standardized to contain 55% kavalactones [82.5 mg kavalactones]) 150 mg.
See Editor's Note No. 21, page 2056.

Kava-77 - Source Naturals
Each softgel contains: Kava Kava root extract (Piper methysticum) (standardized to 55% Kavalactones yielding 75 mg of Kavalactones) 140 mg. In a base of Rice Bran Oil, Lecithin, Silicon Dioxide and Beeswax.

Kavacin - PhytoPharmica
Each capsule contains: Kava root extract (Piper methysticum) 200 mg standardized to contain 30% kavalactones (60 mg per capsule) • Oat Straw extract 10:1 (Avena sativa) 100 mg • Pyridoxine-Alpha-Ketoglutarate (PAK) 50 mg • Pantothenic Acid 50 mg • Nicotinamide 50 mg • Thiamine HCL (Vitamin B1) 25 mg.
See Editor's Note No. 21, page 2056.

KaValerian Caplet - Leiner Health Products
Each caplet contains: Magnesium Citrate 10 mg • Chamomile extract (Matricaria recutita) flower 50 mg • Kava Kava extract (Piper methysticum) root 75 mg • Lecithin 15 mg • Valerian extract (Valeriana officinalis) root 200 mg. Other Ingredients: Dicalcium Phosphate, Cellulose, Stearic Acid, Magnesium Stearate, Dextrin, Silicon Dioxide, Dextrose, Sodium Carboxymethylcellulose, Sodium Citrate.

Kavatime - Bodyonics, Ltd.
Each tablet contains: Kava Kava Root (Piper Methysticum) 350 mg • Kava Kava Powdered Extract 150 mg • Herbolics Support Complex 50 mg: Barley Malt Flour, Brewers Yeast (saccharomyces cerevisiae), Hops (humulus lupulus), Ginger root extract (zingiber officinale). Other Ingredients: Calcium Phosphate, Magnesium Stearate, Gelatin.

KavaTone - Enzymatic Therapy
Each capsule contains: Kava root extract (Piper methysticum) (standardized to contain 30% Kavalactones 60 mg per capsule) 200 mg • Oat Straw extract 10:1 (Avena sativa) 100 mg • Pyridoxine-Alpha-Ketoglutarate (PAK) 50 mg • Pantothenic Acid 50 mg, Nicotinamide 50 mg • Thiamin HCl (Vitamin B1) 25 mg.

Kavatrol - Natrol
Each capsule contains: Kava root extract (30% Kavalactones) 200 mg • In an exclusive base of complementary herbs: Passion flower, Chamomile flower, Hops flower, Schizandra fruit. Other Ingredients: Magnesium Stearate, Silicon Dioxide, Gelatin.

Kelp - Jamieson
Each tablet contains: Pacific Kelp 650 mg (Iodine from Kelp not less than 650 mcg).

Keto Pro - MET-Rx - Rexall - Sundown
Metamyosyn V.4 (unique blend of Milk Protein Isolates, Caseinate, Whey Protein Concentrate, Glutamine, Calcium-B-Hydroxy B-Methylbutyrate Monohydrate, Lactoferrin) • Medium Chain Triglycerides • Natural & Artifical Flavor • Cellulose Gum • Maltodextrin • Dipotassium Phosphate • Potassium Chloride • Potassium Citrate • Carrageenan • Salt • Sodium Citrate • Sucrolose.

KetoCal - SHS North America
Each 100 mL of powder contains: Vitamin A 253 IU • Vitamin D (as vitamin D3) 41.6 IU • Vitamin E 2.2 IU • Vitamin K 8 mcg • Thiamin 0.13 mg • Riboflavin 0.13 mg • Vitamin B6 0.13 mg • Vitamin B12 0.26 mcg • Niacin 1.5 mg • Folic Acid 38 mcg • Pantothenic Acid 0.52 mg • Biotin 2.5 mcg • Vitamin C 12 mg • Choline 96 mg • Inositol 27 mg • Calcium 160 mg • Phosphorous 130 mg • Magnesium 22 mg • Iron 2.2 mg • Zinc 1.2 mg • Manganese 0.32 mg • Copper 120 mcg • Iodine 16.4 mcg • Molybdenum 5.2 mcg • Chromium 3.8 mcg • Selenium 6.8 mcg • Sodium 60 mg • Potassium 216 mg • Chloride 100 mg. Ingredients: Hydrogenated Soybean Oil, Dry Whole Milk, Refined Soybean Oil, Soy Lecithin, Corn Syrup Solids, Tripotassium Citrate, Tricalcium Citrate, Potassium Chloride, Tricalcium Phosphate, Choline Bitartrate, Magnesium Hydrogen Phosphate, Calcium Phosphate, Magnesium Acetate, Trisodium Citrate, M-Inositol, L-Isoleucine, L-Tryptophan, Ethyl Vanillin (artificial flavor), L-Ascorbic Acid, Ferrous Sulfate, Aspartame (artificial sweetener), L-Carnitine, Taurine, Zinc Sulfate, DL-Alpha Tocopheryl, Nicotinamide, Manganese Sulfate, Calcium-D-Pantothenate, Copper Sulfate, Beta Carotene (artificial color), Thiamin Hydrochloride, Pyridoxine Hydrochloride, Riboflavin, Vitamin A Acetate, Folic Acid, Chromium Sulfate, Potassium Iodide, Sodium Molybdate, Sodium Hydrogen Selenite, Phylloquinone, D-Biotin, Vitamin D3, Cyanocobalamin.

Key To Sun - Nikken Inc.
Two tablets contain: Chitin Chitosan Powder 300 mg. Other Ingredients: Dextrin, Crystalline Cellulose, Magnesium Stearate.

Key-E Vitamin E 200 IU - J. R. Carlson Laboratories, Inc.
Each tablet contains: Vitamin E (as d-alpha tocopheryl succinate) 200 IU.

KIC Fuel - TwinLab
Each capsule contains: KIC 500 mg.

Kid Vits - Now
Two tablets contain: Beta-Carotene 4000 IU • Vitamin A (as Palmitate) 1000 IU • Vitamin B1 (Thiamine HCL) 3 mg • Vitamin B2 (Riboflavin) 3.4 mg • Vitamin B3 (Niacinamide) 20 mg • Vitamin B5 (Pantothenic Acid) 15 mg • Vitamin B6 (Pyridoxine HCL) 4 mg • Vitamin B12 (Cyanocobalamin) 10 mcg • Biotin 100 mcg • Folic Acid 400 mcg • Vitamin C (Ascorbic Acid, Calcium Ascorbate) 120 mg • Vitamin D (Cholecalciferol) 200 IU • Vitamin E (d-Alpha Tocopheryl Succinate) 30 IU • Calcium (Carbonate, Ascorbate) 30 mg • Magnesium (Oxide, Amino Acid Chelate) 20 mg • Zinc (Amino Acid Chelate) 5 mg • Iron (Ferrochel Iron Bisglycinate) 5 mg • Copper (Amino Acid Chelate) 0.2 mg • Iodine (Kelp) 75 mcg • Manganese (Amino Acid Chelate) 1 mg • Selenium (Amino Acid Chelate) 10 mcg • Chromium (Chelavite) 60 mcg • Molybdenum (Amino Acid Chelate) 15 mcg • Acerola 25 mg • Bioflavonoids (40 % Hesperidin) 25 mg • Choline 10 mg • Inositol 10 mg • PABA 4 mg.

Kid-Alert - The Herbalist
Ginkgo fresh leaf (Ginkgo biloba) • Gotu Kola fresh herb (Hydrocotyle asiatica) • Lemon Balm fresh leaf (Melissa officinalis) • St. John's Wort fresh flower tops (Hypericum perf.) • Siberian Ginseng fresh-dried root (Eleuthero sent.). In a base of kosher glycerine, distilled water, and Grapefruit seed extract.

Kidalin Adult Formula - Herbs, Etc.
Catnip leaf • Damiana • Kola Nut • Lavender flowers • Chamomile flowers • Periwinkle herb • Lemon Balm • Licorice root • Oat seed • Grain Alcohol.

Kidalin Child Formula - Herbs, Etc.
Catnip leaf • Damiana • Kola Nut • Lavender flowers • Chamomile flowers • Periwinkle herb • Lemon Balm • Licorice root • Oat seed • Grain Alcohol • Vegetable Glycerin • Orange peel oil • Natural Flavorings.

KidCalm St. John's Wort Complex - Enzymatic Therapy
Two capsules contain: Magnesium (Krebs Cycle Chelate) 50 mg • Vitamin B6 (Pyridoxal-5-Phosphate) 15 mg • Zinc (Krebs Cycle chelate) 15 mg. Other Ingredients: St. John's Wort extract (Hypericum perforatum) standardized to contain 0.3% Hypericin, verified by HPLC 100 mg • Valerian root extract (Valerian officinalis) standardized to contain a minimum of 0.8% Valerenic acids 100 mg • GABA (Gamma-Aminobutyric Acid) 100 mg • L-Tyrosine 100 mg • Kava root extract (Piper methysticum) standardized to contain 30% Kavalactones 50 mg • Melissa extract (Melissa officinalis) standardized to contain a minimum of 5% Rosmarinic Acid 50 mg • Grape seed (PCO) extract standardized to contain 95% Procyanidolic Oligomers (PCOs) 20 mg.

Kid-Ease **-** The Herbalist
Lemon Balm fresh leaf (Melissa officinalis) Valerian fresh root (Valeriana officinalis) • St. John's Wort fresh flower tops (Hypericum perf.). In a base of kosher glycerine and Grapefruit seed extract.

Kidney Bladder Formula **-** Nature's Way
Two capsules contain: Proprietary formula: Cramp bark • Ginger • Goldenseal root • Juniper berries • Marshmallow root • Parsley herb • Uva Ursi leaves. Other Ingredients: Gelatin.

Kidney Blend **-** The Herbalist
Dandelion root • Burdock seed • Uva Ursi leaf • Corn Silk • Echinacea root • St. John's Wort flower • Yarrow flower • Cayenne pepper.

Kidney Factors **-** Michael's Naturopathic Programs
Three tablets contain: Vitamin D (as calciferol) 300 IU • Niacin (as niacinamide) 60 mg • Vitamin B6 (as pyridoxine) 6 mg • Vitamin B12 (as cobalamin) 30 mcg • Calcium (as calcium amino acid chelate) 75 mg • Magnesium (as magnesium amino acid chelate) 150 mg • Proprietary Blend 2640 mg: Celery seed (apium graveolens), Gravel root (eupatorium purpureum), Hydrangea root (hydrangea arborescens), Juniper berry (juniperus communis), Glutamine (as L-glutamine), Glycine (as L-glycine), Parsley leaf (petroselinum sativum), Buchu leaf (barosma betulina), Uva ursi leaf (arctostaphylos uva ursi), Bromelain (from pineapple). Other Ingredients: Dicalcium Phosphate, Maltodextrin, Magnesium Stearate, Stearic Acid.

Kidney Plus **-** The Herbalist
Uva Ursi leaf • Juniper berry • Buchu leaf • Echinacea root • Pipsissewa leaf • St. John's Wort flower • Yarrow flower • Cayenne pepper.

Kidney Tea: Soothing Diuretic Tea **-** The Herbalist
Marshmallow root • Juniper berry • Plantain leaf • Dandelion root • Parsley root • Mullein leaf • Horsetail herb • Nettles leaf • Rosehips.

Kidney/Urinary Tract **-** Enzymes, Inc.
Each capsule contains: Vitamin A (100% as Beta Carotene from Dunalelia) 4500 IU • Proprietary Herbal Blend 342 mg: Uva Ursi leaves extract, Cornsilk extract, Wild Hydrangea root extract, Goldenrod leaves extract • Protease 75 mg. Other Ingredients: Cellulose, Water.

Kidneycare **-** PhysioLogics
Two capsules contain: Potassium 50 mg • Dandelion root 300 mg • Astragalus root (70% Polysaccharides, 175 mg) 250 mg • Corn silk 150 mg • Yarrow 150 mg.

Kidney-Liver Complex **-** Enzymatic Therapy
Two capsules contain: Kidney-Liver Complex (Predigested Soluble concentrate) 500 mg • Artichoke extract (Cynara solymus) standardized to contain 15% Caffeylquinic Acids 100 mg • Multi-Glandular Complex 100 mg: Raw Liver, Raw Lung, Raw Pancreas, Raw Heart, Raw Kidney, Raw Spleen, Raw Brain.
See Editor's Note No. 21 and No. 31.

Kids Be Well **-** The Herbalist
Astragalus fresh root (Astragalus membranaceous) • Echinacea fresh root (Echinacea angustifolia) • Lemon Balm fresh leaf (Melissa officinalis) • St. John's Wort fresh flower tops (Hypericum perf.) • Ginkgo fresh leaf (Ginkgo biloba). In a base of kosher glycerine and grapefruit seed extract.

Kid's Choice: Versatile Herbal for Children **-** The Herbalist
Echinacea root • Lemon Balm leaf • Goldenseal root.

KidSoothe **-** PhytoPharmica
Two capsules contain: Vitamin B6 (pyridoxal-5-phosphate) 15 mg • Magnesium (Krebs cycle chelate) 50 mg • Zinc (Krebs cycle chelate) 15 mg • St. John's Wort (Hypericum perforatum) flower head extract (standardized to contain a minimum of 0.3% hypericin and 4% hyperforin) 100 mg• Valerian (Valeriana officinalis) root extract (standardized to contain a minimum of 0.8% valerinic acids) 100 mg • GABA (Gamma-aminobutyric acid) 100 mg • L-Tyrosine 100 mg • Kava (Piper methysticum) root extract (standardized to contain 30% kavalactones) 50 mg • Melissa (Melissa officinalis) leaf extract (standardized to contain a minimum of 5% rosmarinic acid) 50 mg • Grape Seed (PCO) extract (standardized to contain 95% procyanidolic oligomers [PCOs]) 20 mg.
See Editor's Note No. 21, page 2056.

Kinder Love Children's Multivitamin **-** Dial Herbs
Vitamin A • Vitamin C • Vitamin B from Yeast extract • Vitamin E • Thiamin • Niacin • Vitamin B6 • Calcium • Phosphorus • Magnesium • Aqueous extract from: Carrots, Anise, Licorice root, Milfoil herb, Horsetail herb, Chamomile flowers, Peppermint Leaves, Watercress, Wheat Germ, Coriander seeds, Nettles, Spinach, Orange peel • Orange juice • Pear juice concentrate • Malt extract • Yeast extract • Maple Syrup • Honey • Rose Hip extract • Wheat Germ extract • Natural Flavor.

Kindervital **-** Flora, Inc.
Vitamin A • Vitamin B Complex • Vitamin C • Vitamin D • Vitamin E.

Kinder-Vites **-** Atrium Inc.
Two chewable tablets contain: Vitamin A (Palmitate) 2500 IU • Vitamin D (as Vitamin D3) 200 IU • Vitamin E 10 IU • Vitamin K 10 mcg • Vitamin B1 3.2 mg • Vitamin B2 3 mg • Vitamin B6 3.2 mg • Vitamin B12 10 mcg • Vitamin C 100 mg • Niacinamide 13.5 mg • Folic Acid 200 mcg • Pantothenic Acid 5 mg • Biotin 60 mcg. Minerals: Calcium 12 mg • Magnesium 3.2 mg • Manganese 2.5 mg • Copper 100 mcg • Zinc 8 mg • Iron 12 mg • Iodine 100 mcg • Selenium 10 mcg • Chromium 10 mcg • Molybdenum 5 mcg • Vanadium 5 mcg • Citrus Bioflavonoids, Rutin, & Hesperidin 60 mg • Choline 10 mg • Inositol 2 mg • PABA 10 mg. Formulated in a base of pleasant tasting, natural source flavoring & excipients.

Kinerase Cream **-** Valeant Pharmaceuticals International
N(6)furfuryladenine (0.1%) • Purified Water • Propylene Glycol • Stearic Acid • Isopropyl Palmitate • Glyceryl Stearate • Laureth 23 Cetyl Alcohol • Safflower oil • Stearyl Alcohol • Soy Sterol • Panthenol • Aloe Vera gel • Hydrolyzed Elastin • Dimethicone • Methylparaben • Propylparaben • Imidazolidinyl Urea • Carbomer • Triethanolamine • Sodium Hydroxide • Ascorbic Acid.

Kinerase Intensive Eye Cream **-** Valeant Pharmaceuticals International
Purified Water • Glyceryl Stearate • Laureth-23 • Isopropyl Palmitate • Propylene Glycol • Stearic Acid • Cetyl Alcohol • Carthamus Tinctorius seed oil (safflower) • Soya Sterol • Stearyl Alcohol • Dimethicone • Imidazolidinyl Urea • Citric Acid • Sodium Hydroxide • Methylparaben • Soluble Collagen • Carbomer • N(6)furfuryladenine • Panthenol • Propylparaben • Triethanolamine • Ascorbic Acid • Hydrolyzed Elastin • Aloe Barbadensis leaf juice.

Kinerase Lotion **-** Valeant Pharmaceuticals International
Purified Water • Glycerin • Stearyl Alcohol • Glyceryl Stearate • PEG-100 Stearate • Safflower Oil • Octyl Hydroxystearate • Cetyl Alcohol • Aloe Barbadensis gel • Dimethicone • Diazolidinyl Urea • Carbomer • Methylparaben • Soy Sterol • Triethanolamine • Panthenol • Propylparaben • Tocopheryl Acetate • Sodium Hydroxide • Ascorbic Acid • Retinyl Palmitate • Cholecalciferol • Corn Oil • N(6)furfuryladenine.

Kinoko **-** Quality of Life Labs
Four capsules contain: AHCC Proprietary Blend 1000 mg: Mushroom Mycelia extract, Candelilla Wax, Cyclodextrin, Microcrystalline Cellulose. Other Ingredients: Silica, Gelatin, Glycerin.

Kinotakara **-** K-Link International
Each packet contains: Tourmaline • Chitosan • Wood Vinegar • Pearl powder • Silica • Dextrin • Glycol.

Kira **-** Lichtwer Pharma US
Each tablet contains: St. John's Wort (Hypericum perforatum, extract LI 160, standardized to contain 0.3% hypericin) 300 mg. Other Ingredients: Sucrose, Lactose, Talc, Powdered Cellulose, Hydroxypropyl Methylcellulose, Polyethylene Glycol, Castor Oil, Magnesium Stearate, Polyvinylpyrrolidone (pvp), Silicon Dioxide, Gelatin, Titanium Dioxide, Carnauba Wax.

Kirkland Signature B-50 Formula **-** Kirkland
Each tablet contains: Vitamin C (from ascorbic acid) 500 mg • Vitamin E (from DL-alpha tocopheryl acetate) 30 IU • Thiamin (vitamin B1, from thiamin mononitrate) 50 mg • Riboflavin (vitamin B2) 50 mg • Niacin (from niacinamide) 50 mg • Vitamin B6 50 mg • Folate (folic acid) 400 mcg • Vitamin B12 (from cyanocobalamin) 50 mcg • Biotin 300 mcg • Pantothenic Acid (from D-calcium pantothenate) 50 mg • Iron (as ferrous fumarate) 18 mg • Zinc (as zinc oxide) 15 mg • Selenium (as sodium selenate) 25 mcg • Copper (as cupric sulfate) 2 mg. Other Ingredients: Calcium Carbonate, Dibasic Calcium Phosphate, Corn Starch, Cellulose Gel, Gelatin, Maltodextrin, Hydroxypropyl Methylcellulose, Crospovidone, Croscarmellose Sodium, Magnesium Stearate, Silicon Dioxide, Polyethylene Glycol.
See Editor's Note No. 45, page 2058.

Kirkland Signature Calcium with Vitamin D **-** Kirkland
Each tablet contains: Vitamin D (as cholecalciferol) 200 IU • Calcium (as calcium carbonate) 500 mg. Other Ingredients; Maltodextrin, Hydroxypropyl Methylcellulose, Talc, Pregelatinized Starch, Croscarmellose Sodium, Acacia, Hydroxypropyl Cellulose, Silicon Dioxide, Titanium Dioxide, Magnesium Stearate, Polysorbate 80, Yellow 5 Lake, Blue 1 Lake, Polyethylene Glycol 3350, Povidone, Sodium Citrate.
See Editor's Note No. 45, page 2058.

Kirkland Signature Calcium, Vitamin D, Magnesium & Zinc **-** Kirkland
Each tablet contains: Vitamin D 134 IU • Calcium (from calcium carbonate) 334 mg • Magnesium (from magnesium oxide) 134 mg • Zinc (from zinc oxide) 5 mg • Copper (from cupric oxide) 0.66 mg • Manganese (from manganese sulfate) 1.2 mg • Boron (from sodium borate) 168 mcg. Other Ingredients: Maltodextrin, Croscarmellose Sodium, Hydroxypropyl Methylcellulose, Titanium Dioxide, Magnesium Stearate, Polyethylene Glycol, Silicon Dioxide, Triethyl Citrate, Polysorbate 80.
See Editor's Note No. 45, page 2058.

Kirkland Signature Chewable Children's **-** Kirkland
Each tablet contains: Vitamin A (from vitamin A acetate, beta carotene) 5000 IU • Vitamin C (from sodium ascorbate, ascorbic acid) 250 mg • Vitamin D (from ergocalciferol) 400 IU • Vitamin E (from D-alpha tocopheryl acetate) 30 IU • Thiamin (vitamin B1,from thiamine mononitrate) 1.7 mg • Riboflavin (vitamin B2) 1.7 mg • Niacin 20 mg • Vitamin B6 2 mg • Folic Acid 400 mcg • Vitamin B12 (from cyanocobalamin) 6 mcg • Biotin (USP method 2) 40 mcg • Pantothenic Acid (from D-calcium pantothenate) 10 mg • Calcium (from tricalcium phosphate, calcium silicate) 200 mg • Phosphorus (from dicalcium phosphate) 100 mg • Iodine 150 mcg • Magnesium (from magnesium oxide) 20 mg • Zinc (from zinc oxide) 15 mg • Copper (from cupric oxide) 2 mg. Other Ingredients: Sorbitol, Dicalcium Phosphate, Mannitol, Natural & Artificial Flavors (cherry, grape, orange), Mono- & Diglycerides, Magnesium Stearate, Stearic Acid, Corn Starch, Paritally Hydrogenated Soybean Oil, Sucralose (SPLENDA brand), Gelatin, Red 40 Lake, Orange Juice Powder, Yellow 6 Lake, Lactose, Blue 2 Lake.
See Editor's Note No. 45, page 2058.

Kirkland Signature Chewable Vitamin C 500 mg **-** Kirkland
Each tablet contains: Vitamin C (from sodium ascorbate, ascorbic acid) 500 mg. Other Ingredients: Sorbitol, Natural Orange Juice Powder, Natural and Artificial Flavors, Magnesium Stearate, Sucrose, Sucralose, Yellow No. 6 Lake.
See Editor's Note No. 45, page 2058.

Kirkland Signature Daily Multi Vitamins & Minerals **-** Kirkland
Each tablet contains: Vitamin A (as vitamin A acetate) 5000 IU • Vitamin C (as ascorbic acid) 120 mg • Vitamin D 400 IU • Vitamin E (as DL-alpha tocopheryl acetate) 60 IU • Vitamin K (as phylloquinone) 25 mcg • Thiamin (vitamin B1, as thiamin mononitrate) 1.5 mg • Riboflavin (vitamin B2) 1.7 mg • Niacin (as niacinamide) 20 mg • Vitamin B6 (as pyridoxine hydrochloride) 2 mg • Folate (folic acid) 400 mcg • Vitamin B12 (as cyanocobalamin) 6 mcg • Biotin 30 mcg • Pantothenic Acid (as D-calcium pantothenate) 10 mg • Calcium 162 mg • Iron (as ferrous fumarate) 18 mg • Phosphorus 109 mg • Iodine (as potassium iodide) 150 mcg • Magnesium (as magnesium oxide) 100 mg • Zinc (as zinc oxide) 22.5 mg • Selenium (as selenium dioxide) 45 mcg • Copper (as copper oxide) 3 mg • Manganese (as manganese sulfate) 2.5 mg • Chromium (as chromium sulfate, chromium chloride) 120 mcg • Molybdenum (as sodium molybdate) 75 mcg • Chloride 72 mg • Potassium (as potassium chloride) 80 mg • Silicon (as sodium metasilicate) 2 mg • Boron (as sodium borate) 150 mcg • Tin (as stannous chloride) 11 mcg • Vanadium (as sodium metavanadate) 10 mcg • Nickel (as nickelous sulfate) 5 mcg • Lutein 275 mcg. Other Ingredients: Dibasic Calcium Phosphate, Cellulose Gel, Gelatin, Croscarmellose Sodium, Crospovidone, Magnesium Stearate, Hydroxypropyl Methylcellulose, Silicon Dioxide, Corn Starch, Corn Oil, Polyethylene Glycol, Modified Food Starch.
See Editor's Note No. 45, page 2058.

Kirkland Signature Daily Multi-Vitamin **-** Pharmavite Corp.
Each tablet contains: Vitamin A (25% as beta carotene) 10000 IU • Vitamin C 120 mg • Vitamin D 400 IU • Vitamin E 60 IU • Vitamin K 25 mcg • Thiamin 1.5 mg • Riboflavin 1.7 mg • Niacin 20 mg • Vitamin B-6 2 mg • Folic Acid 400 mcg • Vitamin B-12 6 mcg • Biotin 30 mcg • Pantothenic Acid 10 mg • Calcium 162 mg • Iron 9 mg • Phosphorus 109 mg • Iodine 150 mcg • Magnesium 100 mg • Zinc 22.5 mg • Selenium 45 mcg • Copper 3 mg • Manganese 2.5 mg • Chromium 100 mcg • Molybdenum 25 mcg • Chloride 36.3 mg • Potassium 40 mg • Nickel 5 mcg • Tin 10 mcg • Silicon 2 mg • Vanadium 10 mcg • Boron 150 mcg.

Kirkland Signature High Potency Calcium Vitamin D, Magnesium & Zinc **-** Kirkland
Each tablet contains: Vitamin D (as cholecalciferol) 134 IU • Calcium (as calcium carbonate) 334 mg • Magnesium (as magnesium oxide) 134 mg • Zinc (as zinc oxide) 5 mg • Copper (as cupric oxide) 0.66 mg • Manganese (as manganese sulfate) 1.2 mg • Boron (as sodium borate) 168 mcg. Other Ingredients: Maltodextrin, Starch, Hydroxypropyl Methylcellulose, Propylene Glycol, Acacia, Talc, Titanium Dioxide, Croscarmellose Sodium, Hydroxypropyl Cellulose, Silicon Dioxide, Polysorbate 80, Magnesium Stearate, Polyethylene Glycol 3350, Povidone.
See Editor's Note No. 45, page 2058.

Kirkland Signature Mature Adults Daily Multi **-** Kirkland
Each tablet contains: Vitamin A (50% as beta carotene, 50% as vitamin A acetate) 5000 IU • Vitamin C (as ascorbic acid) 60 mg • Vitamin D 400 IU • Vitamin E (as DL-alpha tocopheryl acetate) 60 IU • Vitamin K (as phylloquinone) 10 mcg • Thiamin (vitamin B1, as thiamin mononitrate) 1.5 mg • Riboflavin (vitamin B2) 1.7 mg • Niacin (as niacinamide) 20 mg • Vitamin B6 (as pyridoxine hydrochloride) 3 mg • Folate (folic acid) 400 mcg • Vitamin B12 (as cyanocobalamin) 30 mcg • Biotin 30 mcg • Pantothenic Acid (as D-calcium pantothenate) 10 mg • Calcium (as calcium carbonate) 200 mg • Phosphorus 48 mg • Iodine (as potassium iodide) 150 mcg • Magnesium (as magnesium oxide) 100 mg • Zinc (as zinc oxide) 15 mg • Selenium (as sodium selenate) 20 mcg • Copper (as copper oxide) 2 mg • Manganese (as manganese sulfate) 3.5 mg • Chromium (as chromium chloride) 150 mcg • Molybdenum (as sodium molybdate) 160 mcg • Chloride 72 mg • Potassium (as potassium chloride) 80 mg • Boron (as sodium borate) 300 mcg • Nickel (as nickelous sulfate) 5 mcg • Silicon (as sodium metasilicate) 2 mg • Vanadium (as sodium metavanadate) 10 mcg • Lutein 275 mcg. Other

Ingredients: Dibasic Calcium Phosphate, Cellulose Gel, Gelatin, Croscarmellose Sodium, Magnesium Stearate, Hydroxypropyl Methylcellulose, Silicon Dioxide, Corn Starch, Modified Food Starch, Corn Oil, Polyethylene Glycol.
See Editor's Note No. 45, page 2058.

Kirkland Signature Natural Fish Oil Concentrate **-** Kirkland
Each softgel contains: Natural Fish Oil Concentrate 1000 mg: EPA (eicosapentaenoic acid) 180 mg, DHA (docosahexaenoic acid) 120 mg. Other Ingredients: Gelatin, Glycerin, D-Alpha Tocopherol.
See Editor's Note No. 45, page 2058.

Kirkland Signature Vitamin C 1000 mg **-** Kirkland
Each tablet contains: Vitamin C (from ascorbic acid, rose hips, hesperidin complex, acerola, lemon bioflavonoids complex, rutin) 1000 mg • Citrus Bioflavonoids Complex 100 mg. Other Ingredients: Microcrystalline Cellulose, Corn Starch, Sodium Starch Glycollate, Magnesium Stearate, Hydroxypropyl Methylcellulose, Stearic Acid, Silicon Dioxide, Carnauba Wax, Polyethylene Glycol.
See Editor's Note No. 45, page 2058.

Kirkland Signature Vitamin C 1000 mg with Rose Hips **-** Kirkland
Each tablet contains: Vitamin C 1000 mg • Citrus Bioflavonoids complex 100 mg. Other Ingredients: Microcrystalline Cellulose, Corn Starch, Rose Hips, Sodium Starch Glycollate, Magnesium Stearate, Hydroxypropyl Methylcellulose, Stearic Acid, Silicon Dioxide, Carnauba Wax, Polyethylene Glycol, Acerola, Lemon Bioflavonoids Complex.
See Editor's Note No. 45, page 2058.

Kirkland Signature Vitamin E 1000 I.U. **-** Kirkland
Each softgel contains: Vitamin E (from DL-alpha tocopheryl acetate) 1000 IU. Other Ingredients: Gelatin, Glycerin, Vegetable Oil.
See Editor's Note No. 45, page 2058.

Kirkland Signature Vitamin E 400 I.U. **-** Kirkland
Each softgel contains: Vitamin E (as DL-alpha tocopheryl acetate) 400 IU. Other Ingredients: Gelatin, Glycerin, Water.
See Editor's Note No. 45, page 2058.

KLB6 Grapefruit Diet **-** Puritan's Pride
Four tablets contain: Grapefruit extract 800 mg • Glucomannan 800 mg • Vitamin B6 20 mg • Lecithin 200 mg • Kelp 75 mg • Cider Vinegar 100 mg • Uva Ursi 25 mg • L-Phenylalanine 25 mg.

KlenzTea (World's Best Internal Klenz) **-** Nature's Medicine Corporation
Buckthorn bark • Chamomile flower • Cinnamon bark • Fennel seeds • Ginger root • Milk Thistle • Natural Lemon flavor • Cat's Claw bark • Peppermint leaf • Rose Hip fruit • Senna leaf • Passion fruit • Uva Ursi leaf.

K-Mag Aspartate **-** Source Naturals
Each tablet contains: Potassium (from 565.7 mg of Potassium Aspartate HCl) 99 mg • Magnesium (from 1,027.4 mg of Magnesium Aspartate HCl) 75 mg.

K-Mag C **-** Source Naturals
Each tablet contains: Potassium (Citrate and Ascorbate) 99 mg • Magnesium (Malate and Ascorbate) 75 mg • Vitamin C (Magnesium and Potassium Ascorbates) 500 mg.

K-Mag KG **-** Source Naturals
Each tablet contains: Potassium (from 285 mg Potassium alpha-Ketoglutarate) 99 mg • Magnesium (from 715 mg Magnesium alpha-Ketoglutarate) 100 mg.

Knock Out **-** Schiff
Each tablet contains: Melatonin 3 mg • Valerian extract (valerian officinalis, root) 100 mg • Valerenic Acid 0.8 mg • GABA (gamma aminobutyric acid) 100 mg • L-Theanine 50 mg • Vitamin B6 0.5 mg • Calcium 200 mg • Magnesium 10 mg • Glycine 40 mg.
See Editor's Note No. 26, page 2056.

Koflet **-** The Himalaya Drug Company (Himalaya Heal
Each lozenge contains: Khadira (acacia catechu) 35 mg • Lavanga (syzygium aromaticum) 20 mg • Haritaki (terminalia chebula) 25 mg • Ela (elattaria cardamomum) 2.5 mg • Tvak (cinnamomum zeylanicum) 2.5 mg • Trikatu 9 mg: Piper Nigrum, Piper Longum, Zingiber Officinale.

Koflet Syrup **-** The Himalaya Drug Company (Himalaya Heal
Each 1 tsp (5 mL) serving contains: Madhu (mel despumatum syn. mel depuratum, purified) 1.25 mg • Guggulu (balsamodendron mukul syn. commiphora wightii, purified) 35 mg • Draksha (vitis vinifera) 35 mg • Vishnupriya (ocimum sanctum, syn. o.tenuiflorum) 25 mg • Jufa (hyssopus officinalis) 25 mg • Guduchi (tinospora cordifolia) 20 mg • Vasaka (adhatoda vasica syn. a.zeylanica) 15 mg • Jaatipatree (myristica fragrans, mace) 15 mg • Yashti-Madhu (glycyrrhiza glabra) 10 mg • Gojihva (onosma bracteatum) 10 mg • Neelapuspha (viola odorata) 10 mg • Triphala 9 mg: Emblica Officinalis, Terminalia Chebula, Terminalia Bellirica • Trikatu 9 mg: Piper Nigrum, Piper Longum, Zingiber Officinalis • Vidanga (embelia ribes) 8 mg • Kantakari (solanum xanthocarpum syn. s.surattense) 8 mg • Taja (cinnamomum cassia) 8 mg • Navasagara (ammonii chloridum) 3 mg.

Kong **-** KMS
Two tablets contain: Damiana leaf powder 400 mg • Ashwaganda root powder 200 mg • Catuaba bark powder 220 mg • Tribulus fruit extract (20% steroid saponina) 200 mg • Muira Puama root powder 200 mg • Horny Goat Weed powder 300 mg • Suma root powder 150 mg • Passion Flower powder 100 mg • Dutch Cocoa powder 100 mg • Yohimbe bark powder 70 mg. Other Ingredients: Microcrystalline Cellulose (plant fiber), Dicalcium Phosphate, Croscarmellose Sodium, Stearic Acid, Magnesium Stearate, Silica, Pharmaceutical Glaze, Talc.

Korean Ginseng - Basic Nutrition **-** GNC
Each capsule contains: Korean Ginseng root powder 648 mg. Other Ingredients: Gelatin.

Korean Ginseng 100 mg **-** Nature's Bounty
Each capsule contains: Korean Ginseng root (Panax ginseng, standardized to contain 7% ginsenosides, 7 mg) 100 mg. Other Ingredients: Maltodextrin, Cellulose (plant origin), Gelatin, Vegetable Magnesium Stearate, Silica.

Korean Ginseng Rush **-** GNC
Each capsule contains: Korean Ginseng root 500 mg • Guarana seed extract (Paullinia cupana) 95 mg. Other Ingredients: Gelatin.

Korean Ginseng Standardized **-** Sundown
Each capsule contains: Korean (Asian) Ginseng root extract (standardized to 7% ginsenosides, 7 mg) 100 mg. Other Ingredients: Gelatin, Natural Vegetable Fiber.

Korean Red Ginseng **-** Jamieson
Each caplet contains: Calcium 65 mg • Korean Red Ginseng root (Panax Ginseng) 4% ginsenosides saponins 250 mg.

Korean White Ginseng **-** Nature's Way
Two capsules contain: Korean Ginseng root 1.02 g. Other Ingredients: Gelatin, Magnesium stearate.

Krebs Calcium-Magnesium Chelate **-** Enzymatic Therapy/PhytoPharmica
Each tablet contains: Calcium (chelated with citrate, fumarate, malate, succinate, alpha ketoglutarate [CFMSA chelate]) 200 mg • Magnesium (as CFMSA chelate) 120 mg. Other Ingredients: Stearic Acid, Cellulose, Magnesium Stearate, Silicon Dioxide.
See Editor's Note No. 21, page 2056.

Krebs Cycle Chelates (Vegetarian) **-** Enzymatic Therapy
Four tablets contain: Calcium (chelated with citrate, fumarate, malate, succinate, alpha ketoglutarate [CFMSA chelate]) 600 mg • Iron (as CFMSA chelate) 5 mg • Iodine (from marine organic minerals) 100 mcg • Magnesium (as CFMSA chelate) 400 mg • Zinc (as CFMSA chelate) 15 mg • Selenium (as CFMSA chelate) 15 mg •

Copper (as CFMSA chelate) 1 mg • Manganese (as CFMSA chelate) 2 mg • Chromium (as CFMSA chelate) 100 mcg • Molybdenum (as CFMSA chelate) 25 mcg • Potassium (as CFMSA chelate) 99 mg • Boron (as CFMSA chelate) 4 mg • Vanadium (as CFMSA chelate) 50 mcg. Other Ingredients: Cellulose, Modified Cellulose Gym, Stearic Acid, Silicon Dioxide, Magnesium Stearate, Modified Cellulose, Maltodextrin.

Krebs Ionized Calcium **-** PhytoPharmica
Two tablets contain: Calcium 250 mg.
See Editor's Note No. 21, page 2056.

Krebs Ionized Chelates **-** PhytoPharmica
Four tablets contain: Calcium (chelated (Krebs) with citrate, fumarate, malate, succinate, alpha-ketoglutarate; CFMSA chelate) 600 mg • Iron (CFMSA chelate) 5 mg • Iodine (from marine organic minerals) 100 mcg • Magnesium (CFMSA chelate) 400 mg • Zinc (CFMSA chelate) 15 mg • Selenium (CFMSA chelate) 75 mcg • Copper 1 mg (CFMSA chelate) • Manganese (CFMSA chelate) 2 mg • Chromium (CFMSA chelate) 100 mcg • Molybdenum (CFMSA chelate) 25 mcg • Potassium (CFMSA chelate) 99 mg • Boron (CFMSA chelate) 4 mg • Vanadium (CFMSA chelate) 50 mcg.

Krebs Ionized Zinc **-** PhytoPharmica
Each tablet contains: Zinc 15 mg.
See Editor's Note No. 21, page 2056.

Krebs Magnesium-Potassium Chelates **-** PhytoPharmica
Each tablet contains: Magnesium (as chelated (Krebs) with citrate, fumarate, malate, succinate, and alpha ketoglutarate) 250 mg • Potassium (as chelated (Krebs) with citrate, fumarate, malate, succinate, and alpha ketoglutarate) 100 mg.

Kudja **-** HerbaSway
Kudzu • Ginkgo Biloba • Blackberry • Green Tea • HerbaSwee (Cucurbitaceae fruit).

Kwai ACE **-** Lichtwer Pharma
Each tablet contains: Dried Garlic (guaranteed 0.6% allicin yield, 1800 mcg) 300 mg • Vitamin A 450 mcg • Vitamin C 80 mg • Vitamin E 20 mg.

Kwai Every Day **-** Lichtwer Pharma
Each tablet contains: Garlic clove powder 450 mg (allium sativum L). Other Ingredients: Maltitol, Hydroxypropyl Methylcellulose, Calcium Carbonate, Cellulose, Silica, Acacia, Magnesium Stearate, Carnauba Wax.

Kwai Heart Fit **-** Lichtwer Pharma
Each tablet contains: Garlic powder sucrose 300 mg • Vitamin C (Ascorbic Acid Sorbitol) 80 mg • Vitamin E (Tocopherol Acetate) 20 IU • Vitamin A (Acetate) 2640 IU. Other Ingredients: Talc, Corn Starch, Hydroxypropylmethylcellulose, Polivinylpyrrolidone, Silicon Dioxide, Stearic Acid, Castor oil, Magnesium Stearate, Powdered Cellulose, Glucose Syrup, Titanium Dioxide, Carnauba Wax, Bees Wax, Riboflavin, Beta-Carotene.

Kwai Odor-Free Garlic **-** Lichtwer Pharma
Each tablet contains: Dried Garlic clove powder (yielding 900 mcg of allicin) 150 mg. Other Ingredients: Hydroxypropylmethylcellulose, Silicon Dioxide, Maltitol, Magnesium Stearate, Magnesium Silicate, Carnauba Wax, Powdered Cellulose, Castor Oil, Gum Arabic.

Kwai One-A-Day **-** Lichtwer Pharma
Each tablet contains: Dried Garlic (guaranteed 0.6% allicin yield, 1800 mcg) 300 mg.

Kwai Original **-** Lichtwer Pharma
Each tablet contains: Dried Garlic (guaranteed 0.6% allicin yield, 600 mcg) 100 mg.

Kwik Size XXXL **-** Labrada Bodybuilding Nutrition
Each serving contains: Kwik Carb (Unique blend of Maltodextrin & Polydextrose) • Kwik Pro (Unique blend of cross flow ultrafiltered Whey Protein Concentrate, Calcium Caseinate, Specially Extracted & Spray-Dried Soy Protein Concentrate) • Cocoa powder (dutch processed) • Natural & Artificial flavors • Vitamin & Mineral Blend • Xanthan Gum • Dipotassium Phosphate • Aspartame • Peptigen (proprietary blend of Alpha Amylase, Malt Diatase, Protease, Lactase) • Medium Chain Triglycerides.

Kyno-H **-** Harcourt & Johnston
Each capsule contains: Adenosine Monophosphate (AMP) 370 mg • 3-0-Methal-Chiroinositol 50 mg • Potassium Phosphate 275 mg • Magnesium Gluconate 30 mg • Cnidium Monnier 3.5 mg • Selenium 0.007 mg • Vitamin B5 (pantothenic acid) 14 mg • Vitamin B12 0.00625 mg.

Kyo-Chlorella **-** Wakunaga of America
Each six tablets contain: 100% pure broken cell wall Chlorella powder 3 g.

Kyo-Chrome Aged Garlic Extract Cholesterol Formula **-** Wakunaga of America
Two capsules contain: Aged Garlic extract powder 400 mg • Niacin 20 mg • Chromium (as Chromium Picolinate) 200 mcg. Other Ingredients: Microcrystalline Cellulose, Magnesium Stearate (vegetable source).

Kyo-Dophilus L. Acidophilus; B. Bifidum; B. Longum **-** Wakunaga of America
Each capsule contains: L. Acidophilus [Lactobacillus Acidophilus], B. Bifidum [Bifidobacterium Bifidum], and B. Longum [Bifidobacterium Longum] 1.5 billion cells. Other Ingredients: Vegetable Starch Complex.

Kyo-Green **-** Wakunaga of America
Each teaspoon contains: Kyo-Green Proprietary Blend 2.5 g • Barley Grass Powder • Cooked Brown Rice • Wheat Grass Powder • Bulgarian Chlorella • Pacific Kelp.

Kyolic **-** Wakunaga of America
Each caplet contains: Aged Garlic extract powder 600 mg. Other Ingredients: Microcrystalline Cellulose • Magnesium Stearate • Silicon Dioxide.
See Editor's Note No. 44, page 2058.

Kyolic Aged Garlic Extract Enriched with Vitamin B1 and B12 **-** Wakunaga of America
Each capsule contains: Vitamin B1 (thiamine hydrochloride) 8 mg • Vitamin B12 (cyanocobalamin) 1 mcg. Other Ingredients: Aged Garlic Extract, Liver Extract, Water, Residual Alcohol from extraction.
See Editor's Note No. 14.

Kyolic Aged Garlic Extract Garlic Plus **-** Wakunaga of America
Two capsules (or tablets) contain: Aged Garlic extract powder 540 mg • Brewer's Yeast 54 mg • Kelp 18 mg. Other Ingredients: Whey, Brewer's Yeast, Alginic Acid (seaweed), Kelp, Collodial Silica, Magnesium Stearate (vegetable source).

Kyolic Aged Garlic Extract Kyolic HI-PO **-** Wakunaga of America
Two capsules (or tablets) contain: Aged Garlic extract powder (bulb) 600 mg. Other Ingredients: Whey, Alginic Acid (seaweed), Silica, Cellulose, Magnesium Stearate (vegetable source).

Kyolic Aged Garlic Extract Plus Enzyme **-** Wakunaga of America
Two tablets contain: Aged Garlic powder 700 mg • KYOLIC Enzyme Complex (Amylase, Protease, Cellulose, and Lipase from Aspergillus oryzae and A. niger) 60 mg • Rice Protein-Calcium Complex 40 mg. Other Ingredients: Alginic Acid (seaweed), Colloidal Silica, and Magnesium Stearate (vegetable source).

Some Brand Name Natural Products - What they Contain

www.NaturalDatabase.com contains MANY more listings than appear here.

Kyolic Aged Garlic Extract Plus Lecithin **-** Wakunaga of America
Two capsules contain: Aged Garlic extract powder (bulb) 600 mg • Lecithin 380 mg. Other Ingredients: Silica, Magnesium Stearate (vegetable source).

Kyolic Aged Garlic Extract Vitamin A, C, E, Selenium **-** Wakunaga of America
Two capsules contain: Vitamin A (from 12 mg of beta-carotene) 20000 IU • Vitamin C (calcium ascorbate) 240 mg • Vitamin E (d-alpha-tocopheryl succinate) 120 IU • Selenium (L-selenomethionine) 50 mcg • Aged Garlic extract powder (bulb) 400 mg • Green Tea powder (leaf) 89 mg. Other Ingredients: Silica, Magnesium Stearate (vegetable source).

Kyolic Aged Garlic Extract Vitamin C, Astragalus **-** Wakunaga of America
Two capsules contain: Vitamin C (Ester C) 210 mg • Calcium (citrate polyascorbate) 46 mg • Aged Garlic extract powder (bulb) 440 mg • Astragalus extract powder (root) 200 mg. Other Ingredients: Calcium Citrate, Magnesium Stearate (vegetable source).

Kyolic Aged Garlic Extract Vitamin E, Cayenne, Hawthorn Berry **-** Wakunaga of America
Two capsules contain: Vitamin E (d-alpha-tocopheryl succinate) 200 IU • Aged Garlic extract powder (bulb) 600 mg • Hawthorn berry (fruit) 100 mg • Cayenne Pepper (fruit) 20 mg. Other Ingredients: Cellulose, Magnesium Stearate (vegetable source), Silica.

Kyolic brand **-** Wakunaga of America
Garlic.

Kyolic Cardio Logic **-** Wakunaga of America
Each capsule contains: Vitamin E (as d-alpha-tocopheryl acid succinate) 50 IU • Vitamin B6 5 mg • Folate (as folic acid) 200 mcg • Vitamin B12 100 mcg • Aged Garlic bulb extract powder 200 mg • L-Carnitine 30 mg • Coenzyme Q10 30 mg • Alpha-Lipoic Acid 30 mg. Other Ingredients: Cellulose, Colloidal Silica, Magnesium Stearate (vegetable source).

Kyolic Echinacea Aged Garlic Extract **-** Wakunaga of America
Two capsules contain: Aged Garlic powder (bulb) 600 mg • Echinacea extract powder (root) 100 mg. Other Ingredients: Cellulose (pine), Magnesium Stearate (vegetable source).

Kyolic Estro Logic **-** Wakunaga of America
Each capsule contains: Black Cohosh root extract (standardized to 2.5% triterpene glycosides) 100 mg • Soybean Isoflavones (seed) (standardized to 40% isoflavones) 50 mg • Wild Yam root extract (standardized to 6% total saponins) 33.3 mg • Sage leaf extract 25 mg • Chaste Tree berry extract 12.5 mg • Vervain leaf extract 12.5 mg • Astragalus root extract 12.5 mg • Motherwort leaf extract 12.5 mg. Other Ingredients: Cellulose, Silica, Magnesium Stearate (vegetable source).

Kyolic Formula 100 **-** Wakunaga of America
Two capsules contain: Aged Garlic extract powder (bulb) 600 mg. Other Ingredients: Cellulose, Magnesium Stearate (vegetable source).

Kyolic Liquid Aged Garlic Extract **-** Wakunaga of America
Each 1/4 tsp serving contains: Aged Garlic extract (bulb) 1 mL. Other Ingredients: Water, Residual Alcohol from Extraction.

Kyolic Neuro Logic **-** Wakunaga of America
Two capsules contain: Folate (as folic acid) 200 mcg • Vitamin B12 100 mcg • Aged Garlic bulb powder 400 mg • Lecithin 200 mg • Ginkgo Biloba leaf extract 60 mg • Phosphatidylserine (30%) 50 mg • Acetyl-L-Carnitine 25 mg. Other Ingredients: Cellulose, Colloidal Silica, Magnesium Stearate (vegetable source).

Kyolic One Per Day **-** Life Extension
Each caplet contains: Aged Garlic bulb powder 1000 mg. Other Ingredients: Cellulose, Silica, Magnesium Stearate (vegetable source).

Kyolic Prosta Logic **-** Wakunaga of America
Each capsule contains: Zinc (as Zinc Picolinate) 7.5 mg • Saw Palmetto berry extract 160 mg • Aged Garlic bulb extract powder 100 mg • Pumpkin seed oil extract 50 mg • Pygeum Africanum bark extract 50 mg • Lycopene (as tomato oleoresin) 2.5 mg. Other Ingredients: Wheat Germ Oil, Beeswax, Soft Gelatin Capsule.

Kyolic Reserve Aged Garlic Extract **-** Wakunaga of America
Each capsule contains: Aged Garlic extract powder (bulb) 600 mg. Other Ingredients: Vegetable Protein, Magnesium Stearate (vegetable source), Silica.

Kyolic-EPA Aged Garlic Extract **-** Wakunaga of America
Two capsules contain: EPA (eicosapentaenoic acid) 560 mg • DHA (docosahexaenoic acid) 240 mg • Aged Garlic powder 240 mg • Vitamin E (mixed tocopherol) 10 mg. Other Ingredients: Glycerin, Soft Gelatin Capsule.

L & V Formula **-** Dial Herbs
Wild Lettuce • Valerian • Wood Betony.

L.B.T. Caps: Lower Bowel Tonic **-** The Herbalist
Cascara Sagrada fresh-dried bark (rhamnus purshiana) • Barberry root bark (berberis vulgaris) • Fennel fresh-dried seed (foeniculum vulgare) • Bayberry fresh-dried root bark (myrica cerifera) • Ginger fresh root (zingiber officinale) • Turkey Rhubarb fresh-dried root (rheum palmatum) • Lobelia fresh-dried herb (lobelia inflata) • Cayenne fresh-dried pepper (capsicum annum).

Lactase Enzyme **-** Nature's Way
Three capsules contain: Lactase enzyme 690 mg. Other Ingredients: Gelatin, Magnesium stearate, Maltodextrin.

Lactobacillus Acidophilus Milk-Base **-** Nature's Life
Each capsule contains: Lactobacillus species (Combined L. Acidophilus, L. Bulgaricus & L. Caucasious) 250 mg.

Lactobacillus Acidophilus Milk-Free **-** Nature's Life
Each capsule contains: Lactobacillus acidophilus 500 mg.

LactoCalcium brand **-** Cyvex Nutrition, Inc.
Essential Milk Minerals containing <25% Calcium.
See Editor's Note No. 44, page 2058.

Lactoferrin with Colostrum **-** The Vitamin Shoppe
Each capsule contains: Lactoferrin (from whey) 100 mg • Colostrum (from bovine) providing 20% immunoglobulins 250 mg • Lysozyme (from whey) 5 mg.

Lactoviden ID **-** Metagenics
Each capsule contains: Proprietary Blend 15 billion live oragnisms: Lactobacillus Acidophilus NCFM Strain, Lactobacillus Salivarius Ls-33, Lactobacillus Paracasei Lpc-37, Lactobacillus Plantarum Lp-115, Streptococcus Thermophilus St-21.

Lady V **-** Ultra-V
Three capsules contain: Vitamin D (as Cholecalciferol) 21 IU • Niacin (as Niacinamide) 20 mg • Vitamin B6 (as Pyridoxine HCl) 2.4 mg • Folic Acid (as Folacin) 6.4 mg • Vitamin B12 (as Cyancolalamine) 6 mg • Avena Sativa extract 10:1 150 mg • Kava Kava 10 mg • Guarana 300 mg • White Willow bark 10 mg • Muira Puama 4:1 20 mg • St. John's Wort 250 mg • Siberian Ginseng 35:1 30 mg • Ginkgo Biloba 40 mg • Cordyceps 100 mg • Damiana 20 mg • L-Taurine 200 mg.

Lakota Joint Care Formula **-** Teton Tasunke Pejuta, Inc.
Elk Velvet Antler • Collagen Type II • Hyaluronic Acid • Neutrophils • Pantocrine • Alkaline Phosphatase • Bone Morphogenetic Protein • Glucosamine Sulfate • Herparan Sulfate • Dermatan Sulfate • Keratan Sulfate •Chondroitin Sulfate • Glucosamine Hydrochloride •Sulfur • Uronic Acid • Boswellia Serrata •White Willow bark • Yucca root •Sarsaparilla •Feverfew • Devil's Claw • L-Proline • Bromelain

•Omega 3 & 6 fatty acids • All Essential Amino Acids • Calcium •Iron •Phosphorus •Zinc.
See Editor's Note No. 4 and No. 17.

Land, Lake & Sea **-** Great Life Labs
Two tablets contain: Vitamin A (as beta-carotene and as mixed carotenoids from D. salina algae) 5000 IU • Vitamin C (as ascorbic acid) 100 mg • Vitamin D (as cholecalciferol) 400 IU • Vitamin E (as DL-alpha-tocopheryl acetate) 50 IU • Thiamin (as thiamin mononitrate) 10 mg • Riboflavin (riboflavin) 10 mg • Niacin (niacin) 25 mg • Vitamin B6 (as pyridoxine hydrochloride) 5 mg • Folate (as folic acid) 400 mcg • Vitamin B12 (as cyanocobalamin) 25 mcg • Biotin (as biotin) 300 mcg • Pantothenic Acid (as calcium pantothenate) 10 mg • Calcium (as dibasic calcium phosphate) 225 mg • Iodine (from sea kelp (ascophyllum nodosum)) 150 mcg • Magnesium (as magnesium oxide) 25 mg • Zinc (as zinc citrate) 7.5 mg • Selenium (as selenomethionine) 70 mcg • Copper (as copper gluconate) 1 mg • Manganese (as manganese gluconate) 2 mg • Chromium (as niacin bound dinicotinate glycinate) 120 mcg • Molybdenum (as molybdenum chelate) 75 mcg • Pine bark (pinus strobus) and Grape seed (vitis vinifera) 50/50 blend 50 mg • Fruit and Vegetable Phytonutrient Concentrate Blend 500 mg: Alfalfa sprouts, Asparagus, Broccoli, Brussels sprouts, Cabbage, Cauliflower, Garlic, Kale, Mustard Greens, Soybean, Spinach, Papaya, Pineapple, Cantaloupe, Carrot, Cherry, Grapefruit, Lemon, Orange, Peach, Pear, Red Grape, Red Pepper, Strawberry, Tomato, Yellow Squash, Wheat Grass • Shiitake mushroom 10 mg • California Blue Green Algae (spirulina pratensis) 50 mg • Bulgarian Green Algae (chlorella pyrinoides) 50 mg • Dunaliella Red Algae (dunaliella salina) 20 mg • Phenalgin extract of Cystoseira Canariensis (1% phlorotannin) 50 mg • Maine Coast Sea Kelp (ascophyllum nodosum) 37.25 mg • Irish Moss extract (chondrus crispus) 5 mg. Other Ingredients: Cellulose, Croscarmellose Sodium, Vegetable Stearic Acid, Vegetable Magnesium Stearate, Silica, Pharmaceutical Glaze.

L-Arginine **-** Allergy Research Group
Each capsule contains: L-Arginine 500 mg. Other Ingredients: Cellulose, Silicon Dioxide, Stearic Acid.

L-Arginine **-** NutriCology
Each capsule contains: L-Arginine 500 mg. Other Ingredients: Cellulose, Silicon Dioxide, Stearic Acid.

L-Arginine **-** PhysioLogics
Each capsule contains: L-Arginine 500 mg. Other Ingredients: Gelatin, Vegetable Magnesium Stearate, Silica.

L-Arginine 500 - GNC A-Z **-** GNC
Each capsule contains: L-Arginine 500 mg. Other Ingredients: Gelatin.

L-Arginine 500 mg **-** Nature's Bounty
Each capsule contains: L-Arginine 500 mg. Other Ingredients: Gelatin, Vegetable Magnesium Stearate, Silica.

L-Arginine/L-Ornithine 500/250 mg **-** Solgar
Each vegicap contains: L-Arginine 500 mg • L-Ornithine (as l-ornithine HCl) 250 mg. Inactive Ingredients: Vegetable Cellulose, Vegetable Magnesium Stearate, Silica, Vegetable Glycerin, Water.

Lauricidin (monolaurin) **-** Med-Chem Labs
Each pellet contains: Highly purified Monolaurin lipid.

Lava **-** Universal
Each 83 g serving contains: Creatine Monohydrate 5.5 g • Chromium 75 mcg • Glutamine 2.5 g • Taurine 1.2 g • Sodium 180 mg • Potassium 360 mg. Ingredients: Ultra & Micro-Filtrated Whey Protein Concentrate (Containing Whey Peptide-Rich Lactoglobulins, Lactalbumin, Immunoglobulins & Lactoferrin) • GlycoCarb Complex (Dextrose & Glucose Polymers) • Maltodextrin • 100% Pure Creatine Monohydrate • Glutamine • Taurine • Magnesium Oxide • Disodium Phosphate • Potassium Phosphate • Fruit Flavor • Lecithin • Ascorbic Acid • Vitamin E Succinate • Niacin • Citric Acid • Aspartame • Carmine (for color) • Chromium (GTF).

Laxaco **-** Jamieson
Each capsule contains: Calcium (as Calcium Sulfate) 25 mg • Senna leaf (Cassia senna L.) 240 mg • Cascara Sagrada bark (Rhamnus purshiana DC) 150 mg.

Laxaco - Herbal Laxative Formula **-** Jamieson
Each capsule contains: Cascara Sagrada 150 mg • Senna Leaves 240 mg.

LaxaColon **-** DreamPharm
Each capsule contains: Proprietary Blend: Senna leaf, Aloe, Prune powder.

LaxActin **-** Nature's Plus
Each capsule contains: Cascara Sagrada (Rhamnus purshiana bark) (standardized 25-30% Hydroxyanthracene derivatives - HAD) 100 mg • Passion Flower [(Passiflora incarnata flower) standardized 3.5-4% Flavonoids] 100 mg • Senna [(Cassia senna leaf) standardized 5% Sennosides] 50 mg.

Laxaherb **-** Dial Herbs
Cascara Sagrada • Buckthorn • Ginger • Bayberry • Goldenseal • Raspberry • Fennel • Lobelia • Rhubarb.

L-Carnitine - Basic Nutrition **-** GNC
Each capsule contains: L-Carnitine (as L-Carnitine Fumarate) 250 mg. Other Ingredients: Gelatin, Magnesium Stearate.

L-Carnitine **-** Metabolic Response Modifiers
Each capsule contains: L-Carnitine 500 mg • Vitamin B5 15 mg • Vitamin B6 5 mg.

L-Carnitine **-** New Hope Health Products
Each capsule contains: L-Carnitine 500 mg • Vitamin B5 15 mg • Vitamin B6 5 mg.

L-Carnitine **-** Olympian Labs
Two capsules contain: L-Carnitine Fumarate 1000 mg.

L-Carnitine **-** Source Naturals
Each capsule contains: L-Carnitine 250 mg.

L-Carnitine **-** Swanson
Two capsules contain: L-Carnitine (from tartrate and free-form) 500 mg.

L-Carnitine (250 mg) **-** Allergy Research Group
Each tablet contains: L-Carnitine 250 mg. Other Ingredients: Cellulose, Dicalcium Phosphate, Silicon Dioxide, Magnesium Stearate, Stearic Acid.

L-Carnitine (250 mg) **-** NutriCology
Each tablet contains: L-Carnitine 250 mg. Other Ingredients: Cellulose, Dicalcium Phosphate, Silicon Dioxide, Magnesium Stearate, Stearic Acid.

L-Carnitine (500 mg) **-** Allergy Research Group
Each tablet contains: L-Carnitine 500 mg. Other Ingredients: Cellulose, Dicalcium Phosphate, Silicon Dioxide, Magnesium Stearate, Stearic Acid.

L-Carnitine 250 - GNC A-Z **-** GNC
Each capsule contains: L-Carnitine (as L-carnitine fumarate) 250 mg. Other Ingredients: Gelatin.

L-Carnitine 250 MG **-** PhysioLogics
Each capsule contains: L-Carnitine (as l-carnitine fumarate) 250 mg. Other Ingredients: Gelatin, Rice Powder, Silica, Vegetable Magnesium Stearate.

L-Carnitine 500 **-** Optimum Nutrition
Each tablet contains: Calcium (as dicalcium phosphate) 96 mg • Phosphorus (as dicalcium phosphate) 74 mg • L-Carnitine (as L-

carnitine tartrate) 500 mg. Other Ingredients: Pharmaceutical Glaze, Stearic Acid, Silica, Magnesium Stearate, Croscarmellose Sodium (disintegrant).

L-Carnitine 500 - GNC A-Z - GNC
Each capsule contains: L-carnitine (as L-carnitine L-tartrate) 500 mg. Other Ingredients: Gelatin.

L-Carnitine 500 MG - PhysioLogics
Each tablet contains: L-Carnitine 500 mg. Other Ingredients: Cellulose (plant origin), Dicalcium Phosphate, Vegetable Stearic Acid, Silica, Croscarmellose, Cellulose Coating, Vegetable Magnesium Stearate, Titanium Dioxide Color, Food Glaze, Magnesium Silicate, Vanillin.

L-Citruline - NutriCology
Each 1-1/4 tsp (3 g) serving contains: L-Citruline 3 g.

L-Citrulline - Allergy Research Group
Each 1-1/4 tsp (3 g) serving contains: L-Citrulline 3 g.

L-Cysteine 500 - GNC
Each tablet contains: L-Cysteine 500 mg. Other Ingredients: Cellulose, Dicalcium Phosphate.

LDL-RX - Athletic Technologies Inc.
Two capsules contain: Red Yeast Rice 1000 mg • Niacin 50 mg • Guggulipids 50 mg • Beta-Sisterol 50 mg • Capiscum 50 mg • Garlic 50 mg • Lecithin 200 mg.

Lean "4" - The Vitamin Shoppe
Each six tablets contain: Lecithin 1200 mg • Vitamin B6 (pyridoxine HCl) 50 mg • Iodine (kelp) 210 mcg • Cider Vinegar Powder 240 mg • Grapefruit Powder 300 mg.

Lean & Clean - The Sports Nutrition Source, Inc.
Each capsule contains: Proprietary Blend 470 mg: Papaya fruit, Echinacea root, Black Walnut leaves, Fennel seeds, Parsley plant, Norwegian Kelp plant, Safflower flowers, Burdock root, Chickweed herb, Hawthorn berries, Cayenne fruit.

Lean Body - Labrada Bodybuilding Nutrition
LeanPro: Cross flow ultrafiltered Whey Protein concentrate, ion exchange Whey Protein isolate, cross flow microfiltered Whey Protein isolate, hydrolyzed Whey Protein isolate peptides, Milk Protein isolate, Caseinate, L-Glutamine, Taurine, Magnesium Alpha Keto Glutarate • Maltodextrin • Vitamin and Mineral Blend: Dicalcium Phosphate, Magnesium Oxide, Ascorbic Acid, Vitamin E Acetate, Niacinamide, Electrolytic Iron, Zinc Oxide, Sodium Chloride, D-Calcium Pantothenate, Pyridoxine HCl, Copper Gluconate, Manganese Citrate, Vitamin A Acetate, Thiamine Mononitrate, Riboflavin, Folic Acid, Manganese Sulfate, Potassium Iodide, Chromium Picolinate, Cholecalciferol, Sodium Molybdate, Cyanocobalamin, Sodium Selenite • Natural & Artificial Flavors • Polydextrose • Medium Chain Triglycerides • Xanthan Gum • Cellulose Gum • Aspartame.

Lean Connection - The Coral Connection
Three capsules contain: Calcium (as hydroxycitrate) 165 mg • Chromium (as polynicotate) 133 mcg • Potassium (as hydroxycitrate) 240 mg • Garcinia Cambogia fruit extract 1500 mg • (-) Hydroxycitric Acid 900 mg • Gymnema Sylvestre leaf extract 133 mg • Gymnemic Acids 33 mg • Phaseolamin 2250 330 mg • Green Tea (50% polyphenols) 180 mg • Oat Bran 105 mg • Psyllium husk 105 mg. Other Ingredients: Hydroxypropyl Cellulose, Glycerine, Magnesium Stearate, Silicon Dioxide.

Lean Dreams - The Sports Nutrition Source, Inc.
Each tablet contains: Vitamin B-6 (Pyridoxine) 15 mg • Niacin (niacinamide) 50 mg • L-Ornithine 500 mg • L-Glycine 667 mg • Valerian root extract 150 mg • Hops powder 20 mg.

Lean Formula with Advantra Z - USANA Health Sciences
Two tablets contain: Sour Orange Extract (Citrus Aurantium L. fruit) 650 mg • Green Tea Extract (Camellia Sinensis Kuntze leaf) 50 mg • Guarana Extract (Paullinia Cupana Bonpl. & Kunth. fruit) 50 mg • Cayenne (Capsicum Annum L. fruit) 30 mg. Other Ingredients: Microcrystalline Cellulose, Croscarmellose Sodium, Ascorbyl Palmitate, Collodial Silicon Dioxide, Dextrin, Dextrose.
See Editor's Note No. 40, page 2058.

Lean Gainer - Champion Nutrition
Each serving contains: Peptol-C: Whey Protein Concentrate, Creatine Monohydrate, Amino Acids, L-Leucine, L-Glutamine • Metabarb-V (blend of Simple & Complex Carbohydrates containing Glucose Polymers & Whey) • Low Fat Cocoa powder •Natural & Artificial Flavors • Metavite IV (Vitamin-Mineral Complex) • FIBR3: Cellulose, Oat Fiber, Psyllium husks • Aspartame • Succinate ETF: Potassium Succinate, L-Glutamic Acid, Inosine, Magnesium Succinate, Calcium Succinate • Bromelain •Papain • Defatted Peanut Flour •Sunette (Brand of Acesulfame-K) • Vanadyl Polynicotinate. Contains Phenylalanine.

Lean Image Carb Blocker - Pro Star International
Two tablets contain: Wheat Amylase Inhibitor 10 mg • Pro Carb Blend 300 mg: Gymnema Sylvestre leaf and extract, Fenugreek seed, Lycium berry, Vanadium (from vanadyl sulfate) • Banaba leaf extract (1% corosolic acid) 16 mg. Other Ingredients: Dicalcium Phosphate, Microcrystalline Cellulose, Croscarmellose Sodium, Stearic Acid, Magnesium Stearate, Silica, Pharmaceutical Glaze.
See Editor's Note No. 37, page 2057.

Lean Machine - The Sports Nutrition Source, Inc.
Two scoops contain: Sodium 85 mg • Potassium 85 mg • Protein 37 g • Creatine Monohydrate 3000 mg • L-Glutamine 2000 mg • Methylsulfonylmethane 1000 mg • Glucosamine Sulfate 500 mg • Chondroitin Sulfate 350 mg • White Willow Bark extract 75 mg • Ascorbic Acid 100 mg • Bromelain 100 mg.
See Editor's Note No. 15, page 2055.

Lean System 7 - PPI, Inc.
Three capsules contain: Yerba Mate leaves (ilex paraguanensis) 500 mg • Guarana seed extract (paullinia cupana, standardized to 22% alkaloids as caffeine, 154 mg) 700 mg • Citrus Aurantium fruit extract (standardized for 6% synephrine, 18 mg) 300 mg • ForsLean Coleus Forskohlii root extract (standardized for 20% forskolin, 30 mg) 150 mg • 7-Keto (3-acetyl-7-oxo-dehydroepiandrosterone) 50 mg • Dandelion leaf and root powder (taraxacum officinale) 250 mg • Bioperine Piper Nigrum fruit (98% piperine, 4.9 mg) 5 mg.
See Editor's Note No. 40, page 2058.

Lean Tabs - Fizogen
Three tablets contain: Dexafenadrine (hybrid thermogenic fusion) 785 mg: Caffeine Anhydrous, Green Tea extract, Yerba Mate root extract, Green Coffee bean extract, Cordia Salicifolia extract, Cocoa extract, Taurine, Citrus Naringin, Vinpocetine • Hydropropol (water removal complex) 462 mg: Horse Tail extract, Dandelion root extract, Uva Ursi extract • Carboxen (cabo-metabolic driving agent) 250 mg: Garcinia Cambogia extract (HCA), L-Carnitine • C-AMP SCB (cyclic AMP triggering agent) 140 mg: Clary Sage extract, Bergenin • Myotonal (muscle tone enhancer) 130 mg: Mucuna Pruriens extract, Cyanotis Vaga extract, Rhodiola Rosea extract • Neurotrol (appetite controlling blend) 130 mg: Hoodia Gordonii cactus extract, Caralluma cactus extract, Simthin Jojoba seed extract, Griffonia Simplicifolia seed extract • Tetravlain (thyroid T3/T4 secretagogue) 130 mg: L-Tyrosine, Olive leaf extract, Guggulsterones E&Z • Degestol (hyper digestive fusion) 75 mg: Terminalia Chebula fruit extract, Terminalia Belerica fruit extract, Emblica Officinalis fruit extract • Egc-Heat (thermobolic accelerator) 67 mg: Evodium extract, Ginger root extract, Cayenne extract.

Lean Tea Complex - Optimum Nutrition
Each capsule contains: Green Tea leaf extract (camellia sinensis, standardized to 20% caffeine & 35% EGCG, epigallo-catechin-gallate) 700 mg • Black Tea powdered leaf 10 mg • Oolong Tea powdered leaf 10 mg • Bioperine Piper Nigrum fruit extract (standardized to 95% piperine) 5 mg. Other Ingredients: Gelatin, Magnesium Stearate.

LeanFire **-** InStone Nutrition
Three capsules contain: Vitamin C 120 mg • L-Tyrosine 650 mg • Green Tea 300 mg • Caffeine Anhydrous 300 mg • Evo-Lean Blend 255 mg: Rhodiola Rosea root, Evodia Rutaecarpa, E & Z Guggulsterones • 7-Keto 50 mg. Other Ingredients: Gelatin, Silicon Dioxide, Magnesium Stearate.

Learner's Edge Pure Kids **-** Integrative Therapeutics
Three capsules contain: Selenium (from l-selenomethionine) 25 mcg • Milk Thistle seed extract (silybum marianum, 80% silymarin) 150 mg • NAC (as n-acetyl-l-cysteine) 25 mg • D-Glucarate Calcium D-glucarate 100 mg • Trimethylglycine (as betaine) 150 mg • Alpha-Ketoglutaric Acid 250 mg • Taurine 100 mg • L-Glutathione, reduced 25 mg • L-Methionine 100 mg • Choline (from choline bitartrate) 100 mg • MSM (methylsulfonylmethane) 100 mg. Other Ingredients: Microcrystalline Cellulose, Ascorbyl Palmitate, Capsule (gelatin, water).

Learner's Edge System ChildEssence **-** Integrative Therapeutics
Four capsules contain: Vitamin A (67% from retinyl acetate & 33% as natural beta-carotene with mixed carotenoids) 7500 IU • Vitamin C (as ascorbic acid) 200 mg • Vitamin D (as cholecalciferol) 200 IU • Vitamin E (from natural mixed tocopherols) 100 IU • Thiamin (from thiamine pyrophosphate) 10 mg • Riboflavin (as riboflavin-5'-phosphate) 10 mg • Niacin (as niacinamide) 40 mg • Vitamin B6 (from pyridoxal-5'-phosphate) 25 mg • Folate (as folic acid) 200 mcg • Vitamin B12 (as methylcobalamin) 200 mcg • Biotin 100 mcg • Pantothenic Acid (from calcium pantothenate) 20 mg • Calcium (50% from calcium glycinate, 50% from calcium citrate/malate complex) 200 mg • Iron (from ferrous succinate) 10 mg • Iodine (from potassium iodide) 150 mcg • Magnesium (50% from magnesium glycinate and 50% from calcium citrate/malate complex) 200 mg • Zinc (from zinc sulfate) 7.5 mg • Selenium (from l-selenomethionine) 30 mcg • Chromium (from chromium nicotinate) 50 mcg • Molybdenum (from molybdenum citrate) 25 mcg • Citrus Bioflavonoids 25 mg. Other Ingredients: Microcrystalline Cellulose, Ascorbyl Palmitate, Capsule (gelatin & water).

Learner's Edge System DigestRight **-** Integrative Therapeutics
Two capsules contain: Proprietary Enzyme Blend 315 mg: Protease (provides dipeptidylpeptidase IV, exopeptidase, endopeptidase, peptide peptidohydrolase activity) 14,500 USP/20,200 PC/34,300 HUT/2000 CFAU, Amylase 6700 USP/6000 DU/6000, Lipase 630 LU/300 LU, Lactase 2400 LacU, Cellulase 124 CU, Phytase 0.64 PU, Sucrase (invertase) 300 INVU, Maltase (malt diastase) 10,800 DP. Other Ingredients: Microcrystalline Cellulose, Ascorbyl Palmitate, Capsule (gelatin, water).

Learner's Edge System ImmunoKids **-** Integrative Therapeutics
Three capsules contain: Vitamin C (as ascorbic acid) 500 mg • Calcium (from calcium magnesium phytate) 65 mg • Zinc (from zinc sulfate) 10 mg • IP-6 (inositol hexaphosphate, from calcium magnesium phytate) 400 mg • Inositol 110 mg • Leucoselect Phytosome 83 mg: Grape seed Polyphenols (including procanidolic oligomers (vitis vinifera)) 26 mg, Phosphatidylcholine (from soy bean) 55 mg • Pine bark extract (pinus maritima, 95% polyhenols, including procyanidolic oligomers) 25 mg • Savantero Cat's Claw bark extract (uncaria tomentosa, 1.3% pentacyclic oxindole alkaloids, free of tetracyclic oxindole alkaloids) 10 mg • Aloe Vera inner leaf gel powder 20 mg • Citrus Bioflavonoids 50 mg • Monolaurin (as glyceryl monolaurate) 10 mg. Other Ingredients: Microcrystalline Cellulose, Ascorbyl Palmitate, Capsule (gelatin & water).

Learner's Edge System Learner's Edge **-** Integrative Therapeutics
Three capsules contain: Vitamin E (from d-alpha tocopheryl succinate) 10 IU • DMAE (as dimethylaminoethanol bitartrate) 200 mg • L-Theanine 25 mg • Acetyl-L-Carnitine (from acetyl l-carnitine HCl) 300 mg • L-Carnosine 400 mg • Vitaline Coenzyme Q10 Blend (coenzyme Q10 as ubiquinone 30 mg) 175 mg • Ginkgo Biloba leaf extract (24% flavone glycosides, 6% terpene lactones) 50 mg • American Ginseng root extract (panax quinquefolium, 5% ginsenosides) 200 mg. Other Ingredients: Microcrystalline Cellulose, Ascorbyl Palmitate, Micosolle (vegetable fatty acids, silicon dioxide, magnesium sulfate), Capsule (gelatin, water).

Leci-Choline brand **-** Degussa Food Ingredients/BL BioActives
PhosphatidylCholine.
See Editor's Note No. 44, page 2058.

Leci-Plus **-** Atrium Inc.
Each capsule contains: Raw Unbleached Lecithin 650 mg • Choline Bitartrate 50 mg • Inositol 50 mg • Biotin 60 mcg • Niacinamide 30 mg • Vitamin B6 2 mg • Magnesium Glycero Phosphate 100 mg • Magnesium 12 mg • Phosphorus 16 mg.

Leci-PS brand **-** Degussa Food Ingredients/BL BioActives
PhosphatidylSerine.
See Editor's Note No. 44, page 2058.

Lecithin **-** Health Center for Better Living
"Rich source of choline, a B-complex nutrient," HCBL Lecithin derived from soybeans

Lecithin **-** Jamieson
Each capsule contains: Lecithin derived from Pure Soy 1200 mg.

Leci-Thin **-** Nature's Plus
Each wafer contains: Lecithin 1500 mg derived from natural Soybean, rich in Choline, Inositol & Phosphorus • Wheat Bran 500 mg • Vegetable Cellulose 200 mg • Protein, vegetable soy & peanut 150 mg. Made from the finest quality Lecithin, containing 95% Soy Phosphatides. In an all natural base of carob, coconut & vanilla bean.

Lecithin **-** Now
Four softgels contain: Phosphatidyl Choline 560 mg • Phosphatidyl Ethanolamine 128 mg • Phosphatidyl Inositol 16 mg. Other Ingredients: Soybean Lecithin, Gelatin, Glycerine, Water.

Lecithin & Milk powder **-** Nature's Life
Two heaping tablespoons contain: Linoleic Acid (omega-6) 3681 mg • Linolenic Acid (omega-3) 438 mg • Oleic Acid (omega-9) 575 mg • Palmitic Acid 1269 mg • Stearic Acid 288 mg • Phosphatidyl Choline 2.8g • Phosphatidyl Ethanolamine 2.5 g • Phosphatidyl Inositol 1.8 g • Choline 378 mg • Inositol 275 mg • Calcium 132 mg • Iron 1 mg • Magnesium 11 mg • Phosphorus 471 mg • Potassium 276 mg • Sodium 57 mg • Alanine 103 mg • Arginine 137 mg • Aspartic Acid 213 mg • Cysteine 11 mg • Glutamic Acid 779 mg • Glycine 68 mg • Histidine (essential amino acid) 99 mg • Isoleucine (essential amino acid) 216 mg • Leucine (essential amino acid) 334 mg • Lysine (essential amino acid) 270 mg • Methionine (essential amino acid) 110 mg • Phenylalanine (essential amino acid) 190 mg • Proline 407 mg • Serine 209 mg • Threonine (essential amino acid) 148 mg • Tryptophan (essential amino acid) 49 mg • Tyrosine 209 mg • Valine (essential amino acid) 243 mg.

Lecithin Choline **-** PhysioLogics
Each softgel contains: Phosphatidyl Choline (from soy lecithin concentrate 1200 mg) 420 mg. Other Ingredients: Gelatin, Glycerin.

Lecithin Plus **-** GNC
Two capsules contain: Niacin 20 mg • Chromium (as chromium picolinate) 200 mcg • Garlic powder (allium sativum) 500 mg •Phosphatidyl Choline (as liquid soy lecithin) 141 mg. Other Ingredients: Gelatin, Soybean oil, Glycerin, Caramel Color, Titanium Dioxide.

Lecithin-E **-** Nutrilite
Each tablet contains: Lecithin (from Soybean Oil) 290 mg • Vitamin E 30 IU.

Leg Cramps Ointment **-** Hyland's
Active Ingredients: Aconitum Nap. 3X • Arnica Montana 3X • Ledum Pal. 3X • Magnesia Phosphorica 10X • Rhus Toxicodendron 6X • Viscum. Album 3X. Inactive Ingredients: Olive Oil N.F., Stearyl Alcohol, Natural Wintergreen Oil, Kokam Butter, Glyceryl Monostearate, Soy Lecithin, Methylparaben, Propylparaben, Butylparaben.
See Editor's Note No. 1, page 2053.

Leg Cramps with Quinine **-** Hyland's
Two tablets contain: Cinchona Officinalis 3X (quinine) • Viscum Album 3X • Gnaphalium Polycephalum 3X • Rhus Toxicodendron 6X • Aconitum Napellus 6X • Ledum Palustre 6X • Magnesia Phosphorica 6X. Base: Lactose NF.
See Editor's Note No. 1, page 2053.

Leg Vein Essentials **-** Swanson
Two time-release capsules contain: Vitamin C (as calcium ascorbate) 120 mg • Horse Chestnut extract (22% escin) 400 mg • Butcher's Broom extract (10% saponins calculated as ruscogenin) 150 mg • Gotu Kola extract (10% asiaticosides) 100 mg • Hesperidin (40% bioflavonoids) 100 mg • Bilberry extract (25% anthocyanidins) 20 mg • Grapeseed extract (90%-95% proanthocyanidins) 20 mg • Hawthorn berry extract (2% vitexin-2' rhamnosides) 20 mg.

Leg Veins Formula **-** Nature's Way
Two capsules contain: Butcher's Broom root 200 mg • Cayenne pepper fruit 50 mg • Dandelion leaf 250 mg • Grape seed dried extract 37.5 mg • Horse chestnut dried extract 200 mg • Prickly Ash bark 100 mg • Vitamin C (Ascorbic Acid) 30 mg. Other Ingredients: Gelatin, Magnesium Stearate, Millet.

Leg-Aid **-** Futurebiotics
Two capsules contain: Niacin (as flush free niacin) 20 mg • MSM (methyl-sulfonyl-methane) 400 mg • Citrus Bioflavonoids 220 mg • Glucosamine sulfate 400 mg • Grape Seed powder extract (standardized for 95% (24 mg) proanthocyanidins) 25 mg • Horse Chestnut (standardized at 18-22% (50-62 mg) aescin) 280 mg • Butcher's Broom root powder 200 mg • Prickly Ash bark powder 125 mg • Ginkgo Biloba leaf powder 30 mg. Other Ingredients: Magnesium stearate, Gelatin, Water.

Lemon-Lime Multi-Vitamin For Adults **-** LiFizz Effervescent Vitamins
Each tablet contains: Magnesium 80 mg • Calcium 200 mg • Zinc 5 mg • Iron 6 mg • Vitamin A 5000 IU • Vitamin E 15 IU • Vitamin C 60 mg • Vitamin B2 (Riboflavin) 1.7 mg • Vitamin B6 (Pyridoxine) 2 mg • Vitamin B12 (Cyanocobalamin) 6 mcg • Vitamin B1 (Thiamin) 1.5 mg • Niacin (Vitamin PP or B3) 20 mg • Pantothenic Acid 10 mg • Free Folic Acid 400 mcg • Biotin 300 mcg • Vitamin D 400 IU.

Leptoprin **-** A.G. Waterhouse
Two capsules contain: Calcium (amino acid chelate) 264 mg • Vitamin B6 25 mg • Leptoprin Proprietary Blend 989 mg: Acetylsalicyclic Acid 324 mg, Caffeine (34 mg from standardized kola nut 280 mg) 200 mg • Green Tea leaf extract (standardized for polyphenols/catechins content), L-Tyrosine, Kelp (0.15% iodine 100 mg), Ephedrine Alkaloids (exclusive 10% extract from whole plant ma huang 200 mg) 20 mg, Cayenne fruit. Other Ingredients: Rice Flour.

Leptoprin-SD - A.G. Waterhouse
Two capsules contain: Niacin 20 mg • Calcium (as calcium amino acid chelate) 39 mg • Copper (from copper amino acid chelate) 0.5 mg • Leptoprin-SD Proprietary Blend 1188 mg: Yerba Mate leaf standardized extract (SE), Guarana seed SE, Caffeine, Damiana leaf SE, L-Tyrosine, Acetylsalicylic Acid 81 mg, Green Tea leaf SE, Kola Nut SE, Eucommia bark, Schizonepeta Spica SE, Piper Nigrum fruit, Hoelen, Polygonum root, Turmeric rhizome.

Leptoprin-SF **-** A.G. Waterhouse
Two capsules contain: Calcium (amino acid chelate) 132 mg • Leptoprin-SF Proprietary Blend 1493.5 mg: Calcium Phosphate, Commiphora Mukul extract, Garcinia Cambogia (HCA 125 mg), L-Tyrosine, Acetylsalicylic Acid 162.5 mg, Dipotassium Phosphate, Sodium Phosphtae, Disodium Phosphate, Phosphatidyl Choline, Scutellaria root, Bupleurum root, Epimedium herb. Other Ingredients: Rice Flour.

Level 90 Blood Sugar Stabilizer **-** Market America, Inc.
Two tablets contain: Niacin 7 mg • Niacinamide 10 mg • Magnesium (oxide) 17 mg • Chromium (amino acid chelate) 100 mcg • Cyanocobalamin (vitamin B12) 50 mcg • Glucomannan (amorphophallus tuber extract) 175 mg • L-Glutamic Acid 100 mg • L-Carnitine 50 mg • Coenzyme Q10 10 mg • Vanadium (amino acid chelate) 15 mcg. Other Ingredients: Microcrystalline Cellulose, Stearic Acid, Magnesium Stearate, Silicon Dioxide, Croscarmellose Sodium, Dicalcium Phosphate.

L-Glutamine **-** PhysioLogics
Each tablet contains: L-Glutamine 500 mg. Other Ingredients: Cellulose (plant origin), Dicalcium Phosphate, Hydroxypropyl Cellulose, Vegetable Stearic Acid, Povidone, Silica, Croscarmellose, Vegetable Magnesium Stearate, Cellulose Coating.

L-Glutamine (500 mg) **-** NutriCology
Each capsule contains: L-Glutamine 500 mg. Other Ingredients: Cellulose, Stearic Acid.

L-Glutamine 1000 - GNC A-Z **-** GNC
Each tablet contains: L-glutamine 1000 mg. Other Ingredients: Dicalcium Phosphate, Cellulose.

L-glutamine 1000 mg (Now Sports) **-** Now
Each capsule contains: L-Glutamine (free-form) 1 g. Other Ingredients: Gelatin (capsule), Stearic Acid, Magnesium Stearate, Silica.

L-Glutamine 500 - GNC A-Z **-** GNC
Each capsule contains: L-Glutamine 500 mg. Other Ingredients: Dicalcium Phosphate, Gelatin.

L-Glutamine Free Form Vegetarian (Now Sports) **-** Now
Each 1/4 level tsp serving contains: L-Glutamine 750 mg.

L-Glutamine Plus **-** Atrium Inc.
Each tablet contains: L-Glutamine (an essential amino acid) 300 mg • L-Tryosine (an essential amino acid) 100 mg • Raw Bovine Adrenal concentrate 50 mg • Calcium Ascorbate (Vitamin C) 100 mg.
See Editor's Note No. 14.

L-Glutamine Powder **-** PhysioLogics
Each level teaspoon (3.3 g) contains: L-Glutamine 3.3 g.

LHB (Lipase Herbal Blend) **-** Global Health Trax
Each capsule contains: Chromium (as chromium picolinate, chromium polynicotinate) 50 mcg • Garcinia (whole plant) 125 mg • Bladderwrack (algae) 38 mg • California Nettles (whole plant) 38 mg • Plantain leaf 38 mg • Northern Prickly Ash bark 38 mg • Nature's Turn Enzyme Blend 73 mg: Protease 4.5 (30,000 HUT), Lipase (200 FCCLU), Amylase (3000 DU), Cellulase • Fenugreek seed 20 mg. Other Ingredients: Soy Lecithin Oil Blend, Gelatin, Water.

Libilov for Men **-** Nutrica, Inc.
Each tablet contains: Tribulus Terrestris leaf extract 250 mg • Ginkgo Biloba leaf extract 20 mg. Other Ingredients: Corn Starch, Hydroxypropyl Methylcellulose (HPMC), Colloidal Silicon Dioxide, Microcrystalline Cellulose, Dibasic Calcium Phosphate Dihydrate, Croscarmellose Sodium, Methyl Paraben, Propyl Paraben, Magnesium Stearate, Titanium Dioxide, Talc, Polyethylene Glycol.

Libilov with L-Arginine **-** Nutrica, Inc.
Each tablet contains: Tribulus Terrestris leaf extract 250 mg • Gingko Biloba leaf extract 20 mg • L-Arginine 250 mg. Other Ingredients: Corn Starch, Hydroxypropyl Methylcellulose (HPMC), Colloidal Silicon Dioxide, Microcrystalline Cellulose, Dibasic Calcium Phosphate Dihydrate, Croscarmellose Sodium, Methyl Paraben,

Propyl Paraben, Magnesium Stearate, Titanium Dioxide, Talc, Polyethylene Glycol.

Lice Treatment & Prevention: Herbal Hair Oil **-** The Herbalist
Pure essential oils of Rosemary • Lavender • Bay • Sage • Formulated with botanical extracts of Nettles leaf • Burdock root • Red Clover blossom • Chaparral leaf. In a base of cold-pressed oils of Sweet Almond and Jojoba.

Licorice **-** Nature's Way
Three capsules contain: Licorice root 1.35 g. Other Ingredients: Gelatin.

Licorice Garlic **-** Atrium Inc.
Each capsule contains: Licorice root 250 mg • Garlic 260 mg.

Life Essentials Dietary Supplement **-** Pharmanex
Each capsule contains: Vitamin A (as vitamin A palmitate, 29% as beta carotene from dunaliella salina) 3500 IU • Vitamin C (as ascorbic acid, acerola cherry extract) 70 mg • Vitamin D (as cholecalciferol) 200 IU • Vitamin E (as d-alpha tocopheryl succinate, beta, gamma, delta tocopherols) 30 IU • Thiamin (as thiamine mononitrate) 0.75 mg • Riboflavin 0.85 mg • Niacin (as niacinamide) 10 mg • Vitamin B-6 (as pyridoxine hydrochloride, pyridoxal-5-phosphate) 1 mg • Folic Acid 200 mcg • Vitamin B-12 (as cyanocobalamin) 3 mcg • Biotin 75 mcg • Pantothenic Acid (as D-calcium pantothenate) 5 mg • Calcium (as calcium carbonate, calcium chelate) 100 mg • Iron (as iron chelate) 1.5 mg • Iodine (as potassium iodide) 37.5 mcg • Magnesium (as magnesium chelate, magnesium citrate, magnesium oxide) 50 mg • Zinc (as zinc chelate) 7.5 mg • Selenium (as L-selenomethionine) 17.5 mcg • Copper (as copper chelate) 1 mg • Manganese (as manganese chelate) 1.75 mg • Chromium (as chromium chelate) 60 mcg • Molybdenum (as molybdenum chelate) 37.5 mcg • Potassium (as potassium chloride) 40 mg • Boron (as boron citrate) 0.5 mg • Horsetail extract 75 mg.

Life Extension 7-Keto DHEA **-** Life Extension
Each capsule contains: 7-Keto DHEA (3-acetyl-7-oxo-dehydroepiandrosterone) 25 mg. Other Ingredients: Rice Flour, Gelatin.

Life Extension Mix Caps **-** Life Extension
Fourteen capsules contain: Vitamin A (50% as natural D. salina beta-carotene/mixed carotenoids, 50% as acetate) 10,000 IU • Alpha-Carotene 89 mcg • Zeaxanthin 18 mcg • Cryptoxanthin 24 mcg • Lutein 12 mcg • Vitamin C (as ascorbic acid, calcium ascorbate, ascorbyl palmitate, magnesium ascorbate, niacinamide ascorbate, acerola juice powder) 2605 mg • Vitamin D (D3, as cholecalciferol) 400 IU • Vitamin E (as natural d-alpha tocopheryl succinate) 400 IU • Thiamine (vitamin B1, as thiamine hydrochloride) 125 mg • Riboflavin (vitamin B2, with riboflavin 5-phosphate coenzyme 2 mg) 50 mg • Niacin (vitamin B3, as 53% niacinamide, 40% niacin, 7% niacinamide ascorbate) 187 mg • Vitamin B6 (as pyridoxine HCl with pyridoxal 5' phosphate coenzyme 2.5 mg) 100 mg • Folic Acid 800 mcg • Vitamin B12 (as 42% cyanocobalamin, 42% hydroxylcobalamin, 14% ion exchange resin) 600 mcg • Biotin 3000 mcg • Pantothenic Acid (as d-calcium pantothenate with pantethine 5 mg) 600 mg • Calcium (as calcium ascorbate, calcium pantothenate, calcium d-glucarate) 227 mg • Iodine (as potassium iodine) 75 mg • Magnesium (oxide 260.96 elemental, citrate 15.66 elemental, aspartate 19.62 mg elemental, glycinate 11.74 mg elemental, taurinate 7.83 mg elemental, arginate 5.87 mg elemental, ascorbate 3.40 mg elemental) 325 mg • Zinc (as methionate, zinc succinate) 35 mg • Selenium (as 50% se-methylselenocysteine, 25% selenomax, l-selenomethionine in a base of dicalcium phosphate, 25% sodium selenate) 200 mcg • Copper (as copper amino acid chelate) 1 mg • Manganese (as manganese gluconate) 3 mg • Chromium (as chromium polynicotinate) 200 mcg • Molybdenum (as sodium molybdate) 125 mcg • Potassium (as potassium chloride, aspartate) 37.4 mg • Lysine (as l-lysine HCl) 500 mg • N-Acetyl-Cysteine (NAC) 600 mg • Taurine 500 mg • Choline (as choline bitartrate) 117.5 mg • Inositol 250 mg • Phosphatidylcholine (from soy) 150 mg • Bromelain (from pineapple, 2400 GDU per gram) 15 mg • Para-Aminobenzoic Acid (PABA) 200 mg • Trimethylglycine (TMG, as betaine anhydrous, from sugar beets) 100 mg • Bilberry berry extract (baccinium myrtillus, standardized for 25% anthocyanidins 7.5 mg) 30 mg • Citrus Bioflavonoid complex (hesperidin, citrus aurantium 470 mg, naringin 140 mg, naringenin 7-b-rutinoside/others 10 mg) 1300 mg • Ascorbyl Palmitate (fat soluble vitamin C) 250 mg • Ginger root extract (zingiber officinale, 5% gingerols 10 mg) 200 mg • Grapeseed extract (vitis vinifera, inner core of fruit, 95% proanthocyanidins 23.75 mg) 25 mg • Grape extract (vitis vinifera L.) 25 mg providing the following typical profile of active ingredients: proanthycyanidins [95%, includes dimeric procyanidins 1.25 mg] 23.75 mg, anthocyanidins [5%] 1.25 mg, trans-resveratrol >500 ppm, cis-resveratrol <100 ppm) 25 mg • Milk Thistle seeds extract (silybum marianus, standardized for 85% silymarin 85 mg) 100 mg • Dilaurylthiodipropionate 25 mg • Thiodiproprionic Acid 25 mg • Acerola juice powder extract 1:4 (malpighia punicifolia l.) 300 mg • Alpha-Carotene 1000 IU • Broccoli concentrate complex (proprietary blend: broccoli concentrate, calcium d-glucarate, providing sulphoraphane 1.5 mg) 500 mg • Calcium D-Glucarate 200 mg • Boron (as boron citrate/asparate/glycinate) 3 mg • Labiatae plants extract (from rosemary, thyme, sage) 300 mg • Typical Profile (to equal 4.5-8.5% total flavones, 13.5-25.5 mg): Apigenin-7-Glucoside (3.5-5%) 10.5-15 mg, Apigenin (0.0-1%) 0-3 mg, Luteolin (0.5-1%) 1.5-3 mg, Other Flavones (0.5-1.5%) 1.4-4.5 mg • Lutein (purified concentrate from marigold flowers, tagetes erecta, providing zeaxanthin 99 mcg) 15 mg • Lycopene (from tomato skin extract) 3 mg • Raspberry leaf extract (rubus idaeus, standardized for 38.45% ellagic acid 50 mg) 130 mg. Other Ingredients: Magnesium Stearate. See Editor's Note No. 40, page 2058.

Life Extension Mix Powder w/Stevia **-** Life Extension
Fourteen capsules contain: Vitamin A (50% as natural D. salina beta-carotene/mixed carotenoids, 50% as acetate) 10,000 IU • Alpha-Carotene 89 mcg • Zeaxanthin 18 mcg • Cryptoxanthin 24 mcg • Lutein 12 mcg • Vitamin C (as ascorbic acid, calcium ascorbate, ascorbyl palmitate, magnesium ascorbate, niacinamide ascorbate, acerola juice powder) 2605 mg • Vitamin D (D3, as cholecalciferol) 400 IU • Vitamin E (as natural d-alpha tocopheryl succinate) 400 IU • Thiamine (vitamin B1, as thiamine hydrochloride) 125 mg • Riboflavin (vitamin B2, with riboflavin 5-phosphate coenzyme 2 mg) 50 mg • Niacin (vitamin B3, as 53% niacinamide, 40% niacin, 7% niacinamide ascorbate) 187 mg • Vitamin B6 (as pyridoxine HCl with pyridoxal 5' phosphate coenzyme 2.5 mg) 100 mg • Folic Acid 800 mcg • Vitamin B12 (as 42% cyanocobalamin, 42% hydroxylcobalamin, 14% ion exchange resin) 600 mcg • Biotin 3000 mcg • Pantothenic Acid (as d-calcium pantothenate with pantethine 5 mg) 600 mg • Calcium (as calcium ascorbate, calcium pantothenate, calcium d-glucarate) 227 mg • Iodine (as potassium iodine) 75 mg • Magnesium (oxide 260.96 elemental, citrate 15.66 elemental, aspartate 19.62 mg elemental, glycinate 11.74 mg elemental, taurinate 7.83 mg elemental, arginate 5.87 mg elemental, ascorbate 3.40 mg elemental) 325 mg • Zinc (as methionate, zinc succinate) 35 mg • Selenium (as 50% se-methylselenocysteine, 25% selenomax, l-selenomethionine in a base of dicalcium phosphate, 25% sodium selenate) 200 mcg • Copper (as copper amino acid chelate) 1 mg • Manganese (as manganese gluconate) 3 mg • Chromium (as chromium polynicotinate) 200 mcg • Molybdenum (as sodium molybdate) 125 mcg • Potassium (as potassium chloride, aspartate) 37.4 mg • Lysine (as l-lysine HCl) 500 mg • N-Acetyl-Cysteine (NAC) 600 mg • Taurine 500 mg • Choline (as choline bitartrate) 117.5 mg • Inositol 250 mg • Phosphatidylcholine (from soy) 150 mg • Bromelain (from pineapple, 2400 GDU per gram) 15 mg • Para-Aminobenzoic Acid (PABA) 200 mg • Trimethylglycine (TMG, as betaine anhydrous, from sugar beets) 100 mg • Bilberry berry extract (baccinium myrtillus, standardized for 25% anthocyanidins 7.5 mg) 30 mg • Citrus Bioflavonoid complex (hesperidin, citrus aurantium 470 mg, naringin 140 mg, naringenin 7-b-rutinoside/others 10 mg) 1300 mg • Ascorbyl Palmitate (fat soluble vitamin C) 250 mg •

BRAND NAMES

Ginger root extract (zingiber officinale, 5% gingerols 10 mg) 200 mg • Grapeseed extract (vitis vinifera, inner core of fruit, 95% proanthocyanidins 23.75 mg) 25 mg • Grape extract (vitis vinifera L.) 25 mg providing the following typical profile of active ingredients: proanthycyanidins [95%, includes dimeric procyanidins 1.25 mg] 23.75 mg, anthocyanidins [5%] 1.25 mg, trans-resveratrol >500 ppm, cis-resveratrol <100 ppm) 25 mg • Milk Thistle seeds extract (silybum marianus, standardized for 85% silymarin 85 mg) 100 mg • Dilaurylthiodipropionate 25 mg • Thiodiproprionic Acid 25 mg • Acerola juice powder extract 1:4 (malpighia punicifolia l.) 300 mg • Alpha-Carotene 1000 IU • Broccoli concentrate complex (proprietary blend: broccoli concentrate, calcium d-glucarate, providing sulphoraphane 1.5 mg) 500 mg • Calcium D-Glucarate 200 mg • Boron (as boron citrate/asparate/glycinate) 3 mg • Labiatae plants extract (from rosemary, thyme, sage) 300 mg • Typical Profile (to equal 4.5-8.5% total flavones, 13.5-25.5 mg): Apigenin-7-Glucoside (3.5-5%) 10.5-15 mg, Apigenin (0.0-1%) 0-3 mg, Luteolin (0.5-1%) 1.5-3 mg, Other Flavones (0.5-1.5%) 1.4-4.5 mg • Lutein (purified concentrate from marigold flowers, tagetes erecta, providing zeaxanthin 99 mcg) 15 mg • Lycopene (from tomato skin extract) 3 mg • Raspberry leaf extract (rubus idaeus, standardized for 38.45% ellagic acid 50 mg) 130 mg. Other Ingredients: Stevia, Natural Orange Color, Lecithin Powder.
See Editor's Note No. 40, page 2058.

Life Extension Mix Tabs **-** Life Extension
Nine tablets contain: Vitamin A (50% as natural D. salina beta-carotene/mixed carotenoids, 50% as acetate) 10,000 IU • Alpha-Carotene 89 mcg • Zeaxanthin 18 mcg • Cryptoxanthin 24 mcg • Lutein 12 mcg • Vitamin C (as ascorbic acid, calcium ascorbate, ascorbyl palmitate, magnesium ascorbate, niacinamide ascorbate, acerola juice powder) 2605 mg • Vitamin D (D3, as cholecalciferol) 400 IU • Vitamin E (as natural d-alpha tocopheryl succinate) 400 IU • Thiamine (vitamin B1, as thiamine hydrochloride) 125 mg • Riboflavin (vitamin B2, with riboflavin 5-phosphate coenzyme 2 mg) 50 mg • Niacin (vitamin B3, as 53% niacinamide, 40% niacin, 7% niacinamide ascorbate) 187 mg • Vitamin B6 (as pyridoxine HCl with pyridoxal 5' phosphate coenzyme 2.5 mg) 100 mg • Folic Acid 800 mcg • Vitamin B12 (as 42% cyanocobalamin, 42% hydroxylcobalamin, 14% ion exchange resin) 600 mcg • Biotin 3000 mcg • Pantothenic Acid (as d-calcium pantothenate with pantethine 5 mg) 600 mg • Calcium (as calcium ascorbate, calcium panothenate, calcium d-glucarate) 227 mg • Iodine (as potassium iodine) 75 mg • Magnesium (oxide 260.96 elemental, citrate 15.66 elemental, aspartate 19.62 mg elemental, glycinate 11.74 mg elemental, taurinate 7.83 mg elemental, arginate 5.87 mg elemental, ascorbate 3.40 mg elemental) 325 mg • Zinc (as methionate, zinc succinate) 35 mg • Selenium (as 50% se-methylselenocysteine, 25% selenomax, l-selenomethionine in a base of dicalcium phosphate, 25% sodium selenate) 200 mcg • Copper (as copper amino acid chelate) 1 mg • Manganese (as manganese gluconate) 3 mg • Chromium (as chromium polynicotinate) 200 mcg • Molybdenum (as sodium molybdate) 125 mcg • Potassium (as potassium chloride, aspartate) 37.4 mg • Lysine (as l-lysine HCl) 500 mg • N-Acetyl-Cysteine (NAC) 600 mg • Taurine 500 mg • Choline (as choline bitartrate) 117.5 mg • Inositol 250 mg • Phosphatidylcholine (from soy) 150 mg • Bromelain (from pineapple, 2400 GDU per gram) 15 mg • Para-Aminobenzoic Acid (PABA) 200 mg • Trimethylglycine (TMG, as betaine anhydrous, from sugar beets) 100 mg • Bilberry berry extract (baccinium myrtillus, standardized for 25% anthocyanidins 7.5 mg) 30 mg • Citrus Bioflavonoid complex (hesperidin, citrus aurantium 470 mg, naringin 140 mg, naringenin 7-b-rutinoside/others 10 mg) 1300 mg • Ascorbyl Palmitate (fat soluble vitamin C) 250 mg • Ginger root extract (zingiber officinale, 5% gingerols 10 mg) 200 mg • Grapeseed extract (vitis vinifera, inner core of fruit, 95% proanthocyanidins 23.75 mg) 25 mg • Grape extract (vitis vinifera L.) 25 mg providing the following typical profile of active ingredients: Proanthocyanidins (95%, includes dimeric procyanidins 1.25 mg) 23.75 mg, Anthocyanidins (5%) 1.25 mg, Trans-Resveratrol >500 ppm, Cis-Resveratrol <100 ppm • Milk Thistle seeds extract (silybum marianus, standardized for 85% silymarin 85 mg) 100 mg • Dilaurylthiodipropionate 25 mg • Thiodiproprionic Acid 25 mg • Acerola juice powder extract 1:4 (malpighia punicifolia l.) 300 mg • Alpha-Carotene 1000 IU • Broccoli concentrate complex (proprietary blend: broccoli concentrate, calcium d-glucarate, providing sulphoraphane 1.5 mg) 500 mg • Calcium D-Glucarate 200 mg • Boron (as boron citrate/asparate/glycinate) 3 mg • Labiatae plants extract (from rosemary, thyme, sage) 300 mg • Typical Profile (to equal 4.5-8.5% total flavones, 13.5-25.5 mg): Apigenin-7-Glucoside (3.5-5%) 10.5-15 mg, Apigenin (0.0-1%) 0-3 mg, Luteolin (0.5-1%) 1.5-3 mg, Other Flavones (0.5-1.5%) 1.4-4.5 mg • Lutein (purified concentrate from marigold flowers, tagetes erecta, providing zeaxanthin 99 mcg) 15 mg • Lycopene (from tomato skin extract) 3 mg • Raspberry leaf extract (rubus idaeus, standardized for 38.45% ellagic acid 50 mg) 130 mg. Other Ingredients: Microcrystalline Cellulose, Stearic Acid, Magnesium Stearate, Croscarmellose Sodium, Silica, Pharmaceutical Glaze.
See Editor's Note No. 40, page 2058.

Life Extension One-Per-Day Tablets **-** Life Extension
Each tablet contains: Vitamin A (as beta-carotene 20, as palmitate 80%) 5000 IU • Vitamin C (as niacinamide and calcium ascorbates, ascorbic acid) 500 mg • Vitamin D (as cholecalciferol) 200 IU • Vitamin E (as D-alpha-tocopheryl succinate) 200 IU • Thiamine (vitamin B1, as thiamine HCl) 75 mg • Riboflavin (vitamin B2) 50 mg • Niacin (vitamin B3, as niacinamide ascorbate) 50 mg • Vitamin B6 (as pyridoxine HCl) 75 mg • Folate (as folic acid) 800 mcg • Vitamin B12 (as cyanocobalamin) 300 mcg • Pantothenic Acid (as D-calcium pantothenate) 100 mg • Calcium (from D-calcium pantothenate, calcium ascorbate) 20 mg • Iodine (from Atlantic kelp) 150 mcg • Magnesium (as magnesium oxide) 100 mg • Zinc (as OptiZinc R zinc DL-methionine complex) 30 mg • Selenium (as L-selenomethionine) 100 mcg • Manganese (as manganese gluconate) 2 mg • Chromium (as chromium polynicotinate) 200 mcg • Molybdenum (as molybdenum amino acid chelate) 100 mcg • Potassium (as potassium citrate) 25 mg • Alpha-Carotene 50 mcg • Boron (as boron amino acid chelate) 3 mg • Choline (bitartrate) 22.9 mg • Inositol 50 mg • Xantopina R plus Lutein extract (from marigold cempasuchil flowers (tagetes erectus L.) standardized for 40% lutein (5 mg), 4% zeaxanthin (0.5 mg)) 12.5 mg • Lycopene (as Lyc-O-Mato tomato extract) 2 mg • PABA (para-aminobenzoic acid) 2 mg • Biotin 300 mcg. Other Ingredients: Dicalcium Phosphate, Microcrystalline Cellulose, Maltodextrin, Stearic Acid, Magnesium Stearate, Croscarmellose Sodium, Silicon Dioxide, Purified Water, Methylcellulose, Propylene Glycol.

Life Extension Two-Per-Day Tablets **-** Life Extension
Two tablets contain: Vitamin A (as beta-carotene 20, as palmitate 80%) 5000 IU • Vitamin C (as niacinamide and calcium ascorbates, ascorbic acid) 500 mg • Vitamin D (as cholecalciferol) 400 IU • Vitamin E (as D-alpha-tocopheryl succinate) 200 IU • Thiamine (vitamin B1, as thiamine HCl) 75 mg • Riboflavin (vitamin B2) 50 mg • Niacin (vitamin B3, as niacinamide ascorbate) 50 mg • Vitamin B6 (as pyridoxine HCl) 75 mg • Folate (as folic acid) 800 mcg • Vitamin B12 (as cyanocobalamin) 300 mcg • Biotin 300 mcg • Pantothenic Acid (as D-calcium pantothenate, calcium ascorbate) 20 mg • Iodine (from Atlantic kelp) 150 mcg • Magnesium (as magnesium oxide) 100 mg • Zinc (as OptiZinc zinc DL-methionine complex) 30 mg • Selenium (as L-selenomethionine) 100 mcg • Manganese (as manganese gluconate) 2 mg • Chromium (as chromium polynicotinate) 200 mcg • Molybdenum (as molybdenum amino acid chelate) 100 mcg • Potassium (as potassium citrate) 25 mg • Alpha-Carotene 50 mcg • Boron (as boron amino acid chelate) 3 mg • Choline (bitartrate) 22.9 mg • Inositol 50 mg • Xantopina plus Lutein extract (from marigold cempasuchil flowers (tagetes erectus L.), standardized for 40% lutein (5 mg), 4% zeaxanthin (0.5mg)) 12.5 mg • Lycopene (as Lyc-O-Mato tomato extract) 2 mg • PABA (para-aminobenzoic acid) 30 mg. Other Ingredients: Dicalcium Phosphate, Microcrystalline Cellulose, Maltodextrin, Stearic Acid, Magnesium Stearate, Croscarmellose Sodium, Silicon Dioxde, Purified Water, Methylcellulose, Propylene Glycol.

Life Force Multiple **-** Source Naturals
Two tablets contain: Vitamin A (beta carotene) 7500 IU • Vitamin A (palmitate) 5000 IU • Total Vitamin A activity 12500 IU • Vitamin B-1 (thiamin) 50 mg • Vitamin B-2 (riboflavin) 50 mg • Niacinamide 35 mg • Niacin 15 mg • Vitamin B-5 (pantothenic acid) 50 mg • Vitamin B-6 (pyridoxine HCl) 50 mg • Vitamin B-12 (cyanocobalamin) 100 mcg • Biotin 150 mcg • Folic Acid 400 mcg • Vitamin C (ascorbic acid crystals, ascorbyl palmitate) 500 mg • Vitamin D-3 (cholecalciferol) 200 IU • Vitamin E D-alpha Tocopheryl (natural) 200 IU • Boron (amino acid chelate) 2 mg • Calcium (chelate, citrate, malate) 100 mg • Chromium (ChromeMate yeast-free polynicotinate) 100 mcg • Copper (sebacate) 1 mg • Iodine (from kelp) 100 mcg • Iron (fumarate) 6 mg • Magnesium (chelate, citrate, oxide) 100 mg • Manganese (citrate) 3 mg • Molybdenum (amino acid chelate) 100 mcg • Potassium (citrate) 50 mg • Selenium (L-Selenomethionine and sodium selenite) 100 mcg • Zinc (citrate and OptiZinc monomethionine) 15 mg. Other Ingredients: Coenzyme Q10 (ubiquinone) 20mg, Alpha-Lipoic Acid (thioctic acid) 25 mg, N-Acetyl Cysteine 100 mg, DMAE (bitartrate) 30 mg, Silymarin (milk thistle seed extract) 60 mg, Ginkgo Biloba 24% (50:1 extract) 20 mg, Choline (bitartrate) 50 mg, Inositol 50mg , Hawthorn berry 75 mg, Turmeric root 75 mg, Bilberry fruit extract standardized to 25% anthocyanidins 10 mg, Proanthodyn (grape seed extract) 25 mg, L-Tyrosine 50 mg, Methylsulfonylmethane 25 mg, Bioperine 3 mg.

Life Force Multiple No Iron **-** Source Naturals
Two tablets contain: Vitamin A (beta carotene) 7500 IU • Vitamin A (palmitate) 5000 IU • Total Vitamin A activity 12500 IU • Vitamin B-1 (thiamin) 50 mg • Vitamin B-2 (riboflavin) 50 mg • Niacinamide 35 mg • Niacin 15 mg • Vitamin B-5 (pantothenic acid) 50 mg • Vitamin B-6 (pyridoxine HCl) 50 mg • Vitamin B-12 (cyanocobalamin) 100 mcg • Biotin 150 mcg • Folic acid 400 mcg • Vitamin C (ascorbic acid crystals, ascorbyl palmitate) 500 mg • Vitamin D-3 (cholecalciferol) 200 IU • Vitamin E D-alpha Tocopheryl (natural) 200 IU • Boron (amino acid chelate) 2 mg • Calcium (chelate, citrate, malate) 100 mg • Chromium (ChromeMate yeast-free polynicotinate) 100 mcg • Copper (sebacate) 1 mg • Iodine (from kelp) 100 mcg • Magnesium (chelate, citrate, oxide) 100 mg • Manganese (citrate) 3 mg • Molybdenum (amino acid chelate) 100 mcg • Potassium (citrate) 50 mg • Selenium (L-Selenomethionine and sodium selenite) 100 mcg • Zinc (citrate and OptiZinc monomethionine) 15 mg. Other Ingredients: Coenzyme Q10 (ubiquinone) 20mg, Alpha-Lipoic Acid (thioctic acid) 25 mg, N-Acetyl Cysteine 100 mg, DMAE (bitartrate) 30 mg, Silymarin (milk thistle seed extract) 60 mg, Ginkgo Biloba 24% (50:1 extract) 20 mg, Choline (bitartrate) 50 mg, Inositol 50mg , Hawthorn berry 75 mg, Turmeric root 75 mg, Bilberry fruit extract standardized to 25% anthocyanidins 10 mg, Proanthodyn (grape seed extract) 25 mg, L-Tyrosine 50 mg, Methylsulfonylmethane 25 mg, Bioperine 3 mg.

Life Minerals **-** Source Naturals
Four tablets contain: Calcium (Citrate, Fumarate, Malate, Succinate and alpha-Ketoglutarate) 480 mg • Magnesium (Citrate, Fumarate, Malate, Succinate and alpha-Ketoglutarate) 480 mg • Potassium (Citrate, Malate, Fumarate, Succinate, and alpha-Ketoglutarate) 99 mg • Zinc (OptiZinc Zinc Monomethionine 20 mg and Ascorbate 10 mg) 30mg • Chromium (ChromeMate GTF Chromium Polynicotinate) 300 mcg • Selenium (Selenomethionine and Sodium Selenite) 200 mcg • Iron (Fumarate, Citrate and Succinate) 15 mg • Boron(Amino Acid Chelate) 3 mg • Silica (Horsetail Silica extract) 4.5 mg • Iodine (from Kelp) 150 mcg • Copper (Sebacate) 2 mg • Molybdenum (Chelate) 300 mcg • Vitamin B-6 (Pyridoxine HCl) 10 mg • Vitamin C (Zinc and Manganese Ascorbates) 78 mg • Vitamin D-3 (Cholecalciferol) 200 IU.

Life Minerals-No Iron **-** Source Naturals
Four tablets contain: Calcium (Citrate, Fumarate, Malate, Succinate and alpha-Ketoglutarate) 480 mg • Magnesium (Citrate, Fumarate, Malate, Succinate and alpha-Ketoglutarate) 480 mg • Potassium (Citrate, Malate, Fumarate, Succinate, and alpha-Ketoglutarate) 99 mg • Zinc (OptiZinc Zinc Monomethionine 20 mg and Ascorbate 10 mg) 30 mg • Chromium (ChromeMate GTF Chromium Polynicotinate) 300 mcg • Selenium (Selenomethionine and Sodium Selenite) 200 mcg • Boron (Amino Acid Chelate) 3 mg • Silica (Horsetail Silica extract) 4.5 mg • Iodine (from Kelp) 150 mcg • Copper (Sebacate) 2 mg • Molybdenum (Chelate) 300 mcg • Vitamin B-6 (Pyridoxine HCl) 10 mg • Vitamin C (Zinc and Manganese Ascorbates) 78 mg • Vitamin D-3 (Cholecalciferol) 200 IU.

Life Spark **-** Source Naturals
Four tablets contain: Vitamin B1 (Thiamin) 30 mg • Vitamin B2 (Riboflavin) 30 mg • Vitamin B3 (Niacin 25 mg and Niacinamide 125 mg) 150 mg • Vitamin B5 (Pantothenic Acid) 100 mg • Vitamin B6 (Pyridoxine HCl) 25 mg • Vitamin B12 (Cyanocobalamin) 100 mcg • Vitamin E (D-Alpha Tocopheryl) (Natural) 150 IU • Magnesium (Oxide, Citrate) 250 mg • Potassium (Citrate) 99 mg • Glycine 500 mg • Tyrosine 250 mg • Coenzyme Q10 (Ubiquinone) 50 mg • Alpha-Lipoic Acid 25 mg • Herbal Blend 1170 mg: Siberian Ginseng, Panax Ginseng, Polygonum Multiflori (Fo Ti), Cyperus, Panax Ginseng extract, Tien Chi, and Siberian Ginseng extract.

LifeGuard Advanced Antioxidant **-** Starlight International
Each two tablets contain: Vitamin A (as beta carotene) 5000 IU • Vitamin C (as asorbic acid) 300 mg • Vitamin E (as d-alpha tocopheryl succintate) 30 IU • Zinc (as zinc picolinate) 50 mg • Selenium (as sodium selenite) 60 mcg • Bilberry extract 4:1 (vaccinium myrtillus, fruit) 400 mg • Green Tea extract 4:1 (carmellia sinensis, leaf) 150 mg • Turmeric (curcuma longa, rhizome) 150 mg • Pine Bark extract (pinus strobus, bark) 40 mg • Ginkgo Biloba extract (leaf) 24% Ginkgo flavone glycosides, 6% terpene lactones 20 mg • Garlic (allim salivum, root) deodorized 10 mg • Echinacea purpurea (plant) 10 mg • Goldenseal (hydrastis caradensis, plant) 2 mg. Inactive Ingredients: Croscarmellose Sodium, Dicalcium Phosphate, Hydroxpropylcellulose, Stearic Acid, Magnesium Stearate, Microcrystalline Cellulose, Calcium Carbonate, Calcium Sulfate, Silicon Dioxide, Dextrin, Dextrose, Lecithin, Sodium Citrate.

LifeGuard Cholesterol Control **-** Starlight International
Two tablets contain: Red Rice Yeast (Monascus purpureus, Plant) 800 mg • Fo-Ti (Polygonum multiforum, Plant) 50 mg • Soy 80 mg • Beta Sitosterol 100 mg • English Hawthorn (Crataegus laevigata, Fruit) 30 mg. Other Ingredients: Calcium Carbonate, Microcrystalline Cellulose, Stearic Acid, Croscarmellose Sodium, Magnesium Stearate, Silicon Dioxide, Hydroxypropylcellulose, Dextrin, Dextrose, Lecithin, Sodium Citrate.

LifeGuard Joint Formula **-** Starlight International
Three tablets contain: Manganese (as manganese ascorbate) 6 mg • Glucosamine HCl 750 mg • Chondroitin Sulfate, 95% 250 mg • MSM (methyl-sulfonyl-methane) 100 mg • Sulfate (sodium-sulfate) 30 mg • Turmeric, 90% curcumin (curcuma longa, root) 25 mg • Boswellia Serrata extract, 65% (boswellic acid, trunk) 25 mg. Other Ingredients: Dicalcium Phosphate, Microcrystalline Cellulose, Stearic Acid, Croscarmellose Sodium, Silicon Dioxide, Magnesium Stearate, Dextrin, Dextrose, Lecithin, Sodium Carboxymethylcellulose, Sodium Citrate.
See Editor's Note No. 15, page 2055.

LifeGuard Junior **-** Starlight International
Each two tablets contain: Vitamin A (as beta carotene) 1000 IU • Vitamin C (as sodium ascorbate) 100 mg • Vitamin E (as d-alpha tocopheryl acetate) 20 IU • Bilberry extract 4:1 (vaccinium myrtillus, fruit) 100 mg • Vegetable complex (tomato, carrot, cabbage, broccoli, and green pepper powder) 100 mg • Acerola (malpighia glabra, fruit) 75 mg • Rosehips powder (rosa canina, fruit) 25 mg • Grape Seed extract, 95% flavanols (vitis vinifera seed) 2 mg.

LifePak Prenatal **-** Pharmanex
Each packet contains: Vitamin/phytonutrient capsule: Vitamin A (vitamin A palmitate, 50% as beta carotene from dunaliella salina) 5000 IU • Vitamin C (calcium ascorbate) 150 mg • Vitamin D (D3, cholecalciferol) 200 IU • Vitamin E (D-alpha tocopheryl succinate) 75 IU • Vitamin K (K1, phytonadione) 20 mcg • Thiamin (thiamine

mononitrate) 1.7 mg • Riboflavin (riboflavin) 2 mg • Niacin (niacin, niacinamide) 20 mg • Vitamin B6 (pyridoxine hydrochloride) 2.5 mg • Folate (folic acid) 400 mcg • Vitamin B12 (cyanocobalamin) 8 mcg • Biotin (biotin) 150 mcg • Pantothenic Acid (D-calcium pantothenate) 10 mg • Inositol 250 mcg • Lutein (from marigold flower extract) 1 mg • Lycopene (from tomato extract) 0.5 mg. Mineral capsules (2): Calcium (calcium carbonate, calcium citrate, calcium chelate) 325 mg • Iron (iron chelate) 15 mg • Iodine (potassium iodide) 37.5 mcg • Magnesium (magnesium aspartate, magnesium oxide, magnesium chelate) 175 mg • Zinc (zinc chelate) 10 mg • Selenium (1-selenomethionine) 35 mcg • Copper (copper chelate) 1 mg • Manganese (manganese chelate) 1.5 mg • Chromium (chromium chelate) 90 mcg • Molybdenum (molybdenum chelate) 37.5 mcg • Inositol 250 mcg • Lycopene (from tomato extract) 0.5 mg • Lutein (from marigold flower extract) 1 mg • Boron (as boron citrate) 1.5 mg • Silicon (sodium metasilicate) 1.5 mg • Vanadium (vanadyl sulfate) 10 mcg. Other Ingredients: Maltodextrin, Sodium Carboxymethylcellulose, Magnesium Stearate.

LifePak Prime - Pharmanex
Each packet contains: Vitamin capsule: Vitamin A (as vitamin A palmitate, 83% as beta carotene from palm fruit and blakeslea trispora extracts) 7500 IU • Vitamin C (as calcium ascorbate) 250 mg • Vitamin D (as cholecalciferol) 300 IU • Vitamin E (as D-alpha tocopheryl acetate, beta, gamma, delta tocopherols, tocotrienols) 150 IU • Vitamin K (as phytonadione) 20 mcg • Thiamin 3.75 mg • Riboflavin (as riboflavin) 4.25 mg • Niacin (as niacin, niacinamide) 20 mg • Vitamin B6 (as pyridoxine hydrochloride) 5 mg • Folate (as folic acid) 300 mcg • Vitamin B12 (as cyanocobalamin) 30 mcg • Biotin (as biotin) 150 mcg • Pantothenic Acid (as D-calcium pantothenate) 15 mg • Calcium (as calcium carbonate, calcium ascorbate, tricalcium phosphate, calcium propionate) 500 mg • Phosphorus (as tricalcium phosphate) 100 mg • Iodine (as potassium iodide) 50 mcg. Mineral capsules (3): Magnesium (as magnesium chelate, magnesium oxide) 250 mg • Zinc (as zinc chelate) 10 mg • Selenium (as L-selenomethionine, sodium selenite) 70 mcg • Copper (as copper chelate) 0.5 mg • Manganese (as manganese chelate) 1 mg • Chromium (as chromium chelate) 100 mcg • Molybdenum (as molybdenum chelate) 37.5 mcg • Polyphenol and Flavonoid blend 100 mg • Catechins from Camellia Sinensis leaf extract (20:1) 45 mg • Grape seed extract (min. 92% polyphenols) 25 mg • Quercetin 25 mg • Citrus Bioflavonoids (from citrus fruits) 12.5 mg • Isoflavones (from soy extract) 2.5 mg • Glucosamine Hydrochloride 100 mg • Alpha-Lipoic Acid 25 mg • N-Acetyl-L-Cysteine 25 mg • Milk Thistle fruit extract (silybum marianum 80% silymar) 25 mg • Ginkgo Biloba 27/7 leaf extract (ginkgo biloba) 20 mg. Phytonutrient Capsule: Coenzyme Q-10 (ubiquinone) 10 mg • Inositol (as inositol) 5 mg • Silicon (as sodium metasilicate) 5 mg • Reduced L-Glutathione 5 mg • Lycopene (as lycopene) 2.5 mg • Alpha-Carotene (from palm fruit extract) 1 mg • Lutein (from marigold flower extract) 1 mg • Boron (as boron citrate) 1.5 mg • Vanadium (as vanadyl sulfate) 10 mcg. Other Ingredients: Gelatin, Microcrystalline Cellulose, Magnesium Stearate, Silicon Dioxide.

LifePak Teen - Pharmanex
Two capsules contain: Vitamin A (as vitamin A palmitate, 50% as beta carotene from blakeslea trispora) 5000 IU • Vitamin C (as calcium ascorbate) 100 mcg • Calcium (as calcium carbonate, calcium ascorbate) 250 mg • Iron (as iron chelate) 4.5 mg • Vitamin D (as cholecalciferol) 200 IU • Vitamin E (as mixed natural tocopherols) 50 IU • Vitamin K1 (as phytonadione) 20 mcg • Thiamin (as thiamine mononitrate) 1.5 mg • Riboflavin (as riboflavin) 1.7 mg • Niacin (as niacin, niacinamide) 20 mg • Vitamin B6 (as pyridoxine hydrochloride) 5 mg • Folate (as folic acid) 200 mcg • Vitamin B12 (as cyanocobalamin) 15 mcg • Biotin (as biotin) 150 mcg • Pantothenic Acid (as D-calcium pantothenate) 15 mg • Iodine (as potassium iodide) 37.5 mcg • Magnesium (as magnesium oxide, magnesium chelate) 100 mg • Zinc (as zinc chelate) 7.5 mg • Selenium (as L-selenomethionine, sodium selenite) 35 mcg • Copper (as copper chelate) 1 mg • Manganese (as manganese chelate) 2 mg • Chromium (as chromium chelate) 60 mcg • Molybdenum (as molybdenum chelate) 60 mcg • Boron (as boron citrate) 1.5 mg • Silicon (as sodium metasilicate) 1.5 mg • Vanadium (as vanadyl sulfate) 10 mcg. Other Ingredients: Microcrystalline Cellulose, Sodium Carboxymethyl Cellulose, Magnesium Stearate, Silicon Dioxide.

LifePak Trim (LifePak and TrimPak) - Pharmanex
Each LifePak packet contains: Vitamin A (as vitamin A palmitate, 6250 as beta carotene from palm fruit and blakeslea trispora extracts) 1250 IU • Vitamin C (as calcium ascorbate) 250 mg • Vitamin D (as cholecalciferol) 200 IU • Vitamin E (as D-alpha tocopheryl acetate, beta, gamma, delta tocopherols, tocotrienols) 150 IU • Vitamin K (as phytonadione) 20 mcg • Thiamin (as thiamine mononitrate) 2.75 mg • Riboflavin (as riboflavin) 4.25 mg • Niacin (as niacin, niacinamide) 20 mg • Vitamin B6 (as pyridoxine hydrochloride) 5 mg • Folate (as folic acid) 300 mcg • Vitamin B12 (as cyanocobalamin) 15 mcg • Biotin (as biotin) 150 mcg • Pantothenic Acid (as D-calcium pantothenate) 15 mg • Calcium (as calcium carbonate, calcium ascorbate, calcium propionate) 250 mg • Iodine (as potassium iodide) 50 mcg • Magnesium (as magnesium chelate, magnesium oxide) 125 mg • Zinc (as zinc chelate) 7.5 mg • Selenium (as L-selenomethionine, sodium selenite) 70 mcg • Copper (as copper chelate) 0.5 mg • Manganese (as manganese chelate) 1 mg • Chromium (as chromium chelate) 100 mcg • Molybdenum (as molybdenum chelate) 37.5 mcg. Each TrimPak packet contains: Chromium (as chromium chelate, chromium picolinate) 100 mcg • Garcinia Cambogia with Hydroxy Citric Acid 375 mg • Chitosan (from shellfish) PolmerPlex 1000 mg. Other Ingredients: Calcium Carbonate, Sodium Carboxymethylcellulose, Cellulose Powder, Magnesium Stearate, Maltodextrin.

Life's Greens - Puritan's Pride
Each scoop (8.8 g) contains: Green Organic Gluten-Free Grasses: Wheat Grass powder 350 mg • Barley grass powder 350 mg • Alfalfa grass powder 350 mg • Oat grass powder 350 mg. Blue-Green And Sea Algae: Spirulina 1,000 mg • Chlorella (cracked-cell) 350 mg • Dunaliella salina 40 mg • Nova Scotia Dulse 30 mg. Adapogenic And Support Herbs: Licorice root 100 mg • Siberian Ginseng (Eleuthrococcus senticosus) 60 mg • Suma (Pfaffia paniculata) 60 mg • Astragalus membraneceus 60 mg • Echinacea purpurea 60 mg • Powdered Ginger root 5 mg. Nutrient-Rich Superfoods: Lecithin 99% oil-free 2,000 mg • Wheat sprout powder 350 mg • Acerola berry juice powder 200 mg • Beet juice powder 200 mg • Spinach octacosanol 150 mg • Royal Jelly (5% 10-HDA) 150 mg • Bee Pollen 150 mg • Vitamin E (d'alpha tocopheryl succinate) 100 IU. Dairy-Free Probiotic Cultures (Total count, Non-dairy culture: 5.0 billion): Lactoacillus group (L. rhamnosus A, L. rhamnosus B, L. acidophilus, L. casei, L. delbrueckii subsp. bulgaricus) 3.5 billion • Bifidobacterium group (B. longum, B. breve) 1.0 billion • Streptococcus salivarius subsp. thermophilus 500 million. Natural Fibers: Flaxseed meal 500 mg • Apple Pectin and fiber 500 mg • Fructooligosaccharides (FOS) 500 mg. Standardized Bioflavonoid Extracts: Milk Thistle extract (silybum marianum: standardized for 80% silymarin) 60 mg • Ginkgo Biloba extract (standardized for 6% terpene: lactones & 24 % ginkgo flavoglycosides) 20 mg • Green Tea catechins (standadized for 60% catechins) 20 mg • Grape pip extract (92% proanthocyanidins) 20 mg • Bilberry extract (standardized to 25% anthocyanidins) 20 mg.

Lifezyme - Digestive Enzyme Complex - Life Extension
Each tablet contains: Acidophilus 75 mg • Bromelain 115 mg • Pepsin 30 mg • Papaya 105 mg • Malt Diastase 30 mg • Cellulase 10 mg • Lactase 2 mg • Amylase 15 mg • Protease 10 mg • Lipase 100 mg.

Lift Visage - Jevene
Aloe Vera • Aluminum Silicate • BHT • Ceteareth 20 • Cetearyl Alcohol • Cetyl Alcohol • Diazolidinyl Urea • Dimethicone • EDTA • Fragrance • Glycerin • Glyceryl Stearate • Glycolic Acid • Jojoba oil • Lactic Acid • Methylparaben • Mineral oil • Octyl Methoxycinnamate • PEG-40 Stearate • Potassium Hydroxide • Propylene Glycol •

Propylparaben • Salicylic Acid • Sodium Borate • Tocopheryl Acetate • Water • Xanthan Gum.

Liga-Pane **-** Nutri-Quest Rx
Each tablet contains: Shark Cartilage 50 mg • N-Acetyl Glucosamine 10 mg • Bromelain 10 mg • Valerian 50 mg • Feverfew 150 mg • Passion Flower 50 mg • Scullcap 25 mg • White Willow 100 mg • Magnesium Citrate 150 mg • Calcium Lactate 100 mg • Kava Kava 15 mg • Tumeric 10 mg • Vitamin B6 10 mg • Oregano 10 mg • Marjoram 10 mg • Thyme 10 mg • Basil powder 10 mg • Ginger 10 mg • Suma 10 mg • Manganese Chelate 15 mg • Molybdenum Chelate 50 mcg.

Light & Fit Energy Shake (Chocolate) **-** Earthrise Nutritionals, Inc.
Isolated Soy Protein • Rice Maltodextrin • Dutch processed Cocoa • Acacia Gum • Sucanat organic unrefined Sugar Cane juice • Natural Flavors • Tribasic Calcium Phosphate • Magnesium Oxide • Earthrise Spirulina • Soy Fiber • Dipotassium Phosphate • Xanthan Gum • Potassium Citrate • Soy Lecithin • Lemon Bioflavonoids • Microcrystalline Cellulose • Celluose Gum • Choline Bitartrate • Bee Pollen • Vitamin C (ascorbic acid) • Inositol • Stevia • Vitamin E (D-alpha tocopherol succinate) • Apple Pectin • Rice Bran • Oat Fiber • Genestra powdered whole Beer concentrate • Papain • Bromelain • Vitamin B3 (niacinamide) • Hesperidin complex • Rutin • Magna Sweet Licorice extract • PABA (para amino benzoic acid) • Zinc Oxide • Manganese Sulfate • Vitamin A Palmitate • D-Calcium Pantothenate • Ferrous Fumarate • Copper Sulfate • Vitamin B6 (pyridoxine HCl) • Vitamin B2 (riboflavin) • Vitamin B1 (thiamin HCl) • Grapefruit extract • Vitamin D (D3, cholecalciferol) • Folic Acid • Biotin • Chromium Chloride • Potassium Iodide • Sodium Molybdate • Sodium Selenite • Vitamin K • Vitamin B12 (cyanocobalamin).

Light & Fit Energy Shake (Vanilla) **-** Earthrise Nutritionals, Inc.
Isolated Soy Protein • Rice Maltodextrin • Acacia Gum • Sucanat organic unrefined Sugar Cane juice • Natural Flavors • Tribasic Calcium Phosphate • Magnesium Oxide • Earthrise Spirulina • Soy Fiber • Potassium Phosphate • Xanthan Gum • Potassium Citrate • Soy Lecithin • Lemon Bioflavonoids • Microcrystalline Cellulose • Celluose Gum • Choline Bitartrate • Bee Pollen • Vitamin C (ascorbic acid) • Inositol • Stevia • Vitamin E (D-alpha tocopherol succinate) • Apple Pectin • Rice Bran • Oat Fiber • Genestra powdered whole Beer concentrate • Papain • Bromelain • Vitamin B3 (niacinamide) • Hesperidin complex • Rutin • Magna Sweet Licorice extract • PABA (para amino benzoic acid) • Zinc Oxide • Manganese Sulfate • Vitamin A Palmitate • D-Calcium Pantothenate • Ferrous Fumarate • Copper Sulfate • Vitamin B6 (pyridoxine HCl) • Vitamin B2 (riboflavin) • Vitamin B1 (thiamin HCl) • Grapefruit extract • Vitamin D (D3, cholecalciferol) • Folic Acid • Biotin • Chromium Chloride • Potassium Iodide • Sodium Molybdate • Sodium Selenite • Vitamin K • Vitamin B12 (cyanocobalamin).

Light Appetite Formula **-** Earthrise Nutritionals, Inc.
Three caplets contain: Vitamin A 100 IU • Vitamin C 30 mcg • Thiamin 1.5 mg • Riboflavin 1.7 mg • Niacin 20 mg • Vitamin B6 30 mg • Vitamin B12 15 mcg • Calcium 20 mcg • Iron 1 mg • Iodine 225 mcg • Chromium 50 mcg • Sodium 24 mg • Potassium 26 mg • Proprietary Blend: Earthrise Spirulina, Natural Alfalfa Powder, Soy Lecithin, Apple Cider Vinegar, Sea Kelp, Bladderwrack, Plantain, L-Phenylalanine, Bromelain, Ascorbic Acid, Pyridoxine HCl, Gymnema Sylvester, Thiamin Mononitrate, Chromium Picolinate, Cyanocobalamin. Other Ingredients: D-Calcium Phosphate, Glyceryl Monostearate, Magnesium Stearate, Silica.

Lightly Salted Soynuts - Revival **-** Physicians Laboratories
Each 1/6 cup contains: Certified Isoflavone 10 mg. Other Ingredients: Soy Protein (whole roasted soybeans), Soybean Oil, Salt.

Line Assist Creme **-** Aspen Group, Inc.
Each gram contains: Tocopheryl Acetate 1% • Panthenol 1% • Ascorbyl Palmitate 0.3% • Water • Diisopropyl Adipate • Cetearyl Alcohol • Potassium Cetyl Phosphate • Retinyl Palmitate • Palmitate • Tocopherol • Dimethicone • Carbomer • Ammonium Hydroxide • Quaternium-15 • Disodium EDTA.

Liniment Virtue **-** Blessed Herbs
St. John's Wort flower • Comfrey root • Angelica root • Valerian root • Lobelia herb • Ginger root • Calendula flower • Arnica flower & herb • Cayenne pepper • Essential oils of Myrrh, Hyssop, Rosemary, Lavender & German Chamomile • Grain alcohol & Distilled Water.

Lioness Women's Sexual Libido Enhancer **-** Universal Products
Three capsules contain: Tribulus 667 mg • Muira Puama 427 mg • Catuaba bark 352 mg • Androstenedione 127 mg • L-Arginine 127 mg • Ginseng (Korean) 60 mg • Avena Sativa 60 mg • Natural Vitamin E 37 IU. Other Ingredients: Magnesium Stearate, Gelatin.
See Editor's Note No. 47, page 2058.

LipidEnz **-** Enzymes, Inc.
Each capsule contains: Chromium (50% from Chromium Polynicotinate and 50% from Chromium Picolinate) 100 mcg • Proprietary Blend 500 mg: Garcinia fruit rind extract, Garlic concentrate, Guggulipids extract, Globe Artichoke leaf extract • n-zimes Proprietary Blend 181 mg: Lipase, pHysioProtease. Other Ingredients: Cellulose, Water.

Lipo 6 **-** Nutrex, Inc.
Two liqui-caps contain: Synephrine HCl 20 mg • synthetic 99% Guggulsterones Z&E 1:1 20 mg • Yohimbe HCl 3 mg • Caffeine Anhydrous USP 200 mg • Bioperine Black Pepper extract 5 mg. Other Ingredients: Sesame Oil, Oleic Acid, Gelatin.
See Editor's Note No. 21, page 2056.

Lipo 6 Ephedra Free **-** Nutrex, Inc.
Two capsules contain: Citrus Aurantium 335 mg (total amines 7.5%, individual amines: synephrine 6%, N-methyl tyramine 0.9-1.6%, tyramine 0.2-0.4%, hordenine 0.2-0.4%, octopamine 0.2-0.4%) • Caffeine anhydrous USP 200 mg• Yohimbe HCl 250 mg • Coleus Forskohlii (standardized to 20% forskolin) 100 mg • Carnitrex L-Carnitine 100 mg • Bioperine Black Pepper extract 5 mg. Other Ingredients: Gelatin, L-Tartrate, Maltodextrin, Magnesium Stearate.
See Editor's Note No. 40, page 2058.

Lipo Trim **-** Now
Three tablets contain: Choline 1000 mg • Inositol 1000 mg • L-Methionine 500 mg • Taurine 250 mg • L-Carnitine 100 mg • Pyridoxine (B6) 10 mg • Chromium Picolinate 200 mcg.

Lipo-AMP **-** E'OLA
Each 0.7 mL spray contains: Vitamin B12 10 mcg • Proprietary Blend 188 mg: Ephedra (branch) Extract, Guarana (seed) Extract, Caffeine, Stevia (leaf) Extract, White Willow Bark Extract, Atractylodes (herb) Extract, Licorice (root) Extract, Dimethyl Amino Ethanol Bitartrate, Dibencozide. Other Ingredients: Purified Water, Fructose, Hydrochloric Acid, Natural and Artificial Peppermint Flavor, Lecithin, Potassium Sorbate, Sodium Benzoate.
See Editor's Note No. 30, page 2056.

Lipo-Complex **-** Progressive Labs
Each capsule contains: Pancreatic enzyme concentrate 400 mg (equivalent in enzymatic activity to 4X USP) • Pepsin 1:3000 (from Pepsin 1:10,000) 100 mg • Green Beet leaf powder 100 mg • Raw Liver concentrate 10 mg • Ox bile 10 mg..
See Editor's Note No. 14, page 2055.

Lipodrene **-** High Tech Pharmaceuticals
Each tablet contains: Proprietary Blend 660 mg: Sida Cordifolia leaves extract (supplying 25 mg ephedrine group alkaloides), Citrus Aurantium fruit 10%, Caffeine 100 mg, 5-Hydroxytryptophan (5HTP), Melatonin (5-methoxytryptamine), Green Tea leaves extract,

Cassia Nomame whole plant, Hoodia cactus 12:1 extract, Yohimbe bark 8% extract, Naringen fruit.
See Editor's Note No. 21 and No. 40, pages 2056 and 2058.

Lipodrene-SR **-** High Tech Pharmaceuticals
Each tablet contains: Proprietary Blend 272.5 mg: Citrus Aurantium fruit (12.5 mg synephrine), Hoodia cactus extract, Cassia Nomame extract, 6,6 Dihydroxy Bergaottin fruit, Yohimbe bark extract (1 mg yohimbe alkaloids), Naringen fruit, Commiphora Mukul root/resin, Coleus Forskolin root, Pilocarpus, Jaborandi leaves extract, L050 Hydroxy Tryptophan, 5-Hydroxy Tryptamine HCl • Caffeine (anhydrous) 75 mg • Thermo-RX Complex 250 mg: Green Tea leaves RM7343 extract, Acacia leaves 70% extract, Theobroma, Cocoa seed extract, Phenylethylamine HCl.
See Editor's Note No. 40, page 2058.

Lipoflavonoid **-** Numark Laboratories
Three caplets contain: Vitamin C 300 mg • Thiamine 1 mg • Riboflavin 1 mg • Niacin 10 mg • Vitamin B6 1 mg • Vitamin B12 5 mcg • Pantothenic Acid 5 mg • Choline 334 mg • Bioflavonoids 300 mg • Inositol 334 mg.

Lipoicare **-** PhysioLogics
Each capsule contains: Taurine 200 mg • Alpha-Lipoic Acid 25 mg • Calendula flower, Marigold (5% Lutein 3 mg; > 0.22% Zeaxanthin, 0.13 mg) 60 mg.

LipoKinetix **-** Syntrax Innovations
Each capsule contains: Phenylpropanolamine (PPA) 25 mg • Caffeine 100 mg • Yohimbine 3 mg • Diiodothyronine 100 mg • Sodium Usniate 100 mg.
See Editor's Note No. 11, page 2055.

Liposin **-** Metabolic Nutrition
Each capsule contains: Chitosan, pH modified 3000 mg • Psyllium husk 600 mg • Ascorbic acid 600 mg • L-Carnitine 450 mg • Glucomannan 150 mg.
See Editor's Note No. 37, page 2057.

Lipo-THIN **-** E'OLA
Each 0.7 mL spray contains: Chromium (as Chromium Chloride) 200 mcg • Proprietary Blend 132 mg: L-Carnitine, Green Tea (leaf) Extract, Dibencozide. Other Ingredients: Purified Water, Glycerin, Fructose, Polyglyceryl-10 Oleate, Hydroxylated Soy Lecithin, Potassium Sorbate, Natural and Artificial Flavors.

LipoTrol **-** Advocare International
Two caplets contain: Pyridoxine (as HCl) 2 mg • Zinc (as monomethionine - OptiZinc) 1 mg • Chromium (as polynicotinate - ChromeMate) 50 mcg • Garcinia extract (fruit - Garcinia cambogia) 1000 mg • Tulsi extract (leaf - ocimum sanctum) 25 mg • Taurine 25 mg • Beta-Sitosterol 12.5 mg • L-Carnitine 12.5 mg • Gymnema extract (leaf - gymnema sylvestre) 5 mg • Vanadium (as bis-maltolato-oxovanadium) 100 mcg. Other Ingredients: Dicalcium Phosphate, Silicon Dioxide, Cellulose, Stearic Acid, Magnesium Stearate.

Lipotrope **-** Progressive Labs
Each capsule contains: Vitamin C 50 mg • Vitamin B6 5 mg • Folate (folic acid) 200 mcg • Vitamin B12 200 mcg • Pantothenic Acid 60 mg • Magnesium Aspartate 25 mg • Milk Thistle (Silybum marianum) 100 mg • Choline Bitartrate 150 mg • Inositol 75 mg • Betaine HCl 60 mg • DL-Methionine 50 mg • Black Radish (Raphanus nigra) 50 mg • Green Beet leaf powder 50 mg • Celandine (Chelidonium majus) 15 mg • Chionanthus (Chionanthus virginica) 15 mg • PABA 25 mg.

Lipotropic Action **-** Puritan's Pride
Each capsule contains: Iodine (as potassium iodide) 25 mcg • Magnesium (as magnesium amino acid chelate) 8.3 mg • Selenium (as selenomethionine) 0.33 mcg • Manganese (as manganese amino acid chelate) 1.6 mg • Molybdenum (as molybdenum amino acid chelate) 8.33 mg • Potassium (as potassium amino acid chelate) 16.5 mg • Boron (as boron chelate) 0.33 mcg • Vanadium (as vanadium amino acid chelate) 0.33 mcg • Choline Bitartrate 35.46 mg • Inositol 25 mg • Ginger (zingiber officinale) root 25 mg • L-Methionine 16.67 mg • L-Carnitine (as L-carnitine fumarate) 16.67 mg • Beta Sitosterol 16.67 mg • Dandelion root (taraxacum officinale) 12.5 mg • Barberry (berberis vulgaris) root 12.5 mg • Turmeric (curcuma longa) root 12.5 mg • Milk Thistle (silybum marianum) seed 12.5 mg • Cinnamon (cinnamonum verum) bark 12.5 mg • Siberian Ginseng (eleutherococcus senticosus) root 8.33 mg • Gotu Kola (centella asiatica) aerial 8.33 mg • Fo-Ti (polygonum multiflorum) root 8.33 mg • Cayenne pepper (capsicum annuum) fruit 4.16 mg • DigeZyme enzyme complex: Anylase (1:2,000), Neutral Protease, Cellulase, Galactohydrolase Lactase, Lipase 50 mg.

Lipotropic Complex **-** Nature's Life
Three tablets contain: L-Methionine (Free-Form Amino Acid) 1000 mg • Choline (from 2040 mg Choline Bitartrate) 1000 mg • Inositol 1000 mg • Betaine HCl (Sugar Beets) 250 mg • Milk Thistle (Silybum marianum) 50 mg • Vitamin B6 (Pyridoxine Hydrochloride) 10 mg • L-Taurine (Free-Form Amino Acid) 10 mg • L-Carnitine (Free-Form Amino Acid) 10 mg • Lecithin (Soy) (61% Phosphatides) 10 mg • Beet root powder (Beta vulgaris rubra) 5 mg • Dandelion root powder (Taraxacum officinale) 5 mg • Culvers root powder (Leptandra virginica) 5 mg • Apple Cider Vinegar 5 mg • Barberry root bark (Berberis vulgaris) 5 mg • Chromium (Nutrition 21 Picolinate) 25 mcg.

Lipotropic Complex - Tyler **-** Integrative Therapeutics
Two capsules contain: Vitamin B6 (as pyridoxine hydrochloride USP) 25 mg • Folic Acid USP 100 mcg • Vitamin B12 (as cyanocobalamin USP) 25 mcg • Magnesium (as magnesium aspartate, oxide USP) 34 mg • L-Methionine USP 333 mg • Choline (as choline bitartrate) 192 mg • Black Radish root (Raphanus sativus-niger) 133 mg • Beet leaf (Beta vulgaris) 133 mg • Inositol 125 mg • Fringe Ttree root bark (Chionanthus virginicus) 100 mg • Dandelion root (Taraxacum officinale) 100 mg • Milk Thistle seed (silybum marianum) 100 mg • Celandine aerial parts extract (Chelidonium majus, 2.3% alkaloids) 37 mg • Ox Bile extract 25 mg • Milk Thistle seed extract (Silybum marianum, 80% silymarin) 12.7 mg. Other Ingredients: Ascorbyl Palmitate, Gelatin, Water.
See Editor's Note No. 14.

Lipotropic Fuel **-** TwinLab
Five capsules contain: Choline 500 mg • Inositol 250 mg • L-Methionine 100 mg • Vitamin B12 100 mcg • Betaine 100 mg • L-Carnitine 100 mg • Milk Thistle extract (standardized for 80% Silymarin) 500 mg • Natural Vitamin E (Succinate) 400 IU • Vitamin C 1000 mg • Vitamin B1 25 mg • N-Acetyl Cysteine (NAC) 250 mg • L-Glutathione 100 mg • Vitamin B2 25 mg • Selenium (from Selenomethionine) 150 mcg • Zinc (from Zinc Mono-Methionine) 15 mg.

Lipotropic Plus **-** Vitamin Express
Three tablets contain: Niacin (as nicotinic acid) 100 mg • Vitamin B12 (as cobalamin) 50 mcg • Betaine HCL 50 mg • Choline (as choline bitartrate) 450 mg • Clove 90 mg • DL-Methionine 1000 mg • Hawthorn Berry 30 mg • Inositol 1000 mg • Liver (from desiccated whole liver) 6 mg • Yucca 30 mg. Other Ingredients: Calcium Phosphate, Calcium Stearate, Cellulose, Lecithin, Silica, Stearic Acid.
See Editor's Note No. 14.

Lipovarin **-** Sterling-Grant Laboratories
Three tablets contain: Metabromine fruit extract (theobroma cacao, 6% theobromine 20 mg) 330 mg • 6% Theobromine 20 mg • Advantra Z Citrus Aurantium (10% total amines 35 mg) 350 mg • Green Tea leaf extract (camellia sinensis, 30% tea polyphenols 30 mg, 20% tea catechins 20 mg) 100 mg • Serotain (18.5% 5-hydroxytryptophan 45 mg) 250 mg • Caffeine 200 mg • Glucuronolactone 300 mg • Taurine 200 mg • L-Carnitine L-Tartrate 15 mg • 7-Keto (7-keto-dehydroepiandrosterone acetate) 50 mg • Coral Calcium 200 mg.
See Editor's Note No. 40, page 2058.

Some Brand Name Natural Products - What they Contain

www.NaturalDatabase.com contains MANY more listings than appear here.

BRAND NAMES

Lipovitan B3 Energy Drink **-** Taisho Pharmaceutical CA. Inc.
Carbonated Water • Sugar • Citric Acid • Taurine • Artificial Flavor • Sodium Citrate • Anhydrous Caffeine • Royal Jelly extract • Niacinamide • Riboflavin - 5 - Phosphorous (sodium) • Pyridoxine Hydrochloride • Thiamine Mononitrate.

Lipozyme **-** Young Living Essential Oils
Each capsule contains: Proprietary Blend: Lipase, Bee Pollen, Pancreatin, Tarragon Oil, Ginger Oil, Peppermint Oil, Juniper Oil, Fennel Oil, Lemongrass Oil, Anise Oil, Patchouli Oil.

Liqua B Complex 50 - GNC A-Z **-** GNC
Each capsule contains: Vitamin E (as d-alpha tocopherol) 2 IU • Thiamin (as thiamin mononitrate) 50 mg • Riboflavin 50 mg • Niacin (as niacinamide) 50 mg • Vitamin B6 (as pyridoxine hydrochloride) 50 mg • Folate (folic acid, folacin) 400 mcg • Vitamin B12 (as cyanocobalamin) 50 mcg • Biotin 50 mcg • Pantothenic Acid (as calcium d-pantothenate) 50 mg • Choline Bitartrate 50 mg • Inositol 50 mcg • Para-aminobenzoic Acid (PABA) 50 mg. Other Ingredients: Soybean Oil, Gelatin, Glycerin, Lecithin, Caramel Color, Titanium Dioxide, Korean Ginseng (panax ginseng).

Liqua Thin **-** E'OLA
Each 10 drops contain: Chromium 200 mcg • Proprietary Blend 155 mg: L-Carnitine, Green Tea (leaf) extract, Atractylodes (herb) extract, Choline Bitartrate, Dibencozide. Inactive Ingredients: Water, Hydrochloric Acid, Citric Acid, Glycerine, Sodium Benzoic Acid.

Liqui Lea **-** Shaklee
Each 1 tsp serving (5 mL) contains: Vitamin A (as vitamin A palmitate) 5000 IU • Vitamin D (as cholecalciferol) 400 IU • Vitamin E (as D-A-tocopheryl acetate) 15 IU • Thiamin (as thiamin hydrochloride) 2.1 mg • Riboflavin (as riboflavin sodium phosphate) 1.8 mg • Niacin (as niacinamide) 20 mg • Vitamin B6 (as pyridoxine hydrochloride) 2 mg • Vitamin B12 (as cyanocobalamin) 9 mcg • Biotin (as D-biotin) 300 mcg • Pantothenic Acid (as D-panthenol) 5 mg • Iron (as ferric ammonium citrate) 18 mg. Other Ingredients: Sorbitol, Natural Flavor, Glycerin, Purified Water, Sesame Oil, Soy Lecithin, Gum Ghatti, Citric.

Liquid Aminos **-** Puritan's Pride
Each softgel contains: L-Alanine 30 mg • L-Arginine 54 mg • L-Aspartic Acid 83 mg • L-Cysteine 10 mg • L-Glutamic Acid 145 mg • L-Glycine 33 mg • L-Histidine 20 mg • L-Isoleucine 35 mg • L-Leucine 60 mg • L-Lysine 59 mg • L-Methionine 9 mg • L-Phenylalanine 41 mg • L-Proline 38 mg • L-Serine 39 mg • L-Threonine 32 mg • L-Tryptophan 7 mg • L-Tyrosine 22 mg • L-Valine 33 mg.

Liquid Anti-Oxidant **-** Natrol
Two teaspoons (10 ml) contain: Anti-Oxidant Vitamins & Trace Minerals: Vitamin A (beta carotene) 10000 IU • Vitamin C (Calcium ascorbate) 500 mg • Vitamin E (acetate) 200 IU • Selenium (monomethionine) 90 mcg • Advanced Flavonoids: GP Complex+ 80 mg • Rutin, Quercetin, & Hesperidin 10 mg • Tropical fruit extracts from: Acerola, Cashew fruit, Passion fruit, Orange, Lime & Mango in a specially formulated base of: Purified Water, Brown Rice Syrup, Honey & Citric Acid.

Liquid B-Complex **-** GNC
Each dropperful (1 ml) contains: Riboflavin (as riboflavin-5-phosphate) 1.7 mg • Vitamin B6 (as pyrifoxine hydrochloride) 2 mg • Vitamin B12 (as cyanocobalamin) 1000 mcg • Pantothenic acid (as dexpanthenol) 30 mg. Other Ingredients: Purified Water, Glycerin, Fructose, Sorbitol, Natural Orange, Lemon, and Lime Flavors, Citric Acid, Stevia, Sodium Benzoate.

Liquid Calcium **-** Nature's Bounty
Three softgels contain: Vitamin A (as Retinyl Palmitate) 825 IU • Vitamin D (as Cholecalciferol) 180 IU • Calcium (as Calcium Carbonate) 600 mg. Other Ingredients: Soybean Oil, Gelatin, Glycerin, Lecithin, Titanium Dioxide Color.

Liquid Calcium Magnesium - NF Formulas **-** Integrative Therapeutics
Each tablespoon (15 mL) contains: Vitamin D (as ergocalciferol) 100 IU • Calcium (as calcium carbonate) 500 mg • Magnesium (as magnesium oxide) 500 mg • Boron (as boron oxide) 250 mcg. Other Ingredients: Deionized Water, Glycerin, Cellulose Gum, Methyl Paraben, Propyl Paraben, Ethyl Vanillin.

Liquid Calcium Magnesium Citrate **-** Puritan's Pride
Each teaspoon (15 ml) contains: Calcium (Citrate, Lactate, Gluconate) 600 mg • Magnesium (Citrate) 300 mg • Vitamin D (Cholecalciferol) 400 IU.

Liquid Children's Multiple **-** Natrol
Two teaspoons contain: Essential Vitamins: Vitamin A (beta carotene) 2,500 IU • Vitamin C (calcium ascorbate & ascorbic acid) 100 mg • Vitamin D (as Vitamin D3) (calciferol) 400 IU • Vitamin E (Acetate) 30 IU • Thiamine (Vitamin B1) 1 mg • Riboflavin (Vitamin B2) 1 mg • Niacin (Niacinamide) 12 mg • Vitamin B6 (pyridoxine HCl) 1.4 mg • Vitamin B12 (cyanocobalamin) 2.5 mcg • Pantothenic Acid (calcium d-pantothenate) 6 mg • Folic Acid 100 mcg • Biotin 20 mcg • Flavonoid: Hesperidin, Acerola, Cashew fruit, Passion fruit, Orange & Lime 10 mg • Tropical fruit extracts from: Lemon, Orange, Lime, Mango • Other extracts from: natural Vanilla Bean extract • Herbal extracts: Anise Seed, Licorice root, Millefolium plant, Horsetail Grass plant, Chamomile leaf & flowers, Peppermint leaf, Nettles plant, Spinach leaf & Sodium Benzoate (0.1% added to help protect flavor). In a base of Purified Water, Brown Rice Syrup, Glycerine & Citric Acid.

Liquid Children's Multi-Vitamin **-** Natrol
Two teaspoons (10 ml) contain: Essential Vitamins: Vitamin A (beta carotene) 2500 IU • Vitamin C (calcium ascorbate & ascorbic acid) 100 mg • Vitamin D (as Vitamin D3) (calciferol) 400 IU • Vitamin E (Acetate) 30 IU • Vitamin B1 (Thiamine) 1 mg • Vitamin B2 (Riboflavin) 1 mg • Niacin (Niacinamide) Vitamin B3 12 mg • Vitamin B6 (pyridoxine HCl) 1.4 mg • Vitamin B12 (cyanocobalamin) 2.5 mcg • Pantothenic Acid (calcium d-pantothenate) 6 mg • Folic Acid 100 mcg • Biotin 20 mcg • Flavonoid: Hesperidin 10 mg • Tropical fruit extracts from: Lemon, Orange, Lime, Mango • Other extracts from: natural Vanilla Bean extract • Herbal extracts: Anise Seed, Licorice root, Millefolium plant, Plantain root, Horsetail Grass plant, Chamomile leaf & flowers, Peppermint leaf, Nettles plant, Spinach leaf & Sodium Benzoate (0.1% added to help protect flavor). In a base of: Purified Water, Brown Rice Syrup, Glycerine & Citric Acid.

Liquid Colloidal Mineral Energy **-** World Nutrition
Each fluid ounce contains: Magnesium 100 mg • Calcium 25 mg • Potassium 15 mg • Manganese 5 mg • Silica 1100 mcg • Selenium 50 mcg • Chromium 50 mcg • Vitamin B12 1000 mcg • Biotin 200 mcg • 72 Polycolloidal Mineral Blend (including aluminum) Approximately 1.7 ppm: Antimony, Arsenic, Barium, Beryllium, Bismuth, Boron, Bromine, Cadmium, Cerium, Cesium, Chloride, Cobalt, Copper, Dysprosium, Erbium, Europium, Fluoride, Gadolinium, Gallium, Germanium, Gold, Hafnium, Holmium, Indium, Iodine, Iridium, Iron, Lanthanum, Lead, Lithium, Lutetium, Mercury, Molybdenum, Neodymium, Osmium, Palladium, Phosphorus, Platinum, Praseodymium, Rhenium, Rhodium, Rubidium, Ruthenium, Samarium, Scandium, Silver, Sodium, Strontium, Sulfur, Tantalum, Tellurium, Terbium, Thalium, Thorium, Thulium, Tin, Titanium, Tungsten, Vanadium, Ytterbium, Yttrium, Zirconium. Other Ingredients: Purified Water, Sorbitol, Magnesium Citrate/Gluconate/Sulfate, Polycolloid Minerals (calcium sulfate, diatomaceous earth), Citric Acid, Calcium Citrate/Levulinate, Natural Flavor, Zinc Gluconate/Citrate, Sodium Benzoate (as a preservative), Caramel Color, Manganese Citrate/Sulfate, Potassium Gluconate/Citrate/Chloride, Sodium Metasilicate, Cyanocobalamin, Chromium Picolinate/Chloride, Biotin, Selenium Complex (selenomethionine, sodium selenite).

Liquid Coral Calcium - Utrition Inc.
Each fluid ounce contains: Vitamin D (cholecalciferol) 400 IU • Coral Calcium 1000 mg • Magnesium (citrate) 200 mg • Manganese (gluconate) 1 mg • Boron (sodium bicarbonate) 2 mg • Lysine 10 mg. Other Ingredients: Purified Water, Glycerin USP (vegetable), Crystalline Fructose, Citric Acid, Natural Flavors, Colloidal Silver, Xanthan Gum, Potassium Benzoate, Potassium Sorbate, Stevia Extract.

Liquid Ester-C - Natrol
Two teaspoons (10 ml) contain: Vitamin C (from Ester-C calcium ascorbate) 250 mg • Calcium (from Ester-C calcium ascorbate) 25 mg • Pure Bioflavonoids containing: Rutin, Quercetin, & Hesperidin 10 mg • Tropical fruit extracts from: Acerola, Cashew fruit, Passion fruit, Orange, Lime & Mango. In a specially formulated base of: Purified Water, Brown Rice Syrup, Honey, natural Vanilla Bean extract, Citric Acid & Sodium Benzoate (0.1% added to help protect flavor).

Liquid Iron Ferrochel - Natrol
Four teaspoons (20 mL) contain: Iron & Vitamins: Iron (Ferrochel chelate) 14.5 mg • Vitamin C (Calcium Ascorbate) 100 mg • Vitamin B1 (Thiamine) 1 mg • Vitamin B6 (Pyridoxine HCl) 2 mg • Vitamin B12 (Cyanocobalamin) 3 mcg • Niacinamide 13 mg • Herbal extracts: Nettles, Kelp, Spinach, Yarrow, Angelica, Horsetail Grass, Siberian Ginseng, Yellow Dock, Burdock root, Pau D'Arco, Rose Hips & Alfalfa • Tropical fruit extracts from: Acerola, Pineapple, Cashew fruit, Passion fruit, Lime & Mango. In a specially formulated base of: Purified Water, Brown Rice Syrup, Honey & natural fruit flavors.

Liquid Joint Repair (Pineapple/Orange Flavor) - Utrition Inc.
Two tablespoons contain: Sodium 30 mg • Vitamin C 60 mg • Glucosamine Sulfate 2000 mg • Chondroitin Sulfate 1200 mg • Opti-Methyl Sulfonyl Methane 500 mg. Other Ingredients: Purified Water, Fructose, Citric Acid, Collagen, Red Beet Color, Natural Flavors, Potassium Citrate, Potassium Benzoate, Potassium Sorbate.
See Editor's Note No. 15, page 2055.

Liquid Kalm With Kava Kava root extract - Natrol
Two teaspoons (10 ml) contain: Guaranteed Potency Herbal extracts: Kava Kava root extract standardized to contain 30% Kavalactones 25 mg • Passion flower Herb extract standardized to Contain 3.5% Isovitexin 20 mg • Chamomile flower extract standardized to Contain 0.5% Apigenin 25 mg • Hops Cone extract standardized to Contain 0.35% Flavonoids 25 mg • Vitamin: Vitamin B6 2 mg • Herbal extract blend: Lemon Balm leaf, Oat Straw, Marjoram leaf, Cowslip herb, Rosemary leaf, Scullcap herb. Other ingredients: Honey & Brown Rice Syrup, natural Lemon & Ginger flavor, Cashew fruit & Passion fruit powder, Citric Acid, Sodium Benzoate (0.1% added to protect flavor).

Liquid L-Carnitine 1000 - Optimum Nutrition
Each 2 tbsp (30 mL) serving contains: L-Carnitine 1000 mg • Pantothenic Acid (from D-calcium pantothenic acid) 20 mg.

Liquid Liver Extract - Enzymatic Therapy
Two softgels contain: Vitamin B12 (as cyanocobalamin) 200 mcg • Iron 2 mg • Liquid Liver Fractions (predigested soluble concentrate) 1100 mg. Other Ingredients: Soybean Oil, Gelatin, Glycerin, Lecithin, Caramel Color, Beeswax, Titanium Dioxide Color.
See Editor's Note No. 14.

Liquid Molybdenum - NutriCology
Each drop contains: Molybdenum (as ammonium molybdate) 25 mcg. Other Ingredients: Distilled Water.

Liquid Multi Colloidal Minerals - GNC
Two tablespoons contain: Deionized/Distilled Water, Colloidal Mineral Clay, Methylparaben, Antimony, Barium, Beryllium, Bismuth, Boron, Calcium, Cerium, Cesium, Chromium, Cobalt, Copper, Dysprosium, Erbium, Europium, Gadolinium, Gallium, Gold, Hafnium, Holmium, Indium, Iridium, Iron, Lanthanum, Lithium, Lutetium, Magnesium, Manganese, Molybdenum, Neodymium, Nickel, Niobium, Palladium, Platinum, Phosphorus, Potassium, Praseodymium, Rhenium, Rhodium, Rubidium, Ruthenium, Samarium, Scandium, Selenium, Silica, Silver, Sulfur, Tantalum, Tellurium, Terbium, Thallium, Thorium, Thulium, Titanium, Tungsten, Uranium, Vanadium, Ytterbium, Yttrium, Zinc, Zirconium.

Liquid Multi-Vitamin - Puritan's Pride
Each tablespoonful (15 ml) contains: Vitamin A (as Retinyl Palmitate) 5,000 IU • Vitamin C (as Ascorbic Acid) 250 mg • Vitamin D (as Cholecalciferol) 400 IU • Vitamin E (as d-Alpha Tocopheryl plus Mixed Tocopherols) 125 IU • Thiamin (Vitamin B1; as Thiamine Mononitrate) 25 mg • Riboflavin (Vitamin B2; as Riboflavin-5'-Phosphate Sodium) 25 mg • Niacin (as Niacinamide) 150 mg • Vitamin B-6 (as Pyridoxine Hydrochloride) 50 mg • Folic Acid 400 mcg • Vitamin B-12 (as Cyanocobalamin) 50 mcg • Biotin (as D-Biotin) 50 mcg • Pantothenic Acid (as Dexpanthenol) 150 mg • PABA (Para-Aminobenzoic Acid) 25 mg • Choline Bitartrate 200 mg • Inositol 100 mg.

Liquid Multi-Vitamin - Natrol
Two teaspoons (10 ml) contain: Vitamins & Minerals: Vitamin A (beta carotene) 10000 IU • Vitamin C (Calcium Ascorbate) 200 mg • Vitamin D (cholecalciferol) 400 IU • Vitamin E (Acetate) 100 IU • Vitamin B1 (Thiamine) 7.5 mg • Vitamin B2 (Riboflavin) 8.5 mg • Niacin (Niacinamide) Vitamin B3 20 mg • Vitamin B6 (Pyridoxine HCl) 17 mg • Vitamin B12 (cyanocobalamin) 50 mcg • Pantothenic Acid (calcium d-pantothenate) 50 mg • Inositol 25 mg • Folic Acid 400 mcg • Biotin 300 mcg. Advanced Flavonoids: GP Flavonoids Complex+ 50 mg • Rutin, Quercetin, & Hesperidin 10 mg • Herbal extracts: Nettles, Kelp, Parsley, Ginger, Oats, Alfalfa, Hops, Peppermint, Rose Hips, Spinach & Echinacea, Natural Vanilla Bean flavor, natural Ginger flavor • Tropical fruit extracts from: Acerola, Pineapple, Cashew fruit, Passion fruit, Mango, Orange, Lime & Lemon. In a Specially Formulated Base of: Purified Water, Brown Rice Syrup, Honey, Glycerine, Citric Acid, Sodium Benzoate to help protect flavor, Milk Thistle & Citrus fruits.

Liquid NewBust (Liquid New Bust) - Tiger-One.com
Water • Saw Palmetto • Extra Virgin Olive Oil • Dong Quai • Damiana • Glycerin • Foenugreek seed • Blessed Thistle • Violet • Wild Yam • Fennel Seed • Althea root • Cumin seed • Hops.
See Editor's Note No. 17, page 2055.

Liquid Propolis Extract With Herbs - TwinLab
Ten drops contain: Propolis 500 mg • Proprietary Herbal Blend 500 mg: Golden Seal root, Echinacea root, Myrrh, Black Walnut leaves, Marshmallow root, Licorice root, Garlic, Capsicum.

Liquid Speed - Unknown
Unknown.
See Editor's Note No. 49, page 2059.

Liquid Stevia - Physicians Laboratories
Each 1/8 teaspoon contains: Stevia Rebaudiana Bertoni leaves 15 mg.

Liquid Vitamin B-12 - GNC A-Z - GNC
Each dropperful (1ml) contains: Vitamin B12 (as cyanocobalamin) 1000 mcg. Other Ingredients: Purified Water, Propylene Glycol, Sorbitol, Natural Cherry Flavor, Methylparaben, Stevia, Propylparaben.

Lithinase - Progressive Labs
Each capsule contains: Lithium Amino Acid Chelate 25 mg • Elemental Lithium 50 mcg • Pea powder 25 mg • Buckwheat 25 mg • Millet flour 25 mg • Lentil powder 25 mg (carefully dried to preserve their natural nutrient content).

Lithium Orotate - Life Link
Each tablet contains: Lithium Orotate (elemental lithium 5.8 mg) 135 mg.

Little One Children's Multiple **-** Metabolic Products
Each tablet contains: Vitamin A (Palmitate) 2500 IU • Vitamin A (Natural Mixed Carotenoids) 2500 IU • Vitamin C (Hypoallergenic from Beet sugar and Ascorbyl Palmitate) 100 mg • Vitamin E (D-Alpha, Natural) 60 IU •Vitamin B1 (Thiamin Mononitrate) 5 mg • Vitamin B2 (Riboflavin) 5 mg • Vitamin B3 (Niacinamide) 25 mg • Vitamin B5 (D-Calcium Pantothenate) 25 mg • Vitamin B6 (Pyridoxine) 5 mg • Vitamin B12 (Cyanocobalamin) 10 mcg • Folic Acid 400 mcg • Biotin 300 mcg • Vitamin D (Cholecalciferol) 400 IU • Iron (Carbonyl) 9 mg • Iodine (K-Iodine) 100 mcg • Copper (Gluconate) 2 mg • Manganese (Gluconate) 1 mg • Zinc (Citrate) 15 mg • Molybdenum (Sodium Molybdate) 25 mcg • Chromium (GTF-Polynicotinate) 100 mcg • Selenium (L-Selenomethionine, Sodium Selenite) 100 mcg.

Liv. 52 **-** The Himalaya Drug Company (Himalaya Heal
Each tablet contains: Himsra (capparis spinosa) 65 mg • Kasani (cichorium intybus) 65 mg • Mandur Bhasma (ferric oxide calx) 33 mg • Kakamachi (solanum nigrum) 32 mg • Arjuna (terminalua arjuna) 32 mg • Kasamarda (cassia occidentalis) 16 mg • Biranjasipha (achillea millefolium) 16 mg • Jhavuka (tamarix gallica) 16 mg.

Liv. 52 DS **-** The Himalaya Drug Company (Himalaya Heal
Each tablet contains: Himsra (capparis spinosa) 130 mg • Kasani (cichorium intybus) 130 mg • Mandur Bhasma (ferric oxide calx) 66 mg • Kakamachi (solanum nigrum) 64 mg • Arjuna (terminalia arjuna) 64 mg • Kasamarda (cassia occidentalis) 32 mg • Biranjasipha (achillea millefolium) 32 mg • Jhavuka (tamarix gallica) 32 mg.

Liv. 52 Syrup **-** The Himalaya Drug Company (Himalaya Heal
Each 1 tsp (5 mL) serving contains: Himsra (capparis spinosa) 17 mg • Kasani (cichorium intybus) 17 mg • Kakamachi (solanum nigrum) 8 mg • Arjuna (terminalia arjuna) 8 mg • Kasamarda (cassia occidentalis) 4 mg • Biranjasipha (achillea millefolium) 4 mg • Jhavuka (tamarix gallica) 4 mg.

Livaplex **-** Standard Process, Inc.
Each capsule contains: Proprietary Blend 598 mg: Bovine Liver extract, Spanish Black Radish (root), Bovine Liver, Calcium Lactate, Beet (root), Carrot (root), Tillandsia Usneoides, Dried Beet (leaf) juice, Betaine Hydrochloride, Magnesium Citrate, Choline Bitartrate, Soy (bean), Oat Flour, Bovine Kidney, Bovine Prostate, Bovine Adrenal extract, Defatted Wheat (germ), Bovine Liver Fat extract, Bovine Orchic extract, Ascorbic Acid, Flaxseed Oil extract, Mixed Tocopherols • Gelatin • Zinc Liver Chelate 5.5 mg • Iron Liver Chelate 2.7 mg • Water • Potassium Bicarbonate • Calcium Stearate • Niacinamide 2.8 mg • Copper Liver Chelate 109 mcg • Colors • Pyridoxine Hydrochloride 0.8 mg • Vitamin A Palmitate 1260 IU • Prolamine Iodine (zein) 9.6 mcg.

Liv-A-Tox **-** Enzymatic Therapy
Three tablets contain: Vitamin A (from fish liver oil) 4500 IU • Vitamin C (ascorbic acid and from rose hips) 25 mg • Niacin 40 mg • Vitamin B12 (as cyanocobalamin) 3 mcg • Biotin 200 mcg • Sodium 5 mg • Choline Bitartrate 850 mg • Red Beet root 300 mg • L-Methionine 250 mg • Barberry bark of root (berberis vulgaris) 150 mg • Boldo leaf extract (peumus boldus, 2:1) 150 mg • Celandine whole plant (chelidonium majus) 135 mg • Fringe Tree bark (chionanthus virginicus) 135 mg • Ox Bile extract 90 mg • Betaine HCl 75 mg • Inositol 50 mg. Other Ingredients: Cellulose, Calcium Carbonate, Stearic Acid, Modified Cellulose Gum, Silicon Dioxide, Magnesium Stearate, Chlorophyll Color, Anise Oil.
See Editor's Note No. 14.

Live Calm Sleep Deep **-** Cocoon Nutrition
Each capsule contains: L-Tetrahydropalmatine (Rotundine) 30 mg • Magnesium Chloride 12.6 mg. Other Ingredients: Microcrystalline Cellulose.

Liver **-** Nutrivention
Each tablet contains: Inositol 100 mg • Choline Bitartrate 100 mg • Vitamin E 50 IU • Vitamin B1 10 mg • Niacin 10 mg • Pantothenic Acid 10 mg • Vitamin A (Beta Carotene) 500 IU • Vitamin B12 100 mcg • Vitamin K 15 mcg • Lecithin 300 mg • Milk Thistle (Cardus marianus) 200 mg • Dandelion root 200 mg • Burdock root 50 mg • L-Methionine 50 mg • L-Theronine 30 mg • Yellow Dock 25 mg • Butternut root bark 25 mg.

Liver - BioSet **-** Enzymes, Inc.
Each capsule contains: Vitamin C (100% from Acerola Cherries) 8.5 mg • Proprietary Herbal Blend 421 mg: Milk Thistle seed extract, Chinese Thoroughwax root extract, Beet root extract, Rehmannia root extract, Rice Bran, Dandelion root extract, Safflower petals powder • Proprietary Enzyme Blend 65 mg: pHysioProtease, CereCalase. Other Ingredients: Plant Cellulose, Water.

Liver Chelate **-** Atrium Inc.
Each tablet contains: Ferrous Fumarate as Chelated Proteinates 55 mg • Copper 1 mg • Folic Acid 40 mcg • Vitamin B12 20 mcg • Raw Liver concentrate (not an extract) of Bovine source 190 mg.
See Editor's Note No. 14.

Liver DTX Complex **-** Shaklee
Three caplets contain: Milk Thistle extract (Silybum marianum) seed 300 mg • DTX Enhanced Proprietary Blend 900 mg: Schizandra extract (Schizandra chinensis) fruit, Dandelion extract (Taraxacum officinale) root and leaf, Reishi Mushroom extract (Ganoderma lucidum) cap and stalk, Turmeric extract (Curcuma longa) rhizome, Artichoke extract (Cynara scolymus) leaf. Other Ingredients: Maltodextrin, Cellulose, Acacia Gum, CrosCarmellose Sodium, Silicon Dioxide.

Liver Essentials **-** Swanson
Two capsules contain: Milk Thistle seed extract (85% silymarin) 350 mg • Dandelion root 170 mg • Burdock root 120 mg • Parsley root 120 mg • Picroliv Picrorhiza Kurroa 100 mg • Black Radish root 70 mg • N-Acetyl Cysteine 50 mg • Trimethylglycine (as betaine anhydrous) 50 mg • Alpha Lipoic Acid 20 mg.

Liver Extract **-** PhytoPharmica
Two softgels contain: Iron 2 mg • Liquid Liver Fractions (predigested soluble concentrate) 1100 mg • Sodium 5 mg • Vitamin B12 (as cyanocobalamin) 200 mcg. Other Ingredients: Soybean Oil, Gelatin, Glycerin, Lecithin, Beeswax, Caramel Color, Titanium Dioxide Color.
See Editor's Note No. 14.

Liver Extract with Eleuthero **-** PhytoPharmica
Two softgels contain: Eleuthero root 20:1 extract (eleutherococcus senticosus, standardized to contain a minimum of 0.5% eleutheroside E) 50 mg • Iron 2 mg • Liquid Liver Fractions (predigested soluble concentrate) 1100 mg • Sodium 5 mg • Vitamin B12 (as cyanocobalamin) 200 mcg. Other Ingredients: Soybean Oil, Gelatin, Glycerin, Lecithin, Beeswax, Caramel Color, Titanium Dioxide color.
See Editor's Note No. 14.

Liver Guard **-** Source Naturals
Two tablets contain: Vitamin B1 (Thiamin) 7.5 mg • Vitamin B2 (Riboflavin) 7.5 mg • Niacinamide and Niacin 50 mg • Vitamin B5 (Pantothenic Acid) 15 mg • Vitamin B6 (Pyridoxine HCl) 10 mg • Vitamin B12 (Cyanocobalamin) 25 mcg • Folic Acid 200 mcg • Vitamin C (Ascorbic Acid and Zinc Ascorbate) 527 mg • Fat-Soluble Vitamin C (from 238 mg of Ascorbyl Palmitate) 100 mg • Vitamin E (D-Alpha Tocopheryl) (Natural) 75 IU • Magnesium (Oxide, Malate) 60 mg • Potassium (Citrate) 49.5 mg • Selenium (as L-Selenomethionine) 50 mcg • Zinc (OptiZinc Zinc Monomethionine 10 mg and Zinc Ascorbate 5 mg) 15 mg • Silymarin (from Milk Thistle seed extract) 200 mg • N-Acetyl Cysteine 200 mg • Dandelion root extract 125 mg • • Turmeric extract (95% Curcumin) 76 mg • Choline (Bitartrate) 50 mg • Inositol 50 mg • Alpha-Lipoic Acid (Thioctic acid) 25 mg • Coenzyme Q10 (Ubiquinone) 12.5 mg.

Liver Health - Wellzymes - Enzymes, Inc.
Two capsules contain: n-zimes Proprietary Enzyme Blend 64 mg: pHysioProtease (177,600 pHysio-U), CereCalse Plus • Proprietary Herbal Blend 380 mg: Milk Thistle seed extract (standardized to contain 80% silymarin), Beet root extract (equivalent to 400 mg raw herb), Schizandra fruit extract (equivalent to 320 mg raw herb), Rice Bran, Dandelion root extract (equivalent to 80 mg raw herb), Turmeric root extract (standardized to contain 95% curcumin). Other Ingredients: Plant Cellulose, Water.

Liver Maintenance Formula - PhysioLogics
Each capsule contains: Dandelion root (taraxacum officinale) 50 mg • Milk Thistle seed (silybum marinum, standardized to contain 80% silymarin, 80 mg) 100 mg • Alpha Lipoic Acid 75 mg • Trimethyl Glycine 175 mg • N-Acetyl Cysteine 100 mg. Other Ingredients: Gelatin, Rice Powder, Silica, Vegetable Magnesium Stearate.

Liver Performance - Metabolic Response Modifiers
Each capsule contains: N-Acetyl-Cysteine (NAC) 400 mg • Alpha Lipoic Acid 100 mg • Choline Bitartrate 100 mg • Silymarin (32 mg of milk thistle extract standardized to 80% silymarin) 100 mg • Picrorhiza Kurroa 25 mg • Andographis Paniculata 25 mg • Vitamin E 40 IU • Vitamin B12 (methylcobalamin) 20 mcg.

Liver, Organic Glandular - NutriCology
Each capsule contains: Liver tissue (bovine) 500 mg. Other Ingredients: Silicon Dioxide, Magnesium Stearate.
See Editor's Note No. 14.

Liver-Enhancer - HerbaSway
Reishi • Poria • Cordyceps • Maitake • Shiitake • Hericium • Schisandra • Lycium • Milk Thistle • Blackberry • HerbaSwee (Cucurbitaceae fruit).

LiveRx - Metabolic Response Modifiers
Each capsule contains: N-Acetyl-Cysteine (NAC) 400 mg • Alpha Lipoic Acid 100 mg • Choline 100 mg • Silymarin 100 mg • Picrorhiza kurroa 25 mg • Andrographis Paniculata 25 mg • Vitamin E 40 IU • Vitamin B12 (methylcobalamin) 20 mcg.

Living B Complex - Garden of Life, Inc.
Three caplets contain: Thiamine (vitamin B1) 9 mg • Riboflavin (vitamin B2) 10 mg • Niacin (vitamin B3) 60 mg • Vitamin B6 12 mg • Folic Acid 800 mcg • Vitamin B12 500 mcg • Biotin 300 mcg • Pantothenic Acid 60 mg • Inositol 50 mg • PABA (para-aminobenzoic acid) 10 mg • Choline 30 mg • Poten-Zyme Superfood Blend (25-1) 1650 mg: Brown Rice Bran, Spirulina, Alfalfa grass juice • Poten-Zyme 11 "No Stress" Blend 900 mg: Rhodiola Rosea, Ganoderma Lucidum, Grifola Frondosa, Lentinula Edodes, Agaricus Blazei, Trametes Versicolor, Cordyceps Sinensis, Hericium Erinaceus, Poria Cocos, Tremella Fuciformia, Polyporus Umbellatus, Blakesleo Trispora. Other Ingredients: Cellulose, Stearates (vegetable source).

Living Calcium Homeostatic Calcium - Garden of Life, Inc.
Three caplets contain: Calcium 600 mg • Vitamin C 60 mg • Vitamin D 400 IU • Iodine 150 mcg • Magnesium 150 mg • Zinc 6 mg • Copper 1 mg • Manganese 2 mg • Silica 90 mg • Boron 2 mg • Organic Trace Mineral Blend 1050 mg • Poten-Zyme Organic Green Food Blend (25-1) 930 mg: Alfalfa grass juice, Barley grass juice, Wheat grass juice, Oat grass juice, Rye grass juice • Poten-Zyme Ocean Vegetable Blend 300 mg: Ecloria Radiata, Ascophyllum Nodosum, Laminaria Japonica, Macrocystis Pyrifera, Alaria Esculenta. Other Ingredients: Cellulose, Stearates (vegetable source).

Living Energy - Futurebiotics
Four tablets contain: Chlorella 500 mg • Bee Pollen 1000 mg • Ginseng 4:1 extract equivalent to 250 mg • Royal Jelly (freeze dried) 25 mg • Schizandra 4:1 extract equivalent to 250 mg • Astragalus 4:1 extract equivalent to 250 mg • Spirulina 500 mg • Alfalfa juice concentrate 1200 mg.

Living Multi Iron Free Formula with Homeostatic Nutrients - Garden of Life, Inc.
Nine caplets contain: Vitamin A (beta carotene) 15,000 IU • Vitamin C 225 mg • Vitamin D 400 IU • Vitamin E 225 IU • Vitamin K 60 mcg • Thiamine (vitamin B1) 9 mg • Riboflavin (vitamin B2) 10 mg • Niacin (vitamin B3) 60 mg • Vitamin B6 12 mg • Vitamin B12 500 mcg • Biotin 300 mcg • Pantothenic Acid 60 mg • Calcium 250 mg • Iodine 150 mcg • Magnesium 150 mg • Zinc 15 mg • Selenium 200 mcg • Copper 200 mcg • Manganese 3 mg • Chromium 200 mcg • Potassium 99 mg • Molybdenum 100 mcg • Boron 1 mg • Vanadium 100 mcg • Inositol 50 mg • PABA (para-aminobenzoic acid) 10 mg • Choline 30 mg • Bioflavonoids 100 mg • Lycopene 5 mg • Lutein 5 mg • Alpha Lipoic Acid 150 mg • Poten-Zyme 20 Antioxidant Veggie Juice Blend (25-1) 3150 mg: Alfalfa grass, Barley grass, Wheat grass, Rye grass, Oat grass, Broccoli, Cauliflower, Kale, Collard Greens, Brussels Sprouts, Carrot, Beet, Spinach, Parsley, Cucumber, Asparagus, Celery, Cabbage, Onion, Garlic • Organic Trace Mineral Blend 2900 mg • Poten-Zyme 9 Ocean Vegetable Blend 2000 mg: Spirulina Platensis, Chlorella Vulgaris, Lithothamnion Calcereum, Dunaliella Salina, Ecloria Radiata, Ascophyllum Nodosum, Laminaria Japonica, Macrocystis Pyrifera, Alaria Esculenta • Poten-Zyme 23 Antioxidant Fruit Blend (60-1) 1800 mg: Acerola Cherry, Blueberry (fruit, leaf), Pomegranate, Apple (fruit, skin), Black Currant, Apricot, Nectarine, Prune, White Cherry, Elderberry, Grape (fruit, seed, skin, leaf), Peach, Mango, Strawberry, Raspberry, Blackberry, Orange, Grapefruit, Lemon, Lime, Cranberry, Pineapple, Papaya • Poten-Zyme 11 Tonic Mushroom Blend 800 mg: Ganoderma Lucidum, Grifola Frondosa, Lentinula Edodes, Agaricus Blazei, Trametes Versicolor, Cordyceps Sinensis, Hericium Erinaceus, Poria Cocos, Tremella Fuciformia, Polyporus Umbellatus, Blakesleo Trispora • Poten-Zyme 6 Botanical Blend (40-1) 250 mg: Rhododendron Caucasicum, Yucca, Rosemary, Ginger, Turmeric, Wild Oregano. Other Ingredients: Cellulose, Stearates (vegetable source).

Living Multi Optimal Formula - Garden of Life, Inc.
Nine caplets contain: Vitamin A (beta carotene) 15,000 IU • Vitamin C 225 mg • Vitamin D 400 IU • Vitamin E 225 IU • Vitamin K 60 mcg • Thiamine (vitamin B1) 9 mg • Riboflavin (vitamin B2) 10 mg • Niacin (vitamin B3) 60 mg • Vitamin B12 500 mcg • Biotin 300 mcg • Pantothenic Acid 60 mg • Calcium 250 mg • Iron 9 mg • Iodine 150 mcg • Magnesium 150 mg • Zinc 15 mg • Selenium 200 mcg • Copper 200 mcg • Manganese 3 mg • Chromium 200 mcg • Potassium 99 mg • Molybdenum 100 mcg • Boron 1 mg • Vanadium 100 mcg • Inositol 50 mg • PABA (para-aminobenzoic acid) 10 mg • Choline 30 mg • Bioflavonoids 100 mg • Lycopene 5 mg • Lutein 5 mg • Alpha Lipoic Acid 150 mg • Poten-Zyme 20 Antioxidant Veggie Juice Blend (25-1) 3150 mg: Alfalfa grass, Barley grass, Wheat grass, Rye grass, Oat grass, Broccoli, Cauliflower, Kale, Collard Greens, Brussels Sprouts, Carrot, Beet, Spinach, Parsley, Cucumber, Asparagus, Celery, Cabbage, Onion, Garlic • Organic Trace Mineral Blend 2900 mg • Poten-Zyme 9 Ocean Vegetable Blend 2000 mg: Spirulina Platensis, Chlorella Vulgaris, Lithothamnion Calcereum, Dunaliella Salina, Ecloria Radiata, Ascophyllum Nodosum, Laminaria Japonica, Macrocystis Pyrifera, Alaria Esculenta • Poten-Zyme 23 Antioxidant Fruit Blend (60-1) 1800 mg: Acerola Cherry, Blueberry (fruit, leaf), Pomegranate, Apple (fruit, skin), Black Currant, Apricot, Nectarine, Prune, White Cherry, Elderberry, Grape (fruit, seed, skin, leaf), Peach, Mango, Strawberry, Raspberry, Blackberry, Orange, Grapefruit, Lemon, Lime, Cranberry, Pineapple, Papaya • Poten-Zyme 11 Tonic Mushroom Blend 800 mg: Ganoderma Lucidum, Grifola Frondosa, Lentinula Edodes, Agaricus Blazei, Trametes Versicolor, Cordyceps Sinensis, Hericium Erinaceus, Poria Cocos, Tremella Fuciformia, Polyporus Umbellatus, Blakesleo Trispora • Poten-Zyme 6 Botanical Blend (40-1) 250 mg: Rhododendron Caucasicum, Yucca, Rosemary, Ginger, Turmeric, Wild Oregano. Other Ingredients: Cellulose, Stearates (vegetable source).

Living Multi Optimal Men's Formula with Homeostatic Nutrients - Garden of Life, Inc.
Six caplets contain: Vitamin A (beta carotene) 10,000 IU • Vitamin C

50 mg • Vitamin D 400 IU • Vitamin E 225 IU • Vitamin K 60 mcg • Thiamine (vitamin B1) 9 mg • Riboflavin (vitamin B2) 10 mg • Niacin (vitamin B3) 60 mg • Vitamin B6 12 mg • Folic Acid 800 mcg • Vitamin B12 500 mcg • Biotin 300 mcg • Pantothenic Acid 60 mg • Calcium 250 mg • Iron 9 mg • Iodine 150 mcg • Magnesium 150 mg • Zinc 20 mg • Selenium 200 mcg • Copper 200 mcg • Manganese 3 mg • Chromium 200 mcg • Potassium 99 mg • Molybdenum 100 mcg • Boron 1 mg • Vanadium 100 mcg • Inositol 50 mg • PABA (para-aminobenzoic acid) 10 mg • Choline 30 mg • Bioflavonoids 100 mg • Lycopene 5 mg • Lutein 5 mg • Alpha Lipoic Acid 150 mg • Poten-Zyme 20 Antioxidant Veggie Juice Blend (25-1) 750 mg: Alfalfa grass, Barley grass, Wheat grass, Rye grass, Oat grass, Broccoli, Cauliflower, Kale, Collard Greens, Brussels Sprouts, Carrot, Beet, Spinach, Parsley, Cucumber, Asparagus, Celery, Cabbage, Onion, Garlic • Organic Trace Mineral Blend 800 mg • Poten-Zyme 9 Ocean Vegetable Blend 2050 mg: Spirulina Platensis, Chlorella Vulgaris, Lithothamnion Calcereum, Dunaliella Salina, Ecloria Radiata, Ascophyllum Nodosum, Laminaria Japonica, Macrocystis Pyrifera, Alaria Esculenta • Poten-Zyme 23 Antioxidant Fruit Blend (60-1) 1650 mg: Acerola Cherry, Blueberry (fruit, leaf), Pomegranate, Apple (fruit, skin), Black Currant, Apricot, Nectarine, Prune, White Cherry, Elderberry, Grape (fruit, seed, skin, leaf), Peach, Mango, Strawberry, Raspberry, Blackberry, Orange, Grapefruit, Lemon, Lime, Cranberry, Pineapple, Papaya • Poten-Zyme 11 Tonic Mushroom Blend 750 mg: Ganoderma Lucidum, Grifola Frondosa, Lentinula Edodes, Agaricus Blazei, Trametes Versicolor, Cordyceps Sinensis, Hericium Erinaceus, Poria Cocos, Tremella Fuciformia, Polyporus Umbellatus, Blakesleo Trispora • Poten-Zyme 5 Botanical Blend (40-1) 100 mg: Yucca, Rosemary, Ginger, Turmeric, Wild Oregano • Poten-Zyme 5 Men's Herbal Blend (40-1) 1075 mg: Maca, Rhodiola Rosea, Rhododendron Caucasicum, Bee Pollen, Aralia Racemosa. Other Ingredients: Cellulose, Stearates (vegetable source).

Living Multi Optimal Women's Formula with Homeostatic Nutrients - Garden of Life, Inc.
Six caplets contain: Vitamin A (beta carotene) 10,000 IU • Vitamin C 150 mg • Vitamin D 400 IU • Vitamin E 225 IU • Vitamin K 60 mcg • Thiamine (vitamin B1) 9 mg • Riboflavin (vitamin B2) 10 mg • Niacin (vitamin B3) 60 mg • Vitamin B6 12 mg • Folic Acid 800 mcg • Vitamin B12 500 mcg • Biotin 300 mcg • Pantothenic Acid 60 mg • Calcium 250 mg • Iron 18 mg • Iodine 75 mcg • Magnesium 150 mg • Zinc 15 mg • Selenium 200 mcg • Copper 200 mcg • Manganese 3 mg • Chromium 200 mcg • Potassium 99 mg • Molybdenum 100 mcg • Boron 1 mg • Vanadium 100 mcg • Inositol 50 mg • PABA (para-aminobenzoic acid) 10 mg • Choline 30 mg • Bioflavonoids 100 mg • Lycopene 5 mg • Lutein 5 mg • Alpha Lipoic Acid 150 mg • Poten-Zyme 20 Antioxidant Veggie Juice Blend (25-1) 900 mg: Alfalfa grass, Barley grass, Wheat grass, Rye grass, Oat grass, Broccoli, Cauliflower, Kale, Collard Greens, Brussels Sprouts, Carrot, Beet, Spinach, Parsley, Cucumber, Asparagus, Celery, Cabbage, Onion, Garlic • Organic Trace Mineral Blend 800 mg • Poten-Zyme 9 Ocean Vegetable Blend 1975 mg: Spirulina Platensis, Chlorella Vulgaris, Lithothamnion Calcereum, Dunaliella Salina, Ecloria Radiata, Ascophyllum Nodosum, Laminaria Japonica, Macrocystis Pyrifera, Alaria Esculenta • Poten-Zyme 23 Antioxidant Fruit Blend (60-1) 1650 mg: Acerola Cherry, Blueberry (fruit, leaf), Pomegranate, Apple (fruit, skin), Black Currant, Apricot, Nectarine, Prune, White Cherry, Elderberry, Grape (fruit, seed, skin, leaf), Peach, Mango, Strawberry, Raspberry, Blackberry, Orange, Grapefruit, Lemon, Lime, Cranberry, Pineapple, Papaya • Poten-Zyme 11 Tonic Mushroom Blend 750 mg: Ganoderma Lucidum, Grifola Frondosa, Lentinula Edodes, Agaricus Blazei, Trametes Versicolor, Cordyceps Sinensis, Hericium Erinaceus, Poria Cocos, Tremella Fuciformia, Polyporus Umbellatus, Blakesleo Trispora • Poten-Zyme 5 Botanical Blend (40-1) 100 mg: Yucca, Rosemary, Ginger, Turmeric, Wild Oregano • Poten-Zyme 5 Women's Herbal Blend (40-1) 1075 mg: Maca, Rhodiola Rosea, Rhododendron Caucasicum, Aralia Racemosa, Schizandra. Other Ingredients: Cellulose, Stearates (vegetable source).

Living Vitamin C - Garden of Life, Inc.
Three caplets contain: Vitamin C 500 mg • Bioflavonoids 150 mg • Poten-Zyme Whole Food Vitamin C Blend 2100 mg: Acerola Cherry, Camu Camu (myrciaria dubla), Indian Gooseberry (emblic officinalis) • Poten-Zyme Organic Whole Citrus Blend 750 mg: Orange, Grapefruit, Lemon, Lime (fruit, pulp, peel, seeds) • Poten-Zyme Organic Green Blend (25-1) 450 mg: Alfalfa grass juice, Wheat Grass juice, Oat grass juice, Barley grass juice, Rye grass juice • Organic Trace Mineral Blend 450 mg • Poten-Zyme Organic Fermented Fruit Blend 150 mg: Raspberry, Strawberry, Blueberry, Blackberry, Prune, Grape (fruit, skin, seeds). Other Ingredients: Cellulose, Stearates (vegetable source).

Livr D-Tox - Nutri-Quest Rx
Each tablet contains: Glucuronic Acid 10 mg • Liver 5 mg • Vitamin A 1000 IU • Vitamin C 25 mg • Vitamin B1 5 mg • Vitamin E 10 IU • Black Currant seed oil 5 mg • Cellulase 50 mg • Amylase 50 mg • Lipase 50 mg • Protease 50 mg • Lipoic Acid 2 mg • Phosphatidyl Choline 5.75 mg • Choline Bitartrate 15 mg • DL-Methionine 5 mg • Calcium Chelate 50 mg • Magnesium 50 mg • Zinc Chelate 5 mg • Selenium Chelate 25 mcg • Manganese 1 mg • Milk Thistle 100 mg • Silymarin 5 mg • Garlic 50 mg • Beet root 25 mg • Beet leaf 25 mg. See Editor's Note No. 14.

Liv-R-Actin Milk Thistle Blend in Vegetarian Capsules - Nature's Plus
Two Vegicaps contain: Herbal Blend, 600 mg: Dandelion, Barberry, Goldenseal, Wild Oregon Grape & Celery seed 600 mg • Milk Thistle extract, providing 70%, 98 mg of the active flavonoid Silymarin 140 mg.

Livral - AIE Pharmaceuticals
Each capsule contains: Proprietary Blend 750 mg: Milk Thistle extract, Phyllanthus amarus, Dandelion root (taraxacum officinale), Grape seed extract (vitis vinifera), Artichoke, Choline, Inositol.

Livral Complex - AIE Pharmaceuticals
Each capsule contains: Proprietary Blend 750 mg: Milk Thistle extract, Phyllanthus Amarus, Dandelion root (taraxacum officinale), Cat's Claw bark, Licorice root, Tribulus terrestris, Culver's root, Oregon Grape root, Yellow Dock, Burdock root, Echinacea root, Grape seed extract (vitis vinifera), Artichoke, Catechin.

L-Lysine - PhysioLogics
Each tablet contains: L-Lysine (as l-lysine hydrochloride) 500 mg. Other Ingredients: Cellulose (plant origin), Food Glaze, Croscarmellose, Vegetable Magnesium Stearate, Silica, Magnesium Silicate.

L-Lysine - NutriCology
Each capsule contains: L-Lysine 500 mg. Other Ingredients: Cellulose, Silicon Dioxide, Stearic Acid.

L-Lysine 1000 - GNC A-Z - GNC
Each tablet contains: L-lysine (as L-Lysine Monohydrochloride) 1000 mg. Other Ingredients: Povidone.

L-Lysine 500 - GNC A-Z - GNC
Each tablet contains: L-lysine (as L-Lysine Monohydrochloride) 500 mg. Other Ingredients: Cellulose.

L-Lysine 500 mg - Rexall - Sundown
Each caplet contains: L-Lysine HCl 500 mg. Other Ingredients: Microcrystalline Cellulose, Hydrogenated Cottonseed Oil, Croscarmellose Sodium.

L-Lysine Plus - Atrium Inc.
Each tablet contains: L-Lysine HCL (an essential amino acid) 500 mg • Ascorbic Acid (Vitamin C) 100 mg.

L-Methionine - NutriCology
Each capsule contains: L-Methionine 500 mg. Other Ingredients: Cellulose, Stearic Acid.

Lobelia and Cayenne **-** Dial Herbs
Lobelia • Cayenne.

Lobelia Herb, 425 mg **-** Nature's Way
Each capsule contains: Lobelia (stem, leaf, flower) 425 mg. Other Ingredients: Gelatin, Magnesium Stearate.

Lomatium-Goldenseal Virtue **-** Blessed Herbs
Lomatium root • Astragalus root • Osha root • Echinacea Angustifolia root • Goldenseal root • Siberian Ginseng root • Licorice root • Reishi mycelium • Shitake mycelium • Grain alcohol & Distilled Water.

Longdan Xie Gan Wan **-** KwangChow First Chinese Medicine Factory
Unknown.
See Editor's Note No. 46, page 2058.

Longdan Ziegan Wan **-** China Beijing Tong-Ren Tang
Unknown.
See Editor's Note No. 46, page 2058.

Longest Living Acidophilus **-** Futurebiotics
Each capsule contains: Acidophilus fortified with Rhamnosus, encapsulated in a base of Rice powder & Beet fiber. 1 billion Live Organisms per capsule.

Longevinex **-** Resveratrol Partners, LLC
Each capsule contains: Proprietary Longevinex Blend 100 mg: providing not less than 15 mg Resveratrol from Giant Knotweed leaf extract (polygonum cuspidatum), Red Grape skin extract (vitas vinifera) • Quercetin 75 mg • Phytic Acid 25 mg • Lecithin 100 mg. Other Ingredients: Gelatin.

Longe-Vit-E **-** Holista
Each capsule contains: Vitamin C (Ester-C) 250 mg • Beta Carotene 10000 IU • Vitamin E (d-alpha tocopherol) 200 IU • Selenium 50 mcg • Vitamin B6 25 mg • Magnesium 50 mg • Manganese 1.5 mg • Copper 1.0 mg.

Longevity **-** Young Living Essential Oils
Clove Oil • Orange Oil • Thyme Oil • Frankincense Oil.

Longevity 2AEP + HGHR **-** Urban Nutrition Inc
Three capsules contain: Calcium 2-AEP (2-amino ethanol phosphate; 50 mg elemental calcium) 510 mg • Magnesium 2-AEP (32 mg elemental calcium) 510 mg • Potassium 2-AEP (43 mg elemental calcium) 255 mg • HGHR (human growth hormone releaser): Anterior Pituitary gland 75 mg, L-Arginine 45 mg • L-Glutamine 45 mg • L-Lysine 45 mg • L-Tyrosine 15 mg. Other Ingredients: Duratex, Pure Food Glaze, Avicel, Magnesium Stearate, Cab-O-Sil.
See Editor's Note No. 14.

Longevity Crystal **-** Sante International
Each tablet contains: Herbal Extract-Based Blend 500 mg: Gynostemma Pentaphyllum, Crataegus Pinnatifida (hawthorn leaves/ berries), Camellia Sinensis (green tea).

Longevity Signal A.M. Formula **-** Oasis Wellness Network
Each capsule contains: N-Acetyl-Cysteine 100 mg • Acetyl-L-Carnitine 60 mg • Alpha Lipoic Acid 50 mg • Chlorella powder (whole plant) 50 mg • Fo-Ti root extract 50 mg • Wolfberry fruit extract 50 mg • MaxCell Proprietary Blend 25 mg: Zisyphus Jujube, Piper Nigrum, Aloe Vera, Glycyrrhiza Glabra • 7-Keto DHEA 15 mg • DHEA 7.5 mg. Other Ingredients: Cellulose, Dicalcium Phosphate, Magnesium Stearate, Silica.

Longevity Signal P.M. Formula **-** Oasis Wellness Network
Each capsule contains: Wolfberry fruit extract 200 mg • Chlorella powder (whole plant) 150 mg • Fo-Ti root extract 100 mg • N-Acetyl-Cysteine 50 mg • Alpha Lipoic Acid 50 mg • MaxCell Proprietary Blend 25 mg: Zisyphus Jujube, Piper Nigrum, Aloe Vera, Glycyrrhiza Glabra • DIM (diindolylmethane) 25 mg • Active Aloe (200:1) 20 mg • 7-Keto DHEA 12.5 mg • DHEA 5 mg • R5P (riboflavin-5-phosphate) 3 mg • P5P (pyridoxal-5-phosphate) 3 mg • Methylcobalamin 800 mcg. Other Ingredients: Cellulose, Dicalcium Phosphate, Magnesium Stearate, Silica.

Longs Natural Magnesium 250 mg **-** Longs
Each tablet contains: Magnesium (as magnesium oxide) 250 mg. Other Ingredients: Cellulose, Talc, Sodium Starch Gycolate, Starch, Silicon Dioxide, Croscarmellose Sodium, Polyethylene Glycol, Kelp, Magnesium Stearate.

Long-Term Adrenal **-** Enzymes, Inc.
Each capsule contains: Vitamin C (100% from Acerola Cherries) 10 mg • Proprietary Herbal Blend 385 mg: Codonopsis root extract, Chinese Thoroughwax root extract, Rice Bran, Astragalus root extract • Proprietary Enzyme Blend 80 mg: pHysioProtease, CereCalase. Other Ingredients: Plant Cellulose, Water.

Looking Young **-** FreeLife International
Two caplets contain: Vitamin A (100% from beta-carotene, alpha-carotene, cryptoxanthin, zeaxanthin, lutein) 2500 IU • Vitamin C (from glycosyl flavonebound isoascorbic acids 130 mg) 100 mg • Vitamin E (as natural d-alpha-tocopheryl succinate) 30 IU • Biotin 100 mcg • Pantothenic Acid (as D-calcium pantothenate) 10 mg • Calcium (from calcium hydrogen phosphate) 150 mg • Zinc (as patented OptiZinc zinc monomethionine) 5 mg • Manganese (as patented Chelazome glycine amino acid chelate) 2.5 mg • Glucosamine / Aloe Mucopolysaccharides Complex 1000 mg: Glucosamine Hydrochloride, Vegetable Beta-Polysaccharides, Aloe Vera 40x concentrate • Microencapsulated Lactobacillus Sporogenes 100 million cells • Catalase 1000 units • Proprietary Blend 130 mg: Ascorbic Acid, Sodium Isoascorbate, Citrus Glycosyl Flavones (cirantin, isosakuranetin-7-beta-uritinoside, narirutin, eriocitrin, noblietin, tangeretin, heptamethoxyflavone) • Sea Vegetable Marine Protein/Fiber concentrate (from Irish moss and algae extract) 100 mg • Red Grape skin standardized extract 100 mg • MSM (methylsulfonylmethane) 100 mg • Purified Soy Phosphatides 100 mg • Proprietary Blend 100 mg: RNA (ribonucleic acid), DNA (deoxyribonucleic acid) complex. Proprietary Blend 2500 Units: Soy Polysaccharides, Plant Enzymes. Proprietary Blend 50 mg: Artichoke leaf standardized extract (2% cynarin), Chamomile flower, Citrus Pectin, Gentian root, Milk Thistle seed, Wild Yam root • Silica (colloidal, from N. Atlantic Sea kelp) 30 mg. Other Ingredients: Calcium Hydrogen Phosphate, Cellulose, Vegetable Stearic Acid, Calcium Carbonate, Vegetable Magnesium Stearate, Calcium Silicate, Vita-Coat (vegetable resin, alpha-lipoic acid).

Love Bites **-** Nature's Plus
Each tablet contains: Vitamin A (as beta carotene) 5000 IU • Vitamin C (as ascorbic acid) 75 mg • Vitamin D (as ergocalciferol) 400 IU • Vitamin E (as d-alpha tocopheryl acetate) 30 IU • Vitamin B1 (as thiamine HCl) 5 mg • Vitamin B2 (as riboflavin) 5 mg • Niacin (as niacinamide) 10 mg • Vitamin B6 (as pyridoxine HCl) 5 mg • Folate (as folic acid) 10 mcg • Vitamin B12 (as cyanocobalamin) 10 mcg • Biotin 50 mcg • Pantothenic Acid (as calcium pantothenate) 10 mg • Calcium (as gluconate) 20 mg • Iron (as gluconate) 10 mg • Iodine (from kelp) 100 mcg • Magnesium (as gluconate) 10 mg • Zinc (as gluconate) 3 mg • Manganese (as gluconate) 2 mg • Potassium (as gluconate) 4 mg • Choline (as bitartrate) 2 mg • Inositol 2 mg • PABA (para-aminobenzoic acid) 0.6 mg.

Love-Berries **-** Nature's Plus
Each pill contains: Cranberry concentrate 45X 200 mg • Vitamin C corn free 60 mg. Sweetened with VitaSweet.

Low Thyroid **-** Enzymes, Inc.
Each capsule contains: Proprietary Herbal Blend 390 mg: Bladderwrack kelp extract, Rice Bran, Coleus root extract, Ginger root extract, Black Currant seed extract • Proprietary Herbal Blend 115 mg: pHysioProtease, CereCalase. Other Ingredients: Plant Cellulose, Water.

Low-Carb Apple Autumn Frost - Revival **-** Physicians Laboratories
Each bar contains: Certified Isoflavone 160 mg. Other Ingredients:

Soy Protein Isolate, Rice Starch, Brown Rice Flour, Vegetable Protein, Whey Protein Isolate, Maltitol, Fractionated Palm Kernel Oil, Maltodextrin, Nonfat Yogurt Powder, Partially-Hydrogenated Palm oil, Calcium Caseinate, Soy Lecithin, Lactic Acid, Acesulfame K, Vanilla, Sulfite-Free Apples, Natural and Artificial Flavor, Glycerin, Corn Syrup Solids, Cinnamon, Potassium Sorbate, Citric Acid, Sucralose.

Low-Carb Chocolate Raspberry Zing - Revival **-** Physicians Laboratories
Each Bar Contains: Certified Isoflavone 160 mg. Other Ingredients: Soy Protein Isolate, Rice Starch, Brown Rice Flour, Vegetable Protein, Whey Protein Isolate, Maltitol, Fractionated Palm Kernel Oil, Cocoa (processed with alkali), Partially-Hydrogenated Palm Oil, Soy Lecithin, Acesulfame K, Vanilla, Lactitol, Palm Kernel Oil, Polydextrose, Oat fiber, Dried Strawberries, Dried Raspberries, Natural and Artificial Flavors, Citric Acid, Vegetable Juice Coloring, Malic Acid, Glycerin, Corn Syrup Solids, Potassium Sorbate, Sucralose.

LPC **-** OSMO Therapy
Each capsule contains: Lysophosphatidyl Choline 300 mg.

LPC Serum **-** The Vitamin Factory
Each 1 oz serving contains: Pycnogenol • Vitamin C.

L-Pyroglutamic Acid **-** Source Naturals
Each tablet contains: L-Pyroglutamic acid 1,000 mg.

L-Theanine **-** FoodScience of Vermont
Each capsule contains: L-Theanine (Suntheanine brand) 200 mg. Other Ingredients: Rice Flour, Vegetable Stearate, Gelatin, Water.

L-Theanine **-** PhysioLogics
Each capsule contains: L-Theanine 100 mg. Other Ingredients: Cellulose (plant origin), Dicalcium Phosphate, Gelatin, Vegetable Magnesium Stearate, Magnesium Silicate, Silica.

L-Theanine **-** PhytoPharmica
Each capsule contains: L-Theanine 100 mg. Other Ingredients: Cellulose, Gelatin, Magnesium Stearate, Titanium Dioxide Color.

L-Tyrosine **-** NutriCology
Each capsule contains: L-Tyrosine 500 mg. Other Ingredients: Cellulose, Silicon Dioxide, Stearic Acid.

L-Tyrosine 500 **-** GNC
Each tablet contains: L-Tyrosine 500 mg. Other Ingredients: Cellulose, Acacia.

Lukol **-** The Himalaya Drug Company (Himalaya Heal
Each tablet contains: Dhataki (woodfordia fruticosa) 40 mg • Kokilaksha (hygrohila auriculata syn. asteracantha longifolia) 40 mg • Shatavari (asparagus racemosus) 40 mg • Sarpagandha (rauwolfia serpentina) 20 mg • Punarnava (boerhaavia diffusa) 10 mg • Vasaka (adhatoda zeylanica) 20 mg • Puga (areca catechu) 20 mg • Jatiphalam (myristica fragrans) 16 mg • Ela (elattaria cardamomum) 11 mg • Nagkesara (mesua ferrea) 11 mg • Jeeraka (cuminum cyminum) 10 mg • Chandana (santalum album) 10 mg • Bilva (aegle marmelos) 5 mg • Sunthi (zingiber officinale) 5 mg • Triphala 5 mg: Emblica Officinalis, Terminalia Chebula, Terminalia Bellirica • Maricha (piper nigrum) 5 mg • Hyamarka (wrightia tinctoria) 5 mg • Guggulu (commiphora wightii) 5 mg • Palasa (butea frondosa syn. b.monosperma) 4 mg • Shilajeet (mineral pitch, purified) 9 mg • Praval Bhasma (coral calx) 7 mg • Loh Bhasma (iron calx) 5 mg • Trivang 5 mg: Lead (naga), Tin (vanga), Zinc (yasada).

Lukol DS **-** The Himalaya Drug Company (Himalaya Heal
Each tablet contains: Dhataki (woodfordia fruticosa) 80 mg • Kokilaksha (hygrophila auriculata syn. asteracantha longifolia) 80 mg • Shatavari (asparagus racemosus) 80 mg • Sarpagandha (rauwolfia serpentina) 40 mg • Punarnava (boerhaavia diffusa) 20 mg • Vasaka (adhatoda zeylanica) 20 mg • Puga (areca catechu) 40 mg • Jatiphalam (myristica fragrans) 32 mg • Ela (elattaria cardamomum) 22 mg • Nagkesara (mesua ferrea) 22 mg • Jeeraka (cuminum cyminum) 20 mg • Chandana (santalum album) 20 mg • Bilva (aegle marmelos) 10 mg • Sunthi (zingiber officinale) 10 mg • Triphala 10 mg: Emblica Officinalis, Terminalia Chebula, Terminalia Bellirica • Maricha (piper nigrum) 10 mg • Hyamaraka (wrightia tinctoria) 10 mg • Guggulu (commiphora wightii) 10 mg • Palasa (butea frondosa syn. b.monosperma) 8 mg • Shilajeet (mineral pitch, purified) 18 mg • Praval Bhasma (coral calx) 14 mg • Loh Bhasma (iron calx) 10 mg • Trivang 10 mg: Lead (naga), Tin (vanga), Zinc (yasada).

Lullaby Nighttime Formula **-** Starlight International
Each two tablets contain: Niacin (Niacinamide) 50 mg • Vitamin B6 (pyridoxine HCl) 20 mg • Calcium (as calcium lactate) 10 mg • Magnesium (as magnesium oxide) 114 mg • Kava Kava extract, 4:1 (piper methysticum, root) 200 mg • Valerian extract, 4:1 (valeriana officinalis, root) 150 mg • Lemon Balm (melissa officinalis, leaf) 150 mg • Passion Flower (passiflora incarnata, plant) 150 mg • Melatonin 5 mg. Inactive Ingredients: Dicalcium Phosphate, Microcrystalline Cellulose, Stearic Acid, Gum Acacia, Croscarmellose Sodium, Silicon Dioxide, Magnesium Stearate, Pharmaceutical Glaze, Ethylcellulose, Dextrin, Dextrose, Lecithin, Sodium Citrate.

Luna Chai Tea **-** Clif Bars
Ingredients: Soy Protein Isolate • Rice Flour • Malt Extract • Rolled Oats • Roasted Soybean • Soy Flour • Milled Flaxseed • Brown Rice Syrup • Evaporated Cane Juice • Fractionated Palm Kernel Oil • Soy Flour • Soy Lecithin • Soy Milk • Green Tea Extract • Ground Ginger • Green Tea Leaves • Cloves • Anise • Cinnamon • Cardamom • Sea Salt • Natural Flavors.

Luna Cherry Covered Chocolate **-** Clif Bars
Ingredients: Soy Protein Isolate • Rice Flour • Cocoa • Rolled Oats • Roasted Soybean • Milled Flaxseed • Brown Rice Syrup • Evaporated Cane Juice • Fractionated Palm Kernel Oil • Soy Flour • Soy Lecithin • Oat Flour • Beet Juice (for coloring) • Dried Plums • Cherries • Sea Salt • Natural Flavors.

Luna Chocolate Pecan Pie **-** Clif Bars
Ingredients: Soy Protein Isolate • Rice Flour • Malt Extract • Rolled Oats • Roasted Soybean • Soy Flour • Milled Flaxseed • Brown Rice Syrup • Pecans • Sea Salt • Cinnamon • Evaporated Cane Juice • Fractionated Palm Kernel Oil • Decaffeinated Green Tea Extract • Cocoa • Soy Lecithin • Natural Flavors.

Luna Chocolate Peppermint Stick **-** Clif Bars
Ingredients: Soy Protein Isolate • Rice Flour • Cocoa • Rolled Oats • Roasted Soybean • Milled Flaxseed • Brown Rice Syrup • Evaporated Cane Juice • Fractionated Palm Kernel Oil • Soy Flour • Soy Lecithin • Peppermint Oil • Oat Flour • Sea Salt • Natural Flavors • Red Cabbage extract (for coloring) • Sunflower Oil • Unsweetened Chocolate • Salt • Baking Soda.

Luna Key Lime Pie **-** Clif Bars
Ingredients: Soy Protein Isolate • Rice Flour • Malt Extract • Rolled Oats • Soy Protein Isolate • Soybean • Soy Flour • Milled Flaxseed • Brown Rice Syrup • Evaporated Cane Juice • Fractionated Palm Kernel Oil • Oat Fiber • Oat Flour • Gum Arabic • Citric Acid • Soy Lecithin • Sea Salt • Green Tea Extract • Soy Milk • Natural Flavors • Freeze-dried Lime • Spinach Extract.

Luna LemonZest **-** Clif Bars
Ingredients: Soy Protein Isolate • Rice Flour • Malt Extract • Rolled Oats • Roasted Soybean • Soy Flour • Milled Flaxseed • Brown Rice Syrup • Evaporated Cane Juice • Fractionated Palm Kernel Oil • Oat Fiber • Oat Flour • Gum Arabic • Citric Acid • Lemon Oil • Soy Lecithin • Soy Milk • Decaffeinated Green Tea Extract • Sea Salt • Natural Flavors.

Luna Nuts Over Chocolate **-** Clif Bars
Ingredients: Soy Protein Isolate • Rice Flour • Malt Extract • Rolled Oats • Roasted Soybean • Soy Flour • Milled Flaxseed • Brown Rice Syrup • Evaporated Cane Juice • Fractionated Palm Kernel Oil •

Peanut Flour • Peanut Butter • Cocoa • Soy Lecithin • Soy Milk • Decaffeinated Green Tea Extract • Sea Salt • Natural Flavors.

Luna Orange Bliss - Clif Bars
Ingredients: Soy Protein Isolate • Rice Flour • Malt Extract • Rolled Oats • Soy Protein Isolate • Soybean • Soy Flour • Milled Flaxseed • Brown Rice Syrup • Evaporated Cane Juice • Fractionated Palm Kernel Oil • Oat Fiber • Oat Flour • Citric Acid • Gum Arabic • Soy Lecithin • Paprika Extract • Salt • Sea Salt • Green Tea Extract • Soy Milk • Natural Flavors • Annatto.

Luna Peanut Butter 'N Jelly - Clif Bars
Ingredients: Soy Protein Isolate • Rice Flour • Malt Extract • Cocoa • Rolled Oats • Roasted Soybean • Milled Flaxseed • Brown Rice Syrup • Evaporated Cane Juice • Fractionated Palm Kernel Oil • Soy Flour • Soy Lecithin • Sunflower Oil • Oat Flour • Beet Juice (for coloring) • Strawberry Puree • Cranberries • Apple Juice • Blueberry Juice • Blueberry Extract • Peanut Butter • Peanut Flour • Glucose • Pectin • Citric Acid • Sea Salt • Natural Flavors.

Luna Sesame Raisin Crunch - Clif Bars
Ingredients: Soy Protein Isolate • Rice Flour • Malt Extract • Rolled Oats • Roasted Soybean • Soy Flour • Milled Flaxseed • Brown Rice Syrup • Raisins • Toasted Sesame Seeds • Dry Roasted Sunflower Seeds • Decaffeinated Green Tea Extract • Sea Salt • Natural Flavors.

Luna S'mores - Clif Bars
Ingredients: Soy Protein Isolate • Rice Flour • Malt Extract • Rolled Oats • Roasted Soybean • Soy Flour • Milled Flaxseed • Brown Rice Syrup • Evaporated Cane Juice • Fractionated Palm Kernel Oil • Soy Flour • Soy Lecithin • Oat Fiber • Oat Flour • Gum Arabic • Decaffeinated Green Tea Extract • Sea Salt • Natural Marshmallow & Graham Cracker Flavors • Citric Acid • Cocoa.

Luna Sweet Dreams - Clif Bars
Ingredients: Soy Protein Isolate • Rice Flour • Cocoa • Rolled Oats • Roasted Soybean • Milled Flaxseed • Brown Rice Syrup • Evaporated Cane Juice • Fractionated Palm Kernel Oil • Soy Flour • Soy Lecithin • Peanuts • Defatted Peanut Flour • Sea Salt • Natural Flavors.

Luna Toasted Nuts 'N Cranberry - Clif Bars
Ingredients: Soy Protein Isolate • Rice Flour • Malt Extract • Rolled Oats • Roasted Soybean • Soy Flour • Milled Flaxseed • Brown Rice Syrup • Cashews • Almonds • Pumpkin Seeds • Cranberries • Apple Juice • Decaffeinated Green Tea Extract • Natural Flavors.

Luna Tropical Crisp - Clif Bars
Ingredients: Soy Protein Isolate • Rice Flour • Malt Extract • Rolled Oats • Roasted Soybean • Soy Flour • Milled Flaxseed • Brown Rice Syrup • Evaporated Cane Juice • Fractionated Palm Kernel Oil • Soy Flour • Soy Lecithin • Soy Milk • Toasted Coconut • Coconut Milk Powder • Dried Pineapple • Decaffeinated Green Tea Extract • Freeze-Dried Pineapple • Natural Flavors.

Lung Health - Wellzymes - Enzymes, Inc.
Two capsules contain: n-zimes Proprietary Enzyme Blend 84 mg: pHysioProtease (213,120 pHysio-U), Amylase, CereCalse Plus • Proprietary Herbal Blend 350 mg: Thyme herb extract (equivalent to 520 mg raw herb), Mullein leaf extract (equivalent to 400 mg raw herb), Great Plantain leaf extract (equivalent to 160 mg raw herb), Acerola Cherries extract (standardized to contain 17% Vitamin C), Quercetin, Rice Bran. Other Ingredients: Plant Cellulose, Water.

Lung Support Formula - Gero Vita International
Astragalus membranaceus • Cordyceps sinensis • Ophiopogon japonicus.

Lung Tan Xie Gan pills - Kwangchow Pharmaceutical Industry Co
Unknown.
See Editor's Note No. 46, page 2058.

Lung-Mend - The Herbalist
Elecampane root • Grindelia herb • Pleurisy root • Butterbur root • Marshmallow root • Usnea lichen • Yerba Santa leaf • Lobelia leaf • Yerba Mansa root.

Lungs - Enzymes, Inc.
Two capsules contain: Vitamin C (100% from Acerola Cherries) 17 mg • Proprietary Herbal Blend 490 mg: Mullein herb extract, Thyme herb extract, Sundew herb extract, Ginkgo Biloba leaf extract, Green Tea extract • Proprietary Enzyme Blend 440 mg: Amylase, pHysioProtease. Other Ingredients: Plant Cellulose, Water.

Luprinol - Klein-Becker
Two capsules contain: Ephedrine alkaloids (from standardized whole plant Ma Huang extract 200 mg) 20 mg • Caffeine (34 mg from standardized Kola nut 280 mg) 200 mg • Acetylsalicylic acid 324 mg • DHEA 8.4 mg • Schizonepeta (spica) 250 mg. Other Ingredients: Rice Flour.

Lustre - Source Naturals
Six tablets contain: Vitamin A (Beta Carotene) 15000 IU • Vitamin A (Palmitate) 5000 IU • Vitamin B1 (Thiamin) 10 mg • Vitamin B2 (Riboflavin) 10 mg • Niacinamide 30 mg • Vitamin B5 (Calcium D-Pantothenate) 50 mg • Vitamin B6 (Pyridoxine HCl) 20 mg • Vitamin B12 (Cyanocobalamin) 30 mcg • Biotin 2000 mcg • Folic Acid 800 mcg • Vitamin C (Magnesium, Zinc and Manganese Ascorbates) 1000 mg • Vitamin E (D-Alpha Tocopheryl)(Natural) 200 IU • Copper (Sebacate) 1.5 mg • Magnesium (Ascorbate) 59 mg • Silica (Horsetail Silica Extract) 36 mg • Manganese (Ascorbate) 6 mg • Selenium (as L-Selenomethionine and Sodium Selenite) 200 mcg • L-Proline 600 mg • Inositol 500 mg • L-Cysteine (HCl) 400 mg • Choline (Bitartrate) 100 mg • L-Methionine 100 mg • N-Acetyl Cysteine 100 mg • PABA (Para Amino Benzoic Acid) 100 mg.

Lutein - NSI - Nutraceutical Sciences Institute
Each softgel contains: Lutein 20 mg.

Lutein - PhysioLogics
Each softgel contains: Lutein 20 mg. Other Ingredients: Corn Oil, Gelatin, Glycerin, Yellow Beeswax, Lecithin.

Lutein - Sundown
Each softgel contains: Lutein 6 mg • Healthy Eye Blend 2.3 mg: Bilberry fruit extract 4:1, Spinach leaf, Zeaxanthin. Other Ingredients: Rice Bran Oil, Gelatin, Glycerin, Corn Oil, Water.

Lutein & Bilberry Complex - PhysioLogics
Each capsule contains: Lutein (containing naturally occurring zeaxanthin) 6 mg • Bilberry fruit extract (vacciunum myrtillus, standardized to contain 25% anthocyanosides) 20 mg. Other Ingredients: Dicalcium Phosphate, Cellulose (plant origin), Gelatin, Vegetable Stearic Acid, Silica, Vegetable Magnesium Stearate.

Lutein & Zeaxanthin Complex - Vitamin World
Each softgel contains: Vitamin A (as beta carotene) 14,320 IU • Vitamin C (as ascorbic acid) 226 mg • Vitamin E (as DL-alpha tocopherol acetate) 200 IU • Zinc (as zinc oxide) 34.8 mg • Copper (as copper oxide) 0.8 mg • Lutein 4 mg • Zeaxanthin 172 mcg. Other Ingredients: Soybean Oil, Gelatin, Glycerin, Partially Hydrogenated Corn Oil, Corn Oil, Soy Lecithin, Titanium Dioxide Color, Yellow 6 Lake, Red 40 Lake, Blue 1 Lake.

Lutein 20 mg - Allergy Research Group
Each softgel contains: Vitamin E (as mixed tocopherols) 1 IU • Lutein 20 mg • Zeaxanthin 900 mcg. Other Ingredients: Safflower Oil, Yellow Beeswax, Corn Oil.

Lutein 20 mg - NutriCology
Each softgel contains: Vitamin E (as mixed tocopherols) 1 IU • Lutein 20 mg • Zeaxanthin 900 mcg. Other Ingredients: Safflower Oil, Yellow Beeswax, Corn Oil.

***Lutein 20 mg Natural Carotenoid* -** Puritan's Pride
Each softgel contains: Lutein 20 mg. Other Ingredients: Corn Oil, Gelatin, Glycerin, Yellow Beeswax, Lecithin.

***Lutein 20 mg Natural Carotenoid* -** Nature's Bounty
Each softgel contains: Lutein 20 mg. Other Ingredients: Corn Oil, Gelatin, Glycerin, Yellow Beeswax, Lecithin.

***Lutein 6 mg Natural Carotenoid - Puritan's Pride* -** Puritan's Pride
Each softgel contains: Lutein 6 mg. Other Ingredients: Corn Oil, Gelatin, Glycerin, Beeswax.

***Lutein 6 mg Natural Carotenoid* -** Nature's Bounty
Each softgel contains: Lutein 6 mg. Other Ingredients: Corn Oil, Gelatin, Glycerin, Yellow Beeswax.

***Lutein i care* -** Nature's Life
Each capsule contains: Lutein (FloraGLO) [from Marigold petals (Tagetes erecta)] 5 mg • Beta Carotene [(Dunaliella salina) equivalent to 5000 IU Vitamin A] 3 mg • Other naturally occurring carotenoids in D. salina: Zeaxanthin (T. erecta, D. salina) 370 mcg • Alpha Carotene 106 mcg • Cryptoxanthin 20 mcg • Zinc (Gluconate) 5 mg • Copper (Gluconate) 2.5 mg.

***Lutein Plus* -** Puritan's Pride
Each capsule contains: Lutein (with 240-600 mcg Zeaxanthin) 6 mg • In a 330 mg base of: Spinach, Blueberry Powder and Bilberry extract.

***Lutein Rx-Eye* -** Nature's Plus
Each capsule contains: Vitamin A (as beta carotene) 20,000 IU • Vitamin C (as ascorbic acid, ascorbyl palmitate) 500 mg • Vitamin E (as d-alpha tocopheryl succinate) 200 mg • Vitamin B2 (as riboflavin) 25 mg • Zinc (as monomethionine) 20 mg • Selenium (as amino acid complex) 50 mcg • Chromium (as polynicotinate) 120 mcg • Citrus Bioflavonoid Complex 125 mg • MSM (methylsulfonylmethane) 100 mg • Lutein (active carotenoid from marigold flower extract) 20 mg • Bilberry (vaccinium myrtillus fruit, standardized 25% [5 mg] anthocyanosides) 20 mg • L-Glutathione (free form amino acid) 5 mg • Zeaxanthin (active carotenoid from marigold flower extract) 876 mcg.

***Lutein Z* -** Jamieson
Each capsule contains: Lutein and Zeaxanthin Complex (derived from Marigold flowers) 50 mg • CyanoSome 3 Botanical Complex 4600 mg: European Grape Seed 2500 mg, Ginkgo Biloba Leaf 2000 mg, Bilberry Fruit 100 mg, Green Tea Extract 2.5 mg.

***Lutein-20* -** DreamPharm
Each capsule contains: Lutein (5% powder containing zeaxanthin, extracted from marigold flower) 20 mg • Vitamin C 60 mg • Buckwheat powder 500 mg.

***Lutein-6* -** DreamPharm
Two capsules contain: Lutein (5% powder containing zeaxanthin, extracted from marigold flower) • Vitamin C 60 mg. Other Ingredients: Buckwheat Powder.

***Lycobeads brand* -** H. Reisman Corporation
Lycopene.
See Editor's Note No. 44, page 2058.

***Lyc-o-matic 15 mg* -** Natrol
Each tablet contains: Calcium (as calcium carbonate) 46 mg • Lycopene (from natural tomato powder, tomato extract) 15 mg • Tomato powder 535 mg. Other Ingredients: Cellulose, Stearic Acid, Cellulose Gum, Silica, Magnesium Stearate.

***LYC-O-MATO 15 mg Soft Gel Capsules (Olive oil)* -** Healthy Origins
Each softgel contains: Lyc-O-Mato 250 mg • Vitamin A (as natural beta-carotene) 333 IU • Vitamin E (as d-alpha tocopherol) 5.5 IU • Lycopene 15 mg • Phytoene 1 mg • Phytofluene 1 mg • Phytosterols 1 mg. Other Ingredients: Olive Oil, Gelatin, Glycerin, Purified Water, Annatto.

***LYC-O-MATO 15 mg Soft Gel Capsules (Soybean oil)* -** Healthy Origins
Each softgel contains: Lyc-O-Mato 250 mg • Vitamin A (as natural beta-carotene) 333 IU • Vitamin E (as d-alpha tocopherol) 5.5 IU • Lycopene 15 mg • Phytoene 1 mg • Phytofluene 1 mg • Phytosterols 1 mg. Other Ingredients: Soybean Oil, Gelatin, Glycerin, Purified Water, Annatto.

***LYC-O-MATO 5 mg Soft Gel Capsules (Soybean oil)* -** Healthy Origins
Each softgel contains: Lycopene 5 mg. Other Ingredients: Soybean Oil, Gelatin, Glycerin, Purified Water, Annatto.

***Lyc-O-Mato brand* -** LycoRed Natural Products Industries, Ltd
Tomato extract.
See Editor's Note No. 44, page 2058.

***LYC-O-MATO Clinical Trio (Olive oil)* -** Healthy Origins
Each softgel contains: Lyc-O-Mato 250 mg • Vitamin A (as natural beta-carotene) 333 IU • Vitamin E (as d-alpha tocopherol) 200 IU • Selenium 100 mcg • Lycopene 15 mg • Phytoene 1 mg • Phytofluene 1 mg • Phytosterols 1 mg. Other Ingredients: Gelatin, Glycerin, Olive Oil, Purified Water, Annatto.

***LYC-O-MATO PLUS Seleno Excell Soft Gel Capsules* -** Healthy Origins
Each softgel contains: Lyc-O-Mato 250 mg • Vitamin A (as natural beta-carotene) 333 IU • Seleno Excell Selenium 100 mcg • Vitamin E (as d-alpha tocopherol) 5.5 IU • Lycopene 15 mg • Phytoene 1 mg • Phytofluene 1 mg • Phytosterols 1 mg. Other Ingredients: Soybean Oil, Gelatin, Glycerin, Purified Water, Annatto.

***Lycopene* -** Quest
Each capsule contains: Lyc-o-Mato brand Lycopene 5000 mcg. Other Ingredients: Rice Bran Oil, Sunflower Oil, Vegetable Stearin, Beeswax, Lecithin.

***Lycopene* -** Olympian Labs
Two capsules contain: Tomato Lycopene 300 mg • Vegetable Enzymes (amylase, lipase, protease) 100 mg.

***Lycopene* -** NSI - Nutraceutical Sciences Institute
Each softgel contains: Lycopene 15 mg • Rice Bran oil 231 mg.

***Lycopene* -** PhysioLogics
Each softgel contains: Lycopene 10 mg. Other Ingredients: Soybean Oil, Gelatin, Beeswax / Soybean Oil Mixture, Glycerin.

***Lycopene* -** Nature's Life
Each capsule contains: Lycopene 6 mg • Carrot Carotenoids 2 mg providing: Beta Carotene (Vitamin A equivalent 2500 IU) 1500 mcg, Alpha Carotene (Vitamin A equivalent 417 IU) 500 mcg, Phytoene 39 mcg, Phytofluene 13 mcg.

***Lycopene* -** EcoNugenics
Each softgel contains: Lycopene 15 mg • Tomato Lipids 205 mg. Other Ingredients: Rice Bran Oil, Gelatin, Glycerin, Water, Triglycerides, Beeswax, Silica.

***Lycopene 10 mg* -** Puritan's Pride
Each softgel contains: Lycopene 10 mg.

***Lycopene 5 mg* -** Puritan's Pride
Each softgel contains: Lycopene 5 mg.

***Lycopene Softgels* -** Optimum Nutrition
Each softgel contains: Lycopene 5 mg. Other Ingredients: Gelatin, Soybean Oil, Glycerine, Vegetable Oil, Yellow Beeswax.

Lycopene-Rich Tomato Concentrate - Jamieson
Each caplet contains: Organic Ripe Tomato Concentrate 100 mg • Lycopene Nutritional Factor 10 mg.

Lycosoy - TwinLab
Two softgels contain: Vitamin D 400 IU • Vitamin E 200 IU • Selenium 200 mcg • Omega-3 Fish Oil conc. 460 mcg • Soy Bean extract 150 mg • Lycopene 5 mg • Green Tea leaf extract 2 mg.

Lymph - Enzymes, Inc.
Each capsule contains: Proprietary Herbal Blend 390 mg: Burdock root extract, Wild Indigo root extract, Cleavers herb extract, Yellow Dock root extract, Figwort herb powder • Proprietary Enzyme Blend 110 mg: pHysioProtease, Amylase, Lipase, CereCalase. Other Ingredients: Plant Cellulose, Water.

Lymphatone - The Herbalist
Echinacea root • Red root • Cleavers herb • Yellow Dock root • Burdock root • Wild Indigo root • Poke root.

Lympho-Clear - Enzymatic Therapy
Each capsule contains: Red Clover extract 4:1 (Trifolium pratense) 200 mg • Burdock root extract 4:1 (Arctium lappa) 200 mg • Oregon Grape root extract 6:1 (Berberis aquifolium) 100 mg • Licorice root extract (Glycyrrhiza glabra) standardized to contain 5% Glycyrrhizic Acid 50 mg • Goldenseal root extract (Hydrastis canadensis) standardized to contain 5% total Alkaloids including: Berberine, Hydrastine & Canadine 50 mg.

Lymph-Spleen Soluble Fractions - PhytoPharmica
Each capsule contains: Lymph-Spleen Complex (predigested soluble concentrate) 250 mg • Multi-Glandular Complex 100 mg: Raw Liver, Raw Lung, Raw Pancreas, Raw Heart, Raw Kidney, Raw Spleen & Raw Brain. All organs and glands derived from bovine sources except raw pancreas (porcine).
See Editor's Note No. 21 and No. 31.

Lyprinol - Tyler Encapsulations
Two softgel capsules contain: Marine Lipid extract from Perna Canaliculus 100 mg. Other Ingredients: Olive Oil, D-Alpha Tocopherol, Gelatin, Sorbitol, Glycerin.

Lysozyme Plus - Atrium Inc.
Each tablet contains: Pancreatin (maximum strength) 200 mg • Papain 100 mg • Bromelain 75 mg • Rutin 60 mg • Trypsin 35 mg • Thymus 35 mg • Amylase 15 mg • Lipase 15 mg • Lysozyme 10 mg • Cellulase 2 mg • Zinc Gluconate 4 mg • a-Chymotrypsin 1 mg.
See Editor's Note No. 14.

M.C.H.C. Capsules - Progressive Labs
Each capsule contains: Calcium 250 mg, from 500 mg M.C.H.C. 125 mg, from 500 mg Calcium Citrate 125 mg • Iron (from M.C.H.C.) 0.3 mg • Vitamin K 20 mcg • Phosphorus (from M.C.H.C) 65 mg • Magnesium (from M.C.H.C.) 4 mg • Zinc (from M.C.H.C.) 0.075 mg • Copper (from M.C.H.C.) 0.01 mg • Manganese (from M.C.H.C.) 0.045 mg • Potassium (from M.C.H.C.) 0.035 mg • Protein (from M.C.H.C. as collagen glycosaminoglycans) 125 mg • Boron (as boron aspartate) 0.75 mg • Fluorapatite (from M.C.H.C.) 31 mcg • Silicon (from M.C.H.C.) 19 mcg • Strontium (from M.C.H.C.) 10 mcg.

M.C.H.C. Tablets - Progressive Labs
Each tablet contains: Calcium (elemental) 250 mg, from 500 mg M.C.H.C. 125 mg, from 500 mg. Calcium Citrate 125 mg • Iron (from M.C.H.C.) 0.3 mg • Vitamin K 20 mcg • Phosphorum (from M.C.H.C.) 65 mg • Magnesium (from M.C.H.C.) 4 mg • Zinc (from M.C.H.C.) 0.075 mg • Copper (from M.C.H.C.) 0.01 mg • Manganese (from M.C.H.C.) 0.045 mg • Potassium (from M.C.H.C.) 0.035 mg • Protein (from M.C.H.C. as collagen glycosaminoglycans) 125 mg • Boron (as aspartate) 750 mcg • Fluorapatite (from M.C.H.C.) 31 mcg • Silicon (from M.C.H.C.) 19 mcg • Strontium (from M.C.H.C.) 10 mcg.

M.V. Teen - Futurebiotics
100% or more of the USRDA for 16 vitamins and minerals, 100 mcg of chromium and selenium.

M1T - Higher Power
Each capsule contains: Methyl-1-Testosterone 5 mg. Other Ingredients: Maltodextrin, Magnesium Stearate, Gelatin.

Maca - Source Naturals
Three tablets contain: Maca root extract (MacaPure) (Lepidium meyenii) Standardized to 0.6% macamides and macaenes yielding 4.5 mg macamides and macaenes 750 mg.

Macaroni - Revival - Physicians Laboratories
Two Ounces Contain: Certified Isoflavone 15 mg. Ingredients: Soy Protein Isolate, Niacin, Iron (Ferrous Sulfate), Thiamin Mononitrate, Riboflavin, Folic Acid.

Macerat Drainer Elixir - PhytoPharma
Aqueous extracts blend: Anis seeds, Bardane root, Birch leaves, Black Currant leaves, Black Radish, Cherry stems, Commen, Dandelion roots and leaves, Fennel seeds, Fumitory, Green Tea, Heather, Mint, Nettle, Parsley, Sage, Watercress.

Macerat Purgative Elixir - PhytoPharma
Aqueous extracts blend: Artichoke, Black Radish, Camu Cane, Cardamon, Celery, Chrysantellum Indicum, Muscade.

MacroForce Plus C - ImmuDyne, Inc.
Each capsule contains: Vitamin C (as Calcium Ascorbate) 394 mg • Calcium (as Calcium Carbonate) 44 mg • Beta-1,3-D-glucan (from cell walls of yeast, Saccharomyces cerevisiae) 7.5 mg.

Macro-Min - Atrium Inc.
Each tablet contains: Calcium Aspartate 600 mg • Magnesium Gluconate 300 mg • Potassium Aspartate 88.3 mg • Manganese Aspartate 50 mg • Vitamin D (as Vitamin D3) 250 IU.

Macro-Mineral Complex - Advocare International
Two caplets contain: Calcium (as citrate and hydroxyapatite) 220 mg • Magnesium (as amino acid chelate and ascorbate) 200 mg • Vitamin D (as ergocalciferol) 40 IU • Vitamin C (as magnesium ascorbate) 60 mg • Pyridoxine (as HCl) 3 mg • Manganese (as amino acid chelate) 1 mg • Zinc (as monomethionine, OptiZinc brand) 2 mg • Copper (as amino acid chelate) 200 mcg • Silicon (as amino acid chelate) 300 mcg • Boron (as amino acid chelate) 200 mcg • Potassium Bicarbonate 500 mg • Shave Grass herb extract (equisetum arvense) 50 mg • Green Tea leaf extract (camellia sinensis) 50 mg • Ginger root extract (zingiber officinale) 25 mg. Other Ingredients: Dicalcium Phosphate, Silicon Dioxide, Cellulose, Stearic Acid, Magnesium Stearate.

Macu Care - PhysioLogics
Each capsule contains: Taurine 200 mg • Calendula flower (calendula officinalis, 5% lutein, 3 mg, 0.22% zeaxanthin, 132 mcg) 60 mg • Alpha Lipoic Acid 25 mg • Mixed Xanthophylis (from calendula flower) 2 mg. Other Ingredients: Rice Powder, Gelatin, Vegetable Magnesium Stearate, Silica.

Macula Support Drops - Natural Ophthalmics
Active Ingredients: Calcarea Fluorica HPUS 10x • Calcarea Phosphorica HPUS 10x • Kali Phosphoricum HPUS 6x • Natrum Muriaticum HPUS 6x • Carboneum Sulphuratum HPUS 6x. Inactive Ingredients: Sterile Water, Sodium Chloride, Sodium Citrate, Citrate, Polysorbate 80.

Macular Guardian - Clinician's Choice
Two tablets contain: Vitamin A (as retinyl acetate) 2000 IU • Vitamin C (as ascorbic acid) 120 mg • Vitamin E (as dl-alpha tocopheryl acetate) 200 IU • Riboflavin 6 mg • Selenium (as selenomethionine) 40 mcg • Manganese (as amino acid chelate) 10 mg • Eyebright Herb 200 mg • RoseOx (patented, standardized process for an extract of Rosemary) 100 mg • Ascorbyl Palmitate 20 mg • L-Lysine HCl 20 mg • Lutein 12 mg • L-Glutathione 10 mg • Lycopene 10 mg • Beta-

Carotene 6 mg • Proprietary blend 8 mg: Cruciferex, Carrot Powder, Citrus Bioflavonoid Complex, Bilberry, Zeaxanthin.

MaculaRx Plus - ScienceBased Health
Two capsules contain: Vitamin A (50% from retinyl palmitate and 50% from beta carotene) 2500 IU • Vitamin C (from ascorbic acid) 250 mg • Vitamin E (as d-alpha tocopheryl succinate) 200 IU • Zinc (from zinc ascorbate) 40 mg • Selenium (from selenium amino acid chelate) 35 mcg • Copper (from copper gluconate) 1 mg • Other Carotenoids (Xanthophylls) 7.875 mg • Lutein 7.5 mg • Zeaxanthin 375 mcg. Other Ingredients: Gelatin, Water, Rice Flour.

MacuVision - Health Smart Vitamins
Two capsules contain: Taurine 400 mg • Calendula (5% Lutein, 6 mg; >0.22% Zeaxanthin, 264 mcg) 120 mg • Alpha-Lipoic Acid 50 mg.

Mag Link - Pain & Stress Center
Two tablets contain: Calcium (Calcium Carbonate) 225 mg • Magnesium (Magnesium Chloride Hexahydrate) 130 mg • Chloride 375 mg.

Magic Cigarettes - Alternative Cigarettes Inc
Each cigarette contains: Marshmallow • Yerba Santa • Damiana • Passion Flower • Jasmine • Ginseng. Regular and menthol are available.
See Editor's Note No. 6, page 2053.

Magma Plus - Green Foods Corp.
Each 5.3 oz jar contains: Proprietary Blend 150 g: Young Barley Grass powdered juice, Carrot, Wheat Grass, Alfalfa, Lettuce, Cabbage, Daikon Radish, Bean Sprouts, Celery, Tomato, Spinach, Kale, Maltodextrin, Lecithin, Honey, Bee Pollen, Royal Jelly, Apple, Banana, Pineapple, Papaya, Mango, Raspberry, Chicory root extract, Wheat Germ extract, L. Bifidus, L. Acidophilus, L. Planatarum, Spirulina, Chlorella, Licorice root extract, Coix extract, Vitamin E, Acerola extract, Brown Rice, Red Beet extract, Milk Thistle extract, Echinacea Purpurea extract, Siberian Ginseng extract, American Ginseng extract, Astragalus extract, Aloe Vera, Green Tea extract, Ginger root extract, Stevia extract, Reishi Mushroom extract, Cayenne Pepper, Garlic, Cat's Claw extract, Yucca root extract, Ginkgo Biloba extract, Garcinia Cambogia extract, Glucomannan, Bilberry extract, Grape Seed extract, Lipase, Amylase, Protease.

Magna Pac Daily Basics - Swanson
Each packet (three softgels, five tablets) contains: Vitamin A (as beta-carotene) 25000 IU • Vitamin C USP (as ascorbic acid) 1 g • Vitamin D (from fish liver oil) 400 IU •Vitamin E (as d-alpha tocopheryl acetate) 400 IU • Thiamin (as thiamin HCl; vitamin B-1) 50 mg • Riboflavin (vitamin B-2) 50 mg • Niacin (as niacinamide) 50 mg • Vitamin B-6 (as pyridoxine HCl) 50 mg • Folic Acid USP 40 mcg • Vitamin B-12 (as Cyanocobalamin) 50 mcg • Biotin USP 50 mcg • Pantothenic Acid (as d-calcium pantothenate) 50 mg • Calcium (500 mg from oyster shell, 500 mg from carbonate, aspartate, citrate) 1 g • Iron (from Albion amino acid chelate) 18 mg • Iodine (from kelp) 150 mcg • Magnesium (from magnesium oxide) 250 mg • Zinc 50 mg • Selenium (from selenomethionine) 50 mcg • Copper 2 mg • Manganese 10 mg • Chromium 50 mcg •Potassium (from potassium proteinate) 99 mg • Lecithin 1.2 g • 72 Trace Mineral compound 72 mg • Betaine HCl 50 mg • Choline (as choline bitartrate) 50 mg • Inositol FCC 50 mg • PABA (para-aminobenzoic acid) 50 mg • Rose Hips (from concentrate) 50 mg.

Magna Pac for Cardio - Swanson
Each packet (four capsules, three softgels) contains: Vitamin E (as d-alpha tocopherol from mixed tocopherols) 400 IU • Thiamin (as thiamin HCl; vitamin B-1) 100 mg • Riboflavin (vitamin B-2) 100 mg • Niacinamide USP 100 mg • Vitamin B-6 USP (as pyridoxine HCl) 100 mg • Folic Acid 400 mcg • Vitamin B-12 USP (as cyanocobalamin) 100 mcg • Biotin USP 100 mcg • Pantothenic Acid (as d-calcium pantothenate) 100 mg • Flaxseed Oil 1 g • Trimethylglycine (as betaine anhydrous) 1 g • Standardized Hawthorn berry extract (1.8% vitexin-2' rhamnosides) 250 mg • Hawthorn berry powder 250 mg • Choline (as choline bitartrate) 100 mg • Inositol 100 mg • PABA (para-aminobenzoic acid) 100 mg • Coenzyme Q10 30 mg • Garlic (500:1 concentrate equal to 500 mg of fresh garlic) 1 mg.

Magna Pac for Joints - Swanson
Each packet (seven capsules, one softgel) contains: Manganese (Albion amino acid chelate) 40 mg • Glucosamine Sulfate (2KCl) 1.5 g • Borage Oil (24% GLA) 1 g • Chondroitin Sulfate 1 g • OptiMSM (methylsulfonylmethane) 1 g • Boswellia Serrata powder 300 mg • Boswellia Serrata (65% boswellic acid) 200 mg • Optimum Abzorption Complex Proprietary Blend: Ginger (root), Piper longum, Piper nigrum 45 mg.
See Editor's Note No. 15, page 2055.

Magna Pac for Menopause - Swanson
Each packet (six capsules, two softgels) contains: Vitamin C (ascorbic acid) 1 g • Vitamin E (as d-alpha tocopherol from mixed tocopherols) 400 IU • Borage Oil (24% GLA) 1 g • Black Cohosh powder 860 mg • SoyLife Soy extract (3% soy isoflavones) 750 mg • Dong Quai herb powder 300 mg • Licorice root extract (15% glycyrrhizic acid) 300 mg • Dong Quai extract (1% ligustilides) 200 mg • Licorice root powder 170 mg • Rose Hips (from concentrate) 60 mg • Black Cohosh (5% triterpene glycosides calculated as 27-deoxyactein) 40 mg.

Magna Pac for Prostate - Swanson
Each packet (five capsules, one tablet) contains: Vitamin E (as d-alpha tocopherol from mixed tocopherols) 400 IU • Zinc (from zinc gluconate) 50 mg • Selenium (L-selenomethionine) 50 mcg • Pumpkin Seed oil 1 g • Saw Palmetto (25% fatty acids) 1 g • Pygeum powder 400 mg • Beta Sitosterol (Cholestatin) 120 mg • Pygeum extract (6.5% phytosterols) 100 mg • Lycopene (Lyc-O-Mato) 5 mg.

Magna Rx+ - NEP Products
Each tablet contains: Pygeum Africanum bark 250 mg • Maca root (lepidium meyenii) 125 mg • Horny Goat Weed (epimedium sagittatum) 75 mg • Oat Straw 75 mg • Catuaba 50 mg • Oriental Ginseng root 50 mg • L-Arginine 50 mg • Stinging Nettle leaf 37.5 mg • Cayenne fruit 25 mg • Muira Puama whole herb 25 mg • Orchic substance 25 mg • Oyster extract 25 mg • Tribulus Terrestris L (aerial parts) 25 mg • Smilax Officinalis root 12.5 mg • Astragalus root 10 mg • Licorice root 10 mg • Pumpkin seed 10 mg • Boron (as boron citrate) 1 mg.

MagnaCal - Holista
Each capsule contains: Calcium from citrate (equivalent to 625 mg) 125 mg • Magnesium from oxide (equivalent to 206 mg) 125 mg • Vitamin D (as Vitamin D3) 100 IU.

Magnesium - PhysioLogics
Each caplet contains: Magnesium (as magnesium oxide) 250 mg. Other Ingredients: Dicalcium Phosphate, Cellulose (plant origin), Starch, Magnesium Silicate, Cellulose Coating, Vegetable Magnesium Stearate.

Magnesium - Source Naturals
Each tablet contains: Magnesium (from 500 mg of magnesium amino acid chelate) 100 mg.

Magnesium 100 mg - Jamieson
Each tablet contains: Magnesium 100 mg.

Magnesium 100mg - Sundown
Four caplets contain: Magnesium (as magnesium oxide, magnesium gluconate) 400 mg. Other Ingredients: Microcrystalline Cellulose, Crospovidone, Silica, Lactose, Hydroxypropyl Methyl-Cellulose, Titanium Dioxide (color), Magnesium Stearate, Triacetin, Stearic Acid.

Magnesium 250 - GNC
Each tablet contains: Magnesium (as magnesium oxide and magnesium gluconate) 250 mg. Other Ingredients: Dicalcium Phosphate, Cellulose.

Magnesium 250 mg - Nature Made
Each tablet contains: Magnesium (from magnesium oxide) 250 mg. Other Ingredients: Cellulose Gel, Croscarmellose Sodium, Magnesium Stearate.
See Editor's Note No. 45, page 2058.

Magnesium 250 mg (Inspired by Nature) - Puritan's Pride
Each tablet contains: Magnesium (as magnesium oxide) 250 mg. Other Ingredients: Cellulose (plant origin), Vegetable Stearic Acid, Vegetable Magnesium Stearate, Silica.

Magnesium 50 mg - Jamieson
Each tablet contains: Magnesium 50 mg.

Magnesium 500 - GNC A-Z - GNC
Each capsule contains: Magnesium (as magnesium oxide) 500 mg. Other Ingredients: Gelatin.

Magnesium 500 mg - Puritan's Pride
Each tablet contains: Magnesium (as magnesium oxide) 500 mg. Other Ingredients: Cellulose (plant origin), Starch, Magnesium Silicate, Cellulose Coating, Titanium Dioxide Color, Vegetable Magnesium Stearate.

Magnesium Caps - TwinLab
Each hard gelatin capsule contains: Elemental Magnesium (from magnesium oxide and magnesium aspartate) 400 mg.

Magnesium Chelate - PhysioLogics
Each caplet contains: Calcium (as dicalcium phosphate, calcium stearate) 15 mg • Magnesium (as magnesium glycinate, magnesium oxide) 200 mg. Other Ingredients: Cellulose (plant origin), Crocarmellose, Silica, Vegetable Stearic Acid, Cellulose Coating.

Magnesium Complex - Klaire Laboratories
Each capsule contains: Magnesium Glycinate (Amino Acid Chelate) 100 mg.

Magnesium Malate - Source Naturals
Each tablet contains: Magnesium Malate 1000mg • Malic Acid 825 mg • Magnesium 152 mg.

Magnesium Multi-Min - Nutri-Quest Rx
Each tablet contains: As an Aspartic Acid Chelate (amino acid Chelate): Phosphorus 10 mg • Calcium 100 mg • Magnesium 500 mg • Iron 5 mg • Potassium 200 mg • Zinc 30 mg • Copper 250 mcg • Manganese 30 mg • Chromium 500 mcg • Molybdenum 10 mcg • Selenium 25 mcg • Vanadium 60 mcg • Silicon 0.33 mcg • Lithium 0.05 mcg.

Magnesium-Potassium Aspartate - The Vitamin Shoppe
Magnesium 100 mg • Potassium 100 mg.

Maharishi Amrit Kalash Ambrosia - Maharishi Ayurveda Products
Meda Milkweed • Black Musale • Heart-Leaved Moonseed • East Indian Globe Thistle • Butterfly Pea • Licorice • Vanda Orchid • Elephant Creeper • Indian Wild Pepper.

Maharishi Amrit Kalash Nectar - Maharishi Ayurveda Products
Whole Cane Sugar • Indian Gooseberry • Indian Gallnut • Ghee • Honey • Cardamom • Cinnamon • Dried Catkins • Indian Pennywort • Cyperus • Nutgrass • White Sandalwood • Aloeweed • Butterfly Pea • Shoe Flower • Licorice • Turmeric. Processed in the aqueous extract of: Castor root • Country Mallow • Thatch Grass • Eragrostis cynosuroides • Sugar Cane • Indian Asparagus • Spreading Hogweed • Giant Potato • Winter Cherry • Indian Kudju • Trumpet flower • Premna Integrifolia • Desmodium gangeticum • Uraria picta • Yellow-berried Night Shade • Small Caltrops • Phaseolus trilobus • Teramnus labialis • Bengal Quince • Cashmere bark.
See Editor's Note No. 39, page 2058.

Maharishi Amrit Kalash Sugar-Free Nectar - Maharishi Ayurveda Products
Indian Gooseberry • Indian Gallnut • Cardamom • Cinnamon • Dried Catkins • Indian Pennywort • Cyperus • Nutgrass • White Sandalwood • Aloeweed • Butterfly Pea • Shoe Flower • Licorice • Turmeric. Processed in the aqueous extract of: Castor root • Country Mallow • Thatch Grass • Eragrostis Cynosuroides • Sugar Cane • Indian Asparagus • Spreading Hogweed • Giant Potato • Winter Cherry • Indian Kudju • Trumpet flower • Premna Integrifolia • Desmodium gangeticum • Uraria picta • Yellow-berried Night Shade • Small Caltrops • Phaseolus trilobus • Teramnus labialis • Bengal Quince • Cashmere bark.
See Editor's Note No. 39, page 2058.

Maitake Supreme - Gaia Herbs
Each capsule contains: Maitake Mushroom (grifola frondosa) patented, Alcohol-Free concentrated extract 30 mg • Vitamin C Alcohol-Free concentrated extract 50 mg. Other Ingredients: Vegetable Glycerin, Vegetable Gelatin (capsule).

MaitakeGold 404 Capsules - Natural Factors
Each capsule contains: MaitakeGold 404 powdered extract 15 mg • Multi Mycelia Blend 85 mg: Shiitake, Agaricus Blazei, Schizophyllum Commune, Cordyceps Sinensi, Tremella Fuciformis, Ganoderma Lucidum, Coriolus Versicolor, Pria Cocos, Hericum Einaceus, Grifola Frondosa. Other Ingredients: Rice Powder, Gelatin Capsule (gelatin, purified water), Magnesium Stearate (vegetable grade).

MaitakeGold 404 Drops - Natural Factors
Seven tenths milliliters contain: Vitamin C (as ascorbic acid) 21 mg • MaitakeGold 404 powdered extract 23 mg. Other Ingredients: Vegetable Glycerin, Water.

Male Activator - The Sports Nutrition Source, Inc.
Two capsules contain: Niacin 20 mg • Wild Oats extract 200 mg • Yohimbe bark 250 mg • Damiana leaves 150 mg • Siberian Ginseng root 100 mg • Bee Pollen 100 mg • Cordyceps Mushroom 50 mg • Cayenne 50 mg.

Male Advantage - Body Wise International, Inc.
Three capsules contain: Zinc (Krebs Cycle Chelate) 15 mg • Saw Palmetto berry fruit extract 4:1 (Equivalent to 1000 mg Saw Palmetto) 250 mg • Kava Kava root 250 mg • Alpha-Ketoglutaric Acid 200 mg • Flaxseed 100 mg • Pumpkin seed 75 mg • Korean Ginseng root 75 mg • Siberian Ginseng root 75 mg • Turmeric root extract (95% Curcumin) 50 mg • Damiana leaf 50 mg • L-Alanine 50 mg • L-Glutamic Acid 50 mg • Glycine 50 mg • Pygeum Africana Bark wet extract 150:1 50 mg • Gotu Kola whole plant 50 mg • Bromelain 50 mg. Inactive Ingredients: Gelatin, Magnesium Stearate, Cellulose, Dicalcium Phosphate, Silicon Dioxide.

Male Drive - Dial Herbs
Vitamin E • Yohimbe • Green Oats • Zinc • Siberian Ginseng • l-Histidine. In a base of Velvet Antler, Rehmanniae, Cormus Wolfberries, Astragalus seed, Epimedii, Vaccriae, Cyperi.

Male Formula - 4 Life
Each capsule contains: Damiana leaf 85 mg • Sarsaparilla root 80 mg • Siberian Ginseng root 57 mg • Saw Palmetto fruit 55 mg • Pumpkin seed 55 mg • Male Proprietary Extract Blend 45 mg: Pumpkin seed extract, Muira Puama bark extract, Saw Palmetto frui), Sarsaparilla root extract, Damiana leaf extract • Pygeum bark (pygeum africanum, 25% phytosterols) 23 mg. Other Ingredients: Gelatin Capsule, Magnesium Stearate.

Male Formula - Oasis Wellness Network
Each tablet contains: Calcium 25 mg • Vitamin E (as d-alpha tocopherol acetate) 50 IU • Selenium (yeast) 25 mcg • L-Glutamine 200 mg • MaxCell Proprietary Blend 125 mg: Zisyphus Jujube, Piper Nigrum, Aloe Vera, Glycyrrhiza Glabra • Glucosamine Sulfate 100 mg • Epimedium Grandiflorum leaf extract 100 mg • Tribulus Terrestris fruit extract 75 mg • American Ginseng root extract 50 mg •

Lycopene 2.5 mg. Other Ingredients: Cellulose, Stearic Acid, Calcium Sulfate, Magnesium Stearate, Silica.

Male Fuel **-** TwinLab
Six capsules contain: Yohimbe bark extract (standardized for Yohimbine) 800 mg • L-Arginine HCl 2800 mg • Ginkgo Biloba extract (standardized for 24% flavonoid glycosides) 60 mg • Natural Vitamin E 400 IU • Zinc (from Zinc Picolinate) 30 mg • L-Tyrosine 100 mg • Vitamin B6 50 mg • Choline Bitartrate 200 mg • Vitamin B5 (Pantothenic Acid) 100 mg • Saw Palmetto (Serenoa repens) extract 120 mg • Phytosterol Complex (providing Beta-Sitosterol 60 mg) 120 mg.

Male Multi Vitamins **-** Health Center for Better Living
Each tablet contains: Vitamin A (as retinyl palmitate and 50% from beta-carotene) 5,000 IU • Vitamin C (as ascorbic acid) 150 mg • Vitamin D (as cholecalciferol) 100 IU • Vitamin E (as dl-alpha-tocopheryl acetate) 50 IU • Vitamin K (as phytonadione) 10 mcg • Thiamin (as thiamin HCl) 10 mg • Riboflavin 10 mg • Niacin (as niacinamide) 30 mg • Vitamin B6 (as pyridoxine HCl) 5 mg • Folate (as folic acid) 100 mcg • Vitamin B12 (as cyanocobalamin) 10 mcg • Biotin 100 mcg• Pantothenic Acid (as D-calcium patothenate) 5 mg • Calcium (as calcium carbonate and dicalcium phosphate) 150 mg • Iodine (from Kelp) 50 mcg • Magnesium (as magnesium oxide) 25 mg • Zinc (as zinc citrate) 5 mg • Selenium (as selenomethionine) 100 mcg • Copper (as copper oxide) 1 mg • Manganese (as manganese sulfate) 1 mg • Chromium (as chromium dinicotinate glycinate) 100 mcg • Molybdenum (as sodium molybdate) 20 mcg • Boron (as boron chelate) 300 mcg • Grape seed extract (40% proanthocyanidins) 10 mg • Citrus bioflavonoids complex 15 mg • Rutin 10 mg • Silica (from horsetail herb) 5 mg • Montmorillonite (source of 72 trace minerals) 25 mg • Octacosanol (from rice bran) 2 mg • Saw palmetto berry 50 mg.

Male Performax **-** PhysioLogics
Each capsule contains: Muira Puama root (ptychopetalum olacoides, from 4:1 extract) 500 mg • Korean Ginseng root (panax ginseng, standardized to contain 14% ginsenosides, 3.5 mg) 25 mg • Ginkgo Biloba leaf extract (standardized to contain 24% ginkgo flavonglycosides, 3.2 mg, 6% terpenes, 0.8 mg) 13.3 mg. Other Ingredients: Rice Powder, Gelatin, Vegetable Magnesium Stearate, Silica.

Male Potential **-** Health Smart Vitamins
Each capsule contains: Muira Puama bark 500 mg • Oriental Ginseng (root, Panax ginseng; 14% ginsenosides, 3.5 mg) 25 mg • Ginkgo leaf (24 % ginkgo glavonglycosides 3.2 mg; 6% terpene lactones, 0.8 mg) 13 mg.

Male Power **-** Futurebiotics
Panax Ginseng (Active Standardized Ginsenosides) 5 mg • Siberian Ginseng (50:1 extract from) 750 mg • Avena Sativa (Wild Oats, extract from) 200 mg • Smilax (Sarsaparilla) 200 mg • Saw Palmetto (extract from) 200 mg • Mexican Yam (extract from) 200 mg • Polygonum Multiflorum (extract from) 250 mg • Astragalus (extract from) 250 mg • Schizandra (extract from) 250 mg • Alfalfa 500 mg • Licorice Root (extract from) 500 mg • Muira Puama 150 mg • Deer Antler 50 mg • Kelp 150 mg • Spirulina 100 mg • Black Cohosh 100 mg • Mullein 100 mg • Ginger 35 mg • Bee Pollen 500 mg • Royal Jelly 30 mg • Vitamin B12 500 mcg • Zinc (Citrate) 25 mg • Glandulars: • Pancreas 100 mg • Orchic 90 mg • Thymus 90 mg • Adrenal 80 mg • Heart 75 mg • Lymph 35 mg • Prostate 35 mg • Spleen 20 mg • Pituitary 15 mg.
See Editor's Note No. 14.

Male Response **-** Source Naturals
Three tablets contain: Vitamin E (as Natural D-Alpha Tocopheryl) 100 IU • Vitamin B6 (Pyridoxine HCl) 25 mg • Pantothenic Acid (Vitamin B5) 50 mg • Zinc (as OptiZinc Monomethionine) 15 mg • Selenium (as L-Selenomethionine and Selenium Chelate) 150 mcg • Copper (as Copper Sebacate) 1 mg • Tribulus leaf, stem and flower (Yielding 200 mg of Furostanol Saponins) 500 mg • Maca root extract (Lepidium Meyenii) 300 mg • Yohimbe bark standardized extract 4% (Yielding 9 mg of Yohimbine) 225 mg • Muira Puama stem extract 200 mg • Oat Straw leaf extract (Avena sativa) 200 mg • Siberian Ginseng root 200 mg • Damiana leaf and stem 200 mg • Saw Palmetto berry 200 mg • Mexican Sarsaparilla root 200 mg • Ashwagandha root 150 mg • Panax Ginseng root standardized extract 8% (Yielding 8 mg of Ginsenosides) 100 mg • Ginkgo Biloba leaf extract (50:1) (Yielding 14 mg of Ginkgo Flaconglycosides) 60 mg • Stinging Nettle root extract (16:1) 60 mg • Ginger root 60 mg.

Male Vigor - Wellzymes **-** Enzymes, Inc.
Two capsules contain: Vitamin E (from d-Alpha Tocopheryl Acid Succinate) 40 IU • Zinc (from Zinc Citrate) 14 mg • n-zimes Proprietary Enzyme Blend 32 mg: pHysioProtease, CereCalase Plus • Proprietary Herbal Blend 320 mg: Panax Ginseng root extract (standardized to contain 8% ginsenosides), Damiana leaf extract (equivalent to 400 mg raw herb), Yohimbe bark extract (standardized to contain 3% yohimbine), Ginkgo Biloba leaf extract (standardized to contain 24% flavonoid glycosides), Rice Bran. Other Ingredients: Plant Cellulose, Water.

Malic Acid + **-** PhysioLogics
Each capsule contains: Magnesium (as magnesium oxide, magnesium aspartate) 100 mg • Potassium (as potassium aspartate) 10 mg • Malic Acid 250 mg • Coenzyme Q10 15 mg. Other Ingredients: Rice Powder, Gelatin, Vegetable Magnesium Stearate, Silica.

Malic Acid Plus **-** Pain & Stress Center
Two capsules contain: Malic Acid 800 mg • Boswellia 300 mg • Magnesium 100 mg • Chromium Picolinate 50 mcg • Vitamin C 10 mg • Vitamin B6 5 mg.

Malic Acid+ **-** PhysioLogics
Each capsule contains: Magnesium (Oxide, Aspartate) 100 mg • Potassium (Aspartate) 10 mg • Malic Acid 250 mg • Coenzyme Q10 15 mg.

Maltsupex **-** Wallace Laboratories
Each level scoop contains: Malt Soup Extract derived from natural barley malt 8 g.

Manganese **-** Source Naturals
Each tablet contains: Manganese (from 150 mg of manganese amino acid chelate) 15 mg.

Manganese - GNC A-Z **-** GNC
Each tablet contains: Manganese (as manganese gluconate) 10 mg. Other Ingredients: Dicalcium Phosphate, Cellulose.

Manganese Extra **-** Olympian Labs
Each capsule contains: Manganese Chelate 30 mg • Huckleberry 100 mg • Blueberry 100 mg • Lady Slipper 50 mg • Black Walnut 50 mg.

Mangaplex **-** Progressive Labs
Each tablet contains: Vitamin C (ascorbic acid) 80 mg • Vitamin D (as Vitamin D3) (cholecalciferol) 50 IU • Vitamin E (d-alpha tocopheryl succinate) 10 IU • Thiamin HCl (Vitamin B1) 5 mg • Vitamin B6 (pyridoxine HCl) 10 mg • Vitamin B12 (cyanocobalamin) 10 mcg • Calcium (calcium lactate 175 mg) 26 mg • Manganese (manganese sulfate 200 mg) 73 mg • Choline Bitartrate 30 mg • Bioflavonoids 20 mg • Horsetail 100 mg • Rose Hips 5 mg • Green Pea concentrate 200 mg • Raw Liver concentrate 10 mg.
See Editor's Note No. 14.

MannaBar Protein Formula **-** Mannatech
Each bar contains: Solnuts Soybeans, Soya, toasted Soya pieces • roasted Cashew Butter with Safflower oil • Rice Syrup (partially polished brown rice, koji, water) • Isolated Soy Protein • Dried Apricots • Dried Cranberries (sweetened with apple juice) • Date paste • Natural Vegetable Glycerin • Raspberry flavor • Energy Smart (fruit juice, natural grain dextrins) • Honey Granola: quick Oats, Canola Oil, Honey, Lecithin • Supro Plus Nuggets (isolated soy protein, rice flour, malt, salt) • Pear juice concentrate • Nonfat dry milk solids • Rolled Oats • Flax seed • Whey Protein concentrate •

Wheat Bran • Calcium Caseinate • Ambrotose complex (naturally occurring plant saccharides including freeze-dried aloe vera gel extract - Manapol powder) • Phytosterols from Wild Yam root • Phyt•Aloe flash-dried complex: Broccoli, Brussels Sprouts, Cabbage, Carrot, Cauliflower, Garlic, Kale, Onion, Tomato, Turnip, Papaya, Pineapple • Citric Acid • Natural Flavoring.

MannaBAR, Vanilla Yogurt-Coated Apple Crunch **-** Mannatech
Each bar contains: Coating: dehydrated Cane juice, fractionated Palm Kernel Oil, nonfat Milk powder, Yogurt powder, Lactic Acid, Soy Lecithin, natural Vanilla • Dry Roasted Soybeans • Toasted Cashew Butter with Safflower oil • Dried Apple Pieces • Rice Syrup (partially polished brown rice, koji, water) • Isolated Soy Protein • Date Paste • Natural Vegetable Glycerin • Honey Granola: quick Oats, Canola Oil, Honey, Lecithin • Energy Smart (fruit juice, natural grain dextrins) • Apple Flavor • Supro Plus Nuggets (isolated soy protein, rice flour, malt, salt) • Rolled Oats • Apple Juice Concentrate • Nonfat Dry Milk Solids • Flax Seed • Whey Protein Concentrate • Wheat Bran • Calcium Caseinate • Natural Flavoring • Cinnamon • Ambrotose Complex (naturally occurring plant saccharides including freeze-dried aloe vera inner leaf gel extract - Manapol powder) • Phytosterols from Wild Yam Root • Phyt•Aloe dehydrated Complex: Broccoli, Brussels Sprouts, Cabbage, Carrot, Cauliflower, Garlic, Kale, Onion, Tomato, Turnip, Papaya, Pineapple.

Manna-C **-** Mannatech
Two capsules contain: Vitamin C (from Acerola fruit) 53 mg • Proprietary Blend Ambrotose Complex (patent pending) 84 mg: Arabinogalactan (larix decidua gum), Manapol Aloe Vera gel extract (inner leaf gel), Gum Ghatti, Gum Tragacanth • Herbal Blend 398 mg: Boneset (aerial part), Lemon Verbena (leaves), Sage (leaves), Catnip (aerial part), Peppermint (leaves), Yarrow (flowers), Horehound (aerial part). Other Ingredients: Gelatin, Sodium Starch Glycolate, Stearic Acid.

MannaCLEANSE **-** Mannatech
Two caplets contain: Proprietary Fiber Blend 750 mg: Oat fiber, Black Currant fiber, Psyllium (seed husk), Carrageenan, Glucomannan • Essential Oils/Botanical Blend 145 mg: Fenugreek (seed), Fennel (seed), Ginger (root), Rosemary (leaves), Neroli Orange (blossom), Peppermint (leaves) • Fatty Acid Blend 120 mg: Flax (seed), Sodium Caprylate, Rice (bran), Lecithin, Borage (seed) • Flora Growth Promotants 80 mg: Inulin-Oligosaccharide Complex, Beta-Glucans • Probiotic Flora Blend 24 mg: Lactobacillus Sporogenes, L. Acidophilus, L. Plantarum, L. Casei, Bifidobacterium Bifidum • Enzyme Blend 20 mg: Amylase, Protease, Lactase, Lipase, Cellulase • Ambrotose Complex (patent pending) 2 mg: Arabinogalactan (larix decidua gum), Manapol Aloe Vera gel extract (inner leaf gel), Gum Ghatti, Gum Tragacanth. Other Ingredients: Dibasic Calcium Phosphate, Microcrystalline Cellulose, Croscarmellose Sodium, Stearic Acid, Silicon Dioxide, Magnesium Stearate, Natural Flavor. Film Coat Ingredients: Hydroxypropyl Methycellulose, Hydroxypropyl Cellulose, Polyethylene Glycol.

Mannatonin **-** Mannatech
Each tablet contains: Melatonin 1 mg • Proprietary Blend Ambrotose Complex (patent pending) 10 mg: Naturally Occurring Plant Saccharides (including freeze-dried aloe vera inner leaf gel extract - manapol powder) • Valerian root 100 mg • Lecithin 50 mg. Other Ingredients: Dibasic Calcium Phosphate, Microcrystalline Cellulose, Tribasic Calcium Phosphate, Molasses, Wheat Germ, Croscarmellose Sodium, Magnesium Stearate, Silicon Dioxide, Calcium Silicate, Coating (shellac, talc, gelatin, sucrose, calcium sulfate, kaolin, titanium dioxide, carnauba wax).

Marine Beta Carotene **-** Jarrow Formulas
Each softgel contains: Beta Carotene (from Dunaliella salina) (Equivalent to 25000 IU of pro Vitamin A) activity 15 mg • Vitamin E 5 IU. Other Ingredients: Soybean Oil, Lecithin.

Marine Beta Carotene 25000 IU **-** Nature's Life
Each capsule contains: Beta Carotene (Dunaliella salina) (Vitamin A equivalent 25000 IU) (Other natural Carotenoids occuring in D. Salina) 15 mg • Alpha Carotene 500 mcg • Cryptoxanthin 130 mcg • Zeaxanthin 100 mcg • Lutein 86 mcg. Vitamin E (d-Alpha Tocoherol) 1.5 IU.

Marine Carotene **-** The Vitamin Shoppe
Each softgel contains: Natural Beta-Carotene 15 mg (equivalent to 25,000 IU Vitamin A activity) providing other naturally occurring Carotenoids: Alpha-carotene, Lutein, Cryptoxanthin, and Zeaxanthin.

Marine Omega **-** Pharmanex
Two softgels contain: Vitamin E (as natural mixed tocopherols) 10 IU • Marine Lipid concentrate 2000 mg • Omega 3 Fatty Acids 100 mg: EPA 300 mg, DHA 200 mg, Other Omega 3 Fatty Acids • NKO Krill oil 100 mg. Other Ingredients: Gelatin, Glycerin, Purified Water, Natural Lemon Oil, Vanillin.

Marshmallow **-** Nature's Way
Two capsules contain: Marshmallow root 910 mg. Other Ingredients: Gelatin.

Marshmallow Krunch - Revival **-** Physicians Laboratories
Each Bar Contains: Certified Isoflavone 160 mg. Ingredients: Corn syrup, Sugar, Corn starch, Water, Gelatin, Artificial Flavoring, Soy Protein Isolate, Rice flour, Malt, Salt, Glycerin, Sunflower oil, Soy Lecithin.

Martrim **-** VitaStore
Cayenne • Ginseng (Siberian) • Guarana (Paullinia Cupana) • Gymnema Sylvestre • Kelp • Phenylalanine • Pullulan • Sidacordifilia Extract • Zingiber • Vitamin A • Vitamin B1 • Vitamin B6 • Vitamin B12 • Vitamin C • Vitamin D • Vitamin E (d-alpha tocopherol) • Folic Acid • Iodine (Kelp) • Niacin • d-Biotin • Pantothenic Acid • Potassium Gluconate.

Masculex **-** Enzymatic Therapy
Two capsules contain: Vitamin E (D-Alpha Tocopherol) 100 IU. Other Ingredients: Muira Puama Powdered extract 6:1 (Ptychopetalum olacoides) 250 mg • Liquid Liver Fractions (predigested soluble concentrate) 250 mg • Wheat Germ oil concentrate 100 mg • Beta-Sitosterol 100 mg • Mexican Damiana leaves extract (Tunera diffusa) 100 mg • Saw Palmetto Berry extract (Serenoa repens) standardized to contain 85%-95% fatty acids & biologically active sterols 40 mg • Cola Nut extract (Cola nitida) (contains 4.8 mg Caffeine) 40 mg • Panax ginseng extract standardized to contain 7% Saponins (calculated as Ginsenoside Rg1) 40 mg • Ginkgo Biloba leaves extract (Ginkgo biloba folia) standardized to contain 24% ginkgoflavonglycosides 20 mg.
See Editor's Note No. 14.

Masculex for Men **-** Enzymatic Therapy
Each two softgel capsules contain: Vitamin E (as d-alpha tocopherol) 100 IU • Liquid Liver Fractions (predigested soluble concentrate) 250 mg • Muira Puama (ptychopetalum olacoides, root extract 6:1) 250 mg • Wheat Germ Oil 100 mg • Beta-Sitosterol 100 mg • Damiana (turnera diffusa, leaf extract 5:1) 100 mg • Saw Palmetto (serenoa repens, berrry extract standardized to contain 88-95% fatty acids, 0.2-0.4% total sterols, 0.1-0.3% beta-sitosterol) 40 mg • Cola (cola nitida, nut extract containing 4.8 mg caffeine) 40 mg • Korean Ginseng (panax ginseng, root extract standardized to contain a minimum of 7% ginsenosides) 40 mg • Ginkgo (ginkgo biloba, leaf extract standardized to contain 24% ginkgoflavonglycosides, 6% terpene lactones, and 2% bilobalide) 20 mg.

MascuPlex **-** PhytoPharmica
Two softgel capsules contain: Cola nut extract (cola nitida, standardized to contain 4.8 mg caffeine) 40 mg • Damiana leaf 5:1 extract (turnera diffusa) 100 mg • Ginkgo leaf extract (ginkgo biloba, standardized to contain 24% ginkgoflavonglycosides, 6% terpene lactones, and 2% bilobalide) 20 mg • Liquid Liver Fractions (predigested soluble concentrate) 250 mg • Muira Puama root 6:1

extract (ptychopetalum olacoides) 250 mg • Panax Ginseng root extract (standardized to contain a minimum of 7% ginsenosides) 40 mg • Proprietary Phytosterol Blend 100 mg: Beta Sitosterol, Campesterol, Stigmasterol • Saw Palmetto berry extract (standardized to contain 85-95% fatty acids, 0.2-0.4% total sterols, and 0.1-0.3% beta sitosterol) 40 mg • Vitamin E (as D-alpha tocopherol) 100 IU • Wheat Germ oil 100 mg.
See Editor's Note No. 14.

Mass Action - MET-Rx **-** Rexall - Sundown
Each serving contains: Micronized Creatine 5 g • HMB 1.5 g • Trimethylglycine (TMG) 500 mg • Improved Nutrient Uptake. Ingredients: Glucose • Creatine Monohydrate • HMB • Trimethylglycine • Natural & Artificial Flavors • Beta Carotene & Beet juice powder for colors • Xanthan Gum • Aspartame.

Mass Fuel **-** TwinLab
High Biological-Quality Milk & Egg Proteins • Branched Chain Amino Acids (L-Leucine, L-Isoleucine & L-Valine) • L-Glutamine • Alpha-Ketoglutarates • Keto-Isocaproate (KIC) • L-Ornithine Alpha-Ketoglutarate • L-Carnitine • Creatine Monohydrate • High Potencies Of Vitamins & Minerals • Potassium 2000 mg • Chromium 300 mcg (from patented Chromic Fuel Chromium Picolinate).

Masters **-** Pharmanex
Two capsules contain: Vitamin A (100% as Beta-Carotene)(Beta-Carotene, Dunaliella Salina) 3750 IU • Vitamin C (as Ascorbic Acid) 150 mg • Vitamin D (as Vitamin D3)(as Cholecalciferol) 200 IU • Vitamin E (as d-Alpha Tocopheryl Succinate) 150 IU • Riboflavin (as Riboflavin) 0.85 mg • Vitamin B6 (as Pyridoxine Hydrochloride) 1 mg • Folate (as Folic Acid) 200 mcg • Vitamin B12 (as Cyanocobalamin) 3 mcg • Calcium (Calcium Carbonate, Calcium Chelate, Calcium Citrate) 250 mg • Magnesium (Magnesium Oxide, Magnesium Chelate) 100 mg • Zinc (Zinc Chelate) 7.5 mg • Chromium (Chromium Chelate, Chromium Picolinate) 100 mcg • Korean Panax Ginseng with Ginsenosides 25 mcg • Siberian Ginseng extract with Eleutherosides 25 mg • Ginkgo Biloba Powder with Ginkgoflavonglycosides 20 mg • Echinacea Purpurea Powder with Echinacosides 20 mg • Cranberry Concentrate with Quinnic Acid 12.5 mg • Bilberry Powder with Anthocyanosides 10 mg.

Mathake Herb Tea **-** NutriCology
Each bag contains: Mathake herb (teminalia catappa).

Matrixx **-** Allergy Research Group
Two capsules contain: Vitamin C (as ascorbic acid) 33 mg • Vitamin E (as D-alpha-tocopheryl acid succinate) 55 IU • Calcium (calcium citrate) 27 mg • Magnesium (as magnesium citrate) 40 mg • Zinc (as zinc citrate) 4 mg • Selenium (as sodium selenite/selenomethionine) 33 mcg • Copper (as copper sebacate) 0.27 mg • Manganese (as manganese citrate) 4.7 mg • Molybdenum (as sodium molybdate) 330 mcg • Boron (as boron citrate) 1.2 mg • N-Acetyl-D-Glucosamine 67 mg • Chondroitin Sulfate 130 mg • Glucosamine Sulfate 500 mg • L-Lysine 67 mg • L-Proline 107 mg • Hawthorne dried extract (crataegus oxyacantha) 295 mg • Horsetail dried extract (equisetum arvense) 6.7 mg • Bromelain 10 mg. Other Ingredients: Cellulose, Magnesium Stearate, Ethyl Vanillin.

Mature Woman - Wellzymes **-** Enzymes, Inc.
Two capsules contain: Vitamin E (from d-Alpha Tocopheryl Acid Succinate) 20 IU • n-zimes Proprietary Enzyme Blend 36 mg: pHysioProtease (94,720 pHysio-U), CereCalase Plus • Proprietary Herbal Blend 386 mg: Black Cohosh root extract (standardized to contain 2.5% triterpene glycosides), Deglycyrrhizinized Licorice root extract (equivalent to 400 mg of raw herb), St. John's Wort herb extract (standarized to contain 0.3% hypericin), Rice Bran, Soy Isoflavone extract (standardized to contain 23% genistein & 18% daidzein). Other Ingredients: Plant Cellulose, Water.

Max GLA **-** PhysioLogics
Each softgel contains: Linolenic Acid 375 mg • Gamma-Linolenic Acid (GLA) 229 mg • Oleic Acid 190 mg • Palmitic Acid 114 mg • Stearic Acid 41 mg • Palmitoleic Acid 3 mg.

Maxadrine with Ephedra **-** D & E Pharmaceuticals
Two capsules contain: Pantothenic Acid 40 mg • Citrus Aurantium (standardized to 4% synephrine) 125 mg • Ma Huang plant (standardized to 12.5 mg ephedrine) 208 mg • Guarana seed extract (standardized to 200 mg caffeine) 910 mg • White Willow bark extract (standardized to 15 mg salicin) 105 mg • Acetyl L-Carnitine 100 mg • L-Tyrosine 80 mg • Ginger root 50 mg. Other Ingredients: Calcium Phosphate, Talc, Gelatin, Magnesium Stearate.
See Editor's Note No. 30, page 2056.

Maxativa **-** Futurebiotics
Two tablets contain: Oat extract (4:1) 300 mg • Nettles extract (4:1) 150 mg • Glycine 100 mg • Vitamin C 100 mg • Smilax-Ginseng-Damiana Complex 400 mg • Bee Pollen (Lyophilized) 350 mg • Zinc (Oxide, Gluconate) 15 mg • Royal Jelly (Lyophilized) 45 mg • Niacinamide 15 mg.

MaxEPA **-** Puritan's Pride
Each softgel contains: Eicosapentaenoic Acid (EPA) 180 mg • Docosahexaenoic Acid (DHA) 120 mg. Contains not less than 30% Omega-3 polyunsaturates.

MaxEPA 1000 mg **-** Nature's Life
Each capsule contains: MaxEPA 1000 mg providing the following naturally occuring essential nutrients: EPA (Eicosapentaneoic Acid) 180 mg • DHA (Docosahexaenoic Acid) 180 mg • Vitamin E (d-Alpha Tocopherol) 30 IU. In a natural base of certified organic Safflower oil.

Maxi B-Caps with Taurine **-** Country Life
Each capsule contains: Thiamin (vitamin B1, as thiamine HCl, thiamine cocarboxylase) 25 mg • Riboflavin (vitamin B2, as riboflavin, riboflavin 5' phosphate) 25 mg • Niacin (as 52% niacinamide & 48% niacin) 50 mg • Vitamin B6 (as pyridoxine HCl, pyridoxide alpha-ketoglutarate, pyridoxal 5' phosphate) 63.75 mg • Folic Acid 800 mcg • Vitamin B12 (as dibencozide) 500 mcg • d-Biotin 300 mg • Pantothenic Acid (as d-calcium pantothenate, pantethine) 200 mg • Inositol 100 mg • Taurine (free form) 100 mg • Choline (from 100 mg of choline bitartrate) 46 mg • PAK (pyridoxine alpha-ketoglutarate) 25 mg • PABA (para-aminobenzoic acid) 25 mg. Inactive Ingredients: Cellulose, Magnesium Stearate, Silica.

Maxi-Complete **-** Atrium Inc.
Each tablet contains: Vitamin A Palmitate 10000 IU • Vitamin D (as Vitamin D2 Fish oil) 400 IU • Vitamin B1 Thiamine HCL 10 mg • Vitamin B2 Riboflavin 10 mg • Vitamin B6 Pyridoxine HCL 10 mg • Vitamin B12 Cyanocobalamin 15 mcg • Vitamin C Ascorbic Acid 150 mg • Vitamin E Acetate 60 IU • Biotin 6 mcg • Niacin-Niacinamide 50 mg • Pantothenic Acid 25 mg • Folic Acid 400 mcg • Calcium Amino Acid Chelate 30 mg • Iodine 100 mcg • Iron Amino Acid Chelate 50 mg • Magnesium Amino Acid Chelate 20 mg • Manganese Amino Acid Chelate 6 mg • Phosphorus 20 mg • Zinc Amino Acid Chelate 5 mg • Choline Bitartrate 100 mg • Inositol 100 mg • PABA 30 mg • Rutin 25 mg. In a base of Alfalfa, Bone Meal, Bromelain, Kelp, Papaya, Rose Hips.

Maximum Anti-Oxidant Formula **-** Nature's Bounty
Two tablets contain: Vitamin A (as Beta Carotene) 15000 IU • Vitamin C (as Calcium Ascorbate and Ascorbyl Palmitate) 500 mg • Vitamin E (as d-Alpha Tocopheryl Succinate) 400 IU • Zinc (as Zinc Picolinate) 7.5 mg • Selenium (as L-Selenomethionine) 50 mcg • Copper (as Copper Lysinate) 1 mg • Manganese (as Manganese Arginate) 2.5 mg • Coenzyme Q-10 1000 mcg • Pycnogenol 3000 mcg • Quercetin 15 mg • Citrus Bioflavonoid Complex 50 mg • L-Glutathione 1000 mcg • N-Acetyl Cysteine 5000 mcg • L-Cysteine Hydrochloride 50 mg • Green Tea extract aerial 500 mcg • Echinacea root 25 mg • Bilberry leaf 25 mg • Schizandra berry 25 mg • Barley Juice powder 2 mg • Broccoli powder 2.5 mg • Spirulina 2 mg • Chlorella 2.5 mg • Citrus Fiber 50 mg. Other Ingredients: Cellulose, Dicalcium Phosphate, Vegetable Stearic Acid, Food Glaze, Magnesium Silicate, Vegetable Magnesium Stearate, Silica, Croscarmellose.

Maximum Anti-Oxidant Formula - Vegetarian - Puritan's Pride
Two tablets contain: Vitamin A (as beta carotene) 15,000 IU • Vitamin C (as calcium ascorbate & ascorbyl palmitate) 500 mg • Vitamin E (as d-alpha tocopheryl succinate) 400 IU • Selenium (as l-selenomethionine) 50 mcg • Coenzyme Q10 1000 mcg • Pycnogenol 3000 mg • Quercetin 15 mg • Citrus Bioflavonoids Complex 50 mg • L-Glutathione 1000 mcg • N-Acetyl-Cysteine 5000 mcg • L-Cysteine HCl 50 mg • Copper (as copper lysinate) 1 mg • Manganese (as manganese arginate) 2.5 mg • Zinc (as zinc picolinate) 7.5 mg • Green Tea extract 500 mcg • Echinacea 25 mg • Bilberry 25 mg • Schizandra 25 mg. In a natural base of Broccoli powder 2.5 mg, Spirulina 2 mg, Chlorella 2.5 mg, Barley juice powder 2 mg, and Citrus fiber 50 mg.

Maximum Fat Burners - Optimum Nutrition
Citrimax 500 mg • L-Carnitine • Choline • Inositol • Methionine.

Maximum Strength Flex-A-Min Glucosamine, Chondroitin, MSM - Arthritis Research Corp.
Three tablets contain: Glucosamine Sulfate 1500 mg • Chondroitin Sulfate 1200 mg • MSM 500 mg. Other Ingredients: Cellulose, Vegetable Magnesium Stearate, Silica, Titanium Dioxide Color.
See Editor's Note No. 15, page 2055.

Maximum Strength Glucosamine Chondroitin - Puritan's Pride
Three tablets contain: Glucosamine Hydrochloride 1500 mg • Chondroitin Sulfate 1200 mg.
See Editor's Note No. 15, page 2055.

Maxine Gentle Iron-Free - Country Life
Each two capsules contain: Vitamin A (as beta-carotene, natural mixed carotenoids, retinyl palmitate) 5000 IU • Vitamin C (as calcium ascorbate, potassium ascorbate, ascorbyl palmitate, magnesium ascorbate) 300 mg • Vitamin D (as ergocalciferol) 200 IU • Vitamin E (as d-alpha tocopheryl acid succinate) 200 IU • Vitamin K (as phytonadione) 50 mcg • Thiamin (vitamin B1 as thiamine HCl) 25 mg • Riboflavin (vitamin B2) 25 mg • Niacin 30 mg • Vitamin B6 200 mg • Folic Acid 800 mcg • Vitamin B12 (as cyanocobalamin) 500 mcg • d-Biotin 300 mcg • Pantothenic Acid (as d-calcium pantothenate) 200 mg • Calcium (as calcium hydroxyapatite, tricalcium phosphate, ascorbate, citrate) 200 mg • Phosphorous (as calcium hydroxyapatite) 84 mg • Iodine (from kelp) 225 mcg • Magnesium (as rice chelate, oxide, ascorbate) 300 mg • Zinc (as zinc monomethionine) 15 mg • Selenium (as l-selenomethionine) 100 mcg • Copper (as citrate) 1 mg • Manganese (as citrate) 5 mg • Chromium (as chromium picolinate) 100 mcg • Molybdenum (as molybdenum citrate) 50 mcg • Potassium (as potassium citrate, ascorbate) 99 mg • Inositol 100 mg • L-Tyrosine (free form) 100 mg • Chaste Berry extract (4:1) 50 mg • Choline (from 100 mg choline bitartrate) 45 mg • PABA (para-aminobenzoic acid) 30 mg • Ashwagandha extract (8:1, root) 25 mg • Grape Skin extract 25 mg • Grape Seed extract 25 mg • Enzyme Blend 25 mg: Papain 10525 PU, Lipase 300 LU, Protease 12 SAPU, Lactase 7 LACU, Alpha-Galactosidase 3 AGSU, Phytase 3 PHU, Bromelain 1 STU, Alpha-Amylase 1 SKBU • Marigold extract 20 mg • Black Pepper extract (bioprene) 2 mg • Boron (as boron citrate) 1 mg • Vanadium (from 2.8 mg of BGOV) 500 mcg. Inactive Ingredients: Cellulose, Silica, Gum Acacia, Magnesium Stearate.

Maxi-Sorb Carni Q-Gel + E - Country Life
Each softgel contains: Vitamin C (as ascorbyl palmitate) 12 mg • Vitamin E (as dl-alpha tocopherol) 75 IU • L-Carnitine (from 440 mg of l-carnitine fumerate) 250 mg • Coenzyme Q10 30 mg. Inactive Ingredients: Medium Chain Triglycerides, Polysorbate 80, Triacetin, Lecithin, Gelatin, Glycerin, Sorbitol, Purified Water, Annatto Seed Extract Color, Carob Extract Color (pod), Beeswax, Titanium Dioxide Color.

Maxi-Sorb CoQ10 with 150 IU of Vitamin E - Country Life
Each softgel contains: Vitamin E (as dl-tocopheryl acetate) 150 IU • Coenzyme Q-10 60 mg. Inactive Ingredients: Polysorbate 80, Gelatin, Medium Chain Triglycerides, Glycerin, Lecithin, Sorbitol, Triacetin, Purified Water, Titanium Dioxide, Color, Annatto Seed Extract Color.

Maxogenol - Nutraceutics Corp.
Two caplets contain: Proprietary Blend 300 mg: Grape Seed Extract, Grape Skin Extract, Green Tea Extract, Coastal White Pine Extract, Bilberry, Alpha Tocotrienol, Gamma Tocotrienol, Carotinoids, Co Enzyme Q6-10.

MaxoPlex - Pharmessen
Each capsule contains: Cinnamon leaf oil (cinnamomum zeylanicum) 3.5 mg • Mountain Savory oil (satureja montana) 3.5 mg • Clove oil (eugenia caryophyllata, bud) 3.5 mg • Thymus Capitatus oil (headed savory) 1.75 mg. Other Ingredients: Methylcellulose, Avicel, Olive Oil, Aerosil (food grade certified), Capsule (100% vegetarian, certified Kosher & Pareve, and Halal).

MBX (Meta-Burn Xtreme) - Metabolic Response Modifiers
Each capsule contains: Caffeine (USP) 90 mg • 1R, 2S-norephedrine (HCl) 25 mg • Coleus Forskohlii (20% forskolin) 25 mg • Naringin 5 mg • Yohimbine (HCl) 2.75 mg.

MCHC Calcium - Progressive Labs
Each capsule contains: Vitamin D (D3, as cholecalciferol) 100 IU • Vitamin K (phytonadione) 20 mcg • Calcium (elemental from microcrystalline calcium hydroxyapatite - MCHC - 500 mg, calcium citrate 500 mg) 250 mg • Phosphorus (from MCHC) 65 mg • Magnesium (from MCHC) 4 mg • Zinc (from MCHC) 0.075 mg • Copper (from MCHC) 0.01 mg • Manganese (from MCHC) 0.045 mg • Potassium (from MCHC) 0.035 mg • Protein (from MCHC as collagen glycosaminoglycans) 125 mg • Boron (as aspartate) 750 mg • Fluorapatite (from MCHC) 31 mg • Silicon (from MCHC) 19 mg • Strontium (from MCHC) 10 mcg. Other Ingredients: Magnesium Stearate, Gelatin.

MCH-Cal - Natrol
Two capsules contain: Vitamin D (as Cholecalciferol) 200 IU • Calcium (as calcium hydroxyapatite) 125 mg • Magnesium (as Magnesium oxide) 300 mg. Other Ingredients: Magnesium Stearate, Silicon Dioxide, Gelatin.

MCT Fuel (Emulsified Medium-Chain Triglycerides) - TwinLab
Emulsified Medium Chain Triglycerides (MCTs) • Emulsified Vitamin E. Contains: 100% natural Orange flavor & small amounts of Lecithin & Apple Pectin.

MD6 - BioTest Laboratories, LLC
Two capsules contain: L-Tyrosine 200 mg • Alpha Lipoic Acid 200 mg • Caffeine 100 mg • 5hydroxy L-Tryptophan 25 mg • Yohimbe HCl 5 mg • Ephedra Sinica extra 335 mg. Other Ingredients: Gelatin, Magnesium Stearate, Cellulose.
See Editor's Note No. 21 and No. 30.

Meal Replacement for the Best Shape of Your Life - MET-Rx - Rexall - Sundown
Each powdered packet contains: Extreme Chocolate: Glutamine 6 g • METAMYOSYN: Milk Protein Isolates, Caseinate, Glutamine, Whey Protein Concentrate, Egg White • Maltodextrin • Dutch Cocoa (alkali processed) • Vitamins & Minerals: Dicalcium Phosphate, Potassium Chloride, Dipotassium Phosphate, Potassium Citrate, Salt, Sodium Citrate, Magnesium Oxide, Choline Bitartrate, Ascorbic Acid, d-Alpha-Tocopheryl Acetate, Ferrous Fumarate, Niacinamide, Vitamin A Palmitate, Zinc Oxide, Calcium Pantothenate, Vitamin K, Manganese Sulfate, Vitamin D (as Vitamin D3), Copper Sulfate, Pyridoxine Hydrochloride, Riboflavin, Thiamine Hydrochloride, Chromium Picolinate, Cobalamin Concentrate (Vitamin B12), Folic

Acid, Biotin, Sodium Molybdate, Sodium Selenite, Potassium Iodide • Natural & Artificial Flavors • Partially Hydrogenated Coconut oil • Corn Syrup Solids • Cellulose Gum • Xanthan Gum • Aspartame • Carrageenan • Beta Carotene • Acesulfame Potassium • Lecithin • Mono & Diglycerides. Original: Calories 260 • Protein 37 g • Carbohydrates 24 g •Fat 2 g. Ingredients: METAMYOSYN: Unique blend of Milk Protein Isolates, Caseinate, Glutamine, Whey Protein Concentrate, Egg White, Maltodextrin • Vitamins & Minerals: Dicalcium Phosphate, Potassium Chloride, Dipotassium Phosphate, Potassium Citrate, Salt, Sodium Citrate, Magnesium Oxide, Choline Bitartrate, Ascorbic Acid, d-Alpha-Tocopheryl Acetate, Ferrous Fumarate, Niacinamide, Vitamin A Palmitate, Zinc Oxide, Calcium Pantothenate, Vitamin K, Manganese Sulfate, Vitamin D (as Vitamin D3), Copper Sulfate, Pyridoxine Hydrochloride, Riboflavin, Thiamine Hydrochloride, Chromium Picolinate, Cobalamin Concentrate (Vitamin B12), Folic Acid, Biotin, Sodium Molybdate, Sodium Selenite, Potassium Iodide • Natural & Atrificial Flavors • Corn Syrup Solids • Cellulose Gum • Xanthan Gum • Aspartame • Carrageenan • Beta Carotene • Acesulfame Potassium • Lecithin • Mono & Diglycerides. White Chocolate Mocha: Calories 250 • Protein 37 g • Carbohydrates 22 g • Fat 2 g. Ingredients: METAMYOSYN: Unique blend of Milk Protein Isolates, Caseinate, Glutamine, Whey Protein Concentrate, Egg White, Maltodextrin •Vitamins & Minerals: Dicalcium Phosphate, Potassium Chloride, Dipotassium Phosphate, Potassium Citrate, Salt, Sodium Citrate, Magnesium Oxide, Choline Bitartrate, Ascorbic Acid, d-Alpha-Tocopheryl Acetate, Ferrous Fumarate, Niacinamide, Vitamin A Palmitate, Zinc Oxide, Calcium Pantothenate, Vitamin K, Manganese Sulfate, Vitamin D (as Vitamin D3), Copper Sulfate, Pyridoxine Hydrochloride, Riboflavin, Thiamine Hydrochloride, Chromium Picolinate, Cobalamin Concentrate (Vitamin B12), Folic Acid, Biotin, Sodium Molybdate, Sodium Selenite, Potassium Iodide • Natural & Artificial Flavors • Soluble Coffee • Dutch Cocoa (alkali processed) • Partially Hydrogenated Coconut oil • Corn Syrup Solids • Cellulose Gum • Xanthan Gum • Aspartame • Carrageenan • Beta Carotene • Acesulfame Potassium • Lecithin • Mono & Diglycerides.

Meal Shakes - Bavarian Cocoa - Shaklee
Nonfat Dry Milk, Fructose, Acacia Gum, Calcium Sodium Caseinate, Lowfat Cocoa Processed with Alkali, Maltodextrin, Natural Flavors, Magnesium Oxide, Soy Lecithin, Xanthan Gum, Ascorbic Acid, Selenium Yeast, Chromium Yeast, Ferrous Fumarate, D-alpha Tocopheryl Acetate, Molybdenum Yeast, Niacinamide, Vitamin A Palmitate, Zinc Oxide, Copper Gluconate, Calcium Pantothenate, Manganese Sulfate, Vitamin B12, Pyridoxine Hydrochloride, Vitamin D, Thiamin Mononitrate, Folic Acid, Biotin, Riboflavin, Potassium Iodide.

Meal Shakes - French Vanilla - Shaklee
Nonfat Dry Milk, Fructose, Maltodextrin, Acacia Gum, Calcium Sodium Caseinate, Natural Flavors, Magnesium Oxide, Soy Lecithin, Xanthan Gum, Ascorbic Acid, Selenium Yeast, Chromium Yeast, Ferrous Fumarate, D-alpha Tocopheryl Acetate, Molybdenum Yeast, Niacinamide, Vitamin A Palmitate, Zinc Oxide, Copper Gluconate, Calcium Pantothenate, Manganese Sulfate, Vitamin B12, Pyridoxine Hydrochloride, Vitamin D, Thiamin Mononitrate, Folic Acid, Biotin, Riboflavin, Potassium Iodide.

Mederma - Merz Pharmaceuticals
Purified Water • PEG-4 • Onion (Allium cepa) extract • Xanthan Gum • Allantoin • Fragrance • Methylparaben • Sorbic Acid.

Medicated Cold Sore Balm w/Bee Propolis - Thayers Natural Pharmaceuticals
Camphor • Peppermint Oil (menthol source). A gentle base of Castor Oil, Beeswax, Wheat Germ Oil, Carnuba Palm Wax, Lanolin, Propolis, Vitamin E.

MediHerb Albizia 1:2 - Standard Process, Inc.
Each 5 mL serving contains: Albizia 1:2 extract 5 mL. Other Ingredients: Purified Water, 25% alcohol.

MediHerb Albizia Complex - Standard Process, Inc.
Each tablet contains: Baikal Skullcap root 3:1 extract (from scutellaria baicalensis) 800 mg • Albizia bark 4:1 extract (from albizia lebbek) 800 mg • Feverfew leaf powder (tanacetum parthenium) 50 mg • Calcium 40 mg. Other Ingredients: Calcium Acid Phosphate, Cellulose, Sodium Starch Glycollate, Silica, Hypromellose, Magnesium Stearate.

MediHerb Aloe Vera 4.5:1 - Standard Process, Inc.
Each 25 mL serving contains: Aloe Vera leaf (from aloe barbadensis, 4.5:1, containing acemannan 281 mg) 25 mL • Stevia leaf 1:2 extract (from stevia rebaudiana leaf 250 mg) 500 mcL. Other Ingredients: Natural Citrus Flavors, Purified Water.

MediHerb Andrographis Complex - Standard Process, Inc.
Each tablet contains: Echinacea root 4:1 extract (from echinacea angustifolia 500 mg) 125 mg • Holy Basil leaf 4:1 extract (from ocimum tenuiflorum 500 mg) 125 mg • Andrographis herb 10:1 extract (from andrographis paniculata 1 g, containing andrographolide 10 mg) 100 mg • Holy Basil leaf essential oil (ocimum tenuiflorum) 10 mg • Calcium 40 mg. Other Ingredients: Calcium Acid Phosphate, Cellulose, Hypromellose, Silica, Sodium Starch Glycollate, Magnesium Stearate.

MediHerb Ashwaganda 1:2 - Standard Process, Inc.
Each 5 mL serving contains: Ashwaganda root 1:2 extract (from withania somnifera root 2.5 g) 5 mL. Other Ingredients: Purified Water, 45% Alcohol.

MediHerb Astragalus 1:2 - Standard Process, Inc.
Each 5 mL serving contains: Astragalus root 1:2 extract (from astragalus membranaceus 2.5 g,) 5 mL. Other Ingredients: Purified Water, 25% Alcohol.

MediHerb Astragalus Complex - Standard Process, Inc.
Each tablet contains: Astragalus root 4:1 extract (from astragalus membranaceus 850 mg) 212.5 mg • Echinacea root 6:1 extract (from echinacea purpurea 650 mg) 108.3 mg • Eleuthero root 10:1 extract (from eleutherococcus senticosus 750 mg, containing eleutheroside E 570 mcg) 75 mg • Calcium 40 mg. Other Ingredients: Cellulose, Calcium Acid Phosphate, Silica, Sodium Starch Glycollate, Hypromellose, Magnesium Stearate.

MediHerb Bacopa 1:2 - Standard Process, Inc.
Each 5 mL serving contains: Bacopa herb 1:2 extract (from bacopa monnieri 2.5 g) 5 mL. Other Ingredients: Purified Water, 25% Alcohol.

MediHerb Bacopa Complex - Standard Process, Inc.
Each tablet contains: Schisandra fruit 4:1 extract (from schisandra chinensis 650 mg) 162.5 mg • Eleuthero root 10:1 extract (from eleutherococcus senticosus 500 mg, containing eleutheroside E 380 mcg) 50 mg • Bacopa herb 50:1 extract (from bacopa monnieri herb 1.5 g, containing bacosides 15 mg) 30 mg • Rosemary oil 10 mg • Calcium 40 mg. Other Ingredients: Calcium Acid Phosphate, Cellulose, Hypromellose, Magnesium Stearate, Silica, Sodium Starch Glycollate.

MediHerb Baical Skullcap 1:2 - Standard Process, Inc.
Each 5 mL serving contains: Baikal Skullcap root 1:2 extract (from scutallaria baicalensis root 2.5 g) 5 mL. Other Ingredients: Purified Water, 60% alcohol.

MediHerb Bilberry 1:1 - Standard Process, Inc.
Each 5 mL serving contains: Bilberry fruit fresh 1:1 extract (from vaccinium myrtillus fruit fresh 5 g) 5 mL. Other Ingredients: Purified Water, 25% Alcohol.

MediHerb Bilberry 6000mg - Standard Process, Inc.
Each tablet contains: Bilberry fruit fresh 100:1 extract (from vaccinium myrtillus fruit fresh 6 g, containing anthocyanosides 15 mg) 60 mg • Calcium 20 mg. Other Ingredients: Calcium Acid Phosphate, Cellulose, Magnesium Stearate, Sodium Starch Glycollate, Silica.

MediHerb Black Cohosh 1:2 **-** Standard Process, Inc.
Each 2.5 mL serving contains: Black Cohosh root 1:2 extract (from cimicifuga racemosa 1.25 g) 2.5 mL. Other Ingredients: Purified Water, 60% Alcohol.

MediHerb Black Haw 1:2 **-** Standard Process, Inc.
Each 5 mL serving contains: Black Haw bark 1:2 extract (from viburnum prunifolium 2.5 g) 5 mL. Other Ingredients: Purified Water, 30% Alcohol.

MediHerb Black Walnut Hulls 1:10 **-** Standard Process, Inc.
Each 5 mL serving contains: Black Walnut hulls 1:10 extract (from juglans nigra 500 mg) 5 mL. Other Ingredients: Purified Water, 60% Alcohol.

MediHerb Bladderwrack 1:1 **-** Standard Process, Inc.
Each 5 mL serving contains: Bladderwrack herb 1:1 extract (from fucus vesiculosus 5 g) 5 mL. Other Ingredients: Purified Water, 25% Alcohol.

MediHerb Blue Cohosh 1:2 **-** Standard Process, Inc.
Each 2.5 mL serving contains: Blue Cohosh root 1:2 extract (from caulophyllum thalictroides 1.25 g) 2.5 mL. Other Ingredients: Purified Water, 70% alcohol.

MediHerb Boswellia Complex **-** Standard Process, Inc.
Each tablet contains: Boswellia gum resin 4:1 extract (from boswellia serrata 1.2 g, containing boswellic acids 180 mg) 300 mg • Celery seed fruit 6:1 extract (from apium graveolens 1 g) 166.7 mg • Ginger rhizome 5:1 extract (from zingiber officinales 300 mg) 60 mg • Turmeric rhizome 25:1 extract (from curcuma longa 2 g, containing curcuminoids 70.4 mg) 80 mg • Calcium 40 mg. Other Ingredients: Calcium Acid Phosphate, Cellulose, Hypromellose, Magnesium Stearate, Silica, Sodium Starch Glycollate.

MediHerb Broncafect **-** Standard Process, Inc.
Two tablets contain: Licorice root 3.5:1 extract (from glycyrrhiza glabra 1.5 g) 428.6 mg • Pleurisy root 4:1 extract (from asclepias tuberosa 750 mg) 187.5 mg • Echinacea Purpurea root 6:1 extract (from echinacea purpurea 750 mg) 125 mg • White Horehound herb 4:1 extract (from marrubium vulgare 360 mg) 90 mg • Ginger rhizome 5:1 extract (from zingiber officinale 360 mg) 72 mg • Thyme oil 20 mg • Calcium 80 mg. Other Ingredients: Calcium Acid Phosphate, Hypromellose, Silica, Sodium Starch Glycollate, Magnesium Stearate, Cellulose.

MediHerb Broncafect Phytosynergist **-** Standard Process, Inc.
Each 5 mL serving contains: Echinacea root 1:2 extract (from echinacea angustifolia 500 mg) 1 mL • Licorice root 1:1 extract (from glycyrrhiza glabra 1 g) 1 mL • Pleurisy root 1:2 extract (from asclepias tuberosa 500 mg) 1 mL • Thyme leaf 1:2 extract (from thymus vulgaris 500 mg) 1 mL • Ginger rhizome 1:2 extract (from zingiber officinale 250 mg) 500 mcL • White Horehound herb 1:2 extract (from marrubium vulgare 250 mg) 500 mcL. Other Ingredients: Purified Water, 43% Alcohol.

MediHerb Buchu 1:2 **-** Standard Process, Inc.
Each 5 mL serving contains: Buchu leaf 1:2 extract (from barosma betulina 2.5 g) 5 mL. Other Ingredients: Purified Water, 60% Alcohol.

MediHerb Bugleweed 1:2 **-** Standard Process, Inc.
Each 5 mL serving contains: Bugleweed herb extract (from lycopus virginicus 2.5 g, 1:2) 5 mL. Other Ingredients: Purified Water, 25% Alcohol.

MediHerb Bupleurum 1:2 **-** Standard Process, Inc.
Each 5 mL serving contains: Bupleurum root 1:2 extract (from bupleurum falcatum 2.5 g) 5 mL. Other Ingredients: Purified Water, 45% Alcohol.

MediHerb Burdock 1:2 **-** Standard Process, Inc.
Each 5 mL serving contains: Burdock root 1:2 extract (from arctium lappa 2.5 g) 5 mL. Other Ingredients: Purified Water, 25% Alcohol.

MediHerb Burdock Complex **-** Standard Process, Inc.
Each tablet contains: Burdock root powder (arctium lappa) 242 mg • Sheep Sorrel herb powder (rumex acetosella) 130 mg • Slippery Elm stem bark powder (ulmus rubra) 32 mg • Rhubarb root powder (rheum palmatum) 8 mg • Calcium 40 mg. Other Ingredients: Calcium Acid Phosphate, Cellulose, Hypromellose, Magnesium Stearate, Silica, Sodium Starch Glycollate.

MediHerb Calendula 1:2 **-** Standard Process, Inc.
Each 5 mL serving contains: Calendula flower 1:2 extract (from calendula officinalis 2.5 g) 5 mL. Other Ingredients: Purified Water, 90% Alcohol.

MediHerb Californian Poppy 1:2 **-** Standard Process, Inc.
Each 5 mL serving contains: California Poppy herb 1:2 extract (from eschscholtzia californica 2.5 g) 5 mL. Other Ingredients: Purified Water, 45% Alcohol.

MediHerb Capsella Complex Phytosynergist **-** Standard Process, Inc.
Each 5 mL serving contains: Dong Quai root 1:2 extract (from angelica sinensis 750 mg) 1.5 mL • False Unicorn root 1:2 extract (from chamaelirium luteum 625 mg) 1.25 mL • Shepherd's Purse herb 1:2 extract (from capsella bursa-pastoris 625 mg) 1.25 mL • White Peony root 1:2 extract (from paeonia lactiflora root 500 mg) 1 mL. Other Ingredients: Purified Water, 40% Alcohol.

MediHerb Cat's Claw 1:2 **-** Standard Process, Inc.
Each 5 mL serving contains: Cat's Claw inner bark 1:2 extract (from uncaria tomentosa 2.5 g) 5 mL. Other Ingredients: Purified Water, 60% Alcohol.

MediHerb Cat's Claw Complex **-** Standard Process, Inc.
Each tablet contains: Cat's Claw inner stem bark 5:1 extract (from uncaria tomentosa 1.5 g) 300 mg • Pau d'Arco inner stem bark 5:1 extract (from tabebuia avellanedae 500 mg) 100 mg • Echinacea root 6:1 extract (from echinaca purpurea 500 mg) 83.3 mg • Calcium 40 mg. Other Ingredients: Calcium Acid Phosphate, Cellulose, Hypromellose, Magnesium Stearate, Silica, Sodium Starch Glycollate.

MediHerb Celery Seed 1:2 **-** Standard Process, Inc.
Each 5 mL serving contains: Celery seed fruit 1:2 extract (from apium graveolens 2.5 g) 5 mL. Other Ingredients: Purified Water, 60% Alcohol.

MediHerb Chamomile High Grade 1:2 **-** Standard Process, Inc.
Each 5 mL serving contains: Chamomile flower 1:2 extract (from matricaria recutita 2.5 g, containing bisabolol 2 mg) 5 mL. Other Ingredients: Purified Water, 60% Alcohol.

MediHerb Chaste Tree **-** Standard Process, Inc.
Each tablet contains: Chaste Tree fruit 6:1 extract (from vitex agnus-castus 500 mg) 83.3 mg • Calcium 60 mg. Other Ingredients: Calcium Acid Phosphate, Cellulose, Hypromellose, Magnesium Stearate, Silica, Sodium Starch Glycollate.

MediHerb Chaste Tree 1:2 **-** Standard Process, Inc.
Each 1 mL serving contains: Chaste Tree fruit 1:2 extract (from vitex agnus-castus 500 mg) 1 mL. Other Ingredients: Purified Water, 60% Alcohol.

MediHerb Cinnamon Quills 1:2 **-** Standard Process, Inc.
Each 5 mL serving contains: Cinnamon quills stem bark 1:2 extract (from cinnamomum zeylanicum 2.5 g) 5 mL. Other Ingredients: Purified Water, 70% Alcohol.

MediHerb Cleavers 1:2 **-** Standard Process, Inc.
Each 5 mL serving contains: Cleavers herb 1:2 extract (from galium aparine 2.5 g) 5 mL. Other Ingredients: Purified Water, 25% Alcohol.

MediHerb Colax - Standard Process, Inc.
Each tablet contains: Cascara stem bark 4:1 extract (from rhamnus purshiana 560 mg) 140 mg • Dandelion root 4:1 extract (from taraxacum officinale 375 mg) 93.75 mg • Yellow Dock root 4:1 extract (from rumex crispus 375 mg) 93.75 mg • Dill seed 4:1 extract (from anethum graveolens 375 mg) 93.75 mg • Chamomile flower 4:1 extract (from matricaria recutita 280 mg) 70 mg • Calcium 40 mg. Other Ingredients: Calcium Acid Phosphate, Cellulose, Hypromellose, Magnesium Stearate, Silica, Sodium Starch Glycollate.

MediHerb Coleus 1:1 - Standard Process, Inc.
Each 5 mL serving contains: Coleus Forskohlii root 1:1 extract (from coleus forskholii 5 g, containing forskolin 12.5 mg) 5 mL. Other Ingredients: Purified Water, 50% Alcohol.

MediHerb Corn Silk 1:1 - Standard Process, Inc.
Each 5 mL serving contains: Corn Silk styles and stigma 1:1 extract (from zea mays 5 g) 5 mL. Other Ingredients: Purified Water, 25% Alcohol.

MediHerb Cramp Bark 1:2 - Standard Process, Inc.
Each 5 mL serving contains: Cramp bark 1:2 extract (from viburnum opulus 2.5 g) 5 mL. Other Ingredients: Purified Water, 30% Alcohol.

MediHerb Cramplex - Standard Process, Inc.
Two tablets contain: Corydalis tuber 5:1 extract (from corydalis ambigua 1.2 g) 240 mg • Raspberry leaf 4:1 extract (from rubus ideaus 800 mg) 200 mg • Wild Yam root and rhizome 4:1 extract (from dioscorea villosa 800 mg) 200 mg • Cramp Bark stem bark 5:1 extract (from viburnum opulus 800 mg) 160 mg • Ginger rhizome 6:1 extract (from zingiber officinalis 800 mg) 133.3 mg • Calcium 124 mg. Other Ingredients: Calcium Acid Phosphate, Cellulose, Silica, Sodium Starch Glycollate, Magnesium Stearate, Hypromellose.

MediHerb Cranberry Complex - Standard Process, Inc.
Each tablet contains: Buchu leaf 4:1 extract (from barosma betulina 600 mg) 150 mg • Crataeva stem bark 8:1 extract (from crataeva nurvula 1 g) 125 mg • Uva Ursi leaf 4:1 extract (from arctostaphylos uva-ursi 500 mg) 125 mg • Cranberry fruit juice concentrate 25:1 (from vaccinium macrocarpon fruit fresh 2.5 g) 100 mg. Other Ingredients: Calcium Acid Phosphate, Cellulose, Hypromellose, Magnesium Stearate, Silica, Sodium Starch Glycollate.

MediHerb Cranesbill Root 1:2 - Standard Process, Inc.
Each 5 mL serving contains: Cranesbill root 1:2 extract (from geranium maculatum 2.5 g) 5 mL. Other Ingredients: Purified Water, 45% Alcohol.

MediHerb Damiana 1:2 - Standard Process, Inc.
Each 5 mL serving contains: Damiana leaf 1:2 extract (from turnera diffusa 2.5 g) 5 mL. Other Ingredients: Purified Water, 60% Alcohol.

MediHerb Dandelion Leaves 1:1 - Standard Process, Inc.
Each 5 mL serving contains: Dandelion leaf 1:1 extract (from taraxacum officinale 5 g) 5 mL. Other Ingredients: Purified Water, 25% Alcohol.

MediHerb Dandelion Root 1:2 - Standard Process, Inc.
Each 5 mL serving contains: Dandelion root 1:2 extract (from taraxacum officinale 2.5 g) 5 mL. Other Ingredients: Purified Water, 25% Alcohol.

MediHerb DermaCo - Standard Process, Inc.
Each tablet contains: Oregon Grape root and rhizome 4:1 extract (from berberis aquifolium (mahonia aquifolium) 360 mg) 90 mg • Sarsaparilla root and rhizome 4:1 extract (from smilax ornata 360 mg) 90 mg • Cleavers herb 5:1 extract (from galium aparine 360 mg) 72 mg • Burdock root 4:1 extract (from arctium lappa 270 mg) 67.5 mg • Yellow Dock root 4:1 extract (from rumex crispus 270 mg) 40 mg • Calcium 40 mg. Other Ingredients: Calcium Acid Phosphate, Cellulose, Hypromellose, Magnesium Stearate, Silica, Sodium Starch Glycollate.

MediHerb DiaCo Phytosynergist - Standard Process, Inc.
Each 5 mL serving contains: Echinacea root 1:2 extract (from echinacea angustifolia 500 mg) 1 mL • Elder flower 1:2 extract (from sambucus nigra 500 mg) 1 mL • Lime flower 1:2 extract (from tilia species 500 mg) 1 mL • Yarrow herb 1:2 extract (from achillea millefolium 500 mg) 1 mL • Ginger rhizome 1:2 extract (from zingiber officinale 250 mg) 500 mcL • Licorice root 1:1 extract (from glycyrrhiza glabra 500 mg) 500 mcL. Other Ingredients: Purified Water, 43% Alcohol.

Mediherb DiGest - Standard Process, Inc.
Each tablet contains: Dandelion root 4:1 extract (from taraxacum officinale 500 mg) 125 mg • Tangerine fruit peel 5:1 extract (from citrus reticulata 500 mg) 100 mg • Milk Thistle fruit 70:1 extract (from silybum marianum 2.1 g, containing flavanolignans calculated as silybin 24 mg) 30 mg • Ginger rhizome 5:1 extract (from zingiber officinale 100 mg) 20 mg • Gentian root 5:1 extract (from gentiana lutea 100 mg) 20 mg • Tangerine fruit peel oil (citrus reticulata) 12.5 mg • Chamomile flower essential oil (matricaria recutita) 5 mg • Calcium 52 mg. Other Ingredients: Cellulose, Calcium Acid Phosphate, Silica, Sodium Starch Glycollate, Hypromellose, Magnesium Stearate.

MediHerb DiGest Phytosynergist - Standard Process, Inc.
Each 5 mL serving contains: Chamomile flower 1:2 extract (from matricaria recutita 750 mg) 1.5 mL • Dandelion root 1:2 extract (from taraxacum officinale 500 mg) 1.5 mL • Echinacea root 1:2 extract (from echinacea angustifolia 500 mg) 1 mL • Milk Thistle seed 1:1 extract (from silybum marianum 1 g) 1 mL • Gentian root 1:2 extract (from gentiana lutea 100 mg) 200 mcL. Other Ingredients: Purified Water, 43% Alcohol.

MediHerb Dong Quai - Standard Process, Inc.
Each tablet contains: Dong Quai root 4:1 extract (from angelica sinensis 1 g) 250 mg • Calcium 20 mg. Other Ingredients: Calcium Acid Phosphate, Cellulose, Silica, Sodium Starch Glycollate, Hypromellose, Magnesium Stearate.

MediHerb Dong Quai 1:2 - Standard Process, Inc.
Each 5 mL serving contains: Dong Quai root 1:2 extract (from angelica sinensis 2.5 g) 5 mL. Other Ingredients: Purified Water, 45% Alcohol.

MediHerb Echinacea Premium - Standard Process, Inc.
Each tablet contains: Echinacea root 4:1 extract (from echinacea angustifolia 600 mg, containing aklylamides 2 mg) 150 mg • Echinacea root 6:1 extract (from echinacea purpurea 675 mg, containing alkylamides 2.1 mg) 112.5 mg • Calcium 60 mg. Other Ingredients: Calcium Acid Phosphate, Cellulose, Silica, Sodium Starch Glycollate, Hypromellose, Magnesium Stearate.

MediHerb Echinacea Purpurea 1:2 - Standard Process, Inc.
Each 5 mL serving contains: Echinacea Purpurea root 1:2 extract (from echinacea purpurea 2.5 g) 5 mL. Other Ingredients: Purified Water, 60% Alcohol.

MediHerb Echinacea Purpurea 1:3 Glycetract - Standard Process, Inc.
Each 5 mL serving contains: Echinacea Purpurea root 1:3 extract (from echinacea purpurea 1.67 g) 5 mL. Other Ingredients: Purified Water, Glycerol, Potassium Sorbate.

MediHerb Echincea Premium Blend 1:2 - Standard Process, Inc.
Each 5 mL serving contains: Echinacea root 1:2 extract (from echinacea purpurea 1.5 g) 3 mL • Echinacea root 1:2 extract (from echinacea angustifolia 1 g, total alkylamides from both extracts 7.5 mg) 2 mL. Other Ingredients: Purified Water, 60% Alcohol.

MediHerb Eleuthero - Standard Process, Inc.
Each tablet contains: Eleuthero root 10:1 extract (from eleutherococcus senticosus 1.25 g, containing eleutheroside E 950

mcg) 125 mg • Calcium 20 mg. Other Ingredients: Calcium Acid Phosphate, Cellulose, Magnesium Stearate, Sodium Starch Glycollate.

MediHerb Eleuthero 1:2 **-** Standard Process, Inc.
Each 5 mL serving contains: Eleuthero 1:2 extract (from eleutherococcus senticosus 2.5 g, containing eleutheroside E 2.5 mg) 5 mL. Other Ingredients: Purified Water, 25% Alcohol.

MediHerb Euphrasia Complex **-** Standard Process, Inc.
Each tablet contains: Eyebright herb 4:1 extract (from euphrasia officinalis 650 mg) 162.5 mg • Golden Rod herb 4:1 extract (from solidago virgaurea 650 mg) 162.5 mg • Echinacea purpurea root 6:1 extract (from echinacea purpurea 370 mg) 61.67 mg • Golden Seal root and rhizome 3:1 extract (from hydrastis canadensis 125 mg) 41.67 mg • Cayenne fruit 4:1 extract (from capsicum annuum 10 mg) 2.5 mg • Calcium 60 mg. Other Ingredients: Calcium Acid Phosphate, Cellulose, Hypromellose, Magnesium Stearate, Silica, Sodium Starch Glycollate.

MediHerb Evening Primrose Oil **-** Standard Process, Inc.
Each capsule contains: Evening Primrose Oil (from oenothera biennis seed, containing gamma-linolenic acid 100 mg) 1 g. Other Ingredients: Gelatin.

MediHerb Eyebright 1:2 **-** Standard Process, Inc.
Each 5 mL serving contains: Eyebright herb 1:2 extract (from euphrasia officinalis 2.5 g) 5 mL. Other Ingredients: Purified Water, 45% Alcohol.

MediHerb Fe-Max Iron Tonic **-** Standard Process, Inc.
Each 5 mL serving contains: Iron (from ferrous gluconate) 5 mg • Vitamin C (ascorbic acid) 25 mg • Vitamin B6 (pyridoxine hydrochloride) 2.5 mg • Vitamin B2 (riboflavin) 2.5 mg • Vitamin B1 (thiamine hydrochloride) 2.5 mg • Folic Acid 150 mcg • Vitamin B12 (cyanocobalamin) 1.5 mcg • Codonopsis root 1:2 extract (from codonopsis pilosula 500 mg) 1 mL • Nettle leaf 1:2 extract (from urtica dioica 500 mg) 1 mL • Ashwaganda root 2:1 extract (from withania somnifera 500 mg) 1 mL • Vervain herb 2:1 extract (from verbena officinalis 250 mg) 500 mcL • Licorice root 2:1 extract (from glycrrhiza glabra 500 mg) 143 mg • Ginger rhizome 1:2 extract (from zingiber officinale 50 mg) 100 mcL • Stevia leaf 1:2 extract (from stevia rebaudiana 50 mg) 100 mcL. Other Ingredients: Glycerol, Purified Water, Fruit & Vegetable Juices: Beet Root, Grape, Pear, Apple, Carrot, Lemon.

MediHerb Feverfew **-** Standard Process, Inc.
Each tablet contains: Feverfew leaf powder (tanacetum parthenium, containing parthenolide 900 mcg) 150 mg • Calcium 60 mg. Other Ingredients: Calcium Acid Phosphate, Cellulose, Sodium Starch Glycollate, Silica, Magnesium Stearate.

MediHerb Ganoderma & Shiitake **-** Standard Process, Inc.
Each tablet contains: Shiitake mushroom 4:1 extract (from lentinula edodes 800 mg) 200 mg • Reishi mushroom 66:1 extract (from ganoderma lucidum 6.6 g) 100 mg • Calcium 60 mg. Other Ingredients: Calcium Acid Phosphate, Cellulose, Sodium Starch Glycollate, Silica, Hypromellose, Magnesium Stearate.

MediHerb Garlic 1:1 **-** Standard Process, Inc.
Each 5 mL serving contains: Garlic bulb fresh 1:1 extract (from allium sativum 5 g) 5 mL. Other Ingredients: Purified Water, 45% Alcohol.

MediHerb Garlic 5000mg **-** Standard Process, Inc.
Each tablet contains: Garlic bulb 6.5:1 extract (from allium sativum 1.04 g, containing alliin 4.3 mg) 160 mg • Allium Sativum bulb powder (containing alliin 1.4 mg) 100 mg • Calcium 20 mg. Other Ingredients: Calcium Acid Phosphate, Cellulose, Hypromellose, Magnesium Stearate, Enteric Coating, Sodium Starch Glycollate.

MediHerb Gentian 1:2 **-** Standard Process, Inc.
Each 1 mL serving contains: Gentian root 1:2 extract (from gentiana lutea 500 mg) 1 mL. Other Ingredients: Purified Water, 45% Alcohol.

MediHerb Ginger 1:2 **-** Standard Process, Inc.
Each 2.5 mL serving contains: Ginger rhizome 1:2 extract (from zingiber officinale 1.25 g) 2.5 mL. Other Ingredients: Purified Water, 90% Alcohol.

MediHerb Ginkgo 2:1 **-** Standard Process, Inc.
Each 1 mL serving contains: Ginkgo leaf 2:1 extract (from ginkgo biloba 2 g, containing ginkgo flavone glycosides 9.6 mg) 1 mL. Other Ingredients: Purified Water, 50% Alcohol.

MediHerb Ginkgo 2000mg **-** Standard Process, Inc.
Each tablet contains: Ginkgo Biloba leaf 50:1 extract (from ginkgo biloba 2 g, containing ginkgo flavone glycosides 10.68 mg, containing ginkgolides and bilobalide 2.68 mg) 40 mg • Calcium 40 mg. Other Ingredients: Calcium Acid Phosphate, Cellulose, Magnesium Stearate, Sodium Starch Glycollate.

MediHerb Globe Artichoke 1:2 **-** Standard Process, Inc.
Each 5 mL serving contains: Globe Artichoke leaf 1:2 extract (from cynara scolymus 2.5 g) 5 mL. Other Ingredients: Purified Water, 60% Alcohol.

MediHerb Golden Seal 1:3 **-** Standard Process, Inc.
Each 5 mL serving contains: Golden Seal root and rhizome 1:3 extract (from hydrastis canadensis 1.67 g, containing hydrastine 40 mg and berberine 40 mg) 5 mL. Other Ingredients: Purified Water, 45% Alcohol.

MediHerb Golden Seal 500mg **-** Standard Process, Inc.
Each tablet contains: Golden Seal root and rhizome 3:1 extract (from hydrastis canadensis 500 mg) 166.7 mg • Calcium 40 mg. Other Ingredients: Calcium Acid Phosphate, Cellulose, Hypromellose, Magnesium Stearate, Silica, Sodium Starch Glycollate.

MediHerb Gotu Kola 1:2 **-** Standard Process, Inc.
Each 5 mL serving contains: Gotu Kola herb 1:2 extract (from centella asiatica 2.5 g) 5 mL. Other Ingredients: Purified Water, 45% Alcohol.

MediHerb Grindelia 1:2 **-** Standard Process, Inc.
Each 5 mL serving contains: Grindelia herb 1:2 extract (from grindelia camporum 2.5 g) 5 mL. Other Ingredients: Purified Water, 60% Alcohol.

MediHerb Gymnema 1:1 **-** Standard Process, Inc.
Each 5 mL serving contains: Gymnema leaf 1:1 extract (from gymnema sylvestre 5 g) 5 mL. Other Ingredients: Purified Water, 25% Alcohol.

MediHerb Gymnema 4g **-** Standard Process, Inc.
Each tablet contains: Gymnema Sylvestre leaf 10:1 extract (from gymnema sylvestre 4 g, containing gymnemic acids 100 mg) 400 mg • Calcium 60 mg. Other Ingredients: Calcium Acid Phosphate, Cellulose, Hypromellose, Magnesium Stearate, Enteric Coating, Sodium Starch Glycollate.

MediHerb Hawthorn **-** Standard Process, Inc.
Each tablet contains: Hawthorn herb flowering top 3:1 extract (from crataegus monogyna 1 g, containing vitexin-2-rhamnoside 6.68 mg and catechin polymers 15 mg) 334 mg • Calcium 60 mg. Other Ingredients: Calcium Acid Phosphate, Cellulose, Hypromellose, Magnesium Stearate, Sodium Starch Glycollate.

MediHerb Hawthorn Berries 1:2 **-** Standard Process, Inc.
Each 5 mL serving contains: Hawthorn fruit 1:2 extract (from crataegus monogyna 2.5 g, containing oligomeric procyanidins 26 mg) 5 mL. Other Ingredients: Purified Water, 45% Alcohol.

MediHerb Herbal Throat Spray Phytosynergist **-** Standard Process, Inc.
Four sprays contain: Echinacea root 1:2 extract (from echinacea angustifolia 10 mg) 20 mcL • Calendula flower 1:2 extract (from calendula officinalis 10 mg) 20 mcL • Marshmallow root 1:5 extract (from althaea officinalis 40 mg) 200 mcL • Sage herb 1:2 extract

(from salvia officinalis 30 mg) 60 mcL • Myrrh resin 1:5 extract (from commiphora mol-mol stem oleo-gum-resin 1 mg) 5 mcL • Clove oil (syzgium aromaticum) 1.25 mcL. Other Ingredients: Glycerol, Menthol, Propyl Hydroxybenzoate, Methyl Hydroxybenzoate, Purified Water, 16.25% Ethanol.

MediHerb HiPep Phytosynergist - Standard Process, Inc.
Each 5 mL serving contains: Licorice root 1:1 extract (from glycyrrhiza glabra 1.5 g) 1.5 mL • Meadowsweet herb 1:2 extract (from filipendula ulmaria 625 mg) 1.25 mL • Chickweed fresh herb succus (from stellaria media 1 g) 1 mL • Echinacea root 1:2 extract (from echinacea angustifolia 375 mg) 750 mcL • Golden Seal root and rhizome 1:3 extract (from hydrastis canadensis 167 mg) 500 mcL. Other Ingredients: Purified Water, 34% Alcohol.

MediHerb Horsechestnut 1:2 - Standard Process, Inc.
Each 5 mL serving contains: Horse Chestnut seed 1:2 extract (from aesculus hippocastanum 2.5 g) 5 mL. Other Ingredients: Purified Water, 35% Alcohol.

MediHerb HorseChestnut Complex - Standard Process, Inc.
Each tablet contains: Butcher's Broom root and rhizome 4:1 extract (from ruscus aculeatus 800 mg, containing ruscogenin 20 mg) 200 mg • Horse Chestnut seed 6:1 extract (from aesculus hippocastanum 1.2 g, containing escin 40 mg) 200 mg • Ginkgo Biloba leaf 50:1 extract (from ginkgo biloba 1.5 g, containing ginkgo flavone glycosides 7.3 mg and ginkgolides and bilobalide 1.8 mg) 30 mg • Calcium 20 mg. Other Ingredients: Calcium Acid Phosphate, Cellulose, Hypromellose, Magnesium Stearate, Silica, Sodium Starch Glycollate, Enteric Coating.

MediHerb Horsetail 1:2 - Standard Process, Inc.
Each 5 mL serving contains: Horsetail herb 1:2 extract (from equisetum arvense 2.5 g) 5 mL. Other Ingredients: Purified Water, 25% Alcohol.

MediHerb Hydrangea 1:2 - Standard Process, Inc.
Each 5 mL serving contains: Hydrangea root 1:2 extract (from hydrangea arborescens 2.5 g) 5 mL. Other Ingredients: Purified Water, 45% Alcohol.

MediHerb Jamaican Dogwood 1:2 - Standard Process, Inc.
Each 5 mL serving contains: Jamaican Dogwood root bark 1:2 extract (from piscidia erythrina 2.5 g) 5 mL. Other Ingredients: Purified Water, 60% Alcohol.

MediHerb Korean Ginseng 1:2 - Standard Process, Inc.
Each 2.5 mL serving contains: Korean Ginseng main root 1:2 extract (from Panax ginseng 1.25 g, containing ginsenosides as Rg1 and Rb1 27.5 mg) 2.5 mL. Other Ingredients: Purified Water, 60% Alcohol.

MediHerb Licorice 1:1 - Standard Process, Inc.
Each 2.5 mL serving contains: Licorice root 1:1 extract (from glycyrrhiza glabra 2.5 g) 2.5 mL. Other Ingredients: Purified Water, 20% Alcohol.

MediHerb Licorice High Grade 1:1 - Standard Process, Inc.
Each 2.5 mL serving contains: Licorice root 1:1 extract (from glycyrrhiza glabra 2.5 g, containing glycyrrhizin 75 mg) 2.5 mL. Other Ingredients: Purified Water, 20% Alcohol.

MediHerb LivCo - Standard Process, Inc.
Each tablet contains: Schisandra fruit (4:1 extract from schisandra chinensis fruit 1 g) 250 mg • Rosemary leaf (5:1 extract from rosmarinus officinalis leaf 500 mg) 100 mg •Milk Thistle seed (70:1 extract from silybum marianum seed 2 g, containing flavanoligans calc. as silybin 24 mg) 28.6 mg • Calcium 20 mg. Inactive Ingredi ents: Calcium Acid Phosphate, Cellulose, Sodium Starch Glycollate, Hypromellose, Magnesium Stearate.

MediHerb Livton Complex - Standard Process, Inc.
Each tablet contains: Globe Artichoke leaf 4:1 extract (from cynara scolymus 800 mg) 200 mg • Dandelion root 4:1 extract (from taraxacum officinale 400 mg) 100 mg • Milk Thistle fruit 70:1 extract (from silybum marianum 7 g, containing flavanolignans calculated as silybin 84 mg) 100 mg • Greater Celandine herb 5:1 extract (from chelidonium majus 200 mg) 50 mg • Fringe Tree root bark 5:1 extract (from chionanthus virginicus 160 mg) 32 mg • Calcium 40 mg. Other Ingredients: Calcium Acid Phosphate, Cellulose, Hypromellose, Magnesium Stearate, Silica, Sodium Starch Glycollate.

MediHerb Marshmallow root 1:5 Glycetract - Standard Process, Inc.
Each 5 mL serving contains: Marshmallow root 1:5 extract (from althaea officinalis root 1 g) 5 mL. Other Ingredients: Purified Water, Glycerol, Citrus Seed Extract.

MediHerb Milk Thistle 1:1 - Standard Process, Inc.
Each 5 mL serving contains: Milk Thistle seed 1:1 extract (from silybum marianum 5 g, containing flavanolignans calculated as silybin 125 mg) 5 mL. Other Ingredients: Purified Water, 70% Alcohol.

MediHerb Milk Thistle 1:1 Glycetract - Standard Process, Inc.
Each 5 mL serving contains: Milk Thistle seed 1:1 extract (from silybum marianum 5 g, containing flavanolignans calculated as silybin 50 mg) 5 mL. Other Ingredients: Purified Water, Glycerol, Citrus Seed Extract.

MediHerb Mistletoe 1:2 - Standard Process, Inc.
Each 5 mL serving contains: Mistletoe herb 1:2 extract (from viscum album 2.5 g) 5 mL. Other Ingredients: Purified Water, 45% Alcohol.

MediHerb Motherwort 1:2 - Standard Process, Inc.
Each 5 mL serving contains: Motherwort herb 1:2 extract (from leonurus cardiaca 2.5 g) 5 mL. Other Ingredients: Purified Water, 25% Alcohol.

MediHerb Nettle Leaf 1:2 - Standard Process, Inc.
Each 5 mL serving contains: Nettle leaf 1:2 extract (from urtica dioica 2.5 g) 5 mL. Other Ingredients: Purified Water, 25% Alcohol.

MediHerb Nettle Root 1:2 - Standard Process, Inc.
Each 5 mL serving contains: Nettle root 1:2 extract (from urtica dioica 2.5 g) 5 mL. Other Ingredients: Purified Water, 25% Alcohol.

MediHerb Nevaton - Standard Process, Inc.
Each tablet contains: Schisandra fruit 4:1 extract (from schisandra chinensis 675 mg) 168.8 mg • Damiana leaf 4:1 extract (from turnera diffusa 625 mg) 156.3 mg • Skullcap herb 4:1 extract (from scutellaria lateriflora 500 mg) 125 mg • St. John's Wort herb flowering top 6:1 extract (from hypericum perforatum 750 mg, containing hypericins 413 mcg) 125 mg • Calcium 40 mg. Other Ingredients: Calcium Acid Phosphate, Cellulose, Hypromellose, Magnesium Stearate, Silica, Sodium Starch Glycollate.

MediHerb Oats Seed 1:1 - Standard Process, Inc.
Each 5 mL serving contains: Oats seed 1:1 extract (from avena sativa 5 g) 5 mL. Other Ingredients: Purified Water, 25% Alcohol.

MediHerb Oregon Grape 1:2 - Standard Process, Inc.
Each 5 mL serving contains: Oregon Grape root and rhizome 1:2 extract (from berberis aquifolium (mahonia aquifolium) 2.5 g) 5 mL. Other Ingredients: Purified Water, 25% Alcohol.

MediHerb Pasque Flower 1:2 - Standard Process, Inc.
Each 2.5 mL serving contains: Pasque Flower herb 1:2 extract (from anemone pulsatilla 1.25 g) 2.5 mL. Other Ingredients: Purified Water, 25% Alcohol.

MediHerb Pau d'Arco 1:2 - Standard Process, Inc.
Each 5 mL serving contains: Pau d'Arco bark 1:2 extract (from tabebuia avellanedae 2.5 g) 5 mL. Other Ingredients: Purified Water, 45% Alcohol.

Some Brand Name Natural Products - What they Contain

www.NaturalDatabase.com contains MANY more listings than appear here.

MediHerb Poke Root 1:5 - Standard Process, Inc.
Each 1 mL serving contains: Poke Root root 1:5 extract (from phytolacca decandra 200 mg) 1 mL. Other Ingredients: Purified Water, 45% Alcohol.

MediHerb Prickly Ash 1:2 - Standard Process, Inc.
Each 2.5 mL serving contains: Prickly Ash bark 1:2 extract (from zanthoxylum clava-herculis 1.25 g) 2.5 mL. Other Ingredients: Purified Water, 45% Alcohol.

MediHerb PulmaCo - Standard Process, Inc.
Each tablet contains: Chinese Skullcap root 3:1 extract (from scutellaria baicalensis 500 mg) 166.7 mg • Malabar Nut Tree leaf 5:1 extract (from adhatoda vasica 750 mg) 150 mg • Grindelia herb 4:1 extract (from grindelia camporum 300 mg) 75 mg • Turmeric rhizome 25:1 extract (from curcuma longa 1 g, containing curcuminoids 38 mg) 40 mg • Ginkgo leaf 50:1 extract (from ginkgo biloba 1 g, containing ginkgo flavonglycosides 4.8 mg) 20 mg • Sweet Fennel seed essential oil (foeniculum vulgare) 5 mg • Calcium 40 mg. Other Ingredients: Cellulose, Calcium Acid Phosphate, Silica, Sodium Starch Glycollate, Hypromellose, Magnesium Stearate.

MediHerb Red Clover 1:2 - Standard Process, Inc.
Each 5 mL serving contains: Red Clover flower 1:2 extract (from trifolium pratense 2.5 g) 5 mL. Other Ingredients: Purified Water, 25% Alcohol.

MediHerb Rehmannia 1:2 - Standard Process, Inc.
Each 5 mL serving contains: Rehmannia root 1:2 extract (from rehmannia glutinosa 2.5 g) 5 mL. Other Ingredients: Purified Water, 25% Alcohol.

MediHerb Rehmannia Complex - Standard Process, Inc.
Each tablet contains: Rehmannia root 2.5:1 extract (from rehmannia glutinosa 350 mg) 140 mg • Bupleurum root 4.5:1 extract (from bupleurum falcatum 700 mg) 155.5 mg • Hemidesmus root 5:1 extract (from hemidesmus indicus 500 mg) 100 mg • Feverfew leaf and stem 3:1 extract (from tanacetum parthenium 165 mg) 55 mg • Calcium 59 mg. Other Ingredients: Cellulose, Calcium Hydrogen Phosphate, Silica, Sodium Starch Glycollate • Magnesium Stearate.

MediHerb ResCo - Standard Process, Inc.
Each tablet contains: Licorice root 3.5:1 extract (from glycyrrhiza glabra 500 mg) 142.9 mg • Mullein leaf 4:1 extract (from verbascum thapsus 470 mg) 117.5 mg • Euphorbia herb 4:1 extract (from euphorbia hirta 280 mg) 70 mg • Grindelia herb 4:1 extract (from gindelia camporum 280 mg) 70 mg • Ginger rhizome 5:1 extract (from zingiber officinale 180 mg) 36 mg • Fennel oil (fruit essential oil, foeniculum vulgare) 12 mg • Thyme oil (leaf essential oil, from thymus vulgaris) 12 mg • Calcium 40 mg. Other Ingredients: Calcium Acid Phosphate, Cellulose, Hypromellose, Magnesium Stearate, Silica, Sodium Starch Glycollate.

MediHerb ResCo Phytosynergist - Standard Process, Inc.
Each 5 mL serving contains: Mullein leaf 1:2 extract (from verbascum thapsus 625 mg) 1.25 mL • Licorice root 1:1 extract (from glycyrrhiza glabra 1 g) 1 mL • Elecampane root 1:2 (from inula helenium 375 mg) 750 mcL • Euphorbia herb 1:2 extract (from euphorbia hirta 375 mg) 750 mcL • Grindelia herb 1:2 extract (from grindelia camporum 375 mg) 750 mcL • Ginger rhizome 1:2 extract (from zingiber officinale 250 mg) 500 mcL • Fennel oil (foeniculum vulgare) 15 mcL. Other Ingredients: Purified Water, 46% Alcohol.

MediHerb Sage 1:2 - Standard Process, Inc.
Each 5 mL serving contains: Sage herb 1:2 extract (from salvia officinalis 2.5 g) 5 mL. Other Ingredients: Purified Water, 60% Alcohol.

MediHerb Saligesic - Standard Process, Inc.
Each tablet contains: White Willow stem bark 20:1 extract (from salix spp 8 g, containing salicin 60 mg) 400 mg • Calcium 30 mg.

MediHerb Sarsaparilla 1:2 - Standard Process, Inc.
Each 5 mL serving contains: Sarsaparilla root and rhizome 1:2 extract (from smilax ornata 2.5 g) 5 mL. Other Ingredients: Purified Water, 45% Alcohol.

MediHerb Saw Palmetto 1:2 - Standard Process, Inc.
Each 5 mL serving contains: Saw Palmetto fruit 1:2 extract (from serenoa serrulata 2.5 g) 5 mL. Other Ingredients: Purified Water, 45% Alcohol.

MediHerb Schisandra 1:2 - Standard Process, Inc.
Each 5 mL serving contains: Schisandra fruit 1:2 extract (from schisandra chinensis 2.5 g) 5 mL. Other Ingredients: Purified Water, 45% Alcohol.

MediHerb Serenoa Complex - Standard Process, Inc.
Each capsule contains: Saw Palmetto fruit 10:1 extract (from serenoa serrulata 1.6 g, containing serenoa serrulata fatty acids 144 mg) 160 mg. Other Ingredients: Pumpkin Seed Oil, Soya Oil, Gelatin, Glycerol.

MediHerb Silymarin - Standard Process, Inc.
Each tablet contains: Milk Thistle fruit 70:1 extract (from silybum marianum 14 g, containing flavonolignans calculated as silybin 168 mg) 200 mg • Calcium 20 mg. Other Ingredients: Calcium Acid Phosphate, Cellulose, Sodium Starch Glycollate, Silica, Magnesium Stearate.

MediHerb Skullcap 1:2 - Standard Process, Inc.
Each 5 mL serving contains: Skullcap 1:2 extract (from scutellaria lateriflora 2.5 g) 5 mL. Other Ingredients: Purified Water, 45% Alcohol.

MediHerb St. John's Wort 1.8g - Standard Process, Inc.
Each tablet contains: St. John's Wort herb flowering top 6:1 extract (from hypericum perforatum 1.8 g, containing hypericins 990 mcg and hyperforin 9 mg) 300 mg • Calcium 60 mg. Other Ingredients: Calcium Acid Phospahte, Cellulose, Hypromellose, Magnesium Stearate, Silica, Sodium Starch Glycollate.

MediHerb St. John's Wort 1:2 - Standard Process, Inc.
Each 5 mL serving contains: St. John's Wort herb flowering top 1:2 extract (from hypericum perforatum 2.5 g, containing hypericins 1 mg) 5 mL. Other Ingredients: Purified Water, 45% Alcohol.

MediHerb St. John's Wort High Grade 1:2 - Standard Process, Inc.
Each 5 mL serving contains: St. John's Wort flowering herb 1:2 extract (from hypericum perforatum 2.5 g, containing hypericins 2 mg) 5 mL. Other Ingredients: Purified Water, 60% Alcohol.

MediHerb Thyroid Complex - Standard Process, Inc.
Each tablet contains: Bladderwrack whole plant 3.5:1 extract (from fucus vesiculosus 1.05 g, containing iodine 600 mcg) 300 mg • Withania (ashwaganda) root 5:1 extract (from withania somnifera 600 mg) 120 mg • Bacopa herb 50:1 extract (from bacopa monnieri 2.5 g, containing bacosides 25 mg) 50 mg • Calcium 52 mg. Other Ingredients: Calcium Acid Phosphate, Cellulose, Sodium Starch Glycollate, Hypromellose, Silica, Magnesium Stearate.

MediHerb Tienchi Ginseng 1:2 - Standard Process, Inc.
Each 5 mL serving contains: Tienchi Ginseng root 1:2 extract (from Panax notoginseng 2.5 g) 5 mL. Other Ingredients: Purified Water, 45% Alcohol.

MediHerb Tribulus - Standard Process, Inc.
Each tablet contains: Tribulus herb 4.5:1 extract (from tribulus terrestris 2.79 g, containing furostanol saponins 100 mg) 620 mg • Calcium 24 mg. Other Ingredients: Calcium Acid Phosphate, Cellulose, Hypromellose, Magnesium Stearate, Sodium Starch Glycollate.

MediHerb Turmeric 1:1 **-** Standard Process, Inc.
Each 5 mL serving contains: Turmeric rhizome 1:1 extract (from curcuma longa 5 g) 5 mL. Other Ingredients: Purified Water, 45% Alcohol.

MediHerb UriCo Phytosynergist **-** Standard Process, Inc.
Each 5 mL serving contains: Couch Grass rhizome 1:1 extract (from agropyron repens 1.5 g) 1.5 mL • Echinacea root 1:2 extract (from echinacea angustifolia 625 mg) 1.25 mL • Licorice root 1:1 extract (from glycyrrhiza glabra 1.25 mg) 1.25 mL • Buchu leaf 1:2 extract (from barosma betulina 500 mg) 1 mL. Other Ingredients: Purified Water, 36% Alcohol.

MediHerb Uva Ursi 1:2 **-** Standard Process, Inc.
Each 5 mL serving contains: Uva Ursi leaf 1:2 extract (from arctostaphylos uva-ursi 2.5 g) 5 mL. Other Ingredients: Purified Water, 45% Alcohol.

MediHerb Valerian 1:2 **-** Standard Process, Inc.
Each 5 mL serving contains: Valerian root 1:2 extract (from valeriana officinalis 2.5 g) 5 mL. Other Ingredients: Purified Water, 45% Alcohol.

MediHerb Valerian Complex **-** Standard Process, Inc.
Each tablet contains: Spiny Jujube seed 5:1 extract (from zizyphus spinosa 900 mg) 180 mg • Valerian root and rhizome 5:1 extract (from valeriana officinalis 700 mg) 140 mg • Passion Flower herb 5:1 extract (from passiflora incarnata 500 mg) 100 mg • Calcium 40 mg. Other Ingredients: Calcium Acid Phosphate, Hypromellose, Magnesium Stearate, Silica, Sodium Starch Glycollate.

MediHerb Vitanox **-** Standard Process, Inc.
Each tablet contains: Rosemary leaf 5:1 extract (from rosmarinus officinalis 1 g) 200 mg • Green Tea 6:1 extract (From camelia sinensis 1g, containing catechins 83.35 mg) 166.7 mg • Turmeric rhizome 25:1 extract (from curcuma longa 2 g, containing curcuminoids 70.4 mg) 80 mg • Grape seed 120:1 extract (from vitis vinifera 6 g, containing procyanidins 42.5 mg) 50 mg • Calcium 40 mg. Other Ingredients: Calcium Acid Phosphate, Cellulose, Hypromellose, Magnesium Stearate, Silica, Sodium Starch Glycollate.

MediHerb White Peony 1:2 **-** Standard Process, Inc.
Each 5 mL serving contains: White Peony root 1:2 extract (from paeonia lactiflora 2.5 g) 5 mL. Other Ingredients: Purified Water, 45% Alcohol.

MediHerb Wild Yam 1:2 **-** Standard Process, Inc.
Each 5 mL serving contains: Wild Yam root and rhizome 1:2 extract (from discorea villosa 2.5 g, containing steroidal saponins as dioscin 75 mg) 5 mL. Other Ingredients: Purified Water, 60% Alcohol.

MediHerb Wild Yam Complex **-** Standard Process, Inc.
Each tablet contains: False Unicorn root 4:1 extract (from chamaelirium luteum 360 mg) 90 mg • Wild Yam root and rhizome 4:1 extract (from discorea villosa 360 mg) 90 mg • Sage herb 5:1 extract (from salvia officinalis 290 mg) 58 mg • Korean Ginseng root 5:1 extract (from Panax ginseng 75 mg, containing ginsenosides as Rg1 and Rb1 1.4 mg) 15 mg • St. John's Wort herb flowering top 6:1 extract (from hypericum perforatum 360 mg, containing hypericins 198 mcg) 60 mg • Calcium 60 mg. Other Ingredients: Calcium Acid Phosphate, Cellulose, Hypromellose, Magnesium Stearate, Silica, Sodium Starch Glycollate.

MediHerb Withania Complex **-** Standard Process, Inc.
Each tablet contains: Licorice root 3.5:1 extract (from glycyrrhiza glabra 750 mg) 214 mg • Withania (ashwaganda) root 5:1 extract (from withania somnifera 950 mg) 190 mg • Skullcap herb 4:1 extract (from scutellaria lateriflora 470 mg) 117.5 mg • Korean Ginseng root 5:1 extract (from Panax ginseng 100 mg, containing ginsenosides as Rg1 and Rb1 1.86 mg) 20 mg • Calcium 40 mg. Other Ingredients: Calcium Acid Phosphate, Cellulose, Silica, Sodium Starch Glycollate, Hypromellose, Magnesium Stearate.

MediHerb Withania Complex Phytosynergist **-** Standard Process, Inc.
Each 5 mL contains: Korean Ginseng root (5:1 extract from panax ginseng root 125 mg containing ginsenosides as Rg1 and Rb1 2.32 mg) 25 mg • Ashwaganda root (1:2 extract from withania somnifera root 1.25 g) 2.5 mL • Skullcap herb (1:2 extract from scutellaria lateriflora herb 625 mg) 1.25 mL • Licorice root (1:1 extract from glycyrrhiza glabra root 1 g) 1 mL. Inactive Ingredients: Purified Water, 41% Alcohol.

MediHerb Wormwood 1:5 **-** Standard Process, Inc.
Each 1 mL serving contains: Wormwood herb 1:5 extract (from artemisia absinthium 200 mg) 1 mL. Other Ingredients: Purified Water, 45% Alcohol.

MediHerb Wormwood Complex **-** Standard Process, Inc.
Each tablet contains: Stemona root 3:1 extract (from stemona sessilifolia 1000 mg) 333 mg • Black Walnut green hulls 4:1 extract (from juglans nigra 100 mg) 25 mg • Wormwood herb 4:1 extract (from artemisia absinthium 100 mg) 25 mg • Clove oil 20 mg • Calcium 18 mg. Other Ingredients: Cellulose, Silica, Calcium Acid Phosphate, Sodium Starch Glycollate, Hypromellose, Magnesium Stearate.

MediHerb Yellow Dock 1:2 **-** Standard Process, Inc.
Each 5 mL serving contains: Yellow Dock root 1:2 extract (from rumex crispus 2.5 g) 5 mL. Other Ingredients: Purified Water, 25% Alcohol.

MediTropin **-** Nutraceutics Corp.
Three effervescent tablets contain: Proprietary Blend Glycoamino Acid Complex 6230 mg: Symbiotropin, Anterior Pituitary Peptides (porcine), Protein Growth Factors, GHRH Decapeptides (porcine) • Polyose Complex (mono, poly and oligo saccharides) 3075 mg. Other Ingredients: Citric Acid, Potassium Bicarbonate, Glucose, L-Glutamine, L-Arginine, L-Pyroglutamate, Sodium Bicarbonate, L-Lysine Monohydrochloride, L-Leucine, Glycine, Polyethylene Glycol, Sodium Carbonate, Mixed Berry Flavor, L-Tyrosine, Gamma Aminobutyric Acid, Inositol Hexanicotinate, Sodium Benzoate Powder.

Meditropin Anti-Aging Therapy with Symbiotropin Plus + **-** Nutraceutics Corp.
Three effervescent tablets contain: Glycoamino Acid Proprietary Complex 6230 mg: Symbiotropin, Anterior Pituitary Peptides (porcine), Protein Growth Factors, GHRH Decapeptides (porcine) • Polyose complex 3075 mg: Monosaccharides, Polysaccharides, Oligosaccharides. Other Ingredients: Citric Acid, Potassium Bicarbonate, Glucose, L-Glutamine, L-Arginine, L-Pyrogluatamate, Sodium Bicarbonate, L-Lysine Monohydrochloride, L-Leucine, Glycine, Polyethylene Glycol, Sodium Carbonate, Mixed Berry Flavor, L-Tyrosine, Gamma Aminobutyric Acid, Inositol Hexanicotinate, Sodium Benzoate Powder.

Medphen **-** Olympian Labs
Six capsules contain: Proprietary Blend 3000 mg: Green Tea extract, Garcinia Cambogia, Ginger, Mustard Seed, Cayenne, Astragalus, White Willow Bark, Uva Ursi, Siberian Ginseng, Gotu Kola.

Medroid **-** Sports One
19-Nor-4-Androstenediol • 19-Norandrostenedione • Androstenedione • 4-Androstenediol • 5-Androstenediol • Tribulus Terrestris • Acetyl-L-Carnitine • Thermogenic Formula using a proprietary half-life enzymatic conversion excelerator. Capsule 1: Tribulus Terrestris 250 mg, 5-Androstene-3B,17B-Diol 50 mg. Capsule 2: Androstenedione 100 mg, Acetyl L-Carnitine 100 mg, 4-Androstene-3, 17-Diol 100 mg. Capsule 3 (Proprietary half-life excelerator): Ma Huang herb 10:1 extract, Green Tea leaf 10:1 extract, White Willow bark, Secret Half Life Enzymatic Conversion Excelerator. Capsule 4: 5-Androstene-3B,17B-Diol 50 mg, 19-Nor-4-Androstene-3B, 17B-Diol 50 mg, 19-Norandrostenedione 100 mg.
See Editor's Note No. 47, page 2058.

Mega B-125 **-** The Vitamin Shoppe
Each sustained-release tablet contains: Vitamin B1 (thiamin) 125 mg • Vitamin B2 (riboflavin) 125 mg • Vitamin B6 (pyridoxine HCl) 125 mg • Vitamin B12 (cobalamin concentrate) 125 mcg • Niacinamide 125 mg • Folic Acid 400 mcg • Pantothenic Acid (D-calcium pantothenate) 125 mg • D-Biotin 125 mcg • Choline Bitartrate 125 mg • Inositol 125 mg • PABA 125 mg. In a base of Alfalfa, Watercress, Parsley, and Rice Concentrate.

Mega Cal - Calcium and Magnesium with Zinc **-** Jamieson
Each tablet contains: Elemental Calcium 333 mg • Elemental Magnesium 167 mg • Elemental Zinc Gluconate 20 mg.

Mega Cal - Calcium with Vitamin D **-** Jamieson
Each caplet contains: Elemental Calcium 650 mg • Vitamin D 200 IU.

Mega Cal - Calcium/Magnesium with Vitamin D **-** Jamieson
Each caplet contains: Elemental Calcium 333 mg • Elemental Magnesium 167 mg • Vitamin D 133 IU.

Mega Cal - Chewable Calcium 350 mg **-** Jamieson
Each tablet contains: Elemental Calcium 350 mg.

Mega Cal Calcium **-** Jamieson
Each tablet contains: Elemental Calcium 650 mg.

Mega Cal Calcium - Chewy Swiss Chocolate **-** Jamieson
Each square contains: Elemental Calcium 650 mg • Vitamin D (as Vitamin D3) Cholecalciferol 200 IU.

Mega Cal Calcium and Magnesium **-** Jamieson
Each caplet contains: Elemental Calcium (from microbound formula of carbonate and Krebs cycle sources of Citrate, Fumarate, Malate, Succinate, and Glutamate) 333 mg • Elemental Magnesium (from Oxide and Krebs cycle sources of Citrate, Fumarate, Malate, Succinate, and Glutamate) 167 mg.

Mega Cal Calcium Citrate with Vitamin D **-** Jamieson
Each caplet contains: Elemental Calcium (from Calcium Citrate) 250 mg • Vitamin D (as Vitamin D3 Cholecalciferol) 50 IU.

Mega C-B-R **-** Source Naturals
Each tablet contains: Vitamin C (as ascorbic acid) 1000 mg • Calcium (from citrus bioflavonoid complex) 125 mg • Citrus Bioflavonoid Complex 500 mg • Rutin 52 mg • Hesperidin Complex 50 mg • Acerola 10 mg.

Mega C-Complex 1000 **-** The Vitamin Shoppe
Each tablet contains: Vitamin C (fortified with rose hips) 1000 mg • Citrus Bioflavonoids 500 mg • Hesperidin Complex 50 mg • Rutin 50 mg • Acerola 10 mg.

Mega Chromic Fuel (Chromium Picolinate) 500 mcg **-** TwinLab
Each capsule contains: Trivalent Chromium (from Pure Crystalline Chromium Picolinate) 500 mcg.

Mega Chromium Picolinate **-** Source Naturals
Each tablet contains: Trivalent Chromium (from Chromax brand of yeast-free Chromium Picolinate) 300 mcg.

Mega CoQ10 **-** TwinLab
Each capsule contains: Coenzyme Q10 30 mg.

Mega CoQ10 300 mg **-** Life Extension
Each softgel contains: Coenzyme Q10 (Japanese pharmaceutical grade) 300 mg • Rice Bran oil 475 mg • Rosemary extract 3 mg. Other Ingredients: Gelatin, Glycerin, Water, Beeswax, Lecithin.

Mega Creatine Fuel **-** TwinLab
Each capsule contains: University-Tested Pure Creatine Monohydrate 1200 mg.

Mega Diet Caps **-** Puritan's Pride
Three capsules contain: Ma Huang extract (standardized for 6% Ephedra) 334 mg •Guarana extract (standardized for 22% caffeine) 910 mg • Citrimax (Garcinia Cambogia-Hydroxycitrate) 500 mg •Chromium (Picolinate) 200 mcg •L-Carnitine 100 mg •Potassium Phosphate 50 mg •Magnesium Phosphate 50 mg •Green Tea 10 mg •Citrus Bioflavonoids 10 mg •Ginger root 10 mg •Cayenne 10 mg. See Editor's Note No. 21 and No. 30.

Mega Fat Burners **-** Optimum Nutrition
Two tablets contain: Calcium (as dicalcium phosphate) 241 mg • Phosphorus (as dicalcium phosphate) 186 mg • Chromium (as chromium picolinate) 400 mcg • Garcinia rind extract (garcinia cambogia, standardized to 50% hydroxycitric acid) 500 mg • L-Carnitine (as L-carnitine tartrate) 100 mg • Choline (as choline bitartrate) 400 mg • Inositol 200 mg. Other Ingredients: Pharmaceutical Glaze, Stearic Acid, Croscarmellose Sodium, Magnesium Stearate, Silica.

Mega G **-** CCA Industries, Inc.
Each caplet contains: Grapefruit extract 75 mg • Glucomannan (konjac root) 600 mg • Gymnema Sylvestre (25% standardized) 50 mg. Other Ingredients: Microcrystalline Cellulose, Calcium Carbonate, Stearic Acid, Magnesium Stearate, Croscarmellose.

Mega Glucosamine 750 **-** Swanson
Each capsule contains: Glucosamine Sulfate (2KCI) 750 mg.

Mega Manna 500 mg **-** Nature's Life
Each capsule contains: Glucomannan (Amorphophallus konjac) 500 mg.

Mega Mind **-** Source Naturals
Four tablets contain: Vitamin B1 (Thiamin) 500 mg • Vitamin B2 (Riboflavin) 50 mg • Vitamin B3 (150 mg Niacinamide and 50 mg Niacin) 200 mg • Vitamin B5 (Pantothenic Acid) 50 mg • Vitamin B6 (Pyridoxine HCl) 50 mg • Vitamin B12 (Cyanocobalamin) 50 mcg • Folic Acid 800 mcg • Biotin 500 mcg • Vitamin C (Calcium and Zinc Ascorbates) 197 mg • Calcium (Ascorbate, Carbonate, Malate, Succinate) 100 mg • Magnesium (Malate, Succinate, Taurinate, Oxide) 200 mg • Zinc (Ascorbate) 10 mg • Manganese (Citrate) 5 mg • L-Pyroglutamic Acid 1000 mg • L-Glutamine 500 mg • DMAE (Bitartrate) 160 mg • Acetyl L-Carnitine 400 mg • N-Acetyl L-Tyrosine 300 mg • Taurine (Magnesium Taurinate) 198 mg • Ginkgo Biloba 24% with a Proanthocyanidolic value of 95 (50:1 Extract) 120 mg • Proanthodyn (from Grape Seed extract) 100 mg • GABA (Gamma Amino Butyric Acid) 100 mg • Coenzyme Q10 (Ubiquinone) 15 mg • Alpha-Lipoic Acid (Thioctic Acid) 15 mg.

Mega Mineral Plus **-** Global Health Trax
One tablespoon (16 fl oz) contains: Vitamin D (as cholecalciferol) 200 IU • Calcium (as calcium citrate, tricalcium phosphate) 600 mg • Magnesium (as magnesium citrate) 200 mg • Zinc (as zinc gluconate) 5 mg • Selenium (as selenium amino acid chelate) 25 mcg • Manganese (as manganese gluconate) 2.5 mg • Chromium (as chromium polynicotinate) 125 mcg • Molybdenum (as sodium molybdate) 62.5 mcg • Potassium (as potassium citrate) 50 mg • Boron (as boron amino acid chelate) 1 mg • Chondroitin Sulfate 37.5 mg • Glucosamine Sulfate 75 mg • Silica (from nyacol silica) 200 mg • Glucono Delta Lactone (GDL) 1000 mg • Trace Mineral Blend (from sea mineral salts) 1750 mg. Other Ingredients: Purified Water, Glycerin, Natural Orange Flavor, Natural Vanilla Flavor, Vegetable Gum, Sucralose, Potassium Sorbate, Sodium Benzoate.
See Editor's Note No. 15, page 2055.

Mega Minerals **-** Nature's Life
Four capsules contain: Boron (Citrate) 1 mg • Calcium (Carbonate, Citrate/Malate) 1000 mg • Chromium (Picolinate {US Patent #33988}, Polynicotinate) 200 mcg • Copper (Glyconate, Citrate) 1 mg • Iodine (Kelp) 25 mcg • Iron (Fumerate, Peptonate) 15 mg • Magnesium (Oxide, Citrate) 500 mg • Manganese (Citrate) 10 mg • Molybdenum (Sodium Molybdate) 20 mcg • Potassium (Citrate) 99 mg • Selenium (l-Selenomethionine) 100 mcg • Silicon Dioxide

BRAND NAMES

20 mg • Vanadium (Vanadyl Sulfate) 20 mcg • Zinc (Picolinate, Citrate) 15 mg • Vitamin D (as Vitamin D3) (Cholecalciferol) 200 IU • Betaine HCl 100 mg • Glutamic Acid 100 mg.

Mega N-R-G Thirty **-** Progressive Labs
Four tablets contain: Vitamin A (50% as beta carotene) 15000 IU • Vitamin C 600 mg • Vitamin D (as Vitamin D3) 100 IU • Vitamin E 200 IU • Thiamin (Vitamin B1) 25 mg • Riboflavin (Vitamin B2) 15 mg • Niacin (Vitamin B3) 50 mg • Niacinamide (Vitamin B3) 100 mg • Vitamin B6 25 mg • Folate (folic acid) 400 mcg • Vitamin B12 100 mcg • Biotin 300 mcg • Pantothenic Acid (as calcium pantothenate) 250 mg • Calcium (as aspartate) 120 mg • Iodine (from kelp) 150 mcg • Magnesium (as aspartate) 120 mg • Zinc Gluconate 15 mg • Selenium (as aspartate) 200 mcg • Manganese (as aspartate) 2 mg • Chromium (as aspartate) 200 mcg • Potassium (as aspartate) 9.9 mg • Choline 100 mg • Inositol 100 mg • Bioflavonoids 300 mg • PABA 100 mg • L-Methionine 75 mg • L-Lysine 75 mg.

Mega Once-A-Day **-** Progressive Labs
Each tablet supplies: Vitamin A (as palmitate and beta carotene) 25000 IU • Vitamin C 250 mg • Vitamin D 500 IU • Vitamin E 150 IU • Thiamin (Vitamin B1) 75 mg • Riboflavin (Vitamin B2) 75 mg • Niacinamide 75 mg • Vitamin B6 (pyridoxine) 75 mg • Folate (folic acid) 400 mcg • Vitamin B12 (cyanocobalamin) 75 mcg • Biotin 75 mcg • Pantothenic Acid 75 mg • Calcium (amino acid chelate) 50 mg • Iron (amino acid chelate) 10 mg • Iodine (from kelp) 225 mcg • Magnesium (amino acid chelate) 7 mg • Zinc (amino acid chelate) 15 mg • Selenium (amino acid chelate) 15 mcg • Copper (amino acid chelate) 25 mcg • Manganese (amino acid chelate) 6 mg • Silicon (amino acid chelate) 15 mg • Chromium (amino acid chelate) 10 mg • Molybdenum (amino acid chelate) 5 mcg • Potassium 10 mg • Boron (as boron gluconate) 750 mcg • Choline Bitartrate 75 mg • Inositol 75 mg • Para Amino Benzoic Acid (PABA) 75 mg • Betaine HCl 25 mg • Glutamic Acid HCl 25 mg • Rutin 25 mg • Lemon bioflavonoid complex 25 mg • Hesperidin complex 25 mg. Natural base of: Oat fiber, Alfalfa, Lecithin, Parsley, Bee Pollen, Royal Jelly, and Albumin.

Mega Pak Multiple **-** Nature's Life
Each packet of nine capsules contains: Vitamin A (Fish Liver oil) 7500 IU • Beta Carotene (equivalent to 7500 IU Vitamin A) 4.5 mg • Vitamin B1 (Thiamine HCl) 100 mg • Vitamin B2 (Riboflavin) 100 mg • Vitamin B6 (Pyridoxine HCl) 100 mg • Vitamin B12 (Cobalamin) 100 mcg • Folic Acid 400 mcg • Niacinamide 100 mg • Pantothenic Acid (d-Calcium Pantothenate) 100 mg • Choline (Bitartrate) 100 mg • Inositol 100 mg • Biotin (d-Biotin) 100 mcg • PABA (Para Aminobenzoic Acid) 100 mg • Vitamin C 1000 mg • Lemon Bioflavonoids Complex (TESTLAB) 25 mg • Rose Hips (Rosa canina)15 mg • Acerola (Malpighia glabra) 5 mg • Hesperidin Conplex (Citrus) 5 mg • Rutin (Saphora japonica) 5 mg • Vitamin E (d-Alpha Tocopherol, Beta, Delta & Gamma Tocopherols) 400 IU • Boron (Citrate) 1 mg • Calcium (Carbonate, Citrate/Malate) 1000 mg • Chromium (Picolinate, Polynicotinate) 200 mcg • Copper (Gluconate, Citrate) 1 mg • Iodine (Kelp) 25 mcg • Iron (Fumerate, Peptonate) 15 mg • Magnesium (Oxide, Citrate) 500 mg • Manganese (Citrate) 10 mg • Molybdenum (Sodium Molybdate) 20 mcg • Potassium (Citrate) 99 mg • Selenium (l-Selenomethionine) 100 mcg • Silicon Dioxide 20 mg • Vanadium (Vanadyl Sulfate) 20 mcg • Zinc (Picolinate • Citrate) 15 mg • Vitamin D (as Vitamin D3) (Cholecalciferol) 200 IU • Betaine HCl 100 mg • Glutamic Acid HCl 100 mg • Bromelain (Proteolytic Enzyme from Pineapple, activity: 225 MCU) 250 mg • Papain (Proteolytic Enzyme from Papaya, acivity 17.5 MCU) 250 mg. In a natural base of Lecithin, Rice Bran & Soy oil.

Mega Plus **-** Swanson
Each tablet contains: Vitamin A (from fish liver oil) 10,000 IU • Vitamin C USP (as ascorbic acid) 250 mg • Vitamin D (from fish liver oil) 400 IU • Vitamin E (as d-alpha tocopheryl succinate) 100 IU • Thiamin USP (as thiamin HCl; vitamin B-1) 75 mg • Riboflavin USP (vitamin B-2) 75 mg • Niacinamide 100 mg • Vitamin B-6 (as pyridoxine HCl) 75 mg • Folic Acid USP 400 mcg • Vitamin B-12 (as cyanocobalamin) 250 mcg • Biotin 150 mcg • Pantothenic Acid (as d-calcium pantothenate) 100 mg • Calcium (from bone meal) 150 mg • Iron (as ferrous fumarate) 18 mg • Phosphorus (from bone meal) 72 mg • Iodine (from kelp) 225 mcg • Magnesium (from magnesium oxide) 75 mg • Zinc (from zinc gluconate) 10 mg • Selenium (from amino acid chelate) 50 mcg • Copper (from copper gluconate) 2 mg • Manganese (from manganese carbonate sulfate) 7 mg • Chromium (from amino acid chelate) 20 mcg • Choline (as choline bitartrate) 100 mg.

Mega Potency Fat Burner **-** Optimum Nutrition
L-Carnitine • Citrimax Chromium Picolinate • Chromium Polynicotinate.

Mega Primrose **-** Source Naturals
Each softgel contains: Evening Primrose Oil 1300 mg.

Mega Soy Extract **-** Life Extension
Two capsules contain: Soybean powdered extract 270 mg (standardized to supply genistein/isoform genistin 51.6 mg, Daidzein/isoform daidzin 50 mg, Glycitein/isoform glycitin 9.4 mg). Other Ingredients: Gelatin, Water.

Mega Vim - Level 4 Potency Multivitamin **-** Jamieson
Each caplet contains: Vitamin A (from Acetate) 5000 IU • Beta Carotene 1500 IU • Vitamin D 400 IU • Vitamin C 250 mg • Vitamin E 150 IU • Vitamin B1 75 mg • Vitamin B2 75 mg • Vitamin B3 (No Flush Niacinamide) 75 mg • Vitamin B5 75 mg • Vitamin B6 75 mg • Vitamin B12 75 mg • Folic Acid 400 mcg • Biotin 75 mcg • Calcium 150 mg • Iron 4 mg • Copper 1 mg • Iodine 0.1 mg • Magnesium 75 mg • Zinc 10 mg • Vanadium 1 mcg • Molybdenum 1mcg • Lutein 300 mcg • Lycopene 300 mcg • Ginseng 10 mg • Soy Phosphotidyl Complex 5 mg • Digestive Enzyme Absorption Factors derived from: Peppermint, Bromelaine, Papain, Amylase, Lipase, Cellulose 4000 mg.

Mega Vim 75 **-** Jamieson
Each caplet contains: Vitamin A (from Acetate) 8500 IU • Beta-Carotene (Provitamin A) 1500 IU • Vitamin D 400 IU • Vitamin C (Ascorbic Acid) 250 mg • Vitamin E (from Succinate) 150 IU • Vitamin B1 (Thiamin Mononitrate) 75 mg • Vitamin B2 (Riboflavin) 75 mg • Vitamin B6 (Pyridoxine HCl) 75 mg • Vitamin B12 (Cyanocobalamin) 75 mcg • Niacinamide 75 mg • Vitamin B5 (Pantothenic Acid from Calcium D-Pantothenate) 75 mg • Biotin (D-Biotin) 75 mcg • Folic Acid 0.4 mg • Chelated Calcium, Calcium (Carbonate) 130 mg • Chelated Iron 4 mg • Chelated Copper 1 mg • Iodine (from Kelp) 0.15 mg • Chelated Magnesium, Magnesium (Oxide) 50 mg • Chelated Manganese 0.61 mg • Chelated Zinc 1.5 mg • Chelated Potassium 2 mg • Chelated Chromium 10 mcg • Chelated Selenium 10 mcg • Choline Bitartrate 75 mg • Inositol 75 mg.

Mega Vita Gel **-** Puritan's Pride
Two softgels contain: Vitamin A (as fish liver oil and 40% beta carotene) 10,000 IU • Vitamin C (as ascorbic acid and rose hips) 300 mg • Vitamin D (as fish liver oil) 400 IU • Vitamin E (as mixed tocopherols) 300 IU • Thiamin (Vitamin B1; as thiamine mononitrate) 50 mg • Riboflavin (Vitamin B2) 50 mg • Niacin (as niacinamide) 50 mg • Vitamin B6 (as pyridoxine hydrochloride) 50 mg • Folic Acid 400 mcg • Vitamin B12 (as cyanocobalamin) 50 mcg • Biotin (as d-biotin) 50 mcg • Pantothenic Acid (as d-calcium pantothenate) 50 mg • Calcium (as calcium carbonate and dicalcium phosphate) 200 mg • Iron (as ferrous fumarate) 15 mg • Phosphorus (as dicalcium phosphate) 50 mg • Iodine (as kelp) 150 mcg • Magnesium (as magnesium oxide) 50 mg • Zinc (as zinc citrate) 15 mg • Selenium (as selenium yeast) 25 mcg • Copper (as copper gluconate) 2 mg • Manganese (as manganese carbonate) 10 mg • Chromium (as chromium picolinate) 3.1 mcg • Potassium (as potassium citrate) 30 mg • Boron (as boron amino acid chelate) 1 mg • Rutin 10 mg • Citrus Bioflavonoids 30 mg • PABA 50 mg • Royal Jelly 5 mg • Choline Bitartrate 50 mg • Inositol 50 mcg • Garlic oil 135 mg • Lecithin 80 mg • Octacosanol 10 mcg • RNA 2 mg • DNA 2 mg • Coenzyme Q10 100 mcg.

Mega Vita Liquid - Puritan's Pride
Each 15ml tablespoonful contains: Vitamin A (as retinyl palmitate) 5,000 IU • Vitamin C (as ascorbic acid) 250 mg • Vitamin D (as cholecaliferol) 400 IU • Vitamin E (as d-alpha tocopherol plus mixed tocopherols) 125 IU • Thiamin (Vitamin B1) (as thiamine mononitrate) 25 mg • Riboflavin (Vitamin B2) (as Riboflavin 5'-Phosphate Sodium) 25 mg • Niacin (as niacinamide) 150 mg • Vitamin B6 (as pyridoxine hydrochloride) 50 mg • Folic Acid 400 mcg • Vitamin B12 (as cyanocobalamin) 50 mcg • Biotin (as d-biotin) 50 mcg • Pantothenic Acid (as dexpanthenol) 150 mg • PABA (para-aminobenzoic acid) 25 mg • Choline Bitartrate 200 mg • Inositol 100 mg.

Mega Vita Min for Teens - Puritan's Pride
Three tablets contain: Vitamin A (100% as beta carotene) 5, 000 IU • Vitamin C (as ascorbic acid) 350 mg • Vitamin D (as cholecalciferol) 400 IU • Vitamin E (as d-alpha tocopheryl succinate) 30 IU • Vitamin K (as phytonadione) 10 mcg • Thiamin (Vitamin B1; as thiamine mononitrate) 4.5 mg • Riboflavin (Vitamin B2) 5.1 mg • Niacin (as niacinamide) 20 mg • Vitamin B6 (as pyridoxine hydrochloride) 6 mg • Folic Acid 400 mcg • Vitamin B12 (as cyanocobalamin) 1 mcg • Biotin (as d-biotin) 45 mcg • Pantothenic Acid (as d-calcium pantothenate) 10 mg • Calcium (as dicalcium phosphate and calcium citrate) 100 mg • Iron (as ferrous fumarate) 18 mg • Phosphorus (as dicalicum phosphate) 20 mg • Iodine (as potassium iodide) 150 mcg • Magnesium (as Magnesium oxide) 50 mg • Zinc (as zinc oxide) 15 mg • Selenium (as selenium yeast) 5 mcg • Copper (as copper sulfate) 2 mg • Manganese (as manganese sulfate) 2 mg • Chromium (as GTF chromium yeast) 20 mcg • Molybdenum (as molybdenum yeast) 20 mcg • Choline (as choline bitartrate) 50 mcg • Inositol 50 mcg. Other Ingredients: Cellulose (Plant Origin), Vegetable Stearic Acid, Cellulose Coating, Croscarmellose, Silica, Guar Gum, Mannitol.

Mega Vita Min for Women - Puritan's Pride
Two tablets contain: Vitamin A (as retinyl palmitate and beta carotene) 10,000 IU • Vitamin C (as ascorbic acid and rose hips) 250 mg • Vitamin D (as cholecalciferol) 400 IU • Vitamin E (as d-alpha tocopheryl acetate) 125 IU • Thiamin (Vitamin B1) 80 mg • Riboflavin (Vitamin B2) 80 mg • Niacin 80 mg • Vitamin B6 80 mg • Folic Acid 400 mcg • Vitamin B12 80 mcg • Biotin 300 mcg • Pantothenic Acid 80 mg • Calcium (as calcium carbonate and calcium phosphate) 500 mg • Iron 15 mg • Phosphorus 225 mg • Iodine 150 mcg • Magnesium 200 mg • Zinc 15 mg • Selenium 100 mcg • Copper 2 mg • Manganese 2 mg • Chromium 100 mcg • Molybdenum 25 mcg • Chloride 10 mg • Potassium 10 mg • Boron 2 mg • Silica 2 mg • Cranberry 25 mg • Deordorized Garlic (Allium sativum) bulb 25 mg • Dong Quai (Angelica sinensis) root 25 mg • Black Cohosh (Cimicifuga racemosa) root 25 mg • Red Clover (Trifolium pratense) blossom 25 mg • Wild Yam (Discorea villosa) root 25 mg • Vitex extract (Vitex agnus castus) fruit 25 mg • Chamomile (Matricaria chamomilla) flower 25 mg • Soy isoflavones 25 mg • Ipriflavone 25 mg • Bee Pollen 25 mg • Royal Jelly 5 mg • Barley Grass 5 mg • Choline 10 mg • Inositol 10 mg • Para Aminobenzoic acid 10 mg • Rutin 25 mg • Citrus Bioflavonoids Complex 25 mg • Hesperine Complex 5 mg • Betaine Hydrochloride 25 mg • Coenzyme Q10 500 mcg • Pycnogenol (Pinus maritima) bark 500 mcg.

Mega-16 Permathene Maximum Strength - CCA Industries, Inc.
Each tablet contains: Phenylpropanolamine HCl 75 mg. Other Ingredients: Croscarmellose, D&C Yellow #10, Dicalcium Phosphate, FD&C Blue #1, FD&C Yellow #6, Lactose, Magnesium Stearate, Methylcellulose , Microcrystalline Cellulose, Stearic Acid, Titanium Dioxide.

Mega-Cal Calcium 650 mg - Jamieson
Each caplet contains: Vitamin D (as Cholecalciferol) 200 IU • Calcium (as Calcium Carbonate, Calcium Citrate, Calcium Fumarate, Calcium Malate, Calcium Succinate, Calcium Glutamate) 650 mg.

Mega-Energy - Puritan's Pride
Two tablets contain: Total Carbohydrate 1 g • Calcium 67 mg • Sodium 10 mg • Guarana extract 8:1 seed 225 mg • Kola Nut extract 8:1 seed 200 mg • Royal Jelly 65 mg • Korean Ginseng extract 15:1 root 64 mg • Gotu Kola extract 6:1 aerial parts 23 mg • Alfalfa Parsley blend (Alfalfa aerial parts, Parsley leaf) 16 mg • Barley Grass aerial parts 16 mg • Bee Pollen 16 mg • Disodium Inosinate 16 mg • Suma root 16 mg • Wheat Grass aerial parts 16 mg • Beta-Sitosterol 8.8 mg • Stigmasterol 4 mg • Campesterol 3.2 mg • Octacosanol 1 mg.

Mega-Kid Multiple - Source Naturals
Two tablets contain: Vitamin A (beta-carotene) 6000 IU • Vitamin B-1 (thiamin) 3 mg • Vitamin B-2 (riboflavin) 3 mg • Niacinamide 10 mg • Vitamin B-5 (calcium D-Pantothenate) 8 mg • Vitamin B-6 (pyridoxine HCl) 3 mg • Vitamin B-12 (cyanocobalamin) 10 mcg • Biotin 100 mcg • Folic acid 200 mcg • Vitamin C (calcium and manganese ascorbates) 200 mg • Vitamin D-3 (cholecalciferol) 400 IU • Vitamin E (natural D-alpha) 30 IU • Vitamin K (phytonadione) 20 mcg • Calcium (ascorbate) 21.28 mg • Chromium (ChromeMate yeast-free polynicotinate) 10 mcg •

MegaMind - Source Naturals
DMAE • Acetyl L-Carnitine • GABA • Pyroglutamic • Ginkgo • Lipoic • CoQ10.

MegaMuscle - Life Extension
Six tablets contain: L-Arginine 5000 mg • L-Ornithine 2500 mg • Vitamin C 200 mg • Hypothalamus Gland 10x 50 mg • Pituitary Gland 10x 50 mg • Vitamin B6 20 mg.

MegaNutrition - DreamPharm
Each tablet contains: Vitamin A 560 IU • Beta-Carotene 470 IU • Vitamin D 38 IU • Vitamin E Succinate 40 IU • Ascorbic Acid (vitamin C) 18 mg • Thiamin 5 mg • Riboflavin 4 mg • Pyridoxine 6 mg • Niacin 4 mg • Niacinamide 4 mg • Di-Calcium Phosphate 10.3 mg • Vitamin B12 6.5 mg • Folic Acid 12.5 mg • Biotin 4.8 mg • Choline 10 mg • Inositol 1.3 mg • Para-Aminobenzoic Acid 11.3 mg • Calcium 250 mg • Magnesium 60 mg • Iron 2.5 mg • Iodine 1.5 mcg • Copper 40 mcg • Zinc 3.5 mg • Chromium 4 mcg • Selenium 1.3 mcg • Potassium 15 mg • Manganese 1.5 mg • Pancreatin 25.2 mg • Pancrillipase 6.3 mg • Bromelain 3.8 mg • Ox Bile extract 12.5 mg • Glutamic Acid 10 mg • Cellulose 127 mg • Hydrogenated Vegetable oil 54 mg • Silica 21 mg • Magnesium Stearate 5 mg.
See Editor's Note No. 14.

Mega-Stress Complex - Nature's Plus
Each tablet contains: Vitamin C with Rose Hips 500 mg • Pantothenic Acid 200 mg • Niacinamide 125 mg • Inositol 100 mg • Vitamin B6 (Pyridoxine HCL) 100 mg • Calcium amino acid chelate/complex 100 mg • Vitamin B1 (Thiamine) 60 mg • Vitamin B2 (Riboflavin) 60 mg • Valerian root 50 mg • Magnesium amino acid chelate/complex 50 mg • Choline (Bitartrate) 32 mg • PABA (Para-aminobenzoic acid) 30 mg • Chamomile 25 mg • Zinc amino acid chelate/complex 25 mg • Folic Acid 400 mcg • Vitamin B12 from Cobalamin 250 mcg • Biotin 75 mcg.

MegaTropin - Urban Biologics
Each packet contains: Vitamin C 100 mg • Niacin 50 mg • Vitamin B6 8 mg • Glycoamine Acid-Glucose Complex 2197 mg • Novel Polyose Complex 2030 mg • Megatropin Amino Acid Complex 7450 mg: Glycine, L-Glutamine, L-Arginine, L-Lysine, GABA, Pyroglutamic Acid, L-Ornithine, L-Tyrosine • Mucuna Pruriens 200 mg • Colostrum 100 mg • Alpha GPC 100 mg • Milk Thistle 4:1 extract 70 mg • 5-HTP 50 mg. Other Ingredients: Natural Flavors, Sodium Bicarbonate, Potassium Bicarbonate, Beta Carotene Color.

Megavital Forte - Futurebiotics
One tablet contains: Vitamin C 60 mg • Vitamin B1 (thiamin HCl) 10 mg • Vitamin B2 (riboflavin) 10 mg • Niacinamide 25 mg • Vitamin E 15 IU • Vitamin B6 (pyridoxine Hcl) 10 mg • Folic Acid 400 mcg •

Vitamin B12 (cyanocobalamin) 50 mcg • Magnesium (oxide, gluconate) 25 mg • Zinc (gluconate) 15 mg • Biotin 201 mcg • Pantothenic Acid 20 mg • Choline Bitartrate 100 mg • Inositol 40 mg • Iodine (potassium iodide) 180 mcg • Sodium Phosphate 500 mcg • Phosphatidylcholine (55% strength) 50 mg • Papain 15 mg • Lecithin 25 mg • Selenium (yeast) 100 mcg • Chromium (polynicotinate) 25 mcg • Betaine HCl 25 mg. In a biological base containing a special blend of: Selenium Rich Yeast, Soy protein, Power Green complex (Barley grass, Chlorella, Alfalfa juice concentrate) & Para Amino Benzoic Acid (PABA).

Mega-Vita-Min - Puritan's Pride
Each tablet contains: Vitamin A (as Retinyl Palmitate) 8,000 IU • Vitamin C (as Ascorbic Acid) 250 mg • Vitamin D (as Cholecalciferol) 400 IU • Vitamin E (as d-Alpha Tocopheryl Acetate) 125 IU • Thiamin (Vitamin B-1; as Thiamine Mononitrate) 80 mg • Riboflavin (Vitamin B-2) 80 mg • Niacin (as Niacinamide) 80 mg • Vitamin B-6 (as Pyridoxine Hydrochloride) 80 mg • Folic Acid 400 mcg • Vitamin B-12 (as Cyanoccobalamin) 80 mcg • Biotin 80 mcg • Pantothenic Acid (as-d-Calcium Panothenate) 80 mg • Calcium (as Calcium Carbonate) 8 mg • Iron (as Ferrous Gluconate) 2 mg • Iodine (as Kelp) 150 mcg • Magnesium (as Magnesium Oxide) 6 mg • Zinc (as Zinc Gluconate) 1.4 mg • Selenium (as Sodium Selenate) 25 mcg • Copper (as Copper Gluconate) 0.07 mg • Manganese (as Manganese Gluconate) 0.12 mg • Chromium (as Chromium Picolinate) 25 mcg • Molybdenum (as Sodium Molybdate) 25 mcg • Potassium (as Potassium Gluconate) 1.6 mg • Boron (as Sodium Borate) 0.5 mg • Choline Bitartrate 80 mg • Inositol 80 mg • PABA 80 mg • Rutin 30 mg • Citrus Bioflavonoid Complex 25 mg • Hesperidin Complex 5 mg • Betaine Hydrochloride 25 mg • Coenzyme Q-10 500 mcg • Deodorized Garlic 1 mg • Korean Ginseng 1 mg • Pycnogenol 500 mcg.

Mega-Vita-Min Multiple - Nature's Life
Each tablet contains: Beta Carotene (Vitamin A equivalent to 5000 IU) 3 mg • Vitamin B1 (Thiamine HCl) 10 mg • Vitamin B2 (Riboflavin) 10 mg • Vitamin B6 (Pyridoxine HCl) 10 mg • Vitamin B12 (Cobalamin concentrate) 100 mcg • Niacin 10 mg • Pantothenic Acid (D-Calcium Pantothenate) 20 mg • Folic Acid 400 mcg • Choline (Bitartrate) 90 mg • Inositol 90 mg • Biotin (D-Biotin) 50 mcg • PABA (Para Aminobenzoic Acid) 20 mg • Lemon Bioflavonoids Complex (Testlab) 15mg • Vitamin C 100 mg • Vitamin E (d-Alpha Tocopherol mixed with Tocopherols) 10 IU • Boron (Full-Ranged Amino Acid Chelated) 25 mg • Calcium (Full-Ranged Amino Acid Chelated) 50 mg • Chromium (Nutrition 21 Picolinate) 50 mcg • Copper (Full-Ranged Amino Acid Chelated) 200 mcg • Iodine (Icelandic Kelp) 225 mcg • Magnesium (Full-Ranged Amino Acid Chelated) 50 mg • Manganese (Full-Ranged Amino Acid Chelated) 2 mg • Molybdenum (Proteinate) 25 mcg • Phosphorus (Full-Ranged Amino Acid Chelated & Complexed) 19 mg • Potassium (Proteinate) 15 mg • Selenium (Nutrition 21 Selenomethionine) 25 mcg • Silicon (Dioxide) 25 mcg • Vanadium (Full-Ranged Amino Acid Chelated) 25 mcg • Zinc (Nutrition 21 Picolinate) 2 mg • Betaine HCl 30 mg • Nucleic Acids (RNA & DNA from Yeast) 30 mg • CoQ10 (Co-Enzyme Ubiquione) 500 mcg, Essential Fatty Acids (Soy, Spirulina) 25 mg • Super Green Pro 96 (Soy Protein Super Food) 330 Mg. In a natural base containing: Rose Hips concentrate, Acerola, Rutin, Hesperidin, Lecithin, Milk-Free Lactobacillus Acidophilus, Alfalfa leaf, Watercress, Parsley, "72 Trace Minerals", Rice Bran, Spirulina, Barley Green, Psyllium, Apple Pectin, Oat Bran, Bromelain, Papain, Chlorella & Chlorophyll.

Mega-Vite 85 Multiple - Source Naturals
Each tablet contains: Vitamin A (palmitate 10000 IU, beta carotene 2000 IU) 12000 IU • Vitamin C (calcium, zinc and manganese ascorbates) 250 mg • Vitamin B-1 (thiamin) 85 mg • Vitamin B-2 (riboflavin) 85 mg • Niacinamide 85 mg • Vitamin B-6 (pyridoxine HCl) 85 mg • Folic acid 420 mcg • Vitamin B-12 (cyanocobalamin) 85 mcg • Biotin 85 mcg • Vitamin B-5 (calcium D-Pantothenate) 85 mg • Vitamin D-3 (cholecalciferol) 400 IU • Vitamin E (D-alpha tocopheryl) 100 IU • Calcium (ascorbate, citrate) 30 mg • Iron (fumarate) 12 mg • Iodine (from kelp) 150 mcg • Magnesium (citrate, oxide) 20 mg • Zinc (ascorbate) 15 mg • Copper (sebacate) 1 mg • Potassium (citrate) 10 mg • Manganese (ascorbate) 6 mg • Chromium (amino acid chelate) 100 mcg • Selenium (amino acid chelate) 50 mcg • Molybdenum (amino acid chelate) 100 mcg • Boron (amino acid chelate) 1 mg. Other Ingredients: PABA (para amino benzoic acid) 85 mg, Choline Bitartrate 85 mg, Inositol 85 mg, Bioflavonoid complex 25 mg, Rutin 20 mg, Hesperidin complex 5 mg.

Mega-Vites 75 - The Vitamin Shoppe
Each tablet contains: Vitamin D 400 IU • Vitamin A Activity 10000 IU • Vitamin C 250 mg • Vitamin E 150 IU • Vitamin B1 75 mg • Vitamin B2 75 mg • Vitamin B6 75 mg • Vitamin B12 75 mcg • Niacinamide 75 mg • PABA 75 mg • Pantothenic Acid 75 mg • Choline Bitartrate 75 mg • Inositol 75 mg • D-Biotin 75 mcg • Folic Acid 400 mcg • Rutin 25 mg • Citrus Bioflavonoid Complex 5 mg • Hesperidin 5 mg • Betaine Hydrochloride 25 mg • L-Glutamic Acid 25 mg • Iodine 150 mcg • Calcium 50 mg • Potassium 10 mg • Iron 10 mg • Magnesium 10 mg • Manganese 6.1 mg • Zinc 15 mg • Chromium 10 mcg • Selenium 10 mcg.

Mega-Zyme - Enzymatic Therapy
Two tablets contain: Pancreatic Enzymes 10X full strength, undiluted & uncut 325 mg: Units of Activity: Protease 96580, Amylase 98780, Lipase 24496 • Trypsin 75 mg • Papain 50 mg • Bromelain (1200 MCU) 50 mg • Amylase 10 mg • Lipase 10 mg • Lysozyme 10 mg • Chymotrypsin 2 mg. Potency levels found at time of manufacturing. In a base of other proteolytic enzymes in a special Bicarbonate Complex.
See Editor's Note No. 14.

Mela-Cal - Melaleuca
Two tablets contain: Vitamin C 30 mg • Vitamin D 400 IU • Calcium 650 mg • Phosphorous 493 mg • Magnesium 158 mg.

Melatonex - SunSource - Chattem, Inc.
Each tablet contains: Vitamin B6 (as pyridoxine hydrochloride) 10 mg • Calcium 31 mg • Iron 1 mg Melatonin 3 mg.
See Editor's Note No. 26, page 2056.

Melatonin - Basic Nutrition - GNC
Each tablet contains: Vitamin B6 (as Pyridoxine Hydrochloride) 2 mg • Melatonin 3 mg. Other Ingredients: Dicalcium Phosphate, Cellulose.
See Editor's Note No. 26, page 2056.

Melatonin - BioDynamax
Each capsule contains: Melatonin 3 mg.
See Editor's Note No. 16, page 2055.

Melatonin - Life Extension
Each capsule contains: Melatonin (pure pharmaceutical grade) 3 mg.
See Editor's Note No. 26, page 2056.

Melatonin - Metabolic Response Modifiers
Each capsule contains: Melatonin (5-methoxy-tryptamine) 3 mg.
See Editor's Note No. 16, page 2055.

Melatonin - New Hope Health Products
Each capsule contains: Melatonin (5-methoxy-tryptamine) 3 mg.
See Editor's Note No. 16, page 2055.

Melatonin - NutriCology
Each capsule contains: Melatonin 1.3 mg. Other Ingredients: Cellulose, Stearic Acid.
See Editor's Note No. 26, page 2056.

Melatonin - Olympian Labs
Each capsule contains: Melatonin 3 mg.
See Editor's Note No. 16, page 2055.

Melatonin - Optimum Nutrition
Each tablet contains: Melatonin 3 mg.
See Editor's Note No. 16, page 2055.

Some Brand Name Natural Products - What they Contain

www.NaturalDatabase.com contains MANY more listings than appear here.

Melatonin 1 mg **-** Nature's Bounty
Each tablet contains: Melatonin (as N-acetyl-5-methoxytryptamine) 1 mg. Other Ingredients: Dicalcium Phosphate, Cellulose (plant origin), Vegetable Stearic Acid, Croscarmellose, Vegetable Magnesium Stearate.
See Editor's Note No. 26, page 2056.

Melatonin 1 mg **-** PhysioLogics
Each tablet contains: Melatonin (as n-acetyl-5-methoxytryptamine) 1 mg. Other Ingredients: Dicalcium Phosphate, Cellulose (plant origin), Vegetable Stearic Acid, Croscarmellose, Vegetable Magnesium Stearate.

Melatonin 1 Sublingual **-** GNC
Each tablet contains: Melatonin 1 mg. Other Ingredients: Sorbitol, Mannitol, Natural Flavor.
See Editor's Note No. 26, page 2056.

Melatonin 3 **-** GNC
Each tablet contains: Vitamin B6 (as pyridoxine hydrochloride) 2 mg • Melatonin 3 mg. Other Ingredients: Dicalcium Phosphate, Cellulose.
See Editor's Note No. 26, page 2056.

Melatonin 3 mg **-** Nature's Bounty
Each tablet contains: Melatonin (as N-acetyl-5-methoxytryptamine) 3 mg. Other Ingredients: Dicalcium Phosphate, Cellulose (plant origin), Vegetable Magnesium Stearate, Vegetable Stearic Acid, Silica, Croscarmellose.
See Editor's Note No. 26, page 2056.

Melatonin 3 mg **-** PhysioLogics
Each tablet contains: Melatonin (as n-acetyl-5-methoxytryptamine) 3 mg. Other Ingredients: Dicalcium Phosphate, Cellulose (plant origin), Vegetable Magnesium Stearate, Vegetable Stearic Acid, Silica, Croscarmellose.

Melatonin 3 MG **-** Schiff
Each tablet contains: Vitamin B6 (as pyridoxine hydrochloride) 10 mg • Calcium (as calcium carbonate) 86 mg • Melatonin 3 mg. Other Ingredients: Cellulose, Croscarmellose Sodium, Magnesium Stearate.
See Editor's Note No. 26, page 2056.

Melatonin 3 mg **-** TwinLab
Each tablet contains: Melatonin 3 mg.
See Editor's Note No. 26, page 2056.

Melatonin 3 mg **-** Vitamin World
Each tablet contains: Melatonin (as N-acetyl-5-methoxytryptamine) 3 mg. Other Ingredients: Dicalcium Phosphate, Cellulose (plant origin), Vegetable Magnesium Stearate, Vegetable Stearic Acid, Silica, Croscarmellose.

Melatonin 3 mg (Inspired by Nature) **-** Puritan's Pride
Each tablet contains: Melatonin (as N-acetyl-5-methoxytryptamine) 3 mg. Other Ingredients: Dicalcium Phosphate, Cellulose (plant origin), Vegetable Magnesium Stearate, Vegetable Stearic Acid, Silica, Croscarmellose.

Melatonin 3 Timed Release - GNC A-Z **-** GNC
Each tablet contains: Melatonin 3 mg. Other Ingredients: Dicalcium Phosphate, Cellulose.
See Editor's Note No. 26, page 2056.

Melatonin 500 mcg **-** Nature's Way
Each lozenge contains: Melatonin 500 mcg. Other Ingredients: Magnesium Stearate, Sorbitol.
See Editor's Note No. 16, page 2055.

Melatonin Caps **-** TwinLab
Each capsule contains: Melatonin 3 mg. Other Ingredients: Potato Starch, Cellulose, Gelatin, Purified Water, Magnesium Stearate, MCT.
See Editor's Note No. 26, page 2056.

Melatonin Controlled Release 2 mg **-** TwinLab
Each tablet contains: Melatonin 2 mg.
See Editor's Note No. 26, page 2056.

Melatonin Forte **-** PhytoPharmica
Two capsules contain: Kava (Piper methysticum) root extract (standardized to contain 30% kavalactones) 210 mg • Valerian (Valeriana officinalis) root extract (standardized to contain a minimum of 0.8% valerenic acids) 150 mg • Melatonin 500 mcg.
See Editor's Note No. 21, page 2056.

Melatonin PM Complex **-** Anabolic Laboratories
Each tablet contains: Melatonin 1 mg • Vitamin B6 (pyridoxine HCl) 5 mg • Vitamin B2 (riboflavin) 3 mg • Vitamin B3 (niacinamide) 10 mg • Vitamin B12 (ion-exchange resin) 12.5 mcg • Calcium (lactate) 40 mg • Magnesium (oxide) 30 mg • Chinese Herbal Complex 195 mg: Valerian Root extract, Ziziphus Spinosa seed, Salviae Miltiorrhiza root, Succinum (Amber), Biotae Orientalis seed, Coptis Chinensis rhizome, Chamomile flower, Hops Strobile, Passion Flower, Skullcap herb. Other Ingredients: Cellulose, Stearic Acid, Magnesium Stearate, Vanillin, Vegetable Oil, Silica.
See Editor's Note No. 16, page 2055.

Melatonin Spray **-** Nature's Plus
Each spray contains: Melatonin (N-Acetyl-5-Methoxytryptamine) 1.5 mg • GABA (Gamma Aminobutyric Acid) 2500 mcg • Pyridoxal-5-Phosphate (P5P) 2500 mcg. In a proprietary liposomal complex of Essential Metabolic Factors, Purified Water, Vegetable Glycerine, Purified Lecithin, Citrus seed extract (Citrus sinensis), Vitamin E & natural Peppermint flavor.
See Editor's Note No. 16, page 2055.

Melatonin Tablets, Accurate Release, 1 mg **-** Nature's Bounty
Each tablet contains: Melatonin (n-Acetyl-5 Methoxytryptamine) 1 mg. Other Ingredients: Dicalcium Phosphate, Microcrystalline, Cellulose, Vegetable Magnesium Stearate, Croscarmellose Sodium.
See Editor's Note No. 26, page 2056.

Melatonin Tablets, Accurate Release, 200 mcg **-** Nature's Bounty
Each tablet contains: Pure Melatonin 200 mcg.
See Editor's Note No. 26, page 2056.

Melatonin Time Release - 1 mg **-** Natrol
Each tablet contains: Calcium (as Dicalcium Phosphate) 40 mg • Melatonin 1 mg. Other Ingredients: Time Release Agent (Hydrogenated Vegetable Oil), stearic acid, silica, magnesium stearate.
See Editor's Note No. 26, page 2056.

Melatonin Time Release - 3 mg **-** Natrol
Each tablet contains: Calcium (as Calcium Carbonate) 63 mg • Melatonin 3 mg. Other Ingredients: Cellulose, silica, stearic acid, cellulose gum, magnesium stearate.
See Editor's Note No. 26, page 2056.

Melatonin Ultra **-** FreeLife International
One-half teaspoon contains: Proprietary Blend 400 mg: Fructose, Dextrates, Sorbitol, Natural Orange/Lemon Flavor, Polynesian Kava root extract, German Chamomile leaf extract, European Hops extract (strobile), English Lemon Balm leaf powder, Japanese Peppermint leaf Powder, North American Scullcap (aerial parts), European Valerian root extract • Melatonin (n-acteyl-5-methoxytryptamine) 1 mg. Other Ingredients: Silicon Dioxide, Magnesium Stearate, RapidSorb (exclusive flavoring and transport system).

MeltRX 24 Ultra **-** Unknown
Two capsules contain: Vitamin B6 (as pyridoxal-5-phosphate) 5 mg • Vitamin B12 (as methylcobalamin) 25 mcg • Manganese (as manganese sulfate) 3 mg • Chromium (as chromium dinicotinate glycinate) 150 mcg • Meltpro Proprietary Blend 1499 mg: Glucomannan (from konjac root), Cocoa extract (standardized for theobromine), Green Tea leaf extract (standardized for EGCG and polyphenols), Hoodia Gordonii cactus stem 20:1 extract, Nut Grass

extract (cyperus rotundus, standardized for octopamine), 5-HTP (from griffonia simplicifolia seed), Coleus Forskolin tubers extract, Alpha-Lipoic Acid (standardized for thioctic acid), Banaba leaf extract (lagerstromia speciosa, standardized for corosolic acid), Naringin (from grapefruit rind), Vanadium (as vanadyl sulfate), Bioperine Black Pepper extract. Other Ingredients: Dicalcium Phosphate, Microcrystalline Cellulose, Croscarmellose Sodium, Stearic Acid, Magnesium Stearate, Silica, Pharmaceutical Glaze.

***Mel-Vita* - Melaleuca**
Three tablets contain: Vitamin A 10,000 IU • Vitamin C 135 mg • Vitamin D 250 IU • Vitamin E 30 IU • Vitamin K 25 mcg • Thiamin 15 mg • Riboflavin 17 mg • Niacin 75 mg • Vitamin B6 21 mg • Folate 400 mcg • Vitamin B12 15 mcg • Biotin 30 mcg • Pantothenic Acid 18 mg • Calcium 250 mg • Iron 18 mg • Phosphorous 192 mg • Iodine 150 mcg • Magnesium 240 mg • Zinc 15 mg • Selenium 200 mcg • Copper 3 mg • Manganese 5 mg • Chromium 15 mcg • Molybdenum 200 mcg • Potassium 45 mg.

***MemorAble* - Resource Wellness**
Two softgels contain: Vitamin B6 (Pyridoxine HCl) 2 mg • Vitamin B12 (Cyanocobalamin) 6 mcg • Ginkgo Biloba extract (leaves) 120 mg • Lecithin 1200 mg. Other Ingredients: Gelatin, Soybean Oil, Glycerin, Beeswax, Titanium Dioxide, FD&C Yellow No. 6, FD&C Red No. 40, FD&C Blue No. 1.

***MemorActin* - Nature's Plus**
Two capsules contain: Phosphatidylcholine 250 mg • Inositol 125 mg • Ginkgo Biloba leaf (standardized 24% Ginkgo Flavone-Glycosides, 6% Terpene Lactones) 100 mg • Vitamin C corn free 100 mg • Pantothenic Acid (Calcium Pantothenate) 50 mg • Phosphatidylserine 25 mg • Bilberry (Vaccinium myrtillus fruit) standardized 25% Anthocyanosides 10 mg • Beta Carotene pro-Vitamin A (supplying 10000 IU of Vitamin A activity) 6 mg • Coenzyme Q10 (Ubiquinone) 2.5 mg.

***Memorall* - PharmAssure**
Each softgel contains: Vitamin E 50 IU • Huperzine A 50 mcg. Other Ingredients: Soybean Oil, Gelatin, Glycerin, Caramel Color, Titanium Dioxide.

***Memorall (Preventive Nutrition)* - GNC**
Two softgels contain: Vitamin A (as beta-carotene) 2333 IU • Vitamin C (as ascorbic acid) 60 mg • Vitamin E (as D-alpha tocopheryl acetate) 30 IU • Folate, Folic Acid, Folacin 400 mcg • Vitamin B12 (as cyanocobalamin) 12 mcg • EPA (eicosapentaenoic acid, as fish body oil) 200 mg • DHA (docosahexaenoic acid, as fish body oil) 150 mg • Ginkgo Biloba leaves extract 120 mg • Phosphatidyl Serine (as soy lecithin) 25 mg • Coenzyme Q-10 10 mg • Citrus Bioflavonoids 10 mg • Huperzine A 100 mcg. Other Ingredients: Soybean Oil, Gelatin, Glycerin, Caramel Color, Titanium Dioxide.

***Memory 2000* - Natural Balance**
Two tablets contain: Niacin 40 mg • Ginkgo leaf standardized extract 120 mg • Phosphatidylserine 100 mg • DMAE 100 mg • Acetyl-L-Carnitine 20 mg • Vinpocetine 5 mg.

***Memory Formula* - Youngevity**
Ginkgo biloba leaf • Gotu Kola herb • Cayenne pepper • Siberian Ginseng • Magnesium • Lecithin • L-Glutamine • L-Tyrosine • Vitamin B6 • Vitamin B3 • Vilcabamba Mineral Essence: Potassium, Calcium, Magnesium, Zinc, Chromium, Selenium, Iron, Copper, Molybdenum, Vanadium, Iodine, Cobalt, Manganese.

***Memory Mate* - FreeLife International**
Each caplet contains: Thiamin (as thiamin hydrochloride) 3 mg • Folate (as folic acid) 200 mcg • Vitamin B12 (cyanocobalamin) 12 mcg • Pantothenic Acid (as D-calcium pantothenate) 25 mcg • Zinc (as zinc citrate) 5 mg • Brahmi leaf and stem standardized extract (bacopa monniera, 20% bacosides A & B) 100 mg • Herbal Brain Factors Proprietary Blend 150 mg: Fo-ti root, Ginger root, Gotu Kola leaf, Schizandra berry, Eleuthero root • Soy Activation Complex 50 mg: Phosphatidylcholine, Phosphatidylinositol, Phosphatidylethanolamine, Phosphatidylcephalin, Phosphatidylserine • DMAE (dimethylaminoethanol bitartrate) 75 mg • Ginkgo Biloba leaf standardized extract (27% ginkgo flavonglycosides, 7% sesquiterpene lactones) 60 mg • L-Glutamine 50 mg • Vinpocetine 5 mg • Huperzine A (from huperzia serrata whole plant) 100 mcg • UltraSoy Delivery System Soy Polysaccharides and Plant Enzymes 2500 units. Other Ingredients: Calcium Hydrogen Phosphate, Cellulose, Cellulose Gum, Vegetable Stearic Acid, Silica, Calcium Silicate, Vegetable Magnesium Stearate, Vita-Coat (vegetable resin, alpha-lipoic acid).

***Memory Power* - The Vitamin Shoppe**
Two tablets contain: Ginkgo Biloba extract standardized to contain 24% ginkgoflavonglycosides • L-Phenylalanine • L-Glutamine • RNA • Choline • Gotu Kola • Lecithin • Ginkgo Biloba leaf powder.

***Memory Support Complex* - Leiner Health Products**
Each caplet contains: Vitamin B12 (Cyanocobalamin) 6 mcg • Ginkgo Biloba extract (Ginkgo biloba) leaf 60 mg • Gotu Kola extract (Centella asiatica) leaf 10 mg • Phosphatidylserine 25 mg • Phosphatidylserine complex 83 mg. Other Ingredients: Calcium Carbonate, Maltodextrin, Cellulose, Silicon Dioxide, Polyethylene Glycol 3350, Croscarmellose Sodium, Tricalcium Phosphate, Crospovidone, Magnesium Stearate, Hydroxypropyl Methycellulose, Resin, Hydroxypropyl Cellulose, Polysorbate 80.

***Memorya* - HerbaSway**
Ginkgo Biloba • Dong Quai • Kudzu • Rehmannia • Panax Ginseng • Schisandra • Knotweed • Blackberry • HerbaSwee (Cucurbitaceae fruit).

***Men Plus Ester C* - Nutrivention**
Two tablets contain: Vitamin C 300 mg • Vitamin E 200 IU • Choline Bitartrate 150 mg • Inositol 150 mg • Niacinamide 150 mg • Pantothenic Acid 150 mg • Essential Fatty Acids 100mg • Vitamin A 1500 IU • Vitamin B6 75 mg • Vitamin B2 75 mg • Vitamin B1 75 mg • Vitamin D 1000 IU • Biotin 500 mcg • Vitamin B12 500 mcg • Folic Acid 400 mcg • Iodine (Kelp) 150 mcg • Saw Palmetto berry 200 mg • Sarsaparilla 200 mg • Bioflavonoids 150 mg.

***Men-Applause* - The Herbalist**
Dong Quai root • Black Cohosh root • Chaste Tree berry • Siberian Ginseng root • Oat seed • Wild Yam root.

***Menastil* - Claire Ellen**
Active Ingredient: Calendula Oil 1X. Inactive Ingredients: Menthyl Acetate, Beta-Pinene, Alpha-Pinene, Coriander Oil, Rosemary Oil, Pennyroyal Oil, White Camphor, Cornmint Oil, Almond Oil, Orange Oil, Mineral Oil.
See Editor's Note No. 1, page 2053.

***MenoCare* - The Himalaya Drug Company (Himalaya Heal**
Each tablet contains: Proprietary Blend 900 mg: Cinnamon (cinnamonum cassia), Haritaki (terminalia chebula), Ashwagandha (withania somnifera), Licorice (glycyrrhiza glabra), Arjuna (terminalia arjuna), Shatavari (asparagus racemosus), Asoka Tree (saraca indica), Gotu Kola (centella asiatica).

***MenoEase* - Wellness for Women**
Each capsule contains: Black Cohosh (5% triterpene glycosides calculated as 27-deoxyactein) 20 mg • Black Cohosh powder 430 mg.

***Menofem* - Vitamin Plus Company**
HGH Somatotropin • Liver • Pituitary L.A. • Estrone • Black Cohosh extract (cimicifuga racemosa) • Red Clover extract (trifolium pratense) • L-Arginine • L-Glutamine • Glycine • L-Histidine • L-Isoleucine • L-Leucine • L-Lysine • L-Methionine • L-Ornithine • L-Phenylalanine • L-Threonine • L-Tryptophan • L-Valine.

***Menoflash* - Olympian Labs**
Two capsules contain: Black Cohosh extract 100 mg. In a base of Dong Quai, Siberian Ginseng, and Passion Flower.

Menopace Tablets **-** Vitabiotics
Each tablet contains: Vitamin A (2500 IU) 750 mcg • Vitamin D (200 IU) 5 mcg • Vitamin E (natural source) 30 mg • Vitamin C 45 mg • Vitamin B1 (thiamin) 10 mg • Vitamin B2 (riboflavin) 5 mg • Vitamin B3 (niacin) 20 mg • Vitamin B6 (pyridoxine HCl) 40 mg • Folic Acid 500 mcg • Vitamin B12 (cyanocobalamin) 9 mcg • Biotin 30 mcg • Pantothenic Acid 30 mg • PABA (para-aminobenzoic acid) 25 mg • Iron 6 mg • Magnesium 100 mg • Zinc 15 mg • Iodine 225 mcg • Manganese 2 mg • Copper 1 mg • Chromium 50 mcg • Selenium 100 mcg • Soy Isoflavone extract 20 mg: Diadzein 1.1 mg, Glycetine 0.77 mg, Genistein 0.33 mg, Boron 2 mg.

Menopausal Formula **-** Nature's Herbs
Each capsule contains: Dong Quai 75 mg • Siberian Ginseng 100 mg.

Menopause **-** Nutrivention
Each tablet contains: Pantothenic Acid 50 mg • Vitamin B6 50 mg • Vitamin C 50 mg • Vitamin E 100 IU • PABA 50 mg • Calcium 50 mg • Iodine (Kelp) 150mcg • Borage GLA concentrate 150 mg • Mexican Wild Yam root 150 mg • Chaste Tree berry 150 mg • Dong Quai root 150 mg • Licorice root 100 mg • Unicorn root 100 mg • Black Cohosh root 50 mg • Passion flower 50 mg.

Menopause Balance Complex **-** Shaklee
Two capsules contain: Black Cohosh extract (Cimifuga racemosa) root (Standardized to contain 2.5% total triterpene glycosides as 27-deoxyactein) 80 mg • Soy Isoflavones 30 mg • Flaxseed extract (Linum usitatissimum) seed 333 mg • Flaxseed Oil 600 mg • Phytofem Proprietary Blend 100 mg: Dong Quai extract (Angelica sinensis) root, Red Clover extract (Trifolium pratense) herb, Licorice extract (Glycyrrhiza glabra) root. Other Ingredients: Soybean Oil, Beeswax, Soy Lecithin, Ascorbyl Palmitate, Mixed Tocopherols Concentrate, Rosemary Extract, Gelatin, Glycerin, Water, Annatto.

Menopause Formula **-** Pharmanex
Each capsule contains: Isoflavones (from soy extract) 25 mg • L-Theanine extract 70:1 (from camellia sinensis) 50 mg • Black Cohosh root powder 50 mg. Other Ingredients: Gelatin, Microcrystalline Cellulose, Stearic Acid, Silicon Dioxide.

Menopause Formula **-** Pharmanex
Each capsule contains: Isoflavones from Soy extract 25 mg • Kava Lactones (from Kava Kava root extract) 25.5 mg • Black Cohosh root powder 50 mg. Other Ingredients: Calcium Carbonate, Maltodextrin, Magnesium Stearate, Silicon Dioxide.

Menopause Formula **-** Natrol
Three capsules contain: Calcium (as calcium carbonate) 250 mg • Magnesium (as magnesium oxide) 125 mg • Soy Isoflavones 100 mg (genistein (10%) 10 mg) • Kava Kava 100 mg (kavalactones (30%) 30 mg) • Red Raspberry 100 mg • Mexican Wild Yam 50 mg • Licorice root 50 mg • Red Clover 50 mg • Horse Chestnut 50 mg • Dong Quai 50 mg • Black Cohosh root 40 mg • Damiana 30 mg • Vitex (agnus-castus) 25 mg • Gingko Biloba 24:6 25 mg • Gotu Kola 25 mg • Gamma Oryzanol 20 mg. Other Ingredients: Rice powder, Silicon Dioxide, Magnesium Stearate, Gelatin.

Menopause Formula **-** Nature's Life
Four capsules contain: Black Cohosh root extract (Cimicifuga racemosa) (standardized to provide 2.5% or 4 mg Triterpene Glycosides as 27-Deoxyactein) 160 mg • Vitamin C (Calcium Ascorbate) 1200 mg • Vitamin E (d-Alpha Tocopheryl Succinate) 200 IU • Hesperidin (plant source flavonols) 1200 mg • Women's Phyto-Estrogen Blend 100 mg: Soy bean, Wild Yam, Rice Flour, Flax seed & Amaranth.

Menopause Multiple **-** Source Naturals
Six tablets contain: SoyLife genistein-rich Soy concentrate (Yielding 62 mg of Isoflavones: Daidzein 34 mg, Glycitein 20 mg, Genistein 8 mg) • CimiPure Black Cohosh standardized extract 2.5% (Yielding 4 mg Triterpene Glycosides) (Containing 27-Deoxyactein) 160 mg • Vitex extract (Vitex Agnus-Castus) 150 mg • Dong Quai extract (Angelica sinensis) 100 mg • Licorice root extract (Glycyrrhiza glabra) 15 mg • Taurine (Magnesium taurinate) 455 mg • N-Acetyl Cysteine 100 mg • Silymarin (Milk Thistle seed extract) 60 mg • Alpha-Lipoic Acid (Thioctic Acid) 30 mg • Ginkgo Biloba 24% (50:1 Extract) 20 mg • Coenzyme Q10 (Ubiquinone) 15 mg • Vitamin A (Beta Carotene) 13000 IU • Vitamin A (Palmitate) 7000 IU • Vitamin B1 (Thiamin) 50 mg • Vitamin B2 (Riboflavin) 50 mg • Niacinamide 50 mg • Vitamin B5 (Calcium D-Pantothenate) 70 mg • Vitamin B6 (Pyridoxine HCl) 50 mg • Vitamin B12 (Cyanocobalamin) 50 mcg • Biotin 200 mcg • Folic Acid 600 mcg • Vitamin C (Ascorbic Acid, Calcium and Magnesium Ascorbates) 1000 mg • Vitamin D (as Vitamin D3) (Cholecalciferol) 400 IU • Vitamin E (D-Alpha Tocopheryl) (Natural) 400 IU • Boron (Chelate) 3 mg • Calcium (Carbonate, Citrate and Ascorbate) 300 mg • Chromium (ChromeMate Polynicotinate 100 mcg and Chromium Picolinate 100 mcg) 200 mcg • Magnesium (Oxide, Taurinate, Malate, and Ascorbate) 400 mg • Manganese (Citrate) 2 mg • Selenium (L-Selenomethionine) 200 mcg • Zinc (OptiZinc Monomethionine) 12 mg.

Menopause Nutritional System 1 **-** Schiff
Four caplets contain: Vitamin A (as 50% Acetate & 50% Beta Carotene) 5000 IU • Vitamin C (as Ascorbic Acid) 500 mg • Vitamin D (as Cholecalciferol) 200 IU • Vitamin E (as d-Alpha Tocopheryl Succinate) 400 IU • Thiamin (as Thiamin Hydrochloride) 25 mg • Riboflavin 25 mg • Niacin (Niacinamide) 25 mg • Vitamin B6 (as Pyridoxine Hydrochloride) 15 mg • Folate (as Folic Acid) • Vitamin B12 (as Cyanocobolamin) 25 mcg • Biotin 100 mcg • Pantothenic Acid (as d-Calcium Pantothenate) 25 mg • Calcium (as Citrate) 500 mg • Iron (as Ferrous Fumerate) 7.5 mg • Iodine (from Kelp) 75 mcg • Magnesium (as Oxide) 250 mg • Zinc (as Gluconate) 7.5 mg • Selenium (as L-Selenomethionine) 12.5 mg • Copper (as Gluconate) 1 mg • Manganese (as Gluconate) 5 mg • Chromium (as Polynicotinate) 50 mcg. Potassium (as Gluconate) 50 mg • Choline (as Bitartrate) 25 mg • Inositol 25 mg • PABA (Para AminoBenzioc Acid) 25 mg • Boron (as Amino Acid Chelate) 1.5 mg • Bromelain 50 mg • Papain 32.5 mg • Bioflavonoids (from citrus) 400 mg • Rutin 100 mg. Other Ingredients: Cellulose, Maltodextrin, Stearic Acid, Sillica, Magnesium Sterate, Plyethylene Glycol.

Menopause Nutritional System 2 **-** Schiff
Four caplets contain: Fennel (Foeniculum vulgare) fruit 100 mg • Black Cohosh (Cimicifuga racemosa) root 100 mg • Anise (Pimpinella anisum) seed 100 mg • Blessed Thistle (Cnicus benedictus) whole herb 100 mg.

Menopause Support Formula **-** Body Language Vitamin Co.
Each capsule contains: Black Cohosh extract (Cimicifuga racemosa root, standardized to contain 2.5% triterpine glycosides) 200 mg • Dong Quai (Angelica sinensis root) 150 mg • Red Clover extract (Trifolium pratense flower) 75 mg • Novasoy Phytoestrogen extract (yields 32.5 mg soy isoflavones, genistein and dadzein) 70 mg • Wild Yam 50 mg • Chasteree berry (Vitex agnus-cactus fruit) 50 mg • Hops 50 mg • Fenugreek 50 mg • Damiana (Turnera diffusa leaves) 25 mg. Other Ingredients: Vegetable Cellulose Capsule, Rice Powder, Magnesium Stearate.

Menophase **-** Futurebiotics
Complex of 4:1 extracts & powders (equivalent to 1700 mg of raw herbs) 450 mg containing: Foti, Peony Root, Withania Somnifera, Dong Quai, Chinese Sage & Carlina Ancalis • Pantothenic Acid (Vitamin B5) 75 mg • Ribonucleic Acid (RNA) 40 mg • Pyridoxine (Vitamin B6) 15 mg • Zinc (from gluconate) 7.5 mg.

MenoPro **-** HealthMinded
Two capsules contain: Vitamin E 30 IU • Vitamin B6 10 mg • Folic Acid (100%) 400 mcg • Vitamin B12 25 mg • Calcium 500 mg • Magnesium 50 mg • Chromium 200 mcg • MenoPro Propreitary Blend 344.5 mg: Shen Min (he shou wu standardized extract 10%), Wild Yam root, Isoflavones (genestein0rich phytonutrients from soy), Dong Quai extract, Black Cohosh root, Chasteberry standardized extract, Boron Amino Acid Chelate. Other Ingredients: Stearic Acid, Magnesium Stearate.

Menopryn **-** Rx Vitamins
Black Cohosh (standardized) 50 mg • Isoflavone complex.

Menosan **-** The Himalaya Drug Company (Himalaya Heal
Each tablet contains: Ashoka (saraca indica) 130 mg • Shatavari (asparagus racemosus) 110 mg • Kukkutandatvak Bhasma (hen's egg shell calx) 125 mg • Zahar Mohra Bhasma (calx serpentine, magnesium silicate) 125 mg • Haritaki (terminalia chebula) 110 mg • Bala (sida cordifolia) 105 mg • Yashtimadhu (glycyrrhiza glabra) 100 mg • Mandukaparni (centella asiatica) 50 mg • Vasaka (adhatoda vasica) 30 mg • Amalaki (emblica officinalis) 130 mg • Durva (cynodon dactylon) 30 mg • Nagkesara (mesua ferrea) 60 mg • Lajjalu (mimosa pudica) 30 mg • Lodhra (symplocos racemosa) 65 mg • Chandana (santalum album) 65 mg • Anantamul (hemidesmus indicus) 65 mg • Praval Pishti (processed coral) 130 mg • Sourashtri Bhasma (alum) 30 mg • Trinakantamani Pishti 30 mg.
See Editor's Note No. 39, page 2058.

Menovin **-** Biotech Corp.
Two tablets contain: Natural Vitamin E (dl-alpha tocopherol succinate) 30 IU • Vitamin B6 (pyridoxine HCl) 10 mg • Vitamin B12 (cyanocobalamin) 25 mg • Folate (as folic acid) 400 mg • Calcium (as calcium carbonate, dicalcium phosphate) 500 mg • Magnesium (as magnesium oxide, stearate) 50 mg • Chromium (as patented dinicotinate glycinate) 200 mcg • Shen Min (he shou wu, 12:1 standardized extract to 10% chrysophanics, 1.8% anthraquiones) 100 mg • Isoflavones (genestein-rich phytonutrients from soy (glycine max) and kudzu (peuraria)) 50 mg • Black Cohosh root (cimicifuga racemosa, 4:1 standardized extract) 40 mg • Chasteberry (vitex agnus castus, standardized to 5% vitexin) 75 mg • Dong Quai root (angelica sinensis, 4:1 extract) 50 mg • Kava Kava root (piper methysticum, 30% kavalactones) 100 mg • Wild yam root (discorea villosa) 65 mg • Boron (as boron chelates) 2 mg. Other Ingredients: Microcrystalline Cellulose, Croscarmellose Sodium, Stearic Acid, Silica, Magnesium Stearate, Pharmaceutical Glaze.

Men's AM Multi **-** Clinician's Choice
Two tablets contain: Vitamin A (retinyl acetate & 26% as beta-carotene) 3900 IU • Vitamin C (ascorbic acid) 250 mg • Vitamin D (cholecalciferol) 400 IU • Vitamin E (dl-alpha tocopheryl acetate) 150 IU • Thiamin (mononitrate) 1 mg • Riboflavin 1 mg • Niacin (niacinamide) 10 mg • Vitamin B6 (pyridoxine hydrochloride) 1 mg • Folate (folic acid) 200 mcg • Vitamin B12 (cyanocobalamin) 4 mcg • Biotin 210 mcg • Pantothenic Acid (d-calcium pantothenate) 5 mg • Iodine (potassium iodide) 76 mcg • Calcium (amino acid chelate) 4 mg • Magnesium (oxide, amnio acid chelate) 9 mg • Potassium (chloride, amino acid chelate) 12 mg • Zinc (amino acid chelate, gluconate) 2 mg • Selenium (selenomethionine) 100 mcg • Copper (amino acid chelate) 1 mg • Manganese (amino acid chelate) 3 mg • Chromium (nicotinate, amino acid chelate, chelavite, picolinate) 40 mcg • Molybdenum (amino acid chelate) 4 mcg • RoseOx (patented, standardized process for an extract of Rosemary) 50 mg • Citrus Bioflavonoid Complex 10 mg • Saw Palmetto Berries 10 mg • Whole Oats 10 mg • Panax Ginseng Extract 4 mg • Proprietary Blend 12 mg: Gingko Biloba Leaf, Echinacea Angustifolia, Panax Ginseng Root, Bee Pollen, Cruciferex, Grape Powder.

Men's Formula **-** Rexall - Sundown
Two capsules contain: Vitamin A (100% as beta-carotene, 20% of which is from Dunaliella salina algae) 5000 IU • Vitamin D (as cholecalciferol) 40 IU • Vitamin E (as dl-alpha-tocopheryl acetate and d-alpha-tocopheryl succinate) 60 IU • Niacin (as niacinamide) 10 mg • Vitamin B-6 (as pyridoxine HCl and pyridoxal 5-phosphate) 2 mg • Folic Acid 200 mcg • Vitamin B-12 (as cyanocobalamin) 12 mcg • Biotin 50 mcg • Pantothenic Acid (as calcium d-pantothenate) 20 mg • Calcium (as calcium carbonate, calcium malate, calcium citrate, and hydroxyapatite) 100 mg • Magnesium (as magnesium oxide, magnesium citrate and magnesium chelate) 150 mg • Zinc (as zinc chelate, zinc gluconate and zinc citrate) 7.5 mg • Selenium (as L-selenomethionine and sodium selenate) 50 mcg • Copper (as copper chelate, copper citrate, and copper aspartate) 1 mg • Manganese (as manganese chelate and manganese aspartate) 1 mg • Chromium (as chromium chelate, chromium glutathionate and chromium nicotinate) 100 mcg • Molybdenum (as molybdenum aspartate and molybdenum chelate) 25 mcg • Potassium (as potassium chloride, potassium aspartate and potassium citrate) 50 mg • Saw Palmetto fruit 200 mg • Dry Fish Oil (omega-3 fatty acids) 50 mg • L-Arginine 50 mg • Bromelain 25 mg • L-Carnitine 25 mg • L-Glutamine 25 mg • Papain 25 mg • Taurine 25 mg • Coenzyme Q-10 2.5 mg • Glutathione 2.5 mg • Vanadium (as vanadium aspartate and vanadium chelate) 10 mcg • Men's Formula Blend: Nettle aerial parts, Oats, Pumpkin Seed (curcubita pepo), Tomato, Alfalfa Juice Concentrate aerial parts, Spirulina pacifica blue-green algae, Grape Seed extract, Lycopene, Alpha-Lipoic Acid, Lutein 205 mg. Other Ingredients: Gelatin, Maltodextrin, Magnesium Stearate.

Men's Formula 800+ Prostate Support **-** Nature's Life
Two capsules contain: Saw Palmetto berry extract (Serenoa repens B. standardized to 85% Liposterolic Acids equivalent to 1600 mg whole herb) 160 mg • Stinging Nettle plant (Urtica dioica L.) 150 mg • Pygeum africanum H. bark extract (concentrated 130:1; equivalent to 6500 mg whole herb) 50 mg • Beta Sitosterol (Soy oil) 10 mg • Zinc (Gluconate, Citrate, Picolinate) 15 mg • Copper (Gluconate, Citrate) 1 mg • Flax seed oil (Linum usitatissimum L.) 235 mg • (Omegaflo Process Certified Organically Grown) Providing naturally occuring Omega 3 Essential Fatty Acid: Alpha Linolenic Acid 133 mg.

Men's Formula Plus **-** Swanson
Two softgels contain: Zinc (from zinc gluconate) 15 mg • Saw Palmetto extract (85% free fatty acids) 320 mg • Pumpkin Seed oil 80 mg • Lycopene (tomato) 10 mg.

Men's Longevity Essentials Plus **-** EcoNugenics
Six capsules contain: Vitamin A (as beta-carotene, palmitate) 15,000 IU • Vitamin C (as ascorbic acid, calcium ascorbate, magnesium ascorbate) 1000 mg • Vitamin D (as cholecalciferol) 400 IU • Vitamin E (as alpha tocopherol succinate) 400 IU • Vitamin K 80 mcg • Vitamin B1 (as thiamine hydrochloride) 5 mg • Vitamin B2 (as riboflavin-5-phosphate) 10 mg • Vitamin B3 (as niacin, niacinamide) 50 mg • Vitamin B6 (as pyridoxine hydrochloride, pyridoxal-5-phosphate) 22 mg • Folic Acid 800 mcg • Vitamin B12 (as cyanoco-balamin) 50 mcg • Biotin 300 mcg • Vitamin B5 (as calcium pantothenate) 30 mg • Calcium (as citrate, aspartate) 100 mg • Iodine (as potassium iodide) 150 mcg • Magnesium (as oxide, citrate, aspartate) 200 mg • OptiZinc Zinc 15 mg • Selenium (as selenomethionine) 100 mcg • Copper (as sebacate) 2 mg • Manganese (as sulfate) 3 mg • ChromeMate Chromium 120 mcg • Molybdenum (as sodium molybdate) 75 mcg • Potassium (as citrate, aspartate) 30 mg • Men's Longevity Supernutrient Blend 221 mg: Inositol, Taurine, PABA (para-aminobenzoic acid), Phosphatidylcholine, Choline, Acetyl-l-Carnitine, Ginkgo leaf extract, DMAE (2-dimethylaminoethanol bitartrate), Bilberry berry extract, Boron • Men's Longevity Liver Health Blend 170 mg Glycine, Broccoli extract • Garlic bulb concentrate, Milk Thistle seed extract, Turmeric extract, Oregon Grape root • Men's Longevity Antioxidant Blend 145 mg: Alpha-Lipoic Acid, Hesperidin complex, Citrus Bioflavonoid complex, Quercetin, Grape Seed extract, L-Glutathione, Lutein • Men's Longevity Prostate Health Blend 625 mg: Saw Palmetto berry extract, Oat spiklet extract, Korean Ginseng root, Pygeum bark extract, Stinging Nettle herb, Damiana leaf, Pumpkin seed, Lycopene.

Men's Longevity ProstaCare PC **-** EcoNugenics
Six capsules contain: Vitamin C (as ascorbic acid, calcium ascorbate, magnesium ascorbate) 250 mg • Vitamin D (D3, as cholecalciferol) 600 IU • Vitamin E (as D-alpha tocopherol succinate) 400 IU • Zinc (as orotate, methionine) 40 mg • Selenium (as selenomethionine, sodium selenate) 200 mcg • Turmeric rhizome extract (curcuma longa, 95% curcumin) 500 mg • Saw Palmetto berry (serenoa repens, 45%-50% fatty acids, sterols) 360 mg • Stinging Nettle root extract (urtica dioica) 300 mg • Royal Jelly concentrate 250 mg • PectaSol Modified Citrus Pectin 250 mg • Broccoli extract (brassica oleoracea, 22:1) 200 mg • Garlic bulb concentrate (allium sativum) 150 mg • Alpha-Lipoic Acid 150 mg • Calcium D-Glucarate 150 mg •

Quercetin 100 mg • Pumpkin seed extract (curcurbita pepo) 100 mg • Pygeum bark extract (13% sterols) 100 mg • Mushrooms 250 mg: Reishi, Coriolus, Polyporus • L-Glutathione 100 mg • Indole-3-Carbinol 75 mg • Citrus Bioflavonoid complex 50 mg • Green Tea leaf extract (camellia sinensis) 50 mg • Lycopene 30 mg • Lutein 20 mg • Men's Longevity Prostate Protection Blend 330 mg: Heal-All spiklets, Codonopsis root, Smilax Glabra rhizome, Oldelandia Diffusa herb, Job's Tears seed, Eleuthero root • Men's Longevity Prostate Blend 160 mg: Licorice root extract, Laminaria Japonica herb, Sargassum Fusiforme herb • Men's Longevity Liver Care Blend 115 mg: Taraxaci Mongolici herb/root, Baikal Skullcap root, Mum flower, Chinese Thoroughwax root. Other Ingredients: Gelatin, Dicalcium Phosphate, Silica, Magnesium Stearate.

Men's Mood-Enhancer - HerbaSway
St. John's Wort • Ginkgo biloba • He Sho Wu • Horny Goat Weed • Schisandra • Knotweed • Astragalus • Lycium • Skullcap • Blackberry • Bupleurum • HerbaSwee (Cucurbitaceae fruit).

Men's PM Multi - Clinician's Choice
Two tablets contain: Vitamin A (retinyl acetate & 20% as beta-carotene) 1250 IU • Vitamin C (ascorbic acid) 450 mg • Vitamin D (cholecalciferol) 60 IU • Vitamin E (dl-alpha tocopheryl acetate) 150 IU • Thiamin (mononitrate) 0.5 mg • Riboflavin 0.7 mg • Niacin (niacinamide) 10 mg • Vitamin B6 (pyridoxine hydrochloride) 1 mg • Folate (folic acid) 200 mcg • Vitamin B12 (cyanocobalamin) 2 mcg • Biotin 90 mcg • Pantothenic Acid (d-calcium pantothenate) 5 mg • Calcium (carbonate, amino acid chelate) 84 mg • Iodine (potassium iodide) 74 mcg • Magnesium (oxide, amino acid chelate) 20 mg • Potassium (chloride, amino acid chelate) 16 mg • Zinc (oxide, amino acid chelate, gluconate) 32 mg • Selenium (selenomethionine) 100 mcg • Copper (amino acid chelate) 1 mg • Manganese (amino acid chelate) 1 mg • Chromium (nicotinate, picolinate, chelavite, amino acid chelate) 10 mcg • Molybdenum (amino acid chelate) 2 mcg • RoseOx (patented, standardized process for an extract of Rosemary) 50 mg • Citrus Bioflavonoid Complex 10 mg • Chamomile Flowers 10 mg • Passion Flower 10 mg • Valerian Root 10 mg • Mint Leaves 10 mg • Saw Palmetto Berries 10 mg • Whole Oats 10 mg • Hesperidin Complex 4 mg • Proprietary Blend 8 mg: Reishi Mushroom, Shiitake Mushroom, Cruciferex, Grape Powder.

Men's Potency Support - NAI - Natural Alternatives International
Four capsules contain: Maca root (lepidium meyenii) 900 mg • Tribulus Terrestris whole plant 500 mg • Cordyceps mycelia (cordyceps sinensis) 200 mg • Asian Ginseng root (Panax ginseng) 250 mg • Epimedium (epimedium sagittatum) 50 mg • Muira Puama bark (ptychopetalus olacoides) 200 mg.

Men's Prime Multi - Swanson
Each tablet contains: Vitamin A (as beta-carotene) 3000 IU • Vitamin C (as ascorbic acid) 100 mg • Vitamin D (as cholecalciferol) 50 IU • Vitamin E (as d-alpha tocopheryl succinate) 60 IU • Thiamin (as thiamin HCl; vitamin B-1) 5 mg • Riboflavin (vitamin B-2) 5 mg • Vitamin B-6 (as pyridoxine HCl) 5 mg • Folic Acid 200 mcg • Vitamin B-12 (as cyanocobalamin) 5 mcg • Biotin 5 mcg • Pantothenic Acid (as d-calcium pantothenate) 5 mg • Iron (from Albion® amino acid chelate) 5 mg • Iodine (from kelp) 50 mcg • Magnesium (from magnesium oxide) 50 mg • Zinc (from Albion® amino acid chelate) 15 mg • Selenium (from Albion® amino acid chelate) 100 mcg • Chromium (from Albion® amino acid chelate) 25 mcg • Green Tea powder 50 mg • Pygeum powder 50 mg • Saw Palmetto Extract (5% fatty acids) 50 mg • Rutin 25 mg • Muira Puama 20 mg • Tribulus Terrestris (20% saponins) 20 mg • Yohimbe powder (4:1) 20 mg • Korean Ginseng powder (5% ginsenosides) 15 mg • Nettle Concentrate (4:1) 15 mg • Pumpkin Seed powder 15 mg • Inositol 10 mg, Bilberry powder (25% anthocyanidins) 5 mg • Choline (as choline bitartrate) 5 mg • Ginkgo Biloba leaf extract (24% flavone glycosides, 6% terpene lactones) 5 mg • PABA (para-aminobenzoic acid) 5 mg • Coenzyme Q10 2 mg • Lycopene Complex 100 mcg.

Men's Support - Rainbow Light
Each tablet provides: Sarsaparilla root 50 mg • Wild Oat green tops 100 mg • Damiana oxide 100 mg • Kava Kava rhizome 75 mg • Saw Palmetto fruit 50 mg • Pumpkin seed 25 mg • Ginseng 25 mg • Selenium 25 mg • Wood Betony 50 mg • Blue Vervain 50 mg • Ginger rhizome 100 mg • Vitamin A 1000 IU • Vitamin E 25 IU • Zinc 5 mg.

Men's Virility Power - Now
Two capsules contain: Epimedium extract 375 mg • Muira Puama 100 mg • Maca 100 mg • Tribulus extract 75 mg • Panax Ginseng 50 mg • Damiana 50 mg • Ginkgo Biloba 30 mg • Cayenne 25 mg. Other Ingredients: Cellulose, Stearic Acid, Silica, Magnesium Stearate.

MenstraCalm - Jarrow Formulas
Four capsules contain: Vitamin C (calcium acsorbate) 100 mg • Vitamin D 100 IU • Vitamin E (natural d-alpha- tocopheryl succinate) 100 IU • Vitamin B6 (pyridoxine HCl) 25 mg • Folic Acid 200 mcg • Calcium (as calcium citrate) 132 mg • Magnesium (as magnesium oxide) 60 mg • Potassium (as potassium chloride) 99 mg • Dong Quai Root Extract 5:1 (Angelicae sinensis) 500 mg • Xiang Fu Tuber Extract 5:1 (Cyperus rotundus) 500 mg • Shu Di Huang 5:1 (Rehmannia glutinosa) 400 mg • Lindera 5:1 (Lindera strychnifolin) 200 mg • Chaste Tree Fruit Extract 5:1 (vitex agnus-castus) 300 mg • Dandelion Root (Taraxacum officinale) 200 mg.

Menstrual Health Formula - Chinac - Metabolife International, Inc.
Each caplet contains: Lindera Aggregata (lindera) • Leonurus Japonicus (Chinese motherwort) • Angelica Sinensis (dong quai) • Cyperus Rotundus (cyperus) • Corydalis Yanhusuo (corydalis).

Menstru-Care - Natrol
Two tablets contain: Vitamin B12 (as cobalamin) 75 mcg • Folic Acid 100 mcg • Calcium (as calcium carbonate) 299 mg • Iron (as iron glycinate) 30 mg • Chasteberry 75 mg • CrampBark 4:1 (Viburnum opulus) 75 mg • Dong Quai 75 mg, Ferulic Acid (1%) 750 mcg • Uva Ursi 50 mg • Kava Kava 50 mg, Kavalactones (30%) 15 mg • Squaw Vine 50 mg • Black Cohosh 20 mg, Triterpenes (2.5%) 0.5 mg. Other Ingredients: Mono & Di-Glycerides, Stearic Acid, Croscarmellose Sodium, Silicon Dioxide, Magnesium Stearate.

Mental Acuity Formula - PhytoPharmica
Two capsules contain: Alpha Lipoic Acid 600 mg • Bacopa aerial part extract (bacopa monnieri, standardized to contain 20% bacosides) 300 mg • Folic Acid 800 mcg • Ginkgo leaf extract (ginkgo biloba, standardized to contain 24% ginkgoflavonglycosides, 6% terpene lactones, and 2% bilobalide) • Vitamin B12 (as cyanocobalamin) 500 mcg • Vitamin B6 (as pyridoxine HCl) 15 mg. Other Ingredients: Gelatin, Modified Cellulose Gum, Magnesium Stearate, Silicon Dioxide, Titanium Dioxide Color.

Mental Advantage + Ginkgo - PhytoPharmica
Each chewable tablet contains: Plumbum metallicum 8x • Ambra grisea 5x • Kali phosphoricum 5x • Ginkgo 1x • Magnesia muriatica 1x • Magnesia phosphorica 1x.
See Editor's Note No. 1, page 2053.

Mental Clarity - Sundown
Two capsules contain: Ginkgo Biloba leaf extract (standardized to 24% flavonol glycosides 9.6 mg, 6% terpene lactones 2.4 mg) 40 mg • Ginkgo Biloba leaf 400 mg • Herbal Complex Blend 280 mg: Siberian Ginseng root (eleuthero), Bilberry fruit extract (4:1). Other Ingredients: Gelatin.

Mental Edge - Source Naturals
Four tablets contain: Phosphatidyl Choline 350 mg • Choline (Bitartrate) 100 mg • DMAE (Bitartrate) 160 mg • Ginkgo Biloba leaf extract (50:1) 20 mg • Vitamin B1 (Thiamin) 50 mg • Vitamin B2 (Riboflavin) 20 mg • Vitamin B3 (80 mg Niacinamide and 40 mg Niacin) 120 mg • Vitamin B5 (Calcium D-Pantothenate) 120 mg • Vitamin B6 (Pyridoxine HCl) 25 mg • Vitamin B12 (Cyanocobalamin) 50 mcg • Folic Acid 400 mcg • Biotin 50 mcg • Inositol 30 mg

• Vitamin C (Ascorbic Acid, Zinc and Magnesium Ascorbates) 150 mg • Calcium (Citrate) 60 mg • Magnesium (Oxide, Citrate) 120 mg • Potassium (Citrate) 99 mg • Zinc (Ascorbate) 10 mg • Manganese (Ascorbate) 5 mg • L-Pyroglutamic Acid 500 mg • L-Glutamine 500 mg • L-Tyrosine 275 mg • L-Phenylalanine 125 mg • Taurine 100 mg • Herbal Formula 595 mg: Siberian Ginseng 225 mg, Gotu Kola 150 mg, Schizandra 80 mg, Ginger root 80 mg, Cayenne 60 mg.

Mental Focus - Wellzymes - Enzymes, Inc.
Two capsules contain: n-zimes Proprietary Enzyme Blend 34 mg: pHysioProtease (82,880 pHysio-U), CereCalase Plus • Proprietary Herbal Blend 400 mg: Ginkgo Biloba leaf extract (standardized to contain 24% ginkgolides), Gotu Kola herb extract (standardized to contain 10% asiaticosides), Panax Ginseng root extract (standardized to contain 8% ginsenosides), Rice Bran, Water Hyssop herb extract (standardized to contain 20% bacosides). Other Ingredients: Plant Cellulose, Water.

Mentat - The Himalaya Drug Company (Himalaya Heal
Each tablet contains: Brahmi (bacopa monnieri) 136 mg • Manduk Parani (centella asiatica) 70 mg • Ashvagandha (withania somnifera) 52 mg • Vishnukrantha (evolvulus alsinoides) 52 mg • Jatamansi (nardostachys jatamansi) 52 mg • Tagara (valeriana wallichii syn. v.jatamansi) 50 mg • Vidanga (embelia ribes) 50 mg • Vatadha (prunus amygdalus) 50 mg • Vacha (acorus calamus) 42 mg • Haritaki (terminalia chebula) 36 mg • Amalaki (emblica officinalis) 36 mg • Guduchi (tinospora cordifolia) 36 mg • Jyotishmati (celastrus paniculatus) 32 mg • Shyonaka (oroxylum indicum) 32 mg • Brahmi (bacopa monnieri) 80 mg • Kapikachchhu (mucuna pruriens) 18 mg • Ela (elattaria cardamomum) 18 mg • Arjuna (terminalia arjuna) 18 mg • Shatapuspha (foeniculum vulgare) 18 mg • Vidari (ipomoea digitata) 18 mg • Salabmisri (orchis mascula) 18 mg • Sunthi (zingiber officinale) 14 mg • Vibhitaki (terminalia belirica syn. t.bellirica) 14 mg • Jatiphalam (myristica fragrans) 14 mg • Lavanga (syzygium aromaticum) 10 mg • Mukta Pishti (processed pearl) 3 mg.

Mentat Syrup - The Himalaya Drug Company (Himalaya Heal
Each 1 tsp (5 mL) serving contains: Brahmi (bacopa monnieri) 144 mg • Manduk Parani (centella asiatica) 70 mg • Ashvagandha (withania somnifera) 52 mg • Vishnukrantha (evolvulus alsinoides) 52 mg • Jatamansi (nardostachys jatamansi) 52 mg • Tagara (valeriana wallichii syn. v.jatamansi) 50 mg • Vidanga (embelia ribes) 50 mg • Vatadha (prunus amygdalus) 50 mg • Vacha (acorus calamus) 42 mg • Haritaki (terminalia chebula) 36 mg • Amalaki (emblica officinalis) 36 mg • Guduchi (tinospora cordifolia) 36 mg • Jyotishmati (celastrus paniculatus) 32 mg • Shyonaka (oroxylum indicum) 32 mg • Kapikachchhu (mucuna pruriens) 1.8 mg • Ela (elattaria cardamomum) 1.8 mg • Arjuna (terminalia arjuna) 1.8 mg • Shatapuspha (foeniculum vulgare) 1.8 mg • Vidari (ipomoea digitata) 1.8 mg • Salabmisri (orchis mascula) 1.8 mg • Sunthi (zingiber officinale) 1.4 mg • Vibhitaki (terminalia belirica syn. t.bellirica) 1.4 mg • Jatiphalam (myristica fragrans) 1.4 mg • Lavanga (syzygium aromaticum) 1 mg.

Mentharil - PhytoPharmica
Each enteric-coated softgel capsule contains: Peppermint oil extract (mentha piperita, from leaf) 0.2 mL • Rosemary leaf and stem oil extract (rosmarinus officinalis) 0.02 mL • Thyme oil extract (thymus vulgaris, from whole plant) 0.02 mL.

Mephyton (phytonadione) Vitamin K1 - Merck & Co., Inc.
Each tablet contains: Phytonadione 5 mg. Other Ingredients: Acacia, Calcium Phosphate, Collodial Silicon Dioxide, Lactose, Magnesium Stearate, Starch, Talc.

MeraCap Coral Calcium - ccPure
Each capcule contains: Coral powder 600 mg • Calcium Citrate 5 mg • Vitamin D 400 IU. Other Ingedients: Malic Acid, Betaine HCl.

Meso Vision - PhysioLogics
Each softgel contains: Proprietary Blend 20 mg: Lutein, Meso - Zeaxanthin, Zeaxanthin. Other Ingredients: Soybean Oil, Gelatin, Glycerin, Beeswax (yellow).

Mesosilver - Purest Colloids, Inc.
Each 5 mL contains: Colloidal Silver • Deionized Water.

MESO-Tech - MuscleTech
Each packet contains: MesoPro (Whey Protein concentrate, specially filtered & new Ion-Exchanged Whey Protein) • Maltodextrin • Glutamine Blend • natural & artificial Flavors • Cellulose Gums • Vitamin & Mineral Blend • Phenylalanine • Taurine • Guar Gum • Xanthan Gum • Acesulfame Potassium • Aspartame • Carrageenan • Essential Fatty Acid Blend (EFA's): Borage oil, Lecithin, Flax seed oil. Phenylketonurics: Contains Phenylalanine.

MetaBerry - Oasis Wellness Network
Each ounce (30 mL) contains: Fruit Concentrates Blend 0.5 oz: Cranberry, Cherry, Blueberry, Grape • Active Aloe (200:1) 102 mg • Ginkgo Biloba leaf extract (24%) 20 mg • Alpha Lipoic Acid 20 mg • MaxCell Proprietary Blend 5 mg: Zisyphus Jujube, Piper Nigrum, Aloe Vera, Glycyrrhiza Glabra. Other Ingredients: Sodium Benzoate, Potassium Sorbate.

Metabo Taffy Ephedra Free Starch Neutralizer - The Natural One
Each soft chew contains: Phase-2 extract from White Kidney Bean (Phaseolus vulgaris) 500 mg. Other Ingredients: Glucose Syrup, Sucrose, Sweetened Condensed Milk (whole milk, sugar), Palm Kernel Oil, Whey, Chocolate, Mono and Diglycerides, Soya Lecithin, Natural Flavors.

Metabolean - Premier Marketing
Each caplet contains: Ginger • Magnesium • Vitamin E • Zinc • Mahuang • Astragalus • Guarana • Bee Pollen • Chromium Picolinate • Siberian Ginseng • Sarsaparilla • Goldenseal • Nettles • Gotu Kola • Lecithin • Damiana • Royal Jelly • Bladderwrack • Blue Green Algae • Licorice.
See Editor's Note No. 30, page 2056.

Metabolic Action - Puritan's Pride
Each capsule contains: Vitamin B6 (as Pyridoxine Hydrochloride) 10 mg • Vitamin B12 (as Cyanocoballamin) 6.67 mcg • Chromium (as Chromium Picolinate) 66 mcg • PABA (Para-Aminobenzoic Acid) 16.67 mg • Licorice (Glycyrrhiza glabra) root 116.67 mg • Siberian Ginseng (Eleutherococcus senticosus) root 66.67 mg • Bee Pollen 66.67 mg • L-Glutamine 33.33 mg • L-Tyrosine 33.33 mg • DMAE (as Dimethylaminoethanol Bitartrate) 33.33 mg • L-Taurine 33.33 mg • Korean Ginseng (Panax ginseng) root 33.33 mg • Suma (Pfaffia paniculata) root 33.33 mg • Schizandra (Schisandra chinensis) fruit 33.33 mg • Chlorella plant 33.33 mg • Gymnema (Gymnema Sylvestre) leaf 33.33 mg • American Ginseng (Panax quinquefolius) root 16.67 mg.

Metabolic Booster - Pentabosol
Each tablet contains: Vitamin C (as ascorbic acid) 100 mg • Niacin (from 100 mg of inositol hexanicotinate) 80 mg • Vitamin B6 (as pyridoxine HCL) 50 mg • L-Carnitine (as l-carnitine L-tartrate) 20 mg • Glycine 300 mg • Sodium Pyruvate 125 mg. Inactive Ingredients: Dicalcium Phosphate, Microcrystalline Cellulose, Croscarmellose Sodium, Stearic Acid, Magnesium Stearate, Silica, Pharmaceutical Glaze.

Metabolic Digestive Support - Zone Labs
Two capsules contain: Green Tea extract 250 mg • Bromelain (600 GDU) 600 mg • Quercetin 50 mg • M.E. Complex 3000 mcg: Papain, Lipase, Pancreatin, Ajowan extract, Fennel extract, Lactase, Multi Enzyme complex. Other Ingredients: Gelatin, Microcrystalline Cellulose, Magnesium Stearate, Silica.

Some Brand Name Natural Products - What they Contain

www.NaturalDatabase.com contains MANY more listings than appear here.

Metabolic Fat Loss **-** Olympian Labs
Two capsules contain: Chromium Picolinate 100 mcg • L-Carnitine Fumarate 150 mg • Garcinia Cambogia 500 mg • Uva Ursi 150 mg • Vitamin B6 25 mg • White Willow Bark 20 mg. In a natural base of Guarana.

Metabolic Thyrolean **-** ProLab
Each capsule contains: Phosphatidyl Choline 12.5 mg • Calcium Phosphate 125 mg • Dipotassium Phosphate 75 mg • Sodium Phosphate 37.5 mg • Disodium Phosphate 37.5 mg • Gum Guggul extract (Guggelsterone) 125 mg • Garcinia cambogia 125 mg • L-Tyrosine 125 mg.

Metabolife 356 **-** Metabolife International, Inc.
Each tablet contains: Vitamin E 6 IU • Magnesium (as magnesium chelate) 75 mg • Zinc (as zinc chelate) 5 mg • Chromium (as chromium picolinate) 75 mcg • Proprietary Blend: Guarana Concentrate seed (40 mg naturally-occurring caffeine), Ma Huang concentrate aerial part (12 mg naturally-occurring ephedrines), Bee Pollen, Ginseng root, Ginger root, Lecithin, Bovine Complex, Damiana leaf, Sarsaparilla root, Golden Seal aerial part, Nettles leaf, Gotu Kola aerial part, Spirulina Algae, Royal Jelly 728 mg. Other Ingredients: Methocel, Silica, Croscarmellose Sodium, Magnesium Stearate.
See Editor's Note No. 21 and No. 30.

Metabolife Complete **-** Metabolife International, Inc.
Pre-Breakfast & Pre-Lunch Formula: Two caplets contain: Thiamin (as thiamin mononitrate) 1.5 mg • Riboflavin 1.7 mg • Niacin (as niacinamide) 20 mg • Vitamin B6 (as pyridoxine hdyrochloride) 5 mg • Pantothenic Acid (as D-calcium pantothenate) 10 mg • Calcium (as hydroxycitrate and di-calcium phosphate) 115 mg • Chromium (as chromium polynicotinate) 113 mcg • Sodium 60 mg • Potassium 150 mg • Proprietary Blend 1770 mg: Super CitriMax brand Garcinia fruit extract (standardized for hydroxycitric acid), Guarana seed extract (standardized for caffeine). Other Ingredients: Maltodextrin, Modified Cellulose, Caffeine, Dicalcium Phosphate, Stearic Acid, Silica, Dextrin, Dextrose, Lecithin, Sodium Carboxymethylcellulose, Sodium Citrate.
Pre-Dinner Formula: Two caplets contain: Thiamin (as thiamin mononitrate) 1.5 mg • Riboflavin 1.7 mg • Niacin (as niacinamide) 20 mg • Vitamin B6 (as pyridoxine hydrochloride) 5 mg • Pantothenic Acid (as D-calcium pantothenate) 10 mg • Calcium (as hydroxycitrate) 75 mg • Chromium (as chromium polynicotinate) 133 mcg • Sodium 60 mg • Potassium 150 mg • Proprietary Blend 1556 mg: Super CitriMax brand Garcinia fruit extract (Standardized for hydroxycitric acid). Other Ingredients: Modified Cellulose, Maltodextrin, Stearic Acid, Silica, Dexrin, Titanium Dioxide, Polyehtylene Glycol, Lecithin, Dextrose, Sodium Carboxymethylcellulose, FD&C Yellow #5, FD&C Red #40, Sodium Citrate, FD&C Blue #2.

Metabolife Ephedra Free **-** Metabolife International, Inc.
Two tablets contain: Sodium 60 mg • Potassium 30 mg • Calcium 50 mg • Shromium (as chromium picolinate) 150 mcg • Proprietary Blend 1132 mg: Green Tea extract leaf (standardixed for EGCG and total catechins), Super Citrimax Garcinia Cambogia extract fruit (standardized for hydroxycitric acid), Guarana seed extract (standardized for caffeine), Yerba Mate extract leaf (standardized for caffeine). Other Ingredients: Modified Cellulose, Maltodextrin, Caffeine, Dicalcium Phosphate, Stearic Acid, Sodium Bicarbonate, Silica, Dextrin, Citric Acid, Dextrose, Lecithin, Sodium Carboxymethylcellulose, Sodium Citrate.

Metabolife Ultra **-** Metabolife International, Inc.
Two caplets contain: Thiamin (vitamin B1, as thiamin mononitrate) 1.5 mg • Riboflavin (vitamin B2) 1.7 mg • Niacin (vitamin B3, as niacinamide) 20 mg • Vitamin B6 (as pyridoxine hydrochloride) 5 mg • Pantothenic Acid (as d-calcium pantothenate) 10 mg • Calcium (as hydroxycitrate, dicalcium phosphate) 60 mg • Magnesium (as magnesium oxide) 100 mg • Potassium 80 mg • Garcinia fruit extract (standardized for hydroxycitric acid) 850 mg • Proprietary Blend 292 mg: Guarana seed extract (standardized for caffeine 54 mg), Bitter Orange fruit extract (citrus aurantium amara, standardized for synephrine 6.6 mg). Other Ingredients: Modified Cellulose, Maltodextrin, Caffeine, Dicalcium Phosphate, Stearic Acid, Dextrin, Dextrose, Lecithin, Sodium Carboxymethylcellulose, Magnesium Stearate, Sodium Citrate.
See Editor's Note No. 40, page 2058.

Metabolife Ultra Caffeine Free **-** Metabolife International, Inc.
Two caplets contain: Thiamin (vitamin B1, as thiamin mononitrate) 1.5 mg • Riboflavin (vitamin B2) 1.7 mg • Niacin (vitamin B3, as niacinamide) 20 mg • Vitamin B6 (pyridoxine hydrochloride) 5 mg • Pantothenic Acid (as d-calcium pantothenate) 10 mg • Calcium (as hydroxycitrate) 75 mg • Chromium (as chromium picolinate) 133 mcg • Potassium 150 mg. Other Ingredients: Modified Cellulose, Maltodextrin, Stearic Acid, Silica, Dextrin, Titanium Dioxide, Polyethylene Glycol, Lecithin, Dextrose, Sodium Carboxymethylcellulose, FD&C Yellow 5, FD&C Red 40, Sodium Citrate, FD&C Blue 2.

Metabolift **-** TwinLab
Two capsules contain: Ma Huang extract 334 mg • Guarana extract (standardized for 22% Caffeine) 910 mg • Chromium (from Chromic Fuel patented Chromium Picolinate) 200 mg. In a concentrated herbal base of White Willow bark extract & Cayenne.
See Editor's Note No. 30, page 2056.

Metabolift MaHuang Free Formula **-** TwinLab
Two tablets contain: Guarana seed extract (standardized for 22% caffeine) 800 mg • Citrus Aurantium extract (standardized for 6% synephrine alkaloids) 325 mg • Proprietary Blend 360 mg: St. John's Wort (9 mg, standardized for hypericin), L-Phenylalanine, Green Tea leaf extract (standardized for epigallocatechin gallate), Quercetin Dihydrate, Citrus Bioflavonoid Complex (containing naringin), Ginger root, Cayenne fruit.
See Editor's Note No. 40, page 2058.

Metab-O-Lite **-** Richardson Labs
One tablet contains: Vitamin E 6 IU • Magnesium (as Magnesium chelate) 75 mg • Zinc (as Zinc chelate) 5 mg • Chromium (as Chromium Picolinate) 75 mcg • Proprietary Blend 728 mg: Ephedra (Ma Huang) concentrate (aerial part, 12 mg naturally-occurring ephedrines) • Bee Pollen • Siberian Ginseng root • Ginger root • Lecithin • Bovine Cartilage • Damiana leaf • Sarsaparilla root • Goldenseal aerial part • Nettles leaf • Gotu Kola aerial part • Spirulina Algae • Royal Jelly. Other Ingredients: Cellulose, Croscarmellose Sodium, Hydroxypropyl Cellulose, Silica, Hydroxypropyl Methylcellulose, DL-Alpha-Tocopheryl Acetate, Magnesium Stearate, Maltodextrin, PEG.
See Editor's Note No. 30, page 2056.

Metab-O-LITE Ephedra Free **-** Rexall - Sundown
Two caplets contain: Vitamin C 50 mg • Proprietary Blend 1 g: Black Tea Extract (leaf), Caffeine (from guarana extract seed and caffeine), Rutin, Ginger Extract (root), Dill Extract 20:1 (aerial part). Other Ingredients: Dextrose, Microcrystalline Cellulose, Crospovidone, Maltose, Dextrin, Hydroxypropyl Methylcellulose, Titanium Dioxide (color), Magnesium Stearate, PEG, Riboflavin (color), Soy Lecithin, Blue 2 Lake, Yellow 6 Lake, Red 40 Lake.

Metabolol II **-** Champion Nutrition
Each serving contains: Metacarb Plus (complex carbohydrates from corn hybrids) • Peptol PER4 + protein formulation: Enzyme Modified Egg Albumin, Whey Protein Concentrate, Potassium Caseinate, Peptides from Enzyme Modified Lactalbumin, & Pharmaceutical Grade Amino Acids: L-Leucine, L-Isoleucine, L-Valine, L-Cystine, L-Phenylalanine, L-Methionine, L-Threonine, L-Lysine, L-Glutamic Acid • Polylactate • Medium Chain Triglycerides • Metavite bioactive vitamin mineral formula: Calcium Carbonate, Pyridoxine Alpha-Ketoglutarate (PAK), Choline Bitartrate, Inositol, Di-Calcium Phosphate, Calcium Lactate, Calcium Citrate, Magnesium Oxide,

Magnesium Citrate, Zinc Picolinate, Ester-C, (Esterified Calcium Polyascorbate), Potassium Phosphate, D-Alpha Tocopherol Succinate Esterified Zinc Polyascorbate, Molybdenum Aspartate, Iron Succinate, Manganese Citrate, Niacin, Calcium Pantothenate, Copper Glycinate, Chromium-Polynicotinate • Pyridoxal-5-Phosphate • Retinyl Palmitote, Riboflavin-5-Phosphate • Thiamine HCL • D-Biotin • Potassium Iodide • Ergocalciferol • Folic Acid • Cyanocobalamin • Intrinsic Factor Complex • Succinate ETF Complex: Potassium Succinate, Magnesium Succinate, Calcium Succinate, L-Glutamic Acid, Inosine, & Pyridoxine Alpha-Ketoglutarate (PAK) Inosine, Lecithin, Natural Flavors, L-Carnitine, Lipoic Acid, Selenium Aspartate.

Metaboloss **-** NFI Dietary Supplements
Ginger • Magnesium • Vitamin E • Zinc • Ma Huang • Astragalus • Bee Pollen • Chromium Picolinate • Siberian Ginseng • Sarsaparilla • Goldenseal • Nettles • Gotu Kola • Lecithin • Damiana • Royal Jelly • Bladderwrack • Blue Green Algae • Licorice.
See Editor's Note No. 30, page 2056.

MetaboMax **-** Nature's Sunshine
Each tablet contains: Chinese Ephedra (12 mg total ephedra alkaloids) • Bee Pollen • Siberian Ginseng • Ginger • Lecithin • Cordyceps • Kelp • Damiana • Sarsaparilla • Golden Seal • Nettle • Gotu Kola • Spirulina • Royal Jelly.
See Editor's Note No. 30, page 2056.

MetaBoost **-** Advocare International
Two caplets contain: Vitamin C (as potassium/magnesium/sodium ascorbates) 600 mg • Iodine (as potassium iodide) 50 mcg • Guarana extract (seed - paullinia cupana) 150 mg • Oolong Tea extract (leaf - camellia sinensis) 200 mg • Eleuthero extract (root - eleutherococcus senticosus) 50 mg. Other Ingredients: Dicalcium Phosphate, Silicon Dioxide, Cellulose, Stearic Acid, Magnesium Stearate, Vanillin.

Meta-Booster **-** Nu-Creations
Each capsule contains: Vitamin E 6 IU • Magnesium 75 mg • Zinc 5 mg • Chromium Picolinate 75 mcg • Meta-Booster Proprietary Blend 803 mg: Guarana, Ma Huang concentrate, Bee Pollen, Siberian Ginseng, Ginger, Lecithin, Bovine Complex, Damiana, Sarsaparilla, Goldenseal, Canadensis, Nettle, Gotu Kola, Spirulina, Royal Jelly. Other Ingredients: Dicalcium Phosphate, Pharmaceutical Glaze, Magnesium Stearate.
See Editor's Note No. 30, page 2056.

Metabosurge **-** Puritan's Pride
Each tablet contains: Vitamin C (as Ascorbic Acid) 20 mg • Vitamin E (as dl-Alpha Tocopheryl Acetate) 6 IU • Magnesium (as Magnesium Oxide) 75 mg • Zinc (as Zinc Oxide) 5 mg • Chromium (as Chromium Picoline) 75 mcg • Proprietary Blend: Ma Huang (Ephedra sinica) aerial (standardized for 12 mg ephedra alkaloids), Guarana extract, Citrus Aurantium, Bee Pollen, Korean Ginseng, Ginger, Lecithin, White Willow, Damiana, Sarsaparilla, Golden Seal, Nettles, Gotu Kola, Spirulina, Green Tea extract, Bladderwrack extract 750 mg.
See Editor's Note No. 21 and No. 30, page 2056.

Metabosurge Ephedra Free Formula **-** Puritan's Pride
Two tablets contain: Calcium (from hydroxycitrate and dicalcium phosphate) 50 mg • Chromium (as chromium picolinate) 150 mcg • Proprietary Blend 1132 mg: Green Tea leaf extract (camellia sinensis, standardized to contain polyphenols, EGCG, catechins), Super CitriMax Garcinia Cambogia fruit extract (standardized to contain hydroxycitric acid), Guarana bark extract (paullinia cupana, standardized to contain caffeine), Yerba Mate leaf (ilex paraguariensis, standardized to contain caffeine). Other Ingredients: Cellulose, Silica, Vegetable Stearic Acid, Acacia Gum, Vegetable Magnesium Stearate, Cellulose Coating.

Metabotrim **-** Pharmanex
Each capsule contains: Vitamin C (Calcium Ascorbate) 75 mg • Niacin (Niacinamide) 10 mg • Vitamin B6 (Pyridoxine Hydrochloride, Pycodoxal-5-Phosphate) 3 mg • Vitamin B12 (Cyanocobalamin, Dibencozide) 6 mcg • Magnesium (Magnesium Asparate, Magnesium Citrate, Magnesium Chelate) 20 mg • Chromium (Chromium Chelate, Chromium Picolinate) 100 mcg • Potassium (Potassium Asparate, Potassium Citrate) 20 mg • Carnitine (L-Carnitine L-Tartrate) 100 mg. Other Ingredients: Cellulose, Magnesium Stearate, Vanillin, Silicon Dioxide.

MetaboTrim **-** VitaStore
Each tablet contains: Vitamin E 6 IU • Magnesium (as Magnesium Chelate) 75 mg • Zinc (as Zinc Chelate) 5 mg • Chromium (as Chromium Picolinate) 75 mcg. Blended Formula 728 mg: Guarana Concentrate (seed) (40 mg Naturally-occurring caffeine), Ma Huang Concentrate (herb: aerial part) (12 mg naturally-occurring ephedrine), Bee Pollen, Ginseng (root), Lecithin (vitamin), Bovine Complex, Damiana (leaf), Sarsaparilla (root), Goldenseal (aerial part), Nettles (leaf), Gotu Kola (aerial part), Spirulina Algae, Royal Jelly. Other Ingredients: Methocel, Silica, Croscarmellose Sodium, Magnesium Stearate.
See Editor's Note No. 30, page 2056.

MetaBurn **-** Oasis Wellness Network
Each capsule contains: Calcium (from carbonate, citrate) 75 mg • Green Tea leaves extract (70% polyphenols, 25% EGCG, 5% l-theanine) 300 mg • Bitter Orange fruit extract (6% synephrine) 150 mg • BioResponse DIM Complex 50 mg: Starch, Diindolylmethane, D-Alpha-Tocopheryl Succinate, Phosphatidylcholine, Silica • MaxCell Proprietary Blend 12.5 mg: Jujube fruit extract, Black Pepper fruit extract, Aloe Vera dried gel, Chinese Licorice root. Other Ingredients: Magnesium Stearate, Silica, Gelatin.
See Editor's Note No. 40, page 2058.

Meta-Burn **-** Metabolic Response Modifiers
Two capsules contain: Garcinia cambogia (50%) HCA 500 mg • Ma Huang (8% ephedra) 225 mg • Green Tea (50% caffeine) 100 mg • Caffeine (anhydrous) 100 mg • White Willow bark (2%salicylates) 60 mg • Naringin 20 mg • L-Tyrosine 50 mg • Choline bitartrate 100 mg • Chromium (chelate 10%) 200 mcg • Vanadium (sulfate) 3 mg • Alpha Lipoic Acid 50 mg • Vitamin B5 (pantothenic acid) 50 mg • Potassium (phosphate) 74 mg • Iodine (as potassium iodide) 750 mcg • Cayenne Pepper 10 mg.
See Editor's Note No. 30, page 2056.

Meta-Burn EF **-** Metabolic Response Modifiers
Four capsules contain: Garcinia cambogia (50%) HCA 2000 mg • Citrus aurantium (6% synephrine) 350 mg • Green Tea (40% caffeine) 225 mg • Phosphate (potassium phosphate) 124 mg • White Willow bark (1% salicylates) 60 mg • Coleus Forskohlii (10% Forskolin) 50 mg • Naringin 20 mg • Alpha Lipoic Acid 25 mg • Cayenne Pepper 20 mg • Potassium (potassium phosphate) 101 mg • Iodine (Iodine USP) 750 mcg • Chromium (as chelate) 300 mcg.
See Editor's Note No. 40, page 2058.

Meta-CLA **-** E'OLA
Each capsule contains: Tonalin 500 mg • Aloe-Min E'OLA Mineral Blend 25 mg: Active Aloe, Calcium Gluconate Monohydrate.

MetaCort Spray **-** DermaBolics
Five sprays contain: Androstenetrione 100 mg • 7-OXO-DHEA 100 mg. Other Ingredients: Isopropyl Alcohol, Propylene Glycol, Octyl Salicylate, Triglyceride Complex, Water, D-Limonene.

Meta-Dream **-** Meta-Sure Health
Two caplets contain: Potassium (as potassium phosphate) 160 mg • Calcium (as calcium phosphate) 30 mg • Cellulex Blend: Borage extract seed, Bladderwrack extract, Sweet Clover extract, Grape Seed extract, Lecithin (soy), Ginkgo Biloba extract 250 mg • L-Carnitine 25 mg • L-Tyrosine 70 mg • Collagen Complex 120 mg • Valerian powder root 15 mg • Skullcap powder root 10 mg • Passion Flower powder leaf 10 mg • 5-HTP seed 750 mcg • Melatonin 250 mcg.
See Editor's Note No. 16, page 2055.

Metafolin **-** Source Naturals
Each tablet contains: Folate as Metafolin (L-methylfolate) 800 mcg. Other Ingredients: Microcrystalline Cellulose, Stearic Acid, Colloidal Silicon Dioxide.

MetaFuel - Chocolate **-** Oasis Wellness Network
Two scoops (45 g) contain: Vitamin A (as vitamin A palmitate) 2250 IU • Vitamin C (as ascorbic acid) 30 mg • Vitamin D (as cholecalciferol) 180 IU • Vitamin E (as alpha-tocopheryl acetate) 15 IU • Vitamin K (phytonadione) 5 mcg • Thiamin (as thiamin mononitrate) 1 mg • Riboflavin (USP) 1 mg • Niacin (as niacinamide) 9 mg • Vitamin B6 (as pyridoxine hydrochloride) 1 mg • Folic Acid (USP) 180 mcg • Vitamin B12 (as cyanocobalamin) 3 mcg • Biotin (USP) 120 mcg • Pantothenic Acid (as d-calcium pantothenate) 4.5 mg • Calcium 250 mg • Iron 1 mg • Phosphorus 150 mg • Iodine (as potassium iodide) 30 mcg • Magnesium (as magnesium oxide) 80 mg • Zinc (as zinc oxide) 3 mg • Selenium 32 mcg • Copper (as copper sulfate) 0.4 mg • Manganese (as manganese sulfate) 1 mg • Chromium (as chromium polynicotinate) 42 mcg • Molybdenum (as molybdenum glycinate) 19 mcg • Sodium 280 mg • Potassium 640 mg • MaxCell Proprietary Blend 25 mg: Jujube extract, Aloe Vera gel, Black Pepper extract, Chinese Licorice. Other Ingredients: Protein Blend: Whey Protein, Soy Protein Isolate • Dutch Cocoa • Fiber Blend: Cellulose, Gum Acacia, Xanthan Gum, Flax Seed Powder, Cellulose Gum, Oat Fiber • Inulin • High Oleic Safflower Oil • Natural/Artificial Flavors • Lecithin • Enzyme Blend: Protease, Lipase, Cellulase, Amylase, Bromelain, Papain • Sucralose • Stevia Extract.

MetaFuel - Vanilla **-** Oasis Wellness Network
Two scoops (45 g) contain: Vitamin A (as vitamin A palmitate) 2250 IU • Vitamin C (as ascorbic acid) 30 mg • Vitamin D (as cholecalciferol) 180 IU • Vitamin E (as alpha-tocopheryl acetate) 15 IU • Vitamin K (phytonadione) 5 mcg • Thiamin (as thiamin mononitrate) 1 mg • Riboflavin (USP) 1 mg • Niacin (as niacinamide) 9 mg • Vitamin B6 (as pyridoxine hydrochloride) 1 mg • Folic Acid (USP) 180 mcg • Vitamin B12 (as cyanocobalamin) 3 mcg • Biotin (USP) 120 mcg • Pantothenic Acid (as d-calcium pantothenate) 4.5 mg • Calcium 3000 mg • Iron 1 mg • Phosphorus 150 mg • Iodine (as potassium iodide) 30 mcg • Magnesium (as magnesium oxide) 40 mg • Zinc (as zinc oxide) 3 mg • Selenium 32 mcg • Copper (as copper sulfate) 0.4 mg • Manganese (as manganese sulfate) 1 mg • Chromium (as chromium polynicotinate) 42 mcg • Chloride (as potassium chloride) 25 mg • Molybdenum (as molybdenum glycinate) 19 mcg • Sodium 280 mg • Potassium 640 mg • MaxCell Proprietary Blend 25 mg: Jujube extract, Aloe Vera gel, Black Pepper extract, Chinese Licorice. Other Ingredients: Protein Blend: Whey Protein, Soy Protein Isolate • Fiber Blend: Cellulose, Gum Acacia, Xanthan Gum, Flax Seed Powder, Cellulose Gum, Oat Fiber • Inulin • High Oleic Safflower Oil • Natural/Artificial Flavors • Lecithin • Enzyme Blend: Protease, Lipase, Cellulase, Amylase, Bromelain, Papain • Sucralose • Stevia Extract.

MetaGlycemX **-** Metagenics
Two tablets contain: Vitamin C (as ascorbic acid) 300 mg • Vitamin E (as d-alpha-tocopheryl succinate) 200 IU • Thiamin (as thiamin mononitrate) 15 mg • Riboflavin 9 mg • Niacin (as niacinamide) 90 mg • Pantothenic Acid (as d-calcium pantothenate) 30 mg • Vitamin B6 (as pyridoxine hydrochloride) 9 mg • Vitamin B12 (as cyanocobalamin) 150 mcg • Biotin 2 mg • Folate (as folic acid) 400 mcg • Zinc (as zinc glycinate) 9 mg • Copper (as copper lysinate hydrochloride) 0.75 mg • Manganese (as manganese citrate) 1.2 mg • Chromium (as chromium polynicotinate) 600 mcg • Selenium (as selenomethionine) 90 mcg • Vanadium (as vanadyl sulfate) 0.5 mg • Alpha-Lipoic Acid 100 mg • L-Carnosine 50 mg • Taurine 300 mg • Chinese Cinnamon bark (cinnamomum cassia) 500 mg • Catechins 100 mg • Epigallocatechin Gallate (EGCG, from decaffeinated green tea leaf, camellia sinensis) 66.5 mg.

MetaGreens **-** Oasis Wellness Network
Each tablespoon (6 g) contains: Alfalfa juice (organic, 33:1) 1200 mg • Spirulina (organic) 1200 mg • Inulin 1000 mg • Rice Solubles 500 mg • Kamut (whole leaf, organic, 5:1) 416 mg • Barley (whole leaf, organic, 5:1) 416 mg • Oat (whole leaf, organic, 5:1) 416 mg • Pineapple 250 mg • Cruciferous Vegetable Blend 200 mg • L-Glutamine 100 mg • Nopal Cactus 100 mg • Eleuthero extract 100 mg • Kyo-Dophilus 40 mg • Kelp (wildcrafted) 30 mg • Dulse (wildcrafted) 30 mg • Stevia 20 mg • Aloe Vera gel (organic, 200:1) 10 mg • MaxCell Proprietary Blend 10 mg: Zisyphus Jujube, Piper Nigrum, Aloe Vera gel, Glycyrrhiza Glabra.

Meta-HGH **-** E'OLA
One scoop contains: Niacin 16 mg • Proprietary Blend 4.18 g: Glutamine, Glycine, Gum Guggul, Forskolin, E'OLA Mineral Blend.

Metal Magnet **-** PhytoPharmica
Each capsule contains: Proprietary Humifulvate Complex 75 mg: Humic Acid, Fulvic Acid, Phenolic Acid. Other Ingredients: Cellulose, Gelatin, Magnesium Stearate.

Metalogic **-** PhysioLogics
Each capsule contains: Vitamin C (Ascorbic Acid) 250 mg • Zinc 15 mg • Copper (Glycinate) 500 mcg • N-Acetyl cysteine 200 mg • L-Methionine 30 mg • Alpha-Lipoic Acid 25 mg • L-Glutathione 5 mg • Selenium (Selenomethionine) 75 mcg.

Metamucil **-** Proctor & Gamble
Each rounded teaspoon contains: Pure Psyllium Husk Fiber 3.4 g. Other Ingredients: Sucrose.

Metamucil Sugar Free **-** Proctor & Gamble
Each packet contains: Pure Psyllium husk fiber 3.4 g. Other Ingredients: Aspartame, Citric Acid, Flavoring, Maltodextrin, Yellow #6.

MetaPlex **-** Allergy Research Group
Three tablets contain: Vitamin B6 (as pyridoxal-5-phosphate and pyridoxine hydrochloride) 22.5 mg • Calcium (as calcium pyruvate and dicalcium phosphate) 68 mg • Chromium (as chromium nicotinate) 6 mcg • Chitosan 600 mg • L-Carnitine 150 mg • Arthred Hydrolyzed Collagen 450 mg • Garcinia Cambogia fruit extract (75% hydroxycitric acid) 300 mg • Pyruvate (as calcium pyruvate) 320 mg. Other Ingredients: Dicalcium Phosphate, Modified Cellulose, Stearic Acid, Magnesium Stearate, Silicon Dioxide, Ethyl Vanillin.

MetaPower **-** Oasis Wellness Network
Each softgel contains: Vitamin E 6 IU • Marine Lipid oil 1 g • EPA 300 mg • DHA 200 mg • Coenzyme Q10 3.5 mg • Maxcell Powder Proprietary Blend 8.33 mg: Jujube fruit extract, Black Pepper fruit extract, Aloe Vera gel (dried), Chinese Licorice. Other Ingredients: Gelatin, Glycerin, Beeswax, Water, Lecithin, Titanium Dioxide, Chlorophyllin, Beta-Carotene.

Meta-Sitosterol **-** Metagenics
Three tablets contain: Beta-Sitosterol 1000 mg • Campesterol 500 mg • Stigmasterol 275 mg • Other Plant Sterols 225 mg • Folate (as folic acid, L-5-methyl tetrahydrofolate, 5-formyl tetrahydrofolate) 800 mcg.

Meta-Sure Metagizer **-** Meta-Sure Health
One caplet contains: Vitamin E (as d-alpha Tocopheryl) 7 IU • Niacin 5 mg • Vitamin B6 5 mg • Folic Acid 50 mcg • Vitamin B12 10 mcg • Magnesium (as Magnesium Chelate, Magnesium Salicylate) 11 mg • Zinc (as Zinc Chelate) 3 mg • Chromium (as Chromium Aspartate, Chromium Picolinate) 75 mcg • SurePlex Blend: Guarana concentrate seed (contains 46 mg naturally occuring caffeine), Ma Huang concentrate aerial part (contains 12 mg naturally occuring ephedrines), Taurine, Potassium Citrate, Siberian Ginseng root, Spirulina algae, Ginger root, Green Tea concentrate leaf (contains 2 mg naturally occuring caffeine), Lecithin, Farcinia Cambogia concentrate fruit, Bladderwrack leaf, Inositol, Nettle leaf, Royal leaf, Sarsaparilla root, Cayenne fruit, White Willow bark, Naringen fruit, Hawthorne

fruit, L-Methionine, Ginkgo Biloba leaf, Gotu Kola (aerial part) 700 mg. Other Ingredients: Croscarmellose Sodium, Magnesium Stearate, Methocel, Microcrystalline Cellulose, Silica.
See Editor's Note No. 30, page 2056.

Meta-Thin **-** New Hope Health Products
Two capsules contain: Garcinia cambogia (50%) HCA 750 mg • Ma Huang (8% ephedra) 225 mg • Green Tea (50% caffeine) 125 mg • Caffeine (anhydrous) 100 mg • White Willow bark (2% salicylates) 60 mg • Naringin 20 mg • L-Tyrosine 50 mg • Choline bitartrate 100 mg • Chromium (chelate 10%) 200 mcg • Vanadium (sulfate) 3 mg • Alpha-lipoic acid 50 mg • Vitamin B-5 (Pantothenic acid) 50 mg • Potassium (Phosphate) 74 mg • Iodine (as Potassium iodide) 750 mcg • Cayenne Pepper 10 mg.
See Editor's Note No. 30, page 2056.

MetaTox Oral **-** PhysioLogics
Each capsule contains: Vitamin C (Ascorbic Acid) 250 mg • N-Acetylcysteine 200 mg • L-Methionine (Zn/Se Monomethionine) 52.5 mg • Alpha-Lipoic Acid (USP) 5 mg • L-Glutathione (USP) 5 mg • Zinc (as Zinc Monomethionine) 15 mg • Copper (Glycinate) 0.5 mg • Selenium (Methionine) 75 mcg.

Methoxy Complex Caps **-** Optimum Nutrition
Each capsule contains: 5-Methyl-7-Methoxy-Isoflavone 200 mg • 7-Isopropoxyisoflavone (ipriflavone) 150 mg • Grapefruit extract (standardized to 20% naringin) 50 mg. Other Ingredients: Gelatin, Microcrystalline Cellulose, Magnesium Stearate, Silica.

Methoxy-7 **-** BioTest Laboratories, LLC
Two teaspoons contain: 5-Methyl-7-Methoxy-Isoflavone 400 mg • Cholesterol 520 mg. Other Ingredients: Purified Water, Fatty-Acid Ethyl Esters, Polysorbate 60, Lecithin, Natural and Artificial Flavors, Potassium Sorbate, Methyl Paraben, Disodium EDTA, Butylated Hydroxyanisole, Sucralose, Vegetable Gum.

MethOxyvone **-** Metabolic Response Modifiers
Each capsule contains: 5-methyl-7-methoxyisoflavone 150 mg • 7-isopropoxyisoflavone (ipriflavone) 40 mg • Lysophosphatidylcholine 40 mg.

Methyl 1-Test **-** Legal Gear
Each tablet contains: 17-Methyl-1-Androstene-17b-ol-3one 10 mg. Other Ingredients: Microcrystalline Cellulose, Magnesium Stearate, Gelatin.

Methyl 1-Testosterone Xtreme **-** IDS
Each capsule contains: 17-Alpha-Methyl 1-Testosterone 10 mg • Bergamottin (6,7,-dihydroxybergamottin (DHB)) 100 mg • Proprietary Blend 255 mg: Bupleurum, Hoelen, Cayenne • Vitamin B6 2 mg • Vitamin B12 6 mcg • Niacin 20 mg. Other Ingredients: Gelatin, Magnesium Stearate, Silica.

methylCOBALAMIN - 1 mg **-** Source Naturals
Each tablet contains: Vitamin B12 (as methylcobalamin) 1 mg.

methylCOBALAMIN - 5 mg **-** Source Naturals
Each tablet contains: Vitamin B12 (as methylcobalamin) 5 mg.

Mexican Yam Extract **-** Enzymatic Therapy
Two capsules contain: Wild Yam root extract (dioscorea villosa, standardized to contain 10% diosgenin) 480 mg • Adrenal extract (freeze-dried) 200 mg • Beta Sitosterol 42 mg. Other Ingredients: Gelatin, Cellulose, Magnesium Stearate, Titanium Dioxide Color.
See Editor's Note No. 14.

MGN3 (MGN-3, MGN 3) **-** LaneLabs
Two capsules contain: MGN-3 proprietary blend 500 mg: Rice Bran, Hyphomycetes Mycelia extract, Beet Root Fiber, Calcium Phosphate, Silica, Magnesium Stearate, Gelatin, Water, Glycerin.
See Editor's Note No. 9 and No. 21.

Microhydrin **-** Royal BodyCare
Each capsule contains: Silica hydride powder 250 mg • Flanaga Microclusters (Silica, Potassium Carbonate, Magnesium Sulfate) • Rice flour • Rice Bran oil.

Micronized Creatine **-** AST Sports Science
Each 1 tsp serving contains: Creatine Monohydrate 5 g.

Mid-Life **-** Aspen Group, Inc.
Each tablet contains: Cimicifuga Racemosa root and rhizome (the compounds Triterpine Glycosides, standardized at 1 mg) 40 mg.

Midlife Care **-** Health Factor
Each capsule contains: Oat Straw extract (10:1) (Avena sativa) 250 mg • Dong Quai extract (4:1) (Angelica sinensis) 100 mg • Black Cohosh extract (4:1) (Cimicifuga racemosa) 80 mg • Licorice extract (4:1) (Glycyrrhiza glabra) 70 mg • Chasteberry (Vitex agnus-castus) 50 mg • Pomegranate (Punica granatum) 39.5 mg.

Mid-Life Creme **-** Aspen Group, Inc.
Aloe Vera gel in Distilled Water with Catalyst Altered Normalizer • d-Alpha-Tocopherol & mixed Tocopherols • Cetyl Alcohol • Almond oil • Ociyl Palmitate • Panthenol • Peg 8 Stearate • Hydrogenated Vegetable oil • Glycerine • extract of Wild Yam • Micronized Progesterone • Polysorbate 60 • Propylene Glycol • Hyaluronic Acid • oil of Lemon • Keratin • Carbomer 940 • Grapefruit seed extract.

Midnight Stallion **-** NVE Pharmaceuticals
Each capsule contains: Proprietary Blend 250 mg: Ephedra extract (leaves, stems, 25 mg ephedrine group alkaloids), Kola Nut (seeds, <1 mg caffeine group alkaloids), Green Tea (leaves, <1 mg caffeine group alkaloids), Mate (leaves, <1 mg caffeine group alkaloids), Gotu Kola (leaves), Rhodiola (root) • Caffeine (anhydrous) 300 mg • Other Ingredients: Gelatin, Stearic Acid, Magnesium Stearate, Di Basic Calcium Phosphate, Titanium Dioxide, FD&C Blue #1, FD&C Red #40.
See Editor's Note No. 30, page 2056.

Mighty One 3000 **-** Optimum Nutrition
Four scoops (224 g) contain: Proprietary Protein Blend: Whey Protein Concentrate, Soy Protein Isolate • Complex Carbohydrates • Crystalline Fructose • Cocoa • Artificial Flavor • Mighty One Vitamin Mineral Blend: Ascorbic Acid, DL-Alpha Tocopherol Acetate, Ferrous Fumarate, Niacinamide, Vitamin A Palmitate, Potassium Iodide, D-Calcium Pantothenate, Zinc Oxide, Vitamin D (D3), Copper Sulfate, Pyridoxine Hydrochloride, Riboflavin, Thiamin Mononitrate, Folic Acid, Biotin, Cyanocobalamin (vitamin B12).

MigraActin **-** Nature's Plus
Two capsules contain: Feverfew (Tanacetum parthenium leaf) standardized 1.2% Parthenolide 700 mg • Pantothenic Acid 50 mg • Ginkgo Biloba leaf (standardized 24% Ginkgo Flavone-Glycosides, 6% Terpene Lactones) 10 mg • Bioperine (Piper nigrum fruit) standardized 95% 1-Piperoylpiperidine 5 mg • Trimethylglycine (TMG) 5 mg.

Migraban Feverfew **-** Jamieson
Each tablet contains: Dried Feverfew leaf (Tanacetum parthenium L.) (Equivalent to 250 mcg of Parthenolide with a complete active sesquiterpene lactone complex) 125 mg.

Migracare **-** Enzymatic Therapy
Each capsule contains: Feverfew extract (Tanacetum parthenium) standardized to contain 0.6% Parthenolide 100 mg.

MigraDaily **-** NatureWell Inc.
Each tablet contains: Magnesium (as magnesium oxide) 180 mg •Vitamin B-2 (riboflavin) 200 mg •Vitamin B-1 (thiamin) 15 mg •Feverfew extract (leaf, standardized to 0.8% Parthenolide) 25 mg •White Willow extract (bark, standardized to 15% Salacin) 15 mg. Other Ingredients: Cellulose, Silicon Dioxide, Vegetable Stearine, Titanium Dioxide, Magnesium Stearate.

Some Brand Name Natural Products - What they Contain

www.NaturalDatabase.com contains MANY more listings than appear here.

Migra-Ease **-** Optimum Nutrition
Feverfew • White Willow.

MigraHealth **-** Health Assure
Each caplet contains: Riboflavin (vitamin B2) 200 mg • Magnesium (oxide/citrate) 150 mg • Feverfew leaf (Puracol) 50 mg. Other Ingredients: Vegetable Gum, Cellulose, Vegetable Stearine, Silicon Dioxide, Dextrose, Sodium Starch Glycolate, Titanium Dioxide, Caramel, Carmine, Magnesium Stearate.

Migraine Relief **-** Hyland's
Each tablet contains: Glonoinum 12X • Belladonna 6X • Gelsemium 6X • Nux Vomica 6X • Iris Versicolor 6X • Sanguinaria Canadensis 6X. Other Ingredients: Lactose N.F.
See Editor's Note No. 1, page 2053.

Migra-Lieve **-** Natural Science Corp. of America
Two caplets contain: Feverfew Extract (Tanacetum parthenium, standardized to 0.7% Parthenolide) 100 mg • Magnesium (Citrate/Oxide 1:1) 300 mg •Riboflavin (Vitamin B2) 400 mg.

Migra-Min - Wellzymes **-** Enzymes, Inc.
Two capsules contain: n-zimes Proprietary Enzyme Blend 58 mg: pHysio-Protease (142,080 pHysio-U), CereCalase Plus • Proprietary Herbal Blend 390 mg: Feverfew leaf, Feverfew leaf extract (standardized to contain 0.6% parthenolides), Rosemary leaf extract (equivalent to 320 mg raw herb), Passionflower herb extract (equivalent to 160 mg raw herb), Rice Bran. Other Ingredients: Plant Cellulose, Water.

Migraplex **-** PharmAssure
Two tablets contain: Riboflavin (B2) 50mg • Magnesium (as Magnesium stearate) 200 mg • Ginger Root Extract (Zingiber officinale) 150 mg • Feverfew Leaves Extract (Tanacetum parthenium; 0.5% Parthenolide=0.75mg) 150 mg. Other Ingredients: Dicalcium Phosphate, Cellulose.

MigraSpray **-** NatureWell Inc.
Each spray contains: Proprietary Homeopathic Blend: Feverfew (Tanacetum parenthenium, leaves/flowers), 3x Goldenseal (Hydrastis rhizoma, root) 3x, Dandelion (Taraxicum denleonis, root) 3x, Polyporus Officinalis (Polyporus umbellatus, sclerotium) 3x. Inactive Ingredients: Distilled Water, Glycerin, Ascorbic Acid, Potassium Sorbate, Disodium EDTA.
See Editor's Note No. 1, page 2053.

Migraway **-** PhysioLogics
Each capsule contains: Riboflavin (Vitamin B2) 100 mg • Vitamin B6 (as Pyridoxine Hydrochloride) 20 mg • Ginger root (5% Gingerols, 7.5 mg) 150 mg • Feverfew leaf (1.2% Parthenolides, 0.6 mg) 50 mg • White Willow bark (7.5% Salicin, 3.75 mg) 50 mg • Ginkgo leaf (24% Ginkgoflavonglycosides, 9.6 mg; 6% Terpene Lactones, 2.4 mg) 40 mg.

Migra-X **-** Olympian Labs
Two capsules contain: Feverfew extract 600 mg. In a 300 mg natural base of Ginkgo Biloba extract, Gotu Kola, and White Willow Bark.

Migrelief **-** PR Osteo
Two caplets contain: Puracol Feverfew (whole herb and extract) 100 mg • Riboflavin 400 mg • Magnesium 360 mg.

Milagro For Men **-** Changes International, Inc.
Four caplets contain: Zinc (from Zinc Citrate) 30 mg • L-Arginine Hydrochloride 2800 mg • African Yohimbe bark standardized extract (2% yohimbine) (Pausinystalia johimbe) 800 mg • DHEA (Dehydroepiandrosterone) 50 mg • Global Male Herbal Blend 300 mg: Damiana leaf (Turnera aphrodisiaca), Muira Puama bark (Ptychopetalum olacoides), Jamaica Ginger root (Zingiber officinale), Mucuna pruriens seed, Withania somnifera root, Tinospora cordifolia leaf, Licorice root (Glycyrrhiza uralensis), Tribulus terrestris root, Nutmeg fruit (Myristica fragans), Korean Ginseng (Panax ginseng), Siberian Ginseng (Acanthopanax senticosus), Chinese Red Panax Ginseng (Panax ginseng), Manchurian Tienchi Ginseng (Panax notoginseng), Oat Straw (Avena sativa), Stinging Nettle (Urtica dioica). Other Ingredients: Calcium Phosphate, Vegetable Cellulose, Fractionated Vegetable Oil, Silica, and Vita-Lok Vegetable Resin Glaze.

Milagro For Women **-** Changes International, Inc.
Four caplets contain: Vitamin E (as natural D-Alpha Tocopherol Succinate) 400 IU • Soy Phytoestrogens Concentrate (providing 80 mg isoflavones as daidzin and daidzein, genistin and genistein, glycitin and glycetein) 2670 mg • DHEA (Dehydroepiandrosterone) 50 mg • Global Female Herbal Blend 500 mg: Wild Yam (Discorea villosa), Red Clover blossom (Trifolium pratense), Damiana leaf (Turnera aphrodisiaca), Squaw Vine (Mitchella repens), Jamaica Ginger root (Zingiber officinale), Tribulus Terrestris root, Licorice root (Glycyrrhiza uralensis), Fennel seed (Foeniculum vulgare), Magnolia bark (Magnolia officinalis), Korean Ginseng root (Panax ginseng), Siberian Ginseng root (Acanthopanax ginseng), Chinese Red Panax Ginseng root (Panax ginseng), Manchurian Tienchi Ginseng (Panax notoginseng), Black Cohosh root (Cimicifuaga racemosa), Oat Straw (Avena sativa), Stinging Nettle (Urtica dioica).
Inactive Ingredients: Dicalcium Phosphate, Vegetable Cellulose, Fractionated Vegetable Oil, Silica, Vita-Lok.

Mild Child **-** The Herbalist
Catnip leaf • Fennel seed • Chamomile flower • Lemon Balm leaf.

Milk Free Probiotic Acidophilus (Inspired by Nature) **-** Puritan's Pride
Each capsule contains: Lactobacillus blend 40 mg: Lactobacillus Acidophilus, Lactobacillus Rhamnosus, Lactobacillus Bifidus. Other Ingredients: Dicalcium Phosphate, Cellulose (plant origin), Hydroxypropyl Methylcellulose, Vegetable Stearic Acid, Silica, Vegetable Magnesium Stearate.

Milk Thistle - Basic Nutrition **-** GNC
Each capsule contains: Milk Thistle seed extract (Silybum marianum) 200 mg. Other Ingredients: Gelatin, Celulose, Dicalcium Phosphate, Magnesium Stearate.

Milk Thistle **-** BioDynamax
Each tablet contains: Milk Thistle 175 mg.

Milk Thistle **-** Jamieson
Each caplet contains: Milk Thistle 4500 mg.

Milk Thistle **-** Leiner Health Products
Each softgel contains: Milk Thistle extract (Silybum marianum) fruit 150 mg. Other Ingredients: Soybean Oil, Gelatin, Glycerin, Yellow Beeswax, Lecithin, Polysorbate 80, Caramel, Titanium Dioxide, Red 40, Blue 1.

Milk Thistle **-** Pharmanex
Each capsule contains: Milk Thistle seed extract (Silybum marianum) (30:1) 175 mg. Other Ingredients: Rice Flour, Gelatin, Magnesium Stearate, Silicon Dioxide.

Milk Thistle **-** PhysioLogics
Each capsule contains: Milk Thistle seed extract (silybum marianum, standardized to contain a minimum of 80% silymarin) 250 mg. Other Ingredients: Maltodextrin, Gelatin, Magnesium Silicate, Vegetable Magnesium Stearate, Silica.

Milk Thistle **-** Sundown
Each capsule contains: Milk Thistle seed extract (standardized to 80% silymarin 140 mg) 175 mg. Other Ingredients: Gelatin.

Milk Thistle Combination **-** Swanson
Each capsule contains: Milk Thistle seed extract (standardized to 80% silymarin) 175 mg • Dandelion root 85 mg • Black Radish root 60 mg • Burdock root 60 mg • Ginger root 60 mg • Parsley root 35 mg.

Some Brand Name Natural Products - What they Contain

www.NaturalDatabase.com contains MANY more listings than appear here.

BRAND NAMES

Milk Thistle Extract - NSI - Nutraceutical Sciences Institute
Each capsule contains: Milk Thistle (standardized to 80% silymarin) 300 mg.

Milk Thistle Formula - Quest
Each caplet contains: Milk Thistle seed powder (Silybum marianum) (provided by 60 mg of P.E. 1:8) 480 mg • Butternut bark of root powder (Juglans cineraria) 155 mg • Dandelion root powder (Taraxacum oficinale) 155 mg • Licorice root powder (Glycyrrhiza glabra) 40 mg • Wild Yam root powder (Dioscorea villosa) 10 mg. Other Ingredients: Calcium Phosphate, Microcrystalline Cellulose, Vegetable Stearin, Croscarmellose Sodium, Magnesium Stearate (vegetable source).

Milk Thistle Healthy Liver - DreamPharm
Each capsule contains: Milk Thistle seed extract (standardized to 80% silymarin) 200 mg • Artemisia Vulgaris 100 mg • Corydalis Turtschaninovii rhizome 100 mg • Cyperus Rotundus rhizome 100 mg.

Milk Thistle Seed - Gaia Herbs
Milk Thistle seed (Standardized for 80% silymarins) Standardized Full Spectrum 150 mg of extract per capsule. Guaranteed Potency 75 mg of extract per capsule.

Milk Thistle X - Enzymatic Therapy
Two capsules contain: Milk Thistle fruit extract (silybum marianum, standardized to contain 80% silymarin 240 mg, calculated as silybin) 300 mg • Dandelion root extract (taraxacum officinale, 4:1) 20 mg • Artichoke leaf extract (cynara scolymus, standardized to contain 13-18% caffeylquinic acids calculated as chlorogenic acid) 20 mg • Licorice root extract (glycyrrhiza glabra, standardized to contain 5% glycyrrhizic acid) 20 mg. Other Ingredients: Cellulose, Gelatin, Magnesium Stearate, Titanium Dioxide Color, Silicon Dioxide.

Milk Thistle XTRA - Sundown
Two capsules contain: Milk Thistle seed extract (standardized to 80% silymarin 192 mg) 240 mg • XTRA Premium Blend 560 mg: Dandelion root, Fennel seed, Licorice root. Other Ingredients: Gelatin.

Milk-Based Soy-Free Lactobacillus Acidophilus - Nature's Life
Two tablespoons (1 fl.oz or 29.6 ml) contain: Purified Water • Non-fat Milk powder • viable Lactobacillus Acidophilus Culture.

Milk-Zyme - Atrium Inc.
Each capsule contains: Lactase 30 mg • Rennin 10 mg.

Min-Chex - Standard Process, Inc.
Each capsule contains: Bovine Orchic Cytosol extract 95 mg • Niacinamide 25 mg • Vitamin B6 5 mg. Other Ingredients: Calcium lactate, Kelp powder, Vacuum Dried Bovine and Ovine Spleen, Magnesium citrate, Manganese lactate, Bone Liver powder, Vacuum Dried Porcine Stomach, Processed Soy Bean powder, Potassium Para-Aminobenzoate, Pyridoxine Hydrochloride, Defatted Wheat Germ, Vacuum Dried Bovine Brain, and Ascorbic acid.
See Editor's Note No. 31, page 2056.

Mind & Memory - Health Factor
Each capsule contains: Ginkgo Biloba extract (4:1)(standardized extract to 24% Gingkoflavonglycosides) 160 mg • Gotu Kola extract (4:1)(Hydrocotyle asaitica) 150 mg • Rosemary (Rosmarinus officinalis) 150 mg.

MindPrep - HealthMinded
Four capsules contain: Vitamin A (as acetate) 4000 IU • Vitamin C (ascorbic acid) 250 mg • Vitamin D (as cholecalciferol) 100 IU • Vitamin E (as D-alpha tocopheryl succinate) 30 IU • Thiamin (as thiamin mononitrate) 4 mg • Riboflavin (vitamin B2) 2 mg • Niacin (as nicotinic acid) 26 mg • Vitamin B6 (as pyridoxine HCl) 6 mg • Folic Acid 400 mcg • Vitamin B12 (as cyanocobalamin) 20 mcg • Biotin (as triturate) 300 mcg • Pantothenic Acid (as D-calcium pantothenate) 12 mg • Calcium (as citrate) 50 mg • Iron (as fumarate) 6 mg • Magnesium (as oxide) 100 mg • Zinc (as citrate) 10 mg • Selenium (as amino acid chelate) 20 mcg • Copper (as gluconate) 400 mcg • Manganese (as citrate) 2 mg • Chromium (as polynicotinate) 100 mcg • Molybdenum (as amino acid chelate) 10 mcg • Potassium (as citrate) 50 mg • MindPrep Proprietary Blend 704 mg: DMAE (bitartrate), L-Glutamine, Ginkgo Biloba leaf dried extract, Bacopa aerial parts dried extract, L-Pyroglutamic Acid, Phosphatidylserine (from soy lecithin), Fish Oil (30% EPA/DHA), Choline (bitartrate), Inositol, Pyridoxine Alpha Ketoglutarate, Asian Ginseng root dried extract, N-Acetyl-L-Tyrosine, Bilberry fruit dried extract, GABA, Grape skin dried extract, Grape seed dried extract, Vinpocetine (from periwinkle herb dried extract), Trace Mineral Complex, Huperzine-A (from toothed clubmoss whole plant dried extract), Boron (as citrate), Vanadium (as sodium meta-vanadate), Kelp whole thallus. Other Ingredients: Gelatin, Stearic Acid, Magnesium Stearate.

Mineral Milk Powder - Global Health Trax
Each gram contains: Calcium (from coral) 375 mg • Magnesium (from coral) 7 mg.

Minerogen - ANS - Applied Nutrition Sciences
Each capsule contains: Calcium 200 mg • Magnesium 75 mg • Copper 250 mcg • Chromium 25 mcg • Manganese 100 mcg • Molybdenum 50 mcg • Selenium 25 mcg • Potassium 100 mg • Vanadium 25 mcg • Boron 1 mg • Zinc 7.5 mg.

Mintacin - Enzymatic Therapy
Each capsule contains: Simethicone 25 mg. Other Ingredients: Peppermint oil extract (Mentha piperita) 0.2 mL.

Minute Maid Premium Heart Wise - The Coca-Cola Company
Water • Concentrated Orange Juice • Plant Sterols • Vitamin E (alpha-tocopheryl acetate) • Vitamin B6 (pyridoxine hydrochloride) • Vitamin B12 • Beta Carotene.

Mioplex Pure Extract - Boland Naturals, Inc.
Each tablet contains: Proprietary Blend: Bee Pollen, Flower Pollen.

Mirac - Berean Development
Two capsules contain: Vitamin C (as ascorbic acid) 500 mg • Calcium (from calcium carbonate) 78 mg • Sodium 2 mg • Bioflavonoid Complex 500 mg • Bromelain 500 mg. Other Ingredients: Cellulose, Stearic Acid, Croscarmellose Sodium, Silicon Dioxide, Magnesium Stearate.

Mission Prenatal - Mission Pharmacal
Each tablet contains: Vitamin A 4000 IU • Vitamin C 100 mg • Vitamin D (as Vitamin D3) 400 IU • Vitamin B1 4.7 mg • Vitamin B2 2 mg • Vitamin B3 10 mg • Vitamin B6 2.8 mg • Folate 0.4 mg • Vitamin B12 2 mcg • Vitamin B5 1 mg • Calcium 50 mg • Iron 29.5 mg. Other Ingredients: Sugar, Microcrystalline Cellulose, Color, Povidone, Croscarmellose Sodium, Magnesium Stearate, FD & C Red 40 Lake, Food Glaze, Carnauba Wax, Cholecalciferol, White Beeswax, Sodium Benzoate, Cyanocobalamin.

Mission Prenatal FA - Mission Pharmacal
Each tablet contains: Vitamin A 4000 IU • Vitamin C 100 mg • Vitamin D (as Vitamin D3) 400 IU • Vitamin B1 4.7 mg • Vitamin B2 2 mg • Vitamin B3 10 mg • Vitamin B6 10 mg • Folate 0.8 mg • Vitamin B12 2 mcg • Vitamin B5 1 mg • Calcium 50 mg • Iron 29.5 mg • Zinc 15 mg. Other Ingredients: Sugar, Microsrystalline Cellulose, Color, Magnesium Stearate, Croscarmellose Sodium, Povidone, Food Glaze, Blue 1 Lake, Carnauba Wax, Sodium Benzoate, White Beeswax, Cholecalciferol, Cyanocobalamin.

Mission Prenatal HP - Mission Pharmacal
Each tablet contains: Vitamin A 4000 IU • Vitamin C 100 mg • Vitamin D (Vitamin D3; Cholecalciferol) 400 IU • Vitamin B1 4 mg • Vitamin B2 2 mg • Vitamin B3 10 mg • Vitamin B6 20 mg • Folate 0.8 mg • Vitamin B12 (Cyanocobalamin) 2 mcg • Vitamin B5 1 mg • Calcium 50 mg • Iron 29.5 mg. Other Ingredients: Sugar, Microcrystalline Cellulose, Color, Magnesium Stearate, Croscarmellose

Sodium, Povidone, FD & C Yellow 5 Lake, Food Glaze, FD & C Blue 1 Lake, Sodium Benzoate, Carnauba Wax, FD & C Yellow 6 Lake, White Beeswax.

MI-T-Cell **-** Progressive Labs
Each capsule contains: Vitamin C (ascorbyl palmitate) 50 mg • Vitamin E Succinate 30 mg • Thiamin HCl (Vitamin B1) 5 mg • Riboflavin (Vitamin B2) 5 mg • Magnesium (as magnesium malate) 50 mg • L-Glutathione 50 mg • N-Acetyl-Carnitine 30 mg • N-Acetyl Cysteine 50 mg • CoEnzyme Q10 10 mg • Lipoic Acid 50 mg • L-Isoleucine 225 mcg • Red Grape skin (Vitis vinifera) 2% polyphenols 50 mg.

Mixed Greens **-** Health Smart Vitamins
Each capsule contains: Broccoli aerial parts (2% glucosinolates, 2 mg) 100 mg • Tea green, leaf (50% polyphenols, 50 mg) 100 mg • Tomato fruit (1% lycopene, 0.5 mg) 50 mg • Calendula flower (5% lutein, 1.9 mg) 38 mg • Garlic bulb (10,000 mcg allicin/g, 250 mg) 25 mg • Ginger root (5% gingerols, 1.25 mg) 25 mg • Milk Thistle seed (80% silymarin, 20 mg) 25 mg • Red Grape (Vitis vinifera, skin; 30% anthocyanidins, 7.5 mg) 25 mg • Soy Isoflavones bean (5% isoflavones, 1.25 mg) 25 mg • Turmeric root (95% curcumin, 23.75 mg) 25 mg.

Mixed Vegetable Phytonutrients **-** Leiner Health Products
Two tablets contain: Lutein 3000 mcg • Lycopene 1000 mcg • Sulforaphane 33 mcg • Zeaxanthin 150 mcg. Other Ingredients: Calcium Carbonate, Broccoli, Carrot, Spinach, Tomato, Cellulose, Maltodextrin, Gelatin, Lutein/Lycopene Suspension, Sucrose, Starch, Hydroxypropyl Methylcellulose, Titanium Dioxide, Hydroxypropyl Cellulose, Crospovidone, Silicon Dioxide, Pharmaceutical Glaze, Polyethylene Glycol 3350, Ascorbyl Palmitate, Tocopherols, Magnesium Stearate, Polysorbate 80, Yellow 6 Lake, Blue 2 Lake.

Mixed Vegetables **-** Nature's Plus
Three tablets contain: Broccoli floret (Brassica oleracea) naturally rich in sulorophane & indole-3-carbinol equivalent to 10000 mg fresh broccoli 1000 mg • Spinach leaf (Spinacia oleracea) naturally rich in monoterpenes equivalent to 1000 mg fresh Spinach 100 mg • Carrot root (Daucus carota) naturally rich in carotenoids, coumarins & Polyacetylenes equivalent to 1000 mg fresh Carrot 100 mg • Cabbage leaf (Brassica chinensis) naturally rich in Sterols, Phenolic Acids & Indoles equivalent to 1000 mg. fresh Cabbage 100 mg.

MNS Gold **-** Advocare International
Two white packets contain: Vitamin A (as palmitate) 2500 IU • Vitamin A (as beta-carotene) 12,500 IU • Vitamin C (as ascorbic acid/ mineral ascorbates) 600 mg • Vitamin D (as cholecalciferol) 400 IU • Vitamin E (as D-alpha tocopheryl succinate) 150 IU • Thiamine 9 mg • Riboflavin 10.2 mg • Niacin (as niacinamide/niacin) 120 mg • Vitamin B6 (as pyridoxine HCl) 12 mg • Folic Acid 800 mcg • Vitamin B12 (as cyanocobalamin) 36 mcg • Biotin 300 mcg • Pantothenic Acid 40 mg • Calcium (as amino acid chelate) 150 mg • Phosphorus (as amino acid chelate) 100 mg • Iodine (from kelp) 150 mcg • Magnesium (as amino acid chelate/phosphate) 200 mg • Zinc (as zinc monomethionine) 15 mg • Selenium (L-selenomethionine) 80 mcg • Copper (as amino acid chelate) 2 mg • Manganese (as amino acid chelate) 4 mg • Chromium (as chromium polynicotinate) 100 mcg • Molybdenum (as amino acid chelate) 50 mcg • Potassium (as amino acid chelate/phosphate) 100 mg • Inositol 6 mg • Choline (as bitartrate) 60 mg • Boron (as amino acid chelate) 300 mcg • Vanadium (as bis-gylcinate-oxovanadium) 50 mcg • Silicon (as amino acid chelate) 500 mcg • Coenzyme Q-10 150 mcg • Octacosanol 2 mg • Ribonucleic Acid (RNA) 2 mg • Odorless Garlic bulb powder (allium sativum) 50 mg • L-Glutathione 5 mg • Gamma-Oryzanol 5 mg • Citrus Flavonoids 100 mg • Grape Seed extract (vitis vinifera) 5 mg • Milk Thistle fruit extract (silybum marianum) 5 mg • Ginkgo leaf extract (ginkgo biloba) 10 mg • Eicosapentaenoic Acid (from marine lipids) 180 mg • Docosahexaenoic Acid (from marine lipids) 120 mg • D-Limonene powder 300 mg • Grapefruit juice powder 200 mg • 5-Hydroxytryptophan (griffonia simplicifolia seed) 25 mg. Two gold packets contain: Vitamin A (as beta-carotene) 2000 IU • Vitamin C (as ascorbic acid/mineral ascorbates) 600 mg • Niacin (as niacinamide/niacin) 40 mg • Vitamin B6 (as pyridoxine HCl) 4 mg • Iodine (from kelp) 50 mcg • Magnesium (as amino acid chelate/phosphate) 50 mg • Zinc (as zinc monomethionine) 2 mg • Chromium (as chromium polynicotinate) 100 mcg • Potassium (as amino acid chelate/phosphate) 100 mg • Vanadium (as bis-gylcinate-oxovanadium) 200 mcg • Garcinia fruit extract (garcinia cambogia) 2000 mg • Tulsi leaf extract (ocimum sanctum) 50 mg • Taurine 50 mg • Beta-Sitosterol 25 mg • L-Carnitine 25 mg • Gymnema leaf extract (gymnema sylvestre) 10 mg • Oolong Tea leaf extract (camellia sinensis) 200 mg • Guarana seed extract (paullinia cupana) 550 mg • Eleuthero root extract (eleutherococcus senticosus) 50 mg • Green Tea leaf extract (camellia sinensis) 20 mg • Green Orange pericarp extract (citrus aurantium) 1000 mg. Other Ingredients: Dicalcium Phosphate, Silicon Dioxide, Cellulose, Stearic Acid, Magnesium Stearate, Peppermint Extract, Vanillin, Beet Root Powder (for color), Gelatin, Glycerin, Water.
See Editor's Note No. 40, page 2058.

MNS Platinum **-** Advocare International
Two white packets contain: Vitamin A (as palmitate) 2500 IU • Vitamin A (as beta-carotene) 12,500 IU • Vitamin C (as ascorbic acid/ mineral ascorbates) 600 mg • Vitamin D (as cholecalciferol) 400 IU • Vitamin E (as D-alpha tocopheryl succinate) 150 IU • Thiamine 9 mg • Riboflavin 10.2 mg • Niacin (as niacinamide/niacin) 120 mg • Vitamin B6 (as pyridoxine HCl) 12 mg • Folic Acid 800 mcg • Vitamin B12 (as cyanocobalamin) 36 mcg • Biotin 300 mcg • Pantothenic Acid 40 mg • Calcium (as amino acid chelate) 150 mg • Phosphorus (as amino acid chelate) 100 mg • Iodine (from kelp) 150 mcg • Magnesium (as amino acid chelate) 200 mg • Zinc (as zinc monomethionine) 15 mg • Selenium (L-selenomethionine) 80 mcg • Copper (as amino acid chelate) 2 mg • Manganese (as amino acid chelate) 4 mg • Chromium (as chromium polynicotinate) 100 mcg • Molybdenum (as amino acid chelate) 50 mcg • Potassium (as amino acid chelate) 100 mg • Inositol 6 mg • Choline (as bitartrate) 60 mg • Boron (as amino acid chelate) 300 mcg • Vanadium (as bis-gylcinate-oxovanadium) 50 mcg • Silicon (as amino acid chelate) 500 mcg • Coenzyme Q-10 150 mcg • Octacosanol 2 mg • Ribonucleic Acid (RNA) 2 mg • Odorless Garlic powder (allium sativum bulb) 50 mg • L-Glutathione 5 mg • Gamma-Oryzanol 5 mg • Citrus Flavonoids 100 mg • Grape Seed extract (vitis vinifera) 5 mg • Milk Thistle fruit extract (silybum marianum) 5 mg • Ginkgo leaf extract (ginkgo biloba) 10 mg • Eicosapentaenoic Acid (from marine lipids) 180 mg • Docosahexaenoic Acid (from marine lipids) 120 mg. Two platinum packets contain: Vitamin C (as ascorbic acid/mineral ascorbates) 600 mg • Niacin (as niacinamide/niacin) 10 mg • Vitamin B6 (as pyridoxine HCl) 4 mg • Iodine (from kelp) 50 mcg • Zinc (as zinc monomethionine) 2 mg • Chromium (as chromium polynicotinate) 100 mcg • Vanadium (as bis-gylcinate-oxovanadium) 200 mcg • Garcinia fruit extract (garcinia cambogia) 2000 mg • Tulsi leaf extract (ocimum sanctum) 50 mg • Taurine 50 mg • Beta-Sitosterol 25 mg • L-Carnitine (as tartrate) 25 mg • Gymnema leaf extract (gymnema sylvestre) 10 mg • Oolong Tea leaf extract (camellia sinensis) 800 mg • Kola Nut extract (cola acuminata) 500 mg • Guarana seed extract (paullinia cupana) 150 mg • Coleus Forskohlii root extract 30 mg • Resveratrol (from polygonum cuspidatum) 25 mg • Eleuthero root extract (eleutherococcus senticosus) 50 mg • White Willow bark extract (salix alba) 60 mg • L-Tyrosine 800 mg • L-Glutamine 1600 mg. Other Ingredients: Dicalcium Phosphate, Silicon Dioxide, Cellulose, Stearic Acid, Magnesium Stearate, Peppermint Extract, Vanillin, Beet Root Powder (for color), Gelatin, Glycerin, Water.

MNS Yellow **-** Advocare International
Two white packets contain: Vitamin A (as palmitate) 2500 IU • Vitamin A (as beta-carotene) 12,500 IU • Vitamin C (as ascorbic acid/ mineral ascorbates) 600 mg • Vitamin D (as cholecalciferol) 400 IU • Vitamin E (as D-alpha tocopheryl succinate) 150 IU • Thiamine 9 mg • Riboflavin 10.2 mg • Niacin (as niacinamide/niacin) 120 mg • Vitamin B6 (as pyridoxine HCl) 12 mg • Folic Acid 800 mcg • Vitamin B12 (as cyanocobalamin) 36 mcg • Biotin 300 mcg • Pantothenic Acid 40 mg • Calcium (as amino acid chelate) 150 mg •

Phosphorus (as amino acid chelate) 100 mg • Iodine (from kelp) 150 mcg • Magnesium (as amino acid chelate/phosphate) 200 mg • Zinc (as zinc monomethionine) 15 mg • Selenium (L-selenomethionine) 80 mcg • Copper (as amino acid chelate) 2 mg • Manganese (as amino acid chelate) 4 mg • Chromium (as chromium polynicotinate) 100 mcg • Molybdenum (as amino acid chelate) 50 mcg • Potassium (as amino acid chelate/phosphate) 100 mg • Inositol 6 mg • Choline (as bitartrate) 60 mg • Boron (as amino acid chelate) 300 mcg • Vanadium (as bis-gylcinate-oxovanadium) 50 mcg • Silicon (as amino acid chelate) 500 mcg • Coenzyme Q-10 150 mcg • Octacosanol 2 mg • Ribonucleic Acid (RNA) 2 mg • Odorless Garlic bulb powder (allium sativum) 50 mg • L-Glutathione 5 mg • Gamma-Oryzanol 5 mg • Citrus Flavonoids 100 mg • Grape Seed extract (vitis vinifera) 5 mg • Milk Thistle fruit extract (silybum marianum) 5 mg • Ginkgo leaf extract (ginkgo biloba) 10 mg • Eicosapentaenoic Acid (from marine lipids) 180 mg • Docosahexaenoic Acid (from marine lipids) 120 mg. Two yellow packets contain: Vitamin A (as beta-carotene) 2000 IU • Vitamin C (as ascorbic acid/mineral ascorbates) 600 mg • Niacin (as niacinamide/niacin) 40 mg • Vitamin B6 (as pyridoxine HCl) 4 mg • Iodine (from kelp) 50 mcg • Magnesium (as amino acid chelate/phosphate) 100 mg • Zinc (as zinc monomethionine) 2 mg • Chromium (as chromium polynicotinate) 100 mcg • Potassium (as amino acid chelate/phosphate) 200 mg • Vanadium (as bis-gylcinate-oxovanadium) 200 mcg • Garcinia fruit extract (garcinia cambogia) 2000 mg • Tulsi leaf extract (ocimum sanctum) 50 mg • Taurine 50 mg • Beta-Sitosterol 25 mg • L-Carnitine 25 mg • Gymnema leaf extract (gymnema sylvestre) 10 mg • Oolong Tea leaf extract (camellia sinensis) 200 mg • Guarana seed extract (paullinia cupana) 550 mg • Eleuthero root extract (eleutherococcus senticosus) 50 mg • Green Tea leaf extract (camellia sinensis) 20 mg • Cayenne fruit extract (capsicum annuum) 32 mg • Proprietary Blend ThermoGen-HC 224 mg: Gotu Kola (whole plant), Cassia bark, Peppermint leaf, Peppermint stem, Lemon Verbena leaf, Lemon Verbena flower, Chamomile leaf, Chamomile flower, Ginger root, Chinese Licorice root, Sweet Orange peel, Chicory root. Other Ingredients: Dicalcium Phosphate, Silicon Dioxide, Cellulose, Stearic Acid, Peppermint Extract, Vanillin, Gelatin, Glycerin, Water.

Mocha - Revival - Physicians Laboratories
Eight Fluid Ounces Contain: Certified Isoflavone 15 mg. Ingredients: Whole Roasted Soybeans, Natural and Artificial Flavors.

Modified Citrus Pectin Capsules - NutriCology
Three capsules contain: Modified Citrus Pectin 1.5 g.

Modified Citrus Pectin Powder - NutriCology
Each 1 tsp (5 g) serving contains: Modified Citrus Pectin 5 g.

Modrenal GF - PhysioLogics
Three caplets contain: Vitamin B1 (Thiamine HCl) 40 mg • Vitamin B2 (Riboflavin) 30 mg • Vitamin B5 (Calcium Pantothenate) 150 mg • Vitamin B6 (Pyridoxine HCl) 25 mg • Vitamin B12 (Cyanocobalamin) 30 mcg • Vitamin C (Ascorbic Acid) 200 mg • Vitamin E (D-Alpha Tocopherol) 100 IU • Vitamin B3 (Niacinamide) 50 mg • Iron (Ferrous Succinate) 10 mg • Magnesium (Citrate) 200 mg • Calcium (Citrate) 250 mg • Folic Acid 100 mcg • Biotin 20 mcg • Siberian Ginseng (Eleutherococcus senticosus; GPH: 0.3% eleutherosides b & e) 75 mg • Lemon Bioflavonoids 50 mg • Passion Flower 50 mg • Chamomile 50 mg • Skullcap 50 mg • Choline 40 mg • PABA 10 mg • Inositol 10 mg • Chromium GTF (Nicotinate) 250 mcg.

ModuCare Grape Chewabe Tablets - Purity Life International
Each tablet contains: Sterols (from pinus martima, pinus pinaster) 20 mg • Sterolins (from pinus martima, pinus pinaster) 0.2 mg. Other Ingredients: Zylitol (natural birch sweetener), Natural Grape Flavor, Citric Acid, Malic Acid, Inulin, Silicon Dioxide, Magnesium Stearate.

Moducare Sterinol - Essential Phytosterolins, Inc.
Each capsule contains: Plant Sterols 20 mg • Plant Sterolins 200 mcg. Other Ingredients: White Rice Flour, Magnesium Silicate, Gel Cap.

ModuCare Vegetarian Capsules - Purity Life International
Each capsule contains: Sterols (from pinus martima, pinus pinaster) 20 mg • Sterolins (from pinus martima, pinus pinaster) 0.2 mg. Other Ingredients: Rice Flour, Magnesium Silicate, Vegetable Cellulose, Water, Vegetable Glycerin, Silicon.

ModuChol - Purity Life International
Each capsule contains: Phytosterols Esters (from vegetable oil) 650 mg.

ModuProst - Purity Life International
Each capsule contains: Harzol (providing sterols 10 mg, sterolins 0.1 mg) 112 mg • Saw Palmetto extract 150 mg • Nettles extract (1:10) 100 mg • Green Tea 50 mg • Lycopene 0.25 mg.

Moisture Restore Day Protective Lotion (combination to oily) - Nu Skin Enterprises
Water • Octyldodecyl Neopentanoate • Glycerin • Cyclomethicone • Clyceryl Stearate • PEG-100 Stearate • Cetyl Alcohol • Algae extract • Tocopheryl Acetate • Calendula Officinalis flower extract • Anthemis Nobilis flower extract • Tilia Cordata flower extract • Centaurea Cyanus flower extract • Hypericum Perforatum extract • Allantoin • Hydrogenated Lecithin • Dimethicone • Butylene Glycol • Polyacrylamide • Laureth-7 • Disodium EDTA • Myristyl Myristate • C13-14 Isoparrifin • Phenoxyethanol • Chlorphenesin • Propylparaben • Methylparaben • Benzoic Acid • Fragrance.

Moisture Restore Day Protective Lotion (normal to dry) - Nu Skin Enterprises
Water • Octyldodecyl Neopentanoate • Glycerin • Cyclomethicone • Cetyl Alcohol • Glyceryl Stearate • PEG-75 Stearate • Algae extract • Butyrosperum Parkii extract (shea butter) • Oenothera Biennis oil (evening primrose oil) • Tocopheryl Acetate • Calendula Officinalis flower extract • Anthemis Nobilis flower extract • Tilia Cordata flower extract • Centaurea Cyanus flower extract • Chamomilla Recutita flower extract (matricaria) • Hypericum Perforatum extract • Limnanthes Alba seed oil (meadowfoam) • Allantoin • Hydrogenated Lecithin • Dimethicone • Butylene Glycol • Polyacrylamide • Laureth-7 • Ceteth-20 • Steareth-20 • Tetrasodium EDTA • Myristyl Myristate • C13-14 Isoparrifin • Phenoxyethanol • Chlorphenesin • Propylparaben • Methylparaben • Benzoic Acid • Fragrance.

Moisture Restore Intense Moisturizer - Nu Skin Enterprises
Aqua • Aloe Barbadensis • C12-15 Alkyl Benzoate • Glyceryl Stearate • Milk Lipids (lactis lipida) • Cetearyl Alcohol • Butyrospermum Parkii • Butylene Glycol • Caprylic/Capric Triglycerides • Urea • Sodium Behenoyl Lactylate • Glycerin • Pistacia Vera • Helianthus Annuus • Methyl Gluceth-10 • Sodium PCA • Glycine • Alanine • Proline • Serine • Threonine • Lysine • Arginine • Glutamic Acid • Sorbitol • Betaine • Dimethicone • Tocopheryl Acetate • Tocopherol • Parfum • Chlorphenesin • Methylparaben • Disodium EDTA • Propylparaben.

Moisture Therapy Bath - Abra Therapeutics
Sodium Borate • Sodium Sulfate • Sodium Chloride • Sodium Sesquicarbonate • Olive Oil • Essential Oils Blend: Rose, Palmarosa, Olibanum, Chamomile, Peru Balsam, Ylang Ylang • Herbal Extracts Blend: Calendula flower, Kukui nut oil, Aloe Vera gel • Chromium Oxide • Trace Mineral Salts.

Moisturizing Cleansing Creme - Aspen Group, Inc.
Each gram contains: Tocopheryl Acetate 1% • Panthenol 1% • Water • Mineral Oil • Steareth-2 • PPG-15 • Stearyl Ether • Tocopheryl Acetate • Octyl Palmitate • Isoceteth-20 • Cetearyl Octanoate • Carbomer • Dimethicone • Ammonium Hydroxide • Propylene Glycol • Diazolidinyl Urea • Methylparaben • Propylparaben.

Molymin - Progressive Labs
Each capsule contains: Molybdenum (amino acid chelate) 50 mcg • Pea powder 150 mg • Lentil powder 75 mg • Buckwheat 75 mg • Millet flour 75 mg. Carefully dried to preserve their natural trace nutrient content.

***Monolaurin (Coconut Extract)* - Olympia Nutrition**
Coconut extract 300 mg.

***Monolaurin (Lauric Acid) 300 mg* - Ecological Formulas**
Each capsule contains: Lauric Acid (from coconut oil) 300 mg. Base: Inosine 7.5 mg, Calcium (phosphate) 106 mg. Other Ingredients: Dicalcium Phosphate, Cellulose Powder, Silicon Dioxide.

***Monthly Comfort* - Source Naturals**
Six tablets contain: Vitamin A (Palmitate) 6000 IU • Vitamin C (Ascorbic Acid and Zinc Ascorbate) 600 mg • Vitamin E (D-Alpha Tocopheryl) (Natural) 150 IU • Vitamin B1 (Thiamin) 20 mg • Vitamin B2 (Riboflavin) 20 mg • Niacinamide 100 mg • Vitamin B5 (Calcium D-Pantothenate) 30 mg • Vitamin B6 (Pyridoxine HCl) 150 mg • Vitamin B12 (Cyanocobalamin) 30 mcg • Folic Acid 800 mcg • Calcium (Carbonate, Citrate) 200 mg • Chromium (ChromeMate GTF Yeast-Free Polynicotinate) 300 mcg • Magnesium (Oxide, Citrate) 450 mg • Zinc (Ascorbate) 20 mg • Taurine 500 mg • N-Acetyl Cysteine 300 mg • DLPA (DL-Phenylalanine) 250 mg • Choline (Bitartrate) 100 mg • Inositol 100 mg • Herbal Formula 1350 mg • Chasteberry 400 mgl • Dong Quai root 200 mg • Black Cohosh root 175 mg • Blue Cohosh root 175 mg • Silymarin (Milk Thistle seed extract) 100 mg • Cyperus rhizome 100 mg • Dong Quai root extract 100 mg • Dandelion root extract 100 mg.

***Mood Actives* - VitaStore**
Four tablets contain: St. John's Wort (0.3% Hypericin) 450 mg • Kava Kava 325 mg • Ginseng 200 mg • Valerian 200 mg • Licorice Root 150 mg • L-Methionine 100 mg • L-Phenylalanine 200 mg • L-Tyrosine 500 mg • L-Taurine 500 mg • Folic Acid 0.4 mg • Vitamin C 300 mg • Vitamin B6 (Pyridoxine) 4 mg • Vitamin B12 12 mcg • Zinc 50 mg.

***Mood Aid Formula* - Nature's Way**
Each capsule contains: Korean Ginseng dried extract 33.3 mg • L-5 Hydroxytryptophan (Griffonia bean extract) 3.33 mg • Niacin (Vitamin B3) 3.33 mg • Riboflavin (Vitamin B2) 284 mcg • Scullcap herb 100 mg • St. John's Wort dried extract (0.3% Dianthrones measures as Hypercin) 300 mg • Thiamine (Vitamin B1) 350 mcg • Vitamin B12 (Cyanocobalamin) 1 mcg • Vitamin B6 (Pyridoxine HCl) 330 mcg. Other Ingredients: Gelatin, Magnesium Stearate, Millet.

***Mood Balance* - Source Naturals**
Each three tablets contain: Vitamin C (as zinc ascorbate) 54 mg • Thiamin (vitamin B1) 22 mg • Riboflavin (vitamin B2) 25 mg • Niacinamide 50 mg • Vitamin B6 (as pyridoxine HCl) 50 mg • Folate (as folic acid) 400 mcg • Vitamin B12 (as cyanocobalamin) 30 mcg • Biotin 300 mcg • Pantothenic Acid (as calcium d-pantothenate) 25 mg • Magnesium (as magnesium oxide & taurinate) 194 mg • Zinc (zinc ascorbate) 10 mg • Manganese (as manganese citrate) 3 mg • St. John's Wort (0.3%, yielding 2.7 mg hypericin) 900 mg • L-Tyrosine 200 mg • Lemon Balm leaf 100 mg • Valerian root extract 100 mg • L-Phenylalanine 100 mg • Taurine (as magnesium taurinate) 87 mg • Kava root extract (30%, yielding 26 mg kavalactones) 85 mg • DMAE (as bitartrate) 60 mg • N-Acetyl L-Tyrosine 50 mg.

***Mood Enhance - Wellzymes* - Enzymes, Inc.**
Each capsule contains: n-zimes Proprietary Enzyme Blend 15 mg: pHysioProtease (41,440 pHysio-U), CereCalase Plus • Proprietary Herbal Blend 205 mg: St. John's Wort herb extract (standardized to contain 0.3% hypericin), Ginkgo Biloba leaf extract (standardized to contain 24% ginkgolides), Oat Straw extract (equivalent to 200 mg raw herb), Rice Bran. Other Ingredients: Plant Cellulose, Water.

***Mood Enhancer* - Clinician's Choice**
Three tablets contain: Valerian root 300 mg • St. John's Wort extract (std. 0.3% hypericin) 300 mg • Chamomile flowers 300 mg • L-Tyrosine 30 mg • Proprietary Blend 15 mg: Passion Flower, Sage leaves, Isoflavones, Grape powder, Acetyl-L-Carnitine.

***Mood Mender* - Celestial Seasonings**
Two capsules contain: Vitamin B6 (as pyridoxine HCL) 6 mg • Folic Acid 200 mcg • Vitamin B12 (as cyanocobalamin) 12 mcg • Selenium (as methionine chelate) 140 mcg • Chromium (as polynicotinate) 120 mcg • Proprietary Blend 1930 mg: St. John's Wort (leaf,stem,flower), St. John's Wort (standardized extract), Siberian Ginseng (root), Siberian Ginseng (standardized extract). Other Ingredients: May contain one or more of the following: Dicalcium phosphate, gelatin, rice flour, stearic acid, magnesium stearate, and silicon dioxide.

***Mood Support with St. John's Wort* - Natrol**
One capsule contains: Guaranteed Potency St. John's Wort supplying 0.3% Hypericin 300 mg • Ginseng supplying 8% Ginsenosides 100 mg • L-Tyrosine 50 mg • Lemon Balm 25 mg • DMAE (Di Methyl Amino Ethanol Bitartrate) 25 mg • Vitamin E (d-Alpha Tocopheryl Acetate) 30 IU • Folic Acid 400 mcg • Vitamin B12 (Cyanocobal-amin) 50 mcg • Selenium (l-Selenomethionine) 25 mcg. Other Ingredients: Silica, Magnesium Stearate, Gelatin.

***Mood Sync* - Pain & Stress Center**
Each capsule contains: St. John's Wort 175 mg • GABA 125 mg • Taurine 100 mg • Glutamine 75 mg • 5-HTP 25 mg • Vitamin B6 (Pyridoxine HCl) 5 mg.

***MoodPlex* - PharmAssure**
Three capsules contain: St. John's Wort with Flowers Extract (Hypericum perforatum; 0.3% Hypericin=2.7mg) 900 mg • Griffonia Simplicifolia Seed Extract (20% 5-Hydroxy-Tryptopan=20 mg) 100 mg • D,L-Phenylalanine 100 mg. Other Ingredients: Cellulose, Gelatin, Calcium Carbonate.

***MoodPro* - HealthMinded**
Three capsules contain: Vitamin B1 (thiamine) 60 mg • Vitamin B2 (riboflavin) 45 mg • Vitamin B3 (niacin) 30 mg • Vitamin B6 (pyridoxine) 60 mg • Vitamin B9 (folic acid) 390 mcg • Vitamin B12 150 mcg • 5-HTP 30 mg • DHA 60 mg • Ginkgo Biloba 90 mg • St. John's Wort (3%) 900 mg • MoodPro Proprietary Blend 105 mg: Inositol, Calcium Citrate, Ascorbic Acid, Lemon Balm, Basil, Cayenne, Clove Oil. Other Ingredients: Stearic Acid, Magnesium Stearate.

***Mor-Andro 200* - OSMO Therapy**
Each capsule contains: 4-Androstene-3Beta,17Beta-Diol (androdiol) 100 mg • 4-Androstene-3,17-Dione (androstenedione) 100 mg • Elemental Zinc Gluconate 5 mg • Niacin (nicotinic acid) 20 mg.
See Editor's Note No. 47, page 2058.

***More* - Puritan's Pride**
Six tablets contain: Vitamins: Vitamin A 10,000 IU • Vitamin C (w/ Rose Hips) 500 mg • Vitamin D 400 IU •Vitamin E 100 IU • Thiamine (B-1) 10 mg • Riboflavin (B-2) 15 mg • Niacinamide (B-3) 100 mg • Vitamin B-6 10 mg • Vitamin B-12 25 mcg • Biotin 150 mcg • Choline Bitartrate 250 mg • Folic Acid 400 mcg • Inositol 25 mg • PABA 30 mg • Pantothenic Acid 100 mg. Minerals: Calcium 750 mg • Copper 2 mg • Iodine 0.15 mg • Iron 30 mg • Magnesium 40 mg • Manganese 5 mg • Phosphorus 350 mg • Potassium 50 mg • Sodium 0.3 mg • Zinc 30 mg • Trace amounts of chlorine, flourine, sulphur, silicon, molybdenum, boron, etc. Amino Acids (from yeast and liver): Arginine 6.6 mg • Cysteine 2.8 mg • Glutamic Acid 8 mg • Histidine 3.2 mg • Isoleucine 11 mg • Leucine 12.4 mg • Lysine 13 mg • Methionine 4.2 mg • Phenylalanine 7.4 mg • Threonine 2.25 mg • Tyrosine 9.2 mg • Valine 8.8 mg. Additional Ingredients: Algin 150 mg • Bee Pollen 10 mg • Desiccated Liver 100 mg • Hesperidin 25 mg • Lemon Bioflavonoid complex 50 mg • Red Bone Marrow 60 mg • Rutin 40 mg • Yeast 100 mg. Formulated in a natural food base of vegetable concentrate of watercress, tomato, onion, celery, celery seeds and garlic. Plus lecithin, papain, pepsin, chlorophyll, EFA's, and many others.
See Editor's Note No. 14.

More Milk **-** Motherlove Herbal Co.
Each 2 oz bottle contains: Blessed Thistle • Nettles • Fennel seed. In a base of certified kosher alcohol and glycerin.

More Milk Plus **-** Motherlove Herbal Co.
Each 2 oz bottle contains: Fenugreek • Blessed Thistle • Nettles • Fennel seed. In a base of certified kosher alcohol and glycerin.

More Milk Two **-** Motherlove Herbal Co.
Each 2 oz bottle contains: Raspberry leaf • Nettles • Alfalfa. In a base of certified kosher alcohol and glycerin.

More Than A Diet **-** American Health
Three duotabs contain: Chromium (as chromium picolinate and chromium polynicotinate) 100 mcg • Lipoactive Factors Proprietary Blend 344 mg: L-Carnitine Tartrate, Pyruvate, Inositol, Choline Bitartrate, L-Methionine, Lecithin, Phosphatidyl Choline (PC), Phosphatidyl Serine (PS), Taurine, Betaine Hydrochloride, Vanadium (as vanadyl sulfate) • Amino Factors Proprietary Blend 350 mg: Creatine Monohydrate, L-Lysine, L-Leucine, Glycine, Glutathione, L-Phenylalanine, L-Tyrosine • Herbal Thermo Factors Proprietary Blend 232 mg: Capsicum fruit, Ginger root, Licorice root, Mustard seed, Green Tea leaf, American Ginseng root, Cinnamon bark, Korean Ginseng root, Siberian Ginseng root, Piper Longum fruit, Guggulipid, Suma root, Schizandra fruit, Astragalus root, Hawthorn berry, Kola nut seed, Guarana seed • Fiber Factors Proprietary Blend 500 mg: Oat Bran Fiber, Citrus Pectin Fiber, Pulp Cellulose, Vegetable Cellulose, Beet Fiber • Herbal Fluid Factors Proprietary Blend 190 mg: Uva Ursi leaf, Buchu leaf, Couch Grass rhizome, Corn Silk stigma, Hydrangea root, Juniper berry • Essential Fatty Acids Factors Proprietary Blend 90 mg: Gotu Kola (aerial), Milk Thistle seed (silymarin), Chickweed (aerial), Borage seed oil, Black Currant fruit, Primrose seed oil, Flax seed oil, Conjugated Linoleic Acid, Dandelion root • Appetite Factors Proprietary Blend 550 mg: Citrimax HCA (from garcinia cambogia), Chitosan (shellfish fiber), OP's (wheat oligio peptides), Gymnema Sylvestre leaf, Apple Cider Vinegar, Phaseolus Vulgaris pods • Green Super Food Factors Proprietary Blend 500 mg: Spirulina, Chlorella, Barley Grass juice, Wheat Grass, Kelp, Alfalfa leaf • Enzyme Factors Proprietary Blend 220 mg: Coenzyme Q-10, Bromelain, Lipase, Protease, Cellulase, Aspergillus Niger, Aspergillus Oryzae, Fructooligosaccharides (FOS), Pancreatin • Fruit Extract Factors Proprietary Blend 67.5 mg: Apple, Apricot, Banana, Cranberry, Orange, Lemon, Lime, Papaya, Pineapple, Strawberry, Watermelon, Grapeseed (OPC), Grapefruit • Vegetable Extract Factors Proprietary Blend 50 mg: Cabbage, Celery, Broccoli, Brussel Sprouts, Yams, Carrots, Kale, Collard Greens, Spinach, Cauliflower. Other Ingredients: Dicalcium Phosphate, Cellulose (plant origin), Vegetable Magnesium Stearate, Xanthan Gum, Cellulose Coating, Silica.

MotherNature Saw Palmetto Berry Extract **-** Mother Nature
Each softgel contains: Saw Palmetto extract (serenoa repens) 160 mg. Other Ingredients: Olive Oil, Gelatin, Glycerin, Water.

Mother's Milk **-** Traditional Medicinals
Fennel seed • Anise seed • Coriander seed • Spearmint leaf • Lemongrass leaf • Lemon Verbena leaf • Althea root • Blessed Thistle leaf • Fenugreek seed.

Motion Mate **-** Nature's Way
Two capsules contain: Ginger • Hyssop herb • Meadowsweet herb • Peppermint leaves • Red Raspberry leaves. Other Ingredients: Gelatin, Magnesium Stearate, Millet.

Motion Sickness **-** Hyland's
Two tablets contain: Nux Vomica 6X • Tabacum 6X • Petroleum 12X • Cocculus Indicus 30X. Base: Lactose USP.
See Editor's Note No. 1, page 2053.

Motion Sickness Remedy **-** PhytoPharmica
Twenty drops contain: Cocculus indicus 8x • Plumbum aceticum 8x • Argentum nitricum 6x • Glonoinum 6x • Zincum valerianicum 6x • Belladonna 4x • Nux vomica 4x • Pulsatilla 4x • Vinca minor 3x • Artemesia Vulgaris 1x. In a base of 45% USP alcohol by volume.
See Editor's Note No. 1, page 2053.

Mouth-Mend **-** The Herbalist
Echinacea root • Golden Seal root • Myrrh Gum • Propolis • Spilanthes herb • Yerba Mansa root.

Movana **-** Boehringer Ingelheim
Each tablet contains: St. John's Wort flower & leaves extract WS-5572 (Stabilized minimum hyperforin content 3%, Standardized Hypericin content 0.3%) 300 mg. Other Ingredients: Microcrystalline Cellulose • Corn Starch • Croscarmellose Sodium • Hydroxypropyl Methylcellulose, PEG-4000 • Magnesium Stearate • Silicon Dioxide • Ascorbic Acid • Synthetic Iron Oxide • Titanium Dioxide • Talc • Vanillin.

Move Free **-** Schiff
One caplet contains: Glucosamine Complex [Includes: Glucosamine Hydrochloride, N-Acetyl D-Glucosamine, and Glucosamine Sulfate] 500 mg • Chondroitin Sulfate (Bovine Cartilage Sources) 400 mg. Other ingredients: Cellulose, Coating (Titanium Dioxide, Dextrose, Hydroxypropyl methylcellulose, Polyethelyne Glycol, Sodium Carboxymethyl Cellulose, Mineral Oil, Sodium Citrate, Polysorbate 80, Dextrin), Copolyvidone, Silicon Dioxide, Magnesium Stearate.
See Editor's Note No. 15, page 2055.

Move Free Plus Calcium **-** Schiff
Each tablet contains: Vitamin D (as cholecalciferol) 133 IU • Calcium (as calcium carbonate) 167 mg • Proprietary Blend 500 mg: Glucosamine Hydrochloride, N-Acetyl D-Glucosamine, Glucosamine Sulfate (potassium salt) • Chondroitin Sulfate 400 mg. Other Ingredients: Coating (titanium dioxide [color], dextrose, hydrosypropyl cellulose, triacetin, polyethylene glycol), Maltodextrin, Croscarmellose Sodium, Magnesium Stearate.
See Editor's Note No. 15, page 2055.

Move Free Plus MSM **-** Schiff
Four tablets contain: Proprietary Blend 1.5 g: Glucosamine Hydrochloride, N-Acetyl D-Glucosamine, Glucosamine Sulfate • Chondroitin 1.2 g • MSM (methylsulfonylmethane) 1.5 g. Other Ingredients: Cellulose, Coating (titanium dioxide, polydextrose, hydroxypropyl methylcellulose, triacetin, polyethylene glycol), Copolyvidone, Silicon Dioxide, Magnesium Stearate, Potassium Chloride.
See Editor's Note No. 15, page 2055.

Move Free Plus SAMe **-** Schiff
Three tablets contain: Proprietary Blend 1.5 g: N-Acetyl D-Glucosamine, D-Glucosamine Sulfate, D-Glucosamine Hydrochloride • S-Adenosyl-L-Methionine (SAMe, as s-adenosyl-l-methionine disulfate tosylate) 400 mg. Other Ingredients: Cellulose, Hydroxypropyl Methylcellulose Phithalate, Titanium Dioxide, Mannitol, Stearic Acid, Triacetin, Sodium Starch Glycolate, Modified Cellulose Gum, Citric Acid, Silicon Dioxide, Potassium Chloride.

Move Free Triple Strength **-** Schiff
Two gelcaps contain: Proprietary Blend 1.5 g: Glucosamine Hydrochloride, N-Acetyl D-Glucosamine, Glucosamine Sulfate • Chondroitin 1.2 g. Other Ingredients: Gelatin Coating (gelatin, water, glycerin, titanium dioxide, caramel color), Cellulose, Coating (polydextrose, hydroxypropyl methylcellulose, titanium dioxide, polydextrose, triacetin, polyethylene glycol), Copolyvidone, Silicon Dioxide, Magnesium Stearate, Potassium Chloride.
See Editor's Note No. 15, page 2055.

MP Max **-** E'OLA
Two capsules contain: Saw Palmetto (berry) 8:1 604 mg • Proprietary Blend 350 mg: Pumpkin (seed), Pygeum (bark), Tomato (fruit), Nettle (root). Other Ingredients: Gelatin, Millet Flour, Magnesium Stearate, Silicon Dioxide.

MPF **-** Progressive Labs
Six capsules contain: Vitamin A 25000 IU • Vitamin E 180 IU • Folic Acid 780 mcg • Zinc Picolinate 60 mg • L-Glutamine 1500 mg • N-Acetyl Glucosamine 1050 mg • Gamma Oryzanol 360 mg • Cat's Claw (Uncaria tomentosa) 450 mg.

MPRX **-** AST Sports Science
Two capsules contain: Vitamin B6 22 mg • Magnesium (as magnesium salicylate) 100 mg • Pro-Therm Green Tea leaf extract (standardized for epigallocatechin gallate EGCG, l-phenylalanine, l-tyrosine, caffeine as caffeine anhydrous and theobromine HCl) 1400 mg.

MRP-44 **-** Human Development Technologies (HDT)
Each serving contains: L-Glutamine 2 g • Taurine 1 g • MRP1000 (Micro Ultra Filtered Whey Protein concentrate • Egg Albumen • Micro Ultra Filtered Whey Protein Isolate, Ion Exchanged Whey Protein Isolate) • Maltodextrin • natural & artificial flavorings • L-Glutamine • Di-Calcium Phosphate • Taurine • Inulin • Cellulose Gum • Xanthan Gum • Magnesium Oxide • Lecithin • Fructose • Stevia • Acesulfame Potassium • Ascorbic Acid • Vitamin A Acetate • Vitamin E Acetate • Niacinamide • Iron Electrolytic • Zinc Oxide • D-Calcium Pantothenate • Ergocalciferol • Pyridoxine HCL • Copper Gluconate • Riboflavin • Thiamine Mononitrate • Folic Acid • Biotin • Potassium Ionide • Cyanocobalamin.

MSM **-** Enzymatic Therapy
Each tablet contains: MSM (methylsulfonylmethane) 1000 mg. Other Ingredients: Cellulose, Modified Cellulose, Titanium Dioxide Color, Magnesium Stearate, Lecithin, Carnauba Wax.

MSM **-** Metabolic Response Modifiers
Each capsule contains: MSM (methyl-sulfonyl-methane) 750 mg.

MSM **-** Natural Balance
Each tablet contains: MSM (methylsulfonylmethane) 1000 mg. Other Ingredients: Cellulose, Silicon Dioxide, Stearic Acid, Magnesium Stearate.

MSM **-** Nature's Bounty
Each capsule contains: Methylsulfonylmethane (255 mg organic sulfur) 750 mg. Other Ingredients: Dicalcium Phosphate, Gelatin, Vegetable Magnesium Stearate, Silica.

MSM **-** Now
Two capsules contain: Lignisul MSM (methylsulphonylmethane) 2 g. Other Ingredients: Magnesium Stearate, Stearic Acid.

MSM **-** Olympian Labs
Each capsule contains: MSM (methylsulfonylmethane) 500 mg.

MSM **-** PhytoPharmica
Each tablet contains: MSM (methylsulfonylmethane) 1000 mg.

MSM **-** Quest
Each caplet contains: Lignisul brand MSM 1000 mg. Other Ingredients: Croscarmellose Sodium, Silicon Dioxide, and Magnesium Stearate.

MSM **-** Swanson
Two capsules contain: OptiMSM Methylsulfonylmethane 1 g.

MSM **-** Trimedica
Each capsule contains: Methylsulfonylmethane 99.9% • Water 0.1%.

MSM & Glucosamine Cream **-** PhysioLogics
Purified Water • Stearic Acid • MSM (methylsulfonylmethane) • Cetyl Alcohol • Glyceryl Stearate • Polysorbate 80 • Cetearyl Alcohol • Aloe Vera gel (aloe barbadensis, leaf) • Tocopheryl Acetate • Fragrance • Glucosamine Sulfate • Ceteareth-20 • Triethanolamine • Diazolidinyl Urea • Sweet Almond oil (prunus amygdalus dulcus) • Carbomer • Methylparaben • Propylparaben • Sodium Benzoate • Jojoba oil (simmondsia chinensis) • Cayenne extract (capsicum frutescens) • Arnica extract (arnica montana) • Matricaria Recutita extract (chamomilla recutita) • Ginger extract (zingiber officinale) • Comfrey extract (symphytum officinale).

MSM (OptoMSM) **-** NSI - Nutraceutical Sciences Institute
Each capsule contains: MSM (methyl sulfonyl methane, OptiMSM) 1000 mg.

MSM 1000 **-** Aspen Group, Inc.
Each capsule contains: 100% pure MSM (methyl sulfonyl methane) 1000 mg.

MSM 1000 - GNC A-Z **-** GNC
Each capsule contains: MSM (Methylsulfonyl-Methane) 1000 mg. Other Ingredients: Gelatin.

MSM 1000 **-** Jamieson
Each caplet contains: MSM (Methylsulfonylmethane) 1000 mg.

MSM 1000 **-** Jarrow Formulas
Each capsule contains: Methylsulfonylmethane 1000 mg. Other Ingredients: Magnesium Stearate, Gelatin.

MSM 1000 MG **-** PhysioLogics
Each capsule contains: MSM (methylsulfonylmethane, organic sulfur 340 mg) 1000 mg. Other Ingredients: Gelatin, Calcium Stearate.

MSM 1500 - GNC A-Z **-** GNC
Each tablet contains: MSM (methylsulfonyl-methane) 1500 mg. Other Ingredients: Cellulose, Titanium Dioxide, Caramel Color, Imitation Vanilla.

MSM 1500 mg **-** Vitamin World
Each tablet contains: Methylsulfonylmethane 1500 mg. Other Ingredients: Dicalcium Phosphate, Silica, Vegetable Magnesium Stearate, Cellulose Coating.

MSM 500 / Glucosamine 500 - GNC A-Z **-** GNC
Each capsule contains: MSM (Methylsulfonyl-Methane) 500 mg • Glucosamine Sulfate (as D-Glucosamine Sulfate .2KCl) 500 mg. Other Ingredients: Gelatin.

MSM 500 mg **-** PhysioLogics
Each capsule contains: Methylsulfonylmethane (organic sulfur 170 mg) 500 mg. Other Ingredients: Gelatin, Vegetable Magnesium Stearate, Silica.

MSM 500 mg **-** Rexall - Sundown
Two tablets contain: Calcium 36 mg • MSM (methylsulfonylmethane) 1 g. Other Ingredients: Dicalcium Phosphate, Stearic Acid, Silica.

MSM Caps **-** Optimum Nutrition
Each capsule contains: Methylsulfonylmethane (as glucosamine sulfate potassium) 1 g. Other Ingredients: Gelatin, Magnesium Stearate.

MSM cream **-** Vitamin World
Water • MSM (methylsulfonylmethane) • Stearic Acid • Propylene Glycol • Cetyl Alcohol • Glyceryl Stearate • Cetyl Esters • Polysorbate 80 • Quaternium-15 • Triethanolamine • Magnesium Aluminum Silicate • Sunflower oil • Jojoba oil • Sweet Almond oil • Methylparaben • Carbomer • Propylparaben • Disodium EDTA • Panthenol • Hydrolyzed Collagen • Korean Ginseng (panax ginseng) • Tocopheryl Acetate • Cholecalciferol • Rosemary oil • Essential Oil Blend: Lavender oil (lavendula angustifolia), Petitgrain oil (citrus aurantium), Thyme oil (thymus vulgaris), Rosemary oil (rosmarinus officinalis), Chamomile oil (matricaria chamomilla), Sweet Birch oil (betula lenta) • Aloe Vera Gel (aloe barbadensis) • Ginkgo Biloba (ginkgo biloba) • Lecithin • Retinyl Palmitate.

MSM Extra Strength **-** Olympian Labs
Each tablet contains: MSM (methylsulfonylmethane) 1300 mg.

MSM Formula with White Willow **-** Health Smart Vitamins
Two capsules contain: Vitamin C (as ascorbyl palmitate) 30 mg • MSM (methylsulfonylmethane) 500 mg • Chondroitin Sulfate 300 mg

• White Willow bark (3% salicins, 1.5 mg) 50 mg.
See Editor's Note No. 15, page 2055.

MSM Liquid - Trimedica
Each teaspoon contains: MSM 390 mg. Other Ingredients: Purified Water.

MSM Plex - PharmAssure
Each capsule contains: MSM (methyl-sulfonyl-methane) 500 mg • Glucosamine Sulfate 500 mg.

MSM Plus - Progressive Labs
Each capsule contains: Vitamin C (as magnesium ascorbate) 100 mg • Magnesium (as magnesium ascorbate) 7 mg • Methyl Sulfonyl Methane (MSM) 800 mg.

MSM Plus Glucosamine - Optimum Nutrition
Each tablet contains: Methylsulfonylmethane (MSM) 1 g • Glucosamine (as glucosamine sulfate potassium) 500 mg. Other Ingredients: Pharmaceutical Glaze, Stearic Acid, Magnesium Stearate, CrosCarmellose Sodium (disintegrant).

MSM Powder - Vitamin World
One-half teaspoon contains: MSM (methylsulfonylmethane, 1023 mg organic sulfur) 3000 mg. Other Ingredients: Silica.

MSM Powder - Natural Balance
Each teaspoon contains: Vitamin C (as ascorbic acid) 240 mg • MSM (methylsulfonylmethane) 4000 mg. Other Ingredients: Silicon Dioxide.

MSM Rejuvenator - Progressive Labs
Ingredients: Stabilized Aloe Vera gel • Methylsulfonyl Methane • Glycerine • Caprylic/Capric Triglycerides • Jojoba oil • Polyquanterium-32 (colloidal polymers) • Evening Primrose oil • Cetyl Alcohol • Steryl Alcohol • Tetrahexyldecyl Ascorbate (lipid soluble Vitamin C) • Tocopheryl Acetate (Vitamin E) • Ginseng extract • Chamomile extract. Extracts of: Grape seed, Willow bark, Calendula, White Lily, Japanese Green Tea, Gum Mint, Cucumber, Soapbark, Balm of Gilead, Bee Propolis: Betaglucans. Essential oils of: Lemongrass, Rosemary, Sage, Cedarwood, Tetrasodium EDTA, Methylparaben, Propylparben, Diazolidiny Lurea.

MSM Ultra Caplets - FreeLife International
Each caplet contains: Vitamin C (from glycerol flovone-bound ascorbic and isoascorbic acids) 60 mg • Methylsulfonylmethane (MSM) 1000 mg • Proprietary Blend 100 mg: Ascorbic Acid, Isoascorbic Acid, Citrus Glycosyl Flavones (cirantin, isosakuranetin-7-beta-rutinoside, narirutin, eriocitrin, nobiletin, tangeretin, hepatamethoxyflavone). Other Ingredients: Cellulose, Cellulose Gum, Vegetable Stearic Acid, Silica, Vegetable Magnesium Stearate, Vita-Coat (vegetable resin, alpha-lipoic acid).

MSM Ultra Powder - FreeLife International
One-half teaspoon (2.24 g) contains: Vitamin C (from glycosyl flavone-bound ascorbic and isoascorbic acids 200 mg) 120 mg • MSM (methylsulfonylmethane) 2000 mg • Propreitary Blend 200 mg: Ascorbic Acid, Sodium Isoascorbate, Citrus Glycosyl Flavones • Stevia leaf extract (stevia rebaudiana) 40 mg.

MSM with Glucosamine Cream - Vitamin World
Purified Water • Stearic Acid • MSM (methylsulfonylmethane) • Cetyl Alcohol • Glyceryl Stearate • Propylene Glycol • Polysorbate 80 • Cetearyl Alcohol • Aloe Vera Gel (aloe barbadensis leaf) • Tocopheryl Acetate • Fragrance • Glucosamine Sulfate • Ceteareth-20 • Diazolidinyl Urea • Triethanolamine • Sweet Almond oil (prunus amygdalus dulcis) • Carbomer • Methylparaben • Propylparaben • Sodium Benzoate • Jojoba oil (simmondsia chinensis) • Capsicum Frutescens extract • Arnica Montana extract • Chamomilla Recutita extract (matricaria) • Ginger extract (zingiber officinale) • Comfrey extract (symphytum officinale).

MSM with Glucosamine Sulfate - PhytoPharmica
Each capsule contains: Chloride (from glucosamine sulfate) 78 mg • Sodium (from glucosamine sulfate) 50 mg • Stabilized Glucosamine Sulfate 500 mg • MSM (methylsulfonylmethane) 250 mg.

MSM with GS-500 (OptiMSM) - Enzymatic Therapy
Each capsule contains: Chloride (from glucosamine sulfate) 78 mg • Sodium (from glucosamine sulfate) 50 mg • Glucosamine Sulfate (stabilized) 500 mg • MSM (methylsulfonylmethane) 250 mg. Other Ingredients: Gelatin, Magnesium Stearate, Silicon Dioxide, Titanium Dioxide Color.

MSM, Methylsulfonylmethane - Allergy Research Group
Each capsule contains: Methylsulfonylmethane 500 mg • Molybdenum 10 mcg. Other Ingredients: Cellulose, Silicon Dioxide, Stearic Acid.

MSM, Methylsulfonylmethane - NutriCology
Each capsule contains: Methylsulfonylmethane 500 mg • Molybdenum 10 mcg. Other Ingredients: Cellulose, Silicon Dioxide, Stearic Acid.

Mucho Mate - Traditional Medicinals
Green & Roasted Yerba Mate leaf • Ginger rhizome • Lemon peel • natural Lemon flavor • Stevia leaf.

Mucoplex - Progressive Labs
Each capsule contains: Comfrey root (Symphytum officinale) 225 mg • Pepsin (1:3000) 65 mg • Bromelain 50 mg • Raw Duodenum 10 mg.
See Editor's Note No. 14.

Muco-Plex - Enzymatic Therapy
Two tablets contain: Niacin 30 mg • Vitamin B6 (Pyridoxine HCl) 10 mg • Iodine (Potassium Iodide) 75 mcg. Other Ingredients: Marshmallow extract 8:1 (Althea officinalis) mucilage content 30-40% 450 mg • Raw Duodenum Tissue 450 mg • Pancreatic Enzymes 3X 100 mg • L-Methionine 100 mg • Gastric Mucin powder 100 mg • Pepsin 1:10000 65 mg • Pituitary extract 15 mg. In a base of Crude Licorice extract (glycyrrhiza glabra) & derivatives with an organically bound Allantoin-Methionine (comfrey) Complex, Acidophilus, & Aloe Vera.
See Editor's Note No. 14.

Mullein Lobelia - Atrium Inc.
Each capsule contains: Mullein leaves 375 mg • Lobelia 125 mg.

Multi Caps - Progressive Labs
Three capsules contain: Vitamin A 10000 IU • Vitamin C 120 mg • Vitamin D (as Vitamin D3) 400 IU • Vitamin E 15 IU • Thiamin (Vitamin B1) 10 mg • Riboflavin (Vitamin B2) 10 mg • Niacinamide 100 mg • Vitamin B6 10 mg • Folate (folic acid) 400 mcg • Vitamin B12 50 mcg • Biotin 25 mcg • Pantothenic Acid 40 mg • Calcium 200 mg • Iron 15 mg • Magnesium 100 mg • Zinc 15 mg • Selenium 25 mcg • Manganese 20 mg • Iodine 150 mcg • Chromium 20 mcg • Potassium 99 mg • Choline 75 mg • Inositol 75 mg • PABA 30 mg • Citrus bioflavonoids 100 mg • Rutin 25 mg • Hesperidin 25 mg • Glutamic Acid 30 mg • L-Lysine 50 mg • DL-Methionine 50 mg • Pancreatin 60 mg • Bile Salts 5 mg • RNA (Brain) 50 mg • Unsaturated Fatty Acids 50 mg. Other Ingredients: Rose Hips, Ginseng, Goldenseal, Fo Ti Teng, Gotu Kola, Sarsaparilla, Watercress, Kelp, Green Cabbage, Rice polishings, Raw Stomach substance (not an extract), Alfalfa, Parsley, Papaya.
See Editor's Note No. 31, page 2056.

Multi Carotene - Puritan's Pride
Each softgel contains: Beta Carotene (Pro-Vitamin A Activity) 25,000 IU • Alpha-Carotene 1 mg • Lycopene 5 mg • Lutein 6 mg • Zeaxanthin 0.3 mg.

Multi Chelate - Progressive Labs
Six capsules contain: Calcium 500 mg • Iron 15 mg • Magnesium 250 mg • Zinc 10 mg • Iodine 150 mcg • Selenium 25 mcg • Copper 1 mg • Manganese 10 mg • Chromium 50 mcg • Molybdenum 150 mcg • Potassium 99 mg • Vanadium 150 mcg • Silicone 2 mg • Raw Glandular concentrate 200 mg. The raw glandular materal in this

product is prepared by a special process which does not exceed physiological temperature (37 Celcius). Guaranteed free of chemical pesticides and synthetic hormones.
See Editor's Note No. 14, page 2055.

Multi Fiber Complex **-** Naturade
Each capsule contains: Psyllium seed husk 400 mg • Guar Gum 50 mg • Slippery Elm bark 50 mg • Licorice root 50 mg • Apple Pectin 50 mg • Grapefruit Pectin 50 mg • Glucomannan 50 mg. Other Ingredients: Magnesium Stearate, Silicon Dioxide, Gelatin.

Multi for Seniors **-** Health Center for Better Living
Each tablet contains: Vitamin A (as retinyl acetate and beta-carotene) 6,000 IU • Vitamin C (as ascorbic acid) 60 mg • Vitamin D (as cholecalciferol) 400 IU • Vitamin E (as dl-alpha-tocopheryl acetate) 45 IU • Vitamin K (as phytonadione) 10 mcg • Vitamin B1 (as thiamin mononitrate) 1.5 mg • Vitamin B2 (as riboflavin) 1.7 mg • Niacin (as niacinarnide) 20 mg • Vitamin B6 (as pyridoxine HCl) 3 mg • Folate (as folic acid) 200 mcg • Vitamin B12 (as cyanocobalamin) 25 mcg • Biotin 30 mcg • Pantothenic Acid (as D-calcium patothenate) 10 mg • Calcium (as calcium carbonate and dicalcium phosphate) 200 mg • Iron (as ferrous fumarate) 9 mcg • Phosphorus (as dicalcium phosphate) 48 mcg • Iodine (as potassium iodide) 150 mcg • Magnesium (as magnesium oxide) 100 mg • Zinc (as zinc oxide) 15 mg • Selenium (as sodium selenate) 25 mcg • Copper (as cupric oxide) 2 mg • Manganese (as manganese sulfate (2.5 mg) • Chromium (as chromium amino acid chelate) 100 mcg • Molybdenum (as sodium molybdate) 25 mcg • Potassium (as postassium chloride)80 mg • Nickel (as nickelous sulfate) 5 mcg • Silicon (as sodium metasilicate) 10 mcg • Vanadium (as sodium metavanadate) 10 mcg.

Multi Ginseng 1000 mg, Concentrated - GNC Herbal Plus **-** GNC
Each capsule contains: Multi-Ginseng Root (from 50 mg of multi-ginseng extract 20:1) 1000 mg. Other Ingredients: Soybean Oil, Gelatin, Glycerin, Caramel Color, Titanium Dioxide (natural mineral whitener).

Multi Mega Minerals **-** GNC
Two tablets contain: Vitamin D (as cholecalciferol) 400 IU • Calcium (as calcium carbonate) 1000 mg • Iron (as hydrolyzed protein chelate) 18 mg • Iodine (as kelp) 150 mg • Magnesium (as magnesium oxide) 500 mg • Zinc (as hydrolyzed protein chelate) 22.5 mg • Copper (as hydrolyzed protein chelate) 3 mg • Manganese (as hydrolyzed protein chelate) 10 mcg • Chromium (as hydrolyzed protein chelate) 100 mcg • Chloride (as potassium chloride) 90 mg • Potassium (as potassium chloride) 95 mg • Betaine Hydrochloride 100 mg. Other Ingredients: Cellulose.

Multi Mineral Citrate Complete **-** Puritan's Pride
Four capsules contain: Calcium (Citrate, Carbonate, Aspartate) 1000 mg • Magnesium (Citrate, Oxide, Aspartate) 500 mg • Potassium 99 mg • Zinc 50 mg • Iron (Fumarate) 10 mg • Manganese 10 mg • Copper (Gluconate) 2 mg • Selenium (Chelate) 100 mcg • Chromium (Chelate) 200 mcg • Molybdenum (Chelate) 100 mcg • Silica (Chelate) 10 mcg • Boron 3 mg.

Multi Pro 32X **-** AST Sports Science
Each caplet contains: Vitamin A (as beta carotene/vitamin A acetate) 10,000 IU • Vitamin C (as ascorbic acid) 200 mg • Vitamin D (as vitamin D3) 400 IU • Vitamin E (as DL-alpha tocopheryls) 60 IU • Vitamin K 25 mcg • Thiamin 30 mg • Riboflavin 30 mg • Niacin (as niacinamide) 30 mg • Vitamin B6 30 mg • Folic Acid 400 mcg • Vitamin B12 30 mcg • Biotin 60 mcg • Pantothenic Acid 30 mg • Calcium (as di-calcium phosphate) 75 mg • Iron (as ferrous fumarate) 18 mg • Phosphorus (as di-calcium phosphate) 45 mg • Iodine (as potassium iodine) 150 mcg • Magnesium (as magnesium oxide) 100 mg • Zinc (as zinc chelate) 30 mg • Selenium (as selenium chelate) 25 mcg • Copper (as copper chelate) 2 mg • Manganese (as manganese sulfate) 5 mg • Chromium (as chromium chelate) 25 mcg • Molybdenum (as molybdenum chelate) 25 mcg • Chloride (as potassium chloride) 36 mg • Potassium (as potassium chloride) 40 mg • Silicon 30 mg • Tin (as tin chelate) 10 mcg • Vanadium (as vanadium chelate) 10 mcg • Boron (as boron chelate) 150 mcg • Nickel (as nickel chelate) 25 mcg. Other Ingredients: Croscarmellose Sodium, Magnesium Stearate, Microcrystalline Cellulose.

Multi Ultra Mega - GNC A-Z **-** GNC
Each tablet contains: Vitamin A (50% as beta-carotene, 50% as acetate) 10,000 IU • Vitamin C (as ascorbic acid) 200 mg • Vitamin D (as cholecalciferol) 400 IU • Vitamin E (as d-alpha tocopheryl succinate) 100 IU • Thiamin (as thiamin mononitrate) 75 mg • Riboflavin 75 mg • Niacin (as niacinamide) 75 mg • Vitamin B6 (as pyridoxine hydrochloride) 75 mg • Folate, Folic Acid, Folacin, 400 mcg • Vitamin B12 (as cyanocobalamin) 75 mcg • Biotin 75 mcg • Pantothenic Acid (as calcium d-pantothenate) 75 mg • Calcium (as calcium carbonate) 100 mg • Iron (as ferrous fumarate) 18 mg • Iodine (as kelp) 150 mcg • Magnesium (as magnesium oxide) 7 mg • Zinc (as zinc oxide) 15 mg • Selenium (as hydrolyzed protein chelate) 10 mcg • Copper (as copper sulfate) 250 mcg • Manganese (as manganese sulfate) 6 mg • Chromium (as hydrolyzed protein chelate) 10 mcg • Molybdenum (as hydrolyzed protein chelate) 10 mcg • Potassium (as potassium chloride) 10 mg • Boron (as boron citrate) 100 mcg • Silica (as silicon dioxide) 10 mcg • Choline (as choline bitartrate) 35 mg • Inositol 75 mcg • Para-Aminobenzoic Acid (PABA) 75 mg • Trimethylglycine (TMG) 10 mg • Rutin powder 25 mg • Citrus Bioflavonoid Complex (as 6.25 mg citrus bioflavoniod complex 4x) 25 mg • Hesperidin Complex 5 mg • N-Acetyl-L-Cysteine (NAC) 500 mcg • Alpha-Lipoic Acid 1 mg • Green Tea leaves (camellia sinensis). Other Ingredients: Cellulose, Food Glaze, Rose Hips powder (rosina canina), Soy Protein, Papain, Alfalfa powder (medicagn sativa), Watercress powder (nasturtium officinale), Parsley herb powder (petroselinum crispum), Lecithin powder, Whole Brown Rice powder (oryza sativa).

Multi Ultra Mega Gold Timed Release **-** GNC
Two tablets contain: Vitamin A (75% as Betatene beta-Carotene; 25% as Acetate) 20,000 IU • Vitamin C (as Ascorbic Acid) 500 mg • Vitamin D (as Cholecalciferol) 400 IU • Vitamin E (as d-alpha Tocopheryl Succinate) 300 IU • Thiamin (as Thiamin Mononitrate) 100 mg • Riboflavin 100 mg • Niacin (as Niacinamide) 100 mg • Vitamin B6 (as Pyridoxine Hydrochloride) 100 mg • Folate, Folic Acid, Folacin 400 mcg • Vitamin B12 (as Cyanocobalamin) 150 mcg • Biotin 100 mcg • Pantothenic Acid (as Calcium d-Pantothenate) 100 mg • Calcium (as Calcium Carbonate) 50 mg • Iron (as Ferrous Fumarate) 10 mg • Iodine (as Kelp) 100 mcg • Magnesium (as Magnesium Oxide) 50 mg • Zinc (as Zinc Oxide) 15 mg • Selenium (as Selenium Yeast) 150 mcg • Copper (as Cupric Oxide) 2 mg • Manganese (as Manganese Gluconate) 10 mg • Chromium (as GTF Chromium Yeast) 150 mcg • Molybdenum (as Molybdenum Yeast) 150 mcg • Potassium (as Potassium Chloride) 10 mg • Boron (as Boron Gluconate) 1 mg • Chlorine Bitartrate 50 mg • Inositol 25 mg • Para-Aminobenzoic Acid 50 mg • Trimethylglycine (TMG) 25 mg • Citrus Bioflavonoid Complex 25 mg • Rutin powder 10 mg • Hesperidin Complex 5 mg • Quercetin Dihydrate 10 mg • Natural Carotenoid Complex 15 mg • N-Acetyl-L-cysteine (NAC) 10.5 mg • Amylase 10 mg • Lipase 5 mg • Protease 2 mg • Cellulase 5 mg • Lycopene 200 mcg • Alpha-lipoic Acid 4.5 mg • Green Tea leaves (Camellia sinensis) 15 mg. Other Ingredients: Cellulose, Vegetable Acetoglycerides, Titanium Dioxide, Chlorophyll.

Multi Ultra Mega Gold Without Iron **-** GNC
Two tablets contain: Vitamin A (75% as Betatene Beta-Carotene; 25% as Acetate) 20,000 IU • Vitamin C (as Ascorbic Acid) 500 mg • Vitamin D (as Cholecalciferol) 400 IU • Vitamin E (as d-alpha Tocopheryl Succinate) 300 IU • Thiamin (as Thiamin Mononitrate) 100 mg • Riboflavin 100 mg • Niacin (as Niacinamide) 100 mg • Vitamin B6 (as Pyridoxine Hydrochloride) 100 mg • Folate, Folic Acid, Folacin 400 mcg • Vitamin B12 (as Cyanocobalamin) 150 mcg • Biotin 100 mcg • Pantothenic Acid (as Calcium d-Pantothenate) 100 mg • Calcium (as Calcium Carbonate) 50 mg • Iodine (as Kelp) 100 mcg • Magnesium (as Magnesium Oxide) 50 mg • Zinc (as Zinc

Oxide) 15 mg • Selenium (as Selenium Yeast) 150 mcg • Copper (as Cupric Oxide) 2 mg • Manganese (as Manganese Gluconate) 10 mg • Chromium (as GTF Chromium Yeast) 100 mcg • Molybdenum (as Molybdenum Yeast) 150 mcg • Potassium (as Potassium Chloride) 10 mg • Boron (as Boron Gluconate) 1 mg • Chlorine Bitartrate 50 mg • Inositol 25 mg • Para-Aminobenzoic Acid (PABA) 50 mg • Trimethylglycine (TMG) 25 mg • Citrus Bioflavonoid Complex 25 mg • Rutin powder 10 mg • Hesperidin Complex 5 mg • Quercetin Dihydrate 10 mg • Natural Carotenoid Complex 15 mg • N-Acetyl-L-Cysteine (NAC) 10.5 mg • Amylase 10 mg • Lipase 5 mg • Protease 2 mg • Cellulase 5 mg • Lycopene 200 mcg • Alpha-lipoic Acid 4.5 mg • Green Tea leaves (Camellia sinensis) 15 mg. Other Ingredients: Cellulose, Vegetable Actoglycerides, Titanium Dioxide, Chlorophyll.

Multi Ultra Mega Green **-** GNC

Three tablets contain: Vitamin A (75% as beta-Carotene, 25% as Retinyl Acetate) 20,000 IU • Vitamin C (as Ascorbic Acid) 500 mg • Vitamin D (as Cholecalciferol) 400 IU • Vitamin E (as d-alpha Tocopheryl Succinate) 300 IU • Thiamin (as Thiamin Mononitrate) 25 mg • Riboflavin 25 mg • Niacin (as Niacinamide) 25 mg • Vitamin B6 (as Pyridoxine Hydrochloride) 25 mg • Folate, Folic Acid, Folacin 400 mcg • Vitamin B12 (as Cyanocobalamin) 250 mcg • Biotin 50 mcg • Pantothenic Acid (as Calcium d-Pantothenate) 25 mg • Calcium (as Calcium Carbonate and Hydrolyzed Protein Chelate) 50 mg • Iron (as Hydrolyzed Protein Chelate and Ferrous Fumarate) 10 mg • Iodine (as kelp) 100 mcg • Magnesium (as Magnesium Oxide and Hydrolyzed Protein Chelate) 50 mg • Zinc (as Hydrolyzed Protein Chelate) 15 mg • Selenium (as L-Selenomethionine) 50 mcg • Copper (as Cupric Oxide and Hydrolyzed Protein Chelate) 2 mg • Manganese (as Hydrolyzed Protein Chelate) 10 mg • Chromium (as Hydrolyzed Protein Chelate and Chromium Picolinate) 100 mcg • Molybdenum (as Hydrolyzed Protein Chelate) 150 mcg • Spirulina powder 400 mg • Green Tea leaf powder (camellia sinesis) 250 mg • Citrus Bioflavonoid Complex 100 mg • Safflower oil 100 mg • Flaxseed oil 100 mg • Borage oil 100 mg • Wheat Grass powder (Triticum aestivum) 100 mg • Barley Grass powder (Hordeum vulgare) 100 mg • Bee Pollen 100 mg • Trimethylglycine 100 mg • Choline Bitartrate 50 mg • Para Aminobenzoic Acid (PABA) 50 mg • Chlorella powder 50 mg • Siberian Ginseng root powder (Eleutheroccus senticosus) 50 mg • RNA (Yeast Free) 35 mg • Inositol powder 25 mg • Rutin powder 25 mg • Quercetin Dihydrate 25 mg • Oat Bran powder (Avena sativa) 25 mg • Apple Pectin 25 mg • Betaine Hydrochloride 20 mg • Papain 20 mg • Bromelain 20 mg • N-Acetyl L-Cysteine 15 mg • DNA (Yeast Free) 10 mg • Odorless Garlic powder (allium sativum) 10 mg • Echinacea root powder (Echinacea angustifolia) 10 mg • Milk Thistle extract (Silybum marianum) 10 mg • Goldenseal root powder (Hydrastis canadensis) 10 mg • Ginkgo Biloba extract 50:1 (24% Ginkgo Flavone Glycosides = 2.4 mg) 10 mg • Cayenne Pepper powder (Capsicum frutescens) 10 mg • Alpha Lipoic Acid 10 mg • Hesperidin Complex 5 mg • L-Glutathione 5 mg • Alpha Amylase 5 mg • Lipase 5 mg • Carotenoids (as natural carotenoid powder) 4 mg • Cellulase 2.5 mg • Boron (as protein chelate and boron gluconate powder) 1 mg • Silicon 1 mg • Lycopene 500 mcg. Other Ingredients: Maltodextrin, Cellulose, Povidone, Vegetable Acetoglycerides, Titanium Dioxide, Chlorophyll, Rose Hips powder.

Multi Vitamin **-** Oasis Wellness Network

Each tablet contains: Vitamin A (50% palmitate, 50% beta carotene) 2500 IU • Vitamin C (as ascorbic acid, calcium ascorbate) 125 mg • Vitamin D (as cholecalciferol) 200 IU • Vitamin E (as d-alpha-tocopherol acetate) 30 IU • Vitamin B1 (as thiamin mononitrate) 5 mg • Vitamin B2 (as riboflavin) 5 mg • Vitamin B3 (as niacinamide) 8 mg • Vitamin B6 (as pyridoxine HCl) 10 mg • Folate (as folic acid) 200 mcg • Vitamin B12 (as cyanocobalamin) 25 mcg • Biotin 100 mcg • Pantothenic Acid (as calcium pantothenate) 8 mg • Calcium (as calcium and citrate) 75 mg • Iron (as glycinate) 5 mg • Iodine (as potassium iodide) 75 mcg • Magnesium (as magnesium citrate) 50 mg • Zinc (as monomethionine) 8 mg • Selenium (as sodium selenite) 13 mcg • Copper (as amino acid chelate) 1 mg • Manganese (amino acid chelate) 3 mg • Chromium (as yeast) 25 mcg • Molybdenum (as amino acid chelate) 25 mcg • Potassium (as citrate) 38 mg • Choline (as bitartrate) 25 mg • Betaine (as HCl) 13 mg • Inositol 10 mg • Bioflavonoid Complex 18 mg • MaxCell Proprietary Blend 60 mg: Zisyphus Jujube, Piper Nigrum, Aloe Vera gel, Glycyrrhiza Glabra. Other Ingredients: Stearic Acid, Cellulose, Magnesium Stearate, Silicon Dioxide.

Multi Vitamin Energy Plus for Women **-** Futurebiotics

Two tablets contain: Beta Carotene 8500 IU • Vitamin C (Acerola, Ascorbic Acid) 225 mg • Thiamin 12.5 mg • Riboflavin 12.5 mg • Niacinamide 50 mg • Calcium (Phosphate, Carbonate) 625 mg • Iron (Amino Acid Chelate) 8 mg • Vitamin D 400 IU • Vitamin E (Natural Mixed Tocopherols) 30 IU • Vitamin B6 15 mg • Folic Acid 400 mcg • Vitamin B12 30 mcg • Biotin 300 mcg • Pantothenic Acid 25 mg • Para Amino Benzoic Acid (PABA) 85 mg • Choline 150 mg • Inositol 30 mg • Iodine (Kelp) 150 mcg • Magnesium (Oxide, Ascorbate) 150 mg • Zinc (Amino Acid Chelate) 15 mg • Ribonucleic Acid (RNA) 50 mg • Chromium (Polynicotinate) 60 mcg • Potassium (Amino Acid Chelate) 90 mg • Selenium (Selenomethionine) • In a base of Peony Root, Dong Quai, Aloe Vera, Methionine, Chamomile, Rosemary, American Ginseng, Chlorella, Bee Pollen, Sea Vegetable, Dandelion Root, Betaine HCl, Chinese Licorice & Raw Alfalfa Juice Concentrate.

Multi Vitamin/Mineral Formula **-** Body Language Vitamin Co.

Three tablets contain: Beta Carotene 5000 IU • Magnesium 175 mg • Vitamin B1 25 mg • Calcium 200 mg • Vitamin B2 25 mg • Selenium 25 mcg • Vitamin B5 25 mg • Manganese 1mg • Vitamin B6 25 mg • Zinc 5 mg • Niacinamide 25 mg • Iodine 150 mcg • Vitamin B12 12 mcg • Copper 2 mg • Folic Acid 400 mcg • Molybdenum 10 mcg • Vitamin D (as vitamin D3) 400 IU • Vanadium 10 mcg • Vitamin K 25 mcg • Boron 150 mcg • Vitamin E 100 IU • Taurine 250 mg • Vitamin C 100 mg • Choline 105 mg • Biotin 600 mcg • Chromium 25 mcg • Pine Bark extract 10 mg • Potassium Chloride 37.5 mg • Green Tea extract 25 mg • Phosphoglycolipids 100 mg • Inositol 40 mg • Betaine 25 mg • Burdock 50 mg • Horsetail 50 mg • Sage 50 mg.

MultiBite Plus Iron **-** GNC

Each tablet contains: Vitamin A (14% as Beta Carotene, 86% as Retinyl Acetate) 2500 IU • Vitamin C (as sodium ascorbate) 60 mg • Vitamin D (as cholecaliferol) 400 IU • Vitamin E (as d-alpha tocopheryl acetate) 15 IU • Thiamin (as thiamin mononitrate) 1.05 mg • Riboflavin 1.2 mg • Niacin (as niacinamide) 13.5 mg • Vitamin B-6 (as pyridoxine hydrochloride) 1.05 mg • Folic Acid 300 mcg • Vitamin B-12 (as cyanocobalamin) 4.5 mcg • Iron (as carbonyl iron) 15 mg. Other Ingredients: Fructose, Sorbitol, Natural Flavors, Carmine Color.

Multi-Carotene **-** PhysioLogics

Each softgel contains: Beta-Carotene (pro-vitamin A activity) 25,000 IU • Vitamin E (as mixed tocopherols) 3 IU • Alpha-Carotene 1 mg • Lycopene 5 mg • Lutein 6 mg • Zeaxanthin 0.3 mg • Proprietary Blend 5 mg: Carrot, Tomato, Spinach concentrates, Medium Chain Triglycerides (MCT's). Other Ingredients: Gelatin, Glycerin, Beeswax / Soybean Oil Mixture, Lecithin, St. John's Bread Extract, Caramel Color.

Multi-Carotene Antioxidant **-** Nature's Way

Each softgel contains: Alpha Carotene 9900 mcg • Beta Carotene 18600 mcg • Gamma Carotene 1200 mcg • Lycopene 30 mcg.

Multi-Enzyme Formula **-** Puritan's Pride

Each tablet contains: Betaine 200 mg • Pepsin 50 mg • Bromelain 50 mg • Amylase 100 mg • Lipase 25 mg • Cellulase 10 mg • Papain 50 mg • Protease 100 mg • Ox Bile 30 mg • Pancrease Substance 200 mg.

See Editor's Note No. 14.

Multiglan Chelate **-** Atrium Inc.

Six tablets contain: Calcium 500 mg • Magnesium 250 mg • Potassium 99 mg • Manganese 10 mg • Iron 18 mg • Silicon 2 mg • Zinc 15 mg • Iodine (Kelp) 150 mcg • Chromium 200 mcg •

Selenium 25 mcg • Molybdenum 150 mcg • Vanadium 150 mcg • As Chelated Proteinates, together in a base of of Raw Tissue concentrates (not extracts) from: (Spleen 144 mg, Brain 30 mg, Liver 20 mg, Heart 14 mg, Thymus 4 mg, Adrenal 4 mg, Pancreas 4 mg, Duodenum 4 mg, Pituitary 2 mg) 240 mg.
See Editor's Note No. 31, page 2056.

Multiglan Plus **-** Atrium Inc.
Each tablet contains: Spleen 256.5 mg • Brain 67.5 mg • Liver 45 mg • Heart 31.5 mg • Kidney 31.5 mg • Thymus 8 mg • Adrenal 8 mg • Pituitary 2 mg • Pancreas 9 mg • Duodenum 9 mg.
See Editor's Note No. 31, page 2056.

MultiLogics **-** PhysioLogics
Each caplet contains: Vitamin A (83% as beta carotene, 17% as retinyl palmitate) 15,000 IU • Vitamin C (as ascorbic acid) 250 mg • Vitamin D (as cholecalciferol) 400 IU • Vitamin E (as d-alpha tocopherol acetate) 150 IU • Thiamin (vitamin B1, as thiamin mononitrate) 75 mg • Riboflavin (vitamin B2) 75 mg • Niacin (as niacinamide) 75 mg • Vitamin B6 (as pyridoxine hydrochloride) 75 mg • Folic Acid 400 mcg • Vitamin B12 (as cyanocobalamin) 75 mcg • Biotin 300 mcg • Pantothenic Acid (as d-calcium pantothenate) 75 mg • Calcium (as lithothamnium coralloids, dicalcium phosphate) 57 mg • Iron (as iron amino acid chelate) 1 mg • Iodine (as potassium iodide) 150 mcg • Magnesium (as magnesium amino acid chelate, magnesium oxide) 11mg • Zinc (as zinc amino acid chelate) 10 mg • Selenium (as selenomethionate) 25 mcg • Copper (as copper amino acid chelate) 1 mg • Manganese (as manganese amino acid chelate) 1 mg • Chromium (as chromium amino acid chelate) 25 mcg • Molybdenum (as molybdenum amino acid chelate, molybdenum yeast) 27 mcg • Boron (as boron amino benzoic acid chelate) 500 mcg • Inositol 75 mg • PABA (para-aminobenzoic acid) 75 mg • Choline (as choline bitartrate) 31 mg • Betaine Hydrochloride 25 mg • Citrus Bioflavonoids (citrus spp., fruit) 25 mg • Rutin (dimorphandra mollis, fruit) 25 mg • Hesperidin complex (citrus aurandum, citrus spp., fruit) 5 mg. Other Ingredients: Cellulose (plant origin), Croscarmellose, Vegetable Stearic Acid, Silica, Cellulose Coating.

MultiLogics for Children **-** PhysioLogics
Two tablets contain: Vitamin A (as 67% Beta-Carotene, 33% Fish Liver oil) 7500 IU • Vitamin C (as Ascorbic Acid) 180 mg • Vitamin D (as Vitamin D3)(from Fish Liver oil) 200 IU • Vitamin E (as d-Alpha Tocopherol Succinate) 90 IU • Vitamin K (as Phytonadione) 30 mcg • Thiamine (as Thiamine Mononitrate) 3 mg • Riboflavin (Vitamin B2) 3.4 mg • Niacin (as Niacinamide) 20 mg • Vitamin B6 (as Pyridoxine HCl) 4 mg • Folic Acid 400 mcg • Vitamin B12 12 mcg • Biotin 300 mcg • Pantothenic Acid (as d-Calcium Panthothenate) 20 mg • Calcium (as Calcium Citrate-Aspartate Complex) 100 mg • Iron (as Iron Carbonyl) 4.5 mg • Iodine (as Potassium Iodide, Kelp) 75 mcg • Magnesium (as Magnesium Citrate-Aspartate Complex) 100 mg • Zinc (as Amino Acid Zinc Chelate) 5 mg • Selenium (as Amino Acid Selenium Complex) 50 mcg • Copper (as Copper Gluconate) 400 mcg • Manganese (as Amino Acid Manganese Chelate) 1 mg • Chromium (as Chromium Polynicotinate) 50 mcg • Molybdenum (as Amino Acid Molybdenum Chelate) 50 mcg • Black Currant seed 5 mg • Choline (Bitartate) 5 mg • Boron (Aspartate-Citrate) 1 mg.

MultiLogics for Men **-** PhysioLogics
Three tablets contain: Vitamin E (d-alpha tocopherol acetate) 250 IU • Calcium (aquamins, carbonate) 530 mg • Magnesium (amino acid chelate/oxide) 140 mg • Zinc (amino acid chelate) 15 mg • Iron (ferrous bisglycinate) 5 mg • Copper (amino acid chelate) 1 mg • Chromium (amino acid chelate) 175 mcg • Selenium (amino acid complex) 175 mcg • Tomato extract (1% lycopene, 1.6 mg) 160 mg • Saw Palmetto berry (20-25% fatty acids & lipid sterols 15-18.75 mg) 75 mg • Bioflavonoids (citrus spp.) 50 mg • Rutin 50 mg • Hesperidin 50 mg • Green Tea leaf (45% Polyphenols, 22.5 mg) 50 mg • Betaine HCl 50 mg • Ginkgo Biloba leaf (24% ginkgo flavonglycosides, 9.6 mg; 6% terpene lactones, 24 mg) 40 mg • Nettles (1-2% silica, 300-600 mcg) 30 mg • Beta Sitosterol 30 mg • Black Cohosh root (cimicifuga racemosa) 25 mg • Grapeseed extract (vitis vinifera, standardized to contain 50% proanthocyanidins)25 mg • Tomato concentrate (lycopersicon esculentum, equivalent to tomato 108 mg) 10.8 mg • Black Pepper (piper nigrum) 5 mg • Lutein 3 mg • Tomato extract (blakelea trispora, standardized to cotain 3% lycopenes) 1.6 mg. Other Ingredients: Cellulose (plant origin), Croscarmellose, Vegetable Stearic Acid, Polyvinylpyrrolidone, Silica, Vegetable Magnesium Stearate, Cellulose Coating.

MultiLogics for Women **-** PhysioLogics
Three caplets contain: Vitamin E (as d-alpha tocopheryl acetate) 250 IU • Calcium (as lithothamnium coralliodes, calcium carbonate) 530 mg • Iron (as ferrous bisglycinate) 5 mg • Magnesium (as magnesium amino acid chelate, magnesium oxide) 130 mg • Zinc (as zinc amino acid chelate) 15 mg • Selenium (as selenium amino acid chelate) 174 mcg • Copper (as copper amino acid chelate) 1 mg • Chromium (as chromium amino acid chelate) 174 mcg • Boron (as boron amino acid chelate) 500 mcg • Betaine Hydrochloride 50 mg • Citrus Bioflavonoids (fruit) 50 mg • Green Tea extract (Camellia sinensis, leaf, standardized to contain 50% polyphenols 25 mg) 50 mg • Hesperidin Complex (citrus aurantium and citrus spp., fruit) 50 mg • Rutin (dimorphandra mollis, fruit) 50 mg • Ginkgo Biloba extract (leaf, standardized to contain 24% alkaloids 9.6 mg) 40 mg • Black Cohosh (cimicifuga racemosa, root) 25 mg • Chasteberry extract (vitex agnus castus fruit, standardized to contain 0.5% agmisode 1.26 mg) 25 mg • Dong Quai (angelica sinensis root, 1% ligustilides) 25 mg • Grape seed extract (vitis vinifera leaf, standardized to contain 50% proantocyanids 12.5 mg) 25 g • Choline (as choline bitartrate) 20 mg • Kudzu extract (pueraria thomsonii root, standardized to contain 1% daidzein 0.12 mg) 13 mg • Tomato concentrate (lycopersicon esculentum fruit, equivalent to 108 mg of tomato) 11 mg • Black Pepper (piper nigrum fruit) 5 mg • Lutein 3 mg • Lycopene (from tomato, blakeslea trispora, standardized to contain 3% lycopenes 0.02 mg) 2 mg. Other Ingredients: Cellulose, Croscarmellose, Vegetable Stearic Acid, Polyvinylpyrrolidone, Silica, Vegetable Magnesium Stearate, Cellulose Coating, Potassium Amino Acid Chelate.

Multi-Mega Minerals **-** Puritan's Pride
Two tablets contain: Calcium 1,000 mg • Magnesium 500 mg • Iron 30 mg • Manganese 10 mg • Potassium 95 mg • Chromium 100 mcg • Vitamin D 400 IU • Iodine 150 mcg • Copper 3 mg • Zinc 22.5 mg. Other Components: Betaine Hydrochloride 100 mg • Glutamic Acid Hydrochloride 100 mg • Chloride 90 mg.

Multi-Mineral Citrate Complete **-** The Vitamin Shoppe
Eight capsules contain: Calcium 1000 mg • Magnesium 500 mg • Potassium 99 mg • Zinc 50 mg • Boron 3 mg • Copper 2 mg • Selenium 100 mcg • Chromium 200 mcg • Molybdenum 100 mcg • Iron 10 mg • Manganese 10 mg.

Multi-Minerals **-** The Vitamin Shoppe
Three tablets contain: Calcium 1000 mg • Zinc 22.5 • Copper 1 mg • Selenium 50 mcg • Chromium 100 mcg • Vanadium 50 mcg • Glutamic Acid 50 mg • Magnesium 500 mg • Iron 20 mg • Potassium 99 mg • Manganese 5 mg • Boron 3 mg • Molybdenum 50 mcg • Iodine 150 mcg • Vitamin D 200 IU.

Multi-Minerals Complex **-** Schiff
Three tablets contain: Vitamin D (as cholecalciferol) 400 IU • Calcium (as calcium carbonate) 1.2 g • Iron (as ferrous fumarate) 18 mg • Iodine (from kelp) 150 mcg • Magnesium (as magnesium oxide) 600 mg • Zinc (as zinc citrate) 30 mg • Selenium (as l-selenomethionine) 100 mcg • Copper (as copper gluconate) 2 mg • Manganese (as manganese gluconate) 10 mg • Chromium (as amino acid chelate) 100 mcg • Molybdenum (as amino acid chelate) 100 mcg • Potassium (as potassium citrate) 99 mg • Proprietary Mineral Transport Blend 64 mg: Citrates, Fumerates, Succinates, Gluconates, Aspartates, Ascorbates, Amino Acid Chelates, Ketoglutarates, Picolinates • Boron (as boron aspartate) 3 mg. Other Ingredients: Cellulose, Croscarmellose Sodium, Stearic Acid, Coating (methylcellulose polyethylene glycol), Magnesium Stearate.

Some Brand Name Natural Products - What they Contain

www.NaturalDatabase.com contains MANY more listings than appear here.

BRAND NAMES

Multi-mune **-** Purity Life International
Three capsules contain: Vitamin A (as palmitate) 1605 IU • Vitamin C (as calcium ascorbate, magnesium ascorbate) 1 g • Vitamin E (as d-alpha tocopherol succinate) 1000 IU • Vitamin B6 (as pyridoxal-5-phosphate) 45 mg • Magnesium (as glycinate, ascorbate) 100 mg • Zinc (as citrate) 15 mg • Selenium (as selenomethionine) 100 mcg • Coenzyme Q10 (ubiquinone) 30 mg • Reduced L-Gluthione 45 mg • Alpha Lipoic Acid (thioctic acid) 30 mg. Other Ingredients: Gelatin.

Multiple Vitamins & Minerals - Basic Nutrition **-** GNC
Each tablet contains: Vitamin A (as beta-carotene) 5000 IU • Vitamin C (as Ascorbic Acid) 60 mg • Vitamin D (as Cholecalciferol) 400 IU • Vitamin E (as dl-alpha Tocopheryl Acetate) 30 IU • Thiamin (as Thiamin Mononitrate) 1.5 mg • Riboflavin 1. 7 mg • Niacin (as Niacinamide) 20 mg • Vitamin B6 (as Pyridoxine Hydrochloride) 2 mg • Folate, Folic Acid, Folacin 400 mcg • Vitamin B12 (as Cyanocobalamin) 6 mcg • Biotin 30 mcg • Pantothenic Acid (as Calcium d-Pantothenate) 10 mg • Calcium (as Dicalcium Phosphate) 162 mg • Iron (as Carbonyl Iron) 18 mg • Phosphorus (as Cicalcium Phosphate) 100 mg • Iodine (as Potassium Iodine) 150 mcg • Magnesium (as Magnesium Oxide) 100 mg • Zinc (as Zinc Sulfate)15 mg • Selenium (as Sodium Selenate) 20 mg • Copper (as Copper Oxide) 2 mg • Manganese (as Manganese Sulfate) 7.5 mg • Chromium (as Chromium Chloride) 15 mcg • Molybdenum (as Sodium Molybdate) 15 mcg • Nickel (as Nickerl Sulfate) 5 mcg • Tin (as Stannous Chloride) 10 mcg • Silicon (as Sodium MetaSilicate) 2 mg • Vanadium (as Sodium MetaVanadate) 10 mcg • Boron (as Sodium Borate Decahydrate) 150 mcg. Other Ingredients: Cellulose, Vegetable Acetoglycerides, Stearic Acid, Titanium Dioxide.

Multiplex Formula **-** 4 Life
Each capsule contains: Vitamin A (as beta carotene) 5000 IU • Vitamin C (as ascorbic acid) 150 mg • Vitamin E (as D-alpha tocopheryl succinate) 30 IU • Thiamin (as thiamine mononitrate) 15 mg • Riboflavin (Vitamin B2) 17 mg • Niacin (as niacinamide) 33 mg • Vitamin B6 (as pyridoxine HCl) 8 mg • Folic Acid 600 mcg • Vitamin B12 (as cyanocobalamin) 15 mcg • Biotin 300 mcg • Pantothenic Acid (as calcium pantothenate) 22 mg • Zinc (as zinc fluconate) 10 mg • Selenium (as selenomethionine) 60 mcg • Chromium (as chromium picolinate) 75 mcg • Potassium (as potassium citrate) 33 mg • Hawaiian Spirulina Pacifica 90 mg • Citrus Bioflavanoids (from citrus fruit) 40 mg • Choline (as choline bitartrate) 27 mg • Para-Aminobenzoic (PABA) 25 mg • Inositol 24 mg • Lysine (as L-lysine monohydrochloride) 20 mg • Histidine (as L-histidine HCl monohydrate) 18 mg • Isoleucine (as L-isoleucine) 15 mg • Phenylanine (as DL-phenylalanine) 15 mg • Catnip leaf 15 mg • Rose Hips (Rosa canina) fruit 15 mg • English Hawthorn (berry) 10 mg • Licorice (root) 10 mg.

Multi-Quest **-** Nutri-Quest Rx
Three tablets contain: Vitamin A (Palmitate) 2000 IU • Vitamin D (as Vitamin D3) 400 IU • Vitamin E (Succinate) 200 IU • Vitamin C (Sago Palm) 1000 mg • Lemon Bioflavonoids 100 mg • Rutin 25 mg • Hesperidin Complex 50 mg • Vitamin B6 25 mg • Vitamin B1 13 mg • Vitamin B2 10 mg • Niacin 45 mg • Vitamin B12 30 mcg • Pantothenic Acid (Calcium Pantothenate) 50 mg • Folic Acid 200 mcg • Choline Bitartrate 100 mg • Inositol 100 mg • Biotin 400 mcg • PABA 50 mg • L-Glycine 9.66 mg • Calcium Gluconate 15.36 mg • Vitamin F 5 mg • Chlorophyll 16 mg • Calcium Aspartate 500 mg • Magnesium Aspartate 250 mg • Phosphorus Chelate 200 mg • Potassium Proteinate 30 mg • Copper Chelate 1 mg • Zinc Aspartate 5 mg • Manganese Aspartate 15 mg • Molybdenum Chelate 50 mcg • Chromium Chelate 25 mcg • Selenium Chelate 30 mcg • Iodine (kelp) 50 mcg • Sodium Proteinate 30 mcg • Rubidium Chelate 15 mcg • Lithium Chelate 8 mcg • L-Phenylalanine 13 mg • L-Histidine 6 mg • L-Tyrosine 9 mg • L-Lysine 13 mg • L-Valine 15 mg • DL-Methionine 9 mg • L-Isoleucine 13 mg • L-Leucine 18 mg • L-Threonine 9 mg • L-Glutamic Acid 2 mg • Goldenseal root 45 mg • Siberian Ginseng 45 mg • Garlic 40 mg • Tillandsia 30 mg • Rice Bran 176 mg • Almond Meal 150 mg.

Multiron Capsules **-** Vitabiotics
Each capsule contains: Vitamin A 750 mcg • Vitamin B1 (thiamin) 10 mg • Vitamin B2 (riboflavin) 2 mg • Vitamin B3 (niacin) 18 mg • Folic Acid 500 mcg • Vitamin B12 (cyanocobalamin) 10 mcg • Vitamin D 5 mcg • Vitamin B6 (pyridoxine HCl) 5 mg • Pantothenic Acid 4 mg • Vitamin E 5 mg • Vitamin C 30 mg • Iron 18 mg • Iodine 140 mcg • Magnesium 50 mg • Zinc 15 mg • Copper 1 mg • Manganese 2 mg • Selenium 100 mcg • Chromium 50 mg • Ginseng 40 mg • Citrus Bioflavonoids 30 mg.

Multi-Scorb **-** Progressive Labs
Each tablet contains: Vitamin C (as mineral ascorbates) 1000 mg • Calcium (ascorbate) 50 mg • Magnesium (ascorbate) 30 mg • Zinc (ascorbate) 3 mg • Manganese (ascorbate) 3 mg • Potassium (ascorbate) 60 mg • Citrus BioFlavonoid 5X complex 125 mg (as undiluted hesperidin, naringin and rutin).

Multivit Syrup **-** Hadas Natural Products
Vitamin A 2000 IU • Vitamin D (D3) 400 IU • Vitamin B1 1.25 mg • Vitamin B2 1.5 mg • Vitamin B6 1.25 mg • Vitamin B12 1 mcg • Rose Hip extract 100 mg • Folic Acid 75 mcg • Calcium Pantothenate 10 mg • Nicotinamide 12 mg.

Munit-E **-** Holista
Each capsule contains: Beta Carotene 10000 IU • Vitamin A 5000 IU • Vitamin C 500 mg • Vitamin B6 25 mg • Zinc 20 mg • Echinacea (angustifolia/purpurea) 300 mg • Bioflavonoids 100 mg • Garlic 50 mg • Ginger 50 mg.

Muscle **-** Gary Null & Associates (GNA)
Composed of plant sources. Fortified with Methionine, Leucine, Valine, Isoleucine, and Lysine.

Muscle Dynamo **-** Source Naturals
Four tablets contain: Vitamin B1 (Thiamin) 30 mg • Vitamin B2 (Riboflavin) 30 mg • Niacinamide (125 mg) and Niacin (25 mg) 150 mg • Vitamin B5 (Calcium D-Pantothenate) 100 mg • Vitamin B6 (Pyridoxine HCl) 25 mg • Vitamin B12 (Cyanocobalamin) 100 mcg • Folic Acid 400 mcg • Vitamin E D-Alpha Tocopheryl (Natural) 100 IU • Magnesium (Citrate and Succinate) 181 mg • Potassium (Succinate) 99 mg • Calciium (Succinate) 89 mg • Succinate Complex (Magnesium/Calcium/Potassium Succinates) 1,300 mg • Inosine 500 mg • PAK (Pyridoxine alpha-Ketoglutarate) 100 mg • Coenzyme Q10 (Ubiquinone) 30 mg • Alpha-Lipoic Acid (Thioctic Acid) 25 mg • l-Isoleucine 120 mg • L-Leucine 360 mg • L-Valine 120 mg • Glycine 500 mg • L-Tyrosine 150 mg • Korean Ginseng root 250 mg • Siberian Ginseng root extract 100 mg.

Muscle Dynamo II **-** Source Naturals
One oz contains: Vitamin A 1,250 IU • Vitamin C (Ascorbic Acid) 30 mg • Thiamin (Vitamin B1) 380 mcg • Riboflavin (Vitamin B2) 430 mcg • Niacin 20 mg • Calcium 150 mg • Iron 1 mg • Vitamin D 100 IU • Vitamin E 15 IU • Vitamin B6 500 mcg • Folic Acid 100 mcg • Vitamin B12 3 mcg • Phosphorus 150 mcg • Iodine 25 mcg • Magnesium 50 mg • Zinc 7.5 mg • Copper 250 mcg • Biotin 75 mcg • Pantothenic Acid 2.5 mg • Potassium 300 mg • Manganese 2 mg • Chromium 150 mcg • Molybdenum 50 mcg • Selenium 30 mcg.

Muscle Mass **-** Source Naturals
Two tablets contain: Vitamin C (Ascorbic Acid) 50 mg • Vitamin B5 (Calcium D-Pantothenate) 20 mg • Vitamin B6 (Pyridoxine HCl) 20 mg • Iodine (from kelp) 56 mcg. Other Ingredients: Arginine Pyroglutamate 718 mg, L-Lysine HCl 718 mg, L-Ornithine (Ornithine HCl) 200 mg, Branched Chain Amino Acids (BCAAs) 174 mg (L-Leucine 100 mg, L-Isoleucine 30 mg and L-Valine 44 mg), Lipotropic Factors 360 mg (Choline Bitartrate 200 mg, Inositol 100 mg, L-Methionine 30 mg and Betaine HCl 30 mg), Glycine 50 mg, Trans-Ferulic Acid 50 mg, L-Carnitine (L-Carnitine L-Tartrate) 10 mg, Special Herbal Blend 590 mg: Saw Palmetto, Sarsaparilla, Wild Yam Root, Astragalus, Kelp, Ginseng, Pueraria, Licorice Root.

Muscle Milk **-** CytoSport
Two scoops (or one packet) contain: EVOPRO: Micellar Alpha and Beta Caseins and Casseinates, Whey concentrates (alpha-lactalbumin), Whey isolates, Whey peptides, Purified Bovine Colostrum extract (secretory IgA and IGF-1), Glutamine peptides, L-Taurine, Lactoferrin • LEANLIPIDES: Canola oil, BETAPOL Enzyme Engineered Polyunsaturated Long-Chain Vegetable Oils, MCT, L-Carnitine • Maltodextrin • CYTOVITE I Vitamin and Mineral premix: Vitamin A Acetate, Cholecalciferol, D-Alpha-Tocopherol Acetate, Ascorbic Acid, Folate, Thiamine Monohydrate, Riboflavin, Niacinamide, Pyridoxine HCl, Cyanocobalamin, Biotin, Pantothenic Acid, Di-Calcium Phosphate, Potassium Iodide, Potassium Chloride, Ferrous Fumarate, Magnesium Oxide, Copper Gluconate, Zinc Oxide • Gum Arabic • ENDOCREATINE Creatine Precursor: Glycocyamine, Betaine Anhydrous, SAMe (S-adenosylmethionine • Natural and Artificial Flavors • Lecithin • Sucralose.

Muscle Nitrous **-** VPX Sports
Each 10 cc serving contains: A-AKG Arginine Alpha-Ketoglutarate 3000 mg • Magnesium Peroxide (MgO2) 50 mg. Other Ingredients: Highly Purified Water, Lecithin, Propylene Glycol, Polyethylene Glycol, Glycerine, Lipoject Technologies Proprietary Polylipid, Delivery Matrix, Vegetable Gum, Sucralose, Potassium Sorbate, Natural and Artificial Flavors, EDTA, Phosphoric Acid.

MusclEase **-** PhysioLogics
Two capsules contain: Magnesium (as magnesium aspartate) 100 mg • Calcium (as calcium citrate) 45 mg • Valerian root (valeriana officinalis, standardized to contain 0.8% valernic acid, 0.8 mg) 100 mg • Kava Kava root (piper methysticum, standardized to contain 30% kavalactones, 30 mg) 100 mg • Passion Flower plant (passiflora incarmata, standardized to contain 3.5% flavonoids, 3.5 mg) 100 mg. Other Ingredients: Gelatin, Rice Powder, Vegetable Magnesium Stearate, Silica.

MuscleSoothe **-** Vita Pharmica - formerly Neopharmica
Each two tablets contain: Proprietary Blend 2000 mg: San-Qi Ginseng root, Dong-Quai root, Sichuan Teasel rhizome, Safflower Flower, Astilbe Chinensis plant.

MuscleTech **-** MuscleTech
Six capsules contain: Acetyl-L-Carnitine 1000 mg • Glutamine 2000 mg • L-Leucine 1000 mg • L-Valine 250 mg • L-Isoleucine 250 mg • OKG 100 mg • Zinc 60 mg • Taurine 1000 mg.

Mustard Salve **-** Dial Herbs
Mustard • Wintergreen • Comfrey • Arnica • Camphor • Cayenne. In a base of Beeswax , Glycerine & Cold Pressed Olive oil.

MVP **-** Mannatech
Each caplet contains: Ephedrine (from country mallow) 10 mg • Caffeine (from kola nut) 40 mg • Wild Yam root (standardized for phytoserols) • Kola Nut seed • Country Mallow (sida cortifolia aerial) • Atlantic Kelp whole plant •Cayenne Pepper fruit • Ambrotose Complex: naturally occuring plant polysaccharides including freeze-dried Aloe Vera inner leaf gel extract - Manapol powder. Other Ingredients: Cellulose, Calcium Carbonate, Silicon Dioxide, Hydroxypropyl Methylcellulose, Croscarmellose Sodium, Stearic Acid, Magnesium Stearate.
See Editor's Note No. 17 and No. 39.

My Defense **-** Natrol
Three capsules contain: Vitamin C (as calcium ascorbate) 60 mg • Arabinogalactan 1.5 g • Maitake extract (4:1) 50 mg • Cranberry juice powder 250 mg • Astragalus root powder 100 mg • Papain 100 mg. Other Ingredients: Silica, Magnesium Stearate, Gelatin.

My Favorite Multiple — The Pill Companion **-** Natrol
Two tablets contain: Vitamin A (as d-salina beta-carotene) 5000 IU • Vitamin C (as ascorbic acid) 300 mg • Vitamin D (as cholecalciferol) 200 IU • Vitamin E (as d-alpha tocopherol succinate) 30 IU • Vitamin K (as phytonadione) 40 mcg • Thiamin (vitamin B1) 5 mg • Riboflavin (vitamin B2) 5 mg • Niacin (vitamin B3) 20 mg • Vitamin B6 (as pyridoxine HCl) 15 mg • Folic Acid 600 mcg • Vitamin B12 (as cyanocobalamin) 24 mcg • Biotin 150 mcg • Pantothenic Acid (as calcium d-pantothenate) 5 mg • Calcium (as calcium citrate) 100 mg • Iron (as iron amino acid chealate) 4.5 mg • Magnesium (as magnesium oxide) 300 mg • Zinc (as zinc amino acid chelate) 30 mg • Selenium (as selenium amino acid chelate) 35 mcg • Copper (as copper amino acid chelate) 0.5 mg • Manganese (as manganese amino acid chelate) 0.5 mg • Chromium (as chromium picolinate) 60 mcg • Molybdenum (as molybdenum amino acid chelate) 38 mcg • Boron (as boron amino acid chelate) 1 mg • Soy extract 10 mg • Soy Isoflavones 4 mg. Other Ingredients: Cellulose, Stearic Acid, Silica, Cellulose Gum, Magnesium Stearate, Methylcellulose, Glycerine.

My Favorite Multiple Original - Capsules **-** Natrol
Six capsules contain: Vitamin A (as beta carotene & Vitamin A palmitate) 10000 IU • Vitamin C (as calcium ascorbate) 250 mg • Vitamin D (as cholecalciferol) 400 IU • Vitamin E (as d-alpha tocopheryl succinate) 400 IU • Thiamine (as thiamin HCl) (Vitamin B1) 50 mg • Riboflavin (Vitamin B2) 50 mg • Niacin (as niacin & niacinamide) 50 mg • Vitamin B6 (as pyridoxine HCl) 50 mg • Folic Acid 400 mcg • Vitamin B12 (as cyanocobalamin) 50 mcg • Biotin 300 mcg • Pantothenic Acid (as d-calcium pantothenate) 50 mg • Calcium (as calcium carbonate & calcium citrate) 1 g • Iron (as iron glycinate) 18 mg • Iodine (from kelp) 150 mcg • Magnesium (as magnesium citrate & magnesium oxide) 400 mg • Zinc 25 mg • Selenium 200 mcg • Copper 2 mg • Manganese (as manganese gluconate) 2 mg • Chromium 200 mcg • Molybdenum 50 mcg • Potassium (as potassium chloride) 99 mg • Betaine (as betaine TMG trimethylglycine) 300 mg • MultiEnzyme Blend: Amylase, Papain, Protease, Bromelain, Lipase 110 mg • GP Flavonoid Complex + 100 mg extracted from: Rose Hips fruit, Tumeric root, Acerola berries, Bilberry berries, Hawthorne berries, Grape skin, Milk Thistle seed, & Citrus fruit • PABA (as para amino benzoic acid) 50 mg • Choline (as choline bitartrate) 50 mg • Inositol 50 mg • Hesperidin 25 mg • Rutin 25 mg • Siberian Ginseng 4:1 extract root 1 mg • Boron 200 mcg. Other Ingredients: Silicon Dioxide, Magnesium Stearate, Gelatin.

My Favorite Multiple Original - Tablets **-** Natrol
Four tablets contain: Vitamin A (as d-Salina beta carotene & Vitamin A palmitate) 10000 IU • Vitamin C (as calcium ascorbate) 250 mg • Vitamin D (as cholecalciferol) 400 IU • Vitamin E (as d-alpha tocopheryl succinate) 400 IU • Thiamine (as Thiamine HCl) (Vitamin B1) 50 mg • Riboflavin (Vitamin B2) 50 mg • Niacin (as Niacin & Niacinamide) 50 mg • Vitamin B6 (as pyridoxine HCl) 50 mg • Folic Acid 400 mcg • Vitamin B12 (as cyanocobalamin) 50 mcg • Biotin 300 mcg • Pantothenic Acid (as d-calcium pantothenate) 50 mg • Calcium (as calcium carbonate & calcium citrate) 1 g • Iron (as iron glycinate) 18 mg • Iodine (from kelp) 150 mcg • Magnesium (as magnesium citrate & magnesium oxide) 400 mg • Zinc 25 mg • Selenium 200 mcg • Copper 2 mg • Manganese (as manganese gluconate) 2 mg • Chromium 200 mcg • Molybdenum 50 mcg • Potassium (as potassium chloride) 99 mg • Betaine (as betaine TMG trimethylglycine) 300 mg • Multi Enzyme Blend: amylase, papain, protease, bromelain, lipase 110 mg • GP Flavonoid Complex 100 mg extracted from: Rose Hips fruit, Tumeric root, Acerola berries, Bilberry berries, Hawthorne berries, Grape skin, Milk Thistle Seed, & citrus fruit • PABA (as para amino benzoic acid) 50 mg • Choline (as choline bitartrate) 50 mg • Inositol 50 mg • Hesperidin 25 mg • Rutin 25 mg • Siberian Ginseng 4:1 extract root 15 mg • Boron 200 mcg. Other Ingredients: Microcrystalline Cellulose, Mono & Di-Glycerides, Silicon Dioxide, Magnesium Stearate, Stearic Acid, Croscarmellose Sodium.

My Favorite Multiple Prime **-** Natrol
Six capsules contain: Vitamin A (from retinal acetate, 60% beta carotene [from natural carotenoid blend, d-salina]) 7500 IU • Vitamin C (from calcium ascorbate) 180 mg • Vitamin D (as cholecalciferol) 600 IU • Vitamin E (as d-alpha tocopherol succinate) 120 IU • Thiamin (as thiamin HCl, vitamin B1) 3 mg • Riboflavin (vitamin B2) 3.4 mg • Niacin (niacinamide) 40 mg • Vitamin B6 (as pyridoxine HCl) 4 mg • Folic Acid 600 mcg • Vitamin B12 (as

cyanocobalamin) 100 mcg • Biotin 600 mcg • Pantothenic Acid (as d-calcium pantothenate) 20 mg • Calcium (as calcium: citrate, carbonate, ascorbate) 700 mg • Iron (as iron amino acid chelate) 18 mg • Iodine (from kelp) 150 mcg • Magnesium (as magnesium oxide) 400 mg • Zinc (as zinc amino acid chelate) 30 mg • Selenium (as selenium amino acid chelate) 140 mcg • Copper (as copper amino acid chelate) 4 mg • Manganese (as manganese gluconate) 4 mg • Chromium (as chromium amino acid chelate) 120 mg • Molybdenum (as molybdenum amino acid chelate) 75 mcg • Boron (as boron amino acid chelate) 200 mcg • 50+ Supporting Nutrient Blend 580 mg: Coenzyme Q10 30 mg, Glucosamine HCl 500 mg, Acetyl L-Carnitine 25 mg, Green Tea (50% polyphenols) 10 mg, Bilberry extract (25% anthocyanins) 15 mg • Natrol's Ultra Green Blend 100 mg: Alfalfa juice (leaf), Barley grass, Spirulina (algae), Parsley (leaf), Spinach (leaf), Peppermint (leaf), Spearmint (leaf) • Enzyme Blend 100 mg: Amylase, Papain, Protease, Bromelain, Lipase • Carotenoid Blend 75 mg: Tomato, Marigold, Palm Oil • Beta Carotene 1830 mcg • Lutein 630 mcg • Lycopene 360 mcg • Alpha Carotene 120 mcg • Cryptoxanthin 24 mcg • Zeaxanthin 24 mcg • Inositol 5 mg • Choline Bitartrate 5 mg. Other Ingredients: Silica, Magnesium Stearate, Gelatin.

My Favorite Multiple Take One **-** Natrol
One tablet contains: Vitamin A (as beta carotene) 10000 IU • Vitamin C (as calcium ascorbate) 100 mg • Vitamin D (as cholecalciferol) 400 IU • Vitamin E (as d-alpha tocopheryl succinate) 100 IU • Thiamine (as thiamin HCl) (Vitamin B1) 15 mg • Riboflavin (Vitamin B2) 17 mg • Niacin 20 mg • Vitamin B6 (as pyridoxine HCl) 17 mg • Folic Acid 400 mcg • Vitamin B12 (as cyanocobalamin) 50 mcg • Biotin 300 mcg • Pantothenic Acid (as d-calcium pantothenate) 50 mg • Calcium 25 mg • Iron 18 mg • Iodine 150 mcg • Magnesium 10 mg • Zinc 15 mg • Selenium 200 mcg • Copper 2 mg • Manganese 5 mg • Chromium 200 mcg • Molybdenum 50 mcg • Potassium 5 mg • Silica 10 mg • Vanadium 10 mcg • Boron 3 mg • GP Flavonoid Complex + 100 mg, extracted from: Rose Hips fruit, Tumeric root, Acerola berries, Bilberry berries, Hawthorne berries, Grape skin, Milk Thistle Seed & Citrus fruit • UltraGreen Blend concentrate extract 100 mg from: Alfalfa juice leaf, barley grass, spirulina algae, parsley leaf, spinach leaf, peppermint leaf, & spearmint leaf • Lecithin 50 mg • Choline (as choline bitartrate) 50 mg • PABA (as para amino benzoic acid) 25 mg • Inositol 25 mg. Other Ingredients: Mono & Di-Glycerides, Silicon Dioxide, Stearic Acid, Croscarmellose Sodium, Magnesium Stearate.

My Favorite Multiple Take One Without Iron - Tablets **-** Natrol
Each tablet contains: Vitamin A (as beta carotene) 10000 IU • Vitamin C (as calcium ascorbate) 100 mg • Vitamin D (as cholecalciferol) 400 IU • Vitamin E (as d-alpha tocopheryl succinate) 100 IU • Thiamine (as thiamin HCl) (Vitamin B1) 15 mg • Riboflavin (Vitamin B2) 17 mg • Niacin 20 mg • Vitamin B6 (as pyridoxine HCl) 17 mg • Folic Acid 400 mcg • Vitamin B12 (as cyanocobalamin) 50 mcg • Biotin 300 mcg • Pantothenic Acid (as d-calcium pantothenate) 50 mg • Calcium 25 mg • Iodine 150 mcg • Magnesium 10 mg • Zinc 15 mg • Selenium 200 mcg • Copper 2 mg • Manganese 5 mg • Chromium 200 mcg • Molybdenum 50 mcg • Potassium 5 mg • Silica 10 mg • Vanadium 10 mcg • Boron 3 mg • GP Flavonoids 100 mg, extracted from: Rose Hips fruit, Tumeric root, Acerola berries, Bilberry berries, Hawthorne berries, Grape skin, Milk Thistle seed, & Citrus fruit • UltraGreen Blend 100 mg concentrate extract from: Alfalfa juice leaf, Barley grass, Spirulina algae, Parsley leaf, Spinach leaf, Peppermint leaf, & Spearmint leaf • Lecithin 50 mg • Choline (as choline bitartrate) 50 mg • PABA (as para amino benzoic acid) 25 mg • Inositol 25 mg. Other Ingredients: Mono & Di-Glycerides, Silicon Dioxide, Stearic Acid, Croscarmellose Sodium, Magnesium Stearate.

My Favorite Multiple With Coral Calcium & Zeaxanthin **-** Natrol
Two capslues contain: Vitamin A (as retinal acetate, 10% beta carotene) 5000 IU • Vitamin C (as calcium ascorbate) 60 mg • Vitamin D (as cholecalciferol) 400 IU • Vitamin E (as d-alpha tocopheryl succinate) 30 IU • Vitamin K (as phytonadione) 40 mcg • Riboflavin (vitamin B2) 1.7 mg • Niacin (as niacinamide) 20 mg • Vitamin B6 (as pyridoxine HCl) 2 mg • Folic Acid 400 mcg • Vitamin B12 (as cyanocobalamin) 6 mcg • Biotin 300 mcg • Pantothenic Acid 10 mg • Calcium (from coral and calcium ascorbate) 250 mg • Zinc (as zinc oxide) 15 mg • Selenium (as selenium amino acid chelate) 70 mcg • Copper (as copper sulfate) 2 mg • Manganese (as manganese gluconate) 2 mg • Chromium (as chromium picolinate) 120 mcg • Molybdenum (as amino acid chelate) 75 mcg • Boron (as boron amino acid chelate) 200 mcg • Zeaxanthin 2 mg. Other Ingredients: Gelatin, Silica, Magnesium Stearate.

My Favorite Multiple Without Iron - Capsules **-** Natrol
Six capsules contain: Vitamin A (as beta carotene & Vitamin A palmitate) 10000 IU • Vitamin C (as calcium ascorbate) 250 mg • Vitamin D (as cholecalciferol) 400 IU • Vitamin E (as d-alpha tocopheryl succinate) 400 IU • Thiamine (as thiamin HCl) (Vitamin B1) 50 mg • Riboflavin (Vitamin B2) 50 mg • Niacin (as niacin & niacinamide) 50 mg • Vitamin B6 (as pyridoxine HCl) 50 mg • Folic Acid 400 mcg • Vitamin B12 (as cyanocobalamin) 50 mcg • Biotin 300 mcg • Pantothenic Acid (as d-calcium pantothenate) 50 mg • Calcium (as calcium carbonate & calcium citrate) 1 g • Iodine (from kelp) 150 mcg • Magnesium (as magnesium citrate & magnesium, oxide) 400 mg • Zinc 25 mg • Selenium 200 mcg • Copper 2 mg • Manganese (as manganese gluconate) 2 mg • Chromium 200 mcg • Molybdenum 50 mcg • Potassium(as potassium chloride) 99 mg • Betaine (as betaine TMG trimethylglycine) 300 mg • MultiEnzyme Blend 110 mg: amylase, papain, protease, bromelain & lipase • GP Flavonoid Complex + 100 mg extracted from: Rose Hips fruit, Tumeric root, Acerola berries, Bilberry berries, Hawthorne berries, Grape skin, Milk Thistle Seed & Citrus fruit • PABA (as para amino benzoic acid) 50 mg • Choline (as choline bitartrate) 50 mg • Inositol 50 mg • Hesperidin 25 mg • Rutin 25 mg • Siberian Ginseng 4:1 extract root 15 mg • Boron 200 mcg. Other Ingredients: Silicon Dioxide, Magnesium Stearate, Gelatin.

My Favorite Multiple Without Iron - Tablets **-** Natrol
Four tablets contain: Vitamin A (as d-Salina beta carotene & Vitamin A palmitate) 10000 IU • Vitamin C (as calcium ascorbate) 250 mg • Vitamin D (as cholecalciferol) 400 IU • Vitamin E (as d-alpha tocopheryl succinate) 400 IU • Thiamine (as Thiamine HCl) (Vitamin B1) 50 mg • Riboflavin (Vitamin B2) 50 mg • Niacin (as Niacin & Niacinamide) 50 mg • Vitamin B6 (as pyridoxine HCl) 50 mg • Folic Acid 400 mcg • Vitamin B12 (as cyanocobalamin) 50 mcg • Biotin 300 mcg • Pantothenic Acid (as d-calcium pantothenate) 50 mg • Calcium (as calcium carbonate & calcium citrate) 1 g • Iodine (from kelp) 150 mcg • Magnesium (as magnesium citrate & magnesium oxide) 400 mg • Zinc 25 mg • Selenium 200 mcg • Copper 2 mg • Manganese (as manganese gluconate) 2 mg • Chromium 200 mcg • Molybdenum 50 mcg • Potassium (as potassium chloride) 99 mg • Betaine (as betaine TMG trimethylglycine) 300 mg • MultiEnzyme Blend 110 mg consisting of: Amylase, Papain, Protease, Bromelain & Lipase • GP Flavonoid Complex 100 mg extracted from: Rose Hips fruit, Tumeric root, Acerola berries, Bilberry berries, Hawthorne berries, Grape skin, Milk Thistle seed & Citrus fruit • PABA (as para amino benzoic acid) 50 mg • Choline (as choline bitartrate) 50 mg • Inositol 50 mg • Hesperidin 25 mg • Rutin 25 mg • Siberian Ginseng 4:1 extract root 15 mg • Boron 200 mcg. Other Ingredients: Microcrystalline Cellulose, Mono & Di-Glycerides, Silicon Dioxide, Magnesium Stearate, Stearic Acid, Croscarmellose Sodium.

Mycelia Immunity Formula **-** PhysioLogics
Each capsule contains: Mycelia Complex Blend 500 mg: Shiitake Mushroom Mycelia extract, Rice Bran. Other Ingredients: Gelatin, Silica, Vegetable Magnesium Stearate.

MycoCeutics MycoPhyto Complex Capsules **-** EcoNugenics
Six capsules contain: MycoCeutics MycoPhyto Proprietary Blend 3840 mg: Reishi (ganoderma lucidum), Coriolus (coriolus versicolor), Umbellatus (polyporus umbellatus), Agaricus (agaricus blazei),

Cordyceps (cordyceps sinensis), Maitake (grifola frondosa) • Beta-1,3-Glucan (from purified yeast) 100 mg.

MycoCeutics MycoPhyto Complex Powder **-** EcoNugenics
Each heaping scoop (4 g) contains: MycoCeutics MycoPhyto Proprietary Blend 3840 mg: Reishi (ganoderma lucidum), Coriolus (coriolus versicolor), Umbellatus (polyporus umbellatus), Agaricus (agaricus blazei), Cordyceps (cordyceps sinensis), Maitake (grifola frondosa) • Beta-1,3-Glucan (from purified yeast) 100 mg • Beta-Glucan (naturally occurring in the mushrooms) 337 mg.

MycoCeutics Ten Mushroom Formula **-** EcoNugenics
Four Capsules contain: MycoCeutics 10 Mushroom Proprietary Blend 2400 mg: Reishi (ganoderma lucidum), Poria Cocos, Cordyceps (cordyceps sinensis), Tremella Fuciformia, Umbellatus (polyporus umbellatus), Coriolus (coriolus versicolor), Maitake (grifola frondosa), Shitake (lentinula edodes), Wood Ear (auricularia auricula), Hericium Erinaceus • Beta-1,3-Glucan (from purified yeast) 30 mg • Beta-Glucan (naturally occuring in the mushrooms) 275 mg. Other Ingredients: Gelatin, Magnesium Stearate, Silica.

Myelin-MS **-** Olympia Nutrition
Spingomyelin- pharmaceutical grade.

MygraFew Standardized Feverfew Extract **-** Nature's Way
Each tablet contains: Dried Feverfew Extract (leaf, standardized Feverfew Extract delivering 600 mcg parthenolide, 5% parthenolide) 12 mg.

MygrAid Formula **-** Nature's Way
Each capsule contains: Feverfew leaves 100 mg • Feverfew dried extract 33.3 mg • Lavender flower 50 mg • Linden leaf & flower 70 mg • Magnesium Amino Acid Chelate 33.3 mg. Other Ingredients: Gelatin, Magnesium Stearate, Millet.

Mylanta Calci Tabs - Extra Strength **-** Johnson & Johnson
Two tablets contain: Calcium 600 mg. Other Ingredients: Dextrose, Maltodextrin, Microcrystalline Cellulose, Magnesium Stearate, Starch, Cellulose, Citric and Fumaric Acids, Natural and Artificial Flavors, Mineral Oil, Sucrose, FD&C Yellow #6, FD&C Yellow #5, FD&C Blue #1, FD&C Red #27, Ethylmaltol, Crospovidone, Hydroxypropyl Methylcellulose, Stearic Acid.

Mylanta Calci Tabs - Ultra Strength **-** Johnson & Johnson
Two tablets contain: Calcium Carbonate 1000 mg. Other Ingredients: Dextrose, Maltodextrin, Microcrystalline Cellulose, Magnesium Stearate, Starch, Cellulose, Citric and Fumaric Acids, Natural and Artificial Flavors, Mineral Oil, Sucrose, FD&C Yellow #6, FD&C Yellow #5, FD&C Blue #1, FD&C Red #27, Ethylmaltol, Crospovidone, Hydroxypropyl Methylcellulose, Stearic Acid.

Myo-Blast - MyoBlast **-** Cytodyne Technologies
Each two capsules contain: Cystoseira Canariensis (as MyoZap CSP3) 600 mg • Rhodiola Rosea extract (standardized for 5% rosavin) 200 mg • Rhaponticum Carthomoides extract (standardized for 25% 20-hydroxyecdysone) 62.5 mg • Anabolic Amino Acid Complex 485 mg: Taurine, Carnosine, L-Leucine.

Myo-Comp **-** PhytoPharmica
Two tablets contain: Vitamin C (ascorbic acid) 120 mg • Vitamin D (cholecalciferol) 266 IU • Vitamin E (D-alpha tocopheryl succinate) 20 IU • Thiamin (thiamin HCl, vitamin B1) 10 mg • Riboflavin (vitamin B2) 10 mg • Niacin 10 mg • Vitamin B6 (pyridoxine HCl) 12 mg • Vitamin B12 (cyanocobalamin) 20 mcg • Calcium (bone meal) 360 mg • Magnesium (chelate) 60 mg • Manganese (chelate) 3 mg • Potassium Chloride 50 mg • Choline Bitartrate 100 mg • Muscle extract 100 mg • Inositol 100 mg • Betaine HCl 60 mg • Ammonium Chloride 60 mg • RNA powder 6 mg.

Myoplex Lite Nutrition Shake - Chocolate Caramel **-** EAS
Each packet (53 g) contains: Prolean II (whey protein from concentrate/isolate, calcium caseinate, soy protein isolate, l-glutamine, taurine) • Corn Syrup solids • Natural and Artificial Flavors • Vitamin & Mineral Blend: Tricalcium Phosphate, Calcium Citrate, Potassium Chloride, Disodium Phosphate, Magnesium Oxide, Dipotassium Phosphate, Choline Bitartrate, Beta Carotene, Ascorbic Acid, Dl-Alpha Tocopheryl Acetate, Niacinamide, Ferrous Fumarate, Manganese Gluconate, Biotin, Zinc Oxide, Boron Proteinate, Thiamine Hydrochloride, D-Calcium Pantothenate, Vitamin A Palmitate, Copper Sulfate, Chromium Citrate, Pyridoxine Hydrochloride, Riboflavin, Selenium Amino Acid Chelate, Molybdenum Amino Acid Chelate, Folic Acid, Cyanocobalamin, Potassium Iodide • Oat fiber • Cocoa (processed with alkali) • Maltodextrin • Cellulose Gum • Salt • High Oleic Sunflower Oil • Sucralose (Splenda brand) • Mono- and Diglycerides • Soy Lecithin.

Myoplex Lite Nutrition Shake - Chocolate Mint **-** EAS
Each packet (53 g) contains: Prolean II (whey protein from concentrate/isolate, calcium caseinate, soy protein isolate, l-glutamine, taurine) • Corn Syrup solids • Vitamin & Mineral Blend: Tricalcium Phosphate, Calcium Citrate, Potassium Chloride, Disodium Phosphate, Magnesium Oxide, Dipotassium Phosphate, Choline Bitartrate, Beta Carotene, Ascorbic Acid, Dl-Alpha Tocopheryl Acetate, Niacinamide, Ferrous Fumarate, Manganese Gluconate, Biotin, Zinc Oxide, Boron Proteinate, Thiamine Hydrochloride, D-Calcium Pantothenate, Vitamin A Palmitate, Copper Sulfate, Chromium Citrate, Pyridoxine Hydrochloride, Riboflavin, Selenium Amino Acid Chelate, Molybdenum Amino Acid Chelate, Folic Acid, Cyanocobalamin, Potassium Iodide • Oat fiber • Chocolate chips (sugar, partially hydrogenated vegetable oil (palm kernal, cottonseed oil), cocoa (processed with alkali), corn syrup solids, soy lecithin, artifical flavor, salt) • Cellulose Gum • Salt • High Oleic Sunflower Oil • Natural Flavors • Sucralose (Splenda brand) • Mono and Diglycerides • Soy Lecithin.

Myoplex Lite Nutrition Shake - Chocolate Peanut Butter **-** EAS
Each packet (53 g) contains: Prolean II (whey protein from concentrate/isolate, calcium caseinate, soy protein isolate, l-glutamine, taurine) • Corn Syrup solids • Vitamin & Mineral Blend: Tricalcium Phosphate, Calcium Citrate, Potassium Chloride, Disodium Phosphate, Magnesium Oxide, Dipotassium Phosphate, Choline Bitartrate, Beta Carotene, Ascorbic Acid, Dl-Alpha Tocopheryl Acetate, Niacinamide, Ferrous Fumarate, Manganese Gluconate, Biotin, Zinc Oxide, Boron Proteinate, Thiamine Hydrochloride, D-Calcium Pantothenate, Vitamin A Palmitate, Copper Sulfate, Chromium Citrate, Pyridoxine Hydrochloride, Riboflavin, Selenium Amino Acid Chelate, Molybdenum Amino Acid Chelate, Folic Acid, Cyanocobalamin, Potassium Iodide • Oat fiber • Natural and Artificial Flavors • Cocoa (processed with alkali) • Maltodextrin • Cellulose Gum • Salt • High Oleic Sunflower Oil • Natural Flavors • Sucralose (Splenda brand) • Mono- and Diglycerides • Soy Lecithin.

Myoplex Lite Nutrition Shake - Dark Chocolate **-** EAS
Each packet (53 g) contains: Prolean II (whey protein from concentrate/isolate, calcium caseinate, soy protein isolate, l-glutamine, taurine) • Corn Syrup solids • Cocoa (processed with alkali) • Vitamin & Mineral Blend: Tricalcium Phosphate, Calcium Citrate, Potassium Chloride, Disodium Phosphate, Magnesium Oxide, Dipotassium Phosphate, Choline Bitartrate, Beta Carotene, Ascorbic Acid, Dl-Alpha Tocopheryl Acetate, Niacinamide, Ferrous Fumarate, Manganese Gluconate, Biotin, Zinc Oxide, Boron Proteinate, Thiamine Hydrochloride, D-Calcium Pantothenate, Vitamin A Palmitate, Copper Sulfate, Chromium Citrate, Pyridoxine Hydrochloride, Riboflavin, Selenium Amino Acid Chelate, Molybdenum Amino Acid Chelate, Folic Acid, Cyanocobalamin, Potassium Iodide • Oat fiber • Natural and Artificial Flavors • Maltodextrin • Cellulose Gum • Salt • High Oleic Sunflower oil • Sucralose (Splenda brand) • Mono- and Diglycerides • Soy Lecithin.

Myoplex Low Carb-Chocolate Cream **-** Nutripeak
Each packet contains: Protein 50 g • Vitamin A Palmitate (35% as Beta Carotene) 7500 IU • Vitamin D (Cholecalciferol) 400 mg • Niacin (Niacinamide) 10 mg • Biotin 150 mcg • Magnesium Oxide 240 mg • Manganese Sulfate 2 mg • Vitamin C (Ascorbic Acid)

90 mg • Vitamin E (dl-Alpha Tocopheryl Acetate) 45 IU • Vitamin B6 (Pyridoxine Hydrochloride) 1 mg • Pantothenic Acid (D-Calcium Pantothenate) 5 mg • Zinc Oxide 7.5 mg • Chromium Citrate 96 mcg • Calcium (Tricalcium Phosphate and Dipotassium Phosphate) 0.5 mg • Thiamin Hydrochloride 0.75 mcg • Folic Acid 200 mcg • Phosphorus 0.35 g • Selenium Amino Acid Chelate 32 mcg • Molybdenum Amino Acid Chelate 52.5 mcg • Iron (Ferrous Fumarate) 9 mg • Riboflavin 0.83 mg • Vitamin B12 (Cyanocobalamin) 3 mcg • Iodine (Potassium Iodide) 74 mg • Copper Sulfate 1 mg. Other Ingredients: Protein Blend: Calcium Caseinate, Whey Protein Concentrate, Milk Protein Isolate, Whey Protein Isolate, Sodium Caseinate; Dutch Processed Cocoa; Partially Hydrogenated Canola Oil; Corn Syrup Solids; Natural and Artificial Flavors; Fibersol (Maltodextrin); Salt; Soy Lecithin; Aspartame; Xanthan Gum; Cellulose Gum; Medium Chain Triglycerides; Carrageenan; Mono & Diglycerides.

Myoplex Original **-** EAS
Each packet (76 g) contains: MyoPro: Whey Protein concentrate (from specially filtered and ion-exchanged whey protein), Calcium Caseinate, Milk-Protein isolate, Taurine, L-Glutamine, Sodium Caseinate, Egg Albumin, Alpha-Ketoglutaric Acid (AKG) • Calcium Caseinate • Corn Syrup Solids • Maltodextrin • Cocoa • Oat Fiber • Vitamin and Mineral Blend: Dipotassium Phosphate, Potassium Chloride, Magnesium Oxide, Choline Bitartrate, Disodium Phosphate, Beta Carotene, DL-Alpha Tocopheryl Acetate, Potassium Citrate, Ascorbic Acid, Ferrous Fumarate, Manganese Gluconate, Biotin, Tricalcium Phosphate, Niacinamide, Zinc Oxide, D-Calcium Pantothenate, Vitamin A Palmitate, Copper Sulfate, Chromium Citrate, Cyanocobalamin, Selenium Amino Acid Chelate, Molybdenum Amino Acid Chelate, Folic Acid, Pyridoxine Hydrochloride, Riboflavin, Thiamine Hydrochloride, Potassium Iodide • Sunflower oil • Natural and Artificial Flavors • Salt • Sucralose • Mono and Diglcyerides • Medium Chain Triglycerides • Soy Lecithin.

Myoplex Plus - Vanilla **-** EAS
Each 76 gram serving contains: Potassium 550 mg • Fiber < 1 g • Myopro [A unique blend of Whey Protein Isolate from specially filtered & ion-exchanged Whey Protein, Calcium Caseinate, Milk Protein Isolate, Taurine, L-Glutamine, Sodium Caseinate, Egg Albumin, & Calcium Alpha-Ketoglutarate (AKG)] • Maltodextrin • Corn Syrup Solids • Vitamin & Mineral Blend [Potassium Chloride, Disodium Phosphate, Calcium Phosphate, Magnesium Oxide, Potassium Citrate, Potassium Phosphate, Choline Bitartrate, Beta-Carotene, Ascorbic Acid, Dl-Alpha Tocopheryl Acetate, Ferrous Fumarate, Molybdenum Amino Acid Chelate, Boron Proteinate, Manganese Gluconate, Selenium Amino Acid Chelate, Niacinamide, Zinc Oxide, Calcium Pantothenate, Chromium Citrate, Copper Sulfate, Vitamin A Palmitate, Pyridoxine Hydrochloride, Riboflavin, Thiamine Hydrochloride, Vitamin D (as Vitamin D3), Folic Acid, Biotin, Potassium Iodide, & Cyanocobalamin] • Natural & Artificial Flavor •Partially Hydrogenated Canola oil • Aspartame • Citrimax (Garcinia cambogia), Salt • Medium-Chain Triglycerides • Xanthan Gum • Soy Lecithin • Cellulose Gum • Mono & Diglycerides • Borage oil. Contains Phenylalanine.

Myoplex Plus Deluxe **-** EAS
Each 83 g Vanilla serving contains: Choline 100 mg • Molybdenum 50 mcg • Boron 1 mcg • Manganese 400 mcg • Selenium 33 mcg • Chromium 100 mcg • Vanadyl Sulfate 10 mg • Conjugated Linoleic Acid 1000 mg • Sodium RNA 9.5 mg. Ingredients: MyoPro: A proprietary protein blend containing Whey Protein Isolate from ion-exchanged Whey, Milk Protein Isolate, Calcium Caseinate, Sodium Caseinate, & Egg Albumin • Maltodextrin GKG [A proprietary blend containing L-Glutamine, Calcium Alpha-Ketoglutarate (AKG), Taurine, Potassium Chloride, Potassium Phosphate, Magnesium Phosphate, Magnesium Oxide, Sodium RNA, & Manganese Glycinate] • CLA (Calcium Conjugated Linoleic Acid from Sunflower oil) • Natural & Artificial Flavors • Partially Hydrogenated Canola oil • Xanthan Gum • V2G: A proprietary blend containing Taurine, Vanadyl Sulfate, & Sodium Selenate •Vitamin & Mineral Blend [Choline Bitartrate, Beta-Carotene, Ascorbic Acid, Dl-Alpha Tocopheryl Acetate, Ferrous Fumarate, Molybdenum Amino Acid Chelate, Boron Proteinate, Niacinamide, Zinc Oxide, Calcium Pantothenate, Chromium Citrate, Copper Sulfate,Vitamin A Palmitate, Pyridoxine Hydrochloride, Riboflavin, Thiamine Hydrochloride, Vitamin D (as Vitamin D3), Folic Acid, Biotin, Potassium Iodide, & Cyanocobalamin] • Corn Syrup Solids • Salt • Soy Lecithin • Asparatame • Cellulose Gum • Carrageenan • Citrimax (Garcinia cambogia) • Medium-Chain Triglycerides • Mono & Diglycerides • Borage oil. Contains Phenylalanine.

Myoplex Plus Deluxe Bar **-** EAS
Gral & Artificial Flavors • Nonfat Milk • Milk • Cocoa • Unsweetened Chocolate • GKG [A proprietary blend containing L-Glutamine, Calcium Alpha-Ketoglutarate (AKG), Taurine, Potassium Chloride, Potassium Phosphate, Magnesium Oxide, Magnesium Phosphate, Sodium RNA, & Manganese Glycinate] • V2G: A proprietary blend containing Taurine, Vanadyl Sulfate, Sodium Selenate • Vitamin & Mineral Blend [Dicalcium Phosphate, Sodium Ascorbate, Ferric Orthophosphate, Dl-Alpha Tocopherol Acetate, Niacinamide, Zinc Oxide, Copper Gluconate, Calcium Pantothenate, Chromium Citrate, Vitamin A Palmitate, Pyridoxine Hydrochloride, Riboflavin, Thiamine Mononitrate, Folic Acid, Chromium Chloride, Sodium Molybdate, Biotin, Potassium Iodide, Phylloquinone, Cholecalciferol, & Cyanocobalamin] • CLA (Calcium Conjugated Linoleic Acid from Sunflower oil) • Lecithin.

MyoSport **-** Pharmalogic
Each pouch contains: Phosphorous 179 mg • Magnesium 60 mg • Potassium 80 mg • Creatine Monohydrate 10 g. Other Ingredients: Dextrose, SynChros TD (time released creatine monohydrate), Agave Nectar, Pure Creatine Monohydrate, Disaccharide, Cocoa, Saturated Polyglycolysed Glycerides, Lecithin, Sodium Citrate, Magnesium Citrate, Natural Flavors, Artificial Flavors, Disodium Phosphate, Potassium Phosphate, Gum Acacia, Xantham Gum, Guar Gum, Gum Arabic, Silicon Dioxide.

Myostat **-** BioTest Laboratories, LLC
Each capsule contains: CSP-3 (Sulfo-Polysaccharide Extract from Cultured Cystoseria Canariensis) 500 mg. Other Ingredients: Gelatin, Cellulose, Magnesium Stearate.

Myo-Tone **-** Enzymatic Therapy
Each tablet contains: Vitamin D (Fish Liver oil) 133 IU • Vitamin E succinate/Wheat Germ) 10 IU • Calcium (Bone Meal) 180 mg • Manganese (Chelate) 63 mg • Vitamin C (Ascorbic Acid/Rose Hips) 60 mg • Potassium Chloride 50 mg • Magnesium (Chelate) 30 mg • Vitamin B6 (Pyridoxine HCl) 6 mg • Thiamine HCL (Vitamin B1) 5 mg • Niacin 5 mg • Riboflavin (Vitamin B2) 5 mg • Vitamin B12 (Cyanocobalamin) 10 mcg • Other Ingredients: Choline Bitartrate 50 mg • Muscle extract 50 mg • Inositol 50 mg • Betaine HCl 30 mg • Ammonium Chloride 30 mg, RNA Powder 3 mg.
See Editor's Note No. 14.

MyoVive **-** Nutricia
One pack (4 fl oz) contains: Vitamin A 1113 IU • Vitamin C 125 mg • Vitamin D 100 IU • Vitamin E 400 IU • Thiamin (Vitamin B1) 13 mg • Riboflavin (Vitamin B2) 1.5 mg • Niacin (Vitamin B3) 10 mg • Vitamin B6 3 mg • Folic Acid 300 mcg • Vitamin B12 1.5 mcg • Biotin 50 mcg • Pantothenic Acid (Vitamin B5) 2 mg • Calcium 126 mg • Iron 0.4 mg • Phosphorus 74 mg • Iodine 40 mcg • Magnesium 9 mg • Zinc 6 mg • Selenium 20 mcg • Copper 0.6 mg • Manganese 1.2 mg • Chromium 13 mcg • Molybdenum 20 mcg • Chloride 81 mg • Sodium 50 mg • Potassium 300 mg • Cysteine 115 mg • Choline 40 mg • Coenzyme Q10 68 mg • L-Carnitine 1.4 g • Creatine 875 mg • Taurine 1.4 g • Fluoride 0.4 mg.

Myrrh Salve **-** Dial Herbs
Myrrh • White Poplar • Balsam Fir • Black Walnut • Cayenne. In a base of Beeswax, Glycerine & Cold Pressed Olive oil.

Some Brand Name Natural Products - What they Contain

www.NaturalDatabase.com contains MANY more listings than appear here.

Myrrh-Goldenseal Plus Formula - Nature's Way
Two capsules contain: Proprietary formula: Cayenne pepper fruit • Goldenseal root • Myrrh Gum (Oleo-Gum Resin from stems). Other Ingredients: Gelatin.

Myrrh-Prickly Ash Bark Virtue - Blessed Herbs
Echinacea Angustifolia root • Goldenseal root • Myrrh Gum • Propolis • Prickly Ash bark • Grain alcohol & Distilled Water.

NAC 600 - GNC A-Z - GNC
Each capsule contains: N-Acetyl-L-Cysteine 600 mg. Other Ingredients: Gelatin, Cellulose, Dicalcium Phosphate.

NAC 600 & Glutathione 100 - GNC
Each capsule contains: N-Acetyl-L-Cysteine 600 mg • L-Glutathione 100 mg. Other Ingredients: Gelatin.

NAC Fuel - TwinLab
Each capsule contains: Highest Quality Pharmaceutical Grade NAC (N-Acetyl-Cysteine) 600 mg.

N-A-C Sustain - Jarrow Formulas
Each tablet contains: N-Acetyl-L-Cysteine 600 mg. Other Ingredients: Cellulose, Calcium Phosphate, Magnesium Stearate, Silicon Dioxide.

NAC, N-Acetyl-Cysteine - NutriCology
Each tablet contains: N-Acetyl-L-Cysteine 500 mg. Other Ingredients: Dicalcium Phosphate, Cellulose, Magnesium Stearate, Silicon Dioxide, Stearic Acid.

N-Acetyl Cysteine - PhysioLogics
Each capsule contains: N-Acetyl Cysteine 600 mg. Other Ingredients: Maltodextrin, Gelatin, Silica, Vegetable Magnesium Stearate.

N-Acetyl Glucosamine - Allergy Research Group
Each capsule contains: N-Acetyl-D-Glucosamine 500 mg. Other Ingredients: Cellulose, Stearic Acid.

Nails Special Formulation - Vitamin World
Each capsule contains: Vitamin B-6 (as pyridoxine hydrochloride) 6 mg • Magnesium (as magnesium aspartate) 17 mg • Potassium (as potassium aspartate) 45 mg • Amino Acid (from casein) 1500 mg. Other Ingredients: Cellulose (plant origin), Dicalcium Phosphate, Croscamellose, Vegetable Stearic Acid, Polyvinylpyrrolidone, Silica, Cellulose Coating.

NaPCA Moisture Mist - Nu Skin Enterprises
Water (aqua) • Aloe Vera gel • Glycerin • Propylene Glycol • Sodium PCA • Lactic Acid • Citric Acid • Hyaluronic Acid • Sodium Lactate • Niacinamide • Glycine • Inositol • Urea • Fructose • Octyl Methoxycinnamate • Polysorbate 20 • Methylparaben • Diazolidinyl Urea • 2-Bromo-2-Nitropropane-1,3-Diol • Sodium Benzoate.

NaPCA Moisturizer - Nu Skin Enterprises
Water • Aloe Vera gel • Stearic Acid • Propylene Glycol • Glyceryl Stearate SE • Sodium PCA • Tocopheryl Linoleate • Tocopheryl Acetate • Hyaluronic Acid • Algae extract • Sorbitol • Allantoin • Retinyl Palmitate • Cholecalciferol • Royal Jelly • RNA • Octyl Methoxycinnamate • Octyl Stearate • Octyl Palmitate • Dioctyl Adipate • Cetearyl Alcohol • Ceteareth-20 • Carbomer • Triethanolamine • Fragrance • Diazolidinyl Urea • Methylparaben • Propylparaben • Disodium EDTA • Iron Oxides.

Nasal Clear - Wellzymes - Enzymes, Inc.
Three capsules contain: Zinc (from Zinc Citrate) 9 mg • n-zimes Proprietary Enzyme Blend 126 mg: pHysioProtease (257,520 pHysio-U), Peptidase, Amylase, CereCalase Plus • Proprietary Herbal Blend 510 mg: Elder flower ext. (equivalent to 600 mg raw herb), Echinacea Purpurea Angustifolia root ext. (equivalent to 600 mg raw herb), Acerola Cherries ext. (standardized to contain 17% vitamin C), Quercetin, Eyebright herb ext. (equivalent to 180 mg raw herb), Goldenseal root ext. (standardized to contain 5% total alkaloids), Rice Bran. Other Ingredients: Plant Cellulose, Water.

Nasal Spray - NutriBiotic
Contains 0.1% Grapefruit extract, combined with Sodium Ascorbate (buffered Vitamin C).

NatCell Adrenal - Allergy Research Group
Each bottle (7 mL) contains: NatCell Adrenal (bovine aqueous extract) 7 mL.

NatCell Liver - Atrium Biotechnologies
Each 7 mL vial contains: Water • Liver and Mescenchyme extracts of Bovine Embryos.
See Editor's Note No. 14.

Naticor - Generation+
Three vegetable capsules contain: Nattokinase 108 mg • Serrapeptase 45 mg • Protease 72 mg • Lipoic Acid 105 mg. Other Ingredients: Rutoside, Calcium Citrate, Magnesium Citrate, Zinc Methionate.

Natrol High Nutrition - Natrol
Each capsule contains: Vitamin C (as Ascorbic Acid) 60 mg • Niacin (as Niacinamide) (Vitamin B3) 2 mg • Vitamin B6 (as Pyridoxine HCl) 2 mg • Thiamine (Vitamin B1) 1.5 mg • In a specially formulated base containing: Winter Berry root 4:1 • Country Malva leaf 5:1, Siberian Ginseng root, Ginger root, Licorice root. Other Ingredients: Silicon Dioxide, Magnesium Stearate, Gelatin.

Nattokinase - Advanced Orthomolecular Research (AOR)
Each softgel contains: Nattokinase 38 mg. Other Ingredients: Soy, Lecithin, Soybean Oil, Bees Wax, Glycerin Fatty Acid Ester, Gelatin, Glycerin.

Nattokinase - Source Naturals
Two softgels contain: Nattokinase (providing 1440 fibrinolytic units (FU) of activity) 72 mg. Other Ingredients: Soybean Oil, Gelatin, Glycerin, Beeswax, Glycerin Fatty Acid Ester, Soybean Lecithin.

Nattokinase - Springboard
Two capsules contain: Nattokinase 1440 FU (72 mg). Other Ingredients: Soybean Oil, Soybean Lecithin.

Nattokinase 100 MG - Solaray
Each capsule contains: Nattokinase 100 mg. Other Ingredients: Rice Flour, Gelatin Capsule, Cellulose, Glyceryl Triacetate, Magnesium Stearate, Silica.

Nattokinase 100 mg (2,000 FU) - NSI - Nutraceutical Sciences Institute
Each capsule contains: Nattokinase (providing 2000 fibrinolytic units (FU) of activity (NSK-SD)) 100 mg. Other Ingredients: Kosher Gelatin, Cellulose, Magnesium Stearate.

Nattokinase 1500 - Naturally Vitamins
Two tablets contain: Nattokinase (providing 1500 FU, 20,000 FU/gm) 75 mg • Rutin Bioflavonoid Complex (vitamin P) 100 mg. Other Ingredients: Plant Fiber, Modified Cellulose Gum, Colloidal Silica, Vegetable Magnesium Stearate, Vegetable Stearic Acid, pH-Resistant Enteric Coating.

Nattokinase Fibrenase I - NutriCology
Two capsules contain: Nattokinase 276 mg. Other Ingredients: Soybean Oil, Soybean Lecithin, Glycerin Fatty Acid Ester, Beeswax.

Nattokinase Plus - Vesta Pharmaceuticals
Two capsules contain: Vitamin E 400 IU • Nattokinase 200 mg (3600 FU). Other Ingredients: Microcrystalline Cellulose, Magnesium Stearate, Silicon Dioxide.

Nattokinase with Vitamin E - NutriCology
Two capsules contain: Vitamin E (D-alpha-tocopherol) 20 IU • Nattokinase (1600 FU) 80 mg. Other Ingredients: Rice Bran Oil, Lecithin, Yellow Beeswax.

NattoZyme Nattokinase 50 mg - NutriCology
Two vegetarian capsules contain: Nattokinase (2000 FU) 100 mg. Other Ingredients: Cellulose, Magnesium Stearate.

Natura Mix Adult (Caps) - Aboca USA, Inc
Each capsule contains: Asian Ginseng root Whole Phytocomplex Concentrate (WPC) (panax ginseng, standardized to 4% total ginsenosides) 94.5 mg • Royal Jelly (freeze-dried, 10 hydroxydecenoic acid minimum 2%) 94.5 mg • Siberian Ginseng root WPC (eleutherococcus senticosus, standardized to 0.7% eleutherosides B+E) 40.5 mg • Bee Pollen powder 40.5 mg. Other Ingredients: Gelatin (capsule).

Natura Mix Adult (Vials) - Aboca USA, Inc
Each vial contains: Bilberry fruit juice concentrate (vaccinium myrtillus, total anthocyanidins minimum 0.2%) 8.3 g • Acacia Honey 6 g • Royal Jelly (10 hydroxydecenoic acid minimum 1%) 0.5 g • Asian Ginseng root freeze-dried extract (panax ginseng, standardized to 15% total ginsenosides) 0.12 g • Bee Pollen freeze-dried extract 0.03 g • Siberian Ginseng root freeze-dried extract (eleutherococcus senticosus, standardized to 1.5% eleutherosides B+E) 0.023 g • Brewer's Yeast freeze-dried extract 0.027 g.

Natura Mix Child - Aboca USA, Inc
Each vial contains: Acacia Honey 9.9 g • Bilberry fruit juice complex (vaccinium myrtillus, total anthocyanosides minimum 0.2%) 4 g • Royal Jelly (10 hydroxydecenoic acid minimum 1%) 0.5 g • Blackberry fruit juice concentrate (rubus fruticosus) 0.45 g • Acerola fruit freeze-dried extract (malpighia glabra) 0.04 g • Bee Pollen freeze-dried extract 0.04 g • Brewer's Yeast freeze-dried extract 0.02 g. Other Ingredients: Natural Strawberry Flavoring.

Natura Mix Senior - Aboca USA, Inc
Each vial contains: Acacia Honey 7.7 g • Bilberry fruit juice concentrate (vaccinium myrtillus, total anthocyanidins minimum 0.2%) 6.5 g • Royal Jelly (10 hydroxydecenoic acid minimum 1%) 0.5 g • Ginkgo leaf freeze-dried extract (ginkgo biloba, standardized to 1% terpene lactones, 3% ginkgo flavone glycosides) 0.15 g • Bee Pollen freeze-dried extract 0.06 g • Schisandra fruit (schisandra chinensis, standardized to 1% schizandrins) 0.045 g • Acerola fruit freeze-dried extract (malpighia glabra) 0.035 g. Other Ingredients: Natural Lemon Flavoring.

Naturafed - Pacific BioLogic
Angelica root (dahurica) • Peppermint (field mint) • Bupleurum root (natural) • Ligusticum root (cnidium) • Ligusticum root (Chinese) • Astragalus root (Grade 1) • Scute root • Platycodon root • Honeysuckle flower • Schizonepta stem • Gentian root (Chinese) • Ephedra Herba (aerial) • Jasmine fruit (cape) • Magnolia flower • Houtuynia. See Editor's Note No. 30, page 2056.

Natural B Complex - Nutrilite
Each tablet contains: Thiamin 1.2 mg • Riboflavin 1.2 mg • Niacin 6.7 mg • Vitamin B6 1.2 mg • Folic Acid 133.33 mcg • Vitamin B12 2 mcg • Pantothenic Acid 5 mg • Inositol 3.6 mg • Para-aminobenzoic Acid 3 mg.

Natural B-12 with Liver - Leiner Health Products
Each tablet contains: Vitamin B12 (Cyanocobalamin) 1000 mcg. Other Ingredients: Dicalcium Phosphate, Stearic Acid, Liver, Croscarmellose Sodium, Yeast, Silicon Dioxide, Magnesium Stearate.

Natural Balance B-100 Complex - Leiner Health Products
Each tablet contains: Thiamin Mononitrate (Vitamin B1) 100 mg • Riboflavin (Vitamin B2) 100 mg • Vitamin B6 (Pyridoxine Hydrochloride) 100 mg • Niacin 100 mg • Biotin 100 mcg • Vitamin B12 100 mcg • Pantothenic Acid 100 mg • Folate 400 mcg. Other Ingredients: Calcium Carbonate, Cellulose, Maltodextrin, Croscarmellose Sodium, Silicon Dioxide, Polyethylene Glycol 3350, Dicalcium Phosphate, Crospovidone, Tricalcium Phosphate.

Natural Balance B-50 Complex - Leiner Health Products
Each tablet contains: Vitamin B12 50 mcg • Pantothenic Acid (d-Calcium Pantothenate) 50 mg • Thiamin Mononitrate (Vitamin B1) 50 mg • Riboflavin (Vitamin B2) 50 mg • Vitamin B6 (Pyridoxine Hydrochloride) 50 mg • Niacin (Niacinamide) 50 mg • Folate 100 mcg • Biotin 50 mcg. Other Ingredients: Calcium Carbonate, Cellulose, Maltodextrin, Croscarmellose Sodium, Sodium Starch Glycolate, Silicon Dioxide, Polyethylene Glycol 3350, Tricalcium Phosphate.

Natural Balanced B Complex + C - Leiner Health Products
One tablet contains: Vitamin B12 50 mcg • Vitamin C (Ascorbic Acid) 500 mg • Pantothenic Acid (d-Calcium Pantothenate) 50 mg • Thiamin Mononitrate (Vitamin B1) 50 mg • Riboflavin (Vitamin B2) 50 mg • Vitamin B6 (Pyridoxine Hydrochloride) 50 mg • Niacin 50 mg • Biotin 50 mcg • Folate 400 mcg. Other Ingredients: Calcium Carbonate, Yeast, Cellulose, Croscarmellose Sodium, Sodium Starch Glycolate, Silicon Dioxide, Rose Hips, Polyethylene Glycol 3350, Cyanocobalamin.

Natural Bee Pollen - Lichtwer Pharma US
Each tablet contains: Bee Pollen 500 mg. Other Ingredients: Sorbitol, Calcium Carbonate, Sodium Starch Glycolate, Silicon Dioxide, Maltodextrin, Crospovidone, Hydroxypropyl Methylcellulose, Stearic Acid, Hydroxypropyl Cellulose, Magnesium Stearate, Polysorbate 80, Polyethylene Glycol 3350.

Natural Beta Carotene - Leiner Health Products
Each softgel contains: Vitamin A 25000 IU. Other Ingredients: Soybean Oil, Gelatin, Glycerin, Vegetable Oil (Partially Hydrogenated Cottonseed and Soybean oils), Yellow Beeswax, Beta Carotene, Carrot Oil.

Natural Beta Carotene - Vital Nutrients
Each capsule contains: Beta Carotene (natural beta carotene, mixed carotenes, naturally derived from d. salina) 25,000 IU.

Natural Brewer's Yeast - Leiner Health Products
Two tablets contain: Vitamin B1 0.12 mg • Vitamin B2 0.04 mg • Niacin 0.30 mg • Vitamin B6 0.02 mg. Other Ingredients: Brewer's Yeast, Cellulose, Guar Gum, Silicon Dioxide.

Natural Bronchial Syrup - Tom's of Maine
Each teaspoon (5 ml) contains: Thyme extract (Thymus vulgaris L) 190 mg • Pine extract (Pinus strobus L) 125 mg • Marshmallow aqueous extract (Althaea officinalis L) 103 mg • Licorice extract (Glycyrrhiza glabra L) 75 mg. Other Ingredients: Honey, Natural Black Cherry extract, Natural Almond extract, Xanthan Gum, or Natural Benzoic Acid.

Natural Calcium & Magnesium - Leiner Health Products
Each tablet contains: Magnesium Oxide 167 mg • Calcium 334 mg. Other Ingredients: Oyster Shell, Maltodextrin, Cellulose, Talc, may contain less than 2% of Mineral Oil, Soy Fiber, Croscarmellose Sodium, Sodium Starch Glycolate, Crospovidone, Magnesium Stearate, Stearic Acid.

Natural Calcium Magnesium & Zinc - Leiner Health Products
Each tablet contains: Calcium Carbonate 333 mg • Magnesium Oxide 133 mg • Zinc Sulfate 5 mg. Other Ingredients: Maltodextrin, Starch, Cellulose, Croscarmellose Sodium, Tricalcium Phosphate, Talc, Sodium Starch Glyolate, Hydroxypropyl Methylcellulose, Silicon Dioxide, Magnesium Stearate, Hydroxypropyl Cellulose, Egg.

Natural Chewable Acidophilus - Puritan's Pride
Each tablet contains: Lactobacillus Acidophilus 10 mg. Other Ingredients: Sucrose, Dextrose, Sweet Whey, Maltodextrin, Cellulose (Plant Origin), Carrageenan, Dried Banana Powder, Vegetable Magnesium Stearate, Silica, Vanilla Flavor, Malt Flavor.

Natural Coenzyme Q10 - Nature's Bounty
Each softgel contains: Coenzyme Q-10 30 mg. Other Ingredients: Rice Bran Oil, Gelatin, Glycerin, Beeswax, Soybean Oil Mixture, Lecithin.

Natural Curves - Biotech Corp.
Two tablets contain: Proprietary Blend 493 mg: Saw Palmetto berry (sabal serrulata), Damiana leaves (turnera aphrodisiaca), Dong Quai root (angelica sinensis), Dandelion root (taraxacum officinale),

Blessed Thistle leaves (cnicus benedictus), Kava Kava root (piper methysticum), Wild Yam root (dioscorea villosa), Motherwort leaves (leonurus carduaca), Fenugreek seed (trigonella foenum-graecum), Black Cohosh (cimicifuga racemosa), Fennel seed (foeniculum vulgare), Chasteberry root (vitex agnus castus), Panax Ginseng, Soy Isoflavones (glycine max), BioPerine Piper Nigrum. Other Ingredients: Oat Bran Filler, Anise Oil.

Natural Curves Instant Bust Firming Gel **-** Biotech Corp.
Deionized Water • Propylene Glycol • Niacin • Hydroxypropyl Methylcellulose • Polysorbate 20 • Sodium Hydroxide • DMDM Hydantoin • Iodopropynyl Butylcarbamate • Algae extract • Calendula Officinalis flower extract • Benzophenone-4 • Tocopherol • Blue 1 • Red 33.

Natural Dolomite with Bone Meal **-** Puritan's Pride
Six tablets contain: Calcium (from Dolomite and Bone Meal) 1,287 mg • Magnesium (from Dolomite) 303 mg • Phosphorus (from Bone Meal) 294 mg.

Natural E **-** GNC
Each capsule contains: Vitamin E 400 IU. Other Ingredients: Calcium Sulfate, Gelatin.

Natural E 1000 d-alpha Form - GNC A-Z **-** GNC
Each capsule contains: VItamin E (as d-alpha tocopheryl acetate) 1000 IU. Other Ingredients: Gelatin, Soybean Oil, Glycerin.

Natural E 1000 Natural Mixed Tocopherols - GNC A-Z **-** GNC
Each capsule contains: Vitamin E (as d-alpha tocopherols) 1000 IU. Other Ingredients: Soybean Oil, Gelatin, Glycerin.

Natural E 200 - GNC A-Z **-** GNC
Each capsule contains: Vitamin E (as d-alpha tocopherol) 200 IU. Other Ingredients: Gelatin, Soybean Oil, Glycerin.

Natural E 400 IU - GNC A-Z **-** GNC
Each capsule contains: Vitamin E 400 IU. Other Ingredients: Calcium Sulfate, Gelatin.

Natural E 400 Natural Mixed Tocopherols - GNC A-Z **-** GNC
Each capsule contains: Vitamin E (as d-alpha tocopherol) 400 IU. Other Ingredients: Soybean Oil, Gelatin, Glycerin.

Natural E 400 Softgel Capsules - GNC A-Z **-** GNC
Each capsule contains: Vitamin E (as d-alpha tocopheryl acetate) 400 IU. Other Ingredients: Gelatin, Soybean oil, Glycerin.

Natural E 400 with Selenium - GNC A-Z **-** GNC
Each capsule contains: Vitamin E (as d-alpha tocopheryl acetate) 400 IU • Selenium (as yeast) 100 mcg. Other Ingredients: Soybean oil, Gelatin, Glycerin, Carob extract, Titanium Dioxide.

Natural Facelift Capsule **-** Healthy Revelations Inc.
Meadowfoam seed oil (limnanthes alba) • Cyclomethicone • Tocopheryl Acetate • Isopropyl Alcohol • Isostearoyl Hydrolyzed Collagen • Retinyl Palmitate • Placental Lipids • Alcohol • Calendula Officinalis extract • Olive Oil Unsaponifiables • Soybean Oil Unsaponifiables • Wheat Germ Oil Unsaponifiables • Pollen extract • Isodecyl Citrate • Tripropylene Glycol Citrate • Juniperus Communis extract • Rosemary extract (rosmarinus officinalis) • Eucalyptus extract (eucalyptus globules) • Fenugreek extract (trigonella foenum graecum) • Peppermint extract (mentha piperita) • Propylparaben • Salicylic Acid • Clary extract (salvia sclarea) • Bitter Orange extract (citrus aurantium) • Coenzyme Q10 • N-Stearoyl-DL-Sphinganine • Allantoin • Dibutyl Lauroyl Glutamide • FD&C Green #3.

Natural Facelift Facial Mask **-** Healthy Revelations Inc.
Water • Carbomer • Panthenol • Urea • Aloe extract (aloe barbadensis) • Glycerin • Glyceryl Stearate • Glucose • Caprylic/Capric Triglyceride • Hydrolyzed Elastin • Hydrolyzed Collagen • Soluble Collagen • Lactoyl Methylsilanol Elastinate • Hops extract • Placental Enzymes • Dimethylsilanol Hyaluronate • Methylsilanol Hydroxproline Asparate • Licorice extract • Hydrocotyl extract • Butcherbroom extract • Green Tea extract • Coenzyme Q10 • Tocopheryl Acetate • Meadowfoam seed oil • Placental Lipids • Retinyl Palmitate • Ivy extract • Bearberry extract • Glycosaminoglycans • Arnica extract • Juniper extract • Myrrh extract • Sorbitol • Stearic Acid • Polysorbate 60 • PEG 7 Glyceryl Cocoate • Stearyl Alcohol • Coneflower extract • Methylparaben • Horsetail extract • Propylparaben • Niacinamide • PCA Ethyl Cocoyl Arginate • PVM/MA Decadiene Crosspolymer • Cabbage Rose extract • Dibutyl Lauroyl Glumatide • Tocopherol • Ascorbyl Palmitate • Lecithin • Glyceryl Oleate • Citric Acid • Adenosine Phosphate • Adenosine Triphosphate • Propylene Glycol • Fragrance • FD&C Red #40.

Natural Fast Release Lysine **-** Leiner Health Products
Each tablet contains: L-Lysine Monohydrochloride 500 mg. Other Ingredients: Dicalcium Phosphate, Cellulose, Croscarmellose Sodium, Stearic Acid, Silicon Dioxide, Magnesium Stearate.

Natural Fish Oil Concentrate **-** Leiner Health Products
Two softgels contain: Natural Fish Oil concentrate 2000 mg • EPA (Eicosapentaenoic acid) 360 mg • DHA (Docosahexaenoic acid) 240 mg. Other Ingredients: Fish Oil Concentrate, Gelatin, Glycerin, d-Alpha Tocopherol.

Natural Form GH-3 **-** Life Extension
Each tablet contains: DMAE 100 mg • Tyrosine 100 mg • Chondroitin Sulfate 65 mg • PABA (para-aminobenzoic acid) 50 mg • Glutamine 50 mg • Phosphatidyl Choline 50 mg • Taurine 50 mg • Magnesium (carbonate) 50 mg • Ascorbyl Palmitate 50 mg • Ginkgo Biloba 25 mg • Vitamin E 30 mg • Vitamin B6 15 mg • Vitamin B12 1 mg.
See Editor's Note No. 15, page 2055.

Natural Garlic Oil **-** Leiner Health Products
Each softgel contains: Garlic oil 3 mg. Other Ingredients: Vegetable Oil, Gelatin, Glycerin.

Natural Herbal Energizer Caps **-** Leiner Health Products
Each caplet contains: Ginseng concentrate (American Ginseng, Korean Ginseng, Chinese Panax Ginseng) 200 mg • Herbal Blend 740 mg. Other Ingredients: Yerba Mate Extract, Croscarmellose Sodium, Gotu Kola, Guarana Extract, Dicalcium Phosphate, Stearic Acid, Magnesium Stearate, Silicon Dioxide, Cellulose, Hydroxypropyl Methylcellulose, Polyethylene Glycol 3350, Hydroxypropyl Cellulose, Damiana, Fo-Ti, Green Tea Extract, Jamaican Ginger.

Natural High Potency Iron **-** Leiner Health Products
Each softgel contains: Iron (Ferrous Fumarate) 27 mg. Other Ingredients: Vegetable Oil, Gelatin, Vegetable Shortening (Partially hydrogenated Soybean and Palm Oils), Glycerin, Blackstrap Molasses, Yellow Beeswax, Hydrogenated Soybean Oil, Lecithin, Polysorbate 80, Caramel Color, Titanium Dioxide.

Natural High Potency Multivitamin/Mineral **-** Leiner Health Products
Each tablet contains: Thiamin (Vitamin B1) 10 mg • Riboflavin (Vitamin B2) 10 mg • Phosphorus 40 mg • Biotin 10 mcg • Magnesium Oxide 100 mg • Vitamin B12 12 mcg • Vitamin C (Ascorbic Acid)100 mg • Calcium Carbonate 62 mg • Iron (Ferrous Fumarate) 27 mg • Vitamin A 7500 IU • Vitamin B6 3 mg • Selenium 10 mcg • Copper 2 mg • Folate 400 mcg • Iodine 150 mcg • Niacin (Niacinamide) 20 mg • Pantothenic Acid 10 mg • Vitamin D 400 IU • Vitamin E (dl-Alpha Tocopheryl Acetate) 30 IU • Zinc Sulfate 15 mg. Other Ingredients: Dicalcium Phosphate, Cellulose, Gelatin, Starch, Maltodextrin, Croscarmellose Sodium, Sodium Starch Glycolate, Kelp, Silicon Dioxide.

Natural Imperial Ginseng **-** Leiner Health Products
Each tablet contains: Ginseng (Siberian) root 250 mg. Other Ingredients: Dicalcium Phosphate, Hydrogenated Vegetable Oil, Croscarmellose Sodium, Silicon Dioxide, Magnesium Stearate,

Hydroxopropyl Methylcellulose, Hydroxypropyl Cellulose, Pharmaceutical Glaze, Polysorbate 80, Polyethylene Glycol 3350.

Natural Iron-Free Multivitamin/Mineral Formula **-** Leiner Health Products
Each tablet contains: Molybdenum (Sodium Molybdate) 25 mcg • Vitamin K (Phytonadione) 25 mcg • Selenium (Sodium Selenate) 20 mcg • Magnesium Oxide 100 mg • Chromium Chloride 25 mcg • Calcium Carbonate 162 mg • Manganese Sulfate 2.5 mg • Phosphorus 109 mg • Copper (Cupric Oxide) 2 mg • Folate (Folic Acid) 400 mcg • Iodine (Potassium Iodide) 150 mcg • Niacin (Niacinamide) 20 mg • Pantothenic Acid (d-Calcium Pantothenate) 10 mg • Riboflavin (Vitamin B2) 1.7 mg • Thiamin Mononitrate (Vitamin B1) 1.5 mg • Vitamin A Acetate 5000 IU • Vitamin B12 (Cyanocobalamin - USP Method 2) 6 mcg • Vitamin B6 (Pyridoxine Hydrochloride) 2 mg • Vitamin C (Ascorbic Acid) 60 mg • Vitamin D (Ergocalciferol) 400 IU • Vitamin E (dl-Alpha Tocopheryl Acetate) 30 IU • Zinc Oxide 15 mg • Biotin (USP Method 2) 30 mcg • Chloride 36.3 mg • Potassium Chloride 40 mg • Nickel (Nickelous Sulfate) 5 mcg • Silicon 2 mg • Tin (Stannous Chloride) 10 mcg • Vanadium (Sodium Metavanadate) 10 mcg. Other Ingredients: Dicalcium Phosphate, Gelatin, Cellulose, Croscarmellose Sodium, Sodium Starch Glycolate, Hydroxypropyl Methylcellulose, Starch, Sodium Metasilicates & Oxides, Pharmaceutical Glaze, Polyethylene Glycol 3350, Magnesium Stearate, Maltodextrin, Hydroxypropyl Cellulose, Mannitol, Sodium & Potassium Borates, Polysorbate 80, Beta Carotene, Resin.

Natural KLB6 **-** Puritan's Pride
Two softgels contain: Vitamin B6 (Pyridoxine HCl) 7 mg • Lecithin 200 mg • Kelp 50 mg • Cider Vinegar 80 mg.

Natural L-Formula Lysine **-** Leiner Health Products
Each tablet contains: L-Lysine Monohydrochloride 500 mg. Other Ingredients: Cellulose, Polyethylene Glycol 3350, Croscarmellose Sodium, Silicon Dioxide, Magnesium Stearate.

Natural Light **-** Cell Tech
Each capsule contains: Chromium 50 mcg • Proprietary Algae Blend 80 mg: Blue-Green Algae (aphanizomenon flos-aquae), Bladderwrack Algae, Kelp 1:10 extract • Proprietary Enzyme Blend 40 mg: Lipase, Amylase, CereCalase, Protease, Pectinase • Cell Tech Herbal Weight Loss Blend 577 mg: Garcinia rind extract, Kola nut extract (10% caffeine), Gotu Kola (aerial part), Siberian Ginseng root, Fo-ti root, Gymnema sylvestre leaf extract (25% gymnemic acid), St. John's Wort (aerial part), Bitter Orange standardized extract, Guarana 4:1 extract (seed), Hawthorn extract (leaf and flower), Maca root, Green Tea extract 80/60, Cascara Sagrada bark, Ginkgo Biloba leaf 50:1 extract, Ginger (rhizome), White Willow bark, Cayenne Pepper fruit, Chromium Polynicotinate • Lecithin 15 mg. Other Ingredients: Vegetable Cellulose, Rice Bran, Water.
See Editor's Note No. 40, page 2058.

Natural Lutein 6 MG **-** CVS Pharmacy
Each softgel contains: Lutein 6 mg. Other Ingredients: Corn Oil, Gelatin, Glycerin, Yellow Beeswax.

Natural Magnesium **-** Leiner Health Products
Each tablet contains: Magnesium Oxide 250 mg. Other Ingredients: Cellulose, Talc, Sodium Starch Glycolate, Starch, Silicon Dioxide, Croscarmellose Sodium, Polyethylene Glycol, Kelp, Magnesium Stearate.

Natural Man **-** NDS Nutrition
Two capsules contain: Vitamin A (beta carotene with mixed carotenoids) 10,000 IU • Vitamin D (cholecalciferol) 400 IU • Vitamin E (D-alpha tocopheryl) 100 IU • Vitamin K 80 mcg • Vitamin C (calcium ascorbate) 600 mg • Vitamin B1 (thiamine) 50 mg • Vitamin B2 (riboflavin) 49 mg • Vitamin B3 (niacinamide) 50 mg • Vitamin B5 (calcium pantothenate) 50 mg • Vitamin B6 (pyridoxine) 50 mg • Vitamin B12 200 mcg • Biotin 400 mcg • Folic Acid 400 mcg • Calcium (milk calcium complex) 180 mg • Magnesium (citrate) 90 mg • Zinc (aspartate) 30 mg • Copper (gluconate) 2 mg • Iodine (potassium iodine) 150 mcg • Vanadium (asparate) 10 mcg • Boron (aspartate) 250 mcg &#8226 Manganese (citrate) 2 mg • Selenium (methionine) 100 mcg • Molybdenum (aspartate) 75 mcg • Chromium (nicotinate) 100 mcg. Other Ingredients: Brown Rice, Magnesium Stearate, Gelatine, Water.

Natural Menopause Formula **-** Schiff
Three tablets contain: Vitamin K (as phytonadione) 40 mcg • Vitamin B6 (as pyridoxine hydrochloride) 15 mg • Folate (folic Acid, folacin) 400 mcg • Vitamin B12 (as cyanocobalamin) 12 mcg • Calcium (as calcium carbonate) 500 mg • Magnesium (as magnesium oxide) 200 mg • Sage leaf (salvia officinalis) 100 mg • Black Cohosh root standardized extract (cimifuga racemosa, 2.5% triterpenoidglycosides) 80 mg • Soy Isoflavones 50 mg • Boron (as calcium borogluconate) 2 mg • Giant Knotweed root (polygonum cuspidatum, reservatrol 1 mg) 5 mg. Other Ingredients: Microcrystalline Cellulose, Stearic Acid, Croscarmellose Sodium, Hydroxypropyl Methylcellulose, Maltodextrin, Magnesium Stearate, Methylcellulose, Mannitol, Acacia, Polyethylene Glycol, Hydroxypropyl Cellulose.

Natural Multi-Amino Acid (GNC A-Z) **-** GNC
Three capsules contain: L-Alanine 88.7 mg • L-Arginine 80.7 • L-Aspartic Acid 108 mg • L-Cystine 4.6 mg • L-Glutamic Acid 272.7 mg • Glycerine 142.2 mg • L-Histidine 25.6 mg • L-Isoleucine 33.3 mg • L-Leucine 99 mg • L-Lysine 88.3 mg • L-Methionine 29.2 mg • L-Phenylalanine 60 mg • L-Proline 169.8 mg • L-Serine 71.7 mg • L-Threonine 40.1 mg • L-Tryptophan 10.3 mg • L-Tyrosine 49.7 mg • L-Valine 48.4 mg • Hydroxylysine 5.6 mg • Hydroxyproline 78.9 mg • Protein (as calcium caseinate & gelatin) 2 g • Vitamin E (as d-alpha tocopherol) 1.5 IU • Liquid Soy Lecithin 22.5 mg. Other Ingredients: Soybean Oil, Glycerin, Titanium Dioxide.

Natural Oyster Shell Calcium **-** Leiner Health Products
Each tablet contains: Calcium 500 mg. Other Ingredients: Oyster Shell, Maltodextrin, Acacia Gum, Croscarmellose Sodium, Tricalcium Phosphate, Magnesium Stearate.

Natural Oyster Shell Calcium with D **-** Leiner Health Products
Each tablet contains: Vitamin D 200 IU • Calcium 500 mg. Other Ingredients: Oyster Shell, Maltodextrin, Acacia, may contain less than 2% of Cellulose, Mineral Oil, Croscarmellose Sodium, Tricalcium Phosphate, Soy Fiber, Magnesium Stearate, Ergocalciferol, Crospovidone, Stearic Acid.

Natural Potassium Gluconate **-** Leiner Health Products
Each tablet contains: Potassium Gluconate 90 mg. Other Ingredients: Cellulose, Croscarmellose Sodium, Sodium Starch Glycolate, Starch, Polyethylene Glycol 3350, Silicon Dioxide, Magnesium Stearate.

Natural Prostate Formula **-** Life Extension
Each softgel contains: Saw Palmetto berries CO2 extract (serenoa repens) 160 mg • Free Fatty Acids/Sterols (85-95% from saw palmetto extract) 136 mg • Stinging Nettle root extract (urtica dioica) 120 mg • Pygeum bark extract (pygeum africanum) 50 mg • Sterols (from pygeum extract) 6.5 mg • Lycopene (from tomato extract) 5 mg • Boron (from boron citrate, glycinate/aspartate) 1.5 mg • Rosemary extract (rosmarinus officinalis) 400 mcg. Other Ingredients: Gelatin, Pumpkin Seed Oil, Glycerin, Water, Carob.

Natural Quit **-** JBS Natural Products
Denicotizing Formula: Alfalfa leaf • Barberry bark • Buckthorn bark • Burdock root • Cascara Sagrada • Chaparral • Dandelion root • Goldenseal root • Hyssop • Kelp • Oregon Grape root • Pau D'Arco • Prickly Ash • Yellow Dock root • Yucca root. Anti-Addiction Formula: Anise seed • Barberry bark • Bee Pollen • Blue Cohosh root • Catnip herb • Cayenne 40M • Chamomile • Echinacea angustifolia herb • Eleutherococcus • Fennel seed • Gentian root • Gotu Kola • Hops flower • Lemongrass • Licorice root • Lobelia herb • Myrrh gum • Passionflower • Peppermint leaf • Safflower • Sarsaparilla •Skullcap herb • Slippery Elm bark • Valerian root • Wood Betony. Aromatherapy Formula: Camphor • Eucalyptus • Denatured Alcohol 40 • Peppermint • Rosemary • Ylang Ylang.

Natural Radiance Cream - Life Extension
Vitamin A, Vitamin E, Vitamin C, Green Tea extract, Deionized Water, Grape Seed oil, Cetyl Palmitate, Isocetyl Stearate, Glycerin, Cetyl Alcohol, Polyacrylamide, C13-14 Isoparafin, Laureth-7, Phenyl Trimethicone, Dimethicone, Laurether-16.

Natural Relief Cold & Flu Chewable with Zinc - Boericke & Tafel
Each tablet contains: Aconitum Napellus 4X 25 mg • Bryonia Alba 4X 25 mg • Eucalyptus Globulus 2X 10 mg • Eupatorium Perfoliatum 2X 25 mg • Gelsemium Sempervirens 4X 25 mg • Ipecacuanha 3X 25 mg • Phosphorus 6X 25 mg.
See Editor's Note No. 1, page 2053.

Natural Sensation - Strategic Science & Technology
Water • Choline Chloride • L-Arginine • Sodium Chloride • Mineral Oil • Zinc Chloride • Glyceryl Stearate SE • Squalene • Cetyl Alcohol • Magnesium Chloride • Propylene Glycol Stearate SE • Wheat Germ Oil • Glyceryl Stearate • Isopropyl Myristate • Stearyl Stearate • Polysorbate-60 • Propylene Glycol • Oleic Acid • Tocopherol Acetate • Collagen • Sorbitan Stearate • Vitamin A • Vitamin D • Triethanolamine • Methylparaben • Aloe Vera extract • Imidazolidinyl Urea • Propylparaben • BHA.

Natural Source Calcium & Magnesium - Leiner Health Products
Each tablet contains: Magnesium Oxide 167 mg • Calcium Carbonate 333 mg. Other Ingredients: Maltodextrin, Cellulose, Talc, Croscarmellose Sodium, Mineral Oil, Hydroxypropyl Methylcellulose, Soy Polysaccharide, Citric Acid, Starch Silicon Dioxide, Polyethylene Glycol, Magnesium Stearate, Crospovidone, Gum Arabic Stearic Acid.

Natural Source Calcium + Vitamin D - Leiner Health Products
Each tablet contains: Vitamin D (Cholecalciferol) 125 IU • Calcium Carbonate 250 mg. Other Ingredients: Maltodextrin, Talc, Pregelatinized Starch, Croscarmellose Sodium, Acacia, Silicon Dioxide, Magnesium Stearate.

Natural Source Calcium + Vitamin D - Pharmaceutical Grade - Leiner Health Products
Each tablet contains: Calcium Carbonate 500 mg • Vitamin D (Cholecalciferol) 125 IU. Other Ingredients: Maltodextrin, Talc, Pregelatinized Starch, Croscarmellose Sodium, Acacia, Hydroxypropyl Methylcellulose, Silicon Dioxide, Magnesium Stearate, Hydroxypropyl Cellulose, Polysorbate 80, Polyethylene Glycol 3350.

Natural Source Calcium Pharmaceutical Grade - Leiner Health Products
Each tablet contains: Calcium Carbonate 500 mg. Other Ingredients: Maltodextrin, Acacia, Starch, Croscarmellose Sodium, Cellulose, Hydroxypropyl Methylcellulose, Talc, Silicon Dioxide, Mineral Oil, Soy Polysaccharide, Magnesium Stearate, Polyethylene Glycol 3350, Hydroxypropyl Cellulose, Polysorbate 80, Crospovidone, Stearic Acid.

Natural Source Calcium, Magnesium, & Zinc - Leiner Health Products
Each tablet contains: Calcium Carbonate 333 mg • Magnesium Oxide 133 mg • Zinc Sulfate 5 mg. Other Ingredients: Maltodextrin, Cellulose, Croscarmellose Sodium, Talc, Hydroxypropyl Methylcellulose, Acacia, Soy Polysaccharide, Mineral Oil, Silicon Dioxide, Starch, Magnesium Stearate, Stearic Acid, Citric Acid, Sodium Starch Glycolate, Polyethylene Glycol, Hydroxypropyl Cellulose, Polysorbate 80, Crospovidone.

Natural Source DHEA - Life Extension
Each tablet contains: Discorea Villosa (wild yam) 250 mg • GABA (gamma-aminobutyric acid) 75 mg • Alpha Ketoglutaric Acid 75 mg • Glycine 75 mg • Saw Palmetto 75 mg.

Natural Soya Lecithin - Leiner Health Products
Each softgel contains: Soya Lecithin 1200 mg. Other Ingredients: Gelatin, Glycerin.

Natural Sport Creatine Chewable with FOS - Nutraceutical Corp.
Each two wafers contain: Creatine Monohydrate 3 g • Proprietary FOS Fiber Blend (BeFlora) (265 mg Fructo-oligosaccharides) 530 mg. Inactive Ingredients: Guar Gum, Cellulose, Natural Tangerine flavor, Citric Acid, Stearic Acid, Maltose, Natural Orange flavor, Silica, Magnesium Stearate.

Natural Sports Extreme Cordyceps - Nutraceutical Corp.
Each capsule contains: Cordyceps CS-4 mycelial biomass (Cordyceps sinensis) (Minimum 36 mg Cordycepic acid) 525 mg • Cordyceps mycelial biomass (cordyceps sinensis, minimum 10 mg cordydepic acid, minimum 1 mg cordycepin) 100 mg • Reishi mushroom (ganoderma lucidum) 75 mg • Maitake mushroom (grifolia fondosa) 75 mg. Other Ingredients: Gelatin, Magnesium Stearate, Silica, Brown Rice.

Natural Sterol Complex - Universal
Two tablets contain: Mexican Wild Yam root 1000 mg • Smilax officinalis extract 1000 mg • Muira puama 1000 mg • Gotu Kola 515 mg • Boron 3 mg • Gamma Oryzanol 500 mg • Fucosterol 7959 mcg • Beta Sitosterol 5663 mcg • Campesterol 3376 mcg • Stigmasterol 1924 mcg • "other Sterols" 1009 mcg • Bee Pollen 1000 mg • Guarana 500 mg • Korean Ginseng 100 mg • Cytochrome C 100 mg • Dimethylglycine 100 mg • Inosine 100 mg • Royal Jelly 30 mg • Kola Nut 25 mg • Calcium 200 mg • Magnesium 100 mg • Potassium 99 mg • Linoleic Acid 1040 mg • Oleic Acid 698 mg • Palmitic Acid 263 mg • Linoleic Acid 109 mg • Stearic Acid 56 mg • Lignoceric Acid 14 mg • Arachidonic Acid 13 mg • Behenic Acid 6 mg • Myristic Acid 5 mg • Octacosanol 1650 mcg • RNA 60 mg • DNA 30 mg • Capsicum 100 mg • Alfalfa 100 mg • Dandelion root 100 mg • Garlic 100 mg • Yellow Dock 100 mg • Licorice root 100 mg • Hops 100 mg • Milk Thistle 10 mg.

Natural Time Release B-12 - Leiner Health Products
Each tablet contains: Vitamin B12 (Cyanocobalamin) 1000 mcg. Other Ingredients: Dicalcium Phosphate, Hydrogenated Vegetable Oil, Cellulose, Magnesium Stearate, Silicon Dioxide.

Natural Time Release B-6 - Leiner Health Products
Each tablet contains: Vitamin B6 (Pyridoxine Hydrochloride) 200 mg. Other Ingredients: Dicalcium Phosphate, Hydrogenated Vegetable Oil, Silicon Dioxide, Stearic Acid, Magnesium Stearate, Yeast, Rose Hips, Watercress.

Natural Time Release Balanced B-100 - Leiner Health Products
Each tablet contains: Thiamin Mononitrate (Vitamin B1) 100 mg • Riboflavin (Vitamin B2) 100 mg • Vitamin B6 (Pyridoxine Hydrochloride) 100 mg • Niacin (Niacinamide) 100 mg • Biotin 100 mcg • Vitamin B12 100 mcg • Pantothenic Acid 100 mg • Folate 400 mcg. Other Ingredients: Dicalcium Phosphate, Hydrogenated Vegetable Oil, Stearic Acid, Silicon Dioxide, Magnesium Stearate, Resin, Gum Acacia, Wheat Bran, Cellulose, Para Aminobenzoic Acid.

Natural Time Release Balanced B-50 - Leiner Health Products
Each tablet contains: Vitamin B12 50 mcg • Pantothenic Acid (d-Calcium Pantothenate) 50 mg • Thiamin Mononitrate (Vitamin B1) 50 mg • Riboflavin (Vitamin B2) 50 mg • Vitamin B6 (Pyridoxine Hydrochloride) 50 mg • Niacin (Niacinamide) 50 mg • Biotin 50 mcg • Folate 400 mcg. Other Ingredients: Dicalcium Phosphate, Hydrogenated Vegetable Oil, Stearic Acid, Cellulose, Magnesium Stearate, Silicon Dioxide, Resin, Gum Acacia, Hydroxypropyl Cellulose.

Natural Time Release Complete Multivitamin/Mineral **-** Leiner Health Products
Each tablet contains: Selenium 5 mcg • Calcium 62.5 mg • Magnesium 25 mg • Molybdenum 5 mcg • Vitamin B12 35 mcg • Copper 1 mg • Vitamin C (Ascorbic Acid) 250 mg • Chromium 5 mcg • Pantothenic Acid (d-Calcium Pantothenate) 30 mg • Manganese 5 mg • Thiamin Mononitrate (Vitamin B1) 35 mg • Riboflavin (Vitamin B2) 35 mg • Potassium Chloride 99 mg • Vitamin B6 (Pyridoxine Hydrochloride) 35 mg • Niacin 35 mg • Iodine 225 mcg • Vitamin A 7500 IU • Folate 400 mcg • Iron (Ferrous Sulfate) 18 mg • Vitamin D 400 IU • Vitamin E 30 IU • Zinc 15 mg • Biotin 5 mcg. Other Ingredients: Dicalcium Phosphate, Hydrogenated Vegetable Oil, Cellulose, Stearic Acid, Gelatin, Silicon Dioxide, Magnesium Oxide.

Natural Time Release Maximum Choice **-** Leiner Health Products
Two tablets contain: Chloride 18 mg • Potassium 20 mg • Vitamin B12 50 mcg • Vitamin C (Ascorbic Acid) 400 mg • Vitamin E (d-Alpha Tocopheryl Acid Succinate) 200 IU • Pantothenic Acid (d-Calcium Pantothenate) 50 mg • Iron 8.2 mg • Chromium 50 mcg • Selenium 25 mcg • Thiamin Mononitrate (Vitamin B1) 50 mg • Riboflavin (Vitamin B2) 50 mg • Calcium 260 mg • Vitamin B6 (Pyridoxine Hydrochloride) 50 mg • Niacin (Niacinamide) 50 mg • Magnesium Oxide 100 mg • Vitamin A 10000 IU • Molybdenum 15 mcg • Phosphorus 200 mg • Zinc Sulfate 25 mg • Biotin 50 mcg • Copper 3 mg • Iodine 225 mcg • Manganese 3 mg • Folate 400 mcg • Vitamin D 400 IU. Other Ingredients: Dicalcium Phosphate, Hydrogenated Vegetable Oil, Beta Carotene, Stearic Acid.

Natural Time Release Vitamin C with Rose Hips **-** Leiner Health Products
Each tablet contains: Vitamin C 500 mg. Other Ingredients: Dicalcium Phosphate, Hydrogenated Vegetable Oil, Stearic Acid, Rose Hips, Silicon Dioxide, Magnesium Stearate, Starch, Ethylcellulose.

Natural Ultra E 1000 **-** GNC
Each capsule contains: Vitamin A 1000 IU •Vitamin E 1000 IU. Other Ingredients: Soybean oil, Gelatin, Glycerin, Caramel Color, Titanium Dioxide.

Natural Ultra E 400 - GNC A-Z **-** GNC
Each capsule contains: Vitamin A (as beta-carotene) 400 IU •Vitamin E (as d-alpha tocopherol) 400 IU. Other Ingredients: Gelatin, Soybean Oil, Glycerin, Caramel Color, Titanium Dioxide.

Natural Vitamin A **-** Leiner Health Products
Each softgel contains: Vitamin A 8000 IU. Other Ingredients: Vegetable Oil, Gelatin, Glycerin, Fish Liver Oil.

Natural Vitamin A & D (Cod Liver Oil) USP **-** Leiner Health Products
Each softgel contains: Vitamin D 135 IU • Vitamin A 1250 IU. Other Ingredients: Cod Liver Oil, Gelatin, Glycerin, and may contain Water.

Natural Vitamin C with Rose Hips **-** Leiner Health Products
Each tablet contains: Vitamin C 250 mg. Other Ingredients: Ascorbic Acid, Calcium Carbonate, Cellulose, Rose Hips, Silicon Dioxide, Talc, Polyethylene Glycol 3350, Tricalcium Phosphate, Crospovidone, Magnesium Stearate.

Natural Vitamin E - Biodelivery Nutritional Systems **-** Nutritional Therapeutics, Inc.
Each tablet contains: Vitamin E 200 IU • Pantethine (Coenzyme A Precursor) 25 mg • Selenium 12.5 mg • NT Factor tablet base 47.5 mg.

Natural Vitamin E **-** Leiner Health Products
Each softgel contains: Vitamin E (dl-Alpha Tocopheryl Acetate and d-Alpha Tocopherol) 200 IU. Other Ingedients: Gelatin, Glycerin, Vegetable Oil.

Natural Vitamin E **-** NSI - Nutraceutical Sciences Institute
Each softgel contains: Vitamin E 400 IU.

Natural Vitamin E **-** Optimum Nutrition
Each softgel contains: Vitamin E (as D-alpha tocopherol acetate) 400 IU. Other Ingredients: Gelatin, Soy Oil.

Natural Vitamin E **-** Puritan's Pride
Each softgel contains: Vitamin E (as d-alpha tocopheryl acetate) 400 IU. Other Ingredients: Gelatin, Glycerin, Soybean Oil.

Natural Vitamin E **-** Swanson
Eash softgel contains: Natural Vitamin E (as d-alpha tocopheryl acetate) 400 IU.

Natural Vitamin E 400 I.U. **-** Leiner Health Products
Each softgel contains: Vitamin E (dl-Alpha Tocopheryl Acetate and d-Alpha Tocopherol) 400 IU. Other Ingredients: Gelatin, Glycerin, Vegetable Oil.

Natural Vitamin E d-Alpha **-** Leiner Health Products
Each softgel contains: Vitamin E (d-Alpha Tocopheryl Acetate) 400 IU. Other Ingredients: Vegetable Oil, Gelatin, Glycerin, and may contain Water.

Natural Vitamin E Mixed Tocopherols - Basic Nutrition **-** GNC
Each capsule contains: Vitamin E (as d-alpha Tocopherol) 200 IU. Other Ingredients: Soybean Oil, Gelatin, Glycerin.

Natural Whole Herb Saw Palmetto Concentrated Herb 1000 mg **-** Vitamin World
Each softgel contains: Saw Palmetto berry (serenoa repens, from 250 mg of 4:1 extract) 1000 mg. Other Ingredients: Soybean Oil, Gelatin, Glycerin, Yellow Beeswax, Soy Lecithin, Caramel Color.

Natural Woman **-** NDS Nutrition
Three capsules contain: Vitamin A (beta carotene with mixed carotenoids) 10,000 IU • Vitamin D (cholecalciferol) 400 IU • Vitamin E (D-alpha tocopheryl) 100 IU • Vitamin K 80 mcg • Vitamin C (calcium ascorbate) 500 mg • Vitamin B1 (thiamine) 50 mg • Vitamin B2 (riboflavin) 49 mg • Vitamin B3 (niacinamide) 50 mg • Vitamin B5 (calcium pantothenate) 50 mg • Vitamin B6 (pyridoxine) 50 mg • Vitamin B12 200 mcg • Biotin 400 mcg • Folic Acid 400 mcg • Calcium (milk calcium complex) 400 mg • Magnesium (citrate) 200 mg • Iron (fumerate) 10 mg • Zinc (aspartate) 20 mg • Copper (gluconate) 2 mg • Iodine (potassium iodine) 150 mcg • Vanadium (aspartate) 10 mcg • Boron (aspartate) 250 mcg • Manganese (citrate) 2 mg • Selenium (methionine) 100 mcg • Molybdenum (aspartate) 75 mcg • Chromium (nicotinate) 100 mcg. Other Ingredients: Brown Rice, Magnesium Stearate, Gelatine, Water.

Natural Wonder Woman **-** DreamPharm
Two capsules contain: Dong Quai root (angelica sinensis) 300 mg • Black Cohosh root (cimicifuga racemosa) 150 mg • Blue Cohosh root (caulophyllum thalictroides) 100 mg.

Natural Zinc Gluconate **-** Leiner Health Products
Each tablet contains: Zinc Gluconate 50 mg. Other Ingredients: Starch, Croscarmellose Sodium, Sodium Starch Glycolate, Magnesium Stearate.

Naturally Blended Vitamin E - Basic Nutrition **-** GNC
Each capsule contains: Vitamin E (as dl-alpha Tocopheryl Acetate and d-alpha Tocopherol) 400 IU. Other Ingredients: Gelatin, Glycerin.

Naturally Clear Cleansing Scrub **-** Nature's Life
Ingredients: Distilled Water • Niacinamide • Disodium Oleth-3 Sulfosuccinate (derived from coconut oil) • Walnut Shell powder • Cetyl Alcohol (derived from vegetable oils) • Sucrose Cocoate • Apricot Kernel Oil • Citric Acid • Sodium PCA • Aloe Vera gel • Beta Carotene.

Some Brand Name Natural Products - What they Contain
www.NaturalDatabase.com contains MANY more listings than appear here.

Naturally Clear Dietary Supplement **-** Nature's Life
Each two capsules contain: Vitamin A (as palmitate) 5000 IU • Vitamin C (as ascorbic acid and ascorbyl palmitate) 200 mg • Vitamin D (vitamin D3, as cholecalciferol) 133 IU • Vitamin E (as d-alpha tocopheryl succinate) 100 IU • Thiamine (vitamin B1, as thiamine HCl) 5 mg • Riboflavin (vitamin B2) 5 mg • Vitamin B3 (as niacinamide) 10 mg • Vitamin B6 (as pyridoxine HCl) 10 mg • Folic Acid 133 mcg • Vitamin B12 (as cyanacobalamin) 50 mcg • Biotin (as d-biotin) 100 mcg • Pantothenic Acid (as d-calcium pantothenate) 10 mg • Zinc (from zinc picolinate) 15 mg • Selenium (as selenomethionine/sodium selenite) 100 mcg • Copper (from copper gluconate) 1 mg • Chromium (from chromium nicotinate) 100 mcg • Proprietary Blend 840 mg: L-Lysine HCl, L-Arginine, L-Cysteine HCl, L-Glutamine.
Inactive Ingredients: Gelatin Capsule.

Naturally Clear Nourishing Spray **-** Nature's Life
Ingredients: Distilled Water • Niacinamide • Aloe Vera • Sodium PCA.

Naturally Herbal Phen **-** Optimum Nutrition
St. John's Wort • Bitter Orange.
See Editor's Note No. 40, page 2058.

Naturally Inspired Absorbable Calcium with Vitamin D **-** Vitamin World
Two softgels contain: Vitamin D (as cholecalciferol) 100 IU • Calcium (as calcium carbonate) 1000 mg. Other Ingredients: Soybean Oil, Gelatin, Glycerin, Lecithin, Titanium Dioxide Color.

Naturally Inspired B-100 Ultra B-Complex **-** Vitamin World
Each tablet contains: Thiamin (Vitamin B1) (as Thiamine Mononitrate) 100 mg • Riboflavin (Vitamin B2) 100 mg • Niacin (as Niacinamide) 100 mg • Vitamin B6 (as Pyridoxine Hydrochloride) 100 mg •Folic Acid 100 mcg • Vitamin B12 (as Cyanocobalamin) 100 mcg •Biotin (as D-Biotin) 100 mcg •Pantothenic Acid (as D-Calcium Pantothenate) 100 mg • Inositol 100 mg •PABA (Para-Aminobenzoic Acid) 100 mg • Choline Bitartrate 100 mg •Proprietary Blend 5 mg: Parsley leaves powder, Rice Bran defatted powder, Watercress leaves powder, Alfalfa leaves powder, Lecithin granules. Other Ingredients: Cellulose (Plant Origin), Vegetable Stearic Acid, Croscarmellose, Cellulose Coating, Dicalcium Phosphate, Silica, Guar Gum.

Naturally Inspired Black Currant Oil **-** Vitamin World
Each softgel contains: Black Currant seed oil (providing gamma linolenic acid (GLA) 80 mg) 535 mg. Other Ingredients: Gelatin, Glycerin.

Naturally Inspired Borage Oil 1000 mg **-** Vitamin World
Each softgel contains: Borage oil (borago officinalis seed oil) 1000 mg: Gamma Linolenic Acid (GLA) 240 mg, Linoleic Acid (LA) 360 mg. Other Ingredients: Gelatin, Glycerin.

Naturally Inspired C & E **-** Vitamin World
Each softgel contains: Vitamin C (as ascorbic acid and rose hips) 500 mg • Vitamin E (as D-alpha tocopherol plus D-beta, D-gamma and D-delta tocopherols) 400 IU. Other Ingredients: Gelatin, Glycerin, Soybean Oil, Soy Lecithin, Caramel Color, Yellow Beeswax.

Naturally Inspired Chelated Potassium 99 mg **-** Vitamin World
Each caplet contains: Potassium (as potassium gluconate) 99 mg. Other Ingredients: Crospovidone, Vegetable Stearic Acid, Silica, Vegetable Magnesium Stearate, Cellulose Coating.

Naturally Inspired Chelated Zinc Lozenges 23 mg **-** Vitamin World
Each lozenge contains: Zinc (as zinc citrate and zinc gluconate) 23 mg. Other Ingredients: Fructose, Sorbitol, Honey Powder, Vegetable Stearic Acid, Citric Acid, Natural and Artificial Flavors, Silica, Vegetable Magnesium Stearate.

Naturally Inspired Coral Calcium 500 mg **-** Vitamin World
Two capsules contain: Calcium (from 1000 mg of coral calcium) 370 mg. Other Ingredients: Gelatin, Rice Powder, Silica, Vegetable Magnesium Stearate.

Naturally Inspired Delicious Chewable Vitamin C-500 mg with Rose Hips **-** Vitamin World
Each tablet contains: Vitamin C (as sodium ascorbate, ascorbic acid, and rose hips) 500 mg. Other Ingredients: Sugar, Sorbitol, Vegetable Stearic Acid, Natural Orange Flavor, Silica, Vegetable Magnesium Stearate.

Naturally Inspired EPA Natural Fish Oil 1000 mg **-** Vitamin World
Each softgel contains: Vitamin E (as D-alpha tocopherol plus D-beta, D-gamma and D-delta) 1.1 IU • Fish Oil 1000 mg • EPA (eicosapentaenoic acid) 180 mg • DHA (docosahexaenoic acid) 120 mg. Other Ingredients: Gelatin, Glycerin.

Naturally Inspired Ester-C 1000 mg with Bioflavonoids **-** Vitamin World
Each tablet contains: Vitamin C (as Ester-C calcium ascorbate) 1000 mg • Calcium (as Ester-C calcium ascorbate) 110 mg • Citrus Bioflavonoid fruit (citrus spp.) 100 mg • Rutin fruit (dimorphandra mollis) 20 mg • Hesperidin fruit complex (citrus spp.) 20 mg. Other Ingredients: Cellulose (plant origin), Vegetable Stearic Acid, Croscarmellose, Silica, Vegetable Magnesium Stearate, Cellulose Coating.

Naturally Inspired Ester-C 500 mg with Bioflavonoids **-** Vitamin World
Each capsule contains: Vitamin C (from Ester-C calcium ascorbate) 500 mg • Calcium (as Ester-C calcium ascorbate) 55 mg • Citrus Bioflavonoid fruit (citrus sinensis) 100 mg • Rutin fruit (dimorphandra mollis) 5 mg • Hesperidin fruit complex (citrus spp.) 5 mg. Other Ingredients: Gelatin, Cellulose (plant origin), Silica, Vegetable Magnesium Stearate.

Naturally Inspired Evening Primrose Oil 1000 mg **-** Vitamin World
Each softgel contains: Evening Primrose Oil 1000 mg: Cis-Linoleic Acid (LA) 700 mg, Gamma-Linolenic Acid (GLA) 90 mg. Other Ingredients: Gelatin, Glycerin.

Naturally Inspired Evening Primrose Oil 1300 mg **-** Vitamin World
Each softgel contains: Evening Primrose Oil 1300 mg: Cis-Linoleic Acid (LA) 949 mg, Gamma-Linolenic Acid (GLA) 117 mg. Other Ingredients: Gelatin, Glycerin.

Naturally Inspired Evening Primrose Oil 500 mg **-** Vitamin World
Each softgel contains: Evening Primrose Oil 500 mg: Cis-Linoleic Acid 365 mg, Gamma-Linolenic Acid (GLA) 45 mg. Other Ingredients: Gelatin, Glycerin.

Naturally Inspired Herba Vision Lutein and Bilberry Complex **-** Vitamin World
Each capsule contains: Lutein (containing naturally occurring zeaxanthin) 6 mg • Bilberry fruit extract (vaccinium myrtillus, standardized to contain 25% anthocyanosides) 20 mg. Other Ingredients: Dicalcium Phosphate, Cellulose (plant origin), Gelatin, Vegetable Stearic Acid, Silica, Vegetable Magnesium Stearate.

Naturally Inspired High Potency Calcium 600 + Vitamin D with Soy Isoflavones **-** Vitamin World
Two tablets contain: Vitamin D (as cholecalciferol) 400 IU • Calcium (as calcium carbonate) 1200 mg • Soy Isoflavones 50 mg. Other Ingredients: Acacia Gum, Maltodextrin, Croscarmellose, Cellulose Coating, Vegetable Magnesium Stearate.

Naturally Inspired High Potency Magnesium 500 mg - Vitamin World
Each tablet contains: Magnesium (as magnesium oxide) 500 mg. Other Ingredients: Cellulose (plant origin), Starch, Povidone, Magnesium Silicate, Cellulose Coating, Titanium Dioxide Color, Vegetable Magnesium Stearate, Propylene Glycol.

Naturally Inspired L-Arginine 1000 mg - Vitamin World
Each tablet contains: L-Arginine (as arginine hydrochloride) 1000 mg. Other Ingredients: Cellulose (plant origin), Povidone, Vegetable Stearic Acid, Silica, Cellulose Coating, Vegetable Magnesium Stearate.

Naturally Inspired Lutein 20 mg - Vitamin World
Each softgel contains: Lutein 20 mg. Other Ingredients: Corn Oil, Gelatin, Glycerin, Yellow Beeswax, Lecithin.

Naturally Inspired Macu Vision - Vitamin World
Each capsule contains: Taurine 200 mg • Lutein 3 mg • Alpha Lipoic Acid 25 mg. Other Ingredients: Rice Powder, Gelatin, Vegetable Magnesium Stearate, Silica.

Naturally Inspired Magnesium 250 mg - Vitamin World
Each caplet contains: Magnesium (as magnesium oxide) 250 mg. Other Ingredients: Cellulose (plant origin), Starch, Cellulose Coating, Titanium Dioxide Color, Magnesium Silicate, Vegetable Magnesium Stearate.

Naturally Inspired Magnesium Citrate - Vitamin World
Each tablet contains: Magnesium (as magnesium citrate) 100 mg. Other Ingredients: Cellulose (plant origin), Vegetable Stearic Acid, Croscarmellose, Silica, Vegetable Magnesium-Stearate, Cellulose Coating.

Naturally Inspired Mega Vita-Min - Vitamin World
Each tablet contains: Vitamin A (as retinyl palmitate) 8000 IU • Vitamin C (as ascorbic acid and rose hips) 250 mg • Vitamin D (as cholecalciferol) 400 IU • Vitamin E (as D-alpha tocopheryl acetate) 125 IU • Thiamin (vitamin B1, as thiamine mononitrate) 80 mg • Riboflavin (vitamin B2) 80 mg • Niacin (as niacinamide) 80 mg • Vitamin B6 (as pyridoxine hydrochloride) 80 mg • Folic Acid 400 mcg • Vitamin B12 (as cyanocobalamin) 80 mcg • Biotin (as D-biotin) 80 mcg • Pantothenic Acid (as D-calcium pantothenate) 80 mg • Calcium (as calcium carbonate) 8 mg • Iron (as ferrous gluconate) 2 mg • Iodine (as kelp) 150 mcg • Magnesium (as magnesium oxide) 6 mg • Zinc (as zinc gluconate) 1.4 mg • Selenium (as sodium selenite) 25 mcg • Copper (as copper gluconate) 0.07 mg • Manganese (as manganese gluconate) 0.12 mg • Chromium (as chromium picolinate) 25 mcg • Molybdenum (as sodium molybdate) 25 mcg • Potassium (as potassium gluconate) 1.6 mg • Boron (as sodium borate) 0.5 mg • Choline Bitartrate 80 mg • Inositol 80 mg • PABA (para-aminobenzoic acid) 80 mg • Rutin fruit (dimorphandra mollis) 30 mg • Citrus Bioflavonoids fruit (citrus sinensis) 25 mg • Hesperidin fruit (citrus spp.) 5 mg • Betaine Hydrochloride 25 mg • Coenzyme Q-10 500 mg • Deodorized Garlic bulb (allium sativum) 1 mg • Korean Ginseng root (Panax ginseng) 1 mg • Pycnogenol 500 mcg • Proprietary Blend 4 mg: Alfalfa leaf, Watercress, Parsley leaf, Rice Bran, Lecithin. Other Ingredients: Cellulose (plant origin), Vegetable Stearic Acid, Croscarmellose, Silica, Mannitol, Vegetable Magnesium Stearate, Cellulose Coating, Starch.

Naturally Inspired Milk Free ProBiotic Acidophilus - Vitamin World
Each capsule contains: Lactobacillus Blend 40 mg: Lactobacillus Acidophilus, Lactobacillus Rhamnosus, Lactobacillus Bifidus. Other Ingredients: Dicalcium Phosphate, Cellulose (plant origin), Hydroxypropyl Methylcellulose, Vegetable Stearic Acid, Silica, Vegetable Magnesium Stearate.

Naturally Inspired MSM 750 mg - Vitamin World
Each capsule contains: MSM (methylsulfonylmethane, organic sulfur 255 mg) 750 mg • Other Ingredients: Dicalcium Phosphate, Gelatin, Vegetable Magnesium Stearate, Silica.

Naturally Inspired Time Release Mega Vita-Min Long Acting Formula - Vitamin World
Each tablet contains: Vitamin A (as retinyl palmitate) 8000 IU • Vitamin C (as ascorbic acid and rose hips) 250 mg • Vitamin D (as cholecalciferol) 400 IU • Vitamin E (as D-alpha tocopheryl acetate) 125 IU • Thiamin (vitamin B1, as thiamine mononitrate) 80 mg • Riboflavin (vitamin B2) 80 mg • Niacin (as niacinamide) 80 mg • Vitamin B6 (as pyridoxine hydrochloride) 80 mg • Folic Acid 400 mcg • Vitamin B12 (as cyanocobalamin) 80 mcg • Biotin (as D-biotin) 80 mcg • Pantothenic Acid (as D-calcium pantothenate) 80 mg • Calcium (as calcium carbonate) 8 mg • Iron (as ferrous gluconate) 2 mg • Iodine (as kelp) 150 mcg • Magnesium (as magnesium oxide) 6 mg • Zinc (as zinc gluconate) 1.4 mg • Selenium (as sodium selenite) 25 mcg • Copper (as copper gluconate) 0.07 mg • Manganese (as manganese gluconate) 0.12 mg • Chromium (as chromium picolinate) 25 mcg • Molybdenum (as sodium molybdate) 25 mcg • Potassium (as potassium gluconate) 1.6 mg • Boron (as sodium borate) 0.5 mg • Choline Bitartrate 80 mg • Inositol 80 mg • PABA (para-aminobenzoic acid) 80 mg • Rutin fruit (dimorphandra mollis) 30 mg • Citrus Bioflavonoids fruit (citrus sinensis) 25 mg • Hesperidin fruit (citrus spp.) 5 mg • Betaine Hydrochloride 25 mg • Coenzyme Q-10 500 mg • Deodorized Garlic bulb (allium sativum) 1 mg • Korean Ginseng root (Panax ginseng) 1 mg • Pycnogenol 500 mcg • Proprietary Blend 4 mg: Alfalfa leaf, Watercress, Parsley leaf, Rice Bran, Lecithin. Other Ingredients: Methylcellulose, Vegetable Stearic Acid, Silica, Mannitol, Vegetable Magnesium Stearate, Cellulose Coating, Starch.

Naturally Inspired Vitamin C & Zinc Lozenges - Vitamin World
Each lozenge contains: Vitamin C (as ascorbic acid and rose hips) 300 mg • Zinc (as zinc citrate) 7 mg • Natural Food Base 30 mg: Rutin, Hesperidin, Acerola, Citrus Bioflavonoid, Black Currant. Other Ingredients: Sucrose, Dextrose, Maltodextrin, Cottonseed Oil, Starch, Natural Flavor, Vegetable Magnesium Stearate.

Naturally Inspired Vitamin C-1000 mg with Rose Hips - Vitamin World
Each tablet contains: Vitamin C (as ascorbic acid and rose hips) 1000 mg. Other Ingredients: Cellulose (plant origin), Croscarmellose, Vegetable Stearic Acid, Silica, Cellulose Coating, Vegetable Magnesium Stearate.

Naturally Inspired Vitamin C-500 mg with Rose Hips - Vitamin World
Each tablet contains: Vitamin C (as ascorbic acid and rose hips) 500 mg. Other Ingredients: Cellulose (plant origin), Cellulose Coating, Croscarmellose, Vegetable Stearic Acid, Vegetable Magnesium Stearate, Silica.

Naturally Inspired Yeast Free Chromium Picolinate - Vitamin World
Each tablet contains: Chromium (as Chromium Picolinate) 200 mcg. Other Ingredients: Dicalcium Phosphate, Cellulose (Plant Origin), Vegetable Stearic Acid, Silica, Vegetable Magnesium Stearate.

Naturally Inspired Zinc Picolinate 25 mg - Vitamin World
Each caplet contains: Zinc (as zinc picolinate) 25 mg. Other Ingredients: Dicalcium Phosphate, Cellulose (plant origin), Vegetable Stearic Acid, Vegetable Magnesium Stearate.

Naturally Kids' Calcees Chewable Calcium + D - Naturally Vitamins
Each tablet contains: Calcium 300 mg • Vitamin D (cholecalciferol) 50 IU. Other Ingredients: Fruit concentrate, Vanilla powder.

Naturally Lean Matrix - ProLab
Three capsules contain: Proprietary Blend 2 g: 3-Hydroxy-L-Tyrosine from Mucuna Pruriens, Guggul gum resin (E-guggulsterones, Z-guggulsterones), Caffeine, Green Tea leaf extract (epigallocatechin gallate, polyphenols), Coleus Forskohlii root, Naringin, Evodia Rutaecarpa fruit, Chaste Tree berries (Vitex agnus-castus fruit), Bitter

Orange extract (citrus aurantium fruit, synephrine, N-methyl-tyramine, hordenine, octopamine, tyramine). Other Igredients: Gelatin, Silica, Magnesium Stearate.
See Editor's Note No. 40, page 2058.

Naturally Phen **-** Optimum Nutrition
DL-Phenylalanine L-5-Hydroxytryptophan Tyrosine.

Naturally Ripped **-** Optimum Nutrition
Ma Huang • Guarana • L-Carnitine • Chromium Picolinate.
See Editor's Note No. 21 and No. 30, page 2056.

NaturalMax OstiBone **-** NaturalMax - Nutraceutical
Each capsule contains: Calcium (as Calcium Carbonate) 120 mg • Ostivone (as Isoproproxy Isoflavone) 200 mg. Inactive ingredients: Gelatin, Cellulose, Magnesium Stearate.

Natural-Source d-Alpha Vitamin E brand **-** ADM
Vitamin E.
See Editor's Note No. 44, page 2058.

NaturalTrim **-** Starlight International
Each capsule contains: Chromium (as chromium picolinate) 6 mcg • Magnesium Gluconate 7 mg • Calcium Gluconate 5 mg • Ma Huang (ephedra sinica, plant) 275 mg • Total Ephedrine Alkaloids 22 mg • Bladderwrack (fucus vesiculosus, plant) 35 mg • Uva Ursi extract, 4:1 (arctostaphylosuva ursi, leaf) 25 mg • Couch Grass (agropyron repens, rhizome) 8.75 mg • Dandelion (taraxacum officinale, root) 8.75 mg • Hydrangea (hydrangea arborescans, root) 8.75 mg • Nettle (urtica dioica, leaf) 8.75 mg • Buchu (carosma betulina, leaf) 8.75 mg • Parsley extract, 4:1 (petroselinum crispum, leaf) 8 mg • Corn Silk (zea mays, flower pistil) 7 mg • Fumitory (fumaria officinalis, plant) 6 mg • Goldenrod (solidago odora, leaf) 6 mg • English Hawthorn (crataegus laevigata, berry) 5 mg • Licorice (glycyrrhiza glabra, root) 5 mg • Marshmallow (althea officinalis, root) 5 mg • Apple Pectin 5 mg. Other Ingredients: Silicon Dioxide, Magnesium Stearate, Dicalcium Phosphate, Gelatin.
See Editor's Note No. 21 and No. 30.

NaturalTrim Ephedra Free **-** Starlight International
Each capsule contains: Proprietary Blend 520 mg: Guarana seed extract (paullinia cupana, containing 72 mg caffeine), Rhododendron Caucasicum leaf extract, Arctic root (rhodiola rosea), Corn Silk (zea mays, flower pistil), Buchu leaf (agathosma betulina). Other Ingredients: Silicon Dioxide, Magnesium Stearate, Gelatin.

Naturatussin 1 **-** Pacific BioLogic
Platycodon root (balloon flower) • Licorice root • Cynanchum root • Red Date (Chinese jujube) • Sophora root • Burdock fruit (great) • Fritillaria bulb (tendrilled) • Peppermint (field mint) • Ephedra Herba (aerial) • Apricot kernal (northern) • Aster root (purple).
See Editor's Note No. 30, page 2056.

Naturatussin 2 **-** Pacific BioLogic
Houttuynia Herba • Platycodon root (balloon flower) • Hogfennel root (peucedanum) • Aster root (purple) • Honeysuckle flower • Cynanchum root • Trichosanthes fruit peel • Peach kernal • Momordica Fruit (arhat) • Fritillaria bulb (tendrilled) • Burdock fruit (great).

Natura-UR **-** Pacific BioLogic
Angelica root (dahurica) • Citrus peel (tangerine) • Andrographis • Isatis leaves • Licorice root • Scute root • Platycodon root • Honey Suckle flower • Chrysanthemum flower • Forsynthia fruit • Burdock fruit • Notopterygium root & rhizome.

Nature Cleanse BotaniCleanse **-** Nature's Plus
Each tablet contains: Botanical Proprietary Blend 500 mg: Butternut bark (Juglans cinera), Yellow Dock root (Rumex crispus), Blessed Thistle flower (Cnicus benedictus), Red Clover leaf (Trifolium pratense), Clove bud (Eugenia caryophyllata), Milk Thistle seed (Silybum marianum), Uva Ursi leaf (Arctostaphylos uva-ursi), Cranberry fruit (Vaccinium macrocarpon), Ginger root (Zingiber officinale), Cascara Sagrada bark (Rhamnus purshiana) Hibiscus flower (Hibiscus abelmoschus), Juniper berry (Juniperus oxycedrus), Senna leaf (Cassia senna), Slippery Elm bark (Ulmus rubra), Fennel seed (Foeniculum vulgare), Cayenne fruit (Capsicum frutescens), Dandelion root (Taraxacum officinale), Parsley leaf (Petroselinum crispum), Alfalfa leaf (Medicago sativa), Fenugreek seed (Trigonella foenum-graecum), Aloe Vera, Apple Cider Vinegar • Green Food Proprietary Blend 100 mg: Chlorophyll, Chlorella, broken cell Blue-Green Micro-Algae, Spirulina Algae (Spirulina platensis), Irish Moss (Chondrus crispus), Barley Grass juice (Hordeum vulgare), Pacific Kelp (Laminaria) • Vitamin C (corn free) 100 mg.

Nature Cleanse Fiber Diet **-** Nature's Plus
Nine capsules contain: Oat Bran (87% Fiber) 1912.5 mg • Psyllium husks (80% Fiber) 1912.5 mg • Apple pectin (84% Fiber) 180 mg • Vitamin C 157.5 mg • Butcher's Broom (15% Fiber) 135 mg • Bentonite U.S.P. grade 90 mg • Cellulose (100% Fiber) 90 mg • Lactobacillus acidophilus 90 million viable cells 22.5 mg.

Nature Cleanse PuriFiber Internal Cleansing & Revitalizing Powder **-** Nature's Plus
Each teaspoon (3.75g) contains: Fiber Complex 3500 mg containing a proprietary blend of fiber rich concentrates: Psyllium husks (Plantago ovata), Apple pectin (Malus sylvestris), Butcher's Broom rhizome (Ruscus aceleatus), Bentonite, modified citrus pectin, Cellulose, Rice fiber (Oryza sativa), Slippery Elm bark (Ulmus rubra), Oat bran (Avena sativa), Beet juice & fiber (Beta vulgaris), Prune fiber (Prunus) • Chitosan, vegetarian 50 mg • FOS (Fructooligosaccharides) Lactic flora growth accelerant 50 mg • Lipase fat-digesting enzyme 50 mg • Peptide FM bioactive oligopeptide 25 mg • Lactospor micro-encapsulated pure culture of B. Coagulans, provides 1 million viable cells 1.7 mg.

Nature Derm Skin Care System **-** PhytoPharmica
Two capsules contain: Bromelain (1200 MCU/g) 200 mg • Burdock root 4:1 extract (arctium lappa) 10 mg • Calcium (as calcium lactate) 11 mg • Magnesium (as magnesium oxide) 72 mg • Niacin 10 mg • Pantothenic Acid (as clacium D-pantothenate) 10 mg • Potassium (as potassium chloride) 105 mg • Ribonucleic Acid (RNA) 20 mg • Sulfur (sublimed) 25 mg • Thymus 25 mg • Vitamin A (as retinyl acetate) 10,000 IU • Vitamin B12 (as cyanocobalamin) 3 mcg • Vitamin B6 (as pyridoxine HCl) 8 mg • Vitamin C (ascorbic acid) 200 mg • Zinc (as zinc chelate) 30 mg.
See Editor's Note No. 14.

Nature Derm Skin Care System Acne Cream **-** PhytoPharmica
Each application contains: Sulfur 3%. Other Ingredients: Purified Water, Zinc, Sage Extract, Silymarin Phytosome, Hawthorne Extract, Chamomile Extract, 18-Beta-Glycyrrhetinic Acid, Essential Oil of Rosemary, Urea, and Vitamin E (Tocopherol), Natural and Hypoallergenic Fragrance.

Nature Force **-** Rexall - Sundown
Two tablets contain: Vitamin A (100% beta-carotene) 10000 IU • Vitamin C 300 mg • Vitamin E (dl-alpha-tocopheryl acid succinate) 90 IU • Calcium 255 mg • Selenium (from selenium amino acid chelate) 50 mcg • Sodium 5 mg • Nature Force Proprietary Blend: Mixed Berry Skin extract, Alfalfa aerial parts, Tomato, European Wine Grape concentrate (vitis vinifera), Plant Enzymes (glucose oxidase, peroxidase, catalase), Cruciferous Vegetable concentrate (cabbage head, cauliflower flower head, broccoli flower head), Green Tea leaf extract, Garlic, Rose Hips, and Seeds extract (rosa canina), Freeze-Dried Carrot root juice 188 mg. Other Ingredients: Dicalcium Phosphate, Croscarmellose Sodium, Silica, Magnesium Stearate.

Nature Made Adult Multi-Vitamin Chewable **-** Pharmavite Corp.
Each tablet contains: Vitamin A (as beta-carotene) 5000 IU • Vitamin C 250 mg • Vitamin D 400 IU • Vitamin E 30 IU • Thiamin 1.5 mg • Riboflavin 1.7 mg • Niacin 20 mg • Vitamin B6 2 mg • Folic Acid 400 mcg • Vitamin B12 6 mcg • Biotin 40 mcg • Pantothenic Acid 10 mg • Calcium 200 mg • Phosphorous 100 mg • Iodine 150 mcg •

Magnesium 20 mg • Zinc 15 mg • Copper 2 mg • Sodium 15 mg. Inactive Ingredients: Sorbitol, Fructose, Xylitol, Stearic Acid, Mono & Diglycerides of Fatty Acids, Carrageenan, Gelatin, Aspartame, Yellow 6 Lake, Corn Starch, Citric Acid, Natural & Artificial Flavors, Modified Food Starch, Aluminum Oxide, Red 40 Lake.

Nature Made Balanced B-150 Complex **-** Pharmavite Corp.
Each tablet contains: Thiamin mononitrate (Vitamin B1) 150 mg • Riboflavin (Vitamin B2) 150 mg • Niacin (Niacinamide, Vitamin B3) 150 mg • Vitamin B6 (Pyridoxine Hydrochloride) 150 mg • Folate (Folic Acid, Folacin, as Folate) 400 mcg • Vitamin B12 (Cyanocobalamin) 150 mcg • Biotin 150 mcg • Pantothenic Acid 150 mg. Other Ingredients: Dibasic Calcium Phosphate, Hydroxypropyl Methylcellulose, Magnesium Stearate, Polyethylene Glycol, Carnauba Wax.

Nature Made Cal Burst **-** Pharmavite Corp.
Each soft chew contains: Calcium Carbonate (providing Elemental Calcium 500 mg) 1250 mg • Vitamin D 200 IU. Other Ingredients: Corn Syrup, Calcium Carbonate, Sugar, Hydrogenated Coconut Oil, Cocoa (Chocolate Flavor only), Nonfat Dried Milk, Glycerin, Corn Starch, Salt, Lecithin, Natural and Artificial Flavors.

Nature Made Calcium and Magnesium with Zinc **-** Pharmavite Corp.
Each tablet contains: Calcium Carbonate 333 mg • Magnesium Oxide 133 mg • Zinc Sulfate 5 mg. Other Ingredients: Maltodextrin, Croscarmellose Sodium, Silicon Dioxide, Magnesium Stearate, Hydroxypropyl Methylcellulose, Cellulose, Polyethylene Glycol.

Nature Made Glucosamine **-** Nature Made
Each tablet contains: Glucosamine 500 mg.

Nature Made Magnesium 250 mg **-** Pharmavite Corp.
Each tablet contains: Magnesium (as magnesium oxide) 250 mg. Inactive Ingredients: Cellulose, Croscarmellose Sodium, Magnesium Stearate.

Nature Made Rekindle **-** Pharmavite Corp.
Each two tablets contain: Calcium 250 mg • L-Arginine 1250 mg • Asian Ginseng (Korean) root extract 50 mg • Damiana leaf 25 mg • Ginkgo leaf extract 25 mg. Other Ingredients: L-Arginine Hydrochloride, Calcium Carbonate, Cellulose Gel, Hydroxypropyl Methylcellulose, Stearic Acid, Silicon Dioxide, Magnesium Stearate, Titanium Dioxide, Red 40 Lake, Polyethylene Glycol, Triethyl Citrate, Polysorbate 80, Blue 2 Lake.

Nature Made SAM-e **-** Pharmavite Corp.
Two tablets contain: S-adenosylmethionine 400 mg • 4-butanedisulfonate • Cellulose • Sodium Starch Glycolate • Methacrylic Acid Copolymer • Talc • Polyethylene Glycol • Silica • Magnesium Stearate • Polysorbate 80 • Sodium Hydroxide • Iron Oxide • Simethicone.

Nature Made Soy Isoflavones 50 mg **-** Pharmavite Corp.
Each tablet contains: Soy Isoflavones 50 mg. Other Ingredients: Dibasic Calcium Phosphate, Cellulose, Soy Extract, Croscarmellose Sodium, Magnesium Stearate, Silicon Dioxide.

Nature Made Vinpocetine **-** Pharmavite Corp.
Each tablet contains: Vinpocetine 5 mg.

Nature Made Vitamin C - 1000 **-** Pharmavite Corp.
Each tablet contains: Vitamin C 1000 mg. Other Ingredients: Ascorbic Acid, Corn Starch, Cellulose, Magnesium Stearate, Stearic Acid, Silica Gel.

Nature Made Vitamin E **-** Pharmavite Corp.
Each softgel contains: Vitamin E 400 IU. Other Ingredients: Dl-Alpha Tocopheryl Acetate, Gelatin, Glycerin, Water.

Nature's Cure Two-Part Acne Treatment System for Males **-** Nature's Cure
This is a 2 component product that includes tablets and a cream. Each tablet contains: Calendula officinalis (marigold) 6x • Hydrastis canadensis (golden seal) 6x • Juglans regia (walnut) 6x • Antimonium crudum (antimonius sulfide) 12x • Echinacea angustifolia (cone flower) 12x • Ledum palustre (wild rosemary) 12x • Orchitimun (glandular) 12x • Sarsaparilla (wild licorice) 12x • Hepar Sulfuris Calcareum (calcium sulfide) 24x • Carbo Vegetabilis (vegetable carbon) 30x. Other Ingredients: Lactose. The cream contains: Benzoyl Peroxide (5%). Other Ingredients: Purified Water, Carbomer 940, Allantoin, Aloe Vera concentrate, Diazolidinyl Urea, Disodium Edetate, Dioctyl Sodium Sulfosuccinate, Sodium Hydroxide.
See Editor's Note No. 1, page 2053.

Nature's Cure Two-Part Acne Treatment System, Cream, for Females **-** Nature's Cure
Active Ingredients: Benzoyl Peroxide (5%). Inactive Ingredients: Purified Water, Carbomer 940, Alantoin, Aloe Vera concentrate, Diazolidinyl Urea, Disodium Edetate, Dioctyl Sodium Sulfosuccinate, Sodium Hydroxide.

Nature's Cure Two-Part Acne Treatment System, Tablets, for Females **-** Nature's Cure
Each tablet contains: Juglans regia (walnut) 6x • Antimonium Crudum (antimonius sulfide) 12x • Candida albicans (yeast) 12x, 30x, 60x, 200x • Echinacea angustifolia (cone flower) 12x • Kali Bromatum (potassium bromide) 12x • Ledum palustre (wild rosemary) 12x • Oophorunum (glandular) 12x • Hepar Sulfuris Calcareum (calcium sulfide) 24x • Carbo Vegetabilis (vegetable carbon) • Cimicifuga racemosa (black cohosh) 30x • Cistus canadensis (frost weed) 30 x • Graphites (graphite) 30x. Other Ingredients: Lactose.
See Editor's Note No. 1, page 2053.

Nature's Fingerprint - Fingerprint Botanicals **-** GNC
Each capsule contains: Wild Yam root 150 mg • Evening Primrose 90 mg • Chaste Tree berry 50 mg.

Nature's Life Greens - Capsule **-** Nature's Life
Each 500 mg capsule contains: Green Peas (Pisum sativum) • Celery (Apium graveolens) Cabbage (Brassica oleracea capitata) • Cauliflower (Brassica oleracea botrutis) • Broccoli (Brassica oleracea italica) • Spinach (Spinacia oleracea) • Green Bell Peppers (Capsicum frutescens) • Green Onions (Allium cepa) • Hawaiian grown Spirulina plantesis • Parsley (Petroselinum crispum) • Green Chili Peppers (Capsicum annum) • Green Garlic sprouts (Allium sativum) • Jalepeno Peppers (Capsicum annum) • Green Tea leaves (Camellia sinensis) • Alfalfa (Medicago sativa) • Barley Grass (Hordeum vulgare) • Dunaliella salina • Chlorella • Pacific Alaria (Alaria marginata) • Kelp (Laminaria species) • Pacific Nori (Porphyra tenera) Dulse (Phodymenia palmata) • Kombu (Laminaria setchellii) • Sea Lettuce (Ulva lactuca) • Sea Palm (Pastelsi palmaeformis).

Nature's Life Greens - Powder **-** Nature's Life
Five grams of powder contain: Green Peas (Pisum sativum) • Celery (Apium graveolens) Cabbage (Brassica oleracea capitata) • Cauliflower (Brassica oleracea botrutis) • Broccoli (Brassica oleracea italica) • Spinach (Spinacia oleracea) • Green Bell Peppers (Capsicum frutescens) • Green Onions (Allium cepa) • Hawaiian grown Spirulina plantesis • Parsley (Petroselinum crispum) • Green Chili Peppers (Capsicum annum) • Green Garlic sprouts (Allium sativum) • Jalepeno Peppers (Capsicum annum) • Green Tea leaves (Camellia sinensis) • Alfalfa (Medicago sativa) • Barley Grass (Hordeum vulgare) • Dunaliella salina • Chlorella • Pacific Alaria (Alaria marginata) • Kelp (Laminaria species) • Pacific Nori (Porphyra tenera) Dulse (Phodymenia palmata) • Kombu (Laminaria setchellii) • Sea Lettuce (Ulva lactuca) • Sea Palm (Pastelsi palmaeformis).

Nature's Lining **-** LaneLabs
Each chewable tablet contains: Zinc (from PepZin GI zinc-carnosine) 8 mg • L-Carnosine (from PepZin GI zinc-carnosine) 29.5 mg. Other Ingredients: Fructose, Guar Gum, Microcrystalline Cellulose, Magnesium Stearate, Corn Starch, Peppermint Oil.

Nature's Resource Ginkgo Biloba - Pharmavite Corp.
Each capsule contains: Ginkgo Biloba leaf extract (standardized to 24% ginkgo flavone glycosides) 60 mg. Other Ingredients: Rice Flour, Gelatin, Water.

Nature's Way Digestion Formula - Nature's Way
Two capsules contain: Angelica root 90 mg • Barberry bark 135 mg • Beet root 100 mg • Cayenne pepper fruit 25 mg • Dandelion root 315 mg • Fizyme Enzyme Formula 100 mg • Gentian root 135 mg. Other Ingredients: Gelatin, Magnesium Stearate, Millet.

Nature's Way Lycopene - Nature's Way
Each softgel capsule contains: Tomato seed oil standardized to (Lycopene) 5000 mcg • Canola oil • Beeswax • Lecithin • natural Vitamin E (d-Alpha Tocopheryl).

Nature's White Cross - D & E Pharmaceuticals
Each tablet contains: pure Ephedra extract 400 mg.
See Editor's Note No. 30, page 2056.

Nature's Youth HGH - Nature's Youth, LLC
Each 13 g packet contains: Proprietary Amino Acid Blend: Glycine, L-Glutamine, L-Tyrosine, GABA, L-Arginine HCl, L-Lysine HCl, Pyroglutamic Acid • Glycoamino Acid Complex • Glucose Polymers • Anterior Pituitary Peptides • Broad Bean (l-dopa).

Nature-Slim Tea - Triple Leaves Brand
Malva Verticellata.

Naturex Multi II - Swanson
Each capsule contains: Vitamin A (as palmitate) 5000 IU • Vitamin C USP (as ascorbic acid) 150 mg • Vitamin D (as cholecalciferol) 200 IU • Vitamin E (as d-alpha tocopheryl succinate) 75 IU • Thiamin USP (as thiamin HCl; vitamin B-1) 50 mg • Riboflavin (vitamin B-2) 50 mg • Niacinamide 50 mg • Vitamin B-6 (as pyridoxine HCl) 50 mg • Folic Acid 200 mcg • Vitamin B-12 (as cyanocobalamin) 20 mcg • Biotin 25 mcg • Pantothenic Acid (as d-calcium pantothenate) 50 mg • Iron (from ferrous gluconate) 0.5 mg • Iodine (from potassium iodide) 75 mcg • Zinc (from zinc gluconate) 1.5 mg • Selenium (as selenomethionine) 5 mcg • Copper (from copper gluconate) 0.5 mg • Manganese (from manganese gluconate) 0.5 mg • Chromium (from amino acid chelate) 50 mcg • Choline (as choline bitartrate) 25 mg • Inositol 25 mg • PABA (para-aminobenzoic acid) 25 mg • Betaine HCl 12.5 mg • Lemon Bioflavonoid Complex 12.5 mg • L-Glutamic Acid 12.5 mg • Rutin (from buckwheat) 12.5 mg • Hesperidin Complex 2.5 mg.

Natur-Leaf - Lifeline, Inc.
Each caspule contains: Blend of sprout phytochemicals 300 mg: Wild African Potato root • Lupins sprouts • Fenugreek sprouts • Barley sprouts • Wheat sprouts • Soybean sprouts • African Sunflower sprouts. Blend of enzymes 50 mg: Enzyme Mineral blend • Protease • Amylase • Lipase • Cellulase • Sucrase • Maltase • Lactase • Bromelain • Ionic Mineral blend.

Naturvite - Solgar
Each tablet contains: Vitamin B12 (cobalamin) 250 mcg • Vitamin A (palmitate) 10,000 IU • Vitamin D (cholecalciferol) 400 IU • Vitamin B1 (thiamine mononitrate) 25 mg • Vitamin B2 (riboflavin) 25 mg • Vitamin B6 (pyridoxine HCl) 25 mg • Vitamin C (ascorbic acid) 150 mg • Niacinamide 100 mg • Calcium Pantothenate 50 mg • Vitamin E (d-alpha tocopheryl succinate) 25 IU • Biotin 20 mcg • Folic Acid 100 mcg • Iron (gluconate) 6 mg • Iodine (kelp) 100 mcg • Zinc (gluconate) 180 mcg • Calcium (bone meal) 13.5 mg • Magnesium (gluconate) 388 mcg • Copper (gluconate) 35 mcg • Potassium 1.6 mg • Manganese (gluconate) 670 mcg • Choline (bitartrate) 62 mg • Inositol 150 mg • Rutin 25 mg • PABA (para aminobenzoic acid) 25 mg • Citrus Bioflavonoid complex 25 mg • Betaine HCl 25 mg • Hesperidin 5 mg • Desiccated Liver 50 mg • L-Lysine HCl 10 mg. Other Ingredients: Vegetable Cellulose, Silica, Vegetable Stearic Acid, Alfalfa, Acerola, Kelp, Parsley, Rose Hips, Watercress.
See Editor's Note No. 14.

Naudicelle - Key Pharmaceuticals
Each softgel contains: Evening Primrose oil with 10% GLA (gammalinolinic acid).

NeoCell - PhysioLogics
Two tablets contain: Raw Anterior Pituitary Concentrate 25 mg • GABA (gamma-aminobutyric acid) 125 mg • Phytosterol Complex (soy, rice) 100 mg • Soy Phosphatide Complex (24% phosphatidylcholine, 20% phosphatidylethanolamine, 14% phosphatidylinositol, 13% photoglycolipids) 200 mg • DMG Complex 50 mg: Trimethylglycine Hydrochloride, N,N-Dimethylglycine • Amino Acid Complex 700 mg: L-Glycine, L-Lysine Hydrochloride, L-Tyrosine, L-Arginine Hydrochloride, L-Ornithine Hydrochloride, L-Glutamine. Other Ingredients: Lecithin, Cellulose (plant origin), Silica, Vegetable Stearic Acid, Hydroxy Methylcellulose, Croscarmellose, Vegetable Magnesium Stearate, Cellulose Coating.

NeoProstate B-300 - BCN - Beachwood Canyon, Naturally, Ltd.
Each caplet contains: Beta-sitosterol 300 mg • Zinc Citrate 15 mg. Ingredients: Mixed Sterols including Beta-sitosterol (at least 50%), Stig-masterol, Campesterol, Lupeol, Cycloartenon, Famesol, Phytol and Zinc.

Nerve Guard - Flora, Inc.
St. John's Wort.

Nettle - Nature's Way
Two capsules contain: Nettle herb 870 mg. Other Ingredients: Gelatin.

Nettle & Pygeum with Pumpkin - Enzymatic Therapy
Each capsule contains: Nettle root extract 16:1 (Urticae dioica radix) 300 mg • Pumpkin seed oil (Cucurbita pepo) 175 mg • Pygeum africanum extract standardized to contain 13% total sterols 25 mg.

Nettle and Perilla Flavonoid Complex (Allercept 450) - Jamieson
Each caplet contains: 1:6 Urtica Dioica Nettle Leaf Extract, 1:37 Perilla Fruit Extract (Perilla Frutescens) 450 mg.

Nettle-Pygeum Complex - PhytoPharmica
Each capsule contains: Pumpkin seed oil (cucurbita pepo) 175 mg • Pygeum Africanum bark extract (prunus africana, standardized to contain 13% total sterols) 25 mg • Stinging Nettle root 16:1 extract (urtica dioica) 300 mg.

Nettle-Reishi Virtue - Blessed Herbs
Nettle • Reishi mycelium • Chinese Ephedra • Yerba Santa leaf • Propolis • Ginkgo leaf • Licorice root • Grain alcohol & Distilled Water.
See Editor's Note No. 30, page 2056.

Neuragen - Origin BioMedicinals
Geranium Oil extract • Lavender Oil extract • Bergamot Oil extract • Eucalyptus Oil extract • Tea Tree Oil extract.

Neural Support Formula - The Vitamin Factory
Each tablet contains: Vitamin E (d-Alpha Tocopheryl-Succinate) 100 IU • Neuromins (13% DHA powder) 100 mg • Phosphatidylserine Complex 20% 50 mg • Ginkgo Biloba Leaf extract (24/6) 40 mg • Bacopin extract (Bacopa monniera, min. 20% Bacosides) 25 mg • Pycnogenol (Maritime Pine bark extract) 15 mg.

NeuRecover-DA (Depressant Abuse) - Natural Distributors International, Inc.
Six capsules contain: Vitamin A 2000 IU • Vitamin C 600 mg • Vitamin B1 14.5 mg • Vitamin B2 5 mg • Niacin (Niacinamide Ascorbate) 200 mg • Calcium (Chelate) 150 mg • Iron 9 mg • Vitamin E 30 IU • Vitamin B6 18 mg • Folic Acid 0.4 mg • Vitamin B12 0.03 mg • Magnesium 150 mg • Zinc 15 mg • Biotin 0.3 mg • Pantothenic Acid 90 mg • Chromium (Picolinate) 0.06 mg • DL-Phenylalanine 2760 mg • L-Glutamine 150 mg.

BRAND NAMES

NeuRecover-SA (Stimulant Abuse) - Natural Distributors International, Inc.
Six capsules contain: Vitamin C (Ascorbate) 600 mg • Vitamin B1 10 mg • Vitamin B2 15 mg • Niacin (Niacinamide) 100 mg • Calcium (Chelate) 150 mg • Iron 9 mg • Vitamin B6 (Pyridoxal-5-Phosphate) 20 mg • Folic Acid 0.4 mg • Vitamin B12 0.03 mg • Magnesium (Oxide) 150 mg • Zinc (Chelate) 30 mg • Pantothenic Acid 90 mg • Chromium (Picolinate) 0.06 mg • DL-Phenylalanine 1500 mg • L-Tyrosine 900 mg • L-Glutamine 300 mg.

Neuro Care-Rx - Alternecare Health Products
Each capsule contains: Cayenne 125 mg • Ginger 125 mg • St. John's Wort 125 mg • Ginko Biloba 40 mg • Malic Acid 100 mg • Vitamin B3 100 mg • Vitamin C 60 mg • Manganese 10 mg • Copper 1 mg • Vitamin B6 50 mg.

Neuro Guardian - Clinician's Choice
Two tablets contain: Vitamin E (as dl-alpha tocopheryl acetate) 200 IU • Thiamin (as mononitrate) 10 mg • Riboflavin 10 mg • Niacin (as niacinamide) 50 mg • Pantothenic Acid (d-calcium pantothenate) 10 mg • Zinc (as amino acid chelate) 10 mg • Selenium (selenomethionine) 50 mcg • Chromium (as nicotinate, chelavite, picolinate) 100 mcg • Ginkgo Biloba Leaf Extract 4:1 150 mg • Lecithin 100 mg • Natural Beta Carotene 40 mg • Acetyl-L-Carnitine 30 mg • RoseOx (patented, standardized process for an extract of Rosemary) 30 mg • Lecithin (standardized to 30% phosphatidyl serine) 30 mg • Aminogen 20 mg • Cayenne Fruit Powder 200 mg • Choline (as choline bitartrate) 20 mg • L-Tyrosine 20 mg • Proprietary Blend 8 mg: Astragalus, Carrot Powder, Pacific Kelp, Piper Longum Fruit Powder.

Neuro Optimizer - Jarrow Formulas
Four capsules contain: Cytidine 5'-diphoscholine (CDP Choline) 300 mg • Phosphatidyl Serine (PS) 100 mg • Acetyl L-Carnitine 500 mg • L-Glutamine 500 mg • Alpha Lipoic Acid 50 mg • Taurine 500 mg • Phosphatidylcholine 135 mg. Other Ingredients: Tricalcium Phosphate, Silicon Dioxide.

Neuro-Boost Spray - Nature's Plus
Each spray contains: Phosphatidylserine-rich purified Lecithin concentrate supplying Activated Phosphatides 50 mg: Phosphatidylserine (PS) 10 mg, Phosphatidylcholine (PC) 10 mg, Cephalin (Phosphatidylethanolamine) 6 mg, Phosphoinositides 3 mg • DMAE (2-Dimethylaminoethanol Bitartrate) 12.5 mg • N-Acetyl-Tyrosine pharmaceutical grade free form amino acid 5 mg • Pantothenic Acid 5 mg • Korean Ginseng root (Panax ginseng CA Meyer) standardized 15% ginsenosides 5 mg • Chinese Green Tea leaf (Camellia sinensis) standardized 50% polyphenols 5 mg • Chinese Green Tea leaf standardized 24% ginkgo flavone glycosides, 6% terpene lactones 1000 mcg. In a proprietary Liposomal Complex of Essential Metabolic Factors, Purified Water, Vegetable Glycerine, Purified Lecithin, Citrus seed extract (Citrus sinensis), Vitamin E & (natural Root Beer) Sarsaparilla flavor.

Neuro-DHA - Metabolic Response Modifiers
Each sofgel contains: Fish Oil concentrate 500 mg • Min. 50% DHA 250 mg • Max. 20% EPA 100 mg • 20% Mixed fatty acids 100 mg • 10% stearidonic acid 50 mg • Vitamin C (Ascorbyl palmitate) 2 mg • Vitamin E (mixed-tocopherols) 4 mg.

Neurodyne - Life Extension
Each tablet contains: Acetyl Choline (synaptic factor, herbal proteinomeric neuro-transmitter release agent) 10 mg • Guarana (potentiating factor) 775 mg.

NeuroGenic - Nature's Plus
Two tablets contain: Phosphatidyl Choline 250 mg • L-Glutamine (free-form amino acid) 200 mg • Vitamin C (corn free) 150 mg • Pantothenic Acid 100 mg • L-Phenylalanine (free form amino acid) 100 mg • Ginkgo Biloba (standardized 24% ginkgo flavone-glycosides, 6% terpene lactones) 60 mg • Ashwagandha (withania somnifera, standardized 1.5% withanols) 50 mg • Chinese Green Tea (camellian sinensis, standardized 20% polyphenols) 20 mg • Standardized Bilberry (swedish vaccinium myrtillus, standardized 25% anthocyanosides) 15 mg • PAK (pyridoxal alpha-ketoglutarate) 10 mg • Co-Enzyme Q10 (ubiquinone) 5 mg.

Neuro-Max - Olympia Nutrition
Phosphatidylserine 50 mg • Ashwaganda 50 mg • Ginkgo 20 mg • Pregnenolone 25 mg.

Neuro-Max - Metabolic Response Modifiers
Two capsules contain: Phospholipid Complex 500 mg • Ashwaganda extract 100 mg • Ginkgo Biloba extract 40 mg • Pregnenolone 50 mg.

Neuro-Max - New Hope Health Products
Two capsules contain: Phospholipid Complex (containing 100 mg Phosphatidylserine) 500 mg • Ashwagandha Extract 80 mg • Bacopa Monniera Extract 80 mg • Ginkgo Biloba Extract (28/11) 60 mg • Cytidine diphosphate choline 12 mg • Vinpocetine 5 mg • Niacin 10 mg.

Neuro-Max for Children - Dr. Vanessa's
Each three wafers contain: Lecithin 500 mg • Ginkgo Biloba extract (standardized 24%) 100 mg • Grape Seed extract (standardized 95%) 10 mg • Gotu Kola 100 mg • L-Glutamic Acid 100 mg • L-Glutamine 50 mg • Dimethylglycine 50 mg • Phosphatidylserine 25 mg • L-Tyrosine 50 mg • Folic Acid 100 mcg • Biotin 100 mcg • GABA 50 mg • Choline 20 mg • Inositol 20 mg • Vitamin B1 20 mg • Vitamin B2 20 mg • Vitamin B5 20 mg • Vitamin B6 200 mg • Vitamin B12 50 mg. Inactive Ingredients: Fructose, Natural Flavors, Stearic Acid, and Magnesium Stearate.

Neuro-Max II - Metabolic Response Modifiers
Each capsule contains: Phospholipid complex (containing 100 mg Phosphatidlyserine) 500 mg • Ashwagandha extract 80 mg • Ginkgo Biloba extract (28/11) 60 mg • Cytidine diphosphate choline 12 mg • Vinpocetine 5 mg • Niacin 10 mg.

Neuromins - 200 - Martek Biosciences Corp.
Each capsule contains: DHA (docosahexaenoic acid from algae oil) 200 mg. Inactive Ingredients: High Oleic Sunflower Oil, Ascorbyl Palmitate (vitamin C), Mixed Natural Tocopherol (vitamin E), Natural Mixed Carotenoids, Gelatin, Turmeric, Carmine, Water, Glycerine.

Neuromins DHA - Martek Biosciences - Martek Biosciences Corp.
Each capsule contains: DHA (docosahexaenoic acid from algae oil) 100 mg. Inactive Ingredients: High Oleic Sunflower Oil, Ascorbyl Palmitate (vitamin C), Mixed Natural Tocopherol (vitamin E), Natural Mixed Carotenoids, Gelatin, Water, Glycerine.

Neuromins DHA - Nature's Way
Each softgel contains: Neruomins DHA 100 mg. Other Ingredients: Gelatin, Glycerin, Sunflower Oil, Vitamin C, Vitamin E d-alpha tocopheryl, Water.

Neuromins DHA - Source Naturals
Each softgel contains: Docosahexaenoic Acid (DHA) (Derived rom algal oil (oceanic phytophankton), in a base of high-oleic sunflower oil, vitamin C (ascorbyl palmitate) and vitamin E (mixed tocopherols) as antioxidants) 100 mg.

Neuromins DHA brand - Martek Biosciences Corp.
Docosahexaenoic Acid.
See Editor's Note No. 44, page 2058.

Neuromins DHA Chewables - Martek Biosciences Corp.
Each capsule contains: DHA (docosahexaenoic acid from algal oil) 100 mg. Inactive Ingredients: High Oleic Sunflower Oil, Sugar, Yellow Beeswax, Natural Flavor, Ascorbyl Palmitate (Vitamin C), Mixed Natural Tocoperol (Vitamin E), Mixed Carotenoids, Gelatin, Glycerine, Caramel Color, Titanium Dioxinde.

Some Brand Name Natural Products - What they Contain

www.NaturalDatabase.com contains MANY more listings than appear here.

Neuromins for Kids - Martek Biosciences Corp.
Eah capsule contains: DHA (docosahexaenoic acid) 100 mg. Inactive Ingredients: High Oleic Sunflower Oil, Ascorbyl Palmitate, (vitamin C), Mixed Natural Tocopherol (vitamin E), Natural Mixed Carotenoids, Gelatin, Water, Glycerine.

Neuromins PL - Martek Biosciences Corp.
Each capsule contains: DHA (docosahexaenoic acid) 200 mg. Inactive Ingredients: High Oleic Sunflower Oil, Ascorbyl Palmitate (vitamin C), Mixed Natural Tocopherol, Natural Mixed Carotenoids, Gelatin, Turmeric, Carmine, Water, Glycerine.

NeuroSyn - PharmAssure
Two softgel capsules contain: Vitamin E (as Natural d-alpha tocopheryl Acetate) 30 IU • High Choline Soy Lecithin (35% Phosphatidylcholine=175mg) 500 mg • DHA (Docosahexaenioc Acid;as Marine Microalgae Oil) 100 mg • Ginkgo Biloba Leaves Extract (24% Ginkgo Flavonglycosides=28.8mg, 6% Terpene Lactones=7.2mg) 120 mg • Vinpocetine 5 mg. Other Ingredients: Gelatin, Soybean Oil, Glycerin, Caramel Color, Titanium Dioxide (Natural Mineral Whitener).

Neurozan - Vitabiotics
Each capsule contains: Vitamin D (as D3 200 IU) 5 mcg • Vitamin E (natural source) 60 mg • Vitamin C 30 mg • Vitamin B1 (thiamin) 20 mg • Vitamin B2 (riboflavin) 3.2 mg • Vitamin B3 (niacin) 18 mg • Vitamin B6 (pyridoxine HCl) 25 mg • Folacin (as folic acid) 500 mcg • Vitamin B12 (cyanocobalamin) 50 mcg • Pantothenic Acid 12 mg • Iron 7 mg • Zinc 15 mg • Manganese 4 mg • Copper 1.5 mg • Selenium 200 mcg • Chromium 50 mcg • L-Arginine 40 mg • Glutamine 10 mg • Glutathione 5 mg • Omega-3 DHA (docosahexaenoic acid, 50%) 100 mg • Co-enzyme Q10 6 mg • Phosphatidylserine 10 mg • Phosphatidylcholine 10 mg • Natural Mixed Carotenoids 2 mg • Lecithin 17 mg.

Neurozyme - New Chapter, Inc.
Each softgel contains: DHA (Docosahexaenoic acid), supercritical extract (from Arctic fish oil- 100 mg) (DPA min. 10%- 10 mg, EPA min. 5%- 5 mg) 50 mg • Rosemary leaf, supercritical extract (23% total phenolic antioxidants- 7 mg) 30 mg • Ginger (rhizome), certified organic, supercritical extract (minimum 20% pungent compounds- 6 mg, 5% zingiberence- 1.5 mg) 30 mg • Sage leaf, supercritical extract (38%- 42% total phenolic antioxidants- 6 mg) 15 mg • Chamomile flower, supercritical extract (25% alpha-bisabolol -3.8 mg) 15 mg • Clove bud, supercritical extract (65% euaenol -6.5 mg) 10 mg • Potency Assured Extracts, Ginkgo leaf (12% flavone glycosides- 14 mg) 120 mg • Gotu Kola leaf (10% asiaticoside -12 mg, 30% triterpenes- 36 mg) 120 mg • Club Moss, Chinese Huperzia serrata (0.5% Huperzine A -0.3 mg) 60 mg • Ashwaganda root (extract 4:1) 60 mg • Cat's Claw root (extract 4:1) (3% alkaloids- 1.5 mg) 50 mg • Lemon Balm, Melissa officinalis leaf (5% rosemarininc acid- 1.5 mg) 30 mg • Bacopin, Bacopa monniera (Brahil leaf extract), (Bacosides A and B = 20.65%- 6.2 mg), (0.6% alkaloids- 0.2 mg) 30 mg • Paeonia, Eurpoean (extract 5:1) 20 mg • Holy Basil, Ocimum sanctum (leaf) (2.5% ursalic acid- 0.5 mg) 20 mg • Turmeric (rhizome) (7-9% curcumin- 1.6 mg) 20 mg • Red Wine, (30% total polyphenols- 6 mg) 20 mg • Chamomile flower (extract 5:1) 15 mg • Vitamin E 2 UI. Other Ingredients: Olive Oil - certified organic, Yellow Beeswax.

Neutra-Gas - PhytoPharmica
Each capsule contains: Simethicone 25 mg • Peppermint oil extract (Mentha piperita) 0.2 ml. Chlorophyll is used as a natural coloring agent.
See Editor's Note No. 21, page 2056.

New Choice - The Herbalist
Gingko leaf • Gotu Kola herb • Guarana seed • American Ginseng root • Siberian Ginseng root • Jamaican Sarsaparilla root • Kola Nut • Licorice root • Cinnamon bark • Ginger root • Cayenne pepper.

New Life Colostrum - Symbiotics
100% Bovine Colostrum.

New Life Colostrum Capsules - Symbiotics
Two capsules contain: 100% Bovine Colostrum from New Zealand cows 960 mg • Vitamin A 336 IU • Vitamin C 2.8 mg • Iron 1.4 mg • Calcium 10 mg.

New Life Colostrum High-IG - Symbiotics
Two capsules contain: 100% Bovine Colostrum 960 mg • Vitamin A 504 IU • Vitamin C 4.2 mg • Iron 2.1 mg • Calcium 15 mg • Immunoglobulin 288 mg.

New Life Colostrum Powder - Symbiotics
One teaspoon contains: 100% Bovine Colostrum from New Zealand cows 1440 mg • Vitamin A 504 IU • Vitamin C 4.2 mg • Iron 2.1 mg • Calcium 15 mg • Immunoglobulin 246 mg.

New Life Hair - Sundown
Each tablet contains: Vitamin E 5 IU • Niacin (as niacinamide) 15 mg • Folic Acid 400 mcg • Vitamin B12 (as cyanocobalamin) 6 mcg • Pantothenic Acid (as calcium d-pantothenate) 92 mg • Calcium 100 mg • Iron (as ferrous fumarate) 1 mg • Iodine (as potassium iodide) 150 mcg • Zinc (as zinc gluconate) 15 mg • Manganese (as manganese gluconate) 10 mg • Choline (as choline bitartrate) 120 mg • Silica 26 mg. Other Ingredients: Dicalcium Phosphate, Microcrystalline Cellulose, Croscarmellose Sodium, Hydroxypropyl Methylcellulose, Hydrogenated Vegetable Oil, Magnesium Stearate, Pharmaceutical Glaze, Titanium Dioxide, Dl-Alpha-Tocopheryl Acetate, Riboflavin (colorant), PEG, Polysorbate 80, Yellow 6 Lake.

New Man Tea - The Herbalist
Damiana leaf • Fo-ti root • Sassafras bark • Licorice root • Cinnamon bark • Saw Palmetto berry • Sarsaparilla bark • Parsley root • Marshmallow root • Orange peel.

New Phase - SunSource - Chattem, Inc.
Each caplet contains: Proprietary Blend 410 mg: Soy Protein concentrate, standardized Kudzu extract root, standardized Red Clover extract leaf • standardized Chastetree extract berry 75 mg • standardized Black Cohosh extract root 40 mg.

New Woman Tonic - The Herbalist
Chaste Tree berry • Black Cohosh root • Black Haw bark • Motherwort herb • Cramp bark • Skullcap herb • Ginger root.

NewBust (New Bust) - Tiger-One.com
Saw Palmetto • Dong Quai • Damiana • Fenugreek seed • Blessed Thistle • Violet • Wild Yam • Fennel seed • Althea root • Cumin seed • Hops.
See Editor's Note No. 17, page 2055.

NewBust Lotion (New Bust Lotion) - Tiger-One.com
Water • Saw Palmetto • Extra Virgin Olive Oil • Dong Quai • Damiana • Glycerin • Foenugreek seed • Blessed Thistle • Violet • Wild Yam • Fennel seed • Althea root • Cumin seed • Hops.
See Editor's Note No. 17, page 2055.

Nexcite - Nordic Drinks
Each 100 mL serving contains: Carbonated Water 93 g • Sugar 8.5 g • Citric Acid 0.2 g • Damiana (extract) 59 mg • Schizandra (extract) 58 mg • Mate (extract) 57 mg • (Guarana extract) 56 mg • Caffeine 30 mg • Flavoring 23 mg • Ginseng (extract) 18 mg • Sodium benzoate (E211) 15 mg • Colour (E133) 65 pg.

Nexrutine - Solanova
Each capsule contains: Nexrutine (a patent pending plant extract from Phellodendron amurense) 250 mg. Other Ingredients: Snow White Filler, Microcrystalline Cellulose, Magnesium Stearate, Silicon Dioxide, Gelatin, Glycerin, Purified Water.

NFA-500 - Human Development Technologies (HDT)
Each capsule contains: L-Tyrosine 500 mg • Acetylcholine 25 mg • DMAE 25 mg • St. John's Wort 60 mg. Additional Ingredients: DLPA • Ginkgo Biloba • Vitamin B12 • Vitamin B6 • Vitamin B1 • Vitamin C • Copper Sulfate • Folic Acid • Phosphorus • Zinc • Bioperine.

N-FLAM Plus - Nutri-Quest Rx
Each enteric coated tablet contains: Pancreatin 170 mg • Papain 100 mg • Bromelain 80 mg • Trypsin 40 mg (Chymotrypsin 8 mg) • Lipase 15 mg • Amylase 17 mg • Rutin 85 mg • Calf Thymus 45 mg • Zinc Gluconate 4 mg • Partoid concentrate 1 mg.
See Editor's Note No. 14.

NG-Rx - Maxam Nutraceutics
Distilled Water • Microactivated peptite fractions of Phosphatidylcholine, Phosphatidylserine, N-Acetyl-L-Carnitine, DMAE, Acetyl Serine, L-Tyrosine, Amino Acids, Ginkgo extract, and Mucuna extract in a Colloidal Matrix.

Niacin - Leiner Health Products
Each tablet contains: Niacin (Nicotinic acid) 100 mg. Other Ingredients: Lactose, Starch, Stearic Acid, Silicon Dioxide, Magnesium Stearate.

Niacin - Nature's Bounty
Each tablet contains: Niacin 100 mg. Other Ingredients: Cellulose, Dicalcium Phosphate, Vegetable Stearic Acid, Povidone, Vegetable Magnesium Stearate, Silica.

Niacin - PhytoPharmica
Each capsule contains: Niacin (as inositol hexaniacinate) 590 mg. Other Ingredients: Gelatin, Magnesium Stearate, Titanium Dioxide Color, Silicon Dioxide.

Niacin - Source Naturals
Each tablet contains: Niacin 100 mg.

Niacin 250 - GNC A-Z - GNC
Each tablet contains: Niacin 250 mg. Other Ingredients: Dicalcium Phosphate, Cellulose, Whole Brown Rice powder (Oryza sativa).

Niacin 500 - GNC A-Z - GNC
Each tablet contains: Niacin 500 mg. Other Ingredients: Dicalcium Phosphate, Cellulose, Food Glaze, Whole Brown Rice powder (Oryza Sativa).

Niacin 500 mg - Jamieson
Each caplet contains: Niacin 500 mg.

Niacin 500 mg Timed - Rexall - Sundown
Each caplet contains: Niacin 500 mg • Calcium 106 mg. Other Ingredients: Dicalcium Phosphate, Hydroxypropyl Methylcellulose, Hydrogenated Cottonseed Oil, Stearic Acid, Magnesium Stearate.

Niacin Flush Free - Nature's Bounty
Each capsule contains: Niacin (as Inositol Hexanicotinate) 400 mg • Inositol (as Inositol Hexanicotinate) 100 mg. Other Ingredients: Gelatin, Dicalcium Phosphate, Vegetable Magnesium Stearate, Silica.

Niacin Time Release - Puritan's Pride
Each capsule contains: Niacin 250 mg.

Niacin with Cholestatin - Futurebiotics
Each tablet contains: Niacin 400 mg • Cholestatin 400 mg.

Niacin+ - PhysioLogics
Each capsule contains: Niacin (as inositol hexanicotinate) 400 mg • Vitamin C (as magnesium ascorbate) 100 mg • Chromium (as chromium amino acid chelate) 6 mcg. Other Ingredients: Gelatin, Rice Powder, Vegetable Magnesium Stearate, Silica.

Niacinamide - Nature's Bounty
Each tablet contains: Niacin (as Niacinamide) 500 mg. Other Ingredients: Cellulose, Dicalcium Phosphate, Vegetable Stearic Acid, Silica, Vegetable Magnesium Stearate.

Nicodrops - Nicodrops Company
Each 4 g lozenge contains: Peppermint Flavor • Ginseng • Ginseng flavor • Sugar • Corn Syrup • Valerian fluid extract • St. John's wort fluid extract.

Nicodrops - Canada - Nicodrops Company
Each lozenge contains: Medicinal Ingredients: Lobelia aerial parts (Lobelia inflata) 65 mg. Non-medicinal Ingredients: Peppermint flavor, sugar, corn syrup, Ginseng flavor, Gingeng root (Panax japonicum, Valerian root (Valerian officinalis), St. John's Wort flower tops (Hypericum proforatum).

Nico-End - PhytoPharmica
Each tablet contains: Nux vomica 8x • Lobelia 6x • Staphysagria 6x • Tabacum 6x.
See Editor's Note No. 1 and No. 21.

Night Nervine - Grandma's Herbs
Each capsule contains: Proprietary Blend 0.426 g: Hops flower, Valerian root, Blue Vervain herb, Scullcap herb, St. John's Wort herb, Black Cohosh root, Lady's Slipper root, Lily of the Valley herb, Bladdderpod herb, Mistletoe herb, Spearmint root. Other Ingredients: Gelatin.

Night Supply Nourishing Cream - Nu Skin Enterprises
Water (aqua) • Caprylic/Capric Triglycerides • Cyclomethicone • Cetyl Alcohol • Glycerin • Macadamia Ternifolia seed oil • Glyceryl Stearate • Squalane • PEG-75 Stearate • Phosphatidylcholine • Oenothera Biennis oil (evening primrose) • Butyrospermum Parkii extract (shea butter) • Anthemis Nobilis flower extract • Calendula Officinalis flower extract • Tilia Cordata flower extract • Centaurea Cyanus flower extract • Chamomilla Recutita flower extract (matricaria) • Hypericum Perforatum extract • Limnanthes Alba seed oil (meadowfoam) • Hydrogenated Lecithin • Tocopheryl Acetate • Dimethicone • Butylene Glycol • Polyacrylamide • Ceteth-20 • Steareth-20 • C12-14 Isoparaffin • Laureth-7 • Myristyl Myristate • Neopentyl Glycol Diheptanoate • Fragrance (parfum) • Tetrasodium EDTA • Phenoxyethanol • Methylparaben • Isopropylparaben • Butylparaben • Chlorphenesin.

Night Supply Nourishing Lotion - Nu Skin Enterprises
Water (aqua) • Cyclomethicone • Ethoxydiglycol • Glycerin • Panthenol • Caprylic/Capric Triglyceride • Hydrogenated Polyisobutene • Glyceryl Stearate • PEG-100 Stearate • Phosphatidylcholine • Sodium PCA • Tocopheryl Acetate • Carbomer • Didecene • Glycol Stearate • Cetyl Alcohol • Triethanolamine • Fragrance (parfum) • Phenoxyethanol • Methylparaben • Ethylparaben • Propylparaben • Butylparaben.

Night Time Formulation - Olympian Labs
Each capsule contains: Valerian root 200 mg • Passion Flower 200 mg • Skullcap 50 mg • L-Tyrosine 25 mg • Parsley 50 mg • Peppermint 75 mg • Calcium Citrate 80 mg • Pantothenic Acid 20 mg.

NightRest - Source Naturals
Two tablets contain: Melatonin 4 mg • Magnesium (Magnesium Glycinate and Magnesium Taurinate) 200 mg • Glycine (Magnesium Glycinate and Glycine) 502 mg • Taurine (Magnesium Taurinate) 435 mg • Passionflower 120 mg • GABA (Gamma Amino Butyric Acid) 100 mg • Skullcap 70 mg • Chamomile extract (4:1) 60 mg.
See Editor's Note No. 16, page 2055.

NightTime Complex with Melotonin - Pharmanex
Each capsule contains: Valerian root extract 75 mg • Passion Flower extract 37.5 mg • Kava Lactones (from Kava Kava root extract) 7.5 mg • Hops Strobile powder (fruit) 25 mg • Chamomile flower powder 25 mg • Melissa officinalis powder (leaf & flower) 25 mg • Mixed Tocopherols 0.5 mg • Melatonin 0.5 mg. Other Ingredients: Maltodextrin, Magnesium, Silicon Dioxide.
See Editor's Note No. 26, page 2056.

NightTime Formula - Pharmanex
Each capsule contains: Valerian root extract 75 mg • Passion flower extract 37.5 mg • L-Theanine (from camellia sinensis) 25 mg • Hops Strobils fruit powder 25 mg • Chamomile flower powder 25 mg • Lemon Balm powder (melissa officinalis) 25 mg • Melatonin 0.5 mg.

Other Ingredients: Gelatin, Microcrystalline Cellulose, Magnesium Stearate, Silicon Dioxide.
See Editor's Note No. 26, page 2056.

Nighty Night **-** Traditional Medicinals
Passionflower • Spearmint leaf • Chamomile herb • Lemon Verbena leaf • Licorice root • Lilia Star flower • Lemon peel • Lemongrass leaf • Catnip leaf • Hop Strobile.

Niteworks **-** Herbalife
Two scoops (approx. 9.7 g) contains: Vitamin C (ascorbic acid) 500 mg • Vitamin E (d-alpha tocopheryl acetate) 400 IU • Folic Acid (folate & calcium folinate) 400 mcg • Proprietary Blend 5.2 g: L-Arginine, L-Citrulline • Lemon Balm extract 50 mg • Alpha Lipoic Acid 10 mg. Other Ingredients: Natural Flavor, Sucralose.

Nitric Boost **-** Optimum Nutrition
Three caplets contain: Arginine Alpha-Ketoglutarate (A-AKG) 3 g. Other Ingredients: Dicalcium Phosphate, Pharmaceutical Glaze, Microcrystalline Cellulose, Stearic Acid, Solutab, Magnesium Stearate, Silica.

Nitrix **-** BSN Inc.
Three tablets contain: L-Arginine Alpha-Ketoglutarate (AAKG) 3000 mg • CRTS2 (controlled release technology & support system) 1897 mg: Methocel (micro-polymer hydrophilic ether matrix), Phosphoplexx (calcium phosphate, di-potassium phosphate, sodium phosphate), 2CM (dicreatine malate), L-Citruline, NAD (nicotinamide adenine dinucleotide), Folic Acid (folate). Other Ingredients: Magnesium Stearate.

Nitro Fuel (Ion Exchange Whey Protein Powder) **-** TwinLab
Each serving contains: Pure Protein 25 g.

Nitro Fuel (The Ultimate Anti-Catabolic Amino Acid Drink) **-** TwinLab
Protein (Amino Acids) & Carbohydrates • Whey Protein Concentrate [a source of Branched Chain Amino Acids (L-Leucine, L-Isoleucine, L-Valine)] • Chromium Picolinate • Alpha-Ketoglutarates.

NitrOGenX **-** PharmaGenX
Each 4 cc serving contains: L-Arginine Alpha-Ketoglutarate 1500 mg. Other Ingredients: Water, Natural Vegetable Glycerin, Emulsifiers, Phospholipids, Medium Chain Triglycerides, Sucralose, Potassium Sorbate Benzoate, Natural and Artificial Flavors.

Nitro-Tech **-** MuscleTech
Each 28.5 g scoop contains: Vitamin E 30 IU • Vitamin B6 10.5 mg • Folic Acid 400 mcg • Calcium 140 mg • Iron 0.36 mg • Phosphorous 100 mg • Magnesium 50 mg • Sodium 60 mg • Potassium 180 mg. Ingredients: Whey Peptides, Whey Protein Concentrate, Guar Gum, D-Myo-Inositol, Glucomannan, Taurine, Alpha Lipoic Acid, D-Pinitol, Glycosidal Saponins, Folic Acid, Natural & Artificial Flavors, L-Glutamine Peptides, Calcium Alpha Ketoglutarate, Dipotassium Phosphate, Lecithin, Magnesium Oxide, N-Acetyl-Cysteine, dl-Tocopherol Acetate, Acesulfame Potassium, Aspartame, Pyridoxine Hydrochloride.

No. 1 GARLIC PLUS ESTER-C & FOS **-** Dial Herbs
Two capsules contain: Pure-Gar deodorized Garlic concentrate 300 mg • FOS Micro Flora Growth concentrate 300 mg • Vitamin C from Ester-C 200 mg.

No. 56 K KIDNEY **-** Systemic Formulas
Rose Hips • RNA/DNA Kidney Factors • Gelatin • Magnesium Sulfate • Vitamin C • Ch de Bugre • Fish Liver Oil (Source of Vitamins A and D) • Sete Sangrias • Calcium Carbonate • RNA/DNA Adrenal Factors • Hesperidin • Serine • RNA/DNA Thalamus Factors • Tyrosine • Spearmint Oil • Rose Petal Essence • Aloe Vera.
See Editor's Note No. 14.

NO2 **-** Medical Research Institiute (MRI)
Three capsules contain: Arginine Alpha-Ketoglutarate (A-AKG) 3000 mg.

No-Flush Niacin **-** NutriCology
Each capsule contains: Niacin (as inositol hexanicotinate) 430 mg. Other Ingredients: Cellulose, Silicon Dioxide, Stearic Acid.

No-Jet-Lag **-** Global Source
One tablet contains: Arnica Montana (leopard's bane) 30 C • Bellis Perennis (daisy) 30 C • Chamomilla (wild chamomile) 30 C • Ipecacuanha (ipecac) 30 C • Lycopodium (clubmoss) 30 C. Other Ingredients: Sorbitol, Magnesium Stearate, Sterilized Talc.
See Editor's Note No. 1, page 2053.

Noni **-** Source Naturals
Each capsule contains: Hawaiian Noni (Morinda citrifolia) 375 mg.

Non-Stipation Syrup **-** Hadas Natural Products
Sorbitol Syrup • Plums • Figs • Psyllium • Fennel • Caraway • Ginger • Coriander.

Nopal Strepta (Prickly Pear Cactus) **-** Cactu-Life
Each capsule contains: 100% Opuntia Streptacantha 450 mg.

Nopalacrin **-** 4R Health Products
Each capsule contains: Nopal 500 mg.

Nor Stack - Substrate Solutions **-** ErgoPharm
Each tablet contains: 19-Nor-4-Androstenediol 100 mg • 19-Nor-4-Androstenedione 100 mg.

Norabol **-** Mass Quantities, Inc.
Each capsule contains: 19-Nor-4-androstenedione 100 mg • Silymarin 20 mg • Niacin 10 mg • Zinc 5 mg.

NorCycloDiol-4 (Sports One Cycloplex Pro-Hormone) **-** Sports One
Each lozenge contains: Nor-4-Androstenediol Cycloplex (cyclodextrin complex) 10 mg.

NorCycloDione (Sports One Cycloplex Pro-Hormone) **-** Sports One
Each lozenge contains: 19-Nor-4-Androstenedione Cycloplex (cyclodextrin complex) 25 mg.

Nordisk of Denmark Propolis **-** Health From The Sun
Each capsule contains: 50% Propolis • 50% Bee Pollen in a natural mineral base of Calcium Phosphate.

Norexin **-** Biotech Corp.
Two tablets contain: Natural Vitamin E (as d-alpha tocopheryl succinate) 30 IU • Niacin (as niacinamide) 20 mg • Selenium (as selenomethionine) 35 mcg • Chromium (as chromium dinicotinate glycinate) 200 mcg • Ma Huang herb extract (15 mg ephedrine alkaloids) 150 mg • Green Tea leaf extract (VerdOx, yielding 150 mg natural caffeine, 90 mg polyphenols including EGCG) 600 mg • French Grape Seed extract (AdipoVin) 40 mg • Neurothermic Modulator Proprietary Blend 523 mg: Magnesium Citrate, Glycine, L-Theanine.
See Editor's Note No. 21 and No. 30.

Norexin Ephedra Free **-** Biotech Corp.
Two tablets contain: Natural Vitamin E (as natural d-alpha tocopheryl succinate) 30 IU • Niacin (as niacinamide) 20 mg • Magnesium (as magnesium citrate) 50 mg • Selenium (as selenomethionine) 35 mcg • Chromium (as chromium dinicotinate glycinate) 200 mcg • Citrus Aurantium rind (yielding 8 mg of synephrine) 200 mg • VerdOx standardized Green Tea leaf extract (camellia sinensis, yielding 150 mg of natural caffeine and 90 mg of polyphenols, including EGCG) 600 mg • AdipoVin exclusive French Grape seed (vitis vinifera) 40 mg • Neurothermic Modulator Proprietary Blend 523 mg: Magnesium Citrate, Glycine, L-Theanine. Other Ingredients: Dicalcium Phosphate, Microcrystalline Cellulose, Croscarmellose Sodium, Stearic Acid, Magnesium Stearate, Silica, Peppermint Oil (in coating), Calcium Silicate, Pharmaceutical Glaze.
See Editor's Note No. 40, page 2058.

Norexin Slim Sculpt - Biotech Corp.
Each 15 mL serving contains: Chromium from Picolinate 15 mcg • Garcinia Cambogia extract (50% HCA) 50 mg • Conjugated Linoleic Acid 45 mg. Other Ingredients: Purified Water, Hydrolyzed Collagen, Glycerin, Citric Acid, Natural Flavor, Aloe Vera Concentrate, Acesulfame Potassium, Xanthan Gum, Sodium Citrate, Potassium Sorbate, Sodium Benzoate, Ethyl Maltol, Chromium Picolinate, Calcium Pyruvate.

Norwegian Cod Liver Oil - Nature's Bounty
Each softgel contains: Vitamin A (from Cod Liver Oil) 1250 IU • Vitamin D (from Cod Liver Oil) 135 IU. Other Ingredients: Cod Liver Oil, Soybean Oil, Gelatin, Glycerin.

Norwegian Cod Liver Oil - Puritan's Pride
Each softgel contains: Natural Vitamin A 1,250 IU • Natural Vitamin D (from Cod Liver Oil) 135 IU.

Nose & Throat - Enzymes, Inc.
Two capsules contain: Vitamin C (100% from Acerola Cherries) 70 mg • Zinc (100% as Zinc Citrate) 10 mg • Proprietary Herbal Blend 360 mg: Elder Flower tops extract, Garlic bulb extract, Wild Indigo root extract, Quercetin, Grape seed extract • Proprietary Enzyme Blend 320 mg: Amylase, pHysioProtease, Peptidase. Other Ingredients: Plant Cellulose, Water.

NOW Chondroitin Sulfate, Joint Support, 600 mg - Now
Two capsules contain: Sodium 110 mg • Sodium Chondroitin Sulfate (from bovine cartilage) 1200 mg. Other Ingredients: Rice, Flour, Gelatin (capsule), Magnesium Stearate.
See Editor's Note No. 15, page 2055.

NOW Extra Strength Glucosamine & Chondroitin, Joint Support Factors - Now
Three capsules contain: Vitamin B3 (niacinamide) 100 mg • Vitamin B5 (pantothenic acid) 100 mg • Vitamin B6 (pyridoxine HCl) 50 mg • Vitamin C (ascorbic acid) 100 mg • Magnesium (oxide) 200 mg • Zinc (picolinate) 15 mg • Manganese (amino acid chelate) 7 mg • Copper (amino acid chelate) 3 mg • Glucosamine HCl 1000 mg • Boswellin (boswellia serrata standardized extract) 300 mg • Sea Cucumber 150 mg • Bromelain (2000 GDU activity from pineapple) 150 mg • PABA (para-aminobenzoic acid) 100 mg • Alfalfa juice concentrate 100 mg.

NOW Glucosamine Sulfate, 750 mg Complex, Superior Joint Support - Now
Two capsules contain: Potassium (as potassium chloride) 245 mg • Glucosamine Sulfate (from glucosamine potassium sulfate complex 2040 mg) 1500 mg. Other Ingredients: Gelatin (capsule), Magnesium Stearate.

NOW Relora 300mg - Now
Each Vcap contains: Relora Proprietary Blend 300 mg: Magnolia Officinalis, Phellodendron Amurense. Other Ingredients: Rice Flour, Cellulose (capsule), Modified Food and Corn Starch, Silica, Magnesium Stearate (vegetable source).

Now Sports L-Glutamine Powder - Now
Each 1/4 level tsp serving contains: L-Glutamine 750 mg.

NoX2 - Pinnacle
Three tablets contain: Proprietary Blend 3000 mg: Arginine Alpha-Ketoglutarate (A-AKG), Arginine-Ketoisocaproate (A-KIC). Other Ingredients: Beta Cyclodextrin, Cephalins, Xanthan, Inulin, Sorbitol, Calcium Phosphate, Magnesium Stearate, Stearic Acid.

NoX2 Overnight Extender - Pinnacle
Four tablets contain: Citruline-HP (pure l-citruline citrate-malate) 2000 mg • Arginine Alpha-Ketoglutarate (A-AKG) 1500 mg • Arginine-Ketoisocaproate (A-KIC) • Proprietary NoX2 Enhancers 267 mg: Ketoisocaproate Potassium (kIC-K), American Ginseng (Panax quinquefolius), Saw Palmetto (serenoa repens). Other Ingredients: Gama Cyclodextrin, Cephalins, Xanthan, Inulin, Sorbitol, Calcium Phosphate, Magnesium Stearate, Stearic Acid.

NOX3 - Universal
Three tablets contain: NO Complex 3000 mg: Arginine Alpha-Ketoglutarate, Arginine Ketoisocaproate • NO Booster 100 mg: Ornithine Alpha-Ketoglutarate. Other Ingredients: Beta-Cyclodextrin, Calcium Phosphate, Xanthan, Cellulose, Inulin, Magnesium Stearate.

NO-Xplode - BSN Inc.
Each scoop (20.5 g) contains: Vitamin B6 (pyridoxine HCl) 25 mg • Vitamin B12 (cyanocobalamine) 120 mcg • Folic Acid 400 mcg • Magnesium 360 mg • Phosphorus 500 mg • Calcium 75 mg • NO-Xplode Proprietary Blend 20,500 mg: L-Arginine AKG, Citral-M Citruline Malate, L-Citruline AKG, L-Histidine AKG, RC-NOS Rutacarpine 95%, Gynostemma Pentaphyllum (95% gypenosides), NAD (nicotinamide adenine dinuleotide), 2CM Dicreatine Malate, Betapure Trimethylglycine, Glycovol Glycocyamine, GuaniPro Guanidino Proplonic Acid, Cinnulin PF Aqueous Cinnamon extract, Keto-Isocaproate Potassium, L-Tyrosine, Taurine, Endurlac Glucuronolactone, L-Tyrosine AKG, Methylxanthines (caffeine), MCT (medium chain triglycerides), Vinpocetine 99%, Vincamine 99%, Vinburnine 99%, Calcium Phosphate, Magnesium Oxide, Potassium Phosphate, Sodium Phosphate, Potassium Glycerophosphate, Magnesium Glycerophosphate, Glycerola Stearate. Other Ingredients: Maltodextrine, Citric Acid, Sodium Bicarbonate, Lemon Juice Powder, Malic Acid, Potassium Citrate, Natural and Artificial Flavors, Aspartame, Acesulfame Potassium, FD&C Red 40, FD&C Blue 1.

NoxyLane4 - LaneLabs
Four veggie capsules (or two double strength capsules) contain: MGN3 Proprietary Blend (arabinoxylane compound) 1000 mg: Rice Bran, Hyphomycetes Mycelia enzyme from Shiitake mushroom • HAI (heated algal ingredient) Amino Acid extract (from sea algae) <1 mg. Other Ingrediens: Microcrystalline Cellulose, Hypromellose, Magnesium Stearate, Silica.
See Editor's Note No. 21, page 2056.

NOZ - NutraBolics
Nineteen grams contain: Tricreatine Malate 3 g • Arginine Alpha-KetoGlutarate 1 g • R- ALA 100 mg • N-Acetyl-L-Glutamine 1 g • Glycocyamine 1.5 g. Other Ingredients: Designer Complex Carbohydrates, Glucose Polymers (derived from vegetable sources), Sucralose, Natural/Artificial Flavor.

N-R-G Protein Powder - Naturade
Each 1 oz serving contains: Isolated Soy Protein • Calcium Caseinate • Sweet Dairy whey • Carrageenan • Soy Lecithin • Enzymatically Predigested Lactalbumin • Egg albumin • Papain & Natural Vanilla flavor.

NRG-Nature's Raw Guarana Instant Tea - Herbalife
Maltodextrins • Roasted Guarana Seed extract • Pekoe Tea extract • Lemon Peel extract • Citric Acid.

NRG-Nature's Raw Guarana Tablets - Herbalife
Each tablet contains: Guarana powder (contains 4% naturally occuring caffeine) 800 mg.

NSC-100 Immunition Extra Strength - NSC
Each capsule contains: Beta Glucan (MG Beta-1,3/1,6-Glucan) 10 mg.

NSC-24 Allergy Immunition - NSC
Two capsules contain: Beta Glucan (MG Beta-1,3/1,6-Glucan) 3 mg • Vitamin C 300 mg • Quercetin 300 mg • Hydrastus Canadensis 160 mg • Astragalus 60 mg • OPC (grape seed extract) 30 mg • Vitamin A (palmitate) 9000 IU • Beta Carotene 18 mg • Lemon Bioflavonoids 10 mg • Rutin 10 mg • Hesperidin 10 mg • Rose Hips 10 mg • Acerola Cherry 10 mg • Zinc (picolinate) 4 mg.

NSC-24 Caprylic Acid Immunition - NSC
Four gelatin capsules contain: Beta Glucan (Beta-1,3/1,6-Glucan) 4 mg • Caprylic Acid 360 mg.

NSC-24 Circulatory Immunition - NSC
Six capsules contain: Beta Glucan (Beta-1,3/1,6-Glucan) 6 mg • Vitamin C 1568.16 mg • Bromelain 140 mg • Coenzyme Q10 50 mg • Potassium Ascorbate 245.52 mg • Potassium Aspartate 308.88 mg • Magnesium Aspartate 205.92 mg • Magnesium Ascorbate 245.52 mg • L-Lysine 605.88 mg • L-Proline 605.88 mg.

NSC-24 Immunition Original Formula - NSC
Each capsule contains: Beta Glucan (MG Beta-1,3/1,6-Glucan) 3 mg.

N-TENSE - Raintree Nutrition, Inc.
Each capsule contains: Proprietary Blend 650 mg: Graviola, Mullaca, Vassourinha, Espinheira Santa, Mutamba, Bitter Melon, Suma, Cat's Claw.

Nu Colour Eye Makeup Remover - Nu Skin Enterprises
Water • Cyclomethiocone • Cetearyl Octanoate • C13-14 Isoparaffin • PPG-2 Myristyl Ether Propionate • Jojoba oil (buxus chinensis) • Rice bran oil (oryza sativa) • Polyacrylamide • Polysorbate 20 • Laureth-7 • Tocopherol • Tocopheryl Acetate • Bisabolol • Phenoxyethanol • Methylparaben • Butylparaben • Ropylparaben • Ethylparaben.

Nu Knees - The Sports Nutrition Source, Inc.
Three capsules contain: Glucosamine Sulfate 1000 mg • Chondroitin Sulfate 750 mg • MSM 750 mg • White Willow Bark 150 mg • Bromelain 100 mg • Vitamin C 90 mg.
See Editor's Note No. 15, page 2055.

Nu Skin 180 Face Wash (180 Face Wash) - Nu Skin Enterprises
Glycerin • Ascorbic Acid • Sesame oil (sesamum indicum) • C12-15 Alkyl Benzoate • Sodium Cocoyl Isethionate • Hydrogenated Soybean oil • Sodium C14-16 Olefin Sulfonate • Grape seed extract (vitis vinifera) • Ginkgo Biloba • Ginseng extract (Panax ginseng) • Stearyl Glycyrrhetinate • Carbomer • Titanium Dioixde • Fragrance (parfum).

NuBiotic - PhytoPharmica
Each tablet contains: Vitamin A (fish liver oil) 10,000 IU •Vitamin C (ascorbic acid) 200 mg • Vitamin D (fish liver oil) 35 IU • Vitamin B12 (cyanocobalamin) 2.5 mcg • Pantothenic Acid (calcium D-pantothenate) 25 mg •Calcium (lactate) 41 mg •Magnesium (citrate) 6.7 mg • Zinc (gluconate) 10.5 mg • RNA powder 60 mg • Alfalfa (Medicago sativa) leaf and stem juice powder 50 mg • Lemon Bioflavonoids 30 mg •Spleen extract 30 mg • Thymus extract 25 mg • Trace Mineral Concentrate (kelp) 25 mg •Unsaturated free fatty acids (oil of evening primrose) 15 mg • Lung extract 10 mg.
See Editor's Note No. 14 and No. 21, pages 2055 and 2056.

Nucleic Acid with RNA and DNA - Quest
Each tablet contains: RNA (Ribonucleic Acid) 200 mg • DNA (Deoxyribonucleic Acid) 60 mg • Brewer's Yeast 190 mg. Other Ingredients: Dibasic Calcium Phosphate, Microcrystalline Cellulose, Vegetable Stearin, Magnesium Stearate (vegetable source), Silicon Dioxide.

NuFem - Enzymatic Therapy
Each tablet contains: Black Cohosh (standardized to contain 2.5% triterpene glycosides calculated as 27-deocyacetin) 20 mg. Other Ingredients: Microcrystalline Cellulose, Lactose, Stearic Acid, Silicon Dioxide, Potato Starch, Magnesium Stearate.

NuFem Plus Soy - Enzymatic Therapy
Each tablet contains: Black Cohosh (standardized to contain 2.5% triterpene glycosides calculated as 27-deocyacetin) 20 mg • Soy bean extract (standardized to contain 15% isoflavones calculated as genistein and daidzein, non-GMO) 100 mg. Other Ingredients: Microcrystalline Cellulose, Calcium Carbonate, Stearic Acid, Croscarmellose Sodium, Silicon Dioxide, Magnesium Stearate, Water-Soluble Coating (hydroxypropyl methylcellulose, hydroxypropyl cellulose, polyethylene glycol).

NuFem Plus St. John's Wort - Enzymatic Therapy
Each tablet contains: Black Cohosh (standardized to contain 2.5% triterpene glycosides calculated as 27-deocyacetin) 20 mg • St. John's Wort extract (standardized to contain a minimum of 0.3% hypericin and 4% hyperforin) 100 mg. Other Ingredients: Microcrystalline Cellulose, Stearic Acid, Silicon Dioxide, Croscarmellose Sodium, Magnesium Stearate, Water-Soluble Coating (hydroxypropyl methylcellulose, titanium dioxide, polyethylene glycol, maltodextrin, sodium citrate, polysorbate 80, chlorophyll).

Nugest 900 - Nutraceutics Corp.
Purified Water • Ethoxydiglycol • Progesterone USP • C-12-15 • Alkyl Benzoate • Caprylic/Capric Triglyceride • Demasterone (bioactive multi wild yam species complex) • Trans-V-DS (lipo copolymer complex) • Dimethicone • Tocopheryl Acetate • Essence • Methylparaben • Propylparaben • Polysorbate 40 • Imidazolidinyl Urea • Disodium EDTA.

Nugest Serum - Nutraceutics Corp.
Purified Water • Demasterone (bioactive multi wild yam species complex) • Ethoxydiglycol • Protein Oligopeptide Biofactors • Caprylic/Capric Triglyceride • Trans-V-DS (lipo copolymer complex) • Glyceryl Stearate • PEG-100 Stearate • Caprylic/Capric/Stearic Triglyceride • Progesterone USP • Methyl-Paraben • Phenoxyethanol • Diazolidinly Urea • Disodium EDTA • Polysorbate 20 • Sodium Alginate • Essence.

Nugestrone - Nutraceutics Corp.
Aloe Vera • Glycerin • Canola Oil • Stearic Acid • Safflower Oil • Glyceryl Stearate Se • Wild Mexican Yam Extract • Octyl Palmitate • Deionized Water • Cetyl Alcohol • Glyceryl Stearate • PEG-100 Stearate • Progesterone USP • Polysorbate 60 • Sorbitan Sesquioleate • Methyl Glyceth-20 • Imidazolidinyl Urea • DMDM Hydantoin • Methylparaben • Propylparaben • Citric Acid.

NuHair Hair Regrowth Tablets for Men - Biotech Corp.
Two tablets contain: Folate (as folic acid) 800 mcg • Pantothenic Acid (as dicalcium pantothenate) 200 mg • Biotin 1400 mcg • Iodine (from kelp) 150 mg • Zinc (as zinc monomethionine) 15 mg • He Shou Wu (12:1 standardized extract) 450 mg • He Shou Wu root powder (polygonum multiflorum) 870 mg • Shen Min Herb Blend 433 mg: Saw Palmetto berries (sabal serrulata), Beta Sitosterol, Isoflavones (from pueraria lobata root and soybeans) • Silica (from colloidals) 40 mg • BioPerine Piper Nigrum standardized extract 5 mg. Other Ingredients: Microcrystalline Cellulose, Croscarmellose Sodium, Stearic Acid, Magnesium Stearate, Pharmaceutical Glaze.

NuHair Hair Regrowth Tablets for Women - Biotech Corp.
Two tablets contain: Vitamin A (as retinyl palmitate) 5000 IU • Niacin (as nicotinic acid) 20 mg • Vitamin B6 (pyridoxine HCl) 10 mg • Biotin 1400 mcg • Pantothenic Acid 200 mg • He Shou Wu root standardized extract (12:1) 450 mg • Soy Isoflavones (glycine max, from 50 mg 40% standardized soybean extract) 20 mg • Black Cohosh root standardized extract 40 mg • Horse Chestnut standardized extract 50 mg • Hydrolyzed Collagen 250 mg • Silica 100 mg • Gingko Biloba leaf 100 mg • Uva Ursi root standardized extract 50 mg • Burdock root extract (4:1) 25 mg • Cayenne pepper (80,000 scoville heat units) 25 mg • BioPerine Piper Nigrum standardized extract 5 mg. Other Ingredients: Microcrystalline Cellulose, Croscarmellose Sodium, Stearic Acid, Magnesium Stearate, Dicalcium Phosphate, Pharmaceutical Glaze.

NuHair Thinning Hair Serum - Biotech Corp.
Alcohol SD40 • Purified Water • Propylene Glycol • Jojoba oil • Herbal Blend Hair Complex: Henna, Horsetail, Rosemary, Tormentil, Burdock, Honey, Goldenseal • Lecithin • PEG-40 Stearate • Steareth-20 • Tilisina Complex • Cholesterol • Trichopeptide • Retinyl Palmitate • Tocopheryl Acetate • He Shou Wu extract • Saw Palmetto extract • Nettle extract • Propyl Gallate • Biotin • Polysorbate 20 • Chamomile extract • Carbomer • Disodium EDTA • Aminomethyl Propanol • Phenoxyethanol • Methylparaben • Butylparaben • Ethylparaben • Propylparaben.

NuLung **-** The Council On Natural Health
Two tablets contain: Vitamin A (as beta-carotene, with natural mixed carotenoids) 5000 IU • Vitamin C (as ascorbic acid) 100 mg • Vitamin B12 (as cyanocobalamin) 1.25 mcg • Pantothenic Acid (as d-calcium pantothenate) 3.5 mg • Zinc (as zinc gluconate) 0.6 mg • Calcium Lactate 30 mg • Ribonucleic Acid 30 mg • Lemon Bioflavonoid Complex 15 mg • Thymus substance (porcine) 12.5 mg • Chinese Ging Fei Tang Herbal Bland 500 mg: Skullcap root, Gardenia fruit, Dong Quai root, Licorice root, Ophiopogon tuber, Asparagus root, Schisandra berry, Tritillary bulb, Monus root bark, Platycodon root, Hoelen Scierotium, Bamboo stalk (barrbusa brenflora), Jujube date, Citrus peel (citrus leiocarpus) • Jade Windscreen Herbal Blend 50 mg: Atractylodes rhizome, Astragalus root, Ledebourilla root, Ginger root. Bio-active Base Blend 35 mg: Alfalfa leaf, Barley Malt extracts, Wheat Germ, Rose Hips, Lymphatic Substance (bovine), Chlorophyll (from alfalfa leaf). Other Ingredients: Dicalcium Phosphate, Microcrystalline Cellulose, Croscarmellose Sodium, Stearic Acid, Silica, Magnesium Stearate, Pharmaceutical Glaze.
See Editor's Note No. 14.

Nutraceutics ABC & Tea **-** Nutraceutics Corp.
Each tablet contains: Potassium (bicarbonate) 120 mg • Vitamin A (palmitate) 250 IU • Vitamin C (ascorbic acid) 1000 mg • Calcium (carbonate) 70 mg • Thiamine Mononitrate 15 mg • Riboflavin (as 5-phosphate) 16 mg • Niacinamide 50 mg • Pyridoxine HCl 8 mg • Vitamin B12 (cyanocobalamin) 10 mcg • Biotin 150 mcg • Pantothenic Acid (calcium pantothenate) 25 mg • Green Tea extract 70 mg. Other Ingredients: Sorbitol, Citric Acid, Sodium Bicarbonate, Polyethylene Glycol, Natural and Artificial Flavors, Sodium Benzoate, Sodium Carbonate, Sucralose.

NutraFlora Powder **-** Source Naturals
Three tablets contain: NutraFlora Fructooligosaccharides (FOS) 3000 mg.

NutraFloraFOS **-** Natrol
One capsule contains: FOS (Fructooligosaccaharides) 500 mg. Other Ingredients: Magnesium Stearate, Gelatin.

Nutragel **-** Nutraceutics Corp.
Active Ingredients: Purified Water • Dermasterone (bioactive multi wild yam species) • Protein Oligopeptide Biofactors • Caprylic/Capric Triglyceride • Trans-V-DS (lipo copolymer complex). Inactive Ingredients: Methylparaben, Phenoxyethanol, Diazolidinyl Urea, Disodium EDTA, Polysorbate 20, Sodium Alginate.

NutraGreens **-** Earthrise Nutritionals, Inc.
Twenty tablets contain: Vitamin A 5000 IU • Vitamin C 90 mg • Vitamin D 80 IU • Vitamin E (d-alpha-tocopherol acetate) 30 IU • Thiamin (Vitamin B-1) 1.5 mg • Riboflavin (Vitamin B-12) 1.7 mg • Niacin (Vitamin B-3) 20 mg • Vitamin B6 2 mg • Folic Acid 400 mcg • Vitamin B12 7.2 mcg • Biotin 300 mcg • Pantothenic Acid 10 mg • Calcium (Citrate) 24 mg • Iron (Gluconate) 2.7 mg • Iodine (Kelp) 30 mcg • Magnesium (Citrate) 18 mg • Zinc (Methionine) 10 mg • Selenium (Aminoate) 18 mcg • Copper (Gluconate) 1 mg • Manganese (Gluconate) 2 mg • Chromium (Aminoate) 50 mcg • Potassium (Spirulina & Asparatate) 25 mg • Proprietary Blend: Earthrise Spirulina, Lecithin, Natural Apple Concentrate, Prune Powder, Boron (Aminoate), Licorice extract (DGL), Sarsaparilla root, Siberian Ginseng extract (35:1, root), Ginkgo Biloba extract (24% Flavone Glycosides, 6% Terpene Lactones), Milk Thistle extract (80% Silymarin), Royal Jelly, Kelp, Dulse, Astragalus root, Stevia leaf, Ginger root extract (5%), Green Tea extract (50% Polyphenols), Broccoli Powder, Carrot Powder, Beet Powder, Celery Powder, Grape Seed extract (95% OPC), Octacosanol, Pine Bark extract (50% OPC), Cayenne Pepper fruit, Coenzyme Q-10 4242 mg • Proprietary Digestive Complex: Gum Arabic, Lactobacillus acidophilus DDS, Bifidobacterium longum, Aloe Vera, Amylase, Cellulase 253 mg.

NutraJoint Plus Glucosamine **-** KNOX
Each scoop contains: Sodium 30 mg • Protein 9 g • Vitamin C (as ascorbic acid) 60 mg • Vitamin D (as cholecalciferol) 80 IU • Vitamin E (as dl-alpha tocopheryl acetate) 6 IU • Vitamin K (as phytonadione) 16 mcg • Calcium 300 mg • Zinc (as zinc gluconate) 3 mg • Copper (as copper gluconate) 0.4 mg • Manganese (as manganese sulfate) 0.4 mg • Gelatine 10 g • Glucosamine Hydrochloride 1500 mg.

NutraLife - SAMe **-** NutraLife
Each tablet contains: S-Adenosyl-Methionine Tosylate Disulfate 200 mg.

NutraMetrix B Complex Plus **-** Market America, Inc.
Each capful (3.33 g) contains: Vitamin B2 (riboflavin-5-phosphate) 3 mg • Vitamin B12 (cyanocobalamin) 120 mcg • Folic Acid 400 mcg • Potassium (bicarbonate) 94 mg • Magnesium (carbonate) 40 mg. Other Ingredients: Fructose, Glucose, Citric Acid, Maltodextrin, Silica, Pectin, Calcium Sulfate, Natural Lemon-Lime Flavor.

NutraMetrix Blood Sugar Maintenance **-** Market America, Inc.
Each tablet contains: Biotin 1.3 mg • Magnesium (oxide) 67 mg • Zinc (gluconate) 2.5 mg • Chromium (nicotinate) 67 mcg • Glucomannan 400 mg • Alpha-Lipoic Acid 200 mg • Gymnema Sylvestre 133 mg • American Ginseng 33 mg • Vanadium (amino acid chelate) 15 mcg. Other Ingredients: Dicalcium Phosphate, Microcrystalline Cellulose, Stearic Acid, Magnesium Stearate, Croscarmellose Sodium, Silicon Dioxide.

NutraMetrix Calcium Complete **-** Market America, Inc.
Two capfuls (6.67 g) contain: Calcium (carbonate, lactate, phosphate, sulfate, citrate) 750 mg • Magnesium (oxide, carbonate) 200 mg • Manganese (sulfate) 1 mg • Vitamin B2 (riboflavin-5-phosphate) 2 mg • Vitamin C (ascorbic acid) 58 mg • Vitamin D (D3, cholecalciferol) 400 IU • Boron (sodium borate) 1 mg • Potassium (bicarbonate, citrate) 225 mg. Other Ingredients: Fructose, Glucose, Orange Powder, Citric Acid, Apple Pectin, Malic Acid, Natural/Orange Flavor.

NutraMetrix Coenzyme Q10 100 **-** Market America, Inc.
Each capful (3.33 g) contains: Coenzyme Q10 100 mg • Vitamin E (acetate) 200 IU • Lipase 5 mg • Vitamin B2 (riboflavin) 3 mg • Potassium (bicarbonate) 108 mg. Other Ingredients: Fructose, Glucose, Citric Acid, Silica, Calcium Sulfate, Maltodextrin, Natural Lemon-Lime Flavor.

NutraMetrix Digestive Enzymes with Probiotics **-** Market America, Inc.
Each capful (3.33 g) contains: DigeZyme 100 mg: Amylase 2400 U, Protease 600 U, Cellulase 20 U, Lactase 400 U, Lipase 100 U • Maltase 125 MWU • Sucrase 400 SU • Magnesium (carbonate) 24 mg • Potassium (bicarbonate) 88 mg • Lactobacillus Sporogenes (Lactospore) 150,000,000 CFU. Other Ingredients: Fructose, Glucose, Citric Acid, Maltodextrin, Silica, Apple Pectin, Calcium Sulfate, Natural Lemon-Lime Flavor.

NutraMetrix Female Support Formula **-** Market America, Inc.
Two tablets contain: Thiamin HCl (vitamin B1) 20 mg • Riboflavin (vitamin B2) 20 mg • Niacin (vitamin B3) 20 mg • D-Calcium Pantothenate (vitamin B5) 11.8 mg • Pyridoxine HCl (vitamin B6) 10 mg • Folic Acid 400 mcg • Cyanocobalamin (vitamin B12) 200 mcg • D-Alpha-Tocopherol (vitamin E) 50 IU • Soy extract (soy isoflavones, 3%) 200 mg • Dong Quai root 1% extract 200 mg • Evening Primrose oil 200 mg • Wild Yam 180 mg • Black Cohosh root 2.5% extract 160 mg • Chaste berry extract (vitex agnus-castus) 150 mg • Horsetail 150 mg • Red Clover 140 mg • Passiflora 120 mg • Valerian root 120 mg • Sage 100 mg • St. John's Wort 70 mg. Other Ingredients: Dicalcium Phosphate, Microcrystalline Cellulose, Stearic Acid, Magnesium Stearate, Croscarmellose Sodium, Silicon Dioxide.

Some Brand Name Natural Products - What they Contain

www.NaturalDatabase.com contains MANY more listings than appear here.

NutraMetrix Glucosatrin **-** Market America, Inc.
Three tablets contain: Vitamin C (ascorbic acid) 100 mg • Vitamin K (phytonadione) 100 mcg • Zinc (as zinc sulfate) 10 mg • Copper (as copper gluconate) 30 mcg • Manganese (as manganese sulfate) 5 mg • Glucosamine HCl 1500 mg • Scutellaria Baicalensis root (Chinese skullcap) 150 mg • Oleanolic Acid 150 mg • Boswellia Gum resin extract 200 mg • Hops strobile extract 350 mg. Other Ingredients: Microcrystalline Cellulose, Stearic Acid, Croscarmellose Sodium, Magnesium Stearate, Silica, Pharmaceutical Glaze.

NutraMetrix Herbal Antioxidant **-** Market America, Inc.
Two capsules contain: Vitamin A (as beta-carotene) 5000 IU • Vitamin C (as ascorbic acid) 200 mg • Vitamin E (as d-alpha tocopheryl succinate) 30 IU • Selenium (as SelenoExcell (high selenium yeast)) 200 mcg • Green Tea extract 300 mg • Ginkgo Biloba leaf extract (24% ginkgo flavoglycosides/6% terpene lactones) 50 mg • Milk Thistle 50 mg • L-Glutathione 1 mg • Bilberry powder 50 mg. Other Ingredients: Rice Powder, Silica, Magnesium Stearate, Gelatin.

NutraMetrix Isochrome **-** Market America, Inc.
Each capful (3.33 g) contains: Vitamin B2 (riboflavin) 3 mg • Vitamin B6 (pyridoxine HCl) 2 mg • Chromium (picolinate) 100 mcg • Chromium (argininate) 115 mcg • Potassium (bicarbonate) 95 mg • Coenzyme Q10 60 mg • L-Carnitine 20 mg • Lipase 5 mg • Boron (chelate) 2 mg. Other Ingredients: Fructose, Glucose, Citric Acid, Maltodextrin, Silica, Calcium Sulfate, Natural Lemon-Lime Flavor.

NutraMetrix Maximum ORAC Formula **-** Market America, Inc.
Each capful (3.33 g) contains: Potassium (bicarbonate) 125 mg • Vitamin C (ascorbic acid) 100 mg • Cranberry 200 mg • Blueberry 100 mg • Grape 93 mg • Raspberry 90 mg • Elderberry 40 mg • Black Currant 40 mg • Pomegranate 40 mg • Plum 20 mg • Choke Cherry 20 mg • Natural Tocopherol (d-gamma 70%, d-delta 21%, d-alpha 7%, d-beta 2%) 30 mg • Tocotrienols (mixed isomers) 20 mg • Bioperine Black Pepper extract 56 mcg. Other Ingredients: Fructose, Citric Acid, Maltodextrin, Glucose, Silica.

NutraMetrix MPC **-** Market America, Inc.
Two tablets contain: Zinc Citrate 30 mg • Selenium (as selenomethionine) 100 mcg • Saw Palmetto berry (serenoa repens small) 400 mg • Pygeum Africanum bark extract (standardized to contain 14% beta sitosterol and 0.5% docosanol) 100 mg • Prostate Health Proprietary Blend 425 mg: Chrysanthemum flower (dendranthema morifolium tzvel.), San-Qi Ginseng root (Panax notoginseng burk.), Dyer's Woad leaf (isatis indigotica fort.), Baikal Skullcap root (scutellaira baicalensis georgi), Reishi stem (ganoderma lucidum karst), Rhabdosia leaf (rhabdosia rubescens hara), Licorice root (glycyrrhiza uralensis fisch). Other Ingredients: Microcrystalline Cellulose, Stearic Acid, Magnesium Stearate, Silicon Dioxide, Croscarmellose Sodium, Dicalcium Phosphate.

NutraMetrix Multivitamins & Multiminerals With Iron **-** Market America, Inc.
Each capful (3.3 g) contains: Beta-Carotene 10,000 IU • Vitamin B1 2.6 mg • VItamin B2 3 mg • Niacin 40 mg • Pantothenic Acid 20 mg • Vitamin B6 4 mg • Vitamin B12 75 mcg • Folic Acid 400 mcg • Biotin 300 mcg • Vitamin C 150 mg • Vitamin D (D3) 400 IU • Vitamin E (D-alpha-tocopheryl succinate) 66 IU • Vitamin K 100 mcg • Calcium 50 mg • Chromium 120 mcg • Copper 1000 mcg • Iodine 150 mcg • Iron 1.5 mg • Magnesium 25 mg • Potassium 108 mg • Silicon 2 mg • Selenium 55 mcg • Zinc 7.5 mg. Other Ingredients: Fructose, Citric Acid, Orange Fruit Powder, Mandarin Fruit Powder, Malic Acid, Glucose, Natural Orange Flavor, Tricalcium Phosphate, Sucralose.

NutraMetrix Multivitamins & Multiminerals Without Iron **-** Market America, Inc.
Each capful (3.3 g) contains: Beta-Carotene 10,000 IU • Vitamin B1 2.6 mg • Vitamin B2 3 mg • Niacin 40 mg • Pantothenic Acid 20 mg • Vitamin B6 4 mg • Vitamin B12 75 mcg • Folic Acid 400 mcg • Biotin 300 mcg • Vitamin C 150 mg • Vitamin D (D3) 400 IU • Vitamin E (d-alpha-tocopheryl succinate) 66 IU • Vitamin K 100 mcg • Calcium 50 mg • Chromium 120 mcg • Copper 1000 mcg • Iodine 150 mcg • Magnesium 25 mg • Potassium 108 mg • Selenium 55 mcg • Silicon 2 mg • Zinc 7.5 mg. Other Ingredients: Fructose, Citric Acid, Orange Fruit Powder, Mandarin Fruit Powder, Malic Acid, Glucose, Natural Orange Flavor, Tricalcium Phosphate, Sucralose.

NutraMetrix OPC-3 **-** Market America, Inc.
Each capful (3.33 g) contains: Grape seed extract 25 mg • Red Wine extract 25 mg • Pine bark extract 25 mg • Bilberry extract 25 mg • Citrus Bioflavonoids extract 25 mg • Potassium (bicarbonate) 93 mg. Other Ingredients: Fructose, Glucose, Citric Acid, Maltodextrin, Silica, Calcium Sulfate, Pectin.

NutraMetrix Prostate Health Formula **-** Market America, Inc.
Two tablets contain: Zinc Citrate 30 mg • Selenium (as selenomethionine) 100 mcg • Saw Palmetto berry (serenoa repens) 400 mg • Pygeum Africanum bark extract (standardized to contain 14% beta-sitosterol and 0.5% docosanol) 100 mg • Prostate Health Proprietary Blend 425 mg: Chrysanthemum flower (dendranthema morifolium tzvel.), San-Qi Ginseng root (Panax notoginseng burk.), Dyer's Woad leaf (isatis indigotica fort.), Baikal Skullcap root (scutellaria baicalensis georgi), Reishi stem (ganoderma lucidum karst), Rhabdosia leaf (rhabdosia rubescens hara), Licorice root (glycyrrhiza uralensis fisch). Other Ingredients: Microcrystalline Cellulose, Stearic Acid, Magnesium Stearate, Silicon Dioxide, Croscarmellose Sodium, Dicalcium Phosphate.

NutraMetrix Vision Support Formula **-** Market America, Inc.
Each capful (3.33 g) contains: Beta Carotene 5000 IU • Vitamin C (ascorbic acid) 75 mg • Vitamin E (d, l-alpha-tocopheryl acetate) 33 IU • Potassium (bicarbonate) 150 mg • Zinc (lactate) 7 mg • Chromium (arginate) 100 mcg • Copper (gluconate) 100 mcg • Bilberry 50 mg • Taurine 42 mg • Quercetin 25 mg • Eyebright 10 mg • Lutein 7 mg • Lycopene 2 mg • Zeaxanthin 1.4 mg. Other Ingredients: Fructose, Natural Orange Powder, Citric Acid, Natural Orange Flavor, Malic Acid, Calcium Phosphate, Glucose, Silica, Sucralose.

NutraMetrix Vitamin C **-** Market America, Inc.
Each capful (3.33 g) contains: Vitamin C (ascorbic acid) 500 mg • Beta-Carotene (vitamin A precursor) 800 IU • Potassium (bicarbonate) 101 mg. Other Ingredients: Fructose, Glucose, Maltodextrin, Malic Acid, Natural Orange Flavor, Silica, Citric Acid.

Nutramin Body System **-** Informulab
One Capsule contains: Vitamin A (Beta Carotene) 1562 IU • Vitamin C 125 mg • Vitamin E 25 IU • Vitamin B-1 (Thiamine Mononitrate) 2.5 mg • Vitamin B2 (Riboflavin) 2.5 mg • Vitamin B6 (Pyridoxine HCl) 2.5 mg • Vitamin B12 (Cyanocobalamin) 2.5 mcg • Vitamin B3 (Niacinimide) 5 mg • Vitamin B5 (Pantothenic Acid) 10 mg • Vitamin B8 (Folic Acid) 50 mcg • Biotin (Water soluble Vit. B) 12.5 mcg • Vitamin D 50 IU • Calcium (Amino acid chelate) 62.5 mg • Phosphorus (Di-calcium phosphate) 6.25 mg • Magnesium (Amino acid chelate) 37.5 mg • Iron (Amino acid chelate) 2.25 mg • Zinc (Amino acid chelate) 1.875 mg • Manganese (Amino acid chelate) 0.625 mg • Copper (Amino acid chelate) 0.25 mg • Chromium Chelavite 18.75 mcg • Selenium (Amino acid chelate) 0.625 mcg • Potassium (Amino acid chelate) 3.125 mg • Iodine (as Potassium iodine) 18.75 mcg • Horsetail Herb 3.125 mg • White Willow Bark 3.125 mg • Bee Pollen 3.125 mg • Hops Flower 3.125 mg • Licorice Root 3.125 mg • Skullcap 3.125 mg • Valerian 3.125 mg • Garlic (Bulb-odorless) 3.125 mg • Citrus Bioflavonoids 3.125 mg • Rosehips 3.125 mg • Rutin 3.125 mg • Ginseng Root (Siberian) 3.125 mg • Alfalfa Herb 3.125 mg • Ginkgo Leaf 3.125 mg • Hawthorne Berry 3.125 mg • Beet Root 3.125 mg • Cayenne Fruit 3.125 mg • L-Lysine 3.125 mg • L-Proline 3.125 mg • L-Glutamine 3.125 mg • Live Food Enzyme Blend (vegetable source Protease, Lipase and Amylase) 6.25 mg • Pycnogenol 0.25 mg.

***Nutramine* - Calwood Nutritionals**
Each scoop contains: L-Histidine 280 mg • L-Isoleucine 360 mg • L-Leucine 560 mg • L-Lysine 410 mg • L-Methionine 560 mg •L-Phenylalanine 560 mg • L-Threonine 250 mg • L-Tryptophan 130 mg •L-Valine 410 mg.

***Nutramine T* - Calwood Nutritionals**
Two scoops contain: L-Histidine 220 mg • L-Isoleucine 290 mg • L-Leucine 440 mg • L-Lysine 310 mg • L-Methionine 440 mg • L-Phenylalanine 340 mg • L-Threonine 320 mg • L-Tryptophan 120 mg • L-Valine 360 mg • L-Tyrosine 660 mg.

***NutraSleep* - Source Naturals**
Four tablets contain: Niacinamide 10 mg • Vitamin B6 (Pyridoxine HCl) 2 mg • Calcium (citrate and carbonate) 250 mg • Magnesium (citrate, oxide and taurinate) 450 mg • Taurine (Magnesium taurinate) 1000 mg • Inositol 700 mg • GABA (Gamma Amino Butyric Acid) 600 mg • Skullcap 250 mg • Passionflower 200 mg • Valerian root 200 mg • Chamomile extract 100 mg.

***NutraSpray Quercetin* - Source Naturals**
Each spray contains: Quercetin 50 mg.

***Nutri Fiber* - Progressive Labs**
One tablespoon contains: Calcium 10.2 mg • Iron 0.35% • Thiamin (Vitamin B1) 0.36 mg • Riboflavin (Vitamin B2) 0.18 mg • Niacin 1.89 mg • Vitamin B6 1.66 mg • Pantothenic Acid 044 mg • Phosphorus 11.5 mg • Magnesium 31.8 mg • Zinc 2.42 mg • Copper 0.26 mg • Manganese 0.13 mg • Sodium 0.6% • Potassium 34.2 mg • Linolenic Acid (omega 3) 1.36 g.

***Nutri Plex* - The Sports Nutrition Source, Inc.**
One and a half scoops contain: Sodium 200 mg • Potassium 680 mg • Protein 25 g • Vitamin A 2500 IU • Vitamin C 30 mg • Calcium 800 mg • Iron 9 mg • Vitamin D 200 IU • Vitamin E 15 IU • Pantothenic Acid 5 mg • Vitamin B-1 75 mg • Vitamin B-2 85 mg • Vitamin B-3 10 mg • Vitamin B-6 1 mg • Vitamin B-12 3 mcg • Biotin 125 mcg • Zinc 7.5 mcg • Copper 1 mg • Magnesium 200 mg • Manganese 2 mg • Iodine 75 mcg • Phosphorus 160 mg • Selenium 32 mcg • Molybdenum 60 mcg • Chromium 78 mcg.

***Nutri-1000* - The Vitamin Shoppe**
Each tablet contains: Vitamin D 400 IU • Vitamin A 25000 IU • Vitamin C 100 mg • Vitamin E 100 IU • Vitamin B1 100 mg • Vitamin B2 100 mg • Vitamin B6 100 mg • Vitamin B12 100 mcg • Niacinamide 100 mg • PABA 100 mg • Pantothenic Acid 100 mg • Choline 100 mg • Inositol 100 mg • Biotin 100 mcg • Folic Acid 400 mcg • Rutin 25 mg • Citrus Bioflavonoid Complex 25 mg • Hesperidin Complex 5 mg • Betaine Hydrochloride 25 mg • Glutamic Acid 25 mg • Iodine 150 mcg • Calcium 50 mg • Potassium 15 mg • Iron 25 mg • Magnesium 20 mg Manganese 6.1 mg • Zinc 20 mg • Chromium 15 mcg • Selenium 10 mcg. In a whole-food base of rice concentrate, parsley, kelp, alfalfa, green cabbage, acerola, sarsaparilla, watercress, and golden seal.

***Nutri-All Multiple Powder* - Nature's Life**
Each scoop (about 15 g) contains: Vitamin A (Beta Carotene) 20000 IU • Vitamin E (d-Alpha Tocopheryl Acetate) 390 IU • Vitamin B1 (Thiamine Mononitrate) 30 mg • Vitamin B2 (Riboflavin) 30 mg • Vitamin B3 (Niacinamide) 110 mg • Vitamin B6 (Pyridoxine HCl) 30 mg • Vitamin B12 (Cobalamin concentrate) 30 mcg • Folic Acid 400 mcg • Biotin 30 mcg • Pantothenic Acid (d-Calcium Pantothenate) 110 mg • Inositol 110 mg • Choline (Citrate) 110 mg • Vitamin C 510 mg • Lemon Bioflavonoids (TESTLAB 50% Flavonoids) 100 mg • Rutin 30 mg • Boron (Proteinate) 25 mcg • Calcium (Carbonate, Ascorbate, Citrate/Malate) 800 mg • Chromium (Polinicotinate, Aspartate) 60 mcg • Copper (Citrate) 1 mg • Iodine (Kelp) 22.5 mg • Iron (Fumerate) 8 mg • Magnesium (Oxide, Citrate) 400 mg • Manganese (Citrate) 4 mg • Molybdenum (Molybdate) 60 mcg • Potassium (Gluconate) 99 mg • Selenium (Selenomethionine) 60 mcg • Silicone (Dioxide) 10 mg • Zinc (Picolinate) 20 mg. In a natural base of Protein powder, Oat Fiber, Rice Syrup solids, Psyllium husks & natural Orange flavor. Contains 10 mg of naturally occurring Sodium.

***Nutri-All Multiple Softgel* - Nature's Life**
Six softgel capsules contain: Beta Carotene (Vitamin A equivalent 10000 IU) 6 mg • Vitamin A (Fish Liver oil) 10000 IU • Vitamin D (as Vitamin D3) (Cholecalciferol) 400 IU • Vitamin B1 (Thiamine Mononitrate) 80 mg • Vitamin B2 (Riboflavin) 80 mg • Vitamin B3 (Niacinamide) 80 mg • Vitamin B6 (Pyridoxine HCl) 80 mg • Folic Acid 400 mcg • Vitamin B12 (Trituration of concentrate) 100 mcg • Biotin 50 mcg • Pantothenic Acid (d-Calcium Pantothenate) 80 mg • Choline Bitartrate 50 mg • Inositol 50 mg • Vitamin E (d-Alpha Tocopherol) 400 IU • Vitamin C (Ascorbic Acid & Rose Hips) 500 mg • Lemon Bioflavonoids (50% TESTLAB) 50 mg • Rutin Complex (Dimorphandra mollis) 25 mg • Hesperidin Complex (Citrus) 25 mg • Calcium (Carbonate) 1000 mg • Chromium (Picolinate, Nutrition 21) 200 mcg • Copper (Gluconate) 1 mg • Iodine (Potassium Iodide) 225 mcg • Magnesium (Oxide) 600 mg • Manganese (Citrate) 10 mg • Molybdenum (Molybdate) 20 mcg • Potassium (Citrate) 50 mg • Selenium (l-Selenomethionine) 50 mcg • Vanadium (Vanadyl Sulfate) 20 mcg • Zinc (Citrate) 15 mg • Betaine HCl 25 mg • CoEnzyme Q10 5 mg • Chlorophyll (oil-soluble) 100 mg. In a natural base of Safflower oil, Lecithin & Soy.

***NutriBalance Children's Formula* - NutriCology**
Two scoops (5 g) contain: Vitamin A (71% as beta-carotene) 3500 IU • Vitamin E (as d-alpha-tocopheryl acid succinate) 100 IU • Thiamin (as thiamin hydrochloride) 4.5 mg • Riboflavin (as riboflavin-5-phosphate) 4.5 mg • Niacin 15 mg • Vitamin B6 (as pyridoxine hydrochloride and pyridoxal-5-phosphate) 9.3 mg • Folic Acid 40 mcg • Vitamin B12 20 mcg • Biotin 20 mcg • Pantothenic Acid 25 mg • Calcium (as calcium carbonate) 100 mg • Magnesium (as magnesium carbonate) 250 mg • Chromium (as chromium nitrate) 25 mcg • Para-Aminobenzoic Acid 10 mg • Inositol 10 mg • Choline 25 mg • L-Glutamine 1.5 g • Flax meal 500 mg • Stevia leaves, dried extract 10 mg • Soy protein powder 1.5 g • Cellulose 250 mg • Total Count Probiotic Cultures 1 billion: Lactobacillus group (L. rhamnosus A, L. rhamnosus B, L. acidophilus, L. casei, L. bulgaricus) 700 million • Bifidobacterium goup (B. longum, B. breve) 200 million • Streptococcus Thermophilus 100 million.

***NutriBiotic Capsules Plus* - NutriBiotic**
Grapefruit extract • Echinacea extract • Artemisa annua extract.

***NutriBiotic Tablets* - NutriBiotic**
Grapefruit extract 100 mg.

***NutriClean Aloe* - Market America, Inc.**
Two tablets contain: Aloe Ferox leaf 860 mg • Aloe Barbadensis leaf 200 mg. Other Ingredients: Dicalcium Phosphate, Microcrystalline Cellulose, Croscarmellose Sodium, Stearic Acid, Magnesium Stearate, Silica, Pharmaceutical Glaze.

***NutriClean Fiber Powder* - Market America, Inc.**
Each scoop (15.7 g) contains: Vitamin A (as beta-carotene) 2000 IU • L-Glutamine 1000 mg • NutriClean Fiber Blend 13.3 g: Soy Fiber, Soluble Fiber complex, Alfalfa leaf, Beet root fiber, Flax seed fiber, Guar Gum, Inulin, Oat Bran, Psyllium seed husk • Probiotic Blend 1.5 billion CFU: Lactobacillus Acidophilus, Lactobacilllus Plantarum, Lactobacillus Sporogenes (Lactospore brand encapsulated L. sporogenes), Bifidobacterium Bifidum, Lactobacillus Casei. Other Ingredients: Citric Acid, Natural Flavors, Acesulfame Potassium, Silica, Sucralose.

***NutriClean HepatoCleanse* - Market America, Inc.**
Two capsules contain: Proprietary Blend 1260 mg: Milk Thistle seed extract (standardized to 80% silymarin), N-Acetyl-L-Cysteine, Dandelion root, Garlic bulb, Hawthorn berry extract, Schizandra Chinensis fruit and seed extract, Yellow Dock root, Burdock root, Licorice root, Barberry bark, Rosemary leaf, Ginger root, Bayberry root bark, Green Tea leaf extract, Hyssop (aerial parts), Red Clover flower, Curcumin root extract. Other Ingredients: Calcium Sulfate, Gelatin, Magnesium Stearate, Silica.

Some Brand Name Natural Products - What they Contain

www.NaturalDatabase.com contains MANY more listings than appear here.

NutriClean Release **-** Market America, Inc.
Two tablets contain: Proprietary Blend 1160 mg: Rhubarb root, Buckthorn bark, Cascara Sagrada bark extract (20% hydroxyanthrocene derivatives, calculated as cascaroside A), Gentian root, Anise seed, Fennel seed, Black Walnut bark, Oregon Grape root, Scutellaria root extract, Goldenseal aerial parts, Peppermint leaf. Other Ingredients: Dicalcium Phosphate, Microcrystalline Cellulose, Croscarmellose Sodium, Stearic Acid, Silica, Magnesium Stearate, Pharmaceutical Glaze.

Nutri-Cleanse **-** Nu-Creations
Each tablet contains: Aloe Vera resin 430 mg • Aloe Vera leaf 200 mg. Other Ingredients: Anise, Fennel, Psyllium, Rhubarb, Kelp, Flax, Dicalcium Phosphate, Pharmaceutical Glaze, Magnesium Stearate.

Nutri-Fast Trim **-** Nu-Creations
Three tablets contain: Chromium 400 mcg. Other Ingredients: Guar Gum, Gum Karaya, American Desert Herb, Guarana, Korean Ginseng, Bee Pollen, White Willow, Bladderwrack, Gotu Kola, Licorice, Reishi Mushroom, Chickweed, Mate, Gymnema Sylvestis, Fennel, Astragalus, Ginger, Rehmannia, Dicalcium Phosphate, Pharmaceutical Glaze, Magnesium Stearate.

NutriFi **-** Pharmanex
Each teaspoon contains: Oat Fiber • Maltodextrin • Dextrose (Glucose) • Cellulose • Citrus Pectin • Psyllium Fiber • Gum Arabic.

Nutrilite Antioxidant Complex with Pycnogenol **-** Nutrilite
Each capsule contains: Pycnogenol 60 mg • Grape Seed extract 30 mg • Green Tea extract (Decaffeinated) 300 mg • Alpha-Lipoic Acid 45 mg • Glutathione 60 mg • Turmeric extract 75 mg.

Nutrilite Bilberry with Lutein **-** Nutrilite
Each softgel contains: Bilberry extract • Lutein • Zeaxanthin • DHA.

Nutrilite Bio C Plus **-** Nutrilite
Each tablet contains: Vitamin C (from ascorbic acid and acerola concentrate) 250 mg • Calcium (from calcium carbonate and tricalcium phosphate) 50 mg • Acerola concentrates 200 mg: Acerola Cherry fruit extract (malpighia emarginata L.), Maltodextrin, Silicon Dioxide 200 mg • Citrus Multiflavonoid Complex 35 mg: Grapefruit, Mandarin, Lemon (fruit and peel). Other Ingredients: Calcium Carbonate, Microcrystalline Cellulose, Corn Starch, Sodium Carboxymethylcellulose, Tricalcium Phosphate, Hydroxypropyl Methylcellulose, Magnesium Stearate, Maltodextrin, Glycerin.

Nutrilite Black Cohosh and Soy **-** Nutrilite
Each tablet contains: Black Cohosh extract 120 mg • Soy Protein 300 mg • Isoflavones 49.8 mg • Acerola Cherry Concentrate 30 mg • Calcium 60 mg.

Nutrilite Calcium Magnesium Plus **-** Nutrilite
Each tablet contains: Calcium 651 mg • Magnesium 324 mg • Zinc 10 mg • Copper 2 mg • Manganese 2.5 mg • NUTRILITE Alfalfa Concentrate with Phytofactors Plant Compounds.

Nutrilite ChromPic Extra **-** Nutrilite
Each capsule contains: Chromium 300 mcg (providing Chromium picolinate 2400 mcg) • Vanadium 220 mcg • Gymnema sylvestre 100 mcg.

Nutrilite CoEnzyme Q10 Complex **-** Nutrilite
Each capsule contains: CoEnzyme Q10 30 mg • L-Carnitine 100 mg • Taurine 125 mg • Bioflavonoids 25 mg.

Nutrilite Daily Multivitamin and Multimineral **-** Nutrilite
Each tablet contains: Vitamin A (20% as beta carotene) 5000 IU • Vitamin C 90 mg • Vitamin D 400 IU • Vitamin E 30 IU • Vitamin K 80 mcg • Thiamin 2.3 mg • Riboflavin 2.6 mg • Niacin 20 mg • Vitamin B-6 2 mg • Folic Acid 400 mcg • Vitamin B-12 9 mcg • Biotin 300 mcg • Pantothenic Acid 10 mg • Calcium 200 mg • Iron 6 mg • Phosphorus 45 mg • Iodine 150 mcg • Magnesium 100 mg • Zinc 15 mg • Selenium 70 mcg • Copper 2 mg • Manganese 2 mg • Chromium 120 mcg • Molybdenum 75 mcg • Nutrilite concentrate 518 mg.

Nutrilite Double X **-** Nutrilite
Each tablet contains: Vitamin A (75% as beta carotene) 5000 IU • Vitamin C (from ascorbic acid, acerola powder) 250 mg • Vitamin D 200 IU • Vitamin E (d-alpha tocopheryl succinate) 150 IU • Vitamin K (from phytonadione) 40 mcg • Thiamin 12.5 mg • Riboflavin 12.5 mg • Niacin 35 mg • Vitamin B-6 25 mg • Folic Acid 400 mcg • Vitamin B-12 50 mcg • Biotin (from d-biotin) 150 mcg • Pantothenic Acid 25 mg • Calcium (from calcium carbonate) 450 mg • Phosphorous (from calcium phosphate) 10 mg • Iodine 75 mcg • Magnesium (from magnesium oxide) 225 mg • Zinc (from zinc gluconate) 10 mg • Selenium (from sodium selenite) 50 mcg • Copper (from copper gluconate) 1 mg • Manganese (from manganese gluconate) 2.5 mg • Chromium (from chromium chloride) 60 mcg • Molybdenum (from sodium molybdate) 37.5 mcg • Potassium (from potassium chloride) 40 mg • Alpha Lipoic Acid 5 mg • MSM (methylsulfonyl methane) 30 mg • Lycopene 0.5 mg • Lutein 0.5 mg • Quercetin 50 mg • Spirulina 25 mg • Boron (from boron aspartate) 500 mcg • Vanadium (from vanadyl sulfate) 10 mcg. Other Ingredients: Alfalfa extract, Parsley Dehydrate, Acerola concentrate, Citrus Bioflavonoid concentrate, Quercetin, Methylsulfonyl Methane, Brassica concentrate, Horseradish root, Mixed Tocopheryls, Calcium Pantothenate, Pyridoxine Hydrochloride, Niacinamide, Spirulina algae, Thiamine Mononitrate.

Nutrilite Echinacea with Astragalus **-** Nutrilite
Each tablet contains: Echinacea extract 200.1 mg • Astragalus extract 50.1 mg • Chlorella powder 50.1 mg.

Nutrilite Garlic & Licorice **-** Nutrilite
Each tablet contains: Pure concentrated Garlic 1000 mg • Licorice extract 21 mg.

Nutrilite Garlic Heart Care Formula **-** Access Business Group
Two tablets contain: Garlic bulb powder (allium sativum) 600 mg: Alliin (minimum) 13,500 mcg, Allicin yield (minimum 45% of alliin) 6000 mcg • Peppermint leaves extract 30 mg. Other Ingredients: Microcrystalline Cellulose, Stearic Acid, Lac Resin, Natural Peppermint Flavor, Sodium Starch Glycolate, Sodium Carboxymethylcellulose, Silicon Dioxide, Methylcellulose.

Nutrilite Ginkgo Biloba and DHA **-** Nutrilite
Each softgel contains: Standardized Ginkgo Biloba extract 160 mg • DHA 180 mg • Gotu Kola 68 mg.

Nutrilite Glucosamine HCl with Boswellia **-** Nutrilite
Two tablets contain: Glucosamine HCl 750 mg • Boswellia 60 mg • Bromelain 80 mg. Other Ingredients: Nutrilite Acerola Concentrate, Lemon Bioflavonoid Concentrate (with phytonutrients).

Nutrilite IntestiFlora **-** Nutrilite
Each stick pack (1.4 g) contains: Bifidobacterium Longum 500,000,000 CFU • Lactobacillus Acidophilus 500,000,000 CFU • Fructooligosaccharides (FOS) 1 g. Other Ingredients: Coconut and Palm Oil, Gelatin, Glycerin, Lecithin, Citrus Pectin.

Nutrilite Iron-Folic Plus **-** Nutrilite
Each tablet contains: Folic Acid 133 mcg • Calcium (from calcium carbonate) 40 mg • Iron (from spinach concentrate and ferrous fumarate) 15 mg • Spinach concentrate (spinach dehydrate, spinacla oleracea L. leaf and stem, ferrous gluconate) 142 mg. Other Ingredients: Dextrose, Maltodextrin, Microcrystalline Cellulose, Corn Starch, Sodium Carboxymethylcellulose, Hydroxypropyl Methylcellulose, Silicon Dioxide, Magnesium Stearate, Glycerin.

Nutrilite Kids Chewables Multivitamin Multimineral **-** Nutrilite
Each tablet contains: Vitamin A (from vitamin A palmitate and 25% from beta carotene) 2500 IU • Vitamin C (from ascorbic acid and tropical fruit concentrate) 40 mg • Vitamin D (from cholecalciferol)

200 IU • Vitamin E (from D-alpha tocopheryl acid succinate) 20 IU • Vitamin K (from phytonadione) 40 mcg • Thiamin (from thiamin mononitrate) 0.75 mg • Riboflavin (from riboflavin) 0.85 mg • Niacin (from niacinamide) 10 mg • Vitamin B6 (from pyridoxine hydrochloride) 1 mg • Folate (from folic acid) 200 mcg • Vitamin B12 (from cyanocobalamin) 3 mcg • Biotin 150 mcg • Pantothenic Acid (from calcium pantothenate) 5 mg • Calcium (from calcium carbonate) 75 mg • Iron (from ferrous fumarate) 3 mg • Iodine (from potassium iodide) 75 mcg • Magnesium (from magnesium oxide) 38 mg• Zinc (from zinc oxide) 7.5 mg • Selenium (from selenite) 35 mcg • Copper (from cupric oxide) 1 mg • Manganese (from manganese citrate) 1 mg • Chromium (from chromium chloride) 60 mcg • Molybdenum (from sodium molybdate) 38 mcg • Tropical Fruit Concentrate 50 mg: Acerola Cherry fruit extract (malpighia emarginata L.), Passion fruit (passiflora edulis), Pineapple fruit (bromelia ananas), Guava fruit (psidium guajava), Cashew fruit (anacardium occidentale), Maltodextrin, Dextrin. Other Ingredients: Xylitol, Sorbitol, Partially Hydrogenated Soy Oil, Microcrystalline Cellulose, Natural Flavor, Mono and Diglycerides, Dicalcium Phosphate, Silicon Dioxide, Maltodextrin, Magnesium Stearate, Citric Acid, Sodium Carboxymethylcellulose, Carminic Acid (colorant).

Nutrilite LeadingEdge Heart Pack **-** Nutrilite
Each packet contains: CoEnzyme Q10 • Garlic • Licorice • Omega 3 Complex • Natural B Complex.

Nutrilite Milk Thistle and Dandelion **-** Nutrilite
Each tablet contains: Milk Thistle extract (Silybin Extract 228 mg) 468 mg • Dandelion root extract 375 mg • Turmeric extract 225 mg • Lemon Bioflavonoids • Acerola Cherry Concentrate.

Nutrilite Natural B Complex **-** Nutrilite
Each tablet contains: Thiamin 1.2 mg • Riboflavin 1.2 mg • Niacin 6.67 mg • Vitamin B6 1.2 mg • Folic Acid 133.33 mcg • Vitamin B12 2 mcg • Pantothenic Acid 5 mg • Inositol 3.6 mg • Para-Aminobenzoic Acid 3 mg. Other Ingredients: Dicalcium Phosphate, Yeast, Microcrystalline Cellulose, Lactose, Hydroxypropyl Methylcellulose, Calcium Stearate, Silicon Dioxide, Glycerin.

Nutrilite Omega 3 Complex **-** Nutrilite
Each softgel contains: Vitamin E (from mixed tocopherols) 30 IU • Omega-3 Fatty Acids (from salmon and flaxseed oils) 300 mg • Alpha Linolenic Acid (from flaxseed oil) 185 mg • EPA (eicosapentaenoic acid, from salmon oil) 65 mg • DHA (docosahexaenoic acid, from salmon oil) 45 mg. Other Ingredients: Gelatin, Glycerin, Yellow Bees Wax, Soy Lecithin, Soybean Oil, Caramel Color, Lemon Oil.

Nutrilite Parselenium-E **-** Nutrilite
Each tablet contains: Vitamin E (from vitamin E succinate) 400 IU • Calcium (from tricalcium phosphate) 110 mg • Phosphorous (from tricalcium phosphate) 50 mg • Selenium (from selenium yeast) 10 mcg • Parsley leaf, stem concentrate (nasturium spp.) 77 mg. Other Ingredients: Microcrystalline Cellulose, Hydroxypropyl Methylcellulose, Silicon Dioxide, Magnesium Stearate, Modified Cellulose Gum, Glycerin.

Nutrilite Passionflower with Chamomile **-** Nutrilite
Each tablet contains: Passionflower 129.9 mg • Chamomile 81.3 mg • Hops 18.75 mg.

Nutrilite PriMroSe Plus **-** Access Business Group
Each softgel contains: Vitamin A (100% as betacarotene) 100 IU • Evening Primrose Oil (oenothera biennis, seed) 125 mg • Borage Oil (borago officinalis, seed) 125 mg • Ginger extract (zingiber officinale, root) 32 mg • Chasteberry extract (vitus agnus-castus, fruit) 15 mg • Dong Quai extract (angelica sinensis, root) 15 mg • Lemon Bioflavonoid concentrate (citrus limon L., fruit) 25 mg. Other Ingredients: Gelatin, Glycerin, Yellow Beeswax, Soybean Oil, Maltodextrin, Lecithin, Canola Oil, Corn Oil, Natural Caramel Color.

Nutrilite Saw Palmetto with Nettle Root **-** Nutrilite
Each softgel contains: Saw Palmetto 318 mg • Pumpkin Seed Oil 480 mg • Nettle Root 240 mg.

Nutrilite Siberian Ginseng with Ginkgo Biloba **-** Nutrilite
Each capsule contains: Siberian Ginseng extract 200 mg • Ginkgo Biloba extract 133.6 mg • NUTRILITE Acerola Cherry and Citrus Bioflavonoid Concentrates.

Nutrilite St. John's Wort with Lemon Balm **-** Nutrilite
Each capsule contains: St. John's Wort (0.3% Hypericin) 900 mg • Lemon Balm 78 mg • Lemon Bioflavonoid Concentrate 72 mg • Vitamin C (from Acerola Cherry Concentrate) 10 mg.

Nutrilite Trim Advantage Weight Management Support Pack **-** Nutrilite
Each strip containing four capsules contains: Calcium (from oyster shells) 80 mg • Chromium (from chromium picolinate) 100 mcg •Garcinia Cambogia fruit 633 mg •Conjugated Linoleic Acid (from sunflower oil) 600 mg • Kola Nut extract seed 100 mg • L-Carnitine (from l-carnitine fumarate) 100 mg • Lemon Bioflavonoid extract (citrus lemon peel) 106 mg •Parsley dehydrate stem and leaves 66 mg • Gymnema Sylvestre leaves 33 mg • Vanadium (from vanadium glycinate) 6.7 mcg. Inactive Ingredients: Gelatin, Cellulose, Magnesium Stearate, Beeswax, Lecithin, Caramel Coloring.

Nutrilite Triple Guard Echinacea **-** Access Business Group
Three tablets contain: Triple Guard Echinacea Blend 506 mg: Purpurea root and arial parts, Angustifolia root • Citrus Multiflavonoid Complex 100 mg: Grapefruit, Royal Mandarin, Lemon (fruit and peel). Other Ingredients: Corn Starch, Microcrystalline Cellulose, Maltodextrin, Stearic Acid, Sodium Carboxymethyl Cellulose, Silicon Dioxide, Methylcellulose, Glycerin.

Nutrilite Valerian and Hops **-** Access Business Group
Three tablets contain: Standardized Valerian root extract (0.8% valerenic acid) 450 mg • Valerian whole root extract 150 mg • Lemon Balm leaf extract 150 mg • Hops cone extract 100 mg • Citrus Bioflavonoid concentrate 100 mg: Grapefruit, Mandarin, Lemon. Other Ingredients: Microcrystalline Cellulose, Maltodextrin, Corn Starch, Stearic Acid, Sodium Carboxymethylcellulose, Hydroxypropyl Methylcellulose, Silicon Dioxide, Glycerin, Natural Flavor.

Nutrilite Women's GLA Blend with Evening Primrose Oil **-** Nutrilite
Each softgel contains: Evening Primrose • Borage Oil • Black Currant seed oil • Chasteberry • Dong Quai • Ginger Extract.

Nutrimeal - Dutch Chocolate **-** USANA Health Sciences
Two scoops contain: Soy Protein • Dutch Cocoa • High Oleic Sunflower Oil • Gum Arabic • Vitamin and Mineral Blend: Dicalcium Phosphate, Magnesium Phosphate, Dipotassium Phosphate, Niacinamide (Niacin), Ascorbic Acid (Vitamin C), Ferric Orthophosphate, Zinc Oxide, D-Alpha Tocopheryl Acetate (Natural Vitamin E), Vitamin A Palmitate, Riboflavin (Vitamin B2), Pyridoxine Hydrochloride (Vitamin B6), Thiamin Mononitrate (Vitamin B1), Cholecalciferol (Vitamin D3), Folic Acid, Cyanocobalamin (Vitamin B12), Potassium Iodide • Inulin • Corn Syrup Solids • Rice Syrup Solids • Natural and Artificial Flavors • Cellulose • Oat Fiber • Sodium Caseinate (a milk derivative) • Salt • Cellulose Gum • Mono and Diglycerides • Xanthan Gum • Soy Lecithin • Oligofructose.

Nutrimeal - French Vanilla **-** USANA Health Sciences
Two scoops contain: Soy Protein Isolate • Fructose • High Oleic Sunflower Oil • Gum Arabic • Inulin • Corn Syrup Solids • Vitamin and Mineral Blend: Dicalcium Phosphate, Magnesium Phosphate, Dipotassium Phosphate, Niacinamide (Niacin), Ascorbic Acid (Vitamin C), Ferric Orthophosphate, Zinc Oxide, D-Alpha Tocopheryl Acetate (Natural Vitamin E), Vitamin A Palmitate, Riboflavin (Vitamin B2), Pyridoxine Hydrochloride (Vitamin B6), Thiamin Mononitrate (Vitamin B1), Cholecalciferol (Vitamin D3), Folic Acid, Cyanocobalamin (Vitamin B12), Potassium Iodide • Rice Syrup Solids, Natural Flavors • Cellulose • Oat Fiber • Sodium Caseinate (a milk derivative) • Cellulose Gum • Salt • Mono and Diglycerides • Xanthan Gum • Soy Lecithin • Oligofructose.

Some Brand Name Natural Products - What they Contain

www.NaturalDatabase.com contains MANY more listings than appear here.

Nutrimeal - Wild Strawberry **-** USANA Health Sciences
Two scoops contain: Soy Protein Isolate • Fructose • Gum Arabic • Inulin • High Oleic Sunflower Oil • Corn Syrup Solids • Vitamin and Mineral Blend: Dicalcium Phosphate, Magnesium Phosphate, Dipotassium Phosphate, Niacinamide (Niacin), Ascorbic Acid (Vitamin C), Ferric Orthophosphate, Zinc Oxide, D-Alpha Tocopheryl Acetate (Natural Vitamin E), Vitamin A Palmitate, Riboflavin (Vitamin B2), Pyridoxine Hydrochloride (Vitamin B6), Thiamin Mononitrate (Vitamin B1), Cholecalciferol (Vitamin D3), Folic Acid, Cyanocobalamin (Vitamin B12), Potassium Iodide • Natural and Artificial Flavors • Cellulose • Sodium Caseinate (a milk derivative) • Oat Fiber • Beet Juice Powder (color) • Xanthan Gum • Mono and Diglycerides • Salt • Soy Lecithin • Oligofructose.

Nutrimmune Chews **-** Pharmanex
Each chew contains: Colostrum Microfiltrate 500 mg • Calcium 250 mg. Other Ingredients: Vitamin D.

Nutri-Plex **-** Nu-Creations
Three tablets contain: Vitamin A 5000 IU • Vitamin C 180 mg • Vitamin D 400 IU • Vitamin E 50 IU • Vitamin K 80 mcg • Vitamin B1 1.5 mg • Vitamin B2 1.7 mg • Niacin 20 mg • Vitamin B6 2 mg • Folic Acid 400 mg • Vitamin B12 6 mcg • Biotin 300 mcg • Pantothenic Acid 10 mg • Calcium 100 mg • Phosphorus 100 mg • Iodine 100 mcg • Magnesium 150 mcg • Zinc 50 mg • Selenium 15 mg • Copper 70 mcg • Manganese 2 mg • Chromium 2 mg • Molybdenum 400 mcg • Vanadium 75 mcg • Boron 1 mcg • Potassium 79 mg • Choline 10 mg • Inositol 10 mg • Garcinia cambogia 300 mg • Korean Ginseng 100 mg • Siberian Ginseng 200 mg. Other Ingredients: Anise, Fennel, Psyllium, Rhubarb, Kelp, Flax, Dicalcium Phosphate, Pharmaceutical Glaze, Magnesium Stearate.

Nutri-Shield **-** Nu-Creations
Two capsules contain: Vitamin A 25,000 mg • Vitamin C 1000 mg • Vitamin E 400 mg • Vitamin B6 25 mg • Zinc 25 mg • Selenium 100 mg • Copper 2 mg • Chromium 25 mg • Bioflavonoid Complex 150 mg • Rutin 40 mg • Quercetin 10 mg • Superoxide 100 mg • Astragalus 50 mg • Ginkgo biloba 15 mg • Rosemary 50 mg • Alpha Lipoic Acid 20 mg • Silymarin 50 mg • Lutein 6 mg • Spirulina 100 mg • Grape Seed extract 25 mg • Pine Bark extract 25 mg • Coenzyme Q-10 20 mg • L-Glutathione 10 mg • L-Glycerine 100 mg • Siberian Ginseng 50 mg • Reishi Mushroom 50 mg • Curcumin 50 mg. Other Ingredients: Dicalcium Phosphate, Pharmaceutical Glaze, Magnesium Stearate.

Nutrition Bar - Double Chocolate **-** USANA Health Sciences
One bar contains: Protein Blend: Roasted Soybeans, Soy Protein Isolate, Whey Protein Concentrate • High Fructose Corn Syrup • Coating: Sugar, Palm Kernel Oil, Cocoa Powder, Whey Protein, Nonfat Milk Powder, Lecithin, Natural Flavors • Maltitol Syrup • Fructose • Cocoa • Natural Flavors • Lecithin • Palm Kernel Oil.

Nutrition Bar - Peanut Butter Crunch **-** USANA Health Sciences
One bar contains: Protein Blend: Roasted Soybeans, Soy Protein Isolate, Textured Soy Flour, Whey Protein Concentrate • High Fructose Corn Syrup • Coating: Sugar, Palm Kernel Oil, Cocoa Powder, Whey Powder, Nonfat Milk Powder, Lecithin, Natural Flavors • Maltitol Syrup • Fructose • Peanut Flour • Peanut Butter.

Nutrition Warehouse Boron Complex Plus **-** Puritan's Pride
Four capsules contain: Boron 3 mg • MCHA (microcrystalline hydroxyapatite) 2000 mg • Calcium (from MCHA) 520 mg • Phosphorous (from MCHA) 260 mg • Magnesium carbonate elemental 160 mg • Magnesium aspartate elemental 40 mg • Vitamin D (as Vitamin D3) 260 IU • Vitamin K 120 mcg • Manganese 10 mg • Silica 100 mg. Other Ingredients: Magnesium, Potassium, Zinc, Selenium, Manganese, Iron, Collagen, Glycosaminoglycans, substituent Amino Acids.
See Editor's Note No. 21, page 2056.

Nutrition Warehouse Multi Minerals with Boron **-** Puritan's Pride
Three tablets contain: Calcium (Carbonate, Citrate) 1000 mg • Magnesium (Oxide, Citrate) 500 mg • Zinc 22.5 mg • Iron 20 mg • Copper 1 mg • Potassium 99 mg • Manganese 5 mg • Selenium 50 mcg • Chromium (yeast-free) 100 mcg • Molybdenum 50 mcg • Vanadium 50 mcg • Iodine (Kelp) 150 mcg • L-Glutamic Acid (HCL) 50 mg • Vitamin D (Cholecalciferol) 200 IU • Boron Citrate 3 mg.
See Editor's Note No. 21, page 2056.

Nutri-Vit **-** Progressive Labs
One tablespoon (15 ml) contains: Vitamin A 3750 IU • Vitamin C 60 mg • Vitamin D 600 IU • Vitamin E 15 IU • Thiamin (B1) 1.05 mg • Riboflavin (B2) 1.2 mg • Niacin 13.5 mg • Vitamin B6 1.05 mg • Folate (folic acid) 300 mcg • Vitamin B12 4.5 mcg • Biotin 225 mcg • Pantothenic Acid 7.5 mg • Iron 15 mg • Zinc 12 mg.

Nutrizyme - Tyler **-** Integrative Therapeutics
Three capsules contain: Vitamin A (as natural beta-carotene with mixed carotenoids, palmitate) 10,000 IU • Vitamin C (from Poly-C ascorbates) 150 mg • Vitamin D (as cholecalciferol) 50 IU • Vitamin E (as d-alpha tocopheryl succinate) 25 mg • Vitamin K (as phytonadione) 25 mcg • Thiamine (as thiamine hydrochloride) 25 mg • Riboflavin (as riboflavin 12.6 mg, riboflavin-5'-phosphate 5.1 mg) 17.7 mg • Niacin (as Niacinol) 25 mg • Vitamin B6 (as pyridoxine HCl 37.5 mg, pyridoxal-5'-phosphate 5.1 mg) 42.6 mg • Folic Acid 200 mcg • Vitamin B12 (as cyanocobalamin) 100 mcg • Biotin 150 mcg • Pantothenic Acid (as calcium pantothenate) 25 mg • Calcium (as calcium citrate, malate, ascorbate) 200 mg • Magnesium (as magnesium citrate, ascorbate) 200 mg • Zinc (as zinc picolinate, ascorbate) 10 mg • Selenium (as selenium aspartate) 50 mcg • Copper (as copper aspartate) 0.5 mg • Manganese (as manganese aspartate) 5 mg • Chromium (from GlucoChrome) 75 mcg • Molybdenum (as molybdenum aspartate) 25 mcg • Potassium (as potassium citrate, ascorbate) 25 mg • Plant Enzymes 62 mg: Protease (I, II, IV), Amylase, Cellulase (I), Lipase (II), Lactase (II), Sucrase (invertase), Maltase (malt diastase) • Bioflavonoids 37.5 mg • Choline (as choline bitartrate) 25 mg • Inositol 25 mg • Gamma-Oryzanol (from rice bran oil) 20 mg • Rutin 12.5 mg • Pro-Flora 5 mg • L-Glutathione (reduced) 750 mcg • Boron (as boron aspartate, citrate) 0.5 mg • Vanadium (as vanadium aspartate 25 mcg. Other Ingredients: Microcrystalline Cellulose, Gelatin, Water.

NxTrim **-** Nova Pharmaceutical, Inc.
Two tablets contain: Vitamin C (ascorbic acid) 200 mg • Niacin 10 mg • Vitamin B6 (as pyridoxine hydrochloride) 4 mg • Vitamin B12 (as cyanocobalamin) 166 mcg • Calcium (as dibasic calcium phosphate) 55 mg • Chromium (as chromium polynicotinate) 100 mcg • Phenylalanine (as L-phenylalanine hydrochloride) 300 mg • Glutamine (as L-glutamine hydrochloride) 50 mg • Tyrosine (as L-tyrosine hydrochloride) 100 mg • St. John's Wort extract 50 mg • L-Carnitine 20 mg • Korean Ginseng powdered root 70 mg • Uva Ursi powdered leaves 50 mg. Other Ingredients: Whey, Stearic Acid, Magnesium Stearate, Pharmaceutical Glaze.

Nytol **-** GlaxoSmithKline (GSK)
Each capsule contains: Diphenhydramine Hydrochloride 25 mg. Other Ingredients: Corn Starch, Lactose, Microcrystalline Cellulose, Silica, Stearic Acid.

O.U.T. (Ovarian Uterine Tonic) **-** The Herbalist
Chaparral leaf • Pipsissewa leaf • False Unicorn root • Prickly Ash bark • Cramp bark • Licorice root • Saw Palmetto berry • Red Clover blossom.

Oasis A.M. **-** Oasis Wellness Network
Each tablespoon contains: Potassium 42 mg • Protein 1 g • Calcium 28 mg • Iron 1 mg • Siberian Ginseng root extract 58 mg • Gotu Kola extract (whole plant) 48 mg. Other Ingredients: Roasted Carob, Barley, Chicory Root, Almond, Fig, Dates, Natural Coffee Flavor.

Oats-Sculleap Virtue **-** Blessed Herbs
Oats in milk stage • Sculleap • St. John's Wort flower • Lemon Balm • Lavender flower • Rosemary & Blackberry brandy.

Occuplex **-** Puritan's Pride
Eight capsules contain: Vitamin A 32,800 IU • Vitamin C (Ascorbic Acid) 500 mg • Vitamin E (as dl-Alpha Tocopheryl Acetate) 400 IU • Thiamin 20 mg • Riboflavin 25 mg • Niacin (as Niacinamide and Niacin) 60 mg • Vitamin B6 30 mg • Folic Acid 800 mcg • Vitamin B12 50 mcg • Pantothenic Acid 100 mg • Calcium 100 mg • Magnesium 250 mg • Zinc 30 mg • Selenium 200 mcg • Copper 3 mg • Lutein 10 mg • N-Acetyl-Cysteine 250 mg • Bilberry leaf 40 mg • Ginkgo Biloba 24% extract 60 mg • Quercetin 300 mg • L-Taurine 500 mg • L-Methionine 200 mg • Glutamic acid 50 mg • L-Glycine 50 mg.

Octa-Carotene **-** Nature's Plus
Each softgel contains: Vitamin A (as beta-carotene, carrot oil extract) 10,000 IU • Lutein (marigold flower extract) 6 mg • Lycopene 5 mg • Alpha Carotene (carrot oil extract) 1.7 mg • Zeaxanthin (marigold flower extract) 263 mcg • Phytoene (colorless carrot oil extract) 134 mcg • Astaxanthin (Antarctic crustacea extract) 102 mcg • Phytofluene (colorless carrot oil extract) 45 mcg •

OcuActin **-** Nature's Plus
Two capsules contain: Vitamin C corn free 100 mg • Citrus Bioflavonoid Complex 100 mg • Vitamin E natural 50 IU • Zinc (Monomethionine) 30 mg • Bilberry [(Vaccinium myrtillus fruit) standardized 25% Anthocyanosides] 25 mg • Goldenseal [(Hydrastis canadensis root & rhizome) standardized 10% Alkaloids, 5% Hydrastine] 25 mg • Echinacea [(Echinacea angustifolia root & rhizome) standardized 4% Echinacosides] 25 mg • Chinese Green Tea [(Camellia sinensis leaf) decaffeinated, standardized 50% Polyphenols] 25 mg • Grape Seed [(Vitis vinifera) standardized 95% Proanthocyanidins] 10 mg Glutathione (pharmaceutical grade Free Form Amino Acid) 10 mg • Beta Carotene (supplying 15000 IU of Vitamin A activity) 9 mg • Lutein (active Carotenoid from Marigold flower extract) 6 mg • Coenzyme Q10 (Ubiquinone) 5 mg • Copper (Glycinate) 2 mg • Zeaxanthin (active Carotenoid from Marigold flower extract) 263 mcg • Vitamin A (Retinol) 5000 IU • Selenium (Selenomethionine) 50 mcg.

Ocu-Care **-** Nature's Plus
Two tablets contain: Strengthening Nutrients: Bilberry standardized 25% Anthocyanosides 30 mg • Citrus Bioflavonoid Complex supplying: (Active Flavonones with Hesperidin & Eriocitrin 24%, Active Flavonols & Flavones, Pectin, Cellulose & Narigen 20%) 250 mg • Rutin (Saphora japonica) 100 mg. Protectant Nutrients: Pantothenic Acid 100 mg • L-Lysine free form amino acid 50 mg. Antioxidant Nutrients: Beta Carotene pro-Vitamin A, supplying 20000 IU Vitamin A activity • Vitamin A Fish Liver oil 5000 IU • Vitamin E natural 200 IU • NAC (N-Acetyl-Cysteine) 50 mg • Zinc (Monomethionine) 20 mg.

OcuDyne **-** Allergy Research Group
Two capsules contain: Vitamin A (23% as retinyl palmitate and 77% as beta-carotene) 8125 IU • Vitamin C (as ascorbic acid) 125 mg • Vitamin E (as DL-alpha-tocopheryl acetate) 100 IU • Thiamin (as thiamin hydrochloride) 5 mg • Riboflavin 6.25 mg • Niacin (83% as niacinamide) 15 mg • Vitamin B6 (as pyridoxine hydrochloride) 7.5 mg • Folic Acid 200 mcg • Vitamin B12 12.5 mcg • Pantothenic Acid 25 mg • Calcium (as calcium citrate) 25 mg • Magnesium (as magnesium citrate) 62.5 mg • Zinc (as zinc picolinate) 12.5 mg • Selenium (as sodium selenite and selenomethionine) 50 mcg • Copper (as copper sebacate) 0.75 mg • N-Acetyl-L-Cysteine 62.5 mg • Glycine 12.5 mg • L-Methionine 50 mg • Taurine 125 mg • Glutamic Acid 12.5 mg • Quercetin 75 mg • Ginkgo biloba leaves, dried extract 15 mg • Bilberry fresh berries dried extract (vaccinium myrtillus) 10 mg. Other Ingredients: Cellulose, Stearic Acid.

OcuDyne **-** NutriCology
Two capsules contain: Vitamin A (23% as retinyl palmitate and 77% as beta-carotene) 8125 IU • Vitamin C (as ascorbic acid) 125 mg • Vitamin E (as DL-alpha-tocopheryl acetate) 100 IU • Thiamin (as thiamin hydrochloride) 5 mg • Riboflavin 6.25 mg • Niacin (83% as niacinamide) 15 mg • Vitamin B6 (as pyridoxine hydrochloride) 7.5 mg • Folic Acid 200 mcg • Vitamin B12 12.5 mcg • Pantothenic Acid 25 mg • Calcium (as calcium citrate) 25 mg • Magnesium (as magnesium citrate) 62.5 mg • Zinc (as zinc picolinate) 12.5 mg • Selenium (as sodium selenite and selenomethionine) 50 mcg • Copper (as copper sebacate) 0.75 mg • N-Acetyl-L-Cysteine 62.5 mg • Glycine 12.5 mg • L-Methionine 50 mg • Taurine 125 mg • Glutamic Acid 12.5 mg • Quercetin 75 mg • Ginkgo Biloba dried leaves extract 15 mg • Bilberry dried fresh berries extract (vaccinium myrtillus) 10 mg. Other Ingredients: Cellulose, Stearic Acid.

OcuDyne II with Lutein and Added Minerals **-** Allergy Research Group
Two capsules contain: Vitamin A (23% as retinyl palmitate and 77% as beta-carotene) 8125 IU • Vitamin C (as ascorbic acid) 125 mg • Vitamin E (as D-alpha-tocopheryl acid succinate) 50 IU • Thiamin (as thiamin hydrochloride) 5 mg • Riboflavin 6.25 mg • Niacin (86% as niacinamide) 15 mg • Vitamin B6 (as pyridoxine hydrochloride) 7.5 mg • Folic Acid 200 mcg • Vitamin B12 12.5 mcg • Pantothenic Acid 25 mg • Calcium (as calcium citrate) 25 mg • Iodine (as potassium iodide) 5 mcg • Magnesium (as magnesium citrate) 62.5 mg • Zinc (as zinc citrate) 12.5 mg • Selenium (as sodium selenite and selenomethionine) 50 mcg • Copper (as copper sebacate) 0.75 mg • Manganese (as manganese citrate) 2.5 mg • Chromium (as chromium nicotinate) 50 mcg • Molybdenum (as sodium molybdate) 30 mcg • Potassium (as potassium chloride) 25 mg • Boron (as boron citrate) 150 mcg • N-Acetyl-L-Cysteine 62.5 mg • Glycine 12.5 mg • L-Methionine 50 mg • Taurine 125 mg • Glutamic Acid 12.5 mg • Lutein 2.5 mg • Zeaxanthin 125 mcg • Quercetin 75 mg • Horsetail extract (equisetum arvense) 2.5 mg • Ginkgo Biloba leaves extract 15 mg • Bilberry fresh berries extract (vaccinium myrtillus) 10 mg. Other Ingredients: Cellulose, Magnesium Stearate.

OcuDyne II with Lutein and Added Minerals **-** NutriCology
Two capsules contain: Vitamin A (23% as retinyl palmitate and 77% as beta-carotene) 8125 IU • Vitamin C (as ascorbic acid) 125 mg • Vitamin E (as DL-alpha-tocopheryl acetate) 50 IU • Thiamin (as thiamin hydrochloride) 5 mg • Riboflavin 6.25 mg • Niacin (86% as niacinamide) 15 mg • Vitamin B6 (as pyridoxine hydrochloride) 7.5 mg • Folic Acid 200 mcg • Vitamin B12 12.5 mcg • Pantothenic Acid 25 mg • Calcium (as calcium citrate) 25 mg • Iodine (as potassium iodide) 5 mcg • Magnesium (as magnesium citrate) 62.5 mg • Zinc (as zinc citrate) 12.5 mg • Selenium (as sodium selenite and selenomethionine) 50 mcg • Copper (as copper sebacate) 0.75 mg • Manganese (as manganese citrate) 2.5 mg • Chromium (as chromium nicotinate) 50 mcg • Molybdenum (as sodium molybdate) 30 mcg • Potassium (as potassium chloride) 25 mg • Boron (as boron citrate) 150 mcg • N-Acetyl-L-Cysteine 62.5 mg • Glycine 12.5 mg • L-Methionine 50 mg • Taurine 125 mg • Glutamic Acid 12.5 mg • Lutein 2.5 mg • Zeaxanthin 125 mcg • Quercetin 75 mg • Ginkgo Biloba dried leaves extract 15 mg • Bilberry dried fresh berries extract (vaccinium myrtillus) 10 mg. Other Ingredients: Cellulose, Magnesium Stearate.

Ocular Defense **-** PhysioLogics
Two capsules contain: Vitamin A (as 80% beta-carotene, retinyl palmitate) 12,500 IU •Vitamin E (as d-alpha tocopherol succinate) 100 IU •Riboflavin (vitamin B2) 10 mg •Vitamin B6 (as pyridoxine HCl) 10 mg •Zinc (as zinc copper amino acid chelate) 15 mg • Selenium (as selenium amino acid chelate) 50 mcg •Copper (as copper amino acid chelate) 8 mg • Chromium (as chromium amino acid chelate) 100 mcg •Taurine 200 mg •N-Acetyl Cysteine 100 mg • Bilberry fruit extract (vaccinum myrtillus, standardized to contain 25% anthocyanosides) 60 mg •Quercetin root (dimorphandra gardina) 60 mg •L-Glutathione 25 mg. Other Ingredients: Rice Powder, Gelatin, Vegetable Magnesium Stearate, Silica.

Some Brand Name Natural Products - What they Contain

www.NaturalDatabase.com contains MANY more listings than appear here.

Ocular Defense Plus **-** PhysioLogics
Four capsules contain: Vitamin A (as beta-carotene) 40,000 IU • Vitamin C (as ascorbic acid) 1500 mg • Vitamin E (as d-alpha tocopherol succinate) 400 IU • Riboflavin (vitamin B2) 50 mg • Zinc (as zinc picolinate) 25 mg • Selenium (as selenomethionine) 100 mcg • Chromium (as gtf chromium yeast) 200 mcg • Quercetin fruit (from dimorphandra mollis) 100 mg • Bilberry leaf extract (vaccinium myrtillus, standardized to conatin 25% anthocyanosides) 10 mg • Rutin fruit (dimorphandra mollis) 100 mg • Citrus Bioflavonoid fruit complex (citrus sinensis) 250 mg • Taurine 200 mg • N-Acetyl Cysteine 200 mg • L-Glutathione 10 mg • Lutein 20 mg. Other Ingredients: Gelatin, Silica, Vegetable Magnesium Stearate.

Ocu-Plus **-** Aspen Group, Inc.
Two tablets contain: Beta-Carotene 25,000 IU • Vitamin E (d-alpha tocopherol) 400 IU • Vitamin C 1000 mg • Citrus bioflavonoid complex 250 mg • Quercetin 100 mg • Bilberry extract (25% anthocyanosides) 80 mg • Rutin 100 mg • Zinc (gluconate) 50 mg • Copper (gluconate) 2 mg • Selenium (selenomethionine) 50 mcg • N-Acetyl L-Cysteine (glutathione precursor) 200 mg • L-Glutathione 10 mg • Eyebright 50 mg • Alpha-Lipoic Acid 50 mg • Chromium Picolinate 200 mcg • Lutein (containing zeaxanthin) 6 mg • Ginkgo Biloba 25 mg.

OcuPower **-** NSI - Nutraceutical Sciences Institute
Three capsules contain: Vitamin A (retinyl palmitate) 2500 IU • Betatene Natural Mixed Carotenoids 15,000 IU: Beta Carotene, Alpha-Carotene, Lutein, Zeaxanthin, Cryptoxanthin • Lutein (from 200 mg standardized FloraGlo with zeaxanthin) 10 mg • Lycopene (from 12 mg Lyc-O-Mato) 600 mcg • Vitamin B1 (thiamin) 50 mg • Vitamin B2 (riboflavin) 10 mg • Vitamin B3 (niacinamide) 70 mg • Vitamin B5 (d-calcium pantothenate) 50 mg • Vitamin B6 (pyridoxine HCl) 50 mg • Vitamin B12 (methylcobalamin) 500 mcg • Folic Acid (folacin) 800 mcg • Biotin 300 mcg • Vitamin C (Ester-C) 1500 mg • Vitamin D (D3, cholecalciferol) 400 IU • Vitamin E (natural d-alpha, beta, delta, gamma forms) 500 IU • Calcium (from over 1200 mg of citrate, malate, ascorbate) 256 mg • Magnesium (from taurinate, citate) 300 mg • Zinc (L-OptiZinc) 25 mg • Selenium (l-selenomethionine) 200 mcg • Boron (chelate) 2 mg • Copper (chelate) 1 mg • Manganese (chelate) 2 mg • Chromium (glucose tolerance factor ChromeMate) 200 mcg • Iodine (kelp) 75 mcg • Molybdenum (chelate) 75 mcg • BioPerine Black Pepper 5 mg • Enzymes 50 mg: Amylae, Cellulase, Protease, Lipase, Lactase • Citrus Bioflavonoids 250 mg • Quercetin Bioflavonoids 100 mg • Rutin Bioflavonoids 100 mg • Bilberry extract (standardized 25% anthocyanosides) 160 mg • Alpha Lipoic Acid 150 mg • Taurine (magnesium taurate) 900 mg • N-Acetyl-Cysteine 200 mg • L-Glutathione 10 mg • L-Glycine 100 mg.

OcuSense **-** Natrol
Two capsules contain: Vitamin A (from beta-carotene) 5000 IU • Vitamin C (as calcium ascorbate) 60 mg • Vitamin E (as d-alpha tocopheryl succinate) 30 IU • Zinc (as zinc methionate) 15 mg • Selenium (as l-selenomethioine) 70 mcg • Copper (as copper amino acid chelate) 2 mg • Lutein (from marigold flowers) 13 mg • Zeaxanthin (from marigold flowers) 3 mg • Bilberry fruit extract 2 mg • Anthocyanosides 500 mcg • Carrot powder 10 mg • Carotenoid Blend 10 mg: Tomato, Marigold flowers, Palm seed • Beta-Carotene 295 mcg • Alpha-Carotene 19 mcg • Cryptoxanthin 4 mcg. Other Ingredients: Gelatin, Silica, Magnesium Stearate.

Ocuvite **-** Bausch & Lomb
Each tablet contains: Vitamin A (100% as beta carotene) 5000 IU • Vitamin C (ascorbic acid) 60 mg • Vitamin E (dl-alpha tocopherol acetate) 30 IU • Zinc (from zinc oxide) 40 mg • Selenium (from sodium selenate) 40 mcg • Copper (from cupric oxide) 2 mg. Other Ingredients: Dibasic Calcium Phosphate, Microcrystalline Cellulose, Calcium Carbonate, Crospovidone, Hydroxypropyl Methylcellulose, Titanium Dioxide, Silica Gel, Magnesium Stearate, Stearic Acid, FD&C Yellow No. 6, Triethyl Citrate, Polysorbate 80, and Sodium Lauryl Sulfate.

Ocuvite Extra **-** Bausch & Lomb
Each tablet contains: Vitamin A (beta carotene) 1000 IU • Vitamin C (ascorbic acid) 300 mg • Vitamin E (dl-alpha tocopherol acetate) 100 IU • Riboflavin (B2) 3 mg • Niacin (B3, niacinamide) 40 mg • Zinc (from zinc oxide) 40 mg • Selenium (from sodium selenate) 55 mcg • Copper (from cupric oxide) 2 mg • Manganese 5 mg • L-Glutathione 5 mg • Lutein 2 mg. Other Ingredients: Dibasic Calcium Phosphate, Microcrystalline Cellulose, Calcium Carbonate, Crospovidone, Hydroxypropyl Methylcellulose, Titanium Dioxide, Silicon Dioxide, Magnesium Stearate, Stearic Acid, FD&C Yellow No. 6, Triethyl Citrate, Polysorbate 80, Sodium Lauryl Sulfate.

Ocuvite Lutein **-** Bausch & Lomb
Each capsule contains: Vitamin C (ascorbic acid) 60 mg • Vitamin E (dl-alpha tocopherol acetate) 30 IU • Zinc (from zinc oxide) 15 mg • Copper (from cupric oxide) 2 mg • Lutein 6 mg. Other Ingredients: Lactose Monohydrate, Crospovidone, Magnesium Stearate, Silicon Dioxide.

Ocuvite PreserVision **-** Bausch & Lomb
Two tablets contain: Vitamin A (beta-carotene) 14,320 IU • Vitamin C (ascorbic acid) 226 mg • Vitamin E (dl-alpha tocopheryl acetate) 200 IU • Zinc (zinc oxide) 34.8 mg • Copper (cupric acid) 0.8 mg. Other Ingredients: Lactose Monohydrate, Microcrystalline Cellulose, Crospovidone, Stearic Acid, Magnesium Stearate, Silicon Dioxide, Polysorbate 80, Triethyl Citrate, FD&C Red #40.

Odor-Free Imperial Garlic 6500 **-** Vitamin World
Each tablet contains: Garlic bulb powder (allium sativum) 650 mg standardized to contain a minimum: Allicin yield 6500 mcg, total Thiosulfinates yield 6500 mcg, Alliin yield 14,500 mcg, Gamma-Glutamylcysteines 5200 mcg. Other Ingredients: Dicalcium Phosphate, Cellulose (plant origin), Food Glaze, Calcium Carbonate, Croscarmellose, Vegetable Stearic Acid, Hydroxypropyl Methylcellulose, Ttianium Dioxide Color, Magnesium Silicate, Anise Oil (pimpinella anisum, seed).

Odorless Garlic **-** Jamieson
Each capsule contains: Garlic Bulb Powder - equivalent to 500 mg of fresh garlic.

Odorless Garlic **-** Schiff
Each softgel contains: Freeze Dried 5x Garlic bulb powder (allium sativum) 100 mg • Garlic bulb oil (allium sativum) 1 mg • Hawthorne berry (crataegus spp.) 20 mg • Parsley leaf (petroselinum crispum) 10 mg. Other Ingredients: Capsule (gelatin, glycerin, water), Soybean Oil, Hardened Vegetable Oil Coating (cellulose acetate phithalate, food glaze, beeswax, methyl cellulose, ethyl cellulose, acetylated monoglycerides), Lecithin, Titanium Dioxide.

Odorless Garlic 1000 mg **-** Nature's Bounty
Each softgel contains: Odorless Garlic (allium sativum, from 10 mg garlic oil concentrate, equivalent to 1000 mg of fresh garlic bulb) 1000 mg. Other Ingredients: Soybean Oil, Gelatin, Glycerin, Silica.

Ogoplex Pure Extract **-** Boland Naturals, Inc.
Each tablet contains: Proprietary Blend: Bee Pollen, Flower Pollen, Vitamin A, Vitamin E.

OKG Fuel Capsules OKG (L-Ornithine Alphaketoglutarate) **-** TwinLab
Each capsule contians: OKG 650 mg.

OKG Fuel Powder **-** TwinLab
Each teaspoonful contains: OKG 3.5 grams (3500 mg).

Ola Loa **-** Ola Loa, LLC
Each packet contains: Vitamin C (ascorbic acid) 1000 mg • Vitamin B1 (thiamine) 2 mg • Vitamin B2 (riboflavin) 1 mg • Vitamin B3 (niacinamide) 10 mg • Vitamin B6 (pyridoxine) 10 mg • Folic Acid 600 mcg • Vitamin B12 (hydroxycobalamin) 100 mcg • Pantothenic Acid 10 mg • Biotin 100 mcg • Vitamin D (vitamin D3, cholecalciferol) 200 IU • Vitamin E (d-alpha tocopherol acetate) 30 IU • Vitamin K (vitamin K1, phylloquinone) 20 mcg • Coenzyme Q10 25 mg •

Vitamin A 1000 IU • Lipoic Acid 1 mg • Choline Bitartrate 10 mg • Potassium (bicarbonate) 200 mg • Sodium (bicarbonate) 27 mg • Calcium (carbonate/ascorbate) 29 mg • Magnesium (ascorbate) 25 mg • Zinc (picolinate) 5 mg • Manganese (picolinate) 1.5 mg • Copper (aspartate) 500 mcg • Molybdenum (trioxide) 75 mcg • Selenium (selenite) 50 mcg • Chromium (picolinate) 100 mcg • Potassium Iodide 50 mcg • Boron (citrate) 1 mg • N-Acetyl-Cysteine (NAC) 50 mg • Arginine 100 mg • Lysine 100 mg • Glycine 1000 mg • TMG (Betaine) 1000 mg • Glutamine 100 mg • Bromelain 10 mg • Pineapple Bioflavonoids 100 mg. Other Ingredients: Fructose, Citric Acid, Aspartic Acid, Tartaric Acid, Malic Acid, Natural Fruit Flavors, Stevia.

Ola Loa Orange Energy - Ola Loa, LLC
Each packet contains: Vitamin C 1000 mg • Vitamin B1 2 mg • Vitamin B2 1 mg • Vitamin B3 10 mg • Vitamin B6 10 mg • Folic Acid 600 mcg • Vitamin B12 100 mcg • Pantothenic Acid 10 mg • Biotin 100 mcg • Vitamin D (D3) 200 IU • Vitamin E 30 IU • Vitamin K (K1) 20 mcg • Coenzyme Q10 25 mg • Vitamin A 1000 IU • Lipoic Acid 1 mg • Choline Bitartrate 10 mg • Beta Carotene 3333 IU • Potassium (bicarbonate) 200 mg • Sodium (bicarbonate) 27 mg • Calcium (carbonate, ascorbate) 29 mg • Magnesium (ascorbate) 25 mg • Zinc (picolinate) 5 mg • Manganese (picolinate) 1.5 mg • Copper (aspartate) 500 mcg • Molybdenum (trioxide) 75 mcg • Selenium (selenite) 50 mcg • Chromium (picolinate) 100 mcg • Iodide (potassium iodide) 50 mcg • Boron (citrate) 1 mg • N-Acetyl Cysteine (NAC) 50 mg • Arginine 100 mg • Lysine 100 mg • Glycine 1000 mg • TMG - Betaine 1000 mg • Glutamine 100 mg • Bromelain 10 mg • Pineapple Bioflavonoids 100 mg. Other Ingredients: Fructose, Citric Acid, Aspartic Acid, Tartaric Acid, Malic Acid, Natural Fruit Flavors, Stevia.

Ola Loa Orange Repair - Ola Loa, LLC
Each packet contains: Vitamin A (palmitate) 3000 IU • Vitamin A (as beta carotene) 833 IU • Vitamin C 500 mg • Vitamin D (D3, cholecalciferol) 400 IU • Vitamin K 200 mcg • Calcium (carbonate) 25 mg • Magnesium (oxide) 250 mg • Zinc (citrate) 5 mg • Potassium (bicarbonate) 99 mg • Selenium (l-methionine) 50 mcg • Copper (gluconate) 500 mcg • Manganese (gluconate) 3 mg • Molybdenum (amino acid chelate) 200 mcg • Sodium (sodium bicarbonate) 140 mg • Vanadium (vanadyl sulfate) 1 mg • Boron (boron citrate) 500 mcg • Citrus Bioflavonoids 30 mg • Bromelain (from pineapple) 30 mg • Gotu Kola extract 50 mg • Stevia extract 30 mg • Ginger root extract (10:1) 50 mg • L-Glycine 500 mg • Taurine 250 mg • L-Lysine 100 mg • L-Arginine 100 mg • L-Carnitine 100 mg • Glucosamine Sulfate 500 mg • Betaine TMG 500 mg • Inositol Hexanicotinate 100 mg • Calcium Pyruvate 30 mg. Other Ingredients: Fructose, Citric Acid, Natural Orange Flavor.

Olay Essential Bone Health Formula - Avon
Each tablet contains: Vitamin D 200 IU • Calcium (535 mg from calcium carbonate, 65 mg from dibasic calcium phosphate) 600 mg • Phosphorus 50 mg • Magnesium 40 mg. Other Ingredients: Acacia Gum, Hydroxypropyl Methylcellulose, Croscarmellose Sodium, Titanium Dioxide (artificial color), Polyethylene Glycol, Triethyl Citrate, Polysorbate 80, Sodium Citrate, Corn Starch.

Olay Ester-C Alpha Lipoic Collagen Support - Avon
Each tablet contains: Vitamin C Ester-C (calcium ascorbate) 500 mg • Alpha Lipoic Acid 50 mg. Other Ingredients: Cellulose Gel, Croscarmellose Sodium, Magnesium Stearate, Hydroxypropyl Methylcellulose, Titanium Dioxide (artificial color), Yellow 6 Lake, Polyethylene Glycol, Polysorbate 80.

Olay Super B-Stress Defense - Avon
Each tablet contains: Vitamin C 500 mg • Vitamin E 30 IU • Thiamin (vitamin B1) 10 mg • Riboflavin (vitamin B2) 10 mg • Niacin (vitamin B3) 100 mg • Vitamin B6 5 mg • Folate, Folic Acid, Folacin 400 mcg • Vitamin B12 12 mcg • Biotin 100 mcg • Pantothenic Acid 20 mg. Other Ingredients: Gelatin, Corn Starch, Cellulose Gel, Hydroxypropyl Methylcellulose, Polyethylene Glycol.

Olay Vitamin A Retinol/Beta Carotene - Avon
Each softgel contains: Vitamin A (63% as beta carotene) 8000 IU • Vitamin D 200 IU. Other Ingredients: Soybean Oil, Gelatin, Glycerin, Yellow Beeswax, Corn Oil, Cottonseed Oil, Water.

Olay Vitamins - Beauty Nutrients - Avon
Each packet contains: Vitamin A 5000 IU • Vitamin C 120 mg • Vitamin D 400 IU • Vitamin E 460 IU • Thiamin (vitamin B1) 3 mg • Riboflavin (vitamin B2) 3.4 mg • Niacin (vitamin B3) 20 mg • Vitamin B6 4 mg • Folate, Folic Acid, Folacin 400 mcg • Vitamin B12 25 mcg • Biotin 30 mcg • Pantothenic Acid 10 mg • Calcium 250 mg • Phosphorus 48 mg • Iodine 150 mcg • Magnesium 120 mg • Zinc 22 mg • Selenium 50 mcg • Copper 5 mg • Manganese 2 mg • Chromium 120 mcg • Molybdenum 25 mcg • Chloride 72 mg • Potassium 80 mg • Nickel 5 mcg • Silicon 2 mg • Vanadium 10 mcg • Boron 150 mcg • Alpha Lipoic Acid 50 mg • CoEnzyme Q-10 32 mg • Green Tea Leaf extract (polyphenols 25 mg) 50 mg. Other Ingredients: Soybean Oil, Glycerin, Cellulose Gel, Water, Lactose, Hydroxypropyl Methylcellulose, Acacia, Crospovidone, Kelp, Silicon Dioxide, Polyethylene Glycol, Artificial Colors (Titanium Dioxide, Beta Carotene), Corn Starch, Triethyl Citrate, Blue 2 Lake, Red 40 Lake, Yellow 6 Lake, Polysorbate 80, Modified Food Starch, Sodium Borate, Yellow 5 Lake, Lutein, Blue 1 Lake.

OLAY Vitamins Ultra CoQ10 150 mg - Pharmavite Corp.
Each softgel contains: Vitamin E 100 IU • Coenzyme Q10 150 mg. Other Ingredients: Soybean Oil, Gelatin, Glycerin, Sorbitol, Water, Polysorbate 80, Red 40, Titanium Dioxide, Blue 1.

Olde World Icelandic Cod Liver Oil Lemon Mint Flavor - Garden of Life, Inc.
Each teaspoon (5 mL) contains: Vitamin A 4500 IU • Vitamin D 480 IU • Vitamin E 5 IU • Total Omega-3 Fatty Acids 962 mg: DHA 453 mg, EPA 320 mg, Other Omega-3 189 mg. Other Ingredients: Natural Lemon Essence, Natural Mint Essence.

Olimmune - PhysioLogics
Three capsules contain: Licorice DGL (1% Glycyrrhizin, 7.6 mg) 760 mg • Astragalus (70% Polysaccharides, 140 mg) 200 mg • Ligusticum 200 mg • N-Acetyl-Cysteine (NAC) 135 mg • Olive leaf extract (17% Oleuropein, 17 mg) 100 mg.

Olive Leaf - Jamieson
Each caplet contains: European Concentrate Olive Leaf 1250 mg.

Olive Leaf Extract - Olympian Labs
Each capsule contains: Olive Leaf extract 500 mg.

Olive Leaf Extract - Swanson
Each capsule contains: Olive leaf extract (15% oleuropein) 500 mg.

Olive Leaf Extract with Hawthorn - PhytoPharmica
Two capsules contain: Olive leaf extract (olea europaea, standardized to contain 17%-23% oleuropein) 500 mg • Hawthorn leaf and flower extract (crataegus oxyacantha, standardized to contain 1.8% vitexin-2'-rhamnoside) 300 mg.

Olive Leaf Plus - Health Smart Vitamins
Four capsules contain: Echinacea Blend: Echinacea purpurea root, leaf, Echinacea angustifolia root (4% total phenolic compounds, 10 mg) 1000 mg • Olive leaf, (Olea europaea: 17% oleuropein, 136 mg) 800 mg • Una de Gato inner bark, (Uncaria tomentosa; 2% oxindole alkaloids 1.3 mg) 80 mg.

Olivenol Capsules - CreAgri
Each capsule contains: Proprietary Organic Olive oil extract (containing polyphenols, including 5 mg Hidrox hydroxytyrosol) 300 mg. Other Ingredients: Maltodextrin, Cellulose (plant fiber), 100% Vegetarian Capsule.

Olivenol Tablets - CreAgri
Each tablet contains: Proprietary Olive oil Water Blend (containing polyphenols, including 5 mg Hidrox hydroxytyrosol) 300 mg. Other Ingredients: Calcium Carbonate, Maltodextrin, Microcrystalline

Cellulose, Stearic Acid, Silicon Dioxide, Croscarmellose Sodium, Magnesium Stearate, Dextrin, Dextrose, Lecithin, Sodium Carboxymethylcellulose, Sodium Citrate.

Olympian Energy - Olympian Labs
Two capsules contain: Eleutherococcus Senticosus 200 mg • Gotu Kola (centellia asiatica) 200 mg • Guarana (paullinia cupana) 200 mg • Kola nut (cola acuminata) 200 mg • Korean Ginseng (panax ginseng) 200 mg • Cayenne (capsicum annum) 20 mg • Vitamin B6 (pyridoxine HCl) 10 mg.

Oly-Zymes - Olympian Labs
Each capsule contains: Proprietary Blend: Amylase, Protease, Lipase 200 mg.

Omega 3 Fatty Acids - Trader Joe's
EPA (eicosapentaenoic acid) 300 mg • DHA (docosahexaenoic acid) 200 mg.

Omega 3 Fish Oils - Olympian Labs
Each softgel contains: Marine Lipid concentrate 1000 mg • EPA (eicosapentaenoic acid) 180 mg • DHA (docasahexaenoic acid) 120 mg • Vitamin E (d-alpha tocopherol) 1 mg.

Omega 3-6-9 - The Vitamin Shoppe
Two softgels contain the Omega 3-6-9 essential fatty acids from 100% pure cold-pressed vegetable seed oils of: Borage 500 mg • Flaxseed 150 mg • Safflower 50 mg • Canola 200 mg • Olive 100 mg. Plus 150 mg of Omega-3 components (EPA-DHA) naturally present in Salmon Oil, providing the following: A/Gamma Linolenic Acid (Omega-3) 220 mg • Linoleic Acid (Omega-6) 290 mg • Oleic Acid (Omega-9) 306 mg.

Omega Complete - Body Wise International, Inc.
Each two capsules contain: EPA (eicosapentaenoic acid) 300 mg • DHA (docosahexaenoic acid) 200 mg • Other Omega-3 Fatty Acids 80 mg • GLA (gamma linolenic acid) 36 mg • Other Omega-6 Fatty Acids 74 mg • Omega-9 Fatty Acids 150 mg • Basil Oil (Ocimum basilicum) 10 mg • Thyme Oil (Thymus vulgaris) 10 mg • Turmeric Oil (Curcuma longa) 10 mg • Proprietary Blend 6 mg: Rosemary extract, Ascorbyl Palmitate, Natural Tocopherols.

Omega III Essential Fatty Acids - Nature's Life
Three capsules contain: Eicosapentaenoic Acid (EPA) (Fish Body oils) 540 mg • Docosahexaenoic Acid (DHA) (Fish Body oils) 360 mg • Garlic extract (1000:1)(Allium sativum) 150 mg • Vitamin C (Ascorbate Palmitate) 10 mg • Vitamin E (d-Alpha Tocopherol) 30 IU. In a natural base of certified organic Safflower oil.

Omega Protect - Jamieson
Each capsule contains: Flax Oil 400 mg • Borage Oil 400 mg • Fish Oil 400 mg • Natural Vitamin E 10 IU • Alpha Linolenic Acid 53% 12 mg • Eicosapentaenoic (EPA) 18% 72 mg • Docosahexaenoic (DHA) 12% 48 mg • Linoleic Acid 207 mg • Gamma Linolenic Acid 18% 76 mg • Oleic Acid 173 mg.

Omega Woman - Nordic Naturals
Two softgels contain: Vitamin E (mixed tocopherols) 30 IU • EPA (eicosapentaenoic acid) 36 mg • DHA (docosahexaenoic acid) 24 mg • Evening Primrose Oil 800 mg • GLA (gamma linolenic acid) 82 mg. Other Ingredients: Purified Deep Sea Fish Oil, Soft Gel Capsule, (gelatin, water, glycerin, natural lemon oil), Antioxidant Blend (lecithin, ascorbyl palmitate).

Omega-3 - Natrol
Two softgels contain: Omega-3 Fish Oil 2 g • EPA (eicosapentaenoic acid, 18%) 360 mg • DHA (docosahexaenoic acid, 12%) 240 mg. Other Ingredients: Gelatin, Glycerin, Mixed Tocopherols (natural).

Omega-3 Complex - PhysioLogics
Each softgel contains: Fish Oil 1000 mg: EPA (eicosapentaenoic acid) 180 mg, DHA (docosahexaenoic acid) 120 mg. Other Ingredients: Gelatin, Glycerin.

Omega-3 Complex 1200 MG - PhysioLogics
Each softgel contains: Fish Oil 1200 mg: EPA (eicosapentaenoic acid) 216 mg, DHA (docosahexaenoic acid) 144 mg. Other Ingredients: Gelatin, Glycerin.

Omega-3 Complex HP - PhysioLogics
Each softgel contains: Fish Oil 1000 mg: EPA (eicosapentaenoic acid) 300 mg, DHA (docosahexaenoic acid) 200 mg. Other Ingredients: Gelatin, Glycerin.

Omega-3 Glucosamine - Natrol
Three softgels contain: Glucosamine HCl 1.5 g • Chondroitin Sulfate 100 mg • Fish Oil concentrate 1 g • EPA (eicosapentaenoic acid) 300 mg • DHA (docosapentaenoic acid) 200 mg • Borage Oil 500 mg • GLA (gamma-linolenic acid) 95 mg. Other Ingredients: Soybean Lecithin, Natural Tocopherol, Beeswax, Gelatin, Glycerin, Purified Water, Caramel, Carob.
See Editor's Note No. 15, page 2055.

Omega-H3 Capsules - Vitabiotics
Each capsule contains: Betacarotene 5 mg • Vitamin A 750 mcg • Vitamin D 5 mcg • Vitamin B1 (thiamin) 20 mg • Vitamin B2 (riboflavin) 5 mg • Vitamin B3 (nicotinamide) 25 mg • Calcium Pantothenate 10 mg • Vitamin B6 (pyridoxine HCl) 10 mg • Vitamin B12 (cyanocobalamin) 9 mcg • Biotin 30 mcg • Folic Acid 500 mcg • Vitamin C 60 mg • Vitamin E 20 mg • PABA (para-aminobenzoic acid) 30 mg • Pollen extract 2 mg • Lecithin 40 mg • Wheat Germ Oil 100 mg • Cod Liver Oil 50 mg • Omega-3 Oil 50 mg • Ginseng 4 mg • L-Lysine 40 mg • Methionine 60 mg • Zinc 15 mg • Manganese 2 mg • Inositol 30 mg • Iron 15 mg • Iodine 150 mcg • Copper 2 mg • Magnesium 30 mg • Selenium 100 mcg • Chromium 50 mcg • Molybdenum 50 mcg • Garlic 20 mg • Rutin 10 mg.

OmegaPlex - Advocare International
Three softgels contain: Vitamin E (as D-alpha tocopherol) 15 IU • Eicosapentaenoic Acid (from marine lipids) 900 mg • Docosahexaenoic Acid (from marine lipids) 600 mg. Other Ingredients: Gelatin, Water, Glycerin.

OmegaTru Organic Flaxseed Oil - Swanson
Each tablespoon (1/2 oz) contains: Alpha Linolenic Acid 7 g • Linoleic Acid 2 g • Oleic Acid 2.8 g.

Omega-Zyme (-Zyme) Digestive Enzyme Blend Caplets - Garden of Life, Inc.
Each caplet contains: Proprietary N•zimes Blend 535 mg: Protease blend 74,750 HUT, Bromelain 230,000 FCCPU, Papain 287,500 FCCPU, Lipase 3450 FCCLU, Amylase 23,000 DU, Glucoamylase 30 AGU, Malt Diastase 193 DP, Invertase 64 SU, Lactase 863 ALU, Alpha-Galactosidase 504 GaLU, Cellulase 690 CU, Pectinase 16 endo-PG, Xylanase 575 XU, CereCalase 115 MU • Poten-Zyme Botanical Blend 300 mg: Ginger, Cat's Claw, Yucca juice, Turmeric, Live Probiotic cultures, Barley Grass juice. Other Ingredients: Cellulose, Stearates (vegetable source).

Omega-Zyme (-Zyme) Digestive Enzyme Blend Powder - Garden of Life, Inc.
Each scoop contains: Proprietary N•zimes Blend 500 mg: Protease blend 65,000 HUT, Bromelain 200,000 FCCPU, Papain 250,000 FCCPU, Lipase 3000 FCCLU, Amylase 20,000 DU, Glucoamylase 25.8 AGU, Malt Diastase 168 DP, Invertase 56 SU, Lactase 750 ALU, Alpha-Galactosidase 438 GaLU, Cellulase 1500 CU, Pectinase 14 endo-PG, Xylanase 500 XU, CereCalase 100 MU • Soluble extract of Rice Bran 400 mg.

Omnigest EZ - SunSource - Chattem, Inc.
Each caplet contains: Plant-source Digestive Enzymes 230 mg: Acid Protease 340 APU, Amylase 3400 SKB, Cellulase 5400 C,-ASE, Glucoamylase 22 AG, Lactase 3000 FCC LacU, Lipase 2250 LU, Nautral Protease 11,000 HUT.

O'My O Clitoral Stimulating Gel - O'My Products, Inc.
Water • Vegetable Glycerin • Grapefruit seed extract • Hemp seed oil • Benzyl Nicotinate • Sodium Benzoate • Potassium Sorbate • Menthol • L-Arginine • Aminophylline • Citric Acid.

Oncolyn - Sante International
Each tablet contains: Herbal Extract-Based Blend 750 mg: Gynostemma Pentaphyllum, Crataegus Pinnatifida (hawthorn leaves/ berries), Camellia Sinensis (green tea).

Oncotax - American Metabolic Institute
Unknown.
See Editor's Note No. 19, page 2056.

Oncovite - Mission Pharmacal
Each tablet contains: Vitamin A 9,000 IU • Vitamin C 500 mg • Vitamin D (as Vitamin D3) 400 IU • Vitamin E 100 IU • Thiamine 0.34 mg • Riboflavin 0.5 mg • Niacin 5 mg • Vitamin B6 25 mg • Folate 0.4 mg • Vitamin B12 1.6 mcg • Pantothenic Acid 2.3 mg • Zinc 7.5 mg. Other Ingredients: Microcrystalline Cellulose, Color, Acrylic Resin, Croscarmellose Sodium, Magnesium Silicate, Magnesium Stearate, Ethylcellulose, Silicon Dioxide, Polyethylene Glycol, Food Glaze, Ethyl Vanallin, Cholecalciferol, Cyanocobalamin.

One Daily - The Vitamin Shoppe
Each tablet contains: Vitamin A 10000 IU • Vitamin D (as Vitamin D3) 400 IU • Vitamin C 100 mg • Citrus Bioflavonoids 25 mg • Rutin 5 mg • Hesperidin Complex 5 mg • Vitamin E 150 IU • Vitamin B1 25 mg • Vitamin B2 25 mg • Vitamin B6 25 mg • Vitamin B12 100 mcg • Calcium Pangamate 25 mg • Pantothenic Acid 25 mg • Biotin 50 mcg • Folic Acid 400 mcg • Niacinamide 25 mg • Inositol 25 mg • Choline 25 mg • PABA 25 mg • Calcium 100 mg • Magnesium 50 mg • Potassium 25 mg • Manganese 5 mg • Zinc 15 mg • Iron 18 mg • Selenium 50 mcg • GTF Chromium 50 mcg • Iodine 150 mcg • Copper 2 mg • Molybdenum 100 mcg • Vitamin K 25 mcg • SOD 25 mcg • Octacosanol 100 mcg • L-Carnitine 5 mg • CoQ10 10 mcg • GLA 5 mg • Korean Ginseng 10 mg • Bee Pollen 10 mg • Royal Jelly 5 mg • Betaine HCl 10 mg • Pepsin 10 mg • Bromelain 10 mg • Papain 10 mg • Lecithin 25 mg • L-Glutathione 5 mg • L-Cysteine 5 mg • L-Methionine 5 mg • EPA & DHA 50 mg.

One Daily - Leiner Health Products
Each tablet contains: Folate (Folic Acid) 400 mcg • Niacin (Niacinamide) 20 mg • Pantothenic Acid (d-Calcium Pantothenate) 10 mg • Riboflavin (Vitamin B2) 1.7 mg • Thiamin Mononitrate (Vitamin B1) 1.5 mg • Vitamin A Acetate 5000 IU • Vitamin B12 (Cyanocobalamin - USP Mehtod 2) 6 mcg • Vitamin B6 (Pyridoxine Hydrochloride) 2 mg • Vitamin C (Ascorbic Acid) 60 mg • Vitamin D (Ergocalciferol) 400 IU • Vitamin E (dl-Alpha Tocopheryl Acetate) 30 IU. Other Ingredients: Calcium Carbonate, Gelatin, Maltodextrin, Hydroxypropyl Methylcellulose, Starch, Cellulose, Croscarmellose Sodium, Sodium Starch Glycolate, Silicon Dioxide, Hydroypropyl Cellulose, Red 40 Lake, Polyethylene Glycol 3350, Pharmaceutical Glaze, Magnesium Stearate, Polysorbate 80, Resin, Titanium Dioxide, Povidone, Beta Carotene.

One Daily + Minerals - Leiner Health Products
Each tablet contains: Chromium Yeast 10 mcg • Magnesium Hydroxide100 mg • Selenium Yeast 10 mcg • Calcium 130 mg • Molybdenum Yeast 10 mcg • Manganese Sulfate 2.5 mg • Copper (Cupric Sulfate) 2 mg • Folate (Folic Acid) 400 mcg • Iodine (Potassium Iodide) 150 mcg • Iron (Ferrous Fumarate) 18 mg • Niacin (Niacinamide) 20 mg • Pantothenic Acid (d-Calcium Pantothenate) 10 mg • Riboflavin (Vitamin B2) 1.7 mg • Thiamin Mononitrate (Vitamin B1) 1.5 mg • Vitamin A Acetate 5000 IU • Vitamin B12 (Cyanocobalamin - USP Method 2) 6 mcg • Vitamin B6 (Pyridoxine Hydrochloride) 2 mg • Vitamin C (Ascorbic Acid) 60 mg • Vitamin D (Ergocalciferol) 400 IU • Vitamin E (dl-Alpha Tocopheryl Acetate) 30 IU • Zinc Sulfate 15 mg • Biotin (USP Method 2) 30 mcg • Phosphorus 100 mg • Chloride 34 mg • Potassium Chloride 37.5 mg. Other Ingredients: Dicalcium Phosphate, Gelatin, Pregelatinized Starch, Cellulose, Sodium Starch Glycolate, Hydroxypropyl Methylcellulose, Croscarmellose Sodium, Silicon Dioxide, Tricalcium Phosphate, Red 40 Lake, Polyethylene Glycol 3350, Hydroxypropyl Cellulose, Pharmaceutical Glaze, Magnesium Stearate, Crospovidone, Polysorbate 80, Titanium Dioxide, Beta Carotene, Resin, Povidone.

One Daily 50+ - Leiner Health Products
Each tablet contains: Vitamin B12 (Cyanocobalamin - USP Method 2) 30 mcg • Thiamin Mononitrate (Vitamin B1) 4.5 mg • Vitamin B6 (Pyridoxine Hydrochloride) 6 mg • Magnesium Hydroxide 100 mg • Vitamin K (Phytonadione) 20 mcg • Manganese Sulfate 4 mg • Riboflavin (Vitamin B2) 3.4 mg • Vitamin C (Ascorbic Acid) 120 mg • Vitamin E (dl-Alpha Tocopheryl Acetate) 60 IU • Chromium Chloride 180 mcg • Pantothenic Acid (d-Calcium Pantothenate) 15 mg • Selenium (Sodium Molybdate) 105 mcg • Zinc Sulfate 22.5 mg • Molybdenum (Sodium Molybdate) 93.75 mcg • Calcium Carbonate 120 mg • Copper (Cupric Sulfate) 2 mg • Folate (Folic Acid) 400 mcg • Iodine (Potassium Iodide) 150 mcg • Niacin (Niacinamide Ascorbate) 20 mg • Vitamin A Acetate 5000 IU • Vitamin D (Cholecalciferol) 400 IU • Biotin (USP Method 2) 30 mcg • Chloride 34 mg • Potassium Chloride 37.5 mg. Other Ingredients: Starch, Cellulose, Dicalcium Phosphate, Maltodextrin, Hydroxypropyl Methylcellulose, Croscarmellose Sodium, Gelatin, Titanium Dioxide, Calcium Silicate, Crospovidone, Pharmaceutical Glaze, Magnesium Stearate, Hydroxypropyl Cellulose, Resin, Mannitol, Polyethylene Glycol 3350, Polysorbate 80, Yellow 6 Lake, Blue 2 Lake, Beta Carotene.

One Daily Men's Formula - Leiner Health Products
Each tablet contains: Magnesium Hydroxide 100 mg • Manganese Sulfate 3.5 mg • Riboflavin (Vitamin B2) 2.55 mg • Thiamin Mononitrate (Vitamin B1) 2.25 mg • Vitamin B12 (Cyanocobalamin - USP Mehtod 2) 9 mcg • Vitamin B6 (Pyridoxine Hyrochloride) 3 mg • Vitamin C (Ascorbic Acid) 90 mg • Vitamin E (dl-Alpha Tocopheryl Acetate) 45 IU • Chromium Chloride 150 mcg • Selenium (Sodium Selenate) 87.5 mcg • Copper (Cupric Sulfate) 2 mg • Folate (Folic Acid) 400 mcg • Iodine (Potassium Iodide) 150 mcg • Molybdenum (Sodium Molybdate) 75 mcg • Niacin (Niacinamide Ascorbate) 20 mg • Pantothenic Acid (d-Calcium Pantothenate) 10 mg • Vitamin A 5000 IU • Vitamin D (Cholecalciferol) 400 IU • Zinc Sulfate 15 mg • Chloride 34 mg • Potassium Chloride 37.5 mg. Other Ingredients: Starch, Cellulose, Dicalcium Phosphate, Gelatin, Croscarmellose Sodium, Hydroxypropyl Methylcellulose, Calcium Silicate, Crospovidone, Hydroxypropyl Cellulose, Pharmaceutical Glaze, Polyethylene Glycol 3350, Yellow 6 Lake, Titanium Dioxide, Resin, Beta Carotene, Polysorbate 80.

One Daily Multiple - Nature's Life
Each capsule contains: Beta Carotene (Vitamin A equivalent to 10000 IU) 6 mg • Vitamin D (as Vitamin D3) (Cholecalciferol) 200 IU • Vitamin E (d-Alpha Tocopheryl Succinate) 100 IU • Vitamin B1 (Thiamine Mononitrate) 25 mg • Vitamin B2 (Riboflavin & Riboflavin 5'-Phosphate) 25 mg • Vitamin B6 Pyridoxine HCl & Pyridoxine 5'-Phosphate) 25 mg • Niacinamide 50 mg • Vitamin B12 (Cyancobalamin) 100 mcg • Folic Acid 400 mcg • Pantothenic Acid (d-Calcium Pantothenate) 50 mg • Biotin (d-Biotin) 300 mcg • Choline (Bitartrate) 25 mg • Inositol 25 mg • PABA (Para Aminobenzoic Acid) 25 mg • Vitamin C 100 mg • Boron (Citrate) 50 mcg • Calcium (Carbonate, Citrate/ Malate) 50 mg • Chromium (Picolinate) 100 mcg • Copper (Gluconate, Citrate) 1 mg • Magnesium (Oxide,Citrate) 10 mg • Manganese (Gluconate) 5 mg • Molybdenum (Sodium Molybdate) 150 mcg • Potassium (Chloride) 5 mg • Selenium (Selenomethionine) 100 mcg • Silicon (Dioxide) 10 mg • Vanadium(Vandyl Sulfate) 25 mcg • Zinc (Picolinate) 15 mg.

One Daily with Calcium, Iron, & Zinc - Leiner Health Products
Each tablet contains: Calcium Carbonate 45 mg • Iron (Ferrous Fumarate) 27 mg • Folate (Folic Acid) 400 mcg • Niacin (Niacinamide) 20 mg • Pantothenic Acid (d-Calcium Pantothenate) 10 mg • Riboflavin (Vitamin B2) 1.7 mg • Thiamin Mononitrate (Vitamin

B1) 1.5 mg • Vitamin A Acetate 5000 IU • Vitamin B12 (Cyanocobalamin - USP Method 2) 6 mcg • Vitamin B6 (Pyridoxine Hydrochloride) 2 mg • Vitamin C (Ascorbic Acid) 60 mg • Vitamin D (Cholecalciferol) 400 IU • Vitamin E (dl-Alpha Tocopheryl Acetate) 30 IU • Zinc Oxide 15 mg. Other Ingredients: Maltodextrin, Gelatin, Hydroxypropyl Methylcellulose, Croscarmellose Silicon Dioxide, Propylene Glycol, Titanium Dioxide, Hydroxypropyl Cellulose, Polyethylene Glycol 3350, Pharmaceutical Glaze, Starch, Magnesium Stearate, Yellow 5 Lake, Yellow 6 Lake, Polysorbate 80, Beta Carotene, Povidone, Resin.

One Daily without Iron **-** The Vitamin Shoppe
Each tablet contains: Vitamin A 10000 IU • Vitamin D (as Vitamin D3) 400 IU • Vitamin C 100 mg • Citrus Bioflavonoids 25 mg • Rutin 5 mg • Hesperidin Complex 5 mg • Vitamin E 150 IU • Vitamin B1 25 mg • Vitamin B2 25 mg • Vitamin B6 25 mg • Vitamin B12 100 mcg • Calcium Pangamate 25 mg • Pantothenic Acid 25 mg • Biotin 50 mcg • Folic Acid 400 mcg • Niacinamide 25 mg • Inositol 25 mg • Choline 25 mg • PABA 25 mg • Calcium 100 mg • Magnesium 50 mg • Potassium 25 mg • Manganese 5 mg • Zinc 15 mg • Selenium 50 mcg • GTF Chromium 50 mcg • Iodine 150 mcg • Copper 2 mg • Molybdenum 100 mcg • Vitamin D 25 mcg • SOD 25 mcg • Octacosanol 100 mcg • L-Carnitine 5 mg • CoQ10 10 mcg • GLA 5 mg • Korean Ginseng 10 mg • Bee Pollen 10 mg • Royal Jelly 5 mg • Betaine HCl 10 mg • Pepsin 10 mg • Bromelain 10 mg • Papain 10 mg • Lecithin 25 mg • L-Glutathione 5 mg • L-Cysteine 5 mg • L-Methionine 5 mg • EPA & DHA 50 mg.

One Step **-** Progressive Labs
Each level scoop (approx 31 g) contains: Vitamin A 5000 IU • Ester C Vitamin C 177 mg • Vitamin D 200 IU • Vitamin E Succinate 70 IU • Vitamin K 40 mcg • Thiamin (vitamin B1) 3 mg • Riboflavin (vitamin B2) 3 mg • Niacinamide (vitamin B3) 13 mg • Vitamin B6 (pyridoxine HCl) 30 mg • Folate (folic acid) 446 mcg • Vitamin B12 250 mcg • Biotin 150 mcg • Pantothenic Acid 23 mg • Colloidal Calcium 326 mg • Iron 3 mg • Phosphorus 266 mg • Iodine 38 mcg • Colloidal Magnesium 255 mg • Zinc (as ascorbate) 8 mg • Selenium 40 mcg • Copper (as amino acid chelate) 2 mg • Manganese (as ascorbate) 6 mg • Chromium (as nicotinate) 100 mcg • Molybdenum 13 mg • Chloride 175 mg. Other Ingredients: Arcon VF Hypoallergenic, Predigested Soy Protein concentrate, Rice bran, Lecithin, Glucosamine HCl, Nopal (detoxifier and sugar regulator), MSM (methyl sulfonyl methane), Beta 1,3 Glucans, Inulin, Gamma Oryzanol, L-Glutamine, L-Ornithine, L-Taurine, CitriMax, Globulin Protein, Ascorbic Acid, Trimethylglycine, Citrus Bioflavonoid 5X complex, Aloe Isolate, Pantothenic Acid, Inositol, Creatine Pyruvate, Siberian Ginseng extract, Betatene (lycopene and mixed carotenoids), Alpha Lipoic Acid, Borage Oil, NovaSoy Soy Isoflavones, Gugulipid Extract, Leci-PS Phosphatidylserine, Beta Carotene, L-Glutathione, Quercetin, Seleno-L-Methionine, Atlantic Sea Kelp, Lutein, Pyridoxal-5-Phosphate, Ginkgo Biloba leaf extract, Grape seed extract, Grape skin extract, Bioperine Black Pepper extract, Mixed Tocotrienols, Coenzyme Q10, Pycnogenol, Boron, Natural Vanilla and other Natural Flavors, Stevia.

One-A-Day 50 Plus Formula **-** Bayer
Each tablet contains: Vitamin A 5000 IU • Vitamin C 120 mg • Vitamin D 400 IU • Vitamin E 60 IU • Vitamin K 20 mcg • Thiamin (B1) 4.5 mg • Riboflavin (B2) 3.4 mg • Niacin 20 mg • Vitamin B6 6 mg • Folic Acid 400 mcg • Vitamin B12 30 mcg • Biotin 30 mcg • Pantothenic Acid 15 mg • Calcium (elemental) 120 mg • Iodine 150 mcg • Magnesium 100 mg • Zinc 22.5 mg • Selenium 105 mcg • Copper 2 mg • Manganese 4 mg • Chromium 180 mcg • Molybdenum 93.75 mcg • Chloride 34 mg • Potassium 37.5 mg.

One-A-Day Active Formula **-** Bayer
Each tablet contains: Vitamin A 5000 IU • Vitamin C 120 mg • Vitamin D 400 IU • Vitamin E 60 IU • Vitamin K 25 mcg • Thiamin (vitamin B1) 4.5 mg • Riboflavin (vitamin B2) 5.1 mg • Niacin 40 mg • Vitamin B6 6 mg • Folic Acid 400 mcg • Vitamin B12 18 mcg • Biotin 40 mcg • Pantothenic Acid 10 mg • Calcium (elemental) 110 mg • Iron 9 mg • Phosphorus 48 mg • Iodine 150 mcg • Magnesium 40 mg • Zinc 15 mg • Selenium 45 mcg • Copper 2 mg • Manganese 2 mg • Chromium 100 mcg • Molybdenum 25 mcg • Chloride 180 mg • Potassium 200 mg • Nickel 5 mcg • Tin 10 mcg • Silicon 6 mg • Vanadium 10 mcg • Boron 150 mcg • American Ginseng standardized extract (Panax quinquefolius, root) 55 mg.

One-A-Day Bedtime & Rest **-** Bayer
Each two tablets contain: Calcium 450 mg • Magnesium 80 mg • Lecithin 20 mg • Kava Kava Standardized extract (Piper methysticum) root 100 mg • Valerian Standardized extract (Valeriana officinalis) root 200 mg • Rosemary Standardized extract (Rosmannus officinalis) leaf 10 mg.
See Editor's Note No. 21, page 2056.

One-A-Day Bone Strength **-** Bayer
Each tablet contains: Vitamin D 100 IU • Calcium (precipitated) 500 mg • Soy Standardized extract (Glycine max or spp.) bean 28 mg.
See Editor's Note No. 21, page 2056.

One-A-Day Cholesterol Health **-** Bayer
Each two tablets contain: Vitamin E 200 IU • Lecithin 100 mg • Garlic (Allium sativum) freeze dried/bulb 30 mg • Soy Standardized extract (Glycine max or spp.) bean 140 mg.
See Editor's Note No. 21, page 2056.

One-A-Day Cold Season **-** Bayer
Each tablet contains: Vitamin C 500 mg • Zinc 7.5 mg • Echinacea Standardized extract (Echinacea purpurea) whole plant/root 50 mg.
See Editor's Note No. 21, page 2056.

One-A-Day Energy Formula **-** Bayer
Each tablet contains: Thiamin (B1) 2.25 mg • Niacin 20 mg • Vitamin B6 3 mg • Folic Acid 200 mcg • Pantothenic Acid 10 mg • Chromium (as Picolinate) 100 mcg • Ginseng Standardized extract (Panax ginseng) root 200 mg.

One-A-Day Maximum Formula **-** Bayer
Each tablet contains: Vitamin A Acetate 5000 IU • Vitamin C (Ascorbic Acid) 60 mg • Vitamin D 400 IU • Vitamin E Acetate 30 IU • Vitamin K (Phytonadione) 25 mcg • Thiamin Mononitrate 1.5 mg • Riboflavin (Vitamin B2) 1.7 mg • Niacin (Vitamin B3) 20 mg • Vitamin B6 (Pyridoxine Hydrochloride) 2 mg • Folate (Folic Acid, Folacin) 400 mcg • Vitamin B12 6 mcg • Biotin 30 mcg • Pantothenic Acid (Calcium Pantothenate) 10 mg • Calcium Carbonate 162 mg • Iron (Ferrous Fumarate) 18 mg • Phosphorus 109 mg • Iodine (Potassium Iodide) 150 mcg • Magnesium Hydroxide 100 mg • Zinc Sulfate15 mg • Selenium (Sodium Selenate) 20 mcg • Copper (Cupric Sulfate) 2 mg • Manganese 3.5 mg • Chromium Chloride 65 mcg • Molybdenum (Sodium Molybdate) 160 mcg • Chloride 72 mg • Potassium Chloride 80 mg • Nickel (Nickelous Sulfate) 5 mcg • Tin (Stannous Chloride)10 mcg • Silicon (Sodium Metasilicate) 2 mg • Vanadium (Sodium Metavanadate) 10 mcg • Boron (Disodium Borate) 150 mcg. Other Ingredients: Cellulose, Modified Cellulose Gum, Gelatin, Citric Acid, Hydroxypropyl Methylcellulose, Magnesium Stearate, Artificial Color, Silicon Dioxide, Disodium Borate, Beta Carotene.

One-A-Day Memory & Concentration **-** Bayer
Each tablet contains: Vitamin B6 1 mg • Vitamin B12 3 mcg • Choline 60 mg • Ginkgo Standardized extract (Ginkgo biloba) leaf 60 mg.

One-A-Day Menopause Health **-** Bayer
Each tablet contains: Vitamin E 15 IU • Calcium (precipitated) 250 mg • Lecithin 15 mg • Black Cohosh Standardized extract (Cimicifuga racemosa) root 10 mg • Soy Standardized extract (Glycine max or spp.) bean 42 mg.
See Editor's Note No. 21, page 2056.

One-A-Day Men's Health Formula **-** Bayer
Each tablet contains: Vitamin A (vitamin A acetate, 14% as beta carotene) 3500 IU • Vitamin C (ascorbic acid, ascorbyl palmitate) 90 mg • Vitamin D (ergocalciferol) 400 IU • Vitamin E (DL-alpha

tocopherol acetate) 45 IU • Vitamin K (phytonadione) 20 mcg • Thiamin (B1, thiamine mononitrate) 1.2 mg • Riboflavin (B2) 1.7 mg • Niacin (B3, niacinamide) 16 mg • Vitamin B6 (pyridoxine hydrochloride) 3 mg • Folate, Folic Acid, Folacin 400 mcg • Vitamin B12 (cyanocobalamin) 18 mcg • Biotin 30 mcg • Pantothenic Acid (D-calcium pantothenate) 5 mg • Calcium (elemental, calcium carbonate) 210 mg • Magnesium (magnesium oxide) 120 mg • Zinc (zinc oxide) 15 mg • Selenium (sodium selenate) 105 mcg • Copper (cupric oxide) 2 mg • Manganese (manganese sulfate) 2 mg • Chromium (chromium chloride) 120 mcg • Potassium (potassium chloride) 100 mg • Lycopene (lycopersicon esculentum fruit) 0.6 mg. Other Ingredients: Cellulose, Gelatin, Croscarmellose Sodium, Acacia, Dicalcium Phosphate, Stearic Acid, Silicon Dioxide, Dextrin, Magnesium Stearate, Starch, Calcium Silicate, Sucrose, Mannitol, Hydroxypropyl Methylcellulose, Resin, Dextrose, Lecithin, Sodium Carboxymethylcellulose, Sodium Ascorbate, Sodium Citrate.

***One-A-Day Prostate Health* - Bayer**
Two softgels contain: Zinc Gluconate 15 mg • Pumpkin Seed Oil Standardized extract 80 mg • Saw Palmetto Standardized extract (Serenoa repens) berry 320 mg. Other Ingredients: Gelatin, Glycerin, Vegetable Oil, Beeswax, Lecithin, Titanium Dioxide, FD&C Red #40 (Tartrazine), FD&C Yellow #6, FD&C Blue #1, FD&C Yellow #5 (Tartrazine).

***One-A-Day Tension & Mood* - Bayer**
Each tablet contains: Vitamin C 60 mg • Thiamin (B1) 1.125 mg • Niacin 10 mg • Folic Acid 100 mcg • Pantothenic Acid 5 mg • Lecithin 15 mg • Kava Kava Standardized extract (Piper methysticum) rhizome/root 100 mg • St. John's Wort Standardized extract (Hypericum perforatum) leaves/flowers 225 mg.
See Editor's Note No. 21, page 2056.

***One-A-Day Women's Formula* - Bayer**
Each tablet contains: Vitamin A 2500 IU • Vitamin C 60 mg • Vitamin D 400 IU • Vitamin E 30 IU • Thiamin (Vitamin B1) 1.5 mg • Riboflavin (Vitamin B2) 1.7 mg • Niacin 10 mg • Vitamin B6 2 mg • Folic Acid 400 mcg • Vitamin B12 6 mcg • Pantothenic Acid 5 mg • Calcium (elemental) 450 mg • Iron 18 mg • Magnesium 50 mg • Zinc 15 mg.

***OneSource* - Health Smart Vitamins**
Each caplet contains: Vitamin D (as cholecalciferol) 400 IU • Vitamin A (as 60% retinyl acetate, 40% beta-carotene) 5,000 IU • Vitamin C (as ascorbic acid) 60 mg • Vitamin E (as dl-alpha-tocopheryl acetate) 30 IU • Vitamin K (phytonadione) 25 mcg • Thiamin (as thiamin mononitrate) 1.5 mg • Riboflavin 1.7 mg • Niacin (as niacinamide) 20 mg • Vitamin B6 (as pyridoxine HCl) 2 mg • Folate (as folic acid) 400 mcg • Vitamin B12 (as cyanocobalamin) 6 mcg • Biotin 30 mcg • Pantothenic Acid (as D-calcium pantothenate) 10 mg • Calcium (dicalcium phosphate) 162 mg • Iron (as ferrous fumarate) 18 mg • Phosphorus (as dicalcium phosphate) 125 mg • Iodine (as potassium iodide) 150 mcg • Magnesium (as 90% magnesium oxide, 10% magnesium amino acid chelate) 100 mg • Zinc (as zinc amino acid chelate) 15 mg • Selenium (as selenomethionine) 20 mcg • Copper (as copper sulfate) 2 mg • Manganese (as maganese sulfate) 2.5 mg • Chromium (as chromium picolinate) 25 mcg • Molybdenum (as sodium molybdenate) 25 mcg • Chloride (as potassium chloride) 36 mg • Potassium (as potassium chloride) 40 mg • Silica (as silica dioxide) 2 mg • Boron (as sodium borate) 150 mcg • Tin (as stannous chloride) 10 mcg • Vanadium (as vanadium amino acid chelate) 10 mcg • Nickel (as nickel sulfate) 5 mcg.

***OPCs+95 - 100 mg* - Jarrow Formulas**
Each softgel contains: Grape Seed extract (100:1, 95% polyphonols) 100 mg. Inactive Ingredients: Rice Powder, Magnesium Stearate, Gelatin.

***OPCs+95 - 50 mg* - Jarrow Formulas**
Each softgel contains: Grape Seed extract (100:1, 95% polyphonols) 50 mg. Inactive Ingredients: Rice Powder, Magnesium Stearate, Gelatin.

***Ophthacare* - The Himalaya Drug Company (Himalaya Heal**
Yawani (carum copticum syn. trachyspermum ammi) • Vibhitaki (terminalia belerica syn. t.bellirica) • Amalaki (emblica officinalis) • Haridra (curcuma longa) • Vishu Priya (ocimum sanctum syn. o.tenuiflorum) • Satapatri (rosa damascena syn. r.centifolia) • Karpoora (cinnamomum camphora) • Madhu (mel despumatum syn. mel despumatum, purified) • Phenyl Mercuric Nitrate (as preservative).

***Ophthaplus* - Atrium Inc.**
Each tablet contains: Raw Eye concentrate 120 mg • Raw Brain concentrate 20 mg • Eyebright 150 mg • Rutin 125 mg • Hesperidin Complex 20 mg.
See Editor's Note No. 31, page 2056.

***OptaFlex brand* - Cargill Health & Food Technologies**
Chondroitin.
See Editor's Note No. 44, page 2058.

***Optein* - Solgar**
Each level scoop (35 grams) contains: Vitamin A (3600 IU palmitate 18%, 1400 IU as natural beta carotene from Dunaliella salina) 5000 IU • Vitamin C (as L-ascorbic-acid) 45 mg • Vitamin D (as cholecalciferol) 300 IU • Vitamin E (as D-alpha tocopheryl acetate) 23 IU • Thiamin (as thiamin mononitrate) 1.1 mg • Riboflavin 1.3 mg • Niacin (as niacinamide) 15 mg • Vitamin B6 (as pyridoxine hydrochloride) 1.5 mg • Folic Acid 300 mcg • Vitamin B12 (as cyanocobalamin) 5 mcg • Biotin (as D-biotin) 200 mcg • Pantothenic Acid (as D-calcium pantothenate) 7.5 mg • Calcium (as calcium carbonate, calcium from proteinate) 200 mg • Iron (as reduced iron, iron from proteinate) 9 mg • Iodine (as potassium iodide, brown seaweed extract) 115 mcg • Magnesium (as magnesium oxide, magnesium from proteinate) 100 mg • Zinc (as zinc oxide) 11 mg • Selenium (selenium from proteinate) 14 mcg • Copper (as copper gluconate) 1.5 mg • Manganese (as manganese from proteinate) 0.4 mg • Chromium (as chromium polynicotinate) 24 mcg • Molybdenum (molybdenum from proteinate) 15 mcg • Sodium 120 mg • Potassium (from malted oat cereal solids) 70 mg • Lecithin (from lecithin oil) 500 mg • Dried Red Beet powder 50 mg • Dried Broccoli powder (Brassica aleracea) aerial 50 mg • Dried Carrot powder (Daucus carota) root 40 mg • Spirulina powder 50 mg • Alfalfa Sprouts powder (Medicago sativa) aerial 50 mg • Kamut Grass powder (triticum durham egyptum) aerial 50 mg • Wheat Grass powder (Tritizum vulgare) aerial 50 mg • Barley Grass powder (Hordeum vulgare) aerial 50 mg • Reishi Mushroom extract (Ganoderma lucidum) 20 mg • Maitake Mushroom extract (Gifola frondosa) 20 mg • Shiitake Mushroom powder (Lentinus edodes) 20 mg • Brown Seaweed Extract 30 mg • Isoflavones from Soy concentrate 20 mg • Octacosanol (from wheat germ oil) 250 mcg • Lactoferrins 10 mg • Glutamine Peptides 100 mg • Astragalus extract (Astragalus membranaceus) root 20 mg • Schisandra extract (Schizandra chinensis) fruit 20 mg • American Ginseng extract (Panax quinquefolium) root 20 mg • Siberian Ginseng extract (Acanthopanax seticosus) root 20 mg • Korean Ginseng extract (Panax ginseng) root 20 mg • Rhodiola extract (Rhodiola rosea) root 20 mg • Elderberry extract (Sambucus nigra, canadensis) berry 20 mg • Fruit Polyphenols (from apple, apricot, nectarine, cherry, prune, pomegranate) 20 mg • Beta Glucan (from oat fiber) 25 mg • Dried Colostrum powder 50 mg • Cytidine Monophosphate 5 mg • Adenosine Monophosphate 5 mg • Uridine Monophosphate 5 mg • Guanosine Monophosphate 5 mg • Phosphatidylcholine (from lecithin oil) 100 mg • Phosphatidylinositol (from lecithin oil) 20 mg. Other Ingredients: Malted Oat Cereal Solids, Crystalline Fructose, Soy Protein Isolate, Whey Protein Isolate, Whey Protein Concentrate, Dried Malt, Oat Fiber, Natural Chocolate Flavor, Dutch Cocoa, Soy Concentrate, Apple Fiber, Gum Arabic, Apple Pectin, Dried Cream, Black Currant Fiber, Lemon Fiber, Rice Fiber Concentrate, Fruit Concentrate.

***Opti Fuel (The Ultimate Metabolic Optimizer)* - TwinLab**
Each serving contains: Pharmaceutical Grade Pep-Tide Bonded & Free Amino Acids [derived from the natural Pancreatic digests of

Whey Protein (Lactalbumin) & Egg White Protein (Albumin)] 15 g • Branched Chain Amino Acids (L-Leucine, L-Isoleucine & L-Valine) • Carbohydrates & Medium Chain Triglycerides (MCTs) • High Potency Metabolic Activator Vitamins & Minerals • Electro-Lytes • Antioxidants • Stress B Complex • Lipotropic Factors • Methyl Donors • TMG (Trimethylglycine) • Siberian Ginseng • Octacosanol • Gamma-Oryzanol & Synergistic Metabolic Optimizers (such as Inosine) • L-Carnitine • CoQ10 • Lipoic Acid • Pantetheine • Pyridoxine-Alpha-Ketoglutarate • Soluble Potassium Phosphate & Mineral Succinates • Aspartates • Citrates • Fumarates • Malates • Alpha-Ketoglutarates.

***Opti Fuel 2* - TwinLab**
Each serving contains: Carbohydrates (derived primarily from Glucose Polymers & Glucose with small amounts of 100% Pure Crystalline Fructose) 100 g • Predigested Whey Protein • Extra Branched Chain Amino Acids (L-Leucine, L-Isoleucine, L-Valine) • Vitamin C • Vitamin E • Beta-Carotene • Other Important Antioxidant Nutrients such as: Selenium, Coenzyme Q10 & Alpha Lipoic Acid, High Potency B Complex Vitamins, Calcium, Magnesium, Potassium, Zinc & Chromium Picolinate • Carni Fuel (L-Carnitine Magnesium Citrate). All predigested for easier digestion & assimilation.

***Optiflora Prebiotic Complex* - Shaklee**
Each teaspoon (4 g) contains: Dietary fiber 3 g • Optiflora Proprietary Prebiotic Blend 3 g: Inulin, Fructooligosaccharides (FOS) • Mixed tocopherols 32 mg. Other Ingredients: Fructose, Maltodextrin, Natural Flavors.

***Optiflora Probiotic Complex* - Shaklee**
Each capsule contains: Bifidobacterium longum 250 million • Lactobacillus acidophilus 250 million. Other Ingredients: Palm Oil, Gelatin, Glycerin, Soy Lecithin, Pectin.

***Opti-Lean* - Optimum Nutrition**
Citrimax™ 500 mg • High Quality Protien 20 g • Carbohydrates 20 g.

***Optimal Performance* - Rexall - Sundown**
Each tablet contains: Zinc (as zinc gluconate) 7.5 mg • Spirulina (spirulina pacifica) 125 mg • Bee Pollen 100 mg • Royal Jelly 100 mg • Siberian Ginseng root 75 mg • Octacosanol 0.5 mg. Other Ingredients: Corn Syrup solids, Croscarmellose Sodium, Alfalfa leaf, Hydrogenated Vegetable Oil, Silica, Magnesium Stearate.

***Opti-Men* - Optimum Nutrition**
Two tablets contain: Vitamin A (as CaroCare natural mixed carotenoids) 7500 IU • Vitamin C (as ascorbic acid) 300 mg • Vitamin D (as cholecalciferol) 200 IU • Vitamin E (as D-alpha tocopheryl succinate) 200 IU • Vitamin K (as phytonadione) 75 mcg • Thiamin (as thiamin hydrochloride) 30 mg • Riboflavin 30 mg • Niacin (as niacinamide) 30 mg • Vitamin B6 (as pyridoxine hydrochloride) 30 mg • Folic Acid 400 mcg • Vitamin B12 (as cyanocobalamin) 100 mcg • Biotin 250 mcg • Pantothenic Acid (as D-calcium pantothenate) 30 mg • Calcium (as calcium carbonate, citrate) 200 mg • Iodine (as kelp) 150 mcg • Magnesium (as magnesium oxide, aspartate) 100 mg • Zinc (as zinc citrate) 30 mg • Selenium (as selenomethionine) 70 mcg • Copper (as copper gluconate) 2 mg • Manganese (as manganese gluconate) 5 mg • Chromium (as chromium GTF) 120 mcg • Molybdenum (as molybdenum AA chelate) 80 mcg • Raw Oyster concentrate 50 mg • Saw Palmetto powdered berries 100 mg • Pygeum Africanum powdered bark 70 mg • Damiana powdered leaf 100 mg• Nettles powdered leaf 30 mg • Lycopene (as LYC-O-MATO natural tomato lycopene) 250 mcg • Alpha-Carotene 140 mcg • Cryptoxanthin 34 mcg • Zeaxanthin 28 mcg • Lutein 250 mcg • Alpha Lipoic Acid 25 mg • Citrus Bioflavonoids fruit 70 mg • Grape Seed extract (vitis vinifera, standardized to 95% polyphenols) 25 mg • Deodorized Garlic powdered bulb 50 mg • Ginkgo Biloba powdered leaf 70 mg • Korean Ginseng powdered root 100 mg • PABA (para-aminobenzoic acid) 10 mg • Choline (as choline bitartrate) 10 mg • Inositol 10 mg. Other Ingredients: Stearic Acid, Hydroxy Propyl Methyl Cellulose, Calcium Phosphate, Croscarmellose Sodium (disintegrant), Gelatin, Magnesium Stearate, Gum Acacia, Silica.

***OptimEyes* - Body Wise International, Inc.**
Three tablets contain: Beta Carotene (Dunaliella salina algae) 9 mg (Equivalent to Vitamin A 15000 IU) • Vitamin C (as Ascorbic Acid) 1000 mg • Vitamin E (as D-Alpha Tocopheryl Succinate and Mixed Tocopherols-Alpha, Beta, Gamma and Delta) 100 IU • Zinc (Krebs Cycle Chelate) 20 mg • Selenium (as L-Selenomethionine) 250 mcg • Copper (Krebs Cycle Chelate) 2 mg • Taurine 500 mg • N-Acetyl-L-Cysteine 200 mg • Bilberry fruit extract 100:1 (25% Anthocyanidins) 80 mg • Ginkgo Biloba leaf extract 50:1 (24% Flavonglycosides) 60 mg • Alpha Lipoic Acid 25 mg • Lutein 6 mg.

***Optimized Lecithin 500* - GNC**
Each capsule contains: Vitamin E (as d-alpha tocopherol) 5 IU • Lecithin (as liquid soy lecithin) 500 mg. Other Ingredients: Gelatin, Glycerin, Rosemary oil (Rosmarinus offcinalis).

***OptiMSM brand* - Cardinal Nutrition**
Methysulfonylmethane.
See Editor's Note No. 44, page 2058.

***Optimum Nutrition* - Optimum Nutrition**
Hawthorn Berry • Garlic Extract.

***Optimum Omega* - Pharmanex**
Each capsule contains: Vitamin E (as d-Alpha Tocopheryl Acetate) 5 IU • Marine Lipid Concentrate 1000 mg (Omega 3 Fatty Acids: EPA 180 mg, DHA 120 mg, Other Omega 3 Fatty Acids 50 mg) • Deodorized Garlic Oil 1 mg. Other Ingredients: Gelatin, Glycerin, Purified Water.

***Optimune* - Rx Vitamins**
Pharmaceutical Grade Arabinogalactan 250 mg • Phosphoric Nucleotides 4000 mcg.

***Opti-Pro Meal* - Optimum Nutrition**
Two heaping scoops (73 g) contain: Proprietary Nitroplex Protein Blend: Whey Protein Concentrate, Calcium Caseinate, Egg Albumen, Whey Protein Isolate • Proprietary Polysaccharide Matrix: Maltodextirn, Cellulose Gum, Xanthan Gum, Corn Syrup Solids, Amylopectin (waxy corn starch), High Amylose Corn Starch • Cocoa • Vitaplus Blend: Calcium Citrate, DiPotassium Phosphate, Magnesium Oxide, DiCalcium Phosphate, Choline Bitartrate, Potassium Chloride, Ascorbic Acid, DL-Alpha Tocopheryl Acetate, Ferrous Fumarate, Niacinamide, Vitamin A Palmitate, Zinc Oxide, Potassium Iodide, D-Calcium Pantothenate, Phytonadione, Copper Sulfate Pentahydrate, Manganese Sulfate, Cholecalciferol, Pyridoxine Hydrochloride, Molybdenum Glycinate, Riboflavin, Thiamin Mononitrate, Selenium Glycinate, Chromium Picolinate, Folic Acid, Biotin, Cyanocobalamin • Natural and Artificial Flavor • Medium Chain Triglycerides • Canola oil • Aspartame • Soy Lecithin • Acesulfame Potassium.

***Opti-Pro Meal Bars* - Optimum Nutrition**
Each bar (75 g) contains: Corn Syrup • Protein Blend: Soy Protein Isolate, Whey Protein Isolate, Calcium Caseinate • Milk Chocolate (sugar, palm kernal oil, non-fat dry milk solids, cocoa powder, salt) • Cocoa • Maltodextrin • Raisins • Fructose • Glycerol • Lecithin • Inulin • Artificial Flavor • Vitamin/Mineral Blend: Magnesium Oxide, Ascorbic Acid, Chromium GTF Polynicotinate, Niacinamide, Biotin, D-Alpha Tocopheryl Succinate, Vitamin A Palmitate, Copper Gluconate, Zinc Oxide, D-Calcium Pantothenate, Cholecalciferol, Folic Acid, Pyridoxine Hydrochloride, Riboflavin, Thiamin Mononitrate, Cyanocobalamin • Carbogen • Aminogen.

***OptiSight* - Advocare International**
Two capsules contain: Zinc (as monomethionine OptiZinc) 3 mg • Vitamin C (as potassium ascorbate) 60 mg • Lutein (as esters from tagetes sp.) 20 mg • Zeaxanthin (as free-form and esters from tagetes sp.) 2 mg • Astaxanthin (from Haematococcus sp.) 10 mg • Bilberry

extract (fruit - vaccinium myrtillus) 150 mg • Alpha-Lipoic Acid 50 mg • N-Acetyl Cysteine 75 mg • Taurine 200 mg • Mixed Tocotrienols (from seed - glycine max) 30 mg •Curcumin extract (root - curcuma longa) 50 mg • L-Glutathione 5 mg • Beta-Carotene (from D. salina mixed carotenoids) 1.5 mg. Other Ingredients: Silicon Dioxide, Magnesium Stearate, Gelatin.

Opti-Soy **-** Optimum Nutrition
Each scoop (32 g) contains: Non-GMO Soy Protein Isolate • Vitamin/ Mineral Blend: Calcium Citrate, Magnesium Oxide, Ascorbic Acid, D-Alpha Tocopheryl Succinate (natural vitamin E), Niacinamide, Maltodextrin, D-Calcium Pantothenate, Molybdenum Amino Acid Chelate, Zinc Oxide, Selenomethionine, Vitamin A Palmitate, Riboflavin, Thiamin Mononitrate, Manganese Sulfate, Pyridoxine Hydrochloride (vitamin B6), Folic Acid, Chromium Picolinate, Potassium Iodide, Cyanocobalamin • Cocoa • Natural and Artificial Flavor • Salt • Sucralose.

OptiVision **-** PhysioLogics
Two capsules contain: Vitamin A (Beta-Carotene) 10000 IU • Vitamin A (Palmitate) 2500 IU • Taurine 200 mg • Bilberry (GPH: 36% anthocyanosides) 100 mg • Vitamin E (D-Alpha Tocopherol) 100 IU • N-Acetylcysteine 100 mg • Quercetin (GPH: 98% Bioflavonoids) 50 mg • Glutathione 25 mg • Vitamin B2 (Riboflavin) 10 mg • Vitamin B6 (Pyridoxine HCl) 10 mg • Zinc (Glycinate) 15 mg • Copper (Glycinate) 2 mg • Chromium (Niacin/Glycine Chelate) 100 mcg • Selenium (Selenomethionine) 50 mcg.

OptiVision Forte **-** Similasan
Four caplets contain: Vitamin A (45% (1,650 IU) as Beta Carotene) 3,650 IU • Vitamin C 150 mg • Vitamin D (cholecalciferol) 200 IU • Vitamin E (d-alpha tocopheryl acetate) 75 IU • Thiamin (Vitamin B-1) 25 mg • Riboflavin (Vitamin B-2) 38 mg • Niacin 20 mg • Vitamin B6 (from 25 mg pyridoxyl-5 phosphate) 17 mg • Folic Acid 400 mcg • Vitamin B12 (dibencozide) 84 mcg • Biotin 100 mcg • Pantothenic Acid (from d-calcium panthothenate) 25 mg • Calcium (rice protein chelate) 75 mg • Magnesium (rice protein chelate) 75 mg • Zinc (rice protein chelate) 19 mg • Selenium (rice protein chelate) 50 mcg • Manganese (rice protein chelate) 10 mg • Chromium (rice protein chelate) 25 mcg • Bioflavinoids (citrus) 75 mg • Alpha-Lipoic Acid 30 mg • Lutein (from Calendula officinalis flowers) 5,065 mcg • Coenzyme Q-10 (emulsified) 2.5 mg • Alpha-Carotene 415 mcg • Zeaxanthine 333 mcg • Lycopene 300 mcg • Cryptoxanthine 100 mcg • Proprietary Blend 1130 mg: Eye Bright Herb, Taurine, L-Cysteine, L-Arginine, Cayenne, Garlic Bulb, Ginger Root, Ginkgo Biloba leaf, L-Glutamine, Glycine, Bilberry 5:1 extract, Inositol, L-Histidine, Raw Eye Concentrate, L-Glutathione, Lecithin, and SuperOxide Dismutase (SOD). Other Ingredients: Special Plant Cellulose, Vegtable Stearates, Acacia, Gum Tragacanth, Natural Silica, and Magnesium Stearate.
See Editor's Note No. 14.

Opti-Vites **-** Optimum Nutrition
Each capsule contains: Vitamin A (as beta-carotene, vitamin A palmitate) 5000 IU • Vitamin C (as ascorbic acid) 90 mg • Vitamin D (as cholecalciferol) 400 IU • Vitamin K (as phytonadione) 50 mcg • Thiamin (as thiamin hydrochloride) 2.25 mg • Riboflavin 2.55 mg • Niacin (as niacinamide) 20 mg • Vitamin B6 (as pyridoxine hydrochloride) 3 mg • Biotin 150 mcg • Pantothenic Acid (as D-calcium pantothenate) 10 mg • Calcium (as dicalcium phosphate) 60 mg • Iron (as ferrous fumarate) 3.6 mg • Phosphorus (as dicalcium phosphate) 45 mg • Iodine (as kelp) 150 mcg • Magnesium (as magnesium oxide) 100 mg • Zinc (as zinc citrate) 15 mg • Selenium (as selenomethionine) 87.5 mcg • Copper (as copper AA chelate) 2 mg • Manganese (as manganese gluconate) 1 mg • Chromium (as chromium picolinate) 150 mcg • Molybdenum (as molybdenum AA chelate) 75 mcg • Chloride (as potassium chloride) 63 mg • Potassium (as potassium chloride) 70 mg. Other Ingredients: Gelatin, Magnesium Stearate, Silica.

Opti-Vue **-** The Vitamin Shoppe
Two capsules contain: Vitamin A 10000 IU • Vitamin C 200 mg • Vitamin E 50 IU • Potassium 100 mg • Niacin 30 mg • Zinc 5 mg • Riboflavin 3 mg • Selenium 50 mcg • Lutein 6 mg • Zeaxanthin 240-600 mcg • Eyebright Extract 200 mg • Raw Eye Tissue 160 mg • Raw Muscle Tissue 100 mg • Inositol 100 mg • Alfalfa concentrate 50 mg • Citrus Bioflavonoids 50 mg • Quercetin 200 mg • Rutin 25 mg • Bilberry extract 40 mg • Glutathione 5 mg • N-Acetyl Cysteine 50 mg. In a special food base of rice carrot parsley, and spinach concentrates.
See Editor's Note No. 14.

Opti-Women **-** Optimum Nutrition
Two capsules contain: Vitamin A (as CaroCare natural mixed carotenoids, vitamin A palmitate) 5000 IU • Vitamin C (as ascorbic acid) 250 mg • Vitamin D (as cholecalciferol) 600 IU • Vitamin E (as D-alpha tocopheryl succinate) 100 IU • Vitamin K (as phytonadione) 80 mcg • Thiamin (as thiamin hydrochloride) 20 mg • Riboflavin 20 mg • Niacin (as niacinamide) 20 mg • Vitamin B6 (as pyridoxine hydrochloride) 20 mg • Folic Acid 600 mcg • Vitamin B12 (as cyanocobalamin) 100 mcg • Biotin 250 mcg • Pantothenic Acid (as D-calcium pantothenate) 150 mg • Calcium (as calcium carbonate, citrate) 150 mg • Iron (as iron AA chelate) 18 mg • Iodine (as kelp) 200 mcg • Magnesium (as magnesium aspartate) 75 mg • Zinc (as zinc citrate) 15 mg • Selenium (as selenomethionine) 70 mcg • Copper (as copper gluconate) 2 mg • Manganese (as manganese gluconate) 5 mg • Chromium (as chromium GTF) 120 mcg • Molybdenum (as molybdenum AA chelate) 70 mcg • Ostivone Isopropoxy Isoflavone 10 mg • Soy Isoflavones (as NovaSoy) 2 mg • Lycopene (as LYC-O-MATO natural tomato lycopene) 250 mcg • Alpha-Carotene 93.5 mcg • Zeaxanthin 18.7 mcg • Cryptoxanthin 22.8 mcg • Lutein 250 mcg • Chasteberry 4:1 berry extract (vitus agnus-castus) 50 mg • Grape Seed extract (vitis vinifera, standardized to 95% polyphenols) 10 mg • Dong Quai 4:1 root extract (angelica sinensis) 80 mg • Horse Chestnut root extract (aesculus hippocastanum, standardized to 20% aescin) 25 mg • Butchers Broom powdered root 15 mg • Garcinia rind extract (garcinia cambogia, standardized to 52% HCA) 50 mg • Uva Ursi powdered leaf 50 mg • Alpha Lipoic Acid 20 mg • Deodorized Garlic powdered bulb 10 mg • Citrus Bioflavonoids fruit 10 mg. Other Ingredients: Calcium Phosphate, Gelatin, Magnesium Stearate, Silica.

Optizinc **-** Natrol
One capsule contains: Zinc (Monomethionine) 30 mg. Other Ingredients: Microcrystalline Cellulose, Magnesium Stearate, Gelatin.

OptiZinc brand **-** Cardinal Nutrition
Zinc.
See Editor's Note No. 44, page 2058.

OptiZinc **-** Source Naturals
Each tablet contains: Zinc (from 150 mg of OptiZinc zinc monomethionine) 30 mg • Copper (sebacate) 300 mcg.

Opti-Zyme **-** Changes International, Inc.
One caplet contains: Calcium (from 500 mg Calcium Carbonate) 180 mg • Amylase 4250 DU • Protease 10255 HUT • Cellulase 630 CU • Lactase 350 Lac U • Lipase 65 LU • Invertase 0.6 IAU • Glucoamylase 15 AG • Multi-algae blend: Spirulina algae, Bladderwrack kelp, Klamath Lake algae, Canary Island algae, Chlorella algae, Maine coast kelp, and Sargassi seaweed • Supporting herbal blend: Turmeric rhizome, Fennel seed, Ginger root, and Soy sprouts. Other Ingredients: Vegetable cellulose, Fractionated vegetable oil, Soy polysaccharides, Silica, and Vegetable resin glaze.

Opti-Zyme Pro **-** Changes International, Inc.
One capsule contains: Amylase 3400 SKB • Lipase 2250 LU • Cellulase 5400 C-ase • Protease 10200 HUT • Amyloglucosidase 22 AG • Acid stable protease 340 APU • Invertase 102 Sumner U • Lactase 351 LAU • Lactobacillus acidophilus 100 million CFU • Bifidobacterium bifidum 50 million CFU • Dulse algae 50 mg • Trace mineral complex (Montmorillonite) 100 mg • Spirulina blue-green algae 50 mg • Bromelain 50 mg. Other Ingredients: Gelatin, Calcium Sulfate, Magnesium Stearate, and Silica.

Some Brand Name Natural Products - What they Contain

www.NaturalDatabase.com contains MANY more listings than appear here.

OptOmega **-** USANA Health Sciences
Two teaspoons contain: Certified Organic Cold Pressed Flaxseed, Sunflower Seed, Pumpkin Seed Oil, Mixed Tocopherols, D-Alpha-Tocopherol, Tumeric Extract.

Oraflow Plus **-** Nutrition for Life International
Ten tablets contains: Vitamin A 40,000 IU • Vitamin D 400 IU • Vitamin E 650 IU • Vitamin C 4,500 mg • Folic Acid 400 mcg • Vitamin B1 200 mg • Vitamin B2 (Riboflavin) 30 mg • Niacin 100 mg • Vitamin B6 160 mg • Vitamin B12 200 mcg • Biotin 100 mcg • Pantothenic Acid 3.76 mg • Calcium 300 mg • Iodine 125 mcg • Magnesium 300 mg • Zinc 30 mg • Copper 250 mcg • Potassium 275 mg • Manganese 5 mg • Choline 725 mg • Inositol 40 mg • Chromium 150 mcg • Sodium 15 mg • Selenium 250 mcg • L-Arginine 1 g • L-Methionine 200 mg • N-Acetyl-L-Cysteine 750 mg • Marine Lipids 50 mg • Bioflavonoids 100 mg • PABA 300 mg • Adrenal 50 mg • Spleen 50 mg • Thymus 50 mg • Hawthorne berry 26 mg • Butchers Broom 16 mg.
See Editor's Note No. 14.

Oral Nutrient Chelates **-** Enzymatic Therapy
Six tablets contain: Vitamin C (ascorbic acid) 1.5 g • Niacin (as niacinamide, niacin) 630 mg • Vitamin B6 (as pyridoxine HCl) 150 mg • Calcium (from calcium chloride 291 mg) 105 mg • Iodine (from kelp) 600 mcg • Magnesium (from magnesium orotate 1.8 g, magnesium ascorbate 300 mg) 146 mg • Zinc (from zinc ascorbate 45 mg) 9 mg • Selenium (from selenium ascorbate 30 mg) 300 mcg • Copper (from copper gluconate 750 mcg) 113 mcg • Manganese (from manganese ascorbate) 6 mg • Sodium 5 mg • Potassium (from potassium orotate 150 mg, potassium aspartate 105 mg, potassium phosphate 30 mg, potassium chloride 30 mg) 80 mg • Beta-Sitosterol 450 mg • Taurine 300 mg • Mucopolysaccharide (soluble) 300 mg • Betaine HCl 300 mg • Ammonium Chloride 291 mg • L-Methionine 195 mg • Bromelain (1800 M.C.U./g) 150 mg. Other Ingredients: Cellulose, Fennel (foeniculum vulgare), Stearic Acid, Modified Cellulose Gum, Magnesium Stearate, Silicon Dioxide, Titanium Dioxide Color, Peppermint (mentha x piperita).

Oralmat Drops **-** Schumacher Pharmaceuticals of Melbourne
Each 10 mL contains: Rye (secale cereale) Extract.

Orange Burst **-** Advocare International
Two tablets contain: Vitamin A (as palmitate) 1000 IU • Vitamin C (as ascorbic acid and sodium ascorbate) 450 mg • Vitamin E (as D-alpha tocopheryl succinate) 17.5 IU • Folic Acid 100 mcg • Sodium 5 mg • Mixed Carotenoids (from D. salina) 600 mcg • Grape extract (seed/skin - vitis vinifera, Activin brand) 20 mg. Other Ingredients: Fructose, Xylitol, Stearic Acid, Natural Orange Flavor, Magnesium Stearate, Silicon Dioxide, Guar Gum, Turmeric Extract (for color).

Orange Butterfly **-** Unknown
Unknown.
See Editor's Note No. 49, page 2059.

Organic Alfalfa **-** Jamieson
Each caplet contains: Alfalfa 650 mg.

Organic Flax 1000 **-** Health From The Sun
Two capsules contain: Alpha-Linolenic Acid (ALA) (Omega-3) 1.1 g • Linoleic Acid (Omega-6) 280 mg • Oleic Acid (Omega-9) 290 mg. Ingredients: Certified Organic Flax seed oil, Gelatin, Glycerine, Water, Carob powder.

Organic Flax Oil 1000 mg **-** Nature's Bounty
Each softgel contains: Flax seed oil 1000 mg: Alpha-Linoleic Acid 585 mg, Linoleic Acid 150 mg, Oleic Acid 175 mg, Other Fatty Acids and Phytonutrients 90 mg. Other Ingredients: Gelatin, Glycerin, Caramel Color.

Organic Flax Oil Cold Pressed **-** Nature's Bounty
Each 1 tsp (5 mL) serving contains: Flax seed oil 4650 mg: Alpha-Linolenic Acid 2558 mg, Linoleic Acid 691 mg, Oleic Acid 983 mg, Palmitic Acid 235 mg, Stearic Acid 151 mg.

Organic Flaxseed Oil **-** PhysioLogics
Each softgel contains: Organic Flaxseed oil 1000 mg (typically contains alpha-linolenic acid 585 mg) • Linoleic Acid 150 mg • Oleic Acid 175 mg • Other Fatty Acids, Phytonutrients 90 mg. Other Ingredients: Gelatin, Glycerin, Caramel Color.

Organic Flaxseed Oil **-** Vitamin World
Each 1 tsp (5 mL) serving contains: Organic Flaxseed oil 4650 mg: Alpha-Linolenic Acid 2720 mg, Linoleic Acid 698 mg, Oleic Acid 814 mg, Other Fatty Acids and Phytonutrients 418 mg.

Organic Flaxseed Oil 1000 mg **-** Vitamin World
Each softgel contains: Flaxseed oil 1000 mg: Alpha-Linolenic Acid 585 mg, Linoleic Acid 150 mg, Oleic Acid 175 mg, Other Fatty Acids and Phytonutrients 90 mg. Other Ingredients: Gelatin, Glycerin, Caramel Color.

Organic High Lignan Flaxseed Oil **-** Vitamin World
Each 1 tsp (5 mL) serving contains: Organic high lignan Flaxseed oil 4650 mg: Alpha-Linolenic Acid 2650.5 mg, Linoleic Acid 744 mg, Oleic Acid 837 mg, Palmitic Acid, Stearic Acid 418.5 mg.

Organic Wild Yam Deodorant **-** Avalon
Certified Organic Lavender Floral Water (lavandula officinalis) • Certified Organic Extracts Blend: Wild Yam root (discorea villasa), Echinacea (echinacea purpurea), Golden Seal (hydrastis canadensis), Sage (sage officinales) • Organic Myrrh (comminphora myrrha) • Certified Organic Aloe Barbadensis • Vegetable Cellulose • Grapefruit seed extract (citrus grandis) • Castor oil (ricinus communis) • Tocopherol (vitamin E) • Methyl/Propylparaben • Pure Essential Oils.

Original AntiOx **-** NutriCology
Each capsule contains: Vitamin A (as beta-carotene) 7500 IU • Vitamin C (as ascorbic acid) 45 mg • Vitamin E (as DL-alpha-tocopheryl-acetate) 150 IU • Thiamin (as thiamin hydrochloride) 19 mg • Riboflavin (as riboflavin-5-phosphate) 19 mg • Niacin (as niacinamide) 16.5 mg • Vitamin B6 (as pyridoxal-5-phosphate) 4.5 mg • Pantothenic Acid (as calcium pantothenate) 16.5 mg • Zinc (as zinc sulfate) 11 mg • Selenium (as sodium selenite) 56 mcg • L-Cysteine 75 mg • Glutathione (reduced) 37.5 mg • Trimethylglycine 30 mg. Other Ingredients: Cellulose, Magnesium Stearate, Silicon Dioxide.

Original Roast - Revival **-** Physicians Laboratories
Eight Fluid Ounces Contain: Certified Isoflavone 15 mg. Ingredients: Whole Roasted Soybeans, Natural and Artificial Flavors.

Ornidex **-** Biocodex, Inc.
Each two capsules contain: L-Ornithine 300 mg. Inactive Ingredients: Dibasic Calcium Phosphate, Colloidal Silica, Magnesium Stearate, Hydroxy-proptyl-methyl-cellulose, Titanium Dioxide (E 171).

Orthoflex **-** Pacific BioLogic
Siberian Ginseng • Angelica root (Chinese) • Angelica root (pubescent) • Eucommia bark • Siler root • Cinnamon Twig • Astragalus root (Grade 1) • Homalomena rhizome • Notopterygium root & rhizome • Gentiana root • Pseudoginseng root (whole) • Teasal root • Ginger (Chinese Wild).

OS-Cal **-** SmithKline Beecham
Each tablet contains: Calcium Carbonate 500 mg. Other Ingredients: Dextrose Monohydrate, Maltodextrin, Microcrystalline Cellulose, Magnesium Stearate, Artificial Flavors, Sodium Chloride.

Oscillococcinum (Oscillo) **-** Boiron
Active Ingredients: Anas Barbariae Hepatis et Cordis extractum (duck liver extract) HPUS 200 CK. Inactive Ingredients: Sucrose 0.85 g, Lactose 0.15 g.
See Editor's Note No. 1, page 2053.

Osha-Lomatium Virtue **-** Blessed Herbs
Osha root • Lomatium root • Pau d'Arco bark • Propolis • Shitake mycelium • Echinacea Angustifolia root • Goldenseal root • Licorice root • Grain alcohol & Distilled Water.

Osteo Bi-Flex **-** Rexall - Sundown
Three caplets contain: Sodium 105 mg • Vitamin C 60 mg • Vitamin D 400 IU • Calcium 500 mg • Glucosamine HCl 1500 mg • Chondroitin Sulfate 1200 mg. Other Ingredients: Red Beet Juice powder, Crospovidone, Magnesium Stearate, Croscarmellose Sodium, Silica.
See Editor's Note No. 15, page 2055.

Osteo Bi-Flex: Double Strength Caplets **-** Rexall - Sundown
Three caplets contain: Vitamin C (as ascorbic acid) 60 mg • Manganese (as manganese sulfate) 2 mg • Sodium 105 mg • Glucosamine HCl 1500 mg • Chondroitin Sulfate 1200 mg • Boron (as sodium tetraborate) 3 mg. Other Ingredients: Microcrystalline Cellulose, Sodium Carboxymethylcellulose, Crospovidone, Red 40 Lake, Yellow 5 Lake, Maltodextrin, Magnesium Stearate, Dextrose, Yellow 6 Lake, Soy Lecithin, Sodium Citrate, Blue 1 Lake.
See Editor's Note No. 15, page 2055.

Osteo Bi-Flex: Double Strength Softgels **-** Rexall - Sundown
Three softgels contain: Sodium 100 mg • Glucosamine HCl 1500 mg • Chondroitin Sulfate 1200 mg. Other Ingredients: Soybean Oil, Gelatin, Soy Lecithin, Yellow Beeswax, Silica, Sodium Tripoly-Phosphate, Red 40, Titanium Dioxide (color), Blue 1.
See Editor's Note No. 15, page 2055.

Osteo Bi-Flex: Fast-Acting Caplets **-** Rexall - Sundown
Two caplets contain: Sodium 45 mg • Willow Bark extract (salix spp.) 800 mg • Glucosamine HCl 750 mg • Chondroitin Sulfate 600 mg • Boron 1.5 mg. Other Ingredients: Microcrystalline Cellulose, Hydroxypropyl Methylcellulose, Crospovidone, Boron Amino Acid Chelate (hydrolyzed rice protein, boric acid, glycine, aspartic acid, hydrolyzed soy protein), Pharmaceutical Glaze, Silica, Magnesium Stearate, Titanium Dioxide (color), Yellow 5 Lake, Red 40 Lake, Blue 1 Lake, Yellow 6 Lake, Soy Lecithin.
See Editor's Note No. 15, page 2055.

Osteo Bi-Flex: Performance Caplets **-** Rexall - Sundown
Two caplets contain: Vitamin C (as ascorbic acid) 500 mg • Niacin (as niacinamide) 10 mg • Vitamin B12 (as cyanocobalamin) 10 mcg • Sodium 5 mg • Glucosamine HCl 750 mg • L-Arginine 750 mg • Boron 1.5 mg. Other Ingredients: L-Arginine Monohydrochloride, Microcrystalline Cellulose, Corn Starch, Calcium Silicate, Crospovidone, Boron Amino Acid Chelate (hydrolyzed rice protein, boric acid, glycine, aspartic acid, hydrolyzed soy protein), Hydroxypropyl Methylcellulose, Magnesium Stearate, PEG, Dextrin, Titanium Dioxide (color), Dextrose, Soy Lecithin, Blue 2 Lake, Red 40 Lake, Blue 1 Lake, Yellow 6 Lake.

Osteo Bi-Flex: Plus Calcium Caplets **-** Rexall - Sundown
Three caplets contain: Vitamin C (as ascorbic acid) 60 mg • Vitamin D (as cholecalciferol) 400 IU • Calcium (as calcium carbonate) 500 mg • Sodium 110 mg • Glucosamine HCl 1500 mg • Chondroitin Sulfate 1200 mg. Other Ingredients: Microcrystalline Cellulose, Sodium Carboxymethylcellulose, Crospovidone, Titanium Dioxide (color), Maltodextrin, Magnesium Stearate, Yellow 5 Lake, Dextrose, Soy Lecithin, Sodium Citrate, Red 40 Lake, Blue 1 Lake, Yellow 6 Lake.
See Editor's Note No. 15, page 2055.

Osteo Bi-Flex: Plus MSM Caplets **-** Rexall - Sundown
Four caplets contain: Sodium 115 mg • Glucosamine HCl 1500 mg • Chondroitin Sulfate 1200 mg • Methylsulfonylmethane (MSM) 1000 mg. Other Ingredients: Microcrystalline Cellulose, Sodium Carboxymethylcellulose, Yellow 5 Lake, Crospovidone, Magnesium Stearate, Yellow 6 Lake, Maltodextrin, Dextrose, Soy Lecithin, Sodium Citrate, Red 40 Lake, Blue 1 Lake.
See Editor's Note No. 15, page 2055.

Osteo Bi-Flex: Triple Strength Caplets **-** Rexall - Sundown
Two caplets contain: Vitamin C (as ascorbic acid) 60 mg • Manganese (as manganese sulfate) 2 mg • Sodium 105 mg • Glucosamine HCl 1500 mg • Chondroitin Sulfate 1200 mg • Boron (as sodium tetraborate) 3 mg. Other Ingredients: Microcrystalline Cellulose, Sodium Carboxymethylcellulose, Crospovidone, Red 40 Lake, Yellow 5 Lake, Maltodextrin, Magnesium Stearate, Dextrose, Yellow 6 Lake, Soy Lecithin, Sodium Citrate, Blue 1 Lake.
See Editor's Note No. 15, page 2055.

Osteo Formula **-** Quest
Each tablet contains: Calcium (HVP Chelate) 125 mg • Magnesium (HVP Chelate) 125 mg • Vitamin C 50 mg • Vitamin D (as Vitamin D3) 50 IU • Silicon (HVP Chelate) 125 mcg • N-Acetyl Glucosamine (NAG) 125 mg • Betaine HCl 25 mg. Other Ingredients: Croscarmellose Sodium, Magnesium Stearate (vegetable source), Microcrystalline Cellulose, Vegetable Stearin.

Osteo Guard **-** Clinician's Choice
Four tablets contain: Vitamin C (ascorbic acid) 120 mg • Vitamin D (cholecalciferol) 400 IU • Calcium (carbonate, glycinate, gluconate, citrate, succinate, amino acid chelate, aspartate) 1000 mg • Magnesium (oxide, carbonate, citrate, amino acid chelate) 480 mg • Zinc (amino acid chelate) 10 mg • Manganese (amino acid chelate) 1 mg • L-Glutamic Acid 20 mg • Betaine Hydrochloride 20 mg • Proprietary Blend 20 mg: Piper Longum Fruit, Pacific Kelp, Carrot Powder, Astragalus Membranaceus, Silica (horsetail herb), Boron (boron aspartate).

Osteo Plex **-** Olympian Labs
Four capsules contain: Calcium Citrate 800 mg • Magnesium (oxide) 400 mg • Boron (proteinate) 400 mcg • Zinc (amino acid chelate) 10 mg.

Osteo Protector **-** The Vitamin Shoppe
Each tablet contains: Vitamin D (as cholecalciferol) 100 IU • Calcium (as carbonate, hydroxyapatite) 500 mg • Magnesium (as oxide, citrate) 250 mg • Ipriflavone (7-Isopropoxy Isoflavone (Ostivone)) 200 mg.

Osteo-Aid **-** Futurebiotics
Six capsules contain: Vitamin D 400 IU • Calcium (as calcium citrate) 1000 mg • Magnesium (as magnesium amino acid chelate) 400 mg • Boron (as amino acid chelate) 1.5 mg • Ostivone Ipriflavone (7-isopropoxy isoflavone) 100 mg • Soy Isoflavone extract powder (standardized for 10% (5 mg) phytoestrogen isoflavones) 50 mg. Other Ingredients: Gelatin, Water.

Osteocare **-** Puritan's Pride
Two capsules contain: Vitamin D (as cholecalciferol) 133 IU • Calcium (as calcium citrate) 400 mg • Ipriflavone (as 7-isopropoxy isoflavone) 200 mg.

Osteocare Fizz **-** Vitabiotics
Each tablet contains: Calcium 400 mg • Magnesium 50 mg • Zinc 5 mg • Copper 0.5 mg • Manganese 0.75 mg • Selenium 25 mcg • Vitamin C 60 mg • Vitamin D 2.5 mcg.

Osteocare Liquid **-** Vitabiotics
Two teaspoons contain: Calcium 300 mg • Magnesium 150 mg • Zinc 6 mg • Vitamin D 3.8 mcg.

Osteocare Tablets **-** Vitabiotics
Two tablets contain: Calcium 800 mg • Magnesium 300 mg • Zinc 10 mg • Vitamin D 5 mcg • Manganese 1.5 mg • Selenium 50 mcg • Boron 0.6 mg • Copper 1 mg.

OsteoGuard **-** Advocare International
Four caplets contain: Calcium (as amino acid chelate) 400 mg • Magnesium (as amino acid chelate) 200 mg • Vitamin D (as ergocalciferol) 200 IU • Zinc (as amino acid chelate) 7.5 mg • Copper (as amino acid chelate) 1 mg • Manganese (as amino acid chelate) 800 mcg • Vitamin K (as phytonadione) 80 mcg • Green Tea extract (leaf - camellia sinensis) 50 mg • Ginger extract (root - zingiber officinale) 100 mg • Boron (as amino acid chelate) 1 mg • Silicon (as amino acid chelate) 800 mcg • Ipriflavone (Ostivone) 600 mg. Other Ingredients: Dicalcium Phosphate, Silicon Dioxide, Cellulose, Stearic Acid, Magnesium Stearate.

Some Brand Name Natural Products - What they Contain

www.NaturalDatabase.com contains MANY more listings than appear here.

Osteo-Joint **-** Leiner Health Products
Each caplet contains: Deoiled Lecithin (Glycine max) bean 25 mg • Devil's Claw extract 40 mg • Glucosamine Sulfate powder 500 mg • Methylsulfonylmethane 25 mg • Rice Starch (Oryza sativa) 25 mg. Other Ingredients: Calcium Carbonate, Cellulose, Methylcellulose, Maltodextrin, Deoiled Lecithin, Rice Starch, Silicon Dioxide, Croscarmellose Sodium, Stearic Acid, Dextrin, Crospovidone, Magnesium Stearate.

Osteologic **-** PhysioLogics
Four tablets contain: Vitamin D (as Cholecalciferol) 400 IU • Vitamin K (as Phytonadione) 80 mcg • Vitamin B6 (as Pyridoxine HCl) 2 mg • Folate (Folic Acid) 400 mcg • Pantothenic Acid (as D-Calcium Pantothenate) 10 mg • Calcium (as Calcium Carbonate) 1000 mg • Iodine (from Kelp) 471 mcg • Magnesium (as 58% Magnesium Oxide, 25% Magnesium Glycinate, 17% Magnesium Carbonate) 400 mg • Zinc (as Zinc Citrate) 15 mg • Selenium (from natural salts) 3 mcg • Copper (as Copper Aspartate) 2 mg • Manganese (as mixed Manganese salts) 378 mcg • Chromium (from natural salts) 38 mcg • Molybdenum (from natural salts) 115 mcg • Silicon (as Silicon Dioxide) 20 mg • Boron (as 98% Boron Aspartate, 2% natural salts) 3 mg.

OsteoLogic 2000 **-** PhysioLogics
Three caplets contain: Vitamin D (as cholecalciferol) 400 IU • Vitamin K (as phytonadione) 80 mcg • Calcium (as hydroxyapatite phosphate, dicalcium phosphate) 1020 mg • Phosphorus (as hydroxyapatite phosphate, dicalcium phosphate) 524 mg. Other Ingredients: Cellulose (plant origin), Croscarmellose, Silica, Vegetable Stearic Acid, Cellulose Coating, Vegetable Magnesium Stearate.

OsteoLogic Pro **-** PhysioLogics
Two tablets contain: Vitamin D (as cholecalciferol) 150 IU • Vitamin K (as phytonadione) 28 mcg • Calcium (as calcium citrate, calcium hydroxyapatite, dicalcium phosphate) 400 mg • Phosphorus (as calcium hydroxyapatite, dicalcium phosphate) 112 mg • Magnesium (as magnesium citrate, magnesium oxide) 134 mg • Zinc (as zinc glycinate) 5 mg • Manganese (as manganese amino acid chelate) 0.7 mg • Boron (as boron amino acid chelate) 360 mcg • Silica (as silicon dioxide) 35 mg. Other Ingredients: Cellulose (plant origin), Croscarmellose, Vegetable Stearic Acid, Cellulose Coating, Vegetable Magnesium Stearate.

OsteoMax **-** Nutraceutics Corp.
Each tablet contains: Calcium 500 mg • Magnesium 200 mg • Vitamin D3 200 IU • Lysine (as l-lysine monohydrochloride) 100 mg. Other ingredients: Citric Acid, Calcium Carbonate, Sodium Bicarbonate, Magnesium Oxide, Natural Orange Flavor, Sodium Carbonate, Polysorbate 80.

Osteo-Max **-** Metabolic Response Modifiers
Each capsule contains: Ipriflavone 200 mg • MCHC (yielding 167 mg elemental calcium) 667 mg.

OsteoPeak Men **-** Osteogenic Care Technologies (OST)
Two capsules contain: Vitamin D (as cholecalciferol) 200 IU • Calcium (as calcium citrate) 90 mg • Organic Kosher Certified OsteoPeak Proprietary Blend 250 mg: Rehmannia Glutinosa Libosch, Eleutherococcus Senticosus Max. Other Ingredients: Gelatin Capsule, Organic Maltodextrin.

OsteoPeak Menopause **-** Osteogenic Care Technologies (OST)
Three capsules contain: Vitamin D (as cholecalciferol) 300 IU • Calcium (as calcium citrate) 180 mg • Organic, Kosher Certified OsteoPeak Proprietary Blend 500 mg: Rehmannia Glutinosa Libosch, Eleutherococcus Senticosus Max. Other Ingredients: Gelatin Capsule, Organic Maltodextrin.

OsteoPeak Natural **-** Osteogenic Care Technologies (OST)
Three capsules contain: Organic, Kosher Certified OsteoPeak Proprietary Blend 750 mg: Rehmannia Glutinosa Libosch, Eleutherococcus Senticosus Max. Other Ingredients: Gelatin Capsule, Organic Maltodextrin.

OsteoPeak Osteorus **-** Osteogenic Care Technologies (OST)
Two gummy dinosaurs contain: Vitamin D (as cholecalciferol) 400 IU • Calcium (as tricalcium phosphate) 20 mg • Organic, Kosher Certified OsteoPeak Proprietary Blend 50 mg: Rehmannia Glutinosa Libosch, Eleutherococcus Senticosus Max. Other Ingredients: Organic Sugar, Organic Corn Syrup, Pectin, Fuamric Acid, Citric Acid, Natural Flavors/Colors (turmeric, annatto, black carrot juice concentrate, grape skin extract), Fractionated Coconut Oil, Carnauba Wax.

OsteoPeak Premenopause **-** Osteogenic Care Technologies (OST)
Each capsule contains: Vitamin D (as cholecalciferol) 100 IU • Calcium (as calcium citrate) 55 mg • Organic, Kosher Certified OsteoPeak Proprietary Blend 150 mg: Rehmannia Glutinosa Libosch, Eleutherococcus Senticosus Max. Other Ingredients: Gelatin Capsule, Organic Maltodextrin.

Osteo-Plus **-** Nutri-Quest Rx
Each tablet contains: Boron (special organic complex) 1 mg • Magnesium Chelate 400 mg • Calcium Chelate 100 mg • Calcium Aspartate 100 mg • Calcium Giuconate 50 mg • Calcium (Hydroxyapatite) 156 mg • Calcium (Veal Bone) 39 mg • Red Bone Marrow 10 mg • Calcium Citrate 50 mg • Vitamin C 25 mg • Vitamin D 50 IU • L-Glutamic Acid HCL 15 mg • Betaine HCL 10 mg • Salmiac 10 mg • Parathyroid 2 mg. In a base containing Horsetail Rush (Shave grass), Source of Natural Silicon 15 mg, Calcium Fluoride (Cell Salt) Safflower herb 25 mg.
See Editor's Note No. 14.

Osteoporosis Formula **-** Nature's Life
Each four capsules contain: Calcium (Citrate/Malate, Carbonate) 1000 mg • Magnesium (Oxide, Citrate) 500 mg • Vitamin C (Ascorbic Acid) 40 mg • Betaine HCl 40 mg • Zinc (Picolinate) 15 mg • Manganese (Gluconate) 5 mg • Boron (Citrate) 2 mg • Vitamin K (as Vitamin K1) mg • Copper (Gluconate) 1 mg • Silicon (Dioxide) 1 mg • Vitamin D (as Vitamin D3) (Cholecalciferol) 400 IU. In a natural base of Springtime Horsetail herb (Equisetum arvernse).

OsteoPrime **-** Enzymatic Therapy
Four tablets contain: Vitamin D 200 IU • Calcium (Aspartate, Citrate, Succinate, Fumarate, Carbonate, Lactate, Malate) 600 mg • Magnesium (Aspartate, Oxide) 250 mg • Vitamin C (Ascorbic Acid) 100 mg • Vitamin B6 (Pyridoxine) 25 mg • Niacinamide 20 mg 8 Zinc (Picolinate) 15 mg • Manganese (Aspartate) 15 mg • Thiamine HCl (Vitamin B1) 10 mg • Riboflavin (Vitamin B2) 10 mg • Pantothenic Acid (D-Calcium Pantothenate) 10 mg • Copper (Gluconate) 1.5 mg • Folic Acid 400 mcg • Vitamin K (Phytonadione) 150 mcg • Chromium (Aspartate) 100 mcg • Selenium sodium Selenite) 100 mcg • Molybdenum (Sodium Molybdate) 50 mcg • Vitamin B12 (Cyanocobalamin) 10 mcg. Other Ingredients: Betaine HCl 20 mg • Silicon Sodium Metasilicate 1 mg • Boron (Chelated) 750 mcg • Strontium (Nonradioactice) 500 mcg.

OsteoPrime Fort **-** PhytoPharmica
Four tablets contain: Betaine HCl 20 mg • Boron (as boron Krebs cycle chelates) 2 mg • Calcium (from tricalcium phosphate, clacium carbonate, calcium Krebs cycle chelates, and calcium citrate) 600 mg • Chromium (as chromium aspartate) 200 mcg • Copper (as copper gluconate) 2 mg • Folic Acid 800 mcg • Magnesium (as magnesium oxide and magnesium aspartate) 250 mg • Manganese (as mananese aspartate) 7 mg • Molybdenum (as sodium molybdate) 50 mcg • Niacin (as niacinamide) 50 mg • Pantothenic Acid (as calcium D-pantothenate) 20 mg • Phosphorus (from tricalcium phosphate) 130 mg • Riboflavin (vitamin B2) 20 mg • Selenium (as sodium selenite) 100 mcg • Silicon (as magnesium trisilicate) 1 mg • Strontium (as strontium chloride) 1 mg • Thiamin (as thiamin HCl, vitamin B1) 20 mg • Vitamin B12 (as cyanocobalamin) 20 mcg • Vitamin B6 (as pyridoxine HCl) 25 mg • Vitamin C (ascorbic acid) 100 mg •

Vitamin D (as cholecalciferol) 300 IU • Vitamin K (as phytonadione) 300 mcg • Zinc (as zinc picolinate) 20 mg.

OsteoPure **-** Marathon Nutrifoods
Each two capsules contain: Red Yeast Rice (monascus purpureus went) 200 mg. Inactive Ingredients: Whey, Gelatin, Magnesium Stearate.

OsteoPure + **-** Marathon Nutrifoods
Each two capsules contain: Red Yeast Rice (monascus purpureus went) 200 mg • Pueraria root (pueraria lobata) 300 mg. Inactive Ingredients: Whey, Dicalcium Phosphate, Gelatin, Magnesium Stearate.

OsteoSoy **-** FreeLife International
Four caplets contain: Vitamin D (as cholecalciferol) 125 IU • Vitamin K (as phylloquinone) 30 mcg • Vitamin B6 (as pyridoxine HCl) 5 mg • Folate (as folic acid) 400 mcg • Vitamin B12 (as cyanocobalamin) 25 mcg • Calcium (as hydroxyapatite, calcium hydrogen phosphate, citramal calcium-citrate-malate-glycinate) 1100 mg • Phosphorus (as hydroxyapatite, calcium hydrogen phosphate) 350 mg • Magnesium (as magnesium oxide, chelazome magnesium glycinate, magnesium citrate) 400 mg • Zinc (as chelazome zinc citrate, zinc glycinate) 15 mg • Copper (as chelazome copper glycinate) 1 mg • Manganese (as chelazome manganese glycinate) 2 mg • Chaste berry (from standardized extract 5:1, 5% vitexicarpin, 1% vitricin 50 mg) 250 mg • Dong Quai (from standardized extract 5:1, 10,000 ppm ligustilide 50 mg) 250 mg • Licorice root (from 50 mg standardized extract 4:1, 13% glycyrrihizin 50 mg) 200 mg • Silica (colloidal) 70 mg • Isoflavones (genistein, daidzein, puerarin from kudzu root, soybean) 40 mg • Boron (as boron chelate) 2 mg • Soyatab (caplet disintegration accelerant from soy polysaccharides) 180 mg. Other Ingredients: Cellulose, Cellulose Gum, Vegetable Stearic Acid, Vegetable Magnesium Stearate, Vita-Coat (vegetable resin, alpha-lipoic acid).

Osteosupport **-** Health Factor
Four tablets contain: Calcium (Citrate/Hydroxylapatite) 850 mg • Vitamin D (as Vitamin D3) (Cholecalciferol) 100 IU • Iodine (Kelp) 100 mcg • Magnesium (Citrate) 650 mg • Boron (Citrate) 2 mg • Silicon (Citrate) 500 mcg • Vanadium (Pentoxide) 75 mcg • Betaine HCl 65 mg • Glutamic Acid 65 mg.

Osteo-Support **-** The Vitamin Shoppe
Two tablets contain: Calcium 500 mg • Magnesium 250 mg • Vitamin D 100 IU.

Ostivone **-** PhytoPharmica
Each capsule contains: Ipriflavone (Ostivone brand) 200 mg.

Ostivone **-** Anabolic Laboratories
Each tablet contains: Ipriflavone (ostivone 7-isopropoxy isoflavone) 200 mg.

Ostivone **-** Enzymatic Therapy
Each capsule contains: Ostivone Ipriflavone 200 mg.

Ostivone **-** Natrol
Each capsule contains: 7-Isopropoxy-Isoflavone 100 mg. Other Ingredients: Rice Powder, Magnesium Stearate, Gelatin.

Ostivone **-** Source Naturals
One tablet contains: Ipriflavone (Ostivone) 300 mg.

O-Tropin **-** Orenda International
Active Ingredients: Lipotropin Complex Proprietary Blend 200 mg: Alpha GPC (alpha glycerlphosphoryl choline), GABA (gamma amino butyric acid), Mucuna Pruiens (l-dopa bean extract), Moomiyo extract (Russian mumie) • HGH Stimulator Proprietary Blend 300 mg: Ornithine Alpha Ketoglutarate, L-Glutamine, L-Arginine, L-Lysine, L-Valine, L-Isoleucine, L-Tyrosine, Glycine. Other Ingredients: Purified Water, Lecithin Phospholipids, Sodium Citrate, Citric Acid, Potassium Sorbate, Maltodextrin, Sodium Benzoate, Methylparaben, Natural Flavors, Artificial Flavors.

Ouch Ointment **-** Earth Science
Each 100 mL tube contains: Water • Tea Tree oil • Glyceryl Stearate • Capric Caprylic Triglycerides • Echinacea extract • Witch Hazel extract • Steareth-20 • Glycerine • Calendula extract • Saccharomyces Lysate • St. John's Wort • Dimethicone • Plantain extract • Potassium Sorbate • Sodium Carbomer 940 • Peppermint oil • Mont-Morillonite Clay • Grape extract.

Our Daily Fish **-** Functional Products
Six softgels contain: Vitamin E 0.33 IU • Vitamin B1 0.09 mg • Vitamin B2 0.15 mg • Vitamin B3 3.5 mg • Vitamin B6 0.3 mg • Folic Acid 12 mcg • Pantothenic Acid 0.15 mg • Calcium 260 mg • Iron 1 mg • Phosphorus 200 mg • Iodine 60 mcg • Magnesium 25 mg • Zinc 0.3 mg • Selenium 30 mcg • Copper 0.1 mg • Potassium 250 mg • Arginine 200 mg • Histidine 250 mg • Isoleucine 200 mg • Leucine 30 mg • Lysine 200 mg • Methionine 200 mg • Phenylalanine 200 mg • Threonine 100 mg • Tyrosine 200 mg • Valine 200 mg • Omega 6 Linoleic Acid 300 mg • Omega 3 ALA 85 mg • Omega 3 EPA 230 mg • Omega 3 DHA 450 mg. Ingredients: Fish Oil, Di-Calcium Phosphate, Glycerin (Kosher), Water, Potassium Sulfate, Salmon Oil, Docosahexaenoic Acid, L-Leucine, Linoleic Acid, L-Histidine, L-Arginine, L-Isoleucine, L-Lysine, L-Methionine, L-Phenylalanine, L-Tyrosine, L-Valine, Eicosapentaenoic Acid, Flax Seed Oil, Soybean Lecithin, Safflower Oil, Bees Wax, L-Threonine, Alpha-Linolenic Acid, Magnesium Oxide, Selenium Yeast, Niacinamide, Ferrous Sulfate, Zinc Oxide, Pyridoxine HCl, D-Alpha Tocopherol, Curpric Sulfate, Calcium Phantothenate, Riboflavin, Thiamine HCl, Potassium Iodide, Retinol Palmitate, Folic Acid.

Our Daily Fruit **-** Functional Products
Three softgels contain: Vitamin A 511 IU • Vitamin C 112 mg • Vitamin E 0.36 IU • Vitamin K 10 mcg • Vitamin B1 0.05 mg • Vitamin B2 0.06 mg • Vitamin B3 0.5 mg • Vitamin B6 0.1 mg • Folic Acid 10 mcg • Pantothenic Acid 0.21 mg • Calcium 30 mg • Iron 0.5 mg • Phosphorus 23 mg • Magnesium 20 mg • Zinc 0.17 mg • Copper 0.2 mg • Manganese 0.5 mg • Potassium 250 mg • Omega 6 Linoleic Acid 150 mg • Omega 3 ALA 30 mg. Ingredients: Potassium Sulfate • Gelatin • Vegetable Oil • Safflower Oil • Linoleic Acid • Alpha-Linolenic Acid • Gamma-Linolenic Acid • Glycerin (Kosher) • Ascorbic Acid • Di-Calcium Phosphate • Evening Primrose Oil • Water • Flax Seed Oil • Soybean Lecithin • Bees Wax • Magnesium Oxide • Annatto Seed • Bilberry Extract • Natural Beta Carotene • Ferrous Sulfate • Manganese Sulfate • Phytonadione • Niacinamide • Cupric Sulfate • d-Alpha Tocopheryl • Calcium Pantothenate • Zinc Oxide • Pyridoxine HCl • Riboflavin • Thiamine HCl • Folic Acid.

Our Daily Veggies **-** Functional Products
Three softgels contain: Vitamin A 1916 IU • Vitamin C 39 mg • Vitamin E 0.6 mg • Vitamin K 50 mcg • Vitamin B1 0.12 mg • Vitamin B2 0.1 mg • Vitamin B3 1 mg • Vitamin B6 0.23 • Folic Acid 40 mcg • Pantothenic Acid 0.37 mg • Calcium 88 mg • Iron 2 mg • Phosphorus 70 mg • Magnesium 35 mg • Zinc 0.7 mg • Selenium 10 mcg • Copper 0.1 mg • Manganese 0.5 mg • Potassium 400 mg • Omega 6 Linoleic Acid 670 mg • Omega 3 ALA 100 mg • Omega 3 GLA 20 mg • Soy Isoflavone 0.2 mg • Lutein 0.39 mg • Lycopene 0.18 mg. Ingredients: Safflower Oil, Potassium, Sulfate, Gelatin, Glycerin (Kosher), Di-Calcium Phosphate, Evening Primrose Oil, Flax Seed Oil, Vegetable Oil, Gamma-Linolenic Acid, Alpha-Linolenic Acid, Linoleic Acid, Water, Magnesium Oxide, Soybean Lecithin, Bees Wax, Ascorbic Acid, Tomato Concentrate, Ferrous Sulfate, Natural Beta Carotene, Phytonadione, Selenium Yeast, Lutein, Manganese Sulfate, Lycopene, Niacinamide, Zinc Oxide, D-Alpha Tocopherol, Soy Isoflavone, Calcium Pantothenate, Pyridoxine HCl, Cupric Sulfate, Thiamine HCl, Riboflavin, Folic Acid.

Ovary-Uterus Complex **-** Enzymatic Therapy
Each capsule contains: Ovary-Uterus Complex (predigested Soluble concentrate) 250 mg • Multi-Glandular Complex: Raw Liver, Raw Lung, Raw Pancreas, Raw Heart, Raw Kidney, Raw Spleen, & Raw Brain 100 mg.
See Editor's Note No. 31, page 2056.

Overdrive - Pharmanex
Each capsule contains: Vitamin A (100% as Beta-Carotene from Dunaliella Salina, Beta-Carotene) 2500 IU • Vitamin C (as Ascorbic Acid) 300 mg • Vitamin E (d-Alpha Tocopheryl Succinate) 75 IU • Thiamin (as Thiamine Mononitrate) 0.75 mg • Riboflavin (as Riboflavin) 0.85 mg • Vitamin B6 (as Pyridoxine Hydrochloride) 1 mg • Folate (as Folic Acid) 100 mcg • Vitamin B12 (as Cyanocobalamin) 3 mcg • Pantothenic Acid (as d-Calcium Pantothenate) 5 mg • Magnesium (as Magnesium Asparate, Magnesium Oxide) 60 mg • Selenium (as L-Selenomethionine) 35 mcg • Chromium (as Chromium Chelate, Chromium Picolinate) 100 mcg • Bromelain (from Pineapple extract) 50 mg • Papain (from Papaya extract) 50 mg • Citrus Bioflavonoid Complex 50 mg • Hydromins (from Sea Salt extract) 50 mg • N-Acetyl-L-Cysteine 20 mg • Quercetin 12.5 mg • Grape Seed Extract with Leucoanthocyanin 2.5 mg.

Ox - SAN Nutrition
Three caplets contain: Citruline-Malate 3000 mg • Regall Biosorb 5 mg. Other Ingredients: Cellulose, Stearic Acid, Magnesium Stearate.

Oxy Shield - Futurebiotics
Three tablets contain: Vitamin E (natural d-alpha tocopherol) 400 IU • Beta Carotene 25,000 IU • Vitamin C 1000 mg • N-Acetyl Cysteine 125 mg • Cysteine 125 mg • Zinc (citrate, gluconate) 25 mg • Copper 1 mg • Selenium (selenomethionine) 150 mcg • Garlic (Pure-Gar) 400 mg • Green Tea 400 mg • Rosemary extract 50 mg • Licorice extract 700 mg • Astragalus extract 350 mg • Tricosanthes extract 150 mg • Siberian Ginseng extract 750 mg • Pau D'Arco 50 mg • Cayenne 30 mg • Methionine 50 mg • Red Clover flowers 100 mg • Barley grass powder 100 mg • Chamomile 100 mg • Ribonucleic Acid (RNA) 50 mg • Kelp 100 mg • Iodine (kelp) 150 mcg • Molybdenum 20 mcg.

Oxydrene - Klein-Becker
Two capsules contain: Crenulin-RCC Proprietary Blend 500 mg: Sedum Crenulata root, Hoppophae fruit, Fructus Lychii Chinensis fruit. Other Ingredients: Rice Flour.

Oxy-G2 - Body Wise International, Inc.
Two capsules contain: Beta Carotene (Vitamin A 6250 IU) 3.75 mg • Vitamin C 75 mg • Vitamin E (as d-alpha Tocopheryl Succinate) 30 IU • Pantothenic Acid (from Calcium Pantothenate) 50 mg • Selenium (as L-Selenomethionine) 100 mcg • Molybdenum (Krebs Cycle Chelate) 100 mcg • Organic Germanium 100 mg • Ginkgo Biloba Leaf 100 mg • Milk Thistle Seed Std. Extract (80% Silymarin) 50 mg • Echinacea Purpurea Root 50 mg • Cytochrome C Oxidase 50 mg • Krebs Cycle Chelated Replenished Factors 50 mg • L-Glutathione 50 mg • Ascorbyl Palmitate 50 mg • L-Cysteine 25 mg • L-Tyrosine 25 mg • Pau D'Arco (Taheebo Tea Bark) 25 mg • Chlorophyll 20 mg.

Oxygen Elements Plus - Global Health Trax
Seven drops contain: Global Health Trax Proprietary Blend 326 mg: Ionic Trace Elements, Citric Acid, Gluconic Acid, Rice Vinegar, Hydrogen Sulfate, Purified Water, Amino Acid Blend, Enzyme Blend.

Oxygen Plus - Market America, Inc.
Two capsules contain: Vitamin A (as beta carotene) 5000 IU • Vitamin C (as ascorbic acid) 200 mg • Vitamin E (as d-alpha tocopherol succinate) 30 IU • Selenium (as SelenoPrecise yeast bound selenium) 200 mcg • Green Tea extract 300 mg • Ginko Biloba leaf extract (24% ginko flavoglycosides/6% terpene lactones) 50 mg • Milk Thistle 50 mg • L-Glutathione 1 mg • Bilberry powder 50 mg. Other Ingredients: Rice Powder, Silica, Magnesium Stearate, Gelatin.

Oxy-Moxy - En Garde Health Products
Each twenty drops contain: Proprietary Blend 0.7 g: Deionized Water • Norwegian Seaweed extract from Seawrack & Bladderwrack • Citric Acid • Menthol • Mint leaf extract (Menta viridis).

Oxy-Pro - Progressive Labs
Each capsule contains: Vitamin A (as beta carotene) 12500 IU • Vitamin C 150 mg • Vitamin E (d-alpha tocopheryl succinate) 100 IU • Riboflavin (B2) 12.5 mg • Niacinamide 12.5 mg • Vitamin B6 10 mg • Zinc (as zinc glycinate) 7.5 mg • Selenium (as selenomethionine) 100 mcg • Copper (as copper lysinate) 0.5 mg • Manganese (as manganese glycinate) 4 mg • Molybdenum (as sodium molybdate) 5 mcg • Quercetin 50 mg • N-Acetyl Cysteine 50 mg • Glutathione 2.5 mg.

Oyster Calcium - Puritan's Pride
Each tablet contains: Vitamin A (as Retinyl Acetate) 1600 IU • Vitamin D (as Cholecalciferol) 400 IU • Calcium (as Oyster Shell) 750 mg.

Oyster Calcium - Nature's Bounty
Two tablets contain: Vitamin A (as Retinyl Acetate) 1600 IU • Vitamin D (as Cholecalciferol) 400 IU • Calcium (as Oyster Shell) 750 mg. Other Ingredients: Maltodextrin, Acacia, Cellulose, Croscarmellose, Cellulose Coating, Vegetable Magnesium Stearate.

Oyster Shell Calcium - Nature's Bounty
Each tablet contains: Calcium (as Oyster Shell Powder) 500 mg. Other Ingredients: Maltodextrin, Acacia Gum, Cellulose, Croscarmellose, Cellulose Coating, Vegetable Magnesium Stearate.

Oystercal 500 - Puritan's Pride
Each tablet contains: Calcium (as Calcium Carbonate from Oyster Shell) 500 mg.

Oystercal 500 + D - Puritan's Pride
Each tablet contains: Vitamin D (as Ergocalciferol) 125 IU • Calcium (as Oyster Shell) 500 mg.

PABA - Source Naturals
Each tablet contains: PABA (para-Aminobenzoic Acid) 100 mg.

PABA 500 - GNC A-Z - GNC
Each tablet contains: Para-Aminobenzoic Acid (PABA) 500 mg. Other Ingredients: Cellulose, Whole Brown Rice powder (Oryza Sativa).

Pacific Kelp - Quest
Each tablet contains: Pacific Kelp 650 mg. Other Ingredients: Calcium Carbonate, Silicon Dioxide, Magnesium Stearate (vegetable source).

Padma 28 - Padma A.G.
Each tablet contains: Saussuria 40 mg • Iceland Moss 40 mg • Margosa 35 mg • Myrobalan 30 mg • Red Sandalwood 30 mg • Cardamom 30 mg • Allspice 25 mg • Bengal Quince 20 mg • Potentilla Golden Seal 15 mg • Licorice 15 mg • Ribwort 15 mg • Columbine 15 mg • Knot grass 15 mg • Cloves 12 mg • Gingerlily 10 mg • Heartleaved Sida 10 mg • Valerian 10 mg • Wild Lettuce 6 mg • Marigold 5 mg • Camphor 4 mg • Aconite 1 mg • Calcium sulfate 20 mg • Sorbitol 73 mg • Cilicum dioxide 12 mg.

Padma Basic - EcoNugenics
Two tablets contain: Padma Basic Proprietary Blend 804 mg: Iceland Moss (cetraria islandica L. Ach.), Costus root, Margose fruit (azadirachtaindica A. juss), Cardamom fruit, Red Sandalwood heart wood, Tropical Almond fruit, Allspice fruit, Bengal Quince fruit (aegle marmelos (L.) correa), Calcium Sulfate, Columbine aerial part (aquilegia vulgaris L.), English Plantain aerial part (polygonum aviculare L.), Licorice root, Knotgrass aerial part, Golden Cinquefoil aerial part (potentilla aurea L.), Clove flower, Gingerlily rhizome (hedychium spicatum buch.-Ham.), Heartleaved Sida Cordifolia aerial part (sida cordifolia L.), Valerian root, Lettuce leaf (lactuca sativa L.), Calendula flower, Natural Camphor. Other Ingredients: Sorbitol, Silicon Dioxide.
See Editor's Note No. 39, page 2058.

Pain Away - Dr. Mike's Vitamins
Menthol • Deionized Water • Sesame oil • Canola oil • Borage Seed oil • Ricinoleic Acid (from castor oil) • Emu oil • TEA • MSM • Herbal Extract Blend: Witch Hazel, Feverfew, Marigold, Capsicum, St. John's Wort, Arnica, Rue, Chamomile • Aloe Vera Gel • Carbomer 940 • Methyl Paraben • Propyl Paraben • Fragrance.

Pain Relief Complex **-** Shaklee
Three caplets contain: Boswellia resin extract (boswellia serrata, standardized to 40% totoal boswellic acids) 1000 mg • Safflower flower extract (carthamus tinctorius) 150 mg. Other Ingredients: Microcrystalline Cellulose, Sorbitol, Calcium Stearate, Croscarmellose Sodium.

Pain Stop **-** Flora, Inc.
Willow bark.

PainDefense Joint & Muscle Formula **-** PharmTech
Each capsule contains: Manganese (as manganese citrate) 4 mg • Glucosamine Sulfate (KCl) 500 mg • MSM (methyl-sulfonyl-methane) 250 mg • Panax Notoginseng (50-60 saponins supplying 45% ginsenosides) 50 mg • Chondroitin Complex 140 mg • Collagen Complex 100 mg • Sea Cucumber (25% mucopolysaccharides) 50 mg • Cetyl Myristoleate (CMO) 50 mg • Boswellia Serrate (25% boswellic acid) 50 mg • Bromelain (2400 GDU) 50 mg • White Willow bark (1% salicylates) 40 mg • Turmeric (95% curcuminoids) 34.5 mg.
See Editor's Note No. 15, page 2055.

PainFactor **-** HealthMinded
Water, Glycerin, Glyceryl Stearate, Cetearyl Alcohol, Sodium Stearoyl Lactylate, Caprylic/Capric Triglyceride, Menthol, Dimethicone, PainFactor, Capsicum Frutescens Resin, Phenoxyethanol, Methylparaben, Butylparaben, Ethylparaben, Propylparaben, Propylene Glycol, Diazolidnyl Urea, Mentha Piperita leaf oil (peppermint), Carbomer, Xanthan gum, Tetrasodium EDTA, Tocopheryl Acetate, Sodium PCA, Camellia Sinensis extract, Panax Ginseng root extract, Chamomilla Recutita (matricaria) flower extract, Ginkgo Biloba extract, Aloe Barbadensis leaf juice, Panthenyl Triacetate, Tetrahexyldecyl Ascorbate, Squalane, Retinyl Palmitate, Retinyl.

Pain-Less **-** The Herbalist
White Willow bark • Feverfew herb • Jamaican Dogwood root bark • Black Cohosh root • Passionflower herb • Butterbur root • St. John's Wort flower.

Pain-Less Rub **-** The Herbalist
Oils of Sweet Almond, Aloe Vera, St. John's Wort flower, Calendula flower & Arnica flower • Essential oils of French Lavender, Peppermint, Lemon Grass, Wintergreen, Nutmeg, Bergamot & Camphor • Extracts of Comfrey root, Echinacea root, White Willow bark & Cayenne pepper.

Palmetto Plus **-** USANA Health Sciences
Each capsule contains: Saw Palmetto Extract (Serenoa Repens) fruit standardized to contain a minimum of 85% fatty acids 320 mg • Lycopene (Solanium Lycopersicum) fruit 5 mg • Soy Isoflavones (Glycine Max) seed 25 mg. Other Ingredients: Gelatin, Glycerin, Purified Water, Natural Carob Color, Beeswax, Lecithin, Titanium Dioxide.

Palmitol **-** Flora, Inc.
Saw Palmetto berries • Zinc 50 mg • Vitamin B6 120 mg.

Palmvitee **-** LaneLabs
Two capsules contain: Vitamin E 350 IU (as gamma tocotrienol, alpha tocotrienol, delta tocotrienol, & d-alpha tocopherol). Other Ingredients: Gelatin, water, & glycerin.

Panax Ginseng **-** Pharmanex
Each capsule contains: Ginseng Panax root (5:1) extract (Panax Ginseng C.A. Meyer) 100 mg. Other Ingredients: Rice Flour, Gelatin.

Panax Ginseng Extract **-** Enzymatic Therapy
Each capsule contains: Korean Ginseng root extract (panax ginseng, standardized to contain a minimum of 7% ginsenosides [7 mg]) 100 mg. Other Ingredients: Cellulose, Gelatin, Magnesium Stearate, Titanium Dioxide Color.

Panax Ginseng Phytosome **-** Enzymatic Therapy
Each capsule contains: Korean Ginseng root Phytosome (panax ginseng, bound to phosphatidylcholine) 50 mg. Other Ingredients: Gelatin, Magnesium Stearate, Silicon Dioxide, Titanium Dioxide Color.

Panaxin **-** PhytoPharmica
Each capsule contains: Korean Ginseng (Panax ginseng) root extract (standardized to contain 7% ginsenosides) 100 mg.

Pancreas Chelate Plus **-** Atrium Inc.
Each tablet contains: Zinc (Protein Chelated) 15 mg • Chromium (Protein Chelated) 200 mcg • Pancreas Substance (from total maxi strength Pancreatin 75 mg, Raw Pancreas concentrate 75 mg) 150 mg. To insure the naturally occuring factors as well as the concentrated forms of Lipase & Amylase Enzymes.
See Editor's Note No. 14.

Pancreas Plus **-** Nutri-Quest Rx
Each tablet contains: Pancreatin 270 mg • Pancreas 130 mg [Tissue concentrate (not extract) of Bovine Source]. Natural occuring factors as well as concentrated forms of Protease, Lipase, & Amylase enzymes.
See Editor's Note No. 14.

Pancreas, Organic Glandular (LAMB) **-** NutriCology
Each capsule contains: Pancreas gland, lamb 425 mg. Other Ingredients: Cellulose, Stearic Acid.
See Editor's Note No. 14.

Pancreas, Organic Glandular (PORK) **-** NutriCology
Each capsule contains: Pancreas gland, pork 425 mg. Other Ingredients: Cellulose, Stearic Acid.
See Editor's Note No. 14.

Pancreatic VegEnzymes **-** Pure Encapsulations
Each vegetable capsule contains: Proprietary Blend of Plant Enymes 200 mg (providing 200 PAU): Amylase, Lipase, Protease • Vitamin C (as ascorbyl palmitate) 2 mg.

Pancreatic VegEnzymes L **-** Pure Encapsulations
Each vegetable capsule contains: Proprietary Blend of Plant Enzymes 200 mg (providing 200 PALU): Amylase, Lipase, Protease • Vitamin C (as ascorbyl palmitate) 2 mg.

Pantethine **-** PhytoPharmica
Each tablet contains: Pantethine 300 mg.

Pantethine **-** Puritan's Pride
Each tablet contains: Pantethine 165 mg.

Pantethine Complex **-** The Vitamin Shoppe
Each tablet contains 300 mg of Pantethine Complex supplying: Pantethine (coenzyme A precursor) 150 mg • Pantothenic Acid (d-calcium pantothenate) 150 mg.

Pantothenic Acid **-** Nature's Bounty
Each tablet contains: Pantothenic Acid (as d-Calcium Pantothenate) 200 mg. Other Ingredients: Cellulose, Vegetable Stearic Acid, Starch, Croscarmellose, Silica, Vegetable Magnesium Stearate.

Pantothenic Acid **-** Source Naturals
Each tablet contains: Pantothenic Acid (vitamin B5, as calcium d-pantothenate) 100 mg.

Pantothenic Acid - Allergy Research Group **-** NutriCology
Each capsule contains: Pantothenic Acid (as calcium pantothenate) 500 mg • Calcium (as calcium pantothenate) 42 mg. Other Ingredients: Silicon Dioxide.

Pantothenic Acid 100 mg **-** Puritan's Pride
Each tablet contains: Calcium Pantothenate 109 mg.

Pantothenic Acid 200 mg **-** Puritan's Pride
Each tablet contains: Calcium Pantothenate 218 mg.

Pantothenic Acid 250 - GNC A-Z - GNC
Each tablet contains: Pantothenic Acid (as calcium d-pantothenate) 250 mg. Other Ingredients: Dicalcium Phosphate, Gelatin, Cellulose, Whole Brown Rice powder (Oryza sativa).

Pantothenic Acid 500 - GNC A-Z - GNC
Each capsule contains: Pantothenic Acid 500 mg. Other Ingredients: Gelatin, Cellulose, Whole Brown Rice powder (Oryza sativa).

Papaya - Leiner Health Products
Each tablet contains: Total Carbohydrate 1 g • Papain 10 mg • Papaya fruit powder 250 mg • Pineapple juice solid powder 150 mg. Other Ingredients: Compressible Sugar, Stearic Acid, Mannitol, Cellulose, Magnesium Stearate, Silicon Dioxide, Artificial Pineapple Flavor.

Para Thyrolate - Progressive Labs
Each capsule contains: Calcium 100 mg • Iodine 225 mcg • Phosphorus 40 mg • Parathyroid concentrate 500 mcg • Thyroid concentrate (thyroxin-free) 25 mg. Other Ingredients: Dicalcium Phosphate, Cellulose, Protein Conjugate, Pacific Sea Kelp, Calcium Carbonate, Papain, Guar Gum, Stearic Acid, Gelatin. The glandular material in this product is prepared by a special process which does not exceed physiological temperature (37° C). Guaranteed free of chemical pesticides and synthetic hormones.
See Editor's Note No. 14.

Para-Cid - Atrium Inc.
Each tablet contains: Betaine HCL 250 mg • Pepsin 20 mg. In a slow release matrix.

Paraclear - PhysioLogics
Two capsules contain: Sweet Annie leaf, stem 400 mg • Garlic bulb (10,000 mcg alliin/g, 2 mg) 200 mg • Pau D'Arco bark 200 mg • Goldthread root (10% alkaloids, 15 mg) 150 mg • Black Walnut husk 100 mg • Ficin (from fig) 10 mg. Other Ingredients: Gelatin.

Para-Clens - Nutri-Quest Rx
Each tablet contains: Artemisia Annua 50 mg • Garlic powder 50 mg • Black Walnut 50 mg • Pumpkin seed 50 mg • Oregano oil 1 mg • Tea Tree 2 mg • Grapefruit seed extract 50 mg • Bromelain 50 mg • Papain 50 mg.

ParaFree - Young Living Essential Oils
Sesame Seed Oil • Cumin Oil • Olive Oil • Thyme Oil • Clove • Anise • Nutmeg • Fennel • Vetiver • Idaho Tansy • Melaleuca Alternifolia • Bay Laurel.

ParaNix (World's Best Internal Klenz) - Nature's Medicine Corporation
Black Walnut hulls • Clove buds • Chlorophyll • Diatomaceous Earth • Elecampane plant (inula helenium) • False Unicorn root • Fenugreek seeds • Garlic bulb • Gentian root • Grapefruit seed extract • Hyssop • Myrrh gum • Peppermint leaf • Prickly Ash bark • Pumpkin seeds • Turmeric root • Wormwood • Yellow Dock.

Paraprost - Nikken Kagakusha
Each capsule contains: L-Glutamic Acid 265 mg • L-Alanine 100 mg • Aminoacetic Acid 45 mg.

Para-Relief - Enzymatic Therapy
Two capsules contain: Citricidal extract (citrus paradisi, macfad., grapefruit seed) 100 mg • Goldenseal root (hydrastis canadensis, 5% hydrastine extract) 100 mg • Sweet Annie (artemisia annua, aerial parts) 100 mg • Quassia bark (picrasma excelsa extract 4:1) 100 mg • Black Walnut green outer hull (juglans nigra extract 4:1) 100 mg • Garlic bulb (allium sativum, 0.8% allicin extract) 100 mg • Clove buds (syzygium aromaticum) 100 mg • Pure Plant Enzymes Blend 41 mg: Protease I, II, III (USP XXIII, pH7.5) 3265 USP, FCC IV (pH7.0) 5235 PC, FCC IV (pH4.7) 5440 HUT, Amylase (USP XXI, pH6.8) 3300 USP, FCC IV (pH4.8) 1430 DU, Cellulase II (FCC IV pH4.5) 101 CU, Lipase II (FCC III pH6.5) 43 LU.

Parasillan - Olympian Labs
Each capsule contains: Proprietary Blend 700 mg: Plaintain, Barberry Bark, Chaparral, Citrus Bioflavonoids, Lobelia, Black Walnut, Wormwood, Psyllium Hull, Cayenne Pepper.

Parasites & Worms - Grandma's Herbs
Each capsule contains: Proprietary Blend 0.496 g: Tansy herb, Wormwood leaf, Black Walnut hulls, Garlic herb, Pomegranate rind/bark, Hyssop herb, Pumpkin seed, Blue Vervain herb, Senna leaf, Chaparral herb, Bayberry bark.

Parathyroid - Atrium Inc.
Each tablet contains: Parathyroid (Bovine) 10 mg • Thyroid (Thyroxin free) 30 mg • Stomach (Bovine) 32 mg • Dulse 300 mg • Calcium 50 mg • Phosphorus 22 mg • Vitamin D (as Vitamin D3) 100 IU • Vitamin B12 20 mcg • Folic Acid 440 mcg • Beet 50 mg • Carrot 50 mg. Calcium & Phosphorus from Bone Meal, Beet & Carrot powders, Iodine from Dulse powder.
See Editor's Note No. 14.

Parselenium-E - Nutrilite
Each tablet contains: Vitamin E (d-alpha tocopheryl acid succinate) 400 IU • Selenium 10 mcg. Other Ingredients: Parsley concentrate, Selenium yeast, Tri-calcium Phosphate.

Patented CLAPure CLA - Ultimate Nutrition
Each softgel contains: CLAPure CLA (proprietary blend providing 75-80% conjugated linoleic acid) 1000 mg. Other Ingredients: Gelatin, Glycerin, Natural Caramel Color.

PatentLEAN - Patent Health, LLC
Each capsule contains: 3-acetyl-7-oxo-dehydroepiandrosterone 100 mg.

Pau D'Arco - Source Naturals
Each tablet contains: Pau d'Arco extract (Tabebuia altissima) 500 mg • Pau d'Arco (Inner Bark) 25 mg • Vitamin C (Ascorbic Acid) 10 mg • Pro-Vitamin A (Beta Carotene) 500 IU.

Pau d'Arco-Black Walnut Virtue - Blessed Herbs
Pau d'Arco bark • Usnea lichen • Calendula flower • Echinacea Angustifolia root • Black Walnut hull • Goldenseal root • Myrrh Gum • Grain alcohol & Distilled Water.

PB8 - Nutrition Now
Each two capsules contain: Proprietary Blend 1200 mg: FOS • Lactobacillus acidophilus • Lactobacillus plantarum • Lactobacillus rhamnosus • Lactobacillus casei • Lactobacillus bulgaricus • Streptococcus thermophilus • Bifidobacterium bifidum • Bifidobacterium longum.

PC Calm - High Life Formulas
Three capsules contain: Proprietary Blend 2365 mg: Sterolins (400 mg), Cernitin 63, Scutellaria Baicalensis, Serenoa Repens (standardized 45%), Quercetin, Rabdosia Rubescens, Ganoderma Lucidum, Taraxacum Mongolicum, Isatis Indigotica, Patrinia Villosa, Panax Notoginseng, Oldenlandia Diffusa, Dendranthema Morifolium, Trifolium Pratense (4:1), Glycyrrhiza Uralensis.

PC-55 - LaneLabs
Each 1 tsp serving contains: Phosphatidyl Choline 1.43 g • Choline 210 mg. Other Ingredients: Phosphatidyl Ethanolamine, Inositol Phosphatides, Related Phospholipids.

PCA-Rx - Maxam Nutraceutics
None known.
See Editor's Note No. 41, page 2058.

PC-SPES (PCSPES, PC SPES) - BotanicLab
Each capsule contains: Proprietary Blend 320 mg: Da Qing Ye (Isatis indigotica), Licorice (Glycyrrhiza glabra, Glycyrrhiza uralensis), San Qi (Panax Pseudoginseng), Reishi Mushroom (Ganoderma lucidum), Baikal Skullcap (Scutellaria baicalensis), Chrysanthemum (Dendranthema morifolium), Rabdosia Rubescens,

Saw Palmetto (Serenoa repens).
See Editor's Note No. 7, page 2053.

Peach Drinkable Yogurt **-** Stonyfield Farm
Each 10 fl oz bottle contains: Active Live Cultures: S. Thermophilus • L. Bulgaricus • L. Acidophilus • Bifidus • L. Casei • L. Reuteri. Ingredients: Cultured Pasturized Low Fat Milk • Organic Sugar • Organic Nonfat Dry Milk • Inulin • Pectin • Beet Juice Concentrate • Organic Peach Puree • Natural Flavors.

Peach Stuff **-** Blue Stuff, Inc.
Each jar contains: Whole leaf Aloe Vera concentrate • Purified Water • Glyceryl Stearate • PEG 100 Stearate • Propylene Glycol • Glycerth-26 • Cetyl Alcohol • Stearic Acid • Hydrolyzed Elastin • Hydrolyzed Mucipolysaccharides • Revitalin • Polysorbate-20 • Carbomer-940 • Triethanolamine • Methylparaben • Fragrance • Imidazolidinyl Urean • Propylparaben • Retinol • Tocopherol • FD&C Red No. 33 • FD&C Yellow No. 6.

Peanut Butter Chocolate Pal - Revival **-** Physicians Laboratories
Each Bar Contains: Certified Isoflavone 160 mg. Ingredients: Corn syrup, Corn starch, Water, Gelatin, Artifical Flavoring, Soy Protein Isolate, Rice flour, Malt, Salt, Dry Roasted Peanuts, Glycerin, Cocoa processed with alkali, Chocolate Liquor, Dextrose, Gum Arabic, "High Oleic" Sunflower oil, Natural Flavors, Soy Lecithin.

Peanut Butter Pal - Revival **-** Physicians Laboratories
Each Bar Contains: Certified Isoflavone 160 mg. Ingredients: Corn syrup, Sugar, Corn starch, Water, Gelatin, Soy Protein Isolate, Rice flour, Malt, Salt, Dry Roasted Peanuts, Glycerin, Sunflower oil, Natural and Artificial Flavors, Soy Lecithin.

PectaSol brand **-** EcoNugenics
Modified Citrus Pectin.
See Editor's Note No. 44, page 2058.

PectaSol Modified Citrus Pectin Capsules **-** EcoNugenics
Six capsules contain: PectaSol Modified Citrus Pectin 4.8 g • Dietary Fiber 3.4 g • Sodium 90 mg • Potassium 600 mg.

PectaSol Modified Citrus Pectin Powder **-** EcoNugenics
Each scoop (five grams) contains: PectaSol Modified Citrus Pectin 5 g • Dietary Fiber 3.5 g • Sodium 90 mg • Potassium 600 mg.

Pedi-Active A.D.D. Chewables **-** Nature's Plus
Two tablets contain: LECI-PS (Phosphatidylserine-rich purified Lecithin concentrate) 100 mg • DMAE (2-dimethylaminoethanol bitartrate) 100 mg.

Pedi-Active Spray **-** Nature's Plus
Each spray contains: DMAE (2-Dimethylaminoethanol Bitartrate) 50 mg • LECI-PS Phosphatidylserine-rich purified Lecithin concentrate supplying Activated Phosphatides: [Phosphatidylserine 10 mg, Phosphatidylcholine 10 mg, Cephalin (Phosphatidylethanolamine) 6 mg, Phosphoinositides 3 mg] 50 mg. In a proprietary liposomal complex of Essential Metabolic Factors , Purified Water, Vegetable Glycerine, Purified Lecithin, Citrus seed extract (Citrus sinensis), Vitamin E & natural Wild Berry flavor.

Pedi-ADD **-** Aspen Group, Inc.
Each chewable tablet contains: Phosphatidylserine - Purified Lecithin concentrate supplying Activated Phosphatides 50 mg: Phosphatidylserine 10 mg • Phosphatidylcholine 10 mg • Cephalin (phosphatidylethanolamine) 6 mg • Phosphoinositides 5 mg • DMAE (2-dimethylaminoethanol bitartrate) 50 mg.

PediaLean **-** Klein-Becker
Each capsule contains: Pediatropin Proteinophallus Rivieri / Araceae tuber extract 500 mg.

Pediatric Chewable **-** Clinician's Choice
One tablet contains: Vitamin A (as retinyl acetate & 50% as betacarotene) 2500 IU • Vitamin C (as ascorbic acid & sodium ascorbate) 60 mg • Vitamin D (as cholecalciferol) 200 IU • Vitamin E (as dl-alpha tocopheryl acetate) 15 IU • Thiamin (as mononitrate) 0.75 mg • Riboflavin 0.9 mg • Niacin (as niacinamide) 10 mg • Vitamin B6 (as pyridoxine hydrochloride) 1 mg • Folate (as folic acid) 200 mcg • Vitamin B12 (as cyanocobalamin) 3 mcg • Biotin 30 mcg • Pantothenic Acid (as d-calcium pantothenate) 5 mg • Calcium (as carbonate & gluconate) 85 mg • Iodine (as potassium Iodide) 75 mcg • Magnesium (as oxide) 15 mg • Zinc (as oxide) 7.5 mg • Copper (as cupric oxide) 1 mg • Manganese (as citrate) 0.5 mg • Chromium (as nicotinate) 10 mcg • Molybdenum (sodium molybdate) 5 mcg • Proprietary blend 6 mg: Acerola powdered extract 4:1 • Carrot Powder, Spinach Powder.

Pediatri-Vite **-** Genestra - Seroyal
Each teaspoon (5 mL) contains: Vitamin A (palmitate) 1700 IU • Vitamin D (D3, cholecalciferol) 170 IU • Vitamin E (mixed tocopherols) 10 IU • Vitamin C (ascorbic acid) 50 mg • Thiamin Hydrochloride (vitamin B1) 800 mcg • Riboflavin (vitamin B2) 800 mcg • Niacin (vitamin B3) 4 mg • Pantothenic Acid (d-calcium pantothenate) 2 mg • Pyridoxine Hydrochloride (vitamin B6) 1 mg • Cyanocobalamin (vitamin B12) 10 mcg • Folic Acid 70 mcg • Biotin 70 mcg • Calcium (chloride) 25 mg • Potassium (aspartic acid chelate) 10 mg • Magnesium (aspartic acid chelate) 5 mg • Iron (aspartic acid chelate) 4 mg • Zinc (aspartic acid chelate) 4 mg • Manganese (aspartic acid chelate) 800 mcg • Copper (aspartic acid chelate) 500 mcg • Iodine (potassium iodide) 25 mcg • Molybdenum (aspartic acid chelate) 85 mcg • Vanadium (aspartic acid chelate) 85 mcg • Chromium (chloride) 35 mcg • Selenium (selenomethionine) 35 mcg • Choline (bitartrate) 10 mg • Inositol 800 mcg. Other Ingredients: Natural Cherry Flavor, Fructose.

Pedia-Vit **-** Progressive Labs
Two teaspoons (10 ml) contain: Vitamin A 2500 IU • Vitamin C 40 mg • Vitamin D 400 IU • Vitamin E 10 IU • Thiamin (B1) 0.7 mg • Riboflavin (B2) 0.8 mg • Niacin (B3) 9 mg • Vitamin B6 0.7 mg • Folate (folic acid) 200 mcg • Vitamin B12 3 mcg • Biotin 150 mcg • Pantothenic Acid 5 mg • Iron 10 mg • Zinc 8 mg.

Pedi-Vites Multiple **-** Aspen Group, Inc.
Each tablet contains: Vitamin A Palmitate 180 IU • Vitamin D (as Vitamin D3) 150 IU • Vitamin E 10 IU • Vitamin B1 2 mg • Vitamin B2 2 mg • Vitamin B6 2 mg • Vitamin B12 6 mcg • Vitamin C 60 mg • Niacinamide 5 mg • Folic Acid 100 mcg • Pantothenic Acid 3 mg • Biotin 30 mcg • Calcium (carbonate) 10 mg • Magnesium (gluconate) 2 mg • Manganese (gluconate) 1 mg • Selenium (selenium aspartate) 5 mcg • Chromium (chromium ACP) 5 mcg • Molybdenum (sodium molybdate) 2 mcg • Vanadium (vanadium sulfate) 2 mcg • Chlorophyll 1 mg • Boron (boron citrate) 50 mcg.

Penetran Plus **-** Transdermal Technologies
Active Ingredients: strong Ammonia solution 2.5%. Inactive Ingredients: Allantoin, Ascorbyl Palmitate, Benzethonium Chloride, Cetyl Palmitate, Cold Pressed Lemon Oil, Decanoic Acid Triglyceride, De-Ionized Water, Dexpanthenol, Glycerol Monolaurete, Imidazolinium, Methyl Sulphate, Merguard 1200, Methylsulfonylmethane, Olive Oil, Sorbitan Monopalmitate, Tocopherol Acetate.

Penetrin **-** White-Broadman, Inc.
Each capsule contains: Zinc 10 mg • L-Arginine 1125 mg • Cnidium Monnier extract 30 mg • Xanthoparmelia extract 30 mg • Gamma Amino Butyric Acid 30 mg • Naringh extract 25 mg • Quebracho extract 60 mg.

Penne - Revival **-** Physicians Laboratories
Two Ounces Contain: Certified Isoflavone 15 mg. Ingredients: Soy Protein Isolate, Niacin, Iron (Ferrous Sulfate), Thiamin Mononitrate, Riboflavin, Folic Acid.

Pentabosol Powder **-** Pentabosol
Each 5.3 g scoop contains: Riboflavin 1 mg • Biotin 600 mcg • Chromium Polynicotinate 400 mcg • Proprietary Blend 4510 mg: L-Aspartic Acid, Garcinia Cambogia extract (fruit, 50% (-)

hydroxycitric acid), L-Carnitine Tartrate. Other Ingredients: Guar Gum, Natural & Artificial Flavor, Maltodextrin, Sucralose, Citric Acid.

Pepogest **-** Nature's Way
Each softgel contains: Peppermint oil 0.2 ml • Soybean oil 0.1 ml.

Peppermint Plus **-** Enzymatic Therapy
Each enteric-coated capsule contains: Peppermint oil extract (Mentha piperita) 0.2 ml • Rosemary oil extract (Rosemarinus officinalis) 0.02 ml • Thyme oil extract (Thymus vulgaris) 0.02 ml.

PeppermintZ Intestinal Aid **-** Nature's Life
Each gel contains: Senna leaf (senna alexandria) 400 mg • Peppermint leaf oil (mentha piperita) 180 mg • Caraway seed oil (carum carvi) 50 mg • Proprietary Blend 100 mg: Lemon Balm extract (melissa officinalis), Chamomile flower extract (matricaria chamomilla), Fennel seed extract (foeniculum vulgare), Ginger root extract (zingiber officinale). Inactive Ingredients: Safflower Oil, Enteric Coated Gel Capsule, Beeswax, Lecithin.

PeptiTonic **-** DreamPharm
Each tablets contains: Proprietary Blend: Atractylodes Lanceae Rhizoma, Magnoliae Cortex, Citri Sinensis Exocarpium, Atractylodes Macrocephala Rhizoma, Sclerotium Poriae Cocos, Alismatis Rhizoma, Polyporus Umbellatus, Cinnamomi Cortex, Zingiberis Rhizoma, Zizyphus Jujuba Fructus, Papaya Leaf, Acidophilus, Montmorillanite.

Perfect Antioxidant **-** Sundown
Each caplet contains: Vitamin A (100% as beta-carotene) 7500 IU • Vitamin C (from ascorbic acid, rose hips with seeds) 250 mg • Vitamin E (as dl-alpha-tocopheryl acetate, d-alpha-tocopheryl acid succinate) 200 IU • Calcium (as calcium carbonate) 48 mg • Zinc (as zinc citrate) 7.5 mg • Selenium (as selenium amino acid chelate) 15 mcg • Copper (as cupric sulfate) 1 mg • Manganese (as manganese sulfate) 1.5 mg. Other Ingredients: Microcrystalline Cellulose, Croscarmellose Sodium, Crospovidone, Silica, Hydroxypropyl Methylcellulose, Magnesium Stearate, PEG.

Perfect Cal **-** Futurebiotics
Four tablets contain: Calcium (from Hydroxyappatite crystal) 400 mg • Calcium Complex (Citrate, Carbonate) 600 mg • Magnesium (Citrate, Oxide, Hydroxyappatite) 600 mg • Vitamin D 200 IU • Boron 1.5 mg • Horsetail (from extract) 750 mg.

Perfect Food Original Super Green Formula **-** Garden of Life, Inc.
Two heaping tablespoons (10 g) contain: Perfect Green Blend 5200 mg: 33:1 pure juice concentrates of certified organic Kamut grass, Barley grass, Oat grass, Alfalfa grass, Dandelion grass, Spirulina, Chlorella, Dunalellia, Sea Kelp, Sea Dulse, Sea Vegetables • Perfect Whole Food Matrix 2500 mg: RiceX Solubles, Certified Organic Predigested concentrates of Amaranth, Millet, Buckwheat (containing 22 amino acids, 90 antioxidants, EFAs) • Perfect Seed Blend 1500 mg: Certified Organic raw, naturally stabilized Flax seeds, Chia seeds, Sesame seeds, Sunflower seeds • Perfect Digestion, Detox and Immunity Blend 500 mg: Lactobacillus Acidophilus, L. Bulgaricus, L. Leichmanni, L. Lactis, L. Delbreukii, L. Casei, L. Caucasicus, L. Fermenti, L. Plantarum, L. Brevis, L. Helveticus, Bifidobacterium Bifidum, Bacilus Subtilis, B. Ichenformis, Live Enzymes (protease, amylasae, lipase, cellulase), PhytoSterolins • Perfect Vegetable Blend 300 mg: Certified Organic Carrot, Tomato, Beet, Broccoli, Cauliflower, Kale, Cabbage, Brussles Sprouts, Parsley, Spinach, Asparagus, Celery, Cucumber, Green Bell Pepper, Garlic, Onion, Ginger. Other Ingredients: Cellulose, Vegetable Coating.

Perfect Food Super Green Formula Caplets **-** Garden of Life, Inc.
Five caplets contain: Perfect Green Blend 2600 mg: 100% predigested blend of Barley grass juice, Wheat grass juice, Oat grass juice, Alfalfa grass juice • Perfect Protein-Mineral Blend 1000 mg: 100% pre-digested Spirulina, Chlorella, Dunaleila, Kelp, Dulse • Perfect Whole Food Matrix 1000 mg: 100% pre-digested Flax seeds, Pumpkin seeds, Sesame seeds, Sunflower seeds, Chia seeds, Garbanzo beans, Red Lentils, Miso, Kidney beands, Adzuki beans, Millet, Brown Rice, Maize, Buckwheat (gluten, phytate free) • Perfect Veggie Blend 200 mg: Carrot juice, Beet juice, Tomato juice, Sweet Potato, Broccoli, Kale, Cabbage, Cauliflower, Brussels Sprouts, Parsley, Spinach, Asparagus, Celery, Cucumber, Green Bell Pepper, Garlic, Ginger, Onion • Acerola Cherry 200 mg. Other Ingredients: Cellulose, Vegetable Coating.

Perfect Food Super Green Formula Powder **-** Garden of Life, Inc.
Two heaping tablespoons (10 g) contain: Perfect Green Blend 6000 mg: Barley grass juice, Wheat grass juice, Oat grass juice, Alfalfa grass juice • Perfect Protein-Mineral Blend 2563 mg: 50% predigested blend of Spirulina, Chlorella, Dunaliella, Kelp, Dulse • Perfect Whole Food Matrix 975 mg: 50% pre-digested blend of Brown Rice, Flax seeds, Pumpkin seeds, Sesame seeds, Sunflower seeds, Chia seeds, Garbanzo beans, Red Lentils, Miso, Kidney beans, Adzuki beans, Millet, Buckwheat (gluten free) • Perfect Veggie Blend 250 mg: 50% pre-digested blend of Carrot juice, Beet juice, Tomato juice, Sweet Potato, Broccoli, Kale, Cabbage, Cauliflower, Brussels Sprouts, Parsley, Spinach, Asparagus, Celery, Cucumber, Green Bell Pepper, Garlic, Ginger, Onion • Acerola Cherry 200 mg.

Perfect Meal Shake, Chocolate **-** Advocare International
Each packet contains: L-Lysine 1000 mg • L-Glutamine 500 mg • Choline 5 mg • Inositol 5 mg • Whole Carrot powder 100 mg • Oat Grass powder 100 mg. Other Ingredients: PM-Ultra Protein Complex (modified casein, soy protein powder, whey protein concentrate, dipeptides, tri-peptides), Fructose, Maltodextrin, Cocoa Powder, Purified Cellulose, Canola Oil, Hydrolyzed Guar Gum, Corn Syrup Solids, L-Lysine Monohydrochloride, Potassium Chloride, L-Glutamine, Calcium Carbonate, Magnesium Oxide, Soy Lecithin, Dicalcium Phosphate, Natural Flavors, Artificial Flavors, Carrot Powder, Oat Grass Powder, Lactobacillus Acidophilus, Acesulfame, Medium Chain Triglycerides, Papain, Bromelain, Rice Syrup Solids, Choline Citrate, Ascorbic Acid, Vitamin E Acetate, Inositol, Ferrous Fumarate, Niacinamide, Zinc Oxide, Calcium Pantothenate, Vitamin A Palmitate, Copper Sulfate, Manganese Sulfate, Vitamin D, Pyridoxine Hydrochloride, Riboflavin, Thiamine Mononitrate, Chromium Polynicotinate, Folic Acid, Biotin, Sodium Selenite, Sodium Molybdate, Potasssium Iodide, Vitamin K, Cyanocobalamin.

Perfectil Tablets **-** Vitabiotics
Each tablet contains: Vitamin D 5 mcg • Vitamin E (natural source) 40 mg • Vitamin C 60 mg • Vitamin B1 (thiamin) 8 mg • Vitamin B2 (riboflavin) 4 mg • Vitamin B3 (niacin) 18 mg • Vitamin B6 (pyridoxine HCl) 20 mg • Folic Acid 500 mcg • Vitamin B12 (cyanocobalamin) 9 mcg • Biotin 0.045 mg • Pantothenic Acid 40 mg • Iron 12 mg • Magnesium 75 mg • Zinc 15 mg • Iodine 200 mcg • Manganese 2 mg • Copper 2 mg • Silicon 15 mg • Chromium 50 mcg • Selenium 100 mcg • Cystine 10 mg • Natural Mixed Carotenoids 4 mg • Echinacea extract 195 mg • Burdock extract 80 mg.

Performance Enhancer Creatine Fuel **-** TwinLab
Each capsule contains: Creatine Monohydrate 700 mg.

Performance Gold **-** Advocare International
Two caplets contain: Moomiyo 100 mg • Golden Root extract (root - rhodiola rosea) 25 mg • Siberian Ginseng extract (root - eleutherococcus senticosus) 50 mg • Inosine 500 mg • Enzyme (hydrolyzed whey peptides) 1000 mg. Other Ingredients: Dicalcium Phosphate, Silicon Dioxide, Cellulose, Stearic Acid, Magnesium Stearate.

Perfor-Max **-** Changes International, Inc.
One caplet contains: Grape seed extract (vitis vinifera) 25 mg • Pine bark extract (Pinus pinaster) 25 mg • Turmeric rhisome extract 25 mg • Botanical Blend 50 mg: Green Tea leaf standardized extract (36% catechin & polyphenols), Hawthorn berry standardized extract (5% flavonoid glycosides), and Rosemary leaf extract. Other Ingredients:

Dicalcium Phosphate, Vegetable cellulose, Fractionated vegetable oil, Soy polysaccharides, Silica, and Vegetable resin glaze.

PerforMAXX **-** Optimum Nutrition
Two capsules contain: Vitamin A (as vitamin A acetate, beta carotene) 10,000 IU • Vitamin C (as ascorbic acid) 300 mg • Vitamin D (as cholecalciferol) 300 IU • Vitamin E (as D-alpha tocopheryl succinate) 200 IU • Thiamin (as thiamin mononitrate) 75 mg • Riboflavin 75 mg • Niacin (as niacinamide) 75 mg • Vitamin B6 (as pyridoxine hydrochloride) 7.5 mg • Folic Acid 400 mcg • Vitamin B12 (as cyanocobalamin) 75 mcg • Biotin 75 mcg • Pantothenic Acid (as D-calcium pantothenate) 75 mg • Calcium (as calcium phosphate) 20 mg • Iron (as ferrous fumarate) 9 mg • Iodine (as potassium iodide) 150 mcg • Magnesium (as magnesium oxide, magnesium citrate) 10 mg • Zinc (as zinc oxide, zinc gluconate) 10 mg • Selenium (as selenomethionine) 35 mcg • Copper (as copper gluconate) 1 mg • Manganese (as manganese sulfate) 1 mg • Chromium (as chromium GTF) 60 mcg • Molybdenum (as sodium molybdate) 25 mcg • Potassium (as potassium chloride) 1.8 mg • Proprietary PerforMAXX Blend 334 mg: Inositol, PABA (para-aminobenzoic acid), N-Acetyl Cysteine, Choline (as choline bitartrate), Ginkgo Biloba leaf extract (ginkgo biloba L., standardized to 24% flavone glycosides, 6% terpene lactones), Korean Ginseng root powder, Rutin, Citrus Bioflavonoid powder, Hesperidin complex, Astaxanthin, Boron (as boron citrate), Lycopene, Lutein, Tocotrienols, Alpha Carotene, Cryptoxanthin, Zeaxanthin. Other Ingredients: Gelatin, Microcrystalline Cellulose, Magnesium Stearate, Stearic Acid, Silica.

Peridin-C **-** Beutlich Pharmaceuticals
Each tablet contains: Ascorbic Acid (Vitamin C) 200 mg • Hesperidin Complex (Bioflavonoid) 150 mg • Hesperidin Methyl Chalcone (Bioflavonoid) 50 mg.

Perika St. John's Wort **-** Nature's Way
Each tablet contains: Perika (WS 5572) dried St. John's Wort extract 300 mg.

PermaSlim **-** Momentum
Two capsules contain: Vitamin B12 100 mcg • Vitamin B6 16 mg • Proprietary Blend 600 mg: Citrus Aurantium, Green Tea extract. Other Ingredients: Cellulose, Magnesium Stearate, Silicon Dioxide.
See Editor's Note No. 40, page 2058.

Permathene-16 Maximum Strength Caffeine Free **-** CCA Industries, Inc.
Each tablet contains: Phenylpropanolamine HCl 75 mg. Other Ingredients: Croscarmellose, D&C Yellow #10, Dicalcium Phosphate, FD&C Blue #1, FD&C Yellow #6, Lactose, Magnesium Stearate, Methylcellulose, Microcrystalline Cellulose, Stearic Acid, Titanium Dioxide.

Permeability Factors - Tyler **-** Integrative Therapeutics
Two softgel capsules contain: Vitamin E (as d-alpha tocopheryl acetate) 11 IU • L-Glutamine 500 mg • NAG (n-acetyl glucosamine) 250 mg • Gamma Linolenic Acid (as borage seed oil) 133 mg • Phosphatidylcholine 56 mg. Other Ingredients: Safflower Oil, Lecithin, Beeswax, Gelatin, Glycerin, Titanium Dioxide, Carob.

Persic-GLA **-** Atrium Inc.
Each capsule contains: Borage oil 100 mg • Cold Processed Persic oil yielding to the following Lipid Acids: Referred to as Vitamin F Factors (Oleic 192 mg, Linoleic 109 mg, Gamma Linolenic 30 mg, Palmitic 18 mg, Palmitoleic 5 mg, Stearic 4mg, Linolenic 701 mcg, Heptodecanoic 409 mcg, Arachadic 330 mcg, Arachidonic 111 mcg) 370 mg •Potassium 113 mcg • Sodium 14 mcg • Magnesium 7 mcg • Phosphorus 4 mg •Calcium 4 mcg.

Personal Lubricant with Aloe Vera, Calendula and Vitamin E **-** Transitions for Health, Inc.
Deionized Water • Glycerin • Carbomer • Aloe Vera Gel • Butylene Glycol • Hydroxpropyl Methylcellulose • Calendula Extract • Black Walnut Leaf Extract • Imidazolidinyl Urea • Methylparaben • Allantoin • Citric Acid • Tocopheryl Acetate • Retinyl Palmitate • Squalene.

Petadolex **-** PhytoPharmica
Each softgel contains: Purple Butterbur root extract (petasites hybridus - Petadolex brand, standardized to contain 7.5 mg petasins and to be free of pyrrolizidine alkaloids (PAs)). Other Ingredients: Medium Chain Triglycerides, Gelatin, Glycerin, Water, Riboflavin Color.

Petadolex **-** Weber & Weber
Each capsule contains: Petasites Hybridus extract (butterbur root, 30:1) 50 mg • Petasin and Isopetasin 7.5 mg. Other Ingredients: Natural Coloring, Carmine, Glycerole, Gelatin, Titanoxide.

Petaforce **-** Bioforce Ltd.
Each capsule contains: Butterbur root 30:1 dry extract (petasites hybridus) 25 mg. Other Ingredients: Triglycerides, Gelatin, Glycerol, Sorbitol (from natural plant source), Black and Red Iron Oxides.

Pevonia Anti-Aging Marine Collagen Cream **-** Pevonia Skin Care
Active Ingredients: Collagen • Hyaluronic Acid • Begetal Squalene Oil • Jonquil Essential Oil • Arnica • Micronized Titanium Dioxide.

pH Balance Mattefying Toner (combination to oily skin) **-** Nu Skin Enterprises
Water (aqua) • Hamamelis Virginiana distillate (witch hazel) • Butylene Glycol • Fragaria Vesca fruit (strawberry) • Foeniculum Vulgare fruit extract (fennel) • Copper PCA • Silica • Boron Nitride • Hypericum Perforatum extract • Anthemis Nobilis flower extract • Calendula Officinalis flower extract • Centaurea Cyanus flower extract • Chamomilla Recutita flower extract (matricaria) • Tilia Cordata flower extract • Glycerin • PEG-40 Hydrogenated Castor oil • Fragrance (parfum) • Tetrasodium EDTA • Benzoic Acid • Phenoxyethanol • Chlorphenesin • Methylparaben • Ethylparaben.

pH Balance Toner (normal to dry skin) **-** Nu Skin Enterprises
Water (aqua) • Aloe Barbadensis • Hamamelis Virginiana distillate (witch hazel) • Glycerin • Butylene Glycol • Fragaria Vesca fruit (strawberry) • Camphor • Fucus Vesiculosus extract • Gellidiela Acerosa extract (algae) • Hypnea Musciformis extract • Sargassum Filipendula extract (algae) • Hyaluronic Acid • Sodium PCA • Royal Jelly • Sorbitol • Citric Acid • Triethanolamine • Disodium EDTA • Phenoxyethanol • Methylparaben • Caramel.

PharmaPure PharmaFlex 500 **-** Pure Tek Corp.
Each three tablets contain: Glucosamine 1500 mg • Chondroitin 600 mg • Phellodendron bark extract (Nexrutine) 500 mg.
See Editor's Note No. 15, page 2055.

PharmaPure PharmaFlex 750 **-** Pure Tek Corp.
Each two tablets contain: Glucosamine 1500 mg • Phellodendron bark extract (Nexrutine) 750 mg.

Pharmaton Antistax **-** Boehringer Ingelheim
Each capsule contains: Red Vine leaf extract 180 mg. Other Ingredients: Gelatin, Dried Glucose Syrup, Silicon Dioxide, Talc, Maize Starch, Magnesium Stearate, Colours (E 172, E 171).

Pharmaton Flexium Joint Comfort **-** Boehringer Ingelheim
Two tablets contain: SAM-e (as S-adenosylmethionine 1,4-butanedisulfonate) 400 mg. Other Ingredients: Microcrystalline Cellulose, Sodium Startch Glycolate, Methacrylic Acid Copolymer, Talc, Polyethylene Glycol 6000, Colloidal Silica, Magnesium Stearate, Polysorbate 80, Sodium Hydroxide, Iron Oxide, Simethicone.

Pharmaton Flexium Joint Comfort & Cartilage Renewal **-** Boehringer Ingelheim
Each tablet contain: SAM-e (as S-adenosylmethionine 1,4-butanedisulfonate) 200 mg • Glucosamine HCl 500 mg. Other Ingredients: Microcrystalline Cellulose, Sodium Starch Glycolate, Povidone, Methacrylic Acid Copolymer, Talc, Polyethylene Glycol

6000, Magnesium Stearate, Colloidal Silica, Polysorbate 80, Sodium Hydroxide, Iron Oxide, Simethicone.

Phase 2 **-** Swanson
Two capsules contain: Phaseolamin 2250 Phaseolus vulgaris L. from White Kidney Bean (dried bean fraction) 1 g. Other Ingredients: Gelatin, Magnesium Stearate.

Phase'oLean Forte **-** Life Plus
Each tablet contains: Kidney Bean (Phaseolus vulgaris L.) protein concentrate 500 mg.

PhenCal 106 **-** Great American Nutrition
Six tablets contain: Vitamin B6 (as pyridoxal-5-phosphate) 30 mg • Chromium (as picolinate) 200 mcg • DL-Phenylalanine 2700 mg • L-Tyrosine 300 mg • L-Glutamine 150 mg • L-5-Hydroxytryptophan 15 mg • L-Carnitine 60 mg.

Phen-First **-** Life Extension
Each tablet contains: Ma Huang extract 150 mg • Guarana extract 350 mg • L-Carnitine Fumerate 50 mg • Chromium Picolinate 200 mcg • St. John's Wort 150 mg • Uva Ursi 12.5 mg • Korean Ginseng 12.5 mg • Phenylalanine 12.5 mg • Ginkgo Biloba 12.5 mg • Vitamin B6 5 mg • Vitamin B12 5 mg • Calcium Pyruvate 50 mg • Green Tea extract 12.5 mg.
See Editor's Note No. 30, page 2056.

Phen-Free **-** EAS
Four capsules contain: Caffeine 99 mg • Citrus aurantium 300 mg (Bitter Orange peel standardized to 6% Synephrine) • Yohimbe 100 mg • Cordyceps 500 mg (standardized to 7% Cordyceptic Acid) • L-Tyrosine 500 mg • St. John's Wort 200 Mg (standardized to 0.3% Hypericin) • Cayenne Pepper powder 30 mg.
See Editor's Note No. 40, page 2058.

Phenolox **-** Metabolic Nutrition
Six capsules contain: Green Tea leaf (50%/35%) 1800 mg • Advantra Z Citrus Aurantium (6%) 900 mg • Di Potassium Phosphate 600 mg • L-Carnitine 510 mg • L-Phenylalanine 300 mg • Cayenne pepper extract 300 mg • Coleus Forskohlii (20%) 270 mg • Yohimbe (3%) 180 mg • Chromium Picolinate 750 mcg.
See Editor's Note No. 40, page 2058.

Phen-Rx **-** Athletic Technologies Inc.
Each capsule contains: Magnesium 75 mg • Vitamin E 3 IU • Zinc 1 mg • Chromium Picolinate 10 mcg • Guarana extract (33%) 300 mg • Theobromine 100 mg • Cocoa powder 200 mg • Konjac root 20 mg • Ginger root powder 5 mg • Spirulina 5 mg • Damiana powder 5 mg • Garcinia Cambogia (50% HCA) 5 mg • Gotu Kola 5 mg • Lecithin powder 5 mg.

PhenSafe **-** Applied Nutrition
Three capsules contain: St. John's Wort (.3% hypericin) 300 mg • L-Glutamic Acid HCl 100 mg • B6 Pyridoxine HCl 20 mg • Niacinamide (B3) 10 mg • Zinc 8 mg • Folic Acid 200 mcg • ChromeMate 125 mcg • B12 100 mcg • Selenium 75 mcg. Each serving of the above nutrients is formulated with a special mixture containing these natural ingredients: [Advantra Z (citrus aurantium), Licorice root powder, Ginger root powder, Cayenne powder, Mustard seed powder, Green Tea extract, Fennel seed powder, BioPerine] 640 mg.
See Editor's Note No. 40, page 2058.

Phenyltropic X **-** Mass Quantities, Inc.
Each capsule contains: Proprietary blend 650 mg: Sida Cordifolia • Synepherine • Guarana • White Willow Bark • Commiphora Mukul.
See Editor's Note No. 40, page 2058.

Phoenaz **-** Dazzle, Inc.
Three tablets contain: Vitamin E 60 mg • Vitamin B6 • Calcium carbonate granularV Proprietary Blend 3012 mg: Rye Flour, Malt powder diastatic, Barley Grass, Wheat Grass powder, Blessed Thistle, Wild Yam extract, Corn powder, Damiana leaf powder, Saw Palmetto extract, Soy Isoflavones, European Hops.

Phoenaz **-** Phoenaz, Inc.
Six tablets contain: Calcium (as Calcium Carbonate) 36 mg • Proprietary Blend 520 mg: L-Arginine, Mucuna Pruriens (15% L-Dopa), Ashwaganda, Basil, Alpha GPC, Tribulis Terrestrial extract 40%, Cordyceps Sinesis extract, Optizine. Other Ingredients: Magnesium Stearate, Silicone Dioxide, Gelatin.

Phos Fuel **-** TwinLab
Four capsules contain: Sodium Phosphate (Dibasic) 4000 mg • Potassium Bicarbonate 816 mg • L-Carnosine 50 mg • Lipoic Acid 100 mcg • Vitamin B1 1.5 mg • Vitamin B2 1.9 mg • Vitamin B3 (Niacinamide) 20 mg • Vitamin B6 2 mg • Pantothenic Acid 10 mg • Biotin 300 mcg.

PhosphaGems **-** EAS
Each 42 gram serving contains: Phosphagen (HPCE pure Creatine Monohydrate) 5.2 g • TriCarb Complex (Sucrose, High-Dextrose Corn Syrup & Dextrose) • Phosphagen (HPCE pure Creatine Monohydrate) • Modified Starch • Natural & Artificial Flavor • Disodium Phosphate • Malic Acid • Colored with Cochineal extracts.

Phosphagen **-** EAS
Each 5 gram serving contains: Phosphagen 5 g.

Phosphatide I-C-E **-** Progressive Labs
Each softgel contains: Phosphatidylcholine 420 mg • Phosphatidylethanolamine 210 mg • Phosphatidylinositol 120 mg • Total Phosphatides 750 mg. All phosphatides extracted from soybeans. This product contains the highest known concentration of naturally occuring phosphatides.

Phosphatidyl Choline **-** Source Naturals
Each softgel contains: Soy lecithin 1,200 mg • Phosphatidyl Choline 420 mg.

Phosphatidyl Choline Complex **-** Nature's Life
Each capsule contains: Phosphatidyl Choline Complex (Soy)120 mg. Nutrient profile based on a typical analysis: Phosphatides: Phosphatidyl Choline (contains 65 mg Choline) 420 mg • Phosphatidyl Ethanolamine 108 mg • Phosphatidyl Inositol (contains 6 mg Inositol) 24 mg • Phosphatidic Acid 36 mg. Lipids: Linoleic Acid (Omega-6) 313 mg • Linolenic Acid (Omega-3) 24 mg • Oleic Acid (Omega-9) 73 mg • Palmitic Acid 78 mg • Stearic Acid 24 mg.

Phosphatidyl Serine **-** Progressive Labs
Each softgel contains: Phospholipids: Phosphatidylserine (soy phospholipid) 100 mg • Phosphatidylcholine (soy phospholipid) 45 mg • Phosphatidylethanolamine (soy phospholipid) 10 mg • Phosphatidylinositol (soy phospholipid) 10 mg. Fatty Acids: Linoleic Acid 113 mg • Linolenic Acid 11 mg • Oleic Acid 12 mg • Stearic Acid 1 mg • Palmitic Acid 24 mg • Capric Acid 49 mg • Caprylic Acid 130 mg. Minerals: Phosphorus 8 mg • Potassium 3 mg.

Phosphatidyl Serine 50 - GNC A-Z **-** GNC
Each capsule contains: Phosphatidyl Serine 50 mg. Other Ingredients: Soybean oil, Gelatin, Glycerin.

Phosphatidylserine **-** PhysioLogics
Two capsules contain: Phosphatidylserine Complex 500 mg. Phospholipids: Phosphatidylserine 100 mg • Phosphatidylcholine 100 mg • Phosphatidylethanolamine 60 mg • Phosphatidylinositol 30 mg. Fatty Acids: Linoleic Acid 135 mg • Linolenic Acid 30 mg • Oleic Acid 25 mg • Stearic Acid 15 mg • Palmitic Acid 45 mg. Minerals: Phosphorus 15 mg • Potassium 5 mg.

Phosphatidylserine Complex **-** PhysioLogics
Each softgel contains: Vitamin C (as ascorbic acid) 5 mg • Phospholipid Complex 500 mg: Soy Lecithin standardized to contain 20% phosphatidylserine 100 mg, Phosphatidic Acid, Phosphatidylinositol, Soy Phospholipids/Glycerides, Phosphatidylcholine, Phosphatidylethanolamine. Other Ingredients: Gelatin, Glycerin, Caramel Color, Sorbitol, Titanium Dioxide Color.

Phosphatidylserine Complex **-** NSI - Nutraceutical Sciences Institute
Each softgel contains: Phosphatidylserine 100 mg • Phosphatidylcholine 45 mg • Phosphatidylehtnaolamine 10 mg • Phosphatidylinositol 5 mg.

Phosphatidylserine Complex **-** Solgar
Each tablet contains: Calcium (as dl-calcium phosphate) 40 mg • Phosphatidylserine Complex 500 mg • Phosphatidylserine 100 mg • Phosphatidylcholine 100 mg • Phosphatidylethanolamine 60 mg • Phosphatidylinositol 30 mg.Other Ingredients: Soy Lecithin powder (phosphatidylserine complex), Microcrystalline Cellulose, Dicalcium Phosphate, Vegetable Cellulose, Vegetable Stearic Acid, Vegetable Magnesium Stearate, Silica, Vegetable Glycerin.

Phosphatidylserine Complex **-** The Vitamin Shoppe
Each softgel contains: 500 mg Phospholipids providing 100 mg of Phosphatidylserine and 400 mg other Phospholipids.

Phosphatidylserine Complex With Ginkgo **-** PhysioLogics
Each softgel contains: Vitamin C (as ascorbic acid) 5 mg • Phospholipid Complex from Soy Lecithin 500 mg: standardized to contain 20% Phosphatidylserine 100 mg, Phosphatidic Acid, Phosphatidylinositol, Soy Phospholipids/Glycerides, Phosphatidylcholine, Phosphatidylethanolamine • Ginkgo Biloba extract (standardized to contain 24% ginkgoflavoneglycosides, 7.2 mg) 30 mg. Other Ingredients: Gelatin, Glycerin, Lecithin, Yellow Beeswax, Caramel Color, Sorbitol, Titanium Dioxide Color.

Phospholoba Q10 **-** Olympian Labs
Two capsules contain: Phophatidylserine Complex 500 mg • Ginkgo Biloba 30 mg • Coenzyme Q10 15 mg • Fatty Acids & Minerals 270 mg.

PhosSerine Complex **-** NutriCology
Three softgels contain: Vitamin C (as ascorbic acid) 10 mg • Phosphatidylserine and Lysophosphatidylserine 100 mg • Other Phospholipids and Glycerides 380 mg • Soy Oil 200 mg.

PhysioKids MultiLogics Chewable **-** PhysioLogics
Two tablets contain: Vitamin A (as beta carotene) 5000 IU • Vitamin C (ascorbic acid) 60 mg • Vitamin D (as ergocalciferol) 400 IU • Vitamin E (as d-alpha tocopherol acetate) 30 IU • Thiamin (as thiamine HCl) 1.5 mg • Riboflavin 1.7 mg • Niacin (as niacinamide) 20 mg • Vitamin B6 (as pyridoxine HCl) 2 mg • Folate (folic acid) 10 mcg • Vitamin B12 (as cyanocobalamin) 6 mcg • Biotin 50 mcg • Pantothenic Acid (as calcium pantothenate) 10 mg • Calcium (as calcium amino acid chelate) 20 mg • Iron (as iron amino acid chelate) 5 mg • Iodine (from kelp) 100 mcg • Magnesium (as magnesium amino acid chelate) 10 mg • Zinc (as zinc amino acid chelate) 3 mg • Copper (as copper amino acid chelate) 0.05 mg • Manganese (as manganese amino acid chelate) 0.05 mg • Potassium (as potassium amino acid chelate) 1 mg • Apple (fruit) 50 mg • Papaya (fruit) 50 mg • Pineapple (fruit) 50 mg • Lemon Bioflavonoids 20 mg • Spirulina 20 mg • Sunflower Oil (seed) 20 mg • Rice Bran 10 mg • Beet Greens (leaf) 5 mg • Broccoli (aerial parts) 5 mg • Brown Rice 5 mg • Carrot (root) 5 mg • Dog Rose (rose hips) 5 mg • Mango (fruit) 5 mg • Spinach (leaf) 5 mg • West Indian Cherry (malpighia prunicifolia, fruit) 5 mg • Para-aminobenzoic Acid (PABA) 400 mcg • Choline (as choline bitartrate) 10 mcg • Inositol 10 mcg. Other Ingredients: Fructose, Maple Crystals, Honey, Molasses, Natural Cherry Flavor, Silica, Beet Juice, Magnesium Stearate, Fruit Juices.

PhysioSoy Powder - Chocolate **-** PhysioLogics
Each scoop (31 g) contains: Potassium 180 mg • Dietary Fiber <2g • Protein 25 g • L-Alanine 1035 mg • L-Arginine 1847 mg • L-Aspartic Acid 2826 mg • L-Cysteine 307 mg • L-Glutamic Acid 4646 mg • L-Glycine 1035 mg • L-Histidine 643 mg • L-Isoleucine 1203 mg • L-Leucine 1987 mg • L-Lysine 1539 mg • L-Methionine 307 mg • L-Phenylalanine 1259 mg • L-Proline 1231 mg • L-Serine 1259 mg •L-Threonine 923 mg • L-Tryptophan 335 mg • L-Tyrosine 923 mg • L-Valine 1231 mg • Isoflavone Blend 50 mg: Genistein 30 mg, Daidzein 17 mg, Glycitein 3 mg. Other Ingredients: Isolated Soy Protein, Cocoa Powder, Natural/Artificial Flavors, Soy Lecithin, Acesulfame Potassium, Salt.

PhysioSoy Powder - Natural Flavor **-** PhysioLogics
Each scoop (31 g) contains: Potassium 30 mg • Protein 24 g • L-Alanine 1036 mg • L-Arginine 1848 mg • L-Aspartic Acid 2828 mg • L-Cysteine 308 mg • L-Glutamic Acid 4648 mg • L-Glycine 1036 mg • L-Histidine 644 mg • L-Isoleucine 1204 mg • L-Leucine 1988 mg • L-Lysine 1540 mg • L-Methionine 308 mg • L-Phenylalanine 1260 mg • L-Proline 1232 mg • L-Serine 1260 mg • L-Threonine 924 mg • L-Tryptophan 336 mg • L-Tyrosine 924 mg • L-Valine 1232 mg • Isoflavone Blend 50 mg: Genistein 30 mg, Daidzein 17 mg, Glycitein 3 mg. Other Ingredients: Isolated Soy Protein (with <2% lecithin).

PhysioSoy Powder - Vanilla **-** PhysioLogics
Each scoop (29 g) contains: Potassium 70 mg • Protein 25 g • L-Alanine 1050 mg • L-Arginine 1874 mg • L-Aspartic Acid 2827 mg • L-Cysteine 312 mg • L-Glutamic Acid 4713 mg • L-Glycine 1050 mg • L-Histidine 653 mg • L-Isoleucine 1221 mg • L-Leucine 2016 mg • L-Lysine 1561 mg • L-Methionine 312 mg • L-Phenylalanine 1277 mg • L-Proline 1249 mg • L-Serine 1277 mg • L-Threonine 937 mg • L-Tryptophan 340 mg • L-Tyrosine 937 mg • L-Valine 1249 mg • Isoflavone Blend 50 mg: Genistein 30 mg, Daidzein 17 mg, Glycitein 3 mg. Other Ingredients: Isolated Soy Protein, Natural/Artificial Flavors, Soy Lecithin, Acesulfame Potassium.

PhysioWhey Powder **-** PhysioLogics
Two rounded scoops (28 g) contain: Calcium 70 mg • Phosphorus 70 mg • Magnesium 10 mg • Sodium 55 mg • Potassium 150 mg • L-Glutamine 100 mg • L-Isoleucine 100 mg • L-Leucine 100 mg • L-Valine 100 mg • Stevia leaf extract (stevia rebaudiana) 80 mg. Other Ingredients: Whey Protein Concentrate, Natural Flavors, Fructose, Xanthan Gum.

Phyt•Aloe, Capsules (PhytAloe, Phyt Aloe, Phyt-Aloe) **-** Mannatech
Each capsule contains: Proprietary Blend Phyt Aloe Complex 490 mg: Broccoli, Brussels Sprout, Cabbage, Carrot, Cauliflower, Garlic, Kale, Onion, Tomato, Turnip, Papaya, Pineapple • Ambrotose Complex (patent pending) 50 mg: Arabinogalactan (larix decidua gum), Manapol Aloe Vera gel extract (inner leaf gel), Gum Ghatti, Gum Tragacanth. Other Ingredients: Gelatin, Magnesium Stearate.

PhytAloe, Powder (PhytAloe, Phyt Aloe, Phyt-Aloe) **-** Mannatech
Each one-half teaspoon contains: Proprietary Blend Phyt•Aloe Complex 907 mg: Broccoli, Brussels Sprout, Cabbage, Carrot, Cauliflower, Garlic, Kale, Onion, Tomato, Turnip, Papaya, Pineapple • Ambrotose Complex (patent pending) 93 mg: Arabinogalactan (larix decidua gum), Manapol Aloe Vera gel extract (inner leaf gel), Gum Ghatti, Gum Tragacanth.

Phyto Estrogen Power **-** Nature's Herbs
Four capsules contain: Soy Germ Isoflavone concentrate 1400 mg • Kudzu root extract 100 mg • Certified Potency Korean Ginseng extract 100 mg • Certified Potency Dong Quai extract 100 mg • Mexican Wild Yam extract 100 mg • Boron 3 mg • Natural Vitamin E 800 IU. In a base of Chasteberry powder and Arrowroot.

Phyto Flavonoids **-** Olympia Nutrition
Contains the extracts of Silymarin, Curcumin, Green Tea, Quercetin, Rosemary, Bilberry, Hawthorn, Ginger, Ginkgo Biloba, Bromelain, Cranberry.

Phyto Surge **-** PhytoPharmica
One tablespoon contains: Arsenicum album 6x • Nux vomica 3x • Podophyllum peltatum 3x • Cinchona officinalis 2x • Rhamnus frangula 2x • Artemisia vulgaris 1x • Avena sativa 1x • Cinnamomum 1x • Gentiana lutea 1x • Sterculia acuminata 1x. In a base of 20% USP alcohol by volume.
See Editor's Note No. 1 and No. 21.

Some Brand Name Natural Products - What they Contain

www.NaturalDatabase.com contains MANY more listings than appear here.

Phyto•Bears (Phyto-Bears, Phyto Bears, PhytoBears) **-** Mannatech
Each Phyto-Bear contains: Phyt•Aloe Complex 40 mg: Broccoli, Brussels Sprout, Cabbage, Carrot, Cauliflower, Garlic, Kale, Onion, Tomato, Turnip, Papaya, Pineapple • Ambrotose Complex 4 mg: naturally occurring plant polysaccharides including freeze-dried Aloe Vera inner leaf gel extract - Manapol powder. Other Ingredients: Corn syrup, Sucrose water, Gelatin, Citric acid, Grape juice concentrate, Natural flavors, Natural colors, Olive oil, Beeswax.
See Editor's Note No. 17, page 2055.

Phyto•Bears w/Ambrotose Complex (Phyto-Bears, PhytoBears, Phyto Bears) **-** Mannatech
Each bear contains: Proprietary Blend Phyt Aloe Complex 40 mg: Broccoli, Brussels Sprout, Cabbage, Carrot, Cauliflower, Garlic, Kale, Onion, Tomato, Turnip, Papaya, Pineapple • Ambrotose Complex (patent pending) 4 mg: Naturally Occurring Plant Polysaccharides (including freeze-dried aloe vera inner leaf gel extract - manapol powder). Other Ingredients: Corn Syrup, Sucrose, Water, Gelatin, Citric Acid, Grape Juice Concentrate, Natural Flavors, Natural Colors, Olive Oil, Beeswax.
See Editor's Note No. 17, page 2055.

Phyto-Biotic **-** Enzymatic Therapy
Each capsule contains: Barberry Bark of root extract 6:1 (berberis vulgaris) 200 mg • Oregon Grape root extract 6:1 (berberis aquifolium) 200 mg • Goldenseal root extract (hydrastis canadensis, standardized to contain 5% total alkaloids including berberine, hydrastine & canadine) 50 mg.

Phyto-Clear **-** Phytohealing Inc.
Aloe Vera gel, Huang Lian herb extract, Huang Qin herb extract, Glucose, Cellulose, Thickening Agents.

PhytoDefense **-** GNLD International, LLC.
Each packette contains: Vitamin A (as beta-carotene) 7500 IU • Vitamin C (as ascorbic acid) 100 mg • Vitamin E (as D-alpha-tocopherol) 18 IU • Lycopene 1200 mcg • Lutein / Zeaxanthin 410 mcg • Carotenoid Complex Blend 900 mg: Wild Carrot root oleoresin (daucus carota), Red Bell Pepper fruit oleoresin (capsicum frutescens), Tomato fruit oleoresin (lycopersicon esculentum), Spinach leaves oleoresin (spinacia oleracea), Apricot fruit concentrate (prunus armeniacea), Strawberry fruit concentrate (fragaria vesca), Peach fruit concentrate (prunus persica) • Flavonoid Complex Blend 654 mg: Cranberry fruit extract (vaccinium macrocarpus), Kale leaves concentrate (brassica oleracea acephala), Green Tea leaves extract (camellia sinensis), Beet root concentrate (beta vulgaris), Elderberry fruit extract (sambucus nigra), Red Grape Skin extract (vitis vinifera), Black Grape Skin extract (vitis vinifera), Orange fruit extract (citrus aurantium), Lemon fruit (citrus limon), Grapefruit fruit extract (citrus paradisi) • Cruciferous Complex Blend 525 mg: Soymilk powder, Broccoli leaves extract (brassica oleracea botrytis), Radish root extract (raphanus sativus), Kale leaves extract (brassica oleracea acephala), Orange fruit extract (citrus aurantium), Black Mustard fruit extract (brassica nigra), Licorice root extract (glycyrrhiza glabra), Brown Mustard fruit concentrate (brassica nigra), Watercress leaves and stem concentrate (rorippa nasturtium officinale). Other Ingredients: Microcrystalline Celluose, Gelatin, Olive Oil, Glycerin, Yellow Beeswax, Calcium Carbonate, Purified Water, Lecithin, Sodium Croscarmellose, Stearic Acid, Starch, Silicon Dioxide, Hydroxypropyl Methylcellulose, Soybean Oil, Triacetin, Natural Colors, Simethicone.

Phytodolor **-** PhytoPharmica
Active Ingredients: Common ash (Fraxinus excelsior) bark (4.5:1) 0.20 ml • Aspen (Populus tremula) leaves & bark (4.5:1) 0.60 ml • Goldenrod (Solidago virgaurea) aerial (4.8:1) 0.20 ml. Other Ingredients: Water, Alcohol (45.6%). This patented liquid formula is standardized to contain: Salicin-0.75 mg/ml, Salicylic alcohol-0.042 mg/ml, Isofraxidin-0.015 mg/ml, and Rutin-0.06 mg/ml.
See Editor's Note No. 21, page 2056.

Phytoestrin **-** USANA Health Sciences
Each tablet contains: Soy Isoflavones (Glycine Max) seed 14.0 mg • Black Cohosh extract (Cimicifuga Racemosa) root 50.0 mg • Chasteberry powder (Vitex Agnus-Castus) fruit 50.0 mg • Licorice root extract (Glycyrrhiza Glabrera) 30.0 mg • Dong Quai extract (Angelica Sinensis) root 15.0 mg. Other Ingredients: Dextrose, Ascorbyl Palmitate, Croscarmellose Sodium, Dextrin (Modified Food Starch), Colloidal Silicon Dioxide.

Phytoestrogen Body Cream **-** Transitions for Health, Inc.
Deionized Water • Carbomer • Jojoba Oil • Caprylic / Caprice Triglycerides • Cetyl Ester • Glyceryl Stearate • Ginseng Extract • Glycerin • Peg-100 Stearate • Stearic Acid • Aloe Vera Gel • Hydrolyzed Glycosaminoglycans • Black Walnut Leaf Extract • Black Cohosh Extract • Licorice Root Extract • Chaste Tree Berry Extract • Evening Primrose Oil • Tocopheryl Acetate • Triethanolamine • Imidazolidinyl Urea • Methylparaben • Xanthan Gum • Grape Seed Extract • Red Clover Blossom Extract • Propylparaben • Butylene Glycol • Orange Oil.

Phyto-Estrogen Cream **-** Nature's Herbs
Each ounce contains: Active Ingredients: Liposomal Soy Isoflavone extract 60 mg • Pomegranate seed juice extract 150 mg • Red Clover tops extract 80 mg • Black Cohosh root extract 80 mg • Dong Quai root extract 25 mg. Inactive Ingredients: Purified Water, Lecithin Phospholipid, Aloe Vera Gel, Caprylic/Capric Triglyceride, Glyceryl Stearate, Glycerin, Cetearyl Alcohol, Ceteareth-20, Cetyl Alcohol, Stearic Acid, Tocopheryl Acetate (Natural Vitamin E), Cocoa Butter, Grapefruit seed extract, Methylparaben, Propylparaben, Dowicil, Sorbic Acid, Xanthan Gum, Rosemary Oil, Natural Cherry Almond Fragrance.

Phyto-Flavonoids **-** Futurebiotics
Two capsules contain: Procyanidol • Whole Grape extract* 50 mg • Green Tea powder concentrate 150 mg • Citrus bioflavonoids 500 mg • Rutin 75 mg • Quercetin 150 mg • Soy isoflavone extract 500 mg • Berry blend (Raspberry, Blackberry, Blueberry) 200 mg • Cruciferous Vegetable powder blend 200 mg. *Procyanidol is a concentrated solvent-free grape extract containing high levels of flavonoid polyphenols.

Phyto-Fruit **-** Olympia Nutrition
Guava • Papaya • Mango • Raspberry • Blueberry • Grapefruit • Grape • Ginseng.

PhytoFruit Concentrates **-** Now
Two V Caps contain: Grape seed extract (95% Polyphenols) 20 mg • Concentrated fruit extract powders: Acerola Cherry 50 mg, Cranberry 50 mg, Guava 50 mg, Papaya 50 mg, Raspberry 50 mg, Blueberry 50 mg, Grapefruit 50 mg, Mango 50 mg, Pineapple 50 mg, Strawberry 50 mg • Panax ginseng (5% Ginsenosides) 50 mg • Bromelain (2000 GDU from pineapple) 50 mg • Protease (100 SAP Units) 50 mg • Amylase (3000 DU Units) 50 mg • Lipase (100 LU Units) 50 mg • Cellulase (500 CMC Units) 50 mg.

PhytoGreens **-** Genestra - Seroyal
Each tablespoon contains: Wheat Grass juice 400 mg • Barley Grass juice 400 mg • Alfalfa Grass juice 400 mg • Green Papaya juice 400 mg • Red Beet juice 200 mg • Acerola berry juice 25 mg • Spirulina 1000 mcg • Chlorella 600 mg • Broccoli 600 mg • Cauliflower 600 mg • Lecithin 2000 mg • Phosphatidylcholine 480 mg • Wheat sprout 400 mg • Octacosanol 250 mg • Spinach 250 mg • Dunaliella Salina 50 mg • Dandelion (Iaraxacuru officinale) 50 mg • Celandine (Chelidonium majus) 50 mg • Ginkgo (Ginkgo biloba, 50:1, standardized to 24% ginkgoflavoglycosides, 6% terpene lactones) extract 40 mg • Bilberry (Vaccinium myrtillus, standardized 25% anthocyanins) extract 40 mg • Grape Seed (standardized 85% proanthocyanidins) extract 40 mg • FOS (fructo-oligo-saccharides) 1000 mg • Apple Pectin 25 mg • Bromelain (pineapple) 25 mg • Parsley (Petroselinum sativum) 25 mg • Celery (Apium graveolens) 25 mg • Watercress (Nasturtium officinale) 25 mg • Papain (papaya) 25 mg • Bee Pollen (entomophilous) 200 mg.

***Phytokids Formula* - Body Language Vitamin Co.**
Two chewable tablets contain: Beta Carotene 2500 IU • Magnesium 25 mg • Vitamin B1 1.5 mg • Calcium 50 mg • Vitamin B2 1.7 mg • Selenium 50 mcg • Vitamin B5 10 mg • Manganese 1 mg • Vitamin B6 2 mg • Zinc 5 mg • Niacinamide 10 mg • Iodine 50 mcg • Vitamin B12 6 mcg • Copper 500 mcg • Folic Acid 200 mcg • Molybdenum 2 mcg • Vitamin D (vitamin D3) 400 IU • Vanadium 2 mcg • Vitamin K 80 mcg • Boron 25 mcg • Vitamin E 60 IU • Silica 5 mg • Vitamin C 100 mg • Choline 50 mg • Biotin 200 mcg • Grape Seed extract 1 mg • Pine Bark extract 1 mg • Green Tea extract 20 mg • Flavonoids 50 mg • Lycopene 50 mg • Quercetin 10 mg • Allicin 10 mg • Soy Lecithin 25 mg • Phosphatidylcholine 25 mg.

***Phytolax* - 4 Life**
Each capsule contains: Alder Buckthorn (bark) 100 mg • Cascara Sagrada (bark) 95 mg • Ginger (root) 90 mg • Parsley (leaf) 35 mg • Black Walnut (hull) 30 mg • Frangula extract (bark) 20 mg. Other Ingredients: Xanthum Gum, Gelatin Capsule, Magnesium Stearate.

***PhytoMax* - PhytoPharmica**
Two capsules contain: St. John's Wort (Hypericum perforatum) flower head extract (standardized to contain 0.3% hypericin and 4% hyperforin) 500 mg • Valerian (Valeriana officinalis) root extract (standardized to contain a minimum of 0.8% valerenic acids) 30 mg • Passion Flower (Passiflora incarnata) dried aerial part extract 4:1 30 mg.
See Editor's Note No. 21, page 2056.

***Phytonutritional* - Natural Connections, Inc.**
Each 9500 mg contains: Wheat Grass juice powder 400 mg • Barley Grass juice powder 400 mg • Alfalfa Grass juice powder 400 mg • Green Papaya 400 mg • Blue Green Algae & Spirulina 800 mg • Chlorella (cracked-cell) 800 mg • Broccoli freeze-dried powder 800 mg • Cauliflower freeze-dried powder 800 mg • Lecithin (with phosphatidylcholine) 2000 mg • Wheat Sprout powder (gluten-free) 400 mg • Acerola berry juice powder 300 mg • Beet juice powder 200 mg • Spinach & Octacosanol powder 500 mg • Dunaliella Salina 50 mg • Green Tea extract (60% catechins) 50 mg • Milk Thistle (silybum marianum, 80% silymarin) 50 mg • Ginkgo Biloba (24% ginkgoflavonglycosides, 6% terpenes) 50 mg • Bilberry (25% anthocyanidins) 40 mg • Proanthocyanidins as grape seed extract OPC 85+ and pine bark extract OPC 85 40 mg • Probiotic Cultures (dairy free) 10 billion CFU: L-Acidophilus (DDS-1), L-Rhamnosus, L-Bifidus, S, Lactis, Bifidobacterium longum, B. Bifidim, S. Thermophilus • Fructooligosaccharides (FOS) 1000 mg.
Inactive Ingredients: Apple Pectin, Bromelain (lower stem, pineapple plants, parsley, celery and watercress).

***Phytoslim Active* - Aboca USA, Inc**
Each capsule contains: Bitter Orange young fruit freeze-dried extract (citrus x aurantium, standardized to 5% sinephrine) 242 mg • Green Tea leaf powder (camellia sinensis, standardized to 3% caffeine, to 6% EGCG) 157 mg • Chromium Yeast (saccharomices cerevisiae with chromium, 0.2% organically bound) 25 mg. Other Ingredients: Gelatin (capsule).
See Editor's Note No. 40, page 2058.

***Phytoslim Purifier* - Aboca USA, Inc**
Each tea bag (two grams) contains: Java Tea leaf (orthosiphon stamineus) 0.4 g • Licorice root (glycyrrhiza glabra) 0.4 g • Fennel fruit (foeniculum vulgare) 0.34 g • European Goldenrod flowering top (solidago virgaurea) 0.2 g • Certified Organic Peppermint leaf (mentha piperita) 0.2 g • Certified Organic Dandelion root (taxacum officinale) 0.16 g • Turmeric root (curcuma longa) 0.1 g • Horsetail top (equisetum arvense) 0.1 g • Certified Organic Stinging Nettle leaf (urtica dioica) 0.1 g.

***Phytoslim Reduce* - Aboca USA, Inc**
Each packet contains: Dietary Fiber 2110 mg • Glucomannan micronized tuber (amorphophallus konjac, standardized to 76% fiber) 1500 mg • Tangerine fruit dehydrated juice (citrus reticulata blanco) 1000 mg • Mannite (micronized) 900 mg • Chicory root (cichorium intybus, inulin extracted from the root standardized to 89% fiber) 750 mg • Orange fruit dehydrated juice (citrus sinensis) 500 mg • Psyllium (plantago ovata, micronized, standardized to 98% fiber) 250 mg • Flax seed freeze-dried mucilage (linum usitatissimum) 30 mg • Linden flower freeze-dried mucilage (tilla platyphilos) 30 mg • Marshmallow root freeze-dried mucilage (althaea officinalis) 30 mg. Other Ingredients: Natural Lemon Flavoring.

***Phytosterol Complex* - Progressive Labs**
Each capsule contains: Niacin (vitamin B3) 20 mg • Beta-Sitosterol 106 mg • Campesterol 52 mg • Stigmasterol 42 mg.

***Phytotality* - PhysioLogics**
Each capsule contains: Broccoli extract (2% Glucosinolates, 2 mg) 100 mg •TeaGreen leaf (50 % polyphenols, 50 mg) 100 mg •Tomato extract (1% lycopene, 500 mcg) 50 mg •Calendula flower Marigold (5% Lutein, 150 mcg) 3 mg •Soy Isoflavones extract (5 % Isoflavones, 1.25 mg) 25 mg •Red Grape skin extract (30% Anthocyanidins, 7.5 mg) 25 mg •Garlic bulb (10000 mcg Allicin/g, 250 mcg) 25 mg •Turmeric (95% Curcumin, 1.9 mg) 2 mg •Ginger root (5% Gingerols, 100 mcg) 2 mg •Milk Thistle seed (80% Silymarin, 20 mg)25 mg •Onion 2 mg •Carrot 2 mg •Beet root 2 mg •Celery 2 mg •Leek 2 mg •Garlic 2 mg •Cauliflower 2 mg •Asparagus 2 mg •Broccoli 2 mg •Cabbage 2 mg.

***Phytotality Daily* - PhysioLogics**
Three tablets contain: Vitamin A (100% as beta carotene) 15,000 IU • Vitamin C 1000 mg • Vitamin D 400 IU • Vitamin E 250 IU • Thiamin (vitamin B1) 25 mg • Riboflavin (vitamin B2) 25 mg • Niacin 25 mg • Vitamin B6 25 mg • Folic Acid 400 mcg • Vitamin B12 25 mcg • Biotin 50 mcg • Pantothenic Acid 25 mg • Calcium 250 mg • Iron 15 mg • Iodine 150 mcg • Magnesium 125 mg • Zinc 15 mg • Selenium 25 mcg • Copper 500 mcg • Manganese 4 mg • Chromium 100 mcg • Molybdenum 50 mcg • Potassium 50 mg • Boron 1 mg • Choline Bitartrate 50 mg • Inositol 25 mg • PABA (para-aminobenzoic acid) 25 mg • Citrus Bioflavonoid complex (citrus sinensis) 100 mg • Quercetin (from dimorphandra mollis) 25 mg • Rutin fruit (dimorphandra mollis) 25 mg • Hesperidin Complex 10 mg: Citrus Aurandium, Citrus Spp. • Bromelain (pineapple 2000 GDU/gm) 20 mg • Betaine Hydrochloride 20 mg • Papain (papaya) 20 mg • Amylase 5 mg • Lipase 5 mg • Protease 1 mg • Cellulase 2.5 mg • Proprietary Lactobacillus Blend 25 mg: Lactobacillus Acidophilus, Lactobacillus Bifidus, Lactobacillus Bulgaricus (milk-free: minimum 1 billion viable micro-organisms per gram, at time of manufacture) • Oat Bran husk (avena sativa) 25 mg • Pectin (apple) 25 mg • RNA 35 mg • DNA 10 mg • Carotenoids 10 mg • Chlorophyll 4 mg • Vegetable Oil (borage/sunflower, dry, cold-pressed providing essential fatty acids, GLA) 100 mg • L-Glutathione 5 mg • Spirulina 1000 mg • Wheat Grass juice (dry) 100 mg • Sprouted Barley juice (dry) 100 mg • Flaxseed oil (dry) 100 mg • Chinese Chlorella (broken cell wall) 100 mg • Bee Pollen 100 mg • Eleuthero root (eleutherococcus senticosus) 50 mg • Dehydrated Garlic bulb (allium sativum) 10 mg • Proprietary Herbal Blend 60 mg: Echinacea fruit (echinacea purpurea), Milk Thistle seed (silybum marianum), Goldenseal root (hydrastis canadensis), Ginger root (zingiber officinale), Ginkgo Biloba leaf (ginkgo biloba), Cayenne Pepper fruit (capsicum annuum). Other Ingredients: Silica, Cellulose (plant origin), Acacia Gum, Croscarmellose, Vegetable Stearic Acid, Ferrous Fumarate, Vegetable Magnesium Stearate, Kelp, Sodium Copper Chlorophyllin, Ester-C Cupric Gluconate, Cellulase, Riboflavin 5' Phosphate, Pantethine, Chromium Picolinate, Pyridoxyl 5' Phosphate, Molybdenum Chelates, Coenzyme B12, Calcium Amino Acid Chelates, Calcium Ascorbate, Calcium Aspartate, Calcium Bisglycinate, Calcium Citrate, Calcium Gluconate, Calcium Histidinate, Calcium Ketoglutarate, Calcium Malate, Calcium Spirulina Chelates, Calcium Succinate, Cupric Amino Acid Chelates, Cupric Ascorbate, Cupric Aspartate, Cupric Bisglycinate, Cupric Histidinate, Cupric Ketoglutarate, Cupric Malate, Cupric Spirulina Chelates, Cupric Succinate, Ferrous Amino Acid Chelates, Ferrous Ascorbate, Ferrous Aspartate, Ferrous Bisglycinate, Ferrous Citrate, Ferrous Gluconate, Ferrous Histidinate, Ferrous Ketoglutarate,

Ferrous Malate, Iron Spirulina Chelates, Ferrous Succinate, Magnesium Amino Acid Chelates, Magnesium Ascorbate, Magnesium Aspartate, Magnesium Bisglycinate, Magnesium Citrate, Magnesium Gluconate, Magnesium Histidinate, Magnesium Ketoglutarate, Magnesium Malate, Magnesium Spirulina Chelates, Magnesium Succinate, Manganese Amino Acid Chelates, Manganese Ascorbate, Manganese Aspartate, Manganese Bisglycinate, Manganese Histidinate, Manganese Ketoglutarate, Manganese Malate, Manganese Spirulina Chelates, Manganese Succinate, Potassium Amino Acid Chelates, Potassium Ascorbate, Potassium Aspartate, Potassium Bisglycinate, Potassium Gluconate, Potassium Histidinate, Potassium Ketoglutarate, Potassium Malate, Potassium Spirulina Chelates, Potassium Succinate, Zinc Amino Acid Chelates, Zinc Ascorbate, Zinc Aspartate, Zinc Bisglycinate, Zinc Citrate, Zinc Gluconate, Zinc Histidinate, Zinc Ketoglutarate, Zinc Malate, Zinc Spirulina Chelates, Zinc Succinate, Ergocalciferol.

Phytotality Powder **-** PhysioLogics
Each scoop (9 g) contains: Sodium 35 mg • Potassium 75 mg • Protein 1 g • Vitamin E (as d-alpha tocopheryl acid succinate) 100 IU • Green Organic Gluten-Free Grass Complex: Wheat Grass powder 350 mg, Barley Grass powder 350 mg, Alfalfa Grass powder 350 mg, Oat Grass powder 350 mg • Blue-Green Algae / Sea Algae Complex: Spirulina (arthospire plantensis, microalgae) 1000 mg, Chlorella (chlorella pyrenoidosa, microalgae) 350 mg, Dunaliella Salina 40 mg, Nova Scotia Dulse (palmaria palmata, seaweed) 30 mg • Adaptogenic/Support Herb Complex: Licorice root (glycyrrhiza glabra) 100 mg, Eleuthero root (eltutherococcus senticosus) 60 mg, Suma root (pfaffia paniculata) 60 mg, Astragalus root (astragalus membranaceus) 60 mg, Echinacea leaf (echinacea purpurea) 60 mg, Ginger root (zingiber officinale 5 mg • Nutrient-Rich Superfood Complex: Lecithin (99% oil-free) 2000 mg, Wheat sprout powder 350 mg, Acerola berry juice powder 200 mg, Beet juice powder 200 mg, Spinach Octacosanol 150 mg, Royal Jelly (5% 10-DHA) 150 mg, Bee Pollen 150 mg • Dairy-Free Probiotic Culture Complex 3.5 Billion (total count, non-dairy culture at time of manufacture 5 billion): Lactobacillus Rhamnosus A, Lactobacillus Rhamnosus B, Lactobacillus Acidophilus, Lactobacillus Casei, Lactobacillus Delbrueckii Subsp., Lactobacillus Bulgaricus, Bifidobacterium Longum / Bifidobacterium Breve 1 billion, Streptococcus Salivarius Subsp., Thermophilus 500 million • Natural Fiber Complex: Flaxseed meal 500 mg, Apple Pectin, Apple Fiber 500 mg, Fructooligosaccharides (FOS) 500 mg • Standardized Bioflavonoid Extract Blend: Milk Thistle seed (silybum marianum, standardized for 80% silymarin) 60 mg, Ginkgo Biloba leaf (ginkgo biloba, standardized for 24% ginkgo flavone glycosides) 20 mg, Green Tea Catechins leaf (camellia sinensis, standardized for 60% catechins) 20 mg, Grapeseed (92% proanthocyanidins) 20 mg, Bilberry fruit (myrtilli frucus, standardized to 25% anthocyanidins) 20 mg.

PhytoxyActin **-** Nature's Plus
Two capsules contain: Vitamin C corn free 250 mg • Broccoli [(Brassica oleracea floret) standardized 0.035% Lutein, 0.004% B-Cryptoxanthin, 0.0025% Lycopene, 0.0025% Alpha Carotene, 0.0025% Beta Carotene, 0.004% Sulforaphane] 100 mg • Carrot [(Daucus carota root) standardized 0.003% Lutein, 0.0010% Lycopene, 0.0063% Alpha Carotene, 0.0075% Beta Carotene] 100 mg • Vitamin E natural 100 IU • Spinach [(Spinacia oleracea leaf) standardized 0.0043% Lutein, 0.0024% Lycopene, 0.0043% Beta Carotene, 0.0038% B-Cryptoxanthin] 75 mg • Tomato [(Lycopersicon esculentum fruit) standardized 0.0075% Lutein, 0.0155% Lycopene, 0.0015% Beta Carotene] 75 mg • Echinacea [(Echinacea angustifolia root) standardized 4% Echinacosides] 75 mg • Astragalus [(Astragalus membranaceus root) standardized 0.4% 4'-Hydroxy-3'-Methoxyisoflavone 7-sug] 50 mg • Green Tea [(Camellia sinensis leaf) standardized 50% Polyphenols] 50 mg • Red Wine concentrate alcohol free [(Vitis vinifera fruit) standardized 20% Polyphenols] 50 mg • Turmeric [(Cuizome) standardized 95% Curcumin] 50 mg • Garlic odor-modified [(Allium sativum clove) standardized 0.35% Allicin, 0.65% Allicin, 0.40% Thiosulfinates, 0.085% Allyl Mercaptan] 50 mg • Shiitake Mushroom [(Lentinus edodes mycelia) standardized 3.2% KS-2 Polysaccharides] 25 mg • Grape seed extract [(Vitis vinifera) standardized 95% Proanthocyanidins] 25 mg • Beta Carotene pro-Vitamin A (naturally supplying 25000 IU of Vitamin A activity) 15 mg.

Pick-Me-Up Formula **-** Bee-Alive Inc.
Royal Jelly (non-freeze dried) • Damiana leaf extract • Saw Palmetto fruit extract • Cayenne fruit extract • Asian Ginseng root • Vegetable Glycerin • Clover Honey • Deionized Water • Natural Almond Flavor.

Pilex Ointment **-** The Himalaya Drug Company (Himalaya Heal
Lajjalu (mimosa pudica) • Bhringaraja (eclipta prostrata syn. e.alba) • Nirgundi (vitex negundo) • Zergul (calendula officinalis) • Karpoora (cinnamomum camphora) • Tankana (sodium biborate) • Yashad Bhasma (zinc calx) • Base q.s. ad.

Pilex Tablets **-** The Himalaya Drug Company (Himalaya Heal
Each tablet contains: Guggulu (commiphora wightii syn. balsamodendron mukul) 0.26 mg • Shilajeet (mineral pitch, purified) 32 mg • Nimba seed (melia azadirachta syn. azadiractha indica) 14 mg • Daruharidra (berberis aristata) 64 mg • Amalaki (emblica officinalis) 32 mg • Haritaki (terminalia chebula) 32 mg • Vibhitaki (terminalia bellirica syn. t.belerica) 32 mg • Aragvadha (cassia fistula) 32 mg • Kanchanara (bauhinia variegata) 32 mg • Nagkesara (mesua ferrea) 6 mg.

Pineal Concentrate **-** Progressive Labs
Each capsule contains: Veal bone concentrate 100 mg • Flaxseed oil 20 mg • Pineal concentrate 7 mg • Pituitary concentrate 3 mg. The glandular concentrate in this product is prepared by a special process which does not exceed physiological temperature (37° C). Guaranteed free of chemical pesticides and synthetic hormones.
See Editor's Note No. 14.

Pineal Plus **-** Atrium Inc.
Each tablet contains: Raw Pineal Tissue concentrate (Bovine) 8 mg • Raw Whole Pituitary concentrate (Bovine) 20 mg • Raw Calf Bone concentrate (Bovine) 150 mg • Cold Pressed Flaxseed oil 10 mg.
See Editor's Note No. 14.

Pinna-Cal **-** Changes International, Inc.
Six caplets contain: Vitamin D (as Cholecalciferol) 125 IU • Vitamin K (as Phytonadione) 80 mcg • Calcium (as purified Calcite, Hydroxyapatite, Calcium Citrate, and Calcium Lactate) 1000 mg • Magnesium (as Magnesium Citrate and Oxide) 400 mg • Boron (as Boron Citrate) 2 mg • Ipriflavone 600 mg. Other Ingredients: Vegetable cellulose, Fractionated vegetable oil, Silica, Soy polysaccharides, and Vita-Lok vegetable resin glaze.

Pinnacle 5-HTP Tryptobol **-** Bodyonics, Ltd.
Two capsules contain: Griffonia Simplicifolia (providing 10% (100 mg) 5-HTP (5-Hydroxy-L-Tryptophan)) 1000 mg • Herbolics Support Complex (from Jatoba, Maca, Para Todo, Yerba Mate) 100 mg. Other Ingredients: Calcium Phosphate, Microcrystalline Cellulose, Magnesium Stearate, Gelatin.

Pinnacle Androstat 100 **-** Bodyonics, Ltd.
Each tablet contains Androstenedione 100 mg. Other Ingredients: Calcium Phosphate, Lecithin, Xanthan Gum, Stearic Acid, Magnesium Stearate.
See Editor's Note No. 47, page 2058.

Pinnacle Androstat Pro Six **-** Bodyonics, Ltd.
Each tablet contains: Balanced Andro Complex: 4-androstenediol (4-androstene-3, 17-diol) 125 mg • 4-androstene-3,17-dione (4-androstenedione) 5 mg • 5-androstene-3, 17-dione (5-androstenedione) 5 mg • 5-androstene-3beta,17beta-diol (5-androstenediol) 5 mg • 19-nor-5-androstene-3, 17-diol (19-nor 5-androstendiol) 5 mg. Other Ingredients: Calcium Phosphate, Lecithin, Xanthan Gum, Stearic Acid, Magnesium Stearate.
See Editor's Note No. 47, page 2058.

***Pinnacle Androstat100 Poppers Cool Mint Flavor* -** Bodyonics, Ltd.
Two tablets contain: Balanced Andro Complex: 4-androstene-3, 17-diol (4-androstenediol) 83.33 mg • 4-androstenedione-3,17-dione (4-androstenedione) 3.33 mg • 5-androstene-3, 17-dione (5-androstenedione) 3.33 mg • 5-androstene-3beta,17beta-diol (5-androstenediol) 3.33 mg • 19-nor-5-androstene-3, 17-diol (19-nor 5-androstendiol) 3.33 mg. Other Ingredients: Fructose, Sorbitol, Natural Flavor, Stearic Acid, Magnesium Stearate, Cellulose, Croscarmellose, Sucralose.
See Editor's Note No. 47, page 2058.

***Pinnacle Androstat100 Poppers Licorice Flavor* -** Bodyonics, Ltd.
Two tablets contain: Balanced Andro Complex: 4-androstene-3, 17-diol (4-androstenediol) 83.33 mg • 4-androstene-3,17-dione (4-androstenedione) 3.33 mg • 5-androstene-3, 17-dione (5-androstenedione) 3.33 mg • 5-androstene-3beta,17beta-diol (5-androstenediol) 3.33 mg • 19-nor-5-androstene-3, 17-diol (19-nor 5-androstendiol) 3.33 mg. Other Ingredients: Fructose, Sorbitol, Natural Flavor, Stearic Acid, Magnesium Stearate, Cellulose, Croscarmellose, Sucralose.
See Editor's Note No. 47, page 2058.

***Pinnacle Androstat100 Poppers Wild Berry Flavor* -** Bodyonics, Ltd.
Two tablets contain: Balanced Andro Complex: 4-androstene-3, 17-diol (4-androstenediol) 83.33 mg • 4-androstene-3,17-dione (4-androstenedione) 3.33 mg • 5-androstene-3, 17-dione (5-androstenedione) 3.33 mg • 5-androstene-3beta,17beta-diol (5-androstenediol) 3.33 mg • 19-nor-5-androstene-3, 17-diol (19-nor 5-androstendiol) 3.33 mg. Other Ingredients: Fructose, Sorbitol, Natural Flavor, Stearic Acid, Magnesium Stearate, Cellulose, Croscarmellose, Sucralose.
See Editor's Note No. 47, page 2058.

***Pinnacle Androstat6* -** Bodyonics, Ltd.
Two tablets contain: Balanced Andro Complex: 4-androstene-3, 17-diol (4-androstenediol) 125 mg • 4-androstene-3,17-dione (4-androstenedione) 5 mg • 5-androstene-3, 17-dione (5-androstenedione) 5 mg • 5-androstene-3beta,17beta-diol (5-androstenediol) 5 mg • 19-nor-5-androstene-3, 17-diol (19-nor 5-androstendiol) 5 mg. Other Ingredients: Fructose, Sorbitol, Natural Licorice Flavor, Stearic Acid, Magnesium, Stearate and 100% Natural Beta Cyclodextrins.
See Editor's Note No. 47, page 2058.

***Pinnacle Beta Activated Protein with HMB* -** Bodyonics, Ltd.
Twelve tablets contain: Calcium B-Hydroxy B-Methylbutyrate Monohydrate (HMB) 3 g • Beta Peptide (a proprietary blend of very distinct cosein, whey and aligopeptides) 12 g • Alanine 392 mg • Arginine 419 mg • Aspartic Acid 713 mg • Cystine 74 mg • Glutamic Acid 2806 mg • Glycine 232 mg • Isoleucine (BCAA) 635 mg • Leucine (BCAA) 1044 mg • Lysine 906 mg • Methionine 307 mg • Phenylalanine 556 mg • Proline 1178 mg • Serine 617 mg • Threonine 494 mg • Tryptophan 142 mg • Tyrosine 461 mg • Valine (BCAA) 732 mg. Other Ingredients: Calcium Phosphate, Stearic Acid, Magnesium Stearate, Croscarmellose, Silica.

***Pinnacle BHP-5* -** Bodyonics, Ltd.
Each tablet contains: Hydrolyzed BHP5 (Pregnenolone) 15 mg. Other Ingredients: Calcium Phosphate, Stearic Acid, Magnesium Stearate, Croscarmellose.

***Pinnacle Chrysinex 250* -** Bodyonics, Ltd.
Each tablet contains: Chrysin Complex [Derived from a custonized blend of 98% pure 5,7-Dihydroxyflavone and natural powered extract poplar bud (Populus candicans)] 250 mg • Cruciferous Vegetable Concentrate (Standardized to contain 10% Indole 3-Carbinol) 25 mg. Other Ingredients: Calcium Phosphate, Stearic Acid, Magnesium Stearate, Lecithin, Xanthan Gum.

***Pinnacle Cordyceps 500* -** Bodyonics, Ltd.
Each tablet contains: Dong Chong Zia Cao (Cordyceps sinensis-winter bug, summer herb) • Sha Shen (Adenophora tetraphylla) • WuWei Zi (Schisandra chinensis) • Gan Jiang (Zingiber officinale) • Dahlulin (Dahlia inulin juice concentrate). Other Ingredients: Dicalcium Phosphate, Croscarmellose, Magnesium Stearate, Stearic Acid.

***Pinnacle Crea Glutide 2400* -** Bodyonics, Ltd.
Each tablet contains: Crea-Glutide 2400 mg • Creatine Monohydrate 2 g • Glutamine Peptide 400 mg. Other Ingredients: Calcium Phosphate, Stearic Acid, Magnesium Stearate, Croscarmellose.

***Pinnacle Crea-Glutide* -** Bodyonics, Ltd.
Two tablespoons contains: Dextrose • BioReacted Crea-Glutide Complex • Complex Carbohydrate • Dahlulin (Dry Dahlia Inulin Juice Complex) • Citric Acid • Natural Cranberry Flavor • Xanthan Gum • Stevia Extract • Beet Extract.

***Pinnacle CreaRibose ATP Kichers* -** Bodyonics, Ltd.
Six tablets contain: Creatine Monohydrate 5 grams • D-Ribose 3 grams. Other Ingredients: Magnesium Stearate, Cellulose, Calcium Phosphate, Stearic Acid.

***Pinnacle Fractionized CCK 100* -** Bodyonics, Ltd.
Each tablet contains: Cholecystokinin (CCK) (Derived from a purified blend of edible bovine tissuse fractions, providing 1000 picomotes of standardized Cholecystokinin (CCK) a bioactive substance) 100 mg. Other Ingredients: Calcium Phosphate, Microcrystalline Cellulose, Stearic Acid, Magnesium Stearate, Croscarmellose Silica.
See Editor's Note No. 14.

***Pinnacle Gro Tropin* -** Bodyonics, Ltd.
Three capsules contains: Alpha GPC (Alpha-Glycerylphosarylcholine) 500 mg • AminoGlutein Peptide (standardized to provide 30% Glutamine Peptide) 500 mg • Colostrum (Colostral Isoform Extract) (standardized to provide 1300 nanograms of platelet derived growth factor) 500 mg • Tribulus Terrestris (standardized to provide 40% Furostanol Saponins) 500 mg • Phosphatidyl Serine 500 mcg • Chrysin (98% pure 5,7 Dehydroxyflavone) 750 mcg. Other Ingredients: Magnesium Strearate, Gelatin.

***Pinnacle Horny Goat Weed* -** Bodyonics, Ltd.
Two capsules contain: Horny Goat Weed (Epimedium grandiflorum) standardized 10% Icariin 500 mg • Maca Pure (Lepidium meyenii)standardized to contain 0.6% macamides and macaenes 250 mg • Mucuna pruriens standardized 15% L-Dopa (L-dihydroxyphenylalanine) 33.3 mg • Polypodium vulgare standardized 8% 20-hydroxyecdysone 25 mg. Other Ingredients: Calcium Phosphate, Magnesium Stearate, Gelatin.

***Pinnacle P-ALC 500* -** Bodyonics, Ltd.
Each tablet contains: Phosphorolytic Acetyl L-Carnitine (PALC) (Including Inulin and Succunates) 500 mg. Other Ingredients: Calcium Phosphate, Stearic Acid, Magnesium Stearate, Silica, Croscarmellose.

***Pinnacle PS Complex 500* -** Bodyonics, Ltd.
Each tablet contains: Cephalized PS (Phosphatidyl Serine Complex) (BioActivated Phospholipid fractions standardized to 55% cephalins phosphatidyl serine, choline, inositol and ethanolamine) 500 mg. Other Ingredients: Microcrystalline Cellulose, Calcium Phosphate, Stearic Acid, Magnesium Stearate, Croscarmellose, Silica.

***Pinnacle PYRUVATE 1000* -** Bodyonics, Ltd.
Each tablet contains: Sodium 60 mg • Potassium 40 mg • Calcium 100 mg • Stabilized Trimin Pyruvate Complex 1000 mg (From Calcium, Potassium, and Sodium salts of Pyruvic Acid, plus Dihydroxyacetone. Inulinized in a bioactive complex of Phosphorolytic Dahlia Inulin providing a long chain carbohydrate molecule). Other Ingredients: Calcium Phosphate, Stearic Acid, Magnesium Stearate, Silica, Croscarmellose.

***Pinnacle PYRUVATE 500* -** Bodyonics, Ltd.
Each tablet contains: Sodium 30 mg • Potassium 20 mg • Calcium 50 mg • Stabilized Trimin Pyruvate Complex 500 mg (From Calcium, Potassium, and Sodium salts of Pyruvic Acid, plus Dihydroxyacetone.

Inulinized in a bioactive complex of Phosphorolytic Dahlia Inulin providing a long chain carbohydrate molecule). Other Ingredients: Calcium Phosphate, Stearic Acid, Magnesium Stearate, Silica, Croscarmellose.

Pinnacle SAMe **-** Bodyonics, Ltd.
Each tablet contains SAM-e 200 mg • Vitamin B12 50 mcg • Folic Acid 100 mcg.

Pinnacle Super Crea Glutide A-DS **-** Bodyonics, Ltd.
One scoop contains: Creatine Monohydrate 6 g • Glutamine Peptide 2 g • Taurine 2 g • Dahlulin (Dry Dahlia Inulin Juice Complex) 500 mg • Complex Carbohydrate • Natural Flavor • Xanthan Gum • Stevia Extract • Beta Carotene.

Pinnacle Thermophen **-** Bodyonics, Ltd.
Two tablets contain: St. John's Wort (0.3% hypericin) 150 mg • Citrus Aurantium (Bitter Orange peel) (1.5- 3% synephrine) 200 mg • Kava Kava (40% Kavalactones) 100 mg • Yerba Mate (20% Methylxanthines) 200 mg. Other Ingredients: Calcium Phosphate, Microcrystalline Cellulose, Stearic Acid, Magnesium Stearate, Croscarmellose.
See Editor's Note No. 40, page 2058.

Pinnacle Tribestrol 250 **-** Bodyonics, Ltd.
Two captabs contain: Tribulus Terrestris (providing 40% (100 mg) Furostanol Saponins) 250 mg • Herbolics Support Complex (from Catuaga, Muira Puama, Chachuhuasu, Iporuru) 100 mg. Other Ingredients: Calcium Phosphate, Stearic Acid, Magnesium Stearate, Croscarmellose.

Pinnacle Ultra Strength Volumax Chocolate Flavor **-** Bodyonics, Ltd.
Two scoops contain: Whey Protein Concentrate (Ion Exchange) • Complex Carbohydrate (Maltodextrin) • Creatine Monohydrate • Dutch Cocoa powder • Soy Fiber • Oat Fiber • Natural & Artificial Vanilla Flavor • Glutamine Peptide • Dahluin (Dry Dahlia Inulin Juice Complex) • Whey Protein Hydrolysate • Taurine • Potassium Phosphate • Calcium Phosphate • Magnesium Oxide • Potassium Chloride • Xanthan Gum • Aspartame • Psyllium • Monosodium Phosphate • Ascorbic Acid • Beta Carotene • dl-Alpha Tocopheryl Acetate • Ferrous Fumarate • Niacinamide • Zinc Oxide • Vitamin A Palmitate • D-Calcium Pantothenate • Manganese Sulfate • RNA Powder • Soy Lecithin • Vitamin K (as Vitamin K1) • Copper Sulfate • Pyridoxine Hydrochloride • Riboflavin • Thiamine Hydrochloride • Cyanocobalamin • Vitamin D (as Vitamin D3) • Folic Acid • Chromium Chloride • Biotin • Selenomethionine • Chromium Picolinate • Sodium Molybdate • Potassium Iodide • Sodium Selenate.

Pinnacle Ultra Strength Volumax Vanilla Flavor **-** Bodyonics, Ltd.
Two scoops contain: Whey Protein Concentrate (Ion Exchange) • Complex Carbohydrate (Maltodextrin) • Creatine Monohydrate • Soy Fiber • Oat Fiber • Natural & Artificial Vanilla Flavor • Glutamine Peptide • Dahluin (Dry Dahlia Inulin Juice Complex) • Whey Protein Hydrolysate • Taurine • Potassium Phosphate • Calcium Phosphate • Magnesium Oxide • Potassium Chloride • Xanthan Gum • Aspartame • Psyllium • Monosodium Phosphate • Ascorbic Acid • Beta Carotene • dl-Alpha Tocopheryl Acetate • Ferrous Fumarate • Niacinamide • Zinc Oxide • Vitamin A Palmitate • D-Calcium Pantothenate • Manganese Sulfate • RNA powder • Soy Lecithin • Vitamin K (as Vitamin K1) • Copper Sulfate • Pyridoxine Hydrochloride • Riboflavin • Thiamine Hydrochloride • Cyanocobalamin • Vitamin D (as Vitamin D3) • Folic Acid • Chromium Chloride • Biotin • Selenomethionine • Chromium Picolinate • Sodium Molybdate • Potassium Iodide • Sodium Selenate.

Pinnacle Whey Ahead Chocolate Flavor **-** Bodyonics, Ltd.
One scoop contains: Whey Ahead Complex (a blend of Whey Protein Concentrates and Whey Protein Isolates, and Partially Pre-digested Ion Exchanged Whey Protein Hydrolysates) • Creatine Monohydrate • Glutamin Peptide • Dutch Cocoa Powder • Natural and Artifical Vanilla Flavor • Tourine • Dahlulin (Dry Dahlia Inulin Juice Complex) • Xanthan Gum • Beta Carotene • Aspartame.

Pinnacle Whey Ahead Vanilla Flavored **-** Bodyonics, Ltd.
One scoop contains: Whey Ahead Complex a blend of Whey Protein Concentrates and Whey Protein Isolates and partially Pre-digested Ion Exchanged Whey Protein Hydrolysates • Creatine Monohydrate • Glutamine Peptide • Natural and Artifical Vanilla Flavor • Tourine • Dahlulin (Dry Dahlia Inulin Juice Complex) • Xanthan Gum • Beta Carotene • Aspartame.

Pituitrophin PMG **-** Standard Process, Inc.
Each tablet contains: Proprietary Blend 118 mg: Magnesium Citrate, Bovine Pituitary extract (45 mg). Inactive Ingredients: Calcium (lactate, stearate) 30 mg, Cellulose.

Pizazz **-** Nature's Plus
Each tablespoon contains: L-Phenylalanine free form amino acid 250 mg • Pantothenic Acid 75 mg • Inositol 50 mg • Niacinamide 40 mg • Vitamin B1 (Thiamine) 30 mg • Vitamin B2 (Riboflavin) 30 mg • Vitamin B6 (Pyridoxine HCL) 30 mg • Choline (Bitartrate) 21 mg • Vitamin B12 (from Cobalamin) 100 mcg • Biotin 30 mcg. In a natural high-energy base of Bee Pollen, Ginseng, Gotu Kola, & Fo-Ti. Sweetened with Honey & Blackstrap Molasses.

Plain Soy - Revival **-** Physicians Laboratories
Each Packet Contains: Certified Isoflavone 160 mg. Ingredients: Soy Protein Isolate, Soy Lecithin.

Plant Enzimase **-** Nutri-Quest Rx
Each 360 mg capsule contains: Amylase 4500 DU • Protease 15000 HUT • Lipase 65 IU • Invertase 0.25 IAU • Malt Diastase 150 DPI • Lactase 200 LacU • Cellulase 60 CU. In a base of pure Beet root Fiber.

Plantain Salve **-** Dial Herbs
Plantain • Chickweed • Mint • Comfrey • Oat Straw. In a base of Bees Wax, Glycerine & Cold Pressed Olive oil.

PLUS Herbal-Amino Acid **-** Mannatech
Each caplet contains: Iron 1 mg • Wild Yam (root; standardized for 25 mg phytosterols) 200 mg • L-Glutamic Acid 200 mg • Glycine 200 mg • L-Lysine 200 mg • L-Arginine 100 mg • Beta Sitosterol 25 mg • Proprietary Blend 2.5 mg: Arabinogalactan (larix decidua gum), Manapol Aloe Vera gel extract (inner leaf gel), Gum Ghatti, Gum Tragacanth. Other Ingredients: Microcrystalline Cellulose, Stearic Acid, Croscarmellose Sodium, Silicon Dioxide, Magnesium Stearate, Titanium Dioxide Coating.

PM Evening Activator **-** Slimlife
Two caplets contain: Niacin (as niacinamide) 20 mg • Vitamin B6 (as pyridoxine HCl) 2 mg • Potassium (as gluconate) 100 mg • L-Carnitine HCl 100 mg • Valerian root powder 50 mg. Other Ingredients: Dicalcium Phosphate, Cellulose, Stearic Acid, Magnesium Stearate, Silicone Dioxide, Croscarmellose Sodium, Pharmaceutical Glaze, Talc USP.

PM Menopause Formula **-** PhytoPharmica
PM Formula: Each purple tablet contains: Valerian root extract (valeriana officinalis, standardized to contain a minimum of 0.8% valerenic acids) 200 mg • Hops flower 6.6:1 extract (humulus lupulus) 100 mg • L-Theanine 50 mg • Black Cohosh root and rhizome extract (standardized to contain 2.5% triterpene glycosides calculated as 27-deoxyactein) 20 mg. Other Ingredients: Cellulose, Modified Cellulose, Modified Cellulose Gum, Magnesium Stearate, Carrot and Paprika Extract Color, Lecithin, Carnauba Wax.

PMS **-** Hyland's
Two tablets contain: Viburnum Opulus 2X • Caulophyllum Thalictroides 3X • Cocculus Indicus 3X • Gelsemium Sempervirens 3X. Base: Lactose USP.
See Editor's Note No. 1, page 2053.

BRAND NAMES

PMS Comfort - Wellzymes - Enzymes, Inc.
Two capsules contain: Vitamin E (from d-Alpha Tocopheryl Succinate) 20 IU • n-zimes Proprietary Enzyme Blend 34 mg: pHysioProtease (94,720 pHysio-U), CereCalase Plus • Proprietary Herbal Blend 390 mg: Chasteberry extract (equivalent to 480 mg raw herb), Dong Quai root extract (equivalent to 480 mg raw herb), Cramp Bark extract (equivalent to 360 mg raw herb), Parsley leaf extract (equivalent to 200 mg raw herb), Rice Bran. Other Ingredients: Plant Cellulose, Water.

PMS Escape - Back Bay Scientific
Each packet (50 g) contains: Vitamin C 60 mg • Vitamin B6 0.5 mg • Calcium 50 mg • Magnesium 20 mg. Ingredients: Simple Carbohydrates (dextrose), Complex Carbohydrates (maltodextrin, starch), Citric Acid, Ascorbic Acid, Pyridoxine Hydrochloride, Calcium Lactate, Magnesium Lactate, Natural & Artificial Flavor, FD&C Red #40.

PMS Formula - Nature's Way
Three capsules contain: Black Cohosh root 150 mg • Cramp bark 250 mg • Dandelion leaf 150 mg • L-5 Hydroxytryptophan (Griffonia bean extract) 5 mg • Lobelia herb 150 mg • Magnesium Amino Acid Chelate 50 mg • Niacin (Vitamin B3) 10 mg • Pyridoxine HCL 76 mg • Riboflavin (Vitamin B2) 852 mcg • Thiamine (Vitamin B1) 750 mcg • Vitamin B12 (Cyanocobalamin) 3 mcg. Other Ingredients: Gelatin, Millet.

PMS Formula - The Vitamin Shoppe
Each capsule contains: Vitamin B12 25 mcg • Vitamin B6 10 mg • St. John's Wort 150 mg • Siberian Ginseng 100 mg • Korean Ginseng root 50 mg • Chamomile 100 mg.

PMS Formula - Puritan's Pride
Three tablets contain: Vitamin B-6 354 mg • Folic Acid 400 mcg • Calcium 125 mg • Magnesium 250 mg • Potassium 99 mg • Evening Primrose oil 500 mg • Proprietary Herbal Complex Blend 150 mg: derived from Dong Quai, Black Cohosh, Fo-Ti, Dandelion, Watercress, Parsley, Yellow Dock.

PMS Formula with Indolplex - PhytoPharmica
Two tablets contain: Vitamin D (as cholecalciferol) 250 IU • Calcium (as calcium citrate and calcium carbonate) 200 mg • Iodine (as potassium iodide) 80 mcg • Magnesium (as magnesium aspartate) 100 mg • Chaste Tree (Vitex-agnus castus) berry extract (standardized to contain a minimum of 0.5% agnuside) 20 mg • Diindolylmethane (DIM, as Indolplex brand blend) 14 mg.

PMS Forte - Futurebiotics
Two tablets contain: Thiamin HCl (B1) 12 mg • Riboflavin (B2) 12 mg • Pyridoxine HCl (B6) 65 mg • Niacinamide 50 mg • Vitamin C (ascorbic acid) 60 mg • Dong Quai (extract equal to) 300 mg • Choline Bitartrate 75 mg • Para Amino Benzoic Acid (PABA) 85 mg • Methionine 60 mg • Inositol 50 mg • Iron (ferrous fumarate) 8 mg • Potassium (citrate, gluconate) 60 mg • Magnesium (oxide, amino acid chelate) 350 mg • Vitamin B12 40 mcg • Iodine (potassium, iodide) 150 mcg • Zinc (gluconate) 15 mg • Pantothenic Acid 60 mg • Folic Acid 400 mcg • Calcium (carbonate, phosphate) 300 mg • Vitamin E 30 IU • Ribonucleic Acid (RNA) 40 mg • Biotin 300 mcg. Base: Vitex Agnus Castus, Uva Ursi, Royal Jelly, Raw Alfalfa Juice Concentrate, Cramp Bark, Betaine HCl, Chamomile, Squawvine, American Ginseng Extract, Chinese Licorice, Melissa, Marjoram, Polygonum Multiflorum.

PMS Nutritional Support - NutriCology
Each capsule contains: BioResponse DIM (a patented diindolylmethane complex), Starch, DIM (25% min.), Vitamin E Succinate, Phosphatidylcholine, Silica 75 mg • Green Tea extract (decaffeinated, standardized to 60% catechins) 600 mg • Vitex Agnus-Castus berry extract 20 mg. Other Ingredients: Stearic Acid.

PMS Nutritional Systems Part I - Schiff
Eight softgels contain: Beta Carotene (Vitamin A activity) 15000 IU • Vitamin D 100 IU • Vitamin E (d-Alpha Tocopheryl Acetate) 600 IU • Vitamin C (Ascorbic Acid) 1000 mg • Folic Acid 200 mcg • Thiamine Mononitrate (Vitamin B2) 50 mg • Riboflavin (Vitamin B2) 50 mg • Niacinamide 50 mg • Vitamin B6 (Pyridoxine HCl) 200 mg • Biotin 30 mcg • Pantothenic Acid (d-Calcium Pantothenate) 50 mg • Calcium (Calcium Chlelate) 150 mg • Magnesium (Magnesium Oxide) 300 mg • Iodine (Potassium Iodide) 150 mcg • Iron (Ferrous Chelate) 15 mg • Copper (Cupric Oxide) 0.5 • Zinc (Zinc Gluconate) 25 mg • Choline Bitartrate 500 mg • Manganese (Gluconate) 10 mg • Potassium (Potassuim Chloride) 100 mg • Selenium (Selenium Chelate) 100 mcg • Chromium (Chromium Chelate) 500 mg • Inositol 500 mg • Para Aminobenzoic Acid 50 mg.

PMS Nutritional Systems Part II - Schiff
Each softgel contains: Sarsaparilla root 210 mg • Burdock root 210 mg • Ginger root 70 mg.

PMS Relief Formula - Body Language Vitamin Co.
Each capsule contains: Black Cohosh (Cimicifuga racemosa root, standardized to contain 2.5% triterpine glycosides) 200 mg • Dong Quai (Angelica sinensis root) 200 mg • Wild Yam 100 mg • Chastetree berry (Vitex agnus-castus fruit) 100 mg • Damiana (Turnera diffusa leaves) 50 mg • Red Raspberry 100 mg • Feverfew 150 mcg • Juniper berry 50 mg. Other Ingredients: Vegetable Cellulose Capsule, Rice Powder, Magnesium Stearate.

PMS Symptom Free - Enzymatic Therapy
Two tablets contain: Vitamin D (as cholecalciferol) 250 IU • Calcium (as calcium carbonate, calcium citrate) 200 mg • Iodine (as potassium iodide) 80 mcg • Magnesium (as magnesium aspartate) 100 mg • Chaste Tree berry extract (vitex-agnus castus, standardized to contain 0.5% agnuside) 20 mg • Diindolylmethane (DIM) 14 mg. Other Ingredients: Cellulose, Modified Cellulose, Starch (corn), D-Alpha-Tocopheryl Succinate, Titanium Dioxide Color, Phosphatidylcholine, Lecithin, Silicon Dioxide, Carnauba Wax.

PMS Tea - Traditional Medicinals
One tea bag contains: Dandelion root (Tanaxacum officinale): 500 mg. Other Herbal Ingredients: Roasted Carob pod, Roasted Barley, Roasted Chicory root, Parsley leaf, Oat Straw herb, Nettle leaf, Chickweed herb, Uva Ursi leaf, Cramp bark, Cornsilk style & stigma.

PMSOS - Nature's Herbs
Four capsules contain: Vitamin B6 500 mg • natural Vitamin E (d-Alpha Tocopherol Succinate) 400 IU • Uva Ursi extract (concentrated standardized for 10% Arbutin equivalent to 1200 of dried herb) 400 mg • Valerian root extract (standardized for .72-.88% valernic acid = to 1600 mg of dried herb) 400mg • White Willow bark extract (standardized for 15% salicin - White Willow extract 5:1= to 1600 mg of dried herb) 200 mg • Chasteberry extract (Vitex agnus castus - standardized for 11k ppm Glycosides equivalent to 600 mg of dried herb) 100 mg • Ginger root 305 mg • Dong Quai root 200 mg.

Pneumotrate - Progressive Labs
Each capsule contains: Vitamin A 2500 IU • Beta Carotene 2500 IU • Vitamin C 90 mg • Bovine lung concentrate 200 mg.
See Editor's Note No. 14.

PoisePlus - Atrium Inc.
Six tablets contain: Vitamin A 15000 IU •Vitamin E 140 IU •Vitamin C 1050 mg •Bioflavonoids 300 mg •Chlorophyll (oil) 60 mg •Along with the following Amino Acid chelated minerals: Calcium 500 mg •Magnesium 250 mg •Potassium 99 mg •Manganese 10 mg •Iron 15 mg •Zinc 10 mg •Copper 2 mg •Iodine 150 mcg •Chromium 200 mcg •Selenium 25 mcg •Molybdenum 150 mcg •Vanadium 150 mcg •Silicon 2 mcg. In a base of Raw Bovine Tissue concentrates (not extracts) from the following: (Spleen 150 mg, Brain 30 mg, Liver 25 mg, Heart 15 mg, Kidney 15 mg, Thymus 10 mg, Adrenal 10 mg, Pituitary 10 mg, Pancreas 10 mg, Duodenus 10 mg) 285 mg.
See Editor's Note No. 31, page 2056.

***Poison Ivy/Oak* - Hyland's**
Two tablets contain: Rhus Toxicodendron 6X • Croton Tiglium 6X • Xerophyllum 6X. Base: Lactose USP.
See Editor's Note No. 1, page 2053.

***Pokemon Children's Multiple Vitamin* - Rexall - Sundown**
Each chewable tablet contains: Vitamin A 5000 IU • Vitamin C (as sodium ascorbate and ascorbic acid) 60 mg • Vitamin D (as cholecalciferol) 400 IU • Vitamin E (as dl-alpha tocopheryl acetate) 30 IU • Thiamin (as thiamin mononitrate) 1.5 mg • Riboflavin 1.7 mg • Niacin (as niacinamide) 20 mg • Vitamin B-6 (as pyridoxine HCl) 2 mg • Folic Acid 400 mcg • Vitamin B-12 (as cyanocobalamin) 6 mcg • Biotin 40 mcg • Pantothenic Acid (as calcium d-pantothenate) 10 mg • Calcium 150 mg • Iron (as ferrous sulfate) 18 mg • Phosphorous 80 mg • Iodine (as potassium iodide) 150 mcg • Magnesium (as magnesium oxide) 20 mg • Zinc (as zinc oxide) 15 mg • Copper (as cupric oxide) 2 mg.

***Policosanol* - Life Extension Foundation**
Each tablet contains: Policosanol (enhanced octasanol extract) 10 mg. Other Ingredients: Cellulose, mannitol, hydroxypropylmethylcellulose, citric acid, sodium starch glycolate, polyethylene glycol, croscarmellose sodium, stearic acid, silica, riboflavin.

***Policosanol Cholesterol Complex* - Source Naturals**
Three tablets contain: Vitamin C (as ascorbic acid) 600 mg • Vitamin E (as natural D-alpha-tocopheryl) 200 IU • Niacin (as inositol hexanicotinate) 500 mg • Iodine (from kelp) 150 mcg • Chromium (as chromium picolinate and ChromeMate) 100 mcg • Phytosterols Complex (40% yielding 300 mg beta-sitosterol) 750 mg • Inositol (as inositol hexanicotinate) 640 mg • Garlic powder extract (standardized to 8000 ppm allicin) 600 mg • Turmeric extract (95% curcumin) 526 mg • Artichoke extract (standardized to 2.5% cynarins) 250 mg • Methylmethioninesulfonium Chloride (vitamin U) 200 mg • Green Tea extract 95% 100 mg • Soy Bean concentrate (yielding 40 mg total isoflavones) 100 mg • Guggul Gum resin extract (standardized to 2.5% Gugulipid: guggulsterones Z & E) 100 mg • Ginkgo Biloba leaf 24% (50:1 extract) 60 mg • Dandelion root extract (4:1) 50 mg • Hawthorn berry extract (4:1) 50 mg • Myricetin 30 mg • Policosanol 20 mg. Other Ingredients: Stearic Acid, Modified Cellulose Gum, Hydroxy Propyl Cellulose, Colloidal Silicon Dioxide, Magnesium Stearate.

***Polishing Peel* - Nu Skin Enterprises**
Water (aqua) • Bentonite • Zea Mays starch (corn) • Glycerin • Sorbitol • PEG-40 Hydrogenated Castor oil • Lactobacillus / Cucurbita Pepo fruit ferment extract • Polygonum Cuspidatum root extract • Hamamelis Virginiana water (witch hazel) • Caprylyl Glycol • Polysorbate 80 • Polyvinyl Alcohol • Hexylene Glycol • Ammonium Laureth Sulfate • C20-40 Pareth-10,1,2-Hexanediol • Disodium EDTA • Fragrance (parfum) • Ammonium Silver Zinc Aluminum Silicate • Titanium Dioxide.

***Poly C* - USANA Health Sciences**
Each tablet contains: Vitamin C (as Calcium, Potassium, Magnesium, and Zinc Ascorbates) 600 mg • Citrus Bioflavonoids (Citrus SPP. L.) fruit 65 mg • Rutin 7 mg • Quercetin 3 mg. Other Ingredients: Fumed Silica, Purified Water.

***Polyerga Plus* - Polyerga**
Each tablet contains: Peptides from Porcine Spleen 230 mg. Other Ingredients: Sucrose, Talc, Microcrystalline Cellulose, Calcium Carbonate, Clay, Polyvinyl Pyrrolidone, Powdered Cellulose, Acacia, Shellac, Corn Syrup, Titanium Dioxide, Magnesium Stearate, Cornstarch, Silicon Dioxide, Ferric Oxide, Polyethylene Glycol (MW 6000), Montan Glycol Wax, Castor Oil, Polyoxylated Castor Oil, Sodium Lauryl Sulfate.

***Poly-MVA - PolyMVA* - AMARC Enterprises**
Two teaspoons contain: Proprietary Blend: Palladium, Molybdenum, Ruthenium, Rhodium, Lipoic Acid, Vitamin B1 (HCl), Vitamin B2, Vitamin B12, Vitamin A, Acetyl Cysteine, Formyl Methionine.
See Editor's Note No. 24, page 2056.

***Polyphenon 100 Green Tea Catechin Capsules* - Origin BioMedicinals**
Polyphenon 70 Green Tea extract (100 mg catechins) • Vitamin E (d-alpha-tocopherol) • Soybean Oil • Wheat Germ Oil • Beeswax • Gelatin • Emulsifier.

***Polyphenon Green Tea Acne Cream* - Origin BioMedicinals**
Jojoba Oil • Bees Wax • Lecithin • Ascorbyl Palmitate (vitamin C) • Sorbic Acid • 3% Polyphenon 70 Green Tea extract • 0.5% Salicylic Acid • 0.2% Tea Tree Oil.

***Polyphenon Green Tea Skin Cream* - Origin BioMedicinals**
Jojoba Oil • Aloe Vera • Bees Wax • Lecithin • Polyphenon 70 Green Tea extract • Ascorbyl Palmitate (vitamin C) • Lavender Oil • Tea Tree Oil.

***Polysorbate 80* - The Vitamin Shoppe**
Contains 100% pharmaceutical-grade Polysorbate 80.

***Poly-Vi-Sol Chewable Vitamins* - Mead Johnson Nutritionals**
Each chewable tablet contains: Vitamin A Acetate 2500 IU • Vitamin C (Ascorbic Acid) 60 mg • Vitamin D (Vitamin D3) 400 IU • Vitamin E Acetate 15 IU • Thiamin Mononitrate 1.05 mg • Riboflavin 1.2 mg • Niacin (Niacinamide) 13.5 mg • Vitamin B-6 Hydrochloride 1.05 mg • Folate (Folic Acid) 0.3 mg • Vitamin B-12 4.5 mcg • Iron (Ferrous Fumarate)12 mg • Zinc Oxide 8 mg • Copper (Cupric Oxide) 0.8 mg. Other Ingredients: Dextrates, Sugar, Sodium Ascorbate, Magnesium Stearate, Stearic Acid, Silicon Dioxide, Artificial Flavor and Color (Red 40 Lake), Salt.

***Polyzyme* - Young Living Essential Oils**
Each capsule contains: Proprietary Blend: Protease, Phylase, Peptidase, Papain, Bromelain, Lipase, Anise Oil, Peppermint Oil, Rosemary Oil.

***Pomegranate 250 mg* - Vitamin World**
Each capsule contains: Pomegranate seed (punica granatum) 200 mg • Pomegranate fruit extract (punica granatum, 40% ellagic acid) 50 mg. Other Ingredients: Rice Powder, Gelatin, Vegetable Magnesium Stearate, Silica.

***PomEllagic 70 brand* - Cyvex Nutrition, Inc.**
Pomegranate extract.
See Editor's Note No. 44, page 2058.

***Ponaris Nasal Emollient* - Jamol Laboratories**
Active Ingredients: Pine Oil, Eucalyptus Oil, Peppermint Oil, Cajeput Oil, Cottonseed Oil as iodized organic oils. Total Iodine 0.5%-0.7%.

***POS 1* - Advocare International**
Each caplet contains: Niacin 7 mg • Magnesium (as amino acid chelate) 50 mg • Zinc (as monomethionine, OptiZinc brand) 2 mg • Copper (as amino acid chelate) 167 mcg • Moomiyo 33 mg • L-Arginine 400 mg • L-Ornithine 200 mg • Oatgrass leaf/stem extract (avena sativa) 67 mg • Nettles leaf extract (urtica dioica) 17 mg • Eleuthero root extract (eleutherococcus senticosus) 8 mg • Ashwagandha root extract (withania somnifera) 17 mg • Saw Palmetto berry extract (serenoa repens) 33 mg • Wild Yam root extract (dioscorea villosa) 17 mg • Vanadium (as bis-maltolato-oxovanadium) 67 mcg.

***POS 2 Drink Mix* - Advocare International**
Each pouch contains: Choline 50 mcg • Inositol 50 mg • Vanadium 200 mcg • Boron 250 mcg • Gamma Oryzanol 150 mcg • L-Carnitine 25 mg • Inosine 100 mg • Silicon 1 mg • Creatine 2000 mg • DL-Methionine 250 mg • L-Leucine 200 mg • L-Valine 100 mg • L-Isoleucine 100 mg • Maltodextrin • Fructose • Soy Protein powder • Modified Casein • Cocoa powder • MyoForce: Creatine Monohydrate, Creatine Phosphate, Eleuthero root • Soy Lecithin • Canola oil • Dicalcium Phosphate • Carob powder • Salt • Medium Chain Triglycerides • Magnesium Oxide • Calcium Carbonate • DL-

Methionine • Natural Flavors • Artificial Flavors • L-Leucine • Potassium Chloride • Xanthan Gum • Silicon Dioxide • Guar Gum • Ascorbic Acid • L-Valine • L-Isoleucine • Inosine • Rice Syrup Solids • Fructooligosaccharides • Citrus Pectin • Inositol • Zinc Gluconate • Calcium Pantothenate • L-Carnitine • Niacinamide • Vitamin E Succinate • Beta Carotene • Manganese Sulfate • Ferrous Fumarate • Selenomethionine • Calcium Borate • Copper Gluconate • Pyridoxine Hydrochloride • Riboflavin • Thiamine Hydrochloride • Vanadyl Sulfate • Chromium Polynicotinate (ChromeMate brand) • Cholecalciferol • Papain • Bromelain • Gamma Oryzanol • Folic Acid • Choline Dihydrogen Citrate • Biotin • Sodium Molybdate • Dibencozide • Cyanocobalamin • Potassium Iodide.

POS 3 **-** Advocare International
Each pouch contains: Pure Crystalline Fructose • Maltodextrin • Malic Acid • Dextrose • Magnesium Citrate • Sodium Citrate • Potassium Citrate • Calcium Phosphate • L-Glutamine • Ascorbic Acid • Salt • L-Arginine • Potassium Chloride • Natural Flavors • Beta-Carotene • Beet juice concentrate (for color) • Sucralose • Vegetable Gum • Pyridoxine Alpha-Ketoglutarate • Niacinamide • Calcium Pantothenate • Riboflavin • Thiamine Hydrochloride • Chromium Polynicotinate (ChromeMate brand) • L-Glutathione • Coenzyme Q-10.

POS 4 Arginine Power **-** Advocare International
Each rounded tablespoon contains: Vitamin A (as beta carotene) 1250 IU • Folate 100 mcg • Pantothenic Acid (as calcium salt) 50 mg • Vitamin B12 (as cyanocobalamin) 60 mcg • Chromium (as polynicotinate) 60 mcg • L-Arginine 5 g • -Glycine 1 g • DL-Methionine 150 mg • Choline (as bitartrate) 100 mg.

POS 5 **-** Advocare International
Three caplets contain: B-Hydroxymethylbutyrate 2000 mg • Suma root extract (pfaffia paniculata) 200 mg • Green Tea leaf extract (camellia sinensis) 120 mg • Moomiyo 50 mg • Ashwagandha root extract (withania somnifera) 100 mg. Other Ingredients: Dicalcium Phosphate, Silicon Dioxide, Cellulose, Stearic Acid, Magnesium Stearate.

Positive Thoughts **-** Source Naturals
Three tablets contain: St. John's Wort (Hypericum Perforatum) 900 mg (Yielding 0.3% Hypericin 2.7 mg) • Valerian root extract (Valeriana officinalis) 100 mg (Yielding 0.8% Valerenic Acids 800 mcg) • Kava Root Extract (Piper methysticum) 85 mg (Yielding 30% Kavalactones 25 mg) • Lemon Balm (Melissa officinalis) 100 mg • GABA (Gamma Amino Butyric Acid) 300 mg • Taurine (Magnesium Taurinate) 200 mg • Magnesium (oxide, taurinate) 200 mg • L-Tyrosine 200 mg • N-Acetyl L-Tyrosine 50 mg • L-Phenylalanine 100 mg • DMAE (Dimethylaminoethanol bitartrate) 60 mg • Vitamin C (Zinc ascorbate) 50 mg • Vitamin B1 (Thiamin) 25 mg • Vitamin B2 (Riboflavin) 25 mg • Niacinamide 50 mg • Vitamin B5 (Pantothenic Acid) 25 mg • Vitamin B6 (Pyridoxine HCl) 50 mg • Vitamin B12 (Cyanocobalamin) 25 mg • Biotin 300 mcg • Folic Acid 400 mcg • Manganese (citrate) 3 mg • Zinc (Zinc ascorbate) 10 mg.

Post Laser Surgery **-** Natural Ophthalmics
Active Ingredients: Arnica 12x • Eyebright (euphrasia) 8x • Staphysagria 6x • Aconite 12x • Hypericum 6x. Inactive Ingredients: Sterile Water, Sodium Chloride, Citrates, Polysorbate 80.

Post-Menopausal Formula **-** Oasis Wellness Network
Each tablet contains: Vitamin D (as cholecalciferol) 67 IU • Vitamin E (as d-alpha tocopheryl acetate) 20 IU • MaxCell Proprietary Blend 33 mg: Zisyphus Jujube, Aloe Vera gel, Glycyrrhiza Glabra, Piper Nigrum • Soy Isoflavone extract 8 mg • Black Cohosh root extract 5 mg • Vitamin C (as ascorbyl palmitate) 3 mg • Calcium (as citrate/malate/phosphate) 24 mg • Flax seed powder (deoiled) 133 mg • Wild Yam root extract 100 mg • Dong Quai root extract 67 mg. Other Ingredients: Stearic Acid, Cellulose, Calcium Sulfate, Magnesium Stearate, Silica.

Posture-D **-** Inverness Medical Innovations, Inc.
Each tablet contains: Vitamin D (as cholecalciferol) 125 IU • Calcium (as tribasic) 600 mg. Other Ingredients: Maltodextrin, Croscarmellose Sodium, Cellulose, Hydroxypropyl Methylcellulose, Citric Acid, Starch, Silicon Dioxide, Magnesium Stearate, Titanium Dioxide, Mineral Oil, Polysorbate 80, Sodium Lauryl Sulfate.

Posture-D **-** S.C.P.I.
Two tablets contain: Calcium (as tribasic calcium phosphate) 1200 mg • Vitamin D (as cholecalciferol) 250 IU. Other Ingredients: Dextrose, Carboxymethylcellulose Sodium, Magnesium Stearate, Adipic Acid, Natural & Artificial Flavors, FD&C Red #40 Aluminum Lake, FD&C Blue #2 Aluminum Lake, FD&C Yellow #6 Aluminum Lake.

Potassium - Basic Nutrition **-** GNC
Each tablet contains: Potassium (as Potassium Gluconate) 99 mg. Other Ingredients: Dextrose, Stearic Acid, Silica, Magnesium Stearate.

Potassium **-** Solgar
Each tablet contains: Calcium (as dicalcium phosphate) 70 mg • Potassium (as potassium gluconate) 99 mg. Other Ingredients: Dicalcium Phosphate, Silica, Vegetable Cellulose, Vegetable Magnesium Stearate.

Potassium **-** Source Naturals
Each tablet contains: Potassium (from 495 mg of potassium amino acid chelate) 99 mg.

Potassium & Magnesium Aspartate 250 **-** GNC
Each capsule contains: Magnesium (as Monomagnesium Di-L-Aspartate) 250 mg • Potassium (as Monopotassium Aspartate) 250 mg. Other Ingredients: Gelatin, Cellulose.

Potassium 100 mg Timed Release **-** Jamieson
Each caplet contains: Potassium 100 mg.

Potassium 50 mg **-** Jamieson
Each tablet contains: Potassium (as Potassium Gluconate) 50 mg.

Potassium Caps **-** TwinLab
Each capsule contains: Potassium (from potassium citrate and potassium aspartate) 99 mg. Other Ingredients: Gelatin, Potato Starch, Purified Water, Magnesium Stearate, MCT, Silica.

Potassium Fuel **-** TwinLab
Two capsules contain: Potassium Alpha-Ketoglutarate (supplying Elemental Potassium 99 mg) 325 mg • Magnesium Alpha-Ketoglutarate (supplying Elemental Magnesium 100 mg) 700 mg.

Potassium Gluconate - GNC A-Z **-** GNC
Each tablet contains: Potassium (as potassium gluconate) 99 mg. Other Ingredients: Dextrose.

Potassium Gluconate 550 mg **-** Nature Made
Each tablet contains: Potassium 90 mg • Potassium (from 550 mg potassium gluconate) 90 mg. Other Ingredients: Cellulose Gel, Stearic Acid, Magnesium Stearate, Silicon Dioxide, Croscarmellose Sodium. See Editor's Note No. 45, page 2058.

Potassium Gluconate with Folic Acid **-** Quest
Each tablet contains: Potassium Gluconate 650 mg • Folic Acid 400 mcg. Other Ingredients: Croscarmellose Sodium, Calcium phosphate, Magnesium Stearate (vegetable source), Microcrystalline Cellulose, Vegetable Stearin.

Potassium Plus - Enzymatic Therapy **-** Enzymatic Therapy
Each tablet contains: Potassium (Chloride/Citrate) 99 mg • Magnesium Citrate 10 mg • Magnesium Sulfate 5 mg • Pantothenic Acid (D-Calcium Pantothenate) 5 mg • Vitamin B6 (Pyroxidine HCL) 1 mg. Other Ingredients: Colloidal Alkaline Ash Mineral concentrate: Alfalfa juice concentrate, Sea Plant extract, Bio-Min TR8 (Enzymatic Tract Mineral concentrate), Orange juice concentrate, Banana

concentrate, & Sugar Cane juice concentrate (no sugar) 855 mg, Yucca 25 mg.

Potassium Plus - GNC A-Z - GNC
Two tablets contain: Vitamin A (100% as beta-carotene) 5000 IU • Vitamin C (as ascorbic acid) 60 mg • Riboflavin (B2) 1.7 mg • Pantothenic Acid (as calcium d-pantothenate) 5 mg • Calcium (as calcium carbonate and dicalcium phosphate) 250 mg • Phosphorus (as dicalcium phosphate) 50 mg • Magnesium (as magnesium oxide) 100 mg • Zinc (as zinc citrate) 5 mg • Potassium (as potassium gluconate) 99 mg. Other Ingredients: Cellulose, Titanium Dioxide (natural mineral whitener), Vegetable Acetoglycerides, Rose Hips powder (Rosina canina).

Potassium Plus - Olympian Labs
Each capsule contains: Potassium Gluconate 99 mg • Dandelion 100 mg • Barley Grass 100 mg • Red Clover 50 mg • Basil 50 mg • Mulberry leaf 100 mg • Blessed Thistle 50 mg.

Potassium Plus - PhytoPharmica
Each tablet contains: Colloidal Alkaline Ash Mineral Concentrate 80 mg: Dulse whole plant (palmaria palmata), Orange fruit (citrus sinesis), Banana fruit (musa paradisiaca), Sugarcane stalk concentrate (saccharum officinarum) • Mojave Yucca stem and root (yucca schidgera) 25 mg • Pantothenic Acid (as calcium D-pantothenate) 5 mg • Potassium (as potassium chloride and potassium citrate) 100 mg • Proprietary Trace Mineral Blend 125 mg: Selenium (as selenium yeast, SelenoExcell brand), Silicon (as magnesium trisilicate), Boron (as sodium borate), Nickel (as nickel chelate), Tin (as tin chelate), Molybdenum (as sodium molybdate), Vanadium (as vanadyl sulfate) • Vitamin B6 (as pyridoxine HCl) 1 mg.

Potency Plus - Gero Vita International
Each capsule contains: Morinda Officinalis root extract (5% anthroquinones) 70 mg • Curculigo Orchioides rhizome 8:1 extract 70 mg • Epimedium Grandiflorum leaf extract (5% flavonoids) 70 mg • Rubus Chingii berries extract (12% organic acids) 70 mg • Rehmannia Glutinosa root extract (1% catalpol) 30 mg • Dioscorea Opposita root extract (6% diosgenines) 30 mg • Salvia Miltiorrhiza root 8:1 extract 30 mg • Panax Ginseng root extract (20% ginsenosides) 30 mg • Cinnamomum Cassia bark extract (5% cinnamaldehyde) 30 mg • Ligusticum Chuanxiang rhizome extract (5% ligustrazin) 30 mg. Other Ingredients: Dicalcium Phosphate, Cellulose, Sodium Croscarmellose, Stearic Acid, Silica, Magnesium Stearate, Gelatin, ACF 223.

Potent V with Herbs - Vitamin World
Two tablets contain: Niacin 45 mg • Guarana seed extract (paullinia cupana, standardized to contain 22% caffeine) 300 mg • Yohimbe bark extract (pausinystalia yohimba, standardized to contain 2% yohimbine) 250 mg • Taurine 200 mg • Oats aerial 10:1 extract (avena sativa) 150 mg • Saw Palmetto berry 4:1 extract (serenoa repens) 100 mg • Orchic Substance (raw testicular extract) 50 mg • Ginkgo Biloba leaf extract (ginkgo biloba, standardized to contain 24% ginkgo flavone glycosides) 40 mg • Korean Ginseng root (Panax ginseng) 30 mg. Other Ingredients: Cellulose (plant origin), Dicalcium Phosphate, Croscarmellose, Vegetable Stearic Acid, Acacia Gum, Silica, Vegetable Magnesium Stearate, Polyvinylpyrrolidone, Cellulose Coating.

Power Fuel (Exercise & Recovery Drink) - TwinLab
Each serving contains: Carbohydrates (derived from Glucose Polymers & Glucose with small amounts of Fructose) 100 g • Anticatabolic Branched Chain Amino Acids (L-Leucine, L-Isoleucine, L-Valine) • L-Glutamine & Alpha-Ketoglutarates • Antioxidant Nutrients: Vitamin E, Vitamin C, & Beta-Carotene • B Vitamins • Chromium (from patented Chromic Fuel Chromium Picolinate) • Coenzyme Q10 • L-Carnitine • Potassium • Magnesium • Phosphate & Creatine • Carni Fuel (a preferred form of L-Carnitine & Magnesium).

Power Generation - Rexall - Sundown
Three capsules contain: L-Tyrosine 750 mg • DMAE (as 2-dimethylaminoethanol L-bitartrate) 200 mg • Korean Ginseng extract root (standardized to 7% ginsenosides, 10 mg) 143 mg • Caffeine (as caffeine citrate) 50 mg • Ginkgo Biloba extract leaf (standardized to 24% ginkgo flavone glycosides, 9.6 mg; standardized to 6% terpene lactones, 2.4 mg) 40 mg • Cayenne fruit 30 mg. Other Ingredients: Gelatin, Citric Acid, Maltodextrin, Magnesium Stearate.

Power Herbs Migracin - Nature's Herbs
Each softgel contains: Vitamin E (d-alpha tocopheryl succinate) 400 IU • Magnesium (from magnesium oxide) 200 mg • Feverfew extract (aerial part, standardized for 0.7% sesquiterpene lactones) 10.5 mg • White Willow Bark extract (standardized for 15% salicin) 25 mg • Ginger root extract (standardized for 5% gingerols) 25 mg. Other Ingredients: Soybean Oil, Gelatin, Glycerin, Purified Water, Lecithin, Yellow Beeswax, Titanium Dioxide, Chlorophyll.

Power L-Glutamine Pro - PureForm
Each 5 g serving contains: L-Glutamine (pure pharmaceutical grade) 5 g.

Power Nutrient - Changes International, Inc.
Two tablespoons (1 oz/30 ml) contain: Vitamin A (as 37% Beta-Carotene, 63% Retinyl palmitate) • Vitamin C (as Ascorbic acid) 60 mg • Vitamin D (as Cholecalciferol) 400 IU • Vitamin E (as DL-tocopherol) 30 IU • Thiamin (as Thiamine mononitrate) 1.5 mg • Riboflavin (as Riboflavin monophosphate) 1.7 mg • Niacin (as Niacinamide) 20 mg • Vitamin B6 (as Pyrodoxine HCL) 2 mg • Folate (as Folic acid) 400 mcg • Vitamin B12 (as Cyanocobalamin) 6 mcg • Biotin 300 mcg • Pantothenic acid (Vitamin B5) (as D-calcium pantothenate) 10 mg • Calcium (as Calcium lactate-gluconate) 40 mg • Iron 6 mg. Other Ingredients: Purified water, Fructose, Citric acid, Colloidal mineral blend, Natural Cranberry flavor, Sodium benzoate, Potassium sorbate and Maltodextrin.

Power Nutrient Plus - Changes International, Inc.
One tablespoonful (15 ml) contains: Vitamin A (as 100% Beta-Carotene) 5000 IU • Vitamin C (Ascorbic acid) 60 mg • Vitamin D (as Cholecalciferol) 400 IU • Thiamin (as Thiamin HCl) 1.5 mg • Riboflavin (as Riboflavin-5-phosphate) 1.7 mg • Niacin (as Niacinamide) 5 mg • Vitamin B6 (as Pyridoxine HCl) 2 mg • Folate (Folic acid) 400 mcg • Vitamin B12 (as Cyanocobalamin) 6 mcg • Biotin 300 mcg • Pantothenic acid (as D-calcium pantothenate) 10 mg • Calcium (as Calcium lactate-gluconate) 40 mg • Korean Ginseng root extract 50 mg. Other Ingredients: Purified water, Fructose, Citric acid, Natural flavors, Aloe vera gel, Poly-colloidal organic minerals, Electrolyte complex (Potassium chloride, Magnesium citrate and Sodium citrate), Cellulose gum, Potassium sorbate, and Sodium benzoate.

Power Skin Conditioner - For Men - Jamieson
Aloe Vera Gel • Algae Extract • Royal Jelly • Cucumber • Wheat Amino Acids.

Power Teen - Nature's Plus
Each tablet contains: Vitamin A (67% as beta carotene, 33% as palmitate) 15,000 IU • Vitamin C (as ascorbic acid) 100 mg • Vitamin D (as ergocalciferol) 100 IU • Vitamin E (as d-alpha tocopheryl succinate) 100 IU • Vitamin B1 (as thiamine mononitrate) 50 mg • Vitamin B2 (as riboflavin) 50 mg • Niacin (as niacinamide) 50 mg • Vitamin B6 (as pyridoxine hydrochloride) 50 mg • Folate (as folic acid) 400 mcg • Vitamin B12 (as cyanocobalamin) 2 mcg • Biotin 75 mcg • Pantothenic Acid (as calcium pantothenate) 7 mg • Calcium (as amino acid chealte/complex) 250 mg • Iron (as amino acid chelate) 4.5 mg • Magnesium (as amino acid chelate/complex) 250 mg • Zinc (as amino acid chelate, gluconate) 20 mg • Selenium (as selenomethionine) 75 mcg • Copper (as amino acid chelate) 1 mg • Manganese (as amino acid chelate) 2 mg • Chromium (as chromium polynicotinate) 50 mcg • Molybdenum (as sodium molybdate) 50 mcg • Potassium (as amino acid complex) 20 mg • Proprietary Blend 100 mg: Broccoli, Spinach, Carrot, Spirulina, Chlorella, Evening

Primrose, Black Currant seed • Piper Nigrum fruit (Bioperine, standardized 95% [2.4 mg] 1-piperoylpiperidine) 2.5 mg.

Power Thin **-** Gold Star Nutrition
Ma Huang • Guarana • Magnesium • Chromium • Ginseng • Bladderwrack • Kola Nut • White Willow Bark • Fo-Ti • Ginger root • Gotu Kola • Licorice root • Hawthorne Berries • Saw Palmetto • Ginkgo Biloba • Boron • Spirulina • Potassium Citrate • Vitamin B12 • Folic Acid.
See Editor's Note No. 30, page 2056.

Power V with herbs **-** Nature's Bounty
Two tablets contain: Yohime bark extract (pausinystalie yohimba, standardized to contain 2% yohimbine) 250 mg • Niacin (B3) 45 mg • Oats aerial extract (avena sativa) 150 mg • Ginkgo Biloba leaf extract (ginkgo biloba, standardized to contain 24% ginkgo flavone glycosides) 40 mg • Saw Palmetto berry extract (serenoa repens) 100 mg • Guarana seed extract (paullinia cupana, standardized to contain 22% caffeine) 300 mg • Taurine 200 mg • Siberian Ginseng rot extract (eleutherococcus senticosus) 30 mg • Orchic substance 50 mg.
See Editor's Note No. 14, page 2055.

Power Vitamins for Men **-** Jamieson
Three caplets contain: Vitamin B1 (Thiamine Mononitrate) 20 mg • Vitamin B2 (Riboflavin) 20 mg • Vitamin B6 (Pyrodixine HCl) 20 mg • Niacinamide 150 mg • Vitamin B12 (Cyanocobalamin) 50 mcg • Pantothenic Acid (Calcium D-Panthenate) 30 mg • Folic Acid 0.2 mg • Vitamin A (Acetate) 7500 IU • Beta Carotene (Pro-Vitamin A) 1500 IU • Vitamin D 200 IU • Vitamin E (D-Alpha Tocopheryl Succinate) 30 IU • Vitamin C (Ascorbic Acid) 200 mg • Calcium (Carbonate) 250 mg • Magnesium (Oxide) 100 mg • Potassium 50 mg • Zinc 5 mg • Iodine (Kelp) 15 mg • Selenium 10 mcg • Chromium 10 mcg • Siberian Ginseng root (PE 1:8) 100 mg • Astragalus root (PE 1:4) 50 mg • Codonopsis root 50 mg • Damiana leaves (PE 1:6.5) 50 mg • Licorice root (PE 1:2) 50 mg • Fo-Ti root (PE 1:8) 50 mg • Grape Seed (PE 1:5) 50 mg • Citrus Bioflavonoids 50 mg • European Garlic 80 mg • Spirulina 80 mg • Chlorella 80 mg • Wheat Grass 80 mg • Borage 50 mg • Sunflower Oil 50 mg • Coenzyme Q10 (Ubiquinone) 10 mg • Seed Source Protein (Amaranth, Sunflower, Bean, Quinoa, Diu, Radish) 80 mg • Inositol 20 mg • Dl-Methionine 2.2 mg • Bromelain 48.5 mg • Papain 36.4 mg • Amylase 6.1 mg • Lipase 6.1 mg • Cellulase 3.0 mg.

PowerActin **-** Nature's Plus
Two capsules contain: Korean Ginseng [(Panax ginseng root) standardized 15% Ginsenosides] 250 mg • Siberian Ginseng [(Eleutherococcus senticosus root) standardized 0.8% Eleutherosides] 150 mg • Cayenne [(Capsicum frutescens fruit) standardized 100000 STU] 150 mg • Ashwagandha ([Withania somnifera root) standardized 1.5% Withanolids] 50 mg • Schisandra [(Schisandra chinensis fruit) standardized 9% Schisandrins] 50 mg • Coenzyme Q10 (Ubiquinone) 5 mg • Vitamin B12 (from Cobalamin) 500 mcg.

PoweRelief **-** Pain & Stress Center
Two capsules contain: DLPA (DL-Phenylalanine) 500 mg • GABA 200 mg • Boswellia 300 mg • Passion Flower 150 mg • Magnesium 10 mg • Vitamin B6 4 mg.

PowerKids **-** Advocare International
Two tablets contain: Vitamin A (as palmitate) 500 IU • Vitamin A (as beta-carotene) 5000 IU • Vitamin C (as ascorbic acid) 60 mg • Vitamin D (as ergocalciferol) 200 IU • Vitamin E (as d-alpha tocopheryl succinate) 15 IU • Thiamine (as mononitrate) 1.5 mg • Riboflavin 1.8 mg • Niacin (as niacinamide) 16 mg • Vitamin B6 (as pyridoxine HCl) 2 mg • Folic Acid 200 mcg • Vitamin B12 (as cyanocobalamin) 6 mcg • Biotin 50 mcg • Pantothenic Acid (as calcium pantothenate) 5 mg • Calcium (as amino acid chelate) 50 mg • Iron (as amino acid chelate) 2.5 mg • Iodine (as amino acid chelate) 60 mcg • Magnesium (as amino acid chelate) 50 mg • Zinc (as amino acid chelate) 5 mg • Selenium (as selenomethionine) 35 mcg • Copper (as amino acid chelate) 500 mcg • Manganese (as amino acid chelate) 500 mcg • Chromium (as polynicotinate-ChromeMate) 60 mcg • Molybdenum (as amino acid chelate) 15 mcg • Boron (as amino acid chelate) 100 mcg • Inositol 2.5 mg • Choline (as choline bitartrate) 15 mg • Coenzyme Q-10 50 mcg. Other Ingredients: Fructose, Xylitol, Soybean Oil, Natural Cherry Flavor, Natural Orange Flavor, Stearic Acid, Silicon Dioxide, Magnesium Stearate, Beet Root Powder (for color), Turmeric (for color), Sucralose, Monoammonium Glycyrrhizinate (from licorice), Carrot Powder, Apple Powder.

Pre **-** Pacific BioLogic
Patrina • Peony root (white) • Bupleurum root (natural) • Ligusticum root • Jack-in-the-Pulpit rhizome • Angelica root (Chinese) • Hornet Nest • Vaccaria seeds • Argimony • Cyperus rhizome • Motherwort (Chinese) • Tumeric tuber • Bitter Orange ripened fruit.
See Editor's Note No. 40, page 2058.

Pre-Drinking Formula **-** Sojourn Health
Four capsules contain: Vitamin C (sago palm) 1000 mg • Vitamin D (activated ergosterol) 100 IU • Vitamin E (mixed tocopherols) 400 IU • Vitamin B1 (thiamin HCl) 75 mg • Vitamin B2 (riboflavin) 75 mg • Vitamin B3 (niacinamide) 75 mg • Vitamin B6 (pyridoxine HCl) 75 mg • Folic Acid 400 mcg • VitaminB12 75 mcg • Biotin 200 mcg • Vitamin B5 (pantothenic acid) 75 mg • Calcium (AA chelate) 900 mg • Selenium (AA chelate) 100 mcg • Copper (AA chelate) 1 mg • Proprietary Base 875 mg: Methionine DL, Bioflavonoids, Betaine (HCl), PABA (B10), Choline (bitartrate), Inositol.

PreCare Chewables **-** KV Pharmaceutical Co.
Each tablet contains: Vitamin C (as Ester-C) 50 mg • Calcium (as calcium carbonate) 250 mg • Iron (as MicroMask ferrous fumerate) 40 mg • Vitamin D (vitamin D3, as cholecalciferol) 6 mcg • Vitamin E (as dl-alpha-tocopheryl acetate) 3.5 mg • Vitamin B6 (as pyridoxine HCl) 2 mg • Folic Acid, USP 1 mg • Magnesium (as magnesium oxide, USP) 50 mg • Zinc (as zinc oxide, USP) 15 mg • Copper (as cupric oxide) 2 mg. Inactive Ingredients: Citric Acid, FD&C Yellow No. 6 Lake, Flow Agents, Natural Non-Nutritive Sweetening Agents, Natural and Artificial Flavors.

PreCare Conceive **-** KV Pharmaceutical Co.
Each tablet contains: Vitamin C (as Ester-C) 60 mg • Calcium (as calcium carbonate) 200 mg • Iron (as ferrous fumarate and carbonyl iron) 30 mg • Vitamin E (as dl-alpha-tocopheryl acetate) 30 IU • Thiamine (as thiamine mononitrate) 3 mg • Riboflavin, USP 3.4 mg • Niacin (as niacinamide, USP) 20 mg • Pyridoxine (as pyridoxine HCl, USP) 50 mg • Folic Acid, USP 1 mg • Magnesium (as magnesium oxide) 100 mg • Cyanocobalamin 12 mcg • Zinc (as zinc oxide) 15 mg • Copper (as cupric oxide) 2 mg. Inactive Ingredients: Cellulose Polymers, Flow Agents, Pigment Natural Wax, FD&C Yellow #10 Aluminum Lake, FD&C Yellow #6 Aluminum Lake, Lactose, Other Ingredients.

PreCare Prenatal **-** KV Pharmaceutical Co.
Each caplet contains: Vitamin C (as Ester-C) 50 mg • Calcium (as calcium carbonate) 250 mg • Iron (as ferrous fumerate and carbonyl iron) 40 mg • Vitamin E (as dl-alpha-tocopheryl acetate) 3.5 mg • Vitamin D (vitamin D3, as cholecalciferol) 6 mcg • Thiamine (as thiamine mononitrate, USP) 3 mg • Riboflavin, USP 3.4 mg • Niacin (as niacinamide, USP) 20 mg • Pyridoxine (as pyridoxine HCl, USP) 20 mg • Folic Acid, USP 1 mg • Cyanocobalamin 12 mcg • Magnesium (as magnesium oxide, USP) 50 mg • Zinc (as zinc sulfate, USP) 15 mg • Copper (as cupric sulfate) 2 mg. Inactive Ingredients: Natural Oils, natural Wax, Cellulose Polymers, Flow Agents, FD&C Yellow No. 6 Aluminum Lake, Other Ingredients.

Pregnacare Cream **-** Vitabiotics
Calendula extract (lt. calendula officinalis) • Evening Primrose Oil (lt. oenothera biennis) • Aloe extract (lt. aloe barbadensis) • Allantoin • Pantothenic Acid (as D-panthenol) • Vitamin E (as alpha tocopheryl acetate) • Vitamin C (as sodium ascorbyl phosphate) • Sodium Chloride • Magnesium Sulphate • Zinc Oxide • Menthol.

Pregnacare Tablets **-** Vitabiotics
Each tablet contains: Vitamin D (200 IU) 5 mcg • Vitamin E (natural source) 20 mg • Vitamin C 70 mg • Vitamin B1 (thiamin) 3 mg •

Vitamin B2 (riboflavin) 2 mg • Vitamin B3 (niacin) 20 mg • Vitamin B6 (pyridoxine HCl) 10 mg • Folic Acid 400 mcg • Vitamin B12 (cyanocobalamin) 6 mcg • Betacarotene (natural source) 3 mg • Vitamin K 70 mcg • Iron 20 mg • Magnesium 150 mg • Zinc 15 mg • Iodine 140 mcg • Copper 1 mg.

Pregnancy Tea **-** Traditional Medicinals
Spearmint leaf • Red Raspberry leaf • Lemongrass leaf • Strawberry Leaf • Fennel seed • Nettle leaf • Rose Hip • Alfalfa herb • Lemon Verbena leaf.

Pregnancy-6 Formula (Pregnancy 6) **-** Nature's Way
Each capsule contains Proprietary Formula 425 mg: Black Cohosh root • Blessed Thistle • False Unicorn root • Penny Royal flowering top • Red Raspberry leaves • Squaw Vine vine, leaf, fruit. Other Ingredients: Gelatin.
See Editor's Note No. 8, page 2054.

Pregnenolone **-** Metabolic Response Modifiers
Each capsule contains: Pregnenolone 10 mg.

Pregnenolone - GNC A-Z **-** GNC
Each capsule contains: Pregnenolone 50 mg. Other Ingredients: Cellulose, Gelatin, Calcium Carbonate.

Pregnenolone (100 mg) **-** NutriCology
Each tablet contains: Pregnenolone 100 mg. Other Ingredients: Cellulose, Magnesium Stearate, Silica Gel, Fatty Acids, Silicon Dioxide.

Pregnenolone (50 mg) **-** NutriCology
Each tablet contains: Pregnenolone 50 mg. Other Ingredients: Cellulose, Magnesium Stearate, Silica Gel, Fatty Acids, Silicon Dioxide.

Pregnenolone 30 mg **-** PhysioLogics
Each capsule contains: Pregnenolone 30 mg. Other Ingredients: Dicalcium Phosphate, Cellulose (plant origin), Gelatin, Silica, Vegetable Magnesium Stearate.

Pregnenolone 50 mg **-** PhysioLogics
Each capsule contains: Pregnenolone 50 mg. Other Ingredients: Rice Powder, Gelatin, Vegetable Magnesium Stearate, Silica.

Pregnenolone-15 **-** PhytoPharmica
Each capsule contains: Pregnenolone 15 mg.
See Editor's Note No. 21, page 2056.

Prelief **-** AkPharma Inc.
Two tablets contain: Calcium 130 mg • Phosphorus 100 mg. Other Ingredients: Magnesium Stearate.

Prelieve PMS **-** Boehringer Ingelheim
One mini-tablet contains: Standardized Vitex Agnus-Castus Extract (2:1) (fruit) 20 mg. Other Ingredients: Lactose, magnesium stearate, polyvidone, talc, PEG-100, polymethacrylic acid derivatives, FD&C blue #2, titanium dioxide, synthetic iron oxide.

Pre-Load Creatine Complex **-** Optimum Nutrition
Each scoop (47 g) contains: Creatine Monohydrate 6 g • L-Glutamine 1 g • Taurine 1 g • L-Isoleucine 500 mg • L-Valine 500 mg • L-Arginine 250 mg • L-Glycine 250 mg • Carbogen 200 mg. Other Ingredients: Dextrose, Natural Color, Magnesium Phosphate, Sodium Phosphate, Potassium Phosphate, Citric Acid, Natural Flavor.

Prelox Blue **-** Herbalife
Two tablets contain: Proprietary Blend 1440 mg: L-Arginine HCl, Aspartic Acid, Pycnogenol (dried pine bark extract). Other Ingredients: Microcrystalline Cellulose, Corn Starch, Croscarmellose Sodium, Hypromellose, Magnesium Stearate, Silicon Dioxide, Titanium Dioxide, Triacetin, FD&C Blue #1, FD&C Blue #2.

Premence Capsules **-** Vitabiotics
Each capsule contains: Vitamin A 700 mcg • Vitamin E 30 mg • Vitamin C 60 mg • Vitamin B1 (thiamin) 12 mg • Vitamin B2 (riboflavin) 1.6 mg • Vitamin B3 (niacin) 36 mg • Vitamin B6 (pyridoxine HCl) 10 mg • Folic Acid 400 mcg • Vitamin B12 (cyanocobalamin) 5 mcg • Iron 15 mg • Magnesium 150 mg • Zinc 15 mg • Iodine 100 mcg • Copper 1 mg.

PremensisRx **-** KV Pharmaceutical Co.
Each tablet contains: Vitamin B6 (as pyridoxine HCl) 75 mg • Vitamin B12 (as cyanocobalamin) 12 mcg • Folic Acid, USP 1 mg • Calcium (as calcium carbonate) 200 mg. Inactive Ingredients: Natural Waxes, Cellulose Polymers, FD&C Blue No. 1 Aluminum Lake, FD&C Yellow No. 10 Aluminum Lake, Flow Agents, Other Ingredients.

Premenstra **-** HerbaSway
Dong Quai • Wild Yam • Knotweed • Ginger • Licorice • Blackberry • HerbaSwee (Cucurbitaceae fruit).

Premier One Royal Jelly 2000 **-** Nutraceutical Corp.
Each capsule contains: Royal Jelly 3.5x (equivalent to 2000 mg) 572 mg.

Premium Cleansing Herbs **-** Longevity
Three capsules contain: Riboflavin (vitamin B2) 20 mg • Chelated Minerals Proprietary Blend 318 mg: Potassium, Calcium, Magnesium, Zinc, Chromium, Selenium, Iron, Copper, Molybdenum, Vanadium, Iodine, Cobalt, Manganese • Cascara Sagrada bark (rhamnus purshiana) 300 mg • Yucca root (yucca filimentosa) 300 mg • Fennel Seed fruit (foniclum vulgare) 50 mg • Pau D'arco inner bark (tabebuia avellanedae) 50 mg • Peppermint leaf, top (mentha piperita) 50 mg • Yellowdock root (rumex crispus) 50 mg. Other Ingredients: Gelatin, Rice Flour, Magnesium Stearate (vegetable source), Silicon Dioxide.

Premium Echinacea **-** Holista
Each capsule contains: Echinacea angustifolia (root) from standardized 6.5:1 extract (4% echinacoside) 500 mg.

Premium Echinacea **-** Olympian Labs
Each capsule contains: Premium Echinacea 400 mg.

Premium HGH Precursors **-** Youngevity
Six capsules contain: Vitamin B6 (as pyridoxine hydrochloride) 6 mg • Manganese (as amino acid chelate) 1.5 mg • Chromium (as amino acid chelate) 90 mcg • Arginine (as l-arginine hydrochloride) 300 mg • Glutamine (as l-glutamine) 300 mg • Glycine (as l-glycine) 300 mg • Ornithine (as l-ornithine) 300 mg • Tyrosine (as l-tyrosine) 300 mg • Vilcabamba Mineral Essence Proprietary Blend 300 mg: Potassium, Calcium, Magnesium, Zinc, Chromium, Selenium, Iron, Copper, Molybdenum, Vanadium, Iodine, Cobalt, Manganese • GABA (gamma-aminobutyric acid) 150 mg • Kelp (Laminaria spp., plant) 150 mg. Other Ingredients: Gelatin, Rice Flour, Magnesium Stearate (vegetable source), Silicon Dioxide.

Premium Korean Ginseng **-** Olympian Labs
Each capsule contains: Korean Ginseng 650 mg.

Premium Soy Protein Isolate Powder **-** Puritan's Pride
Each serving approximately contains: Total Isoflavones 60 mg • Genistein 36 mg • Daidzein 21 mg • Glycitein 3 mg.

Premium Super Cell Protector **-** Longevity
Three capsules contain: Chelated Minerals Proprietary Blend 270 mg: Potassium, Calcium, Magnesium, Zinc, Chromium, Selenium, Iron, Copper, Molybdenum, Vanadium, Iodine, Cobalt, Manganese • Grape Seed extract (vitus vinifera, standardized to provide 142.5 mg proanthocyanidins) 150 mg. Other Ingredients: Gelatin, Rice Flour, Magnesium Stearate (vegetable source), Silicon Dioxide.

Pre-Natal **-** Aspen Group, Inc.
Each tablet contains: Vitamin A (from vitamin A acetate & beta carotene) 4000 IU • Vitamin D (cholecalciferol) 400 IU • Vitamin E (d2-alpha tocopherol acetate) 11 mg • Vitamin C (ascorbic acid) 100 mg • Folic acid 0.8 mg • Vitamin B1 (thiamine mononitrate) 1.84 mg • Vitamin B2 (riboflavin) 1.7 mg • Niacinamide 18 mg • Vitamin B6

100 mg • Horsetail grass 100 mg • Hesperidin 50 mg • PABA 30 mg • Rutin 25 mg.

Prenatal Tablets **-** Leiner Health Products
Each tablet contains: Niacin (Niacinamide) 18 mg • Riboflavin (Vitamin B2) 1.7 mg • Vitamin A Acetate 4000 IU • Vitamin B12 (Cyanocobalamin - USP Method 2) 4 mcg • Vitamin E (dl-Alpha Tocopheryl Acetate) 11 IU • Vitamin C (Ascorbic Acid) 100 mg • Zinc Oxide 25 mg • Iron (Ferrous Fumarate) 27 mg • Calcium Sulfate 200 mg • Thiamin Mononitrate (Vitamin B1) 1.84 mg • Vitamin B6 (Pyridoxine Hydrochloride) 2.6 mg • Folate (Folic Acid) 800 mcg • Vitamin D (Ergocalciferol) 400 IU. Other Ingredients: Cellulose, Maltodextrin, Starch, Hydroxypropyl Methylcellulose, Croscarmellose Sodium, Sodium Starch Glycolate, Gelatin, Silicon Dioxide, Tricalcium Phosphate, Polyethylene Glycol 3350, Hydroxypropyl Cellulose, Titanium Dioxide, Magnesium Stearate, Phamaceutical Glaze, Polysorbate 80, Lactose, Yellow 6 Lake, Red 40 Lake, Blue 1 Lake, Beta Carotene, Resin.

Prenatal Vitamins **-** Nature's Bounty
Each tablet contains: Vitamin A (as Retinyl Acetate and Beta Carotene) 4000 IU • Vitamin C (as Ascorbic Acid) 100 mg • Vitamin D (as Cholecalciferol) 400 IU • Vitamin E (as dl-Alpha Tocopheryl Acetate) 11 IU • Thiamin (as Thiamine- Mononitrate) 1.84 mg • Riboflavin (Vitamin B-2) 1.7 mg • Niacin (as Niacinamide) 18 mg • Vitamin B-6 (Pyridoxine Hydrochloride) 2.6 mg • Folic Acid 800 mcg • Vitamin B-12 (as Cyanocobalamin) 4 mcg • Calcium (as Calcium Sulfate) 200 mg • Iron (as Ferrous Fumarate) 27 mg • Zinc (as Zinc Oxide) 25 mg. Other Ingredients: Cellulose, Vegetable Stearic Acid, Croscarmellose, Cellulose Coating, Vegetable Magnesium Stearate, Titanium Dioxide, FD&C Yellow No. 6 Aluminum Lake, FD&C Red No. 40 Aluminum Lake, FD&C Blue No. 1 Aluminum Lake.

Pre-Nate Oil **-** The Herbalist
Herbal oils of Sweet Almond, Safflower, Aloe Vera, Vitamin E, St. John's Wort flower, Calendula flower • Essential oils of French Lavender & Lemon.

Pressur-Lo **-** Futurebiotics
Six tablets contain: Vitamin A (as beta-carotene) 6,000 IU • Vitamin C (as ascorbic acid) 360 mg • Vitamin D (as ergocalciferol) 150 IU • Thiamin 12 mg • Riboflavin 12 mg • Niacin (as niacinamide) 180 mg • Vitamin B6 (as pyridoxine hydrochloride) 12 mg • Vitamin B12 (as cyanocobalamin) 30 mcg • Pantothenic Acid (as calcium pantothenate) 120 mg • Calcium (as calcium carbonate, ascorbate) 480 mg • Magnesium (as magnesium oxide, chloride, citrate) 360 mg • Zinc (as zinc gluconate) 18 mg • Selenium (as selenomethionine) 120 mcg • Manganese (as manganese amino acid chelate) 24 mg • Chromium (as chromium polynicotinate) 180 mcg • Potassium (as potassium chloride, citrate) 330 mg • Garlic bulb powder concentrate 480 mg • Hawthorn berry powder extract (4:1) 282 mg • Horsetail leaf powder 180 mg • Juniper berry powder 180 mg • Valerian root powder 180 mg • Cayenne fruit powder 150 mg • Beta-sitosterol complex 210 mg • Rutin 150 mg • Betaine hydrochloride 150 mg • Taurine 480 mg. Other Ingredients: Cellulose, Stearic Acid, Magnesium Stearate, and Silica.

Prevalin **-** VitaStore
Bee Pollen • Brindal Berry (Hydroxycitric Acid, HCA) • Chromium Picolinate • Ginger • Ginseng • Carnitine • White Willow Bark • Vitamin A • Vitamin B1 • Vitamin B6 • Vitamin B12 • Vitamin C • Vitamin D • Vitamin E (D-Alpha Tocopherol) • Folic Acid • Iodine (Kelp) • Niacin • d-Biotin • Pantothenic Acid • Potassium Gluconate.

Prevent Pro Fiber Formula **-** Deseret Laboratories
Each scoop (6.6 g) contains: Guar Gum, Gum Arabic, Pectin, Locust Bean Gum, Natural Cherry flavor, Citrus flavor enhancer, Beet powder, Maltodextrin, Sucralose, Policosanol 5 mg.

Prevent Spray **-** Xtreme Formulations
Five sprays contain: PREVENT Proprietary Blend 0.875 mL: 3,6,17-Androstenetrione, 4-Hydroxyandrostenedione, Caffeine Anhydrous, (pyridoxine hydrochloride) 2.6 mg • Vitamin B12 (cyanocobalamin) 4 mcg • Calcium (calcium sulfate) 200 mg • Iron (ferrous fumerate) 20 mg • Zinc (zinc oxide) 25 mg.

Pre-Natal **-** Jamieson
Each caplet contains: Vitamin D 1000 IU • Beta Carotene 1800 IU • Vitamin D 200 IU • Vitamin C 150 mg • Vitamin E 30 mg • Vitamin B1 3 mg • Vitamin B2 3.75 mg • Vitamin B6 10 mg • Vitamin B12 10 mcg • Vitamin B3 22 mg • Vitamin B5 10 mg • Biotin 30 mcg • Folic Acid 1 mg • Chelated Calcium 200 mg • Chelated Magnesium 100 mg • Chelated Zinc 20 mg • Chelated Iron 30 mg • Chelated Copper 1 mg • Chelated Chromium 25 mcg • Chelated Manganese 5 mg • Iodine (from kelp) 15 mg. In a base of Rutin, Hesperidin, Acerola, Rosehips, Bioflavonoids, Peppermint, Chamomile, Bromelain, Papain, Amylase, Lipase, Cellulase.

Pre-Natal Caps **-** Now
Four capsules contain: Vitamin A (Beta Carotene) 10000 IU • Vitamin B1 (Thiamine HCL) 5 mg • Vitamin B2 (Riboflavin) 5 mg • Vitamin B3 (Niacinamide) 20 mg • Vitamin B5 (Pantothenic Acid) 20 mg • Vitamin B6 (Pyridoxine HCL) 5 mg • Vitamin B12 (Cyanocobalamin) 20 mcg • Biotin 300 mcg • Folic Acid 800 mcg • Vitamin C (Calcium Ascorbate) 120 mg • Vitamin D (Fish Liver oil) 400 IU • Vitamin E (d-Alpha Tocopheryl Succinate) 150 IU • Vitamin K 80 mcg • Calcium (Carbonate • Ascorbate) 1200 mg • Magnesium (Oxide) 500 mg • Zinc (Amino Acid Chelate) 15 mg • Iron (Bisglycinate) 36 mg • Copper (Amino Acid Chelate) 1 mg • Iodine (Kelp) 150 mcg • Manganese (Amino Acid Chelate) 3.5 mg • Selenium (L-Selenomethionine) 50 mcg • Chromium (Picolinate) 100 mcg • Molybdenum (Amino Acid Chelate) 80 mcg • Potassium (Chloride) 50 mg • Vanadium (Amino Acid Chelate) 25 mcg • Choline 10 mg • Inositol 10 mg • PABA 4 mg.

PreNatal Care **-** Natrol
Three tablets contain: Vitamin A (as Vitamin A palmitate & d-Salina beta carotene) 5000 IU • Vitamin C (calcium ascorbate) 100 mg • Vitamin D (as cholecalciferol) 200 IU • Vitamin E (as d-alpha tocopherol) 100 IU • Vitamin K 25 mcg • Thiamine (Vitamin B1) (as Thiamine HCl) 25 mg • Riboflavin (Vitamin B2) 25 mg • Niacinamide 25 mg • Vitamin B6 (pyridoxine HCl) 25 mg • Folic Acid 800 mcg• Vitamin B12 (as cobalamin) 50 mcg • Biotin 100 mcg • Pantothenic Acid (as calcium pantothenate) 50 mg • Calcium (as calcium carbonate) 250 mg • Iron 25 mg • Iodine (from kelp) 150 mcg • Magnesium (as magnesium oxide) 125 mg • Zinc (as zinc gluconate) 15 mg • Selenium (as l-Selenomethionine) 100 mcg • Copper (copper gluconate) 2 mg • Manganese (as manganese gluconate) 50 mcg • Potassium (as potassium proteinate) 99 mg • DHA (docosahexanoic acid) 100 mg • Choline (as choline bitartrate) 50 mg • Betaine (as betaine HCl) 50 mg • Ginger root extract 50 mg • Inositol 25 mg • PABA (para amino benzoic acid) 25 mg • Red Raspberry extract leaf 15 mg • Rosemary extract leaf 15 mg • Squaw Vine powdered aerial part 15 mg. Other Ingredients: Mono & Di-Glycerides, Microcrystalline Cellulose, Stearic Acid, Silicon Dioxide, Magnesium Stearate.

Prenatal Complex **-** Nature's Plus
Each tablet contains: Vitamin A (as beta carotene) 8000 IU • Vitamin C (as ascorbic acid) 120 mg • Vitamin D (as ergocalciferol) 400 IU • Vitamin E (as d-alpha tocopheryl acetate) 60 IU • Vitamin B1 (as thiamine HCl) 3 mg • Vitamin B2 (as riboflavin) 3.4 mg • Niacin (as niacinamide) 40 mg • Vitamin B6 (as pyridoxine HCl) 4 mg • Folate (as folic acid) 800 mcg • Vitamin B12 (as cyanocobalamin) 12 mcg • Biotin 600 mcg • Pantothenic Acid (as calcium pantothenate) 20 mg • Calcium (as amino acid chelate/complex) 162 mg • Iron (as amino acid chelate/complex) 18 mg • Phosphorous (as amino acid complex) 125 mg • Iodine (from kelp) 300 mcg • Magnesium (as amino acid chelate/complex) 100 mg • Zinc (as gluconate) 7.5 mg • Copper (as gluconate) 4 mg.

Pre-Natal Complex **-** Puritan's Pride
Four capsules contain: Vitamin A (as retinyl acetate) 8,000 IU • Vitamin C (as ascorbic acid) 120 mg • Vitamin D (as cholecalciferol)

400 IU • Vitamin E (as d-alpha tocopheryl acid succinate) 30 IU • Thiamin (Vitamin B1; as thiamine mononitrate) 1.7 mg • Riboflavin (Vitamin B2) 2.0 mg • Niacin (as niacinamide) 20 mg • Vitamin B6 (as pyridoxine hydrochloride) 2.5 mg • Folate (as folic acid) 800 mcg • Vitamin B12 (as cyanocobalamin) 8 mcg • Biotin 300 mcg • Pantothenic Acid (as d-calcium pantothenate) 10 mg • Calcium (as calcium carbonate and calcium citrate) 1,300 mg • Iron (as ferrous fumarate) 28 mg • Iodine (as potassium iodide) 150 mcg • Magnesium (as magnesium oxide) 450 mg • Zinc (as zinc citrate) 15 mg • Selenium (as sodium selenate) 70 mcg • Copper (as cupric gluconate) 2 mg • Manganese (as manganese gluconate) 2 mg • Chromium (as chromium picolinate) 120 mcg • Molybdenum (as sodium molybdate) 75 mcg • Potassium (as potassium chloride and potassium citrate) 10 mg • Choline (as choline bitartrate) 20 mg • Inositol 20 mg • PABA (as Para-Aminobenzoic acid) 2 mg • Cranberry fruit 60 mg • Peppermint Oil 20 mg • Ginger root 20 mg.

Prenatal Daily **-** Health Factor
Three capsules contain: Beta Carotene (pro Vitamin A) 2500 IU • Vitamin A (Acetate) 4000 IU • Vitamin B1 (Thiamine HCl) 10 mg • Vitamin B2 (Riboflavin & R5'P) 10 mg • Vitamin B3 (Niacinamide) 20 mg • Calcium (Ascorbate & Carbonate) 250 mg • Iron (Feronyl) 40 mg • Vitamin D (Ergocalciferol) 400 IU • Vitamin E (d-Alpha Tocopheryl) 100 IU • Vitamin B6 (Pyridoxine HCl & P5'P) 30 mg • Folic Acid 800 mcg • Vitamin B12 (Cobalamin) 100 mcg • Iodine (Potassium Iodide) 150 mcg • Magnesium (Oxide) 125 mg • Zinc (Picolinate) 20 mg • Copper (Citrate) 2 mg • Biotin 300 mcg • Vitamin B5 (Pantothenic Acid) 25 mg • Vitamin B10 (PABA) 25 mg • Vitamin K (Phytonadione) 15 mcg • Choline (Bitartrate) 12.5 mg • Inositol 12.5 mg • Chromium (Nichrome-3) 200 mg • Manganese (Citrate) 7 mg • Selenium (Amino Acid Chelate) 100 mcg • Lemon Bioflavonoids 25 mg • Rutin 5 mg • Hesperidin 5 mg • Lactobacillus Acidophilus (3 billion/gm) 20 mg.

Pre-Natal Formula **-** PhysioLogics
Four capsules contain: Vitamin A (as retinyl acetate) 8000 IU • Vitamin C (as ascorbic acid) 120 mg • Vitamin D (as cholecalciferol) 400 IU • Vitamin E (as d-alpha tocopherol acid succinate) 30 IU • Thiamin (vitamin B1, as thiamine mononitrate) 1.7 mg • Riboflavin (vitamin B2) 2 mg • Niacin (as niacinamide) 20 mg • Vitamin B6 (as pyridoxine hydrochloride) 2.5 mg • Folic Acid 800 mcg • Vitamin B12 (as cyanocobalamin) 8 mcg • Biotin (as d-biotin) 300 mcg • Pantothenic Acid (as d-calcium pantothenate) 10 mg • Calcium (as calcium carbonate and calcium citrate) 1300 mg • Iron (as ferrous fumarate) 28 mg • Iodine (as potassium iodide) 150 mcg • Magnesium (as magnesium oxide) 450 mg • Zinc (as zinc citrate) 15 mg • Selenium (as sodium selenate) 70 mcg • Copper (as cupric gluconate) 2 mg • Manganese (as manganese gluconate) 2 mg • Chromium (as chromium picolinate) 120 mcg • Molybdenum (as sodium molybdate) 75 mcg • Potassium (as potassium chloride and potassium citrate) 10 mg • Choline (as choline bitartrate) 20 mg • Inositol 20 mg • PABA (para-aminobenzoic acid) 2 mg • Cranberry fruit (vaccinium macrocarpon) 60 mg • Peppermint Oil (mentha piperita) 20 mg • Ginger root (zingiber officinale) 20 mg. Other Ingredients: Gelatin, Acacia Gum, Maltodextrin, Vegetable Magnesium Stearate, Silica.

Prenatal Formula **-** Nature Made
Each tablet contains: Vitamin A 4000 IU • Vitamin C 100 mg • Vitamin D 400 IU • Vitamin E 11 IU • Thiamin 1.5 mg • Riboflavin 1.7 mg • Niacin 18 mg • Vitamin B6 2.6 mg • Folate 800 mcg • Vitamin B12 4 mcg • Calcium 20 mg • Iron 27 mg • Zinc 25 mg. Other Ingredients: Cellulose, Acacia, Croscarmellose Sodium, Silicon Dioxide, Corn Starch, Magnesium Stearate, Hydroxypropyl Methylcellulose, Polyethylene Glycol, Peanut Oil.
See Editor's Note No. 45, page 2058.

Prenatal Formulation **-** Olympian Labs
Four tablets contain: Beta Carotene 5000 IU • Vitamin B-1 (thiamine HCl) 1.5 mg • Vitamin B-2 (riboflavin) 1.6 mg • Vitamin B-3 (inositol hexanicotinate) 17 mg • Vitamin B-5 (calcium pantothenate) 10 mg • Vitamin B-6 (pyridoxine HCl) 2.2 mg • Vitamin B-9 (folic Acid) 600 mcg • Vitamin B-12 (cyanocobalamin) 6 mcg • Vitamin C (ascorbic acid) 70 mg • Vitamin D (cholecalciferol) 400 IU • Vitamin E (d-alpha-tocopherol acetate) 30 IU • d-Biotin 300 mcg • Inositol 10 mg • PABA 2 mg • Choline Bitartrate 10 mg • Chromium 25 mcg • Calcium 1200 mg • Copper 2 mg • Iron 30 mg • Magnesium 320 mg • Manganese 2 mg • Potassium 50 mg • Selenium 65 mcg • Zinc 15 mg • Phosphorus 130 mg • Iodine (kelp) 150 mcg.

Prenatal Forte - NF Formulas **-** Integrative Therapeutics
Two tablets contain: Vitamin A (as retinyl acetate, beta-carotene) 3334 IU • Vitamin C (as calcium ascorbate) 166 mg • Vitamin D (as ergocalciferol) 134 IU • Vitamin E (as dl-alpha tocopheryl acetate) 134 IU • Vitamin K (as phytonadione) 10 mcg • Thiamin (as thiamine hydrochloride) 8 mg • Riboflavin 8 mg • Niacin (as niacinamide) 8 mg • Vitamin B6 (as pyridoxine HCl) 16 mg • Folic Acid 267 mcg • Vitamin B12 (as cyanocobalamin) 50 mcg • Biotin 100 mcg • Pantothenic Acid (as calcium pantothenate) 16 mg • Calcium (as calcium carbonate, citrate, and ascorbate) 400 mg • Iron (as iron citrate) 16 mg • Iodine (kelp source, Ascophyllum nodosum) 50 mcg • Magnesium (as magnesium oxide and citrate) 200 mg • Zinc (as zinc citrate) 8 mg • Selenium (as selenium chelate) 34 mcg • Copper (as copper citrate) 1 mg • Manganese (as manganese citrate) 3.4 mg • Chromium (as chromium chelate) 24 mcg • Potassium (as potassium citrate) 34 mg • Citrus Bioflavonoids Complex 66 mg • L-Glutamic Acid HCl 34 mg • Soy Lecithin 34 mg • Alfalfa leaf (Medicago sativa) 26 mg • Raspberry leaf (Rubus idaeus) 26 mg • Yellow Dock root (Rumex crispus) 26 mg • Cranberry fruit extract (Vaccimium macrocarpon, 25:1) 16 mg • Dandelion root (Taraxacum officinale) 16 mg • Papaya leaf (Carica papaya) 16 mg • Stinging Nettle leaf (Urtica diocia) 16 mg • Choline (as choline bitartrate) 8 mg • Inositol 8 mg • Lactobacillus Acidophilus 8 mg • PhytoZyme Enzyme Blend 6 mg: Amylase, Cellulase, Glucoamylase, Invertase, Lipase, Pectinase with Phytase, Protease, Lactase • Hesperidin Complex 4 mg • Rutin 4 mg • Boron (as boron citrate) 84 mcg. Other Ingredients: Microcrystalline Cellulose, Croscarmellose Sodium, Stearic Acid, Silicon Dioxide, Hydroxypropyl Methocellulose, Magnesium Silicate.

Prenatal Multiple **-** Nature's Life
Six capsules contain: Beta Carotene (Vitamin A equivalent to 15000 IU) 9 mg • Vitamin D (Cholecalciferol) 200 IU • Vitamin B1 (Thiamine HCl) 50 mg • Vitamin B2 (Riboflavin) 50 mg • Vitamin B3 (Niacinamide) 50 mg • Vitamin B6 (Pyridoxine HCl) 75 mg • Vitamin B12 (Cyancobalamin concentrate) 50 mcg • Folic Acid 800 mcg • Pantothenic Acid (d-Calcium Pantothenate) 50 mg • Biotin (d-Biotin) 800 mcg • Inositol 50 mg • Choline (Bitartrate) 50 mg • PABA (Para Aminobenzoic Acid) 25 mg • Vitamin C 300 mg • Lemon Bioflavonoids Complex (TESTLAB 50%, Flavonoids, Flavones, Naringen & Eriocitrin) 50 mg • Rutin (Saphora japonica) 25 mg • Vitamin E (d-Alpha Tocopheryl Succinate) 200 IU • Vitamin K (Phylloquinone) 5 mg • Boron (Citrate) 50 mcg • Calcium (Carbonate, Citrate/ Malate) 1000 mg • Chromium (Picolinate, Nutrition 21, US Patent #33988) 200 mcg • Copper (Gluconate, Citrate) 1.5 mg • Iodine (Potassium Iodide) 25 mcg • Iron (Fumarate, Peptonate) 18 mg • Magnesium (Oxide, Citrate) 500 mg • Manganese (Citrate) 10 mg • Molybdenum (Molybdate) 20 mcg • Potassium (Citrate, Iodide) 99 mg • Selenium (l- Selenomethionine) 100 mcg • Silicon (Dioxide) 20 mcg • Vanadium (Vanadyl Sulfate) 20 mcg • Zinc (Picolinate, Methionine) 15 mg • Red Raspberry leaf (Rubus idaeus) 100 mg • Betaine HCl 50 mg.

Prenatal Plus Optizinc **-** Nutrivention
Four tablets contain: Calcium (Chelate) 1200 mg • Magnesium (Chelate) 300 mg • Vitamin C 300 mg • Phosphorus (Chelate) 150 mg • Niacinamide 100 mg • Vitamin E 100 IU • Potassium 99 mg • Vitamin A 1500 IU • Pantothenic Acid 60 mg • Choline Bitartrate 60 mg • Inositol 50 mg • Vitamin B1 50 mg • Iron (Amino Acid Chelate) 45 mg • Vitamin B1 25 mg • Vitamin B2 25 mg • Zinc 25 mg • Manganese (Amino Acid Chelate) 10 mg • Vitamin D 400 IU • Copper 1 mg • Folic Acid 800 mcg • Biotin 300 mcg • Iodine (Kelp) 150 mcg • Chromium 100 mcg • Selenium 100 mcg • Vitamin B12 100 mcg • Vitamin K 100 mcg • Pumpkin seeds 200 mg • Yellow Dock 200 mg • Alfalfa 100 mg • Bioflavonoids 100 mg • Beet tops

1Synephrine HCl, Octopamine HCl, Tyramine HCl. Other Ingredients: Isopropyl Alcohol, Benzyl Alcohol, Water, N-Methyl-2-Pyrrolidinone, Triglyceride Complex, L-Menthol, Laurocapram, Carbomer.

Preventa Tea **-** HerbaSway
Soy • Green Tea • Ginger • Blackberry • HerbaSwee (Cucurbitaceae fruit).

Prevent-X **-** Cambridge Nutraceuticals
Each serving contains: L-Glutamine 10 g • N-Acetyl-Cysteine 4 g • Vitamin A (as mixed carotenoids) 4000 IU • Vitamin C 2000 mg • Vitamin E 700 IU • Folate 300 mcg • Magnesium 300 mg • Selenium 70 mcg • Zinc 10 mg • Copper 0.5 mg.

Previdia **-** Nutrica, Inc.
Each tablet contains: Tribulus Terrestris leaf extract 250 mg • Black Cohosh root extract 50 mg • Calcium 200 mg. Other Ingredients: Corn Starch, High Grade Plant Cellulose (HPMC), Colloidal Silicon Dioxide, Magnesium Stearate, Methyl Paraben, Propyl Paraben, Dibasic Calcium Phosphate Dihydrate, Croscarmellose Sodium, Titanium Dioxide, Talc, Polyethylene Glycol, Usalake FD&C Blue 1.

Pre-Vites **-** Puritan's Pride
Each tablet contains: Vitamin A 2500 IU • Vitamin C 60 mg • Vitamin D 400 IU • Vitamin E 15 IU • Thiamin 1.05 mg • Riboflavin 1.2 mg • Niacin 13.5 mg • Vitamin B6 1.05 mg • Folic Acid 0.3 mg • Vitamin B12 4.5 mcg.

Pre-Vites **-** Nature's Bounty
Each tablet contains: Vitamin A (as Retinyl Acetate) 2500 IU • Vitamin C (as Ascorbic Acid) 60 mg • Vitamin D (as Cholecalciferol) 400 IU • Vitamin E (as d-Alpha Tocopheryl Acetate) 15 IU • Thiamin Mononitrate (Vitamin B1) 1.05 mg • Riboflavin (Vitamin B2) 1.2 mg • Niacin (as Niacinamide) 13.5 mg • Vitamin B-6 (as Pyridoxine Hydrochloride) 1.05 mg • Folic Acid 0.3 mg • Vitamin B-12 (as Cyanocobalamin) 4.5 mcg. Other Ingredients: Sugar, Vegetable Stearic Acid, Natural Orange Flavor, Vegetable Magnesium Stearate, Silica, Mannitol.

Pre-Vites with Iron **-** Nature's Bounty
Each tablet contains: Vitamin A (as Retinyl Acetate) 2500 IU • Vitamin C (as Ascorbic Acid) 60 mg • Vitamin D (as Cholecalciferol) 400 IU • Vitamin E (as d-Alpha Tocopheryl Acetate) 15 IU • Thiamin Mononitrate (Vitamin B1) 0.05 mg • Riboflavin (Vitamin B2) 1.2 mg • Niacin (as Niacinamide) 13.5 mg • Vitamin B6 (as Pyridoxine Hydrochloride) 1.05 mg • Folic Acid 0.3 mg • Vitamin B12 (as Cyanocobalamin) 4.5 mcg • Iron (as Ferrous Fumarate) 7.5 mg. Other Ingredients: Sugar, Vegetable Stearic Acid, Natural Orange Flavor, Vegetable Magnesium Stearate, Silica, Mannitol.

Prima-C **-** PhysioLogics
Each capsule contains: Vitamin C (as Calcium Ascorbate) 500 mg • Calcium (as Calcium Ascorbate) 57 mg • Bioflavonoids (from citrus) 7 mg • Hesperidin 10 mg • Rutin 10 mg.

PrimaCare - Ther-Rx **-** KV Pharmaceutical Co.
Each white softgel capsule contains: AM Regimen: Omega-3 Fatty Acids 150 mg • Linoleic Acid 25 mg • Linolenic Acid 25 mg • Calcium (as calcium carbonate) 150 mg • Vitamin D (vitamin D3, cholecalciferol) 170 IU • Vitamin E (dl-Alpha-Tocopheryl Acetate) 30 IU. Each pink film-coated tablet contains: PM Regimin: Calcium (as calcium carbonate) 250 mg • Vitamin K 90 mcg • Vitamin C (as Ester-C) 100 mg • Vitamin D (vitamin D3, cholecalciferol) 230 IU • Folic Acid USP 1 mg • Thiamine (as thiamine mononitrate, USP) 3 mg • Riboflavin USP 3.4 mg • Niacin (as niacinamide USP) 20 mg • Pyridoxine (as pyridoxine HCl USP) 10 mg • Cyanocobalamin (vitamin B12) 12 mcg • Biotin 35 mcg • Pantothenic Acid 7 mg • Iron (as ferrous fumerate) 30 mg • Zinc (as zinc oxide USP) 13 mg • Copper (as cupric oxide) 1.3 mg • Selenium 75 mcg • Chromium 45 mcg • Molybdenum 50 mcg.

Primaderm **-** Prime Pharmaceutical Corp. (Canadian)
Active Ingredient: Mahonia Aquifolium.

Primal Defense HSO Probiotic Formula Caplets **-** Garden of Life, Inc.
Each caplet contains: Poten-Zyme Superfood Blend 800 mg: Barley grass juice, Oat grass juice, Yucca juice • Ionic Plant Based Minerals 100 mg • HSOs Probiotic Blend 1 billion CFU • Iron (fulvic acid source) 1.8 mg. Other Ingredients: Cellulose, Stearate (vegetable source).

Primal Defense HSO Probiotic Formula Powder **-** Garden of Life, Inc.
Each scoop contains: HSO Probiotic Blend 1 Billion CFU • Poten-Zyme Superfood Blend 800 mg: Dunaliella Salina, Barley grass juice, Oat Grass juice, Yucca juice • Ionic Plant Based Minerals 100 mg • Iron (fulvic acid source) 1.8 mg. Other Ingredients: Cellulose, Stearates (vegetable source).

Primanol Borage Oil **-** Jamieson
Each capsul contains: CIS-Linoleic Acid: from Borage Seed Oil 140.4 mg • CIS-Linoleic Acid: from Sunflower Seed Oil 75.6 • Gamma Linolenic Acid: from Borage Seed Oil 90 mg • Vitamin E (d-Alpha Tocopheryl Acetate) 10 IU.

Primavar **-** Unknown
Each capsule contains: 19-Norandrostenedione 100 mg • 4-Androstenediol 100 mg.

Primavar II **-** Unknown
Each capsule contains: Bolandiol (Norandrostenediol) 100 mg • 4-Androstenediol 100 mg.

PrimaVu Herbal Eye Drops **-** Molecular Health Commerce, Inc.
Matricaria Chamomilla L. tincture (German chamomile) HPUS 3X • Euprhasia Officinalis tincture (eyebright) HPUS 3X.
See Editor's Note No. 1, page 2053.

PrimaVu Herbal Eye Drops Acuta **-** Molecular Health Commerce, Inc.
Euphrasia Officinalis tincture (eyebright) HPUS 3X • Foeniculum Vulgare tincture (fennel) HPUS 3X • Melilotus Officinalis tincture (yellow sweet clover) HPUS 3X.
See Editor's Note No. 1, page 2053.

PrimaVu Herbal Eye Wash – Molecular Health Commerce, Inc.
Euphrasia Officinalis tincture (eyebright) HPUS 4X • Matricaria Chamomilla L. tincture (German chamomile) HPUS 4X.
See Editor's Note No. 1, page 2053.

Prime Advantage Creatine Serum **-** Muscle Marketing USA
Each serving contains: Damiana • Yohimbe • Pygeum africanum • Glucosamine • Vitamin B12.

Prime Dreamz **-** Market America, Inc.
Two tablets contain: Magnesium (as magnesium oxide) 400 mg • Proprietary Herbal Blend 840 mg: Wild Jujube seed extract, Mucuna Pruriens seed extract, Passionflower 4:1 extract (aerial parts), Chamomile flower extract, Hops strobile 4:1 extract (humulus lupulus), Lemon Balm leaf extract, Valerian root extract, Melatonin (3 mg). Other Ingredients: Dicalcium Phosphate, Microcrystalline Cellulose, Croscarmellose Sodium, Stearic Acid, Magnesium Stearate, Silica, Film Coat (hypromellose, hydroxypropyl cellulose, polyethylene glycol, propylene glycol, titanium dioxide, carmine.)

Prime Factor for Men **-** Market America, Inc.
Three tablets contain: Pantothenic Acid (as D-calcium pantothenate) 100 mg • Iodine (from kelp) 75 mcg • Chromium (as chromium dinicotinate glycinate) 50 mcg • Zinc (as zinc arginate) 10 mg • Proprietary Herbal Blend 1571 mg: Silymarin (from milk thistle seed extract), Coleus Forskohlii tuber extract, Fo Ti root extract,

Ashwagandha root extract, Astragalus root extract, Panax Ginseng root, L-Alpha-Glycerylphosphorycholine Hydrate (alpha-GPC), Lycium berry extract, Schizandra berry extract, Gamma-Aminobutyric Acid (GABA), Ornithine Alpha Ketoglutarate, Pregnenolone, Dehydroepiandrosterone (DHEA), Red Date fruit extract, RNA/DNA (from brewer's yeast). Other Ingredients: Dicalcium Phosphate, Guar Gum, Calcium Carbonate, Microcrystalline Cellulose, Stearic Acid, Vegetable Stearin, Citrus Pectin, Magnesium Stearate, Silica, Pharmaceutical Glaze.

Prime Factor for Women **-** Market America, Inc.
Three tablets contain: Pantothenic Acid (as D-calcium pantothenate) 100 mg • Iodine (from kelp) 33 mcg • Chromium (as chromium dinicotinate glycinate) 50 mcg • Zinc (as zinc glycinate) 5 mg • Proprietary Herbal Blend 1720 mg: L-Alpha-Glycerylphosphorycholine Hydrate (alpha-GPC), Silymarin (from milk thistle seed extract), Gamma-Aminobutyric Acid (GABA), Fo Ti root extract, Coleus Forskohlii tuber extract, Ornithine Alpha Ketoglutarate, Dong Quai root, Ashwagandha root extract, Eleuthero root extract, Astragalus root extract, Wild Yam root extract, Lycium berry extract, Red Date fruit, RNA/DNA (from brewer's yeast), Tribulus Terrestris extract (stem and dried fruit), Pregnenolone, Dehydroepiandrosterone (DHEA). Other Ingredients: Dicalcium Phosphate, Guar Gum, Microcrystalline Cellulose, Calcium Carbonate, Stearic Acid, Vegetable Stearin, Citrus Pectin, Magnesium Stearate, Silica, Pharmaceutical Glaze.

Prime Years **-** Schiff
Each softgel contains: Vitamin A (100% as beta carotene) 5000 IU • Vitamin C (as ascorbic acid, niacinamide ascorbate) 100 mg • Vitamin D (as cholecalciferol) 400 IU • Vitamin E (as d-alpha tocopherol) 60 IU • Vitamin K (as phylloquinone) 10 mcg • Vitamin B1 (as thiamin mononitrate) 5 mg • Vitamin B2 (as riboflavin) 5 mg • Vitamin B3 (as niacinamide ascorbate) 20 mg • Vitamin B6 (as pyridoxine hydrochloride) 5 mg • Folate (as folic acid) 400 mcg • Vitamin B12 (as cyanocobalamin) 25 mcg • Biotin 30 mcg • Pantothenic Acid (as d-calcium pantothenate) 20 mg • Calcium (from tricalcium phosphate) 100 mg • Iron (as ferrous chelate) 4 mg • Phosphorus (from tricalcium phosphate) 47 mg • Iodine (from kelp) 150 mcg • Magnesium (as magnesium oxide) 100 mg • Zinc (as zinc oxide) 15 mg • Selenium (from yeast) 20 mcg • Copper (as copper gluconate) 2 mg • Manganese (as manganese gluconate) 3.5 mg • Chromium (from yeast) 130 mcg • Molybdenum (as sodium molybdate) 75 mcg • Potassium (as potassium citrate) 10 mg • DL-Methionine 15 mg • Boron (as boron amino acid chelate) 1 mg. Other Ingredients: Soybean Oil, Softgel (gelatin, glycerin, St. John's bread), Lecithin, Rice Bran, Betaine Hydrochloride, Caramel Color.

Primo GH Stak **-** NutraBolics
Four capsules contain: L-Glutamine 1200 mg • Mucuna Pruriens (15% l-dopa) 100 mg • Colostrum 25% 500 mg • Phosphatidyl Choline 250 mg • Ascorbic Acid 500 mg • Passion Flower extract 400 mg • Schizandra 100 mg.

Primo HGH Stack **-** NutraBolics
Four capsules contain: L-Arginine 800 mg • L-Lysine 800 mg • L-Ornithine 260 mg • IsoLeucine 264 mg • L-Glycine 80 mg • Leucine 264 mg • Vitamin B6 (pyridoxine HCl) 200 mg • Gamma Aminobutyric Acid 400 mg • Valine 264 mg • Passion Flower extract 400 mg • Schizandra 100 mg.

Primobolin **-** National Urological Group
Each capsule contains: Proprietary Blend 550 mg: Epimedium 20% extract, L-Arginine, S-(2-Boeonethy)-L-Cysteine, Xanthoparmelia Scabrosa, Cnidium Monnier, Cistanches 12% extract, L-Citruline, Quebracho 8% extract, Gamma Amino Butyric Acid.

Primrose Oil **-** Atrium Inc.
Each capsule contains: Oil of Evening Primrose 500 mg • Vitamin E (d-Alpha Tocopheryl Acetate) 10 IU • Gamma Linolenic Acid 40 mg • Lenoleic Acid 350 mg.

Pro Blend 55 **-** Human Development Technologies (HDT)
Two scoops contain: Protein Blend of Micro Ultra Filtered Whey Protein concentrate, Egg Albumen, Calcium Caseinate, Micro Ultra Filtered Whey Protein Isolate, Ion Exchanged Whey Protein Isolate, Hydrolyzed Whey Protein Isolate • Natural & artificial Chocolate Flavorings • Acesulfame Potassium • Stevia.

Pro Citravin **-** Unknown
Each tablet contains: Pantothenic Acid (as D-calcium pantothenate) 50 mg • GTF Chromium 60 mcg • Advantra Z Bitter Orange 500 mg • Guarana extract 4:1 (providing 50 mg caffeine) 300 mg • Apple Cider Vinegar 200 mg • Capsicum 50 mg • Ginger root extract 5:1 50 mg • Panax Ginseng root extract 5:1 50 mg. Other Ingredients: Cellulose, Stearic Acid.
See Editor's Note No. 40, page 2058.

Pro Complex APS **-** Optimum Nutrition
Two scoops (68 g) contain: Proprietary Amino Acid Blend 2 g: Glutamine Peptides, L-Leucine, L-Isoleucine, L-Valine • Aminogen 250 mg • Lactase (standardized to 100,000 FCC units/g) 1 mg • Protein Blend: Whey Protein Isolate, Whey Protein Concentrate, Egg Albumen, Whey Peptides • Natural and Artificial Flavor • Lecithin • Vitamin/Mineral Blend: Ascorbic Acid, Chromium GTF Polynicotinate, D-Alpha Tocopheryl Succinate (natural vitamin E), DiCalcium Phosphate, Biotin, Vitamin A Palmitate, Niacinamide, D-Calcium Pantothenate, Cholecalciferol, Folic Acid, Pyridoxine Hydrochloride, Riboflavin, Cyanocobalamin • Acesulfame Potassium, Sucralose.

Pro Complex Bars **-** Optimum Nutrition
Each bar (85 g) contains: Proprietary Blend 50 mg: Glutamine Peptides, L-Leucine, L-Isoleucine, L-Valine, Aminogen • Pro Complex Multi-Protein Blend: Calcium Caseinate, Whey Protein Isolate, Soy Protein Isolate • Glycerine • Maltitol • Coating (maltitol, palm kernal oil, cocoa, whey powder, lecithin, natural flavor) • Filtered Water • Natural Flavor • Lecithin • Peanut Flour • Ground Peanuts • Salt • Vitamin/Mineral Blend: Ascorbic Acid, D-Alpha Tocopheryl Succinate (natural vitamin E), Maltodextrin, Niacinamide, D-Calcium Pantothenate, Pyridoxine Hydrochloride, Chromium Polynicotinate, Riboflavin, Vitamin A Palmitate, Biotin, Folic Acid, Cholecalciferol, Cyanocobalamin • Sucralose • Acesulfame Potassium.

Pro Fuel (Milk & Egg Protein Drink) **-** TwinLab
Each serving contains: Pure Milk & Egg Protein 40 g • Extra Branched Chain Amino Acids (L-Leucine, L-Isoleucine, L-Valine) • L-Glutamine • All Essential Vitamins & Minerals including B Complex Vitamins plus Antioxidant Vitamin C & Vitamin E, Calcium & Magnesium. Patented Chromic Fuel Chromium Picolinate including Potassium, Zinc & Chromium.

Pro Lite **-** Optimum Nutrition
L-Carnitine • Choline • Inositol.

Pro Performance Chewable Creatine Monohydrate Tablets (Lemon-Lime) **-** GNC
Each tablet contains: Creatine Monohydrate 2.5 g. Other Ingredients: Sucrose, Dextrose, Natural Flavors, Beta-Carotene, Riboflavin Color.

Pro Performance Chewable Creatine Monohydrate Tablets (Orange) **-** GNC
Each tablet contains: Creatine Monohydrate 2.5 g. Other Ingredients: Sucrose, Dextrose, Natural Flavors, Beta-Carotene, Riboflavin Color.

Pro Performance Creatine Burst Dietary Supplement (Fruit Punch) **-** GNC
Two scoops (95 g) contain: Vitamin C 250 mg • Riboflavin (B2) 0.85 mg • Vitamin B6 1 mg • Folate, Folic Acid, Folacin 200 mcg • Vitamin B12 3 mcg • Calcium 20 mg • Phosphorus 100 mg • Magnesium 70 mg • Copper 2 mg • Chromium 300 mcg • Potassium 99 mg • Creatine Monohydrate 10 g • Taurine 2 g • L-Serine 1 g • Guanidinoacetate 200 mg. Other Ingredients: Maltodextrin, Natural/

Artificial Flavor, Vitamin/Mineral Blend, Citric Acid, Acesulfame Potassium, Sucralose, FD&C Red #40.

***Pro Performance Weight Gainer 1850, Strawberry Banana* - GNC**
Three cups (400 g) contain: Maltodextrin • Corn Syrup Solids • Protein Blend: Calcium Caseinate, Whey Protein Concentrate, Whey Protein Isolate, Sweet Dairy Whey, Egg Albumen • Fructose, Dextrose, Artificial Banana/Strawberry Flavor • Vitamin/Mineral PreMix: Di-Potassium Phosphate, Magnesium Oxide, Calcium Carbonate, Ascorbic Acid, Ferrous Fumarate, Chromium Polynicotinate, Biotin, D-Alpha Tocopheryl Succinate, Vitamin A Palmitate, Niacinamide, Copper Gluconate, Potassium Iodide, Zinc Oxide, D-Calcium Pantothenate, Selenomethionine, Riboflavin, Folic Acid, Cholecalciferol, Pyridoxine Hydrochloride, Manganese Glycinate, Thiamin Mononitrate, Molybdenum Glycinate, Cyanocobalamin • Guar Gum • Natural Beet Color • Citric Acid • Lecithin • Aminogen • Carbogen.

***Pro-50* - Enzymatic Therapy**
Each capsule contains: Vitamin A (Fish Liver oil) 1500 IU • Zinc (Chelate) 20 mg • Vitamin B6 (Pyridoxine HCL) 10 mg • Other Ingredients: EFA (unrefined Vegetable Lipids) 630 mg • Amino Acid Complex 150 mg • Prostate extract freeze-dried 150 mg • Saw Palmetto Berry extract 4:1 100 mg.
See Editor's Note No. 14.

***ProactEnz* - Enzymes, Inc.**
Each capsule contains: Calcium (from Calcium Citrate) 32 mg • n-zimes pHysioProtease 607 mg. Other Ingredients: Cellulose, Water.

***Pro-Antho Forte* - Progressive Labs**
Each capsule contains: Pycnogenol 10 mg • Grape seed extract (vitis vinifera 5:1 concentrate) 50 mg • Ginkgo leaf extract (Ginkgo biloba, 50:1 concentrate) 20 mg • Green Tea leaf extract (Camellia sinensis, 65% standardized extract) 75 mg • Quercetin 100 mg • Milk Thistle (Silibum marianum, 80% standardized extract) 10 mg.

***Probacillus Plus* - ProJoba**
Each tablet contans: Proprietary Blend 4 billion cells: Lactobacillus Acidophilus, Bifidobacterium Bifidum. Inactive Ingredients: Inositol, Monoatril Glutamas, Ascorbate, Yeast extract, Polysaccharides, Skim Milk Powder, Magnesium Stearate, Dextrose.

***Probiata* - Wakunaga of America**
Each tablet contains: Lactobacillus acidophilus 1 billion live cells in a vegetable starch complex.

***ProBio PCC* - Pharmanex**
Each capsule contains: Lactobacillus Fermentuam P.C.C. 100 mg.

***Probiotic* - Enzymes, Inc.**
Each capsule contains: Proprietary Blend 345 mg: Lactobacillus plantarum, Lactobacillus casei, Bifidobacterium longum, Lactobacillus acidophilus. Other Ingredients: Plant Cellulose, Water.

***Probiotic A.Y.* - Futurebiotics**
Lactobacillus acidophilus 3 billion cells at formulation Fructooligosaccharides (NutraFlora FOS) 600 mg • Inulin FOS 200 mg • Garlic (Pure-Gar 1500TM deodorized concentrate) 75 mg • Pau D'Arco 25 mg • Licorice (4:1 extract) 25 mg • Caprylic Acid (MCT) 100 mg • Echinacea (4:1 extract) 25 mg.

***Probiotic Acidophilus with Pectin (Inspired by Nature)* - Puritan's Pride**
Two capsules contain: Proprietary Blend of Cultures 180 mg: Lactobacillus Acidophilus, L. Brevis, L. Salivarius, L. Helveticus, L. Bulgaricus, Bifidobacterium Bifidum • Citrus Pectin 200 mg. Other Ingredients: Dicalcium Phosphate, Gelatin, Cellulose (plant origin), Silica, Vegetable Magnesium Stearate.

***Probiotic Pearls* - PhytoPharmica**
Each pearl contains: Proprietary Probiotic Blend 1 billion CFU: Lactobacillus Acidophilus, Bifidobacterium Longum. Other Ingredients: Palm Oil, Gelatin, Glycerin, Lecithin, Pectin.

***ProBiotic Restore* - Advocare International**
Two capsules contain: Vitamin A (as beta-carotene) 2000 IU • OptiZinc Zinc (as zinc monomethionine) 1 mg • Lactobacillus Acidophilus 1 billion • Bifidobacterium Bifidum 1 billion • Fructooligosaccharides 500 mg • Moomiyo 50 mg • Aloe Vera rind powder 100 mg. Other Ingredients: Silicon Dioxide, Magnesium Stearate, Gelatin.

***Probiotica* - McNeil Consumer Healthcare**
Each tablet contains: Lactobacillus reuteri 100 million cells. Other Ingredients: Mannitol, Xylitol, Lactulose, Mono- and Diglycerides, Malic Acid, Lemon Flavor, Zein (corn protein), Riboflavin Phosphate (for color).

***Pro-Brom* - Atrium Inc.**
Each tablet contains: Bromelain 100 mg • Papayotin 30 mg.

***Procosa II* - USANA Health Sciences**
Two tablets contain: Manganese (as Manganese gluconate) 2.5 mg • Vitamin C (as Calcium Ascorbate) 150 mg • Glucosamine Sulfate 1000 mg • Silicon (as Amino Acid Complex) 1.5 mg • Turmeric Extract (Curcuma Longal root) 250 mg.

***Procylon (dominor centurion)* – Vision Laboratories**
Two tablets contain: Male Vitality Blend 1150 mg: Korean Ginseng root extract (4% ginsenosides), Yohimbe bark (1% yohimbine alkaloids), Saw Palmetto berry, Damiana leaf, L-Glutamic Acid, L-Lysine HCl, Wild Jujube seed extract, Ginkgo Biloba leaf, L-Arginine HCl, L-Alanine. Other Ingredients: Dicalcium Phosphate, Microcrystalline Cellulose, Toasted Wheat Germ, Croscarmellose Sodium, Stearic Acid, Magnesium Stearate, Silica, Pharmaceutical Glaze.

***Pro-DMG-B15* - PhytoPharmica**
Each capsule contains: Calcium Gluconate 31 mg • Magnesium Aspartate 125 mg • Potassium Aspartate 125 mg • Trimethylglycine (TMG) 100 mg • N,N-Dimethylglycine HCl 100 mg • Glycine 25 mg.
See Editor's Note No. 21, page 2056.

***ProEndorphin* - Nutraceutics Corp.**
Each effervescent sachet contains: Thiamine (as thiamine mononitrate) 15 mg • Riboflavin (as riboflavin phosphate) 16 mg • Niacin 50 mg • Vitamin B6 (as pyridoxine hydrochloride) 41 mg • Vitamin B12 (as cyanocobalamin) 300 mcg • Biotin 150 mcg • Pantothenic Acid (as calcium pantothenate) 48 mg • Novel Polyose Complex 700 mg • P.E. Complex 400 mg: Phenylalanine (as DL phenylalanine), Phenylalanine (as D phenylalanine) • DMAE (2-dimethylaminoethanol bitartrate) 200 mg • Myo-Inositol 100 mg • GNS2 Ginseng extract (panax ginseng, standardized to 20% ginsenosides) 200 mg • NeuroMediating Complex Proprietary Blend 225 mg: Cola Nitida seed, Taurine (as l-taurine). Other Ingredients: Citric Acid, Glucose, Beta Cyclodextrins, Natural Orange, Lemon and Lime Flavor.

***ProEndorphin* - Pharmalogic**
Each sachet contains: Thiamine (as thiamine mononitrate) 15 mg • Riboflavin (as riboflavin phosphate) 16 mg • Niacin 50 mg • Vitamin B6 (as pyridoxine hydrochloride) 41 mg • Vitamin B12 (as cyanocohalamin) 300 mcg • Biotin 150 mcg • Pantothenic Acid (as calcium pantothenate) 48 mg • Novel Polyose Complex 700 mg • Proprietary Blend P.E. Complex 400 mg: Phenylalanine (as dl-phenylalanine), Phenylalanine (as d-phenylalanine) • DMAE (2-dimethylaminoethanol bitartrate) 200 mg • Myo-Inositol 100 mg • GNS2 Ginseng Extract (panax ginseng; standardized to 20% ginsenosides) 200 mg • Proprietary Blend NeuroMediating Complex 225 mg: Cola Nitida (seed), Taurine (as l-taurine). Other Ingredients: Citric Acid, Glucose, Beta Cyclodextrins, Natural Orange, Lemon Flavor, Lime Flavor.

Proenzi 99 (formerly Pro-Enz 99+) - Abundance Marketing
Ephedra stem (Ephedrine) 8 mg • Bladderwrack herb 15 mg • Astragalus root 15 mg • Rehmannia root 10 mg • White Willow bark 10 mg • Siberian Ginseng 10 mg • Kola nut 85 mg • Reishi Mushroom 5 mg • Dandelion root 5 mg • Ginger root 5 mg • Black Pepper extract 2.5 mg. In a base of Green Tea 85 mg • Bee Pollen 10 mg • Chromium (Chloride) 100 mcg • Niacin 1 mg.
See Editor's Note No. 30, page 2056.

Pro-Essence - Flora, Inc.
Burdock root • Juniper Berry • Prickley Ash bark • Slippery Elm bark • Uva Ursi.

ProEstron - Nutraceutics Corp.
Two caplets contain: Proprietary Blend Estrasterone 870 mg: Glycyrrhiza Uralensis (root), Isoflavone Complex, Dong Quai root, Black Cohosh root • Titrated Vitex 500 mg: Vitex Agnus-Castus fruit, Dioscorea root blend. Other Ingredients: Magnesium Stearate, DiCalcium Phosphate, Microcrystalline Cellulose.

Pro-F Complex - PhytoPharmica
Two tablets contain: Vitamin A (Fish Liver oil) 3000 IU • Vitamin D (Fish Liver oil) 100 IU • Calcium (Lactate) 82 mg • Zinc (Chelate) 20 mg • Magnesium (Citrate) 13 mg • Pacific Sea Kelp 200 mg • Ovarian extract 90 mg • Whole Pituitary extract 60 mg • Adrenal extract 60 mg • Uterus extract 60 mg • RNA powder 60 mg. All organs and glands derived from bovine sources.
See Editor's Note No. 14 and No. 21, pages 2055 and 2056.

Profemme - ProJoba
Each tablet contains: Flower Pollen extract WSI 72 mg • Flower Pollen extract LS1 4 mg. Other Ingredients: Microcrystalline Cellulose, Lactose, Magnesium Stearate, Silicon Dioxide, Natural Resin, Polyethylene Glycol, Talc.

Profile 1 - Mannatech
Three tablets contain: Vitamin A 2500 IU • Vitamin B1 27 mg • Vitamin B12 18 mcg • Vitamin B2 24 mg • Vitamin B6 26 mg • Beta Carotene 100 IU • Bioflavonoids 95 mg • Biotin 36 mcg • Vitamin C 187 mg • Choline 19 mg • Vitamin D 400 IU • Vitamin E 30 IU • Folic Acid 400 mcg • Inositol 90 mcg • Vitamin K 90 mcg • Niacinamide 30 mg • PABA 5 mg • Pantothenic Acid 5 mg • Boron 150 mcg • Calcium 10 mg • Copper 20 mcg • GTF Chromium 150 mcg • Iodine 3 mcg • Iron 5 mg • Magnesium 50 mg • Manganese 12 mg • Molybdenum 70 mcg • Potassium 75 mg • Selenium 15 mcg • Silicon 500 mcg • Vanadium 10 mcg • Zinc 7 mg • Ambrotose Complex (naturally occurring plant polysaccharides including freeze-dried Aloe Vera inner leaf gel extract - Manapol powder) 25 mg.
See Editor's Note No. 17, page 2055.

Profile 2 - Mannatech
Three tablets contain: Vitamin A 15000 IU • Vitamin B1 2 mg • Vitamin B12 125 mcg • Vitamin B2 5 mg • Vitamin B6 2 mg • Beta Carotene 5000 IU • Bioflavonoids 56 mg • Biotin 57 mcg • Vitamin C 130 mg • Choline 55 mg • Vitamin D 170 IU • Vitamin E 62 IU • Folic Acid 200 mcg • Inositol 25 mg • Vitamin K 50 mcg • Niacinamide 38 mg • PABA 7 mg • Pantothenic Acid 29 mg • Boron 500 mcg • Calcium 75 mg • Copper 700 mcg • GTF Chromium 50 mcg • Iodine 100 mcg • Iron 2 mg • Magnesium 10 mg • Manganese 2 mg • Molybdenum 70 mcg • Potassium 7 mg • Selenium 15 mcg • Silicon 2.5 mcg • Vanadium 10 mcg • Zinc 15 mg • Ambrotose Complex (naturally occurring plant polysaccharides including freeze-dried aloe Vera inner leaf gel extract - Manapol powder) 25 mg.
See Editor's Note No. 17, page 2055.

Profile 3 - Mannatech
Three tablets contain: Vitamin A 7500 IU • Vitamin B1 7 mg • Vitamin B12 68 mcg • Vitamin B2 8 mg • Vitamin B6 10 mg • Beta Carotene 2500 IU • Bioflavonoids 75 mg • Biotin 52 mcg • Vitamin C 170 mg • Choline 40 mg • Vitamin D 210 IU • Vitamin E 50 IU • Folic Acid 300 mcg • Inositol 20 mcg • Vitamin K 90 mcg • Niacinamide 32 mg • PABA 6 mg • Pantothenic Acid 23 mg • Boron 300 mcg • Calcium 60 mg • Copper 300 mcg • GTF Chromium 80 mcg • Iodine 30 mcg • Iron 3.5 mg • Magnesium 25 mg • Manganese 8 mg • Molybdenum 70 mcg • Potassium 12 mg • Selenium 15 mcg • Silicon 2 mg • Vanadium 10 mcg • Zinc 10 mg • Ambrotose Complex (naturally occurring plant polysaccharides including freeze-dried Aloe Vera inner leaf gel extract - Manapol powder) 25 mg.
See Editor's Note No. 17, page 2055.

Proflavanol - USANA Health Sciences
Each tablet contains: Vitamin C (as calcium, potasium, magnesium and zinc ascorbates) 100 mg • Grape Seed extract 30 mg • Ascorbyl Palmitate 12 mg. Inactive Ingredients: Microcrystalline Cellulose, Croscarmellose Sodium, Pregelatinized Starch, Dextrin, Colloidal Silicon Dioxide, Dextrose.

Proflavanol 90 - USANA Health Sciences
Each tablet contains: Vitamin C (as calcium, potasium, magnesium and zinc ascorbates) 300 mg • Grape Seed extract 90 mg • Ascorbyl Palmitate 12 mg. Inactive Ingredients: Microcrystalline Cellulose, Croscarmellose Sodium, Pregelatinized Starch, Dextrin, Colloidal Silicon Dioxide, Dextrose.

Proflora - BioBotanical Research
Distilled Water • Lactobacillus Acidophilus (whey fermentation) • Bifidobacterium complex • Aloe Vera • Yucca Schidigera • Lactobacillus Salivarius • Chlorophyll • Herba Mentha Piperita • Radix Zingiber Officinalis • Taraxacum Officinale • Viola Odorata.

ProForm Bars, Peanut Chocolate - Advocare International
SusCarb (fructose, maltodextrin, glycerin) • Protein Blend (soy protein isolate, whey protein concentrate, L-glutomine, L-lysine) • Milk Chocolate flavored coating (sugar, palm kernel oil, nonfat milk, cocoa [processed with alkali], dextrose, lecithin, natural flavor) • Water • Crisp Rice (rice flour, malt extract, rice bran) • Cocoa (processed with alkali) • Natural Flavors • Guarana extract • Walnuts • Choline Bitartrate • Kola Nut extract • Taurine • Green Tea extract • Potassium Chloride • Ascorbic Acid • Creatine Monohydrate • Calcium Pantothenate • Salt • Niacinamide • D-Alpha Tocopheryl Succinate • Pyridoxine Hydrochloride • L-Carnitine • Ginkgo Biloba extract • Folic Acid • Riboflavin • Thiamine Hydrochloride • Beta-Carotene • Chromium Polynicotinate (ChromeMate) • Biotin • Cyanocobalamin.

Pro-Gain - Nature's Life
Two scoops (28.35 g) contain: SUPRO brand soy protein isolate containing Lecithin • Whey • Fructose • Non-fat Dry Milk • natural Vanilla Flavor • Yeast • Egg Albumin • Eggshell powder • Kelp • natural Papain Enzyme concentrate • Cobalamin concentrate (B12). Pro-Gain also contains 34 mg of naturally occuring Isoflavones, including 21 mg Genistein & 10 mg Daidzen.

Progensa - Life-Flo
Each ounce contains: Natural Progesterone USP Grade 480 mg. Other Ingredients: Grape seed extract, aloe vera, vitamin E, & primrose.

Pro-Gest - PhytoPharmica
Two tablets contain: Niacinamide 20 mg • Betaine HCl 310 mg • L-Glutamic Acid HCl 310 mg • Bromelain (pineapple whole fruit) 10:1 200 mg • Papain 200 mg • Mylase Lipase 200 mg • Mycozyme (fungal amylase) 50 mg • Ox Bile extract 32 mg • Pancreas extract 32 mg.
See Editor's Note No. 14.

Pro-Gest Body Cream - Transitions for Health, Inc.
Aloe Vera Gel in Distilled Water • D-Alpha Tocopherol and Mixed Tocopherols • Cetyl Alcohol • Almond Oil • Octyl Palmitate • Panthenol • Peg 8 Stearate • Glycerin • USP Progesterone • Polysorbate 60 • Hyaluronic Acid • Oil of Lemon • Keratin • Carbomer 940 • Grapefruit Seed Extract.

Pro-Gest Progesterone Body Cream/ Original Formula - Transitions for Health, Inc.
Deionized Water • Aloe Vera Gel • D-Alpha Tocopherol • Mixed

Tocopherols (Vit. E) • Cetyl Alcohol • Almond Oil • Octyl Palmitate • Panthenol • PEG-8 Stearate • USP Progesterone • Glycerin • Polysorbate 60 • Hyaluronic Acid • Oil of Lemon (Oleum Limonis) • Keratin • Carbomer 940 • Grapefruit Seed Extract (Citrus Grandis).

Pro-Gest Progesterone Cream **-** Transitions for Health, Inc.
Ingredients: Distilled Water • Aloe Barbadensis gel • Tocopheryl Acetate • Cetyl Alcohol • Octyl Palmitate • Sweet Almond oil (prunus amygdalus dulcis) • Panthenol • PEG-8 Stearate • Stearic Acid • Glycerin • USP Progesterone • Polysorbate 60 • Propylene Glycol • Lemon oil (citrus medica limonum) • Carbomer • Methylparaben • Propylparaben • Triethanolamine • Phenoxyethanol.

Progesta Plus **-** Aarisse Health Care
Each 3 oz pump contains: Aloe Vera extract • Shea Butter • Phospholipids/Liposomes • Natural Progesterone USP micronized • Wild Yam extract • Polysaccharides • Evening Primrose Oil • Vitamin E • Allantoin • Potassium Sorbate (fron pears and avocados) • Rosemary Oil • Red Clover Isoflavones.

ProgestaCare **-** Life-Flo
Aloe Vera gel • Caprylic/Capric Triglyceride • natural Progesterone derived from the Mexican Wild Yam root • Evening Primrose oil (Oenothera biennis) • Vitamin E Acetate • Isostearic Acid • Glyceryl Stearate • Siberian Ginseng • Burdock root • Black Cohosh • MSM • Chamomile • Glycerin • Allantoin • Grape seed extract.

Pro-Gest-Ade **-** Enzymatic Therapy
Each tablet contains: Niacinamide 10 mg. Other Ingredients: Betaine HCL 155 mg • Glutamic Acid HCL 155 mg • Bromelain (600 MCU) 100 mg • Papain 100 mg • Mylase (Lipase) 100 mg • Mycozyme (Fungal amylase) 25 mg • Ox Bile extract 16 mg • Pancreas extract 16 mg.
See Editor's Note No. 14.

Progestaroma **-** Global Health Trax
Purified Water • Octyl Palmitate (from palm oil) • Glycerine • Ceteayl Glucoside • Tocopheryl Acetate • Progesterone USP (500 mg/oz) • Cetyl Alcohol (from coconut) • Panthenol • Aloe Vera Gel • Wild Yam extract • Ascorbic Acid • Sodium Hyaluronate • Carbomer • Sodium Hydroxide • Potassium Sorbate • Pure Essential Oils Blend: Sandalwood, Lavender, Orange, Geranium • Grapefruit seed extract.

Progesterone Cream **-** PhysioLogics
Purified Water • Aloe Vera gel • Petrolatum • Tocopheryl Acetate (vitamin E) • Cetearyl Alcohol and Ceteareth-20 • Glyceryl Stearate • C12-15 Alkyl Benzoate • Stearic Acid • Cetyl Alcohol • Glycerin • Progesterone • Triethanolamine • Polysorbate 80 • Keratin Amino Acids • Diazolidinyl Urea • Carbomer • Coconut oil • Almond oil • Grapefruit seed extract (citrus grandis) • Methylparaben • BHA • Lemon oil (citrus medica limonum) • Propylparaben • Panthenol • Sodium Hyaluronate.

Progesterone Cream **-** Source Naturals
Each ounce contains: Natural Progesterone USP from Soy 500 mg. Inactive Ingredients: Purified Water, Aloe Vera Gel, Ceteary1 Glucoside, Caprylic/Capric Triglyceride, Cetyl Alcohol, Glycerin, Wild Yam extract, Tocopheryl Acetate (Natural Vitamin E), Lecithin Phospholipid, Glyceryl Stearate, Jojoba, Squalane, Stearic Acid, Sage leaf extract, Black Cohosh root extract, Ginseng root extract, Marigold tops extract, Grapefruit seed extract, Methylparaben, Propylparaben, Sorbic Acid, Xanthan Gum, Rosemary Oil.

Progesterone Plus Creme **-** Nutri-Quest Rx
Water • Stearic Acid • Cetyl Alcohol • Sesame oil • Progesterone USP (Homeopathic) • Triethanolame • Arnica oil • Evening Primrose oil • Zinc • Copper • Magnesium • Glyconucleopeptides • Peg 10 Soya Sterol • Hydroxyethycellulose • Disodium EDTA • Cetyl Ricinoleate • Canola oil • Wild Yam • Dex - Panthenol (Vitamin B5) • Progesterone USP • Honey • Lecithin • NaPCA • Silicon • Iron • Peg 7 Glycerol Cocoate • Carrot oil • Carbomer • Phenyldimethicone • Sodium Hydroxymethylglycinate.

ProGram16: Chocolate **-** Pharmanex
One bar contains: High Fructose Corn Syrup • Whey Protein Isolate • Soy Protein Isolate • Sugar • Milk Protein Isolate • Cocoa Butter • Unsweetened Chocolate • Lowfat Cocoa (Processed with Alkali) • Milk • Creatine Monohydrate 1 g • Glycerin • Maltodextrin • Dicalcium Phosphate • Natural and Artificial Flavors • Taurine 250 mg • Magnesium Carbonate • Potassium Chloride • Potassium Citrate • Egg Whites • Ascorbic Acid • Lecithin • d-Alpha Tocopherol Acetate • Beta-Carotene • Niacinamide • Calcium Pantothenate • Zinc Oxide • Chromium Chelate • Carbonyl Iron • Copper Gluconate • Manganese Sulfate • Pyridoxine Hydrochloride • Riboflavin • Thiamine Mononitrate • Folate (Folic Acid) • Biotin • Potassium Iodide • Sodium Molybdate • Sodium Selenite • Phytonadine • Cholecalciferol • Cyanocobalamin.

ProGram16: Coconut **-** Pharmanex
Each bar contains: High Fructose Corn Syrup • Whey Protein Isolate • Soy Protein Isolate • Sugar • Partially Defatted Peanut Flour • Milk Protein Isolate • Cocoa Butter • Unsweetened Chocolate • Milk • Creatine Monohydrate 1 g • Glycerin • Natural and Artificial Flavors • Maltodextrin • Dicalcium Phosphate • Potassium Chloride • Taurine 250 mg • Magnesium Carbonate • Egg Whites • Ascorbic Acid • Lecithin • Salt • d-Alpha Tocopherol Acetate • Beta-Carotene • Niacinamide • Calcium Pantothenate • Zinc Oxide • Chromium Chelate • Carbonyl Iron • Copper Gluconate • Manganese Sulfate • Pyridoxine Hydrochloride • Riboflavin • Thiamine Mononitrate • Folate (Folic Acid) • Biotin • Potassium Iodide • Sodium Molybdate • Sodium Selenite • Phytonadine • Cholecalciferol • Cyanocobalamin.

ProGram16: Peanut Butter **-** Pharmanex
Each bar contains: High Fructose Corn Syrup • Whey Protein Isolate • Soy Protein Isolate • Sugar • Partially Defatted Peanut Flour • Milk Protein Isolate • Cocoa Butter • Unsweetened Chocolate • Milk • Creatine Monohydrate 1 g • Glycerin • Maltodextrin • Dicalcium Phosphate • Natural and Artificial Flavors • Taurine 250 mg • Magnesium Carbonate • Potassium Chloride • Egg Whites • Ascorbic Acid • Lecithin • Salt • d-Alpha Tocopherol Acetate • Beta-Carotene • Niacinamide • Calcium Pantothenate • Zinc Oxide • Chromium Chelate • Carbonyl Iron • Copper Gluconate • Manganese Sulfate • Pyridoxine Hydrochloride • Riboflavin • Thiamine Mononitrate • Folate (Folic Acid) • Biotin • Potassium Iodide • Sodium Molybdate • Sodium Selenite • Phytonadine • Cholecalciferol • Cyanocobalamin.

Pro-Guard **-** Nutralife Health & Fitness (NZ) Ltd.
Each tablet contains: Saw Palmetto Fruit 500 mg • Hydrangea Root and Rhiz. 100 mg • Golden Rod Herb 50 mg • Couch Grass Root 200 mg • Horsetail Herb 100 mg • Panax Ginseng Root 100 mg • Zinc Gluconate (Providing 15 mg zinc) 112.5 mg • Magnesium Amino Acid Chelate (Providing magnesium 15 mg) 75 mg • Calcium Ascorbate 250 mg • Pyridoxine Hydrocholoride (Vitamin B6) 15 mg • Glutamine 100 mg • Glycine 100 mg • Alanine 100 mg.

ProHerbs Bone & Joints **-** Mason Vitamins, Inc.
Three tablets contain: Vitamin D (D3) 240 IU • Calcium (as Calcium Carbonate) 1005 mg • Isoflavones as Soy standardized extract 60 mg • Glucosamine Sulfate 510 mg • Chondroitin Sulfate 405 mg • Boron 4.5 mg. Other Ingredients: Croscarmellose Sodium, Hydroxypropylmethylcellulose, Magnesium Stearate, Mineral Oil, Polyethylene Glycol, Stearic Acid, Titanium Dioxide, Sodium Lauryl Sulfate, Iron Oxide.
See Editor's Note No. 15, page 2055.

ProHerbs Breast Health **-** Mason Vitamins, Inc.
Two tablets contain: Vitamin C (as Ascorbic Acid) 200 mg • Selenium (as Selenomethionine) 200 mcg • Broccoli extract (20:1 extract) 170 mg • Curcumin root extract (Curcuma longa standardized to 2% curcuminoids) 600 mg • Genistein from Soy extract 20 mg • Citrus Bioflavonoids 100 mg • Flaxseed powder 400 mg. Other Ingredients: Dicalcium Phosphate, Microcrystalline Cellulose, Croscarmellose Sodium, Stearic Acid, Magnesium Stearate, Hydroxypropylmethylcellulose, Mineral Oil, Triacetin, Titanium Dioxide, FD&C Yellow #6 Lake.

Some Brand Name Natural Products - What they Contain

www.NaturalDatabase.com contains MANY more listings than appear here.

ProHerbs Energy **-** Mason Vitamins, Inc.
Each tablet contains: Thiamin HCl (B1) 25 mg • Riboflavin (B2) 25 mg • Vitamin B6 (Pyridoxine HCl) 25 mg • Vitamin B12 (Cyanocobalamin) 50 mcg • Folic Acid 400 mcg • Korean Ginseng root (Panax Ginseng standardized to 10% ginsenosides) 100 mg • Kola Nut (3:1 extract) (Cola acuminata) 500 mg • Guarana root (Paullina cupana 3:1 extract) 200 mg • Royal Jelly 50 mg. Other Ingredients: Dicalcium Phosphate, Microcrystalline Cellulose, Croscarmellose Sodium, Hydroxypropylmethylcellulose, Magnesium Stearate, Mineral Oil, Stearic Acid, Titanium Dioxide, Triacetin, FD&C Yellow #6 Lake.

ProHerbs Leg Vein & Circulation **-** Mason Vitamins, Inc.
ETwo tablets contain: Vitamin C 240 mg • Green Tea leaves (Camellia sinensis standardized to 50% catechins) 100 mg • Horse Chestnut seed (Aesculus hippocastanum standardized to 18-20% total saponins) 300 mg • Butcher's Broom root (Ruscus aculeatus standardized to 10% saponins) 200 mg • Citrus Bioflavonoid complex 200 mg. Other Ingredients: Dicalcium Phosphate, Croscarmellose Sodium, Mineral Oil, Hydroxypropylmethylcellulose, Magnesium Stearate, Microcrystalline Cellulose, Polyethylene Glycol, Silicon Dioxide, Stearic Acid, Titanium Dioxide, FD&C Red #27 Lake, FD&C Blue #1 Lake.

ProHerbs Memory **-** Mason Vitamins, Inc.
Each tablet contains: Thiamin HCl (B1) 25 mg • Niacin (as Niacinamide) 10 mg • Vitamin B6 (Pyridoxine HCl) 25 mg • Vitamin B12 (Cyanocobalamin) 25 mcg • Ginkgo Biloba extract (Ginkgo biloba leaves standardized to 24% ginkgo flavonoid glycosides & 6% terpene lactones) 120 mg • Memorzine (Huperzia serrata moss extract) 25 mcg • Korean Ginseng (Panax Ginseng root standardized to 4% ginsenosides) 100 mg. Other Ingredients: Dicalcium Phosphate, Microcrystalline Cellulose, Croscarmellose Sodium, Hydroxypropylmethylcellulose, Magnesium Stearate, Mineral Oil, Polyethylene Glycol, Stearic Acid, Titanium Dioxide, Sodium Lauryl Sulfate, FD&C Yellow #10 Lake, FD&C Blue #1 Lake and FD&C Blue #2 Lake.

ProHerbs Prostate **-** Mason Vitamins, Inc.
Two softgels contain: Vitamin E (Dl-Alpha Tocopheryl Acetate) 30 IU • Zinc (as Sulfate) 15 mg • Selenium (as Selenomethionine) 200 mcg • LycoPure (equivalent to 5 mg Lycopene) 71 mg • Saw Palmetto berries (Serenoa repens standardized to 85%-95% free fatty acids) 320 mg • Stinging Nettle root (Urtica dioca L. 2% minimum plant silica) 200 mg • Pumpkin Seed Oil (Cucurbita pepo seeds) 30 mg. Other Ingredients: Soybean Oil, Beeswax, Gelatin, Glycerin, Water, Chlorophyllin, Sodium, Copper, Titanium Dioxide.

ProHerbs Relax & Ease Tension **-** Mason Vitamins, Inc.
Two tablets contain: Thiamine HCl (B1) 50 mg • Riboflavin (B2) 50 mg • Vitamin B6 (Pyridoxine HCl) 50 mg • Vitamin B12 (Cyanocobalamin) 100 mcg • Kava Kava root (Piper methysticum standardized to 30% kavalactones) 300 mg • Passion Flower (Passiflora incarnata standardized to 4% flavonoids) 100 mg • Chamomile flower (Matricaria chamomilla standardized to greater than 1% apigenin) 100 mg. Other Ingredients: Dicalcium Phosphate, Microcrystalline Cellulose, Croscarmellose Sodium, Hydroxypropylmethylcellulose, Magnesium Stearate, Mineral Oil, Polyethylene Glycol, Stearic Acid, Titanium Dioxide, Sodium Lauryl Sulfate, Yellow #6 Lake, FD&C Blue #1 Lake, FD&C Red #40 Lake, FD&C Blue #2 Lake.

ProHerbs Vision Health **-** Mason Vitamins, Inc.
Two tablets contain: Vitamin A (100% Beta Carotene) 2500 IU • Zinc (as Sulfate) 15 mg • Selenium (as Selenomethionine) 200 mcg • Copper (as Cupric Oxide) 2 mg • Bilberry extract (Vaccinium myrtillus fruit standardized to 25% anthocyanidins) 160 mg • Lutein 6 mg • Lycopene 5 mg. Other Ingredients: Dicalcium Phosphate, Microcrystalline Cellulose, Croscarmellose Sodium, Hydroxypropylmethylcellulose, Magnesium Stearate, Mineral Oil, Polyethylene Glycol, Stearic Acid, Titanium Dioxide, Sodium Lauryl Sulfate, FD&C Red #40 Lake, FD&C Blue #1 Lake, FD&C Blue #2 Lake.

PROhGH Sport for Men **-** Nutraceutics Corp.
Each effervescent sachet contains: Symbiotropin Complex 2720 mg: Aminotrope-7, Anterior Pituitary Peptides (porcine) • Novel Polyose Proprietary Complex 1100 mg • Chaperone Molecule Complex 350 mg: Inositol, Tribulus Terrestris. Other Ingredients: Citric Acid, Sodium Bicarbonate, Glucose, L-glutamine, L-Arginine, L-Pyroglutamate, L-Lysine, Glycine, Alpha-Glycerylphosphorylcholine, Gamma Aminobutyric Acid, Mixed Berry Flavor.

PROhGH Sport for Women **-** Pharmalogic
Each sachet contains: Proprietary Blend Symbiotropin 2720 mg: Aminotrope-7, Anterior Pituitary Peptides (porcine) • Novel Polyose Complex 1100 mg • Chaperone Molecule Complex 320 mg: Inositol, Soy Isoflavones. Other Ingredients: Citric Acid, Sodium Bicarbonate, Glucose, L-Glutamine, L-Arginine, L-Pyroglutamate, L-Lysine, Glycine, Alpha-glycerylphosphorylcholine, Gamma Aminobutyric Acid, Mixed Berry Flavor.

ProhGH Symbiotropin **-** Nutraceutics Corp.
Two tablets contain: Glycoamino Acid Complex 4200 mg • Aminotrope-7 Anterior Pituitary Peptides Polyose Complex 2300 mg. Other Ingredients: Citric Acid, Potassium Bicarbonate, Glucose, L-Glutamine, L-Arginine, L-Pyroglutamate, Sodium Bicarbonate, L-Lysine Monohydrochloride, Gamma Aminobutyric Acid, Glycine, Sodium Carbonate, Polyethlene Glycol, Mixed Berry Flavor, Magnesium Stearate, Sodium Benzoate powder.
See Editor's Note No. 14.

PRO-hGH Symbiotropin Growth Hormone Releasing Complex **-** Nutraceutics Corp.
Two tablets contain: Anterior Pituitary Peptides • Aminotrope-7 (a sequenced glycoamino acid complex) 4200 mg • Novel Polyose complex (pharmaceutical mono, poly & oligo saccharides) 2230 mg. All in a base of: L-Glutamine, L-Arginine, L-Pyroglutamate, GABA, L-Glycine, L-Lysine, L-Tyrosine & Vicia Faba Major. Naturally sweetened & flavored.
See Editor's Note No. 14.

Prolab CarbPRO **-** ProLab
Granulated Medium Length Complex Carbohydrates (Maltodextrin) extracted from grains.

ProLab GlutaMASS **-** ProLab
Each capsule contains: L-Glutamine 275 mg • Alpha-Ketoglutaric Acid 250 mg • Taurine 150 mg • Calcium (AKG) 63 mg • Magnesium (oxide) 25 mg • Potassium (citrate) 25 mg • RNA 9.5 mg • Manganese 400 mcg.

ProLab Lean Rx **-** ProLab
Each 72 g packet contains: Protein Blend of Milk Protein Isolates • Caseinates • Whey Protein Concentrates & Egg Whites • Maltodextrin • Cocoa • Natural Flavors • Dicalcium Phosphate • Potassium Chloride • Dipotassium Phosphate • Potassium Citrate • Sodium Chloride • Sodium Citrate • Magnesium Oxide • Medium Chain Triglycerides • Choline Bitartrate • Vegetable Gum • Aspartame • Lecithin • Betaine • Beta Carotene • Manganese Sulfate • Canola oil • Glutamine • Inositol • Vitamin E Acetate • Vitamin B12 • Vitamin A Palmitate • Thiamine • Riboflavin • Vitamin D • Niacin • Pyridoxine HCL • Calcium Pantothenate • Potassium Iodide • Ferrous Gluconate • Copper Gluconate • Zinc Oxide • Biotin • Folic Acid • Selenium Chelate • Molybdenium Yeast • Vitamin K • Paba • Chromium Picolinate.

ProLab MSM **-** ProLab
Each capsule contains: MSM (Methyl-Sulfonyl-Methane) 1000 mg.

ProLab N-Large 2 (N-Large II) **-** ProLab
Each serving (153 g) contains: Maltodextrin • Cross-Flow Micro-Filtered Cold Processed Ion Exchanged Whey • Fructose • Natural Flavoring.

ProLab Stoked **-** ProLab
Each rounded scoop contains: Caffeine 200 mg • Ephedra alkaloids 20 mg • Guarana 10 mg • Green Tea extract 10 mg • White Willow 75 mg. In a base of Yohimbe bark, Quercetin & Citrus aurantium.
See Editor's Note No. 21 and No. 30.

Pro-Life Soy Protein **-** Nature's Life
Two scoops (28.35 g) contain: SUPRO brand soy protein isolate containing Lecithin • natural Vanilla Flavor • natural Papain Enzyme concentrate • Cobalamin concentrate.

Promend **-** The Herbalist
Saw Palmetto berry • Goldenrod flower tops • Echinacea root • Horsetail herb • Plantain herb • Ginger root.

Promensil **-** Novogen
Each tablet contains: Isoflavone Phytoestrogens as Red Clover leaf extract 40 mg. Other Ingredients: Dicalcium phosphate, Microcrystalline cellulose, Hydroxypropyl methylcellulose, Magnesium stearate, Mixed tocopherols, Silica, Soy polysaccharide, Titanium dioxide, Polyethylene glycol, & Organic coloring containing: Red 40, Yellow 6, Yellow 5, Blue 1.

ProMotion **-** Advocare International
Three capsules contain: Glucosamine (as HCl) 1500 mg • Gotu Kola extract (leaf/stem/flower - centella asiatica) 100 mg • Manganese Sulfate (as monohydrate) 10 mg • MSM (methylsulfonyl methane) 100 mg • White Willow bark extract (salix alba) 30 mg. Other Ingredients: Silicon Dioxide, Magnesium Stearate, Gelatin.

ProOmega **-** Nordic Naturals
Each gelcap contains: EPA 173 mg • DHA 123 mg • Other Omega-3 49 mg.

Propalmex Saw Palmetto - SunSource **-** Chattem, Inc.
Each softgel contains: Zinc (as zinc gluconate) 75 mg • Saw Palmetto berry extract 160 mg • Pumpkin Seed Oil extract 40 mg • Lycopene (from Lyc-O-Mato tomato extract) 1.5 mg.

Propax **-** Nutritional Therapeutics, Inc.
Each multipack contains: Vitamin A (as acetate) 4375 IU • Vitamin A (as natural beta-carotene) 3750 IU • Vitamin C (as calcium ascorbate) 150 mg • Vitamin D (as Vitamin D3 cholecalciferol) 32 IU • Vitamin E (as d-alpha tocopherol) 145 IU • Vitamin K (as phytonadione) 2.5 mcg • Vitamin B1 6.25 mg • Vitamin B2 30 mg • Vitamin B3 (as niacinamide) 60 mg • Vitamin B6 (as pyridoxine/P-5-P) 40 mg • Folic Acid (as folate) 200 mcg • Vitamin B12 25 mcg • Biotin 25 mcg • Pantothenic Acid (as d-calcium) 25 mg • Calcium (as phosphate, ascorbate, citrate, sulfate, borogluconate) 360 mg • Iodine (as kelp) 18.75 mcg • Magnesium (as carbonate, oxide, glycinate, sulfate) 160 mg • Zinc (as methionate) 12.5 mg • Selenium (as selenomethionate) 75 mcg • Copper (as tyrosinate) 300 mcg • Manganese (as glycinate) 2.5 mg • Chromium (as nicotinate) 50 mcg • Molybdenum (as glycinate) 20 mcg • Potassium (as citrate) 12.8 mg • DHA (as Docosahexaenoic Acid) 120 mg • EPA (as Eicosopentaenoic Acid) 180 mg • Bioflavonoids (as citrus, rutin, rosehips, quercetin) 165 mg • Boron (as calcium borogluconate) 500 mcg • CoEnzyme Q10 4 mg • Grape Seed Extract 5 mg • Inositol 24 mg • Pantethine (as coenzyme A precursor) 70 mg • Phosphoglycolipids 160 mg • Vanadium (as vanadyl sulfate) 12.5 mcg • Creatine (Monohydrate, Phosphate) 122.5 mg • Alpha-Keto Glutarate 125 mg • Glutathione (as reduced) 5 mg • L-Tyrosine 60 mg • N-Acetyl-L-Cysteine 25 mg • Taurine 110 mg • Green Tea Extract 50 mg • Horsetail (as silica) 12.5 mg • Lactoferrin 4 mg • NT Factor (as tablet base) Proprietary Blend 1400 mg: defatted rice bran, arginine, beet root fiber, black strap molasses, glycine, magnesium sulfate, enriched polyunsaturated phosphatidyl choline (phospholipids), saponin (glycolipids), para-amino benzoate, leek, pantethine (bifidus growth factor), taurine, garlic, calcium borogluconate, omega-6 essential fatty acids, omega-3 essential fatty acids, artichoke, barley malt, potassium citrate, calcium sulfate, spirulina, bromelain, natural vitamin E, calcium ascorbate, alpha-lipoic acid, oligosaccharides, B-6, niacinamide, tocotrienols, riboflavin, inositol, niacin, calcium pantothenate, thiamin, B-12, bifidus, acidophilus, folic acid, chromium picolinate. Other Ingredients: Gelatin (soft gel capsules), microcrystalline cellulose, croscarmellose sodium, vegetable magnesium stearate, silica, water & glycerin.

Propax with NT Factor **-** Pro Health
Each packet contains: Vitamin A (as acetate) 4375 IU • Vitamin A (as natural beta-carotene) 3750 IU • Vitamin C (as calcium ascorbate) 150 mg • Vitamin D (D3, as cholecalciferol) 32 IU • Vitamin E (as d-alpha tocopherol) 145 IU • Vitamin K (phytonadione) 2.5 mcg • Vitamin B1 (as thiamin HCl) 6.25 mg • Vitamin B2 (as riboflavin/ribose-5-phosphate) 30 mg • Vitamin B3 (as niacinamide) 60 mg • Vitamin B6 (as pyridoxine/P-5-P) 40 mg • Folic Acid (as folate) 200 mcg • Vitamin B12 (as cyanocobalamin) 25 mcg • Biotin 25 mcg • Pantothenic Acid (as d-calcium pantothenate) 25 mg • Calcium (as phosphate, ascorbate, citrate, sulfate, borogluconate) 360 mg • Iodine (as kelp) 18.75 mcg • Magnesium (as carbonate, oxide, glycinate, sulfate) 160 mg • Zinc (as methionate) 12.5 mg • Selenium (as selenomethionine) 75 mcg • Copper (as tyrosinate) 300 mcg • Manganese (as glycinate) 2.5 mg • Chromium (as nicotinate) 50 mcg • Molybdenum (as glycinate) 20 mcg • Potassium (as citrate) 12.8 mg • Bioflavonoids (as citrus, rutin, rosehips, quercetin) 165 mg • Boron (as calcium borogluconate) 500 mcg • Co Enzyme Q 10 4 mg • Creatine Monohydrate, Creatine Phosphate 122.5 mg • Grape Seed extract 5 mg • Inositol (inositol/inositol nicotinate) 25 mg • Lactoferrin 4 mg • Pantethine (as coenzyme A precursor) 70 mg • Vanadium (as vanadyl sulfate) 12.5 mcg • Alpha-Keto Glutarate 125 mg • Glutathione (as reduced) 5 mg • L-Tyrosine 60 mg • N-Acetyl-L-Cysteine 25 mg • Taurine 110 mg • Green Tea extract 50 mg • Horsetail (as silica) 12.5 mg • Phosphoglycolipids 160 mg • EPA (as eicosapentaenoic acid) 180 mg • DHA (as docosahexaenoic acid) 120 mg • NT Factor (as tablet base) 1400 mg. Other Ingredients: Gelatin (softgel capsule), Microcrystalline Cellulose, Methylcellulose, Croscarmellose Sodium, Vegetable Magnesium Stearate, Silica, Water, Glycerine.

Prophet 3H (Prophet3H) **-** Prophet 3H
Unknown.
See Editor's Note No. 12, page 2055.

Propo-Mune **-** Atrium Inc.
Each tablet contains: Propolis 5X 92 mg • Thymus 67 mg • Lymph 30 mg • Spleen 25 mg • Brain 25 mg • Folic Acid 400 mcg.
See Editor's Note No. 31, page 2056.

ProPortion Bars - Chocolate Peanut Butter **-** Rexall - Sundown
Each bar contains: Protein 12 g • Vitamin A 2250 IU • Vitamin C 27 mg • Calcium 100 mg • Iron 9 mg • Vitamin D 180 IU • Vitamin E 13.5 IU • Thiamin 0.675 mg • Riboflavin 0.765 mg • Niacin 9 mg • Vitamin B6 0.9 mg • Folate 200 mcg • Vitamin B12 2.7 mcg • Biotin 135 mcg • Pantothenic Acid 4.5 mg • Phosphorus 150 mg • Iodine 67.5 mcg • Magnesium 80 mg • Zinc 6.75 mg • Copper 1 mg • Chromium 52.5 mcg.

Prosina **-** LifeSpan Health Products
Each tablet contains: Beta-Sitosterol 30 mg • Beta-D-Glucosidase 0.1 mg.

Prosplex **-** Olympian Labs
Two capsules contain: Inositol Hexaphosphate 400 mg • Quercetin 200 mg • Saw Palmetto 320 mg • Tomato Lycopene 200 mg • Zinc (gluconate) 10 mg • Pumpkin Seed 10 mg • Pygeum Aficanum 20 mg.

Prosta Glan **-** Progressive Labs
Each capsule contains: Magnesium (as magnesium gluconate) 10 mg • Zinc (as zinc glycinate) 3.3 mg • Raw Bovine prostate concentrate 80 mg • Saw Palmetto 4:1 extract Lipoic Sterolic (Serenoa repens) 100 mg • Pygeum (Prunus africanum) 25 mg • Glutamic Acid 135 mg • Alanine 135 mg • Glycine 135 mg • Uva Ursi leaf (Arctostaphylos uva-ursi) 10 mg • Unsaturated Fatty Acids 10 mg • Pumpkin seed concentrate (Curcurbita pepo) 10 mg • Pollen 5 mg. The glandular

concentrate in this product is prepared by a special process which does not exceed physiological temperature (37° C). Guaranteed free of chemical pesticides and synthetic hormones.
See Editor's Note No. 14.

Prosta Kit **-** Flora, Inc.
Formula 1: Palmitol Saw Palmetto berries • Zinc 50 mg • Vitamin B6 120 mg. Formula 2: Flax-O-Mega cold pressed flax seed oil 1000 mg. Formula 3: Pro-Essence Burdock root • Juniper Berry • Prickly Ash bark • Slippery Elm bark • Uva Ursi.

Prosta Support **-** Nutri-Quest Rx
Each tablet contains: Vitamin C 10 mg • Vitamin B6 10 mg • Vitamin E (Succinate) 5 IU • Zinc Chelate 10 mg • L-Glycine 120 mg • L-Alanine 120 mg • L-Glutamic Acid 120 mg • Saw Palmetto 106 mg • Pygeum africanus extract 10 mg • Pygeum africanus herb 20 mg • Pumpkin seed 200 mg • Stinging Nettle leaves 75 mg • Echinacea 25 mg • Ginkgo Biloba 20 mg • Wild Yam 20 mg • Uva Ursi 10 mg.

Prostabs Plus **-** Futurebiotics
Three tablets contain: Glutamic Acid 390 mg • Glycine 390 mg • Raw Prostate Concentrate 150 mg • Alanine 390 mg • Vitamin B6 7.5 mg • Vitamin C (Ascorbate) 15 mg • Zinc (Gluconate) 30 mg • Magnesium (Oxide) 105 mg • Saw Palmetto Berry Extract (4:1 extract) 300 mg.
See Editor's Note No. 14.

Prosta-Comp **-** Atrium Inc.
Each tablet contains: Saw Palmetto berry extract 100 mg • Pumpkin seed oil extract 50 mg • Pygeum africanum extract 25 mg • Uva Ursi 50 mg • Zinc Gluconate 25 mg • Hydrangea extract 150 mg • Panax ginseng extract 100 mg.

ProstActin **-** Nature's Plus
Two softgels contain: Pygeum [(Prunus africanum bark) standardized 12-13% Phytosterols] 200 mg • Saw Palmetto [(Serenoa repens fruit) standardized 95% Fatty Acids] 80 mg • Glycine (Free form Amino Acid) 50 mg • Alanine (Free Form Amino Acid) 50 mg • Glutamine (Free Form Amino Acid) 50 mg • Turmeric [(Curcuma longa rhizome) standardized 95% Curcumin] 50 mg • Pumpkin Seed oil [(Curcurbita maxima seed) standardized 7% Alpha-Linolenic Acid] 50 mg • Zinc (Zinc Monomethionine) 30 mg • Vitamin E natural 200 IU.

Prost-Actin **-** Nature's Plus
Each tablet contains: Saw Palmetto berries 250 mg • Raw Prostate concentrate 140 mg • Zinc (Monomethionine) 50 mg • Vitamin A (Beta Carotene) 10000 IU • Vitamin E natural 200 IU.
See Editor's Note No. 14.

Prostactive Plus Saw Palmetto **-** Nature's Way
Each softgel contains: Concentrated 12:1 Saw Palmetto Berry Extract 160 mg • Concentrated 10:1 Nettle Root Extract 120 mg.

ProstaGuard **-** PhysioLogics
Each softgel contains: Alphastal Blend 250 mg: Saw Palmetto extract (serenoa repense, berry, standardized to contain 80% fatty acids, sterols), Astaxanthin (from h. pluvialis). Other Ingredients: Gelatin, Glycerin.

Prosta-Health **-** Aarisse Health Care
Each 3 oz. pump contains: Natural Progesterone • Saw Palmetto extract • Red Clover • Damiana • Tribulus Terrestris • Dong Quai • Vitamin A • Vitamin E • Vitamin B5 • Ginseng • Shea Butter • Aloe Vera.

Prostamax Plus **-** Woods Supplements
Each capsule contains: Saw Palmetto extract 150 mg • Cranberry 50 mg • Zinc Gluconate 37.5 mg • Magnesium Oxide 10 mg • Vitamin B6 1.1 mg.

ProstaMed **-** Enzymatic Therapy
Each capsule contains: Saw Palmetto Berry extract 160 mg standardized to contain 85%-95% fatty acids & sterols: 0.15% - 0.3% fatty alcohols, 0.2%-0.4% total sterols, 0.1%-0.3% beta-sitosterol.

Prosta-Metto **-** The Vitamin Shoppe
Each softgel contains: Saw Palmetto extract 160 mg • Pumpkin seed oil 40 mg • Pygeum Africanum extract 10 mg • Bearberry extract 10 mg • Zinc 15 mg • Vitamin B6 5 mg.

Prosta-Metto Saw Palmetto Complex **-** Puritan's Pride
Each softgel contains: Saw Palmetto berry extract (Serenoa repens: Standardized to contain 85-95% fatty acids and biologically active sterol compounds) 80 mg • Pumpkin Seed oil extract (Curburbita pepo) 40 mg • Pygeum Africanum extract 10 mg • Bearberry extract (Uva Ursi) 5 mg.

ProStamina **-** DreamPharm
Two capsules contain: Ginseng radix 30 mg • Angelica Sinensis radix 50 mg • Zingiberis rhizoma 20 mg • Hoelen 40 mg • Licorice root 40 mg • Dioscorea rhizoma 20 mg • Cuscuta semen 30 mg • Schisandra fructus 50 mg • Corni fructus 20 mg • Morindae radix 50 mg • Yohimbe powder 150 mg.

Prosta-Plex **-** Dr. Donsbach
Two capsules contain: Saw Palmetto extract 250 mg • Pygeum extract 7.5 mg • Stinging Nettle extract 100 mg • Zinc gluconate 5 mg.

Prostaprime **-** Puritan's Pride
Each tablet contains: Raw Prostate concentrate 100 mg • Saw Palmetto 100 mg • Pygeum extract 75 mg. Other Ingredients: Golden Rod, Pumpkin Seed Concentrate, Flaxseed Oil, Glycine, Glutamic Acid, and Alanine.
See Editor's Note No. 14.

ProstaPro **-** PhytoPharmica
Each softgel capsule contains: Saw Palmetto berry extract (standardized to contain 85-95% fatty caids, 0.2-0.4% total sterols, and 0.1-0.3% beta sitosterol) 160 mg.

Prosta-Q **-** Farr Laboratories, LLC
Each capsule contains: Zinc (from zinc gluconate) 5 mg • Proprietary Blend [Quercetin, Cranberry (berry), Saw Palmetto (berry), Bromelain, Papain] 540 mg.

Prostasol formerly PC Plus **-** Dr. Donsbach
Two capsules contain: Magnesium (as oxide) 200 mg • Sterolins 400 mg • Quercetin 100 mg • Proprietary Blend 500 mg: Reishi (as ganoderma lucidum), Baikal Skullcap (as scutellaria baicalensis), Rabdosia (as rabdosia rubescens hara), Dyer's Woad (as isatis indigotica fortune), Mum (as dendranthema morifolium tzelev), Saw Palmetto (as serona repens), San-Qi Ginseng (as panax notoginseng), Licorice (as glycyrrhiza glabra L.).

ProstaSoy **-** FreeLife International
Two caplets contain: Zinc (as patented chelazome zinc glycinate) 15 mg • Selenium (as selenomethionine) 100 mcg • Saw Palmetto standardized extract (85%-95% sterols, fatty acids) 320 mg • Proprietary Blend 250 mg: standardized extracts of Soybean, Kudzu root (providing beta sitosterol 60 mg, isoflavones 40 mg) • Proprietary Blend 125 mg: Tomato Lycopene concentrate (2000 mcg/g), Stinging Nettle root 4:1 extract (urtica dioica), African Wild Cherry bark 4:1 extract (pygeum africanum) • Proprietary Blend 2500 Units: Soy Polysaccharides, Plant Enzymes. Other Ingredients: Calcium Hydrogen Phosphate, Cellulose, Vegetable Stearic Acid, Silica, Vegetable Magnesium Stearate, Vita-Coat (vegetable resin, alpha-lipoic acid).

Prostat **-** ProJoba
Each tablet contains: Standardized extract of Graminae Pollen 70 mg • Fat soluble Gramanie extract EA 10 4 mg. Other Ingredients: Microcrystalline Cellulose, Lactose, Magnesium Stearate, Colloidal Silicon Dioxide, Natural Resin, Talc, Propylene Glycol.

Prostata **-** Gero Vita International
Each capsule contains: Urtica Dioica extract 16:1 150 mg • Serenoa Serrulata extract 106 mg • Apis Mellifica 83.33 mg • L-Alanine 66.67 mg • Glycine 66.67 mg • L-Glutamic Acid 66.67 mg • Pygeum Africanum extract 50 mg • Vitamin B6 15 mg • Panax Ginseng

BRAND NAMES

extract 8.33 mg • Zinc Arginate 7.5 mg • Hydrangea extract 5 mg • Copper 0.5 mg • Beta Carotene 8333 IU.

Prostate 5LX **-** New Chapter, Inc.
Two softgels contain: Saw Palmetto berry, extract (85-95% total fatty acids- 272-304 mg) 320 mg • Green Tea leaf, extract (45% polyphenols- 45 mg) 100 mg • Pumpkin Seed Oil 96 mg • Ginger rhizome, certified organic, extract (minimum 20% pungent compounds- 16 mg 5% zingiberene- 4 mg) 80 mg • Urtica root extract (Nettle) hydroalcoholic, 10:1 50 mg • Urtica root extract (Nettle) aqueous, 5:1 50 mg • Selenium, bio-grown 50 mcg • Rosemary leaf and essential oil, extract (23% total phenolic antioxidants- 2.3 mg) 10 mg. Other Ingredients: Olive Oil, Yellow Beeswax, Gelatin, Vegetable Glycerin, Purified Water, Carob.

Prostate Essentials **-** Swanson
Each capsule contains: Zinc (as zinc picolinate) 15 mg • Saw Palmetto extract (20% free fatty acids) 160 mg • Stinging Nettle concentrate 120 mg • Korean Ginseng root 50 mg • Pygeum extract (3% sterols) 50 mg • Pumpkin Seed concentrate 40 mg • Glycine 25 mg • L-Alanine 25 mg • L-Glutamic Acid 25 mg • Beta Sitosterol 20 mg.

Prostate Factors **-** Michael's Naturopathic Programs
Four tablets contain: Vitamin C (as calcium ascorbate) 100 mg • Vitamin E (as D-alpha tocopheryl succinate) 100 IU • Magnesium (as magnesium amino acid chelate) 75 mg • Niacin (as niacinamide) 10 mg • Pantothenic Acid (as calcium pantothenate) 20 mg • Zinc (as zinc monomethionine) 20 mg • Proprietary Blend 1966 mg: Bee Pollen, Alanine (as L-alanine), Parsley leaf (petroselinium sativum), Glutamin (as L-glutamine), Glycine, Echinacea root (echinacea angustifolia), Gravel root (eupatorium purpureum), Soy Isoflavones: Daidzein Glycosides (5.5%), Glycitein Glycosides (3%), Genistein Glycosides (1.9%), Liposterolic extract (from saw palmetto berry), Pygeum bark (pygeum africanum, 1% phytosterols, 250 mcg), Saw Palmetto fruit (serenoa serrulata, 5% fatty acids, 1.3 mg). Other Ingredients: Terra Alba (calcium sulfate), Maltodextrin, Stearic Acid, Magnesium Stearate, Calcium Amino Acid Chelate.

Prostate Formula **-** Life Extension
Each tablet contains: Serenoa Serrulta 100 mg • Pygeum Africanum extract 100 mg • Hydrangea extract 85 mg • Silica 85 mg • L-Alanine 67 mg • Glutamic Acid 68 mg • Glycine 67 mg • Panax Ginseng extract 10 mg • Zinc 10 mg • Vitamin A 10,000 IU • Vitamin E (d-alpha tocopherol) 200 IU.

Prostate Formula **-** Nature's Way
Two capsules contain: Beta Glucan 2.2 mg • Calcium 26 mg • Dandelion leaf 230 mg • Lycopene 2.4 mg • Saw Palmetto dried extract 360 mg • Soy Isoflavone dried extract 25 mg • Zinc (amino acid chelate) 7 mg. Other Ingredients: Gelatin, Magnesium Stearate, Millet, Silica.

Prostate Formula **-** Pharmanex
Each capsule contains: Selenium (as selenium yeast) 100 mcg • Saw Palmetto berry 10:1 extract (sereona repens) 160 mg • Green Tea (camellia sinensis) 85 mg • Lycopene 3 mg. Other Ingredients: Gelatin, Silicon Dioxide, Microcrystalline Cellulose, Magnesium Stearate.

Prostate Formula **-** Youngevity
Saw Palmetto 400 mg • Pygeum bark 80 mg • Pumpkin seed 80 mg • Atractylodes herb • Licorice root 40 mg • Bupleurum root 40 mg • Vitamin E 100 IU • Vitamin C 60 mg • Vitamin B6 4 mg • Vilcabamba Mineral Essence: Potassium, Calcium, Magnesium, Zinc, Chromium, Selenium, Iron, Copper, Molybdenum, Vanadium, Iodine, Cobalt, Manganese.

Prostate Guardian **-** Clinician's Choice
Three tablets contain: Vitamin E (dl-alpha tocopheryl acetate) 150 IU • Zinc (glycinate) 15 mg • Niacin (niacinamide) 15 mg • Pygeum Bark Powder 30 mg • Saw Palmetto Berries 450 mg • Kudzu Root 450 mg • Pumpkin Seeds 360 mg • Panax Ginseng Root 150 mg • Siberian Ginseng Root 150 mg • Oat Straw Extract (10:1) 150 mg • Horny Goat Weed 90 mg • RoseOx (patented, standardized process for an extract of Rosemary) 75 mg • Cayenne Fruit • Proprietary blend 12 mg: Lycopene 1%, Citrus Bioflavonoid Complex, Horsetail Herb, Isoflavones.

Prostate Health **-** Celestial Seasonings
Two capsules contain: Vitamin E (as d-alpha tocopherol acetate) 90 IU • Zinc (as gluconate) 15 mg • Proprietary Blend 1230 mg: Saw Palmetto (berries), Saw Palmetto (standardized extract), Stinging Nettle root (standardized extract). Other Ingredients: (May contain one or more of the following) Dicalcium Phosphate, Gelatin, Rice Flour, Stearic Acid, Magnesium Stearate, and Silicon Dioxide. One servings size is equivalent to: Saw Palmetto 320 mg standardized to 95% fatty acids.

Prostate Health **-** Doctor's A-Z
Each capsule contains: Zinc (as zinc picolinate) 15 mg • Saw Palmetto extract (20% fatty acids) 160 mg • Stinging Nettle concentrate 120 mg • Korean Ginseng root 50 mg • Pygeum extract (3% sterols) 50 mg • Pumpkin Seed concentrate 40 mg • Glycine 25 mg • L-Alanine 25 mg • L-Glutamic Acid 25 mg • Beta Sitosterol 20 mg.

Prostate Health **-** Schiff
Two capsules contain: Vitamin D (as cholecalciferol) 400 IU • Calcium (as calcium silicate, calcium d-glucarate) 29 mg • Zinc (as zinc citrate) 15 mg • Selenium (from high selenium yeast) 70 mcg • Copper (as copper gluconate) 1 mg • Saw Palmetto berry extract (serenoa repens) 667 mg • Free Fatty Acids (from saw palmetto extract) 300 mg • Calcium D-Glucarate 50 mg • Lycopene 12 mg. Other Ingredients: Gelatin, Maltodextrin, Magnesium Stearate, Silicon Dioxide, Titanium Dioxide.

Prostate Health **-** Sundown
Two capsules contain: Zinc (as zinc oxide) 5 mg • Saw Palmetto fruit 450 mg • Herbal Complext Blend 100 mg: Nettle root, Pygeum bark. Other Ingredients: Gelatin.

Prostate Health - Wellzymes **-** Enzymes, Inc.
Three capsules contain: Zinc (from Zinc Citrate) 30 mg • n-zimes Proprietary Enzyme Blend 75 mg: pHysioProtease (213,120 pHysio-U), CereCalase Plus • Proprietary Herbal Blend 495 mg: Saw Palmetto berry extract (standardized to contain 45% fatty acids), Pumpkin seed extract (standardized to contain 25% fatty acids), Pygeum bark extract (equivalent to 1350 mg raw herb), Hydrangea root extract (equivalent to 180 mg raw herb), Rice Bran. Other Ingredients: Plant Cellulose, Water.

Prostate Nutritional Support **-** NutriCology
Two softgels contain: Zinc (as zinc citrate) 10 mg • Pumpkin seed oil 893 mg • Saw Palmetto berry extract (standardized to 85-95% fatty acids) 320 mg • BioResponse DIM 320 mg: Diindolylmethane complex, starch, DIM (25% min.), Vitamin E Succinate, Phosphatidylcholine, Silica • Nettle root extract 16:1 300 mg • Beta-Sitosterol 120 mg • Lycopene 15 mg. Other Ingredients: Yellow Beeswax.

Prostate Support **-** Now
Each gelcap contains: Saw Palmetto • Pygeum • Stinging Nettle • Lycopene. Other Ingredients: Pumpkin seed oil, Zinc & Vitamin B6.

Prostate Support Formula **-** PhysioLogics
Two capsules contain: Zinc (as zinc glycinate) 15 mg • Copper (as copper amino chelate) 2 mg • Vitamin B6 (as pyridoxine HCl) 100 mg • Beta Sitosterol 60 mg • Pygeum bark extract (pygeum africanum, standardized to contain 2.5% phytosterols 5 mg) 100 mg • Pumpkin seed Oil extract (cucurbita pepo) 100 mg • Stinging Nettle leaf (urtica dioica, standardized to contain 1-2% silica, 4-8 mg) 400 mg. Other Ingredients: Gelatin, Rice Powder, Vegetable Magnesium Stearate, Silica.

Prostate-Duo **-** Uronat Nutrition Company, Inc.
Each softgel contains: Saw Palmetto extract (minimun 85% free fatty acids & 5% sterols) 160 mg • Pygeum africanum extract (minimum 13% sterols) 50 mg. Other Ingredients: Gelatin, Glycerin, Pumpkin seed oil, Water, Carob.

Prostatonin **-** PanGeo Health Brands, Inc.
Each capsule contains: Pygeum africanum 25 mg • Nettle Root 300 mg. Other Ingredients: Grape oil, gelatin, triglycerides, glycerol, sorbitol, soya lecithin, synthetic iron oxides, & titanium dioxide.

ProsTect **-** Advocare International
Three capsules contain: Zinc (as monomethionine OptiZinc) 5 mg • Selenium (as selenomethionine) 35 mcg • Vitamin D (as ergocalciferol) 40 IU • Red Clover flower/leaf extract (trifolium pratense) 200 mg • Saw Palmetto berry extract (serenoa repens) 50 mg • Cernitin Flower Pollen Extract 400 mg: Secale Cereale, Zea Mays, Phleum Pratence • Green Tea leaf extract (camellia sinensis) 50 mg • Glycine 200 mg • Tomato fruit extract (lycopene, lycopersicon esculentum) 500 mg. Other Ingredients: Silicon Dioxide, Magnesium Stearate, Gelatin.

Prostenil **-** Aboca USA, Inc
Two capsules contain: Saw Palmetto fruit powder (serenoa repens, standardized to 14% total liposterolic extract) 456 mg • Bearberry leaf freeze-dried extract(arctostaphylos uva-ursi, standardized to 12% arbutin) 60 mg • Stinging Nettle root freeze-dried extract (urtica dioica, standardized to 0.01 scopoletin) 30.6 mg • Echinacea root freeze-dried extract (echinacea pallida standardized to 2% echinacoside) 30 mg • Zinc Yeast (saccharomices cerevisiae, with zinc, 10% organically bound) 22.6 mg. Other Ingredients: Gelatin (capsule), Essential Oils of Cajuput, Italian Cypress.

Prostex **-** Metabolic Products
Two capsules contain: Proprietary Amino Acid blend 810 mg: Glutamic Acid, Alanine, Aminoacetic Acid (glycine). Other Ingredients: Gelatin, Polyethylene glycol 8000.

ProstGard **-** Holista
Each capsule contains: Zinc (from gluconate) 15 mg • Vitamin B6 (pyridoxine HCl) 5 mg • Saw Palmetto (Serenoa repens) extract of berries (10:1) 80 mg • Pumpkin Seed Oil 500 mg.

Prostoid **-** HealthWatchers System
Vitamin C • Vitamin A • Vitamin E • Vitamin B6 • Serenoa Senulata • Pygeum Africanum Extract • Hydrangea Extract • Bee Pollen • Siberian Ginseng Extract • Glutamic Acid • L-Glycine • L-Alanine • Silica • Solidago Fragrans Extract • Zinc • Damiana • Dong Quai • Gotu Kola • Juniper • Copper.

Protagest **-** PhytoPharmica
Three tablets contain: Ammonium Chloride 96 mg • Betaine HCl 975 mg • L-Glutamic Acid HCl 585 mg • Niacin (as niacinamide) 30 mg • Ox Bile extract 45 mg • Pancreatic Enzymez 4X 10 mg • Papain 6X 15 mg • Pepsin 1:3000 292 mg • Potassium (as potassium chloride) 50 mg • Vitamin B6 (as pyridoxine HCl) 1.5 mg.
See Editor's Note No. 14.

Protazyme **-** Enzymatic Therapy
Each tablet contains: Potassium Chloride 32 mg • Niacinamide 10 mg • Vitamin B6 (Pyridoxine HCL) 500 mcg. Other Ingredients: Betaine HCL 325 mg • Glutamic Acid HCL 195 mg • Pepsin 1:10000 97 mg • Ammonium Chloride 32 mg • Papain 6X 30 mg • Ox Bile extract 15 mg • Pancreatic Enzymes 4X 10 mg.
See Editor's Note No. 14.

Protease **-** Enzymes, Inc.
Each capsule contains: Protease 417 mg • Calcium Citrate 45 mg. Other Ingredients: Plant Cellulose, Water.

Protease Plus **-** Enzymes, Inc.
Each capsule contains: Calcium (from Calcium Citrate) 27 mg • pHysioProtease 607 mg. Other Ingredients: Plant Cellulose, Water.

Protector Caps **-** The Vitamin Shoppe
Three capsules contain: Vitamin A (Beta-carotene) 10000 IU • Vitamin E (d-alpha tocopheryl succinate) 200 IU • Ester C 500 mg • Pycnogenol 10 mg • Selenium (L-Selenomethionine) 50 mcg • CoQ10 10 mg • Green Tea extract (30% Polyphenols) 25 mg • Quercetin 25 mg.

Protector SPF 15 **-** Jason
Vitamin C Complex • Beta Hydroxy Acid.

Protein 95 Soy Protein **-** Nature's Life
Two 2 scoops (28.35 g) contain: SUPRO brand Soy Protein Isolate containing Lecithin • natural Vanilla Flavor • natural Papain Enzyme concentrate.

Protein Boost **-** Nutri-Quest Rx
Two tablespoons contain: Alanine 646 mg • Arginine 1190 mg • Aspartic Acid 1853 mg • Cystine 187 mg • Glutamic Acid 3060 mg • Glycine 680 mg • Histidine 408 mg • Isoleucine 765 mg • Leucine 1275 mg • Lysine 986 mg • Methionine 221 mg • Phenylalanine 850 mg • Proline 901 mg • Serine 833 mg • Threonine 612 mg • Tyrosine 629 mg • Valine 782 mg. Ingredients: Isolated Soy Protein, Calcium & Sodium Caseinate, Tri Calcium Phosphate, Lecithin, Soybean oil, Magnesium Oxide, Papain, Ascorbic Acid, Ferrous Fumurate, Kelp, Niacin, Calcium Pantothenate, Vitamin A, Pyridoxine HCL, Thiamine HCL, Riboflavin, Vitamin D & natural Vanilla Flavor. All acids of (L) form.

Protein Cysteine For Hair **-** Life Extension
Each tablet contains: Primary Dried Yeast Blend 500 mg: Histidine, Lysine, Leucine, Tryptophan, Phenylalanine, Methionine, Valine, Threonine, Isoleucine • Proprietary Blend 300 mg: Vitamin B1, Vitamin B2, Niacin, Biotin, Vitamin B6, Folic Acid • Casein 125 mg • L-Cysteine 100 mg • Di-Methione 3 mg. Other Ingredients: Carotene; In 72 Natural-Trace-Mineral Base.

Protein Digestion **-** Enzymes, Inc.
Each capsule contains: Proprietary Enzyme Blend 366 mg: Amylase, Protease, Lipase, Peptidase, Glucoamylase, Cellulase. Other Ingredients: Plant Cellulose, Water.

ProtEnz 375 **-** Enzymes, Inc.
Each capsule contains: n-zimes Protease Blend 625 mg. Other Ingredients: Cellulose, Water.

ProtoChol Chewables - Fields of Nature **-** Inverness Medical Innovations, Inc.
Each tablet contains: Phytosterol Concentrate 400 mg (as Beta-Sitosterol 172 mg, Campesterol 100 mg, Stigmasterol 44 mg). Other Ingredients: Dextrose, Magnesium Stearate, Adipic Acid, Aspartame, Natural and artificial flavors, Artificial colors (FD&C Red No. 40 Lake).

Protogen-A **-** Life Extension
Each tablet contains: Pure Protogen A 250 mg (natural liver base).

Protykin/Resveratrol **-** Natrol
Two capsules contain: Polygonum cuspidatum extract root 50 mg • Trans-Resveratrol 10 mg Total Reservatrols 12 mg • Emodin 5 mg. Other Ingredients: Rice powder, Magnesium Stearate, Gelatin.

Provasca **-** Endomatrix
Each capsule contains: Proprietary Blend 240 mg: Green Seaweed leaf extract powder, L-Arginine (as l-arginine hydrochloride).

Provol **-** Upsher-Smith Laboratories
Each capsule contains: Pygeum africanum bark extract 50 mg.

ProXeed **-** Sigma-Tau Pharmaceuticals, Inc.
Each packet contains: Active Ingredients: L-Carnitine Fumarate 1 g • Fructose • Acetyl L-Carnitine HCL 0.5 g • Citric Acid. Inactive Ingredients: Mannitol, polyethylene glycol, artificial flavorings, povidone, & silicone dioxide.

Proxylon - Syntrax Innovations
Each capsule contains: 7-Isopropoxyisoflavone 250 mg.

PS (Phosphatidylserine) - Metabolic Response Modifiers
Each softgel contains: Phosphatidylserine 100 mg • Other Phospholipids 380 mg • Soy oil 200 mg • Vitamin C 10 mg.

PS 100 - GNC
Each capsule contains: High Serine Soy Lecithin 0.5 g • Phosphatidyl Serine Complex 500 mg • Phosphatidylserine 100 mg • Phosphatidylcholine 45 mg • Phosphatidyethanolamine 10 mg • Phosphatidylinositol 5 mg. Other Ingredients: Gelatin, Glycerin.

PS Memory Care - Rexall - Sundown
Each softgel contains: Phosphatidylserine complex 500 mg Standardized to: Phosphatidylserine 100 mg • Phosphatidylcholine 45 mg • Phosphatidylethanolamine 10 mg • Phosphatidylinositol 5 mg. Other Ingredients: Soya Lecithin, Gelatin, Glycerine, Soybean Oil, Water.

Pseudo Ephedrine 30 mg - D & E Pharmaceuticals
Each tablet contains: Psuedo Ephedrine 30 mg.

Pseudo Ephedrine 60 mg - D & E Pharmaceuticals
Each tablet contains: Pseudo Ephedrine 60 mg.

Psoriacin - Dr. Clayton's Naturals
Each tablet contains: Berberis Aquifolium 3X. Other Ingredients: White Oak bark, Marshmallow root, Mullein leaves, Black Walnut leaves or hulls, Gravel root, Red Clover blossoms, Burdock root, Skullcap.

Psorizide Forte - Loma Lux Laboratories
Each tablet contains: Fumaric Acid 30 mg • Potassium Bromide 22 mg • Nickel Sulfate 2.6 mg. Other Ingredients: Lactose, Magnesium Stearate.

Psycles Female Nutrient Support System - Starlight International
Each two tablets contain: Vitamin B6 (as pyridoxine hydrochloride) 30 mg •Magnesium (as magnesium oxide) 100 mg •Chaste Tree extract 4:1 (vitex agnus-castus, fruit) 200 mg • Black Cohosh extract ,4:1 (cimicifuga racemosa, root) 200 mg •Dong Quai extract, 4:1 (angelica polymorpha, root) 150 mg • Dandelion extract, 4:1 (taraxacum officinale, leaf) 125 mg •Motherwort extract, 4:1 (leonurus cardiaca, herb) 100 mg •Ginger (zingiber officinalis, root) 100 mg •Quercetin 25 mg • Red Raspberry (rubus idaeus, leaf) 2 mg •Stinging Nettle (urtica dioica, leaf) 2 mg • Spirulina 2 mg. Other Ingredients: Maltodextrin, Dicalcium Phosphate, Microcrystalline Cellulose, Croscarmellose Sodium, Stearic Acid, Magnesium Stearate, Silicon Dioxide, Methylcellulose, Microfine Wax, Carbowax.

Psyllium - Metabolic Response Modifiers
Each tablespoon contains: Pysllium husk (4 g dietary fiber) 5 g.

Psyllium (Secrets of the Psyllium & Orange Flavored Psyllium Powder) - Trader Joe's
Psyllium husk fiber • Secrets of the Psyllium 85%: Fiber (per heaping tablespoon) 6 g • Orange flavored Psyllium powder 35%: Fiber (per heaping tablespoon) 3 g.

PTE Support - PhysioLogics
Two capsules contain: Bromelain (2400 GDU) 500 mg • Serratiopeptidase 10 mg.

Pumpkin Seed Extract - Enzymatic Therapy/PhytoPharmica
Each capsule contains: Pumpkin seed extract (cucurbita pepo, 18:1) 300 mg. Other Ingredients: Gelatin, Magnesium Stearate, Silicon Dioxide, Titanium Dioxide Color.
See Editor's Note No. 21, page 2056.

Pumpkin Seed Oil - GNC A-Z - GNC
Each capsule contains: Pumpkin Seed oil 1 g. Other Ingredients: Gelatin, Glycerin.

Pure & Natural Formula - Bee-Alive Inc.
Each 1/5 teaspoon contains: Royal Jelly (non-freeze dried) 1.1 g.

Pure Agility - PhytoPharmica
Three tablets contain: Chloride (from glucosamine sulfate) 234 mg • Chondroitin Sulfate (from marine source, with average molecular weight less than 16,000 daltons) 1200 mg • Glucosamine Sulfate (stabilized) 1500 mg • Sodium 185 mg.

Pure Bovine Cartilage - EcoNugenics
Four capsules contain: Bovine Cartilage 3 g • Calcium 30 mg • Sodium 18 mg. Other Ingredients: Gelatin, Magnesium Stearate, Silica.
See Editor's Note No. 14, page 2055.

Pure Build - PhytoPharmica
Each tablet contains: Indolplex Complex 120 mg: Modified food starch, 25% Diindolylmethane (DIM), D-Alpha-Tocopheryl Succinate, Silicon Dioxide, Phosphatidylcholine.

Pure C Crystals - Nature's Life
Each 1/4 teaspoon contains: Vitamin C (Ascorbic Acid) 1250 mg.

Pure Citrimax - Natrol
One capsule contains: (-) Hydroxycitric Acid 250 mg. Other Ingredients: Gelatin, Magnesium Stearate.

Pure Cleansing Gel (combination to oily skin) - Nu Skin Enterprises
Water (aqua) • Ammonium Lauryl Sulfate • Lauryl Betaine • Sodium Lauroyl Sarcosinate • Glycerin • PEG-120 Methyl Glucose Dioleate • Papain • Citrus Limonum fruit extract (citrus medica limonum, lemon) • Foeniculum Vulgare fruit extract (fennel) • Anthenis Nobilis flower extract • Calendula Officinalis flower extract • Centaurea Cyanis flower extract • Chamomilla Recutita flower extract (matricaria) • Geranium Maculatum extract • Hypericum Perforatum extract • Salvia Officinalis leaf extract (sage) • Sambucus Nigra flower extract • Tilia Cordata flower extract • Carbomer • Butylene Glycol • PVP • Sodium Chloride • Fragrance (parfum) • Tetrasodium EDTA • Benzoic Acid • Phenoxyethanol • Chlorphenesin • Methylparaben.

Pure Core - PhytoPharmica
Three capsules contain: Biotin 150 mcg • Calcium (as calcium lysinate, aspartate, citrate) 150 mg • Choline (as choline bitartrate) 38 mg • Chromium (as chromium glycinate, aspartate, lysinate) 75 mcg • Copper (as copper citrate, aspartate, glycinate, lysinate) 563 mcg • Folic Acid 300 mcg • Inositol 38 mg • Magnesium (as magnesium aspartate, citrate, glycinate, lysinate) 113 mg • Manganese (as manganese aspartate, lysinate, citrate, glycinate) 6 mg • Molybdenum (as molybdenum aspartate, glycinate, lysinate) 38 mcg &#8226 Niacin (as niacinamide, Niacinol brand) 53 mg • Pantothenic Acid (as calcium pantothenate) 150 mg • Potassium (as potassium chloride) 38 mg • Riboflavin (as riboflavin 25 mg, riboflavin-5'-phosphate 10 mg) 26 mg • Selenium (as selenium aspartate, glycinate, lysinate complexes) 38 mcg • Thiamin (as thiamin hydrochloride) 38 mg • Vanadium (as vanadium aspartate, glycinate, lysinate) 38 mcg • Vitamin A (as natural beta carotene with mixed carotenoids) 9375 IU • Vitamin B12 (as cyanocobalamin) 150 mcg • Vitamin B6 (as pyridoxine HCl 50 mg, pyridoxal-5'-phosphate 10 mg) 45 mg • Vitamin C (ascorbic acid) 281 mg • Vitamin E (as D-alpha tocopheryl succinate) 150 IU • Zinc (as zinc picolinate, lysinate, aspartate, glycinate) 9 mg.

Pure Dimension - PhytoPharmica
Three softgels contain: Fish Oil Concentrate 1.5 g: EPA (eicosapentaenoic acid) 210 mg, DHA (docosahexaenoic acid) 125 mg.

Pure Energy - Montana Naturals, Inc.
Each 800 mg caplet contains: Bee Pollen (Apis pollenus) • Dibaxic Calcium Phosphate • Gotu Kola (Centella asiatica) • Siberian Ginseng

(Eleutherococcus senticosus) • Gotu Kola standardized extract • Royal Jelly • Siberian Ginseng standardized extract.

Pure Ephedrene Alkaloid Extract - NVE Pharmaceuticals
Each tablet contains: Ephedra extract (leaves, stems, pure phamaceutical grade, supplying ephedrine alkaloids 24 mg) 240 mg.
See Editor's Note No. 30, page 2056.

Pure Eye Drops - BHI - Heel, Inc.
Active Ingredients: Cochlearia officinalis 5X • Echinacea angustifolia 5X • Euphrasia officinalis 5X • Pilocarpus 5X. Other Ingredient: Saline Solution.
See Editor's Note No. 1, page 2053.

Pure Fuel - PhytoPharmica
Each softgel contains: Eleuthero root 20:1 extract (eleutherococcus senticosus, standardized to contain a minimum of 0.5% eleutheroside E) • Iron 1 mg • Liquid Liver Fractions (predigested soluble concentrate) 550 mg • Vitamin B12 (as cyanocobalamin) 100 mcg.
See Editor's Note No. 14, page 2055.

Pure Relief - Kalchem International
Active Ingredient: Menthol.

Pure Soy Protein Powder - Puritan's Pride
Each scoop (28 g) contains: L-Alanine 1064 mg • L-Arginine 1876 mg • L-Aspartic Acid 2856 mg • L-Cysteine 308 mg • L-Glutamic Acid 4704 mg • L-Glycine 1036 mg • L-Histidine 644 mg • L-Isoleucine 1204 mg • L-Lysine 1540 mg • L-Methionine 336 mg • L-Phenylalanine 1288 mg • L-Proline 1260 mg • L-Serine 1288 mg • L-Threonine 924 mg • L-Tryptophan 308 mg • L-Tyrosine 924 mg • L-Valine 1232 mg.

Pure Symmetry - PhytoPharmica
Each chewable tablet contains: Coenzyme Q10 (ubiquinone 10) 100 mg • Vitamin E (as DL-alpha tocopheryl acetate, D-alpha tocopheryl acetate, and mixed tocopherols) 300 IU.

Pure Vitamin C 500 mg - Nature's Bounty
Each tablet contains: Vitamin C (as ascorbic acid) 500 mg. Other Ingredients: Cellulose (plant origin), Croscarmellose, Vegetable Magnesium Stearate, Silica, Vegetable Stearic Acid.

Pure Vitamin C Capsules - NutriCology
Each capsule contains: Vitamin C (as ascorbic acid) 1000 mg. Other Ingredients: Stearic Acid.

Pure Vitamin C Powder - NutriCology
Each 1/4 tsp (1 g) serving contains: Vitamin C (as ascorbic acid) 1000 mg.

PureChoice Beta-S - Baywood International
Each tablet contains: Calcium (as dl-calcium phosphate) 42 mg •Phosphorus (as dl-calcium phosphate) 26 mg • Beta-Sitosterol complex 300 mg • Pectin (citrus) 30 mg. Other Ingredients: Microcrystalline Cellulose, Lecithin, Silica, Polyvinlyprolidone, Croscarmellose Sodium, Magnesium Stearate, Vinegar (cider).

PureHands Gel - The Himalaya Drug Company (Himalaya Heal
Each 1 mL serving contains: Hrivera (coleus vettiveroides) 35 mg • Dhanyaka (coriandrum sativum) 25 mg • Nimbuka (citrus limon) 25 mg • Ushira (vetiveria zizanioides) 20 mg • Nimba (azadirachta indica) 15 mg. Base: Prasanna (rectified spirit, ethyl alcohol).

Pur-Gar - Now
Each tablet contains: Pur-Gar 600 mg.

Purim - The Himalaya Drug Company (Himalaya Heal
Each tablet contains: Haridra (curcuma longa) 36 mg • Aragvadha (cassia fistula) 36 mg • Bakuchi (psoralea corylifolia) 36 mg • Kushta (saussurea lappa) 36 mg • Katuka (picrorhiza kurroa) 36 mg • Nimba (azadirachta indica syn. melia axadirachta) 32 mg • Guduchi (tinospora cordifolia) 32 mg • Varuna (crataeva magna syn. c.nurvala) 32 mg • Triphala 31 mg: Emblica Officinalis, Terminalia Chebula, Terminalia Bellirica • Vidanga (embelia ribes) 31 mg • Bhringaraja (eclipta alba syn. e.prostrata) 31 mg • Kalamegha (andrographis paniculata) 31 mg.

Puristat Absorb - Abbott Industries
Each tablet contains: Chitosan powder 90% HD 278 mg. Other Ingredients: Dicalcium Phosphate Dihydrate (unmilled), Sweet Dairy Whey SD, Croscarmellose Sodium, Stearic Acid, Magnesium Stearate.

Puristat Boost - Abbott Industries
Two tablets contain: Siberian Ginseng (as Eleuthro L.) root 400 mg. Other Ingredients: Dicalcium Phosphate Dihydrous, Magnesium Stearate, Microcrystalline Cellulose, Silicon Dioxide, Stearic Acid, Sweet Dairy Whey.

Puristat Cleanse - Abbott Industries
Six tablets contain: Cascara Sagrada bark 400 mg • Buckthorn bark 200 mg • Rhubarb root 200 mg • Ginger root 150 mg • Goldenseal herb (aerial parts) 75 mg • Raspberry leaf 75 mg • Fennel seed 75 mg • Cayenne Pepper 25 mg • Mult. Fiber Blend 750 mg: Vegetable Cellulose, Beet fiber, Oat fiber, Pea fiber, Apple Pectin, Citrus Pectin. Other Ingredients: Dicalcium Phosphate, Croscarmellose Sodium, Stearic Acid, Silicon Dioxide, Hydroxypropylmethylcellulose (HPMC).

Puristat Restore - Abbott Industries
Three caplets contain: Lactobacillus Acidophilus & Lactospore 2 billion CFO • Aloe leaf 500 mg • Barberry root 150 mg • Black Radish root 150 mg • Marshmallow root 100 mg • Echinacea herb (aerial parts) 100 mg • Red Clover flower 100 mg • Burdock root 100 mg • Mullein leaf 50 mg • Parsley leaf 50 mg • Wood Betony herb (whole plant) 50 mg • Dandelion root 50 mg • Ginger root 50 mg • Cramp bark 50 mg. Other Ingredients: Magnesium Stearate.

Puritan's Pride One - Puritan's Pride
Each tablet contains: Vitamin A (as Retinyl Palmitate and Beta Carotene) 10,000 IU • Vitamin C (as Ascorbic Acid with Rose Hips) 250 mg • Vitamin D (as Cholecalciferol) 400 IU • Vitamin E (as d-Alpha Tocopheryl Acetate) 30 IU • Thiamin (Vitamin B-1; as Thiamine Hydrochloride) 25 mg • Riboflavin (Vitamin B-2) 25 mg • Niacin (as Niacinamide) 50 mg • Vitamin B-6 (as Pyridoxine Hydrochloride) 50 mg • Folic Acid 400 mcg • Vitamin B-12 (as Cyanocobalamin) 50 mcg • Biotin (as D-Biotin) 50 mcg • Pantothenic Acid (as D-Calcium Pantothenate) 50 mg • Calcium (as Bone Meal) 50 mg • Iron (as Ferrous Fumarate) 10 mg • Phosphorus (as Bone Meal) 23 mg • Iodine (as Potassium Iodide) 150 mcg • Magnesium (as Magnesium Oxide) 100 mg • Zinc (as Zinc Sulfate) 15 mg • Selenium (as Selenium Yeast) 25 mcg • Copper (as Copper Sulfate) 2 mg • Manganese (as Manganese Sulfate) 5 mg • Chromium (as Chromium Chloride) 100 mcg • Molybdenum (as Sodium Molybdate) 15 mcg • Chloride (as Potassium Chloride) 1 mg • Potassium (as Potassium Chloride) 1 mg • PABA (Para-Aminobenzoic Acid) 50 mg • Inositol 15 mg • Choline Bitartrate 15 mg. In a natural base of Bioflavonoids, Rutin, Rose Hips, Yeast, Kelp, and Dolomite.

Puritron - Puritan's Pride
Six tablets contain: Vitamin A (as Fish Liver Oil) 10,000 IU • Vitamin C (as Ascorbic Acid) 300 mg • Vitamin D (as Cholecalciferol) 400 IU • Vitamin E (as d-Alpha Tocopheryl Acetate) 100 IU • Thiamin (Vitamin B-1; as Thiamine Mononitrate) 25 mg • Riboflavin (Vitamin B-2) 25 mg • Niacin (as Niacinamide) 25 mg • Vitamin B-6 (as Pyridoxine Hydrochloride) 25 mg • Folic Acid 400 mcg • Vitamin B-12 (as Cyanocobalamin) 25 mcg • Biotin 150 mcg • Pantothenic Acid (as D-Calcium Pantothenate) 25 mg • Calcium (as Bone Meal) 800 mg • Iron (as Ferrous Gluconate) 30 mg • Phosphorus (as Bone Meal) 400 mg • Iodine (as Kelp) 150 mcg • Magnesium (as Magnesium Oxide) 100 mg • Zinc (as Zinc Gluconate) 30 mg • Selenium (as Selenium Yeast) 25 mcg • Copper (as Copper Gluconate) 1 mg • Manganese (as Manganese Gluconate) 0.07 mg • Potassium (as Potassium Gluconate) 40 mg • Brewer's Yeast 600 mg • Choline

Bitartrate 24 mg • Inositol 36 mcg • PABA (Para-Aminobenzoic Acid) 40 mcg • Rutin 30 mg • Citrus Bioflavonoid complex 30 mg • Hesperidin complex 25 mg • Nucleic Acid 40 mg • Desiccated Liver 100 mg • Red Bone Marrow 60 mg • Lecithin 60 mg • Wheat Germ Oil 20 mg • Papain 20 mg • Rose Hips 1 mg. Brewer's Yeast and Desiccated Liver provide the following Amino Acids per 6 tablets: Alanine 19.3 mg, Arginine 8.1 mg, Aspartic Acid 20.0 mg, Cysteine 2.7 mg, Glutamic Acid 32.8 mg, Glycine 12.8 mg, Histidine 8.0 mg, Isoleucine 13.1 mg, Leucine 21.1 mg, Lysine 21.9 mg, Methionine 5.4 mg, Phenylalanine 12.5 mg, Proline 11.9 mg, Serine 13.6 mg, Threonine 13.2 mg, Tryptophan 3.8 mg, Tyrosine 8.9 mg, Valine 12.6 mg.
See Editor's Note No. 14.

Pycnogenol **-** Leiner Health Products
Each tablet contains: Pycnogenol 50 mg. Other Ingredients: Calcium Carbonate, Maltodextrin, Cellulose, Tricalcium Phosphate, Talc, Polyethylene Glycol 3350, Silicon Dioxide, Crospovidone, Croscarmellose Sodium, Magnesium Stearate.

Pycnogenol **-** Schiff
Each capsule contains: Maritime Pine Bark extract (pinus maritima) 50 mg. Other Ingredients: Maltodextrin, Capsule (gelatin, lauryl sulfate, silicon dioxide), Magnesium Stearate, Silicon Dioxide.

Pycnogenol **-** Now
Each capsule contains: European Pine bark.

Pycnogenol 25 Mg **-** Natrol
One capsule contains: Pine Bark extract 25 mg. Other Ingredients: Microcrystalline Cellulose, Magnesium Stearate, Gelatin.

Pycnogenol 25mg **-** Sundown
Three tablets contain: Vitamin A (100% as beta-carotene) 25,000 IU • Calcium 340 mg • Selenium (as selenium yeast chelate) 100 mg • Maritime Pine bark extract 25 mg • Coenzyme Q-10 10 mg • Grape Seed extract 100 mcg • Whole Food Phytonutrient Blend 120 mg: Broccoli (entire plant), Carrot root, Spinach (entire plant), Tomato fruit. Other Ingredients: Calcium Carbonate, Microcrystalline Cellulose, Croscarmellose Sodium, Magnesium Stearate.

Pycnogenol 50 Mg **-** Natrol
One capsule contains: Pine Bark extract 50 mg. Other Ingredients: Microcrystalline Cellulose, Magnesium Stearate, Gelatin.

Pycnogenol Plus **-** Aspen Group, Inc.
Each capsule contains: Bioflavonoids 200 mg • Grape Seed extract 25 mg • Pycnogenol 25 mg.

Pycnogenol With Citrus Bioflavonoids **-** QualiCeutix
Each tablet contains: Pycnogenol (French martime pine bark extract) 50 mg • Citrus Bioflavonoid complex 250 mg. Other Ingredients: Microcrystalline Cellulose, Dicalcium Phosphate, Stearic Acid, Croscarmellose Sodium, Hydroxypropyl Methylcellulose, Magnesium Stearate, Silicon Dioxide, Polyethlene Glycol.

Pycnogenol with Vitamins C, E, & A **-** Derma E
Pycnogenol • Vitamin C • Vitamin E • Vitamin A.

Pycno-Plus Protection **-** HealthWatchers System
Grape Seed Extract • Pine Bark Pwder Plus • Beta Carotene • Vitamin C • Cat's Claw Powder • Bioflavonoids • Rutin • Acerola.

Pygeum **-** Nature's Way
Each capsule contains: Pygeum bark extract concentrate (standardized to 13% sterols 6.5 mg) 50 mg • Vitamin B6 (Pyridoxine HCl) 12.5 mg • Zinc (Citrate) 15 mg • Copper (Citrate) 1.5 mg • Selenium 50 mcg. In a base of Pumpkin seed oil.

Pyridoxal 5-Phosphate Plus **-** Klaire Laboratories
Each capsule contains: Pyridoxal 5-Phosphate 50 mg • Magnesium (as Magnesium Glycinate Chelate) 100 mg.

Pyridoxine P5P Vitamin B6 **-** NutriCology
Each capsule contains: Vitamin B6 (91% as pyridoxine hydrochloride and 9% as pyridoxal-5-phosphate) 275 mg. Other Ingredients: Cellulose, Stearic Acid, Silicon Dioxide.

Pyruvate **-** Aspen Group, Inc.
Each capsule contains: Calcium Pyruvate 750 mg.

Pyruvate Fuel **-** TwinLab
Each capsule contains: Calcium Pyruvate Monohydrate 750 mg.

Pyruvate Powder **-** Source Naturals
Each capsule contains: Calcium Pyruvate Monohydrate 750 mg.

Pyruvate Power **-** Swanson
Two capsules contain: Calcium (as calcium pyruvate) 244 mg • Pyruvate (as calcium pyruvate) 1.05 g • Cayenne 100 mg.

Pyruvate-C - Richardson Labs **-** Rexall - Sundown
Four caplets contain Pyruvate (Potassium Pyruvate, Calcium Pyruvate) 2 g • Chromium (Picolinate) 400 mcg.

Python **-** Swedish Herbal Institute
One tablet contains: Damiana 100 mg • Gotu Kola 30 mg • Green Oat Straw seeds 100 mg • Muira Puama 100 mg • Saw Palmetto 100 mg • Ginkgo Biloba 30 mg • Siberian Ginseng 200 mg • Korean Ginseng root 200 mg • Guarana seeds 50 mg • Schisandra fruit/seed 100 mg • Stinging Nettle leaf 200 mg • Tribulus Terrestris 250 mg.

Pytodolor **-** Enzymatic Therapy
Each drop contains: Common Ash bark 0.20 ml • Aspen leaves and bark 0.60 ml • Goldenrod aerial 0.20 ml. Other Ingredients: Water, Alcohol 45.6%.

Q-Gel 15 mg **-** Tishcon-GelTec
Each softsule contains: Vitamin E 3 IU • Coenzyme Q-10 15 mg. Other Ingredients: Gelatin, Glycerin, Purified Water, Titanium Dioxide, Annatto Seed Extract, Proprietary Biosolv: Polysorbate 80, Lecithin, Sorbitan Monoleate, Medium Chain Triglycerides.

Q-Gel Brand **-** Tishcon-GelTec
Coenzyme Q10.
See Editor's Note No. 44 and No. 45.

Q-Gel Forte 30 mg **-** Tishcon-GelTec
Each softsule contains: Vitamin E 6 IU • Coenzyme Q-10 30 mg. Other Ingredients: Gelatin, Glycerin, Purified Water, Titanium Dioxide, Annatto Seed Extract, Proprietary Biosolv: Polysorbate 80, Lecithin, Sorbitan Monoleate, Medium Chain Triglycerides.
See Editor's Note No. 45, page 2058.

Q-Gel forte Coenzyme Q10 **-** Solanova
Each softsules contains: Vitamin E (d-alpha tocopherol conc.) 6 IU • Coenzyme Q-10 (ubidecarenone) 30 mg. Other Ingredients: Gelatin, Glycerin, Purified Water, Titanium Dioxide, Annato seed extract, plus a proprietary Bio Solv base (polysorbate 80, lecithin, sorbitan monoleate, medium chain triglycerides).

Q-Gel Ultra **-** Tishcon-GelTec
Each softgel capsule contains: Coenzyme Q-10 60 mg • Vitamin E 150 IU.
See Editor's Note No. 45, page 2058.

Qmelt **-** CVS Pharmacy
Each tablet contains: Natural Coenzyme Q10 60 mg. Other Ingredients: Mannitol, Sorbitol, Citric Acid, Vegetable Stearate, Natural Orange Flavor, Povidone.

Q-Sorb Co Q-10 60 mg Plus Vitamin E **-** Vitamin World
Each capsule contains: Vitamin E (as D-alpha tocopherol acetate) 300 IU • Coenzyme Q-10 120 mg. Other Ingredients: Polysorbate 80, Gelatin, Medium Chain Triglycerides, Glyceryl Tributyrate, Glycerin, Sorbitol, Soy Lecithin, Annatto Extract (color), Titanium Dioxide Color.

Some Brand Name Natural Products - What they Contain

www.NaturalDatabase.com contains MANY more listings than appear here.

Q-Sorb Coenzyme Q-10 **-** Nature's Bounty
Each softgel contains: Coenzyme Q-10 50 mg. Other Ingredients: Rice Bran Oil, Gelatin, Glycerin, Mixture of Beeswax and Soybean Oil, Lecithin, Titanium Dioxide Color.

Q-Sorb Coenzyme Q-10 (120 mg) - Vitamin World **-** VitaStore
Each softgel capsule contains: Coenzyme Q-10 120 mg. Other Ingredients: Rice Bran Oil, Gelatin, Glycerin, Mixture of Beeswax and Soybean Oil, Lecithin, Titanium Dioxide Color.

Q-Sorb Coenzyme Q-10 (30 mg) **-** Vitamin World
Each softgel contains: Q-Sorb Coenzyme Q-10 30 mg. Other Ingredients: Rice Bran Oil, Gelatin, Glycerin, Soy Lecithin, Yellow Beeswax, Titanium Dioxide Color.

Q-Sorb Coenzyme Q-10 (50 mg) **-** Vitamin World
Each softgel contains: Q-Sorb Coenzyme Q-10 50 mg. Other Ingredients: Rice Bran Oil, Gelatin, Glycerin, Soy Lecithin, Yellow Beeswax, Titanium Dioxide Color.

Q-Sorb Coenzyme Q-10 (75 mg) **-** Vitamin World
Each softgel capsule contains: Coenzyme Q-10 75 mg. Other Ingredients: Rice Bran Oil, Gelatin, Glycerin, Mixture of Beeswax and Soybean Oil, Lecithin, Titanium Dioxide Color.

Q-Sorb Coenzyme Q-10 200 mg **-** Puritan's Pride
Each softgel contains: Q-Sorb Coenzyme Q-10 200 mg. Other Ingredients: Rice Bran Oil, Gelatin, Glycerin, Lecithin, Titanium Dioxide Color, Beeswax and Soybean Oil mixture.

Q-Sorb CO-Q-10 120 mg **-** Puritan's Pride
Each softgel contains: Q-Sorb Coenzyme Q-10 120 mg. Other Ingredients: Rice Bran Oil, Gelatin, Glycerin, Soy Lecithin, Yellow Beeswax, Titanium Dioxide Color.

Q-Sorb CO-Q-10 75 mg **-** Puritan's Pride
Each softgel: Q-Sorb Coenzyme Q-10 75 mg. Other Ingredients: Rice Bran Oil, Gelatin, Glycerin, Soy Lecithin, Beeswax and Soybean Oil Mixture, Titanium Dioxide Color.

Quanterra Emotional Balance **-** Warner-Lambert
Each tablet contains: LI 160 WS (hyperforin stabilized) St. John's Wort standardized extract 300 mg.

Quanterra Mental Sharpness, Ginkgo Biloba **-** Warner-Lambert
Each tablet contain: Egb 761 Ginkgo Biloba leaf extract; standardized to 24% Ginkgo flavone glycosides & 6% terpene lactones) 60 mg. Other Ingredients: Lactose, microcrystalline cellulose, maize starch, hydroxypropyl methylcellulose, croscarmellose sodium, polyethylene glycol, magnesium stearate, silicon dioxide, artificial color, talc, ferric oxide, & dimethicone.
See Editor's Note No. 21, page 2056.

Quanterra Prostate, Saw Palmetto **-** Warner-Lambert
Each softgel contains: Saw Palmetto Berry dried extract (Seronoa repens, berry, dried extract) 160 mg. Other Ingredients: Gelatin, Glycerol, & Ferric Oxide.

Quanterra Sinus Defense, Sinupret **-** Warner-Lambert
Each tablet contains: Gentian Root (Gentian lutea) 9 mg •Elder Flower (Sambucus nigra) 29 mg • European Vervain Aerial Parts (Verbena) 29 mg •Primrose Flower (Primula veris) 29 mg • Sorrel Aerial Parts (Rumex acesota) 29 mg. Other Ingredients: Sucrose, talc, lactose monohydrate, calcium carbonate, potato starch, maize starch, maize swell-starch flour, colloidal anhydrous silica, stearic palmitic acid, titanium dioxide, glucose syrup, gelatin, shellac, magnesium oxide, sorbitol, eudragit E 12.5, montan glycol wax, povidone, & castor oil.
See Editor's Note No. 21, page 2056.

Quanterra Sleep Valerian **-** Warner-Lambert
Three tablets contain: Valerian (Valeriana officinalis) root, dried extract 300 mg • Lemon Balm (Melissa officinalis) leaf, dried extract 150 mg. Other Ingredients: Sucrose, Castor Oil, Talc, Methylhydroxypropyl Cellulose, Microcrystalline Cellulose, Crospovidone, Silicon Dioxide, Calcium Carbonate, Polyethylene Glycol, Titanium Dioxide, Eudragit L 30 D, Glucose Syrup, Carmellose Sodium, FD&C Blue No. 2 Aluminum Lake, Magnesium Stearate, Polyvidon, Carnauba Wax, Polysorbate 80.

Quanterra Stomach Comfort, Ginger **-** Warner-Lambert
Two capsules contain: Ginger (Zingiber Officinale, root) 500 mg. Other Ingredients: Gelatin, colloidal anhydrous silica, & sodium laurel sulfate.

QueaseEase **-** Pacific BioLogic
Pinellia rhizome • Citrus peel • Fritillaria bulb • Poria Plant Fungus (hoelen) • Licorice root • Ginger rhizome • Chrysanthemum flower • Astragalus seed • Gastrodia rhizome • Bamboo shavings • Perilla leaf • Peppermint.

Quercetin **-** Metabolic Response Modifiers
Each capsule contains: Quercetin 500 mg.

Quercetin & Vitamin C **-** NSI - Nutraceutical Sciences Institute
Each capsule contains: Vitamin C (ascorbic acid) 700 mg • Quercetin 250 mg.

Quercetin + C **-** Puritan's Pride
Two capsules contain: Quercetin 500 mg • Vitamin C 1400 mg.

Quercetin 300 **-** NutriCology
Each capsule contains: Vitamin C (as calcium ascorbate) 75 mg • Vitamin E (as Dl-alpha-tocopheryl acetate) 70 IU • Quercetin 300 mg. Other Ingredients: Cellulose, Stearic Acid.

Quercetin 500 mg **-** Now
Each Vcap contains: Quercetin (from quercetin dihydrate) 500 mg. Other Ingredients: Cellulose (capsule), Cellulose, Magnesium Stearate (vegetable source).

Quercetin with Bioflavonoids **-** NutriCology
Each capsule contains: Lemon Bioflavonoid complex 400 mg • Quercetin 50 mg • Hesperidin 50 mg • Rutin 50 mg. Other Ingredients: Cellulose, Stearic Acid.

Quercetin-Bromelain **-** Doctor's Best
Each capsule contains: Quercetin 250 mg • Bromelain 125 mg.

Quercezyme-Plus **-** Enzymatic Therapy
Each capsule contain: Vitamin C (Ascorbic Acid) 100 mg • Magnesium (Carbonate) 25 mg. Other ingredients: Bromelain (1800 MCU) 125 mg, Quercetin 125 mg, Mixed Bioflavonoids Complex 50% concentrate 100 mg, L-Cysteine (HCL) 75 mg.

Quick Bust **-** Natural Certified Solutions
Three capsules contain: Fenugreek extract 219 mg • Saw Palmetto 168 mg • Fennel seed 162 mg • L-Tyrosine 135 mg • Mexican Wild Yam 96 mg • Kelp powder 90 mg • Damiana 51 mg • Dong Quai 48 mg • Mother's Wort 48 mg • Black Cohosh extract 45 mg • Avena Sativa 42 mg • Blessed Thistle 39 mg • Humulus Lupulus 30 mg.

Quick Dissolve Maalox **-** Novartis
Each tablet contains: Calcium Carbonate 600 mg. Other Ingredients: Aspartame, Colloidal Silicon Dioxide, Croscarmellose Sodium, Dextrose, Flavors, Magnesium Stearate, Maltodextrin, Mannitol, Pregelatinized Starch, Red #30 Lake.

Quick Dissolve Maalox - Maximum Strength **-** Novartis
Each caplet contains: Calcium Carbonate 1000 mg • Sodium 2 mg. Other Ingredients: Aspartame, Corn Starch, Croscarmellose Sodium, Dextrose, Flavors, Magnesium Stearate, Maltodextrin, Mannitol, Pregelatinized Starch, Silica, Sodium Chloride, Red #30 Lake.

Quick Trim **-** Cybergenics America Co.
Each caplet contains: Complex 1: Guarana seed extract • L-Tyrosine • L-Phenylalanine • Garcinia Cambogia (Citrimax) • Griffonia extract • Kola Nut powder • Chinese Ginseng • Cayenne pepper • Phenalgin • Astragalus root • Cinnamon bark • Green Tea • Pacific Kelp. Complex 2: Lecithin • Ginger • Cascara Sagrada • Buchu leaf extract • Uva Ursi leaf • Juniper berry extract • Choline Bitartrate • Inositol • L-Methionine • Chickweed herb • Red Clover powder • Dandelion root extract • Senna leaf extract • Cynarin complex. Complex 3: Chamomile flower • Valerian root extract • Hawthorne extract • Kava Kava root • Immature Orange peel • Lemon Verbena • Skullcap. Complex 4: Enzyme blend • Magnesium Oxide • Calcium Chelate • Selenium Yeast • Zinccitrata • Zinc Picolinate • Ascorbic Acid • Beta Carotene • Niacin • D Alpha Tocopheryl Acetate • Pyridoxine HCl • Riboflavin • Thiamin HCl • Potassium Iodide • Folic Acid • Cyanocobalamin • Chromium Picolinate • Phytonadione • Cholecalciferol.

Radiant Health Basic Essence EFAs **-** Maximum Efficiency Products
Each capsule contains: Proprietary Blend 725 mg: Essential oils from seeds of Flax, Sunflower, Sesame, Pumpkin, and Borage; and Mixed Tocopherols 725 mg.

Radiant Health Liquid Basic Essence **-** Maximum Efficiency Products
Each bottle contains: Proprietary Blend 8 fl oz: Essential oils from seeds of Flax, Sunflower, Sesame, Pumpkin, and Borage, and Mixed Tocopherols.

Radical Fruits Antioxidant Formula **-** Garden of Life, Inc.
Three caplets contain: Poten-Zyme Grape skin/fruit/seed extract (20:1) 975 mg • Poten-Zyme Raspberry fruit/seed extract (20:1) 585 mg • Poten-Zyme Goat's Milk Whey extract (20:1) 300 mg • Prune extract (60% polyphenols) 198 mg • Poten-Zyme Blueberry extract (20:1) 195 mg • Blueberry leaf extract (20% chlorogenic acid) 102 mg • Pomegranate extract (90% polyphenols, 40% elagic acid) 102 mg • Apple skin extract (80% polyphenols, 5% phloridzine) 99 mg • Grape leaf extract (90% polyphenols, 5% astilbine) 99 mg • Cherry extract (60% polyphenols) 51 mg. Other Ingredients: Cellulose, Stearate (vegetable source).

Radical Raiders **-** Puritan's Pride
Three capsules contain: Vitamin A (beta carotene) 25,000 IU • Vitamin E (d-alpha tocopheryl) 400 IU • Vitamin C (Ester C) 500 mg • Selenium (l-selenomethionine) 50 mcg • Zinc (picolinate) 50 mg • Calcium (Ester C) 50 mg • Coenzyme Q10 3,000 mcg • Pycnogenol 3,000 mcg • Citrus Bioflavonoids complex 50 mg • Quercetin 30 mg • L-Glutathione 1,000 mcg • N-Acetyl-Cysteine 100 mg • Green Tea extract 3,000 mcg • Bilberry extract 30 mg.

Rapid Balance-G.I. **-** DaVinci Laboratories
Each capsule contains: Mannon Oligosaccharides (MOS) 450 mg • Proprietary Probiotic Blend 50 mg: Lactobacillus Acidophilus, Lactobacillus Rhamnosus, Bifidobacterium Tongum (300 million CFU).

Raspberry **-** Natrol
Each single serving contains: Vitamin C (Ascorbic Acid) 250 mg • Acerola berry extract 20 mg • Echinacea (Purpurea extract 16:1) 12.5 mg • White Willow bark 100 mg • Slippery Elm bark 75 mg • Stevia powder 20 mg. Other Ingredients: Lemon Juice powder, Fructose, natural Raspberry flavor, Honey powder, Citric Acid, Natural Elderberry flavor, Calcium Carbonate.

Raspberry Drinkable Yogurt **-** Stonyfield Farm
Each 10 fl oz bottle contains: Active Live Cultures: S. Thermophilus • L. Bulgaricus • L. Acidophilus • Bifidus • L. Casei • L. Reuteri. Ingredients: Cultured Pasturized Low Fat Milk • Organic Sugar • Organic Nonfat Dry Milk • Inulin • Pectin • Beet Juice Concentrate • Carrot Juice Concentrate • Organic Raspberry Puree • Natural Flavors.

Raw Adrenal **-** Enzymatic Therapy
Each two capsules contain: Vitamin C (Ascorbic Acid/Rose Hips) 250 mg • Pantothenic Acid (D-Calcium Pantothenate) 100 mg • Vitamin B6 (Pyridoxine HCL) 50 mg. Other ingredients: L-Tyrosine 250 mg • Betaine 250 mg • Pituitary extract freeze-dried 120 mg • Adrenal extract (Predigested Soluble concentrate*) 400 mg • Adrenal Cortex extract 33 mg. *Free-form concentrate predigested by enzymatic action, creating a highly absorbable form of glandular concentrate containing all the natural principles with a standardized content. All organs & glands derived from bovine sources.
See Editor's Note No. 14.

Raw Adrenal II **-** Enzymatic Therapy
Two tablets contain: Vitamin C (Ascorbic Acid/Rose Hips) 250 mg • Pantothenic Acid (D-Calcium Pantothenate) 250 mg • Vitamin B6 (Pyridoxine HCL) 50 mg. Other ingredients: L-Tyrosine 500 mg • Betaine 250 mg • Pituitary extract freeze-dried 120 mg • Adrenal extract (Predigested Soluble concentrate*) 100 mg • Ginger root extract 6.5:1 (Zingiber officinale) 100 mg • Adrenal Cortex extract 33 mg. *Free-form concentrate predigested by enzymatic action, creating a highly absorbable form of glandular concentrate containing all the natural principles with a standardized content. All organs & glands derived from bovine sources.
See Editor's Note No. 14.

RealSJW **-** Paragon Laboratories
Each tablet contains: St. John's Wort (0.03% Hypericin, 4% min. Hyperforin) 300 mg • Grape Seed extract (LeucoSelect) 1 mg. Other Ingredients: Calcium Phosphate, Dipacic Microcrystalline Cellulose, Vegetable Oil, Croscarmellose Sodium, Magnesium Stearate, Silicon Dioxide.

REBOUND **-** Dynamarketing Group Inc.
Two tablets contain: Fumaric Acid 100 mg • Succinic Acid 250 mg • L-Glutamine 250 mg • L-Cysteine (L-cysteine HCl) 15 mg • Crystal Glucose 250 mg • Young Barley Grass juice powder 75 mg • Vitamin C (calcium ascorbate) 45 mg • Vitamin B1 (thiamine hydrochloride) 2 mg • Vitamin B12 (cyanocobalamin) 1200 mcg • Folic Acid 400 mcg. Other Ingredients: Dextrose, Magnesium Stearate, Stearic Acid, Croscarmellose Sodium, FD&C Blue.

Recall Support **-** The Vitamin Shoppe
Two tablets contain: Ginkgo Biloba Extract 24% ginkgoflavoglycosides 25 mg • Phosphatidylserine 10 mg • L-Phenylalanine 250 mg • L-Glutamine 250 mg • Choline 250 mg • Gotu Kola 200 mg • RNA/DNA 100 mg • Magnesium (citrate, gluconate) 50 mg • Ginseng Extract (Panax Ginseng) 50 mg • B6 10 mg. In a base of Lecithin and Rice concentrate.

Recancostat 400 - Tyler **-** Integrative Therapeutics
Each capsule contains: L-Glutathione (reduced) 400 mg • AnthoRedoxin Proprietary Blend 200 mg: Beet root (Beta vulgaris), Black Currant berry (Ribes nigrum), European Elderberry extract (Sambucus nigra), Bilberry berry extract (Vaccinium mytrillus) • L-Cysteine 80 mg. Other Ingredients: Microcrystalline Cellulose, Ascorbyl Palmitate, Gelatin, Water.

Recovazon **-** Amazon Herb
Dong Quai • Samambaia • Tangerine peel • Aquilaria • Safflower • Manaca • Peach kernel • Dalergia wood • Bitter Orange • Tayuya • Iporuru • Una de Gato.
See Editor's Note No. 40, page 2058.

Red Bull Energy Drink **-** Red Bull N.A., Inc.
Each 250 mL can contains: Carbonated Water • Sucrose • Glucose • Sodium Citrate • Taurine • Glucuronolactone • Caffeine • Inositol • Niacinamide • Calcium Pantothenate • Pyridoxine HCl • Vitamin B12 • Artificial Flavors • Colors.
See Editor's Note No. 42, page 2058.

Red Clover **-** Nature's Way
Each capsule contains: Red Clover blossoms 430 mg. Other Ingredients: Gelatin.

Red Clover Combination - Nature's Way
Each capsule contains: Barberry bark • Buckthorn bark • Burdock root • Cascara Sagrada bark • Echinacea Purpurea stem, leaf, flower • Licorice root • Peach bark • Prickly Ash bark • Red Clover blossoms • Rosemary herb • Sarsaparilla root • Sheep Sorrell. Other ingredients: Gelatin.

Red Clover Extract - Source Naturals
Each tablet contains: Red Clover leaf extract (8%) 500 mg • Calcium 164 mg • Isoflavones 40 mg.

Red Clover Extract Eternal Woman - Source Naturals
Each tablet contains: Red Clover leaf extract (8%) 500 mg • Calcium 164 mg • Isoflavones 40 mg.

Red Clover Support Complex - Puritan's Pride
Each tablet contains: Vitamin E 10 IU • Red Clover extract (Trifolium pratense) aerial (dried weight equivalent) standardized for 40 mg of isoflavone phytoestrogens (naturally contains: genistein, biochanin A, daidzein, formononetin) 200 mg • Soy Isoflavones 40 mg • Black Cohosh extract (Cimicifuga racemosa) root (standarized to contain 2.5% Triterpene) 50 mg • Wild Yam (Dioscorea villosa) root 50 mg • Horse Chestnut extract (Aesculus hippocastanum) seed (standardized to contain 2.5% aescin) 25 mg • Rosemary extract (Rosmarinus officinalis) leaf 15 mg • Silica 25 mg.

Red Dragon Cold & Flu Relief - Jamieson
Each capsule contains: Honeysuckle flower (Lonicera japonica Thunb. PE 1:2) 149.3 mg • Forsythia fruit (Forsythia suspensa Thunb. PE 1:2) 149.3 mg • White Mulberry Leaf (Morus Alba L.PE 1:2) 119.4 mg • Chrysanthemum flower (Chrysanthemum morifolium Ramat PE 1:2) 89.6 mg • Adenophora root (Adenophora Tetraphylla Thunb PE 1:2) 89.6 mg • Schizonepata stem (Schizonepata tenifolia Briq PE 1:2) 89.6 mg • Ningpo Figwort root (Scrophularia ninpoensis Hemsl PE 1:2) 74.6 mg • Great Burdock fruit (Arctium Lappa L PE 1:2) 74.6 mg • Hogfennel root (Peucedanum praeruptorum Dunn PE 1:2) 74.6 mg • Field Mint leaf (Mentha haplocalyx Briq PE 1:2) 44.8 mg • Licorice root (Glycyrrhiza uralensis Fischer PE 1:2) 44.8 mg. (PE = Powdered Extract).

Red Dragon Imperial Ginseng - Jamieson
Each caplet contains: Panax Ginseng (derived from Shiu Chu, Tien Chi and Red Kirin) • 500 mg Roots of: Prince Adenophorae, Salvia, Scrophulara, Codonopsis and Polygonum Ginsengs, Radix Astragail, Canodermae Lucidum, Fructus Lycii Berry.

Red Dragon Imperial Ginseng and Garlic - Jamieson
Each capsule contains: Panax Ginseng (derived from Shiu Chu, Tien Chi and Red Kirin) • Roots of: Prince Adenophorae, Salvia, Scrophulara, Codonopsis and Polygonum Ginseng, Radix Astragail, Canodermae Lucidum, Fructus Lycii Berry 250 mg • Tibetan Plateau Garlic 250 mg.

Red Dragon Imperial Ginseng and Royal Jelly - Jamieson
Each caplet contains: Panax Ginseng (derived from Shiu Chu, Tien Chi and Red Kirin) • Roots of: Prince Adenophorae, Salvia, Scrophulara, Codonopsis and Polygonum Ginseng, Radix Astragail, Canodermae Lucidum, Fructus Lycii Berry 500 mg • Fresh Royal Jelly 250 mg.

Red Dragon Imperial Green Tea - Jamieson
Each tea bag contains: Chinese Green Tea Leaf • Ginger Root • Natural Leechee Fruit Flavour.

Red Dragon Imperial Royal Jelly - Jamieson
Each capsule contains: Pure Royal Jelly concentrate equivalent to fresh Royal Jelly 500 mg.

Red Root-Cleavers Virtue - Blessed Herbs
Nettle • Horsetail Grass • Red Root • Cleavers • Sage leaf • Mullein leaf • Goldenseal root • Poke root • Ginger root • Grain alcohol & Distilled Water.

Red Stuff - Gary Null & Associates (GNA)
Contains a fruit mix including Cranberries, Cherries, Pears, Watermelons, Pink Grapefruit, Lecithin, Apple Pectin, Papayas, and Peaches.

Red Wine Formula - Health Smart Vitamins
Each capsule contains: Tea (green, leaf: 90% polyphenols, 180 mg) 200 mg • Vitis vinifera (grape seed: 95% proanthocyanidins, 95 mg or >260 Porter Value Units) 100 mg • Resveratrol (from Polygonum cuspidatum) 4 mg.

RedLine - VPX Sports
Caffeine Citrate • Caffeine Anhydrous • Evoburn Evodiamine • N-Acetyl-Tyrosine • Yerba Mate • Green Tea • 5-Hydroxy-L-Tryptophan • CAMP (adenosine cyclic 3',5'-monophosphate) • Vinpocetine • Yohimbe HCl • Highly Purified Water • Citric Acid • Carmine Red • Liquid Red • Sucralose • Potassium Sorbate • Natural and Artificial Flavor • Natural Colors.

Reduced L-Glutathione 150 mg - Klaire Laboratories
Reduced L-Glutathione 150 mg.

Reduced L-Glutathione 250 MG - PhysioLogics
Each capsule contains: L-Glutathione (reduced) 250 mg. Other Ingredients: Cellulose (plant origin), Gelatin, Acacia Gum, Vegetable Magnesium Stearate, Silica, Vanilla Flavor.

Reduced L-Glutathione 75 mg - Klaire Laboratories
Reduced L-Glutathione 75 mg.

Regal Pro-Meal - Nature's Life
Two scoops (28.35 g) contain: Supro brand Soy Protein Isolate containing Lecithin • Whey • Fructose • Non-fat Dry Milk • natural Vanilla Flavor • Yeast • Egg Albumin • Eggshell powder • Kelp • natural Papain Enzyme concentrate & Cobalamin concentrate (B12). Regal Pro-Meal also contains 34 mg of naturally occuring Isoflavones including 21 mg Genistein & 10 mg Daidzein.

Regenasure - Cargill Health & Food Technologies
Ingredients: 100% vegetarian Corn-derived Glucosamine.
See Editor's Note No. 43 and No. 44.

RegeniCare - Oasis Wellness Network
Each packet (7 g) contains: Vitamin C (ascorbic acid) 300 mg • Glucosamine Sulfate 1500 mg • MSM (methylsulfonylmethane) 1500 mg • Chondroitin Sulfate 750 mg • Protectin Proprietary Blend 300 mg: Acacia Catechu, Scutellaria Baicalensis • CMO 50 mg • MaxCell Proprietary Blend 20 mg: Zisyphus Jujube, Aloe Vera gel, Piper Nigrum, Glycyrrhiza Glabra. Other Ingredients: Citric Acid, Maltodextrin, Calcium Silicate, Natural Flavors, Stevia.
See Editor's Note No. 15, page 2055.

Regular Vita-Vim - Level 2 Potency Multivitamin - Jamieson
Each caplet contains: Vitamin A (from Acetate) 5000 IU • Beta Carotene 1500 IU • Vitamin D 400 IU • Vitamin C 150 mg • Vitamin E 15 IU • Vitamin B1 2.5 mg • Vitamin B2 2.5 mg • Vitamin B3 (no flush Niacinamide) 25 mg • Vitamin B5 25 mg • Vitamin B6 25 mg • Vitamin B12 25 mg • Folic Acid 400 mcg • Biotin 15 mcg • Calcium 150 mg • Iron 4 mg • Copper 1 mg • Iodine 0.1 mg • Magnesium 75 mg • Zinc 10 mg • Chromium 10 mcg • Selenium 10 mcg • Lutein 300 mcg • Lycopene 300 mcg • Citrus Bioflavonoids 2000 mcg • Soy Phosphotidyl Complex 5 mg • Digestive Enzyme Absorption Factors derived from: Peppermint, Bromelain, Papain, Amylase, Lipase, Cellulose 4000 mg.

Regyon Day - Hadas Natural Products
Each tablet contains: Passiflora Incarnata standardized extract 250 mg • Humulus Lupulus standardized extract 25 mg • Melissa standardized extract 25 mg • Vitamin B1 15 mg • Vitamin B6 15 mg.

Regyon Night - Hadas Natural Products
Each tablet contains: Passiflora Incarnata standardized extract 250 mg • Scutellaria Lateriflora standardized extract 50 mg • Humulus

Lupulus standardized extract 50 mg • Melissa standardized extract 25 mg.

Regyon Syrup - Hadas Natural Products
Each 5 mL serving contains: Orange flavored fructose-glucose syrup • Passiflora standardized extract 250 mg • Humulus Lupulus standardized extract 50 mg • Melissa standardized extract 50 mg.

Rehab Forte - Progressive Labs
Two capsules contain: Vitamin C (ascorbic acid) 500 mg • Niacinamide 200 mg • Vitamin B6 (pyridoxine HCl) 50 mg • Calcium (amino acid chelate) 200 mg • Elemental Calcium 40 mg • Magnesium (amino acid chelate) 100 mg • Elemental Magnesium 20 mg • Zinc (amino acid chelate) 30 mg • Elemental Zinc 7.6 mg • Manganese (amino acid chelate) 50 mg • Elemental Manganese 5 mg • Copper (amino acid chelate) 2 mg • Elemental Copper 0.01 mg • Potassium Sulfate 200 mg • Elemental Potassium 90 mg • Chondroitin Sulfate 50 mg • Lemon bioflavonoids 500 mg • Rutin 50 mg. See Editor's Note No. 15, page 2055.

Rehmannia Complex - Standard Process, Inc.
Each tablet contains: Rehmannia root extract (2.5:1, rehmannia glutinosa 350 mg) 140 mg • Bupleurum root extract (4.5:1, bupleurum falcatum 700 mg) 155.5 mg • Hemidesmus root extract (hemidesmus indicus 500 mg) 100 mg • Feverfew leaf/stem extract (3:1, tanacetum parthenium 165 mg) 55 mg • Calcium 59 mg. Other Ingredients: Cellulose, Calcium Hydrogen Phosphate, Silica, Sodium Starch Glycolate, Magnesium Stearate.

Rehydration - Vidafit
Each serving contains: Thiamine 1 mg • Vitamin A 100 IU • Vitamin C 1 mg • Calcium 20 mg • Iron 0.5 mg • Phosphorus 22 mg • Potassium 30 mg • Sodium 75 mg • Complex Carbohydrates 50 grams.

Reishi 5 - New Chapter, Inc.
Two capsules contain: Vitamin C 60 mg • Ginger extract (rhizome) 5% pungent compounds 50 mg • Mushroom Mycelia Reishi (mycelia), certified organic 200 mg • Shiitake (mycelia), certified organic mushroom extract 200 mg • Reishi (mushroom) minimum 4% triterpenes, 12.5% polysaccharides 40 mg • Maitake (mushroom) minimum 25% total polysaccharides 40 mg • Shiitake (mycelia) LEM, freeze dried, minimum EP3 1.5% PPT1 6% 40 mg • Cordyceps (mycelia) (dong-chong-zia-cao) 4:1 20 mg • Coriolus (mushroom) 8:1 20 mg. Other Ingredients: Vegetable Cellulose.

Reishi Defense - Traditional Medicinals
Red Reishi Mushroom (Ganoderma lucidum) Mycclium & Fruit Body • Ginger rhizome • Astragalus root • Roasted Barley grain • Licorice root • Stevia leaf.

Reishi Extract - Nature's Way
Two capsules contain: Reishi dried extract 376 mg. Other Ingredients: Gelatin, Millet.

ReishiMax GLp - Pharmanex
Each capsule contains: Reishi mushroom 20:1 powdered extract with spores (ganoderma lucidum) 500 mg. Other Ingredients: Gelatin.

Rejoyn Veromax - American MedTech
Two capsules contain: L-Arginine 200 mg • Zizyphi fructus 200 mg • Siberian Ginseng 200 mg • Saw Palmetto 200 mg • Ginkgo Biloba 75 mg • L-Alanine 75 mg • Glutamic Acid 75 mg • L-Lysine 75 mg. Other Ingredients: Pvp, Dicalcium Phosphate, Cellulose, Croscarmellose Sodium, Vegetable sterine, Magnesium stearate, Silicon dioxide and Pharmaceutical glaze.

Reju Veinate - PhysioLogics
Two capsules contain: Vitamin C (as ascorbic acid) 120 mg • Horse Chestnut seed extract (aesculus hippocastanum, standardized to contain 10% aescin, 30 mg) 300 mg • Butcher's Broom aerial parts (ruscus aculeatus, standardized to contain 10% ruscogenin, 20 mg) 200 mg • Gotu Kola aerial parts (centella asiatica) 120 mg • Citrus Bioflavonoids (citrus spp., standardized to contain 29% hesperidin, 23.2 mg) 80 mg • Bilberry fruit (vaccinium myrtillis, standardized to contain 25% anthocyanidins, 10 mg) 40 mg. Other Ingredients: Gelatin, Rice Powder, Vegetable Magnesium Stearate, Silica.

Rejuvenating Cream - Nu Skin Enterprises
Water (aqua) • Aloe Vera gel • Propylene Glycol • Stearic Acid • Cetearyl Alcohol • Ceteareth-20 • Dioctyl Adipate • Octyl Stearate • Octyl Palmitate • Stearamidopropyl Dimethylamine • Ceteth-2 • Glycol Stearate • Glycerin • Tocopheryl Linoleate • Octyl Methoxycinnamate • Hyaluronic Acid • Algae extract • Sorbitol • Hydrolyzed Elastin • Allantoin • Sodium PCA • Retinyl Palmitate • Cholecalciferol • Tocopheryl Acetate • Biotin • Panthenol • Royal Jelly • Citric Acid • RNA • Fragrance (parfum) • Caramel • Triethanolamine • Diazolidinyl Urea • Methylparaben • Propylparaben • Disodium EDTA.

Rejuvenex - Life Extension Foundation
Purified Water • Alkoxylated Diester • Isocetyl Steroyl Stearate • Octyl Salicylate • Glycolic Acid • Cetyl Alcohol • Stearyl Alcohol • Dimethicone • Butyl Methoxydibenzoylmethane • Maleated Soybean oil (ceraphyl NGA) • Potato starch (solanum tuberosum) • Safflower oil (carthamus tinctorius) • Dimethylaminoethanol Bitartrate (DMAE) • Retinyl Palmitate (vitamin A) • Ascorbyl Palmitate (vitamin C) • Sodium Ascorbyl Phosphate (vitamin C) • Tocopheryl Acetate (vitamin E) • Tocopherol (vitamin E) • Alpha-Lipoic Acid • Sodium Hyaluronate • Sodium PCA • RNA • Beta Glucan • Kinetin • Lactic Acid • Allantoin • Panthenol (vitamin B) • Glycerin • Squalane • Zinc Oxide • Ginseng extract (panax ginseng) • Arginine • Aloe Barbadensis gel • Glcyeryl Stearate • PEG-100 Stearate • Phenoxyethanol • Urea • Lavender oil (lavandula angustifolia) • Propylparaben • Methylparaben • Disodium EDTA • Imidazolidinyl Urea • Passion Flower essential oil blend • Ylang Ylang oil (canaga adorata).

Rejuvex - SunSource - Chattem, Inc.
Each caplet contains: Vitamin E (as dl-alpha tocopherol acetate) 30 IU • Thiamin HCl (Vitamin B1) 2 mg • Riboflavin (Vitamin B2) 2 mg • Niacin 10 mg • Vitamin B6 (as pyridoxine hydrochloride) 10 mg • Pantothenic Acid (as d-calcium pantothenate) 10 mg • Magnesium (as magnesium oxide) 500 mg • Selenium (as sodium selenate) 25 mcg • Manganese (as manganese sulfate) 2 mg • Standardized Dong Quai root extract 200 mg • Mammary gland powder 25 mg • Ovary gland powder 19 mg • Uterus gland powder 10 mg • Adrenal gland powder 10 mg • Pituitary gland powder 5 mg • Boron (chelated with citrate & aspartate) 3 mg. Other Ingredients: Microcrystalline Cellulose, Stearic Acid, Silicon Dioxide, Croscarmellose Sodium, Hydroxypropyl Methylcellulose, Magnesium Stearate, Polyethylene Glycol, Mineral oil, Shellac, & Talc.
See Editor's Note No. 14.

Rejuvine - Metabolic Response Modifiers
Two teaspoons contain: DHEA 25 mg • Pregnenolone 25 mg.

Relacore - Carter-Reed Co.
Each capsule contains: Vitamin C 333 mg • Calcium (as carbonate and pantothenate) 21.5 mg • Thiamin (vitamin B1) 5 mg • Riboflavin (vitamin B2) 7 mg • Vitamin B6 17 mg • Vitamin B12 3.5 mcg • Biotin 150 mcg • Pantothenic Acid (as calcium pantothenate) 7.8 mg • Magnesium 67 mg • Relacore Proprietary Blend 266 mg: Magnolia bark SE, Passion Flower herb SE, Scutellaria root SE, Niacinamide, DHEA, Panax Ginseng root, Pinella tuber, Poria fungus, Jujuba fruit, Perilla leaf, Phosphatidylserine.

Relastyl - Nutraceutics Corp.
Water • Butylene Glycol • Hydrogenated Polyisobutene • Glycerin • Tricaprylin • C12-15 Alkyl Benzoate • Cetyl Alcohol • Glyceryl Stearate • Butyrospermum Parkii fruit (shea butter) • PEG-40 Stearate • Sorbitan Stearate • Dimethicone • Carbomer • Polysorbate 20 • Palmitoyl Pentapeptide-3 • Squalane • Biosaccharide Gum-1 • Oenothera Biennis oil (evening primrose) • Hamamelis Virginiana extract (witch hazel) • Cucumis Sativus fruit extract (cucumber) •

Methylparaben • Propylparaben • Phenoxyethanol • Diazolidinyl Urea • Fragrance.

Relax & Sleep **-** Futurebiotics
Two tablets contain: Calcium (as calcium carbonate, phosphate, amino acid chelate) 150 mg • Magnesium (as magnesium oxide, amino acid chelate) 150 mg • Relax & Sleep Blend 860 mg: Valerian root powder, Chamomile flower powder, Hawthorn berry powder, Fennel seed powder, Passion flower powder, Skullcap leaf powder, Hops flower powder, Lemon Balm herb powder, Oat Straw leaf/stem powder, Red Clover herb powder, Catnip leaf powder, Spearmint leaf powder, Vanilla bean powder. Other Ingredients: Dicalcium phosphate, Stearic acid, Magnesium stearate, Silica.

Relax & Sleep Formula 2 **-** Futurebiotics
Two tablets contain: Valerian root - A balanced blend of extract & powder equivalent to dried root 500 mg • Chamomile - A balanced blend of extract & powder equivalent to dried blossoms 250 mg • Magnesium (oxide, amino acid chelate) 150 mg • Calcium (carbonate, phosphate, amino acid chelate) 150 mg. Specially formulated in a base of natural, time-tested herbs (in the form of extracts & powders) including: Hawthorn berry, Fennel, Passion flower, Scullcap, Hops, Lemon Balm, Avena Sativa, Red Clover, Catnip, Spearmint leaves & Vanilla.

Relax Now **-** Health Factor
Each capsule contains: Kava Kava 100 mg • Valerian 100 mg • Scutellaria 100 mg • Passion flower (2:1 extract) 75 mg • Hops 25 mg • Chamomilla 6X • Lady Slipper 3X.

Relax-O-Comp **-** PhytoPharmica
Two tablets contain: Calcium (as calcium citrate) 90 mg • Chamomile flower 4:1 extract (matricaria recutita) 150 mg • Evening Primrose seed oil (oenothera biennis) 20 mg • Hops flower 5:1 extract (humulus lupulus) 60 mg • Magnesium (as magnesium oxide and magnesium gluconate) 105 mg • Niacin (as niacinamide and niacin) 130 mg • Passionflower leaf (passiflora incarnata) 60 mg • Valerian root (valeriana officinalis) 150 mg • Vitamin B6 (as pyridoxine HCl) 20 mg • Vitamin D (as cholecalciferol) 100 IU • Zinc (as zinc chelate) 5 mg.

Relax-U **-** The Herbalist
Valerian root • Skullcap herb • Passionflower herb.

Release Afternoon **-** NDS Nutrition
Each capsule contains: Proprietary Blend 850 mg: Caffeine, L-Tyrosine, Magnesium Salicylate, Theobromine, Guarana, Synephrine, Guggulsterones, Yohimbine 3 mg, Hypericum (using St. John's wort @ 0.3%), Vitamin B12.
See Editor's Note No. 40, page 2058.

Release Evening **-** NDS Nutrition
Each capsule contains: Proprietary Blend 750 mg: Citrin K, Psyllium husk, Valerian root, Ho Shou Wu, Turkey Rhubarb, Cascara Sagrada, Senna extract, Piper Nigrum.

Release Morning **-** NDS Nutrition
Each capsule contains: Proprietary Blend 895 mg: Caffeine, Magnesium Salicylate, Theobromine, Guarana, Synephrine, Guggulsterones, Yohimbine 4.5 mg, Hypericum (using St. John's wort @ 0.3%), Vitamin B12.
See Editor's Note No. 40, page 2058.

Relief Formula **-** Pharmanex
Each capsule contains: MSHA TCM extract 450 mg: Magnolia Biodii flower extract (4:1), Saposhnikovia Divaricata root extract (3:1), Hedysarum Polybotrys root extract (2:1), Atractylodes Macrocephaia root extract (1.5:1).

Relief Plus **-** Health Factor
Each capsule contains: Goldenseal extract (4:1)(Hydrastis canadensis) 125 mg • Chamomile (Matricaria chamomilla) 100 mg • Valerian (Valeriana officinalis) 85 mg • Feverfew (Tanacetum parthenium) 590 mg • Cayenne Pepper 50 mg.

Reliv Arthaffect **-** Reliv International
Each scoop (8.5 g) contains: Arthred (hydrolyzed collagen) • Glucosamine Sulfate • Ginkgo Biloba • Borage Oil Powder • Turmeric • Boswellia Serrata • Ashwagandha • Cat's Claw • Sarsaparilla Root • Licorice Root • Kelp • Burdock Root • Alfalfa • Barley Grass • Echinacea Root • Yucca Extract • Devil's Claw Extract • Bilberry Extract • Celery Seed • Capsicum • Aloe Vera • Bioperine (Piper nigrum extract) • Soy Lecithin.

Reliv Celleboost **-** Reliv International
Two capsules contain: (-)Hydroxycitric Acid 375 mg • Oatrim (Hydrolyzed Oat Flour) 360 mg • Chromium 50 mcg.

Reliv Cellebrate **-** Reliv International
Each scoop contains: (-) Hydroxycitric Acid 375 mg • L-Carnitine 75 mg • Chromium 50 mcg • Choline 50 mg • Inositol 50 mg • Gamma-Linolenic Acid (as Borage Oil Powder) 50 mg • Ginkgo Biloba Leaves 33 mg • Coenzyme Q10 15 mg. Other Ingredients: Maltodextrin, Soy Lecithin, & Quaker Oatrim (Hydrolyzed Oat Flour).

Reliv Classic **-** Reliv International
Each scoop (16 g) contains: Soy Protein Isolate • Soy Flour • Brewer's Yeast • Lecithin • Psyllium Fiber • Dicalcium Phosphate • Ascorbic Acid • Methionine • Potassium Chloride • Magnesium Phosphate • Natural Flavor • Licorice Root • Garlic Rhubarb Root • Rose Hips • Cayenne • Kelp • OptiZinc Brand of Zinc Momomethionine • Ferrous Fumarate • Calcium Pantothenate • Niacinamide • Vitamin E Acetate • Vitamin A Palmitate • Vitamin D • Copper • Gluconate • Papain • Bromelain • Thiamin HCL • Riboflavin • Beta Carotene • Pyridoxine HCL • Biotin • Folic Acid • Potassium Iodine • Vitamin B12 • Soldium Selenite • ChromeMate Brand of Niacin Bound Chromium Polynicotinate.

Reliv FibRestore **-** Reliv International
Each scoop (30 g) contains: Fructose • Fiber Blend: Oat Fiber, Corn Bran, Apple Fiber, Soy Fiber, Pea Fiber, Citrus Fiber, Carrageenan Gum, Guar Gum, Xanthan Gum, Gum Arabic • Maltodextrin • Natural Flavor • Herbal Blend: Oriental Ginseng, Garlic, Cayenne, Licorice Root, Kelp, Rhubarb Root, Hibiscus, Irish Moss, Siberian Ginseng, Aloe Vera Powder, Chicory Root, Dandelion Root, Chamomile Powder, Alfalfa Powder, Pearl Barley, Ginger Root, Celery Seed, Sarsaparilla, Passion Flower, Capsicum Fruit Powder, Fenugreek • Lecithin • Ascorbic Acid • Citric Acid • Beta Carotene • Alpha Tocopheryl Acetate • Pepsin • Papain • Bromelain.

Reliv Innergize! **-** Reliv International
Each scoop (19 g) contains: Fructose • Maltodextrin • Citric Acid • Potassium Citrate • Natural Flavor • Tricalcium Phosphate • Sodium Chloride • Magnesium Oxide • Ascorbic Acid • Beta Carotene • OptiZinc Brand of Zinc Monomethionine • ChromeMate Brand of Niacin Bound Chromium Polynicotinate.

Reliv Now **-** Reliv International
Each scoop (15 g) contains: Whey • Soy Protein Isolate • Fructose • Dicalcium Phosphate • Magnesium Phosphate • Calcium Caseinate • Calcium Carbonate • Natural Flavor • Ascorbic Acid • Potassium Chloride • Lecithin • PABA (para-aminobenzoic acid) • Kelp • OptiZinc Brand of Zinc Monomethionine • Ferrous Fumarate • Calcium Pantothenate • Beta Carotene • Vitamin A Palmitate • Vitamin D (as Vitamin D3) • Thiamin HCL • Riboflavin • Niacinamide • Vitamin E Acetate • Pyridoxine HCL • Folic Acid • Vitamin B12 • Potassium Iodide • Copper Gluconate • Biotin • Sodium Selenite • ChromeMate Brand of Niacin Bound Chromium Polynicotinate • Sodium Molybdate • Vitamin K • Manganese Sulfate • Rutin • Garlic • Cayenne • Butternut Bark • Rhubarb Root • Blue Vervain • Licorice Root • Irish Moss.

Reliv ProVantage **-** Reliv International
Each scoop (26 g) contains: Soy Protein Isolate • Fructose • Medium Chain Triglycerides • Creatine Monohydrate • Tonalin (Conjugated Linoleic Acid-CLA) • Lecithin • L-Arginine • L-Glutamine • L-Leucine • L-Lysine • L-Carnitine • L-Alanine • Glycine • Ornithine

Alpha Ketoglutarate • Coenzyme Q10 • Activin (Grape Seed extract) • Phosphatidylserine & Phosphatidylcholine (as Phosphatidylserine/Phosphatidylcholine Complex) • Bioperine (Piper nigrum extract) • Natural & Artificial Flavors • Alpha-Lipoic Acid

Reliv ReversAge - Reliv International
Each 16 g scoop contains: Proprietary Blend: Aminotrope-7, Anterior Pituitary Peptides (porcine), Alpha Glycerylphosphorycholine, Chaperone Molecule Complex, 7-KETO (3-Acetyl-7-Oxo Dehydroepiandrosterine), S-Adenosyl-L-Methionine, Omega 3 Fatty Acids, Tri Methyl Glycine, Lactobacillus Acidophilus, Bifidobacterium Bifidum, Fructooligosaccharides, Acetyl L-Carnitine 1855 mg • Proprietary Blend 297.5 mg: N-Acetyl Cysteine, Alpha Lipoic Acid, Gluthione, Resveratrol, CoEnzyme Q10 • Proprietary Blend 250 mg: Ginkgo Biloba leaf, Quercetin Dihydrate, Spirulina plant powder, Maca tuber powder, Wild Yam root powder, Chlorella powder, Diosmin, Nettle leaf powder. Inactive Ingredients: Maltodextrin, Fructose, Natural Flavors, Artificial Flavors, Citric Acid, Lecitihin, Xanthan Gum, Potassium Citrate, DiPotassium Phosphate, L-Glutamine, L-Arginine Pyrogluamate, L-Lysine Monochloride, Glycine, Gamma Aminobutyric Acid.

Reliv SoySentials - Reliv International
Each scoop (22 g) contains: Soy Protein Isolate • Fructose • Inulin • Dehydrated Cranberries • Calcium Carbonate • Dicalcium Phosphate • Lactobacillus Acidophilus • Lecithin • Natural & Artifical Flavors • Activin (Grape seed extract) • Protykin (Resveratrol) • Ipriflavone • Black Cohosh Root • Dong Quai Root • Wild Yam • Panax Ginseng • Green Tea Extract • Chasteberry • Horse Chestnut • Nettle Root • Hops • Licorice Root • Coenzyme Q10 • Folic Acid • Ascorbic Acid • Pyridoxine HCL • Alpha Tocopheryl Acetate • Beet Powder • Stevia Extract • Acesulfame Potassium • Alpha Lipoic Acid.

Reliv Ultrim-Plus - Reliv International
Each scoop (28 g) contains: Soy Protein Isolate • Whey • Fructose • Milk Protein • Nonfat Dry Milk • Xanthan Gum • Dicalcium Phosphate • Magnesium Phosphate • Calcium Carbonate • Natural & Artificial Flavor • Ascorbic Acid • Potassium Chloride • Lecithin • Aspartame • PABA (Para-aminobenzoic acid) • Kelp • OptiZinc Brand of Zinc Monomethionine • Ferrous Fumarate • Calcium Pantothenate • Vitamin A Palmitate • Vitamin D (as Vitamin D3) • Thiamin HCL • Riboflavin • Niacinamide • Vitamin E Acetate • Pyridoxine HCL • Folic Acid • Vitamin B12 • Potassium Iodide • Copper Gluconate • Biotin • Sodium Selenite • ChromeMate Brand of Niacin Bound Chromium Polynicotinate • Sodium Molybdate • Vitamin K • Manganese Sulfate • Rutin • Garlic • Cayenne • Butternut Bark • Rhubarb Root • Blue Vervain • Licorice Root • Irish Moss.

Relora - Solanova
Each capsule contains: Relora Magnolia Officinalis & Phellodendron Amurense extract 250 mg. Other Ingredients: Snow White Filler, Magnesium Stearate, Silicon Dioxide, Gelatin, Glycerin, Purified Water.

Relora - Swanson Ultra - Swanson
Each capsule contains: Proprietary Blend 250 mg: Magnolia Officinalis, Phellodendron Amurense. Inactive Ingredients: Gelatin, Microcrystalline Cellulose (plant fiber), Magnesium Stearate.

Remedief - Natrol
Each capsule contains: Boswellia Serrata extract (65% total organic acids) 75 mg • White Willow bark (25% salicylic acid) 160 mg • Phellodendron bark extract (Nexrutine) 75 mg • Kava Kava root extract (30% kavalactones) 100 mg. Inactive Ingredients: Silica, Magnesium Stearate, Gelatin.

Remember When - Bee-Alive Inc.
Two half droppers (2mL) contain: Ginkgo Biloba leaf extract (standardized to 24% flavone glycosides 14.4 mg, 6% terpene lactones 3.6 mg) 60 mg • Rhodiola Rosea root extract 100 mg • Gotu Kola fresh leaf extract 0.17 ml • Royal Jelly (non-freeze dried) 25 mg. Other Ingredients: Vegetable Glycerin, Deionized Water, Clover Honey, Natural Spearmint Flavor, Xanthan Gum.

Remember! Mental Sharpness Formula - Enzymatic Therapy
Each two capsules contain: Vitamin B6 (as pyridoxine HCl) 15 mg • Folic Acid 800 mcg • Vitamin B12 (as cyanocobalamin) 500 mcg • Alpha Lipoic Acid 600 mg • Bacopa (bacopa monnieri, aerial part extract standardized to contain 20% bacosides) 300 mg • Ginkgo (ginkgo biloba, leaf extract standardized to contain 24% ginkgoflavonglycosides, 6% terpene lactones, and 2% bilobalide) 120 mg.

Remi Capsules - MHP
Two capsules contain: Chromium (as picolinate) 100 mcg • Citrus Aurantium extract (6% synephrine) 250 mg • Caffeine (from green tea extract) 100 mg • Theobroma Cacau extract 280 mg. Water Balance Blend: Couchgrass rhizome, Buchu leaf, Uva Ursi leaf, Juniper berry, Hydrangea root, Cornsilk stylus.
See Editor's Note No. 40, page 2058.

Remi Gel - MHP
Purified Water • SD Alcohol 40 • Lipocel 805: 5% Palmaria Palmata extract, 95% Dipropylene Glycol, 1% Laminaria Digitata, 99% Hydroethylcellulose, 0.5% Mannitol • Polysorbate 20 • Lemon peel extract (citrus medica limonum) • Orange extract (citrus aurantium dulcis) • Grapefruit extract (citrus grandis) • Palmarose extract (cymbopogon martini) • Diazolidinyl Urea • Methylparaben • Propylparaben • Tetrasodium EDTA • Citric Acid • FD&C Blue No. 1 • FD&C Red No. 40 • FD&C Yellow No. 5.

Remifemin - PhytoPharmica
Each tablet contains: Black Cohosh (Cimicifuga racemosa) root and rhizome extract (standardized to contain triterpene glycosides [calculated as 27-deoxyactein]) 20 mg.
See Editor's Note No. 21, page 2056.

Remifemin Menopause - GlaxoSmithKline (GSK)
Each tablet contains: Black Cohosh (Cimicifuga racemosa) & rhizome extract (standardized to contain 1 mg of triterpene glycosides calculated as 27-Deoxyacetin) 20 mg. Other Ingredients: Lactose, Cellulose, Potato Starch, Magnesium Stearate, Natural Peppermint Flavor.

Remifemin Plus - Enzymatic Therapy/PhytoPharmica
Each tablet contains: Standardized Cimicifuga racemosa (Black Cohosh) root & rhizome extract (standardized for triterpene glycosides content, calculated as 27-Deoxyactein) 20 mg • St. John's Wort extract standardized to contain hypericin 250 mcg.
See Editor's Note No. 21, page 2056.

Remotiv - Zeller
Each tablet contains: Hypericum extract Ze 117, standardized to a daily amount of 1 mg hypericin (St. John's Wort) 250 mg.

Renalka Syrup - The Himalaya Drug Company (Himalaya Heal
Each 1 tsp (5 mL) serving contains: Gokshura (tribulus terrestris) 50 mg • Varuna (crataeva magna syn. c.nurvala) 50 mg • Sariva (hemidesmus indicus) 50 mg • Musta (cyperus rotundus) 50 mg • Ushira (vetiveria zizanoides) 50 mg • Shatavari (asparagus racemosus) 50 mg • Trikatu 16.5 mg: Piper Nigrum, Piper Longum, Zingiber Officinale • Ela (elattaria cardamomum) 16.5 mg • Kshara Parpati (ammonium chloride, potash alum, potassium nitrate) 75 mg.

Renatrate - Progressive Labs
Each capsule contains: Vitamin A 5000 IU • Vitamin C 90 mg • Bovine kidney concentrate 300 mg. The glandular concentrate in this product is prepared by a special process which does not exceed physiological temperature (37° C). Guaranteed free of chemical pesticides and synthetic hormones.
See Editor's Note No. 14.

Some Brand Name Natural Products - What they Contain

www.NaturalDatabase.com contains MANY more listings than appear here.

Renewal HGH Advanced **-** Always Young
Each spray contains: HGH 9X/30X (somatropin) • Albumin 3C • Colostrum 30C • MSM (methyl-sulfonyl-methane) 9X • Ornithine 9X • Protease 9X • RNA (ribonucleic acid) 9X • Silica 9X • Zinc Sulphate 3C. Inactive Ingredients: Purified Water, 10% USP Alcohol, 8% USP Vegetable Glycerin.
See Editor's Note No. 1, page 2053.

Renewal HGH Workout **-** Always Young
Each spray contains: HGH (somatropin) 9X/12C/30X • IGF-1 (insulin-like growth factor-1) 6X/12X/30X • Growth Factors Elk Velvet Antler 9X/9C • Testosterone 30C/100X/1M • Androstenedione 9C/100X • Creatine Monohydrate 9C/100X • Trans-Ferulic Acid 30C/100X • Amino Acid Complex 10X/30X: L-Arginine Pyroglutimate 30X/30C, L-Carnitine 12X/30X, L-Glutamine 12X/30X, L-Isoleucine 9X, L-Leucine 9X, L-Valine 9X, OKG (ornithine alpha-ketoglutarate) 3C • DHEA (dehydroepiandrosterone) 30X/30C • Hyaluronic Acid 9X/30X/9C • NADH (nicotinamide adenine dinucleotide) 30X/100X/15C • Pituitarium 9X/30X/3C • Pregnenolone 9C/12X • Co-Enzyme A 12C/30X • Protease 9X/100X • Ribose 12C/30C • Trypsin 9X/30C • B Complex 30C/100X • Vitamin E 3C/30X • Boron 30X/30C • Chromium 30X/30C • Germanium 30X • Vanadium 9X/30X/30C • Zinc Sulphate 30X • Trace Minerals 30C/100X. Inactive Ingredients: Purified Water, 10% USP Alcohol, 8% USP Vegetable Glycerin.
See Editor's Note No. 1, page 2053.

Renewal IGF-1 Growth Factor **-** Always Young
Each spray contains: IGF-1 (insulin-like growth factor-1) 12C. Inactive Ingredients: Purified Water, 10% USP Alcohol 8%, USP Vegetable Glycerin.
See Editor's Note No. 1, page 2053.

Renew-U **-** The Herbalist
Milk Thistle seed • Echinacea root • Oregon Grape root • Dandelion herb • Burdock root • Yellow Dock root • Cleavers herb • Wild Indigo root • Ginger root • Fennel seed.

RenuDerm **-** Mellen Nutraceutical Corp.
Each four capsules contain: Vitamin C (as Ester-C) 400 mg • Selenium (sodium selenite) 100 mcg • BioCell Collagen II (chicken-derived) 2000 mg • Chondroitin Sulfate 400 mg • Hyaluronic Acid 200 mg • Alpha Lipoic Acid 100 mg • Tocotrienol (palm-derived) 30 mg • Kelp 75 mg • Bladderwrack 50 mg.
See Editor's Note No. 15, page 2055.

Reosto **-** The Himalaya Drug Company (Himalaya Heal
Each tablet contains: Arjuna (terminalia arjuna) 45 mg • Guggulu (commiphora wightii) 235 mg • Ashvagandha (withania somnifera) 4 5mg • Godanti Bhasma (calcium) 120 mg • Bala (sida cordifolia) 45 mg • Rasna (vanda roxburghii) 50 mg • Kukkutandatvak Bhasma (hen's egg shell calx) 35 mg.
See Editor's Note No. 39, page 2058.

Repagene Emulsion **-** Atrium Inc.
Each teaspoon contains: Squalene 1.5 g (emulsified form).

Repose - SunSource **-** Chattem, Inc.
One caplet contains: Vitamin C (as Calcium Ascorbate) 100 mg • Vitamin B6 (as Pyridoxine HCl) 14 mg • Pantothenic Acid (as D-Calcium Pantothenate) 17 mg • Magnesium (as Magnesium Oxide) 70 mg • Standardized Kava root extract (30% kavalactones) 200 mg • Standardized Siberian Ginseng root extract (0.8% eleutherosides) 65 mg.

Rescue Remedy **-** Bach Flower Essences
Active Ingredients: Rock Rose (Helianthemum nummularium) 5x HPUS • Clematis (clematis vitalba) 5x HPUS • Impatiens (Impatiens glandulifera) 5x HPUS • Cherry Plum (Prunus cerasifera) 5x HPUS • Star of Bethlehem (Ornithogalum umbellatum) 5x HPUS.
See Editor's Note No. 1, page 2053.

Resist **-** Pacific BioLogic
Astragalus root (Grade 1) • Ganoderma Fungus • Codonopsis root • Jujube fruit • Atractylodes (white) rhizome • Peony root (white) • Citrus peel (tangerine) • Cuscuta seeds • Dioscorea root • Schizandra fruit • Licorice root • Milletta root • Platycodon root • Ligustrum fruit • Glehnia root • Rehmannia root (prep.) • Ginger rhizome (fresh).

Resist 2 **-** Pacific BioLogic
Bitter Melon • St. John's Wort • Red Marine Algae • Echinacea Angustifolia • Tumeric rhizome • Licorice root (honey-baked) • Ligustrum root (Chinese) • Citrus peel (tangerine) • Viola (whole plant) • Prunella (selfheal spike) • Trichosanthis root • Knotweed rhizome (bushy) • Aucklandia root.

Respa-Herb **-** Dial Herbs
Ma Huang • Mullein • Goldenseal • Colts Foot • Comfrey • Marshmallow • Lobelia • Cayenne.
See Editor's Note No. 30, page 2056.

Resphora **-** PhysioLogics
Each capsule contains: Tylophora (GPH: 0.1% tylophorine alkaloids) 30 mg • Piper Longum (GPH: 2% piperine) • Picrorhiza Kurroa (GPH: 4% kutkin) 50 mg.

Resphora + **-** PhysioLogics
Each capsule contains: Vitamin C (as ascorbic acid) 150 mg • Long Pepper fruit (piper longum, standardized to contain 1.5% piperine, 1.5 mg) 100 mg • Picrorhiza root (picrorhiza kurroa, standardized to contain 4% kutkin, 2 mg) 50 mg • Quercetin fruit (from dimorphandra mollis) 50 mg • Ginkgo Biloba leaf extract (standardized to contain 24% ginkgo flavone glycosides, 9.5 mg, 6% terpenes, 2.4 mg) • Tylophora leaf (tylophora asthmatica, standardized to contain 0.1% tylophorine alkaloids, 0.3 mg) 30 mg • Serratiopeptidase 7.5 mg. Other Ingredients: Gelatin, Vegetable Magnesium Stearate, Silica.

Respi-Oil **-** The Herbalist
Essential oils of Eucalyptus, Rosemary, Sage, Tea Tree & Nutmeg in a Sweet Almond oil base.

Respir-all **-** Now
Three tablets contain: Vitamin B5 (Pantothenic Acid) 100 mg • Vitamin B6 (Pyridoxine HCL) 20 mg • Vitamin C (as Magnesium Ascorbate) 500 mg • Magnesium (as Magnesium Ascorbate) 40 mg • Zinc (as L-OptiZinc Monomethionine) 10 mg • Quercetin 800 mg • Nettle root extract (Urtica dioica) (standardized 30 ppm Scopoletin) 500 mg • Bromelain (2000 GDU) 500 mg • Licorice root (Glycyrrhiza glabra) 4:1 extract 200 mg.

Respiratory Relief **-** Grandma's Herbs
Each capsule contains: Proprietary Blend .448 g: Mullein leaf, Bayberry bark, Horehound leaf, Bladderpod herb, Heal All herb (prunella vulgaris), Elecampane root, Yerba Santa herb, Plantain herb, Nettle leaf, Coltsfoot powder, Cayenne pepper, Lungwort herb. Other Ingredients: Gelatin.

Respiratory Support Formula **-** PhysioLogics
Two capsules contain: Vitamin C (Ascorbic Acid) 130 mg • Ephedra root, stem (6% total Ephedrine Alkaloids, 12 mg) 200 mg • Lemon Bioflavonoids citrus 66 mg • Pleurisy root 45 mg • Mullein leaf 38 mg • Slippery Elm bark 38 mg • Licorice root 35 mg • Red Clover tops 35 mg • Ginkgo leaf (24% Ginkgo Flavonglycosides, 7.2 mg; 6 % Terpene Lactones, 1.8 mg) 30 mg.
See Editor's Note No. 30, page 2056.

Respi-Tea **-** The Herbalist
Wild Cherry bark • Slippery Elm bark • Coltsfoot leaf • Marshmallow root • Licorice root • Cinnamon bark • Yarrow blossom • Ginger root.

Respitonic **-** The Herbalist
Echinacea root • Golden Seal root • Osha root • Yerba Santa leaf • Horseradish root • Yarrow blossom • Cayenne pepper.

Some Brand Name Natural Products - What they Contain

www.NaturalDatabase.com contains MANY more listings than appear here.

B R A N D N A M E S

Res-Q 1250 **-** N3 Oceanic
Three capsules contain: EPA (Eicosapentaenoic Acid) 1200 mg • DHA (Docosahexaenoic Acid) 900 mg • Other Omega-3 150 mg.

Rest **-** Enzymes, Inc.
Two capsules contain: Calcium (100% as Calcium Citrate) 30 mg • Magnesium (100% as Magnesium Aspartate) 60 mg • Proprietary Herbal Blend 520 mg: Valerian root extract, Passionflower herb extract • pHysioProtease 100 mg. Other Ingredients: Plant Cellulose, Water.

RestEZ **-** Melaleuca
Each capsule contains: Proprietary Blend 385 mg: Valerian root extract (0.8% valerenic acid) • Kava Kava extract (30% kavalactones) • Hops • natural Spearmint powder • Passion Flower extract (4% flavonoids). Inactive Ingredients: Cellulose, Gelatin.

Restful **-** BioDynamax
Two capsules contain: Kava Kava root extract 300 mg • Chamomile 100 mg • Passion flower 100 mg • Calcium 100 mg • Magnesium 50 mg.

Restorative Toner **-** Abra Therapeutics
Deionized Water • Extracts Blend: Elderflower, Calendula, Orange Blossom, Horsetail, Bulgarian Chamomile • Aloe Vera Gel, Sodium PCA, Almond Glycerides • Panthenol • Sea Kelp • Algae extract • Vegetable Glycerin • Sorbitol • Lecithin • Cucumber extract • Vitamin E • Vitamin A • Vitamin C • Chelated Trace Minerals • Essential Oils Blend: Geranium, Ylang Ylang, Clary Sage • Methyl and Propyl Paraben.

Restore-X **-** Cambridge Nutraceuticals
Each serving contains: L-Glutamine 10 g • N-Acetyl-Cysteine 600 mg • L-Arginine (from Zinc Arginate) 140 mg • Vitamin A (as mixed carotenoids) 5000 IU • Vitamin C 500 mg • Vitamin E 200 IU • Thiamin 6 mg • Riboflavin 6.8 mg • Niacin 80 mg • Vitamin B6 8 mg • Pantothenic Acid 40 mg • Magnesium 200 mg • Zinc 20 mg • Selenium 100 mcg • Copper 0.75 mg • Folate 400 mcg • Vitamin B12 50 mcg.

Resveratone **-** Metabolic Response Modifiers
Each capsule contains: Polygonum cuspidatum (yielding 16 mg Resveratrol) 200 mg.

Revenge **-** Champion Nutrition
Each 29 g serving contains: Vitamin C 60 mg • Vitamin E 60 IU • Thiamine 5 mg • Riboflavin 3 mg • Vitamin B6 5 mg • Pantothenic Acid 10 mg • Magnesium 12 mg • Chromium 240 mcg • Potassium 160 mg. Tropical Mango Blast Ingredients: Metacarb VII (proprietary carbohydrate blend which contains Amylopectin Food Starch Modified, Glucose Polymer [Maltodextrin]) • Fructose • Peptol-7 (proprietary Protein-Amino Acid Blend which contains: Whey Protein Concentrate, L-Leucine, Glycine, L-Glutamine, Taurine, L-Isoleucine & L-Valine) • Lactate Blend (Sodium Potassium Lactate, Creatine Lactate, Glycerol Stearate, Magnesium Lactate, Glycerol Lactate) • Glucose (Dextrose) • Natural & Artificial Flavoring • Cellulose • Malic Acid • Trutina Dulcem (Natural Kiwi extract) • Phosphatidylcholine • D-Ribose • Vitamin E Acetate • Talc • Ginseng Root extract • Proteoglycan Support (proprietary blend which includes Glucosamine Hcl & Glucosamine Ascorbate) • Creatine Alpha-Ketoglutarate • Citric Acid • Potassium Phosphate • Guarana seed extract (standardized to 50% Caffeine) • Potassium Citrate • Ascorbic Acid • Quercetin • Willow Bark extract (standardized to 50% Salycin) • Sunett (Acesulfame-K) • Sodium Citrate • Omega-3 Fatty Acids (Fish oil) • Xanthan Gum • Feverfew extract • Vitamin B Blend (Vitamin B1, Vitamin B2, Vitamin B3, Vitamin B5, Vitamin B6, Pantethine) • Curcumin • N-Acetylcysteine • Periwinkle standardized extract • Coenzyme Q10 • Lipoic Acid • Chromium Polynicotinate • Annatto & Carmine (natural colors).

ReVitalize **-** Rx Vitamins
Three purecaps contain: Mixed Carotenoid complex (alpha, beta & gamma carotenes) 25000 IU • Vitamin C (ascorbic acid) 200 mg • Pantothenic Acid (calcium pantothenate) 100 mg • Calcium (amino acid chelate/complex) 50 mg • Magnesium (amino acid chelate/complex) 50 mg • Vitamin B1 (thiamine) 50 mg • Vitamin B2 (riboflavin) 50 mg • Vitamin B3 (niacin) 50 mg • Vitamin B6 (pyridoxine HCl) 50 mg • Citrus Flavonoid complex (active flavonols, flavonones, flavones & naringen-44%) 50 mg • Choline (bitartrate) 50 mg • Inositol 50 mg • Potassium (glycero-phosphate) 25 mg • Zinc (amino acid chelate/complex) 15 mg • Manganese (amino acid chelate/complex) 5 mg • Iron (amino acid chelate/complex) 4.5 mg • Copper (glycinate) 1 mg • Vanadium (as vanadyl sulfate) 1 mg • Vitamin D (calciferol) 400 IU • Vitamin E (d-alpha tocopherol) 200 IU • Folic Acid 400 mcg • Biotin 300 mcg • Iodine (kelp) 150 mcg • Vitamin B12 (cyanocobalamin) 100 mcg • Chromium (polynicotinate) 50 mcg • Selenium (amino acid complex) 50 mcg • Molybdenum (amino acid complex) 20 mcg • Korean Ginseng (Panax ginseng, standardized 5% ginsenosides) 50 mg • Chinese Green Tea extract (Camilla sinensis, standardized 40% polyphenols) 25 mg • Ginkgo Biloba (standardized 24% ginkgoflavoneglycosides, 6% terpene lactones) 10 mg • Bilberry (Vaccinium myrtillus, standardized 25% anthocyanosides) 5 mg • Mahonia Aquifolium (wild grape seed extract, standardized 95-100% leucoanthocyanins) 5 mg • Oleoresin Turmeric (Curcuma longa, standardized 90-95% curcuminoids) 5 mg • Milk Thistle (Silybum marianum, standardized 80% Silymarin) 75 mg • Parsley Leaves (Petroselinum crispum, naturally rich in apiin & luteolin-7-apiolglucoside) 75 mg • Juniper Berries (juniperus communis, naturally rich in glucuronic acid) 50 mg • Celery seed 4x (Aplum graveolens, naturally rich in limonene) 50 mg • Cayenne (Capsicum frutescens, naturally rich in capsaicin) 50 mg • Glucosamine Sulfate (aminomonosaccharide) 30 mg • Borage Seed Oil (Borago officinalis, standardized 25% gamma linolenic acid) 25 mg.

ReVitaMan **-** NorthStar Nutritionals
Each capsule contains: Maca root 67 mg • Muira Puama 167 mg • Catauba bark 33 mg • Ashwagandha powder 33 mg • Gotu Kola herb 14 mg • L-Arginine aspartate 67 mg • Thiamine 3 mg • Riboflavin (vitamin B2) 3 mg • Niacin 7 mg • Vitamin B6 8 mg • Folate 133 mcg • Vitamin B12 33 mg • Pantothenic Acid 8 mg.

RevivAll Classic PhytoSterols & Sterolins **-** Garden of Life, Inc.
Two capsules contain: Whole Food Vitality Blend 1424 mg: 100% pre-digested blend of Sweet Potato, Garbanzo beans, Soy beans, Red Lentils, Adzuki beans, Kidney beans, Brown Rice, Sesame seeds, Flax seeds, Sunflower seeds, Pumpkin seeds • Phytosterol Blend 76 mg: Beta-Sitosterol, Stigmasterol, Campesterol • HSO Probiotic Blend 1.6 billion CFU. Other Ingredients: Cellulose (vegetable source).

RevivAll Female Vitality Formula **-** Garden of Life, Inc.
Four capsules contain: Whole Food Vitality Blend 2000 mg: 100% pre-digested blend of Garbanzo beans, Red Lentils, Soy beans, Flax seeds, Sunflower seeds, Adzuki beans, Kidney beans, Brown Rice • Herbal Vitality Blend 720 mg: 100% pre-digested blend of Sweet Potato, Wild Yam, Dong Quai, Black Cohosh, Licorice, Clover, Horse Chestnut, Chasteberry • Red Clover standardized extract (containing 16% isoflavones) 200 mg • Phytosterol Blend 80 mg: Beta-Sitosterol, Stigmasterol, Campesterol • HSO Probiotic Blend 1.6 Billion CFU. Other Ingredients: Cellulose (vegetable source).

RevivAll Male Vitality Formula **-** Garden of Life, Inc.
Two capsules contain: Whole Food Vitality Blend 1092 mg: 100% pre-digested blend of Garbanzo beans, Red Lentils, Soy beans, Flax seeds, Sunflower seeds, Sesame seeds, Adzuki beans, Kidney beans, Brown rice • Herbal Vitality Blend 200 mg: 100% pre-digested blend of Sweet Potato, Ginger • Cemitin Swedish Flower Pollen extract 132 mg • Phytosterol Blend 76 mg: Beta-Sitosterol, Stigmasterol, Campesterol • HSO Probiotic blend 1.6 billion CFU. Other Ingredients: Cellulose (vegetable source).

Some Brand Name Natural Products - What they Contain

www.NaturalDatabase.com contains MANY more listings than appear here.

Revivogen Bio-Cleansing Shampoo **-** Advanced Skin & Hair Inc
Deionized Water • Decyl Polyglucose • Cocoamphocarboxyglycinate • Cocamide MEA • Aloe Vera • Jojoba oil • Cocoyl Sarcosine • Dimethicone • Ethylene Glycol Stearate • Polyquatrenium-4 • Panthenol (vitamin B5) • Saw Palmetto extract • Niacin (vitamin B3) • Guar gum • Soy Protein • Pyridoxal Hydrochloride • Gamma Linolenic Acid • Linoleic Acid • Zinc Sulfate • Azaleic Acid • Menthol • Benzophnone-4 • Methyl Paraben.

Revivogen Scalp Therapy **-** Advanced Skin & Hair Inc
SD Alcohol-40 • Gamma Linolenic Acid • Alpha Linolenic Acid (GLA & ALA) • Linoleic Acid • Oleic Acid • Azelaic Acid • Saw Palmetto extract • Zinc Sulfate • Vitamin B6 • Ethyl Laurate • Phytol • Beta Sitosterol • Grape seed extract • Procyanidin Oligomers • Niacin (vitamin B3) • Tocopherol Acetate (vitamin E) • EDTA • Purified Water • Perfumes.

Rezoom **-** 4 Life
Each 1/2 oz. serving contains: Vitamin C (as calcium ascorbate, magnesium ascorbate) 6 mg • Thiamin (Vitamin B1) 168 mcg • Riboflavin (Vitamin B2) 189 mcg • Niacin 3.6 mg • Vitamin B6 (as pyridoxine HCl) 225 mcg • Folic Acid 50 mcg • Vitamin B12 (as cyanocobalamin) 0.05 mcg • Pantothenic Acid 0.4 mg • Zinc 50 mcg • Selenium (as selenomethionine) 1 mcg • Chromium (as chromium nicotinate) 2 mcg • Chloride (as sodium chloride) 1 mg • Sodium (as sodium chloride) 1 mg • Potassium (as potassium citrate) 3 mg • Yerba Mate (leaf) 266 mg • Aloe Vera 138 mg • Bio Essential Proprietary Blend 44 mg: Yerba Mate extract (leaf), Astragalus extract (root), English Hawthorn extract (leaf), Sarsaparilla extract (root), Siberian Ginseng extract (root), Yarrow extract (flower), Echinacea Purpurea extract (root), Licorice extract (root), Charparral extract (root), Stillingia extract (root), Korean Ginseng extract (root) • Peppermint extract (leaf) 3 mg • Lime extract (blossom) 2 mg • Lemon Balm extract (peel) 2 mg • Boron 2 mcg. Other Ingredients: Water, Glycerin, High Fructose Corn Syrup, Alcohol, Potassium Sorbate, Sodium Benzoate, Phosphoric Acid, Malic Acid, Lactic Acid.

Rezyme **-** Nature's Secret
Vegetarian Enzyme that contains a proprietary blend of Amylase, Glucoamylase, Cellulase, Lipase, Lactase, Alpha Galactosidase, Bromelain, Papain, Betaine HCl, Gentian, Licorice, and Ginger root. Enzyme Rebuilder, which contains Bitters, Lecithin, L-Glutamine, and Piper longum fruit.

Rheumatex With S.O.D. Catalase **-** Life Extension
Each tablet contains: Superoxide Dismutase 4000 units • Catalase 8000 units • Glutathione Peroxidase 600 units (bovine liver base).

Rhinallergy **-** Boiron
Active Ingredients: Allium Cepa 5 CH 0.5 mg • Ambrosia Artemisiaefolia 5 CH 0.5 mg • Euphraisa Officinalis 5 CH 0.5 mg • Histaminum Muriaticum 9 CH 0.5 mg • Sabadilla 5 CH 0.5 mg • Solidago Virga Aurea 5 CH 0.5 mg. Inactive Ingredients: Lactose, Sucrose, Magnesium Stearate.
See Editor's Note No. 1.

Rhino Acidophilus **-** Dial Herbs
Lactobacillus acidophilus • Bifidobacterium bifidum • Bifidobacterium infantis • FOS, in a base of rice powder & natural flavors • Vitamin C from Ester-C. Flavored & sweetened with all-natural raspberry fruit juice crystals, dextrose & fructose.

Rhino Actalin Bars **-** Nutrition Now
Soy Protein Isolate, Calcium Sodium Caseinate, Whey Protein Concentrate, Glucose, High Fructose Glucose Syrup, Fractionated Vegetable Oils, Turbinado Sugar, Non-Fat Dry Milk, Yogurt Solids, Vanilla, Lecithin, Raisins, Apple Paste, Natural Flavors, Apple Fiber, Graham Flour, and Cinnamon.

Rhino Actalin Dietary Supplement **-** Nutrition Now
Each tablet contains: Magnesium 20 mg • Inosine 50 mg • Phosphatidylserine 50 mg • Amino Acid Blend 50 mg.
See Editor's Note No. 21, page 2056.

Rhino Chewy Vites **-** Dial Herbs
Vitamin A • Vitamin C • Vitamin D • Vitamin E • Vitamin B6 • Vitamin B12 • Calcium • Thiamin • Riboflavin • Folic Acid • Biotin • Pantothenic Acid • Iodine • Magnesium • Zinc • Choline • Inositol • Fruitrim: (Fruit juice, Natural grain dextrins) • Evaporated Cane juice (natural milled sugar) • Gelatin • Lactate • Gluconate • Ascorbic Acid • d-Alpha Tocopheryl Acetate • Citrate Palmitate • Betartrate • Citric Acid • Lactic Acid • Natural Flavors • Natural Colors added including Annatto, Turmeric, Carmine & Grape skin liquid • Lightly polished with Fractionated Vegetable oil (Coconut origin) to prevent sticking • Beeswax.

Rhino Daily Pack **-** Nutrition Now
Two Rhino Vites contain: 100% natural daily multi-vitamin, two Rhino Calcium, one Rhino Ester-C (Vitamin C).

Rhino Echinacea **-** Dial Herbs
Two tablets contain: Echinacea 100 mg • Vitamin C 60 mg. Flavored & sweetened with all natural raspberry fruit juice crystals, dextrose & fructose.

Rhino Echinacea Pops Box **-** Dial Herbs
Each lollipop contains: Isomalt • Maltitol • Citric Acid • Ascorbic Acid 50 mg • Natural Flavor • Color from Beet liquid • Echinacea • Goldenseal • Phosphorus 6x • Drosera 6x • Kali Carbonicum 6x • Belladonna 6x • Rumex Crispus 6x • Hydrastis 6x.
See Editor's Note No. 1, page 2053.

Rhino Ester-C **-** Dial Herbs
Vitamin C from Ester-C • Calcium. Flavored & sweetened with all-natural cherry flavorings, natural fruit flavors, fructose, dextrose & bilberry.

Rhino Support Pack **-** Nutrition Now
Each packet contains: Two Rhino Echinacea, two Rhino Acidophilus, one Rhino Ester-C (Vitamin C).

Rhizinate **-** PhytoPharmica
Two tablets contain: Deglycyrrizinated Licorice root 3:1 extract (DGL, glycyrrhiza glabra) 760 mg • Glycine 100 mg.

Rhizinate - Chocolate-Mint **-** PhytoPharmica
Two tablets contain: Licorice (Glycyrhiza glabra) root extract 4:1 (deglycyrrhizinated) 760 mg • Glycine (amino acid) in a base of fructose 100 mg. Flavored with Dutch Cocoa Powder, Creme Flavor, and Peppermint.

Rhodiola **-** Vitamin World
Each capsule contains: Rhodiola Rosea root extract (rhodiola rosea L., standardized to contain 3% rosavins (4.5 mg), 0.8% salidrosides (1.2 mg)) 150 mg • Rhodiola Rosea (rhodiola rosea L.) 100 mg. Other Ingedients: Gelatin, Cellulose (plant origin), Vegetable Magnesium Stearate, Silica.

RiboCell brand **-** Nutratech
D-Ribose.
See Editor's Note No. 44, page 2058.

Riboflavin **-** PhytoPharmica
Each tablet contains: Riboflavin (vitamin B2) 400 mg.

Rice Bran Oil **-** Progressive Labs
Each tablespoon contains: Rice bran oil 14 g.

RiceMucille **-** NutraCea (formerly NutraStar)
Each 360 g canister contains: Stabailized Rice Bran and Germ.

Rich's MSM Eye and Ear Drops **-** Rich Distributing
Methylsulfonylmethane • Sterilized Activated Water.
See Editor's Note No. 10, page 2055.

Some Brand Name Natural Products - What they Contain

www.NaturalDatabase.com contains MANY more listings than appear here.

Rimostil - Novogen
Each tablet contains: Clovone Isoflavone Proprietary Blend 57 mg: Formononetin, Daidzein, Biochanin A, Genistein. Other Ingredients: Calcium Phosphate, Microcrystalline Cellulose, Soy Polysaccharide, Magnesium Sulfate, Titanium Dioxide.

Ring Stop - NaturalCare
Active Ingredients: Calcarea Carbonica (calcium carbonate) 8X, 30X • Cimicufuga Racemose (black snake root) 3X, 6X, 12X, 30X • Carbo Vegetabilis (vegetable charcoal) 8X, 12X, 30X • Cinchona Officinalis (peruvian bark) 3X, 6X, 30X • Chininum Sulphuricum (sulphite of quinine) 12X, 30X • Coffea Cruda (unroasted coffee) 3X, 12X • Graphites (plumbago) 8X, 12X, 30X • Kali Carbonicum (potassium carbonate) 12X, 30X • Lycopodium (club moss) 6X, 12X, 30X • Natrum Salicylicum (sodium salicylate) 6X • Salicylicum Acidum (salicyclic acid) 6X. Inactive Ingredients: Alpha Lipoic Acid, Butcher's Broom leaf extract, Chinese herbs: Black Sesame seed (hei zhi ma), Cassia bark (gui zhi), Peony root (chi shao), Pueraria (ge gen)(root), Jobs Tears seed (yi yi ten), Ligusticum Wallichii root (chuan xiong) • CoEnzyme Q10, Cyanocobalamin, Folic Acid, Garlic bulb extract (odor-controlled), Ginger (root), Ginkgo Biloba leaf extract 24/6%, Inositol Hexaniacinate, Kelp Extract, L-Arginine Hydrochloride, Magnesium Amino Acid Chelate, Methyl Cobalamin, N-Acetyl-Carnitine HCl, N-Acetylcystine, Pyridoxine HCl, Riboflavin, Thiamine Mononitrate, Vinpocetine, Vitamin A Acetate, Zinc Amino Acid Chelate.
See Editor's Note No. 1, page 2053.

Ring Stop - Dr. Bob Martin's
Active Ingredients: Calcium Carbonate (Calcera carbonics) 8x, 30x • Black Cohosh root (Cimifuga recemose) 3x, 6x, 12x, 30x • Vegetable Charcoal (Carbo vegetabillis) 8x, 12x, 30x • Peruvian Bark (Cinchona officinalis) 3x, 6x, 30x • Sulphite of Quinine (Chininum suphuricum) 12x, 30x • Unroasted Coffee (Coffea cruda) 8x, 12x • Plumbago (Graphites) 8x, 12x, 30x • Potassium Carbonate (Kali carbonicum) 12x, 30x • Club Moss (Lycopodium) 6x, 12x, 30x • Sodium Salicylate (Natrum salicylicum) 6x • Salicylic Acid (Salicylicum acidum) 6x. Other Ingredients: Alpha Lipoic Acid, Beta-Carotene, Chinese Cassia (Gui Zhi, bark), Chinese Peony (Chi Shao, root), Chinese Pueraia (Ge Gen, root), Cyanocobalamin, Folic Acid, Garlic Extract (bulb), Ginger (root), Ginkgo Biloba Extract (leaf), Ipriflavone, Job's Tears (Yi Yi Ren, seed), Kelp, L-Arginine Hydrochloride, Ligusticum Wallchii (Chuan Xiong, root), Magnesium Amino Acid Chelate, Magnolia (Xin Yi Hua, flower), Melatonin, N-Acetylcysteine, Pyridoxine HCl, Vinpocetine, Vitamin A Acetate, Zinc Amino Acid Chelate.
See Editor's Note No. 1, page 2053.

Ripped Fuel - TwinLab
Ma Huang 20 mg • Guarana 200 mg • Chromium 200 mcg • L-Carnitine 100 mg.
See Editor's Note No. 21 and No. 30.

Ripped Fuel - MaHuang Free Formula - TwinLab
Each two capsules contain: Citrus Aurantium extract (standardized for 6% synephrine alkaloids) 325 mg • St. John's Wort extract (aerial parts, standardized for 0.3% hypericin) 300 mg • L-Phenylalanine 50 mg • Guarana seed extract (176 mg of caffeine) 800 mg. Other Ingredients: Thermogenic and Herbal Base Blend: Coleus Forskohlii (pashanabhedi) root extract, Green Tea extract, Citrus Bioflavonoids Complex, Ginger root, Cayenne, Yohimbe bark extract. Inactive Ingredients: Gelatin, Purified Water, MCT, Silica, Vegetable-based Stearic Acid, Magnesium Stearate.
See Editor's Note No. 40, page 2058.

Ripped Fuel (Metabolic Enhancer) - TwinLab
Two capsules contain: Ma Huang extract (standardized for 6% Ephedrine) 334 mg • Guarana extract (standardized for 22% Caffeine) 910 mg • L-Carnitine 100 mg • Chromium (Chromium Picolinate) 200 mcg.
See Editor's Note No. 30, page 2056.

Ripped Fuel Extreme - TwinLab
Two capsules contain: Calcium (from calcium carbonate) 118 mg • Chromium (from chromium polynicotinate) 200 mcg • Proprietary Herbal Extract 125 mg: Baical Skullcap root, Black Catechu bark (standardized for 60% free-b-ring flavonoids and 10% flavans) • Cocoa seed extract (standardized for 10% theobromine as well as caffeine, tyramine and phenylethylamine) 315 mg • Green Tea extract (standardized for 45% epigallocatechin gallate and 6% caffeine) 315 mg • Caffeine (from caffeine anhydrous, green tea leaf extract and cocoa seed extract) 220 mg • L-Carnitine (from L-carnitine L-tartrate) 13 mg • Cayenne fruit extract 50 mg. Other Ingredients: Rice Flour, Gelatin, Purified Water, MCT, Magnesium Stearate, Silica.

Ripping Gel - Urban Biologics
Lecithin • Water (aqua) • Octyl Palmitate • Aminophylline • Fragrance • Vitamin E • Propylene Glycol • BHA • Propyl Gallate • Citric Acid • DMDM Hydantoin • Iodopropynyl Butylcarbamate • Caramel Color.

RiSolubles - NutraCea (formerly NutraStar)
Each 360 g canister contains: Stabilized Rice Bran and Germ.

RM-10 - Garden of Life, Inc.
Two caplets contain: Proprietary Mushroom Blend 1455 mg: Cordyceps Sinensis, Ganoderma Lucidum (reishi), Grifola Frondosa (maitake), Agaricus Blazei, Lentinula Edodes (shiitake), Coriolus Versicolor, Hericium Erinaceus, Polyporus Umbellatus, Tremella Fuciformia, Poria Cocos • Uncaria Tomentosa 330 mg • Aloe Vera extract 15 mg. Other Ingredients: Cellulose, Stearates (vegetable source).

RNA 125 & DNA 125 - GNC
Each tablet contains: RNA (Ribonucleic Acid) 125 mg • DNA (Deoxyribonucleic Acid) 125 mg. Other Ingredients: Dicalcium Phosphate, Cellulose, Food Glaze.

RNA Cream - Life Extension
RNA, PABA, NaPCA, Elastin, Collagen, Safflower oil, Apricot kernal oil, Coconut oil, Vitamin A, Vitamin D, Aloe gel, Squalene, Methylparaben, Propylparaben.

RNA/DNA - Puritan's Pride
Each tablet contains: RNA (Ribonucleic Acid) 100 mg • DNA (Deoxyribonucleic Acid) 100 mg. In a base containing 400 mg of Dried Debittered Brewer's Yeast.

Robert's Complex - Enzymatic Therapy
Each capsule contains: Niacinamide 5 m. Other Ingredients: American Cranesbill (Geranium maculatum) 100 mg • Cabbage extract (Braccica oleracea) 100 mg • Marshmallow extract 4:1 (Althaea officinalis) mucilage content 30-40%) 75 mg • Okra (Hibiscus esculentis) 75 mg • Slippery Elm (Ulma fulva) 75 mg • Duodenal Substance 75 mg • Echinacea root extract (Echinacea angustifolia) standardized to contain greater than 3.5% Echinacosides & 0.65% essential oils 25 mg • Goldenseal root extract (Hydrastis canadensis) standardized to contain 5% total Alkaloids including: Berberine, Hydrastine, & Canadine 25 mg • Pancreatic Enzymes 25 mg.
See Editor's Note No. 14.

Robert's Formula - PhytoPharmica
Two capsules contain: Niacinamide 10 mg • American Cranesbill (Geranium maculatum) root 200 mg • Cabbage (Brassica oleracea) leaf extract 4:1 200 mg • Marshmallow (althaea officinalis) root extract 4.25:1 150 mg •Okra (Abelmoschus esculentis) whole plant 150 mg • Slippery Elm (Ulma fulva) bark 150 mg •Duodenal substance 50 mg •Echinacea (Echinacea angustifolia) root extract (standardized to contain greater than 4% echinacosides) 50 mg • Goldenseal (Hydrastis canadensis) root and rhizome extract 4:1 (standardized to contain 5% total alkaloids including berberine, hydrastine, and canadine) 50 mg • Pancreatic enzymes 50 mg.
See Editor's Note No. 14 and No. 21.

Some Brand Name Natural Products - What they Contain

www.NaturalDatabase.com contains MANY more listings than appear here.

Rockstar **-** Rockstar, Inc.
Each 16 oz can contains: Taurine 1892 mg • Guarana 400 mg • Inositol 50 mg • Carnitine 50 mg • Siberian Ginseng 50 mg • Milk Thistle 40 mg • Ginkgo 30 mg. Ingredients: Carbonated Water, High Fructose Corn Syrup, Dextrose, Citric Acid, Taurine, Natural & Artificial Flavors, Guarana Seed Extract, Ascorbic Acid, Caramel Color, Sodium Benzoate, Potassium Sorbate, Caffeine, L-Carnitine, Inositol, Milk Thistle Extract, Ginkgo Biloba Leaf Extract, Niacin, Calcium Pantothenate, Siberian Ginseng Root Extract, Riboflavin, Pyridoxine Hydrochloride, Cyanocobalamin.

Rogisen **-** Wagner Nutraceuticals
Each caplet contains: Vitamin A (100% as beta-carotene) 5000 IU • Vitamin C (as ascorbic acid) 250 mg • Vitamin E (as dl-alpha-tocopheryl acetate) 100 IU • Zinc (zinc citrate and as zinc oxide) 40 mg • Selenium (as selenium L-methionine complex) 200 mg • Copper (as cupric acid) 2 mg • Rogisen Proprietary Blend 307 mg: Red Wine Grape skin (37% total polyphenols), Orange Bioflavonoids (30%-40% total flavanones, flavonols, flavones), Ginkgo Biloba leaf standardized extract, European Bilberry standardized extract, L-Glutathione, Lutein / Zeaxanthin (active 5:1 ratio). Other Ingredients: Dicalcium Phosphate, Microcrystalline Cellulose, Croscarmellose Sodium, Stearic Acid, Silica, Magnesium Stearate, Film Coat Ingredients (hypromellose, hydroxypropyl cellulose, polyethylene glycol, propylene glycol, titanium dioxide, FD&C yellow #5 lake).

Rolaids - Extra Strength **-** Pfizer, Inc.
Each tablet contains: Calcium Carbonate (providing Calcium 271 mg) 675 mg • Magnesium Hydroxide (providing Magnesium 56 mg) 135 mg •Calcium Carbonate 675 mg •Magnesium Hydroxide 135 mg. Other Ingredients: Dextrose, Magnesium Stearate, Polyethylene Glycol, Pregelatinized Starch, Sucrose.

Roniot Super **-** Hadas Natural Products
Each lozenge contains: Propolis standardized extract 125 mg • Echinacea Purpurea standardized extract 125 mg • Vitamin C 12.5 mg.

Roplex **-** Medspan Laboratories
Each tablet contains: Proprietary Blend 600 mg: Scandenavian Flower Pollen, Saw Palmetto. Other Ingredients: Gelatin, Rice Flour, Dicalcium Phosphate, MCC, Stearic Acid, Crosscarmellose Sodium, Silica, Opedry 2 ns, Magnesium Stearate.

Rosemary **-** Nature's Way
Two capsules contain: Rosemary herb 800 mg. Other Ingredients: Gelatin, Magnesium Stearate.

RoseOx **-** Natrol
One capsule contains: Rosemary dried powdered extract leaf 250 mg. Other Ingredients: Rice powder, Magnesium Stearate, Gelatin.

Rotini - Revival **-** Physicians Laboratories
Two Ounces Contain: Certified Isoflavone 15 mg. Ingredients: Soy Protein Isolate, Niacin, Iron (Ferrous Sulfate), Thiamin Mononitrate, Riboflavin, Folic Acid.

Rovicid **-** Wagner Pharmaceuticals, Inc.
Each tablet contains: Prostate Functional Blend 300 mg: Nettle leaf, Saw Palmetto berry extract, Pygeum bark, Pumpkin seed extract, Swedish Flower Pollen extract, Lycopene • Colon Health Blend 425 mg: Alfalfa leaf, Licorice root, Senna leaf, Ginger root, Psyllium husk, Oat Bran, Fennel seed, Anise seed • Sexual Response Blend 410 mg: Panax Ginseng root extract, Horny Goat Weed extract, L-Arginine HCl, Tribulus Terrestris fruit and root, Maca powder, Catuaba bark extract. Other Ingredients: Dicalcium Phosphate, Microcrystalline Cellulose, Croscarmellose Sodium, Stearic Acid, Magnesium Stearate, Silica, Pharmaceutical Glaze.

Royal Bee Power **-** Nature's Plus
Two tablets contain: Bee Pollen 500 mg • Propolis from extract 500 mg Royal Jelly 50 mg. In a high energy natural base containing Gotu Kola, Ginseng & Fo-Ti.

Royal Brittany Evening Primrose Oil **-** American Health
Each softgel contains: Evening Primrose oil 500 mg: Cis-Linoleic Acid (LA) 350 mg, Gamma-Linolenic Acid (GLA) 350 mg. Other Ingredients: Gelatin, Glycerin.

Royal Jelly **-** DreamPharm
Each capsule contains: Royal Jelly (1.6% extract) 300 mg • Atractylodes Macrocephala 100 mg • Radix Dioscoreae Oppositae 100 mg.

Royaldophilus **-** Young Living Essential Oils
Each capsule contains: Plantain • Lemon Pectin • Magnesium Stearate • 250 Million Lactobacillus and Bifidus Cultures • Gelatin.

RTD 40 Advanced Mega Protein Shake **-** Nutripeak
Each can contains: Protein 40 g • Vitamin A (Retinyl Palmitate) 5000 IU • Vitamin C (Ascorbic Acid) 24 mg • Calcium Caseinate 24 mg • Iron (Ferrous Fumarate) 2.7 mg • Vitamin D (Cholecalciferol) 60 IU • Vitamin E (dl-Alpha Tocopheryl Acetate) 51 IU • Vitamin K (Phytonadione) 8 mcg • Thiamin Mononitrate 0.225 mg • Riboflavin 0.225 mg • Niacin (Niacinamide) 5 mg • Vitamin B6 (Pyridoxine Hydrochloride) 0.3 mg • Folic Acid 100 mcg • Vitamin B12 (Cyanocobalamin) 0.6 mcg • Biotin 45 mcg • Pantothenic Acid (Calcium D-Pantothenate) 1 mg • Phosphorus (Dipotassium Phosphorus and Potassium Triphosphate) 700 mg • Iodine (Potassium Iodide) 15 mcg • Magnesium Oxide 140 mg • Zinc Oxide 4.5 mg • Selenium (Sodium Selenate) 7 mcg • Copper (Cupric Sulfate) 0.2 mg • Manganese Sulfate 0.2 mg • Chromium Picolinate 12 mcg • Molybdenum (Sodium Molybdate) 15 mcg. Other Ingredients: Water; Metamyosyn V4 Protein Blend: Milk Protein Concentrate, Milk Protein Isolate, Calcium Sodium Casseinate, Hydrolyzed Wheat Protein (Gluten), Maltodextrin, High Fat Cocoa (processed with alkali); Sodium Phosphate; Sodium Citrate; Sodium Polyphosphate; Beta Carotene; Natural and Artificial Flavors; Microcrystalline Cellulose, Canola Oil, Soy Lecithin, Citric Acid, Sodium Carboxym-ethylcellulose, Salt, Carrageenan, Sucralose, Polysorbate 80, Dimethylpolysiloxane.

RU-21 **-** Spirit Sciences USA
Two tablets contain: Vitamin C 50 mg • Succinic Acid 200 mg • Fumaric Acid 75 mg • L-Glutamine 200 mg. Other Ingredients: Glucose (Dextrose).

Rubus-Ginger Tea **-** HerbaSway
Ginger • Green Tea • Blackberry • HerbaSwee (Cucurbitaceae fruit).

Rumalaya Cream **-** The Himalaya Drug Company (Himalaya Heal
Karpoora oil (cinnamomum camphora) • Putiha oil (mentah arvensis) • Sarala oil (pinus roxburghii) • Thwak oil (cinnamomum zeylanicum syn. c.verum) • Tila Taila oil (sesamum indicum). Base: q.s. ad.

Rumalaya DS Tablets **-** The Himalaya Drug Company (Himalaya Heal
Each tablet contains: Mahayograj Guggul 0.324 g • Shankh Bhasma (conch shell calx/ash) 130 mg • Shilajeet (mineral pitch, purified) 32 mg • Latakasthuri (abelmoschus moshatus) 20 mg • Swarnamakshik Bhasma (chalcopyrites calx) 10 mg • Maharasnadi Quath 130 mg • Manjishtha (rubia cordifolia) 38 mg • Shigru (moringa pterygosperma) 32 mg • Gokshura (tribulus terrestris) 32 mg.

Rumalaya Forte Tablets **-** The Himalaya Drug Company (Himalaya Heal)
Each tablet contains: Shallaki (boswellia serrata) 240 mg • Guggulu Suddha (commiphora wightii) 200 mg • Rasna (alpinia galanga) 70 mg • Yashti-Madhu (glycyrrhiza glabra) 70 mg • Gokshura (tribulus terrestris) 60 mg • Guduchi (tinospora cordifolia) 60 mg.

Rumalaya Gel **-** The Himalaya Drug Company (Himalaya Heal)
Nirgundi (vitex negundo) 7.5 mg • Devadaru (cedrus deodara) 7.5 mg • Sunthi (zingiber officinale) 7.5 mg • Shallaki (boswellia serrata) 7.5 mg • Pudina (mentha arvensis) 60 mg • Tvak (cinnamomum

zeylanicum) 30 mg • Sarala (pinus roxburghii) 55 mg • Gandhapura Taila (gaultheria fragrantissima) 55 mg • Base q.s. ad 770 mg.

Runners' Shield **-** Source Naturals
Two tablets contain: Vitamin A (Beta Carotene 12,500 IU and Palmitate 5,000 IU) 17,500 IU • Vitamin C (Magnesium Ascorbate, Ascorbic Acid and Manganese Ascorbate) 500 mg • Fat-Soluble Vitamin C (from 186 mg of Ascorbyl Palmitate) 80 mg • Vitamin E (Natural d-alpha) 200 IU • Magnesium (Ascorbate) 30 mg • Zinc (OptiZinc Monomethionine) 15 mg • Manganese (Ascorbate) 5 mg • Copper (Sebacate) 750 mcg • Selenium (Selenomethionine) 100 mcg • Quercetin 200 mg • N-Acetyl-Cysteine 100 mg • Silymarin (Milk Thistle Seed Extract) 50 mg • Ginkgo Biloba extract 24% (50:1) 5 mg • Hawthorn Berry extract (4:1) 150 mg • Rosemary 150 mg • Schizandra 125 mg • Marshmallow root 85 mg • Astragalus 60 mg.

Russian Bear 5000 Weight Gainer **-** Vitol
Three Stage Carbohydrate Mix- (glucose polymers) Containing Complex • Medium Chain and Simple Carbohydrates • Pharmaceutical Grade Protein Blend: Non-Fat Milk Solids, Hydrolyzed Egg White (albumin) • Medium Chain Triglycerides • Vitamin, Mineral, Lipotropic Mixture (which includes Kreb's Cycle complexes) • Yohimbe bark • Eleutherococcus • Crystaline Fructose • Sikadeer Antler powder • Schizandra Chinensis • Inosine HXR • Colostrum • Boron • Chromium Picolinate • Natural Vanilla Flavor.

Rutin 500 mg - GNC A-Z **-** GNC
Each tablet contains: Rutin 500 mg. Other Ingredients: Calcium Sulfate, Cellulose.

Rutozym **-** Wobenzym USA
Two tablets contain: Nattokinase (20,000 IU/gm) 25 mg • Bromelain (2450 GDU/gm) 90 mg • Papain N F (2400 USP units/mg) 100 mg • Rutin Bioflavonoid Copmlex 120 mg • White Willow Bark extract 100 mg. Other Ingredients: Plant Fiber, Povidone, Modified Cellulose Gum, Colloidal Silica, Titanium Dioxide Mineral, Vegetable Stearic Acid, pH Resistant Enteric Coating.

Rx for Life Cellular Essentials Pack (Bio-C) **-** Rexall - Sundown
Each tablet contains: Vitamin C (from ascorbyl palmitate, calcium ascorbate, magnesium ascorbate and ascorbic acid) 300 mg • Citrus Bioflavonoids 75 mg. Other Ingredients: Cellulose, Stearic Acid, Crospovidone, Croscarmellose Sodium, Silica, Magnesium Stearate.

Rx Fuel Bio-Designed Food Formula **-** TwinLab
Two servings contain: Branched Chain Amino Acids (L-Leucine, L-Isoleucine, & L-Valine) • L-Glutamine 1000 mg • L-Carnitine 100 mg • Chromium (from Chromic Fuel Chromium Picolinate) 200 mcg.

Rx-Bone Ostivone **-** Nutritional Dynamics
Two tablets contain: Vitamin D 100 IU • Calcium 1000 mg • Ostivone 200 mg. Other Ingredients: Dicalcium Phosphate, Microcrystalline Cellulose, Silica, Stearic Acid, Pharmaceutical glaze.

S-4 (Sleep Enabler) **-** Oasis Wellness Network
Each capsule contains: Calcium (citrate, carbonate, phosphate) 61 mg • Magnesium (citrate) 11 mg • Niacin (niacinamide ascorbate) 25 mg • Valerian root extract 133 mg • Jujube roasted seed extract 133 mg • MaxCell Proprietary Blend 7 mg: Zisyphus Jujube, Aloe Vera gel, Piper Nigrum, Glycyrrhiza Glabra • Chamomile flower extract 20 mg • Kava Kava root stock extract 7 mg • Melatonin 0.2 mg. Other Ingredients: Cellulose, Magnesium Stearate, Silica.

SAF for Kids **-** Natrol
Six capsules contain: Vitamin C (Ester-C brand) 60 mg • Calcium 100 mg • Vitamin B6 (pyridoxine HCl) 50 mg • Magnesium 50 mg • Additional Ingredients: GABA 800 mg • Glycine 800 mg • Passion flower extract 6:1 500 mg • L-Taurine 500 mg • Other Ingredients: Microcrystalline Cellulose, Magnesium Stearate, Gelatin. SAF Patent #1,540,075.

SAF The Stress Formula **-** Natrol
Four capsules contain: Vitamin C (Ester-C Brand) 100 mg • Thiamine (Vitamin B1) 3 mg • Riboflavin (Vitamin B2) 3.1 mg • Niacin (Niacinamide) 50 mg, • Vitamin B6 (Pyridoxine HCl) 4 mg • Magnesium 100 mg • GABA 650 mg • L-Tyrosine 650 mg • Siberian Ginseng 100 mg • Inositol 100 mg, Patent #4,973,467. Other Ingredients: Calcium Carbonate, Magnesium Stearate, Microcrystalline Cellulose, Gelatin.

Safeway Select Women's One Tablet Multivitamin **-** Safeway, Inc.
Each tablet contains: Vitamin A (50% as beta carotene) 5000 IU • Vitamin C 60 mg • Vitamin D 400 IU • Vitamin E 30 IU • Thiamin 1.5 mg • Riboflavin 1.7 mg • Niacin 20 mg • Vitamin B-6 2 mg • Folate 400 mcg • Vitamin B-12 6 mcg • Pantothenic Acid 10 mg • Calcium 450 mg • Iron 27 mg • Zinc 15 mg.

Sage **-** Motherlove Herbal Co.
Each 2 oz bottle contains: Sage. In a base of certified kosher alcohol and glycerin.

Sage Leaf 285 mg **-** Vitamin World
Each capsule contains: Sage leaf (salvia officinails) 570 mg. Other Ingredients: Gelatin.

Sage Oil **-** Now
100% Pure Sage Oil (Salvia officinalis) USP.

Sage Tincture **-** American Health
100% Organic Sage (Salvia officinalis) tincture. Other Ingredients: R/O Water, 12-24% Alcohol.

Salad-Tabs **-** Wakunaga of America
Two tablets contain: Vitamin A (as palmitate & beta-carotene) 5000 IU • Vitamin C (as asorbic acid) 60 mg • Vitamin D (as cholecalciferol) 400 IU • Vitamin E (as d-alpha-tocopherol acid succinate) 30 IU • Thiamine (vitamin B1) 1.5 mg • Riboflavin (vitamin B2) 1.7 mg • Niacin 20 mg • Vitamin B6 (as pyridoxine hydrochloride) 2 mg • Folate (as folic acid) 400 mcg • Vitamin B12 (as cyanocobalamin) 6 mcg • Biotin 300 mcg • Pantothenic Acid (as calcium pantothenate) 10 mg • Iron (as ferrous fumarate) 18 mg • Iodine (as potassium iodide) 150 mcg • Zinc (as zinc oxide) 15 mg • Copper (as copper gluconate) 2 mg • Manganese (as manganese sulfate) 2 mg • Young Barley and Wheat Grass powder 600 mg • Chlorella 180 mg. Other Ingredients: Cellulose, Silica, Magnesium Stearate (vegetable source).

Salmix Pastilles **-** Functional Products
Each pastille contains: Ammonium Chloride 8 g • Succus Liquorice 12 g. Other Ingredients: Wheat Flour, Saccarose, Medical Coal, Glucose Syrup, Anise Oil, Shellac.

Salmon Oil **-** Puritan's Pride
Two softgels contain: EPA 240 mg • DHA 160 mg.

Salmon Oil - GNC A-Z **-** GNC
Each capsule contains: EPA (Eicosapentaenoic Acid) 180 mg • DHA (Docosahexaenoic Acid) 120 mg. Other Ingredients: Gelatin, Glycerin.

Salmon Oil 1000 mg **-** Jamieson
Each capsule contains: EPA (Eicosapentaenoic Acid) 180 mg • DHA (Docosahexaenoic Acid) 120 mg.

Salmon Oil 500 mg (Inspired by Nature) **-** Puritan's Pride
Two softgels contain: Salmon Oil 1000 mg • Eicosapentaenoic Acid (EPA) 80 mg • Docosahexaenoic Acid (DHA) 120 mg. Other Ingredients: Gelatin, Glycerin.

Salonpas **-** Hisamitsu Pharmaceutical Co., Inc.
Active Ingredients: Methyl Salicylate 132 mg • l-Menthol 120 mg • dl-Camphor 26 mg • Tocopherol Acetate 21 mg.

SaluGuard Tonic for Men **-** Flora, Inc.
Each 20 mL serving contains: Proprietary aqueous extracts blend 662 mg: Bilberry fruit (vaccinium myrtillus) • Pumpkin seed (cucurbita

pepo) • Ginseng root (Panax ginseng) • Nettle herb (urtica dioica) • Saw Palmetto fruit (serenoa serrulata) • Hawthorn berry (crataegus oxyacantha) • Artichoke leaf (cynara scolymus) • Dandelion herb (taraxacum officinale) • Ginkgo leaf (gingko biloba) • Grape Seed extract. Other Ingredients: Pear juice concentrate, Guava pulp, Orange juice concentrate, Mango concentrate, Passion Fruit juice, and Locust seed gum.

***SaluGuard Tonic for Women* - Flora, Inc.**
Each 20 mL contains: Proprietary aqueous extracts blend 518.27 mg: Bilberry fruit (vaccinium myrtillis), Ginseng root (Panax ginseng), Horse Chestnut leaves (hippocastani folium), Green Oat (avena sativa), Hawthorn berry (crataegus oxyacantha), Artichoke leaf (cynara scolymus), Ginkgo leaf (ginkgo biloba), Dandelion herb (taraxacum officinale), Horsetail herb (equisetum pratense), Black Cohosh root (cimicfuga racemosa), Red Clover blossom (trifolium pratense), Grape Seed extract (vitis vinifera). Other Ingredients: Pear Juice Concentrate, Guava Pulp, Orange Juice Concentrate, Mango Concentrate, Passion Fruit Juice, Locust Seed Gum.

***Salusan Herbal Rest* - Flora, Inc.**
St. John's Wort • Passion Flower • Valerian "& other calming herbs."

***Sambu* - Flora, Inc.**
Elderberry.

***Sambucol Black Elder* - Jb Harris**
Each lozenge contains: Vitamin C (as ascorbic acid) 100 mg • Elderberry dried extract (berries) 130 mg. Other Ingredients: Sorbitol, Peppermint extract.

***Sambucol Black Elderberry Extract* - Nature's Way**
Two teaspoons contain: Elderberry extract 3.8 g. Other Ingredients: Glucose Syrup, Raspberry Extract, Honey, Citric Acid, Natural Flavor.

***Sambucol Black Elderberry Sugar Free Extract* - Nature's Way**
Two teaspoons contain: Sambucol patented Black Elderberry extract 3.8 g. Other Ingredients: Citric Acid, Raspberry Extract, Sorbitol, Water.

***Sambucol for Kids* - Nature's Way**
Each 2 tsp serving contains: Proprietary Blend 1.93 g: Echinacea Angustifolia root, Echinacea Purpurea (stem, leaf, flower), Propolis, Sambucol patented Black Elderberry extract. Other Ingredients: Citric Acid, Glucose Syrup, Raspberry extract.

***Sambucol Immune System* - Jb Harris**
Two teaspoons (10 mL) contain: Zinc 10 mg • Vitamin C 100 mg • Proprietary blend 4 g: Elderberry extract (berries), Propolis, Echinacea angustifolia (root), Echinacea purpurea (stems, leaves, flowers). Other Ingredients: Glucose syrup, raspberry extract (berries), honey, citric acid, & natural flavors.

***Sambucol Immune System Formula* - Nature's Way**
Two teaspoons contain: Proprietary Blend 4 g: Echinacea Angustifolia root, Echinacea Purpurea (stem, leaf, flower), Propolis, Sambucol patented Black Elderberry extract • Vitamin C 100 mg • Zinc Gluconate 10 mg. Other Ingredients: Citric Acid, Glucose Syrup, Honey, Raspberry Extract.

***Sambucol Immune System Formula Lozenges* - Nature's Way**
Each lozenge contains: Proprietary Blend: Echinacea Purpurea (stem, leaf, flower), Sambucol patented Black Elderberry extract, Vitamin C, Zinc Gluconate. Other Ingredients: Peppermint Extract, Sorbitol.

***Sambucol Lozenges* - Nature's Way**
Each lozenge contains: Sambucol patented Black Elderberry extract 130 mg • Vitamin C 100 mg. Other Ingredients: Peppermint Extract, Sorbitol.

***Sambucol Original* - Jb Harris**
Each lozenge contains: Black Elder Tree extract (sambucus nigra).

***Sambucol-D (Sugar Free)* - Jb Harris**
Each tablespoon contains: Elderberry juice (Black Elder tree, sambucus nigra 1). Other Ingredients: Liquid sorbitol, water, citric acid, natural flavor, & raspberry.

***SambuGuard* - Flora, Inc.**
Elder flowers (Sambucus nigra) • Elderberries (Sambucus nigra) • Echinacea (Echinacea purpurea plant concentrate 22:1) • Vitamin C (Ascorbic acid) • Acerola Cherry (Malpighia punicifola) fruit powder • Honey.

***SAMe* - Olympian Labs**
Each tablet contains: SAMe (S-adenosyl-L-methionine-tosylate-disulfate) 200 mg.

***SAMe* - Source Naturals**
Two tablets contain: SAMe (S-Adenosyl-L-Methionine) from 800 mg of SAMe Disulfate Tosylate 400 mg.

***SAMe* - Natrol**
Two tablets contain: S-Adenosyl-Methionine (SAMe) (as S-Adenosyl-Methionine Disulfate Ditosylate) 400 mg. Other Ingredients: Cellulose, Mannitol, Hydroxypropyl Methylcellulose Phthalate, Citric Acid, Sodium Starch Glycolate, Glyceryl Triacetate, Croscarmellose Sodium, Stearic Acid, Silica.

***SAM-e* - Quest**
Each caplet contains: S-adenosyl-methionine tosylate (providing 50 mg S-adenosyl-methionine) 100 mg. Other Ingredients: Croscarmellose Sodium, Microcrystalline Cellulose, Calcium Phosphate, Vegetable Stearin, Magnesium Stearate (vegetable source).

***SAM-e* - The Vitamin Shoppe**
Two tablets contain: S-Adenosyl-L-Methionine 400 mg. Other Ingredients: Colloidal Silica, Microcrystalline Cellulose, Sodium Starch Glycolate, Magnesium Stearate, Methacrylic Acid Copolymer, Polyethylene Glycol, Simethicone, Polysorbate 80, Sodium Hydroxide, Magnesium Silicate, Iron Oxide.

***SAM-e* - TwinLab**
Two tablets contain: SAMe (S-adenosylmethionine tosylate) 400 mg. Other Ingredients: Cellulose, Mannitol, Hydroxypropyl Methylcellulose, Citric Acid, Sodium Starch, Glycolate, Glyceryl Triacetate, Croscarmellose Sodium, Stearic Acid.

***Sam-e* - Vitamin World**
Two tablets contain: S-adenosylmethionine 400 mg. Other Ingredients: Cellulose (plant origin), Croscarmellose, Polymethacrylate, Silica, Vegetable Magnesium Stearate, Triethyl Citrate, Vegetable Stearic Acid, Citric Acid, Ascorbic Acid, Riboflavin.

***SAMe 100mg* - GNC**
Each tablet contains: S-Adenosyl-Methionine (SAMe) 100 mg. Other Ingredients: Microcrystalline Cellulose, Magnesium Stearate, Talc, Metacrylic Copolymer.

***Sam-e 200 mg (Inspired by Nature)* - Puritan's Pride**
Two tablets contain: S-Adenosylmethionine 400 mg. Other Ingredients: Cellulose (plant origin), Croscarmellose, Polymethacrylate, Silica, Vegetable Magnesium Stearate, Triethyl Citrate, Vegetable Stearic Acid, Citric Acid, Ascorbic Acid, Riboflavin.

***SAMe Extra Strength Super Size* - Olympian Labs**
Each tablet contains: SAMe (S-adenosyl-L-methionine-tosylate-disulfate) 400 mg.

***SAMe Supersize* - Olympian Labs**
Each tablet contains: SAMe (s-adenosyl-l-methionine-tosylate-disulfate) 200 mg.

***Sandal Turmeric (soap)* - Auromere Ayurvedic Soaps**
Coconut oil • Palmyra oil • Rice Bran oil • Alkali • Water • Hydnocarpus (Cactus) oil • Castor oil • Neem oil • Indian Beech oil • Mohwa (Madhuca Indica) oil • Sesame oil • Sandalwood oil • Neem Bark •

Dhub Grass (Cynodon Dactylon) • Indian Gooseberry (Amla) • Turmeric • Peepal (Bodhi Tree) • Licorice • Celastrus seed • Tulsi (Holy Basil) • Corallacarpus epigaeus • Nutgrass • Zedoary • Indian Madder Root • Costus • Mung Bean • Fenugreek.

Sandelios Beauty Caps **-** Health From The Sun
Each capsule contains: Wheat Germ oil 150 mg • Yeast 50 mg • Vitamin E (d-Alpha Tocopherol) 10 mg • Nicotinamide 10 mg • Vitamin B2 1 mg • Calcium D-Pantothenate 6.5 mg • Vitamin B1 1.2 mg • Vitamin B6 1 mg • Carotin 0.8 mg • D-Biotin 20 mcg • Vitamin B12 2 mcg.

Sandelios Garlic Caps **-** Health From The Sun
Each capsule contains: Garlic oil with Allicin 270 mg.

Sango Caps Coral Calcium **-** The Coral Connection
Two vegetable capsules contain: Coral Calcium Complex (75 trace minerals & elements) 1000 • Calcium (coral calcium/calcium carbonate) 250 mg • Magnesium (coral calcium/magnesium carbonate) 125 mg • Vitamin D (D3) 800 IU • Vitamin E 120 IU • Vitamin C (calcium ascorbate) 60 mg • Chromium (polynicotinate) 120 mcg • Zinc (monomethionine) 15 mg • Iodine (kelp) 15 mcg • Selenium 70 mcg • Copper 2 mg • Manganese 2 mg • Molybdenum 75 mcg • Rubidium (as amino acid chelate) 30 mcg • Vanadium (as amino acid chelate) 60 mcg • Boron (as amino acid chelate) 40 mcg • Silver (as silver nitrate) 10 mcg • Nickel (as amino acid chelate) 20 mcg • Betaine HCl 5 mg • Malic Acid 10 mg.

Sanhelios Circu Caps with Butcher's Broom **-** Health From The Sun
Each capsule contains: natural Rusci Aculeati (Butcher's Broom) extract 75 mg • Rosemary oil 2 mg.

Sanhelios Devil's Claw Caps **-** Health From The Sun
Each capsule contains: natural Devil's Claw extract 120 mg.

Sanhelios Garlic Forte **-** Health From The Sun
Each gelcap contains: Garlic oil, Maceration 2-3:1, 280 mg.

Sanhelios Kalm Caps **-** Health From The Sun
Each capsule contains: Valerian root extract 4:1 150 mg.

Sanhelios Onion Caps **-** Health From The Sun
Each capsule contains: natural etherial Onion oil from Allium Cepa Linne 1.5 mg.

Sanhelios Propolentum Capsules **-** Health From The Sun
Each capsule contains: Propolis 250 mg.

Sanhelios Propolentum Throat Lozenges **-** Health From The Sun
Each lozenge contains: Isomalt 1465 mg • Menthol Crystals 3 mg • Propolis powder 30 mg • Peppermint oil 2 mg.

Sanhelios Prosta Caps **-** Health From The Sun
Each capsule contains: Pumpkin seed oil with Cucurbitin 150 mg • Alpha-Tocopherolacetate equalling 40.8 IU • Vitamin E 30 mg.

Sanhelios Water Caps **-** Health From The Sun
Each capsule contains: natural Juniper berry oil 20 mg.

Satietrol **-** PacificHealth Laboratories, Inc.
Each packet (18 g) contains: Casein from Whey Protein Isolate (enriched with glycomacropeptides) • Potato Fiber • Sunflower Oil • Corn Syrup Solids • Natural & Artificial Flavors • Konjac Flour • Maltodextrin •Guar Gum • Calcium Lactate • Sodium Caseinate • Soy Lecithin •Alfalfa Powder •Monoglycerides • Diglycerides • Dipotassium Phosphate • Sodium Silicoaluminate • Aspartame.

Saventaro **-** Enzymatic Therapy/PhytoPharmica
Each capsule contains: POA Cat's Claw root extract (uncaria tomentosa, pentacyclic chemotype, standardized to contain a minimum of 1.3% pentacyclic oxindole alkaloids) 20 mg. Other Ingredients: Cellulose, Calcium Carbonate, Gelatin, Magnesium Stearate, Silicon Dioxide, Titanium Dioxide Color.

Saw Palmetto - Basic Nutrition **-** GNC
Two capsules contain: Saw Palmetto berry powder (Serenoa repens) 1000 mg. Other Ingredients: Gelatin, Cellulose.

Saw Palmetto **-** EcoNugenics
Each softgel contains: Saw Palmetto extract (85% fatty acids, esterols) 320 mg. Other Ingredients: Gelatin, Glycerin, Water.

Saw Palmetto **-** Gaia Herbs
Saw Palmetto standardized for 90% fatty acids. Standardized Full Spectrum 150 mg of extract per capsule. Guaranteed Potency 75 mg of extract per capsule.

Saw Palmetto **-** Leiner Health Products
Two softgels contain: Saw Palmetto extract (Serenoa repens) berry 160 mg. Other Ingredients: Soybean Oil, Gelatin, Glycerin, Caramel, Titanium Dioxide, Red 40, Blue 1.

Saw Palmetto **-** Metabolic Response Modifiers
Each capsule contains: Saw Palmetto oil (Serenoa repens, containing 85-95% saponins) 160 mg.

Saw Palmetto **-** Natrol
Each softgel contains: Saw Palmetto extract berries (serenoa repens) 160 mg. Other Ingredients: Olive Oil, Glycerin, Gelatin.

Saw Palmetto **-** NSI - Nutraceutical Sciences Institute
Each two softgels contain: Saw Palmetto berry extract 160 mg • Pumpkin seed oil 160 mg.

Saw Palmetto **-** Pharmanex
Each softgel contains: Saw Palmetto berries (10:1) extract (Serenoa repens) 160 mg. Other Ingredients: Olive Oil, Gelatin, Glycerin, Carob.

Saw Palmetto **-** PhysioLogics
Each softgel contains: Saw Palmetto extract (berry, serenoa repens, standardized to contain 85-95% fatty acids, biologically active sterols, 136-152 mg) 160 mg. Other Ingredients: Pure Olive Oil, Gelatin, Glycerin.

Saw Palmetto **-** Puritan's Pride
Each softgel contains: Saw Palmetto extract berry (serenoa repens) 320 mg. Other Ingredients: Gelatin, Glycerin.

Saw Palmetto **-** Smart Basics
Each softgel contains: Saw Palmetto extract berry (Serenoa Repens)160 mg. Other Ingredients: Olive Oil, Gelatin, Glycerin.

Saw Palmetto - Suma Virtue **-** Blessed Herbs
Saw Palmetto berry • Siberian Ginseng root • Jamaican Sarsaparilla root • Suma root • Astragalus root • Damiana • Grain alcohol & Distilled Water.

Saw Palmetto **-** Sundown
Two capsules contain: Saw Palmetto fruit 900 mg. Other Ingredients: Gelatin.

Saw Palmetto **-** Swanson
Each capsule contains: Saw Palmetto berries powder 540 mg.

Saw Palmetto 160 mg **-** Nature's Bounty
Two softgels contain: Saw Palmetto berry extract (serenoa repens, standardized to contain 85-95% fatty acids and biologically active sterols, 136-152 mg) 160 mg. Other Ingredients: Pure Olive Oil, Gelatin, Glycerin.

Saw Palmetto 320 mg Standardized Extract **-** Puritan's Pride
Each softgel contains: Saw Palmetto berry extract (serenoa repens, standardized to contain 85-95% fatty acids and sterols) 320 mg. Other Ingredients: Gelatin, Glycerin.

Saw Palmetto 450 mg Natural Whole Herb **-** Puritan's Pride
Each capsule contains: Saw Palmetto berry (serenoa repens) 450 mg. Other Ingredients: Gelatin.

Some Brand Name Natural Products - What they Contain

www.NaturalDatabase.com contains MANY more listings than appear here.

Saw Palmetto Complex **-** Enzymatic Therapy
Each capsule contains: Saw Palmetto Berry extract standardized to contain 85% to 95% fatty acids & sterols 80 mg • Pumpkin seed oil extract (Cucurbita pepo) 40 mg • Pygeum africanum extract standardized to contain 13% total sterols 10 mg • Bearberry extract (Uva Ursi) standardized to contain 10% Arbutin 5 mg.

Saw Palmetto Complex **-** Jamieson
Each capsule contains: Saw Palmetto Berry 200 mg • Pygeum Bark 7500 mg • Cranberry Fruit 250 mg • Pumpkin Seed Oil 100 mg.

Saw Palmetto Complex **-** Leiner Health Products
Each softgel contains: Zinc Gluconate 7.5 mg • Pumpkin Seed oil extract (Cucurbita pepeo) 40 mg • Saw Palmetto berry extract (serenoa repens) 160 mg. Inactive Ingredients: Gelatin, Glycerin, Vegetable Oil, Beeswax, Lecithin, Titanium Dioxide, Red 40, Yellow 6, Blue 1, Yellow 5.

Saw Palmetto Complex **-** PhytoPharmica
Two softgels contain: Pumpkin seed 2.5:1 extract (cucurbita pepeo) 80 mg • Pygeum bark extract (prunus africana, standardized to contain 12% total sterols calculated as beta sitosterol) 20 mg • Saw Palmetto berry extract (serenoa repens, standardized to contain 85-95% fatty acids, 0.2-0.4% total sterols, and 0.1-0.3% beta sitosterol) 160 mg • Uva-Ursi leaf extract (arctostaphylos uva-ursi, standardized to contain 10% arbutin) 10 mg.

Saw Palmetto Complex **-** Shaklee
Each capsule contains: Saw Palmetto extract (Serenoa repens berry, standardized to contain 85%-95% fatty acids and sterols) 160 mg • Beta Sitosterol (from soybean phytosterols) 15 mg. Other Ingredients: Pumpkin Seed Oil, Soybean Oil, Beeswax, Soy Lecithin, Ascorbyl Palmitate, Mixed Tocopherol Concentrate, Rosemary Extract, Gelatin, Glycerin, Water, Annatto, Caramel, Titanium Dioxide, Turmeric.

Saw Palmetto Complex with Lycopene **-** NutriCology
Two softgels contain: Zinc (as zinc citrate) 10 mg • Pumpkin seed oil 1.5 g • Saw Palmetto berry extract (serenoa repens standardized to 85-95% fatty acids) 320 mg • Beta-Sitosterol 120 mg • Lycopene 15 mg. Other Ingredients: Silicon Dioxide.

Saw Palmetto Extract **-** Jamieson
Each capsule contains: Pumpkin seed oil (Curcubita pepo) 100 mg • Saw Palmetto berry 4:1 extract (Serenoa repens) 50 mg • Pygeum bark 150:1 extract (Pygeum africanum) 50 mg • Cranberry fruit 25:1 extract (Viccinum macrocarpon) 10 mg.

Saw Palmetto Formula **-** Quest
Each caplet contains: Saw Palmetto berry powder (Serenoa serrulate/repens) 110 mg • Corn Silk powder (Zea mays) 110 mg • Pumpkin Seed powder 90 mg • Parsley leaf powder (Petroselinum crispu) 55 mg • Buchu leaf powder (Barosma betulina) 35 mg • Cayenne powder (Capsicum) 35 mg • Kelp powder (Fucus vesiculosis) 35 mg. Other Ingredients: Calcium Phosphate, Microcrystalline Cellulose, Vegetable Stearin, Croscarmellose Sodium, Magnesium Stearate (vegetable source).

Saw Palmetto Male Toner **-** Traditional Medicinals
Hibiscus flower • Saw Palmetto berry • Nettle root • Uva Ursi leaf • Ginger rhizome • Saw Palmetto berry dry extract • Althea root • Rose Hip • natural Lemon flavor • Stevia leaf.

Saw Palmetto Plus **-** Atrium Inc.
Each capsule contains: Saw Palmetto oil (50:1 extract) 160 mg •Olive oil 90 mg.

Saw Palmetto Plus **-** Nature's Bounty
Each softgel contains: Saw Palmetto Complex Blend 95 mg: Saw Palmetto berry extract (serenoa repens, standardized to contain 85-95% free fatty acids and sterols) 80 mg, Pygeum Africanum bark extract (standardized to contain 12% sterols) 10 mg, Bearberry leaf extract (arctostaphylos uva-ursi, standardized to contain 10% arbutin) 5 mg • Pumpkin Seed Oil extract (curcubita pepo) 40 mg. Other Ingredients: Soybean Oil, Gelatin, Glycerin, Lecithin, Silica, Caramel Color, Titanium Dioxide Color.

Saw Palmetto Prostate Health **-** DreamPharm
Each capsule contains: Saw Palmetto fruit 400 mg • Vaccaria Segetalis seeds 50 mg • Dianthus Superbus herb 50 mg • Pumpkin seeds 50 mg • Licorice 50 mg.

Saw Palmetto Standard **-** Sundown
Two softgels contain: Saw Palmetto fruit extract (standardized to 85%-95% fatty acids, 272 mg) 320 mg. Other Ingredients: Gelatin, Glycerin, Water, Titanium Dioxide, Yellow 6 Lake, Red 40 Lake, Blue 2 Lake.

Saw Palmetto Standardized Extract With Pumpkin Seed Oil and Zinc **-** Now
Each softgel contains: Zinc (as zinc gluconate) 30 mg • Saw Palmetto berry extract (serenoa repens, fruit) 160 mg • Pumpkin Seed Oil 1 g. Other Ingredients: Gelatin, Glycerine, Carob, Beeswax, Water.

Saw Palmetto with Lycopene **-** Health Smart Vitamins
Each soft gel contains: Saw Palmetto berry 85-95% fatty acids, 272 mg-304 mg 320 mg • Lycopene (from tomato) 5 mg.

Saw Palmetto XTRA **-** Sundown
Two softgels contain: Vitamin E (as dl-alpha-tocopheryl acetate) 25 IU • Zinc (as zinc oxide) 7.5 mg • Saw Palmetto fruit extract (standardized to 85%-95% fatty acids, 272 mg) 320 mg • XTRA Premium Blend 59 mg: Vitamin E, Nettle root extract (10:1), Beta-Sitosterol, Zinc Oxide. Other Ingredients: Soybean oil, Soy Lecithin, Glycerin, Water, Titanium Dioxide (color), Yellow 6 Lake, Red 40 Lake, Blue 2 Lake.

Say Yes to Beans **-** Nature's Plus
Each Vegicap contains: Legumase (Saccharamyces cerevisae & Aspergillus enzyme complex) 125 mg • Licorice root (Glycyrrhiza glabra) standardized < 2% Glycyrrhizinic acid 75 mg • Ginger root (Zingiber officinale) standardized 5% gingerols 25 mg • Parsley seed (Petroselinum crispum) 20 mg.

SB Normal Stool Formula - Shaman Botanicals **-** P.S. Pharmaceuticals
Each tablet contains: Croton lechleri extract (sap) (standardized to contain 250 mg of SP-303). Other Ingredients: Microcrystalline Cellulose, Coating [Methacrylic Acid Copolymer, Magnesium Silicate, Triethyl Citrate], Glyceryl Monostearate, Sodium Starch Glycolate, Silicon Dioxide.

SBR-Lipocream **-** Ferndale Labs
30 grams contains: White Petrolatum • Purified Water • Mineral Oil • Cetostearyl Alcohol • Ceteth-20 • Methyl Paraben • Citric Acid • Sodium Citrate.

ScalpBlock **-** Biotech Corp.
Octyl Methoxycinnamate • Octocylene • Oxybenzone • Octyl Dodecanol • Butyloctyl Salicylate • Cyclomethicone • C12-15 Alkyl Lactate • PVP/Hexadecene Copolymer • Tocopherol Acetate • Fragrance.

Schisandra **-** Pharmanex
Each capsule contains: Schisandra berry extract (Schisandra chinensis) (10:1) 200 mg. Other Ingredients: Rice Flour, Gelatin, Magnesium Stearate, Silicon Dioxide.

Schoomz **-** Unknown
Unknown.
See Editor's Note No. 49, page 2059.

Sea & Earth **-** The Vitamin Shoppe
Sea-life protein • Vitamin C • Zinc • Silica • Green Tea extract • Red Wine extract • Red Cabbage extract • Grape Juice extract • Pine Bark extract • Citrus Bioflavonoids • Carotene.

Some Brand Name Natural Products - What they Contain

www.NaturalDatabase.com contains MANY more listings than appear here.

BRAND NAMES

Sea Cal Oyster Shell Calcium **-** Nature's Life
Two tablets contain: Calcium (Oyster Shell) 500 mg • Vitamin D (as Vitamin D3) (Cholecaciferol) 250 IU.

Sea Cucumber **-** Futurebiotics
Sea Cucumber 500 mg.

Sea Mussel **-** Futurebiotics
New Zealand Greenshell Mussel 500 mg.

Seacure **-** Proper Nutrition - PNI
Six capsules contain: Vitamin A 157 IU • Calcium 57 mg • Phosphorus 63 mg • Omega-3 32 mg. Ingredients: White Fish, Rosemary extract.

SeaHealth Plus **-** Zone Labs
Aloe Vera • Bladderwrack • Green Sea Lettuce • Irish Moss • Knotted Wrack • Popping Wrack • Purple Laver • Ribbon Kelp • Rockwrack • Sugar Wrack • Purified Water • Grape Seed extract • Wild Blueberry extract • Grape powder • Raspberry extract • Raspberry seed extract • Cranberry powder • Prune powder • Tart Cherry powder • Wild Bilberry extract • Strawberry powder • Dark Sweet Cherry • Honey • Citric Acid • Sodium Benzoate • Potassium Sorbate.

SeaSilver **-** SeaSilver, USA, Inc.
Each 32 ounce bottle contains: Matrix Aloe Vera leaf inner gel (barbadensis miller) • Sealogica Proprietary Blend: Ascophyllum Nodosum, Fucus Vesiculosus, Kelp, Fucus, Chondrus Crispus, Nori, Ulva Latuca • Pau d'Arco inner bark (tabebuia avellanedae) • Juice Concentrate Blend: White Grape, Cranberry, Concord Grape, Black Cherry.
See Editor's Note No. 34, page 2057.

Seasonal Relief **-** Garden of Life, Inc.
Three caplets contain: Wild Oregano concentrate (6% volatile oils) 900 mg • Poten-Zyme Ginger juice extract (20:1) 180 mg • Olive leaf extract (20% oleuropin) 300 mg • Poten-Zyme Horseradish juice extract (20:1) 180 mg • Poten-Zyme Onion juice extract (20:1) 168 mg • Poten-Zyme Peppermint extract 168 mg • Poten-Zyme Yarrow extract 168 mg • Poten-Zyme Elder Flower extract 168 mg • Echinacea Angustifolia extract (24% echinacosides) 99 mg • Elderberry fruit extract (30% anthocyanins) 99 mg • Goldenseal extract (5% hydrastine) 99 mg • Poten-Zyme Garlic juice extract (20:1) 168 mg • Bayberry bark extract (70% myricetin) 24 mg • Lonicera Japonicum extract (40% polyphenols) 18 mg • Poten-Zyme Probiotic Blend 2.4 billion CFU. Other Ingredients: Cellulose, Acacia, Stearates (vegetable source).

SeaVive **-** Proper Nutrition - PNI
Each capsule contains: Vitamin C (L-ascorbic acid) 50 mg • Omega-3 2.1 mg • White Fish (Seacure) 200 mg • Colostrum (casein- & lactose-free, bovine) 200 mg • Beta-1,3-D Glucan 50 mg. Other Ingredients: Gelatin.

Seaweed Virtue **-** Blessed Herbs
Kelp • Bladderwrack • Dulse & "Other Seaweeds as Available" • Grain alcohol & Distilled Water.

Secretagogue-One **-** MHP
Each packet contains: Anterior Pituitary Substance 25 mg • Glycoamino Acid-Glucose Complex 4200 mg • Novel polyose complex 2230 mg • Amino Acid Blend 500 mg • Broad Bean 10 mg. See Editor's Note No. 14.

Sedivitax **-** Aboca USA, Inc
Two capsules contain: Passiflo 2-LMF Passionflower leaf multifraction freeze-dried extract (passiflora incarnata, standardized to 8% total flavonoids) 256 mg • Valerian root Whole Phytocomplex Concentrate (WPC) (valeriana officinalis, standardized to 0.25% total valerenic acids) 192 mg • Lemon Balm leaf WPC (melissa officinalis, standardized to 6.5% rosmarinic acid) 96 mg • California Poppy leaf/flower WPC (eschscholzia californica, standardized to 0.045% protopine) 89.6 mg. Other Ingredients: Gelatin (capsule), Essential Oils Of Lavender, Marjoram.

Sedivitax Drops **-** Aboca USA, Inc
Twenty-five drops contain: Passionflo 2-LMF Passionflower leaf multifraction freeze-dried extract (passiflora incarnata, standardized to 8% total flavonoids) 33.3 mg • Passionflower leaf extract (1:10 in organic grain alcohol 70% by volume, total flavonoids minimum 0.16%) 210.2 mg • Valerian root extract (1:10 in organic grain alcohol 70% by volume, total valerenic acids minimum 0.011%) 210.2 mg • Lemon Balm leaf extract (1:10 in organic grain alcohol 70% by volume, rosmarinic acid minimum 0.28%) 140.1 mg • California Poppy aerial part extract (1:10 in organic grain alcohol 70% by volume, protopine minimum 0.0028% 140.1 mg. Other Ingredients: Essential Oil Of Lavender, Marjoram.

SEE **-** Quantum, Inc.
Each three tablets contain: Bilberry extract 10 mg • Omega-3 Flax Meal (partially defatted) 500 mg • Beta-Carotene (Pro Vitamin A) 25000 IU • Vitamin A (Palmitate) 5000 IU • Vitamin C (Ascorbic Acid) 1000 mg • Natural Vitamin E (D-Alpha Succinate) 200 IU • Citrus Bioflavonoid 250 mg • Vitamin B2 (Riboflavin) 40 mg • Rutin NF (Bioflavonoid) 100 mg • Selenium (Selenomethionine) 100 mcg • Pantothenic Acid (d-Calcium Pantothenate) 40 mg • Chromium (GTF) 200 mcg • Zinc (Citrate) 25 mg • Lutein 5 mg.

Select Herbals Natural Whole Herb Echinacea 400 mg **-** Vitamin World
Each capsule contains: Echinacea (echinacea purpurea, aerial) 400 mg. Other Ingredients: Gelatin.

Select Herbals Natural Whole Herb Saw Palmetto 450 mg **-** Vitamin World
Each capsule contains: Saw Palmetto berry (serenoa repens) 450 mg. Other Ingredients: Gelatin.

Select Herbals Natural Whole Herb Valerian Root 450 mg **-** Vitamin World
Each capsule contains: Valerian root (valeriana officinalis) 450 mg. Other Ingredients: Gelatin.

Selene-E **-** Schiff
Two softgels contain: Vitamin E (as d-alpha tocopherol and non-alpha tocopherols) 200 IU • Selenium (from selenium enriched yeast) 100 mcg • Lecithin 640 mg • Saccharomyces Cerevisiae (yeast, primary) 346 mg. Other Ingredients: Soybean Oil, Softgel (gelatin, glycerin, water), Yellow Beeswax.

Selenium **-** Source Naturals
Each tablet contains: Selenium (yeast free, from 40 mg of L-Selonomethionine) 200 mcg.

Selenium **-** Schiff
Each tablet contains: Selenium (as high selenium yeast) 200 mcg. Other Ingredients: Calcium Carbonate, Cellulose, Coating (dextrin, dextrose, soy lecithin, sodium carboxymethylcellulose, sodium citrate), Croscarmellose Sodium, Magnesium Stearate.

Selenium 100 - GNC A-Z **-** GNC
Each tablet contains: Selenium (as selenium yeast) 100 mcg. Other Ingredients: Cellulose, Dicalcium Phosphate.

Selenium 100 mcg **-** Jamieson
Each tablet contains: Selenium (from Brewer's Yeast) 100 mcg.

Selenium 200 **-** Leiner Health Products
Each tablet contains: Selenium (High Selenium yeast) 200 mcg. Other Ingredients: Calcium Carbonate, Maltodectrin, Cellulose, Croscarmellose Sodium, Tricalcium Phosphate, Crospovidone, Polyethylene Glycol 3350, Silicon Dioxide, Magnesium Stearate, Hydroxypropyl Methylcellulose, Hydroxypropyl Cellulose, Polysorbate 80.

Selenium 200 - GNC A-Z **-** GNC
Each tablet contains: Selenium (as selenomax selenium yeast) 200 mcg. Other Ingredients: Dicalcium Phosphate, Cellulose.

Some Brand Name Natural Products - What they Contain

www.NaturalDatabase.com contains MANY more listings than appear here.

Selenium 200 mcg **-** Nature Made
Each tablet contains: Selenium (from selenium yeast) 200 mcg. Other Ingredients: Dibasic Calcium Phosphate, Cellulose, Stearic Acid, Silicon Dioxide, Hydroxypropyl Methylcelllulose, Magnesium Stearate, Polyethylene Glycol, Carnauba Wax.
See Editor's Note No. 45, page 2058.

Selenium 50 - GNC A-Z **-** GNC
Each tablet contains: Selenium (as selenium yeast) 50 mcg. Other Ingredients: Cellulose, Dicalcium Phosphate.

Selenium 50 mcg **-** Jamieson
Each tablet contains: Selenium (from Brewer's Yeast) 50 mcg.

Selenium 50 mcg - Yeast Free **-** Jamieson
Each caplet contains: Selenium (Proteinate) 50 mcg • Beta-Carotene (Provitamin A) 5000 IU • Vitamin C (Ascorbic Acid) 60 mg • Vitamin E (Natural D-Alpha Tocopheryl Acetate) 10 IU.

Selenium Detoxification Formula - Smokers & Drinkers **-** Life Extension
Each 500 mcg tablet contains: Sodium Selenate 100 mcg • Selenomethionine (yeast free) 50 mcg • Seleno Di- Glutathione 50 mcg • Cysteine 100 mcg • Thiamide 100 mg • Nicotinic Acid 100 mg.

Selenium Solution **-** NutriCology
Each 1/2 tsp (2.5 mL) serving contains: Selenium (as sodium selenite) 100 mcg. Other Ingredients: Distilled Water.

Selenium Tablets **-** Leiner Health Products
Each tablet contains: Selenium Yeast 50 mcg. Other Ingredients: Brewer's Yeast, Dicalcium Phosphate, Cellulose, Stearic Acid, Croscarmellose Sodium, Silicon Dioxide.

Selenomax **-** Source Naturals
Each tablet contains: Selenium (from 100 selenomax high selenium yeast) 100 mcg.

Selenomax brand **-** Nutrition 21
Selenium.
See Editor's Note No. 44, page 2058.

Selenomax Selenium 200 Mcg **-** Nature's Life
Each tablet contains: Selenium (natural food yeast-based) (Nutrition 21 Selenomax) 200 mcg.

Selestro **-** Metagenics
Each tablet contains: Soybean concentrate 100 mg • Total Isoflavones (containing all forms of genistin, daidzin, glycitin) 40 mg • Black Cohosh root/rhizome extract (actaea racemosa, standardized to 2.5% [2 mg] triterpene glycosides as 27-deoxyactein) 80 mg.

Senescegarl **-** Olympian Labs
Three capsules contain: Ginkgo Biloba leaf extract 120 mg • Garlic extract 600 mg • Coenzyme Q10 60 mg • Ascorbic Acid 300 mg • Grape Seed extract 90 mg • Vitamin B-6 (pyridoxine HCl) 30 mg • Zinc (gluconate) 15 mg • Copper (cupric oxide) 1800 mcg • Manganese (manganese sulfate) 1800 mcg.

Senior Moment **-** Nutramax Laboratories, Inc.
Each capsule contains: Cerebral Phospholipids 50 mg: Phosphatidylserine, Phosphatidylethanolamine, and Phosphatidylinositol • Docosahexaenoic acid 40mg. Other Ingredients: Sunflower Oil, Gelatin, Water, Ascorbyl Palmitate, Tocopherols, Titanium dioxide color, FD&C Red #3, Sodium Lauryl sulfate, FD&C Yellow #5, FD&C Blue #1.

Senior-Vites Plus **-** The Vitamin Shoppe
Three tablets contain: Vitamin A Activity 20000 IU • Vitamin D 400 IU • Vitamin C 150 mg • Vitamin E 200 IU • Vitamin B1 35 mg • Vitamin B2 35 mg • Niacinamide 50 mg • Vitamin B6 35 mg • Vitamin B12 50 mcg • Pantothenic Acid 75 mg • Folic Acid 400 mcg • Biotin 300 mcg • PABA 35 mg • Inositol 100 mg • Choline 100 mg • Citrus Bioflavonoids 25 mg • Rutin 25 mg • Glutamine 100 mg • Taurine 100 mg • Glutamic Acid 50 mg • Pancreatin 25 mg • Ox Bile 10 mg • Calcium 100 mg • Magnesium 50 mg • Iron 18 mg • Zinc 15 mg • Manganese 6 mg • Potassium 45 mg • Iodine 225 mcg • Selenium 50 mcg • Chromium 25 mcg • Fo-Ti 50 mg • Gotu Kola 50 mg • Avena Sativa 25 mg • Siberian Ginseng 25 mg • Nettles extract 10 mg.
See Editor's Note No. 14.

Senna Leaves **-** Now
Each capsule contains: Senna leaves (Cassia Angustifolia) 470 mg. Other Ingredients: Gelatin (capsule), Magnesium Stearate.

Sentinel Multi Vitamin **-** Health Center for Better Living
Each tablet contains: Vitamin A (as retinyl acetate and beta-carotene) 5000 IU• Vitamin C (as ascorbic acid) 60 mg • Vitamin D (as cholecalciferol) 400 IU • Vitamin E (as dl-alpha-tocopheryl acetate) 30 IU • Vitamin K (as phytonadione) 25 mcg • Thiamin (as thiamin mononitrate) 1.5 mg • Riboflavin 1.7 mg • Niacin (as niacinamide) 20 mg • Vitamin B6 (as pyridoxine HCl) 2 mg • Folate (as folic acid) 400 mcg • Vitamin B12 (as cyancobalamin) 6 mcg • Biotin 30 mcg • Pantothenic acid (as D-calcium pantothenate) 10 mg • Calcium (as dicalcium phosphate) 162 mg • Iron (as ferrous fumarate) 18 mg • Phosphorus (as dicalcium phosphate) 125 mg • Iodine (as potassium iodide) 150 mcg • Magnesium (as magnesium oxide) 100 mg • Zinc (as zinc oxide) 15 mg • Selenium (as sodium selenate) 25 mcg • Copper (as cupric oxide) 2 mg • Manganese (as manganese sulfate) 2.5 mcg • Chromium (as chromium chloride)• Molybdenum (as sodium moybdate) 25 mcg • Chloride (as potassium choride) 36.3 mg Potassium (as potassium choride) 40 mg • Vanadium (as sodium metavandate) 10 mcg • Tin (as stannous chloride) 10 mcg • Silicon (as sodium metasilicate) 10 mcg • Nickel (as nickelous sulfate) 5 mcg.

Septilin DS **-** The Himalaya Drug Company (Himalaya Heal
Each tablet contains: Guggulu (balsamodendron mukul syn. commiphora wightii, purified) 0.324 g • Shankh Bhasma (conch shell calx/ash) 64 mg • Maharasnadi Quath 130 mg • Guduchi (tinospora cordifolia) 98 mg • Manjishtha (rubia cordifolia) 64 mg • Amalaki (emblica officinalis) 32 mg • Shigru (moringa pterygosperma) 32 mg • Yashti-Madhu (glycyrrhiza glabra) 12 mg.

Septilin Syrup **-** The Himalaya Drug Company (Himalaya Heal
Each 1 tsp (5 mL) serving contains: Guggulu (balsamodendron mukul syn. commiphora wightii, purified) 80 mg • Maharasnadi Quath 30 mg • Manjishtha (rubia cordifolia) 15 mg • Guduchi (tinospora cordifolia) 14 mg • Trikatu 13 mg: Piper Nigrum, Piper Longum, Zingiber Officinale • Kushtah (saussurea lappa) 13 mg • Amalaki (emblica officinalis) 8 mg • Yashti-Madhu (glycyrrhiza glabra) 6 mg.

Seredrin **-** Health Perception
Each tablet contains: Ginkgo Biloba extract with Phytosome 120 mg (standardized to 9.6 mg ginkgo flavoneglycosides, 2.4 mg terpene lactones). Other Ingredients: Microcrystalline Cellulose, Croscarmellose, Magnesium Stearate, Hydroxypropylmethyl Cellulose.

SerenAid **-** Klaire Laboratories
Each capsule contains: Multi-Enzyme Complex (proprietary blend) 317 mg: L-Lysine, Peptidase FP, Papain (sulfite free), Protease, Acid-stable Protease, Lactase.

Serenity **-** Urban Nutrition Inc
Each capsule contains: Lithium Orotate 120 mg (provides elemental lithium 4.6 mg). Other Ingredients: Micro Vortex Enteric Coating.

Serenity with Kava Kava **-** Gaia Herbs
Each capsule contains: Skullcap herb extract (Scutellaria lateriflora) 60 mg • Passionflower vine extract (Passiflora incarnata) 60 mg • Kava Kava rhizome extract (Piper methylsticum) 60 mg • Chamomile flowers extract (Matrica recutita) 45 mg • Wild Oat milky seed extract (Avena sativa) 27 mg • Hops Strobile extract (Humulus lupulus) 24 mg • Mugwort herb extract (Artemesia vulgaris) 15 mg • Peppermint

leaf extract (Mentha piperita) 9 mg. Other Ingredients: Vegetable Glycerin, Vegetable Gelatin (capsule).

Serenoa Repens **-** Progressive Labs
Each softgel contains: Saw Palmetto purified extract (95% free fatty acids) 160 mg • Olive oil 160 mg.

SerenPure brand **-** Soft Gel Technologies, Inc.
Saw Palmetto.
See Editor's Note No. 44, page 2058.

Serious Mass **-** Optimum Nutrition
Two heaping scoops (334 g) contain: Creatine Monohydrate 1 g • L-Glutamine 500 mg • Glutamine Peptides 500 mg • Choline (as choline bitartrate) 250 mg • Inositol 250 mg • PABA (para-aminobenzoic acid) 5 mg • Maltodextrin • Protein Blend: Whey Protein Concentrate, Calcium Caseinate, Egg Albumen, Sweet Dairy Whey • Cocoa • Natural and Artificial Flavor • Vitamin and Mineral Blend: DiPotassium Phosphate, Magnesium Aspartate, DiCalcium Phosphate, Calcium Citrate, Ascorbic Acid, Niacinamide, Zinc Citrate, Beta Carotene, D-Calcium Pantothenate, D-Alpha Tocopheryl Succinate, Selenomethionine, Copper Gluconate, Ferrous Fumarate, Pyridoxine Hydrochloride, Riboflavin, Chromium Polynicotinate, Folic Acid, Biotin, Molybdenum Amino Acid Chelate, Cholecalciferol, Potassium Iodide, Cyanocobalamin • Acesulfame Potassium • Medium Chain Triglycerides.

SeroCalm **-** Directly Young, LLC
Two caplets contain: Calcium (as calcium carbonate) 200 mg • Magnesium (as magnesium oxide) 100 mg • Proprietary Blend 740 mg: L-Tyrosine, Wild Jujube seed extract, Griffonia Simplicifolia seed extract (provides 5-HTP 50 mg), Stinging Nettle leaf extract (provides serotonin 50 mcg). Other Ingredients: Microcrystalline Cellulose, Croscarmellose Sodium, Stearic Acid, Hypromellose, Magnesium Stearate, Silica, Hydroxypropyl Cellulose, Colorants.

SeroSlim **-** Directly Young, LLC
Two caplets contain: Thiamin (as thiamin hydrochloride) 1.5 mg • Riboflavin 1.7 mg • Niacin (as niacinamide) 20 mg • Vitamin B6 (as pyridoxine hydrochloride) 2 mg • Folate (as folic acid) 400 mcg • Vitamin B12 (as cyanocobalamin) 25 mcg • Biotin 300 mcg • Pantothenic Acid (as d-calcium pantothenate) 10 mg • Calcium (as dicalcium phosphate) 20 mg • Chromium (as chromium dinicotinate glycinate) 200 mcg • Proprietary Standardized Extract Blend 800 mg: Green Tea leaf (provides epigallocatechin gallate 90 mg, caffeine 50 mg), Cocoa bean (provides methylxanthines 50 mg), Griffonia Simplicifolia seed (provides 5-HTP 50 mg), Stinging Nettle leaf (provides serotonin 50 mcg). Other Ingredients: Microcrystalline Cellulose, Croscarmellose Sodium, Stearic Acid, Hypromellose, Magnesium Stearate, Silica, Hydroxypropyl Cellulose, Colorants.

Serpina **-** The Himalaya Drug Company (Himalaya Heal
Each tablet contains: Sarpagandha (rauwolfia serpentina) 4 mg.

Serrapeptase (Serraflazyme) **-** Olympia Nutrition
Silk worm enzyme.

Serum C **-** Nutraceutics Corp.
Active Ingredients: L-Ascorbic Acid • Maxogenol (botanical proanthoxidant complex). Inactive Ingredients: Ethoxydiglycol, Butylene Glycol, L-Tyrosine, Fruit & Citric Acid Complex, Phenoxyethanol, Purified Water, Methylparaben.

Sesa Hair Supplement **-** Rani-Pharma Inc.
Mukta Sukti 100 mg • Sudha Shilajeet 100 mg • Rohitak 60 mg • Sudh Bodar 50 mg • Rasayana 90 mg.

Seven Day Souper Cabbage Diet **-** Puritan's Pride
Three capsules contain: 3 Green Onions (organo-sulfurs) • 1 Green Pepper (flavonoids) • 1 small stalk of Celery (polyacetylenes) • 1 whole Tomato (lycopene) • 2 large Carrots (carotenoids) • 1 Zucchini Squash (sulforaphane) • 1 small head of Cabbage (Indole 3 Carbinol: I-3C).

Shake and Bake **-** The Herbalist
Oils of Sweet Almond, Aloe Vera, Safflower, St. John's Wort flower, Calendula flower, & Vitamin E • Extracts of St. John's Wort flower, Calendula flower & Chamomile flower • Essential oils of Sandalwood, Lite Musk, French Vanilla.

Shampoo Stuff **-** Blue Stuff, Inc.
Each 16 oz bottle contains: Whole leaf Aloe Vera concentrate • Purified Water • Tea-Lauryl Sulfate • Lauramide DEA • Pantothenol • Allantoin • Emu oil • Tea Tree oil • Sodium Hexametaphosphate • Methylparaben • Fragrance • Imidazolidinyl Urea • Retinol • Tocopherol • FD&C Blue No. 1 • FD&C Yellow No. 5.

Shape Up! Weight Management Supplement Intensifier for Apple or Pear Body Types **-** CSA Nutraceuticals, LLC
Each packet contains: Vitamin C 750 mg • CoQ10 100 mg • EPA (eicosapentaenoic acid) 300 mg • DHA (docosahexaenoic acid) 200 mg • CLA (conjugated linoleic acid) 2000 mg • Tyrosine 75 mg • L-Theanine 100 mg. Other Ingredients: Microcrystalline Cellulose, Maltodextrin, Gelatin, Tricalcium Phosphate, Magnesium Stearate, Silicon Dioxide, Corn Starch, Carboxymethylcellulose, Natural Color, Glycerin.

Shape Up! Apple Body Types Weight Management Supplement & Complete Multivitamin **-** CSA Nutraceuticals, LLC
Two packets contain: Vitamin A 5000 IU • Vitmain C 500 mg • Vitamin D 400 IU • Vitamin E 200 IU • Vitamin K 80 mcg • Thiamin (B1) 3 mg • Riboflavin (B2) 3.4 mg • Niacin (B3) 40 mg • Vitamin B6 4 mg • Folate, Folic Acid, Folacin 1 mcg • Vitamin B12 1 mcg • Biotin 600 mcg • Pantothenic Acid 20 mg • Calcium 500 mg • Iodine 75 mcg • Magnesium 400 mg • Zinc 30 mg •Selenium 140 mcg • Copper 2 mg • Manganese 2 mg • Chromium 400 mcg • Molybdenum 75 mcg • Vandium 10 mcg • Boron 1 mcg • Garcinia Cambogia fruit 3000 mg • Opuntia Cactus flesh (fics indica) 800 mg • Eleuthero root 100 mg • Kola Nut seed extract 300 mg • L-Carnitine (from l-carnitine tartrate) 100 mg • White Kidney Bean extract 500 mg • Gymnema Sylvestre leaves 300 mg. Other Ingredients: Microcrystalline Cellulose, Stearic Acid, Maltodextrin, Croscarmellose Sodium, Acacia, Magnesium Stearate, Hydroxypropyl Methylcellulose, Corn Starch, Silicone Dioxide, Glycerin, Carnauba Wax, Sodium Starch Glyconate, Corn Syrup Solids, Hydrolized Corn Syrup Solids, Lactose Monohydrate, Carrageenan, Propylene Glycol Alginate.

Shape Up! Complete Nutrition Bar, Chocolate Peanut Butter **-** CSA Nutraceuticals, LLC
Each bar contains: Syrup blend: Corn Syrup, Peanut Butter, Sugar, Hydrogenated Starch, High Fructose Corn Syrup, Salt, Lecithin, Natural Flavor, Carrageenan • Crisps: Soy Protein Isolate, Tapioca Starch, Soy Fiber, Oat Fiber, Rice Flour, Malt extract, Salt • Chocolate Flavored Coating: Lactitol, Fractionated Palm kernal oil, Chicory extract, Cocoa, Sucralose, Salt, Lecithin, Distilled Monoglycerides, Natural Flavor • Sodium Caseinate • Calcium Phosphate • Peanut Flour • Chicory • Partially Hydrolyzed Guar Gum • Acacia • Magnesium Oxide • Salt • Maltodextrin • Natural and Artificial Flavor • Ascorbic Acid (vitamin C) • Ferrous Fumarate • Biotin • Cholecalciferol (vitamin D) • Chromium Chloride • Copper Gluconate • Cyanocobalamin (vitamin B12) • D-Calcium Pantothenate • Dl-Alpha-Tocopheryl Acetate (vitamin E) • Folic Acid • Manganese Sulfate • Niacinamide (vitamin B3) • Phytonadione (vitamin K) • Potassium Iodide • Pyridoxine Hydrochloride (vitamin B6) • Retinyl Palmitate (vitamin A) • Riboflavin (vitamin B2) • Sodium Molybdate • Sodium Selenite • Thiamine Mononitrate (vitamin B1) • Zinc Oxide.

Shape Up! Complete Nutrition Bar, Chocolate Toffee Crunch **-** CSA Nutraceuticals, LLC
Each bar contains: Caramel Syrup: Corn Syrup, Hydrogenated Starch, High Fructose Corn Syrup, Sweetened Condensed Milk, Fractionated Palm Kernal Oil, Butter, Gelatin, Lecithin, Natural Flavor • Crisps: Soy Protein Isolate, Oat Fiber, Tapioca Starch, Rice Flour, Soy Fiber, Malt extract, Salt • Chocolate Flavored Coating: Lactitol, Fraction-

ated Palm Kernal Oil, Chicory extract, Cocoa, Sucralose, Salt, Lecithin, Distilled Monoglycerides, Natural Flavor) • Sodium Caseinate • Partially Hydrolyzed Guar Gum • Calcium Phosphate • Peanut • Chicory • Magnesium Oxide • Maltodextrin • Ascorbic Acid (vitamin C) • Ferrous Fumarate • Biotin • Cholecalciferol (vitamin D) • Chromium Chloride • Copper Gluconate • Cyanocobalamin (vitamin B12) • D-Calcium Pantothenate • Dl-Alpha-Tocopheryl Acetate (vitamin E) • Folic Acid • Manganese Sulfate • Niacinamide (vitamin B3) • Phytonadione (vitamin K) • Potassium Iodide • Pyridoxine Hydrochloride (vitamin B6) • Retinyl Palmitate (vitamin A) • Riboflavin (vitamin B2) • Sodium Molybdate • Sodium Selenate • Thiamine Mononitrate (vitamin B1) • Zinc Oxide.

***Shape Up! Complete Nutrition Bar, Fudge Brownie* - CSA Nutraceuticals, LLC**
Each bar contains: Fudge Syrup: Corn Syrup, Sugar, Hydrogenated Starch, High Fructose Corn Syrup, Fractionated Palm Kernal Oil, Glycerin, Sunflower Oil, Unsweetened Chocolate, Carrageenan, Natural Flavor • Crisps: Soy Protein Isolate, Tapioca Starch, Cocoa Powder, Calcium Carbonate, Oat Fiber, Rice Flour, Malt extract • Chocolate Flavored Coating: Lactitol, Fractionated Palm Kernal Oil, Chicory extract, Cocoa, Sucralose, Salt, Lecithin, Distilled Monoglycerides, Vanilla extract • Peanut • Sodium Caseinate • Partially Hydrolyzed Guar Gum • Calcium Phosphate • Chicory • Chicory extract • Magnesium Oxide • Maltodextrin • Ascorbic Acid (vitamin C) • Ferrous Fumarate • Biotin • Cholecalciferol (vitamin D) • Chromium Chloride • Copper Gluconate • Cyanocobalamin (vitamin B12) • D-Calcium Pantothenate • Dl-Alpha-Tocopheryl Acetate (vitamin E) • Folic Acid • Manganese Sulfate • Niacinamide (vitamin B3) • Phytonadione (vitamin K) • Potassium Iodide • Pyridoxine Hydrochloride (vitamin B6) • Retinyl Palmitate (vitamin A) • Riboflavin (vitamin B2) • Sodium Molybdate • Sodium Selenite • Thiamine Mononitrate (vitamin B1) • Zinc Oxide.

***Shape Up! Complete Nutrition Bar, Oatmeal Raisin* - CSA Nutraceuticals, LLC**
Each bar contains: Syrup Blend: Raisin paste, Malitol syrup, Cocoa butter, High Fructose Corn syrup, Glycerin, Hydrogenated Starch, Molasses, Cinnamon, Caramel Color, Medium Chain Triglycerides, Lecithin • Protein Nuggets: Soy Protein Isolate, Tapioca Starch, Soy Fiber, Salt • Yogurt Coating: Lactitol, Fractionated Palm kernal oil, Nonfat Dry Milk, Chicory extract, Yogurt powder, Distilled Monoglycerides, Sucralose, Soy Lecithin, Vanilla, Salt • Rolled Oats/ Oat Crisps: Oat Fiber, Rice Flour, Malt extract • Calcium Caseinate • Soy Protein Isolate • Milk Protein Isolate • Natural, Artificial Flavor • Magnesium Oxide • Arabic Gum • Maltodextrin • Ascorbic Acid • Ferrous Fumarate • Biotin • Cholecalciferol • Chromium Chloride • Copper Gluconate • Cyanocobalamin • D-Calcium Pantothenate • Dl-Alpha-Tocopheryl Acetate • Folic Acid • Manganese Sulfate • Niacinamide • Phytonadione • Potassium Iodide • Pyridoxine Hydrochloride • Retinyl Palmitate • Riboflavin • Sodium Molybdate • Sodium Selenate • Thiamine Mononitrate • Tricalcium Phosphate • Zinc Oxide • Peanut (possible trace amounts).

***Shape Up! Mix & Drink Nutrition Shake, Authentic Chocolate* - CSA Nutraceuticals, LLC**
Each packet (40 g) contains: Whey Protein Isolate • Nonfat Dry Milk • Alkalyzed Cocoa • Chicory extract • Acacia • Guar Gum • Oat Hull Fiber • Sunflower Oil • Maltodextrin • Cellulose Gel • Trimagnesium Phosphate • Disodium Phosphate • Tricalcium Phosphate • Salt • Carrageenan • Corn Bran • Medium Chain Triglycerides • Soy Lecithin • Cellulose Gum • Xanthan Gum • Sodium Caseinate • Ascorbic Acid • Sucralose • Selenium Yeast • Chromium Yeast • Molybdenum Yeast • D-Alpha-Tocopheryl Acetate • Manganese Gluconate • Copper Citrate • Niacinamide • Zinc Oxide • Electrolyte Iron • Calcium Pantothenate • Pyridoxine Hydrochloride • Vitamin A Palmitate • Riboflavin • Potassium Iodide • Folic Acid • Biotin • Phytonadione • Vitamin D (D3) • Vitamin B12.

***Shape Up! Mix & Drink Nutrition Shake, Genuine Vanilla* - CSA Nutraceuticals, LLC**
Each packet (40 g) contains: Whey Protein Concentrate • Nonfat Dry Milk • Whey Protein Isolate • Chicory extract • Milk Protein Concentrate • Oat Hull Fiber • Acacia • Guar Gum • Sunflower Oil • Maltodextrin • Cellulose Gel • Trimagnesium Phosphate • Disodium Phosphate • Tricalcium Phosphate • Salt • Carrageenan • Corn Bran • Medium Chain Triglycerides • Soy Lecithin • Cellulose Gum • Xanthan Gum • Sodium Caseinate • Ascorbic Acid • Sucralose • Selenium Yeast • Chromium Yeast • Molybdenum Yeast • D-Alpha-Tocopheryl Acetate • Manganese Gluconate • Copper Citrate • Niacinamide • Zinc Oxide • Electrolyte Iron • Calcium Pantothenate • Pyridoxine Hydrochloride • Vitamin A Palmitate • Riboflavin • Potassium Iodide • Folic Acid • Biotin • Phytonadione • Vitamin D (D3) • Vitamin B12.

***Shape Up! Pear Body Types Weight Management Supplement & Complete Multivitamin* - CSA Nutraceuticals, LLC**
Two packets contain: Vitamin A 5000 IU • Vitamin C 500 mg • Vitamin D 400 IU • Vitamin E 200 IU • Vitamin K 80 mcg • Thiamin (B1) 3 mg • Riboflavin (B2) 3.4 mg • Niacin (B3) 40 mg • Vitamin B6 40 mg • Folate, Folic Acid, Folacin 1 mcg • Vitamin B12 1 mcg • Biotin 600 mcg • Pantothenic Acid 20 mg • Calcium 500 mg • Iodine 75 mcg • Magnesium 400 mg • Zinc 30 mg • Selenium 140 mcg • Copper 2 mg • Manganese 2 mg • Chromium 200 mcg • Molybdenum 75 mcg • Boron 1 mcg • Garcinia Cambogia fruit 3000 mg • Opuntia Cactus flesh (fics indica) 800 mg • Eleuthero root 100 mg • Soybean extract 50 mg • Kola Nut seed extract 300 mg • L-Carnitine (from l-carnitine tartrate) 100 mg • Rhodiola Rosea root extract 200 mg • Green Tea leaves extract (camellia sinensis) 1000 mg • EGCG (epigallocatechin gallate, from green tea extract) 270 mg. Other Ingredients: Microcrystalline Cellulose, Stearic Acid, Maltodextrin, Croscarmellose Sodium, Acacia, Magnesium Stearate, Hydroxypropyl Methylcellulose, Corn Starch, Silicone Dioxide, Carnauba Wax, Sodium Starch Glycolate, Hydrogenated Cottonseed Oil, Glycerin, Corn Syrup Solids.

***Shark / Glucosamine Formula* - Health Smart Vitamins**
Three capsules contain: Protein 0.675 g • Calcium (from shark cartilage) 210 mg • Phosphorus (from shark cartilage) 135 mg • Potassium (from glucosamine sulfate) 98 mg • Shark Cartilage 1500 mg • Glucosamine Sulfate 750 mg.

***Shark Cartilage* - Swanson**
Three capsules contain: Shark Cartilage 2.25 g.

***Shark Cartilage* - Olympian Labs**
Each capsule contains: Shark Cartilage 750 mg.

***Shark Cartilage* - Leiner Health Products**
Each capsule contains: Shark Cartilage 500 mg. Other Ingredients: Gelatin, Maltodextrin, Magnesium Stearate, Calcium Carbonate, Sodium Starch Glycolate.

***Shark Cartilage - Basic Nutrition* - GNC**
Each tablet contains: Shark Cartilage powder 750 mg. Other Ingredients: Cellulose, Povidone, Dicalcium Phosphate, Vegetable Acetoglycerides.

***Shark Cartilage Plus* - Life Extension**
Each capsule contains: Shark Cartilage 800 mg • Devil's Claw 35 mg • Black Cohosh 20 mg • Goldenseal 15 mg • L-Histidine 20 mg.

***Shark Energy Drink* - Osotspa Co., Ltd.**
Carbonated Water • Sucrose • Dextrose • Citric Acid • Choline Bitartrate • Natural Caffeine • Inositol • Caramel • Niacinamide • Taurine • Sodium Chloride • Pantothenyl Alcohol • Pyridoxine HCl • Guarana extract • Riboflavin-Phosphate Sodium • Thiamine Mononitrate.

***Shark Oil* - Futurebiotics**
Shark liver oil 460 mg.

Sharp Thinking **-** Changes International, Inc.
Two caplets contain: Ginkgo Biloba leaf standardized extract (24% flavonglycosides, 6% terpene lactones) 120 mg • Huperzine A (from Huperzia serrata extract whole plant) 50 mcg • Green Tea leaf standardized extract (30% polyphenols, 20% methylxanthines) 500 mg • Panax Ginseng root standardized extract (4% ginsenosides) 200 mg • Brahmi leaf standardized extract (10% asiaticosides)(Centella asiatica) 100 mg • Citrus aurantium fruit standardized extract (5-7% alkaloids) 50 mg. Other Ingredients: Dicalcium Phosphate, Vegetable Cellulose, Fractionated vegetable oil, Soy polysaccharides, Silica, and Vegetable resin glaze.
See Editor's Note No. 40, page 2058.

Shen Min **-** Biotech Corp.
Three tablets contain: Shen Min: a proprietary blend of 12:1 standardized He Shou Wu (Fo Ti) root extract and He Shou Wu root powder providing a synergistic complex of chrysophanics and resveratrol 1775 mg • Bioperine Black Pepper (Piper nigrum) 3.0 mg. Other Ingredients: Dicalcium phosphate, Microcrystalline Cellulose, Croscarmellose Sodium, Stearic Acid, Magnesium Stearate, Pharmaceutical glaze.

Shen Min **-** Puritan's Pride
Three tablets contain: Shen Min: a proprietary blend of 12:1 standardized He Shou Wu (Fo Ti) root powder providing a synergistic complex of chrysophanics and resveratrol 1,775 mg • BioPerine black pepper extract (Piper nigrum) 3.0 mg. Other Ingredients: Dicalcium Phosphate, Microcrystalline Cellulose, Croscarmellose Sodium, Stearic Acid, Magnesium Stearate, Pharmaceutical Glaze.

Shen Min Activator with Progestoplex **-** Biotech Corp.
Purified Water • Jojoba oil • Herbal Blend Hair Complex: Henna extract, Horsetail extract, Nettle extract, Chamomile extract, Rosemary extract, Tormentil extract, Burdock extract, Honey extract, Golden Seal root extract • Lecithin • Peg-40 Stearate • Steareth-20 • Cholesterol • Trichopeptide (hydrolyzed keratin) • Lysine Carboxymethyl Cysteinate • Progestoplex Proprietary Blend: Progesterone, Copper Peptide • Retinyl Palmitate • Tocopheryl Acetate • He Shou Wu extract • Saw Palmetto extract • Nettle extract • Propyl Gallate • Biotin • Polysorbate 20 • Chamomile extract • Carbomer • Disodium EDTA • Aminomethyl Propanol • Phenoxyethanol • Methylparaben • Ethylparaben • Propylparaben • Butylparaben.

Shen Min DHT Blocker **-** Biotech Corp.
Each tablet contains: Zinc 10 mg • Selenium 100 mcg • He Shou Wu 100 mg • DHT Block Proprietary Blend 300 mg • Lycopene 2 mg • Isoflavones 20 mg. Other Ingredients: Dicalcium Phosphate, Microcrystalline Cellulose, Hypromellose, Stearic Acid, Vegetable Stearin, Magnesium Stearate, Silica, Calcium Silicate, Pharmaceutical Glaze.

Shen Min Hair Volumizing Serum **-** Biotech Corp.
Aqueous Extracts of Chamomile, Clary Sage, Rosemary, Rhatania root extract, Ginkgo extract • Liposomal Bio-Plex: Hydrolyzed Wheat Protein, Hydrolyzed Wheat Oligosaccharides, Panthenol, Sesame Oil, Lecithin, Retinyl Palmitate, Octyl Methoxycinnamate • Biotin • Carbomer • Henna extract • Methacryl Ethyl Betaine/Acrylates Copolymer • Sodium Hydroxide • Triethyl Citrate • Cyclomethicone • DMDM Hydantoin • Methylparaben • Propylparaben • Dimethicone Copolyol • Disodium EDTA • Fragrance.

Shen Min Hair, Skin & Nails **-** Biotech Corp.
Three tablets contain: Vitamin C (as ascorbic acid) 150 mg • Vitamin D (as cholecalciferol) 400 IU • Thiamin (as thiamine HCl) 10 mg • Riboflavin 10 mg • Vitamin B6 (as pyridoxine HCl) 25 mg • Folate (as folic acid) 400 mcg • Biotin 2000 mcg • Pantothenic Acid (d-calcium pantothenate) 500 mg • Iodine (from kelp) 150 mcg • Zinc (as zinc monomethionine) 5 mg • Selenium (as selenomethionine) 70 mcg • Shen Min (he shou wu standardized to 10% chrysophancis) 150 mg • Shen Min root powder (as he shou wu) 200 mg • Silica (from colloidals) 50 mg • Lecithin (from glycine max, providing 24% phosphatidyl choline and 14% phosphatidyl inositol) 200 mg • Collagen (spray dried) 300 mg • Isoflavones (from glycine max and peuraria lobata) 5 mg • Turmeric rhizome extract (curcuma longa, 92% curcuminoids minimum) 25 mg • Fatty Acids 25 mg • BioPerine Black Pepper extract (piper nigrum) 2.5 mg. Other Ingredients: Microcrystalline Cellulose, Croscarmellose Sodium, Stearic Acid, Magnesium Stearate, Pharmaceutical Glaze.

Shen Min Prostate Health Formula **-** Biotech Corp.
Two tablets contain: Zinc (as zinc citrate, zinc monomethionine) 7.5 mg • Selenium (as selenomethionine) 35 mcg • He Shou Wu root (polygonum multiflorum, 12:1 standardized extract, source of resveratrol and chrysophanics) 100 mg • Saw Palmetto berries (serenoa repens, standardized extract 85%-95% phytosterols) 160 mg • Pumpkin seed extract (curcubito pepo) 80 mg • Pygeum bark (pygeum africanum, 4:1 extract) 75 mg • Isoflavones (from pueraria lobata root standardized extract and soybeans) 10 mg • Tomato concentrate (200 ppm lycopene) 100 mg. Other Ingredients: Dicalcium Phosphate, Microcrystalline Cellulose, Croscarmellose Sodium, Stearic Acid, Magnesium Stearate, Pharmaceutical Glaze.

Shen Min Topical **-** Biotech Corp.
Purified Water • Glycerin (from vegetable) • Jojoba oil • Herbal Blend Complex: Henna, Horsetail, Rosemary, Tormentil, Burdock, Honey, Golden Seal • Lecithin • PEG-40 Stearate • Steareth 20 • Tilisina complex • Cholesterol • Trichopeptide • Hydrolyzed Soy Protein • Retinyl Palmitate • Tocopherol Acetate • He Shou Wu extract • Saw Palmetto extract • Nettle extract • Nicotinic Acid • Pantothenic Acid • Propyl Gallate • Biotin • Chamomile extract • Soap bark extract • Eucalyptus extract • Quaternium-51 • Carbomer • Polysorbate 20 • Phenoxyethanol • Methylparaben • Butylparaben • Ethylparaben • Propylparaben • Aminomethyl Propanol • Disodium EDTA.

Shiitake/Maitake Extract **-** Nature's Way
Each capsule contains: Maitake dried extract 100 mg • Oat grain 200 mg • Shiitake dried extract 100 mg. Other Ingredients: Gelatin, Magnesium stearate, Millet.

Ship-Assure **-** Nature's Plus
Two tablets contain: Ginger root [(Zingiber officinale) standardized 4% Volatile oils] 350 mg • Kava [(Piper methysticum) standardized 29-31% kavalactones] 50 mg • Chamomile flower [(Matricaria recutita) standardized 1% apigenin, 0.5% essential oil] 50 mg • Hops fruit [(Humulus lupulus) standardized 5.2% bitter acids, 4% flavonoids] 50 mg • Siberian Ginseng root [(Eleutherococcus senticosus) standardized 0.8% Eleutherosides] 50 mg • Passion Flower [(Passiflora incarnata) standardized 3.5-4% flavonoids, calculated as isovitexin] 50 mg • Wild Cherry (Prunus virginlana fruit) 50 mg.

SHN Skin-Hair-Nails **-** The Vitamin Shoppe
Three tablets contain: Vitamin A (beta carotene) 10,000 IU • Vitamin C 120 mg • Vitamin B1 10 mg • Vitamin B2 10 mg • Niacinamide 50 mg • Calcium 600 mg • Iron 6 mg • Vitamin D 200 IU • Vitamin E 30 IU • Vitamin B6 10 mg • Folic Acid 400 mcg • Vitamin B12 16 mcg • Phosphorus 300 mg • Iodine (kelp) 225 mcg • Magnesium 200 mg • Zinc 15 mg • Biotin 400 mcg • Pantothenic Acid 30 mg • Choline 150 mcg • Inositol 60 mg • PABA 50 mg • Selenium 25 mcg • Manganese 10 mg • RNA 60 mg • Bioflavonoids 50 mg • Rutin 25 mg • Betaine Hydrochloride 50 mg. In a base of L-Cysteine, Methionine, Gelatin, Papain, Oat Straw, Echinacea, Horse Tail, and Asparagus.

Shogun Imperial Green Tea **-** Green Foods Corp.
Each tablet contains: Green Tea 335 mg.

Short-Term Adrenal **-** Enzymes, Inc.
Each capsule contains: Vitamin C (100% from Acerola Cherries) 4 mg • Proprietary Herbal Blend 365 mg: Siberian Ginseng root extract, Chinese Thoroughwax root extract, Licorice root extract, Rice Bran • n-zimes Proprietary Blend 65 mg: Protease, CereCalase. Other Ingredients: Cellulose, Water.

***Siberian Ginseng* - Gaia Herbs**
Siberian Ginseng standardized for 0.8% eleutherosides B & E. Standardized Full Spectrum 200 mg of extract per capsule. Guaranteed Potency 100 mg of extract per capsule.

***Siberian Ginseng* - Nature's Way**
Three capsules contain: Siberian Ginseng root 1.23 g. Other Ingredients: Gelatin, Magnesium stearate.

***Siberian Ginseng* - Olympian Labs**
Each capsule contains: Siberian Ginseng 500 mg.

***Siberian Ginseng* - Pharmanex**
Each capsule contains: Ginseng, Siberian root extract (Eleutherococcus senticosus Max)(10:1) 150 mg. Other Ingredients: Rice Flour, Gelatin, Magnesium Stearate, Silicon Dioxide.

***Siberian Ginseng* - Quest**
Each capsule contains: Siberian Ginseng 500 mg.

***Siberian Ginseng Extract* - PhytoPharmica**
Each capsule contains: Siberian Ginseng (Eleutherococcus senticosus) root extract 10:1 (standardized to contain greater than 0.5% eleutheroside E) 200 mg.

***Siberian Ginseng Rush* - GNC**
Each capsule contains: Siberian Ginseng root powder (Eleutherococcus) 500 mg • Guarana seed extract (Paullinia cupana) 95 mg. Other Ingredients: Gelatin, Calcium Carbonate, Cellulose.

***Siberian Root 1000 mg, Concentrated - GNC Herbal Plus* - GNC**
Each capsule contains: Siberian Root (eleutherococcus senticosus; from 28.5 mg siberian root extract 35:1) 1000 mg. Other Ingredients: Soybean Oil, Gelatin, Glycerin, Caramel Color, Titanium Dioxide (natural mineral whitener).

***Sil-150* - PhytoPharmica**
Two sofgel capsules contain: Milk Thistle seed extract (silybum marianum, standardized to contain 80% silymarin (240 mg) calculated as silybin) 300 mg.

***Silent Night Formula* - Nature's Way**
Four capsules contain: Proprietary Formula: Hops flower • Scullcap herb • Valerian root. Other Ingredients: Gelatin.

***Silibinin Plus* - Life Extension**
Each capsule contains: Silibinin 266 mg • Silymarin 60 mg. Other Ingredients: Gelatin, Water.

***Silica 10 mg* - Jamieson**
Each caplet contains: Standardized Silica from pure spring Horsetail herb 3080 mg (Equisetum arvense L 770 mg powdered extract 1:4) 10 mg. With natural occurring flavonoids, saponins and minerals.

***Silica Complex* - Puritan's Pride**
Each tablet contains: Calcium (as calcium carbonate and calcium citrate) 200 mg • Magnesium (as magnesium oxide and magnesium citrate) 150 mg • Zinc (as zinc gluconate and zinc citrate) 15 mg • Boron (as Boron Citrate, Boron Glycinate, and Boron Aspartate) 1.5 mg • Betaine (as Betaine Hydrochloride) 38 mg • Horsetail extract (Euisetum arvense) arial (standardized to contain 7% Silica) 500 mg.

***Silica Plus* - Global Health Trax**
One quarter teaspoon contains: Global Health Trax Proprietary Blend 1240 mg: Silica, Ionic Trace Elements, Citric Acid, Gluconic Acid, Rice Vinegar, Hydrogen Sulfate, Purified Water, Amino Acid Blend, Enzyme Blend.

***SiliCare* - Holista**
Each capsule contains Silicon (dioxide) derived from 410 mg 2.9% Spring Horsetail Equisetum arvense extract 5 mg.

***Silver Mineral Water* - WaterOz**
Each bottle contains: Colloidal Silver +/- 100 parts per million • Water.

***Silybin Phytosome* - PhytoPharmica**
Each capsule contains: Silybin phytosome (milk thistle extract) bound to Phosphatidylcholine 120 mg.

***Silymarin* - Aspen Group, Inc.**
Each capsule contains: Silymarin (Milk Thistle, standardized at 80%) 150 mg.

***Silymarin Plus* - Futurebiotics**
Three tablets contain: Milk Thistle seed powder extract (standardized for 80% (420 mg) silymarin) 525 mg • Inositol 240 mg • Choline (as choline bitartrate) 240 mg • Dandelion root powder 300 mg • Alfalfa leaf powder extract 300 mg • Black Radish root powder 300 mg • Beet root powder 300 mg. Other Ingredients: Dicalcium phosphate, Magnesium stearate, Vegetable stearate, Silica, Cellulose.

***Silymarin Plus* - Source Naturals**
Each tablet contains: Silymarin (from Milk Thistle Seed extract) 140 mg • Vitamin C (Ascorbic Acid) 100 mg • Choline (Bitartrate) 50 mg • Inositol 50 mg • Vitamin E (d-alpha tocopheryl natural) 25 IU.

***Simicort* - Enzymatic Therapy**
Active Ingredient: Salicylic Acid 1.8%. Other Ingredients: Purified Water, Organic Fatty Acid Complex (C11-C18), Glyceryl Stearate, Chamomile extract (0.5% Flavonoid Content), 18-Beta-Glycyrrhetinic Acid from Licorice root extract, Allantoin 2.0% from Comfrey root extract, Dimethicone, Vitamin E antioxidant, & Hypoallergenic Fragrance.

***Similase - Tyler* - Integrative Therapeutics**
Two capsules contain: Plant Enzymes 525 mg: Protease (I, II, III, IV), Amylase, Cellulase (I, II), Lipase (I, II), Phytase, Lactase (I, II), Sucrase (invertase), Maltase (malt diastase). Other Ingredients: Microcrystalline Cellulose, Gelatin, Water.

***Simple Cleanse* - PhytoPharmica**
Laxative Formula: Three tablets contain: Magnesium Hydroxide 2600 mg • Proprietary Mucilage Blend 650 mg: Slippery Elm bark (ulmus rubra), Marshmallow root 3.5:1 extract (althaea officinalis), Fenugreek seed 4:1 extract (trigonella foenum-graecum) • Proprietary Soothing Blend 150 mg: Peppermint leaf (mentha x piperita), Fennel seed (foeniculum vulgare), Ginger rhizome extract (zingiber officinale) • Other Ingredients: Cellulose, Modified Cellulose Gum, Modified Cellulose, Magnesium Stearate, Silicon Dioxide, Lecithin, Carnauba Wax. Fiber Formula: Eight capsules contain: Proprietary Fiber Blend 3455 mg: Psyllium husk (plantago ovata), Oat bran (avena sativa), Guar Gum seed extract (cyamposis tetragonoloba), Pectin (from citrus fruit), Marshmallow root 3.5:1 extract (althaea officinalis). Other Ingredients: Cellulose, Gelatin, Magnesium Stearate, Silicon Dioxide.

***Simply Creatine* - PhytoPharmica**
Each 1 1/2 tsp serving (5 g) contains: Creatine Monohydrate 5 g.

***SinEcch* - Alpine Pharmaceuticals**
Each capsule contains: Arnica Montana 12C 500 mg.

***Single Day* - Schiff**
Each tablet contains: Vitamin A (as retinyl palmitate, 10% as beta carotene) 10,000 IU • Vitamin C (as ascorbic acid) 250 mg • Vitamin D (as cholecalciferol) 400 IU • Vitamin E (as d-alpha tocopheryl succinate) 150 IU • Vitamin B1 (as thiamin mononitrate) 75 mg • Vitamin B2 (as riboflavin) 75 mg • Vitamin B3 (as niacinamide) 75 mg • Vitamin B6 (as pyridoxine hydrochloride) 75 mg • Folate (as folic acid) 400 mcg • Vitamin B12 (as cyanocobalamin) 75 mcg • Biotin 75 mcg • Pantothenic Acid (as d-calcium pantothenate) 75 mg • Calcium (as calcium amino acid chelate) 10 mg • Iron (as iron amino acid chelate) 9 mg • Iodine (from kelp) 150 mcg • Magnesium (as magnesium amino acid chelate) 5 mg • Zinc (as zinc amino acid chelate) 5 mg • Selenium (as selenomethionine) 50 mcg • Copper (as

copper amino acid chelate) 25 mcg • Manganese (as manganese amino acid chelate) 600 mcg • Chromium (as chromium polynicotinate) 25 mcg • Potassium (as potassium amino acid chelate) 5 mg • Choline Bitartrate 75 mg • Inositol 75 mg • PABA (para-aminobenzoic acid) 75 mg • Citrus Bioflavonoid Complex 25 mg • Rutin 25 mg • Hesperidin Complex 5 mg. Other Ingredients: Cellulose, Stearic Acid, Magnesium Stearate, Coating (pharmaceutical glaze, ethyl cellulose), Silicon Dioxide, Croscarmellose Sodium.

Single Day Sustained Release **-** Schiff
Each tablet contains: Vitamin A (as retinyl palmitate, 10% as beta carotene) 10,000 IU • Vitamin C (as ascorbic acid) 250 mg • Vitamin D (as cholecalciferol) 400 IU • Vitamin E (as d-alpha tocopheryl succinate) 150 IU • Vitamin B1 (as thiamin hydrochloride) 75 mg • Vitamin B2 (as riboflavin) 75 mg • Niacin 75 mg • Vitamin B6 (as pyridoxine hydrochloride) 75 mg • Folate (as folic acid) 400 mcg • Vitamin B12 (as cyanocobalamin) 75 mcg • Biotin 75 mcg • Pantothenic Acid (as d-calcium pantothenate) 75 mg • Calcium (as calcium amino acid chelate) 10 mg • Iron (as iron amino acid chelate) 9 mg • Iodine (from kelp) 150 mcg • Magnesium (as magnesium amino acid chelate) 5 mg • Zinc (as zinc amino acid chelate) 5 mg • Selenium (as selenomethionine) 50 mcg • Copper (as copper amino acid chelate) 25 mcg • Manganese (as manganese amino acid chelate) 600 mcg • Chromium (as chromium polynicotinate) 25 mcg • Potassium (as potassium amino acid chelate) 5 mg • Choline Bitartrate 75 mg • Inositol 75 mg • PABA (para aminobenzoic acid) 75 mg • Lemon Bioflavonoids 25 mg • Rutin 25 mg • Hesperidin Complex 5 mg. Other Ingredients: Stearic Acid, Methylcellulose, Silicon Dioxide, Magnesium Stearate, Coating (pharmaceutical glaze, ethylcellulose).

Single Herb Extract Bai Ji Li **-** Plum Flower Brand
Blackberry Lily Rhizome 5:1 extract powder (belamcanda chinensis; she gan) 100 g.

SinoFresh Antiseptic Nasal & Sinus Spray **-** SinoFresh Healthcare
Cetylpyridinium Chloride 0.05% • Dibasic Sodium Phosphate • Eucalyptus Oil • Monobasic Sodium Phosphate • Peppermint oil • Polysorbate 80 • Propylene Glycol • Purified Water • Sodium Chloride • Sorbitol solution • Spearmint oil • Wintergreen oil.

Sino-Lung Res-Q **-** Nutri-Quest Rx
Each tablet contains: Lung 35 mg • Thymus 35 mg • Spleen 35 mg • Vitamin C 75 mg • Beta Carotene 12600 IU • Lemon Bioflavonoids 125 mg • Rutin 20 mg • Hesperidin Complex 75 mg • N-Acetyl Cysteine 35 mg • Propolis 20 mg • Cranberry 36 mg • Echinacea 30 mg • Goldenseal 35 mg • Elderberry 10 mg • Scullcap 35 mg.
See Editor's Note No. 14.

SinuCheck **-** Enzymatic Therapy
Each capsule contains: Pseudoephedrine HCl (from ephedra sinensis) 30 mg • Scullcap extract (4:1, scutellaria baicalensis) 100 mg • Chinese Thoroughwax extract (bupleurum falcatum) 100 mg • Chinese Peony extract (4:1, paeonia lactiflora) 100 mg • Dong Quai extract (4:1, angelica sinensis) 100 mg • Licorice root extract (glycyrrhiza glabra, standardized to contain 5% glycyrrhizic acid) 40 mg • Curcuma root extract (curcuma longa, standardized to contain 4% curcumin) 20 mg • Ginger root extract 6.5:1 (zingiber officinale) 20 mg.
See Editor's Note No. 30, page 2056.

SinuClear **-** PhytoPharmica
Each capsule contains: Pseudoephedrine HCl 30 mg (from ephedra sinensis) • Scullcap extract (4:1, scutellaria baicalensis) 100 mg • Chinese Thoroughwax extract (bupleurum falcatum) 100 mg • Chinese Peony extract (4:1, paeonia lactiflora) 100 mg • Dong Quai extract (4:1, angelica sinensis) 100 mg • Licorice root extract (glycyrrhiza glabra, standardized to contain 5% glycyrrhizic acid) 40 mg • Curcuma root extract (curcuma longa, standardized to contain 2.5% curcumin) 20 mg • Ginger root extract (6.5:1, zingiber officinale) 20 mg.
See Editor's Note No. 21 and No. 30, page 2056.

SinuComp **-** PhytoPharmica
Each tablet contains: Cowslip flower (primula veris) 36 mg • Sour Dock aerial part (rumex acetosa) 36 mg • European Elder flower (sambucus nigra) 36 mg • European Vervain (verbena officinalis) 36 mg • Gentian root (gentiana lutea) 12 mg.

SinuFix **-** NaturalCare
Two capsules contain: Vitamin A (as mixed carotenes from dunaliella) 5000 IU • Vitamin C (as ascorbic acid) 250 mg • Vitamin B6 (as pyridoxine HCl) 30 mg • Vitamin B5 (as calcium pantothenate) 100 mg • Zinc (as zinc methionate) 15 mg • Bromelain (1600 MCU) 250 mg • Nettle leaf extract (urtica dioica, 4:1) 200 mg • Wild Mediterranean Oregano leaf extract (4:1) 150 mg • GoldenSeal root 150 mg • Quercetin Bioflavonoid 125 mg • N-Acetylcysteine (NAC) 100 mg • Garlic bulb powder (odor controlled) 100 mg • Echinacea Purpurea/ Angustifolia root extract (4% phenols) 50 mg • Grapefruit seed extract 50 mg • Turmeric root extract (95% curcumin) 50 mg • Peppermint leaf extract (2% essential oil) 50 mg • Cryptoxanthin (from dunaliella) 12 mcg • Zeaxanthin (from dunaliella) 6 mcg. Other Ingredients: Gelatin, Purified Water, Glycerin, Titanium Dioxide.

SinuFix Mist **-** NaturalCare
Active Ingredients: Zinc Gluconate (zincum gluconicum) 2X, 6X • Euphorbium Officinarum 4X, 6X, 12X • Origanum Vulgare (oregano) 3X, 6X • Echinacea Angustifolia (cone flower) 3X, 6X, 12X • Hydrastis Candensis (golden seal) 3X, 6X, 12X • Argentum Metallicum (silver) 8X • Kali Sulphuricum (potassium sulfate) 3X, 6X, 12X • Allium Cepa (red onion) 6X • Ragweed (ambrosia artemisiaefolia) 6X • Calcium Sulfide (hepar sulphuris calcareum) 8X • Potassium Bichromate (kali dichromicum) 6X, 10X • Sanguinaria Canadensis (blood root) 6X • Lemna Minor (duckweed) 3X • Luffa Operculata (luffa fruit) 6X • Pulsatilla (windflower) 3X • Sabadilla (cevadilla seed) 6X • Silicea (silicon dioxide) 8X • Spigelia Anthelmia (pink root) 3X. Other Ingredients: Organically-Grown Aloe Vera Extract, Patented Process Colloidal Silver, Green Tea Extract, Water-Soluble Tea Tree Oil, D-Mannose (natural monosaccharide), Grapefruit Seed Extract 0.1%.
See Editor's Note No. 1, page 2053.

SinuGuard **-** Enzymatic Therapy
Each tablet contains: Cowslip flower (Primula veris) 36 mg • Sour Dock (Rumex acetosa) 36 mg • Elder flower (Sambucus nigra) 36 mg • Verbena (Verbena officinalis) 36 mg • Gentian root (Gentiana lutea) 12 mg.

Sinuplex 120T **-** Metagenics
Each tablet contains: Vitamin C (as ascorbic acid) 150 mg • Quercetin Dihydrate 200 mg • Nettle root 10:1 extract (urtica dioica) 100 mg • Bromelain (2400 GDU/g) 50 mg • N-Acetylcysteine 25 mg.

Sinus **-** nelsons - Nelson Bach USA Ltd.
Active Ingredients: Hydrastis 6c HPUS • Kali bio 6c HPUS • Pulsatilla 6c HPUS • Thuja occ 6c HPUS. Inactive Ingredients: Lactose, Sucrose.
See Editor's Note No. 1, page 2053.

Sinus Ease **-** Nature's Life
Three capsules contain: Bromelain [an enzyme from Pineapple fruit (Ananassa sativa) activity of 1200 mg = 2,880 GDU (4320 MCU)] 1200 mg • Quercetin (a flavonoid from Pilocarpus gaborandi) 300 mg • Vitamin C (Buffered, as Calcium Ascorbic) 133 mg.

Sinus Essentials **-** Swanson
Three capsules contain: Ma Huang (8% ephedra) 252 mg • Fenugreek seed powder 100 mg • Slippery Elm bark 100 mg • Cayenne Pepper 100,000 HU 60 mg • Eucalyptus leaves powder 50 mg • Goldenseal root 50 mg • Aloe Vera leaf powder 25 mg.
See Editor's Note No. 30, page 2056.

Sinus Remedy - PhytoPharmica
Two chewable tablets contain: Kalium bichromicum 5x • Silicea 5x •Mercurius sulphuratus ruber 4x • Kali sulphuricum 4x • Belladonna 3x • Calcarea carbonica 3x •Calcarea fluorica 3x •Hepar sulphuris calcareum 3x • Hydrastis canadensis 3x • Manganum sulphuricum 3x • Sabadilla 3x • Thuja 2x.
See Editor's Note No. 1 and No. 21, pages 2053 and 2056.

SinusHealth - Vita Pharmica - formerly Neopharmica
Each two tablets contain: Proprietary Blend 2500 mg: Baikal Skullcap root, Schizonpeta Tenuifolia, Angelica root, Cinnamon twig, Xanthium Strumarium, Astragalus root.

Sinutone - The Herbalist
Eyebright herb • Golden Seal root • Bayberry root bark • Osha root • Yarrow flower • Horseradish root • Cayenne pepper.

Sinu-X - Olympian Labs
Two capsules contain: Proteolytic Enzymes 150 mg •Spearmint 50 mg •Clove 10 mg •Sea Mussel 50 mg •Zinc Gluconate 20 mg •Echinacea 40 mg •Red Clover 20 mg • Goldenseal 30 mg •Citrus Aurantium 30 mg •Green Tea extract 20 mg.
See Editor's Note No. 40, page 2058.

Sitol - PharmaGen
Each capsule contains: Serenoa repens extract (standardized) 320 mg.

Sitol PA - PharmaGen
Each capsule contains: Serenoa repens extract (standardized) 320 mg • Pygeum africanum extract (standardized) 100 mg.

Skin - Enzymes, Inc.
Each capsule contains: Proprietary Herbal Blend 315 mg: Safflower petals powder, Burdock root extract, Oregon Grape root extract, Dandelion root extract, Calendula flower extract, Black Currant seed extract, Grape seed extract • Proprietary Enzyme Blend 200 mg: Amylase, pHysioProtease, CereCalase, Lipase. Other Ingredients: Plant Cellulose, Water.

Skin Answer - LaneLabs
Willow bark extract • Carbamide • Aloe Vera • Oil of Melaleuca • Menthol • Sandbrier extract (source of glycoalkaloid). Base: Gel.
See Editor's Note No. 9 and No. 21.

Skin Clear - The Herbalist
Echinacea root • Yellow Dock root • Oregon Grape root • Burdock root • Red Clover blossom • Jamaican Sarsaparilla root.

Skin Eternal DMAE Serum - Source Naturals
Deionized water • Propylene Glycol • Polysorbate 80 • Glycerin • DMAE • Vitamin C - Ester (ascorbyl palmitate) • Polyethylene Glycol • MSM (methylsulfonylmethane) • Coconut fragrance • Alpha-Lipoic Acid • Kiwi fragrance • Simethicone • Aloe Vera • Methylparaben • Biotin • Vitamin A Palmitate • Vitamin D (D3) • Vitamin E • Calcium Pantothenate • Coenzyme Q10 • Chamomile flower extract.

Skin Support for Women - Futurebiotics
Two capsules contain: Vitamin A (5000 IU beta carotene, 5000 IU fish liver oil) 10000 IU • Vitamin C (ascorbic acid) 250 mg • Vitamin D (ergocalciferol) 200 IU • Vitamin E (d-alpha tocopherol succinate) 30 IU • Zinc (amino acid chelate) 30 mg • Selenium (amino acid chelate) 100 mcg • Boron (amino acid chelate) 3 mg • MSM (methyl-sulfonyl-methane) 500 mg • Collagen 500 mg • Glucosamine Sulfate 100 mg • Skin Support Herbal Base 200 mg: Citrus Bioflavonoids, Grape Seed extract, Horsetail leaf powder, Papain, Chamomile flower powder, Aloe Vera leaf powder. Other ingredients: Gelatin, Water.

Skin Tone Balancer - Jason
10% Complete Vitamin C Complex with Kojic Ester, beta Hydroxy Acids, and Barberry extract. Super Oxide Dismutase liposome.

Skin, Hair & Nails Formula - Puritan's Pride
Three tablets contain: Vitamin A (as Retinyl Palmitate) 5000 IU • Vitamin C (as Ascorbic Acid) 60 mg • Vitamin D (as Cholecalciferol) 100 IU • Vitamin E (as d-Alpha Tocopheryl Acetate) 15 IU • Thiamin (Vitamin B-1; as Thiamine Hydrochloride) 5 mg • Riboflavin (Vitamin B-2) 5 mg • Niacin (as Niacinamide) 25 mg • Vitamin B-6 (as Pyridoxine Hydrochloride) 5 mg • Folic Acid 200 mcg • Vitamin B-12 (as Cyanocobalamin) 8 mcg • Biotin (as D-Biotin) 200 mcg • Pantothenic Acid (as D-Calcium Pantothentate) 15 mg • Calcium (as Dicalcium Phosphate and Calcium Carbonate) 834 mg • Iron (as Ferrous Gluconate) 3 mg • Phosphorus (as Dicalcium Phosphate) 331 mg • Iodine (as Potassium Iodide) 112.5 mcg • Magnesium (as Magnesium Oxide) 100 mg • Zinc (as Zinc Gluconate) 7.5 mg • Selenium (as L-Selenomethionine) 12.5 mg • Manganese (as Manganese Gluconate) 5 mg • Para-Aminobenzoic Acid 25 mg • Choline Bitartrate 75 mg • Inositol 30 mg • RNA 30 mg • Citrus Bioflavonoid 25 mg • Rutin 12.5 mg • Betaine Hydrochloride 25 mg • Rose Hips 60 mg.

Skin, Hair and Nails - Aspen Group, Inc.
Three tablets contain: Vitamin A 5000 IU • Vitamin C 60 mg • Vitamin B1 5 mg • Riboflavin 5 mg • Niacinamide 25 mg • Calcium 300 mg • Iron 3 mg • Vitamin D 100 IU • Vitamin E 15 IU • Vitamin B6 5 mg • Folic Acid 200 mcg • Vitamin B12 8 mcg • Phosphorus 150 mg • Iodine 112.5 mg • Magnesium 100 mg • Zinc 7.5 mg • Biotin 200 mcg • Pantothenic Acid 15 mg • Choline 75 mg • Inositol 30 mg • PABA 25 mg • Selenium 12.5 mcg • Manganese 5 mg • RNA 30 mg • Bioflavonoids 25 mg • Rutin 12.5 mg • Betaine HCl 25 mg • Horsetail Silica 50 mg.

Skin, Hair and Nails - Wellzymes - Enzymes, Inc.
Three capsules contain: Vitamin A (as Beta Carotene from Dunaliella Algae) 10,500 IU • Zinc (from Zinc Citrate) 15 mg • n-zimes Proprietary Enzyme Blend 75 mg: pHysioProtease (177,600 pHysio-U), CereCalase Plus • Proprietary Herbal Blend 450 mg: Calendula flower extract (standardized to contain 3% lutein), Bladderwrack Kelp extract (equivalent to 450 mg raw herb), Horsetail herb extract (equivalent to 300 mg raw herb), Oregon Grape root extract (equivalent to 240 mg raw herb), Safflower petals, Fo Ti root extract (equivalent to 150 mg raw herb), Rice Bran, Grape seed extract (standardized to contain 95% proanthocyanidins). Other Ingredients: Plant Cellulose, Water.

Skin, Hair, Nails - Natrol
Two capsules contain: Vitamin A (as Vitamin A palmitate) 5000 mg • Vitamin C (ascorbic acid) 100 mg • Vitamin E (as d-alpha tocopherol succinate) 50 IU • Thiamine (Vitamin B1) (as Thiamine HCI) 10 mg • Riboflavin (Vitamin B2) 10 mg • Vitamin B6 (pyridoxine HCI) 20 mg • Vitamin B12 (as cobalamin) 50 mcg • Biotin 500 mcg • Zinc (as zinc oxide) 8 mg • Copper (as amino acid chelate) 2 mg • Manganese (as manganese carbonate) 2 mg • MSM (methyl sulfonyl methane) 250 mg • Trace Mineral Complex 100 mg • Cysteine (as L-cysteine hydrochloride) 75 mg • PABA (para amino benzoic acid) 50 mg • Burdock root 50 mg • Choline (as choline bitartrate) 25 mg • Inositol 25 mg • Silicon (as colloidal silicon) 20 mg • Glutathione (as L-glutathione reduced) 2 mg. Other Ingredients: Rice powder, Magnesium Stearate, Gelatin.

Skindulgence 30-Minute Non-Surgical Facelift Cleanser - Skindulgence
Purified Water • Aloe Vera Gel • Caprylic/Capric Triglyceride • Butylene Glycol • Triethanolamine • Glyceryl Stearate • PEG-100 Stearate • Laureth 4 • Neopentyl Glycol Dicaprylate/Dicaprate • Stearic Acid • C12-15 Alkyl Benzoate • Glyceryl Stearate • Jojoba oil • Cetyl Palmitate • Glycereth-26 • Carbomer • Cyclomethicone • Skindulgence Herbal Blend: Butylene Glycol, Water, Hops extract (humulus lupulus), Rosemary extract (rosemarinum officinalis), Horsetail extract (equistetum arvense), Pine Cone extract (pinus sylvestris), Lemon extract (citrus medica limonum), Borage extract (borago officinalis), Spirulina Maxima extract • Propylene Glycol • Ginkgo Biloba extract • Leucine • Valine • Tyrosine • Arginine • Lysine • Cysteine • Cetyl Alcohol • Stearyl Alcohol • Allantoin • Urea • Tocopheryl Acetate (vitamin E) • Retinol Palmitate (vitamin A) • Jojoba Esters • Polysorbate 20 • Ammonium Lauryl Sulfate •

Tetrasodium EDTA • Diazolidinyl Urea • Methylparaben • Propylparaben • Fragrance.

Skindulgence 30-Minute Non-Surgical Facelift Mask **-** Skindulgence
Acacia Catechu • Purified Water • Aloe Vera Gel (from concentrate) • Corn Starch • Chondrus Crispus (carrageenan) • Polysorbate 20 • Skindulgence Herbal Blend: Butylene Glycol, Water, Hops extract (humulus lupus), Rosemary extract (rosemarinum officinalis), Horsetail extract (equisetum arvense), Pine Cone extract (pinus sylvestris), Lemon extract (citrus medica limonum), Borage extract (borago officinalis), Spirulina Maxima extract • Propylene Glycol • Ginkgo Biloba extract • Leucine • Valine • Tyrosine • Arginine • Lysine • Cysteine • TEA Lauryl Sulfate • Isoceceth-20 • Tetrasodium EDTA • Titanium Dioxide • Diazolidinyl Urea • Methylparaben • Fragrance.

Skindulgence 30-Minute Non-Surgical Facelift Moisturizer **-** Skindulgence
Purified Water • Aloe Vera Gel • Neopentyl Glycol Dicaprylate/Dicaprate • Jojoba oil • Caprylic/Capric Triglyceride • Cetyl Alcohol • Butylene Glycol • Glyceryl Stearate • PEG-100 Stearate • Cetyl Palmitate • Laureth 4 • Skindulgence Herbal Blend: Butylene Glycol, Water, Hops extract (humulus lupus), Rosemary extract (rosmarinus officinalis), Horsetail extract (equisetum arvense), Pine Cone extract (pinus sylvestris), Lemon extract (citrus medica limonum), Borage extract (borago officinalis), Spirulina Maxima extract • Propylene Glycol • Comfrey extract (symphytum officinale) • Plantain extract (plantago ovata) • Hydrolyzed Wheat Protein • Glutamine • Proline • Leucine • Serine • Tocopheryl Acetate (vitamin E) • Retinyl Palmitate (vitamin A) • Sodium Hyaluronate • Panthenol • Allantoin • Glycereth-26 • Glycerin • Carbomer • Triethanolamine • Polysorbate 80 • Xanthan Gum • Tetrasodium EDTA • Ammonium Lauryl Sulfate • Diazolidinyl Urea • Methylparaben • Propylparaben • Fragrance.

SkinGlow **-** NutriCology
Three softgels contain: Hyaluronic Acid powder (9% min. hyaluronic acid) 210 mg. Other Ingredients: Rice Bran Oil, Yellow Beeswax, Titanium Dioxide.

SkinZinc Cream **-** Selfworx
Active Ingredient: Salicylic Acid 2%. Inactive Ingredients: Water, Glyceryl Stearate SE, Propylene Glycol, Glycerin, Mineral oil, Stearic Acid, Ceteareth-20, Cetearyl Alcohol, DMDM Hydantoin, Methylparaben, Propylparaben, Melaleuca Alternifolia (tea tree) leaf oil, Tocopheryl Acetate, Medicago Sativa (alfalfa) extract, Arnica Montana flower extract, Sodium Hydroxide, Epilobium Angustifolium extract (willowherb).

SkinZinc Spray **-** Selfworx
Active Ingredient: Zinc Pyrithione 0.25%. Inactive Ingredients: Water, Glycerine, Propylene, Glycol, Epilobium Angustifolium Extract (Willowherb), Aloe Barbadensis leaf juice, Quarternarium 15.

Sleep Aid **-** nelsons - Nelson Bach USA Ltd.
Active Ingredients: Kali brom 30c HPUS • Coffea cruda 30c HPUS • Passiflora 30c HPUS • Avena 30c HPUS • Alfalfa 30c HPUS • Valeriana 30c HPUS. Inactive Ingredients: Lactose, Sucrose.
See Editor's Note No. 1, page 2053.

Sleep Ease **-** PhytoPharmica
Twenty drops contain: Secale cornutum 4x •Belladonna 3x • Avena sativa 1x • Passiflora incarnata 1x • Valeriana officinalis 1x. In a base of 40% USP alcohol by volume.
See Editor's Note No. 1 and No. 21, pages 2053 and 2056.

Sleep Enhance - Wellzymes **-** Enzymes, Inc.
Two capsules contain: n-zimes Proprietary Enzyme Blend 34 mg: pHysioProtease (94,720 pHysio-U), CereCalase Plus • Proprietary Herbal Blend 410 mg: Valerian root extract (equivalent to 800 mg raw herb), Passionflower herb extract (equivalent to 480 mg raw herb), Wild Lettuce leaf extract (equivalent to 160 mg raw herb), Oat Straw extract (equivalent to 300 mg raw herb), Rice Bran. Other Ingredients: Plant Cellulose, Water.

Sleep Formula **-** Preventive Nutrition
One capsule contains: Kava Kava Root Extract (Piper methysticum; 55% Kavalactones=49.5 mg) 90 mg • Griffonia Seed Extract (20% 5-Hydroxyl-L-Tryptophan=10mg) 50 mg • Melatonin (n-acetyl-5-Methoxytryptamine) 2 mg. Other Ingredients: Polyethylene Glycol, Gelatin, Glycerin, Chlorophyll, Titanium Dioxide (Natural Mineral Whitener).
See Editor's Note No. 16, page 2055.

Sleep Secret **-** SleepSecret
Coffea Cruda 6X • Valeriana Officinalis 6X • Passiflora Incarnata 6X • Magnesia Phosphorica 7X • Medicago Sativa 6X • Avena Sativa 6X. Base: 40% Glycerin, 0.3% Citric Acid, 0.3% Ascorbic Acid, Purified Water, Vanilla Flavoring.
See Editor's Note No. 1, page 2053.

Sleep-Assure **-** Nature's Plus
Each tablet contains: Rapid Release Layer: Melatonin (N-Acetyl-5-Methoxytryptamine) 1.5 mg • GABA (Gamma Aminobutyric Acid) 10 mg • Pyridoxal-5-Phosphate (P5P) 10 mg. Sustained Release Layer: Melatonin (N-Acetyl-5-Methoxytryptamine) 1.5 mg • Herbal Blend containing equal proportions of: [Kava Kava root extract (Piper methysticum) standardized 29-31% kavalactones], Passion Flower extract (Passiflora incarnata) standardized 3.5-4% flavonoids calculated as isovitexin, Valerian root extract (Valeriana officinalis) standardized 1% Valerenic Acid, Chamomile flower (Matricaria recutita) standardized 1% Apigenin 0.5% essential oil] 25 mg.
See Editor's Note No. 16, page 2055.

Sleep-N-Slim **-** Euro Botanicals
L-Glutamine • L-Lysine HCl • Magnesium Citrate • L-Ornithine Glysine • L-Arginine • Collagen • Vitamin B6 (pyridoxine HCl) • L-Carnitine • Vitamin B3 (niacin) • Aloe Vera • Ascorbic Acid • Citric Acid • Sodium Benzoate • Potassium Sorbate • Carrageenan.

SleepRite **-** 4 Life
Each capsule contains: Vitamin B6 (as pyridoxine HCl) 15 mg • Melatonin 2.5 mg • 5-Hydroxytryptophan (Griffonia simplicitolia, seed) 30 mg • Proprietary Blend 215 mg: Valerian (.8% valerinic acid, rood), Kava Kava extract (root), Scullcap (whole herb), Hops (aerial parts), Chamomile (aerial parts).

Sleep-Tite **-** Wellness International Network, Ltd.
Two capsules contain: Herbal Blend (equivalent to 3330 mg of whole herbs) 790 mg: European Valerian root 4:1 extract, Celery seed 4:1 extract, Hops strobile 4:1 extract, Passion flower 4:1 extract, California Poppy 5:1 extract, Chamomile flower 5:1 extract, Chinese Fu Ling 5:1 extract (poria cocos), Kava Kava root 5:1 extract, Feverfew 5:1 extract, Skullcap. Other Ingredients: Dicalcium Phosphate, Micorcrystalline Cellulose, Croscarmellose Sodium, Stearic Acid, Silica, Magnesium Stearate, Sugar Coat (calcium sulfate, sucrose, kaolin, talc, gelatin, shellac, titanium dioxide, anise oil, beeswax, carnauba wax).

Sleepytime Extra **-** Celestial Seasonings
Two capsules contain: Calcium (as carbonate, citrate, and malate) 200 mg • Magnesium (as oxide) 100 mg • Proprietary Blend 800 mg: Valerian (root), Valerian (standardized extract), Kava Kava (root), Kava Kava (standardized extract). Other Ingredients: May contain one or more of the following: Dicalcium phosphate, gelatin, rice flour, stearic acid, spearmint extract, magnesium stearate, and silicon dioxide.

Slender Shaper **-** Pharmagel
E-L-A Complex.

Slender-Mist **-** KareMor International
Vitamin B6 • Pantothenic Acid • Chromium • Hydroxy-Citric Acid • L-Carnitine. Available in Arctic Mint, Berry Supreme, chocolate Fudge, and Tropical Delite.

Some Brand Name Natural Products - What they Contain

www.NaturalDatabase.com contains MANY more listings than appear here.

Slim 7 **-** Swanson
Two tablets contain: Vitamin A (as retinyl palmitate) 1667 IU • Vitamin C (as ascorbic acid) 20 mg • Vitamin E (as d-alpha tocopheryl succinate) 10 IU • Riboflavin (vitamin B-2) 0.6 mg • Niacin 6.6 mg • Vitamin B-6 (as pyridoxine HCl) 0.66 mg • Folic Acid 133.3 mcg • Vitamin B-12 (as cyanocobalamin) 2 mcg • Biotin 100 mcg • Iodine (from kelp) 50 mcg • Selenium (as selenomethionine) 16.6 mcg • Chromium (from Chromax® chromium picolinate) 375 mcg • Chromium (from chromium polynicotinate) 375 mcg • CitriMax™ (Garcinia cambogia fruit extract) 500 mg, (-) Hydroxycitric Acid 250 mg • Proprietary blend of 72 Trace Minerals 200 mg • L-Carnitine (as tartrate) 100 mg • Choline (as choline bitartrate) 67 mg • Green Tea extract (20% polyphenols) 50 mg • Kola Nut extract 50 mg • Capsicum 33.3 mg • Chitosan 33.3 mg • Ginger 33.3 mg • Inositol 33.3 mg • Spirulina 33.3 mg • Betaine HCl 8 mg.

Slim Down Apple Cider Vinegar **-** Jamieson
Each tablet contains: Apple Cider Vinegar Concentrate 500 mg.

Slim Down Bar **-** Jamieson
Each bar contains: Vitamin A 175 RE • Vitamin D 0.44 mcg • Vitamin C (Ascorbic Acid) 8.75 mg • Vitamin E (D-Alpha Acetate) 1.75 mg • Vitamin B1 245 mcg • Vitamin B2 315 mcg • Vitamin B6 315 mcg • Vitamin B12 0.525 mcg • Vitamin B3 1.5 NE • Vitamin B5 1.5 mg • Biotin 21 mcg • Calcium 306 mg • Phosphorus 175 mg • Iron 1.75 mg • Iodide 26.25 mcg • Magnesium 70 mg • Copper 0.26 mg • Zinc 2.45 mg • Manganese 0.79 mg • Selenium (Chelate) 7 mcg • Chromium (Chelate) 7 mcg • Molybdenum (Citrate) 14 mcg • Phaseolamin 2250 tm 100 mg.

Slim Down Carb & Fat Burner **-** Jamieson
Each capsule contains: CitraMax 50% HCA (Hydroxycitric Acid) 125 mg • Advantra Z Citrus Aurantium 125 mg • Kola Nut JKN-10 5 mg. See Editor's Note No. 40, page 2058.

Slim Down CLA 75 - Conjugated Linoleic Acid **-** Jamieson
Each capsule contains: Conjugated Linoleic Acid (pure isometric form) 1000 mg.

Slim Down GTF Chromium 200 mcg **-** Jamieson
Each tablet contains: Chromium (from brewer's yeast) 200 mcg.

Slim Down Natural Source Fibre **-** Jamieson
Each caplet contains: Dietary Fiber (derived from oat grains) 0.5 g.

Slim Essence **-** DreamPharm
Each capsule contains: Senna leaf 150 mg • Persimmon leaf 150 mg • Papaya leaf 100 mg • Orange peel 100 mg • Licorice root 50 mg • Chromium Picolinate 50 mcg.

Slim Form Diet Patch **-** Long Life Services, Inc.
Each 5x5 cm patch contains: Marine Algae • Mannitol • Chlorides • Potassium • Sodium • Magnesium • Amino Acids • Calcium • Glucose • Phosphates • Fucose. The glue contains: Natural Rubber, Natural Lanolin, Natural Parrafin (liquid), Zinc Oxide, Natural Resin.

Slim Smart **-** Health Center for Better Living
Chromium Picolinate 200 mcg; other herbs.

Slim Trim **-** Life Extension
L-Arginine 500 mg • L-Ornithine 250 mg.

Slimmer **-** Dr. Roopas Herbal System
Each capsule contains: Propietary Formula 250 mg: Powder of Cassia Angustifolia, Cinnamomum Tamala, Garcinia Cambogia, Balsamodendron Mukul.

Slimming Formula **-** PhytoPharmica
Each tablet contains: Thyroidinum 8x • Antimonium crudum 3x • Calcarea acetica 2x • Fucus vesiculosus 2x.
See Editor's Note No. 1 and No. 21.

SlimPro **-** HealthMinded
Four capsules contain: Vitamin C 100 mg • Vitamin B6 10 mg • Pantothenic Acid 12 mg • Magnesium 10 mg • Chromium 300 mcg • Garcinia Cambogia extract 200 mg • L-Tyrosine 200 mg • Cocoa extract 200 mg • L-Carnitine Fumarate 120 mg • Theobromine 100 mg • Dimethylaminoethanol (DMAE) 24 mg • SlimPro Proprietary Blend 200 mg: Green Tea extract (decaffeinated, 50% polyphenols), D/L Methionine, Ginger root extract, Quercetin, Bitter Orange extract, White Willow bark extract, Grape seed extract (95% OPC). Other Ingredients: Stearic Acid, Magnesium Stearate.
See Editor's Note No. 40, page 2058.

SlimTrax Forte **-** Pharmessen
Each tablet contains: Proprietary Blend 800 mg: Clove oil (eugenia caryophyllata, leaf), Cinnamon leaf oil (cinnamomum zeylonicum), Olive oil, Microcrystalline Cellulose, Hypromellose, Cab-o-sil, Talcum, Magnesium Stearate.

Slim-Trim **-** Life Extension
Each tablet contains: L-Arginine 500 mg • L-Ornithine 250 mg • Glutathione Peroxidase 600 mg.

Slippery Elm Original Lozenges **-** Thayers Natural Pharmaceuticals
Each lozenge contains: Slippery Elm Bark 150 mg. A soothing base of a natural plant derived sweetener derived from Corn, with Vegetable Stearate as a binder.

Slippery Elm Original Lozenges, Sugar-Free **-** Thayers Natural Pharmaceuticals
Each lozenge contains: Slippery Elm Bark 150 mg. A soothing base of sugar-free Sorbitol (a natural sugar-free sweetener derived from plums, pears, berries, and cherries) with Vegetable Stearate as a binder.

Slippery Elm Tangerine Lozenges with Rose Hips **-** Thayers Natural Pharmaceuticals
Each lozenge contains: Slippery Elm Bark 150 mg • Rose Hips 20 mg • Vitamin C 15 mg. Other Ingredients: Ascorbic Acid. A natural Tangerine flavor in a soothing base of a natural plant derived sweetener derived from Corn, with Vegetable Stearate as a binder.

Slo-Niacin **-** Upsher-Smith Laboratories
Each tablet contains: Niacin 500 mg. Other Ingredients: Cellulose Polymer Derivative, Vegetable Stearine, Magnesium Stearate, Silicon Dioxide, Glyceryl Behenate, FD&C Red #40.

Slow Fe **-** Novartis
Each tablet contains: Dried Ferrous Sulfate USP (160 mg), USP (equivalent to 50 mg). Inactive Ingredients: Cetostearyl Alcohol, Hydroxypropyl Methylcellulose, Lactose, Magnesium Stearate, Polysorbate 80, Talc, Titanium Dioxide, Yellow Iron Oxide, FD&C Blue 32 Aluminum Lake.

Slow-Mag **-** Roberts
Two tablets contain: Calcium (from calcium carbonate) 212 mg • Magnesium 128 mg & Chloride 373 mg (from magnesium chloride hexahydrate) • Cellulose Acetate Phthalate • Pregelatinized Starch • Povidone • Diethylphthalate • Talc • Titanium Dioxide • Magnesium Stearate & FD&C Blue No. 2 Lake.

Slumber **-** Nutrivention
Two tablets contain: Calcium (Amino Acid Chelate) 500 mg • Magnesium (Amino Acid Chelate) 500 mg • Inositol 200 mg • Niacinamide 20 mg • Biotin 100 mcg • Passion flower 200 mg • Blue Vervain 200 mg • Hops 100 mg • Valerian root (Star root) 100 mg • Wild Lettuce 100 mg.

Slumber EZ **-** Bios Biochemicals
Three capsules contain: Thiamin (as thiamin mononitrate) 30 mg • Riboflavin 30 mg • Niacin 30 mg • Vitamin B6 (as pyridoxal 5-phosphate) 15 mg • Magnesium (as magnesium chelate) 90 mg • Molybdenum (as molybdenum chelate) 300 mcg • Proprietary Blend

2160 mg: Glycine, L-Lysine HCl, L-Serine, GABA, Trimethylglycine, 5-HTP. Other Ingredients: Gelatin Capsule, Magnesium Stearate.

SlumberActin **-** Nature's Plus
Three capsules contain: Chamomile [(Matricaria recutita root) standardized 1% Apigenin, 0.5% Essential oil] 200 mg • Valerian [(Valeriana officinalis root) standardized 1% Valernic Acids] 100 mg • Passion Flower [(Passiflora incarnata flower) standardized 3.5-4% Flavonoids] 75 mg • Hops [(Humulus lupulus fruit) standardized 5.2% Bitter Acids, 4% Flavonoids] 75 mg • Kava Kava [(Piper methysticum root) standardized 29-31% Kavalactones] 50 mg • English Hawthorne [(Crataegus laevigata berry) standardized 3.2% Vitexin] 50 mg • Magnesium (Amino Acid Chelate) 50 mg • Calcium (Amino Acid Chelate) 25 mg.

Smart Coffee w/ Ginkgo Biloba **-** Nature's Plus
Each 3 g serving contains: Instant herbal coffee blend: naturally decaffeinated Brazilian coffee (coffea) • Ginkgo Biloba (standardized 24% ginkgo flavone-glycosides, 6% terpene lactones) • Rosemary (Rosmarinus officinalis) • Fo-Ti (Polygonum multiflorum) • Mahonia Aquifolium (wild grape, standardized 95-100% leucoanthocyanidins) • Chinese Apricot (Prunus armeniaca).

Smart Longevity **-** E'OLA
Ten drops contain: Vitamin C (as ascorbic acid) 16 mg • Vitamin E (as dl-alpha tocopheryl acetate) 7 IU • Proprietary Blend 324 mg: Choline Bitartrate, Dimethylaminoethanol Bitartrate, Siberian Ginseng (root), Schizandra (berry), Ginkgo Biloba (leaf). Other Ingredients: Water, Hydrochloric Acid, Sodium Benzoic Acid.

Smart Pill **-** Only Natural, Inc.
Two tablets contain: Ginkgo Biloba leaf extract 10:1 250 mg • Gotu Kola 250 mg • Ginseng 100 mg • Capsicum 50 mg • L-Phenylalanine 200 mg • L-Glutamine 500 mg • L-Tyrosine 200 mg • GABA 300 mg • Vitamin B1 50 mg • Vitamin B3 50 mg • Vitamin B5 100 mg • Vitamin B6 50 mg • Vitamin B12 500 mcg • Folic Acid 200 mcg • Inositol 100 mg • Phosphatidylcholine 500 mg • RNA 100 mg • TMG 50 mg.

Smart Vitamins **-** Jamieson
Each capsule contains: Choline Bitartrate • Molasses cone • L-Glutamine • Brewers Yeast (a natural source of the B complex vitamin family) • Acerola (a natural source of Vitamin C) • Taurine • Kola Nut • Korean Ginseng • Vegetable Magnesium Stearate • Wheat Germ Powder • Silica • Chromium Yeast • Turnera (Damiana aphrodesiaca) • Capsicum (Cayenne) • Ginkgo Biloba • Fo-Ti (Polygonum multiflorum).

Smart Vitamins - Phosphatidyl **-** Jamieson
Each capsule contains: Phosphatidyl Serine 10 mg • Phosphatidyl Choline (Derived from Pure Soy Lechtin) 9 mg • Omega 3 DHA (Derived from North Atlantic Fresh Fish Oil) 3 mg.

Smoke Away Formula 1 **-** The Council On Natural Health
Six tablets contain: Vitamin C (as ascorbic acid) 316 mg • Iron (as ferrous fumarate) 2.4 mg • Iodine (from kelp) 192 mcg • Sodium (as sodium chloride) 25 mg • Proprietary Blend 4000 mg: Alfalfa leaf, Licorice root, Siberian Ginseng root, Cayenne pepper (40,000 scoville heat units), Dandelion root, Echinacea Purpurea (aerial parts), Ginger root, Peppermint leaf, Sarsaparilla root, Buckthorn bark, Burdock root, Hyssop (aerial parts), Lobelia leaf, Passionflower (plant, flower), Cascara Sagrada bark, Oregon Grape root, Barley Grass, Bayberry bark, Golden Seal (aerial parts), Lemon Verbena leaf, Ox bile extract, Safflower seed oil, Elderberry fruit 10:1 extract, Bioperine standardized Black Pepper extract (96-97% piperine). Other Ingredients: Dicalcium Phosphate, Microcrystalline Cellulose, Croscarmellose Sodium, Stearic Acid, Silica, Magnesium Stearate, Pharmaceutical Glaze.
See Editor's Note No. 14.

Smoke Away Formula 2 **-** The Council On Natural Health
Two tablets contain: Vitamin C (as ascorbic acid) 250 mg • Vitamin E (as dl-alpha-tocopheryl acetate) 30 IU • Pantothenic Acid (as d-calcium pantothenate) 10 mg • Selenium (as sodium selenite) 50 mcg • Long Health Blend 250 mg: Red Clover flower, Gotu Kola leaf, Burdock root • L-Glutamine 100 mg • MSM (methylsulfonylmethane) 100 mg • Korean Ginseng root (4% ginsenosides) 100 mg • Milk Thistle seed 100 mg • N-Acetyl-L-Cysteine 50 mg • Smoke Away Blend 100 mg: Rosemary (aerial parts), Thyme leaf, Black Cumin seed • Wild Jujube seed extract 50 mg • 5-HTP 50 mg • Lemon Verbena leaf 25 mg • Quercetin Dihydrate 25 mg. Other Ingredients: Dicalcium Phosphate, Microcrystalline Cellulose, Croscarmellose Sodium, Stearic Acid, Calcium Silicate, Silica, Magnesium Stearate, Pharmaceutical Glaze.

Smoke Free **-** Boericke & Tafel
Each tablet contains: Caladium Seguinum 6X • Daphne Indica 6X • Graphite 12X • Valeriana Officinalis 6X • Lactose (HPU S).
See Editor's Note No. 1, page 2053.

SmokeAway Natural Homeopathic Medicine **-** The Council On Natural Health
Three pellets contain: Tabacum (tobacco) 5C-7C-9C • Lobelia Inflata (Indian tobacco) 5C • Cadmium Sulphuricum (cadmium sulphate) 5C • Nux Vomica (poison nut) 5C • Antimonium Crudum (antimony sulphide) 5C • Caladium Seguinum (American arum) 5C.
See Editor's Note No. 1, page 2053.

Smoke-Less **-** The Herbalist
Lobelia leaf • Milk Thistle seed • Oat seed • Siberian Ginseng root • Licorice root.

Smooth Food 2 **-** New Chapter, Inc.
Three capsules contain: Okra fruit 201 mg • Slippery Elm bark 201 mg • Psyllium husk 159 mg • Licorice root 159 mg • Ginger (rhizome) 159 mg • Marshmallow root 120 mg • Wheat Grass 21 mg • Bio Flora (TM) (100 million probiotic live cells per teaspoon) 21 mg • Chlorella regularis 6 mg • Cayenne fruit 3 mg. Other Ingredients: Vegetable cellulose.

Smooth Move **-** Traditional Medicinals
Sennosides A & B: 20 mg per cup as they naturally occur in Senna leaf (Casala angustifolia) present in the blend. Other Herbal Ingredients: Licorice root, Fennel seed, Orange peel, Cinnamon bark, Coriander seed, Ginger rhizome, natural Orange flavor.

SneezEze **-** EuroPharma
Active Ingredient: Kali Bichromicum (potassium bichromate) 3x. Inactive Ingredient: Cellulose.
See Editor's Note No. 1, page 2053.

Snooze **-** Pacific BioLogic
Valerian root • Dragon Bone (fossilized) • Oyster Shell (untreated) • Mimosa Tree flower • Chamomile • Gotu Kola • Hops • Polygala root • Jujube seed (sour) • Passion flower • Scullcap • Melatonin 1.5 mg per capsule.
See Editor's Note No. 26, page 2056.

Snoreless **-** Nutrition for Life International
Three sprays (approx. 3 mL) contains: Vitamin C 4.5 mg • Vitamin E 7.5 mg • Vitamin B6 3 mg • Olive Oil 210 mg • Sunflower Oil 90 mg • Peppermint Oil 60 mg • Almond Oil 37.5 mg • Sesame Oil 30 mg. Other Ingredients: Purified Water, Glycerine.

SnoreMD **-** Long Life, Inc.
Each caplet contains: Calcium (as dicalcium phosphate) 105 mg • Phosphorus (as dicalcium phosphate) • Proprietary Blend 415 mg: Protease, Amylase, Lipase, Cellulase, Acerola fruit concentarate, Cayenne fruit, Fenugreek seed, Echinacea, Red Clover (aerial part), Yarrow flowers, Eucalyptus leaf, Elderberry flower/fruit. Other Ingredients: Croscarmellose Sodium, Magnesium Stearate, Microcrystalline Cellulose, Polyvinylpyrrolidone, Silica.

Snorenz **-** MedGen, Inc.
Peppermint Oil • Sunflower Oil • Sesame Oil • Olive Oil • Almond Oil.

Some Brand Name Natural Products - What they Contain

www.NaturalDatabase.com contains MANY more listings than appear here.

SnoreStop **-** The Green Pharmacy
Each tablet contains: Nux vomica 4X • Nux vomica 6X • Belladonna 6X • Ephedra vulgaris 6X • Hydrastis canadensis 6X • Kali bichromicum 6X • Teucrium marum 6X • Histaminum hydrochloricum 12X.
See Editor's Note No. 1, page 2053.

Snuffadelic **-** Unknown
Unknown.
See Editor's Note No. 49, page 2059.

Soft Gelatin Multiple **-** Nature's Life
Two capsules contain: Beta Carotene (Vitamin A equivalent 15000 IU) 9 mg • Vitamin A (Fish Liver oil) 10000 IU • Vitamin D (as Vitamin D3) (Cholecalciferol) 400 IU • Vitamin E (d-Alpha Tocopherol) 400 IU • Vitamin C 300 mg • Rose Hips 20 mg • Folic Acid 400 mcg • Vitamin B1 (Thiamine Mononitrate) 50 mg • Vitamin B2 (Riboflavin) 50 mg • Niacinamide 50 mg • Vitamin B6 (Pyridoxine HCl) 50 mg • Vitamin B12 (Cyanocobalamin) 100 mcg • Biotin (d-Biotin) 300 mcg • Pantothenic Acid (d-Calcium Pantothenate) 50 mg • Choline (Bitartrate) 25 mg • Inositol 25 mg • PABA (Para Aminobenzoic Acid) 25 mg • Boron (Calcium Boron Gluconate) 25 mcg • Calcium (Carbonate, Citrate, Aspartate) 200 mg • Chromium (Nutrition 21 Picolinate) 25 mcg • Copper (Gluconate) 2 mg • Iodine (Potassium Iodide) 150 mcg • Iron (Peptonate) 10 mg • Magnesium (Magnesium Oxide) 100 mg • Manganese (Amino Acid Chelate) 15 mg • Molybdenum (Free-Form Amino Acid Chelate) 25 mcg • Potassium (Phosphate & Iodide) 15 mg • Selenium (l-Selenomethionine, yeast-free) 15 mcg • Silicon Dioxide 20 mg • Vanadium (Vanadyl Sulfate) 25 mcg • Zinc (Citrate, Gluconate, Picolinate) 15 mg • Essential Fatty Acids (Safflower oil) 540 mg.

Soft Tissue **-** Enzymes, Inc.
Each capsule contains: Vitamin C (100% from Acerola Cherries) 17 mg • Proprietary Herbal Blend 215 mg: Bladderwrack kelp extract, Quercetin, Tumeric root extract, Cramp bark extract, Corydalis root extract, Grape seed extract • Proprietary Enzyme Blend 227 mg: pHsyioProtease, Peptidase, Bromelain. Other Ingredients: Plant Cellulose, Water.

Solae brand **-** DuPont
Isolated Soy Protein.
See Editor's Note No. 44, page 2058.

Solar Water **-** Unknown
Unknown.
See Editor's Note No. 49, page 2059.

Solaray Continence with Flowtrol **-** Nutraceutical Corp.
Each two capsules contain: Butterbur root extract (Petasites hybridus) (Guaranteed to contain 15 mg sesquiterpenes) 100 mg • Flowtrol Prorietary Blend 870 mg: Cranberry berry extract (Vaccinium macrocarpon as CranActin Cranberry AF Extract), Morinda root extract 5:1, Psoralea fruit extract 5:1, Raspberry fruit extract 5:1 (Rubus chingii), Alpinia oxyphylla fruit and seed extract 5:1, Lobelia (aerial). Inactive Ingredients: Gelatin (capsule), Cellulose, Maltodextrin, Magnesium Stearate, Silica, Magnesium Hydroxide.

Solaray Cordyceps 520 mg **-** Nutraceutical Corp.
Each capsule contains: Cordyceps 520 mg.Inactive Ingredients: Gelatin, Cellulose, & Magnesium stearate.

Solaray DopaBean 333 mg **-** Nutraceutical Corp.
Each capsule contains: Velvet Bean seed extract (Mucuna pruriens) 333 mg • Catecholamines 66 mg • L-dopa 50 mg. Inactive Ingredients: Gelatin (capsule), Rice Flour, Maltodextrin, Magnesium Stearate, Silica, Alpha Galactosidase.

Solaray GP Cordyceps **-** Nutraceutical Corp.
Each two capsules contain: Cordyceps (Cordyceps sinensis) 520 mg.Inactive Ingredients: Gelatin (capsule), Cellulose, Magnesium.

Solaray Indole-3-Carbinol **-** Nutraceutical Corp.
Each capsule contains: Vitamin C (as ascorbic acid) 200 mg • Broccoli 50 mg • Brussel Sprouts 50 mg • Cabbage 50 mg • Cauliflower 50 mg • Kale 50 mg • Indole-3-Carbinol (I3C) 25 mg. Inactive Ingredients: Gelatin (capsule), Magnesium Stearate.

Solaray Pure CoQ-10 **-** Nutraceutical Corp.
Each capsule contains: Coenzyme Q-10 30 mg. Inactive Ingredients: Cellulose, Gelatin (capsule).

Solaray Pure CoQ10-30 **-** Nutraceutical Corp.
Each capsule contains: Coenzyme Q-10 30 mg. Inactive Ingredients: Cellulose, Gelatin.

Solaray Pygeum and Saw Palmetto **-** Nutraceutical Corp.
Each six capsules contain: Vitamin B-6 (as pyridoxine HCl) 20 mg • Zinc (as optizinc) 15 mg • Cranberry extract 800 mg • Saw Palmetto berry oil 320 mg • Pygeum bark extract 100 mg. Inactive Ingredients: Gelatin, Cellulose, Pumpkin Seed, L-Glycerine, Glutamic Acid, L-Alanine, Magnesium Stearate.

Solaray Spectro 3 **-** Nutraceutical Corp.
Each three tablets contain: Vitamin A (from Retinyl Palmitate, and 60% as natural Beta Carotene [Dunaliella salina algae]) 25000 IU • Vitamin C (as natural Ascorbic acid, Rose Hips, Acerola cherry) 1000 mg • Vitamin D (as Cholecalciferol D-3) 400 IU • Vitamin E (as natural d-Alpha Tocopheryl Succinate, d-Alpha Tocopheryl Acetate) 400 IU • Vitamin K 50 mcg • Thiamin (as Thiamine Mononitrate) (Vitamin B1) 25 mg • Riboflavin (Vitamin B2) 25 mg • Niacin (as Niacinamide) 125 mg • Vitamin B6 (as Pyridoxine HCl) 50 mg • Folic Acid 400 mcg • Vitamin B12 (as Cyanocobalamin) 100 mcg • Biotin 300 mcg • Pantothenic Acid (as d-Calcium Pantothenate) 125 mg • Calcium (as Calcium Carbonate, Calcium Amino Acid Chelate) 500 mg • Iron (as Iron Fumarate, Iron Amino Acid Chelate) 18 mg • Phosphorous (as Potassium Phosphate) 23 mg • Iodine (from Kelp) 225 mcg • Magnesium (Magnesium Oxide, Magnesium Amino Acid Chelate) 250 mg • Zinc (as Zinc Citrate, Zinc Picolinate, Zinc Amino Acid Chelate) 15 mg • Selenium (as yeast free I-Selenomethionine) 100 mcg • Copper (as Copper Amino Acid Chelate) 0.5 mg • Potassium (as Potassium Phosphate, Potassium Chloride) 88 mg • Choline Bitartrate 50 mg • Inositol 50 mg • PABA (Para-Aminobenzoic Acid) 30 mg • Lecithin 50 mg • Bioflavonoid concentrate (from Citrus) 150 mg • Rutin concentrate 50 mg • Hesperidin concentrate 50 mg • Pectin 25 mg • Boron (as Tetra-Boron: Boron Citrate, Boron Glycinate, Boron Aspartate, Boron Lysinate) 1.5 mg • Spirulina (Spirulina platensis) 50 mg • Alfalfa juice (aerial) 125 mg • Carrot and Yam concentrate 100 mg • Barley Grass juice concentrate 75 mg • Rosemary leaf extract 25 mg • Aloe Vera gel concentrate 200x (equivalent to 400 mg) 2 mg • Parsley leaf 50 mg • Pancreatin 4x (equivalent to 120 mg) 30 mg • Diatase 20 mg • Papain (from Papaya) 50 mg • Ox Bile extract 20 mg • Glutamic Acid HCl 50 mg • Propolis 2x (equivalent to 50 mg) 25 mg • Royal Jelly 3.5x (equivalent to 14 mg) 4 mg • Bee Pollen. Inactive Ingredients: Cellulose, Stearic Acid, Silica, Siberian Ginseng root, Calcium Phosphate, Whole Rice concentrate, Alfalfa herb, Montmorillonite Clay, Maltodextrin, Natural flavors and Natural food glazed coating.
See Editor's Note No. 14.

Solaray ViraMax **-** Nutraceutical Corp.
Each two capsules contain: Catuaba 500 mg • Yohimbe bark extract (supplying 10 mg of yohimbine) 500 mg • Muira Puama root 250 mg • Peruvian Maca root extract (4:1) 100 mg.

Sollievo **-** Aboca USA, Inc
Each tablet contains: Senna leaf powder (cassia angustifolia, standardized to 2.5% sennosides) 122 mg • Cape Aloe juice (aloe ferox, standardized to 18% aloin A+B) 91.7 mg • Certified Organic Dandelion root powder (taraxacum officinale) 91 mg • Chicory root powder (cichorium intybus) 32 mg • Fennel fruit powder (foeniculum vulgare) 27 mg • Caraway fruit powder (carum carvi) 23 mg • Boldo leaf powder (peumus boldus) 7 mg • Cumin fruit powder (cuminum cyminum) 6 mg. Other Ingredients: Essential Oil of Fennel.

Solo Day Multi Vitamin **-** GNC
Each tablet contains: Vitamin A (29% as beta-carotene, 80% as acetate) 5000 IU • Vitamin C (as ascorbic acid) 60 mg • Vitamin D (as ergocalciferol) 400 IU • Vitamin E (as d-alpha tocopheryl acetate) 30 IU • Vitamin K (as phytonadione) 25 mcg • Thiamin (as thiamin mononitrate) 1.5 mg • Riboflavin 1.7 mg • Niacin (as niacinamide) 20 mg • Vitamin B6 (as pyridoxine hydrochloride) 2 mg • Folate, Folic Acid, Folacin 400 mcg • Vitamin B12 (as cyanocobalamin) 6 mcg • Biotin 30 mcg • Pantothenic Acid (as calcium d-pantothenate) 10 mg • Calcium (as dicalcium phosphate and calcium carbonate) 162 mg • Iron (as ferrous fumarate) 18 mg • Phosphorus (as dicalcium phosphate) 109 mg • Iodine (as potassium iodide) 150 mcg • Magnesium (as magnesium oxide) 100 mg • Zinc (as zinc oxide) 15 mg • Selenium (as sodium selenate) 20 mcg • Copper (as cupric oxide) 2 mg • Manganese (as manganese sulfate) 2 mg • Chromium (as chromium chloride) 120 mcg • Molybdenum (as sodium molybdate) 75 mcg • Chloride (as potassium chloride) 72 mg • Potassium (as potassium chloride) 80 mg • Nickel (as nickel sulfate) 5 mcg • Tin (as stannous chloride) 10 mcg • Vanadium (as sodium meta vanadate) 10 mcg • Boron (as sodium borate) 150 mcg • Silica (as silicon dioxide) 2 mg • Lycopene 300 mcg. Other Ingredients: Cellulose, Vegetable Acetoglycerides, Artificial Color (FD&C Yellow #6), Titanium Dioxide.

Solovites **-** Puritan's Pride
Each tablet contains: Vitamin A 10,000 IU • Vitamin C 200 mg • Vitamin D 400 IU • Vitamin E 30 IU • Thiamin 30 mg • Riboflavin 30 mg • Niacin 30 mg • Vitamin B-6 30 mg • Folic Acid 400 mcg • Vitamin B-12 30 mcg • Biotin 30 mcg • Pantothenic Acid 30 mg • Calcium 60 mg • Iron 18 mg • Phosphorus 30 mg • Iodine 150 mcg • Magnesium 30 mg • Zinc 30 mg • Selenium 25 mcg • Copper 0.5 mg • Manganese 0.6 mg • Chromium 25 mcg • Molybdenum 25 mcg • Potassium 11 mg • PABA (Para-Aminobenzoic Acid) 30 mg • Choline Bitartrate 30 mg • Inositol 30 mcg • Citrus Bioflavonoid complex 25 mg • Betaine Hydrochloride 25 mg. In a base of Alfalfa, Parsley, Oyster Shell, Watercress, Kelp, and Lecithin.

Soluble Enzyme Caps **-** Atrium Inc.
Each capsule contains: Papayotin 110 mg • Pancreatin (Bovine) 90 mg • Calf Thymus (Bovine) 50 mg • Bromelain 50 mg • Lipase 10 mg • Chymotrypsin 15 mg. Lemon flavor.
See Editor's Note No. 14.

Solu-Min **-** Aspen Group, Inc.
Calcium • Phosphorus • Magnesium • Potassium • Sulfur • Iron • Iodine • Copper • Cobalt • Zinc • Chromium • Manganese • Molybdenum • Selenium • Aluminum • Antimony • Barium • Bismuth • Cadmium • Sodium • Cesium • Carbon • Lithium • Nickel • Platinum • Rubidium • Silver • Strontium • Silicon • Tungsten • Tin • Titanium • Tantalum • Thorium • Vanadium • Zirconium • Yttrium. Plus up to 30 other randomly occurring trace minerals in natural combinations.

Somnolin **-** Metagenics
Each tablet contains: L-5 Hydroxytryptophan (L-5-HTP from griffonia simplicifolia) 100 mg • Theanine 100 mg • Vitamin B6 20 mg • Vitamin B12 (as methylcobalamin) 250 mcg • L-5-Methyl Tetrahydrofolate 200 mcg.

Sore Throat Lozenge **-** Jamieson
Each lozenge contains: Slippery Elm bark 50 mg • White Horehound leaves 50 mg • Parsley root 20 mg • Thyme leaves 10 mg • Menthol 5 mg. Other Ingredients: Camphor 50 mcg, Acerola Cherry 40 mg, Sugar, Glucose, Honey, Anise Oil, and natural flavors.

Source of Life Oxygenic **-** Nature's Plus
Three tablets contain: Mixed Wild Berry extract 300 mg: European Red Wine Grape, Bilberry, Blackberry, Black Raspberry, & Red Raspberry (standardized 20% Polyphenols, 4% Anthocyanosides) • Chinese Green Tea extract (standardized 20% Polyphenols) 300 mg • Horseradish concentrate 250 mg • Vitamin C fortified with Rose Hips, Mango, Guava & West Indian Cherry 100 mg • Beta Carotene (Dunaliella salina, Carrot) 2500 IU • Wild Grape seed extract standardized 95-100% Leucoanthocyanins 10 mg • Pycnogenol (Pine bark extract) standardized 85-95% Proanthocyanidins 5 mg. In a whole food base of Broccoli, Spinach, Cauliflower & Beet Greens.

Source of Life Vibra-Gest **-** Nature's Plus
Each vegicap contains: Brown rice fermentation: Amylase, 30000 units/gram 50 mg • Lactase, 1000 units/gram 50 mg • Lipase, 5000 units/gram 50 mg • Cellulase, 5000 units/gram 30 mg • Protease, 100000 units/gram 20 mg • Oxidase, 5000 units/gram 10 mg • Barley malt: Diastase, 1000 units/gram 10 mg • Maltase, 1000 units/gram 10 mg • Sweet potato: Phosphatase, 4000 units/gram 5 mg • Pineapple: Bromelain, 600 GDU/gram 35 mg • Papaya: Papain, 2 million units/gram 30 mg • Carrot powder: Lactobacillus acidophilus 4 billion viable cells/gram 100 mg • Natural cultures: Bifidobacterium longum 1 billion viable cells/gram 50 mg • Lactobacillus bulgaricus 1 billion viable cells/gram 50 mg.

Southern Pecan - Revival **-** Physicians Laboratories
Eight Fluid Ounces Contain: Certified Isoflavone 15 mg. Ingredients: Whole Roasted Soybeans, Natural and Artificial Flavors.

Soy Defense **-** Changes International, Inc.
Two caplets contain: Vitamin E (as D-Alpha-Tocopheryl Succinate and Dl-Alpha-Tocopheryl Acetate) 200 IU • Mixed Soy phytosterols 50 mg • Tri-source isoflavone concentrate [defatted Soy Germ, Red Clover flower, and Kudzu root (providing 40 mg total isoflavones)] 1333 mg • Soy polysaccharides 150 mg. Other Ingredients: Dicalcium Phosphate, Vegetable Cellulose, Fractionated vegetable oil, Silica, Calcium Sulfate, and Vegetable resin glaze.

Soy Essentials **-** Health From The Sun
Four tablets contain: Genistein (Aglycone) 2.88 mg • Daidzein (Aglycone) 2.20 mg • Beta Glucans 7.87 mg. Ingredients: Certified GMO-Free Fermented Soymeal (Soynatto), Microcrystalline Cellulose, Stearic Acid, HPC (cellulose), Croscarmellose Sodium, Magnesium Stearate, Silicon Dioxide, Pharmaceutical Glaze.

Soy Extract **-** Enzymatic Therapy/PhytoPharmica
Each softgel contains: Soybean extract (glycine max, standardized to contain 15% isoflavones calculated as their glycoside forms, genistin/daidzin, non-GMO) 100 mg. Other Ingredients: Soybean Oil, Gelatin, Glycerin, Beeswax, Lecithin.

Soy Force Rx **-** Biotech Corp.
Two tablets contain: Soy Isoflavones 80 mg • Soy Protein Concentrate 500 mg • OPTiSOY Blend 300 mg.

Soy Isoflavone **-** Natrol
Each capsule contains: Soy Isoflavone extract 100 mg containing: Isoflavones (10%) 10 mg • Daidzin & Daidzein (2%) 2 mg • Genistin & Genistein (9%) 9 mg • Glycitin & Glycitein (0.1%) 0.1 mg. Other Ingredients: Rice powder, Magnesium Stearate, Gelatin.

Soy Isoflavone **-** Jamieson
Each capsule contains: Isoflavone Concentrate derived from 125 mg of pure Soy 50 mg.

Soy Isoflavones **-** Olympian Labs
Each capsule contains: Soy Isoflavone dried extract 100 mg.

Soy Isoflavones 40 **-** Pure Encapsulations
Each vegetarian capsule contains: Soy Isoflavone extract (standardized to contain 40% total isoflavones) 100 mg. Other gredients: Hypo-allergenic fiber.

Soy Isoflavones Concentrate Caplet **-** Leiner Health Products
Each caplet contains: Isoflavones - Soy extract 50 mg • Lecithin 15 mg. Other Ingredients: Dicalcium Phosphate, Cellulose, Stearic Acid, Silicon Dioxide, Croscarmellose Sodium, Magnesium Stearate, Dextrin, Dextrose, Sodium Carboxymethylcellulose, Sodium Citrate.

Soy Isoflavones, 50mg **-** Nature Made
Each capsule contains: Soy bean extract 125 mg: Soy Isoflavones 50 mg.

Soy Lecithin Granules - GNC A-Z - GNC
Each tablespoon contains: Soy Lecithin Granules containing: Phosphatidyl Choline 1725 mg • Choline 250 mg.

Soy Lecithin Granules Apple Cinnamon Flavor - GNC
Each Tablespoon contains: Phosphorous 165 mg • Phosphatidyl Choline 1350 mg • Choline 200 mg. Ingredients: Soy Lecithin granules, Dried Apple juice, Dried Apples, Spices.

Soy Miracle Ultimate Antioxidant - FreeLife International
Two caplets contain: ProVitamin A (beta, alpha carotenes) 15,000 IU • Vitamin E (natural d-alpha tocopheryl succinate) 400 IU • Vitamin C (calcium ascorbate) 500 mg • Selenium (l-selenomethionine) 50 mcg • N-Acetyl Cysteine 50 mg • Ultra Soy Complex III 200 mg: standardized Soy kernel concentrate (source of daidzein, saponins), Soybean sprouts concentrate (source of antioxidant enzymes), Pine bark extract, Japanese Grape Seed extract, Glutathione, Red Cabbage, Green Tea, Carrots, Broccoli, Celery, Brussels sprouts, Kale, Cauliflower, Green Onion, Yam • Alfalfa Juice concentrate (medicago sativa) 200 mg • Bilberry extract (vaccinium myrtillis) 25 mg • Citrus Bioflavonoids (citrus limon) 100 mg • Grape Skin extract 50 mg • Ginger (zingiber officinale) 100 mg • Quercetin (sophora japonica) 25 mg • Rutin (sophora japonica) 50 mg • Turmeric (source of curcurmin) 50 mg.

Soy Miracle Ultimate Body Toner - FreeLife International
Two caplets contain: Vitamin B3 (niacinamide) 20 mg • Vitamin B6 (pyridoxine HCl, pyridoxal-5-phosphate) 10 mg • Chromium (yeast-free GTF, picolinate) 200 mcg • Choline Bitartrate 100 mg • Inositol 100 mg • L-Carnitine 50 mg • Methionine 50 mg • Taurine 50 mg • High-Esterase Plant Lipase Enzyme 1500 AP Units • Betaine HCl 100 mg • Panax Ginseng standardized extract (4% ginsenosides) 100 mg • Grapefruit extract (glycinated) 200 mg • Ultra Soy Complex 350 mg: Lecithin, Soy bran, Linoleic Acid, Phosphatidylcholine, Phytosterols (beta sitosterol, campesterol, stigmasterol, fucosterol), Cephalin, Inositol Phosphatides, Phosphatidylserine, Linolenic Acid • Active Herbal Blend 250 mg: Gotu Kola, Uva Ursi, Buchu, Apple Cider Vinegar, Spirulina, Peppermint, Cinnamon, Ginger, Licorice, Cayenne, Chinese Mustard, Spearmint Oil.

Soy Preventive - GNC
Two capsules contain: Vitamin A (100% as Acetate) 5000 IU • Vitamin C (as Ascorbic Acid) 200 mg • Vitamin E (as d-alpha Tocopheryl Succinate) 100 IU • Selenium (as Selenium Yeast) 100 mcg • Soy Isoflavone Concentrate (34% Isoflavones = 8.5 mg) 25 mg. Other Ingredients: Cellulose, Calcium Carbonate, Gelatin.

Soy Protein Chocolate - GNC
One scoop (32g) contains: Isolated Soy Protein • Fructose • Maltodextrin • Cocoa • Natural Flavor • Salt.

Soy Protein Vanilla - GNC
One scoop (32g) contains: Isolated Soy Protein • Fructose • Maltodextrin • Natural Flavor • Salt.

Soya Lecithin 1200 mg - Sundown
Each softgel contains: Soya Lecithin 1200 mg (phospholipids 550 mg). Other Ingredients: Gelatin, Glycerin, Water.

SoyaMax - USANA Health Sciences
Two scoops contain: Potensoy: Soy Protein Isolate, Isoflavine Concentrate • Natural Vanilla Flavor.

Soy-Based Milk-Free Lactobacillus Acidophilus powder - Nature's Life
Each level tablespoon (6 g) contains: A freeze-dried blend of unrefined Apple Juice, Maltodextrin NF, SUPRO brand Soy Protein, pure Crystalline Fructose & our uniquely cultured probiotics Lactobacillus Acidophilus (95%), L. Bulgaricus (3%) & Bifidobacteria Bifidus (2%).

Soygenol 100 - FreeLife International
Each tablet contains: Soygenol 100 [soy-phosphatide-bonded premium Grape Seed OPCs (2:1)] 100 mg • Green Tea leaf standardized extract (30% polyphenols) 100 mg • Ultra Soy Delivery System (Soy polysaccharides and plant enzymes) 5000 Units. Other Ingredients: Calcium Hydrogen Phosphate, Cellulose, Cellulose Gum, Vegetable Stearic Acid, Silica, Vegetable Magnesium Stearate, Calcium Silicate, Vita-Coat (vegetable resin, alpha-lipoic acid).

SoySwee Tea - HerbaSway
Soy • Ginger • Panax Ginseng • Siberian Ginseng • Blackberry • HerbaSwee (Cucurbitaceae fruit).

SP-500 - PhytoPharmica
Each capsule contains: Spleen Polypeptides (a mixture of highly purified bovine-derived spleen polypeptides naturally present in the spleen, including tuftsin, splenopentin, splenin and leukokinin) 375 mg • Goldenseal root extract (Hydrastis canadensis) standardized to contain 5% total alkaloids including Berberine, Hydrastine, and Canadine 125 mg.
See Editor's No. 14 and No. 21.

Spark Drink Mix - Advocare International
Each scoop (0.53 oz/15 g) contains: Vitamin A (as mixed carotenes and vitamin a palmitate) 2500 IU • Vitamin C (as ascorbic acid) 180 mg • Vitamin E (as d-alpha tocopheryl acetate) 30 IU • Thiamine (as HCl) 3 mg • Riboflavin 3.4 mg • Niacin (as niacin and nicinamide) 60 mg • Pyridoxine (as HCl) 15 mg • Vitamin B12 (as cyanocobalamin) 45 mcg • Pantothenic Acid (as calcium pantothenate) 50 mg • Zinc (as monomethionine - OptiZinc) 3 mg • Copper (as glycinate) 200 mcg • Chromium (as polynicotinate - ChromeMate) 24 mcg • Sodium (as phosphate) 20 mg • L-Carnitine (as tartrate) 10 mg • Taurine 200 mg • Gamma-Aminobutyric Acid (GABA) 50 mg • Glycine 100 mg • L-Phenylalanine 500 mg • Ribonucleic Acid 2 mg • Ubiquinone (coenzyme Q-10) 100 mcg • Choline (as citrate and bitartrate) 500 mg • Caffeine 120 mg. Other Ingredients: Maltodextrin, Citric Acid, Natural Flavor, Artificial Flavor, Sucralose, Sodium Phosphate, Silicon Dioxide.

Spark Drink Mix, Cherry - Advocare International
Each scoop (0.53 oz/15 g) contains: Vitamin A (as mixed carotenes and vitamin a palmitate) 2500 IU • Vitamin C (as ascorbic acid) 180 mg • Vitamin E (as d-alpha tocopheryl acetate) 30 IU • Thiamine (as HCl) 3 mg • Riboflavin 3.4 mg • Niacin (as niacin and nicinamide) 60 mg • Vitamin B6 (as pyridoxine HCl) 15 mg • Vitamin B12 (as cyanocobalamin) 45 mcg • Pantothenic Acid (as calcium pantothenate) 50 mg • Zinc (as monomethionine - OptiZinc) 3 mg • Copper (as glycinate) 200 mcg • Chromium (as polynicotinate - ChromeMate) 24 mcg • Sodium (as phosphate) 20 mg • L-Carnitine (as tartrate) 10 mg • Taurine 200 mg • Gamma-Aminobutyric Acid (GABA) 50 mg • Glycine 100 mg • L-Phenylalanine 500 mg • Ribonucleic Acid 2 mg • Coenzyme Q-10 100 mcg • Choline (as citrate and bitartrate) 500 mg • Caffeine 120 mg. Other Ingredients: Maltodextrin, Citric Acid, Natural Flavor, Beet Root Powder (for color), Sucralose, Sodium Phosphate, Silicon Dioxide, Sodium Carboxymethylcellulose.

Speak Easy Throat Spray - The Herbalist
Yerba Mansa root • Echinacea root • Marshmallow root • Propolis • Myrrh Gum • Licorice root in a base of Vegetable Glycerine.

Special B-Complex 50 mg - Nature's Life
Each capsule contains: Vitamin C 50 mg • Vitamin B1 (Thiamine HCl) 50 mg • Vitamin B2 (Riboflavin) 50 mg • Niacinamide 50 mg • Vitamin B6 (Pyridoxine HCl) 50 mg • Folic Acid 800 mcg • Vitamin B12 (Cobalamin concentrate) 50 mcg • Biotin 50 mcg • Pantothenic Acid (d-Calcium Pantothenate) 50 mg • Choline (Choline Bitartrate) 50 mg • Inositol 50 mg • PABA (Para-Aminobenzioc Acid) 50 mg. In a natural base of Rice Bran, Alfalfa, Parsley, Watercress, Rose Hips & Acerola.

Special Delivery B-12 Plus - Bee-Alive Inc.
Each softgel contains: Vitamin B6 (as pyridoxine hydrochloride) 25 mg • Folate (as folic acid) 400 mcg • Vitamin B12 (as cyanocobalamin) 500 mcg • Royal Jelly 25 mg. Other Ingredients: Honey, Gelatin, Glycerin, Sucralose.

Special Two - Now
Two tablets contain: Vitamin A (Beta Carotene) (6 mg) 10000 IU • Vitamin B1 (Thiamine HCL) 50 mg • Vitamin B2 (Riboflavin) 50 mg • Vitamin B3 (Niacinamide) 50 mg • Vitamin B5 (Pantothenic Acid) 50 mg • Vitamin B6 (Pyridoxine HCL) 50 mg • Vitamin B12 (Cyanocobalamin) 100 mcg • Biotin 100 mcg • Folic Acid 400 mcg • Vitamin C (Calcium Ascorbate) 500 mg • Vitamin D (Calciferol) 200 IU • Vitamin E (d-Alpha Succinate) 200 IU • Vitamin K (from green foods) 70 mcg • Calcium (Ascorbate, Carbonate) 100 mg • Magnesium (Oxide , Amino Acid Chelate) 50 mg • Zinc (Amino Acid Chelate) 15 mg • Iron (Amino Acid Chelate) 10 mg • Copper (Amino Acid Chelate) 1 mg • Iodine (Kelp) 150 mcg • Potassium 50 mg • Manganese (Amino Acid Chelate) 5 mg • Selenium (Amino Acid Chelate) 50 mcg • Chromium (Yeast-free GTF) 100 mcg • Molybdenum (Amino Acid Chelate) 50 mcg • Boron (Amino Acid Chelate) 1 mg • Vanadium (Amino Acid Chelate) 50 mcg • Choline (Bitartrate) 50 mg • Inositol 50 mg • PABA 30 mg • Spirulina 250 mg • Chlorella (broken cell wall) 250 mg • Barley grass organic 250 mg • Alfalfa juice concentrate 100 mg • Octacosanol wheat-free 100 mcg • Siberian Ginseng 50 mg • Bioflavonoids (40%) 50 mg • Rutin 25 mg • Psyllium husk fiber 50 mg • Echinacea 50 mg • Apple Pectin 25 mg • Betaine Hydrochloride 25 mg • Glutamic Acid 25 mg • Papain (Papaya) 25 mg • Lipase 10 mg • Amylase 10 mg • Chlorophyll 9 mg • 17 Amino Acids 380 mg derived from Spirulina, Chlorella , Barley grass & Alfalfa juice concentrate. Natural base includes Alfalfa, Rose Hips, Di-Calcium Phosphate, Cellulose, Stearic Acid & natural vegetable protein coating.

Spectra Probiotic with Cofactors - NF Formulas - Integrative Therapeutics
Three capsules contain: Spectra Probiotic Proprietary Blend 600 mg: Lactobacillus Acidophilus, Bifidobacterium Bifidum, Bifidobacterium Infantis, Bifidobacterium Longum, Lactobacillus Blugaricus, Lactobacillus Casei, Lactobacillus Salivarius, Streptococcus Thermophilus • FOS (fructooligosaccharides) 270 mg • NAG (N-acetyl-glucosamine) 105 mg. Other Ingredients: Rice Flour, Gelatin, Water.

Spectrabiotic - Cell Tech
Two capsules contain: Vitamin C (from acerola & rosehips) 75 mg • Vitamin K 4 mcg • Proprietary Blend 559 mg: Lactobacillus Acidophilus, Bifidobacterium Bifidum, Lactobacillus Casei, Lactobacillus Bulgaricus, Lactobacillus Plantarum, Lactobacillus Salivarius, Streptococcus Faecium, Streptococcus Thermophilius, Blue-Green Algae (aphanizomenon flos-aquae) 100 mg, Jerusalem Artichoke root, Lipase, Amylase, Protease, Cellulase. Other Ingredients: Maltodextrin, Vegetarian Capsule (plant fiber, water).

Speman - The Himalaya Drug Company (Himalaya Heal
Each tablet contains: Salabmisri (orchis mascula) 130 mg • Kokilaksha (hygrophila auriculata syn. asteracantha longifolia) 64 mg • Vanya Kahu (lactuca scariola syn. l.serriola) 32 mg • Kapikachchhu (mucuna pruriens) 32 mg • Suvarnavang (mosaic gold, unsublimed tin formulation) 32 mg • Vriddadaru (argyreia speciosa syn. a.nervosa) 32 mg • Gokshura (tribulus terrestris) 64 mg • Jeevanti (leptadenia reticulata) 64 mg • Shaileyam (parmelia perlata) 32 mg.

SPES - BotanicLab
Each capsule contains: Proprietary Blend 300 mg: Pyrola (pyrola rotundifolia L), Agrimony (agrimonia pilosa Ledeb), Corydalis (corydalis yanhusuo W.T. Wang), Reishi (ganoderma lucidum Karst), Rubescens (rabdosia rubescens Hara), Stephania (stephania delavayi Diels), Stephania (stephania sinica Diels), Lycoris (lycoris radiata Herb), Partinia (partrinia heterophylla Bunga), Oriental Ginseng (panax ginseng C.A. Meyer), Pollen (pollen), Prickly Ash (zanthoxylum nitidum DC), Chinese Licorice (glycyrrhiza uralensis Fisch), Cervus (cervus nippon Temmiinck), Broomrape (Ccstanche deserticola Y.C. Ma).
See Editor's Note No. 2, page 2053.

SpiruLEANe - NAI - Natural Alternatives International
Each tablet contains: Proprietary blend 1,545 mg: Ma Huang herb extract (24 mg) • Guarana seed extract (24 mg) • Chromium chelavite (400 mcg) • Spirulina Pacifica • White Willow bark • Green Tea leaf extract • Uva Ursi leaf • Kola Nut seed extract • Bromelain (from pineapple) • Ginger root • Siberian Ginseng root • Ginkgo Biloba leaf extract • Cayenne Pepper • Gotu Kola leaf • Grapefruit seed extract • Royal Jelly • Lecithin.
See Editor's Note No. 30, page 2056.

Spirulina - Earthrise Nutritionals, Inc.
Six tablets contain: Sodium 35 mg • Vitamin A (100% Beta Carotene) 4,000 IU • Calcium 7 mg • Iron 2 mg • Riboflavin 0.06 mg • Niacin 0.35 mg • Potassium 50 mg • Total Carb. 0.5 g • Protein 2 g • Magnesium 7 mg • Thiamin 0.03 mg • Vitamin B12 4.2 mcg • Vitamin K 17 mcg • Phycocyanin 330 mg • Chlorophyll 30 mg • Mixed Carotenoids 8 mg • Gamma Linolenic Acid 30 mg • Sulfolipids 30 mg • Polysaccharides 140 mg.

Spirulina - Jamieson
Each caplet contains: 100% Pure Spirulina Blue-Green Microalgae 500 mg.

Spirulina - Quest
Each capsule contains: Spirulina 500 mg.

Spirulina - Source Naturals
Six tablets contain: Vitamin A (Beta Carotene) 14,000 IU • Vitamin B1 (Thiamin) 100 mcg • Vitamin B2 (Riboflavin) 99 mcg • Niacin 620 mcg • Vitamin B12 (Cobalamin) 6.6 mg • Boron 30 mcg • Iron 3.2 mg • Magnesium 14 mg • Phosphorus 31 mg • Protein 1,800 mg • Phycocyanin 333 mg • Linoleic Acid 33 mg • Gamma-Linolenic Acid (GLA) 30 mg • Omega-3 Fatty Acids 87 mcg • Chlorophyll 23.7 mg • Total Carotenoids 16.2 mg • Superoxide Dismutase (SOD) 1.2 mg.

Spirulina & Chlorella - Earthrise Nutritionals, Inc.
Eight tablets contain: Vitamin A 2900 IU • Vitamin C 30 mg • Vitamin E 0.5 IU Vitamin K 17 mcg • Thiamin 0.04 mg • Riboflavin 0.1 mg • Niacin 0.35 mg • Vitamin B6 0.05 mg • Vitamin B12 2 mcg • Calcium 6 mg • Iron 2 mg • Magnesium 8 mg • Sodium 20 mg Potassium 45 mg 8 Phycocyanin 176 mg • Polysaccharides 75 mg • Chlorophyll 60 mg • Gamma Linolenic Acid 16 mg • Sulfolipids 16 mg • Mixed Carotenoids 8 mg.

Spirulina Bio - Earthrise Nutritionals, Inc.
Six tablets contain: Sodium 35 mg • Vitamin A (100% Beta Carotene) 4,000 IU • Calcium 7 mg • Iron 2 mg • Riboflavin 0.06 mg • Niacin 0.35 mg • Potassium 50 mg • Total Carb. 0.5 g • Protein 2 g • Magnesium 7 mg • Thiamin 0.03 mg • Vitamin B12 4.2 mcg • Vitamin K 17 mcg • Phycocyanin 330 mg • Chlorophyll 30 mg • Mixed Carotenoids 8 mg • Gamma Linolenic Acid 30 mg • Sulfolipids 30 mg • Polysaccharides 140 mg.

Spirulina Bio Powder - Earthrise Nutritionals, Inc.
Three grams contain: Sodium 60 mg • Vitamin A (100% Beta Carotene) 8300 IU • Calcium 12 mg • Iron 3.3 mg • Riboflavin 0.1 mg • Niacin 0.6 mg • Potassium 80 mg • Total Carb. 0.8 g • Protein 3 g • Magnesium 11 mg • Thiamin 0.05 mg • Vitamin B12 7 mcg • Vitamin K 29 mcg • Phycocyanin 550 mg • Chlorophyll 50 mg • Mixed Carotenoids 17 mg • Gamma Linolenic Acid 50 mg • Sulfolipids 50 mg • Polysaccharides 230 mg.

Spirulina Blue Green Algae - Leiner Health Products
Each capsule contains: Spirulina Blue Green Algae (Spirulina pacifica) cell 250 mg. Other Ingredients: Maltodextrin, Gelatin, Cellulose, Magnesium Stearate, Croscarmellose Sodium.

Spirulina Gold - Earthrise Nutritionals, Inc.
Twelve tablets contain: Vitamin A (100% beta carotene) 5000 IU • Calcium 7 mg • Iron 2 mg • Riboflavin 0.306 mg • Niacin 0.35 mg • Zinc 3 mg • Potassium 50 mg • Vitamin C 1.2 mg • Magnesium 7 mg • Thiamin 0.03 mg • Vitamin B12 4.2 mcg • Vitamin K 17 mcg • Phycocyanin 330 mg • Chlorophyll 30 mg • Mixed Carotenoids

10 mg • Gamma Linolenic Acid 30 mg • Sulfolipids 50 mg • Polysaccharides 140 mg.

Spirulina Gold Powder **-** Earthrise Nutritionals, Inc.
Five grams contain: Vitamin A (100% Beta Carotene) 10,000 IU • Vitamin C 2 mg • Vitamin K 29 mcg • Thiamin 0.05mg • Riboflavin 0.1 mg • Niacin 0.6 mg • Vitamin B12 7 mcg • Calcium 12 mg • Iron 3.3 mg • Magnesium 11 mg • Zinc 5 mg • Sodium 80 mg • Potassium 80 mg • Phycocyanin 550 mg • Polysaccharides 230 mg • Sulfolipids 50 mg • Chlorophyll 60 mg • Gamma Linolenic Acid 50 mg • Mixed Carotenoids 18.5 mg.

Spirulina Multiple **-** Source Naturals
Two tablets contain: Spirulina Plankton (Spirulina platensis) 200 mg • Rose Hips 25 mg • Beta Carotene (Pro-Vitamin A) 10,000 IU • Vitamin B1 (Thiamin Mononitrate) 25 mg • Vitamin B2 (Riboflavin) 25 mg • Niacin 25 mg • Vitamin B6 (Pyridoxine HCl) 25 mg • Vitamin B12 (Cobalamin) 100 mcg • Folic Acid 100 mcg • Vitamin C (Ascoribic Acid) 250 mg • Vitamin D (as Vitamin D3) (Cholecalciferol) 400 IU • Vitamin E d-alpha tocopheryl 60 IU • Calcium (Carbonate) 99 mg • Iodine (from Kelp) 150 mcg • Iron (Fumarate) 18 mg • Magnesium (Oxide) 33 mg • Potassium (Chelate) 7.5 mg • Zinc (Citrate) 5 mg.

Spirulina Powder **-** Earthrise Nutritionals, Inc.
Three grams contain: Sodium 60 mg • Vitamin A (100% Beta Carotene) 8,300 IU • Calcium 12 mg • Iron 3.3 mg • Riboflavin 0.1 mg • Niacin 0.6 mg • Potassium 80 mg • Total Carb. .8 g • Protein 3 g • Magnesium 11 mg • Thiamin 0.05 mg • Vitamin B12 7 mcg • Vitamin K 29 mcg • Phycocyanin 550 mg • Chlorophyll 50 mg • Mixed Carotenoids 17 mg • Gamma Linolenic Acid 50 mg • Sulfolipids 50 mg • Polysaccharides 230 mg.

Spirulina Powder **-** Source Naturals
Each teaspoon contains: Vitamin A (Beta Carotene) 42,000 IU • Vitamin B1 (Thiamin) 300 mcg • Vitamin B2 (Riboflavin) 300 mcg • Niacin 2 mg • Vitamin B12 (Cobalamin) 20 mg • Boron 90 mcg • Iron 9.5 mg • Magnesium 43 mg •Phosphorus 93 mg • Protein 5,400 mg • Phycocyanin 1,000 mg • Linoleic Acid 99 mg • Gamma-Linolenic Acid (GLA) 90 mg • Omega-3 Fatty Acids 261 mcg • Chlorophyll 71 mg • Total Carotenoids 48.6 mg • Superoxide Dismutase (SOD) 3.6 mg.

Spirulina- Vegi-Capsules **-** Earthrise Nutritionals, Inc.
Seven Vegi-Capsules Contain: Sodium 35 mg • Vitamin A (100% Beta Carotene) 4,000 IU • Calcium 7 mg • Iron 2 mg • Riboflavin 0.06 mg • Niacin 0.35 mg • Potassium 50 mg • Total Carb. 0.5 mg • Protein 2 g • Magnesium 7 mg • Thiamin 0.03 mg • Vitamin B12 4.2 mcg • Vitamin K 17 mcg • Phycocyanin 330 mg • Chlorophyll 30 mg • Mixed Carotenoids 8 mg • Gamma Linolenic Acid 30 mg • Sulfolipids 30 mg • Polysaccharides 140 mg.

Spirulina Vegi-Capsules **-** Earthrise Nutritionals, Inc.
Three grams contain: Vitamin A 4000 IU • Vitamin K 17 mcg • Thiamin 0.03 mg • Riboflavin 0.06 mg • Niacin 0.35 mg • Vitamin B12 4.2 mcg • Calcium 7 mg • Iron 2 mg • Magnesium 7 mg • Sodium 35 mg • Potassium 50 mg • Phycocyanin 330 mg • Polysaccharides 30 mg • Chlorophyll 30 mg • Gamma Linolenic Acid 30 mg • Mixed Carotenoids 8 mg.

Spirulina+Chlorella **-** Earthrise Nutritionals, Inc.
Eight tablets contain: Sodium 20 mg • Vitamin A (100% Beta Carotene) 2900 IU • Calcium 6 mg • Iron 2 mg • Vitamin E 0.51 IU • Riboflavin 0.1 mg • Niacin 0.35 mg • Protein 2 g • Total Carb. 0.5 g • Potassium 45 mg • Vitamin C 30 mg • Magnesium 8.0 mg • Thiamin 0.04 mg • Vitamin B6 0.05 mg • Vitamin B12 2 mcg • Vitamin K 17 mcg • Phycocyanin 176 mg • Chlorophyll 60 mg • Mixed Carotenoids 8 mg • Gamma Linolenic Acid 16 mg • Sulfolipids 16 mg • Polysaccharides 75 mg.

SPL and PAN **-** Dial Herbs
Chamomile • Dandelion • Goldenseal • Parsley • Uva Ursi • Yellow Dock • Cayenne • Yarrow.

Splash C with Aloe Lemon **-** Pharmanex
Crystalline Fructose • Guam Arabic • Natural Orange Flavors • Citric Acid • Potassium Citrate • Silicon Dioxide • Maltodextrin • Dicalcium Phosphate • Ascorbic Acid • Tricalcium Phosphate • Sodium Chloride (salt) • Oat Fiber • Soy Fiber • Powdered Cellulose • DL-Alpha Tocopheryl Acetate • Beta-Carotene • Aloe Vera concentrate • Folic Acid.

Splash C with Aloe Orange **-** Pharmanex
Crystalline Fructose • Guam Arabic • Natural Orange Flavors • Citric Acid • Potassium Citrate • Silicon Dioxide • Maltodextrin • Dicalcium Phosphate • Ascorbic Acid • Tricalcium Phosphate • Sodium Chloride (salt) • Oat Fiber • Soy Fiber • Powdered Cellulose • DL-Alpha Tocopheryl Aceate • Beta-Carotene • Aloe Vera concentrate • Folic Acid.

Spontane-ES **-** Warner Laboratories
Each tablet contains: Proprietary Blend 325 mg: Epimedium (20% extract, leaves), Xanthoparmelia Scabrosa (lichen), Cnidium Monnier (fruit), Quebracho (8% extract, bark), Ginkgo Biloba (leaves), Mucuna Pruriens (seed), L-Arginine. Other Ingredients: Microcrystalline Cellulose, Magnesium Stearate, Sodium Starch, FD&C Blue #1 Aluminum Lake.

Sport **-** Mannatech
Two capsules contain: Chromium (as chromium picolinate) 200 mcg • Proprietary Blend Sterol Complex 800 mg: Bovine Testes extract 400 mg, Wild Yam (root; standardized for 25 mg phytosterols) 200 mg, Sarsaparilla (root) 200 mg • Boron (as boron citrate) 2 mg • Ambrotose Complex (patent pending) 5 mg: Arabinogalactan (larix decidua gum), Manapol Aloe Vera gel extract (inner leaf gel), Gum Ghatti, Gum Tragacanth. Other Ingredients: Gelatin, Brown Rice Flour, Silicon Dioxide, Magnesium Stearate.

Sport Fuel **-** TwinLab
Six capsules contain: Beta-Carotene (pro-Vitamin A) 25000 IU • Vitamin D (from natural form Vitamin D3) 400 IU • Vitamin C 1000 mg • Natural Vitamin E (Succinate) 800 IU • CoQ10 (Coenzyme Q10) 30 mg • L-Glutathione 100 mg • N-Acetyl Cysteine (NAC) 200 mg • Alpha Lipoic Acid 100 mg • Vitamin B1 (Thiamine) 50 mg • Vitamin B2 (Riboflavin) 50 mg • Vitamin B6 (Pyridoxine) 50 mg • Vitamin B12 (Cobalamin) 100 mg • Folic Acid 400 mcg • Niacinamide 150 mg • Pantothenic Acid 250 mg • Biotin 300 mcg • PABA (Para-Aminobenzoic Acid) 25 mg • Choline Bitartrate 100 mg • Inositol 100 mg • L-Carnitine (from Carni Fuel L-Carnitine Magnesium Citrate) 100 mg • Magnesium (from L-Carnitine Magnesium Citrate, Aspartate, Alpha-Ketoglutarate & Oxide) 600 mg • Potassium (from Potassium Aspartate, Alpha-Ketoglutarate & Citrate) 100 mg • Zinc (from Zinc Picolinate) 30 mg • Manganese (from Manganese Gluconate) 5 mg • Copper (from Copper Gluconate) 2 mg • Iron (from Ferrous Fumarate) 10 mg • Iodine (from Potassium Iodide) 150 mcg • Selenium (from Selenomethionine & Selenate 50/50 mixture) 200 mcg • Chromium (from Chromic Fuel Chromium Picolinate) 400 mcg • Molybdenum (from natural Molybdic Acid) 150 mcg.

Sport Fuel With Iron **-** TwinLab
Six capsules contain: Beta-Carotene (pro-Vitamin A) 25000 IU • Vitamin D (from natural form Vitamin D3) 400 IU • Vitamin C 1000 mg • Natural Vitamin E (Succinate) 800 IU • CoQ10 (Coenzyme Q10) 30 mg • L-Glutathione 100 mg • N-Acetyl Cysteine (NAC) 200 mg • Alpha Lipoic Acid 100 mcg • Vitamin B1 (Thiamine) 50 mg • Vitamin B2 (Riboflavin) 50 mg • Vitamin B6 (Pyridoxine) 50 mg • Vitamin B12 (Cobalamin) 100 mcg • Folic Acid 400 mcg • Niacinamide 150 mg • Pantothenic Acid 250 mg • Biotin 300 mcg • PABA (Para-Aminobenzoic Acid) 25 mg • Choline Bitartrate 100 mg • Inositol 100 mg • L-Carnitine (from Carni Fuel L-Carnitine Magnesium Citrate) 100 mg • Calcium (from Calcium Citrate, Carbonate) 25 mg • Magnesium (from L-Carnitine Magnesium Citrate, Aspartate, Alpha-Ketoglutarate & Oxide) 600 mg • Potassium (from Potassium Aspartate, Alpha-Ketoglutarate & Citrate) 100 mg • Zinc (from Zinc Picolinate) 30 mg • Manganese (from Manganese

Gluconate) 5 mg • Copper (from Copper Gluconate) 2 mg • Iron (from Ferrous Fumarate) 10 mg • Iodine (from Potassium Iodide) 150 mcg • Selenium (from Selenomethionine & Selenate‹50/50 mixture) 200 mcg • Chromium (from Chromic Fuel Chromium Picolinate) 400 mcg • Molybdenum (from natural Molybdic Acid) 150 mcg.

Sport Fuel Without Iron - TwinLab
Six capsules contain: Beta-Carotene (pro-Vitamin A) 25000 IU • Vitamin D (from natural form Vitamin D3) 400 IU • Vitamin C 1000 mg • Natural Vitamin E (Succinate) 800 IU • CoQ10 (Coenzyme Q10) 30 mg • L-Glutathione 100 mg • N-Acetyl Cysteine (NAC) 200 mg • Alpha Lipoic Acid 100 mcg • Vitamin B1 (Thiamine) 50 mg • Vitamin B2 (Riboflavin) 50 mg • Vitamin B6 (Pyridoxine) 50 mg • Vitamin B12 (Cobalamin) 100 mcg • Folic Acid 400 mcg • Niacinamide 150 mg • Pantothenic Acid 250 mg • Biotin 300 mcg • PABA (Para-Aminobenzoic Acid) 25 mg • Choline Bitartrate 100 mg • Inositol 100 mg • L-Carnitine (from Carni Fuel L-Carnitine Magnesium Citrate) 100 mg • Calcium (from Calcium Citrate, Carbonate) 25 mg • Magnesium (from L-Carnitine Magnesium Citrate, Aspartate, Alpha-Ketoglutarate & Oxide) 600 mg • Potassium (from Potassium Aspartate, Alpha-Ketoglutarate & Citrate) 100 mg • Zinc (from Zinc Picolinate) 30 mg • Manganese (from Manganese Gluconate) 5 mg • Copper (from Copper Gluconate) 2 mg • Iodine (from Potassium Iodide) 150 mcg • Selenium (from Selenomethionine & Selenate‹50/50 mixture) 200 mcg • Chromium (from Chromic Fuel Chromium Picolinate) 400 mcg • Molybdenum (from natural Molybdic Acid) 150 mcg.

Sportalyte - Pharmanex
Twenty grams contain: Glucose • Fructose • Maltodextrin • Citric Acid • Natural Flavor • Sodium Chloride • Silicon Dioxide • Sodium Citrate • Magnesium Carbonate • Tricalcium Phosphate • Potassium Citrate • Magnesium Oxide • Ascorbic Acid • d- Alpha Tocopheryl Acetate • Potassium Chloride • Hydromins • Taurine • Fructooligosaccharides.

Sports One DIOL XS - Sports One
Each capsule contains: 4-Androstenediol 100 mg • Nor-4-Androstenediol 100 mg.

Spring Valley Children's Chewables Complete - Leiner Health Products
Each tablet contains: Vitamin A Acetate (as Acetate and Beta Carotene) 5000 IU • Vitamin C (Ascorbic Acid) 60 mg • Vitamin D (Ergocalciferol) 400 IU • Vitamin E (dl-Alpha Tocopheryl Acetate) 30 IU • Thiamin Mononitrate (Vitamin B1) 1.5 mg • Riboflavin (Vitamin B2) 1.7 mg • Niacin (Niacinamide) 20 mg • Vitamin B-6 (Pyridoxine Hydrochloride) 2 mg • Folic Acid 400 mcg • Vitamin B-12 (Cyanocobalamin) 6 mcg • Biotin (USP Method 2) 40 mcg • Pantothenic Acid (d-Calcium Pantothenate) 10 mg • Calcium 100 mg • Iron (Ferrous Fumarate) 18 mg • Phosphorus 100 mg • Iodine (Potassium Iodide) 150 mcg • Magnesium Oxide 20 mg • Zinc Oxide 15 mg • Copper (Cupric Oxide) 2 mg. Other Ingredients: Sorbitol, Dicalcium Phosphate, Magnesium Phosphate, Fructose, Stearic Acid, Mono- & Diglycerides, Xylitol, Gelatin, Sodium Ascorbate, Carrageenan, Aspartame, Citric Acid, Red 40 Lake, Yellow 6 Lake, Starch, Silicon Dioxide, Magnesium Stearate, Blue 2 Lake, Hydroxypropyl Methylcellulose, Resin, Hydroxypropyl Cellulose, Lactose, Polyvinyl Pyrrolidone.

Spring Valley Glucosamine Sulfate - Nature's Bounty
Each capsule contains: Potassium 107 mg • Glucosamine Sulfate (2KCl) 1000 mg. Other Ingredients: Gelatin, Glycerin, Hydroxethyl Methylcellulose, Silica, Vegetable Magnesium Stearate.

Spring Valley Vitamin C with Rose Hips - Leiner Health Products
Each tablet contains: Vitamin C 500 mg. Other Ingredients: Ascorbic Acid, Starch, Cellulose, Rose Hips, Stearic Acid, Silicon Croscarmellose Sodium.

Springs of Life Water Enhancer - Garden of Life, Inc.
Twelve drops contain: Springs of Life Proprietary Blend 489 mg: Purified Water, Seawater extract, Ionic Plant Based Mineral blend, Plant Amino Acid blend, Plant Enzyme blend, Clustered Water concentrate.

SS Cream (SS-Cream) - Cheil Jedang Corporation
70% ethanol extract of Bufonis venenum 10 mg • 100 mg extract of Angelicae gigantic radix, Cistanchis caulis, Torilidis semen, Ginseng radix alba, Zanthoxylli fructos • 10 mg extract of Asiasari radix, Caryophilli flos, Cinnamomi cortex.
See Editor's Note No. 13, page 2055.

St. John's Complex - Body Wise International, Inc.
Each tablet contains: St. John's Wort extract (0.3% Hypericin) 300 mg • Chamomile flowers (Anthemis flores) 25 mg • Passion Flower (Passiflora incarnata) 25 mg.

St. John's Formula - Health Smart Vitamins
Each capsule contains: Vitamin B6 (as pyridoxine hydrochloride) 10 mg • Folate (folic acid) 200 mcg • Vitamin B12 (as cyanocobalamin) 50 mcg • Magnesium (as magnesium oxide) 100 mg • St. John's Wort aerial parts (0.3% hypercins, 0.9 mg) 300 mg • Kava Kava root (30% kavalactones, 22.5 mg) 75 mg • Ginkgo leaf (24% ginkgo flavonglycosides, 9.6 mg; 6% terpene lactone, 2.4 mg) 40 mg.

St. John's Good Mood - Traditional Medicinals
St. John's Wort herb & dry extract • Lemon Balm leaf (Melissa) • Oatstraw herb • Damiana herb • Lavender flower • Berganot herb • Sage leaf • Spearmint leaf • Lemongrass leaf • Licorice root • Rose petals • Stevia leaf.

St. John's Plus - Nutri-Quest Rx
Each tablet contains: St. John's Wort herb 400 mg • Pyridoxal-5-Phosphate 5 mg • Riboflavin (as Riboflavin-5-Phosphate) 5 mg • Folic Acid 100 mcg • Vitamin B1 10 mg • Vitamin B12 250 mcg • Ginkgo Biloba extract 5 mg • Damiana herb 25 mg • Ginkgo Biloba herb 30 mg • Blue Vervain 25 mg • Kava Kava herb 10 mg • Hyssop herb 15 mg • Siberian Ginseng 10 mg • Niacinamide 50 mg • Calcium Citrate 100 mg • Magnesium Citrate 100 mg.

St. John's Plus - Rx Vitamins
Each caplet provides: St. John's Wort flower (Hypericum perforatum, standardized 0.3-0.5 hypericin) 300 mg • Kava root (Piper methylsticum, standardized 29-31% kavalactones) 50 mg • Siberian ginseng root (Eleutherococcus senticosis, standardized 0.8% eleutherosides) 50 mg • Feverfew leaf (Tanacetum parthenium, standardized 0.7% parthenolide) 25 mg • L-Tyrosine (pharmaceutical grade, free form amino acid) 25 mg • Zinc (l-monomethionine) 10 mg • Vitamin B6 (pyridoxine HCl) 5 mg • Vitamin B12 (cyanocobalamin) 10 mcg.

St. John's Plus Kava Kava - Progressive Labs
Each capsule contains: Vitamin B6 (pyridoxine HCl) 25 mg • St. John's Wort 0.3% Hypericin 200 mg • Kava Kava 100 mg.

St. John's Solution - Quantum, Inc.
One softgel contains: St. John's Wort (Hypericum perforatum Standardized 0.3% hypericin) 300 mg.
See Editor's Note No. 21, page 2056.

St. John's Wort - GNC
Each capsule contains: St. John's Wort Herb powder (Hypericum perforatum) 500 mg. Other Ingredients: Gelatin.

St. John's Wort - Celestial Seasonings
Three capsules contain: Proprietary Blend, 1800 mg: St. John's Wort (leaves,stems, flowers), St. John's Wort (standardized extract). Other Ingredients: May contain one or more of the following: Dicalcium phosphate, gelatin, rice flour, stearic acid, magnesium stearate, and silicon dioxide.

Some Brand Name Natural Products - What they Contain

www.NaturalDatabase.com contains MANY more listings than appear here.

St. John's Wort - E'OLA
Two capsules contain: Vitamin C 30 mg • Vitamin D 200 IU • Vitamin B6 20 mg • Folic Acid 200 mcg • Magnesium 40 mg • Chromium 60 mcg • St. John's Wort (3% hypericin) 340 mg • St. John's Wort Herb 100 mg.

St. John's Wort - Gaia Herbs
St. John's Wort standardized for 0.5% hypericins. Standardized Full Spectrum 180 mg of extract per capsule. Guaranteed Potency 90 mg of extract per capsule.

St. John's Wort - Jamieson
Each tablet contains: Vitamin C 2.5 mg • St. John's Wort 4.4:1 extract (Hypericum perforatum L. Aerial parts of flower, stamen and leaf Containing 0.3% hypericin) 225 mg.

St. John's Wort - Leiner Health Products
Each caplet contains: St. John's Wort extract (Hypericum perforatum) herb 330 mg. Other Ingredients: Cellulose, Dicalcium Phosphate, Croscarmellose Sodium, Stearic Acid, Hydroxypropyl Methycellulose, Magnesium Stearate, Silicon Dioxide, Hydroxypropyl Cellulose, Red 40 Lake, Blue 2 Lake, Pharmaceutical Glaze, Polyethylene Glycol 3350, Polysorbate 80, Titanium Dioxide.

St. John's Wort - Metabolic Response Modifiers
Each capsule contains: Hypericum perforatum (0.3% Hypericin) 450 mg.

St. John's Wort - Nature's Way
Two capsules contain: St. John's Wort stem, leaf, flower 600 mg • St. John's Wort (dried extract 0.3% Dianthrones measures as Hypericin) 300 mg. Other Ingredients: Gelatin, Magnesium Stearate, Millet.

St. John's Wort - Pharmanex
Each capsule contains: St. John's Wort flower tops/leaves (Hypericum perforatum 5:1) 300 mg. Other Ingredients: Rice Flour, Gelatin, Magnesium Stearate, Silicon Dioxide.

St. John's Wort - Quest
Each caplet contains: St. John's Wort (Hypericum perfortum) (provided by 300 mg P.E. 1:5 standardized to contain 0.3% Hypercin) 1500 mg. Other Ingredients: Microcrystalline Cellulose, Calcium phosphate, Croscarmellose Sodium Dioxide, Vegetable Stearin, Magnesium Stearate.

St. John's Wort - Swanson - Swanson
Each capsule contains: St. John's Wort powder 375 mg.

St. John's Wort - USANA Health Sciences
Each tablet contains: St. John's wort (standardized extract 0.3% hypericin derivatives by UV analysis) 300 mg. Other Ingredients: Dextrose, Ascorbyl Palmitate, Colloidal Silicon Dioxide, Dextrin (modified food starch), Lecithin, Sodium Citrate.

St. John's Wort + Ginseng Caplet - Leiner Health Products
Each caplet contains: Lecithin 15 mg • Licorice extract (Glycyrrhiza glabra) root 20 mg • Siberian Ginseng extract (Eleutheroxoxxus senticosus) root 50 mg • Siberian Ginseng powder (Eleutherococcus senticosus) root 15 mg • St. John's Wort extract (Hypericum perforatum) aerial parts 300 mg. Other Ingredients: Cellulose, Dicalcium Phosphate, Croscarmellose Sodium, Silicon Dioxide, Stearic Acid, Magnesium Stearate, Hydroxypropyl Methylcellulose, Dextrin.

St. John's Wort + Kava Kava - Leiner Health Products
Each caplet contains: Kava Kava extract (Piper methysticum) root 60 mg • St. John's Wort extract (Hypericum perforatum) aerial parts 300 mg. Other Ingredients: Cellulose, Dicalcium Phosphate, Croscarmellose Sodium, Silicon Dioxide, Stearic Acid, Magnesium Stearate, Dextrin, Dextrose, Lecithin, Sodium Carboxymethylcellulose, Sodium Citrate.

St. John's Wort 1000 mg - GNC Herbal Plus - GNC
Each capsule contains: St. John's Wort Leaves/Flowers (hypericum perforatum; from 166.7 mg of St. John's Wort Herb Extract 6:1) 1000 mg. Other Ingredients: Soybean Oil, Gelatin, Glycerin, Caramel Color, Titanium Dioxide (natural mineral whitener).

St. John's Wort 1000 mg, Concentrated - GNC Herbal Plus - GNC
Each capsule contains: St. John's Wort Leaves/Flowers (hypericum perforatum; from 166.7 mg of St. John's Wort Herb Extract 6:1). Other Ingredients: Soybean Oil, Gelatin, Glycerin, Caramel Color, Titanium Dioxide (natural minerel whitener).

St. John's Wort Blend - VitaStore
Each capsule contains: St. John's Wort (standardized for 0.3% Hypericin) • Kava Kava • Ginkgo Biloba.

St. John's Wort Complete - Futurebiotics
Two capsules contain: Vitamin C (as ascorbic acid) 300 mg • Thiamin 25 mg • Riboflavin 25 mg • Niacin (as niacinamide) 25 mg • Vitamin B6 (as pyridoxine hydrochloride) 25 mg • Folic Acid 400 mcg • Vitamin B12 (as cyanocobalamin) 250 mcg • Biotin 300 mcg • Pantothenic Acid (as calcium pantothenate) 25 mg • St. John's Wort flower powder extract (standardized for 0.3% (0.8 mg) hypericin) 250 mg • Choline (as choline bitartrate) 25 mg • Inositol 25 mg • Para-Aminobenzoic Acid 25 mg • L-Tyrosine 50 mg • L-Phenylalanine 100 mg. Other Ingredients: Gelatin, Water.

St. John's Wort Extract - NSI - Nutraceutical Sciences Institute
Each capsule contains: St. John's Wort extract (standardized to 0.3% hypericin and 3% hyperforin) 450 mg.

St. John's Wort Extract - Enzymatic Therapy
Each capsule contains: St. John's Wort flower head extract (hypericum perforatum, standardized to contain a minimum of 0.3% hypericin, 3% hyperforin) 300 mg. Other Ingredients: Gelatin, Magnesium Stearate, Silicon Dioxide, Titanium Dioxide.

St. John's Wort Forte with Kava - PhytoPharmica
Each capsule contains: St. John's Wort (Hypericum peroratum) flower head extract (standardized to contain a minimum of 0.3% hypericin and 4% hyperforin) 300 mg • Valerian (Valeriana officinalis) root extract (standardized to contain a minimum of 0.8% valerenic acids) 100 mg • Kava (Piper methysticum) root extract (standardized to contain 30% kavalactones) 100 mg.
See Editor's Note No. 21, page 2056.

St. John's Wort Hypericum Perforatum 300 mg - Puritan's Pride
Each capsule contains: St. John's Wort extract (hypericum perforatum, aerial, standardized to contain 0.3% hypericin, 0.9 mg) 300 mg. Other Ingredients: Maltodextrin, Gelatin, Magnesium Silicate, Vegetable Magnesium Stearate, Silica.

St. John's Wort NutraSpray - Source Naturals
Each spray contains: St. John's Wort standardized extract (Hypericum perforatum) 2.7 mg.

St. John's Wort Oil - Blessed Herbs
St. John's Wort flowering tops • organic cold-pressed Olive oil.

St. John's Wort Plus - Aspen Group, Inc.
Each capsule contains: St. John's Wort herb extract standardized to 0.3% Hypericin 300 mg • Kava Kava 100 mg • Vitamin B6 25 mg • Standardized extract St. John's Wort herb extract Hypericum Perforatum.

St. John's Wort Standard Extract, 300mg - Nature Made
Each capsule contains: St. John's Wort aerial part extract 300 mg: Hypericin (by UV) 0.9 mg.

Some Brand Name Natural Products - What they Contain

www.NaturalDatabase.com contains MANY more listings than appear here.

BRAND NAMES

St. John's Wort Supreme **-** Gaia Herbs
St. John's Wort and Kava Kava standardized for 0.5% hypericins and 55% kavalactones. Standardized Full Spectrum 150 mg of extract per capsule. Guaranteed Potency 75 mg of extract per capsule.

St. John's Wort-Go! **-** Wakunaga of America
Each caplet contains: St. John's Wort standardized extract (herb with flower) standardized to 0.3% Hypericin 600 mg. Other Ingredients: Cellulose, Magnesium Stearate (vegetable source), Silica.

St. John's Wort-Kava Kava **-** Futurebiotics
St. John's Wort flower powder extract standardized for 0.3% (0.8 mg) hypericin 250 mg • Kava Kava root powder extract standardized for 30% (30 mg) kavalactones 100 mg. Other ingredients: Gelatin, Water.

Stabilium **-** Smart Basics
Each capsule contains: Predigested Garum Armoricum 105 mg • Virgin Sunflower Oil 83 mg •Soya Lecithin Oil 12 mg.

Stabilium 200 **-** NutriCology
Two capsules contain: Garum Armoricum 210 mg • Virgin Sunflower Oil 170 mg • Lecithin 20 mg.

Stabilized Acidophilus Three Billion **-** Now
Each tablet contains: Lactobacillus Acidophilus 3 billion. Other Ingredients: Anhydrous Dicalcium Phosphate, Microcrystalline Cellulose, Silica, Modified Cellulose Gum, Magnesium Stearate.

Stacker 2 **-** NVE Pharmaceuticals
Each capsule contains: Proprietary Blend 270 mg: Ephedra extract (leaves/stems, 25 mg ephedrine group alkaloids), Kola Nut (seeds, <1 mg caffeine group alkaloids) White Willow bark • Caffeine (anhydrous) 200 mg • Tri-GuggLyptoid Complex 25 mg: Green Tea (leaves, < 1 mg caffeine group alkaloids), Gugglesterone (whole plant), Gymnema (leaves). Other Ingredients: Dextrose, Gelatin, Stearic Acid, Magnesium Stearate, Titanium Dioxide, FD&C Yellow #5, FD&C Yellow #6.
See Editor's Note No. 30, page 2056.

Stacker 2 Ephedra Free **-** NVE Pharmaceuticals
Each capsule contains: Proprietary Blend 196 mg: Kola Nut (seeds, caffeine group alkaloids 3 mg), Citrus Aurantium (fruit, synephrine 2 mg), Cassia Mimosoides extract (leaves/stems/pods), White Willow bark • Caffeine (anhydrous) 200 mg • Tri-GuggLyptoid Complex 25 mg: Green Tea (leaves, <1 mg caffeine group alkaloids), Guggulsterone (whole plant), Gymnema (leaves). Other Ingredients: Dextrose, Gelatin, Stearic Acid, Magnesium Stearate, Titanium Dioxide, FD&C Yellow #5, FD&C Blue #1, FD&C Red #3, FD&C Yellow #6.
See Editor's Note No. 40, page 2058.

Stacker 2 LITE **-** NVE Pharmaceuticals
Each capsule contains: Proprietary Blend 320 mg: Kola Nut (seeds, 4 mg caffeine group alkaloids), Ephedra extract (leaves/stems, 12.5 mg ephedrine group alkaloids), White Willow bark • Caffeine (anhydrous) 100 mg • Tri-GuggLyptoid Complex 25 mg: Green Tea (leaves, <1 mg caffeine group alkaloids), Guggulsterone (whole plant), Gymnema (leaves). Other Ingredients: Dextrose, Gelatin, Stearic Acid, Magnesium Stearate, Titanium Dioxide, FD&C Yellow #5, FD&C Red #3, FD&CRed #40, FD&C Yellow #6.
See Editor's Note No. 30, page 2056.

Stacker 2 Stackerdrene Ephedra Free **-** NVE Pharmaceuticals
Each capsule contains: Magnesium (as magnesium gluconate) 25 mg • Vitamin B6 (as pyridoxine hydrochloride) 6.8 mg • Zinc (as zinc gluconate) 5 mg • Vitamin B12 (as cyanocobalamin) 50 mcg • Proprietary Blend 277 mg: Green Tea leaves extract (60%, polyphenols 120 mg), Grape seed extract (80% of proanthocyanidins), Cactus extract (12:1), Yerba Mate fruit, Guarana seeds • Caffeine Anhydrous 150 mg. Other Ingredients: Gelatin, Di Basic Calcium Phosphate, Stearic Acid, Titanium Dioxide, FD&C Yellow 6, Magnesium Stearate, Dextrose.

Stacker 2 Thermo Infusion Ephedra Free Glucodrene **-** NVE Pharmaceuticals
Two capsules contain: Glucomannan (form amorphophallus konjac root) 1200 mg. Other Ingredients: Gelatin, Microcrystalline Cellulose, Stearic Acid, Magnesium Stearate, Titanium Dioxide, FD&C Yellow 5, FD&C Yellow 6.

Stacker 3 **-** NVE Pharmaceuticals
Each capsule contains: Proprietary Blend 250 mg: Ephedra extract (leaves/stems, 25 mg ephedrine group alkaloids), Kola Nut (seeds, <1 mg caffeine group alkaloids), White Willow bark, Grapefruit extract (fruit), Chitosan (shellfish) • Caffeine (anhydrous) 250 mg • Tri-GuggLyptoid Complex 25 mg: Green Tea (leaves, <1 mg caffeine group alkaloids), Guggulsterone (whole plant), Gymnema (leaves). Other Ingredients: Gelatin, Di Basic Calcium Phosphate, Dextrose, Stearic Acid, Magnesium Stearate, Titanium Dioxide, FD&C Red #3, FD&C Blue #1, FD&C Red #40.
See Editor's Note No. 30, page 2056.

Stacker 3 with Chitosan Ephedra Free Formula **-** NVE Pharmaceuticals
Each capsule contains: Proprietary Blend 225 mg: Kola nut seed (caffeine group alkaloids 4 mg), Cactus extract (whole plant, 12:1), White Willow bark, Grapefruit fruit extract, Chitosan (shellfish) • Caffeine (anhydrous) 250 mg • Tri-Guarcinia3 Complex 25 mg: Green tea leaves (caffeine group alkaloids <1 mg), Guarana seeds, Garcinia fruit. Other Ingredients: Gelatin, Dextrose, Stearic Acid, Magnesium Stearate, Titanium Dioxide, FD&C Red 3, FD&C Blue 1, FD&C Red 40, FD&C Yellow 5.

Stamanex **-** Sterling-Grant Laboratories
Two tablets contain: Niacin 25 mg • Horny Goat Weed (epimedium grandiflorum) 500 mg • Icarin (whole herb) 50 mg • Maca root extract (4:1, lepidium meyenii) • German Tribulus Terrestris fruit extract 250 mg • 70% Furostanolic Saponins Fenusterols (7.5% protodioscin) 150 mg • Avena Sativa extract (10:1, oat straw) 150 mg • Eurycoma Lonifolia (long jack root) 125 mg • Ginko Biloba 75 mg.

Stamina **-** HerbaSway
Horny Goat Weed • Yohimbe • Dong Quai • Knotweed • Panax Ginseng • Licorice • Blackberry • HerbaSwee (Cucurbitaceae fruit).

Stamina 100 **-** Jamieson
Three caplets contain: Vitamin A (as Retinyl Acetate) 7500 IU • Vitamin C (as Ascorbic Acid) 125 mg • Vitamin D (as Cholecalciferol) 200 IU • Vitamin E (as Dl-Alpha Tocopheryl Acetate) 25 IU • Thiamin (as Thiamine Mononitrate) 12.5 mg • Riboflavin (Vitamin B2) 12.5 mg • Niacin (as Nicacinamide) 190 mg • Vitamin B6 (as Pyridoxine Hydrochloride) 12.5 mg • Folate (as Folic Acid) 200 mcg • Vitamin B12 (as Cyanocobalamin) 50 mcg • Pantothenic Acid (as Calcium D-Pantothenate) 30 mg • Calcium (as Calcium Carbonate) 600 mg • Iron (as Ferrous Fumarate) 10 mg • Iodine (as Potassium Iodide) 150 mcg • Magnesium (as Magnesium Oxide) 100 mg • Zinc (as Zinc Gluconate) 5 mg • Selenium (as Seleium Brown Rice Protein Chelate) 12.5 mcg • Manganese (as Manganese Gluconate) 3.5 mg • Chromium (as Chromium Brown Rice Protein Chelate) 10 mcg • Potassium (as Potassium Gluconate) 50 mg.

Stamina Beverage **-** Jamieson
Each bottle contains: Purified Water • Canadian Maple Syrup • Glucose • Natural Lemon and Orange Flavor (Tocopherols, Soybean Oil) • Canadian Ginseng root (Panax Quinquegolium) • Citric Acid • Sodium Benzoate • Xanthan Gum • Caramel (natural color) • Potassium Sorbate.

Standardized Cat's Claw Extract **-** Nature's Way
Each capsule contains: Cat's Claw bark 160 mg • Cat's Claw dried extract 175 mg. Other Ingredients: Gelatin, Millet.

Standardized Chamomile Extract **-** Nature's Way
Each capsule contains: Chamomile flower 220 mg • Chamomile dried extract 125 mg.

Some Brand Name Natural Products - What they Contain

www.NaturalDatabase.com contains MANY more listings than appear here.

Standardized Cider Vinegar with Apple Pectin **-** The Vitamin Shoppe
Each tablet has been standardized to provide 27 mg of acetic acid and 27 mg of apple pectin.

Standardized Feverfew Extract **-** Nature's Way
Each capsule contains: Feverfew leaves (standardized 0.7% Parthenolide) 370 mg.

Standardized Ginkgo Extract **-** Nature's Way
Each capsule contains: Ginkgo Biloba leaf extract; standardized to 24% Ginkgo flavone glycosides & 6% terpene lactones) 60 mg • Gotu Kola stem & leaf 400 mg. Other Ingredients: Gelatin & Millet.

Standardized Kava Extract **-** Nature's Way
Each softgel contains: Concentrated 10:1 Kava Extract (rhizome, standardized to 55% kavalactones) 128 mg.

Standardized Lutein & Bilberry **-** Swanson
Each softgel contains: Bilberry extract (25% anthocyanidins) 20 mg • FloraGLO® Lutein extract (from marigold) 6 mg.

Standardized Milk Thistle - GNC Herbal Plus **-** GNC
Each capsule contains: Milk Thistle Seed Extract (silybum marianum; 80% silymarin = 160 mg) 200 mg. Other Ingredients: Cellulose, Dicalcium Phosphate, Gelatin.

Standardized Saw Palmetto **-** GNC
Each capsule contains: Saw Palmetto berries extract (Serenoa repens; 85% Fatty Acids=136 mg; 0.2% Sterols=0.32 mg) 160 mg. Other Ingredients: Olive Oil, Gelatin, Glycerin, Caramel Color, Titanium Dioxide (natural mineral whitener).

Standardized Saw Palmetto Extract **-** Nature's Way
Each softgel contains: Saw Palmetto extract (berry, standardized to 85-95% Fatty Acids) 160 mg.

Starch Away **-** PhytoPharmica
Each soft chew contains: Phase 2 brand White Kidney bean (phaseolus vulgaris) 500 mg.

Starch Block **-** E'OLA
Each tablet contains: Chromium (as chromium polynicotinate) 100 mcg • Proprietary Blend 300 mg: Kidney Bean extract (10:1), Vanadium (as vanadyl sulfate).

Starch Blocker **-** Whole Health Discount Center
Each vegicap contains: Phaseolamin Phase 2 Phaseolus vulgaris extract • Water extracted from non-GMO White Kidney Beans.

Starch Blocker 1000 **-** R.P.M. Worldwide
Each capsule contains: Legume Protein Concentrate (Phase 2 brand) 500 mg. Other Ingredients: Gelatin, Magnesium Stearate, Stearic Acid, Microcrystalline Cellulose.

Starch Buster **-** Metabolife International, Inc.
Two tablets contain: Kidney Bean extract (Phaseolus vulgaris) 1000 mg. Other Ingredients: Modified Cellulose, Dicalcium Phosphate, Gum Acacia, Sodium Bicarbonate, Stearic Acid, Citric Acid, Dextrin, Dextrose, Lecithin, Sodium Carboxymethylcellulose, Sodium Citrate.

StarPac Daily Complex **-** Starlight International
Each packette contains: Vitamin A (50% as beta carotene and 50% as Vitamin A palmitate) 12,000 IU • Vitamin C (as ascorbic acid) 800 mg • Calcium (as calcium carbonate) 1,000 mg • Vitamin D (as cholecalciferol) 400 IU • Vitamin E (as d-alpha-tocopheryl acetate) 400 IU • Thiamin (as thiamine hydrochloride) 1.5 mg • Riboflavin 1.7 mg • Niacin (as niacinamide) 20 mg • Vitamin B6 (as pyridoxine hydrochloride) 2 mg • Folate (as folic acid) 400 mcg • Vitamin B12 (as cyanocobalamin) 6 mcg • Biotin 300 mcg • Pantothenic Acid (as calcium pantothenate) 10 mg • Iodine (as postassium iodide) 150 mcg • Magnesium (as magnesium oxide) 400 mg • Zinc (as zinc oxide) 15 mg • Selenium (as sodium selenite) 70 mcg • Copper (as copper sulfate) 2 mg • Manganese (as manganese sulfate) 2 mg • Chromium (as chromium picolinatinate) 120 mcg • Molybdenum (as sodium molybdate) 75 mcg • Potassium (as potassium chloride) 50 mg • Omega-3 Fatty Acids (from fish oil) 270 mg • Inositol 50 mg • Omega -6 Fatty Acids (from flaxseed oil) 28 mg • Para-Aminobenzoic Acid 25 mg • Betaine Hydrochloride 20 mg • Bromellain 20 mg • Boron (as boron citrate).

Start-Ups **-** Global Health Trax
Six capsules contain: Chromium (as chromium polynicotinate) 50 mcg • Guggulipid 250 mcg • Rhodiola root 150 mg • Acetyl-L-Carnitine (from hydrochloride) 250 mg • Alpha Lipoic Acid 50 mg • Coleus Forskohlii root 500 mg • Gotu Kola root 350 mg • Astragalus root 250 mg • White Willow bark 250 mg • Green Tea leaf 450 mg • Bitter Orange rind 500 mg • Fructo Oligo Saccharides (FOS) 100 mg • Hydroxycitric Acid (HCA) 1.25 g • Dimethylglycine 30 mg • Rhemannia leaves 250 mg • Lutein 50 mg. Other Ingredients: Methylcellulose, Gelatin.
See Editor's Note No. 40, page 2058.

StayCalm **-** Resource Wellness
Each caplet contains: Vitamin C (Ascorbic Acid) 10 mg • Thiamin Mononitrate 0.25 mg • Vitamin B6 (Pyridoxine HCl) 0.33 mg • Vitamin B12 (Cyanocobalamin) 1 mcg • Calcium 190 mg • St. John's Wort extract aerial parts 300 mg • Valerian root extract (root) 50 mg. Other Ingredients: Dicalcium Phosphate, Microcrystalline Cellulose, Croscarmellose Sodium, Magnesium Stearate, Stearic Acid, Maltodextrin, Silicon Dioxide, Hydroxypropyl Methylcellulose, Hydroxypropyl Cellulose, Polyethylene Glycol.

Steady On **-** Allergy Research Group
Each scoop (20 g) contains: Vitamin A (as beta-carotene) 1680 IU • Vitamin C (as ascorbic acid) 440 mg • Vitamin D (D3) 130 IU • Vitamin E (as mixed tocopherols) 360 IU • Vitamin K 45 mcg • Thiamin (vitamin B1) 22 mg • Riboflavin (vitamin B2) 22 mg • Niacin (as inositol hexanicotinate) 180 mg • Vitamin B6 22 mg • Folic Acid 350 mcg • Vitamin B12 22 mcg • Biotin 130 mcg • Pantothenic Acid 110 mg • Calcium (as calcium citrate/gluconate) 310 mg • Magnesium (as magnesium glycinate/gluconate) 130 mg • Zinc (as zinc arginate) 13 mg • Selenium (as sodium selenite/ selenomethionine) 90 mcg • Copper (as copper glycinate) 0.9 mg • Chromium (as chromium picolinate) 180 mcg • Potassium (as potassium gluconate) 45 mg • Alpha-Carotene 7 mg • Dehydroepiandrosterone (DHEA) 7 mg • Coenzyme Q10 67 mg • Inositol 22 mg • Choline 22 mg • Para-Aminobenzoic Acid 22 mg • Lecithin (26% phosphatidylcholine) 1440 mg • L-Alanine 35 mg • L-Arginine 110 mg • L-Aspartic Acid 95 mg • L-Carnitine 110 mg • L-Cystine 11 mg • L-Glutamine 67 mg • Glycine 67 mg • L-Histidine 22 mg • L-Isoleucine 45 mg • L-Lysine 50 mg • L-Methionine 180 mg • L-Ornithine Hydrochloride 220 mg • L-Phenylalanine 45 mg • L-Proline 45 mg • L-Serine 42 mg • Taurine 670 mg • L-Threonine 45 mg • L-Tyrosine 440 mg • N-Acetyl-L-Cysteine 440 mg • Glutathione (reduced) 110 mg • Pancreatin 13 mg • Papain 22 mg • Bromelain 22 mg • Grape skin extract 220 mg • Garlic (1% allicin) 45 mg • Lutein 1.8 mg • Lycopene 1.3 mg • Eicosapentaenoic Acid (EPA) 160 mg • Docosahexaenoic Acid (DHA) 110 mg • Palmitic Acid 130 mg • Stearic Acid 40 mg • Flax Seed Oil 440 mg • Lipoic Acid 45 mg • Methylsulfonylmethane 45 mg. Other Ingredients: Oat Bran, Rice Bran, Psyllium Bran, Stevia, Apple Fiber, Flavoring.

Sterols/Sterolins **-** Natur-Leaf
Two capsules contain: Proprietary Sterol/Sitosterolin Blend 640 mg: Wild African Potato root, Lupins sprouts, Fenugreek sprouts, Barley sprouts, Wheat sprouts, Soybean sprouts, African Sunflower sprouts • Enzyme/Mineral Blend 60 mg. Other Ingredients: Gelatin (capsule).

Stevia Powder **-** Optimum Nutrition
Each scoop contains: Stevia leaf extract (stevia rebaudiana, standardized to 90% steviosides) 70 mg. Other Ingredients: Maltodextrin, Silica.

Stimulin **-** Naturally Vitamins
Two tablets contain: Calcium (di-calcium phosphate) 100 mg • Magnesium (oxide) 100 mg • Citruline 1875 mg. Other Ingredients: Colloidal Silica, Magnesium Stearate, Cholesterol free stearic acid.

StimuMax for Men **-** Natrol
Proprietary Blend 2.02 g: Maca 4:1 root extract (Lepidium meyenii), Muira Puama 5:1 root extract (Ptychopetalum olacoides), Wild Oats 10:1 extract (Avena sativa), Guarana seed extract (Paullinia Cupana) (20% Caffeine), Korean ginseng root extract (Panax Ginseng), Ginkgo Biloba leaf extract, Epimedium 10% aerial extract (Epimedium grandiflorum). Other Ingredients: Rice powder, Silica, Magnesium Stearate, Gelatin.

StimuMax for Women **-** Natrol
Proprietary Blend 1.90 g: Maca 4:1 root extract (Lepidium meyenii), Muira Puama 5:1 root extract (Ptychopetalum olacoides), Wild Oats 10:1 extract (Avena sativa), Kava Kava standardized root extract (Piper methsyticum), Dong Quai standardized extract (Angelica sinensis), Damiana 4:1 leaf extract (Turnera diffusa), Korean Ginseng root extract (Panax). Other Ingredients: Rice Powder, Silica, Magnesium Stearate, Gelatin.

Stinging Nettle Leaf Extract **-** PhytoPharmica
Two capsules contain: Stinging Nettle (Urtica dioica) leaf extract (standardized to contain 1% silicic acid) 600 mg.

Stomach Calm **-** Enzymes, Inc.
Each capsule contains: n-zimes Proprietary Enzyme Blend 128 mg: Peptidase, Lipase, Amylase, Glucoamylase, Malt Diastase, Lactase, Invertase, alpha-Galactosidase, CereCalase Plus, Cellulase, Xylanase, Pectinase • Proprietary Herbal Blend 355 mg: Marshmallow root extract, Ginger root extract (5% gingerols) plus whole root, Deglycyrrhizinized Licorice root, Papaya leaf, Lavender flower, Rosemary herb. Other Ingredients: Plant Cellulose, Rice Bran, Water, Lecithin.

Stomach Plus **-** Atrium Inc.
Each tablet contains: Raw Stomach concentrate Bovine 323 mg • Folic Acid 100 mcg • Vitamin B12 50 mcg • Glycine 32 mg.
See Editor's Note No. 14, page 2055.

Stomach Soothing Complex **-** Shaklee
Three tablets contain: Peppermint Ginger Proprietary Blend 750 mg: Peppermint powder (Mentha piperita) leaf, Anise powder (Pimpinella anisum) seed, Fennel powder (Foeniculum vulgare) seed, Ginger powder (Zingiber offinale) root • Peppermint Oil (Mentha piperita) leaf 15 mg. Other Ingredients: Cellulose, Fructose, Maltodextrin, Corn Syrup Solids, Microcrystalline Cellulose.

Stomach-Aid **-** Futurebiotics
Two capsules contain: Calcium (carbonate) 200 mg • MSM (methyl-sulfonyl-methane) 300 mg • Ginger (root powder) 400 mg • Peppermint (leaf powder) 100 mg • Bromelain (600 GDU) 100 mg • Pancreatin 4X (Supplying 1600 USP units lipase, 10000 USP units amylase, 10000 USP units protease) 100 mg • Aloe Vera (leaf powder) 50 mg • Papain 50 mg • Stomach Aid Herbal Base 200 mg: Chamomile (flower powder), Catnip (leaf powder), Parsley (leaf powder), Fennel (seed powder). Other Ingredients: Gelatin, Cellulose, Magnesium stearate, Water.
See Editor's Note No. 14, page 2055.

StomachEase **-** Vita Pharmica - formerly Neopharmica
Each two tablets contain: Proprietary Concentrate 1500 mg: Corydalis Tuber, Astragalus root, San-Qi Ginseng root, Chekiang Fritillary bulb, Chinese Licorice root, Gambir leaf and stem, Brown's Lilly bulb, Bletilla Striata, Sepia Esculenta shell.

Stomagic **-** DreamPharm
Two capsules contain: Proprietary Blend: Magnolia Cortex, Citrus Sinensis Exocarpium, Atractylodes Rhizoma, Sclerotium Poria Cocos, Licorice Root, Cinnamomum Cortex, Ginger (zingiber rhizoma), Hawthorn (crataegus fruit), Cyperus Tubercles, Euphoria Longan Arill, Lycium Fruit, Shen Chu Preparation, Lindera Radix, Agastache Herb, Areca Seed, Astragalus Root, Birthwort Root, Cardamom Fruit, Amomum Kravanh (Cluster) Fruit, Coptis Root, Pinellia Root, Curcuma Zedoaria Rhizome, Paeonia Albiflora Radix, Brunoton, Acidophilus, Papaya Leaf.
See Editor's Note No. 46, page 2058.

Stone Root-Corn Silk Virtue **-** Blessed Herbs
Stone root • Gravel root • Hydrangea root • Goldenrod • Corn Silk • Nettle • Grain alcohol & Distilled Water.

Stopsmoking Herbal Tea **-** Health King
Each bag contains: Proprietary Blend: Licorice, Peppermint, Green Tea, Jasmine flower.

Strawberry Drinkable Yogurt **-** Stonyfield Farm
Each 10 fl oz bottle contains: Active Live Cultures: S. Thermophilus • L. Bulgaricus • L. Acidophilus • Bifidus • L. Casei • L. Reuteri. Ingredients: Cultured Pasturized Low Fat Milk • Organic Sugar • Organic Nonfat Dry Milk • Inulin • Pectin • Beet Juice Concentrate • Organic Strawberry Juice from concentrate • Natural Flavors.

Strawberry Smile Fructose - Revival **-** Physicians Laboratories
Each Packet Contains: Certified Isoflavone 160 mg. Ingredients: Soy Protein Isolate, Fructose, Sucrose, Natural and Artificial Flavor, Soy Lecithin, Calcium Phosphate, Beet juice powder, Maltodextrin, Potassium Chloride, Sodium Chloride, Xanthan Gum, Real Strawberry powder, Carboxymethylcellulose, Undegraded Carrageenan.

Strawberry Smile Splenda - Revival **-** Physicians Laboratories
Each Packet Contains: Certified Isoflavone 160 mg. Ingredients: Soy Protein Isolate, Cocoa, Maltodextrin, Calcium Phosphate, Soy Lecithin, Salt, Potassium Chloride, Artificial Flavor, Carrageenan, Carboxymethylcellulose, Xanthan Gum, Sucralose.

Strawberry Smile Unsweetened - Revival **-** Physicians Laboratories
Each Packet Contains: Certified Isoflavone 160 mg. Ingredients: Soy Protein Isolate, Natural and Artificial Flavor, Soy Lecithin, Calcium Phosphate, Beet juice powder, Maltodextrin, Potassium Chloride, Sodium Chloride, Xanthan Gum, Real Strawberry powder, Carboxymethylcellulose, Undegraded Carrageenan.

Strawberry-Apple Lactobacillus Acidophilus **-** Nature's Life
Two tablespoons (1 fl.oz or 29.6 ml) contain: Purified Water • Strawberry concentrate • Unfiltered Apple Juice • Pasteurized Honey • Soy Protein Isolate • Lactobacillus Acidophilus Culture.

ST-Res-Q **-** Nutri-Quest Rx
Each tablet contains: Adrenal 25 mg • Thymus 70 mg • Spleen 20 mg • Stomach 10 mg • Parotid 80 mg (All bovine source) • Vitamin C 175 mg • Vitamin B2 15 mg • Vitamin B6 10 mg • Niacinamide 15 mg • Pantothenic Acid (D-Calcium Pantothenate) 105 mg • Grape seed extract 1 mg • Lemon Bioflavonoids 225 mg • L-Tyrosine 175 mg • Magnesium Oxide 75 mg • Zinc Chelate 5 mg • Chromium Chelate 50 mcg • Potassium Chelate 10 mg • Chlorella 50 mg.
See Editor's Note No. 14, page 2055.

Stress Action **-** Nature's Plus
Two tablets contain: Vitamin C as Mineral Ascorbate 1000 mg • Desiccated Beef Liver 500 mg • Pantothenic Acid (Calcium Pantothenate) 125 mg • Vitamin B1 (Thiamine) 100 mg • Vitamin B2 (Riboflavin) 100 mg•Vitamin B6 (Pyridoxine HCl) 100 mg • Niacinamide 100 mg • Vitamin E natural 100 IU • Choline (Bitartrate) 75 mg • Inositol 75 mg • PABA (Para-aminobenzoic acid) 50 mg • Bee Pollen 50 mg • Ginseng Korean 50 mg • Calcium ascorbate 50 mg • Zinc Ascorbate 25 mg • Magnesium Ascorbate 25 mg • L-Phenylalanine free form amino acid 20 mg • Iron (Gluconate) 20 mg • Potassium (Citrate) 15 mg • L-Cysteine free form amino acid 15 mg • L-Methionine free form amino acid 15 mg • Folic Acid 400 mcg • Vitamin B12 from Cobalamin 250 mcg • Biotin 100 mcg •

Octacosanol 50 mcg • Chromium amino acid chelate 20 mcg • Selenium amino acid complex 10 mcg.
See Editor's Note No. 14, page 2055.

Stress and Tension Formula - Chinac - Metabolife International, Inc.
Each caplet contains: Corydalis yanhusuo (Corydalis) • Angelica dahurica (Fragrant Angelica) • Ligusticum sinense (Sichuan Lovage) • Saposhnikovia divaricata (Siler) • Arctium lappa (Burdock).

Stress Away - Futurebiotics
Two tablets contain: Vitamin C (ascorbic acid/ascorbyl palmitate) 250 mg • Vitamin A (beta carotene) 5000 IU • Vitamin B1 (thiamin) 25 mg • Vitamin B2 (riboflavin) 25 mg • Niacinamide 200 mg • Calcium (phosphate, aspartate) 100 mg • Vitamin B6 5 mg • Folic Acid 400 mcg • Vitamin B12 50 mcg • Iodine (kelp) 75 mg • Magnesium (oxide, amino acid chelate) 100 mg • Zinc (oxide, picolinate) 15 mg • Biotin 300 mcg • Pantothenic Acid 50 mg • Inositol 50 mg • Choline Bitartrate 100 mg • Manganese (amino acid chelate) 3 mg • Chromium (amino acid chelate, polynicotinate) 40 mcg • Para Amino Benzoic Acid (PABA) 50 mg • Valerian 200 mg • Chamomile 100 mg • Skullcap 50 mg • Passion flower 50 mg • Methionine 50 mg • Ribonucleic Acid (RNA) 50 mg.

Stress B Complex - Nature Made
Each tablet contains: Vitamin C 500 mg • Vitamin E 30 IU • Thiamin 10 mg • Riboflavin 10 mg • Niacin 100 mg • Vitamin B6 5 mg • Folic Acid 400 mcg • Vitamin B12 12 mcg • Biotin 45 mcg • Pantothenic Acid 20 mg.
See Editor's Note No. 45, page 2058.

Stress B with C - Nature's Life
Two capsules contain: Vitamin B1 (Thiamine Mononitrate) 50 mg • Vitamin B2 (Riboflavin and Riboflavin 5'-Phosphate) 50 mg • Vitamin B6 (Pyridoxine HCl & Pyridoxal 5'-Phosphate) 50 mg • Vitamin B12 (Cobalamin concentrate) 250 mcg • Niacinamide 100 mg • Folic Acid 400 mcg • Pantothenic Acid (d-Calcium Pantothenate) 250 mg • Biotin (d-Biotin)100 mcg • PABA (Para Aminobenzoic Acid) 50 mg • Choline (Bitartrate) 100 mg • Vitamin C 1000 mg.

Stress B-Complex plus Vitamin C - Optimum Nutrition
Two capsules contain: Vitamin C (as ascorbic acid) 1 g • Thiamin (as thiamin hydrochloride) 50 mg • Riboflavin 50 mg • Niacin (as niacinamide) 100 mg • Vitamin B6 (as pyridoxine hydrochloride) 50 mg • Folic Acid 400 mcg • Vitamin B12 (as cyanocobalamin) 250 mcg • Biotin 100 mcg • Pantothenic Acid (as d-calcium pantothenate) 250 mg • PABA (as para-aminobenzoic acid) 50 mg • Choline (as choline bitartrate) 40 mg • Inositol 100 mg. Other Ingredients: Gelatin, Magnesium Stearate, Silica.

Stress B-Complex with Vitamin C & Zinc - Nature Made
Each tablet contains: Vitamin C (from ascorbic acid) 500 mg • Vitamin E (from DL-alpha tocopheryl acetate) 30 IU • Thiamin (B1, from thiamine mononitrate) 10 mg • Riboflavin (B2) 10 mg • Niacin (B3) 100 mg • Vitamin B6 (from pyridoxine hydrochloride) 50 mg • Folate, Folic Acid, Folacin 400 mcg • Vitamin B12 (from cyanocobalamin) 12 mcg • Biotin 45 mcg • Pantothenic Acid (from D-calcium pantothenate) 20 mg • Zinc (from zinc sulfate) 23.9 mg • Copper (from copper oxide) 3 mg. Other Ingredients: Calcium Carbonate, Cellulose, Magnesium Stearate, Hydroxypropyl Methylcellulose, Stearic Acid, Polyethylene Glycol, Carnauba Wax.
See Editor's Note No. 45, page 2058.

Stress B-Complex with Vitamin C and Iron - Nature Made
Each tablet contains: Vitamin C (from ascorbic acid) 500 mg • Vitamin E (from DL-alpha tocopheryl acetate) 30 IU • Thiamin (from thiamin mononitrate) 10 mg • Riboflavin 10 mg • Niacin (from niacinamide ascorbate) 100 mg • Vitamin B6 (from pyridoxine hydrochloride) 5 mg • Folic Acid 400 mcg • Vitamin B12 (from cyanocobalamin) 12 mcg • Biotin 45 mcg • Pantothenic Acid (from D-calcium pantothenate) 20 mg • Iron (from ferrous fumarate) 18 mg. Other Ingredients: Cellulose, Calcium Carbonate, Gelatin, Croscarmellose Sodium, Corn Starch, Magnesium Stearate, Hydroxypropyl Methylcellulose, Polyethylene Glycol.
See Editor's Note No. 45, page 2058.

Stress Complex - Natrol
Two tablets contain: Thiamin (as thiamin HCl) 20 mg • Riboflavin 20 mg • Niacin (as niacinamide) 20 mg • Vitamin B6 (as pyridoxine HCl) 20 mg • Folic Acid 200 mcg • Vitamin B12 (as cyanocobalamin) 20 mcg • Melatonin 3 mg • Valerian root 5:1 extract 300 mg. Other Ingredients: Cellulose, Stearic Acid, Silica, Cellulose Gum, Magnesium Stearate, Hydroxypropyl Methylcellulose, Polyethylene Glycol, Hydroxypropyl Cellulose.
See Editor's Note No. 26, page 2056, page 2056.

Stress Essentials - PhytoPharmica
Each capsule contains: Vitamin C (Ascorbic Acid & Rose Hips) 100 mg • Calcium (as calcium carbonate and calcium citrate) 50 mg • Magnesium (Oxide) 30 mg • Potassium (Citrate) 25 mg • Pantothenic Acid (D-Calcium Pantothenate) 20 mg • Vitamin B6 (Pyridoxine HCL) 15 mg • Thiamine HCL (Vitamin B1) 12.5 mg • Riboflavin (Vitamin B2) 12.5 mg • Niacin 10 mg • Manganese (Chelate) 5 mg • Zinc (Chelate) 1.5 mg • Biotin 100 mcg • Folic Acid 75 mcg • Vitamin B12 (Cyanocobalamin) 25 mcg • Inositol 50 mg • Siberian Ginseng extract 5:1 (Eleutherococcus senticosus) 50 mg • Valerian extract (Valeriana officinalis; standardized to contain 0.2% to 0.8% valerenic acids) 50 mg • L-Tyrosine 50 mg • Skullcap extract 4:1 (Scutellaria baicalensis) 50 mg • Passion flower extract (Passiflora) 50 mg • Hops extract (Humulus lupulus) 50 mg • PABA (Para-Aminobenzoic Acid) 5 mg.

Stress Fighter - Puritan's Pride
Each tablet contains: Vitamin B1 20 mg • Vitamin B2 15 mg • Vitamin B6 10 mg • Vitamin B12 25 mcg • Folic Acid 400 mcg • Niacinamide 100 mg • Pantothenic Acid 25 mg • Vitamin C 600 mg • Vitamin E 45 IU. Plus valuable minerals such as Zinc, Iron, and Copper.

Stress Formula Calcet Plus - Mission Pharmacal
Each tablet contains: Vitamin A 5000 IU • Vitamin C 500 mg • Vitamin D (as Vitamin D3) 400 IU • Vitamin E 30 IU • Vitamin B1 2.25 mg • Vitamin B2 2.55 mg • Vitamin B3 30 mg • Vitamin B6 3 mg • Folate 0.8 mg • Vitamin B12 9 mcg • Vitamin B5 15 mg • Calcium 160 mg • Iron 18 mg • Zinc 15 mg. Other Ingredients: Sugar, Povidone, Magnesium Stearate, Color, Croscarmellose Sodium, Food Glaze, Carnauba Wax, White Beeswax, Sodium Benzoate, Cyanocobalamin.

Stress Manager - The Council On Natural Health
Two tablets contain: Thiamin (as thiamin HCl) 5 mg • Riboflavin 5 mg • Niacin (as niacinamide) 20 mg • Vitamin B6 (as pyridoxine HCl) 5 mg • Folate (as folic acid) 400 mcg • Vitamin B12 (as cyanocobalamin) 25 mcg • Pantothenic Acid (as d-calcium pantothenate) 10 mg • Kava Kava root 200 mg • Rhodiola Rosea root extract (40% total polyphenols) 10 mg • 5-HTP (from griffonia simplicifolia seeds) 10 mg • Adaptogenic Herbal Blend 150 mg: Ashwagandha root, Astragalus root, Panax Ginseng root, Suma root. Other Ingredients: Dicalcium Phosphate, Microcrystalline Cellulose, Croscarmellose Sodium, Stearic Acid, Silica, Magnesium Stearate, Pharmaceutical Glaze.

Stress Plex - Jamieson
Each tablet contains: Vitamin B1 3 mg • Vitamin B2 2.5 mg • Niacinamide 12 mg • Vitamin B6 3 mg • Vitamin B12 10 mcg • Biotin 10 mcg • Pantothenic Acid 5 mg • Folic Acid 0.05 mg • Vitamin C 250 mg • Zinc 5 mg • Lipotropic Factors: Choline Bitrate 5 mg, Inositol 5 mg.

Stress Plex - Nature's Plus
Two tablets contain: Vitamin C with Rose Hips 500 mg • Pantothenic Acid (Calcium pantothenate) 100 mg • Niacinamide 100 mg • Choline (Bitartrate) 100 mg • Inositol 100 mg • PABA (Para-aminobenzoic acid) 30 mg • Vitamin B1 (Thiamine) 10 mg • Vitamin B2 (Riboflavin) 10 mg • Vitamin B6 (Pyridoxine HCL) 10 mg •Folic

Acid 100 mcg • Vitamin B12 (from Cobalamin) 25 mcg • Biotin 25 mcg. B-Complex vitamins in a fortified rice bran base.

Stress Plus - Now
Each tablet contains: Vitamin B1 (Thiamine) 30 mg • Vitamin B2 (Riboflavin) 30 mg • Vitamin B3 (Niacinamide) 150 mg • Vitamin B6 (Pyridoxine) 30 mg • Vitamin B12 50 mcg • Pantothenic Acid 150 mg • Vitamin C (Ascorbic Acid) 500 mg • Biotin 300 mcg • Folic Acid 400 mcg • Magnesium (Oxide) 100 mg • PABA 40 mg • Choline (Bitartrate) 150 mg • Inositol 150 mg • Valerian root (50 mg of 4:1 extract) 200 mg.

Stress Tab B - Nature's Life
Two tablets contain: Vitamin B1 (Thiamine HCl) 60 mg • Vitamin B2 (Riboflavin) 60 mg • Vitamin B6 (Pyridoxine HCl) 60 mg • Vitamin B12 (Cobalamin concentrate) 60 mcg • Vitamin C 600 mg • Niacin 30 mg • Niacinamide 30 mg • Folic Acid 600 mcg • Pantothenic Acid (d-Calcium Pantothenate) 600 mg • Biotin (d-Biotin) 600 mcg • Choline (Bitartrate) 60 mg • Inositol 60 mg • PABA (Para Aminobenzoic Acid) 60 mg.

Stressease - Jamieson
Each caplet contains: Vitamin B1 35 mg • Vitamin B2 35 mg • Niacinamide 50 mg • Vitamin B6 15 mg • Vitamin B12 30 mcg • Biotin 15 mcg • Vitamin C 500 mg • Vitamin E 30 IU • d-Pantothenic Acid 20 mg • Folic Acid 1 mg • Calcium (Carbonate) 150 mg • Magnesium 75 mg • Zinc 5 mg.

Stress-End - Enzymatic Therapy
Each capsule contains: Vitamin C (Ascorbic Acid/Rose Hips) 100 mg • Calcium (Oyster Shell) 50 mg • Magnesium (Oxide) 30 mg • Potassium (Citrate) 25 mg • Pantothenic Acid (D-Calcium Pantothenate) 20 mg • Vitamin B6 (Pyridoxine HCL) 15 mg • Thiamine HCL (Vitamin B1) 12.5 mg • Riboflavin (Vitamin B2) 12.5 mg • Niacin 10 mg • Manganese (Chelate) 5 mg • Zinc (Chelate) 1.5 mg • Biotin 100 mcg • Folic Acid 75 mcg • Vitamin B12 (Cyanocobalamin) 25 mcg • Other ingredients: Inositol 50 mg • Siberian Ginseng extract 5:1 (Eleutherococcus senticosus) 50 mg • Valerian extract (Valeriana officinalis) standardized to contain 0.2% to 0.8% Valerenic Acids 50 mg • L-Tyrosine 50 mg • Skullcap extract 4:1 (Scutellaria baicalensis) 50 mg • Passion flower extract (Passiflora) 50 mg • Hops extract (Humulus lupulus) 50 mg • PABA (Para-Aminobenzoic Acid) 5 mg.

Stresstabs - Unknown
Each tablet contains: Vitamin C 500 mg • Vitamin E 30 IU • Thiamin 10 mg • Riboflavin 10 mg • Niacinamide 100 mg • Vitamin B6 5 mg • Folic Acid 400 mcg • Vitamin B12 12 mcg • Biotin 45 mcg • Pantothenic Acid 20 mg. Ingredients: Ascorbic Acid • Calcium Carbonate • Cellulose • Niacinamide • dl-Alpha Tocopheryl Acetate (Vitamin E) • Starch • d-Calcium Pantothenate • Hydroxypropyl Methylcellulose • Riboflavin (Vitamin B2) • Thiamine Mononitrate (Vitamin B1) • Dicalcium Phosphate • Pyridoxine Hydrochloride (Vitamin B6) • Silicon Dioxide • Magnesium Stearate • Triethyl Citrate • Stearic Acid • Mineral oil • Folic Acid • Titanium Dioxide • FD&C Yellow #6 Aluminum Lake • Biotin • Cyanocobalamin (Vitamin B12).

Stresstabs + Zinc - Unknown
Each tablet contains: Vitamin C 500 mg • Vitamin E 30 IU • Thiamin 10 mg • Riboflavin 10 mg • Niacinamide 100 mg • Vitamin B6 5 mg • Folic Acid 400 mcg • Vitamin B12 12 mcg • Biotin 45 mcg • Pantothenic Acid 20 mg • Zinc 23.9 mg • Copper 3 mg. Ingredients: Ascorbic Acid • Calcium Carbonate • Cellulose • Niacinamide • dl-Alpha Tocopheryl Acetate (Vitamin E) • Starch • Zinc Oxide • d-Calcium Pantothenate • Hydroxypropyl Methylcellulose • Riboflavin (Vitamin B2) • Thiamine Mononitrate (Vitamin B1) • Dicalcium Phosphate • Pyridoxine Hydrochloride (Vitamin B6) • Silicon Dioxide • Triethyl Stearate • Stearic Acid • Magnesium Stearate • Cupric Oxide • Crospovidone • Providone • Mineral oil • Folic Acid • Titanium Dioxide • FD&C Yellow #6 Aluminum Lake • Biotin • Cyanocobalamin (Vitamin B12).

StriVectin-SD - Klein-Becker
Deionized Water • C12-15 Alkyl Benzoate • Sesame Oil • Caprylic/Capric Triglyceride • Sweet Almond Oil • Cetearyl Olivate • Sorbitan Olivate • Striadil Complex: Phyllanthus Emblica fruit extract, Siegesbeckia Orientalis extract, Polyglyceryl Methyacrylate, Propylene Glycol, Palmitoyl Oligopeptide, Glucosamine HCl, Algae extract, Yeast extract, Urea, Butylene Glycol, Hydrocotyl extract, Coneflower extract, Hydrolyzed Wheat Protein, Hydrolyzed Wheat Starch, Imperata Cylindrica root extract, Bearberry extract, Licorice PTH • Glycerin • PPG-12/SMDI Copolymer • Glyceryl Stearate • PEG-100 Stearate • Cocoa Butter • Stearic Acid • Shea Butter • Tocopheryl Acetate • Mango Butter • Peppermint Oil • Methylparaben • Xanthan Gum • Propylparaben • Triethanolamine • Butylene Glycol • Disodium EDTA • Retinyl Palmitate • Tetrahexyldecyl Ascorbate.

Strixaderm MD - Pure Source
Deionized Water • C12-15 Alkyl Benozate • Sesame oil • Caprylic/Capric/Triglycerides • Almond oil • Cetearyl Olivate • Sorbitan Olivate • Palmitoyl Pentapeptide • Phyllanthus Emblic fruit extract • Siegesbeckia Orietalis extract • Polyglyceryl Methyacrylate • Propylene Glycol• Palmitoyl Oligopeptide • Glucosamine HCl • Algae extract • Stri Vera Blend: Aloe Vera, Yeast extract, Urea, Butylene Glycol, Hydrocotyl extract, Coneflower extract, Hydrolyzed Wheat Protein

Stuart Prenatal Multivitamin/Multimineral Supplement - Integrity Pharmaceutical Corp.
Each tablet contains: Vitamin A Acetate (25% as Beta Carotene) 4000 IU • Vitamin C (Ascorbic Acid) 100 mg • Vitamin D (Cholecalciferol) 400 IU • Vitamin E (dl-Alpha Tocopheryl Acetate) 11 IU • Thiamin Mononitrate (Vitamin B1) 1.8 mg • Riboflavin (Vitamin B2) 1.7 mg • Niacin (Vitamin B3, Niacinamide) 18 mg • Vitamin B6 (Pyridoxine Hydrochloride) 2.6 mg • Folate (Folic Acid, Folacin) 0.8 mcg • Vitamin B12 (Cyanocobalamin) 4 mcg • Calcium Sulfate 200 mg • Iron (Ferrous Fumarate) 27 mg • Zinc Oxide 25 mg. Other Ingredients: Beta Carotene, Croscarmellose Sodium, Hydroxypropyl Methylcellulose, Microcrystalline Cellulose, Pregelatinized Starch, Red Iron Oxide, Titanium Dioxide.

Sublingual B-12 Lozenge Tablets 2500 mcg - Puritan's Pride
Each lozenge contains: Vitamin B-12 2500 mcg.

Sublingual B-12 Lozenge Tablets 500 mcg - Puritan's Pride
Each lozenge contains: Vitamin B-12 500 mcg.

Sublingual B-12 Lozenge Tablets 5000 mcg - Puritan's Pride
Each lozenge contains: Vitamin B-12 5000 mcg.

Sublingual Coenzyme Q10 - Pro Health
Each tablet contains: Coenzyme Q10 (from vegetable/plant lipid) 50 mg. Other Ingredients: Sorbitol, Mannitol, Partially Hydrogenated Vegetable Oil, Natural Citrus Flavor, Mircrocrystalline Cellulose, Silicon Dioxide, Magnesium Stearate, Croscarmellose Sodium, Gelatin.

Sublingual Energy Plus B-12 (1000 mcg) - Pro Health
Each lozenge contains: Folic Acid 100 mcg • Vitamin B12 (as cyanocobalamin) 1 mg. Other Ingredients: Cellulose, Sorbitol, Mannitol, Fructose, Croscarmellose Sodium, Magnesium Stearate (vegetable source), Natural Cherry Flavor.

Sublingual Vitamin B-12 - PhysioLogics
Each tablet contains: Vitamin B12 (as cyanocobalamin) 5000 mcg • Coenzyme B12 (as dibencozide) 100 mcg. Other Ingredients: Sorbitol, Vegetable Stearic Acid, Croscarmellose, Natural Cherry Flavor, Vegetable Magnesium Stearate.

Sugar Metabolism Formula - Pharmacist's Ultimate Health
Two tablets contain: Vitamin B1 (Thiamin) 20 mg • Vitamin B2 (as Riboflavin) 10 mg •Vitamin B5 (as Panthothic Acid) 60 mg • Vitamin B6 (as Pyridoxine HCl) 40 mg •Vitamin C (as Ascorbic Acid) 400 mg •Biotin (Vitamin H) 1 mg • Folate (as Folic Acid) 260 mcg • Chromium (as Picolinate) 133 mcg • Magnesium (as Oxide) 40 mg

BRAND NAMES

•Manganese (as Gluconate) 7 mg •Potassium (as Potassium Chloride) 40 mg • Selenium (as Chleate) 40 mcg •Zinc (as Oxide) 10 mg • Alpha Lipoic Acid 30 mg • Betaine HCl 60 mg •Citrus Bioflavonoids 200 mg •Black Radish powder 120 mg •Beet juice 120 mg •Inositol 80 mg •Blueberry powder std. ext. (4:1) 100 mg •Choline (as Bitartrate) 60 mg • L-Methionine 60 mg • L-Taurine 120 mg.

***Sugar Stopper* - The Sports Nutrition Source, Inc.**
Each capsule contains: Gymnena Sylvestre 300 mg • Chitosan shellfish 100 mg • Garcinia Cambogia 100 mg • Vitamin C 50 mg.

***Sugar/Starch Digestion* - Enzymes, Inc.**
Each capsule contains: Proprietary Enzyme Blend 460 mg: Amylase, Protease, Invertase, Glucoamylase, Lipase, CereCalase, Malt Diastase, Lactase, alpha-Galactosidase, Cellulase, Peptidase. Other Ingredients: Plant Cellulose, Water.

***Sun Pollen* - Futurebiotics**
Cracked Flower Pollen & Pollen Extract.

***Sun Vitamines* - The Fitzpatrick Group, Inc.**
Two capsules contain: Polypodium Leucotomos 240 mg • Green Tea 50 mg • Beta-Carotene 10 mg.

***Sundown CoQ-10 50 Mg* - Rexall - Sundown**
Each softgel contains: Vitamin E (as D-alpha-tocopherol) 5 IU • Coenzyme Q-10 50 mg. Other Ingredients: Soybean Oil, Gelatin, Glycerin, Water, Yellow Beeswax, Titanium Dioxide, Yellow 6 Lake, Red 40 Lake, Blue 1 Lake.

***Sundown CoQ-10 75 Mg* - Rexall - Sundown**
Each softgel contains: Vitamin E (as D-alpha tocopherol) 5 IU • Coenzyme Q-10 75 mg. Other Ingredients: Soybean Oil, Gelatin, Glycerin, Water, Yellow Beeswax, Titanium Dioxide, Yellow 6 Lake, Red 40 Lake, Blue 1 Lake.

***Sundown Echinacea* - Rexall - Sundown**
Each capsule contains: Echinacea Purpurea (aerial parts) 400 mg. Other Ingredients: Gelatin.

***Sundown Zinc Gluconate 50 mg* - Rexall - Sundown**
Each tablet contains: Calcium 56 mg • Zinc (from zinc gluconate and zinc oxide) 50 mg. Other Ingredients: Dicalcium Phosphate, Microcrystalline Cellulose, Croscarmellose Sodium, Hydroxypropyl Methyl-Cellulose, Magnesium Stearate, Titanium Dioxide, PEG, Polysorbate 80.

***Sunkist Vitamin C Citrus Complex* - WN Pharmaceuticals, Ltd.**
Each tablet contains: Vitamin C 250 mg. Other Ingredients: Fructose, Sorbitol, Sucrose, Sodium Ascorbate, Ascorbic Acid, Hydrogenated Soybean Oil, Maltodextrin, Magnesium Stearate, Corn Starch, Hydrogenated Castor oil, Colloidal Silicon Dioxide, Lactose, Natural Flavors, Bioflavonoids.

***SunSpot ES* - LaneLabs**
Water • Aloe Vera • Propylene Glycol • Salicylic Acid • Urea • Carbomer 940 • Tea Tree Oil • Menthol • Glycoalkaloids extract • Imidazolidinylurea.
See Editor's Note No. 21, page 2056.

***Suntheanine brand* – NutriScience Innovations, LLC**
L-Theanine.
See Editor's Note No. 44, page 2058.

***SunVites With Lutein* - Sundown**
Each caplet contains: Vitamin A (20%/1000 IU as beta-carotene) 5000 IU • Vitamin C (as niacinamide ascorbate) 60 mg • Vitamin D (as cholecalciferol) 400 IU • Vitamin E (as DL-alpha tocopheryl acetate) 30 IU • Vitamin K (as phytonadione) 25 mcg • Thiamin (as thiamin mononitrate) 1.5 mg • Riboflavin (vitamin B2) 1.7 mg • Niacin (as niacinamide ascorbate) 20 mg • Vitamin B6 (as pyridoxine HCl) 2 mg • Folic Acid 400 mcg • Vitamin B12 (as cyanocobalamin) 6 mcg • Biotin 30 mcg • Pantothenic Acid (as calcium-D pantothenate) 10 mg • Calcium 170 mg • Iron (as ferrous fumarate) 18 mg • Phosphorus 109 mg • Iodine (as potassium iodide) 150 mcg • Magnesium (as magnesium oxide) 100 mg • Zinc (as zinc oxide) 15 mg • Selenium (as sodium selenate) 20 mcg • Copper (as cupric oxide) 2 mg • Manganese (as manganese sulfate) 2.5 mg • Chromium (chromium chloride) 120 mcg • Molybdenum (as sodium molybdate) 75 mcg • Chloride 36 mg • Potassium (as potassium chloride) 80 mg • Boron (as sodium borate and potassium borate) 150 mcg • Nickel (as nickel sulfate) 5 mcg • Silicon (as silica) 2 mg • Tin (as stannous chloride) 10 mcg • Vanadium (as sodium metavanadate) 10 mcg • Lutein 250 mcg. Other Ingredients: Microcrystalline Cellulose, Gelatin, Hydroxypropyl Methylcellulose, Croscarmellose Sodium, Triacetin, Titanium Dioxide (color), Magnesium Stearate, Corn Starch, Yellow 6 Lake, Retinyl Acetate, PEG.

***Super All-Day Nutricom* - Puritan's Pride**
Each scoop contains: Vitamin A 10,000 IU • Vitamin C 1,000 mg • Vitamin D 500 IU • Vitamin E 400 IU • Vitamin K 5 mcg • Thiamin 25 mg • Riboflavin 25 mg • Niacin 100 mg • Vitamin B-6 25 mg • Biotin 25 mcg • Pantothenic Acid 100 mg • Calcium 500 mg • Iron 18 mg•Phosphorus 200 mg • Iodine 150 mcg • Magnesium 200 mg • Zinc 50 mg • Selenium 50 mcg • Copper 0.2 mg • Manganese 4 mg • Chromium 50 mcg • Molybdenum 50 mcg • Potassium 99 mg • Inositol 100 mg • Choline 100 mg • Para-Aminobenzoic Acid (PABA) 25 mg • Rutin 25 mg • Citrus Bioflavonoids 25 mg • Hesperidin complex 25 mg • Lecithin 350 mg. Typical Amino Acid content per 15 g serving: Alanine 235 mg, Arginine 285 mg, Aspartic Acid 518 mg, Cysteine 27 mg, Glutamic Acid 1,614 mg, Glycine 139 mg, Histidine 212 mg, Isoleucine 458 mg, Leucine 703 mg, Lysine 561 mg, Methionine 216 mg, Phenylalanine 377 mg, Proline 822 mg, Serine 469 mg, Threonine 300 mg, Tryptophan 93 mg, Tyrosine 407 mg, Valine 517 mg.

***Super Anti-OX* - Nutri-Quest Rx**
Each tablet contains: Grape seed extract 20 mg (92-95% Proanthocyanidins) • Zinc (as Ester-C 2 mg) 14 mg • Vitamin C 100 mg • Vitamin E (Succinate) 50 IU • L-Glutathione 2 mg • N-Acetyl Cysteine 5 mg • Magnesium Aspartate 5 mg • Manganese Chelate 1 mg • Selenium Chelate 50 mcg • Chromium Chelate 50 mcg • Milk Thistle 150 mg • Silymarin 5 mg.

***Super Antioxidant* - Health Center for Better Living**
Vitamin C 500 mg • Vitamin E 300 IU.

***Super Antioxidant Capsules* - The Vitamin Shoppe**
Two capsules contain: Vitamin A (beta carotene and mixed carotenoids) 10,000 IU • Vitamin E 200 IU • Vitamin C (Calcium ascorbate) 60 mg • Vitamin B1 25 mg • Vitamin B2 25 mg • Vitamin B3 25 mg • Vitamin B5 25 mg • Vitamin B6 25 mg • Vitamin B12 250 mcg • N-Acetyl Cysteine 50 mg • Glutathione 50 mg • Selenium 75 mcg • Zinc 15 mg • Green Tea Extract (30% Polyphenols) 25 mg • CoQ10 10 mg • Quercetin 25 mg • Alpha Lipoic Acid 10 mg • Garlic (odorless) 100 mg • Grape Seed Extract (minimum 85%-95% proanthocyanidins) 10 mg • Manganese (Gluconate/Citrate) 15 mg

***Super Anti-Oxidant Complex* - Nature's Plus**
Two tablets contain: Vitamin C with Rose Hips 500 mg • Vitamin E natural 200 IU • Vitamin A (Beta Carotene) 10000 IU • Selenium amino acid complex 200 mcg • Chromium amino acid chelate 200 mcg. In a natural base of Carrots, Broccoli, Spinach & Beet Greens.

***Super Antioxidant Formula* - Puritan's Pride**
Each softgel contains: Vitamin E 400 IU • Beta Carotene 25,000 IU • Vitamin C 500 mg • Selenium 50 mcg.

***Super Antioxidant Formula - High Potency* - Nature's Bounty**
Each softgel contains: Vitamin A 25000 IU •Vitamin C (as Ascorbic Acid) 500 mg •Vitamin E (as d-Alpha Tocopherol) 400 IU •Selenium (as Selenium Yeast) 50 mcg. Other Ingredients: Gelatin, Glycerin, Soybean Oil, Soy Lecithin, Beeswax, St. John's Bread extract, Caramel Color.

Super Antioxidant Tablets **-** Clinician's Choice
Two tablets contain: Vitamin C (as ascorbic acid) 120 mg • Vitamin E (as dl-alpha tocopheryl acetate) 200 IU • Zinc (as amino acid chelate) 4 mg • Selenium (selenomethionine) 100 mcg • RoseOx Rosemary extract 200 mg • Schizandra Fruit Powder 100 mg • Grape Powder 60 mg • Ascorbyl Palmitate 20 mg • Proprietary Blend 10 mg: Astragalus, Beta Carotene, Carrot Powder, Coenzyme Q10, Cruciferex, Pycnogenol.

Super Antioxidants **-** Now
Two Vcaps contain: Green Tea extract (Camellia sinensis 40% Catechins) 200 mg • Milk Thistle extract (Silybum marianum 80% Silymarin) 100 mg • Curcumin extract (Curcuma longa min. 90% extract) 100 mg • Quercetin 100 mg • Bromelain from pineapple (2000 GDU) 100 mg • Cranberry powder extract 100 mg • Rosemary extract (Rosmarinus officinalis) 100 mg • Grape seed extract (95% Polyphenols) 30 mg • Ginkgo Biloba extract (24% Ginkgoflavoglycosides) 30 mg • Ginger root (Zingiber officinalis) 30 mg • Hawthorne berry extract (Crataegus oxyacantha 1.8% Vitexin-4"-Rhamnoside) 30 mg • Bilberry extract (Vaccimum myrtillus 25% Anthocyanidins) 20 mg.

Super Antioxidants with Folic Acid **-** Optimum Nutrition
Two capsules contain: Vitamin A (as CaroCare natural mixed carotenoids) 25,000 IU • Vitamin C (as ascorbic acid) 1000 mg • Vitamin E (as D-alpha tocopherol succinate) 400 IU • Folic Acid 400 mcg • Selenium 200 mcg • Alpha-Carotene 490 mcg • Zeaxanthin 94 mcg • Cryptoxanthin 114 mcg • Lutein 72 mcg. Other Ingredients: Gelatin, Microcrystalline Cellulose, Magnesium Stearate, Silica.

Super B Complex 100 **-** The Vitamin Shoppe
Each tablet contains: Vitamin B1 (Thiamin) 100 mg • Vitamin B2 (Riboflavin) 100 mg • Vitamin B6 (Pyridoxine HCl) 100 mg • Vitamin B12 (Cobalamin Concentrate) 100 mcg • Niacinamide 100 mg • Folic Acid 400 mcg • D-Biotin 100 mcg • Choline Bitartrate 100 mg • Inositol 100 mg • Pantothenic Acid (d-calcium pantothenate) 100 mg • PABA 100 mg. In a base of Alfalfa, Watercress, Parsley, Lecithin, and Rice Concentrate.

Super B Complex Vitamins plus Vitamin C **-** Nature's Bounty
Each caplet contains: Vitamin C (as ascorbic acid) 150 mg • Thiamin (vitamin B1, as thiamin mononitrate) 100 mg • Riboflavin (vitamin B2) 20 mg • Niacin (as niacinamide) 25 mg • Vitamin B6 (as pyridoxine hydrochloride) 2 mg • Folic Acid 400 mcg • Vitamin B12 (as cyanocobalamin) 15 mcg • Biotin 5 mcg • Pantothenic Acid (as D-calcium pantothenate) 5.5 mg • Calcium (as dicalcium phosphate) 29 mg • Brewer's Yeast 100 mg. Other Ingredients: Cellulose (plant origin), Croscarmellose, Vegetable Stearic Acid, Stearic Acid, Silica, Vegetable Magnesium Stearate, Cellulose Coating.

Super B-Complex **-** Nature Made
Each tablet contains: Vitamin C 150 mg • Thiamin 100 mg • Riboflavin 20 mg • Niacin 25 mg • Vitamin B6 2 mg • Vitamin B12 15 mcg • Biotin 5 mcg • Pantothenic Acid 5.5 mg • Dried Yeasts 100 mg. Other Ingredients: Dibasic Calcium Phosphate, Cellulose Gel, Croscarmellose Sodium, Corn Starch, Hydroxypropyl Methylcellulose, Magnesium Stearate, Polyethylene Glycol.
See Editor's Note No. 45, page 2058.

Super Biotin 5000 mcg **-** Vitamin World
Each capsule contains: Biotin 5000 mcg. Other Ingredients: Gelatin, Rice Powder, Silica.

Super Blue Stuff **-** Blue Stuff, Inc.
Each jar, bottle, or roll-on contains: Whole leaf Aloe Vera concentrate • Purified Water • MSM • Arnica Extract • SD-Alcohol-40 • Emu Oil • Sorbitol • Menthol • Sodium Chondroitin Sulfate • Glucosamine HCl • Capsicum Oleoresin • Nettle Extract • Coriander Oil • Kava Kava Extract • Extracts of: Blue Bottle, Roman Chamomile, Marigold, Lime tree • Willow Bark Extract • Witch Hazel Extract • Carbomer-940 • Triethanolamine • Fragrance • Ascorbyl Palmitate • FD&C Blue No. 1.
See Editor's Note No. 4 and No. 17.

Super Booster **-** Life Extension
Each softgel contains: Gamma-Tocopherol 210 mg • Gamma-Tocotrienol 35.5 mg • Delta-Tocopherol 78.4 mg • Delta-Tocotrienol 9.3 mg • Alpha-Tocopherol 66.3 mg • Alpha-Tocotrienol 18.5 mg • Beta-Tocopherol 3.5 mg • Lycopene extract (from tomato extract) 10 mg • Lutein extract (from marigold extract) 2.2 mg • Ginkgo extract (28% ginkgo flavone glycosides/7% terpene lactones) 120 mg • Chlorophyllin 100 mg • Vitamin K (K1) 9 mg • Vitamin K (K2) 1 mg • Selenium 200 mcg • Sodium Selenate 50 mcg • Selenomethionine 50 mcg • Methyl-Selenocysteine 100 mcg • Folate (as folic acid) 800 mcg • Vitamin B12 (as cyanocobalamin) 500 mcg • Ascorbyl Palmitate 50 mg • Vitamin C (as calcium ascorbate, ascorbyl palmitate) 90 mg • Vitamin E (as d-alpha tocopherol) 98.8 IU • Calcium (as calcium ascorbate) 10 mg. Other Ingredients: Gelatin, Flaxseed Oil, Glycerine, Purified Water, Yellow Beeswax, Lecithin, Carob Color.

Super Cal Mag Plus **-** Shaklee
Ten tablets contain: Vitamin D (as Cholecalciferol) 400 IU • Vitamin K (as Phytonadione) 40 mcg • Calcium (as Dicalcium phosphate, Calcium carbonate and Calcium citrate) 1200 mg • Phosphorus (as Dicalcium phosphate) 700 mg • Magnesium (as Magnesium oxide) 200 mg • Zinc (as Zinc gluconate) 1.5 mg • Copper (as Copper gluconate) 0.2 mg • Manganese (as Manganese gluconate) 0.2 mg • Sodium 10 mg • Boron (as Boron protein hydrolysate 1 mg. Other Ingredients: Microcrystalline Cellulose, Croscarmellose, Sodium.

Super Calcium 1200 **-** Schiff
Two softgels contain: Vitamin D (as cholecalciferol) 400 IU • Calcium (as calcium carbonate) 1200 mg. Other Ingredients: Vegetable Oil, Gelatin, Glycerin, Lecithin, and Titanium Dioxide.

Super Cal-Mag **-** Nature's Life
Two tablets contain: Calcium (Chelated, Carbonate, Aspartate, Aminoate, Citrate Complex) 1000 mg • Magnesium (Chelated, Oxide, Aspartate, Aminoate, Citrate Complex) 500 mg.

Super Carnosine **-** Life Extension
Each capsule contains: Carnosine 500 mg • Benfotiamine 50 mg • Quercetin (water soluble) 50 mg. Other Ingredients: Magnesium Stearate, Dicalcium Phosphate, Gelatin, Water.

Super Cayenne **-** Swanson
Two capsules contain: Cayenne pepper (100,000 heating units) 450 mg • Ginger root powder 200 mg • Hawthorn berry powder 200 mg • Lecithin granules 50 mg.

Super C-Complex 500 **-** The Vitamin Shoppe
Each tablet contains: Vitamin C (with Rose Hips) 500 mg • Citrus Bioflavonoid Complex 100 mg • Hesperidin Complex 25 mg • Rutin 50 mg • Acerola 1 mg.

Super Chelated Multi-Mineral **-** Puritan's Pride
Three tablets contain: Calcium 750 mg • Phosphorus 300 mg • Magnesium 375 mg • Potassium 99 mg • Manganese 15 mg • Iron 15 mg • Zinc 15 mg • Copper 375 mcg • Iodine 225 mcg • Chromium 30 mcg • Selenium 38 mcg.

Super Chitosan **-** Genesis Nutrition
Two capsules contain: Chitosan 1 g.
See Editor's Note No. 37, page 2057.

Super CitriMax **-** Vitamin World
Two capsules contain: Chromium (as ChromeMate brand chromium polynicotinate) 130 mcg • Gymnema leaf (gymnema sylvestre, standardized to contain 30 mg of gymnemic acid) 130 mg • (-) Hydroxycitric Acid (HCA, provided by 1500 mg of Super CitriMax Plus from garcinia cambogia rind) 900 mg. Other Ingredients: Gelatin, Silica, Magnesium Stearate.

Some Brand Name Natural Products - What they Contain

www.NaturalDatabase.com contains MANY more listings than appear here.

Super CitriMax 750 mg **-** Natural Max
Two tablets contain: Super CitriMax brand Garcinia Cambogia (supplying 750 mg (60%) hydroxycitric acid-HCA) 1250 mg. Other Ingredients: Di-Calcium Phosphate, Cellulose, Stearic Acid, Magnesium Stearate.

Super CitriMax brand **-** InterHealth Nutraceuticals
Hydroxycitric Acid (HCA, extracted from garcinia cambogia fruit). See Editor's Note No. 44, page 2058.

Super CitriMax Clinical Strength brand **-** InterHealth Nutraceuticals
Hydroxycitric Acid (HCA, extracted from garcinia cambogia fruit). See Editor's Note No. 44, page 2058.

Super Climax Cream **-** Media Dreamland Inc.
Organic Damiana leaf (folium terneraceae) • Organic Suma root (radix pfaffiae paniculatae) • Organic Motherwort (herba leonori) • Organic Wild Yam (rhizoma dioscorea villosae) • Organic Ginkgo Biloba • Organic Peppermint leaf (folium menthae piperitae).

Super Coenzyme Q-10 **-** Gary Null & Associates (GNA)
Each tablet contains: Coenzyme Q10 100 mg. Other Ingredients: Dicalcium Phosphate, Cellulose and Modified Cellulose, Stearic Acid, Magnesium Stearate, Silicon Dioxide, Pharmaceutical Glaze.

Super Complete Capsules **-** Ultimate Nutrition
Nine capsules contain: Vitamin A 10000 IU • Vitamin D 400 IU • Vitamin E 400 IU • Vitamin B1 100 mg • Vitamin B2 100 mg • Vitamin B6 100 mg • Vitamin B12 100 mcg • Niacinamide 100 mg • Pantothenic Acid 100 mg • Folic Acid 400 mcg • Biotin 300 mcg • Choline 100 mg • Inositol 100 mg • PABA 100 mg • Vitamin C 1500 mg • Bioflavonoids 250 mg • Rutin 50 mg • Rose Hips powder 20 mg • Hesperidin 20 mg • Acerola Cherry 10 mg • Glutamic Acid HCL 100 mg • Betaine HCl 100 mg • Calcium 1000 mg • Magnesium 500 mg • Iodine 150 mcg • Potassium 95 mg • Iron 30 mg • Zinc 22.5 mg • Manganese 10 mg • Copper 3 mg • Boron 3 mg • Chromium 200 mcg • Selenium 50 mcg.

Super Concentrated Lecithin **-** Jamieson
Each capsule contains: Lecithin in a Super Concentrated form 400 mg. Derived from pure Soy. Standardized to Phosphatidylcholine 140 mg.

Super CoQ10 with Tocotrienols 100 mg **-** Life Extension
Each softgel contains: Coenzyme Q10 (Japanese pharmaceutical grade) 100 mg • Tocomin 30% (palm oil-derived tocotrienol complex) 45 mg • Rice Bran oil 350 mg • Vitamin E 5 IU. Other Ingredients: Gelatin, Glycerin, Water, Beeswax, Lecithin, Rosemary Extract.

Super CoQ10 with Tocotrienols 30 mg **-** Life Extension
Each softgel contains: Coenzyme Q10 (Japanese pharmaceutical grade) 30 mg • Tocomin 30% (palm oil-derived tocotrienol complex) 23 mg • Rice Bran oil 275 mg • Vitamin E 3 IU. Other Ingredients: Gelatin, Glycerin, Water, Beeswax, Lecithin, Rosemary Extract.

Super Cranberry Concentrate **-** Wellness for Women
Each softgel contains: Vitamin C USP (as ascorbic acid) 100 mg • Vitamin E (as dl-alpha tocopheryl acetate) 3 IU • Cranberry juice concentrate, 10:1 (equivalent to 800 mg) 80 mg.

Super Curcumin with Bioperine **-** Life Extension
Each tablet contains: Turmeric root powdered extract (curcuma longa, supplying curcumin 76.1% 685 mg) 900 mg • Demethoxycurcumin (15.7%) 142 mg • Bisdemethoxycurcumin (3.2%) 29 mg • Bioperine Piperine (from black pepper) 5 mg. Other Ingredients: Magnesium Stearate, Gelatin, Water.

Super Detox **-** 4 Life
Two capsules contain: Red Clover 450 mg • Milk Thistle extract (80% silymarin) 200 mg • Calcium d-Glucarate 130 mg • Sulforaphane (from broccoli, 25% DIM) 120 mg • Bupleurum 80 mg • N-Acetyl Cysteine 50 mg • Artichoke (leaf) 50 mg. Other Ingredient: Gelatin Capsule

Super Energy Oil **-** Puritan's Pride
Each softgel contains: Soybean oil 650 mg • Rice Bran oil 228 mg • Wheat Germ oil (cold pressed) 228 mg • Vitamin E (d-alpha tocopherol) 5 IU.

Super Energy Up **-** The Vitamin Shoppe
Each capsule contains: Standardized Panax Ginseng extract, Fo-Ti root, Sukday, Licorice, Lycii Berries, and Damiana leaves in a base of Royal Jelly, Bee Pollen, Vitamin B12, and Octacosanol.

Super Enzymes **-** Now
Each tablet contains: Betaine HCL (from beet molasses) 200 mg • Bromelain (2000 GDU from pineapple) 50 mg • Papain (140 MCU uncoated from papaya) 50 mg • Pancreatin 4x (equivalent to 800 mg) 200 mg supplying: Amylase (20000 USP Units) 100 mg, Protease [Chymotrypsin & Trypsin (20000 USP Units)] 100 mg, Lipase (3400 USP Units) 25 mg • Pepsin Enzymes NF 1:10000 50 mg • Cellulase 10 mg • Ox Bile extract 100 mg • Papaya Enzymes 45 mg • Pineapple Enzymes 45 mg.
See Editor's Note No. 14, page 2055.

Super EPA DHA 500 mg **-** The Vitamin Shoppe
Each softgel contains: Vitamin E (as d-alpha tocopherol) 5 IU • EPA Eicosapentaenoic Acid (as marine fish oil) 300 mg • DHA Docosahexaenoic Acid (as marine fish oil) 200 mg.

Super Flex Joint Formula **-** Natural Balance
Each tablet contains: Vitamin C (as ascorbic acid) 40 mg • Manganese (as chelate) 6.7 mg • Glucosamine (as HCl/sulfate) 500 mg • MSM (methylsulfonylmethane) 333 mg • Boswellia Serrata Gum Resin (extract standardized to 65% total organic acids) 100 mg • Chondroitin Sulfate 50 mg • Ginger root 33 mg • Turmeric (curcumae longae standardized root extract) 15 mg • Polygonum Cuspidatum root (extract standardized to 50% trans-resveratrol) 5.4 mg. Other Ingredients: Microcrystalline Cellulose, Cellulose Gum, Magnesium Stearate, Stearic Acid, Silicon Dioxide.
See Editor's Note No. 15, page 2055.

Super Food **-** Youngevity
Phosphorus • Sulfur • Chloride • Sodium • Vitamin A • Vitamin B1 • Vitamin B2 • Vitamin B3 • Vitamin B5 • Vitamin B6 • Vitamin B12 • Vitamin C • Vitamin D • Vitamin E • Vitamin K • Folic Acid • Biotin • Soy Protein • Soybean Oil • Soy Lecithin • Lactobacillus Acidophilus • FOS • Papaya • Protease • Bromelain • Amylase • Lipase • Cellulase • Soy • Rice • Barley • Oats • Prunes • Citrus • Alfalfa • Capsicum fruit • Chlorella • Garcinia fruit • Licorice.

Super Gainers Fuel **-** TwinLab
Each serving contains: Milk & Egg Proteins 100 g • High Levels of Complex Carbohydrates • Branched Chain Amino Acids (L-Leucine, L-Isoleucine & L-Valine) • L-Glutamine • L-Carnitine • Alpha-Ketoglutarate • Creatine Monohydrate • High Potencies of Vitamins & Minerals including Potassium 2000 mcg & Chromium 600 mcg • Fat 29 g [from Medium Chain Triglycerides (MCTs)]. MCTs are lipids composed of Medium Chain Fatty Acids.

Super Ginseng **-** Dial Herbs
Siberian Ginseng • Korean Ginseng • Brazilian Ginseng • Chinese Ginseng • American Ginseng.

Super GLA/DHA **-** Life Extension
Three softgels contain: Borage seed oil (borago officinalis) 2000 mg • GLA (gamma-linolenic acid) 460 mg • Marine Lipid concentrate 1000 mg • DHA (docosahexaenoic acid) 500 mg • EPA (eicosapentaenoic acid) 125 mg. Other Ingredients: Gelatin, Glycerin, Water, Carob Color, Rosemary Extract.

Super Greens **-** Jamieson
Each 8.5 g serving contains: Lecithin Powder 1220 mg • Concentrated Juice Blend 1710 mg: Alfalfa Leaf, Barley Grass, Buckwheat Seed, Kamut Seed, Red Beet Root, Wheat Grass • Spirulina Blue-Green Algae 1050 mg • Whole Brown Rice Hulls 549 mg • Stevia Root Extract 100 mg • Multi Algae Blend 427 mg: D. Salina Algae,

Nori, Chlorella, Dulse, Kombu, Wakame • Sprouted Multi-Grains 427 mg: Barley Malt Seed, Mung Bean, Soybean, Wheat Berry • Dahlia Tuber and Chicory Root 225 mg • Beet Root Fiber 200 mg • Beta Glucans 200 mg • Soy Fiber 200 mg • Carrot Root Fiber 214 mg • Apple Pectin Fiber 214 mg • Bee Pollen 160 mg • Licorice Root 134 mg Acerola Fruit 134 mg • Astragalus Root 64 mg • Canary Island Brown Algae 50 mg • Sargassi Seaweed 50 mg • Laminaria Seaweed 50 mg • Artichoke Leaf Extract 50 mg • Artichoke Leaf 50 mg • Dahlia Inulin Juice Complex 50 mg • Siberian Ginseng Root 47 mg • Royal Jelly 43 mg • Green Tea Leaf 33 mg • Milk Thistle Seed 32 mg • Jerusalem Artichoke Tuber 25 mg • Ginkgo Biloba Leaf 20 mg • Tomato Fruit 10 mg • Grape Seed Extract 10 mg • Papain Enzyme (from Papaya Fruit) 10 mg • Cellulase Enzyme 10 mg • Bilberry Fruit 11 mg • Natural Spearmint and Wintergreen Flavour.

Super Growth Enhancer **-** Optimum Nutrition
L-Arginine L-Ornithine Vitamin B6 20 mg • Vitamin C 200 mg.

Super Herbal V **-** MD Healthline
Two capsules contain: Yohimbe Bark 250 mg • Damiana Extract 50 mg • Bilberry Powder 100 mg • Gingko Biloba Extract (24%) 60 mg • Siberian Ginseng Extract 100 mg • Schisandra Extract 200 mg • Avena Sativa Extract 10:1 250 mg • Saw Palmetto (30%) 100 mg.

Super Immune **-** Oasis Wellness Network
Each tablet contains: Astragalus Membranaceus root extract 167 mg • Schisandra Chinensis fruit extract 100 mg • MaxCell Proprietary Blend 83 mg: Zisyphus Jujube, Aloe Vera gel, Glycyrrhiza Glabra, Piper Nigrum • L-Arginine (base) 67 mg • Reishi mushroom fruit extract (ganoderma lucidum) 50 mg. Other Ingredients: Stearic Acid, Cellulose, Calcium Sulfate, Magnesium Stearate, Silica.

Super Immuno-Comp **-** Enzymatic Therapy
Two capsules contain: Vitamin A (Beta Carotene) non-toxic form of Vitamin A 5000 IU • Vitamin C (Ascorbic Acid/Rose Hips) 100 mg • Vitamin B6 (Pyridoxine HCl) 5 mg • Zinc (Picolinate) 3 mg • Other Ingredients: Astragalus extract (Astragalus membranaceus) 150 mg • Echinacea extract (Echinacea angustifolia) standardized to contain greater than 3.5% Echinacosides & 0.65% essential oils 150 mg • Goldenseal extract (Hydrastis canadensis) standardized to contain 5% total Alkaloids including: Berberine, Hydrastine & Canadine 150 mg • KS-2 (Peptidomannan Complex) Shiitake Mushroom, a purified extract of Lentinus Edodes 50 mg • Licorice root extract (Glycyrrhiza glabra) standardized to contain 5% Glycyrrhizic Acid 50 mg.

Super Immuno-Tone **-** PhytoPharmica
Two capsules contain: Vitamin A 5000 IU • Vitamin C 100 mg • Vitamin B6 5 mg • Zinc 3 mg • Astragalus extract 150 mg • Echinacea extract 150 mg • Goldenseal extract 150 mg • Shiitake Mushroom (KS-2) 50 mg • Licorice root extract 50 mg.

Super Joints **-** Baywood International
Three caplets contain: Methyll-sulfonyl-methane (LIGNISUL) 1500 MG • Glucosamine (HCl) 1200 mg • Boswellin extract 225 mg • Chondroitin Sulfate 200 mg • Manganese 25 mg • Proprietary Blend 300 mg: Bromelan, Peptizyme SP, Papaine. Other Ingredients: Magnesium Stearate.
See Editor's Note No. 15, page 2055.

Super K with K2 **-** Life Extension
Each softgel contains: Vitamin K (K1) 9 mg • Vitamin K (K2) 1 mg • Medium Chain Triglycerides (MCT oil) 215 mg • Ascorbyl Palmitate (antioxidant) 25 mg. Other Ingredients: Gelatin, Carob, Water.

Super KMH Chromium Liquid **-** Essential Nutrients
Each fluid ounce contains: Potassium 585 mg • Magnesium 50 mg • Calcium 50 mg • Trace Minerals Blend: Aluminum, Antimony, Barium, Beryllium, Bismuth, Boron, Bromine, Cadmium, Calcium, Carbon, Cerium, Cesium, Chlorine, Chromium, Cobalt, Copper, Dysporosium, Erbium, Europium, Fluorine, Gadolinium, Gallium, Germanium, Hafnium, Homium, Hydrogen, Indium, Iodine, Iridium, Iron, Lanthanum, Lithium, Lutetium, Magnesium, Manganese, Molybdenum, Neodymium, Nickel, Niobium, Nitrogen, Oxygen, Palladium, Phosphorus, Potassium, Praseodymium, Rhenium, Thodium, Rubidium, Ruthenium, Samarium, Scandium, Selenium, Silicon, Silver, Sodium, Strontium, Sulfur, Tantalum, Terbium, Thallium, Thorium, Thulium, Tin, Titanium, Tungsten, Vanadium, Ytterbium, Yttrium, Zinc, Zirconium. Herb Blend: Thyme (thymus vulgaris), Senega Snakeroot (polygala senega), Saw Palmetto berries, Sarsaparilla (smilax officinalis), Passion Flower (passiflora incarnata), Licorice root (glycyrrhiza glabra), Horehound root (marrubium), Goldenseal (hydrastis canadensis), Ginseng (panax quinquefolius), Ginkgo (ginkgo biloba), Gentian root (gentiana lutea), Echinacea (echinacea augustifolia), Dandelion root (taraxacum officinalis), Chamomile (matricaria chamomilla), Celery seed (apium gloveclens), Angelica root (angelica archangelica), Alfalfa (medicago sativa).

Super Leci-Thins **-** Nature's Life
Three tablets contain: Lecithin (Soy) 1300 mg • Cider Vinegar 255 mg • Kelp 150 mg • Vitamin B6 (Pyridoxine HCl) 50 mg.

Super Liquid Absorbable Calcium **-** Puritan's Pride
Two softgels contain: Vitamin D (as Cholecalciferol) 100 IU • Calcium (as Calcium Carbonate) 1,000 mg.

Super Lysine Plus+ Cream **-** Quantum, Inc.
L-lysine • Lithium Carbonate 3X • Propolis extract • Calendula Flower extract • Echinacea Flower extract • Zinc Oxide • Goldenseal extract • Vitamin A • Vitamin D • Vitamin E • Cajeput Oil • Tea Tree Oil • Gum Benzoin Tincture. Prepared in a Beeswax and Olive Base.

Super Lysine Plus+ Tablets **-** Quantum, Inc.
Each three tablets contain: L-lysine 1500 mg • Vitamin C (ascorbic acid) 100 mg • Garlic (odorless) 200 mg • Echinacea extract (4:1 PE) 100 mg • Propolis 50 mg • Licorice extract (4:1 PE) 15 mg • Goldenseal root USP (Hydrastis) 15 mg.

Super Male Plex **-** The Vitamin Shoppe
Two tablets contain: Yohimbe extract 10 mg • Raw Testicular 250 mg • Damiana 250 mg • Ginseng (Korean/Siberian) 500 mg • Octacosanol 250 mcg • Vitamin E 250 IU • Histidine 200 mg • Sarsaparilla 100 mg • Saw Palmetto 100 mg • Raw Prostate 100 mg • Bee Pollen 100 mg • Zinc 100 mg • Oyster extract 50 mg • Cayenne 50 mg • Gotu Kola 50 mg • Selenium 50 mcg • Niacin 15 mg • Royal Jelly 5 mg.
See Editor's Note No. 14, page 2055.

Super Male-Plex **-** Puritan's Pride
Two tablets contain: Raw Testicular 250 mg • Damiana 250 mg • Siberian Ginseng 250 mg • Korean Ginseng 250 mg • Octacosanol 250 mcg • Vitamin E 250 IU • Histidine 200 mg • Sarsaparilla 100 mg • Saw Palmetto 100 mg • Raw Prostate 100 mg • Bee Pollen 100 mg • Zinc 30 mg • Oyster extract 50 mg • Cayenne 50 mg • Gotu Kola 50 mg • Selenium 50 mcg • Niacin 15 mg • Royal Jelly 5 mg • Oatstraw 50 mg.
See Editor's Note No. 14, page 2055.

Super Malic **-** Optimox
Six tablets contain: Magnesium (Hydroxide) 300 mg • Malic Acid 1200 mg.

Super Max 1600 Weight Gain **-** Aspen Group, Inc.
Each flavor (vanilla or chocolate) contains: Vitamin C 332 mg • Rose Hips 6.8 mg • Vitamin E 400 IU • Vitamin A 13,332 USP Units • Vitamin D 532 USP Units • Vitamin B1 20 mg • Vitamin B2 16 mg • Vitamin B6 68 mg • Vitamin B12 8 mcg • Niacin 56 mg • Choline 40 mg • Inositol 26.8 mg • Para Aminobenzoic Acid 1600 mg • Pantothenic 132 mg • Biotin 400 mcg • Folic Acid 532 mcg • Rutin 1700 mcg • Glutamic Acid 880 mg • Iodine 200 mcg • Calcium 1280 mg • Phosphorus 1200 mg • Potassium 10 mg • Iron 36 mg • Copper 2800 mg • Magnesium 13.2 mg • Manganese 3200 mg • Zinc 20 mg • Amino Acids: Arginine 7883 mg • Aspartic Acid 220 mg • Alanine 880 mg • Cystine 1100 mg • Glutamic Acid 880 mg • Glycine 1980 mg • Histidine 2332 mg • Isoleucine 7152 mg • Leucine 4840 mg • Lysine 5060 mg • Methionine 1100 mg • Phenylalanine 944 mg •

Proline 328 mg • Serine 4840 mg • Threonine 3300 mg • Tyrosine 220 mg • Tryptophan 880 mg • Valine 4840 mg.

Super Mega Vite II Multiple **-** Nature's Life
Each tablet contains: Beta Carotene (Vitamin A equivalent to 10000 IU) 6 mg • Vitamin B1 (Thiamine HCl) 50 mg • Vitamin B2 (Riboflavin) 50 mg • Niacinamide 75 mg • Pantothenic Acid (Calcium Pantothenate) 75 mg • Vitamin B6 Pyridoxine HCl) 50 mg • Vitamin B12 (Cobalamin concentrate) 250 mcg • Folic Acid 400 mcg • Biotin (d-Biotin) 50 mcg • Choline (Bitartrate) 50 mg • Inositol 50mg • l-Methionine (free form) 25 mg • Vitamin E (d-Alpha Tocopherol plus mixed Tocopherols) 100 IU • Vitamin C 250 mg • Rutin 5 mg • Lemon Bioflavonoids Complex (TESTLAB 50%) 25 mg • Hesperidin Complex 5 mg • Calcium (Carbonate) 100 mg • Chromium (Chelate) 25 mcg • Copper (Chelate) 200 mcg • Iodine (Postassium Idodine) 100 mg • Iron (Chelate) 10 mg • Magnesium (Oxide) 40 mg • Manganese (Chelate) 7 mg • Phosporus (Potassium Phosphate) 45 mg • Potassium (Phosphate, Chloride, Iodide) 67 mg • Selenium (Nutrition 21) (l-Selenomethionine) 10 mcg • Silicon (Dioxide) 20 mg • Zinc (Chelate) 10 mg • Coenzyme Q-10 (Ubiquinone) 500 mcg • Betaine HCl 25 mg • Glutamic Acid HCL 25 mg. In a natural base of "72 Trace Minerals" from an ancient sedimentary sea bed, Chamomile, Rice Bran & Rose Hips.

Super Mega Vite Multiple **-** Nature's Life
Each tablet contains: Vitamin A (Fish Liver oil) 25000 IU • Vitamin D (as Vitamin D3, Cholecalciferol) 400 IU • Vitamin B1 (Thiamine HCl) 30 mg • Vitamin B2 (Riboflavin) 30 mg • Niacinamide 100 mg • Pantothenic Acid (d-Calcium Pantothenate) 100 mg • Vitamin B6 Pyridoxine HCl) 30 mg • Vitamin B12 (Cyanocobalamin) 250 mcg • Folic Acid 400 mcg • PABA (Para Aminobenzoic Acid) 60 mg • Biotin (d-Biotin) 50 mcg • Choline (Choline Bitartrate) 100 mg • Inositol 100 mg • Vitamin E (d-Alpha Tocopheryl Succinate) 100 IU • Vitamin C 250 mg • Lemon Bioflavonoids Complex (50% Total Flavanones) 25 mg • Rutin 25 mg • Hesperidin Complex (50% Total Flavanones) 5 mg • Calcium (Bone Meal) 82.5 mg • Chromium (Chelate) 25 mcg • Copper (Gluconate) 200 mcg • Iodine (Potassium Iodide) 100 mcg • Iron (Ferrous Fumarate) 10 mg • Magnesium (Oxide) 40 mg • Manganese (Gluconate) 7 mg • Phosphorus (Bone Meal) 37.5 mg • Potassium (Iodide) 10 mg • Selenium (Nutrition 21 l-Selenomethionine) 10 mcg • Zinc (Gluconate) 10 mg • Super Oxide Dismutase 30 IU • Betaine HCl 25 mg • Glutamic Acid HCl 25 mg • Methionine 50 mg. In a natural base of Lecithin, Alfalfa, Watercress, Parsley, Duodenal Substance, Rose Hips powder, Chamomile, Molasses, Kale, Cabbage, Goldenseal, Sarsaparilla, "72 Trace Minerals", Pepsin & Kelp.

Super Milk Thistle X **-** PhytoPharmica
Each capsule contains: Milk Thistle fruit extract (silybum marianum) bound to phosphatidylcholine 100 mg • Dandelion root 4:1 extract (taraxacum officinale) 10 mg • Artichoke leaf extract (cynara scolymus, standardized to contain 13%-18% caffeylquinic acids calculated as chlorogenic acid) 40 mg • Licorice root extract (glycyrrhiza glabra, standardized to contain 5% glycyrrhizic acid) 10 mg.

Super MiraForte with Maximum Strength Chrysin **-** Life Extension
Two capsules contain: Zinc (as zinc monomethionine) 7.5 mg • Chrysin 750 mg • Muira Puama (ptychopetalum olacoides) 425 mg • Maca root (lepidium meyenii) 160 mg • Nettle root (urtica dioica) powdered Methanolic extract 141 mg • Ginger root extract (zingiber officinale, rhizome) 25 mg • Piperine (from black pepper) 7.5 mg. Other Ingredients: Gelatin, Water.

Super Multi with Herbs **-** Leiner Health Products
Each tablet contains: Iron (Ferrous Fumarate) 9 mg • Magnesium (Magnesium Oxide) 100 mg • Calcium (Calcium Carbonate) 225 mg • Vitamin B12 (Cyanocobalamin) 12 mcg • Vitamin C (Ascorbic Acid) 120 mg • Vitamin E (dl-Tocopheryl Acetate) 60 IU • Chromium (Chromium Picolinate, Chromium Chloride) 120 mcg • Copper (Cupric Oxide) 2 mg • Folate (Folic Acid) 400 mcg • Iodine (Potassium Iodide) 150 mcg • Manganese (Manganese Sulfate) 2 mg • Molybdenum (Sodium Molybdate) 75 mcg • Niacin (Niacinamide) 20 mg • Pantothenic Acid (d-Calcium Pantothenate) 10 mg • Riboflavin (Vitamin B2) 1.7 mg • Selenium (Sodium Selenate) 70 mcg • Thiamin (Vitamin B1) 1.5 mg • Vitamin A (40% as Beta Carotene) 5000 IU • Vitamin B6 (Pyridoxine Hydrochloride) 2 mg • Vitamin D (Ergocalciferol) 400 IU • Vitamin K (Phytonadione) 80 mcg • Zinc (Zinc Oxide) 15 mg • Biotin (d-Biotin) 30 mcg • Boron (Boron Citrate) 150 mcg • Ginkgo Biloba (Ginkgo biloba) leaf 25 mg • Herbal Complex Blend 25 mg • Siberian Ginseng (Eleutherococcus senticosus) root 25 mg. Other Ingredients: Gelatin, Maltodextrin, Starch, Cellulose, Dicalcium Phosphate, Croscarmellose Sodium, Silicon Dioxide, Polyethylene Glycol 3350, Crospovidone, Tricalcium Phosphate, Hydroxypropyl Methylcellulose, Mannitol, Magnesium Stearate, Pharmaceutical Glaze, Hydroxypropyl Cellulose, Resin, Polysorbate 80.

Super Multi-Pak **-** Optimum Nutrition
Each pak (3 capsules/3 tablets) contains: Vitamin A (as fish liver oil) 10,000 IU • Vitamin C (as ascorbic acid) 1000 mg • Vitamin D (as fish liver oil) 400 IU • Vitamin E (as D-alpha tocopherol succinate) 400 IU • Thiamin (as thiamin hydrochloride) 75 mg • Riboflavin 75 mg • Niacin (as niacinamide) 75 mg • Vitamin B6 (as pyridoxine hydrochloride) 75 mg • Folic Acid 400 mcg • Vitamin B12 (as cyanocobalamin) 75 mcg • Biotin 300 mcg • Pantothenic Acid (as D-calcium pantothenate) 75 mg • Calcium (as calcium carbonate, citrate and dicalcium phosphate) 772 mg • Iron (as iron AA chelate) 9 mg • Phosphorus (as calcium phosphate) 203 mg • Iodine (as kelp) 75 mcg • Magnesium (as magnesium oxide) 250 mg • Zinc (as zinc AA chelate) 15 mg • Selenium (as selenium AA chelate) 56 mcg • Copper (as copper AA chelate) 2 mg • Manganese (as manganese AA chelate) 2 mg • Chromium (as chromium GTF) 96 mcg • Molybdenum (as molybdenum AA chelate) 60 mcg • Chloride (as potassium chloride) 44 mg • Potassium (as potassium chloride) 48.5 mg • Inositol 100 mg • Choline (as choline bitartrate) 100 mg • PABA (as para-aminobenzoic acid) 100 mcg • Lecithin 1200 mg • Citrus Bioflavonoids 100 mg • Rose Hips 10 mg • Betaine (as betaine hydrochloride) 50 mg. Other Ingredients: Pharmaceutical Glaze, Microcrystalline Cellulose, Gelatin, Stearic Acid, Croscarmellose Sodium (disintegrant), Silica.

Super Nails **-** Puritan's Pride
Three tablets contain: Vitamin A (as Fish Liver Oil) 10,000 IU • Vitamin D (as Fish Liver Oil and Cholecalciferol) 400 IU • Riboflavin (Vitamin B2) 50 mg • Folic Acid 200 mcg • Vitamin B12 (as Cyanocobalamin) 100 mcg • Calcium (as Calcium Amino Acid Chelate and Dicalcium Phosphate) 730 mg • Iron (as Iron Amino Acid Chelate) 5 mg • Phosphorus (as Phosphorus Amino Acid Chelate and Dicalcium Phosphate) 372 mg • Magnesium (as Magnesium Amino Acid Chelate) 25 mg • Gelatin 260 mg • Horsetail (Equisetum arvense) stem 250 mg • L-Cysteine 100 mg • DL-Methionine 100 mg • Sulfur (as Potassium Sulfate and from amino acids) 25 mg • Oat Straw (Avena sativa) stem 25 mg • Rice Bran powder 12 mg.

Super Nutrition Power **-** Mascot Enterprise
Deer Velvet • Shark Cartilage • Fish Oil (Salmon) • Royal Jelly • Oyster Extract • Orchic Substance • Siberian Ginseng extract 5:1 • Cinnamon • Garlic • Noni • Muira Puama • Guarana extract 4:1 • Smilax • Avena Sativa 10:1 • Damiana leaf extract 4:1 • Vitamin E • Vitamin C • Vitamin B6 • Boron (Citrate) • Zinc (Sulfate) • Niacinamide.
See Editor's Note No. 14, page 2055.

Super Octacosanol **-** The Vitamin Shoppe
Each softgel contains: Octacosanol 3000 mcg • Wheat Germ Oil 235 mg • Lecithin 9 mg.

Super Odorless Garlic **-** Now
Each capsule contains: odorless Garlic extract 100:1 concentrate (equivalent to 5000 mg fresh Garlic) 50 mg • Hawthorne berry extract (standardized to contain 1.8% Vitexin-2"-Rhamnoside) 100 mg • Hawthorne berry powder 250 mg • Cayenne pepper (40,000 Heat units) 100 mg.

Super Omega 3 **-** Nutri-Quest Rx
Each capsule contains: Natural marine lipid concentrate 1 g • Omega-3 Fatty Acids 110 mg/1 g of Eicosapentaenoic Acid (EPA) • Omega-3 90 mg/1 g of Docosahexaenoic Acid (DHA).

Super Omega-3 Fish Oils **-** Carlson Laboratories
Each capsule contains: Vitamin E (as D-alpha tocopherol) 10 IU • Omega-3 Fatty Acids (from fish oil) 500 mg • DHA (docosahexaenoic acid) 200 mg • EPA (eicosapentaenoic acid) 300 mg.

Super Omega-3 Natural Fish Oil - 1000 mg **-** Vitamin World
Each softgel contains: Fish Oil 1000 mg • EPA (eicosapentaenoic acid) 300 mg • DHA (docosahexaenoic acid) 200 mg. Other Ingredients: Gelatin, Glycerin.

Super Orti Vite **-** Genestra - Seroyal
Each capsule contains: Vitamin A (palmitate) 1250 IU • Beta Carotene 2500 IU • Thiamin Hydrochloride (vitamin B1) 25 mg • Riboflavin (vitamin B2) 15 mg • Niacinamide (vitamin B3) 38 mg • Pantothenic Acid (d-calcium pantothenate) 25 mg • Pyridoxine Hydrochloride (vitamin B6) 15 mg • Pyridoxal 5-Phosphate 500 mcg • Cyanocobalamin (vitamin B12) 25 mcg • Folic Acid 100 mcg • Biotin 75 mcg • Vitamin C (ascorbic acid) 100 mg • Vitamin D (D3, cholecalciferol) 25 IU • Vitamin E (d-alpha tocopherol) 75 IU • Calcium (citrate) 50 mg • Chromium GTF (polynicotinate) 25 mcg • Iodine (potassium iodide) 56 mcg • Iron (aspartic acid chelate) 5 mg • Magnesium (aspartic acid chelate) 20 mg • Manganese (citrate) 5 mg • Potassium (citrate) 5 mg • Selenium (selenomethionine) 25 mcg • Zinc (citrate) 5 mg • Bromelain (pineapple) 5 mg • Choline (bitartrate) 10 mg • Coenzyme Q10 (ubiquinone) 1 mg • Inositol 10 mg • L-Cysteine 10 mg • Non-citrus Bioflavonoids 10 mg • Hesperidin 10 mg • Papain (papaya) 5 mg.

Super Phos 30 **-** Dew's Twenty First Century Products
Ninety drops contain: Phosphorus 360 mg • Inositol 51 mg • Choline Bitartrate 18 mg.

Super Prostate Formula **-** Physician's Choice
Each tablet contains: Soy Phytosterol Complex 660 mg: Beta Sitosterol 300 mg, Campesterol 165 mg, Stigmasterol 138 mg, Brassicasterol 15 mg • Pygeum Africanum extract (standardized, providing 15 mg beta sitosterol) 120 mg • Saw Palmetto extract (standardized) 300 mg • L-Alanine 300 mg • L-Glycine 300 mg • L-Glutamic Acid 300 mg • Stinging Nettles 300 mg • Ginseng 150 mg • Pygeum Africanum powder 48 mg • Lycopene Complex (5% lycopene) 40 mg • Pumpkin seed 30 mg • Zinc (amino acid chelate) 30 mg • PABA 30 mg • Vitamin B6 30 mg • Vitamin A 7500 IU • Vitamin E 30 IU • Piper Nigrum (Bioperine) 2 mg.

Super Q10 **-** Cell Tech
Two softgels contain: Vitamin A (beta-carotene) 4080 IU • Vitamin K 7 mcg • Proprietary Blend 1 g: Flax Seed oil, Blue-Green Algae (aphanizomenon flos-aquae) 170 mg, Coenzyme Q10 60 mg, Essential Oils (rosemary, fennel, ginger, cinnamon), Betatene Carotenoids (d. salina). Other Ingredients: Beeswax (encapsuling aid), Gelatin (gelatin, glycerin, water, carob, titanium dioxide).

Super Salve **-** The Herbalist
Oils of Sweet Almond, St. John's Wort flower, Plantain herb, Calendula flower, & Beeswax • Extracts of Poplar bud, Golden Seal root, Echinacea root, Plantain herb, Comfrey root, Marshmallow root, Yarrow flower.

Super Saw Palmetto **-** Enzymatic Therapy
Each softgel contains: Saw Palmetto berry extract (serenoa repens) 160 mg.

Super Seed Beyond Fiber **-** Garden of Life, Inc.
Two heaping tablespoons contain: Perfect Fiber Blend 18,360 mg: Flax seed meal, whole Chia seed • Poten-Zyme Whole Food Fiber Blend 1500 mg: Flax seeds, Sunflower seeds, Chia seeds, Sesame seeds, Pumpkin seeds, Adzuki beans, Millet, sprouted Quinoa, Garbanzo beans, Buckwheat, sprouted Amaranth, Red Lentils, Kidney beans • Organic Cinnamon 124 mg • Stevia 90% 16 mg • Poten-Zyme Probiotic Blend 1.6 Billion CFU.

Super Silica Complex **-** Futurebiotics
One tablet contains: Calcium (as calcium carbonate, citrate) 200 mg • Magnesium (as magnesium oxide, citrate) 150 mg • Zinc (as zinc gluconate) 15 mg • Betaine hydrochloride 50 mg • Boron 1.5 mg • Horsetail leaf powder extract 275 mg. Other Ingredients: Dicalcium phosphate, Cellulose, Stearic acid, Magnesium stearate.

Super Snooze with Melatonin **-** Puritan's Pride
Each capsule contains: Valerian root 100 mg • Hops 75 mg • Scullcap 75 mg • Chamomile 75 mg • Passion Flower 50 mg • Calcium carbonate 100 mg • Magnesium oxide 50 mg • Inositol 50 mg • L-Taurine 50 mg • Melatonin 3 mg.
See Editor's Note No. 16, page 2055.

Super Sprouts & Algae **-** Cell Tech
Three tablets contain: Vitamin A (beta-carotene) 1845 IU • Vitamin D 24 IU • Vitamin K 8 mcg • Vitamin B12 0.4 mcg • Calcium 60 mg • Iron 0.5 mg • Phosphorus 60 mg • Proprietary Blend 2.4 g: Wheat sprouts, Blue-Green Algae (aphanizomenon flos-aquae) 180 mg, Red Beta Algae (d. salina). Other Ingredients: Dicalcium Phosphate, Glyceryl Monostearate, Croscarmellose Sodium, Silica Dioxide, Magnesium Stearate.

Super Strength Glucosamine Plus CSA **-** Optimum Nutrition
Two tablets contain: Glucosamine Sulfate (as glucosamine sulfate potassium) 1500 mg • Chondroitin Sulfate (as chondroitin sulfate A) 1200 mg. Other Ingredients: Pharmaceutical Glaze, Stearic Acid, Magnesium Stearate, Croscarmellose Sodium (disintegrant), Silica.

Super Stress Formula **-** The Vitamin Shoppe
Two capsules contain: Vitamin C 1000 mg • Vitamin B1 (Thiamin) 50 mg • Vitamin B2 (Riboflavin) 50 mg • Vitamin B6 (Pyridoxine Hcl) 50 mg • Vitamin B12 (Cobalamin) 400 mcg • Niacinamide 100 mg • Folic Acid 400 mcg • Pantothenic Acid 250 mg • Biotin 100 mcg • Choline Bitartrate 100 mg • Inositol 100 mg • PABA 50 mg.

Super Suppositories **-** The Herbalist
Tea Tree Oil • Herbal extracts of Usnea & Calendula in a base of Cocoa Butter & Purified Bees Wax.

Super Vanadyl Fuel **-** TwinLab
Four capsules contain: Vanadyl Sulfate (supplying elemental Vanadium IV 4.87 mg) 25 mg • BMOV [Bis (maltolato) Oxovanadium] (supplying elemental Vanadium IV 320 mcg) 2 mg • Chromium (from Chromic Fuel Chromium Picolinate) 300 mcg • Chromium (from ChromeMate Chromium Nicotinate) 300 mcg • Natural Vitamin E 900 IU • Taurine 1000 mg • Selenium (from Sodium Selenate) 150 mcg • Zinc (from Zinc Picolinate) 30 mg • Manganese (from Manganese Gluconate) 5 mg • Magnesium (from Magnesium Oxide & Aspartate) 400 mg • Biotin 1000 mcg • Niacinamide 100 mg.

Super Vitamin B Complex **-** Schiff
Each tablet contains: Vitamin B1 (as thiamin mononitrate) 30 mg • Vitamin B2 (as riboflavin) 35 mg • Niacin (as niacinamide) 50 mg • Vitamin B6 (as pyridoxine hydrochloride) 15 mg • Folate (as folic acid) 400 mcg • Vitamin B12 (as cyanocobalamin) 100 mcg • Biotin 300 mcg • Pantothenic Acid (as d-calcium pantothenate) 100 mg • Calcium (as dibasic calcium phosphate, d-calcium pantothenate) 37 mg • Choline Bitartrate 50 mg • Inositol 100 mcg • PABA (para-aminobenzoic acid) 50 mg • L-Methionine 25 mcg. Other Ingredients: Cellulose, Coating (hydroxypropyl methylcellulose, carbowax, pharmaceutical glaze shelac, ethyl cellulose), Magnesium Stearate, Croscarmellose Sodium.

Super Vitamin E Creme **-** Aspen Group, Inc.
Each gram contains: Tocopheryl Acetate 25% • Panthenol 1% • Water • Glyceryl Stearate SE • Octyl Palmitate • Isoproyl Palmitate • Propylene Glycol • Cetearyl Alcohol • Cetyl Phosphate • Decyl Oleate

• Aminomethyl Propanol • Carbomer • Allantoin • Diazolidinyl Urea • Methylparaben • Propylparaben.

Super Vita-Vim - Level 3 Potency Multivitamin **-** Jamieson
Each caplet contains: Vitamin A 5000 IU • Beta Carotene 1500 IU • Vitamin C 200 mg • Vitamin D 400 IU • Vitamin E 60 IU • Vitamin B1 30 mg • Vitamin B2 30 mg • Vitamin B3 (No Flush Niacinamide) 50 mg • Vitamin B5 50 mg • Vitamin B6 50 mg • Vitamin B12 50 mg • Folic Acid 400 mcg • Biotin 30 mcg • Calcium 150 mg • Iron 4 mg • Copper 1 mg • Iodine 0.1 mg • Magnesium 75 mg • Zinc 10 mg • Potassium 25 mg • Manganese 1 mg • Chromium 10 mcg • Selenium 10 mcg • Vanadium 1 mcg • Molybdenum 1 mcg • Lutein 300 mcg • Lycopene 300 mcg • Citrus Bioflavonoids 2000 mcg • Ginseng (Canadian) 25 mg • Digestive Enzyme Absorption Factors derived from: Peppermint, Bromelain, Papain, Amylase, Lipase, Cellulose.

Super Vita-Vim with Beta Carotene **-** Jamieson
Each caplet contains: Vitamin A (as Tetinyl Acetate and 15% [1500] IU as Beta-Carotene) 10000 IU • Vitamin C (as Ascorbic Acid) 200 mg • Vitamin D (as Cholecalciferol) 400 IU • Vitamin E (as Dl-Alpha Tocopheryl Acetate) 60 IU • Thiamin (as Thiamine Mononitrate) 30 mg • Riboflavin (Vitamin B2) 30 mg • Niacin (as Niacin and Nicacinamide) 60 mg • Vitamin B6 (as Pyridoxine Hydrochloride) 30 mg • Folate (as Folic Acid) 400 mcg • Vitamin B12 (as Cyanocobalamin) 60 mcg • Biotin 30 mg • Pantothenic Acid (as Calcium D-Pantothenate) 30 mg • Calcium (as Calcium Carbonate) 140 mg • Iron (as reduced Iron) 4 mg • Iodine (from kelp) 100 mcg • Magnesium (as Magnesium Oxide) 100 mg • Zinc (as Zinc Gluconate) 10 mg • Selenium (from yeast) 10 mcg • Copper (as Copper Gluconate) 1 mg • Chromium (as Chromium Rice Protein Chelate) 50 mcg • Potassium (as Potassium Gluconate) 30 mg • Choline Bitartrate 30 mg • Inositol 30 mg • Dl-Methionine 2.2 mg.

Super VM **-** Puritan's Pride
Each tablet contains: Vitamin A (as Retinyl Palmitate) 10,000 IU • Vitamin C (as Ascorbic Acid and Rose Hips) 250 mg • Vitamin D (as Ergocalciferol) 400 IU • Vitamin E (as d-Alpha Tocopheryl Acetate) 150 IU • Thiamin (Vitamin B-1) 60.8 mg • Riboflavin (Vitamin B-2) 75 mg • Niacin (as Niacinamide) 75 mg • Vitamin B-6 (as Pyridoxine Hydrochloride) 61.5 mg • Folic Acid 400 mcg • Vitamin B-12 (as Cyanocobalamin) 75 mcg • Biotin (as D-Biotin) 75 mcg • Pantothenic Acid (as d-Calcium Pantothenate) 75 mg • Calcium (as Calcium Amino Acid Chelate) 50 mg • Iron (as Iron Amino Acid Chelate) 10 mg • Iodine (as Kelp) 150 mcg • Magnesium (as Magnesium Amino Acid Chelate) 25 mg • Zinc (as Zinc Amino Acid Chelate) 15 mg • Selenium (as Sodium Selenate) 10 mcg • Copper (as Cupric Amino Acid Chelate) 0.25 mg • Manganese (as Manganese Amino Acid Chelate) 6.1 mg • Potassium (as Potassium Amino Acid Chelate) 10 mg • PABA (Para-Aminobenzoic Acid) 75 mg • Choline Bitartrate 75 mg • Inositol 75 mg • Rutin 25 mg • Citrus Bioflavonoids 25 mg • Hesperidin 5 mg • Betaine Hydrochloride 25 mg • L-Glutamic Acid 25 mg • Proprietary Blend 3 mg: Alfalfa (leaf), Watercress (plant), Parsley (leaf).

Super Whey Fuel **-** TwinLab
Blend of Three key Whey Proteins: Micro-Filtered & Ion-Exchange Whey Protein Isolate, Modified Molecular Weight & Partially Pre-Digested Whey Protein, & Whey Protein Concentrate enriched with Glutamine, Taurine, Arginine, Leucine, Isoleucine, Valine, Carnitine & Carnosine.

SuperCitriMax **-** Now
Each capsule contains: Calcium (from Citrimax) 90 mg • ChromeMate brand of Chromium (Chromium Polynicotinate) 100 mcg • Iodine (from Kelp) 150 mcg • CitriMax Garcinia cambogia extract 750 mg • Panax ginseng root powder 100 mg.

Super-Green Pro-96 Soy Protein **-** Nature's Life
Two scoops (28.35 g) contain: Full disclosure ingredients: SUPRO brand Soy Protein Isolate (including Lecithin) • Hawaiian Spirulina • natural Vanilla Flavor • Barley Grass • Psyllium seed husks • Apple Pectin • Oat Fiber • Chlorophyll • Lemon Bioflavonoids Complex • Bromelain • Papain • Kelp • Milk-free Lactobacillus acidophilus • Pyridoxine Hydrochloride (Vitamin B6).

Superior Amino 2222 Liquid **-** Optimum Nutrition
Each 4 tbsp (52 mL) serving contains: Proprietary Blend: Hydrolyzed Gelatin, Whey Protein Isolate • Crystalline Fructose • Natural and Artificial Flavors • FD&C Red #40 • Sodium Benzoate • Potassium Sorbate.

Superior Coral Calcium with Magnesium **-** NSI - Nutraceutical Sciences Institute
Two capsules contain: Calcium (from Coral calcium) 700 mg • Magnesium (from Coral calcium and Oxide) 350 mg • Marine Coral (from Okinawa, Japan) 2 g. Other Ingredients: Gelatin, Water, Magnesium Stearate.

Superior EFA Omega-3 **-** NSI - Nutraceutical Sciences Institute
Each softgel contains: Vitamin E (as miexed tocopherols) 3 IU • Fish Oil concentrate 500 mg containing DHA (Docosahexaenoic Acid) 250 mg, EPA (Eicosapentaenoic Acid) 100 mg, other Omega-3 (DPA & ALA) 50 mg.

Superior Kava Kava **-** NutriCology
Each softgel contains: Kava Kava root (piper methysticum forst, minimum 80% kavalactone extract standardized to 75 mg kavalactones). Other Ingredients: Soybean Oil, Beeswax, Glycerin Fatty Acid Ester, Polysorbate 80.
See Editor's Note No. 21, page 2056.

Superior L-Arginine **-** NSI - Nutraceutical Sciences Institute
Each capsule contains: L-Arginine 750 mg.

Superior L-Carnitine Fumerate **-** NSI - Nutraceutical Sciences Institute
Each capsule contains: L-Carnitine (fumerate) 500 mg.

Superior L-Taurine **-** NSI - Nutraceutical Sciences Institute
Each capsule contains: L-Taurine 850 mg. Other Ingredients: Kosher Gelatin (capsule), Magnesium Stearate.

Superior Melatonin **-** NSI - Nutraceutical Sciences Institute
Each capsule contains: Melatonin 3 mg.

Superior One Plus **-** Swanson
Each tablet contains: Vitamin A (as beta-carotene) 25000 IU • Vitamin C USP (as ascorbic acid) 300 mg • Vitamin D (as cholecalciferol) 400 IU • Vitamin E USP (as d-alpha tocopheryl succinate) 15-IU • Thiamin USP (as thiamin HCl; vitamin B-1) 125 mg • Riboflavin (vitamin B-2) 125 mg • Niacinamide 125 mg • Vitamin B-6 USP (as pyridoxine HCl) 125 mg • Folic Acid USP 400 mcg • Vitamin B-12 USP (as cyanocobalamin) 125 mcg • Biotin 125 mcg • Pantothenic Acid USP (as d-calcium pantothenate) 125 mg • Calcium (from calcium carbonate) 75 mg • Iron USP (from ferrous fumarate) 18 mg • Iodine (from kelp) 225 mcg • Magnesium USP (from magnesium oxide) 40 mg • Zinc (from zinc gluconate) 20 mg • Selenium (from yeast) 100 mcg • Manganese USP (from manganese sulfate) 7 mg • Chromium (from yeast) 225 mcg • Inositol 125 mg • Choline (as choline bitartrate) 100 mg • Lemon Bioflavonoid Complex 50 mg • Betaine HCl 30 mg • PABA (para-aminobenzoic acid) 30 mg • Rutin 30 mg, Glutamic Acid HCl 25 mg, Hesperidin Complex 25 mg.

Superior Probiotic **-** NSI - Nutraceutical Sciences Institute
Each enteric coated capsule contains: Bacterial Cultures 50 mg: L. Acidophilus, L. Rhamnosus, S. Thermophilus, L. Bulgaricus.

Superior Selenium **-** NSI - Nutraceutical Sciences Institute
Each capsule contains: Selenium (as selenomethionine) 200 mcg.

Superior Smino 2222 Tabs **-** Optimum Nutrition
Each tablet contains: Whey Protein Concentrate • Soy Protein Isolate • Pharmaceutical Glaze • Stearic Acid • Croscarmellose Sodium •

Silica • Hydrolyzed Whey Peptides • L-Carnitine Tartrate • L-Ornithine Hydrochloride.

Superlax **-** Grandma's Herbs
Each capsule contains: Proprietary Blend 0.476 g: Cascara Sagrada bark, Psyllium seeds, Senna herb, Turkey Rhubarb root, Aloe Vera leaf, Barberry root, Slippery Elm bark. Other Ingredients: Gelatin.

Supra Renal 220 **-** Atrium Inc.
Each tablet contains: Raw Tissue concentrate from Bovine Sources (not extracts): (Adrenal 220 mg & Pituitary 15 mg) 235 mg • Vitamin C 175 mg • Bioflavonoid Complex 45 mg • Pantothenic Acid 70 mg • Methionine 60 mg • Choline 60 mg • Vitamin B1 25 mg • Vitamin B2 25 mg • Vitamin B6 25 mg • Niacinamide 50 mg • Magnesium 100 mg • Folic Acid 400 mcg • RNA 25 mg.
See Editor's Note No. 14, page 2055.

Supraene Creme **-** Atrium Inc.
Two ounces contains: Squalene 30 mg • Triethanolamine 5 mg • Ceresin Wax 5 mg • Glucam F-20 4 mg • Amerchol L-101 2.5 mg • Solulan 16 2.5 mg • Steral 2.5 mg • Cetyl Alcohol 2.5 mg • Carbopol 934 0.5 mg • Methyl Paraben 10 mg • Propyl Paraben 0.05 mg • Distilled Water 45.35 mg.

Suprema C Powder **-** Gary Null & Associates (GNA)
One teaspoon contains: Vitamin C 2500 mg • Selenium 65 mcg • Bioflavonoids 150 mg.

Suprema C Tablets **-** Gary Null & Associates (GNA)
Each tablet contains Vitamin C 500 mg • Selenium 6 mcg • Bioflavonoids 10 mg.

Supreme Greens with MSM capsules **-** Dr. Alex Guerrero
Three capsules contain: Proprietary Blend 1925 mg: Alfalfa leaf (agrimonia eupatoria), Aloe leaf (aloe barbadensis), Barley grass (hordeum vulgare), Barley sprouts (hrodeum vulgare), Beet root (beta vulgaris), Bilberry leaf (vaccinium myrtillus), Broccoli stalk (brassica aleracea italica), Cabbage leaf (brassica aleracea), Carrot stalk (daucus carota), Celery seed (apium graveolens), Cornsilk silk (zea mays), Dandelion leaf (taraxacum officinale), Echinacea herb (echinacea purpurea), Garlic bulb (allium sativum), Ginger root (zingiber officinale), Goldenseal herb (hydrastis canadensis), Grapefruit pectin (citrus paradise), Kale leaf (brassica species), MSM, Okra pulp (abelmoschus esculentus), Parsley leaf (petroselinum sativum), Pau d'Arco bark (tabebuia heptaphylla), Peppermint leaf (mentha piperita), Raspberry berry (rubus idaeus), Rosemary leaf (rosmarinus officinalis), Sage leaf (salvia officinalis), Shavegrass herb (equisetum hyemal), Slippery Elm bark (almus rubra), Spearmint leaf (mentha spicaa), Spinach leaf (spinacea alaracea), Strawberry leaf (fragaria vesca), Watercress herb (nasturtium officinale), Wheatgrass herb (triticum vulgare), White Willow bark (salix alba), Wintergreen leaf (gaultheria procumbens). Other Ingredients: Rice Powder, Magnesium Stearate, Gelatin.

Supreme Greens with MSM powder **-** Dr. Alex Guerrero
Each 1 tsp (2 g) serving contains: Proprietary Blend 2000 mg: Alfalfa leaf (agrimonia eupatoria), Aloe leaf (aloe barbadensis), Barley grass (hordeum vulgare), Barley sprouts (hrodeum vulgare), Beet root (beta vulgaris), Bilberry leaf (vaccinium myrtillus), Broccoli stalk (brassica aleracea italica), Cabbage leaf (brassica aleracea), Carrot stalk (daucus carota), Celery seed (apium graveolens), Cornsilk silk (zea mays), Dandelion leaf (taraxacum officinale), Echinacea herb (echinacea purpurea), Garlic bulb (allium sativum), Ginger root (zingiber officinale), Goldenseal herb (hydrastis canadensis), Grapefruit pectin (citrus paradise), Kale leaf (brassica species), MSM, Okra pulp (abelmoschus esculentus), Parsley leaf (petroselinum sativum), Pau d'Arco bark (tabebuia heptaphylla), Peppermint leaf (mentha piperita), Raspberry berry (rubus idaeus), Rosemary leaf (rosmarinus officinalis), Sage leaf (salvia officinalis), Shavegrass herb (equisetum hyemal), Slippery Elm bark (almus rubra), Spearmint leaf (mentha spicaa), Spinach leaf (spinacea alaracea), Strawberry leaf (fragaria vesca), Watercress herb (nasturtium officinale), Wheatgrass herb (triticum vulgare), White Willow bark (salix alba), Wintergreen leaf (gaultheria procumbens).

Supreme Omega Liquid **-** DaVinci Laboratories
Each 1/2 tsp serving contains: Proprietary Blend 2300 mg: Borage seed oil, Fish oil, Flax seed oil. Other Ingredients: Antioxidant Blend: Rosemary, Mixed Tocopherols, Ascorbyl Palmitate, Citric acid, Natural Cherry Flavor.

Sure Balance **-** Meta-Sure Health
Each two capsules contain: Manganese 2 mg • Vitamin B6 (as pyridoxine HCl) 10 mg • Niacinamide 20 mg • Vitamin C (as ascorbic acid) 60 mg • Folic Acid 400 mcg • Magnesium (as magnesium glycinate) 150 mg • SurePlex Proprietary Blend 300 mg: Red Clover extract (8% isoflavones), Chaste Berry (powder), White Willow bark (1% salicylates), Citrus Flavonoids, Turmeric (95% curcuminoids), L-Taurine • Boron 1 mg • Black Cohosh extract (2.5% triterpenes) 40 mg • Dong Quai (powder) 10 mg • Panax Ginseng (root) 50 mg • Soy Concentrate (40% isoflavones) 85 mg • St. John's Wort (3% hypericin) 75 mg • 5-HTP (griffonia seed) 3 mg.

Surf Buddies CONCENTRATE! **-** PhytoPharmica
Two capsules contain: DMAE (as dimethyalminoethanol bitartrate) 100 mg • L-Theanine 25 mg • N-Acetylcysteine (NAC) 25 mg • Phosphatidylserine (from purified soybean lecithin) 60 mg.

Surf Buddies Daily Multiple **-** PhytoPharmica
Two chewable tablets contain: Bilberry fruit 4:1 extract (vaccinium myrtillus) 2 mg • Biotin 150 mcg • Calcium (from tricalcium phosphate) 100 mg • Chromium (as chromium picolinate) 60 mcg • Cranberry fruit 2:1 extract (vaccinium macrocarpon) 2 mg • European Elder berry 4:1 extract (sambucus nigra) 6 mg • Folic Acid 400 mcg • Iodine (as potassium iodide) 150 mcg • Iron (as ferrous fumarate) 5 mg • Magnesium (as magnesium oxide) 10 mg • Manganese (as magnaese citrate) 1 mg • Niacin (as niacinamide) 5 mg • Pantothenic Acid (as calcium D-pantothenate) 2.5 mg • Phosphorus (as tricalcium phosphate) 50 mg • Riboflavin (vitamin B2) 1.7 mg • Selenium (as L-selenomethionine) 20 mcg • Sour Cherry fruit 10:1 extract (prunus cerasus) 10 mg • Thiamin (as thiamin mononitrate, vitamin B1) 1.5 mg • Vitamin A (as retinyl acetate) 5000 IU • Vitamin B12 (as cyanocobalamin) 6 mcg • Vitamin B6 (as pyridoxine HCl) 1 mg • Vitamin C (ascorbic acid and as calcium ascorbate) 120 mg • Vitamin D (as cholecalciferol) 400 IU • Vitamin E (as D-alpha tocopheryl acid succinate) 30 IU • Vitamin K (as phytonadione) 40 mcg • Zinc (as zinc ascorbate) 5 mg.

Surf Buddies Immune Defense **-** PhytoPharmica
Each chewable tablet contains: European Elder berry 4:1 extract (sambucus nigra) 40 mg • Vitamin A (as beta carotene) 1000 IU • Vitamin B6 (as pyridoxine HCl) 2 mg • Vitamin C (ascorbic acid and as sodium ascorbate) 100 mg • Zinc (as zinc ascorbate) 2 mg.

Swedish Bitters **-** Self Heal Natural Therapies, Ltd.
Aloe • Myrrh • Saffron • Senna leaf • Camphor • Rhubarb root • Zedoary • Manna • Theriaca Venezian • Carline root • Angelica root.

Sweet & Slender **-** Wisdom herbs
Each packet contains: Fructose • Luo Han Guo fruit extract.

Sweet Energy Formula **-** Bee-Alive Inc.
Each teaspoon contains: Royal Jelly (non-freeze dried) 1.06 g. Other Ingredients: Pure Honey.

SweetEase **-** Advocare International
Three capsules contain: L-Arabinose 500 mg • Gymnema extract (leaf - gymnema sylvestre) 200 mg • Dry Bean extract (seed - phaseolus vulgaris) 300 mg • Hibiscus extract (flower - hibiscus sabdariffa) 500 mg • Green Tea extract (leaf - camellia sinensis) 100 mg • Apple extract (fruit - malus sylvestris) 20 mg • Lactobacillus Acidophilus 100 MM • Bifidobacterium Bifidus 100 MM. Other Ingredients: Silicon Dioxide, Magnesium Stearate, Gelatin.

Some Brand Name Natural Products - What they Contain

www.NaturalDatabase.com contains MANY more listings than appear here.

Swiss Herbal **-** The Vitamin Shoppe
Each tablet contains: Senna (Cassia senna) leaves standardized to 3% sennosides 100 mg • Strawberry (Fragaria vesca) leaves 50 mg • Peach (Prunus persica) leaves 50 mg • Anise (Pimpinella anisum) fruit and seeds 50 mg • Cranberry (Vaccinium macrocarpon) fruit 50 mg • Calendula (Calendula officinalis) flower and leaves 25 mg.

Swiss Kriss Tabs **-** Swiss Kriss
Each tablet contains: Finely powdered sun-dried Senna leaves. Other Ingredients: Finely powdered Strawberry Leaves •Peach Leaves •Anise seed •Caraway seed •Hibiscus flowers, Calendula flowers.

Symbiotropin hGH **-** ASN - Advanced Sports Nutrition
Each two tablets contain: Anterior Pituitary Peptides Aminotrope-7 (a sequenced glycoamino acid complex) 4200 mg • Novel Polyose Complex (pharmaceutical mono, poly & oligo saccharides) 2230 mg. In a base of L-Glutamine, L-Arginine, L-Pyroglutamate, GABA, L-Glycine, L-Lysine, L-Tyrosine & Vica faba major, all naturally sweetened & flavored.

Symplex F **-** Standard Process, Inc.
Each tablet contains: Proprietary Blend 138 mg: Magnesium Citrate, Bovine Ovary extract, Bovine Adrenal extract, Bovine Pituitary extract, Bovine Thyroid extract (thyroxine removed). Inactive Ingredients: Calcium (lactate, stearate), Cellulose.

Symplex M **-** Standard Process, Inc.
Each tablet contains: Proprietary Blend 137 mg: Magnesium Citrate, Bovine Orchic extract, Bovine Adrenal extract, Bovine Pituitary extract, Bovine Thyroid extract (thyroxine removed). Other Ingredients: Calcium (lactate, stearate) 20 mg, Cellulose.

Sympt-X Plus **-** Cambridge Nutraceuticals
Each serving contains: Glutamine 10 g • Vitamin A (as mixed carotenoids) 6500 IU • Vitamin C 330 mg • Vitamin E 100 IU • Selenium 50 mcg. Available in 650 g jar and Single Dose Packets.

Synadrene **-** Metaphysics - Pro-Soma Enterprises
Each capsule contains: Citrus Aurantium (bitter orange Peel) 350 mg • Chromium Picolinate 400 mcg.
See Editor's Note No. 40, page 2058.

SynBiotics-1 **-** NutraCea (formerly NutraStar)
Each capsule contains: Stabilized Rice Bran derivative 250 mg • Proprietary Probiotic Blend 250 mg (2.75 billion CFU when shipped): Bifidobacterium Longum, Lactobacillus Rhamnosus A, Lactobacillus Plantarum. Other Ingredients: Maltodextrin, Magnesium Stearate, Hydroxypropylmethyl Cellulose, Metacrylic Acid, Methyl Methacrylate Copolymer.

SynBiotics-2 **-** NutraCea (formerly NutraStar)
Each capsule contains: Stabilized Rice Bran derivative 250 mg • Proprietary Probiotic Blend 250 mg (3 billion CFU when shipped): Bifidobacterium Longum, Lactobacillus Rhamnosus A, Lactobacillus Plantarum. Other Ingredients: Maltodextrin, Magnesium Stearate, Hydroxypropylmethyl Cellulose, Metacrylic Acid, Methyl Methacyrlate Copolymer.

SynBiotics-3 **-** NutraCea (formerly NutraStar)
Each capsule contains: Stabilized Rice Bran derivative 250 mg • Proprietary Probiotic Blend 250 mg (4.5 billion CFU when shipped): Bifidobacterium Longum, Lactobacillus Rhamnosus A, Lactobacillus Plantarum. Other Ingredients: Maltodextrin, Magnesium Stearate, Hydroxypropylmethyl Cellulose, Metacrylic Acid, Methyl Methacrylate Copolymer.

SyneDrex **-** Metabolic Nutrition
Four capsules contain: Advantra Z Citrus Aurantium (30%) 467 mg • Caffeine Anhydrous 700 mg • Green Tea extract (50%/35% polyphenols) 480 mg • Hydroxycitric Acid (garcinia cambogia 50%) 460 mg • Acetyl L-Carnitine 240 mg • L-Tyrosine 320 mg • Glucomannan 800 mg • Naringin 80 mg • Vitamin B6 14 mg • Vitamin B12 400 mcg • Chromium Polynicotinate 700 mcg • 5-HTP 4000 mcg • Simmondsin extract 4000 mcg.
See Editor's Note No. 40, page 2058.

Synephrine 350 mg - GNC Energy **-** GNC
Each capsule contains: Citrus Aurantium Fruit Extract 350 mg. Other Ingredients: Gelatin, Cellulose, Calcium Carbonate.
See Editor's Note No. 40, page 2058.

Synergistic Iron **-** Quest
Each capsule contains: Iron (HVP Chelate) 25 mg • Copper (HVP Chelate) 2 mg • Molybdenum (HVP Chelate) 50 mcg • Vitamin C (Ascorbic Acid) 100 mg • Niacin 10 mg • Vitamin B1 (Thiamine HCl) 5 mg • Vitamin B6 (Pyridoxine HCl) 5 mg • Vitamin B2 (Riboflavin) 2 mg • Pantothenic Acid (d-Calcium Pantothenate) 10 mg • Folic Acid 0.2 mg • Vitamin B12 (Cobalamin) 20 mcg • Biotin 50 mcg. Other Ingredients: Magnesium Stearate (vegetable source), Microcrystalline Cellulose.

Synergistic Magnesium **-** Quest
Each tablet contains: Magnesium (HVP Chelate) 150 mg • Calcium (HVP Chelate) 30 mg • Phosphorus (HVP Complex) 15 mg • Vitamin B6 (Pyridoxine HCl) 20 mg. Other Ingredients: Croscarmellose Sodium, Magnesium Stearate (vegetable source), Microcrystalline Cellulose, Vegetable Stearin.

Synergistic Manganese **-** Quest
Each capsule contains: Manganese (HVP Chelate) 50 mg • Vitamin B1 (Thiamine HCl) 20 mg • Vitamin C 100 mg. Other Ingredients: Magnesium Stearate (vegetable source), Microcrystalline Cellulose.

Synergistic Multiple Mineral **-** Quest
Each tablet contains: Calcium (HVP Chelate) 100 mg • Magnesium (HVP Chelate) 100 mg • Potassium (HVP Chelate) 33 mg • Iron (HVP Chelate) 5 mg • Manganese (HVP Chelate) 5 mg • Zinc (HVP Chelate) 5 mg • Copper (HVP Chelate) 1 mg • Iodine (Potassium Iodide) 50 mcg • Molybdenum (HVP Chelate) 50 mcg • Chromium (HVP Chelate) 10 mcg • Selenium (HVP Complex) 10 mcg. Other Ingredients: Croscarmellose Sodium, Magnesium Stearate (vegetable source), Mircocrystalline Cellulose, Vegetable Stearin.

Synergistic Selenium **-** Quest
Each capsule contains: Selenium (HVP Chelate) 200 mcg • Vitamin E (d-Alpha Tocopheryl Acetate) 25 IU • Vitamin C (Ascorbic Acid) 100 mg. Other Ingredients: Magnesium Stearate (vegetable source), Microcrystalline Cellulose.

Synergistic Zinc **-** Quest
Each tablet contains: Vitamin A (Palmitate) 5000 IU • Zinc (HVP Chelate) 20 mg • Copper (HVP Chelate) 1 mg. Other Ingredients: Calcium Phosphate, Croscarmellose Sodium, Magnesium Stearate (vegetable source), Microcrystalline Cellulose, Vegetable Stearin.

Synergy **-** NSI - Nutraceutical Sciences Institute
Each six capsules contain: Vitamin A (as natural carotenoids beta carotene, alpha carotene, lutein, zeaxanthin, cryptoaxanthin, and palmitate) 5000 IU • Vitamin C (as calcium ascorbate) 500 mg • Vitamin D (vitamin D3 as cholecalciferol) 700 IU • Vitamin E (as d-alpha tocopherol succinate, gamma, delta, and beta) 500 IU • Thiamin (vitamin B1HCl) 50 mg • Riboflavin (vitamin b2) 10 mg • Niacin (vitamin B3) 70 mg • Pyridoxine HCl (vitamin B6) 50 mg • Folic Acid (as folacin) 800 mcg • Vitamin B12 (methylcobalamin) 500 mcg • Biotin 1 mg • Pantothenic Acid (vitamin B5 as d-calcium pantothenate) 50 mg • Calcium from 2,430 mg citrate, malate, and Ester C) 500 mg • Zinc (as l-monomethoinine, OptiZinc) 15 mg • Selenium (selenomethoinine) 200 mcg • Iodine (as kelp) 75 mcg • Magnesium (from 1,190 citrate) 200 mg • Manganese (as chelate, AAC) 2 mg • Chromium (as chromium picolinate, Chromates) 200 mcg • Molybdenum (as chelate, AAC) 75 mcg • Potassium (from 417 mg potassium citrate) 150 mg • Garlic (as aged, odorless, standardized 10,000 ppm allicin) 400 mg • Ginkgo Biloba (gonkoaceace, leaves, standardized 24% ginkgo flavon glycosides, 6% terpene lactones) 60 mg • CoEnzyme Q10 10 mg • Alpha Lipoic Acid 30 mg • Bioflavonoid (Citrus BioComplex Standardized to 50%) 50 mg •

Bioflavonoid as Quercetin 50 mg • Grape seed extract 50 mg • Lutein extract (from 120 mg FloraGLO) 6 mg • Red Wine extract (standardized 30% polyphenols) 50 mg • Green Tea extract (standardized 98% polyphenols, 80% catechins, 45% EGCG) 50 mg • Plant Enzymes (amylase 2,000 SKB HUT, lipase 25 FIP, and lactase 250 ALU) 50 mg • Black Pepper extract (piper nigrum fruit extract, Bipoerine) 5 mg • Inositol 50 mg • Malic Acid (as calcium citrate malate) 367 mg • Copper (as chelate, AAC) 1 mg.

Synerpro Multiple Vitamins & Minerals **-** Nature's Sunshine
Each tablet contains: Vitamin A (beta-carotene) 2,500 IU • Vitamin C 30 mg • Vitamin D 200 IU • Vitamin E (D-alpha tocopherol) 15 IU • Thiamine (vitamin B1) 0.75 mg • Riboflavin (vitamin B2) 0.85 mg • Niacin (as nicotinic acid) 10 mg • Vitamin B6 (pyridoxine HCl) 1 mg • Folate (folic acid) 200 mcg • Vitamin B12 (cyanocobalamin) 3 mcg • Biotin 150 mcg • Pantothenic acid (D-calcium pantothenate) 5 mg • Calcium (D-calcium pantothenate and dicalcium phosphate) 125 mg • Iron (ferrous fumarate) 9 mg • Phosphorus (dicalcium phosphate) 90 mg • Iodine (potassium iodide) 75 mcg • Magnesium (magnesium oxide) 50 mg • Zinc (zinc oxide) 7.5 mg • Selenium (amino acid chelate) 25 mcg • Copper (copper gluconate) 1 mg • Manganese (amino acid chelate) 0.5 mg • Chromium (amino acid chelate) 50 mcg • Molybdenum (amino acid chelate) 38 mcg. Other Ingredients: Broccoli flowers (brassica oleracera), Turmeric root (curcuma longa), Red Beet root (beta vulgaris), Rosemary leaves (rosmarinus officinalis), Wild Carrot root (daucus carota), Tomato fruit (solanum lycopersicum), Chinese Cabbage leaves (brassica rapa), Cabbage leaves (brassica oleracea), Orange Bioflavonoids, Grapefruit Bioflavonoids, Hesperidin, Cellulose (plant fiber), Stearic Acid, Silicon Dioxide (powdered silica).

SynovoDerma **-** Allergy Research Group
Three softgels contain: Hyaluronic Acid powder (9% min. hyaluronic acid) 210 mg. Other Ingredients: Rice Bran Oil, Yellow Beeswax, Titanium Dioxide.

Synthovial 7 **-** Hyalogic LLC
Hyaluronic Acid 2.15 mg.
See Editor's Note No. 38, page 2058.

System 343 **-** Advocare International
Fiber 10: Each pouch (0.7 oz / 20 g) contains: Vitamin A (as beta-carotene) 1000 IU • Vitamin C (as ascorbic acid) 30 mg • Sodium 10 mg • Fructose • Maltodextrin • Citric Acid • Natural Flavors • Artificial Flavors • Acesulfame Potassium • Papaya fruit powder • Prune powder • Rhubarb root extract • Black Walnut hull extract • Licorice root powder • Lactobacillus Acidophilus • Bifidobacterium Bifidum • Digestive Enzyme Complex: Lipase, Cellulase, Protease • Fiber Blend: Psyllium husk, Oats (oat fiber), Carboxymethylcellulose, Guar Gum, Citrus Pectin, Butternut Bark Powder. Herbal Cleanse: Three caplets contain: Vitamin C (as ascorbic acid) 1200 mg • Thiamine (as HCI) 6 mg • Riboflavin 6.8 mg • Niacin/Niacinamide 100 mg • Vitamin B6 (as pyridoxine HCI) 10 mg • Folic Acid 400 mcg • Vitamin B12 (as cyanocobalamin) 30 mcg • Biotin 300 mcg • Pantothenic Acid (as calcium pantothenate) 40 mg • OptiZinc Zinc (as monomethionine) 3 mg • Inositol 5 mg • Taurine 800 mg • System 343 Herbal Concentrate 1350 mg: Wheat Grass juice powder, Cranberry juice powder, Burdock root extract, Senna seed extract, Astragalus root extract, Echinacea Purpurea root extract, Milk Thistle leaf extract, Schisandra fruit extract, Beet root powder, Odorless Garlic bulb powder. Other Ingredients: Dicalcium Phosphate, Silicon Dioxide, Cellulose, Stearic Acid, Magnesium Stearate. ProBiotic Restore: Two capsules contain: Vitamin A (as palmitate) 2000 IU • Vitamin A (as beta-carotene) 2000 IU • OptiZinc Zinc (as monomethionine) 1 mg • Lactobacillus Acidophilus 1 billion • Bifidobacterium Bifidum 1 billion • Fructooligosaccharides 500 mg • Moomiyo 50 mg • Aloe Vera leaf extract 100 mg. Other Ingredients: Silicon Dioxide, Magnesium Stearate, Gelatin.

System D-Tox **-** Nutri-Quest Rx
Six capsules contain: Vitamin A Palmitate 2000 IU • Vitamin C 750 mg • Vitamin B1 20 mg • Niacin 25 mg • Vitamin B12 50 mcg • Folic Acid 300 mcg • Calcium Aspartate 75 mg • Magnesium Glycinate 200 mg • Magnesium Aspartate 100 mg • Chromium Picolinate 50 mcg • Zinc Picolinate 20 mg • N-Acetyl Cysteine 30 mg • L-Glutamine 200 mg • Silymarin extract 5 mg • Quercetin 25 mg • L-Taurine 50 mg • L-Ornithine 20 mg • L-Glutamic Acid 20 mg • L-Carnitine 20 mg • Choline 50 mg • Propolis 20 mg • Yellow Dock 25 mg • Beta Carotene 7500 IU • Vitamin E Succinate Natural 200 IU • Vitamin B2 20 mg • Pyridoxal 5 Phosphate 20 mg • Pantothenic Acid 50 mg • Biotin 200 mcg • Calcium Gluconate 75 mg • Magnesium Citrate 100 mg • Selenomethionine 150 mcg • Manganese Aspartate 5 mg • Molybdenum Citrate 50 mcg • Reduced Glutathione 20 mg • Milk Thistle 50 mg • Beet root 50 mg • Glucaronic Acid 5 mg • L-Glycine 50 mg • L-Methionine 50 mg • L-Arginine 20 mg • L-Tyrosine 20 mg • Inositol 50 mg • Curcumin 5 mg • Chlorophyll 10 mg • Asparagus 15 mg • Dandelion root 25 mg • Siberian Ginseng 30 mg • Broccoli 15 mg • Mullein 25 mg • Co-Enzyme Q-10 1 mg.

Syste-Max (SysteMax) **-** Changes International, Inc.
One heaping teaspoonful (6.8 g) contains: Vitamin A 668 IU • Vitamin C 100 mg • Vitamin E 60 IU • Psyllium seed husk 4000 mg • Soy Germ flour (providing 15 mg of isoflavones) 500 mg • Chitosan 100 mg • Phytosterol complex (providing 43 mg of beta-sitosterol) 100 mg • Oat flour 100 mg.

Sytrinol **-** Source Naturals
Each tablet contains: Calcium 35 mg • Sytrinol (proprietary blend of citrus polymethoxylated flavones and palm tocotrienols) 150 mg. Other Ingredients: Microcrystalline Cellulose, Dibasic Calcium Phosphate, Modified Cellulose Gum, Stearic Acid, Colloidal Dioxide.

Sytropin HGH **-** Speedwinds Nutrition Inc
Alpha GPC • GABA • Glycine • L-Arginine • L-Dopa bean extract • L-Glutamine • L-Isoleucine • L-Tyrosine • L-Valine • L-Lysine • Moomiyo extract • Ornithine Alpha Ketoglutarate. Inactive Ingredients: Deionized Water, Lecithin Phospholipids, Sodium Citrate, Potassium Sorbate, Maltodextrin, Paraben, Citric Acid.

T2 Pro-Thyroid Formula **-** BioTest Laboratories, LLC
Each cap contains: 3;5-diiodo-l-thyronine 50 mcg.

T-5W **-** Dial Herbs
Red Raspberry • Blue Cohosh • Bayberry • Squaw Vine • Blessed Thistle • Ginger • Motherwort • False Unicorn • Wild Yam • Lobelia • Cayenne.

T-ACN **-** Dial Herbs
Black Walnut • Burdock • Chaparral • Yellow Dock • Sassafras • Valerian.

Tadenan **-** European; Not available in the US.
Pygeum africanum extract standardized to contain 14% triterpenes and 0.5% n-docosanol usually in dosages of 100 - 200 mg.

T-AFT **-** Dial Herbs
Wild Lettuce • St. John's Wort • Valerian • Cayenne.

TAG **-** Metabolic Nutrition
Each 2 tsp serving contains: Trans - Alanyl - Glutamine 10 g.

T-AIS **-** Dial Herbs
Rose Hips • Sage • Yarrow • Burdock • Echinacea • Goldenseal • Yellow Dock • Garlic • Nettle • Lemon Grass • White Oak bark • Black Cohosh • Fenugreek • Juniper berry • Oregon Grape • Plantain • Thyme.

T-AKE **-** Dial Herbs
Clove Oil • Oat Straw • Lobelia • Cayenne.

Take 10 Bars, Apple Cinnamon **-** Advocare International
Polydextrose • Dried Apples • Rolled Oats • Raisins • Maltitol Syrup • Figs • Rice Syrup • Oat Fiber • Corn Bran • Glycerin • High Fructose Corn Syrup • Soybean Oil • Natural Flavor • Spice • Arabinogalactan • Fructooligo-Saccharides • Guar Gum • Honey • Sunflower Oil • Sucralose • Soy Lecithin.

Take Control **-** Lipton
Water • Liquid Canola Oil • Vegetable Oil Sterol Esters • Liquid Sunflower Oil • Partially Hydrogenated Soybean Oil • Salt • Whey • Vegetable Mono- and Diglycerides • Potassium Sorbate • Lactic Acid • Calcium Disodium EDTA • Soy Lecithin • Artificial Flavor • Beta Carotene • Vitamin A (Palmitate).

Take Heart **-** Allergy Research Group
Each scoop (20 g) contains: Vitamin A (as beta-carotene) 2000 IU • Vitamin C (as ascorbic acid) 500 mg • Vitamin D (D3) 100 IU • Vitamin E (as D-alpha-tocopherol) 320 IU • Vitamin K 80 mcg • Thiamin (vitamin B1) 30 mg • Riboflavin (vitamin B2) 30 mg • Niacin 160 mg • Vitamin B6 16 mg • Folic Acid 320 mg • Vitamin B12 80 mcg • Biotin 240 mcg • Pantothenic Acid 100 mg • Calcium (as calcium citrate/gluconate) 280 mg • Magnesium (as magnesium glycinate/gluconate) 160 mg • Zinc (as zinc arginate) 12 mg • Selenium (as sodium selenite/selenomethionine) 80 mcg • Copper (as copper glycinate) 0.8 mg • Manganese (as manganese glycinate) 1 mg • Chromium (as chromium polynicotinate) 160 mcg • Molybdenum (as sodium molybdate) 40 mcg • Potassium (as potassium gluconate) 40 mg • Boron (as boron citrate) 0.4 mg • Vanadium (as vanadium pentoxide) 80 mcg • Alpha-Carotene 8 mg • Pregnenolone 6 mg • Dehydroepiandrosterone (DHEA) 6 mg • Coenzyme Q10 60 mg • Inositol 50 mg • Choline 50 mg • Para-Aminobenzoic Acid (PABA) 20 mg • Lecithin (26% phosphatidylcholine) 500 mg • L-Alanine 30 mg • L-Arginine 480 mg • L-Aspartic Acid 85 mg • L-Carnitine 200 mg • L-Cystine 10 mg • L-Glutamine 600 mg • Glycine 30 mg • L-Histidine 20 mg • L-Isoleucine 35 mg • L-Leucine 60 mg • L-Lysine 45 mg • L-Methionine 160 mg • L-Ornithine 200 mg • L-Phenylalanine 38 mg • L-Proline 38 mg • L-Serine 38 mg • Taurine 500 mg • L-Threonine 28 mg • L-Tyrosine 220 mg • L-Valine 40 mg • N-Acetyl-L-Cysteine 200 mg • Glutathione 100 mg • Pancreatin 10 mg • Papain 16 mg • Bromelain 20 mg • Grape skin extract 200 mg • Hawthorn berry extract 200 mg • Garlic (1% allicin) 100 mg • Lutein 2 mg • Lycopene 0.4 mg • Tocotrienols 20 mg • Trimethylglycine 200 mg • Methylsulfonylmethane 80 mg • Eicosapentaenoic Acid (EPA) 145 mg • Docosahexaenoic Acid (DHA) 95 mg • Gamma-Linolenic Acid 90 mg • Linolenic Acid 220 mg • Oleic Acid 85 mg • Palmitic Acid 65 mg • Stearic Acid 25 mg • Flax Seed oil 400 mg • Lipoic Acid 30 mg. Other Ingredients: Oat Bran, Honey Powder, Rice Bran, Psyllium Bran, Apple Fiber, Lemon Flavor, Stevia.

Take Heart II without Hormones **-** Allergy Research Group
Each scoop (20 g) contains: Vitamin A (as beta-carotene) 2000 IU • Vitamin C (as ascorbic acid) 500 mg • Vitamin D (D3) 100 IU • Vitamin E (as D-alpha-tocopherol) 320 IU • Vitamin K 80 mcg • Thiamin (vitamin B1) 30 mg • Riboflavin (vitamin B2) 30 mg • Niacin 160 mg • Vitamin B6 16 mg • Folic Acid 320 mg • Vitamin B12 80 mcg • Biotin 240 mcg • Pantothenic Acid 100 mg • Calcium (as calcium citrate/gluconate) 280 mg • Magnesium (as magnesium glycinate/gluconate) 160 mg • Zinc (as zinc arginate) 12 mg • Selenium (as sodium selenite/selenomethionine) 80 mcg • Copper (as copper glycinate) 0.8 mg • Manganese (as manganese glycinate) 1 mg • Chromium (as chromium polynicotinate) 160 mcg • Molybdenum (as sodium molybdate) 40 mcg • Potassium (as potassium gluconate) 40 mg • Boron (as boron citrate) 0.4 mg • Vanadium (as vanadium pentoxide) 80 mcg • Alpha-Carotene 8 mg • Coenzyme Q10 60 mg • Inositol 50 mg • Choline 50 mg • Para-Aminobenzoic Acid (PABA) 20 mg • Lecithin (26% phosphatidylcholine) 500 mg • L-Alanine 30 mg • L-Arginine 480 mg • L-Aspartic Acid 85 mg • L-Carnitine 200 mg • L-Cystine 10 mg • L-Glutamine 600 mg • Glycine 30 mg • L-Histidine 20 mg • L-Isoleucine 35 mg • L-Leucine 60 mg • L-Lysine 45 mg • L-Methionine 160 mg • L-Ornithine 200 mg • L-Phenylalanine 38 mg • L-Proline 38 mg • L-Serine 38 mg • Taurine 500 mg • L-Threonine 28 mg • L-Tyrosine 220 mg • L-Valine 40 mg • N-Acetyl-L-Cysteine 200 mg • Glutathione 100 mg • Pancreatin 10 mg • Papain 16 mg • Bromelain 20 mg • Grape skin extract 200 mg • Hawthorn berry extract 200 mg • Garlic (1% allicin) 100 mg • Lutein 2 mg • Lycopene 0.4 mg • Tocotrienols 20 mg • Trimethylglycine 200 mg • Methylsulfonylmethane 80 mg • Eicosapentaenoic Acid (EPA) 145 mg • Docosahexaenoic Acid (DHA) 95 mg • Gamma-Linolenic Acid 90 mg • Linolenic Acid 220 mg • Oleic Acid 85 mg • Palmitic Acid 65 mg • Stearic Acid 25 mg • Flax Seed oil 400 mg • Lipoic Acid 30 mg. Other Ingredients: Oat Bran, Honey Powder, Rice Bran, Psyllium Bran, Apple Fiber, Lemon Flavor, Stevia.

T-ALER **-** Dial Herbs
Bayberry • Echinacea • Yarrow • Wild Cherry bark • Cayenne • Goldenseal.

T-ANEM **-** Dial Herbs
Comfrey root • Dandelion • Barberry • Parsley • Yellow Dock • Myrrh • Kelp.

Taraxatone **-** Cytodyne Technologies
Six capsules contain: Vitamin B6 24 mg • Magnesium 8.4 mg • Dandelion leaf powder 1500 mg • Uva Ursi leaf extract 900 mg • Guarana extract 600 mg • Taurine 115 mg.

T-ARTH **-** Dial Herbs
Yucca • Alfalfa • Buckthorn • Burdock • Parsley • Slippery Elm • Yarrow • Cayenne.

Tarvil **-** SHS North America
Each 15 g packet contains: L-Leucine • L-Valine • L-Isoleucine • Sugar • Guar Gum • Artificial Color (beta carotene) • Soy Lecithin • Citric Acid • Artificial Flavor (pineapple) • Artificial Sweetener (Acesulfame K).

T-ASMA **-** Dial Herbs
Blood root • St. John's Wort • Mullein • Comfrey • Saw Palmetto • Wild Cherry bark • Goldenseal • Lobelia • Cayenne.

Taurine (#70620) **-** NutriCology
Each capsule contains: Taurine 500 mg. Other Ingredients: Celluose, Silicon Dioxide, Stearic Acid.

Taurine (#73920) **-** NutriCology
Each capsule contains: Taurine 1000 mg. Other Ingredients: Cellulose, Silicon Dioxide, Stearic Acid.

Taurine 500 - GNC A-Z **-** GNC
Each tablet contains: Taurine 500 mg. Other Ingredients: Dicalcium Phosphate, Cellulose.

Taurox SB 6X Enhanced **-** Allergy Research Group
Active Ingredients: Abies Nigra 6X (14%), 12X (1%), 30X (1%) • Aloe Socotrina 6X (14%), 12X (1%), 30X (1%) • Arnica Montana 6X (14%), 12X (1%), 30X (1%) • Cactus Grandiflora 6X (14%), 12X (1%), 30X (1%) • Lycopodium Clavatum 6X (14%), 12X (1%), 30X (1%) • Tauroxicum (carbobenzoxy beta-alanyl taurine or TAUROX SB) 6X (14%), 12X (1%), 30X (1%) • Calcarea Carbonica 8X (14%), 12X (1%), 30X (1%). Inactive Ingredients: 20% Ethanol, Purified Water.
See Editor's Note No. 1, page 2053.

Taurox SB 7X with Minerals **-** Allergy Research Group
Active Ingredients: Kalir Carbonicum 8X (13%), 12X (1%), 30X (1%) • Phosphoricum Acidum 8X (13%), 12X (1%), 30X (1%) • Selenium Metallicum 8X (13%), 12X (1%), 30X (1%) • Silicea 8X (13%), 12X (1%), 30X (1%) • Tauroxicum (carbobenzoxy beta-alanyl taurine or TAUROX SB) 7X (33&), 12X (1%), 30X (1%) • Zincum Metallicum 8X (13%), 12X (1%), 30X (1%). Inactive Ingredients: 20% Ethanol, Purified Water.
See Editor's Note No. 1, page 2053.

Taurus Male Nutrient Complex **-** Starlight International
Each three tablets contain: Vitamin C (as calcium ascorbate and magnesium ascorbate) 180 mg • Vitamin E - Dry (as d alpha tocopheryl succinate) 75 IU • Vitamin B1 (as thiamine mononitrate) 30 mg • Vitamin B2 (riboflavin) 30 mg • Niacin 15 mg • Vitamin B6 (pyridoxine HCl) 30 mg • Folic Acid 150 mcg • Vitamin B12 (as cyanocobalamin) 30 mcg • Magnesium (as magnesium ascorbate) 18 mg • Potassium (as potassium glycerophosphate) 7.5 mg • Saw Palmetto berry extract, 4:1 (serenoa repens, fruit) 300 mg • Ashwagandha extract, 4:1 (Withania somnifera dunai, root) 300 mg

• He Shou Wu extract, 4:1 (polygonum multiflorum thunb, root) 225 mg • Oriental Ginseng (panax ginseng, root) 150 mg • Kelp 30 mg • Spirulina 30 mg. Inactive Ingredients: Silicon Dioxide, Tricalcium Phosphate, Microcrystalline Cellulose, Hydroxypropylcellulose, Stearic Acid, Rice Flour, Dicalcium Phosphate, Croscarmellose Sodium, Magnesium Stearate, Dextrin , Dextrose, Lecithin, Sodium Citrate, Mono and Diglycerides.

T-BB **-** Dial Herbs
Buckthorn • Yellow Dock • Garlic • Cayenne • Dandelion • Poke root.

T-BC **-** Dial Herbs
White Oak bark • Comfrey • Black Walnut • Marshmallow root • Mullein • Gravel root • Wormwood • Lobelia • Scullcap • Glycerine.

T-BDW **-** Dial Herbs
Corn Silk • Plantain • St. John's Wort • Sanicle • Mullein • Sarsaparilla • Cubeb berries • Watermelon seeds • Cayenne.

T-BF **-** Dial Herbs
Oat Straw • Shavegrass • Comfrey • Slippery Elm • Burdock • Lobelia.

T-CAC **-** Dial Herbs
Buckthorn • Burdock • Chaparral • Dandelion • Cascara Sagrada • Licorice • Red Clover • Barberry.

T-CIRC **-** Dial Herbs
Witch Hazel • Garlic • Ginger • Cayenne.

T-CS **-** Dial Herbs
Bayberry • Myrrh • Echinacea • Goldenseal • Cayenne.

T-DI **-** Dial Herbs
Hyssop • Garlic • Hydrangea • Catnip • Peppermint • Cayenne.

T-DIA **-** Dial Herbs
Yarrow • Juniper berries • Huckleberry • Cayenne • Goldenseal.

T-DREA **-** Dial Herbs
Witch Hazel • Slippery Elm • Ginger • Shepherd's Purse • Raspberry.

T-DRY **-** Dial Herbs
Sage • Yarrow.

T-DTX **-** Dial Herbs
Echinacea • Yellow Dock • Garlic • Lobelia • Cayenne.

Tea Tree Oil **-** Holista
Tea Tree oil (Melaleuca alternifolia) 100% pure.

Tea Tree Oil - Sterisome **-** Jamieson
Contains: 100% Tea Tree Oil (Derived from Australian Melalleuca Alterniflora) 50 ml • Pure Vitamin E Oil (Dl-Alpha Tocopheryl Acetate) 10 IU/50 ml.

T-EC **-** Dial Herbs
Eyebright • Bayberry • Passion flower • Goldenseal • Cayenne.

Teen Advantage Creatine Serum **-** Muscle Marketing USA
Each serving contains: Creatine Monohydrate • Glucosamine • Vitamin B12 • L-Glutamine • Sodium Pyruvate • Royal Jelly • Ginseng • Honey • Natural Glycerine • Natural Flavor • Distilled Water.

Teen Essentials **-** Rexall - Sundown
Two tablets contain: Vitamin A (from retinyl palmitate) 10000 IU • Vitamin C 400 mg • Vitamin D (as cholecalciferol) 400 IU • Vitamin E (as d-alpha-tocopheryl acid succinate and dl-alpha-tocopheryl acetate) 100 IU • Thiamin (as thiamin HCl) 50 mg • Riboflavin (Vitamin B2) 50 mg • Niacin (as niacinamide) 100 mg • Vitamin B-6 (from pyridoxine HCl) 50 mg • Folic Acid 400 mcg • Vitamin B-12 (as cyanocobalamin) 50 mcg • Biotin 150 mcg • Pantothenic Acid (from calcium d-pantothenate) 100 mg • Calcium 200 mg • Iron (from ferrous fumarate) 9 mg • Phosphorus 154 mg • Iodine (from potassium iodide) 75 mg • Magnesium (from magnesium oxide) 100 mg • Zinc (from zinc gluconate) 22 mg • Manganese (from manganese gluconate) 3 mg • Potassium (from potassium gluconate) 90 mg • Choline Bitartrate 100 mg • Para-Aminobenzoic Acid 30 mg • Inositol 10 mg. Other Ingredients: Dicalcium Phosphate, Cellulose, Stearic Acid, Croscarmellose Sodium, Silica, Magnesium Stearate, Hydroxypropyl Methylcellulose, PEG.

Teen Link **-** Pain & Stress Center
Each capsule contains: 5-HTP 25 mg • St. John's Wort 165 mg • GABA 120 mg • Glutamine 100 mg • Taurine 110 mg • Vitamin B6 5 mg.

Teething Gel **-** Hyland's
Calcarea phosphorica as Calcium phosphate 12X HPUS • Chamomilla as Chamomile 6X HPUS • Coffea cruda as Coffee 6X HPUS • Belladonna (Alkaloids 0.0000003%) 6X HPUS. In a base of Deionized Water, Vegetable Glycerin, Hydroxyethyl Cellulose, Methyl Paraben, Propyl Paraben.
See Editor's Note No. 1, page 2053.

Teething Tablets **-** Hyland's
Each tablet contains: Calcarea phosphorica as Calcium Phosphate 3X HPUS • Chamomilla as Chamomile 3X HPUS • Coffea cruda as Coffee 3X HPUS • Belladonna as Alkaloids 0.0003% 3X HPUS. In a base of Lactose NF (Milk Sugar).
See Editor's Note No. 1, page 2053.

Tegreen 97 **-** Pharmanex
Each 250 mg capsule contains a 15:1 extract of Green Tea extract that is standardized to contain a minimum of 97% pure polyphenols including >160 mg of catechins of which >100 mg is EGC.

Ten Mushroom Combination **-** Smart Basics
Each capsule contains: Cordyceps • Reishi • Maitake • Shiitake • Coriolus • Umbellatus Polyporus • Wood Ear • Tremella • Poria • Hericium.

T-ENDO **-** Dial Herbs
Chaparral • Pipsissewa • Licorice • Prickly Ash • Cramp bark • False Unicorn • Saw Palmetto • Red Clover.

Tenshin Essentials Elastase **-** Taiko Healthcare, Inc.
Each tablet contains: Elastase 20 mg. Other Ingredients: Dextran, Talc, Lactose Cellulose, Hydroxy Propyl Cellulose, Silicic Acid Anhydride, Magnesium Stearate, Titanium Dioxide, Methyl-Methacrylate Copolymer, Glycerol Fatty Acid Ester.

Tenshin Essentials Nattokin Plus **-** Taiko Pharmaceutical Co., Ltd.
Each tablet contains: Nattokin (bacillis subtilis) 7 mg • Oligosaccharide 100 mg • Enterocuccuss Faecium 21 mg. Other Ingredients: Vitamin B6, Vitamin B5, Vitamin B3, Vitamin B1, Vitamin C, Starch, Lactose, Glycerol Fatty Acid.

Tenshin Essentials Nattokin Plus Calcium **-** Taiko Pharmaceutical Co., Ltd.
Each tablet contains: Nattokin (bacillis subtilis) 7 mg • Oligosaccharide 100 mg • Calcium 100 mg. Other Ingredients: Vitamin B6, Vitamin B3, Vitamin B1, Vitamin B5, Vitamin C, Starch, Lactose, Glycerol Fatty Acid, Flavoring, Corn Starch.

Tenshin Essentials Nattokin Plus Iron **-** Taiko Pharmaceutical Co., Ltd.
Each tablet contains: Nattokin (bacillis subtilis) 7 mg • Oligosaccharide 100 mg • Iron 9.42 mg. Other Ingredients: Vitamin B6, Vitamin B3, Vitamin B1, Vitamin B5, Vitamin C, Starch, Lactose, Glycerol Fatty Acid.

Tenshin Essentials Nattokin Plus Vitamin C & E **-** Taiko Pharmaceutical Co., Ltd.
Each tablet contains: Nattokin (bacillis subtilis) 7 mg • Oligosaccharide 100 mg • Vitamin C 103 mg • Vitamin E 30 IU. Other Ingredients: Vitamin B6, Vitamin B3, Vitamin B1, Vitamin B5, Starch, Lactose, Glycerol Fatty Acid.

Some Brand Name Natural Products - What they Contain

www.NaturalDatabase.com contains MANY more listings than appear here.

Tenshin Essentials Seirogan - Taiko Pharmaceutical Co., Ltd.
Three tablets contain: Creosote 67 mg • Geranium 75 mg • Phellodendron 75 mg. Other Ingredients: Talc, Calcium Carbonate, Carmellose Calcium.

Tension & stress - nelsons - Nelson Bach USA Ltd.
Active Indredients: Kali phos 6c HPUS • Arnica 6c HPUS. Inactive Ingredients: Lactose, Sucrose.
See Editor's Note No. 1, page 2053.

Tension Tamer Extra - Celestial Seasonings
Two capsules contain: Vitamin B6 (as pyridoxine HCL) 6 mg • Vitamin B12 (as cyanocobalamin) 12 mcg • Magnesium (as ascorbate and oxide) 60 mg • Proprietary Blend 1180 mg: Kava Kava (root), Kava Kava (standardized extract), Chamomile (standardized extract).

Tentex Forte - The Himalaya Drug Company (Himalaya Heal
Each tablet contains: Latakasthuri (abelmoschus moshatus) 10 mg • Ashvagandha (withania somnifera) 65 mg • Vriddadaru (argyreia speciosa syn. a.nervosa) 32 mg • Kapikachchhu (mucuna pruriens) 32 mg • Trivang 32 mg: Lead (naga), Tin (vanga), Zinc (yasada) • Shilajeet (mineral pitch, purified) 32 mg • Kumkuma (crocus sativus) 16 mg • Shudha Kupilu (strychnos nux vomica, detoxified) 16 mg • Makardhwaj (sulphide of mercury) 16 mg • Salabmisri (orchis mascula) 16 mg • Akarakarabha (anacyclus pyrethrum) 16 mg • Bala (sida cordifolia) 16 mg • Shalmali (bombax ceiba) 16 mg • Maricha (piper nigrum) 5 mg.
See Editor's Note No. 39, page 2058.

Tentex Royal - The Himalaya Drug Company (Himalaya Heal
Each capsule contains: Kokilaksha (asteracantha longifolia) 145 mg • Vathada (prunus amygdalus) 126 mg • Sunishannaka (blepharis edulis) 115 mg • Kumkuma (crocus sativus) 14 mg • Gokshura (tribulus terrestris) 100 mg.

T-ER - Dial Herbs
Eyebright • Bayberry • Passion flower • Goldenseal • Cayenne • Mineral Water • Honey.

Testatropinol - ASN - Advanced Sports Nutrition
Each tablet contains: Testatropinol is a 100% natural, non-herbal, non-glandular, synergistic, homeopathic compound, consisting of: Testosterone • Growth Hormone • Adrenalinum • Adrenocorticotropic Hormone • Lutenizing Hormone • Follicle Stimulating Hormone • Thyroid Stimulating Hormone • Progesterone • Estrone.
See Editor's Note No. 1, page 2053.

Testostazine - MedLean
Each tablet contains: Proprietary Blend 1170 mg: Maca root (lepidium meyenii, standardized to 0.6% total glucosinolates), Yerba Mate extract (Ilex paraguariensis leaf, 4:1 extract), N-Acetyl-L-Tyrosine, Blueberry extract (Vaccinium corymbosum leaf, standardized to 25% total polyphenols), Elderberry extract (Sambucus nigra fruit, standardized to 15% total polyphenols, 5% total flavonoids), Pyridoxal-5-Phosphate. Other Ingredients: Rice Flour, Gelatin, Water, Silicon Dioxide.

Testosterone Booster - Life Extension
Each capsule contains: 4- Androstenedione 10 mg • 5- Androstenedione 10 mg • 5- Androstenediol 5 mg • 19-Nor-4- Androstenedione 5 mg • 19-Nor-5- Androstenedione 5 mg • Chrysin 50 mg • Velvet Deer Antler 50 mg.
See Editor's Note No. 47, page 2058.

Testosterone Fuel Booster - TwinLab
Two capsules contain: Natural Testosterone Boosters DHEA (Dehydroepiandrosterone) (Pure Pharmaceutical Grade) 50 mg • Zinc (from Zinc Picolinate) 50 mg • Natural LH Boosters Acetyl-L-Carnitine 500 mg • Tribulus Terrestris extract 150 mg • Natural Aromatase Inhibitor (anti-estrogen) • Novasoy Purified Soy extract (providing 40% isoflavones)(providing isoflavones 80 mg including: Genistein39 mg, Daidzein 34 mg & Glycitein 7 mg) 200 mg • Natural DHT Inhibitors • Saw Palmetto (Serenoa repens) extract 120 mg • Phytosterol Complex (providing 130 mg of Beta-Sitosterol) 250 mg.

Testron SX - Nutraceutics Corp.
Two caplets contain: Boron (chelate) 3 mg • Proprietary Blend TSX Synergistic 1650 mg: Proteusterone (dioscorea machro stachya), Smilex Aristolochiafolii (dried root), Orchic Substance (bovine), Tribulus Terrestris (dried root), Leucine (as l-leucine hydrochloride) • Testrasterone Complex 360 mg: Ptychopetalum olacoides (dried root, dried trunk), Avena sativa (dried leaf and stem), Pfaffia paniculata (dried root), Urtica dioica (dried flowering plant and root).
See Editor's Note No. 14, page 2055.

TestronRX - Nutraceutics Corp.
Two caplets contain: Boron (chelate) 3 mg • TSX Synergisitc Blend 1650 mg: Dioscorea Macrostachya (proteusterone), Smilax Aristolochiaefolii (dried root), Orchic Substance (bovine), Tribulus Terrestris (dried root), Leucine (as l-leucine hydrochloride) • Testrasterone Complex 360 mg: Ptychopetalum Olacoides (dried root, trunk), Avena Sativa (dried leaf, stem), Pfaffia Paniculata (dried root), Urtica Dioica (dried flowering plant, root).
See Editor's Note No. 14, page 2055.

Tetrazene KGM-90 - BioQuest Pharmaceuticals
Two capsules contain: Vitamin B6 2 mg • Biotin 200 mcg • Proprietary Blend 507 mg: KGM-90 super class pharmaceutical grade Glucomannan, Glutamine, Olive leaf extract. Other Ingredients: Magnesium Stearate, Gelatin, Water.

TF Immune Spray - 4 Life
Each spray contains: Transfer Factor XF from Bovine Colostrum 25 mg.

T-FC1 - Dial Herbs
Red Raspberry • Black Cohosh • Lady Slipper • Blessed Thistle • Damiana.

T-FC2 - Dial Herbs
Black Cohosh • Licorice root • Sarsaparilla • Ginseng • Goldenseal.

T-FC3 - Dial Herbs
Black Cohosh • Wood Betony • Blessed Thistle • Chamomile • Fennel • Ginger • Cayenne.

T-FC4 - Dial Herbs
Wood Betony • Sarsaparilla • Valerian • Blessed Thistle • Dandelion • Garlic • Chamomile.

T-FLO - Dial Herbs
Sanicle • Marshmallow • Fennel • Blessed Thistle • Ginger.

T-FVR - Dial Herbs
Peppermint • Garlic • Valerian • Yarrow • Echinacea • Goldenseal • Cayenne • Lobelia.

T-GB - Dial Herbs
Dandelion • Oregon Grape • Rhubarb • Bayberry • Yellow Dock • Lobelia.

T-GS - Dial Herbs
Catnip • Peppermint • Fennel • Cayenne • Lobelia.

T-H - Dial Herbs
White Willow bark • Valerian • Scullcap • Wood Betony.

T-HBP - Dial Herbs
Black Cohosh • Blue Cohosh • Wild Cherry bark.

T-HBRN - Dial Herbs
Sarsaparilla • Thyme • Valerian • Wood Betony • Peppermint • Catnip • White Willow bark.

The Antioxidant Formula - Rx Vitamins
Three capsules contain: Vitamin C (Ascorbate) 500 mg • Beta Carotene 25000 IU • Phytonutrient Blend (Broccoli, Spinach, Tomato) 150 mg • Citrus Bioflavonoid Complex 50 mg • Vitamin E

BRAND NAMES

200 IU • Selenium 50 mcg • Zinc 15 mg • NAC (N-Acetyl-Cysteine) 15 mg • Bilberry 10 mg • L-Glutathione 10 mg • Wild Grape seed extract 10 mg.

The Antioxidant Phyters - The Vitamin Shoppe
Each tablet contains: Green and Red Wine 100 mg • Licorice 100 mg • Pine bark and Grape seed 30 mg • Bilberry 50 mg • Ginkgo Biloba 50 mg • Marigold, Sunflowers 60 mg.

The AstaFactor - Aquasearch
Two softgels contain: Natural Astaxanthin (6 mg total carotenoids) 5 mg. Ingredients: Algal meal (Haematococcus pluvialis), Rice Bran Oil, Natural Gelatin, Beeswax, Natural Vitamin E, Vegetal Glycerin.

The B-Total Solution with Extra B12 - Dial Herbs
Vitamin C • Vitamin B2 • Vitamin B3 • Vitamin B6 • Vitamin B12 • Pantothenic Acid. In a base of Distilled Water, Glycerine, Sorbitol, Sodium Bicarbonate, Citric Acid, Fruit flavors & Sodium Benzoate.

The Fat Metabolizer - The Vitamin Shoppe
Three tablets contain: Elemental Choline (from Choline Bitartrate) 1000 mg • Inositol 100 mg • L-Methionine 500 mg • Taurine 500 mg • Vitamin B6 (Pyridoxine HCl) 30 mg • Betaine HCl 150 mg • Barberry Extract (Berberis vulgaris) 100 mg.

The Fruit Phyters - The Vitamin Shoppe
Two tablets contain: Tomato, Red Grapefruit, Apricot, Watermelon 100 mg • Walnut, Berries, Grape, Apple, Tea • Orange, Lemon, Lime, Grapefruit, Tangerine, Cherry, Tomato, Strawberry 400 mg • Apricot, Cantaloupe, Citrus Fruit 150 mg • Citrus Fruit 100 mg • Papaya, Kiwi, Pineapple 50 mg • Mango, Citrus Fruit 100 mg.

The Greatest Vitamin in the World - The Greatest Vitamin In The World, LLC
Each capsule contains: Opti-Blend Delivery and Digestive Blend 108,918 Active Units: Amylase, Protease I, Protease II, Peptidase, Lipase, Invertase, Cellulase, Lactase, Maltase, Hemi Seb • Stabilized Probiotic Blend 3.510 Billion CFU: DDS-1 Lactobacillus Acidophilus, Bifidobacterium Bifidum, Enterococcus Faecium, Lactobacillus Bulgaricus, Lactobacillus Plantarum, Lactobacillus Salivarius, Streptococus Thermophilus, Bifidobacterium Infantis, Bacillus Caogulans • Calcium (amino acid chelate, dicalcium malate) 1004 mg • Iodine (potassium iodide) 150 mcg • Magnesium (amino acid chelate, oxie, glycyl glutamine) 400 mg • Zinc (amino acid chelate) 15 mg • Iron (Ferrochel, amino acid chelate) 18 mg • Selenium (amino acid complex) 70 mcg • Manganese (amino acid chelate) 2 mg • Copper (amino acid chelate) 2 mg • Chromium (amino acid chelate) 170 mcg • Molybdenum (amino acid chelate) 80 mcg • Potassium (amino acid chelate) 65 mcg • Vitamin A (Betatene, 2.5% beta carotene) 5000 IU • Vitamin C (natural source ascorbic acid) 60 mg • Vitamin E (D-alpha tocopherols from seed oil, Covitol 1185) 30 IU • Biotin 306 mcg • Thiamin (vitamin B1) 1.5 mg • Riboflavin (vitamin B2) 1.7 mg • Niacin (vitamin B3) 20 mg • Pantothenic Acid (vitamin B5) 10 mg • Vitamin B6 2 mg • Folate (folic acid) 400 mcg • Vitamin B12 (cyanocobalamin) 6 mcg • Garlic (pure gar A2000 +A22) 90 mg • Colostrum (Colostrum Gold) 315 mg • Ipriflavone (Ostivone - TSI) 180 mg • Garcinia Cambogia (super citrimax GarcinCambog) 252 mg • Conjugated Linoleic Acid 54 mg • Ginkgo Biloba 45 mg • Lecithin (non GMO) 90 mg • Grape seed extract (95% standardized proanthocyanidins) 45 mg • Pine bark (95% polyphenols) 45 mg • Opti SOD Precursor Blend 405 mcg • Gymnema Sylvestre 135 mg • Milk Thistle 27 mg • Licorice root (declycerinated) 90 mg • Lutein 5.4 mg • Glucosamine Sulfate 2KCl 180 mg • Whole Food Blend 603 mg: Carrot, Wild Yam, Broccoli, Spinach, Tomato, Kale, Nutritional Yeast, Acerola Cherry, Black Currant, Wheat Germ.

The Green Phyters - The Vitamin Shoppe
Two tablets contain: Spirulina 200 mg • Chlorella 200 mg • Barley Juice 200 mg • Wheat Grass 200 mg • Alfalfa Leaf 200 mg • Chlorophyll 200 mg.

The Missing Link: Master Nutrient Formula - Designing Health, Inc.
Each tablespoon contains: Vitamin A (90% as beta carotene) 55 IU • Thiamine (Vitamin B1) 0.1 mg • Calcium 22 mg • Iron 0.7 mg • Omega-3 1000 mg • Omega-6 450 mg • Omega-9 400 mg • Hesperidin 80 mg • Spirulina 8 mg • Kelp (macrocystis pyrifuri)) 6 mg. Other Ingredients: Flax Seed, Blackstrap Molasses, Rice Bran, Nutritional Yeast, Sunflower Seed, Alfalfa, Carrot, Apple, Sesame Seed, Licorice Root, Broccoli, Cherry, Parsely, Sprouted Green Barley, Nettle, Vanilla Bean, Ginger Root, Sage, Rosemary, Garlic, and Yucca Schidigera Extract.

The New AntiOx, Cysteine Free - NutriCology
Each capsule contains: Vitamin A (40% as retinyl palmitate and 60% as beta-carotene) 12,500 IU • Vitamin C (as ascorbyl palmitate) 4 mg • Vitamin E (as DL-alpha-tocopheryl acetate) 100 IU • Thiamin (as thiamin hydrochloride) 10 mg • Riboflavin (80% as riboflavin and 20% as riboflavin-5-phosphate) 12.5 mg • Niacin (50% as niacinamide) 10 mg • Vitamin B6 (80% as pyridoxine hydrochloride and 20% as pyridoxal-5-phosphate) 12.5 mg • Folic Acid 100 mcg • Vitamin B12 (as cyanocobalamin) 100 mcg • Pantothenic Acid (as calcium pantothenate) 12.5 mg • Zinc (as zinc citrate) 7.5 mg • Selenium (87% as sodium selenite and 13% as selenomethionine) 75 mcg • Copper (as copper sebacate) 0.5 mg • Manganese (as manganese citrate) 5 mg • Glutathione (reduced) 50 mg • L-Methionine 50 mg • Taurine 50 mg • Trimethylglycine 50 mg • Proanthocyanidins, as Grape seed extract 12.5 mg • Coenzyme Q10 15 mg • Lipoic Acid 12. 5mg • Ginkgo Biloba extract 20 mg. Other Ingredients: Magnesium Stearate.

The New Grapefruit Diet with Apple Cider Vinegar - Applied Nutrition
Two capsules contain: Vitamin B6 (as pyridoxine HCl) 25 mg • Iodine (kelp) 150 mcg • Chromate Chromium Polynicotinate 200 mcg • Proprietary Blend 774 mg: Soy Lecithin, Grapefruit powder extract, Cider Vinegar powder, Bioperine Black Pepper fruit extract. Other Ingredients: Gelatin, Silica, Magnesium Stearate.

The Ocular Formula - Rx Vitamins
Three capsules contain: Vitamin C (Ascorbate) 200 mg • Citrus Flavonoid Complex 100 mg • Vitamin E 100 IU • Zinc 30 mg • Glutathione 10 mg • Beta Carotene 9 mg • Vitamin A (Retinol) 5000 IU • Selenium 50 mcg • Lutein 6 mg • Zeaxanthin 260 mcg • Bilberry 100 mg • Grape seed 10 mg • Essential Cofactors: CoQ10 5 mg, Copper 3 mg.

The One-Minute Facial - Jason
Seven different Vitamin Cs • Alpha Lipoic Acid.

The Original Happy PMS - Zeller
Purified Water • Stearal Konium Chloride • D-Alpha Tocopherol (vitamin E) • Natural Glycerin • Avocado oil • Natural Progesterone • Aloe Vera oil • Rosemary extract • Vitamin A Palmitate • Carrot oil • Lemon Grass oil.

The Original Hollywood Celebrity Diet Body Slimming & Contouring Creme - Celebrity Products Direct, Inc.
Purified Water • Sesame Seed Oil • Polysorbate 60 • PEG-100 Stearate • Cetyl Alcohol • Caffeine • Dimethicone • Glyceryl Stearate • Phenoxyethanol • Hydro C • Hydroxylated Lecithin • Carbomer • Triethanolamine • Methylparaben • Fragrance • Butylparaben • Theobromine • Vitamin E Acetate • Ethylparaben • Propylparaben.

The Original Hollywood Celebrity Diet Fat Metabolizers - Celebrity Products Direct, Inc.
Each capsule contains: Cocoa extract powder 225 mg • Choline Bitartrate 100 mg • Guarana seed extract 36 mg • Methyl Acetyl Pyruvic Acid 24 mg • Dimethyl Sulfone (MSM) 12 mg • Kava root extract 6 mg • Zhi Shi immature Orange fruit (citri seu ponchi, immaturus) 6 mg • Fennel seed extract 6 mg • White Willow bark extract 18 mg • Proprietary Blend 18 mg: Ginger root powder, L-Aspartic Acid, Gotu Kola, Aloe Vera powder, Garlic, Beet extract

powder, Hawthorn berry powder, Saw Palmetto berry powder, Ginseng root powder, Ginkgo Biloba powder, Bladderwrack, Sea Kelp powder. Other Ingredients: Magnesium Trisilicate, Magnesium Stearate, Natural Gelatin Capsules.
See Editor's Note No. 40, page 2058.

The Original Hollywood Celebrity Diet QuickStart Citrus Juice **-** Celebrity Products Direct, Inc.
Purified Water • Juice Concentrate Blend: Pineapple, Plum, White Grape, Orange, Apple, Lemon • Potassium Citrate (potassium) • Ascorbic Acid (vitamin C) • D-Alpha-Tocopheryl Acetate (vitamin E) • Niacinamide (vitamin B3) • Calcium Pantothenate (vitamin B5) • Beta Carotene • Bilberry extract • Green Tea extract • Ginkgo Biloba extract • Grape Seed extract • Pyridoxine Hydrochloride (vitamin B6) • Riboflavin - 5' Phosphate (vitamin B2) • Thiamine Mononitrate (vitamin B1) • Folic Acid • Cholecalciferol (vitamin D3) • Biotin • Cyanocobalamin (vitamin B12).

The Original Hollywood Celebrity Diet Tea **-** Celebrity Products Direct, Inc.
Each bag (1.8 g) contains: Blackberry leaves • Cassia Angustifolia • Raphamus Sativa • Cassia Tora • Orange peel • Chicory root • Lemon Grass • Lemon peel • Hawthorn berry • Barley • Natural Lemon flavor • Natural Orange flavor.

The Prostate Formula **-** Real Health Laboratories
Three tablets contain: Vitamin D 200.0 IU • Saw Palmetto powder 320.0 mg • Pygeum powder 300.0 mg • Vitamin E 100.0 IU • Stinging Nettle powder 100.0 mg • Vitamin B6 50.00 mg • Pumpkin seed powder 100.0 mg • Zinc 15.0 mg • L-Lysine HCl 250.0 mg • L-Glutamic acid 250.0 mg • Glycine 250.0 mg. Other Ingredients: Dicalcium Phosphate, Hydroxyproplyl Methylcellulose, Microcrystalline Cellulose, Croscarmellose Sodium, Stearic Acid, Polyethylene Glycos, Silica, Titanium Dioxide, Magnesium Stearate, Peppermint oil, Polysorbate 80.

The Sinus Buster **-** SiCap Industries, LLC
Purified Water • Oleoresin Capsicum • Eucalyptus Oil • Rosemary extract • Vitamin C (as ascorbic acid) • Sea Salt.

The Total EFA **-** Health From The Sun
Three capsules contain: Vitamin E 30 IU • Alpha-Linolenic Acid (ALA)(Omega-3) 699 mg • Docosahexaenoic Acid (DHA) (Omega-3) 138 mg • Eicosapentaenoic Acid (EPA)(Omega-3) 216 mg • Gamma Linolenic Acid (GLA)(Omega-6) 288 mg • Lenoleic Acid (Omega-6) 620 mg • Oleic Acid (Omega-9) 520 mg. Ingredients: Certified Organic Flax seed oil, Borage seed oil, Fish oil, Gelatin, Glycerine, Water, Mixed Tocopherols.

The Ultimate Anti-Oxidant Formula **-** Natrol
Two capsules contain: Vitamin A (Beta Carotene from d-Salina) 10000 IU • Vitamin E (d-alpha tocopheryl) 200 IU • Vitamin C (Ester-C Brand) 250 mg • Niacinamide 40 mg • Zinc (Krebs Cycle) 25 mg • Copper (Krebs Cycle) 2 mg • Selenium (Selenomethionine) 125 mcg • Flavonoids, Herbs, & other selected ingredients: Spirulina 300 mg GP Flavonoids Complex+ 200 mg, a 30% guaranteed potency extract of mixed flavonoids extracted from: Rose Hips, Turmeric, Acerola berry, Bilberry, Hawthorne berry, Grape skin, Milk Thistle, & Citrus fruits • Calendula 50 mg • Artichoke extract 10 mg. Other Ingredients: Silicon Dioxide, Magnesium Stearate, Gelatin.

The Ultimate Calcium Formula **-** Roex
Six tablets contain: Calcium (Chelate, Citrate, Hydroxyapatite, Aspartate, Lactate) 1000 mg • Magnesium (Chelate, Oxide, Aspartate) 500 mg • Zinc (Gluconate , Citrate, Aspartate) 15 mg • Manganese 5 mg • Copper 2 mg • Vitamin D (Cholecalciferol) 400 IU • Boron 3 mg • Trace Minerals 25 mg • Silica 150 mg • Selenium 50 mcg • Chromium 50 mcg • Molybdenum 10 mcg.

The Ultimate Natural Facelift Chin & Neck Treatment **-** Healthy Revelations Inc.
Urea • Carbomer • Isopropyl Alcohol • Glyceryl Stearate • Water • Caprylic/Capric Triglyceride • Glycerin • Panthenol • Glucose • Stearic Acid • Horse Chestnut extract (aesculus hippocastanum) • Hydrocotyl extract (centella asiatica) • Green Tea extract (camellia sinensis) • Arnica extract (arnica montana) • Ivy extract (hedera helix) • Yarrow extract (achillea millefolium) • Bladderwrack extract (fucus vesiculosus) • Lactoyl Methylsilanol Elastinate • Methylsilanol Elastinate • Methylsilanol Mannuronate • Hydroiodide T.E.A. • Ginkgo Biloba extract • Polysorbate 60 • PEG-7 Glyceryl Cocoate • Stearyl Alcohol • Sorbitol • Polysorbate 80 • Cetyl Acetate • Acetylated Lanolin Alcohol • Magnesium Aluminum Silicate • Hops extract (humulus lupulus) • Menthol • Aloe extract (aloe barbadensis) • Methylparaben • Camphor • Hydrolyzed Elastin • Hydrolyzed Collagen • Glycosaminoglycans • Saccharide Isomerate • Glycoproteins • Dibutyl Lauroyl Glutamide • Horsetail extract (equisetum arvense) • Propylparaben • Eucalyptus extract (eucalyptus globules) • Adenosine Phosphate • Adenosine Triphosphate • Niacinamide • Placental Enzymes • PVM/MA Decadience Crosspolymer • BHT • Glyceryl Oleate • Ascorbyl Palmitate • Citric Acid • Propylene Glycol • Lecithin • Coenzyme Q10 • Tocopherol • Meadowfoam (limnanthes alba) seed oil • Copper Protein Complex • Rosemary extract (rosmarinus officinalis) • Peppermint extract (mentha piperita) • DMDM Hydantoin • Iodopropynyl Butylcarbamate • Tocopheryl Nicotinate • Fragrance • FD&C Red #40.

The Ultimate Weight Loss & Nutrition System **-** Nature's Secret
Three tablets contain: Vitamin B6 30 mg • Garcinia cambogia extract 600 mg • Pantothenic Acid 100 mg • Magnesium (aspartate) 25 mg • Chromium 300 mcg • Potassium (citrate) 128 mg • L-Carnitine 250 mg • Betaine HCl 100 mg • Lipotropic factors 800 mg • Choline, L-Methionine, Inositol, Lecithin, Triphala powder, Echinacea angustifolia, Cascara sagrada • Astragalus. Thermogenic support factors 757 mg: N-Acetyl Glucosamine, Uva Ursi leaf, Gotu Kola, Siberian Ginseng, L-Glutamine, Parsley leaf, Ginger root, Borage oil, Shave Grass herb, Piper longum, Licorice root. L-Phenylalanine, Corn Silk, Guggulipid, Pacific Kelp, L-Tyrosine, Atractylodes, Bladderwrack, Dulse, Chickweed herb, Dandelion root, Capsicum fruit, Lipase, Mustard seed, Protease, Cellulase.

The Vegi Phyters **-** The Vitamin Shoppe
Two tablets contain: Red, Yellow, and Dark vegetable, Carrots, Kale, Parsley, Spinach, Sweet Potatoes, Turnip Greens, Winter Squash, and Yams 300 mg • Cruciferous Vegetable 300 mg • Horseradish 100 mg • Chili Peppers 100 mg • Cabbage, Brussel Sprouts, Kale, Collard Greens, Broccoli, Mustard Greens 200 mg.

The Vitamin Shoppe Flax Seed Oil 1000 mg **-** The Vitamin Shoppe
Each softgel contains: 1000 mg of 100% pure, organically grown cold-pressed, unrefined virgin flax oil providing the following approximate essential fatty acids: Alpha-Linolenic Acid 550 mg • Linoleic Acid 150 mg • Oleic Acid 190 mg • natural Vitamin E 1 IU.

Thera Zinc Lozenges-Menthol **-** Natrol
One lozenge contains: Vitamin C (as Calcium Ascorbate) 50 mg • Zinc (as Zinc Gluconate) 7.5 mg • Echinacea angustifolia entire plant 10 mg • Bee Propolis 10 mg • Slippery Elm Bark 10 mg • Elderberry 10 mg • Bee Pollen 10 mg. Other Ingredients: Hydrogenated Starch, Hydrolysate, natural Menthol Eucalyptus flavor.

Thera-C 3 Grams Lemon **-** Natrol
One single serving contains: Vitamin C (Ascorbic Acid) 250 mg • Acerola berry extract 20 mg • Echinacea (Purpurea extract 16:1) 12.5 mg • White Willow bark 100 mg • Slippery Elm bark 75 mg • Stevia powder 20 mg. Other Ingredients: Lemon Juice powder, Citric Acid, Menthol from Peppermint, Honey powder, Fructose, Calcium Carbonate.

Theragran Heart Right **-** Bristol-Myers Squibb Co.
Two caplets contain: Vitamin A (8% as Beta-carotene, 2% as Alpha-carotene, Lutein, Lypcopene, Zeaxanthin, Cryptoxanthin 10 mg) 5000 IU • Vitamin C 120 mg • Vitamin D 400 IU • Vitamin E 400 IU • Vitamin K 14 mcg • Thiamin (B1) 3 mg • Riboflavin (B2) 3.4 mg •

Niacin (B3) 20 mg • Vitamin B6 16 mg • Folate, Folic Acid, Folacin 600 mcg • Vitamin B12 30 mcg • Biotin 30 mcg • Pantothenic acid 10 mg • Calcium 55 mg • Iron 4 mg • Iodine 150 mcg • Magnesium 150 mg • Zinc 15 mg • Selenium 70 mcg • Copper 1.5 mg • Manganese 2 mg • Chromium 50 mcg • Molybdenum 75 mcg • Proprietary Blend 10 mg: Beta Carotene, Alpha Carotene, Lutein, Lycopene, Zeaxanthin, Cryptoxanthin.

Theragran-M Advanced **-** Bristol-Myers Squibb Co.
Each caplet contains: Vitamin A Acetate (20% as Beta Carotene) 5000 IU • Vitamin C (Ascorbic Acid) 90 mg • Vitamin D (Vitamin D3) 400 IU • Vitamin E (dl-Alpha Tocopheryl) 60 IU • Vitamin K (Phytonadione) 28 mcg • Thiamin Mononitrate (Vitamin B1) 3 mg • Riboflavin (Vitamin B2) 3.4 mg • Niacin (Vitamin B3, Niacinamide) 20 mg • Vitamin B6 (Pyridoxine Hydrochloride) 6 mg • Folate (Folic acid, Folacin) 400 mcg • Vitamin B12 (Cyanocobalamin) 12 mcg • Biotin 30 mcg • Pantothenic Acid (Calcium Pantothenate) 10 mg • Calcium 40 mg • Iron (Ferrous Fumarate) 9 mg • Phosphorus (Calcium Phosphate) 31 mg • Iodine (Potassium Iodide) 150 mcg • Magnesium Oxide 100 mg • Zinc Oxide 15 mg • Selenium (Sodium Selenate) 70 mcg • Copper (Cupric Sulfate) 2 mg • Manganese Sulfate 2 mg • Chromium Chloride 50 mcg • Molybdenum (Sodium Molybdate) 75 mcg • Chloride 7.5 mg • Potassium Chloride 7.5 mg • Nickel Sulfate 5 mcg • Tin (Stannous Chloride) 10 mcg • Silicon 2 mg • Vanadium (Sodium Metavanadate) 10 mcg • Boron (Sodium Borate) 150 mcg. Other Ingredients: Beta Carotene, Carnauba Wax, Crospovidone, FD&C Blue No.2 Aluminum Lake, FD&C Red No. 40 Aluminum Lake, Flavor, Gelatin, Hydroxypropyl Cellulose, Hydroxypropyl Methylcellulose, Lactose, Magnesium Stearate, Maltodextrin, Microcrystaline Cellulose, Polyethylene Glycol, Polysorbate 80, Potassium Citrate, Povidone, Silica Gel, Stearic Acid, Titanium Dioxide, Triacetin.

Theramune Black Cumin Seed Oil Softgel Capsules **-** Amazing Herbs
Each capsule contains: Black Cumin Seed oil (100% pure) 500 mg.

Theramune Black Seed & Garlic **-** Amazing Herbs
Each capsule contains: Proprietary Blend: Black Seed herb, High Potency Garlic.

Theramune Black Seed Oil **-** Amazing Herbs
Each ounce contains: Black Seed oil (black cumin oil, 100% pure) Which Contains The Following Fatty Acid/Nutrient Blend: Myristic Acid (0.5%), Palmitic Acid (13.7%), Palmitoleic Acid (0.1%), Stearic Acid (2.6%), Oleic Acid (23.7%), Linoleic Acid (Omega-6, 57.9%), Linolenic Acid (Omega-3, 0.2%), Arachidic Acid (1.3%), Protein, Thiamin, Riboflavin, Pyridoxine, Niacin, Folacin, Calcium, Iron, Copper, Zinc, Phosphorus.

Theramune Black Seed Ultimate **-** Amazing Herbs
Each capsule contains: Proprietary Blend: Black Seed, Odorless Garlic extract, Ginger, Cayenne.

Theramune Ginseng Powder **-** Amazing Herbs
Each capsule contains: Proprietary Blend: Black Seed, Korean Ginseng, Siberian Ginseng, American Ginseng.

Theramune Gold **-** Amazing Herbs
Each capsule contains: Proprietary Blend: Echinacea, Goldenseal, Black Seed.

TheraStress liquid **-** Nutriceutical Technologies
Eleuthero root • Schizandra berry • Green Tea extract • Rhodiola root • Garcinia Cambogia • Chinese Ginseng • Reishi mushroom • Stevia herb. Other Ingredients: Vegetable Glycerin, Deionized Water, Natural Flavors.

Theravim-M **-** Puritan's Pride
Each tablet contains: Vitamin A (as retinyl acetate and beta carotene) 5,000 IU • Vitamin C (as ascorbic acid) 90 mg • Vitamin D (as cholecalciferol) 400 IU • Vitamin E (as dl-alpha tocopheryl acetate) 30 IU • Thiamin (Vitamin B1: as thiamine hydrochloride) 3 mg • Riboflavin (Vitamin B2) 3.4 mg • Niacin (as niacinamide) 20 mg • Vitamin B6 (as pyridoxine hydrochloride) 3 mg • Folic Acid 400 mcg • Vitamin B12 (as cyancobalamin) 9 mcg • Biotin (as d-biotin) 30 mcg • Pantothenic Acid (as d-calcium pantothenate) 10 mg • Calcium (as dicalcium phosphate) 40 mg • Iron (ferrous fumarate) 27 mg • Phosphorus (as dicalcium phosphate) 31 mg • Iodine (as potassium iodide) 150 mcg • Magnesium (as magnesium oxide) 100 mg • Zinc (as zinc oxide) 15 mg • Selenium (as sodium selenate) 10 mcg • Copper (as copper sulfate) 2 mg • Manganese (as manganese sulfate) 5 mg • Chromium (as chromium chloride) 15 mcg • Molybdenum (as sodium molybdate) 15 mcg • Chloride (as potassium chloride) 7.5 mg • Potassium (as potassium chloride) 7.5 mg.

Thermadrene **-** SportPharma
Each capsule contains: Ephedra standardized extract 300 mg (equivalent to 24 mg ephedrine) • USP Caffeine 80 mg • Guarana extract 150 mg (equivalent to 15 mg caffeine) • Willow Bark extract 75 mg (natural aspirin, equivalent to less than 5 mg aspirin) • Cayenne 60 mg • Ginger root 40 mg.
See Editor's Note No. 30, page 2056.

Thermic Blast **-** Human Development Technologies (HDT)
Four sprays contain: Caffeine 100 mg • Ephedra extract 8% aerial (Ephedrine 8 mg) 100 mg • Stevia extract 80% leaf (Steviosides 32 mg) 40 mg • White Willow bark 1% bark (Salicin 200 mcg) 20 mg • Green Tea extract 30% leaf (Polyphenols 6 mg) 20 mg • Guarana extract 10% seed (Caffeine 2 mg) 20 mg • Chromium Picolinate 400 mcg. Other Ingredients: Purified Water, Propylene Glycol, natural Cherry & Vanilla Flavors, Polysorbate 20, Benzyl Alcohol, Hydrochloric Acid Lecithin.
See Editor's Note No. 30, page 2056.

Thermicore - MET-Rx **-** Rexall - Sundown
Three capsules contain: Ma Huang extract 250 mg • Caffeine 200 mg • Bitter Orange extract 400 mg. Other Ingredients: Cellulose, Polyvinylpyrrolidone & Gelatin.
See Editor's Note No. 30, page 2056.

Thermo Bond **-** Herbalife
Each tablet contains: Sodium Choleate • Fiber Blend: natural fibers from apple, grains, citrus, & cellulose.

Thermo Cuts **-** Optimum Nutrition
Four capsules contain: Citrimax 2000 mg • MaHuang extract 334 mg • Guarana extract 910 mg • Willow bark extract 100 mg • L-Carnitine 100 mg • Chromium Picolinate 300 mcg.
See Editor's Note No. 30, page 2056.

Thermo DynamX **-** EAS
Three capsules contain: Green Tea Leaf (carnellia sinensis; total catechins 213 mg, epigallocatechin gallates (EGCG) 110) 610 mg • Mate (ilex paraguarensis) leaves and stems 500 mg • Caffeine (from mate, caffeine anhydrous, green tea) 200 mg • Octopamine HCl 200 mg • Synephrine (from citrus aurantium) 20 mg. Other Ingredients: Gelatin, Microcellulose, Magnesium Stearate, Silica.
See Editor's Note No. 40, page 2058.

Thermo Trim **-** Swanson
Three capsules contain: Chromium (chromax chromium picolinate) 200 mcg • Guarana extract (standardized to 22% caffeine) 909 mg • Citrin Garcinia Cambogia extract (50% hydroxycitrate acid) 500 mg • Ma Huang extract (standardized to ephedra alkaloids 20 mg) 334 mg • L-Carnitine (tartrate) 100 mg.
See Editor's Note No. 30, page 2056.

Thermo-Actives **-** Natrol
Each capsule contains: Ginger extract roots (5% gingerols) 150 mg • Sida cordifolia extract (0.8% ephedrine) 100 mg • Mucuna pruriens 5:1 extract 100 mg • Cayenne extract (90000 SHU) 50 mg • Mustard extract seed (50% saponins) 15 mg • Bioperine 4:1 extract 15 mg. Other Ingredients: Rice Powder, Silicon Dioxide, Magnesium Stearate, Gelatin.
See Editor's Note No. 39, page 2058.

ThermoAMP - E'OLA
0.25 mL contains: Proprietary Blend 31 mg: Ephedra extract (branch, ephedra sinesis), White Willow Bark extract (salix alba), Guarana (seed, paullinia cupana) , Atractylodes (herb, atractylodes macrocephala) extract, Licorice (root, glycyrrhiza uralensis), DMAE (dimethyl amino ethenol bitartrate, Vitamin B12 (Dibencozide). Inactive Ingredients: Water, Glycerin, Sodium Benzoic Acid (sodium benzoate), Sorbic Acid (potassium sorbate).
See Editor's Note No. 30, page 2056.

ThermoAMP Herbal Chews - E'OLA
Each chew (8.6 g) contains: Calcium 245 mg • Vitamin B12 20 mcg • Proprietary Blend 31 mg: Ephedra extract (branch, ephedra sinica), White Willow Bark extract (salix alba), Guarana extract (seed, paullinia cupana), Atractylodes extract (herb, atractylodes macrocephala), Licorice root (glcyrrhiza uralensis), DMAE (dimethy amino ethanol bitatrate, Vitamin B12 (dibencozide). Other Ingredients: Corn Syrup, Sweetened Condensed Whole Milk, Sugar, Chocolate, Partially Hydrogenated Soybean Oil, Mono & Diglycerides, Soy Lecithin, Natural & Artificial Flavors.
See Editor's Note No. 30, page 2056.

Thermochrome ephedra free - Market America, Inc.
Two tablets contain: Vitamin C (as ascorbic acid) 100 mg • Vitamin B6 (as pyridoxine HCl) 10 mg • Pantothenic Acid (as dicalcium pantothenate) 12 mg • Magnesium (as magnesium oxide) 10 mg • Chromium (as chromium dinicotinate glycinate and chromium picolinate) 150 mcg • Proprietary Thermobolic Complex 1415 mg: Guarana seed extract (supplying 100 mg caffeine), Citrus Aurantium extract (immature fruit), DL-Phenylalanine, Green Tea leaf standardized extract, Theobroma Cacao standardized extract, Yerba Mate leaf extract, DL-Methionine, Ginger root, Dimethylaminoethanol (DMAE) bitartrate, Grape seed extract, Cinnamon twig extract, Galangal rhizome extract. Other Ingredients: Dicalcium Phosphate, Microcrystalline Cellulose, Croscarmellose Sodium, Stearic Acid, Magnesium Stearate, Silica, Pharmaceutical Glaze.
See Editor's Note No. 40, page 2058.

ThermoDiet for Men - Futurebiotics
Two tablets contain: Spirulina 100 mg • MaHuang (Standardized Extract) 200 mg • Mustard Seed Powder 100 mg • Vitamin C 100 mg • Potassium (Citrate) 99 mg • Magnesium (Aspartate) 50 mg • Chromium (Picolinate) 200 mcg • Kelp 150 mg • Chinese Licorice 250 mg • Smilax.
See Editor's Note No. 30, page 2056.

ThermoDiet For Women - Futurebiotics
Two tablets contain: Spirulina 100 mg • Ma Huang standardized extract 200 mg • Mustard Seed powder 100 mg • Vitamin C 100 mg • Potassium (citrate) 99 mg • Magnesium (aspartate) 50 mg • Chromium (picolinate) 200 mcg • Kelp 150 mg • Peony 250 mg • Foti 250 mg • Dong Quai 250 mg.
See Editor's Note No. 30, page 2056.

Thermo-G - Advocare International
One caplet contains: Vitamin A (as beta-carotene) 1000 IU • Niacin 20 mg • Magnesium (as phosphate) 25 mg • Potassium (as phosphate) 50 mg • Green Orange extract (pericarp - citrus aurantium) 500 mg • Guarana extract (seed - paullinia cupana) 200 mg • Green Tea extract (leaf - camellia sinensis) 10 mg. Other Ingredients: Dicalcium Phosphate, Silicon Dioxide, Cellulose, Stearic Acid, Magnesium Stearate, Beet Root Powder (for color).
See Editor's Note No. 40, page 2058.

Thermogenic Herbal Complex - Starlight International
Each capsule contains: Chromium (as chromium picolinate) 6 mcg • Ma Huang (ephedra sinica, total ephedrine alkaloids 22 mg) 275 mg • Cascara Sagrada bark (rhamnus purshiana) 35 mg • Bladderwrack plant (focus vesiculosus) 35 mg • Uva Ursi leaf extract (4:1, arctostaphylos uva ursi, leaf) 25 mg • Parsley leaf extract, 4:1 (petroselinum crispum) 10 mg • Calcium Gluconate 5 mg • Corn Silk flower pistils (zea mays) 7 mg • Goldenrod leaf (solidago odora) 6 mg • Fumitory Herb aerial parts (fumaria officinalis) 6 mg • Magnesium Gluconate 7 mg • English Hawthorn fruit (crategus laevigata) 5 mg • Licorice root (glycyrrhiza glabra, root) 5 mg • Marshmallow root (athea officinalis) 5 mg • Apple Pectin 5 mg. Other Ingredients: Magnesium Stearate, Silicon Dioxide, Dicalcium Phosphate, Calcium Sulfate.
See Editor's Note No. 30, page 2056.

Thermogenics Original Formula - SilverSage
Each capsule contains: Ephedrine Alkaloids (from standardized ma huang plant extract 310 mg) 25 mg • Caffeine (16.8 mg from standardized bissy nut 140 mg) 50 mg • Acetylsalicylic Acid (aspirin) 110 mg • Proprietary Blend of Synergistic Ingredients 249 mg: Siberian Ginseng root, Schizonepeta Spica extract 5:1, Forsythia fruit extract 5:1, Green Tea leaf extract standardized for Polyphenols/ Catechins content, Cayenne fruit, Ginger root • Vitamin C 50 mg • Pantothenic Acid 25 mg • Zinc amino acid chelate 7 mg • Selenium Amino Acid Chelate 1 mcg • Manganese Amino Acid Chelate 2.5 mg.
See Editor's Note No. 30, page 2056.

ThermoGenics Plus - SilverSage
Each capsule contains: Ephedrine standardized extract (whole ma huang) 14 mg • Caffeine standardized extrac (from bissy nut) • Acetylsalicylic Acid • In a base of Vitamin C, Siberian Ginseng, Green Tea extract (standardized to 50% polyphenols/catechins), Schizonepeta spica extract (5:1), Forsythia fruit extract (5:1), White Willow bark, Cayenne, Pantothenic Acid, Ginger root, Zinc (amino acid chelate), Manganese (amino acid chelate), Selenium (amino acid chelate).
See Editor's Note No. 30, page 2056.

Thermogenics Plus, Stimulant Free - SilverSage
Two capsules contain: Proprietary Phosphosterine Blend 1330 mg: Calcium Phosphate, Commiphora Phytosterol extract, Garcinia Cambogia (HCA 125 mg), L-Tyrosine, Dipotassium Phosphate, Sodium Phosphate, Disodium Phosphate, Phosphatidyl Choline, Scutellaria root, Bupleurum root, Epimedium herb. Other Ingredients: Rice Flour.

Thermogenics Quick Start - SilverSage
Each capsule contains: Ephedrine Alkaloids standardized extract (from ma huang plant 250 mg) 20 mg • Caffeine (26 mg from standardized bissy nut 106 mg) 200 mg • Acetylsalicylic Acid (aspirin) 324 mg • Proprietary Synergistic Blend 198 mg: Siberian Ginseng root, Schizonepeta Spica extract (5:1), Forsythia fruit extract (5:1), Cayenne fruit, Ginger root • Vitamin C 40 mg • Pantothenic Acid 23 mg • Zinc Amino Acid Chelate 14 mg • Selenium Amino Acid Chelate 167 mcg • Manganese Amino Acid Chelate 5 mg.
See Editor's Note No. 30, page 2056.

Thermojetics Beige - Herbalife
Each tablet contains: English Hawthorn berry fruit 80 mg • Alfalfa leaves 70 mg • Parsley leaves 60 mg • Marshmallow root 55 mg •Uva Ursi leaves 50 mg • Cornsilk 50 mg •Magnolia bark 30 mg • Fennel seed 25 mg • Astragalus root 20 mg • Pfaffia root 20 mg • Pau d'Arco bark 20 mg • European Goldenrod leaves 15 mg • Licorice root 15 mg. Other Ingredients: Microcrystaline Cellulose, Tapioca & Corn Starches, Stearic Acid, Cross-linked Sodium Carboxymethylcellulose, Sodium Starch Glyconate, Silicon Dioxide, Magnesium Stearate, Food Grade Shellac, Hydroxypropyl Methylcellulose, Titianium Dioxide, Caramel.

Thermojetics Green Ephedra Free - Herbalife
Each tablet contains: Proprietary Blend: Green Tea extract, Cocoa extract, dried Citrus Aurantium extract (fruit), dried Bitter Orange extract (peel), Yerba Mate. Other Ingredients: Maltodextrin, Corn Starch, Silicon Dioxide, Methylcellulose, Colors, Titanium Dioxide, Sodium Carboxymethyl Cellulose, Hydroxypropylmethyl Cellulose, Magnesium Stearate, Trimethyl Citrate, Black Pepper extract, Flavor.
See Editor's Note No. 40, page 2058.

Thermojetics Green Refresh **-** Herbalife
Each tablet contains: Balu • Yerba Mate extract • Bladderwrack • Meadowsweet • Garcinia Cambogia • Valerian root • Green Tea extract • Fumitory herb • Honeysuckle • FD&C Blue No. 1 Lake.

Thermojetics Herbal Concentrate **-** Herbalife
Each serving contains: Camellia sinensis (Green Tea & Orange Pekoe Tea) extract • Maltodextrin • Fructose • Malva Sylvestris extract • Cardamom extract • Hibiscus extract • Lemon Peel extract.

Thermojetics Original Green **-** Herbalife
Each tablet contains: Calcium (as calcium carbonate) 58 mg • Iodine (from bladderwrack) 30 mg • Chinese Ephedra leaf 140 mg • Yerba Mate leaf 115 mg • Dried MaHuang extract 70 mg • Bladderwrack 40 mg • Valerian root 40 mg • Fumaria Officinalis 30 mg • Dried Salix Purpurea bark extract 30 mg • Chondrus Crispus 5 mg. Other Ingredients: Stearic Acid, Tapioca Starch, Microcrystalline Cellulose, Papain, Cross-linked Sodium Carboxymethylcellulose, Silicon Dioxide, Sodium Starch Glyconate, Magnesium Stearate, Sodium Laurel Sulfate, Food Grade Shellac, Titanium Dioxide, Polyethylene Glycol, Riboflavin, FD&C Blue #1.
See Editor's Note No. 21 and No. 30.

Thermojetics Yellow **-** Herbalife
Each tablet contains: Garcinia (Garcinia Cambogia extract) 400 mg • GTF Chromium (Chomium Polynicotinate) 400 mg.

Thermo-Lift (ThermoLift) **-** Changes International, Inc.
Each caplet contains: Chromium (dinicotinate glycinate, picolinate, niacin bound chromium) 200 mcg • Vanadium (as bis(maltoalto)oxovanadium(iv)) 100 mcg • Ma Huang stem standardized extract (supplying ephedrine alkaloids 25 mg) 310 mg • Thermogenic Herbal Blend 325 mg: Guarana seed standardized extract (20%,supplying caffeine 43 mg), Citrus Peel standardized extract (citrus aurantium, 5-7% alkaloids), White Willow bark, Siberian Ginseng root, Astragalus root, Bee Pollen, Bladderwrack kelp, Ginger root, Gotu Kola leaf, Licorice root, Rehmannia root, Reishi mushroom (fruiting body). Other Ingredients: Dicalcium Phosphate, Vegetable Cellulose, Fractionated Vegetable Oil, Soy Polysaccharides, Silica, Vegetable Resin Glaze.
See Editor's Note No. 30, page 2056.

Thermo-Lift II (ThermoLift II) **-** Changes International, Inc.
Each caplet contains: Niacin 10 mg • Chromium (as Chromium dinicotinate glycinate, Chromium polynicotinate and chromium picolinate) 100 mcg • Vanadium (as Vanadyl sulfate) 50 mcg • Panax Ginseng root standardized extract (8% ginsenosides) 100 mg • Guarana seed standardized extract (20% Caffeine) 225 mg • Yerba Mate leaf standardized extract 100 mg • L-Tyrosine 100 mg • Thermogenic herbal blend 75 mg: Standardized Citrus Peel extract (5% phenethylamines) (Citrus aurantium), Cayenne pepper, Cinnamon bark standardized extract, Ginger root, and White Willow bark • Supporting Herbal Blend 50 mg: Astragalus root, Bladderwrack kelp, Licorice root, Siberian Ginseng root, and Arctic root (Rhodiola rosea) standardized extract. Other Ingredients: Dicalcium phosphate, Vegetable cellulose, Fractionated Vegetable oil, Soy polysaccharides, Silica, and Vegetable resin glaze.
See Editor's Note No. 40, page 2058.

Thermonex Ephedra Free Capsules **-** BSN Inc.
Three capsules contain: L-Tyrosine 300 mg • Caffeine Anhydrous 250 mg • Citrus Aurantium 10% extract (providing synephrine 20 mg) • Naringin 50 mg • Evodiamine 40 mg • Diiodotyrosine 100 mcg • Iodotyrosine 100 mcg • Yerba Mate (25% extract standardized for xanthines) 200 mg • Octopamine HCl 200 mg • Green Tea extract (catachins 243 mg/EGCG 112 mg) 375 mg. Other Ingredients: Magnesium Stearate, Gelatin.
See Editor's Note No. 40, page 2058.

Thermo-Rx **-** Weightlosscontrol
Each capsule contains: Proprietary Blend 565 mg: Sida Cordifolia leaves 25 mg, Ephedrine Group Alkaloids Citrus Aurantium fruit 10 mg, Synephrine Group Alkaloids USP Caffeine 80 mg, Coleus Forskohlii root, Cassia Nomame Green Tea extract, 5-Hydroxytryptophan, 5-Methoxtrytamine.
See Editor's Note No. 40, page 2058.

ThermoSculpt **-** 4 Youthful Health
Four softgels contain: Vitamin B5 (pantothenic acid) 60 mg • Zinc Oxide, 80.3% Zn 40 mg • ChromeMate brand Chromium, 10% Cr 400 mcg • Vanadyl Sulfate, 31.25% 200 mcg • Advantra Z brand Citrus Aurantium 1000 mg: Total Amins 7.5%-8.2%; Synephrine 6%, N-Methyl Tyramine 0.9%-1.6%, Tyramine 0.2%-0.4%, Hordenine 0.2%-0.4%, Octopamine 0.2%-0.4% • Glucosol (corosolic acid) 48 mg.
See Editor's Note No. 40, page 2058.

ThermoSyn **-** PharmAssure
One tablet contains: Chromium (as chromium picolinate) 400 mcg • MaHuang extract (ephedra sinica; 6% ephedrine, 20mcg) 333 mg • Guarana Seed extract (paullinia cupana; 365 caffeine 90mg) 250 mg • Citrus Aurantium fruit extract (4% synephrine, 6mg) 150 mg • White Willow bark extract (salix alba; 15% salicin 15mg) 100 mg. Other Ingredients: Dicalcium Phosphate, Croscarmellose Sodium, Cellulose.
See Editor's Note No. 30, page 2056.

THERMOthin **-** Slimming and Nutrition Consultancy
Each capsule contains: Citrus aurantium • Citrin (HCA) • Guarana • Caffeine • White Willow bark • Chromium • Liquorice extract • Cayenne extract • Siberian Ginseng • Vitamin B6 • Iodine • Betaine HCL.
See Editor's Note No. 40, page 2058.

T-HFV **-** Dial Herbs
Bayberry • Cayenne • Mullein • Lobelia.

ThiaMind **-** Source Naturals
Each tablet contains: Vitamin B1 (Thiamin Mononitrate) 500 mg • Magnesium (Citrate, Malate, Succinate and Oxide) 100 mg.

Thin II **-** E'OLA
Each 0.60 g (Approx. 12 drops) serving contains: Vitamin B12 (as Cyanocobalamin) 20 mcg • Chromium (as Chromium Chloride) 200 mcg • Proprietary Blend 271 mg: Green Tea Extract, Guarana Extract, Caffeine, Kola Nut Extract, Stevia Extract. Other Ingredients: Purified Water, Glycerin, Hydroxylated Lecithin, Benzyl Alcohol, Potassium Sorbate, Potassium Hydroxide.

Thin II Herbal Chews **-** E'OLA
Each 8.6 g chew contains: Calcium 245 • Vitamin B12 20 mcg • Chromium 200 mcg • Proprietary Blend 271 mg: Green Tea extract (Camellia sinensis, leaf), Guarana extract (Paullina cupana, seed), Caffeine, Kola Nut extract (Cola ocuminoto), Stevia extract (stevia reboudiana, leaf). Other Ingredients: Corn Syrup, Sweetened Condensed Whole Milk, Sugar, Chocolate, Partially Hydrogenated Soybean Oil, Mono & Diglycerides, Soy Lecithin, Natural & Artificial Flavors, Maltodextrin.

Thin Spaghetti - Revival **-** Physicians Laboratories
Two Ounces Contain: Certified Isoflavone 15 mg. Ingredients: Soy Protein Isolate, Niacin, Iron (Ferrous Sulfate), Thiamin Mononitrate, Riboflavin, Folic Acid.

Thinfat **-** VPX Sports
Conjugated Linoleic Acid • Triglyceride • Natural Lemon Flavor.

Think Sharp **-** Health Smart Vitamins
Three capsules contain: Vitamin C (ascorbic acid) 250 mg • Thiamin (as thiamin mononitrate) 10 mg • Riboflavin 10 mg • Niacin (as 50% niacinamide, 50% nicotinic acid) 20 mg • Vitamin B6 (as pyridoxine HCl) 10 mg • Folic Acid 400 mcg • Vitamin B12 (as cyanocobalamin) 100 mcg • Biotin 300 mcg • Pantothenic Acid (as calcium pantothenate) 10 mg • Dimethylaminoethanol (DMAE; as Dimethylaminoethanol bitartrate) 500 mg • L-Glutamine 250 mg • L-Pyroglutamic Acid 100 mg • Acetyl-L-carnitine (as Acetyl-L-carnitine HCl) 50 mg.

Think-02 **-** Traditional Medicinals
Contains: Peppermint leaf • Ginkgo leaf and Ginkgo dry leaf extract • Gotu Kola leaf • Sage leaf • Siberian Ginseng root • Lemon Balm leaf • Rosemary leaf • natural Lemon flavor • Stevia leaf.

Thinz Back-To-Nature **-** Alva-Amco Pharmacal Cos., Inc.
Each tablet contains: Phenylpropanolamine HCl 75 mg. Other Ingredients: Apple Powder, Brown Lake Color Blend, Dicalcium Phosphate, D&C Yellow #10, FD&C Yellow #6, Hydroxypropyl Methylcellulose, Magnesium Stearate, Mineral Oil, Oat Bran, Polyethylene Glycol, Titanium Dioxide, Wheat Bran.

Thinz-Span **-** Alva-Amco Pharmacal Cos., Inc.
Each capsule contains: Phenylpropanolamine HCl 75 mg.

Thinzyme **-** General Vitamin
Each tablet contains: Vitamin B6 (pyridoxine HCl) 4 mg • Calcium (carbonatre, aminoate) 108 mg • Choline Bitartrate 300 mg • Dl-Methionine 300 mg • Lecithin (phosphatide-rich soy extract) 10 mg • L-Arginine (free form amino acid) 10 mg • L-Ornithine HCl (free form amino acid) 10 mg • L-Carnitine (l-tartrate) 10 mg • Green Orange (citrus aranthium exocarp extract, standardized 4% synephrine) 100 mg • Super Citrimax (garcinia cambogia exocarp extract, standardized 60% hydroxycitrate) 100 mg • Siberian Ginseng (eleutherococcus senticosis root) 100 mg • Lipase 10 mg. Inactive Ingredients: Dicalcium Phosphate, Microcrystalline Cellulose, Stearic Acid, Pharmaceutical Glaze.
See Editor's Note No. 40, page 2058.

Thisilyn **-** Nature's Way
Each capsule contains: Milk thistle extract (standardized for a flavanoid content of 140 mg silymarin [80%], which includes silybinin, silychristin, and 85 mg of lactose) 175 mg.

ThistleComp **-** PhytoPharmica
Each capsule contains: Artichoke leaves extract (Cynara scolymus) 250 mg • Curcuma root extract (Curcuma longa) 150 mg • Boldo extract (Peumus boldo) 100 mg • Milk Thistle extract (Silybum marianum) (56 mg) calculated as silybin 70 mg.
See Editor's Note No. 21, page 2056.

ThistlePlex **-** Enzymatic Therapy
Each capsule contains: Artichoke leaves extract (Cynara scolymus) standardized to contain 3% Caffeylquinic Acids 250 mg • Curcuma root extract (Curcuma longa) standardized to contain 2.5% Curcumin) 150 mg • Boldo extract (Peumus boldo) standardized to contain 1.52% essential oils) 100 mg • Milk Thistle extract (Silybum marianum) standardized to contain 80% Silymarin (56 mg) calculated as Silybin 70 mg.

ThistleRex **-** PhytoPharmica
Two capsules contain: Artichoke leaf extract (cynara scolymus, standardized to contain 13%-18% caffeylquinic acids) 20 mg • Dandelion root 4:1 exctract (taraxacum officinale) 20 mg • Licorice root and rhizome extract (glycyrrhiza glabra, standardized to contain 5% glycyrrhizic acids) 20 mg • Milk Thistle fruit extract (silybum marianum, standardized to contain 80% silymarin (240 mg) calculated as silybin) 300 mg.

Thistlezyme **-** Olympian Labs
Two capsules contain: Milk Thistle extract (standardized to contain at least 80% Silymarin) 200 mg.

Thorene **-** Thorne Research Inc.
Each capsule contains: Tylophora asthmatica 30 mg • Boswellia serrata extract (60% Boswellin) 150 mg • Piper longa 100 mg • Hesperidin Methyl Chalcone 100 mg.

Three-In-One **-** Changes International, Inc.
Each capsule contains: Vitamin C (as Calcium Ascorbate) 120 mg • Aloe Vera leaf gel 200:1 concentrate 200 mg • Mexican Yam root 4:1 (equivalent to 150 mg) 37.5 mg. Other Ingredients: Gelatin, Maltodextrin, Calcium Sulfate, Magnesium Stearate, and Silica.

ThreeLac **-** Global Health Trax
Each packet contains: Vitamin C 10 mg • Thiamin 0.4 mg • Riboflavin 0.4 mg • Vitamin B6 0.4 mg • Sodium 10 mg. Other Ingredients: Spore Forming Lactic Acid Bacteria (lactobacillus sporogenes), Lemon juice powder, Refined Yeast powder, Castor Oil, Spore Forming Bacteria (bacillus subtills), Lactic Acid Bacteria (streptococcus faecalis).

Throat Coat **-** Traditional Medicinals
Active Ingredient: Slippery Elm bark (ulmus rubra). Inactive Ingredients: Licorice Root, Wild Cherry Bark, Fennel Seed, Cinnamon Bark, Orange Peel, Althea Root.

Throat Spray **-** Botanical Laboratories
Capsicum 6X • Echinacea Angustifolia 1X • Eucalyptus 1X • Kava 1X • Lycopodium Clavatum 4X • Peppermint 6X • Phosphorus 6X • Phytolacca Decandra 3X • Wild Thyme 1X.
See Editor's Note No. 1, page 2053.

T-HRT **-** Dial Herbs
Hawthorne • Lecithin • Tansy • Fenugreek • Garlic • Cayenne.

T-HS **-** Dial Herbs
Ginseng • Damiana • Gotu Kola • Sarsaparilla • Sassafras • Saw Palmetto.

Thyme and Myrrh **-** Dial Herbs
Thyme • Myrrh.

Thymex **-** Standard Process, Inc.
Each tablet contains: Proprietary Blend 195 mg: Bovine Thymus extract (Cytosol), Magnesium citrate. Other Ingredients: Calcium lactate, Cellulose, Calcium stearate, Ascorbic Acid.
See Editor's Note No. 14, page 2055.

Thymucin **-** PhytoPharmica
Two capsules contain: Enzymatic Polypeptide Fractions (Thymus fractions) 750 mg • Astragalus (Astragalus membranaceus) root extract 4-6:1 (standardized to contain 0.5% minimum of the isoflavone 4' hydroxy 3' methoxy isoflavone 7-SUG [GHMIF]) 250 mg.

Thymuplex Capsules **-** Enzymatic Therapy
Four capsules contain: Vitamin A (as beta carotene) 25,000 IU • Vitamin C (ascorbic acid) 250 mg • Vitamin E (as d-alpha tocopheryl acid succinate) 200 IU • Zinc (as zinc krebs cycle chelates) 15 mg • Selenium (as l-selenomethionine) 25 mcg • Proprietary Thymus Polypeptide Fraction/Glandular Complex 935 mg: Thymus Polypeptide fractions, Spleen extract (freeze-dried), Thymus extract, Lymphatic extract (freeze-dried), Bromelain (1200 M.C.U./g), Trypsin, Papain • Echinacea Purpurea root 300 mg • Lysine (as l-lysine HCl) 250 mg • Blue Flag root (iris versicolor) 130 mg • Goldenseal root (hydrastis canadensis) 64 mg. Other Ingredients: Gelatin, Fennel Seed, Magnesium Stearate, Silicon Dioxide, Titanium Dioxide Color.
See Editor's Note No. 14, page 2055.

Thymuplex Tablets **-** Enzymatic Therapy
Two tablets contain: Vitamin A (as beta carotene) 25,000 IU • Vitamin C (ascorbic acid) 250 mg • Vitamin E (as d-alpha tocopheryl acid succinate) 200 IU • Zinc (as zinc krebs cycle chelates) 15 mg • Selenium (as l-selenomethionine) 25 mcg • Proprietary Thymus Polypeptide Fraction/Glandular Complex 935 mg: Thymus Polypeptide fractions, Spleen extract (freeze-dried), Thymus extract, Lymphatic extract (freeze-dried), Bromelain (1200 M.C.U./g), Trypsin, Papain • Echinacea Purpurea root 300 mg • Lysine (as l-lysine HCl) 250 mg • Blue Flag root (iris versicolor) 130 mg • Goldenseal root (hydrastis canadensis) 64 mg. Other Ingredients: Cellulose, Modified Cellulose Gum, Fennel Seed, Modified Cellulose, Magnesium Stearate, Lecithin, Carnauba Wax, Peppermint Leaf.
See Editor's Note No. 14, page 2055.

Thymuril Capsules **-** PhytoPharmica
Four capsules contain: Vitamin A (beta-carotene) 25,000 IU • Vitamin C (ascorbic acid) 250 mg • Vitamin E (D-alpha tocopheryl acetate) 200 IU • Zinc (Krebs chelate) 15 mg • Selenium (L-selenomethionine) chelate 25 mcg • Polypeptide Fractions Thymus Complex (predigested, concentrated soluble extract standardized for peptides and polypeptides with molecular weight less than 10,000 daltons) 935 mg • Echinacea root (echinacea purpurea) 300 mg • L-Lysine (HCl) 250 mg • Blue Flag extract (iris versicolor) 130 mg • Goldenseal root extract (hydrastis canadensis) 64 mg.
See Editor's Note No. 14, page 2055.

Thymuril Tablets **-** PhytoPharmica
Two tablets contain: Blue flag root (iris versicolor) 130 mg • Echinacea Purpurea root 300 mg • Goldenseal root (hydrastis canadensis) 64 mg • Lysine (as L-lysine HCl) 250 mg • Proprietary Thymus Polypeptide/Glandular Complex 935 mg: Thymus Polypeptide fractions, Spleen extract (freeze-dried), Thymus extract, Lymphatic extract (freeze-dried), Bromelain (1200 MCU/g), Trypsin, Papain • Selenium (as L-selenomethionine) 25 mcg • Vitamin A (as beta carotene) 25,000 IU • Vitamin C (ascorbic acid) 250 mg • Vitamin E (as D-alpha tocopheryl acid succinate) 200 IU • Zinc (as zinc Krebs cycle chelates) 15 mg.
See Editor's Note No. 14, page 2055.

Thymus Cream **-** Atrium Inc.
Three fluid ounces contain: Extract of Thymus (Viobin) • Glycerin Hexadecenol • Sodium Laureth Sulfate • Stearic Acid • Methylparaben • Sodium Sulfate • Propylparaben • Natural Fragrance.
See Editor's Note No. 14, page 2055.

T-HYPO **-** Dial Herbs
Licorice • Juniper berry • Wild Yam • Dandelion • Ginger.

Thyrene **-** Metabolic Nutrition
Six capsules contain: Guggulsterone (10%) 900 mg • L-Tyrosine 810 mg • Di Potassium Phosphate 600 mg • Coleus Forskohlii (20%) 260 mg • Sodium Phosphate 240 mg • Di Sodium Phosphate 240 mg • Iodine (organic) 900 mcg.

Thyro Complex **-** Progressive Labs
Each capsule contains: Raw Thyroid concentrate (thyroxin free) 60 mg • Raw Adrenal concentrate 30 mg • Raw Pituitary concentrate 10 mg • Raw Spleen concentrate 10 mg • Kelp 300 mg. This natural product is prepared by a special process which does not exceed physiological temperature (37° C). Guaranteed to be free of chemical pesticides and synthetic hormones.
See Editor's Note No. 14, page 2055.

ThyroFuel **-** E'OLA
Two capsules contain: Proprietary Blend 810 mg: Kelp, Thyroid Extract, Gugulipid Commiphora Mukul Extract, Tyrosine, Gentian (root). Other Ingredients: Gelatin, Rice Flour.

Thyroid & L-Tyrosine Complex **-** Enzymatic Therapy
Each capsule contains: Magnesium (Oxide) 100 mg • Manganese (Chelate) 3 mg • Zinc (Chelate) 3 mg • Copper (Chelate) 150 mcg • Iodine (Kelp) 100 mcg • Molybdenum (Chelate) 50 mcg • Vitamin B12 (Cyanocobalamin) 50 mcg • Other Ingredients: L-Tyrosine 124 mg • Multi-Glandular Complex: Raw Liver, Raw Lung, Raw Pancreas, Raw Heart, Raw Kidney, Raw Spleen, & Raw Brain 35 mg • Thyroid Substance (thyroxin-free) 4X.
See Editor's Note No. 14, page 2055.

Thyroid Complex **-** The Vitamin Shoppe
Each capsule contains: Thiamine (Vitamin B1) 10 mg • Riboflavin (Vitamin B2) 10 mg • Vitamin B6 (as pyridoxine HCl) 10 mg • Vitamin B12 (as cyanocobalamin) 25 mcg • Iodine (from kelp) 150 mcg • Magnesium (as magnesium oxide) 100 mg • Zinc (as zinc chelate) 3 mg • Selenium (as selenium chelate) 70 mcg • Copper (as copper chelate) 150 mcg • Manganese (as manganese chelate) 3 mg • Molybdenum (as molybdenum chelate) 150 mcg • L-Tyrosine 150 mg • Multi Gland Complex (from Bovine Liver, Lung, Pancreas, Heart, Kidney, Spleen, Brain) 35 mg.
See Editor's Note No. 14, page 2055.

Thyroid Essentials **-** Swanson
Each capsule contains: Thiamin USP (as thiamin HCl; vitamin B-1) 25 mg • Riboflavin USP (vitamin B-2) 25 mg • Niacinamide 25 mg • Vitamin B6 (as pyridoxine HCl) 25 mg • Folic Acid 25 mcg • Vitamin B12 (as cyanocobalamin) 25 mcg • Pantothenic Acid (as d-calcium pantothenate) 25 mg • Iodine (from kelp) 100 mcg • Magnesium (from magnesium oxide) 25 mg • Zinc (from zinc oxide) 25 mg • Selenium (as L-selenomethionine) 50 mcg • Copper (from copper gluconate) 2 mg • L-Tyrosine 150 mg • Coleus Forskohlii (18% forskolin) 50 mg.

Thyroid Factors **-** Michael's Naturopathic Programs
Three capsules contain: Vitamin B6 (as pyridoxine) 75 mg • Iodine (from kelp) 450 mcg • Chromium (as chromium polynicotinate) 300 mcg • Manganese (as manganese amino acid chelate) 90 mg • Proprietary Blend 675 mg: Gentian root (gentiana lutea), Irish Moss (whole plant, chondrus crispus), Bladderwrack (whole plant, fucus vesiculosus), Tyrosine (as L-tyrosine). Other Ingredients: Cellulose, Dicalcium Phosphate, Maltodextrin, Magnesium Stearate, Stearic Acid.

Thyroid Support Formula **-** PhysioLogics
Each capsule contains: Riboflavin 20 mg • Niacin (as niacinamide) 20 mg • Vitamin B6 (as pyridoxine hydrochloride) 1 mg • Iodine (from kelp) 110 mcg • Zinc (as zinc gluconate) 5 mg • Copper (as copper glycinate) 300 mcg • Chromium (as chromium chelavite) 75 mcg • L-Tyrosine 300 mg • Coleus Forskohlii leaf (standardized to contain 20% forskholin, 10 mg) 50 mg. Other Ingredients: Gelatin, Rice Powder, Vegetable Magnesium Stearate, Silica.

Thyrosine Complex **-** PhytoPharmica
Two capsules contain: Copper (as copper gluconate) 300 mcg • Iodine (as potassium iodide) 200 mcg • L-Tyrosine 248 mg • Magnesium (as magnesium oxide) 200 mg • Manganese (as manganese gluconate) 2.3 mg • Molybdenum (as sodium molybdate) 100 mcg • Multi-Glandular Copmlex 70 mg: Liver, Lung, Pancreas, Heart, Kidney, Spleen • Thyroid extract (thyroxin-free) 8 mg • Vitamin B12 (as cyanocobalamin) 100 mcg • Zinc (as zinc gluconate) 6 mg.
See Editor's Note No. 31, page 2056.

ThyroStart **-** SilverSage
Two capsules contain: Kelp meal 500 mg • Vitamin C 20 mg • Magnesium 20 mg • L-Tryosine 20 mg • Vitamin B3 20 mg • Vitamin B2 10 mg • Zinc 10 mg • Vitamin B5 10 mg • Horsetail grass 5 mg • Gentian root 5 mg • Blue Flag 5 mg • Nettle leaf herb 5 mg • Radish extract 4:1 5 mg • Parathyroid substance 5 mg • Thymus substance 2.5 mg • Adrenal substance 2.5 mg • Pancreas substance 2.5 mg • Vitamin B6 2 mg • Vitamin B1 1.5 mg • Manganese 1 mg • Copper 0.02 mg • Vitamin A 2000 IU • Beta Carotene 2000 IU • Vitamin E 50 IU • Biotin 50 mcg • Folic Acid 50 mcg • Vitamin B12 10 mcg • Selenium 10 mcg • Molybdenum 10 mcg.
See Editor's Note No. 14, page 2055.

Thyrovarin **-** Klein-Becker
Two capsules contain: Vitamin A 3000 IU • Vitamin C 20 mg • Vitamin E 50 IU • Vitamin B1 1.65 mg • Vitamin B2 10 mg • Vitamin B6 2 mg • Vitamin B9 50 mcg • Vitamin B12 10 mcg • Biotin 50 mcg • Pantothenic Acid 10 mg • Magnesium 20 mg • Zinc 10 mg • Selenium 10 mcg • Copper 20 mcg • Manganese 1 mg • Molybdenum 10 mg • Proprietary Blend 690 mg: Kelp meal (0.15% iodine), L-Tyrosine, Niacinamide, Radish root 4:1 extract, Nettles herb, Horsetail grass stem, Gentian root. Other Ingredients: Rice Flour.

Tiao He Cleanse **-** Nature's Sunshine
Each packet (6 capsules) contains: Chinese Liver Balance (one capsule) 485 mg: Bupleurum root (bupleurum chinense), Peony root (without bark, paeonia officinalis), Typhonium rhizome (typhonium flagelliforme), Cassia Cinnamon twig (cinnamomum cassia), Dong Quai root (angelica polymorpha var. sinensis), Fushen Sclerotium (with root, poria cocos), Scute root (scutellaria baicalensis), Zhishi

fruit (citrus aurantium), Atractylodes rhizome (atractylodes lancea), Ginseng root (panax ginseng), Ginger rhizome (zingiber officinale), Licorice root (glycyrrhiza uralensis). All Cell Detox (one capsule) 475 mg: Gentian root (gentiana lutea), Irish Moss plant (chondrus crispus), Cascara Sagrada bark (rhamnus purhsiana), Golden Seal rhizome (hydrastis canadensis), Fenugreek seed (trigonella foenum-graecum), Slippery Elm bark (ulmus fulva), Safflower flowers (carthamus tinctorius), Black Walnut hulls (juglans nigra), Myrrh gum (commiphora molmol), Yellow Dock root (rumex crispus), Parthenium root (parthenium integrifolium), Oregon Grape root and rhizome (berberis aquifolium), Dandelion root (taraxacum officinale), Uva Ursi leaves (arctostaphylos uva ursi), Chickweed leaves and flowering tops (stellaria media), Catnip aerial parts (nepeta cataria), Cyani flowers (centaurea cyanus). LBS II (one capsule) 425 mg: Cascara Sagrada bark (rhamnus purshiana), Buckthorn bark (rhamnus frangula), Licorice root (glycyrrhiza glabra), Capsicum fruit (capsicum annuum), Ginger rhizome (zingiber officinale), Oregon Grape root and rhizome (berberis aquifolium), Turkey Rhubarb root (rheum officinale), Couch Grass rhizome (agropyron repens), Red Clover flowers (trifolium pratense). One capsule contains: Psyllium hulls (plantago ovata) 465 mg. One capsule contains: Burdock root (arctium lappa) 360 mg. One capsule contains: Black Walnut hulls (juglans nigra) 500 mg. Other Ingredients: Magnesium Stearate (vegetable), Silicon dioxide, Gelatin, Water.
See Editor's Note No. 40, page 2058.

Tiger Vites **-** Body Wise International, Inc.
Two caplets contain: Beta Carotene (Dunaliella Salina Algae) (Equivalent to Vitamin A 5000 IU) 3 mg • Vitamin D (as Vitamin D3) (Cholecalciferol) 200 IU • Vitamin E (d-Alpha Tocopherol Acid Succinate and Mixed Tocopherols Beta, Gamma and Delta) 30 IU • Vitamin C 60 mg • Folic Acid 400 mcg • Vitamin B1 1.5 mg • Vitamin B2 1.7 mg • Vitamin B6 2 mg • Niacin (Niacinamide) 20 mg • Vitamin B12 6 mcg • Pantothenic Acid (d-Calcium Pantothenate) 5 mg • Biotin 150 mcg • Choline (Choline Bitartrate) 10 mcg • Inositol 10 mcg • Calcium (Krebs Cycle Chelate) 50 mg • Magnesium 40 mg • Copper 1 mg • Zinc 7.5 mg • Molybdenum 37.5 mcg • Iodine (Kelp) 75 mcg • Chromium 120 mcg • Selenium (L-Selenomethionine) 17.5 mcg • Manganese 0.5 mg • Potassium 0.5 mg • Iron 1.8 mg • PhytoNutrient Garden Blend* 25 mg • PhytoNutrient Orchard Blend* 25 mg • Pineapple 12.5 mg • Papaya 12.5 mg • Citrus Bioflavonoids 12.5 mg. Other Ingredients: Spirulina, Whole Brown Rice, Spinach, Beet Leaf, Cherry, Rose Hips, Mango.

Tight! **-** SAN Nutrition
Each capsule contains: Thermogenic Proprietary Blend 325 mg: Caffeine anhydrous 99%, Forslean Coleus Forskohlii 10%, Synephrine 96%, Sclareolide 96%, Pure Guggulsterones E & Z 99% 1:1 total mix, Yohimbine 99%, Vinpocetine 99%, Bioperine Black Pepper extract 96%. Other Ingredients: Microcrystalline Cellulose, Gelatin, Red #3, Orange #4.
See Editor's Note No. 40, page 2058.

Tigra Pill **-** Universal Products, Performance Industri
Each tablet contains: Hydrolyzed protein rich in Arginine • D-Alpha-Tocopherol • Aromatic plant extract (Diamiana aphrodisiaca, Dioscorea villosa, Panax Ginseng, Smilax officinalis) • Choline sulfate • Vitamin B3 • Vitamin B1 • Zinc sulfate • Grape Seed extract • Essential oils of Peppermint • Savory • Clove • Magnesium stearate • Carboxymethylcellulosis • Magnesium silicate.

Time Fighters For Men **-** Changes International, Inc.
Four caplets contain: Vitamin A (as Beta-Carotene and mixed carotenoids from D. salina algae) 25000 IU • Vitamin C (as Ascorbic Acid) 500 mg • Vitamin D (as Cholecalciferol) 400 IU •Vitamin E (as Dl-Alpha-Tocopheryl and D-Alpha Tocopheryl Succinate) 200 IU • Vitamin B1 (as Thiamin HCI) 50 mg • Vitamin B2 (as Riboflavin) 50 mg • Niacin (as Niacinamide) 125 mg • Vitamin B6 (as Pyridoxine HCI) 50 mg •Folate (as Folic Acid) 800 mcg •Vitamin B12 (as Cyanocobalamin) 500 mcg • Biotin 300 mcg • Pantothenic acid (as D-Calcium Pantothenate) 50 mg • Calcium (as Calcium Carbonate and Citrate) 400 mg • Iodine (as Potassium Iodide) 150 mcg • Magnesium (as Magnesium Oxide and Aspartate) 500 mg • Zinc (as Zinc Citrate and Picolinate) 50 mg • Selenium (as Selenomethionine) 200 mcg • Copper (as Copper Gluconate) 2 mg • Manganese (as Manganese Gluconate) 2 mg • Chromium (as Chromium Dinicotinate Glycinate) 200 mcg • Molybdenum (as Sodium Molybdate) 150 mcg • Potassium (as Potassium Citrate and Chloride) 10 mg • Life Enhancement Men's Herbal Blend 360 mg: Soybean phytosterol complex (120 mg Beta-Sitosterol), Saw Palmetto berry 4:1 extract, Panax Ginseng extract (4% ginsenosides) • Marigold flower concentrate (2% Lutein) 50 mg • Tomato fruit concentrate (2% Lycopene) 50 mg • Choline Bitartrate 25 mg • Inositol 25 mg • PABA 10 mg • Whole Food Phytonutrient Concentrates 500 mg: Parsley, Dunaliela salina algae, Kale, Spinach, Cantoloupe, Carrot, Papaya, Red Peppers, Tomato, Yellow Squash, Turmeric, Cranberry, Tangerine, Grapefruit, Lemon, Orange, Pineapple, Leek, Onion, Garlic, Raspberry, Green Tea, Alfalfa, Soybean, Cherry, Peach, Pear, Red Grape, Strawberry, Asparagus, Broccoli, Bruessels Sprout, Cabbage, Cauliflower, Mustard Greens. Other Ingredients: Microcrystaline Cellulose, Croscarmellose Sodium, Stearic Acid, Silica, Caramel color, Magnesium Stearate, Vanillin, Pharmaceutical Glaze.

Time Fighters For Women With Iron **-** Changes International, Inc.
Four caplets contain: Vitamin A (as Beta-Carotene and mixed carotenoids from D. salina algae) 25000 IU • Vitamin C (as Ascorbic Acid) 500 mg • Vitamin D (as Cholecalciferol) 800 IU • Vitamin E (as Dl-Alpha-Tocopheryl Acetate and D-Alpha Tocopheryl Succinate) 200 IU • Thiamin (as Thiamin HCl) 25 mg • Riboflavin 25 mg •Niacin (as Niacinamide) 100 mg •Vitamin B6 (as Pyridoxine HCl) 25 mg • Folate (as Folic Acid) 800 mcg • Vitamin B12 (as Cyanocobalamin) 250 mcg • Biotin 300 mcg • Pantothenic Acid (as D-Calcium Pantothenate) 50 mg • Calcium (as Calcium Carbonate and Citrate) 500 mg • Iron (as Ferrous Fumarate) 18 mg • Iodine (as Potassium Iodide) 150 mcg •Magnesium (as Magnesium Oxide and Aspartate) 400 mg •Zinc (as Zinc Citrate and Picolinate) 30 mg •Selenium (as Selenomethionine) 200 mcg • Copper (as Copper Gluconate) 2 mg • Manganese (as Manganese Gluconate) 2 mg • Chromium (as Chromium Dinicotinate Glycinate) 200 mcg • Molybdenum (as Sodium Molybdate) 150 mcg • Potassium (as Potassium Citrate and Chloride) 10 mg • Boron (from Boron Citrate) 3 mg • Marigold flower concentrate (2% Lutein) 50 mg • Tomato fruit concentrate (2% Lycopene) 50 mg • Choline Bitartrate 25 mg • Inositol 25 mg • PABA 10 mg • Life Enhancement Women's Herbal Blend 200 mg : Panax Ginseng root extract, Black Cohosh root, Chaste Tree fruit • Whole Food Phytonutrient Concentrates 500 mg: Parsley, Dunaliela Salina Algae, Kale, Spinach, Cantaloupe, Carrot, Papaya, Tomato, Yellow Squash, Turmeric rhizome, Tangerine, Grapefruit, Lemon, Orange, Red Pepper, Alfalfa, Soybean, Cranberry, Green Tea, Raspberry, Cherry, Peach, Pear, Pineapple, Red Grape, Strawberry, Asparagus spear, Brussesl sprouts, Garlic, Leek, Onion, Broccoli, Cauliflower, Cabbage, Mustard Greens. Other Ingredients: Microcrystalline Cellulose, Croscarmellose Sodium, Stearic Acid, Silica, Magnesium Stearate, Vanillin, and Pharmaceutical Glaze.

Time Fighters For Women Without Iron **-** Changes International, Inc.
Four caplets contain: Vitamin A (as Beta-Carotene and mixed carotenoids from D. salina algae) 25000 IU • Vitamin C (as Ascorbic Acid) 500 mg • Vitamin D (as Cholecalciferol) 800 IU • Vitamin E (as Dl-Alpha-Tocopheryl Acetate and D-Alpha Tocopheryl Succinate) 200 IU • Thiamin (as Thiamin HCI) 25 mg • Riboflavin 25 mg •Niacin (as Niacinamide) 100 mg •Vitamin B6 (as Pyridoxine HCI) 25 mg • Folate (as Folic Acid) 800 mcg • Vitamin B12 (as Cyanocobalamin) 250 mcg • Biotin 300 mcg • Pantothenic Acid (as D-Calcium Pantothenate) 50 mg • Calcium (as Calcium Carbonate and Citrate) 500 mg • Iodine (as Potassium Iodide) 150 mcg •Magnesium (as Magnesium Oxide and Aspartate) 400 mg •Zinc (as Zinc Citrate and Picolinate) 30 mg •Selenium (as Selenomethionine) 200 mcg • Copper (as Copper Gluconate) 2 mg • Manganese (as Manganese Gluconate) 2 mg • Chromium (as Chromium Dinicotinate Glycinate)

200 mcg • Molybdenum (as Sodium Molybdate) 150 mcg • Potassium (as Potassium Citrate and Chloride) 10 mg • Boron (from Boron Citrate) 3 mg • Marigold flower concentrate (2% Lutein) 50 mg • Tomato fruit concentrate (2% Lycopene) 50 mg • Choline Bitartrate 25 mg • Inositol 25 mg • PABA 10 mg • Life Enhancement Women's Herbal Blend 200 mg: Panax Ginseng root extract, Black Cohosh root, Chaste Tree fruit • Whole Food Phytonutrient Concentrates 500 mg: Parsley, Dunaliela Salina Algae, Kale, Spinach, Cantaloupe, Carrot, Papaya, Tomato, Yellow Squash, Turmeric rhizome, Tangerine, Grapefruit, Lemon, Orange, Red Pepper, Alfalfa, Soybean, Cranberry, Green Tea, Raspberry, Cherry, Peach, Pear, Pineapple, Red Grape, Strawberry, Asparagus spear, Brussel sprouts, Garlic, Leek, Onion, Broccoli, Cauliflower, Cabbage, Mustard Greens. Other Ingredients: Microcrystalline Cellulose, Croscarmellose Sodium, Stearic Acid, Silica, Magnesium Stearate, Vanillin, and Pharmaceutical Glaze.

BRAND NAMES

Time Release Athletes Formula **-** Puritan's Pride
Two caplets contain: Vitamin A 10,000 IU • Vitamin C 300 mg • Vitamin D 800 IU • Vitamin E 100 IU • Thiamin (Vitamin B1) 22.25 mg • Riboflavin (Vitamin B2) 25 mg • Niacin 100 mg • Vitamin B6 20.5 mg • Folic Acid 400 mcg • Vitamin B12 100 mcg • Biotin 50 mcg • Pantothenic Acid 25 mg • Calcium 250 mg • Iron 25 mg • Iodine 225 mcg • Magnesium 20 mg • Zinc 50 mg • Selenium (as Yeast) 25 mcg • Copper 0.05 mg • Manganese 5 mg • Chromium 50 mcg • Chloride 240 mg • Sodium 100 mg • Potassium 99 mg • Choline 25 mg • Inositol 25 mg • Lecithin 100 mg • RNA - DNA 25 mg • PABA 25 mg • Bee Pollen 50 mg • Rose Hips 20 mg • Isoleucine 389 mcg • Leucine 610 mcg • Lysine 632 mcg • Methionine 122 mcg • Phenylalanine 337 mcg • Threonine 390 mcg • Valine 500 mcg.

Time Release B-100 Ultra B-Complex **-** Puritan's Pride
Each tablet contains: Thiamin (Vitamin B1; as thiamine mononitrate) 100 mg • Riboflavin (Vitamin B2) 100 mg • Niacin (as niacinamide) 100 mg • Vitamin B6 (as pyridoxine hydrochloride) 100 mg • Folic Acid 100 mcg • Vitamin B12 (as cyanocobalamin) 100 mcg • Biotin (as D-Biotin) 100 mcg • Pantothenic Acid (as D-Calcium Pantothenate) 100 mg • Proprietary Blend 100 mg: Choline Bitartrate, Inositol, PABA (Para-Aminobenzoic Acid), Alfalfa, Watercress, Parsley, Lecithin, and Rice Bran.

Time Release B-50 Vitamin B-Complex **-** Puritan's Pride
Each tablet contains: Thiamin (Vitamin B1; as thiamine mononitrate) 50 mg • Riboflavin (Vitamin B2) 50 mg • Niacin (as niacinamide) 50 mg • Vitamin B6 (as pyridoxine hydrochloride) 50 mg • Folic Acid 100 mcg • Vitamin B12 (as cyanocobalamin) 50 mcg • Biotin (as d-biotin) 50 mcg • Pantothenic Acid (as d-calcium pantothenate) 50 mg • Proprietary Blend 50 mg: Choline Bitartrate, Inositol, PABA (Para-Aminobenzoic Acid), Alfalfa, Watercress, Parsley, Lecithin, and Rice Bran.

Time Release B-Complex + C **-** Puritan's Pride
Each tablet contains: Vitamin C (as Ascorbic Acid and Rose Hips) 200 mg • Thiamin (Vitamin B1; as Thiamine Mononitrate) 10 mg • Riboflavin (Vitamin B2) 10 mg • Niacin (as Niacinamide) 50 mg • Vitamin B6 (as Pyridoxine Hydrochloride) 5 mg • Vitamin B12 (as Cyanocobalamin) 10 mcg • Pantothenic Acid (as D-Calcium Pantothenate) 10 mg.

Time Release Mega Vita-Min **-** Puritan's Pride
Each tablet contains: Vitamin A (as retinyl palmitate) 8000 IU • Vitamin C (as ascorbic acid and rose hips) 250 mg • Vitamin D (as cholecalciferol) 400 IU • Vitamin E (as D-alpha tocopheryl acetate) 125 IU • Thiamin (vitamin B1, as thiamine mononitrate) 80 mg • Riboflavin (vitamin B2) 80 mg • Niacin (as niacinamide) 80 mg • Vitamin B6 (as pyridoxine hydrochloride) 80 mg • Folic Acid 400 mcg • Vitamin B12 (as cyanocobalamin) 80 mcg • Biotin (as D-biotin) 80 mcg • Pantothenic Acid (as D-calcium pantothenate) 80 mg • Calcium (as calcium carbonate) 8 mg • Iron (as ferrous gluconate) 2 mg • Iodine (as kelp) 150 mcg • Magnesium (as magnesium oxide) 6 mg • Zinc (as zinc gluconate) 1.4 mg • Selenium (as sodium selenite) 25 mcg • Copper (as copper gluconate) 0.07 mg • Manganese (as manganese gluconate) 0.12 mg • Chromium (as chromium picolinate) 25 mcg • Molybdenum (as sodium molybdate) 25 mcg • Potassium (as potassium gluconate) 1.6 mg • Boron (as sodium borate) 0.5 mg • Choline Bitartrate 80 mg • Inositol 80 mg • PABA (para-aminobenzoic acid) 80 mg • Rutin fruit (dimorphandra mollis) 30 mg • Citrus Bioflavonoids fruit (citrus sinensis) 25 mg • Hesperidin fruit (citrus spp.) 5 mg • Betaine Hydrochloride 25 mg • Coenzyme Q-10 500 mg • Deodorized Garlic bulb (allium sativum) 1 mg • Korean Ginseng root (Panax ginseng) 1 mg • Pycnogenol 500 mcg • Proprietary Blend 4 mg: Alfalfa leaf, Watercress, Parsley leaf, Rice Bran, Lecithin. Other Ingredients: Methylcellulose, Vegetable Stearic Acid, Silica, Mannitol, Vegetable Magnesium Stearate, Cellulose Coating, Starch.

Time Release Mega Vitamins for the Hair **-** Puritan's Pride
Three tablets contain: Vitamin A (as 100% Beta Carotene) 10,000 IU • Vitamin C (as Ascorbic Acid) 1,000 mg • Thiamin (Vitamin B1; as Thiamine Hydrochloride) 89 mg • Riboflavin (Vitamin B2) 100 mg • Niacin (as niacinamide) 100 mg • Vitamin B6 (as Pyridoxine Hydrochloride) 82 mg • Folic Acid 400 mcg • Vitamin B12 (as Cyanocobalamin) 100 mcg • Biotin 2,000 mcg • Zinc (as Zinc Amino Acid Chelate) 5 mg • Copper (Cupric Sulfate) 2 mg • Choline Bitartrate 500 mg • Inositol 500 mg • PABA (Para-Aminobenzoic Acid) 100 mg • L-Cysteine (as L-Cysteine Hydrochloride) 334 mg.

Time Release Stress B with 500 mg Vitamin C **-** Puritan's Pride
Each tablet contains: Vitamin C (as ascorbic acid) 500 mg • Vitamin B1 (as thiamine hydrochloride) 100 mg • Vitamin B2 (riboflavin) 100 mg • Niacin (as niacinamide) 100 mg • Vitamin B6 (as pyridoxine hydrochloride) 100 mg • Folic Acid 400 mcg • Vitamin B12 (as cyanocobalamin) 500 mcg • Biotin (as D-Biotin) 50 mcg • Pantothenic Acid (as d-calcium pantothenate) 100 mg • Choline Bitartrate 50 mg • Inositol 50 mg • PABA (para-aminobenzoic acid) 50 mg • Citrus Bioflavonoids 50 mg.

Time Release Ultra Man **-** Puritan's Pride
Two tablets contain: Vitamin A (Acetate) 5,000 IU • Vitamin E (d alpha Tocopheryl Acetate) 100 IU • Vitamin C (Ascorbic Acid) 300 mg • Selenium (Selenite) 25 mcg • Citrus Bioflavonoids 25 mg • Superoxide Dismutase (SOD) 10 mcg • Pycnogenol 1 mcg • Biotin 300 mcg • Silica 20 mcg • Inositol 10 mg • L-Cysteine 100 mg • Yohimbe extract 50 mg • Korean Ginseng root 50 mg • Swiss Avena Sativa (Oat Straw) 50 mg • Damiana leaves 50 mg • Muira Puama 50 mg • Nettles leaves 30 mg • Oyster Extract 25 mg • Saw Palmetto berries 50 mg • Prostate glandular 50 mg • Pumpkin Seed 30 mg • Pygeum 25 mg • Golden Seal herb 25 mg • Zinc (Oxide) 2 mg • Vitamin B1 (Thiamine Mononitrate) 30 mg • Vitamin B2 (Riboflavin) 30 mg • Vitamin B3 (Niacin) 30 mg • Vitamin B6 (Pyridoxine Hydrochloride) 30 mg • Vitamin B12 (Cyanocobalamin) 30 mcg • Folic Acid 400 mcg • Pantothenic Acid (Calcium d-Pantothenate) 30 mg • Choline (Choline Bitartrate) 10 mg • PABA (Para Aminobenzoic Acid) 10 mg • Vitamin D (Cholecalciferol) 200 IU • Calcium (Dicalcium Phosphate) 275 mg • Phosphorus (Dicalcium Phosphate) 210 mg • Iodine (Potassium Iodide) 150 mcg • Magnesium (Oxide) 100 mg • Manganese (Gluconate) 5 mg • Potassium (Chloride) 30 mg • Chromium (Picolinate) 50 mcg • Vitamin K (Phytonadione) 25 mcg. In a base of Garlic, Oat Bran, Spirulina, Alfalfa, Parsley, Lecithin, Watercress, Smilax (Sarsaparilla), and Cayenne.
See Editor's Note No. 14, page 2055.

Time Released B Complex Vitamin plus Vitamin C **-** Nature's Bounty
Each tablet contains: Vitamin C (as ascorbic acid and rose hips) 300 mg • Thiamin (vitamin B1, as thiamin mononitrate) 18 mg • Riboflavin (vitamin B2) 10 mg • Niacin (as niacinamide) 50 mg • Vitamin B6 (as pyridoxine hydrochloride) 5 mg • Folic Acid 400 mcg • Vitamin B12 (as cyanocobalamin) 10 mcg • Biotin 50 mcg • Pantothenic Acid (as D-calcium pantothenate) 10 mg. Other Ingredients: Dicalcium Phosphate, Cellulose (plant origin), Cellulose

Coating, Vegetable Stearic Acid, Silica, Vegetable Magnesium Stearate.

Timed Release Vitamin C - Basic Nutrition **-** GNC
Each table contains: Vitamin C (as Ascorbic Acid) 1000 mg • Citrus Bioflavonoids Complex 100 mg. Other Ingredients: Calcium Sulfate, Cellulose, Stearic Acid, Magnesium Stearate, Rose hips, Acerola powder, Hesperidin Complex, Rutin.

Timed Release Vitamin C with Rose Hips - Basic Nutrition **-** GNC
Each tablet contains: Vitamin C (as Ascorbic Acid) 500 mg. Other Ingredients: Dicalcium Phosphate, Cellulose, Food Glaze, Rose hips.

T-ING **-** Dial Herbs
Valerian root • Chamomile • Lobelia • Arnica • Cayenne.

T-JAUN **-** Dial Herbs
Barberry • Chamomile • Dandelion • Horehound • St. John's Wort • Tansy • Wood Betony • Yellow Dock.

T-KB **-** Dial Herbs
Peach bark • Marshmallow • Buchu Leaves • Corn Silk • Echinacea.

T-LB **-** Dial Herbs
Barberry • Cascara Sagrada • Licorice root • Senna Leaves • Red Raspberry • Lobelia • Cayenne.

TLC - Thymic Longevity Compound **-** EcoNugenics
Each packet contains: Purified Thymic Protein 4 mcg. Other Ingredients: Maltodextrin.

T-LS **-** Dial Herbs
Prickly Ash • Sarsaparilla • Poke root • Stillingia • Red Clover • Burdock • Barberry • Peach bark • Licorice root • Chaparral • Echinacea • Cayenne.

T-MEM **-** Dial Herbs
Lady Slipper • Rosemary • Gotu Kola • Borage • Siberian Ginseng • Licorice • Lobelia.

TMG Plus **-** Progressive Labs
Each tablet contains: Trimethylglycine (anhydrous) 500 mg • Vitamin B6 (pyridoxine HCl) 37.5 mg • Vitamin B6 (pyridoxine-5'-phosphate) 7.5 mg • Folate (folic acid) 450 mcg • Vitamin B12 375 mcg • Selenium (from seleno-L-methionine) 7.5 mcg.

T-MISS **-** Dial Herbs
Wild Yam • Ginger • Red Raspberry • Catnip • False Unicorn • Squaw vine.

T-MSLE **-** Dial Herbs
Cleavers • Pleurisy root • Saffron • Valerian root • Yarrow • Bistort • Catnip • Cayenne • Lobelia.

T-MUSCL **-** Dial Herbs
Sarsaparilla • Saw Palmetto • Strawberry.

T-NAUS **-** Dial Herbs
Catnip • Peppermint • Cinnamon • Ginger • Alfalfa • Lobelia.

T-NRV **-** Dial Herbs
Black Cohosh • Blue Cohosh • Blue Vervain • Scullcap • Lobelia.

T-NSU **-** Dial Herbs
Cranesbill • Goldenseal • Marshmallow • Poke root • Echinacea.

Tocotrien-All **-** Natrol
One softgel contains: Tocotrienol Complex 50 mg containing Alpha-tocopherols 30 IU • Gamma-tocotrienols 45 mg • Alpha-tocotrienols 4 mg • Delta-tocotrienols 1 mg. Other Ingredients: Gelatin, Nutriene (Rice oil).

Tocotrienol Antioxidant Complex **-** Source Naturals
Each softgel contains: Vitamin E (as natural d-alpha tocopherol) 100 IU • Total Tocotrienols (yielding gamma tocotrienol 31 mg) 50 mg.

Tocotrienols plus E-100 I.U. **-** The Vitamin Shoppe
Each softgel contains: Vitamin E (as d-alpha, d-gamma, d-beta, d-delta tocopherols) 100 IU • Tocotrienols (NuTriene) (as d-alpha, d-gamma, d-beta, d-delta tocopherols) 35 mg.

Tofupill **-** Se-Cure Pharmaceuticals/Ventiv Health
Each capsule contains: Tofu concentrate 322 mg • Flaxseed 108 mg. Other Ingredients: Cellulose Capsule Shell.

Tomato Lycopene Softgels **-** TwinLab
Each softgel contains: Lycopene (lycopene10, from Lyc-O-Mato natural tomato) 10 mg. Other Ingredients: Rice Bran Oil, Gelatin, Glycerin, Water, MCT, Yellow Beeswax, Silica.

Tomentosin Plus **-** Atrium Inc.
Each capsule contains: Uncaris tomentosa 400 mg • Bromelain 100 mg • Salix alba 50 mg • Curcuma longa 40 mg.

Tonalin **-** Natrol
Each softgel contains: Proprietary Blend 1000 mg: CLA (conjugated linoleic acid), Oleic Acid, Palmitic Acid, Stearic Acid, Linoleic Acid. Other Ingredients: Glycerin, Water, Caramel Powder.

Tonalin 1000 **-** Source Naturals
Three softgels contain: Conjugated Linoleic Acid 2.22 g. Other Ingredients: Gelatin (capsule), Glycerin, Purified Water, Caramel, Titanium Dioxide, Carob.

Tonalin brand **-** Cognis
CLA (conjugated linoleic acid).
See Editor's Note No. 44, page 2058.

Tonalin CLA 1000 Mg **-** Natrol
One softgel contains: Tonalin supplies 60-70% Conjugated Linoleic Acid from Sunflower oil 1000 mg. Other Ingredients: Lecithin, Beeswax, Soybean oil, Gelatin.

Tonalin CLA 750 Mg **-** Natrol
One softgel contains: Tonalin supplies 60-70% Conjugated Linoleic Acid from Sunflower oil 750 mg • Chromium (Picolinate) 75 mcg • ThermoActives Capsicum (200 SCU) 100 mcg • Ginger root 100 mg. Other Ingredients: Lecithin, Beeswax, Soybean oil, Gelatin.

Tonalin CLA for Men **-** Natrol
One capsule contains: Chromium (as Chromium Picolinate) 50 mcg • Sunflower oil 75 mg • CLA • Conjugated Linoleic Acid 150 mg • Alpha Lipoic Acid 8 mg • Vanadyl Sulfate 2 mg • Siberian Ginseng extract root 50 mg • Leucine (as L-Leucine Hydrochloride) 50 mg • Arginine (as L-Arginine Hydrochloride) 50 mg • Isoleucine (as L-Isoleucine Hydrochloride) 12 mg • Valine (as L-Valine Hydrochloride) 25 mg. Other Ingredients: Silicon Dioxide, Magnesium Stearate, Gelatin.

Tonalin XS-CLA **-** NSI - Nutraceutical Sciences Institute
Each softgel contains: Sunflower seed oil 1 g.

Tone 'N' Trim **-** Optimum Nutrition
Citrimax • L-Carnitine • Chromium Picolinate.

Tot Tonic **-** The Herbalist
Echinacea root • Golden Seal root • Lemon Balm herb • Yarrow flower • Yerba Santa leaf.

Total Energy **-** Jamieson
Each caplet contains: Bee Pollen and Royal Jelly (from Organically Monitored Hives) 175 mg • Rocky Mountain Wheat Grass 125 mg • Siberian Ginseng 100 mg • Kola Nut 100 mg.

Total Flora (Total Flora Support) **-** Infinity2
Two capsules contain: Vitamin C (from calcium ascorbate) 60 mg • Manganese (as manganese chelazome) 0.1 mg • Probiotic Blend 260 mg: Lactobacillus Acidophilus 1 billion CFU, Bifidobacterium Bifidum 400 million CFU, Lactobacillus Bulgaricus 200 million CFU, Lactobacillus Plantarum 200 million CFU, Lactobacillus Salivarius 200 million CFU, Streptococcus Thermophilus 200 million

CFU, Lactobacillus Reuteri 40 million CFU, Lactobacillus Brevis 40 million CFU, Bifidobacterium Longum 40 million CFU, Bifidobacterium Infantis 40 million CFU, Lactobacillus Lactis 40 million CFU, Lactobacillus Rhamnosus 200 million CFU • Jerusalem Artichoke (tubers) 60 mg • CAeDS (Chelate Activated Enzyme Delivery System) 40 mg: Amylase, Lipase, Cellulase, Calcium Chelazome, Protease, Zinc Chelazome, Magnesium Chelazome, Manganese Chelazome • Magnesium Glycyl Glutamine (MGG, stabilized glutamine) 10 mg. Other Ingredients: Plant Fiber, Gelatin, Water.

Total Greens **-** Solar Green/Nutraceutical
Four tablets contains: Barley Grass Juice powder (Hordeum vulgare) 600 mg • Wheat Grass (Triticum aestivum) 600 mg • Alfalfa leaf (medicago sativa) 600 mg. Other Ingredients: Cellulose, Stearic Acid, Silica and Magnesium Stearate, Chlorella Broken Cell Algae (chlorella pyrenoidosa), Spirulina (algae pratensis), Norwegian Kelp (fucus vesiculosis).

Total Life Care Nutrition System for Men **-** Rexall - Sundown
Each packet contains: Vitamin A 5000 IU • Vitamin C (as ascorbic acid) 210 mg • Vitamin D (as cholecalciferol) 400 IU • Vitamin E (as dl-alpha-tocopheryl acetate and d-alpha-tocopherol) 100 IU • Thiamin (vitamin B1; as thiamin mononitrate) 1.5 mg • Riboflavin (vitamin B2) 1.7 mg • Niacin (as niacinamide) 20 mg • Vitamin B-6 (as pyridoxine HCl) 11 mg • Folic Acid 1 mg • Vitamin B-12 (as cyanocobalamin) 101 mcg • Pantothenic Acid (as calcium d-pantothenate) 1 mg • Calcium 100 mg • Magnesium (as magnesium oxide) 200 mg • Zinc (as zinc oxide) 5 mg • Selenium (as selenium amino acid chelate) 200 mcg • Fish Oil (EPA [eicosapentaenoic acid] 180 mg, DHA [docosahexaenoic acid] 120 mg) • L-Arginine (L-arginine and L-arginine HCl) 800 mg • Saw Palmetto fruit 450 mg • Calcium D-Glucarate 400 mg • Grape seed extract (vitis vinifera) 60 mg • Nettle root 50 mg • Pygeum (pygeum africanum) 50 mg • Coenzyme Q-10 20 mg.
Inactive Ingredients: Gelatin, Cellulose, Dicalcium Phosphate, Glycerin, White Rice Powder, Croscarmellose Sodium, Calcium Silicate, Water, Hydroxypropyl Methylcellulose, Magnesium Stearate, PEG, Red 40 lake, Retinyl Acetate, Yellow 6 lake, Titanium Dioxide, Polysorbate 80, Blue 2 lake, Beta-carotene.

Total Life Care Nutrition System for Women **-** Rexall - Sundown
One packet contains: Vitamin A 5000 IU • Vitamin C (as ascorbic acid) 410 mg • Vitamin D (as cholecalciferol) 400 IU • Vitamin E (as dl-alpha-tocopheryl acetate and d-alpha-tocopherol) 100 IU • Thiamin (vitamin B1); (as thiamin mononitrate) 1.5 mg • Riboflavin (vitamin B2) 1.7 mg • Niacin (as niacinamide) 20 mg • Vitamin B-6 (as pyridoxine HCl) 11 mg • Folic Acid 1 mg • Vitamin B-12 (as cyanocobalamin) 101 mcg • Pantothenic Acid (as calcium d-pantothenate) 1 mg • Calcium 100 mg • Magnesium (as magnesium oxide) 200 mg • Selenium (as selenium amino acid chelate) 200 mcg • Fish Oil (Eicosapentaenoic Acid [EPA] 180 mg, Docosahexaenoic acid [DHA] 120 mg) 1000 mg • L-Arginine (L-arginine and L-arginine HCl) 800 mg • Calcium D-Glucarate 400 mg • Cranberry fruit juice concentrate 140 mg • Grape seed extract (vitis vinifera) 60 mg • Coenzyme Q-10 20 mg. Other Ingredients: Gelatin, Cellulose, Soybean oil, Glycerin, Dicalcium Phosphate, White Rice Powder, Partially Hydrogenated Soybean Oil, Water, Croscarmellose Sodium, Calcium Silicate, Hydrogenated Soybean Oil, Yellow Beeswax, Hydroxypropyl Methylcellulose, Soy Lecithin, Magnesium Stearate, PEG, Red 40 lake, Retinyl acetate, Silica, Yellow 6 lake, Titanium Dioxide, Polysorbate 80, Blue 2 lake, Beta-carotene.

Total Woman Formula **-** Youngevity
Damiana leaf (Turnera aphrodisiaca) • Dong Quai root (Angelica sinensis) • Saw Palmetto (Serenoa repens) • Fennel seed (Foeniculum vulgare) • Oat Bran (Avena sativa) • Vilcabamba Mineral Essence: Potassium, Calcium, Magnesium, Zinc, Chromium, Selenium, Iron, Copper, Molybdenum, Vanadium, Iodine, Cobalt, Manganese.

Touku Natural Herbal Rheumatic Pills **-** Lishih
Korean Red Ginseng • Bark of Eucommiae • Pseudo Ginseng • Olibanum • Common Myrrh Tree • Starjasmine stem • Radix Astragali • Rhizoma Gastrodiae • Radix Morindae • Clematis root • Rhizoma Ligustici • Angelica root • Radix Dipsaci • Codonoptis Sinensis • Rhizoma Atractylodis Alba • Radix Heraclei • Fructus Chaenomelis • Fructus Liquidambaris • Uncaria Sinensis • Bee Honey.
See Editor's Note No. 46, page 2058.

Toxoid OTC's Toxoid First Aid **-** HealthWatchers System
Zinc (as Zincboracyl crystals) • Menthol • Denatured Ethyl Alcohol 60%.

Toxoid OTC's Toxoid Pain **-** HealthWatchers System
Zinc (as Zincboracyl crystals) • Menthol • Camphor • Fang Fang Extract • Dong Quai Extract • Ling Man Zhin • Qin Jiu Extract.

Toxoid OTC's Toxoid Relief **-** HealthWatchers System
Trace Minerals • Zinc (as Zincboracyl crystals) • Red Cabbage Extract • Aluminum Acetate.

Toxoid OTC's Toxoid Skin **-** HealthWatchers System
Salicylic Acid • Zinc (as Zincoracyl crystals) • Purified Water.

T-PARA **-** Dial Herbs
Wormwood • Black Walnut • Senna • Wild Carrot.

T-PEP **-** Dial Herbs
Gotu Kola • Kelp • Alfalfa • Dandelion • Brigham Tea • Hydrangea • Saffron • Parsley.

T-PERSP **-** Dial Herbs
Pennyroyal • Cayenne • Catnip • Ginger • Chamomile • Mustard.

T-PNF **-** Dial Herbs
Wild Lettuce • Valerian • Scullcap • Blue Vervain • Arnica • Lobelia • Cayenne.

T-PR **-** Dial Herbs
Strawberry • Sassafras • Sarsaparilla • Echinacea • Garlic.

Trace-Min Plus **-** Progressive Labs
Three capsules contain: Vitamin B6 (pyridoxine HCl) 50 mg • Vitamin D (cholecalciferol) 50 IU • Calcium (as calcium carbonate and calcium citrate) 300 mg • Magnesium (as magnesium oxide and magnesium gluconate) 150 mg • Zinc (as zinc gluconate) 15 mg • Manganese (as manganese gluconate) 10 mg • Potassium (as potassium gluconate) 99 mg • Glutamic Acid HCl 325 mg.

Tranquility **-** Nature's Plus
Each tablet contains: Valerian root 200 mg • Magnesium amino acid chelate/complex 200 mg • Calcium Caseinate, amino acid chelate/complex 100 mg • Chamomile 50 mg. In a base of milk protein concentrate (750 mg), containing 10 mg of naturally occuring L-Tryptophan. Yeast free. Sugar & starch free.

Tranquility **-** Wellness International Network, Ltd.
Each capsule contains: Vitamin A (as vitamin A palmitate) 3750 IU • Vitamin C (as ascorbic acid) 30 mg • Vitamin D (as cholecalciferol) 100 IU • Vitamin E (as DL-alpha tocopheryl acetate) 30 IU • Thiamin (as thiamin HCl) 5 mg • Riboflavin 1.6 mg • Niacin (as niacinamide) 18 mg • Vitamin B6 (as pyridoxine HCl) 2 mg • Folic Acid 300 mcg • Vitamin B12 (as cyanocobalamin) 2 mcg • Biotin 30 mcg • Pantothenic Acid (as D-calcium pantothenate) 5 mg • Magnesium (as magnesium amino acid chelate) 2.5 mg • Proprietary Blend 315.2 mg: Glutamic Acid (as isolated soy protein), Choline Bitartrate, Inositol, Lecithin, Ribonucleic Acid (RNA), Valerian root 4:1 extract (valeriana officinalis), Aspartic Acid (as isolated soy protein), Leucine (as isolated soy protein), Arginine (as isolated soy protein), Lysine (as isolated soy protein), Phenylalanine (as isolated soy protein), Serine (as isolated soy protein), Proline (as isolated soy protein), Valine (as isolated soy protein), Isoleucine (as isolated soy protein), Alanine (as isolated soy protein), Glycine (as isolated soy

protein), Threonine (as isolated soy protein), Tyrosine (as isolated soy protein), Histidine (as isolated soy protein), Methionine (as isolated soy protein), Adenosine Triphosphate, Cysteine (as isolated soy protein). Other Ingredients: Talc, Silicon Dioxide, Hydroxypropyl Cellulose.

Transfer Factor **-** 4 Life
Each capsule contains: Transfer Factor E-XF from Bovine Colostrum 300 mg. Other ingredients: Gelatin.

Transfer Factor Cardio **-** 4 Life
Four capsules contain: Vitamin A (as beta carotene) 2500 IU • Vitamin C (as magnesium dehydroascorbate, ascorbyl palmitate and ascorbic acid) 200 mg • Vitamin E (as d-alpha tocopherol succinate) 100 IU • Niacin (as niacinamide) 20 mg • Vitamin B6 (as pyridoxine hydrochloride) 2 mg • Folate (as folic acid) 400 mcg • Vitamin B12 (as cyanocobalamin) 8 mcg • Magnesium (as magnesium: chloride, dehydroascorbate, arginate and lysinate) 180 mg • Zinc (as zinc arginate) 10 mg • Selenium (as selenomethionine) 50 mcg • Copper (as copper glycinate) 2 mg • Potassium (as potassium citrate) 50 mg • Cardio Targeted Transfer Factor (from egg yolk) 200 mg • Proprietary Blend 478 mg: Butcher's Broom root (22% sterolic heterosides), Ginkgo Biloba leaf (24% ginkgo flavone glycosides, 6% terpene lactones), Hawthorn flower and leaf (1.8% rutin), Garlic clove (deodorized), Coenzyme Q10, Red Yeast extract, Resveratrol (from polygonum cuspidatum), Ginger oil. Other Ingredients: Gelatin.

Transfer Factor Chewable **-** 4 Life
Each capsule contains: Transfer Factor E-XF from Bovine Colostrum 200 mg. Other Ingredients: Fructose, Maltose, Sorbitol, Natural Flavors, Stearic and Malic Acids, and Silica.

Transfer Factor Classic **-** 4 Life
Each capsule contains: Transfer Factor XF from Bovine Colostrum 200 mg. Other Ingredients: Gelatin.

Transfer Factor Essentials **-** Pro Health
Two capsules contain: Folic Acid 100 mcg • Vitamin B12 (as cyanocobalamin) 4 mcg • Zinc (as zinc oxide) 5 mg • Selenium (as selenium amino acid chelate) 25 mcg • Transfer Factor Matrix Blend 330 mg: Chicken-derived Transfer Factors, Bovine Colostrum extract containing growth factors, immune components • Beta Glucan 200 mg • Larch Arabinogalactan 333 mg • TMG 375 mg • IP-6 200 mg • Astragalus (1:5 extract) 70 mg. Other Ingredients: Gelatin, Dicalcium Phosphate, Cellulose, Magnesium Stearate, Magnesium Trisilicae, Silica.

Transfer Factor GluCoach **-** 4 Life
Each capsule contains: Chromium 70 mcg • Targeted Transfer Factor from Bovine Colostrum and Egg yolk 50 mg • Pterocarpus Marsupium 200 mg • Fenugreek 50 mg • Momordica Charantia 35 mg • Gymnema Sylvestre 25 mg • Korean Ginseng 20 mg • Alpha Lipoic Acid 30 mg • Vanadium (bis-glycinato oxo vanadium) 150 mg. Other Ingredients: Gelatin.

Transfer Factor Plus **-** 4 Life
One capsule contains: Transfer Factor E-XF from Bovine Colostrum and Egg yolk 150 mg • Proprietary blend 440 mg: IP-6 (inositol hexaphosphate), Soya Bean extract, Cordyceps sinensis (7% cordyceptic acids), Beta Glucan from Baker's Yeast (saacharomyces cerevisiae), Beta Glucan from Oat (avena sativa), Agaricus Blazeii extract, Mannans from Aloe Vera leaf, Maitake mushroom (Grifola frondosa whole plant), Shiitake mushroom (Lentinus edodes whole plant 5:1 extract). Other Ingredients: Gelatin, Lemon Peel.

Transfer Factor ReCall **-** 4 Life
Three capsules contain: Magnesium (as magnesium oxide) 168 mg • Targeted Transfer Factor from Eggs 100 mg • Proprietary Blend 672 mg: Vinpocetine, Huperzine A (Huperzia Serrata extract), Soy Lecithin (30% phosphatidylserine), Glycerophosphocholine, N-Acetyl Tyrosine, N-Acetyl Cysteine, Bacopa Monnieri extract, Lemon Balm extract, Ginkgo Biloba extract (24% ginkgo flavone glycosides, 6% terpene lactones).

Transfer Factor Toothpaste **-** 4 Life
Sorbitol, Deionized Water, Hydrated Silica, Glycerin, Calcium Carbonate, Sodium Lauroyl Sarcosinate, Sodium Bicarbonate, Xylitol, Flavors, Transfer Factor E-XF, Lactoferrin, Carboxymethylcellulose, Titanium Dioxide, Coenzyme Q-10, Stevia, Sodium Benzoate.

Transitions Carbohydrate Absorption Inhibitor **-** Market America, Inc.
Each capsule contains: Magnesium (as magnesium citrate) 50 mg • Chromium (as chromium dinicotinate glycinate) 100 mcg • Wheat Amylase Inhibitor 10 mg • Banaba leaf extract (lagerstroemia speciosa) 16 mg • Vanadium (as vanadium BMOV) 50 mcg • Bitter Melon fruit extract 100 mg. Other Ingredients: Gelatin, Cellulose, Magnesium Stearate, Silica.

Transitions CLA Conjugated Linoleic Acid **-** Market America, Inc.
Four capsules contain: Chromium (from Chromax chromium picolinate) 120 mg • Tonalin CLA (100% pure safflower oil, 2730 mg active CLA) 3500 mg • Caffeine (from guarana seed extract) 200 mg. Other Ingredients: Gelatin, Glycerin, Soybean Oil, Soy Lecithin, Beeswax, Carmine Color, Natural Lemon Flavor.

Transitions Fat Conversion Inhibitor **-** Market America, Inc.
Two tablets contain: Chromium (as chromium dinicotinate glycinate) 67 mcg • Gymnema Sylvestre leaf extract (25% gymnemic acids) 133 mg • Garcinia Cambogia fruit (60% hydroxycitric acid) 1500 mg • Bioperine Black Pepper extract 2.6 mg. Other Ingredients: Dicalcium Phosphate, Microcrystalline Cellulose, Sodium Starch Glycolate, Stearic Acid, Magnesium Stearate, Silica, Pharmaceutical Glaze.

Traumeel Oral Drops **-** Heel, Inc.
Each 100 mL contains: Arnica Montana, Radix 3X 10 mL • Aconitum Napellus 3X 5 mL • Chamomilla 3X 5 mL • Belladonna 4X 5 mL • Symphytum Officinlae 8X 5 mL • Bellis Perennis 2X 2 mL • Calendula Officinalis 2X 2mL • Echinacea Angustifolia 2X 2 mL • Echinacea Purpurea 2X 2mL • Hamamelis Virginiana 2X 2mL • Hypericum Perforatum 3X 2 mL • Millefolium 3X 2 mL • Hepar Suphuris Calcareum 8X 2 mL • Mercurius Solubilis 8X 2 mL • 35% Ethyl Alcohol.
See Editor's Note No. 1, page 2053.

Traumeel Tablets **-** Heel, Inc.
Each tablet contains: Belladonna 4X 75 mg • Arnica Montana, Radix 3X 40 mg • Aconitum Napellus 3X 30 mg • Chamomilla 3X 24 mg • Symphytum Officinale 8X 24 mg • Calendula Officinalis 2X 15 mg • Hamamelis Virginiana 2X 15 mg • Millefolium 3X 15 mg • Hepar Sulphuris Calcareum 8X 15 mg • Mercurius Solubilis 8X 15 mg • Hypericum Perforatum 3X 8 mg • Bellis Perennis 2X 6 mg • Echinacea Angustifolia 2X 6 mg • Echinacea Purpurea 2X 6 mg. Other Ingredients: Lactose Base.
See Editor's Note No. 1, page 2053.

Trenabol-X **-** Higher Power
Each 4 mL serving contains: 1-(5-alpha)-Androsten-17-Beta-0L-3-One 100 mg • 4-Androstene-3,17-Diol 100 mg • 1,4-Androstadienedione 100 mg.

Tres Bien Bars, Crunchy Lemon Burst **-** Advocare International
Each bar contains: Red Clover extract 250 mg • Green Tea extract 100 mg • Phosphatidylcholine 50 mg • Docosahexaenoic Acid [DHA] 30 mg. Other Ingredients: Soy Protein Isolate, High Maltose Corn Syrup, High Fructose Corn Syrup, Sugar, Fractionated Palm Kernel Oil, Toasted Rolled Oats, Rice Syrup, Toasted Soy Pieces, Lemon Juice from Concentrate, Nonfat Milk, Dextrose, Maltodextrin, Crisp Rice (rice flour, rice bran, rosemary extract), Natural Flavor, Tapioca Starch, Red Clover Extract, Nonfat Yogurt Powder (cultured whey, nonfat milk), Soy Lecithin, Soybean Oil, Green Tea Extract, Ascorbic Acid, Pectin, Citric Acid, Guar Gum, Vegetable Oil (algae oil containing docosahexaenoic acid [DHA], ascorbyl palmitate and

tocopherols added to protect flavor), Beta-Carotene, Salt, Titanium Dioxide (added for color), Alpha-Tocopherol Acetate, Honey, Sodium Citrate, Folic Acid, Annatto (added for color).

T-RHU **-** Dial Herbs
Buchu Leaves • Oregon Grape • Cayenne • Black Cohosh • Buckthorn • Burdock • Hydrangea • Lobelia • Nettle • Scullcap • Wild Yam • White Willow bark • Yellow Dock • Arnica.

Tri-40 **-** Progressive Labs
Each capsule contains: Iodine (from kelp) 150 mcg • Thyroid concentrate (thyroxin free) 40 mg • Spleen concentrate 40 mg • Thymus concentrate 40 mg • Pacific Sea Kelp 100 mg. The glandular concentrate in this product is prepared by a special process which does not exceed physiological temperature (37° C). Guaranteed free of chemical pesticides and synthetic hormones.
See Editor's Note No. 14, page 2055.

Tri-Amino Supplement **-** Puritan's Pride
Four tablets contain: L-Arginine Hydrochloride 1447 mg • L-Ornithine Hydrochloride 900 mg • L-Lysine Hydrochloride 1200 mg.

Triax **-** Syntrax Innovations
Each capsule contains: Tiratricol 1 mg. Other ingredients: Barley flour, gelatin, titanium dioxide, red #40, blue #1.

TRIBEST **-** New Hope Health Products
Each capsule contains: Tribulus terrestris (containing Furostanol and Protodioscin) 750 mg.

Tribest **-** Metabolic Response Modifiers
Each capsule contains: Tribulus terrestris (containing Furostanol and Protodioscin) 750 mg.

Tribestan **-** Sopharma
Each tablet contains: Tribestan from Tribulus Terrestris herb.

Tribestrone II **-** ASN - Advanced Sports Nutrition
Each tablet contains: Tribulus Terrestris L. extract 450 mg • Ashwaganda extract 100 mg • Mucuna extract 100 mg • Bioperine standardized extract 1.5 mg.

Tribex **-** BioTest Laboratories, LLC
Four capsules contain: Tribex Full-Spectrum Active Extracts 2000 mg: Tribulus Terrestris, Avena Sativa. Other Ingredients: Gelatin, Cellulose, Magnesium Stearate, FD&C Blue #1, FD&C Red #3, FD&C Red #40, Titanium Dioxide.

Tribulus **-** The Vitamin Shoppe
Each capsule contains: Tribulus Terrestris (fruit, standardized to 20% saponins) 625 mg.

Tribulus 625 Caps **-** Optimum Nutrition
Each capsule contains: Proprietary Tribulus Blend 625 mg: Tribulus Terrestris fruit extract (standardized to 40% furastanol saponins), Tribulus Terrestris powdered aerial parts. Other Ingredients: Gelatin, Silica, Magnesium Stearate.

Tribulus Fuel **-** TwinLab
Each capsule contains: Tribulus Terrestris extract (standardized for 20-29% steroidal saponins) 625 mg.

Tribulus Fuel Stack **-** TwinLab
Two capsules contain: Tribulus Terrestris extract 1250 mg • DHEA (dehydroepiandrosterone) 50 mg.

Tribulus Gold **-** Mass Quantities, Inc.
Each capsule contains: Tribulus extract (standardized 42%) 675 mg.

Tribulus Synergy Male Response Formula **-** Metagenics
Each tablet contains: Proprietary Herbal Extract Blend 500 mg: Tribulus fruit (tribulus terrestris, 7:1 extract, containing saponins), Ashwagandha root (withania somnifera, 5:1 extract, containing withanolides), Cowhage seed (mucuna pruriens, containing naturally occurring levodopa), Sativari root (asparagus racemosus, 4:1 extract, containing saponins).

Triflex Dietary Supplement **-** GNC
Three tablets contain: Glucosamine HCl 1500 mg •Chondroitin Sulfate, Sodium 1200 mg • MSM (Metyhlsulfonylmethane) 900 mg. Ohter Ingredients: Titanium Dioxide.
See Editor's Note No. 15, page 2055.

Tri-Flex Soft Chewables Chocolate **-** GNC
Each chew contains: Glucosamine HCl 500 mg • Chondroitin Sulfate 400 mg • Methylsulfonylmethane (MSM) 25 mg. Ingredients: Corn syrup, Sweetened Condensed Skim Milk, Partially Hydrogenated Soybean oil, Glucosamine HCl, Chondroitin Sulfate, Whey Chocolate liquor, Mono & Diglycerides, Methylsulfonylmethane (MSM), Soy Lecithin, Artificial Flavor.
See Editor's Note No. 15, page 2055.

Triglic-Oil **-** Aboca USA, Inc
Three capsules contain: Fish Oil 930 mg (eicosapentaenoic acid 190 mg, docosahexaenoic acid 480 mg) • Turmeric root extract in Flaxseed oil (1:10) 230 mg. Other Ingredients: Gelatin (capsule), Essential Oils Of Rosemary, Lemon.

Trilean **-** VitaStore
Guarana (Paullinia Cupana) • Glutamine • Fennel • Choline • Spirulina • Hawthorne • Inositol • Bladderwrack • Vitamin A • Vitamin C • Vitamin D • Vitamin E • Vitamin B1 • Vitamin B2 • Vitamin B6 • Vitamin B12 • Folic Acid • Niacin • d-Biotin • Pantothenic Acid • Potassium • Calcium.

Trim Fit with Advantra Z-Tonalin Kit **-** Quest
Six capsules contain: Advantra-ZT Citrus Aurantium (standardized to 4% synephrine) 1050 mg • Green Tea extract (camellia sinensis, P.E. 1:6) 1050 mg • Tonalin (source of conjugated linoleic acid) 900 mg • Kelp (fucus vesiculosus) 300 mg • St. John's Wort extract (hypericum perforatum) 150 mg • Trim-Zyme Enzyme Blend (P.E. 1:5, standardized to 0.3% hypericin) 150 mg: Protease, Lipase, Amylase, Cellulase • Lipoic Acid 30 mg. Other Ingredients: Silicon Dioxide, Magnesium Stearate (vegetable source), Gelatin, Natural Color.
See Editor's Note No. 40, page 2058.

Trim Fit with Advantra Z-Tonalin Kit Phase 2 **-** Quest
Each tablet contains: White Kidney Bean extract 500 mg. Other Ingredients: Calcium Phosphate, Microcrystalline Cellulose, Vegetable Stearin, Croscarmellose Sodium, Ascorbic Acid, Magnesium Stearate (vegetable source), Silicone Dioxide, Methylcellulose Complex (cellcote coating).

Trim Lite **-** Health Smart Vitamins
Three capsules contain: Vitamin C (ascorbic acid) 250 mg • Vitamin E (d-alpha tocopheryl succinate) 150 IU • Vitamin B6 (pyridoxine HCl) 7 mg • Chromium (as chromium nicotinate) 150 mcg • Cola Nut (14% caffeine, 70 mg) 500 mg • Ma Huang root (6% total ephedrine alkaloids, 6 mg) 100 mg • DL-Phenylalanine 75 mg • English Hawthorn leaf & flower (1.8% vitexin, 0.9 mg) 50 mg • l-Carnitine (as L-carnitine tartrate) 30 mg.
See Editor's Note No. 30, page 2056.

Trim4Life Appetite Control Phase II **-** FreeLife International
Each caplet contains: Herbal Energy Standardized Extract Blend 450 mg: Green Tea leaf, Chinese White Ginseng root (panax ginseng), Siberian Eleuthero Ginseng root, Korean Red Ginseng root (panax ginseng), American Five-Leaf Ginseng root (panax quinquefolius), Brazilian Suma Ginseng root (pfaffia paniculata), Central American Osha Ginseng root (ligusticum wallichi), Tibetian Tienchi Ginseng root (panax notoginseng), Manchurian Yellow Ginseng root (caulophyllum thalictrodies), Indian Ashwagandha Ginseng root (withania somnifera), Japanese Ginseng root (panax japonicus), Couchgrass herb, Buchu leaf, Uva Ursi leaf, Juniper berry, Hydrangea root, Cornsilk • Appetite Control Standardized Extract Blend 250 mg: Griffonia seed (griffonia simplicifolia), L-Tyrosine (soy amino acid), standardized Citrus peel extract (citrus aurantium) • Potassium Citrate 50 mg • Vanadium (from glycinate chelate) 50 mcg. Other Ingredients: Calcium Dihydrogen Phosphate, Cellulose, Fractionated

Vegetable Oil, Silica, Vita-coat (protective antioxidant coating system).

Trim4Life Thermogenic Phase 1 - FreeLife International
Each caplet contains: Vitamin B6 (as pyridoxine hydrochloride) 10 mg • Chromium (dinicotinate glycinate) 150 mcg • Thermonutrient Standardized Extract Blend 175 mg: Cinnamon bark, Country Mallow leaf, Piperine extract of Black Pepper • Adrenal Support Standardized Extract Blend 50 mg: Licorice root, Ginger root, Astragalus root. Other Ingredients: Calcium Dihydrogen Phosphate, Cellulose, Fractionated Vegetable Oil, Silica, Vita-Coat (protective antioxidant coating system).
See Editor's Note No. 39, page 2058.

Trimax - Enzymatic Therapy
Each capsule contains: St. John's Wort extract (Hypericum perforatum) standardized to contain 0.15% Hypericins, verified by HPLC 500 mg • Valerian extract (Valeriana officinalis) standardized to contain a minimum of 0.8%, 15 mg • Passionflower extract (Passiflora) 15 mg.

TrimFast (Trim Fast) - Preferred Price Plus
Each capsule contains: Natural Ephedra • White Willow bark • Chromium Polynicotinate.
See Editor's Note No. 30, page 2056.

TrimLife - Proven Health Technologies
Each tablet contains: Vitamin E (as d-alpha tocopheryl succinate) 10 IU • Chromium (from chromium picolinate) 25 mcg • Guarana seed extract 4:1 (contains 100 mg caffeine) 455 mg • L-Tyrosine 167 mg • Ma Huang root standardized extract (8% total alkaloids, contains 10 mg ephedrine) 143 mg • Hydroxy Citric Acid 125 mg • Ginger root 100 mg • Acetyl-L-Carnitine 12.5 mg • Siberian Ginseng roots 10 mg • Capsicum fruit (cayenne pepper, providing approximately 0.126% capsaicin) 1 mg. Other Ingredients: Cellulose, Maltodextrin, Stearic Acid, Croscamellose Sodium, Silicon Dioxide, Magnesium Stearate, Cellulose Film-Coat.
See Editor's Note No. 30, page 2056.

Trim-Plex - Nature's Plus
Three softgels contain: Lecithin (soya) 600 mg • Kelp 300 mg • Apple Cider Vinegar 240 mg • Vitamin B6 (pyridoxine HCl) 50 mg. In a natural blend of Vegetable (soy) oil & Chlorophyll. Sugar & starch free.

TrimSolution Bar - Chocolate - Starlight International
Each bar contains: Starlight Protein Blend: Calcium caseinate, Soy protein isolate, Soy flour, Whey Protein concentrate, nonfat Milk • Rice Syrup • High Fructose Corn Syrup • Confectionary Coating: Sucrose, Fractionated Palm Kernel Oil, Cocoa powder, Whey powder, nonfat Milk, Lecithin, natural Vanilla • Fiber Blend: Guar Gum, Arabic Gum, Soy fiber, Corn bran • Chocolate • Natural Flavors • Garcinia Cambogia • Magnesium carbonate • Glycerin • Phytonutrients: Carrot powder, Spinach powder, Cabbage powder, Tomato powder, Broccoli powder • Ascorbic Acid • dl Alpha Tocopherol Acetate • Vitamin A palmitate • Niacinamide • Omega 3 and 6 Fatty Acids • Zinc oxide • Ferrous Fumarate • Copper gluconate • D-Calcium pantothenate • Schisandra berry extract • Vitamin D3 • Pyridoxine HCl • Riboflavin • Thiamine mononitrate • Vitamin B12 • Canola Oil • Folate • Biotin • Potassium iodide.

TrimSolution Bar - Peanut Butter - Starlight International
Each bar contains: Starlight Protein Blend: Calcium caseinate, Soy protein isolate, Peanut Butter, Soy flour, Whey Protein concentrate, nonfat Milk, defatted Peanut flour • Rice Syrup • High Fructose Corn Syrup • Confectionary Coating: Sucrose, Fractionated Palm Kernel Oil, Cocoa powder, Whey powder, nonfat milk, Lecithin, natural Vanilla • Fiber Blend: Guar Gum, Arabic Gum, Soy fiber, Corn Bran , Oat Bran • Natural Flavors • Tricalcium Phosphate • Garcinia Cambogia • Magnesium carbonate • Glycerin • Phytonutrients: Carrot powder, Spinach powder, Cabbage powder, Tomato powder, Broccoli powder • Ascorbic Acid • dl Alpha Tocopherol Acetate • Vitamin A palmitate • Niacinamide • Omega 3 and 6 Fatty Acids • Zinc oxide • Ferrous Fumarate • Copper gluconate • D-Calcium Pantothenate • Schisandra Berry extract • Vitamin D3 • Pyridoxine Hydrochloride • Riboflavin • Thiamine mononitrate • Vitamin B12 • Canola Oil • Folate • Biotin • Potassium iodide.

TrimSpa - Nutramerica Corp.
Each capsule contains: Chromium (as chromium dinicotinate glycinate) 150 mcg • Vanadium (as vanadium amino acid chelate) 50 mcg • Glucomannan 400 mg • Green Tea leaf extract (60 mg caffeine) 120 mg • Coleus Forskohlii tuber extract (10% forskolin) 250 mg • Sodium Carboxymethylcellulose 100 mg. Other Ingredients: Gelatin, Magnesium Stearate, Silica.

TrimSpa Carb Blocker - Nutramerica Corp.
Two tablets contain: Chromium (as chelavate chromium dinicotinate glycinate) 200 mcg • Phase 2 brand White Kidney bean extract (phaseolus vulgaris) 1000 mg • Vanadium (as vanadium amino acid chelate) 100 mcg. Other Ingredients: Dicalcium Phosphate, Microcrystalline Cellulose, Croscarmellose Sodium, Stearic Acid, Magnesium Stearate, Silica, Pharmaceutical Glaze.
See Editor's Note No. 37, page 2057.

Trimspa Completely Ephedra Free - Nutramerica Corp.
Two tablets contain: Chromium (as chromium dinicotinate glycinate) 150 mcg • Vanadium (as vanadium amino acid chelate) 30 mcg • Glucomannan 400 mg • Sodium Carboxymethylcellulose 100 mg • Citrus Naringinine 10 mg • Glucosamine HCl 100 mg • Cocoa extract (standardized for phenylalanine, tyramine, 10% theobromine) 325 mg • Green Tea extract (40%, standardized for epigallocatechin gallate, polyphenols, 40% caffeine) 250 mg • Hoodia Gordonii cactus (above ground parts) 150 mg. Other Ingredients: Dicalcium Phosphate, Microcrystalline Cellulose, Croscarmellose Sodium, Stearic Acid, Magnesium Stearate.

TrimSpa Fat Blocker - Nutramerica Corp.
Each capsule contains: Vitamin C (as ascorbic acid) 60 mg • Liposan Ultra Chitosan (marine fiber concentrate) 500 mg. Other Ingredients: Calcium Sulfate, Gelatin, Cellulose, Magnesium Stearate, Silica.
See Editor's Note No. 37, page 2057.

Trinovin - Novogen
Each tablet contains: Natural Isoflavones 40 mg. Trinovin is made from red clover, which contains isoflavones (genistein, biochanin, daidzein, formononetin) with a high biochanin content. Other Ingredients: Dicalcium phosphate, Microcrystalline cellulose, Hydroxypropyl methylcellulose, Magnesium stearate, Mixed tocopherols, Silica, Soy polysaccharide, & Natural caramel color.

Triomega Omega-3 Softgels - Pronova Biocare
Each softgel contains: Triomega concentrated Fish oil 800 mg providing: EPA (eicosapentaenoic acid), DHA (docosahexaenoic acid, 62.5% EPA:DHA ratio approximately 2:1 as ethyl esters) 500 mg, total Omega-3 Fatty Acids (71.25%) 570 mg. Other Ingredients: Gelatin, USP Water, Glycerin, Natural Vitamin E (as mixed tocopherols).

Trioxalon 500 - AST Sports Science
Each capsule contains: Tribulus Terrestris extract 500 mg.

Trip2Night - Unknown
Some ingredients include: Ma-huang • Guarana • 5-HTP • Bioperine Black Pepper extract • Indian Bromine • Cinnamon • Cola Nut • Niacin • Fo Ti.
See Editor's Note No. 30 and No. 49.

Trip2night-EF - Unknown
Some ingredients include: Citrus Aurantium • Guarana • 5-HTP • Bioperine Black pepper extract • Indian Bromine • Cinnamon • Cola Nut • Niacin • Fo Ti.
See Editor's Note No. 40 and No. 49.

Triphala - The Himalaya Drug Company (Himalaya Heal
Each capsule contains: Proprietary Blend 250 mg: Emblica officinalis, Terminalia chebula, Terminalia bellirica.

BRAND NAMES

BRAND NAMES

TriPhetamine **-** Pharmalogic
Two caplets contain: Sida Cordifolia Extract (standardized to 6% ephedrine alkaloids) 235 mg • Ma Huang Extract (standardized to 6% ephedrine alkaloids) 100 mg • Caffeinated Green Tea Leaf Extract (standardized to 50% polyphenols; 35% catechins) 200 mg • Cola Nut Extract (seed; standardized to 20% caffeine) 250 mg • Guarana Extract (seed; standardized to 20% caffeine) 250 mg • Caffeine (from caffeine anhydrous) 100 mg • Proprietary Blend 295 mg: L-Tyrosine, DMAE (2-dimethylaminoethanol bitartrate), Hypothalamic Peptides, L-Alanine, Cinnamon Extract (standardized to 5% cinnamonosides). Other Ingredients: Calcium Carbonate, Microcrystalline Cellulose, Stearic Acid, Magnesium Stearate, Titanium Dioxide.
See Editor's Note No. 30, page 2056.

Triple B Super Vision **-** DreamPharm
Each tablet contains: Bilberry fruit (standardized to 20% anthocyanin) 80 mg • Blackberry fruit (standardized to 20% anthocyanin) 60 mg • Blueberry fruit 400 mg • Eyebright herb (euphrasia officinalis) 250 mg • Cassia Obtusifolia seeds 100 mg • Eriocaulon Buergerianum 50 mg • Lutein (5% powder containing zeaxanthin, extracted from marigold flower) 3 mg • Beta-Carotene 600 mcg (100 R.E.).

Triple Cod Liver Oil **-** GNC
Each capsule contains: Vitamin A (as cod liver oil) 1250 IU • Vitamin D (as cod liver oil) 135 IU • Vitamin E (as fish body oil) I IU • EPA (Eicosapentaenoic Acid) 173 mg • DHA (Docosahexaenoic Acid) 120 mg. Other Ingredients: Gelatin, Glycerin.

Triple Defense **-** Olympian Labs
Two capsules contain: Soy Isoflavone dried extract 100 mg • D-Glucarate 400 mg • Lycopene extract (5% Standardized Yielding 30 mg of pure Lycopene) 600 mg • Citrus Bioflavonoids 40 mg.

Triple Delicious High Protein Bar **-** Strength Systems USA
Each bar contains: Protein Blend: Whey Protein Isolate, Hydrolyzed Whey Protein, Calcium Caseinate, Soy Protein Isolate, Whey Protein Concentrate, Milk Protein Concentrate • Maltitol • Water • Glycerine • Hydrolyzed Gelatin • Lactitol • Fractionated Palm Kernal Oil • Almonds • Roasted Soybeans • Non-Fat Milk • Natural and Artificial Flavor • Cocoa • Modified Soybean Oil • Unsweetened Chocolate • Salt • Monoglycerides • Cream • Butter (cream, salt) • Soy Lecithin • Inulin • Sodium Phosphate • Carrageenan • Sucralose • Potassium Sorbate.

Triple Flex **-** Nature Made
Three tablets contain: Sodium 20 mg • Glucosamine Hydrochloride 1500 mg • Chondroitin Sulfate 1200 mg • MSM (methylsulfonylmethane) 375 mg. Other Ingredients: Cellulose Gel, Povidone, Croscarmellose Sodium, Hydroxypropyl Methylcellulose, Magnesium Stearate, Titanium Dioxide, Polyethylene Glycol, Triethyl Citrate, Polysorbate 80, Sodium Citrate.
See Editor's Note No. 15, page 2055.

Triple G Super Health **-** DreamPharm
Two capsules contain: Garlic 300 mg • Ginger 200 mg • Grape Seed extract 100 mg.

Triple Ginseng Rush **-** GNC
Each capsule contains: Korean Ginseng root (Panax ginseng) 200 mg • American Ginseng root extract (Panax quinquefolium) 200 mg • Siberian Ginseng root extract (Eleutherococcus senticosus) 200 mg • Guarana seed extract (Paullinia cupana) 100 mg. Other Ingredients: Gelatin.

Triple Lecithin 1200 **-** GNC
Each capsule contains: Chromium (as chromium picolinate) 100 mcg •High Choline Soy Lecithin (supplying phosphatidyl choline 420 mg) 1200 mg. Other Ingredients: Gelatin, Caramel Color, Titanium Dioxide (natural mineral whitener).

Triple Lecithin 1200 with Phosphatidyl Choline **-** GNC
Each capsule contains: High Choline Lecithin 1200 mg • Phosphatidyl Choline (as soy lecithin) 420 mg. Other Ingredients: Gelatin, Glycerin.

Triple Lecithin 400 **-** GNC
Each capsule contains: Vitamin E (as d-alpha tocopherol) 5 IU • High Choline Soy Lecithin (supplying phosphatidyl choline 140 mg) 400 mg. Other Ingredients: Gelatin, Glycerin, Rosemary oil (rosmariunus officinalis).

Triple Omega 3-6-9 Flax, Fish and Borage Oils **-** Vitamin World
Each softgel contains: Vitamin E (D-alpha tocopherol) 15 IU • Flaxseed Oil 1200 mg • Borage seed oil 1200 mg • Fish Oil (50% omega-3) 1200 mg • Omega-6 Fatty Acids 828 mg • Omega-9 Fatty Acids (oleic acid) 456 mg. Other Ingredients: Gelatin, Glycerin.

Triple Stack **-** Crystal Springs
Each tablet contains: Tribulis 250 mg • DHEA 50 mg • Androstenedione 50 mg • Saw Palmetto 200mg • Pygeum 100 mg.
See Editor's Note No. 47, page 2058.

Triple Strength Glucosamine 750 mg Chondroitin 600 mg **-** Vitamin World
Two caplets contain: Sodium (as chondroitin sulfate) 70 mg • Glucosamine Hydrochloride 1500 mg • Chondroitin Sulfate 1200 mg. Other Ingredients: Crospovidone, Beet Juice, Cellulose, Vegetable Magnesium Stearate.
See Editor's Note No. 15, page 2055.

Triple Whey Fuel **-** TwinLab
Blend of three key Whey Proteins: Micro-Filtered & Ion-Exchange Whey Protein Isolate (with ~57% Beta-Lactoglobulin, ~24% Alpha-Lactalbumin, ~12% Immunoglobulins, ~7% Minor Peptones & Lactoferrin) •modified molecular weight & partially predigested (hydrolyzed) Whey Protein (providing di-, tri-, oligo- & poly-peptides) • Whey Protein Concentrate enriched with Glutamine.

TripleFlex Triple Strength **-** Nature Made
Two caplets contain: Glucosamine Hydrochloride 1.5 g • Chondroitin Sulfate 1.2 g • Methylsulfonylmethane (MSM) 250 mg. Other Ingredients: Croscarmellose Sodium, Beet Powder, Silicon Dioxide, Hydroxypropyl Methylcellulose, Magnesium Stearate, Polyethylene Glycol.

Tropical Fruit Drinkable Yogurt **-** Stonyfield Farm
Each 10 fl oz bottle contains: Active Live Cultures: S. Thermophilus • L. Bulgaricus • L. Acidophilus • Bifidus • L. Casei • L. Reuteri. Ingredients: Cultured Pasturized Low Fat Milk • Organic Sugar • Organic Nonfat Dry Milk • Inulin • Pectin • Pumpkin Juice Concentrate • Carrot Juice Concentrate • Organic Banana Puree • Natural Flavors.

Tropical Noni **-** NutraMed
Morinda citrifolia.

Tropical Ola Loa **-** Ola Loa, LLC
Each packet contains: Vitamin C 1000 mg • Vitamin B1 1 mg • Vitamin B2 1 mg • Vitamin B3 10 mg • Vitamin B6 10 mg • Folic Acid 600 mcg • Vitamin B12 100 mcg • Pantothenic Acid 10 mg • Biotin 100 mcg • Vitamin D (D3) 200 IU • Vitamin E 30 IU • Vitamin K (K1) 20 mcg • Coenzyme Q10 25 mg • Vitamin A 1000 IU • Lipoic Acid 1 mg • Choline Bitartrate 10 mg • Potassium (bicarbonate) 200 mg • Sodium (bicarbonate) 27 mg • Calcium (carbonate, ascorbate) 29 mg • Magnesium (ascorbate) 25 mg • Zinc (picolinate) 1.5 mg • Manganese (picolinate) 1.5 mg • Copper (aspartate) 500 mcg • Molybdenum (trioxide) 75 mcg • Selenium (selenite) 50 mcg • Chromium (picolinate) 100 mcg • Potassium Iodide 50 mcg • Boron (citrate) 1 mg • N-Acetyl Cysteine (NAC) 50 mg • Arginine 100 mg • Lysine 100 mg • Glycine 1000 mg • TMG - Betaine 1000 mg • Glutamine 100 mg • Bromelain 10 mg • Pineapple Bioflavonoids 100 mg. Other Ingredients: Fructose, Citric Acid, Aspartic Acid, Tartaric Acid, Malic Acid, Grape Flavor, Pineapple Strawberry Flavor, Lemon Juice Flavor.

Some Brand Name Natural Products - What they Contain

www.NaturalDatabase.com contains MANY more listings than appear here.

TrueBlue Coral Calcium **-** CFU Distribution Co.
Each capsule contains: Calcium (from coral) 230 mg • Magnesium (from coral & chelated minerals) 51 mg • Vitamin D 400 IU • Malic Acid (from apples) 10 mg • Betaine HCl 5 mg • Vitamin C (as ascorbic acid) 5 mg • 73 Minerals from Coral 370 mg.

Trym Tone 1200 **-** Futurebiotics
Four tablets contain: L-Arginine HCl 2100 mg • L-Glycine 1800 mg • L-Lysine HCl 300 mg • Vitamin C 30 mg • Pyridoxine HCl 15 mg • Chromium (polynicotinate) 75 mcg.

T-SEPT **-** Dial Herbs
Bayberry • Goldenseal • Myrrh • Mineral Water.

T-SHK **-** Dial Herbs
Lobelia • Cayenne • Mineral Water.

T-SKT **-** Dial Herbs
Myrrh • White Poplar bark • Balsam.

T-SLC **-** Dial Herbs
Comfrey • Mullein • Peppermint • Chickweed • Lobelia • Cayenne.

T-SS **-** Dial Herbs
Damiana • Licorice • Ginseng • Passion flower • Cayenne.

T-THD **-** Dial Herbs
Kelp • Parsley • Irish Moss • Cayenne • Licorice • Dulse • Bayberry • Bugleweed.

T-ULC **-** Dial Herbs
Goldenseal • Cayenne • Myrrh • Ginger • Comfrey • Poke root • Yellow Dock.

Tulsi-Neem (soap) **-** Auromere Ayurvedic Soaps
Coconut oil • Palmyra oil • Rice Bran oil • Alkali • Water • Neem oil • Hydnocarpus (cactus) oil • Castor Oil • Tulsi (Holy Basil) • Rose Petals • Zedoary • Turmeric • Fenugreek • Psoralea corlifolia (Babchi Seed) • Peepal (Bodhi Tree) • Alangium salviifolium • Costus • Indian Sarsaparilla • Shiva Neem (variety of Neem) • Hibiscus.

Tum-Ease **-** The Herbalist
Catnip leaf • Fennel seed • Angelica root • Gentian root • Oregon Grape root • Ginger root.

Tumeric Extract **-** Nature's Way
Each capsule contains: Tumeric root 50 mg • Tumeric dried extract 450 mg. Other Ingredients: Cellulose, Gelatin, Silica.

Tums Calcium for Life Bone Health Calcium Supplement **-** GlaxoSmithKline (GSK)
Each tablet contains: Calcium Carbonate 500 mg. Other Ingredients: Sucrose, Corn Starch, Talc, Mineral Oil, Natural and Artificial Flavors, Adipic Acid, Sodium Polyphosphate, Red 40 Lake, Yellow 6 Lake, Yellow 5 Lake, Blue 1 Lake.

Turbo Charge Energy Formula (Ephedra Free) **-** Natural Balance
Each tablet contains: Proprietary Blend 985 mg: Guarana seed extract (contains caffeine), Korean Ginseng root standardized extract, Eleuthero root, Gotu Kola extract (aerial portion), Passion Flower extract (aerial portion), Wood Betony (aerial portion). Other Ingredients: Microcrystalline Cellulose, Silicon Dioxide, Cellulose Gum, Stearic Acid, Magnesium Stearate.

TurboShake, Choc-o-Blast **-** Advocare International
AdvoKids Protein Complex (calcium sodium caseinates, soy protein, L-lysine hydrochloride, whey protein isolate, L-glutamine) • Fructose • Maltodextrin • Cocoa powder • Guar Gum • Medium Chain Triglycerides • Calcium Phosphate • Potassium Chloride • Rice Syrup Solids • Cellulose • Magnesium Oxide • Natural Flavors • Artificial Flavors • Apple powder • Taurine • Calcium Ascorbate • Choline Citrate • Sodium Chloride • Oatgrass powder • Carrot powder • Vitamin E Acetate • Sucralose • Gum Acacia • Silicon Dioxide • Bromelain • Papain • Biotin • Boron Citrate • Niacinamide • Inositol • Folic Acid • Zinc Oxide • Selenomethionine • Copper Gluconate • Calcium Pantothenate • Vitamin A Palmitate • Vitamin K • Cholecalciferol • Chromium Polynicotinate (ChromeMate) • Manganese Carbonate • Pyridoxine Hydrochloride • Lactobacillus Acidophilus • Bifidobacterium Bifidus • Riboflavin • Thiamine Hydrochloride • Cyanocobalamin • Sodium Molybdate • Potassium Iodide.

TurboTrim Plus **-** Trim International
Each tablet contains: MaHuang • Guarana • Chromium Picolinate • Chitosan • Gymnema Sylvestre • Garcinia Cambogia • Vitamin E • Magnesium Chelate • Zinc Chelate • Proprietary Blend: Bee Pollen, Ginseng root, Ginger root, Lecithin, Bovine complex, Damiana herb, Sarsaparilla root, Goldenseal herb, Nettle leaf, Gotu Kola herb, Spirulina, Royal Jelly. Other Ingredients: Di-Calcium Phosphate, Magnesium Stearate, Stearic Acid.
See Editor's Note No. 30, page 2056.

T-VV **-** Dial Herbs
Oat Straw • Buckthorn • Yarrow • Brigham Tea • Witch Hazel • St. John's Wort • Cayenne.

Twinlab B-1 Caps **-** TwinLab
Each capsule contains: Thiamin (from thiamin monoitrate) 100 mg.

Two Trees Slippery Elm Lozenges **-** Thayers Natural Pharmaceuticals
Each lozenge contains: Slippery Elm Bark 150 mg. A pure all-natural Maple Sugar with Vegetable Stearate as a binder.

T-WRT **-** Dial Herbs
Garlic • Celandine • Mullein • Buckthorn.

Ty-Glute **-** Atrium Inc.
Each tablet contains: L-Glutamine 255 mg • L-Tyrosine 155 mg • Vitamin C 150 mg • Adrenal concentrate 45 mg.
See Editor's Note No. 14, page 2055.

T-YI **-** Dial Herbs
Echinacea • Goldenseal • Bayberry • Myrrh • Plantain • Slippery Elm • Wild Carrot.

UC - II **-** PhysioLogics
Each capsule contains: Undenatured Type II Collagen (from UC-II undenatured type II collagen complex 40 mg) 10 mg. Other Ingredients: Potassium Chloride, Cellulose (plant origin).

Udo's Choice Beyond Greens **-** Flora, Inc.
Each 1 tsp serving (8 g) contains: Udo's Choice perfected seed blend: Certified Organic Flax seed, Defatted Flax, Certified Organic Sunflower seed, Defatted Sunflower seed, Certified Organic Sesame seed, Defatted Sesame seed, Rice germ, Bran powder, Oat germ, Bran powder • Pines Barley Grass powder • Cracked Golden Flax seed • Pumpkin seed • Pines Alfalfa Grass powder • Rice bran • Dried Cane juice • Carrot • Soyforce Sprouted Soybeans • Tomato • Pines Oat Grass • Pines Rye Grass • Red Beet • Cinnamon • Peppermint • Ginger • Bilberry leaf • Spirulina • Bee pollen • Dulse • Chlorella • Broccoli • Parsley • Kelp • Hawthorne berry • Milk Thistle • Burdock root • Red Clover • Kale • Licorice root • Chrysanthemum • Yucca • Natural Almond flavor • Lemon Grass • Udo's Choice Digestive Enzyme blend: Protease, Lipase, Amylase, Cellulase, Maltase, Glucoamylase, Invertase, Pectinase, with Phytase, Lactase • Beet juice • American Ginseng • Ginkgo extract • Psyllium • Slippery Elm • Stevia leaf • Artichoke • Dandelion root • Dandelion leaf • Rosemary • Thyme • Sage • Standardized Grape seed extract.

Udo's Choice Fast Food Blend **-** Flora, Inc.
Certified Organic Flax • Sunflower & Sesame seeds • Pines Organic Cereal Grasses • Soyforce Powdered Sprouted Soybeans & "much more."

Udo's Choice Oil Blend **-** Flora, Inc.
Flax oil • Sunflower oil • Sesame oil • Medium Chain Triglycerides • Evening Primrose oil (12.6 mg GLA per tablespoon) • Rice germ &

Bran oil • Soy Lecithin • d-Alpha Tocopherol (natural Vitamin E) • Oat germ & Bran oil.

Udo's Choice Perfect Oil Blend **-** Flora, Inc.
Flax oil • sesame seed oil • Sunflower oil & other unrefined oils • medium triglycerides • Lecithin & d-alpha tocopherol.

Udo's Choice Super 5 **-** Flora, Inc.
Each tablet contains: 1 billion plus viable organisms of Lactobacillus acidophilus DDS-1 • B. bifidum • L. bulgaricus • S. thermophilus & L. salivarius in a base of: (Maltodextrin, Fructose & Ascorbic Acid).

Ultimate Aloe **-** Market America, Inc.
Whole Leaf Aloe Vera Linne gel • Purified Water • Ascorbic Acid • Sodium Benzoate • Potassium Sorbate • Citric Acid • Malic Acid • Caramel.

Ultimate Antioxidant II **-** Gary Null & Associates (GNA)
Three capsules contain: Citrus Bioflavonoid Complex 300 mg • Rutin 25 mg • Bilberry extract 25 mg • Red Wine Concentrate 25 mg • Grape Skin extract 200 mg • China Green Tea 200 mg • Beta Carotene 10000 IU • L-Glutathione 5 mg • L-Cysteine 200 mg • Vitamin C 500 mg • Vitamin E 200 IU • Selenium 10 mcg • Zinc Picolinate 25 mg • CoQ10 10 mg • NAC 25 mg • Alpha Lipoic Acid 100 mg • Ascorbyl Palmitate 100 mg • SOD 25 mg • Vitamin B6 10 mg • Copper Lysinate 2 mg • Taurine 50 mg • Quercetin 50 mg • Pycnogenol 5 mg • Licorice 25 mg • Broccoli 25 mg • Lutein 25 mg • Cabbage 25 mg • Carrot powder 25 mg • Milk Thistle 25 mg.

Ultimate Ascorbate C **-** Source Naturals
Vitamin C (from magnesium, potassium, calcium, zinc, & manganese ascorbates) 1000 mg • Calcium (as calcium ascorbate) 20 mg • Magnesium (as magnesium ascorbate) 32 mg • Zinc (as zinc ascorbate) 3 mg • Manganese (as manganese ascorbate) 1 mg • Potassium (as potassium ascorbate) 90 mg.

Ultimate Balance - Antioxidant Formula **-** Bioadvantex Pharma
Two caplets contain: N-Acetyl Cysteine (NAC) 700 mg • Alpha-Lipoic Acid 200 mg • Milk Thistle seed extract 200 mg

Ultimate Cleanse **-** Nature's Secret
Each tablet contains: Multi-Herb: Alfalfa Leaf • Fenugreek Seed • Ginger Root • Dandelion Root • Fennel Seed • Yarrow Flower • Hawthorne Berries • Horsetail Herb • Licorice Root • Marshmallow Root • Peppermint Leaf • Red Clover Tops • Red Raspberry Leaf • Safflower Oil • Scullcap Herb • Burdock Root • Chickweed Herb • Mullein Leaf • Papaya Leaf • Black Cohosh Root • Cayenne Fruit • Irish Moss • Pacific Kelp • Slippery Elm Bark • Yellow Dock Root • Plantain Herb • Echinacea Angustifolia Extract • Ginkgo Biloba Leaf Extract • Milk Thistle Extract. Multi-Fiber: Cascara Sagrada Bark • Fennel Seed • Psyllium Seed • Ginger Root • Acacia Gum • Alfalfa Leaf • Apple Pectin • Apple Powder • Barley Rice Fiber • Beet Root • Glucomannan • Karaya Gum • Peppermint Leaf • Lemon Peel • Oat Bran • Red Raspberry Leaf • Slippery Elm Bark • Shattered Cell Wall Chlorella • Lactobacillus Acidophilus (dairy free) • Guar Gum.

Ultimate Ester-C **-** Source Naturals
Each two tablets contain: Vitamin C (as magnesium, calcium, potassium, zinc, & manganese ascorbates) 2000 mg • Vitamin D (as cholecalciferol) 85 IU • Calcium (as calcium ascorbate & carbonate) 100 mg • Magnesium (as magnesium ascorbate & oxide) 100 mg • Zinc (as zinc ascorbate) 25 mg • Copper (as copper sebacate) 500 mcg • Manganese (as manganese ascorbate) 5 mg • Potassium (as potassium ascorbate & citrate) 99 mg • Bioflavonoids 250 mg • Rutin 31 mg • Hesperidin 30 mg.

Ultimate Eye Formula **-** Purity Products
Three capsules contain: Vitamin C (magnesium ascorbate) 360 mg • Vitamin E 50 IU • Vitamin B-6 10 mg • Vitamin B-12 500 mcg • Alpha-Lipoic Acid 150 mg • L-Taurine 250 mg • Bilberry fruit extract 120 mg • Lutein 10 mg • Wolfberry fruit powder 25 mg • Pomegranate fruit 50 mg • IP6 (inositol hexaphosphate) 150 mg • Soy Isoflavones 200 mg • Gamma Oryzanol 100 mg.

Ultimate Fiber **-** Nature's Secret
Psyllium husks, Slippery Elm bark, Acidophilus powder, Fructooligosaccharides.

Ultimate Green **-** Nature's Secret
Each packet contain: Shattered Cell Wall Chlorella • Hawaiian Blue-Green Algae • Barley Grass • Wheat Grass • Alfalfa • Spinach.

Ultimate H.A. Formula **-** Purity Products
Three capsules contain: Hyaluronic Acid 150 mg • Chondroitin Sulfate 300 mg • BioCell Collagen II 1500 mg.
See Editor's Note No. 15, page 2055.

Ultimate Iron **-** Enzymatic Therapy
Two softgels contain: Vitamin C (ascorbic acid) 120 mg • Folic Acid 400 mcg • Vitamin B12 (as cyanocobalamin) 200 mcg • Iron (as ferrous succinate) 50 mg • Liquid Liver Fractions (predigested soluble concentrate) 500 mg • Chlorophyll (fat-soluble) 10 mg. Other Ingredients: Soybean Oil, Gelatin, Glycerin, Beeswax, Lecithin.
See Editor's Note No. 14, page 2055.

Ultimate Libido Formula for Women **-** MD Healthline
Two capsules contain: Niacin 40 mg • Yohimbe Bark 500 mg • Dong Quai 150 mg • Sativari (Asparagus racemosus) 150 mg • Ashwagandha 100 mg • L-Tyrosine 100 mg • L-Histidine 66 mg • Tree Peony 4:1 Extract 50 mg • Royal Jelly 50 mg • Wild Yam 10:1 Extract 40 mg • Quebracho Bark 20 mg • Ginger Root 5:1 Extract 20 mg • Sundew 20 mg • Guarana 20 mg • Damiana 20 mg • DHEA 10 mg.

Ultimate Men's Peak Performance **-** Swanson
Each tablet contains: Vitamin E (as d-alpha tocopheryl succinate) 50 IU • Niacin 25 mg • Zinc (from zinc amino acid chelate) 7.5 mg • Yohimbe extract (2% yohimbine alkaloids) 250 mg • Tribulus Terrestris extract (40% steroidal saponins) 125 mg • Avena Sativa wild oats (5:1 extract) 50 mg • Cayenne Pepper 50 mg • Damiana leaf powder 50 mg • Ginger root powder 50 mg • Ginkgo Biloba leaf powder 50 mg • Ginseng extract (5% ginsenosides) 50 mg • Guarana extract (12.5% alkaloids) 50 mg • Hawthorn berry powder 50 mg • L-Arginine HCl 50 mg • Oyster extract 50 mg • Saw Palmetto berry powder 50 mg • Rhodiola Rosea extract (1% rosevin) 25 mg.

Ultimate Multi Plus **-** Nature's Secret
Contains over 90 vitamins, minerals, amino acids, antioxidants, herbs, superfoods, digestive enzymes and Herbalgest.

Ultimate Oil **-** Nature's Secret
Blend of oils that offer a mixture of the essential fatty acids, Omega 3 and Omega 6.

Ultimate Orange Powercaps **-** Next Nutrition
Three softgels contain: Magnesium 9.7 mg • L-Tyrosine 500 mg • Ma Huang whole plant 313 mg • Guarana seed 227 mg •Caffeine 200 mg •Proprietary Blend 100 mg: Sida Cordifolia root, Korean Ginseng root, Green Tea leaf, Coleus Forskohlii root, Orange Peel Bioflavonoids, Grapefruit extract, Cayenne Pepper. Other Ingredients: Soybean Oil, Gelatin, Glycerin Water, Titanium Dioxide, FD&C Yellow 6, FD&C Red 40.
See Editor's Note No. 30, page 2056.

Ultimate Performance Max Protein Bar - Vanilla Almond **-** Rexall - Sundown
Each bar contains: Protein 18 g • Vitamin A (as retinyl palmitate) 2500 IU • Vitamin C 30 mg • Vitamin D (as cholecalciferol) 200 IU • Vitamin E (as dl-alpha-tocopheryl acetate) 15 IU • Thiamin (as thiamine HCl) 0.75 mg • Riboflavin (Vitamin B-2) 0.85 mg • Niacin (as niacinamide) 10 mg • Vitamin B-6 (as pyridoxine HCl) 1 mg • Folic Acid 200 mcg • Vitamin B-12 (as cyanocobalamin) 3 mcg • Biotin 150 mcg • Pantothenic Acid (as calcium d-pantothenate) 5 mg • Calcium 500 mg • Iron (as ferrous fumarate) 9 mg • Phosphorus 700 mg • Iodine (as potassium iodide) 75 mcg • Magnesium (as

magnesium oxide) 200 mg • Zinc (as zinc oxide) 7.5 mg • Copper (as copper gluconate) 1 mg • Chromium (as chromium picolinate) 5 mcg • Sodium 110 mg. Other Ingredients: Brown Rice Syrup, Cocoa Coating (sugar, fractionated palm kernel oil, cocoa powder, whey powder, nonfat dry milk powder, soy lecithin, natural vanilla flavor), Whey Protein Isolate, High Fructose Corn Syrup, Whey Protein Concentrate, Crystaline Fructose, Almond Butter, Natural flavor, Oat Fiber, Dicalcium Phosphate, L-Glutamine, Taurine.

Ultimate Plenamins **-** Rexall - Sundown
Each tablet contains: Vitamin A (from retinyl acetate) 5000 IU • Vitamin C (as niacinamide ascorbate and ascorbic acid) 120 mg • Vitamin D (as cholecalciferol) 400 IU • Vitamin E (as dl-alpha-tocopheryl acetate and d-alpha-tocopheryl acid succinate) 30 IU • Vitamin K (as phytonadione) 25 mcg • Thiamin (as thiamin HCl) 3 mg • Riboflavin (vitamin B-2) 3.4 mg • Niacin (from niacinamide ascorbate) 20 mg • Vitamin B-6 (from pyridoxine HCl) 4 mg • Folic Acid 400 mcg • Vitamin B-12 (as cyanocobalamin) 25 mcg • Biotin 50 mcg • Pantothenic Acid (from d-calcium pantothenate) 10 mg • Calcium (from dicalcium phosphate and calcium carbonate) 200 mg • Iron (from ferrous fumarate) 18 mg • Phosphorus (as dicalcium phosphate) 125 mg • Iodine (from potassium iodide) 150 mcg • Magnesium (from magnesium oxide) 100 mg • Zinc (from zinc sulfate) 15 mg • Selenium (from sodium selenate) 25 mcg • Copper (from cupric oxide) 2 mg • Manganese (from manganese sulfate) 5 mg • Chromium (from chromium chloride) 15 mcg • Molybdenum (from sodium molybdate) 25 mcg • Potassium (from potassium chloride) 30 mg • Vanadium (from vanadium aspartate) 10 mcg • Silicon (from silicon dioxide) 10 mcg • Nickel (from nickel sulfate) 5 mcg • PABA (para-aminobenzoic acid) 1 mg • Choline Bitartrate 1 mg • Inositol 100 mcg • Bee Pollen 25 mg • Siberian Ginseng root 25 mg • Fish Oil (EPA [eicosapentaenoic acid] 18 mg, DHA [docosahexaenoic acid] 12 mg) 100 mg • Plenamin nutritional catalyst base: Rose Hips and seed extract, Kelp, Soy Lecithin, Soy protein isolate, Wheat Germ, Hesperidin, Rutin, Acerola fruit extract, Citrus Bioflavonoids 3.5 mg. Other Ingredients: Cellulose, Croscarmellose sodium, Hydroxypropyl methylcellulose, Magnesium stearate, PEG, Red 40 lake, Blue 2 lake, Titanium dioxide, Polysorbate 80, Beta-carotene.

Ultimate Prostate Formula **-** Purity Products
Three capsules contain: Vitamin E 60 IU • Vitamin B-6 50 mg • Zinc (zinc citrate) 15 mg • Selenium (selenomethionine) 50 mcg • Saw Palmetto extract 575 mg • Pygeum extract 310 mg • Nettle root extract 300 mg • Lycopene 7 mg • L-Alanine 400 mg • Glutamic Acid 400 mg • Glycine 400 mg • Quercetin 100 mg.

Ultimate Prostate Support **-** NorthStar Nutritionals
Each two softgel capsules contain: Saw Palmetto berry extract (85-90% fatty acids) 160 mg • Pygeum Africanum 50 mg • Nettle root extract 150 mg • Lycopene 5 mg • Vitamin E (d-alpha tocopherol, natural) 100 mg • Selenium 5 mcg • Zinc Arginate 7.5 mg.

Ultimate Sleep System **-** Rainbow Light
Two tablets contain: Valerian rhizome (standardized to 0.8% valernic acid) 160 mg • Kava Kava root (standardized to 30% kavalactones) 40 mg • Spirulina 100 mg • 4:1 Custom Herbal extracts: [Valerian rhizome, Hops strobiles, Kava Kava root, Orange oil, Passion flower herb, Valerian oil, Reishi fruiting body (providing 3200 mg herbal powder equivalent)] 800 mg. Nutritional Cofactors: N-Acetyl-L-Carnitine (NAC) 10 mg • Niacin/Niacinamide (Vitamin B3) 115 mg • Magnesium (Oxide, Pyroglutamate) 47.3 mg • Chromium (Polynicotinate) 30 mcg.

Ultimate Wild Yam **-** Swanson
Four tablets contain: Yam extract 12 mg • Avena sativa 2 mg • Camellia sinensis 2 mg • Crataegus oxyacantha 2 mg • Dioscorea Quat 2 mg • Extracts of Barbasco 2 mg • Lactase 2 mg • Licorice root 2 mg • Medicago sativa 2 mg • Prunus SPP 2 mg • Smilax aristolochiaefolia 2 mg • Soy extracts 2 mg.

Ultimate Women's Intimate Performance **-** Swanson
Each tablet contains: Niacin 8.3 mg • Ginseng extract (6% ginsenosides) 100 mg • Avena Sativa oats (5:1 extract) 33.3 mg • Cayenne pepper 33.3 mg • Damiana leaf powder 33.3 mg • Dong Quai extract (1% ligustilides) 33.3 mg • Ginger root powder 33.3 mg • Guarana extract (12.5% alkaloids) 33.3 mg • L-Arginine HCl 33.3 mg • Licorice extract (12% glycyrrhizic acid) 33.3 mg • Muira Puama root 33.3 mg • Agnus Castus (chasteberry) extract (0.5% agnusides) 8.3 mg • Black Cohosh extract (2.5% triterpene glycosides) 8.3 mg • Ovary extract 8.3 mg.
See Editor's Note No. 14, page 2055.

Ultimate Zinc-C Lozenges **-** Now
Each lozenge contains: Vitamin A (from Fish Liver oil) 1000 IU • Vitamin C (as Ascorbic Acid) 150 mg • Zinc (as Zinc Gluconate) 24 mg • Echinacea root powder 100 mg • Bee Propolis 100 mg • Slippery Elm bark powder (Ulmus fulva) 25 mg.

Ultra 30/20 Fish oil **-** Health From The Sun
Two capsules contain: Vitamin E 4 IU • Omega-3 Fatty Acids 1.2 g [EPA (600 mg) DHA (400 mg)]. Ingredients: All natural Fish Body oil concentrate, Gelatin, Glycerine, Mixed Tocopherols.

Ultra Antioxidant **-** Pro Health
Two capsules contain: Vitamin A (as beta carotene, retinyl palmitate) 5000 IU • Vitamin C (as ascorbic acid, Ester C calcium ascorbate) 1000 mg • Vitamin E (as natural d-alpha-tocopheryl succinate) 400 IU • Zinc (as Optizinc) 10 mg • Selenium (as l-selenomethionine) 100 mcg • Alpha Lipoic Acid 100 mg • Green Tea leaf extract (camellia var. sinensis, 75% polyphenols (37.5 mg)) 50 mg • Grapeseed extract (vitis vinifera, inner core of fruit, 95% proanthocyanidins (28.5 mg)) 30 mg • Lutein extract (from marigold flowers, 5% lutein (1.5 mg)) 30 mg • Lycopene extract (from tomatoes as Lycobeads, 1% lycopene (0.3 mg)) 30 mg • N-Acetyl Cysteine 30 mg • Odorless garlic bulb powder (allium sativa) 30 mg • Quercetin Dihydrate 30 mg • L-Glutathione 20 mg • Coenzyme Q10 10 mg. Other Ingredients: Gelatin, Water, Magnesium Stearate, Silicon Dioxide, Hydrolyzed Gelatin, Vegetable Oil and Oleoresin, Sucrose, Corn Starch Water, Ascorbyl Palmitate, Natural Tocopherol.

Ultra B-Complex High Potency with Folic Acid **-** Pro Health
Each capsule contains: Thiamin (vitamin B1, as thiamine HCl) 100 mg • Riboflavin (vitamin B2) 100 mg • Niacin (vitamin B3, as niacinamide) 100 mg • Vitamin B6 (as pyridoxine HCl) 100 mg • Folate (as folic acid) 400 mcg • Vitamin B12 (as cyanocobalamin) 100 mcg • Biotin 100 mcg • Pantothenic Acid (as d-calcium pantothenate) 100 mg • Choline (as choline bitartrate) 47 mg • Inositol 100 mg • PABA (para-aminobenzoic acid) 100 mg. Other Ingredients: Gelatin, Water, Magnesium Stearate, Silicon Dioxide.

Ultra Beauty Formula **-** Leiner Health Products
Two tablets contain: Biotin 266 mcg • Folate 266 mcg • Vitamin E (Mixed Tocopherols) 20 IU • Zinc Gluconate 10 mg • Thiamin (Vitamin B1) 6.6 mg • Calcium Carbonate 400 mg • Riboflavin (Vitamin B2) 6.6 mg • Manganese Oxide 6.6 mg • Vitamin B6 6.6 mg • Magnesium Oxide 133 mg • Vitamin D 133 IU • Iron 4 mg • Selenium 16 mcg • Pantothenic Acid 20 mg • Phosphorus 200 mg • Vitamin B12 10 mcg • Niacin 33 mg • Vitamin A 6666 IU • Vitamin C (Ascorbic Acid) 80 mg • Iodine 150 mcg • Betaine 33 mg • Bioflavonoids 33 mg • Choline Bitartrate 100 mg • Inositol 40 mg • L-Cysteine 680 mcg • PABA 33 mg • Ribonucleic Acid 40 mg • Rutin 16 mg. Other Ingredients: Dicalcium Phosphate, Cellulose, Stearic Acid, Croscarmellose Sodium, Sodium Starch Glycolate. In a base containing: Asparagus, Echinacea, Horsetail, L-Methionine, Gelatin, Oat Straw, and Papain.

Ultra Bone Balance **-** Source Naturals
Four tablets contain: Vitamin C (as Calcium, Magnesium, Manganese Ascorbates) 52 mg • Vitamin D (as Cholecalciferol) 300 IU • Vitamin B6 (as Pyridoxine HCl) 20 mg • Folate (as Folic Acid) 200 mcg • Calcium (as Calcium Carbonate, Citrate, Ethanolamine Phosphate, Malate, Ascorbate) 1200 mg • Magnesium (as Magnesium Oxide,

Citrate, Fumarate, Malate, Ascorbate) 600 mg • Zinc (as Zinc Chelate) 7.5 mg • Copper (as Copper Sebacate) 1 mg • Manganese (as Manganese Ascorbate) 6 mg • Ipriflavone (Ostivone) 600 mg • Genistein Rich Soy concentrate (Yielding 50 mg total isoflavones) 125 mg • Silica (from Horsetail silica extract) 10 mg • Boron (as Boron Chelate) 3 mg.

Ultra Carb **-** Sterling-Grant Laboratories
Two tablets contain: Chromium (as chromium dinicotinate glycinate) 100 mcg • Phaseolamin Northern White Kidney Bean extract 700 mg • Green Tea leaf extract (50% catechins, 35% polyphenols) 200 mg. Other Ingredients: Gelatin, Dicalcium Phosphate, Magnesium Stearate, Silica.

Ultra Carbo Blocker 2000 **-** Tiffin International, Inc.
Each capsule contains: Chromium 100 mcg • Proprietary Blend 200 mg: Phaseolus Vulgaris, Gymnema Sylvestre. Other Ingredients: Gelatin, Sodium Lauryl Sulfate, Colloidal Silicon Dioxide, Purified Water.
See Editor's Note No. 37, page 2057.

Ultra Carbo Blocker 3000 **-** PotentHerbs
Each capsule contains: Chromium (as chromium polynicotinate) 100 mcg • Proprietary Blend 450 mg: Phaseolus Vulgaris (Phase 2), Gymnema Sylvestre. Other Ingredients: Kosher Capsules, Silicon Dioxide.
See Editor's Note No. 37, page 2057.

Ultra Carotenoid Complex **-** The Vitamin Shoppe
Each softgel contains: Phytofluene 0.026 mg • Lycopene (LYC-O-MATO) 5 mg • Lutein 5 mg • Beta-carotene (25000 IU Vitamin A) 15 mg • Alpha-carotene (833 IU Vitamin A) 1 mg • Zeaxanthin 0.24 mg • Phytoene 0.055 mg.

Ultra Cee 500 mg **-** Puritan's Pride
Each capsule contains: Vitamin C 500 mg.

Ultra Chondroitin 600 **-** Nature's Plus
Each protein coated tablet contains: Chondroitin Sulfate A - CSA (Glucuronic, N-Acetyl-D-Galactosamine 4-Sulfate) 600 mg • Bioperine bioavailability enhancing thermonutrient, (95% 1-piperoylpiperdine) 2.5 mg.
See Editor's Note No. 15, page 2055.

Ultra Chroma Slim Plan with Biotrol - Richardson Labs - Rexall - Sundown
Three caplets contain: Manganese (as manganese picolinate) 1.25 mg • Chromium (as chromium picolinate) 200 mcg • Blood Sugar Support blend 10.4 mg: Manganese Picolinate, Chromium Picolinate, Vanadium (as vanadyl sulfate) 60 mcg 10.4 mg • Lipotropic & Metabolic Support blend 1.1 grams: Choline Bitartrate, L-Carnitine Tartrate • Appetite Control & Neurotransmitter Support blend 1.6 grams: Inulin, L-Phenylalanine, St. John's Wort extract leaves & flowers standardized to 0.3% hypercin, Capsicum fruit extract 10:1, Peppermint oil • Energy Support blend 252 mg: Siberian Ginseng root, Calcium Pyruvate. Other Ingredients: Cellulose, Modified Cellulose Gum, Stearic Acid, Silica, Hydroxypropyl Methylcellulose, Magnesium Stearate, Peppermint leaves.

Ultra Chromium GTF **-** Source Naturals
Each tablet contains: Chromium GTF (100 mcg of ChromeMate Chromium Polynicotinate and 100 mcg of Chromium Picolinate) 200 mcg • Niacin (Polynicotinate) 9 mg.

Ultra Chromium Picolinate **-** The Vitamin Shoppe
Each capsule contains: Chromium Picolinate, a compound of yeast-free trivalent chromium and picolinic acid 500 mcg.

Ultra Chromium Picolinate 500 **-** Source Naturals
Each tablet contains: Trivalent Chromium (from Chromax brand of yeast-free chromium picolinate) 500 mcg.

Ultra Colloidal Silver **-** Olympia Nutrition
Deionized Water • Silver (10 ppm).

Ultra CoQ10 **-** Nature's Plus
Each softgel contains: Coenzyme Q10 (ubiquinone) 100 mg.

Ultra Cranberry 1000 **-** Nature's Plus
Each protein coated tablet contains: Cranberry concentrate 45X 1000 mg • Vitamin C corn free 100 mg. In a highly active herbal base of Juniper berries (Juniperus communis), Parsley (Petroselinum crispum), Uva Ursi (Arctostaphylos uva ursi) & Red Clover (Trifolium pratense).

Ultra DHA 50 **-** Health From The Sun
Two capsules contain: Vitamin E 4 IU • Omega-3 Fatty Acids 700 mg [DHA (425 mg) EPA (200 mg)]. Ingredients: All natural Fish Body oil concentrate, Gelatin, Glycerine, Mixed Tocopherols.

Ultra Diet Pep **-** Natural Balance
Each tablet contains: Potassium (as chloride) 50 mg • Vitamin B6 (as pyridoxine HCl) 10 mg • Vitamin B12 (as cyanocobalamin) 6 mcg • Pantothenic Acid (as d-calcium pantothenate) 25 mg • Iodine (from kelp) 80 mcg • DynaChrome Chromium (as arginate/chelidamate) 120 mcg • Proprietary Blend 750 mg: Green Tea leaf extract (contains caffeine), L-Tyrosine, Kelp leaf, Dandelion leaf, Ginger root, Passion flower aerial portion extract. Other Ingredients: Microcrystalline Cellulose, Modified Cellulose Gum, Silicon Dioxide, Stearic Acid, Magnesium Stearate.

Ultra Diet Pep 2000 **-** Natural Balance
Two capsules contain: Vitamin C (ascorbic acid) 30 mg • Vitamin B6 (pyridoxine HCl) 7.5 mg • Pantothenic Acid (d-calcium pantothenate) 25 mg • DynaChrome Chromium (arginate/chelidamate) 100 mcg • Citrin (garcinia cambogia fruit extract standardized to 50% HCA) 750 mg • Proprietary Blend 495 mg: Kola Nut seed extract (contains caffeine), Siberian Ginseng root, Guarana seed extract (contains caffeine), Wild Yam rhizome, Dandelion leaf, standardized Kelp (thallus), Passion flower aerial portion extract, Licorice root, Gotu Kola aerial portion extract • Choline Bitartrate 25 mg • Inositol 25 mg. Other Ingredients: Gelatin, Magnesium Stearate, Silicon Dioxide.

Ultra Diet-Phen **-** Source Naturals
Each two tablets contain: St. John's Wort (Hypericum perforatum) standardized extract 0.3 %, yielding 1.2 of Hypericin 400 mg • Bitter Orange peel standardized extract, yielding 24 mg of Synepherine 570 mg • Green Tea standardized extract, yielidng 40 mg of Polypheols and 10 mg of Caffeine 100 mg • L-Phenylalanine 500 mg • Cayenne fruit 150 mg • Piper nigrum seed 150 mg • Mustard Seed 150 mg • Ginger root 150 mg • Dandelion Leaf 100 mg • Dandelion Root 100 mg • Chromium (300 mcg ChromeMate Polynicotinate and 100 mcg Chromium Picolinate) 400 mcg.
See Editor's Note No. 40, page 2058.

Ultra Diet-Phen Calm Mood Night Formula **-** Source Naturals
Each tablet contains: Vitamin C (as zinc ascorbate) 54 mg • Vitamin B6 (as pyridoxine HCl) 10 mg • Folate (as folic acid) 100 mcg • Magnesium (as magnesium taurinate) 5 mg • Zinc (as zinc ascorbate) 10 mg • St. John's Wort leaf/flower extract (standardized to 0.3% yielding 1.5 mg hypericin) 500 mg • L-Glutamine 150 mg • GABA (gamma amino butyric acid) 50 mg • Valerian root extract (0.8%) 50 mg • Lemon Balm leaf 50 mg • L-Carnitine (as l-carnitine l-tartrate) 25 mg • Taurine (as magnesium taurinate) 22 mg. Other Ingredients: Dibasic Calcium Phosphate, Stearic Acid, Colloidal Silicon Dioxide, Modified Cellulose Gum, Magnesium Stearate.

Ultra Fuel **-** TwinLab
Each 16 ounce serving contains: Carbohydrates 100 g • Carbohydrate & Energy Metabolizers including Chromium • Stress B Vitamins • Vitamin C.

Ultra Garlite **-** Nature's Plus
Each tablet contains: Deodorized Garlic (equivalent to a minimum of 2.5 times its weight in fresh garlic) 1000 mg.

Some Brand Name Natural Products - What they Contain
www.NaturalDatabase.com contains MANY more listings than appear here.

Ultra H-3 **-** Uni Key Health Systems, Inc.
Each tablet contains: Procaine HCl 100 mg • Ascorbic Acid 25 mg • Citric Acid 25 mg • Niacin 16 mg • Folic Acid 0.4 mg • Biotin 0.3 mg • Potassium 11 mg • Magnesium 4 mg • Proprietary Blend 25 mg: Ginkgo Biloba 25:1 standardized extract, Bilberry 25:1 standardized extract.

Ultra Hair **-** Nature's Plus
Two tablets contain: Vitamin C with Rose Hips 500 mg • Pantothenic Acid 500 mg • Inositol 500 mg • Choline (Bitartrate) 210 mg • L-Cysteine free form amino acid 100 mg • Vitamin B6 (Pyridoxine HCL) 100 mg • Vitamin B2 (Riboflavin) 100 mg • PABA (Para-aminobenzoic acid) 100 mg • Vitamin B1 (Thiamine) 30 mg • Niacinamide 30 mg • Zinc (Amino Acid Chelate) 5 mg • Vitamin A (Beta Carotene) 10000 IU • Biotin 2000 mcg • Folic Acid 400 mcg. In a natural base of unsaturated fatty acids from safflower oil, rice bran & spirulina, naturally rich in RNA, DNA, amino acids & trace minerals.

Ultra Harmony - Wise Women Essentials
Purified Water • Wild Yam extract • Chaste Tree berry (vitex) • Apricot kernal oil • Jojoba oil • Aloe Vera • Retinyl Palmitate (vitamin A) • Tocopheryl Acetate (vitamin E) • Calciforal (vitamin D).

Ultra High Carb **-** The Sports Nutrition Source, Inc.
Four level scoops contain: Biotin 300 mcg • Chromium 200 mcg • Vitamin B-1 1.5 mg • Vitamin B-2 1.7 mg • Vitamin B-3 20 mg • Vitamin B-6 2 mg • Pantothenic Acid 100 mg • Vitamin C 60 mg • Potassium (from soluble potassium phosphate) 99 mg • Magnesium (from magnesium succinate) 25 mg.

Ultra Inosine **-** Source Naturals
Two tablets contain: Vitamin C (Potassium and Sodium Ascorbates) 350 mg • Calcium (Carbonate) 100 mg • Vitamin B6 (Pyridoxine HCl) 10 mg • Magnesium (Oxide, Aspartate) 100 mg • Vitamin B5 (Pantothenic Acid) 50 mg • Potassium (Citrate, Ascorbate and Aspartate) 99 mg • Sodium (Ascorbate) 20 mg • Inosine (Pure Crystalline) 1000 mg • Aspartic Acid (Potassium and Magnesium Aspartates and L-Aspartic Acid) 200 mg • Branched Chain Amino Acids (BCAAs) (L-Leucine 100 mg, L-Isoleucine 30 mg, L-Valine 44 mg) 174 mg • L-Carnitine L-Tartrate 20 mg • L-Lysine (HCl) 60 mg • Glycine 60 mg • Bee Pollen 200 mg • Octacosanol 4000 mcg • Spirulina 70 mg • Siberian Ginseng 100 mg • Tienchi Ginseng 100 mg.

Ultra Joint Response **-** Source Naturals
Three tablets contain: Vitamin A 5000 IU • Vitamin C 250 mg • Niacinamide 50 mg • Vitamin B6 12.5 mg • Zinc 15 mg • Selenium 100 mcg • Copper 1 mg • Manganese 10 mg • Molybdenum 130 mcg • MSM 1125 mg • Glucosamine Sulfate 900 mg • Boswellia serrata extract 321 mg • Quercetin 150 mg • Horse Chestnut extract 100 mg • Turmeric root extract 50 mg • Stinging Nettle leaf extract 50 mg • Ashwagandha root extract 50 mg • N-Acetyl Cysteine 50 mg • Sea Cucumber 40 mg • Grape Seed extract 25 mg • Aloe Vera whole leaf concentrate 25 mg • Black Pepper fruit extract 1 mg.

Ultra KLB6 **-** Puritan's Pride
Three tablets contain: Lecithin 1200 mg • Vitamin B6 (Pyridoxine HCl) 50 mg • Kelp powder 100 mg • Cider Vinegar 240 mg.

Ultra Lean **-** Schiff
Two tablets contains: Garcinia cambogia extract (min. 50% HCA) 500 mg • Dandelion Root 4:1 extract (Taraxacum officinate) 100 mg • Horsetail standardized extract (10% silicic acid, 6.3% organic silica - from Springtime Equisetum arvense) 50 mg • Juniper Berries 4:1 extract (Juniper communis) 50 mg • Cayenne (oleoresin capsium 6:1 extract from capsicum frutescens) 25 mg • Betaine HCl 50 mg • Iodine (Norwegian kelp) 150 mcg • Potassium (glycerophosphate) 25 mg • Magnesium (glycinate) 40 mg • Chromium (picolinate) 200 mcg.

Ultra Lipo-Plex **-** Nature's Plus
Two tablets contain: Choline Bitartrate equivalent to 1000 mg of choline 2381 mg • Inositol 1000 mg • L-Methionine free form amino acid 500 mg • Vitamin B6 (Pyridoxine HCL) 100 mg. In a natural herbal base containing Dandelion root, Fennel seed, Barberry bark, Parsley, Capsicum & Ginger.

Ultra Lycopene, Advanced Heart Health Capsules **-** Natrol
Each capsule contains: Vitamin E (as d-alpha-tocopheryl acid succinate) 400 IU • Lycopene (from natural tomato powder) 4 mg. Other Ingredients: Rice Powder, Gelatin.

Ultra Max 46 **-** Puritan's Pride
Each tablet contains: Vitamin A (13% as beta-carotene) 7,500 IU • Vitamin D 400 IU • Vitamin K 10 mcg • Thiamine (Vitamin B-1) 50 mg • Riboflavin (Vitamin B-2) 50 mg • Niacin 50 mg • Vitamin B-6 50 mg • Folic Acid 400 mcg • Vitamin B-12 50 mcg • Biotin 300 mcg • Pantothenic Acid 50 mg • Calcium 106 mg • Iron 9 mg • Iodine 150 mcg • Magnesium 100 mg • Zinc 50 mg • Selenium 50 mcg • Copper 1 mg • Manganese 5 mg • Chromium 50 mcg • Sodium 5 mg • Potassium 50 mg • Choline Bitartrate 50 mg • PABA (para-aminobenzoic acid) 25 mg • Inositol 10 mg.

Ultra Mega - GNC Women's **-** GNC
Two tablets contain: Vitamin A (50% as beta-carotene;50% as retinyl acetate) 10,000 IU • Vitamin C (as ascorbic acid) 200 mg • Vitamin D (as cholecalciferol) 400 IU • Vitamin E (as d-alpha tocopheryl acetate) 100 IU • Vitamin K (as phytonadione) 75 mcg • Thiamin B1 (as thiamin mononitrate) 80 mg • Riboflavin B2 80 mg • Niacin B3 (as niacin and niacinamide) 80 mg • Vitamin B6 (as pyridoxine hydrochloride) 80 mg • Folate (folic acid, folacin) 400 mcg • Vitamin B12 (as cyanocobalamin) 80 mcg • Biotin 80 mcg • Pantothenic Acid (as calcium d-pantothenate) 80 mg • Calcium (as calcium carbonate) 500 mg • Iron (as hydrolyzed protein chelate) 27 mg • Iodine (as kelp) 150 mcg • Magnesium (as magnesium oxide) 200 mg • Zinc (as zinc oxide) 15 mg • Selenium (as hydrolyzed protein chelate) 100 mcg • Copper (as hydrolyzed protein chelate) 2 mg • Manganese (as hydrolyzed protein chelate) 5 mg • Chromium (as hydrolyzed protein chelate) 100 mcg • Molybdenum (as hydrolyzed protein chelate) 50 mcg • Boron (as hydrolyzed protein chelate) 2 mcg • Dong Quai Root Powder (angelica sinensis) 50 mg • Bee Pollen Powder 25 mg • Citrus Bioflavonoids Complex 25 mg • Choline (as choline bitartrate) 10 mg • Cranberry Concentrate (vaccinium macrocarpon) 10 mg • Para-Aminobenzoic Acid 10 mg • Royal Jelly 5 mg • Silica (as hydrolyzed protein chelate) 2 mg • Boron (as hydrolyzed protein chelate) 2 mg • Red Raspberry Leaves (rubus idaeus) 2 mg • Lutein 500 mcg • Inositol 10 mcg. Other Ingredients: Cellulose, Rice Protein Chelate, Titanium Dioxide (natural mineral whitener), Vegetable Acetoglycerides, Rose Hips Powder (rosina canina), Acerola, Chlorophyll.

Ultra Mega Gold Without Iron Timed Release **-** GNC
Two tablets contain: Vitamin A (75% as Betatene Beta-Carotene; 25% as Acetate) 20,000 IU • Vitamin C (as Ascorbic Acid) 500 mg • Vitamin D (as Cholecalciferol) 400 IU • Vitamin E (as d-alpha Tocopheryl Succinate) 300 IU • Thiamin (as Thiamin Mononitrate) 100 mg • Riboflavin 100 mg • Niacin (as Niacinamide) 100 mg • Vitamin B6 (as Pyridoxine Hydrochloride) 100 mg • Folate, Folic Acid, Folacin 400 mcg • Vitamin B12 (as Cyanocobalamin) 150 mcg • Biotin 100 mcg • Pantothenic Acid (as Calcium d-Pantothenate) 100 mg • Calcium (as Calcium Carbonate) 50 mg • Iodine (as Kelp) 100 mcg • Magnesium (as Magnesium Oxide) 50 mg • Zinc (as Zinc Oxide) 15 mg • Selenium (as Selenium Yeast) 150 mcg • Copper (as Cupric Oxide) 2 mg • Maganese (as Manganese Gluconate) 10 mg • Chromium (as GTF Chromium Yeast) 100 mcg • Molybdenum (as Molybdenum Yeast) 150 mcg • Potassium (as Potassium Chloride) 10 mg • Boron (as Boron Gluconate) 1 mg • Chlorine Bitartrate 50 mg • Inositol 25 mg • Para-Aminobenzoid Acid (PABA) 50 mg • Trimethylglycine (TMG) 25 mg • Citrus Bioflavanoid Complex 25 mg • Rutin Powder 10 mg • Hesperidin Complex 5 mg • Quercetin Dihydrate 10 mg • Natural Carotenoid Complex 15 mg • N-Acetyl-L-

Cysteine (NAC) 10.5 mg • Amylase 10 mg • Lipase 5 mg • Protease 2 mg • Cellulase 5 mg • Lycopene 200 mcg • Alpha-lipoic Acid 4.5 mg • Green Tea Leaves (Camellia sinensis) 15 mg. Other Ingredients: Cellulose, Vegetable Actoglycerides, Titanium Dioxide, Chlorophyll.

***Ultra Mega Vite Multiple* - Nature's Life**
Each tablet contains: Vitamin A (Fish Liver oil) 10000 IU • Vitamin D (as Vitamin D3) (Cholecalciferol) 400 IU • Vitamin E (d-Alpha Tocopherol) 200 IU • Vitamin B1 (Thiamine Mononitrate) 100 mg • Vitamin B2 100 mg • Vitamin B3 (Niacinamide) 100 mg • Vitamin B6 (Pyridoxine HCl • Pyridoxal 5'-Phosphate) 100 mg • Vitamin B12 (Cobalamin concentrate) 100 mg • Folic Acid 400 mcg • Biotin 300 mcg • Pantothenic Acid (d-Calcium Pantothenate) 100 mg • Inositol 10 mg • Choline (Bitartrate) 10 mg • PABA (Para Aminobenzoic Acid) 10 mg • Vitamin C 300 mg • Lemon Bioflavonoids (TESTLAB 50% Flavonoids) 50 mg • Rutin 25 mg • Hesperidin Complex (10% Flavonoids) 25 mg • Boron (Citrate) 25 mcg • Calcium (Carbonate, Citrate/Malate) 100 mg • Chromium (Amino-Nicotinate) 100 mcg • Copper (Gluconate, Citrate) 1 mg • Iodine (Potassium) 25 mcg • Iron (Fumerate, Peptonate) 10 mg • Magnesium (Oxide, Citrate) 60 mg • Manganese (Citrate, Gluconate) 5 mg • Molybdenum (Molybdate) 25 mcg • Potassium (Citrate) 15 mg • Selenium (Yeast) 50 mcg • Silicon (Dioxide) 10 mg • Vanadium (Sulfate) 25 mcg • Zinc (Citrate) 20 mg • Chlorophyll 5 mg • Betaine HCl 30 mg • Glutamic Acid HCl 30 mg • Nature's Life Greens 20 mg.

***Ultra Mega without Iron - GNC Women's* - GNC**
Two tablets contain: Vitamin A (50% as beta-carotene; 50% as retinyl acetate) 10,000 IU • Vitamin C (as ascorbic acid) 200 mg • Vitamin D (as cholecalciferol) 400 IU • Vitamin E (as d-alpha tocopheryl acetate) 100 IU • Vitamin K (as phytonadione) 75 mcg • Thiamin B1 (as thiamin mononitrate) 80 mg • Riboflavin B2 (vitamin B2) 80 mg • Niacin B3 (as niacin and niacinamide) 80 mg • Vitamin B6 (as pyridoxine hydrochloride) 80 mg • Folate (folic acid, folacin) 400 mcg • Vitamin B12 (as cyanocobalamin) 80 mcg • Biotin 80 mcg • Pantothenic Acid (as calcium d-pantothenate) 80 mg • Calcium (as calcium carbonate) 500 mg • Iodine (as kelp) 150 mcg • Magnesium (as magnesium oxide) 200 mg • Zinc (as zinc oxide) 15 mg • Selenium (as hydrolyzed protein chelate) 100 mcg • Copper (as hydrolyzed protein chelate) 2 mg • Manganese (as hydrolyzed protein chelate) 5 mg • Chromium (as hydrolyzed protein chelate) 100 mcg • Molybdenum (as hydrolyzed protein chelate) 50 mcg • Boron (as hydrolyzed protein chelate) 2 mcg • Dong Quai Root Powder (angelica sinensis) 50 mg • Bee Pollen Powder 25 mg • Citrus Bioflavonoids Complex 25 mg • Choline (as choline bitartrate) 10 mg • Cranberry Concentrate (vaccinium macrocarpon) 10 mg • Para-Aminobenzoic Acid 10 mg • Royal Jelly 5 mg • Silica (as hydrolyzed protein chelate) 2 mg • Red Raspberry Leaves (rubus idaeus) 2 mg • Lutein 500 mcg • Inositol 10 mcg. Other Ingredients: Cellulose, Rice Protein Chelate, Titanium Dioxide (natural mineral whitener), Vegetable Acetoglycerides, Rose Hips Powder (rosina canino), Acerola, Chlorophyll.

***Ultra Multiple* - Source Naturals**
Six tablets contain: Vitamin A (palmitate 10000 IU and beta carotene 3000 IU) 13000 IU • Vitamin B-1 (thiamin) 100 mg • Vitamin B-2 (riboflavin) 75 mg • Niacinamide 75 mg and Niacin 25 mg 100mg • Vitamin B-5 (calcium D-Pantothenate) 150 mg • Vitamin B-6 (pyridoxine HCl) 125 mg • Vitamin B-12 (cyanocobalamin) 300 mcg • Biotin 150 mcg • Folic acid 420 mcg • Vitamin C (calcium, magnesium and manganese ascorbates) 500 mg • Vitamin D-3 (cholecalciferol) 402 IU • Vitamin E (natural D-alpha succinate) 200 IU • Magnesium (ascorbate, oxide, citrate) 125 mg • Potassium (citrate) 10 mg • Iron (fumarate) 12 mg • Calcium (ascorbate, carbonate, citrate) 125 mg • Zinc (citrate) 15 mg • Manganese (ascorbate) 6 mg • Chromium (ChromeMate polynicotinate) 50 mcg • Copper (sebacate) 250 mcg • Selenium (sodium selenite) 100 mcg • Iodine (from kelp) 225 mcg.

***Ultra Nails* - Nature's Plus**
Two tablets contain: Calcium amino acid chelate/complex 500 mg • Gelatin 260 mg • Horsetail supplying natural silica 250 mg • Phosphorus amino acid complex 200 mg • L-Cysteine free form amino acid 100 mg • L-Methionine free form amino acid 100 mg • Vitamin B2 (Riboflavin) 50 mg • Sulphur from Sulphur containing amino acids 25 mg • Oat straw 25 mg • Magnesium amino acid chelate/complex 25 mg • Iron (Amino Acid Chelate) 5 mg • Vitamin A Fish Liver oil 10000 IU • Folic Acid 200 mcg • Vitamin B12 from Cobalamin 100 mcg • Vitamin D Fish Liver oil 400 IU. In a natural rice bran base, supplying a complete balance of B-Complex vitamins & trace minerals. Yeast free. Sugar & starch free.

***Ultra Omega-3 Fish Oil* - Health From The Sun**
Two capsules contain: Omega-3 Fatty Acids 600 mg [EPA (360) DHA (240 mg)]. Ingredients: All natural Fish Body Oil, Gelatin, Glycerine, Water, Carob powder, Mixed Tocopherols (Vitamin E).

***Ultra Potassium* - Source Naturals**
Each tablet contains: Potassium (citrate, malate, ketoglutarate, fumarate, succinate, asparate, glycinate, and ascorbate) 99 mg.

***Ultra Power Nutrient* - Changes International, Inc.**
One packet (6g) contains: Vitamin A (as Retinyl palmitate with Lemongrass and Beta Carotene) 5000 IU • Vitamin C (as buffered mineral ascorbates) 60 mg • Vitamin D (as Cholecalciferol) 400 IU • Thiamin (Vitamin B1 as Thiamine hydrochloride) 1.5 mg • Riboflavin (Vitamin B2) 1.7 mg • Vitamin B6 (as Pyridoxine hydrochloride) 2 mg • Folate (as Folic acid) 400 mcg • Vitamin B12 (as Cyanocobalamin) 6 mcg • Biotin 300 mcg • Pantothenic acid (Vitamin B5) (as Calcium pantothenate) 10 mg • Calcium (as Calcium citrate ascorbate) 40 mg • Magnesium (as Magnesium citrate ascorbate) 20 mg • Sodium (as Sodium citrate ascorbate) 60 mg • Potassium (as Potassium citrate ascorbate) 200 mg • Sea minerals from Celtic marine algae 10 mg. Other Ingredients: Crystalline fructose, Maltodextrin, Natural citrus flavors, Non-nutritive sweetener.

***Ultra Prenatal Complex* - Nature's Plus**
Two tablets contain: Vitamin A (as beta carotene) 10,000 IU • Vitamin C (as ascorbic acid) 150 mg • Vitamin D (as ergocalciferol) 400 IU • Vitamin E (as d-alpha tocopheryl acetate) 100 IU • Vitamin B1 (as thiamine HCl) 15 mg • Vitamin B2 (as riboflavin) 15 mg • Niacin (as niacinamide) 40 mg • Vitamin B6 (as pyridoxine HCl) 50 mg • Folate (as folic acid) 800 mcg • Vitamin B12 (as cyanocobalamin) 20 mcg • Biotin 600 mcg • Pantothenic Acid (as calcium pantothenate) 25 mg • Calcium (as amino acid chelate/complex) 600 mg • Iron (as amino acid chelate/complex) 36 mg • Phosporous (as amino acid complex) 200 mg • Iodine (from kelp) 225 mcg • Magnesium (as amino acid chelate/complex) 300 mg • Zinc (as amino acid chelate/complex) 15 mg • Manganese (as amino acid chelate/complex) 6 mg • Potassium (as amino acid complex) 6 mg • Choline (as bitartrate) 10 mg • Inositol 10 mg • PABA (para-aminobenzoic acid) 10 mg.

***Ultra Prime Secretagogue HGH Enhancer* - Market America, Inc.**
Each scoop (17.7 g) contains: Folate (as folic acid) 150 mcg • Magnesium (as magnesium citrate) 150 mg • L-Arginine Aspartate 2.5 g • Glycine 4 g • L-Arginine 3 g • Proprietary Blend 3.3 g: L-Glutamine, Colostrum, L-Lysine (as L-lysine HCl), Taurine, RNA/DNA (from brewer's yeast). Other Ingredients: Citric Acid, Malic Acid, Natural Flavors, Beet juice powder, Silica, Glucose Polymers, Ascesulfame Potassium, Sucralose.

***Ultra Prosta-Metto* - The Vitamin Shoppe**
Each softgel contains: Vitamin E 50 IU • Vitamin B6 5 mg • Zinc 15 mg • Saw Palmetto berries 160 mg • Pumpkin seed 40 mg • Pygeum Africanum bark 10 mg • Stinging Nettle leaf 50 mg • Lycopene 2.5 mg.

***Ultra Quercetin - Flavonoid Complex* - Jamieson**
Each caplet contains: Quercetin Pure Flavonoid Active Potency 165 mg • Nettle Leaf Extract 1:6 and Perilla Fruit Extract 1:37 35 mg.

Ultra S **-** E'OLA
1/2 teaspoon contains: Silver 25 mcg.

Ultra Skin **-** Nature's Plus
Two tablets contain: Unsaturated Fatty Acids from natural Safflower oil 500 mg • Vitamin C with Rose Hips 200 mg • Vitamin B2 (Riboflavin) 200 mg • Vitamin B6 (Pyridoxine HCL) 200 mg • Vitamin E natural 200 IU • Niacinamide 150 mg • PABA (Para-Aminobenzoic Acid) 150 mg • Pantothenic Acid 150 mg • Vitamin B1 (Thiamine) 100 mg • Zinc amino acid chelate/complex 50 mg • Vitamin A (Beta Carotene) 25000 IU • Biotin 400 mcg • Folic Acid 100 mcg • Vitamin B12 (from Cobalamin) 100 mcg • Vitamin D (Calciferol) 1000 IU. In a natural base of rice bran & spirulina (naturally rich in RNA, DNA, amino acids & trace minerals).

Ultra Slim Down **-** Jamieson
Carb & Fat Burner: Each capsule contains: CitraMax 50% HCA Hydroxycitric Acid (derived from fruit of garcinia cambogia) 125 mg • Advantra Z Citrus Aurantium (derived from fruit of bitter orange) 125 mg • Kola nut JKN-10 (P.E. 10%) 5 mg. Calorie & Fat Eliminator: Each capsule contains: Natural soluble and insoluble Fibre Complex 343 mg: Derived from Chitosan of North Atlantic Shellfish, Mediterranean Nopal Cactus, and Organic Citrus Orange fruit fibre.
See Editor's Note No. 40, page 2058.

Ultra Stress with Iron **-** Nature's Plus
Each tablet contains: Vitamin C with Rose Hips 500 mg • Pantothenic Acid 200 mg • Vitamin B1 (Thiamine) 125 mg • Vitamin B2 (Riboflavin) 125 mg • Vitamin B6 (Pyridoxine HCL) 125 mg • Niacinamide 125 mg • Inositol 75 mg • PABA (Para-aminobenzoic acid) 50 mg • Choline (Bitartrate) 32 mg • Iron amino acid chelate/complex 20 mg • Vitamin B12 from Cobalamin 500 mcg • Folic Acid 400 mcg • Biotin 125 mcg. B-Complex vitamins in a fortified rice bran base.

Ultra Sugar Control **-** Nature's Plus
Two tablets contain: CITRIMAX (Garcinia cambogia fruit) standardized 50% [-] hydroxycitrate 500 mg • Rehmannia Glutinosa root [naturally rich in Beta-Sitosterol, Catalpol & Aucubin] 400 mg • L-Glutamine pharmaceutical grade free form amino acid 250 mg • L-Alanine pharmaceutical grade free form amino acid 250 mg • Gymnema Sylvestre leaf standardized 75% Gymnemic acids 200 mg • Chromium (Polynicotinate) 500 mcg.

Ultra Vein-Gard **-** NaturalCare
Active Ingredients: Horse Chestnut (aesculus hippocastanum)3X, 6X, 3C • Witch Hazel (hamamelis virginica) 1X, 4X, 3C • Honeybee (apis mellifica) 3X, 6X, 12X, 30X • Wind Flower (pulsatilla) 3X, 6X, 30X • St. Mary's Thistle (carduus marianus) 3X, 6X • Club Moss (lycopodium clavatum) 6X, 30X • Vegetable Charcoal (carbo vegetabilis) 6X, 30X • Ergot (secale cornutum) 3X. Other Ingredients: Aloe Vera Gel, Horse Chestnut Seed Extract (at 20% Escin), Purified Water, Butcher's Broom Extract (at 10% Ruscogenin), Rutin, Gotu Kola Extract (at 10% triterpenoids), Vegetable Glycerin, Glyceryl Stearate (vegetable), Cetyl Alcohol, Cetearyl Alcohol, Caprylic/Capric Triglyceride (from coconut), Stearic Acid (from vegetable oil), Beeswax, Jojoba Oil, Vitamin C (ascorbyl palmitate), Vitamin E (d-alpha tocopherol), Vitamin A (retinyl palmitate), Quercetin, Methyl Glucoses (from fruit), Xanthan Gum, Grapefruit Seed Extract, Rosemary Extract, Neem Oil, Tea Tree Oil, Glycyrrhetinic Acid (from licorice root), St. John's Wort Oil, Lavender Oil.
See Editor's Note No. 1, page 2053.

Ultra Virile-Actin **-** Nature's Plus
Two protein coated tablets contain: Vitamin E natural 200 IU • Korean Ginseng [(Panax ginseng root) standardized 15% Ginsenosides] 100 mg • Siberian Ginseng [Eleutherococcus senticosus root) standardized 0.8% Eleutherosides] 100 mg • Bee Pollen, Spanish 75 mg • Saw Palmetto [(Serenoa repens berry) standardized 35%-45% free fatty acids] 60 mg • Brazilian Muirapuama (Phychopetalum olacoides root & rhizome) 50 mg • L-Histidine, pharmaceutical grade free form amino acid 50 mg • Zinc (Monomethionine) 50 mg • Cayenne [(Capsicum frutescens fruit) standardized 125000 STU/gram] 50 mg • L-Phenylalanine pharmaceutical grade free form amino acid 50 mg • St. John's Wort [(Hypericum perforatum flower) 0.3%-0.5% Hypericin] 50 mg • Royal Jelly 25 mg • L-Carnitine (L-Carnitine-L-Tartrate) 25 mg • Pacific Oyster extract [(Crassostreagis thunberg) naturally rich in trace elements & amino acids] 10 mg • Vitamin B6 (Pyridoxine HCL) 5 mg • Coenzyme Q10 (Ubiquinone) 2500 mcg.

Ultra Vita-Min **-** Puritan's Pride
Each tablet contains: Vitamin A (as retinyl palmitate and beta carotene) 10,000 IU • Vitamin C (as ascorbic acid) 150 mg • Vitamin D (as cholecalciferol) 400 IU • Vitamin E (as d-alpha tocopheryl succinate) 12.5 IU • Thiamin (Vitamin B-1; as thiamine hydrochloride) 25 mg • Riboflavin (Vitamin B-2) 25 mg • Niacin (as niacinamide) 50 mg • Vitamin B6 (pyridoxine hydrochloride) 15 mg • Folic Acid 400 mcg • Vitamin B12 (as cyanocobalamin) 50 mcg • Biotin 1 mcg • Pantothenic Acid (as d-calcium pantothenate) 12.5 mg • Calcium (as oyster shell and bone meal) 60 mg • Iron (as ferrous gluconate) 6.26 mg • Phosphorus (as bone meal) 24.3 mg • Iodine (as potassium iodide) 100 mcg • Magnesium (as magnesium gluconate) 0.42 mg • Zinc (as zinc gluconate) 0.72 mg • Selenium (as sodium selenate) 10 mcg • Copper (as cupric gluconate) 0.035 mg • Manganese (as manganese gluconate) 0.76 mg • Chromium (as chromium picolinate) 2.35 mg • Molybdenum (as sodium molybdate) 10 mcg • Potassium (as potassium gluconate) 0.5 mg • PABA 15 mg • Choline Bitartrate 25 mg • Inositol 25 mg • Boron (as sodium borate) 500 mcg • Betaine Hydrochloride 25 mg • Rose Hips powder 10 mg • Rutin 5 mg • Citrus Bioflavonoids complex 15 mg • Royal Jelly 5 mg • Bee Propolis powder 5 mg • Coenzyme Q10 30 mcg • Octacosanol 50 mcg • Deodorized Garlic powder 10 mg • Ginseng root 15 mg • RNA 2 mg • DNA 2 mg.

Ultra Zinc Lozenge - GNC A-Z **-** GNC
Two lozenges contain: Beta-Carotene 1.2 mg • Vitamin C (ascorbic acid) 200 mg • Zinc (zinc oxide) 20 mg • Copper (copper oxide) 1 mg • Bee Propolis extract 1:5 20 mg • Echinacea Purpurea powder 20 mg. Other Ingredients: Sorbital, Fructose, Stearic Acid, Magnesium Stearate, Citric Acid, Natural Flavors.

UltraAC **-** Great American Nutrition
Four capsules contain: Potassium (as potassium glycerophosphate) 112 mg • Chromium (as chromium picolinate) 200 mcg • Potassium Glycerophosphate 450 mg • DL-Phenylalanine 1000 mg • Zhi Shi fruit (Citrus aurantium (Bitter Orange peel) containing 10 mg synephrine from a 4% standardized extract) 250 mg • Kola Nut nut (Cola acuminata, containing 50 mg caffeine from a 10% standardized extract) 500 mg • Ginger root (Zingiber officinale) 100 mg. Other Ingredients: Rice powder, Magnesium Silicate & Magnesium Stearate.
See Editor's Note No. 40, page 2058.

UltraAP Activated Pyruvate **-** Great American Nutrition
Four capsules contain: Potassium (as potassium glycerophosphate) 125 mg • Potassium Glycerophosphate 500 mg • Caffeine (from caffeine citrate & Kola nut) 150 mg • Zhi Shi fruit (Citrus aurantium (Bitter Orange peel), synephrine from a 4% standardized extract 10 mg) 250 mg • Kola Nut nut (Cola acuminata) 500 mg • Siberian Ginseng root (Eleutherococcus senticosus) 200 mg • Quercetin 100 mg • Jing jie leaves(Schizonepeta divaricata, 5:1 extract) 10 mg • Fang feng leaves (Ledebouriella tenuifolia, 5:1 extract) 10 mg. Other Ingredients: Rice powder, Maltodextrin, Magnesium Silicate and Magnesium Stearate.
See Editor's Note No. 40, page 2058.

Ultra-Cal Night **-** Source Naturals
Four tablets contain: Calcium (Citrate, Carbonate, Malate, Fumarate, Ethanolamine Phosphate, and Ascorbate) 600 mg • Magnesium (Oxide, Citrate, Fumarate, Malate, and Ascorbate) 600 mg • SoyLife Genistein Rich Soy Concentrate (Daidzein 13 mg, Glycitein 9 mg, Genistein 3 mg, total Isoflavones 25 mg) 830 mg • Vitamin C (Magnesium and Calcium Ascorbates, Ascorbic Acid and Manganese

Ascorbate) 285 mg • Vitamin B6 (Pyridoxine HCl) 20 mg • Vitamin D (as Vitamin D3) (Cholecalciferol) 200 IU • Folic Acid 200 mcg • L-Lysine (HCl) 60 mg • Silica (Horsetail Silica Extract) 10 mg • Zinc (Chelate) 7.5 mg • Manganese (Ascorbate) 6 mg • Boron (Amino Acid Chelate) 3 mg • Copper (Sebacate) 1 mg.

Ultra-Eyebright **-** Nutri-Quest Rx
Each tablet contains: Eyebright 100 mg • Bilberry extract 6 mg • Ginkgo Biloba 6 mg • Siberian Ginseng 15 mg • Gymnema sylvestre 100 mg • Tumeric 25 mg • Quercetin 10 mg • Lemon Bioflavonoids 40 mg • Bromelain 30 mg • Pancreatin 30 mg • Papain 30 mg • Trypsin 40 mg (Chymotrypsin 8 mg) • Pancreolipase 15 mg • Amylase-Diastase 15 mg • Ox Bile 30 mg • Betaine HCL 10 mg • Rutin 50 mg • L-Glutathione 2.5 mg • L-Taurine 15 mg • N-Acetyl Cysteine 10 mg • Selenium Chelate 10 mcg • Zinc Chelate 15 mg • Chromium Aspartate 1 mg • Parotid 1 mg • Beta Carotene 1000 IU • Vitamin C 75 mg • Vitamin D 200 IU • Vitamin E (Succinate) 20 IU • Vitamin B2 20 mg • Vitamin B6 10 mg • Folic Acid 50 mcg.
See Editor's Note No. 14, page 2055.

UltraFlax **-** Aidan Products, LLC
Each capsule contains: Omega-3 667 mg • Omega-6 194 mg • Omega-9 218 mg • Flaxseed particulate (containing lignan) 285 mg. Other Ingredients: Gelatin, Carob.

UltraGlycemX **-** Metagenics
Two scoops (50 g) contain: Dietary Fiber 9g • Vitamin A (as retinyl palmitate) 2500 IU • Beta-Carotene (as mixed carotenoids) 2500 IU • Vitamin D 100 IU • Vitamin C (as Ultra Potent-C) 250 mg • Vitamin E (as d-alpha tocopheryl succinate) 200 IU • Thiamin (as thiamin hydrochloride) 1 mg • Riboflavin 1 mg • Niacin (as niacin, niacinamide, niacinamide ascorbate) 39 mg • Pantothenic Acid (as d-calcium pantothenate) 5 mg • Vitamin B6 (as pyridoxine hydrochloride) 1 mg • Vitamin B12 (as cyanocobalamin) 3 mcg • Biotin 5 mg • Folic Acid 200 mcg • Sodium 170 mg • Potassium 580 mg • Calcium (as calcium phosphate) 500 mg • Phosphorus 400 mg • Magnesium (as magnesium citrate) 200 mg • Zinc (as zinc glycinate) 15 mg • Copper (as copper lysinate) 1.5 mg • Manganese (as manganese glycinate) 1 mg • Molybdenum (as molybdenum amino acid chelate) 38 mcg • Chromium (as polynicotinate) 500 mcg • Selenium (as selenomethionine) 150 mcg • Soy Isoflavones 17 mg • Alpha-Lipoic Acid 200 mg • Inositol 100 mg • Vanadium (as vanadyl sulfate) 2.5 mg. Other Ingredients: Soy Protein Isolate (PharmaSoy), Corn Maltodextrin, Modified High Amylose Starch, Rice Polishings, Partially Hydrolyzed Guar Gum, Fructose, Natural Flavors, Locust Bean Gum, Lecithin.

Ultra-Mag **-** Source Naturals
Two tablets contain: Magnesium (citrate, taurinate, glycinate, malate and succinate) 400 mg • Vitamin B-6 (pyridoxine HCl) 50 mg.

Ultramet - Vanilla Flavor **-** Champion Nutrition
Each packet contains: Peptol-EX protein 42 grams including Ion-Exchange Whey Protein Isolate, Calcium Caseinate, Milk Protein Isolate, Potassium Caseinate, Egg Albumen, Whey Protein Concentrate, Sodium Caseinate, L-Glutamine, Taurine, Calcium Alpha-Ketoglutarate & L-Arginine.

Ultra-Pro Training Pak **-** The Sports Nutrition Source, Inc.
One packet of eight tablets contains: Vitamin A 20000 IU •Vitamin C 1000 mg •Vitamin D 200 IU •Vitamin E 400 IU •Thiamin (B-1) 100 mg •Riboflavin (B-2) 120 mg •Niacin 125 mg •Vitamin B-6 100 mg •Biotin 300 mcg •Pantothenic Acid 200 mg •Folic Acid 400 mcg •Vitamin B-12 200 mcg • Calcium 1000 mg •Iron 25 mg •Iodine 150 mcg • Magnesium 600 mg •Zinc 25 mg •Selenium 200 mcg • Copper 500 mcg •Manganese 15 mg •Chromium 100 mcg •Molybdenum 20 mcg •Potassium 99 mg • Rutin 100 mg • Bioflavonoids 100 mg •Gamma Oryzanol 40 mg •Inosine 10 mg •Coenzyme Q10 5 mg •Germanium 100 mcg •PABA 25 mcg •Choline 200 mg • Inositol 100 mg • Bromelain 25 mg • Papain 25 mg •Beta Sisterol 20 mg •L-Carnitine 10 mg •Cayenne 20 mg • Gotu Kola 10 mg • Sarsaparilla 10 mg • Siberian Ginseng 10 mg •L-Leucine 78 mg •L-Isoleucine 48 mg •L-Valine 60 mg • L-Alanine 47 mg •L-Arginine 84 mg •L-Aspartic Acid 77 mg •L-Cystine 14 mg • L-Glutamic Acid 193 mg •L-Glycine 50 mg •L-Histidine 15 mg • L-Lysine 47 mg •L-Methionine 50 mg •L-Ornithine 46 mg • L-Phenylalanine 58 mg • L-Proline 35 mg • L-Serine 47 mg • L-Taurine 50 mg • L-Threonine 35 mg •L-Typtophan 13 mg •L-Tyrosine 53 mg.

Ultrasex **-** Life Extension
Three capsules contain: Yohimbe extract (4:1, equal to 1000 mg) 250 mg • Avena Sativa (wild oats) 200 mg • Siberian Ginseng 200 mg • Damiana 200 mg • Saw Palmetto 200 mg • Sarsaparilla 200 mg • Fo-Ti 100 mg • Ginkgo Biloba 50 mg • Yerba Mate 50 mg • Irish Moss 50 mg • White Yellow 50 mg • Cayenne 25 mg.

Ultra-Zyme **-** Nature's Plus
Two tablets contain: Pancreatin 4X quadruple strength 325 mg, supplying: Amylase 32500 USP Units, Protease (Trypsin & Chymotrypsin) 32500 USP Units, Lipase (Pancreatic lipase) 2600 USP Units • Glutamic Acid HCL 200 mg • Acidophilus (Lactobacillus, Bulgaricus, Bifidus) 150 mg • Ox Bile 120 mg • Bromelain, 1:10, pineapple, 100 mg • Pepsin NF 1:15000 65 mg • Malt Diastase 65 mg • Cellulase • Hemicellulase • 5 mg • Lactase 5 mg. In a natural herbal base of Peppermint, Fennel seed, Ginger & Rosemary.
See Editor's Note No. 14, page 2055.

Umcka ColdCare Alcohol Free Drops **-** Nature's Way
Active Ingredient: Pelargonium sidoides 1x. Other Ingredients: Purified Water, Vegetable-Source Glycerin.
See Editor's Note No. 1, page 2053.

Umcka ColdCare Cherry Syrup **-** Nature's Way
Active Ingredients: Pelargonium sidoides 1x. Other Ingredients: Aronia Juice, Citric Acid, Fructose, Natural Cherry Flavor, Purified Water, Vegetable-source Glycerin.
See Editor's Note No. 1, page 2053.

Umcka ColdCare Menthol Syrup **-** Nature's Way
Active Ingredient: Pelargonium sidoides 1x. Other Ingredients: Alcohol (8.2%), Fructose, Spearmint Flavor, Purified Water, Vegetable-source Glycerin.
See Editor's Note No. 1, page 2053.

Umcka ColdCare Original Drops **-** Nature's Way
Active Ingredient: Pelargonium sidoides 1x. Other Ingredients: Purified Water, Vegetable-Source Glycerin.
See Editor's Note No. 1, page 2053.

Umph **-** Frontsiders, LLC
Each tablet contains: Vitamin B6 0.75 mg • Sodium 188 mg • Potassium 116 mg • Ginseng root (panax) 30 mg • Caffeine 99 mg. Other Ingredients: Citric Acid, Sorbitol, Polyethylene Glycol, Natural Flavors, Acesulfame Potassium.

Una De Gato-Go! Cat's Claw Extract **-** Wakunaga of America
Each capsule contains: Cat's Claw standardized extract (Una De Gato)(bark) 250 mg. Other Ingredients: Cellulose, Colloidal Silica, Magnesium Stearate (vegetable source).

UnDo **-** Lindsey Duncan's Home Nutrition
Blended Fiber Formula: Each tablet contains: Proprietary blend 495 mg: Fiber blend: [Apple pectin, Beet fiber, Barley fiber, Psyllium husk, Karaya Gum, Oat Bran] • Fennel seed • Buckthorn bark • Cascara Sagrada bark • Kava Kava root • Red Raspberry leaf • Ginger root • Capsicum Fruit. Blended Herb Formula: Each tablet contains: Proprietary blend 368 mg: Panax Ginseng root • Ginkgo Biloba leaf extract (50:1) • Garlic bulb • Milk Thistle extract (80% Silymarin) • Echinacea Angustifolia leaf extract (6:1) • Cat's Claw bark • Uva Ursi leaf • Alfalfa leaf • Hawthorn berries • Licorice root • Ginger root • Rosemary leaf • Oregon Grape root • Turmeric root • Dandelion leaf • Burdock root • Yellow Dock root • Mullein leaf • Fenugreek seed • Horsetail herb • Safflower flower • Butcher's Broom root • Red root • Capsicum fruit • Schizandra fruit.

Univase **-** Rocky Fork Formulas
Each tablet contains: Pancreatin 4X (equivalend to 1250 mg) 313 mg • Papain 150 mg • Bromelain 150 mg • Trypsin 125 mg • Alpha-Chymotrypsin 3 mg • Superoxide Dismutase (SOD) 50 mcg • Catalase 200 units • L-Glutathione 10 mg • Lipase 50 mg • Amylase 50 mg • Rutin 100 mg • Lyophilized Calf Thymus 55 mg • Zinc (as gluconate) 1.4 mg.

Univase Forte **-** Rocky Fork Formulas
Each tablet contains: Pancreatin (4X, equivalent to 1250 mg) 313 mg • Papain 150 mg • Bromelain 150 mg • Trypsin 125 mg • Alpha-Chymotrypsin 45 mg • Super Oxide Dismutase (SOD) 50 mcg • Catalase 200 units • L-Glutathione 10 mg • Lipase 50 mg • Amylase 50 mg • Rutin 100 mg • Lyophilized Calf Thymus 55 mg • Zinc (as gluconate) 1.4 mg.
See Editor's Note No. 14, page 2055.

Unsalted Soynuts - Revival **-** Physicians Laboratories
Each 1/6 Cup Contains: Certified Isoflavone 10 mg. Ingredients: Soy Protein (whole roasted soybeans), Soybean Oil.

Up Your Gas (Ma Huang Formula) **-** National Health Products
Each tablet contains: Proprietary Blend 1200 mg: Guarana seed (aullinia cupana) • Ma Huang herb (ephedra sinica, standardized 6% extract) 285 mg • Korean Ginseng root (panax ginseng) • Bee Pollen • Vitamin E (d-alpha-tocopheryl acetate) • Spirulina Blue-Green Algae (spirulina pratensis) • Gotu Kola (centella asiatica) • Inosine • Octacosanol • Pyridoxal-Alpha-Ketoglutarate • Wheat Grass (triticum aestivum) • Cayenne pepper (capsicum frutescens) • Lipoic Acid • Cytochrome C. In Calcium, Magnesium, Potassium Succinate Base.
See Editor's Note No. 21 and No. 30.

Up Your Gas (No Ma Huang) **-** National Health Products
Each tablet contains: Niacin 15 mg • Guarana seed standardized extract (caffeine 90 mg) 450 mg • Kola nut standardized extract (caffeine 10 mg) 50 mg • Yerba Mate leaf 125 mg • Panax Ginseng root standardized ginseng (ginsenosides 8 mg) 100 mg • Herbal Base 65 mg: Gotu Kola leaf, Bee Pollen, Barley Grass, Spirulina, Wheat Grass • Krebs Cycle Chelates 65 mg: Calcium Carbonate, Magnesium Carbonate, Potassium Citrate • Activator Base 25 mg: Cayenne Pepper fruit, Octacosanol, Ginkgo Biloba leaf extract, Inosine, Lipoic Acid. Other Ingredients: Dicalcium Phosphate, Microcrystalline Cellulose, Croscarmellose Sodium, Stearic Acid, Magnesium Stearate, Silica, Pharmaceutical Glaze.

Upper Di-GST **-** Nutri-Quest Rx
Each tablet contains: L-Glutamine 50 mg • Okra 25 mg • Stomach 125 mg • Folic Acid 250 mcg • Vitamin A 1500 IU • Parotid 10 mg • Aloe Vera 5 mg • N-Acetyl Glucosamine 50 mg • Bromelain 25 mg • Duodenum 125 mg • Deglycerrized Licorice root 156 mg • Cabigen extract (Vitamin U) 20 mg • Slippery Elm 25 mg • Magnesium Chelate 75 mg.
See Editor's Note No. 14, page 2055.

UpTime Herbal **-** Uptime Sports Nutrition
Three caplets contain: Vitamin A (beta-carotene) (10% DV) 501 IU • Vitamin C (150% DV) 90 mg • Thiamin (thiamin mononitrate) (100% DV) 1.5 mg • Riboflavin (100% DV) 1.71 mg • Niacin (niacinamide) (225% DV) 45 mg • Vitamin B6 (pyridoxine hydrochloride) (300% DV) 6 mg • Folate (folic acid) (98% DV) 390 mcg • Vitamin B12 (cyanocabalamin) (300% DV) 18 mcg • Pantothenic Acid (Calcium pantothenate) (300% DV) 30 mg • Chromium (aspartate) (250% DV) 300 mcg • Molybdenum (amino acid chelate) (300% DV) 225 mcg • Vanadium (vanadyl sulfate) 2.85 mcg • Herbal Powder Base 1014 mg: Green Tea leaf, Dong Quai, Schisandra berry, Kola Nut seed, Ashwaganda leaf, Organic Bee Pollen, Yerba Mate leaf, Siberian Ginseng root, Papain (from papaya), Long Pepper fruit, Jujube fruit, Gamma Oryzanol, Wild Yam root, White Ginseng root, Fo-ti root, Ligustrum fruit, Astragalus root, Ginger root.

UpTime Nutritional Fitness **-** Uptime Sports Nutrition
Three caplets contain: Vitamin C (as ascorbic acid) (1500% DV) 900 mg • Calcium (as Calcium carbonate) (70% DV) 700 mg • Chromium (as picolinate) (8% DV) 10 mcg • Uptime Power Base: Spirulina Blue Green Algae, Wheat Grass, Alfalfa leaf, Caffeine, Papaya fruit, Silica, Cayenne fruit, Siberian Ginseng extract, Echinacea herb, Ginkgo Biloba extract, Carnitine (tartrate), Coenzyme Q10, Chromium (picolinate) 750 mg.

Urban Air Defense **-** Source Naturals
Two tablets contain: Vitamin A (Beta Carotene 12500 IU and Palmitate 5000 IU) 17500 IU • Vitamin C (Magnesium Ascorbate, Vitamin C and Manganese Ascorbate) 500 mg • Fat-Soluble Vitamin C (from 186 mg of Ascorbyl Palmitate) 80 mg • Vitamin E (D-Alpha Tocopheryl)(Natural) 200 IU • Magnesium (Ascorbate) 30 mg • Zinc (OptiZinc Monomethionine) 15 mg • Manganese (Ascorbate) 5 mg • Copper (Sebacate) 750 mcg • Selenium (as L-Selenomethionine) 100 mcg • Quercetin 200 mg • N-Acetyl Cysteine 100 mg • Silymarin (Milk Thistle seed extract) 50 mg • Ginkgo Biloba extract 24% (50:1) 5 mg • Hawthorn berry 150 mg • Rosemary 150 mg • Schizandra 125 mg • Marshmallow root 85 mg • Astragalus 60 mg.

Urinary & Kidney Care **-** Wellness for Women
Each capsule contains: Vitamin C (as ascorbic acid) 50 mg • Thiamin USP (as thiamin HCl; vitamin B-1) 12.5 mg • Riboflavin (vitamin B-2) 12.5 mg • Niacinamide 12.5 mg • Vitamin B-6 (as pyridoxine HCl) 12.5 mg • Folic Acid 100 mcg • Vitamin B-12 (as cyanocobalamin) 100 mcg • Biotin 12.5 mcg • Pantothenic Acid (as d-calcium pantothenate) 12.5 mg • Potassium (from potassium gluconate and potassium chloride) 99 mg • Cranberry extract (10:1 concentrate) 200 mg • Juniper berry powder 50 mg • Corn Silk 25 mg • Uva Ursi 25 mg • Choline (as choline bitartrate) 12.5 mg • Inositol 12.5 mg • PABA (para-aminobenzoic acid) 12.5 mg.

Urinary Formula **-** Nature's Way
Three capsules contain: Cleavers herb 180 mg • Corn Silk 150 mg • Cranberry concentrate fruit 600 mg • Dandelion leaf 180 mg • Goldenseal stem, leaf, flower 60 mg • Marshmallow root 180 mg. Other Ingredients: Gelatin, Magnesium Stearate, Millet.

Uriphron **-** PhytoPharmica
Two tablets contain: Birch leaf 5.5:1 extract (betula pendula) 218 mg • European Goldenrod aerial part 5.9:1 extract (solidago virgaurea) 272 mg • Java Tea leaf 6.2:1 extract (orthosiphon aristatus) 194 mg.

Uriplex **-** Enzymatic Therapy
Each tablet contains: Goldenrod extract 5.9:1 (Solidago virgaurea) 136 mg • Birch Leaf extract 5.5:1 (Betula pendula) 109 mg • Orthosiphon Leaf extract 6.2:1 (O. aristata) 97 mg.

Usanimals **-** USANA Health Sciences
One tablet contains: Vitamin A (as Beta Carotene) 2500 IU • Vitamin C (as Ascorbic Acid and Calcium Ascorbate) 100 mg • Vitamin D (as Cholecalciferol) 150 IU • Vitamin E (as D-Alpha Tocopheryl Succinate 36 IU • Vitamin K (as Phylloquinone) 10 mcg • Thiamine (as Thiamine Mononitrate) 0.75 mg • Riboflavin 1 mg • Niacin (as Niacinamide) 10 mg • Vitamin B6 (as Pyridoxine Hydrochloride) 1.25 mg • Folate (as Folic Acid) 200 mcg • Vitamin B12 (as Cyanocobalamin) 3 mcg • Biotin 15 mcg • Pantothenic Acid (as D-Calcium Pantothenate) 2.5 mg • Calcium (as Carbonate and Ascorbate) 75 mg • Iodine (as Sodium Iodide) 37.5 mcg • Magnesium (as Oxide and Amino Acid Chelate) 25 mg • Zinc (as Citrate) 2.5 mg • Selenium (as Amino Acid Complex) 10 mcg • Manganese (as Amino Acid Chelate) 0.5 mg • Chromium (as Amino Acid Chelate) 10 mcg • Molybdenum (as Amino Acid Chelate) 12.5 mcg • Hesperidin (Citrus SPP. L.) Fruit 4 mg. Other Ingredients: Xylitol, Natural Flavor Blend, Vegetable-Derived Stearic Acid, Ascorbyl Palmitate, Collodial Silicon Dioxide.

Usnea-Propolis Virtue **-** Blessed Herbs
Usnea lichen • Pau d'Arco bark • Echinacea Angustifolia root • Propolis • Goldenseal root • Myrrh Gum • Grain alcohol & Distilled Water.

Some Brand Name Natural Products - What they Contain

www.NaturalDatabase.com contains MANY more listings than appear here.

U-Tract **-** Progressive Labs
Each level teaspoon contains: Pure Mannoplex D-Alpha-Mannose 1.9 g.

Utrophin PMG **-** Standard Process, Inc.
Each tablet contains: Proprietary Blend 192 mg: Bovine uterus (PMG) extract, Magnesium citrate. Other Ingredients: Calcium Lactate, Cellulose, Calcium stearate.
See Editor's Note No. 14, page 2055.

Uva Ursi Formula **-** Quest
Each caplet contains: Uva Ursi leaf powder (Arctostaphylos uva-ursi) 85 mg • Dandelion root powder (Taraxacum officinale) 60 mg • Gentian root powder (Gentiana lutea) 55 mg • Huckleberry leaf powder (Vaccinium Myrtillus) 55 mg • Parsley leaf powder (Petroselinum crispum) 45 mg • Buchu leaf powder (Barosma betulina) 35 mg • Kelp powder (Fucus vesiculosis) 35 mg • Raspberry leaf powder (Rubus idaeus) 35 mg • Saw Palmetto berry powder (Serenoa serrulata/repens) 35 mg • Bladderwrack powder (Fuccus vesiculosis) 20 mg. Other Ingredients: Calcium Phosphate, Microcrystalline Cellulose, Vegetable Stearin, Croscarmellose Sodium, Magnesium Stearate (vegetable source).

U-Viva Vitamin E (Chewable) **-** Uviva
Each tablet contains: Vitamin E (d-alpha tocopheryl succinate) 400 IU. Other Ingredients: Sucrose, Wheat Starch, Talc Purified, Kaolin, CL 75470, Gelatin.

V12 (V-12) **-** SAN Nutrition
Each 9.5 g serving contains: TriCreatine Malate 3 g • Betaine-Glycocyamine 1.5 g • NitroArginine (arginine alpha-ketoglutarate) 1 g • NAG (N-acetyl-L-glutamine) 1 g • Micronized Taurine 1 g. Other Ingredients: Citric Acid, Natural Flavors, Acesulfame K, Aspartame, Orange Extract Powder, Calcium Silicate.

V2G **-** EAS
Each capsule contains: Vanadyl Sulfate 7.5 mg • Taurine 800 mg • Selenium (Sodium Selenate) 33 mcg.

Vaginitis **-** Hyland's
Two tablets contain: Natrum Muriaticum 12X • Candida Albicans 30X • Kreosotum 12X • Carbolicum Acidum 12X. Base: Lactose.
See Editor's Note No. 1, page 2053.

Vag-Mend **-** The Herbalist
Golden Seal root • Thuja leaf • Usnea lichen • Bayberry root bark • Echinacea root • Red Raspberry leaf.

Valaxin **-** Nutraceutics Corp.
Each caplet contains: Niacinamide 10 mg • Magnesium (as magnesium oxide) 10 mg • Suanzaorentang Extract (dried root) 400 mg • Valeriana Officinalis Extract (dried root) 400 mg • Passiflora Incarnata Extract (aerial parts) 25 mg • Proprietary Blend 150 mg: Bupleurum Chinensis (root), L-Glycine, Gaba (as gamma aminobutyric acid). Other Ingredients: Magnesium Stearate, DiCalcium Phosphate, Microcrystalline Cellulose, FD&C Lake Blue #1, Yellow #6.

Valer-A-Somn **-** PhytoPharmica
Each capsule contains: Valerian extract (Valeriana officinalis) - (standardized to contain 0.2%-0.8% valerenic acids) 150 mg.
See Editor's Note No. 21, page 2056.

Valerian **-** Jamieson
Each capsule contains: Valerian Root 400 mg.

Valerian **-** Leiner Health Products
Two caplets contain: Valerian extract (Valeriana officinalis) root 200 mg. Other Ingredients: Calcium Carbonate, Cellulose, Maltodextrin, Hydroxypropyl Methylcellulose, Silicon Dioxide, Polyethylene Glycol 3350, Croscarmellose Sodium, Hydroxypropyl Cellulose, Pharmaceutical Glaze, Crospovidone, Magnesium Stearate, Blue 1 Lake, Polysorbate 80, Titanium Dioxide, Sodium Citrate.

Valerian **-** Pharmanex
Each capsule contains: Valerian root extract (6:1) (Valerian officinalis) 350 mg. Other Ingredients: Gelatin, Rice Flour, Magnesium Stearate, Silicon Dioxide.

Valerian 400 **-** Enzymatic Therapy
Two capsules contain: Valerian root extract (valeriana officinalis, standardized to contain a minimum of 0.8% valerenic acids) 800 mg. Other Ingredients: Gelatin, Magnesium Stearate, Silicon Dioxide, Titanium Dioxide Color.

Valerian Extract **-** Nature's Way
Two capsules contain: Calcium 30 mg • Valerian Nighttime (dried valerian extract) 220 mg • Valerian root 800 mg. Other Ingredients: Gelatin.

Valerian Nighttime **-** Nature's Way
Each tablet contains: Lemon Balm dried extract 80 mg • Valerian Nighttime (dried valerian extract) 160 mg.

Valerian Plus **-** PhysioLogics
Each capsule contains: Valerian (0.8% Valerenic Acids, 1.52 mg) 190 mg • Chamomile 90 mg • Peppermint 90 mg • Propolis 45 mg • Passion flower 45 mg • American Ginseng 40 mg.

Valerian Root **-** Gaia Herbs
Each capsule contains: Valerian root (standardized for 0.8% valerenic acid, and full spectrum up to 100 mg of extract per capsule) 50 mg.

Valerian Root **-** Olympian Labs
Each capsule contains: Valerian root 500 mg.

Valerian Root 450 mg **-** Puritan's Pride
Each capsule contains: Valerian root (valeriana officinalis) 450 mg. Other Ingredients: Gelatin.

Valerian Root Concentrated Herb 1000 mg **-** Puritan's Pride
Each softgel contains: Valerian root (valeriana officinalis, from 250 mg of 4:1 extract) 1000 mg. Other Ingredients: Soybean Oil, Gelatin, Glycerin, Beeswax / Soybean Oil Mixture, Lecithin, Caramel Color, Titanium Dioxide Color.

Valerian Root Extract, 100mg **-** Nature Made
Two softgels contain: Valerian root extract 200 mg: Valerenic Acid 1.6 mg.

Valerian-400 **-** PhytoPharmica
Two capsules contain: Valerian (Valeriana officinalis) root extract (standardized to contain a minimum of 0.8% valerenic acids) 800 mg.
See Editor's Note No. 21, page 2056.

Valerian-Primrose Virtue **-** Blessed Herbs
Valerian root • Primrose flower & leaf • California Poppy flower & leaf • Hops strobile • Wild Lettuce • Passion flower • Scullcap • Grain alcohol & Distilled Water.

Val-Tran **-** Atrium Inc.
Each tablet contains: Valerian (standardized extract) 100 mg • Vitamin B6 5 mg • Magnesium Gluconate 50 mg • Magnesium Oxide 50 mg. In a base containing Chamomile, Anise & Peppermint.

Vanadyl Factors **-** Olympia Nutrition
Vanadyl Sulfate + 800 mg Taurine.

Vanadyl pH **-** SportPharma
Each capsule contains: Vanadyl Sulfate 7.5 mg.

Vanadyl Plus with Chromium **-** Olympian Labs
Each capsule contains: Chromium Picolinate 200 mcg • Vanadyl Sulfate 10 mg • Niacin 20 mg.

Vanadyl Sulfate **-** Life Extension
Each capsule contains: Vanadyl Sulfate 10 mg • Choline Complex 25 mg.

Vanadyl Sulfate **-** Ultimate Nutrition
Each tablet contains: Vanadyl Sulfate 10 mg.

Vanadyl Sulfate with Niacin **-** Olympian Labs
Each capsule contains: Vanadyl Sulfate 20 mg • Niacin 25 mg.

Vancol (Cholesterol Lowering Plan) **-** Omnicron International
Two chewable tablets contain: Beta Sitosterol 10 mg • Psyllium 200 mg • Chromium from Picolinate 50 mcg with natural Quinone Antioxidants. In a base of Calcium Carbonate & Magnesium Stearate.

Vanilla PerfectRx **-** Nature's Best
Chocolate flavor contains: Perfect Unique Protein Blend (Milk Protein Isolate, Calcium Caseinate, Whey Protein Concentrates, Egg Albumin), Maltodextrin, Potassium Chloride, Potassium Citrate, Sodium Chloride, Sodium Citrate, Dipotassium Phosphate, Natural & Artificial Flavors, Aspartame, Magnesium Oxide, Choline Bitartrate, Cellulose, Ascorbic Acid, d-Alpha Tocopheryl Acetate, Ferrous Fumarate, Niacin, Biotin, Xanthan Gum, Vitamin A Palmitate, Zinc, Oxide, D-Calcium Pantothenate, Vitamin K, Manganese Sulfate, Beta-Carotene, Copper Sulfate, Pyridoxine HCL, Riboflavin, Thiamine HCL, L-Glutamine, Chromium Picolinate, Cobalamin Concentrate (vitamin B12), Vitamin D (as Vitamin D3), Folic Acid, Sodium Molybdate, Potassium Iodide, Sodium Selenite.

Vanilla Phosphagain 2 **-** EAS
Each 59 gram serving contains: Potassium 730 mg • Chromium 50 mcg • Selenium 30 mcg • Manganese 1 mg • Vitamin K 40 mcg • Molybdenum 60 mcg • Choline 80 mg. Ingredients: Nitrogenin 2 proprietary Protein/Nitrogen reinforcing matrix [Milk Protein Isolate, Calcium Caseinate, L-Glutamine, Taurine, Calcium Alpha-Ketoglutarate (AKG) & Egg Albumin] • Phosphagen (HPCE Pure Creatine Monohydrate) • Maltodextrin, Dextrose • Vitamin & Mineral Blend: Potassium Phosphate, Potassium Citrate, Salt, Magnesium Oxide, Choline Bitartrate, Disodium Phosphate, Beta-Carotene, Ascorbic Acid, Dl-Alpha Tocopheryl Acetate, Ferrous Fumarate, Niacin, Zinc Oxide, D-Calcium Pantothenate, Copper Sulfate,Vitamin A Palmitate, Manganese Sulfate, Chromium Citrate, Pyridoxine Hydrochloride, Riboflavin, Thiamine Hydrochloride, Sodium Molybdate, Vitamin D (as Vitamin D3), Folic Acid, Biotin, Potassium Iodide, Sodium Selenate, Vitamin K, & Cyanocobalamin • Corn Syrup Solids • Partially Hydrogenated Canola oil • Xanthan Gum • Natural & Artificial Flavors • Sodium RNA • Soy Lecithin • Aspartame • Carrageenan • Phenylalanine.

Vanilla Pleasure Fructose - Revival **-** Physicians Laboratories
Each Packet Contains: Certified Isoflavone 160 mg. Ingredients: Soy Protein Isolate, Fructose, Sucrose, Calcium Phosphate, Maltodextrin, Soy Lecithin, Salt, Potassium Chloride, Modified Corn Starch, Artificial Flavor, Carrageenan, Carboxymethylcellulose, Xanthan Gum.

Vanilla Pleasure Splenda - Revival **-** Physicians Laboratories
Each Packet Contains: Certified Isoflavone 160 mg. Ingredients: Soy Protein Isolate, Cocoa, Maltodextrin, Calcium Phosphate, Soy Lecithin, Salt, Potassium Chloride, Artificial Flavor, Carrageenan, Carboxymethylcellulose, Xanthan Gum, Sucralose.

Vanilla Pleasure Unsweetened - Revival **-** Physicians Laboratories
Each Packet Contains: Certified Isoflavone 160 mg. Ingredients: Soy Protein Isolate, Maltodextrin, Calcium Phosphate, Soy Lecithin, Salt, Potassium Chloride, Modified Corn Starch, Artificial Flavor, Carrageenan, Carboxymethylcellulose, Xanthan Gum.

VariCare **-** Enzymatic Therapy
Each tablet contains: Butcher's Broom extract (Ruscus aculeatus) standardized to contain 9 - 11% Saponins calculated as Ruscogenin 150 mg • Horse Chestnut extract (Aesculus hippocastanum) standardized to contain 20 - 22% Saponins calculated as Escin 125 mg • Gotu Kola Phytosome (Centella asiatica) standardized to contain 30 - 35% Centella Triterpenes 15 mg.

Varicosin **-** PhytoPharmica
Two tablets contain: Butcher's Broom root and rhizome extract (ruscus aculeatus, standardized to contain 9-11% saponins calculated as ruscogenins) 300 mg • Gotu Kola leaf phytosome (centella asiatica, one part gotu kola extract, standardized to contain 90% centella triterpenes, bound to two parts phosphatidylcholine) 30 mg • Horse Chestnut seed extract (aesculus hippocastanum, standardized to contain 20% triterpene glycosides calculated as escin) 250 mg.

Vascular Complete **-** Rexall - Sundown
Each tablet contains: Vitamin C 33.3 mg • Calcium 260 mg • Sodium 10 mg • Chondroitin Sulfate 66.7 mg • Alpha-Ketoglutaric Acid (from calcium alpha-ketoglutarate) 33.3 mg • Citric Acid 33.3 mg • L-Arginine (from L-arginine HCl) 33.3 mg • L-Lysine (from L-lysine HCl) 33.3 mg • L-Proline 33.3 mg • L-Ornithine (from L-ornithine HCl) 16.7 mg • Choline (from choline bitartrate) 16.7 mg • Silica 7 mg • Vascular Complete base blend: Rose Hips and seeds extract (Rosa canina), Citrus Bioflavonoids, rutin, Hesperidin, Acerola Fruit extract (malpighia punicifolia) 7 mg. Other Ingredients: Calcium Carbonate, Cellulose, Croscarmellose Sodium, Hydroxypropyl Methylcellulose, Talc, Magnesium Stearate, Riboflavin (colorant), Titanium Dioxide, Calcium Sulfate, Polysaccharides.

Vascular Maintenance **-** Enzymes, Inc.
Each capsule contains: Vitamin E (100% from d-Alpha Tocopheryl Acid Succinate) 20 IU • Proprietary Herbal Blend 350 mg: Garlic bulb extract, Guggulipids extract, Lecithin (Soy Phospholipids), Turmeric root extract, Flaxseed oil powder, Globe Artichoke leaf extract • Proprietary Enzyme Blend 150 mg: Lipase, pHysioProtease. Other Ingredients: Plant Cellulose, Water.

Vascular Support Formula **-** The Vitamin Factory
Each tablet contains: Vitamin C (Ascorbic Acid) 500 mg • Pycnogenol (Maritime Pine bark extract) 100 mg.

VasoRect **-** Real Health Laboratories
Each capsule contains: L-Arginine 625 mg • Calcium 12.5 mg.

Vazoplex **-** Gerovicap
Propylene Glycol • Deionized Water • Hydroxyethyl Cellulose • Wild Yam extract • Nicotinate • DHEA • Menthol • L-Arginine • Methylparaben.

Vege Fuel **-** TwinLab
Pure Isolated Soy (All-Vegetable) Protein 100%.

Vege Fuel (Aspartame Free) **-** TwinLab
Pure Isolated Soy (All-Vegetable) Protein 100%.

Veg-Easy **-** Progressive Labs
Two tablets contain: Blend 1400 mg: Broccoli powder • Spirulina • Wheat Grass • Alfalfa powder • Spinach powder • Cabbage powder • Green Tea • Carrot • Barley grass • Parsley • Beet root powder • Kale • Oat fiber medium • Brussels Sprouts • Lipase • Amylase • Protease • Cellulase • Powdered Cellulose • Beet leaf powder • Barley fiber • Oat bran • Lactobacillus Acidophilus • Glucomannan & Calcium Gluconate.

Veg-Enzyme **-** Atrium Inc.
Each capsule contains: Protease Enzymes 150 mg • Amylase Enzymes 140 mg • Lipase Enzymes 25 mg • Cellulase Enzymes 10 mg.

VegeSil **-** Flora, Inc.
Silica extract • Spring Horsetail.

Vegetarian Children's Chewable **-** Nature's Plus
Each tablet contains: Vitamin A (beta carotene) 5000 IU • Vitamin C (with rose hips) 90 mg • Vitamin D (calciferol) 400 IU • Vitamin E (natural) 30 IU • Vitamin B1 (as thiamin HCl) 10 mg • Vitamin B2 (as riboflavin) 10 mg • Niacin (as niacinamide) 20 mg • Vitamin B6 (pyridoxine HCl) 10 mg • Folate (as folic acid) 15 mcg • Vitamin B12 (as cyanocobalamin) 15 mcg • Biotin 50 mcg • Pantothenic Acid 10 mg • Calcium (gluconate) 15 mg • Iron (gluconate) 10 mg • Iodine

BRAND NAMES

(kelp) 0.1 mg • Magnesium (gluconate) 0.25 mg • Zinc (gluconate) 0.25 mg • Manganese (gluconate) 50 mcg • Potassium (gluconate) 1 mg • Choline (as bitartrate) 15 mcg • Inositol 15 mcg • PABA (para-aminobenzoic acid) 0.6 mg.

Vegetarian Digestive Enzymes **-** NSI - Nutraceutical Sciences Institute
Each capsule contains: Protease 82,000 HUT • Amylase 8,000 SKB • Lipase 90 FIP • Cellulase 600 CU • Malt Diastase 215 DP • Invertase 525 SUMNER • Lactase 1,000 ALU • Pectinase 55 ENDO-PG • Alpha Galactosidase 300 GAL.

Vegetarian Enzyme Complex **-** Futurebiotics
Protease 6500 HUT • Amylase 2000 DU • Cellulase 20 CU • Lipase 14.5 LU • Papaya enzyme (papain) 50 mg • Lactase 100 LacU • Alfalfa powder 50 mg • Pineapple enzyme (bromelain) 50 mg • Betaine HCl 3 mg. Enzyme activity is determined & reported according to Standard Food Chemical Codex procedures accepted by the FDA.

Vegetarian Enzyme Complex 50 Plus **-** Futurebiotics
Protease 8000 HUT* • Amylase 4000 DU* • Cellulase 100 CU* • Lipase 40 LU* • Invertase 0.2 IAU* • Lactase 240 LacU* • Papain 10 mg • Maltase 15 AGU* • Gentian root 100 mg • Bromelain 10 mg • Fennel seed 50 mg. *Enzyme activity is determined & reported according to Standard Food Chemical Codex procedures accepted by the FDA.

Vegetarian Glucosamine & MSM **-** Now
Two Vcaps contain: Regenasure Glucosamine HCl (vegetarian source) 1 g • Lignisul MSM (methylsulfonylmethane) 1g. Other Ingredients: Cellulose (capsule), Magnesium Stearate (vegetable source), Stearic Acid (vegetable source), Silica.
See Editor's Note No. 43, page 2058.

Vegetarian Mega Minerals **-** Nature's Life
Two tablets contain: Boron (Citrate) 1 mg • Calcium (Carbonate, Citrate/Malate) 1000 mg • Chromium (Picolinate {US Patent #33,988}, Polynicotinate) 200 mcg • Copper (Glyconate, Citrate) 1 mg • Iodine (Kelp) 25 mcg • Iron (Fumerate, Peptonate) 15 mg • Magnesium (Oxide, Citrate) 500 mg • Manganese (Citrate) 10 mg • Molybdenum (Sodium Molybdate) 20 mcg • Potassium (Citrate) 99 mg • Selenium (l-Selenomethionine) 100 mcg • Silicon Dioxide 20 mg • Vanadium (Vanadyl Sulfate) 20 mcg • Zinc (Picolinate, Citrate) 15 mg • Betaine HCl 100 mg • Glutamic Acid HCl 100 mg.

Vegetarian Super Multi **-** Futurebiotics
Three tablets contain: Vitamin C 500 mg • Beta Carotene 15,000 IU • Vitamin B1 (thiamin) 20 mg • Vitamin B2 (riboflavin) 20 mg • Niacinamide 75 mg • Vitamin D 200 IU • Vitamin E (natural succinate) 100 IU • Vitamin B6 20 mg • Folic Acid 400 mcg • Vitamin B12 100 mcg • Biotin 300 mcg • Pantothenic Acid 50 mg • Inositol 50 mg. Minerals: Calcium: (carbonate, phosphate, ascorbate) 200 mg • Iron (gluconate) 8 mg • Phosphorus 100 mg • Iodine (kelp) 150 mcg • Magnesium: (oxide, ascorbate, amino acid chelate) 25 mcg • Zinc (gluconate, oxide) 25 mg • Copper (gluconate) 1 mg • Selenium (amino acid chelate) 200 mcg • Chromium (amino acid chelate) 200 mcg • Manganese (proteinate) 5 mg • Molybdenum (amino acid chelate) 25 mcg. Other Ingredients: Choline 150 mg • Para Amino Benzoic Acid (PABA) 75 mg • Bioflavonoid complex 100 mg • Sodium Phosphate 1 mg • Methionine 75 mg • Betaine HCl 75 mg • Bromelain 75 mg • RNA/DNA (chlorella) 50 mg • Chlorella 400 mg. Other Ingredients: Sea Vegetable, Ginkgo Biloba, Milk Thistle, Goldenseal, Dandelion, Burdock root, Alfalfa & Horsetail 500 mg.

Veggie Carotenoids **-** Now
Two VCaps contain: natural Beta-Carotene (D. salina) 12 mg/20000 IU • Alpha Carotene (D. salina) 400 mcg containing additional Carotenoids from D. salina algae: Xeaxanthin, Cryptoxanthin, Lycopene & Lutein • Lutein Floraglo Marigolds 3 mg • Lycopene natural source 3 mg • Broccoli concentrate (250 mcg Sulforaphane) 250 mg • Spinach concentrate (75 mcg Lutein) 100 mg • Tomato concentrate (140 mcg Lycopene) 100 mg • Kale powder 50 mg • Cabbage powder 50 mg • Brussels Sprouts powder 50 mg.

Veggie Magma **-** Green Foods Corp.
Each 5.3 oz jar contains: Proprietary Blend 150 g: Powdered Barley Grass juice, Maltodextrin, Alfalfa juice, Carrot juice, Tomato juice, Celery juice, dried Spinach, Cilantro juice, Broccoli juice, Broccoli Sprout juice, dried Green Pepper, Cucumber juice, dried Kale, Red Beet juice, Shiitake extract, Ginger root extract, dried Garlic, Aloe Vera.

Veggies4Life **-** Swanson
Two tablets contain: Alfalfa leaf powder 100 mg • Beet powder 100 mg • Broccoli powder 100 mg • Carrot powder 100 mg • Odor-Controlled Garlic bulb (PureGar® 10,000 ppm allicin potential) 100 mg • Parsley powder 100 mg • Spinach powder 100 mg • Tomato powder 100 mg • Barley Grass powder 50 mg • Cabbage powder 50 mg • Celery Seed powder 50 mg • Kale powder 50 mg • Kelp powder 50 mg • Wheat Grass powder 50 mg • Oregano powder 40 mg.

Vegie-Tabs One **-** Dial Herbs
Parsley • Garlic • Black Walnut hulls • Red Beet • Kelp • Dulse • Wheat bran • Wheat germ • Oat straw • Honey • Spinach • Cabbage • Carrots • Squash • Onion • Broccoli • Yellow Dock • Chickweed • Echinacea • Ginger • Cloves • Alfalfa • Alfalfa seeds • Papaya seeds • Rice Bran Capsicum • Sweet Potato.

Vegie-Tabs Two **-** Dial Herbs
Parsley • Hawthorne • Black Walnut hulls • Red Beet • Kelp • Dulse • Millet • Oat Straw • Honey • Spinach • Cabbage • Carrots • Squash • Onion • Broccoli • Yellow Dock • Chickweed • Echinacea • Alfalfa • Alfalfa seeds • Papaya seeds • Rice Bran • Capsicum • Ginger • Cloves.

Vegiplex **-** HealthWatchers System
Brocolli • Kale • Sprouts • Spinach • Radish • Carrot • Beet • Tomato • Celery • Onion • Leek • Cauliflower • Brussel Sprouts. (All ingredients are whole and powdered.)

Vegzyme **-** Progressive Labs
Each 500 mg capsule contains: Protease 10000 NP Units • Lipase 3600 NL Units • Amylase 4000 NA Units • Cellulase 30 NC Units • Papaya leaf powder 25 mg. Other Ingredients: Plant fiber. All-vegetable source from cultures of Aspergillus Oryzae & Niger & Papaya. Naturally occurring Invertase, Maltase, Beta-Amylase, Hemicellulase, Phosphatase, Peroxidase, Catalase & Hydrolase are also present.

Vein Formula **-** Pharmanex
Each tablet contains: Vitamin C (as Calcium Ascorbate) 60 mg • Grape Seed Extract (as Masquelier's Original OPC's) 75 mg. Other Ingredients: Gelatin, Maltodextrin, Microcrystalline Cellulose, Magnesium stearate, Silicon dioxide.

Vein Guard Horse Chestnut Standardized **-** Sundown
Each capsule contains: Horse Chestnut seed extract (standardized to 18% escin, 54 mg) 300 mg. Other Ingredients: Maltodextrin, Gelatin, Magnesium Stearate.

Vein Support Formula **-** Baywood International
Each tablet contains: Proprietary Flavonoid Blend: Diosmin • Hesperidin 500 mg. Other Ingredients: Microcrystalline Cellulose, Maize Starch, Opadry II Orange, Povidone.

Vein-Gard **-** NaturalCare
Active Ingredients: Horse Chestnut (aesculus hippocastanum)3X, 6X, 3C • Witch Hazel (hamamelis virginica) 1X, 4X, 3C • Honeybee (apis mellifica) 3X, 6X, 12X, 30X • Wind Flower (pulsatilla) 3X, 6X, 30X • St. Mary's Thistle (carduus marianus) 3X, 6X • Club Moss (lycopodium clavatum) 6X, 30X • Vegetable Charcoal (carbo vegetabilis) 6X, 30X • Ergot (secale cornutum) 3X. Other Ingredients: Bromelain (1500 mcu), Vitamin C, Rutin, Horse Chestnut Seed Extract (at 20% escin), Butcher's Broom (at 9-11% ruscogenin), Ginger, Cayenne, Lecithin, Gotu Kola Extract (at 8-10%

triterpenoids), Quercetin, Grape Seed Extract (at 95% proanthocyanidins).
See Editor's Note No. 1, page 2053.

Veinicin **-** Gero Vita International
Each capsule contains: Diosmin Complex (92% diosmin) 450 mg • Hesperidin Complex (98% bioflavonoids). Other Ingredients: Gelatin, Silicon Dioxide, Magnesium Stearate.

Veinish **-** WellQuest International, Inc.
Sesame Oil • Emulsifying Wax • Stearic Acid • Marine Algae • Propylene Glycol • Cetyl Alcohol • Canola Oil • Calendula Oil • Marigold Extract • Chickweed Extract • Lecithin • Essence of Lemon.

VeinTain **-** Resource Wellness
Each caplet contains: Vitamin A 250 IU • Vitamin C 30 mg • Calcium 175 mg • Grape Seed extract 25 mg • Horse Chestnut extract 250 mg. Other Ingredients: Dicalcium Phosphate, Microcrystalline Cellulose, Croscarmellose Sodium, Stearic Acid, Magnesium Stearate, Silicon Dioxide, Hydroxypropyl Methylcellulose, Hydroxypropyl Cellulose, Polyethylene Glycol.

VelvaMax **-** Gold Mountain Trading
Ginseng (Panax Ginseng) • Reishi (Ganoderma lucidum) • Tienchi (Radix Pseudoginseng) • Astragalus (Astragalus membranaceus) • Licorice (Radix glycyrrhizae uralensis).

VenaFit **-** Biotech Corp.
Two tablets contain: Horse Chestnut standardized extract (18%-22% aescin, aesculin free) 280 mg • Niacin (as nicotinic acid) 20 mg • Ginkgo leaf powder 250 mg • Garlic (5:1 standardized extract) 100 mg • Hawthorne berries standardized extract 100 mg • Ginger root powder 100 mg • Citrus Bioflavonoids 100 mg.

Venastat **-** PanGeo Health Brands, Inc.
Each Supro Cap contains: Sustained Release Pellets of Standardized Horse Chestnut seed extract as Triterpene glycosides calculated as Escin (16%) 300 mg. Other Ingredients: Dextrin, Gelatin, Copolyvidone, Talc, Polymethacrylic Acid Derivatives, Titanium Dioxide, Dibutyl Phthalate, Synthetic Iron Oxide.

Venix **-** Pharmanex
Two capsules contain: Triacin, a proprietary blend of 1325 mg: Cs-4 Mushroom Mycelia Cordyceps Sinensis ([Berk.]Sacc.), L-Arginine (as L-Arginine HCL), Ginkgo Biloba leaf extract (50:1). Other Ingredients: Gelatin, Magnesium Stearate, Silicon Dioxide.

Ventilean **-** PharmaGenX
Two LipoGels contain: Guarana 750 mg • Zhi Shi (standardized to 95% synephrine) 20 mg • Vinpocetine • Yohimbe 5.3 mg • Vitamin B1 1.4 mg • Vitamin B2 1.3 mg • Vitamin B6 1.3 mg • Vitamin B12 24 mcg. Other Ingredients: Water, Glycerin, Propylene Glycol, Emulsifiers, Phospholipids, Licorice Flavor, Peppermint Oil, Medium Chain Triglycerides, Sucralose, Aspartame, Cinnamon Oil, Potassium Sorbate, Sodium Benzoate, Phosphoric Acid, Natural and Artificial Colors, Kelp, Sodium Citrate, Sodium Phosphate, Mono Potassium Phosphate, Collagen.
See Editor's Note No. 40, page 2058.

Veromax for Men **-** Veromax International
Each tablet contains: Jujube Dates (Zizyphi fructus) fruit 100 mg • Proprietary Amino Blend: L-Arginine, L-Alanine, Glutamic Acid, Lysine (L-Lysine hydrochloride) 213 mg • Proprietary Herbal Blend: Korean Ginseng root powder, Ginkgo Biloba leaf powder, Saw Palmetto berry powder 238 mg. Other Ingredients: Calcium Carbonate, Microcrystalline Cellulose, Croscarmellose Sodium, Stearic Acid, Silica, Magnesium Stearate, Hydroxypropyl Methylcellulose.

Veromax Sexual Performance Enhancer for Women **-** Nx Nutraceuticals
Each tablet contains: Jujube Dates fruit (zizyphi fructus) 100 mg • Proprietary Amino Potency Power Blend 175 mg: Arginine (as l-arginine hydrochloride), Alanine, Glutamic Acid, Lysine (as l-lysine hydrochloride) • Proprietary Veromax Herbal Blend 177.5 mg: Siberian Ginseng root powder, Ginkgo Biloba leaf powder, Isoflavones (from kudzo root extract). Other Ingredients: Calcium Carbonate, Microcrystalline Cellulose, Croscarmellose Sodium, Stearic Acid, Silica, Magnesium Stearate, Hydroxypropyl Methylcellulose.

Vertigoheel **-** Heel, Inc.
Each 50 mL contains: Cocculus (Indian berries) 4X 35 ml • Conium (Spotted Hemlock) 3x • Ambra (Amber) 6X • Petroleum (Mineral Oil) 8X 5 mg. Contains 35 Vol.% alcohol.
See Editor's Note No. 1, page 2053.

Vertigoheel Tablets **-** Heel, Inc.
Each tablet contains: Cocculus (Indian berries) 4X 210 mg • Conium (Spotted Hemlock) 3X • Ambra (Amber) 6X • Petroleum (Mineral Oil) 8X ana 30 mg.
See Editor's Note No. 1, page 2053.

V-Gel **-** The Himalaya Drug Company (Himalaya Heal
Each 1 gm serving contains: Triphala 4 mg: Emblica Officinalis, Terminalia Chebula, Terminalia Bellirica • Satapatri (rosa damascena syn. r.centifolia) 3.6 mg • Ela (elattaria cardamomum) 3.6 mg • Punarnava (boerhaavia diffusa) 3.6 mg • Shaileyam (parmelia perlata) 2 mg • Nirgundi (vitex negundo) 1.6 mg • Haridra (curcuma longa) 1.6 mg.

VHandC Tabs **-** Dial Herbs
Vinegar • Honey • Cayenne.

Viactiv Soft Calcium Chews **-** Mead Johnson Nutritionals
Each chew contains: Calcium (as calcium carbonate) 500 mg • Vitamin D 100 IU • Vitamin K 40 mcg • Potassium 15 mg • Phosphorus 8 mg • Lactose 0.5 mg • Caffeine 1.14 mg. Other Ingredients: Corn syrup, calcium carbonate, sugar, chocolate, nonfat milk, cocoa butter, salt, soy lecithin, glyceryl monostearate, artificial flavor, carrageenan, & sodium phosphate.

Viacyn **-** Live Well Nutrition, LLC
Two capsules contain: Zinc 50 mg • L-Arginine 250 mg • Catuaba 100 mg • Oatstraw 150 mg • Nettle leaf 75 mg • Tribulus 50 mg • Cayenne 50 mg • Astragalus 25 mg • Sarsaparilla 25 mg • Boron 2 mg • Pumpkin seed 20 mg • Licorice root 20 mg • Siberian Ginseng 125 mg. Other Ingredients: Magnesium Stearate, Gelatin, Water, Epimedium Sagittatum (horny goat weed extract, 20:1), Maca, Orchic Substance, Oyster Meat, Muira Puama.
See Editor's Note No. 14, page 2055.

ViaViente **-** ViaViente
Two tablespoons (25 ml) contain: Proprietary PhytoNectar Blend 13,500 mg: Whole Grape PhytoNectar (vitis vinifera, fruit), Whole leaf Aloe Vera PhytoNectar (aloe barbadensis, inner leaf gel), Apple PhytoNectar (malva pumila, fruit), Morinda Citrifolia PhytoNectar (fruit), Chinese Scullcap PhytoNectar (scutellaria biacalensis, root), Blueberry PhytoNectar (vaccinium spp., fruit), Prune PhytoNectar (prunus domestica, fruit), Cranberry PhytoNectar (vaccinium macrocarpon, fruit), Elderberry PhytoNectar (sambucus cerulea, fruit), Bilberry PhytoNectar (vaccinium myrtillus, fruit), Gentian PhytoNectar (gentiana lutea, root) • Proprietary Vilcabamba Mineral Essence Blend 150 mg: Potassium, Calcium, Magnesium, Zinc, Chromium, Selenium, Iron, Copper, Molybdenum, Vanadium, Iodine, Cobalt, Manganese. Other Ingredients: Vilcabamba Mineral Water, Citric Acid, Natural Flavors, Sodium Benzoate (0.1%), Potassium Sorbate (0.1%).

ViaVita **-** DreamPharm
Two tablets contain: Proprietary Blend: Lecithin (soya), Calcium (carbonate), Citric Acid (anhydrous), Iron (ferrous fumarate), Vitamin B12.

Vibrant Celcaps **-** Vibrant Health
Three celcaps contain: Celadrin Proprietary Blend 1050 mg: Cetyl Myristate, Cetyl Myristoleate, Cetyl Esters. Other Ingredients: Soy Lecithin, Fish Oil.

BRAND NAMES

Vibrant Creme with Celadrin - Vibrant Health
Menthol • Benzyl Alcohol • Butylparaben • Carbomer • Proprietary Cetyl Ester Blend (Celadrin): Cetyl Myristate, Cetyl Oleate • Cetyl Palmitoleate • Cetyl Laurate • Cetyl Myristoleate • Ethylparaben • Glycerin • Glyceryl Stearate • Isobutylparaben • Lecithin • Methylparaben • Olea Europaea fruit oil (olive) • PEG 100 Stearate • Peppermint oil • Phenoxyethanol • Potassium Hydroxide • Propylparaben • Tocopheryl Acetate • Water.

Viga - Health Nutrition (RMA Labs)
Each tablet contains: Yohimbe extract 40 mg • Muira Puama 10 mg • Tribulus Terrestris 40 mg • Ginseng 40 mg • Saw Palmetto 40 mg • Oat straw 10 mg • DHEA 10 mg • Androstenedione 10 mg.
See Editor's Note No. 47, page 2058.

Viga for Women - Health Nutrition (RMA Labs)
Muira Puama • Ginseng • Maca • Wild Yam • Damiana • L-Arginine • Dong Quai • Guarana • Horny Goat Weed • Macuna Prurions extract.

Vigorelle - Leading Edge Herbals
Organic Damiana leaf (folium turneraceae) • Organic Suma root (radix pfaffiae paniculatae) • Organic Motherwort (herba leonori) • Organic Wild Yam (rhizoma dioscorea villosae) • Organic Ginkgo Biloba • Organic Peppermint leaf (folium menthae piperitae).

Vigorex Femme - New Hope Health Products
Each tablet contains: Sabal Serrulata (Saw Palmetto) • Avena Sativa (Common Oats).

Vigorex Forte - New Hope Health Products
Each capsule contains: Avena Sativa Extract 300 mg.

Vigorex forte - Doc Johnson Enterprises
Active Ingredient: Avena sativa 1X. In a base of lactose.
See Editor's Note No. 1, page 2053.

Vigor-Max - Shenlong Natural International, Inc.
Each tablet contains: Epimedium Macranthum 84 mg • Polygonum Multiflorum 72 mg • Ligustrum Lucidum 72 mg • Curculigo Orchioides 54 mg • Panax Ginseng 18 mg.

Vigrex - Puritan's Pride
Each tablet contains: Yohimbe 500 mg • Tribulus Terrestris herb 225 mg • Maca root 200 mg • Muira Puama root 200 mg • Panax Ginseng 150 mg • Ginger extract 100 mg • Citrus Aurantium extract (Bitter Orange) 50 mg • Fructooligosaccharides (FOS) 50 mg • Saw Palmetto (Standardized for 30% fatty acids) 15 mg. Other Ingredients: Dicalcium Phosphate, Cellulose, Magnesium Stearate, Silica, Stearic Acid.
See Editor's Note No. 40, page 2058.

VigRx - Albion Medical
Each capsule contains: Epimedium Sagittatum extract 330 mg • Cuscuta seed 100 mg • Ginkgo Biloba 100 mg • Korean Red Ginseng (panax ginseng) 100 mg • Saw Palmetto (fructus serenoae) 100 mg • Muira Puama extract (4:1) 50 mg. Other Ingredients: MCC, Magnesium Stearate, D-Calcium Phosphate, Croscarmellose Sodium, PVP K90, Silicon Dioxide.

Vimax Pills - PillsExpert.com
Two capsules contain: Vitamin E (as natural d-alpha tocopheryl) 20 IU • Inosine 50 mg • Proprietary Blend 938 mg: Yohimbe bark 4:1, Muira Puama balsam, Deer Antler Velvet, Ginkgo leaf, Damiana leaf, Cayenne fruit, Oats (entire plant), Panax Ginseng root, Tribulus fruit. Other Ingredients: Cellulose, Vegetable Stearate, Silica.

Vinarol - Bionate International
Each tablet contains: VASX Proprietary Blend 500 mg: Cassia tree, Dodder seed, Epimedium, Wolfberry, Saling, Cistanche, Magnolia vine fruit, Red Raspberry, Narrow-leaved Polygala, Rehmannia root, Eucommia bark, Hindo Lotus seed, Bidemate bark, Milk Vetch seed, Cherokee Rose, Arborvitae seed, American Ginseng, Gingko Biloba. Other Ingredients: Microcrystalline Cellulose, Stearic Acid, Silicon Dioxide, Magnesium Stearate, Pharmaceutical Coating.
See Editor's Note No. 25, page 2056.

Vincamine - Source Naturals
Each tablet contains: Vincamine 30 mg.

Vincazine - Smart Basics
Each capsule contains: Vinpocetine 10 mg • (-) Huperzine A 50 mcg.

Vine Essence - Capital United (Beijing) Medical Manufac
Active ingredients: Geranium (Geranium eriostemon) herb, Erycibe (Erycibe obtusifolia Benth.) stem (Ding-Gong-Teng), Chinese Angelica Tree (Aralia chinensis L.) herb, Futokadsura (Piper futokadsura Sieb. Et Zucc.) stem (Hai-Feng-Teng), Oriental (Renshen), Pipefish, Ilicis (Ilex Pubescens Hook et Arn), Kadsura (Kadsura cocchinea [Lem] A.C.) root, Epimedium (Epimedium sagittatum [Sieb. et Zucc.] Maxim.) (Yin-Yang-Huo), Dong-Qaui Root, Homalomeana (Homalomeana sagittaefolia Jungh.) rhizome (Qian-Nian-Jian), Chinese Licorice (Gan-Cao) root, Sichuan Lovage (Chuan-Xiong) rhizome, Morinda (Ba-Ji-Tian), Ligusticum (Gao-Ben) rhizome, Gastrodia (Tian-Ma) rhizome, Sichuan Teasel (Xu-Duan) root, Fo-Ti (He-Shou-Wu) root.
See Editor's Note No. 17, page 2055.

Vinpocetine - PhysioLogics
Each softgel contains: Vinpocetine 10 mg. Other Ingredients: Lecithin, Soybean Oil, Gelatin, Beeswax / Soybean Oil Mixture, Glycerin, Titanium Dioxide Color.

Vinpocetine - Amerifit Nutrition
Each tablet contains: Vinpocetine 5 mg • Green Tea standardized extract 200 mg. Other Ingredients: Dicalcium phosphate, croscarmellose sodium, microcrystalline cellulose, magnesium stearate, silica stearic acid, & pharmaceutical glaze.
See Editor's Note No. 21, page 2056.

Vinpocetine - Source Naturals
Each tablet contains: Vinpocetine 10 mg. Inactive Ingredients: Microcrystalline Cellulose, Stearic Acid, Magnesium.

Vinpo-Zine - Smart Nutrition
Each capsule contains: Vinpocetine 10 mg • Huperzine A 50 mcg.

Viper - Puritan's Pride
Each capsule contains: Kola Nut 175 mg • Oatstraw 150 mg • Nettles 100 mg • Yohimbe 2% extract 50 mg • Siberian Ginseng 50 mg • Horny Goat Weed 20 mg • Catuaba 10 mg • Muira Puama 10 mg • Korean Ginseng 10 mg • Turnera Aphrodisiaca 10 mg • Saw Palmetto 10 mg.

ViraPlex - Enzymatic Therapy
Each tablet contains: Vitamin A (Fish Liver oil) 10000 IU • Vitamin D (Fish Liver oil) 35 IU • Vitamin C (Ascorbic Acid/Rose Hips) 200 mg • Calcium (Lactate) 41 mg • Pantothenic Acid (D-Calcium Pantothenate) 25 mg • Zinc (Gluconate) 10.5 mg • Magnesium (Citrate) 6.7 mg • Vitamin B12 (Cyanocobalamin) 2.5 mcg • Other ingredients: RNA Powder 60 mg • Alfalfa juice powder 50 mg • Lemon Bioflavonoids 30 mg • Spleen extract 30 mg • Thymus extract 25 mg • Trace Mineral concentrate (Kelp) 25 mg • Unsaturated Free Fatty Acids 15 mg • Lung extract 10 mg. In a base of Chlorophyll, Lymph, & Fermentation extract.
See Editor's Note No. 14, page 2055.

Viraplex EB with Elderberrry - Enzymatic Therapy
Each tablet contains: Vitamin A (as acetate) 10,000 IU • Vitamin C (ascorbic acid) 200 mg • Vitamin D (as cholecalciferol) 35 IU • Vitamin B12 (as cyanocobalamin) 50 mcg • Pantothenic Acid (as calcium d-pantothenate) 25 mg • Calcium (as calcium lactate) 41 mg • Magnesium (as magnesium citrate) 6.7 mg • Zinc (as zinc gluconate) 10.5 mg • European Elderberry extract (sambucus nigra, 4:1) 100 mg • Alfalfa aerial part extract (medicago sativa, 10:1) 50 mg • Astragalus root extract (astragalus membranaceus, standardized to contain a minimum of 0.5% 4-hydroxy-3#-methoxyisoflavone-7-glucoside) 50 mg • Mixed Bioflavonoids 50% (from citrus fruits)

30 mg • Proprietary Trace Mineral Blend 24 mg: Selenium (as selenium yeast), Silicon (as magnesium trisilicate), Boron (as sodium borate), Nickel (as nickel chelate). Other Ingredients: Cellulose, Modified Cellulose, Magnesium Stearate, Carnauba Wax, Lecithin.

Virile 1 **-** Biotech Corp.
Two tablets contain: Yohimbine bark (from 540 mg standardized extract) 5.4 mg • Shen Min (from a 4:1 extract) 100 mg • DHEA (dehydroepiandrosterone) 12.5 mg • Pregnenolone (pharmaceutical grade) 2.5 mg • VIRILE 1 FORMULA Proprietary Herb Blend 635 mg: Saw Palmetto berries (4:1 extract), Licorice root (4:1 extract), Muira Puama (4:1 extract), Fennel seed, Damiana leaf, Avena Sativa straw extract, Pygeum bark, Nettle.

Virile V for Him **-** USA Pharmacal Sales
Two tablets contain: Niacin 10 mg •Yohimbe 250 mg •Avena Sativa 150 mg •Androstenedione 100 mg •Saw Palmetto 100 mg •Guarana 300 mg •Taurine 200 mg •Siberian Ginseng 30 mg •Panax Ginseng 30 mg •Tribulus Terrestris 50 mg •Rhodiola Roseo 10 mg •Wild Yam 250 mg •Maca 100 mg •Arginine 100 mg.
See Editor's Note No. 47, page 2058.

Virility Pills VP-RX **-** EyeFive, Inc.
Two capsules contain: Vitamin E (as d-alpha tocopheryl acetate) 20 IU • Soy Protein concentrate 550 mg • Damiana leaf 200 mg • Muira Puama herb (ptychopetalum olacoides) 200 mg • Ginkgo Biloba leaf 120 mg • Panax Ginseng root 120 mg • Tribulus Terrestris herb extract 120 mg • Yohimbe bark extract 4:1 120 mg • Inosine 50 mg • Oat Straw 32 mg • Cayenne fruit 20 mg • Velvet Deer Antler 6 mg. Other Ingredients: Gelatin, Microcrystalline Cellulose, Magnesium Stearate, Silicon Dioxide.

Virility Support Formula **-** The Vitamin Factory
Each tablet contains: Niacin 10 mg • L-Arginine 250 mg • Muirapuama root & bark extract 10:1 100 mg • Yohimbe bark extract (min 1% Yohimbe) 100 mg • Quebracho Branco bark extract (Aspidosperma • min. 6% Quebrachine) 25 mg • Catuaba bark extract 4:1 50 mg • Pycnogenol (Maritime Pine bark extract) 10 mg.

Virility-V **-** Aspen Group, Inc.
Two tablets contain: Yohimbe extract 2% 500 mg • Avena Sativa extract 10.1 150 mg • Androstenedione 90 mg • Saw Palmetto extract 4.1 100 mg • Guarana extract 22% 300 mg • Taurine 200 mg • Siberian Ginseng extract 35.1 30 mg • Tribulus Terrestris extract 40% 50 mg. Other ingredients: Dicalcium Phosphate, Microcrystaline Cellulose, Magnesium Stearte, Stearic Acid.
See Editor's Note No. 47, page 2058.

Virility-V Female **-** Aspen Group, Inc.
Three tablets contain: Vitamin D (as colecalciferol) 21 IU • Niacin (as Niacinamide) 20 mg • Vitamin B6 (as pyridoxine hydrochloride) 2.4 mg • Folic Acid (as folacin) 6.4 mg • Vitamin B12 (as cyanocobalamin) 6 mg. Other Ingredients: Avena Sativa (10:1) 150 mg, Kava Kava (30%) 10 mg, Muira Puama (4:1) 20 mg, St. John's Wort (0.3%) 250 mg, Siberian Ginseng (35:1) 30 mg, Gingko Biloba (24%) 40 mg, Cordyceps 100 mg, Damiana 20 mg, L-Taurine 200 mg.

Virilogarl **-** Olympian Labs
Three capsules contain: Ginkgo Biloba leaf extract 120 mg • Garlic extract 600 mg • L-Arginine 390 mg • Bilberry extract 150 mg • Grape Seed extract 75 mg • Green Tea leaf extract 225 mg.

Virx **-** Nutri-Quest Rx
Each tablet contains: Olive leaf 100 mg • L-Lysine 100 mg • Vitamin C 25 mg • Zinc Chelate 10 mg • Elderberry extract 100 mg • Selenium Chelate 50 mcg • Olive leaf extract 5 mg • Vitamin A 3333.33 IU • Echinacea 100 mg • Goldenseal 50 mg • Astragalus 100 mg • natural Beta Carotene 3333.33 IU.

Vision Answer for Women **-** Doctor's Preferred, Inc. (Phillips Healt
Two softgels contain: Vitamin A (as beta carotene) 250 IU•Vitamin C (as ascorbic acid) 250 mg • Zinc (as chelate) 10 mg • Selenium (as chelate) 50 mcg • Copper (as gluconate) 1000 mcg • Rutin (from pod) 250 mg • Vegetable Blend 134 mg: Green Tea extract, Pine bark extract, Broccoli, Tomato, Carrot, Spinach, Kale, Brussels Sprouts • Grape seed extract 50 mg • Lutein (from marigold flowers) 15 mg • Lycopene (from tomato) 4 mg • Polygonum Cuspidatum root extract 4 mg • Astaxanthin (from algae) 3 mg • Zeaxanthin (from marigold flowers) 3 mg.

Vision Complete **-** Rexall - Sundown
Two capsules contain: Vitamin A (100% as beta-carotene, 60% of which is from dunaliella salina algae) 5000 IU • Vitamin C (as ascorbic acid and ascorbyl palmitate) 60 mg • Vitamin E (as dl-alpha-tocopheryl acetate and d-alpha-tocopheryl succinate) 30 IU • Riboflavin (Vitamin B2) 3.4 mg • Vitamin B-6 (as pyridoxine HCl) 2 mg • Lutein (from marigold flower extract) 5 mg • Bilberry leaf 10 mg • Piperine (from black pepper fruit extract) 4.75 mg • Alpha-Lipoic Acid 10 mg • Glutathione 5 mg • Spinach leaf 20 mg. Other Ingredients: Maltodextrin, Gelatin, Water, Magnesium Stearate.

Vision Essentials **-** Enzymatic Therapy
Each capsule contains: Vitamin A (Beta Carotene) non-toxic form of Vitamin A 5000 IU • Vitamin C (Ascorbic Acid) 100 mg • Riboflavin (Vitamin B2) 5 mg • Other Ingredients: Bilberry extract (Vaccinium myrtillus Fructus) standardized to contain 25% Anthocyanosides (20 mg per capsule) calculated as Anthocyanidins 80 mg.

Vision Formula **-** Nature's Way
Two capsules contain: Bilberry fruit (dried extract 25% Anthocyanins) 50 mg • Biotin (Biotin Triurate) 40 mcg • Cayenne pepper fruit 100 mg • Citrus Bioflavonoids 150 mg • Copper (Amino Acid Chelate) 1 mg • Lutein 6 mg • Niacin (Vitamin B3) 20 mg • Riboflavin (Vitamin B2) 8 mg • Siberian Ginseng root 50 mg • Taurine 150 mg • Tru-OPCs (dried Grape seed extract) 20 mg • Vitamin A (Retinol Palmitate) 2000 IU • Vitamin E (d-Alpha Tocopheryl) 80 IU • Zinc (Amino Acid Chelate) 16 mg. Other Ingredients: Gelatin, Magnesium Stearate, Millet.

Vision Nutrients **-** Puritan's Pride
Each tablet contains: Pro-Vitamin A (Beta Carotene) 5,000 IU • Vitamin E (dl-alpha Tocopheryl) 30 IU • Vitamin C (Ascorbic Acid) 60 mg • Zinc (Zinc Oxide) 40 mg • Copper (Cupric Oxide) 2 mg • Selenium 40 mcg.

Vision Spray **-** Natural Ophthalmics
Three sprays contain: Vitamin A (beta carotene) 500 IU • Vitamin B3 (niacin) 5 mg • Vitamin C (Ester-C) 15 mg • Vitamin E 4 IU • Zinc 5 mg • Lutein (FloraGLO) 10 mg • Zeaxanthin 0.1 mg • Vinpocetine 1 mg • Bilberry extract 5 mg • Eyebright 2 mg • Glutathione 2 mg • Ginkgo Biloba 1 mg • MSM 5 mg • L-Taurine 5 mg • L-Glycine 5 mg • Rutin 5 mg • Quercetin 5 mg. Other Ingredients: Purified Water, Vegetable Glycerin, Aloe Vera, Trace Minerals, Grapefruit Seed extract, Potassium Sorbate, Stevia, Flavorings.

Visionace **-** Vitabiotics
Each tablet contains: Vitamin A (1000 IU) 300 mcg • Vitamin D (100 IU) 2.5 mcg • Vitamin E (natural source) 60 mg • Vitamin C 150 mg • Vitamin B1 (thiamin) 12 mg • Vitamin B2 (riboflavin) 4.8 mg • Vitamin B3 (niacin) 18 mg • Vitamin B6 (pyridoxine HCl) 10 mg • Folacin (as folic acid) 400 mcg • Vitamin B12 (cyanocobalamin) 9 mcg • Pantothenic Acid 20 mg • Iron 6 mg • Magnesium 50 mg • Zinc 15 mg • Iodine 100 mcg • Copper 1 mg • Manganese 4 mg • Selenium 150 mcg • Chromium 50 mcg • Natural Mixed Carotenoids 3 mg • Citrus Bioflavonoids 15 mg • Bilberry extract 60 mg • Lutein Esters 4 mg.

Visionex **-** USANA Health Sciences
Two tablets contain: Vitamin C (as Calcium, Potassium, Magnesium, Zinc Ascorbates) 500 mg • Zinc (as Citrate) 20 mg • Lutein 10 mg • Zeaxanthin 2000 mg • Bilberry Extract (Vaccinium Myrtillus L.) Fruit 50 mg. Other Ingredients: Microcrystalline Cellulose, Croscarmellose Sodium, Ascorbyl Palmitate, Dextrin, Dextrose.

VisionPro **-** HealthMinded
Four capsules contain: Vitamin A 20,000 IU • Vitamin C 200 mg • Vitamin E 440 IU • Calcium 117 mg • Zinc 60 mg • Selenium 20 mcg • Copper 8 mg • Chromium 200 mcg • VisionPro Proprietary Blend 782.5 mg: Citrus Bioflavonoids, L-Taurine, Quercetin, Rutin, Eyebright, N-Acetyl-Cysteine, Bilberry fruit extract, L-Glutathione, Lutein complex, Astaxanthin, Zeaxanthin. Other Ingredients: Stearic Acid, Magnesium Stearate.

Visioplex **-** Progressive Labs
Each capsule contains: Vitamin A (acetate) 937 IU • Vitamin A (beta carotene) 3125 IU • Vitamin C 62.5 mg • Calcium (as calcium citrate) 12.5 mg • Vitamin E (dl-alpha tocopherol) 50 IU • Thiamin (vitamin B1) 2.5 mg • Riboflavin (vitamin B2) 3.1 mg • Niacin 1.25 mg • Niacinamide 6.25 mg • Vitamin B6 (pyridoxine HCl) 3.75 mg • Folate (folic acid) 100 mcg • Vitamin B12 6.25 mcg • Pantothenic Acid 12.5 mg • Magnesium (as magnesium citrate) 31.25 mg • Zinc (as zinc picolinate) 6.25 mg • Selenium (selenomethionine) 25 mcg • Copper (amino acid chelate) 0.375 mg • Raw Eye concentrate 8.75 mg • Eyebright (Euphrasia officinalis) 18.75 mg • Bilberry powder (Vaccinium myrtillis) 5 mg • Ginkgo extract (Ginkgo biloba) 7.5 mg • N-Acetyl-Cysteine (NAC) 31.25 • Quercetin 37.5 mg • Taurine 62.5 mg • L-Methionine 25 mg • Glutamic Acid 6.25 mg • Glycine 6.25 mg.
See Editor's Note No. 14, page 2055.

Visual Eyes **-** Source Naturals
Four tablets contain: Vitamin A (Beta Carotene) 25000 IU • Vitamin A (Palmitate) 7500 IU • Vitamin B2 50 mg • Inositol Hexanicotinate 100 mg • Vitamin C (Magnesium Ascorbate) 1500 mg • Vitamin E (D-Alpha Tocopheryl Succinate) 400 IU • Chromium (ChromeMate Polynicotinate 125 mcg and Chromium Picolinate 125 mcg) 250 mcg • Copper (Sebacate) 1 mg • Magnesium (Ascorbate, Taurinate) 164 mg • Selenium (L-Selenomethionine) 200 mcg • Zinc (Monomethionine) 30 mg • Bilberry extract (Yielding 37 mg of Anthocyanosides)100 mg • Lutein 10 mg • Alpha-Lipoic Acid 25 mg • Ginkgo Biloba 24% (50:1 Extract) 45 mg • Grape Seed extract (Proanthodyn with a Proanthocyanidolic Value of 95) 45 mg • Quercetin 320 mg • N-Acetyl Cysteine 400 mg • Taurine (Magnesium Taurinate) 500 mg • Inositol (Hexanicotinate) 10 mg.

Vita C **-** Shaklee
Each tablet contains: Vitamin C (as Ascorbic acid) 500 mg • Sodium 5 mg. Other Ingredients: Bioflavonoid Complex (Lemon, Orange, Grapefruit, and Hesperidin Complex), Rose Hips, Dicalcium Phosphate, Alginic Acid, Carnauba Wax, Carrageenan, Pectin, Acacia Gum, Guar Gum, Locust Bean Gum, Agar-Agar, Grapefruit Oil.

Vita E **-** Shaklee
Each tablet contains: Vitamin E (as D-alpha tocopheryl acid succinate) 400 IU • Selenium (as Selenium yeast) 10 mcg. Other Ingredients: Dicalcium Phosphate, Silicon Dioxide, Modified Food Starch, Mixed Tocopherol Concentrate, Wheat Germ Flour, Natural Beet Powder.

Vita E Complex **-** Shaklee
Two capsules contain: Vitamin E (as D-alpha Tocopherol concentrate and mixed Tocopherols concentrate) 800 IU • Selenium (as Selenium protein hydrolysate) 130 mcg • Grapeseed extract (Vitis vinifera) seed/skin 76 mg. Other Ingredients: Soybean Oil, Beeswax, Soy Lecithin, Gelatin, Glycerin, Water, Annatto, Caramel.

Vita Fuel With Iron **-** TwinLab
Nine capsules contain: Beta-Carotene (pro-Vitamin A) 25000 IU • Vitamin D (from natural form Vitamin D3) 400 IU • Vitamin C 2000 mg • Natural Vitamin E (Succinate) 800 IU • CoQ10 (Coenzyme Q10) 30 mg • L-Glutathione 100 mg • N-Acetyl Cysteine (NAC) 200 mg • Alpha-Lipoic Acid 100 mcg • Vitamin B1 (Thiamine) 50 mg • Vitamin B2 (Riboflavin) 50 mg • Vitamin B6 (Pyridoxine) 50 mg • Vitamin B12 (Cobalamin) 100 mcg • Niacinamide 75 mg • Pantothenic Acid 100 mg • Folic Acid 800 mcg • Biotin 600 mcg • PABA 10 mg • Choline Bitartrate 100 mg • Inositol 100 mg • L-Carnitine (from Carni Fuel L-Carnitine Magnesium Citrate) 100 mg • Creatine (Monohydrate) 1000 mg • Calcium (from Calcium Citrate & Carbonate) 500 mg • Magnesium (from L-Carnitine Magnesium Citrate, Aspartate, Alpha-Ketoglutarate & Oxide) 500 mg • Potassium (from Potassium Alpha-Ketoglutarate, Citrate & Aspartate) 500 mg • Zinc (from Zinc Picolinate) 50 mg • Manganese (from Manganese Gluconate) 10 mg • Iron (from Ferrous Fumarate) 10 mg • Copper (from Copper Gluconate) 2 mg • Iodine (from Potassium Iodide) 150 mcg • Selenium (from Selenomethionine & Selenate<50/50 mixture) 200 mcg • Chromium (from Chromic Fuel patented Chromium Picolinate) 400 mcg • Molybdenum (from natural Molybdic Acid) 150 mcg.

Vita Fuel Without Iron **-** TwinLab
Nine capsules contain: Beta-Carotene (pro-Vitamin A) 25000 IU • Vitamin D (from natural form Vitamin D3) 400 IU • Vitamin C 2000 mg • Natural Vitamin E (Succinate) 800 IU • CoQ10 (Coenzyme Q10) 30 mg • L-Glutathione 100 mg • N-Acetyl Cysteine (NAC) 200 mg • Alpha-Lipoic Acid 100 mcg • Vitamin B1 (Thiamine) 50 mg • Vitamin B2 (Riboflavin) 50 mg • Vitamin B6 (Pyridoxine) 50 mg • Vitamin B12 (Cobalamin) 100 mcg • Niacinamide 75 mg • Pantothenic Acid 100 mg • Folic Acid 800 mcg • Biotin 600 mcg • PABA 10 mg • Choline Bitartrate 100 mg • Inositol 100 mg • L-Carnitine (from Carni Fuel L-Carnitine Magnesium Citrate) 100 mg • Creatine (Monohydrate) 1000 mg • Calcium (from Calcium Citrate & Carbonate) 500 mg • Magnesium (from L-Carnitine Magnesium Citrate, Aspartate, Alpha-Ketoglutarate & Oxide) 500 mg • Potassium (from Potassium Alpha-Ketoglutarate, Citrate & Aspartate) 500 mg • Zinc (from Zinc Picolinate) 50 mg • Manganese (from Manganese Gluconate) 10 mg • Copper (from Copper Gluconate) 2 mg • Iodine (from Potassium Iodide) 150 mcg • Selenium (from Selenomethionine & Selenate<50/50 mixture) 200 mcg • Chromium (from Chromic Fuel patented Chromium Picolinate) 400 mcg • Molybdenum (from natural Molybdic Acid) 150 mcg.

Vita Lea for Children Fruit **-** Shaklee
Two tablets contain: Vitamin A (as Vitamin A acetate) 2500 IU • Vitamin C (as Ascorbic acid) 60 mg • Vitamin D (as Choloecalciferol) 400 IU • Vitamin E (as D-alpha tocopheryl acetate) 30 IU • Vitamin K (as Phytonadione) 10 mcg • Thiamin (as Thiamin mononitrate) 1.5 mg • Riboflavin 1.7 mg • Niacin (as Niacinamide) 20 mg • Vitamin B6 (as Pyridoxine hydrochloride) 2 mg • Folate (as Folic acid) 400 mcg • Vitamin B12 (as Cyanocobalamin) 6 mcg • Biotin (as D-biotin) 300 mcg • Pantothenic acid (as D-calcium pantothenate) 10 mg • Calcium (as Dicalcium iphosphate) 200 mg • Iron (as Ferrous fumerate) 10 mg • Phosphorus (as Dicalcium phosphate) 160 mg • Iodine (as Potassium iodide) 90 mcg • Magnesium (as Magnesium oxide) 80 mg • Zinc (as Zinc gluconate) 10 mg • Selenium (as trace mineral Protein hydrolysate) 20 mcg • Copper (as Copper oxide) 1 mg • Manganese (as Manganese gluconate) 1.5 mg • Chromium (as trace mineral Protein hydrolysate) 50 mcg • Molybdenum 50 mcg. Other Ingredients: Sorbitol, Fructose, Natural Flavors, Vegetable Juice Extracts (Beet, Carrot, Cabbage) and Annatto, Acacia Gum, Citric Acid, Inositol, Choline Bitartrate, Mixed Tocopherols, Rice Bran Powder, Rose Hips Powder, Alfalfa Powder, Acerola Extract, Grapefruit Bioflavonoid, Hesperidin Complex, Lemon Bioflavonoid, Orange Bioflavonoid, Sea Kelp Powder.

Vita Lea Iron Formula **-** Shaklee
Two tablets contain: Vitamin A (as Vitamin A acetate) 5000 IU • Vitamin C (as Ascorbic acid) 120 mg • Vitamin D (as Cholecalciferol) 400 IU • Vitamin E (as D-alpha tocopheryl acid succinate) 60 IU • Vitamin K (as Phytonadione) 80 mcg • Thiamin (as Thiamin mononitrate) 1.5 mg • Riboflavin 1.7 mg • Niacin (as Niacinamide) 20 mg • Vitamin B6 (as Pyridoxine hydrochloride) 2 mg • Folate (as Folic acid) 400 mcg • Vitamin B12 (as Cyanocobalamin) 6 mcg • Biotin (as D-biotin) 300 mcg • Pantothenic acid (as D-calcium pantothenate) 10 mg • Calcium (as Dicalcium phosphate) 450 mg • Iron (as Ferrous fumarate) 18 mg • Phosphorus (as Dicalcium phosphate) 350 mg • Iodine (as Potassium iodide and sea kelp) 150 mcg • Magnesium (as Magnesium oxide) 200 mg • Zinc (as Zinc

gluconate) 15 mg • Selenium (as trace mineral Protein hydrolysate) 70 mcg • Copper (as Copper gluconate) 2 mg • Manganese (as Manganese gluconate) 3.5 mg • Chromium (as trace mineral Protein hydrolysate) 130 mcg • Molybdenum (as trace mineral Protein hydrolysate) 130 mcg • Sodium 5 mg • Nickel (as trace mineral Protein hydrolysate) 15 mcg • Tin (as trace mineral Protein hydrolysate) 10 mcg • Vanadium (as trace mineral Protein hydrolysate) 2 mcg • Boron (as trace mineral Protein hydrolysate) 1 mg • Silicon (as Silicon dioxide) 2 mg. Other Ingredients: Microcrystalline Cellulose, Hydroxypropyl Methylcellulose, Croscarmellose Sodium, Spirulina, Inositol, Choline Bitartrate, Alfalfa Powder, Grapefruit Bioflavonoid, Hesperidin Complex, Lemon Bioflavonoid, Mixed Tocopherols, Orange Bioflavonoid, Rice Bran Powder, Rose Hips Powder, Acerola Extract, Hydroxylated Soy Lecithin, Carnauba Wax.

Vita Lea No Iron Formula - Shaklee
Two tablets contain: Vitamin A (as Vitamin A acetate) 5000 IU • Vitamin C (as Ascorbic acid) 120 mg • Vitamin D (as Cholecalciferol) 400 IU • Vitamin E (as D-alpha tocopheryl acid succinate) 60 IU • Vitamin K (as Phytonadione) 80 mcg • Thiamin (as Thiamin mononitrate) 1.5 mg • Riboflavin 1.7 mg • Niacin (as Niacinamide) 20 mg • Vitamin B6 (as Pyridoxine hydrochloride) 2 mg • Folate (as Folic acid) 400 mcg • Vitamin B12 (as Cyanocobalamin) 6 mcg • Biotin (as D-biotin) 300 mcg • Pantothenic Acid (as D-calcium pantothenate) 10 mg • Calcium (as Dicalcium phosphate) 450 mg • Phosphorus (as Dicalcium phosphate) 350 mg • Iodine (as Potassium iodide and sea kelp) 150 mcg • Magnesium (as Magnesium oxide) 200 mg • Zinc (as Zinc gluconate) 15 mg • Selenium (as Trace mineral protein hydrolysate) 70 mcg • Copper (as Copper gluconate) 2 mg • Manganese (as Manganese gluconate) 3.5 mg • Chromium (as Trace mineral protein hydrolysate) 130 mcg • Molybdenum (as Trace mineral protein hydrolysate) 160 mcg • Sodium 5 mg • Nickel (as Trace mineral protein hydrolysate) 15 mcg • Tin (as Trace mineral protein hydrolysate) 10 mcg • Vanadium (as Trace mineral protein hydrolysate) 2 mcg • Boron (as Trace mineral protein hydrolysate) 1 mg • Silicon (as Silicon dioxide) 2 mg. Other Ingredients: Microcrystalline Cellulose, Hydroxypropyl Methylcellulose, Croscarmellose Sodium, Spirulina, Inositol, Choline Bitartrate, Alfalfa Powder, Grapefruit Bioflavonoid, Hesperidin Complex, Lemon Bioflavonoid, Mixed Tocopherols, Orange Bioflavonoid, Rice Bran Powder, Rose Hips Powder, Acerola Extract, Hydroxylated Soy Lecithin, Carnauba Wax.

Vita Male - Nutri-Quest Rx
Each tablet contains: Yohimbe bark 250 mg • Damiana 40 mg • Gotu Kola 25 mg • Hawthorne berries 25 mg • Beet root.

Vita-Bears - Melaleuca
Four tablets contain: Vitamin A (as beta-carotene) 5000 IU • Vitamin C 80 mg • Vitamin D 400 IU • Vitamin E 30 IU • Vitamin B1 (thiamine) 2 mg • Vitamin B2 (riboflavin) 2 mg • Niacinamide 20 mg • Vitamin B6 (pyridoxine) 2 mg • Folic Acid 400 mcg • Vitamin B12 (cyanocobalamin) 6 mcg • Biotin 40 mcg • Pantothenic Acid 10 mg • Calcium 10 mg • Iron 18 mg • Phosphorous 40 mg • Iodine 150 mcg • Magnesium 20 mg • Zinc 16 mg • Copper 2 mg • Chromium 10 mcg.

VitaCardia - PhysioLogics
Three capsules contain: Vitamin B6 (as pyridoxine HCl) 10 mg • Folic Acid 810 mcg • Vitamin B12 (as cyanocobalamin) 510 mcg • Magnesium (as magnesium glycinate) 50 mg • Potassium (as potassium chloride) 95 mg • Hawthorn fruit extract (crataegus oxyacantha, standardized to contain 1.8% vitexin, 10.8 mg) 600 mg • Cordyceps (standardized to contain 7% cordyceptic acid, 28 mg) 400 mg • Taurine 200 mg. Other Ingredients: Gelatin, Silica, Vegetable Magnesium Stearate.

Vitacor Plus - Matthias Rath, Inc.
Each tablet contains: Ascorbic Acid 230 mg • Ascorbyl Palmitate 170 mg • Calcium Ascorbate 100 mg • Magnesium Ascorbate 100 mg • Vitamin E (d-Alpha-Tocopherol) 130 IU • Vitamin A (Beta-Carotene) 1665 IU • Vitamin B1 (Thiamine) 7 mg • Vitamin B2 (Riboflavin) 7 mg • Niacin 10 mg • Niacinamide 35 mg • Pantothenic Acid (d-Calcium Pantothenate) 40 mg • Vitamin B6 (Pyridoxal Phosphate) 10 mg • Vitamin B12 (Cyanocobalamin) 20 mcg • Vitamin D (as Vitamin D3) (Cholecalciferol) 130 IU • Folic Acid 90 mcg • Biotin 65 mcg • L-Proline 110 mg • L-Lysine 110 mg • L-Carnitine 35 mg • L-Arginine 40 mg • L-Cysteine 35 mg • Calcium (Glycinate, Ascorbate) 35 mg • Magnesium (Glycinate, Ascorbate) 40 mg • Potassium (Chelate) 20 mg • Zinc (Glycinate) 7 mg • Manganese (Chelate) 1.3 mg • Copper (Glycinate) 330 mcg • Selenium (L-Seleno Methionine) 20 mcg • Chromium (Glycinate) 10 mcg • Molybdenum (Glycinate) 4 mcg • Inositol 35 mg • Coenzyme Q10 7 mg • Phosphorous (Dicalcium Phosphate) 15 mg • Pycnogenol 7 mg • Citrus Bioflavonoids 100 mg • Vitamin E (Beta, Gamma & Delta Tocopherols) 22 mg • Carotenoids (Alpha-Carotene, Lutein, Zeaxanthin, & Cryptoxanthin) 50 mcg.

VitAdvance Immune Advance Formula - Avon
Each tablet contains: Vitamin A (as beta-carotene) 3333 IU • Vitamin C (as ascorbic acid) 200 mg • Vitamin E (as d-alpha tocopheryl acetate) 200 IU • Vitamin B6 (as pyridoxine HCl) 6 mg • Zinc (as zinc gluconate) • Astragalus root extract (astragalus membranaceus, standardized to 0.4% 7-glyco-4'-hydroxy-3'-methyoxyisoflavone) 50 mg • Green Tea leaf extract (camellia sinensis, standardized to 50% polyphenols) 50 mg. Other Ingredients: Microcrystalline Cellulose, Croscarmellose Sodium, Silicon Dioxide, Hydroxypropyl Methylcellulose, Stearic Acid, Titanium Dioxide, Magnesium Stearate, Polyethylene Glycol, Caramel, Riboflavin.

VitAdvance Joint Formula - Avon
Each tablet contains: Vitamin C (as ascorbic acid) 30 mg • Manganese (as manganese gluconate) 1.5 mg • Glucosamine Sulfate powder (includes potassium chloride 125 mg) 500 mg • Devil's Claw (harpagophytum procumbens) root extract (standardized to 2% harpagosides) 150 mg. Other Ingredients: Microcrystalline Cellulose, Croscarmellose Sodium, Stearic Acid, Magnesium Stearate, Hydroxypropyl Methylcellulose, Polyethylene Glycol, Carnauba Wax.

VitAdvance Menopause Support - Avon
Each tablet contains: Calcium (as dicalcium phosphate) 61 mg • Chaste Tree berry fruit (vitex angus-castus, standardized to 0.5% angusides) 50 mg • Black Cohosh roots extract (cimicifuga racemosa, standardized to 2.5% triterpene glycosides) 40 mg • Soy Isoflavones 22.5 mg • Boron (as sodium borate) 1.5 mg. Other Ingredients: Microcrystalline Cellulose, Stearic Acid, Magnesium Stearate, Silicon Dioxide, Hydroxypropyl Methylcellulose, Polyethylene Glycol, Carnauba Wax.

VitAdvance Men's Complete Multivitamin - Avon
Each tablet contains: Vitamin A (as retinyl acetate and 20% (1000 IU) as beta-carotene) 5000 IU • Vitamin C (as ascotbic acid) 90 mg • Vitamin D (as cholecalciferol) 400 IU • Vitamin E (as d-alpha tocopheryl acetate) 45 IU • Vitamin K (as phytonadione) 80 mcg • Thiamin (a thiamin mononitrate) 2.25 mcg • Niacin (as niacinamide) 20 mg • Vitamin B6 (as pyridoxine hydrochloride) 3 mg • Folate (as folic acid) 400 mcg • Vitamin B12 (as cyanocobalamin) 12 mcg • Biotin 60 mcg • Pantothenic Acid (as calcium d-pantothenate) 10 mg • Calcium (as dicalcium phosphate) 100 mg • Iron (as ferrous gluconate) 18 mg • Phosphorous (as dicalcium phosphate) 78 mg • Iodine (as potassium iodide) 150 mcg • Magnesium (as magnesium oxide) 100 mg • Zinc (as zinc gluconate) 15 mg • Selenium (as selenium-brown rice protein chelate) 70 mcg • Copper (as copper gluconate) 2 mg • Manganese (as manganese gluconate) 2 mg • Chromium (as chromium-brown rice protein chelate) 120 mcg • Molybdenum (as molybdenum citrate) 75 mcg • Chloride (as potassium chloride) 72 mg • Potassium (as potassium chloride) 82 mg • Silicon (as silicon dioxide) 2 mg • Lycopene 400 mcg • Lutein 250 mcg • Boron (as sodium borate) 150 mcg • Vanadium (as vanadium citrate) 10 mcg • Tin (as stannous chloride) 10 mcg • Nickel (as nickel sulphate) 5 mcg.
Inactive Ingredients: Microcrystalline Celluslose, Croscarmellose Sodium, Stearic Acid, Magnesium Stearate, Hydroxypropyl Methylcellulose, Titanium Dioxide, Hydroxypropyl Cellulose, Polyethylene Glycol, Caramel, Polysorbate 80, Carnauba Wax, Acetylated Monoglycerides, Xanthan Gum.

VitAdvance Menstrual Comfort I **-** Avon
Each tablet contains: Vitamin B6 (as pyridoxine hydrochloride) 50 mg • Magnesium (as magneisum oxide) 250 mg • Calcium (as dicalcium phosphate) 85 mg • Chaste Tree berry standardized extract (vitex angus-castus, 0.5% angusides) 30 mg. Other Ingredients: Microcrystalline Cellulose, Stearic Acid, Magnesium Stearate, Silicon Dioxide, Hydroxypropyl Methylcellulose, Polyethylene Glycol, Carnauba Wax.

VitAdvance Menstrual Comfort II **-** Avon
Each softgel contains: Vitamin E (as d-alpha tocopheryl acetate) 10 IU • Evening Primrose Oil (cold pressed seeds of oenothera biennis) 500 mg • Fatty Acid Profile: Linoleic Acid (omega 6) 350 mg • Oleic Acid (omega 9) 55 mg • Gamma Linolenic Acid (omega 6) 50 mg • Palmitic Acid 30 mg • Linolenic Acid (omega 3) 12 mg. Other Ingredients: Soybean Oil, Gelatin, Glycerin, Stearic Acid.

VitAdvance Multi-Kids Complete **-** Avon
Each tablet contains: Vitamin A (as retinyl acetate and 5% (250 IU) as beta-carotene) 5000 IU • Vitamin C (as ascorbic acid) 60 mg • Vitamin D (as cholecalciferol) 400 IU • Vitamin E (as d-alpha tocopheryl acetate) 30 IU • Vitamin K (as phytonadione) 80 mcg • Thiamin (as thiamin mononitrate) 1.5 mg • Riboflavin (vitamin B2) 1.7 mg • Niacin (as niacinamide) 20 mg • Vitamin B6 (as pyridoxine hydrochloride) 2 mg • Folate (as folic acid) 400 mcg • Vitamin B12 (as cyanocobalamin) 6 mcg • Biotin 50 mcg • Pantothenic Acid (as calcium d-pantothenate) 10 mg • Calcium (as carbonate) 100 mg • Iron (as ferrous fumerate) 10 mg • Iodine (as potassium iodide) 150 mcg • Magnesium (as magnesium oxide) 20 mg • Zinc (as zinc citrate) 15 mg • Copper (as cupric acid) 2 mg • Manganese (as manganese citrate) 2 mg. Inactive Ingredients: Sorbitol, Fructose, Natural Flavor, Microcrystalline Cellulose, Stearic Acid, Magnesium Stearate, Silicon Dioxide, Carmine (natural colorant), Sucralose.

VitAdvance Restful Sleep **-** Avon
Each tablet contains: Valerian root extract (valeriana officinalis, standardized to 0.8% valerenic acid) 250 mg • Passionflower herb extract (passiflora incarnata, standardized to 4% vitexin) 150 mg. Other Ingredients: Mircrocrystalline Cellulose, Croscarmellose Sodium, Hydroxypropyl Methylcellulose, Stearic Acid, Silicon Dioxide, Titanium Dioxide, Polyethylene Glycol, Magnesium Stearate, Caramel, Peppermint Oil, Riboflavin.

Vita-E **-** Shaklee
Each tablet contains: Vitamin E (as D-alpha tocopheryl acid succinate) 400 IU • Selenium (as selenium yeast) 10 mcg. Other Ingredients: Dicalcium Phosphate, Silicon Dioxide, Modified Food Starch, Wheat Germ Flour, Natural Beet Powder.

VitaGreen **-** Young Living Essential Oils
Each capsule contains: Bee Pollen • Barley Juice Concentrate • Spirulina • Choline Bitartrate • Ginseng • Alfalfa Juice Concentrate • Pacific Kelp • L-Arginine • L-Cysteine • L-Tyrosine • Lemon Oil • Lemongrass Oil • Melissa Oil • Rosemary Oil • Gelatin.

Vital Green **-** Futurebiotics
Ten tablets contain: Alfalfa leaf juice powder concentrate 1350 mg • Barley grass juice powder concentrate 100 mg • Wheat Grass juice powder concentrate 250 mg • Spirulina powder 150 mg • Chlorella powder (broken cell) 150 mg. Other Ingredients: Dicalcium phosphate, Cellulose, Magnesium stearate, Vegetable stearate, Silica.

Vital K + Ginseng Capsules **-** Futurebiotics
Potassium • Calcium • Magnesium • 16 Herbal extracts Plus the Triple Ginseng Action of Korean, Siberian & American Ginseng.

Vital K + Ginseng Extra **-** Futurebiotics
Siberian, Korean, & American Ginseng • "16 Invigorating Herbal extracts" • Potassium • Calcium & Iron found in the Original Vital K.

Vital K Original with Magnesium **-** Futurebiotics
Potassium • Magnesium • Calcium • Iron & "17 Herbal extracts" including the major Chinese adaptogenic herbs: Ginseng, Astragalus, Schizandra & Dong Quai.

Vital Memory **-** TwinLab
Each tablet contains: Vitamin C (from ascorbic acid) 50 mg • Vitamin E (from d-alpha tocopheryl acid succinate) 33.34 IU • Folic Acid 133.34 mcg • Vitamin B12 (from cyanocobalamin) 16.67 mcg • Calcium (from calcium phosphate, carbonate and silicate) 336 mg • Phosphorus (from calcium phosphate) 192 mg • Phosphatidylserine 100 mg • Acetyl L-Carnitine Hydrochloride 50 mg • Alpha Lipoic Acid 16.67 mg. Other Ingredients: Cellulose, Croscarmellose Sodium, Maltodextrin, Vegetable Stearate, Magnesium Stearate, Silica.

Vital PSP+ **-** Healthywise
Each 50 g scoop contains: Proprietary Blend 5000 mg: Alpha-Glycan Polysaccharidepeptides of Rice Flour, Natural Spirulina.

Vital Vein **-** Puritan's Pride
Three capsules contain: Vitamin A 10,000 IU • Vitamin C 250 mg • Vitamin E 100 IU • Magnesium 100 mg • Zinc 3 mg • Selenium 0.42 mcg • Grape Seed extract 15 mg • Gotu Kola herb (centella asiatica) 800 mg • Lecithin 200 mg • Butchers' Broom herb (Ruscus aculeatus) 400 mg • Rutin 125 mg • Spirulina 100 mg • White Oak Bark (Quercus alba) 75 mg • Ginkgo Biloba leaf (Ginkgo biloba) 100 mg • Kelp 100 mg • Bromelain 50 mg • Ginger root (Zingiber officinate) 50 mg • Hawthorn berry (Crataegus laevigata) 50 mg.

Vita-Licious Vitamin Chews **-** Bronson Laboratories
Each chew contains: Vitamin C 500 mg.

Vitaline Chewable CoQ10 (100 mg, maple nut/orange creme/chocolate) **-** PhytoPharmica
Each chewable tablet contains: Coenzyme Q10 (coq10, ubiquinone 10) 100 mg • Vitamin E (as D-alpha tocopheryl acetate) 300 IU.

Vitaline Chewable CoQ10 (200 mg, maple nut) **-** PhytoPharmica
Each chewable tablet contains: Coenzyme Q10 (coq10, ubiquinone 10) 200 mg • Vitamin E (as DL-alpha tocopheryl aceate, D-alpha tocopheryl acetate, and mixed tocopherols) 400 IU.

Vitaline CoQ10 - 100 mg - Chocolate Flavor **-** PhytoPharmica
Each chewable wafer contains: Vitamin E (as dl-alpha tocopheryl acetate, d-alpha tocopheryl acetate, and mixed tocopherals) 300 IU • Coenzyme Q10 (CoQ10; Ubiquinone) certified by Assay 100 mg.

Vitaline CoQ10 - 100 mg - Maple Nut Flavor **-** PhytoPharmica
Each chewable wafer contains: Vitamin E (as dl-alpha tocopheryl acetate, d-alpha tocopheryl acetate, and mixed tocopherols) 300 IU • Coenzyme Q10 (CoQ10; Ubiquinone) certified by Assay 100 mg.

Vitaline CoQ10 - 200 mg - Chocolate Flavor **-** PhytoPharmica
Each chewable wafer contains: Vitamin E (as dl-alpha tocopheryl acetate, d-alpha tocopheryl acetate, and mixed tocopherols) 400 IU • Coenzyme Q10 (CoQ10; Ubiquinone) certified by Assay 200 mg.

Vitaline CoQ10 - 200 mg - Maple Nut Flavor **-** PhytoPharmica
Each chewable wafer contains: Vitamin E (as dl-alpha tocopheryl acetate, d-alpha tocopheryl acetate, and mixed tocopherols) 400 IU • Coenzyme Q10 (CoQ10; Ubiquinone) certified by Assay 200 mg.

Vitaline CoQ10 - 60 mg - Chocolate Flavor **-** PhytoPharmica
Each chewable wafer contains: Vitamin E (as dl-alpha tocopheryl acetate, d-alpha tocopheryl acetate, and mixed tocopherols) 180 IU • Coenzyme Q10 (CoQ10; Ubiquinone) certified by Assay 60 mg.

Vitaline CoQ10 - 60 mg - Maple Nut Flavor **-** PhytoPharmica
Each chewable wafer contains: Vitamin E (as dl-alpha tocopheryl acetate, d-alpha tocopheryl acetate, and mixed tocopherols) 180 IU • Coenzyme Q10 (CoQ10; Ubiquinone) certified by Assay 60 mg.

Vitaline CoQ10, Creatin, and Acetyl-L-Carnitine **-** PhytoPharmica
Each scoop contains: Acetyl-L-Carnitine HCl 2.5 g • Creatine (as creatine pyruvate) 5 g • Natural Coenzyme Q10 (trans-coq10, ubiquinone 10, derived from yeast fermentation) 1.2 g • Vitamine E (as DL-alpha tocopheryl acetate) 1200 IU.

Vitaline L-Carnitine **-** PhytoPharmica
Each caplet contains: L-Carnitine 500 mg.

Vitaliza **-** HerbaSway
Horny Goat Weed • Dong Quai • He Sho Wu • Panax Ginseng • Knotweed • Schisandra • Blackberry • HerbaSwee (Cucurbitaceae fruit).

Vitalize Shampoo **-** Biotech Corp.
Purified Water • Saponified Oils of Coconut Oil and Olive Oil • Vegetable Glycerin • Methylsulfonylmethane (MSM) • Aloe Vera gel • Jojoba oil • PEG-150 Distearate (from plant) • Hydrolyzed Wheat Protein • Natural Essential Oils • Avena Sativa (oat) extract • Citric Acid • Rosemary Oil.

Vitalux AREDS **-** Novartis
Each tablet contains: Beta Carotene (provitamin A) 12,500 IU • Vitamin C (ascorbic acid) 250 mg • Vitamin E (d-alpha tocopheryl acetate) 200 IU • Zinc (zinc gluconate) 40 mg • Copper (HVP chelate) 1 mg • Lutein (supplying 132 mg of Zeaxanthin).

Vitalux with Lutein **-** Novartis
Each tablet contains: Beta-Carotene (provitamin A) 10,000 IU • Vitamin C (ascorbic acid) 300 mg • Vitamin E (acetate) 100 IU • Vitamin B2 (riboflavin) 20 mg • Selenium (HVP chelate) 50 mcg • Zinc (gluconate) 40 mg • Copper (HVP chelate) 2 mg • Lutein 4 mg (supplying 176 mcg of Zeaxanthin) 4 mg. Other Ingredients: Cellulose, Calcium Silicate, Hydroxypropyl Methylcellulose, Stearic Acid, Magnesium Stearate, Silicon Dioxide, Titanium Dioxide, Hydroxypropyl Cellulose, Polyethylene Glycol, Caramel Color, Polysorbate 80, Vegetable Wax, Ethyl Vanillin, Diacetylated Monoglycerides, Xanthan Gum.

Vita-Min **-** Puritan's Pride
Six tablets contain: Vitamin A (as Retinyl Acetate and Beta Carotene) 7,650 IU •Vitamin D (as Cholecalciferol) 200 IU • Vitamin C (as Ascorbic Acid) 200 mg • Vitamin E (as d-Alpha Tocopheryl Acid Succinate) 10 IU • Thiamin (Vitamin B-1; as Thiamine Hydrochloride) 6 mg • Riboflavin (Vitamin B-2) 12 mg • Niacin 3 mg • Vitamin B-6 (as Pyridoxine Hydrochloride) 2 mg • Folic Acid 400 mcg • Vitamin B-12 (as Cyanocobalamin) 5 mcg • Biotin (as D-Biotin) 5 mcg • Pantothenic Acid (as D-Calcium Pantothenate) 0.12 mg • Calcium (as Dicalcium Phosphate) 800 mg • Iron (as Ferrous Gluconate) 14 mg • Phosphorus (as Dicalcium Phosphate) 600 mg • Iodine (as Potassium Iodide) 100 mcg • Magnesium (as Magnesium Oxide) 50 mg • Zinc (as Zinc Sulfate) 0.022 mg • Selenium (as Sodium Selenate) 70 mcg • Copper (as Copper Sulfate) 0.022 mg • Manganese (as Manganese Sulfate) 0.0042 mg • Potassium (as Potassium Chloride and Potassium Iodide) 0.0574 mg • Silicon (as Silicon Dioxide) 0.097 mcg • Boron (as Sodium Borate Decahydrate) 300 mcg • PABA (Para-Aminobenzoic Acid) 37.5 mg • Choline Bitartrate 5.25 mg • Inositol 10 mg • Alfalfa 40 mg • L-Lysine 10 mg • Methionine 1.25 mg • Leucine 4.5 mg • Cysteine 1.25 mg • Isoleucine 4.5 mg • Phenylalanine 2.6 mg • Arginine 1.93 mg • Histidine 1.09 mg • Threonine 2.08 mg • Valine 3.16 mg • Wheat Germ powder 60 mg • Papain 20 mg • Chlorophyll 10 mg • Citrus Bioflavonoid 30 mg • Wheat Germ oil 20 mg • Peppermint leaves 20 mg • Ginkgo Biloba leaf 30 mg • Coenzyme Q-10 30 mcg • Ginseng 12 mg • Deodorized Garlic 12 mg • Echinacea Purpurea 24 mg • Spirulina 12 mg • Chlorella 12 mg • Klamath Lake Blue Green Algae 12 mg • Grapeseed extract complex 200 mcg. In a natural base of Watercress, Parsley, Kelp, and Lecithin.

Vitamin & Aloe Mosturizing Creme **-** Aspen Group, Inc.
Each gram contains: Tocopheryl Acetate 1% • Panthenol 1% • Water • Hydrogenated Polyisobutane • Octyl Methoxycinnamate • Mineral Oil • Ceteraryl Alcohol • Cetyl Phosphate • Dimethicone • Aloe Vera Gel • Aminomethyl Propanol • Fragrance • Carbomer • Propylene Glycol • Diazolidinyl Urea • Methylparaben • Propylparaben.

Vitamin A - Basic Nutrition **-** GNC
Each capsule contains: Vitamin A (as Fish Liver Oil) 10,000 IU. Other Ingredients: Soybean oil, Gelatin, Glycerin.

Vitamin A - In Water Soluble Base **-** Nature's Bounty
Each softgel contains: Vitamin A (as Retinyl Palmitate) 10000 IU. Other Ingredients: Polysorbate 80, Gelatin, Glycerin, Propylene Glycol.

Vitamin A **-** Jamieson
Each capsule contains: Vitamin A (from Halibut liver oil) 10000 IU.

Vitamin A **-** Nature's Bounty
Each softgel contains: Vitamin A (from Fish Liver Oils) 10000 IU. Other Ingredients: Soybean Oil, Gelatin, Glycerin.

Vitamin A **-** Nature's Way
Each softgel contains: Vitamin A (cod liver oil) 10,000 IU. Other Ingredients: Gelatin, Glycerin, Soybean Oil, Water.

Vitamin A **-** Puritan's Pride
Each softgel contains: Vitamin A (as derived from fish liver oils) 10,000 IU.

Vitamin A & D - GNC A-Z **-** GNC
Each capsule contains: Vitamin A (as fish liver oil) 5000 IU • Vitamin D (as fish liver oil) 400 IU. Other Ingredients: Soybean Oil, Gelatin, Glycerin.

Vitamin A & D - Health Smart Vitamins **-** Health Smart Vitamins
Each softgel contains: Vitamin A (from cod liver oil) 10,000 IU • Vitamin D (from cod liver oil) 400 IU.

Vitamin A & D **-** Jamieson
Each capsule contains: Vitamin A (Retinol) 5000 IU • Vitamin D 400 IU.

Vitamin A & D **-** Nature's Bounty
Each tablet contains: Vitamin A (as Retinyl Palmitate) 10000 IU •Vitamin D (as Cholecalciferol) 400 IU. Other Ingredients: Dicalcium Phosphate, Cellulose, Calcium Sulfate, Vegetable Stearic Acid, Cellulose Coating, Vegetable Magnesium Stearate, Silica.

Vitamin A & D **-** Source Naturals
Each tablet contains: vitamin A (as palmitate) 10,000 IU • Vitamin D (as cholecalciferol) 400 IU.

Vitamin A & D Fortified **-** Jamieson
Each capsule contains: Vitamin A 10,000 IU • Vitamin D 400 IU.

Vitamin A 10,000 I.U. **-** Nature Made
Each softgel contains: Vitamin A (from fish liver oil) 10,000 IU. Other Ingredients: Soybean Oil, Gelatin, Glycerin, Water.
See Editor's Note No. 45, page 2058.

Vitamin A 10,000 IU **-** Jamieson
Each capsule contains: Vitamin A Retinol (Derived from fresh, pure fish liver oil) 10,000 IU.

Vitamin A 10,000 IU - GNC A-Z **-** GNC
Each capsule contains: Vitamin A (as fish liver oil) 10,000 IU. Other Ingredients: Soybean Oil, Gelatin, Glycerin.

BRAND NAMES

Vitamin A 8000 IU - Nature Made - Nature Made
Each softgel contains: Vitamin A (from fish liver oil) 8000 IU. Other Ingredients: Soybean Oil, Gelatin, Glycerin, Water.
See Editor's Note No. 45, page 2058.

Vitamin A Cream - Life Extension
Vitamin A, De-Ionized Water, Aloe, Emollients, Cetearyl Alcohol, Methyl Glucose, Sesquisterate, Mink oil, Vitamin D oil (vitamin D2), Vitamin E oil, BHT, BHA, Tea, Sesame oil, Lanolin.

Vitamin A Palmitate - Source Naturals
Each tablet contains: Vitamin A (as palmitate) 10,000 IU.

Vitamin A Retinol - Anti-Aging Moisturizer - Jamieson
Contains: Vitamin A Retinol (Retinyl Palmitate) • SPF Active Ingredients • Aloe Vera Extract • Bee Pollen Extract • Chamomile Extract • Comfrey Extract • Watercress Extract.

Vitamin A Retinol - Night Treatment Moisturizer - Jamieson
Vitamin A Retinol (Retinyl Palmitate) • Tocopheryl Acetate • Aloe Vera Extract • Fennel Extract • Hops Extract • Chamomile Extract • Balm Mint Extract • Mistletoe Extract • Bee Pollen Extract • Jojoba Oil • Wheat Germ Oil • Fructose • Glucose • Sucrose.

Vitamin A Retinyl Palmitate Wrinkle Treatment - Derma E
Vitamin A 10000 IU/100 gm • Vitamin E • Vitamin D • Allantoin.

Vitamin B 100 Complex - Jamieson
Each caplet contains: Thiamin (as Thiamine Mononitrate) 100 mg • Riboflavin (Vitamin B2) 100 mg • Niacin (as Niacinamide) 100 mg • Vitamin B6 (as Pyridoxine Hydrochloride) 100 mg • Folate (as Folic Acid) 400 mcg • Vitamin B12 (as Cyanocobalamin) 100 mcg • Biotin 100 mcg • Pantothenic Acid (as Calcium D-Pantothenate) 100 mg • Calcium 555 mg • Choline Bitartrate 100 mg • Inositol 100 mg.

Vitamin B Complex - NSI - NSI - Nutraceutical Sciences Institute
Each capsule contains: Thiamine HCl (B1) 250 mg • Riboflavin (B2) 10 mg • Niacinamide (B3) 100 mg • Pantothenic Acid (B6) 100 mg • Methylcobalamin (B12) 500 mcg • Folic Acid 800 mcg • Biotin 500 mcg • Vitamin C (magnesium acorbate, Ester C) 100 mg.

Vitamin B Complex - PhysioLogics - PhysioLogics
Each capsule contains: Thiamin (vitamin B1, as thiamin mononitrate) 100 mg • Riboflavin (vitamin B2) 100 mg • Niacin (as niacinamide) 100 mg • Vitamin B6 (as pyrdioxine hydrochloride) 100 mg • Folic Acid 400 mcg • Vitamin B12 (as cyanocobalamin) 100 mcg • Biotin 100 mcg • Pantothenic Acid (as d-calcium pantothenate) 100 mg • Choline Bitartrate 100 mg • PABA (para-aminobenzoic acid) 100 mg • Inositol 100 mg • Proprietary Blend 7.5 mg: Alfalfa, Watercress, Parsley, Lecithin, Rice Bran. Other Ingredients: Gelatin, Vegetable Magnesium Stearate, Silica.

Vitamin B-1 - Nature's Bounty
Each tablet contains: Thiamin (as Thiamine Hydrochloride) 100 mg. Other Ingredients: Dicalcium Phosphate, Cellulose, Vegetable Stearic Acid, Silica, Vegetable Magnesium Stearate.

Vitamin B1 - Source Naturals
Each tablet contains: Thiamin (vitamin B1) 100 mg.

Vitamin B1 100 mg - Jamieson
Each tablet contains: Vitamin B1 (Thiamine Mononitrate) 100 mg.

Vitamin B-1 100 mg - Nature Made
Each tablet contains: Thiamin (B1, from thiamine hydrochloride) 100 mg. Other Ingredients: Dibasic Calcium Phosphate, Cellulose, Magnesium Stearate, Silicon Dioxide.
See Editor's Note No. 45, page 2058.

Vitamin B1 100 mg - Solgar
Each tablet contains: Thiamin (as thiamin HCl, vitamin B1) 100 mg • Calcium (as dicalcium phosphate) 85 mg. Other Ingredients: Microcrystalline Cellulose, Silica, Vegetable Cellulose, Vegetable Stearic Acid, Vegetable Magnesium Stearate.

Vitamin B1 50 mg - Solgar
Each tablet contains: Thiamin (as thiamin HCl, vitamin B1) 50 mg • Calcium (as dicalcium phosphate) 85 mg. Other Ingredients: Dicalcium Phosphate, Vegetable Cellulose, Vegetable Stearic Acid.

Vitamin B-12 - Basic Nutrition - GNC
Each tablet contains: Vitamin B12 (as Cyanocobalamin) 500 mcg. Other Ingredients: Dextrose, Stearic Acid, Magnesium Stearate, Whole Brown rice powder.

Vitamin B12 - Jamieson
Each tablet contains: Vitamin B12 (as Cyanocobalamin) 1200 mcg • Calcium 80 mg.

Vitamin B-12 - Leiner Health Products
Each tablet contains: Vitamin B12 (Cyanocobalamin) 100 mcg. Other Ingredients: Lactose, Starch, Dicalcium Phosphate, Magnesium Stearate, Red 40 Lake.

Vitamin B-12 - Nature's Bounty
Each tablet contains: Vitamin B-12 (as Cyanocobalamin) 100 mcg. Other Ingredients: Dicalcium Phosphate, Cellulose, Vegetable Stearic Acid, Mannitol, Silica, Vegetable Magnesium Stearate.

Vitamin B12 - Source Naturals
Each tablet contains: Vitamin B12 2 mg.

Vitamin B12 100 mcg - Jamieson
Each tablet contains: Vitamin B12 (Cyanocobalamin) 100 mcg.

Vitamin B-12 1000 - GNC
Each tablet contains: Vitamin B12 (as cyanocobalamin) 1000 mcg. Other Ingredients: Dicalcium Phosphate, Cellulose, Whole Brown Rice powder (oryza sativa).

Vitamin B12 1200 mcg - Timed Release - Jamieson
Each tablet contains: Vitamin B12 (Cyanocobalamin) 1200 mcg.

Vitamin B-12 1500 - GNC A-Z - GNC
Each capsule contains: Vitamin B12 (as cyanocobalamin) 1500 mcg. Other Ingredients: Dicalcium Phosphate, Cellulose, Calcium Carbonate, Gelatin.

Vitamin B12 25 mcg - Jamieson
Each tablet contains: Vitamin B12 (Cyanocobalamin) 25 mcg.

Vitamin B12 250 mcg - Jamieson
Each tablet contains: Vitamin B12 (Cyanocobalamin) 250 mcg.

Vitamin B-12 250 mcg - Nature Made
Each tablet contains: Vitamin B12 (from cyanocobalamin) 250 mcg. Other Ingredients: Dibasic Calcium Phosphate, Cellulose, Stearic Acid, Croscarmellose Sodium, Magnesium Stearate.
See Editor's Note No. 45, page 2058.

Vitamin B12 50 mcg - Jamieson
Each tablet contains: Vitamin B12 (Cyanocobalamin) 50 mcg.

Vitamin B-12 500 - GNC A-Z - GNC
Each tablet contains: Vitamin B12 (as cyanocobalamin) 500 mcg. Ingredients: Cyanocobalamin, Dextrose, Dicalcium Phosphate, Whole Brown Rice powder (oryza sativa).

Vitamin B-12 500 mcg - Puritan's Pride
Each tablet contains: Ener-B Vitamin B12 (as cyanocobalamin) 500 mcg. Other Ingredients: Dicalcium Phosphate, Cellulose (plant origin), Croscarmellose, Vegetable Stearic Acid, Silica, Vegetable Magnesium Stearate.

Vitamin B12 500 mcg - Nature Made
Each tablet contains: Vitamin B12 (from cyanocobalamin) 500 mcg. Other Ingredients: Dibasic Calcium Phosphate, Cellulose Gel, Stearic Acid, Croscarmellose Sodium, Magnesium Stearate.
See Editor's Note No. 45, page 2058.

Vitamin B-12 Timed Release 1000 mcg **-** Nature Made
Each tablet contains: Vitamin B12 (cyanocobalamin) 1000 mg. Other Ingredients: Dibasic Calcium Phosphate, Cellulose Gel, Stearic Acid, Magnesium Stearate.

Vitamin B125 **-** Source Naturals
Each tablet contains: Thiamin (vitamin B1) 125 mg • Riboflavin (as vitamin B2) 125 mg • Niacinamide 100 mg • Niacin 25 mg • Vitamin B6 (as pyridoxine HCl) 125 mg • Folate (as folic acid) 400 mcg • Vitamin B12 (as cyanocobalamin) 125 mcg • Biotin 125 mcg • Pantothenic Acid (as calcium d-pantotehnate) 125 mcg • Choline (as choline bitartrate) 125 mcg • Inositol 125 mcg • PABA (para-aminobenzoic acid) 125 mcg.

Vitamin B-2 **-** Nature's Bounty
Each tablet contains: Riboflavin 100 mg. Other Ingredients: Dicalcium Phosphate, Cellulose, Vegetable Stearic Acid, Guar Gum, Croscarmellose, Silica.

Vitamin B2 **-** Source Naturals
Each tablet contains: Riboflavin (vitamin B2) 100 mg.

Vitamin B2 100 mg **-** Jamieson
Each tablet contains: Vitamin B2 (Riboflavin) 100 mg.

Vitamin B-2 50 - GNC A-Z **-** GNC
Each tablet contains: Riboflavin (as vitamin B-2) 50 mg. Other Ingredients: Dicalcium Phosphate, Cellulose, Vegetable Acetoglycerides, Whole Brown Rice powder (oryza sativa).

Vitamin B2 50 mg **-** Solgar
Each tablet contains: Riboflavin (vitamin B2) 50 mg • Calcium (as dicalcium phosphate) 100 mg. Other Ingredients: Dicalcium Phosphate, Vegetable Stearic Acid, Silica, Vegetable Cellulose, Vegetable Magnesium Stearate.

Vitamin B50 Complex **-** Source Naturals
Each tablet contains: Thiamin (vitamin B1) 50 mg • Riboflavin (vitamin B2) 50 mg • Niacinamide 50 mg • Vitamin B6 (as pyridoxine HCl) 50 mg • Folate (as folic acid) 100 mcg • Vitamin B12 (as cyanocobalamin) 50 mcg • Biotin 50 mcg • Pantothenic Acid (as calcium d-pantothenate) 100 mg • Choline (as bitartrate) 50 mg • Inositol 50 mg • PABA (as para amino benzoic Acid) 30 mg.

Vitamin B-50 Complex - Basic Nutrition **-** GNC
Each tablet contains: Thiamin (as Thiamin Mononitrate) 50 mg • Riboflavin 50 mg • Niacin (as Niacinamide) 50 mg • Vitamin B6 (as Pyridoxine Hydrochloride) 50 mg • Folate, Folic Acid, Folacin 400 mg • Vitamin B12 (as Cyanocobalamin) 50 mcg • Biotin 50 mcg • Pantothenic Acid (as Calcium d-Pantothenate) 50 mg • Choline Bitartrate 50 mg • Inositol 50 mcg • Para-aminobenzoic acid (PABA) 50 mcg. Other Ingredients: Dicalcium Phosphate, Cellulose, Magnesium Stearate, Yeast, Alfalfa, Watercress, Parsley, Lecithin, Rice Bran, Vegetable Acetoglycerides.

Vitamin B-6 - Basic Nutrition **-** GNC
Each tablet contains: Vitamin B6 (as Pyridoxine Hydrochloride) 50 mg. Other Ingredients: Dextrose, Stearic Acid, Magnesium Stearate, Cellulose, Whole Brown Rice powder.

Vitamin B6 **-** Jamieson
Each tablet contains: Vitamin B6 (as Pyridoxine Hydrochloride) 100 mg.

Vitamin B-6 **-** Leiner Health Products
Each tablet contains: Vitamin B6 (Pyridoxine Hydrochloride) 100 mg. Other Ingredients: Dicalcium Phosphate, Cellulose, Starch, Croscarmellose Sodium, Polyethylene Glycol 3350, Silicon Dioxide, Magnesium Stearate.

Vitamin B-6 **-** Nature's Bounty
Each tablet contains: Vitamin B-6 (Pyridoxine Hydrochloride) 50 mg. Other Ingredients: Dicalcium Phosphate, Cellulose, Vegetable Stearic Acid, Croscarmellose, Vegetable Magnesium Stearate, Silica.

Vitamin B-6 **-** PhysioLogics
Each tablet contains: Vitamin B6 (as pyridoxine hydrochloride) 100 mg. Other Ingredients: Cellulose (plant origin), Dicalcium Phosphate, Vegetable Stearic Acid, Croscarmllose, Cellulose Coating, Silica, Vegetable Magnesium Stearate.

Vitamin B-6 100 - GNC A-Z **-** GNC
Each tablet contains: Vitamin B6 (as Pyridoxine hydrochloride) 100 mg. Other Ingredients: Dicalcium Phosphate, Whole Brown Rice powder (oryza sativa).

Vitamin B6 100 mg **-** Jamieson
Each tablet contains: Vitamin B6 (Pyridoxine Hydrochloride) 100 mg.

Vitamin B6 100 mg **-** Nature Made
Each tablet contains: Vitamin B6 (from pyridoxine hydrochloride) 100 mg. Other Ingredients: Dibasic Calcium Phosphate, Cellulose Gel, Croscarmellose Sodium, Stearic Acid, Magnesium Stearate. See Editor's Note No. 45, page 2058.

Vitamin B6 100 mg **-** Source Naturals
Each tablet contains: Vitamin B6 (as pyridoxine HCl) 100 mg.

Vitamin B-6 200 - GNC A-Z **-** GNC
Each tablet contains: Vitamin B6 (as pyridoxine hydrochloride) 200 mg. Other Ingredients: Dicalcium Phosphate, Cellulose, Whole Brown Rice powder (oryza sativa).

Vitamin B6 25 mg **-** Jamieson
Each tablet contains: Vitamin B6 (Pyridoxine Hydrochloride) 25 mg.

Vitamin B6 250 mg **-** Jamieson
Each tablet contains: Vitamin B6 (Pyridoxine Hydrochloride) 250 mg.

Vitamin B-6 50 - GNC A-Z **-** GNC
Each tablet contains: Vitamin B6 (as pyridoxine hydrochloride) 50 mg. Other Ingredients: Dextrose, Whole Brown Rice powder (oryza sativa).

Vitamin B6 50 mg **-** Jamieson
Each tablet contains: Vitamin B6 (Pyridoxine Hydrochloride) 50 mg.

Vitamin B-6 50 mg **-** Nature Made
Each tablet contains: Vitamin B6 (from pyridoxine HCl) 50 mg. Other Ingredients: Dibasic Calcium Phosphate, Cellulose, Croscarmellose Sodium, Magnesium Stearate.
See Editor's Note No. 45, page 2058.

Vitamin B6 50 mg **-** Source Naturals
Each tablet contains: Vitamin B6 (as pyridoxine HCl) 50 mg.

Vitamin B6 500 mg Time Release **-** Source Naturals
Each tablet contains: Vitamin B6 (pyridoxine HCl) 500 mg • Calcium 27 mg.

Vitamin B-Complex **-** PhysioLogics
Each capsule contains: Thiamine (as Thiamine Mononitrate) 50 mg • Riboflavin 50 mg • Niacin 55 mg • Pantothenic Acid (as Calcium Pantothenate) 100 mg • Vitamin B6 (as Pyridoxine HCl) 50 mg • Vitamin B12 (as Cyanocobalamin) 50 mcg • Folic Acid 400 mcg • Biotin 300 mcg • Inositol 50 mg • Choline (Bitartrate) 50 mg • PABA 50 mg.

Vitamin C - 1000 **-** Nature's Bounty
Each tablet contains: Vitamin C (as ascorbic acid) 1000 mg. Other Ingredients: Cellulose Plant Origin, Vegetable Magnesium Stearate, Vegetable Stearic Acid, Silica.

Vitamin C - 1000 mg Capsules with Bioflavonoids **-** Puritan's Pride
Each capsule contains: Vitamin C 1000 mg • Bioflavonoids 30 mg.

Vitamin C - 1500 mg Tablets with Rose Hips - Puritan's Pride
Each tablet contains: Vitamin C with Rose Hips 1500 mg.

Vitamin C - 500 mg Tablets with Rose Hips - Puritan's Pride
Each tablet contains: Vitamin C with Rose Hips 500 mg.

Vitamin C - 500 with Rose Hips - Windmill Health Products
Each tablet contains: Vitamin C 500 mg • Ascorbic Acid 500 mg • Rose Hips 30 mg.

Vitamin C - Ascorbic Acid Crystals - Source Naturals
Each one-fourth teaspoon contains: Vitamin C (as ascorbic acid) 1.065 g.

Vitamin C - Basic Nutrition - GNC
Each tablet contains: Vitamin E (as dl-alpha Tocopheryl Acetate) 1000 IU • Vitamin C (as Ascorbic Acid) 500 mg. Other Ingredients: Cellulose, Magnesium Stearate, Stearic Acid.

Vitamin C - CVS Pharmacy
Each tablet contains: Vitamin C 500 mg. Other Ingredients: Ascorbic Acid, Starch, Cellulose, Stearic Acid, Croscarmellose Sodium, Lactose, Magnesium Stearate, Silicon Dioxide.

Vitamin C - Leiner Health Products
Each tablet contains: Vitamin C (Ascorbic Acid) 250 mg. Other Ingredients: Calcium Carbonate, Maltodextrin, Cellulose, Starch, Silicon Dioxide, Stearic Acid, Magnesium Stearate, Sodium Starch Glycolate, Croscarmellose Sodium.

Vitamin C - NSI - Nutraceutical Sciences Institute
Each capsule contains: Vitamin C (ascorbic acid) 1000 mg.

Vitamin C - Optimum Nutrition
Each capsule contains: Vitamin C (as ascorbic acid) 500 mg. Other Ingredients: Microcrystalline Cellulose, Gelatin, Magnesium Stearate.

Vitamin C & Zinc Lozenges - Puritan's Pride
Each lozenge contains: Vitamin C (as Ascorbic Acid and Rose Hips) 300 mg • Zinc (as Zinc Citrate) 7 mg • Natural Food Base 15 mg: Rutin, Hesperidin, Acerola, Citrus Bioflavonoids, Black Currant.

Vitamin C + Echinacea - Leiner Health Products
Each tablet contains: Vitamin C (Ascorbic Acid) 500 mg • Echinacea (Echinacea angustifolia) herb 35 mg • Echinacea (Echinacea angustifolia) root 15 mg • Echinacea (Echinacea purpurea) herb 50 mg. Other Ingredients: Cellulose, Hydroxypropyl Methylcellulose, Croscarmellose Sodium, Magnesium Stearate, Silicon Dioxide, Lemon Bioflavonoids, Rose Hips, Acerola, Hesperidin, Orange Peel, Quercetin, Rutin, Polyethylene Glycol 3350.

Vitamin C 1000 - Olympian Labs
Each capsule contains: Vitamin C 1000 mg •Rose Hips 50 mg •Citrus Bioflavonoids 100 mg.

Vitamin C 1000 - PhysioLogics
Each tablet contains: Vitamin C (Ascorbic Acid) 1000 mg •Bioflavonoids lemon 30 mg.

Vitamin C 1000 mg - Nature Made
Each tablet contains: Vitamin C (from ascorbic acid) 1000 mg. Other Ingredients: Corn Starch, Cellulose, Magnesium Stearate, Stearic Acid, Silica Gel.
See Editor's Note No. 45, page 2058.

Vitamin C 1000 mg - Jamieson
Each caplet contains: Vitamin C (Ascorbic Acid) 1000 mg.

Vitamin C 1000 mg - Timed Release - Jamieson
Each caplet contains: Vitamin C (Ascorbic Acid) 1000 mg.

Vitamin C 1000 mg Timed Release - Jamieson
Each caplet contains: Vitamin C (as Ascorbic Acid) 1000. Other Ingredients: Rutin, Hesperidin, Lemon Bioflavonoids, Acerola, Rosehips.

Vitamin C 1000 mg with Rose Hips - GNC A-Z - GNC
Each tablet contains: Vitamin C 1000 mg. Ingredients: Rose Hips powder, Cellulose, Magnesium Stearate, Dicalcium Phosphate, Food Glaze, Stearic Acid, Silica.

Vitamin C 1000 with Bioflavonoids and Rose Hips - GNC A-Z - GNC
Each tablet contains: Vitamin C (as ascorbic acid) 1000 mg. Other Ingredients: Cellulose, Calcium Sulfate, Rose Hips powder (rosina canina).

Vitamin C 1000 with Rose Hips - Nature's Way
Each capsule contains: Vitamin C 1000 mg. Other Ingredients: Cellulose, Gelatin, Magnesium Stearate, Rose Hips.

Vitamin C 1000MG - Nature Made
Each tablet contains: Vitamin C 1000 mg.
See Editor's Note No. 45, page 2058.

Vitamin C 1500MG with Rose Hips - Nature Made
Each tablet contains: Vitamin C 1500 mg.
See Editor's Note No. 45, page 2058.

Vitamin C 200 mg - The Vitamin Shoppe
Each tablet contains: Vitamin C 200 mg • Citrus Bioflavonoid Complex 20 mg.

Vitamin C 2000 mg with Rose Hips - GNC A-Z - GNC
Each tablet contains: Vitamin C (as ascorbic acid) 2000 mg. Other Ingredients: Cellulose, Rose Hips (rosina canina).

Vitamin C 250MG - Nature Made
Each tablet contains: Vitamin C 250 mg.
See Editor's Note No. 45, page 2058.

Vitamin C 500 mg - Jamieson
Each tablet contains: Vitamin C (as Ascorbic Acid and Sodium Ascorbate) 500 mg • Sodium (as Sodium Ascorbate) 35 mg. Available in Chewable Orange, Grape Juice-Chewable, and Chewable Tropical Fruit flavors.

Vitamin C 500 mg - Citrus Juice - Jamieson
Each tablet contains: Vitamin C (Ascorbic Acid, Sodium Ascorbate) 500 mg.

Vitamin C 500 mg - GNC A-Z - GNC
Each tablet contains: Vitamin C (as ascorbic acid) 500 mg. Other Ingredients: Cellulose.

Vitamin C 500 mg - Grape Juice - Jamieson
Each tablet contains: Vitamin C (Ascorbic Acid, Sodium Ascorbate) 500 mg.

Vitamin C 500 mg - Tangy Orange - Jamieson
Each tablet contains: Vitamin C 500 mg.

Vitamin C 500 mg - Tropical Fruit - Jamieson
Each tablet contains: Vitamin C (Ascorbic Acid, Sodium Ascorbate) 500 mg.

Vitamin C 500 mg Timed Release - Caplets - Jamieson
Each caplet contains: Vitamin C 500 mg.

Vitamin C 500 mg Timed Release - Capsules - Jamieson
Each capsule contains: Vitamin C (Ascorbic Acid) 500 mg.

Vitamin C 500 mg with Rose Hips Timed Release - GNC A-Z - GNC
Each capsule contains: Vitamin C (as ascorbic acid) 500 mg. Other Ingredients: Sucrose, Starch, Gelatin, Food Glaze, Rose Hips powder (rosina canina).

Vitamin C 500 with Bioflavonoids - Nature's Way
Two capsules contain: Citrus Bioflavonoids 600 mg • Vitamin C (ascorbic acid) 1000 mg.

Vitamin C 500 with Rose Hips - GNC A-Z - GNC
Each tablet contains: Vitamin C (as ascorbic acid) 500 mg. Other Ingredients: Dicalcium Phosphate, Cellulose, Rose Hips powder (rosina canina), Food Glaze.

Vitamin C 500MG - Nature Made
Each tablet contains: Vitamin C 500 mg.
See Editor's Note No. 45, page 2058.

Vitamin C 500MG with Rose Hips - Nature Made
Each tablet contains: Vitamin C 500 mg.
See Editor's Note No. 45, page 2058.

Vitamin C Chewable - Leiner Health Products
Each tablet contains: Vitamin C (Ascorbic Acid) 500 mg • Sodium 40 mg • Total Carbohydrate less than 1 g • Sugars less than 1 g. Other Ingredients: Sucrose, Sodium Ascorbate, Stearic Acid, Starch, Natural Flavor, Magnesium Stearate, Silicon Dioxide, Sorbitol, Yellow 6 Lake, Lactose, Ethylmaltol.

Vitamin C Crystals - Puritan's Pride
Each teaspoon contains: Vitamin C 5000 mg.

Vitamin C Crystals Buffered - GNC A-Z - GNC
1/2 Teaspoon contains: Vitamin C (as calcium ascorbate) 2000 mg • Calcium (as calcium ascorbate) 230 mg. Other Ingredients: Calcium Ascorbate.

Vitamin C Crystals with Rose Hips - GNC A-Z - GNC
1/2 Teaspoon contains: Vitamin C (as ascorbic acid) 2000 mg. Other Ingredients: Rose Hips powder.

Vitamin C Moisturizing Lotion - Jamieson
Maleated Soybean Oil • Propylene Glycol • Glycerin • Panthenol • Aloe Barbadenis Gel • SPF Active Ingredients: Octocrylene 7% w/w, Octyl Methoxycinnamate 7% w/w, Oxybenzone 3% w/w.

Vitamin C Plex - Olympian Labs
Each capsule contains: Vitamin C (calcium ascorbate) 500 mg • Calcium (ascorbate) 55 mg • Citrus Bioflavonoid Complex 50 mg • Hesperidin 25 mg • Rutin 20 mg • Ascorbyl Palmitate 10 mg.

Vitamin C Skin Supplement Cream - Orjene
Antioxidants • Vitamin C • Ginkgo Biloba • Germanium • Chamomile.

Vitamin C Solution - Dial Herbs
Vitamin C • Vitamin B3 • Citrus bioflavonoids extract. In a base of Distilled Water, Fructose, Sorbitol, Vegetable Glycerine (kosher), Fruit flavors, Sodium Benzoate & Caramel color.

Vitamin C with Citrus Bioflavonoids & Rose Hips - Optimum Nutrition
Two capsules contain: Vitamin C (as ascorbic acid) 1000 mg • Proprietary Citrus Blend 751 mg: Citrus Bioflavonoids fruit, Rose Hips. Other Ingredients: Gelatin, Magnesium Stearate.

Vitamin C with Echinacea - Holista
Each tablet contains: Vitamin C 500 mg • Echinacea 100 mg.

Vitamin C with Rose Hips 1000 mg, Timed Release - Nature Made
Each tablet contains: Vitamin C (from rose hips) 1000 mg. Other Ingredients: Hydroxypropyl Methylcellulose, Corn Starch, Stearic Acid, Magnesium Stearate, Polyethylene Glycol, Riboflavin, Carnauba Wax.
See Editor's Note No. 45, page 2058.

Vitamin C with Rose Hips 500 mg - Nature Made
Each tablet contains: Vitamin C (from ascorbic acid, rose hips) 500 mg. Other Ingredients: Corn Starch, Cellulose Gel, Croscarmellose Sodium, Stearic Acid, Silicon Dioxide, Magnesium Stearate.
See Editor's Note No. 45, page 2058.

Vitamin C with Rose Hips and Echinacea - PhysioLogics
Each tablet contains: Vitamin C (as ascorbic acid, rose hips (rosa canina)) 500 mg • Echinacea aerial parts, root (echinacea purpurea, echinacea angustifolia) 100 mg. Other Ingredients: Dicalcium Phosphate, Cellulose (plant origin), Vegetable Stearic Acid, Croscarmellose, Silica, Vegetable Magnesium Stearate, Cellulose Coating.

Vitamin C, 500 mg (special) - Nature's Life
Vitamin C (Ascorbic Acid), 500 mg. In a natural base of Rose Hips Powder. Excipients: Cellulose, Magnesium stearate and Micro-Cellulose (tm) coating.

Vitamin C, Hesperidin & Mineral Powder - Wonder Foods
Two grams of powder contain: Ascorbic Acid 800 mg • Calcium Ascorbate 200 mg • Hesperidin 190 mg • Calcium Phosphate 100 mg • Magnesium Phosphate 190 mg • Zinc Sulfate Monohydrate 2.9 mg.

Vitamin C-1000 mg Tablets with Rose Hips (Inspired by Nature) - Puritan's Pride
Each tablet contains: Vitamin C with Rose Hips 1000 mg.

Vitamin C-500 mg Softgels with Rose Hips (Inspired by Nature) - Puritan's Pride
Each softgel contains: Vitamin C with Rose Hips 500 mg. Other Ingredients: Soybean Oil, Gelatin, Lecithin, Beeswax, St. John's Bread extract, Caramel Color.

Vitamin D - Puritan's Pride
Each tablet contains: Vitamin D 400 IU.

Vitamin D - Basic Nutrition - GNC
Each tablet contains: Vitamin D (as Ergocalciferol) 400 IU. Other Ingredients: Dicalcium Phosphate, Cellulose.

Vitamin D 1000 IU - Jamieson
Each tablet contains: Vitamin D (as Cholecaliciferol) 1000 IU • Calcium (as Dicalcium Phosphate) 20 mg • Peanut oil.

Vitamin D 1000 IU - Jamieson
Each tablet contains: Vitamin D 1000 IU.

Vitamin D 400 - GNC A-Z - GNC
Each tablet contains: Vitamin D (as ergocalciferol) 400 IU. Other Ingredients: Dicalcium Phosphate, Cellulose.

Vitamin D 400 IU - Jamieson
Each tablet contains: Vitamin D (as Vitamin D3) 400 IU.

Vitamin E - Olympian Labs
Each capsule contains: Vitamin E (d-alpha tocopherol) 400 IU. In a base of Soybean Oil or Safflower Oil.

Vitamin E - Health Smart Vitamins
Each softgel contains: Vitamin E (as 50% d-alpha tocopherol, 50% dl-alpha tocopheryl acetate) 1,000 IU.

Vitamin E - Nature's Way
Each softgel contains: Vitamin E (d-alpha tocopheryl) 400 IU. Other Ingredients: Gelatin.

Vitamin E - Vitamins.com
Each softgel contains: Vitamin E Complex 400 IU. Other Ingredients: Glycerin, Gelatin.

Vitamin E - A&D Cream - Atrium Inc.
Three ounces contain: Vitamin E 1500 IU • Vitamin A 750 IU • Vitamin D 300 IU. In a Silicone Cream Base: Stearic Acid, Glycerol, Cetyl Alcohol, Beeswax, Apricot Kernel oil, Triethanolamine, Borax, Allantoin, Methyl Parasept.

Vitamin E & Selenium - Swanson
Each softgel contains: Vitamin E (as d-alpha tocopherol) 400 IU • Selenium (as selenomethionine) 50 mcg.

Vitamin E 100 IU - Jamieson
Each capsule contains: Natural Source Vitamin E (D-Alpha Tocopheryl Acetate from Purified Soy Oil) 100 IU.

Vitamin E 1000 IU - Basic Nutrition - GNC
Each capsule contains: Vitamin E (as d-alpha Tocopheryl Acetate) 1000 IU. Other Ingredients: Gelatin, Glycerin.

Vitamin E 1000 IU - GNC A-Z - GNC
Each capsule contains: Vitamin E (as dl-alpha tocopheryl acetate) 1000 IU. Other Ingredients: Gelatin, Glycerin.

Vitamin E 1000 IU - Nature Made
Each softgel contains: Vitamin E (from DL-alpha tocopheryl acetate) 1000 IU. Other Ingredients: Gelatin, Glycerin, Water.
See Editor's Note No. 45, page 2058.

Vitamin E 200 IU - Leiner Health Products
Each softgel contains: Vitamin E (dl-Alpha Tocopheryl Acetate) 200 IU. Other Ingredients: Gelatin, Glycerin, Vegetable Oil.

Vitamin E 200 IU - Jamieson
Each capsule contains: Natural Source Vitamin E (D-Alpha Tocopheryl Acetate from Purified Soy Oil) 200 IU.

Vitamin E 200 IU - Basic Nutrition - GNC
Each capsule contains: Vitamin E (as dl-alpha Tocopheryl Acetate) 200 IU. Other Ingredients: Gelatin, Glycerin.

Vitamin E 200 IU - Chewable - Jamieson
Each tablet contains: Vitamin E (dl-Alpha Tocopheryl Acetate) 200 IU.

Vitamin E 200 IU with Selenium - Jamieson
Each caplet contains: Natural Source Vitamin E (D-Alpha Tocopheryl Acetate) 200 IU • Selenium (from Yeast) 2 mcg.

Vitamin E 2000 IU Moisture Cream - Jamieson
4% Antioxidant Vitamin E • Chamomile.

Vitamin E 30,000 IU Moisture Cream - Jamieson
27% Antioxidant Vitamin E (Tocopheyrl Acetate) with Swiss Alpine Herbs: Fennel, Hops, Chamomile, Balm Mint, Mistletoe.

Vitamin E 400 IU - Jamieson
Each capsule contains: Vitamin E (as D-alpha tocopheryl acetate) 400 IU.

Vitamin E 400 IU - PhytoPharmica
Each softgel capsule contains: Mixed Tocopherols (gamma, delta, alpha, and beta) 50 mg • Vitamin E (as D-alpha tocopherol) 400 IU.

Vitamin E 400 IU (Natural Source) - Jamieson
Each capsule contains: Natural Source Vitamin E (D-Alpha Tocopheryl Acetate from Purified Soy Oil) 400 IU.

Vitamin E 400 IU, Blended - GNC A-Z - GNC
Each capsule contains: Vitamin E (as dl-alpha tocopheryl acetate and d-alpha tocopherol) 400 IU. Other Ingredients: Gelatin, Glycerin.

Vitamin E 400 IU, dl-alpha Form - GNC A-Z - GNC
Each capsule contains: Vitamin E (as dl-alpha tocopheryl acetate) 400 IU. Other Ingredients: Gelatin, Glycerin.

Vitamin E 400 IU, Naturally Blended - GNC A-Z - GNC
Each capsule contains: Vitamin E (as dl-alpha tocopheryl acetate and d-alpha tocopherol) 400 IU. Other Ingredients: Gelatin, Glycerin.

Vitamin E 400 IU, Softgel - GNC A-Z - GNC
Each capsule contains: Vitamin E (as di-alpha tocopheryl acetate). Other Ingredients: Gelatin, Glycerin.

Vitamin E 400IU 294mg - Nature's Sunshine
Each capsule contains: Vitamin E (d-alpha tocopherol) 294 mg (400 IU).

Vitamin E 800 I.U. - Leiner Health Products
Each softgel contains: Vitamin E (dl-Alpha Tocopheryl Acetate) 800 IU. Other Ingredients: Gelatin, Glycerin.

Vitamin E 800 IU - Jamieson
Each capsule contains: Vitamin E (as D-Alpha Tocopheryl Acetate) 800 IU.

Vitamin E Complex - Schiff
Each softgel contains: Vitamin E 400 IU.

Vitamin E Complex - Optimum Nutrition
Each softgel contains: Vitamin E (as D-alpha tocopherol plus D-beta, D-gamma, D-delta tocopherols) 400 IU. Other Ingredients: Gelatin, Soy Oil.

Vitamin E Essential Skin Cream - Orjene
Vitamin E 6000 IU • Vitamin A 20000 USP units • Vitamin D 5000 USP units.

Vitamin E Microtargeted Moisture Oil - Jamieson
Each capsule contains: Grape Seed Oil • Sesame Seed Oil • Coconut Oil • Squalane • Phytosterol • Glycolipids • Tocopheryl Acetate • Chamomile Oil • Tocopheryl Linoleate.

Vitamin E Oil - Orjene
6000 IU of Vitamin E and Vitamin A and Vitamin D.

Vitamin E Oil 28,000 IU - Jamieson
Contains: 100% Vitamin E (Tocopheryl Acetate) 28,000 IU.

Vitamin E Soothing Ointment - Jamieson
Contains: Petrolatum • Mineral Oil • Vitamin E.

Vitamin E Succinate 400 IU - Life Extension Foundation
Each capsule contains: Vitamin E (as d-alpha-tocopheryl succinate) 400 IU. Other Ingredients: Magnesium Stearate, Rice Flour, Gelatin, Water.

Vitamin E Water Dispersible - Leiner Health Products
Each softgel contains: Vitamin E (dl-Alpha Tocopheryl Acetate) 400 IU. Other Ingredients: Gelatin, Polysorbate 80, Glycerin, Soybean Oil.

Vitamin E with Tocotrienols - PhysioLogics
Each softgel contains: Vitamin E (as d-alpha tocopherol) 400 IU • Tocotrienols 35 mg. Other Ingredients: Gelatin, Glycerin.

Vitamin for the Hair - Puritan's Pride
Each tablet contains: Calcium Pantothenate 100 mg • Choline Bitartrate 125 mg • Inositol 50 mg • Niacin (Nicotinic Acid) 35 mg • Para-Aminobenzoic Acid 30 mg • Folic Acid 0.4 mg • Cobalamin (Vitamin B12) 6 mcg • Iron (Ferrous Sulfate) 18 mg • Copper (Copper Gluconate) 2 mg • Iodine (Kelp) 0.15 mg • Manganese (Manganese Gluconate) 5 mg • Protein (from Soy Protein) 100 mg • Zinc (Zinc Gluconate) 15 mg.

Vitamin Foundation Creme - Aspen Group, Inc.
Each gram contains: Tocopheryl Acetate • Panthenol • Water • Octyldodecyl Neopetanoate • Octyl Methoxycinnmate • Cetearyl Alcohol • Cetyl Phosphate • Dimethicone • Beeswax • Carbomer • Aminomethyl Propanol • Propylene Glycol • Diazolidinyl Urea • Methylparaben • Propylparaben.

Vitamin K 100 mcg - GNC A-Z - GNC
Each tablet contains: Vitamin K (as phytonadione) 100 mcg. Other Ingredients: Dicalcium Phosphate, Cellulose.

Vitamin O - R-Garden Internationale
Stabilized Oxygen in a solution of distilled water, Sodium Chloride, and trace minerals.

Vitargo CGL - Nutrex, Inc.
Two level scoops contain: Magnesium 50 mg • Phosphorus 200 mg • Potassium 150 mg • Creatine Monohydrate 10 g • Vitargo (sugar free high molecular weight (500.000-700.000) carbohydrate from Swedish waxy maize starch) 60 mg. Other Ingredients: Natural and

Artificial Flavors, Citric Acid, Osmosis Balancing Electrolytes (dipotassium phosphate, disodium phosphate, dimagnesium phosphate), Silicon Dioxide, Sucralose, FD&C Red 40.

Vitasana **-** Boehringer Ingelheim
Two gelcaps contain: Vitamin A (as beta carotene) 4000 IU • Vitamin C (as ascorbic acid) 120 mg • Vitamin D (as cholecalciferol) 400 IU • Vitamin E (as dl-alpha tocopheryl acetate) 30 IU • Vitamin B1 (as thiamine mononitrate) 2.4 mg • Vitamin B2 (riboflavin) 3.4 mg • Vitamin B3 (niacinamide) 30 mg • Vitamin B6 (as pyridoxine HCl) 4 mg • Folic Acid 400 mcg • Vitamin B12 (as cobalamin conc.) 2 mcg • Calcium (as calcium phosphate) 200 mg • Iron (as ferrous sulfate) 18 mg • Phosphorus (as calcium phosphate) 160 mg • Magnesium (as magnesium oxide) 20 mg • Zinc (as zinc sulfate) 2 mg • Copper (as copper sulfate) 2 mg • Manganese (as manganese sulfate) 2 mg • Standardized G115 Ginseng Extract (from Panax Ginseng, C.A. Meyer, root) 80 mg.

Vitase Digestion Formula **-** Enzymatic Therapy
Two capsules contain: Pure Plant Enzymes Blend 352 mg: Amylase (USP XXI [pH6.8]) 33,000 USP (FCC IV [pH4.8]) 14,300 DU, Protease I,II,III,IV (USP XXIII [pH7.5]) 29,150 USP (FCC IV [pH7.0]) 46,500 PC.. (FCC IV [pH5.7]) 36,150 HUT, Lactase I,II (FCC III [pH4.5]) 840 LacU, Cellulase I (FCC IV[pH4.5]) 142 CU, Lipase II (FCC III [pH6.5]) 215 LU, Maltase (malt diatase) (FCC IV[pH4.6]) 19,650 DP, Sucrase (invertase) (FCC IV[pH4.6]) 240 INVU.

Vita-Smart High Potency Vitamins and Minerals **-** K-mart
Each tablet contains: Vitamin A 8000 IU • Vitamin C 120 mg • Vitamin D 400 IU • Vitamin E 30 IU • Thiamin 5 mg • Riboflavin 5 mg • Niacin 30 mg • Vitamin B-6 5 mg • Folic Acid 400 mcg • Vitamin B-12 10 mcg • Biotin 10 mcg • Pantothenic Acid 10 mg • Calcium 100 mg • Iron 18 mg • Phosphorous 78 mg • Iodine 150 mcg • Magnesium 100 mg • Zinc 15 mg • Copper 2 mg • Chloride 15 mg • Potassium 15 mg.

Vita-Vim **-** Jamieson
Each caplet contains: Vitamin A (as Retinyl Acetate) 10000 IU • Vitamin C (as Ascorbic Acid) 150 mg • Vitamin D (as Cholecalciferol) 400 IU • Vitamin E (as Dl-Alpha Tocopheryl Acetate) 15 IU • Thiamin (as Thiamine Mononitrate) 4.5 mg • Riboflavin (Vitamin B2) 7.5 mg • Niacin (as Niacin and Nicacinamide) 65 mg • Vitamin B6 (as Pyridoxine Hydrochloride) 3 mg • Folate (as Folic Acid) 400 mcg • Vitamin B12 (as Cyanocobalamin) 14 mcg • Biotin 10 mcg • Pantothenic Acid (as Calcium D-Pantothenate) 15 mg • Calcium (as Calcium Carbonate) 130 mg • Iron (as reduced Iron) 4 mg • Iodine (as from Kelp) 100 mcg • Magnesium (as Magnesium Oxide) 100 mg • Zinc (as Zinc Gluconate) 10 mg • Selenium (from yeast) 15 mcg • Copper (as Copper Gluconate) 1 mg • Choline Bitartrate 20 mg • Inositol 20 mg • Dl-Methionine 2.2 mg.

Vita-Vitamin **-** Olympian Labs
Two tablets contain: Vitamin A (palmitate) 5000 IU • Vitamin B-1 (thiamine HCl) 50 mg • Vitamin B-2 (riboflavin) 80 mg • Vitamin B-3 (inositol hexanicotinate) 80 mg • Vitamin B-5 (calcium pantothenate) 80 mg • Vitamin B-6 (pyridoxine HCl) 80 mg • Vitamin B-9 (folic acid) 400 mcg • Vitamin B-12 (cyanocobalamin) 60 mcg • Vitamin C (ascorbic acid) 300 mg • Vitamin D (cholecalciferol) 400 IU • Vitamin E (d-alpha-tocopherol acetate) 100 IU • Alpha Lipoic Acid 10 mg • Betaine HCl 30 mg • Boron 100 mcg • Calcium (citrate and phosphate) 120 mg • Choline Bitartrate 50 mg • Chromium 120 mcg • Citrus Bioflavonoid Complex 30 mg • Coenzyme Q10 10 mg • d-Biotin 300 mcg • Grape Skin extract 50 mg • Hesperidin 5 mg • Inositol 50 mg • Iodine (Kelp) 150 mcg • Lutein/Zeaxanthin 3 mg • Lycopene (100 mg Yielding 5 mg Pure Lycopene) 5 mg • Magnesium (Citrate and Magnesium Oxide) 40 mg • Manganese (Amino Acid Chelate) 2 mg • Molybdenum (Amino Acid Chelate) 75 mcg • PABA 50 mg • Potassium (Amino Acid Chelate) 7 mg • Rutin 30 mg • Selenium (L-Selenomethionine) 50 mcg • Vanadium (Amino Acid Chelate) 5 mcg • Zinc (Amino Acid Chelate) 20 mg. In a Proprietary Base: Barley Grass, Echinacea purpurea, Goldenseal root, Lecithin, Parsley, Pau d' Arco, Rice Bran, and Watercress.

Vitex **-** Pharmanex
Each capsule contains: Vitex fruit 20:1 extract 175 mg. Other Ingredients: Rice flour, Gelatin.

Vitex **-** Puritan's Pride
Each capsule contains: Vitex (Chastetree fruit powder: Vitex agnus-castus) 400 mg.

Vitex Chaste Berry **-** Jamieson
Each capsule contains: Vitex Chaste Berry Formula VH1 (Vitex Agnuscastus, 200 mg powdered extract 1:20) 4000 mg. Derived only from the fruit of the Chaste Berry.

Vitex Extract **-** PhytoPharmica
Each capsule contains: Chaste Tree berry extract (vitex agnus-castus, standardized to contain a minimum of 0.5% agnuside [1,130 mcg per capsule]) 225 mg.

Vitex/Chaste Tree **-** PhysioLogics
Two capsules contain: Vitex (agnus castus, chaste tree fruit powder) 800 mg. Other Ingredients: Gelatin, Calcium Sulfate, Cellulose (plant origin), Vegetable Magnesium Stearate, Silica.

Vit-Min 100+ **-** Now
Each tablet contains: Vitamin A (6 mg Beta-Carotene) 10000 IU • Vitamin A (Acetate) 10000 IU • Vitamin B1 (Thiamine HCL) 100 mg • Vitamin B2 (Riboflavin) 100 mg • Vitamin B3 (Niacinamide) 100 mg • Vitamin B5 (Pantothenic Acid) 100 mg • Vitamin B6 (Pyridoxine HCL) 100 mg • Vitamin B12 (Cyanocobalamin) 100 mcg • Biotin 100 mcg • Folic Acid 400 mcg • Vitamin C (Calcium Ascorbate) 250 mg • Vitamin D (Calciferol) 400 IU • Vitamin E (d-Alpha Tocopheryl Succinate) 150 IU • Calcium (Ascorbate, Carbonate) 50 mg • Magnesium (Oxide • Amino Acid Chelate) 30 mg • Zinc (Amino Acid Chelate) 15 mg • Copper (Amino Acid Chelate) 500 mcg • Iodine (Kelp) 150 mcg • Iron (Amino Acid Chelate) 10 mg • Potassium 10 mg • Manganese (Amino Acid Chelate) 5 mg • Selenium (Amino Acid Chelate) 25 mcg • Chromium (Yeast-free GTF) 100 mcg • Molybdenum (Amino Acid Chelate) 50 mcg • Boron (Amino Acid Chelate) 500 mcg • Vanadium (Amino Acid Chelate) 50 mcg • Choline (Bitartrate) 100 mg • Inositol 100 mg • PABA 50 mg • Rutin 25 mg • Betaine (HCL) 25 mg • Glutamic Acid 25 mg • Spirulina 50 mg • Barley grass organic 50 mg • Citrus Bioflavonoids (40% Hesperidin) 25 mg • Psyllium husk fiber 25 mg. This timed release multiple is formulated in a base of 72 Trace Minerals, Dicalcium Phosphate, Cellulose, Stearic Acid, Silica & natural vegetable protein coating.

Vit-Min 75+ **-** Now
Each tablet contains: Vitamin A (natural Fish Liver oil) 10000 IU • Beta-Carotene (6 mg) 10000 IU • Vitamin B1 (Thiamine HCL) 75 mg • Vitamin B2 (Riboflavin) 75 mg • Vitamin B3 (Niacinamide) 75 mg • Vitamin B5 (Pantothenic Acid) 75 mg • Vitamin B6 (Pyridoxine HCL) 75 mg • Vitamin B12 (Cyanocobalamin) 100 mcg • Biotin 100 mcg • Folic Acid 400 mcg • Vitamin C (Ascorbic Acid) 250 mg • Vitamin D (natural Fish Liver oil) 400 IU • Vitamin E (100% d-Alpha) 150 IU • Calcium (Amino Acid Chelate, Oystershell) 100 mg • Magnesium (Oxide, Amino Acid Chelate) 60 mg • Zinc (Amino Acid Chelate) 15 mg • Copper (Amino Acid Chelate) 1 mg • Iodine (Kelp) 150 mcg • Iron (Amino Acid Chelate) 10 mg • Choline (Bitartrate) 100 mg • Inositol 75 mg • PABA 30 mg • Rutin 25 mg • Citrus Bioflavonoids (40%) 100 mg • Betaine (HCL) 25 mg • Glutamic Acid 25 mg • Potassium (Amino Acid Chelate) 10 mg • Manganese (Amino Acid Chelate) 5 mg • Selenium (Amino Acid Chelate) 25 mcg • Chromium (Yeast-free GTF) 50 mcg • Boron (Amino Acid Chelate) 500 mcg • Molybdenum (Amino Acid Chelate) 50 mcg • Nucleic Acid 50 mg. In a natural base containing Alfalfa, Parsley, Rice polishings, Lecithin & Rose Hips, Dicalcium Phosphate, Cellulose, Stearic Acid & Silica.

BRAND NAMES

Vitox **-** Pharmanex
Two capsules contain: Vitamin A (Vitamin A Palmitate) 3750 IU • Beta-Carotene (Beta-Carotene, Spirulina Pacifica) 6250 IU • Vitamin C (Calcium Ascorbate Complex-Ester-C, Acorbyl Palmitate) 250 mg • Vitamin D (as Vitamin D3, Cholecalciferol) 200 IU • Vitamin E (d-Alpha Tocopheryl Succinate, Beta, Gamma, Delta Tocopherols) 150 IU • Vitamin K (Phylloquinone) 35 mcg • Thiamin (Thiamine Mononitrate) 1.5 mg • Riboflavin (Riboflavin, Riboflavin-5-Phosphate) 1.7 mg • Niacin (Niacinamide Ascorbate) 20 mg • Vitamin B6 (Pyridoxine Hydrochloride, Pyridoxal-5-Phosphate) 2 mg • Folate (Folic Acid) 200 mcg • Vitamin B12 (Cyanocobalamin, Dibencozide) 6 mg • Biotin (Biotin) 150 mcg • Pantothenic Acid (d-Calcium Pantothenate) 25 mg • Calcium (Calcium Carbonate, Calcium Citrate, Calcium Chelate) 250 mg • Iron (Iron Chelate) 3 mg • Magnesium (Magnesium Oxide, Magnesium Citrate, Magnesium Chelate) 100 mg • Zinc (Zinc Chelate) 7.5 mg • Selenium (L-Selenomethionine) 50 mcg • Copper (Copper Chelate) 2.5 mg • Manganese (Manganese Chelate) 2.5 mg • Chromium (Chromium Chelate, Chromium Picolinate) 50 mcg • Boron (Boron) 0.5 mg • Reduced Glutathione 0.5 mg • Leucoanthocyanin (Grape Seed extract) 0.5 mg.

Vitrin **-** Nutraceutics Corp.
Two caplets contain: Vitamin A (20% as b-carotene) 5000 IU • Vitamin C 60 mg • Vitamin D 400 IU • Vitamin E 30 IU • Vitamin K 50 mcg • Vitamin B1 (thiamine) 1.5 mg • Vitamin B2 (riboflavin) 1.7 mg • Niacinamide 20 mg • Vitamin B6 (pyridoxine) 2 mg • Vitamin B12 6 mcg • Folic Acid 400 mcg • Pantothenic Acid 10 mg • Calcium 170 mg • Phosphorus 114 mg • Magnesium 100 mg • Zinc 15 mg • Iodine 150 mcg • Manganese 2 mg • Copper 2 mg • Potassium 80 mg • Chloride 72 mg • Selenium 20 mcg • Chromium 120 mcg • Molybdenum 75 mcg • Boron 150 mcg • Nickel 5 mcg • Silicon 2 mg • Tin 10 mcg • Vanadium 10 mcg • Lutein 250 mcg • Proprietary Blend HiORAC 600 mg: Grape Seed Extract, Dried Apple Juice Concentrate, Dried Orange Juice Concentrate, Dried Pineapple Juice Concentrate, Dried Peach Juice Concentrate, Dried Broccoli Concentrate, Dried Cauliflower Concentrate, Dried Spinach Concentrate, Dried Carrot Concentrate. Other Ingredients: Microcrystalline Cellulose, Gelatin, Crospovidone, Hydroxypropyl Methylcellulose, Starch, Lactose, Sodium Benzoate.

Vitrix **-** Nutrex, Inc.
Six liqui-caps contain: Liquid German Tribulus Terrestris (total saponins 80%, protodioscin 20%) 1000 mg • NTS-5 Liquid Proprietary Phyto-Nutrient Blend 500 mg: Vitex Agnus Castus, Avena Sativa, Epimedium, Eurycomo Longfolia Jack. Other Ingredients: Sesame Oil, Gelatin.

Viva Cell Plus **-** E'OLA
Three capsules contain: Proprietary Blend 2125 mg: Arabinogalactan (larix occidentalis) (tree), Bladderwrack (herb), Pau D'Arco (bark), Cat's Claw (Uncaria Tomentosa) (bark), Astragalus (root), Thymus Gland Extract. Other Ingredients: Rice Flour, Maltodexrin, Magnesium Stearate, Gelatin.

Vivace **-** Veromax International
Each tablet contains: Siberian Ginseng root 100 mg • Ginkgo Biloba leaf 37.5 mg • Jujube Dates (Zizyphi fructus) 100 mg • Isoflavones 40 mg • Proprietary Blend 175 mg: Glutamic acid, L-lysine HCL, L-Alanine. Other Ingredients: Dicalcium Phosphate, Microcrystalline Cellulose, Croscarmellose Sodium, Stearic Acid, Magnesium Stearate, Silicon Dioxide.

Vivarin **-** GlaxoSmithKline (GSK)
Each tablet contains: Caffeine 200 mg. Other Ingredients: Carnauba Wax, Colloidal Silicon Dioxide, FD&C Yellow #10 Lake, Dextrose, FD&C Yellow #6 Lake, Hydroxypropyl Methylcellulose, Magnesium Stearate, Microcrystalline Cellulose, Polyethylene Glycol, Polysorbate 80, Starch, Titanium Dioxide.

Vivaxl **-** Nutraceutics Corp.
Each packet contains: Thiamine (as HCl) 13 mg • Riboflavin (as 5-phosphate) 15 mg • Niacin 50 mg • Pyridoxine (as HCl) 40 mg • Vitamin B12 (cyanocobalamin) 300 mcg • Biotin 150 mcg • Pantothenic Acid (calcium pantothenate) 21 mg • Folic Acid 400 mcg • L-Arginine HCl 2800 mg • DL-Phenylalanine 400 mg • D-Phenylalanine 500 mcg • DMAE (2-dimethylaminoethanol bitartrate) 200 mg • GNS2 Ginseng extract (panax ginseng, standardized to 20% ginsenosides) 200 mg • Kola nut (cola acumenata) 175 mg • Inositol 100 mg • Trimethyl Glycine 100 mg • L-Taurine 50 mg • L-Citruline 50 mg • Sodium (carbonates) 98 mg. Other Ingredients: Dextrose, Citric Acid, Sodium Bicarbonate, Natural/Artificial Flavors, Sodium Carbonate, Sucralose.

VIVEX Beet Root Adjuvant **-** Functional Products
Each capsule contains: Beet Root Powder 435 mg • Celljuvant 4.35 mg. Other Ingredients:Gelatin, Magnesium Stearate.

VIVEX Brain Adjuvant **-** Functional Products
Each capsule contains: Siberian Ginseng Root Extract, Standardized to 0.8% 200 mg • Ginkgo Biloba Extract Standardized to 24% Flavon 50 mg. Other Ingredients: Gelatin, Eleutherococcus Senticosus Radix, Magnesium Stearate.

VIVEX Digestion Adjuvant **-** Functional Products
Each capsule contains: Pancreatin 6x 30 mg • Bromelain (600 GDU) 65 mg • Papain (100) 60 mg • Papaya Leaves 30 mg • Pepsin (1:3000) 60 mg • Betain HCl 55 mg • Bile Salt 30 mg. Other Ingredients: Gelatin, Magnesium Stearate.

VIVEX Heart Adjuvant **-** Functional Products
Three capsules contain: Hawthorn Extract 1.8% Vitexin 1100 mg. Other Ingredients: Gelatin, Crataegi Fructus Pulvis.

VIVEX Immune Adjuvant **-** Functional Products
Each capsule contains: Vitamin C 235 mg • Echinacea Angustifolia Extract, 4% Echinacosides 100 mg • Astragalus Extract 70% Polysaccharides 100 mg • Siberian Ginseng Extract, 0.8% Eleutherosides 50 mg. Other Ingredients: Gelatin, Magnesium Stearate.

VIVEX Joint Adjuvant **-** Functional Products
Two capsules contain: Devil's Claw Root Extract (2% Harpagoside) 850 mg. Other Ingredients: Gelatin, Magnesium Stearate, Harpagophytum Procumbensens.

VIVEX Laxative Adjuvant **-** Functional Products
Each capsule contains: Senna Pods 89 mg • Aloe Juice 78.5 mg • Buckthorn Bark 59.5 mg • Caraway Seed 33.5 mg • Rhubarb Root 26 mg • Fennel Seed 26 mg • Cascara Bark 14 mg. Other Ingredients: Gelatin, Magnesium Stearate.

VIVEX Migra-Feverfew Adjuvant **-** Functional Products
Two capsules contain: Feverfew Extract 66.66 mg. Other Ingredients: Chrysanthenum Partenium Herb, Gelatin, Magnesium Stearate.

VIVEX Mood Adjustment **-** Functional Products
Each capsule contains: St. John's Wort, 0.3% Hypericin 300 mg • Kava Kava Extract, 30% Kavapyrones. Other Ingredients: Gelatin, Kava Kava Radix, Fumed Silica, Magnesium Stearate.

VIVEX Nerve Adjuvant **-** Functional Products
Each capsule contains: Valerian Root 243 mg • Lemon Balm Herb 41 mg • Hops 81 mg • St. John's Wort Tops 81 mg • Chamomile 81 mg • Celljuvant 5.2 mg. Other Ingredients: Gelatin, Kava Kava Radix, Fumed Silica, Magnesium Stearate.

VIVEX Prostate Adjuvant **-** Functional Products
Each capsule contains: Saw Palmetto Extract, 905 Fatty Acids and Sterols 220 mg • Nettle Root Extract, 0.85% Belasitosterols 100 mg • Pumpkin Seed Oil, 90% Fatty Acids and Sterols 50 mg. Other Ingredients: Gelatin, Vegetable Oil, Glycerin (Kosher), Caramel, Soybean, Lecithin, Yellow Bees Wax, Water.

VIVEX Stomach Adjuvant **-** Functional Products
Each capsule contains: Yarrow Herb 61 mg • Chamomile Flower 61 mg • Peppermint Leaves 61 mg • Caraway Seed 61 mg • Ginger Root 61 mg • Thyme Leaves 61 mg • Licorice Root 61 mg. Other Ingredients: Gelatin, Magnesium Stearate.

VIVEX Vein & Artery Adjuvant **-** Functional Products
Each capsule contains: Vitamin E 50 IU • Garlic Powder 970 mg • Celljuvant 9.7 mg. Other Ingredients: Gelatin, Cellulose, Magnesium Stearate.

VIVEX Vitamin Mineral Complex **-** Functional Products
Three capsules contain: Vitamin A 3000 IU • Vitamin C 250 mg • Vitamin E 22 IU • Vitamin B1 10 mg • Vitamin B2 10 mg • Niacinamide 100 mg • Vitamin B6 5 mg • Vitamin B12 0.005 mg • Calcium 80 mg • Iron 17 mg • Magnesium 15 mg • Manganese 0.6 mg • Molybdenum 0.2 mg. Ingredients: Soybean Oil, Gelatin, Ascorbic Acid, Calcium Carbonate, Glycerin (Kosher), Niacinamide, Water, Soybean Lecithin, Ferrous Sulfate, Magnesium Oxide, Bees Wax, d-Alpha Tocopherol, Thiamine HCl, Vitamin A Palmitate, Manganese Gluconate, Molybdenum Glycinate, Cyanocobalamin 1%.

VIVEX Women's Adjuvant **-** Functional Products
Each capsule contain: Vitamin E 42.19 mg • Black Cohosh Root Extract, 2.5% Triterpene Glycosides 500 mg. Other Intredients: Gelatin, Magnesium Stearate.

Volkov's V16 **-** Advocare International
Each wafer contains: Vitamin A (as acetate and beta-carotene) 2000 IU • Vitamin C (as ascorbic acid) 75 mg • Vitamin D (as cholecalciferol) 200 IU • Vitamin E (as acetate) 10 IU • Vitamin K (as phylloquinone) 60 mcg • Thiamine (as mononitrate) 2 mg • Riboflavin 2 mg • Niacin (as niacinamide) 20 mg • Vitamin B6 (as pyridoxine HCl) 2 mg • Folic Acid 200 mcg • Vitamin B12 (as cyanocobalamin) 5 mcg • Biotin 60 mcg • Pantothenic Acid (as calcium pantothenate) 10 mg • Golden Root extract (root - rhodiola rosea) 30 mg • Leuzea extract (root - rhaponticum carthamoides) 20 mg • Wild Schisandra extract (fruit - schisandra chinensis) 10 mg. Other Ingredients: Dextrose, Potassium Bicarbonate, Citric Acid, Sucralose, Natural Flavors.

Volumex **-** Mass Quantities, Inc.
Each rounded teaspoon contains: Creatine Monohydrate 5 grams.

VP2 **-** AST Sports Science
Each serving contains: 100% Hydrolyzed "Oligopeptide" Isolated Whey Protein Fractions consisting of precision engineered Whey Protein Isolate Fractions (Beta-Lactoglobulin, Alpha-Lacalbumin, Immunoglobulin, Proteose-Peptone, Glycomacropeptides (GMP), Bovine Serum Albumin, Lactoferrin, Lactoperoxidase. Lysozyme, Relaxin, Lactollin, & Beta-Microglobulin), natural & artificial Flavors & Aspartame.

V-Pro **-** HealthMinded
Two capsules contain: V-Pro Proprietary Blend 1080 mg: Korean Red Ginseng, Saw Palmetto berry powder, Hawthorn berry, Ginkgo Biloba, Muira Puama powder extract (5:1), Catuaba bark extract (4:1), Cuscuta seed (4:1), Epimedium extract (20:1). Other Ingredients: Stearic Acid, Magnesium Stearate.

VPS Coriolus versicolor **-** JHS Natural Products
Each capsule contains: Coriolus extract 625 mg.

VS-10 Vanadyl Sulfate **-** Optimum Nutrition
Each tablet contains: Vanadyl Sulfate 10 mg.

VSL #3 **-** Questcor Pharmaceuticals
Each packet contains: Yougurt bacteria 450 billion.

VyoPro **-** AST Sports Science
Each serving contains: Fat-Free Whey Protein (L-Glutamine & B Vitamins) 18 g • 100% cool processed, (partially digested) "amino-specific" controlled Chymotrypsin/ Trypsin Hydrolyzed CCTH (Tryptic Hydrolysate) Oligopeptide Whey Protein from "Micro Filtered" & "Stirred-Bed Reactor" Ion-Exchange Whey Protein providing the highest percentage of Oligopeptides along with Di-, Tri-, & Poly-Peptides (multi-spectrum short & long amino acid chains) with specifically tailored & precision engineered molecular weight profiles [isolate fractions 53% Beta-Lactalbumin (molecular weight - MW 18,400 - 36,800D), 24% Alpha-Lactalbumin (MW 14,200) 17% Immunoglobulin (MW 16,000-160,000D) 6% Minor Peptones {lactoferrin, lactoperoxidase, lysozyme, relaxin, lactollin, & Beta-microglobulin (MW 4,000 - 40,000D)}] • Dual Stage Glutamine Composite, consisting of low molecular weight Whey Glutamine Peptides (MW 500 - 10,000) & Microencapsulated Pure Crystalline L-Glutamine • Protein Absorption Enhancing Matrix (Cyanocobalamin, Pyridoxine HCL, Thiamin, Riboflavin, & Calcium Pantothenate) •Natural Flavors • Aspartame.

Walgreens Multiple Vitamins **-** Walgreens
Each tablet contains: Vitamin A 5000 IU • Vitamin C 60 mg • Vitamin D 400 IU • Vitamin E 30 IU • Thiamin 1.5 mg • Riboflavin 1.7 mg • Niacin 20 mg • Vitamin B-6 2 mg • Folic Acid 400 mcg • Vitamin B-12 6 mcg • Pantothenic Acid 10 mg • Iron 18 mg.

Wal-Mart Equate Ultra Dairy Digest **-** Perrigo
Each caplet contains: Lactase 9000 FCC Units. Inactive Ingredients: Dextrates, Microcrystalline Cellulose, Dextrose, Sodium Citrate, Calcium Carbomethylcellulose, Magnesium Stearate, Silicon Dioxide.

Warm Cream **-** Strategic Science & Technology
Water • Choline chloride • L-Arginine • Sodium chloride • Mineral oil • Glyceryl stearate SE • Squalane • Cetyl alcohol • Magnesium chloride • Propylene glycol stearate SE • Wheat germ oil • Glyceryl stearate • Isopropyl myristate • Stearyl stearate • Polysorbate-60 • Propylene gylcol • Oleic acid • Tocopherol acetate • Collagen • Sorbitan stearate • Vitamin A • Vitamin D • Triethanolamine • O capsic • Methylparaben • Aloe vera extract • Imidazolidinyl urea • Propylparaben • BHA.

Water Balance **-** Nutrivention
Three tablets contain: Vitamin B6 (Pyridoxine) 150 mg • Potassium (Amino Acid Complex) 149 mg • Corn Silk (Stigmata maidis) 900 mg • Buchu (Barosma betulina) 600 mg • Elder flowers (Sambuccua canadensis nigra) 300 mg • Hydrangea (Hydrangea arborescens) 300 mg • Uva Ursi (Arctostaphylos uva ursi) 300 mg • Parsley (Petroselinum sativum) 150 mg • Samphire (Crithmum maritimum) 150 mg • Watermelon seed (Citrullus vulgaris) 150 mg.

Water Garden Pycnogenol Skin Lotion **-** Quantum, Inc.
Purified Water • Aloe Vera gel • Propylene Glycol • Hybrid Safflower Oil • Glyceryl Stearate • Stearic Acid • Octyl Palmitate • Sorbitol • Cetyl Alcohol • Tocopherol Acetate (vitamin E) • Panthenol • Allantoin • Sodium PCA • Jojoba Oil • Shea Butter • Kelp extract • Chamomile extract • Calendula extract • Lecithin • Tocopherol • Dimethicone • Triethanolamine • Methylparaben • Propylparaben • Vitamin A • Vitamin D (as Vitamin D3) • Diazolidinyl Urea • Pycnogenol • Super Oxide Dismutase.

Water Garden Pycnogenol Wrinkle Therapy Cream **-** Quantum, Inc.
Deionized Water • Aloe Vera gel • Dioctyl Dodecyl Dodecane Dioate • Propylene Glycol • Dimethicone • Toccopheryl Acetate (vitamin E) • Stearic Acid • Emulsifying Wax • Cetyl Alcohol • Jojoba Oil • Pycnogenol • Lecithin • Panthenol • Allantoin • Extracts of Ginkgo Biloba • Echinacea • Chamomile • Super Oxide Dismutase SOD • Lipoderm • Glyceryl Stearate • Xanthan Gum • Triethanolamine • Methylparaben • Propylparaben • Diazolidinyl Urea • Tocopherol (Vitamin E).

Water Garden Pycnogenol+ **-** Quantum, Inc.
Each tablet contains: Pycnogenol Atlantic Pine Bark extract (Pinus maritma) 30 mg • Grape Seed extract standardized 85% proanthocyanidins (Vinus vinifera) 20 mg.

Water Pill **-** Natrol
Two tablets contain: Vitamin B6 (as Pyridoxine HCl) 150 mg • Potassium (as Potassium Gluconate) 99 mg • Buchu extract leaf 4:1 100 mg • Parsley extract leaf 4:1 100 mg • Uva Ursi extract leaf 4:1 100 mg • Juniper extract berry 4:1 20 mg. Other Ingredients: Calcium Carbonate, Mono & Di-Glycerides, Stearic Acid, Croscarmellose Sodium, Silicon Dioxide, Magnesium Stearate.

Water Pill **-** Puritan's Pride
Two tablets contain: Potassium (as Potassium Gluconate) 40 mg • Buchu (Barosma betulina) leaf (25 mg of Buchu leaves 4:1 extract) 100 mg • Uva Ursi (Arctostaphylos uva-ursi) leaf (33.4 mg of Uva Ursi 3:1 extract) 100 mg • Juniper (Juniperus communis) berry 20 mg • Parsley (Petroselinum crispum) leaf 100 mg.

Weight Gain **-** Vidafit
Each serving contains: Folate 300 mcg • Niacin 16 mg • Pantothenic Acid 5 mg • Riboflavin 1.3 mg • Thiamine 1.2 mg • Vitamin A 3300 IU • Vitamin B12 2.4 mcg • Vitamin B6 1.3 mg • Vitamin C 75 mg • Vitamin D 200 IU • Vitamin E 10 IU • Calcium 500 mg • Chromium 50 mcg • Copper 1 mg • Iodine 150 mcg • Magnesium 420 mg • Phosphorus 500 mg • Potassium 100 mg • Zinc 15 mg • Complex Carbohydrates 13 grams • Soy Protein 7 grams • Whey Protein 13 grams.

Weight Gain Plus Appetite Increaser **-** VitaSalveo
Two capsules contain: Vitamin A Acetate 5000 IU • Ascorbic Acid 30 mg • Vitamin D (D3) 200 IU • Vitamin E 15 IU • Thiamine HCl 2.4 mg • Riboflavin 2.6 mg • Niacinamide 10 mg • Pyridoxine HCl 2.6 mg • Folic Acid 300 mcg • Vitamin B12 6 mcg • D-Calcium 10 mg • Iodine 150 mcg • Phosphorus Proteinate 10 mg • Magnesium Oxide powder 80 mg • Zinc Citrate powder 15 mg • Chromium Chloride 50 mcg • Potassium Chelate 10 mg • Whey Protein 200 mg • Soy Protein (isolated) 150 mg.

Weight Wellness **-** NorthStar Nutritionals
Each capsule contains: Rhodiola Rosea extract 100 mg • Rhododendron Caucasicum extract 50 mg • Blueberry extract 100 mg • Kelp extract 200 mg.

Weightless Cinnamon-Spice **-** Traditional Medicinals
Cinnamon bark • Fennel seed • Roasted Chicory root • Uva Ursi leaf • Cleavers herb • Flax seed • Licorice root • Red Clover top • Clove stem • Star Anise seed • Hibiscus flower • Buchu leaf • Natural Flavors.

Weightless Cranberry **-** Traditional Medicinals
Contains: Hibiscus flower • Roasted Chicory root • Fennel seed • Red Clover top • Uva Ursi leaf • Parsley leaf • Cleavers herb • Cranberry • Other natural flavors.

Weightless Tea **-** Traditional Medicinals
Fennel seed • Hibiscus flower • Lemongrass leaf • Uva Ursi leaf • Lemon Verbena leaf • Flax seed • Spearmint leaf • Cleavers herb • Red Clover top • Parsley leaf • Buchu leaf • Natural flavors.

Welah Mide **-** Shawnee Moon
Buchu leaf • Red Clover • Saw Palmetto • Uva Ursi.

Well Mind **-** NutriCology
Each capsule contains: Zinc (as zinc valerate) 60 mcg • St. John's Wort dried leaves and flowers extract (hypericum perforatum) 125 mg • Kava Kava dried root extract (piper methysticum) 60 mg • Valerian dried root extract 30 mg • Passionflower dried leaves extract (passiflora incarnata) 30 mg • Schizandra dried berries extract (schizandra chinensis) 30 mg • Gotu Kola powdered herb (centella asiatica) 15 mg • Cypripedium dried root extract (cypripedium pubescens) 2.5 mg. Other Ingredients: Cellulose, Magnesium Stearate, Silicon Dioxide.

Wellman Fizz **-** Vitabiotics
Each tablet contains: Vitamin C 30 mg • Vitamin B1 (thiamin) 12 mg • Vitamin B2 (riboflavin) 5 mg • Vitamin B3 (niacin) 27 mg • Vitamin B6 (pyridoxine HCl) 10 mg • Folic Acid 400 mcg • Vitamin B12 (cyanocobalamin) 30 mcg • Biotin 50 mcg • Pantothenic Acid 6 mg • Iron 5 mg • Magnesium 50 mg • Zinc 5 mg • Selenium 30 mcg • L-Tyrosine 20 mg • Siberian Ginseng extract 150 mg • Co-Enzyme Q10 5 mg • L-Carnitine 75 mg.

Wellman Tablets **-** Vitabiotics
Each tablet contains: Vitamin A 750 mcg • Vitamin D 5 mcg • Vitamin E 20 mg • Vitamin C 60 mg • Vitamin B1 (thiamin) 12 mg • Vitamin B2 (riboflavin) 5 mg • Vitamin B3 (niacin) 20 mg • Vitamin B6 (pyridoxine HCl) 9 mg • Folic Acid 500 mcg • Vitamin B12 (cyanocobalamin) 9 mcg • Biotin 0.05 mg • Pantothenic Acid 10 mg • Iron 6 mg • Magnesium 50 mg • Zinc 15 mg • Iodine 150 mcg • Manganese 3 mg • Copper 1.5 mg • Chromium 50 mcg • Selenium 150 mcg • Silicon 10 mg • Arginine 20 mg • Methionine 20 mg • Betacarotene 2 mg • PABA (para-aminobenzoic acid) 20 mg • Ginseng 20 mg • Bioflavonoids 10 mg • Co-Enzyme Q10 2 mg • L-Carnitine 30 mg.

Wellness C-1000 **-** Source Naturals
Each tablet contains: Vitamin C (as ascorbic acid, potassium, magnesium and calcium ascorbates, ascorbyl palmitate, zinc and manganese ascorbates) 1000 mg • Bioflavonoids 100 mg • Ascorbyl Palmitate 60 mg • Rose Hips fruit 25 mg • Rutin 25 mg • Quercetin 25 mg • Grape seed extract (Proanthodyn, with a proanthocyanidolic value of 95) 15 mg • Alpha-Lipoic Acid 10 mg.

Wellness Cell Response **-** Source Naturals
Each capsule contains: Polyvalent Transfer Factor (as colostral fraction with minimum 20 potency units) 5 mg.

Wellness Cold and Flu **-** Source Naturals
Each tablet contains: Echinacea angustifolia 3X • Allium cepa (red onion) 4X • Bryonia alba (white bryony) 4X • Eupatorium perfoliatum (boneset) 4X • Gelsemium sempervirens (yellow jasmine) 4X • Sanguinaria canadensis (blood root) 4X • Kali bichromicum (potassium dichromate) 6X • Phosphorus 6X • Aconitum napellus (monkshood) 12X • Influenzinum 12X.
See Editor's Note No. 1, page 2053.

Wellness Colloidal Silver Liquid **-** Source Naturals
Each two tablespoons contain: Silver 30 ppm.

Wellness Colloidal Silver Nasal Spray **-** Source Naturals
Each spray contains: Silver 30 ppm.

Wellness Colloidal Silver Throat Spray **-** Source Naturals
Each spray contains: Silver 30 ppm.

Wellness Earache **-** Source Naturals
Each tablet contains: Capsicum annuum (Cayenne Pepper) 6X • Silicea (Silica) 6X • Verbascum thapsus (Mullein) 6X • Ferrum phosphoricum (Ferrosoferric Phosphate) 12X • Kali muriaticum (Potassium Chloride) 12X • Aconitum napellus (Aconite) 30X • Belladonna (Nightshade) 30X • Calcarea carbonica (Calcium Carbonate) 30X • Pulsatilla (Wind Flower) 30X.
See Editor's Note No. 1, page 2053.

Wellness Elderberry Extract Liquid **-** Source Naturals
Each teaspoon contains: Elder berry & flower extract (Sambucus nigra) 2 mL.

Wellness Elderberry Extract Tablets **-** Source Naturals
Each three tablets contain: Elder berry and flower (standardized extract yielding 81 mg bioflavonoids and anthocyanins) 1020 mg • Elderberries and flowers 480 mg.

Wellness Formula **-** Source Naturals
Three tablets contain: Vitamin A (Palmitate 4000 IU, Beta Carotene 1000 IU) 5000 IU • Vitamin C (Ascorbic Acid, and Zinc, Calcium, and Magnesium Ascorbates) 1075 mg • Calcium (Ascorbate) 7.5 mg • Copper (Sebacate) 300 mcg • Magnesium (Ascorbate) 3.8 mg • Selenium (Sodium Selenite) 25 mcg • Zinc (Ascorbate) 23 mg • Propolis 324 mg • Propolis extract 126 mg • Garlic clove 360 mg • Boneset leaf 328 mg • Polygonum Odoratum 200 mg • Echinacea

root 196 mg • Echinacea extract 164 mg • Isatis (root and leaf) 159 mg • Horehound stems 150 mg • Bioflavonoids 120 mg • Astragalus root 90 mg • Angelica Archangelica root 87 mg • Mullein leaf 80 mg • Goldenseal root 75 mg • Siberian Ginseng root 66 mg • Hawthorn berry 55 mg • Oregon Grape root 55 mg • Siberian Ginseng extract 54 mg • Pau d'Arco extract 36 mg • Cayenne fruit 30 mg.

Wellness GarliCell **-** Source Naturals
Each tablet contains: Garlic clove 650 mg.

Wellness Herbal Resistance - Alcohol Free **-** Source Naturals
Each half teaspoon contains: Proprietary Extract 1.7 mL: Echinacea (E. purpurea & E. angustifolia standardized extract), Goldenseal root, Yin Chiao formula (lonicera, forsythia, mint, prepared sojae, licorice, schizonepeta phragmitis, platycodon, arctium, lophatherum), Ginger root, Boneset leaf & stem, Siberian Ginseng root, Elderberry flowers, Isatis leaf & root, Horehound aerial parts, Bayberry bark.

Wellness Herbal Resistance Liquid **-** Source Naturals
Each half teaspoon contains: Proprietary Extract 2.5 mL: Echinacea (E. purpurea & E. angustifolia standardized extract), Goldenseal root, Yin Chiao formula (lonicera, forsythia, mint, prepared sojae, licorice, schizonepeta phragmitis, platycodon, arctium, lophatherum), Ginger root, Boneset leaf & stem, Siberian Ginseng root, Elderberry flowers, Isatis leaf & root, Horehound aerial parts, Bayberry bark.

Wellness Larchtree Extract **-** Source Naturals
Each two tablets contain: Larch Tree extract (Larix occidentalis, standardized to 85% arabinogalactans yielding 1.7 grams of arabinogalactans) 2 g • Calcium 91 mg.

Wellness Multiple **-** Source Naturals
Each four tablets contain: Vitamin A (as palmitate 15,000 IU & beta carotene 10,000 IU) 25,000 IU • Vitamin C (as magnesium ascorbate, ascorbic acid, calcium, potassium, zinc & manganese ascorbates) 1000 mg • Vitamin E (as natural d-alpha tocopheryl) 400 IU • Thiamin (vitamin B1) 50 mg • Riboflavin (vitamin B-2) 50 mg • Niacinamide 50 mg • Niacin 25 mg • Vitamin B6 (as pyridoxine HCl) 50 mg • Folate (as folic acid) 400 mcg • Vitamin B12 (as cyanocobalamin) 100 mcg • Biotin 100 mcg • Pantothenic Acid (as calcium d-pantothenate) 50 mg • Calcium (as calcium ascorbate) 25 mg • Magnesium (as magnesium ascorbate) 25 mg • Zinc (as zinc ascorbate) 15 mg • Selenium (as l-selenomethionine [Selenomax] & sodium selenite) 200 mcg • Copper (as copper sebacate) 2 mg • Manganese (as manganese ascorbate) 3 mg • Chromium (as chromium polynicotinate [ChromeMate] & picolinate) 200 mcg • Molybdenum (as molybdenum chelate) 200 mcg • Potassium (as potassium ascorbate) 25 mg • N-Acetyl Cysteine 400 mg • Quercetin 200 mg • whole leaf Aloe Vera concentrate (200:1) 100 mg • Turmeric root extract 100 mg • Milk Thistle seed extract yielding 50 mg silymarin) 60 mg • Choline (as choline bitartrate) 50 mg • Grape seed extract (Proanthodyn, with a proanthocyanidolic value of 95) 50 mg • Inositol 50 mg • Coenzyme Q10 (ubiquinone) 30 mg • Alpha-Lipoic Acid 30 mg • Green Tea leaf extract 20 mg.
Proprietary Blend 1310 mg: Cat's Claw bark, Elderberry flowers, St. John's Wort leaf & flower extract, Reishi Mycelia, Astragalus root, Schizandra fruit, Garlic clove, Maitake Mycelia, Shiitake Mycelia, Elderberry extract, Siberian Ginseng root extract, Atractylodes rhizome.

Wellness Olive Leaf **-** Source Naturals
Each two tablets contain: Olive leaf (standardized extract of olea europaea yielding 75 mg of Oleuropein) 1000 mg.

Wellness Plus Capsules **-** Vista Vitamins
Each packet contains: Vitamin A (as retinyl palmitate) 5000 IU • Vitamin A (as alpha and beta carotene) 2500 IU • Vitamin C (as ascorbic acid) 120 mg • Vitamin D (as cholecalciferol) 400 IU • Vitamin E (as d-alpha tocopheryl acetate) 50 IU • Vitamin K (as phylloquinone) 60 mcg • Thiamin (as thiamin hydrochloride) 12 mg • Riboflavin 13 mg • Niacin (as niacinamide) 16 mg • Vitamin B6 (as pyridoxine hydrochloride) 14 mg • Folic Acid 400 mcg • Vitamin B12 (as methylcobalamin) 120 mcg • Biotin 150 mcg • Pantothenic Acid (as d-calcium pantothenate) 10 mg • Calcium (as calcium amino acid chelate) 150 mg • Iron (as ferrochel ferrous bis-glycine) 4 mg • Iodine (as potassium iodide) 75 mcg • Magnesium (as magnesium amino acid chelate) 100 mg • Zinc (as chelazome amino acid chelate) 11 mg • Selenium (as selenium amino acid complex) 70 mcg • Copper (as chelazome amino acid chelate) 0.45 mg • Manganese (as chelazome amino acid chelate) 1.15 mg • Chromium (as chelavite amino acid chelate) 75 mcg • Molybdenum (as molybdenum amino acid chelate) 22.5 mcg • Potassium (as potassium chloride) 49.5 mg • Boron (as boron amino acid complex) 0.75 mg • Larix occidentalis (arabinogalatans) 250 mg • Lactobacillus sporogenes 5 million. Other Ingredients: Gelatin, Cellulose, Stearic Acid, Silicon Dioxide, Magnesium Stearate, Titanium Dioxide.

Wellness Source **-** HealthWatchers System
Vitamin A • Vitamin D • Vitamin E • Vitamin C • Vitamin B6 • Vitamin B2 • Vitamin B1 • Vitamin B12 • Vitamin U • Bioflavonoids • Choline Bitartrate • Niacin-Niacinamide • Pantothenic Acid • Inositol • Rutin • Papain • PABA • Lecithin • Quercetin • RNA • Hesperidin • DNA • CoQ10 • Folic Acid • Octacosanol • Biotin • Magnesium • Calcium • Zinc • Boron • Potassium • Manganese • Copper • Iodine (Kelp) • Selenium • Chromium.

Wellness Source Booster **-** HealthWatchers System
Beta Carotene • Vitamin E • Vitamin C • Calcium • Magnesium • Choline • Potassium • Silica • Niacinamide.

Wellness Zinc Lozenges **-** Source Naturals
Each lozenge contains: Zinc (as zinc gluconate, ascorbate, & chelate) 23 mg • Vitamin C (as zinc ascorbate) 30 mg.

Wellness Zinc Throat Spray **-** Source Naturals
Each two fluid ounces contain: Vitamin C (as ascorbic acid) 11 mg • Zinc (as zinc gluconate) 23 mg • Echinacea extract 40 mg • Elderberry extract 34 mg.

Wellwoman Capsules **-** Vitabiotics
Each capsule contains: Starflower Oil 100 mg • Evening Primrose Oil 100 mg • Vitamin D (200 IU) 5 mcg • Vitamin E (natural source) 30 mg • Vitamin C 60 mg • Vitamin B1 (thiamin) 10 mg • Vitamin B2 (riboflavin) 5 mg • Vitamin B3 (niacin) 36 mg • Vitamin B6 (pyridoxine HCl) 20 mg • Folic Acid 400 mcg • Vitamin B12 (cyanocobalamin) 20 mcg • Biotin 50 mcg • Pantothenic Acid 6 mg • Vitamin K 90 mcg • Natural Mixed Carotenoids 2 mg • Iron 12 mg • Magnesium 100 mg • Zinc 12 mg • Manganese 2.5 mg • Copper 1.5 mg • Selenium 100 mcg • Chromium 50 mcg • PABA (para-aminobenzoic acid) 30 mg • Citrus Bioflavonoids 10 mg.

Wellwoman Fizz **-** Vitabiotics
Each tablet contains: Vitamin C 30 mg • Vitamin B1 (thiamin) 10 mg • Vitamin B2 (riboflavin) 5 mg • Vitamin B3 (niacin) 27 mg • Vitamin B6 (pyridoxine HCl) 10 mg • Folic Acid 400 mcg • Vitamin B12 (cyanocobalamin) 40 mcg • Biotin 100 mcg • Pantothenic Acid 6 mg • Iron 8 mg • Magnesium 50 mg • Zinc 5 mg • L-Carnitine 100 mg • Gotu Kola extract 40 mg • Guarana extract 150 mcg.

Wheat Germ Oil 1000 mg - GNC A-Z **-** GNC
Each capsule contains: Wheat Germ oil 1 g. Other Ingredients: Gelatin, Glycerin.

Wheat Grass **-** Pines International
Seven tablets (or 1 teaspoon of powder) contain: Protein 860 mg • Chlorophyl 18.5 mg •Biotin 4 mcg •Choline 5 mg •Lutein 1 mg •Lycopene 29 mcg •Vitamin A (beta-carotene) 1668 IU •Vitamin B-1 (thiamine) 11 mcg •Vitamin B-2 (riboflavin) 260 mcg •Vitamin B-3 (niacin) 252 mcg •Vitamin B-5 (pantothenic acid) 36 mcg •Vitamin B-6 (pyridoxine) 39 mcg • Vitamin B-8 (folic acid) 21 mcg •Vitamin B-12 (cobalamin) .05 mcg •Vitamin C 7.5 mg • Vitamin E 320 mcg •Vitamin K 35 mcg •Zeaxanthin 279 mcg • Calcium 15 mg •Cobalt 1.7 mcg •Copper 17 mcg •Iodine 8 mcg •Iron 870 mcg •Magnesium 3.9 mcg •Manganese 240 mcg •Phosphorus 14 mg •Potassium 137 mg •Selenium 3.5 mcg • Sodium 1 mg •Sulfur 10.5 mg • Zinc 62 mcg •Alanine 69 mg •Arginine 66 mg •Aspartic Acid 50 mg •Cystine 11 mg •Glutamic Acid 76 mg • Glycine 49 mg •Histidine 18 mg

•Isoleucine 35 mg •Leucine 72 mg •Lysine 38 mg •Methionine 18 mg •Phenylalanine 36 mg •Proline 46 mg •Serine 31 mg •Threonine 42 mg •Tryptophan 6 mg •Tyrosine 33 mg •Valine 48 mg.

Whey MRP **-** Optimum Nutrition
Each packet (76 g) contains: Protein Blend: Whey Protein Concentrate, Whey Protein Isolate, Hydrolyzed Whey Peptides • Maltodextrin • Gum Blend: Cellulose Gum, Xanthan Gum, Carrageenan • Vitamin/ Mineral Blend: DiMagnesium Phosphate, Calcium Carbonate, TriCalcium Phosphate, Ascorbic Acid, Ferric Orthophosphate, D-Alpha Tocopheryl Acetate, Boron Proteinate, Maltodextrin, Niacinamide, Zinc Oxide, Manganese Sulfate, D-Calcium Pantothenate, Molybdenum AA Chelate, Selenomethionine, Pyridoxine Hydrochloride, Riboflavin, Beta Carotene, Folic Acid, Biotin, Potassium Iodide, Cyanocobalamin • Brown Rice Syrup Solids • Natural & Artificial Flavor • Salt • Sucralose • Acesulfame Potassium • Aminogen • Carbogen • Lactase.

Whey Protein **-** The Sports Nutrition Source, Inc.
Each scoop contains: Sodium 50 mg • Potassium 75 mg • Protein 16 g.

WheyFit 2000 **-** Young Living Essential Oils
Each scoop contains: Whey Protein • Egg Whites • Soy Protein • Lecithin • Fructooligosaccharides (FOS) • Stevia • Blueberry Powder • Strawberry Powder • Blueberry Flavor (liquid) • Natural Flavors • Vanilla Extract • Zinc Citrate • Sodium Selenate • Magnesium Citrate • Citric Acid • Lemon Oil • Enzyme Complex Blend: Amylase, Cellulase, Lactase, Lipase, Natural Protease.

White Stuff **-** Blue Stuff, Inc.
Each 1 oz jar contains: Whole leaf Aloe Vera concentrate • Squalene • Petroleum • Glycerin • Ceresin • Cetyl Dimethicone • Copolyol • Octyl Palmitate • Emu oil • Phenylephrine HCL • Alpha Bisabolol • Grapefruit Seed extract • Fragrance.

White Willow Bark Extract **-** Nature's Way
Each capsule contains: White Willow Bark 250 mg • White Willow Bark, dried extract 200 mg. Other Ingredients: Gelatin.

Whole Body Cleanse **-** PhytoPharmica
Whole Body Cleanse Laxative Formula: Three tablets contain: Magnesium Hydroxide 2600 mg • Proprietary Mucilage Blend 650 mg: Slippery Elm bark (ulmus rubra), Marshmallow root 3.5:1 extract (althaea officinalis), Fenugreek seed 4:1 extract (trigonella foenum-graecum) • Burdock root 3:1 extract (arctium lappa) 300 mg • Proprietary Soothing Blend 150 mg: Peppermint leaf (mentha x piperita), Fennel seed (foeniculum vulgare), Ginger rhizome extract (zingiber officinale) • Red Clover blossom 4:1 extract (trifolium pratense) 100 mg. Other Ingredients: Cellulose, Modified Cellulose Gum, Modified Cellulose, Magnesium Stearate, Silicon Dioxide, Lecithin, Carnauba Wax. Fiber Formula: Eight capsules contain: Proprietary Fiber Blend 3455 mg: Psyllium husk (plantago ovata), Oat bran (avena sativa), Guar Gum seed extract (cyamposis tetragonoloba), Pectin (from citrus fruit), Marshmallow root 3.5:1 extract (althaea officinalis). Other Ingredients: Cellulose, Gelatin, Magnesium Stearate, Silicon Dioxide. Super Milk Thistle: Each softgel contains: Milk Thistle fruit phytosome (silybum marianum, one part milk thistle extract, standardized to contain 80% silymarin, bound to two parts phosphatidylcholine) 100 mg • Artichoke leaf extract (cynara scolymus, standardized to contaon 13-18% caffeylquinic acids calculated as chlorogenic acid) 40 mg • Dandelion root 4:1 extract (taraxacum officinale) 10 mg • Licorice root and rhizome extract (glycyrrhiza glabra, standardized to contain 5% glycyrrhizic acid) 10 mg. Other Ingredients: Soybean Oil, Gelatin, Glycerin, Beeswax, Lecithin.

Whole Heart Multivitamin **-** PhytoPharmica
Two tablets contain: Alpha Lipoic Acid 100 mg • Biooin 300 mcg • Calcium (as calcium carbonate and calcium citrate) 200 mg • Choline Bitartrate 138 mg • Chromium (as chromium picolinate) 100 mcg • Copper (as copper gluconate) 1 mg • Folic Acid 450 mcg • Iodine (as potassium iodide) 150 mcg • Lutein (from calendula officinalis) 750 mcg • Lycopene 3 mg • Magnesium (as magnesium aspartate and magnesium oxide) 125 mg • Manganese (as manganese citrate) 1 mg • Molybdenum (as sodium molybdate) 38 mcg • Niacin (as niacinamide and niacin) 60 mg • Pantothenic Acid (as calcium D-pantothenate) 50 mg • Riboflavin (vitamin B2) 30 mg • Selenium (as L-selenomethionine) 100 mcg • Sodium 5 mg • Thiamin (as thiamin HCl, vitamin B1) 30 mg • Vanadium (as vanadyl sulfate) 50 mcg • Vitamin A (75% as beta carotene and as retinyl acetate) 5000 IU • Vitamin B12 (as cyanocobalamin) 500 mcg • Vitamin B6 (as pyridoxine HCl) 30 mg • Vitamin C (ascorbic acid) 250 mg • Vitamin D (as cholecalciferol) 200 IU • Vitamine E (as D-alpha tocopheryl acid succinate) 200 IU • Zeaxanthin (from calendula officinalis) 33 mcg • Zinc (as zinc gluconate) 15 mg.

Wild Brazilian SUMA-750 **-** Nature's Plus
Each capsule contains: Wild Brazilian SUMA (Pfaffia paniculata [Martius] Kuntze) 750 mg. Naturally rich in the 6 Saponins, Pfaffosides A,B,C,D,E & F - average 6%; 100% pure.

Wild Cherry Syrup **-** Dial Herbs
Wild Cherry bark • Cubeb berry • Mullein • Skunk Cabbage • Lobelia • Honey • Clove.

Wild Cherry Virtue **-** Blessed Herbs
Wild Cherry bark • Plantain leaf • Mullein leaf • Mullein flower • Licorice root • Black Cherry concentrate.

Wild Cherry-Slippery Elm Bark Formula **-** Quest
Each caplet contains: Wild Cherry bark powder (Prunus serotina) 60 mg • Slippery Elm bark powder (Ulmus fulva) 60 mg • Pleurisy Root powder (Asclepias tuberosa) 60 mg • Chickweed powder (Stellaria media) 40 mg • Horehound powder (Marrubium vulgare) 40 mg • Kelp powder (Fucus vesiculosus) 40 mg • Licorice root powder (Glycyrrhiza glabra) 40 mg • Mullein leaf powder (Verbascum thapsus) 40 mg • Cayenne powder (Capsicum minimum) 35 mg • Saw Palmetto berry powder (Serenoa serrulata) 15 mg. Other Ingredients: Calcium Phosphate, Microcrystalline Cellulose, Vegetable Stearin, Croscarmellose Sodium, Magnesium Stearate (vegetable source).

Wild Rose Nerve Formula **-** Dial Herbs
Valerian root • Mistletoe • Scullcap • Hops • Lady Slipper • Passion flower.

Wild Vites **-** Nature's Life
Each tablet contains: Vitamin A (Acetate) 5000 IU • Vitamin D3 (Cholecalciferol) 400 IU • Vitamin E (d-Alpha Tocopheryl acetate) 30 IU • Vitamin C (Ascorbic Acid) 60 mg • Vitamin B1 (Thiamine Monoitrate) 1.5 mg • Vitamin B2 (Riboflavin) 1.7 mg • Vitamin B3 (Niacinamide) 20 mg • Vitamin B5 (Pantothenic Acid) 10 mg • Vitamin B6 Pyridoxine HCl) 2 mg • Vitamin B12 (Cobalamin) 6 mcg • Folic Acid 400 mcg • Biotin 300 mg. In a natural base of low-Glycemic pure Crystalline Fructose & Sorbitol.

Wild Yam **-** Alvin Last
Wild Yam extract • Aloe Vera gel • Soybean Oil • Stearic Acid • Cetyl Alcohol • Triethanolamine • Tocopheryl Acetate • Glycerin • Methylparaben • Propylparaben.

Wild Yam & Progesterone+ **-** Wise Women Essentials
Wild Yam extract • Natural Progesterone USP (origin from wild yam) • Chaste Tree (vitex) • Liposome-Water / Soy Lecithin • Jojoba oil • Squalane (from olives) • Allantoin • Retinyl Palmitate • Ascorbyl Palmitate • Tocopheryl Acetate (liposomes of vitmains A, C and E) • Dong Quai extract • Licorice extract • Black Cohosh extract • Grapefruit seed extract • Ascorbic Acid.

Wild Yam Cream **-** Youngevity
Wild Yam root extract (Dioscorea villosa) • Aloe Vera gel • Natural Emollients and Moisturizers • Avocado oil • Oat oil • Key Lime fragrance • Chamomile (Matricaria chamomilla) • Burdock root (Arctium lappa) • Black Cohosh (Cimicifuga racemosa) • Siberian

Ginseng (Eleutherococcus senticosus) • D-Alpha Tocopherol Acetate • Methylparaben • Propylparaben.

Wild Yam Extract **-** PhytoPharmica
Two capsules contain: Wild (Mexican) Yam (Dioscorea villosa) root extract 10:1 (standardized to contain 10% diosgenin) 480 mg • Adrenal extract (freeze-dried) 200 mg • Beta-sitosterol 42 mg.

Wild Yam Root **-** Nature's Bounty
Two capsules contain: Wild Yam root (Dioscorea Villosa) 810 mg. Other Ingredients: Cellulose, Gelatin, Vegetable Magnesium Stearate, Silica.

Wild Yam/Dong Quai Formula **-** PhysioLogics
Each capsule contains: Dong Quai root extract (angelica sinensis, standardized to contain 1% lingustilides, 2 mg) 200 mg • Wild Yam root extract (dioscorea villosa, standardized to contain 6% saponins, 12 mg) 200 mg • Soybean seed extract (glycine max, standardized to contain 5% isoflavones, 5 mg) 100 mg. Other Ingredients: Gelatin, Rice Powder, Vegetable Magnesium Stearate, Silica.

Wild Yam-False Unicorn Virtue **-** Blessed Herbs
False Unicorn root • Black Haw bark • Wild Yam root • Lobelia • Grain alcohol & Distilled Water.

Winter Wellness **-** Now
Two tablets contain: Vitamin A 5000 IU • Vitamin C 500 mg • Potassium 20 mg • Zinc 15 mg • Bee Propolis 200 mg • Deodorized Garlic Extract 200 mg • Ginger root 200 mg • Oregon Grape root 150 mg • Peptizyme 125 mg • Echinacea angustifolia root extract 100 mg • Elderberry extract 100 mg • Olive leaf extract 100 mg • Quercetin 100 mg • Shitake mushroom extract 100 mg • Reishi mushroom 100 mg • American Ginseng root 100 mg • Licorice root extract 100 mg • Goldenseal root 75 mg • Cayenne pepper 50 mg.

Wobenzym N (Wobenzym-N) **-** Mucos Pharma GMBH & Co
Each tablet contains: Pancreatin 100 mg • Trypsin 24 mg • Chymotrypsin 1 mg • Bromelain 45 mg • Papain 60 mg • Rutoside 50 mg. See Editor's Note No. 18, page 2055.

WomanPrime **-** NutriCology
Each capsule contains: Vitamin A (as vitamin A palmitate) 1250 IU • Vitamin C (as ascorbic acid) 25 mg • Vitamin E (as D-alpha-tocopheryl acid succinate) 125 IU • Vitamin B6 (as pyridoxine hydrochloride) 6.25 mg • Folic Acid 200 mcg • Vitamin B12 5 mcg • Pantothenic Acid (as calcium pantothenate) 70 mg • Magnesium (as magnesium aspartate) 8.25 mg • Selenium (as selenomethionine) 12.5 mcg • Boron (as boron citrate) 250 mcg • Hesperidin 125 mg • PABA (para-aminobenzoic acid) 75 mg • Adrenal 31 mg • Korean Ginseng extract 25 mg • Black Cohosh extract 25 mg. Other Ingredients: Cellulose, Magnesium Stearate, Silicon Dioxide.

Woman's Choice **-** PhytoPharmica
Three capsules contain: Vitamin A (Beta Carotene) - (Non-toxic form of Vitamin A) 16665 IU • Vitamin E (D-Alpha Tocopherol Succinate) 200 IU • Vitamin C (Ascorbic Acid) 200 mg • Magnesium L-Aspartate 150 mg • Pantothenic Acid (D-Calcium Pantothenate) 100 mg • Thiamine HCL (Vitamin B1) 50 mg • Riboflavin (Vitamin B2) 50 mg • Calcium Citrate 50 mg • Iron (Ferrous Succinate) 18 mg • Zinc (Gluconate) 15 mg • Chromium (Polynicotinate) 250 mcg • Folic Acid 100 mcg • Vitamin B12 (Cyanocobalamin) 50 mcg • Selenium (L-Selenomethionine) 50 mcg • Dong Quai extract 4:1 (Angelica sinensis) 75 mg • Licorice root extract (Glycyrrhiza glabra) 60 mg • Milk Thistle extract 50 mg (Silybum marianum) • Black Cohosh extract 4:1 (Cimicifuga racemosa) 30 mg • Chaste Tree berry extract (Vitex agnus-castus) 20 mg • Pyridoxal-5'-Phosphate 10 mg.

Women's AM Multi **-** Clinician's Choice
Two tablets contain: Vitamin A (retinyl acetate & 26% as beta-carotene) 3900 IU • Vitamin C (ascorbic acid) 250 mg • Vitamin D (cholecalciferol) 400 IU • Vitamin E (dl-alpha tocopheryl acetate) 150 IU • Thiamin (mononitrate) 1 mg • Riboflavin 1 mg • Niacin (nianicamide) 10 mg • Vitamin B6 (pyridoxine hydrochloride) 2 mg • Folate (folic acid) 250 mg • Vitamin B12 (cyanocobalamin) 4 mcg • Biotin 200 mcg • Pantothenic Acid (d-calcium pantothenate) 5 mg • Calcium (carbonate, amino acid chelate, ascorbate, aspartate, citrate, gluconate) 220 mg • Iron (amino acid chelate) 12 mg • Iodine (potassium iodide) 76 mcg • Magnesium (oxide, amino acid chelate) 9 mg • Zinc (oxide, amino acid chelate, gluconate) 8 mg • Selenium (selenomethionine) 100 mcg • Copper (amino acid chelate) 1 mg • Manganese (amino acid chelate) 3 mg • Potassium (chloride, amino acid chelate) 12 mg • Chromium (nicotrate, picolinate, chelavite, amino acid chelate) 40 mcg • Molybdenum (amino acid chelate) 4 mcg • RoseOx (patented, standardized process for an extract of Rosemary) 60 mg • Citrus Bioflavonoid Complex 10 mg • Dong Quai 10 mg • Wild Yam 10 mg • Black Currant 10 mg • Red Raspberry Leaf 10 mg • Proprietary Blend 12 mg: Panax Ginseng Extract, Schizandra Fruit, Echinacea Angustifolia, Grape Powder, Bee Pollen, Cruciferex.

Women's Cycle Multivitamins **-** Leiner Health Products
Each caplet contains: Iron (Ferrous Fumarate) 15 mg • Vitamin K (Phytonadione) 65 mcg • Folate (Folic Acid) 300 mcg • Biotin 200 mcg • Molybdenum (Sodium Molybdate) 38 mcg • Niacin (Niacinamide) 8.5 mg • Calcium 160 mg • Vitamin B6 (Pyridoxine Hydrochloride) 3 mg • Vitamin E (dl-Alpha Tocopheryl Acetate) 45 IU • Riboflavin (Vitamin B2) 2.5 mg • Selenium 100 mcg • Thiamin Mononitrate (Vitamin B1) 2 mg • Magnesium Oxide 50 mg • Phosphorus 124 mg • Chromium Chloride 120 mcg • Copper (Cupric Oxide) 2 mg • Iodine 10 mcg • Manganese Sulfate 2 mg • Pantothenic Acid (d-Calcium Pantothenate) 10 mg • Vitamin A Acetate 5000 IU • Vitamin B12 (Cyanocobalamin - USP Method 2) 6 mcg • Vitamin C (Ascorbic Acid) 60 mg • Vitamin D (Ergocalciferol) 400 IU • Zinc Oxide 15 mg • Borage Oil complex (Borage officinalis) seed (Standardized to 10% GLA) 25 mg • Chloride 18 mg • Isoflavones from Soy extract 5 mg • Kelp (Macrocystis pyrifera) frond 5 mg • Lecithin powder (Glycine max) bean 20 mg • Nickel (Nickelous Sulfate) 5 mcg • Potassium Chloride 20 mg • Silicon Dioxide 2 mg • Tin (Stannous Chloride) 10 mcg • Trace Mineral complex 5 mg • Vanadium (Sodium Metavanadate) 10 mcg. Other Ingredients: Dicalcium Phosphate, Cellulose, Gelatin, Stearic Acid, Croscarmellose Sodium, Hydroxypropyl Methylcellulose, Titanium Dioxide, Red Raspberry Powder, Dextrin, Maltodextrin, Mannitol, Hydroxypropyl Cellulose, Polyethylene Glycol, Kelp Powder, Trace Mineral Complex, Starch, Polysorbate 80, Blue 1 Lake, Red 40 Lake, Dextrose.

Women's Exclusive Formula **-** Puritan's Pride
Two tablets contain: Vitamin A 5,000 IU • Vitamin C 60 mg • Vitamin D 400 IU • Vitamin E (as d-Alpha Tocopheryl Acetate) 30 IU • Thiamin (Vitamin B-1) 26.7 mg • Riboflavin (Vitamin B-2) 30 mg • Niacin 30 mg • Vitamin B-6 24.6 mg • Folic Acid 400 mcg • Vitamin B-12 100 mcg • Biotin 30 mcg • Pantothenic Acid 30 mg • Calcium 500 mg • Iron 15 mg • Phosphorus 30 mg • Iodine 150 mcg • Magnesium 250 mg • Zinc 15 mg • Selenium 25 mcg • Copper 0.5 mg • Manganese 5 mg • Chromium 25 mcg • Molybdenum 25 mcg • Potassium 11.5 mg • Inositol 30 mg • Choline Bitartrate 30 mg • PABA (Para-Aminobenzoic Acid) 30 mg • Citrus Bioflavonoids 25 mg • Betaine Hydrochloride 25 mg • L-Cysteine 50 mg • Dong Quai 50 mg • Rose Hips 6 mg.

Women's Formula 1 **-** Rexall - Sundown
Two tablets contain: Vitamin C 67 mg • Vitamin D (as cholecalciferol) 67 IU • Vitamin B-6 (as pyridoxine HCl) 3.3 mg • Folic Acid 100 mcg • Vitamin B-12 (as cyanocobalamin) 3.3 mcg • Calcium (as calcium carbonate, calcium citrate and calciulm gluconate) 333 mg • Iron (as carbonyl iron) 3 mg • Magnesium (as magnesium gluconate and magnesium oxide) 133 mg • Zinc (as zinc gluconate) 3.3 mg • Selenium (as sodium selenate) 16.7 mcg • Copper (as copper gluconate) 0.17 mg • Manganese (as manganese sulfate) 5 mg • Molybdenum (as sodium molybdate) 16.7 mcg • Potassium (as potassium chloride) 35 mg • Boron (as potassium borate and sodium borate) 16.7 mcg • Silica 7 mg • Phytonutrient Vegetable Blend (Broccoli, Carrot, Spinach, Tomato) 40 mg. Other Ingredients:

Cellulose, Croscarmellose Sodium, Hydroxypropyl Methylcellulose, Magnesium Stearate, PEG.

Women's Formula 2 **-** Rexall - Sundown
Two tablets contain: Vitamin C 33 mg • Vitamin D (as cholecalciferol) 67 IU • Vitamin K (as phytonadione) 3.3 mcg • Vitamin B-6 (as pyridoxine HCl) 3.3 mg • Folic Acid 33.3 mcg • Vitamin B-12 (as cyanocobalamin) 6.7 mcg • Calcium (as calcium carbonate, calcium citrate and calciulm gluconate) 400 mg • Iodine (as potassium iodide) 16.7 mcg • Magnesium (as magnesium gluconate and magnesium oxide) 150 mg • Zinc (as zinc gluconate) 1.7 mg • Selenium (as sodium selenate) 16.7 mcg • Copper (as copper gluconate) 0.1 mg • Manganese (as manganese sulfate) 5 mg • Molybdenum (as sodium molybdate) 16.7 mcg • Potassium (as potassium chloride) 35 mg • Boron (as potassium borate and sodium borate) 16.7 mcg • Betaine (as betaine HCl) 33.3 mg • Silica 6.9 mg • Phytonutrient Vegetable Blend (Broccoli, Carrot, Spinach,Tomato) 40 mg. Other Ingredients: Cellulose, Croscarmellose Sodium, Magnesium Stearate, Hydroxypropyl Methylcellulose, PEG.

Women's Formula Plus **-** Rexall - Sundown
Two caplets contain: Calcium 518 mg • Calcium D-Glucarate 400 mg • Women's Nutritional Blend: Flaxseed, Citrus Bioflavonoids, Red Clover (flower head), Soybean (standardized to 3.5% Isoflavones) 176 mg. Other Ingredients: Calcium Carbonate, Cellulose, Croscarmellose Sodium, Stearic Acid, Magnesium Stearate.

Women's Group Formulas Vaginal Lubricant **-** Transitions for Health, Inc.
Deionized Water • Glycerin • Butylene Glycol • Aloe Vera Gel • Citric Acid • Black Cohosh (Cimicifuga racemosa) Extract • Marigold (Calendula officinalis) Extract • Chamomile (Matricaria chamomilla) Extract • Ginseng (Panax ginseng) Extract • Black Walnut (Juglans nigra) Extract • d-alpha Tocopherol and Mixed Tocopherols (Vit. E) • Retinyl Palmitate • Evening Primrose (Oenothera biennis) Oil.

Women's Guardian **-** Clinician's Choice
Two tablets contain: Vitamin B6 (pyridoxine HCl) 2 mg • Pantothenic Acid (calcium pantothenate) 50 mg • Beta-Sitosterol 300 mg • Dong Quai Herb 200 mg • Red Raspberry Leaf 160 mg • Kudzu Root 100 mg • Wild Yam 100 mg • Squaw Vine 50 mg • L-Isoleucine 40 mg • L-Leucine 40 mg • L-Valine 40 mg • Aminogen 20 mg • Black Cohosh Root 20 mg • Evening Primrose 20 mg • Lycopene (1%) 20 mg • Proprietary Blend 12 mg: Lutein (5%), Chamomile Flowers, Passion Flower, Sage Leaves, Isoflavones, Grape Powder.

Women's Liberty **-** Traditional Medicinals
Licorice root • Orange peel • Wild Yam root • Ginger rhizome • Cinnamon bark • Dong Quai root • Clove stem • Fo Ti root • Angelica root.

Women's Longevity Rhythms **-** EcoNugenics
Five capsules contain: Vitamin A (as beta carotene) 5000 IU • Vitamin C (as ascorbic acid) 200 mg • Vitamin D 50 IU • Vitamin E (as d-alpha tocopherol) 150 IU • Vitamin B1 (as thiamine hydrochloride) 40 mg • Vitamin B2 (as riboflavin-5-phosphate) 40 mg • Vitamin B3 (as niacinamide) 125 mg • Vitamin B6 (as pyridoxine hydrochloride) 40 mg • Folic Acid 400 mcg • Vitamin B12 (as cyanocobalamin) 50 mcg • Biotin 200 mcg • Vitamin B5 (as calcium pantothenate) 40 mg • Calcium (as citrate, carbonate, aspartate) 300 mg • Iodine (from kelp) 17.5 mcg • Magnesium (as oxide, citrate, aspartate) 160 mcg • Zinc (as citrate) 15 mg • Selenium (as selenomethionine) 70 mcg • Copper (as sebacate) 1 mg • Manganese (as sulfate) 2 mg • EcoGen Soy Isoflavone concentrate 400 mg • Women's Longevity Blend 350 mg: Dried extracts of Burdock root, Eleuthero root, Blue Cohosh root, Horsetail herb, Alfalfa leaf, Green Tea leaf, Uva Ursi leaf, Thymus Gland extract, Chaste Tree berry (vitex), Cranberry fruit • Chinese Herbal Extract Blend 310 mg: Dong Quai root, White Peony root, Sichuan Lovage root, Poria Cocos, Rehmannia root, Ginseng root, Atractylodes root, Ginger root, Jujube fruit • Royal Jelly 250 mg • MycoCeutics 10 Mushroom Proprietary Blend 100 mg: Reishi (ganoderma lucidum), Poria cocos, Cordyceps (cordyceps sinensis), Tremella Fuciformis, Umbellatus (polyporus umbellatus), Coriolus (coriolus versicolor), Maitake (grifola frondosa), Shitake (lentinula edodes), Wood Ear (auricularia auricula), Hericium Erinaceus • Inositol 50 mg • Choline (as bitartrate) 40 mg • Para-Aminobenzoic Acid (PABA) 40 mg • Citrus Bioflavonoid complex 20 mg • Taurine 10 mg • Beta-1,3-Glucan (from purified yeast, baker's yeast) 5 mg • Boron (as boric acid) 1 mg. Other Ingredients: Gelatin, Cellulose, Silica, Magnesium Stearate.
See Editor's Note No. 14, page 2055.

Women's Longevity Rhythms Gold **-** EcoNugenics
Six capsules contain: Vitamin A (beta-carotene) 5000 IU • Vitamin C (ascorbic acid, corn-free) 200 mg • Vitamin D (ergocalciferol, from fish oil) 100 IU • Vitamin D (D3, cholecalciferol, from fish oil) 50 IU • Vitamin E (d-alpha tocopherol natural) 175 IU • Vitamin B1 (thiamine hydrochloride) 50 mg • Vitamin B2 (riboflavin 5-phosphate) 50 mg • Vitamin B3 (niacinamide) 150 mg • Vitamin B6 (pyridoxine hydrochloride) 50 mg • Folic Acid 0.5 mg • Vitamin B12 (cyanocobalamin) 100 mcg • Biotin 200 mcg • Vitamin B5 (calcium pantothenate) 50 mg • Calcium (as carbonate, citrate, hydroxyapatite, aspartate) 500 mg • Iodine (as kelp) 17.5 mcg • Magnesium (as oxide, citrate, aspartate) 200 mg • Zinc (as citrate) 15 mg • Selenium (as selenomethionine) 80 mcg • Copper (as sebacate) 1.5 mg • Manganese (as sulfate) 4 mg • Chromium (as picolinate, non-yeast) 120 mcg • Chinese Herbal Blend 535 mg: Dried Extracts of Dong Quai, White Peony root, Chinese Yam, Chinese Licorice root, Chinese Hawthorne fruit, Chinese Motherwort herb • Women's Longevity Blend 642 mg: Dried Extracts of Wild Oats, Korean Ginseng root, Black Cohosh root, Burdock root, Chaste Tree berry (vitex), Damiana herb, Ginkgo Biloba leaf (24%), Horsetail herb, Uva Ursi herb • EcoGen Soy Isoflavone concentrate 400 mg • Royal Jelly (freeze dried) 300 mg • MycoCeutics 10 Mushroom Proprietary Blend 300 mg: Reishi (ganoderma lucidum), Poria Cocos, Cordyceps (cordyceps sinensis), Tremella Fuciformis, Umbellatus (polyporus umbellatus), Coriolus (coriolus versicolor), Maitake (grifola frondosa), Shitake (lentinula edodes), Wood Ear (auricularia auricula), Hericium Erinaceus • Inositol 50 mg • Choline (as bitartrate) 50 mg • PABA (para-aminobenzoic acid) 50 mg • N-Acetyl Cysteine 50 mg • Saw Palmetto berry extract 50 mg • Glucosamine Sulfate 50 mg • Hesperidin complex 50 mg • Taurine 50 mg • Beta-1,3-Glucan (from purified yeast) 6 mg • Co-Enzyme Q-10 5 mg • Boron (as boric acid) 2 mg. Other Ingredients: Gelatin, Cellulose, Silica, Magnesium Stearate.

Women's Mood-Enhancer **-** HerbaSway
St. John's Wort • Dong Quai • Rehmannia • Schisandra • Coptis • Ginkgo biloba • Cassia tora • Astragalus • Blackberry • HerbaSwee (Cucurbitaceae fruit).

Women's Nutritional System **-** Rainbow Light
Six tablets contain: Beta Carotene 10000 IU • Vitamin D 400 IU • Vitamin E natural 120 IU • Vitamin K 30 mcg • Thiamin (Vitamin B1) 36 mg • Riboflavin (Vitamin B2) 41 mg • Niacinamide 80 mg • Pantothenic Acid 80 mg • Pyridoxine (Vitamin B6) 48 mg • Folic Acid 800 mcg • Biotin (d-Biotin) 300 mcg • Cyanocobalamin (Vitamin B12) 144 mcg • Vitamin C 500 mg • Calcium (Amino Acid Chelate, Citrate) 200 mg • Magnesium (Amino Acid Chelate, Ascorbate, Oxide) 400 mg • Potassium (Aspartate, Chloride) 99 mg • Manganese (Amino Acid Chelate) 2.5 mg • Iron (Amino Chelate) 22.5 mg • Zinc (Picolinate) 15 mg • Copper (Amino Acid Chelate) 1 mg • GTF Chromium (Polynicotinate) 30 mcg • Selenium (l-Selenomethionine) 40 mcg • Iodine (Kelp) 150 mcg • Molybdenum (Aspartate) 50 mcg • Choline (Bitartrate) 40 mg • Inositol 40 mg • PABA (Para Aminobenzioc Acid) 30 mg • Octacosanol (Spinach) 300 mcg • Black Currant (seed) 30 mg • Bioflavonoids 250 mg • Rutin 20 mg • L-Tyrosine 20 mg • Hesperidin Complex 15 mg • Protease 3600 HUT • Amylase 282 DU • Lipase 3 LU • Cellulase 3.2 CU. Superfood & Herbal Ingredients: Bee Pollen • Spirulina • Lemon juice powder • Wheatgrass • Dong Quai • Barley Grass • Echinacea agustifolia • Reishi (Ling Chi) • Rosemary oil • Blue Cohosh 4:1) 530 mg. Custom

Herbal extracts: Vitex • Red Raspberry • Mulberry • Fo-Ti • Bladderwrack • Tumeric • Peony Cistanche • Cynomorium 270 mg.

Women's PM Multi **-** Clinician's Choice
Two tablets contain: Vitamin A (retinyl acetate & 20% as beta-carotene) 1250 IU • Vitamin C (ascorbic acid) 250 mg • Vitamin D (cholecalciferol) 60 IU • Vitamin E (dl-alpha tocopheryl acetate) 150 IU • Thiamin (mononitrate) 0.5 mg • Riboflavin 0.7 mg • Niacin (niacinamide) 10 mg • Folate (folic acid) 200 mcg • Vitamin B12 (cyanocobalamin) 2 mcg • Biotin 150 mcg • Pantothenic Acid (d-calcium pantothenate) 5 mg • Calcium (amino acid chelate, aspartate, citrate, gluconate) 16 mg • Iron (glycinate) 6 mg • Iodine (potassium iodide) 76 mcg • Magnesium (oxide, amino acid chelate) 20 mg • Potassium (chloride, amino acid chelate, gluconate) 16 mg • Zinc (oxide, amino acid chelate, gluconate) 12 mg • Selenium (selenomethionine) 100 mcg • Copper (amino acid chelate) 1 mg • Manganese (amino acid chelate) 1 mg • Chromium (nicotinate, picolinate, chelavite, amino acid chelate) 10 mcg • Molybdenum (amino acid chelate) 2 mcg • RoseOx (patented, standardized process for an extract of Rosemary) 50 mg • Citrus Bioflavonoid Complex 10 mg • Chamomile Flower 10 mg • Passion Flower 10 mg • Valerian Root 10 mg • Mint Leaves 10 mg • Dong Quai 10 mg • Wild Yam 10 mg • Black Currant 10 mg • Red Raspberry Leaf 10 mg • Hesperidin 4 mg • Proprietary Blend 10 mg: Isoflavones, Echinacea, Milk Thistle Fruit, Cruciferex, Grape Powder.

Women's Prime Multi **-** Swanson
Each tablet contains: Vitamin A (as beta-carotene) 3000 IU • Vitamin C (as ascorbic acid) 100 mg • Vitamin D (as cholecalciferol) 60 IU • Vitamin E (as d-alpha tocopheryl succinate) 60 IU • Thiamin USP (as thiamin HCl; Vitamin B-1) 5 mg • Riboflavin USP (Vitamin B-2) 5 mg • Niacin (as niacinamide) 5 mg • Vitamin B-6 (as pyridoxine HCl) 5 mg • Folic Acid 200 mcg • Vitamin B-12 (as cyanocobalamin) 50 mcg • Biotin 5 mcg • Pantothenic Acid (as d-calcium pantothenate) 5 mg • Calcium (50 mg from calcium citrate, 12 mg from calcium glucarate, 4 mg from calcium phytate) 66 mg • Iron (from Albion amino acid chelate) 5 mg • Iodine (from kelp) 50 mcg • Magnesium (from magnesium oxide) 30 mg • Zinc (from Albion® amino acid chelate) 7.5 mg • Selenium (from Albion amino acid chelate) 100 mcg • Manganese (from Albion® amino acid chelate) 2 mg • Chromium (from Albion amino acid chelate) 25 mcg • Dong Quai powder 50 mg • Green Tea powder 50 mg • Soy powder 50 mg • IP-6 (inositol hexaphosphate)-(from calcium phytate) 25 mg • Korean Ginseng powder (5% ginsenosides) 15 mg • Black Cohosh (2.5% triterpenoids) 10 mg • Choline (as choline bitartrate) 10 mg • GLA (gamma-linolenic acid from borage) 10 mg • Inositol 10 mg • Bilberry powder (25% anthocyanidins) 5 mg • Ginkgo Biloba leaf extract (24% flavon glycosides, 6% terpene lactones) 5 mg • PABA (para-aminobenzoic acid) 5 mg • Rutin (from buckwheat) 5 mg • Coenzyme Q10 2 mg • Boron 1 mg.

Women's Stress System **-** Rainbow Light
Two tablets contain: Vitamin A (Beta Carotene) 250 IU • Vitamin E (d-Alpa Tocopheryl Acetate) 30 IU • Vitamin C (Ascorbic Acid) 120 mg • Magnesium (Citrate) 60 mg • Potassium (Chloride) 40 mg • Niacin-Niacinamide (Vitamin B3) 40 mg • Pantothenic Acid (Vitamin B5) 20 mg • Pyridoxine (Vitamin B6) 10 mg • Zinc (Glycinate) 8 mg • Riboflavin (Vitamin B2) 3 mg • Thiamin (Vitamin B1) 3 mcg • Copper (Glycinate) 750 mcg • Folic Acid 400 mcg • Biotin 300 mcg • Cyanocobalamin (Vitamin B12) 12 mcg • Soy extract 150 mg • Hawaiian Spirulina 70 mg • standardized to 1.5% Isoflavonoids Citrus Bioflavonoids 50 mg • Wheat Grass 80 mg • 4:1 Custom Herbal extracts containing 302 mg: [Siberian Ginseng (Eleuthero root), St. John's Wort herb, Kava root, Codonopsis root, Vitex berry, Lavender oil]. Other Nutritional Ingredients: L-Glutamine 50 mg, L-Taurine 20 mg, Alpha-Lipoic Acid 25 mg, L-Methionine 15 mg, L-Tyrosine 25 mg.

Women's Support Formula **-** PhysioLogics
Each capsule contains: Vitamin E (as d-alpha tocopheryl acetate) 50 IU • Vitamin B6 (as pyridoxine HCl) 25 mg • Folic Acid 200 mcg • Magnesium (as magnesium oxide) 100 mg • Zinc (as zinc amino acid chelate) 3.75 mg • Copper (as copper amino acid chelate) 0.5 mg • Black Cohosh root (cimicifuga racemosa) 100 mg • Chastetree fruit (vitex agnus-castus, standardized to contain 5% flavonoids, 5 mg) 100 mg • Dong Quai root (angelica sinensis, standardized to contain 1% ligustilides) 100 mg • Soy Isoflavones 50 mg • Kava Kava root (piper methysticum, standardized to conatin 30% kavalactones, 7.5 mg) 25 mg. Other Ingredients: Rice Powder, Gelatin, Vegetable Magnesium Stearate, Silica.

XanGo Juice **-** XanGo Corp
Garcinia Mangostana (reconstituted juice from whole fruit) • Apple juice concentrate • Pear juice concentrate • Grape juice concentrate • Pear puree • Blueberry juice concentrate • Raspberry juice concentrate • Strawberry juice concentrate • Cranberry juice concentrate • Cherry juice concentrate • Citric Acid • Natural Flavor • Pectin • Xanthan Gum • Sodium Benzoate • Potassium Sorbate.

Xantrex ThermoGenics Plus Rapid Weight Loss for Men **-** SilverSage
Two capsules contain: Niacin 50 mg • Proprietary Xantrex Blend 1243.5 mg: Yerba Mate bark standardized extract (SE), Caffeine, Guarana seed SE, Damiana leaf/stem SE, Schizonepeta Spica SE, Green Tea leaf SE, Piper Nigrum fruit SE, Tibetan Ginseng root SE, Panax Ginseng root SE, Maca herb SE, Cocoa bean SE, Tribulus Terrestris root SE, Kola Nut SE, Thea Sinensis leaf complex, NADH. Other Ingredients: Rice Flour.

Xantrex ThermoGenics Plus Rapid Weight Loss for Women **-** SilverSage
Two capsules contain: Niacin 50 mg • Proprietary Xantrex Blend 1243.5 mg: Yerba Mate bark standardized extract (SE), Caffeine, Guarana seed SE, Damiana leaf/stem SE, Schizonepeta spica SE, Green Tea leaf SE, Piper Nigrum fruit SE, Tibetan Ginseng root SE, Panax Ginseng root SE, Vitex Agnus Castus fruit SE, Hawthorne berry SE, Sodium Bicarbonate, Kola nut SE, Thea Sinensis leaf complex, NADH. Other Ingredients: Rice Flour.

Xcel Patch **-** Unknown
L-Arginine • Nettle leaf • Cayenne • Muira Puama • Orchic substance • Oyster meat • Tribulus • Zinc • Sarsaparilla • Astragalus • Licorice root • Pumpkin seed • Boron • Pygeum • Maca • Horny Goat Weed • Oat straw • Catuaba.

Xenadrine EFX **-** Cytodyne Technologies
Two capsules contain: Vitamin C 100 mg • Vitamin B6 10 mg • Pantothenic Acid 12 mg • Magnesium 10 mg • Proprietary Thermodyne Complex 1415 mg: Tyroplex proprietary blend of L-Tyrosine and Acetyl L-Tyrosine, Green Tea extract (standardized for EGCG and caffeine), Seropro propreitary Cocoa extract (standardized for phenylethylamine, tyramine and theobromine), Yerba Mate (standardized for caffeine), DL-Methionine, Ginger root (standardized for gingerols), Isotherm proprietary blend of Quercetin and Fisetin, Bitter Orange (standardized for synephrine), DMAE (2-diemthylaminoethanol), Grape Seed extract.
See Editor's Note No. 40, page 2058.

Xenadrine NRG **-** Cytodyne Technologies
Two tablets contain: Vitamin B12 188 mcg • Norambrolide 37.5 mg • Proprietary Thermoxanthin Blend 454 mg: L-Tyrosine, L-Theanine, Yerba Mate leaf, Guarana seed, Cocoa seed, Green Tea leaf, Green Coffee bean extract, infused with natural Caffeine. Other Ingredients: Calcium Phosphate, Cellulose, Sorbitol, Gamma Cyclodextrin, Cephalins, Xanthan, Inulin, Magnesium Stearate, Natural Protective Coating.

Xenadrine RFA-1 **-** Cytodyne Technologies
Two capsules contain: Citrus Aurantium peel (bitter orange, standardized for 4% synephrine) 125 mg • Ma Huang (standardized for 6% ephedrine) 335 mg • Guarana extract (standardized for 22% caffeine) 910 mg • White Willow bark extract (standardized for 15% salicin) 105 mg • Acetyl L-Carnitine 100 mg • L-Tyrosine 80 mg • Ginger root 50 mg • Vitamin B5 (pantothenic acid) 40 mg.
See Editor's Note No. 30, page 2056.

Xomatropin hGH Spray **-** ASN - Advanced Sports Nutrition
Each two part formula contains: Part One: Secreatagoges • GH & IGF-1 Peptides. Part Two: Anti-Soatosatin called Revosatin (a power suppressor of an antagonistic hormone called somatosatin responsible for what is called the negative feedback loop for GH).

XTEND-LIFE Neurological Formula **-** Xtend-Life Nutraceuticals Inc.
Six tablets contain: 5-HTP (5-hydroxytryptophan) 50 mg • Alpha Lipoic Acid 200 mg • Betaine HCl 100 mg • Choline Bitartrate 100 mg • DMAE (dimethylaminoethanol) 275 mg • Huperzine A 300 mcg • Phosphatidyl Choline (as lecithin) 160 mg • Phosphatidyl Serine (phosphatidyl-L-serine) 100 mg • Quercetin 50 mg • Resveratrol 30 mg • SAMe (S-adenosylmethionine) 100 mg • Vinpocetine 15 mg • Acetyl L-Carnitine 150 mg • D-Phenylalanine 80 mg • L-Carnosine 150 mg • L-Carnitine Tartrate 150 mg • L-Glutamine 50 mg • L-Histidine 50 mg • L-Taurine 50 mg • L-Threonine 20 mg • L-Tyrosine 100 mg • L-Valine 50 mg • Amylase 50 mg • Bromelain 50 mg • Biotin 2 mg • Folic Acid 600 mcg • Inositol Hexaphosphate 75 mg • Piperine 10 mg • Selenium 500 mcg • Vitamin B6 20 mg • Vitamin D (D3, as cholecalciferol) 400 IU • Bacopin 50 mg • Bilberry 50 mg • Blueberry 50 mg • Chamomile 50 mg • Dandelion root 100 mg • Ginkgo Biloba 100 mg • Gotu Kola 50 mg • Green Tea 100 mg • Hawthorn berry 50 mg • Hops 60 mg • Passion Flower 50 mg • Pomegranate 80 mg • Grape seed 100 mg • Rhodiola Rosea 100 mg • Rosemary 50 mg • Schizandra 50 mg • Siberian Ginseng 50 mg • Silymarin (milk thistle) 100 mg • Yucca root 50 mg.

XTEND-LIFE Prostate **-** Xtend-Life Nutraceuticals Inc.
Each capsule contains: Saw Palmetto extract 160 mg • Pygeum extract 50 mg • Pumpkin Seed extract 40 mg.

XTEND-LIFE Total Balance **-** Xtend-Life Nutraceuticals Inc.
Each tablet contains: Amino Acid Blend: L-Arginine, Aspartic Acid, L-Glutamic Acid, L-Lysine, Glycine, Tryptophan, L-Phenylalanine, L-Serine, L-Methionine, L-Leucine, L-Isoleucine, L-Alanine, L-Proline, L-Threonine, L-Histidine 200 mg • N-Acetyl L-Tyrosine 20 mg •L-Carnitine 20 mg •L-Glutathione 20 mg •N-Acetyl Cysteine 20 mg •L-Taurine 20 mg • Bromelain 2000 GUI 10 mg •Lipase 10 mg •Catalase 10 mg •Betaine HCl 10 mg • Citrus Bioflavonoids 30 mg •Hesperidin 10 mg •Quercetin 10 mg •Trimethylglycine 15 mg •Inositol 20 mg • N-Acetyl Glucosamine 20 mg •Chondroitin Sulfate 20 mg •MSM (Methyl Sulfonyl Methane) 20 mg •DMAE (Bitartrate) 20 mg •Lutein 2 mg •Lycopene 2 mg •Alpha-Lipoic Acid 10 mg • Rutin 10 mg •Phosphatidyl Choline 25 mg •Choline (Bitartrate) 25 mg •Octacosanol 5 mg •1,3-Beta Glucan 10 mg •Hawthorne berry extract 25 mg • Grape Seed extract 25 mg •Ginkgo Biloba 40 mg •Bilberry extract 20 mg •Whole Leaf Aloe Vera extract 20 mg •Turmeric extract 20 mg •Green Tea extract 60 mg •Silymarin (Milk Thistle Seed extract) 20 mg •Ginger root extract 25 mg • Barley Grass Juice powder 80 mg •Artichoke powder 50 mg •Green Oat Juice powder 50 mg •Beet Juice powder 50 mg •Vitamin A (Beta Carotene) 2500 IU • Vitamin A (Palmitate) 1000 IU •Vitamin B-1 (Thiamin Nitrate) 2 mg • Vitamin B-2 (Riboflavin) 2 mg •Vitamin B-3 (Niacinamide) 12 mg •Vitamin B-5 (d-Pantothenate) 12 mg •Vitamin B-6 (Pyridoxine HCl) 6 mg •Vitamin B-12 (Cyanocobalamin) 24 mcg •Biotin 100 mcg •Folic Acid 200 mcg • Vitamin C 20 mg •Vitamin D (Cholecalciferol) 100 IU •Vitamin E (d-Alpha Tocopheryl) 25 mg •Vitamin K (Phytonadione) 20 mcg •PABA 10 mg •Boron (Chelate) 1 mg • Calcium (Citrate) 50 mg •Chromium (Polynicotinate) 120 mcg •Copper (Gluconate) 150 mcg •Iodine (from Kelp) 50 mcg • Magnesium (Aspartate) 50 mg •Manganese (Chelate) 1.5 mg •Molybdenum 75 mcg •Potassium (Aspartate) 20 mg • Selenium 70 mcg •Vanadium 25 mcg •Zinc (Gluconate) 10 mg. Other Ingredients: Cellulose Powder, Hydroxypropylcellulose, Magnesium Stearate, Silicon Dioxide.
See Editor's Note No. 15, page 2055.

Xtra Advantage Creatine Serum **-** Muscle Marketing USA
Each 5 mL serving contains: Creatine Monohydrate • Glucosamine • L-Glutamine • L-Taurine • L-Carnitine • Magnesium • Zinc • Calcium • Vitamin B12 • Royal Jelly • Ginseng • Honey • Natural Glycerine • Natural Flavor • Distilled Water.

Xtra Fuel **-** TwinLab
Three capsules contain: Guarana extract (standardized for 22% Caffeine) 910 mg • Citrus aurantium extract (Bitter Orange peel standardized for 4% Synephrine) 325 mg • L-Tyrosine 500 mg • Vitamin C 250 mg • Vitamin B6 10 mg • Ginkgo Biloba extract (standardized for 24% flavonoid glycoside) 60 mg • DMAE (2-Dimethylaminoethanol) 100 mg • Vitamin B5 (Pantothenic Acid) 100 mg.
See Editor's Note No. 40, page 2058.

Xtra Strength 5HTP **-** Pro Health
Each capsule contains: 5HTP (5-hydroxy-l-tryptophan, from griffonia seed) 200 mg. Other Ingredients: Gelatin, Rice Flour, Magnesium Trisilicate, Magnesium Stearate.

Xtra-Mineral **-** The Herbalist
Yellow Dock root • Red Raspberry leaf • Nettles leaf • Dandelion root.

Xtreme Cut with Super CitriMax **-** Vitamin World
Two capsules contain: Chromium (as chromium polynicotinate) 120 mcg • (-) Hydroxycitric Acid (HCA, provided by 1500 mg of Super CitriMax Plus brand from garcinia cambogia rind) 825 mg • Guarana bark extract (paullinia cupana, standardized to contain 36% caffeine) 430 mg • Kola Nut seed extract (cola acuminata, standardized to contain 10% caffeine) 320 mg • Gymnema leaf (gymnema sylvestre, standardized to contain 25% gymnemic acid) 120 mg • Black Tea leaf extract (camellia sinensis, stnadardized to contain 60% polyphenols and 15% EGCG) 100 mg • Green Tea leaf extract (camellia sinensis, standardized to contain 90% polyphenols, 45% EGCG and 70% catechins) 100 mg • Caffeine (from guarana, kola nut and tea extracts) 200 mg • Alpha Lipoic Acid 30 mg • L-Carnitine (as carnitine fumarate) 20 mg. Other Ingredients: Gelatin, Vegetable Magnesium Stearate, Silica.

Xtreme Trim **-** Puritan's Pride
Two capsules contain: Pantothenic Acid (as d-calcium pantothenate) 10 mg • Citrus Aurantium extract fruit (standardized for 4% synephrine) 125 mg • Ma Huang extract (Ephedra sinica) leaf (standardized for 6% ephedrine) 335 mg • Guarana extract (Paullinia cupana) seed (standardized for 22% caffeine) 910 mg • White Willow extract (Salix alba) bark (standardized for 15% silicin) 105 mg • Acetyl-L-Carnitine Hydrochloride 50 mg • L-Tyrosine 40 mg • Ginger (zingiber officinale) root 25 mg.
See Editor's Note No. 30, page 2056.

Xtreme Trim Ephedra Free **-** Puritan's Pride
Two capsules contain: Vitamin C (as ascorbic acid) 100 mg • Vitamin B6 (as pyridoxine hydrochloride) 10 mg • Pantothenic Acid (as d-calcium pantothenate) 12 mg • Magnesium (as magnesium oxide) 10 mg • Xtreme Trim Thermo Complex 1415 mg: Yerba Mate leaf extract (standardized for methylxanthines (caffeine)), Green Tea leaf extract (camellia sinensis, standardized for epigallocatechin gallate, caffeine, polyphenols), Metabromine Cocoa extract (standardized for theobromine, caffeine), Bitter Orange fruit extract (citrus aurantium, standardized for synephrine, n-methyltyramine, hordenine, octopamine, tyramine), Tyrosine Complex (l-tyrosine, acetyl l-tyrosine), L-Methionine, Ginger root extract (zingiber officinale), Grape seed extract, Flavone complex (proprietary blend of 3, 3', 4', 5-7-pentahydroxyflavone, 3, 3', 4', 7 tetrahydroxyflavone), DMAE (dimethylaminoethanol). Other Ingredients: Gelatin, Vegetable Magnesium Stearate, Silica.
See Editor's Note No. 40, page 2058.

Xtreme Trim Phase 2 White Kidney Bean Extract **-** Vitamin World
Each tablet contains: Calcium (as dicalcium phosphate) 182 mg • Phase 2 Brand Phaseolus Vulgaris (from white kidney bean extract) 1000 mg. Other Ingredients: Cellulose (plant origin), Croscarmellose,

Vegetable Stearic Acid, Silica, Cellulose Coating, Vegetable Magnesium Stearate.

Xzite Female Sexual Enhancement **-** BJH Laboratories
Each capsule contains: Proprietary Xzite Blend 500 mg: Ligusticom Wallichi 166 mg, Acanthopanax 166 mg, Chrysanthemum 168 mg. Other Ingredients: Rice Protein, Magnesium Stearate (vegetable), Gelatin (capsule).

Yam Extract Plus 30 **-** Atrium Inc.
Each capsule contains: Mexican Yam extract 500 mg • Adrenal Substance (freeze dried) 200 mg.
See Editor's Note No. 14, page 2055.

Yam Extract Plus 30 **-** Aspen Group, Inc.
Each capsule contains: Mexican Yam extract 500 mg • Adrenal substance (freeze dried) 200 mg.
See Editor's Note No. 14, page 2055.

Yamoa Powder **-** Yamoapowder.com
Each capsule contains: Funtumia Elastica Gum Tree powdered bark 500 mg. Other Ingredients: Magnesium Stearate 10 mg.

Yarrow-Pipsissewa Virtue **-** Blessed Herbs
Echinacea Angustifolia root • Yarrow flower • Pipsissewa • Oregon Grape root • Corn Silk • Kava Kava root • Hydrangea root • Grain alcohol & Distilled Water.

Yeast Fighters **-** TwinLab
Five hard gelatin capsules contain: High Potency Freeze Dried Lactobacillus Acidophilus (milk free, supplying 2.5 billion viable cells) 1000 mg • Concentrated Odorless Garlic extract powder (equivalent to 1500 mg of fresh garlic) 100 mg • Natural Caprylic Acid 100 mg • Biotin 900 mcg • Fiber Blend 3000 mg: Psyllium seed husks, Guar Gum, Apple Pectin. Base: Pau d'Arco, Onion, Black Walnut, Echinacea, Golden Seal root.

Yeast Formula **-** PhytoPharmica
Two softgel capsules contain: Goldenseal root and rhizome extract (hydrastis canadensis, standardized to contain 5% total alkaloids including berberine, hydrastine and canadine) 100 mg • Oregano oil of aerial part extract (origanum vulgare) 0.2 mL • Peppermint oil of leaf extract (mentha x piperita) 0.2 mL • Thyme oil of leaf and stem extract (thymus vulgaris) 0.1 mL.

Yeast Raiders **-** Puritan's Pride
Five capsules contain: Vitamin C 60 mg • Biotin 900 mcg • Zinc 10 mg • Selenium 50 mcg • Freeze Dried Lactobacillus Acidophilus 1,000 mg • Concentrated Odorless Garlic extract (equivalent to 1,500 mg of fresh Garlic) 100 mg • Natural Caprylic Acid 100 mg • Fiber Blend: Psyllium seed husks (Plantago ovata), Guar Gum, Apple Pectin 3,000 mg • Barberry (Berberis vulgaris) root 100 mg • Ginger (Zingiber officinale) root 10 mg • Thyme (Thymus vulgaris) herb 10 mg • Cinnamon bark (cinnamomum verum) 10 mg • Proprietary Blend 50 mg: Pau D'Arco, Onion powder, Black Walnut, Echinacea, Goldenseal root.

Yellow Dock **-** Nature's Way
Two capsules contain: Yellow Dock root 1 g. Other Ingredients: Gelatin.

Yellow Swarm **-** NVE Pharmaceuticals
Each capsule contains: Proprietary Blend 261 mg: Ephedra extract (leaves, stems, 25 mg ephedrine group alkaloids), Capsicum Annum (whole pepper), Kola Nut (seeds, <1 mg caffeine group alkaloids), Ginseng (root) • Caffeine (anhydrous) 300 mg • Other Ingredients: Gelatin, Dextrose, Stearic Acid, Magnesium Stearate, Titanium Dioxide, FD&C Red #40, FD&C Blue #1, FD&C Yellow #5, FD&C Yellow #6.
See Editor's Note No. 30, page 2056.

Yerba Manza-Eyebright Virtue **-** Blessed Herbs
Yerba Manza root • Yerba Santa leaf • Usnea lichen • Osha root • Eyebright • Propolis • Goldenseal root • Myrrh Gum • Licorice root • Grain alcohol & Distilled Water.

Yerba Santa-Echinacea Virtue **-** Blessed Herbs
Yerba Santa leaf • Osha root • Usnea lichen • Lomatium root • Pau d'Arco bark • Echinacea Angustifolia root • Goldenseal root • Myrrh Gum • Shitake mycelium • Propolis • Licorice root • Grain alcohol & Distilled Water.

Y-Factors **-** Advocare International
Three capsules contain: Niacin 25 mg • Zinc (as monomethionine OptiZinc) 7.5 mg • Proprietary Blend a-MPC 1130 mg: Yohimbe extract (bark - pausinystalia yohimbe), Saw Palmettto extract (berry - serenoa repens), Pygeum extract (bark - pygeum africanum) • Ginkgo extract (leaf - ginkgo biloba) 120 mg • Cranberry extract (fruit - vaccinium macrocarpon) 100 mg • Swedish Flower pollen extract (cernitin - secale cereal) 100 mg • American Ginseng extract (root - panax quinquefolius) 15 mg. Other Ingredients: Cellulose, Silicon Dioxide, Magnesium Stearate, Gelatin.

Yin-Yang Athletic Tone **-** Flora, Inc.
Chinese Red Ginseng • American Ginseng • Astragalus • Reishi Mushroom • Schisandra • Panax Notoginseng • He Shou Wu • Codonopsis • Lycii berries • Licorice • Rehmania • Du Zhong • Prince Ginseng • Dodder Seed • Asparagus root.

Yin-Yang Beautiful Lady **-** Flora, Inc.
Peony • Schisandra • Lycii berries • Licorice • He Shou Wu • Asparagus root • Noto Ginseng • Dang Gui • Codonopsis • Atractylodes • Poria.

Yin-Yang Crystal Clear Vision **-** Flora, Inc.
Rehmania • Dodder Seed • Lycii berries • Chrysanthemum • He Shou Wu • Poria • Ligusticum • Acorus • Plantago Seeds.

Yin-Yang Golden Passage **-** Flora, Inc.
Curculigo • Epimedii • Morinda root • Dang Gui • Phellodendron bark • Anemarrhena • Schisandra • Lycii berries • He Shou Wu • Licorice.

Yin-Yang Premenstrual Harmony **-** Flora, Inc.
Bupleurum • Dang Gui • Peony • Poria • Atractylodes • Ginger • Licorice • Peppermint • Peony root bark • Cyperus berries • Ligusticum • Citrus Peel.

Yin-Yang Secret of Longevity **-** Flora, Inc.
Chinese Red Ginseng • Astragalus • Noto Ginseng • Reishi Mushroom • Dang gui • Lycii berries • Asparagus root • Licorice • Poria • Prince Ginseng • Rehmania • Ligustrum Fruit • Schisandra • He Shou Wu.

Yin-Yang Tranquil Spirit **-** Flora, Inc.
Zizyphus Jujube seed • Poria • Biota Seed • Anemarrhena • Licorice • Schisandra • Dang Gui.

Yogurt-covered Soynuts - Revival **-** Physicians Laboratories
Each 1/6 Cup Contains: Certified Isoflavone 10 mg. Ingredients: Yogurt Coating (sugar, palm kernel oil, whey powder, yogurt powder, artificial color, lecithin), Soy Protein (whole roasted soybeans), Vanillin, Soybean Oil, Sucrose, Corn Syrup, Tapioca, Dextrin, Confectioner's Glaze.

YoHIMbe **-** HVL
Two capsules contain: Yohimbe 500 mg (Ultra Strength extract 4:1 equivalent to 2000 mg of Yohimbe) • Cellulose • Gelatin • Silica and Magnesium Stearate (vegetable source).

Yohimbe 1111 Caps **-** Optimum Nutrition
Each capsule contains: Yohimbe bark extract (pausinystalie yohimbe, standardized to 2% yohimbine) 1111 mg. Other Ingredients: Gelatin, Magnesium Stearate.

Yohimbe B-12 **-** Puritan's Pride
Each 1 ml serving contains: Yohimbe extract (Pausinystalia yohimbe) bark (dried weight equivalent) 1,000 mg • Co-Enzyme B-12 (as Dibencozide) 5,000 mcg.

Yohimbe Fuel **-** TwinLab
Yohimbine (the active component in Yohimbe bark) 8 mg.

Young Again **-** Aspen Group, Inc.
Four tablets contain: Vitamin A Palmitate 500,000 IU/GR 8000 IU • Niacinamide 80 mg • Vitamin B6 20 mg • Vitamin C (magnesium ascorbate) 400 mg • Vitamin E (succinate) 100 IU • N-Acetyl Glucosamine 160 mg • L-Proline 360 mg • L-Lysine 320 mg • Glucosamine Sulfate 560 mg • Chondroitin Sulfate 160 mg • N-Acetyl Cysteine 120 mg • Quercetin Powder 80 mg • Grape seed extract (proanthodyn) 30 mg • Zinc (gluconate) 12 mg • Manganese Ascorbate 12 mg • Copper (gluconate) 0.5 mg • Selenomethionine 80 mcg.
See Editor's Note No. 15, page 2055.

YourLife Daily Pak Essential **-** Leiner Health Products
Each packet contains: Biotin 60 mcg • Calcium 498 mg • Chloride 72 mg • Chromium 200 mcg • Copper 2.5 mg • Folic Acid (folate) 400 mcg • Iodine 150 mcg • Iron 8 mg • Magnesium 233 mg • Manganese 7.5 mg • Molybdenum 208 mcg • Niacin (vitamin B3) 40 mg • Pantothenic Acid (vitamin B5) 10 mg • Phosphorus 130 mg • Potassium 80 mg • Riboflavin (vitamin B2) 5.1 mg • Selenium 200 mcg • Thiamin (vitamin B1) 4.5 mg • Vitamin A 7500 IU • Vitamin B12 18 mcg • Vitamin B6 6 mg • Vitamin C 620 mg • Vitamin D 400 IU • Vitamin E 460 IU • Vitamin K 80 mcg • Boron 200 mcg • Citrus Bioflavonoids complex 10 mg • Ginkgo Biloba leaf 25 mg • Grape Seed extract (vitis vinefera) 1 mg • Hesperidin complex 5 mg • Kelp frond powder (macrocystis pyrifera) 5 mg • Lecithin 10 mg • Mixed Carotenoids complex 10 mg • Nickel 6.5 mcg • Siberian Ginseng root powder (eleutherococcus senticosus) 25 mg • Silicon 2 mg • Tin 13 mcg • Tocotrienol complex 5 mg • Trace Mineral complex 10 mg • Vanadium 13 mcg. Other Ingredients: Calcium Carbonate, Glucosamine Sulfate, Glucosamine Hydrochloride, Cellulose, Methylcellulose, Maltodextrin, Silicon Dioxide, Hydroxypropyl Methylcellulose, Polyethylene Glycol 3350, Propylene Glycol, Starch, Crospovidone, Croscarmellose Sodium, Acacia.

YourLife Daily Pak Maximum **-** Leiner Health Products
Each packet contains: Zinc 12.5 mg • Biotin 25 mg • Copper 1.5 mg • Iodine 112.5 mg • Manganese 1.5 mg • Vitamin D 200 IU • Vitamin B12 25 mg • Chromium 425 mcg • Vitamin E (dl-alpha tocopheryl acetate) 900 IU • Pantothenic Acid 25 mg • Iron 4.1 mg • Vitamin C (ascorbic acid) 1200 mg •Selenium 12.5 mcg • Thiamin (vitamin B1) 25 mg • Riboflavin (vitamin B2) 25 mg • Calcium Carbonate 130 mg • Vitamin B6 25 mg • Niacin 25 mg • Magnesium 54.55 mg • Folate 400 mg • Vitamin A 5000 IU • Molybdenum 7.5 mcg • Phosphorus 100 mg • Ginseng 250 mg • Inositol 5 mg • PABA 2.5 mg. Other Ingredients: Dicalcium Phosphate, Gelatin, Glycerin, Cellulose, Hydroxypropyl Methylcellulose, Hydrogenated Vegetable Oil, Magnesium Oxide, Starch, Silicon Dioxide, Stearic Acid, Maltodextrin.

YourLife Daily Pak Men's 50+ **-** Leiner Health Products
Each packet contains: Biotin 60 mcg • Calcium 533 mg • Chloride 90 mg • Chromium 200 mcg • Folate (folic acid) 400 mcg • Iodine 150 mcg • Magnesium 267 mg • Manganese 7.5 mg • Molybdenum 200 mcg • Niacin (vitamin B3) 40 mg • Pantothenic Acid (vitamin B5) 10 mg • Phosphorus 130 mg • Potassium 100 mg • Riboflavin (vitamin B2) 5.1 mg • Selenium 200 mcg • Thiamin (vitamin B1) 4.5 mg • Vitamin A 7500 IU • Vitamin B12 30 mcg • Vitamin B6 6 mg • Vitamin C 120 mg • Vitamin D 400 IU • Vitamin E 460 IU • Vitamin K 10 mcg • Zinc 15 mg • Bilberry 25 mg • Bilberry berry extract (vaccinium myrtillus) 500 mcg • Boron 1 mg • Citrus Bioflavonoids complex 5 mg • DHA (docosahexaenoic acid) 500 mcg • Grape Seed extract (vitis vinifera) 1 mg • Hesperidin 10 mg • Korean Ginseng root extract (panax ginseng) 100 mg • Lecithin 5 mg • Lutein 500 mcg • Mixed Carotenoids complex 1 mg • Nickel 6.5 mg • Saw Palmetto berry extract (serenoa repens) 160 mg • Siberian Ginseng root powder (eleutherococcus senticosus) 25 mg • Silicon 2 mg • Tin 13 mcg • Tocotrienol complex 1 mg • Trace Mineral complex 1 mg • Vanadium 13 mcg. Other Ingredients: Gelatin, Cellulose, Maltodextrin, Olive Oil, Glycerin, Croscarmellose Sodium, Hypromellose, Silicon Dioxide, Talc, Crospovidone, Magnesium Stearate, Acacia, Mineral Oil, Corn Starch, Soy Polysaccharide, Polyethylene Glycol, Dextrose, Methylcellulose, Dextrin, Lecithin, Hydroxypropyl Cellulose, Caramel, Pharmaceutical Glaze, Sodium Carboxymethylcellulose, Polysorbate 80, Yellow 6 Lake, Kelp, Stearic Acid, Red 40 Lake, Sodium Lauryl Sulfate, Blue 1 Lake, Carnauba Wax.

YourLife Daily Pak Women's **-** Leiner Health Products
Each packet contains: Vitamin A (Acetate) 2500 IU • Vitamin A (Beta Carotene) 5000 IU • Vitamin C (Ascorbic Acid) 120 mg • Vitamin D (Ergocalciferol) 200 IU • Vitamin E (dl-Alpha Tocopheryl Acetate) 230 IU • Vitamin K (Phytonadione) 10 mcg • Vitamin B1 (Thiamine Mononitrate) 2 mg • Vitamin B2 (Riboflavin) 3 mg • Niacin (Niacinamide) 20 mg • Vitamin B6 (Pyridoxine HCl) 2 mg • Folate (Folic Acid) 400 mcg • Vitamin B12 (Cyanocobalamin) 3 mcg • Biotin (d-Biotin) 30 mcg • Pantothenic Acid (d-Calcium Pantothenate) 10 mg • Calcium (Oyster Shell, Calcium Carbonate, Calcium Phosphate) 725 mg • Iron (Ferrous Fumarate) 4 mg • Phosphorus (Calcium Phosphate) 50 mg • Iodine (Potassium Iodide) 100 mcg • Magnesium (Magnesium Oxide) 100 mg • Zinc (Zinc Oxide) 20 mg • Selenium (Selenium Amino Acid Chelate) 30 mcg • Copper (Copper Oxide) 3 mg • Manganese (Manganese Sulfate) 4 mg • Chromium (Chromium Amino Acid Chelate) 20 mcg • Molybdenum (Molybdenum Amino Acid Chelate) 25 mcg • Chloride (Potassium Chloride) 36 mg • Evening Primrose oil (Evening Primrose Seed) 500 mg. 7 day iron strip contains: Iron (Ferrous Sulfate) 18 mg. Contains colors: Titanium Dioxide, Yellow 6 Lake, Red 40 Lake, Blue 2 Lake.

YourLife Daily Pak Women's 50+ **-** Leiner Health Products
Each packet contains: Biotin 30 mcg • Calcium 1362 mg • Chloride 36.3 mg • Chromium 25 mcg • Copper 2 mg • Folic Acid (folate) 400 mcg • Iodine 150 mcg • Magnesium 100 mg • Manganese 2.5 mg • Molybdenum 25 mcg • Niacin (vitamin B3) 20 mg • Pantothenic Acid (vitamin B5) 10 mg • Phosphorus 109 mg • Potassium 40 mg • Riboflavin (vitamin B2) 1.7 mg • Selenium 20 mcg • Thiamin (vitamin B1) 1.5 mg • Vitamin A 5000 IU • Vitamin B12 6 mcg • Vitamin B6 2 mg • Vitamin C 560 mg • Vitamin D 400 IU • Vitamin E 430 IU • Vitamin K 25 mcg • Zinc 15 mg • Boron 150 mcg • Deoiled Lecithin bean (glycine max) 25 mg • Devil's Claw root extract (harpogophytum procumbens) 40 mg • Glucosamine Sulfate 500 mg • MSM (methylsulfonylmethane) 200 mg • Nickel 5 mcg • Silicon 2 mg • Vanadium 10 mcg. Other Ingredients: Cellulose, Gelatin, Maltodextrin, Glycerin, Soybean Oil, Croscarmellose Sodium, Silicon Dioxide, Hydroxypropyl Methylcellulose, Talc, Yellow Wax, Magnesium Stearate, Stearic Acid, Glycolate, Dextrin, Crospovidone, Hydroxypropyl Cellulose, Polythylene Glycol 3350, Mannitol, Dextrose, Red 40 • Polysorbate 80, Sodium Carboxymethylcellulose, Resin, Blue 1.

YourLife Energy B-Complex **-** Leiner Health Products
Each tablet contains: Biotin 10 mcg • Folic Acid (folate) 100 mcg • Niacin (vitamin B3) 10 mg • Pantothenic Acid (vitamin B5) 10 mg • Riboflavin (vitamin B2) 10 mg • Thiamin (vitamin B1) 10 mg • Vitamin B12 10 mcg • Vitamin B6 10 mg. Other Ingredients: Calcium Carbonate, Maltodextrin, Hydroxypropyl Methylcellulose, Cellulose, Starch, Para-Aminobenzoic Acid, Croscarmellose Sodium, Sodium Starch Glycolate, Silicon Dioxide, Hydroxypropyl Cellulose, Red 40 Lake, Polyethylene Glycol 3350, Magnesium Stearate, Resin, Polysorbate 80, Titanium Dioxide, Povidone, Pharmaceutical Glaze.

YourLife Energy Daily Pak **-** Leiner Health Products
Each packet contains: Biotin 100 mcg • Folic Acid (folate) 400 mcg • Niacin (vitamin B3) 100 mg • Pantothenic Acid (vitamin B5) 100 mg • Riboflavin (vitamin B2) 100 mg • Thiamin (vitamin B1) 100 mg • Vitamin B12 100 mcg • Vitamin B6 100 mg • American Ginseng root extract (panax quinquefolium) 70 mg • Chinese Panax Ginseng root

extract (panax ginseng) 260 mg • Damiana leaf (turmera diffusa) 2 mg • Fo-Ti root (polygonum multiflorum) 2 mg • Gotu Kola whole plant (centella asiatica) 78 mg • Green Tea leaf extract (camellia sinensis, 50% catechins) 2 mg • Jamaican Ginger root (zingiber officinalis) 2 mg • Korean Ginseng root extract (panax ginseng) 70 mg • Yerba Mate leaf extract (ilex paraguariensis) 575 mg. Other Ingredients: Calcium Carbonate, Cellulose, Maltodextrin, Dicalcium Phosphate, Croscarmellose Sodium, Polyethylene Glycol, Magnesium Stearate, Silicon Dioxide, Hydroxypropyl Cellulose, Hypromellose, Crospovidone, Tricalcium Phosphate, Dextrin, Corn Starch, Wheat Bran, Lecithin, Alfalfa Powder, Brewer's Yeast, Para-Aminobenzoic Acid, Parsley Powder, Watercress, Dextrose, Sodium Carboxymethylcellulose, Polysorbate 80, Sodium Citrate.

YourLife Energy Natural Balance B-100 Complex **-** Leiner Health Products
Each tablet contains: Biotin 100 mcg • Folic Acid (folate) 400 mcg • Niacin (vitamin B3) 100 mg • Pantothenic Acid (vitmain B5) 100 mg • Riboflavin (vitamin B2) 100 mg • Thiamin (vitamin B1) 100 mg • Vitamin B12 100 mcg • Vitamin B6 100 mg. Other Ingredients: Calcium Carbonate, Cellulose, Maltodextrin, Croscarmellose Sodium, Silicon Dioxide, Polyethylene Glycol 3350, Dicalcium Phosphate, Crospovidone, Tricalcium Phosphate.

YourLife Energy Natural Balance B-50 Complex **-** Leiner Health Products
Each tablet contains: Biotin 50 mcg • Folic Acid (folate) 100 mcg • Niacin (vitamin B3) 50 mg • Pantothenic Acid (vitamin B5) 50 mg • Riboflavin (vitamin B2) 50 mg • Thiamin (vitamin B1) 50 mg • Vitamin B12 50 mcg • Vitamin B6 50 mg. Other Ingredients: Calcium Carbonate, Cellulose, Maltodextrin, Croscarmellose Sodium, Sodium Starch Glycolate, Silicon Dioxide, Polyethylene Glycol 3350, Tricalcium Phosphate.

YourLife Immune System Natural Vitamin A **-** Leiner Health Products
Each softgel contains: Vitamin A 8000 IU. Other Ingredients: Vegetable Oil, Gelatin, Glycerin, Fish Liver Oil.

YourLife Immune System Natural Vitamin A & D **-** Leiner Health Products
Each softgel contains: Vitamin A (from cod liver oil) 1250 IU • Vitamin D 135 IU. Other Ingredients: Gelatin, Glycerin, Water.

YourLife Specialty Supplements Natural Beta Carotene **-** Leiner Health Products
Each softgel contains: Vitamin A 25,000 IU. Other Ingredients: Soybean Oil, Gelatin, Glycerin, Vegetable Oil (partially hydrogenated cottonseed, soybean oils), Yellow Beeswax, Carrot Oil.

Youth-Assure **-** Nature's Plus
Two tablets contain: Rapid Release Layer: Melatonin (N-Acetyl-5-Methoxytryptamine) 3 mg. Sustained Release Layer: Pregnenolone pharmaceutical grade 50 mg • DHEA pharmaceutical grade Dehydroepiandrosterone 25 mg • LECI-PS, Phosphatidylserine-rich purified Lecithin concentrate supplying Activated Phosphatides: [Phosphatidylserine (PS) 5 mg, Phosphatidylcholine (PC) 5 mg, Cephalin (Phosphatidylethanolamine) 3 mg, Phosphoinositides 1.5 mg] 25 mg.
See Editor's Note No. 16, page 2055.

YST-RES-Q **-** Nutri-Quest Rx
Two tablets contain: Lacto Bacillus 1 million IU • Caprylic Acid 50 mg • Grapefruit seed extract 100 mg • Garlic 25 mg • Berberis aquifolium 100 mg • Aloe Vera 25 mg • Undecenoic Acid 50 mg.

Yucca-AR Formula **-** Nature's Way
Two capsules contain: Proprietary Formula: Black Cohosh root • Black Walnut hulls • Brigham Tea herb • Burdock root • Cayenne pepper fruit • Hydrangea root • Rosemary herb • Sarsaparilla root • Valerian root • Wild Lettuce leaves • Wild Yam root • Yucca stalk. Other Ingredients: Gelatin.

Yunnan Paiyao **-** Yunnan Paiyao Group
Active Ingredients: San-Qi Ginseng root, Herb of Clarke, Chinese Yam root, Wild Yam root, Geranium aerial parts, Lesser Galangal herb, Ox Gallbladder. Inactive Ingredients: Gelatin, Water, FD&C Red No. 40.

Zaizao **-** Balanceuticals
Each capsule contains: Proprietary Blend 500 mg: Herba Hedyotis Diffusae, Radix Sophorae Tonkinenisis, Radix Astragali Seu Hedysari, Aloe, Garlic, Fructus Chebulae, Fructus Chaenomelis, Radix Ginseng, Radix.

Zallnex Male Formula **-** Nutranex
Two capsules contain: Vitamin B6 (pyridoxine HCl) 3 mg • Magnesium (magnesium aspartate) 8.5 mg • Zinc (zinc aspartate) 1.6 mg • Zallouh root (Ferula harmonis L.) 250 mg • Muira Puama bark (pxchopetalum olecosides L.) 250 mg • Arginine HCl 200 mg • Tribulis terrestris L. fruit 100 mg. Other Ingredients: Gelatin (capsules), Rice Flour.

Zamoreve Female Formula **-** Nutranex
Two capsules contain: Vitamin B6 (pyridoxine HCl) 3 mg • Magnesium (magnesium aspartate) 8.5 mg • Zinc (zinc aspartate) 1.6 mg • Zallouh root (Ferula harmonis L) 200 mg • Tribulis terrestris L. fruit 100 mg • Avena sativa L. fruit 100 mg • Nettle root 100 mg. Other Ingredients: Gelatin (capsules), Rice Flour.

Zand Quietussin **-** Botanical Laboratories
Each 1 tsp serving contains: Chinese Fritillaria bulb • Loquat leaf • Mullein leaf • Platycodon Grandiflorum root • Schisandra fruit • Pinellia rhizome • Peucedanum root • Marshmallow root • Trichosanthes root • Licorice root • Horehound herb • Fritillaria Cirrhosa bulb • Scullcap herb • Coptis rhizome.

Zantrex-3 **-** Zoller Laboratories
Two capsules contain: Niacin (vitamin B3) 50 mg • Zantrex-3 Proprietary Blend 1312 mg: Yerba Mate bark standardized extract (SE), Caffeine, Guarana seed SE, Damiana leaf/stem SE, Schizonepeta Spica SE, Green Tea leaf SE, Piper Nigrum fruit SE, Tibetan Ginseng root SE, Panax Ginseng root SE, Maca root SE, Cocoa Nut SE, Kola Nut SE, Thea Sinensis leaf complex. Other Ingredients: Rice Flour.

ZeaVision **-** ZeaVision, LLC
Each capsule contains: Zeaxanthin 10 mg. Inactive Ingredients: Gelatin, Sodium Laurel Sulfate, Cellulose, Vegetable Stearate, Sucrose, Corn Starch, Sodium Ascorbate, Ascorbyl Palmitate, dl-Alpha-Tocopherol, Titanium Dioxide, FD&C Yellow #6, FD&C Red #3.

Zeel Tablets **-** Heel, Inc.
Each tablet contains: Silicea 6X 3 mg • Arnica Montana, Radix 1X 0.6 mg • Rhus Toxicodendron 1X 0.54 mg • Sulphur 6X 0.54 mg • Sanguinaria Canadensis 3X 0.45 mg • Cartilago Suis 4X 0.3 mg • Embryo Totalis Suis 4X 0.3 mg • Funiculus Umbilicalis Suis 4X 0.3 mg • Placenta Suis 4X 0.3 mg • Dulcamara 2X 0.15 mg • Symphytum Officinale 8X 0.15 mg • Coenzyme A 6X 0.03 mg • Lipoicum Acidum 6X 0.03 mg • Nadidum 6X 0.03 mg • Natrum Oxalaceticum 6X 0.03 mg. Other Ingredients: Lactose Base.
See Editor's Note No. 1, page 2053.

Zenibolin **-** Syntrax Innovations
Each .25 mL contains: 19-Nor (5) Androstenediol • Isotonic Saline • Carboxymethylcellulose • Benzyl Alcohol.

ZenMind **-** NutriCology
Two capsules contain: GABA (gamma-aminobutyric acid) 550 mg • L-Theanine 200 mg. Other Ingredients: Silicon Dioxide, Carbowax.

Zero Gravity Weight Management Formula **-** Garden of Life, Inc.
Three caplets contain: Poten-Zyme Organic Grapefruit extract 1320 mg • Sea Vegetable Blend (45% fucoidans) 600 mg: Ecklonia, Ascophyllum Nodosum, Laminaria Japonica, Macrocystis, Alaria •

BRAND NAMES

Rhododendron Caucasicum extract (40% polyphenols) 450 mg • Rhodiola Rosea extract (3% rosavin) 300 mg • Blueberry leaf extract (20% chlorogenic acid) 150 mg • Magnolia extract (60% magnolol) 30 mg • Poten-Zyme Probiotic blend 2.4 Billion CFU. Other Ingredients: Cellulose, Silicon Dioxide (natural source), Stearates (vegetable source).

Zestra Feminine Arousal Fluid - QualiLife Pharmaceuticals
Borage Seed Oil • Evening Primrose Oil • Angelica Extract • Coleus Extract • Vitamin C • Vitamin E • Natural Fragrances.
See Editor's Note No. 29, page 2056.

Zesty Onion & Garlic Soynuts - Revival - Physicians Laboratories
Each 1/6 Cup Contains: Certified Isoflavone 10 mg. Ingredients: Soy Protein (whole roasted soybeans), Soybean Oil, Dehydrated Onion and Garlic, Salt, Dextrose, Corn Starch, Parsley, Natural Flavor.

Zicam Cold Remedy Nasal Spray - Matrixx Initiatives
Active Ingredients: Zinc (zincum gluconium) 2%. Inactive Ingredients: Benzalkonium Chloride, Glycerine, Hydroxyethylcellulose, Purified Water, Sodium Chloride, Sodium Hydroxide.

Zinaxin - FreeLife International
Each softgel contains: Patented Ginger extract EV.EXT 33 (Zingiber officinale) root 255 mg. Other Ingredients: Soybean oil, Silicon Dioxide, Lecithin, Gelatine, Glycerin, Sorbitol, Water, Natural Chlorophyll Complex, Titanium Dioxide (natural mineral color).

Zinaxin (HMP-33) - Eurovita A/S, Denmark
Each capsule contains: Zingiber Officinale Roscoe Extract (HMP-33 Extract) 255 mg. Recommended dosage is 2 capsules per day, in divided doses with liquid for the first month.

Zinaxin Rapid - Eurovita A/S, Denmark
Each capsule contains: Ginger Extract EV.EXT 77 (255 mg is equivalent to approximately 3000 mg of dried ginger rhizome and 1500 mg of dried galanga rhizome) • Sunflower Seed Oil • Gelatin • Glycerol • Beeswax Yellow • Lecithin • Titanium Dioxide • Copper Chlorophyllins. Recommended dosage is 2 capsules daily. Results should become noticeable within 2-4 weeks.

Zinc - Source Naturals
Each tablet contains: Zinc (from 500 mg of zinc amino acid chelate) 50 mg • Copper (from 3.57 mg of copper sebacate) 500 mcg.

Zinc 10 mg - Jamieson
Each tablet contains: Elemental Zinc 10 mg.

Zinc 10 mg - Chelated - Jamieson
Each tablet contains: Elemental Zinc 10 mg. Chelated (microbound) to Amino Acid from organic Soy to aid in Zinc assimilation.

Zinc 100 mg - GNC A-Z - GNC
Each tablet contains: Zinc (as zinc gluconate) 100 mg. Other Ingredients: Cellulose.

Zinc 25 mg - Jamieson
Each tablet contains: Elemental Zinc (gluconate) 25 mg.

Zinc 30 mg - Nature Made
Each tablet contains: Zinc (from zinc gluconate) 30 mg. Other Ingredients: Dibasic Calcium Phosphate, Magnesium Stearate, Croscarmellose Sodium.
See Editor's Note No. 45, page 2058.

Zinc 50 mg - Jamieson
Each tablet contains: Elemental Zinc (gluconate) 50 mg.

Zinc 50 mg - GNC A-Z - GNC
Each tablet contains: Zinc (as zinc gluconate) 50 mg. Other Ingredients: Cellulose.

Zinc 50 mg - Timed Release - Jamieson
Each tablet contains: Zinc (organic gluconate) 50 mg. Prepared in a special time-diffused micro-encapsulation allowing for a gradual release of Zinc over six to eight hours.

Zinc 50MG - Nature Made
Each tablet contains: Zinc 50 mg.
See Editor's Note No. 45, page 2058.

Zinc 60 mg - Nature Made
Each tablet contains: Zinc (from zinc gluconate) 60 mg. Other Ingredients: Dibasic Calcium Phosphate, Cellulose Gel, Stearic Acid, Magnesium Stearate, Croscarmellose Sodium.
See Editor's Note No. 45, page 2058.

Zinc Chewable - Aspen Group, Inc.
Each tablet contains: Amino Acid Chelated Minerals as Zinc 29 mg • Raw Tissue concentrates (bovine source) from: Spleen 29 mg, Brain 8 mg, Liver 5 mg, Heart 4 mg, Kidney 4 mg, Thymus 2 mg, Adrenal 2 mg, Pituitary 1 mg, Duodenum 1 mg.
See Editor's Note No. 31, page 2056.

Zinc Citrate - Quest
Each tablet contains: Zinc (Citrate) 50 mg. Other Ingredients: Croscarmellose Sodium, Calcium Phosphate, Magnesium Stearate (vegetable source), Microcrystalline Cellulose, Silicon Dioxide, Vegetable Stearin.

Zinc for Acne - Puritan's Pride
Two tablets contain: Vitamin A (as Retinyl Palmitate) 1,000 IU • Vitamin C (as Ascorbic Acid and Rose Hips) 150 mg • Vitamin E (as dl-alpha tocopheryl acetate) 50 IU • Vitamin B6 (Pyridoxine Hydrochloride) 20 mg • Zinc (as Zinc Gluconate) 50 mg.

Zinc Lozenge - Nature's Way
Each lozenge contains: Echinacea Purpurea (stem, leaf, flower) 20 mg • Stevia dried extract 3 mg • Vitamin C (ascorbic acid) 100 mg • Zinc Citrate 23 mg. Other Ingredients: French Vanilla flavor, Fructose, Magnesium stearate, Mannitol, Sodium, Sorbitol, Wild Berry flavor.

Zinc Lozenge - Nutri-Quest Rx
Each lozenge contains: Zinc Gluconate 75 mg.

Zinc Lozenges - Futurebiotics
One lozenge contains: Vitamin C (from ascorbic acid) 60 mg • Zinc (as zinc citrate) 15 mg • Herbal Lozenge Blend, 8 mg: Echinacea leaf powder 4:1 extract, Goldenseal root powder 4:1 extract, Elderberry flower powder, Bee Propolis powder, Peppermint leaf powder, Kava Kava root powder. Other Ingredients: Orange crystals, Orange flavor, Magnesium stearate, Stearic acid, Mannitol, Fructose, Cane sugar.

Zinc Lozenges - Jamieson
Each lozenge contains: Vitamin C (as Ascorbic Acid) 50 mg • Zinc (as Zinc Gluconate) 5 mg. Other Ingredients: Eucalyptus, Anise Oil, Menthol, Camphor, Lemon.

Zinc Lozenges - Nature's Life
Each lozenge contains: Zinc (Gluconate) 10 mg • Vitamin C 100 mg • Beta Carotene (equivalent to 500 IU Vitamin A) 300 mcg • Purple Cone Flower root (Echinacea purpurea) 25 mg. In a natural base of low-Glycemic, pure Crystalline Fructose, pasteurized Honey powder, Hydrogenated Vegetable oil, natural Peppermint flavor, Eucalyptus leaf (Eucalyptus globulus) Licorice root (Glycyrrhiza glabra), Goldenseal root (Hydrastis canadensis), Slippery Elm bark (Ulmus ruba), & Fenugreek seed (Trigonella foenum-graecum).

Zinc Lozenges - Oringinal Formula - Jamieson
Each lozenge contains: Zinc Gluconate 35 mg.

Zinc Lozenges - Vitamin C, Anise, Menthol, Camphor, Eucalyptus - Jamieson
Each lozenge contains: Vitamin C (as Ascorbic Acid) 50 mg • Zinc

BRAND NAMES

(as Zinc Gluconate) 5 mg • In a base of Eucalyptus, Anise Oil, Menthol, Camphor, Lemon.

Zinc Lozenges Cherry with Vitamin C and B-6 **-** Leiner Health Products
Each lozenge contains: Vitamin B6 (Pyridoxine Hydrochloride) 5 mg • Vitamin C 60 mg • Zinc 15 mg • Other Ingredients: Sugar, Zinc Aspartate, Stearic Acid, Sodium Ascorbate, Maltodextrin, Ascorbic Acid, Mono- and Diglycerides, Magnesium Stearate, Silicon Dioxide, Aspartame, Red 40 Lake, Artificial Cherry Flavor, Starch. Phenylketonurics: Contains Phenylalanine.

Zinc Lozenges Plus **-** The Vitamin Shoppe
Each lozenge contains: Zinc 24 mg • Echinacea 100 mg • Vitamin C 150 mg • Propolis 100 mg • Vitamin A 1000 IU • Slippery Elm 25 mg. In a base of Golden Seal, Acerola, Fructose Cellulose, with Vanilla and Orange flavor.

Zinc Lozenges with Echinacea and Vitamin C **-** Jamieson
Each lozenge contains: Elemental Zinc (from Zinc Citrate) 5 mg • Vitamin C (Ascorbic Acid) 50 mg • Echinacea (Derived from 12.5 mg root extract, 1:4 of Echinanea Purpurea) 50 mg • Sorbitol • Fructose • Wild Cherry Flavor.

Zinc Lozenges with Vitamin C **-** GNC
Two lozenges contain: Sodium 10 mg • Vitamin C 120 mg (as Ascorbic Acid and Sodium Ascorbate) • Zinc (as Zinc Oxide, Zinc Gluconate). Ingredients: Sorbitol, Lactitol, Cellulose, Natural Flavors, Peppermint oil, Eucalyptus oil, Anise oil, Sucralose, Camphor.

Zinc Lozenges with Vitamin C - Jamieson **-** Jamieson
Each lozenge contains: Elemental Zinc (from Zinc Citrate) 5 mg • Vitamin C (Ascorbic Acid) 50 mg • Echinacea Root (Echinacea Purpurea) 50 mg • Sorbitol • Fructose.

Zinc Magnesium Aspartate - Substrate Solutions **-** ErgoPharm
Three capsules contain: Zinc (as L-OptiZinc & Aspartate) 30 mg • Magnesium (as Aspartate) 450 mg • Vitamin B6 (Pyridoxine Hydrochloride) 10.5 mg. Other Ingredients: Cellulose, Magnesium Stearate, Gelatin.

Zinc Picolinate 30 mg - GNC A-Z **-** GNC
Each tablet contains: Zinc (as zinc picolinate) 30 mg • Copper (as copper gluconate) 2 mg. Other Ingredients: Dicalcium Phosphate, Cellulose, Food Glaze.

Zinc Plex **-** PhysioLogics
Each capsule contains: Zinc (50% as zinc arginine amino acid chelate, 25% as zinc histidinate amino acid chelate, 25% as zinc glycinate) 30 mg • Copper (53% as copper amino acid chelate, 47% as copper lysine amino acid chelate) 2 mg. Other Ingredients: Rice Powder, Gelatin, Silica, Vegetable Magnesium Stearate.

Zinc Plus **-** Olympian Labs
Each capsule contains: Zinc Chelate 30 mg. In a base of Pumpkin Seeds, Kelp, and Dulse.

ZincEchinacea Drops **-** Quantum, Inc.
Each drop contains: Vitamin A acetate 500 IU • Elemental Zinc (Zinc acetate) 14 mg • Echinacea purpurea extract (4:1) 20 mg • Slippery Elm bark (Ulmus fulva) 20 mg • Bee Propolis extract powder (5:1) 5 mg • Goldenseal 2 mg. Other Ingredients: Sugar, Corn Syrup, Natural and Artificial Flavors.

ZincEchinacea Lozenges **-** Quantum, Inc.
Each lozenge contains: Zinc acetate 14 mg • Vitamin A acetate 500 IU • Slippery Elm bark (Ulmus fulva) 20 mg • Echinacea (4:1) 20 mg • Propolis 5 mg. In a base of Goldenseal, Sugar, Dextrose, Fructose.

ZincEchinacea Pops **-** Quantum, Inc.
Each pop contains: Vitamin A acetate 167 IU • Elemental Zinc (Zinc acetate) 5 mg • Echinacea purpurea extract (4:1) 7 mg • Slippery Elm bark 7 mg • Bee Propolis extract powder (5:1) 2 mg • Goldenseal 1 mg. Other Ingredients: Sugar, Corn Syrup, Natural Flavor.

Zing! **-** Health Center for Better Living
Each capsule contains: Siberian Ginseng Root 106 mg • Ginkgo Biloba Leaf 79 mg • Gota Kola Herb 79 mg • Kola Nut 79 mg • Bee Pollen 53 mg • Foti Root 26 mg • Rehmannia Root 26 mg • Spirulina 26 mg.

Zingiforce **-** New Chapter, Inc.
One softgel contains: Ginger (rhizome), certified organic, supercritical extract (minimum 20% pungent compounds- 20 mg, 4% zingiberene- 4 mg) 100 mg • Rosemary leaf & essential oil, supercritical extract (23% total phenolic antioxidants [TPA] - 1.15 mg) 5 mg. Other Ingredients: Olive Oil - certified organic, Yellow Beeswax, Gelatin, Vegetable Glycerin, Purified Water, Carob.

Zinlori 75 **-** Metagenics
Each tablet contains: Zinc Carnosine 75 mg.

ZMA **-** SNAC Systems, Inc.
Each capsule contains: Zinc (Monomethionine/Asparate) 10 mg • Magnesium (Aspartate) 150 mg • Vitamin B6 3.5 mg.

ZMA - Now Sports **-** Now
Three capsules contain: Vitamin B6 15 mg • Magnesium 450 mg • Zinc 30 mg • ZMA (zinc magnesium aspartate) 2.4 g (2400 mg). Other Ingredients: Gelatin (capsule), Magnesium Stearate.

ZMA for Men **-** Optimum Nutrition
Three capsules contain: Zinc (as monomethionine and aspartate) 30 mg • Magnesium (as aspartate) 450 mg • Vitamin B6 (as pyridoxine HCl) 10.5 mg. Other Ingredients: Rice Powder, Gelatin, Magnesium Stearate.

ZMA for Women **-** Optimum Nutrition
Two capsules contain: Zinc (as monomethionine and aspartate) 30 mg • Magnesium (as aspartate) 450 mg • Vitamin B6 (as pyridoxine HCl) 10.5 mg. Other Ingredients: Rice Powder, Gelatin, Magnesium Stearate.

ZMA Rx-Strength **-** Nature's Plus
Three capsules contain: Vitamin B6 (as Pyridoxine HCl) 0.5 mg • Magnesium (as Aspartate) 450 mg • Zinc (As Aspartate/ Monomethionine) 30 mg • ZMA (Proprietary Anabolic Support Factor) 2424 mg.

Z-Mass PM **-** Cytodyne Technologies
Four capsules contain: Vitamin B6 11 mg • Magnesium 450 mg • Zinc 30 mg • Potassium 10 mg • Proprietary Anabolic Herbal Blend 706 mg: Mucuna Pruriens seeds (standardized for L-dopa), Polypodium Vulgare / Suma (root, standardized for 20-hydroxyecdysone).

ZonePerfect Fish Oil Capsules **-** ZonePerfect
Each capsule contains: Molecularly Distilled Fish oil • Natural Vitamin E 20 IU • EPA 160 mg • DHA 107 mg.

Zotrin (Zotril) for Men **-** Klein-Becker
Two caps contain: Proprietary Blend 847.8 mg: Yerba Mate bark (standardized proprietary extract), Guarana seed (standardized proprietary extract), Damiana leaf and stem, Calcium Phosphate, Microcrystalline Cellulose, Magnesium Stearate, Barberry root and bark, L-Tyrosine, Trimethylglycine • Proprietary Blend 158 mg: Schizonepeta (spica), Yucca plant, Passion flower (aerial parts), Panax ginseng root, Maca root, St. John's Wort.

Zotrin (Zotril) for Women **-** Klein-Becker
Two capsules contain: Proprietary Blend 847.8 mg: Yerba Mate bark (standardized proprietary extract), Guarana seed (standardized proprietary extract), Damiana leaf/stem (standardized proprietary extract), Calcium Phosphate, Microcrystallene Cellulose, Magnesium Stearate, Barberry root/bark SE, L-Tyrosine, Trimethylglycine • Proprietary Blend 158 mg: Rosemary leaf/twig SE, Forsythia fruit,

Sage leaf, Black Cohosh root SE, Chasteberry fruit SE, Shisandra herb, Chlorella, St. John's Wort herb SE. Other Ingredients: Rice Flour.

Z-Plex **-** PharmAssure
One softgel capsule contains: Kava Kava Root Extract (Piper methysticum; 55% Kavalactones=55mg) 100 mg • Griffonia Seed Extract (Griffonia simplicifolia; 20% 5-Hydroxy-L-Tryptophan=10mg) 50 mg • Melatonin (N-Acetyl-5-Methoxytryptamine) 2 mg. Other ingredients: Polyethylene Glycol, Gelatin, Glycerin, Chlorophyll, Titanium Dioxide (Natural Mineral Whitener).
See Edior's Note No. 16.

Zyflamend **-** New Chapter, Inc.
Two softgels contain: Rosemary leaf (100 mg supercritical extract and 50 mg extract, 23% total phenolic antioxidants (TPA)-34.5 mg) 150 mg • Turmeric rhizome (10 mg supercritical extract, 45% turmerones-4.5 mg and 100 mg ethanolic extract (7% curcuminoids-7 mg)) 100 mg • Ginger rhizome (54 mg supercritical extract (30% pungent compounds-16.2 mg, 8% zingiberene-4.3 mg) and 46 mg PSE extract (3% pungent compounds-1.4 mg)) 100 mg • Holy Basil leaf extract (2% ursolic acid-2 mg) 100 mg • Green Tea leaf extract (45% polyphenols-45 mg) 100 mg • Hu Zhang root and rhizome extract (polygonum cuspidatum, 8% resveratrol-6.4 mg) 80 mg • Chinese Goldthread root extract (6% berberine-2.4 mg) 40 mg • Barberry root extract (6% berberine-2.4 mg) 40 mg • Oregano leaf supercritical extract (0.8% TPA-0.32 mg) 40 mg • Scutellaria Baicalensis root extract 5:1 20 mg. Other Ingredients: Olive Oil (certified organic), Yellow Beeswax, Gelatin, Vegetable Glycerin, Purified Water, Carob.

Zyflamend PM **-** New Chapter, Inc.
Two softgels contain: Holy Basil leaf, extract (2% ursolic acid- mg) 150 mg • Melissa leaf, extract (1% essential oil- 0.85 mg) (including neral and geranial) 85 mg • Tumeric (rhizome) extract (7% curcumin-7 mg) 100 mg • Scutellaria baicalensis root, extract 5:1 100 mg • Ginger (rhizome) certified organic (post-ethanolic extract) (3% pungent compunds- 1.5 mg) 50 mg • Ginger, SBSC (rhizome), certified organic (minimum 20% pungent compounds 5 mg, 4% zingiberene-1 mg) 25 mg • Chamomile flower, extract (25% alpha-bisabolol- 12.5 mg) 50 mg • Hops (strobiles) ethanolic extract (1.5% xanthohumol- 0.37 mg) 25 mg • Chamomile flower, extract (3% apigeninglycosides- 0.75 mg) 25 mg • Mexican Valerian and Valerian root, extract 30:1 20 mg. Other Ingredients: Olive oil -certified organic, Yellow Beeswax.

Zygest **-** PhysioLogics
Two capsules contain: Zygest Blend 104 mg: Bromelain (from pineapple) 120 GDU, Papain (from papaya fruit) 600,000 FCCPU, Protease 3.0 (from aspergillus oryzae) 10 SAPU, Amylase (from aspergillus oryzae) 400 DU, Lipase (from aspergillus niger 60 FCCLU, Protease 4.5 (from aspergillus oryzae) 400 HUT, Lactase (from aspergillus oryzae) 20 ALU, Cellulase (from trichoderma longbrachiatum) 10 CU, Hemicellulase (from aspergillus niger) 10 HCU. Other Ingredients: Rice Powder, Gelatin, Vegetable Magnesium Stearate, Silica.

Zyladex Plus **-** Medlabs
Each tablet contains: Proprietary Blend 717 mg: Desert Tea, Guarana extract, Hawthorne berry, Citrin, Choline, White Willow bark, Borage seed, Wild Yam, Couch Grass, Hydrangea, Corn Silk, Bucchu, Alisma, Inositol, L-Methionine, L-Carnitine, Chromium picolinate, L-Tyrosine, Vitamin B12, Whey, Croscarmellos, Silica, Steric Acid, Magnesium stearate.

Zylodrine XP **-** Unknown
Each tablet contains: Chromium Picolinate 50 mcg • Betaine 25 mg • Choline complex 25 mg • Korean Ginseng 100 mg • Metabolism Booster Complex 50 mg: L-Phenylalanine 25 mg, L-Tyrosine 25 mg • Cascara Sagrada 25 mg.

Zymatein **-** Metabolic Nutrition
Each scoop (30 g) contains: Micro-Filtered Whey Protein Concentrate • Vitamin Mineral Matrix • Cocoa • Natural Flavors • Nutrient Stabilizers • Sucralose • Sodium Chloride • Digestive Enzyme Complex: Amylase, Cellulase, Lactase, Lipase, Protease.

Zymax **-** HealthWatchers System
Pancreatin • Papain • Rutin • Bromelain • Pancrelipase • Peppermint • Trypsin • Lipase • Amylase • Lysozyme • Cellulase • Chymotrypsin.
See Editor's Note No. 14, page 2055.

ZymaX A.M. Formula **-** Denman Scientific Research
Two tablets contain: Vitamin E 6 IU • Magnesium (magnesium chelate) 75 mg • Zinc (zinc chelate) 5 mg • Chromium (chromium picolinate) 75 mcg • Proprietary Blend 175 mcg: Evening Primrose Oil (contains gamma linolenic acid), Borage seed oil, Bladderwrack extract (dried fucus vesiculosus), Grape Seed extract, Bioflavonoids, Soya Lecithin, Fatty Acids, Dried Sweet Red Clover extract (mellotus officinalis, tri foliumratense, standardized to contain 50 mg methylxanthines) • Proprietary Blend 100 mg: Bee Pollen, Ginseng root, Ginger root, Lecithin, Bovine complex, Damiana leaf, Sarsaparilla root, Golden Seal aerial part, Nettles leaf, Gotu Kola aerial part, Spirulina Algae, Royal Jelly • Proprietary Blend 500 mg: Ma Huang extract (standardized for 15 mg ephedrine), Guarana extract (standardized for 50 mg caffeine), White Willow Bark extract (standardized for 3 mg salicin).
See Editor's Note No. 30, page 2056.

ZymaX Accelerator Formula **-** Denman Scientific Research
Each capsule contains: Garcinia cambogia 500 mg. Inactive Ingredients: Calcium Carbonate, Calcium Phosphate, Cellulose, Gelatin, Stearic Acid, Croscarmellose, and Magnesium Stearate.

ZymaX P.M. Formula **-** Denman Scientific Research
Each tablet contains: Proprietary Blend 400 mg: Evening Primrose oil (contains gamma linolenic oil), Borage (seed oil), Bladderwrack extract, dried Fucus Vesiculosus extract, Grape Seed extract, Bioflavonoids, Soya Lecithin, Fatty Acids, dried sweet Red Clover extract (standardized to contain flavonglycosides), Griffonia simplicifolia (standardized to contain 20 mg 5-HTP).

Zymitol **-** Generation+
Three vegetable capsules contain: Proprietary Blend 2265 mg: Serrapeptase 45 mg, MSM, Protease, Bromelain, Papain, Amylase, Lipase, Alpha Lipoic Acid, Magnesium Citrate, Rutin.

Zypan **-** Standard Process, Inc.
Each two tablets contain: Proprietary Blend 700 mg: Betaine hydrochloride, Pancreas extract (Cytosol), Pancreatin (3X), Fatty Acid, Pepsin (1:10,000), Ammonium chloride, Bovine Spleen, Ovine Spleen. Other Ingredients: Cellulose, Lactose, Calcium stearate.
See Editor's Note No. 14, page 2055.

Zzz (Lipospray) **-** Advocare International
Each full spray contains: Pyridoxine (as HCl) 20 mg • Zinc (as gluconate) 500 mcg • Vitamin E (as acetate) 1.5 IU • Kava Kava extract (root - piper methysticum) 1.5 mg • Melatonin 1.5 mg • 5-Hydroxytryptophan (from seed - griffonia simplicifolia) 20 mg • Stevia extract (leaf - stevia rebaudiana) 7.4 mg. Other Ingredients: Purified Water, Propylene Glycol, Polysorbate-80, Natural Flavors, Hydroxylated Lecithin, Lactic Acid, Potassium Sorbate (as preservative).

Editor's Note No. 1
This is a homeopathic preparation. Homeopathy is a system of medicine established in the 19th century by a German physician named Samuel Hahnemann. Its basic principles are that "like treats like" and "potentiation through dilution." For example, in homeopathy, diarrhea would be treated with an extreme dilution of a substance that normally causes diarrhea when taken in high doses. Practitioners of homeopathy believe that more dilute preparations are more potent. Many homeopathic preparations are so diluted that they contain little or no active ingredient. Therefore, most homeopathic products are not expected to have any pharmacological effects, drug interactions, or other harmful effects. Any beneficial effects are controversial and cannot be explained by current scientific methods.
Dilutions of 1 to 10 are designated by an "X." So a 1X dilution = 1:10, 3X=1:1000; 6X=1:1,000,000. Dilutions of 1 to 100 are designated by a "C." So a 1C dilution = 1:100; 3C = 1:1,000,000. Dilutions of 24X or 12C or more contain zero molecules of the original active ingredient.
Homeopathic products are permitted for sale in the US due to legislation passed in 1938 sponsored by a homeopathic physician who was also a Senator. The law still requires that the FDA allow the sale of products listed in the Homeopathic Pharmacopeia of the United States. However, homeopathic preparations are not held to the same safety and effectiveness standards as conventional medicines.

Editor's Note No. 2
Product Recall: On January 28, 2002, this product was voluntarily withdrawn from the market. Lab testing by the California Department of Health Services discovered amounts of the prescription drug alprazolam (Xanax) in a sample of the product (3576). Advise patients using this product to discontinue taking it.

Editor's Note No. 3
Product Recall: On February 15, 2002, Health Canada required the withdrawal of this product from the market. Lab testing discovered amounts of a drug similar to sidenafil (Viagra) in a sample of the product (7093). Advise patients using this product to discontinue taking it.

Editor's Note No. 4
The potential risk of transmission of bovine spongiform encephalopathy (BSE, mad cow disease) is raising patients' concerns about products containing chondroitin. Chondroitin is produced from bovine trachea. Although bovine trachea tissue does not seem to carry a high risk of BSE disease infectivity, in some cases manufacturing methods might lead to contamination with other diseased animal tissues. So far there are no reports of BSE, or other disease transmission to humans from dietary supplements containing animal materials and the risk of potential disease transmission is thought to be low. The manufacturer of this product reports taking extensive steps to ensure that their chondroitin is not contaminated.

Editor's Note No. 5
Herbal Ecstacy is no longer being produced under an agreement with the FDA. Global World Media now produces Organic Ecstacy which they claim to be ephedra free. The ingredients of Organic Ecstacy are currently unknown.

Editor's Note No. 6
In April 2000, the Federal Trade Commission filed a complaint against manufacturers of natural or herbal cigarettes for making claims that these products were safer than conventional cigarettes. The labeling on these products in now required to state "Herbal cigarettes are dangerous to your health. They produce tar and carbon monoxide." If they use the term "No additives" they must also state "No additives in our tobacco does NOT mean a safer cigarette."

Editor's Note No. 7
Product Recall: On February 8, 2002, this product was voluntarily withdrawn from the market. Lab testing by the California Department of Health Services discovered amounts of the prescription drug warfarin (Coumadin) in a sample of the product (8010). Advise patients using this product to discontinue taking it. On June 1, 2002, BotanicLab closed operations, following product recalls. The future availability of PC-SPES is unknown (8136).
PC-SPES is a combination product containing eight Chinese herbs that has been available commercially since 1996. It is used therapeutically for prostate cancer. "PC" stands for prostate cancer and "spes" is Latin for hope (5548). So far, studies look promising. Preliminary clinical evidence from several small uncontrolled studies and anecdotal reports show that PC-SPES can benefit patients with both hormone-sensitive and hormone-insensitive or refractory prostate cancers. In both groups of patients, PC-SPES can significantly decrease serum prostate-specific antigen (PSA) levels (5122,5548,6284,6286,6483,7785,7786,11764,11765). In patients with hormone-sensitive prostate cancer, PC-SPES can decrease PSA levels by at least 50% in 78-100% of patients (3577,5548,6483,6484,11764,11765). In 56-80% of patients PSA levels become undetectable after approximately 6 months (3577,6484). PC-SPES also seems to significantly decrease PSA in patients with hormone-insensitive prostate cancer. PSA levels decrease more than 50% in about 50-90% of patients after 6 months of treatment

(3577,6286,6483,6484,7786,11764,11765). This effect rapidly reverses when PC-SPES is discontinued; PSA levels may rise dramatically within 2 to 6 weeks; increases up to 1300% can occur in some patients (5548,8137). PC-SPES also seems to cause clinically significant reductions in serum testosterone (5548,6484), improve quality of life, and reduce pain and analgesic use (6286) in patients with prostate cancer.

There is also some evidence that PC-SPES in combination with conventional hormonal therapy for 5 months can improve quality of life, reduce PSA levels, and reduce pain in patients with metastatic prostate cancer (6286). Although PC-SPES does not contain estrogen, the licorice and Panax-pseudoginseng constituents have estrogenic activity. The saw palmetto constituent also inhibits 5-alpha reductase, an enzyme involved in conversion of testosterone to the more biologically active dihydrotestosterone (5548). Laboratory studies on prostate cancer cell lines show PC-SPES might decrease tumor cell proliferation and might induce apoptosis in both hormone sensitive and insensitive cancer cells, indicating that its estrogenic effects are not the sole mechanism of action (6284,6285,6483,7784). However, PC-SPES seems to reduce tumor cell proliferation more in hormone sensitive prostate cancer (6483). Some retrospective research suggests that PC-SPES might be more effective against androgen-independent prostate cancer in older men and in men with a longer duration of initial antiandrogen therapy (7785). Laboratory studies also suggest that PC-SPES might protect prostate cells from cancer. Licorice seems to have antimutagenic activity (7783). Reduction in pain by PC-SPES could result from the antitumor effect or from some of its components with reported anti-inflammatory and analgesic properties: licorice, reishi mushroom, chrysanthemum, and Panax-pseudoginseng (7784).

The composition of PC-SPES has been inconsistent. Various lots of PC-SPES contain differing amounts of phytoestrogens, licochalcone A (a constituent of licorice), and baicalin (a constituent of Baikal scullcap). PC-SPES may also contain diethylstilbestrol, indomethacin, and warfarin (11763).

Although PC-SPES is generally well-tolerated, some side effects are relatively common. Most side effects can be attributed to the estrogenic effects of PC-SPES, similar to those of diethylstilbestrol (DES) (7784,7785). One of the most common side effects is nipple and breast tenderness and breast enlargement. This seems to occur in up to 90% of patients (3577,6483). Other frequently reported side effects include leg cramps, indigestion, nausea, diarrhea, decreased libido, erectile dysfunction, and hot flashes. Other side effects that might occur are reduction in overall body hair, pitting edema, significant drop in lipoprotein a, hypertriglyceridemia, and venous and pulmonary thrombosis (5122,5548,6287,6483,6484,7785,11764,11765).

There is a lot of concern about the potential for thrombosis formation in patients taking PC-SPES. So far, it seems to occur in about 2-4% of patients (3577,6483). Pulmonary embolus has been reported, leading some practitioners to suggest prophylactic anticoagulation (7785,7787). Since PC-SPES has estrogenic effects, there is also some concern that it might interfere with conventional hormone therapies for prostate cancer if used concurrently. In vitro evidence suggests combination therapy of PC-SPES and paclitaxel decreases the effectiveness of paclitaxel therapy alone, in both androgen-independent and androgen-sensitive prostate carcinoma situations (11482). Because of these risks patients should avoid using PC-SPES without the supervision of a healthcare provider. Tell patients not to attempt to self-treat prostate cancer with PC-SPES.

Although PC-SPES might be helpful for some patients, it should only be used in conjunction with a comprehensive treatment plan developed between the patient and oncologist. Clinical trials have used 6-9 capsules daily. Each capsule contains 320 mg of the herbal combination. In some studies patients started with one capsule three times daily during the first week and 2 capsules three times daily during the second week. Then, if this dose was tolerated, it was increased to 3 capsules three times daily. PC-SPES should be taken on an empty stomach and should not be administered concurrently with antacids or other medicines (3577). Depending on the dose required, cost is estimated to range from $162-$486/month (5233).

Editor's Note No. 8

The FDA has recently declared this product as adulterated and misbranded. It is adulterated because it is promoted for use during the last 6 weeks of pregnancy, but contains ingredients that should not be used during any stage or pregnancy. These include black cohosh, blessed thistle, false unicorn root, and pennyroyal. It also contains raspberry leaf which should be avoided during pregnancy unless used under the guidance of a health professional. It is misbranded because its labeling does not state that it should not be used by pregnant women.

Editor's Note No. 9

This product is considered by the FDA to be an unapproved drug due to promotion of the product for the treatment of cancer and other diseases. The manufacturer has been barred from selling these products without first gaining FDA approval as a new drug (12069). The FDA first cited this manufacturer for marketing an unapproved drug in 1999 (387). In June 2000, the manufacturer of this product also settled Federal Trade Commission charges of making unsubstantiated claims for a one million dollar judgment (6999).

Editor's Note No. 10
The manufacturer has voluntarily recalled this product after FDA laboratories found contamination problems. It might be contaminated with yeast and Pseudomonas flourescens. Use of this contaminated product might result in sever eye injury and loss of sight. This product should not be used. People who have used this product should contact their physician or other health care professional.

Editor's Note No. 11
There are serious concerns about the safety of this product. LipoKinetix is marketed for weight loss. However, there is no reliable evidence it works. From July to December 2000 there have been at least seven cases of acute hepatotoxicity in patients taking LipoKinetix. Symptoms including nausea, weakness and fatigue, abdominal pain, and yellowing of the skin usually develop from 2 weeks to 3 months after starting LipoKinetix. Symptoms resolve when it is discontinued (7091). Tell patients not to use this product.

Editor's Note No. 12
The manufacturer refuses to disclose the ingredients of this product. Anecdotal evidence suggests that this product may have induced a seizure in one patient. Patients should be strongly encouraged to avoid using this product until more is known about its contents and safety.

Editor's Note No. 13
There is some evidence that SS Cream can be helpful for premature ejaculation. Applying SS Cream to the glans penis one hour prior to intercourse and washing off immediately before intercourse seems to significantly delay ejaculation compared to placebo. A single application of SS Cream seems to be safe. However, the safety of SS Cream with repeated application is not known. SS Cream seems to be well tolerated, but can sometimes cause sporadic erectile dysfunction, excessively delayed ejaculation, mild pain, and local irritation and burning.

Editor's Note No. 14
There is some concern about the safety of this product because it contains glandular or organ material derived from animals. The concern is that animal materials might be obtained from diseased animals, including those harboring bovine spongiform encephalopathy (BSE, mad cow disease). There are no reports of BSE or other disease transmission to humans from dietary supplements containing glandular or organ material and the risk of potential disease transmission is thought to be low. However, until more is known about the safety of these products, tell patients to avoid this and other supplements containing glandular or organ materials.

Editor's Note No. 15
The potential risk of transmission of bovine spongiform encephalopathy (BSE, mad cow disease) is raising patients' concerns about products containing chondroitin. Chondroitin is produced from bovine trachea. Although bovine trachea tissue does not seem to carry a high risk of BSE disease infectivity, in some cases manufacturing methods might lead to contamination with other diseased animal tissues. So far there are no reports of BSE or other disease transmission to humans from dietary supplements containing animal materials and the risk of potential disease transmission is thought to be low. However, until more is known about the quality of manufacturing practices, tell patients to avoid this product.

Editor's Note No. 16
The potential risk of transmission of bovine spongiform encephalopathy (BSE, mad cow disease) is raising patients' concerns about products containing melatonin. Melatonin is a hormone sometimes harvested from the pineal gland of animals. However, some melatonin products are made synthetically and are free of this potential risk. The manufacturer of this product has not disclosed its source of melatonin. Until more is known, tell patients to avoid this product.

Editor's Note No. 17
The manufacturer of this product refuses to disclose specific details about the ingredients. Because the exact amounts of ingredients are unknown, tell patients to avoid this product.

Editor's Note No. 18
Wobenzym N is promoted for reducing inflammation and edema, and speeding recovery from certain injuries. Often it is used by individuals with arthritis and by athletes, including some professional and Olympic athletes. Enzymes in this product are thought to activate macrophages that attack inflammation-causing circulating immune complexes. Rutoside, and additional ingredient, acts as an antioxidant. To date there is no convincing clinical evidence that Wobenzym is effective for these uses. Because these enzymes do not affect prostaglandin synthesis, Wobenzym N is also promoted to be free of many of the side effects associated with non-steroidal anti-inflammatory drugs (NSAIDS). Adverse reactions reported after oral administration include loose stools, increased gas, and skin reactions. Wobenzym N contains enzymes with fibrinolytic activity and might affect coagulation. It should be used cautiously by people on anticoagulant medications such

as aspirin, clopidogrel (Plavix), dalteparin (Fragmin), enoxaprin (Lovenox), heparin, ticlopidine (Ticlid), warfarin (Coumadin), and others (6060).

Editor's Note No. 19
This product is utilized at the Mexican cancer clinic American Metabolic Institute and promoted by Geronimo Rubio, MD, the clinic's medical director. However, the clinic does not disclose the ingredients of this preparation. Tell patients to avoid this and other products that do not disclose ingredients.

Editor's Note No. 20
This product was recently reformulated. Many of the ingredients increased in strength. For example, amounts of procaine, thiamine, riboflavin, pyridoxine, niacin, and chromium doubled.

Editor's Note No. 21
This product has been discontinued by the manufacturer.

Editor's Note No. 22.
This product and others similar to it have been marketed as an alternative to anabolic steroids for increasing testosterone levels and improving muscle size and strength. So far, evidence indicates that Andro-6 does not increase testosterone levels or significantly improve muscle strength (7514). However, this product, like other products containing androstenedione, has been shown to significantly increase levels of estrogens (7514) and might be associated with estrogenic side effects in men, including acne, behavior changes, sticular atrophy, and gynecomastia (674,6000).

Editor's Note No. 23
Lab testing has discovered amounts of the drug tadalafil (Cialis) in a sample of this product (9605). This drug is a prescription product in many countries and is similar to sildenafil (Viagra). Advise patients using this product to discontinue taking it.

Editor's Note No. 24
Poly-MVA is a combination of minerals, vitamins, and amino acids (hence, the acronym "MVA") that was patented in 1995. It's promoted as a "metalo-vitamin"...as a cancer preventative and as a nontoxic alternative to chemotherapy for treating cancer. There is no reliable clinical research or preclinical research about Poly-MVA...no credible evidence to support anecdotal claims of tumor regression, pain reduction, and prolonged survival in patients with various kinds of cancer. There is no reliable information about potential risks or adverse reactions.
The ingredients of Poly-MVA are a "proprietary blend." Under dietary supplement regulations, the manufacturer is not required to include specific amounts of any ingredient on the product label. Poly-MVA is available as a reddish brown liquid that is mixed with juice or water. Poly-MVA is very expensive...$165 for a 4-ounce bottle, which is less than a one-week supply.

Editor's Note No. 25
Product Recall: On April 4, 2003, this product was voluntarily withdrawn from the market. Lab testing found that it contained the prescription drug sildenafil (Viagra). Advise patients using this product to discontinue taking it.

Editor's Note No. 26
The potential risk of transmission of bovine spongiform encephalopathy (BSE, mad cow disease) is raising patients' concerns about products containing melatonin. Melatonin is a hormone sometimes harvested from the pineal gland of animals. However, the melatonin contained in this product is produced synthetically and is free of this potential risk.

Editor's Note No. 27
This product is not available in the U.S.

Editor's Note No. 28
This product may contain excessive levels of lead. An analysis shows it can contain as much as 2.5 mcg of lead per gram of calcium (9598). Advise patients not to use this product.

Editor's Note No. 29
Using Zestra topically might improve symptoms of female sexual arousal disorder. A small clinical study suggests massaging 0.5 to 1 ml into the external female genitalia, clitoris, labia, and vaginal opening for 3 to 5 minutes prior to intercourse may improve sexual pleasure (11968). More evidence is needed to rate Zestra for this use. Topically, Zestra appears to be safe for short term use (11968,11969). Zestra can cause mild genital burning sensations that last 5 to 30 minutes (11968).

Editor's Note No. 30
This product contains ephedra, also commonly known as ma huang. On December 30, 2003, the FDA announced that it will ban ephedra-containing products in the U.S. This is due to numerous reports that link ephedra use to severe adverse reactions including heart attack, stroke, hypertension, seizure, and others (10055). Advise patients not to use this or other products containing ephedra.

Editor's Note No. 31
There is concern about the safety of this product because it contains glandular or organ material derived from animals. The concern is that animal materials

might be obtained from diseased animals, including those harboring bovine spongiform encephalopathy (BSE, mad cow disease). There are no reports of BSE or other disease transmission to humans from dietary supplements containing glandular or organ material and the risk of potential disease transmission is thought to be low. However, as of July 1, 2004, the FDA has banned all dietary supplements containing brain or spinal cord material from cows over 30 months of age (4953). This product appears to contain brain materials. Tell patients to avoid this and other supplements containing glandular or organ materials.

Editor's Note No. 32
Immunace (Immunance) is a high-dose combination micronutrient product containing vitamins, minerals, and the amino acid cystine. In the recommended daily dose of 2 tablets, some of the ingredients exceed the recommended dietary allowance (RDA) set for healthy people. Some clinical research suggests that this supplement might improve survival of HIV-infected patients with CD4 cell counts below 200 million cells per liter. The mechanism of action is unknown, but seems to be independent of change in CD4 cell count (11348). Immunace (Immunance) is not available in the US, but can be ordered from the UK via the Internet. Tell patients not to attempt to self-treat with Immunace (Immunance). Although Immunace (Immunance) might be helpful for some patients, it should only be used in conjunction with a comprehensive treatment plan developed between the patient and health care provider. Although tablets were used in the study, Immunace (Immunance) is only available in capsule form.

Editor's Note No. 33
In August 2004 the manufacturer of this product was warned by the US Food and Drug Administration (FDA) for making unsubstantiated claims about the benefits of this product. The FDA indicates that claims made in promotional materials such as "controls appetite", "burn calories more efficiently", "controls cortisol levels within a healthy range" and several other claims are false and misleading and therefore the product is misbranded (12141).

Editor's Note No. 34
In March 2004, the US Food and Drug Administration ordered the manufacturer and distributors of SeaSilver to discontinue marketing it and to recall existing product. This is due to their unsubstantiated claims that SeaSilver can treat over 650 diseases including cancer, AIDS, diabetes, heart disease, hepatitis, and many others. Due to these claims this product is considered by the FDA to be a misbranded drug (6814).

Editor's Note No. 35
Juice Plus+ Garden Blend is a commercially available mixed vegetable supplement made from dehydrated juice concentrates. It is used with Juice Plus+ Orchard Blend, a mixed fruit supplement made from dehydrated juice concentrates, to reduce coronary heart disease (CHD) risk. Preliminary clinical evidence from several small studies suggests Juice Plus+ may have pharmacologic activity that could reduce CHD risk (11374,11375,11376,11377). It may lower plasma homocysteine levels, raise plasma antioxidant vitamin and folate levels, and raise serum nitrate and nitrite levels (11374,11375). Juice Plus+ may also improve flow-mediated vasoactivity and reduce oxidative changes in DNA (11376,11377). But there's no reliable evidence showing Juice Plus+ decreases risk of death or cardiovascular events such as stroke or myocardial infarction. Preliminary clinical research trials have used two capsules Juice Plus+ Garden Blend and two capsules Juice Plus+ Orchard Blend divided twice daily (11374,11375,11376,11377).

Editor's Note No. 36
Juice Plus+ Orchard Blend is a commercially available mixed fruit supplement made from dehydrated juice concentrates. It is used with Juice Plus+ Garden Blend, a mixed vegetable supplement made from dehydrated juice concentrates, to reduce coronary heart disease (CHD) risk. Preliminary clinical evidence from several small studies suggests Juice Plus+ may have pharmacologic activity that could reduce CHD risk (11374,11375,11376,11377). It may lower plasma homocysteine levels, raise plasma antioxidant vitamin and folate levels, and raise serum nitrate and nitrite levels (11374,11375). Juice Plus+ may also improve flow-mediated vasoactivity and reduce oxidative changes in DNA (11376,11377). But there's no reliable evidence showing Juice Plus+ decreases risk of death or cardiovascular events such as stroke or myocardial infarction. Preliminary clinical research trials have used two capsules Juice Plus+ Garden Blend and two capsules Juice Plus+ Orchard Blend divided twice daily (11374,11375,11376,11377).

Editor's Note No. 37
On April 1, 2004, the FDA warned the distributor of this product to stop making false and misleading claims about this product's use for weight loss. This and other similar products sometimes claim to block starch, carbohydrates, and calories to help users lose weight without making any lifestyle changes such as calorie restriction or exercise. The FDA indicates that these claims are not supported by reliable scientific evidence (12005).

BRAND NAMES

Editor's Note No. 38
On May 5, 2004, the FDA warned the company that produces this product to stop making false and misleading claims about this product's use. The labeling for this product stated that it provides "cushioning" and "lubrication" for the joints and that it alleviates pain from arthritis and fibromyalgia. The FDA indicates that these claims are not supported by reliable scientific evidence (12029).

Editor's Note No. 39
This product contains country mallow, which is a source of ephedrine. On December 30, 2003, the FDA announced that it will ban ephedrine-containing products such as country mallow and ephedra in the U.S. This is due to numerous reports that link the ephedrine-containing product ephedra to severe adverse reactions including heart attack, stroke, hypertension, seizure, and others (10055). Advise patients not to use this or other products containing ephedrine.

Editor's Note No. 40
This product contains the ingredient synephrine. Synephrine is a stimulant similar to ephedrine, which is contained in the herb ephedra (ma huang). Ephedra products were removed from the U.S. market due to safety concerns. Ephedra is linked to stroke, heart attack, seizure, and other serious side effects.
Many manufacturers have now substituted synephrine in products that used to contain ephedra. These products are typically promoted for weight loss. Many of these products are now labeled as ephedra-free or ma huang-free, but they often still contain the stimulant synephrine. These synephrine-containing products likely have the same risks as the ephedra-containing products.
Synephrine is a constituent of bitter orange (Citrus aurantium). Products that list bitter orange or Citrus aurantium on the label also likely contain synephrine. Advise patients about the potential risks associated with this and other synephrine-containing products.

Editor's Note No. 41
The manufacturer refuses to disclose the ingredients of this product. Because the ingredients are unknown, tell patients to avoid this product.

Editor's Note No. 42
There is preliminary clinical evidence that drinking 250 mL or 1 can of Red Bull Energy Drink might improve anaerobic exercise endurance by 24% and aerobic exercise endurance by 9% in patients on cycle ergometers. Red Bull Energy Drink might also improve subjective mental performance in the areas of concentration, immediate memory recall, and reaction time (11470).

Editor's Note No. 43
This formulation of glucosamine is corn-derived. Most glucosamine products are animal-derived, from the shell of crustaceans. This product may be a safer alternative for people with a shellfish allergy. However, clinical studies have only evaluated glucosamine products derived from shellfish.

Editor's Note No. 44
This is a "branded ingredient." This means that it is an ingredient used in other companies' products. For example, this product might be just one ingredient used in another company's product that contains multiple ingredients. These branded ingredients usually are not available for sale as stand alone products for consumers.

Editor's Note No. 45
This product has been certified by the United States Pharmacopeia (USP) Dietary Supplement Verification Program. This certification ensures that this product contains the ingredients listed on the label and meets USP standards for purity and good manufacturing practices. This certification does not ensure safety or effectiveness. For information about safety, effectiveness, side effects, interactions and other clinical information, click the links for the individual ingredients to review the detailed ingredient monographs. For more information about the USP certification program, visit: http://www.uspverified.org/pinfo/overview.html.

Editor's Note No. 46
This product contains aristolochic acid. The FDA considers all products containing aristolochic acid to be unsafe and adulterated (6118). The FDA intends to automatically detain, without physical examination, any product which contains plants known or suspected to contain aristolochic acid, or which might be adulterated with plants known to contain aristolochic acid. Each detained product will be released only after the responsible party provides direct analytical evidence that it is free of aristolochic acid (6118). Aristolochia is also banned in Germany, Austria, France, Great Britain, Belgium, and Japan (367).
Health Canada, the Canadian health authority, removed five aristolochia-containing Chinese herbal medicine products from sale. The products include Touku Natural Herbal Rheumatic Pills, two brands of Tri-Snakegall & Fritillary Powder, Tracheitis Pills, and Gastropathy Capsules (367).

Editor's Note No. 47
This product contains the ingredient androstenedione. In March 2004, the U.S. Food and Drug Administration told manufacturers of products containing this ingredient to immediately stop distribution. The FDA considers these dietary supplements to be adulterated drugs due

to the lack of historical data regarding dietary use that establishes a reasonable expectation of safety. There are concerns that these products are unsafe. Androstenedione might have potent androgenic effects and lead to serious side effects including impotence, liver problems, and increased cancer risk (12001).

Editor's Note No. 48
The potential risk of transmission of bovine spongiform encephalopathy (BSE, mad cow disease) is raising patients' concerns about products containing chondroitin. Chondroitin is sometimes produced from bovine trachea. However, the chondroitin in this product is not from a bovine source, so this product is free of this potential risk.

Editor's Note No. 49
This product is marketed as a street drug alternative and is claimed to produce a safe legal high. This and other products marketed by Cytotec Solutions have been found to contain high levels of over-the-counter drugs such as diphenhydramine, dextromethorphan, or ephedrine. In some cases, the controlled substances gamma-butyrolactone (GBL) and gamma-hydroxybutyrate (GHB) have been found in these products. The FDA considers these products to be illegal unapproved drugs (12007). Advise patients against using this or other products marketed by Cytotec Solutions.

Editor's Note No. 50
This product is a Bach flower remedy. Bach (pronounced Batch) flower remedies were developed by Dr. Edward Bach in the 1930's. Dr. Bach believed that illnesses are "manifestations of flaws" in one's personality. He believed that a person's own nature, character, and feelings play a key role in the development of diseases. Therefore, Bach flower remedies are often promoted to help mental and emotional problems, rather than to directly treat physical ailments.
Bach flower remedies are produced from a "mother tincture" by adding only a few drops of extract to distilled water, which are then preserved with brandy. Many people often refer to Bach flower remedies as homeopathic products because they are diluted like homeopathic remedies. In fact, Dr. Bach developed the first 7 of his 38 remedies while working at the London Homeopathic Hospital.
Bach flower remedies are often so dilute that they contain little or no detectable amounts of active ingredients. Therefore, just as with homeopathic preparations, Bach flower remedies are not expected to have any beneficial pharmacological effects, or any drug interactions, or side effects.

Therapeutic Efficacy

For more information on any of the natural medicines identified in this list, review the listing for that monograph in the database. Just because a product has a positive effectiveness rating does not mean it is appropriate for all patients. In some cases natural medicines that are rated effective might be unsafe for certain patients due to contraindications, drug interactions, or other reasons.

Abortion
Possibly Effective
Chinese Cucumber Root
Possibly Ineffective
Rosemary

ACE inhibitor-associated cough
Possibly Effective
Iron

Acetaminophen poisoning
Effective
N-Acetyl Cysteine
Possibly Effective
Methionine

Acne
Possibly Effective
Alpha Hydroxy Acids
Bovine Cartilage
Chasteberry
Saccharomyces Boulardii
Tea Tree Oil
Zinc

Acrodermatitis enteropathica
Possibly Effective
Zinc

Acute bronchitis
(see also Bronchitis)
Possibly Ineffective
Vitamin C

Acute myocardial infarction (MI)
[see also Myocardial infarction (MI)]
Possibly Effective
Magnesium

Acute respiratory distress syndrome (ARDS)
[see also Respiratory distress syndrome (RDS)]
Possibly Effective
Borage Seed Oil

Acute respiratory illness (ARI)
Possibly Effective
Ginseng, American

Adjustment disorder with anxious mood
Possibly Effective
Passionflower

Adrenal insufficiency
Possibly Effective
DHEA

Adrenoleukodystrophy and adrenomyeloneuropathy
Likely Ineffective
Lorenzo's Oil

Age-related cognitive impairment
Possibly Effective
Acetyl-L-Carnitine
Citicoline
Phosphatidylserine

Age-related macular degeneration (AMD)
Possibly Effective
Beta-Carotene
DHA (Docosahexaenoic Acid)
Lutein
Vitamin C

Age-related macular degeneration (AMD) (cont.)
Possibly Effective (cont.)
Vitamin E
Zinc
Possibly Ineffective
EPA (Eicosapentaenoic Acid)

Age-related maculopathy
Possibly Effective
Fish Oils

Age-related memory impairment
Possibly Effective
Ginkgo Leaf
Likely Ineffective
Choline

Aging skin
(see also Wrinkled skin)
Possibly Effective
DHEA
Pyruvate

AIDS
(see HIV/AIDS)

AIDS diarrhea-wasting syndrome
Possibly Ineffective
Zinc

AIDS-related diarrhea
(see also HIV/AIDS-related diarrhea)
Possibly Effective
Sangre De Grado

AIDS-related myelopathy
Possibly Effective
SAMe

AIDS-related wasting
(see also HIV/AIDS-related wasting)
Possibly Effective
Hydroxymethylbutyrate (HMB)
L-Arginine
Possibly Ineffective
Medium Chain Triglycerides

Albuminuria
Possibly Effective
Vitamin C

Alcoholism
Possibly Effective
Gamma-Hydroxybutyrate (GHB)

Alcohol-related liver disease
(see also Cirrhosis and Liver disease)
Possibly Ineffective
Alpha-Lipoic Acid

Allergic rhinitis (hayfever)
Possibly Effective
Butterbur
Thymus Extract
Possibly Ineffective
EPA (Eicosapentaenoic Acid)
Grape Seed

Alopecia areata
Possibly Effective
Cedarwood Oil
Lavender
Rosemary
Thyme Oil

Alopecia areata (cont.)
Possibly Ineffective
Zinc

Altitude sickness
Possibly Effective
Ginkgo Leaf

Alzheimer's disease
(see also Dementia)
Possibly Effective
Acetyl-L-Carnitine
Idebenone
Lemon Balm
Niacin and Niacinamide
Phosphatidylserine
Sage
Vitamin E
Possibly Ineffective
5-HTP
Beta-Carotene
Choline
DHEA
Inositol
Vitamin C
Likely Ineffective
Deanol
Lecithin
N-Acetyl Cysteine

Amenorrhea
(see also Menstrual disorders)
Likely Effective
Progesterone

Amyloidosis
Possibly Effective
DMSO (Dimethylsulfoxide)

Amyotrophic lateral sclerosis (ALS, Lou Gehrig's disease)
Possibly Ineffective
Creatine
N-Acetyl Cysteine
Threonine
Transfer Factor
Likely Ineffective
Branched-Chain Amino Acids

Anal fissures
Possibly Effective
Bovine Cartilage

Anal pruritus
Possibly Effective
Bovine Cartilage

Anemia
(see also Hereditary sideroblastic anemia, Iron deficiency anemia, and Pernicious anemia)
Possibly Effective
Vitamin E
Possibly Ineffective
Histidine
Vitamin A

Anemia of chronic disease
Effective
Iron

Angina
(see also Vasospastic angina)
Possibly Effective
L-Arginine
L-Carnitine
N-Acetyl Cysteine
Propionyl-L-Carnitine
Terminalia
Possibly Ineffective
Vitamin E

Angioplasty
Possibly Effective
Fish Oils

Anorexia
Possibly Effective
Branched-Chain Amino Acids

Anorexia nervosa
Possibly Effective
Zinc

Antibiotic-associated diarrhea
Possibly Effective
Lactobacillus
Saccharomyces Boulardii
Yogurt

Antibiotic-induced gastrointestinal adverse effects
Possibly Effective
Bifidobacteria

Antidepressant-induced sexual dysfunction
Possibly Ineffective
Ginkgo Leaf

Antiphospholipid syndrome-associated miscarriage
Possibly Effective
Fish Oils

Anxiety
Likely Effective
Kava
Possibly Effective
St. John's Wort
Valerian

Ariboflavinosis
Effective
Riboflavin

Arrhythmias
(see also Cardiac glycoside-induced arrythmias)
Possibly Effective
Magnesium

Asthma
(see also Exercise-induced asthma)
Possibly Effective
Caffeine
Choline
Forskolin
Lycopene
Magnesium
Thymus Extract
Possibly Ineffective
EPA (Eicosapentaenoic Acid)
Picrorhiza
Yogurt

Atelectasis
Effective
N-Acetyl Cysteine

Atherosclerosis
Possibly Effective
Black Tea
Fish Oils
Garlic
Niacin and Niacinamide
Vitamin C
Possibly Ineffective
Vitamin E

Athlete's Foot
(see Tinae pedis)

Athletic conditioning
Possibly Ineffective
Androstenediol
Boron
Chromium
Chrysin
Likely Ineffective
Androstenedione
Creatine

Athletic performance
Possibly Effective
Caffeine
Creatine
Deanol
Pycnogenol
Possibly Ineffective
Bee Pollen
Branched-Chain Amino Acids
Choline
Cordyceps
Ginseng, Panax
Ginseng, Siberian
Glutamine
L-Tryptophan
Magnesium
Ornithine
Ornithine Ketoglutarate
Pangamic Acid
Likely Ineffective
Coca
Coenzyme Q-10
Glycerol
Inosine
L-Carnitine
Phosphate Salts

Atopic dermatitis (eczema)
Possibly Effective
Bifidobacteria
Lactobacillus
Rice Bran
Possibly Ineffective
Borage Seed Oil
Evening Primrose Oil
Zinc

Atopic disease
Possibly Effective
Lactobacillus
Whey Protein

Atrial fibrillation
Likely Effective
Digitalis
Possibly Effective
Fish Oils

Atrophic acne scars
Possibly Effective
Alpha Hydroxy Acids

Attention deficit disorder (ADD)
Possibly Ineffective
Tyrosine

Attention deficit-hyperactivity disorder (ADHD)
Possibly Effective
Lithium
Zinc
Possibly Ineffective
Caffeine
DHA (Docosahexaenoic Acid)
Evening Primrose Oil
Phenylalanine
Pycnogenol
Tyrosine
Vitamin C

Autism
Possibly Ineffective
Dimethylglycine
Inositol
Pyridoxine
Likely Ineffective
Secretin

Back pain
Possibly Effective
Willow Bark

Bacterial vaginosis
Possibly Effective
Yogurt

Barium enema-related colonic spasm
Possibly Effective
Peppermint Oil

Bee sting allergy
Likely Effective
Bee Venom

Benign prostatic hyperplasia (BPH)
Likely Effective
Beta-Sitosterol
Pygeum
Saw Palmetto
Possibly Effective
African Wild Potato
Rye Grass
Possibly Ineffective
Stinging Nettle Root

Benzodiazepine withdrawal
Possibly Effective
Kava
Melatonin
Possibly Ineffective
Progesterone

Beta blocker-induced dyslipidemia
Possibly Effective
Chromium

Therapeutic Efficacy

For additional data, refer to the database.

Beta-thalassemia
Possibly Effective
Vitamin E
Biliary stones
Possibly Effective
DMSO (Dimethylsulfoxide)
Biotin deficiency
Likely Effective
Biotin
Bipolar disorder
Effective
Lithium
Possibly Effective
Fish Oils
Bladder cancer
Possibly Effective
Green Tea
Vitamin E
Possibly Ineffective
Lycopene
Tomato
Bone substitute
Likely Effective
Coral
Breast cancer
Possibly Effective
Beta-Carotene
Folic Acid
Green Tea
Lentinan
Olive Oil
Soy
Vitamin A
Possibly Ineffective
Black Tea
Coffee
Garlic
Likely Ineffective
Vitamin E
Breast cancer-related hot flashes
Possibly Ineffective
Vitamin E
Breast engorgement
Possibly Effective
Cabbage
Breast pain
(see Mastalgia)
Brittle nails
Possibly Effective
Biotin
Bronchial diagnostic studies
Effective
N-Acetyl Cysteine
Bronchitis
(see also Acute bronchitis and Chronic obstructive bronchitis)
Possibly Effective
N-Acetyl Cysteine
Bronchopulmonary disorders
Effective
N-Acetyl Cysteine
Bronchopulmonary dysplasia
Possibly Effective
Superoxide Dismutase
Possibly Ineffective
Vitamin E
Bruxism
Possibly Ineffective
L-Tryptophan
Burns
Possibly Effective
Chymotrypsin
Honey
Ornithine Ketoglutarate
Zinc
Possibly Ineffective
RNA and DNA
Tannic Acid
Cachexia
Possibly Effective
Adenosine
Fish Oils
Medium Chain Triglycerides
Cancer
(see also various types of Cancer)
Possibly Effective
Beta Glucans
Coriolus Mushroom
Fish Oils
Vitamin C
Possibly Ineffective
Beer
Shark Cartilage
Likely Ineffective
Beta-Carotene
DMSO (Dimethylsulfoxide)
European Mistletoe
Ineffective
Apricot
Cancer-associated neuropathic pain
Possibly Effective
Magnesium
Cardiac arrest
Possibly Ineffective
Magnesium
Cardiac autonomic neuropathy
Possibly Ineffective
Alpha-Lipoic Acid
Cardiac glycoside-induced ventricular arrhythmias
(see also Arrythmias)
Likely Effective
EDTA
Cardiovascular disease
Effective
Oat Bran
Likely Effective
Beer
Wine
Possibly Effective
Alpha-Linolenic Acid
Niacin and Niacinamide
Tomato
Cardiovascular disease (cont.)
Possibly Ineffective
Lycopene
Selenium
Likely Ineffective
Beta-Carotene
Vitamin E
Carpal tunnel syndrome
Possibly Ineffective
Pyridoxine
Cataracts
Effective
Chymotrypsin
Likely Effective
Hyaluronic Acid
Possibly Effective
Lutein
Niacin and Niacinamide
Riboflavin
Thiamine
Tomato
Vitamin A
Possibly Ineffective
Beta-Carotene
Zinc
Cerebellar ataxia
Possibly Effective
5-HTP
Possibly Ineffective
Choline
Cerebral palsy
Possibly Ineffective
Magnesium
Cerebrovascular disease
Possibly Effective
Citicoline
Mesoglycan
Cervical dysplasia
Possibly Effective
Green Tea
Cervical dysplasia (cervical intraepithelial neoplasia, CIN)
Possibly Effective
Indole-3-Carbinol
Chemotherapy extravasation
Possibly Effective
Vitamin E
Chemotherapy toxicity
Possibly Effective
Glutathione
Chemotherapy-induced gastrointestinal (GI) adverse effects
Possibly Ineffective
Vitamin A
Chemotherapy-induced nausea
Possibly Effective
Ginger
Cholera
Possibly Effective
Niacin and Niacinamide
Cholestasis
Possibly Effective
Activated Charcoal

Therapeutic Efficacy

For additional data, refer to the database.

Chronic cerebral ischemia
Possibly Effective
Acetyl-L-Carnitine
Chronic fatigue syndrome (CFS)
Possibly Effective
Magnesium
Possibly Ineffective
Folic Acid
Melatonin
Transfer Factor
Chronic ischemic heart disease
Possibly Effective
Propionyl-L-Carnitine
Chronic obstructive bronchitis
(see also Bronchitis)
Possibly Effective
English Ivy
Chronic obstructive pulmonary disease (COPD)
Possibly Effective
Beta-Carotene
Magnesium
N-Acetyl Cysteine
Chronic pouchitis
Possibly Effective
Bifidobacteria
Lactobacillus
Chronic venous insufficiency
Likely Effective
Horse Chestnut
Possibly Effective
Butcher's Broom
Grape Leaf
Grape Seed
Pycnogenol
Sweet Clover
Circadian rhythm sleep disorders
Likely Effective
Melatonin
Possibly Ineffective
Vitamin B12
Cirrhosis
(see also Alcohol-related liver disease and Liver disease)
Possibly Ineffective
Fish Oils
Cisplatin-induced neurotoxicity
Possibly Effective
Vitamin E
Claudication
Possibly Ineffective
Fish Oils
Clostridium difficile diarrhea
Possibly Effective
Lactobacillus
Saccharomyces Boulardii
Cluster headache
(see also Headache)
Possibly Effective
Magnesium
Melatonin
Coenzyme Q-10 deficiency
Likely Effective
Coenzyme Q-10

Cognitive function
Possibly Effective
Beer
Brahmi
Ginkgo Leaf
Ginseng, Panax
Huperzine A
Iron
Wine
Possibly Ineffective
DHEA
Cognitive impairment
Possibly Effective
Acetyl-L-Carnitine
Cold sores
(see Herpes labialis)
Colorectal adenoma
Possibly Ineffective
Blond Psyllium
Colorectal cancer
Possibly Effective
Beta-Carotene
Calcium
Coffee
Folic Acid
Garlic
Lutein
Olive Oil
Vitamin E
Possibly Ineffective
Barley
Green Tea
Hydrazine Sulfate
Lycopene
Oat Bran
Oats
Rice Bran
Wheat Bran
Colostomy odor
Possibly Ineffective
Chlorophyll
Common cold
Possibly Effective
Andrographis
Echinacea
Vitamin C
Zinc
Concentration, coordination, and endurance
Possibly Effective
Schisandra
Condylomata acuminata
(see Genital warts)
Congestive heart failure (CHF)
Likely Effective
Digitalis
Possibly Effective
Coenzyme Q-10
Creatine
Hawthorn
L-Arginine
L-Carnitine
Propionyl-L-Carnitine
Taurine

Congestive heart failure (CHF) (cont.)
Possibly Effective (cont.)
Terminalia
Possibly Ineffective
Vitamin E
Constipation
Effective
Agar
Black Psyllium
Blond Psyllium
Magnesium
Likely Effective
Alder Buckthorn
Aloe Latex
Cascara
Castor Oil
European Buckthorn
Flaxseed
Glycerol
Olive Oil
Podophyllum
Senna
Possibly Effective
Guar Gum
Inulin
Karaya Gum
Sweet Almond
Wheat Bran
Xanthan Gum
Contraception
Possibly Effective
Castor Seed
Gossypol
Contrast agent-induced nephropathy
Possibly Effective
N-Acetyl Cysteine
Copper deficiency
Likely Effective
Copper
Corneal calcium deposits
Possibly Effective
EDTA
Coronary artery bypass
Possibly Effective
Fish Oils
Coronary artery disease
Possibly Effective
DHA (Docosahexaenoic Acid)
EPA (Eicosapentaenoic Acid)
Magnesium
Ribose
Possibly Ineffective
Folic Acid
Coronary heart disease
Possibly Effective
English Walnut
Fish Oils
Likely Ineffective
EDTA
L-Arginine

Therapeutic Efficacy

For additional data, refer to the database.

Corticosteroid-induced osteoporosis
- *Likely Effective*
  - Calcium
  - Vitamin D

Cough
- *Effective*
  - Camphor

Critical illness (trauma)
- *Possibly Effective*
  - Glutamine

Crohn's disease
- *Possibly Effective*
  - Saccharomyces Boulardii
- *Possibly Ineffective*
  - Glutamine

Cutaneous sporotrichosis
- *Effective*
  - Iodine

Cyclosporine-induced hypertension
- *Possibly Effective*
  - Fish Oils

Cyclosporine-induced nephrotoxicity
- *Possibly Effective*
  - Fish Oils

Cystic fibrosis
- *Effective*
  - N-Acetyl Cysteine
- *Possibly Ineffective*
  - EPA (Eicosapentaenoic Acid)

Cystinuria
- *Possibly Ineffective*
  - Glutamine

Deep vein thrombosis (DVT)
- *Possibly Ineffective*
  - Mesoglycan

Delayed sleep phase syndrome (DSPS)
- *Possibly Effective*
  - Melatonin

Dementia
(see also Alzheimer's disease)
- *Possibly Effective*
  - Ginkgo Leaf
  - Huperzine A
  - Vinpocetine
  - Vitamin E
- *Possibly Ineffective*
  - NADH
  - Vitamin C
- *Likely Ineffective*
  - Lecithin

Dental caries
- *Effective*
  - Fluoride
- *Likely Effective*
  - Xylitol

Dental hypersensitivity
- *Effective*
  - Strontium

Depression
- *Likely Effective*
  - Lithium
  - SAMe
  - St. John's Wort

Depression (cont.)
- *Possibly Effective*
  - 5-HTP
  - EPA (Eicosapentaenoic Acid)
  - Fish Oils
  - Folic Acid
- *Possibly Ineffective*
  - DHA (Docosahexaenoic Acid)
  - Inositol
  - Tyrosine
- *Likely Ineffective*
  - Melatonin

Dermatitis
- *Likely Effective*
  - Lecithin
- *Possibly Ineffective*
  - German Chamomile

Diabetes
- *Possibly Effective*
  - Alpha-Lipoic Acid
  - Beer
  - Blond Psyllium
  - Cassia Cinnamon
  - Chromium
  - Coffee
  - Fenugreek
  - Ginseng, American
  - Ginseng, Panax
  - Glucomannan
  - Guar Gum
  - Magnesium
  - Niacin and Niacinamide
  - Oat Bran
  - Oats
  - Prickly Pear Cactus
  - Soy
  - Vanadium
  - Vitamin D
  - Wine
  - Xanthan Gum
- *Possibly Ineffective*
  - Cranberry
  - DHA (Docosahexaenoic Acid)
  - EPA (Eicosapentaenoic Acid)
  - Garlic
  - Wheat Bran
- *Likely Ineffective*
  - Fish Oils

Diabetic foot ulcers
- *Possibly Effective*
  - Iodine

Diabetic nephropathy
- *Possibly Effective*
  - Cod Liver Oil
  - Fish Oils

Diabetic neuropathy
- *Possibly Effective*
  - Gamma Linolenic Acid
- *Likely Ineffective*
  - Inositol

Diabetic retinopathy
(see also Retinopathy)
- *Possibly Effective*
  - Ginkgo Leaf

Diaper rash
- *Possibly Ineffective*
  - Tannic Acid

Diarrhea
(see also AIDS-related diarrhea, Antibiotic-associated diarrhea, and HIV-related diarrhea)
- *Effective*
  - Pectin
- *Likely Effective*
  - Zinc
- *Possibly Effective*
  - Blond Psyllium
  - Guar Gum
  - Kaolin
  - Lactobacillus
  - Saccharomyces Boulardii
  - Soy
  - Yogurt
- *Possibly Ineffective*
  - Glutamine

Digestive disorders
- *Likely Ineffective*
  - Pancreatin

Digestive tract cancers
- *Possibly Ineffective*
  - Coffee

Doxorubicin-induced cardiac toxicity
- *Possibly Ineffective*
  - N-Acetyl Cysteine

Dry eyes
- *Possibly Effective*
  - Chondroitin Sulfate

Dry mouth
- *Possibly Effective*
  - Betaine Anhydrous

Dry skin
- *Likely Effective*
  - Alpha Hydroxy Acids
  - Lecithin

Duchenne muscular dystrophy
- *Possibly Ineffective*
  - Vitamin E

Dyslexia
- *Possibly Effective*
  - Fish Oils

Dyslipidemia
- *Possibly Effective*
  - Fish Oils
  - Gamma Oryzanol

Dysmenorrhea
- *Possibly Effective*
  - Fish Oils

Therapeutic Efficacy

For additional data, refer to the database.

Dyspepsia
Effective
Calcium
Possibly Effective
Artichoke
Caraway Oil
Peppermint Oil
Turmeric

Dyspraxia
Possibly Effective
Fish Oils
Thyme Oil
Vitamin E

Earwax
Possibly Ineffective
Olive Oil

Eclampsia
Likely Effective
Magnesium

Eczema
(see Atopic dermatitis)

Elevated lead concentrations
Possibly Ineffective
Calcium

Endometrial cancer
Possibly Effective
Fish Oils

Endometrial hyperplasia
Possibly Effective
Progesterone

End-stage renal disease (ESRD)
Effective
L-Carnitine
Likely Effective
Folic Acid
Possibly Effective
N-Acetyl Cysteine
Possibly Ineffective
Blond Psyllium

Enhancing infant development
Possibly Ineffective
Omega-6 Fatty Acids

Epilepsy
Possibly Effective
N-Acetyl Cysteine
Possibly Ineffective
Dimethylglycine

Epithelial growths
Likely Effective
Podophyllum

Erectile dysfunction (ED)
Possibly Effective
DHEA
Ginseng, Panax
L-Arginine
Melanotan-II
Yohimbe

Erythema
Possibly Effective
Vitamin C

Erythropoietic protoporphyria (EPP)
Effective
Beta-Carotene
Possibly Effective
Canthaxanthin

Esophageal Cancer
Possibly Effective
Green Tea

Exercise-induced asthma
(see also Asthma)
Possibly Effective
Beta-Carotene

Exercise-induced muscle soreness
Possibly Ineffective
Soy

Exercise-induced respiratory infections
Possibly Effective
Vitamin C

Extrapyramidal disorders
Likely Ineffective
Lecithin

Extravasation
Possibly Effective
DMSO (Dimethylsulfoxide)

Eye surgery
Likely Effective
Chondroitin Sulfate

Fall prevention
Likely Effective
Vitamin D

Familial hypercholesterolemia
Possibly Effective
Sitostanol
Possibly Ineffective
Garlic

Familial hypophosphatemia
Effective
Vitamin D

Fanconi syndrome
Effective
Vitamin D

Fetal and early infant mortality
Possibly Ineffective
Vitamin A

Fetal bone mineralization
Likely Effective
Calcium

Fibrocystic breast disease
Possibly Effective
Iodine

Fibromyalgia
Possibly Effective
5-HTP
Alpha Hydroxy Acids
Capsicum
Gamma-Hydroxybutyrate (GHB)
Magnesium
SAMe

Fibrosing alveolitis
Possibly Effective
N-Acetyl Cysteine

Flatulence
Possibly Effective
Activated Charcoal

Fluorosis
Possibly Effective
Calcium

Folate deficiency
Effective
Folic Acid

Food allergies
Possibly Effective
Thymus Extract

Fractures
Possibly Effective
Chymotrypsin

Fragile-X syndrome
Likely Ineffective
Folic Acid

Galactosemia
Possibly Effective
Soy

Gallbladder disease
Possibly Effective
Caffeine
Coffee
Vitamin C
Possibly Ineffective
Lecithin
Likely Ineffective
Beta-Sitosterol

Gastric cancer
Possibly Effective
Barley
Beta-Carotene
Garlic
Green Tea
Lentinan
Oat Bran
Oats
Rice Bran
Vitamin C
Wheat Bran

Gastroesophageal cancer
Possibly Effective
Vitamin E

Gastroesophageal reflux disease (GERD)
Effective
Magnesium

Gastrointestinal cancer
Possibly Ineffective
Black Tea

Generalized anxiety disorder (GAD)
Possibly Effective
Passionflower

Genital warts (condylomata acuminata)
Likely Effective
Podophyllum

Gingivitis
Possibly Effective
Zinc
Possibly Ineffective
Fish Oils

CHARTS

Glaucoma
Possibly Effective
Ginkgo Leaf
Marijuana
Glomerulosclerosis
Possibly Effective
Vitamin E
Glucose-6-phosphate dehydrogenase (G6PD) deficiency
Possibly Effective
Vitamin E
Granuloma annulare
Possibly Effective
Vitamin E
Gyrate atrophy of the choroid and retina
Possibly Effective
Creatine
Hangover
Possibly Effective
Prickly Pear Cactus
Possibly Ineffective
Artichoke
Hayfever
(see Allergic rhinitis)
Head and neck cancer
Likely Ineffective
N-Acetyl Cysteine
Vitamin A
Headache
(see also Cluster headache, Migraine headache, Postoperative headache, and Tension headache)
Effective
Caffeine
Hearing loss
Possibly Effective
Magnesium
Heart failure
Possibly Effective
Beer
Wine
Heart transplant
Possibly Effective
Fish Oils
Helicobacter pylori (H pylori)
Possibly Effective
Beer
Lactobacillus
Vitamin C
Wine
Yogurt
Possibly Ineffective
Fish Oils
Garlic
Hemodialysis grafts
Possibly Effective
Fish Oils
Hemorrhagic disease
Effective
Vitamin K
Hemorrhoids
(see also Internal Hemorrhoids)
Possibly Effective
Blond Psyllium
Bovine Cartilage
Diosmin
Wheat Bran
Witch Hazel
Hepatic encephalopathy
Possibly Effective
Branched-Chain Amino Acids
Likely Ineffective
Ornithine Ketoglutarate
Hepatic steatosis
Likely Effective
Choline
Possibly Effective
Lecithin
Hepatitis
Possibly Effective
Schisandra
Taurine
Hepatitis A
Possibly Ineffective
Phosphatidylcholine
Hepatitis B
Possibly Ineffective
Chanca Piedra
Hepatitis C
Possibly Effective
Phosphatidylcholine
Possibly Ineffective
St. John's Wort
Hereditary lactase deficiency
Possibly Effective
Soy
Hereditary sideroblastic anemia
Effective
Pyridoxine
Herpes labialis (cold sores)
Possibly Effective
Lemon Balm
Lysine
Rhubarb
Sage
Possibly Ineffective
Tannic Acid
Tea Tree Oil
Herpes simplex virus (HSV)
Possibly Effective
Sangre De Grado
Zinc
Possibly Ineffective
Echinacea
Herpes simplex virus type 2 (HSV-2)
Possibly Effective
Ginseng, Siberian
Propolis
Herpes zoster (shingles)
Possibly Effective
DMSO (Dimethylsulfoxide)
Papain
Transfer Factor
HIV
(see HIV/AIDS)
HIV transmission
Possibly Effective
Vitamin C
Possibly Ineffective
Vitamin A
HIV/AIDS
Possibly Effective
Beta Glucans
Coenzyme Q-10
Lentinan
Red Yeast
Possibly Ineffective
St. John's Wort
HIV/AIDS-related wasting
(see also AIDS-related wasting)
Possibly Effective
Glutamine
HIV/AIDS-related weight loss
Possibly Effective
Marijuana
Whey Protein
HIV-associated peripheral neuropathy
Possibly Ineffective
Capsicum
HIV-related dementia
Possibly Ineffective
Alpha-Lipoic Acid
HIV-related diarrhea
(see also AIDS-related diarrhea)
Possibly Effective
Saccharomyces Boulardii
Vitamin A
Homocystinuria
Effective
Betaine Anhydrous
Hormone replacement therapy (HRT)
Likely Effective
Progesterone
Hot flashes
(see Menopausal symptoms)
Huntington's disease
Effective
Coenzyme Q-10
Possibly Effective
Vitamin E
Hypercalcemia
Likely Effective
EDTA
Phosphate Salts
Hypercalciuria
Possibly Effective
Potassium
Rice Bran
Hypercholesterolemia
(see also Familial hypercholesterolemia)
Effective
Oat Bran
Likely Effective
Beta-Sitosterol
Blond Psyllium
Flaxseed

Hypercholesterolemia (cont.)
Likely Effective (cont.)
Oats
Red Yeast
Sitostanol
Possibly Effective
Activated Charcoal
Alfalfa
Avocado
Barley
Beta Glucans
Black Psyllium
Calcium
English Walnut
Jiaogulan
Magnesium
Olive Oil
Pectin
Policosanol
Rice Bran
Safflower
Soybean Oil
Sweet Orange
Possibly Ineffective
Amaranth
Cod Liver Oil
Guggul
Inulin
Lecithin
Red Clover

Hyperhomocysteinemia
Likely Effective
Folic Acid
Pyridoxine
Vitamin B12
Possibly Effective
N-Acetyl Cysteine

Hyperkinetic cerebral dysfunction syndrome
Possibly Effective
Pyridoxine

Hyperlipidemia
Effective
Niacin and Niacinamide
Likely Effective
Soy
Possibly Effective
Artichoke
Garlic
Green Tea
Inositol Nicotinate
Yogurt
Likely Ineffective
Kefir

Hyperlipoproteinemia
Possibly Effective
Pantethine

Hyperparathyroidism
Likely Effective
Calcium

Hyperparathyroidism-related bone loss
Possibly Effective
Vitamin D

Hypertension
Possibly Effective
Blond Psyllium
Calcium
Cod Liver Oil
Coenzyme Q-10
Fish Oils
Garlic
Magnesium
Olive Leaf
Olive Oil
Potassium
Pycnogenol
Soy
Stevia
Sweet Orange
Vitamin C
Wheat Bran
Possibly Ineffective
Oats
Vitamin E

Hyperthyroidism
Possibly Effective
L-Carnitine

Hypertriglyceridemia
Likely Effective
Cod Liver Oil
Fish Oils
Possibly Effective
Guar Gum
Inulin
Mesoglycan

Hypocalcemia
Effective
Calcium

Hypogeusia
Possibly Effective
Zinc

Hypoglycemia
Possibly Effective
Chromium

Hypokalemia
Effective
Potassium

Hypomagnesemia
Effective
Magnesium

Hypoparathyroidism
Effective
Vitamin D

Hypophosphatemia
Effective
Phosphate Salts

Hypoprothrombinemia
Effective
Vitamin K

Hypotension
Possibly Effective
Black Tea
Caffeine
Coffee

Hypothyroidism
Possibly Effective
Tiratricol

Idiopathic congestive cardiomyopathy
Possibly Effective
Forskolin

Ifosfamide (Ifex) toxicity
Possibly Effective
N-Acetyl Cysteine

IgA nephropathy
Possibly Effective
Fish Oils

Imerslund-Grasbeck disease
Effective
Vitamin B12

Infectious diarrhea
Possibly Effective
Colostrum

Infertility
Likely Effective
Progesterone
Possibly Effective
Acetyl-L-Carnitine
Chasteberry
L-Carnitine
Vitamin E

Inflammatory bladder disease
Possibly Effective
DMSO (Dimethylsulfoxide)

Inflammatory bowel disease (IBD)
Possibly Ineffective
Zinc

Influenza
Possibly Effective
Elderberry
N-Acetyl Cysteine
Possibly Ineffective
Zinc

Insomnia
Possibly Effective
Melatonin
Passionflower
Valerian

Interferon-related retinopathy
Possibly Ineffective
Vitamin C

Intermittent claudication
Possibly Effective
Ginkgo Leaf
Policosanol
Propionyl-L-Carnitine
Possibly Ineffective
Vitamin E

Internal hemorrhoids
Possibly Effective
Hesperidin

Interstitial cystitis
Effective
DMSO (Dimethylsulfoxide)
Possibly Effective
L-Arginine
Superoxide Dismutase

Intestinal bacterial overgrowth
Possibly Ineffective
Lactobacillus

CHARTS

Therapeutic Efficacy

For additional data, refer to the database.

Intestinal parasitic infection
Possibly Effective
Oregano

Intracranial hemorrhage
Possibly Effective
Vitamin E

Intracranial pressure
Possibly Effective
DMSO (Dimethylsulfoxide)

Intrahepatic cholestasis
Possibly Effective
SAMe

Intrauterine growth
Possibly Ineffective
EPA (Eicosapentaenoic Acid)

Intraventricular hemorrhage
Possibly Effective
Vitamin E

Iron absorption
Likely Effective
Vitamin C

Iron deficiency anemia
Effective
Iron

Irradiated skin
Possibly Ineffective
Pantothenic Acid

Irritable bowel syndrome (IBS)
Possibly Effective
Artichoke
Blond Psyllium
Guar Gum
Lactobacillus
Wheat Bran
Possibly Ineffective
Brahmi

Ischemic reperfusion injury
Possibly Effective
Alpha-Ketoglutarate
Coenzyme Q-10
Vitamin E

Ischemic stroke
(see also Stroke)
Possibly Effective
Calcium
Citicoline

Isolated systolic hypertension
Possibly Effective
Coenzyme Q-10

Itching
(see Pruritus)

Jet lag
Possibly Effective
Melatonin

Kidney disease
Possibly Effective
Soy

Kidney failure
(see Renal failure)

Kidney stones (nephrolithiasis)
Possibly Effective
Black Tea
IP-6
Magnesium

Kidney stones (nephrolithiasis) (cont.)
Possibly Effective (cont.)
Phosphate Salts
Pyridoxine

Labor facilitation
(see also Parturition)
Possibly Ineffective
Raspberry Leaf

Lactose intolerance
Likely Effective
Lactase
Possibly Effective
Soy
Yogurt
Possibly Ineffective
Lactobacillus

L-carnitine deficiency
Effective
L-Carnitine

Lead toxicity
Effective
EDTA
Possibly Effective
Vitamin C

Leg ulcers
Possibly Effective
Glycine

Leprosy
Possibly Effective
Zinc

Lice
Effective
Pyrethrum
Possibly Effective
Quassia

Lithium-induced side effects
Possibly Effective
Inositol

Liver disease
(see also Alcohol-related liver disease and Cirrhosis)
Possibly Effective
SAMe

Lometrexol toxicity
Possibly Ineffective
Folic Acid

Low birth weight
Possibly Effective
L-Carnitine

Lung cancer
Possibly Effective
Lycopene
Pyridoxine
Possibly Ineffective
Garlic
Selenium
Transfer Factor
Vitamin E
Likely Ineffective
Beta-Carotene
Hydrazine Sulfate
N-Acetyl Cysteine

Lymphedema
Possibly Ineffective
Diosmin
Hesperidin

Malaria
Possibly Effective
Vitamin A
Possibly Ineffective
Zinc

Male aging
Possibly Effective
Acetyl-L-Carnitine
Propionyl-L-Carnitine

Malignant melanoma
(see also Skin cancer)
Possibly Ineffective
Transfer Factor

Malnourishment-related diarrhea
Possibly Ineffective
Yogurt

Mandibular alveolitis
Possibly Effective
Bovine Cartilage

Manganese deficiency
Effective
Manganese

Mania
Possibly Effective
Branched-Chain Amino Acids

Mastalgia
Possibly Effective
Evening Primrose Oil
Possibly Ineffective
Fish Oils

Mastodynia
Possibly Effective
Progesterone

McArdle's disease
Possibly Effective
Creatine
Likely Ineffective
Ribose

Measles
Possibly Effective
Vitamin A

Melasma
Possibly Effective
Alpha Hydroxy Acids

Menopausal anxiety
Possibly Effective
Kava

Menopausal symptoms
Possibly Effective
Black Cohosh
DHEA
Flaxseed
Progesterone
Soy
Possibly Ineffective
Dong Quai
Evening Primrose Oil
Ginseng, Panax
Red Clover
Wild Yam

Therapeutic Efficacy

For additional data, refer to the database.

Menorrhagia
(see Menstrual disorders)
Menstrual disorders (amenorrhea, polymenorrhea, oligomenorrhea, menorrhagia)
Possibly Effective
Chasteberry
Mental alertness
Likely Effective
Black Tea
Caffeine
Coffee
Green Tea
Metabolic disorders
Effective
Thiamine
Methotrexate toxicity
Likely Effective
Folic Acid
Migraine headache
(see also Headache)
Effective
Caffeine
Possibly Effective
Butterbur
Coenzyme Q-10
L-Arginine
Magnesium
Olive Oil
Riboflavin
Possibly Ineffective
Fish Oils
Minor bleeding
Possibly Effective
Witch Hazel
Mitochondrial encephalomyopathies
Effective
Coenzyme Q-10
Mitral valve prolapse
Possibly Effective
Magnesium
Morning sickness
Possibly Effective
Ginger
Motion sickness
Possibly Ineffective
Ginger
Multiple sclerosis (MS)
Possibly Effective
Marijuana
Vitamin D
Multisystem organ failure
Likely Ineffective
N-Acetyl Cysteine
Muscle breakdown
Possibly Effective
Branched-Chain Amino Acids
Muscle catabolism
Possibly Effective
Alpha-Ketoglutarate
Muscle cramps
Possibly Effective
Zinc

Muscle strength
Possibly Ineffective
DHEA
Vitamin D
Muscular dystrophy
(see also Myotonic dystrophy)
Possibly Effective
Coenzyme Q-10
Creatine
Myalgia
(see also Pain)
Possibly Ineffective
Bromelain
Fish Oils
Myasthenia gravis
Possibly Effective
Huperzine A
Myoadenylate deaminase deficiency (MAD)
Possibly Effective
Ribose
Myocardial infarction (MI)
[see also Acute myocardial infarction (MI)]
Possibly Effective
Black Tea
Coenzyme Q-10
L-Carnitine
Olive Oil
Likely Ineffective
Superoxide Dismutase
Myocarditis
Possibly Effective
L-Carnitine
Myofascial pain
Possibly Ineffective
L-Tryptophan
Myotonic dystrophy
(see also Muscular dystrophy)
Possibly Ineffective
Vitamin E
Narcolepsy
Effective
Gamma-Hydroxybutyrate (GHB)
Necrotizing enterocolitis (NEC)
Possibly Effective
Bifidobacteria
L-Arginine
Nematodes
Possibly Effective
Costus Root
Neonatal apnea
Possibly Effective
Caffeine
Nephrolithiasis
(see Kidney stones)
Neural tube birth defects
Likely Effective
Folic Acid
Niacin deficiency
Effective
Niacin and Niacinamide

Nicotine withdrawal
Possibly Effective
Melatonin
Night vision
Possibly Ineffective
Bilberry
Nitrate tolerance
Possibly Effective
L-Arginine
Vitamin C
Vitamin E
Likely Ineffective
N-Acetyl Cysteine
Nodulocystic acne
Possibly Effective
Guggul
Obesity
Possibly Effective
5-HTP
Chromium
Conjugated Linoleic Acid
Diacylglycerol
Ephedra
Fish Oils
Possibly Ineffective
Garcinia
Inulin
Obsessive-compulsive disorder (OCD)
Possibly Effective
Inositol
Ocular stress
Possibly Effective
Grape Seed
Onychomycosis
Possibly Effective
Tea Tree Oil
Opiate withdrawal
Possibly Effective
Gamma-Hydroxybutyrate (GHB)
Passionflower
Oral leukoplakia
Possibly Effective
Beta-Carotene
Blue-Green Algae
Green Tea
Oral mucosal lesions
Possibly Ineffective
Vitamin E
Oral mucositis
Likely Effective
Hyaluronic Acid
Possibly Effective
German Chamomile
Glutamine
Iodine
Kaolin
Orlistat (Xenical) side effects
Possibly Effective
Blond Psyllium

Therapeutic Efficacy

For additional data, refer to the database.

Osteoarthritis
Likely Effective
Chondroitin Sulfate
Glucosamine Sulfate
SAMe
Possibly Effective
Avocado
Beta-Carotene
Bovine Cartilage
Bromelain
Camphor
Cat's Claw
Devil's Claw
DMSO (Dimethylsulfoxide)
Glucosamine Hydrochloride
Hyaluronic Acid
Niacin and Niacinamide
Rutin
Soybean Oil
Stinging Nettle
Above Ground Parts
Superoxide Dismutase
Trypsin
Vitamin C
Vitamin E
Possibly Ineffective
Bee Venom
Cod Liver Oil

Osteogenesis imperfecta
Possibly Effective
Vitamin D

Osteomalacia
Effective
Vitamin D

Osteoporosis
(see also Corticosteroid-induced osteoporosis)
Likely Effective
Calcium
Ipriflavone
Vitamin D
Possibly Effective
Evening Primrose Oil
Fish Oils
Fluoride
Magnesium
Manganese
Soy
Strontium
Possibly Ineffective
Flaxseed
Progesterone

Otitis media
Possibly Effective
Xylitol
Possibly Ineffective
Olive Oil

Ovarian cancer
Possibly Effective
Beta-Carotene
Green Tea
Lycopene
Possibly Ineffective
Black Tea

Paget's disease
Possibly Effective
Ipriflavone

Pain
(see also Myalgia)
Effective
Camphor
Procaine
Likely Effective
Capsicum
Possibly Ineffective
Phenylalanine

Painful bony metastases
Effective
Strontium

Palatal myoclonus
Possibly Effective
5-HTP

Pancreatic cancer
Possibly Effective
Folic Acid
Green Tea
Possibly Ineffective
Vitamin E

Pancreatic insufficiency
Effective
Pancreatin

Pancreatitis
Possibly Effective
Chlorophyll

Panic disorder
Possibly Effective
Inositol

Pantothenic acid deficiency
Effective
Pantothenic Acid

Parenteral nutrition
Effective
Soybean Oil

Parkinson's disease
Possibly Effective
Black Tea
Caffeine
Coenzyme Q-10
Coffee
Green Tea
Vitamin E

Paroxysmal supraventricular tachycardia
Effective
Adenosine

Parturition
(see also Labor facilitation)
Possibly Effective
Castor Oil
Possibly Ineffective
Laminaria

Pediatric congestive heart failure
Effective
Coenzyme Q-10

Pellagra
Effective
Niacin and Niacinamide

Peptic ulcers
Possibly Effective
Zinc

Periodontal disease
Likely Ineffective
Coenzyme Q-10

Periodontitis
Possibly Effective
Chitosan

Peripheral arterial disease
Possibly Effective
L-Arginine
Mesoglycan
Vitamin C
Possibly Ineffective
Garlic

Peripheral neuropathy
Possibly Effective
Alpha-Lipoic Acid

Peripheral vascular disease
Possibly Effective
Inositol Nicotinate

Peritoneal dialysis
Possibly Ineffective
Phosphatidylcholine

Pernicious anemia
Effective
Vitamin B12

Pervasive developmental disorder
Likely Ineffective
Secretin

Peyronie's disease
Possibly Effective
Acetyl-L-Carnitine

Pharyngitis
Possibly Effective
Papain

Pharyngotonsillitis
Possibly Effective
Andrographis

Phenylketonuria (PKU)
Effective
Tyrosine

Phenytoin-induced gingival hyperplasia
Possibly Effective
Folic Acid

Photoreactive keratectomy
Possibly Effective
Vitamin A
Vitamin E

Pituitary resistance to thyroid hormone (PRTH)
Likely Effective
Tiratricol

Plastic surgery
Possibly Effective
Chitosan

Pneumonia
Possibly Effective
Zinc
Likely Ineffective
Vitamin A

Therapeutic Efficacy

For additional data, refer to the database.

Poison oak and poison ivy dermatitis
Possibly Effective
Bovine Cartilage

Poisoning
Likely Effective
Activated Charcoal
Possibly Effective
Ipecac

Polycystic ovary syndrome
Possibly Effective
Inositol

Polymenorrhea
(see Menstrual disorders)

Polyneuropathy
Possibly Ineffective
St. John's Wort

Postdural puncture headache
Possibly Effective
Caffeine

Postherpetic neuralgia
Possibly Effective
DMSO (Dimethylsulfoxide)

Post-hysterectomy pain
Possibly Effective
Magnesium

Postoperative headache
Effective
Caffeine

Postoperative infection
Possibly Effective
Beta Glucans

Postoperative nausea
Possibly Effective
Peppermint Oil

Postoperative nausea and vomiting
Possibly Effective
Ginger

Post-partum complications
Possibly Effective
Beta-Carotene
Vitamin A

Post-surgery recovery
Possibly Effective
L-Arginine

Pre-eclampsia
Likely Effective
Magnesium
Possibly Effective
Vitamin C
Vitamin E
Possibly Ineffective
L-Arginine

Pregnancy-induced hypertension
Possibly Ineffective
EPA (Eicosapentaenoic Acid)

Pregnancy-induced leg cramps
Possibly Effective
Magnesium

Pregnancy-induced nausea and vomiting
Possibly Effective
Pyridoxine

Pregnancy-related complications
Possibly Effective
Beta-Carotene
Calcium
Vitamin A

Pregnancy-related gingivitis
Possibly Effective
Folic Acid

Pregnancy-related iron deficiency
Possibly Ineffective
Zinc

Premature ejaculation
Possibly Effective
Angelica Root
Cinnamon Bark
Clove Dried
Flowerbud, Leaf, Stem
Ginseng, Panax

Premenstrual dysphoric disorder (PMDD)
Possibly Effective
L-Tryptophan

Premenstrual syndrome (PMS)
Likely Effective
Calcium
Possibly Effective
Brewer's Yeast
Chasteberry
Ginkgo Leaf
Magnesium
Manganese
Pyridoxine
Vitamin E
Possibly Ineffective
Evening Primrose Oil
Progesterone

Preoperative anxiety and sedation
Possibly Effective
Melatonin

Preterm labor
Possibly Effective
Magnesium

Prickly heat
Possibly Ineffective
Tannic Acid

Prostate cancer
Possibly Effective
Beta-Carotene
Fish Oils
Garlic
Lentinan
Lycopene
Melatonin
Selenium
Soy
Strontium
Tomato
Vitamin E
Possibly Ineffective
Shiitake Mushroom

Prostatitis
Possibly Effective
Quercetin

Prurigo nodularis
Possibly Effective
Capsicum

Pruritus (itching)
(see also Anal pruritis)
Effective
Camphor

Psoriasis
Effective
Vitamin D
Possibly Effective
Aloe Gel
Bovine Cartilage
DHA (Docosahexaenoic Acid)
EPA (Eicosapentaenoic Acid)
Fish Oils
Possibly Ineffective
Zinc

Psoriatic arthritis
Possibly Ineffective
Zinc

Pyridoxine deficiency
Effective
Pyridoxine

Pyridoxine-dependent seizures
Effective
Pyridoxine

Quality of life
Possibly Ineffective
Ginseng, Panax

Radiation
Effective
Iodine

Radiation dermatitis
Possibly Ineffective
Vitamin C

Radiation-induced fibrosis
Possibly Effective
Vitamin E

Raynaud's syndrome
Possibly Effective
Fish Oils
Ginkgo Leaf

Reflex sympathetic dystrophy (RSD)
Possibly Effective
Vitamin C

Renal cell carcinoma
Effective
Shark Cartilage

Renal failure
Effective
Calcium
Possibly Effective
Chitosan

Renal osteodystrophy
Effective
Vitamin D
Possibly Effective
Ipriflavone

Renal transplant
Possibly Effective
L-Arginine

Renal transplant-related bone loss
Possibly Ineffective
Vitamin D
Respiratory congestion
Effective
Iodine
Possibly Effective
Eucalyptus Dried Leaf
Respiratory distress syndrome
[see also Acute respiratory distress syndrome (ARDS)]
Possibly Effective
Inositol
Respiratory infections
Possibly Effective
Lactobacillus
Thymus Extract
Possibly Ineffective
Vitamin E
Retinitis pigmentosa
Possibly Ineffective
Vitamin E
Retinopathy
(see also Diabetic retinopathy)
Possibly Effective
Bilberry
Pycnogenol
Retrolental fibroplasia
Possibly Effective
Vitamin E
Rheumatoid arthritis (RA)
Possibly Effective
Borage Seed Oil
Bovine Cartilage
Cat's Claw
DMSO (Dimethylsulfoxide)
Fish Oils
Olive Oil
Superoxide Dismutase
Thunder God Vine
Vitamin E
Possibly Ineffective
Creatine
Feverfew
Flaxseed Oil
Histidine
New Zealand Green-Lipped Mussel
Selenium
Zinc
Rickets
Effective
Vitamin D
Rotating shift work
Possibly Ineffective
Melatonin
Rotaviral diarrhea
Likely Effective
Lactobacillus
Possibly Effective
Bifidobacteria
Scabies
Ineffective
Pyrethrum
Scarring
Possibly Ineffective
Vitamin E
Schistosomiasis
Possibly Effective
Gotu Kola
Schizophrenia
Possibly Effective
DHEA
Glycine
Lithium
Possibly Ineffective
EPA (Eicosapentaenoic Acid)
Inositol
Likely Ineffective
Choline
Scleroderma
Possibly Ineffective
DMSO (Dimethylsulfoxide)
EDTA
Gamma Linolenic Acid
Para-Aminobenzoic Acid (PABA)
Scurvy
Possibly Effective
Acerola
Seasonal affective disorder (SAD)
Possibly Ineffective
Ginkgo Leaf
Seborrheic dermatitis
Possibly Ineffective
Biotin
Seizures
Possibly Effective
Medium Chain Triglycerides
Sexual arousal
Possibly Ineffective
DHEA
Sexual desire
Possibly Effective
Maca
Sexual dysfunction
Possibly Effective
Yohimbe
Shingles
(see Herpes zoster)
Sickle cell disease
Possibly Effective
Zinc
Sinusitis
Possibly Effective
Cowslip
Elderflower
Gentian
Sorrel
Verbena
Sjogren's syndrome
Possibly Effective
Xanthan Gum
Skin cancer
(see also Malignant melanoma)
Possibly Ineffective
Selenium
Skin flap ischemia
Possibly Effective
DMSO (Dimethylsulfoxide)
Skin infection
Effective
Iodine
Skin irritation
Possibly Effective
Sweet Almond
Witch Hazel
Skin ulceration
Possibly Effective
Honey
Sleep
Possibly Effective
Lemon Balm
Sleep deprivation
Possibly Effective
Tyrosine
Sleep-wake cycle disturbances
Likely Effective
Melatonin
Smoking cessation
Possibly Effective
L-Tryptophan
Likely Ineffective
Lobelia
Solid tumors
Possibly Effective
Melatonin
Sore throat
Possibly Effective
Slippery Elm
Spinal spasticity
Possibly Effective
Threonine
Stroke
(see also Ischemic stroke)
Possibly Effective
Fish Oils
Glycine
Magnesium
Potassium
Sweet Orange
Possibly Ineffective
Beta-Carotene
Folic Acid
Mesoglycan
Pyridoxine
Vitamin B12
Vitamin C
Likely Ineffective
Glycerol
Sulcoplasty
Possibly Effective
Propolis
Sunburn
Effective
Para-Aminobenzoic Acid (PABA)
Possibly Effective
Beta-Carotene
Melatonin

Sunburn (cont.)
Possibly Effective (cont.)
Vitamin C
Vitamin E

Surgery
Possibly Effective
EPA (Eicosapentaenoic Acid)
Glutamine

Surgical recovery
Possibly Effective
RNA and DNA

Systemic lupus erythematosus (SLE)
Possibly Effective
DHEA
Possibly Ineffective
Fish Oils

Systemic lupus erythematosus (SLE) nephritis
Possibly Effective
Flaxseed

Tanning skin
Possibly Effective
Melanotan-II

Tardive dyskinesia
Possibly Effective
Branched-Chain Amino Acids
Melatonin
Pyridoxine
Vitamin E
Possibly Ineffective
Phosphatidylcholine
Likely Ineffective
Deanol

Temporomandibular joint (TMJ) arthritis
Possibly Effective
Glucosamine Sulfate

Tension headache
Possibly Effective
Peppermint Oil
Possibly Ineffective
5-HTP

Thiamine deficiency
Effective
Thiamine

Thrombocytopenia
Possibly Effective
Melatonin

Thyroid cancer
Possibly Effective
Tiratricol

Thyroid conditions
Effective
Iodine

Tick bites
Possibly Effective
Garlic

Tinea corporis
Possibly Effective
Bitter Orange
Garlic

Tinea cruris
Possibly Effective
Bitter Orange
Garlic

Tinea pedis (athlete's foot)
Possibly Effective
Bitter Orange
Garlic
Tea Tree Oil

Tinnitus
Possibly Ineffective
Ginkgo Leaf
Zinc

Tooth retention
Possibly Effective
Calcium

Torsade de pointes
Likely Effective
Magnesium

Tracheostomy care
Effective
N-Acetyl Cysteine

Traveler's diarrhea
Possibly Effective
Bifidobacteria
Lactobacillus
Saccharomyces Boulardii
Sangre De Grado
Possibly Ineffective
Fructo-Oligosaccharides

Tuberculosis
Possibly Ineffective
Beta-Sitosterol

Tyrosinemia
Likely Effective
Vitamin C

Ulcerative colitis
Possibly Effective
Bifidobacteria
Blond Psyllium

Urinary odor
Possibly Effective
Cranberry
Possibly Ineffective
Chlorophyllin

Urinary tract infections (UTIs)
Possibly Effective
Cranberry
Dandelion Entire Plant
Uva Ursi

Urine drug tests
Possibly Ineffective
Goldenseal

Uveitis
Possibly Effective
Vitamin E

Vaginal candidiasis
Possibly Effective
Echinacea
Yogurt

Valproic acid-induced toxicities
Possibly Effective
L-Carnitine

Vasospastic angina
(see also Angina)
Possibly Effective
Magnesium

Venous insufficiency
Possibly Effective
Gotu Kola
Mesoglycan

Venous leg ulcers
Possibly Effective
Zinc

Venous stasis ulcers
Possibly Effective
Adenosine
Diosmin
Hesperidin
Mesoglycan

Vertigo
Possibly Effective
Ginger
Ginkgo Leaf

Vitamin A deficiency
Effective
Vitamin A
Possibly Effective
Zinc

Vitamin B12 deficiency
Effective
Vitamin B12

Vitamin C deficiency
Effective
Vitamin C

Vitamin E deficiency
Effective
Vitamin E

Vitiligo
Possibly Effective
Folic Acid
Phenylalanine
Picrorhiza

Vulval lichen sclerosis
Possibly Ineffective
Progesterone

Vulvovaginitis
Possibly Ineffective
Lactobacillus

Warfarin anticoagulation
Effective
Vitamin K

Water purification
Effective
Iodine

Weight loss
Possibly Effective
Caffeine
Calcium
Pyruvate
Vitamin A
Possibly Ineffective
Blue-Green Algae
Chitosan
Glycerol
Guar Gum

Weight loss (cont.)
Likely Ineffective
Tiratricol
Wilson's disease
Effective
Zinc
Wisdom tooth extraction
Possibly Ineffective
Arnica
Wound healing
Possibly Effective
Magnesium
Trypsin
Wrinkled skin
(see also Aging skin)
Likely Effective
Alpha Hydroxy Acids
Possibly Effective
Vitamin C
Zinc deficiency
Effective
Zinc

Potential Interactions Between Drugs and Natural Medicines

For details on possible interactions between natural medicines and drugs, see the listing for the specific natural medicine in the body of this database. This chart does not contain all theoretical or unknown interactions.

Drug	Natural Medicine
5-HT1 AGONISTS ("Triptans") Some drugs in this category include: Eletriptan (*Relpax*) • Naratriptan (*Amerge*) • Rizatriptan (*Maxalt*) • Sumatriptan (*Imitrex*) • Zolmitriptan (*Zomig*)	St. John's Wort
ACARBOSE (*Precose, Prandase*)	Pancreatin
ACE INHIBITORS (ACEIs) Some drugs in this category include: Captopril (*Capoten*) • Enalapril (*Vasotec*) • Lisinopril (*Prinivil, Zestril*) • Fosinopril (*Monopril*) • Moexipril (*Univasc*) • Perindopril (*Aceon*) • Quinapril (*Accupril*) • Ramipril (*Altace*) • Spirapril (*Renormax*) • Trandolapril (*Mavik*)	Capsicum • Iodine • Laminaria • Lithium • Pomegranate • Potassium
ACENOCOUMAROL (*Sintrom*)	L-Carnitine
ACETAMINOPHEN (*Tylenol*, others)	Cabbage • Glucosamine Sulfate • Vitamin C
ACETYLCHOLINESTERASE (AChE) INHIBITORS Some drugs in this category include: Donepezil (*Aricept*) • Galantamine (*Reminyl*) • Rivastigmine (*Exelon*) • Tacrine (*Cognex*)	Chinese Club Moss • Huperzine A
ACTIVATED CHARCOAL	Ipecac • N-Acetyl Cysteine
ADENOSINE (*Adenocard*)	Black Tea • Caffeine • Cocoa • Coffee • Cola Nut • Green Tea • Guarana • Mate
ALCOHOL (Ethanol)	Acacia • Baikal Skullcap • Black Tea • Butanediol (BD) • Caffeine • Calcium D-Glucarate • Coca • Coffee • Cola Nut • Gamma Butyrolactone (GBL) • Gamma-Hydroxybutyrate (GHB) • Ginseng, Siberian • Green Tea • Guarana • Hops • Indian Snakeroot • Magnolia • Mate • Red Yeast • Ribose • Tansy • Valerian
ALENDRONATE (*Fosamax*)	Coffee • Whey Protein
ALPHA-ADRENERGIC AGONISTS Some drugs in this category include: Pseudoephedrine (*Sudafed*, others) • Phenylephrine • Phenylpropanolamine	Butcher's Broom
ALPHA-ADRENERGIC ANTAGONISTS Some drugs in this category include: Phenoxybenzamine (*Dibenzyline*) • Phentolamine (*Regitine*) • Tamsulosin (*Flomax*) • Terazosin (*Hytrin*) • Prazosin (*Minipress*) • Doxazosin (*Cardura*)	Butcher's Broom
ALPRAZOLAM (*Xanax*)	Kava • St. John's Wort
ALUMINUM	Cherokee Rosehip • Rose Hip • Vitamin C
AMINOGLYCOSIDES Some drugs in this category include: Gentamicin (*Garamycin*) • Amikacin (*Amikin*) • Tobramycin (*Tobrex*)	Magnesium
AMINOLEVULINIC ACID	St. John's Wort
AMINOSALICYLIC ACID (*Paser, Teebacin, Tubasal*)	Procaine
AMIODARONE (*Cordarone*)	Iodine • Pyridoxine
AMITRIPTYLINE (*Elavil*)	St. John's Wort
AMPHETAMINES	Butanediol (BD) • Cola Nut • Gamma Butyrolactone (GBL) • Gamma-Hydroxybutyrate (GHB) • Green Tea • Guarana • Mate
ANASTROZOLE (*Arimidex*)	DHEA

CHARTS

Potential Interactions: Drug/Natural Medicine

For additional data, refer to the database.

Drug	Natural Medicine
ANESTHESIA Some drugs in this category include: Thiopental Sodium (*Pentothal*) • Methohexital Sodium (*Brevital*) • Etomidate (*Amidate*) • Ketamine (*Ketalar*) • Propofol (*Diprivan*) • Nitrous Oxide • Enflurane (*Ethrane*) • Halothane (*Fluothane*) • Methoxyflurane (*Penthrane*) • Sevoflurane (*Ultane*) • Isoflurane (*Forane*) • Desflurane (*Suprane*)	Borage Seed Oil • Cowhage • Evening Primrose Oil • Fever Bark
ANGIOTENSIN RECEPTOR BLOCKERS (ARBs) Some drugs in this category include: Candesartan (*Atacand*) • Eprosartan (*Teveten*) • Irbesartan (*Avapro*) • Losartan (*Cozaar*) • Telmisartan (*Micardis*) • Valsartan (*Diovan*)	Iodine • Potassium
ANTACIDS Some drugs in this category include: Aluminum Hydroxide (*Amphojel*, others) • Calcium Carbonate (*Tums*, others) • Aluminum and Magnesium Hydroxide (*Maalox, Mylanta*)	Aletris • Alpinia • Angelica Herb, Seed • Angelica Root • Aristolochia • Black Mustard Oil • Black Mustard Seed • Blessed Thistle • Calamus • Capsicum • Cinchona • Colombo • Cubebs • Dandelion Entire Plant • Devil's Claw • Gentian • Ginger • Goldenseal • Goldthread • Northern Prickly Ash • Peppermint Oil • Phosphate Salts • Quassia • Southern Prickly Ash • Wormwood Above Ground Parts • Yarrow
ANTIBIOTICS (see also individual listings) Some drugs in this category include: Fluoroquinolones: Ciprofloxacin (*Cipro*) • Levofloxacin (*Levequin*) • Norfloxacin (*Noroxin*) • Ofloxacin (*Floxin*) • Enoxacin (*Penetrex*) • Lomefloxacin (*Maxaquin*) • Trovafloxacin; Alatrofloxacin (*Trovan*) Penicillins: Penicillin (*Bicillin, Veetids*) • Nafcillin (*Unipen*) • Oxacillin (*Bactocill*) • Dicloxacillin (*Dynapen*) • Cloxacillin (*Cloxapen*) • Ampicillin (*Principen*) • Amoxicillin (*Amoxil*) • Amoxicillin;Potassium Clavulanate (*Augmentin*) • Ticarcillin (*Ticar*) • Ticarcillin;Clavulanate (*Timentin*) • Mezlocillin (*Mezlin*) • Piperacillin (*Pipracil*) • Piperacillin;Tazobactam (*Zosyn*) • Carbenicillin (*Geocillin*) Macrolides: Clarithromycin (*Biaxin*) • Azithromycin (*Zithromax*) • Dirithromycin (*Dynabac*) • Erythromycin Base (*E-Mycin, Ery-Tab*) • Erythromycin Ethylsuccinate (*E.E.S.*) Vancomycin (*Vancocin*) Clindamycin (*Cleocin*) Aminoglycosides: Tobramycin (*Nebcin*) • Amikacin (*Amikin*) • Kanamycin (*Kantrex*) • Gentamicin (*Garamycin*) Metronidazole (*Flagyl*) Sulfadiazine • Sulfasoxazole • Sulfamethoxazole (*Gantanol*) • Sulfamethoxazole;Trimethoprim (*Bactrim*) Nitrofurantoin (*Macrodantin*) Tetracycline (*Sumycin*) • Doxycycline (*Vibramycin*) • Minocycline (*Minocin*) Cefpodoxime (*Vantin*) • Cefaclor (*Ceclor*) • Cephalexin (*Keflex*) • Cefadroxil (*Duricef*) • Cephradine (*Velosef*) • Loracarbef (*Lorabid*) • Cefprozil (*Cefzil*) • Cefitbuten (*Cedax*) • Cefdinir (*Omnicef*) • Cephapirin (*Cefadyl*) • Cefazolin (*Ancef*) • Cefoxitin (*Mefoxin*) • Cefuroxime (*Ceftin*) • Cefonicid (*Monocid*) • Ceftriaxone (*Rocephin*) • Cefixime (*Suprax*) • Cefoperazone (*Cefobid*) • Cefotaxime (*Claforan*) • Cefotetan (*Cefotan*) • Ceftazidime (*Fortaz*) • Cefamandole (*Mandol*) • Imipenem;Cilastatin (*Primaxin*) • Aztreonam (*Azactam*)	Bifidobacteria • Lactobacillus • Soy

Potential Interactions: Drug/Natural Medicine For additional data, refer to the database.

Drug	Natural Medicine
ANTICHOLINERGIC DRUGS Some drugs in this category include: Amitriptyline (*Elavil*) • Diphenhydramine (*Benadryl*) • Cyproheptadine (*Periactin*) • Amantadine (*Symmetrel*) • Atropine;Belladonna;Scopolamine (*Donnatal*) • Clozapine (*Clozaril*) • Prochlorperazine (*Compazine*)	Angel's Trumpet • Areca • Belladonna • Calabar Bean • Chinese Club Moss • Deanol • European Mandrake • Henbane • Huperzine A • Iboga • Jimson Weed • Riboflavin (Vitamin B2) • Scopolia
ANTICOAGULANT / ANTIPLATELET DRUGS Some drugs in this category include: Ardeparin (*Normiflo*) • Dalteparin (*Fragmin*) • Danaparoid (*Orgaran*) • Enoxaparin (*Lovenox*) Heparin Antithrombin III (*Thrombate III*) Lepirudin (*Refludan*) Warfarin (*Coumadin*) • Dicumarol • Clopidogrel (*Plavix*) • Cilostazol (*Pletal*) • Dipyridamole (*Persantine*) • Ticlopidine (*Ticlid*) • Tirofiban (*Aggrastat*) • Eptifibatide (*Integrilin*) • Abciximab (*ReoPro*) • Anagrelide (*Agrylin*)	Allspice • Andrographis • Angelica Herb, Seed • Angelica Root • Arnica • Asafoetida • Bishop's Weed • Black Tea Bladderwrack • Bogbean • Boldo • Borage Seed Oil • Bromelain • Buchu • Caffeine • Capsicum • Carrageenan • Cinchona • Clove Dried Flowerbud, Leaf, Stem • Clove Oil • Cod Liver Oil • Coffee • Danshen • Deertongue • DHA (Docosahexaenoic Acid) • Dong Quai • EPA (Eicosapentaenoic Acid) • Epimedium • Evening Primrose Oil • Fenugreek • Feverfew • Fish Oils • Flaxseed • Flaxseed Oil • Forskolin • Gamma Linolenic Acid • Garlic • Ginger • Ginkgo Leaf • Ginseng, Panax • Ginseng, Siberian • Green Tea • Guarana • Guggul • Horse Chestnut • Inositol Nicotinate • IP-6 • Jiaogulan • Kudzu • Mate • Melatonin • Mesoglycan • Nattokinase • Onion • Pantethine • Parsley Leaf, Root • Pau D'arco • Policosanol • Red Clover • Reishi Mushroom • Resveratrol • Safflower • Saw Palmetto • Sea Buckthorn • Sweet Clover • Sweet Vernal Grass • Tiratricol • Turmeric • Vanadium • Vinpocetine • Vitamin E • Willow Bark • Yarrow
ANTICONVULSANTS Some drugs in this category include: Carbamazepine (*Tegretol*) • Clonazepam (*Klonopin*) • Ethosuximide (*Zarontin*) • Gabapentin (*Neurontin*) • Lamotrigine (*Lamictal*) • Levetiracetam (*Keppra*) • Methsuximide (*Celontin*) • Oxcarbazepine (*Trileptal*) • Tiagabine (*Gabitril*) • Topiramate (*Topamax*) • Valproic Acid (*Depakote*) • Zonisamide (*Zonegran*)	Butanediol (BD) • Cedar Leaf • Cedar Leaf Oil • Gamma Butyrolactone (GBL) • Gamma-Hydroxybutyrate (GHB) • Ginkgo Seed • Glutamine • Lithium • Sage • Wormwood Above Ground Parts
ANTIDEPRESSANTS Some drugs in this category include: Bupropion (*Wellbutrin*) Nefazodone (*Serzone*) <u>Tetracyclics</u>: Maprotiline (*Ludiomil*) • Mirtazapine (*Remeron*) Trazodone (*Desyrel*) <u>Monoamine Oxidase Inhibitors</u>: Phenelzine (*Nardil*) • Tranylcypromine (*Parnate*) • Isocarboxazid (*Marplan*) <u>Selective Serotonin Reuptake Inhibitors:</u> Citalopram (*Celexa*) • Fluoxetine (*Prozac*) • Fluvoxamine (*Luvox*) • Paroxetine (*Paxil*) • Sertraline (*Zoloft*) • Venlafaxine (*Effexor*) <u>Tricyclics:</u> Amitriptyline (*Elavil*) • Clomipramine (*Anafranil*) • Amoxapine (*Asendin*) • Desipramine (*Norpramin*) • Doxepin (*Sinequan*) • Imipramine (*Tofranil*) • Nortriptyline (*Pamelor*)	5-HTP • Ergot • Hawaiian Baby Woodrose • Lithium • L-Tryptophan • SAMe • St. John's Wort
ANTIDIABETES DRUGS Some drugs in this category include: Insulin (*Humulin, Novolin, Lantus, Humalog, Novolog*) <u>Biguanides:</u> Metformin (*Glucophage*) <u>Meglitinides:</u> Repaglinide (*Prandin*) • Nateglinide (*Starlix*) <u>Alpha-Glucosidase Inhibitors:</u> Acarbose (*Precose*) • Miglitol (*Glyset*)	Ackee • Agrimony • Aloe Gel • Alpha-Lipoic Acid • Annatto • Baikal Skullcap • Banaba • Barley • Bean Pod • Bilberry • Bitter Melon • Black Mulberry • Black Psyllium • Black Tea • Blond Psyllium • Blue Cohosh • Blueberry • Branched-Chain Amino Acids • Bugleweed • Burdock • Caffeine • Cassia Auriculata • Cassia Cinnamon • Chanca Piedra • Chinese Cucumber Root • Cinnamon Bark • Cocoa • Coffee • Cola Nut • Corn Silk • Country Mallow • Cowhage • Cumin • Damiana • Dandelion Entire Plant • Devil's Claw • Devil's Club • Ephedra • Eucalyptus Dried Leaf • Fenugreek • Flaxseed •

Potential Interactions: Drug/Natural Medicine

For additional data, refer to the database.

Drug	Natural Medicine
ANTIDIABETES DRUGS (cont.) Sulfonylureas: Chlorpropamide (*Diabinese*) • Glimepiride (*Amaryl*) • Glipizide (*Glucotrol*) • Glyburide (*DiaBeta, Glynase, Micronase*) • Tolbutamide (*Orinase*) Thiazolidinediones: Pioglitazone (*Actos*) • Rosiglitazone (*Avandia*)	Fo-Ti • Ginger • Ginseng, American • Ginseng, Panax • Ginseng, Siberian • Glucomannan • Glucosamine Hydrochloride • Glucosamine Sulfate • Goat's Rue • Green Tea • Guar Gum • Guarana • Gymnema • Horse Chestnut • Hydrazine Sulfate • Inositol Nicotinate • Juniper • Kudzu • Lycium • Madagascar Periwinkle • Maitake Mushroom • Marshmallow • Mate • Melatonin • Myrrh • N-Acetyl Glucosamine • Niacin and Niacinamide • Olive Leaf • Olive Oil • Onion • Ribose • Sage • Solomon's Seal • Spinach • Stevia • Stinging Nettle Above Ground Parts • Tiratricol • Vanadium • Xanthan Gum
ANTIFUNGALS Some drugs in this category include: Ciclopirox (*Loprox*) • Griseofulvin (*Grisactin, Gris-PEG*) • Terbinafine (*Lamisil*) • Clotrimazole (*Lotrimin, Mycelex*) • Fluconazole (*Diflucan*) • Itraconazole (*Sporanox*) • Ketoconazole (*Nizoral*) • Miconazole (*Desenex, Monistat*) • Terconazole (*Terazol*) • Amphotericin B (*Amphotec*) • Nystatin (*Mycostatin*)	Brewer's Yeast • Saccharomyces Boulardii
ANTIGOUT DRUGS Some drugs in this category include: Allopurinol (*Zyloprim*) • Probenecid (*Benemid*) • Colchicine	Adenosine
ANTIHYPERTENSIVE DRUGS Some drugs in this category include: Beta-Adrenergic Blockers: Atenolol (*Tenormin*) • Labetalol (*Normodyne*) • Metoprolol (*Lopressor*) • Nadolol (*Corgard*) • Propranolol (*Inderal*) Calcium Channel Blockers: Amlodipine (*Norvasc*) • Diltiazem (*Cardizem*) • Felodipine (*Plendil*) • Nifedipine (*Adalat, Procardia*) • Verapamil (*Calan*) Antiadrenergic Agents: Reserpine • Methyldopa (*Aldomet*) • Clonidine (*Catapres*) • Guanfacine (*Tenex*) • Guanabenz (*Wytensin*) Alpha-1 Adrenergic Blockers: Doxazosin (*Cardura*) • Prazosin (*Minipress*) • Terazosin (*Hytrin*) Angiotensin II Receptor Antagonists: Irbesartan (*Avapro*) • Losartan (*Cozaar*) • Valsartan (*Diovan*) Angiotensin-Converting Enzyme Inhibitors: Benazepril (*Lotensin*) • Captopril (*Capoten*) • Enalapril (*Vasotec*) • Fosinopril (*Monopril*) • Lisinopril (*Prinivil*) • Quinapril (*Accupril*) • Ramipril (*Altace*)	Andrographis • Asafoetida • Betony • Blue Cohosh • Carrageenan • Cat's Claw • Cod Liver Oil • Coenzyme Q-10 • Coltsfoot • Corn Silk • Devil's Claw • DHA (Docosahexaenoic Acid) • EPA (Eicosapentaenoic Acid) • Epimedium • European Mistletoe • Fish Oils • Ginger • Goldenseal • L-Arginine • Licorice • Lycium • Olive Leaf • Periwinkle • Pomegranate • Reishi Mushroom • Stevia • Stinging Nettle Above Ground Parts • Theanine • Verbena • Wild Carrot • Yohimbe
ANTIMITOTIC CHEMOTHERAPY Some drugs in this category include: Etoposide (*VePesid*) • Teniposide (*Vumon*) • Vinblastine (*Velban*) • Vincristine (*Oncovin*) • Vinorelbine (*Navelbine*)	Glucosamine Hydrochloride • Glucosamine Sulfate
ANTIPSYCHOTIC DRUGS Some drugs in this category include: Benzisoxazoles: Risperidone (*Risperdal*) Dibenzapines: Clozapine (*Clozaril*) • Loxapine (*Loxitane*) • Olanzapine (*Zyprexa*) • Quetiapine (*Seroquel*) • Ziprasidone (*Geodon*) Thioanthenes: Thiothixene (*Navane*) Phenylbutylpiperadines: Haloperidol (*Haldol*) Phenothiazines: Chlorpromazine (*Thorazine*) • Fluphenazine (*Prolixin*) • Mesoridazine (*Serentil*) • Perphenazine (*Trilafon*) • Thioridazine (*Mellaril*) • Trifluoperazine (*Stelazine*)	Butanediol (BD) • Chasteberry • Cowhage • Gamma Butyrolactone (GBL) • Gamma-Hydroxybutyrate (GHB) • Ginseng, American • Ginseng, Panax • Green Tea • Indian Snakeroot • Phenylalanine

Potential Interactions: Drug/Natural Medicine
For additional data, refer to the database.

Drug	Natural Medicine
ANTITHYROID DRUGS Some drugs in this category include: Methimazole (*Tapazole*) • Potassium Iodide (*SSKI, Pima*) • Propylthiouracil; PTU	Iodine
AROMATASE INHIBITORS Some drugs in this category include: Anastrozole (*Arimidex*) • Exemestane (*Aromasin*) • Letrozole (*Femara*)	Chrysin
ARTEMETHER (*Artenam, Paluther*)	Grapefruit • Grapefruit Seed Extract
ASPIRIN	Beer • Cherokee Rosehip • Kudzu • Meadowsweet • Onion • Parsley Leaf, Root • Ribose • Rose Hip • Vitamin C • Willow Bark • Wine • Wintergreen Oil
BARBITURATES Some drugs in this category include: Pentobarbital (*Nembutal*) • Phenobarbital • Primidone (*Mysoline*) • Secobarbital (*Seconal*)	Beer • Cedarwood • Ginger • Indian Snakeroot • Lavender • Magnolia • Marijuana • Passionflower • St. John's Wort • Wine • Yarrow
BENZODIAZEPINES Some drugs in this category include: Alprazolam (*Xanax*) • Lorazepam (*Ativan*) • Clonazepam (*Klonopin*) • Clorazepate (*Tranxene*) • Chlordiazepoxide (*Librium*) • Diazepam (*Valium*) • Estazolam (*Prosom*) • Flurazepam (*Dalmane*) • Midazolam (*Versed*) • Oxazepam (*Serax*) • Quazepam (*Doral*) • Triazolam (*Halcion*) • Temazepam (*Restoril*)	Ashwagandha • Baikal Skullcap • Beer • Butanediol (BD) • Gamma Butyrolactone (GBL) • Gamma-Hydroxybutyrate (GHB) • German Chamomile • Grapefruit • Grapefruit Seed Extract • L-Tryptophan • Magnolia • Melatonin • Valerian • Wine
BETA-ADRENERGIC AGONISTS Some drugs in this category include: Albuterol (*Ventolin*) • Metaproterenol (*Alupent*) • Terbutaline (*Brethine*) • Isoproterenol (*Isuprel*)	Cocoa
BETA-CAROTENE (*Solatene*)	Pectin
BISPHOSPHONATES Some drugs in this category include: Alendronate (*Fosamax*) • Etidronate (*Didronel*) • Pamidronate (*Aredia*) • Risedronate (*Actonel*) • Tiludronate (*Skelid*)	Calcium • Dolomite • Iron • Magnesium
BUSPIRONE (*BuSpar*)	Ginkgo Leaf • Grapefruit • Grapefruit Seed Extract
CAFFEINE (*NoDoz, Stay Alert, Vivarin*)	Ginseng, Panax • Grapefruit • Grapefruit Seed Extract • Melatonin
CALCIUM CHANNEL BLOCKERS Some drugs in this category include: Amlodipine (*Norvasc*) • Diltiazem (*Cardizem*) • Felodipine (*Plendil*) • Isradipine (*DynaCirc*) • Nicardipine (*Cardene*) • Nifedipine (*Procardia, Adalat*) • Nisoldipine (*Sular*) • Verapamil (*Calan*)	Calcium • Forskolin • Grapefruit • Grapefruit Seed Extract • Hawthorn • Lithium • Magnesium • Pangamic Acid • Stevia
CALCIUM SUPPLEMENTS (*Citracal, Caltrate, Os-Cal, Titrilac*)	Lily-of-the-Valley • Lysine • Oleander • Pheasant's Eye • Squill • Strophanthus • Wallflower
CARBAMAZEPINE (*Tegretol*)	Adenosine • Black Psyllium • Blond Psyllium • Cassia Auriculata • Cinchona • Grapefruit • Grapefruit Seed Extract
CARBIDOPA (*Lodosyn*)	5-HTP
CARVEDILOL (*Coreg*)	Grapefruit • Grapefruit Seed Extract
CEFAMANDOLE (*Mandol*)	Beer • Wine
CEFOPERAZONE (*Cefobid*)	Beer • Wine
CELIPROLOL (*Celicard*)	Sweet Orange
CHEMOTHERAPY Some drugs in this category include: Alkyl Sulfonates: Busulfan (*Myleran*) Triazines: Dacarbazine (*DTIC-Dome*) Nitrogen Mustards: Chlorambucil (*Leukeran*) • Cyclophosphamide (*Cytoxan*) • Ifosfamide (*Ifex*) • Melphalan (*Alkeran*)	Alpha-Lipoic Acid • Coenzyme Q-10 • Glutamine • N-Acetyl Glucosamine • Vitamin C (Ascorbic Acid) • Vitamin E

CHARTS

Potential Interactions: Drug/Natural Medicine

For additional data, refer to the database.

Drug	Natural Medicine
CHEMOTHERAPY (cont.) Nitrosoureas: Carmustine, BCNU (*Gliadel*) • Lomustine (*CeeNu*) • Streptozocin (*Zanosar*) Platinum Coordination Complex: Carboplatin (*Paraplatin*) • Cisplatin (*Platinol*) Hydroxyurea (*Hydrea*) Folic Acid Analogs: Methotrexate (*Rheumatrex*) Pyrimidine Analogs: Cytarabine ARA-C (*Cytosar-U*) • Fluorouracil, 5-FU (*Efudex*) • Gemcitabine (*Gemzar*) Purine Analogs: Cladribine (*Leustatin*) • Fludarabine (*Fludara*) • Mercaptopurine (*Purinethol*) • Pentostatin (*Nipent*) • Thioguanine Vinca Alkaloids: Vinblastine (*Velban*) • Vincristine (*Oncovin*) Taxoids: Paclitaxel (*Taxol*) • Docetaxel (*Taxotere*) Anthracyclines: Daunorubicin (*DaunoXome*) • Doxorubicin (*Adriamycin*) • Idarubicin (*Idamycin*) • Valrubicin (*Valstar*)	
CHLORAL HYDRATE (*Aquachloral*)	Clary Sage • Lavender
CHLORAMPHENICOL (*Chloromycetin*)	Dibencozide • Iron • Vitamin B12
CHLORPROPAMIDE (*Diabinese*)	Beer • Prickly Pear Cactus • Solomon's Seal • Wine
CHLORZOXAZONE (*Parafon Forte, Paraflex*)	Watercress
CHOLESTYRAMINE (*Questran*)	Phosphate Salts • Tiratricol
CHOLINE MAGNESIUM TRISALICYLATE (*Trilisate*)	Cherokee Rosehip • Meadowsweet • Ribose • Rose Hip • Vitamin C • Willow Bark
CHOLINERGIC DRUGS Some drugs in this category include: Bethanechol (*Urecholine*) • Echothiophate (*Phospholine Iodide*) • Neostigmine (*Prostigmin*) • Physostigmine (*Antilirium*) • Pyridostigmine (*Mestinon*) • Succinylcholine (*Anectine*)	Areca • Chinese Club Moss • Huperzine A • Iboga
CIMETIDINE (*Tagamet*)	Black Tea • Cocoa • Coffee • Cola Nut • Green Tea • Guarana • Mate
CIPROFLOXACIN (*Cipro*)	Fennel Fruit, Seed • Yogurt
CISAPRIDE (*Propulsid*)	Beer • Grapefruit • Grapefruit Seed Extract • Wine
CISPLATIN (*Platinol-AQ*)	Zinc
CLOMIPRAMINE (*Anafranil*)	Grapefruit • Grapefruit Seed Extract
CLONIDINE (*Catapres*)	Yohimbe
CLOZAPINE (*Clozaril*)	Black Tea • Caffeine • Cocoa • Coffee • Cola Nut • Glycine • Green Tea • Guarana • Hawaiian Baby Woodrose • Mate
CNS DEPRESSANTS Some drugs in this category include: Secobarbital (*Seconal*) • Pentobarbital (*Nembutal*) • Clonazepam (*Klonopin*) • Diazepam (*Valium*) Midazolam (*Versed*) • Zolpidem (*Ambien*) • Zaleplon (*Sonata*) • Hydroxyzine (*Atarax*) • Temazepam (*Restoril*) • Flurazepam (*Dalmane*) • Triazolam (*Halcion*) • Lorazepam (*Ativan*) • Estazolam (*Prosom*) • Secobarbital (*Seconal*) • Phenobarbital (*Luminal*)	Ashwagandha • Baikal Skullcap • Beer • Bitter Almond • Butanediol (BD) • Calamus • Calendula • California Poppy • Capsicum • Catnip • Celery • Cowslip • Elecampane • Gamma Butyrolactone (GBL) • Gamma-Hydroxybutyrate (GHB) • German Chamomile • Ginseng, Siberian • Goldenseal • Gotu Kola • Hawthorn • Hops • Hydrazine Sulfate • Jamaican Dogwood • Kava • Lavender • L-Tryptophan • Lemon Balm • Magnolia • Marijuana • Marsh Tea • Melatonin • Motherwort • Passionflower • Sage • Sassafras • Shepherd's Purse • Stinging Nettle Above Ground Parts • Sweet Bay • Valerian • Wild Lettuce • Wine • Yerba Mansa
COCAINE	Capsicum • Cola Nut • Green Tea • Guarana • Mate

Potential Interactions: Drug/Natural Medicine

For additional data, refer to the database.

Drug	Natural Medicine
COLCHICINE	Autumn Crocus
COLESTIPOL (*Colestid*)	Phosphate Salts
CONTRACEPTIVE DRUGS Some drugs in this category include: Ethinyl Estradiol and Levonorgestrel (*Alesse, Levlen, Triphasil*, others) • Ethinyl Estradiol and Norethindrone (*Brevicon, Demulen, Loestrin, Ortho Novum*, others)	Alfalfa • Anise • Black Tea • Caffeine • Chasteberry • Cocoa • Coffee • Cola Nut • Fennel Fruit, Seed • Fish Oils • Garlic • Green Tea • Guarana • Kudzu • Mate • Melatonin • Red Clover • Saw Palmetto • St. John's Wort
CORTICOSTEROIDS Some drugs in this category include: Beclomethasone (*Beclovent*) • Betamethasone (*Valisone*) • Budesonide (*Rhinocort*) • Cortisone (*Cortone*) • Dexamethasone (*Decadron*) • Fludrocortisone (*Florinef*) • Flunisolide (*Aerobid*) • Fluocinonide (*Lidex*) • Fluticasone (*Flovent*) • Hydrocortisone (*Cortef*) • Methylprednisolone (*Medrol*) • Prednisolone (*Prelone*) • Prednisone (*Orasone, Deltasone*) • Triamcinolone (*Kenalog*)	Alder Buckthorn • Aloe Latex • Butternut • Cascara • Castor Oil • Cesium • Corn Silk • DHEA • Gamboge • Horsetail • Licorice • Lily-of-the-Valley • Pheasant's Eye • Rhubarb • Squill • Strophanthus • Wallflower
CORTISONE (*Cortisone Acetate*)	Para-Aminobenzoic Acid (PABA)
CYCLOPHOSPHAMIDE (*Cytoxan*)	Astragalus • Cordyceps
CYCLOSPORINE (*Neoral, Sandimmune*)	Garlic • Grapefruit • Grapefruit Seed Extract • Peppermint Oil • Red Yeast • St. John's Wort • Wine
CYPROHEPTADINE (*Periactin*)	Hawaiian Baby Woodrose
CYTOCHROME P450 1A1 (CYP1A1) SUBSTRATES Some drugs in this category include: Chlorzoxazone • Theophylline • Bufuralol	Nutmeg and Mace
CYTOCHROME P450 1A2 (CYP1A2) SUBSTRATES Some drugs in this category include: Clozapine (*Clozaril*) • Cyclobenzaprine (*Flexeril*) • Fluvoxamine (*Luvox*) • Haloperidol (*Haldol*) • Imipramine (*Tofranil*) • Mexiletine (*Mexitil*) • Olanzapine (*Zyprexa*) • Pentazocine (*Talwin*) • Propranolol (*Inderal*) • Tacrine (*Cognex*) • Theophylline • Zileuton (*Zyflo*) • Zolmitriptan (*Zomig*)	Cabbage • Chrysin • Diindolylmethane • Ginkgo Leaf • Ginseng, Siberian • Grape Fruit, Skin • Indole-3-Carbinol • Ipriflavone • Kava • Methoxylated Flavones • Nutmeg and Mace • St. John's Wort
CYTOCHROME P450 2B1 (CYP2B1) SUBSTRATES	Nutmeg and Mace
CYTOCHROME P450 2B2 (CYP2B2) SUBSTRATES	Nutmeg and Mace
CYTOCHROME P450 2B6 (CYP2B6) SUBSTRATES Some drugs in this category include: Ketamine (*Ketalar*) • Phenobarbital (*Luminal*) • Orphenadrine (*Norflex*) • Secobarbital (*Seconal*) • Dexamethasone (*Decadron*)	Licorice
CYTOCHROME P450 2C19 (CYP2C19) SUBSTRATES Some drugs in this category include: Amitriptyline (*Elavil*) • Clomipramine (*Anafranil*) • Cyclophosphamide (*Cytoxan*) • Diazepam (*Valium*) • Lanzoprazole (*Prevacid*) • Omeprazole (*Prilosec*) • Lansoprazole (*Protonix*) • Phenytoin (*Dilantin*) • Phenobarbital (*Luminal*)	Kava
CYTOCHROME P450 2C9 (CYP2C9) SUBSTRATES Some drugs in this category include: Celecoxib (*Celebrex*) • Diclofenac (*Voltaren*) • Fluvastatin (*Lescol*) • Glipizide (*Glucotrol*) • Ibuprofen (*Advil, Motrin*) • Irbesartan (*Avapro*) • Losartan (*Cozaar*) • Phenytoin (*Dilantin*) • Piroxicam (*Feldene*) • Tamoxifen (*Nolvadex*) • Tolbutamide (*Tolinase*) • Torsemide (*Demadex*) • Warfarin (*Coumadin*)	Cranberry • Ginkgo Leaf • Ginseng, Siberian • Ipriflavone • Kava • Lycium • Milk Thistle • St. John's Wort
CYTOCHROME P450 2D6 (CYP2D6) SUBSTRATES Some drugs in this category include: Amitriptyline (*Elavil*) • Codeine • Desipramine (*Norpramin*) • Flecainide (*Tambocor*) • Haloperidol (*Haldol*) • Imipramine (*Tofranil*) • Metoprolol (*Lopressor, Toprol XL*) • Ondansetron (*Zofran*) • Paroxetine (*Paxil*) • Risperidone (*Risperdal*) • Tramadol (*Ultram*) • Venlafaxine (*Effexor*)	Ginkgo Leaf • Ginseng, Panax • Ginseng, Siberian • Kava
CYTOCHROME P450 3A4 (CYP3A4) INDUCERS Some drugs in this category include: Aminoglutethimide (*Cytadren*) • Aprepitant (*Emend*) • Carbamazepine (*Tegretol*) • Dexamethasone (*Dexone, Hexadrol*) • Efavirenz (*Sustiva*) • Ethosuximide (*Zarontin*) •	Comfrey

CHARTS

Potential Interactions: Drug/Natural Medicine

For additional data, refer to the database.

Drug	Natural Medicine
CYTOCHROME P450 3A4 (CYP3A4) INDUCERS (cont.) Glucocorticoids • Glutethimide (*Doriden*) • Griseofulvin (*Fulvicin, Grisactin*) • Modafinil (*Provigil*) • Nafcillin (*Nallpen, Unipen*) • Nevirapine (*Viramune*) • Oxcarbazepine (*Trileptal*) • Phenobarbital (*Luminal*) • Phenytoin (*Dilantin, Phenytek*) • Primidone (*Mysoline*) • Rifabutin (*Mycobutin*) • Rifampin (*Rifadin, Rimactane*) • Rifapentine (*Priftin*)	
CYTOCHROME P450 3A4 (CYP3A4) INHIBITORS Some drugs in this category include: Clarithromycin (*Biaxin*) • Erythromycin • Itraconazole • Ketoconazole • Cimetidine • Nefazodone (*Serzone*) • Indinavir (*Crixivan*) • Nelfinavir (*Viracept*) • Saquinavir (*Invirase*)	Ergot • Red Yeast
CYTOCHROME P450 3A4 (CYP3A4) SUBSTRATES Some drugs in this category include: Alprazolam (*Xanax*) • Amlodipine (*Norvasc*) • Clarithromycin (*Biaxin*) • Cyclosporine (*Sandimmune*) • Erythromycin • Lovastatin (*Mevacor*) • Ketoconazole (*Nizoral*) • Itraconazole (*Sporanox*) • Fexofenadine (*Allegra*) • Triazolam (*Halcion*) • Verapamil (*Calan, Isoptin*)	American Elder • Bishop's Weed • Bitter Orange • Cat's Claw • DHEA • Echinacea • Garlic • German Chamomile • Ginkgo Leaf • Ginseng, Siberian • Goldenseal • Grapefruit • Grapefruit Seed Extract • Kava • Licorice • Lime Fruit, Peel • Milk Thistle • Peppermint Oil • Red Clover • Resveratrol • St. John's Wort • Valerian • Wild Cherry
DAPSONE (*Avlosulfon*)	Para-Aminobenzoic Acid (PABA)
DEXAMETHASONE (*Decadron*)	Country Mallow • Ephedra
DEXTROMETHORPHAN (*Robitussin DM,* and others)	5-HTP • Bitter Orange • Ergot • Grapefruit • Hawaiian Baby Woodrose • Lithium • L-Tryptophan • SAMe • St. John's Wort
DIGOXIN (*Lanoxin*)	Alder Buckthorn • Aloe Latex • Apple Cider Vinegar • Black Hellebore • Black Psyllium • Black Root • Blond Psyllium • Blue Flag • Butternut • Calotropis • Canadian Hemp • Cascara • Castor Oil • Cereus • Colocynth • Danshen • Digitalis • European Buckthorn • Fo-Ti • Gamboge • Ginseng, Siberian • Gossypol • Greater Bindweed • Hawthorn • Hedge Mustard • Horsetail • Indian Snakeroot • Jalap • Khella • Laminaria • Licorice • Lily-of-the-Valley • Manna • Mexican Scammony Root • Oleander • Pangamic Acid • Pectin • Pheasant's Eye • Pleurisy Root • Procaine • Quassia • Rhubarb • Sarsaparilla • Senna • Squill • St. John's Wort • Strophanthus • Swamp Milkweed • Uzara • Wahoo • Wallflower • Wheat Bran • Yellow Dock
DILTIAZEM (*Cardizem*)	Guggul
DIPYRIDAMOLE (*Persantine*)	Adenosine • Black Tea • Caffeine • Cocoa • Coffee • Cola Nut • Green Tea • Guarana • Mate
DISULFIRAM (*Antabuse*)	Beer • Black Tea • Caffeine • Cocoa • Coffee • Cola Nut • Green Tea • Guarana • Kombucha Tea • Marijuana • Mate • Wine
DIURETIC DRUGS Some drugs in this category include: Thiazides: Indapamide (*Lozol*) • Chlorothiazide (*Diuril*) • Hydrochlorothiazide (*Esidrix, Hydrodiuril,* others) • Chlorthalidone (*Hygroton*) • Metolazone (*Zaroxolyn*) Loop Diuretics: Bumetanide (*Bumex*) • Ethacrynic Acid (*Edecrin*) • Furosemide (*Lasix*) • Torsemide (*Demadex*)	Alder Buckthorn • Aloe Latex • Apple Cider Vinegar • Birch • Black Hellebore • Black Root • Bladderwrack • Blue Flag • Butternut • Calotropis • Canadian Hemp • Cascara • Castor Oil • Cesium • Colocynth • Corn Silk • Cowslip • Digitalis • EDTA • European Buckthorn • Figwort • Fo-Ti • Gamboge • Goldenrod • Gossypol • Greater Bindweed • Hedge Mustard • Horsetail • Indian Snakeroot • Jalap • Juniper • Licorice • Lily-of-the-Valley • Lovage • Manna • Mexican Scammony Root • Oleander • Parsley Leaf, Root • Parsley Seed • Pheasant's Eye • Pleurisy Root • Podophyllum • Quassia • Rhubarb • Senna • Squill • Stone Root • Strophanthus • Swamp Milkweed • Uzara • Wahoo • Wallflower • Yellow Dock
DOPAMINE AGONISTS Some drugs in this category include: Bromocriptine (*Parlodel*) • Carbidopa (*Lodosyn*) • Carbidopa;Levodopa (*Sinemet*) • Pergolide (*Permax*) • Pramipexole (*Mirapex*) • Ropinirole (*Requip*)	Black Horehound • Chasteberry

CHARTS

Potential Interactions: Drug/Natural Medicine	For additional data, refer to the database.
Drug	**Natural Medicine**
EPHEDRINE	Black Tea • Caffeine • Coffee • Cola Nut • Green Tea • Guarana • Indian Snakeroot • Mate
ERGOT DERIVATIVES Some drugs in this category include: Bromocriptine (*Parlodel*) • Caffeine;Ergotamine (*Cafergot*) • Dihydroergotamine (*D.H.E.*) • Ergotamine (*Ergostat*) • Methylergonovine (*Methergine*) • Methysergide (*Sansert*)	Country Mallow • Ephedra • Ergot
ERGOTAMINE (*Ergomar*)	Cocoa
ERYTHROMYCIN (*E.E.S., E-Mycin, PCE*)	Beer • Grapefruit • Wine
ESTRADIOL	Vitamin C
ESTROGENS (*Estrace, Estratest, Menogen, Ogen, Premarin*)	Acerola • Alfalfa • Androstenediol • Androstenedione • Anise • Black Tea • Boron • Caffeine • Calcium • Chasteberry • Cherokee Rosehip • Cocoa • Coffee • Cola Nut • Dolomite • Fennel Fruit, Seed • Grapefruit • Grapefruit Seed Extract • Green Tea • Guarana • Kudzu • Licorice • Mate • Milk Thistle • Pleurisy Root • Pregnenolone • Progesterone • Red Clover • Rose Hip • Saw Palmetto • Soy • Wild Carrot
ETHACRYNIC ACID (*Edecrin*)	Licorice
ETOPOSIDE (*VePesid*)	Grapefruit
EXEMESTANE (*Aromasin*)	DHEA
EZETIMIBE (*Zetia*)	Beta-Sitosterol
FELODIPINE (*Plendil*)	Bitter Orange • Wine
FENFLURAMINE (*Pondimin*)	St. John's Wort
FEXOFENADINE (*Allegra*)	Apple • Grapefruit • St. John's Wort • Sweet Orange
FLUCONAZOLE (*Diflucan*)	Black Tea • Caffeine • Cocoa • Coffee • Cola Nut • Green Tea • Guarana • Mate
FLUMAZENIL (*Romazicon*)	Melatonin
FLUOXETINE (*Prozac*)	Ginkgo Leaf (Ginkgo Leaf Extract) • Marijuana
FLUPHENAZINE (*Prolixin*)	Acerola • Cherokee Rosehip • Rose Hip • Vitamin C
FLUVOXAMINE (*Luvox*)	Caffeine • Coffee • Cola Nut • Green Tea • Guarana • Mate • Melatonin
FOSPHENYTOIN (*Cerebyx*)	Folic Acid
FULVESTRANT (*Faslodex*)	DHEA
FUROSEMIDE (*Lasix*)	Germanium • Ginseng, Panax • Licorice
GEMFIBROZIL (*Lopid*)	Red Yeast
GLUCURONIDATED DRUGS Some drugs in this category include: Acetaminophen (*Tylenol*) • Estrogens (*Estrace, Premarin*, others) and Oral Contraceptives • Entacapone (*Comtan*) • Irinotecan (*Camptosar*) • Atorvastatin (*Lipitor*) • Diazepam (*Valium*) • Digoxin • Lamotrigine (*Lamictal*) • Lorazepam (*Ativan*) • Lovastatin (*Mevacor*) • Meprobamate • Morphine • Oxazepam (*Serax*)	Cabbage • Calcium D-Glucarate • Chrysin • Milk Thistle
GRISEOFULVIN (*Fulvicin*)	Beer • Wine
GUANABENZ (*Wytensin*)	Yohimbe
GUANETHIDINE (*Ismelin*)	Cowhage
H2-BLOCKERS Some drugs in this category include: Famotidine (*Pepcid*) • Ranitidine (*Zantac*) • Nixatidine (*Axid*) • Cimetidine (*Tagamet*)	Aletris • Alpinia • Angelica Herb, Seed • Angelica Root • Aristolochia • Beer • Black Mustard Oil • Black Mustard Seed • Blessed Thistle • Calamus • Capsicum • Cinchona • Colombo • Cubebs • Dandelion Entire Plant • Devil's Claw • Gentian •

CHARTS

Potential Interactions: Drug/Natural Medicine

For additional data, refer to the database.

Drug	Natural Medicine
H2-BLOCKERS (cont.)	Ginger • Goldenseal • Goldthread • Northern Prickly Ash • Peppermint Oil • Quassia • Southern Prickly Ash • Wine • Wormwood Above Ground Parts • Yarrow
HALOPERIDOL (*Haldol*)	Butanediol (BD) • Gamma Butyrolactone (GBL) • Gamma-Hydroxybutyrate (GHB) • Scotch Broom Herb
HEPARIN	Vitamin C
HEPATOTOXIC DRUGS Some drugs in this category include: Amphotericin B (*Fungizone*) • Azathioprine (*Imuran*) • Carbamazepine (*Tegretol*) • Disulfiram (*Antabuse*) • Felbamate (*Felbatol*) • Flutamide (*Eulexin*) • Hydroxychloroquine (*Plaquenil*) • Indinavir (*Crixivan*) • Interferon (*Roferon, Intron, Wellferon*) • Itraconazole (*Sporanox*) • Leflunomide (*Arava*) • Methotrexate (*Rheumatrex*) • Procainamide (*Procan*) • Rosiglitazone (*Avandia*) • Stavudine, d4T (*Zerit*) • Tacrine (*Cognex*) • Terbinafine (*Lamisil*) • Ticlopidine (*Ticlid*) • Tolcapone (*Tasmar*) • Zalcitabine, ddC (*Hivid*)	Beer • Bishop's Weed • Black Cohosh • Borage Flower, Dried Above Ground Parts • Chaparral • Comfrey • Kava • Khella • Sweet Clover • Vitamin A • Wine
HEXOBARBITAL	Greek Sage
HEXOBARBITONE	Clary Sage
HMG-CoA REDUCTASE INHIBITORS ("Statins") Some drugs in this category include: Atorvastatin (*Lipitor*) • Fluvastatin (*Lescol*) • Lovastatin (*Mevacor*) • Pravastatin (*Pravachol*) • Simvastatin (*Zocor*)	Beta-Carotene • Grapefruit • Grapefruit Seed Extract • Inositol Nicotinate • Niacin and Niacinamide • Red Yeast • Selenium • Vitamin C • Vitamin E
IBUPROFEN	Tamarind
IMATINIB (*Gleevec*)	St. John's Wort
IMMUNOSUPPRESSANTS Some drugs in this category include: Azathioprine (*Imuran*) • Basiliximab (*Simulect*) • Cyclosporine (*Neoral, Sandimmune*) • Daclizumab (*Zenapax*) • Muromonab-CD3 (*OKT3*) • Mycophenolate (*CellCept*) • Prednisone (*Orasone, Deltasone*) • Sirolimus (*Rapamune*) • Tacrolimus (*FK506, Prograf*)	Andrographis • Ashwagandha • Astragalus • Beta Glucans • Cat's Claw • Echinacea • European Mistletoe • Ginseng, Panax • Ipriflavone • Jiaogulan • Kefir • Lactobacillus • Larch Arabinogalactan • Melatonin • Picrorhiza • Pycnogenol • Thunder God Vine • Thymus Extract • Yogurt
INDINAVIR (*Crixivan*)	Bitter Orange • Milk Thistle
INJECTABLE DRUGS	DMSO (Dimethylsulfoxide)
INSULIN	Apple Cider Vinegar • Burdock • Chromium • DHEA • EDTA • Ginkgo Leaf • Ginseng, Panax • Gymnema • Licorice • Ribose • Solomon's Seal
IRINOTECAN (*Camptosar*)	St. John's Wort
ITRACONAZOLE (*Sporanox*)	Grapefruit
IVERMECTIN	Sweet Orange
KANAMYCIN	Calcium D-Glucarate
LACTULOSE	Glutamine
LETROZOLE (*Femara*)	DHEA
LEVODOPA	Branched-Chain Amino Acids • Indian Snakeroot • Iron • Kava • Phenylalanine • Pyridoxine • SAMe • Tyrosine • Whey Protein
LEVODOPA/CARBIDOPA (*Sinemet*)	Octacosanol
LEVOTHYROXINE (*Levothroid, Levoxyl, Synthroid*, and others)	Calcium • Celery • Colloidal Silver • Dolomite • Horseradish • Iron • Red Yeast
LITHIUM (*Eskalith, Lithobid*)	Black Psyllium • Black Tea • Bladderwrack • Blond Psyllium • Caffeine • Cocoa • Coffee • Cola Nut • Dandelion Entire Plant • Green Tea • Guarana • Iodine • Mate

CHARTS

Potential Interactions: Drug/Natural Medicine

For additional data, refer to the database.

Drug	Natural Medicine
LOOP DIURETICS Some drugs in this category include: Bumetanide (*Bumex*) • Ethacrynic Acid (*Edecrin*) • Furosemide (*Lasix*)	Lithium
LOSARTAN (*Cozaar*)	Grapefruit
LOVASTATIN (*Mevacor*)	Pectin
MACROLIDE ANTIBIOTICS Some drugs in this category include: Azithromycin (*Zithromax*) • Clarithromycin (*Biaxin*) • Dirithromycin (*Dynabec*) • Erthromycin (*E.E.S.*, E-*Mycin*, *Ery-Tab*)	Black Hellebore • Digitalis • Hedge Mustard • Lily-of-the-Valley • Oleander • Swamp Milkweed • Uzara • Wahoo
MEPERIDINE (*Demerol*)	5-HTP • Ergot • Hawaiian Baby Woodrose • Lithium • L-Tryptophan • SAMe • St. John's Wort
METFORMIN (*Glucophage*)	Beer • Quillaia • Raspberry Leaf • Water Avens • Wine
METHOTREXATE (*MTX*, *Rheumatrex*)	Folic Acid
METHYLDOPA (*Aldomet*)	Cowhage • Iron • Lithium
METHYLPREDNISOLONE (*Adlone, A-Methapred, depMedalone, Depoject, Medrol, Solu-Medrol*)	Grapefruit
METHYLXANTHINES Some drugs in this category include: Caffeine (*NoDoz, Vivarin*) • Theophylline (*Slo-Bid, Theo-Dur, Theolair*)	Adenosine • Country Mallow • Ephedra • Lithium
METOCLOPRAMIDE (*Reglan*)	Chasteberry
METRONIDAZOLE (*Flagyl*)	Beer • Wine
MEXILETINE (*Mexitil*)	Caffeine • Cocoa • Coffee • Cola Nut • Green Tea • Guarana • Mate
MIDAZOLAM (*Versed*)	Bitter Orange • Echinacea
MONOAMINE OXIDASE INHIBITORS (MAOIs) Some drugs in this category include: Phenelzine (*Nardil*) • Tranylcypromine (*Parnate*)	5-HTP • Anise • Bitter Orange • Black Tea • Brewer's Yeast • Caffeine • Calamus • Cereus • Cocoa • Coffee • Cola Nut • Country Mallow • Cowhage • Ephedra • Ergot • Ginseng, American • Ginseng, Panax • Green Tea • Guarana • Hawaiian Baby Woodrose • Hydrazine Sulfate • Indian Snakeroot • Lithium • L-Tryptophan • Mate • Phenylalanine • SAMe • Scotch Broom Flower • Scotch Broom Herb • St. John's Wort • Wine • Yohimbe
MORPHINE (*Kadian, MS Contin, MSIR, Oramorph, Roxanol*)	Oat Above Ground Parts • Oats
MYCOPHENOLATE MOFETIL (*CellCept*)	Iron
NALOXONE (*Narcan*)	Butanediol (BD) • Fever Bark • Gamma Butyrolactone (GBL) • Gamma-Hydroxybutyrate (GHB) • Yohimbe
NARCOTIC DRUGS Some drugs in this category include: Acetaminophen;Oxycodone (*Percocet*) • Acetaminophen;Propoxyphene (*Darvocet*) • Aspirin;Oxycodone (*Percodan*) • Fentanyl (*Duragesic*) • Hydromorphone (*Dilaudid*) • Meperidine (*Demerol*) • Methadone (*Methadose, Dolophine*) • Morphine (*MS Contin, Roxanol*) • Oxycodone (*OxyContin*) • Propoxyphene (*Darvon*) • Sufentanil (*Sufenta*)	Beer • Butanediol (BD) • Gamma Butyrolactone (GBL) • Gamma-Hydroxybutyrate (GHB) • Meadowsweet • St. John's Wort • Sweet Bay • Wine
NEFAZODONE (*Serzone*)	St. John's Wort
NEPHROTOXIC DRUGS Some drugs in this category include: Carbamazepine (*Tegretol*) • Diclofenac (*Voltaren*) • Diflunisal (*Dolobid*) • Ganciclovir (*Cytovene*) • Gatifloxacin (*Tequin*) • Interferon • Meloxicam (*Mobic*) • Spironolactone (*Aldactone*) • Tacrolimus (*Prograf*) • Valacyclovir (*Valtrex*) • Amphotericin B (*Fungizone*) • Cisplatin (*Platinol*) • Cyclosporine (*Neoral*) • Enalapril (*Vasotec*) • Nafcillin (*Unipen*) • Tobramycin (*Nebcin*)	Creatine
NIACIN (*Niacor, Niaspan, Nicobid, Slo-Niacin*)	Beta-Carotene • Red Yeast • Selenium • Vitamin C • Vitamin E

Potential Interactions: Drug/Natural Medicine

For additional data, refer to the database.

Drug	Natural Medicine
NICOTINE (*Habitrol, Nicoderm, Nicorette, Nicotrol, Prestep*)	Blue Cohosh • Cola Nut • Green Tea • Guarana • Mate
NIFEDIPINE (*Adalat, Procardia*)	Coca
NIFEDIPINE GITS (*Procardia XL*)	Melatonin
NITRATES Some drugs in this category include: Isosorbide Dinitrate (*Isordil*) • Isosorbide Mononitrate (*Imdur*) • Nitroglycerin (*Nitrostat*)	Forskolin • Hawthorn • L-Arginine
NITROGLYCERIN (*Minitran, Nitrek, Nitrostat*)	N-Acetyl Cysteine
NMDA ANTAGONISTS	Threonine
NON-NUCLEOSIDE REVERSE TRANSCRIPTASE INHIBITORS (NNRTIs) Some drugs in this category include: Nevirapine (*Viramune*) • Delavirdine (*Rescriptor*) • Efavirenz (*Sustiva*)	Garlic • St. John's Wort
NONSTEROIDAL ANTI-INFLAMMATORY DRUGS (NSAIDs) Some drugs in this category include: Diclofenac (*Voltaren*) • Etodolac (*Lodine*) • Flurbiprofen (*Ansaid*) • Ibuprofen (*Motrin*) • Indomethacin (*Indocin*) • Ketoprofen (*Orudis*) • Ketorolac (*Toradol*) • Meclofenamate; Mefenamic Acid (*Ponstel*) • Nabumetone (*Relafen*) • Naproxen (*Naprosyn*) • Oxaprozine (*Daypro*) • Piroxicam (*Feldene*) • Sulindac (*Clinoril*)	Beer • Borage Seed Oil • Chromium • Feverfew • Gossypol • Lithium • Wine
NORTRIPTYLINE (*Pamelor, Aventyl*)	St. John's Wort
ORAL DRUGS	Acacia • Activated Charcoal • Agar • Alder Buckthorn • Algin • Aloe Latex • American Chestnut • Barley • Bistort • Black Psyllium • Black Walnut • Blond Psyllium • Butternut • Carrageenan • Cascara • Castor Oil • Coffee Charcoal • DMSO (Dimethylsulfoxide) • European Buckthorn • European Chestnut • European Mandrake • Fenugreek • Flaxseed • Glucomannan • Guar Gum • Iceland Moss • Jalap • Kaolin • Karaya Gum • Larch Arabinogalactan • Marshmallow • Mexican Scammony Root • Mormon Tea • Oats • Pinus Bark • Pomegranate • Quillaia • Quince • Raspberry Leaf • Rhatany • Rhubarb • Rice Bran • Slippery Elm • Sorrel • Tannic Acid • Tragacanth • Water Avens • Willow Bark
OXAZEPAM (*Serax*)	Cabbage
PAROXETINE (*Paxil*)	St. John's Wort
PENICILLAMINE (*Cuprimine*)	Colloidal Silver • Copper • Iron • Zinc
PENTAZOCINE (*Talwin*)	5-HTP • Ergot • Hawaiian Baby Woodrose • Lithium • L-Tryptophan • SAMe • St. John's Wort
P-GLYCOPROTEIN SUBSTRATES Some drugs in this category include: Etoposide (*VePesid*) • Paclitaxel (*Taxol*) • Vinblastine (*Velban*) • Vincristine (*Oncovin*) • Ketoconazole • Itraconazole • Amprenavir (*Agenerase*) • Indinavir (*Crixivan*) • Nelfinavir (*Viracept*) • Squinavir (*Fortovase, Invirase*) • Cimetidine • Ranitidine • Diltiazem • Verapamil • Corticosteroids • Erythromycin • Fexofenadine (*Allegra*) • Cyclosporine • Loperamide (*Imodium*) • Quinidine	St. John's Wort
PHENACETIN	Grape Fruit, Skin
PHENOBARBITAL (*Luminal*)	Cinchona • Folic Acid • Nutmeg and Mace • Pyridoxine • St. John's Wort • Vitamin D
PHENOTHIAZINES Some drugs in this category include: Thioridazine (*Mellaril*) • Mesoridazine (*Serentil*) • Trifluoperazine (*Stelazine*) • Chlorpromazine (*Thorazine*) • Fluphenazine (*Prolixin*)	Black Tea • Coffee • Evening Primrose Oil • Fever Bark • Gamma Linolenic Acid • Lithium • L-Tryptophan • Yohimbe
PHENPROCOUMON	St. John's Wort

Potential Interactions: Drug/Natural Medicine

For additional data, refer to the database.

Drug	Natural Medicine
PHENYLPROPANOLAMINE (*Propagest, Rhindecon*)	Black Tea • Caffeine • Cocoa • Coffee • Cola Nut • Green Tea • Guarana • Mate
PHENYTOIN (*Dilantin*)	Beer • Black Pepper and White Pepper • Folic Acid • Indian Long Pepper • Peony Root • Pyridoxine • St. John's Wort • Vitamin D • Wine
PHOTOSENSITIZING DRUGS Some drugs in this category include: Acyclovir (*Zovirax*) • Amitriptyline (*Elavil*) • Azithromycin (*Zithromax*) • Captopril (*Capoten*) • Carbamazepine (*Tegretol*) • Chloroquine (*Aralen*) • Chlorthiazide (*Diuril*) • Chlorpromazine (*Thorazine*) • Ciprofloxacin (*Cipro*) • Dantrolene (*Dantrium*) • Dapsone • Divalproex (*Depakote*) • Oral Contraceptives • Felbamate (*Felbatol*) • Fluorouracil (*Efudex, Carac*) • Flutamide (*Eulexin*) • Furosemide (*Lasix*) • Glipizide (*Glucotrol*) • Glyburide (*Micronase*) • Hydroxychloroquine (*Plaquenil*) • Isotretinoin (*Accutane*) • Methoxsalen (*Oxsoralen*) • Minocycline (*Minocin*) • Phenobarbital • Promethazine (*Phenergan*) • Quinidine (*Quinidex*) • Sulfamethoxazole;Trimethoprim (*Bactrim, Septra*) • Tacrolimus (*Prograf*) • Tolbutamide (*Orinase*) • Trazodone (*Desyrel*) • Tretinoin (*Retin-A*) • Valproic Acid (*Depakene*)	Alfalfa • Angelica Root • Arrach • Bergamot Oil • Bishop's Weed • Celery • Chenopodium Oil • Chlorophyll • Khella • Lime Oil • Masterwort • Rue • St. John's Wort • Wild Carrot
POTASSIUM SUPPLEMENTS	Laminaria
POTASSIUM-SPARING DIURETICS Some of the drugs in this category include: Amiloride (*Midamor*) • Triamterene (*Dyrenium*) • Spironolactone (*Aldacton*)	Dandelion Above Ground Parts • Dandelion Entire Plant • Dolomite • Iodine • Laminaria • Magnesium • Morinda • Potassium • Zinc
PRAVASTATIN (*Pravachol*)	Beta-Sitosterol
PRAZIQUANTEL (*Biltricide*)	Grapefruit
PREDNISOLONE (*Pediapred*)	Cordyceps
PRIMIDONE (*Mysoline*)	Folic Acid
PROBENECID (*Benemid*)	Riboflavin
PROCYCLIDINE (*Kemadrin*)	Areca
PROGESTIN	Pregnenolone
PROPRANOLOL (*Inderal*)	Black Pepper and White Pepper • Guggul • Indian Long Pepper • Indian Snakeroot • Ribose
PROTEASE INHIBITORS (PIs) Some drugs in this category include: Indinavir (*Crixivan*) • Nelfinavir (*Viracept*) • Squinavir (*Invirase*)	St. John's Wort • Vitamin C
PROTON PUMP INHIBITORS (PPIs) Some drugs in this category include: Esomeprazole (*Nexium*) • Lansoprazole (*Prevacid*) • Omeprazole (*Prilosec*) • Pantoprazole (*Protonix*) • Rabeprazole (*Aciphex*)	Aletris • Alpinia • Angelica Herb, Seed • Angelica Root • Aristolochia • Black Mustard Oil • Black Mustard Seed • Blessed Thistle • Calamus • Capsicum • Cinchona • Colombo • Cubebs • Dandelion Entire Plant • Devil's Claw • Gentian • Ginger • Goldenseal • Goldthread • Northern Prickly Ash • Peppermint Oil • Quassia • Southern Prickly Ash • Wormwood Above Ground Parts • Yarrow
PYRIMETHAMINE (*Daraprim*)	Folic Acid
QT INTERVAL-PROLONGING DRUGS Some drugs in this category include: • Amitriptyline • Clarithromycin (*Biaxin*) • Erythromycin • Quinidine • Sotalol (*Betapace*) • Thioridazine • Indapamide (*Lozol*) • Risperidone (*Risperdal*) • Moxifloxacin (*Avelox*) • Ziprasidone (*Geodon*)	Country Mallow • Ephedra
QUINIDINE (*Quinidex*)	Cinchona • Grapefruit • Grapefruit Seed Extract • Pheasant's Eye • Scopolia • Scotch Broom Herb • Squill • Strophanthus • Wallflower
QUININE	Black Hellebore • Cinchona • Digitalis • Hedge Mustard • Lily-of-the-Valley • Oleander • Strophanthus • Swamp Milkweed • Uzara • Wahoo • Wallflower

Potential Interactions: Drug/Natural Medicine

For additional data, refer to the database.

Drug	Natural Medicine
QUINOLONE ANTIBIOTICS Some drugs in this category include: Ciprofloxacin (*Cipro*) • Gatifloxacin (*Tequin*) • Levofloxacin (*Levaquin*) • Moxifloxacin (*Avelox*) • Norfloxacin (*Noroxin*) • Ofloxacin (*Floxin*) • Trovafloxacin (*Trovan*)	Black Tea • Caffeine • Calcium • Cocoa • Coffee • Cola Nut • Colloidal Silver • Dolomite • Green Tea • Guarana • Iron • Magnesium • Manganese • Mate • Quercetin • Whey Protein • Zinc
RESERPINE	Country Mallow • Ephedra • St. John's Wort
RETINOIDS Some drugs in this category include: Adapelene (*Differin*) • Isotretinoin (*Isotrex*) • Tretinon (*Retin-A, Retinova*)	Vitamin A
RILUZOLE (*Rilutek*)	Black Tea • Caffeine • Coffee • Cola Nut • Green Tea • Guarana • Mate
RISPERIDONE (*Risperdal*)	Hawaiian Baby Woodrose
RITONAVIR (*Norvir*)	Butanediol (BD) • Gamma Butyrolactone (GBL) • Gamma-Hydroxybutyrate (GHB)
SALSALATE (*Disalcid*)	Meadowsweet • Ribose • Rose Hip • Vitamin C • Willow Bark
SAQUINAVIR (*Fortovase, Invirase*)	Butanediol (BD) • Gamma Butyrolactone (GBL) • Gamma-Hydroxybutyrate (GHB) • Garlic • Grapefruit • Grapefruit Seed Extract
SCOPOLAMINE (*Transderm Scop*)	Alpha-GPC • Grapefruit
SEIZURE THRESHOLD LOWERING DRUGS Some of the drugs in this category include: Anesthetics (Propofol, others) • Antiarrhythmics (Mexiletine) • Antibiotics (Amphotericin, Penicillin, Cephalosporins, Imipenem) • Antidepressants (Bupropion, others) • Antihistamines (Cyproheptadine, others) • Immunosuppressants (Cyclosporin) • Narcotics (Fentanyl, others) • Stimulants (Methylphenidate, others) • Theophylline	Ginkgo Leaf • Ginkgo Seed
SERTRALINE (*Zoloft*)	St. John's Wort
SILDENAFIL (*Viagra*)	Grapefruit • L-Arginine
SIMVASTATIN (*Zocor*)	St. John's Wort
SKELETAL MUSCLE RELAXANTS Some drugs in this category include: Baclofen (*Lioresal*) • Botulinum Toxin Type A (*Botox*) • Chlorzaoxazone (*Parafon Forte*) • Cyclobenzaprine (*Flexeril*) • Dantrolene (*Dantrium*) • Metaxalone (*Skelaxin*) • Orphenadrine (*Norflex*)	Butanediol (BD) • Gamma Butyrolactone (GBL) • Gamma-Hydroxybutyrate (GHB) • Lithium • Magnesium • Procaine
SOTALOL (*Betapace*)	Calcium • Dolomite
STIMULANT DRUGS Some drugs in this category include: Pemoline (*Cylert*) • Methylphenidate (*Ritalin*) • Fenfluramine (*Pondimin*) • Dextroamphetamine (*Dexedrine*) • Dexfenfluramine (*Redux*) • Caffeine (*NoDoz*) • Pseudoephedrine	Bitter Orange • Black Tea • Caffeine • Coffee • Ergot • Fever Bark • Ginseng, American • Ginseng, Panax • Indian Snakeroot • Peyote • Theanine • Tiratricol • Yohimbe
STIMULANT LAXATIVES Some drugs in this category include: Senna (*Senokot*) • Bisacodyl (*Dulcolax*)	Alder Buckthorn • Aloe Latex • Black Hellebore • Butternut • Calotropis • Cascara • Castor Oil • Digitalis • Fo-Ti • Gamboge • Gossypol • Hedge Mustard • Jalap • Lily-of-the-Valley • Mexican Scammony Root • Oleander • Pheasant's Eye • Rhubarb • Squill • Strophanthus • Swamp Milkweed • Uzara • Wahoo • Wallflower
SUCCINYLCHOLINE	Procaine
SULFONAMIDE ANTIBIOTICS Some drugs in this category include: Sulfamethoxazole;Trimethoprim (*Bactrim*) • Sulfacetamide (*Sodium Sulamyd*) • Sulfisoxazole (*Gantrisin*)	Beer • Para-Aminobenzoic Acid (PABA) • Procaine • Wine
SYRUP OF IPECAC	Activated Charcoal
TACROLIMUS (*Prograf, Protopic*)	St. John's Wort
TAMOXIFEN (*Nolvadex*)	Anise • DHEA • Fennel Fruit, Seed • Kudzu • Red Clover • Soy

CHARTS

Potential Interactions: Drug/Natural Medicine

For additional data, refer to the database.

Drug	Natural Medicine
TERBINAFINE (*Lamisil*)	Black Tea • Caffeine • Coffee • Cola Nut • Green Tea • Guarana • Mate
TERFENADINE (*Seldane*)	Grapefruit • Grapefruit Seed Extract
TESTOSTERONE	Androstenediol • Pregnenolone
TETRACYCLINES (*Sumycin*)	Black Hellebore • Bromelain • Calcium • Colloidal Silver • Digitalis • Dolomite • Hedge Mustard • Iron • Lily-of-the-Valley • Magnesium • Manganese • Oleander • Pectin • Swamp Milkweed • Uzara • Vitamin A • Wahoo • Whey Protein • Yogurt • Zinc
THEOPHYLLINE (*Theo-Dur*)	Black Pepper and White Pepper • Black Tea • Caffeine • Capsicum • Cocoa • Coffee • Cola Nut • Gossypol • Grapefruit • Green Tea • Guarana • Indian Long Pepper • Ipriflavone • Marijuana • Mate • St. John's Wort
THIAZIDE DIURETICS Some drugs in this category include: Chlorothiazide (*Diuril*) • Metolazone (*Zaroxolyn*)	Calcium • Dolomite • Ginkgo Leaf • Lithium • Pangamic Acid • Vitamin D • Zinc
THROMBOLYTIC DRUGS (*tPA*, *Alteplase*)	Mesoglycan • Potato
THYROID HORMONE Some drugs in this category include: Levothyroxine (*Synthroid, Levothroid, Levoxyl*)	Ashwagandha • Bladderwrack • Bugleweed • Guggul • Laminaria • Shepherd's Purse • Tiratricol • Tyrosine
TOLBUTAMIDE (*Orinase*)	Beer • Wine
TOPICAL DRUGS	DMSO (Dimethylsulfoxide)
TRAMADOL (*Ultram*)	5-HTP • Ergot • Hawaiian Baby Woodrose • Lithium • L-Tryptophan • SAMe • St. John's Wort
TRANSDERMAL NICOTINE (*Nicoderm*, *Nicotrol*)	Inositol Nicotinate • Niacin And Niacinamide
TRAZODONE (*Desyrel*)	Ginkgo Leaf
TRIAZOLAM (*Halcion*)	DHEA
TRICYCLIC ANTIDEPRESSANTS (TCAs) Some drugs in this category include: Amitriptyline (*Elavil*) • Clomipramine (*Anafranil*) • Desipramine (*Norpramin*) • Doxepin (*Sinequan*) • Imipramine (*Tofranil*) • Nortriptyline (*Pamelor*) • Protriptyline (*Vivactil*)	Black Tea • Coffee • Cowhage • Indian Snakeroot • Scopolia • Yohimbe
VERAPAMIL (*Calan*, *Covera*, *Isoptin*, *Verelan*)	Black Tea • Caffeine • Cocoa • Coffee • Cola Nut • Guarana • Mate • Melatonin
WARFARIN (*Coumadin*)	Acerola • Alfalfa • Avocado • Beer • Black Psyllium • Blond Psyllium • Boldo • Cabbage • Cherokee Rosehip • Chlorella • Chondroitin Sulfate • Coenzyme Q-10 • Corn Silk • Cranberry • Danshen • Devil's Claw • Dong Quai • EDTA • Fenugreek • Garlic • Ginkgo Leaf • Ginseng, American • Ginseng, Panax • Glucosamine Hydrochloride • Glucosamine Sulfate • Grape Seed • Grapefruit • Grapefruit Seed Extract • Great Plantain • Green Tea • L-Carnitine • Lycium • N-Acetyl Glucosamine • Papaya • Rose Hip • Smartweed • Soy • Spinach • St. John's Wort • Stinging Nettle Above Ground Parts • Vinpocetine • Vitamin A • Vitamin C • Vitamin E • Vitamin K • Watercress • Wine • Wintergreen Oil

Potential Interactions Between Natural Medicines and Drugs

For details on possible interactions between natural medicines and drugs, see the listing for the specific natural medicine in the body of this database. This chart does not contain all theoretical or unknown interactions.

Natural Medicine	Drug
5-HTP	Antidepressant Drugs • Carbidopa (*Lodosyn*) • Dextromethorphan (*Robitussin DM*, others) • Meperidine (*Demerol*) • Monoamine Oxidase Inhibitors (MAOIs) • Pentazocine (*Talwin*) • Tramadol (*Ultram*)
Acacia	Alcohol (Ethanol) • Oral Drugs
Acerola	Estrogens • Fluphenazine (*Prolixin*) • Warfarin (*Coumadin*)
Ackee	Antidiabetes Drugs
Activated Charcoal	Oral Drugs • Syrup of Ipecac
Adenosine	Antigout Drugs • Carbamazepine (*Tegretol*) • Dipyridamole (*Persantine*) • Methylxanthines
Agar	Oral Drugs
Agrimony	Antidiabetes Drugs
Alder Buckthorn	Corticosteroids • Digoxin (*Lanoxin*) • Diuretic Drugs • Oral Drugs • Stimulant Laxatives
Aletris	Antacids • H2-Blockers • Proton Pump Inhibitors (PPIs)
Alfalfa	Contraceptive Drugs • Estrogens • Photosensitizing Drugs • Warfarin (*Coumadin*)
Algin	Oral Drugs
Allspice	Anticoagulant/Antiplatelet Drugs
Aloe Gel	Antidiabetes Drugs
Aloe Latex	Corticosteroids • Digoxin (*Lanoxin*) • Diuretic Drugs • Oral Drugs • Stimulant Laxatives
Alpha-GPC	Scopolamine
Alpha-Lipoic Acid	Antidiabetes Drugs • Chemotherapy
Alpinia	Antacids • H2-Blockers • Proton Pump Inhibitors (PPIs)
American Chestnut	Oral Drugs
American Elder	Cytochrome P450 3A4 (CYP3A4) Substrates
Andrographis	Anticoagulant/Antiplatelet Drugs • Antihypertensive Drugs • Immunosuppressants
Androstenediol	Estrogens • Testosterone
Androstenedione	Estrogens
Angelica Herb, Seed	Antacids • Anticoagulant/Antiplatelet Drugs • H2-Blockers • Proton Pump Inhibitors (PPIs)
Angelica Root	Antacids • Anticoagulant/Antiplatelet Drugs • H2-Blockers • Photosensitizing Drugs • Proton Pump Inhibitors (PPIs)
Angel's Trumpet	Anticholinergic Drugs
Anise	Contraceptive Drugs • Estrogens • Monoamine Oxidase Inhibitors (MAOIs) • Tamoxifen (*Nolvadex*)
Annatto	Antidiabetes Drugs
Apple	Fexofenadine (*Allegra*)
Apple Cider Vinegar	Digoxin (*Lanoxin*) • Diuretic Drugs • Insulin
Areca	Anticholinergic Drugs • Cholinergic Drugs • Procyclidine
Aristolochia	Antacids • H2-Blockers • Proton Pump Inhibitors (PPIs)
Arnica	Anticoagulant/Antiplatelet Drugs
Arrach	Photosensitizing Drugs
Asafoetida	Anticoagulant/Antiplatelet Drugs • Antihypertensive Drugs

Potential Interactions: Natural Medicine/Drug

For additional data, refer to the database.

Natural Medicine	Drug
Ashwagandha	Benzodiazepines • CNS Depressants • Immunosuppressants • Thyroid Hormone
Astragalus	Cyclophosphamide • Immunosuppressants
Autumn Crocus	Colchicine
Avocado	Warfarin (*Coumadin*)
Baikal Skullcap	Alcohol (Ethanol) • Antidiabetes Drugs • Benzodiazepines • CNS Depressants
Banaba	Antidiabetes Drugs
Barley	Antidiabetes Drugs • Oral Drugs
Bean Pod	Antidiabetes Drugs
Beer	Aspirin • Barbiturates • Benzodiazepines • Cefamandole (*Mandol*) • Cefoperazone (*Cefobid*) • Chlorpropamide (*Diabinese*) • Cisapride (*Propulsid*) • CNS Depressants • Disulfiram (*Antabuse*) • Erythromycin • Griseofulvin (*Fulvicin*) • H2-Blockers • Hepatotoxic Drugs • Metformin (*Glucophage*) • Metronidazole (*Flagyl*) • Narcotic Drugs • Nonsteroidal Anti-Inflammatory Drugs (NSAIDs) • Phenytoin (*Dilantin*) • Sulfonamide Antibiotics • Tolbutamide (*Orinase*) • Warfarin (*Coumadin*)
Belladonna	Anticholinergic Drugs
Bergamot Oil	Photosensitizing Drugs
Beta Glucans	Immunosuppressants
Beta-Carotene	HMG-CoA Reductase Inhibitors ("Statins") • Niacin
Beta-Sitosterol	Ezetimibe (*Zetia*) • Pravastatin (*Pravachol*)
Betony	Antihypertensive Drugs
Bifidobacteria	Antibiotic Drugs
Bilberry	Antidiabetes Drugs
Birch	Diuretic Drugs
Bishop's Weed	Anticoagulant/Antiplatelet Drugs • Cytochrome P450 3A4 (CYP3A4) Substrates • Hepatotoxic Drugs • Photosensitizing Drugs
Bistort	Oral Drugs
Bitter Almond	CNS Depressants
Bitter Melon	Antidiabetes Drugs
Bitter Orange	Cytochrome P450 3A4 (CYP3A4) Substrates • Dextromethorphan (*Robitussin DM*, and others) • Felodipine (*Plendil*) • Indinavir (*Crixivan*) • Midazolam (*Versed*) • Monoamine Oxidase Inhibitors (MAOIs) • Stimulant Drugs
Black Cohosh	Hepatotoxic Drugs
Black Hellebore	Digoxin (*Lanoxin*) • Diuretic Drugs • Macrolide Antibiotics • Quinine • Stimulant Laxatives • Tetracycline Antibiotics
Black Horehound	Dopamine Agonists
Black Mulberry	Antidiabetes Drugs
Black Mustard Oil	Antacids • H2-Blockers • Proton Pump Inhibitors (PPIs)
Black Mustard Seed	Antacids • H2-Blockers • Proton Pump Inhibitors (PPIs)
Black Pepper And White Pepper	Phenytoin (*Dilantin*) • Propranolol (*Inderal*) • Theophylline
Black Psyllium	Antidiabetes Drugs • Carbamazepine (*Tegretol*) • Digoxin (*Lanoxin*) • Lithium • Oral Drugs • Warfarin (*Coumadin*)
Black Root	Digoxin (*Lanoxin*) • Diuretic Drugs

CHARTS

Potential Interactions: Natural Medicine/Drug For additional data, refer to the database.	
Natural Medicine	**Drug**
Black Tea	Adenosine (*Adenocard*) • Alcohol (Ethanol) • Anticoagulant/Antiplatelet Drugs • Antidiabetes Drugs • Cimetidine (*Tagamet*) • Clozapine (*Clozaril*) • Contraceptive Drugs • Dipyridamole (*Persantine*) • Disulfiram (*Antabuse*) • Ephedrine • Estrogens • Fluconazole (*Diflucan*) • Lithium • Monoamine Oxidase Inhibitors (MAOIs) • Phenothiazines • Phenylpropanolamine • Quinolone Antibiotics • Riluzole (*Rilutek*) • Stimulant Drugs • Terbinafine (*Lamisil*) • Theophylline • Tricyclic Antidepressants (TCAs) • Verapamil (*Calan*, *Covera*, *Isoptin*, *Verelan*)
Black Walnut	Oral Drugs
Bladderwrack	Anticoagulant/Antiplatelet Drugs • Diuretic Drugs • Lithium • Thyroid Hormone
Blessed Thistle	Antacids • H2-Blockers • Proton Pump Inhibitors (PPIs)
Blond Psyllium	Antidiabetes Drugs • Carbamazepine (*Tegretol*) • Digoxin (*Lanoxin*) • Lithium • Oral Drugs • Warfarin (*Coumadin*)
Blue Cohosh	Antidiabetes Drugs • Antihypertensive Drugs • Nicotine
Blue Flag	Digoxin (*Lanoxin*) • Diuretic Drugs
Blueberry	Antidiabetes Drugs
Bogbean	Anticoagulant/Antiplatelet Drugs
Boldo	Anticoagulant/Antiplatelet Drugs • Warfarin (*Coumadin*)
Borage Flower, Dried Above Ground Parts	Hepatotoxic Drugs
Borage Seed Oil	Anesthesia • Anticoagulant/Antiplatelet Drugs • Nonsteroidal Anti-Inflammatory Drugs (NSAIDs)
Boron	Estrogens
Branched-Chain Amino Acids	Antidiabetes Drugs • Levodopa
Brewer's Yeast	Antifungals • Monoamine Oxidase Inhibitors (MAOIs)
Bromelain	Anticoagulant/Antiplatelet Drugs • Tetracycline Antibiotics
Buchu	Anticoagulant/Antiplatelet Drugs
Bugleweed	Antidiabetes Drugs • Thyroid Hormone
Burdock	Antidiabetes Drugs • Insulin
Butanediol (BD)	Alcohol (Ethanol) • Amphetamines • Anticonvulsants • Antipsychotic Drugs • Benzodiazepines • CNS Depressants • Haloperidol (*Haldol*) • Naloxone (*Narcan*) • Narcotic Drugs • Ritonavir (*Norvir*) • Saquinavir (*Fortovase*, *Invirase*) • Skeletal Muscle Relaxants
Butcher's Broom	Alpha-Adrenergic Agonists • Alpha-Adrenergic Antagonists
Butternut	Corticosteroids • Digoxin (*Lanoxin*) • Diuretic Drugs • Oral Drugs • Stimulant Laxatives
Cabbage	Acetaminophen (*Tylenol*, others) • Cytochrome P450 1A2 (CYP1A2) Substrates • Glucuronidated Drugs • Oxazepam (*Serax*) • Warfarin (*Coumadin*)
Caffeine	Adenosine (*Adenocard*) • Alcohol (Ethanol) • Anticoagulant/Antiplatelet Drugs • Antidiabetes Drugs • Clozapine (*Clozaril*) • Contraceptive Drugs • Dipyridamole (*Persantine*) • Disulfiram (*Antabuse*) • Ephedrine • Estrogens • Fluconazole (*Diflucan*) • Fluvoxamine (*Luvox*) • Lithium (*Eskalith*) • Mexiletine (*Mexitil*) • Monoamine Oxidase Inhibitors (MAOIs) • Phenylpropanolamine • Quinolone Antibiotics • Riluzole (*Rilutek*) • Stimulant Drugs • Terbinafine (*Lamisil*) • Theophylline • Verapamil (*Calan*, *Covera*, *Isoptin*, *Verelan*)
Calabar Bean	Anticholinergic Drugs
Calamus	Antacids • CNS Depressants • H2-Blockers • Monoamine Oxidase Inhibitors (MAOIs) • Proton Pump Inhibitors (PPIs)

CHARTS

Potential Interactions: Natural Medicine/Drug For additional data, refer to the database.

Natural Medicine	Drug
Calcium	Bisphosphonates • Calcium Channel Blockers • Estrogens • Levothyroxine (*Synthroid*, *Levothroid*, *Levoxyl*, and others) • Quinolone Antibiotics • Sotalol (*Betapace*) • Tetracycline Antibiotics • Thiazide Diuretics
Calcium D-Glucarate	Alcohol (Ethanol) • Glucuronidated Drugs • Kanamycin
Calendula	CNS Depressants
California Poppy	CNS Depressants
Calotropis	Digoxin (*Lanoxin*) • Diuretic Drugs • Stimulant Laxatives
Canadian Hemp	Digoxin (*Lanoxin*) • Diuretic Drugs
Capsicum	ACE Inhibitors (ACEIs) • Antacids • Anticoagulant/Antiplatelet Drugs • CNS Depressants • Cocaine • H2-Blockers • Proton Pump Inhibitors (PPIs) • Theophylline
Carrageenan	Anticoagulant/Antiplatelet Drugs • Antihypertensive Drugs • Oral Drugs
Cascara	Corticosteroids • Digoxin (*Lanoxin*) • Diuretic Drugs • Oral Drugs • Stimulant Laxatives
Cassia Auriculata	Antidiabetes Drugs • Carbamazepine (*Tegretol*)
Cassia Cinnamon	Antidiabetes Drugs
Castor Oil	Corticosteroids • Digoxin (*Lanoxin*) • Diuretic Drugs • Oral Drugs • Stimulant Laxatives
Catnip	CNS Depressants
Cat's Claw	Antihypertensive Drugs • Cytochrome P450 3A4 (CYP3A4) Substrates • Immunosuppressants
Cedar Leaf	Anticonvulsants
Cedar Leaf Oil	Anticonvulsants
Cedarwood	Barbiturates
Celery	CNS Depressants • Levothyroxine (*Synthroid*, *Levothroid*, *Levoxyl*, and others) • Photosensitizing Drugs
Cereus	Digoxin (*Lanoxin*) • Monoamine Oxidase Inhibitors (MAOIs)
Cesium	Corticosteroids • Diuretic Drugs
Chanca Piedra	Antidiabetes Drugs
Chaparral	Hepatotoxic Drugs
Chasteberry	Antipsychotic Drugs • Contraceptive Drugs • Dopamine Agonists • Estrogens • Metoclopramide (*Reglan*)
Chenopodium Oil	Photosensitizing Drugs
Cherokee Rosehip	Aluminum • Aspirin • Choline Magnesium Trisalicylate (*Trilisate*) • Estrogens • Fluphenazine (*Prolixin*) • Warfarin (*Coumadin*)
Chinese Club Moss	Acetylcholinesterase (AChE) Inhibitors • Anticholinergic Drugs • Cholinergic Drugs
Chinese Cucumber Root	Antidiabetes Drugs
Chlorella	Warfarin (*Coumadin*)
Chlorophyll	Photosensitizing Drugs
Chondroitin Sulfate	Warfarin (*Coumadin*)
Chromium	Insulin • Nonsteroidal Anti-Inflammatory Drugs (NSAIDs)
Chrysin	Aromatase Inhibitors • Cytochrome P450 1A2 (CYP1A2) Substrates • Glucuronidated Drugs
Cinchona	Antacids • Anticoagulant/Antiplatelet Drugs • Carbamazepine (*Tegretol*) • H2-Blockers • Phenobarbital (*Luminal*) • Proton Pump Inhibitors (PPIs) • Quinidine • Quinine

CHARTS

Potential Interactions: Natural Medicine/Drug

For additional data, refer to the database.

Natural Medicine	Drug
Cinnamon Bark	Antidiabetes Drugs
Clary Sage	Chloral Hydrate • Hexobarbitone
Clove Dried Flowerbud, Leaf, Stem	Anticoagulant/Antiplatelet Drugs
Clove Oil	Anticoagulant/Antiplatelet Drugs
Coca	Alcohol (Ethanol) • Nifedipine
Cocoa	Adenosine (*Adenocard*) • Antidiabetes Drugs • Beta-Adrenergic Agonists • Cimetidine (*Tagamet*) • Clozapine (*Clozaril*) • Contraceptive Drugs • Dipyridamole (*Persantine*) • Disulfiram (*Antabuse*) • Ergotamine (*Ergomar*) • Estrogens • Fluconazole (*Diflucan*) • Lithium • Mexiletine (*Mexitil*) • Monoamine Oxidase Inhibitors (MAOIs) • Phenylpropanolamine • Quinolone Antibiotics • Theophylline • Verapamil (*Calan, Covera, Isoptin, Verelan*)
Cod Liver Oil	Anticoagulant/Antiplatelet Drugs • Antihypertensive Drugs
Coenzyme Q-10	Antihypertensive Drugs • Chemotherapy • Warfarin (*Coumadin*)
Coffee	Adenosine (*Adenocard*) • Alcohol (Ethanol) • Alendronate (*Fosamax*) • Anticoagulant/Antiplatelet Drugs • Antidiabetes Drugs • Cimetidine (*Tagamet*) • Clozapine (*Clozaril*) • Contraceptive Drugs • Dipyridamole (*Persantine*) • Disulfiram (*Antabuse*) • Ephedrine • Estrogens • Fluconazole (*Diflucan*) • Fluvoxamine (*Luvox*) • Lithium • Mexiletine (*Mexitil*) • Monoamine Oxidase Inhibitors (MAOIs) • Phenothiazines • Phenylpropanolamine • Quinolone Antibiotics • Riluzole (*Rilutek*) • Stimulant Drugs • Terbinafine (*Lamisil*) • Theophylline • Tricyclic Antidepressants (TCAs) • Verapamil (*Calan, Covera, Isoptin, Verelan*)
Coffee Charcoal	Oral Drugs
Cola Nut	Adenosine (*Adenocard*) • Alcohol (Ethanol) • Amphetamines • Antidiabetes Drugs • Cimetidine (*Tagamet*) • Clozapine (*Clozaril*) • Cocaine • Contraceptive Drugs • Dipyridamole (*Persantine*) • Disulfiram (*Antabuse*) • Ephedrine • Estrogens • Fluconazole (*Diflucan*) • Fluvoxamine (*Luvox*) • Lithium • Mexiletine (*Mexitil*) • Monoamine Oxidase Inhibitors (MAOIs) • Nicotine • Phenylpropanolamine • Quinolone Antibiotics • Riluzole (*Rilutek*) • Terbinafine (*Lamisil*) • Theophylline • Verapamil (*Calan, Covera, Isoptin, Verelan*)
Colloidal Silver	Levothyroxine • Penicillamine • Quinolone Antibiotics • Tetracycline Antibiotics
Colocynth	Digoxin (*Lanoxin*) • Diuretic Drugs
Colombo	Antacids • H2-Blockers • Proton Pump Inhibitors (PPIs)
Coltsfoot	Antihypertensive Drugs
Comfrey	Cytochrome P450 3A4 (CYP3A4) Inducers • Hepatotoxic Drugs
Copper	Penicillamine
Cordyceps	Cyclophosphamide • Prednisolone
Corn Silk	Antidiabetes Drugs • Antihypertensive Drugs • Corticosteroids • Diuretic Drugs • Warfarin (*Coumadin*)
Country Mallow	Antidiabetes Drugs • Dexamethasone (*Decadron*) • Ergot Derivatives • Methylxanthines • Monoamine Oxidase Inhibitors (MAOIs) • QT Interval-Prolonging Drugs • Reserpine
Cowhage	Anesthesia • Antidiabetes Drugs • Antipsychotic Drugs • Guanethidine (*Ismelin*) • Methyldopa (*Aldomet*) • Monoamine Oxidase Inhibitors (MAOIs) • Tricyclic Antidepressants (TCAs)
Cowslip	CNS Depressants • Diuretic Drugs
Cranberry	Cytochrome P450 2C9 (CYP2C9) Substrates • Warfarin (*Coumadin*)
Creatine	Nephrotoxic Drugs
Cubebs	Antacids • H2-Blockers • Proton Pump Inhibitors (PPIs)

Potential Interactions: Natural Medicine/Drug

For additional data, refer to the database.

Natural Medicine	Drug
Cumin	Antidiabetes Drugs
Damiana	Antidiabetes Drugs
Dandelion Above Ground Parts	Potassium-Sparing Diuretics
Dandelion Entire Plant	Antacids • Antidiabetes Drugs • H2-Blockers • Lithium • Potassium-Sparing Diuretics • Proton Pump Inhibitors (PPIs)
Danshen	Anticoagulant/Antiplatelet Drugs • Digoxin (*Lanoxin*) • Warfarin (*Coumadin*)
Deanol	Anticholinergic Drugs
Deertongue	Anticoagulant/Antiplatelet Drugs
Devil's Claw	Antacids • Antidiabetes Drugs • Antihypertensive Drugs • H2-Blockers • Proton Pump Inhibitors (PPIs) • Warfarin (*Coumadin*)
Devil's Club	Antidiabetes Drugs
DHA (Docosahexaenoic Acid)	Anticoagulant/Antiplatelet Drugs • Antihypertensive Drugs
DHEA	Anastrozole (*Arimidex*) • Corticosteroids • Cytochrome P450 3A4 (CYP3A4) Substrates • Exemestane (*Aromasin*) • Fulvestrant (*Faslodex*) • Insulin • Letrozole (*Femara*) • Tamoxifen (*Nolvadex*) • Triazolam (*Halcion*)
Dibencozide	Chloramphenicol
Digitalis	Digoxin (*Lanoxin*) • Diuretic Drugs • Macrolide Antibiotics • Quinine • Stimulant Laxatives • Tetracycline Antibiotics
Diindolylmethane	Cytochrome P450 1A2 (CYP1A2) Substrates
DMSO (Dimethylsulfoxide)	Injectable Drugs • Oral Drugs • Topical Drugs
Dolomite	Bisphosphonates • Estrogens • Levothyroxine (*Synthroid*, *Levothroid*, *Levoxyl*, and others) • Potassium-Sparing Diuretics • Quinolone Antibiotics • Sotalol (*Betapace*) • Tetracycline Antibiotics • Thiazide Diuretics
Dong Quai	Anticoagulant/Antiplatelet Drugs • Warfarin (*Coumadin*)
Echinacea	Cytochrome P450 3A4 (CYP3A4) Substrates • Immunosuppressants • Midazolam (*Versed*)
EDTA	Diuretic Drugs • Insulin • Warfarin (*Coumadin*)
Elecampane	CNS Depressants
EPA (Eicosapentaenoic Acid)	Anticoagulant/Antiplatelet Drugs • Antihypertensive Drugs
Ephedra	Antidiabetes Drugs • Dexamethasone (*Decadron*) • Ergot Derivatives • Methylxanthines • Monoamine Oxidase Inhibitors (MAOIs) • QT Interval-Prolonging Drugs • Reserpine
Epimedium	Anticoagulant/Antiplatelet Drugs • Antihypertensive Drugs
Ergot	Antidepressant Drugs • Cytochrome P450 3A4 (CYP3A4) Inhibitors • Dextromethorphan (*Robitussin DM*, and others) • Ergot Derivatives • Meperidine (*Demerol*) • Monoamine Oxidase Inhibitors (MAOIs) • Pentazocine (*Talwin*) • Stimulant Drugs • Tramadol (*Ultram*)
Eucalyptus Dried Leaf	Antidiabetes Drugs
European Buckthorn	Digoxin (*Lanoxin*) • Diuretic Drugs • Oral Drugs
European Chestnut	Oral Drugs
European Mandrake	Anticholinergic Drugs • Oral Drugs
European Mistletoe	Antihypertensive Drugs • Immunosuppressants
Evening Primrose Oil	Anesthesia • Anticoagulant/Antiplatelet Drugs • Phenothiazines
Fennel Fruit, Seed	Ciprofloxacin (*Cipro*) • Contraceptive Drugs • Estrogens • Tamoxifen (*Nolvadex*)

CHARTS

Potential Interactions: Natural Medicine/Drug For additional data, refer to the database.

Natural Medicine	Drug
Fenugreek	Anticoagulant/Antiplatelet Drugs • Antidiabetes Drugs • Oral Drugs • Warfarin (*Coumadin*)
Fever Bark	Anesthesia • Naloxone (*Narcan*) • Phenothiazines • Stimulant Drugs
Feverfew	Anticoagulant/Antiplatelet Drugs • Nonsteroidal Anti-Inflammatory Drugs (NSAIDs)
Figwort	Diuretic Drugs
Fish Oils	Anticoagulant/Antiplatelet Drugs • Antihypertensive Drugs • Contraceptive Drugs
Flaxseed	Anticoagulant/Antiplatelet Drugs • Antidiabetes Drugs • Oral Drugs
Flaxseed Oil	Anticoagulant/Antiplatelet Drugs
Folic Acid	Fosphenytoin (*Cerebyx*) • Methotrexate (*MTX, Rheumatrex*) • Phenobarbital (*Luminal*) • Phenytoin (*Dilantin*) • Primidone (*Mysoline*) • Pyrimethamine (*Daraprim*)
Forskolin	Anticoagulant/Antiplatelet Drugs • Calcium Channel Blockers • Nitrates
Fo-Ti	Antidiabetes Drugs • Digoxin (*Lanoxin*) • Diuretic Drugs • Stimulant Laxatives
Gamboge	Corticosteroids • Digoxin (*Lanoxin*) • Diuretic Drugs • Stimulant Laxatives
Gamma Butyrolactone (GBL)	Alcohol (Ethanol) • Amphetamines • Anticonvulsants • Antipsychotic Drugs • Benzodiazepines • CNS Depressants • Haloperidol (*Haldol*) • Naloxone (*Narcan*) • Narcotic Drugs • Ritonavir (*Norvir*) • Saquinavir (*Fortovase, Invirase*) • Skeletal Muscle Relaxants
Gamma Linolenic Acid	Anticoagulant/Antiplatelet Drugs • Phenothiazines
Gamma-Hydroxybutyrate (GHB)	Alcohol (Ethanol) • Amphetamines • Anticonvulsants • Antipsychotic Drugs • Benzodiazepines • CNS Depressants • Haloperidol (*Haldol*) • Naloxone (*Narcan*) • Narcotic Drugs • Ritonavir (*Norvir*) • Saquinavir (*Fortovase, Invirase*) • Skeletal Muscle Relaxants
Garlic	Anticoagulant/Antiplatelet Drugs • Contraceptive Drugs • Cyclosporine (*Neoral, Sandimmune*) • Cytochrome P450 3A4 (CYP3A4) Substrates • Non-Nucleoside Reverse Transcriptase Inhibitors (NNRTIs) • Saquinavir (*Fortovase, Invirase*) • Warfarin (*Coumadin*)
Gentian	Antacids • H2-Blockers • Proton Pump Inhibitors (PPIs)
German Chamomile	Benzodiazepines • CNS Depressants • Cytochrome P450 3A4 (CYP3A4) Substrates
Germanium	Furosemide (*Lasix*)
Ginger	Antacids • Anticoagulant/Antiplatelet Drugs • Antidiabetes Drugs • Antihypertensive Drugs • Barbiturates • H2-Blockers • Proton Pump Inhibitors (PPIs)
Ginkgo Leaf (Ginkgo Leaf Extract)	Anticoagulant/Antiplatelet Drugs • Buspirone (*Buspar*) • Cytochrome P450 1A2 (CYP1A2) Substrates • Cytochrome P450 2C9 (CYP2C9) Substrates • Cytochrome P450 2D6 (CYP2D6) Substrates • Cytochrome P450 3A4 (CYP3A4) Substrates • Fluoxetine (*Prozac*) • Insulin • Seizure Threshold Lowering Drugs • Thiazide Diuretics • Trazodone (*Desyrel*) • Warfarin (*Coumadin*)
Ginkgo Seed	Anticonvulsants • Seizure Threshold Lowering Drugs
Ginseng, American	Antidiabetes Drugs • Antipsychotic Drugs • Monoamine Oxidase Inhibitors (MAOIs) • Stimulant Drugs • Warfarin (*Coumadin*)
Ginseng, Panax	Anticoagulant/Antiplatelet Drugs • Antidiabetes Drugs • Antipsychotic Drugs • Caffeine • Cytochrome P450 2D6 (CYP2D6) Substrates • Furosemide (*Lasix*) • Immunosuppressants • Insulin • Monoamine Oxidase Inhibitors (MAOIs) • Stimulant Drugs • Warfarin (*Coumadin*)
Ginseng, Siberian	Alcohol (Ethanol) • Anticoagulant/Antiplatelet Drugs • Antidiabetes Drugs • CNS Depressants • Cytochrome P450 1A2 (CYP1A2) Substrates • Cytochrome P450 2C9 (CYP2C9) Substrates • Cytochrome P450 2D6 (CYP2D6) Substrates • Cytochrome P450 3A4 (CYP3A4) Substrates • Digoxin (*Lanoxin*)

CHARTS

Potential Interactions: Natural Medicine/Drug

For additional data, refer to the database.

Natural Medicine	Drug
Glucomannan	Antidiabetes Drugs • Oral Drugs
Glucosamine Hydrochloride	Antidiabetes Drugs • Antimitotic Chemotherapy • Warfarin (*Coumadin*)
Glucosamine Sulfate	Acetaminophen (*Tylenol*, others) • Antidiabetes Drugs • Antimitotic Chemotherapy • Warfarin (*Coumadin*)
Glutamine	Anticonvulsants • Chemotherapy • Lactulose
Glycine	Clozapine (*Clozaril*)
Goat's Rue	Antidiabetes Drugs
Goldenrod	Diuretic Drugs
Goldenseal	Antacids • Antihypertensive Drugs • CNS Depressants • Cytochrome P450 3A4 (CYP3A4) Substrates • H2-Blockers • Proton Pump Inhibitors (PPIs)
Goldthread	Antacids • H2-Blockers • Proton Pump Inhibitors (PPIs)
Gossypol	Digoxin (*Lanoxin*) • Diuretic Drugs • Nonsteroidal Anti-Inflammatory Drugs (NSAIDs) • Stimulant Laxatives • Theophylline
Gotu Kola	CNS Depressants
Grape Fruit, Skin	Cytochrome P450 1A2 (CYP1A2) Substrates • Phenacetin
Grape Seed	Warfarin (*Coumadin*)
Grapefruit	Artemether (*Artenam, Paluther*) • Benzodiazepines • Buspirone (*Buspar*) • Caffeine • Calcium Channel Blockers • Carbamazepine (*Tegretol*) • Carvedilol (*Coreg*) • Cisapride (*Propulsid*) • Clomipramine (*Anafranil*) • Cyclosporine (*Neoral, Sandimmune*) • Cytochrome P450 3A4 (CYP3A4) Substrates • Dextromethorphan (*Robitussin DM*, and others) • Erythromycin • Estrogens • Etoposide (*Vepesid*) • Fexofenadine (*Allegra*) • HMG-CoA Reductase Inhibitors ("Statins") • Itraconazole (*Sporanox*) • Losartan (*Cozaar*) • Methylprednisolone • Praziquantel (*Biltricide*) • Quinidine • Saquinavir (*Fortovase, Invirase*) • Scopolamine • Sildenafil (*Viagra*) • Terfenadine (*Seldane*) • Theophylline • Warfarin (*Coumadin*)
Grapefruit Seed Extract	Artemether (*Artenam, Paluther*) • Benzodiazepines • Buspirone (*Buspar*) • Caffeine • Calcium Channel Blockers • Carbamazepine (*Tegretol*) • Carvedilol (*Coreg*) • Cisapride (*Propulsid*) • Clomipramine (*Anafranil*) • Cyclosporine (*Neoral, Sandimmune*) • Cytochrome P450 3A4 (CYP3A4) Substrates • Estrogens • HMG-CoA Reductase Inhibitors ("Statins") • Quinidine • Saquinavir (*Fortovase, Invirase*) • Terfenadine (*Seldane*) • Warfarin (*Coumadin*)
Great Plantain	Warfarin (*Coumadin*)
Greater Bindweed	Digoxin (*Lanoxin*) • Diuretic Drugs
Greek Sage	Hexobarbital
Green Tea	Adenosine (*Adenocard*) • Alcohol (Ethanol) • Amphetamines • Anticoagulant/Antiplatelet Drugs • Antidiabetes Drugs • Antipsychotic Drugs • Cimetidine (*Tagamet*) • Clozapine (*Clozaril*) • Cocaine • Contraceptive Drugs • Dipyridamole (*Persantine*) • Disulfiram (*Antabuse*) • Ephedrine • Estrogens • Fluconazole (*Diflucan*) • Fluvoxamine (*Luvox*) • Lithium • Mexiletine (*Mexitil*) • Monoamine Oxidase Inhibitors (MAOIs) • Nicotine • Phenylpropanolamine • Quinolone Antibiotics • Riluzole (*Rilutek*) • Terbinafine (*Lamisil*) • Theophylline • Warfarin (*Coumadin*)
Guar Gum	Antidiabetes Drugs • Oral Drugs
Guarana	Adenosine (*Adenocard*) • Alcohol (Ethanol) • Amphetamines • Anticoagulant/Antiplatelet Drugs • Antidiabetes Drugs • Cimetidine (*Tagamet*) • Clozapine (*Clozaril*) • Cocaine • Contraceptive Drugs • Dipyridamole (*Persantine*) • Disulfiram (*Antabuse*) • Ephedrine • Estrogens • Fluconazole (*Diflucan*) • Fluvoxamine (*Luvox*) • Lithium • Mexiletine (*Mexitil*) • Monoamine Oxidase Inhibitors (MAOIs) • Nicotine • Phenylpropanolamine • Quinolone Antibiotics • Riluzole (*Rilutek*) • Terbinafine (*Lamisil*) • Theophylline • Verapamil (*Calan, Covera, Isoptin, Verelan*)

Potential Interactions: Natural Medicine/Drug For additional data, refer to the database.

Natural Medicine	Drug
Guggul	Anticoagulant/Antiplatelet Drugs • Diltiazem (*Cardizem*) • Propranolol (*Inderal*) • Thyroid Hormone
Gymnema	Antidiabetes Drugs • Insulin
Hawaiian Baby Woodrose	Antidepressant Drugs • Clozapine (*Clozaril*) • Cyproheptadine • Dextromethorphan (*Robitussin DM*, and others) • Meperidine (*Demerol*) • Monoamine Oxidase Inhibitors (MAOIs) • Pentazocine (*Talwin*) • Risperidone (*Risperdal*) • Tramadol (*Ultram*)
Hawthorn	Calcium Channel Blockers • CNS Depressants • Digoxin (*Lanoxin*) • Nitrates
Hedge Mustard	Digoxin (*Lanoxin*) • Diuretic Drugs • Macrolide Antibiotics • Quinine • Stimulant Laxatives • Tetracycline Antibiotics
Henbane	Anticholinergic Drugs
Hops	Alcohol (Ethanol) • CNS Depressants
Horse Chestnut	Anticoagulant/Antiplatelet Drugs • Antidiabetes Drugs
Horseradish	Levothyroxine (*Synthroid*, *Levothroid*, *Levoxyl*, others)
Horsetail	Corticosteroids • Digoxin (*Lanoxin*) • Diuretic Drugs
Huperzine A	Acetylcholinesterase (AChE) Inhibitors • Anticholinergic Drugs • Cholinergic Drugs
Hydrazine Sulfate	Antidiabetes Drugs • CNS Depressants • Monoamine Oxidase Inhibitors (MAOIs)
Iboga	Anticholinergic Drugs • Cholinergic Drugs
Iceland Moss	Oral Drugs
Indian Long Pepper	Phenytoin (*Dilantin*) • Propranolol (*Inderal*) • Theophylline
Indian Snakeroot	Alcohol (Ethanol) • Antipsychotic Drugs • Barbiturates • Digoxin (*Lanoxin*) • Diuretic Drugs • Ephedrine • Levodopa • Monoamine Oxidase Inhibitors (MAOIs) • Propranolol (*Inderal*) • Stimulant Drugs • Tricyclic Antidepressants (TCAs)
Indole-3-Carbinol	Cytochrome P450 1A2 (CYP1A2) Substrates
Inositol Nicotinate	Anticoagulant/Antiplatelet Drugs • Antidiabetes Drugs • HMG-CoA Reductase Inhibitors ("Statins") • Transdermal Nicotine (*Nicoderm*, *Nicotrol*)
Iodine	ACE Inhibitors (ACEIs) • Amiodarone (*Cordarone*) • Angiotensin Receptor Blockers (ARBs) • Antithyroid Drugs • Lithium • Potassium-Sparing Diuretics
IP-6	Anticoagulant/Antiplatelet Drugs
Ipecac	Activated Charcoal
Ipriflavone	Cytochrome P450 1A2 (CYP1A2) Substrates • Cytochrome P450 2C9 (CYP2C9) Substrates • Immunosuppressants • Theophylline
Iron	Bisphosphonates • Chloramphenicol • Levodopa • Levothyroxine (*Levothroid*, *Levoxyl*, *Synthroid*, and others) • Methyldopa (*Aldomet*) • Mycophenolate Mofetil (*CellCept*) • Penicillamine • Quinolone Antibiotics • Tetracycline Antibiotics
Jalap	Digoxin (*Lanoxin*) • Diuretic Drugs • Oral Drugs • Stimulant Laxatives
Jamaican Dogwood	CNS Depressants
Jiaogulan	Anticoagulant/Antiplatelet Drugs • Immunosuppressants
Jimson Weed	Anticholinergic Drugs
Juniper	Antidiabetes Drugs • Diuretic Drugs
Kaolin	Oral Drugs
Karaya Gum	Oral Drugs
Kava	Alprazolam (*Xanax*) • CNS Depressants • Cytochrome P450 1A2 (CYP1A2) Substrates • Cytochrome P450 2C19 (CYP2C19) Substrates • Cytochrome P450 2C9 (CYP2C9) Substrates • Cytochrome P450 2D6 (CYP2D6) Substrates • Cytochrome P450 3A4 (CYP3A4) Substrates • Hepatotoxic Drugs • Levodopa

CHARTS

Potential Interactions: Natural Medicine/Drug

For additional data, refer to the database.

Natural Medicine	Drug
Kefir	Immunosuppressants
Khella	Digoxin (*Lanoxin*) • Hepatotoxic Drugs • Photosensitizing Drugs
Kombucha Tea	Disulfiram (*Antabuse*)
Kudzu	Anticoagulant/Antiplatelet Drugs • Antidiabetes Drugs • Aspirin • Contraceptive Drugs • Estrogens • Tamoxifen (*Nolvadex*)
Lactobacillus	Antibiotic Drugs • Immunosuppressants
Laminaria	ACE Inhibitors (ACEIs) • Digoxin (*Lanoxin*) • Potassium Supplements • Potassium-Sparing Diuretics • Thyroid Hormone
Larch Arabinogalactan	Immunosuppressants • Oral Drugs
L-Arginine	Antihypertensive Drugs • Nitrates • Sildenafil (*Viagra*)
Lavender	Barbiturates • Chloral Hydrate • CNS Depressants
L-Carnitine	Acenocoumarol (*Sintrom*) • Warfarin (*Coumadin*)
Lemon Balm	CNS Depressants
Licorice	Antihypertensive Drugs • Corticosteroids • Cytochrome P450 2B6 (CYP2B6) Substrates • Cytochrome P450 3A4 (CYP3A4) Substrates • Digoxin (*Lanoxin*) • Diuretic Drugs • Estrogens • Ethacrynic Acid (*Edecrin*) • Furosemide (*Lasix*) • Insulin
Lily-of-the-Valley	Calcium Supplements • Corticosteroids • Digoxin (*Lanoxin*) • Diuretic Drugs • Macrolide Antibiotics • Quinine • Stimulant Laxatives • Tetracycline Antibiotics
Lime Fruit, Peel	Cytochrome P450 3A4 (CYP3A4) Substrates
Lime Oil	Photosensitizing Drugs
Lithium	ACE Inhibitors (ACEIs) • Anticonvulsants • Antidepressant Drugs • Calcium Channel Blockers • Dextromethorphan (*Robitussin DM*, others) • Loop Diuretics • Meperidine (*Demerol*) • Methyldopa (*Aldomet*) • Methylxanthines • Monoamine Oxidase Inhibitors (MAOIs) • Nonsteroidal Anti-Inflammatory Drugs (NSAIDs) • Pentazocine (*Talwin*) • Phenothiazines • Skeletal Muscle Relaxants • Thiazide Diuretics • Tramadol (*Ultram*)
Lovage	Diuretic Drugs
L-Tryptophan	Antidepressant Drugs • Benzodiazepines • CNS Depressants • Dextromethorphan (*Robitussin DM*, others) • Meperidine (*Demerol*) • Monoamine Oxidase Inhibitors (MAOIs) • Pentazocine (*Talwin*) • Phenothiazines • Tramadol (*Ultram*)
Lycium	Antidiabetes Drugs • Antihypertensive Drugs • Cytochrome P450 2C9 (CYP2C9) Substrates • Warfarin (*Coumadin*)
Lysine	Calcium Supplements
Madagascar Periwinkle	Antidiabetes Drugs
Magnesium	Aminoglycoside Antibiotics • Bisphosphonates • Calcium Channel Blockers • Potassium-Sparing Diuretics • Quinolone Antibiotics • Skeletal Muscle Relaxants • Tetracycline Antibiotics
Magnolia	Alcohol (Ethanol) • Barbiturates • Benzodiazepines • CNS Depressants
Maitake Mushroom	Antidiabetes Drugs
Manganese	Quinolone Antibiotics • Tetracycline Antibiotics
Manna	Digoxin (*Lanoxin*) • Diuretic Drugs
Marijuana	Barbiturates • CNS Depressants • Disulfiram (*Antabuse*) • Fluoxetine (*Prozac*) • Theophylline (*Theo-Dur*, *Slo-Bid*)
Marsh Tea	CNS Depressants
Marshmallow	Antidiabetes Drugs • Oral Drugs
Masterwort	Photosensitizing Drugs

Potential Interactions: Natural Medicine/Drug

For additional data, refer to the database.

Natural Medicine	Drug
Mate	Adenosine (*Adenocard*) • Alcohol (Ethanol) • Amphetamines • Anticoagulant/Antiplatelet Drugs • Antidiabetes Drugs • Cimetidine (*Tagamet*) • Clozapine (*Clozaril*) • Cocaine • Contraceptive Drugs • Dipyridamole (*Persantine*) • Disulfiram (*Antabuse*) • Ephedrine • Estrogens • Fluconazole (*Diflucan*) • Fluvoxamine (*Luvox*) • Lithium (*Eskalith*) • Mexiletine (*Mexitil*) • Monoamine Oxidase Inhibitors (MAOIs) • Nicotine • Phenylpropanolamine • Quinolone Antibiotics • Riluzole (*Rilutek*) • Terbinafine (*Lamisil*) • Theophylline • Verapamil (*Calan, Covera, Isoptin, Verelan*)
Meadowsweet	Aspirin • Choline Magnesium Trisalicylate (*Trilisate*) • Narcotic Drugs • Salsalate (*Disalcid*)
Melatonin	Anticoagulant/Antiplatelet Drugs • Antidiabetes Drugs • Benzodiazepines • Caffeine • CNS Depressants • Contraceptive Drugs • Flumazenil (*Romazicon*) • Fluvoxamine (*Luvox*) • Immunosuppressants • Nifedipine GITS (*Procardia XL*) • Verapamil (*Calan, Covera, Isoptin, Verelan*)
Mesoglycan	Anticoagulant/Antiplatelet Drugs • Thrombolytic Drugs
Methoxylated Flavones	Cytochrome P450 1A2 (CYP1A2) Substrates
Mexican Scammony Root	Digoxin (*Lanoxin*) • Diuretic Drugs • Oral Drugs • Stimulant Laxatives
Milk Thistle	Cytochrome P450 2C9 (CYP2C9) Substrates • Cytochrome P450 3A4 (CYP3A4) Substrates • Estrogens • Glucuronidated Drugs • Indinavir (*Crixivan*)
Morinda	Potassium-Sparing Diuretics
Mormon Tea	Oral Drugs
Motherwort	CNS Depressants
Myrrh	Antidiabetes Drugs
N-Acetyl Cysteine	Activated Charcoal • Nitroglycerin
N-Acetyl Glucosamine	Antidiabetes Drugs • Chemotherapy • Warfarin (*Coumadin*)
Nattokinase	Anticoagulant/Antiplatelet Drugs
Niacin and Niacinamide (Vitamin B3)	Antidiabetes Drugs • HMG-CoA Reductase Inhibitors ("Statins") • Transdermal Nicotine (*Nicoderm, Nicotrol*)
Northern Prickly Ash	Antacids • H2-Blockers • Proton Pump Inhibitors (PPIs)
Nutmeg and Mace	Cytochrome P450 1A1 (CYP1A1) Substrates • Cytochrome P450 1A2 (CYP1A2) Substrates • Cytochrome P450 2B1 (CYP2B1) Substrates • Cytochrome P450 2B2 (CYP2B2) Substrates • Phenobarbital (*Luminal*)
Oat Above Ground Parts	Morphine
Oats	Morphine • Oral Drugs
Octacosanol	Levodopa/Carbidopa (*Sinemet*)
Oleander	Calcium Supplements • Digoxin (*Lanoxin*) • Diuretic Drugs • Macrolide Antibiotics • Quinine • Stimulant Laxatives • Tetracycline Antibiotics
Olive Leaf	Antidiabetes Drugs • Antihypertensive Drugs
Olive Oil	Antidiabetes Drugs
Onion	Anticoagulant/Antiplatelet Drugs • Antidiabetes Drugs • Aspirin
Pancreatin	Acarbose (*Precose, Prandase*)
Pangamic Acid	Calcium Channel Blockers • Digoxin (*Lanoxin*) • Thiazide Diuretics
Pantethine	Anticoagulant/Antiplatelet Drugs
Papaya	Warfarin (*Coumadin*)
Para-Aminobenzoic Acid (PABA)	Cortisone (*Cortisone Acetate*) • Dapsone (*Avlosulfon*) • Sulfonamide Antibiotics
Parsley Leaf, Root	Anticoagulant/Antiplatelet Drugs • Aspirin • Diuretic Drugs
Parsley Seed	Diuretic Drugs

Potential Interactions: Natural Medicine/Drug

For additional data, refer to the database.

Natural Medicine	Drug
Passionflower	Barbiturates • CNS Depressants
Pau d'Arco	Anticoagulant/Antiplatelet Drugs
Pectin	Beta-Carotene • Digoxin (*Lanoxin*) • Lovastatin (*Mevacor*) • Tetracycline Antibiotics
Peony Root	Phenytoin (*Dilantin*)
Peppermint Oil	Antacids • Cyclosporine (*Neoral, Sandimmune*) • Cytochrome P450 3A4 (CYP3A4) Substrates • H2-Blockers • Proton Pump Inhibitors (PPIs)
Periwinkle	Antihypertensive Drugs
Peyote	Stimulant Drugs
Pheasant's Eye	Calcium Supplements • Corticosteroids • Digoxin (*Lanoxin*) • Diuretic Drugs • Quinidine • Stimulant Laxatives
Phenylalanine	Antipsychotic Drugs • Levodopa • Monoamine Oxidase Inihibtors (MAOIs)
Phosphate Salts	Antacids • Cholestyramine (*Questran*) • Colestipol (*Colestid*)
Picrorhiza	Immunosuppressants
Pinus Bark	Oral Drugs
Pleurisy Root	Digoxin (*Lanoxin*) • Diuretic Drugs • Estrogens
Podophyllum	Diuretic Drugs
Policosanol	Anticoagulant/Antiplatelet Drugs
Pomegranate	ACE Inhibitors (ACEIs) • Antihypertensive Drugs • Oral Drugs
Potassium	ACE Inhibitors (ACEIs) • Angiotensin Receptor Blockers (ARBs) • Potassium-Sparing Diuretics
Potato	Thrombolytic Drugs
Pregnenolone	Estrogens • Progestin • Testosterone
Prickly Pear Cactus	Chlorpropamide (*Diabinese*)
Procaine	Aminosalicylic Acid • Digoxin (*Lanoxin*) • Skeletal Muscle Relaxants • Succinylcholine • Sulfonamide Antibiotics
Progesterone	Estrogens
Pycnogenol	Immunosuppressants
Pyridoxine (Vitamin B6)	Amiodarone (*Cordarone*) • Levodopa • Phenobarbital (*Luminal*) • Phenytoin (*Dilantin*)
Quassia	Antacids • Digoxin (*Lanoxin*) • Diuretic Drugs • H2-Blockers • Proton Pump Inhibitors (PPIs)
Quercetin	Quinolone Antibiotics
Quillaia	Metformin (*Glucophage*) • Oral Drugs
Quince	Oral Drugs
Raspberry Leaf	Metformin (*Glucophage*) • Oral Drugs
Red Clover	Anticoagulant/Antiplatelet Drugs • Contraceptive Drugs • Cytochrome P450 3A4 (CYP3A4) Substrates • Estrogens • Tamoxifen (*Nolvadex*)
Red Yeast	Alcohol (Ethanol) • Cyclosporine (*Neoral, Sandimmune*) • Cytochrome P450 3A4 (CYP3A4) Inhibitors • Gemfibrozil (*Lopid*) • HMG-CoA Reductase Inhibitors ("Statins") • Levothyroxine (*Synthroid*, *Levothroid*, *Levoxyl*, and others) • Niacin
Reishi Mushroom	Anticoagulant/Antiplatelet Drugs • Antihypertensive Drugs
Resveratrol	Anticoagulant/Antiplatelet Drugs • Cytochrome P450 3A4 (CYP3A4) Substrates
Rhatany	Oral Drugs
Rhubarb	Corticosteroids • Digoxin (*Lanoxin*) • Diuretic Drugs • Oral Drugs • Stimulant Laxatives

Potential Interactions: Natural Medicine/Drug For additional data, refer to the database.

Natural Medicine	Drug
Riboflavin (Vitamin B2)	Anticholinergic Drugs • Probenecid (*Benemid*)
Ribose	Alcohol (Ethanol) • Antidiabetes Drugs • Aspirin • Choline Magnesium Trisalicylate (*Trilisate*) • Insulin • Propranolol (*Inderal*) • Salsalate (*Disalcid*)
Rice Bran	Oral Drugs
Rose Hip	Aluminum • Aspirin • Choline Magnesium Trisalicylate (*Trilisate*) • Estrogens • Fluphenazine (*Prolixin*) • Salsalate (*Disalcid*) • Warfarin (*Coumadin*)
Rue	Photosensitizing Drugs
Saccharomyces Boulardii	Antifungals
Safflower	Anticoagulant/Antiplatelet Drugs
Sage	Anticonvulsants • Antidiabetes Drugs • CNS Depressants
SAMe	Antidepressant Drugs • Dextromethorphan (*Robitussin DM*, and others) • Levodopa • Meperidine (*Demerol*) • Monoamine Oxidase Inhibitors (MAOIs) • Pentazocine (*Talwin*) • Tramadol (*Ultram*)
Sarsaparilla	Digoxin (*Lanoxin*)
Sassafras	CNS Depressants
Saw Palmetto	Anticoagulant/Antiplatelet Drugs • Contraceptive Drugs • Estrogens
Scopolia	Anticholinergic Drugs • Quinidine • Tricyclic Antidepressants (TCAs)
Scotch Broom Flower	Monoamine Oxidase Inhibitors (MAOIs)
Scotch Broom Herb	Haloperidol (*Haldol*) • Monoamine Oxidase Inhibitors (MAOIs) • Quinidine
Sea Buckthorn	Anticoagulant/Antiplatelet Drugs
Selenium	HMG-CoA Reductase Inhibitors ("Statins") • Niacin
Senna	Digoxin (*Lanoxin*) • Diuretic Drugs
Shepherd's Purse	CNS Depressants • Thyroid Hormone
Slippery Elm	Oral Drugs
Smartweed	Warfarin (*Coumadin*)
Solomon's Seal	Antidiabetes Drugs • Chlorpropamide (*Diabinese*) • Insulin
Sorrel	Oral Drugs
Southern Prickly Ash	Antacids • H2-Blockers • Proton Pump Inhibitors (PPIs)
Soy	Antibiotic Drugs • Estrogens • Tamoxifen (*Nolvadex*) • Warfarin (*Coumadin*)
Spinach	Antidiabetes Drugs • Warfarin (*Coumadin*)
Squill	Calcium Supplements • Corticosteroids • Digoxin (*Lanoxin*) • Diuretic Drugs • Quinidine • Stimulant Laxatives
St. John's Wort	5-HT1 Agonists (*Triptans*) • Alprazolam (*Xanax*) • Aminolevulinic Acid • Amitriptyline (*Elavil*) • Antidepressant Drugs • Barbiturates • Contraceptive Drugs • Cyclosporine (*Neoral, Sandimmune*) • Cytochrome P450 1A2 (CYP1A2) Substrates • Cytochrome P450 2C9 (CYP2C9) Substrates • Cytochrome P450 3A4 (CYP3A4) Substrates • Dextromethorphan (*Robitussin DM*, and others) • Digoxin (*Lanoxin*) • Fenfluramine (*Pondimin*) • Fexofenadine (*Allegra*) • Imatinib (*Gleevec*) • Irinotecan (*Camptosar*) • Meperidine (*Demerol*) • Monoamine Oxidase Inhibitors (MAOIs) • Narcotic Drugs • Nefazodone (*Serzone*) • Non-Nucleoside Reverse Transcriptase Inhibitors (NNRTIs) • Nortriptyline (*Pamelor, Aventyl*) • P-Glycoprotein Substrates • Paroxetine (*Paxil*) • Pentazocine (*Talwin*) • Phenobarbital (*Luminal*) • Phenprocoumon • Phenytoin (*Dilantin*) • Photosensitizing Drugs • Protease Inhibitors (PIs) • Reserpine • Sertraline (*Zoloft*) • Simvastatin (*Zocor*) • Tacrolimus (*Prograf, Protopic*) • Theophylline • Tramadol (*Ultram*) • Warfarin (*Coumadin*)
Stevia	Antidiabetes Drugs • Antihypertensive Drugs • Calcium Channel Blockers

Potential Interactions: Natural Medicine/Drug

For additional data, refer to the database.

Natural Medicine	Drug
Stinging Nettle Above Ground Parts	Antidiabetes Drugs • Antihypertensive Drugs • CNS Depressants • Warfarin (*Coumadin*)
Stone Root	Diuretic Drugs
Strophanthus	Calcium Supplements • Corticosteroids • Digoxin (*Lanoxin*) • Diuretic Drugs • Quinidine • Quinine • Stimulant Laxatives
Swamp Milkweed	Digoxin (*Lanoxin*) • Diuretic Drugs • Macrolide Antibiotics • Quinine • Stimulant Laxatives • Tetracycline Antibiotics
Sweet Bay	CNS Depressants • Narcotic Drugs
Sweet Clover	Anticoagulant/Antiplatelet Drugs • Hepatotoxic Drugs
Sweet Orange	Celiprolol (*Celicard*) • Fexofenadine (*Allegra*) • Ivermectin
Sweet Vernal Grass	Anticoagulant/Antiplatelet Drugs
Tamarind	Ibuprofen
Tannic Acid	Oral Drugs
Tansy	Alcohol (Ethanol)
Theanine	Antihypertensive Drugs • Stimulant Drugs
Threonine	NMDA Antagonists
Thunder God Vine	Immunosuppressants
Thymus Extract	Immunosuppressants
Tiratricol	Anticoagulant/Antiplatelet Drugs • Antidiabetes Drugs • Cholestyramine (*Questran*) • Stimulant Drugs • Thyroid Hormone
Tragacanth	Oral Drugs
Turmeric	Anticoagulant/Antiplatelet Drugs
Tyrosine	Levodopa • Thyroid Hormone
Uzara	Digoxin (*Lanoxin*) • Diuretic Drugs • Macrolide Antibiotics • Quinine • Stimulant Laxatives • Tetracycline Antibiotics
Valerian	Alcohol (Ethanol) • Benzodiazepines • CNS Depressants • Cytochrome P450 3A4 (CYP3A4) Substrates
Vanadium	Anticoagulant/Antiplatelet Drugs • Antidiabetes Drugs
Verbena	Antihypertensive Drugs
Vinpocetine	Anticoagulant/Antiplatelet Drugs • Warfarin (*Coumadin*)
Vitamin A	Hepatotoxic Drugs • Retinoids • Tetracycline Antibiotics • Warfarin (*Coumadin*)
Vitamin B12	Chloramphenicol
Vitamin C (Ascorbic Acid)	Acetaminophen (*Tylenol*, others) • Aluminum • Aspirin • Chemotherapy • Choline Magnesium Trisalicylate (*Trilisate*) • Estradiol • Fluphenazine (*Prolixin*) • Heparin • HMG-CoA Reductase Inhibitors ("Statins") • Niacin • Protease Inhibitors (PIs) • Salsalate (*Disalcid*) • Warfarin (*Coumadin*)
Vitamin D	Phenobarbital (*Luminal*) • Phenytoin (*Dilantin*) • Thiazide Diuretics
Vitamin E	Anticoagulant/Antiplatelet Drugs • Chemotherapy • HMG-CoA Reductase Inhibitors ("Statins") • Niacin • Warfarin (*Coumadin*)
Vitamin K	Warfarin (*Coumadin*)
Wahoo	Digoxin (*Lanoxin*) • Diuretic Drugs • Macrolide Antibiotics • Quinine • Stimulant Laxatives • Tetracycline Antibiotics
Wallflower	Calcium Supplements • Corticosteroids • Digoxin (*Lanoxin*) • Diuretic Drugs • Quinidine • Quinine • Stimulant Laxatives

Potential Interactions: Natural Medicine/Drug

For additional data, refer to the database.

Natural Medicine	Drug
Water Avens	Metformin (*Glucophage*) • Oral Drugs
Watercress	Chlorzoxazone (*Parafon Forte, Paraflex*) • Warfarin (*Coumadin*)
Wheat Bran	Digoxin (*Lanoxin*)
Whey Protein	Alendronate (*Fosamax*) • Levodopa • Quinolone Antibiotics • Tetracycline Antibiotics
Wild Carrot	Antihypertensive Drugs • Estrogens • Photosensitizing Drugs
Wild Cherry	Cytochrome P450 3A4 (CYP3A4) Substrates
Wild Lettuce	CNS Depressants
Willow Bark	Anticoagulant/Antiplatelet Drugs • Aspirin • Choline Magnesium Trisalicylate (*Trilisate*) • Oral Drugs • Salsalate (*Disalcid*)
Wine	Aspirin • Barbiturates • Benzodiazepines • Cefamandole (*Mandol*) • Cefoperazone (*Cefobid*) • Chlorpropamide (*Diabinese*) • Cisapride (*Propulsid*) • CNS Depressants • Cyclosporine (*Neoral, Sandimmune*) • Disulfiram (*Antabuse*) • Erythromycin • Felodipine (*Plendil*) • Griseofulvin (*Fulvicin*) • H2-Blockers • Hepatotoxic Drugs • Metformin (*Glucophage*) • Metronidazole (*Flagyl*) • Monoamine Oxidase Inhibitors (MAOIs) • Narcotic Drugs • Nonsteroidal Anti-Inflammatory Drugs (NSAIDs) • Phenytoin (*Dilantin*) • Sulfonamide Antibiotics • Tolbutamide (*Orinase*) • Warfarin (*Coumadin*)
Wintergreen Oil	Aspirin • Warfarin (*Coumadin*)
Wormwood Above Ground Parts	Antacids • Anticonvulsants • H2-Blockers • Proton Pump Inhibitors (PPIs)
Xanthan Gum	Antidiabetes Drugs
Yarrow	Antacids • Anticoagulant/Antiplatelet Drugs • Barbiturates • H2-Blockers • Proton Pump Inhibitors (PPIs)
Yellow Dock	Digoxin (*Lanoxin*) • Diuretic Drugs
Yerba Mansa	CNS Depressants
Yogurt	Ciprofloxacin (*Cipro*) • Immunosuppressants • Tetracycline Antibiotics
Yohimbe	Antihypertensive Drugs • Clonidine (*Catapres*) • Guanabenz (*Wytensin*) • Monoamine Oxidase Inhibitors (MAOIs) • Naloxone (*Narcan*) • Phenothiazines • Stimulant Drugs • Tricyclic Antidepressants (TCAs)
Zinc	Cisplatin (*Platinol-AQ*) • Penicillamine • Potassium-Sparing Diuretics • Quinolone Antibiotics • Tetracycline Antibiotics • Thiazide Diuretics

Drug Influences on Nutrient Levels and Depletion

Some medications can affect the levels of certain nutrients in the body. There is considerable interest in using nutritional supplements to counteract these possible drug-induced "nutrient depletions." The chart below shows the current scientific understanding of these relationships, and suggested actions.

DRUGS (Includes some representative U.S. and Canadian Brand Names.)	NUTRIENT DEPLETED	POSSIBLE MECHANISM	COMMENTS & REFERENCES
ANTI-INFECTIVES			
ANTIBIOTICS			
Antibiotics - General: Cephalosporins, Fluoroquinolones, Isoniazid, Macrolides, Penicillins, Sulfonamides, Tetracyclines, Trimethoprim/Sulfamethoxazole	Dibencozide Niacin and Niacinamide Pantothenic Acid (B5) Pyridoxine (B6) Riboflavin (B2) Thiamine (B1) Vitamin B12 Vitamin K	Destruction of normal intestinal microflora may lead to decreased production of various B vitamins and vitamin K. Some cephalosporins interfere directly with vitamin K-dependant clotting factor production.	The intestinal microflora is reduced by antibiotics. However, the B vitamins are mainly obtained from the diet, and any changes in their production by intestinal bacteria is unlikely to be clinically significant.[4434-43,6243,9502,9530] Reduction in vitamin K-dependant clotting factor production may be significant in people with other risk factors for low vitamin K levels. Monitor these patients closely.[4437,4439,7135,9502,11513-6]
	Folic Acid	Disruption of normal intestinal microflora decreases enterohepatic circulation and reabsorption of folic acid, and may reduce synthesis. Trimethoprim inhibits conversion of folic acid to its active form.	Folic acid synthesized by intestinal microflora probably doesn't contribute significantly to overall folate status, and supplements aren't necessary with normal courses of antibiotics.[2677,4436,4437,6243] Prolonged courses of high-dose trimethoprim rarely cause megaloblastic anemia, and folic acid supplements have been used to prevent this. However, some evidence suggests folic acid supplements can reduce the efficacy of trimethoprim. Avoid supplements unless recommended by a physician.[4468,7857,7859,7862,7875]
Aminoglycosides: Amikacin (*Amikin*) Gentamicin (*Garamycin*) Kanamycin (*Kantrex*) Netilmicin (*Netromycin*) Streptomycin Tobramycin (*Nebcin*)	Magnesium Potassium	Increased urinary excretion, associated with drug-induced renal damage.	Monitor patients for electrolyte disturbances and declining renal funciton. Give intravenous electrolyte replacement if necessary.[15]
Fluoroquinolones: Ciprofloxacin (*Cipro*), Enoxacin (*Penetrex*), Gatifloxacin (*Tequin*), Levofloxacin (*Levaquin*), Lomefloxacin (*Maxaquin*), Moxifloxacin (*Avelox*), Norfloxacin (*Noroxin*), Ofloxacin (*Floxin*), Sparfloxacin (*Zagam*), Trovafloxacin (*Trovan*)	Calcium Iron Magnesium Zinc	Formation of insoluble complexes (prevents absorption of both nutrient and fluoroquinolone).	Significant effects on levels of these nutrients are unlikely when fluoroquinolones are taken at least 2 hours before, or 4-6 hours after calcium/iron/magnesium/zinc-containing foods or supplements.[828,2682,4412,4531]
Neomycin (*Mycifradin*)	Beta-Carotene Dibencozide Vitamin A Vitamin B12	Reduced absorption.	Not clinically significant with short-term use of neomycin.[3046,5916,8434,10565-6]

Drug Influences on Nutrient Levels and Depletion

Some medications can affect the levels of certain nutrients in the body. There is considerable interest in using nutritional supplements to counteract these possible drug-induced "nutrient depletions." The chart below shows the current scientific understanding of these relationships, and suggested actions.

DRUGS (Includes some representative U.S. and Canadian Brand Names.)	NUTRIENT DEPLETED	POSSIBLE MECHANISM	COMMENTS & REFERENCES
ANTI-INFECTIVES (cont.)			
Penicillins (sodium-containing): Carbenicillin (*Geocillin*), Mezlocillin (*Mezlin*), Penicillin G sodium (*Pfizerpen*), Piperacillin (*Pipracil*), Ticarcillin (*Ticar*)	Potassium	Large sodium load is presented to the kidneys, resulting in sodium reabsorption and potassium excretion.	Monitor potassium levels, and give supplements or switch to a different antibiotic if necessary.[9519]
Tetracyclines: Tetracycline (*Achromycin V, Panmycin, Robitet, Robicaps, Sumycin, Teline, Tetracap, Tetracyn, Tetralan*), Demeclocycline (*Declomycin*), Doxycycline (*Bio-Tab, Doryx, Doxy Caps, Doxychel, Doxychel Hyclate, Monodox, Periostat, Vibra-Tabs, Vibramycin*), Minocycline (*Dynacin, Vectrin*), Oxytetracycline (*Terramycin, Uri-Tet*)	Calcium Iron Magnesium Zinc	Formation of insoluble complexes (prevents absorption of both nutrient and tetracycline). Doxycycline does not reduce zinc absorption.	Significant effects on levels of these nutrients are unlikely when tetracyclines are taken at least 2 hours before, or 4-6 hours after calcium/iron/magnesium/zinc-containing foods or supplements.[9,4412,4531,4549-50]
	Potassium	Increased renal excretion associated with nephropathy.	Due to a toxic degradation product in outdated tetracyclines. Avoid outdated drugs.[4425]
ANTIFUNGALS			
Amphotericin B (*Abelcet, AmBisome, Amphocin, Amphotec, Fungizone*)	Magnesium Potassium	Increased urinary excretion, associated with drug-induced renal damage.	Monitor patients for electrolyte disturbances and declining renal function. Give intravenous electrolyte replacement if necessary.[15]
Fluconazole (*Diflucan*)	Potassium	Increased urinary excretion, associated with drug-induced renal damage.	Monitor potassium levels and renal function in people on prolonged fluconazole therapy, and in those with other risk factors for hypokalemia.[9519]
ANTIMALARIALS			
Pyrimethamine (*Daraprim*)	Folic Acid	Folate antagonism. Binds to dihydrofolate reductase, preventing conversion of folic acid to its active form.	At lower pyrimethamine doses, the need for supplementation has not been adequately studied. Advise patients to maintain good dietary folate intake. People receiving larger pyrimethamine doses (those required to treat toxoplasmosis), should receive folinic acid (leucovorin) to prevent megaloblastic anemia. Avoid folic acid (antagonizes therapeutic effects of pyrimethamine).[4532,9380]
Quinacrine	Riboflavin (B2)	Can interfere with conversion to the active form flavin adenine dinubleotide (FAD).	May cause riboflavin deficiency. Clinical significance is not known.[505,10522]

CHARTS

Drug Influences on Nutrient Levels and Depletion

Some medications can affect the levels of certain nutrients in the body. There is considerable interest in using nutritional supplements to counteract these possible drug-induced "nutrient depletions." The chart below shows the current scientific understanding of these relationships, and suggested actions.

DRUGS (Includes some representative U.S. and Canadian Brand Names.)	NUTRIENT DEPLETED	POSSIBLE MECHANISM	COMMENTS & REFERENCES
ANTI-INFECTIVES (cont.)			
ANTIPROTAZOALS			
Pentamidine (*NebuPent, Pentacarinat, Pentam 300*)	Folic Acid	Weak folate antagonist, preventing conversion of folic acid to its active form.	Rare cases of megaloblastic anemia, but only with prolonged parenteral therapy. Folic acid supplements are usually not necessary.[9378]
	Magnesium	Increased urinary excretion, associated with drug-induced renal damage.	Monitor serum magnesium levels and give oral or intravenous supplements as needed.[8872,9618,9619]
ANTIRETROVIRALS			
Zidovudine (AZT, *Combivir, Retrovir*)	Copper Dibencozide L-carnitine Vitamin B12	Some HIV patients taking zidovudine have subnormal copper, L-carnitine, and vitamin B12 levels. Mechanism unknown.	Preliminary evidence suggests lower copper levels are not harmful and supplements shouldn't be used.[4986,8970] Consider L-carnitine supplements only if clinical judgement warrants it.[3617] Preliminary data suggests vitamin B12 supplements aren't helpful.[10532-3]
ANTITUBERCULOSIS AGENTS			
Aminosalicylic Acid (para-aminosalicylic acid, *Paser*)	Folic Acid	Inhibits absorption in the gastrointestinal tract.	May worsen the folic acid deficiency associated with tuberculosis. Recommend supplements if diet is folate-deficient.[9363,9388,9395-7]
	Iron	Reduced gastrointestinal absorption.	Monitor for signs and symptoms of iron deficiency and give supplements if needed.[9574]
	Dibencozide Vitamin B12	Reduced gastrointestinal absorption.	Monitor vitamin B12 levels if treatment lasts more than one month.[4558,9395,9397]
Cycloserine (*Seromycin*)	Folic Acid	Possibly reduces absorption or increases metabolism.	Rare cases of megaloblastic anemia reported, but usually with other factors contributing to folate deficiency. Recommend supplements only if dietary intake is deficient.[4531,4536,9363]
Isoniazid (*Laniazid*, INH)	Pyridoxine (B6)	Interferes with pyridoxine metabolism.	Patients receiving > 10 mg/kg/day of INH should be supplemented with 50 - 100 mg of pyridoxine per day.[4481-2]
	Niacin and Niacinamide	Isoniazid inhibits the conversion of tryptophan to niacin.	Might induce pellagra, particularly in poorly nourished patients.[4865-6]

CHARTS

Drug Influences on Nutrient Levels and Depletion

Some medications can affect the levels of certain nutrients in the body. There is considerable interest in using nutritional supplements to counteract these possible drug-induced "nutrient depletions." The chart below shows the current scientific understanding of these relationships, and suggested actions.

DRUGS (Includes some representative U.S. and Canadian Brand Names.)	NUTRIENT DEPLETED	POSSIBLE MECHANISM	COMMENTS & REFERENCES
ANTI-INFECTIVES (cont.)			
ANTITUBERCULOSIS AGENTS (cont.)			
Rifampin (*Rifadin, Rimactane, Rofact)*	Vitamin D	Increased vitamin D metabolism.	There is no consensus that vitamin D supplementation is always required. Give supplements of this vitamin only if clinical judgment warrants it.[4514]
	Vitamin K	Possibly decreased gastrointestinal absorption, destruction of vitamin K-producing bacteria, and interference with regeneration of vitamin K from inactive metabolite.	Consider supplements in people with other risk factors for vitamin K deficiency.[11517-8]
ANTIVIRALS			
Foscarnet (*Foscavir)*	Magnesium	Chelation and increased excretion.	Monitor magnesium levels and give supplements as necessary.[8869,9617]
ANTIGOUT/ANTIRHEUMATIC			
Aspirin, other salicylates	Folic Acid	Decreases protein binding and serum levels.	Folic acid appears to be redistributed rather than lost from the body. Red blood cell folate levels are normal. Supplements are not needed.[9351,9360]
	Iron	Mucosal damage and GI bleeding, even if asymptomatic, can cause chronic blood loss.	Monitor for signs and symptoms of anemia. Encourage intake of iron-fortified foods since supplements may exacerbate GI irritation.[8888,9515,9576-7]
	Vitamin C (ascorbic acid)	Increases urinary excretion.	Deficiency of vitamin C is unlikely. Only consider supplementation with long-term therapy and symptoms of deficiency.[3046]
Colchicine	Beta-Carotene	Reduced absorption.	Colchicine 1-2 mg/day doesn't affect beta-carotene serum levels, but higher doses may. Give supplements only if clinical judgement warrants it.[4543,5921]
	Dibencozide Vitamin B12	Decreases intestinal absorption of vitamin B12.	There is limited evidence that people on colchicine may have reduced levels of vitamin B12. Give supplements of this vitamin only if clinical judgment warrants it.[4543-5,5921]

Drug Influences on Nutrient Levels and Depletion

Some medications can affect the levels of certain nutrients in the body. There is considerable interest in using nutritional supplements to counteract these possible drug-induced "nutrient depletions." The chart below shows the current scientific understanding of these relationships, and suggested actions.

DRUGS (Includes some representative U.S. and Canadian Brand Names.)	NUTRIENT DEPLETED	POSSIBLE MECHANISM	COMMENTS & REFERENCES
ANTIGOUT/ANTIRHEUMATIC (cont.)			
Methotrexate (*Rheumatrex*)	Folic Acid	Folate antagonism. Binds to dihydrofolate reductase, preventing conversion of folic acid to its active form.	In people taking long-term, low-dose methotrexate for rheumatoid arthritis or psoriasis, reduced folate levels increase the risk of side effects. Recommend folic acid 1 mg/day, especially in people with a low dietary folate intake or who are experiencing side effects. This doesn't reduce the efficacy of methotrexate in these conditions.[768,2162,4492-4,4546,9369,9418-9] People taking methotrexate for cancer should avoid folic acid supplements unless recommended by their oncologist, since they may interfere with the anticancer effects.[9420]
Nonsteroidal Anti-inflammatory Drugs (NSAIDS): Diclofenac (*Voltaren*), Etodolac (*Lodine*), Fenoprofen (*Nalfon*), Flurbiprofen (*Ansaid*), Ibuprofen (*Advil, Motrin*, etc), Indomethacin (*Indocin*), Ketoprofen (*Orudis, Oruvail*), Ketorolac (*Toradol*), Meclofenamate, Mefenamic acid (*Ponstel*), Meloxicam (*Mobic*), Nabumetone (*Relafen*), Naproxen (*Anaprox, Naprosyn, Naprelan*), Oxaprozin (*Daypro*), Piroxicam (*Feldene*), Sulindac (*Clinoril*), Tolmetin (*Tolectin*)	Iron	Mucosal damage and GI bleeding, even if asymptomatic, can cause chronic blood loss.	Monitor for signs and symptoms of anemia. Encourage intake of iron-rich foods since supplements may exacerbate GI irritation.[8888,9515,9576-7]
Penicillamine (*Cuprimine, Depen*)	Copper Iron Magnesium Pyridoxine (B6) Zinc	Pyridoxine - inactivates pyridoxal-5'-phosphate, increasing pyridoxine requirements. Copper, Iron, Magnesium, Zinc – Forms chelation complexes in the GI tract. Decreases absorption of these elements.	Magnesium, pyridoxine, zinc - The need for supplementation has not been adequately studied. Give supplements of these nutrients only if clinical judgment warrants it.[4453,4531,4534,9630] Copper, Iron - Supplements may reverse taste loss associated with penicillamine treatment of rheumatoid arthritis. Separate copper or iron and penicillamine administration by at least 2 hours.[4453,4531,4534,9630]

CHARTS

Drug Influences on Nutrient Levels and Depletion

Some medications can affect the levels of certain nutrients in the body. There is considerable interest in using nutritional supplements to counteract these possible drug-induced "nutrient depletions." The chart below shows the current scientific understanding of these relationships, and suggested actions.

DRUGS (Includes some representative U.S. and Canadian Brand Names.)	NUTRIENT DEPLETED	POSSIBLE MECHANISM	COMMENTS & REFERENCES
CARDIOVASCULAR			
ANTIHYPERTENSIVES			
Hydralazine (*Apresoline*)	Pyridoxine (B6)	Inactivates pyridoxal-5'-phosphate, increasing pyridoxine requirements.	The need for supplementation has not bee adequately studied. Give supplements of pyridoxine only if clinical judgment warrants it.[4453,4531,4533]
Captopril (*Capoten*)	Zinc	Captopril increases urinary elimination of zinc.	Clinical significance is unknown.[25,26,6543]
CARDIAC GLYCOSIDES			
Digoxin (*Lanoxicaps, Lanoxin*)	Magnesium	Limits reabsorption of magnesium in the renal tubule, leading to magnesium excretion.	Low magnesium levels can increase the risk of arrhythmias. Hypomagnesemia more likely with concurrent diuretic use. Monitor magnesium levels as clinical judgment warrants and give supplements if necessary.[4556,9613,9631]
CHOLESTEROL-REDUCING DRUGS			
HMG CoA Reductase Inhibitors ("Statins"): Atorvastatin (*Lipitor*) Fluvastatin (*Lescol*) Lovastatin (*Mevacot*) Pravastatin (*Pravachol*) Simvastatin (*Zocor*)	Coenzyme Q-10	HMG CoA reductase inhibitors block synthesis of mevalonic acid, which is a precursor of coenzyme Q10. Therefore, production of coenzyme Q10 is decreased.	Serum levels of coenzyme Q-10 are reduced but muscle levels are not affected. Therefore, this is probably not clinically significant.[3367,3370,4404-10,8915,12099]
Cholestyramine (*LoCHOLEST, Prevalite, Questran*)	Beta-Carotene Folic Acid Dibencozide Iron Niacin and Niacinamide Vitamins A, B12, D, E, K	All nutrients – Reduces gastrointestinal absorption.	It is likely that cholestyramine does bind with some of these nutrients but there has never been clinical proof that supplements are necessary. Supplementation may be valuable in some patients. Separate dosing times of cholestyramine and supplements as much as possible.[4454-9,9566,10542-3,10562,10566-9]
	Calcium	Cholestyramine decreases absorption of vit D, which also leads to reduced calcium absorption.	Taking over 32 g-day of cholesyramine or >2 years could result in vit D and calcium deficiency and related complications. Supplemental vit D and calcium may be necessary.[4458,5655,5809,5838]
	Magnesium	Reduces absorption and increases urinary magnesium excretion.	Magnesium deficiency had not been reported. Supplements aren't likely to be needed.[9566,9627]
Colestipol (*Colestid*)	Beta-Carotene Dibencozide Folic Acid Iron Niacin and Niacinamide Vitamins A, B12, D, E, K	All nutrients – Reduces gastrointestinal absorption.	It is possible that supplementation with folic acid and vitamin D may be appropriate. In some cases it may be appropriate to supplement all nutrients depleted by colestipol.[4460-1]

Drug Influences on Nutrient Levels and Depletion

Some medications can affect the levels of certain nutrients in the body. There is considerable interest in using nutritional supplements to counteract these possible drug-induced "nutrient depletions." The chart below shows the current scientific understanding of these relationships, and suggested actions.

DRUGS (Includes some representative U.S. and Canadian Brand Names.)	NUTRIENT DEPLETED	POSSIBLE MECHANISM	COMMENTS & REFERENCES
CARDIOVASCULAR (cont.)			
CHOLESTEROL-REDUCING DRUGS (cont.)			
Gemfibrozil (*Lopid*)	Vitamin E	Gemfibrozil can decrease vitamin E serum levels.	The clinical significance is unknown.[4096]
DIURETICS			
Loop Diuretics: Bumetanide (*Bumex, Burinex),* Ethacrynic acid (*Edecrin*), Furosemide (*Lasix*), Torsemide (*Demadex*)	Calcium Folic Acid Magnesium Potassium Sodium Thiamine (B1) Zinc	Increased urinary excretion.	Electrolyte disturbances more likely with higher doses. Hypokalemia and hypomagnesemia occur most commonly. May need to use potassium and/or magnesium supplements, or add a potassium-sparing diuretic (which will also spare magnesium).[4412,9613-4,9622] Thiamine deficiency may occur in elderly people with poor dietary intake who are on high doses of diuretics (e.g. > 80 mg furosemide/day) for several months. Thiamine deficiency may worsen heart failure. Supplement of 200mg/day has improved cardiac function in some thiamine-deficient people on diuretics, but there isn't enough data to recommend routine use.[1286,10507-9] The need for folic acid supplementation has not been adequately studied.[1898]
Thiazide and Thiazide Derivatives: Bendroflumethiazide (*Naturetin*), Benzthiazide (*Exna*), Chlorothiazide (*Diuril*), Chlorthalidone (*Hygroton, Thalitone*), Hydrochlorothiazide (*Esidrix, Hydrodiuril, Oretic*), Hydroflumethiazide (*Diucardin, Saluron*), Indapamide (*Lozide, Lozol),* Methyclothiazide (*Aquatensen, Enduron*), Metolazone (*Mykrox, Zaroxolyn*), Polythiazide (*Renese*), Quinethazone (*Hydromox*), Trichlormethiazide (*Diurese, Metahydrin, Naqua*)	Folic Acid Magnesium Potassium Sodium Thiamine (B1) Zinc	Increased urinary excretion.	Electrolyte disturbances are more likely with higher doses. Hypokalemia and hypomagnesemia occur most commonly. May need to use potassium and/or magnesium supplements, or add a potassium sparing diuretic (which will also spare magnesium).[4412,9613-4,9622] The need for folic acid supplementation has not been adequately studied.[1898] Thiamine deficiency may occur in elderly people with poor dietary intake who are on high doses of diuretics for several months. Thiamine deficiency may worsen heart failure. Supplement of 200 mg/day has improved cardiac function in some thiamine-deficient people on diuretics, but there isn't enough data to recommend routine use.[1283-6,10506-9]

Drug Influences on Nutrient Levels and Depletion

Some medications can affect the levels of certain nutrients in the body. There is considerable interest in using nutritional supplements to counteract these possible drug-induced "nutrient depletions." The chart below shows the current scientific understanding of these relationships, and suggested actions.

DRUGS (Includes some representative U.S. and Canadian Brand Names.)	NUTRIENT DEPLETED	POSSIBLE MECHANISM	COMMENTS & REFERENCES
CARDIOVASCULAR (cont.)			
DIURETICS (cont.)			
Triamterene (*Dyrenium*)	Folic Acid	Reduces absorption of folic acid and prevents its conversion to the active form.	The need for supplementation has not been adequately studied. Give supplements of this vitamin only if dietary intake is inadequate.[4425,4536-7,9375]
CENTRAL NERVOUS SYSTEM			
ANTICONVULSANTS			
Carbamazepine (*Atretol, Epitol, Tegretol*)	Folic Acid	Two mechanisms have been proposed: Induction of hepatic microsomal enzymes leading to increased folic acid metabolism and decreased intestinal absorption.	Megaloblastic anemia due to folic acid deficiency hasn't been reported with carbamazepine. Low folic acid levels might contribute to mental changes in some people on carbamazepine, but folic acid supplements may worsen seizure control. Advise patients to consult their physician before starting folic acid supplements.[4426-9,9359]
	Vitamin D Calcium	Increases the rate of vitamin D metabolism leading to decreased levels of various forms of vitamin D. Decreased vitamin D levels reduce calcium absorption.	Hypocalcemia and osteomalacia have occurred for 6 months or longer that they should have their vitamin D and calcium levels checked, and that they may need supplements.[4430-1]
	Vitamin K	Induction of liver enzymes may increase vitamin K metabolism, producing a significant decrease in vitamin K levels in neonates, who haven't built up stores of the vitamin.	Increases risk of neonatal intracranial hemorrhage. Women who need to take carbamazepine during pregnancy should take vitamin K, 10-20 mg/day, during the last month of pregnancy. The baby should receive vitamin K immediately after delivery.[11521-5]
Phenytoin (*Dilantin*), Fosphenytoin (*Cerebyx*)	Folic Acid	Reduced absorption, increased metabolism, and increased demand for folate as a coenzyme for induced hepatic enzymes.	Folic acid supplements may reduce phenytoin side effects, but can also reduce phenytoin serum levels and may independently worsen seizure control. Advise patients to consult a physician before starting folic acid supplements.[4427,4471,4477,4536,9354-9]
	Thiamine (B1)	Mechanism unknown.	Thiamine deficiency might contribute to neurologic side effects, but there's insufficient evidence to recommend supplements.[10510-2]
	Dibencozide Vitamin B12	Reduces absorption of vitamin B12.	This may contribute to the megaloblastic anemia, primarily caused by folate deficiency. Monitor vitamin B12 and folate if symptoms of anemia develop.[7843,10502-5]

CHARTS

Drug Influences on Nutrient Levels and Depletion

Some medications can affect the levels of certain nutrients in the body. There is considerable interest in using nutritional supplements to counteract these possible drug-induced "nutrient depletions." The chart below shows the current scientific understanding of these relationships, and suggested actions.

DRUGS (Includes some representative U.S. and Canadian Brand Names.)	NUTRIENT DEPLETED	POSSIBLE MECHANISM	COMMENTS & REFERENCES
CENTRAL NERVOUS SYSTEM (cont.)			
ANTICONVULSANTS (cont.)			
Phenytoin (*Dilantin*), Fosphenytoin (*Cerebyx*) (Cont.)	Vitamin D Calcium	Increases the rate of vitamin D metabolism leading to decreased levels of various forms of vitamin D. Phenytoin may also increase the renal excretion of polar vitamin D metabolites. Decreased vitamin D levels reduce calcium absorption.	Hypocalcemia and osteomalacia have occurred with long-term anticonvulsant therapy. Advise patients taking phenytoin for 6 months or longer that they should have their vitamin D and calcium levels checked, and that they may need supplements.[2675]
	Vitamin K	Induction of liver enzymes may increase vitamin K metabolism, producing a significant decrease in vitamin K levels in neonates, who haven't built up stores of the vitamin.	Increases risk of neonatal intracranial hemorrhage. Women who need to take these anticonvulsants during pregnancy should take vitamin K, 10-20 mg/day, during the last month of pregnancy. The baby should receive vitamin K immediately after delivery.[11521-5]
Phenobarbital (*Luminal, Solfoton*) Primidone (*Mysoline*)	Folic Acid	Reduced absorption, increased metabolism, and increased demand for folate as a coenzyme for induced hepatic enzymes.	Reduced folic acid levels due to treatment with phenobarbital or primidone occasionally lead to megaloblastic anemia, and may contribute to neurological side effects and mental changes. However, folic acid supplements can worsen seizure control. Advise patients to consult a physician before starting folic acid supplements.[4427,4530,4536,9357-9]
	Dibecozide Vitamin B12	Reduced absorption	Unknown whether this is clinically significant.[7843,10502-5]
	Vitamin D Calcium	Increases the rate of vitamin D metabolism leading to decreased levels of various forms of vitamin D. Decreased vitamin D levels reduce calcium absorption.	Hypocalcemia and osteomalacia have occurred with long-term anticonvulsant therapy. Advise patients taking phenobarbital or primidone for 6 months or longer that they should have their vitamin D and calcium levels checked, and that they may need supplements.[2675]
	Vitamin K	Induction of liver enzymes may increase vitamin K metabolism, producing a significant decrease in vitamin K levels in neonates, who haven't built up stores of the vitamin.	Increases risk of neonatal intracranial hemorrhage. Women who need to take these anticonvulsants during pregnancy should take vitamin K, 10-20 mg/day, during the last month of pregnancy. The baby should receive vitamin K immediately after delivery.[11521-5]

CHARTS

Drug Influences on Nutrient Levels and Depletion

Some medications can affect the levels of certain nutrients in the body. There is considerable interest in using nutritional supplements to counteract these possible drug-induced "nutrient depletions." The chart below shows the current scientific understanding of these relationships, and suggested actions.

DRUGS (Includes some representative U.S. and Canadian Brand Names.)	NUTRIENT DEPLETED	POSSIBLE MECHANISM	COMMENTS & REFERENCES
CENTRAL NERVOUS SYSTEM (cont.)			
ANTICONVULSANTS (cont.)			
Valproic Acid (*Depakene, Depakote*)	Folic Acid	Reduced levels occur occasionally but mechanism is unclear.	Symptomatic folic acid deficiency has not been reported. Avoid supplements since they may worsen seizure control.[4427-8,9355-6,9359]
	L-Carnitine	Affects carnitine metabolism in the mitochondria of cells, forming valproylcarnitine which is excreted in the urine.	Recommend L-carnitine supplements in some subgroups of patients. See footnote at the end of the chart.[4523-9,5798]
PHENOTHIAZINES			
Chlorpromazine (*Thorazine*)	Riboflavin (B2)	Interference with conversion to active form of vitamin; increased renal excretion.	These effects occur in animals, but there isn't enough data in humans to recommend supplements.[10515,10518-21]
ANTI-DIABETICS			
Metformin (*Glucophage*)	Dibencozide Folic Acid Vitamin B12	Causes malabsorption of dietary vitamin B12 and possibly folic acid.	The *Glucophage* package insert recommends obtaining hematological parameters annually and obtaining B12 at 2-3 year intervals in patients at increased risk for B12 deficiency. Symptomatic folic acid deficiency is unlikely.[9366-8] Give supplements only if clinical judgment warrants it.[32,4490-1,8834,9520-9]
	Thiamine	Might reduce thiamine activity.	Theoretically, reducing thiamine activity could result in more pyruvate entering the Kreb's cycle and being converted to lactic acid. This might be associated with metformin-related lactic acidosis. But this has not been substantiated.[9536,11466]

CHARTS

Drug Influences on Nutrient Levels and Depletion

Some medications can affect the levels of certain nutrients in the body. There is considerable interest in using nutritional supplements to counteract these possible drug-induced "nutrient depletions." The chart below shows the current scientific understanding of these relationships, and suggested actions.

DRUGS (Includes some representative U.S. and Canadian Brand Names.)	NUTRIENT DEPLETED	POSSIBLE MECHANISM	COMMENTS & REFERENCES
GASTROINTESTINALS			
ANTACIDS			
Aluminum Salts (*Amphojel, Alternajel, Basaljel,* etc), Magnesium Salts (*Mag-Ox, Milk of Magnesia,* etc), Aluminum Salt/Magnesium Salt mixtures (*Maalox,* etc)	Calcium Phosphate Salts	Aluminum salts bind phosphate in the gastrointestinal tract. This reduces phosphate levels, which induces movement of calcium from bones into the blood, increasing urinary calcium excretion. High serum magnesium levels can increase urinary calcium excretion.	Prolonged administration of large doses of antacids may lead to hypocalcemia and/or hypophosphatemia. Avoid prolonged administration of large doses.[3371,4400,5979]
	Chromium	Antacids may reduce chromium absorption from the gastrointestinal tract.	Unlikely to be clinically significant.[7135]
	Folic Acid	Increased intestinal pH produced by antacids may reduce folic acid absorption.	Long-term use of large doses of antacids can cause folate depletion if dietary intake is very low. Most people don't need supplementation.[2677,8441]
	Iron	Increased gastric pH reduces iron solubility and absorption.	Separate dosing times as much as possible. Monitor for adequate response to iron.[3046,3072]
GI ANTI-INFLAMMATORIES			
Sulfasalazine (*Azulfidine, Salazopyrin)*	Folic Acid	Interferes with breakdown of dietary folate to its active form. Can also cause hemolysis, which increases folate requirements for red blood cell formation.	Decreased folate levels may lead to megaloblastic anemia, hyperhomocysteinemia, and an increased risk of colon cancer. Recommend that patients increase their dietary folate intake if possible, or take a supplement, especially if they have other factors contributing to folate deficiency.[2677,4515-7,4536,4560,9353,9376-7,9379]
HISTAMINE-2 BLOCKERS			
H2 Blockers: Cimetidine (*Tagamet*), Famotidine (*Pepcid*), Nizatidine (*Axid*), Ranitidine (*Zantac*)	Calcium	Absorption of some calcium supplements, especially the carbonate salt, is decreased by increased gastric pH.	There isn't any evidence of a clinically significant effect on calcium levels.[2738,4330-1,5060]
	Chromium Folic Acid	Chromium and folic acid absorption from the gastrointestinal tract may be decreased by increased pH.	The clinical significance of the effect on chromium absorption isn't known.[7135] A significant effect on folic acid levels is unlikely unless dietary intake is very low.[4483,8441]
	Dibencozide Iron Vitamin B12	May decrease iron and vitamin B12 absorption from the gastrointestinal tract.	The need for iron and vitamin B12 supplementation hasn't been adequately studied. Depletion may be significant in people with inadequate dietary intake, poor stores of iron and B12, or continuous intake of H2 blockers for more than 2 years. Monitor for anemia and give supplements if clinical judgement warrants it.[4483,4539,8876,9578]

CHARTS

Drug Influences on Nutrient Levels and Depletion

Some medications can affect the levels of certain nutrients in the body. There is considerable interest in using nutritional supplements to counteract these possible drug-induced "nutrient depletions." The chart below shows the current scientific understanding of these relationships, and suggested actions.

DRUGS (Includes some representative U.S. and Canadian Brand Names.)	NUTRIENT DEPLETED	POSSIBLE MECHANISM	COMMENTS & REFERENCES
GASTROINTESTINALS (cont.)			
LAXATIVES			
Mineral Oil	Beta-Carotene Calcium Vitamins A, D, E, K	Decreases gastrointestinal absorption.	May be avoided by limiting duration of use to less than 4 months.[4454,4495-6]
Sodium phosphates (*Fleet Phospho-Soda*)	Magnesium Potassium	Increased loss of electrolytes from gastrointestinal tract.	High doses (such as those used for preoperative bowel cleansing) can cause severe electrolyte disturbances. Avoid high doses and monitor electrolyte levels in the elderly and others with risk factors for hypomagnesemia or hypokalemia.[8877,9531,9615-6]
Stimulant Laxatives: Senna (*Senexon, Senolax, Senokot, Senna-Gen, Senokotxtra, Black-Draught, Gentlax, Dr. Caldwell Senna, Fletcher's Castoria, Dosalax*), Bisacodyl Tablets (*Bisacodyl, Uniserts, Bisco-Lax, Correctol, Dulcagen, Dulcolax, Feen-a-mint, Fleet Laxative*)	Calcium Potassium Sodium Vitamin D	Calcium and Vitamin D - Decreases gastrointestinal absorption. Sodium and Potassium – Increases gastrointestinal losses.	Excessive use of stimulant laxatives may result in depletion of these essential elements and vitamin D. Limit to short-term use of recommended doses.[506,4425] Hypokalemia has been reported in patients undergoing short-term bowel-cleansing regimens. Use caution in patients who may be predisposed to hypokalemia (i.e. aggressive diuretic therapy). Give supplements of potassium if clinical judgment warrants it.[4411-2]
PANCREATIC ENZYMES			
Pancreatin (*Donnazyme, Pancrezyme*) Pancrelipase (*Cotazym, Creon, Pancrease, Ultrase, Viokase*)	Folic Acid Iron	Forms complexes with folic acid/iron in the gastrointestinal tract, reducing absorption.	Supplements may be needed with prolonged pancreatic enzyme therapy.[9374,9575,9585]
PROTON PUMP INHIBITORS			
Proton Pump Inhibitors: Lansoprazole (*Prevacid*), Omeprazole (*Losec, Prilosec*), Rabeprazole (*Aciphex*), Pantoprazole (*Pantoloc, Protonix*)	Beta-Carotene Calcium Chromium Dibencozide Folic Acid Iron Vitamin B12	May decrease beta carotene, calcium, chromium, folic acid, iron and vitamin B12 absorption from the gastrointestinal tract, due to increased pH.	There isn't any evidence of a clinically significant effect on calcium levels.[2738,5060] A significant effect on folic acid levels is unlikely unless dietary intake is very low.[4483,8441] The clinical significance of the effect on beta-carotene, chromium, iron, and vitamin B12 absorption isn't known. Give supplements of these vitamins and minerals only if clinical judgement warrants it.[31,4483,4539,7135,8876,9578]

CHARTS

Drug Influences on Nutrient Levels and Depletion

Some medications can affect the levels of certain nutrients in the body. There is considerable interest in using nutritional supplements to counteract these possible drug-induced "nutrient depletions." The chart below shows the current scientific understanding of these relationships, and suggested actions.

DRUGS (Includes some representative U.S. and Canadian Brand Names.)	NUTRIENT DEPLETED	POSSIBLE MECHANISM	COMMENTS & REFERENCES
HORMONES			
Corticosteroids [Glucocorticoids]: **Short-acting** Cortisone (*Cortone*), Hydrocortisone [Cortisol] (*Cortef, Hydrocortone*) **Intermediate-acting** Prednisone (*Deltasone, Meticorten, Orasone, Panasol-S*), Prednisolone (*Delta-Cortef, Prelone, Pediapred*), Triamcinolone (*Aristocort, Atolone, Kenacort*), Methylprednisolone (*Medrol*) **Long-acting** Dexamethasone (*Decadron, Dexameth, Dexone*), Betamethasone (*Celestone*)	Calcium (Indirectly – Vitamin D)	Calcium – Increases renal calcium excretion and decreases intestinal calcium absorption. Vitamin D - Depletion of calcium by steroids creates a greater need for vitamin D, which is necessary for appropriate GI absorption of calcium.	Steroid-induced osteoporosis, and the associated increase in fracture risk, are well-recognized consequences of long-term administration of corticosteroids, in doses equivalent to prednisone 7.5 mg/day or higher. Recommend patients maintain a calcium intake of 1500 mg/day. Monitor serum calcium levels regularly. Vitamin D supplements may also be needed.[1832,4462-7]
	Chromium	Increases renal excretion of chromium, possibly leading to chromium deficienc, which may contribute to cortisteroid-induced hyperglycemia.	The need for chromium supplementation has not been adequately studied. Give supplements only if clinical judgement warrants it.[5039]
	Magnesium	Drug-induced bone loss releases magnesium from bone and increases urinary excretion.	Serum magnesium levels are usually not affected and no supplements are needed.[9507-9,9628-9]
	Potassium	Corticosteroids cause sodium retention, resulting in compensatory renal potassium excretion.	Hypokalemia is dose-dependent and more common with steroids having high mineralocorticoid activity (hydrocortisone, cortisone, fludrocortisone, prednisone, prednisolone). Monitor potassium levels with chronic therapy. If necessary, give supplements, or switch to a steroid with no mineralocorticoid activity (betamethasone, dexamethasone, methylprednisolone, triamcinolone).[4425,4453]
	Strontium	Might increase urinary excretion of strontium.	Dose adjustments for strontium might be necessary.[11405]

CHARTS

Drug Influences on Nutrient Levels and Depletion

Some medications can affect the levels of certain nutrients in the body. There is considerable interest in using nutritional supplements to counteract these possible drug-induced "nutrient depletions." The chart below shows the current scientific understanding of these relationships, and suggested actions.

DRUGS (Includes some representative U.S. and Canadian Brand Names.)	NUTRIENT DEPLETED	POSSIBLE MECHANISM	COMMENTS & REFERENCES
HORMONES (cont.)			
Estrogens: (*Alora, Cenestin, Climara, Estinyl, Estrace, Estraderm, Estratab, FemPatch, Menest, Ogen, Premarin, Premphase, Prempro, Vivelle*)	Folic Acid	Folic Acid - possibly reduced absorption, increased excretion, increased protein binding and induction of liver enzymes which use folate.	Folic acid supplements should be considered only in people with a very low dietary intake, or with other conditions which contribute to folate deficiency.[4459,4498,7843-4,9371-3]
	Strontium	Might decrease urinary excretion of strontium.	Dose adjustments fro strontium might be necessary.[11405]
Estrogen-containing oral contraceptives	Magnesium	Magnesium – shift from plasma to other tissues.	Monitor magnesium levels in people with other risk factors for hypomagnesemia.[9621,9638-40]
	Pyridoxine (B6)	Pyridoxine – interference with metabolism.	Although there is much talk about giving pyridoxine supplements to people on estrogens, the need for this hasn't been proven.[4459,4470,4498,4547-8]
	Riboflavin (B2)	Riboflavin - possibly reduced absorption or interference with conversion to active form.	Riboflavin supplements aren't necessary unless dietary intake is inadequate.[4548,9373,10523-7,10536]
	Vitamin A	Vitamin A - Estrogens stimulate production of retinol binding protein, increasing amount of vitamin removed from liver storage and carried in blood.	Vitamin A supplements might help maintain liver stores, but the need for this hasn't been proven.[9373,9505,10523,10548]
	Dibencozide Vitamin B12	Vitamin B12 - reduced protein binding, leading to increased tissue uptake.	Vitamin B12 supplements aren't necessary.[4498,4547,7843,9371-3,9505,10123]
	Vitamin C (ascorbic acid)	Vitamin C - possibly increased elimination.	Data is limited, but vitamin C supplements probably aren't necessary.[11875-6]
Androgens	Strontium	Might decrease urinary excretion of strontium.	Dose adjustments for strontium might be necessary.[11405]
Levothyroxine	Calcium	Increase bone turnover which may increase urinary calcium losses.	Calcium loss is unlikely to be clinically significant with doses of thyroid hormones used to treat hypothyroidism. Check thyroid function tests to ensure patients are not receiving excessive thyroid hormone doses, which may increase calcium losses.[27,28,2684-5,2695,2697-8,2721]

Drug Influences on Nutrient Levels and Depletion

Some medications can affect the levels of certain nutrients in the body. There is considerable interest in using nutritional supplements to counteract these possible drug-induced "nutrient depletions." The chart below shows the current scientific understanding of these relationships, and suggested actions.

DRUGS (Includes some representative U.S. and Canadian Brand Names.)	NUTRIENT DEPLETED	POSSIBLE MECHANISM	COMMENTS & REFERENCES
MISCELLANEOUS			
Cyclosporine (*Neoral, Sandimmune*)	Magnesium	Increased urinary excretion probably associated with drug-induced renal damage.	Monitor serum magnesium levels.[9117,9632-3]
Nitrous oxide (N_2O)	Dibencozide Vitamin B12	Inactivates the cobalamin form of vitamin B12.	Deficiency symptoms may occur after a single dose of nitrous oxide in people with pre-existing, subclinical deficiency. Check B12 levels before using N_2O anesthesia in people with risk factors for vitamin B12 deficiency.[9527,9532]
Orlistat (*Xenical*)	Beta-Carotene Vitamin E Vitamin A Vitamin D Vitamin K	Beta-Carotene - Decreases the absorption of beta-carotene supplements by 30%. Vitamin E - Decreases the absorption of vitamin E supplements by 60%. Vitamin A, vitamin D, and vitamin K - Possibly decreases the absorption from the gastrointestinal tract.	Recommend people on orlistat also take a multivitamin supplement. Separate administration of orlistat and beta-carotene, vitamin A, vitamin D, vitamin E, and vitamin K supplements by 2-hours to avoid this interaction.[1725-7,1730,6001,9595,10570-1]
Tacrolimus (FK506, *Prograf*)	Magnesium	Reduced renal tubular reabsorption leads to increased excretion of magnesium.	Hypomagnesemia occurs in a significant proportion of patients. Monitor levels and give supplements as necessary.[8900,9620]
RESPIRATORY			
Beta-2-Agonists: Albuterol (salbutamol, *Proventil, Ventolin*), Bitolterol (*Tornalate*), Isoetharine, Levalbuterol (*Xopenex*), Metaproterenol (*Alupent*), Pirbuterol (*Maxair*), Salmeterol (*Serevent*), Terbutaline (*Brethine*)	Magnesium Potassium	Intracellular shift of magnesium and potassium.	May contribute to arrhythmias, especially at high doses and in people with other risk factors. Monitor electrolyte levels during acute use of high doses (e.g. in preterm labor or acute asthma attacks), and in people with other risk factors. With chronic use of beta-2-agonists, electrolyte levels may return to baseline.[2644,6203,6205,6209,6210,6217,7001,8880-6,8889-91,9507,9517,9534,9599,9641]
Methylxanthines	Potassium	Possibly increased intracellular uptake.	Risk for hypokalemia is dose-dependent. Monitor potassium levels in people on high doses or with other risk factors.[9534,9537-9]
Theophylline (*Slobid, Theo-24, Theo-Dur, Theolair*)	Pyridoxine (B6)	Interferes with pyridoxine metabolism.	Studies of the use of pyridoxine supplements with theophylline have given conflicting results. Give supplements of this vitamin only if clinical judgment warrants it.[4522,7064-6]

Drug Influences on Nutrient Levels and Depletion

Some medications can affect the levels of certain nutrients in the body. There is considerable interest in using nutritional supplements to counteract these possible drug-induced "nutrient depletions." The chart below shows the current scientific understanding of these relationships, and suggested actions.

DRUGS (Includes some representative U.S. and Canadian Brand Names.)	NUTRIENT DEPLETED	POSSIBLE MECHANISM	COMMENTS & REFERENCES
ANTICANCER DRUGS			
Aldesleukin (interleukin-2, IL-2, *Proleukin*)	Magnesium	Intracellular shift of magnesium.	Supplements usually not needed - serum magnesium levels normalize after course complete.[8874]
Amifostine (*Ethyol*)	Magnesium	Increased urinary excretion.	This is usually only a transient effect, with levels returning to baseline in 24 hours.[9625]
Cisplatin (*Platinol-AQ*), Carboplatin (*Paraplatin*)	Magnesium	Increased urinary excretion probably associated with drug-induced renal damage.	Hypomagnesemia worsens with repeated courses of treatment, and is more severe with cisplatin. Monitor magnesium levels and give supplements as necessary.[9626]
Doxorubicin (*Adriamycin, Rubex, Doxil*)	Riboflavin	Formation of inactive complexes, interference with binding and conversion to active form, increased renal excretion.	This might contribute to doxorubicin toxicity, but it isn't known if riboflavin supplements are helpful.[9533,10528-30]
Fluorouracil (5-FU, *Adrucil*)	Thiamine (B1)	Interference with activation, increased breakdown.	There isn't sufficient data to recommend routine use of supplements.[10522-4]

Footnote: Oral L-carnitine supplementation is strongly suggested for the following groups: patients with certain secondary carnitine deficiency syndromes; symptomatic VPA-associated hyperammonemia; multiple risk factors for VPA-associated hepatotoxicity; infants and young children taking VPA. An oral L-carnitine dosage of 100 mg/kg/day, up to a maximum of 2 g/day has been recommended.

CHARTS

(1S)-1,2,4/3,5,6-inositol .... see INOSITOL
(1S)-inositol .... see INOSITOL
(3 beta)-3-hydroxypregn-5-en-20-one .... see PREGNENOLONE
(3-carboxy-2-hydroxypropyl) trimethylammonium hydroxide inner salt .... see L-CARNITINE
(3-carboxy-2-hydroxy-propyl) trimethylammonium hydroxide inner salt acetate .... see ACETYL-L-CARNITINE
(Beta-hydroxyethyl) trimethylammonium hydroxide .... see CHOLINE
(Dimethylamino) acetic acid ..... see DIMETHYLGLYCINE
(R)-(3-carboxy-2-hydroxypropyl) trimethylammonium hydroxide .... see L-CARNITINE
(R)-3-hydroxy-4-trimethylammonio-butyrate .... see L-CARNITINE
(Z,Z,Z)-octadeca-6,9,12-trienoic acid .... see GAMMA LINOLENIC ACID
1 alpha (OH)D3 .... see VITAMIN D
1,2,3,4,5,6-cyclohexanehexol .... see INOSITOL
1,2,3-propanetriol .... see GLYCEROL
1,2,5/3,4,6-inositol .... see INOSITOL
1,25-dihydroxycholecalciferol .... see VITAMIN D
1,2-butanolide .... see GAMMA BUTYROLACTONE (GBL)
1,2-diglyceride .... see DIACYLGLYCEROL
1,2-dithiolane-3-pentanoic acid .... see ALPHA-LIPOIC ACID
1,2-dithiolane-3-valeric acid ..... see ALPHA-LIPOIC ACID
1,3,7-trimethylxanthine .... see CAFFEINE
1,3-diglyceride .... see DIACYLGLYCEROL
1,4-BD .... see BUTANEDIOL (BD)
1,4-butanediol .... see BUTANEDIOL (BD)
1,4-butylene glycol .... see BUTANEDIOL (BD)
1,4-dihydroxybutane .... see BUTANEDIOL (BD)
1,4-tetramethylene glycol .... see BUTANEDIOL (BD)
1-3,1-6-beta-glucan .... see BETA GLUCANS
1-alpha-hydroxycholecalciferol .... see VITAMIN D
1-isothiocyanate-4-methyl-sulfonyl butane .... see SULFORAPHANE
1-octacosanol .... see OCTACOSANOL
13-docosenoic acid .... see LORENZO'S OIL
17 beta-(1-ketoethyl)-delta 5-androsten-3 beta-ol .... see PREGNENOLONE
2(3H)-furanone di-dihydro .... see BUTANEDIOL (BD)
2(3H)-furanone dihydro .... see GAMMA BUTYROLACTONE (GBL)
.... see ACETYL-L-CARNITINE
2,3 dihydro furanone .... see GAMMA BUTYROLACTONE (GBL)
2,3-dimethoxy-5-methyl-6-(10-hydroxydecyl)-1,4-benzoquinone. .... see IDEBENONE
2,3-diphosphoglycerate .... see INOSINE
2,6-di-tert-butyl-P-creosol .... see BHT (BUTYLATED HYDROXYTOLUENE)
2-(acetyloxy)-3-carboxy-N,N,N-trimethyl-1-propanaminium inner salt ....
2-acetamido-2-deoxyglucose .... see N-ACETYL GLUCOSAMINE
2-amino-2-deoxy-beta-D-glucopyranose .... see GLUCOSAMINE HYDROCHLORIDE, GLUCOSAMINE SULFATE
2-amino-2-deoxyglucose hydrochloride .... see GLUCOSAMINE HYDROCHLORIDE
2-amino-2-deoxyglucose sulfate .... see GLUCOSAMINE SULFATE
2-amino-3-(4-hydroxyphenyl) propionic acid .... see TYROSINE
2-amino-3-methylbutanoic acid .... see BRANCHED-CHAIN AMINO ACIDS
2-amino-3-methylvaleric acid .... see BRANCHED-CHAIN AMINO ACIDS
2-amino-4-methylvaleric acid .... see BRANCHED-CHAIN AMINO ACIDS
2-amino-5-guanidinopentanoic acid .... see L-ARGININE
2-aminoethane sulfonic acid .... see TAURINE
2-diethylaminoethyl P-aminobenzoate monohydrochloride .... see PROCAINE
2-dimethyl aminoethanol .... see DEANOL
2-hydroxypropionic acid ... see ALPHA HYDROXY ACIDS
2-methyl-3-phytyl-1,4-naphthoquinone ...... see VITAMIN K
2-oxoglutaric acid .... see ALPHA-KETOGLUTARATE
2-oxopentanedoic acid .... see ALPHA-KETOGLUTARATE
2-oxopropanoate .... see PYRUVATE
2-oxypropanoic acid .... see PYRUVATE
20-dione .... see PROGESTERONE
22,23-dihydrostigmasterol .... see BETA-SITOSTEROL
24-alpha-ethylcholestanol .... see SITOSTANOL
24-beta-ethyl-delta-5-cholesten-3beta-ol .... see BETA-SITOSTEROL
24-ethyl-cholesterol .... see BETA-SITOSTEROL
25-hydroxycholecalciferol .... see VITAMIN D
3'S-astaxanthin .... see ASTAXANTHIN
3,3',4'5,7-penthydroxyflavone .... see QUERCETIN
3,3',5-triiodothyroacetic acid .... see TIRATRICOL
3,3'-diindolylmethane .... see DIINDOLYLMETHANE
3,3'-dihydroxy-4,4'-diketo-beta-carotene .... see ASTAXANTHIN
3,4,3',4'-hydroxyl-benzopyranol[5,4,3-c,d,e][1]benzopyrn-6-6'-dione .... see ELLAGIC ACID
3,4',5-stilbenetriol .... see RESVERATROL
3,4',5-trihydroxystilbene .... see RESVERATROL
3,5,4'-trihydroxystilbene .... see RESVERATROL
3,5,6,7,8,3',4'-heptamethoxyflavone .... see METHOXYLATED FLAVONES
3-acetyl-7-oxo-dehydroepiandrosterone .... see 7-KETO-DHEA
3-beta,5-alpha-stigmastan-3-ol .... see SITOSTANOL
3-beta-acetoxy-androst-5-ene-7,17-dione .... see 7-KETO-DHEA
3-beta-stigmast-5-en-3-ol .... see BETA-SITOSTEROL
3-carboxy-2-hydroxy-N,N,N-trimethyl-1-propanaminium inner salt .... see L-CARNITINE
3-dehydroretinol .... see VITAMIN A
3-hydroxy-4-N-trimethylaminobutyrate .... see L-CARNITINE
3-hydroxybutyric acid lactone .... see GAMMA BUTYROLACTONE (GBL)
3-hydroxymethyl indole .... see INDOLE-3-CARBINOL
3-pyridine carboxamide .... see NIACIN AND NIACINAMIDE (VITAMIN B3)
32-C .... see POLICOSANOL
3R,3'R-astaxanthin .... see ASTAXANTHIN
3R,3'S-astaxanthin .... see ASTAXANTHIN
3S .... see ASTAXANTHIN
4,4-diketo-beta-carotene .... see CANTHAXANTHIN
4-AD .... see ANDROSTENEDIOL

INDEX

4-amino-2-methyl-1-naphthol .... see VITAMIN K
4-aminobenzoic acid .... see PARA-AMINOBENZOIC ACID (PABA)
4-androstene-3,17-dione .... see ANDROSTENEDIONE
4-androstene-3,6,17-trione ..... see ANDROSTENETRIONE
4-androstene-3beta,17beta-diol .... see ANDROSTENEDIOL
4-androstenediol .... see ANDROSTENEDIOL
4-butanolide ..... see GAMMA BUTYROLACTONE (GBL)
4-butyrolactone .... see GAMMA BUTYROLACTONE (GBL)
4-hydroxy butyrate .... see GAMMA-HYDROXYBUTYRATE (GHB)
4-hydroxybutanoic acid lactone .... see GAMMA BUTYROLACTONE (GBL)
4-hydroxybutyric acid .... see GAMMA-HYDROXYBUTYRATE (GHB)
4-pregnene-3 .... see PROGESTERONE
5'-cytidine diphosphate choline .... see CITICOLINE
5,6,7,3',4'-pentamethoxyflavone .... see METHOXYLATED FLAVONES
5,6,7,8,3',4'-hexamethoxyflavone .... see METHOXYLATED FLAVONES
5,6,7,8,4'-pentamethoxyflavone .... see METHOXYLATED FLAVONES
5,7-chrysin .... see CHRYSIN
5,7-dihydroxyflavone .... see CHRYSIN
5-(1,2-dithiolan-3-yl) valeric acid .... see ALPHA-LIPOIC ACID
5-AD .... see ANDROSTENEDIOL
5-androsten-3-beta-17-one-DHEA .... see 7-KETO-DHEA
5-androstene-3beta,17beta-diol .... see ANDROSTENEDIOL
5-androstenediol .... see ANDROSTENEDIOL
5-HTP .... see 5-HTP
5-hydroxytryptophan .... see 5-HTP
5-N-ethylglutamine .... see THEANINE
6,8-dithiooctanoic acid .... see ALPHA-LIPOIC ACID
6,8-thioctic acid .... see ALPHA-LIPOIC ACID
6,9-dihydro-9-B-D-ribofuranosyl-1H-puin-6-one .... see INOSINE
6-furfurylaminopurine .... see KINETIN
6-oxo .... see ANDROSTENETRIONE
7-isopropoxy isoflavone .... see IPRIFLAVONE
7-keto-DHEA .... see 7-KETO-DHEA
7-ODA .... see 7-KETO-DHEA
7-oxo-dehydroepiandrosterone-3-acetate .... see 7-KETO-DHEA
7-oxo-DHEA .... see 7-KETO-DHEA
7-oxo-DHEA-acetate .... see 7-KETO-DHEA
9-B-D-ribofuranosylhypoxanthine .... see INOSINE
A-beta-carotene .... see BETA-CAROTENE
A-chymotrypsin .... see CHYMOTRYPSIN
A-ketoglutaric acid .... see ALPHA-KETOGLUTARATE
A-lan-thus .... see TREE OF HEAVEN
A-lipoic acid .... see ALPHA-LIPOIC ACID
A5MP .... see ADENOSINE
Aamalaki .... see INDIAN GOOSEBERRY
Aaron's Rod .... see GOLDENROD, HOUSELEEK, MULLEIN
ABA .... see PARA-AMINOBENZOIC ACID (PABA)
Abelmoschus moschatus .... see AMBRETTE
Abelmosk .... see AMBRETTE
Abies alba .... see FIR, FIR NEEDLE OIL
Abies alba f. pendula .... see FIR, FIR NEEDLE OIL
Abies alba f. pyramidalis .... see FIR, FIR NEEDLE OIL
Abies balsamea .... see CANADA BALSAM
Abies excelsa .... see HEMLOCK SPRUCE
Abies gmelinii .... see LARCH ARABINOGALACTAN
Abies sachalinensis .... see FIR NEEDLE OIL
Abies sibirica .... see FIR NEEDLE OIL
Abokado .... see AVOCADO
Abrojos .... see PUNCTURE VINE
Abrus precatorius .... see PRECATORY BEAN
ABSCESS ROOT .... see ABSCESS ROOT
Absinth .... see WORMWOOD above ground parts
Absinthe .... see WORMWOOD above ground parts
Absinthii Herba ...... see WORMWOOD above ground parts
Absinthites .... see WORMWOOD above ground parts
Absinthium .... see WORMWOOD above ground parts
ABUTA .... see ABUTA
Abyssinian Myrrh .... see MYRRH
Abyssinian Tea .... see KHAT
ACACIA .... see ACACIA
Acacia Catechu Heartwood Extract .... see CATECHU
Acacia farnesiana .... see CASSIE ABSOLUTE
Acacia senegal .... see ACACIA
Acacia smallii .... see CASSIE ABSOLUTE
Acacia verek .... see ACACIA
Acanthopanax senticosus .... see GINSENG, SIBERIAN
ACE .... see ADRENAL EXTRACT
Acedera comun .... see SORREL
Acer rubrum .... see RED MAPLE
ACEROLA .... see ACEROLA
Acetate Replacing Factor .... see ALPHA-LIPOIC ACID
Acetyl Carnitine .... see ACETYL-L-CARNITINE
Acetylcysteine .... see N-ACETYL CYSTEINE
Acetylformic Acid .... see PYRUVATE
Acetylglucosamine .... see N-ACETYL GLUCOSAMINE
ACETYL-L-CARNITINE .... see ACETYL-L-CARNITINE
Acetyl-levocarnitine .... see ACETYL-L-CARNITINE
Ache des Marais .... see CELERY
Achilee .... see YARROW
Achillea .... see YARROW
Achillea borealis .... see YARROW
Achillea lanulosa .... see YARROW
Achillea magna .... see YARROW
Achillea millefolium .... see YARROW
Achillea ptarmica .... see SNEEZEWORT
Achiote .... see ANNATTO
Achiotillo .... see ANNATTO
Achweed .... see GOUTWEED
Acidophilus .... see LACTOBACILLUS
Acidophilus Milk .... see YOGURT
Acidulated Phosphate Fluoride .... see FLUORIDE
ACKEE .... see ACKEE
Ackerkraut .... see AGRIMONY
ACONITE .... see ACONITE
Aconiti tuber .... see ACONITE
Aconitum napellus .... see ACONITE
Aconitum sp. .... see ACONITE
Acorus americanus .... see CALAMUS
Acorus calamus .... see CALAMUS
Acorus gramineus .... see CALAMUS
Acorus sp. .... see CALAMUS
Acrid Crowfoot .... see BUTTERCUP
Acrid Lettuce .... see WILD LETTUCE
Actaea alba .... see WHITE COHOSH

INDEX

Actaea macrotys .... see BLACK COHOSH
Actaea pachypoda .... see WHITE COHOSH
Actaea racemosa .... see BLACK COHOSH
Actaea rubra .... see WHITE COHOSH
Actinidia chinensis .... see KIWI
ACTIVATED CHARCOAL .... see ACTIVATED CHARCOAL
Activin .... see GRAPE seed
Aculiee .... see YARROW
Adam's Apple .... see LIME fruit, peel; LIME OIL
Adam's Flannel .... see MULLEIN
Adam's Needle .... see YUCCA
Adaptogen .... see JIAOGULAN
Adder's Eyes .... see SCARLET PIMPERNEL
Adder's Root .... see ARUM
Adderwort .... see BISTORT
Ademetionine .... see SAMe
Adenine Nucleoside .... see ADENOSINE
Adenine Riboside .... see ADENOSINE
ADENOSINE .... see ADENOSINE
Adenosine Diphosphate .... see ADENOSINE
Adenosine Monophosphate .... see ADENOSINE
Adenosine Phosphate .... see ADENOSINE
Adenosine Triphosphate .... see ADENOSINE
Adenosine-5-monophosphate .... see ADENOSINE
Adenosylcobalamin .... see DIBENCOZIDE
Adenosylmethionine .... see SAMe
Adermine Hydrochloride .... see PYRIDOXINE (VITAMIN B6)
Adiantifolia .... see GINKGO leaf (GINKGO leaf extract)
Adiantum capillus-veneris .... see MAIDENHAIR FERN
Adiantum pedatum .... see MAIDENHAIR FERN
Adiptam .... see BURNING BUSH leaf
Adonis Herba .... see PHEASANT'S EYE
Adonis vernalis .... see PHEASANT'S EYE
ADP .... see ADENOSINE
Adrenal Complex .... see ADRENAL EXTRACT
Adrenal Cortex Extract .... see ADRENAL EXTRACT
ADRENAL EXTRACT .... see ADRENAL EXTRACT
Adrenal Factors .... see ADRENAL EXTRACT
Adrenal Substance .... see ADRENAL EXTRACT
ADRUE .... see ADRUE
ADT .... see ANDROSTENETRIONE
Adulsa .... see MALABAR NUT
AE-941 .... see SHARK CARTILAGE
Aegle marmelos .... see BAEL
Aegopodium podagraria .... see GOUTWEED
Aesculus hippocastanum .... see HORSE CHESTNUT
Aetheroleum pelargonii .... see ROSE GERANIUM OIL
Aethusa cynapium .... see FOOL'S PARSLEY
AFA .... see BLUE-GREEN ALGAE
Aframomum melegueta .... see GRAINS OF PARADISE
African Chillies .... see CAPSICUM
African Civet .... see CIVET
African Coffee Tree .... see CASTOR OIL, CASTOR seed
African Cucumber .... see BITTER MELON
African Ginger .... see GINGER
African Marigold .... see TAGETES
African Myrrh .... see MYRRH
African Pepper .... see CAPSICUM
African Plum Tree .... see PYGEUM
AFRICAN WILD POTATO .... see AFRICAN WILD POTATO
AG .... see LARCH ARABINOGALACTAN
AGA .... see AGA
AGAR .... see AGAR
Agar-agar .... see AGAR
Agarweed .... see AGAR
Agathosma betulina .... see BUCHU
Agathosma crenulata .... see BUCHU
Agathosma serratifolia .... see BUCHU
Aged Garlic Extract .... see GARLIC
Agnolyt .... see CHASTEBERRY
Agnus Castus .... see CHASTEBERRY
Agracejo .... see EUROPEAN BARBERRY
Agriao .... see WATERCRESS
Agrimonia eupatoria .... see AGRIMONY
Agrimonia odorata .... see AGRIMONY
Agrimonia procera .... see AGRIMONY
Agrimoniae Herba .... see AGRIMONY
AGRIMONY .... see AGRIMONY
Agromonia .... see AGRIMONY
Agropyron .... see WHEATGRASS
Agropyron firmum .... see WHEATGRASS
Agropyron repens .... see WHEATGRASS
Agrostemma githago .... see CORN COCKLE
Ague .... see ALETRIS
Ague Tree .... see SASSAFRAS
Agueweed .... see BONESET
AHA .... see ALPHA HYDROXY ACIDS
Ahuacate .... see AVOCADO
Ail .... see GARLIC
Ailanthus altissima .... see TREE OF HEAVEN
Ailanthus cacodendron .... see TREE OF HEAVEN
Ailanthus giraldii .... see TREE OF HEAVEN
Ailanthus glandulosa .... see TREE OF HEAVEN
Ailanthus vilmoriniana .... see TREE OF HEAVEN
Ailanto .... see TREE OF HEAVEN
Airelle .... see BILBERRY
Ajagandha .... see ASHWAGANDHA
Ajamoda .... see CELERY
Ajava Seeds .... see BISHOP'S WEED
Ajenjo .... see WORMWOOD above ground parts
Ajenuz .... see BLACK SEED
Ajmaline .... see INDIAN SNAKEROOT
Ajo .... see GARLIC
Ajowan .... see BISHOP'S WEED
Ajowan Caraway .... see BISHOP'S WEED
Ajowan Seed .... see BISHOP'S WEED
Ajowanj .... see BISHOP'S WEED
Ajuga .... see BUGLE
Ajuga chamaepitys .... see GROUND PINE
Ajuga reptans .... see BUGLE
Ak .... see CALOTROPIS
Akada .... see CALOTROPIS
Akarakarabha .... see PELLITORY
Akee .... see ACKEE
AKG .... see ALPHA-KETOGLUTARATE
Aki .... see ACKEE
Akschota .... see ENGLISH WALNUT
ALA .... see ALPHA-LINOLENIC ACID, ALPHA-LIPOIC ACID
Alant .... see ELECAMPANE
Alarka .... see CALOTROPIS
ALC .... see ACETYL-L-CARNITINE
Alcachofa .... see ARTICHOKE
Alcacuz .... see LICORICE
Alcanna .... see HENNA

INDEX

Alcar .... see ACETYL-L-CARNITINE
Alcaucil .... see ARTICHOKE
Alcazuz .... see LICORICE
Alcea rosea .... see HOLLYHOCK
ALCHEMILLA .... see ALCHEMILLA
Alchemilla alpina .... see ALPINE LADY'S MANTLE
Alchemilla arvensis .... see PARSLEY PIERT
Alchemilla occidentalis .... see PARSLEY PIERT
Alchemilla vulgaris .... see ALCHEMILLA
Alchemilla xanthochlora .... see ALCHEMILLA
Alchemillae Alpinae Herba .... see ALPINE LADY'S MANTLE
Alchornea castaneifolia .... see IPORURU
Alcohol .... see BEER, WINE
ALDER BUCKTHORN .... see ALDER BUCKTHORN
Alder Dogwood .... see ALDER BUCKTHORN
Alehoof .... see GROUND IVY
ALETRIS .... see ALETRIS
Aletris farinosa .... see ALETRIS
Aleurites cordatus .... see TUNG SEED
Aleurites javanicus .... see TUNG SEED
Aleurites moluccanus .... see TUNG SEED
Aleurites pentaphyllus .... see TUNG SEED
Aleurites remyi .... see TUNG SEED
Aleurites trilobus .... see TUNG SEED
Alexandrian Senna .... see SENNA
Alexandrian-laurel .... see LAURELWOOD
Alexandrinische Senna .... see SENNA
Alexandrinischer Lorbeer .... see LAURELWOOD
Alfacalcidol .... see VITAMIN D
Alfa-ecdysone .... see ECDYSTERONE
ALFALFA .... see ALFALFA
Algerian Geranium Oil .... see ROSE GERANIUM OIL
ALGIN .... see ALGIN
Alginates .... see ALGIN
Alhandal .... see COLOCYNTH
Alholva .... see FENUGREEK
Alhucema .... see LAVENDER
Alisma .... see WATER PLANTAIN
Alisma orientale .... see WATER PLANTAIN
Alisma plantago-aquatica .... see WATER PLANTAIN
Alisma plantago-aquatica subsp. orientale .... see WATER PLANTAIN
Alkanet .... see ALKANNA
ALKANNA .... see ALKANNA
Alkanna lehmanii .... see ALKANNA
Alkanna Radix .... see ALKANNA
Alkanna tinctoria .... see ALKANNA
Alkanna tuberculata .... see ALKANNA
All Rac-alpha-tocopherol .... see VITAMIN E
All-heal .... see EUROPEAN MISTLETOE, SELF-HEAL, VALERIAN
Alligator Pear .... see AVOCADO
Allii cepae bulbus .... see ONION
Allii sativi bulbus .... see GARLIC
Allium .... see GARLIC
Allium cepa .... see ONION
Allium sativum .... see GARLIC
Allium schoenoprasum .... see CHIVE
Allium sibiricum .... see CHIVE
Allium ursinum .... see BEAR'S GARLIC
Allseed Nine-joints .... see KNOTWEED
ALLSPICE .... see ALLSPICE
All-trans Lycopene .... see LYCOPENE
Almond .... see SWEET ALMOND
Almond Oil .... see SWEET ALMOND
Alnus barbata .... see BLACK ALDER
Alnus glutinosa .... see BLACK ALDER
Alnus serrulata .... see SMOOTH ALDER
Aloe .... see ALOE gel, ALOE latex
Aloe africana .... see ALOE gel, ALOE latex
Aloe arborescens .... see ALOE gel, ALOE latex
Aloe arborescens natalenis .... see ALOE gel
Aloe barbadensis .... see ALOE gel, ALOE latex
Aloe Capensis .... see ALOE gel, ALOE latex
Aloe Dried Juice from Leaf .... see ALOE latex
Aloe Ferox .... see ALOE gel, ALOE latex
Aloe frutescens .... see ALOE gel, ALOE latex
ALOE gel .... see ALOE gel
Aloe indica .... see ALOE gel, ALOE latex
Aloe Juice .... see ALOE latex
ALOE latex .... see ALOE latex
Aloe natalenis .... see ALOE gel, ALOE latex
Aloe perfoliata .... see ALOE gel
Aloe perryi .... see ALOE gel, ALOE latex
Aloe spicata .... see ALOE gel, ALOE latex
Aloe supralaevis .... see ALOE gel, ALOE latex
Aloe ucriae .... see ALOE gel, ALOE latex
Aloe Vera .... see ALOE gel, ALOE latex
Aloe Yucca .... see YUCCA
Aloerot .... see ALETRIS
Aloysia citrodora .... see LEMON VERBENA
Aloysia triphylla .... see LEMON VERBENA
Alpenkraut .... see HEMP AGRIMONY
Alpha-amino-4-imidazole propanoic acid .... see HISTIDINE
Alpha-aminohydrocinnamic acid .... see PHENYLALANINE
Alpha-chymotrypsin .... see CHYMOTRYPSIN
Alpha-glycerylphosphorylcholine .... see ALPHA-GPC
ALPHA-GPC .... see ALPHA-GPC
Alpha-hydroxyethanoic acid .... see ALPHA HYDROXY ACIDS
Alpha-keto acid .... see PYRUVATE
ALPHA-KETOGLUTARATE .... see ALPHA-KETOGLUTARATE
Alpha-ketoglutaric acid .... see ALPHA-KETOGLUTARATE
Alpha-ketopropionic acid .... see PYRUVATE
ALPHA-LINOLENIC ACID .... see ALPHA-LINOLENIC ACID
ALPHA-LIPOIC ACID .... see ALPHA-LIPOIC ACID
Alpha-lipoic acid extract .... see ALPHA-LIPOIC ACID
Alpha-tocopherol .... see VITAMIN E
ALPHA HYDROXY ACIDS .... see ALPHA HYDROXY ACIDS
Alpha Ketoglutaric Acid .... see ALPHA-KETOGLUTARATE
Alpha KG .... see ALPHA-KETOGLUTARATE
Alpha Linolenic Acid .... see ALPHA-LINOLENIC ACID
Alpha Lipoic Acid .... see ALPHA-LIPOIC ACID
Alpha Tocopherol Acetate .... see VITAMIN E
Alpha Tocopheryl Acetate .... see VITAMIN E
Alpha Tocotrienol .... see VITAMIN E
ALPINE CRANBERRY .... see ALPINE CRANBERRY
ALPINE LADY'S MANTLE .... see ALPINE LADY'S MANTLE
ALPINE RAGWORT .... see ALPINE RAGWORT

Alpine Strawberry .... see STRAWBERRY
ALPINIA .... see ALPINIA
Alpinia officinarum .... see ALPINIA
Alquitran de Enebro .... see CADE OIL
Alraunwurzel .... see EUROPEAN MANDRAKE
Alsine media .... see CHICKWEED
Alstonia Bark .... see FEVER BARK
Alstonia constricta .... see FEVER BARK
Altamisa .... see FEVERFEW
Alteia .... see MARSHMALLOW
Althaea ficifolia .... see HOLLYHOCK
Althaea officinalis .... see MARSHMALLOW
Althaea rosea .... see HOLLYHOCK
Althaea taurinensis .... see MARSHMALLOW
Althaeae Folium .... see MARSHMALLOW
Althaeae Radix .... see MARSHMALLOW
Althea .... see MARSHMALLOW
Althea Rose .... see HOLLYHOCK
Aluminum Phosphate .... see PHOSPHATE SALTS
Amachazuru .... see JIAOGULAN
Amalaki .... see INDIAN GOOSEBERRY
Amangura .... see ASHWAGANDHA
Amanita muscaria .... see AGA
Amantilla .... see VALERIAN
AMARANTH .... see AMARANTH
Amaranthus frumentaceus .... see AMARANTH
Amaranthus hypochondriacus .... see AMARANTH
Amaranthus leucocarpus .... see AMARANTH
Amargo .... see QUASSIA
Amber .... see ST. JOHN'S WORT
Amber Touch-and-heal .... see ST. JOHN'S WORT
Amblabaum .... see INDIAN GOOSEBERRY
Ambreine .... see LABDANUM
Ambretta .... see AMBRETTE
AMBRETTE .... see AMBRETTE
Ambroise .... see WOOD SAGE
AMERICAN ADDER'S TONGUE .... see AMERICAN ADDER'S TONGUE
American Arborvitae .... see CEDAR leaf, CEDAR LEAF OIL
American Aspen .... see ASPEN
American Aspidium .... see MALE FERN
AMERICAN BITTERSWEET .... see AMERICAN BITTERSWEET
AMERICAN CHESTNUT .... see AMERICAN CHESTNUT
American Cone Flower .... see ECHINACEA
American Corn Mint .... see JAPANESE MINT
American Cranberry .... see CRANBERRY
American Dill .... see DILL above ground parts, DILL seed
AMERICAN DOGWOOD .... see AMERICAN DOGWOOD
American Dwarf Palm Tree .... see SAW PALMETTO
AMERICAN ELDER .... see AMERICAN ELDER
American Elderberry .... see AMERICAN ELDER
American Ginseng .... see GINSENG, AMERICAN
American Greek Valerian .... see ABSCESS ROOT
AMERICAN HELLEBORE .... see AMERICAN HELLEBORE
American Indigo .... see WILD INDIGO
American Ipecacuanha .... see INDIAN PHYSIC
AMERICAN IVY .... see AMERICAN IVY
American Liverleaf .... see LIVERWORT
American Mandrake .... see PODOPHYLLUM
AMERICAN MISTLETOE .... see AMERICAN MISTLETOE
American Mullein .... see MULLEIN
American Nightshade .... see POKEWEED berry, POKEWEED root
AMERICAN PAWPAW .... see AMERICAN PAWPAW
American Pennyroyal .... see PENNYROYAL leaf, PENNYROYAL OIL
American Saffron .... see SAFFLOWER
AMERICAN SPIKENARD .... see AMERICAN SPIKENARD
American Spinach .... see POKEWEED berry, POKEWEED root
American Storax .... see STORAX
American Valerian .... see NERVE ROOT
American Veratrum .... see AMERICAN HELLEBORE
American White Hellebore .... see AMERICAN HELLEBORE
AMERICAN WHITE POND LILY .... see AMERICAN WHITE POND LILY
American Woodbine .... see AMERICAN IVY
American Wormgrass .... see PINK ROOT
Amibiasine .... see MANGOSTEEN
Amino Monosaccharide .... see GLUCOSAMINE HYDROCHLORIDE, GLUCOSAMINE SULFATE
Aminoacetic Acid .... see GLYCINE
Aminobenzoate Potassium .... see PARA-AMINOBENZOIC ACID (PABA)
Aminobenzoic Acid .... see PARA-AMINOBENZOIC ACID (PABA)
Aminoethanesulfonate .... see TAURINE
Amla .... see INDIAN GOOSEBERRY
Ammi .... see KHELLA
Ammi daucoides .... see KHELLA
Ammi glaucifolium .... see BISHOP'S WEED
Ammi majus .... see BISHOP'S WEED
Ammi visnaga .... see KHELLA
Ammocallis rosea .... see MADAGASCAR PERIWINKLE
Amomum cardamomum .... see CARDAMOM
Amomum melegueta .... see GRAINS OF PARADISE
Amomum zedoaria .... see ZEDOARY
Amomum zingiber .... see GINGER
Amoraciae Rusticanae Radix .... see HORSERADISH
Amorphophallus konjac .... see GLUCOMANNAN
Amorphophallus rivieri .... see GLUCOMANNAN
AMP .... see ADENOSINE
Amukkirag .... see ASHWAGANDHA
Amygdala amara .... see BITTER ALMOND
Amygdala dulcis .... see SWEET ALMOND
Amygdaloside .... see APRICOT
Amygdalus armeniaca .... see APRICOT
Amygdalus communis .... see BITTER ALMOND
Amygdalus dulcis .... see BITTER ALMOND
Amyris kataf .... see MYRRH
Anabaena sp. .... see BLUE-GREEN ALGAE
Anacardium occidentale .... see CASHEW
Anacyclus pyrethrum .... see PELLITORY
Anagallis arvensis .... see SCARLET PIMPERNEL
Anamirta cocculus .... see LEVANT BERRY
Anamirta paniculata .... see LEVANT BERRY
Ananas ananas .... see BROMELAIN
Ananas comosus .... see BROMELAIN
Ananas duckei .... see BROMELAIN

Ananas sativus ... see BROMELAIN
Anas barbaria ... see OSCILLOCOCCINUM
Anas barbariae ... see OSCILLOCOCCINUM
Anas moschata ... see OSCILLOCOCCINUM
Anashca ... see MARIJUANA
Anatherum zizanioides ... see VETIVER
Anchi Ginseng ... see GINSENG, AMERICAN
Anchusa ... see ALKANNA
Anchusa bracteolata ... see ALKANNA
Anchusa tuberculata ... see ALKANNA
Andira araroba ... see GOA POWDER
ANDIROBA ... see ANDIROBA
Andiroba-saruba ... see ANDIROBA
ANDRACHNE ... see ANDRACHNE
Andrachne aspera ... see ANDRACHNE
Andrachne cordifolia ... see ANDRACHNE
Andrachne phyllanthoides ... see ANDRACHNE
Andro ... see ANDROSTENEDIONE
Androdiol ... see ANDROSTENEDIOL
ANDROGRAPHIS ... see ANDROGRAPHIS
Andrographis paniculata ... see ANDROGRAPHIS
Andrographolide ... see ANDROGRAPHIS
Andropogon citratus ... see LEMONGRASS
Andropogon flexuosus ... see LEMONGRASS
Andropogon nardus ... see CITRONELLA OIL
Andropogon odoratus ... see VETIVER
Andropogon sorghum ... see BROOM CORN
Androst-4-ene-3,6,17-trione ... see ANDROSTENETRIONE
Androst-4-ene-3,17-dione ... see ANDROSTENEDIONE
Androstene ... see ANDROSTENEDIONE
ANDROSTENEDIOL ... see ANDROSTENEDIOL
ANDROSTENEDIONE ... see ANDROSTENEDIONE
ANDROSTENETRIONE ... see ANDROSTENETRIONE
Anemia californica ... see YERBA MANSA
Anemone a Lobes Aigus ... see LIVERWORT
Anemone acutiloba ... see LIVERWORT
Anemone americana ... see LIVERWORT
Anemone d'Amerique ... see LIVERWORT
Anemone groenlandica ... see GOLDTHREAD
Anemone hepatica ... see LIVERWORT
Anemone nemorosa ... see WOOD ANEMONE
Anemone nigricans ... see PULSATILLA
Anemone pratensis ... see PULSATILLA
Anemone pulsatilla ... see PULSATILLA
Anemone serotina ... see PULSATILLA
Anemopsis californica ... see YERBA MANSA
Anethi Fructus ... see DILL seed
Anethi Herba ... see DILL above ground parts
Anethum foeniculum ... see FENNEL fruit, seed; FENNEL OIL
Anethum graveolens ... see DILL above ground parts, DILL seed
Anethum piperitum ... see FENNEL fruit, seed
Anethum sowa ... see DILL above ground parts, see DILL seed
Aneurine Hydrochloride ... see THIAMINE (VITAMIN B1)
Angel Tulip ... see JIMSON WEED
Angelica ... see ANGELICA herb, seed; ANGELICA root
Angelica archangelica ... see ANGELICA herb, seed; ANGELICA root
Angelica atropurpurea ... see ANGELICA root
Angelica curtisi ... see ANGELICA root
ANGELICA herb, seed ... see ANGELICA herb, seed
Angelica levisticum ... see LOVAGE
Angelica officinalis ... see ANGELICA herb, seed; ANGELICA root
Angelica polymorpha var. sinensis ... see DONG QUAI
Angelica pubescens ... see ANGELICA root
ANGELICA root ... see ANGELICA root
Angelica rosaefolia ... see ANGELICA root
Angelica sinensis ... see DONG QUAI
Angelica sylvestris ... see ANGELICA root
Angelica Tree ... see NORTHERN PRICKLY ASH
Angelicae ... see ANGELICA herb, seed
Angelicae Fructus ... see ANGELICA herb, seed
Angelicae Herba ... see ANGELICA herb, seed
Angelicin ... see BETA-SITOSTEROL
ANGEL'S TRUMPET ... see ANGEL'S TRUMPET
Angled Loofah ... see LUFFA
ANGOSTURA ... see ANGOSTURA
Angostura trifoliata ... see ANGOSTURA
Angurate ... see MENTZELIA
Angustura ... see ANGOSTURA
Anhydrous Aluminum Silicates ... see COLLOIDAL MINERALS
Anhydrous Caffeine ... see CAFFEINE
Aniba duckei ... see BOIS DE ROSE OIL
Aniba rosaeodora ... see BOIS DE ROSE OIL
Animal Charcoal ... see ACTIVATED CHARCOAL
Anis des Vosges ... see CARAWAY dried fruit, seed
ANISE ... see ANISE
Aniseed ... see ANISE
Aniseed Stars ... see STAR ANISE
Anisi Fructus ... see ANISE
Anisi Stellati Fructus ... see STAR ANISE
ANNATTO ... see ANNATTO
Annona cherimola ... see GRAVIOLA
Annona macrocarpa ... see GRAVIOLA
Annona muricata ... see GRAVIOLA
Annona triloba ... see AMERICAN PAWPAW
Annotta ... see ANNATTO
Annual Mugwort ... see SWEET ANNIE
Annual Wormwood ... see SWEET ANNIE
Antelaea azadirachta ... see NEEM
Antennaria dioica ... see CAT'S FOOT
Antennariase Dioicae Flos ... see CAT'S FOOT
Anthemis grandiflorum ... see CHRYSANTHEMUM
Anthemis nobilis ... see ROMAN CHAMOMILE
Anthemis pyrethrum ... see PELLITORY
Anthemis stipulacea ... see CHRYSANTHEMUM
Anthoxanthum odoratum ... see SWEET VERNAL GRASS
Anthriscus cerefolium ... see CHERVIL
Anthriscus longirostris ... see CHERVIL
Antialopecia Factor ... see INOSITOL
Antiberiberi Factor ... see THIAMINE (VITAMIN B1)
Antiberiberi Vitamin ... see THIAMINE (VITAMIN B1)
Anti-Blacktongue Factor ... see NIACIN AND NIACINAMIDE (VITAMIN B3)
Antineuritic Factor ... see THIAMINE (VITAMIN B1)
Antineuritic Vitamin ... see THIAMINE (VITAMIN B1)
Antipellagra Factor ... see NIACIN AND NIACINAMIDE (VITAMIN B3)
Antiscorbutic Vitamin ... see VITAMIN C (ASCORBIC ACID)
Antitumor Angiogenesis Factor (Anti-TAF) ... see BOVINE CARTILAGE

Antixerophthalmic Vitamin .... see VITAMIN A
Anurine .... see THIAMINE (VITAMIN B1)
Aonla .... see INDIAN GOOSEBERRY
Aortic GAGs .... see MESOGLYCAN
Aortic Glycosaminoglycans .... see MESOGLYCAN
Aphanes arvensis .... see PARSLEY PIERT
Aphanizomenon Flos-aquae ..... see BLUE-GREEN ALGAE
Apii Fructus .... see CELERY
Apis cerana .... see BEESWAX
Apis mellifera .... see BEE VENOM, BEESWAX, HONEY, ROYAL JELLY
Apis Venenum Purum .... see BEE VENOM
Apitoxin .... see BEE VENOM
Apium carvi .... see CARAWAY dried fruit, seed; CARAWAY OIL
Apium crispum .... see PARSLEY leaf, root
Apium graveolens .... see CELERY
Apium petroselinum .... see PARSLEY leaf, root; PARSLEY seed
Aplotaxis lappa .... see COSTUS OIL, COSTUS root
Apocynum cannabinum .... see CANADIAN HEMP
Apothecary Rose .... see ROSE HIP
APPLE .... see APPLE
Apple Acid .... see ALPHA HYDROXY ACIDS
APPLE CIDER VINEGAR .... see APPLE CIDER VINEGAR
APRICOT .... see APRICOT
Apricot Vine .... see PASSIONFLOWER
Aqua pimentae .... see ALLSPICE
Aqueous Liver Extract .... see LIVER EXTRACT
Aquilegia vulgaris .... see COLUMBINE
Ara-6 .... see LARCH ARABINOGALACTAN
Arabian Myrrh .... see MYRRH
Arabian-tea .... see KHAT
Arabic Gum .... see ACACIA
Arabinogalactan .... see LARCH ARABINOGALACTAN
Arachis .... see PEANUT OIL
Arachis hypogaea .... see PEANUT OIL
Aralia Pseuodoginseng .... see PANAX PSEUDOGINSENG
Aralia racemosa .... see AMERICAN SPIKENARD
Arandano americano .... see CRANBERRY
Arandano trepador .... see CRANBERRY
Aranuel .... see BLACK SEED
Araoba .... see GOA POWDER
Arberry .... see UVA URSI
Arborvitae .... see CEDAR leaf, CEDAR LEAF OIL
Arbre fricasse .... see ACKEE
Arbutus Uva-ursi .... see UVA URSI
Archangel .... see WHITE DEAD NETTLE FLOWER
Archangelica officinalis .... see ANGELICA herb, seed; ANGELICA root
Archangle .... see BUGLEWEED
Arcostaphylos .... see UVA URSI
Arctic Root .... see ROSEROOT
Arctium .... see BURDOCK
Arctium lappa .... see BURDOCK
Arctium minus .... see BURDOCK
Arctium tomentosum .... see BURDOCK
Arctostaphylos Uva-ursi .... see UVA URSI
ARECA .... see ARECA
Areca Catechu .... see ARECA
Areca Nut .... see ARECA
ARENARIA RUBRA .... see ARENARIA RUBRA
Arg .... see L-ARGININE
Argasse .... see SEA BUCKTHORN
Argilla .... see KAOLIN
Arginine .... see L-ARGININE
Arginine HCl .... see L-ARGININE
Arginine Hydrochloride .... see L-ARGININE
Argousier .... see SEA BUCKTHORN
Argyreia nervosa ...... see HAWAIIAN BABY WOODROSE
Argyreia speciosa ..... see HAWAIIAN BABY WOODROSE
Arishta .... see NEEM
ARISTOLOCHIA .... see ARISTOLOCHIA
Aristolochia auricularia .... see ARISTOLOCHIA
Aristolochia clematitis .... see ARISTOLOCHIA
Aristolochia fangchi .... see ARISTOLOCHIA
Aristolochia heterophylla .... see ARISTOLOCHIA
Aristolochia kwangsiensis .... see ARISTOLOCHIA
Aristolochia moupinensis .... see ARISTOLOCHIA
Aristolochia reticulata .... see ARISTOLOCHIA
Aristolochia serpentaria .... see ARISTOLOCHIA
Arjuna .... see TERMINALIA
Arka .... see CALOTROPIS
Armeniaca .... see APRICOT
Armeniaca vulgaris .... see APRICOT
Armoise .... see WORMWOOD above ground parts
Armoise capillaire .... see YIN CHEN
Armoise commune .... see MUGWORT
Armoracia lopathifolia .... see HORSERADISH
Armoracia rusticana .... see HORSERADISH
Armstrong .... see KNOTWEED
ARNICA .... see ARNICA
Arnica cordifolia .... see ARNICA
Arnica Flos .... see ARNICA
Arnica Flower .... see ARNICA
Arnica fulgens .... see ARNICA
Arnica latifolia .... see ARNICA
Arnica montana .... see ARNICA
Arnica sororia .... see ARNICA
Arnikablüten .... see ARNICA
Arnotta .... see ANNATTO
Aromatic Sumac .... see SWEET SUMACH
ARRACH .... see ARRACH
Arrow Bamboo .... see BAMBOO
ARROWROOT .... see ARROWROOT
Arrowwood .... see ALDER BUCKTHORN, WAHOO
Arruda bravam .... see JABORANDI
Arruda do Mato .... see JABORANDI
Arryan .... see CHEKEN
Arsesmart .... see SMARTWEED
Artemisia .... see MUGWORT, WORMWOOD above ground parts, WORMWOOD OIL
Artemisia absinthium .... see WORMWOOD above ground parts, WORMWOOD OIL
Artemisia annua .... see SWEET ANNIE
Artemisia capillaris .... see YIN CHEN
Artemisia cina .... see WORMSEED
Artemisia dracunculus .... see TARRAGON
Artemisia glauca .... see TARRAGON
Artemisia scoparia .... see YIN CHEN
Artemisia vulgaris .... see MUGWORT
Artemisiae Vulgaris Herba .... see MUGWORT
Artemisiae Vulgaris Radix .... see MUGWORT
Artemisinin .... see SWEET ANNIE
Artesian absinthium .... see WORMWOOD above ground parts

INDEX

Arthritica ... see COWSLIP
Artichaut commun ... see ARTICHOKE
ARTICHOKE ... see ARTICHOKE
Artichoke Extract ... see ARTICHOKE
Artichoke Leaf ... see ARTICHOKE
Artichoke Leaf Extract ... see ARTICHOKE
Artischocke ... see ARTICHOKE
ARUM ... see ARUM
Arum maculatum ... see ARUM
Arundinaria japonica ... see BAMBOO
Arundo phragmites ... see REED HERB
Arundo vulgaris ... see REED HERB
Arusa ... see MALABAR NUT
Asafetida ... see ASAFOETIDA
ASAFOETIDA ... see ASAFOETIDA
Asan ... see ASHWAGANDHA
ASARABACCA ... see ASARABACCA
Asaroun ... see ASARABACCA
Asarum ... see ASARABACCA
Asarum europaeum ... see ASARABACCA
Asclepias incarnata ... see SWAMP MILKWEED
Asclepias procera ... see CALOTROPIS
Asclepias tuberosa ... see PLEURISY ROOT
Asclepias vincetoxicum ... see GERMAN IPECAC
Ascophyllum nodosum ... see ALGIN, BLADDERWRACK
Ascorbate ... see VITAMIN C (ASCORBIC ACID)
Ascorbic Acid ... see VITAMIN C (ASCORBIC ACID)
Ascorbyl Palmitate ... see VITAMIN C (ASCORBIC ACID)
Asgand ... see ASHWAGANDHA
Asgandh ... see ASHWAGANDHA
Asgandha ... see ASHWAGANDHA
ASH ... see ASH
Ashagandha ... see ASHWAGANDHA
Ashangee ... see BUGLEWEED
Ashe Juniper ... see CEDARWOOD
Ashvagandha ... see ASHWAGANDHA
Ashwaganda ... see ASHWAGANDHA
ASHWAGANDHA ... see ASHWAGANDHA
Ashweed ... see GOUTWEED
Asian Ginseng ... see GINSENG, PANAX
Asiatic Ginseng ... see GINSENG, PANAX
Asimina triloba ... see AMERICAN PAWPAW
Asoda ... see ASHWAGANDHA
Aspalathus contaminatus ... see RED BUSH TEA
Aspalathus linearis ... see RED BUSH TEA
Asparagi Rhizoma Root ... see ASPARAGUS
ASPARAGUS ... see ASPARAGUS
Asparagus longifolius ... see ASPARAGUS
Asparagus officinalis ... see ASPARAGUS
Aspartate Chelated Minerals ... see ASPARTATES
Aspartate Mineral Chelates ... see ASPARTATES
ASPARTATES ... see ASPARTATES
Aspartic Acid ... see ASPARTATES
ASPEN ... see ASPEN
Asperge ... see ASPARAGUS
Asperula odorata ... see SWEET WOODRUFF
Aspidosperma Quebracho-blanco ... see QUEBRACHO
Asplenium scolopendrium ... see HARTSTONGUE
Ass Ear ... see COMFREY
Assant ... see ASAFOETIDA
Ass's Foot ... see COLTSFOOT
ASTAXANTHIN ... see ASTAXANTHIN
Aster helenium ... see ELECAMPANE
Aster officinalis ... see ELECAMPANE
Asthma Weed ... see LOBELIA
Asthmaplant ... see EUPHORBIA
Astragali ... see ASTRAGALUS
ASTRAGALUS ... see ASTRAGALUS
Astragalus gummifer ... see TRAGACANTH
Astragalus membranaceus ... see ASTRAGALUS
Astragalus mongholicus ... see ASTRAGALUS
Asundha ... see ASHWAGANDHA
Asvagandha ... see ASHWAGANDHA
Aswagandha ... see ASHWAGANDHA
Atasi ... see FLAXSEED, FLAXSEED OIL
Athenon ... see GLYCINE
Athyrium filix-femina ... see LADY FERN
Atlantic Yam ... see WILD YAM
Atmagupta ... see COWHAGE
Atomic number 3 ... see LITHIUM
Atomic number 5 ... see BORON
Atomic number 9 ... see FLUORIDE
Atomic number 12 ... see MAGNESIUM
Atomic number 19 ... see POTASSIUM
Atomic number 20 ... see CALCIUM
Atomic number 23 ... see VANADIUM
Atomic number 24 ... see CHROMIUM
Atomic number 25 ... see MANGANESE
Atomic number 26 ... see IRON
Atomic number 29 ... see COPPER
Atomic number 30 ... see ZINC
Atomic number 32 ... see GERMANIUM
Atomic number 34 ... see SELENIUM
Atomic number 38 ... see STRONTIUM
Atomic number 53 ... see IODINE
Atomic number 55 ... see CESIUM
ATP ... see ADENOSINE
Atropa acuminata ... see BELLADONNA
Atropa belladonna ... see BELLADONNA
Aubepine ... see HAWTHORN
Auckland Costus ... see COSTUS OIL, COSTUS root
Aucklandia costus ... see COSTUS OIL, COSTUS root
Augentrostkraut ... see EYEBRIGHT
August Flower ... see GUMWEED
Aurantii pericarpium ... see BITTER ORANGE
Australian febrifuge ... see FEVER BARK
Australian Fever Bush ... see FEVER BARK
Australian Quinine ... see FEVER BARK
Australian Tea Tree Oil ... see TEA TREE OIL
AUTUMN CROCUS ... see AUTUMN CROCUS
Autumn Crocus ... see AUTUMN CROCUS, SAFFRON
Autumn Monkshood ... see ACONITE
Ava ... see KAVA
Ava Pepper ... see KAVA
Ava Root ... see KAVA
Avarada ... see ASHWAGANDHA
Avaram ... see CASSIA AURICULATA
Avari Panchaga Choornam ... see CASSIA AURICULATA
Aveleira ... see HAZELNUT
Avelinier ... see HAZELNUT
Avellano ... see HAZELNUT
Avena byzantina ... see OAT above ground parts, OAT BRAN, OAT STRAW, OATS
Avena Fructus ... see OATS
Avena orientalis ... see OAT above ground parts, OAT BRAN, OAT STRAW, OATS
Avena sativa ... see OAT above ground parts, OAT BRAN, OAT STRAW, OATS

INDEX

Avena volgensis .... see OAT above ground parts, OAT BRAN, OAT STRAW, OATS
Avenae Herba .... see OAT above ground parts
Avenae stramentum .... see OAT STRAW
AVENS .... see AVENS
Avian Heart and Liver .... see OSCILLOCOCCINUM
Avian Liver Extract .... see OSCILLOCOCCINUM
AVOCADO .... see AVOCADO
Avocato .... see AVOCADO
Awa .... see KAVA
Axerophtholum .... see VITAMIN A
Axjun Argun .... see TERMINALIA
AY-27255 .... see VINPOCETINE
Ayak chichira .... see MACA
Ayegreen .... see HOUSELEEK
Ayron .... see HOUSELEEK
Ayuk Willku .... see MACA
Ayurvedic Ginseng .... see ASHWAGANDHA
Azadirachta indica .... see NEEM
Azafron .... see SAFFRON
Azarum .... see ASARABACCA
Azeda-brava .... see SORREL
Aztec Marigold .... see TAGETES
Azucacaa .... see STEVIA
B .... see BORON
B Complex .... see VITAMIN B12
B Complex Vitamin .... see FOLIC ACID, NIACIN AND NIACINAMIDE (VITAMIN B3), PANTOTHENIC ACID (VITAMIN B5), PYRIDOXINE (VITAMIN B6), RIBOFLAVIN (VITAMIN B2), THIAMINE (VITAMIN B1), VITAMIN B12
B(t) Factor .... see L-CARNITINE
B. Bifidum .... see BIFIDOBACTERIA
B-12 .... see VITAMIN B12
B-alanyl Histidine .... see CARNOSINE
B-alanyl-L-histidine .... see CARNOSINE
B-DPNH .... see NADH
B-hydroxy B-methylbutyrate monohydrate .... see HYDROXYMETHYLBUTYRATE (HMB)
B-hydroxy-N-trimethyl aminobutyric acid .... see L-CARNITINE
B-stosterol 3-B-D-glucoside .... see BETA-SITOSTEROL
B-sitosterolin .... see BETA-SITOSTEROL
B6 .... see PYRIDOXINE (VITAMIN B6)
BA JI TIAN .... see BA JI TIAN
Ba Ji Tian .... see BA JI TIAN, MORINDA
Baby Hawaiian Woodrose .... see HAWAIIAN BABY WOODROSE
Baby Woodrose .... see HAWAIIAN BABY WOODROSE
Bac Ngu Vi Tu .... see SCHISANDRA
Baccae .... see ELDERBERRY
Bach .... see CALAMUS
Bachelor's Buttons .... see FEVERFEW
Backache Root .... see MARSH BLAZING STAR
Bacopa .... see BRAHMI
Bacopa monniera .... see BRAHMI
Bacopa monnieri .... see BRAHMI
Bacterial Polysaccharide .... see XANTHAN GUM
Badama .... see BITTER ALMOND
Badiana .... see STAR ANISE
Badijamun .... see JAMBOLAN bark
BAEL .... see BAEL
Bahama cascarilla .... see CASCARILLA
Bahera .... see TERMINALIA
Bahia Powder .... see GOA POWDER
Bahira .... see TERMINALIA
Bai Dou Kou .... see CARDAMOM
Bai Guo Ye .... see GINKGO leaf (GINKGO leaf extract)
Bai Qu Cai ...... see GREATER CELANDINE dried above ground parts
Baiguo .... see GINKGO seed
BAIKAL SKULLCAP .... see BAIKAL SKULLCAP
Baikal Skullcap Root .... see BAIKAL SKULLCAP
Baises de Sureau .... see ELDERBERRY
Baker's Yeast .... see BREWER'S YEAST
Bal .... see MYRRH
Bala .... see COUNTRY MALLOW
Bala Harade .... see TERMINALIA
Bald-faced Hornet .... see BEE VENOM
Baldrian .... see VALERIAN
Baldrianwurzel .... see VALERIAN
Balera .... see TERMINALIA
Ballota .... see BLACK HOREHOUND
Ballota nigra .... see BLACK HOREHOUND
Balm .... see LEMON BALM
Balm of Gilead .... see CANADA BALSAM, POPLAR
Balm of Gilead Fir .... see HEMLOCK SPRUCE
Balmony .... see TURTLE HEAD
Balsam .... see CANADA BALSAM, COPAIBA BALSAM, OREGON FIR BALSAM, PERU BALSAM, TOLU BALSAM
Balsam Canada .... see CANADA BALSAM
Balsam Fir .... see CANADA BALSAM, HEMLOCK SPRUCE
Balsam Fir Canada .... see CANADA BALSAM
Balsam Fir Oregon .... see OREGON FIR BALSAM
Balsam of Fir .... see CANADA BALSAM
Balsam of Peru .... see PERU BALSAM
Balsam of Tolu .... see TOLU BALSAM
Balsam Oregon .... see OREGON FIR BALSAM
Balsam Pear .... see BITTER MELON
Balsam Peru .... see PERU BALSAM
Balsam Poplar Buds .... see POPLAR
Balsam styracis .... see STORAX
Balsam Tolu .... see TOLU BALSAM
Balsam-apple .... see BITTER MELON
Balsambirne .... see BITTER MELON
Balsamina foemina .... see JEWELWEED
Balsamo .... see BITTER MELON
Balsamodendron myrrha .... see MYRRH
Balsamodendrum habessinicum .... see MYRRH
Balsamodendrum mukul .... see GUGGUL
Balsamodendrum myrrha .... see MYRRH
Balsamodendrum wightii .... see GUGGUL
Balsamum peruvianum .... see PERU BALSAM
Balsamum styrax liquidus .... see STORAX
Balsamum tolutanum .... see TOLU BALSAM
Balsam-weed .... see JEWELWEED
Balucanat .... see TUNG SEED
BAMBOO .... see BAMBOO
Ban Xia .... see PINELLIA TERNATA
BANABA .... see BANABA
Banafshah .... see SWEET VIOLET
Band Man's Plaything .... see YARROW
Baneberry .... see BLACK COHOSH, WHITE COHOSH
Banha .... see PINELLIA TERNATA

INDEX

Banji ... see MARIJUANA
Banksia abyssinica ... see KOUSSO
Bannal ... see SCOTCH BROOM flower, SCOTCH BROOM herb
Bantu Tulip ... see AFRICAN WILD POTATO
Baptisia tinctoria ... see WILD INDIGO
Baptista ... see WILD INDIGO
Bara Nimbu ... see LIME fruit, peel; LIME OIL
Baraka ... see BLACK SEED
Barbados Cherry ... see ACEROLA
Barbary-fig Cactus ... see PRICKLY PEAR CACTUS
Barbasco ... see CANELLA, WILD YAM
Barberry ... see OREGON GRAPE
Barberry Matrimony Vine ... see LYCIUM
Barber's Brush ... see TEAZLE
Bardana ... see BURDOCK
Bardanae Radix ... see BURDOCK
Bardane ... see BURDOCK
Bariar ... see COUNTRY MALLOW
Bari-sanuf ... see FENNEL fruit, seed
BARLEY ... see BARLEY
Barosma betulina ... see BUCHU
Barosma crenulata ... see BUCHU
Barosma serratifolia ... see BUCHU
Barosmae Folium ... see BUCHU
Barrenwort ... see EPIMEDIUM
Barweed ... see CLIVERS
Basam ... see SCOTCH BROOM herb
Basidiomycetes Polysaccharide ... see GENISTEIN COMBINED POLYSACCHARIDE
BASIL ... see BASIL
Basil Thyme ... see CALAMINT
Basilici Herba ... see BASIL
Basket Willow ... see WILLOW BARK
Basking Shark Liver Oil ... see SHARK LIVER OIL
Bassora tragacanth ... see KARAYA GUM
Basswood ... see LINDEN CHARCOAL, LINDEN dried flower, LINDEN dried leaf, LINDEN dried sapwood
Bastard Cinnamon ... see CASSIA CINNAMON
Bastard Ginseng ... see CODONOPSIS
Bastard Mahogany ... see ANDIROBA
Bastard Saffron ... see SAFFLOWER
Batavia Cassia ... see CINNAMON bark
Batavia Cinnamon ... see CINNAMON bark
Batchelor's Buttons ... see BUTTERCUP, CORNFLOWER
Bauchweh ... see YARROW
Baurenlilien ... see WHITE LILY
Bay ... see SWEET BAY
Bay Laurel ... see SWEET BAY
Bay Leaf ... see SWEET BAY
Bay Tree ... see SWEET BAY
Bay Willow ... see WILLOW BARK
BAYBERRY ... see BAYBERRY
Bayberry ... see BAYBERRY, SWEET GALE
BCAA ... see BRANCHED-CHAIN AMINO ACIDS
BC-PS ... see PHOSPHATIDYLSERINE
BD ... see BUTANEDIOL (BD)
Bdellium ... see MYRRH
BDO ... see BUTANEDIOL (BD)
Bead Tree ... see NEEM
Bead Vine ... see PRECATORY BEAN
Bean Herb ... see SUMMER SAVORY
BEAN POD ... see BEAN POD
Bean Trifoil ... see LABURNUM
Bear Grass ... see YUCCA
Bear Root ... see OSHA
Bearberry ... see UVA URSI
Bearbind ... see GREATER BINDWEED
Beard Moss ... see USNEA
Bearded Darnel ... see TAUMELLOOLCH
Beargrape ... see UVA URSI
BEAR'S GARLIC ... see BEAR'S GARLIC
Bear's Grape ... see POKEWEED berry, POKEWEED root, UVA URSI
Bear's Paw ... see MALE FERN
Bear's Weed ... see YERBA SANTA
Bear's-bind ... see GREATER BINDWEED
Bearsgrape ... see UVA URSI
Beaumont Root ... see BLACK ROOT
Beaver Poison ... see WATER HEMLOCK
Beaver Tree ... see MAGNOLIA
Beccabunga ... see BROOKLIME
Bedstraw ... see CLIVERS
Bedumil ... see VITAMIN B12
Bee Balm ... see OSWEGO TEA
Bee Glue ... see PROPOLIS
Bee Nettle ... see WHITE DEAD NETTLE FLOWER
Bee Plant ... see BORAGE flower, dried above ground parts
BEE POLLEN ... see BEE POLLEN
Bee Pollen Extract ... see BEE POLLEN
Bee Propolis ... see PROPOLIS
Bee Saliva ... see ROYAL JELLY
Bee Spit ... see ROYAL JELLY
Bee Sting Venom ... see BEE VENOM
BEE VENOM ... see BEE VENOM
Beebread ... see BORAGE flower, dried above ground parts; RED CLOVER
Beeflower ... see WALLFLOWER
Beefsteak Plant ... see PERILLA
BEER ... see BEER
Bee's Wax ... see BEESWAX
Beesnest Plant ... see WILD CARROT
BEESWAX ... see BEESWAX
BEET ... see BEET
Beg Kei ... see ASTRAGALUS
Beggar's Blanket ... see MULLEIN
Beggar's Buttons ... see BURDOCK
Beggarweed ... see DODDER, KNOTWEED
Beggary ... see FUMITORY
Behada ... see TERMINALIA
Bei Chai Hu ... see BUPLEURUM
Bei Qi ... see ASTRAGALUS
Bei Wu Wei Zi ... see SCHISANDRA
Bejunco de Cerca ... see ABUTA
Bel ... see BAEL
Beleric Myrobalan ... see TERMINALIA
Belgium Valerian ... see VALERIAN
Belladone ... see BELLADONNA
BELLADONNA ... see BELLADONNA
Belladonna ... see BELLADONNA, SCOPOLIA
Belladonna scopola ... see SCOPOLIA
Bellflower ... see CODONOPSIS
Bellis perennis ... see WILD DAISY
Benedict's Herb ... see AVENS
Bengal Quince ... see BAEL
Benibana Flower ... see SAFFLOWER

INDEX

Benibana Oil ... see SAFFLOWER
Bennet's Root ... see AVENS
Benzoe ... see BENZOIN
BENZOIN ... see BENZOIN
Berberidis Cortex ... see EUROPEAN BARBERRY
Berberidis Fructus ... see EUROPEAN BARBERRY
Berberidis Radicis Cortex ... see EUROPEAN BARBERRY
Berberidis Radix ... see EUROPEAN BARBERRY
Berberis aquifolium ... see OREGON GRAPE
Berberis diversifolia ... see OREGON GRAPE
Berberis jacquinii ... see EUROPEAN BARBERRY
Berberis nervosa ... see OREGON GRAPE
Berberis repens ... see OREGON GRAPE
Berberis sanguinea ... see EUROPEAN BARBERRY
Berberis sonnei ... see OREGON GRAPE
Berberis vulgaris ... see EUROPEAN BARBERRY
Berberitze ... see EUROPEAN BARBERRY
Berberry ... see EUROPEAN BARBERRY
Berbis ... see EUROPEAN BARBERRY
Bergamot ... see BERGAMOT OIL
BERGAMOT OIL ... see BERGAMOT OIL
Bergamot Orange ... see BERGAMOT OIL
Bergamota ... see BERGAMOT OIL
Bergamotier ... see BERGAMOT OIL
Bergamoto ... see BERGAMOT OIL
Bergamotte ... see BERGAMOT OIL
Bergamotto Bigarade Orange ... see BERGAMOT OIL
Bergwohlverleih ... see ARNICA
Berro ... see WATERCRESS
Berro di Agua ... see WATERCRESS
Besenginaterkraut ... see SCOTCH BROOM flower
Besom ... see SCOTCH BROOM herb
Beta-1,3-D-glucan ... see BETA GLUCANS
Beta-1-6,1,3-beta-glucan ... see BETA GLUCANS
Beta-alanyl-L-histidine ... see CARNOSINE
BETA-CAROTENE ... see BETA-CAROTENE
Beta-D-fructofuranosidase ... see FRUCTO-OLIGOSACCHARIDES
Beta-D-ribofuranose ... see RIBOSE
Beta-ecdysone ... see ECDYSTERONE
Beta-galactosidase ... see LACTASE
Beta-glucans ... see BETA GLUCANS
Beta-glycans ... see BETA GLUCANS
Beta-hydroxy beta-methylbutyric acid ... see HYDROXYMETHYLBUTYRATE (HMB)
Beta-hydroxy-beta-methylbutyrate ... see HYDROXYMETHYLBUTYRATE (HMB)
Beta-hydroxy-gamma-trimethylammonium butyrate ... see L-CARNITINE
Beta-phenyl-alanine ... see PHENYLALANINE
Beta-sitostanol ... see SITOSTANOL
BETA-SITOSTEROL ... see BETA-SITOSTEROL
Beta-sitosterol Glucoside ... see BETA-SITOSTEROL
Beta-sitosterol Glycoside ... see BETA-SITOSTEROL
Beta-tocopherol ... see VITAMIN E
Beta 1,3 Glucans ... see BETA GLUCANS
BETA GLUCANS ... see BETA GLUCANS
Beta Glycans ... see BETA GLUCANS
Beta Sitosterin ... see BETA-SITOSTEROL
Beta Sitosterol ... see BETA-SITOSTEROL
Beta Tocotrienol ... see VITAMIN E
Beta vulgaris ... see BEET
Beta(2-1)fructans ... see INULIN
Beta,beta-carotene-4,4-dione ... see CANTHAXANTHIN
Beta,epsilon-carotene-3,3'-diol ... see LUTEIN
Betaine ... see BETAINE ANHYDROUS, BETAINE HYDROCHLORIDE
BETAINE ANHYDROUS ... see BETAINE ANHYDROUS
Betaine HCl ... see BETAINE HYDROCHLORIDE
BETAINE HYDROCHLORIDE ... see BETAINE HYDROCHLORIDE
Betel Nut ... see ARECA
Betel Quid ... see ARECA
BETH ROOT ... see BETH ROOT
Betonica officinalis ... see BETONY
BETONY ... see BETONY
Betula ... see BIRCH
Betula alba ... see BIRCH
Betula alnus ... see BLACK ALDER
Betula glutinosa ... see BLACK ALDER
Betula pendula ... see BIRCH
Betula pubescens ... see BIRCH
Betula verrucosa ... see BIRCH
Betulae Folium ... see BIRCH
BGA ... see BLUE-GREEN ALGAE
Bhang ... see MARIJUANA
BHT (BUTYLATED HYDROXYTOLUENE) ... see BHT (BUTYLATED HYDROXYTOLUENE)
Bhunimba ... see ANDROGRAPHIS
Bi Bo ... see INDIAN LONG PEPPER
Bi Ji ... see BA JI TIAN
Bianco Spino ... see HAWTHORN
Bibernellkraut ... see PIMPINELLA above ground parts
Bible Frankincense ... see FRANKINCENSE
Biblical Mint ... see ENGLISH HORSEMINT
Bidara ... see ANDROGRAPHIS
Bidens tripartita ... see BURR MARIGOLD
Bifido ... see BIFIDOBACTERIA
BIFIDOBACTERIA ... see BIFIDOBACTERIA
Bifidobacteria bifidus ... see BIFIDOBACTERIA
Bifidobacterium ... see BIFIDOBACTERIA
Bifidobacterium adolescentis ... see BIFIDOBACTERIA
Bifidobacterium bifidum ... see BIFIDOBACTERIA
Bifidobacterium breve ... see BIFIDOBACTERIA
Bifidobacterium infantis ... see BIFIDOBACTERIA
Bifidobacterium lactis ... see BIFIDOBACTERIA
Bifidobacterium longum ... see BIFIDOBACTERIA
Bifidum ... see BIFIDOBACTERIA
Big Marigold ... see TAGETES
Bignonia heptaphylla ... see PAU D'ARCO
Bignonia sempervirens ... see GELSEMIUM
Bihara ... see TERMINALIA
Bija ... see ANNATTO
Bijapura ... see LIME fruit, peel; LIME OIL
BILBERRY ... see BILBERRY
Bilberry Fruit ... see BILBERRY
Bilberry Leaf ... see BILBERRY
Biletan ... see ALPHA-LIPOIC ACID
Bilva ... see BAEL
Bilwa ... see BAEL
Biobran ... see MGN-3
Bioelectrical Minerals ... see COLLOIDAL MINERALS
Bioflavonoid Concentrate ... see GRAPEFRUIT SEED EXTRACT
Biota orientalis ... see ORIENTAL ARBORVITAE
BIOTIN ... see BIOTIN
Biowater ... see WILLARD WATER

Birangasifa .... see YARROW
Birangasipha .... see YARROW
Biranjasipha .... see YARROW
BIRCH .... see BIRCH
Birch Sugar .... see XYLITOL
Bird Bread .... see COMMON STONECROP
Bird Pepper .... see CAPSICUM
Birdlime Mistletoe .... see EUROPEAN MISTLETOE
Bird's Eye Maple .... see RED MAPLE
Bird's Foot .... see FENUGREEK
Bird's Nest Root .... see WILD CARROT
Bird's Tongue .... see ASH, KNOTWEED
Birdweed .... see KNOTWEED
Birthroot .... see BETH ROOT
Birthwort .... see ARISTOLOCHIA
Bis-carboxyethyl germanium sesquioxide .... see GERMANIUM
Bis-pantothenamidoethyl disulfide .... see PANTETHINE
Bischofskrautfruchte .... see KHELLA
Biscuits .... see TORMENTIL
Bishop Wort .... see BETONY
Bishop's Elder .... see GOUTWEED
Bishop's Flower .... see BISHOP'S WEED
BISHOP'S WEED .... see BISHOP'S WEED
Bishop's Weed .... see BISHOP'S WEED, KHELLA
Bishop's Weed Fruit .... see KHELLA
Bishopsweed .... see GOUTWEED
Bishopswort .... see BETONY, GOUTWEED
Bissy Nut .... see COLA NUT
BISTORT .... see BISTORT
BITTER ALMOND .... see BITTER ALMOND
Bitter Almond Oil .... see BITTER ALMOND
Bitter Apple .... see BITTER MELON, COLOCYNTH
Bitter Ash .... see WAHOO
Bitter Bark .... see CASCARA
Bitter Buttons .... see TANSY
Bitter Candytuft .... see CLOWN'S MUSTARD PLANT
Bitter Cucumber .... see BITTER MELON, COLOCYNTH
Bitter Damson .... see SIMARUBA
Bitter Fennel .... see FENNEL fruit, seed
Bitter Gourd .... see BITTER MELON
Bitter Herb .... see CENTAURY, TURTLE HEAD
Bitter Lettuce .... see WILD LETTUCE
BITTER MELON .... see BITTER MELON
BITTER MILKWORT .... see BITTER MILKWORT
Bitter Nightshade .... see BITTERSWEET NIGHTSHADE
BITTER ORANGE .... see BITTER ORANGE
Bitter Redberry .... see AMERICAN DOGWOOD
Bitter Root .... see CANADIAN HEMP, GENTIAN
Bitter Stick .... see CHIRATA
Bitter Winter .... see PIPSISSEWA
Bitter Wintergreen .... see PIPSISSEWA
Bitter Wood .... see QUASSIA
Bitter-Ash .... see QUASSIA
Bitterbark .... see FEVER BARK
Bittergurke .... see BITTER MELON
Bitterstick .... see CHIRATA
Bittersweet .... see BITTERSWEET NIGHTSHADE
BITTERSWEET NIGHTSHADE .... see BITTERSWEET NIGHTSHADE
Bitterwood .... see QUASSIA
Bitterwort .... see GENTIAN
Bixa orellana .... see ANNATTO
Bizzom .... see SCOTCH BROOM herb
BLACK ALDER .... see BLACK ALDER
Black Balsam .... see PERU BALSAM
Black Berry .... see BLACKBERRY
Black Bindweed .... see BLACK BRYONY
BLACK BRYONY .... see BLACK BRYONY
Black Caraway .... see BLACK SEED
Black Catechu .... see CATECHU
Black Cherry .... see WILD CHERRY
Black Choke .... see WILD CHERRY
BLACK COHOSH .... see BLACK COHOSH
Black Cumin .... see BLACK SEED
BLACK CURRANT .... see BLACK CURRANT
Black Cutch .... see CATECHU
Black Date .... see JUJUBE
Black Dogwood .... see ALDER BUCKTHORN
Black Elder .... see ELDERBERRY, ELDERFLOWER
Black Elderberry .... see ELDERBERRY
Black Ginger .... see GINGER
Black Grape Raisins .... see GRAPE fruit, skin
BLACK HAW .... see BLACK HAW
BLACK HELLEBORE .... see BLACK HELLEBORE
BLACK HOREHOUND .... see BLACK HOREHOUND
Black Leaf Tea .... see BLACK TEA
BLACK MULBERRY .... see BLACK MULBERRY
Black Mustard .... see BLACK MUSTARD seed
BLACK MUSTARD OIL .... see BLACK MUSTARD OIL
BLACK MUSTARD seed .... see BLACK MUSTARD seed
BLACK NIGHTSHADE .... see BLACK NIGHTSHADE
BLACK PEPPER AND WHITE PEPPER .... see BLACK PEPPER AND WHITE PEPPER
BLACK PSYLLIUM .... see BLACK PSYLLIUM
BLACK ROOT .... see BLACK ROOT
Black Root .... see BLACK ROOT, COMFREY
Black Sampson .... see ECHINACEA
BLACK SEED .... see BLACK SEED
Black Snakeroot .... see BLACK COHOSH
Black Stinking Horehound .... see BLACK HOREHOUND
Black Susans .... see ECHINACEA
Black Tang .... see BLADDERWRACK
BLACK TEA .... see BLACK TEA
BLACK WALNUT .... see BLACK WALNUT
Black Whortles .... see BILBERRY
Black-berried Alder .... see ELDERBERRY, ELDERFLOWER
BLACKBERRY .... see BLACKBERRY
Blackeye Root .... see BLACK BRYONY
Black-Eyed Susan .... see PRECATORY BEAN
Blackhaw .... see BLACK HAW
Blackthorn .... see BLACKTHORN berry, BLACKTHORN flower
BLACKTHORN berry .... see BLACKTHORN berry
BLACKTHORN flower .... see BLACKTHORN flower
Blackthorn Fruit .... see BLACKTHORN berry
Blackwort .... see COMFREY
Bladder Fucus .... see BLADDERWRACK
Bladder Wrack .... see BLADDERWRACK
Bladderpod .... see LOBELIA
BLADDERWORT .... see BLADDERWORT
BLADDERWRACK .... see BLADDERWRACK
Blanc Poivre .... see BLACK PEPPER AND WHITE PEPPER
Blanket Herb .... see MULLEIN
Blanket Leaf .... see MULLEIN
Blasentang .... see BLADDERWRACK

INDEX

Blatterdock .... see BUTTERBUR
Blazing Star .... see ALETRIS, FALSE UNICORN, MARSH BLAZING STAR
Bleaberry .... see BILBERRY
Bleached Beeswax .... see BEESWAX
Bleeding Heart .... see NERVE ROOT, TURKEY CORN, WAHOO
Blessed Milk Thistle .... see MILK THISTLE
BLESSED THISTLE .... see BLESSED THISTLE
Blighia sapida .... see ACKEE
Blind Nettle .... see WHITE DEAD NETTLE FLOWER
Blind Weed .... see SHEPHERD'S PURSE
Blisterweed .... see BUTTERCUP
Blond Plantago .... see BLOND PSYLLIUM
BLOND PSYLLIUM .... see BLOND PSYLLIUM
Blonde Psyllium .... see BLOND PSYLLIUM
Blood Elder .... see DWARF ELDER
Blood Hilder .... see DWARF ELDER
Blood of the Dragon .... see SANGRE DE GRADO
Blood Root .... see BLOODROOT
Blood Vine .... see FIREWEED
Bloodroot .... see BLOODROOT, TORMENTIL
Bloodwood .... see LOGWOOD
Bloodwort .... see BLOODROOT, YARROW
Blooming Sally .... see FIREWEED, PURPLE LOOSESTRIFE
Blowball .... see DANDELION above ground parts, DANDELION entire plant
Blue Balm .... see OSWEGO TEA
Blue Barberry .... see OREGON GRAPE
Blue Bells .... see ABSCESS ROOT
Blue Cap .... see CORNFLOWER
Blue Centaury .... see CORNFLOWER
Blue Chamomile .... see GERMAN CHAMOMILE
BLUE COHOSH .... see BLUE COHOSH
Blue Curls .... see SELF-HEAL
BLUE FLAG .... see BLUE FLAG
Blue Flag .... see BLUE FLAG, ORRIS
Blue Ginseng .... see BLUE COHOSH
Blue Gum .... see EUCALYPTUS dried leaf
Blue Mallee .... see EUCALYPTUS dried leaf
Blue Mallee Oil .... see EUCALYPTUS OIL
Blue Mallow .... see MALLOW leaf
Blue Mallow Flower .... see MALLOW flower
Blue Monkshood Root .... see ACONITE
Blue Nightshade .... see BITTERSWEET NIGHTSHADE
Blue Pimpernel .... see SKULLCAP
Blue Sailors .... see CHICORY
Blue Skullcap .... see SKULLCAP
Blue Vervain .... see VERBENA
BLUEBERRY .... see BLUEBERRY
Blueberry .... see BILBERRY, BLUEBERRY
Bluebonnet .... see CORNFLOWER
Bluebottle .... see CORNFLOWER
Bluebow .... see CORNFLOWER
Bluebuttons .... see FIELD SCABIOUS
BLUE-GREEN ALGAE .... see BLUE-GREEN ALGAE
Blue-Green Micro-Algae .... see BLUE-GREEN ALGAE
Blunt .... see MARIJUANA
BNADH .... see NADH
Bobbins .... see ARUM
Bockshornklee .... see FENUGREEK
Bockshornsame .... see FENUGREEK
Bofareira .... see CASTOR OIL, CASTOR seed
BOG BILBERRY .... see BOG BILBERRY
Bog Myrtle .... see SWEET GALE
Bog Rhubarb .... see BUTTERBUR
BOGBEAN .... see BOGBEAN
Bogshorns .... see BUTTERBUR
Bohnenkraut .... see SUMMER SAVORY
BOIS DE ROSE OIL .... see BOIS DE ROSE OIL
Bois Douleur .... see MORINDA
Bol .... see MYRRH
Bola .... see MYRRH
Boldea fragrans .... see BOLDO
Boldine .... see BOLDO
BOLDO .... see BOLDO
Boldo Folium .... see BOLDO
Boldoak Boldea .... see BOLDO
Boldus .... see BOLDO
Boldus Boldus .... see BOLDO
Boletus Versicolor .... see CORIOLUS MUSHROOM
Bolivian Coca .... see COCA
Bolus Alba .... see KAOLIN
Bombus terrestis .... see BEE VENOM
Bonduc .... see DIVI-DIVI
Bone Meal .... see CALCIUM
BONESET .... see BONESET
Bonnet Bellflower .... see CODONOPSIS
Bonplandia trifoliata .... see ANGOSTURA
Bookoo .... see BUCHU
Boor Tree .... see ELDERBERRY, ELDERFLOWER
Borage .... see BORAGE flower, dried above ground parts
BORAGE flower, dried above ground parts .... see BORAGE flower, dried above ground parts
Borage Oil .... see BORAGE SEED OIL
BORAGE SEED OIL .... see BORAGE SEED OIL
Borago .... see BORAGE flower, dried above ground parts
Borago officinalis .... see BORAGE flower, dried above ground parts, BORAGE SEED OIL
Borate .... see BORON
Borates .... see BORON
Borbonia pinifolia .... see RED BUSH TEA
Borforsin .... see FORSKOLIN
Boric Acid .... see BORON
Boric Anhydride .... see BORON
Boric Tartrate .... see BORON
Borneo-mahogany .... see LAURELWOOD
BORON .... see BORON
Boswellia .... see INDIAN FRANKINCENSE
Boswellia carteri .... see FRANKINCENSE
Boswellia sacra .... see FRANKINCENSE
Boswellia serrata .... see INDIAN FRANKINCENSE
Boswellin .... see INDIAN FRANKINCENSE
Boswellin Serrata Resin .... see INDIAN FRANKINCENSE
Bottle Brush .... see HORSETAIL
Bouncing Bess .... see RED-SPUR VALERIAN
Bouncing-bet .... see RED SOAPWORT
Bountry .... see ELDERBERRY, ELDERFLOWER
Bourbon Geranium Oil .... see ROSE GERANIUM OIL
Bourbon Vanilla .... see VANILLA
Bouillon Blanc .... see MULLEIN
BOVINE CARTILAGE .... see BOVINE CARTILAGE
Bovine Colostrum .... see COLOSTRUM
Bovine Cortex Phosphatidylserine .... see PHOSPHATIDYLSERINE
Bovine Dialyzable Leukocyte Extract .... see TRANSFER FACTOR

INDEX

Bovine Dialyzable Transfer Factor .... see TRANSFER FACTOR
Bovine Immunoglobulin .... see COLOSTRUM
Bovine Lactoferrin .... see LACTOFERRIN
Bovine Orchic Extract .... see ORCHIC EXTRACT
Bovine Phosphatidylserine .... see PHOSPHATIDYLSERINE
Bovine Spleen .... see SPLEEN EXTRACT
Bovine Testicle Extract .... see ORCHIC EXTRACT
Bovine Tracheal Cartilage .... see BOVINE CARTILAGE
Bovine Transfer Factor .... see TRANSFER FACTOR
Bovine Whey Protein Concentrate .... see WHEY PROTEIN
Bovis and Soldier .... see RED-SPUR VALERIAN
Bovista .... see PUFF BALL
Bowman's Root .... see BLACK ROOT, INDIAN PHYSIC
Box Holly .... see BUTCHER'S BROOM
Box Tree .... see AMERICAN DOGWOOD
Boxberry .... see WINTERGREEN leaf, WINTERGREEN OIL
BOXWOOD .... see BOXWOOD
Boxwood .... see AMERICAN DOGWOOD, BOXWOOD
Boxwood Extract .... see BOXWOOD
Brahma-buti .... see GOTU KOLA
Brahma-manduki .... see GOTU KOLA
BRAHMI .... see BRAHMI
Brahmi .... see BRAHMI, GOTU KOLA
Brake Root .... see LADY FERN
Bramble .... see BLACKBERRY
Bran .... see WHEAT BRAN
BRANCHED-CHAIN AMINO ACIDS .... see BRANCHED-CHAIN AMINO ACIDS
Branching Phytolacca .... see POKEWEED berry, POKEWEED root
Brandlattich .... see COLTSFOOT
Brandy Mint .... see PEPPERMINT leaf
Brassica alba .... see WHITE MUSTARD
Brassica nigra .... see BLACK MUSTARD OIL, BLACK MUSTARD seed
Brassica oleracea .... see CABBAGE
Brassica oleracea var. capitata .... see CABBAGE
Brauneria angustifolia .... see ECHINACEA
Brauneria pallida .... see ECHINACEA
Brayera anthelmintica .... see KOUSSO
Brazil Powder .... see GOA POWDER
Brazil Root .... see IPECAC
Brazilian Cherimoya .... see GRAVIOLA
Brazilian Cocoa .... see GUARANA
Brazilian Ginseng .... see SUMA
Brazilian Ipecac .... see IPECAC
Brazilian Mahogany .... see ANDIROBA
Brazilian Paw Paw .... see GRAVIOLA
Brazilian Rhatany .... see RHATANY
Brechnusssamen .... see NUX VOMICA
Breeam .... see SCOTCH BROOM herb
Brewer's Yeast (Hansen CBS 5926) .... see SACCHAROMYCES BOULARDII
BREWER'S YEAST .... see BREWER'S YEAST
Brideweed .... see YELLOW TOADFLAX
Bridewort .... see MEADOWSWEET
Brigham Tea .... see MORMON TEA
Brindal Berry .... see GARCINIA
Brindle Berry .... see GARCINIA
British Indian Lemongrass .... see LEMONGRASS
British Myrrh .... see SWEET CICELY
British Tobacco .... see COLTSFOOT
Brittle Willow .... see WILLOW BARK
Broad-leafed Laurel .... see MOUNTAIN LAUREL
Broad-leaved Dock .... see YELLOW DOCK
Broad-leaved Garlic .... see BEAR'S GARLIC
BROMELAIN .... see BROMELAIN
Bromelains .... see BROMELAIN
Bromelainum .... see BROMELAIN
Bromelia ananas .... see BROMELAIN
Bromelia comosa .... see BROMELAIN
Bromelin .... see BROMELAIN
Brook Mint .... see JAPANESE MINT
BROOKLIME .... see BROOKLIME
Brook-tongue .... see WATER HEMLOCK
Broom .... see SCOTCH BROOM herb
BROOM CORN .... see BROOM CORN
Broom Flower .... see DYER'S BROOM
Broom Tops .... see SCOTCH BROOM flower
Browme .... see SCOTCH BROOM herb
Brown Algae .... see LAMINARIA
Brown Psyllium .... see BLACK PSYLLIUM
Brownwort .... see SELF-HEAL
Bruchkraut .... see RUPTUREWORT
Brugmansia suaveolens .... see ANGEL'S TRUMPET
Bruisewort .... see COMFREY, WILD DAISY
Brum .... see SCOTCH BROOM herb
Brunfelsia hopeana .... see MANACA
Brunfelsia uniflora .... see MANACA
Brunnenkresse .... see WATERCRESS
Brushes and Combs .... see TEAZLE
BRYONIA .... see BRYONIA
Bryonia alba .... see BRYONIA
Bryonia cretica .... see BRYONIA
Bryoniae Radix .... see BRYONIA
BSP .... see NATTOKINASE
BTC .... see BOVINE CARTILAGE
Bucco .... see BUCHU
BUCHU .... see BUCHU
Buchweizen .... see BUCKWHEAT
Buck Qi .... see ASTRAGALUS
Buckbean .... see BOGBEAN
Buckels .... see COWSLIP
Buckeye .... see HORSE CHESTNUT
Buckhorn .... see BUCKHORN PLANTAIN
BUCKHORN PLANTAIN .... see BUCKHORN PLANTAIN
Buckthorn .... see ALDER BUCKTHORN, CASCARA, EUROPEAN BUCKTHORN, SEA BUCKTHORN
Buckthorn Berry .... see EUROPEAN BUCKTHORN
Bucku .... see BUCHU
BUCKWHEAT .... see BUCKWHEAT
Buckwheat Pollen .... see BEE POLLEN
Bud .... see MARIJUANA
Buddhist Rosary Bead .... see PRECATORY BEAN
Budwood .... see AMERICAN DOGWOOD
Buergeria salicifolia .... see MAGNOLIA
Bugbane .... see AMERICAN HELLEBORE, BLACK COHOSH
BUGLE .... see BUGLE
Bugle .... see BUGLE, GROUND PINE
Bugle Weed .... see BUGLEWEED
BUGLEWEED .... see BUGLEWEED
Bugloss .... see BORAGE SEED OIL

INDEX

Bugula .... see BUGLE
Bugwort .... see BLACK COHOSH
BULBOUS BUTTERCUP .... see BULBOUS BUTTERCUP
Bulgarian Chlorella .... see CHLORELLA
Bulgarian Green Algae .... see CHLORELLA
Bulgarian Yogurt .... see YOGURT
Bull Balls Extract .... see ORCHIC EXTRACT
Bullock's Eye .... see HOUSELEEK
Bull's Eyes .... see MARSH MARIGOLD
Bullsfoot .... see COLTSFOOT
Bullwort .... see BISHOP'S WEED
Bumblebee Venom .... see BEE VENOM
BUPLEURUM .... see BUPLEURUM
Bupleurum chinense .... see BUPLEURUM
Bupleurum exaltatum .... see BUPLEURUM
Bupleurum falcatum .... see BUPLEURUM
Bupleurum fruticosum .... see BUPLEURUM
Bupleurum longifolium .... see BUPLEURUM
Bupleurum multinerve .... see BUPLEURUM
Bupleurum octoradiatum .... see BUPLEURUM
Bupleurum rotundifolium .... see BUPLEURUM
Bupleurum scorzonerifolium .... see BUPLEURUM
Burage .... see BORAGE SEED OIL
BURDOCK .... see BURDOCK
Burn Plant .... see ALOE latex
Burnet Saxifrage .... see BURNING BUSH leaf, BURNING BUSH root, PIMPINELLA above ground parts, PIMPINELLA root
Burning Bush .... see BURNING BUSH leaf, BURNING BUSH root, WAHOO
BURNING BUSH leaf .... see BURNING BUSH leaf
BURNING BUSH root .... see BURNING BUSH root
BURR MARIGOLD .... see BURR MARIGOLD
Burr Seed .... see BURDOCK
Burrage ..... see BORAGE flower, dried above ground parts; BORAGE SEED OIL
Burren Myrtle .... see BILBERRY
Burrwort .... see BUTTERCUP
Bursae Pastoris Herba .... see SHEPHERD'S PURSE
Bursting Heart .... see WAHOO
Bush Tree .... see BOXWOOD
Butane-1,4-diol .... see BUTANEDIOL (BD)
BUTANEDIOL (BD) .... see BUTANEDIOL (BD)
BUTCHER'S BROOM .... see BUTCHER'S BROOM
Butcher's-broom .... see BUTCHER'S BROOM, SCOTCH BROOM flower
Butter and Eggs .... see YELLOW TOADFLAX
Butter Bur .... see BUTTERBUR
Butter Daisy .... see OX-EYE DAISY
Butter Rose .... see COWSLIP
BUTTERBUR .... see BUTTERBUR
Butterburr .... see BUTTERBUR
BUTTERCUP .... see BUTTERCUP
Butter-dock .... see BUTTERBUR
Buttered Hayhocks .... see YELLOW TOADFLAX
Butterfly Dock .... see BUTTERBUR
Butterfly Weed .... see PLEURISY ROOT
Butternussbaum .... see BUTTERNUT
BUTTERNUT .... see BUTTERNUT
Butterweed .... see CANADIAN FLEABANE
Button Snakeroot .... see MARSH BLAZING STAR
Buttonhole .... see HARTSTONGUE
Buttons .... see TANSY
Butua .... see ABUTA
Butylated Hydroxytoluene .... see BHT (BUTYLATED HYDROXYTOLUENE)
Butylene Glycol .... see BUTANEDIOL (BD)
Butylhydroxytoluene .... see BHT (BUTYLATED HYDROXYTOLUENE)
Butyrolactone .... see GAMMA BUTYROLACTONE (GBL)
Butyrolactone Gamma .... see GAMMA BUTYROLACTONE (GBL)
Buxaceae .... see BOXWOOD
Buxus .... see BOXWOOD
Buxus chinensis .... see JOJOBA
Buxus colchica .... see BOXWOOD
Buxus hyrcana .... see BOXWOOD
Buxus sempervirens .... see BOXWOOD
Ca .... see CALCIUM
Caa-he-e .... see STEVIA
Ca-a-jhei .... see STEVIA
Ca-a-yupi .... see STEVIA
CABBAGE .... see CABBAGE
Cabbage Palm .... see SAW PALMETTO
Cabernet Franc .... see GRAPE fruit, skin
Cabernet Sauvignon .... see GRAPE fruit, skin
Cabra .... see CAPERS
Cacao .... see COCOA
Cachou .... see CATECHU
Cactus Flowers .... see PRICKLY PEAR CACTUS
Cactus Fruit .... see PRICKLY PEAR CACTUS
Cactus grandiflorus .... see CEREUS
Cactus Pear Fruit .... see PRICKLY PEAR CACTUS
CADE OIL .... see CADE OIL
Caesalpinia bonduc .... see DIVI-DIVI
Caesalpinia bonducella .... see DIVI-DIVI
Caesalpinia crista .... see DIVI-DIVI
Caesium .... see CESIUM
Cafe .... see COFFEE
CAFFEINE .... see CAFFEINE
Caffeine and Sodium Benzoate .... see CAFFEINE
Caffeine Anhydrous .... see CAFFEINE
Caffeine Citrate .... see CAFFEINE
Cairina moschata .... see OSCILLOCOCCINUM
Caje Oil .... see NIAULI OIL
CAJEPUT OIL .... see CAJEPUT OIL
Cajeputi aetheroleum .... see CAJEPUT OIL
Cajuput .... see CAJEPUT OIL
CALABAR BEAN .... see CALABAR BEAN
CALAMINT .... see CALAMINT
Calamintha hortensis .... see SUMMER SAVORY
Calamintha montana .... see WINTER SAVORY
Calamintha nepeta .... see CALAMINT
CALAMUS .... see CALAMUS
Calamus Draco .... see DRAGON'S BLOOD
Calanolide .... see LAURELWOOD
Calcifediol .... see VITAMIN D
Calcii pantothenas .... see PANTOTHENIC ACID (VITAMIN B5)
Calcipotriene .... see VITAMIN D
Calcitriol .... see VITAMIN D
CALCIUM .... see CALCIUM
Calcium Acetate .... see CALCIUM
Calcium Ascorbate .... see VITAMIN C (ASCORBIC ACID)

Calcium Aspartate .... see CALCIUM
Calcium Carbonate .... see CALCIUM
Calcium Carbonate Matrix .... see CORAL
Calcium Chelate .... see CALCIUM
Calcium Chloride .... see CALCIUM
Calcium Citrate .... see CALCIUM
CALCIUM D-GLUCARATE .... see CALCIUM D-GLUCARATE
Calcium Disodium Edathamil .... see EDTA
Calcium Disodium Edetate .... see EDTA
Calcium Disodium EDTA .... see EDTA
Calcium Disodium Versenate .... see EDTA
Calcium Edetate .... see EDTA
Calcium EDTA .... see EDTA
Calcium Glucarate .... see CALCIUM D-GLUCARATE
Calcium Gluconate .... see CALCIUM
Calcium Lactate .... see CALCIUM
Calcium Lactogluconate .... see CALCIUM
Calcium Orotate .... see CALCIUM
Calcium Pangamate .... see PANGAMIC ACID
Calcium Pantothenate .... see PANTOTHENIC ACID (VITAMIN B5)
Calcium Phosphate .... see CALCIUM, PHOSPHATE SALTS
Calcium Pyruvate .... see PYRUVATE
CALENDULA .... see CALENDULA
Calendula officinalis .... see CALENDULA
Caley Pea .... see LATHYRUS
Calgam .... see PANGAMIC ACID
Calico Bush .... see MOUNTAIN LAUREL
California Buckthorn .... see CASCARA
California Fern .... see HEMLOCK
California Poppies .... see CALIFORNIA POPPY
CALIFORNIA POPPY .... see CALIFORNIA POPPY
Callicocca ipecacuanha .... see IPECAC
Calluna vulgaris .... see HEATHER
Calluna Vulgaris Flos .... see HEATHER
Callunae Vulgaris Herba .... see HEATHER
Calomba Root .... see COLOMBO
Calophyllum inophyllum .... see LAURELWOOD
CALOTROPIS .... see CALOTROPIS
Calotropis procera .... see CALOTROPIS
Caltha palustris .... see MARSH MARIGOLD
Caltrop .... see PUNCTURE VINE
Calumba .... see COLOMBO
Calumbo Root .... see COLOMBO
Calves' Snout .... see YELLOW TOADFLAX
Calystegia sepium .... see GREATER BINDWEED
Calzin .... see GRAPE fruit, skin
Camboge .... see GAMBOGE
Cambogia gummi-guta .... see GARCINIA
Camellia sinensis .... see BLACK TEA, GREEN TEA
Camellia thea .... see BLACK TEA, GREEN TEA
Camellia theifera .... see BLACK TEA, GREEN TEA
Cammock .... see SPINY RESTHARROW
Camolea .... see MEZEREON
Camomilla .... see GERMAN CHAMOMILE
Camomille allemande .... see GERMAN CHAMOMILE
CAMPHOR .... see CAMPHOR
Camphor of the Poor .... see GARLIC
Camphor Tree .... see CAMPHOR
Camphora .... see CAMPHOR
Canada Balsam .... see CANADA BALSAM, HEMLOCK SPRUCE
Canada Pitch .... see PINUS BARK
Canada Root .... see PLEURISY ROOT
Canada Tea .... see WINTERGREEN leaf, WINTERGREEN OIL
Canada Turpentine .... see CANADA BALSAM
Canadian Balsam .... see CANADA BALSAM
Canadian Beaver .... see CASTOREUM
CANADIAN FLEABANE .... see CANADIAN FLEABANE
Canadian Ginseng .... see GINSENG, AMERICAN
Canadian Goldenrod .... see GOLDENROD
Canadian Hemlock .... see PINUS BARK
CANADIAN HEMP .... see CANADIAN HEMP
Canadian Horseweed .... see CANADIAN FLEABANE
Canadian Mint .... see JAPANESE MINT
Canadian Trailing Arbutus .... see CANADIAN FLEABANE
Canadian-fleabane .... see CANADIAN FLEABANE
CANAIGRE .... see CANAIGRE
Cananga odorata forma. genuina .... see YLANG YLANG OIL
Cananga odorata forma. macrophylla .... see CANANGA OIL
CANANGA OIL .... see CANANGA OIL
Canangium odoratum forma. genuina .... see YLANG YLANG OIL
Canangium odoratum forma. macrophylla .... see CANANGA OIL
Canard de Barbarie .... see OSCILLOCOCCINUM
Canarium commune .... see ELEMI
Canarium indicum .... see ELEMI
Canarium luzonicum .... see ELEMI
Canarywood .... see MORINDA
Cancer Jalap .... see POKEWEED berry, POKEWEED root
Candleberry .... see BAYBERRY, TUNG SEED
Candleberry Tree .... see TUNG SEED
Candleflower .... see MULLEIN
Candlenut .... see TUNG SEED
Candlewick .... see MULLEIN
Candytuft .... see CLOWN'S MUSTARD PLANT
CANELLA .... see CANELLA
Canella alba .... see CANELLA
Canella winteriana .... see CANELLA
Cankerroot .... see GOLDTHREAD
Cankerwort .... see DANDELION above ground parts, DANDELION entire plant, TANSY RAGWORT
Cannabis .... see MARIJUANA
Cannabis sativa .... see MARIJUANA
Cannelier de Ceylan .... see CINNAMON bark
Cannelli Beans .... see BEAN POD
CANTHAXANTHIN .... see CANTHAXANTHIN
Canthaxanthine .... see CANTHAXANTHIN
Canton Cassia .... see CASSIA CINNAMON
Cao Mahuang .... see EPHEDRA
Cao Ma-huang .... see EPHEDRA
Capdockin .... see BUTTERBUR
Cape Aloe .... see ALOE latex
Cape Gooseberry .... see WINTER CHERRY
Cape Periwinkle .... see MADAGASCAR PERIWINKLE
CAPERS .... see CAPERS
Capillary Wormwood .... see YIN CHEN
Capim Doce .... see STEVIA
Capim-Cidrao .... see LEMONGRASS
Capparis rupestris .... see CAPERS

INDEX

Capparis spinosa .... see CAPERS
Cappero .... see CAPERS
Capsaicin .... see CAPSICUM
Capsella .... see SHEPHERD'S PURSE
Capsella Bursa-pastoris .... see SHEPHERD'S PURSE
CAPSICUM .... see CAPSICUM
Capsicum annuum .... see CAPSICUM
Capsicum baccatum .... see CAPSICUM
Capsicum chinense .... see CAPSICUM
Capsicum Fruit .... see CAPSICUM
Capsicum Frutescens .... see CAPSICUM
Capsicum pubscens .... see CAPSICUM
Caramuru .... see CATUABA
Carapa .... see ANDIROBA
Carapa guianensis .... see ANDIROBA
CARAWAY dried fruit, seed .... see CARAWAY dried fruit, seed
CARAWAY OIL .... see CARAWAY OIL
Carbenia benedicta .... see BLESSED THISTLE
Carbon .... see ACTIVATED CHARCOAL
Carbonaceous Activated Water .... see WILLARD WATER
Carboxyethylgermanium sesquioxide .... see GERMANIUM
Card Thistle .... see TEAZLE
CARDAMOM .... see CARDAMOM
Cardo .... see ARTICHOKE
Cardo de Comer .... see ARTICHOKE
Cardo Santo .... see BLESSED THISTLE
Cardomomi Fructus .... see CARDAMOM
Cardon d'Espagne .... see ARTICHOKE
Cardoon .... see ARTICHOKE
Cardui Mariae Fructus .... see MILK THISTLE
Cardui Mariae Herba .... see MILK THISTLE
Carduus .... see BLESSED THISTLE
Carduus benedictus .... see BLESSED THISTLE
Carduus marianus .... see MILK THISTLE
Carex arenaria .... see GERMAN SARSAPARILLA
Carica papaya .... see PAPAIN, PAPAYA
Carica peltata .... see PAPAYA
Carica posoposa .... see PAPAYA
Caricae Fructus .... see FIG
Caricae Papayae Folium .... see PAPAYA
Caricis Rhizoma .... see GERMAN SARSAPARILLA
Carilla Gourd .... see BITTER MELON
CARLINA .... see CARLINA
Carlina acaulis .... see CARLINA
Carlinae Radix .... see CARLINA
Carline Thistle .... see MUGWORT
Carmantina .... see ANDROGRAPHIS
Carnitine .... see L-CARNITINE
Carnitine Acetyl Ester .... see ACETYL-L-CARNITINE
Carnitor .... see L-CARNITINE
CARNOSINE .... see CARNOSINE
CAROB .... see CAROB
Carolina Pink .... see PINK ROOT
Carolina Vanilla .... see DEERTONGUE
Caroline Jasmine .... see GELSEMIUM
Carony Bark .... see ANGOSTURA
Carophyll Red .... see CANTHAXANTHIN
Carosella .... see FENNEL fruit, seed
Carotenes .... see BETA-CAROTENE
Carotenoids .... see BETA-CAROTENE
Carotte a Moreau .... see WATER HEMLOCK
Carpenter's Herb .... see BUGLE, SELF-HEAL
Carpenter's Square .... see FIGWORT
Carpenter's Weed .... see SELF-HEAL, YARROW
Carphephorus odoratissimus .... see DEERTONGUE
CARRAGEENAN .... see CARRAGEENAN
Carrageenin .... see CARRAGEENAN
Carragheenan .... see CARRAGEENAN
Carrot Weed .... see HEMLOCK
Cartagena Ipecac .... see IPECAC
Carthamus tinctorius .... see SAFFLOWER
Carum .... see BISHOP'S WEED
Carum carvi .... see CARAWAY dried fruit, seed; CARAWAY OIL
Carum petroselinum .... see PARSLEY leaf, root; PARSLEY seed
Carum velenovskyi .... see CARAWAY dried fruit, seed
Carvacrol .... see OREGANO
Carvi Fructus .... see CARAWAY dried fruit, seed
Caryophylli .... see CLOVE dried flowerbud, leaf, stem
Caryophyllum .... see CLOVE OIL
Caryophyllus .... see CLOVE dried flowerbud, leaf, stem; CLOVE OIL
Caryophyllus aromaticus .... see CLOVE dried flowerbud, leaf, stem; CLOVE OIL
Cascabela thevetia .... see OLEANDER
CASCARA .... see CASCARA
Cascara Sagrada .... see CASCARA
CASCARILLA .... see CASCARILLA
Caseweed .... see SHEPHERD'S PURSE
CASHEW .... see CASHEW
Cashou .... see CATECHU
Casse .... see SENNA
Cassia .... see CASSIA CINNAMON
Cassia acutifolia .... see SENNA
Cassia angustifolia .... see SENNA
Cassia aromaticum .... see CASSIA CINNAMON
CASSIA AURICULATA .... see CASSIA AURICULATA
Cassia Bark .... see CASSIA CINNAMON
Cassia Cinnamon .... see CASSIA CINNAMON
Cassia lanceolata .... see SENNA
Cassia lignea .... see CASSIA CINNAMON
Cassia senna .... see SENNA
CASSIE ABSOLUTE .... see CASSIE ABSOLUTE
Cassis .... see BLACK CURRANT
Castanea americana .... see AMERICAN CHESTNUT
Castanea dentata .... see AMERICAN CHESTNUT
Castanea sativa .... see EUROPEAN CHESTNUT
Castanea vesca .... see EUROPEAN CHESTNUT
Castanea vulgaris .... see EUROPEAN CHESTNUT
Castaneae Folium .... see EUROPEAN CHESTNUT
Castor .... see CASTOR OIL, CASTOR seed
Castor Bean .... see CASTOR seed
Castor canadensis .... see CASTOREUM
Castor Fiber .... see CASTOREUM
CASTOR OIL .... see CASTOR OIL
Castor Oil Plant .... see CASTOR OIL
CASTOR seed .... see CASTOR seed
CASTOREUM .... see CASTOREUM
Catalonina Jasmine .... see JASMINE
Catalyst Altered Water .... see WILLARD WATER
Catarrh Root .... see ALPINIA
Catchfly .... see CANADIAN HEMP
Catchweed .... see CLIVERS
CATECHU .... see CATECHU
Catechu nigrum .... see CATECHU
Caterpillar Fungus .... see CORDYCEPS

INDEX

Catha edulis .... see KHAT
Catharanthus .... see MADAGASCAR PERIWINKLE
Catharanthus roseus ....
.... see MADAGASCAR PERIWINKLE
Catmint .... see CATNIP
Catnep .... see CATNIP
CATNIP .... see CATNIP
Catrix .... see BOVINE CARTILAGE
Catrix-S .... see BOVINE CARTILAGE
CAT'S CLAW .... see CAT'S CLAW
Cat's Ear Flower .... see CAT'S FOOT
CAT'S FOOT .... see CAT'S FOOT
Catsfoot .... see GROUND IVY
Cat's-head .... see PUNCTURE VINE
Cat's-paw .... see GROUND IVY
Catswort .... see CATNIP
CATUABA .... see CATUABA
Catuaba casca .... see CATUABA
Caulophyllum .... see BLUE COHOSH
Caulophyllum thalictroides .... see BLUE COHOSH
Caulophyllum Tree .... see LAURELWOOD
Cavinton .... see VINPOCETINE
Cayenne .... see CAPSICUM
Cayenne Rosewood Oil .... see BOIS DE ROSE OIL
CDP-choline .... see CITICOLINE
CDS .... see CHONDROITIN SULFATE
Ce Bai .... see ORIENTAL ARBORVITAE
Ceanothus americanus .... see NEW JERSEY TEA
Ceanothus intermedius .... see NEW JERSEY TEA
Cedar .... see CEDAR leaf, CEDARWOOD
CEDAR leaf .... see CEDAR leaf
CEDAR LEAF OIL .... see CEDAR LEAF OIL
CEDARWOOD .... see CEDARWOOD
CEDARWOOD OIL .... see CEDARWOOD OIL
Cedarwood Oil Texas .... see CEDARWOOD OIL
Cedoaria .... see ZEDOARY
Cedro .... see ANDIROBA
Celandine ....
..... see GREATER CELANDINE dried above ground parts; see GREATER CELANDINE rhizome, root
Celandine Herb ....
...... see GREATER CELANDINE dried above ground parts
Celandine Root ....
.... see GREATER CELANDINE rhizome, root
Celastrus edulis .... see KHAT
Celastrus scandens .... see AMERICAN BITTERSWEET
CELERY .... see CELERY
Celery Fruit .... see CELERY
Celery Seed .... see CELERY
Celery-leafed crowfoot ....
.... see POISONOUS BUTTERCUP
Cemphire .... see CAMPHOR
Centaurea cyanus .... see CORNFLOWER
Centaurea segetum .... see CORNFLOWER
Centaurium erythraea .... see CENTAURY
Centaurium minus .... see CENTAURY
Centaurium umbellatum .... see CENTAURY
CENTAURY .... see CENTAURY
Centella .... see GOTU KOLA
Centella asiatica .... see GOTU KOLA
Centella coriacea .... see GOTU KOLA
Centellase .... see GOTU KOLA
Centinode .... see KNOTWEED
Centranthus ruber .... see RED-SPUR VALERIAN
Centraria .... see ICELAND MOSS
Centroporus squamosus .... see SHARK LIVER OIL
Cephaelis acuminata .... see IPECAC
Cephaelis ipecacuanha .... see IPECAC
Cephalin .... see PHOSPHATIDYLSERINE
Cerasee .... see BITTER MELON
Cerasomal-cis-9-cetylmyristoleate ....
.... see CETYLATED FATTY ACIDS
Cerasus laurocerasus .... see CHERRY LAUREL WATER
Cerasus vulgaris .... see SOUR CHERRY
Ceratonia siliqua .... see CAROB
Cerbera thevetia .... see OLEANDER
Cereal Fiber .... see BARLEY, OAT BRAN, OATS, RICE BRAN, WHEAT BRAN
CEREUS .... see CEREUS
Cereus grandiflorus .... see CEREUS
Cerezo Acido .... see SOUR CHERRY
Cerisier Acide .... see SOUR CHERRY
Cervus elaphus .... see DEER VELVET
Cervus nippon .... see DEER VELVET
CESIUM .... see CESIUM
Cesium Chloride .... see CESIUM
Cesium-137 .... see CESIUM
Cetoal .... see ZEDOARY
Cetorhinus maximus .... see SHARK LIVER OIL
Cetraria islandica .... see ICELAND MOSS
Cetyl Laureate .... see CETYLATED FATTY ACIDS
Cetyl Myristate .... see CETYLATED FATTY ACIDS
Cetyl Myristoleate .... see CETYLATED FATTY ACIDS
Cetyl Oleate .... see CETYLATED FATTY ACIDS
Cetyl Palmitate .... see CETYLATED FATTY ACIDS
Cetyl Palmitoleate .... see CETYLATED FATTY ACIDS
Cetylated Fatty Acids ..... see CETYLATED FATTY ACIDS
Cetylated Monounsaturated Fatty Acids ....
.... see CETYLATED FATTY ACIDS
Cetylmyristoleate .... see CETYLATED FATTY ACIDS
Cevitamic Acid .... see VITAMIN C (ASCORBIC ACID)
Ceylon Cinnamon .... see CINNAMON bark
Ceylon Citronella .... see CITRONELLA OIL
Ceylon Citronella Grass .... see LEMONGRASS
Ceylonzimt .... see CINNAMON bark
Ceylonzimtbaum .... see CINNAMON bark
Chaat .... see KHAT
Chai-jen-shen .... see PANAX PSEUDOGINSENG
Chamaelirium carolianum .... see FALSE UNICORN
Chamaelirium luteum .... see FALSE UNICORN
Chamaemelum nobile .... see ROMAN CHAMOMILE
Chamaenerion angustifolium .... see FIREWEED
Chamaesyce hirta .... see EUPHORBIA
Chamerion angustifolium .... see FIREWEED
Chamomile .... see GERMAN CHAMOMILE, ROMAN CHAMOMILE
Chamomilla .... see GERMAN CHAMOMILE, ROMAN CHAMOMILE
Chamomilla recutita .... see GERMAN CHAMOMILE
Chamomillae Ramane Flos .... see ROMAN CHAMOMILE
Champagne Of Life .... see KOMBUCHA TEA
CHANCA PIEDRA .... see CHANCA PIEDRA
Chancapiedra .... see CHANCA PIEDRA
Chanca-piedra blanca .... see CHANCA PIEDRA
Chandana .... see WHITE SANDALWOOD wood
Chandana Oil .... see WHITE SANDALWOOD OIL
Chandrika .... see FENUGREEK, INDIAN SNAKEROOT
Chanvrin .... see HEMP AGRIMONY

INDEX

CHAPARRAL .... see CHAPARRAL
Charas .... see MARIJUANA
Charcoal .... see ACTIVATED CHARCOAL
Chardonnay .... see GRAPE fruit, skin
Charity .... see JACOB'S LADDER
Charnuska .... see BLACK SEED
Chaste Berry .... see CHASTEBERRY
Chaste Tree .... see CHASTEBERRY
Chaste Tree Berry .... see CHASTEBERRY
CHASTEBERRY .... see CHASTEBERRY
Chastetree .... see CHASTEBERRY
CHAULMOOGRA .... see CHAULMOOGRA
Cheat .... see TAUMELLOOLCH
Chebulic Myrobalan .... see TERMINALIA
Checkerberry ..... see SQUAWVINE, WINTERGREEN leaf, WINTERGREEN OIL
Cheese Fruit .... see MORINDA
Cheese Rennet .... see LADY'S BEDSTRAW
Cheese Renning .... see LADY'S BEDSTRAW
Cheeseflower .... see MALLOW flower
Cheiranthus cheiri .... see WALLFLOWER
Chekan .... see CHEKEN
CHEKEN .... see CHEKEN
Chelated Boron .... see CHELATED MINERALS
Chelated Calcium .... see CHELATED MINERALS
Chelated Chromium .... see CHELATED MINERALS
Chelated Cobalt .... see CHELATED MINERALS
Chelated Copper .... see CHELATED MINERALS
Chelated Iron .... see CHELATED MINERALS
Chelated Magnesium .... see CHELATED MINERALS, MAGNESIUM
Chelated Manganese .... see CHELATED MINERALS
CHELATED MINERALS .... see CHELATED MINERALS
Chelated Molybdenum .... see CHELATED MINERALS
Chelated Potassium .... see CHELATED MINERALS
Chelated Selenium .... see CHELATED MINERALS
Chelated Trace Minerals .... see CHELATED MINERALS
Chelated Vanadium .... see CHELATED MINERALS
Chelated Zinc .... see CHELATED MINERALS
Chelidonii .... see GREATER CELANDINE dried above ground parts
Chelidonii Herba .... see GREATER CELANDINE dried above ground parts
Chelidonium majus .... see GREATER CELANDINE dried above ground parts; GREATER CELANDINE rhizome, root
Chelone .... see TURTLE HEAD
Chelone glabra .... see TURTLE HEAD
Chenopodium ambrosioides .... see CHENOPODIUM OIL
Chenopodium anthelminticum .... see CHENOPODIUM OIL
CHENOPODIUM OIL .... see CHENOPODIUM OIL
Chenopodium vulvaria .... see ARRACH
CHEROKEE ROSEHIP .... see CHEROKEE ROSEHIP
CHERRY LAUREL WATER .... see CHERRY LAUREL WATER
CHERVIL .... see CHERVIL
Chervis .... see SKIRRET
Chestnut .... see HORSE CHESTNUT
Chi Hu .... see BUPLEURUM
CHICKEN COLLAGEN .... see CHICKEN COLLAGEN
Chicken Collagen Type II .... see CHICKEN COLLAGEN
Chicken Toe .... see CORAL ROOT
Chickling Vetch .... see LATHYRUS
Chick-pea .... see LATHYRUS
CHICKWEED .... see CHICKWEED
CHICORY .... see CHICORY
Chicory Extract .... see INULIN
Chicory Inulin .... see INULIN
Chicory Inulin Hydrolysate .... see FRUCTO-OLIGOSACCHARIDES
Chiendent Odorant .... see VETIVER
Ch'ih Shen .... see DANSHEN
Child Pick-a-back .... see CHANCA PIEDRA
Children's Bane .... see WATER HEMLOCK
Chili Pepper .... see CAPSICUM
Chimaphila .... see PIPSISSEWA
Chimaphila corymbosa .... see PIPSISSEWA
Chimaphila umbellata .... see PIPSISSEWA
Chimarrao .... see MATE
Chimney-sweeps .... see BUCKHORN PLANTAIN
Chin Cups .... see CUPMOSS
China Bark .... see QUILLAIA
China Clay .... see KAOLIN
China Gooseberry .... see KIWI
China Root .... see ALPINIA, WILD YAM
Chinarinde .... see CINCHONA
China-wood oil .... see TUNG SEED
Chinchilla Enana .... see TAGETES
Chinese Almond .... see APRICOT
Chinese Angelica .... see DONG QUAI
Chinese Anise .... see STAR ANISE
Chinese Arborvitae .... see ORIENTAL ARBORVITAE
Chinese Boxthorn .... see LYCIUM
Chinese Cinnamon .... see CASSIA CINNAMON
Chinese Club Moss .... see CHINESE CLUB MOSS
Chinese Cornbind .... see FO-TI
Chinese Cucumber .... see CHINESE CUCUMBER fruit, CHINESE CUCUMBER root, CHINESE CUCUMBER seed
CHINESE CUCUMBER fruit .... see CHINESE CUCUMBER fruit
CHINESE CUCUMBER root .... see CHINESE CUCUMBER root
CHINESE CUCUMBER seed .... see CHINESE CUCUMBER seed
Chinese Date .... see JUJUBE
Chinese Ephedra .... see EPHEDRA
Chinese Gelatin .... see AGAR
Chinese Ginger .... see ALPINIA
Chinese Ginseng .... see GINSENG, PANAX
Chinese Goldthread .... see GOLDTHREAD
Chinese Gooseberry .... see KIWI
Chinese Joint-fir .... see EPHEDRA
Chinese Jujube .... see JUJUBE
Chinese Knotweed .... see FO-TI
Chinese Lantern .... see WINTER CHERRY
Chinese Licorice .... see LICORICE
Chinese Mint .... see JAPANESE MINT
Chinese Mint Oil .... see JAPANESE MINT
Chinese Parsley .... see CORIANDER
Chinese Privet .... see GLOSSY PRIVET
Chinese Rhubarb .... see RHUBARB
Chinese Rosehip .... see CHEROKEE ROSEHIP
Chinese Scholartree .... see PAGODA TREE
Chinese Scullcap .... see BAIKAL SKULLCAP
Chinese Senega .... see SENEGA
Chinese Skullcap .... see BAIKAL SKULLCAP

Chinese Snake Gourd ..... see CHINESE CUCUMBER fruit, CHINESE CUCUMBER root, CHINESE CUCUMBER seed
Chinese Star Anise ..... see STAR ANISE
Chinese Sumach ..... see TREE OF HEAVEN
Chinese Tea ..... see GREEN TEA
Chinese Thoroughwax ..... see BUPLEURUM
Chinese Wolfberry ..... see LYCIUM
Chinese Wormwood ..... see SWEET ANNIE
Chinesischer limonenbaum ..... see SCHISANDRA
Ching-hao ..... see SWEET ANNIE
Chinli-chih ..... see BITTER MELON
Chintul ..... see ADRUE
Chinwood ..... see YEW
Chionanthus ..... see FRINGETREE
Chionanthus virginicus ..... see FRINGETREE
CHIRATA ..... see CHIRATA
Chirayta ..... see CHIRATA
Chirbhita ..... see PAPAYA
Chiretta ..... see ANDROGRAPHIS, CHIRATA
Chitosamine ..... see GLUCOSAMINE HYDROCHLORIDE, GLUCOSAMINE SULFATE
CHITOSAN ..... see CHITOSAN
Chitosan Ascorbate ..... see CHITOSAN
Chittem Bark ..... see CASCARA
Chiu ..... see YIN CHEN
CHIVE ..... see CHIVE
Chives ..... see CHIVE
CHLORELLA ..... see CHLORELLA
Chlorella pyrenoidosa ..... see CHLORELLA
Chlorella vulgaris ..... see CHLORELLA
CHLOROPHYLL ..... see CHLOROPHYLL
Chlorophyll a ..... see CHLOROPHYLL
Chlorophyll b ..... see CHLOROPHYLL
Chlorophyll c ..... see CHLOROPHYLL
Chlorophyll d ..... see CHLOROPHYLL
CHLOROPHYLLIN ..... see CHLOROPHYLLIN
Chocola ..... see COCOA
Chocolate Root ..... see WATER AVENS
Choke Cherry ..... see WILD CHERRY
Cholecalciferol ..... see VITAMIN D
CHOLINE ..... see CHOLINE
Choline Alphoscerate ..... see ALPHA-GPC
Choline Bitartrate ..... see CHOLINE
Choline Chloride ..... see CHOLINE
Chondrodendron tomentosum ..... see PAREIRA
Chondroitin ..... see CHONDROITIN SULFATE
Chondroitin 4-sulfate ..... see CHONDROITIN SULFATE
Chondroitin 6-sulfate ..... see CHONDROITIN SULFATE
Chondroitin Polysulfate ..... see CHONDROITIN SULFATE
CHONDROITIN SULFATE ..... see CHONDROITIN SULFATE
Chondroitin Sulfate B ..... see CHONDROITIN SULFATE
Chondroitin Sulfate C ..... see CHONDROITIN SULFATE
Chondroitin Sulphate A Sodium ..... see CHONDROITIN SULFATE
Chondrus crispus ..... see CARRAGEENAN
Chondrus Extract ..... see CARRAGEENAN
Chongras ..... see POKEWEED berry, POKEWEED root
Chop Nut ..... see CALABAR BEAN
Chosen-gomischi ..... see SCHISANDRA
Chota-chand ..... see INDIAN SNAKEROOT
Christe Herbe ..... see BLACK HELLEBORE
Christmas Flower ..... see POINSETTIA
Christmas Rose ..... see BLACK HELLEBORE
Christmas Rose Plant ..... see BLACK HELLEBORE
Christ's Spear ..... see ENGLISH ADDER'S TONGUE
Christ's Thorn ..... see HOLLY
Chromic Chloride ..... see CHROMIUM
CHROMIUM ..... see CHROMIUM
Chromium 3+ ..... see CHROMIUM
Chromium Acetate ..... see CHROMIUM
Chromium Chloride ..... see CHROMIUM
Chromium III ..... see CHROMIUM
Chromium III Picolinate ..... see CHROMIUM
Chromium Nicotinate ..... see CHROMIUM
Chromium Picolinate ..... see CHROMIUM
Chromium Polynicotinate ..... see CHROMIUM
Chromium Trichloride ..... see CHROMIUM
Chromium Tripicolinate ..... see CHROMIUM
Chrysanthemi Vulgaris Flos ..... see TANSY
Chrysanthemi Vulgaris Herba ..... see TANSY
CHRYSANTHEMUM ..... see CHRYSANTHEMUM
Chrysanthemum cinerariifolium ..... see PYRETHRUM
Chrysanthemum leucanthemum ..... see OX-EYE DAISY
Chrysanthemum morifolium ..... see CHRYSANTHEMUM
Chrysanthemum parthenium ..... see FEVERFEW
Chrysanthemum sinense ..... see CHRYSANTHEMUM
Chrysanthemum stipulaceum ..... see CHRYSANTHEMUM
Chrysanthemum vulgare ..... see TANSY
Chrysatobine ..... see GOA POWDER
CHRYSIN ..... see CHRYSIN
Chrysopogon zizanioides ..... see VETIVER
Chua ..... see AMARANTH
Chuan Dang ..... see CODONOPSIS
Chuan Xin Lian ..... see ANDROGRAPHIS
Chuan Xin Lin ..... see ANDROGRAPHIS
Chuan-wu ..... see ACONITE
Chuchuhuasha ..... see CATUABA
Chuchupate ..... see OSHA
Church Broom ..... see TEAZLE
Church-flower ..... see MADAGASCAR PERIWINKLE
Churnstaff ..... see YELLOW TOADFLAX
CHYMOTRYPSIN ..... see CHYMOTRYPSIN
Chymotrypsin A ..... see CHYMOTRYPSIN
Chymotrypsin B ..... see CHYMOTRYPSIN
Chymotrypsinum ..... see CHYMOTRYPSIN
CI Food Orange 8 ..... see CANTHAXANTHIN
Ci Wu Jia ..... see GINSENG, SIBERIAN
Cichorii Herba ..... see CHICORY
Cichorii Radix ..... see CHICORY
Cichorium intybus ..... see CHICORY
Cicuta bulbifera ..... see WATER HEMLOCK
Cicuta californica ..... see WATER HEMLOCK
Cicuta douglasii ..... see WATER HEMLOCK
Cicuta mackenzieana ..... see WATER HEMLOCK
Cicuta maculata ..... see WATER HEMLOCK
Cicuta occidentalis ..... see WATER HEMLOCK
Cicuta vagans ..... see WATER HEMLOCK
Cicuta virosa ..... see WATER HEMLOCK
Cider Vinegar ..... see APPLE CIDER VINEGAR
CIGUATERA ..... see CIGUATERA
Ciguatera Poisoning ..... see CIGUATERA
Cilantro ..... see CORIANDER
Cimicifuga ..... see BLACK COHOSH
Cimicifuga racemosa ..... see BLACK COHOSH
Cinchol ..... see BETA-SITOSTEROL

CINCHONA ... see CINCHONA
Cinchona calisaya ... see CINCHONA
Cinchona carabayensis ... see CINCHONA
Cinchona ledgeriana ... see CINCHONA
Cinchona officinalis ... see CINCHONA
Cinchona pubescens ... see CINCHONA
Cinchona succirubra ... see CINCHONA
Cineraria maritima ... see DUSTY MILLER
Cinnamomi Cassiae Cortex ... see CASSIA CINNAMON
Cinnamomum ... see CASSIA CINNAMON, see CINNAMON bark
Cinnamomum aromaticum ... see CASSIA CINNAMON
Cinnamomum camphora ... see CAMPHOR
Cinnamomum cassia ... see CASSIA CINNAMON
Cinnamomum verum ... see CINNAMON bark
Cinnamomum zeylanicum ... see CINNAMON bark
Cinnamon ... see CASSIA CINNAMON, CINNAMON bark
CINNAMON bark ... see CINNAMON bark
Cinnamon Flos ... see CASSIA CINNAMON
Cinnamon Sedge ... see CALAMUS
Cinnamon Wood ... see SASSAFRAS
Cinquefoil ... see EUROPEAN FIVE-FINGER GRASS, TORMENTIL
Cique Vireuse ... see WATER HEMLOCK
Cis-1,2,3,5-trans-4,6-cyclohexanehexol ... see INOSITOL
Cis-9,trans-11 conjugated linoleic acid ... see CONJUGATED LINOLEIC ACID
Cis-9-cetylmyristoleate ... see CETYLATED FATTY ACIDS
Cis-9-octadecenoic acid ... see LORENZO'S OIL
Cis-hexahydro-2-oxo-1H-thieno[3,4-d]-imidazole-4-valeric acid ... see BIOTIN
Cis-resveratrol ... see RESVERATROL
Cissampelos pareira ... see ABUTA
Ciste ... see LABDANUM
Cistus canadensis ... see FROSTWORT
Cistus creticus ... see LABDANUM
Cistus incanus ... see LABDANUM
Cistus ladanifer ... see LABDANUM
Cistus ladaniferus ... see LABDANUM
Cistus polymorphus ... see LABDANUM
Cistus villosus ... see LABDANUM
CITICOLINE ... see CITICOLINE
Citrated Caffeine ... see CAFFEINE
Citri sinensis ... see SWEET ORANGE
Citric Acid ... see ALPHA HYDROXY ACIDS
Citronella ... see LEMONGRASS, STONE ROOT
CITRONELLA OIL ... see CITRONELLA OIL
Citrullus colocynthis ... see COLOCYNTH
Citrus acida ... see LIME fruit, peel; LIME OIL
Citrus amara ... see BITTER ORANGE
Citrus aurantifolia ... see LIME fruit, peel; LIME OIL
Citrus aurantium ... see BITTER ORANGE
Citrus aurantium var. bergamia ... see BERGAMOT OIL
Citrus aurantium var. dulcis ... see SWEET ORANGE
Citrus aurantium var. sinensis ... see SWEET ORANGE
Citrus bergamia ... see BERGAMOT OIL
Citrus bigarradia ... see BITTER ORANGE
Citrus Bioflavones ... see METHOXYLATED FLAVONES
Citrus Bioflavonoids ... see DIOSMIN, HESPERIDIN, METHOXYLATED FLAVONES, QUERCETIN, RUTIN
Citrus decumana ... see GRAPEFRUIT, GRAPEFRUIT OIL, GRAPEFRUIT SEED EXTRACT
Citrus Flavones ... see METHOXYLATED FLAVONES
Citrus Flavonoids ... see METHOXYLATED FLAVONES
Citrus grandis Extract ... see GRAPEFRUIT SEED EXTRACT
Citrus lima ... see LIME fruit, peel; LIME OIL
Citrus limetta var. aromatica ... see LIME fruit, peel; LIME OIL
Citrus limon ... see LEMON
Citrus limonum ... see LEMON
Citrus macracantha ... see SWEET ORANGE
Citrus maxima ... see GRAPEFRUIT, GRAPEFRUIT OIL, GRAPEFRUIT SEED EXTRACT
Citrus medica var. acida ... see LIME fruit, peel; LIME OIL
Citrus paradisi ... see GRAPEFRUIT, GRAPEFRUIT OIL, GRAPEFRUIT SEED EXTRACT
Citrus Polymethoxylated Flavones ... see METHOXYLATED FLAVONES
Citrus Seed Extract ... see GRAPEFRUIT SEED EXTRACT
Citrus sinensis ... see SWEET ORANGE
Citrus vulgaris ... see BITTER ORANGE
Civan percemi ... see YARROW
Cives ... see CHIVE
CIVET ... see CIVET
Civettictis civetta ... see CIVET
Ciwujia ... see GINSENG, SIBERIAN
CLA ... see CONJUGATED LINOLEIC ACID
Cladonia pyxidata ... see CUPMOSS
CLA-FFA ... see CONJUGATED LINOLEIC ACID
CLA-free fatty acid ... see CONJUGATED LINOLEIC ACID
Clarified Honey ... see HONEY
Clary ... see CLARY SAGE
CLARY SAGE ... see CLARY SAGE
Clary Wort ... see CLARY SAGE
CLA-triacylglycerol ... see CONJUGATED LINOLEIC ACID
Claviceps purpurea ... see ERGOT
Clay Suspension Products ... see COLLOIDAL MINERALS
Clear Eye ... see CLARY SAGE
Cleavers ... see CLIVERS
Cleaverwort ... see CLIVERS
CLEMATIS ... see CLEMATIS
Clematis ... see CLEMATIS, WOODBINE
Clematis recta ... see CLEMATIS
Clematis virginiana ... see WOODBINE
Clematis vitalba ... see TRAVELER'S JOY
Clerodendranthus spicatus ... see JAVA TEA
Clerodendrum spicatum ... see JAVA TEA
Climbing Knotweed ... see FO-TI
Clinopodium nepeta ... see CALAMINT
CLIVERS ... see CLIVERS
Clotbur ... see BURDOCK
Clot-bur ... see MULLEIN
Cloud Mushroom ... see CORIOLUS MUSHROOM
Clous de Girolfe ... see CLOVE dried flowerbud, leaf, stem; CLOVE OIL
Clove ... see CLOVE dried flowerbud, leaf, stem;
CLOVE dried flowerbud, leaf, stem ... see CLOVE dried flowerbud, leaf, stem

Clove Flower .... see CLOVE dried flowerbud, leaf, stem
Clove Garlic .... see GARLIC
CLOVE OIL .... see CLOVE OIL
Clove Pepper .... see ALLSPICE
Clovone .... see RED CLOVER
Clown's Lungwort .... see MULLEIN
CLOWN'S MUSTARD PLANT .... see CLOWN'S MUSTARD PLANT
CLUB MOSS .... see CLUB MOSS
Clustered Wintercherry .... see ASHWAGANDHA
Clutia eluteria .... see CASCARILLA
CM .... see CETYLATED FATTY ACIDS
CMO .... see CETYLATED FATTY ACIDS
Cnici Benedicti Herba .... see BLESSED THISTLE
Cnicus .... see BLESSED THISTLE
Cnicus benedictus .... see BLESSED THISTLE
CO Q10 .... see COENZYME Q-10
Coachweed .... see CLIVERS
Coakum .... see POKEWEED berry, POKEWEED root
Coakum-chorngras .... see POKEWEED berry, POKEWEED root
Coastal Douglas Fir .... see OREGON FIR BALSAM
Cobalamin .... see VITAMIN B12
Cobalamin Enzyme .... see DIBENCOZIDE
Cobalamins .... see VITAMIN B12
Cobamamide .... see DIBENCOZIDE
Cobamin .... see VITAMIN B12
Cobnut .... see HAZELNUT
COCA .... see COCA
Cocaine Plant .... see COCA
Cocash Weed .... see GOLDEN RAGWORT
Cocculus .... see LEVANT BERRY
Cocculus indicus .... see LEVANT BERRY
Cocculus lacunosus .... see LEVANT BERRY
Cocculus palmatus .... see COLOMBO
Cocculus suberosus .... see LEVANT BERRY
Cochin Ginger .... see GINGER
Cochin Lemongrass .... see LEMONGRASS
Cochlearia armoracia .... see HORSERADISH
Cochlearia officinalis .... see SCURVY GRASS
COCILLANA .... see COCILLANA
Cockle .... see CORN COCKLE
Cockle Buttons .... see BURDOCK
Cocklebur .... see AGRIMONY, BURDOCK
Cockspur Rye .... see ERGOT
Cockup Hat .... see QUEEN'S DELIGHT
Cocky Baby .... see ARUM
Coco Palm .... see COCONUT OIL
COCOA .... see COCOA
Cocoa Bean .... see COCOA
Cocoa Butter .... see COCOA
Cocoa Oleum .... see COCOA
Cocoa Seed .... see COCOA
Cocoa Semen .... see COCOA
Cocoa Testae .... see COCOA
COCONUT OIL .... see COCONUT OIL
Coconut Palm .... see COCONUT OIL
Cocos nucifera .... see COCONUT OIL
Cocowort .... see SHEPHERD'S PURSE
Coculus fructus .... see LEVANT BERRY
COD LIVER OIL .... see COD LIVER OIL
Cod Liver Oil .... see COD LIVER OIL, FISH OILS
Cod Oil .... see COD LIVER OIL
CODONOPSIS .... see CODONOPSIS
Codonopsis pilosula .... see CODONOPSIS
Codonopsis pilosula modesta .... see CODONOPSIS
Codonopsis tangshen .... see CODONOPSIS
Codonopsis tubulosa .... see CODONOPSIS
Coenzyme 1 .... see NADH
Coenzyme B-12 .... see DIBENCOZIDE
COENZYME Q-10 .... see COENZYME Q-10
Coenzyme R .... see BIOTIN
Coffea arabica .... see COFFEE, COFFEE CHARCOAL
Coffea arnoldiana .... see COFFEE
Coffea bukobensis .... see COFFEE
Coffea canephora .... see COFFEE, COFFEE CHARCOAL
Coffea liberica .... see COFFEE, COFFEE CHARCOAL
Coffea robusta .... see COFFEE
COFFEE .... see COFFEE
COFFEE CHARCOAL .... see COFFEE CHARCOAL
Cognassier .... see QUINCE
Coing .... see QUINCE
Cokan .... see POKEWEED berry, POKEWEED root
Cola acuminata .... see COLA NUT
Cola nitida .... see COLA NUT
COLA NUT .... see COLA NUT
Colchicum .... see AUTUMN CROCUS
Colchicum autumnale .... see AUTUMN CROCUS
Colchicum speciosum .... see AUTUMN CROCUS
Colchicum vernum .... see AUTUMN CROCUS
Cold-pressed grapefruit oil .... see GRAPEFRUIT OIL
Coleus barbatus .... see FORSKOLIN
Coleus forskohlii .... see FORSKOLIN
Colewort .... see AVENS, CABBAGE
Colforsin .... see FORSKOLIN
Colic Root .... see ALETRIS, ALPINIA, MARSH BLAZING STAR, WILD YAM
Colinsonia .... see STONE ROOT
Collagen Hydrolysate .... see GELATIN
Colle du Japon .... see AGAR
Collinsonia canadensis .... see STONE ROOT
COLLOIDAL MINERALS .... see COLLOIDAL MINERALS
COLLOIDAL SILVER .... see COLLOIDAL SILVER
Colloidal Silver Protein .... see COLLOIDAL SILVER
Colloidal Trace Minerals .... see COLLOIDAL MINERALS
COLOCYNTH .... see COLOCYNTH
Colocynth Pulp .... see COLOCYNTH
Colocynthidis Fructus .... see COLOCYNTH
Colocynthis vulgaris .... see COLOCYNTH
COLOMBO .... see COLOMBO
Color Index No. 40850 .... see CANTHAXANTHIN
Colorado Cough Root .... see OSHA
COLOSTRUM .... see COLOSTRUM
Colour Index No. 40850 .... see CANTHAXANTHIN
COLTSFOOT .... see COLTSFOOT
Coltstail .... see CANADIAN FLEABANE
COLUMBINE .... see COLUMBINE
Comb Flower .... see ECHINACEA
Combretum .... see OPIUM ANTIDOTE
Combretum micranthum .... see OPIUM ANTIDOTE
Combucha Tea .... see KOMBUCHA TEA
COMFREY .... see COMFREY
Cominho Negro .... see BLACK SEED
Commiphora .... see MYRRH
Commiphora abyssinica .... see MYRRH
Commiphora erythraea .... see MYRRH
Commiphora habessinica .... see MYRRH

INDEX

Commiphora kataf .... see MYRRH
Commiphora madagascariensis .... see MYRRH
Commiphora molmol .... see MYRRH
Commiphora mukul .... see GUGGUL
Commiphora myrrha .... see MYRRH
Commiphora wightii .... see GUGGUL
Common Alder .... see BLACK ALDER
Common Ash .... see ASH
Common Barberry .... see EUROPEAN BARBERRY
Common Basil .... see BASIL
Common Bean .... see BEAN POD
Common Bearberry .... see UVA URSI
Common Borage .... see BORAGE flower, dried above ground parts
Common Bugloss .... see BORAGE flower, dried above ground parts
Common Centaury .... see CENTAURY
Common Cherry Laurel ... see CHERRY LAUREL WATER
Common Chicory Root .... see CHICORY
Common Comfrey .... see COMFREY
Common Condorvine .... see CONDURANGO
Common Dandelion .... see DANDELION above ground parts, DANDELION entire plant
Common Dubbletjie .... see PUNCTURE VINE
Common Elder .... see ELDERFLOWER
Common Elderberry .... see AMERICAN ELDER
Common Fennel .... see FENNEL fruit, seed
Common Figwort .... see FIGWORT
Common Groundsel .... see GROUNDSEL
Common Guelder-rose .... see CRAMP BARK
Common Hoarhound .... see WHITE HOREHOUND
Common Hops .... see HOPS
Common Jasmine .... see JASMINE
Common Juniper Berry .... see JUNIPER
Common Lavender .... see LAVENDER
Common Melilot .... see SWEET CLOVER
Common Nettle .... see STINGING NETTLE above ground parts, STINGING NETTLE root
Common Nightshade .... see BITTERSWEET NIGHTSHADE
Common Oak .... see OAK bark
Common Oleander .... see OLEANDER
Common Parsley .... see PARSLEY leaf, root; PARSLEY seed
Common Peony .... see PEONY flower, PEONY root
Common Periwinkle .... see PERIWINKLE
Common Plantain .... see GREAT PLANTAIN
Common Polypod .... see LADY FERN
Common Ragwort .... see TANSY RAGWORT
Common Reed .... see REED HERB
Common Rue .... see RUE
Common Sage .... see SAGE
Common Sandspurry .... see ARENARIA RUBRA
Common Sassafras .... see SASSAFRAS
Common Shrubby Everlasting .... see IMMORTELLE, SANDY EVERLASTING
Common Sorrel .... see WOOD SORREL
COMMON STONECROP .... see COMMON STONECROP
Common Thyme ..... see THYME flower, leaf; THYME OIL
Common Valerian .... see VALERIAN
Common Vanilla .... see VANILLA
Common Verbena .... see VERBENA
Common Vervain .... see VERBENA
Common Wormwood .... see WORMWOOD above ground parts
Common Yarrow .... see YARROW
Common Yew .... see YEW
Compass Plant .... see ROSEMARY
Compass Weed .... see ROSEMARY, ROSINWEED
Compound Q .... see CHINESE CUCUMBER fruit, CHINESE CUCUMBER root, CHINESE CUCUMBER seed
Condensed Tannins .... see PYCNOGENOL
CONDURANGO .... see CONDURANGO
Condurango Cortex .... see CONDURANGO
Coneflower .... see ECHINACEA
Conium .... see HEMLOCK
Conium maculata .... see HEMLOCK
Conium maculatum .... see HEMLOCK
CONJUGATED LINOLEIC ACID .... see CONJUGATED LINOLEIC ACID
Consolida regalis .... see DELPHINIUM
Consolidae Radix .... see COMFREY
Consound .... see COMFREY
Constancy .... see LILY-OF-THE-VALLEY
Consumptive's Weed .... see YERBA SANTA
Continental Tea .... see LABRADOR TEA
Contrayerba .... see CONTRAYERVA
CONTRAYERVA .... see CONTRAYERVA
Convallaria .... see LILY-OF-THE-VALLEY
Convallaria Herba .... see LILY-OF-THE-VALLEY
Convallaria majalis .... see LILY-OF-THE-VALLEY
Convall-lily .... see LILY-OF-THE-VALLEY
Convolvulus nervosus .... see HAWAIIAN BABY WOODROSE
Convolvulus orizabensis .... see MEXICAN SCAMMONY ROOT
Convolvulus purga .... see JALAP
Convolvulus speciosus .... see HAWAIIAN BABY WOODROSE
Convolvulus superbus .... see MEXICAN SCAMMONY ROOT
Conyza canadensis .... see CANADIAN FLEABANE
Cool Tankard .... see BORAGE flower, dried above ground parts
COOLWORT .... see COOLWORT
Coon Root .... see BLOODROOT
Copaiba .... see COPAIBA BALSAM
COPAIBA BALSAM .... see COPAIBA BALSAM
Copaiba oleoresin .... see COPAIBA BALSAM
Copaifera langsdorffii .... see COPAIBA BALSAM
Copaifera officinalis .... see COPAIBA BALSAM
Copaifera reticulata .... see COPAIBA BALSAM
Copaiva .... see COPAIBA BALSAM
Copal Tree .... see TREE OF HEAVEN
Copalm .... see STORAX
COPPER .... see COPPER
Copperose .... see CORN POPPY
Coptide .... see GOLDTHREAD
Coptis .... see GOLDTHREAD
Coptis chinensis .... see GOLDTHREAD
Coptis deltoidea .... see GOLDTHREAD
Coptis groenlandica .... see GOLDTHREAD
Coptis teeta .... see GOLDTHREAD
Coptis teetoides .... see GOLDTHREAD

Coptis trifolia .... see GOLDTHREAD
Coquerest .... see WINTER CHERRY
CORAL .... see CORAL
Coral Calcium .... see CORAL
Coral Peony .... see PEONY flower, PEONY root
CORAL ROOT .... see CORAL ROOT
Coralberry .... see WHITE COHOSH
Coralline Hydroxyapatite .... see CORAL
Corallorhiza odontorhiza .... see CORAL ROOT
CORDYCEPS .... see CORDYCEPS
Cordyceps sinensis .... see CORDYCEPS
CORIANDER .... see CORIANDER
Coriandri Fructus .... see CORIANDER
Coriandrum sativum .... see CORIANDER
Coridothymus capitatus .... see SPANISH ORIGANUM OIL
Coriolus .... see CORIOLUS MUSHROOM
CORIOLUS MUSHROOM .... see CORIOLUS MUSHROOM
Coriolus versicolor .... see CORIOLUS MUSHROOM
CORKWOOD TREE .... see CORKWOOD TREE
Corn Campion .... see CORN COCKLE
CORN COCKLE .... see CORN COCKLE
Corn Flower .... see CORNFLOWER
Corn Horsetail .... see HORSETAIL
Corn Mint .... see JAPANESE MINT
CORN POPPY .... see CORN POPPY
Corn Rose .... see CORN COCKLE, CORN POPPY
CORN SILK .... see CORN SILK
Corn Sugar Gum .... see XANTHAN GUM
Cornel .... see AMERICAN DOGWOOD
Cornelian Tree .... see AMERICAN DOGWOOD
CORNFLOWER .... see CORNFLOWER
Cornmint Oil .... see JAPANESE MINT
Cornsilk .... see CORN SILK
Cornu Cervi Parvum .... see DEER VELVET
Cornus florida .... see AMERICAN DOGWOOD
Corona de Cristo .... see PASSIONFLOWER
Corona Solis .... see SUNFLOWER OIL
Corossol epineux .... see GRAVIOLA
Corossolier .... see GRAVIOLA
Corosolic Acid .... see BANABA
Corpus Luteum Hormone .... see PROGESTERONE
Cortex cinnamomi .... see CASSIA CINNAMON
Corydalis .... see CORYDALIS
Corydalis cava .... see CORYDALIS
Corydalis tuberosa .... see CORYDALIS
Corylus avellana .... see HAZELNUT
Corylus heterophylla .... see HAZELNUT
Corynanthe johimbi .... see YOHIMBE
Corynanthe yohimbi .... see YOHIMBE
Cossoo .... see KOUSSO
Costus .... see COSTUS OIL, COSTUS root
COSTUS OIL .... see COSTUS OIL
COSTUS root .... see COSTUS root
COTTON .... see COTTON
Cotton Dawes .... see CUDWEED
Cotton Root .... see COTTON
Cotton Weed .... see CUDWEED
Cottonseed Oil .... see GOSSYPOL
Couchgrass .... see WHEATGRASS
Coudrier .... see HAZELNUT
Coughroot .... see BETH ROOT
Coughweed .... see GOLDEN RAGWORT
Coughwort .... see COLTSFOOT
Couhage .... see COWHAGE
Coumarouna Odorata .... see TONKA BEAN
COUNTRY MALLOW .... see COUNTRY MALLOW
Country Walnut .... see TUNG SEED
Covanamilpori .... see INDIAN SNAKEROOT
Cow Cabbage .... see AMERICAN WHITE POND LILY, MASTERWORT
Cow Clover .... see RED CLOVER
Cow Grass .... see KNOTWEED
Cow Milk Colostrum .... see COLOSTRUM
Cow Parsnip .... see MASTERWORT
Cowbane .... see WATER HEMLOCK
Cowberry .... see ALPINE CRANBERRY
COWHAGE .... see COWHAGE
Cowitch .... see COWHAGE
COWSLIP .... see COWSLIP
Cowslip .... see COWSLIP, MARSH MARIGOLD
CPS .... see CHONDROITIN SULFATE
Cr .... see CHROMIUM, CREATINE
Cr III .... see CHROMIUM
Cr3+ .... see CHROMIUM
Crab's Eye .... see PRECATORY BEAN
Crabwood .... see ANDIROBA
Crack Willow .... see WILLOW BARK
CRAMP BARK .... see CRAMP BARK
Crampweed .... see POTENTILLA
CRANBERRY .... see CRANBERRY
Crape Myrtle .... see BANABA
Crataegi Flos .... see HAWTHORN
Crataegi Folium .... see HAWTHORN
Crataegi Folium Cum Flore .... see HAWTHORN
Crataegi Fructus .... see HAWTHORN
Crataegus cuneata .... see HAWTHORN
Crataegus kulingensis .... see HAWTHORN
Crataegus laevigata .... see HAWTHORN
Crataegus monogyna .... see HAWTHORN
Crataegus oxyacantha .... see HAWTHORN
Crataegus pinnatifida .... see HAWTHORN
Crawley .... see CORAL ROOT
Crawley Root .... see CORAL ROOT
Crawlgrass .... see KNOTWEED
Creat .... see ANDROGRAPHIS
CREATINE .... see CREATINE
Creatine Monohydrate .... see CREATINE
Creeper .... see AMERICAN IVY
Creeping Barberry .... see OREGON GRAPE
Creeping Charlie .... see GROUND IVY
Creeping Jenny .... see MONEYWORT
Creeping Joan .... see MONEYWORT
Creeping Tom .... see COMMON STONECROP
Creosote Bush .... see CHAPARRAL
Crepe Myrtle .... see BANABA
Crescione di Fonte .... see WATERCRESS
Cresson au Poulet .... see WATERCRESS
Cresson de Fontaine .... see WATERCRESS
Cresson d'Eau .... see WATERCRESS
Crest Marine .... see SAMPHIRE
Crewel .... see COWSLIP
Crithmum maritimum .... see SAMPHIRE
Croci Stigma .... see SAFFRON
Crocus .... see AUTUMN CROCUS
Crocus sativus .... see SAFFRON
Crosswort .... see BONESET
Croton .... see CROTON SEEDS

INDEX

Croton eluteria .... see CASCARILLA
Croton lechleri .... see SANGRE DE GRADO
CROTON SEEDS .... see CROTON SEEDS
Croton tiglium .... see CROTON SEEDS
Crow Corn .... see ALETRIS
Crowberry .... see POKEWEED berry, POKEWEED root
Crowfoot .... see BULBOUS BUTTERCUP, WOOD ANEMONE
Crown-of-the-field .... see CORN COCKLE
Crude Chrysarobin .... see GOA POWDER
Crystalline DMSO .... see MSM (METHYLSULFONYLMETHANE)
Cs .... see CESIUM
CS .... see CHONDROITIN SULFATE
Cs-4 .... see CORDYCEPS
CSA .... see CHONDROITIN SULFATE
CSC .... see CHONDROITIN SULFATE
CsCl .... see CESIUM
CSE .... see GRAPEFRUIT SEED EXTRACT
Cu .... see COPPER
Cubeb Berries .... see CUBEBS
Cubeba .... see CUBEBS
Cubeba officinalis .... see CUBEBS
CUBEBS .... see CUBEBS
Cuckoo Bread .... see WOOD SORREL
Cuckoo Buds .... see BULBOUS BUTTERCUP
Cuckoo Flower .... see SALEP
Cuckoo Pint .... see ARUM
Cuckowes Meat .... see WOOD SORREL
Cucumis colocynthis .... see COLOCYNTH
Cucumis pepo .... see PUMPKIN
Cucurbita galeottii .... see PUMPKIN
Cucurbita mammeata .... see PUMPKIN
Cucurbita pepo .... see PUMPKIN
Cucurbitea Peponis Semen .... see PUMPKIN
Cuddy's Lungs .... see MULLEIN
CUDWEED .... see CUDWEED
Cudweed .... see CAT'S FOOT, CUDWEED
Cuivre .... see COPPER
Cukilanarpak .... see DEVIL'S CLUB
Culveris Root .... see BLACK ROOT
Culvers .... see BLACK ROOT
Culver's Physic .... see BLACK ROOT
Culver's Root .... see BLACK ROOT
Culverwort .... see COLUMBINE
Cumaru .... see TONKA BEAN
CUMIN .... see CUMIN
Cumin des Pres .... see CARAWAY dried fruit, seed
Cuminum cyminum .... see CUMIN
Cuminum odorum .... see CUMIN
Cummin .... see CUMIN
Cundeamor .... see BITTER MELON
CUP PLANT .... see CUP PLANT
Cupania sapida .... see ACKEE
CUPMOSS .... see CUPMOSS
Cup-puppy .... see CORN POPPY
Cupreol .... see BETA-SITOSTEROL
Cupressus sempervirens .... see CYPRESS
Cupric Oxide .... see COPPER
Curbana .... see CANELLA
Curcuma .... see JAVANESE TURMERIC, TURMERIC
Curcuma aromatica .... see TURMERIC
Curcuma domestica .... see TURMERIC
Curcuma longa .... see TURMERIC
Curcuma xanthorrhiza .... see JAVANESE TURMERIC
Curcuma zedoaria .... see ZEDOARY
Curcumae Longae Rhizoma .... see TURMERIC
Curcumae xanthorrhizae rhizoma .... see JAVANESE TURMERIC
Curcumin .... see TURMERIC
Curdwort .... see LADY'S BEDSTRAW
Cure-all .... see LEMON BALM, WATER AVENS
Curled Dock .... see YELLOW DOCK
Curled Mint .... see SPEARMINT
Curly Dock .... see YELLOW DOCK
Cursed Crowfoot .... see POISONOUS BUTTERCUP
Cuscus .... see VETIVER
Cuscus Grass .... see VETIVER
Cuscuta chinensis .... see DODDER
Cuscuta epithymum .... see DODDER
Cuscutae .... see DODDER
Cusparia .... see ANGOSTURA
Cusparia Bark .... see ANGOSTURA
Cusparia febrifuga .... see ANGOSTURA
Cusparia trifoliata .... see ANGOSTURA
Custard Apple .... see AMERICAN PAWPAW
Cutch .... see CATECHU, WHEATGRASS
Cutweed .... see BLADDERWRACK
Cyamopsis psoraloides .... see GUAR GUM
Cyamopsis tetragonoloba .... see GUAR GUM
Cyani Blossoms .... see CORNFLOWER
Cyani Flos .... see CORNFLOWER
Cyani Flowers .... see CORNFLOWER
Cyani Petals .... see CORNFLOWER
Cyanobacteria .... see BLUE-GREEN ALGAE
Cyanocobalamin .... see VITAMIN B12
Cyanocobalaminum .... see VITAMIN B12
CYCLAMEN .... see CYCLAMEN
Cyclamen europaeum .... see CYCLAMEN
Cyclamen purpurascens .... see CYCLAMEN
Cyclohexitol .... see INOSITOL
Cycobemin .... see VITAMIN B12
Cydonia oblongata .... see QUINCE
Cydonia vulgaris .... see QUINCE
Cymbidium odontorhizum .... see CORAL ROOT
Cymbopogon afronardus .... see CITRONELLA OIL
Cymbopogon citratus .... see LEMONGRASS
Cymbopogon flexuosus .... see LEMONGRASS
Cymbopogon nardus .... see CITRONELLA OIL
Cymbopogon validus .... see CITRONELLA OIL
Cymbopogon winterianus .... see CITRONELLA OIL
Cynanchum vincetoxicum .... see GERMAN IPECAC
Cynara cardunculus .... see ARTICHOKE
Cynara scolymus .... see ARTICHOKE
Cynoglossi Herba .... see HOUND'S TONGUE
Cynoglossi Radix .... see HOUND'S TONGUE
Cynoglossum officinale .... see HOUND'S TONGUE
Cynosbatos .... see ROSE HIP
Cyperus articulatus .... see ADRUE
Cyperus corymbosus .... see ADRUE
CYPRESS .... see CYPRESS
Cypress Powder .... see ARUM
CYPRESS SPURGE .... see CYPRESS SPURGE
Cypripedium .... see NERVE ROOT
Cypripedium calceolus .... see NERVE ROOT
Cypripedium parviflorum .... see NERVE ROOT
Cypripedium pubescens .... see NERVE ROOT
Cystadane .... see BETAINE ANHYDROUS

Cyste .... see LABDANUM
Cytidine 5'-diphosphocholine .... see CITICOLINE
Cytisi Scoparii Flos .... see SCOTCH BROOM flower
Cytisi Scoparii Herba .... see SCOTCH BROOM herb
Cytisus alschingeri .... see LABURNUM
Cytisus laburnum .... see LABURNUM
Cytisus scoparius .... see SCOTCH BROOM flower, SCOTCH BROOM herb
D-alpha-tocopherol .... see VITAMIN E
D-alpha-tocopheryl .... see VITAMIN E
D-alpha-tocopheryl acetate .... see VITAMIN E
D-alpha-tocopheryl succinate .... see VITAMIN E
D-beta-tocopherol .... see VITAMIN E
D-biotin .... see BIOTIN
D-bis-(N-pantothenyl-B-aminoethyl)-disulfide .... see PANTETHINE
D-calcium pantothenate .... see PANTOTHENIC ACID (VITAMIN B5)
D-carnitine .... see L-CARNITINE
D-chiro-inositol .... see INOSITOL
D-chiro-inositol, synonym (+)-chiroinositol .... see INOSITOL
D-delta-tocopherol .... see VITAMIN E
D-gamma-tocopherol .... see VITAMIN E
D-glucarate (GA) .... see CALCIUM D-GLUCARATE
D-glucaro-1,4-lactone (1,4 GL) .... see CALCIUM D-GLUCARATE
D-glucosamine .... see GLUCOSAMINE SULFATE
D-glucosamine HCl .... see GLUCOSAMINE HYDROCHLORIDE
D-pantethine .... see PANTETHINE
D-panthenol .... see PANTOTHENIC ACID (VITAMIN B5)
D-pantothenic acid .... see PANTOTHENIC ACID (VITAMIN B5)
D-pantothenyl alcohol .... see PANTOTHENIC ACID (VITAMIN B5)
D-phenylalanine .... see PHENYLALANINE
D-ribose .... see RIBOSE
D-tocopherol .... see VITAMIN E
D-tocopheryl acetate .... see VITAMIN E
Da Huang .... see RHUBARB
DA QING YE .... see DA QING YE
Da Zao .... see JUJUBE
Dadima .... see POMEGRANATE
Daemonorops Draco .... see DRAGON'S BLOOD
DAFFODIL .... see DAFFODIL
DAG .... see DIACYLGLYCEROL
Dage of Jerusalem .... see LUNGWORT
Dagger Plant .... see YUCCA
Daggers .... see ORRIS
Dahlia Extract .... see INULIN
Dahlia Inulin .... see INULIN
Daidzein .... see KUDZU, RED CLOVER, SOY
Daisy .... see TANSY
Dalmatian Sage .... see SAGE
Dalmation Insect Flowers .... see PYRETHRUM
Dalmation Pellitory .... see PYRETHRUM
Dambrose .... see INOSITOL
DAMIANA .... see DAMIANA
Damiana aphrodisiaca .... see DAMIANA
Damiana Herb .... see DAMIANA
Damiana Leaf .... see DAMIANA
Dan Shen .... see DANSHEN
Dancing Mushroom .... see MAITAKE MUSHROOM
Dandelion .... see DANDELION above ground parts, DANDELION entire plant
DANDELION above ground parts .... see DANDELION above ground parts
DANDELION entire plant .... see DANDELION entire plant
Dandelion Herb .... see DANDELION above ground parts
Dandelion Root .... see DANDELION entire plant
Danewort .... see DWARF ELDER
Dang Gui .... see ANGELICA root, DONG QUAI
Danggui .... see DONG QUAI
Dangshen .... see CODONOPSIS
DANSHEN .... see DANSHEN
Dan-shen .... see DANSHEN
Daphne .... see MEZEREON, SWEET BAY
Daphne mezereum .... see MEZEREON
Daphne Willow .... see WILLOW BARK
Dark Catechu .... see CATECHU
Darnel .... see TAUMELLOOLCH
Darri .... see BROOM CORN
DATE PALM .... see DATE PALM
Datura .... see JIMSON WEED
Datura inermis .... see JIMSON WEED
Datura stramonium .... see JIMSON WEED
Datura suaveolens .... see ANGEL'S TRUMPET
Datura tatula .... see JIMSON WEED
Daucus .... see WILD CARROT
Daucus carota subsp. carota .... see WILD CARROT
Daucus visagna .... see KHELLA
Dead Man's Bells .... see DIGITALIS
Dead Tongue .... see HEMLOCK WATER DROPWORT
Deadly Nightshade .... see BELLADONNA, BITTERSWEET NIGHTSHADE
Deaf Nettle .... see WHITE DEAD NETTLE FLOWER
DEANOL .... see DEANOL
Deanol aceglumate .... see DEANOL
Deanol acetamidobenzoate .... see DEANOL
Deanol benzilate .... see DEANOL
Deanol bisorcate .... see DEANOL
Deanol cyclohexylpropionate .... see DEANOL
Deanol hemisuccinate .... see DEANOL
Deanol pidolate .... see DEANOL
Deanol tartrate .... see DEANOL
Death-of-man .... see WATER HEMLOCK
Deep Sea Shark Liver Oil .... see SHARK LIVER OIL
Deer Antler .... see DEER VELVET
Deer Antler Velvet .... see DEER VELVET
Deer Balls .... see PUFF BALL
Deer Musk .... see MUSK
DEER VELVET .... see DEER VELVET
Deerberry .... see SQUAWVINE, WINTERGREEN leaf, WINTERGREEN OIL
Deernut .... see JOJOBA
Deer's Tongue .... see DEERTONGUE
DEERTONGUE .... see DEERTONGUE
Dehydroepiandrosterone .... see DHEA
Dehydroretinol .... see VITAMIN A
Delicate Bess .... see RED-SPUR VALERIAN
Delphinii Flos .... see DELPHINIUM
DELPHINIUM .... see DELPHINIUM
Delphinium consolida .... see DELPHINIUM
Delphinium staphisagria .... see STAVESACRE
Delta-tocopherol .... see VITAMIN E
Delta 5-pregnen-3 beta-ol-20-one .... see PREGNENOLONE

INDEX

Delta Tocotrienol .... see VITAMIN E
Demon Chaser .... see ST. JOHN'S WORT
Denatured Collagen .... see GELATIN
Dendranthema grandiflorum ...... see CHRYSANTHEMUM
Dendranthema morifolium .... see CHRYSANTHEMUM
Dentidia nankinensis .... see PERILLA
Deoxynucleic Acid .... see RNA AND DNA
Deoxyribonucleic Acid .... see RNA AND DNA
Derriere Dos .... see CHANCA PIEDRA
Des Dos .... see CHANCA PIEDRA
Desert Herb .... see EPHEDRA
Desert Tea .... see MORMON TEA
Devil Tree .... see FEVER BARK
Devil's Apple .... see JIMSON WEED, PODOPHYLLUM
Devil's Bit .... see FEVER BARK, PREMORSE
Devil's Bite .... see AMERICAN HELLEBORE
Devil's Bite Prairie-pine ...... see MARSH BLAZING STAR
Devil's Bones .... see WILD YAM
Devil's Bush .... see GINSENG, SIBERIAN
Devil's Cherries .... see BELLADONNA
DEVIL'S CLAW .... see DEVIL'S CLAW
Devil's Claw Root .... see DEVIL'S CLAW
DEVIL'S CLUB .... see DEVIL'S CLUB
Devil's Darning Needle .... see WOODBINE
Devil's Dung .... see ASAFOETIDA
Devil's Eye .... see HENBANE
Devil's Fuge .... see EUROPEAN MISTLETOE
Devil's Guts .... see DODDER
Devil's Head .... see YELLOW TOADFLAX
Devil's Herb .... see BELLADONNA
Devil's Nettle .... see YARROW
Devil's Plaything .... see YARROW
Devil's Ribbon .... see YELLOW TOADFLAX
Devil's Root .... see PEYOTE
Devil's Shrub .... see GINSENG, SIBERIAN
Devil's Trumpet .... see ANGEL'S TRUMPET, JIMSON WEED
Devil's Turnip .... see BRYONIA
Devil's Vine .... see GREATER BINDWEED
Devil's-bit .... see ALETRIS
Devil's-thorn .... see PUNCTURE VINE
Devil's-weed .... see PUNCTURE VINE
Dew Plant .... see SUNDEW
Dewberry .... see BLACKBERRY
Dexpanthenol .... see PANTOTHENIC ACID (VITAMIN B5)
Dexpanthenolum .... see PANTOTHENIC ACID (VITAMIN B5)
DHA (DOCOSAHEXAENOIC ACID) .... see DHA (DOCOSAHEXAENOIC ACID)
Dhanburua .... see INDIAN SNAKEROOT
Dhanyaka .... see CORIANDER
Dhar-bu .... see SEA BUCKTHORN
DHEA .... see DHEA
Di-isopropylamine Dichloroacetate .... see PANGAMIC ACID
Di Gu Pi .... see LYCIUM
DIACYLGLYCEROL .... see DIACYLGLYCEROL
Diacylglycerol Oil .... see DIACYLGLYCEROL
Dialyzable Leukocyte Extract .... see TRANSFER FACTOR
Dialyzable Transfer Factor .... see TRANSFER FACTOR
DIBENCOZIDE .... see DIBENCOZIDE
Dibutylated Hydroxytoluene .... see BHT (BUTYLATED HYDROXYTOLUENE)
Di-calcium Phosphate .... see CALCIUM
Dicentra cucullaria .... see TURKEY CORN
Dictamnus albus .... see BURNING BUSH leaf, BURNING BUSH root
Dictamnus caucasicus .... see BURNING BUSH leaf, BURNING BUSH root
Dictamnus fraxinellus .... see BURNING BUSH leaf, BURNING BUSH root
Dictamo Blanco .... see BURNING BUSH leaf
Dicylglycerol Oil .... see DIACYLGLYCEROL
Didin .... see MYRRH
Didthin .... see MYRRH
Dietary Fiber .... see BARLEY, BLACK PSYLLIUM, BLOND PSYLLIUM, GUAR GUM, LARCH ARABINOGALACTAN, OAT BRAN, OATS, RICE BRAN, WHEAT BRAN
DIGITALIS .... see DIGITALIS
Digitalis lanata .... see DIGITALIS
Digitalis purpurea .... see DIGITALIS
Diglyceride .... see DIACYLGLYCEROL
Digupi .... see LYCIUM
Dihe .... see BLUE-GREEN ALGAE
Dihydro-2(3H)-furanone .... see GAMMA BUTYROLACTONE (GBL)
Dihydro-beta-sitosterol .... see SITOSTANOL
Dihydrotachysterol .... see VITAMIN D
Dihydroxysuccinic Acid .... see ALPHA HYDROXY ACIDS
DIINDOLYLMETHANE ...... see DIINDOLYLMETHANE
Dill .... see DILL above ground parts, DILL seed
DILL above ground parts .... see DILL above ground parts
Dill Herb .... see DILL above ground parts
DILL seed .... see DILL seed
Dill Weed .... see DILL above ground parts
Dillweed .... see DILL above ground parts
Dilly .... see DILL above ground parts, DILL seed
DIM .... see DIINDOLYLMETHANE
Dimethyl Glycine .... see DIMETHYLGLYCINE
Dimethyl Sulfone .... see MSM (METHYLSULFONYLMETHANE)
Dimethyl Sulfoxide .... see DMSO (DIMETHYLSULFOXIDE)
Dimethyl Sulphoxide .... see DMSO (DIMETHYLSULFOXIDE)
Dimethylaminoethanol .... see DEANOL
Dimethylethanolamine .... see DEANOL
DIMETHYLGLYCINE .... see DIMETHYLGLYCINE
Dimethylis Sulfoxidum .... see DMSO (DIMETHYLSULFOXIDE)
Dimethylsulfone .... see MSM (METHYLSULFONYLMETHANE)
Dimethylsulfoxide .... see DMSO (DIMETHYLSULFOXIDE)
Dioscorea .... see WILD YAM
Dioscorea communis .... see BLACK BRYONY
Dioscorea composita .... see WILD YAM
Dioscorea floribunda .... see WILD YAM
Dioscorea hirticaulis .... see WILD YAM
Dioscorea macrostachya .... see WILD YAM
Dioscorea mexicana .... see WILD YAM
Dioscorea tepinapensis .... see WILD YAM
Dioscoreae .... see WILD YAM
Diosma .... see BUCHU
Diosma crenulata .... see BUCHU

INDEX

Diosma serratifolia ..... see BUCHU
Diosmetin ..... see DIOSMIN
DIOSMIN ..... see DIOSMIN
Dipsacus fullonum ..... see TEAZLE
Dipsacus sylvestris ..... see TEAZLE
Dipteryx odorata ..... see TONKA BEAN
Discorea villosa ..... see WILD YAM
Dishcloth Sponge ..... see LUFFA
Disodium Edathamil ..... see EDTA
Disodium Edetate ..... see EDTA
Disodium EDTA ..... see EDTA
Disodium Ethylenediamine Tetraacetic Acid ..... see EDTA
Disodium Tetraacetate ..... see EDTA
Dita Bark ..... see FEVER BARK
Ditch Reed ..... see REED HERB
Dittany ..... see BURNING BUSH leaf, BURNING BUSH root
Divale ..... see BELLADONNA
DIVI-DIVI ..... see DIVI-DIVI
Divine Mexican Mint ..... see DIVINER'S SAGE
Diviner's Mint ..... see DIVINER'S SAGE
DIVINER'S SAGE ..... see DIVINER'S SAGE
Divinorin ..... see DIVINER'S SAGE
Divinorin A ..... see DIVINER'S SAGE
DL-alpha-tocopherol ..... see VITAMIN E
DL-alpha-tocopheryl ..... see VITAMIN E
DL-alpha-tocopheryl acetate ..... see VITAMIN E
DL-carnitine ..... see L-CARNITINE
DL-methionine ..... see METHIONINE
DL-phenylalanine ..... see PHENYLALANINE
DL-tocopherol ..... see VITAMIN E
DLE ..... see TRANSFER FACTOR
DLPA ..... see PHENYLALANINE
DMAE ..... see DEANOL
DMG ..... see DIMETHYLGLYCINE
DMSO (DIMETHYLSULFOXIDE) ..... see DMSO (DIMETHYLSULFOXIDE)
DMSO2 ..... see MSM (METHYLSULFONYLMETHANE)
DNA ..... see RNA AND DNA
Docosahexaenoic Acid ..... see DHA (DOCOSAHEXAENOIC ACID)
Doctor Oje ..... see FICIN
DODDER ..... see DODDER
Dodder of Thyme ..... see DODDER
Dog-banana ..... see AMERICAN PAWPAW
Dog-bur ..... see HOUND'S TONGUE
Dog-tree ..... see AMERICAN DOGWOOD
Dog Fish Liver Oil ..... see SHARK LIVER OIL
Dog Grass ..... see WHEATGRASS
Dog Parsley ..... see FOOL'S PARSLEY
Dog Poison ..... see FOOL'S PARSLEY
Dog Rose ..... see ROSE HIP
Dog Standard ..... see TANSY RAGWORT
Dog Wood ..... see ALDER BUCKTHORN
Dogbane ..... see CANADIAN HEMP
Doggies ..... see YELLOW TOADFLAX
Dog's Arrach ..... see ARRACH
Dog's Tongue ..... see HOUND'S TONGUE
Dog's Tooth Violet ..... see AMERICAN ADDER'S TONGUE
Dogwood ..... see AMERICAN DOGWOOD
Dogwood Bark ..... see CASCARA
Dolichos hirsutus ..... see KUDZU
Dolichos lobatus ..... see KUDZU
Dolichos psoraloides ..... see GUAR GUM
Dolichos soja ..... see SOY, SOYBEAN OIL
Dolloff ..... see MEADOWSWEET
Doll's Eye ..... see WHITE COHOSH
DOLOMITE ..... see DOLOMITE
Dolomitic Limestone ..... see DOLOMITE
Dong Chong Xia Cao ..... see CORDYCEPS
Dong Qua ..... see DONG QUAI
DONG QUAI ..... see DONG QUAI
Dongqingzi ..... see GLOSSY PRIVET
Donnerkraut ..... see HEMP AGRIMONY
Doorweed ..... see KNOTWEED
Dope ..... see MARIJUANA
Dorstenia contrayerva ..... see CONTRAYERVA
Dostenkraut ..... see HEMP AGRIMONY, OREGANO
Dotriacontanol ..... see POLICOSANOL
Douglas Fir ..... see OREGON FIR BALSAM
Douglas Spruce ..... see OREGON FIR BALSAM
Downy Birch ..... see BIRCH
Drachenkraut ..... see HEMP AGRIMONY
Draconis resina ..... see DRAGON'S BLOOD
Dracontium ..... see SKUNK CABBAGE
Dracontium foetidum ..... see SKUNK CABBAGE
Dracorubin ..... see DRAGON'S BLOOD
Drago ..... see SANGRE DE GRADO
Dragon Root ..... see ARUM
Dragon-Bushes ..... see YELLOW TOADFLAX
DRAGON'S BLOOD ..... see DRAGON'S BLOOD
Dragon's Blood ..... see DRAGON'S BLOOD, HERB ROBERT, SANGRE DE GRADO
Dragon's-blood Palm ..... see DRAGON'S BLOOD
Dragonwort ..... see BISTORT
Drake ..... see TAUMELLOOLCH
Draksha ..... see GRAPE fruit, skin
Drimia indica ..... see SQUILL
Drimia maritima ..... see SQUILL
Drimys chilensis ..... see WINTER'S BARK
Drimys winteri ..... see WINTER'S BARK
Dromiceius novahollandiae ..... see EMU OIL
Dropberry ..... see SOLOMON'S SEAL
Dropsy Plant ..... see LEMON BALM
Dropwort ..... see MEADOWSWEET
Drosera ..... see SUNDEW
Drosera anglica ..... see SUNDEW
Drosera intermedia ..... see SUNDEW
Drosera longifolia ..... see SUNDEW
Drosera ramentacea ..... see SUNDEW
Drosera rotundifolia ..... see SUNDEW
Drudenfuss ..... see EUROPEAN MISTLETOE
Drug Centaurium ..... see CENTAURY
Drunken Sailor ..... see RED-SPUR VALERIAN
Dry Ground Cranberry ..... see ALPINE CRANBERRY
Dryopteris filix-mas ..... see MALE FERN
Duboisia myoporoides ..... see CORKWOOD TREE
Duck Liver Extract ..... see OSCILLOCOCCINUM
Duck's Foot ..... see PODOPHYLLUM
DUCKWEED ..... see DUCKWEED
Dudgeon ..... see BOXWOOD
Duffle ..... see MULLEIN
Dukong Anak ..... see CHANCA PIEDRA
Dulcarara ..... see BITTERSWEET NIGHTSHADE
Dumb Nettle ..... see WHITE DEAD NETTLE FLOWER
Dumpling Cactus ..... see PEYOTE
Dun Daisy ..... see OX-EYE DAISY

Dungkulcha .... see JIAOGULAN
Durfa Grass .... see WHEATGRASS
Durian Benggala .... see GRAVIOLA
Durmast Oak .... see OAK bark
Durri .... see BROOM CORN
DUSTY MILLER .... see DUSTY MILLER
Dutch Agrimony .... see HEMP AGRIMONY
Dutch Eupatoire Commune .... see HEMP AGRIMONY
Dutch Myrtle .... see SWEET GALE
Dutch Rushes .... see HORSETAIL
Dutch Tonka .... see TONKA BEAN
Dutchman's Breeches .... see TURKEY CORN
Dwale .... see BELLADONNA
Dwarf Bay .... see MEZEREON
Dwarf Bilberry .... see BILBERRY
Dwarf Carline .... see CARLINA
DWARF ELDER .... see DWARF ELDER
Dwarf Flax .... see MOUNTAIN FLAX
Dwarf Mallow .... see MALLOW leaf
Dwarf Marigold .... see TAGETES
DWARF PINE NEEDLE .... see DWARF PINE NEEDLE
Dwarf-pine .... see PINE
Dwayberry .... see BELLADONNA
Dyeberry .... see BILBERRY
DYER'S BROOM .... see DYER'S BROOM
Dyer's Bugloss .... see ALKANNA
Dyer's Greenwood .... see DYER'S BROOM
Dyer's Madder .... see MADDER
Dyer's Saffron .... see SAFFLOWER
Dyer's Weed .... see DYER'S BROOM
Dyer's Whin .... see DYER'S BROOM
Dyer's Woad .... see DA QING YE
Dysentery Bark .... see SIMARUBA
Dysentery Weed .... see CUDWEED
E-zhu .... see ZEDOARY
E161 .... see CANTHAXANTHIN
E967 .... see XYLITOL
Eagle-vine Bark .... see CONDURANGO
Early Fumitory .... see CORYDALIS
Early Goldenrod .... see GOLDENROD
Earlyflowering .... see PERIWINKLE
Earth-nut .... see PEANUT OIL
Earth Gall .... see AMERICAN HELLEBORE
Earth Smoke .... see FUMITORY
Earthbank .... see TORMENTIL
East India Catarrh Root .... see ALPINIA
East India Root .... see ALPINIA
East Indian Almond .... see CASHEW
East Indian Balmony .... see CHIRATA
East Indian Lemongrass .... see LEMONGRASS
East Indian Sandalwood .... see WHITE SANDALWOOD wood
East Indian Sandalwood Oil .... see WHITE SANDALWOOD OIL
Easter Flower .... see POINSETTIA, PULSATILLA
Easter Giant .... see BISTORT
Easter Mangiant .... see BISTORT
Eastern Arborvitae ... see CEDAR leaf, CEDAR LEAF OIL
Eastern Burning Bush .... see WAHOO
Eastern Fir .... see CANADA BALSAM
Eastern Hemlock .... see PINUS BARK
Eastern Mistletoe .... see AMERICAN MISTLETOE
Eastern Red Cedar .... see CEDARWOOD
Eastern White Cedar .... see CEDAR leaf, CEDAR LEAF OIL
Eberesche .... see MOUNTAIN ASH
Ebereschenbeeren .... see MOUNTAIN ASH
Eberwurz .... see CARLINA
Eburnamenine-14-carboxylic acid .... see VINPOCETINE
Ecdisten .... see ECDYSTERONE
Ecdysone .... see ECDYSTERONE
ECDYSTERONE .... see ECDYSTERONE
ECHINACEA .... see ECHINACEA
Echinacea angustifolia .... see ECHINACEA
Echinacea pallida .... see ECHINACEA
Echinacea purpurea .... see ECHINACEA
Echinaceawurzel .... see ECHINACEA
Echinopanax horridus .... see DEVIL'S CLUB
Echte Kamille .... see GERMAN CHAMOMILE
Ecorce de Quina .... see CINCHONA
Ecuadorian Sarsaparilla .... see SARSAPARILLA
Edamame .... see SOY
Edible Burdock .... see BURDOCK
EDTA .... see EDTA
EGCG .... see GREEN TEA
Egg Lecithin .... see LECITHIN
Eggs and Bacon .... see YELLOW TOADFLAX
Eggs and Collops .... see YELLOW TOADFLAX
Egyptian Alcee .... see AMBRETTE
Egyptian Privet .... see HENNA
Ehrenpreiskraut .... see VERONICA
Eichenrinde .... see OAK bark
Eicosapentaenoic Acid .... see EPA (EICOSAPENTAENOIC ACID)
Eight-horned Anise .... see STAR ANISE
Eight Horns .... see STAR ANISE
Einbeere .... see HERB PARIS
Eira-caa .... see STEVIA
Eisenkraut .... see VERBENA
Ela .... see CARDAMOM
Elder .... see ELDERBERRY
Elder Berry .... see ELDERBERRY
Elder Flower .... see AMERICAN ELDER
ELDERBERRY .... see ELDERBERRY
Elderberry .... see AMERICAN ELDER, ELDERBERRY
ELDERFLOWER .... see ELDERFLOWER
Eldrin .... see RUTIN
ELECAMPANE .... see ELECAMPANE
Elemental Copper .... see COPPER
Elemental Iron .... see IRON
ELEMI .... see ELEMI
Elemi Oleoresin .... see ELEMI
Elemi Resin .... see ELEMI
Elephant-climber .... see HAWAIIAN BABY WOODROSE
Elephant Creeper .... see HAWAIIAN BABY WOODROSE
Elephant's Gall .... see ALOE latex
Elettaria cardamomum .... see CARDAMOM
Eleuthero Ginseng .... see GINSENG, SIBERIAN
Eleutherococci Radix .... see GINSENG, SIBERIAN
Eleutherococcus .... see GINSENG, SIBERIAN
Eleutherococcus senticosus .... see GINSENG, SIBERIAN
Elfdock .... see ELECAMPANE
Elfwort .... see ELECAMPANE
Elichrysum orientale .... see SANDY EVERLASTING
Elichrysum stoechas .... see SANDY EVERLASTING
Elk Antler .... see DEER VELVET
Elk Antler Velvet .... see DEER VELVET
ELLAGIC ACID .... see ELLAGIC ACID
Ellanwood .... see ELDERBERRY, ELDERFLOWER

INDEX

Ellhorn ... see ELDERBERRY, ELDERFLOWER
ELM BARK ... see ELM BARK
Eltroot ... see GOUTWEED
Elymus repens ... see WHEATGRASS
Elytrigia repens ... see WHEATGRASS
Emblic ... see INDIAN GOOSEBERRY
Emblic myrobalan ... see INDIAN GOOSEBERRY
Emblica ... see INDIAN GOOSEBERRY
Emblica officinalis ... see INDIAN GOOSEBERRY
Emetic Herb ... see LOBELIA
Emperor ... see GRAPE fruit, skin
Emu ... see EMU OIL
EMU OIL ... see EMU OIL
Enada ... see NADH
Enchanter's Plant ... see VERBENA
Enebro ... see JUNIPER
ENGLISH ADDER'S TONGUE ... see ENGLISH ADDER'S TONGUE
English Alder ... see BLACK ALDER
English Chamomile ... see ROMAN CHAMOMILE
English Cowslip ... see COWSLIP
English Goatweed ... see GOUTWEED
English Green Valerian ... see JACOB'S LADDER
English Hawthorn ... see HAWTHORN
ENGLISH HORSEMINT ... see ENGLISH HORSEMINT
ENGLISH IVY ... see ENGLISH IVY
English Lavender ... see LAVENDER
English Mandrake ... see BRYONIA
English Morello ... see SOUR CHERRY
English Oak ... see OAK bark
English Plantain ... see BUCKHORN PLANTAIN
English Sarsaparilla ... see TORMENTIL
English Tea ... see BLACK TEA
English Tonka ... see TONKA BEAN
ENGLISH WALNUT ... see ENGLISH WALNUT
English Watercress ... see HEDGE MUSTARD
English Yew ... see YEW
Englishman's Foot ... see BLOND PSYLLIUM
Enocianina ... see GRAPE fruit, skin
EPA (EICOSAPENTAENOIC ACID) ... see EPA (EICOSAPENTAENOIC ACID)
Epazote ... see CHENOPODIUM OIL
EPHEDRA ... see EPHEDRA
Ephedra distachya ... see EPHEDRA
Ephedra equisetina ... see EPHEDRA
Ephedra gerardiana ... see EPHEDRA
Ephedra intermedia ... see EPHEDRA
Ephedra nevadensis ... see MORMON TEA
Ephedra shennungiana ... see EPHEDRA
Ephedra sinensis ... see EPHEDRA
Ephedra sinica ... see EPHEDRA
Ephedra vulgaris ... see EPHEDRA
Ephedrae Herba ... see EPHEDRA
Epigaea repens ... see TRAILING ARBUTUS
Epigallo Catechin Gallate ... see GREEN TEA
Epilobium angustifolium ... see FIREWEED
Epilobium spicatum ... see FIREWEED
EPIMEDIUM ... see EPIMEDIUM
Epimedium acuminatum ... see EPIMEDIUM
Epimedium brevicornum ... see EPIMEDIUM
Epimedium grandiflorum ... see EPIMEDIUM
Epimedium grandiflorum f. flavescens ... see EPIMEDIUM
Epimedium koreanum ... see EPIMEDIUM
Epimedium pubescens ... see EPIMEDIUM
Epimedium sagittatum ... see EPIMEDIUM
Epimedium wushanense ... see EPIMEDIUM
Epine Blanche ... see HAWTHORN
Epine de Mai ... see HAWTHORN
Epine-vinette ... see EUROPEAN BARBERRY
EPO ... see EVENING PRIMROSE OIL
Epsom Salts ... see MAGNESIUM
Equisetum ... see HORSETAIL
Equisetum arvense ... see HORSETAIL
Equisetum telmateia ... see HORSETAIL
Eranda ... see CASTOR OIL, CASTOR seed
Erandachirbhita ... see PAPAYA
Erba da Cartentieri ... see YARROW
Erba da Falegname ... see YARROW
Ergocalciferol ... see VITAMIN D
ERGOT ... see ERGOT
Erica vulgaris ... see HEATHER
Eriffe ... see CLIVERS
Erigeron canadensis ... see CANADIAN FLEABANE
Eringo ... see ERYNGO above ground parts, ERYNGO root
Eriodictyon ... see YERBA SANTA
Eriodictyon californicum ... see YERBA SANTA
Eriodictyon glutinosum ... see YERBA SANTA
Erucic Acid ... see LORENZO'S OIL
Erva Doce ... see STEVIA
Eryngii Herba ... see ERYNGO above ground parts
Eryngii Radix ... see ERYNGO root
Eryngium campestre ... see ERYNGO above ground parts, see ERYNGO root
Eryngium maritimum ... see ERYNGO above ground parts, ERYNGO root
Eryngium yuccifolium ... see ERYNGO above ground parts, ERYNGO root
Eryngo ... see ERYNGO above ground parts, ERYNGO root
ERYNGO above ground parts ... see ERYNGO above ground parts
ERYNGO root ... see ERYNGO root
Eryngo-leaved Liverwort ... see ICELAND MOSS
Erysimum ... see HEDGE MUSTARD
Erysimum cheiri ... see WALLFLOWER
Erysimum officinale ... see HEDGE MUSTARD
Erythraea centaurium ... see CENTAURY
Erythrina piscipula ... see JAMAICAN DOGWOOD
Erythronium ... see AMERICAN ADDER'S TONGUE
Erythronium americanum ... see AMERICAN ADDER'S TONGUE
Erythroxylum catuaba ... see CATUABA
Erythroxylum coca ... see COCA
Erythroxylum novogranatense ... see COCA
Eschscholzia californica ... see CALIFORNIA POPPY
Escine ... see HORSE CHESTNUT
Esere Nut ... see CALABAR BEAN
Espigon ... see PUNCTURE VINE
Espino armarillo ... see SEA BUCKTHORN
Espino cambron ... see EUROPEAN BARBERRY
Espino Falso ... see SEA BUCKTHORN
Espresso ... see COFFEE
Esrar ... see MARIJUANA
Essential Fatty Acid ... see ALPHA-LINOLENIC ACID
Estoraque Liquido ... see STORAX
Estragon ... see TARRAGON
Eternal Flower ... see IMMORTELLE, SANDY EVERLASTING

Ethanol .... see BEER, WINE
Ethyl Apovincaminate .... see VINPOCETINE
Ethyl Dihydroxypropyl Aminobenzoate .... see PARA-AMINOBENZOIC ACID (PABA)
Ethyl Eicosapentaenoic Acid .... see EPA (EICOSAPENTAENOIC ACID)
Ethyl Ester .... see VINPOCETINE
Ethylapovincaminoate .... see VINPOCETINE
Ethylenediamine Tetraacetic Acid .... see EDTA
Eucalypti Folium .... see EUCALYPTUS dried leaf
Eucalyptus .... see EUCALYPTUS dried leaf
Eucalyptus bicostata .... see EUCALYPTUS dried leaf, EUCALYPTUS OIL
EUCALYPTUS dried leaf .... see EUCALYPTUS dried leaf
Eucalyptus fruticetorum .... see EUCALYPTUS dried leaf, EUCALYPTUS OIL
Eucalyptus globulus .... see EUCALYPTUS dried leaf, EUCALYPTUS OIL
Eucalyptus odorata .... see EUCALYPTUS dried leaf, EUCALYPTUS OIL
EUCALYPTUS OIL .... see EUCALYPTUS OIL
Eucalyptus polybractea .... see EUCALYPTUS dried leaf, EUCALYPTUS OIL
Eucalyptus smithii .... see EUCALYPTUS dried leaf, EUCALYPTUS OIL
Eucalyptusblatter .... see EUCALYPTUS dried leaf
Euchema sp. .... see CARRAGEENAN
Eugenia aromatica .... see CLOVE dried flowerbud, leaf, stem; CLOVE OIL
Eugenia caryophyllata .... see CLOVE dried flowerbud, leaf, stem; CLOVE OIL
Eugenia caryophyllus .... see CLOVE dried flowerbud, leaf, stem; CLOVE OIL
Eugenia chequen .... see CHEKEN
Eugenia cumini .... see JAMBOLAN bark, JAMBOLAN seed
Eugenia jambolana .... see JAMBOLAN bark, JAMBOLAN seed
Eugenia pimenta .... see ALLSPICE
Euonymus atropurpureus .... see WAHOO
Eupatoriadelphus purpureus .... see GRAVEL ROOT
Eupatorium .... see HEMP AGRIMONY
Eupatorium cannabinum .... see HEMP AGRIMONY
Eupatorium perfoliatum .... see BONESET
Eupatorium purpureum .... see GRAVEL ROOT
Eupatorium rebaudianum .... see STEVIA
EUPHORBIA .... see EUPHORBIA
Euphorbia capitulata .... see EUPHORBIA
Euphorbia cyparissias .... see CYPRESS SPURGE
Euphorbia hirta .... see EUPHORBIA
Euphorbia pilulifera .... see EUPHORBIA
Euphorbia poinsettia .... see POINSETTIA
Euphorbia pulcherrima .... see POINSETTIA
Euphraisia Eye Bright .... see EYEBRIGHT
Euphrasia officinalis .... see EYEBRIGHT
Euphrasiae Herba .... see EYEBRIGHT
Eurixor .... see EUROPEAN MISTLETOE
European Alder .... see BLACK ALDER, ELDERBERRY, ELDERFLOWER
European Angelica .... see ANGELICA root
European Ash .... see ASH
European Aspen .... see ASPEN
European Aspidium .... see MALE FERN
EUROPEAN BARBERRY .... see EUROPEAN BARBERRY
European Beaver .... see CASTOREUM
European Bitter Polygala .... see BITTER MILKWORT
European Black Alder .... see BLACK ALDER
European Black Currant .... see BLACK CURRANT
EUROPEAN BUCKTHORN .... see EUROPEAN BUCKTHORN
EUROPEAN CHESTNUT .... see EUROPEAN CHESTNUT
European Cranberry-bush .... see CRAMP BARK
European Cranberry .... see CRANBERRY
European Dill .... see DILL above ground parts, DILL seed
European Elder Flower .... see ELDERFLOWER
European Elder Fruit .... see ELDERBERRY
European Elderberry .... see ELDERBERRY
European Filbert .... see HAZELNUT
EUROPEAN FIVE-FINGER GRASS .... see EUROPEAN FIVE-FINGER GRASS
European Goldenrod .... see GOLDENROD
European Hazel .... see HAZELNUT
European Hellebore .... see WHITE HELLEBORE
European Hops .... see HOPS
European Linden .... see LINDEN CHARCOAL, LINDEN dried flower, LINDEN dried leaf, LINDEN dried sapwood
EUROPEAN MANDRAKE .... see EUROPEAN MANDRAKE
EUROPEAN MISTLETOE .... see EUROPEAN MISTLETOE
European Mountain-ash .... see MOUNTAIN ASH
European Mullein .... see MULLEIN
European Oregano .... see OREGANO
European Pasqueflower .... see PULSATILLA
European Pennyroyal .... see PENNYROYAL leaf, PENNYROYAL OIL
European Peony .... see PEONY flower, PEONY root
European Ragwort .... see TANSY RAGWORT
European Sanicle .... see SANICLE
European Senega .... see BITTER MILKWORT
European Squill .... see SQUILL
European Vervain .... see VERBENA
European Water Hemlock .... see WATER HEMLOCK
European White Hellebore .... see WHITE HELLEBORE
European Wild Pansy .... see HEART'S EASE
Eurphrasia rostkoviana .... see EYEBRIGHT
EVENING PRIMROSE OIL .... see EVENING PRIMROSE OIL
Evening Trumpet Flower .... see GELSEMIUM
Evergreen .... see PERIWINKLE
Evergreen Snakeroot .... see BITTER MILKWORT
Everlasting .... see CUDWEED, SANDY EVERLASTING
Everlasting Friendship .... see CLIVERS
Everlasting Pea .... see LATHYRUS
Evernia prunastri .... see OAK MOSS
Eve's Cups .... see PITCHER PLANT
Ewe Daisy .... see TORMENTIL
Exogonium purga .... see JALAP
Expressed Almond Oil .... see SWEET ALMOND
Expressed Grapefruit Oil .... see GRAPEFRUIT OIL
Extrait de Pepins de Raisin .... see GRAPE seed
Exwort .... see BUTTERBUR
Eye Balm .... see GOLDENSEAL
Eye Bright .... see EYEBRIGHT
Eye Root .... see GOLDENSEAL
EYEBRIGHT .... see EYEBRIGHT

Eyebright .... see EYEBRIGHT, CLARY SAGE
Eyrnigium planum .... see ERYNGO above ground parts, ERYNGO root
F .... see FLUORIDE
Fa-tha-lai-jone .... see ANDROGRAPHIS
Faba calabarica .... see CALABAR BEAN
Faex medicinalis .... see BREWER'S YEAST
Fagopyrum esculentum .... see BUCKWHEAT
Fagopyrum sagittatum .... see BUCKWHEAT
Fagopyrum tataricum .... see BUCKWHEAT
Fagopyrum vulgare .... see BUCKWHEAT
Fagus castanea .... see EUROPEAN CHESTNUT
Fagus procera .... see EUROPEAN CHESTNUT
Fairy Bells .... see WOOD SORREL
Fairy Cap .... see DIGITALIS
Fairy Caps .... see COWSLIP
Fairy Finger .... see DIGITALIS
Fairy Flax .... see MOUNTAIN FLAX
Fairy Herb .... see JIAOGULAN
Fairywand .... see FALSE UNICORN
Fake Saffron .... see SAFFLOWER
Fall Crocus .... see AUTUMN CROCUS
False Bittersweet .... see AMERICAN BITTERSWEET
False Box .... see AMERICAN DOGWOOD
False Cinnamon .... see CASSIA CINNAMON
False Coltsfoot .... see ASARABACCA
False Grapes .... see AMERICAN IVY
False Hellebore .... see AMERICAN HELLEBORE, PHEASANT'S EYE
False Indigo .... see WILD INDIGO
False Jacob's Ladder .... see ABSCESS ROOT
False Jasmine .... see GELSEMIUM
False Pareira .... see ABUTA
False Parsley .... see WATER HEMLOCK
False Saffron .... see SAFFLOWER
FALSE UNICORN .... see FALSE UNICORN
False Valerian .... see GOLDEN RAGWORT
Farberrote .... see MADDER
Farberwaid .... see DA QING YE
Farfarae Folium Leaf .... see COLTSFOOT
Farmer's Lily .... see WHITE LILY
Fatsia .... see DEVIL'S CLUB
Fatsia horrida .... see DEVIL'S CLUB
Fe .... see IRON
Featerfoiul .... see FEVERFEW
Featherfew .... see FEVERFEW
Featherfoil .... see FEVERFEW
Feigen .... see FIG
Feijao Macaco .... see COWHAGE
Feldkamille .... see GERMAN CHAMOMILE
Fellen .... see BITTERSWEET NIGHTSHADE
Fellonwood .... see BITTERSWEET NIGHTSHADE
Felon Herb .... see MUGWORT
Felonwort .... see BITTERSWEET NIGHTSHADE
Feltwort .... see MULLEIN
Female Regulator .... see GOLDEN RAGWORT
Fen Ke .... see KUDZU
Fenge .... see KUDZU
Fennel .... see FENNEL fruit, seed; FENNEL OIL
Fennel Flower .... see BLACK SEED
FENNEL fruit, seed .... see FENNEL fruit, seed
FENNEL OIL .... see FENNEL OIL
FENUGREEK .... see FENUGREEK
Fer .... see IRON
Fermented Dairy Product .... see KEFIR
Fermented Genistein .... see GENISTEIN COMBINED POLYSACCHARIDE
Fermented Isoflavone .... see GENISTEIN COMBINED POLYSACCHARIDE
Fermented Milk .... see KEFIR
Fermented Soybeans .... see NATTOKINASE
Ferrous Carbonate Anhydrous .... see IRON
Ferrous Fumarate .... see IRON
Ferrous Gluconate .... see IRON
Ferrous Pyrophosphate .... see IRON
Ferrous Sulfate .... see IRON
Ferrula .... see SUMBUL
Ferula Assa-foetida .... see ASAFOETIDA
Ferula foetida .... see ASAFOETIDA
Ferula galbaniflua .... see GALBANUM
Ferula gummosa .... see GALBANUM
Ferula pseudalliacea .... see ASAFOETIDA
Ferula rubricaulis .... see ASAFOETIDA
Ferula sumbul .... see SUMBUL
Fetid Nightshade .... see HENBANE
Feuille de Luzerne .... see ALFALFA
Feuilles d'Alchemille .... see ALCHEMILLA
Feuilles la Fievre .... see CHANCA PIEDRA
FEVER BARK .... see FEVER BARK
Fever Grass .... see LEMONGRASS
Fever Plant .... see EVENING PRIMROSE OIL
Fever Root .... see CORAL ROOT, WATER HEMLOCK
Fever Tree .... see EUCALYPTUS dried leaf
Fever Twig .... see BITTERSWEET NIGHTSHADE
FEVERFEW .... see FEVERFEW
Fevertree .... see EUCALYPTUS dried leaf
Feverwort .... see BONESET
Ficaria .... see LESSER CELANDINE
Fichtennadelöl .... see FIR NEEDLE OIL
FICIN .... see FICIN
Ficus anthelminthica .... see FICIN
Ficus carica .... see FIG
Ficus glabrata .... see FICIN
Ficus insipida .... see FICIN
Fiddlehead Fern .... see OSTRICH FERN
Fieberbaumblatter .... see EUCALYPTUS dried leaf
Fieberrinde .... see CINCHONA
Field Balm .... see CATNIP
Field Horsetail .... see HORSETAIL
Field Lady's Mantle .... see PARSLEY PIERT
Field Melilot .... see SWEET CLOVER
Field Mint Oil .... see JAPANESE MINT
Field Pansy .... see HEART'S EASE
Field Pumpkin .... see PUMPKIN
FIELD SCABIOUS .... see FIELD SCABIOUS
Field Scorpion Grass .... see FORGET-ME-NOT
Field Seven .... see PANAX PSEUDOGINSENG
Field Sorrel .... see YELLOW DOCK
Fieldhove .... see COLTSFOOT
FIG .... see FIG
FIGWORT .... see FIGWORT
Figwort .... see FIGWORT, LESSER CELANDINE
Filaginella uliginosa .... see CUDWEED
Filipendula .... see MEADOWSWEET
Filipendula ulmaria .... see MEADOWSWEET
Filuis Ante Patrem .... see COLTSFOOT
Finbar .... see SEA BUCKTHORN
Finnochio .... see FENNEL fruit, seed

INDEX

FIR .... see FIR
FIR NEEDLE OIL .... see FIR NEEDLE OIL
Fir Tree .... see FIR, HEMLOCK SPRUCE
FIREWEED .... see FIREWEED
Fish Berries .... see LEVANT BERRY
Fish Killer .... see LEVANT BERRY
Fish Mint .... see SPEARMINT
Fish Oil .... see COD LIVER OIL
Fish Oil Fatty Acid .... see DHA (DOCOSAHEXAENOIC ACID), EPA (EICOSAPENTAENOIC ACID)
FISH OILS .... see FISH OILS
Fish Poison Bark .... see JAMAICAN DOGWOOD
Fish Wood .... see WAHOO
Fishfudle .... see JAMAICAN DOGWOOD
Fish-poison Tree .... see JAMAICAN DOGWOOD
Fitch .... see BLACK SEED
Fitolaca .... see POKEWEED berry, POKEWEED root
Five-finger Blossom .... see EUROPEAN FIVE-FINGER GRASS
Five-finger Fern .... see MAIDENHAIR FERN
Five-fingered Root .... see HEMLOCK WATER DROPWORT
Five-flavor-fruit .... see SCHISANDRA
Five-flavor-seed .... see SCHISANDRA
Five Fingers .... see EUROPEAN FIVE-FINGER GRASS
Five Leaves .... see AMERICAN IVY
Fixed Almond Oil .... see SWEET ALMOND
FL-113 .... see IPRIFLAVONE
Flag Lily .... see ORRIS
Flaggon .... see ORRIS
Flagroot .... see CALAMUS
Flake Manna .... see MANNA
Flame Seedless .... see GRAPE fruit, skin
Flannelflower .... see MULLEIN
Flapperdock .... see BUTTERBUR
Flat-podded Vetch .... see LATHYRUS
Flavin .... see RIBOFLAVIN (VITAMIN B2)
Flavine .... see RIBOFLAVIN (VITAMIN B2)
Flavone X .... see CHRYSIN
Flavonoid .... see CHRYSIN, DIOSMIN, HESPERIDIN, QUERCETIN, RUTIN, METHOXYLATED FLAVONES
Flax .... see SENEGA
Flax Oil .... see FLAXSEED OIL
Flax Seed .... see FLAXSEED
Flax Seed Oil .... see FLAXSEED OIL
Flax Weed .... see RUPTUREWORT
FLAXSEED .... see FLAXSEED
FLAXSEED OIL .... see FLAXSEED OIL
Flaxweed .... see YELLOW TOADFLAX
Flea Wort .... see CANADIAN FLEABANE
Fleaseed .... see BLACK PSYLLIUM
Fleawort .... see BLACK PSYLLIUM
Fleischfarbige .... see PASSIONFLOWER
Flesh and Blood .... see TORMENTIL
Fleur de Camomile .... see GERMAN CHAMOMILE
Fleur de Camomille Romaine .... see ROMAN CHAMOMILE
Fleur de la Passion .... see PASSIONFLOWER
Fleur de Pied de Chat .... see SANDY EVERLASTING
Fleurs d'Arnica .... see ARNICA
Fliggers .... see ORRIS
Flirtwort Midsummer Daisy .... see FEVERFEW
Flor de Passion .... see PASSIONFLOWER
Florence Fennel .... see FENNEL fruit, seed
Florentine Iris .... see ORRIS
Flores Anthemidis .... see ROMAN CHAMOMILE
Flores Caryophylli .... see CLOVE OIL
Flores Caryophyllum .... see CLOVE dried flowerbud, leaf, stem
Florist's Chrysanthemum .... see CHRYSANTHEMUM
Flos Magnoliae .... see MAGNOLIA
Flower Velure .... see COLTSFOOT
Flowering Ammi .... see BISHOP'S WEED
Flowering Ash .... see MANNA
Flowering Sally .... see PURPLE LOOSESTRIFE
Flowering Willow .... see FIREWEED
Flowering Wintergreen .... see BITTER MILKWORT
Flowery Knotweed .... see FO-TI
Fluelli .... see YELLOW TOADFLAX
Fluffweed .... see MULLEIN
FLUORIDE .... see FLUORIDE
Fluorophosphate .... see FLUORIDE
Flux Root .... see PLEURISY ROOT
Fly-catcher .... see PITCHER PLANT
Fly-trap .... see CANADIAN HEMP, PITCHER PLANT
Fly Agaric .... see AGA
FO-TI .... see FO-TI
Fo-ti-tient .... see FO-TI
Foal's Foot .... see COLTSFOOT
Foalswort .... see COLTSFOOT
Foam Flower .... see COOLWORT
Fodder Beet .... see BEET
Foeniculi antheroleum .... see FENNEL OIL
Foeniculum capillaceum .... see FENNEL fruit, seed; FENNEL OIL
Foeniculum officinale .... see FENNEL fruit, seed; FENNEL OIL
Foeniculum piperitum .... see FENNEL fruit, seed; FENNEL OIL
Foeniculum vulgare .... see FENNEL fruit, seed; FENNEL OIL
Foenugraeci Semen .... see FENUGREEK
Foenugreek .... see FENUGREEK
Folacin .... see FOLIC ACID
Folate .... see FOLIC ACID
Folia Vitis Viniferae .... see GRAPE leaf
FOLIC ACID .... see FOLIC ACID
Food of the Gods .... see ASAFOETIDA
Fool's-cicely .... see FOOL'S PARSLEY
FOOL'S PARSLEY .... see FOOL'S PARSLEY
Forest Mushroom .... see SHIITAKE MUSHROOM
FORGET-ME-NOT .... see FORGET-ME-NOT
Forskohlii .... see FORSKOLIN
FORSKOLIN .... see FORSKOLIN
FOS .... see FRUCTO-OLIGOSACCHARIDES
Fossil Tree .... see GINKGO leaf (GINKGO leaf extract), GINKGO seed
Foti .... see FO-TI
Foxberry .... see ALPINE CRANBERRY
Foxglove .... see DIGITALIS
Fox's-brush .... see RED-SPUR VALERIAN
Fox's Clote .... see BURDOCK
Fragaria collina .... see STRAWBERRY
Fragaria insularis potentilla vesca .... see STRAWBERRY
Fragaria vesca .... see STRAWBERRY
Fragaria virginiana .... see STRAWBERRY

Fragaria viridis ... see STRAWBERRY
Fragariae Folium ... see STRAWBERRY
Fragrant Agrimony ... see AGRIMONY
Fragrant Sumac ... see SWEET SUMACH
Fragrant Valerian ... see VALERIAN
Framboise ... see RASPBERRY leaf
Frangula ... see ALDER BUCKTHORN
Frangula alnus ... see ALDER BUCKTHORN
Frangula purshiana ... see CASCARA
Frangulae Cortex ... see ALDER BUCKTHORN
FRANKINCENSE ... see FRANKINCENSE
Frauenmantelkraut ... see ALCHEMILLA
Fraxinella ... see BURNING BUSH leaf, BURNING BUSH root
Fraxinus americana ... see ASH
Fraxinus excelsior ... see ASH
Fraxinus ornus ... see MANNA
Free Base Glycine ... see GLYCINE
French Honeysuckle ... see GOAT'S RUE
French Lavender ... see LAVENDER
French Lilac ... see GOAT'S RUE
French Marigold ... see TAGETES
French Marine Pine Bark Extract ... see PYCNOGENOL
French Maritime Pine Bark Extract ... see PYCNOGENOL
French Psyllium ... see BLACK PSYLLIUM
French Thyme ... see THYME flower, leaf
French Willow ... see FIREWEED
Freshwater Green Algae ... see CHLORELLA
Freshwater Seaweed ... see CHLORELLA
Friar's Cowl ... see ARUM
Frijol de Soya ... see SOY
Fringe Tree ... see FRINGETREE
FRINGETREE ... see FRINGETREE
Frogsfoot ... see BULBOUS BUTTERCUP
Frogwort ... see BULBOUS BUTTERCUP
Frost Plant ... see FROSTWORT
Frostweed ... see FROSTWORT
FROSTWORT ... see FROSTWORT
Fructooligosaccarides ... see FRUCTO-OLIGOSACCHARIDES, INULIN
FRUCTO-OLIGOSACCHARIDES ... see FRUCTO-OLIGOSACCHARIDES
Fructo-oligosaccarides ... see FRUCTO-OLIGOSACCHARIDES, INULIN
Fructus Cortex ... see ENGLISH WALNUT
Fructus Lycii ... see LYCIUM
Fructus Lycii Berry ... see LYCIUM
Fructus Rosae Laevigatae ... see CHEROKEE ROSEHIP
Fruit de Celeri ... see CELERY
Fruits de Khella ... see KHELLA
Fu Ling ... see PORIA MUSHROOM
Fucostanol ... see SITOSTANOL
Fucus ... see BLADDERWRACK
Fucus vesiculosus ... see BLADDERWRACK
Fuga daemonum ... see ST. JOHN'S WORT
Fum ... see ASAFOETIDA
Fumaria officinalis ... see FUMITORY
Fumiterry ... see FUMITORY
FUMITORY ... see FUMITORY
Fumus ... see FUMITORY
Funffing ... see AGRIMONY
Funffingerkraut ... see AGRIMONY
Fungus japonicus ... see KOMBUCHA TEA
Furze ... see DYER'S BROOM
Fusanum ... see WAHOO
FuShen ... see PORIA MUSHROOM
Fusoria ... see WAHOO
Fytic Acid ... see IP-6
G Salt ... see GLYCINE
G6S ... see GLUCOSAMINE SULFATE
GABA (GAMMA-AMINOBUTYRIC ACID) ... see GABA (GAMMA-AMINOBUTYRIC ACID)
Gadrose ... see WAHOO
GAG ... see CHONDROITIN SULFATE
Gaga ... see MARIJUANA
Gaglee ... see ARUM
Gagroot ... see LOBELIA
Galactosaminoglucuronoglycan Sulfate ... see CHONDROITIN SULFATE
Galanga ... see ALPINIA
Galangal ... see ALPINIA
Galangal Root ... see ALPINIA
Galangin Flavanone ... see CHRYSIN
GALBANUM ... see GALBANUM
Galbanum Gum ... see GALBANUM
Galbanum Gum Resin ... see GALBANUM
Galbanum Oleogum Resin ... see GALBANUM
Galbanum Oleoresin ... see GALBANUM
Galbanum Resin ... see GALBANUM
Galega bicolor ... see GOAT'S RUE
Galega officinalis ... see GOAT'S RUE
Galega patula ... see GOAT'S RUE
Galegae Officinalis Herba ... see GOAT'S RUE
Galeopsidis Herba ... see HEMPNETTLE
Galeopsis ochroleuca ... see HEMPNETTLE
Galeopsis segetum ... see HEMPNETTLE
Galgant ... see ALPINIA
Galii Odorati Herba ... see SWEET WOODRUFF
Galipea officinalis ... see ANGOSTURA
Galium aparine ... see CLIVERS
Galium odorata ... see SWEET WOODRUFF
Galium verum ... see LADY'S BEDSTRAW
Gall Weed ... see GENTIAN
Gallium ... see CLIVERS
Gallwort ... see YELLOW TOADFLAX
Gambierdiscus toxicus (dinoflagellate) ... see CIGUATERA
Gambodia ... see GAMBOGE
GAMBOGE ... see GAMBOGE
Gamma Amino Butyric Acid ... see GABA (GAMMA-AMINOBUTYRIC ACID)
GAMMA BUTYROLACTONE (GBL) ... see GAMMA BUTYROLACTONE (GBL)
Gamma Hydrate ... see GAMMA-HYDROXYBUTYRATE (GHB)
Gamma Hydroxybutyrate Sodium ... see GAMMA-HYDROXYBUTYRATE (GHB)
Gamma Hydroxybutyric Acid ... see GAMMA-HYDROXYBUTYRATE (GHB)
Gamma Hydroxybutyric Acid Lactone ... see GAMMA BUTYROLACTONE (GBL)
GAMMA LINOLENIC ACID ... see GAMMA LINOLENIC ACID
Gamma Linolenic Acid (GLA) ... see EVENING PRIMROSE OIL, GAMMA LINOLENIC ACID
GAMMA ORYZANOL ... see GAMMA ORYZANOL
Gamma Tocotrienol ... see VITAMIN E
Gamma-aminobutyric acid ... see GABA (GAMMA-AMINOBUTYRIC ACID)

INDEX

Gamma-alutamylcysteinylglycine ...... see GLUTATHIONE
Gamma-glutamylethylamide ...... see THEANINE
GAMMA-HYDROXYBUTYRATE (GHB) ...... see GAMMA-HYDROXYBUTYRATE (GHB)
Gamma-L-glutamyl-L-cysteinylglycine ...... see GLUTATHIONE
Gamma-OH ...... see GAMMA-HYDROXYBUTYRATE (GHB)
Gamma-OZ ...... see GAMMA ORYZANOL
Gamma-tocopherol ...... see VITAMIN E
Gamma-trimethyl-beta-acetylbutyrobetaine ...... see ACETYL-L-CARNITINE
Gamolenic Acid ...... see GAMMA LINOLENIC ACID
Gan Cao ...... see LICORICE
Gan Zao ...... see LICORICE
Gandana ...... see YARROW
Gandapura ...... see AMBRETTE
Gandharva Hasta ...... see CASTOR OIL, CASTOR seed
Ganga ...... see MARIJUANA
Gange ...... see KUDZU
Ganoderma lucidum ...... see REISHI MUSHROOM
Gao Liang ...... see ALPINIA
Garacilaria confervoides ...... see AGAR
Garance ...... see MADDER
GARCINIA ...... see GARCINIA
Garcinia cambogia ...... see GARCINIA
Garcinia gummi-guta ...... see GARCINIA
Garcinia hanburyi ...... see GAMBOGE
Garcinia mangostana ...... see MANGOSTEEN
Garden Angelica ...... see ANGELICA root
Garden Artichoke ...... see ARTICHOKE
Garden Asparagus ...... see ASPARAGUS
Garden Balsam ...... see JEWELWEED
Garden Basil ...... see BASIL
Garden Beet ...... see BEET
Garden Burnet ...... see GREATER BURNET
Garden Chamomile ...... see ROMAN CHAMOMILE
Garden Chervil ...... see CHERVIL
GARDEN CRESS ...... see GARDEN CRESS
Garden Fennel ...... see FENNEL fruit, seed
Garden Fern ...... see OSTRICH FERN
Garden Heliotrope ...... see VALERIAN
Garden Lavender ...... see LAVENDER
Garden Marigold ...... see CALENDULA
Garden Marjoram ...... see MARJORAM
Garden Mint ...... see SPEARMINT
Garden Nightshade ...... see BLACK NIGHTSHADE
Garden Parsley ...... see PARSLEY leaf, root; PARSLEY seed
Garden Pepper ...... see CAPSICUM
Garden Rhubarb ...... see RHUBARB
Garden Rue ...... see RUE
Garden Sage ...... see SAGE
Garden Sorrel ...... see SORREL
Garden Thyme ...... see THYME flower, leaf
Garden Valerian ...... see VALERIAN
GARDEN VIOLET ...... see GARDEN VIOLET
Garden Violet .... see GARDEN VIOLET, SWEET VIOLET
Gardenin D ...... see METHOXYLATED FLAVONES
Gargaut ...... see ALPINIA
Garget ...... see POKEWEED berry, POKEWEED root
Garijara ...... see WILD CARROT
GARLIC ...... see GARLIC
Garlic Clove ...... see GARLIC
Garlic Sage ...... see WOOD SAGE
Gartenmajoran ...... see MARJORAM
Gas Black ...... see ACTIVATED CHARCOAL
Gas Plant ...... see BURNING BUSH leaf, BURNING BUSH root
Gat ...... see KHAT
Gatten ...... see WAHOO
Gatter ...... see WAHOO
Gattilier ...... see CHASTEBERRY
Gaultheria Oil ...... see WINTERGREEN OIL
Gaultheria procumbens ...... see WINTERGREEN leaf, WINTERGREEN OIL
Gay-feather ...... see MARSH BLAZING STAR
Gayfeather ...... see MARSH BLAZING STAR
GBL ...... see GAMMA BUTYROLACTONE (GBL)
GCP ...... see GENISTEIN COMBINED POLYSACCHARIDE
Ge ...... see GERMANIUM
Ge Gen ...... see KUDZU
Ge-132 ...... see GERMANIUM
Ge-Oxy 132 ...... see GERMANIUM
Gea ...... see KAVA
Gegen ...... see KUDZU
Geissrautenkraut ...... see GOAT'S RUE
GELATIN ...... see GELATIN
Gelatine ...... see GELATIN
Gelidiella acerosa ...... see AGAR
Gelidium amanasii ...... see AGAR
Gelidium cartilagineum ...... see AGAR
Gelidium crinale ...... see AGAR
Gelidium divaricatum ...... see AGAR
Gelidium pacificum ...... see AGAR
Gelidium vagum ...... see AGAR
Gelosa ...... see AGAR
Gelsemii Rhizoma ...... see GELSEMIUM
Gelsemin ...... see GELSEMIUM
GELSEMIUM ...... see GELSEMIUM
Gelsemium nitidum ...... see GELSEMIUM
Gelsemium sempervirens ...... see GELSEMIUM
Gelsemiumwurzelstock Jessamine ...... see GELSEMIUM
Gemeine Schafgarbe ...... see YARROW
Gemeiner Beifuss ...... see MUGWORT
Gemeiner Wasswedost ...... see HEMP AGRIMONY
Gemnema melicida ...... see GYMNEMA
Gemuseartischocke ...... see ARTICHOKE
General Plantain ...... see GREAT PLANTAIN
Genet ...... see SPANISH BROOM
Genet a Balais ...... see SCOTCH BROOM flower
Genievre ...... see JUNIPER
Genista andreana ...... see SCOTCH BROOM flower, SCOTCH BROOM herb
Genista juncea ...... see SPANISH BROOM
Genista tinctoria ...... see DYER'S BROOM
Genistein ...... see RED CLOVER, SOY
GENISTEIN COMBINED POLYSACCHARIDE ...... see GENISTEIN COMBINED POLYSACCHARIDE
Genistein Polysaccharide ...... see GENISTEIN COMBINED POLYSACCHARIDE
GENTIAN ...... see GENTIAN
Gentiana ...... see GENTIAN
Gentiana acaulis ...... see GENTIAN
Gentiana chirata ...... see CHIRATA
Gentiana chirayita ...... see CHIRATA
Gentiana kochiana ...... see GENTIAN

INDEX

Gentiana lutea ... see GENTIAN
Gentianae Radix ... see GENTIAN
Geranium robertianum ... see HERB ROBERT
GERMAN CHAMOMILE ... see GERMAN CHAMOMILE
GERMAN IPECAC ... see GERMAN IPECAC
German Lactucarium ... see WILD LETTUCE
German Rue ... see RUE
GERMAN SARSAPARILLA ... see GERMAN SARSAPARILLA
GERMANDER ... see GERMANDER
GERMANIUM ... see GERMANIUM
Germanium Lactate Citrate ... see GERMANIUM
Gero-vita ... see PROCAINE
Gerovital ... see PROCAINE
Gerovital-H3 ... see PROCAINE
Geum ... see AVENS
Geum rivale ... see WATER AVENS
Geum urbanum ... see AVENS
Gewurznelken Nagelein ... see CLOVE dried flowerbud, leaf, stem; CLOVE OIL
GH-3 ... see PROCAINE
GHB ... see GAMMA-HYDROXYBUTYRATE (GHB)
Ghoda Asoda ... see ASHWAGANDHA
Ghrita-kumari ... see ALOE gel, ALOE latex
Gi ... see KAVA
Giant Fennel ... see ASAFOETIDA
Giant Reed ... see REED HERB
Grifolan (GRN) ... see BETA GLUCANS
Gigartina mamillosa ... see CARRAGEENAN
Gillenia ... see INDIAN PHYSIC
Gillenia trifoliata ... see INDIAN PHYSIC
Gill-go-by-the-hedge ... see GROUND IVY
Gill-go-over-the-ground ... see GROUND IVY
Gillyflower ... see WALLFLOWER
Ginepro ... see JUNIPER
Gingembre ... see GINGER
GINGER ... see GINGER
Ginger Root ... see GINGER
Ginjeira ... see SOUR CHERRY
Ginkgo ... see GINKGO leaf (GINKGO leaf extract), GINKGO seed
Ginkgo Biloba ... see GINKGO leaf (GINKGO leaf extract), GINKGO seed
Ginkgo Folium ... see GINKGO leaf (GINKGO leaf extract)
GINKGO leaf (GINKGO leaf extract) ... see GINKGO leaf (GINKGO leaf extract)
GINKGO seed ... see GINKGO seed
Ginseng ... see GINSENG, AMERICAN; GINSENG, PANAX; GINSENG, SIBERIAN
Ginseng Asiatique ... see GINSENG, PANAX
Ginseng Radix ... see GINSENG, PANAX
Ginseng Root ... see GINSENG, AMERICAN; GINSENG, PANAX; GINSENG, SIBERIAN
GINSENG, AMERICAN ... see GINSENG, AMERICAN
GINSENG, PANAX ... see GINSENG, PANAX
GINSENG, SIBERIAN ... see GINSENG, SIBERIAN
Ginsterkraut ... see SCOTCH BROOM flower
Giroflier ... see WALLFLOWER
GL701 ... see DHEA
GLA ... see GAMMA LINOLENIC ACID
Gladdon ... see CALAMUS
Gladyne ... see ORRIS
Glandular ... see ADRENAL EXTRACT
Glechoma hederacea ... see GROUND IVY
Glicerol ... see GLYCEROL
GLN ... see GLUTAMINE
Globe Amaranth ... see BUTTERCUP
Globe Artichoke ... see ARTICHOKE
Globe Crowfoot ... see GLOBE FLOWER
GLOBE FLOWER ... see GLOBE FLOWER
Globe Ranunculus ... see GLOBE FLOWER
Globe Trollius ... see GLOBE FLOWER
Glockenbilsenkraut ... see SCOPOLIA
Glossy Buckthorn ... see ALDER BUCKTHORN
GLOSSY PRIVET ... see GLOSSY PRIVET
Glucerite ... see GLYCEROL
GLUCOMANNAN ... see GLUCOMANNAN
Gluconolactone ... see ALPHA HYDROXY ACIDS
Glucosamine ... see GLUCOSAMINE SULFATE
Glucosamine HCl ... see GLUCOSAMINE HYDROCHLORIDE
GLUCOSAMINE HYDROCHLORIDE ... see GLUCOSAMINE HYDROCHLORIDE
Glucosamine N-acetyl ... see N-ACETYL GLUCOSAMINE
GLUCOSAMINE SULFATE ... see GLUCOSAMINE SULFATE
Glucosamine Sulphate ... see GLUCOSAMINE SULFATE
Glucose Tolerance Factor ... see CHROMIUM
Glucose Tolerance Factor-Cr ... see CHROMIUM
Glucose-6-phosphate ... see GLUCOSAMINE HYDROCHLORIDE, GLUCOSAMINE SULFATE
Glucose-6-sulfate ... see GLUCOSAMINE SULFATE
Glucose-6-sulphate ... see GLUCOSAMINE SULFATE
Glutamate ... see GLUTAMINE
Glutamic Acid ... see GLUTAMINE
Glutaminate ... see GLUTAMINE
GLUTAMINE ... see GLUTAMINE
GLUTATHIONE ... see GLUTATHIONE
Glycerin ... see GLYCEROL
GLYCEROL ... see GLYCEROL
Glycerol Trierucate Oil ... see LORENZO'S OIL
Glycerol Trioleate Oil ... see LORENZO'S OIL
Glycerolum ... see GLYCEROL
Glycerophosphorylcholine ... see ALPHA-GPC
Glyceryl Alcohol ... see GLYCEROL
Glyceryl Paraaminobenzoate ... see PARA-AMINOBENZOIC ACID (PABA)
GLYCINE ... see GLYCINE
Glycine abrus ... see PRECATORY BEAN
Glycine gracilis ... see SOY, SOYBEAN OIL
Glycine hispida ... see SOY, SOYBEAN OIL
Glycine max ... see SOY, SOYBEAN OIL
Glycine soja ... see SOY, SOYBEAN OIL
Glycoaminoglycan ... see HYALURONIC ACID
Glycocoll ... see GLYCINE
Glycolic Acid ... see ALPHA HYDROXY ACIDS
Glycosaminoglycan Polysulphuric Acid Complex ... see BOVINE CARTILAGE
Glycosaminoglycans ... see MESOGLYCAN
Glycosthene ... see GLYCINE
Glycyrrhiza ... see LICORICE

Glycyrrhiza glabra ... see LICORICE
Glycyrrhiza glabra typica ... see LICORICE
Glycyrrhiza glabra var. glandulifera ... see LICORICE
Glycyrrhiza glabra violacea ... see LICORICE
Glycyrrhiza uralensis ... see LICORICE
Gnaphalium angustifolium ... see SANDY EVERLASTING
Gnaphalium dioicum ... see CAT'S FOOT
Gnaphalium italicum ... see SANDY EVERLASTING
Gnaphalium orientale ... see SANDY EVERLASTING
Gnaphalium stoechas ... see SANDY EVERLASTING
Gnaphalium uliginosum ... see CUDWEED
GOA POWDER ... see GOA POWDER
Goat Colostrum ... see COLOSTRUM
Goathead ... see PUNCTURE VINE
Goatnut ... see JOJOBA
Goat's Arrach ... see ARRACH
Goat's Leaf ... see HONEYSUCKLE
Goat's Pod ... see CAPSICUM
GOAT'S RUE ... see GOAT'S RUE
Goat's Rue Herb ... see GOAT'S RUE
Goat's Thorn ... see TRAGACANTH
Goatweed ... see ST. JOHN'S WORT
Gobo ... see BURDOCK
God's-hair ... see HARTSTONGUE
Goji ... see LYCIUM
Goji Berry ... see LYCIUM
Goji Juice ... see LYCIUM
Gokhru ... see PUNCTURE VINE
Gokshura ... see PUNCTURE VINE
Gold Chain ... see COMMON STONECROP
Gold Cup ... see BUTTERCUP
Gold Thread ... see GOLDTHREAD
Gold-bloom ... see CALENDULA
Goldcup ... see BULBOUS BUTTERCUP
Golden Chain ... see LABURNUM
Golden Daisy ... see OX-EYE DAISY
Golden Groundsel ... see GOLDEN RAGWORT
Golden Moss ... see COMMON STONECROP
GOLDEN RAGWORT ... see GOLDEN RAGWORT
Golden Root ... see ROSEROOT
Golden Seal ... see GOLDENSEAL
Golden Senecio ... see GOLDEN RAGWORT
Golden Trumpet ... see CATUABA
GOLDENROD ... see GOLDENROD
Goldenroot ... see GOLDENSEAL
GOLDENSEAL ... see GOLDENSEAL
Goldenseal ... see GOLDENSEAL, OX-EYE DAISY
Goldenthread ... see GOLDTHREAD
Goldilocks ... see IMMORTELLE, SANDY EVERLASTING
Goldsiegel ... see GOLDENSEAL
GOLDTHREAD ... see GOLDTHREAD
Gomishi ... see SCHISANDRA
Gomme Arabique ... see ACACIA
Gomme de Senegal ... see ACACIA
Gommelaque ... see SHELLAC
Gomphrena paniculata ... see SUMA
Goniopora sp. ... see CORAL
Gonolobus condurango ... see CONDURANGO
Goose Grass ... see CLIVERS, POTENTILLA
Goose Tansy ... see POTENTILLA
Goosebill ... see CLIVERS
Goosefoot ... see ARRACH
Goosewort ... see POTENTILLA
Gorikapuli ... see GARCINIA
Gosling Weed ... see CLIVERS
Gossypium herbaceum ... see COTTON, GOSSYPOL
Gossypium hirsutum ... see COTTON, GOSSYPOL
GOSSYPOL ... see GOSSYPOL
Gota Kola ... see GOTU KOLA
Gotu Cola ... see GOTU KOLA
GOTU KOLA ... see GOTU KOLA
Gou Qi Zi ... see LYCIUM
Goudron de Cade ... see CADE OIL
Gouqizi ... see LYCIUM
Gout Herb ... see GOUTWEED
Goutberry ... see BLACKBERRY
GOUTWEED ... see GOUTWEED
Goutwort ... see GOUTWEED
GPC ... see ALPHA-GPC
Gracemere-pear ... see PRICKLY PEAR CACTUS
Graine de Lin ... see FLAXSEED, FLAXSEED OIL
GRAINS OF PARADISE ... see GRAINS OF PARADISE
Grains of Paradise ... see CAPSICUM, GRAINS OF PARADISE
Graminis Rhizoma ... see WHEATGRASS
Granada ... see POMEGRANATE
Grano Turco ... see BUCKWHEAT
Grape ... see GRAPE fruit, skin; GRAPE leaf; GRAPE seed
Grape Bark ... see COCILLANA
Grape Fruit ... see GRAPE fruit, skin
GRAPE fruit, skin ... see GRAPE fruit, skin
Grape Juice ... see GRAPE fruit, skin
GRAPE leaf ... see GRAPE leaf
Grape Leaf Extract ... see GRAPE leaf
GRAPE seed ... see GRAPE seed
Grape Seed Extract ... see GRAPE seed
Grape Seed Oil ... see GRAPE seed
Grape Skin ... see GRAPE fruit, skin
Grape Skin Extract ... see GRAPE fruit, skin
GRAPEFRUIT ... see GRAPEFRUIT
Grapefruit Extract ... see GRAPEFRUIT SEED EXTRACT
GRAPEFRUIT OIL ... see GRAPEFRUIT OIL
GRAPEFRUIT SEED EXTRACT ... see GRAPEFRUIT SEED EXTRACT
Grapefruit Seed Glycerate ... see GRAPEFRUIT SEED EXTRACT
Grapes ... see GRAPE fruit, skin
Grapeseed ... see GRAPE seed
Grapple Plant ... see DEVIL'S CLAW
Grass ... see MARIJUANA, SWEET VERNAL GRASS
Grass Myrtle ... see CALAMUS
Grass Pollen ... see RYE GRASS
Grass Pollen Extract ... see RYE GRASS
Gratiola ... see HEDGE-HYSSOP
Gratiola officinalis ... see HEDGE-HYSSOP
Gravel Plant ... see TRAILING ARBUTUS
GRAVEL ROOT ... see GRAVEL ROOT
GRAVIOLA ... see GRAVIOLA
Gray Beard Tree ... see FRINGETREE
Gray Ephedra ... see MORMON TEA
Gray Nicker ... see DIVI-DIVI
Greasewood ... see CHAPARRAL
Great Bur ... see BURDOCK
Great Burdocks ... see BURDOCK

Great Morel .... see BELLADONNA
Great Ox-eye .... see OX-EYE DAISY
GREAT PLANTAIN .... see GREAT PLANTAIN
Great Raifort .... see HORSERADISH
Great Stinging Nettle .... see STINGING NETTLE above ground parts, STINGING NETTLE root
Great Willowherb .... see FIREWEED
GREATER BINDWEED .... see GREATER BINDWEED
GREATER BURNET .... see GREATER BURNET
Greater Burnet-saxifrage .... see PIMPINELLA root
Greater Celandine .... see GREATER CELANDINE dried above ground parts; GREATER CELANDINE rhizome, root
GREATER CELANDINE dried above ground parts .... see GREATER CELANDINE dried above ground parts
GREATER CELANDINE rhizome, root .... see GREATER CELANDINE rhizome, root
Greater Plantain .... see GREAT PLANTAIN
Grecian Laurel .... see SWEET BAY
Greek Clover .... see FENUGREEK
Greek Hay .... see FENUGREEK
Greek Hay Seed .... see FENUGREEK
Greek Oregano .... see GREEK SAGE
GREEK SAGE .... see GREEK SAGE
Green Alga .... see CHLORELLA
Green Algae .... see CHLORELLA
Green Arrow .... see YARROW
Green Bean .... see BEAN POD
Green Bell Pepper .... see CAPSICUM
Green Broom .... see DYER'S BROOM
Green Chili Pepper .... see CAPSICUM
Green Dragon .... see TRAGACANTH
Green Endive .... see WILD LETTUCE
Green Ginger .... see WORMWOOD above ground parts
Green Hellebore .... see AMERICAN HELLEBORE
Green Lipped Mussel .... see NEW ZEALAND GREEN-LIPPED MUSSEL
Green Mint .... see SPEARMINT
Green Oil of Charity .... see ENGLISH ADDER'S TONGUE
Green Onion .... see ONION
Green Orange .... see BITTER ORANGE
Green Ozier .... see AMERICAN DOGWOOD
Green Sauce .... see WOOD SORREL
GREEN TEA .... see GREEN TEA
Green Veratrum .... see AMERICAN HELLEBORE
Green Wolf's Foot .... see BUGLEWEED
Greenweed .... see DYER'S BROOM
Grenadier .... see POMEGRANATE
Griffe du Chat .... see CAT'S CLAW
Griffe du Diable .... see DEVIL'S CLAW
Grifola .... see MAITAKE MUSHROOM
Grifola frondosa .... see MAITAKE MUSHROOM
Grindella .... see GUMWEED
Grindelia camporum .... see GUMWEED
Grindelia robusta .... see GUMWEED
Grindelia squarrosa .... see GUMWEED
Grindeliae Herba .... see GUMWEED
Griottier .... see SOUR CHERRY
Grip Grass .... see CLIVERS
Grisset .... see SEA BUCKTHORN
Groats .... see OATS
GroPCho .... see ALPHA-GPC
Groseillier de Ceylan .... see INDIAN GOOSEBERRY
Grosse Kamille .... see ROMAN CHAMOMILE
Grosse Moosbeere .... see CRANBERRY
Ground Apple .... see ROMAN CHAMOMILE
Ground Berry .... see WINTERGREEN leaf, WINTERGREEN OIL
Ground Elder .... see GOUTWEED
Ground Furze .... see SPINY RESTHARROW
Ground Glutton .... see GROUNDSEL
Ground Holly .... see PIPSISSEWA
GROUND IVY .... see GROUND IVY
Ground Laurel .... see TRAILING ARBUTUS
Ground Lemon .... see PODOPHYLLUM
Ground Lily .... see BETH ROOT
GROUND PINE .... see GROUND PINE
Ground Raspberry .... see GOLDENSEAL
Ground Thistle .... see CARLINA
Groundbread .... see CYCLAMEN
Groundnuts .... see PEANUT OIL
GROUNDSEL .... see GROUNDSEL
Grundy Swallow .... see GOLDEN RAGWORT, GROUNDSEL
GS .... see GLUCOSAMINE SULFATE
GSE .... see GRAPEFRUIT SEED EXTRACT
GSH .... see GLUTATHIONE
GTF .... see CHROMIUM
GTF-Cr .... see CHROMIUM
Gua Lou .... see CHINESE CUCUMBER fruit
Gua Luo Ren .... see CHINESE CUCUMBER seed
Guaiac .... see GUAIAC WOOD resin, wood
Guaiac Heartwood .... see GUAIAC WOOD resin, wood
GUAIAC WOOD resin, wood .... see GUAIAC WOOD resin, wood
Guaiacum .... see GUAIAC WOOD resin, wood
Guaiacum guatemalense .... see GUAIAC WOOD resin, wood
Guaiacum officinale .... see GUAIAC WOOD resin, wood
Guaiacum sanctum .... see GUAIAC WOOD resin, wood
Guajaci Lignum .... see GUAIAC WOOD resin, wood
Guanabana .... see GRAVIOLA
Guanavana .... see GRAVIOLA
Guapi .... see COCILLANA
Guar Flour .... see GUAR GUM
GUAR GUM .... see GUAR GUM
GUARANA .... see GUARANA
Guarea guara .... see COCILLANA
Guarea guidonia .... see COCILLANA
Guarea rusbyi .... see COCILLANA
Guarea spiciflora .... see COCILLANA
Guarea trichilioides .... see COCILLANA
Guatemala Lemongrass .... see LEMONGRASS
Gubak .... see ANDROGRAPHIS, ARECA
Guelder Rose .... see CRAMP BARK
Guflatich .... see COLTSFOOT
Guggal .... see GUGGUL
GUGGUL .... see GUGGUL
Guggul Gum Resin .... see GUGGUL
Guggulipid .... see GUGGUL
Guggulsterone .... see GUGGUL
Guggulu .... see GUGGUL
Guggulu suddha .... see GUGGUL
Guigai .... see GINSENG, PANAX
Guilandina bonduc .... see DIVI-DIVI
Guilandina bonducella .... see DIVI-DIVI

INDEX

Guindo .... see SOUR CHERRY
Guinea Corn .... see BROOM CORN
Guinea Grains .... see GRAINS OF PARADISE
Guinea Rush .... see ADRUE
Guinea Sorrel .... see HIBISCUS
Gul-khair .... see MALLOW flower, MALLOW leaf
Gully Gum .... see EUCALYPTUS dried leaf
Gully Gum Oil .... see EUCALYPTUS OIL
Gum Acacia .... see ACACIA
Gum Arabic .... see ACACIA
Gum Benjamin .... see BENZOIN
Gum Benzoin .... see BENZOIN
Gum Bush .... see YERBA SANTA
Gum Camphor .... see CAMPHOR
Gum Dragon .... see TRAGACANTH
Gum Guggal .... see GUGGUL
Gum Guggulu .... see GUGGUL
Gum Ivy .... see ENGLISH IVY
Gum Myrrh .... see MYRRH
Gum Plant .... see COMFREY, YERBA SANTA
Gum Senegal .... see ACACIA
Gum Tragacanth .... see TRAGACANTH
Gum Tree .... see EUCALYPTUS dried leaf, STORAX
Gum Weed .... see GUMWEED
Gummae Mimosae .... see ACACIA
Gummi Tragacanthae .... see TRAGACANTH
Gummigutta .... see GAMBOGE
GUMWEED .... see GUMWEED
Gumweed Herb .... see GUMWEED
Gurmar .... see GYMNEMA
Gur-mar .... see GYMNEMA
Gurmarbooti .... see GYMNEMA
Guru Nut .... see COLA NUT
Gutta Cambodia .... see GAMBOGE
Gutta Gamba .... see GAMBOGE
Guttagamba .... see GAMBOGE
Gworo .... see COLA NUT
GYMNEMA .... see GYMNEMA
Gymnema sylvestre .... see GYMNEMA
Gynocardia Oil .... see CHAULMOOGRA
Gynostemma .... see JIAOGULAN
Gynostemma pedatum .... see JIAOGULAN
Gynostemma pentaphyllum .... see JIAOGULAN
Gypsophila paniculata .... see WHITE SOAPWORT
Gypsophilae Radix .... see WHITE SOAPWORT
Gypsy Flower .... see HOUND'S TONGUE
Gypsy Weed .... see BUGLEWEED, VERONICA
Gypsy's-rose .... see FIELD SCABIOUS
Gypsywort .... see BUGLEWEED
Haagdorn .... see HAWTHORN
Haba Soya .... see SOY
Hackmatack .... see CEDAR leaf, CEDAR LEAF OIL
Haematoxylum campechianum .... see LOGWOOD
Haematoxylum lignum .... see LOGWOOD
Hagedorn .... see HAWTHORN
Hagenia abyssinica .... see KOUSSO
Hag's Taper .... see MULLEIN
Hai Ba Ji .... see MORINDA
Hair of Venus .... see MAIDENHAIR FERN
Hairy Mint .... see WILD MINT
Hallelujah .... see WOOD SORREL
Hallfoot .... see COLTSFOOT
Hamamelis .... see WITCH HAZEL
Hamamelis virginiana .... see WITCH HAZEL
Hamburg Parsley .... see PARSLEY leaf, root
Handflower .... see WALLFLOWER
Hansen CBS 5926 .... see SACCHAROMYCES BOULARDII
Happy Major .... see BURDOCK
Hara .... see TERMINALIA
Harada .... see TERMINALIA
Haravi .... see CARAWAY dried fruit, seed
Hardback .... see STONE ROOT
Hardhack .... see STONE ROOT
Hardhay .... see ST. JOHN'S WORT
Hardock .... see BURDOCK
Hardy Fern .... see OSTRICH FERN
Harebur .... see BURDOCK
Hare's Beard .... see MULLEIN
Hare's Ear Root .... see BUPLEURUM
Haridra .... see TURMERIC
Haritaki .... see TERMINALIA
Harnblumen .... see SANDY EVERLASTING
HARONGA .... see HARONGA
Haronga madagascariensis .... see HARONGA
Harongabladder Leaf .... see HARONGA
Harongarinde Bark .... see HARONGA
Harpagophyti Radix .... see DEVIL'S CLAW
Harpagophytum .... see DEVIL'S CLAW
Harpagophytum procumbens .... see DEVIL'S CLAW
Harthorne .... see HAWTHORN
Hartogia betulin .... see BUCHU
Hart's Tree .... see SWEET CLOVER
Hart's Truffle Puffball .... see PUFF BALL
Hartshorn .... see EUROPEAN BUCKTHORN
HARTSTONGUE .... see HARTSTONGUE
Harungana madagascariensis .... see HARONGA
Harunganae Madagascariensis Cortex Bark .... see HARONGA
Harunganae Madagascariensis Folium Leaf .... see HARONGA
Haselnuss .... see HAZELNUT
Haselstrauch .... see HAZELNUT
Hasenklee .... see YELLOW LUPIN
Hash .... see MARIJUANA
Hashish .... see MARIJUANA
Hauhechelwurzel .... see SPINY RESTHARROW
Haw .... see HAWTHORN
HAWAIIAN BABY WOODROSE .... see HAWAIIAN BABY WOODROSE
HAWTHORN .... see HAWTHORN
Hawthorn Extract .... see HAWTHORN
Hawthorn Flower .... see HAWTHORN
Hawthorn Fruit .... see HAWTHORN
Hawthorn Leaf .... see HAWTHORN
Hawthorne .... see HAWTHORN
Hay Flower .... see SWEET CLOVER
Haymaids .... see GROUND IVY
Hayriffe .... see CLIVERS
Hayruff .... see CLIVERS
Hazel .... see HAZELNUT, WITCH HAZEL
Hazel Alder .... see SMOOTH ALDER
Hazel Nut .... see HAZELNUT
HAZELNUT .... see HAZELNUT
Hazelwort .... see ASARABACCA
HCA .... see GARCINIA
He Shou Wu .... see FO-TI
He Zi .... see TERMINALIA

Headache ... see CORN POPPY
Headsman ... see BUCKHORN PLANTAIN
Headwark ... see CORN POPPY
Heal-All ... see FIGWORT, SELF-HEAL, STONE ROOT
Healing Herb ... see COMFREY
Health Inca Tea ... see COCA
Heart of the Earth ... see SELF-HEAL
Heartleaf ... see COUNTRY MALLOW
HEART'S EASE ... see HEART'S EASE
Heated Oyster Shell-Seaweed Calcium ... see CALCIUM
HEATHER ... see HEATHER
Heaven Tree ... see TREE OF HEAVEN
Heavy Kaolin ... see KAOLIN
Hebanthe eriantha ... see SUMA
Hebanthe paniculata ... see SUMA
Hedeoma pulegioides ... see PENNYROYAL leaf, PENNYROYAL OIL
Hedera helix ... see ENGLISH IVY
Hedera senticosa ... see GINSENG, SIBERIAN
Hedera taurica ... see ENGLISH IVY
Hederae Helicis Folium ... see ENGLISH IVY
Hedge Bindweed ... see GREATER BINDWEED
Hedge Convolvulus ... see GREATER BINDWEED
Hedge Fumitory ... see FUMITORY
Hedge Hyssop ... see HEDGE-HYSSOP
Hedge Lily ... see GREATER BINDWEED
HEDGE MUSTARD ... see HEDGE MUSTARD
Hedge Nettles ... see BETONY
Hedge Taper ... see MULLEIN
Hedge-burs ... see CLIVERS
Hedgeheriff ... see CLIVERS
Hedgehog ... see ECHINACEA
HEDGE-HYSSOP ... see HEDGE-HYSSOP
Hedgemaids ... see GROUND IVY
Hedgethorn ... see HAWTHORN
Hediondilla ... see CHAPARRAL
Hedysarum tuberosum ... see KUDZU
Heeng ... see ASAFOETIDA
Heerabol ... see MYRRH
Hei Zao ... see JUJUBE
Helenium grandiflorum ... see ELECAMPANE
Helianthemum canadense ... see FROSTWORT
Helianthi Annui Oleum ... see SUNFLOWER OIL
Helianthus annuus ... see SUNFLOWER OIL
Helichrysum ... see SANDY EVERLASTING
Helichrysum angustifolium ... see SANDY EVERLASTING
Helichrysum arenarium ... see IMMORTELLE
Helichrysum italicum ... see SANDY EVERLASTING
Helichrysum orientale ... see SANDY EVERLASTING
Helichrysum stoechas ... see SANDY EVERLASTING
Helixor ... see EUROPEAN MISTLETOE
Helleborus niger ... see BLACK HELLEBORE
Hellweed ... see DODDER
Helmet Flower ... see SKULLCAP
Helonias ... see FALSE UNICORN
Helonias dioica ... see FALSE UNICORN
Helonias lutea ... see FALSE UNICORN
Hemicellulose Complex with Arabinoxylane ... see MGN-3
HEMLOCK ... see HEMLOCK
Hemlock Bark ... see PINUS BARK
Hemlock Gum ... see PINUS BARK
HEMLOCK SPRUCE ... see HEMLOCK SPRUCE
Hemlock Spruce ... see HEMLOCK SPRUCE, PINUS BARK
HEMLOCK WATER DROPWORT ... see HEMLOCK WATER DROPWORT
Hemlocktanne ... see PINUS BARK
Hemp ... see MARIJUANA
HEMP AGRIMONY ... see HEMP AGRIMONY
Hemp Tree ... see CHASTEBERRY
HEMPNETTLE ... see HEMPNETTLE
Hemprichia erythraea ... see MYRRH
Hen Bell ... see HENBANE
Hen of the Woods ... see MAITAKE MUSHROOM
HENBANE ... see HENBANE
Hendibeh ... see CHICORY
HENNA ... see HENNA
Henna ... see ALKANNA, HENNA
Hennae Folium ... see HENNA
Henne ... see HENNA
Hens and Chickens ... see HOUSELEEK
Heparinoid Fraction ... see MESOGLYCAN
Heparinoids ... see MESOGLYCAN
Hepatica nobilis var. acuta ... see LIVERWORT
Hepatica nobilis var. obtusa ... see LIVERWORT
Hepatici Noblis Herba ... see LIVERWORT
Hepatique a Lobes Aigus ... see LIVERWORT
Hepatique d'Amerique ... see LIVERWORT
Heps ... see ROSE HIP
Heptacosanol ... see POLICOSANOL
Heptamethoxyflavones ... see METHOXYLATED FLAVONES
Heracleum lanatum ... see MASTERWORT
Heracleum maximum ... see MASTERWORT
Heracleum montanum ... see MASTERWORT
Heracleum sphondylium ... see MASTERWORT
Heracleum sphondylium subsp. montanum ... see MASTERWORT
Herbe-chapeau ... see CONTRAYERVA
Herb-of-grace ... see RUE
Herb-of-the-Virgin ... see DIVINER'S SAGE
Herb-Paris ... see HERB PARIS
Herb Bennet ... see AVENS
Herb Gerard ... see GOUTWEED
Herb Louisa ... see LEMON VERBENA
Herb Margaret ... see OX-EYE DAISY
Herb of Grace ... see VERBENA
Herb of the Cross ... see VERBENA
HERB PARIS ... see HERB PARIS
Herb Perter ... see COWSLIP
HERB ROBERT ... see HERB ROBERT
Herb Trinity ... see LIVERWORT
Herb Two-pence ... see MONEYWORT
Herba ... see SWEET VIOLET
Herba de la Pastora ... see DAMIANA
Herba de María ... see DIVINER'S SAGE
Herba Dictamni Herba ... see BURNING BUSH leaf, BURNING BUSH root
Herba epimedii ... see EPIMEDIUM
Herba eupatoriae ... see AGRIMONY
Herba fumariae ... see FUMITORY
Herba malvae ... see MARSHMALLOW
Herbal Ecstasy ... see EPHEDRA
Herbe aux Charpentiers ... see YARROW
Herbe d'Absinthe ... see WORMWOOD above ground parts
Herbe d'Aigremoine ... see AGRIMONY

INDEX

Herbe de Hogweed .... see SCOTCH BROOM flower
Herbe de Sainte Cunegonde .... see HEMP AGRIMONY
Herbe de Saint-Guillaume .... see AGRIMONY
Herbe d'Euphraise .... see EYEBRIGHT
Herbygrass .... see RUE
Hercules Woundwort .... see SELF-HEAL
Herniaria glabra .... see RUPTUREWORT
Herniaria hirsuta .... see RUPTUREWORT
Herniariae Herba .... see RUPTUREWORT
Herniary .... see RUPTUREWORT
Herpestis monniera .... see BRAHMI
Hervea .... see MATE
Heshouwu .... see FO-TI
HESPERIDIN .... see HESPERIDIN
Hexacosanol .... see POLICOSANOL
Hexacosanol (26-C) .... see OCTACOSANOL
Hexahydroxycyclohexane .... see INOSITOL
Hexamethoxyflavones .... see METHOXYLATED FLAVONES
Hexanicotinoyl Inositol .... see INOSITOL NICOTINATE
Hexanicotinyl cis-1,2,3-5-trans-4,6-cyclohexane .... see INOSITOL NICOTINATE
Hexenbesen .... see EUROPEAN MISTLETOE
HIBISCUS .... see HIBISCUS
Hibiscus abelmoschus .... see AMBRETTE
Hibiscus sabdariffa .... see HIBISCUS
Hieracium pilosella .... see MOUSE EAR
Hierba Carmin .... see POKEWEED berry, POKEWEED root
Hierba de la Virgen .... see DIVINER'S SAGE
Hierba de San Juan .... see MUGWORT
Hierba Pastel .... see DA QING YE
Hierba Santa .... see YERBA SANTA
High Balm .... see OSWEGO TEA
High Mallow .... see MALLOW flower, MALLOW leaf
High pH Therapy .... see CESIUM
Highbush Blueberry .... see BLUEBERRY
High-bush Cranberry .... see CRAMP BARK
Highwaythorn .... see EUROPEAN BUCKTHORN
Higtaper .... see MULLEIN
Hilberry .... see WINTERGREEN leaf, WINTERGREEN OIL
Hillside Blueberry .... see BLUEBERRY
Himalayan Ginseng .... see PANAX PSEUDOGINSENG
Himalayan Mayapple .... see PODOPHYLLUM
Himalayan Rhubarb .... see RHUBARB
Himsra .... see CAPERS
Hind Heal .... see TANSY, WOOD SAGE
Hind's Tongue .... see HARTSTONGUE
Hing Hua .... see SAFFLOWER
Hini .... see BLACK ROOT
Hip .... see ROSE HIP
Hip Fruit .... see ROSE HIP
Hip Sweet .... see ROSE HIP
Hipberry .... see ROSE HIP
Hippocastani Cortex .... see HORSE CHESTNUT
Hippocastani Flos .... see HORSE CHESTNUT
Hippocastani Folium .... see HORSE CHESTNUT
Hippocastani Semen .... see HORSE CHESTNUT
Hippophae Rhamnoides .... see SEA BUCKTHORN
Hipposelinum levisticum .... see LOVAGE
Hirala .... see TERMINALIA
Hirshklee .... see HEMP AGRIMONY
Hissopo .... see HYSSOP
HISTIDINE .... see HISTIDINE
Hive Dross .... see PROPOLIS
Hive Vine .... see SQUAWVINE
HL-362 .... see FORSKOLIN
HMB .... see HYDROXYMETHYLBUTYRATE (HMB)
Ho-no-ki .... see MAGNOLIA
Ho Shou Wu .... see FO-TI
Hoarhound .... see BUGLEWEED, WHITE HOREHOUND
Hoary Plantain .... see BUCKHORN PLANTAIN
Hock-heal .... see SELF-HEAL
Hockle Elderberry .... see LEVANT BERRY
Hoelen .... see PORIA MUSHROOM
Hog Apple .... see MORINDA, PODOPHYLLUM
Hog Bean .... see HENBANE
Hog Gum .... see TRAGACANTH
Hogberry .... see UVA URSI
Hogweed .... see CANADIAN FLEABANE, KNOTWEED, MASTERWORT, SCOTCH BROOM flower, SCOTCH BROOM herb
Hojas de la Pastora .... see DIVINER'S SAGE
Hoku-gomishi .... see SCHISANDRA
Holcus bicolor .... see BROOM CORN
Holligold .... see CALENDULA
Holly-leaved Berberis .... see OREGON GRAPE
Holly .... see HOLLY, PIPSISSEWA
Holly Barberry .... see OREGON GRAPE
Holly Bay .... see MAGNOLIA
Holly Mahonia .... see OREGON GRAPE
HOLLYHOCK .... see HOLLYHOCK
Hollyhock Flower .... see HOLLYHOCK
Holm .... see HOLLY
Holme Chase .... see HOLLY
Holunderbeeren .... see ELDERBERRY
Holy Herb .... see YERBA SANTA
Holy Rope .... see HEMP AGRIMONY
Holy Thistle ..... see BLESSED THISTLE, MILK THISTLE
Holy Tree .... see HOLLY, NEEM
Holy Weed .... see YERBA SANTA
Holywort .... see VERBENA
Honduran Sarsaparilla .... see SARSAPARILLA
HONEY .... see HONEY
Honey Bee Milk .... see ROYAL JELLY
Honey Bee Pollen .... see BEE POLLEN
Honey Plant .... see LEMON BALM
Honey Suckle .... see HONEYSUCKLE
Honeybee Pollen .... see BEE POLLEN
Honeybee Venom .... see BEE VENOM
Honeybloom .... see CANADIAN HEMP
HONEYSUCKLE .... see HONEYSUCKLE
Hong Qu .... see RED YEAST
Hong Shen .... see GINSENG, PANAX
Hong Zao .... see JUJUBE
Honghua .... see SAFFLOWER
Honig .... see HONEY
HOODIA .... see HOODIA
Hoodia Cactus .... see HOODIA
Hoodia Extract .... see HOODIA
Hoodia gordonii .... see HOODIA
Hoodia Gordonii Cactus .... see HOODIA
Hoodia P57 .... see HOODIA
Hoodwort .... see SKULLCAP
Hop Fruit .... see ROSE HIP
Hop Strobile .... see HOPS

INDEX

Hop Strobili ... see HOPS
Hopfenzapfen ... see HOPS
HOPS ... see HOPS
Hordeum ... see BARLEY
Hordeum distychum ... see BARLEY
Hordeum vulgare ... see BARLEY
Horehound ... see WHITE HOREHOUND
Horns of Gold ... see DEER VELVET
Hornseed ... see ERGOT
Horny Goat Weed ... see EPIMEDIUM
Horse Balm ... see STONE ROOT
Horse Blobs ... see MARSH MARIGOLD
HORSE CHESTNUT ... see HORSE CHESTNUT
Horse Daisy ... see OX-EYE DAISY
Horse Gowan ... see OX-EYE DAISY
Horse Tongue ... see HARTSTONGUE
Horse Willow ... see HORSETAIL
Horsebane ... see HEMLOCK WATER DROPWORT, WATER FENNEL
Horse-elder ... see ELECAMPANE
Horsefly Weed ... see WILD INDIGO
Horsefoot ... see COLTSFOOT
Horseheal ... see ELECAMPANE
Horsehoof ... see COLTSFOOT
HORSEMINT ... see HORSEMINT
HORSERADISH ... see HORSERADISH
HORSETAIL ... see HORSETAIL
Horseweed ... see STONE ROOT
Horsewood ... see CANADIAN FLEABANE
Hoshouwu ... see FO-TI
Hot Pepper ... see CAPSICUM
Hou Po ... see MAGNOLIA
Hou Po Hua ... see MAGNOLIA
Houblon ... see HOPS
HOUND'S TONGUE ... see HOUND'S TONGUE
Hound's Tongue ... see DEERTONGUE, HOUND'S TONGUE
Houndsbane ... see WHITE HOREHOUND
Houndsberry ... see BLACK NIGHTSHADE
Houpu ... see MAGNOLIA
HOUSELEEK ... see HOUSELEEK
HP-200 ... see COWHAGE
Hsia Ts'ao Tung Ch'ung ... see CORDYCEPS
Hsiang-dan ... see ALOE latex
Hu Huang Lian ... see PICRORHIZA
Hu Lu Ba ... see FENUGREEK
Hua Gu ... see SHIITAKE MUSHROOM
Huacatay ... see TAGETES
Huang Ken ... see DANSHEN
Huang Lian ... see GOLDTHREAD
Huang Qi ... see ASTRAGALUS
Huang Qin ... see BAIKAL SKULLCAP
Huangquin ... see BAIKAL SKULLCAP
Huang-t'eng ken ... see THUNDER GOD VINE
Huantli ... see AMARANTH
Huanuco Coca ... see COCA
Huckleberry ... see BILBERRY
Huile de Bourrache ... see BORAGE SEED OIL
Huile d'Onagre ... see EVENING PRIMROSE OIL
Huisache ... see CASSIE ABSOLUTE
Hulm ... see HOLLY
Hulver Bush ... see HOLLY
Hulver Tree ... see HOLLY
Human Dialyzable Leukocyte Extract ... see TRANSFER FACTOR
Human Transfer Factor ... see TRANSFER FACTOR
Humic Shale ... see COLLOIDAL MINERALS
Hummingbird Tree ... see TURTLE HEAD
Humulus lupulus ... see HOPS
Hungarian Chamomile ... see GERMAN CHAMOMILE
Hungarian Pepper ... see CAPSICUM
Hungarian Silver Linden ... see SILVER LINDEN
Huntsman's Cup ... see PITCHER PLANT
Huo Xiang ... see PATCHOULY OIL
HupA ... see HUPERZINE A
Huperazon ... see CHINESE CLUB MOSS
Huperzia serrata ... see CHINESE CLUB MOSS
Huperzine ... see HUPERZINE A
HUPERZINE A ... see HUPERZINE A
Hurtleberry ... see BILBERRY
Hurtsickle ... see CORNFLOWER
Husked Nut ... see EUROPEAN CHESTNUT
Hwanggi ... see ASTRAGALUS
Hwanggum ... see BAIKAL SKULLCAP
Hyaluran ... see HYALURONIC ACID
Hyaluronan ... see HYALURONIC ACID
Hyaluronate ... see HYALURONIC ACID
Hyaluronate Sodium ... see HYALURONIC ACID
HYALURONIC ACID ... see HYALURONIC ACID
Hydnocarp ... see CHAULMOOGRA
Hydnocarpus ... see CHAULMOOGRA
Hydnocarpus anthelminthicus ... see CHAULMOOGRA
Hydnocarpus kurzii ... see CHAULMOOGRA
Hydnocarpus sp. ... see CHAULMOOGRA
HYDRANGEA ... see HYDRANGEA
Hydrangea arborescens ... see HYDRANGEA
Hydrastis ... see GOLDENSEAL
Hydrastis canadensis ... see GOLDENSEAL
Hydrated Aluminum Silicate ... see KAOLIN
Hydrazine ... see HYDRAZINE SULFATE
HYDRAZINE SULFATE ... see HYDRAZINE SULFATE
Hydrocotyle ... see GOTU KOLA
Hydrocotyle Asiatica ... see GOTU KOLA
Hydrocotyle Asiatique ... see GOTU KOLA
Hydrogen Fluoride ... see FLUORIDE
Hydrolyzed Collagen Protein ... see GELATIN
Hydrolyzed Gelatin ... see GELATIN
Hydrolyzed Liver Extract ... see LIVER EXTRACT
Hydrolyzed Soy Protein ... see SOY
Hydrolyzed Spleen Extract ... see SPLEEN EXTRACT
Hydroxocobalamin ... see VITAMIN B12
Hydroxocobalaminum ... see VITAMIN B12
Hydroxocobemine ... see VITAMIN B12
Hydroxyacetic Acid ... see ALPHA HYDROXY ACIDS
Hydroxyapatite ... see CALCIUM
Hydroxycaprylic Acid ... see ALPHA HYDROXY ACIDS
Hydroxycitrate ... see GARCINIA
Hydroxycitric Acid ... see GARCINIA
Hydroxydecyl Benzoquinone ... see IDEBENONE
Hydroxyecdysterone ... see ECDYSTERONE
HYDROXYMETHYLBUTYRATE (HMB) ... see HYDROXYMETHYLBUTYRATE (HMB)
Hydroxypropionic Acid ... see ALPHA HYDROXY ACIDS
Hydroxysuccinic Acid ... see ALPHA HYDROXY ACIDS
Hyoscyami Folium ... see HENBANE
Hyoscyamus niger ... see HENBANE
Hypereikon ... see ST. JOHN'S WORT
Hyperici Herba ... see ST. JOHN'S WORT
Hypericum ... see ST. JOHN'S WORT

Hypericum perforatum ... see ST. JOHN'S WORT
Hyperimmune Bovine Colostrum ... see COLOSTRUM
Hypoxanthine Riboside ... see INOSINE
Hypoxanthosine ... see INOSINE
Hypoxis hemerocallidea ... see AFRICAN WILD POTATO
Hypoxis Plant ... see AFRICAN WILD POTATO
Hypoxis rooperi ... see AFRICAN WILD POTATO
Hysope officinale ... see HYSSOP
HYSSOP ... see HYSSOP
Hyssopus officinalis ... see HYSSOP
I ... see IODINE
I3C ... see INDOLE-3-CARBINOL
Iandirova ... see ANDIROBA
Iberis amara ... see CLOWN'S MUSTARD PLANT
Iberis coronaria ... see CLOWN'S MUSTARD PLANT
IBOGA ... see IBOGA
Ice Vine ... see PAREIRA
Iceland Lichen ... see ICELAND MOSS
ICELAND MOSS ... see ICELAND MOSS
Ichthyomethia piscipula ... see JAMAICAN DOGWOOD
Ici Fructus ... see CAPSICUM
Iconyl ... see GLYCINE
IDEBENONE ... see IDEBENONE
Idrocotyle ... see GOTU KOLA
Idrossocobalamina ... see VITAMIN B12
Igelkopfwurzel ... see ECHINACEA
IGNATIUS BEAN ... see IGNATIUS BEAN
Ilex ... see MATE
Ilex aquifolium ... see HOLLY
Ilex opaca ... see HOLLY
Ilex paraguariensis ... see MATE
Ilex vomitoria ... see HOLLY
Illicium ... see STAR ANISE
Illicium verum ... see STAR ANISE
Imber ... see GINGER
Imlee ... see TAMARIND
Immortality Herb ... see JIAOGULAN
IMMORTELLE ... see IMMORTELLE
Impatiens ... see JEWELWEED
Impatiens balsamina ... see JEWELWEED
Impatiens biflora ... see JEWELWEED
Impatiens capensis ... see JEWELWEED
Impatiens giorgii ... see JEWELWEED
Impatiens pallida ... see JEWELWEED
In Chen ... see YIN CHEN
Inca Health Tea ... see COCA
Inca Tea ... see COCA
Inchinko ... see YIN CHEN
Inchin-ko-to ... see YIN CHEN
Indhana ... see WORMWOOD above ground parts
India Root ... see ALPINIA
Indian-fig Prickly Pear Cactus ... see PRICKLY PEAR CACTUS
Indian-gooseberry ... see INDIAN GOOSEBERRY
Indian-hemp ... see CANADIAN HEMP
Indian Almond ... see TERMINALIA
Indian Apple ... see PODOPHYLLUM
Indian Arrowroot ... see WAHOO, ZEDOARY
Indian Arrowwood ... see WAHOO
Indian Bael ... see BAEL
Indian Balm ... see BETH ROOT
Indian Balsam ... see PERU BALSAM
Indian Bark ... see MAGNOLIA
Indian Bdellium-tree ... see GUGGUL
Indian Bead ... see PRECATORY BEAN
Indian Belladonna ... see BELLADONNA
Indian Berry ... see LEVANT BERRY
Indian Bolonong ... see CHIRATA
Indian Bread ... see PORIA MUSHROOM
Indian Chocolate ... see WATER AVENS
Indian Cluster Bean ... see GUAR GUM
Indian Corn ... see CORN SILK
Indian Cress ... see NASTURTIUM, WATERCRESS
Indian Dye ... see GOLDENSEAL
Indian Echinacea ... see ANDROGRAPHIS
Indian Elm ... see SLIPPERY ELM
INDIAN FRANKINCENSE ... see INDIAN FRANKINCENSE
Indian Gentian ... see CHIRATA
Indian Ginseng ... see ASHWAGANDHA
INDIAN GOOSEBERRY ... see INDIAN GOOSEBERRY
Indian Guar Plant ... see GUAR GUM
Indian Gum ... see CUP PLANT
Indian Head ... see ECHINACEA
Indian Hippo ... see INDIAN PHYSIC
Indian Jointfir ... see EPHEDRA
Indian Lilac ... see NEEM
INDIAN LONG PEPPER ... see INDIAN LONG PEPPER
Indian Mulberry ... see BA JI TIAN, MORINDA
Indian Olibanum ... see INDIAN FRANKINCENSE
Indian Parsley ... see OSHA
Indian Pennywort ... see GOTU KOLA
INDIAN PHYSIC ... see INDIAN PHYSIC
Indian Physic ... see CANADIAN HEMP, INDIAN PHYSIC
Indian Pink ... see PINK ROOT
Indian Plant ... see BLOODROOT, GOLDENSEAL
Indian Plantago ... see BLOND PSYLLIUM
Indian Podophyllum ... see PODOPHYLLUM
Indian Poke ... see AMERICAN HELLEBORE
Indian Red Paint ... see BLOODROOT
Indian Rhubarb ... see RHUBARB
Indian Root ... see AMERICAN SPIKENARD
Indian Saffron ... see SAFFRON, TURMERIC
Indian Sage ... see BONESET
Indian Senna ... see SENNA
Indian Shamrock ... see BETH ROOT
INDIAN SNAKEROOT ... see INDIAN SNAKEROOT
Indian Squill ... see SQUILL
Indian Tobacco ... see LOBELIA
Indian Tragacanth ... see KARAYA GUM
Indian Tumeric ... see GOLDENSEAL
Indian Valerian ... see VALERIAN
Indian Walnut ... see TUNG SEED
Indian Water Navelwort ... see GOTU KOLA
Indian-laurel ... see LAURELWOOD
Indigo Broom ... see WILD INDIGO
Indischer Wassernabel ... see GOTU KOLA
INDOLE-3-CARBINOL ... see INDOLE-3-CARBINOL
Indole-3-methanol ... see INDOLE-3-CARBINOL
Inkberry ... see POKEWEED berry, POKEWEED root
Inorganic Germanium ... see GERMANIUM
Inose ... see INOSITOL
INOSINE ... see INOSINE
Inosite ... see INOSITOL
INOSITOL ... see INOSITOL
Inositol Hexaniacinate ... see INOSITOL NICOTINATE
Inositol Hexanicotinate ... see INOSITOL NICOTINATE

INDEX

Inositol Hexaphosphate .... see IP-6
Inositol Monophosphate .... see INOSITOL
Inositol Niacinate .... see INOSITOL NICOTINATE
INOSITOL NICOTINATE .... see INOSITOL NICOTINATE
Insam .... see GINSENG, PANAX
Intoxicating Long Pepper .... see KAVA
Intoxicating Pepper .... see KAVA
Intrachol .... see CHOLINE
Intralipid .... see SOYBEAN OIL
Inula .... see ELECAMPANE
Inula helenium .... see ELECAMPANE
INULIN .... see INULIN
Inulin Hydrolysate .... see FRUCTO-OLIGOSACCHARIDES
IODINE .... see IODINE
IP-6 .... see IP-6
Ipe .... see PAU D'ARCO
Ipe Roxo .... see PAU D'ARCO
IPECAC .... see IPECAC
Ipecacuanha .... see IPECAC
Ipes .... see PAU D'ARCO
Ipomoea .... see MEXICAN SCAMMONY ROOT
Ipomoea orizabensis .... see MEXICAN SCAMMONY ROOT
Ipomoea purga .... see JALAP
Ipomoea superba .... see MEXICAN SCAMMONY ROOT
Ipomoea tyrianthina .... see MEXICAN SCAMMONY ROOT
Iporoni .... see IPORURU
Iporuro .... see IPORURU
IPORURU .... see IPORURU
IPRIFLAVONE .... see IPRIFLAVONE
Ipurosa .... see IPORURU
Ipururo .... see IPORURU
Iris .... see BLUE FLAG, ORRIS
Iris caroliniana .... see BLUE FLAG
Iris florentina .... see ORRIS
Iris germanica .... see ORRIS
Iris germanica var. florentina .... see ORRIS
Iris junonia .... see ORRIS
Iris pallida .... see ORRIS
Iris versicolor .... see BLUE FLAG
Iris virginica .... see BLUE FLAG
Irish Broom .... see SCOTCH BROOM herb
Irish Broom Tops .... see SCOTCH BROOM flower
Irish Moss .... see CARRAGEENAN
Irish Moss Extract .... see CARRAGEENAN
Irish Potato .... see POTATO
IRON .... see IRON
Iron EDTA .... see EDTA
Isatis indigotica .... see DA QING YE
Isatis tinctoria .... see DA QING YE
Iscador .... see EUROPEAN MISTLETOE
Iso-ascorbic acid .... see VITAMIN C (ASCORBIC ACID)
Isoflavone .... see KUDZU, LICORICE, RED CLOVER
Isoflavone Combined Polysaccharide .... see GENISTEIN COMBINED POLYSACCHARIDE
Isoinokosterone .... see ECDYSTERONE
Isoleucine .... see BRANCHED-CHAIN AMINO ACIDS
Isorel .... see EUROPEAN MISTLETOE
Ispaghula .... see BLOND PSYLLIUM
Ispagol .... see BLOND PSYLLIUM
Italian Fitch .... see GOAT'S RUE
Italian Jasmine .... see JASMINE
Italian Limetta .... see LIME fruit, peel; LIME OIL
Itchweed .... see AMERICAN HELLEBORE
Ivy .... see AMERICAN IVY, ENGLISH IVY
Ivy-leafed cyclamen .... see CYCLAMEN
Jaatipatree .... see NUTMEG AND MACE
JABORANDI .... see JABORANDI
Jaborandi Pepper .... see INDIAN LONG PEPPER
Jack-jump-about .... see GOUTWEED
Jack-of-the-buttery .... see COMMON STONECROP
JACOB'S LADDER .... see JACOB'S LADDER
Jacob's Ladder .... see JACOB'S LADDER, LILY-OF-THE-VALLEY
Jacob's Staff .... see MULLEIN
Jacob's Sword .... see ORRIS
Jaffa Orange .... see SWEET ORANGE
Jaguar Gum .... see GUAR GUM
Jalanimba .... see BRAHMI
JALAP .... see JALAP
Jalap ..... see JALAP, POKEWEED berry, POKEWEED root
Jalapa .... see JALAP
Jalape .... see JALAP
Jalnaveri .... see BRAHMI
Jamaica Dogwood .... see JAMAICAN DOGWOOD
Jamaica Ginger .... see GINGER
Jamaica Mignonette .... see HENNA
Jamaica Pepper .... see ALLSPICE
Jamaica Sorrel .... see HIBISCUS
JAMAICAN DOGWOOD .... see JAMAICAN DOGWOOD
Jamaican Quassia .... see QUASSIA
Jamaican Sarsaparilla .... see SARSAPARILLA
Jambolan .... see JAMBOLAN bark, JAMBOLAN seed
JAMBOLAN bark .... see JAMBOLAN bark
JAMBOLAN seed .... see JAMBOLAN seed
Jambu .... see JAMBOLAN bark
Jambul .... see JAMBOLAN bark, JAMBOLAN seed
James' Tea .... see MARSH TEA
Jamestown Weed .... see JIMSON WEED
Jamguarandi .... see JABORANDI
Jamum .... see JAMBOLAN bark, JAMBOLAN seed
Japanaese Lantern .... see WINTER CHERRY
Japanese Arrowroot .... see KUDZU
Japanese Belladonna .... see SCOPOLIA
Japanese Epimedium .... see EPIMEDIUM
Japanese Ginseng .... see GINSENG, PANAX
Japanese Honeysuckle .... see HONEYSUCKLE
Japanese Isinglas .... see AGAR
JAPANESE MINT .... see JAPANESE MINT
Japanese Pagoda Tree .... see PAGODA TREE
Japanese Silver Apricot .... see GINKGO leaf (GINKGO leaf extract), GINKGO seed
Japanese Tea .... see GREEN TEA
Japanese Whitebark Magnolia .... see MAGNOLIA
Jarilla .... see CHAPARRAL
JASMINE .... see JASMINE
Jasminum grandiflorum .... see JASMINE
Jasminum officinale .... see JASMINE
Jateorhiza columba .... see COLOMBO
Jateorhiza miersii .... see COLOMBO
Jateorhiza palmata .... see COLOMBO
Jati .... see JASMINE
Jatikosha .... see NUTMEG AND MACE

INDEX

Jatipatra ... see NUTMEG AND MACE
Jatipatri ... see NUTMEG AND MACE
Jatiphala ... see NUTMEG AND MACE
Jatiphalam ... see NUTMEG AND MACE
Jatropha moluccana ... see TUNG SEED
Jaundice Berry ... see EUROPEAN BARBERRY
Jaundice Root ... see GOLDENSEAL
Java ... see COFFEE
Java Citronella ... see CITRONELLA OIL
Java Coca ... see COCA
Java Pepper ... see CUBEBS
Java Plum ... see JAMBOLAN bark, JAMBOLAN seed
JAVA TEA ... see JAVA TEA
Java Turmeric ... see JAVANESE TURMERIC
JAVANESE TURMERIC ... see JAVANESE TURMERIC
Jeeraka ... see CUMIN
Jen-shen ... see GINSENG, PANAX
Jequirity Bean ... see PRECATORY BEAN
Jequirity Seed ... see PRECATORY BEAN
Jersey Tea ... see NEW JERSEY TEA
Jesuit Tea ... see CHENOPODIUM OIL
Jesuit's Balsam ... see COPAIBA BALSAM
Jesuit's Bark ... see CINCHONA
Jesuit's Tea ... see MATE
Jethi-madh ... see LICORICE
Jewel Balsam Weed ... see JEWELWEED
Jewel Weed ... see JEWELWEED
JEWELWEED ... see JEWELWEED
Jew's Harp Plant ... see BETH ROOT
Jew's Myrtle ... see BUTCHER'S BROOM
Jia Renshen ... see PANAX PSEUDOGINSENG
Jia Yang ... see POPLAR
Jiang ... see GINGER
Jiao Gu Lan ... see JIAOGULAN
JIAOGULAN ... see JIAOGULAN
JIMSON WEED ... see JIMSON WEED
Jinsao ... see GINSENG, PANAX
Jintsam ... see GINSENG, PANAX
Jinyingzi ... see CHEROKEE ROSEHIP
Jinyinhua ... see HONEYSUCKLE
Joe Pye ... see GRAVEL ROOT
Joe-pye Weed ... see GRAVEL ROOT
Johimbi ... see YOHIMBE
Johnny-jump-up ... see HEART'S EASE
Joint ... see MARIJUANA
Joint Fir ... see EPHEDRA
Jointed Flat Sedge ... see ADRUE
Joint-podded Charlock ... see WILD RADISH
JOJOBA ... see JOJOBA
Joshua Tree ... see YUCCA
Ju Hua ... see CHRYSANTHEMUM
Juarandi ... see JABORANDI
Jufa ... see HYSSOP
Juglandis ... see ENGLISH WALNUT
Juglandis Folium ... see ENGLISH WALNUT
Juglans ... see ENGLISH WALNUT
Juglans cinerea ... see BUTTERNUT
Juglans nigra ... see BLACK WALNUT
Juglans regia ... see ENGLISH WALNUT
JUJUBE ... see JUJUBE
Jujube Plum ... see JUJUBE
Jujubi ... see JUJUBE
Jumbul ... see JAMBOLAN bark, JAMBOLAN seed
Jungle Weed ... see OPIUM ANTIDOTE
JUNIPER ... see JUNIPER
Juniper Tar Oil ... see CADE OIL
Juniperi Fructus ... see JUNIPER
Juniperus ashei ... see CEDARWOOD OIL
Juniperus communis ... see JUNIPER
Juniperus mexicana ... see CEDARWOOD OIL
Juniperus oxycedrus ... see CADE OIL
Juniperus sabina ... see SAVIN TOPS
Juniperus virginiana ... see CEDARWOOD, CEDARWOOD OIL
Juno's Tears ... see VERBENA
Jupiter's Bean ... see HENBANE
Jupiter's Beard ... see HOUSELEEK, RED-SPUR VALERIAN
Jupiter's Eye ... see HOUSELEEK
Jupiter's Nut ... see EUROPEAN CHESTNUT
Justicia adhatoda ... see MALABAR NUT
Justicia paniculata ... see ANDROGRAPHIS
Ju-zhong ... see SAW PALMETTO
K ... see POTASSIUM
K1 ... see VITAMIN K
K2 ... see VITAMIN K
K3 ... see VITAMIN K
K4 ... see VITAMIN K
Kaa Jhee ... see STEVIA
Kadaya ... see KARAYA GUM
Kadeol ... see CADE OIL
Kadira ... see KARAYA GUM
Kadsura chinensis ... see SCHISANDRA
Kaffree Tea ... see RED BUSH TEA
Kairata ... see CHIRATA
Kajuputi leucadendra ... see CAJEPUT OIL
Kakamachi ... see BLACK NIGHTSHADE
Kalahari Cactus ... see HOODIA
Kalahari Diet ... see HOODIA
Kalajaji ... see BLACK SEED
Kalajira ... see BLACK SEED
Kalamegha ... see ANDROGRAPHIS
Kale ... see CABBAGE
Kalidruma ... see TERMINALIA
Kalmia latifolia ... see MOUNTAIN LAUREL
Kalmus ... see CALAMUS
Kalonji ... see BLACK SEED
Kalpa Herbal Tea ... see CASSIA AURICULATA
KAMALA ... see KAMALA
Kamani Punna ... see LAURELWOOD
Kamcela ... see KAMALA
Kameela ... see KAMALA
Kamillen ... see GERMAN CHAMOMILE
Kana ... see INDIAN LONG PEPPER
Kanaje Hindi ... see ASHWAGANDHA
Kankusta ... see GARCINIA
Kansas Snakeroot ... see ECHINACEA
Kanya ... see ALOE gel, ALOE latex
Kao ... see KAVA
KAOLIN ... see KAOLIN
Kapikachchhu ... see COWHAGE
Karavella ... see BITTER MELON
Karaya ... see KARAYA GUM
KARAYA GUM ... see KARAYA GUM
Kardone ... see ARTICHOKE
Karela ... see BITTER MELON
Kargasok Tea ... see KOMBUCHA TEA
Kariyat ... see ANDROGRAPHIS

Karkade ... see HIBISCUS
Karpasa ... see COTTON, GOSSYPOL
Karpoora ... see CAMPHOR
Karshaphala ... see TERMINALIA
Kasani ... see CHICORY
Kastanienblaetter ... see EUROPEAN CHESTNUT
Kasturidana ... see AMBRETTE
Kasturilatika ... see AMBRETTE
Kat ... see KHAT
Kathilla ... see BITTER MELON
Katila ... see KARAYA GUM
Katki ... see PICRORHIZA
Katsenpfotchenbluten ... see CAT'S FOOT
Katuka ... see PICRORHIZA
Katuko ... see PICRORHIZA
Katurohini ... see PICRORHIZA
Katuvira ... see CAPSICUM
Katvi ... see PICRORHIZA
Katzenkrat ... see YARROW
Katzenpfotchenbluten ... see SANDY EVERLASTING
Kaunch ... see COWHAGE
KAVA ... see KAVA
Kava Pepper ... see KAVA
Kava Root ... see KAVA
Kavain ... see KAVA
Kavapipar ... see KAVA
Kawa Kawa ... see KAVA
Kawa Pepper ... see KAVA
Kawanch ... see COWHAGE
Kawapfeffer ... see KAVA
Kawaratake ... see CORIOLUS MUSHROOM
Kawara-yomogi ... see YIN CHEN
KEFIR ... see KEFIR
Kefir Cheese ... see KEFIR
Kefir Grains ... see KEFIR
Kefir Yogurt ... see KEFIR
Keiri ... see WALLFLOWER
Kelp ... see BLADDERWRACK, LAMINARIA
Kelpware ... see BLADDERWRACK
Kelp-ware ... see BLADDERWRACK
Kephalin ... see PHOSPHATIDYLSERINE
Kerala ... see BITTER MELON
Kermesbeere ... see POKEWEED berry, POKEWEED root
Kew ... see KAVA
Kew Tree ... see GINKGO leaf (GINKGO leaf extract), GINKGO seed
Key Flower ... see COWSLIP
Key Lime ... see LIME OIL
Key of Heaven ... see COWSLIP
KH-3 ... see PROCAINE
Khadira ... see CATECHU
Khair ... see CATECHU
Khareti ... see COUNTRY MALLOW
Kharjura ... see DATE PALM
Khartoum Senna ... see SENNA
Khas-khas ... see VETIVER
KHAT ... see KHAT
KHELLA ... see KHELLA
Khella Fruit ... see KHELLA
Khellin ... see KHELLA
Kher ... see ACACIA
Khurasani-ajavayan ... see HENBANE
Khus-khus Grass ... see VETIVER
Khus Khus ... see VETIVER
Kidney Root ... see GRAVEL ROOT
Kidney Wort ... see LIVERWORT
Kif ... see MARIJUANA
Kijitsu ... see BITTER ORANGE
Kiln-dried Allspice ... see ALLSPICE
Kinerase ... see KINETIN
Kinetase ... see KINETIN
KINETIN ... see KINETIN
King of Bitters ... see ANDROGRAPHIS
King of Mushrooms ... see MAITAKE MUSHROOM
Kingcups ... see MARSH MARIGOLD
Kings and Queens ... see ARUM
King's Clover ... see SWEET CLOVER
King's Crown ... see ROSEROOT
King's Cup ... see BULBOUS BUTTERCUP
King's Cure ... see PIPSISSEWA
King's Cureall ... see EVENING PRIMROSE OIL, PIPSISSEWA
Kinnikinnik ... see UVA URSI
Kirata ... see CHIRATA
Kirta ... see ANDROGRAPHIS
Kita-gomishi ... see SCHISANDRA
Kiwach ... see COWHAGE
KIWI ... see KIWI
Kiwi Fruit ... see KIWI
Klamath Blue/Green Algae ... see BLUE-GREEN ALGAE
Klamath Weed ... see ST. JOHN'S WORT
Klapperschlangen ... see SENEGA
Kleine Kamille ... see GERMAN CHAMOMILE
Kn ... see KINETIN
Knackweide ... see WILLOW BARK
Knautia arvensis ... see FIELD SCABIOUS
Knee Holly ... see BUTCHER'S BROOM
Kneeholm ... see BUTCHER'S BROOM
Knight's Spur ... see DELPHINIUM
Knitback ... see COMFREY
Knitbone ... see COMFREY
Knob Grass ... see STONE ROOT
Knob Root ... see STONE ROOT
Knobweed ... see STONE ROOT
Knot Grass ... see KNOTWEED
Knotgrass ... see KNOTWEED
Knotted Marjoram ... see MARJORAM
Knotted Wrack ... see BLADDERWRACK
Knotty Brake ... see MALE FERN
KNOTWEED ... see KNOTWEED
Knotweed Herb ... see KNOTWEED
Kojo-kon ... see RESVERATROL
Kola Nut ... see COLA NUT
Koloquinthen ... see COLOCYNTH
Kombe ... see STROPHANTHUS
Kombe-strophanthus Seeds ... see STROPHANTHUS
Kombu ... see LAMINARIA
Kombucha Mushroom Tea ... see KOMBUCHA TEA
KOMBUCHA TEA ... see KOMBUCHA TEA
Konjac ... see GLUCOMANNAN
Konjac Mannan ... see GLUCOMANNAN
Kooso ... see KOUSSO
Korean Ginseng ... see GINSENG, PANAX
Korean Panax Ginseng ... see GINSENG, PANAX
Korean Red Ginseng ... see GINSENG, PANAX
Koriander ... see CORIANDER
Kosho ... see BLACK PEPPER AND WHITE PEPPER
Kosso ... see KOUSSO

INDEX

KOUSSO ... see KOUSSO
Kraftwurz ... see ARNICA
Krameria ... see RHATANY
Krameria argentea ... see RHATANY
Krameria iluca ... see RHATANY
Krameria lappacea ... see RHATANY
Krameria triandra ... see RHATANY
Kranbeere ... see CRANBERRY
Krestin ... see CORIOLUS MUSHROOM
Kreuzdornbeeren ... see EUROPEAN BUCKTHORN
Krishan Jeeraka ... see CARAWAY dried fruit, seed
Krishna ... see BLACK PEPPER AND WHITE PEPPER
Krishnajiraka ... see CARAWAY dried fruit, seed
Kua ... see ZEDOARY
Kuandong Hua ... see COLTSFOOT
Kudsu ... see KUDZU
KUDZU ... see KUDZU
Kudzu Vine ... see KUDZU
Kuguazi ... see BITTER MELON
K'u-kua ... see BITTER MELON
Kukui ... see TUNG SEED
Kullo ... see KARAYA GUM
Kumari ... see ALOE gel, ALOE latex
Kumkuma ... see SAFFRON
Kummel ... see CARAWAY dried fruit, seed
Kummich ... see CARAWAY dried fruit, seed
Kunigundendraut ... see HEMP AGRIMONY
Kuntze Saloop ... see SASSAFRAS
Kuru ... see PICRORHIZA
Kus es Salahin ... see KHAT
Kushta ... see COSTUS OIL, COSTUS root
Kushtha ... see COSTUS OIL, COSTUS root
Kustumburi ... see CORIANDER
Kuth ... see COSTUS OIL, COSTUS root
Kuthmithi ... see ASHWAGANDHA
Kutki ... see PICRORHIZA
Kwaao Khruea ... see KUDZU
Kwassan ... see KOMBUCHA TEA
Kydney Root ... see GRAVEL ROOT
Kyunchinho ... see YIN CHEN
L Arginine ... see L-ARGININE
L(+)-2-aminoglutaramic acid ... see GLUTAMINE
L(+)-ornithine Alpha-ketoglutarate ... see ORNITHINE KETOGLUTARATE
L-2,5-diaminovaleric acid ... see ORNITHINE
L-2,6-diaminohexanoic acid ... see LYSINE
L-2-amino-3-(1H-imidazol-4-yl) propionic acid ... see HISTIDINE
L-2-amino-3-(indole-3-yl) propionic acid ... see L-TRYPTOPHAN
L-2-amino-4-(methylthio) butyric acid ... see METHIONINE
L-3-hydroxy-4-(trimethylammonium)-butyrate ... see L-CARNITINE
L-5 HTP ... see 5-HTP
L-5 Hydroxytryptophan ... see 5-HTP
L-5-aminorvaline ... see ORNITHINE
L-75-1362B ... see FORSKOLIN
L-acetylcarnitine ... see ACETYL-L-CARNITINE
L-alpha-glycerylphosphorylcholine ... see ALPHA-GPC
L-ARGININE ... see L-ARGININE
L-arginine HCl ... see L-ARGININE
L-arginine Hydrochloride ... see L-ARGININE
L-arginine-HCl ... see L-ARGININE
L-ascorbic acid ... see VITAMIN C (ASCORBIC ACID)
L-CARNITINE ... see L-CARNITINE
L-carnitine propionyl ... see PROPIONYL-L-CARNITINE
L-carnosine ... see CARNOSINE
L-cysteine ... see N-ACETYL CYSTEINE
L-glutamic acid ... see GLUTAMINE
L-glutamic acid 5-amide ... see GLUTAMINE
L-glutamine ... see GLUTAMINE
L-glutathione ... see GLUTATHIONE
L-glycine ... see GLYCINE
L-histidine ... see HISTIDINE
L-isoleucine ... see BRANCHED-CHAIN AMINO ACIDS
L-leucine ... see BRANCHED-CHAIN AMINO ACIDS
L-lysine ... see LYSINE
L-methionine ... see METHIONINE
L-ornithine ... see ORNITHINE
L-ornithine alpha-ketoglutarate ... see ORNITHINE KETOGLUTARATE
L-phenylalanine ... see PHENYLALANINE
L-selenomethionine ... see SELENIUM
L-taurine ... see TAURINE
L-theanine ... see THEANINE
L-threonine ... see THREONINE
L-trypt ... see L-TRYPTOPHAN
L-tryptophan ... see L-TRYPTOPHAN
L-tyrosine ... see TYROSINE
L-valine ... see BRANCHED-CHAIN AMINO ACIDS
L. acidophilus ... see LACTOBACILLUS
L. amylovorus ... see LACTOBACILLUS
L. brevis ... see LACTOBACILLUS
L. bulgaricus ... see LACTOBACILLUS
L. casei ... see LACTOBACILLUS
L. crispatus ... see LACTOBACILLUS
L. delbrueckii ... see LACTOBACILLUS
L. fermentum ... see LACTOBACILLUS
L. gallinarum ... see LACTOBACILLUS
L. johnsonii ... see LACTOBACILLUS
L. johnsonii LC-1 ... see LACTOBACILLUS
L. plantarum ... see LACTOBACILLUS
L. reuteri ... see LACTOBACILLUS
L. sporogenes ... see LACTOBACILLUS
La Hembra ... see DIVINER'S SAGE
LABDANUM ... see LABDANUM
Labrador Tea ... see LABRADOR TEA
LABURNUM ... see LABURNUM
Laburnum Anagyroides ... see LABURNUM
Lac ... see SHELLAC
Lacca ... see SHELLAC
Laccifer lacca ... see SHELLAC
Laciniaria spicata ... see MARSH BLAZING STAR
LACTASE ... see LACTASE
Lactic Acid ... see ALPHA HYDROXY ACIDS
Lacto Bacillus ... see LACTOBACILLUS
Lactobacilli ... see LACTOBACILLUS
LACTOBACILLUS ... see LACTOBACILLUS
Lactobacillus acidophilus ... see LACTOBACILLUS
Lactobacillus amylovorus ... see LACTOBACILLUS
Lactobacillus brevis ... see LACTOBACILLUS
Lactobacillus bulgaricus ... see LACTOBACILLUS
Lcatobacillus casei ... see LACTOBACILLUS
Lactobacillus crispatus ... see LACTOBACILLUS
Lactobacillus delbrueckii ... see LACTOBACILLUS
Lactobacillus fermentum ... see LACTOBACILLUS
Lactobacillus gallinarum ... see LACTOBACILLUS

INDEX

Lactobacillus GG .... see LACTOBACILLUS
Lactobacillus johnsonii .... see LACTOBACILLUS
Lactobacillus plantarum .... see LACTOBACILLUS
Lactobacillus reuteri .... see LACTOBACILLUS
Lactobacillus rhamnosus .... see LACTOBACILLUS
Lactobacillus rhamnosus GG .... see LACTOBACILLUS
Lactobacillus sporogenes .... see LACTOBACILLUS
LACTOFERRIN .... see LACTOFERRIN
Lactoflavin .... see RIBOFLAVIN (VITAMIN B2)
Lactuca virosa .... see WILD LETTUCE
Lactucarium .... see WILD LETTUCE
Ladder-to-Heaven .... see LILY-OF-THE-VALLEY
Ladies' Delight .... see HEART'S EASE
Ladies' Seal .... see BRYONIA
Lady Bleeding .... see AMARANTH
LADY FERN .... see LADY FERN
Lady of the Meadow .... see MEADOWSWEET
LADY'S BEDSTRAW .... see LADY'S BEDSTRAW
Lady's Mantle .... see ALCHEMILLA
Lady's Nightcap .... see GREATER BINDWEED
Lady's Purse .... see SHEPHERD'S PURSE
Lady's Seals .... see SOLOMON'S SEAL
Lady's Slipper .... see NERVE ROOT
Lady's Thimble .... see DIGITALIS
Lady's Thistle .... see MILK THISTLE
Ladysmock .... see ARUM
Lady's-seal .... see BLACK BRYONY
Laetrile .... see APRICOT
Lagerstroemia flos-reginae .... see BANABA
Lagerstroemia speciosa .... see BANABA
Lai Margose .... see BITTER MELON
Lakritze .... see LICORICE
Lamb Mint .... see PEPPERMINT leaf, SPEARMINT
Lambkill .... see MOUNTAIN LAUREL
Lamb's Quarters .... see BETH ROOT
Lamb's Tongue .... see AMERICAN ADDER'S TONGUE
Lamii Albi Flos .... see WHITE DEAD NETTLE FLOWER
LAMINARIA .... see LAMINARIA
Laminaria digitata .... see ALGIN, LAMINARIA
Laminaria japonica .... see LAMINARIA
Lamium Album .... see WHITE DEAD NETTLE FLOWER
Lamp Black .... see ACTIVATED CHARCOAL
Land Whin .... see SPINY RESTHARROW
Langer Pfeffer .... see INDIAN LONG PEPPER
Languas officinarum .... see ALPINIA
Langwort .... see BUTTERBUR, WHITE HELLEBORE
Lan-hiqui .... see SANGRE DE GRADO
Laniqui .... see SANGRE DE GRADO
Lapacho .... see PAU D'ARCO
Lapacho colorado .... see PAU D'ARCO
Lapacho morado .... see PAU D'ARCO
Lappa .... see BURDOCK
Larch .... see LARCH ARABINOGALACTAN
LARCH ARABINOGALACTAN .... see LARCH ARABINOGALACTAN
Larch Gum .... see LARCH ARABINOGALACTAN
LARCH TURPENTINE .... see LARCH TURPENTINE
Large Cranberry .... see CRANBERRY
Large Fennel .... see FENNEL fruit, seed
Large Indian Civet .... see CIVET
Large-leaved Germander .... see WOOD SAGE
Larix .... see LARCH ARABINOGALACTAN
Larix dahurica .... see LARCH ARABINOGALACTAN
Larix decidua .... see LARCH TURPENTINE
Larix europaea .... see LARCH TURPENTINE
Larix gmelinii var. gmelinii .... see LARCH ARABINOGALACTAN
Larix occidentalis .... see LARCH ARABINOGALACTAN
Lark Heel .... see DELPHINIUM
Lark's Claw .... see DELPHINIUM
Lark's Toe .... see DELPHINIUM
Larkspur .... see DELPHINIUM
Larkspur Lion's Mouth .... see YELLOW TOADFLAX
Larrea divaricata .... see CHAPARRAL
Larrea mexicana .... see CHAPARRAL
Larrea tridentata .... see CHAPARRAL
Larreastat .... see CHAPARRAL
Lasuna .... see GARLIC
Latakasthuri .... see AMBRETTE
Latakasturi .... see AMBRETTE
Lathakasthuri .... see AMBRETTE
LATHYRUS .... see LATHYRUS
Lathyrus cicera .... see LATHYRUS
Lathyrus clymenum .... see LATHYRUS
Lathyrus hirsutus .... see LATHYRUS
Lathyrus incanus .... see LATHYRUS
Lathyrus odoratus .... see LATHYRUS
Lathyrus pusillus .... see LATHYRUS
Lathyrus sativus .... see LATHYRUS
Lathyrus sylvestris .... see LATHYRUS
Laurel .... see MOUNTAIN LAUREL, SWEET BAY
Laurel Camphor .... see CAMPHOR
Laurel Willow .... see WILLOW BARK
LAURELWOOD .... see LAURELWOOD
Laurocerasus Leaves .... see CHERRY LAUREL WATER
Laurocerasus officinalis .... see CHERRY LAUREL WATER
Laurocerasus ottinii .... see CHERRY LAUREL WATER
Laurocerasus vulgaris .... see CHERRY LAUREL WATER
Laurus albida .... see SASSAFRAS
Laurus camphora .... see CAMPHOR
Laurus Cinnamomum .... see CINNAMON bark
Laurus nobilis .... see SWEET BAY
Laurus persea .... see AVOCADO
Laurus winteriana .... see CANELLA
Lavandula angustifolia .... see LAVENDER
Lavandula dentata .... see LAVENDER
Lavandula latifolia .... see LAVENDER
Lavandula officinalis .... see LAVENDER
Lavandula pubescens .... see LAVENDER
Lavandula spica .... see LAVENDER
Lavandula stoechas .... see LAVENDER
Lavandula vera .... see LAVENDER
Lavanga .... see CLOVE dried flowerbud, leaf, stem, CLOVE OIL
LAVENDER .... see LAVENDER
LAVENDER COTTON .... see LAVENDER COTTON
Lavose .... see LOVAGE
Lawsonia alba .... see HENNA
Lawsonia inermis .... see HENNA
Layor Carang .... see AGAR
LC-1 .... see LACTOBACILLUS
Leaves of the Virgin Shepherdess .... see DIVINER'S SAGE
Leberbluemchenkraut .... see LIVERWORT
Leberkraut .... see HEMP AGRIMONY
Leche de Higueron .... see FICIN
Leche de Oje .... see FICIN
LECI PS .... see PHOSPHATIDYLSERINE
LECITHIN .... see LECITHIN

INDEX

Lecithin Phosphatidylserine .... see PHOSPHATIDYLSERINE
Ledi Palustris Herba .... see MARSH TEA
Ledum groenlandicum .... see LABRADOR TEA
Ledum latifolium .... see LABRADOR TEA
Ledum palustre .... see MARSH TEA
Legalon .... see MILK THISTLE
Legume .... see BEAN POD, CALABAR BEAN, LABURNUM, PRECATORY BEAN, SOY, SOYBEAN OIL, TONKA BEAN
Lei Gong Teng .... see THUNDER GOD VINE
Lei-kung T'eng .... see THUNDER GOD VINE
Leimmistel .... see EUROPEAN MISTLETOE
Leinsamen .... see FLAXSEED
Lemna minor .... see DUCKWEED
LEMON .... see LEMON
LEMON BALM .... see LEMON BALM
LEMON VERBENA .... see LEMON VERBENA
Lemon Walnut .... see BUTTERNUT
LEMONGRASS .... see LEMONGRASS
Lemon-scented Verbena .... see LEMON VERBENA
Lent Lily .... see DAFFODIL
Lenticus edodes .... see LENTINAN, SHIITAKE MUSHROOM
LENTINAN .... see LENTINAN
Lentinan .... see LENTINAN, BETA GLUCANS
Lentinan edodes .... see LENTINAN, SHIITAKE MUSHROOM
Lentinula .... see SHIITAKE MUSHROOM
Lentinula edodes .... see LENTINAN, SHIITAKE MUSHROOM
Lentinus edodes .... see SHIITAKE MUSHROOM
Lentisk .... see MASTIC
Leontodon taraxacum .... see DANDELION above ground parts, DANDELION entire plant
Leontopodium .... see ALCHEMILLA
Leonuri Cardiacae Herba .... see MOTHERWORT
Leonurus .... see MOTHERWORT
Leonurus cardiaca .... see MOTHERWORT
Leopard's Bane .... see ARNICA
Leopard's Foot .... see MARSH MARIGOLD
Lepidium meyenii .... see MACA
Lepidium peruvianum .... see MACA
Lepidium sativum .... see GARDEN CRESS
Leptandra virginica .... see BLACK ROOT
Lesser calamint .... see CALAMINT
LESSER CELANDINE .... see LESSER CELANDINE
Lesser Centauru .... see CENTAURY
Lesser Dodder .... see DODDER
Lesser Galangal .... see ALPINIA
Lesser Hemlock .... see FOOL'S PARSLEY
Lesser Periwinkle .... see PERIWINKLE
Lettsomia nervosa .... see HAWAIIAN BABY WOODROSE
Lettuce Opium .... see WILD LETTUCE
Leucine .... see BRANCHED-CHAIN AMINO ACIDS
Leucoanthocyanidins .... see PYCNOGENOL
Leucoanthocyanin .... see GRAPE seed
Levacecarnine .... see ACETYL-L-CARNITINE
Levant .... see WORMSEED
LEVANT BERRY .... see LEVANT BERRY
Levant Nut .... see LEVANT BERRY
Levant Salep .... see SALEP
Levant Storax .... see STORAX
Levistici Radix .... see LOVAGE
Levisticum officinale .... see LOVAGE
Levocarnitine .... see L-CARNITINE
Levoglutamide .... see GLUTAMINE
Levoglutamine .... see GLUTAMINE
Levo-histidine .... see HISTIDINE
Levure de Biere .... see BREWER'S YEAST
Li .... see LITHIUM
LI 132 .... see HAWTHORN
Lian Fang .... see LOTUS flower
Lian Xu .... see LOTUS flower
Lian Zi .... see LOTUS seed
Liatris .... see DEERTONGUE
Liatris callilepis .... see MARSH BLAZING STAR
Liatris spicata .... see MARSH BLAZING STAR
Lichen islandicus .... see ICELAND MOSS
Lichen Oak Moss .... see OAK MOSS
Lichwort .... see PELLITORY-OF-THE-WALL
LICORICE .... see LICORICE
Licorice Root .... see LICORICE
Life Everlasting .... see CAT'S FOOT
Life of Man .... see AMERICAN SPIKENARD
Life Root .... see ALPINE RAGWORT, GOLDEN RAGWORT
Life-giving Vine of Peru .... see CAT'S CLAW
Life-of-man .... see AMERICAN SPIKENARD
Liferoot .... see ALPINE RAGWORT, GOLDEN RAGWORT
Light Kaolin .... see KAOLIN
Lignum rhodium .... see ROSEROOT
Ligusticum levisticum .... see LOVAGE
Ligusticum porteri .... see OSHA
Ligustilides .... see DONG QUAI
Ligustro .... see GLOSSY PRIVET
Ligustrum .... see GLOSSY PRIVET
Ligustrum Fruit .... see GLOSSY PRIVET
Ligustrum lucidum .... see GLOSSY PRIVET
Lilium candidum .... see WHITE LILY
Lilium martagon .... see MARTAGON
Lily .... see LILY-OF-THE-VALLEY
Lily of the Desert .... see ALOE latex
LILY-OF-THE-VALLEY .... see LILY-OF-THE-VALLEY
Lime .... see LIME fruit, peel
Lime Blossom .... see LINDEN dried flower
Lime Flower .... see LINDEN dried flower
LIME fruit, peel .... see LIME fruit, peel
LIME OIL .... see LIME OIL
Lime Tree .... see LINDEN CHARCOAL, LINDEN dried flower, LINDEN dried leaf, LINDEN dried sapwood
Limette .... see LIME fruit, peel
Limette Turanj .... see LIME OIL
Limon .... see LEMON
Limonia aurantiifolia .... see LIME fruit, peel; LIME OIL
Limonnik Kitajskij .... see SCHISANDRA
Linaria vulgaris .... see YELLOW TOADFLAX
Linden .... see LINDEN dried flower, LINDEN dried leaf, LINDEN dried sapwood, LINDEN CHARCOAL
LINDEN CHARCOAL .... see LINDEN CHARCOAL
LINDEN dried flower .... see LINDEN dried flower

INDEX

LINDEN dried leaf ... see LINDEN dried leaf
LINDEN dried sapwood ... see LINDEN dried sapwood
Linden Tree ... see LINDEN dried flower
Linden Wood ... see LINDEN dried sapwood
Ling ... see HEATHER
Ling Chih ... see REISHI MUSHROOM
Ling Zhi ... see REISHI MUSHROOM
Lingen ... see ALPINE CRANBERRY
Lingenberry ... see ALPINE CRANBERRY
Lingon ... see ALPINE CRANBERRY
Lingonberry ... see ALPINE CRANBERRY
Lingum Vitae ... see GUAIAC WOOD resin, wood
Lini Semen ... see FLAXSEED
Linoleic Acid ... see CONJUGATED LINOLEIC ACID, EVENING PRIMROSE OIL, FLAXSEED OIL
Linseed ... see FLAXSEED
Linseed Oil ... see FLAXSEED OIL
Lint Bells ... see FLAXSEED
Linum ... see FLAXSEED
Linum catharticum ... see MOUNTAIN FLAX
Linum crepitans ... see FLAXSEED, FLAXSEED OIL
Linum humile ... see FLAXSEED, FLAXSEED OIL
Linum usitatissimum ... see FLAXSEED, FLAXSEED OIL
Lion's Ear ... see MOTHERWORT
Lion's Foot ... see ALCHEMILLA
Lion's Mouth ... see DIGITALIS
Lion's Tail ... see MOTHERWORT
Lion's Tooth ... see DANDELION above ground parts, DANDELION entire plant
LIPASE ... see LIPASE
Lipoic Acid ... see ALPHA-LIPOIC ACID
Lipoicin ... see ALPHA-LIPOIC ACID
Lipositol ... see INOSITOL
Lipotropic Factor ... see CHOLINE
Lippia citrodora ... see LEMON VERBENA
Lippia triphylla ... see LEMON VERBENA
Lipstick Tree ... see ANNATTO
Liquid Amber ... see STORAX
Liquid Liver Extract ... see LIVER EXTRACT
Liquid Oxygen ... see VITAMIN O
Liquid Storax ... see STORAX
Liquidambar macrophylla ... see STORAX
Liquidambar orientalis ... see STORAX
Liquidambar styraciflua ... see STORAX
Liquiritiae Radix ... see LICORICE
Liquirizia ... see LICORICE
Liquorice ... see LICORICE
LITHIUM ... see LITHIUM
Lithium Carbonate ... see LITHIUM
Lithium Citrate ... see LITHIUM
Lithium Orotate ... see LITHIUM
Lithospermum lehmanii ... see ALKANNA
Little Dragon ... see TARRAGON
Little Pollom ... see BITTER MILKWORT
Live Culture Yogurt ... see YOGURT
Liveforever ... see HOUSELEEK
Liver ... see LIVER EXTRACT
Liver Concentrate ... see LIVER EXTRACT
LIVER EXTRACT ... see LIVER EXTRACT
Liver Factors ... see LIVER EXTRACT
Liver Fractions ... see LIVER EXTRACT
Liver Hydrolysate ... see LIVER EXTRACT
Liver Lily ... see ORRIS
Liver Oil ... see COD LIVER OIL
Liver Substance ... see LIVER EXTRACT
Liverleaf ... see LIVERWORT
Liverweed ... see LIVERWORT
LIVERWORT ... see LIVERWORT
Liverwort ... see AGRIMONY, LIVERWORT
Liverwort-leaf ... see LIVERWORT
Lizard's Tail ... see YERBA MANSA
Lizzy-run-up-the-hedge ... see GROUND IVY
LNA ... see ALPHA-LINOLENIC ACID
Lobaria pulmonaria ... see LUNGMOSS
LOBELIA ... see LOBELIA
Lobelia inflata ... see LOBELIA
Lobelie ... see LOBELIA
Lobster Flower Plant ... see POINSETTIA
Lobsterplant ... see POINSETTIA
Lochnera rosea ... see MADAGASCAR PERIWINKLE
Locoweed ... see JIMSON WEED
Locust Bean ... see CAROB
Locust Pods ... see CAROB
LOGWOOD ... see LOGWOOD
Lolium temulentum ... see TAUMELLOOLCH
Long Birthwort ... see ARISTOLOCHIA
Long Pepper ... see INDIAN LONG PEPPER, KAVA
Long Purples ... see PURPLE LOOSESTRIFE
Long-chain Oligosaccharides ... see INULIN
Longwort ... see MULLEIN
Lonicera ... see HONEYSUCKLE
Lonicera aureoreticulata ... see HONEYSUCKLE
Lonicera caprifolia ... see HONEYSUCKLE
Lonicera japonica ... see HONEYSUCKLE
Lonicera marilandica ... see PINK ROOT
Loofa ... see LUFFA
Loofah ... see LUFFA
LOOSESTRIFE ... see LOOSESTRIFE
Loosestrife ... see LOOSESTRIFE, PURPLE LOOSESTRIFE
Lophophora williamsii ... see PEYOTE
Lorbeerweide ... see WILLOW BARK
Lords and Ladies ... see ARUM
LORENZO'S OIL ... see LORENZO'S OIL
Lotus ... see LOTUS flower, LOTUS seed
LOTUS flower ... see LOTUS flower
LOTUS seed ... see LOTUS seed
Louisa ... see LEMON VERBENA
Louisiana Long Pepper ... see CAPSICUM
Louisiana Sport Pepper ... see CAPSICUM
Louseberry ... see LEVANT BERRY
Lousewort ... see STAVESACRE
LOVAGE ... see LOVAGE
Love Apple ... see TOMATO
Love Bean ... see PRECATORY BEAN
Love in a Mist ... see BLACK SEED
Love in Winter ... see PIPSISSEWA
Love Leaves ... see BURDOCK
Love Parsley ... see LOVAGE
Love-lies-bleeding ... see AMARANTH
Lovely Bleeding ... see AMARANTH
Love-man ... see CLIVERS
Low Balm ... see OSWEGO TEA
Low Chamomile ... see ROMAN CHAMOMILE
Lowbush Blueberry ... see BLUEBERRY
Lowbush Cranberry ... see ALPINE CRANBERRY
LPC ... see PROPIONYL-L-CARNITINE

Lu Rong .... see DEER VELVET
Lu Song Guo .... see IGNATIUS BEAN
Lucerne .... see ALFALFA
Lucky Bean .... see PRECATORY BEAN
Luei Gong Gen .... see GOTU KOLA
LUFFA .... see LUFFA
Luffa acutangula .... see LUFFA
Luffa aegyptiaca .... see LUFFA
Luffa cylindrica .... see LUFFA
Luffaschwamm .... see LUFFA
Lu-hui .... see ALOE latex
Luma chequen .... see CHEKEN
Lungenkraut .... see LUNGWORT
LUNGMOSS .... see LUNGMOSS
LUNGWORT .... see LUNGWORT
Lungwort .... see LUNGMOSS, LUNGWORT
Luoling .... see MORINDA
Lupin Jaune .... see YELLOW LUPIN
Lupinus luteus .... see YELLOW LUPIN
Lupuli Strobulus .... see HOPS
Lurk-in-the-ditch .... see PENNYROYAL leaf, PENNYROYAL OIL
Lustwort .... see SUNDEW
Luteal Hormone .... see PROGESTERONE
LUTEIN .... see LUTEIN
Luteohormone .... see PROGESTERONE
Lutine .... see PROGESTERONE
Lycii Berries .... see LYCIUM
LYCIUM .... see LYCIUM
Lycium barbarum .... see LYCIUM
Lycium chinense .... see LYCIUM
LYCOPENE .... see LYCOPENE
Lycoperdon sp. .... see PUFF BALL
Lycopersicon esculentum .... see TOMATO
Lycopi Herba .... see BUGLEWEED
Lycopodium .... see CLUB MOSS
Lycopodium clavatum .... see CLUB MOSS
Lycopus americanus .... see BUGLEWEED
Lycopus europaeus .... see BUGLEWEED
Lycopus virginicus .... see BUGLEWEED
Lyngbya wollei .... see BLUE-GREEN ALGAE
Lys .... see LYSINE
Lysimachia nummularia .... see MONEYWORT
Lysimachia vulgaris .... see LOOSESTRIFE
LYSINE .... see LYSINE
Lysine Hydrochloride .... see LYSINE
Lysine Monohydrochloride .... see LYSINE
Lythrum .... see PURPLE LOOSESTRIFE
Lythrum salicaria .... see PURPLE LOOSESTRIFE
M Mei Gee .... see SCHISANDRA
Ma Bian Cao .... see VERBENA
Ma Huang .... see EPHEDRA
Ma Huang Root .... see EPHEDRA
MACA .... see MACA
Maca Maca .... see MACA
Macambo .... see CANELLA
Mace .... see NUTMEG AND MACE
Macis .... see NUTMEG AND MACE
Mackerel Mint .... see SPEARMINT
Macochihua .... see IPORURU
Macrocystis pyrifera .... see ALGIN
Macrotys .... see BLACK COHOSH
Mad Weed .... see SKULLCAP
Madagascar Cinnamon .... see CINNAMON bark
Madagascar Lemongrass .... see LEMONGRASS
MADAGASCAR PERIWINKLE .... see MADAGASCAR PERIWINKLE
Madagascar Vanilla .... see VANILLA
Mad-apple .... see JIMSON WEED
MADDER .... see MADDER
Mad-dog Skullcap .... see SKULLCAP
Mad-dog Weed .... see WATER PLANTAIN
Madecassol .... see GOTU KOLA
Madelonitrile .... see APRICOT
Madhunashini .... see GYMNEMA
Madhura .... see DILL above ground parts, DILL seed
Madnep .... see MASTERWORT
Madonna Lily .... see WHITE LILY
Madre Selva .... see PASSIONFLOWER
Madrepora sp. .... see CORAL
Madreselva .... see HONEYSUCKLE
Magadhi .... see INDIAN LONG PEPPER
Magdalena .... see MADAGASCAR PERIWINKLE
Maggi Plant .... see LOVAGE
Magnesia .... see MAGNESIUM
MAGNESIUM .... see MAGNESIUM
Magnesium Aspartate .... see MAGNESIUM
Magnesium Carbonate .... see MAGNESIUM
Magnesium Chloride .... see MAGNESIUM
Magnesium Citrate .... see MAGNESIUM
Magnesium Gluconate .... see MAGNESIUM
Magnesium Hydroxide .... see MAGNESIUM
Magnesium Lactate .... see MAGNESIUM
Magnesium Orotate .... see MAGNESIUM
Magnesium Oxide .... see MAGNESIUM
Magnesium Pyruvate .... see PYRUVATE
Magnesium Sulfate .... see MAGNESIUM
Magnesium Trisilicate .... see MAGNESIUM
MAGNOLIA .... see MAGNOLIA
Magnolia biondii .... see MAGNOLIA
Magnolia conspicua .... see MAGNOLIA
Magnolia denudata .... see MAGNOLIA
Magnolia emargenata .... see MAGNOLIA
Magnolia fargesii .... see MAGNOLIA
Magnolia glauca .... see MAGNOLIA
Magnolia heptaperta .... see MAGNOLIA
Magnolia hypoleuca .... see MAGNOLIA
Magnolia nicholsoniana .... see MAGNOLIA
Magnolia obovata .... see MAGNOLIA
Magnolia officinalis .... see MAGNOLIA
Magnolia proctoriana .... see MAGNOLIA
Magnolia salicifolia .... see MAGNOLIA
Magnolia sargentiana .... see MAGNOLIA
Magnolia sprengeri .... see MAGNOLIA
Magnolia taliensis .... see MAGNOLIA
Magnolia Vine .... see SCHISANDRA
Magnolia virginiana .... see MAGNOLIA
Magnolia wilsonii .... see MAGNOLIA
Magnolia yulan .... see MAGNOLIA
Mahajambu .... see JAMBOLAN bark
Mahogany .... see ANDIROBA, LAURELWOOD
Mahonia aquifolium .... see OREGON GRAPE
Mahonia diversifolia .... see OREGON GRAPE
Mahonia nervosa .... see OREGON GRAPE
Mahonia repens .... see OREGON GRAPE
Mahonia sonnei .... see OREGON GRAPE
Mahuanggen .... see EPHEDRA
Mai Ya .... see BARLEY

Maiden Fern .... see MAIDENHAIR FERN
MAIDENHAIR FERN .... see MAIDENHAIR FERN
Maidenhair Tree .... see GINKGO leaf (GINKGO leaf extract), GINKGO seed
Maidis Stigma .... see CORN SILK
Maid's Hair .... see LADY'S BEDSTRAW
Maino .... see MACA
Maitake .... see MAITAKE MUSHROOM
MAITAKE MUSHROOM ... see MAITAKE MUSHROOM
Maize Pollen .... see BEE POLLEN
Maize Silk .... see CORN SILK
Majoran .... see MARJORAM
Majorana Aetheroleum Oil .... see MARJORAM
Majorana Herb .... see MARJORAM
Majorana hortensis .... see MARJORAM
Majorana majorana .... see MARJORAM
Maka .... see MACA
Makombu Thallus .... see LAMINARIA
MALABAR NUT .... see MALABAR NUT
Malabar Tamarind .... see GARCINIA
MALE FERN .... see MALE FERN
Malic Acid .... see ALPHA HYDROXY ACIDS
Mallaguetta Pepper .... see GRAINS OF PARADISE
Mallards .... see MARSHMALLOW
Mallotus philippensis .... see KAMALA
Mallow .... see MALLOW flower, MALLOW leaf
MALLOW flower .... see MALLOW flower
MALLOW leaf .... see MALLOW leaf
Malohu .... see KAVA
Malpighia glabra .... see ACEROLA
Malpighia punicifolia .... see ACEROLA
Maluk .... see KAVA
Malus sylvestris .... see APPLE, APPLE CIDER VINEGAR
Malva .... see HOLLYHOCK
Malva Flower .... see HOLLYHOCK
Malva mauritiana .... see MALLOW flower, MALLOW leaf
Malva neglecta .... see MALLOW leaf
Malva rotundifolia .... see MALLOW leaf
Malva sylvestris ...... see MALLOW flower, MALLOW leaf
Malvae Arboreae Flos .... see HOLLYHOCK
Malvae Flos .... see MALLOW flower
Malvae Folium .... see MALLOW leaf
Mamaerie .... see PAPAYA
MANACA .... see MANACA
Manchurian Fungus .... see KOMBUCHA TEA
Manchurian Mushroom Tea .... see KOMBUCHA TEA
Mandragora .... see EUROPEAN MANDRAKE
Mandragora officinarum .... see EUROPEAN MANDRAKE
Mandragora vernalis .... see EUROPEAN MANDRAKE
Mandragore .... see EUROPEAN MANDRAKE
Mandrake .... see EUROPEAN MANDRAKE, PODOPHYLLUM
Manduk Parani .... see GOTU KOLA
Mandukaparni .... see GOTU KOLA
Mang Cut .... see MANGOSTEEN
MANGANESE .... see MANGANESE
Manganese Amino Acid Chelate .... see MANGANESE
Manganese Aminoate .... see MANGANESE
Manganese Ascorbate .... see MANGANESE
Manganese Aspartate Complex .... see MANGANESE
Manganese Chloride .... see MANGANESE
Manganese Chloridetetrahydrate .... see MANGANESE
Manganese Dioxide .... see MANGANESE
Manganese Gluconate .... see MANGANESE
Manganese Sulfate .... see MANGANESE
Manganese Sulfate Monohydrate .... see MANGANESE
Manganese Sulfate Tetrahydrate .... see MANGANESE
Manganum .... see MANGANESE
Mangel .... see BEET
Manggis .... see MANGOSTEEN
Manggistan .... see MANGOSTEEN
Mangold .... see BEET
Mangosta .... see MANGOSTEEN
Mangostan .... see MANGOSTEEN
Mangostana .... see MANGOSTEEN
Mangostana cambogia .... see GARCINIA
Mangostanier .... see MANGOSTEEN
Mangostao .... see MANGOSTEEN
MANGOSTEEN .... see MANGOSTEEN
Mangostier .... see MANGOSTEEN
Mangoustanier .... see MANGOSTEEN
Mangouste .... see MANGOSTEEN
Manguita .... see MANGOSTEEN
Manila Elemi .... see ELEMI
MANNA .... see MANNA
Manna Ash .... see MANNA
Mannentake .... see REISHI MUSHROOM
Manzanilla .... see GERMAN CHAMOMILE, ROMAN CHAMOMILE
Manzanita .... see UVA URSI
Maori Kava .... see KAVA
Mapato .... see RHATANY
Maracuja .... see PASSIONFLOWER
Maranhao Jaborandi .... see JABORANDI
Maranta .... see ARROWROOT
Maranta arundinacea .... see ARROWROOT
Marcory .... see QUEEN'S DELIGHT
Marginal Fern .... see MALE FERN
Margosa .... see NEEM
Marguerite .... see OX-EYE DAISY
Marian Thistle .... see MILK THISTLE
Maricha .... see BLACK PEPPER AND WHITE PEPPER
Mariendistel .... see MILK THISTLE
Marienmantel .... see ALCHEMILLA
Marigold .... see CALENDULA, TAGETES
Marigold of Peru .... see SUNFLOWER OIL
Mariguana .... see MARIJUANA
Marihuana .... see MARIJUANA
MARIJUANA .... see MARIJUANA
Marine Oils .... see FISH OILS
Marjolaine .... see MARJORAM
MARJORAM .... see MARJORAM
Markweed .... see POISON IVY
Marmelo .... see QUINCE
Marron Europeen .... see HORSE CHESTNUT
Marrubii Herba .... see WHITE HOREHOUND
Marrubium .... see WHITE HOREHOUND
Marrubium vulgare .... see WHITE HOREHOUND
Marsdenia cundurango .... see CONDURANGO
Marsdenia reichenbachii .... see CONDURANGO
MARSH BLAZING STAR .... see MARSH BLAZING STAR
Marsh Citrus .... see MARSH TEA
MARSH MARIGOLD .... see MARSH MARIGOLD
Marsh Mint .... see WILD MINT
Marsh Penny .... see GOTU KOLA
MARSH TEA .... see MARSH TEA

INDEX

Marsh Trefoil see BOGBEAN
MARSHMALLOW see MARSHMALLOW
MARTAGON see MARTAGON
Mary Jane see MARIJUANA
Mary Thistle see MILK THISTLE
Marybud see CALENDULA
Maryland Pink see PINK ROOT
Master of the Wood see SWEET WOODRUFF
MASTERWORT see MASTERWORT
Masterwort see GOUTWEED, MASTERWORT
MASTIC see MASTIC
Mastich see MASTIC
Mastix see MASTIC
Mastranzo see WHITE HOREHOUND
MATE see MATE
Mate de Coca see COCA
Mate Folium see MATE
Matricaire see GERMAN CHAMOMILE
Matricaria chamomilla see GERMAN CHAMOMILE
Matricaria eximia see FEVERFEW
Matricaria morifolia see CHRYSANTHEMUM
Matricaria parthenium see FEVERFEW
Matricaria recutita see GERMAN CHAMOMILE
Matricariae Flos see GERMAN CHAMOMILE
Matrimony Vine see LYCIUM
Matsbouza see SCHISANDRA
Matsuhodo see PORIA MUSHROOM
Matteuccia struthiopteris see OSTRICH FERN
Matto Grosso Ipecac see IPECAC
Maudlin Daisy see OX-EYE DAISY
Maudlinwort see OX-EYE DAISY
Mauls see MALLOW flower
May see HAWTHORN
May Bells see LILY-OF-THE-VALLEY
May Lily see LILY-OF-THE-VALLEY
Mayapple see PODOPHYLLUM
Maybush see HAWTHORN
Mayflower see COWSLIP
Maypop see PASSIONFLOWER
Maypop Passion Flower see PASSIONFLOWER
Maythorn see HAWTHORN
MCT see MEDIUM CHAIN TRIGLYCERIDES (MCT)
Meadow-wart see MEADOWSWEET
Meadow Anenome see PULSATILLA
Meadow Buttercup see BUTTERCUP
Meadow Cabbage see SKUNK CABBAGE
Meadow Clover see RED CLOVER
Meadow Lily see WHITE LILY
Meadow Queen see MEADOWSWEET
Meadow Routs see MARSH MARIGOLD
Meadow Runagates see MONEYWORT
Meadow Saffran see AUTUMN CROCUS
Meadow Sage see SAGE
Meadow Windflower see PULSATILLA
Meadowbloom see BULBOUS BUTTERCUP, BUTTERCUP
MEADOWSWEET see MEADOWSWEET
Mealy Kudzu see KUDZU
Mechoacan see JALAP
Medhika see FENUGREEK
Medicago see ALFALFA
Medicago sativa see ALFALFA
Medicinal Charcoal see ACTIVATED CHARCOAL
Medicinal Rhubarb see RHUBARB
Medicinal Yeast see BREWER'S YEAST
Mediterranean Bay see SWEET BAY
Mediterranean Oregano see OREGANO
Mediterranean Squill see SQUILL
MEDIUM CHAIN TRIGLYCERIDES (MCT) see MEDIUM CHAIN TRIGLYCERIDES (MCT)
Meerdorn see SEA BUCKTHORN
Meereiche see BLADDERWRACK
Meerrettich see HORSERADISH
Mehlbeebaum see HAWTHORN
Mehndi see HENNA
Meidorn see HAWTHORN
Mejorana see MARJORAM
Mel see HONEY, MELATONIN
Melaleuca leucadendra see CAJEPUT OIL
Melaleuca alternifolia see TEA TREE OIL
Melaleuca Oil see TEA TREE OIL
Melaleuca quinquenervia see CAJEPUT OIL
Melaleuca viridiflora see NIAULI OIL
Melampode see BLACK HELLEBORE
MELANOTAN-II see MELANOTAN-II
MELATONIN see MELATONIN
Melegueta Pepper see GRAINS OF PARADISE
Meletin see QUERCETIN
Melia azadirachta see NEEM
Melilot see SWEET CLOVER
Meliloti Herba see SWEET CLOVER
Melilotus see SWEET CLOVER
Melilotus altissimus see SWEET CLOVER
Melilotus arvensis see SWEET CLOVER
Melilotus macrorrhizus see SWEET CLOVER
Melilotus officinalis see SWEET CLOVER
Melilotus vulgaris see SWEET CLOVER
Melissa see LEMON BALM
Melissa nepeta see CALAMINT
Melissa officinalis see LEMON BALM
Melissa pulegioides see PENNYROYAL leaf, PENNYROYAL OIL
Melissae Folium see LEMON BALM
Melissenblatt see LEMON BALM
Melon Tree see PAPAYA
Melonenbaumblaetter see PAPAYA
Membranous Milk Vetch see ASTRAGALUS
Membrillo see QUINCE
Memeniran see CHANCA PIEDRA
Menadiol Acetate see VITAMIN K
Menadione see VITAMIN K
Menaquinone see VITAMIN K
Mendee see HENNA
Mengkudu see MORINDA
Menhaden Oil see FISH OILS
Meniran see CHANCA PIEDRA
Menispermum cocculus see LEVANT BERRY
Menispermum columba see COLOMBO
Menispermum lacunosum see LEVANT BERRY
Menispermum palmatum see COLOMBO
Menkoedoe see MORINDA
Menta de Gato see CATNIP
Mentha aquatica see WILD MINT
Mentha arvensis aetheroleum see JAPANESE MINT
Mentha arvensis var. piperascens see JAPANESE MINT
Mentha cablin see PATCHOULY OIL
Mentha canadensis see JAPANESE MINT
Mentha cordifolia see SPEARMINT

Mentha crispa .... see SPEARMINT
Mentha lavanduliodora .... see PEPPERMINT leaf, PEPPERMINT OIL
Mentha longifolia .... see ENGLISH HORSEMINT
Mentha palustris .... see WILD MINT
Mentha piperita .... see PEPPERMINT leaf, PEPPERMINT OIL
Mentha pulegium .... see PENNYROYAL leaf, PENNYROYAL OIL
Mentha spicata .... see SPEARMINT
Mentha sylvestris .... see ENGLISH HORSEMINT
Mentha viridis .... see SPEARMINT
Menthae piperitae aetheroleum .... see PEPPERMINT OIL
Menthae Piperitae Folium .... see PEPPERMINT leaf
Menthe Poivree .... see PEPPERMINT leaf, PEPPERMINT OIL
MENTZELIA .... see MENTZELIA
Mentzelia cordifolia .... see MENTZELIA
Menyanthes .... see BOGBEAN
Menyanthes trifoliata .... see BOGBEAN
Merasingi .... see GYMNEMA
Mercurialis annua .... see MERCURY HERB
MERCURY HERB .... see MERCURY HERB
Merlot .... see GRAPE fruit, skin
Meruk .... see KAVA
Mescal Buttons .... see PEYOTE
Mescaline .... see PEYOTE
Meseter .... see MANGOSTEEN
Meshashringi .... see GYMNEMA
Meso-inositol .... see INOSITOL
Meso-inositol Hexanicotinate .... see INOSITOL NICOTINATE
Meso-xylitol .... see XYLITOL
MESOGLYCAN .... see MESOGLYCAN
Mespilus laevigata .... see HAWTHORN
Metavanadate .... see VANADIUM
Methi .... see FENUGREEK
METHIONINE .... see METHIONINE
Methoxyflavones .... see METHOXYLATED FLAVONES
METHOXYLATED FLAVONES .... see METHOXYLATED FLAVONES
Methyl Sulfone .... see MSM (METHYLSULFONYLMETHANE)
Methyl Sulphoxide .... see DMSO (DIMETHYLSULFOXIDE)
Methylated Phosphatidylethanolamine .... see CHOLINE
Methylcobalamin .... see VITAMIN B12
Methylphytyl Naphthoquinone .... see VITAMIN K
Methyl-sulfonyl-methane .... see MSM (METHYLSULFONYLMETHANE)
Methylxanthine .... see CAFFEINE
Mexican Chilies .... see CAPSICUM
Mexican Damiana .... see DAMIANA
Mexican Flame Leaf .... see POINSETTIA
Mexican Marigold .... see TAGETES
Mexican Sage .... see DIVINER'S SAGE
Mexican Sage Incense .... see DIVINER'S SAGE
Mexican Sanguinaria .... see KNOTWEED
Mexican Sarsaparilla .... see SARSAPARILLA
MEXICAN SCAMMONY ROOT .... see MEXICAN SCAMMONY ROOT
Mexican Tea .... see CHENOPODIUM OIL
Mexican Valerian .... see VALERIAN
Mexican Vanilla .... see VANILLA
Mexican Yam .... see WILD YAM
Mexico Weed .... see CASTOR OIL, CASTOR seed
MEZEREON .... see MEZEREON
MFP .... see FLUORIDE
Mg .... see MAGNESIUM
MGN-3 .... see MGN-3
Microalgae .... see ASTAXANTHIN
Microcystis aeruginosa .... see BLUE-GREEN ALGAE
Microcystis wesenbergii .... see BLUE-GREEN ALGAE
Middle Comfrey .... see BUGLE
Middle Confound .... see BUGLE
Miel Blanc .... see HONEY
Mignonette Tree .... see HENNA
Milefolio .... see YARROW
Milfoil .... see YARROW
Milik .... see KAVA
Milium nigricans .... see BROOM CORN
Milk Ipecac .... see BETH ROOT, CANADIAN HEMP
Milk of Magnesia .... see MAGNESIUM
MILK THISTLE .... see MILK THISTLE
Milk Thistle Fruit .... see MILK THISTLE
Milk Thistle Seed .... see MILK THISTLE
Milk Vetch .... see ASTRAGALUS
Milk Willow-herb .... see PURPLE LOOSESTRIFE
Milkweed .... see CANADIAN HEMP
Milkwort .... see SENEGA
Mill Mint .... see CALAMINT
Mill Mountain .... see MOUNTAIN FLAX
Millefeuille .... see YARROW
Millefolii Flos .... see YARROW
Millefolii Herba .... see YARROW
Millefolium .... see YARROW
Millegoglie .... see YARROW
Millepertuis .... see ST. JOHN'S WORT
Mimosa catechu .... see CATECHU
Mimosa farnesiana .... see CASSIE ABSOLUTE
Mimosa senegal .... see ACACIA
Mineral Aspartates .... see ASPARTATES
Mineral-Amino Acid Complex .... see CHELATED MINERALS
Minor Centaury .... see CENTAURY
Mint Oil .... see JAPANESE MINT
Minzol .... see JAPANESE MINT
Miraa .... see KHAT
Miracle Grass .... see JIAOGULAN
Miracle Plant .... see ALOE latex, GYMNEMA
Mirchi .... see CAPSICUM
Mirobalano .... see INDIAN GOOSEBERRY
Mirobalanus embilica .... see INDIAN GOOSEBERRY
Miso .... see SOY
Mistlekraut .... see EUROPEAN MISTLETOE
Mistletein .... see EUROPEAN MISTLETOE
Mistletoe .... see AMERICAN MISTLETOE, EUROPEAN MISTLETOE
Mitchella repens .... see SQUAWVINE
Mitoquinone .... see COENZYME Q-10
Mitrewort .... see COOLWORT
Mixed Fruit Acid .... see ALPHA HYDROXY ACIDS
Mixed Tocopherols .... see VITAMIN E
Mixed Vespids .... see BEE VENOM
Mizibcoc .... see DAMIANA
Mizu-garashi .... see WATERCRESS
MLT .... see MELATONIN
Mn .... see MANGANESE

INDEX

Moccasin Flower .... see NERVE ROOT
Mocha .... see COFFEE
Mockeel Root .... see WATER HEMLOCK
Mohave Yucca .... see YUCCA
Mokko .... see COSTUS OIL, COSTUS root
Mokkou .... see COSTUS OIL, COSTUS root
Momordica charantia .... see BITTER MELON
Momordica murcata .... see BITTER MELON
Momordique .... see BITTER MELON
Monarda .... see OSWEGO TEA
Monarda didyma .... see OSWEGO TEA
Monarda lutea .... see HORSEMINT
Monarda punctata .... see HORSEMINT
Monascus .... see RED YEAST
Monascus purpureus .... see RED YEAST
Monazol .... see GLYCINE
MONEYWORT .... see MONEYWORT
Mongolian Ephedra .... see EPHEDRA
Mongolian Larch .... see LARCH ARABINOGALACTAN
Mongolian Larchwood .... see LARCH ARABINOGALACTAN
Mongolian Milk .... see ASTRAGALUS
Moniera cuneifolia .... see BRAHMI
Monkey Flower .... see NERVE ROOT, YELLOW TOADFLAX
Monkey Nuts .... see PEANUT OIL
Monkey's Bench .... see MAITAKE MUSHROOM
Monk's Pepper .... see CHASTEBERRY
Monkshood .... see ACONITE
Monkshood Tuber .... see ACONITE
Mono-carboxymethylated chitosan .... see CHITOSAN
Monofluorophosphate .... see FLUORIDE
Monohydroxysuccinic Acid .... see ALPHA HYDROXY ACIDS
Mono-sulfated saccharide .... see GLUCOSAMINE SULFATE
Monounsaturated Fatty Acid .... see OLIVE OIL
Montmorency Cherry .... see SOUR CHERRY
Moon Daisy .... see OX-EYE DAISY
Moon Flower .... see OX-EYE DAISY
Moon Penny .... see OX-EYE DAISY
Moor Grass .... see POTENTILLA
Moosbeere .... see BOG BILBERRY
Moose Elm .... see SLIPPERY ELM
Moosebeere .... see CRANBERRY
Mora de la India .... see MORINDA
Morella caroliniensis .... see BAYBERRY
Morella cerifera .... see BAYBERRY
Morella pensylvanica .... see BAYBERRY
Morello Cherry .... see SOUR CHERRY
MORINDA .... see MORINDA
Morinda .... see BA JI TIAN, MORINDA
Morinda citrifolia .... see MORINDA
Morinda officinalis .... see BA JI TIAN
Morinda Root .... see BA JI TIAN
Morindae officinalis .... see BA JI TIAN
Morindae Radix .... see BA JI TIAN
MORMON TEA .... see MORMON TEA
Moroccan Geranium Oil .... see ROSE GERANIUM OIL
Mortal .... see BITTERSWEET NIGHTSHADE
Mortification Root .... see MARSHMALLOW
Morus nigra .... see BLACK MULBERRY
Moschus moschiferus .... see MUSK
Mosquito Plant .... see PENNYROYAL leaf, PENNYROYAL OIL
Moss Cranberry .... see ALPINE CRANBERRY
Mossberry .... see CRANBERRY
Moth Herb .... see MARSH TEA
Mother of Rye .... see ERGOT
Mother of Thyme .... see WILD THYME
Mother's-heart .... see SHEPHERD'S PURSE
MOTHERWORT .... see MOTHERWORT
Mountain-grape .... see OREGON GRAPE
Mountain-sweet .... see NEW JERSEY TEA
MOUNTAIN ASH .... see MOUNTAIN ASH
Mountain Balm .... see CALAMINT, OSWEGO TEA, YERBA SANTA
Mountain Box .... see UVA URSI
Mountain Cranberry .... see UVA URSI
Mountain Damson .... see SIMARUBA
Mountain Everlasting .... see CAT'S FOOT
MOUNTAIN FLAX .... see MOUNTAIN FLAX
Mountain Geranium .... see HERB ROBERT
Mountain Grape .... see EUROPEAN BARBERRY
Mountain Hydrangea .... see HYDRANGEA
Mountain Ivy .... see MOUNTAIN LAUREL
MOUNTAIN LAUREL .... see MOUNTAIN LAUREL
Mountain Lovage .... see OSHA
Mountain Mint .... see CALAMINT, OREGANO, OSWEGO TEA
Mountain Pink .... see TRAILING ARBUTUS
Mountain Polygala .... see SENEGA
Mountain Radish .... see HORSERADISH
Mountain Savory Oil .... see WINTER SAVORY
Mountain Sorrel .... see WOOD SORREL
Mountain Strawberry .... see STRAWBERRY
Mountain Tea .... see WINTERGREEN leaf, WINTERGREEN OIL
Mountain Tobacco .... see ARNICA
Mouse Antialopecia Factor .... see INOSITOL
MOUSE EAR .... see MOUSE EAR
Mouse Ear .... see CUDWEED, MOUSE EAR
Mousetail .... see COMMON STONECROP
Mousse d'Irlande .... see CARRAGEENAN
Mouth-smart .... see BROOKLIME
Mouth Root .... see GOLDTHREAD
MSI-1256F .... see SHARK CARTILAGE
MSM (METHYLSULFONYLMETHANE) .... see MSM (METHYLSULFONYLMETHANE)
MT-II .... see MELANOTAN-II
Mu Xiang .... see COSTUS OIL, COSTUS root
Mucara .... see KARAYA GUM
Mucopolysaccharide .... see MESOGLYCAN
Mucuna .... see COWHAGE
Mucuna hirsuta .... see COWHAGE
Mucuna pruriens .... see COWHAGE
Mucuna pruriens var. hirsuta .... see COWHAGE
Mucuna prurient .... see COWHAGE
Mudar Bark .... see CALOTROPIS
Muder Yercum .... see CALOTROPIS
Mugrela .... see BLACK SEED
Muguet .... see LILY-OF-THE-VALLEY
MUGWORT .... see MUGWORT
Mugwort .... see MUGWORT, TARRAGON
MUIRA PUAMA .... see MUIRA PUAMA
Muirapuama .... see MUIRA PUAMA
Mukul Myrrh Tree .... see GUGGUL
Mulberry .... see BLACK MULBERRY, MORINDA
Mulhathi .... see LICORICE

INDEX

MULLEIN ... see MULLEIN
Multiflora Preparata ... see FO-TI
Mum ... see CHRYSANTHEMUM
Munchausia speciosa ... see BANABA
Munjariki ... see BASIL
Murillo Bark ... see QUILLAIA
Muscadier ... see NUTMEG AND MACE
Muscatel Sage ... see CLARY SAGE
Muscovy Duck ... see OSCILLOCOCCINUM
Mushroom of Immortality ... see REISHI MUSHROOM
Mushroom of Spiritual Potency ... see REISHI MUSHROOM
MUSK ... see MUSK
Musk Deer ... see MUSK
Musk Root ... see SUMBUL
Musk Seed ... see AMBRETTE
Muskadana ... see AMBRETTE
Muskat ... see GRAPE seed
Muskatbuam ... see NUTMEG AND MACE
Muskatnuss ... see NUTMEG AND MACE
Muskmallow ... see AMBRETTE
Muskrat Weed ... see WATER HEMLOCK
Musquash Root ... see WATER HEMLOCK
Mustard ... see BLACK MUSTARD seed
Mustard Oil ... see BLACK MUSTARD OIL
Mustelia eupatoria ... see STEVIA
Muster John Henry ... see TAGETES
Mutton Chops ... see CLIVERS
Muzei Ma Huang ... see EPHEDRA
Myo-inositol ... see INOSITOL
Myo-inositol Hexa-3-pyridine-carboxylate ... see INOSITOL NICOTINATE
Myosotis arvensis ... see FORGET-ME-NOT
Myrica ... see BAYBERRY
Myrica caroliniensis ... see BAYBERRY
Myrica cerifera ... see BAYBERRY
Myrica gale ... see SWEET GALE
Myrica heterophylla ... see BAYBERRY
Myrica pensylvanica ... see BAYBERRY
Myrica pumila ... see BAYBERRY
Myristica ... see NUTMEG AND MACE
Myristica fragrans ... see NUTMEG AND MACE
Myristica officinalis ... see NUTMEG AND MACE
Myristicae Aril ... see NUTMEG AND MACE
Myristicae Semen ... see NUTMEG AND MACE
Myrobalan ... see TERMINALIA
Myrobalan Emblic ... see INDIAN GOOSEBERRY
Myrobalanus bellirica ... see TERMINALIA
Myrobroma fragrans ... see VANILLA
Myrospermum pereirae ... see PERU BALSAM
Myroxylan balsamum ... see TOLU BALSAM
Myroxylan toluiferum ... see TOLU BALSAM
Myroxylon balsamum ... see TOLU BALSAM
Myroxylon pereirae ... see PERU BALSAM
MYRRH ... see MYRRH
Myrrhis odorata ... see SWEET CICELY
Myrti aetherolum ... see MYRTLE
Myrti Folium ... see MYRTLE
Myrtilli Fructus ... see BILBERRY
Myrtle ... see MADAGASCAR PERIWINKLE, MYRTLE, PERIWINKLE
Myrtle Flag ... see CALAMUS
Myrtle Flower ... see ORRIS
Myrtle Sedge ... see CALAMUS
Myrtus ... see CHEKEN
Myrtus chequen ... see CHEKEN
Myrtus communis ... see MYRTLE
Myrtus leucadendra ... see CAJEPUT OIL
Mysteria ... see AUTUMN CROCUS
Mystyldene ... see EUROPEAN MISTLETOE
N,O-sulfated chitosan ... see CHITOSAN
N-(2-furanylmethyl)-1H-purin-6-amine ... see KINETIN
N(6)furfuryladenine ... see KINETIN
N-(aminoiminomethyl)-N methyl glycine ... see CREATINE
N,N-dimethylaminoacetic acid ... see DIMETHYLGLYCINE
N,N-dimethylglycine ... see DIMETHYLGLYCINE
N-3 Fatty Acid ... see ALPHA-LINOLENIC ACID COD LIVER OIL, DHA (DOCOSAHEXAENOIC ACID), EPA (EICOSAPENTAENOIC ACID), FISH OILS
N-3 Polyunsaturated Fatty Acid ... see ALPHA-LINOLENIC ACID, FISH OILS
N-6 ... see OMEGA-6 FATTY ACIDS
N-6 EFAs ... see OMEGA-6 FATTY ACIDS
N-6 Essential Fatty Acids ... see OMEGA-6 FATTY ACIDS
N-9 Fatty Acid ... see OLIVE OIL
Nabin Chanvandi ... see ANDROGRAPHIS
NAC ... see N-ACETYL CYSTEINE
N-ACETYL CYSTEINE ... see N-ACETYL CYSTEINE
N-acetyl D-glucosamine ... see N-ACETYL GLUCOSAMINE
N-ACETYL GLUCOSAMINE ... see N-ACETYL GLUCOSAMINE
N-acetyl L-cysteine ... see N-ACETYL CYSTEINE
N-acetyl-5-methoxytryptamine ... see MELATONIN
N-acetyl-B-cysteine ... see N-ACETYL CYSTEINE
N-acetyl-carnitine ... see ACETYL-L-CARNITINE
N-ACETYL-CYSTEINE ... see N-ACETYL CYSTEINE
N-acetyl-D-glucosamine ... see N-ACETYL GLUCOSAMINE
N-acetyl-L-carnitine ... see ACETYL-L-CARNITINE
N-acetyl-L-cysteine ... see N-ACETYL CYSTEINE
N-carboxybutyl chitosan ... see CHITOSAN
N-methylsarcosine ... see DIMETHYLGLYCINE
N-octacosanol ... see OCTACOSANOL
NAD ... see NADH
NADH ... see NADH
NAG ... see N-ACETYL GLUCOSAMINE
Nagadamni ... see MUGWORT
Naked Ladies ... see AUTUMN CROCUS
N-amidinosarcosine ... see CREATINE
Nan Shanzha ... see HAWTHORN
Nangka Blanda ... see GRAVIOLA
Nangka Londa ... see GRAVIOLA
Nanny Bush ... see BLACK HAW
Nanwuweizi ... see SCHISANDRA
Narcissus pseudonarcissus ... see DAFFODIL
Narrow Dock ... see YELLOW DOCK
Narrow-leaved Purple Cone Flower ... see ECHINACEA
Nasilord ... see WATERCRESS
Nasturtii Herba ... see WATERCRESS
NASTURTIUM ... see NASTURTIUM
Nasturtium armoracia ... see HORSERADISH
Nasturtium officinale ... see WATERCRESS

INDEX

Natto ... see SOY
Natto Extract ... see NATTOKINASE
NATTOKINASE ... see NATTOKINASE
Natural DHEA ... see WILD YAM
Nature's Viagra ... see PUNCTURE VINE
Naughty Man's Cherries ... see BELLADONNA
Navel Orange ... see SWEET ORANGE
Navy Bean ... see BEAN POD
Nebraska Fern ... see HEMLOCK
Neckweed ... see BROOKLIME
Nectar of the Gods ... see GARLIC
Neelapushpa ... see SWEET VIOLET
NEEM ... see NEEM
Nees ... see CASSIA CINNAMON
Neli ... see INDIAN GOOSEBERRY
Nelumbo caspica ... see LOTUS flower, LOTUS seed
Nelumbo komarovii ... see LOTUS flower, LOTUS seed
Nelumbo nelumbo ... see LOTUS flower, LOTUS seed
Nelumbo nucifera ... see LOTUS flower, LOTUS seed
Nelumbo speciosum ... see LOTUS flower, LOTUS seed
Neopicrorhiza scrophulariiflora ... see PICRORHIZA
Neovastat ... see SHARK CARTILAGE
Nepal Ginseng ... see PANAX PSEUDOGINSENG
Nepeta cataria ... see CATNIP
Nepeta hederacea ... see GROUND IVY
Nerium indicum ... see OLEANDER
Nerium odorum ... see OLEANDER
Nerium oleander ... see OLEANDER
Neroli Oil ... see BITTER ORANGE
NERVE ROOT ... see NERVE ROOT
Netchweed ... see ARRACH
Nettle ... see STINGING NETTLE above ground parts, STINGING NETTLE root
Neuromins ... see DHA (DOCOSAHEXAENOIC ACID)
Neustanthus chinensis ... see KUDZU
Nevada Ephedra ... see MORMON TEA
NEW JERSEY TEA ... see NEW JERSEY TEA
NEW ZEALAND GREEN-LIPPED MUSSEL ... see NEW ZEALAND GREEN-LIPPED MUSSEL
Ngu Mei Gee ... see SCHISANDRA
Nhau ... see MORINDA
NIACIN AND NIACINAMIDE (VITAMIN B3) ... see NIACIN AND NIACINAMIDE (VITAMIN B3)
Niando ... see IPORURU
Niauli aetheroleum ... see NIAULI OIL
NIAULI OIL ... see NIAULI OIL
Nicamid ... see NIACIN AND NIACINAMIDE (VITAMIN B3)
Nicaragua Ipecac ... see IPECAC
Nichol Seeds ... see DIVI-DIVI
Nicosedine ... see NIACIN AND NIACINAMIDE (VITAMIN B3)
Nicotinamide ... see NIACIN AND NIACINAMIDE (VITAMIN B3)
Nicotinic Acid ... see NIACIN AND NIACINAMIDE (VITAMIN B3)
Nicotinic Acid Amide ... see NIACIN AND NIACINAMIDE (VITAMIN B3)
Nicotylamidum ... see NIACIN AND NIACINAMIDE (VITAMIN B3)
Nigella sativa ... see BLACK SEED
Nigelle de Crete ... see BLACK SEED
Night Blooming Cereus ... see CEREUS
Night Willow-herb ... see EVENING PRIMROSE OIL
Nightshade ... see JIMSON WEED
Nikkar Nuts ... see DIVI-DIVI
Nim ... see NEEM
Nimb ... see NEEM
Nimba ... see NEEM
Nimbaka ... see LEMON
Nimbuka ... see LEMON
Nindo ... see HONEYSUCKLE
Nine Hooks ... see ALCHEMILLA
Ninety-knot ... see KNOTWEED
Ning Xia Gou Qi ... see LYCIUM
Ninjin ... see GINSENG, PANAX
Nira-brahmi ... see BRAHMI
Niruri ... see CHANCA PIEDRA
Nisha ... see TURMERIC
NK ... see NATTOKINASE
Noah's Ark ... see NERVE ROOT
Nobiletin ... see METHOXYLATED FLAVONES
Noble Laurel ... see SWEET BAY
Noble Yarrow ... see YARROW
No-flush Niacin ... see INOSITOL NICOTINATE
Nogal Americano ... see BLACK WALNUT
Nogal Ceniciento ... see BUTTERNUT
Nogueira-Preta ... see BLACK WALNUT
Noisetier ... see HAZELNUT
Noix Muscade ... see NUTMEG AND MACE
Nokyong ... see DEER VELVET
Nonacosanol ... see POLICOSANOL
Noni ... see BA JI TIAN, MORINDA
Nono ... see MORINDA
Nonu ... see MORINDA
Noon Kie Oo Nah Yeah ... see SQUAWVINE
Nopal ... see PRICKLY PEAR CACTUS
Nopol ... see PRICKLY PEAR CACTUS
North American Ginseng ... see GINSENG, AMERICAN
NORTHERN PRICKLY ASH ... see NORTHERN PRICKLY ASH
Northern Schisandra ... see SCHISANDRA
Northern White Cedar ... see CEDAR leaf, CEDAR LEAF OIL
Norway Pine ... see HEMLOCK SPRUCE
Norway Spruce ... see FIR, HEMLOCK SPRUCE
Nosebleed ... see YARROW
Noyer Cerdre ... see BUTTERNUT
Noyer Noir ... see BLACK WALNUT
NSC-763 ... see DMSO (DIMETHYLSULFOXIDE)
NSC-9704 ... see PROGESTERONE
Nu Zhen ... see GLOSSY PRIVET
Nu Zhen Zi ... see GLOSSY PRIVET
Nucleic Acid ... see RNA AND DNA
Nucleotides ... see RNA AND DNA
Nuez Moscada ... see NUTMEG AND MACE
NUTMEG AND MACE ... see NUTMEG AND MACE
Nutmeg Flower ... see BLACK SEED
Nux Moschata ... see NUTMEG AND MACE
NUX VOMICA ... see NUX VOMICA
Nuzhenzi ... see GLOSSY PRIVET
Nymphaea maximilianii ... see AMERICAN WHITE POND LILY
Nymphaea nelumbo ... see LOTUS flower, LOTUS seed
Nymphaea odorata ... see AMERICAN WHITE POND LILY
Nymphaea rosea ... see AMERICAN WHITE POND LILY

INDEX

NZGLM .... see NEW ZEALAND GREEN-LIPPED MUSSEL
O-sulfated N-acetylchitosan .... see CHITOSAN
Oak .... see OAK bark
OAK bark .... see OAK bark
Oak Fern .... see LADY FERN
Oak Lungs .... see LUNGMOSS
OAK MOSS .... see OAK MOSS
Oat .... see OAT above ground parts, OAT BRAN, OAT STRAW, OATS
OAT above ground parts .... see OAT above ground parts
OAT BRAN .... see OAT BRAN
Oat Fruit .... see OATS
Oat Grain .... see OATS
Oat Herb .... see OAT above ground parts
OAT STRAW .... see OAT STRAW
Oatmeal .... see OATS
OATS .... see OATS
Oblepikha .... see SEA BUCKTHORN
Occidental Ginseng .... see GINSENG, AMERICAN
Ocimum aristatum .... see JAVA TEA
Ocimum basilicum .... see BASIL
Ocimum frutescens .... see PERILLA
OCTACOSANOL .... see OCTACOSANOL
Octacosanol .... see OCTACOSANOL, POLICOSANOL
Octacosyl Alcohol .... see OCTACOSANOL
Octyl Diemthyl PABA .... see PARA-AMINOBENZOIC ACID (PABA)
Oderwort .... see BISTORT
Oenanthe aquatica .... see WATER FENNEL
Oenanthe crocata ... see HEMLOCK WATER DROPWORT
Oenothera biennis .... see EVENING PRIMROSE OIL
Oenothera muricata .... see EVENING PRIMROSE OIL
Oenothera purpurata .... see EVENING PRIMROSE OIL
Oenothera rubricaulis .... see EVENING PRIMROSE OIL
Oenothera suaveolens .... see EVENING PRIMROSE OIL
Ofbit .... see PREMORSE
Ogi .... see ASTRAGALUS
Ogon .... see BAIKAL SKULLCAP
Oil Nut .... see BUTTERNUT
Oil of Cade .... see CADE OIL
Oil of Clove .... see CLOVE OIL
Oil of Juniper Tar .... see CADE OIL
Oil of Melaleuca .... see TEA TREE OIL
Oil of Oregano .... see OREGANO
Oje .... see FICIN
Ojo de Pajaro .... see PRECATORY BEAN
OKG .... see ORNITHINE KETOGLUTARATE
Okra .... see AMBRETTE
Old Maid .... see MADAGASCAR PERIWINKLE
Old Man .... see ROSEMARY
Old Man's Beard .... see FRINGETREE, TRAVELER'S JOY, USNEA, WOODBINE
Old Man's Night Cap .... see GREATER BINDWEED
Old Man's Pepper .... see YARROW
Old Man's Root .... see AMERICAN SPIKENARD
Old Woman's Broom .... see DAMIANA
Olea europaea .... see OLIVE leaf, OLIVE OIL
Oleae Folium .... see OLIVE leaf
OLEANDER .... see OLEANDER
Oleanderblatter .... see OLEANDER
Oleandri folium .... see OLEANDER
Oleic Acid .... see LORENZO'S OIL
Oleovitamin A .... see VITAMIN A
Oleum Bergamotte .... see BERGAMOT OIL
Oleum Cadinum .... see CADE OIL
Oleum Chaulmoograe .... see CHAULMOOGRA
Oleum Geranii .... see ROSE GERANIUM OIL
Oleum Juniperi Empyreumaticum .... see CADE OIL
Oleum Melaleucae .... see TEA TREE OIL
Olibanum .... see FRANKINCENSE
Oligofructose .... see FRUCTO-OLIGOSACCHARIDES
Oligomeric Proanthocyanidins .... see GRAPE seed, PYCNOGENOL
Oligomeric Procyanidins .... see GRAPE seed
Oligosaccharides .... see FRUCTO-OLIGOSACCHARIDES, INULIN
Olivae Oleum .... see OLIVE OIL
Olive .... see OLIVE leaf, OLIVE OIL
OLIVE leaf .... see OLIVE leaf
OLIVE OIL .... see OLIVE OIL
Olivier .... see OLIVE leaf
Omega 3 Fatty Acid .... see ALPHA-LINOLENIC ACID, COD LIVER OIL, DHA (DOCOSAHEXAENOIC ACID), EPA (EICOSAPENTAENOIC ACID), FISH OILS
Omega 6 Oils .... see OMEGA-6 FATTY ACIDS
OMEGA-6 FATTY ACIDS .... see OMEGA-6 FATTY ACIDS
Omega-9 Fatty Acid .... see OLIVE OIL
Omicha .... see SCHISANDRA
Omum .... see BISHOP'S WEED
Onagra biennis .... see EVENING PRIMROSE OIL
One-berry .... see HERB PARIS, SQUAWVINE
Oneseed Hawthorn .... see HAWTHORN
ONION .... see ONION
Ononidis Radix .... see SPINY RESTHARROW
Ononis spinosa .... see SPINY RESTHARROW
Onopordum acanthium .... see SCOTCH THISTLE
Ontario Ginseng .... see GINSENG, AMERICAN
OPC .... see GRAPE seed, PYCNOGENOL
Ophioglossum vulgatum .... see ENGLISH ADDER'S TONGUE
Ophioxylon serpentinum .... see INDIAN SNAKEROOT
OPI .... see PRICKLY PEAR CACTUS
OPIUM ANTIDOTE .... see OPIUM ANTIDOTE
Oplopanax horridus .... see DEVIL'S CLUB
Opobalsam .... see TOLU BALSAM
Opopanax .... see MYRRH
Opossum Tree .... see STORAX
Opuntia .... see PRICKLY PEAR CACTUS
Opuntia cardona .... see PRICKLY PEAR CACTUS
Opuntia ficus .... see PRICKLY PEAR CACTUS
Opuntia ficus-indica .... see PRICKLY PEAR CACTUS
Opuntia hyptiacantha .... see PRICKLY PEAR CACTUS
Opuntia lasciacantha .... see PRICKLY PEAR CACTUS
Opuntia macrocentra .... see PRICKLY PEAR CACTUS
Opuntia megacantha .... see PRICKLY PEAR CACTUS
Opuntia puberula .... see PRICKLY PEAR CACTUS
Opuntia streptacantha .... see PRICKLY PEAR CACTUS
Opuntia velutina .... see PRICKLY PEAR CACTUS
Opuntia violacea .... see PRICKLY PEAR CACTUS
Oraches .... see ARRACH
Oranda-garashi .... see WATERCRESS
Orange .... see SWEET ORANGE

Orange Milkweed .... see PLEURISY ROOT
Orange Mullein .... see MULLEIN
Orange Root .... see GOLDENSEAL
Orange Swallow Wort .... see PLEURISY ROOT
Orchanet .... see ALKANNA
Orchic .... see ORCHIC EXTRACT
Orchic Concentrate .... see ORCHIC EXTRACT
ORCHIC EXTRACT .... see ORCHIC EXTRACT
Orchic Factors .... see ORCHIC EXTRACT
Orchic Substance .... see ORCHIC EXTRACT
Orchid .... see SALEP
Orchis morio .... see SALEP
Ordeal Bean .... see CALABAR BEAN
OREGANO .... see OREGANO
Oregano Oil .... see OREGANO
Oregon Balsam .... see OREGON FIR BALSAM
Oregon Barberry .... see OREGON GRAPE
OREGON FIR BALSAM .... see OREGON FIR BALSAM
OREGON GRAPE .... see OREGON GRAPE
Oregon Grape .... see EUROPEAN BARBERRY, OREGON GRAPE
Oregon Grape-holly .... see OREGON GRAPE
Organic Germanium .... see GERMANIUM
Organy .... see OREGANO
Orgotein .... see SUPEROXIDE DISMUTASE
ORIENTAL ARBORVITAE .... see ORIENTAL ARBORVITAE
Oriental Ginseng .... see GINSENG, PANAX
Origan de Marais .... see HEMP AGRIMONY
Origani Vulgaris Herba .... see OREGANO
Origano .... see OREGANO
Origanum .... see OREGANO
Origanum majorana .... see MARJORAM
Origanum Oil .... see SPANISH ORIGANUM OIL
Origanum vulgare .... see OREGANO
Orizaba Jalap .... see MEXICAN SCAMMONY ROOT
Ormenis nobilis .... see ROMAN CHAMOMILE
Ornicetil .... see ORNITHINE KETOGLUTARATE
ORNITHINE .... see ORNITHINE
Ornithine Alpha Ketoglutarate .... see ORNITHINE KETOGLUTARATE
ORNITHINE KETOGLUTARATE .... see ORNITHINE KETOGLUTARATE
Orozuz .... see LICORICE
ORRIS .... see ORRIS
Orthosiphon .... see JAVA TEA
Orthosiphon aristatus .... see JAVA TEA
Orthosiphon stamineus .... see JAVA TEA
Orthosiphonis Folium .... see JAVA TEA
Orthovanadate .... see VANADIUM
Ortie .... see STINGING NETTLE above ground parts
Oryza sativa .... see RICE BRAN
Oryzanol .... see GAMMA ORYZANOL
Oscillo .... see OSCILLOCOCCINUM
OSCILLOCOCCINUM .... see OSCILLOCOCCINUM
OSHA .... see OSHA
Osier .... see AMERICAN DOGWOOD
Osier Rouge .... see WILLOW BARK
Osmunda struthiopteris .... see OSTRICH FERN
Osterick .... see BISTORT
OSTRICH FERN .... see OSTRICH FERN
OSWEGO TEA .... see OSWEGO TEA
Otaheite Walnut .... see TUNG SEED
Ou-gon .... see BAIKAL SKULLCAP
Our Lady's Flannel .... see MULLEIN
Our Lady's Keys .... see COWSLIP
Our Lady's Mint .... see SPEARMINT
Our Lady's Tears .... see LILY-OF-THE-VALLEY
Our Lady's Thistle .... see MILK THISTLE
Our-Lord's-candle .... see YUCCA
Ovoester .... see ASTAXANTHIN
Ovolecithin .... see LECITHIN
Owler .... see BLACK ALDER
OX-EYE DAISY .... see OX-EYE DAISY
Oxadoddy .... see BLACK ROOT
Oxalis acetosella .... see WOOD SORREL
Oxalis montana .... see WOOD SORREL
Oxerutin .... see RUTIN
Oxeye .... see PHEASANT'S EYE
Oxitriptan .... see 5-HTP
Ox's Tongue .... see BORAGE flower, dried above ground parts
Oxycoccus hagerupii .... see CRANBERRY
Oxycoccus macrocarpos .... see CRANBERRY
Oxycoccus microcarpus .... see CRANBERRY
Oxycoccus palustris .... see CRANBERRY
Oxycoccus quadripetalus .... see CRANBERRY
Oxykrinin .... see SECRETIN
Oyster Shell Calcium .... see CALCIUM
P. Ternata .... see PINELLIA TERNATA
P57 .... see HOODIA
P-aminobenzoic acid .... see PARA-AMINOBENZOIC ACID (PABA)
PABA .... see PARA-AMINOBENZOIC ACID (PABA)
Pachyrhizus thunbergianus .... see KUDZU
Pacific Valerian .... see VALERIAN
Pacific Yew .... see YEW
Padamate O .... see PARA-AMINOBENZOIC ACID (PABA)
Padang-Cassia .... see CINNAMON bark
Paddock-pipes .... see HORSETAIL
Paeonia .... see PEONY flower, PEONY root
Paeonia caucasica .... see PEONY flower, PEONY root
Paeonia mascula .... see PEONY flower, PEONY root
Paeonia officinalis .... see PEONY flower, PEONY root
Paeoniae Flos .... see PEONY flower
Paeoniae Radix .... see PEONY root
Pagla-ka-dawa .... see INDIAN SNAKEROOT
PAGODA TREE .... see PAGODA TREE
Pahari Pudina .... see SPEARMINT
Paigle .... see COWSLIP
Paigle Peggle .... see COWSLIP
Paintedleaf .... see POINSETTIA
Pakistani Ephedra .... see EPHEDRA
Pale Coneflower .... see ECHINACEA
Pale Gentian .... see GENTIAN
Pale Mara .... see FEVER BARK
Pale Psyllium .... see BLOND PSYLLIUM
Pali-mara .... see FEVER BARK
Palma Christi .... see CASTOR OIL, CASTOR seed
Palmier Nain .... see SAW PALMETTO
Palo de Santa Maria .... see LAURELWOOD
Palo Maria .... see LAURELWOOD
Palsy Root .... see MARSH MARIGOLD
Palsywort .... see COWSLIP
Panama Bark .... see QUILLAIA
Panama Ipecac .... see IPECAC
Panang Cinnamon .... see CINNAMON bark

Panax ginseng .... see GINSENG, PANAX
Panax Horridum .... see DEVIL'S CLUB
Panax notoginseng .... see PANAX PSEUDOGINSENG
PANAX PSEUDOGINSENG .... see PANAX PSEUDOGINSENG
Panax quinquefolius .... see GINSENG, AMERICAN
Panax schinseng .... see GINSENG, PANAX
PANCREATIN .... see PANCREATIN
Pancreatinum .... see PANCREATIN
Pancreatis pulvis .... see PANCREATIN
PANGAMIC ACID .... see PANGAMIC ACID
Panicum caffrorum .... see BROOM CORN
Pansy .... see HEART'S EASE
PANTETHINE .... see PANTETHINE
Pantetina .... see PANTETHINE
Panthenol .... see PANTOTHENIC ACID (VITAMIN B5)
Pantomin .... see PANTETHINE
Pantosin .... see PANTETHINE
PANTOTHENIC ACID (VITAMIN B5) .... see PANTOTHENIC ACID (VITAMIN B5)
Pantothenol ..... see PANTOTHENIC ACID (VITAMIN B5)
Pantothenylol .... see PANTOTHENIC ACID (VITAMIN B5)
Papagallo .... see POINSETTIA
PAPAIN .... see PAPAIN
Papainum Crudum .... see PAPAIN
Paparaminta .... see PEPPERMINT leaf, see PEPPERMINT OIL
Papaver rhoeas .... see CORN POPPY
Papaw .... see PAPAYA
PAPAYA .... see PAPAYA
Papaya carica .... see PAPAYA
Papayas .... see PAPAYA
Paperbark Tree Oil .... see CAJEPUT OIL
Papoose Root .... see BLUE COHOSH
Pappelknospen .... see POPLAR
Paprika .... see CAPSICUM
PARA-AMINOBENZOIC ACID (PABA) .... see PARA-AMINOBENZOIC ACID (PABA)
Paradisapfel .... see GRAPEFRUIT
Paradise Tree .... see TREE OF HEAVEN
Paraguay Tea .... see MATE
Paraguayan Sweet Herb .... see STEVIA
Parapetalifera betulina .... see BUCHU
Parapetalifera crenulata .... see BUCHU
Parapetalifera odorata .... see BUCHU
Parapetalifera serrata .... see BUCHU
Parapetalifera serratifolia .... see BUCHU
Parasigaya .... see HENBANE
PAREIRA .... see PAREIRA
Pareira .... see ABUTA, PAREIRA
Paricalcitol .... see VITAMIN D
Parietaria officinalis .... see PELLITORY-OF-THE-WALL
Paris quadrifolia .... see HERB PARIS
Pariswort .... see BETH ROOT
Parsley .... see PARSLEY leaf, root; PARSLEY seed
Parsley Breakstone .... see PARSLEY PIERT
Parsley Fern .... see TANSY
Parsley Fruit .... see PARSLEY seed
PARSLEY leaf, root .... see PARSLEY leaf, root
Parsley Piercestone .... see PARSLEY PIERT
PARSLEY PIERT .... see PARSLEY PIERT
PARSLEY seed .... see PARSLEY seed
Parsnip .... see PARSNIP above ground parts, PARSNIP root
PARSNIP above ground parts .... see PARSNIP above ground parts
PARSNIP root .... see PARSNIP root
Parson and Clerk .... see ARUM
Parthenocissus quinquefolia .... see AMERICAN IVY
Partridge Berry .... see WINTERGREEN leaf, WINTERGREEN OIL
Partridgeberry .... see ALPINE CRANBERRY, SQUAWVINE
Pas d'Ane .... see COLTSFOOT
Pas Diane .... see COLTSFOOT
Pasania Fungus .... see SHIITAKE MUSHROOM
Pasqueflower .... see PULSATILLA
Passe Flower .... see PULSATILLA
Passiflora .... see PASSIONFLOWER
Passiflora incarnata .... see PASSIONFLOWER
Passiflorae Herba .... see PASSIONFLOWER
Passiflore .... see PASSIONFLOWER
Passiflorina .... see PASSIONFLOWER
Passion Flower .... see PASSIONFLOWER
Passion Vine .... see PASSIONFLOWER
Passionaria .... see PASSIONFLOWER
Passionblume .... see PASSIONFLOWER
PASSIONFLOWER .... see PASSIONFLOWER
Passionflower Herb .... see PASSIONFLOWER
Passionsblumenkraut .... see PASSIONFLOWER
Password .... see COWSLIP
Pastel des Teinturiers .... see DA QING YE
Pastinaca sativa .... see PARSNIP above ground parts, PARSNIP root
Pastinacae Herba .... see PARSNIP above ground parts
Pastinacae Radix .... see PARSNIP root
Patacon .... see ABUTA
Patalagandhi .... see INDIAN SNAKEROOT
Patchouli .... see PATCHOULY OIL
Patchouly .... see PATCHOULY OIL
PATCHOULY OIL .... see PATCHOULY OIL
Patience Dock .... see BISTORT
Pattens and Clogs .... see YELLOW TOADFLAX
PAU D'ARCO .... see PAU D'ARCO
Pau de Arco .... see PAU D'ARCO
Pau de Reposta .... see CATUABA
Pau-azeitona .... see MORINDA
Paullinia .... see GUARANA
Paullinia cupana .... see GUARANA
Paullinia sorbilis .... see GUARANA
Paul's Betony .... see BUGLEWEED
Pausinystalia johimbe .... see YOHIMBE
Pausinystalia yohimbe .... see YOHIMBE
Pauson .... see BLOODROOT
Pawpaw .... see AMERICAN PAWPAW
PCO .... see GRAPE seed, PYCNOGENOL
Pea Tree .... see LABURNUM
Peachwood .... see LOGWOOD
Peagle .... see COWSLIP
PEANUT OIL .... see PEANUT OIL
PEAR .... see PEAR
Pearl Barley .... see BARLEY
PECTIN .... see PECTIN
Pectinic Acid .... see PECTIN
Pedlar's Basket .... see YELLOW TOADFLAX
Pedunculate Oak .... see OAK bark
Pegu Catechu .... see CATECHU
Pegwood .... see WAHOO

INDEX

Pelargonium graveolens .... see ROSE GERANIUM OIL
Pelargonium Oil .... see ROSE GERANIUM OIL
Pelican Flower .... see ARISTOLOCHIA
Pellagra Preventing Factor .... see NIACIN AND NIACINAMIDE (VITAMIN B3)
PELLITORY .... see PELLITORY
PELLITORY-OF-THE-WALL .... see PELLITORY-OF-THE-WALL
Pellote .... see PEYOTE
Pennyroyal .... see PENNYROYAL leaf, PENNYROYAL OIL
PENNYROYAL leaf .... see PENNYROYAL leaf
PENNYROYAL OIL .... see PENNYROYAL OIL
Pennywort .... see YELLOW TOADFLAX
Pensee Sauvage .... see HEART'S EASE
Penta Tea .... see JIAOGULAN
Pentamethoxyflavones .... see METHOXYLATED FLAVONES
Pentaptera arjuna .... see TERMINALIA
Pentaptera glabra .... see TERMINALIA
Peony .... see PEONY flower, PEONY root
PEONY flower .... see PEONY flower
PEONY root .... see PEONY root
Pepe .... see BLACK PEPPER AND WHITE PEPPER
Pepino Montero .... see BITTER MELON
Pepo .... see PUMPKIN
Pepper .... see BLACK PEPPER AND WHITE PEPPER
Pepper-and-salt .... see SHEPHERD'S PURSE
Pepper Bark .... see WINTER'S BARK
Pepper Extract .... see BLACK PEPPER AND WHITE PEPPER
Pepper Plant .... see BLACK PEPPER AND WHITE PEPPER
Pepper Wood .... see NORTHERN PRICKLY ASH
Peppercorn .... see BLACK PEPPER AND WHITE PEPPER
Peppermint .... see PEPPERMINT leaf, PEPPERMINT OIL
PEPPERMINT leaf .... see PEPPERMINT leaf
PEPPERMINT OIL .... see PEPPERMINT OIL
Pepperrot .... see HORSERADISH
Pereira Brava .... see PAREIRA
Pericarpium .... see SWEET ORANGE
PERILLA .... see PERILLA
Perilla arguta .... see PERILLA
Perilla frutescens .... see PERILLA
Perilla nankinensis .... see PERILLA
Perilla ocymoides .... see PERILLA
Periploca sylvestris .... see GYMNEMA
PERIWINKLE .... see PERIWINKLE
Periwinkle .... see MADAGASCAR PERIWINKLE, PERIWINKLE
Perna canaliculus .... see NEW ZEALAND GREEN-LIPPED MUSSEL
Persea americana .... see AVOCADO
Persea gratissima .... see AVOCADO
Persea leiogyna .... see AVOCADO
Persea persea .... see AVOCADO
Persely .... see PARSLEY leaf, root
Persian Lilac .... see NEEM
Persian Willow .... see FIREWEED
Persil .... see PARSLEY leaf, root; PARSLEY seed
Personata .... see BURDOCK
PERU BALSAM .... see PERU BALSAM
Peru-apple .... see JIMSON WEED
Peruvian Balsam .... see PERU BALSAM
Peruvian Bark .... see CINCHONA
Peruvian Coca .... see COCA
Peruvian Ginseng .... see MACA
Peruvian Rhatany .... see RHATANY
Petasites .... see BUTTERBUR
Petasites Flower .... see BUTTERBUR
Petasites hybridus .... see BUTTERBUR
Petasites Leaf .... see BUTTERBUR
Petasites officinalis .... see BUTTERBUR
Petasites Rhizome .... see BUTTERBUR
Petasites Root .... see BUTTERBUR
Petasitidis Folium .... see BUTTERBUR
Petasitidis hybridus .... see BUTTERBUR
Petasitidis Rhizoma .... see BUTTERBUR
Peter's Cress .... see SAMPHIRE
Petersylinge .... see PARSLEY leaf, root
Petite Sirah .... see GRAPE fruit, skin
Petroselini Fructus .... see PARSLEY seed
Petroselini Herba .... see PARSLEY leaf, root
Petroselinum crispum .... see PARSLEY leaf, root; PARSLEY seed
Petroselinum hortense .... see PARSLEY leaf, root; PARSLEY seed
Petroselinum sativum .... see PARSLEY leaf, root; PARSLEY seed
Petroselinum vulgare .... see PARSLEY leaf, root
Petrosilini Radix .... see PARSLEY leaf, root
Pettigree .... see BUTCHER'S BROOM
Petty Morel .... see BLACK NIGHTSHADE
Petty Mugget .... see LADY'S BEDSTRAW
Petty Mulleins .... see COWSLIP
Petty Whin .... see SPINY RESTHARROW
Pettymorell .... see AMERICAN SPIKENARD
Peucedanum graveolens .... see DILL above ground parts, DILL seed
Peumus boldus .... see BOLDO
Peumus fragrans .... see BOLDO
Pewterwort .... see HORSETAIL
PEYOTE .... see PEYOTE
Pfaffia .... see SUMA
Pfaffia paniculata .... see SUMA
Pfeffer .... see BLACK PEPPER AND WHITE PEPPER
Pferdefut .... see COLTSFOOT
PGG Glucan .... see BETA GLUCANS
Phaca membranacea .... see ASTRAGALUS
Phadena .... see JAMBOLAN bark
Phalaris zizanioides .... see VETIVER
Phaseoli Fructus .... see BEAN POD
Phaseolus max Soja hispida .... see SOY, SOYBEAN OIL
Phaseolus vulgaris .... see BEAN POD
PHEASANT'S EYE .... see PHEASANT'S EYE
PHENYLALANINE .... see PHENYLALANINE
Philanthropium .... see BURDOCK
Phoenix dactylifera .... see DATE PALM
Phoradendron flavescens .... see AMERICAN MISTLETOE
Phoradendron leucarpum .... see AMERICAN MISTLETOE
Phoradendron macrophyllum .... see AMERICAN MISTLETOE
Phoradendron serontium .... see AMERICAN MISTLETOE
Phoradendron tomentosum .... see AMERICAN MISTLETOE
PHOSPHATE SALTS .... see PHOSPHATE SALTS
Phosphatidyl Choline .... see PHOSPHATIDYLCHOLINE

Phosphatidyl Serine .... see PHOSPHATIDYLSERINE
PHOSPHATIDYLCHOLINE .... see PHOSPHATIDYLCHOLINE
PHOSPHATIDYLSERINE .... see PHOSPHATIDYLSERINE
Phragmites .... see REED HERB
Phragmites australis .... see REED HERB
Phragmites communis .... see REED HERB
Phragmites longivalvis .... see REED HERB
Phragmites vulgaris .... see REED HERB
Phyllanthus emblica .... see INDIAN GOOSEBERRY
Phyllanthus niruri .... see CHANCA PIEDRA
Phylloquinone .... see VITAMIN K
Physalis alkekengi .... see WINTER CHERRY
Physalis somnifera .... see ASHWAGANDHA
Physic Root .... see BLACK ROOT
Physostigma venenosum .... see CALABAR BEAN
Physotigma .... see CALABAR BEAN
Phytic Acid .... see IP-6
Phytoestrogen .... see ALFALFA; ANISE; BLACK COHOSH; DONG QUAI; FENNEL fruit, seed; FENNEL OIL; FLAXSEED; GINSENG, SIBERIAN; LICORICE; RED CLOVER; RESVERATROL; SOY; WILD YAM
Phytolacca americana .... see POKEWEED berry, POKEWEED root
Phytolacca Berry .... see POKEWEED berry, POKEWEED root
Phytolacca decandra .... see POKEWEED berry, POKEWEED root
Phytomenadione .... see VITAMIN K
Phytonadione .... see VITAMIN K
Phytoprogestin .... see OREGANO
Phytostanol .... see SITOSTANOL
Phytosterols .... see BETA-SITOSTEROL
Pica Pica .... see COWHAGE
Picea abies .... see FIR, FIR NEEDLE OIL, HEMLOCK SPRUCE
Picea aetheroleum .... see FIR NEEDLE OIL, HEMLOCK SPRUCE
Picea excelsa .... see FIR; FIR NEEDLE OIL; HEMLOCK SPRUCE
Picea turiones recentes .... see HEMLOCK SPRUCE
Piceae aetheroleum .... see FIR NEEDLE OIL
Piceae turiones recentes .... see FIR
Pickaway Anise .... see WAFER ASH
Pick-pocket .... see SHEPHERD'S PURSE
Picrasma .... see QUASSIA
Picrasma excelsa .... see QUASSIA
PICRORHIZA .... see PICRORHIZA
Picrorhiza kurroa .... see PICRORHIZA
Picrorhiza scrophulariiflora .... see PICRORHIZA
Pie Cherry .... see SOUR CHERRY
Pierce-stone .... see SAMPHIRE
Pigeonberry .... see POKEWEED berry, POKEWEED root
Pigeon's Grass .... see VERBENA
Pigeonweed .... see VERBENA
Pignut .... see JOJOBA
Pigrush .... see KNOTWEED
Pigweed .... see GOUTWEED, KNOTWEED
Pigwood .... see WAHOO
Pilewort .... see AMARANTH, BULBOUS BUTTERCUP, LESSER CELANDINE
Piliolerial .... see PENNYROYAL leaf, PENNYROYAL OIL
Pillbearing Spurge .... see EUPHORBIA
Pilocarpus microphyllus .... see JABORANDI
Pilosella officinarum .... see MOUSE EAR
Pilot Plant .... see CUP PLANT
Pilot Weed .... see ROSINWEED
Pimela luzonica .... see ELEMI
Pimenta .... see ALLSPICE, BLACK PEPPER AND WHITE PEPPER
Pimenta dioica .... see ALLSPICE
Pimenta officinalis .... see ALLSPICE
Pimenta-longa .... see INDIAN LONG PEPPER
Pimento .... see ALLSPICE, CAPSICUM
Pimento Oil .... see ALLSPICE
Pimento Water .... see ALLSPICE
Pimienta .... see BLACK PEPPER AND WHITE PEPPER
Pimpernell .... see PIMPINELLA above ground parts, PIMPINELLA root
Pimpinella .... see PIMPINELLA above ground parts, PIMPINELLA root
PIMPINELLA above ground parts .... see PIMPINELLA above ground parts
Pimpinella anisum .... see ANISE
Pimpinella magna .... see PIMPINELLA above ground parts, PIMPINELLA root
Pimpinella major ..... see PIMPINELLA above ground parts, PIMPINELLA root
PIMPINELLA root .... see PIMPINELLA root
Pimpinella saxifraga .... see PIMPINELLA above ground parts, PIMPINELLA root
Pimpinellae Herba .... see PIMPINELLA above ground parts
Pimpinellae Radix .... see PIMPINELLA root
Pin Heads .... see GERMAN CHAMOMILE
Pinag .... see ARECA
PINE .... see PINE
Pine Bark .... see PYCNOGENOL
Pine Bark Extract .... see PYCNOGENOL
Pine Needle Oil .... see SCOTCH PINE NEEDLE
Pine Oils .... see SCOTCH PINE NEEDLE
Pine Pollen .... see BEE POLLEN
Pineal Hormone .... see MELATONIN
Pineapple Enzyme .... see BROMELAIN
PINELLIA TERNATA .... see PINELLIA TERNATA
Pinellia Tuber .... see PINELLIA TERNATA
Pinellia tubifera .... see PINELLIA TERNATA
Piney .... see PEONY flower, PEONY root
Pini Atheroleum .... see SCOTCH PINE NEEDLE
Pini Turiones .... see PINE
PINK ROOT .... see PINK ROOT
Pinkroot .... see PINK ROOT
Pinlag .... see ARECA
Pin-ma Ts'ao .... see DANSHEN
Pinto Bean .... see BEAN POD
Pinus abies .... see FIR; FIR NEEDLE OIL; HEMLOCK SPRUCE
Pinus australis .... see TURPENTINE OIL
Pinus balsamea .... see CANADA BALSAM
PINUS BARK .... see PINUS BARK
Pinus larix .... see LARCH TURPENTINE
Pinus marittima .... see PYCNOGENOL

INDEX

Pinus montana .... see DWARF PINE NEEDLE
Pinus mugo .... see DWARF PINE NEEDLE
Pinus mugo var. pumilio .... see DWARF PINE NEEDLE
Pinus palustris .... see TURPENTINE OIL
Pinus pinaster ..... see PYCNOGENOL, TURPENTINE OIL
Pinus pumilio .... see DWARF PINE NEEDLE
Pinus sylvestris .... see PINE, SCOTCH PINE NEEDLE
Pinus viminalis .... see FIR, FIR NEEDLE OIL, HEMLOCK SPRUCE
Piper .... see BLACK PEPPER AND WHITE PEPPER
Piper cubeba .... see CUBEBS
Piper longum .... see INDIAN LONG PEPPER
Piper methysticum .... see KAVA
Piper nigrum .... see BLACK PEPPER AND WHITE PEPPER
Piperine .... see BLACK PEPPER AND WHITE PEPPER
Pipiltzintzintli .... see DIVINER'S SAGE
Pippali .... see INDIAN LONG PEPPER
Pipperidge .... see EUROPEAN BARBERRY
Piprage .... see EUROPEAN BARBERRY
PIPSISSEWA .... see PIPSISSEWA
Piratancara .... see CATUABA
Piripiri .... see ADRUE
Piscidia communis .... see JAMAICAN DOGWOOD
Piscidia erythrina .... see JAMAICAN DOGWOOD
Piscidia piscipula .... see JAMAICAN DOGWOOD
Pissenlit .... see DANDELION above ground parts, DANDELION entire plant
Pistacia lentiscus .... see MASTIC
PITCHER PLANT .... see PITCHER PLANT
Pitirishi .... see CHANCA PIEDRA
Pituri .... see CORKWOOD TREE
Pix Cadi .... see CADE OIL
Pix Juniper .... see CADE OIL
Pix Liquida .... see PINE
Pix Oxycedri .... see CADE OIL
Plant-derived Liquid Minerals .... see COLLOIDAL MINERALS
Plant Estrogen .... see SOY
Plant of Immortality .... see ALOE latex
Plant Protease Concentrate ...... see BROMELAIN, PAPAIN
Plant Stanol .... see SITOSTANOL
Plant Stanol Esters .... see SITOSTANOL
Plant Sterols .... see BETA-SITOSTEROL
Plantaginis Lanceolatae Herba .... see BUCKHORN PLANTAIN
Plantaginis Ovatae Semen .... see BLOND PSYLLIUM
Plantaginis Ovatae Testa .... see BLOND PSYLLIUM
Plantago decumbens .... see BLOND PSYLLIUM
Plantago fastigiata .... see BLOND PSYLLIUM
Plantago insularis .... see BLOND PSYLLIUM
Plantago ispaghula .... see BLOND PSYLLIUM
Plantago lanceolata .... see BUCKHORN PLANTAIN
Plantago major .... see GREAT PLANTAIN
Plantago ovata .... see BLOND PSYLLIUM
Plantago psyllium .... see BLACK PSYLLIUM
Plantain .... see BLACK PSYLLIUM, BUCKHORN PLANTAIN
Platycladus orientalis .... see ORIENTAL ARBORVITAE
PLC .... see PROPIONYL-L-CARNITINE
Plectranthus barbatus .... see FORSKOLIN
Pleurisy .... see PLEURISY ROOT
PLEURISY ROOT .... see PLEURISY ROOT
Plumrocks .... see COWSLIP
PMF .... see METHOXYLATED FLAVONES
Pocan .... see POKEWEED berry, POKEWEED root
Pockwood .... see GUAIAC WOOD resin, wood
Podophylli Pelati Resina .... see PODOPHYLLUM
Podophylli Pelati Rhizoma .... see PODOPHYLLUM
PODOPHYLLUM .... see PODOPHYLLUM
Podophyllum emodi .... see PODOPHYLLUM
Podophyllum hexandrum .... see PODOPHYLLUM
Podophyllum peltatum .... see PODOPHYLLUM
Poet's Jessamine .... see JASMINE
Pogostemon cablin .... see PATCHOULY OIL
Pogostemon heyneanus .... see PATCHOULY OIL
Pogostemon patchouly .... see PATCHOULY OIL
Pohl .... see MANACA
POINSETTIA .... see POINSETTIA
Poinsettia pulcherrima .... see POINSETTIA
Poison-hemlock .... see HEMLOCK
Poison Ash .... see FRINGETREE
Poison Black Cherries .... see BELLADONNA
Poison Flag .... see ORRIS
Poison Fool's Parsley .... see HEMLOCK
POISON IVY .... see POISON IVY
Poison Lettuce .... see WILD LETTUCE
Poison Nut .... see NUX VOMICA
Poison Parsnip .... see WATER HEMLOCK
Poison Tobacco .... see HENBANE
Poison Vine .... see POISON IVY
Poisonberry .... see BLACK NIGHTSHADE, LEVANT BERRY
POISONOUS BUTTERCUP .... see POISONOUS BUTTERCUP
Poivre .... see BLACK PEPPER AND WHITE PEPPER
Poivre Long .... see INDIAN LONG PEPPER
Poivre Noir .... see BLACK PEPPER AND WHITE PEPPER
Poke .... see POKEWEED berry, POKEWEED root
Poke Root .... see POKEWEED root
Pokeberry .... see POKEWEED berry, POKEWEED root
Pokeweed .... see POKEWEED berry, POKEWEED root
POKEWEED berry .... see POKEWEED berry
POKEWEED root .... see POKEWEED root
Polar Plant .... see CUP PLANT, ROSEMARY, ROSINWEED
Polecatbush .... see SWEET SUMACH
Polecatweed .... see SKUNK CABBAGE
Polemonium caeruleum .... see JACOB'S LADDER
Polemonium reptans .... see ABSCESS ROOT
Poleo .... see JAPANESE MINT
POLICOSANOL .... see POLICOSANOL
Pollen .... see BEE POLLEN
Pollen d'Abeille .... see BEE POLLEN
Poly-[1-6]-beta-D-glucopyranosyl-[1-3]-beta-D-glucopyranose .... see BETA GLUCANS
Polygala amara .... see BITTER MILKWORT
Polygala glomerata .... see SENEGA
Polygala japonica .... see SENEGA
Polygala reinii .... see SENEGA
Polygala senega .... see SENEGA
Polygala tenuifolia .... see SENEGA
Polygalae Radix .... see SENEGA
Polygonatum multiflorum .... see SOLOMON'S SEAL
Polygoni Avicularis Herba .... see KNOTWEED
Polygonum .... see FO-TI
Polygonum aviculare .... see KNOTWEED

INDEX

Polygonum bistorta ... see BISTORT
Polygonum hydropiper ... see SMARTWEED
Polygonum multiflorum ... see FO-TI
Polygonum tataricum ... see BUCKWHEAT
Polymethoxylated Flavones ... see METHOXYLATED FLAVONES
Poly-NAG ... see N-ACETYL GLUCOSAMINE
Polypodium filix-femina ... see LADY FERN
Polyporus ... see PORIA MUSHROOM
Polyporus versicolor ... see CORIOLUS MUSHROOM
Polysaccharide Krestin ... see CORIOLUS MUSHROOM
Polysaccharide Peptide ... see CORIOLUS MUSHROOM
Polysaccharide-K ... see CORIOLUS MUSHROOM
Polystictus versicolor ... see CORIOLUS MUSHROOM
Polyunsaturated Fatty Acids ... see COD LIVER OIL, OMEGA-6 FATTY ACIDS
POMEGRANATE ... see POMEGRANATE
Pomelo ... see GRAPEFRUIT, GRAPEFRUIT OIL
Pond Lily ... see AMERICAN WHITE POND LILY
Poogiphalam ... see ANDROGRAPHIS, ARECA
Poolroot ... see SANICLE
Poor Man's Parmacettie ... see SHEPHERD'S PURSE
Poor Man's Treacle ... see GARLIC
Poor Man's Weatherglass ... see SCARLET PIMPERNEL
Popinac Absolute ... see CASSIE ABSOLUTE
POPLAR ... see POPLAR
Popotillo ... see EPHEDRA, MORMON TEA
Poppy California ... see CALIFORNIA POPPY
Populi Cortex ... see ASPEN
Populi Folium ... see ASPEN
Populi gemma ... see POPLAR
Populus balsamifera ... see POPLAR
Populus canadensis ... see POPLAR
Populus candicans ... see POPLAR
Populus euramericana ... see POPLAR
Populus marilandica ... see POPLAR
Populus serotina ... see POPLAR
Populus tacamahacca ... see POPLAR
Populus tremula ... see ASPEN
Populus tremuloides ... see ASPEN
Porcelain Clay ... see KAOLIN
Poria ... see PORIA MUSHROOM
Poria cocos ... see PORIA MUSHROOM
PORIA MUSHROOM ... see PORIA MUSHROOM
Porites sp. ... see CORAL
Porteranthus trifoliatus ... see INDIAN PHYSIC
Porter's Licorice Root ... see OSHA
Portland Arrowroot ... see ARUM
Pot ... see MARIJUANA
Pot Barley ... see BARLEY
Pot Marigold ... see CALENDULA
POTASSIUM ... see POTASSIUM
Potassium Acetate ... see POTASSIUM
Potassium Bicarbonate ... see POTASSIUM
Potassium Chloride ... see POTASSIUM
Potassium Citrate ... see POTASSIUM
Potassium Gluconate ... see POTASSIUM
Potassium Iodide ... see IODINE
Potassium Phosphate ... see PHOSPHATE SALTS, POTASSIUM
Potassium Pyruvate ... see PYRUVATE
POTATO ... see POTATO
Potency Wood ... see MUIRA PUAMA
POTENTILLA ... see POTENTILLA
Potentilla ... see POTENTILLA, TORMENTIL
Potentilla anserina ... see POTENTILLA
Potentilla erecta ... see TORMENTIL
Potentilla reptans ... see EUROPEAN FIVE-FINGER GRASS
Potentilla tormentilla ... see TORMENTIL
Potentilla virginiana ... see STRAWBERRY
Potentilla viridis ... see STRAWBERRY
Poterium officinale ... see GREATER BURNET
Poverty Weed ... see OX-EYE DAISY
Povidone Iodine ... see IODINE
Prairie Dock ... see CUP PLANT
Prairie Grub ... see WAFER ASH
Prasterone ... see DHEA
Prayer Beads ... see PRECATORY BEAN
Prayer Head ... see PRECATORY BEAN
Prebiotic ... see FRUCTO-OLIGOSACCHARIDES, INULIN
PRECATORY BEAN ... see PRECATORY BEAN
Predigested Spleen Extract ... see SPLEEN EXTRACT
Predigested Thymus Extract ... see THYMUS EXTRACT
Pregnancy Hormone ... see PROGESTERONE
Pregnanedione ... see PROGESTERONE
PREGNENOLONE ... see PREGNENOLONE
Prele ... see HORSETAIL
PREMORSE ... see PREMORSE
Premorse scaboius ... see PREMORSE
Pretty Betsy ... see RED-SPUR VALERIAN
Prick Madam ... see COMMON STONECROP
Prickly Ash ... see NORTHERN PRICKLY ASH, SOUTHERN PRICKLY ASH
Prickly Eleutherococcus ... see GINSENG, SIBERIAN
PRICKLY PEAR CACTUS ... see PRICKLY PEAR CACTUS
Prickly Yellow Wood ... see SOUTHERN PRICKLY ASH
Prickwood ... see WAHOO
Pride of China ... see NEEM
Pride-of-India ... see BANABA
Prideweed ... see CANADIAN FLEABANE
Priest's Crown ... see DANDELION above ground parts, DANDELION entire plant
Primrose ... see COWSLIP, EVENING PRIMROSE OIL
Primula ... see COWSLIP
Primula elatior ... see COWSLIP
Primula officinalis ... see COWSLIP
Primula veris ... see COWSLIP
Prince's Feather ... see AMARANTH, POTENTILLA
Prince's Pine ... see PIPSISSEWA
Privet ... see GLOSSY PRIVET
Proacemic Acid ... see PYRUVATE
Proanthodyn ... see GRAPE seed
Probiotics ... see BIFIDOBACTERIA, LACTOBACILLUS, SACCHAROMYCES BOULARDII, YOGURT
PROCAINE ... see PROCAINE
Procaine Hydrochloride ... see PROCAINE
Processed Bovine Cartilage ... see BOVINE CARTILAGE
Procyandiol Oligomers ... see PYCNOGENOL
Procyanidin Oligomers ... see PYCNOGENOL
Procyanidolic Oligomers ... see GRAPE seed
Procyanodolic Oligomers ... see PYCNOGENOL
Progestational Hormone ... see PROGESTERONE
PROGESTERONE ... see PROGESTERONE

INDEX

Progesteronum .... see PROGESTERONE
PROPIONYL-L-CARNITINE ....
.... see PROPIONYL-L-CARNITINE
PROPOLIS .... see PROPOLIS
Propolis Balsam .... see PROPOLIS
Propolis Resin .... see PROPOLIS
Propolis Wax .... see PROPOLIS
Proteinase .... see TRYPSIN
Proteolytic Enzyme .... see TRYPSIN
Protykin .... see RESVERATROL
Provitamin A .... see BETA-CAROTENE
Pruche de l'Est .... see PINUS BARK
Prunella .... see SELF-HEAL
Prunella vulgaris .... see SELF-HEAL
Pruni Spinosae Fructus .... see BLACKTHORN berry
Pruni Spinosae Llos .... see BLACKTHORN flower
Prunus africana .... see PYGEUM
Prunus amygdalus .... see BITTER ALMOND
Prunus amygdalus dulcis .... see SWEET ALMOND
Prunus armeniaca .... see APRICOT
Prunus cerasus .... see SOUR CHERRY
Prunus communis .... see BITTER ALMOND
Prunus dulcis .... see BITTER ALMOND
Prunus dulcis var. amara .... see BITTER ALMOND
Prunus grandifolia .... see CHERRY LAUREL WATER
Prunus laurocerasus .... see CHERRY LAUREL WATER
Prunus serotina .... see WILD CHERRY
Prunus spinosa .... see BLACKTHORN berry, BLACKTHORN flower
Prunus virginiana .... see WILD CHERRY
Prunus vulgaris .... see SOUR CHERRY
PS .... see PHOSPHATIDYLSERINE
Pseudoginseng Root .... see PANAX PSEUDOGINSENG
Pseudosasa japonica .... see BAMBOO
Pseudotsuga douglasii .... see OREGON FIR BALSAM
Pseudotsuga menziesii .... see OREGON FIR BALSAM
Pseudotsuga mucronata .... see OREGON FIR BALSAM
Pseudotsuga taxifolia .... see OREGON FIR BALSAM
Psi-psi-carotene .... see LYCOPENE
PSK .... see CORIOLUS MUSHROOM
Psoralea linearis .... see RED BUSH TEA
Psoralea tetragonoloba .... see GUAR GUM
Psoriacin .... see BOVINE CARTILAGE
Psoriacin-T .... see BOVINE CARTILAGE
PSP .... see CORIOLUS MUSHROOM
Psychotria ipecacuanha .... see IPECAC
Psyllion .... see BLACK PSYLLIUM
Psyllios .... see BLACK PSYLLIUM
Psyllium .... see BLOND PSYLLIUM
Psyllium afra .... see BLACK PSYLLIUM
Psyllium arenaria .... see BLACK PSYLLIUM
Psyllium indica .... see BLACK PSYLLIUM
Psyllium Seed .... see BLACK PSYLLIUM
Ptarmigan Berry .... see UVA URSI
PtdSer .... see PHOSPHATIDYLSERINE
Ptelea trifoliata .... see WAFER ASH
Pterocarpus santalinus .... see RED SANDALWOOD
Pteroylglutamic Acid .... see FOLIC ACID
Pteroylmonoglutamic Acid .... see FOLIC ACID
Pteroylpolyglutamate .... see FOLIC ACID
Ptychopetali lignum .... see MUIRA PUAMA
Ptychopetalum olacoides .... see MUIRA PUAMA
Ptychopetalum uncinatum .... see MUIRA PUAMA
Public House Plant .... see ASARABACCA
Pudding Grass .... see PENNYROYAL leaf, PENNYROYAL OIL
Pudina .... see JAPANESE MINT
Pueraria .... see KUDZU
Pueraria candollei .... see KUDZU
Pueraria hirsuta .... see KUDZU
Pueraria lobata .... see KUDZU
Pueraria lobata var. chinensis .... see KUDZU
Pueraria mirifica .... see KUDZU
Pueraria montana var. lobata .... see KUDZU
Pueraria montana var. thomsonii .... see KUDZU
Pueraria pseudohirsuta .... see KUDZU
Pueraria Root .... see KUDZU
Pueraria thomsonii .... see KUDZU
Pueraria thunbergiana .... see KUDZU
Pueraria tuberosa .... see KUDZU
Puerto Rican Cherry .... see ACEROLA
PUFAs .... see FISH OILS, OMEGA-6 FATTY ACIDS
PUFF BALL .... see PUFF BALL
Puga .... see ARECA
Pukeweed .... see LOBELIA
Pulegium .... see PENNYROYAL leaf, PENNYROYAL OIL
Pulegium vulgare .... see PENNYROYAL leaf, PENNYROYAL OIL
Pulmonaria officinalis .... see LUNGWORT
Pulmonariae Herba .... see LUNGWORT
PULSATILLA .... see PULSATILLA
Pulsatilla nigricans .... see PULSATILLA
Pulsatilla pratensis .... see PULSATILLA
Pulsatilla vulgaris .... see PULSATILLA
Pumacuchu .... see RHATANY
Pumilio Pine .... see PINE
PUMPKIN .... see PUMPKIN
Pumpkin Seed .... see PUMPKIN
PUNCTURE VINE .... see PUNCTURE VINE
Puncturevine .... see PUNCTURE VINE
Punica granatum .... see POMEGRANATE
Punk Tree .... see CAJEPUT OIL
Punnanga .... see LAURELWOOD
Pupurweide .... see WILLOW BARK
Purging Flax .... see MOUNTAIN FLAX
Purging Thorn .... see SEA BUCKTHORN
Purines .... see RNA AND DNA
Purple Boneset .... see GRAVEL ROOT
Purple Clover .... see RED CLOVER
Purple Cockle .... see CORN COCKLE
Purple Cone Flower .... see ECHINACEA
Purple Foxglove .... see DIGITALIS
Purple Lapacho .... see PAU D'ARCO
Purple Leptandra .... see BLACK ROOT
PURPLE LOOSESTRIFE .... see PURPLE LOOSESTRIFE
Purple Medick .... see ALFALFA
Purple Mulberry .... see BLACK MULBERRY
Purple Osier .... see WILLOW BARK
Purple Osier Willow .... see WILLOW BARK
Purple Passion Flower .... see PASSIONFLOWER
Purple Pitcher Plant .... see PITCHER PLANT
Purple Rocket .... see FIREWEED
Purple Side-saddle Flower .... see PITCHER PLANT
Purple Turk's Cap Lily .... see MARTAGON
Purple Willow-herb .... see PURPLE LOOSESTRIFE
Purpursonnenhutkraut .... see ECHINACEA
Purpursonnenhutwurzel .... see ECHINACEA

Purshiana Bark .... see CASCARA
P'u-t'ao .... see BITTER MELON
Putcha-pat .... see PATCHOULY OIL
Putiha .... see JAPANESE MINT, SPEARMINT
Putikaranja .... see DIVI-DIVI
PYCNOGENOL .... see PYCNOGENOL
Pygenol .... see PYCNOGENOL
PYGEUM .... see PYGEUM
Pygeum africanum .... see PYGEUM
Pyinma .... see BANABA
PYRETHRUM .... see PYRETHRUM
Pyrethrum cinerariifolium .... see PYRETHRUM
Pyrethrum parthenium .... see FEVERFEW
Pyridoxal Phosphate .... see PYRIDOXINE (VITAMIN B6)
Pyridoxal-5-phosphate .... see PYRIDOXINE (VITAMIN B6)
Pyridoxamine .... see PYRIDOXINE (VITAMIN B6)
PYRIDOXINE (VITAMIN B6) .... see PYRIDOXINE (VITAMIN B6)
Pyridoxine HCl .... see PYRIDOXINE (VITAMIN B6)
Pyridoxine Hydrochloride .... see PYRIDOXINE (VITAMIN B6)
Pyrimidines .... see RNA AND DNA
Pyroleum juniperi .... see CADE OIL
Pyroleum oxycedri .... see CADE OIL
Pyrus asiae-mediae .... see PEAR
Pyrus aucuparia .... see MOUNTAIN ASH
Pyrus balansae .... see PEAR
Pyrus bourgaeana .... see PEAR
Pyrus communis .... see PEAR
Pyrus cydonia .... see QUINCE
Pyrus domestica .... see PEAR
Pyrus elata .... see PEAR
Pyrus medvedevii .... see PEAR
PYRUVATE .... see PYRUVATE
Pyruvic Acid .... see PYRUVATE
Q .... see GLUTAMINE
Qian Ceng Ta .... see CHINESE CLUB MOSS
Qing Hao .... see SWEET ANNIE
Qinghao .... see SWEET ANNIE
Qinghaosu .... see SWEET ANNIE
Quack Grass .... see WHEATGRASS
Quaker .... see ARUM
Quaker Bonnet .... see SKULLCAP
Quaker Buttons .... see NUX VOMICA
Quaking Aspen .... see ASPEN
QUASSIA .... see QUASSIA
Quassia amara .... see QUASSIA
Quassia Bark .... see QUASSIA
Quassia simarouba .... see SIMARUBA
Quebra Pedra .... see CHANCA PIEDRA
QUEBRACHO .... see QUEBRACHO
Quebracho Blanco .... see QUEBRACHO
Quebrachol .... see BETA-SITOSTEROL
Quebrapedra .... see CHANCA PIEDRA
Queen Anne's Lace .... see WILD CARROT
Queen of Fruits .... see MANGOSTEEN
Queen of the Meadow .... see GRAVEL ROOT, MEADOWSWEET
Queen's Crape Myrtle .... see BANABA
QUEEN'S DELIGHT .... see QUEEN'S DELIGHT
Queen's Root .... see QUEEN'S DELIGHT
QUERCETIN .... see QUERCETIN
Quercetin-3-rhamnoglucoside .... see RUTIN
Quercetin-3-rutinoside .... see RUTIN
Quercus alba .... see OAK bark
Quercus cortex .... see OAK bark
Quercus Marina .... see BLADDERWRACK
Quercus pedunculata .... see OAK bark
Quercus petraea .... see OAK bark
Quercus robur .... see OAK bark
Quercus sessiliflora .... see OAK bark
Quick-in-the-hand .... see JEWELWEED
Quickbeam .... see MOUNTAIN ASH
QUILLAIA .... see QUILLAIA
Quillaja .... see QUILLAIA
Quillaja saponaria .... see QUILLAIA
Quimotripsina .... see CHYMOTRYPSIN
QUINCE .... see QUINCE
Quing Dai .... see DA QING YE
Quinina Criolla .... see CHANCA PIEDRA
Quinine .... see CINCHONA
Quinine Creole .... see CHANCA PIEDRA
Quitch Grass .... see WHEATGRASS
Quitte .... see QUINCE
Quittenbaum .... see QUINCE
Qut .... see KHAT
Rabbiteye Blueberry .... see BLUEBERRY
Rabbits .... see YELLOW TOADFLAX
Rabo de Gato .... see HYSSOP
Raccoon Berry .... see PODOPHYLLUM
Race Ginger .... see GINGER
Racine de Carline Acaule .... see CARLINA
Racine de Guimauve .... see MARSHMALLOW
Racine d'Echininacea .... see ECHINACEA
Radicula nasturtium .... see WATERCRESS
Radis .... see RADISH
RADISH .... see RADISH
Radix Anchusae .... see ALKANNA
Radix Cardopatiae .... see CARLINA
Radix Chamaeleontis Albae .... see CARLINA
Radix Codonopsis .... see CODONOPSIS
Radix Ginseng Rubra .... see GINSENG, PANAX
Radix Pimpinelle Franconiae .... see MASTERWORT
Radix Polygoni Multiflori .... see FO-TI
Radix Polygoni Shen Min .... see FO-TI
Radix Puerariae .... see KUDZU
Rag Paper .... see MULLEIN
Ragged Cup .... see CUP PLANT
Ragweed .... see TANSY RAGWORT
Ragwort .... see GOLDEN RAGWORT, TANSY RAGWORT
Rainbow Weed .... see PURPLE LOOSESTRIFE
Raisin d'Amerique .... see POKEWEED berry, POKEWEED root
Raisin d'Ours .... see UVA URSI
Raisins .... see GRAPE fruit, skin
Raiz Para Los Dientes .... see RHATANY
Rajajambu .... see JAMBOLAN bark
Rajani .... see TURMERIC
Rakta Khakasa .... see CORN POPPY
Rakta-posta .... see CORN POPPY
Ramdana .... see AMARANTH
Ram-goat Rose .... see MADAGASCAR PERIWINKLE
Rami Buah .... see CHANCA PIEDRA
Ramp .... see ARUM
Ramsons .... see BEAR'S GARLIC
Ramsted .... see YELLOW TOADFLAX

INDEX

Ramsthorn .... see EUROPEAN BUCKTHORN
Ranawara .... see CASSIA AURICULATA
Ranunculus .... see LESSER CELANDINE
Ranunculus acris .... see BUTTERCUP
Ranunculus bulbosus .... see BULBOUS BUTTERCUP
Ranunculus ficaria .... see LESSER CELANDINE
Ranunculus friesianus .... see BUTTERCUP
Ranunculus sceleratus .... see POISONOUS BUTTERCUP
Raphani Sativi Radix .... see RADISH
Raphanus raphanistrum .... see WILD RADISH
Raphanus sativus .... see RADISH
Rasna .... see ALPINIA
Raspberry .... see RASPBERRY leaf
RASPBERRY leaf .... see RASPBERRY leaf
Ratanhiae Radix .... see RHATANY
Ratanhiawurzel .... see RHATANY
Rattle Pouches .... see SHEPHERD'S PURSE
Rattle Root .... see BLACK COHOSH
Rattle Top .... see BLACK COHOSH
Rattlebush .... see WILD INDIGO
Rattlesnake Root .... see BETH ROOT, BLACK COHOSH, SENEGA
Rattlesnake Violet .... see AMERICAN ADDER'S TONGUE
Rattleweed .... see BLACK COHOSH
Rauschpfeffer .... see KAVA
Raute .... see RUE
Rauvolfia serpentina .... see INDIAN SNAKEROOT
Rauwolfae Radix .... see INDIAN SNAKEROOT
Rauwolfia .... see INDIAN SNAKEROOT
Rauwolfia serpentina .... see INDIAN SNAKEROOT
Rauwolfiawurzel .... see INDIAN SNAKEROOT
Raw Liver .... see LIVER EXTRACT
Raw Spleen .... see SPLEEN EXTRACT
Ray-grass .... see TAUMELLOOLCH
Red .... see DANSHEN
Red-Ink Plant .... see POKEWEED berry, POKEWEED root
Red American Ginseng .... see CANAIGRE
Red Baneberry .... see WHITE COHOSH
Red Bay .... see MAGNOLIA
Red Bearberry .... see UVA URSI
Red Beet .... see BEET
Red Berry .... see GINSENG, AMERICAN
Red Bilberry .... see ALPINE CRANBERRY
Red Bush .... see RED BUSH TEA
RED BUSH TEA .... see RED BUSH TEA
Red Cabbage .... see CABBAGE
Red Cedarwood .... see CEDARWOOD
Red Cherry .... see SOUR CHERRY
Red Chickweed .... see SCARLET PIMPERNEL
Red Cinchona Bark .... see CINCHONA
RED CLOVER .... see RED CLOVER
Red Cockscomb .... see AMARANTH
Red Cole .... see HORSERADISH
Red Date .... see JUJUBE
Red Elm .... see SLIPPERY ELM
Red Fir .... see OREGON FIR BALSAM
Red Ginseng .... see GINSENG, PANAX
Red Globe .... see GRAPE fruit, skin
Red Gum .... see EUCALYPTUS dried leaf, STORAX
Red Indian Paint .... see BLOODROOT
Red Juniper .... see CEDARWOOD
Red Lapacho .... see PAU D'ARCO
Red Legs .... see BISTORT
Red Malaga .... see GRAPE fruit, skin
RED MAPLE .... see RED MAPLE
Red Morocco .... see PHEASANT'S EYE
Red Pepper .... see CAPSICUM
Red Periwinkle .... see MADAGASCAR PERIWINKLE
Red Pimpernel .... see SCARLET PIMPERNEL
Red Plant .... see POKEWEED berry, POKEWEED root
Red Poppy .... see CORN POPPY
Red Puccoon .... see BLOODROOT
Red Raspberry .... see RASPBERRY leaf
Red Rhatany .... see RHATANY
Red Rice Yeast .... see RED YEAST
Red River Snakeroot .... see ARISTOLOCHIA
Red Robin .... see KNOTWEED
Red Root .... see BLOODROOT, NEW JERSEY TEA
Red Rot .... see SUNDEW
Red Sage .... see DANSHEN, GERMAN SARSAPARILLA
RED SANDALWOOD .... see RED SANDALWOOD
Red Sanderswood .... see RED SANDALWOOD
Red Saunders .... see RED SANDALWOOD
RED SOAPWORT .... see RED SOAPWORT
Red Spur Valerian .... see RED-SPUR VALERIAN
Red Squill .... see SQUILL
Red Sunflower .... see ECHINACEA
Red Tea .... see HIBISCUS
Red Thyme Oil .... see THYME OIL
Red Valerian .... see RED-SPUR VALERIAN
Red Vine Leaf AS 195 .... see GRAPE leaf
Red Vine Leaf Extract .... see GRAPE leaf
Red Weed .... see POKEWEED berry, POKEWEED root
Red Wheatgrass .... see GERMAN SARSAPARILLA
Red Whortleberry .... see ALPINE CRANBERRY
RED YEAST .... see RED YEAST
Red Yeast Rice .... see RED YEAST
Redberries .... see ALPINE CRANBERRY
Redberry .... see UVA URSI
Redroot .... see NEW JERSEY TEA
RED-SPUR VALERIAN .... see RED-SPUR VALERIAN
Reduced DPN .... see NADH
Reduced Nicotinamide Adenine Dinucleotide .... see NADH
Reed .... see REED HERB
REED HERB .... see REED HERB
Reglisse .... see LICORICE
Regliz .... see LICORICE
Reifweide .... see WILLOW BARK
Reishi .... see REISHI MUSHROOM
Rei-shi .... see REISHI MUSHROOM
REISHI MUSHROOM .... see REISHI MUSHROOM
Ren Dong .... see HONEYSUCKLE
Ren Shen .... see GINSENG, AMERICAN; GINSENG, PANAX
Renshen .... see GINSENG, AMERICAN; GINSENG, PANAX
Renxian .... see GINSENG, PANAX
Requia .... see ANDIROBA
Reseda .... see HENNA
Reshira .... see VETIVER
Resin Tolu .... see TOLU BALSAM
Resina Tolutana .... see TOLU BALSAM
Restharrow .... see SPINY RESTHARROW
RESVERATROL .... see RESVERATROL
Retinispora juniperoides .... see ORIENTAL ARBORVITAE
Retinoids .... see VITAMIN A
Retinol .... see VITAMIN A

Retinol Acetate .... see VITAMIN A
Retinol Palmitate .... see VITAMIN A
Retinyl Acetate .... see VITAMIN A
Retinyl Palmitate .... see VITAMIN A
Reunion Vanilla .... see VANILLA
RGH-4405 .... see VINPOCETINE
Rhamni Cathartica Fructus .... see EUROPEAN BUCKTHORN
Rhamni Purshianae Cortex .... see CASCARA
Rhamnol .... see BETA-SITOSTEROL
Rhamnus cathartica .... see EUROPEAN BUCKTHORN
Rhamnus frangula .... see ALDER BUCKTHORN
Rhamnus purshiana .... see CASCARA
Rhamnus zizyphus .... see JUJUBE
Rhatanhia .... see RHATANY
Rhatania .... see RHATANY
RHATANY .... see RHATANY
Rhei .... see RHUBARB
Rhei Radix .... see RHUBARB
Rheum .... see RHUBARB
Rheum australe .... see RHUBARB
Rheum cultorum .... see RHUBARB
Rheum emodi .... see RHUBARB
Rheum hybridum .... see RHUBARB
Rheum officinale .... see RHUBARB
Rheum palmatum .... see RHUBARB
Rheum rhabarbarum .... see RHUBARB
Rheum rhaponticum .... see RHUBARB
Rheum tanguticum .... see RHUBARB
Rheumatism Root .... see WILD YAM
Rheumatism Weed .... see PIPSISSEWA
Rhizoma Dioscoreae .... see WILD YAM
Rhizoma Iridis .... see ORRIS
Rhizome di Kava-kava .... see KAVA
Rhizome Galangae .... see ALPINIA
Rhodiola .... see ROSEROOT
Rhodiola rosea .... see ROSEROOT
Rhododendri Ferruginei Folium .... see RUSTY-LEAVED RHODODENDRON
Rhododendron ferrugineum .... see RUSTY-LEAVED RHODODENDRON
Rhododendron groenlandicum .... see LABRADOR TEA
Rhododendron palustre .... see MARSH TEA
Rhododendron tomentosum var. tomentosum .... see MARSH TEA
Rhoeados Flos .... see CORN POPPY
RHUBARB .... see RHUBARB
Rhus aromatica .... see SWEET SUMACH
Rhus cacodendron .... see TREE OF HEAVEN
Rhus canadensis .... see SWEET SUMACH
Rhus radicans .... see POISON IVY
Rhus toxicodendron .... see POISON IVY
Ribes Nero .... see BLACK CURRANT
Ribes Nigri Folium .... see BLACK CURRANT
Ribes nigrum .... see BLACK CURRANT
Ribgrass .... see BUCKHORN PLANTAIN
RIBOFLAVIN (VITAMIN B2) .... see RIBOFLAVIN (VITAMIN B2)
Riboflavine .... see RIBOFLAVIN (VITAMIN B2)
Ribonucleic Acid .... see RNA AND DNA
RIBOSE .... see RIBOSE
Ribwort .... see BUCKHORN PLANTAIN
Ribwort Plantain .... see BUCKHORN PLANTAIN
RICE BRAN .... see RICE BRAN
Rice Bran Oil .... see RICE BRAN
Ricebran Oil .... see RICE BRAN
Rich Weed .... see STONE ROOT
Richleaf .... see STONE ROOT
Richmond .... see SOUR CHERRY
Ricin .... see CASTOR seed
Ricinus communis .... see CASTOR OIL, CASTOR seed
Ricinus sanguines .... see CASTOR OIL, CASTOR seed
Ringworm Powder .... see GOA POWDER
Rio Ipecac .... see IPECAC
Ripplegrass .... see BUCKHORN PLANTAIN
Rittersspornblüten .... see DELPHINIUM
RNA .... see RNA AND DNA
RNA AND DNA .... see RNA AND DNA
Robbia .... see MADDER
Robin-run-in-the-grass .... see CLIVERS
Robin-run-in-the-hedge .... see GROUND IVY
Rock-rose .... see FROSTWORT
Rock-up-hat .... see ECHINACEA
Rock Brake .... see LADY FERN
Rock Cranberry .... see ALPINE CRANBERRY
Rock Fern .... see MAIDENHAIR FERN
Rock of Polypody .... see LADY FERN
Rock Parsley .... see PARSLEY leaf, root
Rockberry .... see UVA URSI
Rockrose .... see LABDANUM
Rockweed .... see BLADDERWRACK
Rockwrack .... see BLADDERWRACK
Rodia Riza .... see ROSEROOT
Roga Mari .... see YARROW
Rokitnik .... see SEA BUCKTHORN
Rokujo .... see DEER VELVET
Roman-coriander .... see BLACK SEED
ROMAN CHAMOMILE .... see ROMAN CHAMOMILE
Roman Cumin .... see CARAWAY OIL
Roman Laurel .... see SWEET BAY
Roman Motherwort .... see MOTHERWORT
Romarin Sauvage .... see MARSH TEA
Römische Kamille .... see ROMAN CHAMOMILE
Ronce d'Amerique .... see CRANBERRY
Rooibos .... see RED BUSH TEA
Rooibos Tea .... see RED BUSH TEA
Root of the Holy Ghost .... see ANGELICA root
Rooted Sage .... see DANSHEN
Rorippa armoracia .... see HORSERADISH
Rorippa nasturtium .... see WATERCRESS
Rosa alba .... see ROSE HIP
Rosa camellia .... see CHEROKEE ROSEHIP
Rosa canina .... see ROSE HIP
Rosa centifolia .... see ROSE HIP
Rosa cherokeensi .... see CHEROKEE ROSEHIP
Rosa chinensis .... see CHEROKEE ROSEHIP
Rosa damascena .... see ROSE HIP
Rosa de Castillo .... see ROSE HIP
Rosa gallica .... see ROSE HIP
Rosa indica .... see CHEROKEE ROSEHIP
Rosa laevigata .... see CHEROKEE ROSEHIP
Rosa lutetiana .... see ROSE HIP
Rosa nivea .... see CHEROKEE ROSEHIP
Rosa pomifera .... see ROSE HIP
Rosa provincialis .... see ROSE HIP
Rosa roulettii .... see CHEROKEE ROSEHIP
Rosa rugosa .... see ROSE HIP
Rosa sinica .... see CHEROKEE ROSEHIP

Rosa ternata .... see CHEROKEE ROSEHIP
Rosa villosa .... see ROSE HIP
Rosae Pseudofructus Cum Semen .... see ROSE HIP
Rosary Pea .... see PRECATORY BEAN
Rose-a-rubie .... see PHEASANT'S EYE
Rose-colored Silkweed .... see SWAMP MILKWEED
Rose Apple .... see JAMBOLAN bark, JAMBOLAN seed
Rose Bay .... see OLEANDER
Rose Bay Willow .... see FIREWEED
ROSE GERANIUM OIL .... see ROSE GERANIUM OIL
ROSE HIP .... see ROSE HIP
Rose Hip with Seed .... see ROSE HIP
Rose Hips .... see ROSE HIP
Rose Laurel .... see MOUNTAIN LAUREL, OLEANDER
Rose Mallow .... see HOLLYHOCK
Rose Root .... see ROSEROOT
Rose Root Extract .... see ROSEROOT
Rose Willow .... see AMERICAN DOGWOOD
Roseau Commun .... see REED HERB
Rosebay .... see RUSTY-LEAVED RHODODENDRON
Rosebay Willow .... see FIREWEED
Rosehips .... see ROSE HIP
Roselle .... see HIBISCUS
ROSEMARY .... see ROSEMARY
Rosenoble .... see FIGWORT
Rosenroot .... see ROSEROOT
ROSEROOT .... see ROSEROOT
Rosewood Oil .... see BOIS DE ROSE OIL
Rosin Rose .... see ST. JOHN'S WORT
Rosin Weed .... see GUMWEED
ROSINWEED .... see ROSINWEED
Rosinweed .... see CUP PLANT, ROSINWEED
Rosmarinus officinalis .... see ROSEMARY
Roter Sonnenhut .... see ECHINACEA
Roter Wasserhanf .... see GRAVEL ROOT
Rotten Cheese Fruit .... see MORINDA
Rottlera Tinctoria .... see KAMALA
Rou Gui .... see CASSIA CINNAMON
Roucou .... see ANNATTO
Round-leafed Sundew .... see SUNDEW
Round-leaved Hepatica .... see LIVERWORT
Round-lobe Hepatica .... see LIVERWORT
Round Buchu .... see BUCHU
Roupellia grata .... see STROPHANTHUS
Rowan Tree .... see MOUNTAIN ASH
Roxanthin Red 10 .... see CANTHAXANTHIN
Royal Jasmine .... see JASMINE
ROYAL JELLY .... see ROYAL JELLY
RRR-alpha-tocopherol .... see VITAMIN E
Rubbed Thyme .... see THYME flower, leaf
Rubi Fruticosi Folium .... see BLACKBERRY
Rubi Fruticosi Radix .... see BLACKBERRY
Rubi Idaei Folium .... see RASPBERRY leaf
Rubia .... see MADDER
Rubia tinctorum .... see MADDER
Rubiae Tinctorum Radix .... see MADDER
Rubus .... see RASPBERRY leaf
Rubus affinis .... see BLACKBERRY
Rubus buschii .... see RASPBERRY leaf
Rubus fruticosus .... see BLACKBERRY
Rubus idaeus .... see RASPBERRY leaf
Rubus plicatus .... see BLACKBERRY
Rubus strigosus .... see RASPBERRY leaf
Rubywood .... see RED SANDALWOOD
Ruda .... see QUASSIA, RUE
RUE .... see RUE
Rue officinale .... see RUE
Ruibarbo Caribe .... see MORINDA
Rum Cherry Bark .... see WILD CHERRY
Rumalon .... see BOVINE CARTILAGE
Rumex .... see YELLOW DOCK
Rumex acetosa .... see SORREL
Rumex aquaticus .... see WATER DOCK
Rumex crispus .... see YELLOW DOCK
Rumex hymenosepalus .... see CANAIGRE
Rumex obtusifolius .... see YELLOW DOCK
Rumput Roman .... see YIN CHEN
Run-by-the-ground .... see PENNYROYAL leaf, PENNYROYAL OIL
Running Box .... see SQUAWVINE
Running Jenny .... see MONEYWORT
RUPTUREWORT .... see RUPTUREWORT
Rusci Aculeati .... see BUTCHER'S BROOM
Rusci Aculeati Rhizoma .... see BUTCHER'S BROOM
Ruscus aculeatus .... see BUTCHER'S BROOM
Rusmari .... see ROSEMARY
Russian Krainer Tollkraut .... see SCOPOLIA
Russian Licorice .... see LICORICE
Russian Penicillin .... see PROPOLIS
Russian Root .... see GINSENG, SIBERIAN
Rust Treacle .... see GARLIC
Rust-red Rhododendron .... see RUSTY-LEAVED RHODODENDRON
RUSTY-LEAVED RHODODENDRON .... see RUSTY-LEAVED RHODODENDRON
Ruta graveolens .... see RUE
Rutae Folium .... see RUE
Rutae Herba .... see RUE
RUTIN .... see RUTIN
Rutine .... see RUTIN
Rutinum .... see RUTIN
Rutland Beauty .... see GREATER BINDWEED
Rutosid .... see RUTIN
Rutoside .... see RUTIN
Rutosidum .... see RUTIN
Rye .... see RYE GRASS
RYE GRASS .... see RYE GRASS
Rye Grass Pollen .... see RYE GRASS
Rye Grass Pollen Extract .... see RYE GRASS
Rye Pollen Extract .... see RYE GRASS
S-adenosyl Methionine .... see SAMe
S-adenosyl-L-methionine .... see SAMe
S-adenosylmethionine .... see SAMe
S. Boulardii .... see SACCHAROMYCES BOULARDII
S.O.D. .... see SUPEROXIDE DISMUTASE
Sabal .... see SAW PALMETTO
Sabal Fructus .... see SAW PALMETTO
Sabal serrulata .... see SAW PALMETTO
Sabina .... see SAVIN TOPS
Sabline Rouge .... see ARENARIA RUBRA
Saccharomyces .... see SACCHAROMYCES BOULARDII
SACCHAROMYCES BOULARDII .... see SACCHAROMYCES BOULARDII
Saccharomyces cervisiae .... see BREWER'S YEAST
Saccharomyces Cerevisiae Hansen CBS 5926 .... see SACCHAROMYCES BOULARDII
Sacha Foster .... see CHANCA PIEDRA
Sacred Bark .... see CASCARA

INDEX

Sacred Herb .... see YERBA SANTA
Sacred Mushroom .... see PEYOTE
Sadgrantha .... see CALAMUS
Sadi .... see DIVINER'S SAGE
Sadilata .... see ANDROGRAPHIS
SAFFLOWER .... see SAFFLOWER
SAFFRON .... see SAFFRON
Saffron Crocus .... see SAFFRON
Saffron Marigold .... see TAGETES
Safran .... see SAFFRON
Sagackhomi .... see UVA URSI
SAGE .... see SAGE
Sage of Bethlehem .... see SPEARMINT
Sage of the Seers .... see DIVINER'S SAGE
Sagrada Bark .... see CASCARA
Sahlep .... see SALEP
Sailor's Tobacco .... see MUGWORT
Saint Ignatius-beans .... see IGNATIUS BEAN
Sakau .... see KAVA
Salad Chervil .... see CHERVIL
Salad Oil .... see OLIVE OIL
Salai Guggal .... see INDIAN FRANKINCENSE
SALEP .... see SALEP
Salicare .... see PURPLE LOOSESTRIFE
Salicis Cortex .... see WILLOW BARK
Salisburia adiantifolia .... see GINKGO leaf (GINKGO leaf extract)
Salix alba .... see WILLOW BARK
Salix daphnoides .... see WILLOW BARK
Salix fragilis .... see WILLOW BARK
Salix pentandra .... see WILLOW BARK
Salix purpurea .... see WILLOW BARK
Sallow Thorn .... see SEA BUCKTHORN
Salmon Oil .... see FISH OILS
Saloop .... see SALEP
Salsaparilha .... see SARSAPARILLA
Salsepareille .... see SARSAPARILLA
Salsify .... see COMFREY
Salt-rheum Weed .... see TURTLE HEAD
Salvia .... see DIVINER'S SAGE
Salvia bowleyana .... see DANSHEN
Salvia divinorum .... see DIVINER'S SAGE
Salvia fruticosa .... see GREEK SAGE
Salvia lavandulaefolia .... see SAGE
Salvia miltiorrhiza .... see DANSHEN
Salvia officinalis .... see SAGE
Salvia przewalskii .... see DANSHEN
Salvia Root .... see DANSHEN
Salvia sclarea .... see CLARY SAGE
Salvia triloba .... see GREEK SAGE
Salvia yunnanensis .... see DANSHEN
Salvinorin .... see DIVINER'S SAGE
Salvinorin A .... see DIVINER'S SAGE
SAM-e .... see SAMe
Sambilata .... see ANDROGRAPHIS
Sambrani Chettu .... see BRAHMI
Sambuci Sambucus .... see ELDERBERRY
Sambucus ...... see AMERICAN ELDER, ELDERFLOWER
Sambucus canadensis .... see AMERICAN ELDER
Sambucus ebulus .... see DWARF ELDER
Sambucus nigra ...... see ELDERBERRY, ELDERFLOWER
Samch'il .... see PANAX PSEUDOGINSENG
SAMe .... see SAMe
Samento .... see CAT'S CLAW
Samm al Ferakh .... see ASHWAGANDHA
Sammy .... see SAMe
SAMPHIRE .... see SAMPHIRE
Sampier .... see SAMPHIRE
San Qi .... see PANAX PSEUDOGINSENG
San Qui .... see PANAX PSEUDOGINSENG
Sand Plantain .... see BLOND PSYLLIUM
Sand Sedge .... see GERMAN SARSAPARILLA
Sandalwood .... see WHITE SANDALWOOD wood
Sandalwood Padauk .... see RED SANDALWOOD
Sandberry .... see UVA URSI
Sanddorn .... see SEA BUCKTHORN
Sanderswood .... see WHITE SANDALWOOD OIL
Sandriedgraswurzelstock .... see GERMAN SARSAPARILLA
Sandwort .... see ARENARIA RUBRA
SANDY EVERLASTING .... see SANDY EVERLASTING
Sang ...... see GINSENG, AMERICAN; GINSENG, PANAX
Sangre de Drago .... see SANGRE DE GRADO
Sangre de Dragon .... see SANGRE DE GRADO
SANGRE DE GRADO .... see SANGRE DE GRADO
Sangree Root .... see ARISTOLOCHIA
Sangrel .... see ARISTOLOCHIA
Sangue de Agua .... see SANGRE DE GRADO
Sangue de Drago .... see SANGRE DE GRADO
Sanguinaria .... see BLOODROOT
Sanguinaria canadensis .... see BLOODROOT
Sanguinary .... see SHEPHERD'S PURSE, YARROW
Sanguis draconis .... see DRAGON'S BLOOD
Sanguisorba .... see GREATER BURNET
Sanguisorba carnea .... see GREATER BURNET
Sanguisorba officinalis .... see GREATER BURNET
Sanguisorba polygama .... see GREATER BURNET
SANICLE .... see SANICLE
Sanicula europaea .... see SANICLE
Saniculae Herba .... see SANICLE
Sanshichi .... see PANAX PSEUDOGINSENG
Santa Maria .... see FEVERFEW
Santal Oil .... see WHITE SANDALWOOD OIL
Santali Lignum Albi .... see WHITE SANDALWOOD wood
Santali Lignum Rubrum .... see RED SANDALWOOD
Santalum album .... see WHITE SANDALWOOD OIL, WHITE SANDALWOOD wood
Santolina .... see LAVENDER COTTON
Santolina chamaecyparissus ...... see LAVENDER COTTON
Santonica .... see WORMSEED
Sanuf .... see FENNEL fruit, seed
Saponaria officinalis .... see RED SOAPWORT
Saponariae Rubrae Radix .... see RED SOAPWORT
Sappan .... see RED SANDALWOOD
Sarapin .... see PITCHER PLANT
Sardian Nut .... see EUROPEAN CHESTNUT
Sarothamnus scoparius .... see SCOTCH BROOM flower, SCOTCH BROOM herb
Sarothamnus vulgaris .... see SCOTCH BROOM flower, SCOTCH BROOM herb
Sarpagandha .... see INDIAN SNAKEROOT
Sarracenia purpurea .... see PITCHER PLANT
Sarrasin .... see BUCKWHEAT
Sarsa .... see SARSAPARILLA
SARSAPARILLA .... see SARSAPARILLA
Sarsaparillae Radix .... see SARSAPARILLA
Sarsaparillewurzel .... see SARSAPARILLA
Sasa japonica .... see BAMBOO

INDEX

Sasha Foster .... see CHANCA PIEDRA
SASSAFRAS .... see SASSAFRAS
Sassafras albidum .... see SASSAFRAS
Sassafras officinale .... see SASSAFRAS
Sassafras variifolium .... see SASSAFRAS
Sassafrax .... see SASSAFRAS
Satahva .... see DILL above ground parts, DILL seed
Satan's Apple .... see EUROPEAN MANDRAKE
Satapatri .... see ROSE HIP
Satapatrika .... see ROSE HIP
Sati .... see ZEDOARY
Sativari .... see ASPARAGUS
Satureja calamintha .... see CALAMINT
Satureja capitata .... see SPANISH ORIGANUM OIL
Satureja hortensis .... see SUMMER SAVORY
Satureja montana .... see WINTER SAVORY
Satureja nepeta .... see CALAMINT
Satureja obovata .... see WINTER SAVORY
Satyrion .... see SALEP
Sauerdorn .... see EUROPEAN BARBERRY
Sauerkirsche .... see SOUR CHERRY
Sauerkirschenbaum .... see SOUR CHERRY
Sauge .... see SAGE
Saussurea costus .... see COSTUS OIL, COSTUS root
Saussurea lappa .... see COSTUS OIL, COSTUS root
Sauvignon Blanc .... see GRAPE fruit, skin
Savin .... see SAVIN TOPS
SAVIN TOPS .... see SAVIN TOPS
Savine .... see SAVIN TOPS
Savory .... see SUMMER SAVORY, WINTER SAVORY
SAW PALMETTO .... see SAW PALMETTO
Saw Palmetto Berry .... see SAW PALMETTO
Sawi .... see MARIJUANA
Saxifrage .... see PIMPINELLA above ground parts, PIMPINELLA root
Saxifrax .... see SASSAFRAS
Saynt Johannes Wort .... see ST. JOHN'S WORT
Scabiosa arvensis .... see FIELD SCABIOUS
Scabiosa succisa .... see PREMORSE
Scabish .... see EVENING PRIMROSE OIL
Scabwort .... see ELECAMPANE
Scaldweed .... see DODDER
Scale Insect .... see SHELLAC
Scaley Dragon's Claw .... see CORAL ROOT
Scandix cerefolium .... see CHERVIL
Scarlet Berry .... see BITTERSWEET NIGHTSHADE
Scarlet Monarda .... see OSWEGO TEA
SCARLET PIMPERNEL .... see SCARLET PIMPERNEL
Scarlet Sage .... see SAGE
Sceau d'Or .... see GOLDENSEAL
Sceitbezien .... see SEA BUCKTHORN
Scented Fern .... see TANSY
SC-FOS .... see FRUCTO-OLIGOSACCHARIDES
Schilf .... see REED HERB
SCHISANDRA .... see SCHISANDRA
Schisandra Berry .... see SCHISANDRA
Schisandra chinensis .... see SCHISANDRA
Schisandra chinensis var. rubriflora .... see SCHISANDRA
Schisandra splenanthera .... see SCHISANDRA
Schisandrae .... see SCHISANDRA
Schizandra .... see SCHISANDRA
Schizandrae .... see SCHISANDRA
Schizophyllan .... see BETA GLUCANS
Schmallblaettrige Kegelblumenwurzel .... see ECHINACEA
Schmallblaettriger Sonnenhut .... see ECHINACEA
Schollkraut .... see GREATER CELANDINE dried above ground parts
Schwarze Walnuss .... see BLACK WALNUT
Schwarzkümmel .... see BLACK SEED
Schweintang .... see BLADDERWRACK
Scilla .... see SQUILL
Scilla indica .... see SQUILL
Scilla maritima .... see SQUILL
Sclerotium Poriae Cocos .... see PORIA MUSHROOM
Sclerutin .... see RUTIN
Scoke .... see POKEWEED berry, POKEWEED root
Scolopendrium vulgare .... see HARTSTONGUE
Scoparium .... see SCOTCH BROOM herb
Scoparius .... see SCOTCH BROOM flower, SCOTCH BROOM herb
Scopola .... see SCOPOLIA
SCOPOLIA .... see SCOPOLIA
Scopolia carniolica .... see SCOPOLIA
Scopoliae Rhizoma .... see SCOPOLIA
Scotch Barley .... see BARLEY
Scotch Broom .... see SCOTCH BROOM flower, SCOTCH BROOM herb
SCOTCH BROOM flower .... see SCOTCH BROOM flower
SCOTCH BROOM herb .... see SCOTCH BROOM herb
Scotch Fir .... see PINE
Scotch Heather .... see HEATHER
Scotch Mercury .... see DIGITALIS
Scotch Pine .... see PINE
SCOTCH PINE NEEDLE .... see SCOTCH PINE NEEDLE
Scotch Quelch .... see WHEATGRASS
SCOTCH THISTLE .... see SCOTCH THISTLE
Scouring Rush .... see HORSETAIL
Scraperoot .... see OREGON GRAPE
Scratchweed .... see CLIVERS
Scrophula Plant .... see FIGWORT
Scrophularia .... see FIGWORT
Scrophularia marilandica .... see FIGWORT
Scrophularia nodosa .... see FIGWORT
Scrubby Grass .... see SCURVY GRASS
Scubby Trefoil .... see WAFER ASH
Scullcap .... see BAIKAL SKULLCAP, SKULLCAP
SCURVY GRASS .... see SCURVY GRASS
Scurvy Grass .... see SCURVY GRASS, WATERCRESS
Scurvy Root .... see ECHINACEA
Scute .... see BAIKAL SKULLCAP
Scutellaria baicalensis .... see BAIKAL SKULLCAP
Scutellaria lateriflora .... see SKULLCAP
Scutellaria macrantha .... see BAIKAL SKULLCAP
Scutelluria .... see SKULLCAP
Se .... see SELENIUM
Sea Ash .... see SOUTHERN PRICKLY ASH
Sea Buckhorn .... see SEA BUCKTHORN
SEA BUCKTHORN .... see SEA BUCKTHORN
Sea Coral .... see CORAL
Sea Fennel .... see SAMPHIRE
Sea Girdles .... see LAMINARIA
Sea Grape .... see EPHEDRA
Sea Holly .... see ERYNGO above ground parts, ERYNGO root
Sea Holme .... see ERYNGO above ground parts, ERYNGO root
Sea Hulver .... see ERYNGO above ground parts, ERYNGO root

INDEX

Sea Onion ... see SQUILL
Sea Parsley ... see LOVAGE
Sea Sedge ... see GERMAN SARSAPARILLA
Sea Squill Bulb ... see SQUILL
Sea Wormwood ... see WORMSEED
Seabuckthorn ... see SEA BUCKTHORN
Seagirdle Thallus ... see LAMINARIA
Sealroot ... see SOLOMON'S SEAL
Sealwort ... see SOLOMON'S SEAL
Seaweed ... see CHLORELLA
Seawrack ... see BLADDERWRACK
Secale cereale ... see RYE GRASS
Secale cornutum ... see ERGOT
SECRETIN ... see SECRETIN
Sedum acre ... see COMMON STONECROP
Sedum rhodiola ... see ROSEROOT
Sedum rosea ... see ROSEROOT
See Bright ... see CLARY SAGE
Seed-free Bean Pods ... see BEAN POD
Seed on the Leaf ... see CHANCA PIEDRA
Seedorn ... see SEA BUCKTHORN
Segg ... see ORRIS
Sehydrin ... see HYDRAZINE SULFATE
Selada-air ... see WATERCRESS
Selagine ... see HUPERZINE A
Selenicereus grandiflorus ... see CEREUS
Selenite ... see SELENIUM
SELENIUM ... see SELENIUM
Selenium Dioxide ... see SELENIUM
Selenized Yeast ... see SELENIUM
Selenomethionine ... see SELENIUM
SELF-HEAL ... see SELF-HEAL
Self-heal ... see SANICLE, SELF-HEAL
Selleriefruchte ... see CELERY
Selleriesamen ... see CELERY
Semen Anisi ... see ANISE
Semen Cumini Pratensis ... see CARAWAY dried fruit, seed
Semen Nelumbinis ... see LOTUS seed
Semences de Carvi ... see CARAWAY dried fruit, seed
Sementah ... see MANGOSTEEN
Semetah ... see MANGOSTEEN
Seminole Bead ... see PRECATORY BEAN
Sempervivum tectorum ... see HOUSELEEK
Sena Alejandrina ... see SENNA
Senaga Snakeroot ... see SENEGA
Sene d'Egypte ... see SENNA
Seneca ... see SENEGA
Seneca Snakeroot ... see SENEGA
Senecio aureus ... see GOLDEN RAGWORT
Senecio cineraria ... see DUSTY MILLER
Senecio Herb ... see ALPINE RAGWORT
Senecio jacobaea ... see TANSY RAGWORT
Senecio nemorensis ... see ALPINE RAGWORT
Senecio vulgaris ... see GROUNDSEL
SENEGA ... see SENEGA
Senega Snakeroot ... see SENEGA
Senegalia senegal ... see ACACIA
Seneka ... see SENEGA
Seng ... see GINSENG, PANAX
Sengreen ... see HOUSELEEK
SENNA ... see SENNA
Senna alexandrina ... see SENNA
Senna auriculata ... see CASSIA AURICULATA
Sennae Folium ... see SENNA
Sennae Fructus ... see SENNA
Sennae Fructus Acutifoliae ... see SENNA
Sennae Fructus Angustifolia ... see SENNA
Septfoil ... see TORMENTIL
Serenoa repens ... see SAW PALMETTO
Serenoa serrulata ... see SAW PALMETTO
Seriphidium cinum ... see WORMSEED
Serpentaria ... see ARISTOLOCHIA, MONEYWORT
Serpentine-wood ... see INDIAN SNAKEROOT
Serpent's Tongue ... see AMERICAN ADDER'S TONGUE, ENGLISH ADDER'S TONGUE
Serpyllum ... see WILD THYME
Serratula spicata ... see MARSH BLAZING STAR
Seso Vegetal ... see ACKEE
Sessile Oak ... see OAK bark
Seven Barks ... see HYDRANGEA
Seville Orange ... see BITTER ORANGE
SFN ... see SULFORAPHANE
Shaddock Oil ... see GRAPEFRUIT OIL
Shallaki ... see INDIAN FRANKINCENSE
Shallot ... see ONION
Shamrock ... see WOOD SORREL
Shang ... see GINSENG, AMERICAN
Shangzhou Zhiqiao ... see BITTER ORANGE
Shanzha ... see HAWTHORN
SHARK CARTILAGE ... see SHARK CARTILAGE
Shark Cartilage Extract ... see SHARK CARTILAGE
Shark Cartilage Powder ... see SHARK CARTILAGE
SHARK LIVER OIL ... see SHARK LIVER OIL
Sharp-lobe Hepatica ... see LIVERWORT
Shatapuspha ... see FENNEL fruit, seed
Shatavari ... see ASPARAGUS
Shati ... see ZEDOARY
Shatter Stone ... see CHANCA PIEDRA
Shave Grass ... see HORSETAIL
She Gen Mu ... see INDIAN SNAKEROOT
Sheep Laurel ... see MOUNTAIN LAUREL
Sheep Sorrel ... see YELLOW DOCK
Sheep-lice ... see HOUND'S TONGUE
Sheggs ... see ORRIS
Shelf Fungi ... see MAITAKE MUSHROOM
SHELLAC ... see SHELLAC
Shellflower ... see TURTLE HEAD
Shen Min ... see FO-TI
Sheng Shai Shen ... see GINSENG, PANAX
Shepherd's Barometer ... see SCARLET PIMPERNEL
Shepherd's Club ... see MULLEIN
Shepherd's Heart ... see SHEPHERD'S PURSE
Shepherd's Knapperty ... see TORMENTIL
Shepherd's Knot ... see TORMENTIL
Shepherd's Needle ... see SWEET CICELY
SHEPHERD'S PURSE ... see SHEPHERD'S PURSE
Shepherd's Purse Herb ... see SHEPHERD'S PURSE
Shepherd's Scrip ... see SHEPHERD'S PURSE
Shepherd's Sprout ... see SHEPHERD'S PURSE
Shepherd's Staff ... see MULLEIN
Shepherd's Thyme ... see WILD THYME
Shi Liu Gen Pi ... see POMEGRANATE
Shi Liu Pi ... see POMEGRANATE
Shield Fern ... see MALE FERN
Shigoka ... see GINSENG, SIBERIAN
Shih Yin Ch'en ... see YIN CHEN
Shiitake ... see SHIITAKE MUSHROOM
SHIITAKE MUSHROOM ... see SHIITAKE MUSHROOM

INDEX

Shikha-mula .... see WILD CARROT
Shisandra .... see SCHISANDRA
Shitake .... see SHIITAKE MUSHROOM
Shivaphala .... see ANDROGRAPHIS, BAEL
Sho-saiko-to .... see BUPLEURUM
Shoe .... see NERVE ROOT
Shoga .... see GINGER
Shore Cranberry .... see ALPINE CRANBERRY
Short Buchu .... see BUCHU
Short Chain Fructo-Oligosaccharides .... see FRUCTO-OLIGOSACCHARIDES
Shou-wu .... see FO-TI
Shou-wu-pian .... see FO-TI
Shovelweed .... see SHEPHERD'S PURSE
Shoyu .... see SOY
Shrubby Hare's-ear .... see BUPLEURUM
Shu-wei Ts'ao .... see DANSHEN
Shuang Sui Ma Huang .... see EPHEDRA
Shudha Kupilu .... see NUX VOMICA
Siberian Beaver .... see CASTOREUM
Siberain Ginseng .... see GINSENG, SIBERIAN
Sicilian Thyme .... see SPANISH ORIGANUM OIL
Sickle-leaf Hare's-ear .... see BUPLEURUM
Sicklewort .... see BUGLE, SELF-HEAL
Siclewort .... see SELF-HEAL
Sida Cordifolia .... see COUNTRY MALLOW
Side-saddle Plant .... see PITCHER PLANT
Sigualuo .... see LUFFA
Silberdistelwurz .... see CARLINA
Silberweide .... see WILLOW BARK
Silerkraut .... see ALCHEMILLA
Silky Cornel .... see AMERICAN DOGWOOD
Silky Loofah .... see LUFFA
Silphium laciniatum .... see ROSINWEED
Silphium perfoliatum .... see CUP PLANT
Silver Birch .... see BIRCH
Silver in Suspending Agent .... see COLLOIDAL SILVER
Silver Leaf .... see QUEEN'S DELIGHT
Silver Lime .... see SILVER LINDEN
SILVER LINDEN .... see SILVER LINDEN
Silver Protein .... see COLLOIDAL SILVER
Silverhull Buckwheat .... see BUCKWHEAT
Silver-morning-glory .... see HAWAIIAN BABY WOODROSE
Silverweed .... see JEWELWEED, POTENTILLA
Silybin .... see MILK THISTLE
Silybum .... see MILK THISTLE
Silybum marianum .... see MILK THISTLE
Silymarin .... see MILK THISTLE
Simarouba .... see SIMARUBA
Simarouba amara .... see SIMARUBA
SIMARUBA .... see SIMARUBA
Simmondsia californica .... see JOJOBA
Simmondsia chinensis .... see JOJOBA
Simpler's Joy .... see VERBENA
Simson .... see GROUNDSEL
Sinapis alba .... see WHITE MUSTARD
Sinapis Albae Semen .... see WHITE MUSTARD
Sinapis nigra .... see BLACK MUSTARD OIL, BLACK MUSTARD seed
Sine Semine .... see BEAN POD
Sinensetin .... see METHOXYLATED FLAVONES
Singer's Plant .... see HEDGE MUSTARD
Singletary Pea .... see LATHYRUS
Sinsemilla .... see MARIJUANA
Sisymbrium nasturtium .... see WATERCRESS
Sisymbrium officinale .... see HEDGE MUSTARD
SITOSTANOL .... see SITOSTANOL
Sitosterin .... see BETA-SITOSTEROL
Sitosterol .... see BETA-SITOSTEROL
Sitosterolins .... see BETA-SITOSTEROL
Sitosterols .... see BETA-SITOSTEROL
Sium douglasii .... see WATER HEMLOCK
Sium sisarum .... see SKIRRET
SJW .... see ST. JOHN'S WORT
Ska Maria .... see DIVINER'S SAGE
Ska Maria Pastora .... see DIVINER'S SAGE
Skewerwood .... see WAHOO
SKIRRET .... see SKIRRET
Skoke .... see POKEWEED berry, POKEWEED root
Skullcap .... see BAIKAL SKULLCAP, SKULLCAP
SKUNK CABBAGE .... see SKUNK CABBAGE
Skunkbrush .... see SWEET SUMACH
Skunkweed .... see SKUNK CABBAGE
Slave Wood .... see SIMARUBA
Slipper Root .... see NERVE ROOT
Slipper Weed .... see JEWELWEED
SLIPPERY ELM .... see SLIPPERY ELM
Slippery Root .... see COMFREY
Sloe .... see BLACKTHORN berry
Sloe Berry .... see BLACKTHORN berry
Sloe Flower .... see BLACKTHORN flower
Slough-heal .... see SELF-HEAL
Small Cranberry .... see CRANBERRY
Small Hemlock .... see FOOL'S PARSLEY
Small Nettle .... see STINGING NETTLE above ground parts, STINGING NETTLE root
Small Periwinkle .... see PERIWINKLE
Small Radish .... see RADISH
Small Spikenard .... see AMERICAN SPIKENARD
Smallage .... see CELERY, LOVAGE
Smallpox Plant .... see PITCHER PLANT
Smallwort .... see LESSER CELANDINE
Smart Weed .... see SMARTWEED
SMARTWEED .... see SMARTWEED
Smell Fox .... see WOOD ANEMONE
Smellage .... see LOVAGE
Smilax .... see SARSAPARILLA
Smilax aristolochiaefolia .... see SARSAPARILLA
Smilax febrifuga .... see SARSAPARILLA
Smilax medica .... see SARSAPARILLA
Smilax officinalis .... see SARSAPARILLA
Smilax ornata .... see SARSAPARILLA
Smilax regelii .... see SARSAPARILLA
Smooth-leaved Elm .... see ELM BARK
SMOOTH ALDER .... see SMOOTH ALDER
Smooth Hydrangea .... see HYDRANGEA
Smooth Lawsonia .... see HENNA
Smooth Loofah .... see LUFFA
Smut Rye .... see ERGOT
Snake Berry .... see BITTERSWEET NIGHTSHADE
Snake Butter .... see SHIITAKE MUSHROOM
Snake Leaf .... see AMERICAN ADDER'S TONGUE
Snake Lily .... see ORRIS
Snake Root .... see SENEGA
Snake Weed .... see WATER HEMLOCK
Snakeberry .... see WHITE COHOSH

Snakebite ... see BETH ROOT, BLOODROOT
Snakehead ... see TURTLE HEAD
Snakeroot ... see ARISTOLOCHIA, ASARABACCA, BITTER MILKWORT, BLACK COHOSH, ECHINACEA, WATER HEMLOCK
Snakeweed ... see ARISTOLOCHIA, BISTORT, EUPHORBIA
Snap Bean ... see BEAN POD
Snapdragon ... see YELLOW TOADFLAX
Snapping Tobacco Wood ... see WITCH HAZEL
Sneezeweed ... see SNEEZEWORT
SNEEZEWORT ... see SNEEZEWORT
Snow Rose ... see RUSTY-LEAVED RHODODENDRON
Snowball Bush ... see CRAMP BARK
Snowdrop Tree ... see FRINGETREE
Snowflower ... see FRINGETREE
Soap Tree ... see QUILLAIA
Soap Tree Bark ... see QUILLAIA
Soapbark ... see QUILLAIA
Soapweed ... see YUCCA
Soapwort ... see RED SOAPWORT, WHITE SOAPWORT
SOD ... see SUPEROXIDE DISMUTASE
Sodium 4-hydroxybutyrate ... see GAMMA-HYDROXYBUTYRATE (GHB)
Sodium Alginate ... see ALGIN
Sodium Ascorbate ... see VITAMIN C (ASCORBIC ACID)
Sodium Borate ... see BORON
Sodium Edetate ... see EDTA
Sodium Fluoride ... see FLUORIDE
Sodium Gamma-hydroxybutyrate ... see GAMMA-HYDROXYBUTYRATE (GHB)
Sodium Hyaluronate ... see HYALURONIC ACID
Sodium Monofluorophosphate ... see FLUORIDE
Sodium Oxybate ... see GAMMA-HYDROXYBUTYRATE (GHB)
Sodium Oxybutyrate ... see GAMMA-HYDROXYBUTYRATE (GHB)
Sodium Phosphate ... see PHOSPHATE SALTS
Sodium Pyruvate ... see PYRUVATE
Sodium Usniate ... see USNEA
Sodom-apple ... see CALOTROPIS
Soja ... see SOY
Soja max ... see SOY, SOYBEAN OIL
Sojabohne ... see SOY
Solanum dulcamara ... see BITTERSWEET NIGHTSHADE
Solanum nigrum ... see BLACK NIGHTSHADE
Solanum tuberosum ... see POTATO
Soldiers ... see PURPLE LOOSESTRIFE
Soldier's Herb ... see BUCKHORN PLANTAIN
Soldier's Wound Wort ... see YARROW
Solidago canadensis ... see GOLDENROD
Solidago gigantea ... see GOLDENROD
Solidago longifolia ... see GOLDENROD
Solidago serotina ... see GOLDENROD
Solidago virgaurea ... see GOLDENROD
SOLOMON'S SEAL ... see SOLOMON'S SEAL
Solsequia ... see MARSH MARIGOLD
Soma ... see AGA
Somalien Myrrh ... see MYRRH
Sonnenhutwurzel ... see ECHINACEA
Sophora japonica ... see PAGODA TREE
Sophorin ... see RUTIN
Sophretin ... see QUERCETIN
Sorb Apple ... see MOUNTAIN ASH
Sorbi Acupariae Fructus ... see MOUNTAIN ASH
Sorbus aucuparia ... see MOUNTAIN ASH
Sorghum ... see BROOM CORN
Sorghum bicolor ... see BROOM CORN
Sorghum vulgare ... see BROOM CORN
Sorosi ... see BITTER MELON
SORREL ... see SORREL
Sorrel ... see SORREL, YELLOW DOCK
Sorrel Dock ... see SORREL
Sotapa ... see DILL above ground parts, DILL seed
Soudan Coffee ... see COLA NUT
SOUR CHERRY ... see SOUR CHERRY
Sour Dock ... see SORREL, YELLOW DOCK
Sour Orange ... see BITTER ORANGE
Sour Sop ... see GRAVIOLA
Sour Trefoil ... see WOOD SORREL
Souring Rush ... see HORSETAIL
Soursop ... see GRAVIOLA
South African Star Grass ... see AFRICAN WILD POTATO
Southern Bayberry ... see BAYBERRY
Southern Black Haw ... see BLACK HAW
Southern Ginseng ... see JIAOGULAN
SOUTHERN PRICKLY ASH ... see SOUTHERN PRICKLY ASH
Southern Schisandra ... see SCHISANDRA
Southern Wax Myrtle ... see BAYBERRY
Southernwood Root ... see CARLINA
Sow Berry ... see EUROPEAN BARBERRY
Sowa ... see DILL above ground parts, DILL seed
Sowbread ... see CYCLAMEN
SOY ... see SOY
Soy ... see SOY, SOYBEAN OIL
Soy Bean Lecithin ... see LECITHIN
Soy Bean Oil ... see SOYBEAN OIL
Soy Fiber ... see SOY
Soy Isoflavone Polysaccharide ... see GENISTEIN COMBINED POLYSACCHARIDE
Soy Lecithin ... see LECITHIN
Soy Milk ... see SOY
Soy Phosphatidylserine ... see PHOSPHATIDYLSERINE
Soy Protein ... see SOY
Soy Protein Extract ... see SOY
Soya ... see SOY
Soya Lecithin ... see LECITHIN
Soya Oil ... see SOYBEAN OIL
Soybean ... see SOY, SOYBEAN OIL
Soybean Curd ... see SOY
Soybean Lecithin ... see LECITHIN
SOYBEAN OIL ... see SOYBEAN OIL
Soybeans ... see SOYBEAN OIL
Soyca ... see SOYBEAN OIL
Soy-PS ... see PHOSPHATIDYLSERINE
SP 303 ... see SANGRE DE GRADO
Spadic ... see COCA
Spanish Bayonet ... see YUCCA
SPANISH BROOM ... see SPANISH BROOM
Spanish Chestnut ... see EUROPEAN CHESTNUT, HORSE CHESTNUT
Spanish Jasmine ... see JASMINE
Spanish Lavender ... see LAVENDER
Spanish Licorice ... see LICORICE
Spanish Origanum ... see SPANISH ORIGANUM OIL
SPANISH ORIGANUM OIL ... see SPANISH ORIGANUM OIL

INDEX

Spanish Pimienta ... see ALLSPICE
Spanish Psyllium ... see BLACK PSYLLIUM
Spanish Saffron ... see SAFFRON
Spanish Sage ... see SAGE
Spanish Thyme ... see SPANISH ORIGANUM OIL; THYME flower, leaf; THYME OIL
Spanish Vetchling ... see LATHYRUS
Spargelkraut ... see ASPARAGUS
Spargelwurzelstock ... see ASPARAGUS
Sparrow Grass ... see ASPARAGUS
Sparrow Tongue ... see KNOTWEED
Spartium junceum ... see SPANISH BROOM
Spartium scoparium ... see SCOTCH BROOM flower, SCOTCH BROOM herb
Spathyema foetidus ... see SKUNK CABBAGE
SPEARMINT ... see SPEARMINT
Speckled Jewels ... see JEWELWEED
Speedwell ... see BROOKLIME, VERONICA
Spergularia rubra ... see ARENARIA RUBRA
SPG ... see BETA GLUCANS
Spiceberry ... see WINTERGREEN leaf, WINTERGREEN OIL
Spigelia marilandica ... see PINK ROOT
Spignet ... see AMERICAN SPIKENARD
Spike Lavender ... see LAVENDER
Spiked Loosestrife ... see PURPLE LOOSESTRIFE
Spikenard ... see AMERICAN SPIKENARD
SPINACH ... see SPINACH
Spinacia inermis ... see SPINACH
Spinacia oleracea ... see SPINACH
Spinacia spinosa ... see SPINACH
Spinaciae Folium ... see SPINACH
Spinatblatter ... see SPINACH
Spindle Tree ... see WAHOO
Spiny Dogfish Shark ... see SQUALAMINE
SPINY RESTHARROW ... see SPINY RESTHARROW
Spiraea trifoliata ... see INDIAN PHYSIC
Spiraea ulmaria ... see MEADOWSWEET
Spiraeae Flos ... see MEADOWSWEET
Spire Mint ... see SPEARMINT
Spireae Herba ... see MEADOWSWEET
Spirit Plant ... see REISHI MUSHROOM
Spirits of Turpentine ... see TURPENTINE OIL
Spirogermanium ... see GERMANIUM
Spirulina ... see BLUE-GREEN ALGAE
Spirulina maxima ... see BLUE-GREEN ALGAE
Spirulina pacifica ... see BLUE-GREEN ALGAE
Spirulina platensis ... see BLUE-GREEN ALGAE
Spitzwegerichkraut ... see BUCKHORN PLANTAIN
Spleen ... see SPLEEN EXTRACT
Spleen Concentrate ... see SPLEEN EXTRACT
SPLEEN EXTRACT ... see SPLEEN EXTRACT
Spleen Factors ... see SPLEEN EXTRACT
Spleen Peptides ... see SPLEEN EXTRACT
Spleen Polypeptides ... see SPLEEN EXTRACT
Splenopentin ... see SPLEEN EXTRACT
Spogel ... see BLOND PSYLLIUM
Sponge Cucumber ... see LUFFA
Sponsa Solis ... see MARSH MARIGOLD
Spoon Laurel ... see MOUNTAIN LAUREL
Spoonwood ... see KAMALA
Spoonwort ... see SCURVY GRASS
Spotted Cowbane ... see WATER HEMLOCK
Spotted Elder ... see WITCH HAZEL
Spotted Hemlock ... see HEMLOCK, WATER HEMLOCK
Spotted Monarda ... see HORSEMINT
Spotted Parsley ... see WATER HEMLOCK
Spotted Thistle ... see BLESSED THISTLE
Spotted Touch-me-not ... see JEWELWEED
Spotted Wintergreen ... see PIPSISSEWA
Spring Grass ... see SWEET VERNAL GRASS
Spruce ... see FIR, HEMLOCK SPRUCE
Spruce Fir ... see FIR, HEMLOCK SPRUCE
Spumonto ... see KOMBUCHA TEA
Spurge Flax ... see MEZEREON
Spurge Laurel ... see MEZEREON
Spurge Olive ... see MEZEREON
Spurred Rye ... see ERGOT
SPV 30 ... see BOXWOOD
SQ-9453 ... see DMSO (DIMETHYLSULFOXIDE)
SQUALAMINE ... see SQUALAMINE
Squalus acanthias ... see SHARK CARTILAGE, SHARK LIVER OIL, SQUALAMINE
Squaw Balm ... see PENNYROYAL leaf, PENNYROYAL OIL
Squaw Berry ... see SQUAWVINE
Squaw Root ... see BLACK COHOSH, BLUE COHOSH
Squaw Tea ... see MORMON TEA
Squaw Vine ... see SQUAWVINE
Squaw Weed ... see ALPINE RAGWORT, GOLDEN RAGWORT
Squawbush ... see SWEET SUMACH
Squawmint ... see PENNYROYAL leaf, PENNYROYAL OIL
SQUAWVINE ... see SQUAWVINE
Squawweed ... see ALPINE RAGWORT, GOLDEN RAGWORT
SQUILL ... see SQUILL
Squirrel Corn ... see CORYDALIS, TURKEY CORN
Sr ... see STRONTIUM
Sri Lanka Cinnamon ... see CINNAMON bark
SSG ... see BETA GLUCANS
St. Anthony's Turnip ... see BULBOUS BUTTERCUP
St. Barbara's Hedge Mustard ... see HEDGE MUSTARD
St. Bartholemew's Tea ... see MATE
St. Benedict Thistle ... see BLESSED THISTLE
St. James' Tea ... see LABRADOR TEA
St. James' Weed ... see SHEPHERD'S PURSE
St. James' Wort ... see TANSY RAGWORT
St. John's Bread ... see CAROB
St. John's Herb ... see HEMP AGRIMONY
St. John's Plant ... see MUGWORT
ST. JOHN'S WORT ... see ST. JOHN'S WORT
St. Josephwort ... see BASIL
St. Mary Thistle ... see MILK THISTLE
St. Mary's Seal ... see SOLOMON'S SEAL
ST-200 ... see ACETYL-L-CARNITINE
Stabilized Liquid Oxygen ... see VITAMIN O
Stabilized Oxygen ... see VITAMIN O
Stabilized Rice Bran ... see RICE BRAN
Stable strontium ... see STRONTIUM
Stachys betonica ... see BETONY
Stachys officinalis ... see BETONY
Staff Vine ... see BITTERSWEET NIGHTSHADE
Stag Bush ... see BLACK HAW
Staggerweed ... see DELPHINIUM, TURKEY CORN
Staggerwort ... see TANSY RAGWORT
Stag's Horn ... see CLUB MOSS

Stammerwort ... see TANSY RAGWORT
Standardized Extract of Grapefruit ... see GRAPEFRUIT SEED EXTRACT
Stannous Fluoride ... see FLUORIDE
STAR ANISE ... see STAR ANISE
Star Chickweed ... see CHICKWEED
Starbloom ... see PINK ROOT
Star-bu ... see SEA BUCKTHORN
Starch Blocker ... see BEAN POD
Starchwort ... see ARUM
Starflower ... see BORAGE SEED OIL
Stargrass ... see ALETRIS
Starweed ... see CHICKWEED
Starwort ... see ALETRIS, FALSE UNICORN
Staunchweed ... see YARROW
Stave Oak ... see OAK bark
Stave Wood ... see SIMARUBA
STAVESACRE ... see STAVESACRE
Stay Plough ... see SPINY RESTHARROW
Stellaria ... see ALCHEMILLA
Stellaria media ... see CHICKWEED
Stemless Carlina Root ... see CARLINA
Stemless Gentian ... see GENTIAN
Sterculia acuminata ... see COLA NUT
Sterculia Gum ... see KARAYA GUM
Sterculia nitida ... see COLA NUT
Sterculia tragacantha ... see KARAYA GUM
Sterculia urens ... see KARAYA GUM
Sterculia villosa ... see KARAYA GUM
Sterinol ... see BETA-SITOSTEROL
Sterolins ... see BETA-SITOSTEROL
Sterretjie ... see AFRICAN WILD POTATO
STEVIA ... see STEVIA
Stevia eupatoria ... see STEVIA
Stevia purpurea ... see STEVIA
Stevia rebaudiana ... see STEVIA
Stevoside ... see STEVIA
Sthula Tvak ... see CASSIA CINNAMON
Stick-a-back ... see CLIVERS
Stickwort ... see AGRIMONY, WOOD SORREL
Stigma Maydis ... see CORN SILK
Stigmastanol ... see SITOSTANOL
Stillingia ... see QUEEN'S DELIGHT
Stillingia sylvatica ... see QUEEN'S DELIGHT
Stillingia tenuis ... see QUEEN'S DELIGHT
Stinging Nettle ... see STINGING NETTLE above ground parts, STINGING NETTLE root
STINGING NETTLE above ground parts ... see STINGING NETTLE above ground parts
STINGING NETTLE root ... see STINGING NETTLE root
Stingless Nettle ... see WHITE DEAD NETTLE FLOWER
Stinking Arrach ... see ARRACH
Stinking Balm ... see PENNYROYAL leaf, PENNYROYAL OIL
Stinking Benjamin ... see BETH ROOT
Stinking Goosefoot ... see ARRACH
Stinking Motherwort ... see ARRACH
Stinking Nanny ... see TANSY RAGWORT
Stinking Nightshade ... see HENBANE
Stinking Prairie Bush ... see WAFER ASH
Stinking Roger ... see TAGETES
Stinking Rose ... see GARLIC
Stinking Tommy ... see SPINY RESTHARROW
Stinking Willie ... see TANSY
Stinktree ... see TREE OF HEAVEN
Stinkweed ... see JIMSON WEED
Stinkwort ... see JIMSON WEED
Stinky Bob ... see HERB ROBERT
Stizolobium hirsutum ... see COWHAGE
Stone Breaker ... see CHANCA PIEDRA
Stone Oak ... see OAK bark
STONE ROOT ... see STONE ROOT
Stonebreaker ... see CHANCA PIEDRA
STORAX ... see STORAX
Storkbill ... see HERB ROBERT
Stractan ... see LARCH ARABINOGALACTAN
Strained Honey ... see HONEY
Stramonium ... see JIMSON WEED
Strangle Tare ... see DODDER
Straw ... see OAT STRAW
STRAWBERRY ... see STRAWBERRY
Strawberry Bush ... see WAHOO
Strawberry Tomato ... see WINTER CHERRY
Strawberry Tree ... see WAHOO
String Bean ... see BEAN POD
String of Sovereigns ... see MONEYWORT
Stringy Bark Tree ... see EUCALYPTUS dried leaf
Strong-scented Lettuce ... see WILD LETTUCE
STRONTIUM ... see STRONTIUM
Strontium Chloride ... see STRONTIUM
Strontium Citrate ... see STRONTIUM
Strontium Ranelate ... see STRONTIUM
Strontium-89 Chloride ... see STRONTIUM
Strophanthi Grati Semen ... see STROPHANTHUS
Strophanthi Kombe Semen ... see STROPHANTHUS
STROPHANTHUS ... see STROPHANTHUS
Strophanthus gratus ... see STROPHANTHUS
Strophanthus kombe ... see STROPHANTHUS
Strophanthus Seeds ... see STROPHANTHUS
Strychni Semen ... see NUX VOMICA
Strychnos ignatii ... see IGNATIUS BEAN
Strychnos nux-vomica ... see NUX VOMICA
Strychnos Seed ... see NUX VOMICA
Strychnos tieute ... see IGNATIUS BEAN
Stubwort ... see WOOD SORREL
Styphnolobium japonicum ... see PAGODA TREE
Styrax ... see STORAX
Styrax benzoin ... see BENZOIN
Styrax paralleloneurum ... see BENZOIN
Subholz ... see LICORICE
Subtilisin NAT ... see NATTOKINASE
Succory ... see CHICORY
Sudanese Tea ... see HIBISCUS
Sugandhapatra ... see EUCALYPTUS dried leaf
Sugandhimula ... see VETIVER
Sugar Maple ... see RED MAPLE
Sugar Pods ... see CAROB
Sugarbeet ... see BEET
Suikazura ... see HONEYSUCKLE
Sulfated Monosaccharide ... see GLUCOSAMINE SULFATE
Sulfated N-carboxymethylchitosan ... see CHITOSAN
Sulfated O-carboxymethylchitosan ... see CHITOSAN
Sulfated Saccharide ... see GLUCOSAMINE SULFATE
Sulfomucopolysaccharide ... see MESOGLYCAN
Sulfonyl Sulfur ... see MSM (METHYLSULFONYLMETHANE)

Sulforafane ... see SULFORAPHANE
SULFORAPHANE ... see SULFORAPHANE
Sulphated Monosaccharide ... see GLUCOSAMINE SULFATE
Sulphinybismethane ... see DMSO (DIMETHYLSULFOXIDE)
Sulphorafane ... see SULFORAPHANE
Sultanas ... see GRAPE fruit, skin
SUMA ... see SUMA
Suma ... see ECDYSTERONE, SUMA
Sumaruba ... see SIMARUBA
Sumatra Benzoin ... see BENZOIN
SUMBUL ... see SUMBUL
SUMMER SAVORY ... see SUMMER SAVORY
Sumpfporst ... see MARSH TEA
Sun Drop ... see EVENING PRIMROSE OIL
Sun Rose ... see FROSTWORT
SUNDEW ... see SUNDEW
Sunflower ... see SUNFLOWER OIL
SUNFLOWER OIL ... see SUNFLOWER OIL
Sunflower Seed Oil ... see SUNFLOWER OIL
Sunkfield ... see EUROPEAN FIVE-FINGER GRASS
Sunthi ... see GINGER
Supari ... see ANDROGRAPHIS, ARECA
Super Dioxide Dismutase ... see SUPEROXIDE DISMUTASE
SUPEROXIDE DISMUTASE ... see SUPEROXIDE DISMUTASE
Surasa ... see BASIL
Surelle ... see WOOD SORREL
Surinam Quassia ... see QUASSIA
Surinam Wood ... see QUASSIA
Sushavi ... see BITTER MELON
Svetajiraka ... see CUMIN
Swallow Wort ... see GERMAN IPECAC, PLEURISY ROOT
Swamp Cabbage ... see SKUNK CABBAGE
Swamp Cedar ... see CEDAR leaf, CEDAR LEAF OIL
Swamp Dogwood ... see AMERICAN DOGWOOD, WAFER ASH
Swamp Laurel ... see MAGNOLIA
Swamp Maple ... see RED MAPLE
SWAMP MILKWEED ... see SWAMP MILKWEED
Swamp Root ... see YERBA MANSA
Swamp Sassafras ... see MAGNOLIA
Swamp Silkweed ... see SWAMP MILKWEED
Swamp Tea ... see MARSH TEA
Sweating Plant ... see BONESET
Sweatroot ... see ABSCESS ROOT
Sweet-cus ... see SWEET CICELY
Sweet-fern ... see SWEET CICELY
Sweet-humlock ... see SWEET CICELY
Sweet-smelling Trefoil ... see HEMP AGRIMONY
Sweet Acacia ... see CASSIE ABSOLUTE
SWEET ALMOND ... see SWEET ALMOND
Sweet Almond Oil ... see SWEET ALMOND
SWEET ANNIE ... see SWEET ANNIE
Sweet Balm ... see LEMON BALM
Sweet Bark ... see CASCARILLA
Sweet Basil ... see BASIL
Sweet Bay ... see MAGNOLIA, SWEET BAY
Sweet Bracken ... see SWEET CICELY
Sweet Broom ... see BUTCHER'S BROOM
Sweet Bugle ... see BUGLEWEED
Sweet Calamus ... see CALAMUS
Sweet Cane ... see CALAMUS
Sweet Chamomile ... see ROMAN CHAMOMILE
Sweet Chervil ... see SWEET CICELY
Sweet Chestnut ... see EUROPEAN CHESTNUT
SWEET CICELY ... see SWEET CICELY
Sweet Cinnamon ... see CALAMUS
SWEET CLOVER ... see SWEET CLOVER
Sweet Cumin ... see ANISE
Sweet Dock ... see BISTORT
Sweet Elder ... see AMERICAN ELDER, ELDERFLOWER
Sweet Elm ... see SLIPPERY ELM
Sweet False Chamomile ... see GERMAN CHAMOMILE
Sweet Fennel ... see FENNEL fruit, seed
Sweet Flag ... see BLUE FLAG, CALAMUS
SWEET GALE ... see SWEET GALE
Sweet Grass ... see CALAMUS
Sweet Gum ... see STORAX
Sweet Herb of Paraguay ... see STEVIA
Sweet Leaf of Paraguay ... see STEVIA
Sweet Lucerne ... see SWEET CLOVER
Sweet Mandulin ... see HEMP AGRIMONY
Sweet Marjoram ... see MARJORAM
Sweet Mary ... see LEMON BALM
Sweet Melilot ... see SWEET CLOVER
Sweet Myrtle ... see CALAMUS
Sweet Oil ... see OLIVE OIL
SWEET ORANGE ... see SWEET ORANGE
Sweet Pea ... see LATHYRUS
Sweet Pepper ... see CAPSICUM
Sweet Root ... see CALAMUS, LICORICE
Sweet Rush ... see CALAMUS
Sweet Scented Cactus ... see CEREUS
Sweet Sedge ... see CALAMUS
Sweet Slumber ... see BLOODROOT
SWEET SUMACH ... see SWEET SUMACH
Sweet Vernal ... see PHEASANT'S EYE
SWEET VERNAL GRASS ... see SWEET VERNAL GRASS
SWEET VIOLET ... see SWEET VIOLET
Sweet Violet Herb ... see SWEET VIOLET
Sweet Violet Root ... see SWEET VIOLET
Sweet Weed ... see MARSHMALLOW
Sweet Wood Bark ... see CASCARILLA
SWEET WOODRUFF ... see SWEET WOODRUFF
Sweet Wormwood ... see SWEET ANNIE
Sweethearts ... see CLIVERS
Sweetleaf ... see STEVIA
Sweets ... see SWEET CICELY
Swertia chirata ... see CHIRATA
Swertia chirayita ... see CHIRATA
Swine Snout ... see DANDELION above ground parts, DANDELION entire plant
Swinebread ... see CYCLAMEN
Swine's Grass ... see KNOTWEED
Swiss Mountain Pine ... see PINE
Swynel Grass ... see KNOTWEED
Sycocarpus rusbyi ... see COCILLANA
Symphytum officinale ... see COMFREY
Symphytum Radix ... see COMFREY
Symplocarpus foetidus ... see SKUNK CABBAGE
Synephrine ... see BITTER ORANGE
Synkfoyle ... see EUROPEAN FIVE-FINGER GRASS

INDEX

Syrian Tragacanth .... see TRAGACANTH
Syxygii Cumini Cortex .... see JAMBOLAN bark
Syxygii Cumini Semen .... see JAMBOLAN seed
Syzygium aromaticum .... see CLOVE dried flowerbud, leaf, stem; CLOVE OIL
Syzygium cumini .... see JAMBOLAN bark, JAMBOLAN seed
Syzygium jambolanum .... see JAMBOLAN bark, JAMBOLAN seed
Tabasco Pepper .... see CAPSICUM
Tabebuia avellanedae .... see PAU D'ARCO
Tabebuia heptaphylla .... see PAU D'ARCO
Tabebuia impetiginosa .... see PAU D'ARCO
Tabebuia ipe .... see PAU D'ARCO
Tabebuia palmeri .... see PAU D'ARCO
Tabernanthe iboga .... see IBOGA
Table Grapes .... see GRAPE fruit, skin
Tag Alder .... see SMOOTH ALDER
Tagara .... see VALERIAN
TAGETES .... see TAGETES
Tagetes erecta .... see TAGETES
Tagetes glandulifera .... see TAGETES
Tagetes minuta .... see TAGETES
Tagetes patula .... see TAGETES
Taheebo .... see PAU D'ARCO
Taheebo Tea .... see PAU D'ARCO
Tahiti Vanilla .... see VANILLA
Tahitian Noni Juice .... see MORINDA
Tahitian Vanilla .... see VANILLA
Tailapatra .... see EUCALYPTUS dried leaf
Tailed Chubebs .... see CUBEBS
Tailed Pepper .... see CUBEBS
Taja .... see CASSIA CINNAMON
Takila .... see ANDROGRAPHIS
Talepetrako .... see GOTU KOLA
Talewort ..... see BORAGE flower, dried above ground parts
Tall Buttercup .... see BUTTERCUP
Tall Melilot .... see SWEET CLOVER
Tall Nasturtium .... see WATERCRESS
Tall Speedwell .... see BLACK ROOT
Tall Veronica .... see BLACK ROOT
Tallow Shrub .... see BAYBERRY
Tamalaka .... see CHANCA PIEDRA
TAMARIND .... see TAMARIND
Tamarindo .... see TAMARIND
Tamarindus indica .... see TAMARIND
Tame Withy .... see FIREWEED
Tamus .... see BRYONIA
Tamus communis .... see BLACK BRYONY
Tamus edulis .... see BLACK BRYONY
Tan Kue Bai Zhi .... see DONG QUAI
Tan Xiang .... see WHITE SANDALWOOD wood
Tanaceti parthenii .... see FEVERFEW
Tanacetum boreale .... see TANSY
Tanacetum cinerariifolium .... see PYRETHRUM
Tanacetum parthenium .... see FEVERFEW
Tanacetum vulgare .... see TANSY
Tang .... see BLADDERWRACK
Tang Kuei .... see DONG QUAI
Tangantangan Oil Plant .... see CASTOR OIL, CASTOR seed
Tangeretin .... see METHOXYLATED FLAVONES
Tanner's Bark .... see OAK bark
Tanner's Cassia .... see CASSIA AURICULATA
Tanner's Oak .... see OAK bark
TANNIC ACID .... see TANNIC ACID
Tan-shen .... see DANSHEN
TANSY .... see TANSY
Tansy Flower .... see TANSY
Tansy Herb .... see TANSY
TANSY RAGWORT .... see TANSY RAGWORT
Tantusara .... see ARECA
Tar Weed .... see GUMWEED
Taraktogenos kurzii .... see CHAULMOOGRA
Taraxaci Herba .... see DANDELION above ground parts
Taraxacum .... see DANDELION above ground parts, DANDELION entire plant
Taraxacum dens-leonis .... see DANDELION above ground parts
Taraxacum officinale .... see DANDELION above ground parts, DANDELION entire plant
Taraxacum vulgare .... see DANDELION above ground parts, DANDELION entire plant
Tare .... see TAUMELLOOLCH
Target-leaved Hibiscus .... see AMBRETTE
TARRAGON .... see TARRAGON
Tart Cherry .... see SOUR CHERRY
Tartaric Acid .... see ALPHA HYDROXY ACIDS
Tarweed .... see YERBA SANTA
Tasmanian Blue Gum .... see EUCALYPTUS dried leaf
Taso-ho-hua .... see THUNDER GOD VINE
Taspine .... see SANGRE DE GRADO
Tatuaba .... see CATUABA
TAUMELLOOLCH .... see TAUMELLOOLCH
TAURINE .... see TAURINE
Tausendaugbram .... see YARROW
Taxus baccata .... see YEW
Taxus brevifolia .... see YEW
TC-80 .... see IPRIFLAVONE
Tchaad .... see KHAT
T'chai from the Sea .... see KOMBUCHA TEA
TCV-3b .... see VINPOCETINE
Tea .... see BLACK TEA, GREEN TEA
Tea Green .... see GREEN TEA
TEA TREE OIL .... see TEA TREE OIL
Teaberry .... see WINTERGREEN leaf, WINTERGREEN OIL
Teamster's Tea .... see EPHEDRA, MORMON TEA
Teasel .... see BONESET, TEAZLE
TEAZLE .... see TEAZLE
Tecoma impetiginosa .... see PAU D'ARCO
Tecoma ipe .... see PAU D'ARCO
Tecuitlatl .... see BLUE-GREEN ALGAE
Teinturiere .... see POKEWEED berry, POKEWEED root
Tempeh .... see SOY
Temu Kuning .... see ZEDOARY
Temu Lawak .... see JAVANESE TURMERIC
Temu Lawas .... see JAVANESE TURMERIC
Temu Putih .... see ZEDOARY
Terebinthina Laricina .... see LARCH TURPENTINE
Terebinthina Veneta .... see LARCH TURPENTINE
Terebinthinae aetheroleum .... see TURPENTINE OIL
TERMINALIA .... see TERMINALIA
Terminalia arjuna .... see TERMINALIA
Terminalia bellirica .... see TERMINALIA

INDEX

Terminalia chebula .... see TERMINALIA
Tetracosanol .... see POLICOSANOL
Tetracosanol (24-C) .... see OCTACOSANOL
Tetrahydro-2-furanone ....
.... see GAMMA BUTYROLACTONE (GBL)
Tetramethoxyflavones ....
.... see METHOXYLATED FLAVONES
Tetramethylene Glycol .... see BUTANEDIOL (BD)
Tetramethylene-1,4-diol .... see BUTANEDIOL (BD)
Tetratriacontanol .... see POLICOSANOL
Tetterberry .... see BRYONIA
Tetterwort .... see BLOODROOT, GREATER CELANDINE dried above ground parts
Teucrium chamaedrys .... see GERMANDER, GROUND PINE
Teucrium scordium .... see WATER GERMANDER
Teucrium scorodonia .... see WOOD SAGE
Tewon Lawa .... see JAVANESE TURMERIC
Texas Cedarwood .... see CEDARWOOD
Texas Snakeroot .... see ARISTOLOCHIA
Texturized Vegetable Protein .... see SOY
TF .... see TRANSFER FACTOR
TFd .... see TRANSFER FACTOR
Thalictroc .... see HEDGE MUSTARD
The Roman Plant .... see SWEET CICELY
Thea bohea .... see BLACK TEA, GREEN TEA
Thea sinensis .... see BLACK TEA, GREEN TEA
Thea viridis .... see BLACK TEA, GREEN TEA
Theanine .... see THEANINE
Theobroma .... see COCOA
Theobroma cacao .... see COCOA
Theobroma sativum .... see COCOA
Theobromine .... see COCOA
Thevetia neriifolia .... see OLEANDER
Thevetia peruviana .... see OLEANDER
Thiamin .... see THIAMINE (VITAMIN B1)
Thiamin Chloride .... see THIAMINE (VITAMIN B1)
Thiamin Hydrochloride ..... see THIAMINE (VITAMIN B1)
THIAMINE (VITAMIN B1) ....
.... see THIAMINE (VITAMIN B1)
Thiamine Chloride .... see THIAMINE (VITAMIN B1)
Thiamine Hydrochloride ....
.... see THIAMINE (VITAMIN B1)
Thiaminium Chloride Hydrochloride ....
.... see THIAMINE (VITAMIN B1)
Thick-leaved Pennywort .... see GOTU KOLA
Thimbleberry .... see BLACKBERRY
Thioctacid .... see ALPHA-LIPOIC ACID
Thioctan .... see ALPHA-LIPOIC ACID
Thioctic Acid .... see ALPHA-LIPOIC ACID
Thlaspi bursa-pastoris .... see SHEPHERD'S PURSE
Thomas Balsam .... see TOLU BALSAM
Thompson Seedless .... see GRAPE fruit, skin
Thormantle .... see TORMENTIL
Thorn-apple .... see JIMSON WEED
Thorny Bearer of Free Berries ....
.... see GINSENG, SIBERIAN
Thorny Burr .... see BURDOCK
Thoroughwax .... see BUPLEURUM
Thoroughwort .... see BONESET, HEMP AGRIMONY
Thor's Beard .... see HOUSELEEK
Thousand-leaf .... see YARROW
Three Seven .... see PANAX PSEUDOGINSENG
Three-leafed Ivy .... see POISON IVY
Three-leafed Nightshade .... see BETH ROOT
Three-leaved Grass .... see WOOD SORREL
Three-leaved Hop Tree .... see WAFER ASH
Three-lobe Sage .... see GREEK SAGE
Threewingnut .... see THUNDER GOD VINE
THREONINE .... see THREONINE
Throat Root .... see WATER AVENS
Throatwort .... see DIGITALIS, FIGWORT
Throw-wort .... see MOTHERWORT
Thuga .... see CEDAR leaf
Thuja .... see CEDAR leaf, CEDAR LEAF OIL
Thuja occidentalis .... see CEDAR leaf, CEDAR LEAF OIL
Thuja Oil .... see CEDAR LEAF OIL
Thuja orientalis .... see ORIENTAL ARBORVITAE
THUNDER GOD VINE .... see THUNDER GOD VINE
Thunder Plant .... see HOUSELEEK
Thwak .... see CINNAMON bark
Thyme .... see THYME flower, leaf; THYME OIL
Thyme Aetheroleum .... see THYME OIL
THYME flower, leaf .... see THYME flower, leaf
THYME OIL .... see THYME OIL
Thyme-leave Gratiola .... see BRAHMI
Thymi Herba .... see THYME flower, leaf
Thymic Extract .... see THYMUS EXTRACT
Thymomodulin .... see THYMUS EXTRACT
Thymosin .... see THYMUS EXTRACT
Thymostimulin .... see THYMUS EXTRACT
Thymus .... see THYMUS EXTRACT
Thymus-derived Polypeptides ..... see THYMUS EXTRACT
Thymus Acid Lysate Derivative ....
.... see THYMUS EXTRACT
Thymus capitatus .... see SPANISH ORIGANUM OIL
Thymus Complex .... see THYMUS EXTRACT
Thymus Concentrate .... see THYMUS EXTRACT
THYMUS EXTRACT .... see THYMUS EXTRACT
Thymus Factors .... see THYMUS EXTRACT
Thymus Polypeptides .... see THYMUS EXTRACT
Thymus serpyllum .... see WILD THYME
Thymus Substance .... see THYMUS EXTRACT
Thymus vulgaris ..... see THYME flower, leaf; THYME OIL
Thymus zygis .... see THYME flower, leaf; THYME OIL
Tian Hua Fen .... see CHINESE CUCUMBER root
Tian Qi .... see PANAX PSEUDOGINSENG
Tiarella cordifolia .... see COOLWORT
Tickleweed .... see AMERICAN HELLEBORE
Tickweed .... see PENNYROYAL leaf, PENNYROYAL OIL
Tiglium .... see CROTON SEEDS
Tiglium Seeds .... see CROTON SEEDS
Tilia argentea .... see SILVER LINDEN
Tilia cordata .... see LINDEN CHARCOAL, LINDEN dried flower, LINDEN dried leaf, LINDEN dried sapwood
Tilia grandifolia .... see LINDEN CHARCOAL, LINDEN dried flower, LINDEN dried leaf, LINDEN dried sapwood
Tilia parvifolia .... see LINDEN CHARCOAL, LINDEN dried flower, LINDEN dried leaf, LINDEN dried sapwood
Tilia platyphyllos .... see LINDEN CHARCOAL, LINDEN dried flower, LINDEN dried leaf, LINDEN dried sapwood
Tilia rubra .... see LINDEN CHARCOAL, LINDEN dried flower, LINDEN dried leaf, LINDEN dried sapwood

INDEX

Tilia tomentosa ... see SILVER LINDEN
Tilia ulmifolia ... see LINDEN CHARCOAL, LINDEN dried flower, LINDEN dried leaf, LINDEN dried sapwood
Tiliae Carbo ... see LINDEN CHARCOAL
Tiliae Flos ... see LINDEN dried flower
Tiliae Folium ... see LINDEN dried leaf
Tiliae Lignum ... see LINDEN dried sapwood
Tiliae Tormentosae Flos ... see SILVER LINDEN
Tilki Uzumu ... see HERB PARIS
Tindved ... see SEA BUCKTHORN
Tinnevelly Senna ... see SENNA
Tipton Weed ... see ST. JOHN'S WORT
TIRATRICOL ... see TIRATRICOL
TMG ... see BETAINE ANHYDROUS, BETAINE HYDROCHLORIDE
To-nezumimochi ... see GLOSSY PRIVET
Toadpipe ... see HORSETAIL, YELLOW TOADFLAX
Tocopherol ... see VITAMIN E
Tocopheryl Acetate ... see VITAMIN E
Tocopheryl Acid Succinate ... see VITAMIN E
Tocopheryl Succinate ... see VITAMIN E
Tocotrienol ... see VITAMIN E
Tocotrienol Concentrate ... see VITAMIN E
Tofu ... see SOY
Toge-banreisi ... see GRAVIOLA
Tohai ... see KHAT
Tohat ... see KHAT
Tolu ... see TOLU BALSAM
TOLU BALSAM ... see TOLU BALSAM
Toluifera balsamum ... see TOLU BALSAM
Toluifera pereirae ... see PERU BALSAM
Toluiferum Balsamum ... see TOLU BALSAM
Tom Rong ... see GAMBOGE
TOMATO ... see TOMATO
Tonga ... see KAVA
Tonka ... see TONKA BEAN
TONKA BEAN ... see TONKA BEAN
Tonka Seed ... see TONKA BEAN
Tonquin Bean ... see TONKA BEAN
Tonquin Musk ... see MUSK
Toothache Bark ... see NORTHERN PRICKLY ASH
Toothache Tree ... see SOUTHERN PRICKLY ASH
Toothpick Ammi ... see KHELLA
Toothpick Plant ... see KHELLA
Torch Weed ... see MULLEIN
Torches ... see MULLEIN
TORMENTIL ... see TORMENTIL
Tormentilla ... see TORMENTIL
Tormentillae Rhizoma ... see TORMENTIL
Toronja ... see GRAPEFRUIT
Torquin Bean ... see TONKA BEAN
Touchi ... see SOY
Touch-me-not ... see GINSENG, SIBERIAN; JEWELWEED
Toute Epice ... see BLACK SEED
Toxicodendron altissimum ... see TREE OF HEAVEN
Toxicodendron pubescens ... see POISON IVY
Toxicodendron quercifolium ... see POISON IVY
Toxicodendron radicans ... see POISON IVY
Toxicodendron toxicarium ... see POISON IVY
Toywort ... see SHEPHERD'S PURSE
Trackleberry ... see BILBERRY
TRAGACANTH ... see TRAGACANTH
Tragacanth Gum ... see TRAGACANTH
TRAILING ARBUTUS ... see TRAILING ARBUTUS
Trailing Mahonia ... see OREGON GRAPE
Trailing Swamp Cranberry ... see CRANBERRY
Trailing Tansy ... see POTENTILLA
Trametes versicolor ... see CORIOLUS MUSHROOM
Trans-10,cis-12 conjugated linoleic acid ... see CONJUGATED LINOLEIC ACID
TRANSFER FACTOR ... see TRANSFER FACTOR
Trans-resveratrol ... see RESVERATROL
TRAVELER'S JOY ... see TRAVELER'S JOY
Traveler's Joy ... see TRAVELER'S JOY, WOODBINE
Travmulsion ... see SOYBEAN OIL
Tree Moss ... see OAK MOSS, USNEA
TREE OF HEAVEN ... see TREE OF HEAVEN
Tree of Life ... see CEDAR leaf, CEDAR LEAF OIL
Tree's Dandruff ... see USNEA
Trefoil ... see LIVERWORT, RED CLOVER
Trembling Aspen ... see ASPEN
Triac ... see TIRATRICOL
Triacontanol (30-C) ... see OCTACOSANOL
Triacylglycerol lipase ... see LIPASE
Tribule Terrestre ... see PUNCTURE VINE
Tribulis ... see PUNCTURE VINE
Tribulus ... see PUNCTURE VINE
Tribulus terrestris ... see PUNCTURE VINE
Tricalcium Phosphate ... see CALCIUM
Tricholomopsis edodes ... see LENTINAN, SHIITAKE MUSHROOM
Trichosanthes ... see CHINESE CUCUMBER fruit, CHINESE CUCUMBER root, CHINESE CUCUMBER seed
Trichosanthes Fruit Peel ... see CHINESE CUCUMBER fruit
Trichosanthes japonica ... see CHINESE CUCUMBER fruit, CHINESE CUCUMBER root, CHINESE CUCUMBER seed
Trichosanthes kirilowii ... see CHINESE CUCUMBER fruit, CHINESE CUCUMBER root, CHINESE CUCUMBER seed
Trifolium ... see RED CLOVER
Trifolium macrorrhizum ... see SWEET CLOVER
Trifolium officinale ... see SWEET CLOVER
Trifolium pratense ... see RED CLOVER
Trigonella ... see FENUGREEK
Trigonella foenugraecum ... see FENUGREEK
Trigonella foenum-graecum ... see FENUGREEK
Triiodothyroacetic Acid ... see TIRATRICOL
Trilisa odoratissima ... see DEERTONGUE
Trillium erectum ... see BETH ROOT
Trimethyl Chitosan Chloride ... see CHITOSAN
Trimethyl Glycine ... see BETAINE ANHYDROUS, BETAINE HYDROCHLORIDE
Trimethylethanolamine ... see CHOLINE
Trimethylglycine ... see BETAINE ANHYDROUS, BETAINE HYDROCHLORIDE
Trimethylglycine Anhydrous ... see BETAINE ANHYDROUS
Trimethylglycine Hydrochloride ... see BETAINE HYDROCHLORIDE
Tripsin ... see TRYPSIN
Tripterygium wilfordii ... see THUNDER GOD VINE

Trisodium Ethylenediamine Tetraacetic Acid ...... see EDTA
Triticum .... see WHEATGRASS
Triticum aestivum .... see WHEAT BRAN
Triticum firmum .... see WHEATGRASS
Triticum repens .... see WHEATGRASS
Trivalent Chromium .... see CHROMIUM
Troene de Chine .... see GLOSSY PRIVET
Trollius europaeus .... see GLOBE FLOWER
Trompillo .... see COCILLANA
Tropaeolum majus .... see NASTURTIUM
Tropical Almond .... see TERMINALIA
True Angostura .... see ANGOSTURA
True Bay .... see SWEET BAY
True Chamomile .... see GERMAN CHAMOMILE
True Ivy .... see ENGLISH IVY
True Lavender .... see LAVENDER
True Saffron .... see SAFFRON
True Sage .... see SAGE
True Senna .... see SENNA
True Unicorn Root .... see ALETRIS
Trueno .... see GLOSSY PRIVET
Trumpet Bush .... see PAU D'ARCO
Trumpet Flower .... see GELSEMIUM
Trumpet Weed .... see GRAVEL ROOT
Truxillo Coca .... see COCA
TRYPSIN .... see TRYPSIN
Tryptophan .... see L-TRYPTOPHAN
Tschambucco .... see KOMBUCHA TEA
Tschut .... see KHAT
Tsubo-kusa .... see GOTU KOLA
Tsuga canadensis .... see PINUS BARK
Tsuru-kokemomo .... see CRANBERRY
Tu Si Zi .... see DODDER
Tuber Root .... see PLEURISY ROOT
Tuckahoe .... see PORIA MUSHROOM
Tuftsin .... see SPLEEN EXTRACT
Tumba .... see COLOCYNTH
TUMERIC .... see TURMERIC
Tuna Cardona .... see PRICKLY PEAR CACTUS
Tung .... see TUNG SEED
TUNG SEED .... see TUNG SEED
Tungchian .... see GOTU KOLA
Tun-hoof .... see GROUND IVY
Turangi-ghanda .... see ASHWAGANDHA
Turanj .... see LIME fruit, peel
Turi Hutan .... see CHANCA PIEDRA
Turkey Claw .... see CORAL ROOT
TURKEY CORN .... see TURKEY CORN
Turkey Grass .... see VERBENA
Turkey Rhubarb .... see RHUBARB
Turkey Tail .... see CORIOLUS MUSHROOM
Turk's Cap .... see MARTAGON
TURMERIC .... see TURMERIC
Turmeric .... see TURMERIC, ZEDOARY
Turmeric Root .... see GOLDENSEAL, TURMERIC
Turnera diffusa .... see DAMIANA
Turnera diffusa var. aphrodisiaca .... see DAMIANA
Turnera microphylla .... see DAMIANA
Turnerae Diffusae Folium .... see DAMIANA
Turnerae Diffusae Herba .... see DAMIANA
Turnhoof .... see GROUND IVY
Turnip Radish .... see RADISH
Turpentine .... see TURPENTINE OIL
TURPENTINE OIL .... see TURPENTINE OIL
Turpentine Weed .... see CUP PLANT
TURTLE HEAD .... see TURTLE HEAD
Turtlebloom .... see TURTLE HEAD
Tussilage .... see COLTSFOOT
Tussilago farfara .... see COLTSFOOT
Tussilago hybrida .... see BUTTERBUR
Tvak .... see CINNAMON bark
Twinberry .... see SQUAWVINE
Twitchgrass .... see WHEATGRASS
Two-eyed Berry .... see SQUAWVINE
Twopenny Grass .... see MONEYWORT
Tyosen-azami .... see ARTICHOKE
Type II Collagen .... see CHICKEN COLLAGEN
Tyr .... see TYROSINE
TYROSINE .... see TYROSINE
Tyrosinum .... see TYROSINE
Tzu Tan-ken .... see DANSHEN
Ubidecarenone .... see COENZYME Q-10
Ubiquinol .... see COENZYME Q-10
Ubiquinone .... see COENZYME Q-10
Udakiryaka .... see DIVI-DIVI
Ugragandha .... see CALAMUS
Ulmus fulva .... see SLIPPERY ELM
Ulmus minor .... see ELM BARK
Ulmus rubra .... see SLIPPERY ELM
Umbellate Wintergreen .... see PIPSISSEWA
Umbrella Leaves .... see BUTTERBUR
Una de Gato .... see CAT'S CLAW
Uncaria guianensis .... see CAT'S CLAW
Uncaria procumbens .... see DEVIL'S CLAW
Uncaria tomentosa .... see CAT'S CLAW
Undi .... see LAURELWOOD
Unsaturated Fatty Acid .... see OLIVE OIL
Untouchable .... see GINSENG, SIBERIAN
Upas .... see COCILLANA
Upright Virgin's Bower .... see CLEMATIS
Upstart .... see AUTUMN CROCUS
Ura .... see MORINDA
Uragoga granatensis .... see IPECAC
Uragoga ipecacuanha .... see IPECAC
Urginea indica .... see SQUILL
Urginea maritima .... see SQUILL
Urginea scilla .... see SQUILL
Urtica .... see STINGING NETTLE above ground parts, STINGING NETTLE root
Urtica diocia .... see STINGING NETTLE above ground parts, STINGING NETTLE root
Urtica urens .... see STINGING NETTLE above ground parts, STINGING NETTLE root
Urticae Herba et Folium .... see STINGING NETTLE above ground parts
Urticae Radix .... see STINGING NETTLE root
Ushana .... see INDIAN LONG PEPPER
Ushira .... see VETIVER
USNEA .... see USNEA
Usnea barbata .... see USNEA
Usnea florida .... see USNEA
Usnea hirta .... see USNEA
Usnea Lichen .... see USNEA
Usnea plicata .... see USNEA
Usnic Acid .... see USNEA
Ussuri .... see GINSENG, SIBERIAN

INDEX

Ussurian Thorny Pepperbrush .... see GINSENG, SIBERIAN
Utricularia vulgaris .... see BLADDERWORT
Uva de Raposa .... see HERB PARIS
UVA URSI .... see UVA URSI
Uvae Ursi Folium .... see UVA URSI
UZARA .... see UZARA
Uzarae Radix .... see UZARA
V .... see VANADIUM
Vaccinium altomontanum .... see BLUEBERRY
Vaccinium amoenum .... see BLUEBERRY
Vaccinium angustifolium .... see BLUEBERRY
Vaccinium ashei .... see BLUEBERRY
Vaccinium brittonii .... see BLUEBERRY
Vaccinium constablaei .... see BLUEBERRY
Vaccinium corymbosum .... see BLUEBERRY
Vaccinium gaultherioides .... see BOG BILBERRY
Vaccinium hagerupii .... see CRANBERRY
Vaccinium lamarckii .... see BLUEBERRY
Vaccinium macrocarpon .... see CRANBERRY
Vaccinium microcarpum .... see CRANBERRY
Vaccinium myrtillus .... see BILBERRY
Vaccinium occidentale .... see BOG BILBERRY
Vaccinium oxycoccos .... see CRANBERRY
Vaccinium pallidum .... see BLUEBERRY
Vaccinium palustre .... see CRANBERRY
Vaccinium pensylvanicum .... see BLUEBERRY
Vaccinium uliginosum .... see BOG BILBERRY
Vaccinium vacillans .... see BLUEBERRY
Vaccinium virgatum .... see BLUEBERRY
Vaccinium vitis-idaea .... see ALPINE CRANBERRY
Vacha .... see CALAMUS
Valencia Orange .... see SWEET ORANGE
VALERIAN .... see VALERIAN
Valeriana .... see VALERIAN
Valeriana edulis .... see VALERIAN
Valeriana jatamansii .... see VALERIAN
Valeriana officinalis .... see VALERIAN
Valeriana Rhizome .... see VALERIAN
Valeriana rubra .... see RED-SPUR VALERIAN
Valeriana sitchensis .... see VALERIAN
Valeriana wallichii .... see VALERIAN
Valerianae Radix .... see VALERIAN
Valeriane .... see VALERIAN
Valine .... see BRANCHED-CHAIN AMINO ACIDS
Vanadate .... see VANADIUM
VANADIUM .... see VANADIUM
Vanadium Pentoxide .... see VANADIUM
Vanadyl .... see VANADIUM
Vanadyl Sulfate .... see VANADIUM
Vanatulasi .... see BASIL
VANILLA .... see VANILLA
Vanilla fragrans .... see VANILLA
Vanilla Leaf .... see DEERTONGUE
Vanilla planifolia .... see VANILLA
Vanilla Plant .... see DEERTONGUE
Vanilla tahitensis .... see VANILLA
Vanilla Trilisa .... see DEERTONGUE
Vanillin .... see VANILLA
Vapor .... see FUMITORY
Varech .... see BLADDERWRACK
Varnish Tree .... see TREE OF HEAVEN, TUNG SEED
Varvara .... see BASIL
Vatadha .... see BITTER ALMOND
Vataireopsis araroba .... see GOA POWDER
Vathada .... see BITTER ALMOND
Vatya .... see COUNTRY MALLOW
Vayambur .... see CALAMUS
Vegetable Antimony .... see BONESET
Vegetable Caterpillar .... see CORDYCEPS
Vegetable Gelatin .... see AGAR
Vegetable Mercury .... see MANACA, PODOPHYLLUM
Vegetable Pepsin .... see PAPAIN
Vegetable Sponge .... see LUFFA
Vegetable Sulfur .... see CLUB MOSS
Vegetable Tallow .... see BAYBERRY
Vegilecithin .... see LECITHIN
Vellaja .... see BLACK PEPPER AND WHITE PEPPER
Vellorita .... see AUTUMN CROCUS
Velvet Antler .... see DEER VELVET
Velvet Bean .... see COWHAGE
Velvet Dock .... see ELECAMPANE
Velvet Flower .... see AMARANTH
Velvet Leaf .... see PAREIRA
Velvet of Young Deer Horn .... see DEER VELVET
Velvet Plant .... see MULLEIN
Velvetleaf .... see ABUTA
Venastat .... see HORSE CHESTNUT
Venetian Turpentine .... see LARCH TURPENTINE
Venostasin Retard .... see HORSE CHESTNUT
Venostat .... see HORSE CHESTNUT
Venus' Basin .... see TEAZLE
Venus' Hair .... see MAIDENHAIR FERN
Venus' Shoe .... see NERVE ROOT
Veratro Verde .... see AMERICAN HELLEBORE
Veratrum album .... see WHITE HELLEBORE
Veratrum eschscholtzii .... see AMERICAN HELLEBORE
Veratrum lobelianum .... see WHITE HELLEBORE
Veratrum luteum .... see FALSE UNICORN
Veratrum viride .... see AMERICAN HELLEBORE
Verbasci Flos .... see MULLEIN
Verbascum densiflorum .... see MULLEIN
Verbascum phlomides .... see MULLEIN
Verbascum thapiforme .... see MULLEIN
Verbascum thapsus .... see MULLEIN
VERBENA .... see VERBENA
Verbena officinalis .... see VERBENA
Verbena triphylla .... see LEMON VERBENA
Verbenae Herba .... see VERBENA
Vernicia cordata .... see TUNG SEED
Vernis de Japon .... see TREE OF HEAVEN
VERONICA .... see VERONICA
Veronica beccabunga .... see BROOKLIME
Veronica Herb .... see VERONICA
Veronica officinalis .... see VERONICA
Veronica virginica .... see BLACK ROOT
Veronica Virginica Root .... see BLACK ROOT
Veronicae Herba .... see VERONICA
Veronicastrum virginicum .... see BLACK ROOT
Verrucaria .... see MARSH MARIGOLD
Vervain .... see VERBENA
Verveine Citronelle .... see LEMON VERBENA
Vespula maculata .... see BEE VENOM
VETIVER .... see VETIVER
Vetivergras .... see VETIVER
Vetiveria zizanioides .... see VETIVER
Vibhitaki .... see TERMINALIA
Viburnum .... see BLACK HAW

Viburnum alnifolium .... see HYDRANGEA
Viburnum americanum .... see HYDRANGEA
Viburnum lentago .... see BLACK HAW
Viburnum opulus .... see CRAMP BARK
Viburnum prunifolium .... see BLACK HAW
Viburnum rufidulum .... see BLACK HAW
Vidhara .... see HAWAIIAN BABY WOODROSE
Vinca minor .... see PERIWINKLE
Vinca rosea .... see MADAGASCAR PERIWINKLE
Vincae Minoris Herba .... see PERIWINKLE
Vincetoxicum hirundinaria .... see GERMAN IPECAC
Vincetoxicum officinale .... see GERMAN IPECAC
Vine Bower .... see WOODBINE
Vine of Mount Ida .... see ALPINE CRANBERRY
Vine-of-Sodom .... see COLOCYNTH
Vinettier .... see EUROPEAN BARBERRY
Vinpocetin .... see VINPOCETINE
VINPOCETINE .... see VINPOCETINE
Viola .... see HEART'S EASE
Viola odorata ..... see GARDEN VIOLET, SWEET VIOLET
Viola tricolor .... see HEART'S EASE
Violae Odoratae Rhizoma .... see SWEET VIOLET
Violae Tricoloris Herba .... see HEART'S EASE
Violet .... see SWEET VIOLET
Violet Bloom .... see BITTERSWEET NIGHTSHADE
Violet Willow .... see WILLOW BARK
Virginia Cedarwood .... see CEDARWOOD
Virginia Creeper .... see AMERICAN IVY
Virginia Serpentary .... see ARISTOLOCHIA
Virginia Snakeroot .... see ARISTOLOCHIA
Virginia Water Horehound .... see BUGLEWEED
Virginian Poke .... see POKEWEED berry, POKEWEED root
Virginian Prune .... see WILD CHERRY
Virginian Strawberry .... see STRAWBERRY
Virgin's Bower .... see WOODBINE
Visci .... see EUROPEAN MISTLETOE
Visci Albi Folia .... see EUROPEAN MISTLETOE
Visci Albi Fructus .... see EUROPEAN MISTLETOE
Visci Albi Herba .... see EUROPEAN MISTLETOE
Visci Albi Stipites .... see EUROPEAN MISTLETOE
Viscum album .... see EUROPEAN MISTLETOE
Vishamushti .... see NUX VOMICA
Vishani .... see GYMNEMA
Visnaga .... see KHELLA
Visnaga Fruit .... see KHELLA
Visnagae .... see KHELLA
Visnagafruchte .... see KHELLA
Visnagin .... see KHELLA
Vitacarn .... see L-CARNITINE
Vitadurin .... see VITAMIN B12
VITAMIN A .... see VITAMIN A
Vitamin A1 .... see VITAMIN A
Vitamin A2 .... see VITAMIN A
Vitamin B(t) .... see L-CARNITINE
Vitamin B(t) Acetate .... see ACETYL-L-CARNITINE
Vitamin B1 .... see THIAMINE (VITAMIN B1)
Vitamin B2 .... see RIBOFLAVIN (VITAMIN B2)
Vitamin B3 .... see NIACIN AND NIACINAMIDE (VITAMIN B3)
Vitamin B5 ...... see PANTOTHENIC ACID (VITAMIN B5)
Vitamin B6 .... see PYRIDOXINE (VITAMIN B6)
Vitamin B8 .... see INOSITOL
Vitamin B9 .... see FOLIC ACID
Vitamin B10 .... see PARA-AMINOBENZOIC ACID (PABA)
VITAMIN B12 .... see VITAMIN B12
Vitamin B15 .... see PANGAMIC ACID
Vitamin B17 .... see APRICOT
VITAMIN C (ASCORBIC ACID) .... see VITAMIN C (ASCORBIC ACID)
VITAMIN D .... see VITAMIN D
VITAMIN E .... see VITAMIN E
Vitamin G .... see RIBOFLAVIN (VITAMIN B2)
Vitamin H .... see BIOTIN, PARA-AMINOBENZOIC ACID (PABA)
VITAMIN K .... see VITAMIN K
Vitamin K1 .... see VITAMIN K
VITAMIN O .... see VITAMIN O
Vitamin PP .... see NIACIN AND NIACINAMIDE (VITAMIN B3)
Vitaminum A .... see VITAMIN A
Vitellin .... see LECITHIN
Vitex .... see CHASTEBERRY
Vitex agnus-castus .... see CHASTEBERRY
Vitis coignetiae .... see GRAPE seed
Vitis pentaphylla .... see JIAOGULAN
Vitis vinifera .... see GRAPE fruit, skin; GRAPE leaf; GRAPE seed; WINE
Viverra civetta .... see CIVET
Vizra Ufar .... see ANDROGRAPHIS
Vogelknoeterichkraut .... see KNOTWEED
Vogelmistel .... see EUROPEAN MISTLETOE
Volatile Almond Oil .... see BITTER ALMOND
Vomit Wort .... see LOBELIA
Vriddadaru .... see HAWAIIAN BABY WOODROSE
Vrikshamla .... see GARCINIA
Vysorel .... see EUROPEAN MISTLETOE
W Factor .... see BIOTIN
W-3 Fatty Acid .... see DHA (DOCOSAHEXAENOIC ACID), EPA (EICOSAPENTAENOIC ACID), FISH OILS
Wacholderbeeren .... see JUNIPER
Wacholderteer .... see CADE OIL
WAFER ASH .... see WAFER ASH
WAHOO .... see WAHOO
Wake Robin .... see ARUM, BETH ROOT
Waldmeister .... see SWEET WOODRUFF
Walewort .... see DWARF ELDER
Wall Germander .... see GERMANDER
Wall Ginger .... see COMMON STONECROP
WALLFLOWER .... see WALLFLOWER
Wallflower .... see CANADIAN HEMP, WALLFLOWER
Wallpepper .... see COMMON STONECROP
Wallstock-gillofer .... see WALLFLOWER
Wallwort .... see COMFREY
Walnussblätter .... see ENGLISH WALNUT
Walnussfrüchtschalen .... see ENGLISH WALNUT
Walnut .... see ENGLISH WALNUT
Walnut Fruit .... see ENGLISH WALNUT
Walnut Hull .... see ENGLISH WALNUT
Walnut Leaf .... see ENGLISH WALNUT
Walpole Tea .... see NEW JERSEY TEA
Wandering Jenny .... see MONEYWORT
Wandering Tailor .... see MONEYWORT
Wang Sun .... see HERB PARIS
Warnera .... see GOLDENSEAL
Wartwort .... see CUDWEED

Wasp Venom .... see BEE VENOM
Wasserkresse .... see WATERCRESS
Wasser-schierling .... see WATER HEMLOCK
Wasshanf .... see HEMP AGRIMONY
Wateorhiza palmata .... see COLOMBO
Water-cup .... see PITCHER PLANT
Water-holly .... see OREGON GRAPE
Water Agrimony .... see BURR MARIGOLD
WATER AVENS .... see WATER AVENS
Water Blobs .... see MARSH MARIGOLD
Water Bugle .... see BUGLEWEED
Water Cabbage .... see AMERICAN WHITE POND LILY
Water Chisch .... see WATER AVENS
WATER DOCK .... see WATER DOCK
Water Dragon .... see MARSH MARIGOLD
Water Dropwort .... see WATER FENNEL
WATER FENNEL .... see WATER FENNEL
Water Flag .... see BLUE FLAG, ORRIS
Water Flower .... see WATER AVENS
WATER GERMANDER .... see WATER GERMANDER
Water Gourd .... see LUFFA
WATER HEMLOCK .... see WATER HEMLOCK
Water Hoarhound .... see BUGLEWEED
Water Horehound .... see BUGLEWEED
Water Lemon .... see PASSIONFLOWER
Water Lily .... see AMERICAN WHITE POND LILY
Water Maudlin .... see HEMP AGRIMONY
Water Mint .... see WILD MINT
Water Nymph .... see AMERICAN WHITE POND LILY
Water of Pimento .... see ALLSPICE
Water Pepper .... see SMARTWEED
Water Pimpernel .... see BROOKLIME
Water Pink .... see TRAILING ARBUTUS
WATER PLANTAIN .... see WATER PLANTAIN
Water Purslane .... see BROOKLIME
Water Shamrock .... see BOGBEAN
WATERCRESS .... see WATERCRESS
Waterhemp .... see HEMP AGRIMONY
Waterkres .... see WATERCRESS
Wax Bean .... see BEAN POD
Wax Cluster .... see WINTERGREEN leaf, WINTERGREEN OIL
Wax Dolls .... see FUMITORY
Wax Myrtle .... see BAYBERRY
Waxberry .... see BAYBERRY
Waxwork .... see AMERICAN BITTERSWEET
Waythorn .... see EUROPEAN BUCKTHORN
Weather Plant .... see PRECATORY BEAN
Weaver's Broom .... see SPANISH BROOM
Weed .... see MARIJUANA
Weeping Ash .... see ASH
Weibe Senfsamen .... see WHITE MUSTARD
Weidenrinde .... see WILLOW BARK
Weissdorn .... see HAWTHORN
Wermut .... see WORMWOOD above ground parts
Wermutkraut .... see WORMWOOD above ground parts
West Indian Cherry .... see ACEROLA
West Indian Dogwood .... see JAMAICAN DOGWOOD
West Indian Lemongrass .... see LEMONGRASS
Western-huckleberry .... see BOG BILBERRY
Western Larch .... see LARCH ARABINOGALACTAN
Western Shisandra .... see SCHISANDRA
Western Yew .... see YEW
Westwood-pear .... see PRICKLY PEAR CACTUS
Weyl Ash .... see GOUTWEED
WHEAT BRAN .... see WHEAT BRAN
WHEATGRASS .... see WHEATGRASS
WHEY PROTEIN .... see WHEY PROTEIN
Whig Plant .... see ROMAN CHAMOMILE
White Archangel .... see WHITE DEAD NETTLE FLOWER
White Ash .... see ASH, GOUTWEED
White Baneberry .... see WHITE COHOSH
White Bay .... see MAGNOLIA
White Beeswax .... see BEESWAX
White Birch .... see BIRCH
White Bole .... see KAOLIN
White Bryony .... see BRYONIA
White Cabbage .... see CABBAGE
White Cedar .... see CEDAR leaf, CEDAR LEAF OIL
White Cinnamon .... see CANELLA
WHITE COHOSH .... see WHITE COHOSH
White Daisy .... see OX-EYE DAISY
WHITE DEAD NETTLE FLOWER .... see WHITE DEAD NETTLE FLOWER
White Dragon Flower .... see ORRIS
White Fringe .... see FRINGETREE
White Ginseng .... see GINSENG, PANAX
White Gum .... see STORAX
WHITE HELLEBORE .... see WHITE HELLEBORE
WHITE HOREHOUND .... see WHITE HOREHOUND
White Kidney Bean .... see BEAN POD
White Laurel .... see MAGNOLIA
WHITE LILY .... see WHITE LILY
WHITE MUSTARD .... see WHITE MUSTARD
White Pepper .... see BLACK PEPPER AND WHITE PEPPER
White Pond Lily .... see WHITE LILY
White Potato .... see POTATO
White Quebracho .... see QUEBRACHO
White Root .... see PLEURISY ROOT
White Rot .... see GOTU KOLA
White Sandalwood .... see WHITE SANDALWOOD OIL, WHITE SANDALWOOD wood
WHITE SANDALWOOD OIL .... see WHITE SANDALWOOD OIL
WHITE SANDALWOOD wood .... see WHITE SANDALWOOD wood
White Saunders .... see WHITE SANDALWOOD wood
White Saunders Oil .... see WHITE SANDALWOOD OIL
WHITE SOAPWORT .... see WHITE SOAPWORT
White Sorrel .... see WOOD SORREL
White Spruce Oil .... see FIR NEEDLE OIL
White Squill .... see SQUILL
White Thyme Oil .... see THYME OIL
White Walnut .... see BUTTERNUT
White Wax .... see BEESWAX
White Waxtree .... see GLOSSY PRIVET
White Weed .... see OX-EYE DAISY
White Willow .... see WILLOW BARK
White Willow Bark .... see WILLOW BARK
White Wood .... see CANELLA
White-faced Hornet .... see BEE VENOM
Whitehorn .... see HAWTHORN
Whitetube Stargrass .... see ALETRIS
Whole Adrenal Extract .... see ADRENAL EXTRACT
Whorlywort .... see BLACK ROOT
Whortleberry .... see BILBERRY

Wickup ... see FIREWEED
Wicopy ... see FIREWEED
Wiesen-feldkummel ... see CARAWAY dried fruit, seed
Wiesensauerampfer ... see SORREL
Wigandia californicum ... see YERBA SANTA
Wild Agrimony ... see POTENTILLA
Wild Angelica ... see ANGELICA root
Wild Balsam ... see JEWELWEED
Wild Bergamot ... see HORSEMINT
Wild Black Cherry ... see WILD CHERRY
Wild Boar Fruit ... see ROSE HIP
WILD CARROT ... see WILD CARROT
Wild Carrot ... see HEMLOCK, WATER HEMLOCK, WILD CARROT
Wild Celandine ... see JEWELWEED
Wild Celery Root ... see OSHA
Wild Chamomile ... see GERMAN CHAMOMILE
WILD CHERRY ... see WILD CHERRY
Wild Chicory ... see CHICORY
Wild Cinnamon ... see CANELLA
Wild Clover ... see RED CLOVER
Wild Coleus ... see PERILLA
Wild Cotton ... see CANADIAN HEMP
Wild Crane's-bill ... see HERB ROBERT
Wild Cucumber ... see BITTER MELON
Wild Cumin ... see CARAWAY OIL
Wild Curcuma ... see GOLDENSEAL
WILD DAISY ... see WILD DAISY
Wild Dill ... see WATER HEMLOCK
Wild Endive ... see DANDELION above ground parts, DANDELION entire plant
Wild Fennel ... see FENNEL fruit, seed
Wild Garlic ... see BEAR'S GARLIC
Wild Gentian ... see GENTIAN
Wild Germander ... see GERMANDER
Wild Ginger ... see ASARABACCA
Wild Gourd ... see COLOCYNTH
Wild Hops ... see BRYONIA
Wild Hydrangea ... see HYDRANGEA
Wild Ice Leaf ... see MULLEIN
WILD INDIGO ... see WILD INDIGO
Wild Iris ... see ORRIS
Wild Laburnum ... see SWEET CLOVER
Wild Lady's Slipper ... see JEWELWEED
Wild Lemon ... see PODOPHYLLUM
WILD LETTUCE ... see WILD LETTUCE
Wild Liquorice ... see SPINY RESTHARROW
Wild Mandrake ... see PODOPHYLLUM
Wild Marjoram ... see OREGANO
Wild Mexican Yam ... see WILD YAM
WILD MINT ... see WILD MINT
Wild Mint ... see ENGLISH HORSEMINT, WILD MINT
Wild Nard ... see ASARABACCA
Wild Nep ... see BRYONIA
Wild Oat Herb ... see OAT above ground parts
Wild Pansy ... see HEART'S EASE
Wild Parsnip ... see WATER HEMLOCK
Wild Passion Flower ... see PASSIONFLOWER
Wild Pea ... see LATHYRUS
Wild Pepper ... see GINSENG, SIBERIAN; MEZEREON
Wild Pine ... see MORINDA
Wild Plum Flower ... see BLACKTHORN flower
WILD RADISH ... see WILD RADISH
Wild Red American Ginseng ... see CANAIGRE
Wild Red Desert Ginseng ... see CANAIGRE
Wild Rosemary ... see MARSH TEA
Wild Snowball ... see NEW JERSEY TEA
Wild Strawberry ... see STRAWBERRY
Wild Sunflower ... see ELECAMPANE
WILD THYME ... see WILD THYME
Wild Tobacco ... see LOBELIA
Wild Vanilla ... see DEERTONGUE
Wild Vine ... see BRYONIA
Wild Woodbine ... see AMERICAN IVY
Wild Woodvine ... see AMERICAN IVY
Wild Wormwood ... see MUGWORT
WILD YAM ... see WILD YAM
WILLARD WATER ... see WILLARD WATER
Williard's Water ... see WILLARD WATER
WILLOW BARK ... see WILLOW BARK
Willow Herb ... see FIREWEED
Willow Sage ... see PURPLE LOOSESTRIFE
Willowherb ... see FIREWEED
Wind Flower ... see PULSATILLA, WOOD ANEMONE
Wind Root ... see PLEURISY ROOT
WINE ... see WINE
Wine Grapes ... see GRAPE fruit, skin
Wineberry ... see BILBERRY
Wingseed ... see WAFER ASH
Winter Bloom ... see WITCH HAZEL
WINTER CHERRY ... see WINTER CHERRY
Winter Cherry ... see ASHWAGANDHA, WINTER CHERRY
Winter Clover ... see SQUAWVINE
Winter Marjoram ... see OREGANO
Winter Pink ... see TRAILING ARBUTUS
WINTER SAVORY ... see WINTER SAVORY
Wintera ... see WINTER'S BARK
Wintera aromatica ... see WINTER'S BARK
Winterana canella ... see CANELLA
Wintergreen ... see PERIWINKLE, WINTERGREEN leaf, WINTERGREEN OIL
WINTERGREEN leaf ... see WINTERGREEN leaf
WINTERGREEN OIL ... see WINTERGREEN OIL
Winterlien ... see FLAXSEED
WINTER'S BARK ... see WINTER'S BARK
Winter's Cinnamon ... see WINTER'S BARK
Wintersweet ... see OREGANO
Wisconsin Ginseng ... see GINSENG, AMERICAN
Witch Grass ... see WHEATGRASS
WITCH HAZEL ... see WITCH HAZEL
Witch Meal ... see CLUB MOSS
Witchazel ... see WITCH HAZEL
Witchen ... see MOUNTAIN ASH
Witches' Pouches ... see SHEPHERD'S PURSE
Witch's Bells ... see DIGITALIS
Withania ... see ASHWAGANDHA
Withania somnifera ... see ASHWAGANDHA
Wogon ... see BAIKAL SKULLCAP
Wolfberry ... see LYCIUM
Wolfiporia cocos ... see PORIA MUSHROOM
Wolf's Bane ... see ARNICA
Wolf's Claw ... see CLUB MOSS
Wolfsbane ... see ACONITE
Wolfstrapp ... see BUGLEWEED
Wolly Foxglove ... see DIGITALIS
Woman's Long Hair ... see USNEA
Wonder Bulb ... see AUTUMN CROCUS

INDEX

Wonder Tree .... see CASTOR OIL, CASTOR seed
Wood-rose .... see HAWAIIAN BABY WOODROSE
WOOD ANEMONE .... see WOOD ANEMONE
Wood Betony .... see BETONY
Wood Gum .... see LARCH ARABINOGALACTAN
WOOD SAGE .... see WOOD SAGE
Wood Sanicle .... see SANICLE
WOOD SORREL .... see WOOD SORREL
Wood Sour .... see WOOD SORREL
Wood Spider .... see DEVIL'S CLAW
Wood Strawberry .... see STRAWBERRY
Wood Sugar .... see LARCH ARABINOGALACTAN
Wood Vine .... see BRYONIA
Wood Waxen .... see DYER'S BROOM
Woodbind .... see ENGLISH IVY
WOODBINE .... see WOODBINE
Woodbine .... see GELSEMIUM, HONEYSUCKLE, WOODBINE
Woodruff .... see SWEET WOODRUFF
Woody .... see BITTERSWEET NIGHTSHADE
Woody Climber .... see AMERICAN IVY
Woody Nightshade .... see BITTERSWEET NIGHTSHADE
Woolen .... see MULLEIN
Woolly Morning Glory .... see HAWAIIAN BABY WOODROSE
Woolly Parsnip .... see MASTERWORT
Woolly Thistle .... see SCOTCH THISTLE
Woolmat .... see HOUND'S TONGUE
Wordward .... see SWEET WOODRUFF
Worm Seed .... see WORMSEED
Wormgrass .... see PINK ROOT
WORMSEED .... see WORMSEED
Wormwood .... see WORMWOOD above ground parts, WORMWOOD OIL
WORMWOOD above ground parts .... see WORMWOOD above ground parts
WORMWOOD OIL .... see WORMWOOD OIL
Wound Wort .... see YARROW
Woundwort .... see GOLDENROD, SELF-HEAL
WS 1442 .... see HAWTHORN
Wu Jia Pi .... see GINSENG, SIBERIAN
Wu Ning .... see MORINDA
Wu Wei Zi .... see SCHISANDRA
Wu-jia .... see GINSENG, SIBERIAN
Wundkraut .... see ARNICA, WORMWOOD above ground parts
Wurzelstock .... see KAVA
Wuweizi .... see SCHISANDRA
Wymote .... see MARSHMALLOW
Xango .... see MANGOSTEEN
Xango Juice .... see MANGOSTEEN
Xanthan .... see XANTHAN GUM
XANTHAN GUM .... see XANTHAN GUM
Xanthomonas campestris .... see XANTHAN GUM
Xanthophyll .... see LUTEIN
Xanthoxylum .... see NORTHERN PRICKLY ASH, SOUTHERN PRICKLY ASH
Xhoba .... see HOODIA
Xi Yang Shen .... see GINSENG, AMERICAN
Xi Zang Hu Huang Lian .... see PICRORHIZA
Xian Ling Pi .... see EPIMEDIUM
Xianxao .... see JIAOGULAN
Xiwuweizi .... see SCHISANDRA
Xue Jie .... see DRAGON'S BLOOD
Xue Zhi Kang .... see RED YEAST
Xylit .... see XYLITOL
Xylite .... see XYLITOL
XYLITOL .... see XYLITOL
Xylo-pentane-1,2,3,4,5-pentol .... see XYLITOL
Xysmalobium undulatum .... see UZARA
Yadake .... see BAMBOO
Yagona .... see KAVA
Yam .... see WILD YAM
Yangona .... see KAVA
Yaqona .... see KAVA
YARROW .... see YARROW
Yashtimadhu .... see LICORICE
Yashti-madhu .... see LICORICE
Yashti-madhuka .... see LICORICE
Yavani .... see BISHOP'S WEED
Yavatikta .... see ANDROGRAPHIS
Yaw Root .... see QUEEN'S DELIGHT
Yeast-derived Beta Glucan .... see BETA GLUCANS
Yege .... see KUDZU
Yellow-jacket Venom .... see BEE VENOM
Yellow Astringent .... see EPHEDRA
Yellow Bark .... see CASCARA
Yellow Beeswax .... see BEESWAX
Yellow Beet .... see BEET
Yellow Broom .... see WILD INDIGO
Yellow Bugle .... see GROUND PINE
Yellow Chaste Weed .... see IMMORTELLE, SANDY EVERLASTING
Yellow Cleavers .... see LADY'S BEDSTRAW
YELLOW DOCK .... see YELLOW DOCK
Yellow Flag .... see ORRIS
Yellow Galium .... see LADY'S BEDSTRAW
Yellow Gentian .... see GENTIAN
Yellow Ginseng .... see BLUE COHOSH
Yellow Hornet .... see BEE VENOM
Yellow Horse .... see EPHEDRA
Yellow Indian Paint .... see GOLDENSEAL
Yellow Indigo .... see WILD INDIGO
Yellow Iris .... see ORRIS
Yellow Jasmine .... see GELSEMIUM
Yellow Jessamine Root .... see GELSEMIUM
YELLOW LUPIN .... see YELLOW LUPIN
Yellow Melilot .... see SWEET CLOVER
Yellow Oleander .... see OLEANDER
Yellow Paint .... see GOLDENSEAL
Yellow Pheasant's Eye .... see PHEASANT'S EYE
Yellow Puccoon .... see GOLDENSEAL
Yellow Rod .... see YELLOW TOADFLAX
Yellow Root .... see GOLDENSEAL
Yellow Sandalwood ..... see WHITE SANDALWOOD wood
Yellow Sandalwood Oil .... see WHITE SANDALWOOD OIL
Yellow Saunders .... see WHITE SANDALWOOD wood
Yellow Saunders Oil ..... see WHITE SANDALWOOD OIL
Yellow Snakeleaf .... see AMERICAN ADDER'S TONGUE
Yellow Snowdrop .... see AMERICAN ADDER'S TONGUE
Yellow Starwort .... see ELECAMPANE
Yellow Sweet Clover .... see SWEET CLOVER
YELLOW TOADFLAX .... see YELLOW TOADFLAX
Yellow Vine .... see THUNDER GOD VINE
Yellow Water Dropwort .... see HEMLOCK WATER DROPWORT
Yellow Wax .... see BEESWAX

Yellow Willowherb .... see LOOSESTRIFE
Yellow Wood .... see NORTHERN PRICKLY ASH
Yellowdock .... see YELLOW DOCK
Yellowroot .... see GOLDTHREAD
Yellows .... see BUTTERCUP, NERVE ROOT
Yellowweed .... see BUTTERCUP
Yemen Myrrh .... see MYRRH
Yerba Buena .... see SPEARMINT
Yerba de Maria .... see DIVINER'S SAGE
Yerba Dulce .... see STEVIA
YERBA MANSA .... see YERBA MANSA
Yerba Manza .... see YERBA MANSA
Yerba Mate .... see MATE
YERBA SANTA .... see YERBA SANTA
YEW .... see YEW
YIN CHEN .... see YIN CHEN
Yin Ch'en .... see YIN CHEN
Yin Ch'en Hao .... see YIN CHEN
Yin Du Zhang Ya Cai .... see CHIRATA
Yin Yang Huo .... see EPIMEDIUM
Yinhsing .... see GINKGO leaf (GINKGO leaf extract), GINKGO seed
Ylang Ylang .... see YLANG YLANG OIL
YLANG YLANG OIL .... see YLANG YLANG OIL
Yoghurt .... see YOGURT
Yogourt .... see YOGURT
YOGURT .... see YOGURT
YOHIMBE .... see YOHIMBE
Yohimbehe .... see YOHIMBE
Yohimbehe Cortex .... see YOHIMBE
Yohimbine .... see YOHIMBE
Yongona .... see KAVA
Yougurt .... see YOGURT
Youthwort .... see MASTERWORT, SUNDEW
Ysop .... see HYSSOP
YUCCA .... see YUCCA
Yucca aloifolia .... see YUCCA
Yucca angustifolia .... see YUCCA
Yucca arborescens .... see YUCCA
Yucca brevifolia .... see YUCCA
Yucca filamentosa .... see YUCCA
Yucca glauca .... see YUCCA
Yucca mohavensis .... see YUCCA
Yucca schidigera .... see YUCCA
Yucca whipplei .... see YUCCA
Yuma .... see WILD YAM
Yun Mu Xiang .... see COSTUS OIL, COSTUS root
Yun-Zhi .... see CORIOLUS MUSHROOM
Zacate Violeta .... see VETIVER
Zaffer .... see SAFFLOWER
Zafran .... see SAFFLOWER
Zanthoxylum .... see NORTHERN PRICKLY ASH, SOUTHERN PRICKLY ASH
Zanthoxylum americanum .... see NORTHERN PRICKLY ASH
Zanthoxylum clava-herculis .... see SOUTHERN PRICKLY ASH
Zanzibar Pepper .... see CAPSICUM
Zao .... see JUJUBE
Zappania citrodora .... see LEMON VERBENA
Zea .... see CORN SILK
Zea mays .... see CORN SILK
Zeaxanthin .... see LUTEIN
Zedoaire .... see ZEDOARY
Zedoaria .... see ZEDOARY
Zedoarie Rhizoma .... see ZEDOARY
ZEDOARY .... see ZEDOARY
Zergul .... see CALENDULA
Zhi Qiao .... see BITTER ORANGE
Zhi Shi .... see BITTER ORANGE
Zhi Tai .... see RED YEAST
Zhihe Shou Wu .... see FO-TI
Zhong Mahuang .... see EPHEDRA
Zi Shou Wu .... see FO-TI
Zibeth .... see CIVET
Zimbluten .... see CASSIA CINNAMON
Zimbro .... see JUNIPER
ZINC .... see ZINC
Zinc Acetate .... see ZINC
Zinc Acexamate .... see ZINC
Zinc Aspartate .... see ZINC
Zinc Citrate .... see ZINC
Zinc Gluconate .... see ZINC
Zinc Methionine .... see ZINC
Zinc Monomethionine .... see ZINC
Zinc Oxide .... see ZINC
Zinc Picolinate .... see ZINC
Zinc Pyrithione .... see ZINC
Zinc Sulfate .... see ZINC
Zingiber officinale .... see GINGER
Zingiber Officinalis .... see GINGER
Zingiberis Rhizoma .... see GINGER
Zira .... see CUMIN
Zitter-pappel .... see ASPEN
Zitwer .... see ZEDOARY
Zitwerwirtzelstock .... see ZEDOARY
Ziziphus jujuba .... see JUJUBE
Ziziphus sativa .... see JUJUBE
Ziziphus spinosa .... see JUJUBE
Ziziphus vulgaris .... see JUJUBE
Ziziphus zizyphus .... see JUJUBE
Zizyphus .... see JUJUBE
Zn .... see ZINC
Zoom .... see GUARANA
Zygophyllum tridentatum .... see CHAPARRAL
Zyzyphus jujube .... see JUJUBE

INDEX

Call, fax, or email your comments. Thanks!

"Tell the Editors..."

This *Database* is constantly evolving. Our research and editorial team analyzes new studies and updates the Web version of this *Database* every day. We view our work as similar to a clearing house of information on natural medicines. If you spot a statement that needs to be updated, use this form to communicate directly with the editors. Feel free to mail, email, or fax your comments. We appreciate your help!

1. What part of the *Database* are you commenting about?

Page # ______________________ Section ______________________

____

2. What wording should be added?

Please be specific about the exact wording you are proposing. Use additional pages if needed.

____

____

____

____

3. What wording should be deleted?

Please tell us which words you think should be removed.

____

____

____

4. What reference citations support this change?

Please give us specific reference citations. We base entries into this *Database* on reliable studies published in peer-reviewed professional literature. Please give enough information for us to find the reference.

____

____

5. How can we contact you?

Name ____

Address ____

Phone ______________________ Email ______________________

NATURAL MEDICINES
COMPREHENSIVE DATABASE

For your convenience, fax to (209)472-2249.
Call (209)472-2244 • mail@naturaldatabase.com
Visit us online at www.naturaldatabase.com
3120 W. March Lane, PO Box 8190, Stockton, CA 95208

Now You Can Offer the *Consumer Version* on YOUR Website

The *Consumer Version* of the *Database* provides comprehensive, consumer-friendly information online.

Your organization can license the *Consumer Version* for users to access from YOUR website.

Our editors update the *Consumer Version* along with the *Professional Version*...so the info in each is consistent. The two versions go hand in hand.

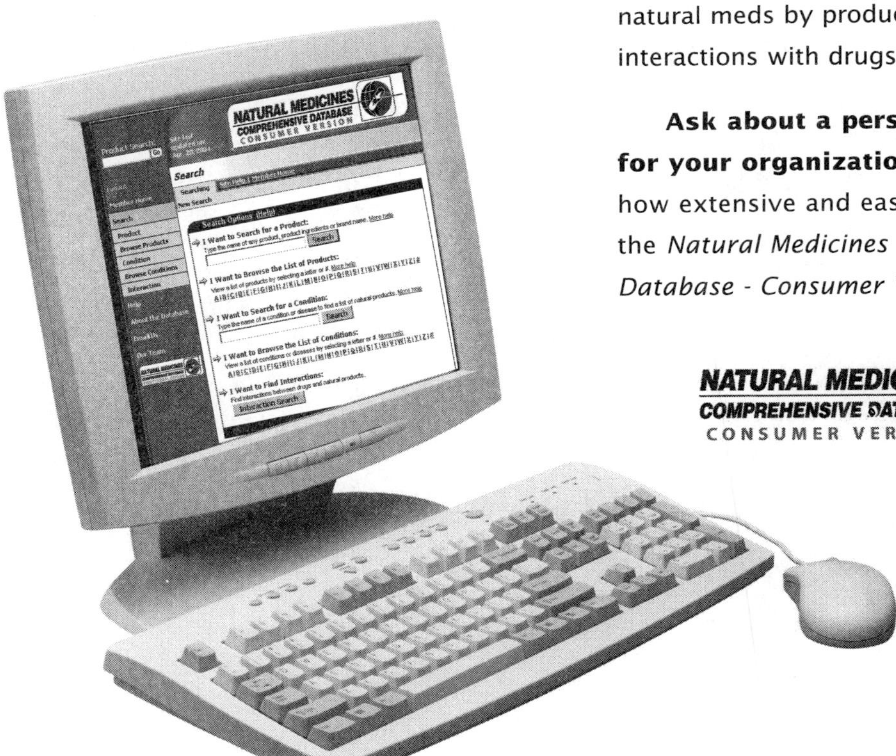

Patients appreciate having reliable information in an easy-to-understand format.

Patients who use the *Consumer Version* can find thousands of product names. Patients will also be thrilled to find more info on dietary and sports supplements, brand names, and ingredients.

All the information is written with the patient's needs and questions in mind. Patients can easily search for more info on natural meds by product, condition, and interactions with drugs they are taking.

Ask about a personalized demo for your organization to see firsthand how extensive and easy it is to use the *Natural Medicines Comprehensive Database - Consumer Version*.

NATURAL MEDICINES
COMPREHENSIVE DATABASE
CONSUMER VERSION

NATURAL MEDICINES
COMPREHENSIVE DATABASE

For your convenience, call (209) 472-2244.
Fax (209) 472-2249 • mail@naturaldatabase.com
Visit us online at www.naturaldatabase.com
3120 W. March Lane, PO Box 8190, Stockton, CA 95208

Order Additional Copies

☐ **Yes, START MY NEW SUBSCRIPTION.** ***BONUS: Online CE FREE with Web Access.***

- ☐ Book . . . . $92 ($131 CAN)
- ☐ One year Web Access to www.naturaldatabase.com (single-user price) . . . . . $92 ($131 CAN)
- ☐ Book + Web Combo: One year web access (single-user price) plus book . . . $132 ($171 CAN)
- ☐ PDA Version . . . . $92 ($131 CAN)
- ☐ PDA Version (if ordered with Book or Web). . . . .$59.80 ($87 CAN)

☐ **Yes, EXTEND MY EXISTING SUBSCRIPTION.** ***BONUS: Online CE FREE with Web Access.***

- ☐ Send me a new edition of the Book when it is published . . . . $92 ($131 CAN)
- ☐ Add one year Web Access to www.naturaldatabase.com (single-user price) . . $92 ($131 CAN)
- ☐ Book + Web Combo: One year web access (single-user price) plus book . . $132 ($171 CAN)
- ☐ PDA Version . . . . $92 ($131 CAN)
- ☐ PDA Version (if ordered with Book or Web). . . . . $59.80 ($87 CAN)

☐ I want Continuing Education credits. Send me two CE Booklets. Four credits per booklet.

If current subscriber, two (2) Booklets are . . . . $19 ($32.60 CAN)
If not current subscriber, two (2) Booklets are . . . . $75 ($116.30 CAN)

For the book only, please add:

In California, add 7.75% sales tax . . . . $ ________
Shipping in U.S. . . . . FREE
Shipping in Canada . . . . $19 CAN
Shipping outside of North America. . . . . $18 US

TOTAL . . . .$ ________

Website users will have an opportunity to agree to the license agreement on the website, or get a full refund.

Name ____________________ Degree ________ Member # (optional) ________
Address ________________________________
City ____________________ State/Province ________ Zip Code ________
Email ____________________ Phone ________________

☐ Payment enclosed (please make check payable to *Natural Database*).

☐ Charge my VISA, MasterCard, American Express, or Discover Card.
Card No. ____________________ Exp. Date ________

☐ Bill my business or institution with this Purchase Order # ________________

NATURAL MEDICINES
COMPREHENSIVE DATABASE

For fastest ordering, call (209) 472-2244.
Fax (209) 472-2249 • mail@naturaldatabase.com
Visit us online at www.naturaldatabase.com
3120 W. March Lane, PO Box 8190, Stockton, CA 95208

Order Additional Copies

☐ **Yes, START MY NEW SUBSCRIPTION.** ***BONUS: Online CE FREE with Web Access.***

- ☐ Book . . . . $92 ($131 CAN)
- ☐ One year Web Access to www.naturaldatabase.com (single-user price) . . . . . $92 ($131 CAN)
- ☐ Book + Web Combo: One year web access (single-user price) plus book . . . $132 ($171 CAN)
- ☐ PDA Version . . . . $92 ($131 CAN)
- ☐ PDA Version (if ordered with Book or Web). . . . . $59.80 ($87 CAN)

☐ **Yes, EXTEND MY EXISTING SUBSCRIPTION.** ***BONUS: Online CE FREE with Web Access.***

- ☐ Send me a new edition of the Book when it is published . . . . $92 ($131 CAN)
- ☐ Add one year Web Access to www.naturaldatabase.com (single-user price) . . $92 ($131 CAN)
- ☐ Book + Web Combo: One year web access (single-user price) plus book . . $132 ($171 CAN)
- ☐ PDA Version . . . . $92 ($131 CAN)
- ☐ PDA Version (if ordered with Book or Web). . . . . $59.80 ($87 CAN)

☐ I want Continuing Education credits. Send me two CE Booklets. Four credits per booklet.

If current subscriber, two (2) Booklets are . . . . $19 ($32.60 CAN)
If not current subscriber, two (2) Booklets are . . . . $75 ($116.30 CAN)

For the book only, please add:

In California, add 7.75% sales tax . . . . $ ________
Shipping in U.S. . . . . FREE
Shipping in Canada . . . . $19 CAN
Shipping outside of North America. . . . . $18 US

TOTAL . . . . $ ________

Website users will have an opportunity to agree to the license agreement on the website, or get a full refund.

Name ______________________ Degree ________ Member # (optional) ________
Address ______________________
City ______________________ State/Province ________ Zip Code ________
Email ______________________ Phone ______________________

☐ Payment enclosed (please make check payable to *Natural Database*).

☐ Charge my VISA, MasterCard, American Express, or Discover Card.
Card No. ______________________ Exp. Date ________

☐ Bill my business or institution with this Purchase Order # ______________________

NATURAL MEDICINES COMPREHENSIVE DATABASE

For fastest ordering, call (209) 472-2244.
Fax (209) 472-2249 • mail@naturaldatabase.com
Visit us online at www.naturaldatabase.com
3120 W. March Lane, PO Box 8190, Stockton, CA 95208